VOLUME 2

Wintrobe's
CLINICAL HEMATOLOGY

FIFTEENTH EDITION

VOLUME 2

Wintrobe's CLINICAL HEMATOLOGY

FIFTEENTH EDITION

Editors

Robert T. Means, Jr., MD, MACP
Professor of Internal Medicine
Clinical Professor of Pathology
James H. Quillen College of Medicine
East Tennessee State University
Johnson City, Tennessee

George M. Rodgers, MD, PhD
Professor of Medicine
Department of Medicine/Hematology
University of Utah Health Sciences Center
Salt Lake City, Utah

Bertil Glader, MD, PhD
Stanford Medicine Professor of Pediatric
   Hematology/Oncology
Professor of Pathology (by courtesy)
Medical Director, RBC Special Studies Lab
Stanford University School of Medicine
Stanford, California

Daniel A. Arber, MD
Donald West and Mary Elizabeth King Professor
   and Chair
Department of Pathology
University of Chicago
Chicago, Illinois

Frederick R. Appelbaum, MD
Deputy Director
Fred Hutchinson Cancer Research Center
Professor
University of Washington School of Medicine
Seattle, Washington

Angela Dispenzieri, MD
Serene and Francis C. Durling Professor of Medicine
Division of Hematology and Division of Clinical Chemistry
Departments of Internal Medicine and Laboratory Medicine
Mayo Clinic
Rochester, Minnesota

Todd A. Fehniger, MD, PhD
Professor of Medicine
Division of Oncology
Department of Medicine
Washington University School of Medicine
Saint Louis, Missouri

Laura C. Michaelis, MD
Armand J. Quick Professor of Medicine
Chief, Division of Hematology/Oncology
Medical College of Wisconsin
Milwaukee, Wisconsin

John P. Leonard, MD
Senior Associate Dean for Innovation and Initiatives
Richard T. Silver Distinguished Professor of Hematology
   and Medical Oncology
Weill Department of Medicine
Weill Cornell Medicine
New York Presbyterian Hospital
New York, New York

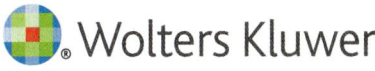

Philadelphia • Baltimore • New York • London
Buenos Aires • Hong Kong • Sydney • Tokyo

Acquisitions Editor: Joe Cho
Associate Director of Content Development: Anne Malcolm
Development Editor: Eric McDermott
Editorial Coordinator: Remington Fernando
Editorial Assistant: Kristen Kardoley
Marketing Manager: Kirsten Watrud
Production Project Manager: Frances Gunning
Manager, Graphic Arts & Design: Stephen Druding
Manufacturing Coordinator: Lisa Bowling
Prepress Vendor: TNQ Technologies

Fifteenth edition

Copyright © 2024 Wolters Kluwer.

Copyright © 1942, 1946, 1951, 1956, 1961, 1967, 1971, 1974, 1981 Lea & Febiger; Copyright © 1993, Williams & Wilkins; Copyright © 1999, 2004, 2009 Lippincott Williams & Wilkins; Copyright © 2014, Lippincott Williams & Wilkins, a Wolters Kluwer business. Copyright © 2019 Wolters Kluwer.

All rights reserved. This book is protected by copyright. No part of this book may be reproduced or transmitted in any form or by any means, including as photocopies or scanned-in or other electronic copies, or utilized by any information storage and retrieval system without written permission from the copyright owner, except for brief quotations embodied in critical articles and reviews. Materials appearing in this book prepared by individuals as part of their official duties as U.S. government employees are not covered by the above-mentioned copyright. To request permission, please contact Wolters Kluwer at Two Commerce Square, 2001 Market Street, Philadelphia, PA 19103, via email at permissions@lww.com, or via our website at shop.lww.com (products and services). 4/2023

9 8 7 6 5 4 3 2 1

Printed in Mexico.

Library of Congress Cataloging-in-Publication Data

ISBN-13: 978-1-975184-69-8

Cataloging in Publication data available on request from publisher.

This work is provided "as is," and the publisher disclaims any and all warranties, express or implied, including any warranties as to accuracy, comprehensiveness, or currency of the content of this work.

This work is no substitute for individual patient assessment based on healthcare professionals' examination of each patient and consideration of, among other things, age, weight, gender, current or prior medical conditions, medication history, laboratory data, and other factors unique to the patient. The publisher does not provide medical advice or guidance, and this work is merely a reference tool. Healthcare professionals, and not the publisher, are solely responsible for the use of this work, including all medical judgments, and for any resulting diagnosis and treatments.

Given continuous, rapid advances in medical science and health information, independent professional verification of medical diagnoses, indications, appropriate pharmaceutical selections and dosages, and treatment options should be made, and healthcare professionals should consult a variety of sources. When prescribing medication, healthcare professionals are advised to consult the product information sheet (the manufacturer's package insert) accompanying each drug to verify, among other things, conditions of use, warnings, and side effects and identify any changes in dosage schedule or contraindications, particularly if the medication to be administered is new, infrequently used, or has a narrow therapeutic range. To the maximum extent permitted under applicable law, no responsibility is assumed by the publisher for any injury and/or damage to persons or property, as a matter of products liability, negligence law or otherwise, or from any reference to or use by any person of this work.

shop.lww.com

Contents

VOLUME 1

Part 1 — LABORATORY HEMATOLOGY

Chapter 1	**Examination of the Blood and Bone Marrow** *Kristi J. Smock*	1
Chapter 2	**Clinical Flow Cytometry** *Anna Porwit*	18
Chapter 3	**Cytogenetics** *Patricia T. Greipp, Jess F. Peterson, Linda B. Baughn, and Min Fang*	48
Chapter 4	**Molecular Diagnosis in Hematology** *Bing Melody Zhang and James L. Zehnder*	61

Part 2 — THE NORMAL HEMATOLOGIC SYSTEM

SECTION 1 — HEMATOPOIESIS — 69

Chapter 5	**Origin and Development of Blood Cells** *Daniel K. Borger and Robert T. Means Jr.*	69

SECTION 2 — THE ERYTHROCYTE — 93

Chapter 6	**The Birth, Life, and Death of Red Blood Cells: Erythropoiesis, the Mature Red Blood Cell, and Cell Destruction** *John G. Quigley, Robert T. Means Jr., and Bertil Glader*	93

SECTION 3 — GRANULOCYTES AND MONOCYTES — 136

Chapter 7	**Neutrophilic Leukocytes** *Laura G. Schuettpelz and Daniel C. Link*	136
Chapter 8	**The Human Eosinophil** *Manali Mukherjee, Parameswaran Nair, and Paige Lacy*	168
Chapter 9	**Mast Cells and Basophils: Ontogeny, Characteristics, and Functional Diversity** *A. Dean Befus, Marianna Kulka, Kelly M. McNagny, and Judah A. Denburg*	196
Chapter 10	**Monocytes, Macrophages, and Dendritic Cells** *Matthew Collin, Venetia Bigley, and Florent Ginhoux*	208

SECTION 4 — THE LYMPHOCYTES — 233

Chapter 11	**Lymphocytes and Lymphatic Organs** *Christopher Y. Park and Matthew M. Klairmont*	233

Chapter 12	**B Lymphocytes** *Jeffrey J. Bednarski II*	267
Chapter 13	**T Lymphocytes** *Justin C. Boucher, Rawan G. Faramand, and Marco L. Davila*	288
Chapter 14	**Natural Killer and Innate Lymphoid Cells** *Matthew R. Lordo, Todd A. Fehniger, Bethany L. Mundy-Bosse, and Aharon G. Freud*	309
Chapter 15	**Major Histocompatibility Complex** *Qiuheng Jennifer Zhang, Michelle Hickey, Maxim Rosario, Nwe Nwe Soe, Carrie L. Butler, Rebecca A. Sosa, J. Michael Cecka, and Elaine F. Reed*	322
Chapter 16	**Complement System** *Robert A. Brodsky and Evan M. Braunstein*	338
SECTION 5	**HEMOSTASIS**	356
Chapter 17	**Megakaryocytes** *William Vainchenker, Najet Debili, and Hana Raslova*	356
Chapter 18	**Platelet Structure** *Elisabeth M. Battinelli and Katie Maurer*	391
Chapter 19	**Platelet Function in Hemostasis and Thrombosis** *David C. Calverley*	402
Chapter 20	**Blood Coagulation and Fibrinolysis** *Stephen J. Everse, Thomas Orfeo, Kathleen E. Brummel-Ziedins, and Kenneth G. Mann*	427
Chapter 21	**Endothelium: Angiogenesis and the Regulation of Hemostasis** *George M. Rodgers*	531

Part 3 — TRANSFUSION MEDICINE

Chapter 22	**Red Cell, Platelet, and White Cell Antigens** *Eric A. Gehrie, Heather M. Smetana, and Paul M. Ness*	540
Chapter 23	**Transfusion Medicine** *Mrigender Singh Virk, Suchitra Pandey, and Jennifer Andrews*	558

Part 4 — DISORDERS OF RED BLOOD CELLS

SECTION 1	**INTRODUCTION**	600
Chapter 24	**Anemia: General Considerations** *Robert T. Means Jr., and Bertil Glader*	600
SECTION 2	**DISORDERS OF IRON METABOLISM**	628
Chapter 25	**Iron Deficiency and Related Disorders** *Elizabeta Nemeth, Marie Hollenhorst, and Lawrence T. Goodnough*	628
Chapter 26	**Sideroblastic Anemias** *Mark D. Fleming*	656
Chapter 27	**Hemochromatosis** *James C. Barton and Charles J. Parker*	678
Chapter 28	**Porphyrias** *Makiko Yasuda, John D. Phillips, and Robert J. Desnick*	702

SECTION 3	**HEMOLYTIC ANEMIA**	726
Chapter 29	**Hereditary Spherocytosis, Hereditary Elliptocytosis, and Other Disorders Associated With Abnormalities of the Erythrocyte Membrane** *Patrick G. Gallagher and Bertil Glader*	726
Chapter 30	**Hereditary Hemolytic Anemias Due to Red Blood Cell Enzyme Disorders** *Rachael F. Grace and Bertil Glader*	749
Chapter 31	**Autoimmune Hemolytic Anemia** *Richard C. Friedberg and Clara Lo*	770
Chapter 32	**Paroxysmal Nocturnal Hemoglobinuria** *Charles J. Parker and Russell E. Ware*	792
Chapter 33	**Acquired Nonimmune Hemolytic Disorders** *Robert T. Means Jr., and Bertil Glader*	821
SECTION 4	**HEREDITARY DISORDERS OF HEMOGLOBIN STRUCTURE AND SYNTHESIS**	833
Chapter 34	**Sickle Cell Anemia and Other Sickling Syndromes** *Parul Rai, Jane Silva Hankins, and Jeremie E. Estepp*	833
Chapter 35	**Thalassemia Syndromes: Quantitative Disorders of Globin Chain Synthesis** *Eugene Khandros and Janet L. Kwiatkowski*	883
Chapter 36	**Hemoglobins With Altered Oxygen Affinity, Unstable Hemoglobins, M-Hemoglobins, and Dyshemoglobinemias** *Madeleine Verhovsek and Martin H. Steinberg*	933
SECTION 5	**OTHER RED CELL DISORDERS**	945
Chapter 37	**Megaloblastic Anemias: Disorders of Impaired DNA Synthesis** *Sally P. Stabler*	945
Chapter 38	**Inherited Aplastic Anemia Syndromes Germline** *Nina Weichert-Leahey and Akiko Shimamura*	974
Chapter 39	**Acquired Aplastic Anemia** *Amy E. DeZern and Robert A. Brodsky*	995
Chapter 40	**Red Cell Aplasia: Acquired and Congenital Disorders** *Anupama Narla, Jeffrey M. Lipton, and Robert T. Means Jr.*	1008
Chapter 41	**Congenital Dyserythropoietic Anemias** *Theodosia A. Kalfa, Bertil Glader, and Gary Kupfer*	1020
Chapter 42	**Anemia of Inflammation and of Systemic Disorders** *Robert T. Means Jr.*	1033
Chapter 43	**Anemias During Pregnancy and the Postpartum Period** *Robert T. Means Jr.*	1047
Chapter 44	**Anemias Unique to the Fetus and Neonate** *Robert D. Christensen and Robin K. Ohls*	1053
Chapter 45	**Erythrocytosis** *Robert T. Means Jr., and Bertil Glader*	1070

VOLUME 2

Part 5 — DISORDERS OF HEMOSTASIS AND COAGULATION

SECTION 1 — INTRODUCTION ... 1080

Chapter 46 — Diagnostic Approach to the Bleeding Disorders ... 1080
George M. Rodgers

SECTION 2 — THROMBOCYTOPENIA ... 1095

Chapter 47 — Thrombocytopenia: Pathophysiology and Classification ... 1095
George M. Rodgers

Chapter 48 — Thrombocytopenia Caused by Immunologic Platelet Destruction ... 1097
David C. Calverley, Christopher McKinney, and Christiane D. Thienelt

Chapter 49 — Thrombotic Thrombocytopenic Purpura, Hemolytic-Uremic Syndrome, and Related Disorders ... 1123
Han-Mou Tsai

Chapter 50 — Miscellaneous Causes of Thrombocytopenia ... 1153
Archana M. Agarwal, and George M. Rodgers

Chapter 51 — Bleeding Disorders Caused by Vascular Abnormalities ... 1162
George M. Rodgers

Chapter 52 — Thrombocytosis and Essential Thrombocythemia ... 1175
Tsewang Tashi and George M. Rodgers

Chapter 53 — Qualitative Disorders of Platelet Function ... 1182
Emanuela Falcinelli, Loredana Bury, and Paolo Gresele

SECTION 3 — COAGULATION DISORDERS ... 1202

Chapter 54 — Inherited Coagulation Disorders ... 1202
Ming Y. Lim and George M. Rodgers

Chapter 55 — Acquired Coagulation Disorders ... 1241
George M. Rodgers and Ming Y. Lim

SECTION 4 — THROMBOSIS ... 1276

Chapter 56 — Thrombosis and Antithrombotic Therapy ... 1276
Stacy A. Johnson and George M. Rodgers

Part 6 — DISORDERS OF LEUKOCYTES, IMMUNODEFICIENCY, AND THE SPLEEN

Chapter 57 — Diagnostic Approach to Tissue Examination and Testing ... 1321
Aaron C. Shaver and Adam C. Seegmiller

Chapter 58 — Neutropenia ... 1331
Nathalie Javidi-Sharifi and Nancy Berliner

Chapter 59 — Qualitative Disorders of Leukocytes ... 1344
Laura C. Michaelis

Chapter 60 — Lysosomal Abnormalities of the Monocyte-Macrophage System: Gaucher and Niemann-Pick Diseases ... 1359
Margaret M. McGovern and Robert J. Desnick

Chapter 61 — Langerhans Cell Histiocytosis ... 1364
Amit Rajaram and Michael M. Henry

Chapter 62	**Pathology of Langerhans Cell Histiocytosis and Other Histiocytic Proliferations** Andrew L. Feldman	1376
Chapter 63	**Infectious Mononucleosis and Other Epstein-Barr Virus–Related Disorders** Laura F. Walsh and Richard F. Ambinder	1382
Chapter 64	**Primary Immunodeficiency Diseases** Troy R. Torgerson	1393
Chapter 65	**Human Immunodeficiency Virus Infection** Ariela Noy and Roy M. Gulick	1409
Chapter 66	**Disorders of the Spleen** William C. Chapman Jr., and William C. Chapman	1423
Chapter 67	**Tumors of the Spleen** Daniel A. Arber	1437

Part 7 — HEMATOLOGIC MALIGNANCIES

SECTION 1 — GENERAL ASPECTS — 1444

Chapter 68	**Hematopoietic Neoplasms: Principles of Pathologic Diagnosis** Daniel A. Arber	1444
Chapter 69	**Principles of Targeted Therapies for Hematologic Malignancies** Nitin Jain, Shilpa Paul, Naveen Pemmaraju, and Varsha Gandhi	1454
Chapter 70	**Infectious Complications in Hematologic Malignancies** Markus Plate, Alexander Drelick, and Michael J. Satlin	1468
Chapter 71	**Immunotherapy** Trisha R. Berger and Marcela V. Maus	1494
Chapter 72	**Gene Therapy for Hematopoietic Stem Cell Disorders** Andre Larochelle	1522

SECTION 2 — THE ACUTE LEUKEMIAS — 1562

Chapter 73	**Molecular Genetics of Acute Leukemia** Ridas Juskevicius, Utpal P. Davé, and Mary Ann Thompson	1562
Chapter 74	**Diagnosis and Classification of the Acute Leukemias and Myelodysplastic Syndromes** Daniel A. Arber and Attilio Orazi	1595
Chapter 75	**Acute Lymphoblastic Leukemia in Adults** Ehab Atallah and Kristen O'Dwyer	1608
Chapter 76	**Acute Myeloid Leukemia in Adults** Ashkan Emadi and Maria R. Baer	1627
Chapter 77	**Acute Lymphoblastic Leukemia in Children** Maureen M. O'Brien, Alix E. Seif, and Stephen P. Hunger	1667
Chapter 78	**Acute Myeloid Leukemia in Children** Jennifer L. Kamens, Danielle Shin, and Norman Lacayo	1694
Chapter 79	**Acute Promyelocytic Leukemia** Yasmin M. Abaza, Martin S. Tallman, and Jessica K. Altman	1721
Chapter 80	**Myelodysplastic Syndromes** Namrata S. Chandhok and Mikkael A. Sekeres	1737
Chapter 81	**Clonal Hematopoiesis of Indeterminate Potential and Myeloid Diseases** Mrinal M. Patnaik and Pinkal Desai	1754

SECTION 3	MYELOPROLIFERATIVE DISORDERS	1763
Chapter 82	**Pathology of the Myeloproliferative Neoplasms** *Tracy I. George and Devon S. Chabot-Richards*	1763
Chapter 83	**Chronic Myeloid Leukemia** *Ehab Atallah and Michael W. Deininger*	1782
Chapter 84	**Polycythemia Vera** *Laura C. Michaelis and Robert T. Means Jr.*	1808
Chapter 85	**Myelofibrosis** *Andrew T. Kuykendall, Srdan Verstovsek, Eric Padron, and Rami Komrokji*	1821
Chapter 86	**Eosinophilic Neoplasms and Hypereosinophilic Syndrome** *Jason Gotlib*	1836
Chapter 87	**Systemic Mastocytosis** *Dean D. Metcalfe, Jonathan J. Lyons, and Jason Gotlib*	1849
SECTION 4	**LYMPHOPROLIFERATIVE DISORDERS**	**1866**
Chapter 88	**Diagnosis and Classification of Lymphomas** *Pedro Horna, Ji Yuan, and Rebecca L. King*	1866
Chapter 89	**Molecular Genetic Aspects of Non-Hodgkin Lymphomas** *Annette S. Kim, Scott B. Lovitch, and Mark A. Murakami*	1900
Chapter 90	**Non-Hodgkin Lymphoma in Adults** *Tarsheen K. Sethi, Shalin Kothari, Erin Mulvey, Francine Foss, John P. Leonard, and John P. Greer*	1942
Chapter 91	**Non-Hodgkin Lymphoma in Children** *Nitya Gulati and Lisa Giulino-Roth*	1991
Chapter 92	**Chronic Lymphocytic Leukemia** *Sameer A. Parikh, Saad S. Kenderian, Neil E. Kay, and James B. Johnston*	2010
Chapter 93	**Hairy Cell Leukemia** *James B. Johnston, Graeme R. Quest, and Michael R. Grever*	2049
Chapter 94	**Cutaneous T-Cell Lymphoma: Mycosis Fungoides and Sézary Syndrome** *John A. Zic, Francine Foss, Eva Niklinska, and Jeff P. Zwerner*	2072
Chapter 95	**Hodgkin Lymphoma in Adults** *Reid W. Merryman and Ann LaCasce*	2116
Chapter 96	**Hodgkin Lymphoma in Children** *Christine Moore Smith and Debra L. Friedman*	2133
SECTION 5	**PLASMA CELL DYSCRASIAS**	**2144**
Chapter 97	**Practical Approach to the Evaluation of Monoclonal Gammopathies** *Taxiarchis Kourelis and Francis K. Buadi*	2144
Chapter 98	**Molecular Genetic Aspects of Plasma Cell Disorders** *Peter Leif Bergsagel, Linda B. Baughn, Dragan Jevremovic, and Yan Asmann*	2152
Chapter 99	**Monoclonal Gammopathy of Undetermined Significance and Smoldering Multiple Myeloma** *S. Vincent Rajkumar, Robert A. Kyle, and Ronald S. Go*	2160
Chapter 100	**Multiple Myeloma** *Wilson I. Gonsalves, Prashant Kapoor, and Shaji K. Kumar*	2175
Chapter 101	**Immunoglobulin Light Chain Amyloidosis** *Morie A. Gertz, Eli Muchtar, and Angela Dispenzieri*	2238

Chapter 102	**Waldenström Macroglobulinemia** *Stephen M. Ansell and Rafael Fonseca*	2267
Chapter 103	**Monoclonal Gammopathies of Clinical Significance** *Angela Dispenzieri, David Dingli, and Rahma Warsam*	2276

Part 8 — HEMATOPOIETIC CELLULAR THERAPY

Chapter 104	**Hematopoietic Cell Transplantation** *Rachel B. Salit and Frederick R. Appelbaum*	2297
Chapter 105	**Hematopoietic Cell Transplantation for Nonmalignant Disorders** *Mark C. Walters and Nahal Rose Lalefar*	2314
Chapter 106	**Hematopoietic Cell Transplantation for Hematologic Malignancies** *Bhagirathbhai Dholaria, Jennifer Marvin-Peek, and Bipin N. Savani*	2335
Chapter 107	**Graft-vs-Host Disease and Graft-vs-Tumor Response** *Joseph Pidala, Brian C. Betts, Frederick L. Locke, and Claudio Anasetti*	2355
Chapter 108	**Late Effects After Hematopoietic Cell Transplantation** *Paul A. Carpenter*	2371
	Index	I-1

Part 5

DISORDERS OF HEMOSTASIS AND COAGULATION

Section 1 ■ INTRODUCTION

Chapter 46 ■ Diagnostic Approach to the Bleeding Disorders
GEORGE M. RODGERS

INTRODUCTION

Except for that which occurs during menstruation, spontaneous bleeding is abnormal. Surprisingly, little blood is lost, even after large injuries, because of the efficiency with which vascular integrity is normally maintained and the rapidity with which it is restored after injury. In general, these phenomena reflect the functional effectiveness of normal hemostasis (see Chapters 19-21). It must be recognized, however, that the adequacy of hemostasis is only relative, and despite the presence of normal vessels, platelets, and coagulation factors, bleeding can occur as the result of localized pathologic processes (structural bleeding).

The 11 chapters in Part 5 deal with disorders that result from abnormalities of the hemostatic process. This chapter is a summary of the diagnostic approach to these disorders and includes a brief discussion of laboratory methods for their study. In subsequent chapters, individual disorders are considered in six categories: thrombocytopenia (Chapters 47-50), bleeding disorders caused by vascular abnormalities (Chapter 51), thrombocytosis (Chapter 52), disorders of platelet function (Chapter 53), inherited coagulation disorders (Chapter 54), and acquired coagulation disorders (Chapter 55). The pathophysiology of thrombosis and the principles of antithrombotic therapy are summarized in Chapter 56.

CLINICAL EVALUATION OF THE BLEEDING PATIENT

A careful evaluation of the patient presenting with a bleeding disorder can often provide valuable clues as to whether the abnormality resides in the vessels, platelets, or the process of blood coagulation; a carefully obtained history can usually establish whether the disorder is inherited or acquired; and the physical examination may reveal findings such as the characteristic skin lesions of hereditary hemorrhagic telangiectasia, which alone may provide the diagnosis of a previously perplexing bleeding problem. Results of the clinical evaluation should lead to a rational and efficient laboratory investigation.

It is important to ask specific questions about bleeding because people with normal hemostasis may believe they bleed excessively.[1] Certain questions may discriminate between those with normal and those with abnormal hemostasis, including whether excessive bleeding occurs after tooth extraction or small cuts, whether spontaneous bruising or muscle bleeding occurs, or whether the patient has ever been transfused or treated with blood products.[1]

Bleeding assessment tools have been developed to identify patients with a likely bleeding disorder. Unfortunately, the bleeding assessment tool developed by the International Society of Thrombosis and Haemostasis does not identify patients at increased risk for future bleeding.[2]

MANIFESTATIONS OF DISORDERED HEMOSTASIS

Certain signs and symptoms are virtually diagnostic of disordered hemostasis. They can be divided arbitrarily into two groups: those seen more often in disorders of blood coagulation and those most commonly noted in disorders of the vessels and platelets. The clinical findings that are most valuable in distinguishing between these two broad categories are summarized in *Table 46.1*. Although these criteria are relative, they provide valuable clues to the probable diagnosis if they are applied to the predominant clinical features in a given patient.

Bleeding Into Skin and Soft Tissues

Petechiae are characteristic of an abnormality of the vessels or the platelets, such as thrombocytopenia, and are exceedingly rare in the coagulation disorders. These lesions are small capillary hemorrhages ranging from the size of a pinhead to much larger (*Figure 46.1*). They characteristically develop and regress in crops and are most conspicuous in areas of increased venous pressure, such as the dependent parts of the body and areas subjected to pressure or constriction from girdles or stockings. In patients with scurvy, petechiae may be distributed around hair follicles in the "saddle area" of the thighs and buttocks (see Figure 51.4). Petechiae must be distinguished from small telangiectasias and angiomas; vascular structures such as telangiectasias or angiomas blanch with pressure, whereas petechiae do not.

Petechiae are commonly associated with multiple superficial ecchymoses, which usually develop without perceptible trauma but seldom spread into deeper tissues. Small isolated ecchymoses are commonly noted in apparently normal women, especially on the legs, and in small children.

Table 46.1. Clinical Distinction Between Disorders of Vessels or Platelets and Disorders of Blood Coagulation

Finding	Disorders of Coagulation	Disorders of Platelets or Vessels
Petechiae	Rare	Characteristic
Deep dissecting hematomas	Characteristic	Rare
Superficial ecchymoses	Common; usually large and solitary	Characteristic; usually small and multiple
Hemarthrosis	Characteristic	Rare
Delayed bleeding	Common	Rare
Bleeding from superficial cuts and scratches	Minimal	Persistent; often profuse
Sex of patient	80%-90% of inherited forms occur only in male patients	Relatively more common in females
Positive family history	Common	Rare (except von Willebrand disease and hereditary hemorrhagic telangiectasia)

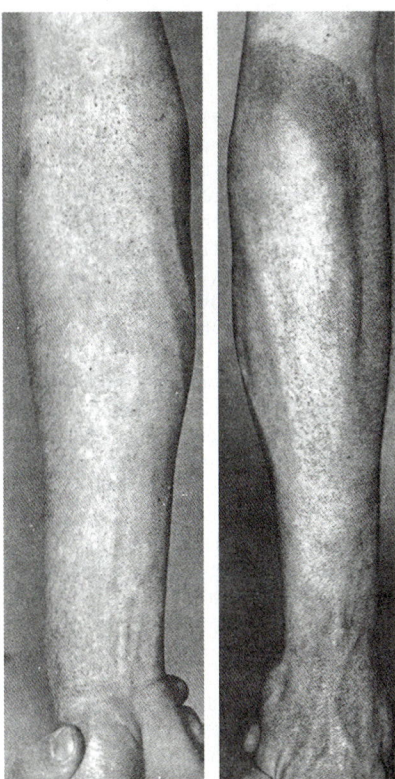

FIGURE 46.1 Diffuse petechial rash induced by a tourniquet in a patient with chronic idiopathic thrombocytopenic purpura (platelet count = $40 \times 10^9/L$).

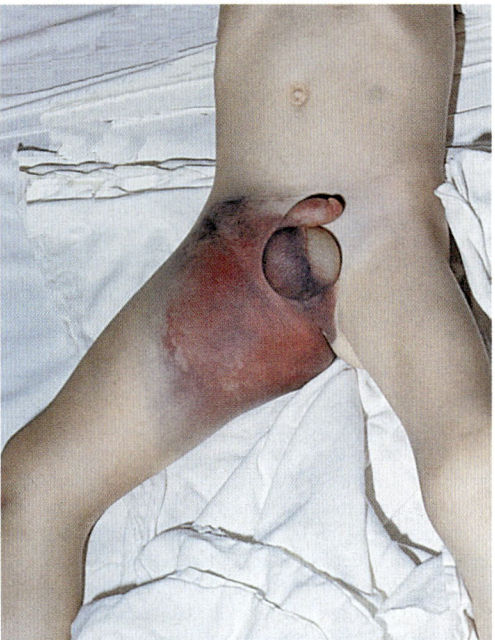

FIGURE 46.2 Large dissecting hematoma of thigh in a patient with hemophilia. The lesion resulted from a slight bump to the inguinal area and spread to involve the entire thigh. (Courtesy of Dr John Lukens.)

Although large superficial ecchymoses may be seen in association with the coagulation disorders, the most characteristic lesion is the large spreading hematoma (*Figure 46.2*). Such hematomas may arise spontaneously or after trivial trauma and often spread to involve an entire limb by dissecting within muscles and deep fascial spaces, often with minimal discoloration of the overlying skin.

Hemarthrosis

Hemorrhage into synovial joints is virtually diagnostic of a severe inherited coagulation disorder, most commonly hemophilia A or hemophilia B, and is rare in disorders of the vessels and platelets or in acquired coagulation disorders. This disabling problem often develops with pain and swelling as chief symptoms, but without discoloration or other external evidence of bleeding (see Figure 54.2). Subperiosteal hemorrhages in children with scurvy and swollen painful joints that may develop in some patients with allergic purpura occasionally may be confused with hemarthrosis.

Traumatic Bleeding

The unavoidable traumas of daily life and even minor surgical procedures are a greater challenge to hemostasis than any test yet developed in the laboratory. In contrast to "spontaneous" bleeding manifestations, bleeding after trauma in a person with a hemorrhagic diathesis differs in a quantitative way from that which would normally be expected in terms of the amount, duration, and magnitude of the inciting trauma. Such variables are extremely difficult to assess accurately by taking the patient's history. The amount of blood lost may be exaggerated by the patient. The need for transfusions and the number administered may serve as a rough guide. The patient's statement concerning the duration of bleeding is more reliable. Detailed inquiry as to past injuries and operations must be made because the patient is likely to forget procedures or injuries that were uncomplicated and to dwell on those in which bleeding was a problem. Whether reoperation was required for prolonged bleeding after tooth extraction or other minor surgical procedures may be helpful in identifying a patient with abnormal hemostasis.

In individuals with a coagulation disorder, the onset of bleeding after trauma is often delayed. For example, bleeding after a tooth extraction may stop completely, only to recur in a matter of hours and to persist despite the use of styptics, vasoconstrictors, and packing. The temporary hemostatic adequacy of the platelet plug despite defective blood coagulation may explain this phenomenon of delayed bleeding. In contrast, posttraumatic or postoperative surgical bleeding in thrombocytopenic patients is usually immediate in onset, as a rule responds to local measures, and is rarely as rapid or voluminous as that encountered in patients with coagulation disorders. However, it may persist for hours or days after surprisingly small injuries.

The response to trauma is an excellent screening test for the presence of an inherited hemorrhagic disorder, and a history of surgical procedures or significant injury without abnormal bleeding is equally good evidence against the presence of such a disorder. The removal of molar teeth is a major challenge to hemostasis, as is a tonsillectomy, and it is a rare hemophiliac, however mildly affected, who can withstand these procedures without excessive bleeding.

Miscellaneous Bleeding Manifestations

Although structural causes for bleeding (such as polyps, varices, and tumors) are commonly seen in patients with hematuria, hematemesis, and melena, bleeding from these sites may also be associated with both platelet-type and coagulation disorders. Severe menorrhagia may be the sole symptom of women with von Willebrand disease (vWD), mild thrombocytopenia, or autosomally inherited coagulation disorders. Recurrent gastrointestinal bleeding or epistaxis in the absence of other bleeding manifestations is common in hereditary hemorrhagic telangiectasia. A coagulation disorder or a disorder of platelet function should be considered if protracted hematuria is the only symptom.

Bleeding into serous cavities and internal fascial spaces often occurs in patients with inherited coagulation disorders and may create serious diagnostic problems. In hemophilia, retroperitoneal hemorrhage or bleeding into the psoas sheath may mimic appendicitis, and hemorrhage into the bowel wall may be confused with intestinal obstruction. Signs and symptoms simulating a variety of acute intra-abdominal disorders may also be seen in association with allergic purpura. The coexistence of bleeding and thromboembolic phenomena or bleeding from previously intact venipuncture sites is suggestive of disseminated intravascular coagulation (DIC). Protracted wound healing, wound dehiscence, and abnormal scar formation have been described in inherited afibrinogenemia, the dysfibrinogenemias, and factor XIII deficiency.[3] Hemoptysis is rarely associated with hemorrhagic disorders.

CLINICAL FEATURES OF INHERITED BLEEDING DISORDERS

An inherited bleeding disorder is suggested by the onset of bleeding symptoms in infancy and childhood, a positive family history (particularly if it reveals a consistent genetic pattern), and laboratory evidence of a single or an isolated abnormality, most commonly the deficiency of a single coagulation factor.

Age at Onset: Bleeding in the Neonate

Birth and the neonatal period provide unique challenges to the hemostatic mechanism,[4] and bleeding during the first month of life is often the first evidence of an inherited disorder of hemostasis. Small cephalohematomas and petechiae are common in the newborn as a result of the trauma of delivery. Large cephalohematomas that progressively increase in size may result from hemophilia but are more common in association with acquired bleeding disorders such as hemorrhagic disease of the newborn (see Chapter 55). Bleeding from the umbilical stump and after circumcision is common in acquired coagulation disorders, and it also occurs in the inherited coagulation disorders.[5] In the evaluation of bleeding in the neonate, the clinician should remember that hematochezia and hematemesis may originate from swallowed blood of maternal origin. Simple tests to distinguish such maternal blood from fetal blood have been described.[5]

Many infants with inherited coagulation disorders do not bleed significantly in the neonatal period. Less than one-third of patients with hemophilia A and hemophilia B and only 10% of those with other inherited coagulation disorders have hemorrhagic symptoms during the first week of life. In such patients, the disorder may become clinically silent for a time. Hematomas may first be seen only when the child becomes active. Hemarthrosis commonly does not develop until a child is 3 or 4 years of age.

A mild inherited hemorrhagic disorder may be difficult to distinguish from the insidious onset of an acquired defect. Patients with mild inherited coagulation disorders may enter adult life before characteristic bleeding manifestations occur. These patients and those with some forms of inherited thrombocytopenia and disordered platelet function often describe a history of posttraumatic bruising and hematoma formation that they have come to accept as normal. In hereditary hemorrhagic telangiectasia, the lesions become more prominent with advancing age and may not be symptomatic until middle age. Similarly, in patients with Ehlers-Danlos syndrome, bleeding may not be a problem until adult life.

Family History

The family history is of great importance in the evaluation of bleeding disorders. In disorders inherited as autosomal dominant traits with characteristic symptoms and high penetrance, such as hereditary hemorrhagic telangiectasia, an accurate pedigree spanning several generations can often be obtained. The presence of typical bleeding manifestations in male siblings and maternal uncles is virtually diagnostic of X-linked recessive inheritance, which characterizes hemophilia A and hemophilia B. In such X-linked traits, the family history may also be helpful in a negative sense—that is, it may clearly exclude the disorder in certain offspring, such as the sons of a known hemophiliac. Details of the various genetic patterns that may be encountered are discussed in the chapters that deal with these conditions.

The limitations of the family history, however, are greater than is commonly realized. Hearsay history is difficult to evaluate, and it is often impossible to assess the significance of easy bruising or to differentiate between manifestations of a generalized bleeding disorder and more common localized lesions, such as peptic ulcer and uterine leiomyomas. A negative family history is of no value in excluding an inherited coagulation disorder in an individual patient. As many as 30% to 40% of patients with hemophilia A have a negative family history.[6] The family history is usually negative in the autosomal recessive traits, and consanguinity, which is commonly present in these kindreds, is notoriously difficult to document or exclude.

CLINICAL FEATURES OF ACQUIRED BLEEDING DISORDERS

Generalized bleeding may be a prominent feature of a wide variety of acquired disorders that encompass virtually the entire field of medicine. Bleeding manifestations are usually less severe than in the inherited forms, and the clinical picture is often dominated by evidence of the underlying disorder rather than by bleeding alone. In the neonate, for example, DIC is usually associated with significant complications such as sepsis, hypoxia, acidosis, or problems related to prematurity. The physician should suspect sepsis or occult thrombosis in any sick neonate with unexplained thrombocytopenia.[5] Multiple hemostatic defects are commonly present in patients with acquired hemorrhagic diseases, which often include thrombocytopenia and significant coagulation abnormalities. In contrast, a single abnormality is usually found in patients with inherited hemorrhagic disorders.

In general, the emphasis of the study of the acquired bleeding disorders should be on the patient, not on the laboratory. A thorough history and the physical examination often reveal the cause of thrombocytopenia, such as a drug or acute leukemia. In most vascular disorders, including Bateman purpura, allergic purpura, scurvy, and amyloidosis, the history and physical examination are of primary diagnostic importance, and the laboratory has little to offer.

Drug History

The importance of exhaustive interrogation regarding drug use and chemical exposure cannot be overemphasized. The list of drugs associated with thrombocytopenia (see Table 48.6) or vascular purpura grows longer each year. Less common but more serious is drug-induced aplastic anemia, which may present initially with bleeding. Many commonly used drugs, notably aspirin, impair platelet function and produce abnormal findings on laboratory tests, which often lead to expensive and unnecessary additional laboratory studies. The same drugs may provoke bleeding when administered to patients with pre-existing hemostatic defects, such as hemophilia A. Drug ingestion may also produce coagulation abnormalities, and drugs that potentiate or antagonize the anticoagulant effects of coumarin derivatives may lead to bleeding or erratic laboratory control. The surreptitious ingestion of such agents is not uncommon.

Results of various coagulation tests may be abnormal in a surprisingly large percentage of hospitalized patients because of heparin that is administered therapeutically or is used in small amounts to maintain the patency of indwelling venous catheters, venous pressure lines, arteriovenous shunts, and various pumps and infusion machines. The partial thromboplastin time (PTT), in particular, may be greatly prolonged in patients who have received even a minute amount of this anticoagulant. Such coagulation abnormalities are often confused with DIC, inhibitors of factor VIII, and other serious coagulation disorders, and they commonly lead to repeated, and usually useless, coagulation studies. A thorough bedside inventory is often required to find out that heparin is indeed responsible. Prolongation of the thrombin time associated with a normal reptilase time, or direct assay of heparin, provides laboratory evidence of heparin contamination.

LABORATORY METHODS FOR STUDY OF HEMOSTASIS AND BLOOD COAGULATION

The interpretation of the most commonly used tests and the range of values obtained in normal subjects with representative techniques are summarized in *Table 46.2*. Definitive coagulation methods usually require a specially equipped laboratory and trained personnel and are discussed here from a general standpoint only.

Tests of Vascular and Platelet Phases
Bleeding Time

Older studies using the bleeding time test supported the view that this test might be helpful in predicting bleeding in individual patients.[11] More recent studies suggest that a bleeding time result is determined

Table 46.2. Interpretation of Common Tests of Hemostasis and Blood Coagulation

Test	Normal Range[a] (±2 SD)	Common Causes of Abnormalities

Platelet count
  Phase microscopy
  (automated)
	140,000-440,000/μL
	177,000-406,000/μL
		Thrombocytopenia, thrombocytosis

Partial thromboplastin time (activated)[b]	26-36 s[c,7]	Deficiencies or inhibitors of prekallikrein; high-molecular-weight kininogen; factors XII, XI, IX, VIII, X, and V; prothrombin or fibrinogen; lupus inhibitors; heparin; warfarin
Prothrombin time[b]	12.0-15.5 s[c,8]	Deficiencies or inhibitors of factors VII, X, and V; prothrombin or fibrinogen; dysfibrinogenemia; lupus inhibitors; heparin; warfarin
Thrombin time[b]	14.7-19.5 s	Afibrinogenemia, dysfibrinogenemia, hypofibrinogenemia, and hyperfibrinogenemia; inhibitors of thrombin (heparin or direct thrombin inhibitors) or fibrin polymerization (fibrin degradation products, paraproteins)
Fibrinogen assay[b]	150-430 mg/dL[9]	Afibrinogenemia, dysfibrinogenemia, and hypofibrinogenemia; inhibitors of thrombin or fibrin polymerization
Factor VIII assay[b]	50-150 U/dL	Hemophilia A and von Willebrand disease; acquired antibodies to factor VIII
Fibrin degradation product assay	0-5 μg/mL[10]	Disseminated intravascular coagulation; fibrinogenolysis; thrombolytic drugs, liver disease; dysfibrinogenemia
D-dimer assay	0-0.4 μg/mL	Disseminated intravascular coagulation, recent surgery, pregnancy, thromboembolism, thrombolytic therapy

[a]Normal range in the University of Utah Coagulation Laboratory.
[b]Tests affected by heparin.
[c]Significant variations depending on reagents and technique.

not only by platelet count and function but also by hematocrit,[12] certain components of the coagulation mechanism,[13,14] skin quality,[15] and technique.[16] A careful analysis of this literature indicates that there is no correlation between a skin template bleeding time and certain visceral bleeding times[16,17] and that no correlation exists between preoperative bleeding time results and surgical blood loss or transfusion requirements.[18]

A clinical outcomes study reported that discontinuation of the bleeding time in a major academic medical center had no detectable adverse clinical impact.[19] A position paper of the College of American Pathologists and the American Society of Clinical Pathologists concluded that the bleeding time was not effective as a screening test and that a normal bleeding time does not exclude a bleeding disorder.[20] Patients thought to have a platelet-type bleeding disorder based on their personal or family history (or both) should be evaluated for vWD and the inherited qualitative platelet disorders, using recommended assays discussed in the section on Platelet Function Assays. Newer assays that may be useful in screening patients for platelet dysfunction are also discussed in the section on New Assays of Platelet Function.

Platelet Enumeration

Platelets are considerably more difficult to count than erythrocytes or leukocytes. This difficulty is to be expected in view of the small size of these cells and their tendency to adhere to foreign surfaces and to aggregate when activated.

An estimate of platelet counts in a well-prepared blood smear by an experienced observer is a valuable check on the platelet count as determined by any method. In general, when a blood smear is examined at ×100 power, each platelet counted/field represents approximately 10,000 platelets × 10^9/L. Consequently, a normal blood smear should demonstrate, on average, at least 14 platelets per high-power field.

Instruments for totally automated platelet counting are widely used. Details of automated cell counters are discussed in Chapter 1. When automated methods are used, various nontechnical factors may produce falsely low platelet counts.[21] These factors include platelet agglutinins,[22] abnormal amounts of plasma proteins in various paraproteinemias, previous contact of platelets with foreign surfaces such as dialysis membranes,[23] large or giant platelets, platelet satellitism,[24] lipemia,[25] and ethylenediaminetetraacetic acid–induced platelet clumping,[26] a phenomenon that may produce platelet clumps of sufficient size to artifactually increase the leukocyte count.[27] Spuriously high platelet counts may result from the presence of microspherocytes,[28] fragments of leukemic or red blood cells,[29] and Pappenheimer bodies.[30] Special technical modifications may be required to eliminate or minimize these artifacts to obtain accurate platelet counts.

Platelet Volume Measurements

The widespread availability of particle counters in the clinical laboratory permits the accurate measurement of platelet volume on a routine basis. Mean platelet volume (MPV) is increased in disorders associated with accelerated platelet turnover as the result of large numbers of megathrombocytes[31] or in patients with Bernard-Soulier syndrome. Normal or decreased values for MPV are usually obtained in patients with disorders associated with deficient platelet production, in some patients with sepsis,[32] and in people with certain big spleen syndromes.[33]

Some authors suggest that increased MPV provides evidence of accelerated platelet production and may be interpreted in the same way as the reticulocyte count. The method is difficult to standardize, however, and when determined on routinely collected specimens by automated counters, it is affected by numerous variables pertaining to specimen collection, anticoagulant, temperature, and duration of storage.[34] In view of these problems and the difficulty in interpreting platelet size heterogeneity under normal and abnormal conditions,[35] these measurements should be interpreted with caution.

A more reliable marker for measuring increased platelet turnover is the immature platelet fraction, a parameter reported routinely in most automated CBC instruments. Immature platelets can be a useful marker of thrombopoietic activity.[36]

Platelet Function Assays

Since the 1960s, light transmission platelet aggregation using platelet-rich plasma has been the "gold standard" method to assess platelet function. This method uses aggregometers, which are modified nephelometers that permit measurement of changes in optical density of a platelet suspension under conditions of constant temperature and continuous agitation (*Figure 46.3*). Most instruments measure a combination of light scatter and absorption. Instruments have been developed that permit both nephelometric and photometric measurements and the simultaneous measurement of aggregation and nucleotide release.[37]

Platelet aggregation is usually studied in suspensions of citrated platelet-rich plasma, in which the size and dimensions of the stirring bar, variations in plasma citrate concentration attributable to variations in hematocrit, the pH, and the nature of the buffers are important variables. Platelet suspensions are usually prepared by differential centrifugation, but methods that use albumin density gradient centrifugation

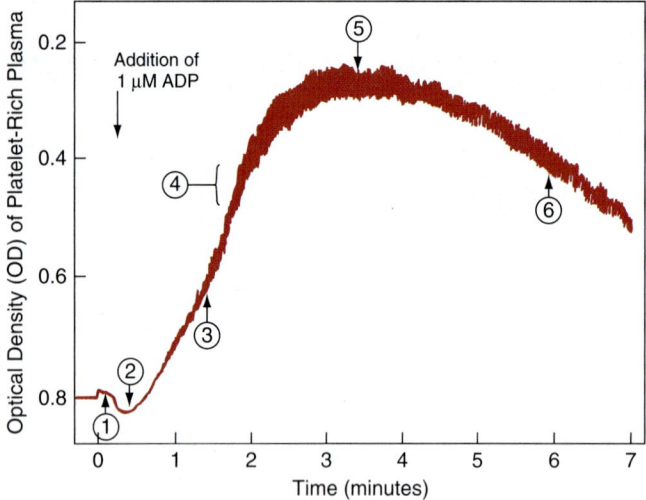

FIGURE 46.3 The interpretation of aggregometer tracings. Tracing of platelet aggregation produced by a low concentration of adenosine diphosphate, illustrating normal changes in optical density (OD)—that is, (1) a slight decrease caused by dilution with aggregating agent; (2) a transient increase caused by initial platelet swelling or shape change; (3) a rapid progressive decrease as platelet aggregates form, the size of which is roughly proportional to the amplitude of the oscillations in the tracing (4). The OD then reaches a nadir (5) from which maximal aggregation as a percentage of the initial OD may be calculated as follows: maximal aggregation (%) = OD at T0 − minimum OD/OD at T0. After this (6), a slow increase in OD caused by disaggregation occurs under some conditions.

and gel filtration have also been described.[38] Methods for the study of platelet aggregation in whole blood[39,40] have also been described. Interfaced computer systems have been developed for calculating and expressing platelet function data.[41]

Adenosine diphosphate (ADP) in concentrations of 5 µM/L or higher produces platelet aggregation directly that is independent of the release of platelet-contained ADP.[42] Various other aggregating agents act mainly by inducing the release reaction, such as a suspension of connective tissue particles (collagen), epinephrine and norepinephrine, and thrombin. With epinephrine (5 µM/L), a weak primary aggregating effect can usually be clearly distinguished from the subsequent release reaction, which produces a secondary wave of aggregation. Such primary and secondary waves of aggregation may also be seen with carefully titrated amounts of ADP (0.2-1.5 µM/L).[42] *Ristocetin* is an antibiotic that induces platelet agglutination (platelet metabolic activity not required) in the presence of von Willebrand factor (vWF). Patients deficient in vWF (vWD) or in the receptor for vWF (Bernard-Soulier syndrome) have an abnormal ristocetin response. Ristocetin is tested in concentrations of 0.6 to 1.2 mg/mL; the lower concentrations are helpful in identifying specific variants of vWD, type 2B, and platelet-type vWD (see Chapters 53 and 54).

The release reaction is measured only indirectly by routine aggregometry—that is, the aggregation associated with the release of ADP from the platelets (release-induced aggregation or secondary aggregation). Methods for the quantitation of various substances released from platelets have been described. For example, the amounts of ADP or serotonin released/unit of time serve as indices of dense body release[43]; the amount of various hydrolytic enzymes or platelet factor 4 released is a measure of the extent of α-granule release.[44] Suggested guidelines for standardization of platelet aggregation methods have been proposed.[45-47]

Sensitive methods have been developed for the determination of platelet-derived substances in plasma that may serve as markers of intravascular platelet activation, including platelet factor 4, β-thromboglobulin, stable prostaglandins (6-keto prostaglandin $F_{1\alpha}$ and thromboxane A_2), and leukotrienes.[47] These measurements may have diagnostic value in thromboembolic disorders and syndromes characterized by intravascular platelet aggregation.

New Assays of Platelet Function

An appreciation of the limitations of the bleeding time test has led to the development of newer assays to evaluate platelet function.[48] Some of these are point-of-care tests. The clinical use and predictive value of these tests to identify patients with hemostatic disorders remain to be established. One assay, the platelet function analyzer (PFA-100 or PFA-200), has been well investigated, and many published reports using this assay are available. In this method, citrated blood samples are exposed to high shear rates in a capillary flowing through an aperture within a membrane coated with collagen and either ADP or epinephrine.[49] The closure time to hemostatic plug formation within the aperture is the end point of the test. A large study using the PFA-100 found that prolonged closure times could be attributed to specific quantitative or qualitative abnormalities in platelet function or vWF (or both) in 93% of patients tested.[50] However, the International Society on Thrombosis and Haemostasis has taken the position that the PFA-100 is insufficiently sensitive and specific to be used as a screening device for platelet disorders.[51] It has been suggested that optimal use of the PFA in evaluation of hemostasis would use an algorithmic approach, evaluating not only PFA closure times but also a complete blood count, blood smear, and assays for vWD and platelet aggregation to further evaluate abnormal closure times. An addition to the PFA repertoire is the INNOVANCE PFA P2Y test (PFA-200) designed to assess P2Y12-receptor blockade.

Several additional platelet function assays are available on the market, although they are not as well studied as the PFA-100.[52] The ICHOR II-Plateletworks system (Helena Laboratories, Beaumont, TX) compares impedance-derived platelet counts in samples with and without added platelet agonists to assess platelet function. This system has historically been used to evaluate cardiopulmonary bypass patients but more recently has been applied to patients undergoing coronary stent placement. The Impact-R (Matis Medical, Beersel, Belgium) is an automated cone-and-plate research analyzer that assesses platelet adhesion and aggregation on a polystyrene surface under laminar flow conditions. The VerifyNow system analyzes platelet agonist–induced aggregation of fibrinogen-coated microparticles to assess platelet function. Agonist cartridges are designed to evaluate the effects of aspirin, clopidogrel, and GP IIb/IIIa platelet receptor inhibitor administration on platelet function. Platelet mapping, a modification of thromboelastography, measures the platelet contribution to clot strength in the presence of specific agonists.[53] To date, none of these platelet function assays has been sufficiently validated to warrant routine clinical use.[52,54,55]

Tests of Coagulation Phase

In general, meticulous performance of coagulation tests is more important than the exact technique chosen. Blood samples obtained by traumatic venipunctures or from indwelling catheters are often inadequate for coagulation studies.[56] A poorly collected blood sample is a far more common cause of inaccurate results than is technical error.

All coagulation tests are performed on citrated plasma, most commonly obtained using blue-top vacuum blood collection tubes that pull in nine parts of blood to one part citrate. The International Society for Thrombosis and Haemostasis recommends the routine use of 3.2% sodium citrate. A pool of freshly frozen citrated plasma from several normal donors is a suitable control for screening procedures in most laboratories. Lyophilized control plasma and borderline abnormal control plasmas are available commercially to standardize coagulation assays and to provide reference standards.

The citrate ion does not enter the erythrocyte. Consequently, the plasma citrate concentration is abnormally high when blood with a high hematocrit (>55%) is collected in usual concentrations of this anticoagulant. This may produce artifactual prolongation of one-stage screening tests of coagulation, such as the PTT.[57] To obtain interpretable data on such samples, tubes containing citrate concentrations appropriate for the hematocrit must be prepared by removing an aliquot of the citrate anticoagulant contained in standard blue-top tubes.

Activated Partial Thromboplastin Time

The activated PTT is a simple test of the intrinsic and common pathways of coagulation. When a mixture of plasma and a phospholipid platelet

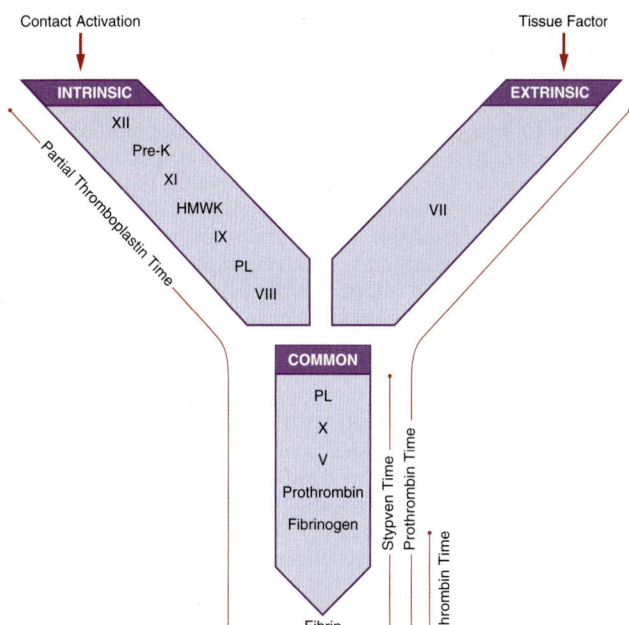

FIGURE 46.4 **The interpretation of common screening tests of blood coagulation.** Coagulation factors are indicated within arrow-shaped blocks, which represent the major pathways of coagulation. Screening tests are indicated at the side of these blocks in relation to pathways and coagulation factors measured by each. HMWK, high-molecular-weight kininogen; PL, phospholipid; pre-K, prekallikrein.

substitute is recalcified, fibrin forms at a normal rate only if the factors involved in the intrinsic pathway (prekallikrein, high-molecular-weight kininogen, and factors XII, XI, IX, and VIII) and in the common pathway (factors X and V, prothrombin, and fibrinogen) are present in normal amounts (*Figure 46.4*). Platelet substitutes of various kinds may be used, such as chloroform extract of brain[58] and other crude cephalin fractions as well as soybean phosphatides (inosithin). In the PTT, such platelet substitutes are provided in excess and the test is unaffected by the count of platelets remaining in the plasma (unless the sample contains antiphospholipid antibodies). Platelet substitutes are only partial thromboplastins, however, and they are incapable of activating the extrinsic pathway, which requires complete tissue thromboplastin (tissue factor). Thus, the PTT bypasses the extrinsic pathway and is unaffected by a deficiency of factor VII. The PTT assay is used to detect factor deficiency, screen for the lupus anticoagulant, and monitor heparin anticoagulation.

The PTT is somewhat more sensitive to deficiencies of factors VIII and IX than to deficiencies of factors XI and XII or factors involved in the common pathway,[7,59] but with most techniques, the test usually yields abnormal results if the plasma level of any of the essential factors is <15% to 30% of the normal value. The PTT thus detects some mild coagulation disorders. However, the ability to detect mild factor deficiency is reagent-dependent, and certain PTT reagents may not detect factor deficiency as low as 5% to 10%.[60] As is the case with all one-stage tests, the PTT may be shortened by high levels of a single factor, most commonly factor VIII. Thus, a short PTT may signify any of the various hypercoagulable states (see Chapter 56),[61] and high levels of any of the factors involved in the intrinsic or common pathways of coagulation may mask deficiencies of other factors.[62]

In the original method, contact activation was provided by the glass tube, but the addition of activators, such as ellagic acid, or particulate silicates, such as celite or kaolin, provides more optimal and standardized contact activation and represents a significant improvement over the original nonactivated test.[63,64] The PTT is the routine assay currently used to evaluate intrinsic coagulation. The PTT of plasma deficient in prekallikrein (Fletcher factor) is abnormal when it is determined by standard methods using particulate activators such as celite or kaolin.[65] This abnormality is minimized or abolished by protracted contact activation (15 minutes,[66] as compared with 2-3 minutes used in the standard technique). The PTT may yield normal results in prekallikrein deficiency when soluble activators such as ellagic acid are used.[66] A large pediatric reference interval study found no significant differences between adult PTT values and those of children aged 7 to 17 years.[67]

Increased PTT values may suggest a bleeding disorder, whereas shortened PTT values have been found to be independent predictors of an increased risk of death, thrombosis, bleeding, and morbidity.[61,68] The use of the PTT in the control of heparin therapy and in the detection of the lupus anticoagulant is discussed in Chapters 56 and 55, respectively.

Prothrombin Time

The production of fibrin by means of the extrinsic and common pathways (*Figure 46.4*) requires tissue factor and factor VII, in addition to factors X and V, prothrombin, and fibrinogen. These pathways are measured by the prothrombin time (PT),[8,69,70] in which plasma is recalcified in the presence of excess tissue factor. This test does not require contact activation and bypasses the intrinsic pathway and the factors involved therein. Because tissue thromboplastins contain phospholipids that act as platelet substitutes, the test is unaffected by platelet counts. Of the five coagulation factors measured by the PT (factors V, VII, and X; prothrombin; and fibrinogen), three (prothrombin and factors VII and X) are vitamin K-dependent and are decreased by coumarin-like drugs. As a result, the PT is the test most widely used for controlling oral anticoagulation with warfarin therapy. The PT is usually prolonged if the plasma levels of any of the requisite factors are <10% of normal, and it is more sensitive to deficiencies of factors VII and X than to deficiencies of fibrinogen and prothrombin. The PT is also prolonged by inhibitors of any of the essential factors and by heparin (unless heparin neutralizers are present in the PT reagent), but it is less sensitive to the anticoagulant action of heparin than is the PTT. A large pediatric reference interval study found that children aged 7 to 17 years have PT values ~1 second longer than normal adults.[67]

Various modified techniques and thromboplastins,[71] including recombinant human thromboplastins,[72] have been developed to improve the use of the PT in the control of coumarin anticoagulant therapy (see Chapter 56). Use of the international normalized ratio in monitoring oral anticoagulation therapy is the recommended format (discussed in Chapter 56). The PT performed with bovine brain thromboplastin is abnormal in patients with certain genetic variants of factor IX deficiency but is normal in patients with the more common form of this disorder. The venom of the Russell viper contains an enzyme that initiates coagulation by the direct activation of factor X and does not require factor VII. The one-stage "prothrombin time" performed with this venom (the Stypven time) thus distinguishes between deficiency of factor VII and deficiency of factor X (*Figure 46.4*).

Assay of Plasma Fibrinogen

Several accurate methods are available for the quantitative assay of plasma fibrinogen, a measurement of great clinical importance that should be available in all laboratories. Fibrinogen may be converted into fibrin, which is quantitated by gravimetric, nephelometric,[73] or chemical[9] methods. An immunologic[74] method has also been described. Kinetic techniques based on the thrombin time, however, are simple to perform, and they have been widely adopted.[75] Both gravimetric methods and those based on the thrombin time underestimate fibrinogen in the presence of high concentrations of fibrin (fibrinogen) degradation products (FDPs); technical modifications designed to avoid these problems have been proposed.[76] Some nephelometric methods appear to be minimally affected by FDP. Modified methods that eliminate interference by heparin,[77] as well as automated techniques, have been described. Marked differences in fibrinogen levels obtained by gravimetric and immunologic methods and those obtained by functional techniques are found in patients with the inherited dysfibrinogenemias. Reference values to identify patients with dysfibrinogenemia have been reported.[78]

Thrombin Time and Related Techniques

When thrombin is added to plasma, the time required for clot formation is a measure of the rate at which fibrin forms (*Figure 46.4*). This test (thrombin time) yields abnormal results when the fibrinogen level is <70 to 100 mg/dL, but it is unaffected by the levels of any of the other coagulation factors[79]; it is greatly prolonged by heparin. The thrombin time may also be prolonged by a qualitatively abnormal fibrinogen (dysfibrinogen), elevated levels of FDPs, certain paraproteins, and hyperfibrinogenemia. The thrombin time and modifications thereof are technically simple, can be performed quickly, and are valuable, particularly in the diagnosis of DIC. The reptilase clotting time is similar to the thrombin time in principle, but coagulation induced by this enzyme, which is prepared from snake venom, is unaffected by the presence of heparin.

Tests for Fibrin (Fibrinogen) Degradation Products and D-Dimer

FDPs are protein fragments of varying sizes that result from the proteolytic action of plasmin on fibrin or fibrinogen (see Chapter 20).[80] Plasma levels of these fragments are commonly increased in association with DIC and fibrinogenolysis, disorders in which their presence is of considerable diagnostic significance. Quantitative assays for FDP are based on several principles, such as the agglutination of latex particles coated with antifibrinogen antibody,[10] immunodiffusion,[81] and red cell hemagglutination inhibition.[82] Serum containing rheumatoid factor[10] or residual fibrinogen may yield false-positive results in some assays.[83]

None of the aforementioned methods distinguish between FDPs and fibrinogen degradation products; to make this distinction, measurement of the DD-dimer or even more sophisticated methods are required.[84] Extremely sensitive methods for the measurement of fibrinopeptides and specific FDP, such as the DD-dimer,[85] DDE-trimer, or B-β 15-42–related peptide, are useful as indices of DIC and as markers of subtle activation of coagulation in vivo (see Chapter 55).

Unpolymerized fibrin monomer is commonly present in the blood of patients with DIC. Various techniques (paracoagulation techniques) for demonstrating such monomers have been described; these range from the ethanol gelation test,[86] which is insensitive, to various protamine gelation techniques,[87] which are highly sensitive but nonspecific. All of these assays to diagnose DIC have been supplanted by the D-dimer test.[85] The use of D-dimer tests to exclude venous thromboembolism is discussed in Chapter 56.

Tests for Factor XIII Activity

The principle of the factor XIII screening test is that clots cross-linked by factor XIII resist denaturation by high concentrations of urea or acid. Deficiency of factor XIII results in premature clot lysis.[3] Patient plasma is recalcified to induce a clot; the clot is then suspended in 5 mol/L urea (or 1% monochloroacetic acid) for 24 hours. Clot stability is examined visually after 24 hours of incubation. Because this assay is a screening test, abnormal results should be repeated and confirmed using a quantitative factor XIII method, such as measuring factor XIII–dependent incorporation of labeled amines into substances such as fibrinogen or casein.[88]

Tests for Fibrinolysis

The plasma euglobulin fraction contains plasminogen activators and fibrinogen. Most of the major antiplasmins are removed in the pseudoglobulin supernatant fluid. The rate of lysis of a fibrin clot prepared from the euglobulin fraction (the euglobulin clot lysis time) thus provides a measure of fibrinolysis in the absence of major inhibitors and is a measure of the activity of plasminogen activators.[89]

Tests for fibrinogenolysis and assays for individual components of the fibrinolytic enzyme system, including plasminogen,[90] free plasmin,[91] and antiplasmins, are available. Routine coagulation assays for plasminogen activators and plasminogen activator inhibitors typically involve enzyme-linked immunosorbent assay methods.[92,93] Blood collection methods, timing, processing, and determination of assay-specific reference ranges are critically important in accurate evaluation of fibrinolysis parameters.[92,93]

Moderate concentrations of ε-aminocaproic acid (4×10^{-4} mol/L) inhibit plasminogen activators but not free plasmin. Thus, a shortened euglobulin lysis time in the presence of such concentrations of ε-aminocaproic acid indicates the presence of free plasmin, as in association with fibrinogenolysis (see Chapter 55).

Bioassays for Coagulation Factors

Bioassays for coagulation factors are usually based on the familiar screening tests, such as the PT and PTT. In principle, the extent to which an unknown sample corrects the abnormality in plasma with a known deficiency is assumed to be proportional to the content of the deficient factor in the sample. The results of coagulation assays may be expressed in terms of units, which equal the amount of a given factor that is present in 1 mL of normal pooled or reference plasma. Alternatively, plasma levels of various factors may be expressed as a percentage of normal. Thus, plasma levels of various coagulation factors typically range from 50 to 150 U/dL, or 50% to 150% of normal.

One-stage methods for factors VIII and IX, which are based on the PTT and use substrate plasma from patients with severe inherited deficiencies (<1% of normal) of these factors, are somewhat simpler to perform than comparable two-stage methods. However, two-stage methods are more specific than one-stage methods, particularly in patients with intravascular coagulation and liver disease,[94] presumably because the two-stage methods are less affected by the presence of activated coagulation factors or traces of thrombin that increase the activity of factors V and VIII. One study found that, for detecting low factor VIII levels, the clot-based assay was better than the chromogenic assay, whereas for elevated factor VIII levels, the chromogenic assay was preferred.[95] Plasmas deficient in specific factors are available commercially. Details of coagulation assay methodology have been summarized.[96]

Tests for Inhibitors of Coagulation

Abnormalities in any test of coagulation, if caused by deficiency of an essential factor, are corrected by the addition of small amounts of normal plasma. If the abnormality is caused by the presence of one of the various inhibitors of coagulation rather than a deficiency of an essential factor, the opposite is true: small amounts of the patient's plasma impair coagulation in normal samples. These tests are called *mixing studies* or *inhibitor screens*. This phenomenon is the essence of all screening tests for inhibitors, most of which are based on one-stage coagulation techniques, such as the PT and PTT.[97] The presence of heparin may be confirmed in various ways, including the use of thrombin time and reptilase time assays, correction by protamine sulfate, or direct assays for activity of heparin or low-molecular-weight heparin.[96]

Tests for Physiologic Inhibitors of Coagulation

Several methods have been described for the assay of physiologic inhibitors of coagulation,[98] such as antithrombin,[99] heparin cofactor II, protein C,[98,100] and protein S.[101,102] Both immunologic and functional assays are available for many of these components.[98] Quantitative assays of such physiologic inhibitors may yield valuable information in patients with certain thromboembolic disorders (see Chapter 56).

Automated Coagulation Methods

Numerous instruments are available to detect automatically the end point of blood coagulation. These devices operate on a variety of principles: mechanical detection of the onset of fibrin formation, photometric recording of clot opacity, or the rate of fibrin polymerization. Such instruments are helpful in the performance of one-stage screening tests, such as the PT and PTT, especially if a large number of tests must be done daily.

Totally automated methods for performing coagulation tests are widely used. Automated instrument platforms have been developed to perform a large variety of coagulation methods with significant cost savings, permitting more laboratories to do comprehensive coagulation testing.[103] A College of American Pathologists website has summarized coagulation instrumentation (www.cap.org; see Online Product Guides at the CAP Today link).

Thromboelastography and *thromboelastometry* are coagulation methodologies that monitor viscoelastic changes in whole-blood clots during blood coagulation and fibrinolysis. Three versions of viscoelastic monitors are currently available on the market and have been increasingly adopted for use by trauma and cardiovascular services, primarily to guide transfusion practices. Different thromboelastograms are described in association with various bleeding disorders and hypercoagulable states.[104] This is not a commonly used methodology to diagnose coagulation abnormalities in laboratories. Its primary use is as a point-of-care instrument in the surgical setting.[48] A 2015 Cochrane Systematic Review concluded that there were insufficient data to support the use of thromboelastography or thromboelastometry to diagnose trauma-induced coagulopathy.[105] A 2016 update of a Cochrane Systematic Review evaluating the use of thromboelastography or thromboelastometry to monitor hemostatic treatment in adults or children found that there was low quality of evidence supporting the use of either method for the management of bleeding patients.[106] Although these methodologies may be helpful in blood product management, there are limited data that they improve key clinical outcomes.[107]

The activated clotting time (ACT) is a whole-blood clotting assay now used primarily as a point-of-care test. The ACT measures the clotting time for a whole-blood sample after addition of particulate (contact) activators such as kaolin or celite; thus, this assay measures the intrinsic pathway of coagulation. The ACT is used mostly to monitor anticoagulation in the setting of cardiopulmonary bypass, cardiac catheterization, or dialysis. The ACT is preferable to the PTT in certain settings that require high-dose heparin, such as cardiopulmonary bypass.[108]

Chromogenic and Fluorometric Techniques

Artificial peptides release chromogenic substances or fluorophores when they are enzymatically cleaved.[109] The hydrolysis of such peptides by activated coagulation factors provides a novel means for assessing various coagulation reactions.[110] Such chromogenic and fluorometric techniques have been developed for the assay of numerous coagulation and fibrinolytic analytes. These methods appear to be intrinsically more precise and may be less time consuming than traditional coagulation methods, and instruments designed specifically for their performance are available. Chromogenic and fluorometric assays are expensive, however, and are currently used mainly in research and in large reference coagulation laboratories.

INITIAL LABORATORY EVALUATION

Primary Screening Tests

The initial laboratory study of the bleeding patient should be guided by the information obtained from the clinical evaluation. In many cases, however, the routine use of a small battery of screening tests has merit because it usually saves time, and the results direct the course of further study. It is generally agreed that the most essential information can usually be obtained from the three tests summarized in *Table 46.3*, which, in view of their availability, simplicity, and low cost, are well suited to serve as primary screening tests. The platelet count provides the most reliable and reproducible test of primary hemostasis. The PTT measures all of the coagulation factors involved in the intrinsic and common pathways (*Figure 46.4*) and is generally accepted as the best single screening test for disorders of blood coagulation. When supplemented with the PT, which assesses the extrinsic as well as the common pathway, the abnormality can be usually localized to one of the three pathways and the factors involved therein (*Figure 46.4* and *Table 46.3*). The results of these three tests thus provide a presumptive diagnosis, which can then be clarified further by the confirmatory methods summarized in the next section. The bleeding time test has been omitted from this evaluation because of its nonspecificity in the general clinical setting.[16,20] The definitive laboratory diagnosis of individual bleeding disorders is discussed in Chapters 47 to 55.

It is important to realize that patients with mild bleeding disorders (factor VIII, IX, or XI deficiency) may have normal PTT values, because most PTT reagents do not detect mild deficiency states (factor levels of 20%-30%).[60] Consequently, if the clinical suspicion is high, specific factor assays for these disorders should be performed, even if the initial evaluation suggested in *Table 46.3* is not productive.

CONFIRMATORY TESTS

Thrombocytopenia

Thrombocytopenia, like anemia, is a symptom, not a diagnosis. It is the most common of the acquired bleeding disorders. Additional laboratory tests are usually not indicated merely to confirm the presence of thrombocytopenia (*Table 46.3*) but are helpful in establishing the mechanism for thrombocytopenia. It is useful, however, to examine the thrombocytopenic patient's blood smear to exclude pseudothrombocytopenia, which may be seen in a small number of patients.[22,23] The differential diagnosis of thrombocytopenia is discussed at length in Chapters 47 to 50. One approach to evaluating thrombocytopenia is shown in *Figure 46.5*.

von Willebrand Disease

vWD is the result of an abnormality in primary hemostasis combined with mild to moderate deficiency of factor VIIIc (see Chapter 54). In the classic case, the results of screening tests reveal a normal platelet count and a prolonged PTT (*Table 46.3*). In many patients, however, the PTT will be normal. Furthermore, the results of all of the laboratory tests tend to fluctuate from time to time.[111] If the clinical suspicion is high, initial laboratory studies directed at excluding vWD should be performed because vWD is more common than the inherited disorders of platelet function (*Figure 46.6*). Useful tests include bioassay of factor VIII (VIIIc), immunoassay of vWF antigen, and measurement of ristocetin cofactor activity. In many cases, the diagnosis of vWD requires repeated testing.

Another available test to evaluate patients for vWD is multimeric analysis of vWF. Patient plasma is separated by agarose electrophoresis, and vWF is identified by immunologic methods. The patient's multimeric pattern is compared with that of normal plasma. A more detailed description of this test is given in Chapter 54.

Qualitative Platelet Disorders

Symptoms of mucocutaneous bleeding in the presence of a normal count of platelets and normal results of coagulation tests (*Table 46.3*) are presumptive evidence of a disorder of platelet function (see Chapter 53). Inherited forms are uncommon, but bleeding caused by platelet dysfunction may be an important complication in patients with various acquired disorders, such as uremia. Commonly available confirmatory tests occasionally provide useful information regarding platelet dysfunction. Various morphologic abnormalities of the platelets may be seen on the blood smear. Strikingly large platelets are characteristic of certain inherited disorders, such as Bernard-Soulier syndrome. A markedly elevated platelet count is present in the myeloproliferative disorder, essential thrombocytosis.

Definitive methods for the study of platelet dysfunction are time consuming and technically difficult. The absence of platelet aggregation by ADP, collagen, and epinephrine is characteristic of Glanzmann thrombasthenia. Deficient secondary wave aggregation is associated with various disorders of the release reaction, such as inherited deficiency of storage nucleotides, uremia, and aspirin ingestion. Abnormal responses to ristocetin indicate vWD or Bernard-Soulier syndrome.

Disorders of the Intrinsic Pathway of Coagulation

Disorders of the intrinsic pathway of coagulation are characterized by a prolonged PTT and a normal PT (*Table 46.3*). Inherited forms include deficiencies of factor VIII or IX (hemophilia A and hemophilia B), prekallikrein, high-molecular-weight kininogen, factor XI, or factor XII (*Figure 46.7*). Factor XII (Hageman factor) deficiency and deficiencies of prekallikrein or high-molecular-weight kininogen can be excluded readily because they are not associated with excessive clinical bleeding. Distinguishing between deficiencies of factors VIII, IX, and XI is done by performing specific assays for these factors. Screens (mixing studies) should also be performed to exclude

Table 46.3. Profiles of Hemostasis Screening Tests in Patients With Bleeding Disorders

Prothrombin Time	Activated Partial Thromboplastin Time	Platelet Count	Differential Diagnosis
↑	—	—	Common
			Acquired factor VII deficiency (early liver disease, early vitamin K deficiency, early warfarin therapy)
			Rare
			Factor VII inhibitor, dysfibrinogenemia, some cases of DIC, inherited factor VII deficiency, certain factor X variants
—	↑	—	Common
			Deficiency or inhibitor of factor VIII, IX, or XI; vWD; heparin
			Rare
			Lupus inhibitor with qualitative platelet defect, certain factor X variants
↑	↑	—	Common
			Vitamin K deficiency, liver disease, warfarin, heparin, superwarfarin
			Rare
			Deficiency or inhibitor of factor X or V, prothrombin, or fibrinogen; lupus inhibitor with hypoprothrombinemia; DIC; dysfibrinogenemia; primary fibrinolysis
↑	↑	↓	Common
			DIC, liver disease
			Rare
			Heparin therapy with associated thrombocytopenia
—	—	↓	Common
			Increased platelet destruction, decreased platelet production, hypersplenism, hemodilution
			Rare
			Certain inherited platelet disorders (Wiskott-Aldrich syndrome, Bernard-Soulier syndrome)
—	—	↑	Myeloproliferative disorders
—	—	—	Common
			Mild vWD, acquired qualitative platelet disorders (uremia, antiplatelet medications)
			Rare
			Inherited qualitative platelet disorders, vascular disorders, fibrinolytic disorders, factor XIII deficiency, autoerythrocyte sensitization, dysfibrinogenemia, mild factor deficiency (VIII, IX, and XI), disorders of platelet procoagulant activity

The differential diagnosis of bleeding disorders suggested by results of the PT, PTT, and platelet count is listed for each profile. This table includes the differential diagnosis of hemostasis screening test results in patients with a history of bleeding. Consideration of patients with abnormal coagulation tests and negative bleeding histories is not included in this table.
Abbreviations: —, normal; ↑, increased; ↓, decreased; DIC, disseminated intravascular coagulation; vWD, von Willebrand disease.
Modified with permission from Rodgers GM. Common clinical bleeding disorders. In: Boldt DH, ed. *Update on Hemostasis*. Churchill Livingstone; 1990;75-120. Copyright © Dr. David H. Boldt.

antibodies to the intrinsic factor under study. If a factor VIII inhibitor is identified, the titer should be quantitated (see Chapter 55). An algorithm approach for evaluating bleeding patients with an isolated, prolonged PTT is shown in *Figure 46.8*.

Acquired coagulation disorders associated with a prolonged PTT and a normal PT include the lupus inhibitor and antibodies to factor VIII. Prolongation of the PTT is commonly the result of heparin administration or poorly collected blood samples.

Disorders of the Common Pathway of Coagulation

Prolongation of the PTT and PT in a patient with an inherited bleeding disorder indicates a deficiency of one of the factors in the common pathway—factor X, factor V, prothrombin, fibrinogen, or a dysfibrinogen (*Table 46.3* and *Figure 46.7*). Such isolated deficiencies are exceedingly rare. On the other hand, deficiency of one or more of these factors is associated with additional abnormalities in the intrinsic and extrinsic pathways in many of the common acquired coagulation disorders, such as vitamin K deficiency, liver disease, and DIC. A prolonged PT usually suggests an acquired disorder (excluding the rare cases of inherited factor VII deficiency) and is usually associated with a complex abnormality involving multiple pathways, such as DIC.

When confronted with this combination of findings, the first step should be to exclude or to identify an abnormality of fibrinogen. This may be accomplished by determination of the plasma fibrinogen level and tests for increased amounts of D-dimer or FDP. The most helpful ancillary procedures are the platelet count and examination of the blood smear for schistocytes. The laboratory findings characteristic of DIC are summarized in Chapter 55.

Inherited disorders associated with a low fibrinogen level include afibrinogenemia, hypofibrinogenemia, and dysfibrinogenemia (see Chapter 54). Inherited deficiencies of factor V, factor X, and prothrombin can be diagnosed by specific factor assays.

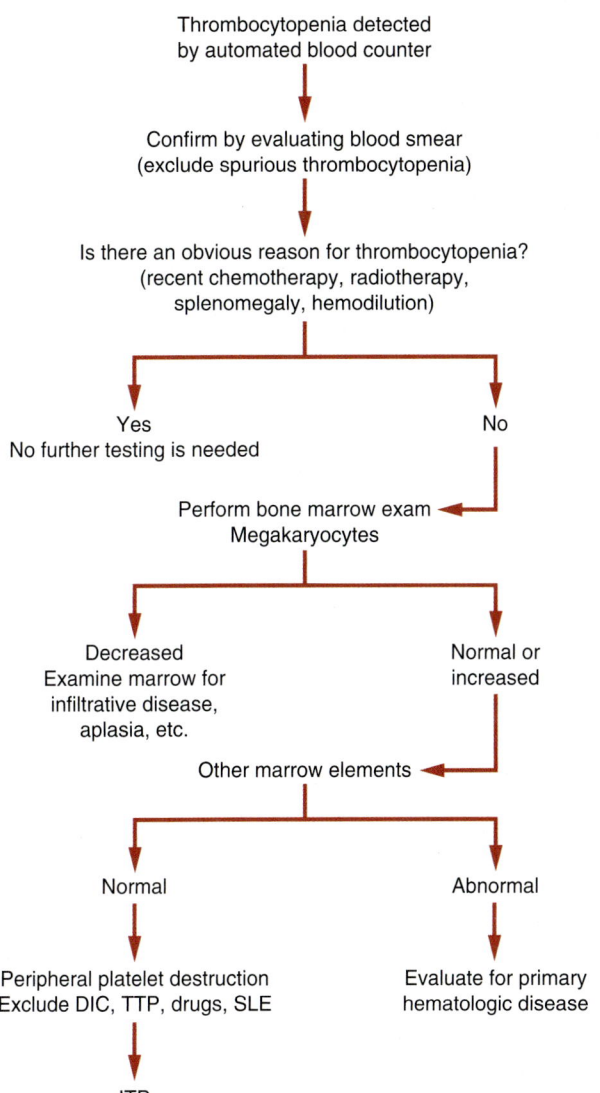

FIGURE 46.5 An approach for evaluation of thrombocytopenia. Idiopathic thrombocytopenic purpura (ITP) is a diagnosis of exclusion. DIC, disseminated intravascular coagulation; SLE, systemic lupus erythematosus; TTP, thrombotic thrombocytopenic purpura. (Redrawn from Kjeldsberg C, ed. *Practical Diagnosis of Hematologic Disorders.* 4th ed. ASCP Press; 2006:319. Copyright © 2006 by American Society for Clinical Pathologists.)

Disorders of the Extrinsic Pathway of Coagulation

A prolonged PT and a normal PTT (*Table 46.3*) suggest an isolated deficiency of factor VII, which is rare and may be the result of an inherited or an acquired abnormality (*Figures 46.7* and *46.9*). Less commonly, inhibitors of factor VII have been reported (see Chapter 55). In addition, certain cases of DIC or dysfibrinogenemia may present with isolated prolonged PT values.[112] Because factor VII is essential only in the tissue factor–activated extrinsic pathway of coagulation, the Stypven time is normal in patients with factor VII deficiency.

Disorders in Which Results of Primary Screening Tests Are Normal

Screening tests usually yield normal results in patients with bleeding disorders related to vascular abnormalities (*Tables 46.3* and *46.4*). The diagnosis is usually made from the associated clinical findings that are often characteristic, such as the skin lesions of hereditary hemorrhagic telangiectasia, allergic purpura, scurvy, and Bateman purpura. The results of screening tests are also normal in factor XIII (fibrin-stabilizing factor) deficiency, a disorder in which the diagnosis is made by the demonstration of characteristic clot solubility in urea or monochloroacetic acid.

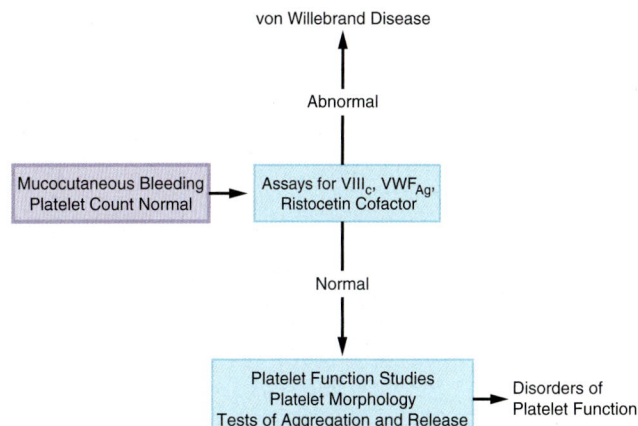

FIGURE 46.6 Laboratory diagnosis of von Willebrand disease (vWD) and platelet dysfunction. The initial evaluation reveals mucocutaneous bleeding symptoms in a patient with a normal platelet count (block on left). In vWD, the partial thromboplastin time may also be prolonged because of deficiency of factor VIIIc. Additional tests (blocks) and a suggested sequence for their performance are indicated as a flow diagram. Some patients with vWD may have normal assays for factor VIIIc, von Willebrand factor Ag (vWF$_{Ag}$), and ristocetin cofactor activity. These patients may be diagnosed by abnormal ristocetin-induced platelet agglutination when aggregation studies are performed, by measuring collagen-binding activity, or by multimeric analysis of vWF. For patients with normal studies for vWD and platelet dysfunction who are strongly suspected of having an inherited disorder, von Willebrand studies should be repeated.

Although abnormal in the typical case, the results of screening tests may be normal or equivocal in patients with mild coagulation disorders (including heterozygous carriers), certain disorders of platelet function, mild forms of vWD, and dysfibrinogenemia or abnormal fibrinolysis.[95,113] More definitive tests are required to establish the diagnosis in these patients (*Table 46.4*). An increasing number of reports have indicated that many bleeding patients with normal screening studies have disorders of platelet procoagulant activity, such as Scott syndrome.[114]

There are patients with a significant bleeding history in whom the results of detailed studies of hemostasis and blood coagulation are normal. Some have disorders of hemostasis that cannot be detected by methods currently available. The clinical management of these cases requires great care, and the fact that a clear-cut history of bleeding is always more significant than negative laboratory data cannot be overemphasized.

PREOPERATIVE HEMOSTASIS EVALUATION

The value of obtaining routine screening tests before surgical procedures has been debated for years.[115] The screening tests for hemostasis are not totally satisfactory in detecting all mild hemostatic defects. Nevertheless, routine preoperative laboratory screening is of great value in certain high-risk patients who have disorders that predispose them to unexpected postsurgical bleeding, even from limited biopsy procedures. Important in this category are patients with liver disease, biliary obstruction, renal disease (particularly if complicated by azotemia), myelofibrosis, polycythemia vera, and other myeloproliferative disorders, particularly those associated with thrombocytosis and those with paraproteinemias. Included in this list should be all patients scheduled to undergo procedures involving the use of extracorporeal circulatory devices.

One approach to the question of preoperative hemostasis screening tests is to balance the financial costs of laboratory testing with the extent of surgery to be performed and with the amount of bleeding that can be safely tolerated. This approach makes the patient's hemostasis history

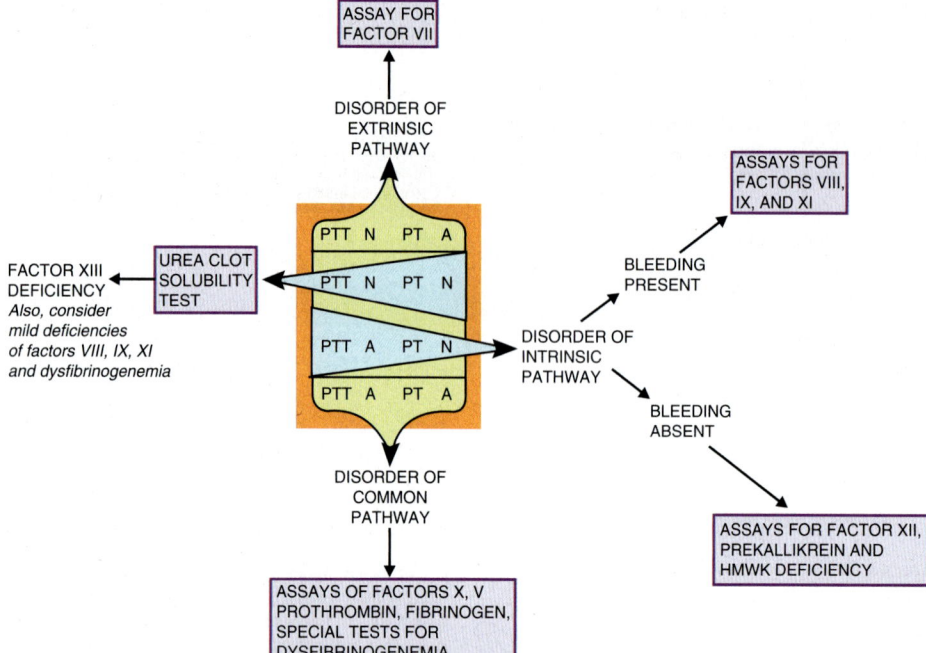

FIGURE 46.7 Laboratory diagnosis of inherited coagulation disorders. Results of primary screening tests of coagulation (activated partial thromboplastin time [PTT], prothrombin time [PT]) are summarized in the center block. Additional tests (blocks) and a suggested sequence for their performance are presented as a flow diagram. A more complete list of the differential diagnosis of bleeding disorders is presented in *Table 46.3*. A, abnormal; HMWK, high-molecular-weight kininogen; N, normal.

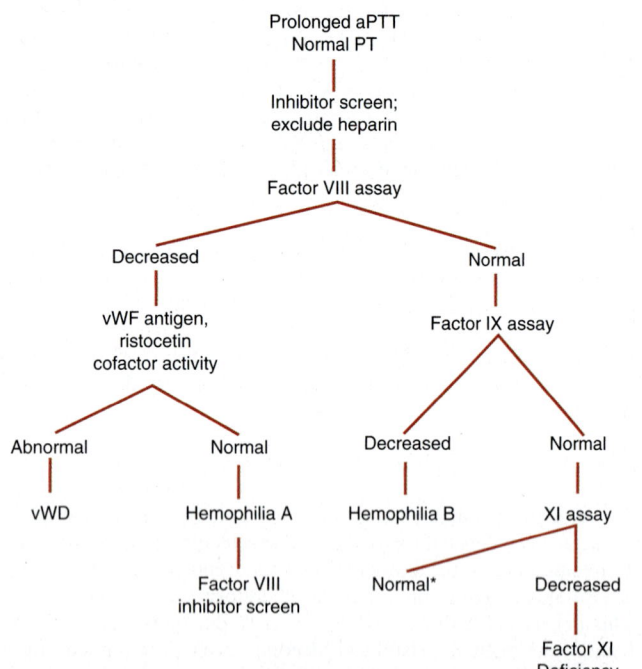

FIGURE 46.8 Evaluation of a patient with bleeding and an isolated, prolonged partial thromboplastin time (PTT). Asterisk indicates that patients with clinical bleeding but normal studies should be evaluated further for lupus anticoagulants associated with either platelet dysfunction or thrombocytopenia. PT, prothrombin time; vWD, von Willebrand disease; vWF, von Willebrand factor. (Redrawn from Kjeldsberg CR, Perkins SL, eds. *Practical Diagnosis of Hematologic Disorders.* 5th ed. ASCP Press; 2010:349. Copyright © 2010 by American Society for Clinical Pathologists.)

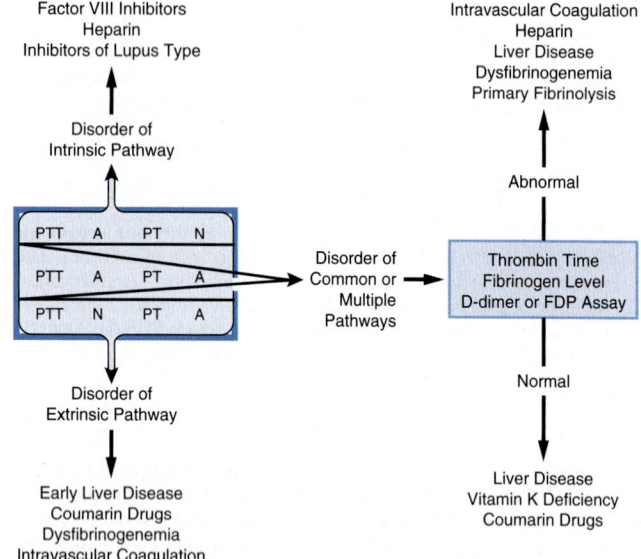

FIGURE 46.9 Laboratory diagnosis of acquired coagulation disorders. Results of primary screening tests of coagulation (partial thromboplastin time [PTT], prothrombin time [PT]) are summarized in the left-side block. Additional tests (right-side block) and a suggested sequence for their performance are presented as a flow diagram. Because of the complexity of acquired coagulation disorders and great variations in the results of laboratory tests that may be encountered in the various disorders and in individual patients, this diagram should be regarded as a general guide only. A more complete list of the differential diagnosis of bleeding disorders is presented in *Table 46.3*. A, abnormal; FDP, fibrin degradation products; N, normal.

Table 46.4. Bleeding Disorders in Which the Results of Primary Screening Tests May Be Normal

von Willebrand Disease
Mild inherited coagulation disorders, particularly factor XI deficiency
Heterozygous carriers of inherited coagulation disorders
Factor XIII (fibrin-stabilizing factor) deficiency
Some forms of dysfibrinogenemia
Disordered platelet function, particularly deficient release reaction; Scott syndrome
Hereditary hemorrhagic telangiectasia
Allergic and other vascular purpuras
α_2-Plasmin inhibitor deficiency
Elevated levels of plasminogen activator
Psychogenic purpura (autoerythrocyte sensitization)

Table 46.5. Guidelines for Preoperative Hemostasis Evaluation

Level	Bleeding History	Surgical Procedure	Recommended Hemostasis Evaluation
I	Negative	Minor	None
II	Negative	Major	Platelet count, PTT
III	Equivocal	Major, involving hemostatic impairment	PT, PTT, platelet count, factor XIII assay, FDP
IV	Positive	Major or minor	Level III tests; if negative, then factors VIII, IX, and XI assays, thrombin time, α_2-antiplasmin assay; consider von Willebrand disease and platelet aggregation testing; consider specific tests for uncommon disorders listed in *Table 46.3*

Information in this table is a revision based on the suggested preoperative guidelines for hemostasis testing by Rapaport.[115] The bleeding time is omitted as a hemostasis test because of more recent appreciation of its weakness as a useful test. The FDP test screens for abnormal fibrinolysis. Comprehensive testing should be performed on level IV patients. Abbreviations: FDP, fibrin degradation products; PT, prothrombin time; PTT, partial thromboplastin time.
Modified from Rodgers GM. Preoperative hemostasis screening. In: Kjeldsberg CR, Perkins SL, eds. *Practical Diagnosis of Hematologic Disorders*. 5th ed. ASCP Press; 2010:373. Copyright © 2010 by American Society for Clinical Pathologists.

particularly important. Patients scheduled for minor surgical procedures (dental and skin biopsy) do not need routine hemostasis screening tests if they have a negative history. In contrast, patients undergoing neurosurgery or other procedures that may induce a hemostatic defect (use of a bypass pump) or patients with a positive bleeding history need a hemostasis evaluation by the laboratory. *Table 46.5* summarizes the recommendations of Rapaport in evaluating preoperative patients.[115]

EVALUATION OF THE NEONATE

Laboratory investigation of hemostasis and blood coagulation in the neonate and infant differs from that just outlined in several respects.[116] First, the quantity of blood that can be obtained is limited, and often, the venipuncture is difficult. Second, in terms of adult norms, the results of some tests are abnormal, even in healthy full-term infants (*Table 46.6*). Such physiologic abnormalities are presumably the result of deficiencies of the vitamin K–dependent factors and of additional abnormalities in the contact phase of coagulation and in the thrombin-fibrinogen reaction.[4,117]

The PT may be prolonged but is often normal if vitamin K is administered to the infant or mother.[117] Abnormalities of the thrombin time and the PTT are present in many normal neonates. These findings usually disappear within 2 to 6 months.[4] These abnormalities and moderate deficiencies of the vitamin K–dependent factors (prothrombin; factors VII, IX, and X; and proteins C and S) are more pronounced in the premature than in the full-term infant, and they are inversely proportional to gestational age and birth weight. Levels of factors VIII and V as well as antithrombin may be low in extremely premature infants.[118] Factor VIII levels and the ratio of vWF_{Ag} to VIIIc are higher in term infants than in adults or older children.

Levels of factor V are normal in both neonates and thriving premature infants.[117,119] Levels of antithrombin and other physiologic inhibitors of coagulation and of factor XIII are below adult norms in term neonates.[120] Significant abnormalities of platelet aggregation and of the results of other platelet function tests may be seen in normal neonates.[121] The newborn is also abnormally susceptible to drugs that impair platelet function, including those transferred placentally from the mother. The platelet count in term infants, as well as in thriving premature infants, is within the range found in adults and older children. *Table 46.6* summarizes coagulation reference ranges in newborns, children, and adults.

Table 46.6. Age-Related Coagulation Reference Values in Newborns, Children, and Adults

Coagulation Tests	Age								
	3 days[a]	1-12 months[a]	1-5 years[a]	7-9 years[b,c]	10-11 years[b,c]	12-13 years[b,c]	14-15 years[b,c]	16-17 years[b,c]	Adult[b,c]
Fibrinogen (g/L)	2.83-4.01	0.82-3.83	1.62-4.01	1.98-4.13	1.97-4.10	2.15-3.78	2.04-3.92	2.08-4.38	2.11-4.41
Prothrombin (U/mL)	0.50-0.73	0.62-1.03	0.70-1.09	0.78-1.25	0.78-1.20	0.72-1.23	0.75-1.35	0.77-1.30	0.86-1.50
Factor V (U/mL)	0.92-1.54	0.94-1.41	0.67-1.27	0.69-1.32	0.66-1.36	0.66-1.35	0.61-1.29	0.65-1.31	0.62-1.40
Factor VII (U/mL)	0.67-1.07	0.83-1.60	0.72-1.50	0.67-1.45	0.71-1.63	0.78-1.60	0.74-1.80	0.63-1.63	0.80-1.81
Factor VIII (U/mL)	0.83-2.74	0.54-1.45	0.36-1.85	0.76-1.99	0.80-2.09	0.72-1.98	0.69-2.37	0.63-2.21	0.56-1.91
Factor IX (U/mL)	0.44-0.97	0.43-1.21	0.44-1.27	0.70-1.33	0.72-1.49	0.73-1.52	0.80-1.61	0.86-1.76	0.78-1.84
Factor X (U/mL)	0.46-0.75	0.77-1.22	0.72-1.25	0.74-1.30	0.70-1.34	0.69-1.33	0.63-1.46	0.74-1.46	0.81-1.57
Factor XI (U/mL)	0.24-0.79	0.62-1.25	0.65-1.62	0.70-1.38	0.66-1.37	0.68-1.38	0.57-1.29	0.65-1.59	0.56-1.53
vWF$_{Ag}$ (U/mL)	—	—	—	0.62-1.80[d]	0.63-1.89[d]	0.60-1.89[d]	0.57-1.99[d]	0.50-2.05[d]	0.52-2.14[d]
R:Cof (U/mL)	—	—	—	0.52-1.76	0.60-1.95	0.50-1.84	0.50-2.03	0.49-2.04	0.51-2.15
Antithrombin (U/mL)	0.60-0.89	0.72-1.34	1.01-1.31	0.90-1.35	0.90-1.34	0.90-1.32	0.90-1.31	0.87-1.31	0.76-1.28
Protein C (U/mL)	0.24-0.51	0.28-1.24	0.50-1.34	0.70-1.42	0.68-1.43	0.66-1.62	0.69-1.70	0.70-1.71	0.83-1.68
Protein S[e] (U/mL)	0.33-0.67	0.29-1.62	0.67-1.36	M 0.66-1.40	0.65-1.39	0.72-1.39	0.68-1.45	0.77-1.67	0.66-1.43
				F 0.62-1.51	0.65-1.42	0.70-1.40	0.55-1.45	0.51-1.47	0.57-1.31
Plasminogen (U/mL)	—	—	—	0.76-1.16	0.74-1.17	0.66-1.14	0.71-1.24	0.75-1.32	0.71-1.44
α$_2$-Antiplasmin (U/mL)	—	—	—	0.88-1.47	0.90-1.44	0.87-1.42	0.83-1.36	0.77-1.34	0.82-1.33

PT and PTT values are not shown because these values depend on reagent selection. Adult values represent those of the University of Utah Medical Center Hemostasis and Thrombosis Laboratory. There are no data for children aged 6 years.
Abbreviation: vWF$_{Ag}$, von Willebrand factor Ag.
[a]Monagle P, Barnes C, Ignjatovic V, et al. Developmental haemostasis. Impact for clinical haemostasis laboratories. *Thromb Haemost.* 2006;95:362-372.
[b]Flanders MM, Crist RA, Roberts WL, Rodgers GM. Pediatric reference intervals for seven common coagulation assays. *Clin Chem.* 2005;51:1738-1742.
[c]Flanders MM, Phansalkar AR, Crist RA, et al. Pediatric reference intervals for uncommon bleeding and thrombotic disorders. *J Pediatr.* 2006;149:275-277.
[d]Results are of antigenic assays; all other results are of functional assays.
[e]Gender-specific reference ranges are given for protein S for children aged 7 to 9 years and older.

References

1. Wahlberg T, Blomback M, Hall P, Axelsson G. Application of indicators, predictors and diagnostic indices in coagulation disorders. *Methods Inf Med.* 1980;19:194-200.
2. Fasulo MR, Biguzzi E, Abbattista M, et al. The ISTH bleeding assessment tool and the risk of future bleeding. *J Thromb Haemost.* 2018;16:125-130.
3. Lorand L, Losowsky MS, Miloszewski KJ. Human factor XIII: fibrin-stabilizing factor. *Prog Hemost Thromb.* 1980;5:245-290.
4. Oski FA, Naiman JL. *Hematologic Problems in the Newborn.* WB Saunders; 1966.
5. Glader BE, Buchanan GR. The bleeding neonate. *Pediatrics.* 1976;58:548-555.
6. Biggs R, MacFarlane RG. Haemophilia and related conditions: a survey of 187 cases. *Br J Haematol.* 1958;4:1-27.
7. Goulian M, Beck WS. The partial thromboplastin time test. *Am J Clin Pathol.* 1965;44:97-103.
8. Quick AJ. Determination of prothrombin. *Am J Med Sci.* 1935;190:501-511.
9. Ratnoff OD, Menzie C. A new method for the determination of fibrinogen in small samples of plasma. *J Lab Clin Med.* 1951;37:316-320.
10. Marder VJ, Cruz GO, Schumer BR. Evaluation of a new anti-fibrinogen-coated latex particle agglutination test in the measurement of serum fibrin degradation products. *Thromb Haemost.* 1977;37:183-191.
11. Day HJ, Rao AK. Evaluation of platelet function. *Semin Hematol.* 1986;23:89-101.
12. Livio M, Gotti E, Marchesi D. Uraemic bleeding: role of anaemia and beneficial effect of red cell transfusions. *Lancet.* 1982;2:1013-1015.
13. Weiss HJ, Rogers J. Fibrinogen and platelets in the primary arrest of bleeding. Study in two patients with congenital afibrinogenemia. *N Engl J Med.* 1971;285:369-374.
14. Breederveld K, van Royen EA, ten Cate JW. Severe factor V deficiency with prolonged bleeding time. *Thromb Diath Haemorrh.* 1974;32:538-548.
15. Evensen SA, Myhre L, Stormorken H. Haemostatic studies in osteogenesis imperfecta. *Scand J Haematol.* 1984;33:177-179.
16. Rodgers RP, Levin J. A critical reappraisal of the bleeding time. *Semin Thromb Hemost.* 1990;16:1-144.
17. O'Laughlin JC, Hoftiezer JW, Mahoney JP, Ivey KJ. Does aspirin prolong bleeding from gastric biopsies in man? *Gastrointest Endosc.* 1981;27:1-5.
18. Lind SE. The bleeding time does not predict surgical bleeding. *Blood.* 1991;77:2547-2552.
19. Lehman CM, Blaylock RC, Alexander DP, Rodgers GM. Discontinuation of the bleeding time test without detectable adverse clinical impact. *Clin Chem.* 2001;47:1204-1211.
20. Peterson P, Hayes TE, Arkin CF, et al. The preoperative bleeding time test lacks clinical benefit. *Arch Surg.* 1998;133:134-139.
21. Manthorpe R, Kofod B, Wiik A, et al. Pseudothrombocytopenia. In vitro studies on the underlying mechanism. *Scand J Haematol.* 1981;26:385-392.
22. Onder O, Weinstein A, Hoyer LW. Pseudothrombocytopenia caused by platelet agglutinins that are reactive in blood anticoagulated with chelating agents. *Blood.* 1980;56:177-182.
23. Lindsay RM, Koens F, Linton AL. An evaluation of the Coulter thrombocounter in counting platelets before and after contact with foreign surfaces and its use in tests of platelet retention. *J Lab Clin Med.* 1975;86:863-872.
24. Kjeldsberg CR, Hershgold EJ. Spurious thrombocytopenia. *JAMA.* 1974;227:628-630.
25. Nicholls PD. Erroneous platelet counts on the Coulter Model S Plus counter after correction for hyperlipaemia. *Med Lab Sci.* 1983;40:69-71.
26. Payne BA, Pierre RV. Pseudothrombocytopenia: a laboratory artifact with potentially serious consequences. *Mayo Clin Proc.* 1984;59:123-125.
27. Savage RA. Pseudoleukocytosis due to EDTA-induced platelet clumping. *Am J Clin Pathol.* 1984;81:317-322.
28. Akwari AM, Ross DW, Stass SA. Spuriously elevated platelet counts due to microspherocytosis. *Am J Clin Pathol.* 1982;77:220-221.
29. Armitage JO, Goeken JA, Feagler JR. Spurious elevation of platelet count in acute leukemia. *JAMA.* 1978;239:433-434.
30. Morton BD, Orringer EP, LaHart L, Stass SA. Pappenheimer bodies. An additional cause for a spurious platelet count. *Am J Clin Pathol.* 1980;74:310-311.
31. Trowbridge EA, Martin JF. The platelet volume distribution: a signature of the prethrombotic state in coronary artery disease? *Thromb Haemost.* 1987;58:714-717.
32. Bessman JD, Gardner FH. Platelet size in thrombocytopenia due to sepsis. *Surg Gynecol Obstet.* 1983;156:177-180.

33. Karpatkin S, Freedman ML. Hypersplenic thrombocytopenia differentiated from increased peripheral destruction by platelet volume. *Ann Intern Med.* 1978;89:200-203.
34. Milton JG, Yung W, Frojmovic MM. Dependence of platelet volume measurements on heterogeneity of platelet morphology. *Biophys J.* 1981;35:257-261.
35. Roper-Drewinko PR, Drewinko B, Corrigan G, et al. Standardization of platelet function tests. *Am J Hematol.* 1981;11:183-203.
36. Corpataux N, Franke K, Kille A, et al. Reticulated platelets in medicine: current evidence and further perspectives. *J Clin Med.* 2020;9:3737.
37. Feinman RD, Lubowsky J, Charo I, Zabinski MP. The lumi-aggregometer: a new instrument for simultaneous measurement of secretion and aggregation by platelets. *J Lab Clin Med.* 1977;90:125-129.
38. Walsh PN, Mills DC, White JG. Metabolism and function of human platelets washed by albumin density gradient separation. *Br J Haematol.* 1977;36:281-296.
39. Challen A, Branch WJ, Cummings JH. Quantitation of platelet mass during aggregation in the electronic (Wellcome) whole-blood aggregometer. *J Pharmacol Methods.* 1982;8:115-122.
40. Ingerman-Wojenski CM, Silver MJ. A quick method for screening platelet dysfunctions using the whole-blood lumi-aggregometer. *Thromb Haemost.* 1984;51:154-156.
41. Miller JL. Platelet function testing: an improved approach utilizing lumi-aggregation and an interactive computer system. *Am J Clin Pathol.* 1984;81:471-476.
42. Hardisty RM, Hutton RA, Montgomery D, et al. Secondary platelet aggregation: a quantitative study. *Br J Haematol.* 1970;19:307-319.
43. Weiss HJ, Chervenick PA, Zalusky R, Factor A. A familial defect in platelet function associated with impaired release of adenosine diphosphate. *N Engl J Med.* 1969;281:1264-1270.
44. Niewiarowski S, Lowery CT, Hawiger J, et al. Immunoassay of human platelet factor 4 (PF4, antiheparin factor) by radial immunodiffusion. *J Lab Clin Med.* 1976;87:720-733.
45. Zhou L, Schmaier AH. Platelet aggregation testing in platelet-rich plasma. Description of procedures with the aim to develop standards in the field. *Am J Clin Pathol.* 2005;123:172-183.
46. Cattaneo M, Cerletti C, Harrison P, et al. Recommendations for the standardization of light transmission aggregometry: a consensus of the working party from the platelet physiology subcommittee of SSC/ISTH. *J Thromb Haemost.* 2013;11:1183-1189.
47. Israels SJ. Laboratory testing for platelet function disorders. *Int J Lab Hematol.* 2015;37(suppl 1):18-24.
48. Harrison P, Lordkipanidzé M. Testing platelet function. *Hematol Oncol Clin North Am.* 2013;27:411-441.
49. Kundu SK, Heilmann EJ, Sio R, et al. Description of an in vitro platelet function analyzer-PFA-100. *Semin Thromb Hemost.* 1995;21:106-112.
50. Ortel TL, James AH, Thames EH, et al. Assessment of primary hemostasis by PFA-100 analysis in a tertiary care center. *Thromb Haemost.* 2000;84:93-97.
51. Hayward CP, Harrison P, Cattaneo M, Ortel TL, Rao AK. Platelet physiology subcommittee of the scientific and standardization committee of the international society on thrombosis and haemostasis. Platelet function analyzer (PFA)-100 closure time in the evaluation of platelet disorders and platelet function. *J Thromb Haemost.* 2006;4:312-319.
52. Bennett ST, Lehman CM, Rodgers GM, eds. *Practical Handbook of Laboratory Hemostasis for Pathologists.* 2nd ed. Springer; 2015.
53. Kwak YL, Kim JC, Choi YS, Yoo KJ, Song Y, Shim JK. Clopidogrel responsiveness regardless of the discontinuation date predicts increased blood loss and transfusion requirement after off-pump coronary artery bypass graft surgery. *J Am Coll Cardiol.* 2010;56:1994-2002.
54. Breet NL, van Werkum JW, Bouman HJ, et al. Comparison of platelet function tests in predicting clinical outcome in implantation. *JAMA.* 2010;303:754-762.
55. Gurbel PA, Mahla E, Tantry US. Peri-operative platelet function testing: the potential for reducing ischaemic and bleeding risks. *Thromb Haemost.* 2011;106:248-252.
56. Jacobsson B, Nilsson IM. Catheter material and blood coagulation studies in vitro. *Scand J Haematol.* 1969;6:386-394.
57. Koepke JA, Rodgers JL, Ollivier MJ. Pre-instrumental variables in coagulation testing. *Am J Clin Pathol.* 1975;64:591-596.
58. Bell WN, Alton HG. A brain extract as a substitute for platelet suspensions in the thromboplastin generation test. *Nature.* 1954;174:880-881.
59. Nye SW, Graham JB, Brinkhous KM. The partial thromboplastin time as a screening test for the detection of latent bleeders. *Am J Med Sci.* 1962;243:279-287.
60. Martin BA, Branch DW, Rodgers GM. The preparation of a sensitive partial thromboplastin reagent from bovine brain. *Blood Coagul Fibrinolysis.* 1992;3:287-294.
61. Tripodi A, Chantarangkul V, Martinelli I, et al. A shortened activated partial thromboplastin time is associated with the risk of venous thromboembolism. *Blood.* 2004;104:3631-3634.
62. Edson JR, Krivit W, White JG. Kaolin partial thromboplastin time: high levels of procoagulants producing short clotting times or masking deficiencies of other procoagulants or low concentrations of anticoagulants. *J Lab Clin Med.* 1967;70:463-470.
63. Proctor RR, Rapaport SI. The partial thromboplastin time with kaolin. *Am J Clin Pathol.* 1961;36:212-219.
64. Robbins JA, Rose SD. Partial thromboplastin time as a screening test. *Ann Intern Med.* 1979;90:796-797.
65. Margolis J. Initiation of blood coagulation by glass and related surfaces. *J Physiol.* 1957;137:95-109.
66. Hattersley PG, Hayse D. The effect of increased contact activation time on the activated partial thromboplastin time. *Am J Clin Pathol.* 1976;66:479-482.
67. Flanders MM, Crist RA, Roberts WL, Rodgers GM. Pediatric reference intervals for seven common coagulation assays. *Clin Chem.* 2005;51:1738-1742.
68. Reddy NM, Hall SW, MacKintosh FR. Partial thromboplastin time. Prediction of adverse events and poor prognosis by low abnormal values. *Arch Intern Med.* 1999;159:2706-2710.
69. Quick AJ. Determination of prothrombin. *Proc Soc Exp Biol Med.* 1939;42:788-789.
70. Quick AJ. On the quantitative estimation of prothrombin. *Am J Clin Pathol.* 1945;15:560-566.
71. Boekhout-Mussert MJ, vander Kolk-Schaap PJ, Hermans J, Loeliger EA. Prospective double-blind clinical trial of bovine, human, and rabbit thromboplastins in monitoring long-term oral anticoagulation. *Am J Clin Pathol.* 1981;75:297-303.
72. Tripodi A, Chantarangkul V, Braga M, et al. Results of a multicentre study assessing the status of a recombinant thromboplastin. *Thromb Haemost.* 1994;72:261-267.
73. Ellis BC, Stransky A. A quick and accurate method for the determination of fibrinogen in plasma. *J Lab Clin Med.* 1961;58:477-488.
74. Feinberg JG. A new quantitative method for antigen-antibody titration in gels. *Nature.* 1956;177:530-531.
75. Koepke JA. Standardization of fibrinogen assays. *Scand J Haematol Suppl.* 1980;37:130-138.
76. Alving BM, Bell WR. Methods for correcting inhibitory effects of fibrinogen degradation products in fibrinogen determinations. *Thromb Res.* 1976;9:1-8.
77. Saleem A, Krieg AF, Fretz K. Improved micromethod for plasma fibrinogen unaffected by heparin therapy. *Am J Clin Pathol.* 1975;63:426-433.
78. Rodgers GM, Garr SB. Comparison of functional and antigenic fibrinogen values from a normal population. *Thromb Res.* 1992;68:207-210.
79. Jim RT. A study of the plasma thrombin time. *J Lab Clin Med.* 1957;50:45-60.
80. Marder VJ, Matchett MO, Sherry S. Detection of serum fibrinogen and fibrin degradation products. *Am J Med.* 1971;51:71-82.
81. Thomas DP, Niewiarowski S, Myers AR, et al. A comparative study of four methods for detecting fibrinogen degradation products in patients with various diseases. *N Engl J Med.* 1970;283:663-668.
82. Merskey C, Kleiner GJ, Johnson AJ. Quantitative estimation of split products of fibrinogen in human serum, relation to diagnosis and treatment. *Blood.* 1966;28:1-18.
83. Rutstein JE, Holahan JR, Lyons RM, Pope RM. Rheumatoid factor interference with the latex agglutination test for fibrin degradation products. *J Lab Clin Med.* 1978;92:529-535.
84. Edgington TS. Fibrinogen and fibrin degradation products: their differentiation. *Thromb Haemost.* 1975;34:671-676.
85. Johnson ED, Schell JC, Rodgers GM. The D-dimer assay. *Am J Hematol.* 2019;94:833-839.
86. Breen FA, Tullis JL. Ethanol gelation: a rapid screening test for intravascular coagulation. *Ann Intern Med.* 1968;69:1197-1206.
87. Gurewich V, Hutchinson E. Detection of intravascular coagulation by a serial-dilution protamine sulfate test. *Ann Intern Med.* 1971;75:895-902.
88. Francis JL. The detection and measurement of factor XIII activity: a review. *Med Lab Sci.* 1980;37:137-147.
89. Lowe ML, Cannon DC. Improved method for euglobulin clot lysis time. *Clin Biochem.* 1975;8:206-212.
90. Wu KK, Jacobsen CD, Hoak JC. Highly sensitive method for the assay of plasminogen. *J Lab Clin Med.* 1973;81:484-488.
91. Moroz LA, Gilmore NJ. A rapid and sensitive 125I-fibrin solid-phase fibrinolytic assay for plasmin. *Blood.* 1975;46:543-553.
92. Chandler WL, Schumer G, Stratton JR. Optimum conditions for the stabilization and measurement of tissue plasminogen activator in human plasma. *J Lab Clin Med.* 1989;113:362-371.
93. Angleton P, Chandler WL, Schmer G. Diurnal variation of tissue-type plasminogen activator and its rapid inhibitor (PAI-1). *Circulation.* 1989;79:101-106.
94. Rogers JS, Eyster ME. Relationship of factor VIII-like antigen (VIII AGN) and clot promoting activity (VIII AHF) as measured by one- and two-stage assays in patients with liver disease. *Br J Haematol.* 1976;34:655-661.
95. Chandler WL, Ferrell C, Lee J, Tun T, Kha H. Comparison of three methods for measuring factor VIII levels in plasma. *Am J Clin Pathol.* 2003;120:34-39.
96. Rodgers GM. Inherited coagulation disorders. In: Kjeldsberg CR, Perkins SL, eds. *Practical Diagnosis of Hematologic Disorders.* 5th ed. ASCP Press; 2010;345-356.
97. Schleider MA, Nachman RL, Jaffe EA, Coleman M. A clinical study of the lupus anticoagulant. *Blood.* 1976;48:499-509.
98. Rodgers GM, Chandler WL. Laboratory and clinical aspects of inherited thrombotic disorders. *Am J Hematol.* 1992;41:113-122.
99. Buller HR, ten Cate JW. Acquired antithrombin III deficiency: laboratory diagnosis, incidence, clinical implications, and treatment with antithrombin III concentrate. *Am J Med.* 1989;87(suppl 3B):44S-48S.
100. Marler RA, Adcock DM. Clinical evaluation of protein C: a comparative review of antigenic and functional assays. *Hum Pathol.* 1989;20:1040-1047.
101. Comp PC. Measurement of the natural anticoagulant protein S: how and when. *Am J Clin Pathol.* 1990;94:242-243.
102. Edson JR, Vogt JM, Huesman DA. Laboratory diagnosis of inherited protein S deficiency. *Am J Clin Pathol.* 1990;94:176-186.
103. Flanders MM, Crist R, Safapour S, Rodgers GM. Evaluation and performance characteristics of the STA-R coagulation analyzer. *Clin Chem.* 2002;48:1622-1624.
104. Zuckerman L, Cohen E, Vagher JP, et al. Comparison of thromboelastography with common coagulation tests. *Thromb Haemost.* 1981;46:752-756.
105. Hunt H, Stanworth S, Curry N, et al. Thromboelastography (TEG) and rotational thromboelastometry (ROTEM) for trauma induced coagulopathy in adult trauma patients with bleeding. *Cochrane Database Syst Rev.* 2015;2015:CD010438.
106. Wikkelsø A, Wetterslev J, Møller AM, Afshari A. Thromboelastography (TEG) or thromboelastometry (ROTEM) to monitor haemostatic treatment versus usual care in adults or children with bleeding. *Cochrane Database Syst Rev.* 2016;2016:CD007871.

107. Amgalan A, Allen T, Othman M, Ahmadzia HK. Systematic review of viscoelastic testing (TEG/ROTEM) in obstetrics and recommendations from the women's SSC of the ISTH. *J Thromb Haemost*. 2020;18:1813-1838.
108. Olson JD, Arkin CF, Brandt JT, et al. Laboratory monitoring of unfractionated heparin therapy. *Arch Pathol Lab Med*. 1998;122:782-798.
109. Fareed J, Messmore HL, Bermes EW. New perspectives in coagulation testing. *Clin Chem*. 1980;26:1380-1391.
110. Huseby RM, Smith RE. Synthetic oligopeptide substrates: their diagnostic application in blood coagulation, fibrinolysis, and other pathologic states. *Semin Thromb Hemost*. 1980;6:173-314.
111. Abildgaard CF, Suzuki Z, Harrison J, et al. Serial studies in von Willebrand disease: variability versus "variants". *Blood*. 1980;56:712-716.
112. Colman RW, Robboy SJ, Minna JD. Disseminated intravascular coagulation: a reappraisal. *Annu Rev Med*. 1979;30:359-374.
113. Bachman F. Diagnostic approach to mild bleeding disorders. *Semin Hematol*. 1980;17:292-305.
114. Solum NO. Procoagulant expression in platelets and defects leading to clinical disorders. *Arterioscler Thromb Vasc Biol*. 1999;19:2841-2846.
115. Rapaport SI. Preoperative hemostatic evaluation: which tests, if any? *Blood*. 1983;61:229-231.
116. Buchanan GR. Coagulation disorders in the neonate. *Pediatr Clin North Am*. 1986;33:203-220.
117. Aballi AM, de Lamerens S. Coagulation changes in the neonatal period and in early infancy. *Pediatr Clin North Am*. 1962;9:785-817.
118. Barnard DR, Simmons MA, Hathaway WE. Coagulation studies in extremely premature infants. *Pediatr Res*. 1979;13:1330-1335.
119. Holmberg L, Henriksson P, Ekelund H, Astedt B. Coagulation in the human fetus. Comparison with term newborn infants. *J Pediatr*. 1974;85:860-864.
120. Mahasandana C, Hathaway WE. Circulating anticoagulants in the newborn: relation to hypercoagulability and the idiopathic respiratory distress syndrome. *Pediatr Res*. 1973;7:670-673.
121. Mull MM, Hathaway WE. Altered platelet function in newborns. *Pediatr Res*. 1970;4:229-237.

Section 2 ■ THROMBOCYTOPENIA

Chapter 47 ■ Thrombocytopenia: Pathophysiology and Classification

GEORGE M. RODGERS

PATHOPHYSIOLOGY

Thrombocytopenia may be defined as a subnormal number of platelets in the circulating blood. It is the most common cause of abnormal bleeding. Despite the number and diversity of disorders that may be associated etiologically, thrombocytopenia results from only four processes: artifactual thrombocytopenia, deficient platelet production, accelerated platelet destruction, and abnormal distribution or pooling of the platelets within the body (*Figure 47.1*). The changes in the basic parameters of thrombopoiesis that are characteristic of each of these processes are summarized in *Table 47.1*.

Artifactual Thrombocytopenia

Artifactual thrombocytopenia, or falsely low platelet counts, occurs ex vivo when platelets are not counted accurately. This mechanism should be considered in patients who have thrombocytopenia but no petechiae or ecchymoses. Although inaccurate counting may occur in the presence of giant platelets[1] or with platelet satellitism,[2] the most common cause of artifactual thrombocytopenia is platelet clumping (pseudothrombocytopenia).[3] Platelet clumping in pseudothrombocytopenia appears to be caused by anticoagulant-dependent platelet agglutinins that are immunoglobulins (Igs) of IgG, IgA, or IgM subtypes. Although clumping is most commonly seen when blood is collected into ethylenediaminetetraacetic acid anticoagulant, other anticoagulants may cause clumping, even hirudin or Phe-Pro-Arg chloromethyl ketone.[4] Platelet clumping is also time dependent and varies with the type of instrumentation used for automatic counting.[4] There is evidence that the autoantibodies bind to glycoprotein IIb/IIIa,[5] and in one study, there was over 80% concordance between the presence of anticardiolipin antibody and platelet agglutinins in individual patient plasmas.[6] These autoantibodies have no known associations with disease or drugs and have been noted in some patients for over 10 years.[7]

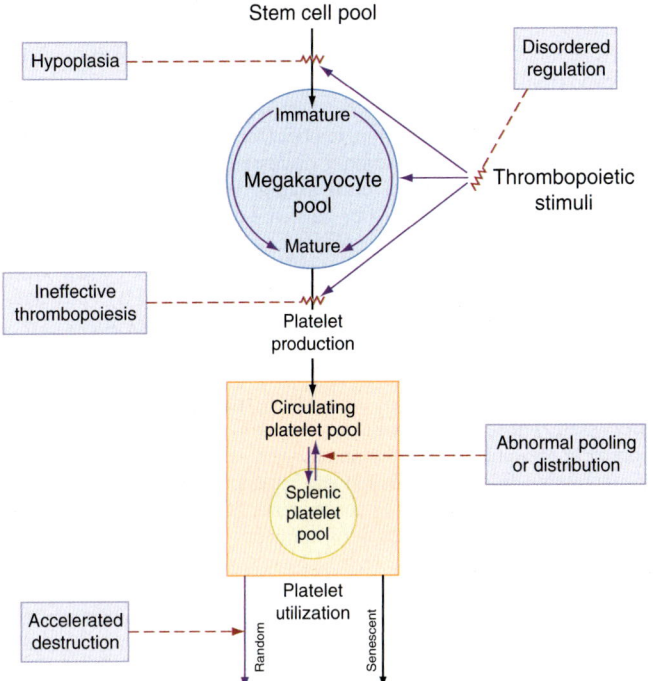

FIGURE 47.1 Pathophysiology of thrombocytopenia. A simplified diagram of the biodynamics of the megakaryocyte-platelet system (solid lines) and the mechanisms (dashed lines) by which pathologic processes (shaded blocks) produce thrombocytopenia.

Table 47.1. Thrombokinetic Patterns in Various Forms of Thrombocytopenia

	Decreased Production		Accelerated Destruction[c]	Abnormal Pooling
Measurement	Hypoproliferation or Hypoplasia[a]	Ineffective Thrombopoiesis[b]		
Total megakaryocyte mass[d]	Decreased	Increased	M increased	V increased
Megakaryocyte number	Decreased	M increased	Increased	V increased
Megakaryocyte volume	Increased	Normal or V decreased	Increased	V increased
Platelet turnover rate or production rate[e]	Decreased	Decreased	Increased	V increased
Total platelet mass	Decreased	Decreased	Decreased	? Normal
Splenic platelet pool	Decreased	Decreased	Decreased[f]	Increased
Platelet survival	Normal	V shortened	Shortened	V shortened

Abbreviations: ?, possibly; M, markedly; V, variably.
Based on Harker LA. Megakaryocyte quantitation. *J Clin Invest.* 1968;47:452-457; Harker LA. Thrombokinetics in idiopathic thrombocytopenic purpura. *Br J Haematol.* 1970;19:95-104; Harker LA, Finch CA. Thrombokinetics in man. *J Clin Invest.* 1969;48:963-974.
[a]Includes myelophthisic processes.
[b]Mainly in megaloblastic hematopoiesis; component of accelerated destruction present in some cases.
[c]Minor component of ineffective thrombopoiesis present in some cases.
[d]Equated to total thrombopoiesis.
[e]Equated to effective thrombopoiesis.
[f]Not representative of sequestered antibody-sensitized platelets.

Accelerated Platelet Destruction

Accelerated platelet destruction is the most common cause of thrombocytopenia. It leads to stimulation of thrombopoiesis and, consequently, to an increase in the number, size, and rate of maturation of the precursor megakaryocytes (*Figure 47.1*).[8] When the rate of platelet destruction exceeds this compensatory increase in platelet production, thrombocytopenia develops. "Compensated" platelet destruction without thrombocytopenia may also occur in patients with prosthetic heart valves and idiopathic thrombocytopenic purpura after splenectomy.[9-11]

Platelet destruction may result from both intracorpuscular defects and extracorpuscular abnormalities. Intracorpuscular defects are rare but have been demonstrated in certain forms of hereditary thrombocytopenia, such as Wiskott-Aldrich syndrome (see Chapter 50).[12] In such disorders, the survival of affected platelets is shortened in the circulation of both the patient and normal recipients. Platelets injured by either intracorpuscular or extracorpuscular processes are usually removed from the circulation by the spleen, liver, and reticuloendothelial system. Platelet destruction most often is the result of extracorpuscular factors; various immunologic phenomena are the most common. Immunologic platelet destruction is discussed in Chapter 48.

Platelet consumption in intravascular thrombi or on damaged endothelial surfaces is another cause of thrombocytopenia. This occurs in disseminated intravascular coagulation (see Chapter 55) and thrombotic thrombocytopenic purpura (see Chapter 49) and other microangiopathic processes. Thrombocytopenia caused by other nonimmunologic platelet destruction is discussed in Chapter 50.

Deficient Platelet Production

Deficient platelet production may result from any of a number of processes. Those that depopulate the stem cell or megakaryocyte compartments are the most common, such as marrow injury by myelosuppressive drugs or irradiation and aplastic anemia. Deficient platelet production may also be the consequence of disordered proliferation within a precursor compartment of normal or even increased size. For example, in disorders characterized by megaloblastic hematopoiesis, hypertrophy of the precursor compartment occurs in response to thrombopoietic stimuli, but thrombopoiesis is ineffective and platelet production is insufficient. Rarely, abnormalities of the processes that normally regulate thrombopoiesis appear to underlie deficient platelet production, such as deficiency of thrombopoietin and cyclic thrombocytopenia.

Abnormal Pooling

Abnormal pooling or abnormal in vivo distribution of an essentially normal total platelet mass may produce thrombocytopenia. This type of thrombocytopenia is seen in the various disorders associated with splenomegaly (see Chapter 50), in which platelet production is normal or even increased, but most of the platelets are sequestered in the vastly enlarged extravascular splenic pool. Thrombocytopenia may also be caused by dilution of platelets when patients are massively transfused during blood loss. A discussion of various forms of thrombocytopenia attributable to deficient or ineffective thrombopoiesis or abnormal platelet pooling is included in Chapter 50.

CLASSIFICATION

A classification of thrombocytopenia based on pathophysiologic criteria is presented in *Table 47.2*. It should be recognized that multiple pathogenetic factors may simultaneously or sequentially play a role in the production of thrombocytopenia.

Bone marrow evaluation and measurement of serum thrombopoietin concentrations or reticulated platelets (immature platelet fraction) may elucidate the pathophysiology of thrombocytopenia in various disease states and determine the mechanism of thrombocytopenia in individual patients. Measurement of the percentage of reticulated platelets identifies platelets that have recently been released from the bone marrow. There is an increased percentage of reticulated platelets in patients with thrombocytopenia caused by increased destruction and a normal to reduced percentage of reticulated platelets in patients with deficient production.[13,14] The sensitivity and specificity of this method of distinguishing between these categories is reported to be more than 95%.[15]

Table 47.2. Pathophysiologic Classification of Thrombocytopenia

Artifactual Thrombocytopenia
Platelet clumping caused by anticoagulant-dependent immunoglobulin (pseudothrombocytopenia)
Platelet satellitism
Giant platelets

Decreased Platelet Production (see Chapter 50)
Hypoplasia of megakaryocytes
Ineffective thrombopoiesis
Disorders of thrombopoietic control
Hereditary thrombocytopenias

Increased Platelet Destruction
Caused by immunologic processes (see Chapter 48)
- Autoimmune
  - Idiopathic
  - Secondary: infections, pregnancy, collagen vascular disorders, lymphoproliferative disorders, drugs, miscellaneous
- Alloimmune
  - Neonatal thrombocytopenia
  - Posttransfusion purpura

Caused by nonimmunologic processes
- Thrombotic microangiopathies
  - Disseminated intravascular coagulation (see Chapter 55)
  - Thrombotic thrombocytopenic purpura (see Chapter 49)
  - Hemolytic-uremic syndrome (see Chapter 49)

Platelet damage by abnormal vascular surfaces (see Chapter 50)
Miscellaneous (see Chapter 50)
- Infection
- Massive blood transfusions

Abnormal Platelet Distribution or Pooling (see Chapter 50)
Disorders of the spleen (neoplastic, congestive, infiltrative, infectious, of unknown cause)
Hypothermia
Dilution of platelets with massive transfusions

References

1. Kjeldsberg CR, Hershgold EJ. Spurious thrombocytopenia. *JAMA*. 1974;227:628-630.
2. Bizzaro N. Platelet satellitosis to polymorphonuclears: cytochemical, immunological, and ultrastructural characterization of eight cases. *Am J Hematol*. 1991;36:235-242.
3. Gowland E, Kay HE, Spillman JC, et al. Agglutination of platelets by a serum factor in the presence of EDTA. *J Clin Pathol*. 1969;22:460-464.
4. Schrezenmeier H, Müller H, Gunsilius E, et al. Anticoagulant-induced pseudothrombocytopenia and pseudoleukocytosis. *Thromb Haemost*. 1995;73:506-513.
5. Pegels JG, Bruynes EC, Engelfriet CP, et al. Pseudothrombocytopenia: an immunologic study on platelet antibodies dependent on ethylene diamine tetra-acetate. *Blood*. 1982;59:157-161.
6. Bizzaro N, Brandalise M. EDTA-dependent pseudothrombocytopenia: association with antiplatelet and antiphospholipid antibodies. *Am J Clin Pathol*. 1995;103:103-107.
7. Bizzaro N. EDTA-dependent pseudothrombocytopenia: a clinical and epidemiologic study of 112 cases, with 10-year follow-up. *Am J Hematol*. 1995;50:103-109.
8. Harker LA. Megakaryocyte quantitation. *J Clin Invest*. 1968;47:452-457.
9. Harker LA. Thrombokinetics in idiopathic thrombocytopenic purpura. *Br J Haematol*. 1970;19:95-104.
10. Branehög I. Platelet kinetics in idiopathic thrombocytopenic purpura (ITP) before and at different times after splenectomy. *Br J Haematol*. 1975;29:413-426.
11. Hope AF, Heyns AD, Lötter MG, et al. Kinetics and sites of sequestration of indium 111-labeled human platelets during cardiopulmonary bypass. *J Thorac Cardiovasc Surg*. 1981;81:880-886.
12. Harker LA, Finch CA. Thrombokinetics in man. *J Clin Invest*. 1969;48:963-974.
13. Rinder HM, Munz UJ, Ault KA, et al. Reticulated platelets in the evaluation of thrombocytopenic disorders. *Arch Pathol Lab Med*. 1993;117:606-610.
14. Watanabe K, Takeuchi K, Kawai Y, et al. Automated measurement of reticulated platelets in estimating thrombopoiesis. *Eur J Haematol*. 1995;54:163-171.
15. Richards EM, Baglin TP. Quantitation of reticulated platelets: methodology and clinical application. *Br J Haematol*. 1995;91:445-451.

Chapter 48 ■ Thrombocytopenia Caused by Immunologic Platelet Destruction

DAVID C. CALVERLEY • CHRISTOPHER MCKINNEY • CHRISTIANE D. THIENELT

INTRODUCTION

Immune thrombocytopenia (ITP) occurs when platelets undergo premature destruction as a result of autoantibody or immune complex deposition on their membranes. Although this disorder was previously known as *idiopathic thrombocytopenic purpura*, it is now correctly termed ITP because this nomenclature more clearly reflects the immune-mediated mechanism of the disease.[1] In this chapter, both primary and secondary types of ITP are discussed (*Table 48.1*). Human immunodeficiency virus (HIV)-related autoimmune thrombocytopenia, which is also in major part a result of the deposition of autoantibody or immune complexes, or both, on the platelet surface, is discussed in Chapter 65.

The diagnosis of ITP is primarily a diagnosis of exclusion, because currently available clinical assays for platelet-associated antibodies or serum antiplatelet antibodies/immune complexes are neither specific nor sensitive enough for routine clinical use. These disorders are characterized by peripheral thrombocytopenia (confirmed by examination of the peripheral smear), with a normal or increased number of megakaryocytes present on bone marrow examination, and absence of splenomegaly. Those patients who have no identifiable underlying cause, which might include infections, collagen vascular diseases, lymphoproliferative disorders (chronic lymphocytic leukemia or lymphoma), or drugs, are diagnosed as primary ITP. In some instances, ITP may be the presenting manifestation of an underlying disease, and additional manifestations appear weeks to months later.

PRIMARY IMMUNE THROMBOCYTOPENIA

Primary ITP refers to thrombocytopenia in which apparent exogenous etiologic factors are lacking and in which diseases known to be associated with secondary thrombocytopenia have been excluded. This syndrome has been recently reviewed.[2-6]

Acute ITP and chronic ITP differ in incidence, prognosis, and therapy (*Table 48.2*). These differences illustrate the wide spectrum of disorders that, by definition, are included in the syndrome, but many clinicians have long believed that acute ITP and chronic ITP are fundamentally different disorders.

Nomenclature

ITP has previously been called idiopathic thrombocytopenic purpura, immune thrombocytopenic purpura, or autoimmune thrombocytopenic purpura. These terms have been replaced by immune thrombocytopenia to reflect the known autoantibody mechanism and absence of purpura in some patients. Primary ITP is defined as a platelet count of less than 100,000/µL in the absence of other causes or disorders that may be associated with thrombocytopenia.[1] The threshold of 100,000/µL is based partly on the observation that patients presenting with a platelet count between 100,000 and 150,000/µL have only a 6.9% chance of developing a persistent count of less than 100,000/µL over 10 years of follow-up. In addition, both the physiologic thrombocytopenia associated with pregnancy and healthy members of certain non-Western ethnic groups may both be considered to have normal values between 100,000 and 150,000/µL.[1]

Incidence

The annual incidence of ITP in the United States is estimated to be 1.6 per 10,000.[7] *Acute ITP*, defined as thrombocytopenia occurring for <6 months and usually resolving spontaneously, most often affects children and young adults. The incidence peaks in the winter and spring, following the incidence of viral infections.[8,9] Acute ITP is most common between 2 and 6 years of age. Approximately 10% to 20% of children with acute ITP develop the chronic variety.[10-13] Chronic ITP, lasting >6 months and requiring therapy to improve the thrombocytopenia, occurs most commonly in adults. In chronic ITP in adults, the median age is usually 40 to 45 years,[14,15] although in one large series of patients, 74% of 934 cases were younger than age 40 years (range, 16-87 years).[16] More recently, the duration of ITP has been reclassified as newly diagnosed (<3 months), persistent (3-12 months), or chronic (>12 months).[5] The persistent ITP category was created to reflect the fact that up to an additional 25% of patients may experience platelets recovery between 7 and 12 months from diagnosis.[10] The ratio of females to males is nearly 1:1 in acute ITP[9,17,18] and is historically considered to be 2 to 3:1 in chronic ITP,[17,18] although more recent surveillance data have challenged the idea of ITP being predominantly a disease of young women; rather, the disorder was reported to show a progressive increase in incidence with age and a gender balance in the older population. In this analysis of 1169 Maryland patients with primary ITP, there was a predominance of males in childhood and of females in the middle-adult years, with an overall prevalence ratio of 1.9 for females to males.[19]

Pathophysiology

The syndrome of ITP is caused by platelet-specific autoantibodies that bind to autologous platelets, which are then rapidly cleared from the

Table 48.1. Immune Thrombocytopenia

Primary
Secondary
Infections
Collagen vascular diseases
Lymphoproliferative disorders
Solid tumors
Drugs
Primary immunodeficiencies and immune dysregulatory disorders
Miscellaneous

Table 48.2. Features of Acute and Chronic Immune Thrombocytopenia

Feature	Acute ITP	Chronic ITP
Peak age of incidence	Children, 2-6 y	Adults, 31-64 y
Sex predilection	None	3:1 female to male
Antecedent infection	Common 1-3 wk before	Unusual
Onset of bleeding	Abrupt	Insidious
Hemorrhagic bullae in mouth	Present in severe cases	Usually absent
Platelet count	<20,000/µL	30,000-80,000/µL
Eosinophilia and lymphocytosis	Common	Rare
Duration	2-6 wk; rarely longer	Months or years
Spontaneous remissions	Occur in 80% of cases	Uncommon

Abbreviation: ITP, immune thrombocytopenia.

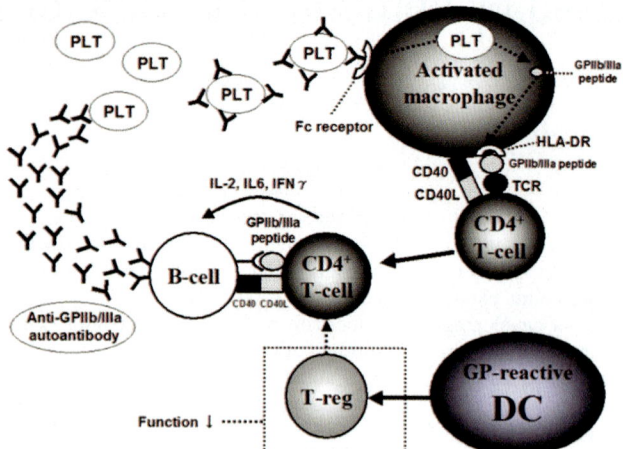

FIGURE 48.1 Pathogenesis of immune thrombocytopenia (ITP). Activated macrophages in the reticuloendothelial system transfer the antigenic information such as GPIIb/IIIa peptide to autoreactive CD4+ T cells. Autoreactive CD4+ T cells and antibody-producing B cells maintain antiplatelet autoantibody production in patients with ITP. There exists a continuous pathogenic loop in ITP. T_reg in ITP has less functional strength than it used to. DC, dendritic cell; GP, glycoprotein; PLT, platelet; T-reg, regulatory T cell; TCR, T-cell receptor. (From Nomura S. Advances in diagnosis and treatments for immune thrombocytopenia. *Clin Med Insights Blood Disord.* 2016;9:15-22. Copyright © 2016 SAGE Publications. Reprinted by permission of SAGE Publications, Inc.)

circulation by the mononuclear phagocyte system via macrophage Fcγ receptors predominantly in the spleen and liver[20] (*Figures 48.1* and *48.2*). The ITP antibody does not fix complement in vitro when tested by the usual techniques, but activation of components of complement on the platelet surface may be demonstrated[21,22] (*Figure 48.2*).

An array of diverse immunologic perturbations involving T and B lymphocytes, dendritic cells, plasma cells, and macrophages may contribute to different extents to the pathophysiology of primary ITP. These in turn lead to both shortened platelet survival and inhibition of platelet production. Given this pathogenic diversity, it has been suggested that primary ITP is not a specific disorder but a "syndrome" with broadly categorized immune tolerance defects.[23] These authors speculate that lessons learned from secondary forms of ITP suggest that primary ITP is equally heterogeneous. As such, the pathogenesis of childhood ITP or ITP that follows viral infections such as cytomegalovirus (CMV), varicella zoster, or *Helicobacter pylori*, or COVID-19[24] infections is less complex and affects primarily peripheral immune tolerance in the setting of immune stimulation in response to a transient antigenic stimulus. It is more likely to respond more readily to therapy or remit spontaneously. In contrast, ITP pathogenesis involving a differentiation block or loss of central tolerance (e.g., in hematologic malignancies or autoimmune disease) is multifaceted, involving a largely autoreactive lymphocyte repertoire that is able to reconstitute quickly after therapy, and therefore often refractory or only transiently responsive to treatment. In these cases, combination therapy that targets more than one aspect of the faulty immune response may be effective because additional cell types are involved in disease pathogenesis.[23]

A compensatory increase in platelet production takes place in most patients in response to the autoantibody-mediated platelet destruction described previously. In others, however, platelet production appears to be impaired as a result of either intramedullary destruction of antibody-coated platelets by marrow macrophages or the inhibition of megakaryopoiesis. Autoantibodies from patients with ITP have been shown to inhibit production of megakaryocytes in vitro, and megakaryocyte apoptosis has also been observed in this setting.[25-27] Turnover studies have shown platelet production to be reduced or inappropriately normal in around two-thirds of patients with ITP.[28,29] In one study, megakaryocytes were small in patients with anti-gpIb/V/IX autoantibodies and increased in size and cytoplasmic area in patients with anti-gpIIb/IIIa autoantibodies, suggesting that the anti-gpIIb/IIIa autoantibody impairs platelet production.[30] Megakaryocyte colony formation (colony-forming unit megakaryocyte) is increased in acute ITP.[31,32] In chronic ITP, decreased megakaryocyte colony formation has been reported.[33]

Consistent with findings of inappropriately low platelet production in ITP, plasma levels of endogenous thrombopoietin (TPO) have not been found to be elevated in ITP.[34,35] This differs from impaired platelet production settings such as following chemotherapy.[34-36] Once TPO is produced, circulating TPO levels are regulated by the volume of the total platelet mass. Platelets and megakaryocytes contain high-affinity TPO (c-Mpl) receptors that bind and clear TPO from the circulation, directly determining the circulating TPO concentration.[37] When the platelet count is normal, high-affinity TPO receptors on the platelets clear most of the TPO and produce a normal plasma TPO concentration, thereby providing basal stimulation of bone marrow megakaryocytes and a normal rate of platelet production. When platelet production and the platelet count are transiently low as in chemotherapy-associated impaired marrow function, the overall clearance of TPO mediated by megakaryocyte and platelet TPO receptors is reduced, sequentially increasing the plasma TPO concentration and then megakaryocyte and platelet production.[34,35]

Platelet Antibodies

In 1951, Harrington and colleagues first reported that the infusion of plasma from patients with ITP predictably induced thrombocytopenia in normal recipients.[38] Shulman and colleagues then demonstrated that the responsible factor was an immunoglobulin (Ig) of the IgG class that was species specific and could be removed from serum by absorption to and elution from normal human platelets.[39] In addition, the platelet-depressing factor produced effects in vivo that were quantitatively and qualitatively similar to those produced by known platelet antibodies. In 1982, van Leeuwen first identified platelet membrane glycoprotein IIb/IIIa as a dominant antigen by demonstrating that the autoantibodies eluted from ITP platelets bound to normal platelets but not to platelets from patients with Glanzmann thrombasthenia.[40] Increased quantities of IgG have been demonstrated on the platelet surface in ITP, and the rate of platelet destruction is proportional to levels of such platelet-associated Ig.[41,42] Autoantibodies are readily found in plasma or platelet eluate in patients with active disease but are infrequently found in patients in remission.[43,44] Disappearance of the antibodies correlates with the appearance of normal platelet counts.[43]

The antiplatelet antibodies and platelet antigens involved in ITP have been extensively studied (*Table 48.3*). Antiplatelet autoantibodies bind to many of the major platelet membrane glycoproteins through

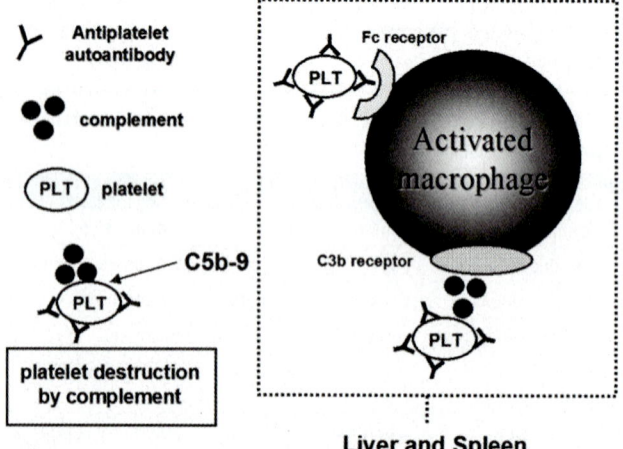

FIGURE 48.2 Mechanisms leading to thrombocytopenia. Human macrophages express Fc receptor that binds IgG specifically. Liver and spleen are dominant organs for the clearance of IgG-coated platelets. There is also direct cytotoxicity by complement such as C5b-9. (From Nomura S. Advances in diagnosis and treatments for immune thrombocytopenia. *Clin Med Insights Blood Disord.* 2016;9:15-22. Copyright © 2016 SAGE Publications. Reprinted by permission of SAGE Publications, Inc.)

Table 48.3. Characteristics of Platelet Autoantibodies in Primary Immune Thrombocytopenia

		Comments
Ig subtype	IgG, IgA, IgM[a]	IgG and IgA have equal frequency
Antigen specificity	gpIIb/IIIa, Ib/V/IX	Most common antigens
	gpIa/IIa, IV	Never only antigen if positive
	Granule membrane protein-140	One patient reported
	Glycosphingolipid	Rare; unclear pathogenetic importance
	Cardiolipin	Common; unclear pathogenetic importance
Presence of antibody		
Plasma	85% of patients	
Platelet eluate	75% of patients	
Complement fixation by antibody	Rare	Unresolved importance
Circulating immune complexes	Rare	Unresolved importance

Abbreviations: gp, glycoprotein; Ig, immunoglobulin.
[a]IgM is never present as the only antiplatelet Ig in an individual patient.

the Fab portion of the molecule[45,46] (*Figure 48.3*). Platelet gpIIb/IIIa was the first platelet antigen detected, and microtiter assays using platelet monoclonal antibodies to gpIb and gpIIb/IIIa later demonstrated that platelet autoantibodies bind to both major platelet membrane glycoproteins.[47-49] Serum autoantibodies can react with IIb or IIIa or the intact IIb/IIIa complex.[49-60] Platelet autoantibody binding to gpIbα has been reported, but data indicate that the majority of Ib/V/IX autoantibodies are directed to the complex.[61,62] Some autoantibodies react with gpIV and $\alpha_2\beta_1$, although the plasma from these patients usually also contains autoantibodies reacting with one of the other two major platelet membrane antigens.[62] Serum antibodies to P-selectin (CD62P) and $\alpha_v\beta_3$ have been detected as well, but their clinical significance is unknown.[63,64]

Antibodies in ITP sera have also been demonstrated to bind to glycosphingolipids[65,66] and cardiolipin.[67-70] Although two studies identified antiphospholipid antibodies (lupus anticoagulant activity or anticardiolipin antibodies) in 46% and 38%, respectively, of patients with ITP at diagnosis, there was little clinical evidence that they played a role in the pathogenesis of the disease or affected outcome.[71,72]

The presence of antibodies against multiple antigens is seen in most patients.[73] Once destruction of platelets within antigen-presenting cells occurs, this generates a series of neoantigens, which in turn results in sufficient antibody to cause thrombocytopenia. This phenomenon is termed *epitope spread*.[74] Plasma autoantibodies and autoantibodies eluted from platelets in the same patient may have slight differences in antigen specificities within a membrane glycoprotein complex.[54] There is evidence from two studies that the specific β_3 antigen epitope in any given patient to which anti-gpIIIa autoantibodies are directed may influence the clinical presentation and course of the disease.[54,75] Whether these findings can be generalized to other ITP autoantibody epitopes is unknown.

Autoantibodies bind to platelets and cause thrombocytopenia primarily by shortening platelet survival. However, rare autoantibodies have also been reported that bind to glycoproteins and activate platelets.[76-80] In addition, one patient with an anti-gpIIIa antibody was reported to have developed an antibody-related defect in aggregation and adhesion.[81]

The incidence of serum autoantibodies to platelet gpIIb/IIIa is the same in the acute and chronic forms of childhood ITP (68% vs 62%, respectively).[82] The presence of anti-gpIIb/IIIa, therefore, does not predict which children will develop the chronic form of the disease, and, in fact, these data provide evidence that the mechanism may be the same in both acute and chronic forms of ITP.

Cell-Mediated Immunity

While autoantibodies are considered the diagnostic hallmark of ITP, T cells are also implicated in antibody production and thrombocytopenia. Along these lines, although it is unclear how B- and T-cell tolerance is perturbed in primary or secondary ITP, different theories have been proposed that include a diversity of different autoimmune mechanisms, including the existence of tolerance checkpoint defects.[23] Implicated T-cell changes have included (1) excessive activation and proliferation of platelet antigen-reactive cytotoxic T cells, (2) production of abnormal helper T cells (T_H), and (3) abnormalities in the number and function of regulatory T cells (T_{regs}).[83-88] Several studies have supported polarization of T_H cells in the immune response in patients with chronic ITP[85,86,88] and have suggested a peripheral regulatory mechanism controlling these glycoprotein-reactive T cells is necessary to prevent autoimmunity (*Figure 48.1*).[87,89]

Impaired Platelet Production

Studies have shown that the extent of platelet production impairment in ITP is variable between patients and that this may contribute to why up to one-third do not respond or respond and later relapse in response to splenectomy or other therapy directed at reducing platelet clearance.[23] Plasma samples from different patients with ITP vary in their ability to inhibit megakaryocyte production in vitro, and in vivo platelet autoantibodies may also impair megakaryocyte development, induce apoptosis, impede platelet release from megakaryocytes, or promote phagocytosis within the bone marrow.[25,29] The pathophysiologic roles of the known immune system aberrations associated with primary ITP such as antibody or cell-mediated marrow apoptosis is a largely unexplored field at the present time.[27]

Other pathophysiologic mechanisms seen in primary ITP include impaired regulation of B-cell development[90] along with the role of the spleen in both antibody production and opsonized platelet clearance that is mediated through the low-affinity IgG binding FcγRII and FcγRIII receptors (*Figure 48.2*).

Clinical Picture
Immune Thrombocytopenia in Children

The clinical course of ITP in children varies from the typical clinical course in adults, with a sudden onset of symptomatic severe thrombocytopenia frequently followed by spontaneous resolution being more typical in children (*Table 48.2*). The annual incidence of pediatric ITP is estimated to be between 1.9 and 6.4 per 100,000/year.[91] In children under 6 years, the incidence of ITP is higher in males than in females. In older children, however, the incidence is higher in females.[92] The onset of severe thrombocytopenia is frequently preceded by an illness, immunization, or allergic reaction.[93] In a population-based study from the United Kingdom, 88.5% of pediatric patients with ITP had a single infection and 5.8% had two different infections in the 8 weeks preceding the ITP diagnosis.[92] A preceding infection was more commonly documented in patients under 2 years of age.[92] Upper respiratory infections are the most common infections reported in patients who go on to develop ITP.[92,94] The vaccine most commonly associated with ITP is the measles-mumps-rubella vaccine, and ITP is unlikely to develop after other early childhood vaccines. In older children, there is a possible association of ITP with hepatitis A, varicella, and tetanus-diphtheria-acellular vaccines.[95]

Pediatric ITP is most common in children between the ages of 2 and 5 years; however, ITP occurs in all pediatric age groups. Otherwise healthy children typically present with an acute appearance of petechiae and purpura over the preceding 24 to 48 hours.[96] Platelet count at diagnosis is typically less than 10 to 20 × 10^9/L.[96,97] Lymphadenopathy or hepatosplenomegaly are atypical features of pediatric ITP, although a spleen tip is sometimes palpable.[97,98] The

AUTOANTIBODIES

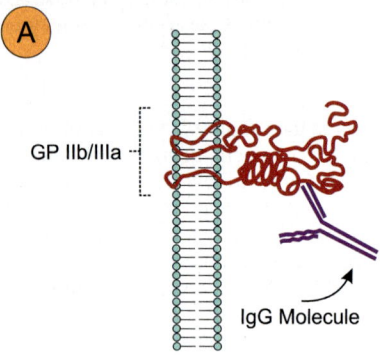

DRUG-DEPENDENT ANTIBODIES

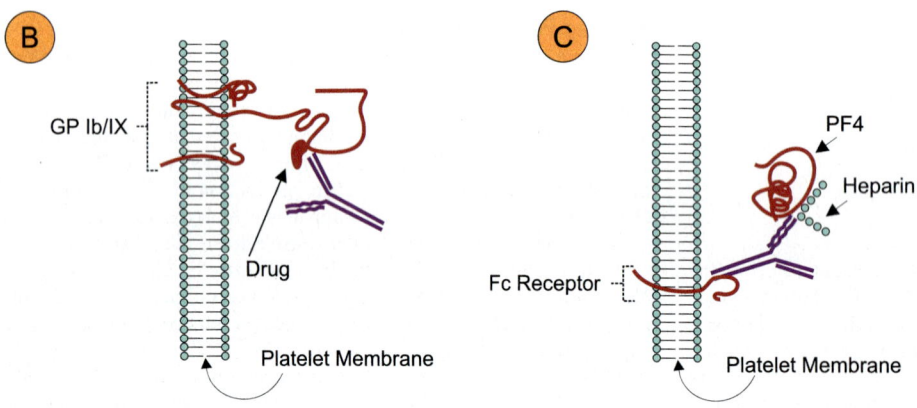

ALLOANTIBODIES

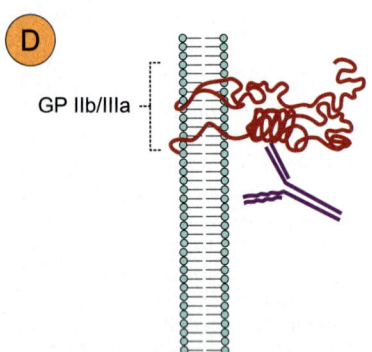

FIGURE 48.3 **Types of antibody-mediated platelet destruction. A,** Platelet autoantibodies bind to variable external and internal platelet epitopes. **B,** Quinine/quinidine-dependent antibodies. The antibody target is a complex of drug and glycoprotein (GP) (usually gpIb/V/IX or gpIIb/IIIa). **C,** Heparin-dependent antibodies. The antigen-antibody complex (target: platelet factor 4 [PF4]/heparin) activates platelets by the binding of immunoglobulin G (IgG) to Fc γRIIA on platelets. **D,** Platelet alloantibodies bind to platelet tertiary conformational epitopes on the platelet membrane. (Modified with permission from Kelton JG. The serologic investigation of patients with autoimmune thrombocytopenia. *Thromb Haemost.* 1995;74(1):228-233. Copyright © Georg Thieme Verlag KG.)

complete blood count should be otherwise normal, although anemia may be present if there is significant bleeding.[97] It is important to obtain detailed medical and family histories in order to exclude congenital thrombocytopenic disorders such as MYH9 macrothrombocytopenias, Bernard-Soulier syndrome, gray platelet syndrome, or Wiskott-Aldrich syndrome.[97] Despite the severity of thrombocytopenia, a minority (2.9%) of pediatric patients with acute ITP develop severe hemorrhage (defined by the Intercontinental Childhood ITP Study Group as epistaxis, melena, menorrhagia, and/or intracranial hemorrhage [ICH]).[99] ICH occurred in one case (0.15%) in this series.

Acute ITP in pediatric patients is generally self-limited, and at least two-thirds of patients will achieve a complete remission (defined as a platelet count greater than 150×10^9/L within 6 months of initial diagnosis and without need for ongoing platelet-directed therapy).[97] The outcome of acute pediatric ITP does not appear to be affected by initial treatment.[100] The number of children with platelet counts less than 20×10^9/L decreases with time. In a Swiss-Canadian retrospective analysis of 554 children with acute ITP, only 6% of children had platelet counts of less than 20×10^9/L at 12 months from diagnosis.[101] Spontaneous remission and short duration of ITP (<2 weeks) has been associated with abrupt onset of bleeding symptoms and age of onset of ≤10 years.[102]

Immune Thrombocytopenia in Adults

In adults, the onset of the chronic form of the disorder is usually insidious (*Table 48.2*). A long history of hemorrhagic symptoms of mild to moderate severity is often described by the patient, but antecedent infections or fever is uncommon. Patients with chronic ITP usually have a fluctuating clinical course. Episodes of bleeding may last days or weeks and may be intermittent or even cyclic. Spontaneous remissions are very uncommon in adults, with an estimated occurrence of <5%.[17,18,103-105] Most spontaneous remissions occur early; however, remissions have been described after 6 months in a small number of patients.[17] Relapses in some cases are associated with vaccination.[106] Often, the clinical course is surprisingly benign. Why some develop recurrent epistaxis, frequent ecchymoses, or other bleeding manifestations at platelet counts between 5 and 20 × 10^9/L, whereas others rarely bleed at these levels is unknown. One common manifestation that is reported in 22% to 39% of surveyed patients with primary ITP is marked fatigue associated with severe thrombocytopenia, and no biochemical explanation for this has been forthcoming.[107,108]

Bleeding Manifestations

The hemorrhagic manifestations of ITP are of the purpuric type. Patients with only ecchymoses and petechiae have "dry" purpura; those with mucous membrane bleeding in addition to skin manifestations have "wet" purpura.[109] Platelet counts are usually lower and the complication rates higher in those with wet purpura. In a series of 712 patients reported by the Israeli ITP study group, 82% of all patients had bleeding limited to the skin, although 43% of adult women reported menometrorrhagia.[110]

In general, the severity and frequency of hemorrhagic manifestations correlate with the platelet count.[111] Bleeding after trauma without spontaneous hemorrhage is usual in mildly affected patients with platelet counts >30,000/μL. Thrombocytopenia associated with counts between 10,000 and 30,000/μL results in spontaneous hemorrhagic manifestations of varying severity, such as ecchymoses and petechiae. Patients with platelet counts <10,000/μL are at risk for serious morbidity and mortality from bleeding, although the mortality rate is actually quite low.[112] Patients who have an increased risk of bleeding include those with a history of bleeding, those with additional bleeding diatheses, and patients >60 years of age.[14,112] Older patients have also been reported to have an increased incidence of major, life-threatening bleeding.[14,113,114]

Skin and Mucous Membranes

Spontaneous bleeding into the skin in the form of petechiae is characteristic. These lesions are minute, red to purple hemorrhages that range in size from that of a pinpoint to that of a pinhead (*Figure 48.4*). They are flat, do not blanch with pressure, and appear and regress, often in crops, over a period of days. They are most conspicuous in areas of vascular stasis, such as the areas below tourniquet sites, the dependent portions of the body (especially around the ankles), and areas subjected to constriction from belts or stockings, as well as on skin surfaces over bony prominences. The presence of petechiae on the face and neck is unusual, except as the result of coughing.

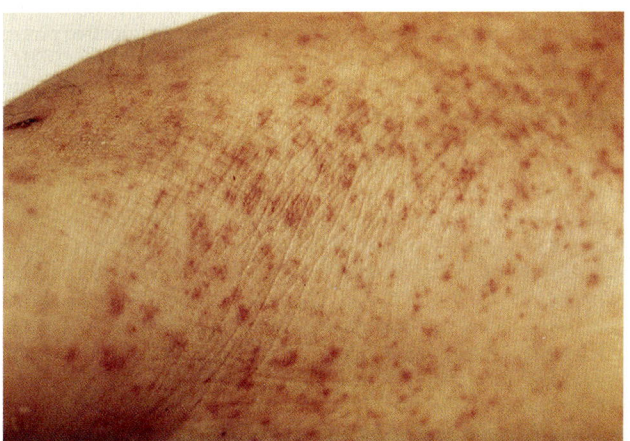

FIGURE 48.4 Petechiae. Pinpoint, nonblanching erythematous capillary bleeding sites are most common in dependent body areas or pressure points.

Ecchymoses may develop on any skin surface. In ITP, they are seldom associated with subcutaneous hematomas and infrequently spread or dissect into deeper or adjacent structures. Large, purple, superficial ecchymoses may be seen, particularly on the back and thighs. Circular ecchymoses often surround even atraumatic venipuncture sites, but external bleeding from such sites is uncommon. Hemorrhagic vesicles or bullae may be seen inside the mouth and on other mucous surfaces. The bullae probably are the result of severe acute thrombocytopenia rather than a specific feature of any particular pathogenetic form.

Gingival bleeding and epistaxis are common. The latter usually responds for a time to conservative measures, such as nasal packing or tamponade, often to recur intermittently. Epistaxis may originate from lesions resembling petechiae in the nasal mucosa. Such lesions may also be found in the mucous membranes of the throat and mouth, sometimes in the absence of cutaneous hemorrhage. In many patients, discrete bleeding points cannot be identified.

The genitourinary tract is a frequent site of bleeding. Menorrhagia may be the only symptom of ITP and may appear for the first time at puberty. Hematuria also is a common symptom, the blood coming from the kidneys, the bladder, or the urethra, although bleeding into the kidney parenchyma is rare. Gastrointestinal bleeding is usually manifested by melena or, less often, by hematemesis.

Central Nervous System

ICH is the most serious complication of ITP. Fortunately, it is rare, affecting 1% to 2% or less of patients with severe thrombocytopenia.[9,115] The hemorrhages are usually subarachnoid, often multiple, and vary in size from petechiae to large extravasations of blood. Numerous small hemorrhages are often seen in the retina; subconjunctival hemorrhage may also occur.

Bleeding After Trauma

Excessive bleeding often follows tooth extractions, tonsillectomy, or other operations or injuries and may first suggest the diagnosis of ITP. In contrast to the hereditary coagulation disorders, such traumatic bleeding is seldom voluminous or rapid. Slow persistent oozing may occur after trivial cuts, razor nicks, and scratches. Delayed bleeding and spontaneous hemarthrosis, which are characteristic of the hereditary coagulation disorders, are extremely rare in ITP.

Laboratory Findings
Blood

The mean platelet count of patients at the time of diagnosis of ITP is 25,000 to 30,000, and severe thrombocytopenia (<10,000) is frequently seen.[115,116] Abnormalities in platelet size and morphologic appearance are common. The platelets are often abnormally large (3-4 μm in diameter) and reveal more than normal variation in size and shape. Abnormally small platelets and platelet fragments ("microparticles") are also evident and may represent the equivalent of microspherocytes and schistocytes.[117-120] Although megakaryocyte fragments may be apparent in routine blood smears, quantitative studies reveal subnormal numbers of these fragments.[121]

Estimates of mean platelet volume (MPV) and the extent of platelet size heterogeneity (platelet distribution width) by means of automated particle counters may, if present, provide useful information in the evaluation of patients with ITP.[122] The presence of numerous megathrombocytes results in high MPV values.[123] Platelet distribution width is also increased, presumably reflecting an abnormal degree of platelet anisocytosis.[107] The exact mechanism underlying such megathrombocytosis is still uncertain, but it may be the result of accelerated platelet production in response to platelet destruction. When MPV is increased in patients with ITP, it is typically inversely correlated in a nonlinear manner with the platelet count. In contrast, low MPV values have been reported in association with big spleen syndromes[107] and some myeloproliferative disorders, after chemotherapy with cytotoxic drugs, and in patients with septic thrombocytopenia.[124]

Significant abnormalities in the other blood counts should prompt a thorough evaluation for other causes of thrombocytopenia because these findings are unusual in ITP. Anemia, if present, is proportional to the extent of blood loss and is usually normocytic. If bleeding has been severe and long-standing, iron deficiency anemia may occur. Occasionally, recent severe hemorrhage may produce reticulocytosis and moderate macrocytosis. Antiplatelet antibodies in patients with ITP do not usually cross-react with erythrocytes, although erythrocyte fragmentation, presumably the result of weak complement activation, may occur.[119] Patients may also have a positive direct Coombs test and autoimmune hemolytic anemia; the combination is known as *Evans syndrome*.[125,126]

The total leukocyte count and the differential count are usually normal. Eosinophilia has been noted, particularly in children, but this finding is by no means consistent. Lymphocytosis with abnormal cells resembling those characteristic of infectious mononucleosis has also been reported.[127,128]

Tests of hemostasis and blood coagulation reveal only changes attributable to thrombocytopenia. The results of tests of blood coagulation, including prothrombin time, partial thromboplastin time, and fibrinogen, are normal in patients with uncomplicated ITP. Slight increases in the levels of fibrinogen degradation products have been demonstrated in the plasma of some patients with ITP.[124] Plasma levels of glycocalicin, a portion of platelet membrane gpIb, may be high in patients with ITP and other forms of platelet destruction. As noted previously, concentrations of thrombopoietin are not significantly increased in ITP.

Bone Marrow

ITP causes no characteristic bone marrow changes; therefore, bone marrow examination should not be routine. The American Society of Hematology (ASH) guidelines for management of ITP recommend against bone marrow biopsy in both children and adults with history, physical examination, complete blood count, and peripheral smear typical of ITP.[5] However, bone marrow aspiration may be helpful in the differential diagnosis of ITP in patients who have atypical findings that may suggest some of these other etiologies. In children, atypical findings include fever, bone or joint pain, family history of low platelets or easy bruising, risk factors for HIV infection, skeletal or soft tissue morphologic abnormalities, nonpetechial rash, lymphadenopathy, or an abnormal hemoglobin, white blood cell count, or white cell morphology.[5] A marrow is not indicated in children prior to initiation of corticosteroid treatment or in those who fail intravenous immunoglobulin (IVIG) therapy.[5] Studies have demonstrated that the yield of bone marrow examination to rule out acute leukemia in a patient presenting with typical findings of ITP is low.[129] In adults, there is no evidence for an age threshold at which a bone marrow examination is required.

In patients with ITP, alterations in the bone marrow are usually limited to the megakaryocytes, although normoblastic hyperplasia may develop as a result of blood loss. The leukocytes are essentially normal with the exception of occasional eosinophilia.[130]

Megakaryocytes are usually increased in size[131] and are increased or normal in number,[132,133] the numbers correlating roughly with the MPV. Morphologic abnormalities of these giant cells are present in most patients with ITP. "Smooth" forms with single nuclei, scanty cytoplasm, and relatively few granules are common. Presumably, they represent the results of markedly accelerated platelet production and the presence of many young forms.[134,135] The changes just summarized are similar to those found in most forms of thrombocytopenia caused by accelerated platelet destruction and are not characteristic or diagnostic of ITP.

Antiplatelet Antibodies

Primary ITP is a diagnosis of exclusion and relies on clinical impression. A number of different types of antiplatelet antibody tests have been developed and reported through the years.[41,136-143] Most of these tests were quite cumbersome and therefore never became available for routine testing. These tests measured different types of Ig, including serum antiplatelet antibodies, platelet-associated surface Ig, or total platelet Ig and are now regarded as unreliable.[5,144] The platelet Ig is released, along with other α-granule proteins, such as platelet factor 4 and β-thromboglobulin, during platelet activation and secretion. It is presumed that some of these released proteins bind to the platelet surface. These observations make it difficult to use either the platelet-associated IgG assays or the total platelet Ig assays for the diagnosis of ITP.[145] Future direction might include the use of flow cytometry in the diagnosis and follow-up of autoimmune thrombocytopenia.[146]

Diagnosis

Primary ITP is a diagnosis of exclusion in children and adults in which the causes of secondary ITP are ruled out. A careful history, physical examination, and review of the complete blood count and peripheral blood smear remain the key components of diagnosis of primary ITP. There is insufficient evidence to suggest the routine use of antiplatelet, antiphospholipid, and antinuclear antibodies; thrombopoietin levels; or platelet parameters obtained on automatic analyzers.[5] If during treatment or monitoring atypical features develop in adults such as one or multiple cytopenias, lymphadenopathy, fevers, night sweats, and significant involuntary weight loss, then the diagnosis of ITP should be reassessed. Hepatitis C and HIV serology should both be obtained in adults with suspected primary ITP because treatment of these disorders would typically be expected to favorably alter the course of secondary disease.

Differential Diagnosis

The initial step in the evaluation of a thrombocytopenic patient is inspection of the peripheral blood smear to confirm the decreased platelet count.[147] Thrombocytopenia may be produced artifactually by clumping of the platelets in the blood sample caused by ethylenediaminetetra acetic acid–associated platelet agglutinins (pseudothrombocytopenia),[148,149] or the platelets may be unavailable for counting because they are bound in rosette formation to the surface of white blood cells in the venous blood sample ("platelet satellitism").[150,151]

As already noted, the diagnosis of ITP is a diagnosis of exclusion based on a demonstration of peripheral thrombocytopenia, with a history, physical examination, and complete blood count that do not suggest another cause for the thrombocytopenia. Although a spleen tip is sometimes palpable in children[7,98] splenomegaly otherwise suggests that the thrombocytopenia may be a result of hypersplenism related to the presence of a separate underlying disease associated with splenic enlargement.

The initial manifestations of acute leukemia, myelodysplastic syndrome,[152,153] myelophthisic processes, and aplastic anemia may mimic ITP. These other types of underlying hematologic disorders are suggested by anemia out of proportion to blood loss and by changes in the leukocytes not attributable to either hemorrhage or complicating infection. Although not routinely recommended for the diagnosis of ITP, as noted previously, bone marrow aspiration may be helpful in the differential diagnosis of ITP of patients who have atypical findings that may suggest some of these other etiologies.

The presence of schistocytes in the blood smear suggests that thrombocytopenia may be associated with a microangiopathic process (see Chapter 49). In thrombotic thrombocytopenic purpura (TTP) or hemolytic uremic syndrome (HUS), thrombocytopenia is associated with laboratory manifestations of hemolysis, including elevated levels of lactate dehydrogenase and indirect bilirubin.[154] Patients may also have transient, multifocal neurologic signs or symptoms, renal insufficiency, and/or fever in TTP, or renal insufficiency alone in HUS. After a diagnosis of ITP, the next essential step is to distinguish between primary and secondary forms of ITP such as HIV, hepatitis C, or *H. pylori* infections; collagen vascular diseases such as systemic lupus erythematosus (SLE); lymphoproliferative disorders such as chronic lymphocytic leukemia; and drug ingestion. As already noted, the ASH guidelines recommend considering testing all adults with a new diagnosis of ITP for hepatitis C and HIV because treatment plans differ in these settings.[5] The importance of careful inquiry regarding drug ingestion or exposure to toxic substances cannot be overemphasized, because thrombocytopenia attributable to drugs or toxins is often indistinguishable from ITP.[155] The development of thrombocytopenia in an adult, in particular, should arouse suspicion of a pharmacologic etiology, because many of the drugs associated with thrombocytopenia are used more often by adults than by children. It is also essential to eliminate the possibility that the thrombocytopenia is secondary to heparin administration. ITP may be produced by heparin administered in any dose and by any route of administration, including heparin-bonded catheters.[156] Finally, the antiphospholipid antibody syndrome is a disorder that may be associated with thrombocytopenia. In the usual case, this presentation may be associated with thromboembolic manifestations, anticardiolipin antibodies, and coagulation inhibitors of the lupus type (see Chapter 55).

Treatment of Primary Immune Thrombocytopenia

Many of the treatment recommendations for ITP are based on expert opinion rather than high-level evidence from randomized controlled trials. The ASH has published a practice guideline on ITP.[5,157,158] The reader is referred to this practice guideline for specific questions regarding the treatment of patients with ITP.

Children

Childhood ITP is usually benign and self-limited. Therefore, treatment is not required for most patients. Treatment is reserved for patients with severe thrombocytopenia (<20,000/µL) and moderate to severe bleeding (Buchanan and Adix bleeding score ≥ 3-high),[159] patients with diminished healthcare-related quality of life, or patients who remain thrombocytopenic for >3 to 12 months (Table 48.4).[160] Treatment guidelines recommend observation for all children with no or mild bleeding, regardless of platelet count.[5] Although the greatest fear in the acute form is ICH, several large studies show that even with low platelet counts (<30,000/µL) life-threatening bleeding and ICH are rare (<0.5%).[99,160,161]

Treatment guidelines for pediatric ITP recommend first-line treatment with steroids preferentially over a single dose of IVIG (0.8-1 g/kg) for patients with non-life-threatening bleeding.[5] Treatment with IVIG did not show any appreciable benefit in terms of durable response, remission rates, prevention of bleeding complications, or mortality in these patients.[162-164] In pediatric patients, short courses of prednisone lasting less than 1 week are recommended in lieu of longer steroid courses or repeated courses of dexamethasone owing to the high likelihood of spontaneous remission, low incidence of severe bleeding complications, and tolerability of steroid-related side effects in growing children.[5,165] Several multicenter randomized trials have been performed in high-risk patients with acute ITP to define whether treatment is associated with a prompt increase in platelet counts. These clinical trials demonstrated that treatment with either oral prednisone or IVIG was associated with a more rapid rise in platelet count to >20,000/µL than either no therapy or treatment with anti-D.[166,167] Only IVIG shortened the time to reach a platelet count >50,000/µL. Children with platelet counts <10,000/µL or counts of 10,000 to 29,000/µL and mucosal bleeding were studied in a prospective randomized clinical trial, and IVIG raised platelet counts faster than three corticosteroid regimens.[168] Therefore, IVIG should be preferentially used if a rapid rise in platelet count is desired.

Treatment of children who develop persistent ITP or are unresponsive to initial treatment is evolving. A trial of thrombopoietin receptor agonists is now preferred over rituximab or splenectomy. Splenectomy is considered an option of last resort, and many experts recommend delaying splenectomy for at least 12 months given the frequency of spontaneous remission.[5] Both eltrombopag and romiplostim have a US Food and Drug Administration (FDA) indication for treatment of chronic ITP in pediatric patients as young as 1 year of age.[169] In phase I/II trials, 88% of pediatric patients receiving romiplostim maintained a platelet count of >50,000/µL for a median of 7 weeks as compared with those receiving placebo.[170] In the eltrombopag trials, 40% of pediatric patients receiving eltrombopag maintained a platelet count of >50,000/µL for at least 6 weeks as compared with those receiving placebo.[171] A multicenter retrospective study of TPO-RA use in pediatric patients demonstrated that 40% of patients receiving TPO-RAs maintained a stable response (platelet count > 50,000/µL) with consistent dosing.[169] This study also noted that almost 20% of patients taking the TPO-RAs had acute ITP.[169] The advantages of the TPO-RAs, including desirable safety profiles, lack of immune suppression, and convenience of the medications make them attractive agents in pediatric ITP; however, the optimal use and timing of TPO-RAs in pediatric ITP warrants further study.

Rituximab treatment can be used in children with refractory ITP. Response rates in pediatric populations can be as high as 63.8% and prior steroid responsiveness is a main predictor of pediatric rituximab response (87.5% in steroid-responsive patients vs 48% in steroid-nonresponsive patients).[172] Therefore, rituximab may be considered as an alternative to splenectomy in children with chronic ITP or in patients with persistent bleeding despite first-line treatments.[5] High-dose dexamethasone (0.6 mg/kg/d) may also be considered in patients who are unresponsive to initial therapy based on small studies showing a 25% response rate in refractory patients.[173]

Adults

Patients with chronic ITP may have mild thrombocytopenia that can be followed without treatment. The incidence of bleeding is correlated with the platelet count; therefore, patients with platelet counts >50,000/µL rarely have spontaneous bleeding and may require treatment only if extensive operative procedures are planned. Patients with platelet counts <20,000 to 30,000/µL or significant mucosal membrane bleeding with platelet counts <50,000/µL are usually treated[5] (Table 48.4 and Figure 48.5).

No prospective studies on long-term prognosis of ITP after treatment are reported. However, it has been reported that most adult patients have a good response to treatment (without necessarily returning to normal platelet counts) and have no excess mortality when compared with the general population.[174] A small group of patients who had severe thrombocytopenia after 2 years of primary and secondary therapies had a mortality risk of 4.2 (95% confidence interval, 1.7-10.0) resulting from both bleeding and infectious complications related to therapy.

Thirty percent of patients with ITP in reported series are >45 years of age.[130,175] However, these patients may be more refractory to therapy[113] and appear to have a higher incidence of hemorrhagic complications than younger patients.[14] Guthrie and colleagues reported a 52% incidence of life-threatening or fatal bleeding in their series of 40 patients over 45 years old.[113] This risk of fatal bleeding in patients with platelet counts that are chronically <30,000/µL is estimated at 0.4% per year for patients <40 years old and 13.0% per year for patients >60 years old.[176]

First-Line Treatment

Initial treatment for adult patients with newly diagnosed ITP is typically steroids. Other options that increase the platelet count rapidly

Table 48.4. Recommendations for Initial Treatment of Immune Thrombocytopenia Patients With Platelet Counts <20,000 to 30,000/µL

	Children	Adults
Asymptomatic	None	Steroids (preferred) or IVIG
Minor purpura	None	Steroids (preferred) or IVIG
Mucosal membrane bleeding that may require clinical intervention	IVIG or steroids	IVIG and/or steroids
Severe, life-threatening bleeding	Steroids and IVIG Hospitalization Consider platelet transfusion and other measures	Steroids and IVIG Hospitalization Consider platelet transfusion and other measures

Abbreviation: IVIG, intravenous immunoglobulin.
The current ASH guidelines recommend treatment for adults with platelet counts of <30,000/µL.

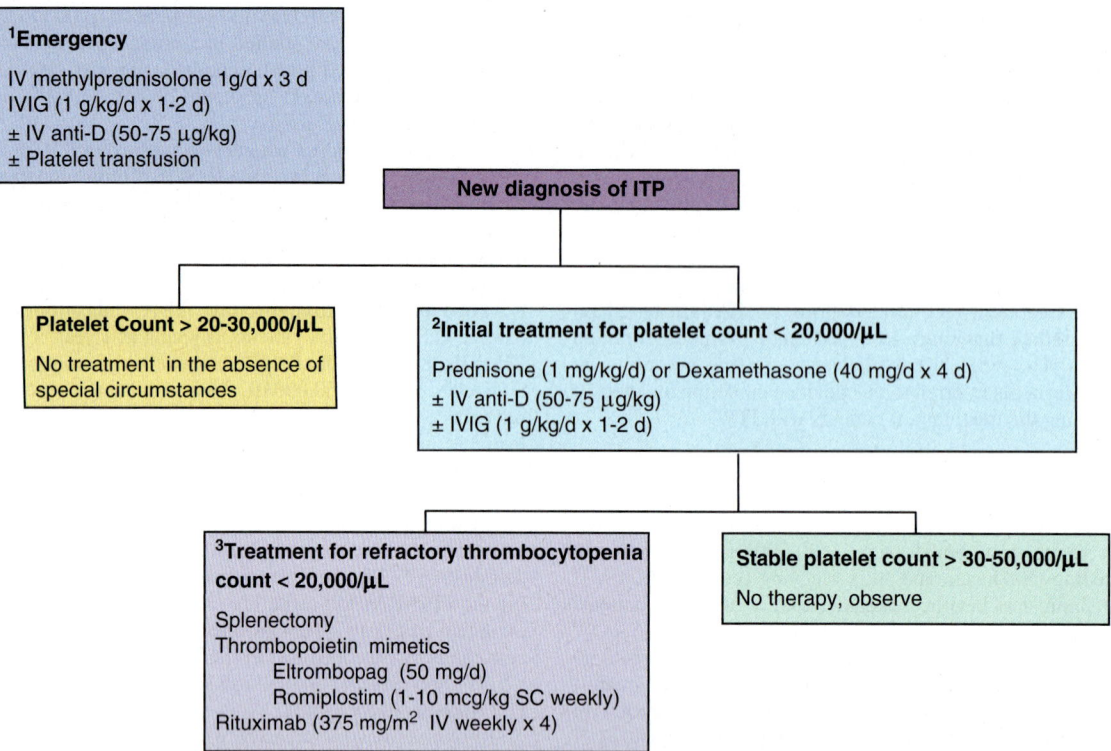

FIGURE 48.5 Therapy of adult immune thrombocytopenia (ITP). (*1*) Minimal emergency therapy for severe or life-threatening bleeding includes intravenous (IV) methylprednisolone and intravenous immunoglobulin (IVIG). Intravenous anti-D and platelet transfusions may be given as needed. All three modalities given prior to transfusions may help preserve platelet longevity in the circulation, and repeated or continuous platelet transfusions may be required in urgent situations. (*2*) Initial treatment of ITP typically consists of steroids (prednisone or dexamethasone) with the goal of attaining a platelet count of >30,000/μL and cessation of bleeding. IVIG or anti-D may be used if steroids are contraindicated or the patient has persistent thrombocytopenia despite steroids. IVIG can be used concurrently with corticosteroids if a more rapid increase in platelet count is required. (*3*) Thrombocytopenia recurs in most adults as corticosteroids are tapered and longer tapering courses are preferred to shorter courses or IVIG. Treatment options for refractory ITP include splenectomy (if there is relapse after gradual corticosteroid tapering or daily required prednisone dose to maintain platelet count >30,000/μL is contraindicated or exceeds 10 mg every second day), rituximab (if there is relapse after one line of therapy such as corticosteroids, IVIG, or splenectomy), or thrombopoietin mimetics (if there is relapse after splenectomy or splenectomy is contraindicated and there is relapse after at least one other therapy such as corticosteroids or IVIG). (Modified from Neunert C, Terrell DR, Arnold DM, et al. The American Society of Hematology 2019 evidence-based practice guideline for immune thrombocytopenia. *Blood*. 2019;3:3829-3866; Cines DB, Bussel JB. How I treat idiopathic thrombocytopenic purpura (ITP). *Blood*. 2005;106:2244-2251.)

Table 48.5. Therapeutic Agents and Their Dosing Schedules

Agent	Dose and Schedule
Anti-D immunoglobulin	50-75 μg/kg IV, repeated at 3-wk intervals as indicated
Cyclophosphamide	150 mg daily for up to 8 wk
Colchicine	200 mg daily for up to 4 wk
Dexamethasone	40 mg daily for 4 d, repeated every 14 d for 4 cycles
Danazol	400 mg twice daily for 1 mo or longer
Eltrombopag	50 mg daily. Must be continued indefinitely
Fostamatinib	100 mg twice daily, increase to 150 mg twice daily based on platelet response
Intravenous immunoglobulin	1 g/kg IV for 1-2 d, repeated every 2-4 wk as indicated
Prednisone	1 mg/kg daily for up to 28 d, then taper to lowest dose possible
Rituximab	375 mg/m^2 IV weekly for 4 doses
Romiplostim	1-10 μg/kg subcutaneous injection weekly. Start at 1 μg/kg and titrate based on platelet count. Must be continued indefinitely
Vincristine	2 mg at 5-7 d intervals for 2 or more doses
Vinblastine	7.5 mg at 5-7 d intervals for 3 or more doses

Abbreviation: IV, intravenous.
Modified from Narang M, Penner JA, Williams D. Refractory autoimmune thrombocytopenic purpura: responses to treatment with a recombinant antibody to lymphocyte membrane antigen CD20 (rituximab). *Am J Hematol*. 2003;74(4):263-267. Copyright © 2003 Wiley-Liss, Inc., A Wiley Company. Reprinted by permission of John Wiley & Sons, Inc.

include IVIG and anti-D. The most recent ASH guideline recommends use of these alternative first-line therapies in patients with contraindications to steroids.[5] Patients with life-threatening bleeding may require parenteral glucocorticoids and IVIG followed by platelet transfusions,[177] plasmapheresis,[178] or even emergency splenectomy as first-line treatment. Standard ITP treatments and their dosing schedules are shown in *Table 48.5*.

Steroids

Steroids are the conventional first-line therapy for adult ITP. Dameshek first reported his experience with prednisone therapy in 1958,[179] when 30 consecutive patients with acute ($N = 11$) or chronic ($N = 19$) ITP were treated with 20 to 150 mg/d of prednisone. Twenty-two of the patients demonstrated an increase in platelet count to normal after an average interval of 22 days and were then maintained on 2.5 to 15.0 mg/d of prednisone. In eight patients, prednisone was discontinued without relapse.

Numerous retrospective studies of steroid treatment in both children and adults with ITP have been reported.[17,18,98,103-105,110,130,175,180-183] The criteria for inclusion of patients in the individual studies and the criteria for response to treatment vary significantly among the reports; therefore, it is difficult to combine the data accurately. However, some useful observations can be made. Complete (CR) and partial (>50,000/μL) responses (PR) in patients treated with prednisone (usually, 1 mg/kg/d as starting dose) average 65% to 85%, but sustained responses after discontinuation of the drug occur in only 25% or less of patients.[184,185] Platelet counts usually increase within 1 week in responding patients and have usually reached peak values by 2 to 4 weeks. Patients who have not had any response by 4 weeks are unlikely to respond to prednisone and should therefore be considered for other forms of treatment. No pretreatment patient characteristics have predicted a patient's response to steroids.

Several prospective randomized prednisone-based trials in patients with ITP have been reported. Bellucci and colleagues randomized patients between low- (0.25 mg/kg/d) and high- (1.0 mg/kg/d) dose prednisone for 3 weeks, with taper and discontinuation by the end of the fourth week.[186] If bleeding continued, the drug could be increased from low dose to high dose, or a second 4-week course could be given. CR, defined as a platelet count > 100,000/μL for at least 6 months, was seen in 74% of children and 41% of adults. CRs or PRs occurred in 83% of children and 59% of adults. No significant differences were seen between low- and high-dose regimens in either age group. Mazzucconi and colleagues randomized patients between prednisone 0.5 mg/kg/d and 1.5 mg/kg/d.[187] The response rates in adults were not significantly different between patients treated with low- versus high-dose steroids: 30% and 34% CR, respectively. In children, however, the rates were 64% for low-dose versus 81% for high-dose prednisone. Therefore, there is evidence to support the use of lower doses of steroids in adults than have conventionally been used at the beginning of treatment. However, based on the opinion of an expert panel convened by the ASH, high-dose prednisone (1 mg/kg/d) is recommended as appropriate initial treatment in patients with ITP with platelets <30,000/μL, including asymptomatic patients.[5,157,158]

Another prospective randomized, controlled trial compared prednisone (1 mg/kg/d) with IVIG (400 mg/kg/d for 4 days) or to both in a small number of patients.[188] A platelet count >50,000/μL was achieved in 82%, 54%, and 92% of patients, respectively. The median times to peak platelet counts were 8.5, 7.0, and 7.0 days. These authors concluded that there was no advantage for IVIG over conventional corticosteroid treatment. In another randomized control trial, platelet counts >50,000/μL were achieved more quickly in patients receiving IVIG than in those receiving intravenous methylprednisolone, but long-term outcomes were the same.[189]

There are several studies that have evaluated the role of high-dose dexamethasone in the initial treatment of ITP. This protocol was initially developed because of concern regarding long-term side effects of daily prednisone use. Initial trials showed that using 40 mg of dexamethasone daily for 4 consecutive days results in an initial response in 85% of patients.[190,191] Additional work has shown that repeating dexamethasone bursts may provide long-term disease control in some patients. Mazzucconi and colleagues treated newly diagnosed patients with ITP with dexamethasone 40 mg daily for 4 days, repeating these cycles every 14 days for 4 cycles.[192] A total of 85% of patients responded, with 65% achieving a CR. Relapse-free survival at 15 months was 81%, indicating that many of these patients may be long-term responders.

Until recently there have been conflicting opinions regarding the choice of prednisone versus dexamethasone for first-line treatment of ITP. The writers of the 2011 ASH guidelines favor longer-term prednisone over dexamethasone,[5] but other experts in the field think that either is reasonable.[193] The first randomized trial in this setting recently demonstrated improved overall initial response, CR, and time to response among 192 newly diagnosed adult patients with ITP given either high-dose dexamethasone 40 mg daily for 4 days or prednisone 1 mg/kg daily for 4 weeks.[194] Sustained response rates were similar (40.0% vs 41.2%), and dexamethasone was better tolerated.

The mechanism of action of steroids in ITP involves both direct and indirect effects on thrombocytopenia. Steroids ameliorate thrombocytopenia directly by several mechanisms. Steroids may (a) decrease consumption of antibody-coated platelets by the spleen[195,196] or bone marrow, (b) reduce antibody production by the spleen,[95,197] (c) decrease antibody production by the bone marrow,[198] and/or (d) increase marrow platelet production by undetermined mechanisms.[199]

There is little doubt that corticosteroids in high doses ameliorate splenic sequestration of antibody-coated platelets. Corticosteroids decrease antibody-coated red blood cell sequestration in guinea pig spleens by decreasing Fcγ receptor proteins on macrophages,[200] and in vivo and in vitro data support a similar action of steroids in humans.[91,92,195,201,202] Corticosteroids also decrease monocyte Fc receptors in autoimmune hemolytic anemia.[203] This downregulation of monocyte/macrophage Fc receptors may account for the early effects of steroid treatment on platelet counts. Chronic corticosteroid treatment is associated with a decrease in antibody production, but this usually occurs after several weeks of high-dose steroids. Steroid treatment also results in increased platelet production in some patients with ITP,[199] an effect that may be secondary to reduction of the antiplatelet Ig effect on thrombopoiesis, reduction in intramedullary destruction of antibody-coated platelets before their release into the circulation, or decreased antibody synthesis by bone marrow lymphocytes.

In addition to these direct effects on thrombocytopenia, steroids also act on endothelial cells to reduce bleeding. Experimental evidence indicates that thinning of the endothelium with development of endothelial fenestrations occurs in both animal models and humans with ITP, suggesting that platelets play a role in normal endothelial homeostasis.[204,205] Clinically, steroids are known to ameliorate the purpuric bleeding in patients with ITP before the platelet count actually increases. Experimentally, investigators have demonstrated that 3 days after steroid therapy in rabbits and 4 days after steroid therapy in patients, the endothelial thinning reverts toward normal, providing a scientific explanation for this clinical observation.[205,206] This endothelial effect may in part be explained by the observation that, when endothelial cells are cultured with steroids, cell morphology is altered, with greater confluence and increased protein synthesis and content.[207]

Intravenous Immunoglobulin

The intravenous administration of polyvalent Ig (IVIG), first used in 1981,[208] may induce remissions in patients with life-threatening bleeding or in patients with refractory ITP. IVIG therapy has proved most effective in infants and small children,[209,210] an age group in which the response is difficult to evaluate because of the frequency of spontaneous remissions. In adults, this regimen has produced relatively less impressive long-term results,[211-214] although an occasional patient enters complete remission after the initial treatment and a series of booster doses.[215-218] In a review of 28 published reports of IVIG in 282 adults, 64% of patients had a peak platelet count >100,000/μL and 83% had peak platelet counts >50,000/μL[219] after the initial infusion. Platelets may begin to rise after 2 days and usually reach peak levels by 1 week after treatment.

Regimens of 400 mg/kg/d for 5 days vs 1000 mg/kg/d for either 1 or 2 days[220,221] have been equally effective in randomized trials, and doses of 0.5 g/kg are as effective as 1.0 g/kg for maintenance therapy.[222] These doses produce significant increases in serum and platelet levels of IgG.[210,215,217] In a randomized controlled trial, one dose of 1000 mg/kg was superior to 500 mg/kg in raising platelet counts to >80,000/μL by day 4.[221] Most of these patients were being prepared for splenectomy or delivery. One protocol that utilized concurrent IVIG (1 g/kg) and platelet transfusion (1 pheresis unit every 8 hours) resulted in over 60% of patients achieving a platelet count over 50,000/uL after 24 hours.[222]

Several mechanisms are thought to be involved in the beneficial effects of IVIG. They include Fc receptor blockade of reticuloendothelial cells,[215,217,223-226] effects on B cells and antibodies,[227-232] and anti-inflammatory effects.[233,234] No evidence exists that reduction of antiplatelet antibodies accounts for the acute effects of therapy.[233]

Therapy with IVIG remains expensive. The rapid nature of the response to treatment makes it an ideal agent for treatment of patients for life-threatening bleeding or before surgery[235,236]; however, the role of IVIG in long-term therapy remains uncertain. The major side effect of treatment is headache, although some patients also develop fever, myalgias, and skin rashes.[235] There are also reports of acute renal failure occurring in up to 7% of patients, especially older patients and those with diabetes, or baseline increases in creatinine (or both).[237,238] The patients may be oliguric, and most demonstrate peak creatinine levels by day 5 after the IVIG infusion. Hemodialysis may be required acutely, and several patients required chronic dialysis. The volume of fluid required for IVIG administration can also be a major problem in some older patients with comorbidities such as congestive heart failure.

Anti-D

Intravenous Rho (D) immune globulin (anti-D) has been studied in children and adult ITP as an alternative to IVIG.[239-241] The mechanism of action is unknown; however, it is believed that the antibody coats the red blood cells of Rh-positive patients and either blocks the reticuloendothelial clearance of platelets or modulates the immune system, resulting in an increase in the platelet count.[241,242] Although infusion of both IVIG and anti-D slow the Fcγ-receptor–mediated destruction of antibody-coated platelets, responses to anti-D appear to uniquely correlate with polymorphisms specific to the FcγRIIa and FcγRIIIa receptors.[243] This is characterized by increases in the plasma levels of IL-6, tumor necrosis factor-α, monocyte-chemoattractant protein-1, and IL-10 that are specific to IV anti-D infusions compared with IVIG.

Children respond better than adults, and nonsplenectomized patients respond better than splenectomized patients to anti-D.[242,244] The platelet count does not begin to increase for 48 to 72 hours, so it may not be as effective for the treatment of life-threatening bleeding compared with IVIG. The effect lasts for several weeks to a month, and patients respond well to retreatment. They may respond to intramuscular injections given weekly as maintenance.[245] Occasionally, patients have a sustained remission.[246] Most patients exhibit a modest decrease in hemoglobin, and most have subclinical signs of mild hemolysis,[244] with decreased haptoglobin, increased lactate dehydrogenase, and increased indirect bilirubin. Red cell survival is only modestly reduced.[247] No correlation has been found between the amount of hemolysis and the platelet response, leading some investigators to question the proposed effect on reticuloendothelial blockade.[248] Reinfusion of autologous red blood cells that have been opsonized with anti-D has produced both complete and partial remissions in a small number of patients, even after splenectomy.[249] With respect to anti-D dosing, early studies in adults receiving 25 to 50 μg/kg/d showed an increase in platelet count of >20,000/μL in 79% of patients. However, the platelet count did not increase for >72 hours, which made this treatment approach less efficient for bleeding patients.[250] More recent studies have shown a more rapid increase in the platelet count within 24 hours and a longer duration of the increase when using a higher dose of 75 μg/kg compared with 50 μg/kg.[251]

Anti-D therapy now carries a black box warning that requires observation of the patient for 8 hours after administration because of the risk of intravascular hemolysis and disseminated intravascular coagulation.[252] Although either IVIG or anti-D is appropriate as a first-line ITP treatment if corticosteroids are contraindicated, the latter should be used with caution given these recent FDA warnings of severe hemolysis, and its use is not recommended in those with bleeding causing a decline in hemoglobin, evidence of autoimmune hemolysis, renal function abnormalities, and current or recent significant infection, especially Epstein-Barr virus. During the postinfusion period it has been recommended that clinicians monitor for any evidence of severe hemolysis by obtaining a complete blood count and urinalysis and perform further testing as necessary.[253]

Rituximab

The addition of rituximab has been evaluated in adults to provide intensification of upfront therapy. In two randomized trials of dexamethasone alone versus dexamethasone and rituximab weekly for 4 weeks, it was found that sustained platelet counts were achieved more frequently in the latter versus former groups.[254,255] A third study found daily low-dose rituximab (100 mg) given concurrently for 4 days with dexamethasone 40 mg led to a high sustained remission rate of 76.2%.[256] Greater evidence is needed to determine the role of rituximab in this setting.[257]

Treatment of Chronic Primary Immune Thrombocytopenia

Many adult patients with ITP, even if they initially respond to steroids, will develop chronic ITP. Chronic ITP is defined as ITP lasting longer than 12 months.[1] Patients who are asymptomatic and have platelet counts between 30,000 and 50,000/μL may be managed with careful observation.[157,185] Symptomatic patients with platelet counts <30,000/μL who had an initial response to steroids can be retreated with prednisone and then tapered to find the minimum dose that can maintain the patient hemorrhage free, even if the platelet count is not >30,000/μL. If patients can be maintained on 10 mg every other day, additional treatment may not be indicated. Some patients observed for years with platelet counts of 10,000/μL have had no significant bleeding other than ecchymoses or petechiae, even without steroid therapy.[258] Splenectomy has been the traditional therapy for refractory cases of ITP. There are more options now with accumulating evidence regarding the role of rituximab and thrombopoiesis-stimulating agents.

Splenectomy

Patients with severe thrombocytopenia (<10,000/μL) who do not respond to steroids (administered for up to 4 weeks) or who relapse during steroid tapering and patients with platelet counts of <30,000/μL for periods of up to 3 months should be considered for splenectomy. Most patients demonstrate a response to steroids within 2 to 4 weeks, but a late response is rarely seen. Based on updated ASH guidelines, it is now recommended to delay splenectomy at least 1 year after diagnosis because of the potential for spontaneous remission in the first year. In addition, a course of rituximab is recommended prior to splenectomy.[5] Sustained CRs to splenectomy (variously defined as platelet counts of 100,000-150,000/μL) have been reported in 50% to 80% of patients, depending on the series.[258-271] After the operation, the platelet count may increase rapidly, often within 24 to 48 hours, and may reach levels as high as 1 million/μL or even higher in approximately 10 days.[98] Operative mortality is <1%, and perioperative bleeding is rare.[17,18,99,103,104] Platelet transfusions are usually given only if the patient has bleeding after the spleen has been removed. Postsplenectomy infections are also rare, especially if patients have received immunization to encapsulated organisms (*Streptococcus pneumoniae*, *Haemophilus influenzae*, and *Neisseria meningitidis*) before splenectomy. Laparoscopic splenectomies in patients with ITP are as successful as conventional splenectomies, although patients occasionally may require conversion to an open procedure.[272,273] Therapeutic responses are also reported when splenic ultrasound,[273] splenic radiation,[274,275] or partial splenic embolization[276] was used instead of splenectomy.

Patients who do not respond to splenectomy or who relapse after an initial response to splenectomy should be considered for investigation related to the presence of accessory spleens.[268,277-281] The incidence of accessory spleens found at the time of the original splenectomy ranges from 15% to 20%.[263,268] The incidence of accessory spleens in patients who relapse after splenectomy may be as high as 50%,[130,269,270] and, surprisingly, the majority of these patients demonstrate postsplenectomy changes (ie, Howell-Jolly bodies) on their peripheral blood smears. Relapse secondary to an accessory spleen may occur weeks to years after the initial splenectomy. Scanning methods have varying sensitivities; conventional ^{99m}technetium scans, ^{99m}technetium scans using heat-denatured red blood cells, or computed tomography scans can be used. Accessory spleens as small as 0.5 cm have been found when[106] indium scans were performed preoperatively, and isotope detector probes were used intraoperatively to detect all accessory splenic tissue.[263] A review of 56 published cases demonstrated a 73% excellent therapeutic response and a 27% moderate response to accessory splenectomy.[263]

The effectiveness of splenectomy in the therapy for ITP is attributed to removal of the organ that is primarily responsible for the destruction of antibody-sensitized platelets. The increase in platelet count correlates with an increase in platelet survival, whereas platelet production remains unchanged.[199] The removal of the spleen may also result in a reduction of antibody production, but this effect is probably of minimal significance in view of the immediate favorable responses to splenectomy. No factors have consistently predicted a response to splenectomy; age, concentration of platelet-associated IgG, the time between diagnosis and splenectomy, the patient's response to steroids, IVIG or intravenous anti-D, and the peak postoperative platelet count have all been studied.[262,282-286] The site of platelet sequestration, based on preoperative[51] chromium- and[111] indium-labeled platelet survival studies, may be predictive of response,[266,287] but these techniques are seldom used.

Rituximab

Rituximab, an anti-CD20 monoclonal antibody, has produced 6-month platelet counts >50,000/μL in approximately 40% to 60% of patients.[288-292] Response rates, unfortunately, wane over time, and a durable response of 21% to 26% 5 years after infusion is typical,[293] implying rituximab is not a curative therapy. Rituximab causes selective B-cell lysis in vitro and B-cell depletion in vivo.[294] Involved mechanisms of action include apoptosis, antibody-dependent cell-mediated cytotoxicity, and/or complement-dependent cytotoxicity. Recovery of B-cell counts usually occurs by 6 to 12 months after completion of treatment.

Most of the patients in the studies of rituximab in ITP had relapsed or refractory disease, and some had undergone splenectomy. The majority of studies have used the standard treatment dose of 375 mg/m^2 weekly for four weekly doses[292]; however, published reports have shown that lower doses can be effective as well.[295] The side effects were mild and seen most commonly after the first infusion. The long-term safety profile of rituximab is felt to be favorable, although hepatitis B reactivation is a recognized complication necessitating documentation of negative serology prior to initiation. Only one case of progressive multifocal leukoencephalopathy, a rare but fatal consequence of rituximab administration, has been reported in a patient with ITP.[296] There are two different response patterns, early versus late.[297] Patients with an early response to four weekly infusions had an increasing platelet count after the first or second infusion and peaked between weeks 6 and 10. Late responders had no rise in their platelet count during treatment but increased their platelet count between weeks 6 and 8, with the peak occurring shortly thereafter. In one study, the B-cell count in patients who responded was lower than in patients who did not have a response.[291]

A meta-analysis of studies employing rituximab in the treatment of refractory/relapsed patients consisted of 299 patients described in 15 reports.[298] The overall response rate was 55%, of which 38% of patients achieved a CR, which was defined as a platelet count of at least 100,000 to 150,000/μL. In addition, 17% of the patients achieved a PR, which was defined as a platelet count of >50,000 and <100,000/μL. The median duration of response was 74 weeks (24-120 weeks) and in PR patients 55 weeks (12-160 weeks). CR in splenectomized patients (62%) was higher than in nonsplenectomized patients (available from five studies, n = 126).[278] Another meta-analysis showed similar results with 43.6% of patients achieving a CR (>150,000/μL) and 62.5% of patients achieving a PR (>50,000/μL).[292] A more recent meta-analysis of 5 randomized trials of 467 nonsplenectomized adults comparing rituximab with corticosteroids, IVIG, and/or anti-D globulin demonstrated a platelet count of 100,000/μL or higher at 6 months in 46.8% versus 32.5%, respectively.[299]

Longer-term studies have shown that prolonged disease responses are less common. A recent update from the French multicenter registry study of 248 adults with ITP treated with rituximab showed that at 60 months follow-up, 73 (29.4%) patients had a sustained response.[300] The incidence of severe infections was 2/100 patient-years.

Notably, 24 patients with an initial response and then relapse received retreatment with rituximab, with a response of 92% and longer duration of response in 54%. As a result of its safety profile and its sustained response, rituximab could be an effective and safe option for retreatment, which would serve to confirm an earlier observation.[301]

Thrombopoiesis-Stimulating Agents

Thrombopoiesis-stimulating agents (thrombopoietin mimetics) are another treatment option for management of refractory ITP. There are now three available thrombopoiesis-stimulating agents approved for ITP, eltrombopag, romiplostim, and avatrombopag. Patients to consider for this drug class include those needing bridge therapy (e.g., before surgery), those needing to avoid immunosuppression associated with splenectomy or rituximab, or those with relapse after splenectomy or after at least one other therapy such as corticosteroids or IVIG with splenectomy contraindicated. Six large randomized-controlled trials using one of the two agents (eltrombopag, romiplostim) showed 50% to 90% response rates with good safety and tolerability and durable long-term responses in 40% to 60% patients. Treatment with TPO agonists led to reduced bleeding complications and decreased need for concomitant or rescue medication. Only a small number of patients developed moderate-severe reticulin fibrosis; however, this is usually reversed after discontinuation of the TPO-RA.[302-305]

Eltrombopag, an oral agent, is a peptide that interacts with the transmembrane domain of the thrombopoietin receptor, thereby stimulating differentiation and proliferation of megakaryocytes in the bone marrow. In a 2009 study, 114 patients with refractory ITP were randomized to eltrombopag versus placebo in a 2:1 randomization.[302] After 6 weeks of follow-up, 59% of patients in the eltrombopag arm versus 16% in the placebo arm had achieved a platelet count >50,000, and less bleeding was observed in the eltrombopag arm. Platelet counts dropped again within 2 weeks of discontinuing therapy. A 2011 phase III study (RAISE) in patients with chronic ITP showed similar results.[306]

The open-label EXTEND study enrolled 302 patients with a median duration of 2.37 years (2 days-8.76 years). Median platelet counts increased to 50×10^9/L or more by week 2 and were sustained throughout the treatment period. Overall, 259 patients (85.8%) achieved a response (platelet count ≥ 50×10^9/L at least once in the absence of rescue), and 133 (52%) of 257 patients achieved a continuous response of 25 weeks or longer. Rates of thromboembolic events (6%) and hepatobiliary adverse events (15%) did not increase with treatment duration past 1 year. EXTEND demonstrated that long-term use of eltrombopag was effective in maintaining platelet counts of 50×10^9/L or more and reducing bleeding in most patients with ITP of more than 6 months' duration. Important adverse events (e.g., thrombosis, hepatobiliary, and bone marrow fibrosis) were infrequent.[307]

Similar results have been seen with romiplostim, an injectable thrombopoietin mimetic that is given once per week. It is a peptide (peptibody) that binds to the thrombopoietin receptor. In a randomized study published in 2008, patients with ITP were randomized in a 2:1 fashion to romiplostim versus placebo.[308] In splenectomized and nonsplenectomized patients, 79% and 88% of patients receiving romiplostim achieved a platelet count >50,000. Only a very low number of patients in the placebo arm achieved this threshold (14% of nonsplenectomized patients, 0% of splenectomized patients). This correlated with decreased use of other ITP therapies. The most common side effects are arthralgias, fatigue, and nausea. Serious adverse events are rare and, like eltrombopag, can include bone marrow reticulin and thrombosis. Additional trials have shown that romiplostim is safe and effective for prolonged use[309] and that decreased bleeding is observed in patients receiving romiplostim due to higher platelet counts.[310] With prolonged use, patients do still require regular platelet monitoring because the dose required may vary over time.[309] As with eltrombopag, indefinite treatment is required because platelet counts fall quickly when treatment is discontinued. Long-term figures on both agents suggest the response in platelet counts can be maintained.[310,311]

Avatrombopag is an oral TPO receptor agonist with the advantage of absorption being unaffected by food. It is currently FDA approved in chronic ITP based on a phase 3 trial[312] as well as in thrombocytopenia in chronic liver disease prior to a scheduled procedure. Avatrombopag is begun 10 to 13 days prior to the scheduled procedure. Patients should undergo the procedure 5 to 8 days after the last avatrombopag dose.[313]

Recent expert guidelines recommend a TPO agonist or splenectomy in adults with ITP lasting >3 months who are corticosteroid dependent or have no response to corticosteroids.[5] This recommendation also reflects the need for patient preferences and values in the decision process.

Fostamatinib

Fostamatinib is an oral spleen tyrosine kinase (Syk)-inhibitor, which was approved for ITP in 2018. In ITP, antiplatelet antibodies bind via the Fc region to Fc-gamma receptors on macrophages, which then activates the syk signaling pathway that initiates phagocytosis of platelets.

Therefore, syk inhibition has been a therapeutic target. Fostamatinib was studied in two identical, 24-week, randomized, double-blinded, placebo-controlled phase 3 multicenter studies and showed a stable response in 17% patients on fostamatinib vs. 2% of patients on placebo ($P < .001$) and clinically meaningful overall platelets response (>50 K/µL) in 43% of patients on fostamatinib vs 14% on placebo ($P = .0006$).[314]

The baseline ITP duration was 8 years and median platelet count was 16,000/µL. Prior treatment included TPO agents (47%), splenectomy (35%), and rituximab (32%).

Twenty-seven (19%) patients achieved a stable response with median duration of >28 months and a median platelet count of 89,000/µL. Sixty-four (44%) patients achieved an overall response including stable responders with a median platelet count of 63,000/µL and a median response duration >28 months. Twenty-four of 71 (34%) patients who had failed TPO agents achieved overall responses to fostamatinib. Almost half of the patients achieved an overall response, and most of these maintained their responses for >2 years.[315]

Immunosuppressive Drugs

Immunosuppressive therapy for ITP has yet to be evaluated thoroughly; the overall effectiveness of these potent drugs is variable, and remissions achieved have been short-lived. Poor results were reported in children.[316] Favorable results are, nevertheless, noteworthy, because they were obtained in refractory patients who had not responded to splenectomy or steroids.[317]

Among the multiple immunosuppressive agents studied over decades in the ITP second-line setting, mycophenolate mofetil and dapsone have been investigated in 11 larger, more modern cohorts.[108] Three studies of 83 refractory patients treated with mycophenolate mofetil reported response rates of 52% to 69% (platelets > 30,000-50,000/µL), which lasted up to a median of 24 weeks in one of the studies. Treatment was reported as well tolerated in general. A review of 8 published case series of dapsone with more than 10 patients in refractory ITP revealed an overall platelet response rate of 40% to 62% in children and adults, with responses tending to persist if the drug was continued. Mild dose-dependent hemolysis is reported in up to 20% of dapsone users, and its use is contraindicated in patients with glucose-6-phosphate-dehydrogenase deficiency.

Preliminary reports of successful treatment in refractory patients have been published using high-dose methylprednisolone[235,318] and cyclophosphamide-based combination chemotherapy.[319] Cyclophosphamide alone, either daily oral or pulse intravenous therapy, induced remissions in 16% to 55% of patients.[18,317,320-322] However, this drug must be administered for several weeks before the platelet count rises and often must be continued for an indefinite period to maintain the remission, and side effects such as leukopenia and alopecia are often significant. Azathioprine, cyclosporin A, mycophenolate mofetil, actinomycin, and other immunosuppressive agents, either alone or in combination with corticosteroids, have variable success.[323-329] Vincristine and vinblastine, administered intravenously at weekly intervals, may be as effective as cyclophosphamide but act more rapidly, often increasing the platelet count within 7 days.[330-333] In addition to their suppressive effects on cellular and humoral immune responses, these agents increase platelet production in both animals and normal human subjects.[334,335] In ITP, their mechanism of action has been postulated to be inhibition of microtubule-dependent events required for monocyte-macrophage function.[336,337]

In a recently reported case-control study of 37 patients with ITP with no response to a median of 10.5 prior treatment lines (including splenectomy, rituximab, or TPO receptor agonists), it was found when compared with a historical cohort of 183 "typical" patients with ITP that they had an overrepresentation of secondary ITP (35%) and monoclonal gammopathy of uncertain significance (20%).[338] Only 1 of 14 responded to immunosuppressive therapy alone, whereas 7 of 10 responded to a combination of this class of agents with a TPO agonist that lasted a median of 15 months. It was concluded that combining immunosuppressant therapy with a TPO receptor agonist may be a relevant option for these challenging patients that carry high morbidity and mortality.

Other Proposed Therapies

A number of other therapies have been reported to be successful in single case reports or in small series of patients. Danazol, an attenuated androgen, has been effective in increasing platelet counts in patients with ITP in doses ranging from 50[339] to 800 mg/d.[340-342] The mechanism of action is postulated to be a danazol-induced reduction of Fc receptors on phagocytic cells.[343] Long-term results indicate a final response rate of >40% at a median follow-up of 10 years with a reasonable safety profile.[344] Recombinant α-interferon can increase platelet counts in up to 50% of patients when injected subcutaneously three times a week, and some responses were durable after stopping treatment.[345,346]

A recent review of the approach to refractory ITP in adults and children who do not respond to, cannot tolerate, or are unwilling to undergo splenectomy includes a three-tiered approach to those who require therapy to increase the platelet count to a safe level.[347] Tier 1 options include low-dose prednisone (≤5 mg daily), rituximab, and TPO agonists. Once these are all tried, tier 2 options include immunosuppressive agents (6-MP, azathioprine, cyclosporine A, cyclophosphamide, danazol, dapsone, mycophenolate mofetil, vinca alkaloids) that the authors often prescribe concurrently with a tier 1 agent or a second tier 2 agent with a different mechanism of action. Tier 3 agents are of uncertain benefit and/or high toxicity (e.g., ATRA, colchicine).

Supportive Measures

Physical activity should be restricted to minimize the hazards of trauma, particularly head injury. Drugs, such as nonsteroidal anti-inflammatory drugs, that impair platelet function should be avoided. Blood loss should be treated as indicated, and platelet concentrates should be administered in the presence of significant bleeding.[347] However, transfusions typically produce only a slight and transient increase in the platelet count, no doubt because of the rapidity with which they are destroyed in vivo.[348] Platelet transfusions, nevertheless, may produce some increase in platelet numbers in many patients,[349,350] often diminish bleeding for a time, and can be effective in the management of serious complications such as subarachnoid hemorrhage. They should be reserved for such life-threatening emergencies or for the immediate preoperative treatment of patients with serious hemorrhage before splenectomy. A single large dose of IVIG followed by a platelet transfusion can be effective in arresting hemorrhage in some critically ill patients.[236] In most patients with platelet counts >50,000/µL, preoperative platelet transfusions are not indicated. Platelet transfusions should be avoided in patients with chronic ITP because of subsequent development of alloantibodies. Anovulatory hormones are useful when menorrhagia is a major complaint. Because of the risk of septicemia, polyvalent pneumococcal vaccine, H. influenzae B vaccine, and quadrivalent meningococcal polysaccharide vaccine should be administered at least 2 weeks before elective splenectomy in both adults and children.[351]

Immune Thrombocytopenia in Pregnancy

Both ITP and non-ITP thrombocytopenia may occur during pregnancy.[352,353] Thrombocytopenia was present in 7% of women when they were admitted to hospital for a full-term delivery in a prospective 7-year study of 15,741 mothers and 15,932 newborns.[353-355] Most platelet counts were between 100,000 and 150,000/µL, and 1% of women had platelet counts <100,000/µL. Thrombocytopenia was detected incidentally in the majority of women, and only 0.01% of their infants had fetal platelet counts <50,000/µL. None of the infants had hemostatic impairment, and most mothers had normal or near-normal platelet counts by discharge. If the mothers had an obstetric or medical complication, the incidence of thrombocytopenia (<50,000/µL) in the infants was 0.35%. It is unclear when the incidental thrombocytopenia (called *physiologic or gestational thrombocytopenia*) developed during pregnancy, and the etiology of this mild abnormality may include hemodilution and accelerated clearance. Antiplatelet antibody testing was not sufficiently specific to differentiate patients with gestational thrombocytopenia from those with ITP.[356] Among those with maternal thrombocytopenia, 74% have incidental thrombocytopenia and only 4% have ITP.[357] It is therefore recommended that healthy pregnant women with a platelet count of 80,000 to 150,000/μL require no specific investigations or treatment at delivery and the mode of delivery should be determined only by obstetric indications.[5] A diagnosis of gestational thrombocytopenia is unlikely if platelets are under 50,000/μL, and an alternative etiology should be sought for platelets <80,000/μL.[358] Evaluation of thrombocytopenia presenting in the first or early second trimester is similar to that in nonpregnant patients with review of the peripheral blood smear and assessments for thyroid, liver, viral, and potential autoimmune disorders such as autoimmune hemolysis, and lupus. Primary ITP is the most common cause of maternal thrombocytopenia in this time period.

A retrospective 11-year analysis of obstetric patients with ITP examined 92 women with ITP during 119 pregnancies.[359] For most women, the pregnancy was uneventful, although women had moderate to severe bleeding in 25 pregnancies (21.5%). Women in 37 pregnancies received treatment to increase platelet counts. During delivery, 44 women received epidural analgesia without complications, with most having a platelet count between 50,000 and 149,000/μL. Most deliveries were vaginal (82.4%). Bleeding was uncommon at delivery. In most settings epidural analgesia is held if platelets are less than 80,000 to 90,000/μL.

Platelet autoantibodies in pregnant patients with ITP cross the placenta and can produce thrombocytopenia and clinical bleeding in the infant. During pregnancy, both maternal and infant health must be considered, and management of women with ITP diagnosed before or during pregnancy is therefore more difficult.[357-359] Women with severe ITP should be treated with IVIG or the lowest dose of steroids needed to maintain a platelet count >30,000/μL, which is considered safe until approaching term when the counts need to be monitored more closely in anticipation of delivery.[360] Although 30,000/μL is considered reasonable, there is no available evidence to support specific "safe" platelet count thresholds in the ante- or peripartum periods.[5] It should be noted that, when mothers have been treated during pregnancy, changes in their platelet counts do not correlate with the fetal platelet counts when these have been sampled before and after treatment.[361] IVIG and steroids both increase platelet counts with similar efficacy and relatively little toxicity for the mother or neonate.[362] When betamethasone or placebo was given for 4 weeks before delivery in a randomized trial, no differences were seen in either the maternal or infant platelet counts or the incidence of bleeding at delivery.[363] Splenectomy during pregnancy may have higher complication rates, but it is not contraindicated. IVIG with or without concurrent platelet transfusions can be used before elective delivery to increase the platelet count rapidly. The safety of other forms of therapy used in nonpregnant patients with ITP is uncertain. Use of anti-D immune globulin, cyclosporine, and rituximab have all been reported with good outcomes but cannot be routinely recommended.[360]

At the time of delivery, it must be decided whether to deliver the infant by cesarean section or by vaginal delivery. When 474 infants were analyzed from series reported over a 20-year period, 10% of infants had platelet counts between 50,000 and 100,000/μL and 15% had platelet counts < 50,000/μL.[364] ICH occurred in 3%, but no significant association existed between ICH and mode of delivery. More recent data indicate that morbidity and mortality in infants with neonatal thrombocytopenia are lower than originally reported. Burrows and Kelton published a systematic review of pregnancy in patients with ITP, selecting only those series with more than 10 patients and those that included fetal platelet counts and infant outcome.[365] They reported 288 live births and an incidence of fetal thrombocytopenia of 10% with platelet counts < 50,000/μL and 4% with platelet counts < 20,000/μL. There were no deaths and no cases of ICH, and there was no difference in morbidity between cesarean sections and vaginal births. During the decade from 1990 to 2000, these cumulative totals from 13 prospective studies were 9% and 4%.[357] Minor bleeding complications occurred in 3% of infants, and 2% had major bleeding complications.

Many studies have been done to determine maternal characteristics that may correlate with severe thrombocytopenia in the newborn[357] and to help with decisions regarding method of delivery. To date, only the birth of a previously affected older sibling correlates with the incidence of neonatal thrombocytopenia. Other variables that were analyzed, such as the mother's platelet count or prior splenectomy, were predictive in some studies but not in others.

SECONDARY AUTOIMMUNE THROMBOCYTOPENIC PURPURA

Autoimmune thrombocytopenia can be associated with drugs and with several common diseases (ie, collagen vascular disease, infections, lymphoproliferative disorders, and Graves disease). Secondary ITP is discussed separately because of its unique features and the issues of diagnosis and management. ITP associated with HIV infection is discussed in Chapter 65.

Autoimmune Thrombocytopenia Secondary to Drugs

Numerous drugs have been associated with ITP. In some cases, the evidence associating a given drug with ITP is circumstantial. However, a systematic review is available in which specific criteria were established to determine the likelihood of drug-induced ITP caused by specific drugs (*Table 48.6*).[155,357,366,367] The most common drugs with level 1 evidence are quinidine, quinine, rifampin, trimethoprim-sulfamethoxazole, danazol, methyldopa (Aldomet), acetaminophen, and digoxin. The most common drugs with level 2 evidence are gold, procainamide, carbamazepine, hydrochlorothiazide, ranitidine, and chlorpropamide. Heparin, which causes ITP in as many as 1% of patients, is discussed in Chapter 56.

Pathophysiology

Drug-induced platelet antibodies are the result of an idiosyncratic reaction that develops in only a small percentage of patients exposed to a drug. This ranges from an estimated 38 cases per 1 million exposures for trimethoprim-sulfamethoxazole to as many as 1 in 100 patients for gold salts and 3 in 100 patients for true immune-mediated heparin-induced thrombocytopenia.[368,369] It is not clear whether there are predisposing risk factors for most of the drugs that cause ITP, although evidence suggests that the risk of developing antibodies to gold salts depends on host human leukocyte antigen (HLA) type, with the majority of patients studied expressing HLA-DR3 antigen.[370]

Drug-induced antibodies may be complement- or noncomplement-activating antibodies that react with platelets, either in the absence (autoantibodies) or in the presence of drugs. The most completely studied antibodies are those that develop in response to quinidine/quinine and heparin.[45] Most nonheparin drug–induced antibodies bind specifically to platelet membrane glycoproteins in the IIb/IIIa or the Ib/V/IX complex through the Fab portion of the antibody molecule (*Figure 48.3B*). In contrast, antibodies to heparin bind to a heparin–platelet factor 4 complex, and the immune complex then binds to the platelet membrane via the Fc portion of the antibody molecule (*Figure 48.3C*).

Most of the drug-induced antibodies are developed in response to the parent drug, and drug-dependent antibodies can be demonstrated in a variety of in vitro tests. In some cases, however, these tests are negative when the parent compound is present but positive if known metabolites are used instead of the parent compound. Antibodies against drug metabolites have been reported with acetaminophen, para-aminosalicylic acid, naproxen, and trimethoprim-sulfamethoxazole.

Clinical Features

Drug-induced thrombocytopenia is associated with a heterogeneous clinical picture and varying degrees of bleeding. Thrombocytopenia and bleeding usually appear abruptly and may be severe. Mucosal membrane bleeding from all sites and oral hemorrhagic bullae may occur, and patients often develop fever, chills, nausea, vomiting, and fatigue as part of a prodrome to the bleeding.

Severe thrombocytopenia usually develops within hours in sensitized patients ingesting quinidine or quinine; however, a minimum of 6 to 7 days is required to initiate a primary immune response in individuals taking the drug for the first time. Some patients do not develop thrombocytopenia for months or years, a characteristic that seems to be more dependent on the host than the type of drug. The amount of drug required to cause thrombocytopenia is quite variable; however, even the amount of quinine present in a gin and tonic cocktail (15 mg) is sufficient to produce severe thrombocytopenia and bleeding in a patient who has been previously sensitized to quinine ("cocktail purpura").[371] After the drug is stopped, platelet counts return to normal within days and are usually normal by 1 week. Thrombocytopenia induced by gold salts resolves more slowly, usually over weeks or months, because gold remains in the tissues.

Diagnosis

It is often difficult to make a definite diagnosis of drug-associated ITP because either the patient has taken the medication intermittently or a hospitalized patient is receiving more than one drug that may cause thrombocytopenia. Although it may be possible to demonstrate drug-dependent antibodies against the parent drug or its metabolites, this type of testing is beyond the scope of hospital laboratories. The readministration of the suspected drug in an attempt to confirm an etiologic relationship is not recommended as a routine diagnostic measure. Most of the level 1 drugs listed in *Table 48.6* were demonstrated to cause immune-mediated thrombocytopenia because of patient response to an inadvertent in vivo challenge.

A detailed history, including all prescribed drugs, over-the-counter medications, and any herbal supplements, is of great benefit. Complete data from all English-language articles describing patients with assumed drug-induced thrombocytopenia have been cataloged on the Internet (http://www.ouhsc.edu/platelets/ditp.html).

Treatment

Ordinarily, no therapy is needed, because withdrawal of the offending drug is followed by recovery. IVIG and plasmapheresis may be helpful if life-threatening bleeding occurs. Many patients are treated with corticosteroids, and a normal platelet count is usually restored within 1 week. The major exception is gold-induced thrombocytopenia, which may persist for weeks or even months. British anti-Lewisite (dimercaprol) may accelerate the excretion of gold and speed recovery.[372]

Autoimmune Thrombocytopenia in Systemic Lupus Erythematosus

Thrombocytopenia may complicate collagen vascular diseases and other disorders associated with disordered immunologic responses such as thymoma[373] and myasthenia gravis.[374-376] In most instances, the ITP in SLE appears to result from immunologic platelet injury and is identical to primary ITP in most respects.

From 5% to 15% of patients with ITP fulfill the criteria for diagnosis of SLE at the time of presentation.[377,378] Other patients have a positive antinuclear antibody test when they are first diagnosed with ITP, and a small number of them may develop SLE within several years. Patients with high-titer antinuclear antibody in a speckled pattern and antibodies against native DNA and other nuclear antigens are most likely to develop SLE.[379-382] SLE is a chronic and debilitating disease, so it is important to identify such patients so therapy can be directed at all aspects of the autoimmune disease.

ITP in patients with SLE may be the result of either specific platelet autoantibodies or immune complex deposition on platelets. Only a few studies have been reported in which the newest platelet antigen–capture autoantibody tests have been used, and in these patients, platelet autoantibodies to platelet membrane glycoproteins have been detected.[383-386] Thrombocytopenia correlates with SLE disease activity[376] but not the presence of antiphospholipid antibodies.[387-389] These antibodies, which may be present in SLE or in otherwise healthy patients, also bind to platelet membrane gpIIb/IIIa or Ib/IX/V.[386,387,390] It is unclear, however, whether they are specific to these glycoproteins or cross-reactive.

Table 48.6. Drugs Associated With Immune Thrombocytopenia and Criteria for Their Classification

Level 1[a]		Level 2[b]
Acetaminophen	Iopanoic acid	Acetazolamide
Alprenolol	Isoniazid	Ampicillin
Aminoglutethimide	Levamisole	Captopril
Aminosalicylic acid	Linezolid	Carbamazepine
	Lithium	
Amiodarone	Meclofenamate	Chlorpropamide
		Filgrastim (G-CSF)
Amphotericin B	Mesalamine	Fluconazole
Amrinone	Methicillin	Glibenclamide
Atorvastatin	Methyldopa (Aldomet)	Gold
	Methylprednisolone	
Cephalothin	Minoxidil	Hydrochlorothiazide
Chlorothiazide	Nalidixic acid	Ibuprofen
Chlorpromazine	Naphazoline	Oxyphenbutazone
Cimetidine	Nitroglycerine	Oxytetracycline
Danazol	Novobiocin	Phenytoin
	Orofiban	
Deferoxamine	Oxprenolol	Procainamide
Diatrizoate meglumine/ diatrizoate sodium	Pentoxifylline	Ranitidine
	Piperacillin	Sulindac
Diazepam	Quinidine	Ticlopidine
Diazoxide	Quinine	Trastuzumab
Diclofenac	Rifampin	
Diethylstilbestrol	Sulfasalazine	
Difluoromethylornithine	Sulfisoxazole	
Digoxin	Tamoxifen	
Ethambutol	Thiothixene	
Haloperidol	Tolmetin	
Indinavir	Trimethoprim-sulfamethoxazole	
Interferon-α	Vancomycin	

Criteria
1. The candidate drug preceded thrombocytopenia, and recovery from thrombocytopenia was complete and sustained after the drug was discontinued.
2. The candidate drug was the only drug used before the onset of thrombocytopenia, or other drugs were continued or reintroduced after discontinuation of the candidate drug with a sustained normal platelet count.
3. Other etiologies for thrombocytopenia were excluded.
4. Reexposure to the candidate drug resulted in recurrent thrombocytopenia.

Modified from publications by George JN, Raskob GE, Shah SR, et al. Drug-induced thrombocytopenia: a systematic review of published case reports. *Ann Intern Med.* 1998;129:886-890; Blanchette VS, Luke B, Andrew M, et al. A prospective, randomized trial of high-dose intravenous immune globulin G therapy, oral prednisone therapy, and no therapy in childhood acute immune thrombocytopenic purpura. *J Pediatr.* 1993;123:989-995; Gill KK, Kelton JG. Management of idiopathic thrombocytopenic purpura in pregnancy. *Semin Hematol.* 2000;37:275-289; Webert KE, Mittal R, Sigouin C, et al. A retrospective 11-year analysis of obstetric patients with idiopathic thrombocytopenic purpura. *Blood.* 2003;102:4306-4311; Silver RM, Branch W, Scott JR. Maternal thrombocytopenia in pregnancy: time for a reassessment. *Am J Obstet Gynecol.* 1995;173:479-482.
[a]Level 1 evidence met criteria 1 to 4.
[b]Level 2 evidence met criteria 1 to 3.

Patients with ITP and SLE should be treated the same as patients with primary ITP, even though there are conflicting reports on the success rate of splenectomy in this population.[391,392] *Rituximab* is often preferred to splenectomy because it may also be used to treat other manifestations of SLE.

Autoimmune Thrombocytopenia in Hepatitis C

A number of studies have suggested an association between hepatitis C virus (HCV) infection and ITP either as a consequence of interferon therapy or in the setting of chronic infection without therapy.[393,394] One of the largest studies included 120,691 US veterans with chronic HCV who were matched with 454,905 controls.[395] HCV was associated with ITP in both treated and untreated patients. Corticosteroids may increase the platelet count in HCV-associated ITP, but it will also increase viral load. IVIG may result in a short-lived platelet count increase and is recommended as the initial treatment for HCV-ITP along with antiviral therapy (with close monitoring of the platelet count if interferon is included).[5] Splenectomy is also effective for HCV-associated ITP.[5] It is recommended that any pharmacologic management of thrombocytopenia in HCV-associated ITP that is being considered should be in concert with a hepatology or infectious disease provider.

Immune Thrombocytopenia in Other Disorders

ITP has been reported in association with a number of other medical conditions, including infections, neoplasms, and thyroid disease, and it is unknown whether this increased platelet destruction involves antibody binding, immune complex deposition, and/or antibody-mediated complement activation.

ITP has been documented in patients with infectious mononucleosis, cytomegalovirus, varicella zoster,[396-399] tuberculosis,[400] COVID,[24] and HIV infections (discussed in Chapter 65). ITP is associated with *H. pylori*, particularly in Europe and Japan and other countries with a high background prevalence of *H. pylori*. Platelet counts may or may not normalize with treatment directed only at *Helicobacter*.[401-410] The ASH guidelines recommend that *H. pylori* infection be considered in all adults with ITP for whom eradication therapy would be undertaken if testing were positive. Routine *H. pylori* testing is not recommended for children because the incidence of *H. pylori* infection is similar between patients with persistent and chronic ITP and the general population.[5]

ITP is a well-known complication of chronic lymphocytic leukemia,[411] although it is not as frequent as autoimmune hemolytic anemia in these patients. It has also been reported in patients with other lymphoproliferative disorders, including Hodgkin disease.[412-414] Thrombocytopenia in patients with a variety of solid tumors has also been thought to most likely be immune mediated.[415-417]

Thrombocytopenia may accompany Graves disease and Hashimoto thyroiditis,[418-420] but it is not certain that it is immunologically mediated. Platelet-associated IgG has been increased when studied,[420] but there may also be an element of enhanced reticuloendothelial phagocytosis.

ALLOIMMUNE THROMBOCYTOPENIA

Platelets express membrane-associated epitopes as a result of polymorphisms in discrete regions of the platelet membrane surface glycoproteins.[421] No natural antibodies to human platelet antigens are known. Acquired platelet alloantibodies are of clinical importance in three circumstances: (a) Neonatal alloimmune thrombocytopenia (NAIT), which is the result of the placental transfer of alloantibodies formed by the mother to incompatible fetal platelet antigens[422]; (b) posttransfusion purpura (PTP), a rare disorder in which the transfusion of platelet-containing blood products provokes the formation of alloantibodies that act as autoantibodies[423]; and (c) passive transfer of platelet alloantibodies after transfusion from a multiparous or multiply transfused donor.[424-427]

Neonatal Alloimmune Thrombocytopenia
Pathophysiology

NAIT was first described in 1962 in otherwise normal infants of healthy mothers as TTP caused by destruction of fetal platelets by maternal antibodies.[428] Several prospective studies have implicated maternal alloimmunization to platelet-specific paternal antigens.[429,430] Thus, as a consequence of the inheritance by the fetus of platelet antigens lacking in the mother, alloantibodies are formed in the maternal circulation and cross the placenta, producing the leading cause of severe thrombocytopenia in the fetus[431] (*Figure 48.6*).

Alloimmunization to platelet antigens can occur at any time during the first pregnancy and recurs in >80% of patients during subsequent pregnancies.[432] However, alloimmunization can develop following exposure to fetal blood during infant delivery, leading to cases of NAIT in subsequent pregnancies.[433] Antibodies can be detected as early as the 19th week, and thrombocytopenia has been found in utero by 20 weeks' gestation.[434] However, not all mothers who lack the antigens present on fetal platelets develop antibodies, and not all fetuses and neonates develop thrombocytopenia despite maternal antibody development.[430]

The most commonly formed antibodies are directed against human platelet antigen (HPA)-1a (Pl^{A1},Zw^A) or HPA-5b (Br^a, Zav, Hc), with more than 95% of the serologically confirmed cases caused by antigen alloimmunization against HPA-1, -2, -3, -5, and -15.[429,430,435] One large study examined maternal sera for platelet-reactive antibodies in mothers of infants suspected of NAIT and found maternal HPA-1a alloimmunization accounted for 79% of confirmed NAIT cases.[436] Other antigens less commonly detected have also been found to be responsible for cases of NAIT.[429,430,436-447] These antigens are present on several platelet membrane glycoproteins (GPs), including GPIb-V-IX, GPIIb/IIIa, and CD109, and they interact with protein components of blood vessel walls, the extracellular matrix, and other coagulation factors.[436,448] The overwhelming majority of platelet polymorphisms found are caused by a single base-pair mutation leading to a single amino acid substitution in the polypeptide chain of the specific glycoprotein.[435] Rarely, HLA antibodies are responsible[429,449]; however, alloimmunization against low-frequency HPA and HLA antigens accounts for a small proportion of cases.[438] ABO antigen incompatibility has also been implicated in cases of NAIT.[425] It is known that platelets express A and B surface antigens in small quantities, and maternal anti-B IgG antibodies have been shown to be causal.[450]

HPA-1 mismatch is present in 1 in 50 births, yet NAIT occurs in only 1 in 1000 to 2000 births.[429,431,434,440] Maternal HLA class II determinants appear to be important. A high incidence of maternal allotypes HLA-DR3 and HLA-DRw52a has been demonstrated in mothers alloimmunized to fetal alloantigen HPA-1,[429,449] and a high

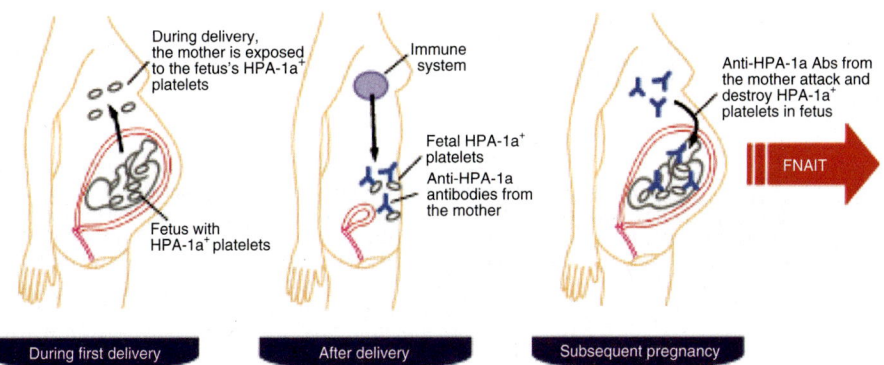

FIGURE 48.6 Pathophysiology of antibody development. HPA, human platelet antigen. (Reprinted from Podolak-Dawidziak M. Megakaryocyte progenitors in immune thrombocytopenic purpura/ITP. *Thromb Res.* 1991;62(1-2):93-96. Copyright © 1991 by Elsevier Ireland. With permission.)

incidence of HLA-DR6 has been reported in mothers sensitized to PLA-5b.[430] Interestingly, a large prospective study showed that infants born to women who were sensitized to class I HLA antigens were unaffected and showed no correlation between antibody development and infant platelet count.[451]

Clinical Features

Infants with NAIT are born with signs and symptoms of severe thrombocytopenia, including petechiae, purpura, and bleeding, and are at risk for significant morbidity and mortality.[452,453] Thrombocytopenia is usually present at birth, but the platelet count may fall further during the postpartum period. ICH occurs in 10% to 30% of infants, with up to three-quarters of the episodes occurring in utero.[454,455] Risk for development of ICH is likely related to gestational age of the infant and severity of thrombocytopenia. ICH in a previous infant, especially that which occurred antenatally, is the only predictor for ICH recurrence in subsequent pregnancies.[455,456] Over 75% of ICH cases occur after 20 weeks of gestation and 54% occur prior to 28 weeks of gestation.[457] An overall mortality rate of 6% to 14% has been reported.[436,440,441] Thrombocytopenia usually resolves after 10 to 14 days. Platelet antibody titers during the second half of the pregnancy appear to correlate with the risk of thrombocytopenia or bleeding, or both, in NAIT.[452,458]

Laboratory Diagnosis

When infants are born with isolated thrombocytopenia with platelet counts <20,000 μL, NAIT must be suspected, especially during the first pregnancy. Unfortunately, the first indication of NAIT is usually following birth when the newborn presents with the clinical symptoms previously described. Investigators have looked at screening mothers found to be HPA-1a antibody negative during various stages of gestation in an attempt to identify at-risk infants and to reduce morbidity and mortality.[459] To date, the best positive predictive factor of NAIT is the mother's anti-HPA-1a antibody level during pregnancy, with the antibody titer inversely proportional to the neonatal platelet count.[460] Maternal plasma should be studied with paternal or neonatal platelets as targets; maternal (antigen-negative) platelets and paternal plasma are appropriate negative controls. NAIT is diagnosed when platelet antigen incompatibility is found between the parents, maternal antipaternal platelet antibodies are present, and the antibody detected corresponds to the incompatibility of platelet antigens that have been noted. However, confirmed cases of NAIT using serologic diagnostic modalities are made in less than half of the cases.[437] Maternal autoantibodies might not be detected in cases where the mother has a history of autoimmune thrombocytopenia or is thrombocytopenic.[438]

Treatment

Aggressive treatment of severely thrombocytopenic infants is indicated, especially if clinical signs and symptoms of bleeding are present. Immediate treatment with platelet transfusions to obtain a platelet count > 25,000 to 30,000 μL will reduce the likelihood of severe bleeding complications.[461-463] Higher platelet transfusion thresholds of 50,000/μL or higher have been associated with increased rates of mortality and severe bleeding in preterm infants in a recent prospective randomized clinical trial in patients with severe thrombocytopenia.[462] Platelets, ideally, should be ABO compatible, CMV negative, volume reduced (if indicated), and irradiated. Therapy should not be delayed if only random (nonmatched) donor platelets are available.[461] While HPA-selected platelet transfusion results in a higher platelet increment, random-donor platelets have been shown to yield an adequate platelet increment of >30,000/μL.[462] HPA 1a–negative and HPA 5b–negative donor platelets are available but may be in short supply or difficult to quickly obtain. Also, maternal platelets are antigen negative and can be obtained by pheresis, then concentrated, irradiated, washed, and transfused. IVIG may be given concomitantly with a platelet transfusion to potentially subdue the antibody response and prolong platelet survival.[432] The dose of IVIG varies from 0.4 to 2 g/kg given once per day over 1 to 5 days.[432,464] A recent meta-analysis of 754 infants did not demonstrate a clear benefit of IVIG administration on platelet count increment with about one-third of patients receiving IVIG.[463] A treatment guideline for infants with suspected NAIT was proposed in a recent study (Figure 48.7).[465]

Prevention of NAIT: In women with no personal or family history of NAIT, screening by platelet typing is not currently recommended and has not been widely adopted.[432,466] Maternal platelet antigen typing has been recommended for those with a sister whose pregnancy was complicated by NAIT or if personal or family history is suggestive of NAIT (e.g., neonatal thrombocytopenia of undetermined origin or fetal or neonatal ICH of undetermined origin). In these cases, maternal and paternal platelet typing is performed simultaneously in order to look for incompatibility in the platelet HLA-1 antigen system. Screening studies to detect neonatal thrombocytopenia during the first pregnancy have been limited to patients with known PL^{A1} incompatibility and an HLA allotype associated with an increased incidence of antibody formation.[429] However, after the birth of one child with NAIT, subsequent pregnancies should be evaluated antenatally.

When maternal and paternal platelet typing document a risk of NAIT, after the index case over 85% of that couples' subsequent fetuses will be at risk for NAIT. In the absence of any intervention, thrombocytopenia in the second affected fetus is always as severe as or more severe than in the previous fetus/infant.[467] Because of the high risk of in utero bleeding, the majority of which includes ICH, initiating therapy antenatally, rather than waiting until birth, has become standard. Previously, it was recommended that fetal platelet typing[443-446] and platelet counts should be obtained at 18 to 20 weeks' gestation.[447] Because the use of serial fetal blood sampling procedures is clearly associated with an increased risk of fetal morbidity and mortality, some practitioners prefer to avoid performing fetal blood sampling and choose to treat empirically. The precise role of

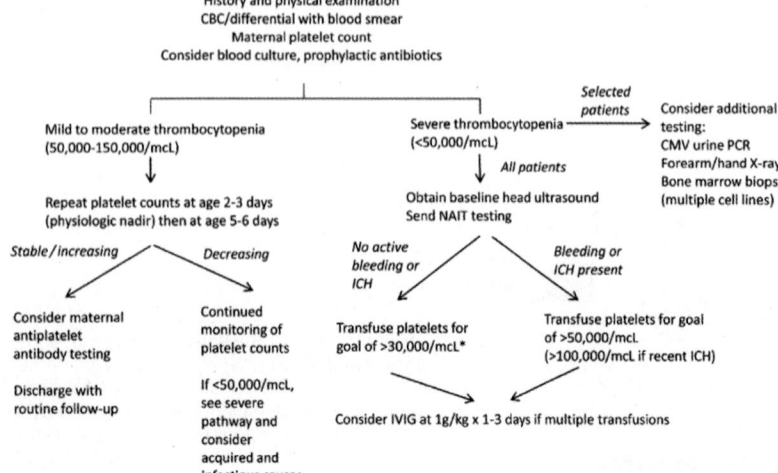

FIGURE 48.7 Proposed schema for infants with suspected neonatal alloimmune thrombocytopenia (NAIT). CBC, complete blood count; CMV, cytomegalovirus; ICH, intracranial hemorrhage; IVIG, intravenous immunoglobulin; PCR, polymerase chain reaction. (Adapted with permission of SLACK Incorporated from Sillers L, Van Slambrouck C, Lappin-Carr G. Neonatal thrombocytopenia: etiology and diagnosis. *Pediatr Ann.* 2015;44(7):e175-e180; permission conveyed through Copyright Clearance Center, Inc.)

this invasive procedure remains to be determined, and overall, the practice has diminished.[432,468,469] A risk-stratified approach should be considered in each case (*Figure 48.8*).[470] The father's HPA genotype can also be used to determine if the infant has a possibility of inheriting an implicated antigen (*Figure 48.9*).[470] In an infant at risk for NAIT, the severity of the disease can be estimated by testing the strength of the anti-HPA antibody present in the mother's serum or by the severity of thrombocytopenia in an affected sibling.[438] If upon testing platelet incompatibility is noted and the infant is thrombocytopenic, maternal treatment should be instituted and maintained during the pregnancy.[435,471] Maternal treatment options include IVIG, corticosteroids, intrauterine platelet transfusion, and early delivery.[432,470] Combination therapy with IVIG plus steroids may lead to higher platelet counts in women with a previous child with ICH or a current fetus with platelet counts <20,000 μL[454]; however, the recent literature suggests a stratified treatment approach for each case.[470] Fetal platelet transfusions have been advocated. However, because of the risk of fetal mortality, this has become a therapy of last resort, to be used only if IVIG or prednisone is ineffective.[472] Monitoring for development of ICH is recommended every 4 weeks starting at about 16 to 20 weeks' gestation.[473,474] There is no consensus on whether fetuses affected by NAIT or at risk for NAIT should be delivered by cesarean section.[475] Several studies have suggested elective delivery via caesarian section at 37 to 38 weeks' gestation for high-risk pregnancies, whereas others have recommended that vaginal delivery be allowed only in those with fetal platelet counts > 50,000 μL.[432,468,472]

Studies of the cost-effectiveness of empiric maternal treatment versus treatment directed by fetal blood sampling favored empiric treatment, decreasing perinatal deaths, although increasing the number of infants with long-term neurologic deficits.[469] Follow-up studies of children after antenatal treatment for alloimmune thrombocytopenia show that general health and neurodevelopmental outcome is comparable with that of the general population. However, significantly more infections and hearing problems were observed in children who were not exposed to maternal IVIG treatment in comparison with children who were exposed to IVIG treatment or the normal population.[476]

Posttransfusion Purpura

Alloantibodies that develop as a result of frequent transfusions are responsible for the destruction of the transfused platelets. Rarely, however, severe thrombocytopenia in the recipient—that is, destruction of host platelets—is produced by the transfusion of incompatible platelets, and this potentially fatal reaction is known as PTP.[256,257,477]

Over 250 cases of PTP have been reported since the initial description in 1961. PTP is characterized by abrupt onset of severe thrombocytopenia and bleeding that occurs approximately 1 week following a blood transfusion. Timing of onset together with primarily mucocutaneous bleeding and presence of potent HPA-specific antibodies are diagnostic of PTP; however, the diagnosis is a clinical one and physicians must consider this diagnosis in any patient who develops thrombocytopenia within 3 to 14 days after transfusion. PTP most often occurs after transfusion of packed red blood cells but has been described after whole blood, platelets, and plasma are given.[478] While leukoreduction of whole blood reduced platelet contamination 100-fold,[479] the recent reemergence of use of whole blood may lead to increased exposure to platelet antigen with an increase in PTP.

The syndrome occurs most commonly in multiparous women who have been sensitized by pregnancy; however, previously transfused patients may also develop PTP. The antibody most commonly develops against PL^{A1} (HPA-1a) in PL^{A2} (HPA-1b) homozygous recipients, but the Bak (HPA-3a/HPA-3b), Pen (HPA-4a/HPA-4b), Br (HPA-5a/HPA-5b), and Nak^a polymorphisms have been implicated as well[256,257,423,479-482] (*Table 48.7*).

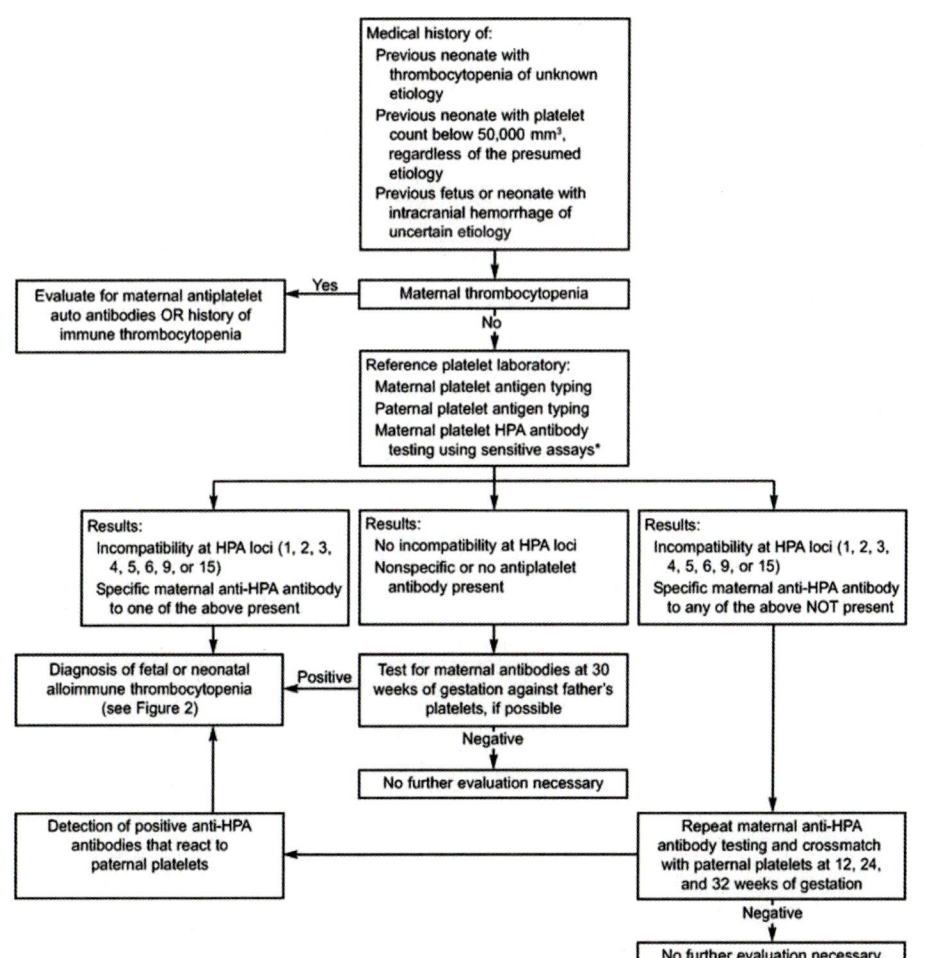

FIGURE 48.8 Risk-stratified approach and management stratum to maternal workup in neonatal alloimmune thrombocytopenia. HPA, human platelet antigen. (Reprinted with permission from Pacheco LD, Berkowitz RL, Moise KJ Jr, et al. Fetal and neonatal alloimmune thrombocytopenia: a management algorithm based on risk stratification. *Obstet Gynecol*. 2011;118(5):1157-1163. Copyright © 2011 by The American College of Obstetricians and Gynecologists.)

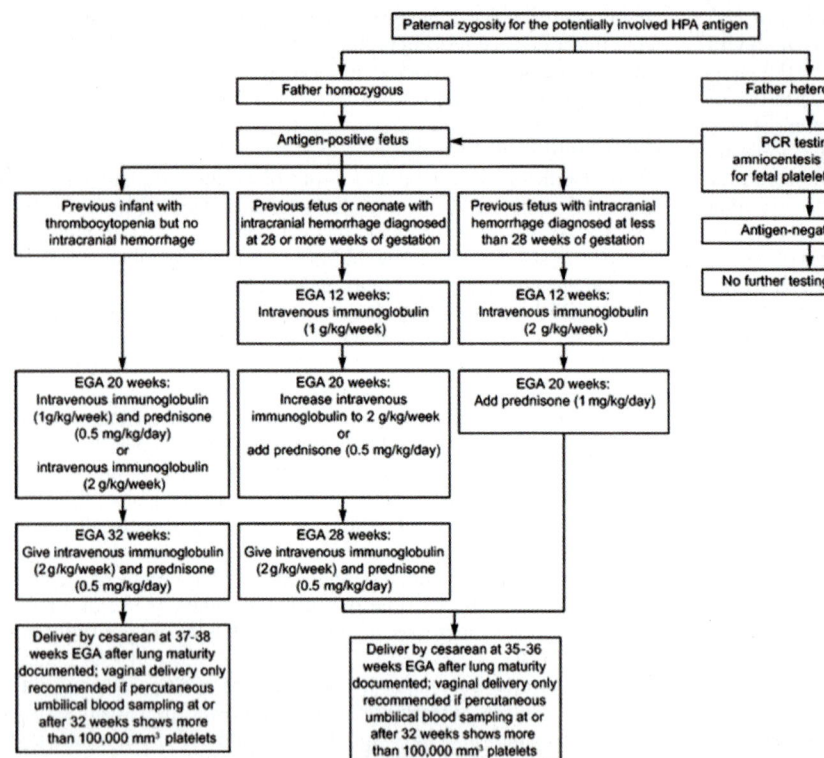

FIGURE 48.9 Risk-stratified approach and management stratum to paternal zygosity in neonatal alloimmune thrombocytopenia (NAIT). CVS, chorionic villus sampling; EGA, estimated gestational age; HPA, human platelet antigen; PCR, polymerase chain reaction. (Reprinted with permission from Pacheco LD, Berkowitz RL, Moise KJ Jr, et al. Fetal and neonatal alloimmune thrombocytopenia: a management algorithm based on risk stratification. *Obstet Gynecol*. 2011;118(5):1157-1163. Copyright © 2011 by The American College of Obstetricians and Gynecologists.)

The pathophysiology of this rare but severe thrombocytopenia is still uncertain, but several hypotheses have been proposed: (a) autologous platelets are destroyed because of binding of immune complexes to their surface; (b) recipient platelets acquire the phenotype of the donor's platelets because they bind soluble antigens from the transfused blood product, and the platelets are then destroyed by alloantibodies; and (c) exposure to foreign platelets in transfused products induces the formation of autoantibodies to the recipient's platelets.[423,483,484]

PTP is self-limited, resolving within 1 to 3 weeks in most patients. Treatment with IVIG, plasmapheresis, and steroids may shorten the period of thrombocytopenia. IVIG 1 g/kg daily for 2 days is much more preferable because, although plasmapheresis is effective in many patients,[478,485-487] both it and steroids take two or more weeks to act and pheresis requires central venous access with large-bore catheters, which places the patient in danger of significant bleeding.[488-492] Platelet transfusions should be reserved for life-threatening hemorrhage, because patients often develop a febrile reaction and an increase in platelet count is infrequent.

References

1. Rodeghiero F, Stasi R, Gernsheimer T, et al. Standardization of terminology, definitions and outcome criteria in immune thrombocytopenic purpura of adults and children: report from an international working group. *Blood*. 2009;113:2386-2393.
2. George JN. Management of immune thrombocytopenia-something old, something new. *N Engl J Med*. 2010;363:1959-1961.
3. Tolti LJ, Arnold DM. Pathophysiology and management of chronic immune thrombocytopenia: focusing on what matters. *Br J Haematol*. 2010;152:52-60.
4. Bussel JB. Traditional and new approaches to the management of immune thrombocytopenia: issues of when and who to treat. *Hematol Oncol Clin North Am*. 2009;23:1329-1341.
5. Neunert C, Terrell DR, Arnold DM, et al. The American Society of Hematology 2019 evidence-based practice guideline for immune thrombocytopenia. *Blood*. 2019;3:3829-3866.
6. Provan D, Stasi R, Newland A, et al. International consensus report on the investigation and management of primary immune thrombocytopenia. *Blood*. 2010;115:168-186.
7. George J, Harake M, Aster R. Thrombocytopenia due to enhanced platelet destruction by immunologic mechanisms. In: Beutler E, Lichtman MA, Coller BS, Kipps TJ, eds. *Williams Hematology*. 5th ed. McGraw-Hill; 1995:1315-1355.
8. Lusher JM, Zuelzer WW. Idiopathic thrombocytopenic purpura in childhood. *J Pediatr*. 1966;68:971-979.
9. Lusher JM, Iyer R. Idiopathic thrombocytopenic purpura in children. *Semin Thromb Hemost*. 1977;3:175-199.
10. Imbach P, Kuhne T, Müller D, et al. Childhood ITP: 12 months follow-up data from the prospective registry 1 of the Intercontinental Childhood ITP Study Group (ICIS). *Pediatr Blood Cancer*. 2006;46:351-356.
11. Heitink-Polle KMJ, Uiterwaal CSPM, Porcelijn L, et al. Intravenous immunoglobulin vs observation in childhood immune thrombocytopenia: a randomized controlled trial. *Blood*. 2018;132:883-891.
12. Rosthøj S, Rajantie J, Treutiger I, et al. Duration and morbidity of chronic ITP in children: five-year Follow-up of a Nordic cohort. *Acta Paediatr*. 2012;101:761-766.
13. Neunert CE, Buchanan GR, Imbach P, et al. Bleeding manifestations and management of children with persistent and chronic immune thrombocytopenia: data from the Intercontinental Cooperative ITP Study Group (ICIS). *Blood*. 2013;121:4457-4462.
14. Cortelazzo S, Finazzi G, Buelli M, et al. High risk of severe bleeding in aged patients with chronic idiopathic thrombocytopenic purpura. *Blood*. 1991;77:31-33.
15. Stasi R, Stipa E, Masi M, et al. Long-term observation of 208 adults with chronic idiopathic thrombocytopenic purpura. *Am J Med*. 1995;98:436-442.
16. Pizzuto J, Ambriz R. Therapeutic experience on 934 adults with idiopathic thrombocytopenic purpura: multicentric trial of the Cooperative Latin American Group on Hemostasis and Thrombosis. *Blood*. 1984;64:1179-1183.

Table 48.7. Platelet Alloantigens Implicated in the Development of Posttransfusion Purpura

Serologic Designation	Alternative Designation	Phenotype Frequency	Antigen Location
PL^{A1} (HPA-1a)	Zw^a	0.96-0.99	gpIIIa
PL^{A2} (HPA-1b)	Zw^b	0.27	gpIIIa
Bak^a (HPA-3a)	Lek^a	0.78-0.89	gpIIb
Bak^b (HPA-3b)	Lek^b	0.50-0.70	gpIIb
Pen^a (HPA-4a)	Yuk^b	0.99	gpIIIa^a
Pen^b (HPA-4b)	Yuk^a	0.01	gpIIIa^a
Br^b (HPA-5a)	Zav^b	0.99	gpIa
Br^a (HPA-5b)	Zav^a	0.18-0.20	gpIa

Abbreviations: gp, glycoprotein; HPA, human platelet alloantigen.
Modified from McCrae KR, Herman JH. Posttransfusion purpura: two unusual cases and a literature review. *Am J Hematol*. 1996;52(3):205-211. Copyright © 1996 Wiley-Liss, Inc. Reprinted by permission of John Wiley & Sons, Inc.
^{a}Antigen appears to be distinct from PL^{A1} (HPA-1a).

17. Choi SI, McClure PD. Idiopathic thrombocytopenic purpura in childhood. *Can Med Assoc J.* 1967;97:562-568.
18. Komrower GM, Watson GH. Prognosis in idiopathic thrombocytopenic purpura of childhood. *Arch Dis Child.* 1954;29:502.
19. Segal JB, Powe NR. Prevalence of immune thrombocytopenia: analyses of administrative data. *J Thromb Haemost.* 2006;4:2377-2383.
20. Kiefel V, Santoso S, Mueller-Eckhardt C. Serological, biochemical, and molecular aspects of platelet autoantigens. *Semin Hematol.* 1992;29:26-33.
21. Horstman L, Jy W, Schultz DR, et al. Complement-mediated fragmentation and lysis of opsonized platelets: gender differences in sensitivity. *J Lab Clin Med.* 1994;123:515-525.
22. Nomura S, Yanabu M, Soga T, et al. Analysis of idiopathic thrombocytopenic purpura patients with antiglycoprotein IIb/IIIa or Ib autoantibodies. *Acta Haematol.* 1991;86:25-30.
23. Cines DB, Bussel JB, Liebman HA. The ITP syndrome: pathogenic and clinical diversity. *Blood.* 2009;113:6511-6521.
24. Mahevas M, Moulis G, Andres E, et al. Clinical characteristics, management and outcome of COVID19-associated immune thrombocytopenia: a French multicentre series. *Br J Haematol.* 2020;190:e224-e229.
25. McMillan R, Wang L, Tomer A, Nichol J, Pistillo J. Suppression of in vitro megakaryocyte production by antiplatelet autoantibodies from adult patients with chronic ITP. *Blood.* 2004;103:1364-1369.
26. Chang M, Nakagawa PA, Williams SA, et al. Immune thrombocytopenic purpura (ITP) plasma and purified ITP monoclonal autoantibodies inhibit megakaryocytopoiesis in vitro. *Blood.* 2003;102:887-895.
27. Houwerzijl EJ, Blom NR, van der Want JJ, et al. Ultrastructural study shows morphologic features of apoptosis and para-apoptosis in megakaryocytes from patients with idiopathic thrombocytopenic purpura. *Blood.* 2004;103:500-506.
28. Heyns Adu P, Badenhorst PN, Lotter MG, et al. Platelet turnover and kinetics in immune thrombocytopenic purpura: results with autologous 111In-labeled platelets and homologous 51Cr-labeled platelets differ. *Blood.* 1986;67:86-92.
29. Ballem PJ, Segal GM, Stratton JR, et al. Mechanisms of thrombocytopenia in chronic autoimmune thrombocytopenic purpura: evidence of both impaired platelet production and increased platelet clearance. *J Clin Invest.* 1987;80:33-40.
30. Hasegawa Y, Nagasawa T, Kamoshita M, et al. Effects of anti-platelet glycoprotein Ib and/or IIb/IIIa autoantibodies on the size of megakaryocytes in patients with immune thrombocytopenia. *Eur J Haematol.* 1995;55:152-157.
31. de Alarcon PA, Mazur EM, Schmeider JA. In vitro megakaryocytopoiesis in children with acute idiopathic thrombocytopenic purpura. *Am J Pediatr Hematol Oncol.* 1987;9:212-218.
32. Podolak-Dawidziak M. Megakaryocyte progenitors in immune thrombocytopenic purpura/ITP. *Thromb Res.* 1991;62:93-96.
33. Abgrall JF, Berthou C, Sensebe L, et al. Decreased in vitro megakaryocyte colony formation in chronic idiopathic thrombocytopenic purpura. *Br J Haematol.* 1993;85:803-804.
34. Emmons RV, Reid DM, Cohen RL, et al. Human thrombopoietin levels are high when thrombocytopenia is due to megakaryocyte deficiency and low when due to increased platelet destruction. *Blood.* 1996;87:4068-4071.
35. Ichikawa N, Ishida F, Shimodaira S, et al. Regulation of serum thrombopoietin levels by platelets and megakaryocytes in patients with aplastic anaemia and idiopathic thrombocytopenic purpura. *Thromb Haemostasis.* 1996;76:156-160.
36. Nichol JL. Thrombopoietin levels after chemotherapy and in naturally occurring human diseases. *Curr Opin Hematol.* 1998;5:203-208.
37. Scheding S, Bergmann M, Shimosaka A, et al. Human plasma thrombopoietin levels are regulated by binding to platelet thrombopoietin receptors in vivo. *Transfusion.* 2002;42:321-327.
38. Harrington WJ, Minnich V, Hollingsworth JW, Moore CV. Demonstration of a thrombocytopenic factor in the blood of patients with thrombocytopenic purpura. *J Lab Clin Med.* 1951;38:1-10.
39. Shulman NR, Marder VJ, Weinrach RS. Similarities between known antiplatelet antibodies and factor responsible for thrombocytopenia in idiopathic thrombocytopenic purpura. *Ann N Y Acad Sci.* 1965;124:499.
40. Van Leeuwen EF, van der Ven JT, Engelfriet CP, von dem Borne AE. Specificity of autoantibodies in autoimmune thrombocytopenia. *Blood.* 1982;59:23-26.
41. Dixon R, Rosse W, Ebbert L. Quantitative determination of antibody in idiopathic thrombocytopenic purpura: correlation of serum and platelet bound antibody with clinical response. *N Engl J Med.* 1975;292:230-236.
42. Kernoff LM. Influence of the amount of platelet-bound IgG on platelet survival and the site of sequestration in autoimmune thrombocytopenia. *Blood.* 1980;55:730-733.
43. Berchtold P, Wenger M. Autoantibodies against platelet glycoproteins in autoimmune thrombocytopenic purpura: their clinical significance and response to treatment. *Blood.* 1993;81:1246-1250.
44. Hou M, Stockelberg D, Kutti J, Wadenvik H. Antibodies against platelet GPIb/IX, GPIIb/IIIa, and other platelet antigens in chronic idiopathic thrombocytopenic purpura. *Eur J Hematol.* 1995;55:307-314.
45. Kelton JG. The serologic investigation of patients with autoimmune thrombocytopenia. *Thromb Haemostasis.* 1995;74:228-233.
46. Hou M, Stockelberg D, Kutti J, Wadenvik H. Fab-mediated binding of glycoprotein Ib/IX and IIb/IIIa specific antibodies in chronic idiopathic thrombocytopenic purpura. *Br J Haematol.* 1995;91:944-950.
47. Woods VL, Oh E, Mason D, McMillan R. Autoantibodies against the platelet glycoprotein IIb/IIIa complex in patients with chronic ITP. *Blood.* 1984;63:368-375.
48. Woods VL, Kurata Y, Montgomery RR, et al. Autoantibodies against platelet glycoprotein Ib in patients with chronic immune thrombocytopenic purpura. *Blood.* 1984;64:156-160.
49. Beardsley DS, Spiegel JE, Jacobs MM, et al. Platelet membrane glycoprotein IIIa contains target antigens that bind antiplatelet antibodies in immune thrombocytopenias. *J Clin Invest.* 1984;74:1701-1707.
50. Tsubakio T, Tani P, Woods VL, McMillan R. Autoantibodies against platelet GPIIb/IIIa in chronic ITP react with different epitopes. *Br J Haematol.* 1987;67:345-348.
51. Tomiyama Y, Kurata Y, Mizutani H, et al. Platelet glycoprotein IIb as a target antigen in two patients with chronic idiopathic thrombocytopenic purpura. *Br J Haematol.* 1987;66:535-538.
52. Tomiyama Y, Kurata Y, Shibata Y, et al. Immunochemical characterization of an autoantigen on platelet glycoprotein IIb in chronic ITP: comparison with the Baka alloantigen. *Br J Haematol.* 1989;71:77-83.
53. Fujisawa K, O'Toole TE, Tani P, et al. Autoantibodies to the presumptive cytoplasmic domain of platelet glycoprotein IIIa in patients with chronic immune thrombocytopenic purpura. *Blood.* 1991;77:2207-2213.
54. Fujisawa K, Tani P, O'Toole TE, et al. Different specificities of platelet-associated and plasma autoantibodies to platelet GPIIb-IIIa in patients with chronic immune thrombocytopenic purpura. *Blood.* 1992;79:1441-1446.
55. Fujisawa K, Tani P, McMillan R. Platelet-associated antibody to glycoprotein IIb/IIIa from chronic immune thrombocytopenic purpura patients often binds to divalent cation-dependent antigens. *Blood.* 1993;81:1284-1289.
56. Bowditch RD, Tani P, McMillan R. Reactivity of autoantibodies from chronic ITP patients with recombinant glycoprotein IIIa peptides. *Br J Haematol.* 1995;91:178-184.
57. Hou M, Stockelberg D, Kutti J, Wadenvik H. Glycoprotein IIb/IIIa autoantigenic repertoire in chronic idiopathic thrombocytopenic purpura. *Br J Haematol.* 1995;91:971-975.
58. Kuwana M, Kaburaki J, Kitasato H, et al. Immunodominant epitopes on glycoprotein IIb-IIIa recognized by autoreactive T cells in patients with immune thrombocytopenic purpura. *Blood.* 2001;98:130-139.
59. Kosugi S, Tomiyama Y, Honda S, et al. Platelet-associated anti-GPIIb-IIIa autoantibodies in chronic immune thrombocytopenic purpura recognizing epitopes close to the ligand-binding site of glycoprotein (GP) IIb. *Blood.* 2001;98:1819-1827.
60. McMillan R, Lopez-Dee J, Loftus JC. Autoantibodies to αIIbβ3 in patients with chronic immune thrombocytopenic purpura bind primarily to epitopes on αIIbβ. *Blood.* 2001;97:2171-2172.
61. Kiefel V, Santoso S, Kaufmann E, Mueller-Eckhardt C. Autoantibodies against platelet glycoprotein Ib/IX: a frequent finding in autoimmune thrombocytopenic purpura. *Br J Haematol.* 1991;79:256-262.
62. He R, Reid DM, Jones CE, Shulman NR. Extracellular epitopes of platelet glycoprotein Ibα reactive with serum antibodies from patients with chronic idiopathic thrombocytopenic purpura. *Blood.* 1995;86:3789-3796.
63. Bierling P, Bettaieb A, Fromont P, et al. Anti-GMP 140 (CD62) autoantibody in a patient with autoimmune thrombocytopenia. *Br J Haematol.* 1994;87:631-633.
64. Kosugi S, Tomiyama Y, Honda S, et al. Anti-αvβ3 antibodies in chronic immune thrombocytopenia. *Thromb Haemostasis.* 2001;85:36-41.
65. van Vliet HH, Kappers-Klune MC, van der Hel JW, Abels J. Antibodies against glycosphingolipids in sera of patients with idiopathic thrombocytopenic purpura. *Br J Haematol.* 1987;67:103-108.
66. Koerner TAW, Weinfeld HM, Bullard LSB, Williams LCJ. Antibodies against platelet glycosphingolipids: detection in serum by quantitative HPTLC-autoradiography and association with autoimmune and alloimmune processes. *Blood.* 1989;74:274-284.
67. Harris EN, Asherson RA, Gharavi AE, et al. Thrombocytopenia in SLE and related autoimmune disorders: association with anticardiolipin antibody. *Br J Haematol.* 1985;59:227-230.
68. Nomura S, Yanabu M, Fukuroi T, et al. Anti-phospholipid antibodies bind to platelet microparticles in idiopathic (autoimmune) thrombocytopenic purpura. *Ann Haematol.* 1992;65:46-49.
69. Nomura S, Yanabu M, Miyake T, et al. Relationship of microparticles with β2-glycoprotein I and P-selectin positivity to anticardiolipin antibodies in immune thrombocytopenic purpura. *Ann Haematol.* 1995;70:25-30.
70. Arfors L, Winiarski J, Lefvert AK. Prevalence of antibodies to cardiolipin in chronic ITP and reactivity with platelet membranes. *Eur J Haematol.* 1996;56:230-234.
71. Stasi R, Stipa E, Masi M, et al. Prevalence and clinical significance of elevated antiphospholipid antibodies in patients with idiopathic thrombocytopenic purpura. *Blood.* 1994;84:4203-4208.
72. Diz-Kucukkaya R, Hacihanefioglu A, Yeneral M, et al. Antiphospholipid antibodies and antiphospholipid syndrome in patients presenting with immune thrombocytopenic purpura: a prospective cohort study. *Blood.* 2001;98:1760-1764.
73. He BR, Reid DM, Jones CE, Shulman NR. Spectrum of Ig classes, specificities, and titers of serum antiglycoproteins in chronic idiopathic thrombocytopenic purpura. *Blood.* 1994;83:1024-1032.
74. Cines DB, Blanchette VS. Immune thrombocytopenic purpura. *N Engl J Med.* 2002;346:995-1008.
75. Nardi MA, Liu LX, Karpatkin S. GPIIIa-(49-66) is a major pathophysiologically relevant antigenic determinant for anti-platelet GPIIIa of HIV-1 related immunologic thrombocytopenia. *Proc Natl Acad Sci U S A.* 1997;94:7589-7594.
76. Sugiyama T, Okuma M, Ushikubi F, et al. A novel platelet-aggregating factor found in a patient with defective collagen-induced platelet aggregation and autoimmune thrombocytopenia. *Blood.* 1987;69:1712-1720.
77. Yanabu M, Nomura S, Fukuroi T, et al. Synergistic action in platelet activation induced by an antiplatelet autoantibody in ITP. *Br J Haematol.* 1991;78:87-93.
78. Yanabu M, Nomura S, Fukuroi T, et al. Platelet activation induced by an antiplatelet autoantibody against CD9 antigen and its inhibition by another autoantibody in immune thrombocytopenic purpura. *Br J Haematol.* 1993;84:694-701.

79. Hashimoto Y, Tanabe J, Mohri H, Ohkubo T. Autoimmune antibody in a patient with idiopathic thrombocytopenic purpura reacted to the platelet low molecular weight glycoproteins and activated platelets. *Am J Clin Pathol.* 1994;101:370-374.
80. Deckmyn H, DeReys S. Functional effects of human antiplatelet antibodies. *Semin. Thromb Haemostasis.* 1995;21:46-59.
81. Balduini CL, Bertolino G, Noris P, et al. Defect of platelet aggregation and adhesion induced by autoantibodies against platelet glycoprotein IIIa. *Thromb Haemostasis.* 1992;68:208-213.
82. Taub JW, Warrier I, Holtkamp C, et al. Characterization of autoantibodies against the platelet glycoprotein antigens IIb/IIIa in childhood idiopathic thrombocytopenia purpura. *Am J Hematol.* 1995;48:104-107.
83. Ware RE, Howard TA. Phenotypic and clonal analysis of T lymphocytes in childhood immune thrombocytopenic purpura. *Blood.* 1993;82:2137-2142.
84. Semple JW, Milev Y, Cosgrove D, et al. Differences in serum cytokine levels in acute and chronic autoimmune thrombocytopenic purpura: relationship to platelet phenotype and antiplatelet T-cell reactivity. *Blood.* 1996;87:4245-4254.
85. Olsson B, Andersson PO, Jernås M, et al. T-cell-mediated cytotoxicity toward platelets in chronic idiopathic thrombocytopenic purpura. *Nat Med.* 2003;9:1123-1124.
86. Wang TT, Zhao H, Ren H, et al. Type 1 and type 2 T-cell profiles in idiopathic thrombocytopenic purpura. *Haematologica.* 2005;90:914-923.
87. Zhang XL, Peng J, Sun JZ, et al. De novo induction of platelet-specific $CD4^+CD25^+$ regulatory T cells from $CD4^+CD25^-$ cells in patients with chronic thrombocytopenic purpura. *Blood.* 2009;113:2568-2577.
88. Ji X, Zhang L, Peng J, Hou M. T cell immune abnormalities in immune thrombocytopenia. *J Hematol Oncol.* 2014;7:72-77.
89. Bao W, Bussel JB, Heck S, et al. Improved regulatory T-cell activity in patients with chronic immune thrombocytopenia treated with thrombopoietic agents. *Blood.* 2010;116:4639-4645.
90. McKenzie CGJ, Guo L, Freedman J, et al. Cellular immune dysfunction in immune thrombocytopenia (ITP). *Br J Haematol.* 2013;163:10-23.
91. Terrell DR, Beebe LA, Vesely SK, Neas BR, Segal JB, George JN. The incidence of immune thrombocytopenic purpura in children and adults: a critical review of published reports. *Am J Hematol.* 2010;85:174-180.
92. Yong M, Schoonen WM, Li L, et al. Epidemiology of paediatric immune thrombocytopenia in the general practice research database. *Br J Haematol.* 2010;149:855-864.
93. Nugent DJ. Immune thrombocytopenic purpura of childhood. *Hematology Am Soc Hematol Educ Program.* 2006;2006:97-103.
94. Shad AT, Gonzalez CE, Sandler SG. Treatment of immune thrombocytopenic purpura in children: current concepts. *Paediatr Drugs.* 2005;7:325-336.
95. O'Leary ST, Glanz JM, McClure DL, et al. The risk of immune thrombocytopenic purpura after vaccination in children and adolescents. *Pediatrics.* 2012;129:248-255.
96. British Committee for Standards in Haematology General Haematology Task Force. Guidelines for the investigation and management of idiopathic thrombocytopenic purpura in adults, children and in pregnancy. *Br J Haematol.* 2003;120:574-596.
97. Blanchette V, Bolton-Maggs P. Childhood immune thrombocytopenic purpura: diagnosis and management. *Pediatr Clin North Am.* 2008;55:393-420. ix.
98. McWilliams NB, Mauer HM. Acute idiopathic thrombocytopenic purpura in children. *Am J Hematol.* 1979;7:87-96.
99. Neunert CE, Buchanan GR, Imbach P, et al. Severe hemorrhage in children with newly diagnosed immune thrombocytopenic purpura. *Blood.* 2008;112:4003-4008.
100. Kuhne T, Imbach P, Bolton-Maggs PH, et al. Newly diagnosed idiopathic thrombocytopenic purpura in childhood: an observational study. *Lancet.* 2001;358:2122-2125.
101. Imbach P, Akatsuka J, Blanchette V, et al. Immunthrombocytopenic purpura as a model for pathogenesis and treatment of autoimmunity. *Eur J Pediatr.* 1995;154:S60-S64.
102. Yacobovich J, Revel-Vilk S, Tamary H. Childhood immune thrombocytopenia—who will spontaneously recover? *Semin Hematol.* 2013;50(suppl 1):S71-S74.
103. Jacobs P, Wood L, Dent DM. Results of treatment in immune thrombocytopenia. *Q J Med.* 1986;58:153-165.
104. den Ottolander JJ, Gratama JW, de Koning J, Brand A. Long-term follow-up study of 168 patients with immune thrombocytopenia: implications for therapy. *Scand J Haematol.* 1984;32:101-110.
105. Ikkala E, Kivilaakso E, Kotilainen M, Hastbacka J. Treatment of idiopathic thrombocytopenic purpura in adults: long-term results in a series of 41 patients. *Ann Clin Res.* 1978;10:83-86.
106. Kelton JG. Vaccination-associated relapse of immune thrombocytopenia. *JAMA.* 1981;245:369-371.
107. Karpatkin S, Freedman ML. Hypersplenic thrombocytopenia differentiated from increased platelet destruction by platelet volume. *Ann Intern Med.* 1978;89:200-203.
108. Grace RF, Neunert C. Second-line therapies in immune thrombocytopenia. *Hematology.* 2016;2016:698-706.
109. Crosby WH. Wet purpura, dry purpura. *JAMA.* 1975;232:744-745.
110. Ben-Yehuda D, Gillis S, Eldor A. Israeli ITP Study Group. Clinical and therapeutic experience in 712 Israeli patients with idiopathic thrombocytopenic purpura. *Acta Haematol.* 1994;91:1-6.
111. Lacey JV, Penner JA. Management of idiopathic thrombocytopenic purpura in the adult. *Semin. Thromb Haemostasis.* 1977;3:160-174.
112. Schattner E, Bussel J. Mortality in immune thrombocytopenic purpura: report of seven cases and consideration of prognostic indicators. *Am J Hematol.* 1994;46:120-126.
113. Guthrie TH, Brannan DP, Prisant LM. Idiopathic thrombocytopenic purpura in the older adult patient. *Am J Med Sci.* 1988;296:17-21.
114. Linares M, Cervero A, Colomina P, et al. Chronic idiopathic thrombocytopenic purpura in the elderly. *Acta Haematol.* 1995;93:80-82.
115. Kuhne T, Berchtold W, Michaels LA, et al. Newly diagnosed immune thrombocytopenia in children and adults: a comparative prospective observational registry of the Intercontinental Cooperative Immune Thrombocytopenia Study Group. *Haematologica.* 2011;96:1831-1837.
116. Wong GC, Lee LH. A study of idiopathic thrombocytopenic purpura (ITP) patients over a ten-year period. *Ann Acad Med Singapore.* 1998;27:789-793.
117. Jy W, Horstman LL, Arce M, Ahn YS. Clinical significance of platelet microparticles in autoimmune thrombocytopenias. *J Lab Clin Med.* 1992;119:334-345.
118. Khan I, Zucker-Franklin D, Karpatkin S. Microthrombocytosis and platelet fragmentation associated with idiopathic/autoimmune thrombocytopenic purpura. *Br J Haematol.* 1975;31:449-460.
119. Zucker-Franklin D, Karpatkin S. Red-cell and platelet fragmentation in idiopathic thrombocytopenic purpura. *N Engl J Med.* 1977;297:517-523.
120. Zucker-Franklin D. Clinical significance of platelet microparticles. *J Lab Clin Med.* 1992;119:321-322.
121. Ikkala E, Suhonen O. Circulating megakaryocytes in immune thrombocytopenias. *Ann Clin Res.* 1972;4:1-6.
122. Nelson RB, Kehl D. Electronically determined platelet indices in thrombocytopenic patients. *Cancer.* 1981;48:954-956.
123. Garg SK, Lackner H, Karpatkin S. The increased percentage of megathrombocytes in various clinical disorders. *Ann Intern Med.* 1972;77:361-369.
124. Bessman JD, Gardner FH. Platelet size in thrombocytopenia due to sepsis. *Surg Gynecol Obstet.* 1983;156:177-180.
125. Evans RS, Takahashi K, Duane RT, et al. Primary thrombocytopenic purpura and acquired hemolytic anemia. *Arch Intern Med.* 1951;87:48-65.
126. Pegels JG, Helmerhorst FM, van Leeuwen EF, et al. The Evans syndrome: characterization of the responsible autoantibodies. *Br J Haematol.* 1982;51:445-450.
127. Rosenberg A, Van Slyck EJ. A syndrome resembling infectious mononucleosis after splenectomy for idiopathic thrombocytopenic purpura. *Ann Intern Med.* 1965;63:965-971.
128. Tager MJ, Klinghoffer KA. Acute thrombocytopenic purpura hemorrhagica with lymphocytosis; report of a case. *Ann Intern Med.* 1943;18:96.
129. Calpin C, Dick P, Poon A, Feldman W. Is bone marrow aspiration needed in acute childhood idiopathic thrombocytopenic purpura to rule out leukemia? *Arch Pediatr Adolesc Med.* 1998;152:345-347.
130. DiFino SM, Lachant NA, Kirshner JJ, Gottlieb AJ. Adult idiopathic thrombocytopenic purpura: clinical findings and response to therapy. *Am J Med.* 1980;69:430-442.
131. Harker LA. Megakaryocyte quantitation. *J Clin Invest.* 1968;47:452-457.
132. Harker LA, Finch CA. Thrombokinetics in man. *J Clin Invest.* 1969;48:963-974.
133. Louwes H, Lathori OAZ, Vellenga E, et al. Platelet kinetic studies in patients with idiopathic thrombocytopenic purpura. *Am J Med.* 1999;106:430-434.
134. Pisciotta AV, Stefanini M, Dameshek W. Studies on platelets. X. Morphologic characteristics of megakaryocytes by phase contrast microscopy in normals and in patients with idiopathic thrombocytopenic purpura. *Blood.* 1953;8:703-723.
135. Queisser U, Queisser W, Spiertz B. Polyploidization of megakaryocytes in normal humans, in patients with idiopathic thrombocytopenia and with pernicious anemia. *Br J Haematol.* 1971;20:489-501.
136. Luiken GA, McMillan R, Lightsey AL, et al. Platelet-associated IgG in immune thrombocytopenic purpura. *Blood.* 1977;50:317-325.
137. LoBuglio AF, Court WS, Vinocur L, et al. Use of a 125I-labeled antihuman IgG monoclonal antibody to quantify platelet-bound IgG. *N Engl J Med.* 1983;309:459-463.
138. Sugiura K, Steiner M, Baldini MG. Platelet antibody in idiopathic thrombocytopenic purpura. *J Lab Clin Med.* 1980;96:640-653.
139. Karpatkin M, Siskind GW, Karpatkin S. The platelet factor 3 immunoinjury technique re-evaluated. Development of a rapid test for antiplatelet antibody. Detection in various clinical disorders, including immunologic drug-induced and neonatal thrombocytopenias. *J Lab Clin Med.* 1977;89:400-408.
140. Cines DB, Schreiber AD. Immune thrombocytopenia. Use of a Coombs antiglobulin test to detect IgG and C3 on platelets. *N Engl J Med.* 1979;300:106-111.
141. Hirschman RJ, Shulman NR. The use of platelet serotonin release as a sensitive method for detecting anti-platelet antibodies and plasma anti-platelet factor in patients with idiopathic thrombocytopenic purpura. *Br J Haematol.* 1973;24:793-802.
142. Mueller-Eckhardt C, Kayser W, Mersch-Baumert K, et al. The clinical significance of platelet-associated IgG: a study on 298 patients with various disorders. *Br J Haematol.* 1980;46:123-131.
143. Hegde UM, Ball S, Zuiable A, Roter BLT. Platelet associated immunoglobulins (PAIgG and PAIgM) in autoimmune thrombocytopenia. *Br J Haematol.* 1985;59:221-226.
144. Chong BH, Ho SJ. Autoimmune thrombocytopenia. *J Thromb Haemost.* 2005;3:1763-1772.
145. George JN. Platelet immunoglobulin G: its significance for the evaluation of thrombocytopenia and for understanding the origin of α-granule proteins. *Blood.* 1990;76:859-870.
146. Tomer A. Flow cytometry for the diagnosis of autoimmune thrombocytopenia. *Curr Hematol Rep.* 2006;5:64-69.
147. Nilsson T, Norberg B. Thrombocytopenia and pseudothrombocytopenia: a clinical and laboratory problem. *Scand J Haematol.* 1986;37:341-346.
148. Casonato A, Bertomoro A, Pontara E, et al. EDTA dependent pseudothrombocytopenia caused by antibodies against the cytoadhesive receptor of platelet gpIIb-IIIa. *J Clin Pathol.* 1994;47:625-630.
149. Bizzaro N. EDTA-dependent pseudothrombocytopenia: a clinical and epidemiological study of 112 cases, with 10-year follow-up. *Am J Hematol.* 1995;50:103-109.
150. Bizzaro N. Platelet satellitosis to polymorphonuclears: cytochemical, immunological, and ultrastructural characterization of eight cases. *Am J Hematol.* 1991;36:235-242.

151. Bizzaro N, Goldschmeding R, von dem Borne AE. Platelet satellitism is Fc gamma RIII (CD16) receptor-mediated. *Am J Clin Pathol.* 1995;103:740-744.
152. Menke DM, Colon-Otero G, Cockerill KJ, et al. Refractory thrombocytopenia: a myelodysplastic syndrome that may mimic immune thrombocytopenic purpura. *Am J Clin Pathol.* 1992;98:502-510.
153. Najean Y, Lecompte T. Chronic pure thrombocytopenia in elderly patients. *Cancer.* 1989;64:2506-2510.
154. George JN. How I treat patients with thrombotic thrombocytopenic purpura: 2010. *Blood.* 2010;116:4060-4069.
155. George JN, Raskob GE, Shah SR, et al. Drug-induced thrombocytopenia: a systematic review of published case reports. *Ann Intern Med.* 1998;129:886-890.
156. Laster J, Silver D. Heparin-coated catheters and heparin-induced thrombocytopenia. *J Vasc Surg.* 1988;7:667-672.
157. George JN, Woolf SH, Raskob GE, et al. Idiopathic thrombocytopenic purpura: a practice guideline developed by explicit methods for the American Society of Hematology. *Blood.* 1996;88:3-40.
158. The American Society of Hematology ITP practice guideline panel. Diagnosis and treatment of idiopathic thrombocytopenic purpura: recommendations of the American Society of Hematology. *Ann Intern Med.* 1997;126:319-326.
159. Schoettler ML, Graham D, Tao W, et al. Increasing observation rates in low-rsk pediatric immune thrombocytopenia using a standardized clinical assessment and management plan (SCAMP). *Pediatr Blood Cancer.* 2017;64. doi: 10.1002/pbc.26303
160. Rosthoj S, Hedlund-Treutiger I, Rajantie J, et al. Duration and morbidity of newly diagnosed idiopathic thrombocytopenic purpura in children: a prospective Nordic study of an unselected cohort. *J Pediatr.* 2003;143:302-307.
161. Kuhne T, Buchanan GR, Zimmerman S, et al. A prospective comparative study of 2540 infants and children with newly diagnosed idiopathic thrombocytopenic purpura (ITP) from the intercontinental childhood IP study group. *J Pediatr.* 2003;143:605-608.
162. Rosthoj S, Nielsen S, Pedersen FK. Randomized trial comparing intravenous immunoglobulin with methylprednisolone pulse therapy in acute idiopathic thrombocytopenic purpura. Danish I.T.P. StudyGroup. *Act Paediatr.* 1996;85:910-915.
163. Celik M, Bulbul A, Adogan G, et al. Comparison of anti-D immunoglobulin, methylprednisolone, or intravenous immunogloblin therapy in newly diagnosed pediatric immune thrombocytopenic purpura. *J Thromb Thrombolysis.* 2013;35:228-233.
164. Imbach P, Wagner HP, Berchtold W, et al. Intravenous immunoglobulin versus oral corticosteroids in acute immune thrombocytopenic purpura in childhood. *Lancet.* 1985;2:464-468.
165. Benesch M, Kerbl R, Lackner H, et al. Low-dose versus high-dose immunoglobulin for primary treatment f acute immune thrombocytopenic purpura in children: results o a prospective, randomized single-center trial. *J Pediatr Hematol Oncol.* 2003;25:797-800.
166. Blanchette VS, Luke B, Andrew M, et al. A prospective, randomized trial of high-dose intravenous immune globulin G therapy, oral prednisone therapy, and no therapy in childhood acute immune thrombocytopenic purpura. *J Pediatr.* 1993;123:989-995.
167. Blanchette V, Imbach P, Andrew M, et al. Randomized trial of intravenous immunoglobulin G, intravenous anti-D, and oral prednisone in childhood acute immune thrombocytopenic purpura. *Lancet.* 1994;344:703-707.
168. Fujisawa K, Iyori H, Ohkawa H, et al. A prospective randomized trial of conventional, dose-accelerated corticosteroids and intravenous immunoglobulin in children with newly diagnosed idiopathic thrombocytopenic purpura. *Int J Haematol.* 2000;72:376-383.
169. Neunert C, Despotovic J, Haley K, et al. Thrombopoietin receptor agonist use in children: data from the pediatric ITP consortium of North America ICON2 study. *Pediatr Blood Cancer.* 2016;63:1407-1413.
170. Bussel JB, Buchanan GR, Nugent DJ, et al. A randomized, double-blind study of romiplostim to determine its safety and efficacy in children with immune thrombocytopenia. *Blood.* 2011;118:28-36.
171. Grainger JD, Locatelli F, Chotsampancharoen T, et al. Eltrombopag for children with chronic immune thrombocytopenia (PETIT2): a randomised, multicentre, placebo-controlled trial. *Lancet.* 2015;386:1649-1658.
172. Grace RF, Bennett CM, Ritchey AK, et al. Response to steroids predicts response to rituximab in pediatric chronic immune thrombocytopenia. *Pediatr Blood Cancer.* 2012;58:221-225.
173. Hedlund-Treutiger I, Henter JI, Elinder G. Randomized study of IVIg and high-dose dexamethasone therapy for children with chronic idiopathic thrombocytopenic purpura. *J Pediatr Hematol Oncol.* 2003;25:139-144.
174. Portielje JEA, Westendorp RGJ, Kluin-Nelemans HC, et al. Morbidity and mortality in adults with idiopathic thrombocytopenic purpura. *Blood.* 2001;97:2549-2554.
175. Jiji RM, Firozvi T, Spurling CL. Chronic idiopathic thrombocytopenic purpura: treatment with steroids and splenectomy. *Arch Intern Med.* 1973;132:380-383.
176. Cohen YC, Djulbegovic B, Shamai-Lubovitz O, et al. The bleeding risk and natural history of idiopathic thrombocytopenic purpura in patients with persistent low platelet counts. *Arch Intern Med.* 2000;160:1630-1638.
177. Baumann MA, Menitove JE, Aster RH, Anderson T. Urgent treatment of idiopathic thrombocytopenic purpura with single-dose gammaglobulin infusion followed by platelet transfusion. *Ann Intern Med.* 1986;104:808-809.
178. Flick JT, Grush O, Morgan S, et al. Case report: the role of apheresis in the support of life-threatening ITP relapse. *Am J Med Sci.* 1987;294:444-447.
179. Dameshek W, Rubio F, Mahoney JP, et al. Treatment of idiopathic thrombocytopenic purpura (ITP) with prednisone. *JAMA.* 1958;166:1805-1815.
180. Thompson RL, Moore RA, Hess CE, et al. Idiopathic thrombocytopenic purpura: long-term results of treatment and the prognostic significance of response to corticosteroids. *Arch Intern Med.* 1972;130:730-734.
181. Bunting WL, Kiely JM, Campbell DC. Idiopathic thrombocytopenic purpura: treatment in adults. *Arch Intern Med.* 1961;108:733-738.
182. Carpenter AF, Wintrobe MW, Fuller EA, et al. Treatment of idiopathic thrombocytopenic purpura. *JAMA.* 1959;171:1911-1916.
183. Shashaty GG, Rath CE. Idiopathic thrombocytopenic purpura in the elderly. *Am J Med Sci.* 1978;276:263-267.
184. Berchtold P, McMillan R. Therapy of chronic idiopathic thrombocytopenic purpura in adults. *Blood.* 1989;74:2309-2317.
185. George JN, El-Harake MA, Raskob GE. Chronic idiopathic thrombocytopenic purpura. *N Engl J Med.* 1994;331:1207-1211.
186. Bellucci S, Charpak Y, Chastang C, Tobelem G; the Cooperative Group on Immune Thrombocytopenic Purpura. Low doses v conventional doses of corticoids in immune thrombocytopenic purpura (ITP): results of a randomized clinical trial in 160 children, 223 adults. *Blood.* 1988;71:1165-1169.
187. Mazzucconi GB, Francesconi M, Fidani P, et al. Treatment of idiopathic thrombocytopenic purpura (ITP): results of a multicentric protocol. *Haematologica.* 1985;70:329-336.
188. Jacobs P, Wood L, Novitzky N. Intravenous gammaglobulin has no advantages over oral corticosteroids as primary therapy for adults with immune thrombocytopenia: a prospective randomized clinical trial. *Am J Med.* 1994;97:55-59.
189. Godeau B, Chevret S, Varet B, et al. Intravenous immunoglobulin or high-dose methylprednisolone, with or without oral prednisone, for adults with untreated severe autoimmune thrombocytopenic purpura: a randomized, multicentre trial. *Lancet.* 2002;359:23-29.
190. Cheng Y, Wong RS, Soo YO, et al. Initial treatment of immune thrombocytopenic purpura with high dose dexamethasone. *N Engl J Med.* 2003;349:831-836.
191. Andersen JC. Response of resistant idiopathic thrombocytopenic purpura to pulsed high-dose dexamethasone therapy. *N Engl J Med.* 1994;330:1560-1564.
192. Mazzucconi MG, Fazi P, Bernasconi S, et al. Therapy with high-dose dexamethasone (HD-DXM) in previously untreated patients affected by idiopathic thrombocytopenic purpura: a GIMEMA experience. *Blood.* 2007;109:1401-1407.
193. George JN. Sequence of treatments for adults with primary immune thrombocytopenia. *Am J Hematol.* 2012;87:S12-S15.
194. Wei Y, Ji X, Wang Y, et al. High-dose dexamethasone vs prednisone for treatment of adult immune thrombocytopenia: a prospective multicenter randomized trial. *Blood.* 2016;127:296-302.
195. Handin RI, Stossel TP. Effect of corticosteroid therapy on the phagocytosis of antibody-coated platelets by human leukocytes. *Blood.* 1978;51:771-779.
196. Verp M, Karpatkin S. Effect of plasma, steroids, or steroid products on the adhesion of human opsonized thrombocytes to human leukocytes. *J Lab Clin Med.* 1975;85:478-486.
197. Fujisawa K, Tani P, Piro L, McMillan R. The effect of therapy on platelet-associated autoantibody in chronic immune thrombocytopenic purpura. *Blood.* 1993;81:2872-2877.
198. McMillan R, Longmire R, Yelenosky R. The effect of corticosteroids on human IgG synthesis. *J Immunol.* 1976;116:1592-1595.
199. Gernsheimer T, Stratton J, Ballem PJ, Slichter SJ. Mechanisms of response to treatment in autoimmune thrombocytopenic purpura. *N Engl J Med.* 1989;230:974-980.
200. Atkinson JP, Frank MM. Complement-independent clearance of IgG-sensitized erythrocytes: inhibition by cortisone. *Blood.* 1974;44:629-637.
201. Branehog I, Weinfeld A. Platelet survival and platelet production in idiopathic thrombocytopenic purpura (ITP) before and during treatment with cortico-steroids. *Scand J Haematol.* 1974;12:69-79.
202. Greendyke RM, Bradley EM, Swisher SN. Studies of the effects of administration of ACTH and adrenal corticosteroids on erythrophagocytosis. *J Clin Invest.* 1965;44:746-753.
203. Fries LF, Brickman CM, Frank MM. Monocyte receptors for the Fc portion of IgG increase in number in autoimmune hemolytic anemia and other hemolytic states and are decreased by glucocorticoid therapy. *J Immunol.* 1983;131:1240-1245.
204. Kitchens CS, Weiss L. Ultrastructural changes of endothelium associated with thrombocytopenia. *Blood.* 1975;46:567-578.
205. Kitchens CS, Pendergast JF. Human thrombocytopenia is associated with structural abnormalities of the endothelium that are ameliorated by glucocortico-steroid administration. *Blood.* 1986;67:203-206.
206. Kitchens CS. Amelioration of endothelial abnormalities by prednisone in experimental thrombocytopenia in the rabbit. *J Clin Invest.* 1977;60:1129-1134.
207. Maca RD, Fry GL, Hoak JC. The effects of glucocorticoids on cultured human endothelial cells. *Br J Haematol.* 1978;38:501-509.
208. Imbach P, Barandun S, d'Apuzzo V, et al. High-dose intravenous gammaglobulin for idiopathic purpura in childhood. *Lancet.* 1981;1:1228-1231.
209. Warrier I, Lusher JM. Intravenous gamma globulin treatment for chronic idiopathic thrombocytopenic purpura in children. *Am J Med.* 1984;76:193-198.
210. Warrier IA, Lusher JM. Intravenous gammaglobulin (Gamimune) for treatment of chronic idiopathic thrombocytopenic purpura (ITP): a two-year follow-up. *Am J Hematol.* 1986;23:323-328.
211. Korninger C, Panzer S, Graninger W, et al. Treatment of severe chronic idiopathic thrombocytopenic purpura in adults with high-dose intravenous immunoglobulin. *Scand J Haematol.* 1985;34:128-132.
212. Uchino H, Yasunaga K, Akatsuka JI. A cooperative clinical trial of high-dose immunoglobulin therapy in 177 cases of idiopathic thrombocytopenic purpura. *Thromb Haemostasis.* 1984;51:182-185.
213. Oral A, Nusbacher J, Hill JB, Lewis JH. Intravenous gamma globulin in the treatment of chronic idiopathic thrombocytopenic purpura in adults. *Am J Med.* 1984;76:187-192.
214. Godeau B, Lesage S, Divine M, et al. Treatment of adult chronic autoimmune thrombocytopenic purpura with repeated high-dose intravenous immunoglobulin. *Blood.* 1993;82:1415-1421.

215. Bierling P, Divine M, Farcet JP, et al. Persistent remission of adult chronic autoimmune thrombocytopenic purpura after treatment with high-dose intravenous immunoglobulin. *Am J Hematol.* 1987;25:271-275.
216. Bussel JB, Kimberly RP, Inman RD, et al. Intravenous immunoglobulin treatment of chronic idiopathic thrombocytopenic purpura. *Blood.* 1983;62:480-486.
217. Bussel JB, Pham LC, Aledort L, Nachman R. Maintenance treatment of adults with chronic refractory immune thrombocytopenic purpura using repeated intravenous infusions of gammaglobulins. *Blood.* 1988;72:121-127.
218. Bussel JB, Pham LC. Intravenous treatment with gammaglobulin in adults with immune thrombocytopenic purpura: a review of the literature. *Vox Sang.* 1987;52:206-211.
219. Carroll RR, Noyes WD, Kitchens CS. High-dose intravenous immunoglobulin therapy in patients with immune thrombocytopenic purpura. *JAMA.* 1983;249:1748-1750.
220. Kurlander R, Coleman RE, Moore J, et al. Comparison of the efficacy of a two-day and a five-day schedule for infusing intravenous gamma globulin in the treatment of immune thrombocytopenic purpura in adults. *Am J Med.* 1987;83(suppl 4A):17-24.
221. Godeau B, Caulier MT, Decuypere L, et al. Intravenous immunoglobulin for adults with autoimmune thrombocytopenic purpura: results of a randomized trial comparing 0.5 and 1 g/kg b.w. *Br J Haematol.* 1999;107:716-719.
222. Bussel JB, Fitzgerald-Pedersen J, Feldman C. Alternation of two doses of intravenous gammaglobulin in the maintenance treatment of patients with immune thrombocytopenic purpura: more is not always better. *Am J Hematol.* 1990;33:184-188.
223. Spahr JE, Rodgers GM. Treatment of immune-mediated thrombocytopenia purpura with concurrent intravenous immunoglobulin and platelet transfusion: a retrospective review of 40 patients. *Am J Hematol.* 2007;83:122-125.
224. Newland AC. Annotation: the use and mechanisms of action of intravenous immunoglobulin – an update. *Br J Haematol.* 1989;72:301-305.
225. Fehr J, Hofmann V, Kappeler U. Transient reversal of thrombocytopenia in idiopathic thrombocytopenic purpura by high dose intravenous gamma globulin. *N Engl J Med.* 1982;306:1254-1258.
226. Kimberly RP, Salmon JE, Bussel JB, et al. Modulation of mononuclear phagocyte function by intravenous γ-globulin. *J Immunol.* 1984;132:745-750.
227. Saleh M, Court W, Huster M, et al. Effect of commercial immunoglobulin G preparation on human monocyte Fc-receptor dependent binding of antibody coated platelets. *Br J Haematol.* 1988;68:47-51.
228. Dammacco F, Iodice G, Campobasso N. Treatment of adult patients with idiopathic thrombocytopenic purpura with intravenous immunoglobulin: effects on circulating T cell subsets and PWM-induced antibody synthesis in vitro. *Br J Haematol.* 1986;62:125-135.
229. Winiarski J, Kreuger E, Ejderhamn J, Holm G. High dose intravenous IgG reduces platelet associated immunoglobulins and complement in idiopathic thrombocytopenic purpura. *Scand J Haematol.* 1983;31:342-348.
230. Delfraissy JF, Tchernia G, Laurian Y, et al. Suppressor cell function after intravenous gammaglobulin treatment in adult chronic idiopathic thrombocytopenic purpura. *Br J Haematol.* 1985;60:315-322.
231. Tsubakio T, Kurata Y, Katagiri S, et al. Alteration of T cell subsets and immunoglobulin synthesis in vitro during high dose γ-globulin therapy in patients with idiopathic thrombocytopenic purpura. *Clin Exp Immunol.* 1983;53:697-702.
232. Berchtold P, Dale GL, Tani P, McMillan R. Inhibition of autoantibody binding to platelet glycoprotein IIb/IIIa by anti-idiotypic antibodies to intravenous immunoglobulin. *Blood.* 1989;74:2414-2417.
233. Williams Y, Lynch S, McCann S, et al. Correlation of platelet Fc γRIIA polymorphism in refractory idiopathic (immune) thrombocytopenic purpura. *Br J Haematol.* 1998;101:779-782.
234. Barbano G, Saleh MN, Mori PG, et al. Effect of intravenous gammaglobulin on circulating and platelet bound antibody in immune thrombocytopenia. *Blood.* 1989;73:662-665.
235. Samuelsson A, Towers TL, Ravetch JV. Anti-inflammatory activity of IVIG mediated through the inhibitory Fc receptor. *Science.* 2001;291:484-486.
236. von dem Borne AE, Vos JJ, Pegels JG, et al. High dose intravenous methylprednisolone or high dose intravenous gammaglobulin for autoimmune thrombocytopenia. *Br Med J (Clin Res Ed).* 1988;296:249-250.
237. Spahr JE, Rodgers GM. Treatment of immune-mediated thrombocytopenia purpura with concurrent intravenous immunoglubulin and platelet transfusion: a retrospective review of 40 patient. *Am J Hematol.* 2008;83:122-125.
238. Sati HIA, Ahya R, Watson HG. Incidence and associations of acute renal failure complicating high-dose intravenous immunoglobulin therapy. *Br J Haematol.* 2001;113:556-557.
239. Gupta N, Ahmed I, Nissel-Horowitz S, et al. Intravenous immunoglobulin-associated acute renal failure. *Am J Hematol.* 2001;66:151-152.
240. Salama A, Kiefel V, Amberg R, Mueller-Eckhardt C. Treatment of autoimmune thrombocytopenic purpura with rhesus antibodies [Anti-Rho (D)]. *Blut.* 1984;49:29-35.
241. Salama A, Mueller-Eckhardt C. Use of Rh antibodies in the treatment of autoimmune thrombocytopenia. *Transfus Med Rev.* 1992;6:17-25.
242. Andrew M, Blanchette VS, Adams M, et al. A multicenter study of the treatment of childhood chronic idiopathic thrombocytopenic purpura with anti-D. *J Pediatr.* 1992;120:522-527.
243. Scaradavou A, Woo B, Woloski BMR, et al. Intravenous anti-D treatment of immune thrombocytopenic purpura: experience in 272 patients. *Blood.* 1997;89:2689-2700.
244. Cooper N, Heddle NM, deHaas M, et al. Intravenous anti-D and IV immunoglobulin achieve acute platelet increases by different mechanisms: modulation of cytokine and platelet responses to IV anti-D by FcγRIIa and FcγRIIIa polymorphisms. *Br J Haematol.* 2004;124:511-518.
245. Becker T, Kuenzlen E, Salama A, et al. Treatment of childhood idiopathic thrombocytopenic purpura with Rhesus antibodies (anti-D). *Eur J Pediatr.* 1986;145:166-169.
246. Gringeri A, Cattaneo M, Santagostino E, Mannucci PM. Intramuscular anti-D immunoglobulins for home treatment of chronic immune thrombocytopenic purpura. *Br J Haematol.* 1992;80:337-340.
247. Cooper N, Woloski BMR, Fodero EM, et al. Does treatment with intermittent infusions of intravenous anti-D allow a proportion of adults with recently diagnosed immune thrombocytopenic purpura to avoid splenectomy? *Blood.* 2002;99:1922-1927.
248. Salama A, Kiefel V, Mueller-Eckhardt C. Effect of IgG anti-Rho (D) in adult patients with chronic autoimmune thrombocytopenia. *Am J Hematol.* 1986;22:241-250.
249. Panzer S, Grumayer ER, Haas OA, et al. Efficacy of rhesus antibodies (anti-Rho [D]) in autoimmune thrombocytopenia: correlation with response to high dose IgG and the degree of hemolysis. *Blut.* 1986;52:117-121.
250. Ruiz-Arguelles GJ, Apreza-Molina MG, Perez-Romano B, Ruiz-Arguelles A. The infusion of anti-RhO-(D) opsonized erythrocytes may be useful in the treatment of patients, splenectomized or not, with chronic, refractory autoimmune thrombocytopenic purpura—a prospective study. *Am J Hematol.* 1993;43:72-73.
251. Bussell JB, Graziano JN, Kimberly JN, et al. Intravenous anti-D treatment of immune thrombocytopenic purpura: analysis of efficacy, toxicity and mechanism of effect. *Blood.* 1991;77:1884-1893.
252. Newman GC, Novoa MV, Fodero EM, et al. A dose of 75 μg/kg/d of IV anti-D increases the platelet count more rapidly and for a longer period of time than does 50 μg/kg/d in adults with immune thrombocytopenic purpura (ITP). *Br J Haematol.* 2001;112:1076-1078.
253. Gaines AR. Disseminated intravascular coagulation associated with acute hemoglobinemia or hemoglobinuria following Rho (D) immune globulin administration for immune thrombocytopenic purpura. *Blood.* 2005;106:1532-1537.
254. Despotovic J, Lambert MP, Herman J, et al. RhIG for the treatment of immune thrombocytopenia: consensus and controversy (CME). *Transfusion.* 2012;52:1126-1136.
255. Zaja F, Baccarani M, Mazza P, et al. Dexamethasone plus rituximab yields higher sustained response rates than dexamethasone monotherapy in adults with primary immune thrombocytopenia. *Blood.* 2010;115:2755-2762.
256. Gudbrandsdottir S, Birgens HS, Frederiksen H, et al. Rituximab and dexamethasone vs dexamethasone monotherapy in newly diagnosed patients with primary immune thrombocytopenia. *Blood.* 2013;121:197.
257. Vogelsang G, Kickler TS, Bell WR. Post-transfusion purpura: a report of five patients and a review of the pathogenesis and management. *Am J Hematol.* 1986;21:259-267.
258. Chapman JF, Murphy MF, Berney SI, et al. Post-transfusion purpura associated with anti-Bak^a and anti-PL^{A2} platelet antibodies and delayed hemolytic transfusion reactions. *Vox Sang.* 1987;52:313-317.
259. Picozzi VJ, Roeske WR, Creger WP. Fate of therapy failures in adult idiopathic thrombocytopenic purpura. *Am J Med.* 1980;69:690-694.
260. Brown DN, Elliott RHE. The results of splenectomy in thrombocytopenic purpura. *JAMA.* 1936;107:1781-1788.
261. Eliason EL, Ferguson LK. Splenectomy in purpura hemorrhagica. *Ann Surg.* 1932;96:801-829.
262. Wintrobe MM, Hanrahan EM, Thomas CB, et al. Purpura haemorrhagica with special reference to course and treatment. *JAMA.* 1937;109:1170-1176.
263. Kernoff LM, Malan E. Platelet antibody levels do not correlate with response to therapy in idiopathic thrombocytopenic purpura. *Br J Haematol.* 1983;53:559-562.
264. Akwari OE, Itani KMF, Coleman RE, Rosse WF. Splenectomy for primary and recurrent immune thrombocytopenic purpura. *Ann Surg.* 1987;206:529-541.
265. Schwartz SI, Hoepp LM, Sachs S. Splenectomy for thrombocytopenia. *Surgery.* 1980;88:497-506.
266. Mintz SJ, Petersen SR, Cheson B, et al. Splenectomy for immune thrombocytopenic purpura. *Arch Surg.* 1981;116:645-650.
267. Gugliotta L, Isacchi G, Guarini A, et al. Chronic idiopathic thrombocytopenic purpura (ITP): site of platelet sequestration and results of splenectomy. *Scand J Haematol.* 1981;26:407-412.
268. Brennan MF, Rappeport JM, Moloney WC, Wilson RE. Correlation between response to corticosteroids and splenectomy for adult idiopathic thrombocytopenic purpura. *Am J Surg.* 1975;129:490-492.
269. Chirletti P, Cardi M, Barillari P, et al. Surgical treatment of immune thrombocytopenic purpura. *World J Surg.* 1992;16:1001-1005.
270. Fabris F, Zanatta N, Casonata A, et al. Response to splenectomy in idiopathic thrombocytopenic purpura: prognostic value of the clinical and laboratory evaluation. *Acta Haematol.* 1989;81:28-33.
271. Gibson J, May J, Rickard KA, et al. Management of splenectomy failures in chronic immune thrombocytopenic purpura: role of accessory splenectomy. *Aust N Z J Med.* 1986;16:695-698.
272. Naouri A, Feghali B, Chabal J, et al. Results of splenectomy for idiopathic thrombocytopenic purpura. *Acta Haematol.* 1993;89:200-203.
273. Szoid A, Schwartz J, Abu-Abeid S, et al. Laparoscopic splenectomies for idiopathic thrombocytopenic purpura: experience of 60 cases. *Am J Hematol.* 2000;63:7-10.
274. Kathouda N, Grant SW, Mavor E, et al. Predictors of response after laparoscopic splenectomy for immune thrombocytopenic purpura. *Surg Endosc.* 2001;15:484-488.
275. Calverley DC, Jones GW, Kelton JG. Splenic radiation for corticosteroid-resistant immune thrombocytopenia. *Ann Intern Med.* 1992;116:977-981.
276. Caulier MT, Darloy F, Rose C, et al. Splenic irradiation for chronic autoimmune thrombocytopenic purpura in patients with contra-indications to splenectomy. *Br J Haematol.* 1995;91:208-211.
277. Miyazaki M, Itoh H, Kaiho T, et al. Partial splenic embolization for the treatment of chronic idiopathic thrombocytopenic purpura. *AJR Am J Roentgenol.* 1994;163:123-126.
278. Wallace D, Fromm D, Thomas D. Accessory splenectomy for idiopathic thrombocytopenic purpura. *Surgery.* 1982;91:134-136.

279. Ambriz P, Munoz R, Quintanar E, et al. Accessory spleen complicating response to splenectomy for idiopathic thrombocytopenic purpura. *Radiology.* 1985;155:793-796.
280. Verheyden CN, Beart RW, Clifton MD, Phyliky RL. Accessory splenectomy in management of recurrent idiopathic thrombocytopenic purpura. *Mayo Clin Proc.* 1978;53:442-446.
281. Massey MD, Stevens JS. Residual spleen found on denatured red blood cell scan following negative colloid scans. *J Nucl Med.* 1991;32:2286-2287.
282. Facon T, Caulier MT, Fenaux P, et al. Accessory spleen in recurrent chronic immune thrombocytopenic purpura. *Am J Hematol.* 1992;41:184-189.
283. Julia A, Araguas C, Rossello J, et al. Lack of useful clinical predictors of response to splenectomy in patients with chronic idiopathic thrombocytopenic purpura. *Br J Haematol.* 1990;76:250-255.
284. Ruivard M, Caulier MT, Vantelon JM, et al. The response to high-dose intravenous immunoglobulin or steroids is not predictive of outcome after splenectomy in adults with autoimmune thrombocytopenic purpura. *Br J Haematol.* 1999;105:1130-1132.
285. Choi CW, Kim BS, Seo JH, et al. Response to high-dose intravenous immune globulin as a valuable factor predicting the effect of splenectomy in chronic idiopathic thrombocytopenic purpura patients. *Am J Hematol.* 2001;66:197-202.
286. Fabris F, Tassan T, Ramon R, et al. Age as the major predictive factor of long-term response to splenectomy in immune thrombocytopenic purpura. *Br J Haematol.* 2001;112:637-640.
287. Bussel JB, Kaufman CP, Ware RE, Woloski BM. Do the acute platelet responses of patients with immune thrombocytopenic purpura (ITP) to IV anti-D and to IV gammaglobulin predict response to subsequent splenectomy? *Am J Hematol.* 2001;67:27-33.
288. Najean Y, Dufour V, Rain JD, Toubert ME. The site of platelet destruction in thrombocytopenic purpura as a predictive index of the efficacy of splenectomy. *Br J Haematol.* 1991;79:271-276.
289. Stasi R, Pagano A, Stipa E, et al. Rituximab chimeric anti-CD20 monoclonal antibody treatment for adults with chronic idiopathic thrombocytopenic purpura. *Blood.* 2001;98:952-957.
290. Saleh MN, Moore M, Feinberg B, et al. A pilot study of anti-CD20 MOAB rituximab in patients with refractory immune thrombocytopenia. *Semin Oncol.* 2000;27(6 suppl 12):99-103.
291. Cooper N, Feuerstein M, Bussel JB. The use of rituximab, a chimeric anti-CD20 monoclonal antibody, in adults with refractory immune thrombocytopenic purpura. *Blood.* 2001;98:521.
292. Grillo-Lopez AJ, Hendrick C, Rashford M, et al. Rituximab: ongoing and future clinical development. *Semin Oncol.* 2002;29:105-112.
293. Arnold DM, Dentali F, Crowther MA, et al. Systemic review: efficacy and safety of rituximab for adults with idiopathic thrombocytopenic purpura. *Ann Intern Med.* 2007;146:25-33.
294. Patel VL, Mahévas M, Lee SY, et al. Outcomes 5 years after response to rituximab therapy in children and adults with immune thrombocytopenia. *Blood.* 2012;119(25):5989-5995.
295. Cooper N, Stasi R, Cunningham-Rundles S, et al. The efficacy and safety of B-cell depletion with anti-CD20 monoclonal antibody in adults with chronic immune thrombocytopenic purpura. *Br J Haematol.* 2004;125:232-239.
296. Zaja F, Vianelli N, Volpetti S, Battista ML, et al. Low-dose rituximab in adult patients with primary immune thrombocytopenia. *Eur J Haematol.* 2010;85:329-334.
297. Carson KR, Evens AM, Richey EA, et al. Progressive multifocal leukoencephalopathy after rituximab therapy in HIV-negative patients: a report of 57 cases form the Research on Adverse Drug Events and Reports project. *Blood.* 2009;113:4834-4840.
298. Stasi R, Stipa E, Forte V, et al. Variable patterns of response to rituximab treatments in adults with chronic idiopathic thrombocytopenic purpura. *Blood.* 2002;99:3872-3873.
299. Ramanarayanan J, Brodzik F, Czuczman MS, et al. Efficacy and safety of rituximab in the treatment of refractory/relapsed idiopathic thrombocytopenic purpura (ITP): results of a meta-analysis of 299 patients [abstract]. *Blood.* 2006;108:1076.
300. Deshayes S, Khellaf M, Zarour A, et al. Long-term safety and efficacy of rituximab in 248 adults with immune thrombocytopenia: results at 5 year from the French prospective registry ITP-Ritux. *Am J Hematol.* 2019;94:1314-1324.
301. Patel V, Mihatov N, Cooper N, et al. Long-term Follow-up of patients with immune thrombocytopenic purpura (ITP) whose initial response to Rituximab lasted a minimum of 1 year. *Blood.* 2006;108:479.
302. Arnold DM, Heddle NM, Carruthers J, et al. A pilot randomized trial of adjuvant rituximab or placebo for nonsplenectomized patients with immune thrombocytopenia. *Blood.* 2012;119:1356-1362.
303. Bussel JB, Provan D, Shamsi T, et al. Effect of eltrombopag on platelet counts and bleeding during the treatment of chronic idiopathic thrombocytopenic purpura: a randomised, double-blind, placebo-controlled trial. *Lancet.* 2009;373:641-648.
304. Kuter DJ, Mufti GJ, Bain BJ, et al. Evaluation of bone marrow reticulin formation in chronic immune thrombocytopenia patients treated with romiplostim. *Blood.* 2009;114:3748-3756.
305. Kuter DJ, Bussel JB, Newland A, et al. Long-term treatment with romiplostim in patients with chronic immune thrombocytopenia: safety and efficacy. *Br J Haematol.* 2013;161:411-423.
306. Chang G, Saleh MN, Marcher C, et al. Eltrombopag for management of chronic immune thrombocytopenia (RAISE): a 6-month, randomized, phase 3 study. *Lancet.* 2011;377:393-402.
307. Wong RSM, Saleh MN, Khelif A, et al. Safety and efficacy of long-term treatment of chronic/persistent ITP with eltrombopag: final results of the EXTEND study. *Blood.* 2017;121:537-545.
308. Kuter DJ, Bussel JB, Lyons RM, et al. Efficacy of romiplostim in patients with chronic immune thrombocytopenic purpura: a double-blind, randomised controlled trial. *Lancet.* 2008;371:395-403.
309. Khellaf M, Michel M, Quittet P, et al. Romiplostim safety and efficacy for immune thrombocytopenia in clinical practice: 2-year results of 72 adults in a romiplostim compassionate-use program. *Blood.* 2011;118:4338-4345.
310. Bussel JB, Kuter DJ, Pullarkat V, et al. Safety and efficacy of long-term treatment with romiplostim in thrombocytopenic patients chronic ITP. *Blood.* 2009;113:2161-2171.
311. Kuter DJ, Rummel M, Boccia R, et al. Romiplostim or standard of care in patients with immune thrombocytopenia. *N Engl J Med.* 2010;363:1889-1899.
312. Jurczak W, Chojnowski K, Mayer J, et al. Phase 3 randomised study of avatrombopag, a novel thrombopoietin receptor agonist for the treatment of chronic immune thrombocytopenia. *Br J Haematol.* 2018;183:479-490.
313. Terrault N, Chen YC, Izumi N, et al. Avatrombopag before procedures reduces need for Platelet transfusions in patients with chronic Liver disease and Thrombocytopenia. *Gastroenterology.* 2018;155:705-708.
314. Bussel, Arnold DM, Grossbard E, et al. Fostamatinib for the treatment of adult persistent and chronic immune thrombocytopenia: results of two phase 3, randomized, placebo-controlled trials. *Am J Hematol.* 2018;93:921-930.
315. Bussel J, Arnold DM, Boxer MA, et al. long-term fostamatinib treatment of adults with immune thrombocytopenia during the phase 3 clinical trial program. *Am J Hematol.* 2019;94:546-553.
316. Joseph A, Evans DIK. Immunosuppressive treatment of idiopathic thrombocytopenic purpura in children. *Acta Paediatr Scand.* 1982;71:467-469.
317. Finch SC, Castro O, Cooper M, et al. Immunosuppressive therapy of chronic thrombocytopenic purpura. *Am J Med.* 1974;56:4-12.
318. Godeau B, Zini JM, Schaeffer A, Bierling P. High-dose methylprednisolone is an alternative treatment for adults with autoimmune thrombocytopenic purpura refractory to intravenous immunoglobulins and oral corticosteroids. *Am J Hematol.* 1995;48:282-284.
319. Figueroa M, Gehlsen J, Hammond D, et al. Combination chemotherapy in refractory immune thrombocytopenic purpura. *N Engl J Med.* 1993;328:1226-1229.
320. Laros RK, Penner JA. "Refractory" thrombocytopenic purpura treated successfully with cyclophosphamide. *JAMA.* 1971;215:445-449.
321. Verlin M, Laros RK, Penner JA. Treatment of refractory thrombocytopenic purpura with cyclophosphamide. *Am J Hematol.* 1976;1:97-104.
322. Reiner A, Gernsheimer T, Slichter SJ. Pulse cyclophosphamide therapy for refractory autoimmune thrombocytopenic purpura. *Blood.* 1995;85:351-358.
323. Bouroncle BA, Doan CA. Refractory idiopathic thrombocytopenic purpura treated with azathioprine. *N Engl J Med.* 1966;275:630-635.
324. Bouroncle BA, Doan CA. Treatment of refractory idiopathic thrombocytopenic purpura. *JAMA.* 1969;207:2049-2052.
325. Hilgartner MW, Lanzkowsky P, Smith CH. The use of azathioprine in refractory thrombocytopenic purpura in children. *Acta Paediatr Scand.* 1970;59:409-415.
326. Quiquandon I, Fenaux P, Caulier MT, et al. Re-evaluation of the role of azathioprine in the treatment of adult chronic idiopathic thrombocytopenic purpura: a report on 53 cases. *Br J Haematol.* 1990;74:223-228.
327. Kappers-Klune MC, Van't Veer MB. Cyclosporin A for the treatment of patients with chronic idiopathic thrombocytopenic purpura refractory to corticosteroids or splenectomy. *Br J Haematol.* 2001;114:121-125.
328. Ahn YS, Harrington WJ, Steelman RC, Eytel CS. Vincristine therapy of idiopathic and secondary thrombocytopenias. *N Engl J Med.* 1974;291:376-380.
329. Colovic M, Suvajdzic N, Colovic N, et al. Mycophenolate mophetil therapy form chronic immune thrombocytopenic purpura resistant to steroids, immunosuppresants, and/or splenectomy in adults. *Platelets.* 2011;22:153-156.
330. Manoharan A. Slow infusion of vincristine in the treatment of idiopathic thrombocytopenic purpura. *Am J Hematol.* 1986;21:135-138.
331. Manoharan A. Targeted-immunosuppression with vincristine infusion in the treatment of immune thrombocytopenia. *Aust N Z J Med.* 1991;21:405-407.
332. Sultan Y, Delobel J, Jeanneau C, Caen JP. Effect of periwinkle alkaloids in idiopathic thrombocytopenic purpura. *Lancet.* 1971;1:496-497.
333. Aisenberg AC, Wilkes B. Studies on the suppression of immune response by the periwinkle alkaloids vincristine and vinblastine. *J Clin Invest.* 1964;43:2394-2403.
334. Robertson JH, McCarthy GM. Periwinkle alkaloids and the platelet-count. *Lancet.* 1969;2:353-355.
335. Hwang YF, Hamilton HE, Sheets RF. Vinblastine-induced thrombocytosis. *Lancet.* 1969;2:1075-1076.
336. Owellen RJ, Owens AH, Donigian DW. The binding of vincristine, vinblastine and colchicine to tubulin. *Biochem Biophys Res Commun.* 1972;47:685-691.
337. Paulson JC, McClure WO. Inhibition of axoplasmic transport by colchicine, podophyllotoxin, and vinblastine: an effect on microtubules. *Ann N Y Acad Sci.* 1975;253:517-527.
338. Mahévas M, Gerfaud-Valentin M, Moulis G, et al. Characteristics, outcome, and response to therapy of multirefractory chronic immune thrombocytopenia. *Blood.* 2016;128:1625-1630.
339. Mylvaganam R, Ahn YS, Garcia RO, et al. Very low dose danazol in idiopathic thrombocytopenic purpura and its role as an immune modulator. *Am J Med Sci.* 1989;298:215-220.
340. Ahn YS, Harrington WJ, Simon SR, et al. Danazol for the treatment of idiopathic thrombocytopenic purpura. *N Engl J Med.* 1983;308:1396-1399.
341. Buelli M, Cortelazzo S, Viero P, et al. Danazol for the treatment of idiopathic thrombocytopenic purpura. *Acta Haematol.* 1985;74:97-98.
342. Ahn YS, Mylvaganam R, Garcia RO, et al. Low-dose danazol therapy in idiopathic thrombocytopenic purpura. *Ann Intern Med.* 1987;107:177-181.
343. Schreiber AD, Chien P, Tomaski A, Cines DB. Effect of danazol in immune thrombocytopenic purpura. *N Engl J Med.* 1987;316:503-508.
344. Maloisel F, Andrès E, Zimmer J, et al. Danazol therapy in patients with chronic idiopathic thrombocytopenic purpura; long-term results. *Am J Med.* 2004;116:590-594.

345. Donato H, Kohan R, Picon A, et al. Alpha-interferon therapy induces improvement of platelet count in children with chronic idiopathic thrombocytopenic purpura. *J Pediatr Hematol Oncol*. 2001;23:598-603.
346. Proctor SJ. Alpha interferon therapy in the treatment of idiopathic thrombocytopenic purpura. *Eur J Cancer*. 1991;27:S63-S68.
347. Cucker A, Neunert CE. How I treat refractory immune thrombocytopenia. *Blood*. 2016;128:1547-1554.
348. Kahn RA. Clinical evaluation of platelet transfusions in thrombocytopenic patients: methods and interpretation. *Vox Sang*. 1981;40(suppl 1):87-97.
349. Zucker MB, Lundberg A. Platelet transfusions. *Anesthesiology*. 1966;27:385-398.
350. Carr JM, Kruskall MS, Kaye JA, Robinson SH. Efficacy of platelet transfusions in immune thrombocytopenia. *Am J Med*. 1986;80:1051-1054.
351. Mourtzoukou EG, Pappas G, Peppas G, Falagas ME. Vaccination of asplenic or hyposplenic adults. *Br J Surg*. 2008;95:273-280.
352. Kaplan C, Forestier F, Dreyfus M, et al. Maternal thrombocytopenia during pregnancy: diagnosis and etiology. *Semin Thromb Haemost*. 1995;21:85-94.
353. McCrae KR, Samuels P, Schreiber AD. Pregnancy-associated thrombocytopenia: pathogenesis and management. *Blood*. 1992;80:2697-2714.
354. Burrows RF, Kelton JG. Incidentally detected thrombocytopenia in healthy mothers and their infants. *N Engl J Med*. 1988;319:142-145.
355. Burrows RF, Kelton JG. Thrombocytopenia at delivery: a prospective survey of 6715 deliveries. *Am J Obstet Gynecol*. 1990;162:731-734.
356. Burrows RF, Kelton JG. Fetal thrombocytopenia and its relation to maternal thrombocytopenia. *N Engl J Med*. 1993;329:1463-1466.
357. Lescale KB, Eddleman KA, Cines DB, et al. Antiplatelet antibody testing in thrombocytopenic pregnant women. *Am J Obstet Gynecol*. 1996;174:1014-1018.
358. Gill KK, Kelton JG. Management of idiopathic thrombocytopenic purpura in pregnancy. *Semin Hematol*. 2000;37:275-289.
359. Webert KE, Mittal R, Sigouin C, et al. A retrospective 11-year analysis of obstetric patients with idiopathic thrombocytopenic purpura. *Blood*. 2003;102:4306-4311.
360. Silver RM, Branch W, Scott JR. Maternal thrombocytopenia in pregnancy: time for a reassessment. *Am J Obstet Gynecol*. 1995;173:479-482.
361. Gernsheimer TB. Congenital and acquired bleeding disorders in pregnancy. *Hematology*. 2016;2016:232-235.
362. Kaplan C, Daffos F, Forestier F, et al. Fetal platelet counts in thrombocytopenic pregnancy. *Lancet*. 1990;336:979-982.
363. Sun D, Shehata N, Ye XY, et al. Corticosteroids compared with intravenous immune globulin for the treatment of immune thrombocytopenia in pregnancy. *Blood*. 2016;128:1329-1335.
364. Christiaens GC, Nieuwenhuis HK, von dem Borne AE, et al. Idiopathic thrombocytopenic purpura in pregnancy: a randomized trial on the effect of antenatal low dose corticosteroids on neonatal platelet count. *Br J Obstet Gynaecol*. 1990;97:893-898.
365. Burrows RF, Kelton JG. Pregnancy in patients with idiopathic thrombocytopenic purpura: assessing the risks for the infant at delivery. *Obstet Gynecol Surv*. 1993;48:781-788.
366. Rizvi MA, Kojouri K, George JN. Drug-induced thrombocytopenia: an updated systematic review. *Ann Intern Med*. 2001;134:346.
367. Swisher KK, Li X, Vesely SK, George JN. Drug-induced thrombocytopenia: an updated systematic review, 2008. *Drug Saf*. 2009;32:85-86.
368. Nguyen L, Reese J, George JN. Drug-induced thrombocytopenia: an updated systematic review, 2010. *Drug Saf*. 2011;34:437-438.
369. Kaufman DW, Kelly JP, Johannes CB, et al. Acute thrombocytopenic purpura in relation to the use of drugs. *Blood*. 1993;82:2714-2718.
370. Girolami B, Prandoni P, Stefani PM, et al. The incidence of heparin-induced thrombocytopenia in hospitalized medical patients treated with subcutaneous unfractionated heparin: a prospective cohort study. *Blood*. 2003;101:2955-2999.
371. Belkin GA. Cocktail purpura: an unusual case of quinine sensitivity. *Ann Intern Med*. 1967;66:583-586.
372. Wooley PH, Griffin J, Panayi GS, et al. HLA-DR antigens and toxic reaction to sodium aurothiomalate and D-penicillamine in patients with rheumatoid arthritis. *N Engl J Med*. 1980;303:300-302.
373. Pedersen-Bjergaard U, Anderson M, Hansen PB. Drug-specific characteristics of thrombocytopenia caused by non-cytotoxic drugs. *Eur J Clin Pharmacol*. 1998;54:701-706.
374. Kobayashi H, Kitano K, Ishida F, et al. Aplastic anemia and idiopathic thrombocytopenic purpura with antibody to platelet glycoprotein IIb/IIIa following resection of malignant thymoma. *Acta Haematol*. 1993;90:42-45.
375. Bowen LM, Williams DM. Association of myasthenia gravis and idiopathic thrombocytopenic purpura. *South Med J*. 1981;74:513-514.
376. Anderson MJ, Woods VL, Tani P, et al. Autoantibodies to platelet glycoprotein IIb/IIIa and to the acetylcholine receptor in a patient with chronic idiopathic thrombocytopenic purpura and myasthenia gravis. *Ann Intern Med*. 1984;100:829-831.
377. Jansen PHP, Renier WO, deVaan G, et al. Effect of thymectomy on myasthenia gravis and autoimmune thrombocytopenic purpura in a 13-year-old girl. *Eur J Pediatr*. 1987;146:587-589.
378. Panzer S, Penner E, Graninger W, et al. Antinuclear antibodies in patients with chronic idiopathic autoimmune thrombocytopenia followed 2-30 years. *Am J Hematol*. 1989;32:100-103.
379. Nossent JC, Swaak AJG. Prevalence and significance of haematological abnormalities in patients with systemic lupus erythematosus. *Q J Med*. 1991;291:605-612.
380. Anderson MJ, Peebles CL, McMillan R, Curd JG. Fluorescent antinuclear antibodies and anti-SS-A/Ro in patients with immune thrombocytopenia subsequently developing systemic lupus erythematosus. *Ann Intern Med*. 1985;103:548-550.
381. Kurata Y, Miyagawa S, Kosugi S, et al. High-titer antinuclear antibodies, anti-SSA/Ro antibodies and antinuclear RNP antibodies in patients with idiopathic thrombocytopenic purpura. *Thromb Haemostasis*. 1994;71:184-187.
382. Perez HD, Katler E, Embury S. Idiopathic thrombocytopenic purpura with high-titer, speckled pattern antinuclear antibodies: possible marker for systemic lupus erythematosus. *Arthritis Rheum*. 1985;28:596-597.
383. Miescher PA, Tucci A, Beris P, Favre H. Autoimmune hemolytic anemia and/or thrombocytopenia associated with lupus parameters. *Semin Hematol*. 1992;29:13-17.
384. Kurata Y, Hayashi S, Kosugi S, et al. Elevated platelet-associated IgG in SLE patients due to anti-platelet antibody: differentiation between autoantibodies and immune complexes by ether elution. *Br J Haematol*. 1993;85:723-728.
385. Berchtold P, Harris JP, Tani P, et al. Autoantibodies to platelet glycoproteins in patients with disease-related immune thrombocytopenia. *Br J Haematol*. 1989;73:365-368.
386. Macchi L, Rispal P, Clofent-Sanchez G, et al. Anti-platelet antibodies in patients with systemic lupus erythematosus and the primary antiphospholipid antibody syndrome: their relationship with the observed thrombocytopenia. *Br J Haematol*. 1997;98:336-341.
387. Pujol M, Ribera A, Vilardell M, et al. High prevalence of platelet autoantibodies in patients with systemic lupus erythematosus. *Br J Haematol*. 1995;89:137-141.
388. Averbuch M, Koifman B, Levo Y. Lupus anticoagulant, thrombosis and thrombocytopenia in systemic lupus erythematosus. *Am J Med Sci*. 1987;293:1-5.
389. Out HJ, deGroot PG, van Vliet M, et al. Antibodies to platelets in patients with antiphospholipid antibodies. *Blood*. 1991;77:2655-2659.
390. Godeau B, Piette JC, Fromont I, et al. Specific antiplatelet glycoprotein autoantibodies are associated with the thrombocytopenia of primary antiphospholipid syndrome. *Br J Haematol*. 1997;98:873-879.
391. Fabris F, Steffan A, Cordiano I, et al. Specific antiplatelet antibodies in patients with antiphospholipid antibodies and thrombocytopenia. *Eur J Haematol*. 1994;53:232-236.
392. Coon WW. Splenectomy for cytopenias associated with systemic lupus erythematosus. *Am J Surg*. 1988;155:391-394.
393. Hall S, McCormick JL, Griepp PR, et al. Splenectomy does not cure the thrombocytopenia of systemic lupus erythematosus. *Ann Intern Med*. 1985;102:325-328.
394. Pivetti S, Novarino A, Merico F, et al. High prevalence of autoimmune phenomena in hepatitis C virus antibody positive patients with lymphoproliferative and connective tissue disorders. *Br J Haematol*. 1996;95:204-211.
395. Pawlotsky JM, Bouvier M, Fromont P, et al. Hepatitis C virus infection and autoimmune thrombocytopenic purpura. *J Hepatol*. 1995;23:635-639.
396. Chiao EY, Engels EA, Kramer JR, et al. Risk of immune thrombocytopenic purpura and autoimmune hemolytic anemia among 120 908 US veterans with hepatitis C virus infection. *Arch Intern Med*. 2009;169:357-363.
397. Kappers-Klunne MC, van Vliet HHDM. IgM and IgG platelet antibodies in a case of infectious mononucleosis and severe thrombocytopenia. *Scand J Haematol*. 1984;32:145-148.
398. Kahane S, Dvilansky A, Estok L, et al. Detection of anti-platelet antibodies in patients with idiopathic thrombocytopenic purpura (ITP) and in patients with rubella and herpes group viral infections. *Clin Exp Immunol*. 1981;44:49-56.
399. Ellman L, Carvalho A, Jacobson BM, Colman RW. Platelet autoantibody in a case of infectious mononucleosis presenting as thrombocytopenic purpura. *Am J Med*. 1973;55:723-726.
400. Krishnamurthy M, Lee CK, Dosik H. Case report: infectious mononucleosis and severe thrombocytopenia. *Am J Med Sci*. 1976;272:221-224.
401. Al-Majed SA, Al-Momen AK, Al-Kassimi FA, et al. Tuberculosis presenting as immune thrombocytopenic purpura. *Acta Haematol*. 1995;94:135-138.
402. Gasbarrini A, Franceschi F, Tartaglione R, et al. Regression of autoimmune thrombocytopenia after eradication of *Helicobacter pylori*. *Lancet*. 1998;352:878.
403. Grimaz S, Damiani D, Brosolo P, et al. Resolution of thrombocytopenia after treatment for *Helicobacter pylori*: a case report. *Haematologica*. 1999;84:283-284.
404. Tohda S, Ohkusa T. Resolution of refractory idiopathic thrombocytopenic purpura after eradication of *Helicobacter pylori*. *Am J Hematol*. 2000;65:329-330.
405. Emilia G, Longo G, Luppi M, et al. *Helicobacter pylori* eradication can induce platelet recovery in idiopathic thrombocytopenic purpura. *Blood*. 2001;97:812-814.
406. Bussel JB. *Novel Approaches to Management of Immune Thrombocytopenic Purpura: Results of Recent Trials. American Society of Hematology Education Book*. American Society of Hematology; 2001;282-293.
407. Jarque I, Andreu R, Llopis I, et al. Absence of platelet response after eradication of *Helicobacter pylori* infection in patients with chronic idiopathic purpura. *Br J Haematol*. 2001;115:1002-1003.
408. Stasi R, Sarpartwari A, Segal JB, et al. Effects of eradication of *Helicobacter pylori* infection in patients with immune thrombocytopenic purpura: a systemic review. *Blood*. 2009;113:1231-1240.
409. Arnold DM, Bernotas A, Nazi I, et al. Platelet count response to *H. pylori* treatment in patients with immune thrombocytopenia with and without *H pylori* infection: a systemic review. *Haematologica*. 2009;94:850-856.
410. Jackson SC, Beck P, Buret AG, et al. Long term platelet responses to *Helicobacter pylori* eradication in Canadian patients with immune thrombocytopenic purpura. *Int J Hematol*. 2008;88:212-218.
411. Ebbe S, Wittels B, Dameshek W. Autoimmune thrombocytopenic purpura ("ITP" type) with chronic lymphocytic leukemia. *Blood*. 1962;19:23-37.
412. Hassidim K, McMillan R, Conjalka MS, Morrison J. Immune thrombocytopenic purpura in Hodgkin disease. *Am J Hematol*. 1979;6:149-153.
413. Waddell CC, Cimo PL. Idiopathic thrombocytopenic purpura occurring in Hodgkin disease after splenectomy: report of two cases and review of the literature. *Am J Hematol*. 1979;7:381-387.
414. Xiros N, Binder T, Anger B, et al. Idiopathic thrombocytopenic purpura and autoimmune hemolytic anemia in Hodgkin's disease. *Eur J Haematol*. 1988;40:437-441.

415. Kaden BR, Rosse WF, Hauch TW. Immune thrombocytopenia in lymphoproliferative disorders. *Blood.* 1979;53:545-551.
416. Schwartz KA, Slichter SJ, Harker LA. Immune-mediated platelet destruction and thrombocytopenia in patients with solid tumors. *Br J Haematol.* 1982;51:17-24.
417. Kim HD, Boggs DR. A syndrome resembling idiopathic thrombocytopenic purpura in 10 patients with diverse forms of cancer. *Am J Med.* 1979;67:371-377.
418. Valenta LJ, Treadwell T, Berry R, Elias AN. Idiopathic thrombocytopenic purpura and Graves disease. *Am J Hematol.* 1982;12:69-72.
419. Adrouny A, Sandler RM, Carmel R. Variable presentation of thrombocytopenia in Grave's disease. *Arch Intern Med.* 1982;142:1460-1464.
420. Hymes K, Blum M, Lackner H, Karpatkin S. Easy bruising, thrombocytopenia, and elevated platelet immunoglobulin G in Graves' disease and Hashimoto's thyroiditis. *Ann Intern Med.* 1981;94:27-30.
421. Bizzaro N. Familial association of autoimmune thrombocytopenia and hyperthyroidism. *Am J Med.* 1992;39:294-298.
422. Newman PJ. Nomenclature of human platelet alloantigens: a problem with the HPA system? *Blood.* 1994;83:1447-1451.
423. Goldman M, Filion M, Proulx C, et al. Neonatal alloimmune thrombocytopenia. *Transfus Med Rev.* 1994;8:123-131.
424. McCrae KR, Herman JH. Posttransfusion purpura: two unusual cases and a literature review. *Am J Hematol.* 1996;52:205-211.
425. Warkentin TE, Smith JW, Hayward CP, et al. Thrombocytopenia caused by passive transfusion of anti-glycoprotein Ia/IIa alloantibody (anti-HPA-5b). *Blood.* 1992;79:2480-2484.
426. Ballem PJ, Buskard NA, Decary F, Doubroff P. Post-transfusion purpura secondary to passive transfer of anti-P1A1 by blood transfusion. *Br J Haematol.* 1987;66:113-114.
427. Nijjar TS, Bonacosa IA, Israels LG. Severe acute thrombocytopenia following infusion of plasma containing anti P1A1. *Am J Hematol.* 1987;25:219-221.
428. Scott EP, Moilan-Bergeland J, Dalmasso AP. Posttransfusion thrombocytopenia associated with passive transfusion of a platelet-specific antibody. *Transfusion.* 1988;28:73-76.
429. Shulman N, Aster R, Pearson H, et al. Immunoreactions involving platelets. *J Clin Invest.* 1962;41(5):1059-1069.
430. Blanchette VS, Chen L, de Friedberg ZS, et al. Alloimmunization to the PLA-1 antigen: results of a prospective study. *Br J Haematol.* 1990;74:209-215.
431. Panzer S, Auerbach L, Cechova E, et al. Maternal alloimmunization against fetal platelet antigens: a prospective study. *Br J Haematol.* 1995;90:655-660.
432. Sainio S, Jarvenpaa AL, Renlund M, et al. Thrombocytopenia in term infants: a population-based study. *Obstet Gynecol.* 2000;95:441-446.
433. Mcquilten ZK, Wood EM, Savoia H, Cole S. A review of pathophysiology and current treatment for neonatal alloimmune thrombocytopenia (NAIT) and introducing the Australian NAIT registry. *Aust N Z J Obstet Gynaecol.* 2011;51:191-198.
434. Stuge TB, Skogen B, Ahlen MT, Husebekk A, Urbaniak SJ, Bessos H. The cellular immunobiology associated with fetal and neonatal alloimmune thrombocytopenia. *Transfus Apher Sci.* 2011;45(1):53-59.
435. Kaplan C, Daffos F, Forestier F, et al. Management of alloimmune thrombocytopenia: antenatal diagnosis and in utero transfusion of maternal platelets. *Blood.* 1988;72:340-343.
436. Ghevaert C, Rankin A, Huiskes E, et al. Alloantibodies against low-frequency human platelet antigens do not account for a significant proportion of cases of feto-maternal alloimmune thrombocytopenia: evidence from 1054 cases. *Transfusion.* 2009;49(10):2084-2089.
437. Newman PJ, Derbes RS, Aster RH. The human platelet alloantigens, PlA1 and PlA2 are associated with a leucine33/proline33 amino acid polymorphism in membrane glycoprotein IIIa, and are distinguishable by DNA typing. *J Clin Invest.* 1989;83:1778-1781.
438. Curtis B, Fick A, Lochowicz A, et al. Neonatal alloimmune thrombocytopenia associated with maternal-fetal incompatibility for blood group B. *Transfusion.* 2008;48(2):358-364.
439. Noris P, Simsek S, de Bruijne-Admiraal LG, et al. Max[a], a new low frequency platelet-specific antigen localized on glycoprotein IIb, is associated with neonatal alloimmune thrombocytopenia. *Blood.* 1995;86:1019-1026.
440. von dem Borne AE, van Leeuwen EF, von Riesz LE, et al. Neonatal alloimmune thrombocytopenia: detection and characterization of the responsible antibodies by the platelet immunofluorescence test. *Blood.* 1981;57:649-656.
441. Mueller-Eckhardt C, Kiefel V, Grubert A, et al. 348 cases of suspected neonatal alloimmune thrombocytopenia. *Lancet.* 1989;1:363-366.
442. Kaplan C, Morel-Kopp MC, Kroll H, et al. HPA-5b (Br(a)) neonatal alloimmune thrombocytopenia: clinical and immunological analysis of 39 cases. *Br J Haematol.* 1991;78:425-429.
443. Mueller-Eckhardt C, Becker T, Weisheit M, et al. Neonatal alloimmune thrombocytopenia due to fetomaternal Zwb incompatibility. *Vox Sang.* 1986;50:94-96.
444. Mueller-Eckhardt C. Annotation: post-transfusion purpura. *Br J Haematol.* 1986;64:419-424.
445. McFarland JG, Blanchette V, Collins J, et al. Neonatal alloimmune thrombocytopenia due to a new platelet-specific alloantibody. *Blood.* 1993;81:3318-3323.
446. McFarland JG, Aster RH, Bussel JB, et al. Prenatal diagnosis of neonatal alloimmune thrombocytopenia using allele-specific oligonucleotide probes. *Blood.* 1991;78:2276-2282.
447. Glade-Bender J, McFarland JG, Kaplan C, et al. Anti-HPA-3A induces severe neonatal alloimmune thrombocytopenia. *J Pediatr.* 2001;138:862-867.
448. Berry JE, Murphy CM, Smith GA, et al. Detection of Gov system antibodies by MAIPA reveals an immunogenicity similar to the HPA-5 alloantigens. *Br J Haematol.* 2000;110:735-742.
449. Curtis BR, Edwards JT, Hessner MJ, Klein JP, Aster RH. Blood group A and B antigens are strongly expressed on platelets of some individuals. *Blood.* 2000;96:1574-1581.
450. Clemetson KJ. Platelets and primary haemostasis. *Thromb Res.* 2012;129(3):220-224.
451. Valentin N, Vergracht A, Bignon JD, et al. HLA-DRw52a is involved in alloimmunization against PL-A1 antigen. *Hum Immunol.* 1990;27:73-79.
452. King KE, Kao KJ, Bray PF, et al. The role of HLA antibodies in neonatal thrombocytopenia: a prospective study. *Tissue Antigens.* 1996;47:206-211.
453. Williamson LM, Hackett G, Rennie J, et al. The natural history of fetomaternal alloimmunization to the platelet-specific antigen HPA-1a (Pl[A1], Zw[a]) as determined by antenatal screening. *Blood.* 1998;92:2280-2287.
454. Bussel JB. Alloimmune thrombocytopenia in the fetus and newborn. *Semin Thromb Hemost.* 2001;27:245-252.
455. Doughty HA, Murphy MF, Metcalfe P, Waters AH. Antenatal screening for fetal alloimmune thrombocytopenia: the results of a pilot study. *Br J Haematol.* 1995;90:321-325.
456. Delbos F, Bertrand G, Croisille L, et al. Fetal and neonatal alloimmune thrombocytopenia: predictive factors of intracranial hemorrhage. *Transfusion.* 2016;56:59-66.
457. Tiller H, Kamphuis MM, Flodmark O, et al. Fetal intracranial haemorrhages caused by fetal and neonatal alloimmune thrombocytopenia: an observational cohort study of 43 cases from an international multicentre registry. *BMJ Open.* 2013;3:e002490. doi: 10.1136/ bmjopen-2012-002490
458. Bussel JB, Berkowitz RL, Hung C, et al. Intracranial hemorrhage in alloimmune thrombocytopenia: stratified management to prevent recurrence in the subsequent affected fetus. *Am J Obstet Gynecol.* 2010;203(2):135.e1-135.e14.
459. Ohto H, Yamaguchi T, Takeuchi C, et al. Anti-HPA-5b induced neonatal alloimmune thrombocytopenia: antibody titre as a predictor. *Br J Haematol.* 2000;110:223-227.
460. Skogen B, Killie MK, Kjeldsen-Kragh J, et al. Expert Review of Hematology prevention Reconsidering fetal and neonatal alloimmune thrombocytopenia with a focus on screening and prevention. *Expert Rev Hematol.* 2010;3(5):559-566.
461. Jaegtvik S, Husebekk A, Aune B, et al. Neonatal alloimmune thrombocytopenia due to anti-HPA l a antibodies; the level of maternal antibodies predicts the severity of thrombocytopenia in the newborn. *Br J Obstet Gynaecol.* 2000;107:691-694.
462. Curley A, Stanworth SJ, Willoughby K, et al. Randozmied trail of platelet-transfusion thresholds in neonates. *NEJM.* 2019;380:242.
463. Baker JM, Shehata N, Bussel J, et al. Postnatal intervention for the treatment of FNAIT: a systematic review. *J Perinatol.* 2019;39:1329-1339.
464. Kiefel V, Bassler D, Kroll H, et al. Antigen-positive platelet transfusion in neonatal alloimmune thrombocytopenia (NAIT). *Blood.* 2006;107:3761-3763.
465. Bussel J. Diagnosis and management of the fetus and neonate with alloimmune thrombocytopenia. *Thromb Haemostasis.* 2009;7(suppl 1):253-257.
466. Sillers L, Van Slambrouck C, Lappin-Carr G. Neonatal thrombocytopenia: etiology and diagnosis. *Pediatr Ann.* 2015;44(7):e175-e180.
467. Tiller H, Killie MK, Skogen B, et al. Neonatal alloimmune thrombocytopenia in Norway: poor detection rate with nonscreening versus a general screening program. *BJOG.* 2009;116:594-598.
468. Birchall JE, Murphy MF, Kaplan C, et al. European collaborative study of the antenatal management of feto-maternal alloimmune thrombocytopenia. *Br J Haematol.* 2003;122:275-288.
469. Berkowitz RL, Kolb EA, McFarland JG, et al. Parallel randomized trials of risk-based therapy for fetal alloimmune thrombocytopenia. *Obstet Gynecol.* 2006;107:91-96.
470. Thung SF, Grobman WA. The cost effectiveness of empiric intravenous immunoglobulin for the antepartum treatment of fetal and neonatal alloimmune thrombocytopenia. *Am J Obstet Gynecol.* 2005;193:1094-1099.
471. Pacheco LD, Berkowitz RL, Moise KJ, Jr, et al. Fetal and neonatal alloimmune thrombocytopenia: a management algorithm based on risk stratification. *Obstet Gynecol.* 2011;118:1157-1163.
472. Davoren A, Curtis BR, Aster RH, et al. Human platelet antigen-specific alloantibodies implicated in 1162 cases of neonatal alloimmune thrombocytopenia. *Transfusion.* 2004;44:1220-1225.
473. Kovanlikaya A, Tiwari P, Buseel JB, et al. Imaging and management of fetuses and neonatas with alloimmune thrombocytopenia. *Pediatr Blood Cancer.* 2017;64:e26690.
474. Winkelhorst D, Murphy MF, Greinacher A, et al. Antenatal management in fetal and neonatal alloimmune thrombocytopenia: a systematic review. *Blood.* 2017;129:1538-1547.
475. Rayment R, Brunskill SJ, Soothill PW, et al. Antenatal interventions for fetomaternal alloimmune thrombocytopenia (review). *Cochrane Database Syst Rev.* 2011;2011(5):CD004226.
476. van den Akker E, Oepkes D, Brand A, Kanhai HH. Vaginal delivery of fetuses at risk of alloimmune thrombocytopenia? *BJOG.* 2006;113:781-783.
477. Radder CM, de Haan MJ, Brand A, et al. Follow up of children after antenatal treatment for alloimmune thrombocytopenia. *Early Hum Dev.* 2004;80:65-76.
478. Shulman NR, Aster RH, Leitner A, Hiller MC. Immunoreactions involving platelets. V. Post-transfusion purpura due to complement-fixing antibody against a genetically controlled platelet antigen. A proposed mechanism for thrombocytopenia and its relevance in "autoimmunity." *J Clin Invest.* 1961;40:1597-1620.
479. Prowse CV, Hornsey VS, Drummond O, et al. Preliminary assessment of whole-blood, red-cell and platelet- leucodepleting filters for possible induction of prion release by leucocyte fragmentation during room temperature processing. *Br J Haemat.* 1999;106:240-147.
480. Cimo PL, Aster RH. Post-transfusion purpura: successful treatment by exchange transfusion. *N Engl J Med.* 1972;287:290-292.
481. Keimowitz RM, Collins J, Davis K, Aster RH. Post-transfusion purpura associated with alloimmunization against the platelet-specific antigen, Bak[a]. *Am J Hematol.* 1986;21:79-88.
482. Kickler TS, Herman JH, Furihata K, et al. Identification of Bak[a], a new platelet-specific antigen associated with posttransfusion purpura. *Blood.* 1988;71:894-898.

483. Christie DJ, Pulkrabek S, Putnam JL, et al. Post-transfusion purpura due to an alloantibody reactive with glycoprotein Ia/IIa (anti-HPA-5b). *Blood*. 1991;77:2785-2789.
484. Bierling P, Godeau B, Fromont P, et al. Posttransfusion purpura-like syndrome associated with CD36 (Nak[a]) isoimmunization. *Transfusion*. 1995;35:777-782.
485. Taaning E, Tonnesen F. Pan-reactive platelet antibodies in post-transfusion purpura. *Vox Sang*. 1999;76:120-123.
486. Lucas GF, Pittman SJ, Davies S, et al. Post-transfusion purpura (PTP) associated with anti-HPA-1a, anti-HPA-2b and anti-HPA-3a antibodies. *Transfus Med*. 1997;7:295-299.
487. Gerstner JB, Smith MJ, Davis KD, et al. Post-transfusion purpura: therapeutic failure of PL[A1]-negative platelet transfusion. *Am J Hematol*. 1979;6:71-75.
488. Laursen B, Morling N, Rosenkvist J, et al. Post-transfusion purpura treated with plasma exchange by Haemonetics Cell Separator. *Acta Med Scand*. 1978;203:539-543.
489. Lau P, Sholtis CM, Aster RH. Post-transfusion purpura: an enigma of alloimmunization. *Am J Hematol*. 1980;9:331-336.
490. Becker T, Panzer S, Maas D, et al. High-dose intravenous immunoglobulin for post-transfusion purpura. *Br J Haematol*. 1985;61:149-155.
491. Berney SI, Metcalfe P, Wathen NC, Waters AH. Post-transfusion purpura responding to high dose intravenous IgG: further observations on pathogenesis. *Br J Haematol*. 1985;61:627-632.
492. Glud TK, Rosthøj S, Jensen MK, et al. High-dose intravenous immunoglobulin for post-transfusion purpura. *Scand J Haematol*. 1983;31:495-500.

Chapter 49 ■ Thrombotic Thrombocytopenic Purpura, Hemolytic-Uremic Syndrome, and Related Disorders

HAN-MOU TSAI

The various forms of thrombocytopenia discussed in this chapter often share the common features of concurrent hemolysis with characteristic schistocytes on blood smears (microangiopathic hemolytic anemia [MAHA]) (*Figure 49.1*). It is believed that hemolysis with schistocytes results from mechanical injury of the red blood cells by abnormal levels of shear stress in the circulation.

Fragmentation of the red blood cells occurs in two types of mechanical injury: vascular devices such as prosthetic heart valves, ventricular assist devices (VADs), and extracorporeal membrane oxygenator; and arteriolar stenosis. In patients without vascular devices, fragmentation of the red blood cells signifies stenosis in the arteriolar microvasculature. This is because wall shear stress, as determined by flow rate, the inverse of the luminal diameter to the third order, and blood viscosity, is at its highest in the arterioles (e.g., 86 ± 17 dyne/cm^2 systolic in the first-order retinal arterioles)[1] and may be further increased to exceed the threshold level of instantaneous red cell fragmentation (1500 dynes/cm^2)[2] when the vascular lumen is narrowed (e.g., by more than 62%). Stenosis of large arteries usually causes clinically apparent ischemic organ dysfunction before it is sufficiently severe to cause significant red cell fragmentation. The shear stress profile in the venules and veins is too low to cause red cell fragmentation even in the presence of stenosis.

A classification of the disorders that may be associated with the syndrome of MAHA and thrombocytopenia is listed in *Table 49.1*. In this classification, based on the types of the pathologic lesions (*Figure 49.2*), thrombotic microangiopathy (TMA) is only one of the five different types of pathology that are associated with the syndrome of MAHA and thrombocytopenia.

ACQUIRED THROMBOTIC THROMBOCYTOPENIC PURPURA

Pathology

The pathology of thrombotic thrombocytopenic purpura (TTP), as first described by Moschcowitz in 1925,[3] is quite distinctive. It is characterized by widespread hyaline thrombi in the terminal arterioles and capillaries, accompanied by no or little evidence of endothelial injury or inflammation (*Figure 49.2A*). The thrombi are present most extensively in the heart, pancreas, spleen, kidney, adrenal gland, and brain (mainly cerebral cortex) and are composed primarily of platelets and von Willebrand factor (vWF) (*Figure 49.2B*).[4-6] Small amounts of fibrin may be present surrounding or sometimes penetrating the amorphous or granular material. Glomerular microthrombi are usually spotty, and cortical necrosis of the kidney is uncommon in TTP. Fibrinoid necrosis and vascular or perivascular inflammatory cell infiltration are characteristically absent or minimal.

In chronic cases, the thrombi may be infiltrated by fibroblasts or converted to subendothelial deposits by reactive endothelial cells. Pseudoaneurysmal dilatation may also be present upstream of the stenosis or occlusion.

In some reports, the lesions of TTP were shown to include prominent injury of endothelial cells. A review of the clinical and pathologic features in those reports suggests that the patients likely had Shiga toxin–associated hemolytic-uremic syndrome (STX-HUS) or atypical hemolytic-uremic syndrome (AHUS) instead of TTP.

Pathogenesis

TTP was first described as a clinicopathologic syndrome of MAHA, thrombocytopenia, and widespread hyaline thrombi in arterioles and capillaries of unknown etiology and pathogenesis.

In practice, to make the diagnosis of TTP without tissues for pathology, a pentad of MAHA, thrombocytopenia, neurologic deficits, renal abnormalities, and fever was proposed. The pentad was subsequently reduced to the triad of MAHA, thrombocytopenia, and neurologic deficits and then the diad of MAHA and thrombocytopenia. The main reason for the shift was the recognition that many patients of TTP first present with the syndrome of diad before advancing to the syndromes of triad and pentad.

Because delay in diagnosis and treatment may expose the patient to the risk of serious complications and even death, a patient presenting with the diad of MAHA and thrombocytopenia is presumed to have TTP and promptly treated with plasma exchange.

This practice gradually leads to the common but incorrect belief that the syndrome of MAHA and thrombocytopenia constitutes the diagnosis of TTP. This equation of TTP with the syndrome of diad, triad, or pentad ignores the fact that these syndromes may result from other disorders with vastly different pathogenesis and pathology (*Table 49.1*). The misconception led to the common practice of treating all patients with any of the syndromes as cases of TTP, sometimes with disastrous outcomes. It also contributes to confusion in the literature, as clinical cases or case series comprise variable mixes of TTP and other causes of the syndrome.

On the other hand, some patients with TTP may present with complications of thrombosis such as focal neurologic deficits without MAHA and/or thrombocytopenia. The correct diagnosis of TTP is delayed for these patients until both MAHA and thrombocytopenia become overt later.

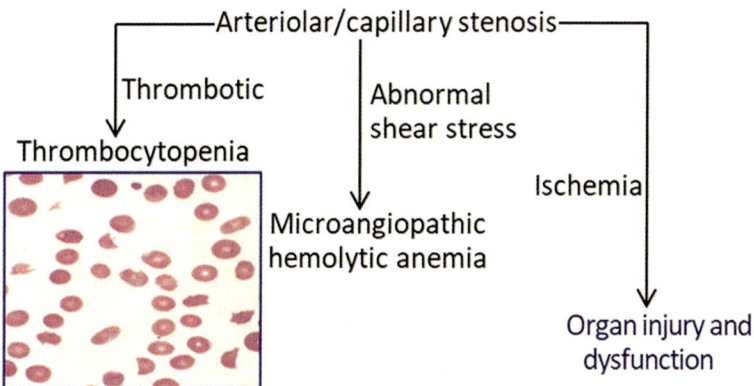

FIGURE 49.1 Arteriolar and capillary stenosis is the pathologic basis for the syndrome of microangiopathic hemolytic anemia and thrombocytopenia.

Table 49.1. A Pathological Classification of the Syndrome of MAHA and Thrombocytopenia

Pathology	Disorders	Major Pathogenetic Process
vWF-rich platelet thrombosis	Thrombotic thrombocytopenic purpura (TTP)	Activation of circulating vWF by shear stress under conditions of severe ADAMTS13 deficiency
Thrombotic microangiopathy (TMA) (endothelial injury)	STX-associated HUS	STX-mediated endothelial injury
	Atypical HUS	Uncontrolled complement activation on endothelial surface
	Pneumococcal HUS	T-activation (exposure of Thomsen–Friedenreich antigen)
	Anti-VEGF drugs	Depletion of VEGF signaling
	Other drugs	Undetermined
	Antiphospholipid syndrome	Undetermined
	DGKE nephropathy	Phosphokinase C activation
	Cobalamin C disease	High homocysteine plasma level (presumed)
Fibrin-rich platelet thrombosis	Disseminated intravascular coagulopathy	Intravascular activation of the coagulation cascade
	CAPS, HITT, PNH	Intravascular activation of platelet and/or coagulation
	HELLP syndrome of pregnancy	Hepatic sinusoidal injury (presumed)
Vasculitis/vasculopathy	Immune or immune complex vasculitis, renal scleroderma	Anti-vessel Ab or deposition of immune complexes
	RMSF, anthrax, fungemia, viremia	Infection of the vessel wall
	Malignant hypertension	Physical injury[a]
Intravascular clusters of neoplastic cells	"Tumor cell embolism"	Intravascular proliferation and dissemination of neoplastic cells

Abbreviations: Ab, antibody; ADAMTS13, A Disintegrin And Metalloprotease with ThromboSpondin type 1 repeats, member 13; CAPS, catastrophic antiphospholipid syndrome; DGKE, diacylglycerol kinase epsilon; HELLP, hemolysis, elevated liver enzymes and low platelet count; HITT, heparin-induced thrombocytopenia and thrombosis; HUS, hemolytic-uremic syndrome; MAHA, microangiopathic hemolytic anemia; PNH, paroxysmal nocturnal hemoglobinuria; RMSF, Rocky Mountain spotted fever; STX, Shiga toxin; TMA, thrombotic microangiopathy; VEGF, vascular endothelial growth factor; vWF, von Willebrand factor.
[a]Some cases of "malignant hypertension" have been found to be atypical HUS with TMA.

The discovery of A Disintegrin And Metalloprotease with ThromboSpondin type 1 repeats, member 13 (ADAMTS13) and its deficiency in TTP resolves these dilemmas.[7-9] It is now recognized that TTP is a disorder with propensity to vWF-platelet thrombosis when ADAMTS13 is very low (<10% of normal), due to inhibitory antibodies (Abs) of ADAMTS13 in the acquired form of TTP and genetic mutations of ADAMTS13 in the hereditary form of the disease.

ADAMTS13 is synthesized primarily in the stellate cells of the liver.[10,11] ADAMTS13 may also be expressed, albeit at much lower levels by at least one to two orders, in the spleen and other organs. The localization of its biosynthesis to the stellate cells instead of hepatocytes may account for the lack of correlation between ADAMTS13 deficiency and liver failure. In fact, the stellate cells react to liver injury by activation and proliferation. The synthesis of ADAMTS13 may be downregulated by cytokines, such as interferon-γ, tumor necrosis factor (TNF)-α, and interleukin (IL)-4.[12]

Expression of ADAMTS13 has been described in the renal glomerular podocytes and endothelial cells.[13,14] The ADAMTS13 expressed in renal glomeruli may cleave vWF before the protease is neutralized by inhibitory auto-Abs. This process may explain why renal injury tends to be milder in acquired TTP than in hereditary TTP (hTTP).

Rather than a syndrome, TTP is now considered a disease with propensity to intravascular vWF-platelet thrombosis due to ADAMTS13 deficiency (Table 49.2). Consistent with this pathogenetic approach, STX-HUS and AHUS are also defined as diseases rather than syndromes. To avoid confusion, TMA only refers to the pathologic syndrome resulting from endothelial injury.

This pathogenetic scheme of classification distinguishes TTP from other causes of the syndrome of MAHA and thrombocytopenia. Furthermore, since it does not rely on the presence of thrombocytopenia and MAHA, the new definition of TTP encompasses patients with atypical presentations, such as stroke or myocardial infarction with no MAHA, with or without thrombocytopenia.

Awareness of this history of evolution in terminology is critical when one reviews the literature of TTP, HUS, and TMA, as these diagnostic terms were often loosely used to include various mixtures of disorders and the findings are not directly comparable.

Causes of ADAMTS13 Deficiency

In most cases of TTP, inhibitory auto-Abs of ADAMTS13 cause severe deficiency (<10% of normal) of the protease.[7] In a small number of patients, the deficiency is the consequence of homozygous or compound heterozygous mutations of the ADAMTS13 gene.[7-9]

The ADAMTS13 activity level is also decreased in various inflammatory conditions, with its magnitude of decrease often correlating with the severity of inflammation. The decrease in these conditions by itself is insufficiently severe to cause platelet aggregation and thrombosis. Nevertheless, such a decrease may precipitate vWF-platelet aggregation and thrombosis in patients with preexisting ADAMTS13 mutations or inhibitors, giving rise to the appearance that these conditions "cause" TTP.

Indeed, TTP does relapse following vaccinations.[15,16] Such exacerbation of subclinical TTP may also account for some of the "de novo" TTP cases reported after pneumococcal or COVID-19 vaccination or infection.[17-24]

ADAMTS13 activity is less stable in pathologic blood samples. Improper handling of the test blood samples may yield falsely low ADAMTS13 levels.

Inhibitory Antibodies of ADAMTS13

In patients with acquired TTP, which accounts for >95% of TTP cases, deficiency of ADAMTS13 results from inhibitory Abs to the ADAMTS13 protease. It is speculated that an otherwise innocuous infection, via antigenic mimicry, may trigger an autoimmune reaction to ADAMTS13 in genetically susceptible individuals. Indeed, 10% to 40% of TTP patients exhibit positive autoimmune reactions to other targets such as nuclear antigens, suggesting they have constitutional defects in immune regulation.

Ticlopidine and HIV infection are two conditions that are associated with an increased risk of acquired TTP. Ticlopidine therapy increases the risk of acquired TTP by 50- to 300-fold.[25,26] The disease typically presents between 2 and 8 weeks after institution of ticlopidine therapy.

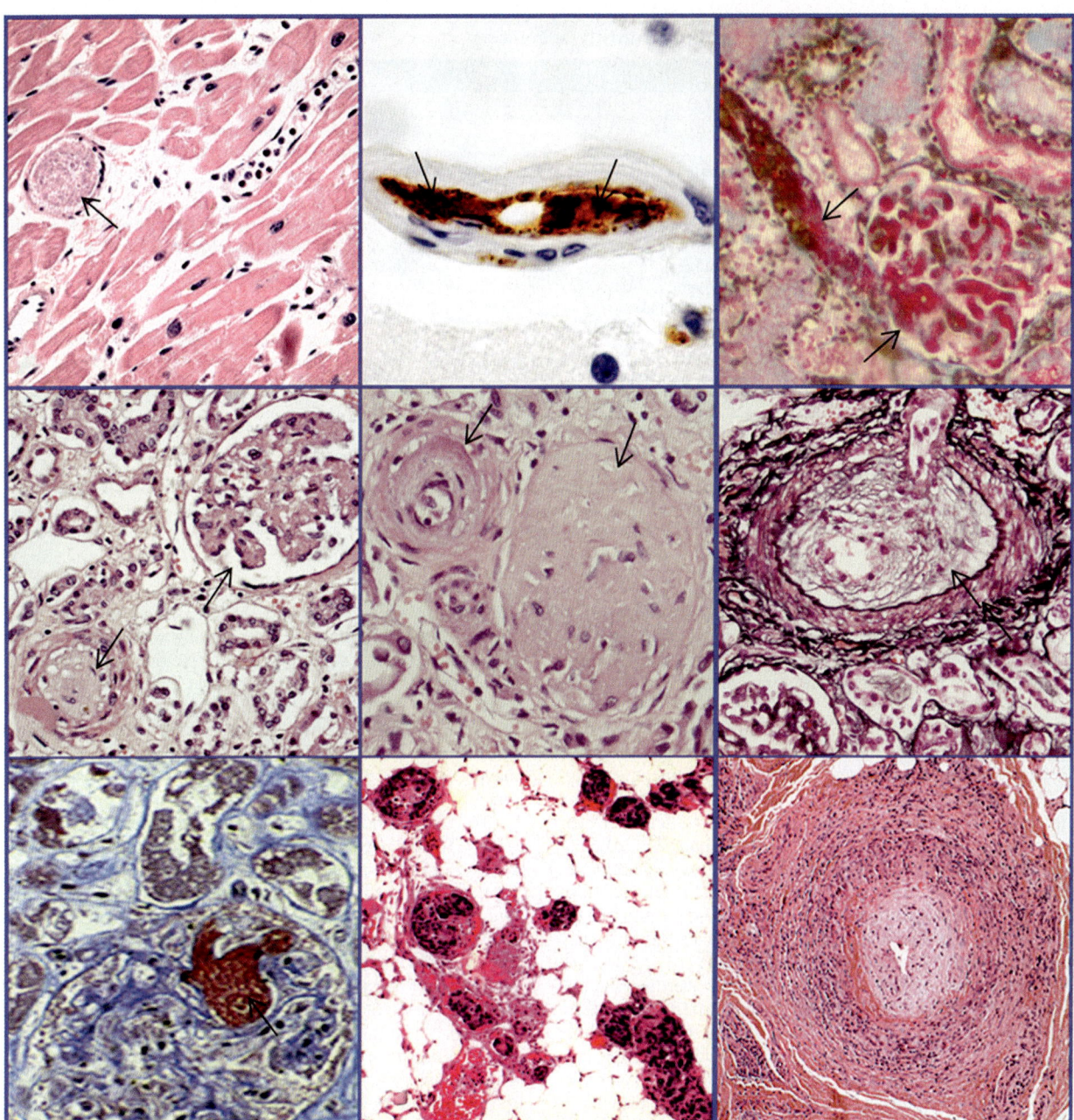

FIGURE 49.2 **Histopathology and histochemistry of TTP and other disorders associated with MAHA.** A, TTP (heart); B, TTP (brain); C, (STX-HUS) (kidney); D-F, AHUS (kidney); G, DIC (kidney); H, metastatic tumor cell clusters in the microvasculature of bone marrow; I, proliferative vasculitis of lupus causing microvascular stenosis (soft tissue). The endothelial cells and the vessel wall are intact in TTP. All are H&E stains except B (immunohistochemical stain for vWF, brown), C and G (fibrin stain of Carstair), and F (Jones silver stain). AHUS, atypical hemolytic-uremic syndrome; DIC, disseminated intravascular coagulation; MAHA, microangiopathic hemolytic anemia; STX-HUS, Shiga toxin–associated hemolytic-uremic syndrome; TTP, thrombotic thrombocytopenic purpura; vWF, von Willebrand factor.

It responds to plasma exchange and discontinuation of the culprit drug, and generally does not recur after ticlopidine is discontinued. Another antiplatelet thienopyridine, clopidogrel, has also been implicated, but never confirmed in causing acquired TTP.[26,27]

HIV infection has been associated with acquired TTP. It is estimated that the risk of having aTTP is increased by nearly 40-fold among patients not being treated with antiretroviral therapy.[28] This higher risk may be a part of the predisposition to autoimmunity in association with untreated HIV infection.

Characteristics of the Inhibitors

In most TTP patients, the levels of ADAMTS13 inhibitors are low (<10 Bethesda U/mL)[29] and often further decrease to undetectable levels after a few weeks or months. This decrease is critical for remission of TTP. Occasionally, the inhibitor level may persist or surge to very high levels, resulting in refractory disease or a fatal outcome.[30]

The ADAMTS13 inhibitors of TTP are primarily immunoglobulin G (IgG), with IgA and IgM Abs detectable less frequently.[31] The VH1-69 germline heavy-chain gene appears to be used most frequently in producing the ADAMTS13 Abs.[32] All four subclasses of IgG have been detected, although IgG4 appears to be the most prevalent, detectable in greater than 90% of patients according to one study.

Targets of the ADAMTS13 Inhibitors

ADAMTS13, comprising 1427 amino acid residues, belongs to the ADAMTS metalloprotease family that shares a conserved domain

Table 49.2. Diagnostic Terms: Historical and Current Definitions

Term	Historical	Current
TMA	Synonymous with the syndrome of • MAHA and thrombocytopenia, • TTP, or • The pathology of microvascular thrombosis	Endothelial injury in small arteries, arterioles, and capillaries, often with thrombosis at sites of endothelial disruption, but with no or little inflammatory cell infiltration
TTP	The syndrome of • MAHA and thrombocytopenia with the pathology of hyaline thrombi in arterioles and capillaries of multiple organs, • MAHA and thrombocytopenia (diad), • Diad and neurologic deficits (triad), or • Triad, renal abnormalities and fever (pentad)	Propensity to vWF-platelet thrombosis in arterioles and capillaries due to severe deficiency of ADAMTS13 caused by inhibitory antibodies (acquired TT) or genetic mutations (hereditary TTP)
STX-HUS	The syndrome of • Renal failure, MAHA, and thrombocytopenia following a prodrome of hemorrhagic diarrhea (typical HUS, D + HUS), or • The above after infection with Shiga toxin–producing microorganisms	The pathology of TMA and its clinical manifestations following infection with a Shiga toxin–producing microorganism
AHUS	The syndrome of renal failure, MAHA, and thrombocytopenia in children without a prodrome of hemorrhagic diarrhea or infection with Shiga toxin–producing microorganisms	Propensity to TMA and other complications due to defective regulation of the alternative complement pathway

Abbreviations: ADAMTS13, A Disintegrin And Metalloprotease with ThromboSpondin type 1 repeats, member 13; AHUS, atypical hemolytic-uremic syndrome; MAHA, microangiopathic hemolytic anemia; STX-HUS, Shiga toxin–associated HUS; TMA, thrombotic microangiopathy; TTP, thrombotic thrombocytopenic purpura; vWF, von Willebrand factor.

structure of metalloprotease (MP)-disintegrin (Dis)-thrombospondin type 1 repeat (TSR)-cysteine–rich (Cys) and spacer (Spa) domains. ADAMTS13 contains seven additional TSR downstream of the Spa domain, followed by two unique CUB (complement C1r/C1s, Uegf, Bmp1) domains (Figure 49.3).[9]

The metalloprotease domain of ADAMTS13 contains a catalytic 224–HEIGHSFGLEHD–235 module characteristic of the ADAMTS protease family (conserved residues are underlined). Structural analysis has identified three surface exosites of ADAMTS13 in the Dis-Spa region that react with discrete epitopes of the vWF A2 sequence near and downstream of the Tyr1605-Met1606 scissile bond.[33,34] Another exosite in the TSR5-CUB region of ADAMTS13 may interact with a constitutively exposed epitope in the N-terminal D4-CK region of vWF. This C-terminal binding may facilitate the interactions of the exosites upstream. The exosite binding greatly enhances the efficiency of catalytic reaction between ADAMTS13 and vWF.

The inhibitory Abs of TTP target the exosites rather than the catalytic site of ADAMTS13. ADAMTS13 variants truncated upstream of the Cys-Spa domains exhibit markedly decreased but detectable vWF cleaving activity that is not suppressible by inhibitors of patients with TTP,[35] indicating that the Cys-Spa region is an integral part of the ADAMTS13 epitope that reacts with the inhibitors of TTP patients.

However, recombinant ADAMTS13 fragments comprising the Cys-Spa sequence do not exhibit binding with TTP inhibitors until the sequence is extended upstream to include the distal part of the metalloprotease domain, suggesting that TTP inhibitors likely target a spatial epitope of ADAMTS13 rather than a short peptide sequence, or the target peptide sequence may be cryptic in certain constructs. Recombinant ADAMTS13 variants not suppressible by TTP inhibitors may be exploited therapeutically to circumvent the obstacle of inhibitory Abs in patients with acquired TTP.

The CUB domains at the C-terminus are found to be inhibitory of ADAMTS13 cleavage of abbreviated vWF peptide substrates such as VWF115 (comprising residues 1554-1668 of the full-length vWF peptide). Presumably, when the C-terminus sequence is not interacting with vWF D4-CK region (Figure 49.3, ❶), it is bent over to interact with a certain sequence in the Spa domain (Figure 49.3, ❶). In this closed conformation of ADAMTS13, as suggested by atomic force microscopy findings,[36] the exosites in the Dis-Spa domains are less available for interaction with the exosites in VWF A2 domain (Figure 49.3, ❷).[37] This binding facilitates the cleavage of the Y1605-M1606 bond by the Zn^{++}-catalytic sequence of ADAMTS13 (Figure 49.3, ❸). The blocking phenomenon by CUB domains is abolished when the spacer domain sequence is mutated (as in the gain-of-function [GoF]

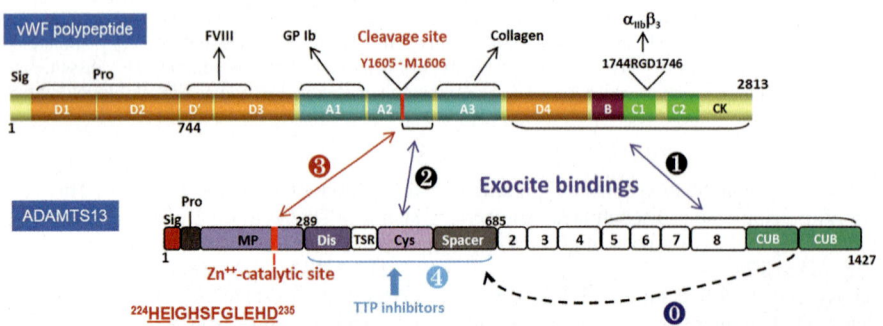

FIGURE 49.3 Domain structures of vWF and ADAMTS13 and their interactions. The domain locations of their functional epitopes and the $zinc^{++}$-catalytic consensus sequence of ADAMTS13 are depicted. Native state ADAMTS13 exists in a closed conformation in which the CUB domains are bent over to mask the spacer domain (❶). In the presence of vWF, exosite binding (❶) occurs constitutively. This binding transforms ADAMTS13 to an open conformation. Exosite binding (❷) occurs only when the sequence in the A2 domain downstream of the scissile bond Tyr1605-Met1606 is exposed by shear stress. The exosite bindings help orient the Zn^{++}-catalytic site to attack the scissile bond of vWF (❸). The inhibitors of TTP patients target the exosites of ADAMTS13 downstream of the MP domain (❹), thereby preventing exosite binding (❷) while it maintains ADAMTS13 in its open conformation even when there is no exosite binding (❶). ADAMTS13, A Disintegrin And Metalloprotease with ThromboSpondin type 1 repeats, member 13; GP, glycoprotein; MP, metalloprotease; thrombotic thrombocytopenic purpura (TTP); vWF, von Willebrand factor.

variant with R568K/F592Y/R660K/Y661F/Y665F mutations),[38] or when the CUB domains are deleted.[37] The closed conformation of ADAMTS13 in the absence of vWF D4-CK may explain why, compared to CUB-truncated ADAMTS13, full-length ADAMTS13 is less effective in cleaving abbreviated vWF peptide substrate, yet more effective in cleaving vWF multimers.

Compared to wild-type ADAMTS13, the GoF variant exhibits nearly half of the Km (~2-fold binding propensity) but similar $k$cat (catalytic rate) against an abbreviated vWF peptide, VWF115.[37] In contrast, ADAMTS13 truncated at the TSR2 domain exhibits a similar Km but higher $k$cat against a shorter vWF peptide (VWF73).[39] Overall, truncation of either vWF or ADAMTS13 may alter its overall conformation and hence their modes of interaction. The proteolytic activities of ADAMTS13 variants determined using abbreviated vWF peptide substrates need to be corroborated with their activities against vWF multimers.

The ADAMTS13 GoF variant, with its epitope for interaction with the CUB domain sequence abolished by the introduced mutations, exists in open conformation. Yet it is not susceptible to inhibition by TTP inhibitors, because the mutations also abolish the epitopes recognized by the inhibitory Abs of acquired TTP. The GoF variant would seem a good therapeutic candidate for acquired TTP. Nevertheless, its effect on fibrin stability may be an obstacle.[40]

Some studies have found that TTP Abs may also target other epitopes downstream of the Cys-Spa domain. However, it is unclear whether these Abs contribute to ADAMTS13 deficiency in TTP patients.[41]

ADAMTS13 Mutations

DNA sequence analysis reveals that hTTP patients have compound heterozygous or, less commonly, homozygous mutations of the ADAMTS13 gene on chromosome 9q34.[9] More than 100 mutations, including nonsense, missense, frame-shifting insertion or deletion, and splicing mutations, have been detected in patients with hTTP.

Only a few mutations have been detected recurrently in seemingly unrelated families. One mutation, 4143insA, has been detected in at least 15 patients in central-northern Europe, Turkey, and Australia that appear to share a common haplotype.[42]

More than 25 polymorphisms have also been detected in the coding sequence of ADAMTS13. One polymorphism, P475S, common among Japanese (5%), Koreans (4%), and Chinese (1%), makes the ADAMTS13 variant more susceptible to inhibition by urea,[43-45] which is used in some ADAMTS13 assays.[8] Urea-based assays yield falsely low ADAMTS13 activity levels in individuals with the P475S polymorphism.[46] Certain cis-combinations of polymorphisms or mutation-polymorphism may result in severe ADAMTS13 deficiency.[47]

Animal Models of ADAMTS13 Deficiency

Animal models of severe ADAMTS13 deficiency have been created in mice by inactivation of the ADAMTS13 gene and in baboons by infusion of an inhibitory ADAMTS13 Ab.[48-50] In both models, thrombi comprising vWF and platelets, similar to the lesions of TTP, are found in arterioles. The findings in these animal models support the role of ADAMTS13 deficiency in causing microvascular thrombosis of TTP. Nevertheless, some mouse strains are phenotypically free of thrombosis. The difference in phenotypic severity among the mouse strains highlights the importance of epistasis in which the composition of other genes affects the expression of a molecularly or genetically defined disease.

Other Pathogenic Mechanisms of Thrombotic Thrombocytopenic Purpura

Over the years, various hypotheses have been proposed to explain the thrombosis of TTP, including defects in fibrinolytic activity or prostacyclin homeostasis, increased circulating thrombomodulin (THBD), abnormal tissue plasminogen activator or plasminogen activator inhibitor-1 levels, antiendothelial cell antibodies, immune complexes, platelet aggregating proteins, anti-CD36 Abs, calcium-dependent cysteine proteases, endothelial cell apoptotic factors, and activation of the complement system.[51-57] These observed changes were preliminary, not specific for TTP, or represented secondary changes.

Pathophysiology

Historically, two broad schemes were proposed to account for the thrombosis in TTP: endothelial cell injury and uncontrolled platelet aggregation. The predominance of vWF and platelets in the thrombi and the integrity of vascular endothelial cells in pathologic lesions suggest that thrombosis results from dysregulation of the vWF-platelet interaction.

Indeed, when ADAMTS13 is severely deficient, vWF is activated by shear stress at levels comparable to those in the arteriolar circulation.[7] The activated vWF may cause intravascular platelet aggregation and thrombosis seen in TTP.

vWF, a plasma glycoprotein derived primarily from vascular endothelial cells, is best known for its unique capability to support platelet adhesion and aggregation under high–shear stress conditions. vWF is synthesized in vascular endothelial cells as a disulfide-bonded polymer, yet it is found to exist as a series of multimers in the circulation (*Figure 49.4*, upper panel).[58] Deficiency in vWF or a decrease of the large multimers causes defective hemostasis and platelet-type bleeding diathesis in patients with von Willebrand disease.

For many years, vWF posed four enigmas. Firstly, little was known about how the multimers were generated. Secondly, vWF coexists with platelets without causing platelet aggregation in normal circulation. However, as soon as it adheres to the vessel wall, vWF begins to support platelet adhesion and aggregation. Shear stress promotes the adhesion and aggregation of platelets mediated by vWF.[59] Thirdly, the size of the multimers is a major determinant of vWF hemostatic activity, although all multimers contain the epitopes necessary for binding with platelet receptors.[58] Fourthly, fragments of the vWF peptides resulting from cleavage at the Tyr1605-Met1606 peptide bond of the A2 domain are present in normal plasma,[60] yet no protease activity is detectable in test tubes.

These enigmas were unraveled when it was discovered that a hitherto unknown plasma metalloprotease, ADAMTS13, converted the endothelial vWF polymer to multimers in the plasma by cleavage at the Tyr1605-Met1606 bond (*Figure 49.4*, lower panel). The protease evades detection in vitro because it only cleaves vWF under conditions of shear stress.[61] Furthermore, in the absence of ADAMTS13, shear stress alters the vWF conformation to an active form for supporting platelet adhesion.[7,62]

Under static conditions vWF exists in a compact configuration,[63] with its cleavage sites and platelet binding sites cryptic. This explains why in test tubes, vWF is not susceptible to cleavage by ADAMTS13 and is also inactive in causing platelet aggregation. High levels of shear stress as exist in the arteriolar circulation induce a conformational change of vWF, exposing its binding sites for platelet receptors (*Figure 49.5A*).[64]

Hence, due to its responsiveness to shear stress, vWF is uniquely capable of supporting platelet adhesion and aggregation under conditions of high shear stress. Furthermore, large multimers are hemostatically more effective than small multimers because their larger molecular sizes make them more responsive to shear stress.[63]

In the circulation, cleavage of vWF by ADAMTS13 occurs whenever its cleavage sites are exposed by shear stress (*Figure 49.5B*) at levels encountered in the arterioles (~65 or higher dynes/cm^2). The vWF scissile bond and the exosite binding sites of the vWF A2 domain (*Figure 49.3*), normally cryptic, are exposed by tensile force to initiate interaction with ADAMTS13. The process of proteolysis is repeated during each cycle of transit through the arteriolar circulation. This process of proteolysis prevents the activation of vWF by shear stress in the circulation to cause platelet aggregation while it converts vWF from a large polymer to a series of multimers (*Figure 49.5B*).

With ADAMTS13 deficiency, this proteolytic regulation of vWF activation does not occur in TTP. Instead, ADAMTS13 deficiency leads to unfolding and activation of vWF by shear stress. The activated vWF binds to the platelet glycoprotein 1b/IX/V receptor, resulting

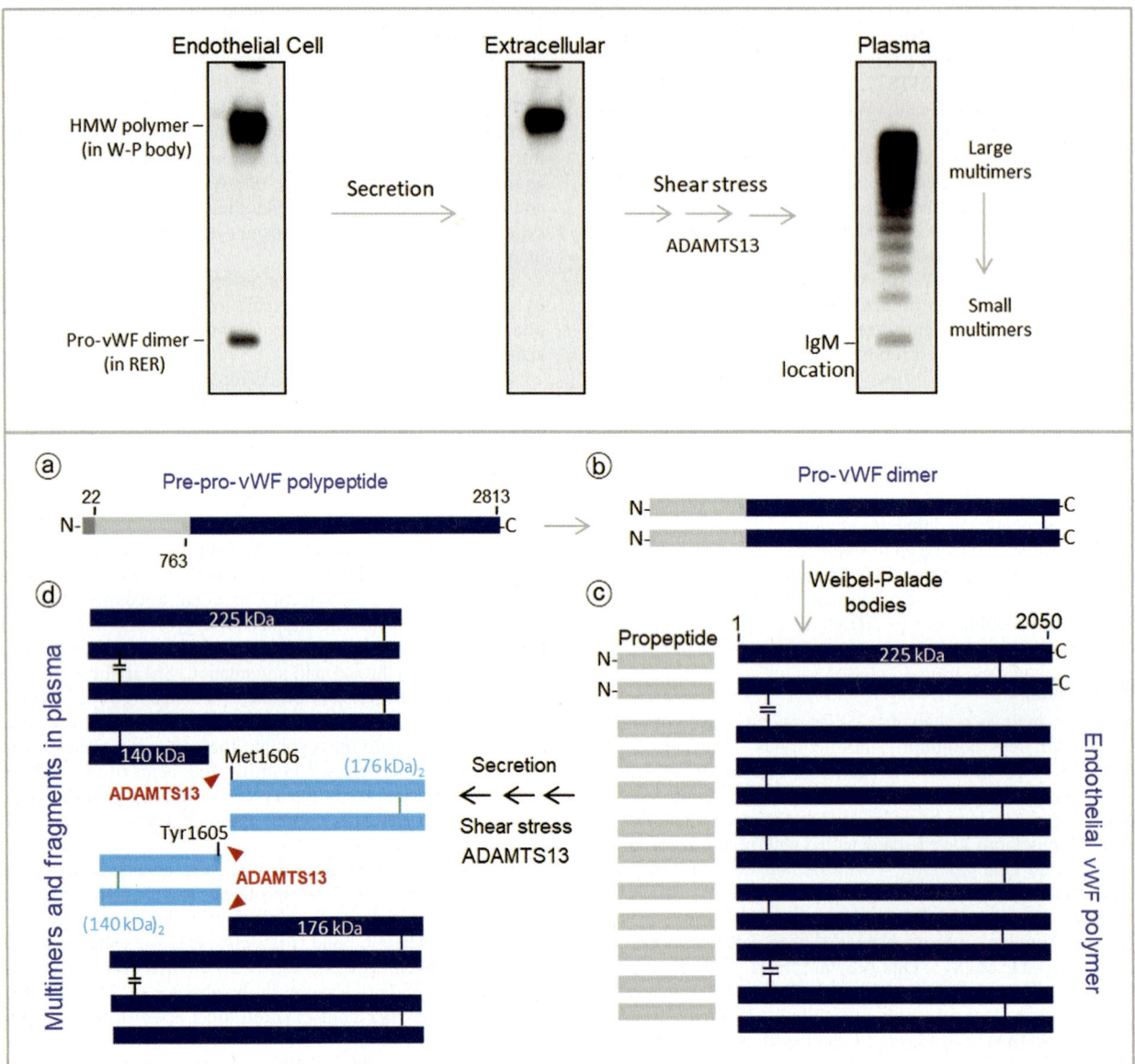

FIGURE 49.4 ADAMTS13 and the generation of vWF multimers. Upper panel: Molecular forms of vWF in endothelial cells and plasma as analyzed with SDS-agarose gel electrophoresis and visualized with radiolabeled antibodies to vWF. In vascular endothelial cells, vWF exists in two forms, a dimer of pro-vWF polypeptide in the RER and a polymer of mature vWF polypeptide in the Weibel-Palade (W-P) body. Only the vWF polymer is secreted. Under the high-shear stress conditions of arterioles, the vWF polymer is cleaved by ADAMTS13, repeated at each cycle of transit, to become a series of multimers in normal plasma. Lower panel: a schematic depiction of vWF biosynthesis and proteolysis. A, Newly synthesized pre-pro-vWF. B, In the RER, dimers of pro-vWF are formed via disulfide bonding near the C-terminus. C, In Weibel-Palade bodies, a vWF polymer is formed through disulfide bonding near the N-terminus of vWF dimers while the propeptide is cleaved. D, Upon secretion from endothelial cells and exposure to high levels of shear stress, the vWF polymer is repeatedly cleaved by ADAMTS13 at the Tyr1605-Met1606 bond, generating a series of multimers. Dimers of the 140 and 176 kDa fragments (in light blue) are the smallest forms detectable in normal plasma. ADAMTS13, A Disintegrin And Metalloprotease with ThromboSpondin type 1 repeats, member 13; HMW, high-molecular-weight; Ig, immunoglobulin; RER, rough endoplasmic reticulum; SDS, sodium dodecyl sulfate; vWF, von Willebrand factor.

in vWF-platelet aggregation and microvascular thrombosis (*Figure 49.5C*). This explains why severe deficiency of ADAMTS13 can lead to arteriolar thrombosis characteristic of TTP.

Serial investigations of patients with TTP reveal that vWF-platelet aggregation and thrombosis do not occur until the plasma ADAMTS13 activity level is less than 10% of normal. On the other hand, a patient with ADAMTS13 activity less than 10% may be asymptomatic and have a normal platelet count. This is because activation of vWF requires shear stress at ~65 dynes/cm^2 or higher,[64] a level that may not be achieved in some individuals.[1] Furthermore, certain plasma components such as thrombospondin and others can modify the proteolysis of vWF by ADAMTS13 under conditions of shear stress.[65] vWF-platelet aggregation and thrombosis may be triggered in these patients by an increase in the circulatory shear stress, a change in the plasma environments, and/or a further decrease of the protease level due to inflammation or increased ADAMTS13 inhibitors.

Conformation of von Willebrand Factor and Its Interaction With ADAMTS13

The vWF polypeptide comprises a series of homologous domains. The ADAMTS13 cleavage site, Tyr1605-Met1606, of vWF is located in the A2 domain, which is sandwiched between the A1 domain that contains the epitopes interacting with platelet glycoprotein receptor Ib/IV/V and the A3 domain where a collagen binding epitope is located (*Figure 49.3*). This topographic arrangement facilitates the regulation of platelet thrombus formation because cleavage of vWF at the A2

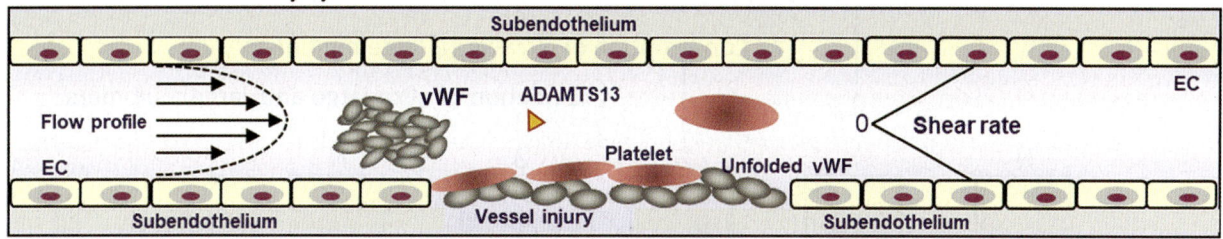

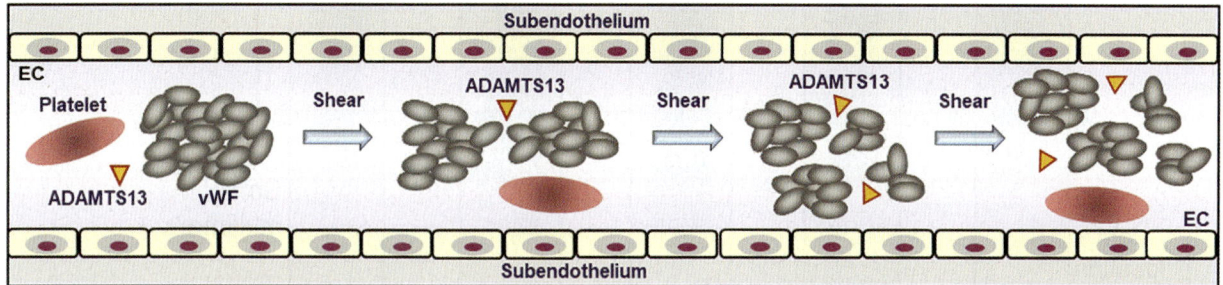

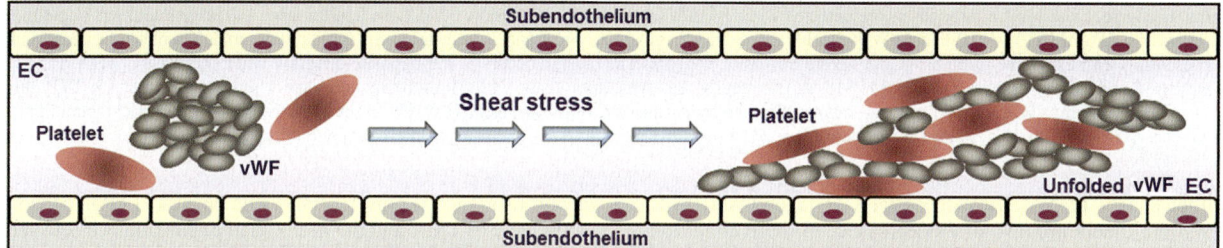

FIGURE 49.5 ADAMTS13 deficiency leads to vWF-platelet aggregation and thrombosis in TTP. A, The responsiveness of vWF to shear stress allows it to be activated at sites of microvascular injury to support platelet adhesion and aggregation. B, In the circulation, activation of vWF and platelet thrombosis is prevented by ADAMTS13, which cleaves vWF whenever its cleavage sites are exposed by shear stress. This process, repeated with each cycle of transit through the arteriolar microcirculation, maintains vWF in its compact, inactive configuration while its size progressively becomes smaller. C, In the absence of ADAMTS13, vWF is relentlessly activated by shear stress, leading to vWF activation, vWF-platelet aggregation, and microvascular thrombosis of TTP. Thrombosis increases the shear stress in the microcirculation, leading to further cycles of vWF-platelet aggregation. ADAMTS13, A Disintegrin And Metalloprotease with ThromboSpondin type 1 repeats, member 13; TTP, thrombotic thrombocytopenic purpura; vWF, von Willebrand factor. (Reprinted by permission from Springer: Tsai HM. Acquired thrombotic thrombocytopenic purpura. In: Rodgers G. ed. *ADAMTS13: Biology and Disease*. Springer; 2015:91-128. Copyright © 2015 Springer International Publishing Switzerland.)

domain disengages the platelet from the vessel wall. Structural analysis confirms that shear stress induces vWF cleavage by altering the conformation of vWF.[64,66] Narrow-angle neutron scattering studies of vWF in guanidine hydrochloride, which also promotes vWF cleavage by ADAMTS13,[67] or after exposure to shear stress, show that conformational change at the subdomain level is sufficient for proteolysis to occur.[68,69] Unfolding of vWF to extended configurations at the multimeric level as depicted in *Figure 49.5* is not necessary for proteolysis.

Alteration of von Willebrand Factor Multimers in TTP

The involvement of vWF in the pathophysiology of TTP was first suggested by the discovery that ultra-large multimers were present in plasma samples from patients with chronic relapsing TTP (a clinical phenotype of hTTP) during remission.[70] Infusion of normal plasma decreased the largest multimers, suggesting a vWF "depolymerase" is missing in the plasma of chronic relapsing TTP. It was postulated that vWF-platelet thrombosis occurs in chronic relapsing TTP because the ultra-large vWF multimers are hyperactive. However, this scheme does not explain why ultra-large multimers are detected during remission while both ultra-large and normal multimers are often missing when the patients present with profound thrombocytopenia (*Figure 49.6*, lane 3).

The complexity of vWF multimer changes in TTP reflects two opposite dynamic processes in patients with ADAMTS13 deficiency. On the one hand, ADAMTS13 deficiency leads to the appearance of ultra-large multimers because there is less proteolysis. On the other hand, the activation of vWF by shear stress leads to the consumption and depletion of vWF, which begins with the largest forms because their larger sizes make them more responsive to shear stress.

As a consequence, three types of abnormal vWF multimeric patterns are observed in TTP. A shift of vWF to ultra-large forms is detectable when ADAMTS13 activity is <20% to 30% (the sensitivity of detection depends on the agarose gel concentration); at this stage, no platelet thrombosis occurs (*Figure 49.6*, lane 1). The ultra-large and large multimers are partially depleted when ADAMTS13 is <10% and vWF-platelet aggregation begins to occur (*Figure 49.6*, lane 2). The ultra-large multimers are depleted and the large multimers are further decreased in patients presenting with extensive thrombosis and severe thrombocytopenia (*Figure 49.6*, lane 3).

Each vWF multimeric pattern in TTP represents a snapshot of the balance of two processes acting in opposite directions. Transition from one multimer pattern to another occurs during the course of the disease, reflecting the balance between diminished vWF proteolysis and increased vWF-platelet aggregation.

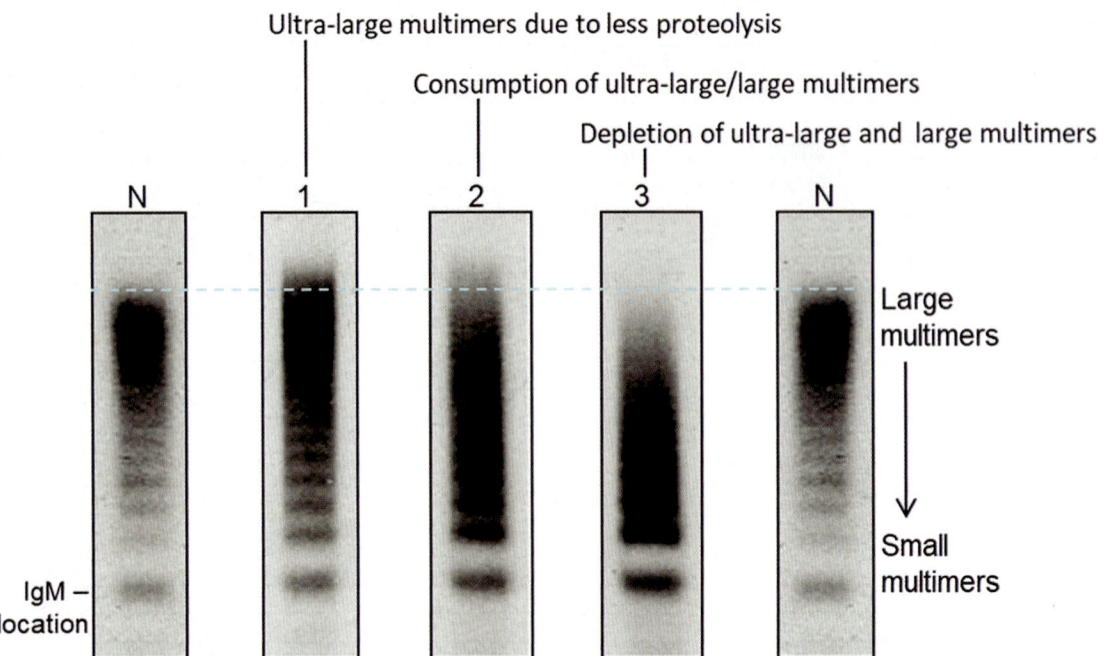

FIGURE 49.6 vWF multimers in TTP. The change of the plasma vWF multimer profile is dynamic in TTP, reflecting the consequences of ADAMTS13 deficiency, which shifts vWF to larger sizes, and vWF-platelet thrombosis, which consumes largest forms of vWF. Three types of vWF abnormalities can be detected in TTP during its course. Lane 1, ultra-large forms are detected when ADAMTS13 activity is <20% to 30%. Lane 2, ultra-large and large multimers begin to decrease from the top when ADAMTS13 is <10% and vWF-platelet aggregation begins to occur. Lane 3, ultra-large and large multimers are depleted or decreased in TTP patients presenting with extensive thrombosis and severe thrombocytopenia. The change occurs in the opposite direction when the plasma ADAMTS13 activity level is increased with plasma exchange. ADAMTS13, A Disintegrin And Metalloprotease with ThromboSpondin type 1 repeats, member 13; TTP, thrombotic thrombocytopenic purpura; vWF, von Willebrand factor. (Adapted by permission from Springer: Tsai HM. Acquired thrombotic thrombocytopenic purpura. In: Rodgers G. eds. *ADAMTS13: Biology and Disease*. Springer; 2015:91-128. Copyright © 2015 Springer International Publishing Switzerland.)

In other causes of MAHA such as STX-HUS and AHUS, the large vWF multimers are also often decreased. In these conditions, the decrease in large multimers is due to excessive cleavage of vWF by ADAMTS13 under conditions of abnormal shear stress created by arteriolar stenosis or thrombosis.[5] Ultra-large multimers are not seen in these causes of MAHA because it is uncommon that the plasma ADAMTS13 activity is below 20% to 30%.

Ultra-large multimers may appear in conditions without ADAMTS13 deficiency, as are observed following infusion of desmopressin.[71] Desmopressin infusion does not decrease the plasma ADAMTS13 activity, nor does it grossly affect the shear stress profile in the circulation. It is assumed that ultra-large multimers appear because desmopressin increases secretion of vWF from endothelial cells in vasculature with lower levels of shear stress and hence are less proteolyzed by ADAMTS13.

Distinction Between TTP the Disease and Its Complications

The new pathogenetic definition of TTP allows the diagnosis of the disease in patients without symptoms, MAHA and/or thrombocytopenia. An individual with autoimmune inhibitors or genetic mutations of ADAMTS13 is considered to have the disease of TTP even when the person is completely asymptomatic and has no MAHA or thrombocytopenia. Such an asymptomatic individual is at risk of developing vWF-platelet thrombosis, thrombocytopenia, MAHA, and organ dysfunctions, either spontaneously or upon exposure to triggering conditions such as infection, vaccination, inflammation, intravenous radio-contrast agents, surgery, trauma, or pregnancy. These patients require management of their TTP disease to prevent its complications.

Clinical Features

The incidence of TTP is estimated to be 1.74 to 14.5 cases per 10^6 population annually.[72,73] The broad range of the observed incidence rates likely reflects differences in study design, diagnostic criteria, demographics, and most importantly, the prevalence rate of HIV infection in the population. Incidence rate estimates based on databases of health insurance claims are unreliable because TTP is coded nondescriptively as TMA and the health plan population is a selected group of the population in general.

Acquired TTP primarily affects adolescents and adults, with median and mode ages between 30 and 40 years, although it may occasionally affect children <10 years of age. In most clinical series, the female-to-male ratio is 2 to 3:1 or higher. Among patients with HIV infection, there is no apparent gender imbalance.[72]

In a typical case, the course of acquired TTP begins with the appearance of ADAMTS13 inhibitory antibodies, which progressively decrease the plasma ADAMTS13 activity level. Ultra-large multimers are detected when the ADAMTS13 activity is below 20% to 30%. Thrombosis may begin to occur when ADAMTS13 is less than 10% of normal, eventually leading to thrombocytopenia, MAHA, and dysfunction of the brain and other organs (*Figure 49.7*).

Serial monitoring of patients with a history of acquired TTP suggests that the plasma ADAMTS13 activity level may trend downward, with some fluctuation, for weeks to months before decreasing to less than 10% of normal and causing thrombosis. Initially, microvascular thrombosis occurs without thrombocytopenia and MAHA, although it may cause vague, ill-defined symptoms. Occasionally, it may present as transient ischemic attack or stroke if thrombosis happens to affect a vital area of the brain. Thrombocytopenia is detected when thrombosis is widespread and platelet consumption exceeds compensatory platelet production.

The state of thrombocytopenia without overt hemolytic anemia may last for days to months. Such patients may be incorrectly given the diagnosis of immune thrombocytopenic purpura. The course of TTP at this stage is not invariably downhill; some patients may spontaneously revert to a normal platelet count.

MAHA is apparent when abnormal shear stress due to arteriolar thrombosis is sufficient to cause fragmentation of the red blood cells. Confusion and seizures typically present later, when microvascular thrombosis is widespread in the brain, accompanied with evident thrombocytopenia and MAHA.

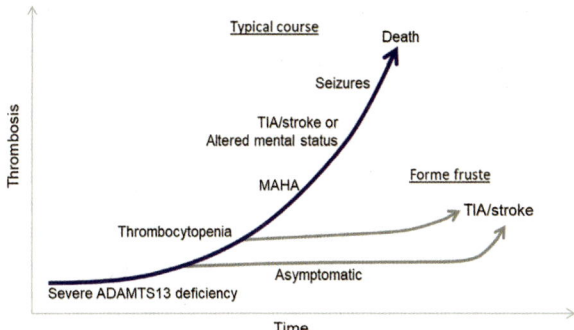

FIGURE 49.7 Typical and atypical presentations of TTP. As the inhibitor level increases and ADAMTS13 level decreases, von Willebrand factor (vWF)-platelet thrombosis may begin to occur when the ADAMTS13 activity level decreases below the threshold of 10%. In a typical course, TTP evolves progressively from asymptomatic thrombocytopenia to MAHA, fleeting neurologic deficits, stroke, altered mental status, seizures, and death if it is not treated. Other ischemic complications such as myocardial injury or infarction and abdominal pain due to pancreatitis or intestinal ischemia may also occur. Occasionally, a patient may be encountered at the stage of thrombocytopenia when a complete blood count is ordered for other reasons and is mistakenly given the diagnosis of idiopathic thrombocytopenic purpura. TTP may also present atypically, with stroke or myocardial infarction presenting before thrombocytopenia or MAHA ensues. ADAMTS13, A Disintegrin And Metalloprotease with ThromboSpondin type 1 repeats, member 13; MAHA, microangiopathic hemolytic anemia; TTP, thrombotic thrombocytopenic purpura.

Many of the patients have no apparent antecedent illness before noticing ill-defined symptoms such as dizziness and fatigue that are often considered inconsequential or "viral infection," until more alarming complications such as petechiae, pallor, profound fatigue, focal neurologic deficits, syncope, confusion, and/or seizures ensue. Less frequently, a patient may present with abdominal pain, anorexia, nausea, or vomiting, with or without pancreatitis, chest pain from myocardial ischemia or infarction, and even sudden death.

Hematuria is a frequent finding. However, overt renal failure causing oliguria, anuria, fluid retention, electrolyte abnormalities, and/or uremia is uncommon in acquired TTP. The serum creatinine level only increases minimally. When overt renal failure occurs in a patient with acquired TTP, it should prompt a search for a separate cause.

Some patients present with complications of TTP after exposure to conditions such as fever, infection, vaccination, inflammation, intravenous radio-contrast agents, surgery, trauma, and pregnancy, giving rise to the appearance that these conditions cause TTP. In fact, these conditions merely trigger the development of vWF-platelet thrombosis in patients with preexisting and subclinical ADAMTS13 deficiency.

Mechanistically, vWF-platelet thrombosis may be triggered in patients with TTP via an increase in the shear stress profile in the circulation, which is determined by cardiac output, blood pressure, and heart rate; further decrease of an already low plasma ADAMTS13 level to below the threshold level necessary to prevent vWF activation; an increase in platelet reactivity; and/or an increase of vWF secretion from vascular endothelial cells. Changes in the levels of thrombospondin[65] and other plasma components may also affect the proteolysis of vWF by ADAMTS13 under conditions of shear stress.

Diagnosis of Thrombotic Thrombocytopenic Purpura

The diagnosis of TTP proceeds in three steps: the possible diagnosis of TTP is raised, the diagnosis of TTP is confirmed, and acquired TTP is distinguished from hTTP (Table 49.3).

TTP is most commonly suspected in patients presenting with the diad of MAHA and thrombocytopenia. The diagnosis should also be suspected in patients presenting with unexplained thrombocytopenia, especially if there is a history of TTP, symptoms or signs of brain or myocardial ischemia; and in patients presenting with brain or heart ischemia without common risk factors of cardiovascular disease.

ADAMTS13 Tests

The diagnosis of TTP requires confirmation with ADAMTS13 tests. The tests include ADAMTS13 activity and ADAMTS13 inhibitors. Some laboratories may also perform enzyme-linked immunosorbent assay (ELISA) for ADAMTS13 antibodies. The ELISA tests may yield 5% to 10% falsely positive results unless special steps are included to eliminate false positivity.

ADAMTS13 antigen test is generally unnecessary and unhelpful for the diagnosis of TTP. Preferably, blood samples for ADAMTS13 tests are obtained before any transfusion of blood products, when the platelet count is low and not rising, or is normal but decreasing.

Table 49.3. Thrombotic Thrombocytopenic Purpura (TTP): Principles of Diagnosis

When TTP should be suspected:
• Microangiopathic hemolytic anemia (MAHA) and thrombocytopenia
• Thrombocytopenia and a history of TTP
• Thrombocytopenia of unknown etiology, especially if associated with
• Unusual symptoms (headache, confusion)
• Fleeting ischemia, stroke or myocardial Infarction
• Fleeting neurologic deficits, stroke or myocardial infarction, with no common risk factors
Confirming the diagnosis of TTP: Plasma ADAMTS13 activity assay is essential
• Do the test preferably when platelet count is low and not rising, or normal but decreasing
• ADAMTS13 activity <10%: Diagnostic of TTP
• ADAMTS13 > 10%:
• Platelet count is low and not rising, or normal but decreasing: TTP is excluded as the cause of the thrombocytopenia
• Platelet count is normal, or low but rising: TTP is not excluded
• Repeat the test when the platelet count is decreasing or low and not rising
Distinction between acquired and hereditary TTP
• Acquired TTP: Positive inhibitors of ADAMTS13
• A negative inhibitor test does not exclude acquired TTP
• A positive ADAMTS13 antibody is unreliable for diagnosis of acquired TTP[a]
• ADAMTS13 increase is less than expected after plasma exchange or infusion
• ADAMTS13 increased to >10% during remission without plasma therapy
• Hereditary TTP: Negative inhibitor tests and
• Presentation during infancy with no HIV infection
• Increase and decrease of ADAMTS13 activity as expected after plasma infusion or exchange
• Partial or severe ADAMTS13 deficiency in parents and/or children

Abbreviation: ADAMTS13, A Disintegrin And Metalloprotease with ThromboSpondin type 1 motif, member 13.
[a]Unless the test is run with a proper control to exclude antibodies of the ELISA components.

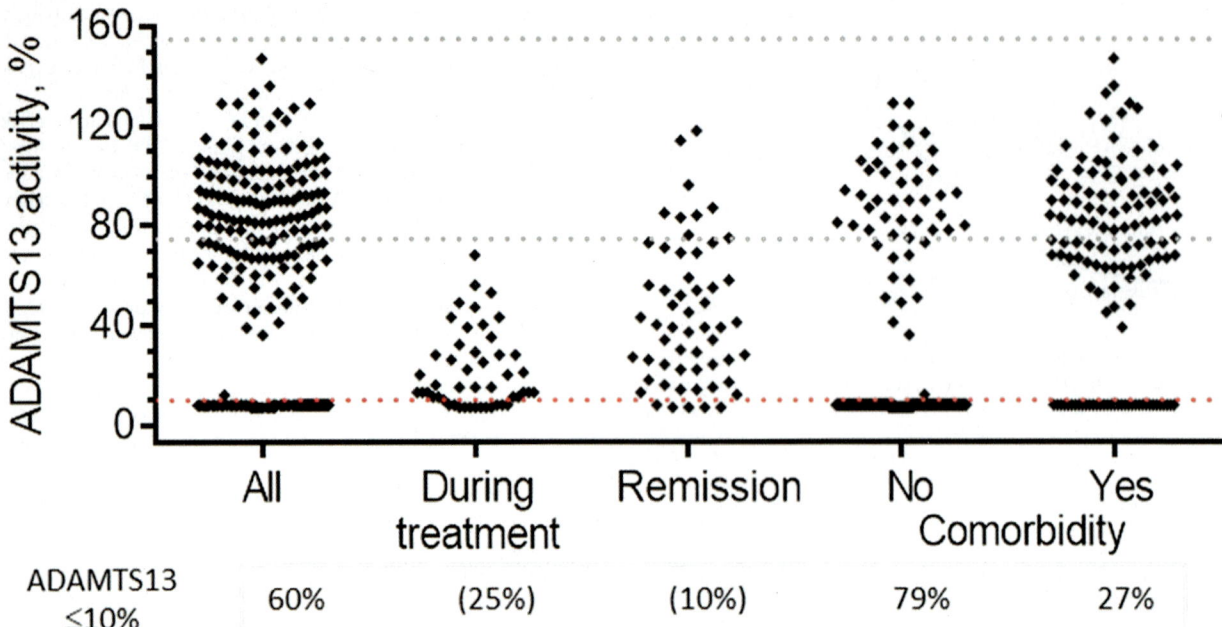

FIGURE 49.8 **The ADAMTS13 activity level distinguishes TTP from other causes of MAHA and thrombocytopenia.** Patients (365 cases) investigated for thrombocytopenia and MAHA segregate in two nonoverlapping groups based on their plasma ADAMTS13 activity levels. Severe ADAMTS13 deficiency (<10% of normal, 11% in one) is detected in 219 patients (60%) of the entire group, 184 cases (79%) of the subgroup of 234 patients without comorbidity, and only 35 (27%) of the subgroup of 131 patients with comorbid conditions such as recent intravenous radiocontrast media, surgery, pancreatitis, HIV infection, drugs, lupus, lupus anticoagulants, or other autoimmune disorders ($P < .001$ by Chi-square test). ADAMTS13 activity remains less than 10% in 25% of the samples obtained after receiving plasma or blood transfusion and in 9% of the samples obtained during remission. In samples, the ADAMTS13 level is less than 20% (mean − 3 standard deviations of the non-TTP group) and is, therefore, likely diagnostic of TTP in 36% and 22% of the cases, respectively. Because the study includes many referral cases and subgroup analysis, the actual percentages may differ in practice. The two upper dotted lines encompass the normal range of plasma ADAMTS13 activity for the assay used. The lowest line indicates the 10% threshold for active thrombosis. ADAMTS13, A Disintegrin And Metalloprotease with ThromboSpondin type 1 repeats, member 13; MAHA, microangiopathic hemolytic anemia; TTP, thrombotic thrombocytopenic purpura.

A plasma ADAMTS13 activity <10% of normal is diagnostic of TTP (*Figure 49.8*). Occasionally, faulty sample handling or laboratory technical mishaps may yield falsely low results. ADAMTS13 activity >10% does not exclude the diagnosis of TTP if the blood sample is obtained when the platelet count is low but rising, or stable in the normal range (*Table 49.3*).

Once the diagnosis of TTP is confirmed, the next step is to distinguish between acquired TTP and hTTP. A positive ADAMTS13 inhibitor test indicates that the patient has acquired TTP. However, a negative test result does not exclude the diagnosis of acquired TTP because the test is only positive in 80% to 90% among those presenting with acute symptoms.

ADAMTS13 antibody test by ELISA is more sensitive, yielding positive results in more than 90% to 95% of the cases. Nevertheless, a positive ADAMTS13 antibody ELISA test result is not diagnostic of acquired TTP unless an appropriate control is performed in the laboratory to exclude false-positive reactions caused by Abs against the components used in the ELISA test.

For patients with negative ADAMTS13 inhibitor tests, the distinction between acquired and hTTP is not straightforward. A patient is likely to have acquired TTP if the magnitude of ADAMTS13 activity increases is less than expected after plasma infusion or exchange, or the plasma ADAMTS13 activity is >10% during remission without plasma therapy.

On the other hand, the patient is likely to have hTTP if the disease presents during the neonatal period in the absence of HIV infection; the parents and/or children are partially or severely deficient in ADAMTS13 activity; or the ADAMTS13 level increases and decreases as expected after plasma infusion or exchange (e.g., 7.5 mL/kg fresh-frozen plasma for an individual with plasma volume of 45 mL/kg is expected to raise the ADAMTS13 by 14%, with a half-life of 1-3 days). Detection of homozygous or compound heterozygous pathogenic mutations of the ADAMTS13 gene supports the diagnosis of hTTP. Nevertheless, detected novel variants are often of uncertain significance without time-consuming expression studies.

Other Laboratory Findings

Common laboratory findings include thrombocytopenia; hemolysis with increased reticulocytes, lactate dehydrogenase (LDH), and indirect bilirubin; undetectable or decreased haptoglobin; and the presence of schistocytes on blood smear. "Schistocyte"-like cells may be seen in severe megaloblastic anemia, myelodysplastic syndrome with or without HIV infection, and hereditary pyropoikilocytosis.

Hematuria and proteinuria reflect renal glomerular thrombosis. The increase in the creatinine level is minimal in most cases. This is consistent with the pathologic findings that the kidney is focally affected and its architecture is well preserved in TTP patients at autopsy.

Overt renal failure causing hypertension, fluid retention, electrolyte derangement, oliguria, or anuria only occurs when there is a concurrent renal disease. On the other hand, acute and chronic renal failure may occur in patients with hTTP.[74]

Imaging studies such as computed tomography (CT) or magnetic resonance imaging (MRI) are often requested for neurologic dysfunction. In most cases, the studies yield negative results or only reveal subtle ischemic changes.

Occasionally, a TTP patient may present with macrovascular ischemic strokes detectable by conventional imaging studies. It is speculated that in such cases, the macrovascular thrombosis results from vessel wall injury of a large artery due to thrombosis in its vasa vasorum.

The literature includes reports of "TTP" case series with a high percentage showing abnormal CT or MRI findings. However, a review of these cases reveals that most of these patients likely had STX-HUS or AHUS rather than TTP.

Abnormal electrocardiograms with nonspecific ST-T wave changes and elevated creatinine phosphokinase or troponin levels are common. As in strokes, thrombosis may affect a large coronary artery, leading to myocardial infarctions. Cardiac arrhythmia is uncommon. Electromechanical dissociation, heart failure with elevated BNP (NT-ProBNP) with or without decreased ejection fraction, or pulmonary infiltrates or hemorrhage occur in advanced, preterminal cases.

The amylase and lipase levels may be elevated. Abnormal liver function is rare. Abdominal CT scans may detect focal pancreatitis, intestinal wall, or mesenteric stranding due to ischemia or infarction.

Differential Diagnosis

Although the diagnosis of TTP depends on the demonstration of severe ADAMTS13 deficiency, it is essential to exclude other causes of MAHA and thrombocytopenia listed in *Table 49.1*, as TTP may coexist with STX-HUS, AHUS, or other conditions.[75-77] Such dual diagnosis would not have been possible using the old syndrome-based scheme of disease classification.

A complete history and physical examination should be supplemented with appropriate laboratory tests such as stool cultures, ELISA, or polymerase chain reaction (PCR) tests for Shiga toxins in the stool; blood or viral cultures or PCR analysis for pneumococcal or other bacterial or viral infections if clinically warranted; autoimmune serology tests for lupus, scleroderma, antiphospholipid antibodies, and related autoimmune disorders; coagulation profile such as prothrombin time, activated partial thromboplastin time, fibrinogen, D-dimer, and additional clotting factor assays as needed for disseminated intravascular coagulopathy; MRI with T2-FLAIR for mental status changes; CT scan or other imaging studies and tissue biopsies for metastatic neoplasm; platelet factor 4/heparin Abs and serotonin-release assay for patients being treated with heparin; and flow cytometry for paroxysmal nocturnal hemoglobinuria (PNH).

Importantly, advanced renal failure, hypertension, and complications of abnormal vascular permeability such as brain edema, pleural or pericardial effusions, pulmonary edema, acute respiratory distress syndrome, ascites, and anasarca are uncommon in TTP. Any of these complications in a patient with the diagnosis should prompt the consideration of other disorders.

Scoring systems have been developed to assist the diagnosis of TTP and determination of its prognosis.[78-80] These scoring systems were developed and validated primarily by analysis of patients who were referred for plasma exchange for suspected TTP. Few patients presenting atypically were included in the development or validation of the scores. Furthermore, TTP patients with comorbidities are likely to have features that affect their scores.

In practice, the performance of the scoring systems is often less than desirable, especially for incipient cases and patients with comorbidities or more than one cause of MAHA and thrombocytopenia (e.g., TTP presenting with thrombocytopenia only, with thrombocytopenia and stroke or myocardial infarction, with liver disease and high INR (international normalized ratio) or MCV (mean corpuscular volume), with renal failure due to another condition, or after hematopoietic stem cell therapy; TTP and active cancer; TTP and AHUS; and TTP and STX-HUS).

Management and Prognosis

Historically, the goal of TTP management focused on induction of clinical remission, using the platelet count as a surrogate parameter to objectively follow its activity. Among the various empiric treatment modalities, plasma exchange was the most effective, leading to remission in ~80% to 90% of the cases. However, the remaining 10% to 20% of the cases are either refractory to the treatment and succumb to the disease, or cannot be weaned off the treatment. A small fraction of the cases die due to delay in diagnosis and treatment, complications of the treatment, or an unrelated comorbidity. With more patients surviving the initial episode, it is increasingly recognized that relapse is a common problem (*Figure 49.9*, upper panel).

With the discovery of ADAMTS13 autoimmunity as its pathogenetic mechanism, it is now possible to manage acquired TTP more rationally by focusing on three pathogenetic targets: severe ADAMTS13 deficiency, vWF-platelet aggregation and thrombosis, and autoimmune inhibitors of ADAMTS13 (*Table 49.4*). The goals of treatment not only should include remission but also prevention of relapse. The current principles of managing acquired TTP are depicted in *Table 49.5*.

Plasma Therapy

Before plasma exchange or infusion was introduced in the 1970s,[81,82] more than 90% of patients died after presenting with symptomatic acquired TTP. With plasma exchange or plasma infusion, a mortality rate of 10% to 20% and 40% to 50% is expected, respectively.[83]

Plasma exchange is typically performed daily at 1 to 1.5 total plasma volumes until the platelet count is normal in at least two consecutive tests and then gradually tapered to ensure the platelet count is stable before the therapy is discontinued. It is believed that plasma exchange therapy replenishes the deficient ADAMTS13. Removal of antibodies may be contributory to its therapeutic effect.

Plasma infusion has the advantage that it does not require a large venous catheter and special equipment and can be started quickly. Its efficacy is limited by fluid overload. For acquired TTP, plasma infusion is used primarily as an emergent substitute until plasma exchange is instituted.

Cryoprecipitate-depleted plasma has been advocated as a more effective alternative of fresh-frozen plasma because it lacks large vWF multimers. However, fresh-frozen plasma and cryoprecipitate-depleted plasma are not different in their ADAMTS13 activity levels. In fact, two small randomized controlled trials have failed to demonstrate superiority of cryoprecipitate-depleted plasma as the replacement fluid.

Serial analysis shows that the plasma ADAMTS13 activity level often fluctuates in the first several weeks before it gradually stabilizes to a steady-state level. This explains why the response to plasma therapy may be unsteady for weeks to months and why it is important to closely monitor the blood cell counts when and after plasma exchange therapy is tapered.

ADAMTS13 levels persistently less than 10% of normal at the end of plasma therapy indicate a high risk of early relapse. On the other hand, a measurable ADAMTS13 level at the end of plasma therapy does not preclude the possibility of relapse. Serial platelet counts and ADAMTS13 activity level are essential for early detection of relapses.

Remission has been reported in patients with chronic or subacute courses and some Jehovah witness patients without using fresh-frozen plasma.[84,85] With newly available treatment modalities, it is anticipated that more patients may achieve remission without plasma exchange.

Immunosuppressive Therapy

Acquired TTP is an autoimmune disease that seldom goes away. Plasma therapy does not address the autoimmune nature of the disease nor does it prevent its relapse.

Patients with acquired TTP are able to achieve sustained remission primarily because the intensity of autoimmunity spontaneously alleviates, allowing the recovery of the ADAMTS13 activity above the threshold level. However, the plasma ADAMTS13 level remains decreased in many patients during remission (*Figure 49.8*). Relapses may occur later even in those whose ADAMTS13 level reaches the normal range. Overall, nearly 90% of the patients will experience at least one relapse in 7 years (*Figure 49.9*, upper panel). Some patients develop repeated relapses or refractory disease after years of quiescence.

For patients who cannot be weaned off plasma exchange as a result of persistent ADAMTS13 deficiency, depletion of B cells with rituximab, a chimeric monoclonal antibody to CD20, induces clinical remission in approximately 75% to 90% of the patients.[86-89] Rituximab increases the ADAMTS13 level by suppressing the ADAMTS13 inhibitors. A small increase in the ADAMTS13 activity level above 10% is sufficient to induce clinical remission, allowing the patient to be weaned off plasma therapy. Rituximab is less effective in patients with high ADAMTS13 inhibitor levels.

Early rituximab may decrease the risk of immediate relapse in patients with severe ADAMTS13 deficiency.[84,90-92] Rituximab may also be used preemptively to avert relapses in patients exhibiting a trend of declining ADAMTS13 activity levels during remission.[93]

Among patients treated for relapsing TTP, the efficacy of rituximab lasts for several months to a few years, with median remission duration of approximately 2.5 years (*Figure 49.9*, lower panel).

Patients with acquired TTP should have their plasma ADAMTS13 activity monitored monthly during remission. Rituximab retreatment when their plasma ADAMTS13 activity begins to show a steady trend of decline toward 20% to 40% may reverse the downward trend before

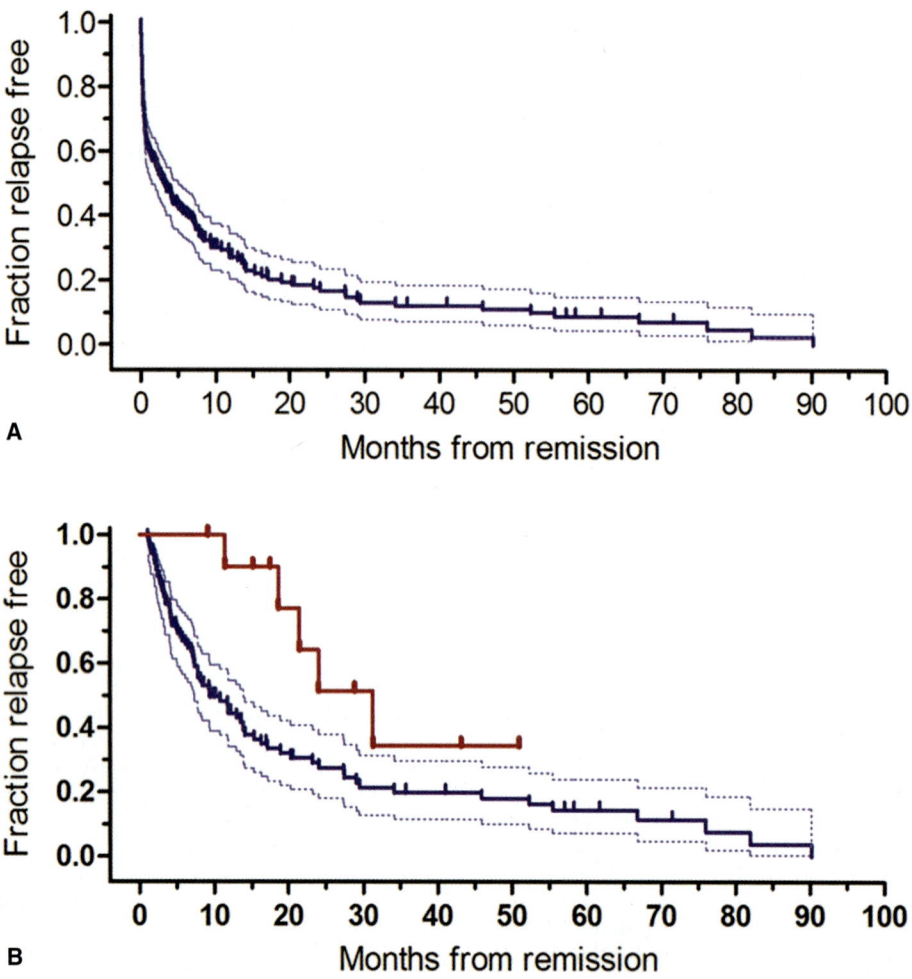

FIGURE 49.9 Relapse-free survival after plasma exchange for an acute episode of TTP, with or without rituximab treatment. A, Relapse-free survival after 182 episodes of acquired TTP. Remission is defined as two consecutive normal platelet counts. HIV-infected patients accounted for nine of the episodes. Only three of the censored events were death. Relapses occurring after rituximab therapy are excluded for this analysis. The median duration of relapse-free survival is only 3.2 months. B, Comparison of relapse-free survival of 11 cases who were treated with rituximab with those of 105 cases who were not treated with rituximab. To account for the delay in the effect of rituximab, only relapses occurring at least 4 weeks after remission are included in this analysis. Rituximab increases the median duration of relapse-free survival from 9.4 to 31.3 months; however, 65% of the patients experienced relapse by 3 years. Dashed lines encompass the 95% confidence intervals. (Reprinted by permission from Springer: Tsai HM. Acquired thrombotic thrombocytopenic purpura. In: Rodgers G. ed. *ADAMTS13: Biology and Disease*. Springer; 2015:91-128. Copyright © 2015 Springer International Publishing Switzerland.)

it further decreases to cause relapse. With such a strategy, patients can remain in remission for many years (*Figure 49.10*). The schedule of ADAMTS13 monitoring and the threshold ADAMTS13 activity level for preemptive rituximab retreatment may be modified based on the test turnaround time, with threshold set higher for slow turnarounds.

Major side effects of rituximab include allergic reactions and reactivation or exacerbation of viral infections such as hepatitis B and occasional cases of progressive multifocal leukoencephalopathy. Prophylaxis as determined by HBV infection status is essential.

Rituximab is primarily distributed intravascularly. Hence, after each total plasma exchange, its concentration decreases by ~65%.[94] No studies have examined how the removal of rituximab by plasma exchange may affect its therapeutic effects. Among patients treated with another monoclonal antibody eculizumab for AHUS, concurrent plasma exchange delays the response of the disease to the treatment.[95] Empirically, TTP patients on plasma exchange are treated with additional doses of rituximab to reach a total of eight doses or four doses after plasma exchange is discontinued.

Rituximab depletes B cells but has no effect on plasma cells, which do not express CD20. The response of acquired TTP to rituximab treatment may be delayed or inadequate if plasma cells, which may last for a long time,[96] continue to produce ADAMTS13 inhibitors.

Bortezomib, a proteasome inhibitor, may be used to deplete plasma cells in patients with no or inadequate response to rituximab.[97] However, the experience of using bortezomib for aTTP remains quite limited. The reported cases often received less than four doses of rituximab during plasma exchange and hence might have responded to additional rituximab treatments without bortezomib.

Other immunosuppressive therapies that have been used in TTP include corticosteroids, vincristine, cyclophosphamide, azathioprine, and cyclosporine. In particular, corticosteroids are often used for the autoimmune nature of TTP, presumably to augment the immunosuppressive effect of rituximab, albeit without concrete supporting evidence. Long-term corticosteroid therapy is often associated with serious side effects. The other immunosuppressive therapies are generally slow in action, less predictable in effectiveness, and/or more likely to cause serious side effects.

Splenectomy has been used for patients who are unable to wean off plasma exchange or experience frequent relapses even before the autoimmune nature of acquired TTP was discovered.[98] The efficacy of rituximab and caplacizumab and concerns of its long-term adverse effects, such as severe infections, venous thromboembolism, and possibly neoplastic diseases,[99] diminish the indication of splenectomy for acquired TTP.

Table 49.4. Therapeutic Targets and Treatment Options for TTP

Target	Treatment	Comment
ADAMTS13 deficiency	**Plasma exchange (PEx)**	aTTP: autoimmunity not addressed hTTP: only for patients intolerant of plasma volume Invasive and technically demanding
	Plasma infusion	Predictable response for hTTP Used for aTTP only before PEx is available
	rADAMTS13	In clinical trial (for hereditary TTP, NCT03393975)
ADAMTS13 autoimmunity	**Rituximab**	Highly effective in promoting remission and delaying relapse Response is neither immediate nor indefinite
	Bortezomib	As a supplement to rituximab, to deplete "long-living plasma cells" Anecdotal case reports only
	Splenectomy	Invasive, with unpredictable response Long-term adverse effects
	Corticosteroids, cyclophosphamide, azathioprine, vincristine, calcineurin inhibitors	Less effective than rituximab Risk of serious side effects after long-term use
vWF-platelet thrombosis	**Caplacizumab**	Inhibits vWF-platelet aggregation Promotes TTP remission Exacerbation, if vWF is not fully suppressed High relapse risk, if stopped before ADAMTS13 > 10% Increased risk of serious bleeding Thrombocytosis and thromboembolism Not cost-effective when used as in clinical trials
	Antiplatelet drugs (dextran, aspirin, dipyridamole, $P2Y_{12}$ receptor antagonists)	Modest suppression of vWF-platelet binding Rarely used
	N-acetylcysteine (NAC)	Large doses are needed to "depolymerize" vWF Anecdotal case reports only

Abbreviation: ADAMTS13, A Disintegrin And Metalloprotease with ThromboSpondin type 1 repeat, member 13.
Major treatment options are in bold; aTTP, acquired thrombotic thrombocytopenic purpura; hTTP, hereditary thrombotic thrombocytopenic purpura; rADAMTS13, recombinant ADAMTS13; vWF, von Willebrand factor.

Table 49.5. Principles of Managing Acquired Thrombotic Thrombocytopenic Purpura (aTTP)

Goals: To Achieve Clinical Remission and Prevent Relapse

To raise ADAMTS13 above 10%
- Plasma exchange, daily until two consecutive normal platelet counts, then taper
  - Indicated for most patients with acquired TTP presenting with acute symptoms
  - In selected patients, remission may be achieved with rituximab ± prednisone ± caplacizumab, e.g., patients with intermittent TIA, mild-moderate thrombocytopenia ± mild hemolysis, or contraindications of plasma therapy.
- Plasma infusion: only used before plasma exchange is available

- To suppress the ADAMTS13 inhibitors
  - Rituximab: promotes and prolongs the duration of clinical remission, not indefinitely
    - Before treatment: Check and monitor HBV infection status to determine the need of prophylaxis
    - Initiate rituximab treatment as soon as aTTP is confirmed
      - Eight doses during plasma exchange; or four doses after discontinuation of plasma exchange
    - Retreatment, guided by serial ADAMTS13 activity, for long-term remission (*Figure 49.10*)
  - High-dose corticosteroids: often used in conjunction with plasma exchange for aTTP
    - Efficacy is unproven with concurrent rituximab
    - Long-term use often leads to unacceptable side effects
  - Bortezomib: may supplement the effect of rituximab by depleting long-living plasma cells; not necessary for most cases

- To block vWF-platelet aggregation and thrombosis
  - Caplacizumab accelerates remission; not cost-effective when used as in the clinical trial
    - Bleeding, exacerbation during treatment, relapse, thromboembolism, and high cost
    - Bleeding and relapse:
      - Avoid in patients without ADAMTS13 confirmation
      - Check ADAMTS13 activity twice or once weekly
      - Discontinue the treatment when ADAMTS13 is stably >15%-20%
    - Exacerbation: check vWF ristocetin cofactor activity or ristocetin-induced platelet aggregation in patients with comorbidities to help ensure adequacy of vWF suppression
    - Thromboembolism:
      - Consider prophylactic anticoagulation during platelet recovery
      - Monitor D-dimer during platelet recovery; anticoagulation therapy for rising D-dimer levels

Abbreviations: ADAMTS13, A Disintegrin and Metalloprotease with ThromboSpondin type 1 repeat, member 13; TIA, transient ischemic attack; vWF, von Willebrand factor.

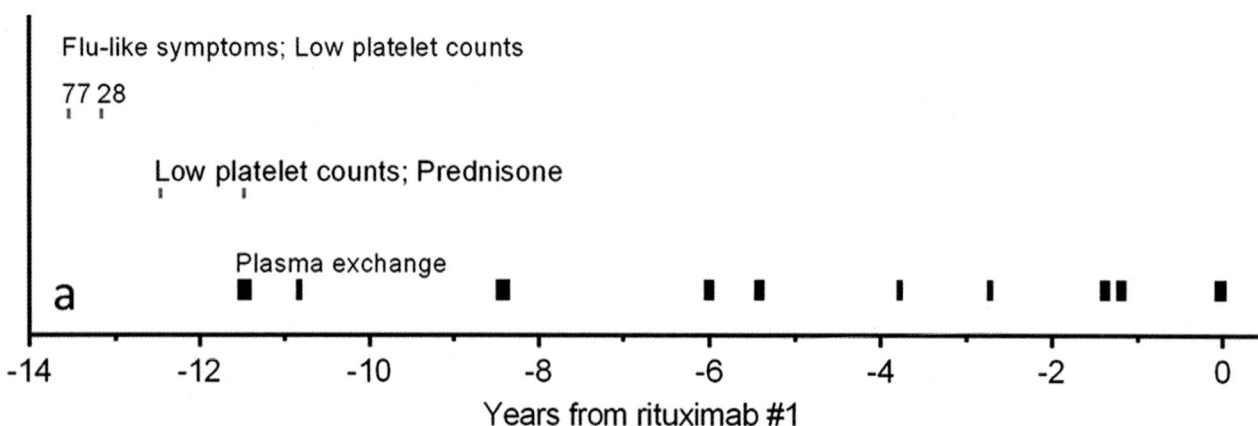
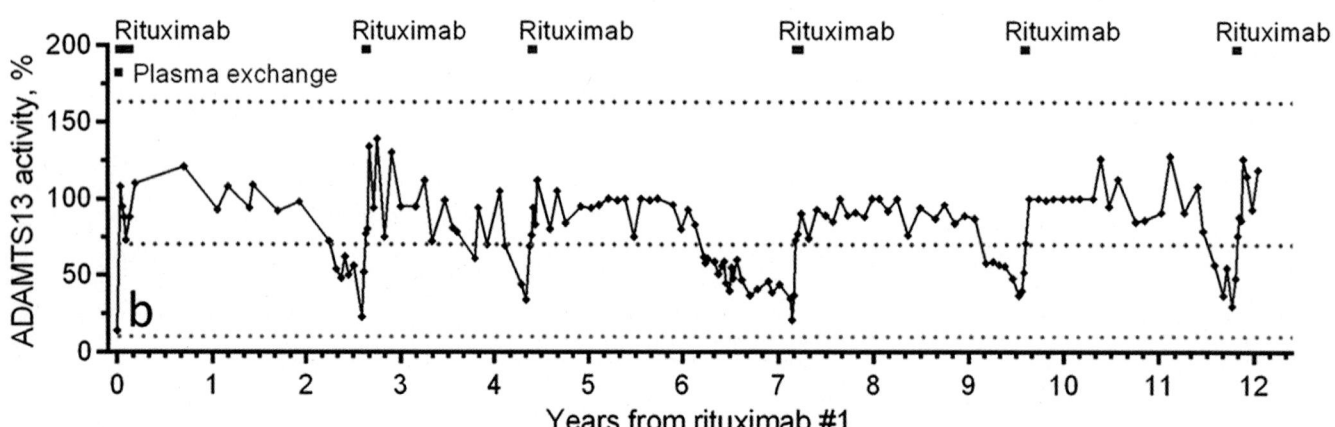
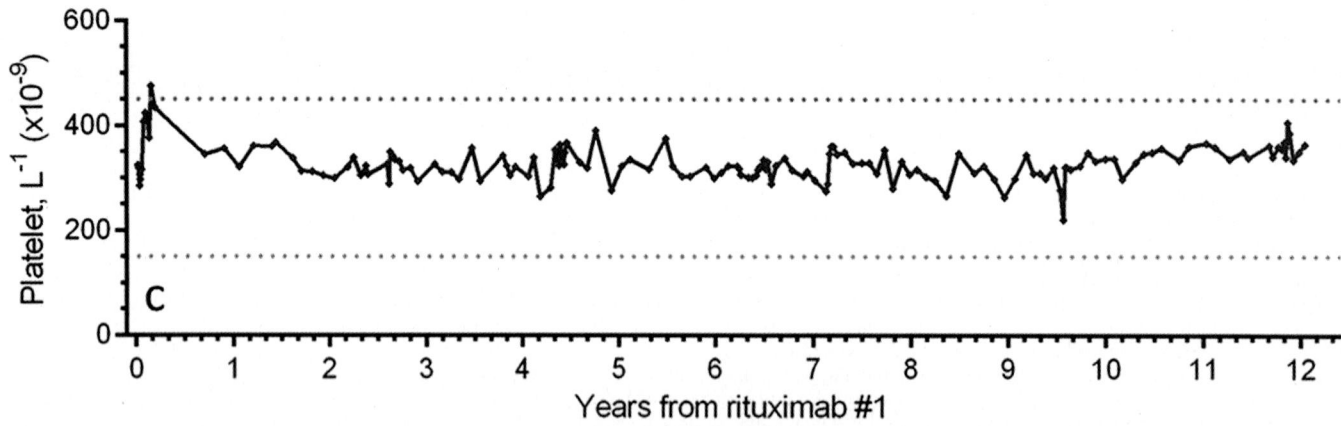

FIGURE 49.10 ADAMTS13-guided rituximab therapy prevents the relapse of TTP. This patient initially presented with thrombocytopenia and was treated as ITP with prednisone before the correct diagnosis of TTP was recognized nearly 2 years later. She required 10 courses of plasma exchange therapy for her relapses of TTP in the subsequent 11.5 years before she was treated with rituximab and started monthly ADAMTS13 testing. She required five additional courses of rituximab during this period, when the ADAMTS13 activity level trended toward 30% at intervals between 2 and 2.5 years. With this strategy, she has been in clinical and hematological remission and ongoing. ADAMTS13, A Disintegrin And Metalloprotease with ThromboSpondin type 1 repeats, member 13; TTP, thrombotic thrombocytopenic purpura; ITP, idiopathic thrombocytopenic purpura. (Reprinted by permission from Springer: Tsai HM. Acquired thrombotic thrombocytopenic purpura. In: Rodgers G. ed. *ADAMTS13: Biology and Disease.* Springer; 2015:91-128. Copyright © 2015 Springer International Publishing Switzerland.)

Caplacizumab

Caplacizumab, a humanized bivalent nanobody that blocks the vWF A1 domain from interacting with platelet receptor glycoprotein 1b-IX-V, promotes recovery and decreases the rate of exacerbation of acquired TTP during its treatment.[93] However, there is a high risk of recurrence if the treatment is discontinued before plasma ADAMTS13 activity is stably >10% of normal.

Caplacizumab treatment increases the risk of bleeding, which was serious in more than 10% of the cases in the clinical trial. Caplacizumab treatment is also associated with high risk of thromboembolism, affecting 12% of the case in one series.[100] It remains to be determined whether the high risk of thromboembolism was related to thrombocytosis (19 cases, 21%).

Caplacizumab has been found to be too costly for its benefit.[101] The unfavorable cost vs effectiveness may be improved by limiting its use only to ADAMTS13-test confirmed cases, especially those with higher risks of death, early institution of rituximab therapy in patients with no contraindications of its use to promote suppression of ADAMTS13 inhibitors, and monitoring of vWF activity in patients with comorbidity for any necessary dosage adjustment to prevent exacerbation. Monitoring of the plasma ADAMTS13 activity once to twice weekly may help ensure that caplacizumab is only used for as long as it is needed (Table 49.5), instead of following a fixed schedule. Caplacizumab treatment should be individualized and discontinued when ADAMTS13 is stably >15% to 20%. Based on the published protease data, caplacizumab use was unnecessarily prolonged in more than 30% of the patients at 2 weeks and in more than 50% of the patients at a fixed duration of 4 weeks.[100]

Other Treatment Options

Antiplatelet drugs such as dextran, aspirin, and dipyridamole were the most commonly used treatments of TTP before the era of plasma therapy. These drugs as well as $P2Y_{12}$ ADP receptor antagonists such as clopidogrel are not effective inhibitors of vWF-platelet aggregation.

N-acetylcysteine, a disulfide reducing agent primarily used for acetaminophen overdose, chronic obstructive pulmonary disease, and cystic fibrosis, has been used in some cases of refractory TTP. It is assumed that N-acetylcysteine may prevent platelet aggregation by reducing the size of vWF multimers. However, massive doses of N-acetylcysteine may be required.[102] Its efficacy at the commonly used dosage remains to be validated.

Recombinant ADAMTS13 is undergoing clinical trials for hTTP. Recombinant ADAMTS13 proteins, especially the variants that are not suppressible by inhibitors of acquired TTP,[35,38] have the potential of replacing fresh-frozen plasma therapy for acquired TTP.

Preventing Relapse and Death From TTP

Death of TTP patients may be classified into three types, with each requiring different strategies for prevention: (1) death of TTP, usually from neurologic or cardiac failure, can be early (within a week of presentation), late (beyond 1 week), or during a relapse; (2) death related to medical procedures, such as bleeding and infectious complications associated with central venous catheters; and (3) death from unrelated disorders.

A patient presenting with acquired TTP may have very advanced organ dysfunction that causes death before plasma therapy can be initiated or begins to increase the plasma ADAMTS13 activity. Prompt diagnosis and treatment are essential for minimizing early deaths. Conceivably, caplacizumab may be at its best use for such patients to prevent early deaths. However, serious bleeding may be a concern, especially if the diagnosis turns out to not be TTP. Recombinant ADAMTS13 variant proteins with deleted or mutations in the Spa domain, if available, may have the potential of preventing early deaths.

Late TTP death usually results from persistence or exacerbation of ADAMTS13 autoimmunity. Early institution of rituximab, supplemented with caplacizumab for patients with overt organ dysfunction, may help minimize the risk of such deaths.

TTP deaths at relapse are mostly caused by delay in diagnosis or treatment. Such events should be minimized by appropriate planning at the time of discharge. The platelet count should be monitored daily, with the test interval gradually increased based on the platelet counts and the results of serial ADAMTS13 activity tests, which is tested twice weekly, gradually increased to once monthly. The patients should be advised against traveling to locations where expertise in the diagnosis and treatment of TTP is not readily available.

Patients without contraindications should be treated with rituximab as early in the course as possible. The total doses should be eight during plasma exchange or four doses after discontinuation of plasma exchange. Periodic courses of rituximab therapy for downward trending of ADAMTS13 activity during remission may help reduce the risk of relapse (Figure 49.10) and TTP death.

A policy of placing central venous catheters and performing plasma exchange therapy only by specialized teams helps decrease the risk of therapy-related death in TTP patients. Attention to associated medical conditions is essential to decrease the risk of death from other causes.

ADAMTS13 Tests and the Management of TTP

ADAMTS13 activity assays are not only essential for diagnosis of TTP but also quite helpful in assisting management of plasma exchange therapy and relapse prevention (Table 49.6).

In general, vWF-platelet aggregation does not occur when ADAMTS13 activity is >10% of normal. Thus, in a patient with persistent thrombocytopenia or declining platelet counts, an ADAMTS13 activity >10% of normal precludes TTP as the cause of the low or decreasing platelet count and requires a search for other causes.

During remission, persistently low (<10%) ADAMTS13 levels connote a high risk of immediate or impending relapse. To allow a margin of safety, the threshold level of ADAMTS13 activity for initiating a course of rituximab therapy is set higher (e.g., 20%-40%, depending on the test turnaround time).

Hereditary Thrombotic Thrombocytopenic Purpura

Also known as Schulman-Upshaw syndrome or chronic relapsing TTP,[103,104] hTTP, due to homozygous or more commonly double heterozygous mutations, is rare, accounting for <1% to 5% of all TTP cases. Because the diagnosis is often not recognized in milder cases, the prevalence rate may be higher than presently appreciated.

The severity of hTTP is quite variable (Table 49.7). In severe cases, hTTP has its initial manifestations during the neonatal period, but may not be recognized until later in life.[105,106] Milder cases may present with thrombotic complications or have their disease recognized in adulthood or old age. Some women are given the diagnosis of ITP for thrombocytopenia, with the diagnosis of hTTP only suspected and confirmed during pregnancy. Some of these patients have siblings who died before birth, presumably due to hTTP complications.

In a typical severe case, the affected neonate is born with meconium stain or presents within a few hours after birth with neonatal

---

Table 49.6. ADAMTS13 Activity Level Assists the Management of TTP

- During therapy to achieve remission
  - Distinction between refractory TTP and other causes of thrombocytopenia
    - ADAMTS13 > 10%: Consider other causes of thrombocytopenia (e.g., drug- or heparin-Induced thrombocytopenia, sepsis, HIV Infection)
- During remission
  - ADAMTS13 assay at the end of plasma therapy provides a baseline for reference
    - ADAMTS13 activity <30%: rituximab therapy to increase the level above 30%
  - ADAMTS13 assay monthly, with the test interval revised as needed
    - A clear trend of decrease toward 20%-40% suggests impending relapse
    - Preemptive rituximab therapy may prevent relapse (Figure 49.10)

Abbreviations: ADAMTS13, A Disintegrin And Metalloprotease with ThromboSpondin type 1 repeats, member 13; TTP, thrombotic thrombocytopenic purpura.

Table 49.7. Clinical Features and Management of Hereditary TTP

Phenotypic severity: variable
- Thrombosis: neonatal, childhood, adulthood, or asymptomatic
- Siblings with the same genetic Mutations may Vastly Differ in Phenotypic severity
- Residual ADAMTS13 activity level is not the sole determinant of the phenotypic severity

Manifestations of thrombosis due to genetic ADAMTS13 deficiency
- Neonatal presentations are often unrecognized:
  - Stillbirth, meconium aspiration, jaundice, stroke, altered mental status, and/or seizures
  - Thrombocytopenia and MAHA are not invariably present
- Neurological abnormalities: focal deficits (stroke or TIA), altered mental status, seizures
- Renal injury is common without maintenance plasma therapy
  - Acute renal failure: at least once in ~10%; chronic renal injury: ~10%
- Other less common complications: pancreatitis, myocardial injury or infarction

Clinical course:
- Broad spectrum: frequent, intermittent, occasional, asymptomatic
- Common triggers: fever, infection, vaccination, inflammation, intravenous radiocontrast agents, surgery, trauma, pregnancy
  - Inconspicuous inflammation such as chronic cholecystitis (due to pigment gallstones of chronic subclinical hemolysis) may transform the course from an uneventful one to one with frequent episodes of thrombosis, only to be calmed down after cholecystectomy

Management
- Goals
  - Prevention of thrombocytopenia, MAHA, and acute/chronic brain, heart, kidney injury
- Acute: Fresh-frozen plasma (5-7.5 mL/kg) is effective for control of acute episodes
  - Plasma exchange is only used for patients intolerant of the plasma volume
- Long-term:
  - History of thrombosis: Fresh-frozen plasma (~7.5 mL/kg) every 2 wk
    - Adjustment based on symptoms, CBC, and renal function
  - No history of thrombosis:
    - Patients may be resistant to regular plasma infusion therapy
    - Frequent monitoring of CBC may unmask periods of subclinical thrombocytopenia and strengthen the indication for regular plasma therapy.
    - Alternative: event-directed prophylactic plasma therapy before or immediately upon exposure to triggers

Abbreviations: ADAMTS13, A Disintegrin And Metalloprotease with ThromboSpondin type 1 repeats, member 13; CBC, complete blood count; MAHA, microangiopathic hemolytic anemia; TIA, transient ischemic attack; TTP, thrombotic thrombocytopenic purpura.

distress and jaundice, with or without thrombocytopenia. Anemia may not be severe, and schistocytes on blood smears may be overlooked. Occasionally, serious complications such as seizures and reduced level of mental alertness may occur.

TTP symptoms and signs improve immediately with transfusion of whole blood, platelet concentrates, or exchange transfusion, performed unknowingly for anemia, thrombocytopenia, or hyperbilirubinemia. Because there are no inhibitors, a small amount of normal plasma is often sufficient to alleviate vWF-platelet thrombosis. Consequently, the neonates may be discharged from the hospital without a correct diagnosis, only to present with complications of the disease weeks or years later.

The variability of phenotypic severity also is observed in siblings with the same mutations and in the same individuals at different time periods of their life. The genetic basis of epistasis is mostly unknown. The factors for temporal variability usually include fever, infection, inflammation, vaccination, surgery, and pregnancy. Some of the conditions may be quite subtle, such as chronic cholecystitis with pigmented gallstones due to long-term subclinical hemolysis. Removal of the triggers such as cholecystectomy may help calm down the clinical course.

The thrombotic process may cause focal neurologic deficits, seizures, pancreatitis, or renal failure.[107,108] Among the patients not receiving maintenance plasma infusion, approximately 10% of the cases develop at least one episode of acute renal failure requiring dialysis during their course.[74] Acute renal failure is reversible if it is promptly treated with plasma infusion or exchange. Chronic renal failure occurs in approximately 10% of the patients not being regularly treated with plasma infusion, conceivably a cumulative result of subclinical ischemic injury to the kidney.

The propensity for acute and chronic renal disease in hTTP is quite different from its rarity in aTTP. It is speculated that in aTTP, local expression of ADAMTS13 in renal glomerular podocytes and endothelial cells[13] may provide protection against vWF-platelet aggregation before its activity is neutralized by inhibitors. Such protection is not present in patients with hTTP. Occasionally, renal failure may occur because the patient has concurrent AHUS.[76]

In hTTP, vWF-platelet thrombosis responds readily to infusion of fresh-frozen plasma. One infusion of fresh-frozen plasma at 7.5 mL/kg of body weight increases the plasma ADAMTS13 activity from <10% to ~14% for an individual with a plasma volume of 45 mL/kg. This is sufficient to suppress vWF-platelet thrombosis and alleviate TTP symptoms and signs for approximately 2 weeks but may need to be repeated.

Plasma exchange therapy is used only when the patients are intolerant of plasma volume. For patients allergic to fresh-frozen plasma, factor VIII concentrates that contain ADAMTS13 such as Koate-DVI (9.1 U/mL) may be used.[109]

For long-term management, patients with frequent vWF-platelet thrombosis require maintenance fresh-frozen plasma infusion to suppress thrombosis. The regimen of maintenance plasma therapy should be tailored to prevent not only symptoms and thrombocytopenia but also progression of neurologic or renal dysfunction. Most patients require ~7.5 mL/kg fresh-frozen plasma per 45 mL/kg plasma volume every 2 weeks to achieve these goals. Larger volumes may not be tolerated.

Neurologic, mental, and renal functions; complete blood count (CBC); and urinalysis are monitored before each treatment and the regimen is adjusted as needed to ensure that it is adequate to prevent not only acute episodes but also chronic organ injuries.

For patients who never experience any TTP-related symptoms, the choice is less straightforward. The patients may be reluctant to go on long-term plasma therapy. Frequent monitoring of CBC may unmask periods of asymptomatic thrombocytopenia and strengthen the indication of long-term prophylaxis. At least, the patients should be advised to have prophylactic plasma therapy during high-risk periods such as fever, infection, vaccination, surgery, intravenous radiocontrast agents, and pregnancy, and have immediate access to expert assessment for symptoms and signs suggesting the possibility of TTP thrombosis.

Thrombotic Thrombocytopenic Purpura and Pregnancy

An association between pregnancy and acquired TTP has long been suspected, but never confirmed. Because TTP affects women in their reproductive years, it may occur coincidentally during pregnancy. Patients presenting with acquired TTP during pregnancy should be treated with plasma exchange, with tapering of the treatment guided by serial platelet counts and ADAMTS13 levels.

The benefit of rituximab and caplacizumab treatments should be weighed against the uncertainty of their impacts on the pregnancy. Postmarketing data indicate that rituximab is detectable in the serum of infants exposed to the drug in utero. B cell depletion may occur but generally lasts less than 6 months. Anecdotally, rituximab has been used during pregnancy, and no other apparent adverse consequences have been reported. Caplacizumab may increase the risk of bleeding in the fetus, neonate, and mother. Thus, therapeutic decisions should be based on a full discussion with the patient regarding the potential benefits and risks.

A more challenging issue is counseling and management of women with a history of acquired TTP who desire pregnancy. During pregnancy the ADAMTS13 level progressively decreased, to approximately 70% at uncomplicated term and nearly down to 35% if the pregnancy is complicated by preeclampsia or the *h*emolysis, *e*levated *l*iver enzymes, and *l*ow *p*latelet count (HELLP) syndrome.[110,111] Pregnancy also increases plasma vWF levels. Therefore, pregnancy may lead to exacerbation of thrombosis in patients with preexisting TTP. Thrombosis caused by severe ADAMTS13 deficiency increases maternal and fetal morbidities and mortalities.

For women with a history of acquired TTP, counseling on the risk of TTP relapse should begin before conception. If the patient decides to proceed and the plasma ADAMTS13 activity level is decreased, rituximab is an option to increase the ADAMTS13 activity to its highest level before conception. Serial monitoring of ADAMTS13 levels is essential during pregnancy. Whenever ADAMTS13 decreases to 20% to 40% of normal, rituximab therapy should be considered to prevent its further decrease and relapse of TTP.

Women with hTTP should continue regular plasma therapy, or initiate the treatment if she is not already having it. The usual regimen of ~7.5 mL/kg per 45 mL/kg plasma volume every 2 weeks should be titrated to prevent thrombocytopenia and thrombosis.

Some women with milder forms of hTTP may become pregnant with the disease undiagnosed. These patients may develop thrombocytopenia that may be incorrectly attributed to gestational or immune thrombocytopenia, only to develop more serious TTP exacerbation or fetal complications later. A high index of suspicion and liberal use of ADAMTS13 tests may help identify such patients before serious complications occur.

SHIGA TOXIN–ASSOCIATED HEMOLYTIC-UREMIC SYNDROME

First described by Gasser et al in 1955,[112] typical hemolytic-uremic syndrome (HUS) refers to the symptom constellation of acute renal failure, microangiopathic hemolysis, and thrombocytopenia following a bout of hemorrhagic diarrhea. Typical HUS or D(iarrhea)+ HUS, now more appropriately known as STX-HUS (*Table 49.2*), is the most common cause of acute renal failure in children and often draws public attention during outbreaks of foodborne illnesses.

Etiology

Globally, the incidence rate of Shiga toxin–producing *Escherichia coli* (STEC) gastroenteritis (1990-2012) was estimated at 43.1 cases/10^5 population, with HUS developing in 0.14%; and end-stage renal disease, in 6.9% of the HUS cases.[113] Nevertheless, both rates of STX-EC infection and HUS varied broadly, ranging from 1.4/10^5 to 152.6/10^5 and from 0.03% to 0.33%, respectively.

Serotype O157:H7 is the most common cause of STX-HUS. STEC of non-O157 serotypes and even *Shigella dysenteriae* serotype I have also been implicated in causing the syndrome of HUS.

The offending organisms share the capacity of producing powerful Shiga toxins, which are encoded by phage DNA and comprise several genotypes.[114] Most HUS cases are caused by Shiga toxin genotype 2 or 1 + 2. With more laboratories adopting the Shiga toxin ELISA or PCR, increasing numbers of non-O157 *E. coli* serotypes, such as O26:H11, O103:H2, O111:H8, and O145:H28, are detected.

E. coli O104:H4 that caused the outbreaks in Germany, France, and other countries in 2011 evolved from an unusual progenitor of enteroaggregative *E. coli* through acquisition of a STX 2-encoding prophage and a plasmid encoding a CTX-M-15 extended-spectrum β-lactamase gene.[115] It caused bloody diarrhea less frequently, yet was associated with a higher rate of HUS whose demographic was dominated by adults rather than young children. Hence, neurologic involvement was also common.

Many strains of STEC have not been associated with hemorrhagic diarrhea or HUS, indicating that other virulence factors are also critical for pathogenesis. The expression of additional genes on a chromosomal locus of enterocyte effacement pathogenicity island, including intimin encoded by the eae gene, has a strong association with the risk of HUS.[116] Nevertheless, *E. coli* O104:H4 (2011) lacked the common pathogenicity gene eae although it did harbor other genes such as *aggR*, *aap*, *aatA*, and *aggA*. STEC is one of the surveillance infections conducted by the Centers for Disease Control and Prevention's Foodborne Disease Active Surveillance Network (FoodNet).

With the exception of *E. coli* O104:H4 (2011), STEC usually has a reservoir in the intestine of ruminant animals such as cattle and is transmitted by meat, milk, or water contaminated with ruminant feces. Most cases of STX-HUS result from ingestion of contaminated food, such as beef, leafy vegetables, dairy, fruits, nuts, sprouts, poultry, or water. Other modes of transmission include direct animal contacts at farms and person-to-person contact during the acute diarrheal phase.

Very low infectious doses (<100 organisms) are sufficient to cause disease. Outbreaks account for only 20% of the cases. Approximately 50% of the cases occur during the summer months.

Pathology

The pathology of STX-HUS is TMA, which is quite different from that of TTP. It is dominated by glomerular endothelial cell swelling or necrosis and subendothelial expansion in the kidney arterioles and small arteries.[117,118] Fibrin-platelet thrombi are commonly present in glomerular loops and hila and may be seen extending into small- and medium-sized arteries, including the interlobular arteries (*Figure 49.2C*). Neutrophil infiltration may be present. Extensive thrombosis may result in renal cortical infarcts.

Other organs such as brain, heart, intestinal tract, and pancreas may also be affected, either with edema due to abnormal vascular permeability or with ischemic injury due to microvascular stenosis or thrombosis.

Pathophysiology

It is believed that the pathology of TMA is a consequence of the cytotoxic effect of Shiga toxins on vascular endothelial cells (*Figure 49.11*).[119,120] However, binding of the toxins to other types of cells may also contribute to severity of disease.

A Shiga toxin molecule comprises an A-subunit and a pentameric B-subunit. The toxin molecule binds via its B-subunit pentamer to globotriaosylceramide (Gb3) expressed on the membrane lipid rafts of renal microvascular endothelial and other types of cells. This binding is followed by internalization of the A-subunit via endocytosis. After proteolysis by a furin-like protease, a smaller fragment of the A-subunit is generated that is capable of disrupting the 60S ribosomes, blocking protein synthesis in the target cells.

The sensitivity of endothelial cells to Shiga toxins is determined primarily by the level of Gb3 expression, which may be enhanced by cytokines such as IL-1 and TNF-α released upon exposure to endotoxins.[120]

Additional studies suggest that Shiga toxins may also alter the expression of vasoactive factors (e.g., endothelin-1, CXCR4/SDF-1, Ang-2/Ang-1 ratio), adhesive proteins (e.g., vWF, $\alpha_v\beta_3$, PCAM-1, and

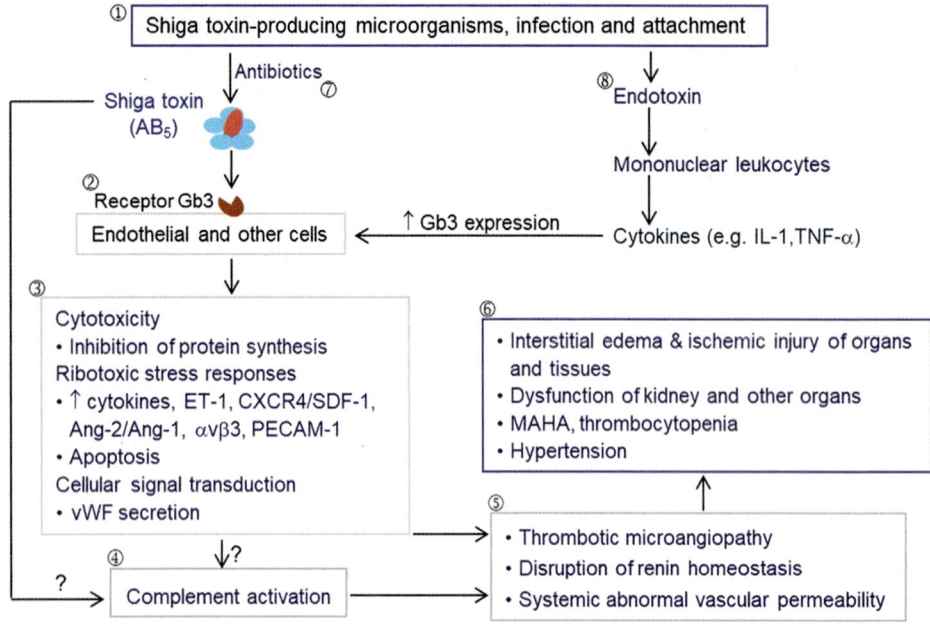

FIGURE 49.11 **Pathophysiology of STX-HUS.** Major determinants include bacterial virulence that influence the amount of STXs entering the circulation (①), the expression of globotriaosylceramide (Gb3) receptors on endothelial and other cells (②), cellular changes following the toxin-Gb3 binding (③), possible activation of the complement system (④), and endothelial injury/thrombosis and vasomotor dysregulation (⑤), leading to the clinical expression of STX-HUS (⑥). Release of Shiga toxin and expression of Gb3 receptor may be increased by use of certain antibiotics (⑦) and bacterial endotoxin (⑧), respectively. IL, interleukin; MAHA, microangiopathic hemolytic anemia; NO, nitric oxide; STX-HUS, Shiga toxin–associated hemolytic-uremic syndrome; TNF, tumor necrosis factor.

P-selectin), cytokines, and chemokines, and induce cellular apoptosis in a process of ribotoxic response.[121-124] Binding of the B-subunit may induce a cytoplasmic signal transduction and the secretion of vWF from endothelial cell Weibel-Palade bodies.[125] STXs may also activate the alternative complement pathway,[126] and the CXCR4/stromal cell–derived factor 1 (SDF-1) pathway, which may cause abnormal endothelial permeability, thereby contributing to some of the serious complications of STX-HUS.[127]

Overall, the most prominent cellular effects of STXs are endothelial cell swelling and necrosis and abnormal vascular permeability. Endothelial cell disruption exposes the underlying thrombogenic glomerular basement membrane, triggering the activation of the coagulation cascade and subsequent thrombosis. Thrombosis leads to ischemic organ injury, thrombocytopenia, and abnormal shear stress, which, in turn, may cause red cell fragmentation and hemolysis. Vascular stenosis may also result from endothelial swelling and subendothelial expansion. Activation of CXCR4/SDF-1 and the complement system may also increase vascular permeability, resulting in interstitial edema of brain and other organs and tissues, pleural or pericardial effusions, ascites, and anasarca.

Clinical Presentation

The spectrum of illness following ingestion of STEC ranges from no symptoms to self-limited enterocolitis, HUS, and death. After STEC infection, diarrhea and other gastrointestinal symptoms develop between 1 and 120 days (median, 3-4 days, with the exception of 8 days after *O104:H4* [2011] infection). The diarrhea may turn bloody 1 to 3 days later.

Symptoms and signs of HUS begin to manifest as the diarrhea begins to improve, approximately 6 to 9 days after the first symptoms. Risk factors for HUS after infection with STEC include young or old age, bloody diarrhea, long duration of diarrhea, elevated leukocyte count, and use of antidiarrheal drugs and certain antibiotics.[128]

The onset of hemolysis and renal failure may be dramatic, with sudden pallor, abdominal pain, vomiting, and the appearance of dark red or nearly black urine. These manifestations may quickly lead to oliguria or even anuria. On the other hand, mild or incomplete HUS with thrombocytopenia but no anemia or azotemia is almost as frequent as the complete form of HUS.

Extrarenal complications occur in approximately 50% of patients and may include hypertension, pancreatitis, glucose intolerance, colonic necrosis and perforation, myocardial dysfunction, congestive heart failure, pericardial or pleural effusion, pulmonary edema, and acute respiratory distress syndrome.[129]

Neurologic complications, including lethargy, irritability, transient paralysis, stroke, seizures, and coma, are the most serious and may result from cerebral edema. Hemorrhagic or thrombotic stroke may also occur. Elderly individuals, especially frail nursing home residents, are more likely to experience cardiovascular and neurologic complications and death.[130]

Laboratory Findings

Hematologic findings are similar to those of TTP, although the severity of thrombocytopenia is more variable and often does not correlate with the severity of renal dysfunction. The anemia is also variable, but may be quite severe and is accompanied by hemoglobinemia and polymorphonuclear leukocytosis.

The prothrombin time and partial thromboplastin time are usually normal or minimally prolonged. However, fibrin degradation products or D-dimer tests are frequently elevated.[131] Serum haptoglobin levels are typically undetectable. The bilirubin level is usually elevated, as are liver transaminases and amylase.[132] The blood urea nitrogen and serum creatinine levels may be quite high. The urine usually contains hemoglobin and hemosiderin in addition to albumin. Microscopically, erythrocytes, leukocytes, and casts are seen.

CT and MRI studies of the brain in patients with neurologic complications may reveal various abnormalities, including restricted water diffusion, edema or posterior reversible encephalopathy syndrome (PRES), contrast enhancement, or hemorrhage in the basal ganglia, thalamus, cerebellum, or brainstem.[133] Brain findings are most commonly due to abnormal vascular permeability, which often resolve on follow-up examinations, and are not necessarily associated with a poor long-term neurologic outcome.

With rare exception, patients with STX-HUS have normal or slightly to moderately decreased ADAMTS13 activity levels and no inhibitory antibodies.[5] Large vWF multimers may be decreased because abnormal shear stress created by microvascular thrombosis not only fragments red blood cells but also augments proteolysis of vWF by ADAMTS13.

Diagnosis, Management, and Prognosis

Conventionally, *E. coli* O157:H7 is detected by plating fresh feces on sorbitol-MacConkey agar. Direct detection of Shiga toxins by ELISA or PCR analysis is more sensitive and has shorter turnaround times. The latter tests also detect non-O157:H7 serotypes.[134]

No specific treatment is available for STX-HUS. Avoidance of antidiarrhea medications and maintenance of good hydration before oliguria ensues may decrease the subsequent severity of renal failure.[135] Careful control of the blood pressure and the judicious use of packed red cell and platelet transfusions appear to constitute the safest and most effective approach to the management of HUS.

Because of its excellent results achieved in the treatment of TTP and difficulty in distinguishing HUS from TTP, plasma exchange is often used to treat patients with STX-HUS, although the evidence in support of this practice remains circumstantial in both children as well as in adults.[136-138]

The benefit or harm of antibiotics for enterocolitis due to *E. coli* infection has been controversial. Antibiotics such as beta-lactams and trimethoprim/sulfamethoxazole may increase the risk of HUS following STEC infection, whereas others such as fosfomycin may decrease this risk if the treatment is started early in the course of the enteric illness.[139] Anti–Shiga toxin antibody-containing bovine colostrum, Shiga toxin binding agent (Synsorb Pk: a silicon dioxide-based agent), and a monoclonal antibody against Shiga toxin (urtoxazumab) were investigated in clinical trials of individuals with STEC gastroenteritis. None of the interventions showed a significant reduction in the rate of HUS.[140]

Dialysis is required in approximately 50% of patients with STX-HUS. The usual indications for dialysis support include fluid overload unresponsive to diuretics, a rapidly rising creatinine value, anuria for more than 24 hours, severe electrolyte imbalance, and serious clinical signs of uremia.

Recently, based on laboratory observations of complement activation by Shiga toxins and endothelial P-selectin,[141] eculizumab, a humanized monoclonal antibody targeting C5 approved for treatment of PNH and AHUS, was used in some patients with severe STX-HUS, reportedly with prompt improvement in clinical status.[142,143] Optimism is tempered by lack of published results from two clinical trials of eculizumab for STX-HUS (NCT01410916 and NCT02205541), completed in 2012 and 2018, respectively.

Direct person-to-person transmission occurs during the acute diarrheal phase. In some cases, excretion of the microorganisms may persist for several months. Contact isolation and frequent hand washing are essential to minimize the spread of infection.

The overall case fatality rate in children with STX-HUS is 12% (range 0%-30%). The majority of patients recover without serious consequences. Long-term renal injury such as decreased glomerular filtration rate, proteinuria, hypertension, or renal failure may be present in as many as one of every four survivors.[144,145] Some patients may develop irritable bowel syndrome.[146] A previous report of increased gestational hypertension has not been validated.[147] A few patients may require long-term dialysis or renal transplantation therapy. Posttransplant recurrence of TMA should prompt investigation for possibility of AHUS.[148]

ATYPICAL HEMOLYTIC-UREMIC SYNDROME

AHUS originally referred to the triad of acute renal failure, MAHA, and thrombocytopenia in children without a prodrome of hemorrhagic diarrhea or another apparent cause. Defective regulation of the alternative complement pathway has been found in most cases of conventionally defined AHUS.[148] It is now recognized that AHUS may present in adulthood as frequently as in childhood.

Defective regulation of the alternative complement pathway is also found in some of the patients with HUS following bone marrow/hematopoietic stem cell therapy and women with pregnancy-associated HUS.[149] Some of the patients with the "HUS due to malignant hypertension" may have AHUS instead as the cause of hypertension, MAHA and thrombocytopenia.[150,151]

Because of overlapping clinical features of MAHA and thrombocytopenia, AHUS, especially of adult cases, often were not distinguished from TTP. In fact, many of the so-called "TTP without severe ADAMTS13 deficiency" cases really had AHUS instead. Interpretation of reports in the literature is difficult when the case definitions do not provide a clear distinction of the various diagnoses under the umbrella of "TTP," "TTP/HUS," or "TMA."

The conventional approach of relying on syndromes for diagnosis is unworkable. The definitions of AHUS, TTP, STX-HUS, and TMA, past and present, are depicted in *Table 49.2*. Importantly, with the new definitions, the diagnosis of AHUS, TTP, or STX-HUS does not require the presence of MAHA or thrombocytopenia. Occasionally, a patient may have more than one of these disorders.

Pathology

Although AHUS and TTP share the common features of thrombocytopenia and MAHA and both are often referred to as "thrombotic microangiopathy (TMA)" in the literature, they differ vastly in pathology.

In AHUS, the affected glomerular capillaries, arterioles, and interlobular small arteries typically exhibit endothelial cell swelling or necrosis and subendothelial expansion due to edema and/or fibroblast proliferation and collagenous deposition, often but not invariably accompanied by thrombosis (*Figure 49.2D-F*).[152] The glomerular tufts may show mesangiolysis, double basement membranes, mesangial cell proliferation with expansion of the matrix, and/or interstitial fibrosis. The lesions often include admixtures of acute and chronic changes in AHUS, suggesting that antecedent subclinical injury is common even in patients at their first presentation. This contrasts with the primarily acute changes of TMA in STX-HUS.

The most common pathology of AHUS beyond the kidney is interstitial edema in the brain, pulmonary alveoli, bronchial airways, gastrointestinal tracts, mesentery, pancreas, and cutaneous soft tissues. Fluid accumulation may be present in the pericardial, alveolar, pleural, and peritoneal spaces. These changes, uncommon in TTP, result from abnormal vascular permeability. The pathology of TMA as seen in the kidney is often absent or minimal outside the kidney.

Pathogenesis

The complement system, an important component of the innate host defense against invading microorganisms, may be triggered by immune complexes or microbial mannose (classic and lectin pathways). The alternative pathway, via complement factors B, D, and P (CFB, CFD, and CFP), amplifies complement activation by promoting the generation of alternative C3b and C5b convertases (*Figure 49.12*). Complement factor H (CFH), complement factor I (CFI), membrane cofactor protein (MCP, i.e., CD46), and THBD are all involved in regulating the self-perpetuating complement activation of the alternative pathway, especially on endothelial surfaces.

Genetic mutations of regulators or activators of the alternative pathway are detected in approximately 40% to 75% of AHUS patients, with a higher prevalence among patients with a family history (~75%) than in those without a family history (~40%). The molecular defects include inactivating mutations of *CFH* (25%), *CD46*, *CFI*, and *THBD* (5%-10% each); GoF mutations of activators *C3* (5%-10%) and *CFB* (a few pedigrees).[153-155] Additionally, antibodies to CFH are detected in 5% to 10% of the cases, often with concurrent homozygous or heterozygous genomic deletion of CFH-related protein 1 (*CFHR1*).[156,157]

Certain genetic lesions are a major determinant of the prognosis of AHUS. The long-term survival rate without advanced renal failure is only 20% to 30% for patients with *CFH* mutations and approximately 80% to 90% for patients with *MCP* mutations. However, the genetics of AHUS is quite complex. More than one mutation is detected in 10% to 40% of the patients. More than 50% of patients with *CFI* mutations have concurrent mutations affecting other complement activator or regulatory proteins. Concurrence mutations increase the risk of serious AHUS complications.[158]

In some pedigrees, complications of AHUS only occur in individuals with more than one variant.[159] Analysis of single-nucleotide polymorphisms (SNPs) of complement activators and regulators further shows that the risk of AHUS is significantly increased or decreased with certain SNPs and haplotypes of *CFH, CD46, CFHR2, CFHR4*, and intergenic complement receptor 1 *(CR1)-CD46* among patients with mutations of *CFH, CD46*, and/or *CFI*.[160] Laboratory studies also demonstrate that certain combinations of common variants (complotype) of the complement activators and regulators may increase the risk of the disease.[161]

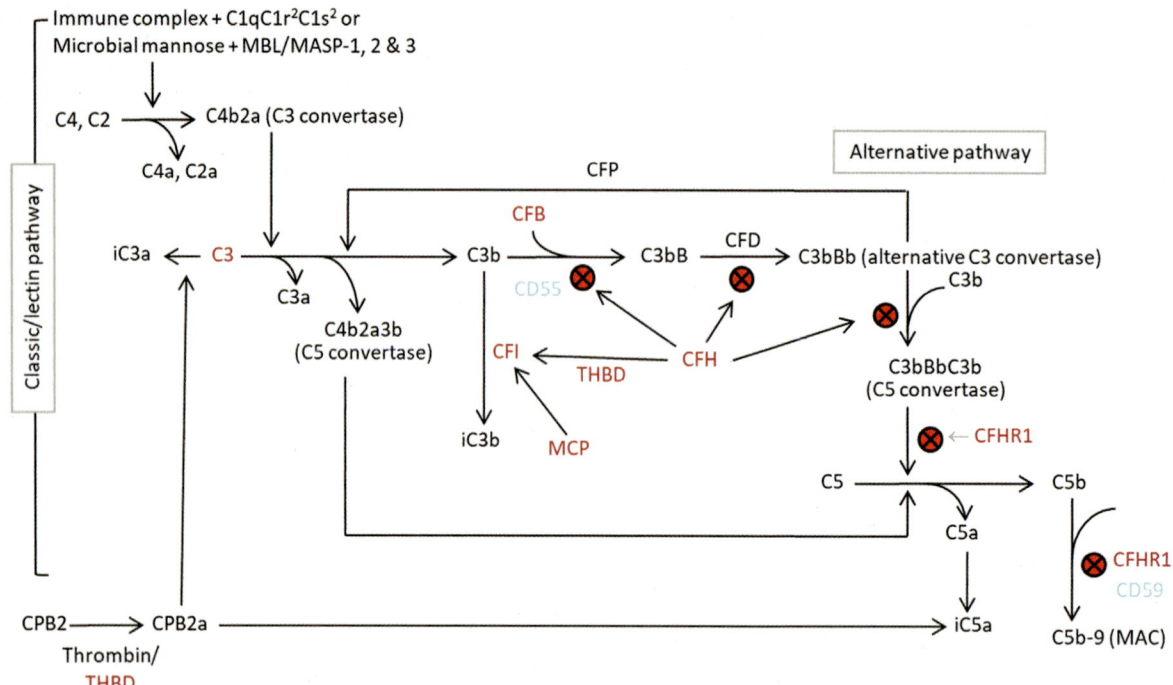

FIGURE 49.12 The complement system and its regulation. The alternative pathway self-perpetually produces alternative C3 and C5 convertases via CFP. Hence, regulators help terminate its activity. The scheme highlights the regulators and activators (in red) whose mutation or deletion has been associated with AHUS. Regulators deficient in PNH are also shown (light blue). These include CFH, CFI, MCP, THBD, and CFHR1; and activators C3 and factor B. Defective regulation of the alternative pathway may also result from antibodies to CFH. Homozygous or heterozygous genomic deletion of CFHR1 is found in many patients with AHUS due to antibodies of CFH or CFI mutations. AHUS, atypical hemolytic-uremic syndrome; CFH, complement factor H; CFHR1, complement factor H–related protein 1; CFB, complement factor B; CFI, complement factor I; CFP, complement factor P; CPB2, carboxypeptidase B2; MAC, membrane attack complex; MCP, membrane cofactor protein; PNH, paroxysmal nocturnal hemoglobinuria; THBD, thrombomodulin.

CFHR1-5 are the products of a series of genes located immediately downstream of the *CFH* gene in a region of chromosome 1q containing multiple retrotransposon sequences. The high level of sequence identity among these retrotransposons favors genomic rearrangements through nonallelic homologous recombination, resulting in genomic deletions, most commonly of *CFHR3-CFHR1* that is strongly associated with aHUS due to anti-CFH auto-Abs, and hybrid genes of *CFH/CFHR3* or *CFH/CFHR1*.[162] The fusion proteins may cause aHUS by acting as antagonists of CFH.

Genomic deletion of *CFHR1* is detected only ~3% of the control population, but is present in 28% of AHUS patients.[161,163,164] Intriguingly, further analysis reveals that genomic *CFHR1* deletion is present in 90% of AHUS patients with CFH auto-Abs and 20% of patients with *CFI* mutations, but is not different from its background prevalence among patients with other or no detectable mutations.[165] *CFHR1* deletion markedly increases the severity of AHUS in patients with *CFI* mutations.[158,165] The presence of CFHR1 protein may alleviate the severity of AHUS by blocking the binding between CFH and its Abs in autoimmune AHUS patients.[155,166]

Overall, the regulation of the alternative complement pathway is redundant. Hence, it often takes more than one genetic variant to be pathogenic. On the other hand, some genetic variants may dampen instead of augment the pathogenic effects of other variants.

A consequence of this genetic complexity is that AHUS is transmitted as an autosomal dominant trait, but with variable penetrance, which is greater than 50% with *CFH* and *MCP* mutations, but lower with mutations of the other proteins.

Pathophysiology

The clinical features of AHUS are the consequence of uncontrolled complement activation on endothelial surfaces, which causes endothelial injury and the pathology of TMA in the kidney and abnormal vascular permeability in various organs and tissues.

When the complement system is activated, defective regulation of the alternative pathway leads to unrelenting generation of complement activation products, most importantly membrane attack complex (MAC, C5b-9) and anaphylatoxins C3a and C5a. Because MAC is cell membrane bound, it causes injury of vascular endothelial cells and the pathology of TMA at the sites of complement activation. In contrast, C3a and C5a may enter the circulation to induce secretion of histamine and other vasoactive mediators from basophils and mast cells, leading to abnormal vascular permeability in retina and various other tissues and organs. The clinical manifestations of AHUS include thrombocytopenia, MAHA, hypertension, renal failure, and extrarenal complications of abnormal vascular permeability (*Figures 49.13* and *49.14*).

Thrombocytopenia occurs when consumption of platelets exceeds thrombocytopoiesis. MAHA is caused by mechanical injury of the red blood cells under conditions of abnormal shear stress created by arteriolar thrombosis, and/or endothelial cell swelling and subendothelial edema, fibroblastic proliferation, and/or collagen deposition (*Figure 49.2E* and *F*). Rapid changes in these pathologic changes may account for the instability of the blood pressure, a common feature of AHUS.

Renal function impairment may result from ischemia due to arteriolar stenosis or thrombosis as well as direct injury by MAC. Extrarenal complications and anasarca are believed to be the consequence of abnormal vascular permeability induced by anaphylatoxins released from the kidney where complement activation occurs. Hence, extrarenal complications are often ameliorated when the kidney is nonfunctioning (end-stage renal disease) but recur after the patient undergoes kidney transplantation.

The multitude of pathophysiologic pathways explains why thrombocytopenia, MAHA, hypertension, renal failure, and extrarenal complications are often discordant during the course of AHUS.

Other Phenotypes of Complement Dysregulation

The renal pathology of mesangiocapillary or membranoproliferative glomerulonephropathy (MPGN) comprises three subgroups based on

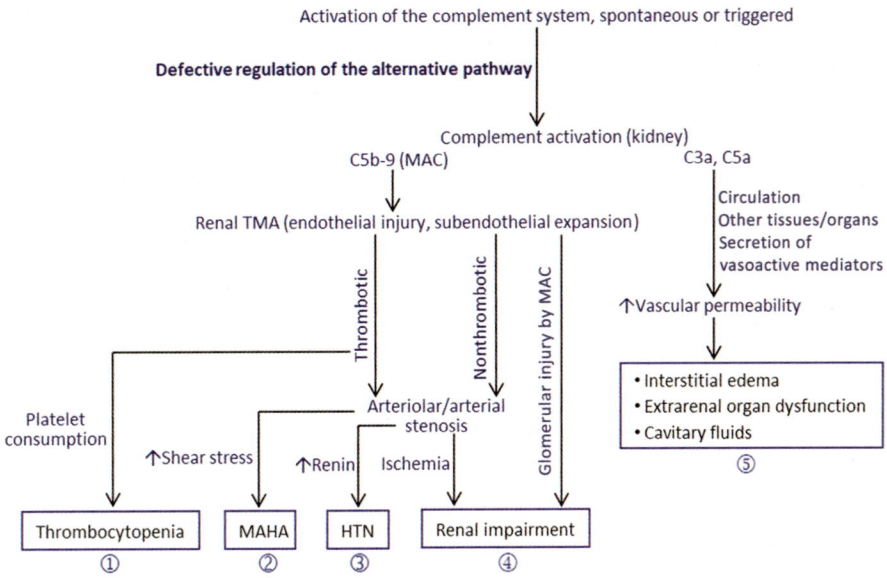

FIGURE 49.13 **Pathophysiology of atypical hemolytic-uremic syndrome.** Defective regulation of the alternative complement pathway in the kidney can lead to persistent generation of C5b-9 (membrane attack complex, MAC), which causes endothelial injury, resulting in thrombosis and thrombocytopenia (①). Thrombotic and nonthrombotic subendothelial expansion can lead to arteriolar/arterial stenosis, creating abnormally high levels of shear stress to hemolyze RBC (microangiopathic hemolytic anemia, MAHA, ②), dysregulated renin secretion and hypertension (HTN, ③), and renal ischemic injury (④). MAC may also directly cause glomerular injury. C3a and C5a, released in the circulation, may induce secretion of vasoactive mediators from basophils and tissue mast cells, thereby increasing vascular permeability, interstitial edema and various extrarenal dysfunctions (⑤), including brain edema, heart failure, and noncardiogenic pulmonary edema. TMA, thrombotic microangiopathy.

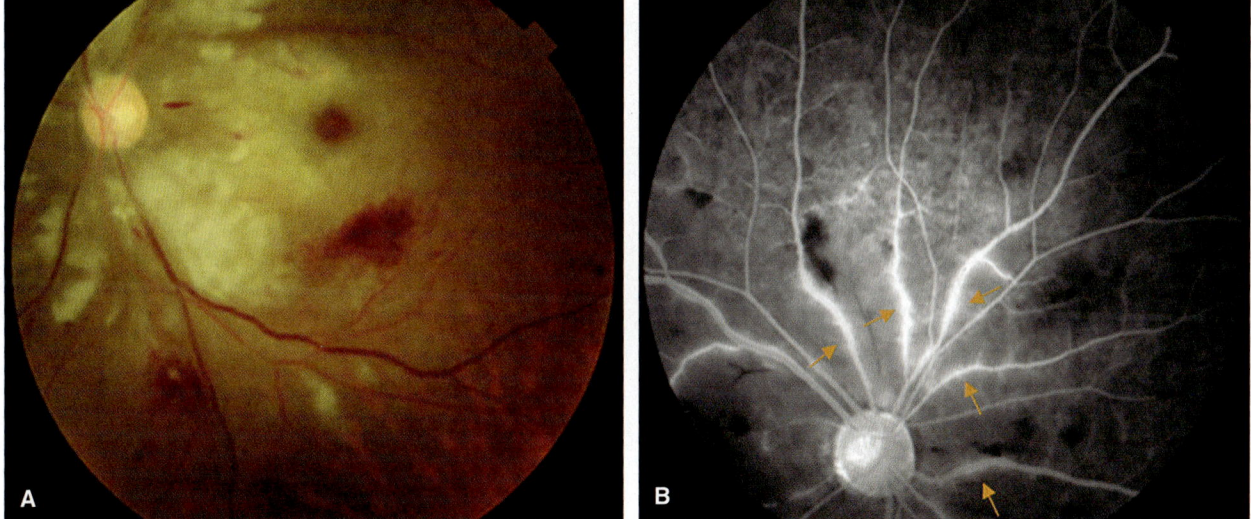

FIGURE 49.14 **Retinopathy and abnormal vascular permeability in atypical hemolytic-uremic syndrome.** A, Purtscher-like retinopathy. B, Fluorescence angiography showing transudation of the fluorescent dye from the arterioles (arrows).

the presence of immunoglobulin by immunohistochemistry (Ig-MPGN) or dense deposits of C3d in the glomerular basement membrane under electron microscopy (dense deposit disease), or the absence of both (C3 glomerulonephritis [C3GN]).[167] The pathology of C3GN may be quite similar to that of AHUS without thrombosis. This overlap in pathology may account for some reported cases of "MPGN," "C3G," or "C3GN" in association with mutations more typical for AHUS.

Similar overlap also occurs with diacylglycerol kinase epsilon (*DGKE*) mutations, which have been detected in patients given the diagnosis of "MPGN" or "AHUS."[168,169]

Genetic analysis reveals that age-related macular degeneration (AMD) may be associated with defective alternative complement regulation in some cases.[170] The connection between AMD and AHUS is best illustrated by *CFH* R1210C, which is associated with a nearly complete penetrance of AMD, yet only a 30% penetrance of AHUS.[170,171] Furthermore, most patients with CFH R1210C-positive AHUS have additional pathogenic genetic variants that affect the regulation of the alternative complement pathway. Hence, a likely scenario is that genetic variants that only mildly affect the alternative complement pathway may cause the phenotype of AMD. Overt AHUS only occurs when the defect is more profound due to additional genetic variants. On the other hand, advanced AMD is associated with decreased estimated glomerular filtration rate (eGFR, <60 mL/min/1.73 m^2) and hypertension,[172] suggesting subclinical renal injury due to defective complement regulation may occur in AMD with subtle defects in complement regulation. The propensity of complement dysregulation to affect retina is consistent with frequent Purtscher-like retinopathy observed in AHUS patients (*Figure 49.14*).

Uncontrolled complement activation also underlies the mechanism of hemolysis in patients with PNH.[173] More than 20 cases of CFI deficiency have been described from 19 pedigrees with increased risk of pyogenic infection.[174]

Clinical Features

The prevalence of AHUS has been estimated at 3 per million children. Newly diagnosed AHUS is likely to be as common as TTP in adults. Both males and females are equally affected.

The onset of an acute AHUS crisis may occur after exposure to an apparent trigger of complement activation, such as fever, infection, vaccination, surgery, trauma, inflammation, pancreatitis, intravenous contrast agents, or pregnancy. Sometimes, the trigger may not be obvious. In severe cases, pathologic complement activation occurs relentlessly, requiring long-term maintenance therapy.

Although renal failure, MAHA, and thrombocytopenia are its best-known features, AHUS is a systemic disease affecting multiple organs. The complications of AHUS comprise five pathophysiologic categories (*Figure 49.13*). All five categories should be included in the assessment of the disease. No single category provides a full representation of the disease.

Renal Injury

Proteinuria, hematuria, and renal function impairment are common. Hematuria is microscopic in most cases but may be gross occasionally. The severity of renal failure is variable. Some patients may present with very mild elevation of creatinine initially, and others present with anuric renal failure requiring dialysis support. During its course, renal injury may continue to occur with or without thrombocytopenia and/or MAHA.

Hypertension

Hypertension is common with AHUS. It may be severe and labile and difficult to control with antihypertensive drugs, presumably reflecting the varying severity of arteriolar stenosis that affects renin secretion from the juxtaglomerular apparatus. Some patients present with hypertension, along with symptoms of extrarenal complications, for years before the conventional triad of renal failure, MAHA, and thrombocytopenia becomes apparent.[151] Severe unstable hypertension may contribute to the development of intracranial hemorrhage.

AHUS may also present as "gestational hypertension" and may be mistaken to be preeclampsia or preeclampsia/HELLP (hemolysis, elevated liver enzymes, and low platelet count) syndrome during pregnancy.[175] Since the complement system is activated in preeclampsia/HELLP syndrome, its transition to AHUS in genetically susceptible women may pose challenge in diagnosis and management.

Abnormal Vascular Permeability

The extrarenal complications of AHUS are primarily a result of abnormal vascular permeability (*Figure 49.14*). Lesions of TMA are absent or inconspicuous in extrarenal organs and tissues at autopsy. Furthermore, extrarenal complications are often ameliorated in patients with complete renal failure with no or little residual function, suggesting that abnormal vascular permeability in extrarenal organs is the consequence of complement activation in functioning kidneys. In accord with this scheme, the complications of abnormal vascular permeability often reappear when the patients undergo kidney transplantations.

Extrarenal complications are a major source of morbidity and mortality in AHUS. Some patients have extrarenal complications along with hypertension that wax and wane for months to years before they present with overt renal failure, thrombocytopenia, and MAHA.

Neurologic symptoms and signs are often associated with posterior reversible encephalopathy syndrome (PRES) on MRI with T2-FLAIR or brain edema in advanced cases. Focal neurologic deficits may occur, but they are not as frequent as with TTP. Visual defects may be associated with Purtscher-like retinopathy, with fluorescence angiography showing abnormal permeability (*Figure 49.14*). Brain edema may cause abrupt clinical deterioration due to brainstem herniation.

Chest pain, cough, dyspnea, and respiratory failure may result from bronchial wall inflammation, thickening, alveolar edema, pleural and pericardial effusion, and/or cardiac failure on imaging studies. Acute deterioration of respiratory or cardiac failure or arrhythmia may cause sudden death.

Gastrointestinal complications, such as abdominal pain, anorexia, and nausea, are the most common initial symptoms. Vomiting and diarrhea with or without blood are less common. Imaging studies may reveal ascites, pancreatic swelling, and edematous thickening of the mesentery and intestinal wall.

Soft-tissue swelling such as puffy face, limb swelling, or anasarca is often incorrectly attributed to renal failure but does not improve with dialysis.

MAHA and Thrombocytopenia

MAHA and thrombocytopenia are both quite variable in severity. Thrombocytopenia and MAHA are indicative of active disease. However, injury of the kidney and other organs may occur while the platelet count and hemoglobin level are normal or only mildly decreased. Petechiae or other bleeding symptoms may occur but are uncommon.

Diagnosis

The diagnosis of AHUS is most commonly suspected in patients presenting with the triad of renal failure, MAHA, and thrombocytopenia. AHUS should also be suspected in patients without the triad (*Table 49.8*).

No simple tests are presently available for direct assessment of the regulation of the alternative complement regulation. The C3 level is decreased in approximately 30% to 50% of the patients. The C4 level is decreased in less than 10% of the cases. These changes are not specific for AHUS. In patients with mutations of *CFH* or *CFI*, the antigen levels of the affected proteins are decreased in approximately 30% of the cases.

A kidney biopsy is often necessary to assist the differential diagnosis, unless there are contraindications to the procedure. In patients with kidney biopsy showing TMA, the diagnosis of aHUS is presumed after other causes of TMA (*Table 49.1*) are excluded. The confidence of the diagnosis is further strengthened if immunostaining detects C5b-9 deposits on endothelial cell surfaces.[176]

Genetic analysis and ELISA for anti-CFH are often requested. Positive genetic test results support the diagnosis of aHUS for patients with consistent symptoms and signs. However, the results may detect novel variants of undetermined significance. Negative molecular results do not exclude the diagnosis of AHUS.

Measurement of C5b-9 deposits on static or ADP-stimulated microvascular endothelial cells after the cell culture is incubated with patient's serum may support the diagnosis of excessive complement activation and reflect the pathophysiologic status of the disease.[177] However, the test requires cultured endothelial cells that are not readily available in clinical laboratories. The performance of the test also needs to be more broadly validated.

In patients without contraindications such as uncontrolled infection and not being treated with plasma exchange, therapeutic diagnosis with one or two test doses of eculizumab may help determine if the condition is mediated by complement activation. In AHUS, the platelet count should begin to show steady increase by day 3 and normalize by day 7.[95] Labile blood pressures should be stabilized and extrarenal complications due to abnormal vascular permeability should be improved in 1 to 2 weeks. Concurrent plasma exchange or comorbidities may delay or affect the expected responses, making determination of therapeutic effects less reliable.

Management

Historically, AHUS patients were treated with plasma exchange. This practice was an extension of plasma exchange therapy for TTP, which was in fact the diagnosis given to most adult AHUS patients until recent years.

Empirically, the efficacy of plasma exchange or plasma infusion is unpredictable. It ranges from good response and remission with

Table 49.8. Diagnosis of Atypical Hemolytic-Uremic Syndrome (AHUS)

When AHUS should be suspected
- Renal failure and unexplained thrombocytopenia ± MAHA
- TMA in kidney biopsy
- Hypertension, uncontrollable or with progressive renal failure
- Symptoms of abnormal vascular permeability
  - Unexplained PRES on MRI with T2-FLAIR
  - Edema of brain, bronchial wall, pulmonary alveoli, intestinal wall, pancreas, mesentery, and/or soft tissues
- Renal failure of undetermined etiology, prior to kidney transplant
- Onset, persistence or worsening "HELLP" or "Preeclampsia/eclampsia" after delivery

Confirming the diagnosis of AHUS
- TMA in kidney biopsy
  - Exclude other causes of TMA (*Table 49.1*)
  - Immunostaining for C5b-9 deposits on endothelial cells if available
- Genetic analysis and anti-CFH test:
  - Genes: *CFH, CD46, CFI, C3, CFB, THBD*, and *CFHR1-R3*
  - Conventional sequencing with MLPA or next generation sequencing, targeted panel
  - Positive in 50%-75% of the cases; negative tests do not exclude AHUS
  - Pathogenicity of novel variants is often uncertain
- Soluble C5b-9 or amount of C5b-9 on microvascular endothelial cells after incubation with patient's serum
  - Specificity and sensitivity to be validated; cell cultures not easily standardized
- Therapeutic diagnosis with eculizumab:
  - Platelet count should normalize before the second weekly dose
  - Extrarenal complications improved and blood pressure stabilized in 1-2 wk
  - Exceptions: concurrent plasma exchange, comorbidities

Abbreviations: CFB, complement factor B; CFH, complement factor H; CFI, complement factor I; CFHR, complement factor H–related protein; MAHA, microangiopathic hemolytic anemia; MLPA, multiplex ligation-dependent probe amplification; PRES, posterior reversible encephalopathy syndrome; THBD, thrombomodulin; TMA, thrombotic microangiopathy.
aOther non-AHUS genes such as diacylglycerol kinase epsilon (*DGKE*), methylmalonic aciduria and homocystinuria, Cb1C type (*MMACHC*), and plasminogen (*PLG*) are often included.

or without subsequent relapses, to partial response with subsequent deterioration and even no response. Some patients respond to plasma therapy but cannot be weaned off the treatment without immediate deterioration. Furthermore, when the platelet count is normalized and plasma therapy is discontinued, as is the accepted practice in the management of TTP, many patients go on to develop end-stage renal disease months or years later, without ever experiencing an overt relapse. The worsening of renal failure is most likely the result of persistent low-grade renal injury. Retrospective analysis shows that with plasma exchange as the mainstay of treatment, the dialysis-free survival rate was approximately 50% or lower. Now, plasma therapy is only used for AHUS when anticomplement therapy is unavailable.

Anticomplement Therapy

A major advance in the treatment of AHUS is eculizumab, a humanized monoclonal Ab to C5 originally approved in 2007 for the treatment of PNH. Eculizumab has been approved since 2011 for the treatment of pediatric and adult AHUS. In clinical trials, patients without identifiable mutations also responded to eculizumab, confirming that negative genetic studies do not exclude the diagnosis of AHUS.[178] This was followed by ravulizumab, a bioengineered version of eculizumab with a longer half-life.[179,180]

With eculizumab therapy, normalization of the platelet count and resolution of extrarenal complications are expected within 1 to 2 weeks,[95,179,180] unless the patient has other disorders for their persistence or is being treated with plasma exchange. The recovery of hemolysis may be delayed by a few weeks. Worsening of kidney function is not expected, although its recovery may be very slow and often incomplete in adult cases.[95] The current principles of management for patients with AHUS are summarized in *Table 49.9*.

The aims of eculizumab therapy for AHUS include resolution of thrombocytopenia and MAHA, stabilization of the blood pressure, recovery or stabilization of the kidney and other organ functions, and prevention of acute relapses and death.

Because sudden death is a risk of AHUS, especially in patients with extrarenal complications of abnormal vascular permeability, eculizumab should be instituted as soon as possible without waiting for confirmation of the diagnosis by molecular testing. Anticomplement therapy also should not be delayed for patients with deteriorating renal function or severe uncontrollable hypertension.

Two Asian polymorphisms of complement C5 (R885H and R885C) disrupt the eculizumab target epitope on C5 and its inhibition of C5 activation.[181] Eculizumab is ineffective for patients with PNH with one of these polymorphisms. It is conceivable that eculizumab is also ineffective for AHUS patients with the same polymorphisms. Such patients may be candidates for clinical trials or compassionate use of alternative inhibitors of C5 (e.g., crovalimab, effective against R885H in vitro), C3 (e.g., pegcetacoplan, approved for PNH), or CFD.[182-185] CH50, AH50, functional C5 assay, or free C5 may be used to check the adequacy of anticomplement therapy. Eculizumab should be started only when active infections are under control, with exceptions such as COVID-19. Eculizumab is generally well tolerated with minor adverse reactions. However, eculizumab may predispose patients to fulminant *Neisseria meningitidis* infections. Patients should have meningococcal vaccination and take prophylactic antibiotics for at least until 2 weeks after the vaccination. Patients should also carry an identification card to facilitate emergency management of any infectious complications. Concern of serious infection has prompted recommendation of long-term prophylactic antibiotic therapy, or to have a valid antibiotic prescription immediately available. Vaccination against *Streptococcus pneumoniae* and *Haemophilus influenzae* type b should also be considered, especially for children. Consult CDC ACIP for updated immunization information (https://www.immunize.org/clinic/vaccine-recommendations.asp).

Eculizumab has been used in a limited number of patients during pregnancy with no apparent adverse effects in the mother and fetus.[186] However, animal studies using a mouse analogue of eculizumab at 2 to 8 times the human dose showed increased rates of developmental abnormalities and fetal death.[187] Eculizumab should only be used during pregnancy when the benefit justifies the potential risk to the fetus on a case-by-case basis.

Ravulizumab is a humanized monoclonal antibody derived from eculizumab by substitution of amino acid residues in its complementarity determining region and Fc sequences to promote dissociation with C5 at pH 6.0 and efficacy of binding with neonatal type Fc receptor (FcRn). These changes increase the terminal half-life to ~51.8 days from ~11 days.[179] Thus, ravulizumab may be administered every 8 weeks (4 weeks for small children BW < 20 kg) instead of every 2 weeks.

Anticomplement therapy is initiated with eculizumab when the diagnosis or indication of long-term treatment is uncertain. It may be

Table 49.9. Atypical Hemolytic-Uremic Syndrome (AHUS): Principles of Management

Anticomplement therapy with eculizumab; switched to ravulizumab for long-term treatment	
• Plasma exchange is only used when anticomplement therapy is unavailable	
• Prophylaxis of fulminant sepsis	
• Control of active infections before initiation of anticomplement therapy	
• Vaccination vs *Neisseria meningitidis* for all, and *Streptococcus pneumoniae* and *Haemophilus influenzae* type b (Hib) for children and possibly for adults	
• Prophylactic antibiotics for at least two weeks after vaccination	
Treatment should be instituted as soon as possible for patients with deteriorating renal function, complications due to abnormal vascular permeability, or severe uncontrollable hypertension	
• Delay in treatment may increase the risk of serious complications such as irreversible renal failure, intracranial hemorrhage, brain herniation, and even sudden death	
Responses to anticomplement therapy may help determine the validity of diagnosis (*Table 49.8*)	
• Assess symptoms and monitor blood pressure daily	
• CBC, LDH, haptoglobin, and kidney function daily at least during the first week of treatment	
• Platelet count begins to steadily increase by day 3, normalizing by day 7	
• Renal recovery is variable, may not be apparent for weeks, but continue slowly for >1 y	
• Concurrent plasma exchange or comorbidities may delay or affect the expected responses to eculizumab treatment	
Tapering and discontinuation of eculizumab treatment in selected patients	
• Patients without a clear indication for long-term treatment such as a history of relapse, or symptoms, signs and/or unstable blood pressure before the next scheduled dose	
• Taper only after renal function has reached maximal recovery	
• Taper slowly—increase the treatment interval by 1-2 d every 2-4 wk	
• Daily recording of symptoms and blood pressures	
• CBC, LDH, haptoglobin and kidney function weekly, gradually increased to every 2-4 wk	
• Immediate access to expert evaluation and treatment for any suspicion of relapse	
Patients who are not on long-term anticomplement therapy	
• Prophylactic anticomplement therapy for triggering conditions (infection, vaccination, inflammation, surgery, trauma, intravenous radiocontrast agents, and pregnancy)	
Patients requiring dialysis for advanced renal failure	
• Check glomerular filtration rate to confirm the lack of renal function	
• Extrarenal complications of abnormal vascular permeability may still occur if there is residual renal function	
• Avoid renal transplantation to allow anticomplement therapy for at least 6-12 mo till maximal renal function recovery	
• Avoid relatives as the donor for renal transplantation	
• Start anticomplement therapy preoperatively (if not already being treated)	
• Continue anticomplement therapy indefinitely after renal transplantation, except for	
• Patients with isolated *MCP* (*CD46*) mutation	
• Combined kidney-liver transplantation	

Abbreviations: CBC, complete blood count; LDH, lactate dehydrogenase; *MCP*, membrane cofactor protein.

switched to ravulizumab when the diagnosis is established and long-term treatment is expected.

In clinical trials, ravulizumab generally provides comparable improvement in hematologic and renal functions.[188-190] However, incomplete suppression of free C5 and deterioration of renal function may occur, highlighting the importance of checking CH50, AH50, C5 functional, or free C5 to ensure adequate therapeutic suppression of complement activation.

Long-Term Management

A major challenge in the management of aHUS is the unpredictability of long-term course. Some patients with aHUS remain free of symptoms with stable renal function for many years without any treatment after their single episodes. For such patients, the merit of long-term maintenance therapy is questionable. However, it is not possible to reliably identify such patients a priori.

Eculizumab treatment should be continued to allow time for maximal kidney function recovery, often for more than 6 to 12 months. Long-term anticomplement treatment is indicated if the patients experience symptoms, unstable blood pressures and/or elevated CH50/AH50 (total and alternative complement functional assays) before the next scheduled doses. For such patients, the treatment interval should be decreased to control the symptoms and stabilize the blood pressure. In general, long-term treatment is indicated for patients with relapses or with chronic changes in renal biopsy. Patients who do not have any of these indications may be candidates for tapering of eculizumab treatment (*Table 49.9*). The patients should have immediate access to expert evaluation whenever a relapse is suspected. Anticomplement therapy should be immediately available when retreatment is indicated.

For patients with AHUS in association with antibodies to CFH, immunosuppressive therapy with corticosteroids, cyclophosphamide, mycophenolate, or rituximab has been tried and even advocated to suppress the antibody level. However, suppression of CFH antibody, even if successful, often does not last indefinitely. It is unknown whether monitoring of anti-CFH antibody or CFH protein level will detect impending relapse in such patients. For patients with anti-CFH, the pros and cons of long-term eculizumab therapy vs immunosuppressive drugs such as rituximab should be carefully evaluated for individual cases.

Renal Transplantation

Owing to high rates of disease recurrence, AHUS patients, except those with mutations of membrane proteins such as MCP as the sole cause, have a very high risk (>80%-90%) of graft failure following kidney transplantation. Anticomplement therapy prevents recurrence of TMA in the graft. Hence, kidney transplantation is no longer a contraindication for AHUS patients as it once was. However, preoperative evaluation and planning are essential.

Patients undergoing kidney transplantation for end-stage renal disease of unknown etiology should have molecular testing to evaluate the possibility of AHUS as the cause of their renal failure, even for those with no history of MAHA and thrombocytopenia. For patients with a positive result of AHUS molecular testing, eculizumab therapy should be started prior to the operation and continued postoperatively to prevent complement activation and recurrence of TMA.[191]

Negative genetic and CFH Ab ELISA results do not exclude AHUS. Patients with negative diagnostic test results should be closely monitored during and after the operation for early detection of any complement activation and AHUS disease activity.

Previously, combined kidney and liver transplantation was performed on patients with end-stage renal disease due to AHUS, based on the rationale that restoration of normal CFH in the circulation by the transplanted liver would prevent recurrence of AHUS and renal graft failure. However, this procedure was associated with a very high risk of morbidity and mortality.[192] Anticomplement therapy during the perioperative period may help prevent complications resulting from excessive complement activation.[193] The pros and cons of liver or combined kidney and liver transplantation need to be weighed against those of long-term anticomplement therapy without liver transplantation.

Patients with AHUS solely caused by mutations of membrane proteins, such as *MCP*, are expected to be cured, at least from the renal perspective, by a kidney allograft. Nevertheless, graft failure may occur if the donor is a family member who happens to also carry the molecular trait. Owing to the incomplete phenotypic expression of AHUS, healthy family members of AHUS patients may carry the same mutations and should not be the organ donors. Relapse of TMA and graft failure may also occur if the patient carries additional identified or unidentified mutations.

Prognosis

Historically, approximately 10% to 30% of AHUS patients treated with plasma exchange died during their acute presentation.[155,194] The overall risk of death or end-stage renal failure was approximately 60% by 1 to 2 years. Most deaths were caused by extrarenal complications such as brain edema, respiratory failure, or heart failure. The risk was the highest (70%-80%) for patients with *CFH* mutations, compound mutations, or *CFI* mutation with *CFHR1* deletion, and the lowest mortality (10%-20%) was observed in patients with *MCP* mutations only.

Anticomplement therapy resolves and prevents acute crisis of AHUS. Properly executed, anticomplement therapy should also prevent progression of renal failure. Death, advanced renal failure, and other complications due to AHUS may still occur if diagnosis or treatment is delayed or there are comorbidities. Death occasionally occurs due to uncontrolled or fulminant infection.

OTHER CAUSES OF MICROANGIOPATHIC HEMOLYTIC ANEMIA

The syndrome of MAHA and thrombocytopenia may occur in patients with various clinical conditions. ADAMTS13 tests are indicated for all patients presenting with MAHA and thrombocytopenia to exclude the diagnosis of TTP.

After TTP is excluded, there are three types of associations (Table 49.10). In the first group, the clinical conditions may trigger the activation of the complement system, thereby resulting in the pathology of TMA and the manifestation of AHUS in individuals with preexisting defects in the regulation of the alternative complement pathway. In the second group, the conditions may lead to certain types of pathology (Table 49.1) that create abnormal intravascular shear stress and fragmentation of the red blood cells. In the third group, the conditions and MAHA are both the consequence of an underlying disorder that requires laboratory investigation for diagnosis.

MAHA and thrombocytopenia in patients with certain other conditions may result via more than one type of pathology (Table 49.11). For patients with renal injury, a kidney biopsy is often indicated for differential diagnosis.

In some patients of HSCT, myeloablation or infection may trigger AHUS due to preexisting genetic defects in the regulation of the alternative complement pathway. On the other hand, among patients who do not require long-term anti–graft-vs-host disease (anti-GVHD) therapy after HSCT, anti-ADAMTS13 inhibitors or anti-CFH antibodies may appear, resulting in acquired TTP or AHUS, a few months to over 1 year after the anti-GVHD treatment is discontinued.

PLATELET AND RED CELL DAMAGE BY ABNORMAL VASCULAR SURFACES

Platelets are subject to damage by interactions with "nonphysiologic" surfaces within the vascular system. Pathologic alterations of vessels that may produce such platelet damage include stenotic and roughened heart valves,[195] extensive atherosclerosis, metastatic cancer, and kidney disease associated with severe vascular changes in renal vessels.[196] An increasing number of surgical techniques involve the

Table 49.10. Clinical Conditions and the Likely Mechanisms of MAHA and Thrombocytopenia (Excluding TTP*)

Comorbid Condition	Cause or Mechanism	Confirmation of Diagnosis
Group 1: Triggering conditions		
Infection, vaccination, inflammation, trauma, surgery, or intravenous contrast agents	Triggers of complement activation may cause TMA in patients with defective complement regulation	AHUS genetic panel, CFH Ab Anti-C5 therapeutic diagnosis
Group 2: Etiologies with specific pathology		
Streptococcus pneumoniae *Clostridium perfringens* *Vibrio cholerae*	TMA due to Thomsen-Friedenreich (T) activation by microbial neuraminidases	RBC phenotyping with T-Ag binding lectins
Anti-VEGF drugs	TMA due to deprivation of VEGF	Drug discontinuation Kidney biopsy
Other drugs	TMA due to unknown mechanisms	
Heparin exposure	Heparin-induced thrombocytopenia with microvascular thrombosis	Heparin/PF4 Ab Serotonin release assay
Group 3: Syndromes due to a particular type of etiology		
Prodrome of diarrhea, often hemorrhagic	Shiga toxin-associated HUS	Shiga toxin analysis
Abdominal pain, bloody diarrhea, normal renal function	Paroxysmal nocturnal hemoglobinuria with mesenteric microvascular thrombosis	PNH flow cytometry
Fever, skin rashes, history of exposure	Vasculitis of *Rickettsia rickettsii* (Rocky Mountain spotted fever) or *Bacillus anthracis* (anthrax)	Serology, blood culture, tissue biopsy

Abbreviations: AHUS, atypical hemolytic-uremic syndrome; CFH, complement factor H; HUS, hemolytic-uremic syndrome; MAHA, microangiopathic hemolytic anemia; PF4, platelet factor 4; PNH, paroxysmal nocturnal hemoglobinuria; TMA, thrombotic microangiopathy; TTP, thrombotic thrombocytopenic purpura; VEGF, vascular endothelial growth factor.

Table 49.11. Comorbid Conditions With More Than One Potential Mechanism of MAHA and Thrombocytopenia (Excluding TTP*)

Comorbidity	Differential Diagnosis	Comments
Autoimmunity (ANA, ANCA, antiphospholipid Ab)	• Vasculitis or vasculopathy • Fibrin-platelet thrombosis (CAPS) • TMA of unknown pathogenesis • AHUS	• Biopsy is often indicated for differential diagnosis • Empiric anti-C5 for TMA, or mTOR inhibitors for vasculopathy
HIV infection	• Vasculitis of fungemia or viremia • TMA of unknown pathogenesis • AHUS	• Exclude or treat infection • Empiric anti-C5 for TMA after exclusion of infection
Hematopoietic stem cell therapy	• Vasculitis of fungemia or viremia • TMA due to myeloablative or anti-GVHD drugs • AHUS	• Exclude or treat infection • Adjust anti-GVHD regimen • Empiric anti-C5 after exclusion of other causes
Solid organ transplant	• Vasculitis of fungemia or viremia • Anti-rejection drugs • Severe rejection reaction • AHUS	• Exclude or treat infection • Adjust anti-rejection regimen • Biopsy for severe rejection vs TMA • Empiric anti-C5 therapy
Malignant hypertension or hypertensive crisis	• Severe hypertension causing endothelial injury • AHUS with severe hypertension	• Anti-hypertensive treatment • Kidney biopsy • Empiric anti-C5 therapy for TMA
Pregnancy	• Preeclampsia/HELLP syndrome • AHUS	• Termination of pregnancy • Empiric anti-C5 therapy for prominent renal failure, extrarenal complications of abnormal vascular permeability, or onset/persistence/worsening after delivery
Neoplastic disease	• Drug-induced TMA • Intravascular metastasis • AHUS	• Discontinue culprit drugs • Kidney biopsy • Bone marrow or tissue biopsy • Empiric anti-C5 for TMA after other causes are excluded

*ADAMTS13 test for all cases.
Abbreviations: AHUS, atypical hemolytic-uremic syndrome; ANA, antinuclear antibody; ANCA, antineutrophil cytoplasmic antibodies; CAPS, catastrophic antiphospholipid syndrome; GVHD, graft-vs-host disease; HELLP, hemolysis elevated liver enzymes and low platelet; MAHA, microangiopathic hemolytic anemia; mTOR, mammalian target of rapamycin; TMA, thrombotic microangiopathy; TTP, thrombotic thrombocytopenic purpura.

implantation of devices containing foreign material within the vascular system. Such circulatory prostheses include cardiac valves, vascular grafts or stents of many types, indwelling catheters,[197] intra-aortic balloon pumps,[198] extracorporeal membrane oxygenator (ECMO),[199] and VAD.[200] Vast efforts have been made to render such materials nonthrombogenic, but most of these devices produce varying degrees of platelet destruction as well as hemolysis.[201]

Cardiopulmonary bypass surgery may create a condition of bleeding diathesis. The factors contributing to bleeding are multifactorial, including surgical/vascular factors, dilution of clotting factors and platelets, inadequate neutralization of heparin, platelet dysfunction,[202] and enhanced fibrinolysis. Hemodilution leads to a rapid reduction in the platelet count and clotting factors by as much as 50% shortly after cardiopulmonary bypass surgery begins. Thromboelastography is used to monitor the adequacy of heparin neutralization and occurrence of excessive fibrinolysis. Platelets are activated and partially degranulated, This may contribute to platelet functional defects.[202,203]

Efforts to minimize platelet and coagulation abnormalities in association with cardiac surgery include higher heparin doses to suppress thrombin generation,[204,205] heparin-coated circuit,[205] miniaturized closed circuit,[206] and off-pump operations.[207] Avoidance of cardiotomy suction, perhaps in combination with a direct thrombin inhibitor such as bivalirudin or argatroban as the anticoagulant, may help minimize activation of the coagulation system.[208]

Bleeding is often reduced by infusion of normal platelets if there is thrombocytopenia or 1-deamino-8-D-arginine vasopressin for platelet dysfunction. If there is evidence of fibrinolysis, epsilon aminocaproic acid or tranexamic acid may help control bleeding.[209-213] Aprotinin is associated with a higher risk of end-organ damage.[214] Nitric oxide plus iloprost may reduce the deleterious effects of cardiopulmonary bypass on platelets and even reduce postoperative bleeding.[215]

Coronary stents are associated with platelet adhesion, activation, and aggregation that may contribute to intra-stent thrombosis. This is best controlled with dual antiplatelet drugs such as aspirin plus either clopidogrel or prasugrel,[216] usually for 6 to 15 months, until the stents are endothelialized. Surface endothelialization may be delayed in drug-eluting stents but promoted by surface modification and texturing.[217] Vascular factors such as calcification and progression of atherosclerosis and physical factors such as vessel-stent size mismatch may also contribute to the risk of thrombosis.

Red cell fragmentation and intravascular hemolysis is common in patients with left ventricular assist device (LVAD), ECMO, or prosthetic heart valves. In such patients, monitoring of plasma hemoglobin concentration is recommended. An increase in plasma hemoglobin level may herald intradevice thrombosis or dehiscence.

In patients with LVAD, particularly of the nonpulsatile type, analysis of vWF may show a decrease in the normal large multimers, creating a pattern similar to type 2A von Willebrand disease. Similar vWF multimer changes are also found in patients with aortic valve stenosis.[218] The vWF changes alone may not be sufficient to cause bleeding; yet, they may contribute to the bleeding diathesis induced by anticoagulation or antiplatelet therapy, thrombocytopenia, platelet function defects, and, most critically, angiodysplasia of the gastrointestinal tract.

Both LVAD and aortic valve stenosis are associated with angiodysplasia.[219,220] The association of gastrointestinal bleeding with aortic stenosis is often referred to as Heyde syndrome.[221] Efforts to replace the missing large vWF multimers have been futile. Instead, angiodysplasia resolves after replacement of the diseased aortic valve.[222] For LVAD, the risk of gastrointestinal bleeding is nearly 10-fold higher with nonpulsatile than with pulsatile ventricular devices.[219] Aortic stenosis and nonpulsatile LVAD share the common feature of narrow pulse pressures. It is assumed that narrow pulse pressures may promote angiodysplasia throughout the digestive tract,[223] presumably due to persistent dilatation of the precapillary sphincters and activation of the angiogenesis signaling cascade via the hypoxia-inducible factor-1α/angiopoietin-2 pathway. In a retrospective review with multivariate-adjusted Cox regression, the use of digoxin, an inhibitor of HIF-1α synthesis, was associated with an 80% reduction in the risk of gastrointestinal bleeding due to angiodysplasia, but no difference in non-angiodysplasia bleeding.[224]

MISCELLANEOUS FORMS OF NONIMMUNOLOGIC PLATELET DESTRUCTION

In patients hospitalized for burns, the platelet count follows a distinct course—decreasing by 50% to a nadir of ~150 × 10^9/L by day 3, followed by increasing to a peak of ~650 × 10^9/L by day 15, before declining to the normal upper normal limit of ~400 × 10^9/L by 4 weeks.[225] The mechanism of platelet count decrease soon after burn injury is not determined, but likely results from entrapment of platelets in thermally injured vessels. It is not associated with decreased megakaryocytes in the bone marrow or disseminated intravascular coagulation.[226] A lower peak level is associated with a higher mortality, independent of age, % burn surface area, and sepsis.

Thrombocytopenia has been well described after hepatic cryotherapy.[227,228] After hepatic cryotherapy, platelets primarily accumulate within the cryolesion, presumably due to vascular and platelet cryoinjury, with the magnitude of decrease relating to the extent of hepatocellular injury. Thrombocytopenia may also occur with therapeutic hypothermia.[229,230] Platelet activity is sensitive to low temperature. In vitro, shear-induced platelet aggregation is progressively increased as the temperature decreases below 35 °C.[231]

Certain drugs may produce thrombocytopenia by nonimmunologic mechanisms. Ristocetin, an antituberculous agent no longer used clinically, promotes the attachment of vWF to platelet receptor glycoprotein Ib/IX and initiates platelet-platelet aggregation. Type 2B- or pseudo–von Willebrand disease, characterized by platelet aggregation induced in vitro with low concentrations of ristocetin, may present with thrombocytopenia, presumably due to shear-induced vWF-platelet aggregation in vivo.

Oxaliplatin commonly causes thrombocytopenia due to bone marrow toxicity. Occasionally drug-dependent immune thrombocytopenia may occur.[232] After repeated treatment cycles, oxaliplatin may cause prolonged thrombocytopenia due to portal hypertension and splenomegaly, a consequence of oxaliplatin-induced hepatic sinusoidal injury and fibrosis.[233] Protamine may produce transient thrombocytopenia due to reversible accumulation of platelets in the liver without affecting survival.[234]

References

1. Nagaoka T, Yoshida A. Noninvasive evaluation of wall shear stress on retinal microcirculation in humans. *Invest Ophthalmol Vis Sci.* 2006;47:1113-1119.
2. Leverett LB, Hellums JD, Alfrey CP, Lynch EC. Red blood cell damage by shear stress. *Biophys J.* 1972;12:257-273.
3. Moschcowitz E. An acute febrile pleiochromic anemia with hyaline thrombosis of the terminal arterioles and capillaries: an undescribed disease. *Proc NY Pathol Soc.* 1924;1924:21-24.
4. Asada Y, Sumiyoshi A, Hayashi T, Suzumiya J, Kaketani K. Immunohistochemistry of vascular lesion in thrombotic thrombocytopenic purpura, with special reference to factor VIII related antigen. *Thromb Res.* 1985;38:469-479.
5. Tsai HM, Chandler WL, Sarode R, et al. von Willebrand factor and von Willebrand factor-cleaving metalloprotease activity in *Escherichia coli* O157:H7-associated hemolytic uremic syndrome. *Pediatr Res.* 2001;49:653-659.
6. Hosler GA, Cusumano AM, Hutchins GM. Thrombotic thrombocytopenic purpura and hemolytic uremic syndrome are distinct pathologic entities. A review of 56 autopsy cases. *Arch Pathol Lab Med.* 2003;127:834-839.
7. Tsai HM, Lian EC. Antibodies to von Willebrand factor-cleaving protease in acute thrombotic thrombocytopenic purpura. *N Engl J Med.* 1998;339:1585-1594.
8. Furlan M, Robles R, Galbusera M, et al. von Willebrand factor-cleaving protease in thrombotic thrombocytopenic purpura and the hemolytic-uremic syndrome. *N Engl J Med.* 1998;339:1578-1584.
9. Levy GG, Nichols WC, Lian EC, et al. Mutations in a member of the ADAMTS gene family cause thrombotic thrombocytopenic purpura. *Nature.* 2001;413:488-494.
10. Zhou W, Inada M, Lee TP, et al. ADAMTS13 is expressed in hepatic stellate cells. *Lab Invest.* 2005;85:780-788.
11. Uemura M, Tatsumi K, Matsumoto M, et al. Localization of ADAMTS13 to the stellate cells of human liver. *Blood.* 2005;106:922-924.
12. Cao WJ, Niiya M, Zheng XW, Shang DZ, Zheng XL. Inflammatory cytokines inhibit ADAMTS13 synthesis in hepatic stellate cells and endothelial cells. *J Thromb Haemost.* 2008;6:1233-1235.
13. Manea M, Kristoffersson A, Schneppenheim R, et al. Podocytes express ADAMTS13 in normal renal cortex and in patients with thrombotic thrombocytopenic purpura. *Br J Haematol.* 2007;138:651-662.
14. Turner N, Nolasco L, Tao Z, Dong JF, Moake J. Human endothelial cells synthesize and release ADAMTS-13. *J.Thromb.Haemost.* 2006;4:1396-1404.
15. Brodin-Sartorius A, Guebre-Egziabher F, Fouque D, et al. Recurrent idiopathic thrombotic thrombocytopenic purpura: a role for vaccination in disease relapse? *Am J Kidney Dis.* 2006;48:e31-e34.
16. Sissa C, Al-Khaffaf A, Frattini F, et al. Relapse of thrombotic thrombocytopenic purpura after COVID-19 vaccine. *Transfus Apher Sci.* 2021;60:103145.
17. Kojima Y, Ohashi H, Nakamura T, et al. Acute thrombotic thrombocytopenic purpura after pneumococcal vaccination. *Blood Coagul Fibrinolysis.* 2014;25:512-514.
18. Tehrani HA, Darnahal M, Vaezi M, Haghighi S. COVID-19 associated thrombotic thrombocytopenic purpura (TTP); A case series and mini-review. *Int Immunopharmacol.* 2021;93:107397.
19. Kirpalani A, Garabon J, Amos K, et al. Thrombotic thrombocytopenic purpura temporally associated with BNT162b2 vaccination in an adolescent successfully treated with caplacizumab. *Br J Haematol.* 2021;196(1):e11-e14.
20. Al-Ahmad M, Al-Rasheed M, Shalaby NAB. Acquired thrombotic thrombocytopenic purpura with possible association with AstraZeneca-Oxford COVID-19 vaccine. *EJHaem.* 2021;2(3):534-536.
21. Waqar SHB, Khan AA, Memon S. Thrombotic thrombocytopenic purpura: a new menace after COVID bnt162b2 vaccine. *Int J Hematol.* 2021;114(5):626-629.
22. Chamarti K, Dar K, Reddy A, et al. Thrombotic thrombocytopenic purpura presentation in an elderly gentleman following COVID vaccine circumstances. *Cureus.* 2021;13:e16619.
23. Yocum A, Simon EL. Thrombotic thrombocytopenic purpura after Ad26.COV2-S vaccination. *Am J Emerg Med.* 2021;49:441.e3-441.e4.
24. de Bruijn S, Maes MB, De Waele L, Vanhoorelbeke K, Gadisseur A. First report of a de novo iTTP episode associated with an mRNA-based anti-COVID-19 vaccination. *J Thromb Haemost.* 2021;19:2014-2018.
25. Bennett CL, Weinberg PD, Rozenberg-Ben-Dror K, et al. Thrombotic thrombocytopenic purpura associated with ticlopidine. A review of 60 cases. *Ann Intern Med.* 1998;128:541-544.
26. Tsai HM, Rice L, Sarode R, Chow TW, Moake JL. Antibody inhibitors to von Willebrand factor metalloproteinase and increased binding of von Willebrand factor to platelets in ticlopidine-associated thrombotic thrombocytopenic purpura. *Ann Intern Med.* 2000;132:794-799.
27. Bennett CL, Connors JM, Carwile JM, et al. Thrombotic thrombocytopenic purpura associated with clopidogrel. *N Engl J Med.* 2000;342:1773-1777.
28. Tsai HM. Acquired thrombotic thrombocytopenic purpura—a disease due to inhibitors of ADAMTS13. In Rodgers GM (ed.), *ADAMTS13—Biology and Disease*, Springer, 2015;Chapter 6:91-128.
29. Tsai HM, Li A, Rock G. Inhibitors of von Willebrand factor-cleaving protease in thrombotic thrombocytopenic purpura. *Clin Lab.* 2001;47:387-392.
30. Tsai HM. High titers of inhibitors of von Willebrand factor-cleaving metalloproteinase in a fatal case of acute thrombotic thrombocytopenic purpura. *Am J Hematol.* 2000;65:251-255.
31. Ferrari S, Mudde GC, Rieger M, et al. IgG subclass distribution of anti-ADAMTS13 antibodies in patients with acquired thrombotic thrombocytopenic purpura. *J Thromb Haemost.* 2009;7:1703-1710.
32. Pos W, Luken BM, Hovinga JA, et al. VH1-69 germline encoded antibodies directed towards ADAMTS13 in patients with acquired thrombotic thrombocytopenic purpura. *J Thromb Haemost.* 2009;7:421-428.
33. Akiyama M, Takeda S, Kokame K, Takagi J, Miyata T. Crystal structures of the noncatalytic domains of ADAMTS13 reveal multiple discontinuous exosites for von Willebrand factor. *Proc Natl Acad Sci USA.* 2009;106:19274-19279.
34. Crawley JT, de GR, Xiang Y, Luken BM, Lane DA. Unraveling the scissile bond: how ADAMTS13 recognizes and cleaves von Willebrand factor. *Blood.* 2011;118:3212-3221.
35. Zhou W, Dong L, Ginsburg D, Bouhassira EE, Tsai HM. Enzymatically active ADAMTS13 variants are not inhibited by anti-ADAMTS13 autoantibodies: a novel therapeutic strategy? *J Biol Chem.* 2005;280:39934-39941.
36. Yu S, Liu W, Fang J, et al. AFM imaging reveals multiple conformational states of ADAMTS13. *J Biol Eng.* 2019;13:9.
37. South K, Luken BM, Crawley JT, et al. Conformational activation of ADAMTS13. *Proc Natl Acad Sci USA.* 2014;111:18578-18583.
38. Jian C, Xiao J, Gong L, et al. Gain-of-function ADAMTS13 variants that are resistant to autoantibodies against ADAMTS13 in patients with acquired thrombotic thrombocytopenic purpura. *Blood.* 2012;119:3836-3843.
39. Zhou W, Bouhassira EE, Tsai HM. An IAP retrotransposon in the mouse ADAMTS13 gene creates ADAMTS13 variant proteins that are less effective in cleaving von Willebrand factor multimers. *Blood.* 2007;110:886-893.
40. South K, Freitas MO, Lane DA. Conformational quiescence of ADAMTS-13 prevents proteolytic promiscuity. *J Thromb Haemost.* 2016;14:2011-2022.
41. Zheng XL, Wu HM, Shang D, et al. Multiple domains of ADAMTS13 are targeted by autoantibodies against ADAMTS13 in patients with acquired idiopathic thrombotic thrombocytopenic purpura. *Haematologica.* 2010;95:1555-1562.
42. Schneppenheim R, Kremer Hovinga JA, Becker T, et al. A common origin of the 4143insA ADAMTS13 mutation. *Thromb Haemost.* 2006;96:3-6.
43. Akiyama M, Kokame K, Miyata T. ADAMTS13 P475S polymorphism causes a lowered enzymatic activity and urea lability in vitro. *J Thromb Haemost.* 2008;6:1830-1832.
44. Jang MJ, Kim NK, Chong SY, et al. Frequency of Pro475Ser polymorphism of ADAMTS13 gene and its association with ADAMTS-13 activity in the Korean population. *Yonsei Med J.* 2008;49:405-408.
45. Ruan C, Dai L, Su J, Wang Z, Ruan C. The frequency of P475S polymorphism in von Willebrand factor-cleaving protease in the Chinese population and its relevance to arterial thrombotic disorders. *Thromb Haemost.* 2004;91:1257-1258.

46. Kokame K, Matsumoto M, Soejima K, et al. Mutations and common polymorphisms in ADAMTS13 gene responsible for von Willebrand factor-cleaving protease activity. *Proc Natl Acad Sci USA.* 2002;99:11902-11907.
47. Plaimauer B, Fuhrmann J, Mohr G, et al. Modulation of ADAMTS13 secretion and specific activity by a combination of common amino acid polymorphisms and a missense mutation. *Blood.* 2006;107:118-125.
48. Banno F, Kokame K, Okuda T, et al. Complete deficiency in ADAMTS13 is prothrombotic, but it alone is not sufficient to cause thrombotic thrombocytopenic purpura. *Blood.* 2006;107:3161-3166.
49. Feys HB, Roodt J, Vandeputte N, et al. Thrombotic thrombocytopenic purpura directly linked with ADAMTS13 inhibition in the baboon (*Papio ursinus*). *Blood.* 2010;116:2005-2010.
50. Motto DG, Chauhan AK, Zhu G, et al. Shigatoxin triggers thrombotic thrombocytopenic purpura in genetically susceptible ADAMTS13-deficient mice. *J Clin Invest.* 2005;115:2752-2761.
51. Burns ER, Zucker-Franklin D. Pathologic effects of plasma from patients with thrombotic thrombocytopenic purpura on platelets and cultured vascular endothelial cells. *Blood.* 1982;60:1030-1037.
52. Hori Y, Wada H, Mori Y, et al. Plasma sFas and sFas ligand levels in patients with thrombotic thrombocytopenic purpura and in those with disseminated intravascular coagulation. *Am J Hematol.* 1999;61:21-25.
53. Kelton JG, Moore JC, Murphy WG. The platelet aggregating factor(s) of thrombotic thrombocytopenic purpura. *Prog Clin Biol Res.* 1990;337:141-149.
54. Leung DY, Moake JL, Havens PL, Kim M, Pober JS. Lytic anti-endothelial cell antibodies in haemolytic-uraemic syndrome. *Lancet.* 1988;2:183-186.
55. Schultz DR, Arnold PI, Jy W, et al. Anti-CD36 autoantibodies in thrombotic thrombocytopenic purpura and other thrombotic disorders: identification of an 85 kD form of CD36 as a target antigen. *Br J Haematol.* 1998;103:849-857.
56. Siddiqui FA, Lian EC. Platelet-agglutinating protein P37 from a thrombotic thrombocytopenic purpura plasma forms a complex with human immunoglobulin G. *Blood.* 1988;71:299-304.
57. Tandon NN, Rock G, Jamieson GA. Anti-CD36 antibodies in thrombotic thrombocytopenic purpura. *Br J Haematol.* 1994;88:816-825.
58. Ruggeri ZM, Zimmerman TS. The complex multimeric composition of factor VIII/von Willebrand factor. *Blood.* 1981;57:1140-1143.
59. Weiss HJ, Turitto VT, Baumgartner HR. Effect of shear rate on platelet interaction with subendothelium in citrated and native blood. I. Shear rate: dependent decrease of adhesion in von Willebrand's disease and the Bernard-Soulier syndrome. *J Lab Clin Med.* 1978;92:750-764.
60. Dent JA, Berkowitz SD, Ware J, Kasper CK, Ruggeri ZM. Identification of a cleavage site directing the immunochemical detection of molecular abnormalities in type IIA von Willebrand factor. *Proc Natl Acad Sci USA.* 1990;87:6306-6310.
61. Tsai HM, Sussman II, Nagel RL. Shear stress enhances the proteolysis of von Willebrand factor in normal plasma. *Blood.* 1994;83:2171-2179.
62. Tsai HM. Von Willebrand factor, ADAMTS13, and thrombotic thrombocytopenic purpura. *J Mol Med.* 2002;80:639-647.
63. Marchant RE, Barb MD, Shainoff JR, et al. Three dimensional structure of human fibrinogen under aqueous conditions visualized by atomic force microscopy. *Thromb Haemost.* 1997;77:1048-1051.
64. Schneider SW, Nuschele S, Wixforth A, et al. Shear-induced unfolding triggers adhesion of von Willebrand factor fibers. *Proc Natl Acad Sci USA.* 2007;104:7899-7903.
65. Bonnefoy A, Daenens K, Feys HB, et al. Thrombospondin-1 controls vascular platelet recruitment and thrombus adherence in mice by protecting (sub)endothelial VWF from cleavage by ADAMTS13. *Blood.* 2006;107:955-964.
66. Siedlecki CA, Lestini BJ, Kottke-Marchant KK, et al. Shear-dependent changes in the three-dimensional structure of human von Willebrand factor. *Blood.* 1996;88:2939-2950.
67. Tsai HM, Sussman II, Ginsburg D, et al. Proteolytic cleavage of recombinant type 2A von Willebrand factor mutants R834W and R834Q: inhibition by doxycycline and by monoclonal antibody VP-1. *Blood.* 1997;89:1954-1962.
68. Singh I, Shankaran H, Beauharnois ME, et al. Solution structure of human von Willebrand factor studied using small angle neutron scattering. *J Biol Chem.* 2006;281:38266-38275.
69. Singh I, Themistou E, Porcar L, Neelamegham S. Fluid shear induces conformation change in human blood protein von Willebrand factor in solution. *Biophys J.* 2009;96:2313-2320.
70. Moake JL, Rudy CK, Troll JH, et al. Unusually large plasma factor VIII:von Willebrand factor multimers in chronic relapsing thrombotic thrombocytopenic purpura. *N Engl J Med.* 1982;307:1432-1435.
71. Ruggeri ZM, Mannucci PM, Lombardi R, Federici AB, Zimmerman TS. Multimeric composition of factor VIII/von Willebrand factor following administration of DDAVP: implications for pathophysiology and therapy of von Willebrand's disease subtypes. *Blood.* 1982;59:1272-1278.
72. Dobson CE, Tsai HM. HIV infection increases the risk of thrombotic thrombocytopenic purpura. *J Thromb Circ.* 2018;4:127-123. doi:10.4172/2572-9462.1000127.
73. Terrell DR, Williams LA, Vesely SK, et al. The incidence of thrombotic thrombocytopenic purpura-hemolytic uremic syndrome: all patients, idiopathic patients, and patients with severe ADAMTS-13 deficiency. *J Thromb Haemost.* 2005;3:1432-1436.
74. Tsai HM. The kidney in thrombotic thrombocytopenic purpura. *Minerva Med.* 2007;98:731-747.
75. Veyradier A, Brivet F, Wolf M, et al. Total deficiency of specific von Willebrand factor-cleaving protease and recovery following plasma therapy in one patient with hemolytic-uremic syndrome. *Hematol J.* 2001;2:352-354.
76. Noris M, Bucchioni S, Galbusera M, et al. Complement factor H mutation in familial thrombotic thrombocytopenic purpura with ADAMTS13 deficiency and renal involvement. *J Am Soc Nephrol.* 2005;16:1177-1183.
77. Tsai E, Chapin J, Laurence JC, Tsai HM. Use of eculizumab in the treatment of a case of refractory, ADAMTS13-deficient thrombotic thrombocytopenic purpura: additional data and clinical follow-up. *Br J Haematol.* 2013;162:558-559.
78. Bentley MJ, Lehman CM, Blaylock RC, Wilson AR, Rodgers GM. The utility of patient characteristics in predicting severe ADAMTS13 deficiency and response to plasma exchange. *Transfusion.* 2010;50:1654-1664.
79. Benhamou Y, AssiÃ© C, Boelle PY, et al. Development and validation of a predictive model for death in acquired severe ADAMTS13 deficiency-associated idiopathic thrombotic thrombocytopenic purpura: the French TMA Reference Center experience. *Haematologica.* 2012;97:1181-1186.
80. Bendapudi PK, Hurwitz S, Fry A, et al. Derivation and external validation of the PLASMIC score for rapid assessment of adults with thrombotic microangiopathies: a cohort study. *Lancet Haematol.* 2017;4:e157-e164.
81. Bukowski RM, King JW, Hewlett JS. Plasmapheresis in the treatment of thrombotic thrombocytopenic purpura. *Blood.* 1977;50:413-417.
82. Byrnes JJ, Khurana M. Treatment of thrombotic thrombocytopenic purpura with plasma. *N Engl J Med.* 1977;297:1386-1389.
83. Rock GA, Shumak KH, Buskard NA, et al. Comparison of plasma exchange with plasma infusion in the treatment of thrombotic thrombocytopenic purpura. Canadian Apheresis Study Group. *N Engl J Med.* 1991;325:393-397.
84. Tsai HM, Shulman K. Rituximab induces remission of cerebral ischemia caused by thrombotic thrombocytopenic purpura. *Eur J Haematol.* 2003;70:183-185.
85. Galindo-Calvillo CD, RodrÃ CS, GÃ³mez-De LA, TarÃ L, GÃ³mez-Almaguer D. Treating thrombotic thrombocytopenic purpura without plasma exchange during the COVID-19 pandemic. A case report and a brief literature review. *Transfus Apher Sci.* 2021;60:103107.
86. Gutterman LA, Kloster B, Tsai HM. Rituximab therapy for refractory thrombotic thrombocytopenic purpura. *Blood Cells Mol Dis.* 2002;28:385-391.
87. Chemnitz J, Draube A, Scheid C, et al. Successful treatment of severe thrombotic thrombocytopenic purpura with the monoclonal antibody rituximab. *Am J Hematol.* 2002;71:105-108.
88. Yomtovian R, Niklinski W, Silver B, Sarode R, Tsai HM. Rituximab for chronic recurring thrombotic thrombocytopenic purpura: a case report and review of the literature. *Br J Haematol.* 2004;124:787-795.
89. Elliott MA, Heit JA, Pruthi RK, et al. Rituximab for refractory and or relapsing thrombotic thrombocytopenic purpura related to immune-mediated severe ADAMTS13-deficiency: a report of four cases and a systematic review of the literature. *Eur J Haematol.* 2009;83:365-372.
90. Fakhouri F, Vernant JP, Veyradier A, et al. Efficiency of curative and prophylactic treatment with rituximab in ADAMTS13-deficient thrombotic thrombocytopenic purpura: a study of 11 cases. *Blood.* 2005;106:1932-1937.
91. Galbusera M, Bresin E, Noris M, et al. Rituximab prevents recurrence of thrombotic thrombocytopenic purpura: a case report. *Blood.* 2005;106:925-928.
92. Scully M, McDonald V, Cavenagh J, et al. A phase 2 study of the safety and efficacy of rituximab with plasma exchange in acute acquired thrombotic thrombocytopenic purpura. *Blood.* 2011;118:1746-1753.
93. Tsai H. New concepts of thrombotic thrombocytopenic purpura and a strategy to prevent its relapse. *J Hematol Thromboembolic Dis* 2014;2:157-167.
94. McDonald V, Manns K, MacKie IJ, Machin SJ, Scully MA. Rituximab pharmacokinetics during the management of acute idiopathic thrombotic thrombocytopenic purpura. *J Thromb Haemost.* 2010;8:1201-1208.
95. Tsai HM, Kuo E. Eculizumab therapy leads to rapid resolution of thrombocytopenia in atypical hemolytic uremic syndrome. *Adv Hematol.* 2014;2014:295323.
96. Bhoj VG, Arhontoulis D, Wertheim G, et al. Persistence of long-lived plasma cells and humoral immunity in individuals responding to CD19-directed CAR T-cell therapy. *Blood.* 2016;128:360-370.
97. Shortt J, Oh DH, Opat SS. ADAMTS13 antibody depletion by bortezomib in thrombotic thrombocytopenic purpura. *N Engl J Med.* 2013;368:90-92.
98. Aqui NA, Stein SH, Konkle BA, Abrams CS, Strobl FJ. Role of splenectomy in patients with refractory or relapsed thrombotic thrombocytopenic purpura. *J Clin Apheresis.* 2003;18:51-54.
99. Kristinsson SY, Gridley G, Hoover RN, Check D, Landgren O. Long-term risks after splenectomy among 8,149 cancer-free American veterans: a cohort study with up to 27 years follow-up. *Haematologica.* 2014;99:392-398.
100. Coppo P, Bubenheim M, Azoulay E, et al. A regimen with caplacizumab, immunosuppression, and plasma exchange prevents unfavorable outcomes in immune-mediated TTP. *Blood.* 2021;137:733-742.
101. Goshua G, Sinha P, Hendrickson JE, et al. Cost effectiveness of caplacizumab in acquired thrombotic thrombocytopenic purpura. *Blood.* 2021;137:969-976.
102. Shortt J, Opat SS, Wood EM. N-Acetylcysteine for thrombotic thrombocytopenic purpura: is a von Willebrand factor-inhibitory dose feasible in vivo? *Transfusion.* 2014;54:2362-2363.
103. Schulman I, Pierce M, Lukens A, Currimbhoy Z. Studies on thrombopoiesis. I. A factor in normal human plasma required for platelet production; Chronic thrombocytopenia due to its deficiency. *Blood.* 1960;16:943-957.
104. Upshaw JD, Jr. Congenital deficiency of a factor in normal plasma that reverses microangiopathic hemolysis and thrombocytopenia. *N Engl J Med.* 1978;298:1350-1352.
105. Jubinsky PT, Moraille R, Tsai HM. Thrombotic thrombocytopenic purpura in a newborn. *J Perinatol.* 2003;23:85-87.
106. Schiff DE, Roberts WD, Willert J, Tsai HM. Thrombocytopenia and severe hyperbilirubinemia in the neonatal period secondary to congenital thrombotic thrombocytopenic purpura and ADAMTS13 deficiency. *J Pediatr Hematol Oncol.* 2004;26:535-538.
107. Veyradier A, Obert B, Haddad E, et al. Severe deficiency of the specific von Willebrand factor-cleaving protease (ADAMTS 13) activity in a subgroup of children with atypical hemolytic uremic syndrome. *J Pediatr.* 2003;142:310-317.
108. Tsai HM. Mechanisms of microvascular thrombosis in thrombotic thrombocytopenic purpura. *Kidney Int Suppl.* 2009;112:S11-S14.

109. Peyvandi F, Mannucci PM, Valsecchi C, et al. ADAMTS13 content in plasma-derived factor VIII/von Willebrand factor concentrates. *Am J Hematol*. 2013;88:895-898.
110. Lattuada A, Rossi E, Calzarossa C, Candolfi R, Mannucci PM. Mild to moderate reduction of a von Willebrand factor cleaving protease (ADAMTS-13) in pregnant women with HELLP microangiopathic syndrome. *Haematologica*. 2003;88:1029-1034.
111. Sanchez-Luceros A, Farias CE, Amaral MM, et al. von Willebrand factor-cleaving protease (ADAMTS13) activity in normal non-pregnant women, pregnant and post-delivery women. *Thromb Haemost*. 2004;92:1320-1326.
112. Gasser C, Gautier E, Steck A, et al. Hamolytisch-uramische sydrome: bilaterale Nierenrindennekrosen bei akutenerworbenen hamolytischen anamien. *Schweiz Med Wochenshr*. 1955;85:905-909.
113. Majowicz SE, Scallan E, Jones-Bitton A, et al. Global incidence of human Shiga toxin-producing *Escherichia coli* infections and deaths: a systematic review and knowledge synthesis. *Foodborne Pathog Dis*. 2014;11:447-455.
114. Tarr PI, Gordon CA, Chandler WL. Shiga-toxin-producing *Escherichia coli* and haemolytic uraemic syndrome. *Lancet*. 2005;365:1073-1086.
115. Kampmeier S, Berger M, Mellmann A, Karch H, Berger P. The 2011 German enterohemorrhagic Escherichia coli O104:H4 outbreak—the danger is still out there. *Curr Top Microbiol Immunol*. 2018;416:117-148.
116. Joseph A, Rafat C, Zafrani L, et al. Early differentiation of shiga toxin-associated hemolytic uremic syndrome in critically ill adults with thrombotic microangiopathy syndromes. *Crit Care Med*. 2018;46:e904-e911.
117. Habib R. Pathology of the hemolytic uremic syndrome. In: Kaplan BS, Trompeter RS, Moake JL, eds. *Hemolytic Uremic Syndrome and Thrombotic Thrombocytopenic Purpura*. Vol 10. Marcel Dekker; 1992:315-353.
118. Inward CD, Howie AJ, Fitzpatrick MM, et al. Renal histopathology in fatal cases of diarrhoea-associated haemolytic uraemic syndrome. British Association for Paediatric Nephrology. *Pediatr Nephrol*. 1997;11:556-559.
119. Obrig TG, Del Vecchio PJ, Brown JE, et al. Direct cytotoxic action of Shiga toxin on human vascular endothelial cells. *Infect Immun*. 1988;56:2373-2378.
120. Louise CB, Obrig TG. Shiga toxin-associated hemolytic-uremic syndrome: combined cytotoxic effects of Shiga toxin, interleukin-1 beta, and tumor necrosis factor alpha on human vascular endothelial cells in vitro. *Infect Immun*. 1991;59:4173-4179.
121. Morigi M, Galbusera M, Binda E, et al. Verotoxin-1-induced up-regulation of adhesive molecules renders microvascular endothelial cells thrombogenic at high shear stress. *Blood*. 2001;98:1828-1835.
122. Jandhyala DM, Ahluwalia A, Obrig T, Thorpe CM. ZAK: a MAP3Kinase that transduces Shiga toxin- and ricin-induced proinflammatory cytokine expression. *Cell Microbiol*. 2008;10:1468-1477.
123. Cherla RP, Lee SY, Mulder RA, Lee MS, Tesh VL. Shiga toxin 1-induced proinflammatory cytokine production is regulated by the phosphatidylinositol 3-kinase/Akt/mammalian target of rapamycin signaling pathway. *Infect Immun*. 2009;77:3919-3931.
124. Lee SY, Lee MS, Cherla RP, Tesh VL. Shiga toxin 1 induces apoptosis through the endoplasmic reticulum stress response in human monocytic cells. *Cell Microbiol*. 2008;10:770-780.
125. Huang J, Haberichter SL, Sadler JE. The B subunits of Shiga-like toxins induce regulated VWF secretion in a phospholipase D1-dependent manner. *Blood*. 2012;120:1143-1149.
126. Orth D, Khan AB, Naim A, et al. Shiga toxin activates complement and binds factor H: evidence for an active role of complement in hemolytic uremic syndrome. *J Immunol*. 2009;182:6394-6400.
127. Petruzziello-Pellegrini TN, Marsden PA. Shiga toxin-associated hemolytic uremic syndrome: advances in pathogenesis and therapeutics. *Curr Opin Nephrol Hypertens*. 2012;21:433-440.
128. McGannon CM, Fuller CA, Weiss AA. Different classes of antibiotics differentially influence shiga toxin production. *Antimicrob Agents Chemother*. 2010;54:3790-3798.
129. Brandt JR, Fouser LS, Watkins SL, et al. *Escherichia coli* O 157:H7-associated hemolytic uremic syndrome after ingestion of contaminated hamburgers. *J Pediatr*. 1994;125:519-526.
130. Carter AO, Borczyk AA, Carlson JA, et al. A severe outbreak of *Escherichia coli* O157:H7--associated hemorrhagic colitis in a nursing home. *N Engl J Med*. 1987;317:1496-1500.
131. Chandler WL, Jelacic S, Boster DR, et al. Prothrombotic coagulation abnormalities preceding the hemolytic-uremic syndrome. *N Engl J Med*. 2002;346:23-32.
132. Tapper D, Tarr P, Avner E, Brandt J, Waldhausen J. Lessons learned in the management of hemolytic uremic syndrome in children. *J Pediatr Surg*. 1995;30:158-163.
133. Steinborn M, Leiz S, Rudisser K, et al. CT and MRI in haemolytic uraemic syndrome with central nervous system involvement: distribution of lesions and prognostic value of imaging findings. *Pediatr Radiol*. 2004;34:805-810.
134. Gould LH, Bopp C, Strockbine N, et al. Recommendations for diagnosis of shiga toxin--producing *Escherichia coli* infections by clinical laboratories. *MMWR Recomm Rep (Morb Mortal Wkly Rep)*. 2009;58:1-14.
135. Grisaru S, Xie J, Samuel S, et al. Associations between hydration status, intravenous fluid administration, and outcomes of patients infected with shiga toxin-producing *Escherichia coli*: a systematic review and meta-analysis. *JAMA Pediatr*. 2017;171:68-76.
136. Loirat C, Sonsino E, Hinglais N, et al. Treatment of the childhood haemolytic uraemic syndrome with plasma. A multicentre randomized controlled trial. The French Society of Paediatric Nephrology. *Pediatr Nephrol*. 1988;2:279-285.
137. Rizzoni G, Claris-Appiani A, Edefonti A, et al. Plasma infusion for hemolytic-uremic syndrome in children: results of a multicenter controlled trial. *J Pediatr*. 1988;112:284-290.
138. Dundas S, Murphy J, Soutar RL, et al. Effectiveness of therapeutic plasma exchange in the 1996 Lanarkshire *Escherichia coli* O157:H7 outbreak. *Lancet*. 1999;354:1327-1330.
139. Kakoullis L, Papachristodoulou E, Chra P, Panos G. Shiga toxin-induced hemolytic uraemic syndrome and the role of antibiotics: a global overview. *J Infect*. 2019;79:75-94.
140. Imdad A, Mackoff SP, Urciuoli DM, et al. Interventions for preventing diarrhoea-associated haemolytic uraemic syndrome. *Cochrane Database Syst Rev*. 2021;7:CD012997.
141. Morigi M, Galbusera M, Gastoldi S, et al. Alternative pathway activation of complement by Shiga toxin promotes exuberant C3a formation that triggers microvascular thrombosis. *J Immunol*. 2011;187:172-180.
142. Dinh A, Anathasayanan A, Rubin LM. Safe and effective use of eculizumab in the treatment of severe Shiga toxin Escherichia coli-associated hemolytic uremic syndrome. *Am J Health Syst Pharm*. 2015;72:117-120.
143. Lapeyraque AL, Malina M, Fremeaux-Bacchi V, et al. Eculizumab in severe shiga-toxin-associated HUS. *N Engl J Med*. 2011;364:2561-2563.
144. Gagnadoux MF, Habib R, Gubler MC, Bacri JL, Broyer M. Long-term (15-25 years) outcome of childhood hemolytic-uremic syndrome. *Clin Nephrol*. 1996;46:39-41.
145. Garg AX, Suri RS, Barrowman N, et al. Long-term renal prognosis of diarrhea-associated hemolytic uremic syndrome: a systematic review, meta-analysis, and meta-regression. *JAMA*. 2003;290:1360-1370.
146. Marshall JK. Post-infectious irritable bowel syndrome following water contamination. *Kidney Int Suppl*. 2009;112:S42-S43.
147. Nevis IF, Sontrop JM, Clark WF, et al. Hypertension in pregnancy after *Escherichia coli* O157:H7 gastroenteritis: a cohort study. *Hypertens Pregnancy*. 2013;32:390-400.
148. Alberti M, Valoti E, Piras R, et al. Two patients with history of STEC-HUS, posttransplant recurrence and complement gene mutations. *Am J Transplant*. 2013;13:2201-2206.
149. Fakhouri F, Roumenina L, Provot F, et al. Pregnancy-associated hemolytic uremic syndrome revisited in the era of complement gene mutations. *J Am Soc Nephrol*. 2010;21:859-867.
150. Tsai HM. Atypical hemolytic uremic syndrome: beyond hemolysis and uremia. *Am J Med*. 2019;132:161-167.
151. Tsai HM. Does anticomplement therapy have a role in the management of malignant hypertension? *J Clin Hypertens*. 2016;18:359-360.
152. Taylor CM, Chua C, Howie AJ, Risdon RA. Clinico-pathological findings in diarrhoea-negative haemolytic uraemic syndrome. *Pediatr Nephrol*. 2004;19:419-425.
153. Le QM, Roumenina L, Noris M, Fremeaux-Bacchi V. Atypical hemolytic uremic syndrome associated with mutations in complement regulator genes. *Semin Thromb Hemost*. 2010;36:641-652.
154. Maga TK, Nishimura CJ, Weaver AE, Frees KL, Smith RJ. Mutations in alternative pathway complement proteins in American patients with atypical hemolytic uremic syndrome. *Hum Mutat*. 2010;31:E1445-E1460.
155. Noris M, Caprioli J, Bresin E, et al. Relative role of genetic complement abnormalities in sporadic and familial aHUS and their impact on clinical phenotype. *Clin J Am Soc Nephrol*. 2010;5:1844-1859.
156. Dragon-Durey MA, Sethi SK, Bagga A, et al. Clinical features of anti-factor H autoantibody-associated hemolytic uremic syndrome. *J Am Soc Nephrol*. 2010;21:2180-2187.
157. Moore I, Strain L, Pappworth I, et al. Association of factor H autoantibodies with deletions of CFHR1, CFHR3, CFHR4, and with mutations in CFH, CFI, CD46, and C3 in patients with atypical hemolytic uremic syndrome. *Blood*. 2010;115:379-387.
158. Bienaime F, Dragon-Durey MA, Regnier CH, et al. Mutations in components of complement influence the outcome of Factor I-associated atypical hemolytic uremic syndrome. *Kidney Int*. 2010;77:339-349.
159. Esparza-Gordillo J, Jorge EG, Garrido CA, et al. Insights into hemolytic uremic syndrome: segregation of three independent predisposition factors in a large, multiple affected pedigree. *Mol Immunol*. 2006;43:1769-1775.
160. Ermini L, Goodship TH, Strain L, et al. Common genetic variants in complement genes other than CFH, CD46 and the CFHRs are not associated with aHUS. *Mol Immunol*. 2012;49:640-648.
161. Heurich M, Martinez-Barricarte R, Francis NJ, et al. Common polymorphisms in C3, factor B, and factor H collaborate to determine systemic complement activity and disease risk. *Proc Natl Acad Sci USA*. 2011;108:8761-8766.
162. Feitz WJC, van de Kar NCAJ, Orth-Höller D, van den Heuvel LPJW, Licht C. The genetics of atypical hemolytic uremic syndrome. *Med Genet*. 2018;30:400-409.
163. Zipfel PF, Edey M, Heinen S, et al. Deletion of complement factor H-related genes CFHR1 and CFHR3 is associated with atypical hemolytic uremic syndrome. *PLoS Genet*. 2007;3:e41.
164. Jozsi M, Licht C, Strobel S, et al. Factor H autoantibodies in atypical hemolytic uremic syndrome correlate with CFHR1/CFHR3 deficiency. *Blood*. 2008;111:1512-1514.
165. Dragon-Durey MA, Blanc C, Marliot F, et al. The high frequency of complement factor H related CFHR1 gene deletion is restricted to specific subgroups of patients with atypical haemolytic uraemic syndrome. *J Med Genet*. 2009;46:447-450.
166. Strobel S, Abarrategui-Garrido C, Fariza-Requejo E, et al. Factor H-related protein 1 neutralizes anti-factor H autoantibodies in autoimmune hemolytic uremic syndrome. *Kidney Int*. 2011;80:397-404.
167. Kaartinen K, Safa A, Kotha S, Ratti G, Meri S. Complement dysregulation in glomerulonephritis. *Semin Immunol*. 2019;45:101331.
168. Lemaire M, Frémeaux-Bacchi V, Schaefer F, et al. Recessive mutations in DGKE cause atypical hemolytic-uremic syndrome. *Nat Genet*. 2013;45:531-536.

169. Ozaltin F, Li B, Rauhauser A, et al. DGKE variants cause a glomerular microangiopathy that mimics membranoproliferative GN. *J Am Soc Nephrol.* 2013;24:377-384.
170. Martinez-Barricarte R, Pianetti G, Gautard R, et al. The complement factor H R1210C mutation is associated with atypical hemolytic uremic syndrome. *J Am Soc Nephrol.* 2008;19:639-646.
171. Raychaudhuri S, Iartchouk O, Chin K, et al. A rare penetrant mutation in CFH confers high risk of age-related macular degeneration. *Nat Genet.* 2011;43:1232-1236.
172. Weiner DE, Tighiouart H, Reynolds R, Seddon JM. Kidney function, albuminuria and age-related macular degeneration in NHANES III. *Nephrol Dial Transplant.* 2011;26:3159-3165.
173. Richards SJ, Dickinson AJ, Cullen MJ, et al. Presentation clinical, haematological and immunophenotypic features of 1081 patients with GPI-deficient (paroxysmal nocturnal haemoglobinuria) cells detected by flow cytometry. *Br J Haematol.* 2020;189:954-966.
174. Vyse TJ, Spath PJ, Davies KA, et al. Hereditary complement factor I deficiency. *QJM.* 1994;87:385-401.
175. Tsai HM, Kuo E. From gestational hypertension and preeclampsia to atypical hemolytic uremic syndrome. *Obstet Gynecol.* 2016;127:907-910.
176. Magro CM, Momtahen S, Mulvey JJ, et al. Role of the skin biopsy in the diagnosis of atypical hemolytic uremic syndrome. *Am J Dermatopathol.* 2015;37:349-356.
177. Galbusera M, Noris M, Gastoldi S, et al. An ex vivo test of complement activation on endothelium for individualized eculizumab therapy in hemolytic uremic syndrome. *Am J Kidney Dis.* 2019;74:56-72.
178. Legendre CM, Licht C, Muus P, et al. Terminal complement inhibitor eculizumab in atypical hemolytic-uremic syndrome. *N Engl J Med.* 2013;368:2169-2181.
179. Sheridan D, Yu ZX, Zhang Y, et al. Design and preclinical characterization of ALXN1210: a novel anti-C5 antibody with extended duration of action. *PLoS One.* 2018;13:e0195909.
180. Rondeau E, Scully M, Ariceta G, et al. The long-acting C5 inhibitor, Ravulizumab, is effective and safe in adult patients with atypical hemolytic uremic syndrome naive to complement inhibitor treatment. *Kidney Int.* 2020;97:1287-1296.
181. Nishimura J, Yamamoto M, Hayashi S, et al. Genetic variants in C5 and poor response to eculizumab. *N Engl J Med.* 2014;370:632-639.
182. Hillmen P, Szer J, Weitz I, et al. Pegcetacoplan versus eculizumab in paroxysmal nocturnal hemoglobinuria. *N Engl J Med.* 2021;384:1028-1037.
183. Barratt J, Weitz I. Complement factor D as a strategic target for regulating the alternative complement pathway. *Front Immunol.* 2021;12:712572.
184. Hoy SM. Pegcetacoplan: first approval. *Drugs.* 2021;81:1423-1430.
185. Risitano AM, Marotta S, Ricci P, et al. Anti-complement treatment for paroxysmal nocturnal hemoglobinuria: time for proximal complement inhibition? A position paper from the SAAWP of the EBMT. *Front Immunol.* 2019;10:1157.
186. UKTIS. *Use of Eculizumab in Pregnancy*; 2021. www.medicinesinpregnancy.org/bumps/monographs/USE-OF-ECULIZUMAB-IN-PREGNANCY/
187. Food and Drug Administration. *Eculizumag Prescribing Information*; 2007. https://www.accessdata.fda.gov/drugsatfda_docs/label/2011/125166s172lbl.pdf
188. Barbour T, Scully M, Ariceta G, et al. Long-term efficacy and safety of the long-acting complement C5 inhibitor ravulizumab for the treatment of atypical hemolytic uremic syndrome in adults. *Kidney Int Rep.* 2021;6:1603-1613.
189. Tanaka K, Adams B, Aris AM, et al. The long-acting C5 inhibitor, ravulizumab, is efficacious and safe in pediatric patients with atypical hemolytic uremic syndrome previously treated with eculizumab. *Pediatr Nephrol.* 2021;36:889-898.
190. Gackler A, Schonermarck U, Dobronravov V, et al. Efficacy and safety of the long-acting C5 inhibitor ravulizumab in patients with atypical hemolytic uremic syndrome triggered by pregnancy: a subgroup analysis. *BMC Nephrol.* 2021;22:5.
191. Weitz M, Amon O, Bassler D, Koenigsrainer A, Nadalin S. Prophylactic eculizumab prior to kidney transplantation for atypical hemolytic uremic syndrome. *Pediatr Nephrol.* 2011;26:1325-1329.
192. Saland JM, Ruggenenti P, Remuzzi G. Liver-kidney transplantation to cure atypical hemolytic uremic syndrome. *J Am Soc Nephrol.* 2009;20:940-949.
193. Fayek SA, Allam SR, Martinez E, et al. Atypical hemolytic uremic syndrome after kidney transplantation: lessons learned from the good, the bad, and the ugly. A case series with literature review. *Transplant Proc.* 2020;52:146-152.
194. Fremeaux-Bacchi V, Fakhouri F, Garnier A, et al. Genetics and outcome of atypical hemolytic uremic syndrome: a nationwide French series comparing children and adults. *Clin J Am Soc Nephrol.* 2013;8:554-562.
195. Jacobson RJ, Rath CE, Perloff JK. Intravascular haemolysis and thrombocytopenia in left ventricular outflow obstruction. *Br Heart J.* 1973;35:849-854.
196. Appel GB, Pirani CL, D'Agati V. Renal vascular complications of systemic lupus erythematosus. *J Am Soc Nephrol.* 1994;4:1499-1515.
197. Kim YL, Richman KA, Marshall BE. Thrombocytopenia associated with Swan-Ganz catheterization in patients. *Anesthesiology.* 1980;53:261-262.
198. Vonderheide RH, Thadhani R, Kuter DJ. Association of thrombocytopenia with the use of intra-aortic balloon pumps. *Am J Med.* 1998;105:27-32.
199. Plotz FB, van OW, Bartlett RH, Wildevuur CR. Blood activation during neonatal extracorporeal life support. *J Thorac Cardiovasc Surg.* 1993;105:823-832.
200. Velik-Salchner C, Maier S, Innerhofer P, et al. An assessment of cardiopulmonary bypass-induced changes in platelet function using whole blood and classical light transmission aggregometry: the results of a pilot study. *Anesth Analg.* 2009;108:1747-1754.
201. Bick RL. Hemostasis defects associated with cardiac surgery, prosthetic devices, and other extracorporeal circuits. *Semin Thromb Hemost.* 1985;11:249-280.
202. Rinder CS, Mathew JP, Rinder HM, et al. Modulation of platelet surface adhesion receptors during cardiopulmonary bypass. *Anesthesiology.* 1991;75:563-570.
203. Wenger RK, Lukasiewicz H, Mikuta BS, Niewiarowski S, Edmunds LH, Jr. Loss of platelet fibrinogen receptors during clinical cardiopulmonary bypass. *J Thorac Cardiovasc Surg.* 1989;97:235-239.
204. Despotis GJ, Joist JH. Anticoagulation and anticoagulation reversal with cardiac surgery involving cardiopulmonary bypass: an update. *J Cardiothorac Vasc Anesth.* 1999;13:18-29.
205. Kutay V, Noyan T, Ozcan S, et al. Biocompatibility of heparin-coated cardiopulmonary bypass circuits in coronary patients with left ventricular dysfunction is superior to PMEA-coated circuits. *J Card Surg.* 2006;21:572-577.
206. Castiglioni A, Verzini A, Pappalardo F, et al. Minimally invasive closed circuit versus standard extracorporeal circulation for aortic valve replacement. *Ann Thorac Surg.* 2007;83:586-591.
207. Lo B, Nierich AP, Kalkman CJ, Fijnheer R. Relatively increased von Willebrand factor activity after off-pump coronary artery bypass graft surgery. *Thromb.Haemost.* 2007;97:21-26.
208. Koster A, Yeter R, Buz S, et al. Assessment of hemostatic activation during cardiopulmonary bypass for coronary artery bypass grafting with bivalirudin: results of a pilot study. *J Thorac Cardiovasc Surg.* 2005;129:1391-1394.
209. Salzman EW, Weinstein MJ, Weintraub RM, et al. Treatment with desmopressin acetate to reduce blood loss after cardiac surgery. A double-blind randomized trial. *N Engl J Med.* 1986;314:1402-1406.
210. Despotis GJ, Levine V, Saleem R, Spitznagel E, Joist JH. Use of point-of-care test in identification of patients who can benefit from desmopressin during cardiac surgery: a randomised controlled trial. *Lancet.* 1999;354:106-110.
211. Levi M, Cromheecke ME, de JE, et al. Pharmacological strategies to decrease excessive blood loss in cardiac surgery: a meta-analysis of clinically relevant endpoints. *Lancet.* 1999;354:1940-1947.
212. Munoz JJ, Birkmeyer NJ, Birkmeyer JD, O'Connor GT, Dacey LJ. Is epsilon-aminocaproic acid as effective as aprotinin in reducing bleeding with cardiac surgery? a meta-analysis. *Circulation.* 1999;99:81-89.
213. Ray MJ, O'Brien MF. Comparison of epsilon aminocaproic acid and low-dose aprotinin in cardiopulmonary bypass: efficiency, safety and cost. *Ann Thorac Surg.* 2001;71:838-843.
214. Mangano DT, Tudor IC, Dietzel C. The risk associated with aprotinin in cardiac surgery. *N Engl J Med.* 2006;354:353-365.
215. Chung A, Wildhirt SM, Wang S, Koshal A, Radomski MW. Combined administration of nitric oxide gas and iloprost during cardiopulmonary bypass reduces platelet dysfunction: a pilot clinical study. *J Thorac Cardiovasc Surg.* 2005;129:782-790.
216. Wiviott SD, Braunwald E, McCabe CH, et al. Prasugrel versus clopidogrel in patients with acute coronary syndromes. *N Engl J Med.* 2007;357:2001-2015.
217. Jana S. Endothelialization of cardiovascular devices. *Acta Biomater.* 2019;99:53-71.
218. Gill JC, Wilson AD, Endres-Brooks J, Montgomery RR. Loss of the largest von Willebrand factor multimers from the plasma of patients with congenital cardiac defects. *Blood.* 1986;67:758-761.
219. Crow S, John R, Boyle A, et al. Gastrointestinal bleeding rates in recipients of nonpulsatile and pulsatile left ventricular assist devices. *J Thorac Cardiovasc Surg.* 2009;137:208-215.
220. Greenstein RJ, McElhinney AJ, Reuben D, Greenstein AJ. Colonic vascular ectasias and aortic stenosis: coincidence or causal relationship? *Am J Surg.* 1986;151:347-351.
221. Heyde EC. Gastrointestinal bleeding in aortic stenosis. *N Engl J Med.* 1958;259:196.
222. King RM, Pluth JR, Giuliani ER. The association of unexplained gastrointestinal bleeding with calcific aortic stenosis. *Ann Thorac Surg.* 1987;44:514-516.
223. Tsai HM. von Willebrand factor, shear stress, and ADAMTS13 in hemostasis and thrombosis. *ASAIO J.* 2012;58:163-169.
224. Vukelic S, Vlismas PP, Patel SR, et al. Digoxin is associated with a decreased incidence of angiodysplasia-related gastrointestinal bleeding in patients with continuous-flow left ventricular assist devices. *Circ Heart Fail.* 2018;11:e004899.
225. Marck RE, Montagne HL, Tuinebreijer WE, Breederveld RS. Time course of thrombocytes in burn patients and its predictive value for outcome. *Burns.* 2013;39:714-722.
226. Eurenius K, Mortensen RF, Meserol PM, Curreri PW. Platelet and megakaryocyte kinetics following thermal injury. *J Lab Clin Med.* 1972;79:247-257.
227. Pistorius GA, Alexander C, Krisch CM, et al. Local platelet trapping as the cause of thrombocytopenia after hepatic cryotherapy. *World J Surg.* 2005;29:657-660.
228. Goodie DB, Horton MD, Morris RW, Nagy LS, Morris DL. Anaesthetic experience with cryotherapy for treatment of hepatic malignancy. *Anaesth Intensive Care.* 1992;20:491-496.
229. Straub A, Krajewski S, Hohmann JD, et al. Evidence of platelet activation at medically used hypothermia and mechanistic data indicating ADP as a key mediator and therapeutic target. *Arterioscler Thromb Vasc Biol.* 2011;31:1607-1616.
230. Ranucci M, Carlucci C, Isgrà G, et al. Hypothermic cardiopulmonary bypass as a determinant of late thrombocytopenia following cardiac operations in pediatric patients. *Acta Anaesthesiol Scand.* 2009;53:1060-1067.
231. Zhang JN, Wood J, Bergeron AL, et al. Effects of low temperature on shear-induced platelet aggregation and activation. *J Trauma.* 2004;57:216-223.
232. Tam EL, Draksharam PL, Park JA, Sidhu GS. Acute immune-mediated thrombocytopenia due to oxaliplatin and irinotecan therapy. *Case Rep Oncol Med.* 2019;2019:4314797.
233. Jardim DL, Rodrigues CA, Novis YAS, Rocha VG, Hoff PM. Oxaliplatin-related thrombocytopenia. *Ann Oncol.* 2012;23:1937-1942.
234. Heyns AD, Lotter MG, Badenhorst PN, et al. Kinetics and in vivo redistribution of (111)Indium-labelled human platelets after intravenous protamine sulphate. *Thromb Haemost.* 1980;44:65-68.

Chapter 50 ■ Miscellaneous Causes of Thrombocytopenia

ARCHANA M. AGARWAL • GEORGE M. RODGERS

INTRODUCTION

This chapter summarizes the miscellaneous forms of congenital and acquired thrombocytopenia (Table 50.1), including thrombocytopenia attributable to deficient platelet production, associated with abnormal platelet pooling in the spleen, and resulting from dilution with massive transfusions.

CONGENITAL/HEREDITARY THROMBOCYTOPENIA

Hereditary thrombocytopenias are a heterogeneous group of rare disorders that may be inherited as an autosomal dominant trait, an autosomal recessive trait, or an X-linked recessive trait. It accounts for approximately 2.7 in 100,000 cases.[1] Bleeding can be mild, and in some instances the affected family members are virtually asymptomatic, being identified only through incidental platelet counts or family studies after the identification of the propositus. It is important to recognize these mild forms of familial thrombocytopenia because, although they may resemble autoimmune thrombocytopenic purpura, patients do not respond to steroid treatment or intravenous immunoglobulin, and this therapy may be harmful. With the advent of whole exome sequencing and whole genome sequencing, novel genes have been described that could account for at least 50% to 60% of the inherited forms of congenital thrombocytopenia.[1-3] At least 42 different genes have been implicated that have roles in megakaryocytic differentiation, maturation, and platelet production.[4,5] Owing to wide heterogeneity and overlap, there is no consensus on their classification and many different categories of classification, for example, based on size of the platelets, clinical features, inheritance pattern, and associated diseases, have been proposed. Table 50.2 shows the classification based on size.

Another proposed classification is based on the platelet's pathogenic mechanism: 1. defective megakaryocytic maturation, 2. defective platelet production/increased clearance, and 3. unknown causes. The common genes involved in the above classification are shown in Table 50.3.

Defective megakaryocytic maturation: This could be due to defective differentiation of megakaryocytes and is characterized by decrease or absence of megakaryocytes in bone marrow or altered maturation of megakaryocytes leading to normal or increased numbers in bone marrow. Approximately eight of them are due to transcription factors responsible for megakaryopoiesis and include *RUNX1*, *GATA1*, *ETV6*, *HOXA11*, *MECOM*, *FLI1*, *GFI1B*, and *IKZF5*. FLI1 activates the transcription of several other genes, for example, *MPL*, *ITGA2B*, *GP9*, *GP1BA*, and *PF4*. The *GATA1* and *GF1B* genes also control red blood cell (RBC) production, while *RUNX1* and *ETV6* mutations are associated with predisposition to myeloid disorders. Thrombopoietin gene (*THPO*) and thrombopoietin receptor gene (*c-mpl/MPL*) are causative of THPO-related thrombocytopenia and congenital amegakaryocytic thrombocytopenia (CAMT). The *FYB* gene codes for the cytoskeletal protein, and *RBM8A* gene codes for the protein of the exon-junction complexes.

Defective platelet production/clearance: Most of these forms are associated with large platelets. Genes involved here mainly take part in actomyosin or microtubular cytoskeletal system, for example, *MYH9*, *ACTN1*, *FLNA*, *TPM4*, *TRPM7*, or *TUBB1*. Mutations are also seen in the genes in major membrane glycoprotein (GP) complexes, GP1B/IX/V and GP11B/IIIA.

Classic Inherited Thrombocytopenia
Congenital Amegakaryocytic Thrombocytopenia

The presence of severe thrombocytopenia, absence of megakaryocytes in the bone marrow, and absence of any physical anomaly in an infant characterize CAMT.[6] Patients with CAMT have markedly elevated serum levels of thrombopoietin (TPO)[7] and mutations in the *c-mpl* gene. Multiple mutations in the *c-mpl* gene have been reported, including deletions, nonsense mutations, and missense mutations. Owing to these mutations, the cells cannot bind TPO, leading to higher levels of TPO. Many of the patients studied are compound heterozygotes with

Table 50.1. Miscellaneous Causes of Thrombocytopenia

Congenital thrombocytopenia
Autosomal recessive thrombocytopenias
Congenital amegakaryocytic thrombocytopenia
Thrombocytopenia with absent radius (TAR) syndrome
Bernard-Soulier syndrome
Autosomal dominant thrombocytopenias
MYH9-related disorder
May-Hegglin anomaly
Sebastian anomaly
Fechtner anomaly
Epstein anomaly
Familial platelet disorder with predisposition to myeloid disorders
Mediterranean macrothrombocytopenia
Paris-Trousseau syndrome (in association with deletion of *FLI1* gene)
Autosomal dominant thrombocytopenia with ANKRD26 gene mutation (THC2)
Gray platelet syndrome
Amegakaryocytic thrombocytopenia with radial-ulnar synostosis (ATRUS) syndrome
Variant von Willebrand disease (type 2b and platelet type) (see Chapter 54)
X-linked thrombocytopenia
X-linked microthrombocytopenia (*WAS* gene mutation)
X-linked macrothrombocytopenia with dyserythropoiesis (*GATA-1* mutation)
Others
22q11 deletion syndrome (DiGeorge Syndrome)
Acquired Thrombocytopenia
Thrombocytopenia caused by deficient platelet production
Acquired pure amegakaryocytic thrombocytopenic purpura
Chemical and physical agents that produce generalized bone marrow suppression
Drugs that selectively suppress the megakaryocyte
Drugs that cause ineffective thrombopoiesis
Thrombocytopenia caused by abnormal platelet pooling
Thrombocytopenia caused by hypothermia
Thrombocytopenia associated with infections
Thrombocytopenia associated with viral infections
Thrombocytopenia associated with bacterial and protozoal infections
Thrombocytopenia after massive blood transfusions

Table 50.2. Classification of Inherited Thrombocytopenia by Platelet Size (MPV)

Low MPV	Normal MPV	Increased MPV
Wiskott-Aldrich syndrome	ATRUS syndrome	MYH9-related disorders
	Thrombocytopenia with absent radius syndrome	Mediterranean macrothrombocytopenia
	Congenital amegakaryocytic thrombocytopenia	Bernard-Soulier syndrome
	Familial platelet disorder with predisposition to AML	GATA-1 mutation
	THC2	Gray platelet syndrome
	X-linked thrombocytopenia with GATA-1 mutation	Paris-Trousseau syndrome
		vWD type 2B
		Platelet-type vWD
		22q11 deletion syndrome

GATA-1 mutation platelets may have normal or increased MPV.
AML, acute myelocytic leukemia; ATRUS, amegakaryocytic thrombocytopenia with radial-ulnar synostosis; MPV, mean platelet volume; THC2, autosomal dominant thrombocytopenia with incomplete megakaryocyte differentiation and linkage to chromosome 10; vWD, von Willebrand disorder.
Adapted from Drachman JG, Inherited thrombocytopenia: when a low platelet count does not mean ITP. *Blood.* 2004;103:390-398; Lambert MP. What to do when you suspect an inherited platelet disorder. *Hematology Am Soc Hematol Educ Program.* 2011;2011:377-383.

Table 50.3. Classification of Congenital Thrombocytopenia Based on Pathogenic Mechanism With Selected Genes Involved

Defective Megakaryocytic Maturation	Defective Platelet Production and Clearance	Unknown Causes
THPO, MPL, HOXA11, MECOM, FLI1, RUNX1, GATA1, GF1B, ETV6, ANKRD26, FYB, IKZF5, MPL, NBEAL2, RBM8A	MYH9, FLNA, DIAPH1, TUBB1, GPIBA, GPIBB, GPIX, VWF, ACTB, ACTN1, ARPC1B, CYCS, ITGA2B, ITGB3, KDSR, MPIG68, PRKACG, STIM1, TRPM7, TPM, WAS	ABCGS, ABCG8, GNE, SRC, PTPRJ

one mutation inherited from each parent.[8-10] Because patients with CAMT develop progressive bone marrow aplasia during the course of the disease, it is likely that Mpl signaling is essential for the production of mature megakaryocytes as well as maintenance of the hematopoietic stem cell population and proliferation.[11]

Further subgrouping of patients with CAMT into two groups has been proposed based on their clinical course: group CAMT I, with a more severe type of thrombocytopenia with constantly low platelet counts and an early onset of pancytopenia, and group CAMT II, which is characterized by a transient increase in platelet counts during the first year of life and a later development of pancytopenia.[9] The type of *mpl* mutation determines the clinical course of CAMT; a total loss of the TPO receptor due to homozygous nonsense mutations, deletions, and frameshift mutations causes the more severe form of disease found in patients with CAMT I. In contrast, the transient increase in platelet counts and the later development of pancytopenia in patients with homozygous or compound heterozygous missense mutations are the result of a residual function of the TPO receptor.[10,12] Hematopoietic stem cell transplant is the only curative treatment for these patients, and matched sibling transplants have been successful.

Thrombocytopenia With Absent Radius Syndrome

The thrombocytopenia with absent radius (TAR) syndrome is a congenital malformation syndrome characterized by bilateral absence of the radii but with thumbs present, hypomegakaryocytic thrombocytopenia, and a number of additional features including skeletal and cardiac anomalies.[13,14] Among the skeletal anomalies, bilateral absence of the radii may be accompanied by ulnar or humeral anomalies, and the most severe cases exhibit phocomelia. Lower limb involvement is variable and includes dislocation of the patella and/or of the hips, absent tibiofibular joint, and lower limb phocomelia. Among the cardiac anomalies, tetralogy of Fallot and atrial septal defects are common.[15,16] Studies have noted a high incidence (62%) of cow's milk intolerance, which presents as persistent diarrhea and failure to thrive.

These patients have elevated serum TPO levels and normal *c-mpl* and *HOX* genes. However, they have a profound defect in megakaryocyte differentiation and platelet production and no response of megakaryocytes to TPO. Although specific microdeletion of chromosome 1q21.1 has been reported in the majority of individuals with TAR syndrome, it is not the disease-causing mutation.[17] Biallelic variants of the *RBM8A* gene with the association of a null allele and a hypomorphic noncoding variant have found to be the cause of TAR syndrome.[18] *RBM8A* controls the production of the protein Y14, and its low level is responsible for low platelets.[17]

Diagnosis is rarely difficult because of obvious morphologic abnormalities in association with thrombocytopenia. Prenatal diagnosis has been described by ultrasonographic detection of morphologic abnormalities and detection of low fetal platelet counts.[19-22] Congenital rubella and some variants of Fanconi syndrome as well as syndromes with malformations of the upper limb should be excluded. Platelet counts gradually increase during the first 2 years of life. The degree of thrombocytopenia is usually greatest at the time of birth; platelet transfusions are frequently required and are effective. Thrombocytopenia becomes less severe during the first year of life, and most affected individuals with TAR do not require platelet transfusions after infancy.[15,23]

Bernard-Soulier Syndrome

Bernard-Soulier syndrome is an autosomal recessive bleeding disorder associated with deficiency of platelet membrane proteins GPIb, GPIX, and GPV. This results in abnormal platelet interaction with ligands of these receptor proteins, which include thrombin, von Willebrand factor (vWF), P-selectin, and leukocyte integrin $\alpha_M\beta_2$, in addition to causing thrombocytopenia. Autosomal dominant forms have also been described. This topic is described in more detail in Chapter 53.

MYH9-Related Disorders

A group of autosomal dominant macrothrombocytopenias caused by mutations in the *MYH9* gene with variable penetrance and expression has been defined.[24-27] These include May-Hegglin anomaly, Sebastian syndrome, Epstein syndrome, and Fechtner syndrome. These disorders are defined by the presence of mutations involving the *MYH9* gene located at chromosome 22q12.3–13.1 and include single nucleotide changes, in-frame deletions or duplications, and frameshift and nonsense mutations.[28] The *MYH9* gene encodes nonmuscle myosin heavy chain IIA (NMMHC-IIA).[29] NMMHC-IIA is part of the nonmuscle myosin IIA hexamer that is a component of the contractile cytoskeleton in megakaryocytes, platelets, and other tissues. Thrombocytopenia is usually mild and derives from complex defects of megakaryocyte maturation and platelet formation. More specifically, these mutations likely affect the platelet release from the mature megakaryocytes.[30] All of these *MYH9* gene mutation–related disorders have macrothrombocytopenia and leukocyte inclusion bodies (Döhle body–like inclusions) and can have various combinations of hereditary nephritis, deafness, and cataracts (Table 50.4). Sometimes, the inclusions are rarely appreciated on conventional May-Grunwald-Giemsa staining, especially in patients with mutations at codon 702 because of their low RNA content. These cases can be diagnosed by the use of immunofluorescence assays.[31] Thrombocytopenia is generally mild to moderate. Peripheral blood smears reveal enlarged platelets with frequent giant platelets.

Table 50.4. Syndromes Caused by *MYH9* Gene Defects

Syndrome	Macrothrombocytopenia	Döhle-Like Bodies	Nephritis	Deafness	Cataracts
May-Hegglin	Yes	Yes	No	No	No
Sebastian	Yes	Yes	No	No	No
Fechtner	Yes	Yes	Yes	Yes	Yes
Epstein	Yes	Yes	Yes	Yes	No

Clinically, patients have a mild platelet-type bleeding disorder. May-Hegglin anomaly and Sebastian syndrome both have macrothrombocytopenia and granulocyte inclusions, but ultrastructural analysis of the Döhle-like inclusions demonstrates diagnostic differences between these two syndromes, and both types of inclusions can also be distinguished from Döhle bodies seen in acute infection. Patients with Fechtner syndrome and Epstein syndrome have hearing disability and nephritis. In Fechtner syndrome, cataracts are also present.[32] These two disorders result from allelic mutations at amino acid 702, which cause conformational changes to the myosin head.[25,28,33,34] Diagnosis is suggested by detection of macrothrombocytopenia and the presence of one or more of the above-mentioned clinical features. Döhle-like inclusion bodies within neutrophils on May-Grünwald-Giemsa–stained peripheral blood are highly suggestive of an *MYH9*-related disorder. Abnormal staining of neutrophil inclusions with anti-NMMHC-IIA may offer greater sensitivity. Definitive diagnosis requires the demonstration of a causative mutation within the *MYH9* gene.[25] Treatment options for bleeding include platelet transfusion, allogeneic stem cell transplantation, or use of a thrombopoietic drug (eltrombopag).[35,36]

Platelet-type von Willebrand disease is another autosomal dominant disorder associated with hereditary thrombocytopenia, characterized by abnormal binding of large vWF multimers to platelets. This intrinsic platelet defect results in mild thrombocytopenia, increased ristocetin-induced platelet aggregation, and a selective loss of high-molecular-weight vWF multimers from the plasma. This disorder resembles type 2b von Willebrand disease (see Chapter 54).

Familial Platelet Disorder With Predisposition to Myeloid Malignancy

Familial platelet disorder (FPD) with predisposition to myelodysplastic syndrome/acute myelogenous leukemia is an autosomal dominant disorder usually related to defects in transcription factors required during early stages of megakaryocytic maturation and is characterized by moderate thrombocytopenia, a defect in platelet function, and predisposition to develop myeloid malignancies.[37] The defect in platelet function is manifested by prolonged bleeding times and abnormal platelet aggregation. Bone marrow from affected patients shows decreased megakaryopoiesis. One of the first genes associated with FPD was germline heterozygous mutations in the hematopoietic transcription factor AML1, also known as RUNX1/CBFA2 by linkage analysis of several pedigrees.[38] These mutations include missense, frameshift, and nonsense mutations and a large intragenic deletion. Normal megakaryopoiesis requires TPO binding to the Mpl receptor. In FPD, RUNX1 mutation leads to diminished Mpl receptor expression, resulting in impaired TPO signaling leading to thrombocytopenia. Germline mutations have also been identified in *ANKRD26* gene, particularly in the 5′ untranslated region (UTR) region in patients with autosomal dominant thrombocytopenia along with myelodysplastic syndromes.[39] This disorder is characterized by moderate thrombocytopenia, and mild bruising, but absence of major bleeding even with minor surgery and childbirth, suggesting that the residual platelets have normal hemostatic function. However, platelets are deficient in GPIa and α-granule content. Morphologically, the platelets appear normal. Bone marrow examination reveals impaired megakaryocyte maturation and small megakaryocytes. Serum TPO level is only moderately elevated and is usually lower than expected for the degree of thrombocytopenia.[39,40] This is one of the most prevalent forms of inherited thrombocytopenia ranging from 10% to 17% of all inherited cases. Most common mutations are single nucleotide variants in the 5′UTR of the *ANKRD26* gene. This disorder also predisposes to increased likelihood of myelodysplastic syndrome/acute myeloid leukemia, and affected patients should be recommended for genetic counseling.

Germline mutations in the ETV6 gene has also been shown to be associated with thrombocytopenia and predisposition to hematological malignancy including acute lymphoblastic leukemia.[41,42]

Mediterranean Macrothrombocytopenia

A relatively common and mild form of macrothrombocytopenia has been described in a group of 145 apparently healthy subjects from Italy and the Balkan peninsula. Because this abnormality was not detected in control subjects from northern Europe, the condition was named Mediterranean macrothrombocytopenia.[43] Linkage analysis localized the gene mutation to the short arm of chromosome 17, in an interval containing the *GPIbα* gene. GPIbα, together with other proteins, constitutes the plasma vWF receptor, which is altered in Bernard-Soulier syndrome. Sequencing of the gene identified a mutation of GPIbα (Ala156Val) shared by 10 of 12 pedigrees studied.[44] These data demonstrate that, for most families with Mediterranean thrombocytopenia, the genotype and phenotype are equivalent to that of a carrier of Bernard-Soulier syndrome. Clinically, patients have a mild bleeding diathesis, usually diagnosed after incidental discovery of thrombocytopenia. Peripheral blood shows platelets that are larger than normal.

Paris-Trousseau Syndrome (in Association With Deletion of the FLI1 Gene)

Paris-Trousseau syndrome (PTS) is an inherited disorder characterized by several congenital anomalies including dysmegakaryopoiesis with two morphologically distinct populations of megakaryocytes and giant α-granules in a low percentage of platelets. These features occur in association with deletion of the long arm of chromosome 11 at 11q23.3 (which includes the *FLI1* gene), a region that is also deleted in Jacobsen syndrome (a variant form of PTS). Clinical features include a combination of mild to moderate psychomotor retardation, trigonocephaly, facial dysmorphism, cardiac defects, and thrombocytopenia.[45] Hematologic history, biologic data, and ultrastructural and molecular investigations were reported from a case series of 10 patients.[46] Thrombocytopenia is chronic, with mild clinical bleeding. Peripheral blood smears and electron microscopy show abnormal platelets with giant granules. Bone marrow findings consist of dysmegakaryopoiesis with many micromegakaryocytes. Abnormal α-granules are not seen in the bone marrow and cultured megakaryocytes. Platelets have a normal lifespan in the circulation. The number of megakaryocytes in the bone marrow is increased, accompanied by impaired maturation. Together these findings suggest that platelet release is substantially impaired. PTS occurs as a result of hemizygous loss of the *FLI1* transcription factor gene, which has been shown to be critical for megakaryocyte differentiation and release of platelets. *FLI1* shows monoallelic expression during a brief window in megakaryocyte differentiation. This monoallelic expression explains the dominant inheritance pattern of PTS despite the presence of one normal *FLI1* allele.[47,48]

Gray Platelet Syndrome

The gray platelet syndrome for which both autosomal recessive and autosomal dominant inheritance have been described is characterized by macrothrombocytopenia with bleeding tendency, myelofibrosis, and classical abnormal platelet morphology.[49] The α-granules are absent or greatly reduced, giving the platelets a gray color on Wright-Giemsa stain. The α-granules are the principal storage site for hemostatic proteins such as fibrinogen, vWF, thrombospondin, and factor V and for growth factors such as platelet-derived growth factor and transforming growth factor-β.[50] One result of absence of α-granules is a continued leakage of growth factors and cytokines into the marrow, causing myelofibrosis. Homozygous or compound heterozygous mutations in the NBEAL2 gene cause gray platelet syndrome.[51] NBEAL2 is a scaffolding protein involved in α-granule ontogeny.[51]

Amegakaryocytic Thrombocytopenia With Radial-Ulnar Synostosis Syndrome in Association With HOXA11 and MECOM Mutation

Homeobox genes encode regulatory proteins that are critical to bone morphogenesis as well as hematopoietic differentiation and proliferation.[52] This defect is the first reported germline HOX gene mutation associated with a human nonneoplastic hematologic disorder and only the third HOX gene implicated in a human disorder.[53] HOXA11 is suggested to be endogenously expressed in very early hematopoietic precursor cells and involved in regulation of megakaryocytic differentiation.[54] Heterozygosity mutations has also been described in the MECOM gene (MDS1 and EV1 complex) in few Japanese children.[55] Clinical features are variable and include CAMT, aplastic anemia, proximal radial-ulnar synostosis, clinodactyly, syndactyly, hip dysplasia, bone marrow failure, and sensorineural hearing loss.[55-57] Platelet transfusions are effective as initial symptomatic management. The only definitive treatment is hematopoietic stem cell transplantation.[58]

X-Linked Microthrombocytopenia (WAS Gene Mutation)

Wiskott-Aldrich syndrome (WAS), originally described in 1937, is now known as an X-linked hereditary disorder associated with combined immunodeficiency, thrombocytopenia, small platelets, eczema, and an increased risk of autoimmune disorders and cancers. It has a broad range of phenotypes.[59] At one end of the clinical spectrum, patients exhibit platelet abnormalities only, and at the other end, patients manifest thrombocytopenia, eczema, and immune abnormalities with progressive T-cell lymphopenia, and increased susceptibility to infection. The severe form of WAS and its milder manifestations X-linked thrombocytopenia and X-linked neutropenia are caused by mutations in the gene WAS, located at Xp11.22–p11.23 and cloned in 1994.[60-63] The WAS gene is composed of 12 exons and encodes a polypeptide of 502 amino acids. Most mutations consist of single-nucleotide substitutions, small insertions and deletions, and splice-site mutations, and these are distributed throughout the coding region and the intron-exon junctions.[64] Even within families, the same genotype can be associated with varying phenotypes. The mature WASP contains numerous protein-interacting domains and appears to provide a critical link between the cellular cytoskeleton and signal transduction pathways. WASP is a key regulator of actin polymerization in hematopoietic cells. It has five well-defined domains that are involved in signaling, cell locomotion, and immune synapse formation. WASP facilitates the nuclear translocation of nuclear factor κB and has been shown to play an important role in lymphoid development and in the maturation and function of myeloid monocytic cells.[65]

Megakaryocyte mass is normal or increased in WAS. Platelet differentiation and production are normal, and platelets produced in vitro are normal in size. These observations suggest that increased destruction in the spleen is responsible for both the thrombocytopenia and decreased platelet size. Management of patients with WAS is challenging; however, early diagnosis is very important for prophylaxis and treatment.[66] Prophylactic antibiotics and platelet transfusion are conventional treatment. Intravenous immune globin is indicated in patients with significant antibody deficiency. The only curative therapy remains hematopoietic stem cell transplantation, which corrects both thrombocytopenia and immunodeficiency. Gene therapy is another potentially curative option and has been under investigation for a while. The first few retroviral trials showed initial improvement of symptoms but were complicated by leukemia later on.[67,68] Lentiviral-based gene therapy trials have shown encouraging results in seven[69] and eight patients[70] who are still alive.

X-Linked Macrothrombocytopenia With Dyserythropoiesis Associated With GATA-1 Mutation

The X-linked gene GATA-1 regulates the expression of a large number of genes in multiple cell types.[71,72] GATA-1 transcription factor contains both DNA binding and transactivation activity within three functional domains: two zinc fingers (known as the N-finger and the C-finger) and an N-terminal activation domain. The C-finger is responsible for binding of GATA-1 to typical GATA-binding sites (WGATAR consensus). The N terminus of GATA-1 constitutes an activation domain, as defined by the ability of this region to confer transcriptional activation in reporter assays in fibroblasts.[73] Taken together, these domains act in a manner similar to a multitude of transcription factors that bind DNA and activate transcription of target genes. In addition to binding DNA, the N finger has a second essential function, recruitment of the cofactor Friend of GATA-1 (FOG-1).[74] FOG-1, as is GATA-1, is primarily expressed in hematopoietic cells and is absolutely essential for the development of RBCs and megakaryocytes. It regulates expression of several genes such as GP1BA, GP1BB, ITGA2B, PF4, MPL, and NFE2, and in erythropoiesis, HBB, ALAS1, and BCL2L1. Several families with germline mutations of GATA-1 that cause X-linked disorders have been described, and all mutations cluster in the N-terminal zinc finger.[75,76]

GATA-1 mutation–associated thrombocytopenia is clinically distinguished from WAS by the presence of large or normal-sized platelets and the absence of immunodeficiency, eczema, and lymphomas.[77] Thrombocytopenia is more severe (10,000-40,000/μL). Clinically, bleeding and bruising in affected individuals are severe, and platelet aggregation studies have shown that platelet function is also diminished.[78] The bone marrow is hypercellular, with dysplastic features in the erythroid and megakaryocytic lineages.[79]

Others

22q11.2 Deletion Syndrome (DiGeorge Syndrome)

This relatively common genetic disorder occurs in 1:4000 live births and is associated with, in addition to thrombocytopenia, cardiac abnormalities, velofacial anomalies, hypocalcemia, immune defects, and a variety of other features.[80] One particular gene in the region of 22q11-TBX1 is likely responsible for cardiac defects.[80] The macrothrombocytopenia seen in this disorder is mild.[77]

ACQUIRED THROMBOCYTOPENIA

Deficient Platelet Production

Deficient platelet production may result from three mechanisms: Hypoplasia or suppression of the precursor megakaryocytes; ineffective thrombopoiesis despite a normal precursor mass; or, rarely, deficiency or aberration of thrombopoietic control mechanisms.

Acquired Amegakaryocytic Thrombocytopenic Purpura

Acquired amegakaryocytic thrombocytopenic purpura (AATP) is a rare cause of thrombocytopenia associated with decreased or absent megakaryocytes in otherwise normal bone marrow. The prevalence is possibly higher than reported, as many cases are underdiagnosed or misdiagnosed as immune thrombocytopenia.

The differential diagnosis of patients with severe thrombocytopenia and isolated amegakaryocytosis includes a misdiagnosis of immune thrombocytopenic purpura, as mentioned above; ethanol use or drug ingestion; immune suppression associated with diseases such as systemic lupus erythematosus; and prodromal manifestations of acquired aplastic anemia, myelodysplastic disorders, or acute leukemia.[81] Thrombocytopenia and amegakaryocytosis caused by chemotherapy or postradiation therapy should be apparent.

The pathogenesis of AATP is uncertain. AATP can occur individually or as a component of aplastic anemia secondary to exposure to environmental agents such as viruses (cytomegalovirus [CMV], parvovirus B19) and certain toxins such as benzene.[82] Both cell-mediated suppression of megakaryopoiesis and the role of humoral immunity in AATP have been proposed, but the exact role of either remains unclear. A marked increase of T-activated suppressor cells (CD8+/DR+) in association with AATP has been reported.[83] AATP has also been associated with high levels of anti-TPO IgG antibodies.[84] No cytogenetic abnormality has been shown to be consistently associated with AATP.[85] A defect in cytokine-mediated regulation of megakaryopoiesis is another proposed mechanism leading to AATP, but conclusive data are lacking.

Patients with AATP do not have a palpable spleen. The platelets are usually small or normal in size. An increased mean red cell volume is a common finding. In most patients, an etiology cannot be determined, and empirical therapy is necessary. Platelet transfusions should be used to treat bleeding and may be required prophylactically in some patients. Although there are occasional spontaneous remissions, most sustained remissions have occurred in patients receiving immunosuppressive therapy. Treatment with intravenous immunoglobulin, prednisone, cyclophosphamide, and vincristine has not been efficacious in AATP. Myeloablative chemotherapy (busulfan and cyclophosphamide) followed by allogeneic bone marrow transplant from a fully HLA-matched sibling is effective.[86] Antithymocyte globulin (ATG) alone,[87] rituximab,[88] azathioprine,[89] and cyclosporine alone or in combination with ATG, have been shown to be very effective in treatment of AATP.[90] The availability of thrombopoietic drugs,[91] eltrombopag and romiplostim, has been shown to be effective[92-94] and may offer another treatment option for patients with AATP. Progression to aplastic anemia and rarely into MDS have been seen.[93]

Chemical and Physical Agents That Produce Generalized Bone Marrow Suppression

Ionizing radiation, alkylating agents, antimetabolites, and cytotoxic drugs may produce thrombocytopenia as the result of predictable suppression of the marrow. The mechanisms by which these agents act are well defined, and thrombocytopenia is a common complication when they are used in immunosuppression and cancer chemotherapy. In addition, many drugs, such as chloramphenicol, produce marrow hypoplasia as a result of idiosyncratic reactions. The pathophysiology in these cases is poorly understood.

Agents that produce thrombocytopenia may damage other bone marrow precursors as well as megakaryocytes, and the usual picture is one of diffuse bone marrow hypoplasia and pancytopenia. Rarely, only thrombocytopenia may be present. Platelets often are the last cell type to return to normal after recovery from bone marrow hypoplasia; in some patients, thrombocytopenia may persist indefinitely.

Drugs That Selectively Suppress the Megakaryocyte

Chlorothiazides. Chlorothiazides and various congeners may produce thrombocytopenia by one of at least two mechanisms: by the formation of platelet antibodies or by a poorly understood suppression of thrombopoiesis.[95] The latter action is by far the most common. Evidence of marrow suppression is largely indirect. Serologic tests for platelet antibodies usually yield negative results. Diminution in the number of megakaryocytes has been observed in infants born of mothers who were taking these drugs, but few instances of megakaryocytic hypoplasia have been documented in adults. Mild asymptomatic thrombocytopenia may occur in as many as 25% of patients taking these agents, an observation that implies that thrombocytopenia may be a pharmacologic rather than an idiosyncratic effect. Recovery from thrombocytopenia associated with the use of thiazide drugs is slow, and thrombocytopenia usually can be reproduced only by readministration of the drug for a protracted period.

Estrogens. Estrogenic hormones appear to affect platelet kinetics in animals both by facilitating reticuloendothelial phagocytosis and by impairing thrombopoiesis. Neither effect has been convincingly demonstrated in humans, but several instances of "amegakaryocytic" thrombocytopenia have been reported after the administration of diethylstilbestrol. In one patient, thrombocytopenia recurred when the hormone was readministered.[96]

Ethanol. Ethanol can suppress platelet production, a phenomenon that may be a common cause of mild thrombocytopenia in the alcoholic patient. Platelet counts <100,000/μL occur in as many as 26% of acutely ill alcoholics.[97] The experimental administration of ethanol produces thrombocytopenia with decreased platelet survival and platelet turnover.[94] Bleeding is rare, and when ethanol is withdrawn, the platelet count begins to increase in 2 to 3 days and returns to normal or supranormal levels in 2 to 3 weeks.[98] Several patients developed venous thromboembolic disease when platelet counts reached values >500,000/μL.[99]

Pathophysiologic studies in alcohol-induced thrombocytopenia reveal accelerated platelet destruction and a subnormal compensatory increase in thrombopoiesis. Platelet function abnormalities have also been described. The bone marrow usually reveals normal numbers of megakaryocytes. Studies using mice and guinea pig megakaryocytes demonstrate that the effect of ethanol is primarily on the maturing megakaryocytes, a finding consistent with ineffective thrombopoiesis.[100] Several cases of bone marrow hypoplasia secondary to consumption of excessive alcohol have also been described. Colony-forming unit granulocyte-macrophage–derived colony formation in one of these patients was inhibited by much lower concentrations of ethanol than that of normal volunteers.[101]

Drugs That Cause Ineffective Thrombopoiesis. Ineffective thrombopoiesis may play a role in several different types of thrombocytopenia. Thrombocytopenia is a consistent feature of megaloblastic hematopoiesis that results from deficiency of vitamin B_{12} or folic acid. It is analogous to ineffective erythropoiesis, which is also characteristic of the megaloblastic anemias. Platelet production, whether calculated per megakaryocyte or per nuclear unit, is diminished. Although the number of megakaryocytes increases in response to thrombopoietic stimuli, the normal concomitant increase in their volume does not occur.

Thrombocytopenia Caused by Abnormal Platelet Pooling

The splenic pool normally contains approximately one-third of the total platelet mass, and this pool may increase in size as a result of disorders that are associated with splenomegaly, such as chronic liver disease with portal hypertension, sarcoidosis and other granulomatous infections, Gaucher and other lipid-storage diseases, leukemias and lymphomas, and Felty syndrome.[99,102,103] This shift of platelets into the spleen may result in thrombocytopenia in the circulating blood despite a normal or even increased total platelet mass. The clinical picture in hypersplenic thrombocytopenia is usually dominated by the underlying disease, and numerous other hematologic abnormalities, such as neutropenia, anemia, and coagulation defects, may also be present.

The pathophysiology of thrombocytopenia in disorders associated with splenomegaly is not completely understood. It is hypothesized that the splenic pool increase may occur because of very slow passage of platelets through the tortuous splenic vasculature. The platelets in the splenic pool are in equilibrium with the circulating pool and can be mobilized with an infusion of epinephrine or during plateletpheresis.[104,105] This is in contrast to the irreversible thrombocytopenia caused by splenic removal of damaged or antibody-coated platelets in disorders such as autoimmune thrombocytopenic purpura. There is some evidence for accelerated platelet destruction in many instances of thrombocytopenia associated with disorders of the spleen.[106] The usual laboratory findings are pancytopenia with mild thrombocytopenia and a normal or moderately increased number of megakaryocytes in the bone marrow. Platelet counts in cirrhotic patients have been as low as 20,000/μL, although thrombocytopenia of this severity is uncommon. Patients with hypersplenism have smaller platelets than those with autoimmune thrombocytopenia, so platelet sizing may provide a means of differentiating between thrombocytopenia related primarily to immunologic platelet destruction and that related to big-spleen syndromes. In general, the severity of the thrombocytopenia correlates poorly with the size of the spleen, but it is nonetheless difficult to entertain a diagnosis of thrombocytopenia caused by abnormal splenic platelet pooling in the absence of significant splenic enlargement.

Therapy is seldom indicated for thrombocytopenia alone, but splenectomy, embolic occlusion of the splenic vasculature, and splenic damage secondary to infusion of radiolabeled particles can improve the thrombocytopenia and sometimes alleviate the pancytopenia completely.[107] Patients with thrombocytopenia secondary to cirrhosis with portal hypertension may benefit from portocaval shunts or transjugular intrahepatic portosystemic shunts.[108]

Thrombocytopenia Caused by Hypothermia

In humans, mild reversible thrombocytopenia is a predictable consequence of surgical hypothermia below 25 °C.[109] Thrombocytopenia has also been noted after hypothermia caused by environmental exposure.[17]

Adhesion of platelets to subendothelium is mediated through an interaction of the platelet GP Ib-IX-V complex and subendothelial vWF. The GP Ib-IX-V complex comprises four transmembrane polypeptide chains, GPIbα, GPIbβ, GPIX, and GPV. Lipid rafts (also known as glycolipid-enriched membranes) are dynamic assemblies of cholesterol and sphingolipids that are more ordered in structure than the rest of the plasma membrane.[110] Receptor clustering is an essential feature of signaling through lipid rafts and occurs in platelet membrane at lower temperatures.[111] A subset of the GP Ib-IX-V complex is constitutively associated with lipid rafts in unstimulated platelets.[112] Upon exposure to cold, the cooled platelets irreversibly reorganize vWF receptors (the [GPIb$\alpha\beta$IX]$_2$V complex) into clusters on the platelet surface. The hepatic macrophage integrin receptor Mac-1 (CD11b/CD18) recognizes clustered GPIbα, leading to phagocytosis of cooled platelets. Cooling, however, does not grossly impair the interaction between GPIb and activated vWF, implying that the hemostatic and clearance functions of GPIb are distinct.[113]

Thrombocytopenia Associated With Infections

Purpura was recognized as a manifestation of pestilential fevers 2000 years ago. Several factors are now known to cause bleeding in association with infections, of which thrombocytopenia is the most common.

Thrombocytopenia Associated With Viral Infections

Viruses may produce thrombocytopenia by several different mechanisms: impaired platelet production as a result of invasion of megakaryocytes by the virus, impaired platelet production caused by toxic effects of viral proteins on progenitor cells, viral-induced hemophagocytosis, destruction of circulating platelets by the virus, and increased platelet destruction caused by binding of viral-induced autoantibodies or viral antigen-antibody complexes.

The administration of live measles vaccine produced significant yet subclinical thrombocytopenia in most normal children.[114] Degenerating vacuolated megakaryocytes were evident 3 days after administration of the vaccine. The nadir of the platelet count occurred 7 days after vaccination. There are now several reports of thrombocytopenia occurring after immunization with measles-mumps-rubella vaccine, monovalent measles vaccine, and measles-mumps vaccine.[115] Thrombocytopenia has been severe (<20,000/µL), and some patients have had significant hemorrhagic complications. The majority of the patients have been <2 years of age, but the age range was 1 to 40 years.[116] Thrombocytopenia after vaccination for hepatitis A and B and varicella has also been noted.[117-119] Children with neonatal infections with mumps and rubella are often thrombocytopenic,[120] and hepatomegaly and splenomegaly may also be present. CMV infection is usually asymptomatic in immunocompetent adults. However, there are reports of severe thrombocytopenia and even thrombocytopenia with hemolysis.[121] It is unclear whether the thrombocytopenia is caused by a direct cytopathologic effect of the virus on megakaryocytes, viral-induced hemophagocytosis, or immunologic destruction.

Parvovirus B19 is the etiologic agent responsible for erythema infectiosum. It is also cytotoxic to erythroid progenitors and can cause aplastic crises in patients with hemolytic anemia and chronic bone marrow failure in immunocompromised hosts. Thrombocytopenia may occur in some of these patients, and recent studies demonstrate cytotoxic effects of viral nonstructural-1 proteins on megakaryocytes.[122]

Thrombocytopenia has been reported following the administration of adenoviral gene transfer vectors.[123] The interaction between adenovirus and platelets leads to platelet activation and rapid exposure of P-selectin on the platelet surface. Adenovirus also activates endothelial cells either directly or indirectly through activated platelets. It is followed by increases in total amounts of vWF and of ultralarge vWF multimers in plasma as well as an increase in the number of circulating endothelial cell–derived microparticles. Endothelial cell activation and the associated upregulation of adhesion molecules (VCAM-1) contribute to leukocyte and/or platelet leukocyte aggregate rolling and transendothelial migration, a critical process for tissue macrophage influx. This is followed by removal of activated platelets by tissue macrophages.

An ongoing pandemic due to novel coronavirus disease (COVID-19) caused by severe acute respiratory syndrome corona virus (SARS-CoV-2) has been shown to be associated with thrombocytopenia. Although the incidence is variable, mild thrombocytopenia is seen in almost one-third of the cases.[124] Idiopathic thrombocytopenic purpura (ITP) defined as platelet count <100 × 10^9/L was seen in approximately 45 cases of new-onset ITP in a systematic review.[124] A majority of the cases were seen in elderly with few exceptions of pediatric cases. Usually, a short course of glucocorticoids or intravenous immune globulin is effective in these conditions.[124] ITP has also been reported after COVID 19 vaccination.[124-126]

Thrombocytopenia Associated With Bacterial and Protozoal Infections

Thrombocytopenia commonly is associated with septicemia resulting from both gram-negative and gram-positive bacteria. This complication is particularly common in infants and children, and the presence of unexplained thrombocytopenia, particularly in this age group, should always alert the physician to the possibility of septicemia. The etiology of thrombocytopenia may be multifactorial. Thrombocytopenia may be caused by disseminated intravascular coagulation (DIC), and the diagnosis of DIC may be apparent when coagulation studies are performed. Thrombocytopenia has also been described in patients with gram-negative or gram-positive septicemia, and 46% of these patients had elevated platelet-associated immunoglobulin G without evidence of DIC. These studies were interpreted as demonstrating the presence of platelet destruction caused by splenic destruction of immune complex–coated platelets. These data must be reinterpreted with third-generation immune complex capture assays that can better define platelet autoantibodies and immune complexes.

Platelet adherence to damaged vascular surfaces may also account for thrombocytopenia in certain bacterial infections, such as meningococcemia. Endotoxins, exotoxins, or platelet-activating factor may damage platelets, resulting in increased clearance. Patients with sepsis syndrome may develop hemophagocytic histiocytosis with phagocytosis of platelets, white cells, and platelets in bone marrow histiocytes.[127]

Thrombocytopenia may also be caused by direct platelet toxicity caused by the microorganism. Thrombocytopenia occurs in >80% of patients with malaria, and platelets from patients with malaria have been demonstrated to contain plasmodia.[128] Significant ultrastructural changes in platelets of patients with malaria are present, and the extent of abnormal findings correlates with the level of parasitemia.[129]

The pathophysiology of thrombocytopenia in malaria has recently been studied in a mouse model of experimental malaria induced by *Plasmodium berghei*. Signaling through multipotent immunomodulator CD40L and its receptor CD40, expressed on activated platelets, initiates the caspase cascade, resulting in apoptosis of the platelet and the formation of platelet microparticles.[130] Early depletion of platelets leads to an altered immune response with significantly decreased levels of proinflammatory cytokines, such as interferon-γ and interleukin (IL) 2, as well as increased levels of IL-10, indicating a role for platelets in the regulation of pathogenic cytokines and cell-mediated immune responses.[131] Cell-mediated rather than the humoral immune response has been shown to play a major role in development of thrombocytopenia.[132]

Theoretically, any bacterial or protozoal infection can be associated with thrombocytopenia that is caused by one of the mechanisms hypothesized in this chapter. There are reports of thrombocytopenia in Lyme disease and *Mycoplasma pneumoniae* infections, a manifestation of these infections that appears to be uncommon.[133,134]

Patients with thrombocytopenia associated with infection should be tested for the presence of DIC. The most important therapy for infection-related thrombocytopenia is that directed at the underlying infection. Platelet transfusions, with or without intravenous IgG, can be used to control bleeding until antimicrobial therapy is effective.

Thrombocytopenia After Massive Blood Transfusion

Massive blood transfusion is defined as complete replacement of a patient's blood volume within 24 hours, usually 10 units of packed RBCs for an average-sized adult. Because packed RBCs do not contain a significant number of functional platelets and do not replace labile clotting factors, there has been concern about the incidence of developing hemostatic abnormalities and clinical bleeding in patients given only packed RBCs.

Some studies demonstrate a correlation between the number of units of packed RBCs transfused and both reduction in platelet counts ("dilutional thrombocytopenia") and increases in prothrombin and partial thromboplastin times. However, significant changes (platelets, 50,000-100,000/μL) are not apparent until patients have received >15 units of blood.[135,136] *Severe thrombocytopenia*, defined as a platelet count <50,000/μL, is most common in patients receiving >20 units of blood.[137] Microvascular bleeding occurs in 20% to 60% of patients who are massively transfused, but neither the platelet count nor changes in coagulation studies can be used to predict which patients will bleed.[135] Although bleeding appears to be more dependent on thrombocytopenia than on coagulation abnormalities, prophylactic administration of platelets was no more effective than equivalent volumes of prophylactic fresh-frozen plasma infusions in preventing bleeding.[136] Therefore, it is recommended that platelet and plasma replacement during massive transfusions be guided by serial monitoring of platelet counts, prothrombin time, and partial thromboplastin time and that platelet counts be kept >75,000/μL and prothrombin time and partial thromboplastin time <1.5 times normal. The coagulopathy associated with massive blood transfusion is discussed further in Chapter 55.

References

1. Balduini CL, Pecci A, Noris P. Inherited thrombocytopenias: the evolving spectrum. *Hämostaseologie*. 2012;32:259-270.
2. Johnson B, Doak R, Allsup D, et al. A comprehensive targeted next-generation sequencing panel for genetic diagnosis of patients with suspected inherited thrombocytopenia. *Res Pract Thromb Haemost*. 2018;2:640-652.
3. Mekchay P, Ittiwut C, Ittiwut R, et al. Whole exome sequencing for diagnosis of hereditary thrombocytopenia. *Medicine (Baltim)*. 2020;99:e23275.
4. Noris P, Pecci A. Hereditary thrombocytopenias: a growing list of disorders. *Hematology Am Soc Hematol Educ Program*. 2017;2017:385-399.
5. Bury L, Falcinelli E, Gresele P. Learning the ropes of platelet count regulation: inherited thrombocytopenias. *J Clin Med*. 2021;10(3):533.
6. Freedman MH, Estrov Z. Congenital amegakaryocytic thrombocytopenia: an intrinsic hematopoietic stem cell defect. *Am J Pediatr Hematol Oncol*. 1990;12:225-230.
7. Muraoka K, Ishii E, Tsuji K, et al. Defective response to thrombopoietin and impaired expression of c-mpl mRNA of bone marrow cells in congenital amegakaryocytic thrombocytopenia. *Br J Haematol*. 1997;96:287-292.
8. Ihara K, Ishii E, Eguchi M, et al. Identification of mutations in the c-mpl gene in congenital amegakaryocytic thrombocytopenia. *Proc Natl Acad Sci U S A*. 1999;96:3132-3136.
9. Ballmaier M, Germeshausen M, Schulze H, et al. c-mpl mutations are the cause of congenital amegakaryocytic thrombocytopenia. *Blood*. 2001;97:139-146.
10. Germeshausen M, Ballmaier M. CAMT-MPL: congenital Amegakaryocytic Thrombocytopenia caused by MPL mutations—heterogeneity of a monogenic disorder—comprehensive analysis of 56 patients. *Haematologica*. 2021;106(9):2439-2448.
11. Ng AP, Kauppi M, Metcalf D, et al. Mpl expression on megakaryocytes and platelets is dispensable for thrombopoiesis but essential to prevent myeloproliferation. *Proc Natl Acad Sci U S A*. 2014;111:5884-5889.
12. Germeshausen M, Ballmaier M, Welte K. MPL mutations in 23 patients suffering from congenital amegakaryocytic thrombocytopenia: the type of mutation predicts the course of the disease. *Hum Mutat*. 2006;27:296.
13. Hall JG, Levin J, Kuhn JP, Ottenheimer EJ, van Berkum KA, McKusick VA. Thrombocytopenia with absent radius (TAR). *Medicine (Baltim)*. 1969;48:411-439.
14. Shaw S, Oliver RA. Congenital hypoplastic thrombocytopenia with skeletal deformaties in siblings. *Blood*. 1959;14:374-377.
15. Hedberg VA, Lipton JM. Thrombocytopenia with absent radii. A review of 100 cases. *Am J Pediatr Hematol Oncol*. 1988;10:51-64.
16. Greenhalgh KL, Howell RT, Bottani A, et al. Thrombocytopenia-absent radius syndrome: a clinical genetic study. *J Med Genet*. 2002;39:876-881.
17. Albers CA, Paul DS, Schulze H, et al. Compound inheritance of a low-frequency regulatory SNP and a rare null mutation in exon-junction complex subunit RBM8A causes TAR syndrome. *Nat Genet*. 2012;44:435-439.
18. Boussion S, Escande F, Jourdain AS, et al. TAR syndrome: clinical and molecular characterization of a cohort of 26 patients and description of novel noncoding variants of RBM8A. *Hum Mutat*. 2020;41:1220-1225.
19. Weinblatt M, Petrikovsky B, Bialer M, Kochen J, Harper R. Prenatal evaluation and in utero platelet transfusion for thrombocytopenia absent radii syndrome. *Prenat Diagn*. 1994;14:892-896.
20. Donnenfeld AE, Wiseman B, Lavi E, Weiner S. Prenatal diagnosis of thrombocytopenia absent radius syndrome by ultrasound and cordocentesis. *Prenat Diagn*. 1990;10:29-35.
21. Boute O, Depret-Mosser S, Vinatier D, et al. Prenatal diagnosis of thrombocytopenia-absent radius syndrome. *Fetal Diagn Ther*. 1996;11:224-230.
22. Tongsong T, Sirichotiyakul S, Chanprapaph P. Prenatal diagnosis of thrombocytopenia-absent-radius (TAR) syndrome. *Ultrasound Obstet Gynecol*. 2000;15:256-258.
23. Geddis AE. Inherited thrombocytopenias: an approach to diagnosis and management. *Int J Lab Hematol*. 2013;35:14-25.
24. D'Apolito M, Guarnieri V, Boncristiano M, Zelante L, Savoia A. Cloning of the murine non-muscle myosin heavy chain IIA gene ortholog of human MYH9 responsible for May-Hegglin, Sebastian, Fechtner, and Epstein syndromes. *Gene*. 2002;286:215-222.
25. Seri M, Cusano R, Gangarossa S, et al. Mutations in MYH9 result in the May-Hegglin anomaly, and Fechtner and Sebastian syndromes. The May-Hegglin/Fechtner syndrome consortium. *Nat Genet*. 2000;26:103-105.
26. Kelley MJ, Jawien W, Ortel TL, Korczak JF. Mutation of MYH9, encoding non-muscle myosin heavy chain A, in May-Hegglin anomaly. *Nat Genet*. 2000;26:106-108.
27. Kelley MJ, Jawien W, Lin A, et al. Autosomal dominant macrothrombocytopenia with leukocyte inclusions (May-Hegglin anomaly) is linked to chromosome 22q12-13. *Hum Genet*. 2000;106:557-564.
28. Dong F, Li S, Pujol-Moix N, et al. Genotype-phenotype correlation in MYH9-related thrombocytopenia. *Br J Haematol*. 2005;130:620-627.
29. Seri M, Pecci A, Di Bari F, et al. MYH9-related disease: May-Hegglin anomaly, Sebastian syndrome, Fechtner syndrome, and Epstein syndrome are not distinct entities but represent a variable expression of a single illness. *Medicine (Baltim)*. 2003;82:203-215.
30. Balduini CL, Pecci A, Savoia A. Recent advances in the understanding and management of MYH9-related inherited thrombocytopenias. *Br J Haematol*. 2011;154:161-174.
31. Savoia A, De Rocco D, Panza E, et al. Heavy chain myosin 9-related disease (MYH9 -RD): neutrophil inclusions of myosin-9 as a pathognomonic sign of the disorder. *Thromb Haemostasis*. 2010;103:826-832.
32. Saito H, Kunishima S. Historical hematology: May-Hegglin anomaly. *Am J Hematol*. 2008;83:304-306.
33. Pecci A, Panza E, Pujol-Moix N, et al. Position of nonmuscle myosin heavy chain IIA (NMMHC-IIA) mutations predicts the natural history of MYH9-related disease. *Hum Mutat*. 2008;29:409-417.
34. Heath KE, Campos-Barros A, Toren A, et al. Nonmuscle myosin heavy chain IIA mutations define a spectrum of autosomal dominant macrothrombocytopenias: May-Hegglin anomaly and Fechtner, Sebastian, Epstein, and Alport-like syndromes. *Am J Hum Genet*. 2001;69:1033-1045.
35. Pecci A, Gresele P, Klersy C, et al. Eltrombopag for the treatment of the inherited thrombocytopenia deriving from MYH9 mutations. *Blood*. 2010;116:5832-5837.
36. Bastida JM, Gonzalez-Porras JR, Rivera J, Lozano ML. Role of thrombopoietin receptor agonists in inherited thrombocytopenia. *Int J Mol Sci*. 2021;22(9):4330.
37. Nurden AT, Nurden P. Inherited thrombocytopenias: history, advances and perspectives. *Haematologica*. 2020;105:2004-2019.
38. Jongmans MC, Kuiper RP, Carmichael CL, et al. Novel RUNX1 mutations in familial platelet disorder with enhanced risk for acute myeloid leukemia: clues for improved identification of the FPD/AML syndrome. *Leukemia*. 2010;24:242-246.
39. Noris P, Perrotta S, Seri M, et al. Mutations in ANKRD26 are responsible for a frequent form of inherited thrombocytopenia: analysis of 78 patients from 21 families. *Blood*. 2011;117:6673-6680.
40. Drachman JG, Jarvik GP, Mehaffey MG. Autosomal dominant thrombocytopenia: incomplete megakaryocyte differentiation and linkage to human chromosome 10. *Blood*. 2000;96:118-125.
41. Noetzli L, Lo RW, Lee-Sherick AB, et al. Germline mutations in ETV6 are associated with thrombocytopenia, red cell macrocytosis and predisposition to lymphoblastic leukemia. *Nat Genet*. 2015;47:535-538.

42. Melazzini F, Palombo F, Balduini A, et al. Clinical and pathogenic features of ETV6-related thrombocytopenia with predisposition to acute lymphoblastic leukemia. *Haematologica*. 2016;101:1333-1342.
43. Behrens WE. Mediterranean macrothrombocytopenia. *Blood*. 1975;46:199-208.
44. Savoia A, Balduini CL, Savino M, et al. Autosomal dominant macrothrombocytopenia in Italy is most frequently a type of heterozygous Bernard-Soulier syndrome. *Blood*. 2001;97:1330-1335.
45. Grossfeld PD, Mattina T, Lai Z, et al. The 11q terminal deletion disorder: a prospective study of 110 cases. *Am J Med Genet A*. 2004;129A:51-61.
46. Favier R, Jondeau K, Boutard P, et al. Paris-Trousseau syndrome: clinical, hematological, molecular data of ten new cases. *Thromb Haemostasis*. 2003;90:893-897.
47. Raslova H, Komura E, Le Couedic JP, et al. FLI1 monoallelic expression combined with its hemizygous loss underlies Paris-Trousseau/Jacobsen thrombopenia. *J Clin Invest*. 2004;114:77-84.
48. Shivdasani RA. Lonely in Paris: when one gene copy isn't enough. *J Clin Invest*. 2004;114:17-19.
49. Nurden AT, Nurden P. The gray platelet syndrome: clinical spectrum of the disease. *Blood Rev*. 2007;21:21-36.
50. Harrison P, Cramer EM. Platelet alpha-granules. *Blood Rev*. 1993;7:52-62.
51. Kahr WH, Hinckley J, Li L, et al. Mutations in NBEAL2, encoding a BEACH protein, cause gray platelet syndrome. *Nat Genet*. 2011;43:738-740.
52. Mark M, Rijli FM, Chambon P. Homeobox genes in embryogenesis and pathogenesis. *Pediatr Res*. 1997;42:421-429.
53. Thompson AA, Nguyen LT. Amegakaryocytic thrombocytopenia and radio-ulnar synostosis are associated with HOXA11 mutation. *Nat Genet*. 2000;26:397-398.
54. Horvat-Switzer RD, Thompson AA. HOXA11 mutation in amegakaryocytic thrombocytopenia with radio-ulnar synostosis syndrome inhibits megakaryocytic differentiation in vitro. *Blood Cells Mol Dis*. 2006;37:55-63.
55. Niihori T, Ouchi-Uchiyama M, Sasahara Y, et al. Mutations in MECOM, encoding oncoprotein EVI1, cause radioulnar synostosis with amegakaryocytic thrombopenia. *Am J Hum Genet*. 2015;97:848-854.
56. Thompson AA, Woodruff K, Feig SA, Nguyen LT, Schanen NC. Congenital thrombocytopenia and radio-ulnar synostosis: a new familial syndrome. *Br J Haematol*. 2001;113:866-870.
57. Germeshausen M, Ancliff P, Estrada J, et al. MECOM-associated syndrome: a heterogeneous inherited bone marrow failure syndrome with amegakaryocytic thrombocytopenia. *Blood Adv*. 2018;2:586-596.
58. Bolton-Maggs PH, Chalmers EA, Collins PW, et al. A review of inherited platelet disorders with guidelines for their management on behalf of the UKHCDO. *Br J Haematol*. 2006;135:603-633.
59. Bosticardo M, Marangoni F, Aiuti A, Villa A, Grazia Roncarolo M. Recent advances in understanding the pathophysiology of Wiskott-Aldrich syndrome. *Blood*. 2009;113:6288-6295.
60. Devriendt K, Kim AS, Mathijs G, et al. Constitutively activating mutation in WASP causes X-linked severe congenital neutropenia. *Nat Genet*. 2001;27:313-317.
61. Derry JM, Kerns JA, Weinberg KI, et al. WASP gene mutations in Wiskott-Aldrich syndrome and X-linked thrombocytopenia. *Hum Mol Genet*. 1995;4:1127-1135.
62. Derry JM, Ochs HD, Francke U. Isolation of a novel gene mutated in Wiskott-Aldrich syndrome. *Cell*. 1994;78:635-644.
63. Ancliff P, Blundell MP, Gale RE, et al. Activating mutations in the Wiskott-Aldrich syndrome protein may define a sub-group of severe congenital neutropenia (SCN) with specific and unusual laboratory features. *Blood*. 2001;98:493.
64. Jin Y, Mazza C, Christie JR, et al. Mutations of the Wiskott-Aldrich Syndrome Protein (WASP): hotspots, effect on transcription, and translation and phenotype/genotype correlation. *Blood*. 2004;104:4010-4019.
65. Ochs HD, Thrasher AJ. The Wiskott-Aldrich syndrome. *J Allergy Clin Immunol*. 2006;117:725-738. quiz 39.
66. Thrasher AJ. New insights into the biology of Wiskott-Aldrich syndrome (WAS). *Hematology Am Soc Hematol Educ Program*. 2009;2009:132-138.
67. Braun CJ, Boztug K, Paruzynski A, et al. Gene therapy for Wiskott-Aldrich syndrome--long-term efficacy and genotoxicity. *Sci Transl Med*. 2014;6:227ra33.
68. Boztug K, Schmidt M, Schwarzer A, et al. Stem-cell gene therapy for the Wiskott-Aldrich syndrome. *N Engl J Med*. 2010;363:1918-1927.
69. Morris EC, Fox T, Chakraverty R, et al. Gene therapy for Wiskott-Aldrich syndrome in a severely affected adult. *Blood*. 2017;130:1327-1335.
70. Ferrua F, Cicalese MP, Galimberti S, et al. Lentiviral haemopoietic stem/progenitor cell gene therapy for treatment of Wiskott-Aldrich syndrome: interim results of a non-randomised, open-label, phase 1/2 clinical study. *Lancet Haematol*. 2019;6:e239-e53.
71. Wall L, deBoer E, Grosveld F. The human beta-globin gene 3' enhancer contains multiple binding sites for an erythroid-specific protein. *Genes Dev*. 1988;2:1089-1100.
72. Tsai SF, Martin DI, Zon LI, D'Andrea AD, Wong GG, Orkin SH. Cloning of cDNA for the major DNA-binding protein of the erythroid lineage through expression in mammalian cells. *Nature*. 1989;339:446-451.
73. Martin DI, Orkin SH. Transcriptional activation and DNA binding by the erythroid factor GF-1/NF-E1/Eryf 1. *Genes Dev*. 1990;4:1886-1898.
74. Tsang AP, Fujiwara Y, Hom DB, Orkin SH. Failure of megakaryopoiesis and arrested erythropoiesis in mice lacking the GATA-1 transcriptional cofactor FOG. *Genes Dev*. 1998;12:1176-1188.
75. Songdej N, Rao AK. Hematopoietic transcription factor mutations: important players in inherited platelet defects. *Blood*. 2017;129:2873-2881.
76. Nichols KE, Crispino JD, Poncz M, et al. Familial dyserythropoietic anaemia and thrombocytopenia due to an inherited mutation in GATA1. *Nat Genet*. 2000;24:266-270.
77. Drachman JG. Inherited thrombocytopenia: when a low platelet count does not mean ITP. *Blood*. 2004;103:390-398.
78. Hollanda LM, Lima CS, Cunha AF, et al. An inherited mutation leading to production of only the short isoform of GATA-1 is associated with impaired erythropoiesis. *Nat Genet*. 2006;38:807-812.
79. Zucker J, Temm C, Czader M, Nalepa G. A child with dyserythropoietic anemia and megakaryocyte dysplasia due to a novel 5'UTR GATA1s splice mutation. *Pediatr Blood Cancer*. 2016;63:917-921.
80. McDonald-McGinn DM, Sullivan KE. Chromosome 22q11.2 deletion syndrome (DiGeorge syndrome/velocardiofacial syndrome). *Medicine (Baltim)*. 2011;90:1-18.
81. Hoffman R. Acquired pure amegakaryocytic thrombocytopenic purpura. *Semin Hematol*. 1991;28:303-312.
82. Bhattacharyya J, Kumar R, Tyagi S, Kishore J, Mahapatra M, Choudhry VP. Human parvovirus B19-induced acquired pure amegakaryocytic thrombocytopenia. *Br J Haematol*. 2005;128:128-129.
83. Benedetti F, de Sabata D, Perona G. T suppressor activated lymphocytes (CD8+/DR+) inhibit megakaryocyte progenitor cell differentiation in a case of acquired amegakaryocytic thrombocytopenic purpura. *Stem Cell*. 1994;12:205-213.
84. Shiozaki H, Miyawaki S, Kuwaki T, Hagiwara T, Kato T, Miyazaki H. Autoantibodies neutralizing thrombopoietin in a patient with amegakaryocytic thrombocytopenic purpura. *Blood*. 2000;95:2187-2188.
85. Agarwal N, Spahr JE, Werner TL, Newton DL, Rodgers GM. Acquired amegakaryocytic thrombocytopenic purpura. *Am J Hematol*. 2006;81:132-135.
86. Lonial S, Bilodeau PA, Langston AA, et al. Acquired amegakaryocytic thrombocytopenia treated with allogeneic BMT: a case report and review of the literature. *Bone Marrow Transplant*. 1999;24:1337-1341.
87. Trimble MS, Glynn MF, Brain MC. Amegakaryocytic thrombocytopenia of 4 years duration: successful treatment with antithymocyte globulin. *Am J Hematol*. 1991;37:126-127.
88. Deeren D, Dorpe JV. Effective use of rituximab for acquired amegakaryocytic thrombocytopenia. *Am J Hematol*. 2010;85:977-978.
89. Chang H, Tang TC. Successful treatment of amegakaryocytic thrombocytopenia with azathioprine. *Acta Haematol*. 2011;126:135-137.
90. Quintas-Cardama A. Acquired amegakaryocytic thrombocytopenic purpura successfully treated with limited cyclosporin A therapy. *Eur J Haematol*. 2002;69:185-186.
91. Bussel JB, Kuter DJ, George JN, et al. AMG 531, a thrombopoiesis-stimulating protein, for chronic ITP. *N Engl J Med*. 2006;355:1672-1681.
92. Zimmerman BS, Marcellino B, El Jamal SM, Renteria AS. Acquired amegakaryocytic thrombocytopenia as a rare cause of thrombocytopenia during pregnancy. *BMJ Case Rep*. 2019;12(6):e230361.
93. Novotny JP, Kohler B, Max R, Egerer G. Acquired amegakaryocytic thrombocytopenic purpura progressing into aplastic anemia. *Prague Med Rep*. 2017;118:147-155.
94. Cowan DH. Thrombokinetic studies in alcohol-related thrombocytopenia. *J Lab Clin Med*. 1973;81:64-76.
95. Kutti J, Weinfeld A. The frequency of thrombocytopenia in patients with heart disease treated with oral diuretics. *Acta Med Scand*. 1968;183:245-250.
96. Cooper BA, Bigelow FS. Thrombocytopenia associated with the administration of diethylstilbestrol in man. *Ann Intern Med*. 1960;52:907-909.
97. Cowan DH. Effect of alcoholism on hemostasis. *Semin Hematol*. 1980;17:137-147.
98. Cowan DH, Hines JD. Thrombocytopenia of severe alcoholism. *Ann Intern Med*. 1971;74:37-43.
99. Heyns AD, Lotter MG, Badenhorst PN, van Reenen O, Pieters H, Minnaar PC. Kinetics and fate of (111)Indium-oxine labelled blood platelets in asplenic subjects. *Thromb Haemostasis*. 1980;44:100-104.
100. Levine RF, Spivak JL, Meagher RC, Sieber F. Effect of ethanol on thrombopoiesis. *Br J Haematol*. 1986;62:345-354.
101. Nakao S, Harada M, Kondo K, Mizushima N, Matsuda T. Reversible bone marrow hypoplasia induced by alcohol. *Am J Hematol*. 1991;37:120-123.
102. Queisser U, Queisser W, Spiertz B. Polyploidization of megakaryocytes in normal humans, in patients with idiopathic thrombocytopenia and with pernicious anaemia. *Br J Haematol*. 1971;20:489-501.
103. Aster RH. Pooling of platelets in the spleen: role in the pathogenesis of "hypersplenic" thrombocytopenia. *J Clin Invest*. 1966;45:645-657.
104. Peters AM, Klonizakis I, Lavender JP, Lewis SM. Use of 111Indium-labeled platelets to measure spleen function. *Br J Haematol*. 1980;46:587-593.
105. Wadenvik H, Kutti J. The effect of an adrenaline infusion on the splenic blood flow and intrasplenic platelet kinetics. *Br J Haematol*. 1987;67:187-192.
106. Lee EJ, Schiffer CA. Evidence for rapid mobilization of platelets from the spleen during intensive plateletpheresis. *Am J Hematol*. 1985;19:161-165.
107. Pinca A, Di Palma A, Soriani S, et al. Effectiveness of partial splenic embolization as treatment for hypersplenism in thalassaemia major: a 7-year follow up. *Eur J Haematol*. 1992;49:49-52.
108. Pursnani KG, Sillin LF, Kaplan DS. Effect of transjugular intrahepatic portosystemic shunt on secondary hypersplenism. *Am J Surg*. 1997;173:169-173.
109. Chan KM, Beard K. A patient with recurrent hypothermia associated with thrombocytopenia. *Postgrad Med J*. 1993;69:227-229.
110. Simons K, Ikonen E. Functional rafts in cell membranes. *Nature*. 1997;387:569-572.
111. Tablin F, Wolkers WF, Walker NJ, et al. Membrane reorganization during chilling: implications for long-term stabilization of platelets. *Cryobiology*. 2001;43:114-123.
112. Shrimpton CN, Borthakur G, Larrucea S, Cruz MA, Dong JF, Lopez JA. Localization of the adhesion receptor glycoprotein Ib-IX-V complex to lipid rafts is required for platelet adhesion and activation. *J Exp Med*. 2002;196:1057-1066.
113. Josefsson EC, Gebhard HH, Stossel TP, Hartwig JH, Hoffmeister KM. The macrophage alphaMbeta2 integrin alphaM lectin domain mediates the phagocytosis of chilled platelets. *J Biol Chem*. 2005;280:18025-18032.

114. Oski FA, Naiman JL. Effect of live measles vaccine on the platelet count. *N Engl J Med*. 1966;275:352-356.
115. Nieminen U, Peltola H, Syrjala MT, Makipernaa A, Kekomaki R. Acute thrombocytopenic purpura following measles, mumps and rubella vaccination. A report on 23 patients. *Acta Paediatr*. 1993;82:267-270.
116. Beeler J, Varricchio F, Wise R. Thrombocytopenia after immunization with measles vaccines: review of the vaccine adverse events reporting system (1990 to 1994). *Pediatr Infect Dis J*. 1996;15:88-90.
117. Poullin P, Gabriel B. Thrombocytopenic purpura after recombinant hepatitis B vaccine. *Lancet*. 1994;344:1293.
118. Meyboom RH, Fucik H, Edwards IR. Thrombocytopenia reported in association with hepatitis B and A vaccines. *Lancet*. 1995;345:1638.
119. Myllyla G, Vaheri A, Vesikari T, Penttinen K. Interaction between human blood platelets, viruses and antibodies. IV. Post-Rubella thrombocytopenic purpura and platelet aggregation by Rubella antigen-antibody interaction. *Clin Exp Immunol*. 1969;4:323-332.
120. Cooper LZ, Green RH, Krugman S, Giles JP, Mirick GS. Neonatal thrombocytopenic purpura and other manifestations of rubella contracted in utero. *Am J Dis Child*. 1965;110:416-427.
121. van Spronsen DJ, Breed WP. Cytomegalovirus-induced thrombocytopenia and haemolysis in an immunocompetent adult. *Br J Haematol*. 1996;92:218-220.
122. Murray JC, Morad AB, Pierce MA, Mihm S. Thrombocytopenia accompanying early postnatal infection by human parvovirus B19. *Am J Hematol*. 1995;49:360.
123. Varnavski AN, Calcedo R, Bove M, Gao G, Wilson JM. Evaluation of toxicity from high-dose systemic administration of recombinant adenovirus vector in vector-naive and pre-immunized mice. *Gene Ther*. 2005;12:427-436.
124. Bhattacharjee S, Banerjee M. Immune thrombocytopenia secondary to COVID-19: a systematic review. *SN Compr Clin Med*. 2020;2(11):1-11.
125. Akiyama H, Kakiuchi S, Rikitake J, et al. Immune thrombocytopenia associated with Pfizer-BioNTech's BNT162b2 mRNA COVID-19 vaccine. *IDCases*. 2021;25:e01245.
126. Shah SRA, Dolkar S, Mathew J, Vishnu P. COVID-19 vaccination associated severe immune thrombocytopenia. *Exp Hematol Oncol*. 2021;10:42.
127. Stephan F, Thioliere B, Verdy E, Tulliez M. Role of hemophagocytic histiocytosis in the etiology of thrombocytopenia in patients with sepsis syndrome or septic shock. *Clin Infect Dis*. 1997;25:1159-1164.
128. Fajardo LFTC. Malarial parasites withing human platelets. *JAMA*. 1974;229:1205.
129. el-Shoura S. Falciparum malaria in naturally infected humans. III. Platelet ultrastructural alterations during thrombocytopenia. *Virchows Arch B Cell Pathol Incl Mol Pathol*. 1993;63:257-262.
130. Piguet PF, Kan CD, Vesin C. Thrombocytopenia in an animal model of malaria is associated with an increased caspase-mediated death of thrombocytes. *Apoptosis*. 2002;7:91-98.
131. van der Heyde HC, Gramaglia I, Sun G, Woods C. Platelet depletion by anti-CD41 (alphaIIb) mAb injection early but not late in the course of disease protects against Plasmodium berghei pathogenesis by altering the levels of pathogenic cytokines. *Blood*. 2005;105:1956-1963.
132. Gramaglia I, Sahlin H, Nolan JP, Frangos JA, Intaglietta M, van der Heyde HC. Cell- rather than antibody-mediated immunity leads to the development of profound thrombocytopenia during experimental Plasmodium berghei malaria. *J Immunol*. 2005;175:7699-7707.
133. Ballard HS, Bottino G, Bottino J. The association of thrombocytopaenia and Lyme disease. *Postgrad Med J*. 1994;70:285-287.
134. Pugliese A, Levchuck S, Cunha BA. Mycoplasma pneumoniae induced thrombocytopenia. *Heart Lung*. 1993;22:373-375.
135. Harrigan C, Lucas CE, Ledgerwood AM, Walz DA, Mammen EF. Serial changes in primary hemostasis after massive transfusion. *Surgery*. 1985;98:836-844.
136. Reed RL, IInd, Ciavarella D, Heimbach DM, et al. Prophylactic platelet administration during massive transfusion. A prospective, randomized, double-blind clinical study. *Ann Surg*. 1986;203:40-48.
137. Leslie SD, Toy PT. Laboratory hemostatic abnormalities in massively transfused patients given red blood cells and crystalloid. *Am J Clin Pathol*. 1991;96:770-773.

Chapter 51 ■ Bleeding Disorders Caused by Vascular Abnormalities

GEORGE M. RODGERS

INTRODUCTION

This chapter discusses causes of bleeding that are not the result of thrombocytopenia, coagulation factor deficiency, or qualitative platelet defects. Bleeding disorders caused by these various "vascular" abnormalities represent a heterogenous group of diseases, and in considering the differential diagnosis, it is convenient to consider cutaneous causes, connective tissue abnormalities, vascular lesions, and intravascular causes.

CLINICAL APPROACH TO THE PATIENT

The initial approach to the bleeding patient is discussed in Chapter 46. When considering "vascular" causes of bleeding, the appearance of the lesions (petechiae vs more extensive ecchymosis, size, shape, color), location and pattern of involvement, associated features (fever, ulcers, scars, livedo reticularis), and the clinical setting are helpful clues. *Table 51.1* lists some common physical finding patterns helpful in considering the differential diagnosis of vascular disorders.

Purpura is the term used to describe the skin lesions that develop when red blood cells extravasate from capillaries. Purpura refers to either pinpoint lesions called petechiae or more widespread lesions known as ecchymoses. True purpura does not blanch with pressure.

MECHANICAL PURPURA

External pressure such as blunt trauma results in ecchymoses when the force is sufficient to disrupt vascular integrity and allow extravasation of red blood cells. The size of the resulting lesion is dependent on the durability of the tissue traumatized, the vascularity of the region, the density of the surrounding tissue, and the time elapsed.[1,2] The extent of bruising can increase over time, and tracking through tissue planes can occur, resulting in bruises in areas remote from the area of trauma.[3] The color of the lesion is in part dependent on the location of the red cells—lesions near the surface have a more reddish color, and deeper lesions appear bluish. This finding is due to optical scattering in the dermis and the fact that blue wavelengths scatter and reflect more than red.[4]

Mechanical purpura can be seen on occasion with minor trauma such as blood pressure cuff monitoring in anticoagulated patients[2] or even vigorous scratching. Young adults playing active sports such as basketball can develop calcaneal petechiae resulting from relatively minor, but repetitive, heel trauma.[5] Periorbital, face, or neck purpura can occur after a sudden increase in intravascular pressure with a Valsalva maneuver[6] and has been described after bungee jumping.[7]

Suction purpura occurs when negative pressure is applied to the skin in sufficient force to result in extravasation of erythrocytes. Young healthy people develop petechiae with 350 to 400 mm Hg negative pressure, but the required amount of pressure to induce purpura decreases with age to as low as 100 mm Hg.[8] The application of rubber suction devices to the forehead can result in circumscribed purpura. This seems to occur mostly when new parents apply children's suction toys to their foreheads and has been termed *cyclops purpura*.[9] A similar, relatively common cause of suction purpura is seen in adolescents who place a drinking glass over their chin and suck out the air to form a vacuum, ultimately causing chin or perioral purpura.[10]

Larger ecchymotic areas may also demonstrate other patterns that can be a clue to underlying pathology. The well-known Cullen sign refers to bluish discoloration around the umbilicus, and Grey-Turner sign is flank ecchymosis. Both may indicate hemorrhagic pancreatitis or a rectus sheath hematoma.[11] Scrotal ecchymosis may be a clue to intraperitoneal hemorrhage, and perianal ecchymosis has been described as a manifestation of aneurysmal rupture into the sigmoid mesocolon.[12] "Raccoon eyes" and mastoid ecchymosis (Battle sign) may indicate a basilar skull fracture after head trauma.[13]

STRUCTURAL MALFORMATIONS OF VESSELS

Hereditary Hemorrhagic Telangiectasia

Hereditary hemorrhagic telangiectasia (HHT) was first described in 1864 by Sutton[14] and later recognized and reported by Rendu,[15] Osler,[16] and Weber,[17] and it is thus also known as Osler-Weber-Rendu syndrome. It is an autosomal dominant disorder characterized by multiple telangiectatic lesions involving the skin and mucous membranes associated with epistaxis and other bleeding complications. HHT has an estimated prevalence of 1 in 8000,[18] with complete penetrance by 40 years of age.[19]

Genetic studies have identified several mutations responsible for the vascular malformations. Mutations in the endoglin gene on chromosome 9 (HHT1) or in the activin receptor–like kinase (*ALK1*) gene on chromosome 12 (HHT2) account for ~85% of the cases. Currently more than 500 mutations in the *ALK1* or endoglin gene have been identified, and each family studied appears to have a unique mutation.[18] Endoglin is an integral membrane glycoprotein expressed on endothelial cells in arterioles, venules, and capillaries. This glycoprotein and *ALK1* serve as a binding protein for transforming growth factor-β (TGF-β). TGF-β regulates many transcriptional targets and plays a crucial role in vascular development and homeostasis. Other mutations seen with HHT include mutations in the *SMAD4* gene associated with juvenile polyposis and HHT[20] and the *GDF2* gene.[21]

Ultrastructural analysis of cutaneous HHT lesions suggests that postcapillary venule dilation is the earliest identifiable morphologic abnormality.[22,23] As the venules enlarge, they become convoluted and interconnect with arterioles through capillary segments. The capillary segments eventually disappear, and direct arteriolar-venular communications are established. An infiltrate of mononuclear cells appears in the perivascular region of the HHT lesions.

The bleeding manifestations are thought to occur because of mechanical fragility of these vessels. Common abnormalities in the hemostatic system do not seem to represent a major factor in the underlying bleeding tendency. Patients with HHT manifest a variety of other complications including shunting, emboli, and thrombosis.

Clinical Manifestations

The cutaneous lesions usually appear in affected persons by 40 years of age, and they increase in number with age. The lesions measure 1 to 3 mm in diameter and are sharply demarcated in appearance (*Figure 51.1*). They blanch with pressure, but the blanching may be incomplete as a result of "strangulation" of coiled loops of vessels.[24,25] The telangiectatic lesions are most commonly found on the face, lips, nares, tongue, nail beds, and hands. Some patients have only a few lesions, necessitating a thorough search in anyone suspected of having HHT. Bleeding

Table 51.1. Common Physical Findings and Associations of Vascular Disorders

Pattern and Usual Location	Etiology	Associated Features
Subconjunctival and axillary petechiae	Fat emboli	Dyspnea
Periorbital, facial, and neck petechiae	Valsalva maneuvers	
Periorbital ecchymosis ("black eye")	Trauma; in penetrating globe injuries without periorbital trauma, suggests posterior rupture	
"Raccoon eyes"	Basilar skull fracture	
"Battle sign" (mastoid ecchymosis)	Basilar skull fracture	
Palatal petechiae	Viral upper respiratory infection	
Ecchymosis of limbs and face of infant	AIHE	Inflammatory edema
Eyelid and periorbital edema and purpura, often after dependency; purpura in other areas with minimal trauma	Amyloid	
Glove and stocking petechiae with areas of confluence and sharp line of demarcation between normal and abnormal areas	PPGSS	
Palm and sole petechiae	Rat bite fever and other infections	
Purpuric lesions on the forearm in elderly patients	Solar or steroid purpura	
Bluish discoloration of the umbilicus (Cullen sign)	Hemorrhagic pancreatitis or rectus sheath hematoma	
Flank ecchymosis (Grey-Turner sign)	Hemorrhagic pancreatitis	
Periumbilical purpura with "thumbprint" signing	*Strongyloides* infection	
Scrotal/perineal ecchymosis	Intraperitoneal hemorrhage or iliac aneurysmal rupture (rupture into sigmoid mesocolon)	
Telangiectatic lesions along the face, lips, nares, tongue, and nail beds	HHT	
Lower extremity palpable, nonblanching purpura	Vasculitis	
Perifollicular lower extremity, with areas of confluence	Scurvy	Gingival, intramuscular bleeds
Urticarial lesions followed by purpura	Urticarial vasculitis	
Proximal thigh involvements often with a "kissing" or symmetric lesion	Calciphylaxis	
Mucosal oozing and easy bruising	EDS	Skin hyperextensibility, joint immobility
Hemorrhagic bulla	Bacterial infections (*Clostridium*, *Vibrio*, *Aeromonas*); hypersensitivity to insect bites, snakebites; pemphigus	
"Tram lines"	Blunt force with cylindrical or linear object	
"Ring" bruises	Blunt force with circular end or sphere; may also be seen in normal bruise resolution	

Abbreviations: AIHE, acute infantile hemorrhagic edema; EDS, Ehlers-Danlos syndrome; HHT, hereditary hemorrhagic telangiectasia; PPGSS, papular-purpuric gloves and socks syndrome.

from these cutaneous telangiectasias is uncommon and rarely of clinical importance.

Epistaxis is the presenting complaint in up to 90% of patients with HHT. This symptom results from bleeding telangiectatic lesions over the inferior turbinates and nasal septum. Symptoms usually occur before 35 years of age and are highly variable. Some patients have severe symptoms, often requiring inpatient treatment, transfusions, or chronic iron replacement therapy, and surgery.[25]

Pulmonary arteriovenous malformations (PAVMs) occur in 30% of patients with HHT, and 85% to 90% of people with PAVM are found to have HHT.[22,24-26] Genetic linkage studies have found that patients with endoglin mutations have significantly higher rates of PAVMs (40%) than patients with HHT having other mutations (14%).[27,28] The PAVMs are primarily located in the lower lung lobes and are multiple. These PAVMs may result in a significant right-to-left shunt, and patients may develop dyspnea, cyanosis, clubbing, fatigue, decreased exercise tolerance, migraine headaches, and polycythemia. Paradoxic emboli can occur and result in brain abscesses, transient ischemic attacks, and strokes. These lesions may also bleed and result in hemoptysis or hemothorax; pregnant women with PAVMs appear to be at increased risk.[29] A chest radiograph may detect a coin lesion but often misses smaller lesions. Physiologic tests such as measuring O_2 saturation in the supine and standing positions (on room air and 100% O_2) can detect the positional change in shunting and can be used to screen patients for PAVMs. However, the best screening test for PAVM appears to be contrast echocardiography.[30] Patients with a positive screening test should undergo an unenhanced spiral computed tomography (CT) to confirm and further characterize the PAVM.[31]

Approximately 20% of patients with HHT develop significant upper and lower gastrointestinal (GI) tract hemorrhage. Approximately 40% of the bleeding episodes occur from upper GI tract lesions, whereas only 10% occur in the colon, and a full half are indeterminate after evaluation.[25] Spontaneous regression of

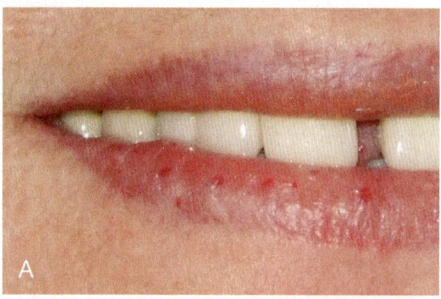
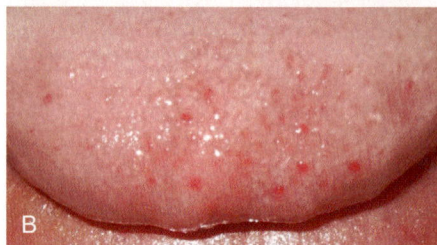

FIGURE 51.1 **Telangiectases in hereditary hemorrhagic telangiectasia (HHT).** Telangiectasias of (A) the lips and (B) the mucous membranes (here the tongue) are typical in the autosomal HHT, which frequently presents with nosebleeds and possibly severe gastrointestinal, pulmonary, or cerebral hemorrhages. Life-threatening lung hemorrhages, resulting from arteriovenous malformations, are a serious complication in pregnancy. HHT is caused by mutations in genes involved in the transforming growth factor-β (TGF-β) signaling cascade (e.g., ENG, ALK1, and SMAD4). (Reprinted with permission from Schaaf CP, Zschocke J, Potocki L. *Human Genetics*. Wolters Kluwer; 2011. Figure 20-4.)

Table 51.2. Curacao Criteria for the Diagnosis of HHT

Epistaxis—spontaneous and recurrent
Telangiectasias—multiple, at characteristic sites (lips, oral cavity, fingers, nose)
Visceral lesions—with or without bleeding (gastrointestinal, pulmonary, cerebral, hepatic)
Positive family history—a first-degree relative with HHT

The presence of three of the above criteria indicate definite HHT; the presence of two criteria are suspicious for HHT. Abbreviation: HHT, hereditary hemorrhagic telangiectasia. Adapted from Shovlin CL, Guttmacher AE, Buscarini E, et al. Diagnostic criteria for hereditary hemorrhagic telangiectasia (Rendu–Osler–Weber syndrome). *Am J Med Genet*. 2000;91(1):66-67. Copyright © 2000 Wiley-Liss, Inc. Reprinted by permission of John Wiley & Sons, Inc.

Management

Asymptomatic patients with HHT should be screened with a thorough history, careful physical examination, complete blood count, liver function tests, serum ferritin, and stool guaiac studies. A brain MRI to screen for cerebral AVMs is recommended, and contrast echocardiography to screen for PAVMs should be performed in all patients at least once after the age of 10 years. Children younger than 10 years should be screened with oxygen saturations in the sitting and supine positions every 1 to 2 years, with further testing for saturations <97%.[29] Hepatic AVM screening is recommended, and ultrasound is the preferred study.[32]

Recurrent epistaxis can be a perplexing problem. Prophylactic measures include humidification and saline nose drops. Nasal trauma from vigorous nose blowing, straining, and finger manipulation should be avoided. Antihistamines should also be avoided to prevent drying of the nasal mucosa. Mild bleeding can be treated with absorptive packing and direct pressure. Cautery is commonly used to stop persistent bleeding, but repeated cauterizations can result in necrosis and septal perforation and should be avoided.[37] The neodymium:yttrium-aluminum-garnet (Nd:YAG) laser system has been shown to be an effective treatment of epistaxis. Argon plasma coagulation also appears promising, and application of topical estrogens may be useful.[38] Arterial embolization or ligation is effective in some patients. Septal dermoplasty is a technique of removing diseased nasal mucosa and the subepithelial telangiectasias and replacing abnormal tissue with an enduring barrier. In refractory cases, nasal closure surgery (Young procedure) may be required.[39] The use of estrogen and ε-aminocaproic acid is discussed in the following section.

PAVMs are treated with transcatheter embolotherapy[40] to diminish the risk of paradoxic emboli and other complications. PAVMs with feeder artery diameters >3 mm should be treated. This procedure is effective in decreasing the right-to-left shunt and improving oxygen saturation, and it has a low complication rate. In cases in which embolotherapy is technically difficult, surgical resection should be used. After embolotherapy or surgery, small AVMs may enlarge and become clinically significant. For this reason, patients should undergo screening helical CT scans every 5 years.[22] Because brain abscesses and septic emboli occur in 1% to 20% of patients with HHT and PAVM, these patients should receive prophylactic antibiotic therapy before dental or surgical procedures.[41]

Bleeding GI vascular malformations can be treated with endoscopic thermal devices including bipolar electrocautery and laser techniques. The mucosa coagulates and sloughs, leaving a small ulcer in the place of the vascular lesion.[42] The ulcer re-epithelializes over the next few days. These treatments are rarely effective for the long term, however, because new lesions continue to develop and small intestinal lesions are not accessible. Estrogen and progesterone have been effective in decreasing the bleeding episodes.

Cerebral AVMs have been treated with surgery, stereotactic radiosurgery, and embolotherapy. A follow-up angiogram should

GI bleeding is rare, and steady progression or chronic intermittent bleeding is the norm.

Hepatic involvement occurs in 70% of patients, but symptoms and complications are rare.[32] Patients may have hepatomegaly, a hepatic bruit or thrill, or elevated liver function studies.[33] Types of intrahepatic shunting include hepatic artery to hepatic vein (arteriovenous), hepatic artery to portal vein (arterioportal), and portal vein to hepatic vein (portovenous). These shunts can lead to clinical complications of high-output heart failure, portal hypertension, encephalopathy, biliary ischemia, and nodular regenerative hyperplasia. Nodular regenerative hyperplasia is found with a 100-fold increased prevalence compared with the general population and along with portal hypertension can lead to a misdiagnosis of cirrhosis (pseudocirrhosis).[32] It is important to consider this diagnosis in the setting of a liver mass, because biopsy should generally be avoided when suspected. In addition, if patients with known focal nodular hyperplasia are being treated with estrogen or progesterone therapy, close monitoring is indicated with discontinuation of hormones in the case of symptomatic tumor enlargement.[32] Hepatic AVMs can be detected by dynamic CT,[33] color Doppler ultrasound, magnetic resonance imaging (MRI)/magnetic resonance angiography, or celiac angiography.

The neurologic manifestations of HHT result from PAVM in up to two-thirds of cases.[22] The remaining neurologic symptoms are the result of cerebrovascular telangiectasias, AVMs, aneurysms, and cavernous hemangiomas. Of the patients, 10% to 20% with HHT have cerebral arteriovenous malformation (AVM), but only 10% of people who have cerebral AVM are found to have HHT.[34] The cerebral AVMs are often multiple.[34] The annual risk of bleeding from cerebral AVM is low, reported as 0.41% to 0.72%/year (compared with 2%-4% risk for sporadic, non-HHT AVM).[34,35] MRI is recommended for detecting these lesions.[29]

The clinical diagnostic criteria (Curacao criteria) are listed in Table 51.2.[36] Genetic testing is available; consultation with a medical geneticist is recommended.

be repeated at 1 year, followed by periodic MRI. Hepatic malformations resulting in high-output heart failure, portal hypertension, or cholangitis should be treated with intensive medical management. Refractory cases have been treated with transcatheter embolization, but the complication rate is significant.[43] The mortality rate of this procedure in HHT has been calculated to be as high as 25% to 40%.[42] Consensus recommendations suggest that the procedure should be used only "as a last resort in patients who are not candidates for liver transplant" and should be absolutely avoided in patients with biliary signs or symptoms.[33] Other treatments that have been successfully used include hepatic artery ligation for localized vascular malformations[42] and liver transplant in patients with extensive lesions.[44] A recent update of HHT management guidelines has been published.[45]

Medical Therapy

Observations in the 1950s that epistaxis decreased during pregnancy and increased after menopause led to the use of estrogens as therapy for HHT. Estrogens in large doses result in metaplasia of the nasal mucosa, resulting in thick layers of squamous epithelium, and electron microscopy studies indicated that estrogen reestablished endothelial cell continuity.[46] A small randomized trial of 3 months' duration showed no benefit in reducing the number of bleeding episodes with estradiol valerate.[47] However, another author reported 100% success in an uncontrolled series of 67 consecutively treated patients who continued with high-dose estrogen therapy.[46] Several case reports and one small randomized controlled trial evaluated the use of low-dose estrogen-progesterone combination therapy in patients with severe GI bleeding. The bleeding episodes and transfusion requirements significantly diminished in treated patients.[48] Patients on tamoxifen have also been noted in case reports to have decreased episodes of bleeding. Clinical trials demonstrated that both oral tranexamic acid and low-dose thalidomide were effective in reducing epistaxis episodes.[49,50]

Numerous case reports and trials describe regression of telangiectatic lesions and decreased bleeding in patients treated with interferon, sirolimus, and bevacizumab,[51-53] suggesting a possible role for angiogenic inhibitors in managing HHT. Bevacizumab is now recommended to treat patients with HHT who fail antifibrinolytic therapy and cautery.[45]

Virtually all patients with HHT have iron deficiency anemia that requires more than oral iron replacement. Patients with significant blood loss and anemia who do not respond to or do not tolerate maximal doses of oral iron should be given intravenous (IV) iron therapy.[54] Several products are available for parenteral iron therapy: low-molecular-weight iron dextran, iron gluconate, iron sucrose, ferric carboxymatose, ferumoxytol, and ferric derisomaltose. With the currently available options for iron replacement in anemic patients with HHT, red cell transfusion should rarely be necessary.

Genetic counseling should be part of the treatment, and referral to a designated HHT center should be considered in most cases. Twenty-six US and Canadian HHT centers currently exist and are listed on the HHT Foundation International, Inc website (www.hht.org). Additional centers exist in Europe, South America, Israel, and Asia. Recent reviews summarize all aspects of HHT diagnosis and management.[45,55]

Vascular Malformations

Vascular malformations result from abnormal angiogenic development. The underlying molecular genetics of angiogenesis are complex (see Chapter 21). Mutations in angiogenic pathways can result in a variety of malformations, including capillary or venous angiomas, cerebral cavernous malformations (CCMs), and AVMs, either as isolated or multifocal lesions. Bleeding problems occur from rupture or leakage from these vascular anomalies, and the clinical sequelae depend on their location. Kasabach-Merritt phenomenon and its coagulopathy are discussed in Chapter 55.

Skin lesions are the most common vascular malformations and include a variety of birthmarks. Hemoptysis can result from pulmonary vascular anomalies including AVM and a rare disease known as pulmonary capillary hemangiomatosis. Hematuria may rarely be due to genitourinary AVMs or hemangiomas.

GI bleeding may be due to vascular malformations such as the blue rubber nevus syndrome, gastric antral vascular ectasia, telangiectasias, and AVM. GI angiodysplastic lesions deserve special attention, given their frequency. They appear to be due to degenerative dysplasia and are the most frequent cause of obscure GI bleeding. The cause is thought to be intermittent obstruction of the submucosal veins where they penetrate the muscular layers of the colon, ultimately leading to dilated, tortuous submucosal veins and venules.[56] Small intestinal angiodysplastic lesions can be particularly hard to detect, but capsule endoscopy can facilitate this diagnosis. Endoscopic-based therapy or surgery may be required for treatment. This disorder is frequently associated with aortic stenosis, and there are reports of cessation of bleeding after aortic valve repair. Up to 20% of patients with von Willebrand disease have GI bleeding associated with angiodysplasia.[57] Continuous estrogen-progestin treatment is not useful in the prevention of rebleeding from GI angiodysplasia.[58]

Central nervous system vascular lesions include AVMs, berry aneurysms, and cavernomas. Bleeding from these lesions may account for 30% of spontaneous intraparenchymal lobar bleeds.[59] Autopsy studies show the presence of intracranial aneurysms in 1% to 5% of the adult population, and 20% to 50% of these aneurysms rupture. They are sporadically acquired, but patients with autosomal dominant polycystic kidney disease may have up to a 40% incidence. Histologically, there is a decrease in the tunica media causing structural defects, leading to aneurysmal dilatation at branch points at the base of the brain. Rupture leads to subarachnoid hemorrhage, with symptoms ranging from headache and nuchal rigidity to drowsiness, stupor, and coma.[60]

CCMs are vascular lesions characterized by abnormally enlarged capillary cavities without intervening brain parenchyma. The most common presentation is with seizures and cerebral hemorrhage. Sporadic and familial forms exist, with the familial form showing autosomal dominant inheritance with incomplete penetrance. The familial forms usually have multiple CCM lesions. Three CCM loci have been identified, and the clinical and neuroradiologic features compared.[61]

Patients with brain AVMs present between the ages of 10 and 40 years. The risk of bleeding in patients with untreated AVMs is 2.8% per year but varies between 1% in low-risk patients to 30% in high-risk patients.[62] The defects in abnormal blood vessel architecture may be reversible by statin therapy.[63,64]

Other Vasculopathies

Amyloidosis

Patients with multiple myeloma or systemic amyloidosis may have light chain deposits in the cutaneous blood vessels. These vessels are particularly fragile, and purpura can occur as a result of minor trauma ("pinch purpura"). The eyelids and periorbital regions are particularly prone to developing purpura (*Figure 51.2*), and a classic sign is postproctoscopic periorbital purpura occurring after proctoscopies (for diagnostic rectal biopsies done in the past) or after Valsalva maneuvers. Purpura also commonly develops in other flexural skin areas such as the nasolabial folds, neck, axillae, and umbilicus.[65] Biopsies of the cutaneous vascular lesions demonstrate amyloid deposits in the dermis and subcutaneous tissues, and inflammatory cells are scarce.

Moyamoya Disease

Moyamoya disease is a chronic cerebral vasculopathy initially described in Japan. The disease is characterized by occlusion of the terminal portion of the internal carotid arteries or the proximal aspects of the middle or anterior cerebral arteries. An abnormal vascular network of collaterals develops in the regional area of occlusion. Cerebral infarcts are common in children, but adults have a higher propensity for intracranial hemorrhage. The risk of bleeding appears to be highest

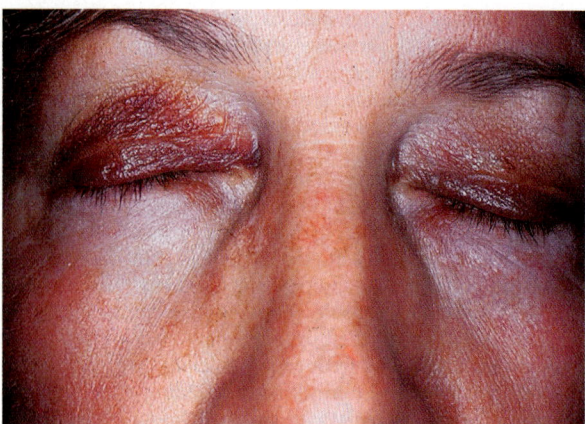

FIGURE 51.2 Periorbital purpura in a 58-year-old woman with immunoglobulin A κ plasma cell dyscrasia associated with secondary amyloidosis. (This photograph was kindly provided by Drs Theresa Scholz and Pamela Nemzer, Department of Dermatology, University of Utah Health Sciences Center.)

in adult Asians. The etiology is unknown, and diagnosis rests on characteristic angiographic findings.[66]

Cerebral Small Vessel Disease

Cerebral small vessel disease usually refers to arterioles <100 μm in size consisting of an internal elastic membrane and a tunica media one to two layers thick, or small arteries measuring 100 to 400 μm in size with tunica media composed of smooth muscle cells three to four layers thick. These vessels are usually end arteries. A constellation of syndromes is now recognized as causing cerebral small vessel disease, and these are mostly characterized by recurrent ischemic strokes with progressive cognitive impairment. Bleeding, however, is a recognized complication of most of these disorders, and it is important to recognize that many disorders have a substantially increased risk of bleeding with anticoagulants.

Degenerative cerebral microangiopathy is characterized by lipohyalinosis of small vessels associated with aging and increasing in severity with vascular risk factors such as hypertension, diabetes, and hyperhomocystinemia. The vessel walls thicken due to sclerosis, hyalinosis, and lipid deposition. Most of the bleeding appears to occur at or near the bifurcation of affected arteries where prominent degeneration of the media and smooth muscles is most appreciated. Occlusion leads to lacunar infarcts, and rupture can lead to cerebral microbleeds and lobar intracranial hemorrhages.

Cerebral amyloid angiopathy typically presents with lobar hemorrhages in patients older than 70 years and is due to several types of mutations that lead to the accumulation of β-amyloid material in the media and adventitia of small cortical and leptomeningeal vessels. This leads to a "vessel in vessel" appearance on pathology studies. Because of the higher risk of bleeding, strict avoidance of anticoagulation and antiplatelet agents is recommended.

Cerebral autosomal dominant arteriopathy with stroke and ischemic leukoencephalopathy (CADASIL) is a cerebral vasculopathy occurring in patients usually between the ages of 40 and 60 years. Patients present with subcortical strokes and a slowly progressive dementia and may have mood disorders, migraine headaches, and, in the later stages, pseudobulbar palsy. The diagnosis is suggested by a characteristic finding of widespread leukoencephalopathy on MRI. White matter lesions located in the temporal poles of the brain are considered pathognomonic for CADASIL syndrome.[67] Cerebral microbleeds are found in 31% to 69% of patients with CADASIL syndrome, and intracranial hemorrhaging occurs in 25% of patients.[68] The vascular defect lies in the smooth muscle cells, with electron microscopy showing exocytosis of granular osmophilic material from the vascular smooth muscle cells and pericytes. Mutations in *NOTCH3* are thought to be causal.[69]

BLEEDING DUE TO DISORDERS OF PERIVASCULAR TISSUE

Ehlers-Danlos Disease

The Ehlers-Danlos syndromes (EDSs) are a group of rare connective tissue disorders caused by abnormalities of collagen synthesis or processing. The prevalence is estimated to be 1 in between 10,000 and 20,000 births. An updated classification system has identified 13 types of EDSs and their genetic defects.[70] The clinical features include hyperextensible, fragile skin associated with joint hypermobility. The majority of patients with EDS also report a history of excessive bruising and bleeding.[71] Other bleeding manifestations may include subcutaneous nodular hematomas, mucosal oozing after dental procedures, hemoptysis, and GI bleeding. In most patients, screening tests show no hemostatic abnormalities, and the bleeding is thought to result from abnormalities in the perivascular collagen, leading to fragility of the subcutaneous vessels. However, several authors have noted abnormal platelet function studies, as well as factor deficiencies in individual patients.[71,72]

Certain types of EDS have an increased risk of major bleeding. In particular, vascular EDS (type IV) has unique clinical features of interest to hematologists. This disorder is due to quantitative or qualitative defects in type 3 collagen, which is particularly abundant in the arterial wall[73-75] and intestine. Patients with this disorder are prone to develop arterial aneurysms and dissections, significant bleeding from spontaneous rupture of medium-sized abdominal arteries, and intestinal rupture.

In addition to vascular abnormalities, patients with vascular EDS have characteristic facial features (prominent eyes, thin nose, small lips, and lobeless ears)[76] and thin translucent skin with a conspicuous venous network. Patients usually have minimal joint hypermobility (often limited to the hands) or skin hyperextensibility. Median life expectancy is 48 years with one-fourth of the patients developing complications by age 20 years and 80% developing complications by age 40 years.[77] The diagnosis can be confirmed by skin fibroblast cultures with biochemical analysis of type 3 collagen with or without screening for *COL3A1* mutations. If vascular EDS is suspected but the above-mentioned test results are negative, patients should be screened for TGF-β receptor gene mutations, because clinical features overlap with those of Loeys-Dietz syndrome (see section Loeys-Dietz syndrome).

Patients with EDS, particularly vascular EDS, should generally avoid contact sports and isometric exercise and are advised to avoid medications with antiplatelet properties.[74] Arterial rupture should be considered in the differential diagnosis when these patients present with new-onset symptoms such as abdominal pain. Diagnostic procedures that involve arterial puncture are relatively contraindicated because of a high incidence of complications.[74,78] If surgery is mandatory, extreme care should be used in the manipulation of vascular tissues. Postpartum hemorrhage is a major risk for pregnant patients with EDS, and the management of pregnancy has been reviewed in case reports.[79] Patients with vascular EDS can develop uterine or vessel rupture in the peripartum period and should be followed in high-risk centers.[77] Genetic counseling and referral to the Ehlers-Danlos National Foundation (www.ednf.org) should be considered.

Marfan Syndrome

Marfan syndrome is a genetic disorder with characteristic ocular, skeletal, and cardiovascular abnormalities, affecting 1 in 5000 individuals. Easy bruisability has been reported but does not seem to be a major feature of the Marfan syndrome.[80] However, the risk of postpartum hemorrhage is reported to be increased.[81]

The basic defect is due to a mutated fibrillin gene on chromosome 15.[82] Fibrillin is a component of extracellular microfibrils associated with elastin and is necessary for connecting and anchoring tissue. Fibrillin was recently found to be important as a TGF-β receptor–binding protein, holding TGF-β in an inactive complex. Dietz's group discovered that blocking TGF-β in affected mice prevents some of the developmental abnormalities (including aneurysms), suggesting that certain clinical manifestations are due to excess levels of TGF-β.[83] Further studies, in fact, showed that some families diagnosed with Marfan syndrome and familial thoracic aneurysms have a missense mutation in the TBF-β receptor 2, and this syndrome is now known as the Loeys-Dietz syndrome.[83,84]

Loeys-Dietz Syndrome

The pathogenesis of Loeys-Dietz syndrome has been described.[85] Patients with Loeys-Dietz syndrome have a phenotype characterized by hypertelorism, bifid uvula or cleft palate, and arterial tortuosity with vascular aneurysms, resulting in dissections and arterial rupture. The natural history of Loeys-Dietz varies from Marfan syndrome and EDS, with median survival of 37 years (vs 48 and 70 years, respectively), but with a much lower complication rate after vascular surgery.

Osteogenesis Imperfecta

Osteogenesis imperfecta (OI) is an autosomal dominant disease characterized by brittle bones with pathologic fractures as a result of a deficiency in bone matrix. Approximately 95% of cases are caused by mutations in the genes *COLA1* and *COLA2*, which code for the pro-α1(1) and pro-α2(2) peptides of type 1 collagen.[86] Eight clinical types of OI are currently recognized.[86] Approximately 25% of patients have been noted to bruise easily; this tendency appears to vary with the clinical type.[87] Skin contains predominantly type 1 collagen, and bruising is thought to be the result of defective supporting structures. The ecchymoses are generally mild and insignificant compared with the broader clinical picture. Excessive bleeding from wound sites after surgery has also been described.[88] Recombinant factor VIIa and desmopressin have been reported to be useful in postoperative bleeding in case reports.[89,90] The Osteogenesis Imperfecta Foundation can be accessed at http://www.oif.org.

Pseudoxanthoma Elasticum

Pseudoxanthoma elasticum is an inherited connective tissue disorder that results in calcification of elastic fibers,[91] especially in the internal elastic lamina of medium-sized arteries. The basic genetic defect is now known to be a variety of loss-of-function mutations in the gene encoding the transmembrane transporter protein ABC-C6. Mutations result in mineralization of affected peripheral tissues.[92]

Patients with pseudoxanthoma elasticum have skin that becomes grooved and thickened over time and has been described as resembling Moroccan leather.[93] Other cutaneous features include the development of yellow cutaneous plaques, usually in the neck or axillary region or in other flexural sites. Cardiovascular disease results from calcification of the arterial internal elastic lamina. Criteria for the diagnosis of pseudoxanthoma elasticum have been published.[91] Bleeding can result when the calcified vessels rupture. The manifestations include bruising, epistaxis, and bleeding from the uterus, bladder, and joints. GI bleeding occurs in 13% of patients, usually between 20 and 30 years of age, and is usually of gastric origin. Treatment should include the avoidance of gastric irritants and careful control of hypertension and hypercholesterolemia. Regular ophthalmology evaluations are also recommended, as is the avoidance of antiplatelet agents and trauma. First-degree relatives should be screened. The National Association for Pseudoxanthoma Elasticum can be contacted at napeusa.com.

Scurvy

Humans require vitamin C in the diet to promote the peptidyl hydroxylation of procollagen. In the absence of vitamin C, collagen strands are weakened as a result of abnormal triple helical structures. The abnormal collagen results in defective perivascular supportive tissues, which predispose to capillary fragility and delayed wound healing.[94,95]

The clinical manifestations of scurvy depend on the severity of vitamin C deficiency. Patients classically develop perifollicular petechiae (*Figure 51.3*).[94] The petechiae can coalesce and form purpura, particularly in a "saddle" distribution, and patients may develop gingival or intramuscular hemorrhage. Up to 75% of patients have a multifactorial normochromic, normocytic anemia. Other manifestations include peripheral edema and fatigue.

Patients at risk for scurvy include elderly edentulous patients who cook for themselves, alcoholics, mentally ill patients, and people on unusual diets. The treatment is replacement of ascorbic acid in doses of 200 mg/d.[94,96]

Steroid-Induced Purpura

Patients on chronic steroids develop thinning of the connective tissues, and minor trauma can result in extensive purpura, especially in older patients. Avoidance of trauma is the best prophylaxis for bleeding in these patients.

Solar Purpura

Senile purpura or solar purpura is a common phenomenon first described in 1817 by Bateman. The lesions are typically located on the extensor surfaces of the forearms and dorsum of the hands and occur without recognized preceding trauma (*Figure 51.4*).[97] The prevalence in hospitalized patients older than 65 years is approximately 5%, but it increases exponentially with age to include up to 30% of men 90 years or older.[98] The skin in elderly people is thin as a result of loss of subcutaneous fat and changes in both the amount and quality of collagen. Skin lesions are thought to develop by incidental lateral displacement of slack skin with resulting capillary shearing. The lesions tend to last longer than other purpuric lesions and do not generally undergo the changes in hue that other ecchymotic lesions do.[97] Hemostasis tests are normal, and no treatment other than reassurance is indicated.

VASCULITIS

The nomenclature of the vasculitides is quite confusing, but an international consensus conference has developed a system based on vessel size. This classification system recommends abandoning the term *hypersensitivity vasculitis* in favor of *microscopic polyangiitis* for small vessel vasculitides with few or no immune complexes and *cutaneous leukocytoclastic* vasculitis for small vessel vasculitis with isolated skin involvement.[99]

Cutaneous Leukocytoclastic Vasculitis

Leukocytoclastic vasculitis is characterized by immune complex deposition in postcapillary venules resulting in an inflammatory infiltrate, red cell extravasation, fibrinoid necrosis of the vessel wall, and fragmentation of nuclei (leukocytoclasis). The lesions typically develop 7 to 10 days after exposure to the offending antigen.

Palpable purpura is the classic clinical finding associated with cutaneous small vessel vasculitis. The lesions are the result of extravasation of erythrocytes into the inflamed dermis; therefore, the

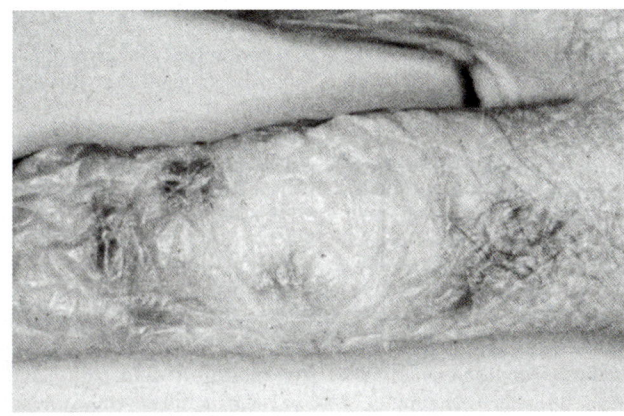

FIGURE 51.3 Perifollicular hemorrhages and corkscrew hairs in a patient with scurvy. (Reprinted from Ghorbani AJ, Eichler C. Scurvy. *J Am Acad Dermatol*. 1994;30(5 Pt 2):881-883. Copyright © 1994 Elsevier. With permission.)

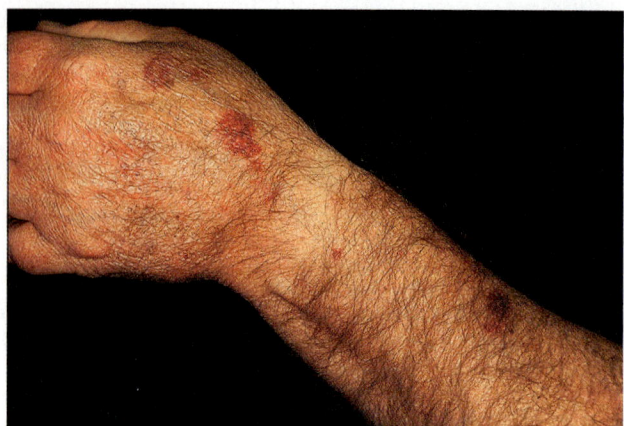

FIGURE 51.4 Senile purpura (also known as Bateman purpura) in a 70-year-old man. (This photograph was kindly provided by Dr Kappa Meadows, Department of Dermatology, University of Utah Health Sciences Center.)

Table 51.3. Etiologies of Leukocytoclastic Vasculitis

Underlying Disorders
Malignancy (leukemia, lymphoma, myeloma, cryoglobulinemia)
Autoimmune disease (systemic lupus, ulcerative colitis, periarteritis nodosa, Sjögren syndrome, viral hepatitis, primary biliary cirrhosis, etc)
Infections (viral, bacterial, mycobacterial, fungal)
Drugs/Chemicals
Penicillin, aspirin, phenothiazines, tetracycline, retinoids, colony-stimulating factors, contrast dye, insecticides, herbicides
Idiopathic

lesions do not blanch with pressure. The lesions range in size from pinpoint to several centimeters in diameter and are most prominent on the lower legs. The diagnosis should be confirmed by skin biopsy. Evaluation for the etiologic agent can be challenging and requires a detailed history to identify causative agents (*Table 51.3*).[100,101]

Antineutrophil Cytoplasmic Antibody–Positive Vasculitis

A major advance in understanding and classifying the vasculitides has been the recognition of anti–neutrophil cytoplasmic antibodies (ANCAs) in specific vasculitic syndromes. Patients with ANCA-associated small vessel vasculitis include three major categories, which are histologically identical. Speed in the diagnosis of ANCA-associated small vessel vasculitis is critical, because early treatment with immunosuppressive drugs can prevent life-threatening organ damage.[100]

Wegener granulomatosis is distinguished by necrotizing granulomatous inflammation and pulmonary, upper respiratory, and renal involvement. Vascular inflammation in these areas can cause epistaxis, hemoptysis, and hematuria. Churg-Strauss disease is defined by the presence of necrotizing granulomas with asthma and eosinophilia. Vasculitis primarily affects the nerves, GI tract, and skin. Microscopic polyangiitis is recognized by the characteristic histology with the absence of asthma and granulomas. This vasculitis typically occurs in men older than 50 years. Prodromal symptoms include fever, myalgias, and arthralgias. Microhematuria, proteinuria, and oliguric renal failure may develop, and 30% to 40% of patients develop cutaneous lesions (splinter hemorrhages, palpable purpura). Pulmonary involvement occurs in one-third of patients.

Cryoglobulinemia

Essential cryoglobulinemic vasculitis is a vasculitis with cryoglobulin immune deposits. Cryoglobulins are immunoglobulins (Igs) that form a precipitate in cooled serum. They were first described by Wintrobe and Buell in 1933.[102] The cryoglobulins can precipitate in dermal vessels and result in leukocytoclastic vasculitis[103] and palpable purpura. When the cryocrit is significantly elevated (e.g., in lymphoproliferative diseases), hyaline thrombi can form and result in vasculopathy without associated vasculitis.[103]

Clinically, patients develop crops of purpuric macules, papules, and patches most prominently over the lower extremities that are occasionally associated with burning or pruritus. Cutaneous infarcts and petechiae are also occasionally present. Only rarely are these symptoms precipitated by exposure to cold; more commonly, prolonged standing or exercise is the inciting event. Systemic manifestations of cryoglobulinemia include arthralgias, asthenia, neuropathy, and renal disease.[103] Cryoglobulinemia is further discussed in Chapter 103.

Hypergammaglobulinemic Purpura

Hypergammaglobulinemic purpura (HP) is a syndrome first described by Waldenström in 1943; this disorder is characterized by polyclonal hypergammaglobulinemia associated with recurrent attacks of palpable or nonpalpable purpura.[104] The syndrome has a marked predilection for women. The onset is often in the third and fourth decades of life, but young children and octogenarians have also been reported to develop this syndrome. The attacks of purpura are often sudden in onset and sometimes occur after prolonged standing, exercise, dancing, wearing tight-fitting clothes (e.g., jeans), and alcohol ingestion. Some patients have premonitory symptoms such as stinging, itching, or mild pain before the development of purpura. The purpura typically involves the lower extremities and is palpable in approximately 75% of cases.[105] Associated systemic symptoms include arthralgias (particularly adjacent to the purpura), low-grade fever, and lower extremity edema. The purpura usually resolves over 2 to 10 days. Recurrences are common but highly variable. Some patients have up to four attacks per week; others have only rare recurrences.[105]

HP can be divided into primary and secondary forms. Primary HP occurs with no underlying disease process; secondary HP is identified when the typical symptoms of HP develop in patients with underlying diseases such as Sjögren syndrome, systemic lupus erythematosus, or other autoimmune, inflammatory, or neoplastic diseases.[105] The purpuric lesions can occur years before or after the diagnosis of autoimmune disease.

A prospective, nonrandomized trial of 17 patients suggests that milder cases respond to indomethacin or hydroxychloroquine (200 mg twice daily) and more severe cases respond to prednisone at doses more than 20 mg/d.[105] Plasmapheresis results in only temporary relief of symptoms.[106]

Urticarial Vasculitis

Patients who present with purpura after resolution of urticaria may have urticarial vasculitis. Typically, the urticarial lesions burn, sting, or itch and last longer than 24 hours. The trunk and proximal extremities are affected more than the distal extremities. Residual hyperpigmentation may be present after resolution of the skin lesions. The pathogenesis appears to be due to immune complexes that activate complement and lead to mast cell degranulation. Patients with normal complement levels usually have minimal, if any, systemic involvement, whereas patients with depressed complement levels may have more severe disease.[107] Hypocomplementemic urticarial vasculitis is due to anti-C1q precipitins.

Acute Infantile Hemorrhagic Edema

Acute infantile hemorrhagic edema is a leukocytoclastic vasculitis confined to the skin in infants 4 to 24 months of age. Patients present with the dramatic onset of ecchymotic purpura involving the limbs and face, with inflammatory edema in an otherwise healthy child. Spontaneous and complete resolution occurs in 1 to 3 weeks. Pathology shows leukocytoclastic vasculitis. Perivascular IgA deposits are often identified, and some authors consider this disorder to be a variant of Henoch-Schönlein purpura (HSP).[108]

Henoch-Schönlein Purpura

HSP is an acute vasculitic syndrome with features of colicky abdominal pain, nephritis, arthritis, and palpable purpura. The manifestations of the syndrome were initially described by Schönlein in 1837 and further developed by Henoch in 1874.[109,110] The disease occurs primarily in children, with a peak incidence occurring between 4 and 11 years of age. There appears to be a seasonal variation, with most reported cases occurring from fall to spring and a paucity of cases in the summer.[109,111] Many of the cases occur after upper respiratory infections. This space-time clustering suggests a possible role for an infectious agent in precipitating the disease. Other infections, medications, insect bites, and malignancy have also been described as potential precipitating factors.

Biopsies of the superficial dermis and bowel in HSP show an acute vasculitis of precapillary arterioles and postcapillary venules. Immunofluorescent staining commonly shows IgA deposits in the walls of the arterioles of both the involved and noninvolved skin.[112] In patients with renal involvement, a proliferative and necrotizing vasculitis is described and IgA deposits are found in the glomerular mesangium.[113] Circulating immune complexes containing IgA are detected in approximately 70% of patients shortly after the onset of purpura, followed by the appearance of complement and IgA, IgM, and IgG immune complexes later in the disease course.[114]

The onset of symptoms is usually acute, with fever and palpable purpura involving the extremities and buttocks.[109,110] The purpuric lesions appear in symmetric crops with a predilection for extensor surfaces of the extremities (*Figure 51.5*). They are most abundant around the knees, ankles, and elbows.[110] A transient oligoarticular arthritis involving the large joints occurs in approximately 40% of cases, and the pain is often out of proportion to the physical findings. Renal involvement is manifest as proteinuria or hematuria. The renal abnormalities are almost always transient in younger children, but up to 20% to 25% of older children and adults have progressive renal disease.[109,115]

Diffuse, crampy abdominal pain occurs in more than one-third of the cases and may occur before the characteristic purpura. The abdominal pain can be severe enough to mimic a surgical abdomen and appears to be due to submucosal bleeding, edema, and ulcerations. Because abdominal pain is common, it is important to be aware that rare complications requiring surgery do occur and include intussusception, perforation, and bowel necrosis.[116] GI bleeding presenting as melena or hematochezia can occur and is occasionally severe. Scrotal involvement is not uncommon, affecting up to 20% of males, and can mimic testicular torsion.[117]

Criteria for the classification of HSP have been published.[109] The presence of two of the following four criteria can usually accurately differentiate HSP from other forms of vasculitis: palpable purpura, age of onset 20 years or younger, acute abdominal pain, and biopsy showing granulocytes in the walls of arterioles or venules. A biopsy is not required in children with the classic presentation of HSP. The prognosis depends in part on the age at presentation. Children usually recover completely from HSP, but relapses may occur over a 3- to 6-week period before complete resolution of symptoms.[109] Adults have more severe disease at presentation, with a worse renal prognosis.[118]

Supportive care alone is used to treat mild cases. Steroids may be useful to alleviate symptoms in severe cases but do not prevent renal complications from developing.[119] Nonsteroidal anti-inflammatory drugs are beneficial for symptom relief in some patients, and plasmapheresis is of reported use with renal involvement.[120] IV IgG is effective in treating gastrointestinal symptoms of HSP.[121]

Serum Sickness

Serum sickness is a specific clinical syndrome with systemic features and immune complex–induced vasculitis. The clinical syndrome typically occurs 7 to 12 days after administration of heterologous serum. The features include fever, urticaria, palpable purpura or other rash, and lymphadenopathy.[122] The purpura is caused by immune complex deposition, and skin biopsies show a necrotizing angiitis. Drugs such as cefaclor, penicillin, hydralazine, sulfonamides, and thiazide diuretics have been associated with serum sickness–like reactions.

PURPURA ASSOCIATED WITH INFECTION

Infectious agents can cause petechiae, purpura, and diffuse bleeding manifestations through a variety of mechanisms including disseminated intravascular coagulation, vasculitis, septic emboli, vascular toxins, and direct vascular or endothelial invasion.[123] Certain clinical syndromes in the latter two categories are considered here. Septic emboli are briefly discussed under the section on vascular obstruction.

Acute Febrile Illness With Petechiae

Petechiae are often associated with acute febrile illnesses in children and immediately raise the concern for possible meningococcemia. Although a florid meningococcal infection may be instantly recognizable, children who present with small skin hemorrhages and fever, but who are not acutely ill, can be a diagnostic challenge. Petechiae that are present only above the nipple line in the distribution of the superior vena cava are often due to the coughing or vomiting that accompanies the acute infection. Bacterial agents such as streptococcal infections, pneumococcus, and *Haemophilus influenzae* may cause fever and petechiae. Viral illnesses due to enterovirus and adenovirus are well-known causes of fever and petechiae as well.[124]

Papular-Purpuric Gloves and Socks Syndrome

Patients with sharply demarcated purpura involving the hands and feet may have a syndrome known as papular-purpuric "gloves and socks" syndrome, as shown in *Figure 51.6*. This syndrome was initially described in 1990[125] and has been confirmed in several other reports.[126] Patients are usually adolescents or young adults who present in the spring or summer with pruritic edema and erythema of the hands and feet. Petechiae and confluent purpura follow, with a relatively sharp demarcation at the wrists and ankles. Oral mucosal involvement is common, and patients may have other systemic signs or symptoms including lymphadenopathy, fever, elevated liver function studies, and cytopenias. Rare presentations may include a perioral petechial rash or more generalized petechial eruption. The syndrome is self-limited and usually resolves within 1 to 2 weeks. The etiologic agent is usually parvovirus B19,[127] but cytomegalovirus, hepatitis B, measles, rubella, and human herpesvirus 6 have also been implicated.

Rickettsial Diseases

Rickettsial infection results in damage to the endothelial cell with a characteristic multifocal lymphohistiocytic immune response causing increased vascular permeability, decreased perfusion, and activation of coagulation.

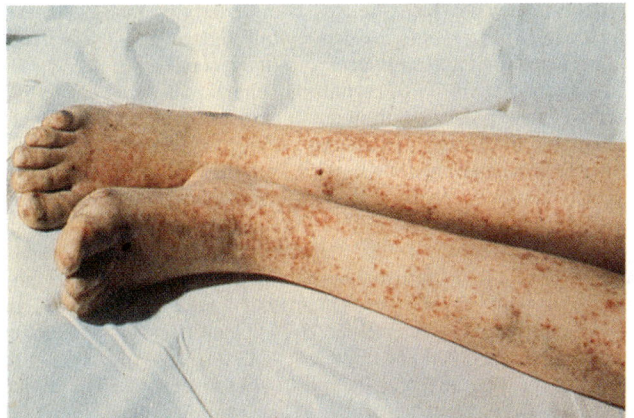

FIGURE 51.5 Lower extremity palpable purpura in a patient with Henoch-Schönlein purpura. (Reprinted from Van Hale HM, Gibson LE, Schroeter AL. Henoch-Schönlein vasculitis: direct immunofluorescence study of uninvolved skin. *J Am Acad Dermatol*. 1986;15(4 Pt 1):665-670. Copyright © 1986 Elsevier. With permission.)

Rocky Mountain spotted fever is transmitted by the bite of ixodid ticks and, therefore, has a peak incidence in the United States in May, June, and July. The incubation period is 2 to 14 days (mean, 7 days), and symptoms usually include the sudden onset of fever, chills, headache, and myalgia. A pink macular rash develops on the wrists, hands, and ankles and spreads to cover most of the body. After 2 to 7 days, the lesions become petechial, and hemorrhagic areas may coalesce to form large areas of ecchymosis. The major complications are a result of vascular injury, and multiple organs may become involved. Diagnosis is based on serologic studies showing a rise in antibody titers or biopsy of the skin lesions with immunofluorescent identification of the organisms. Treatment is with a tetracycline or chloramphenicol.

Other rickettsial diseases such as Mediterranean spotted fever, Asian tick typhus, and Queensland tick typhus are generally milder and have an eschar (tache noire) at the site of the primary tick bite. The treatment is the same as that for Rocky Mountain spotted fever.[128]

Hemorrhagic Fever Viruses

The hemorrhagic fever viruses are a diverse group of small RNA viruses with a lipid envelope. The clinical presentations vary, but symptoms usually begin with fever, headache, and myalgias progressing to generalized malaise. These symptoms last 3 to 4 days and are followed by petechiae, mucosal bleeding, and GI tract hemorrhage. However, infection of the endothelium may be common to all,[129] and direct disruption of endothelial cells may occur. Some of the viruses have almost no cytopathologic effect; however, others are highly destructive to the endothelial cells. Activation of immune cells with the release of cytokines and chemokines that target endothelial cells is another suggested mechanism of damage.[130] Release of tissue factor from damaged cells can trigger coagulation abnormalities,[131] and varying degrees of thrombocytopenia and disseminated intravascular coagulation are present and contribute to the bleeding diathesis.

A high index of suspicion is required to diagnose hemorrhagic fever virus. Risk factors for naturally occurring cases include foreign travel, handling of animal carcasses, contact with sick animals or people, and arthropod bites within 21 days of the onset of symptoms. Lack of identifiable risk factors should raise the suspicion of a bioterrorist attack.[132]

PURPURA ASSOCIATED WITH VASCULAR OBSTRUCTION

Although oversimplified, it is often convenient to think of some disorders as causing purpura by intravascular obstruction with subsequent hemorrhage due to necrosis, vasculitic injury, or consumptive coagulopathy. *Table 51.4* lists disorders that can be grouped together as causing abruptly decreased blood flow with subsequent bleeding. Note that cold agglutinins are not included because necrosis and bleeding are not expected complications.

Cryofibrinogenemia

Cryofibrinogens are cold-precipitable plasma proteins that dissolve as plasma is rewarmed. The proteins are distinct from cryoglobulins, which precipitate on cooling of serum (after the plasma proteins have been removed). Approximately 3% to 13% of hospitalized patients have detectable cryofibrinogens when appropriate assays are used.[133] Cryofibrinogens can be associated with underlying malignancies or inflammatory processes (secondary cryofibrinogenemia) or be present as an isolated finding (essential cryofibrinogenemia).

Although patients with cryofibrinogenemia are often asymptomatic, they may present with symptoms of lower extremity or acral ulcers, cold intolerance, cutaneous purpura, livedo reticularis, gangrene, or Raynaud phenomenon.[134] Paradoxic bleeding may occur and appears to be proportional to the cryocrit.[135] The cutaneous lesions develop as a result of fibrin thrombi obstructing the small and medium-sized dermal vessels.[134] Leukocytoclastic vasculitis has also been described.[136] To measure cryofibrinogens, blood should be anticoagulated with ethylenediaminetetraacetic acid, citrate, or oxalate. The sample should be maintained at 37 °C until centrifuged, and the separated plasma should be chilled at 4 °C for 72 hours. Chilling the sample in this way increases the sensitivity for detection. The cryocrit is expressed as a percentage of the plasma sample volume.

Cryofibrinogenemia may be asymptomatic and require no treatment. Mild cases can be treated with avoidance of cold and procedures that include cooling. Patients with more severe symptoms are usually treated with streptokinase, other fibrinolytic agents, or plasmapheresis. A small clinical trial and case reports have suggested that stanozolol,

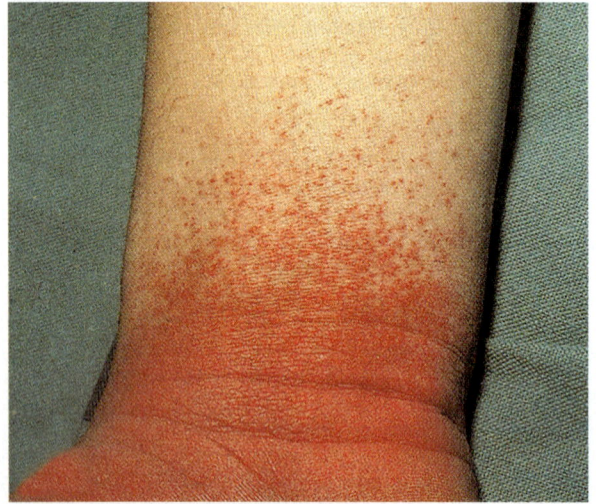
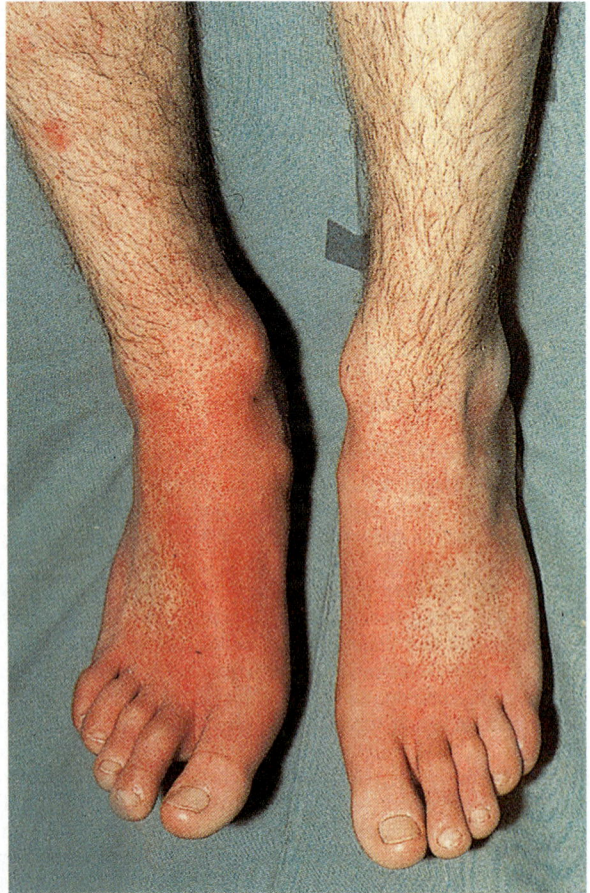

FIGURE 51.6 Skin lesions of hands (A) and feet (B) associated with **papular-purpuric gloves and socks syndrome.** (Reprinted from Harms M, Feldmann R, Saurat JH. Papular-purpuric "gloves and socks" syndrome. *J Am Acad Dermatol.* 1990;23(5 Pt 1):850-854. Copyright © 1990 Elsevier. With permission.)

Table 51.4. Classification of Bleeding Disorders Associated With Vascular Obstruction

Vascular Obstruction Component	Disease Examples
Thrombus	Warfarin-induced skin necrosis, disseminated intravascular coagulation
Emboli	
Thromboemboli	Atrial fibrillation
Septic emboli	Endocarditis
Marantic emboli	Sterile endocarditis
Cholesterol emboli	Invasive vascular procedures, warfarin blue-toe syndrome
Immunoglobulins	Waldenström macroglobulinemia, myeloma
Plasma Proteins	Cryoglobulinemia
Fibrin	Cryofibrinogenemia
Red cells	Polycythemia
Platelets	Thrombocytosis, heparin-induced skin necrosis
Fat	Fat emboli syndrome

an androgenic steroid with fibrinolytic activity, can produce excellent results.[134,137] Immunosuppressant agents have been reported to be effective in some patients.

Cholesterol Embolization Syndrome

Cholesterol embolization syndrome is an increasingly recognized disorder caused by dislodged cholesterol crystals from atherosclerotic plaques. This occurs after vascular procedures or can be due to warfarin (blue-toe syndrome) and results in renal insufficiency, peripheral emboli, and possibly GI or central nervous system involvement. Livedo reticularis is the most common skin finding and can be best appreciated with the patient in the upright position. Cyanosis, purpura, ulcers, and gangrene can all occur.[138] Biopsies of the cutaneous lesions, including livedo reticularis, demonstrate thrombi with cholesterol "clefts," because the cholesterol is dissolved during fixation.

PURPURA ASSOCIATED WITH SKIN DISEASES

Pigmented Purpuric Dermatitis

Pigmented purpuric eruptions encompass a group of related skin diseases that have in common the clinical appearance of red-brown skin pigmentation (caused by hemosiderin deposits) associated with purpura or petechiae. These lesions tend to develop on the lower extremities of middle-aged people and are usually chronic. Histologically, there is a mononuclear upper dermal infiltrate without evidence of leukocytoclasis. Extravasated red blood cells are present around the capillaries, and hemosiderin deposits are found in older lesions. Six skin diseases are commonly classified as pigmented purpura. In Schamberg progressive pigmentary dermatosis, the lesions appear as orange-brown patches of skin with "cayenne pepper spots" at the borders or within the lesion (*Figure 51.7*). Majocchi purpura annularis is distinguished by an annular 0.5- to 2.0-cm patch of reddish-brown macules. Eczematoid-like purpura has a seasonal pattern and appears as pinpoint lesions that spread rapidly over 2 to 4 weeks and develop a slight scale. The lesion in pigmented purpura lichenoid dermatitis (Gougerot-Blum purpura) is a reddish-brown macule with telangiectasias. These lesions tend to coalesce and form plaques. Itching purpura presents with an acute onset of pigmented macules associated with severe pruritus. Lastly, lichen aureus is described as "grouped copper-orange to purple lichenoid papules forming an irregular, usually singular, plaque."[139] The etiology of pigmented purpura is unknown, but some degree of venous stasis is apparent in many patients and may

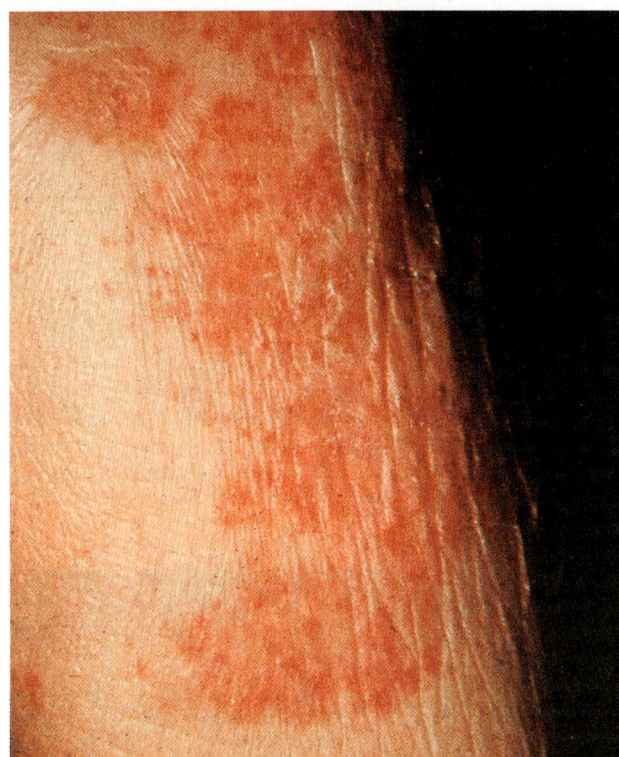

FIGURE 51.7 Skin lesions associated with Schamberg progressive pigmentary dermatosis. Note the irregular patches of punctate hemorrhagic lesions with yellow-brown discoloration of hemosiderin deposits. (Reprinted with permission from Shrertz EF. Pigmented purpuric eruptions. *Semin Thromb Hemost.* 1984;10(3):190-195. Copyright © Georg Thieme Verlag KG.)

be a factor in its development. The importance of these lesions is to differentiate them from other causes of chronic purpura with hemosiderin deposits such as purpura associated with abnormal proteins. The lesions may clear in up to two-thirds of patients with long-term follow-up.[140]

Pigmented purpuric eruptions have been described in children[141] (*Figure 51.8*) and may be familial. Treatment in the past has been with fluorinated steroids, but recently, psoralen plus ultraviolet light of A wavelength has been found to be effective in some cases.

Drug Reactions

Drug reactions can cause nonthrombocytopenic purpura by a number of different mechanisms, including leukocytoclastic vasculitis, serum sickness, and, occasionally, a pigmented purpura. Some of the drugs associated with pigmented purpuric dermatosis include acetaminophen, aspirin, glipizide, hydralazine, meprobamate, dipyridamole, creatine, thiamine, interferon, injected medroxyprogesterone acetate, and infliximab.[142] A fixed drug reaction can occur, with an isolated purpuric-appearing lesion occurring in a location without preceding trauma (*Figure 51.9*).

PSYCHOGENIC PURPURA

Autoerythrocyte Sensitization

Autoerythrocyte sensitization is a rare disorder characterized by recurrent spontaneous ecchymotic lesions in patients with otherwise normal hemostasis. The syndrome was first described in 1955 by Gardner and Diamond after their discovery that intradermal injections of autologous red blood cells reproduced the skin lesion.[143] Since the original description, more than 200 cases have been described, with the largest series collected by Ratnoff.[144] Agle and Ratnoff made the important clinical association of this phenomenon with patients who have significant emotional and psychiatric problems.[145]

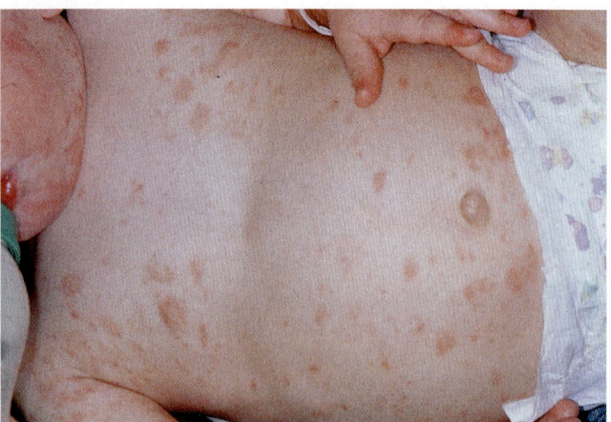

FIGURE 51.8 Pigmented purpura in a child. (This photograph was kindly provided by Drs Payem Tristani-Firouzi and Sheryll Vanderhooft, Department of Dermatology, University of Utah Health Sciences Center.)

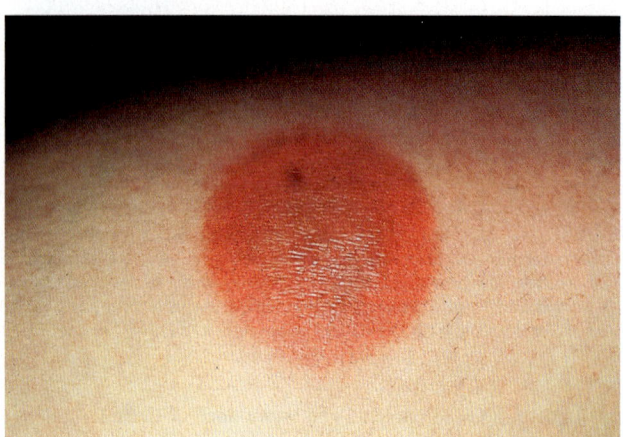

FIGURE 51.9 A fixed drug eruption lesion. This 30-year-old woman developed the thigh lesion after taking ibuprofen. (This photograph was kindly provided by Dr Pamela Nemzer, Department of Dermatology, University of Utah Health Sciences Center.)

The cutaneous lesions are usually preceded by localized symptoms, including pain and a burning or stinging sensation in the involved area. The area then becomes erythematous, raised, and warm, and within hours, ecchymoses occur in the inflamed area. The ecchymoses can range in size from 1 to 2 cm to extensive involvement of the trunk or an extremity. The erythema and swelling usually subside within 48 hours of the development of ecchymoses. The lesions can recur weeks to years later. The ecchymotic lesions are usually only one symptom among many. Patients commonly have systemic symptoms including headaches, paresthesias, syncopal episodes, abdominal pain, nausea, vomiting, chest pain, dyspnea, dysuria, and arthralgia.

Psychogenic purpura typically affects adolescent to middle-aged women who have significant underlying emotional problems. Patients are commonly found to suffer from depression, anxiety, and inability to handle hostile feelings, as well as hysterical and masochistic character traits. They have often sustained significant physical and emotional trauma in the past, and up to two-thirds of the patients describe significant emotional stress present at the time the initial purpuric lesions develop.

The skin lesions can classically be reproduced in some patients with the intradermal injection of 0.1 mL autologous whole blood, packed red blood cells, or red cell stroma. However, this test has limited sensitivity, and most authorities recommend using clinical criteria to diagnose this disorder. No specific therapy is of proven value in psychogenic purpura. Psychotherapy appears to be beneficial in some younger patients but is less effective in the older population.[146,147]

Factitious Purpura

Self-inflicted ecchymoses can be difficult to diagnose. This disorder should be considered when there is a clear secondary gain present, when the lesions only occur in accessible areas, or when ecchymotic lesions assume unusual shapes. Circular, well-circumscribed lesions around the upper limbs and breasts may be a result of sucking of the skin.

Religious Stigmata

Purpuric religious stigmata are bruises that allegedly occur spontaneously and resemble the wounds of the crucified body of Christ. The phenomenon usually occurs in women, and many have belonged to a religious order. The etiology is unknown.[144]

References

1. Simpson K, Knight B. *Types of injury and wounds.* In: *Forensic Medicine.* Edward Arnold; 1985:48-70.
2. Pedley CF, Bloomfield RL, Colflesh MJ, Rodriguez-Porcel M, Porcel MR, Novikov SV. Blood pressure monitor–induced petechiae and ecchymosis. *Am J Hypertens.* 1994;7:1031-1032.
3. Stephenson T, Bialas Y. Estimation of the age of bruising. *Arch Dis Child.* 1996;74:53-55.
4. Bohnert M, Baumgartner R, Pollak S. Spectrophotometric evaluation of the color of intra- and subcutaneous bruises. *Int J Leg Med.* 2000;113:343-348.
5. Casas JG, Woscoff A. Letter. Calcaneal petechiae. *Arch Dermatol.* 1974;109:571.
6. Pierson JC, Suh PS. Powerlifter's purpura: a Valsalva–associated phenomenon. *Cutis.* 2002;70:93-94.
7. Amgwerd MG. Acute venous stasis in the area of the head after bungee-jumping. A report of two cases. [Article in German]. *Unfallchirurg.* 1995;98:447-448.
8. Gough KR. Capillary resistance to suction in hypertension. *Br Med J.* 1962;1:21-24.
9. Fisher AA. Suction purpura. Part 1. "Sucker daddy" or "cyclops purpura." *Cutis.* 1992;49:393-394.
10. Metzker A, Merlob P. Suction purpura. *Arch Dermatol.* 1992;128:822-824.
11. Guthrie CM, Stanfey HA. Rectus sheath haematoma presenting with Cullen's sign and Grey–Turner's sign. *Scott Med J.* 1996;41:54-55.
12. Ratzan RM, Donaldson MC, Foster JH, Walzak MP. The blue scrotum sign of Bryant: a diagnostic clue to ruptured abdominal aortic aneurysm. *J Emerg Med.* 1987;5:323-329.
13. Herbella FA, Mudo M, Delminti C, Braga FM, Del Grande JC. "Raccoon eyes" (periorbital hematoma) as a sign of skull base fracture. *Injury.* 2001;32:745-747.
14. Sutton HG. Epistaxis as an indication of impaired nutrition and of degeneration of the vascular system. *Med Mirror.* 1864;1:786.
15. Rendu M. Epistaxis repetees chez un sujet porteur de petis angiomes cutanes et muquenx. *Bull Mem Soc Med Hop Paris.* 1896;13:731-733.
16. Osler W. On a family form of recurring epistaxis associated with multiple telangiectasias of the skin and mucous membranes. *Bull Johns Hopkins Hosp.* 1901;12:333-337.
17. Weber FP. Multiple hereditary developmental angiomata (telangiectases) of the skin and mucous membranes associated with recurring haemorrhages. *Lancet.* 1907;2:160-162.
18. Giordano P, Nigro A, Lenato GM, et al. Screening for children of families with Rendu–Osler–Weber disease: from geneticist to clinician. *J Thromb Haemost.* 2006;4:1237-1245.
19. Plauchu H, de Chadarevian JP, Bidean A, Robert JM. Age-related clinical profile of hereditary hemorrhagic telangiectasia in an epidemiologically recruited population. *Am J Med Genet.* 1989;32:291-297.
20. Gallione CJ, Repetto GM, Legius E, et al. A combined syndrome of juvenile polyposis and hereditary haemorrhagic telangiectasia associated with mutations in MADH4 (SMAD4). *Lancet.* 2004;363:852-859.
21. Shovlin CL, Simeoni I, Downes K, et al. Mutational and phenotypic characterization of hereditary hemorrhagic telangiectasia. *Blood.* 2020;136:1907-1918.
22. Guttmacher AE, Marchuk DA, White RI, Jr. Hereditary hemorrhagic telangiectasia. *N Engl J Med.* 1995;333:918-924.
23. Braverman IM, Keh A, Jacobsen BS. Ultrastructure and three-dimensional organization of the telangiectasias of hereditary hemorrhagic telangiectasia. *J Invest Dermatol.* 1990;95:422-427.
24. Porteous ME, Burn J, Proctor SJ. Hereditary haemorrhagic telangiectasia: a clinical analysis. *J Med Genet.* 1992;29:527-530.
25. Reilly PJ, Nostrant TT. Clinical manifestations of hereditary hemorrhagic telangiectasia. *Am J Gastroenterol.* 1984;79:363-367.
26. Kjeldsen AD, Oxhoj H, Andersen PE, Green A, Vase P. Prevalence of pulmonary arteriovenous malformations (PAVMS) and occurrence of neurologic symptoms in patients with hereditary hemorrhagic telangiectasia (HHT). *J Intern Med.* 2000;248:255-262.
27. Haitjema T, Westermann CJ, Overtoom TT, et al. Hereditary hemorrhagic telangiectasia (Osler-Weber-Rendu disease): new insights in pathogenesis, complications and treatment. *Arch Intern Med.* 1996;156:714-719.
28. McAllister KA, Lennon F, Bowles-Biesecker B, et al. Genetic heterogeneity in hereditary hemorrhagic telangiectasia: possible correlation with clinical phenotype. *J Med Genet.* 1994;31:927-932.
29. Bayrak-Toydemir P, Mao R, Lewin S, McDonald J. Hereditary hemorrhagic telangiectasia: an overview of diagnosis and management in the molecular era for clinicians. *Genet Med.* 2004;6:175-191.

30. Nanthakumar K, Graham AT, Robinson TI, et al. Contrast echocardiography for detection of pulmonary arteriovenous malformations. *Am Heart J.* 2001;141:243-246.
31. Remy J, Remy-Jardin M, Giraud F, Wattinne L. Angioarchitecture of pulmonary arteriovenous malformations: clinical utility of three dimensional helical CT. *Radiology.* 1994;191:657-664.
32. Buscarini E, Plauchu H, Garcia-Tsao G, et al. Liver involvement in hereditary hemorrhagic telangiectasia: consensus recommendations. *Liver Int.* 2006;26:1040-1046.
33. Bernard G, Mion F, Henry L, Plauchu H, Paliard P. Hepatic involvement in hereditary hemorrhagic telangiectasia: clinical, radiological and hemodynamic studies of 11 cases. *Gastroenterology.* 1993;105:482-487.
34. Willemse RB, Johannes JM, Westerman CJ, Overtoom TT, Mauser H, Wolbers JG. Bleeding risk of cerebrovascular malformations in hereditary hemorrhagic telangiectasia (HHT). *J Neurosurg.* 2000;92:779-784.
35. Maher CO, Piepgras DG, Brown RD, Jr, Friedman JA, Pollock BE. Cerebrovascular manifestations in 321 cases of hereditary hemorrhagic telangiectasia. *Stroke.* 2001;32:877-882.
36. Shovlin CL, Guttmacher AE, Buscarini E, et al. Diagnostic criteria for hereditary hemorrhagic telangiectasia (Rendu-Osler-Weber syndrome). *Am J Med Genet.* 2000;91:66-67.
37. Rebeiz EE, Bryan DJ, Ehrlichman RJ, Shapshay SM. Surgical management of life-threatening epistaxis due to Osler-Weber-Rendu disease. *Ann Plast Surg.* 1995;35:208-213.
38. Bergler W, Sadick H, Gotte K, Riedel F, Hörmann K. Topical estrogens combined with argon plasma coagulation in the management of epistaxis in hereditary hemorrhagic telangiectasia. *Ann Otol Rhinol Laryngol.* 2002;111(3 pt 1):222-228.
39. Sena ES, Cardoso C, Silva A, Abrunhosa J, Almeida E Sousa C. Nasal closure for the treatment of epistaxis secondary to hereditary hemorrhagic telangiectasia. *Acta Otorrinolaringol Esp.* 2016;67(6):345-348.
40. Lee DW, White RI, Jr, Egglin TK, et al. Embolotherapy of large pulmonary arteriovenous malformations: long-term results. *Ann Thorax Surg.* 1997;64:930-940.
41. Mohler ER, Monahan B, Canty MD, Flockhart DA. Cerebral abscess associated with dental procedure in hereditary hemorrhagic telangiectasia. *Lancet.* 1991;338:508-509.
42. Buchi KN. Vascular malformations of the gastrointestinal tract. *Surg Clin North Am.* 1992;72:559-570.
43. Whiting JH, Jr, Morton KA, Datz FL, Patch GG, Miller FJ, Jr. Embolization of hepatic arteriovenous malformations using radiolabeled and non-radiolabeled polyvinyl alcohol sponge in a patient with hereditary hemorrhagic telangiectasia: case report. *J Nucl Med.* 1992;33:260-262.
44. Bauer T, Britton P, Lomas D, Wight DG, Friend PJ, Alexander GJ. Liver transplantation for hepatic arteriovenous malformation in hereditary hemorrhagic telangiectasia. *J Hepatol.* 1995;22:586-590.
45. Faughnan ME, Mager JJ, Hetts SW, et al. Second international guidelines for the diagnosis and management of hereditary hemorrhagic telangiectasia. *Ann Intern Med.* 2020;173:989-1001.
46. Harrison DF. Use of estrogen in treatment of familial hemorrhagic telangiectasia. *Laryngoscope.* 1982;92:314-320.
47. Vase P. Estrogen treatment of hereditary hemorrhagic telangiectasia. A double-blind controlled clinical trial. *Acta Med Scand.* 1981;209:393-396.
48. van Cutsem E, Rutgeerts P, Vantrappen G. Treatment of bleeding gastrointestinal malformations with oestrogen-progesterone. *Lancet.* 1990;335:953-955.
49. Geisthoff UW, Seyfert UT, Kubler M, Bieg B, Plinkert PK, König J. Treatment of epistaxis in hereditary hemorrhagic telangiectasia with tranexamic acid-a double-blind placebo-controlled cross-over phase IIIB study. *Thromb Res.* 2014;134:565-571.
50. Invernizzi R, Quaglia F, Klersy C, et al. Efficacy and safety of thalidomide for the treatment of severe recurrent epistaxis in hereditary haemorrhagic telangiectasia: results of a non-randomized, single-centre, phase 2 study. *Lancet Haematol.* 2015;2:e465-e473.
51. Wheatley-Price P, Shovlin C, Chao D. Interferon for metastatic renal cell cancer causing regression of hereditary hemorrhagic telangiectasia. *J Clin Gastroenterol.* 2005;39:344-345.
52. Skaro AI, Marotta PJ, McAlister VC. Regression of cutaneous and gastrointestinal telangiectasia with sirolimus and aspirin in a patient with hereditary hemorrhagic telangiectasia. *Ann Intern Med.* 2006;144:226-227.
53. Al-Samkari H, Kasthuri RS, Parambil JG, et al. An international, multicenter study of intravenous bevacizumab for bleeding in hereditary hemorrhagic telangiectasia. *Haematologica.* 2020;106(8):2161-2216.
54. Silverstein SB, Rodgers GM. Parenteral iron therapy options. *Am J Hematol.* 2004;76:74-78.
55. Geisthoff UW, Nguyen HL, Roth A, Seyfert U. How to manage patients with hereditary haemorrhagic telangiectasia. *Br J Haematol.* 2015;171:443-452.
56. Sharma R, Gorbien MJ. Angiodysplasia and lower gastrointestinal tract bleeding in elderly patients. *Arch Intern Med.* 1995;155:807-812.
57. Randi AM. Endothelial dysfunction in von Willebrand disease: angiogenesis and angiodysplasia. *Thromb Res.* 2016;141(suppl 2):S55-S58.
58. Junquera F, Feu F, Papo M, et al. A multicenter, randomized clinical trial of hormonal therapy in the prevention of rebleeding from gastrointestinal angiodysplasia. *Gastroenterology.* 2001;121:1073-1079.
59. Barnes B, Cawley CM, Barrow DL. Intracerebral hemorrhage secondary to vascular lesions. *Neurosurg Clin N Am.* 2002;13:289-297.
60. Brisman JL, Sony JK, Newell DW. Cerebral aneurysms. *N Engl J Med.* 2006;335:928-939.
61. Zafar A, Quadri SA, Farooqui M, et al. Familial cerebral cavernous malformations. *Stroke.* 2019;50:1294-1301.
62. Friedlander RM. Clinical practice. Arteriovenous malformation of the brain. *N Engl J Med.* 2007;356:2704-2712.
63. Patterson C. Torturing a blood vessel. *Nat Med.* 2009;15:137-138.
64. Zhou Z, Tang AT, Wong WY, et al. Cerebral cavernous malformations arise from endothelial gain of MEKK3-KLF2/4 signaling. *Nature.* 2016;532:122-126.
65. Williams JT, Arrington J,IIIrd, Gruber HM. Purpura as the presenting sign of an internal disease. Multiple myeloma. *Arch Dermatol.* 1993;129:775-776.
66. Berry JA, Cortez V, Toor H, et al. Moyamoya: an update and review. *Cureus.* 2020;12:e10994.
67. Ringelstein EB, Nabavi DG. Cerebral small vessel disease: cerebral microangiopathies. *Curr Opin Neurol.* 2005;18:179-188.
68. Choi JC, Kang SY, Kang JH, Park JK. Intracerebral hemorrhages in CADASIL. *Neurology.* 2006;67:2042-2044.
69. Mizuno T, Mizuta I, Watanabe-Hosomi A, et al. Clinical and genetic aspects of CADASIL. *Front Aging Neurosci.* 2020;12:91. doi: 10.3389/fnagi.2020.00091
70. Malfait F, Francomano C, Byers P, et al. The 2017 international classification of the Ehlers-Danlos syndromes. *Am J Med Genet C Semin Med Genet.* 2017;175C:8-26.
71. Anstey A, Mayne K, Winter M, Van de Pette J, Pope FM. Platelet and coagulation studies in Ehlers-Danlos syndrome. *Br J Dermatol.* 1991;125:155-163.
72. Jesudas R, Chaudhury A, Laukaitis CM. An update in the new classification of Ehlers-Danlos syndrome and review of the causes of bleeding in this population. *Haemophilia.* 2019;25:558-566.
73. De Paepe A. Ehlers-Danlos syndrome type IV. Clinical and molecular aspects and guidelines for diagnosis and management. *Dermatology.* 1994;189(suppl 2):21-25.
74. Lum YW, Brooke BS, Black JH,IIIrd. Contemporary management of vascular Ehlers-Danlos syndrome. *Curr Opin Cardiol.* 2011;26:494-501.
75. Byers PH, Belmont J, Black J, et al. Diagnosis, natural history, and management of vascular Ehlers-Danlos syndrome. *Am J Med Genet C Semin Med Genet.* 2017;175C:40-47.
76. De Paepe A, Malfait F. Bleeding and bruising in patients with Ehlers-Danlos syndrome and other collagen vascular disorders. *Br J Haematol.* 2004;127:491-500.
77. Pepin M, Schwarze U, Superti-Furga A, Byers PH. Clinical and genetic features of Ehlers-Danlos syndrome type IV, the vascular type. *N Engl J Med.* 2000;342:673-680.
78. Mattar SG, Kumar AG, Lumsden AB. Vascular complication in Ehlers-Danlos syndrome. *Am Surg.* 1994;60:827-831.
79. Weinbaum PJ, Cassidy SB, Campbell WA, et al. Pregnancy management and successful outcome of Ehlers-Danlos syndrome type IV. *Am J Perinatol.* 1987;4:134-137.
80. Pyeritz RE, McKusick VA. The Marfan syndrome: diagnosis and management. *N Engl J Med.* 1979;300:772-777.
81. Irons DW, Pollard KP. Post-partum haemorrhage secondary to Marfan's disease of the uterine vasculature. *Br J Obstet Gynaecol.* 1993;100:279-281.
82. Cañadas V, Vilacosta I, Bruna I, Fuster V. Marfan syndrome. Part 1: pathophysiology and diagnosis. *Nat Rev Cardiol.* 2010;7:256-265.
83. Loeys BL, Schwarze U, Holm T, et al. Aneurysm syndromes caused by mutations in the TGF-β receptor. *N Engl J Med.* 2006;355:788-798.
84. Gelb BD. Marfan's syndrome and related disorders—more tightly connected that we thought. *N Engl J Med.* 2006;355:841-842.
85. Van Hemelrijk C, Renard M, Loeys B. The Loeys-Dietz syndrome: an update for the clinician. *Curr Opin Cardiol.* 2010;25:546-551.
86. Van Dijk FS, Pals G, Van Rijn RR, Nikkels PG, Cobben JM. Classification of osteogenesis imperfecta revisited. *Eur J Med Genet.* 2010;53:1-5.
87. Falvo KA, Root L, Bullough PG. Osteogenesis imperfecta: clinical evaluation and management. *J Bone Joint Surg Am.* 1974;56:783-793.
88. Edge G, Okafor B, Fennelly ME, Ransford AO. An unusual manifestation of bleeding diathesis in a patient with osteogenesis imperfecta. *Eur J Anaesthesiol.* 1997;14:215-219.
89. Kastrup M, von Heymann C, Hotz H, et al. Recombinant factor VIIa after aortic valve replacement in a patient with osteogenesis imperfecta. *Ann Thorac Surg.* 2002;74:910-912.
90. Keegan MT, Whatcott BD, Harrison BA. Osteogenesis imperfecta, perioperative bleeding and desmopressin. *Anesthesiology.* 2002;97:1011-1013.
91. Uitto J, Bercovitch L, Terry SF, Terry PF. Pseudoxanthoma elasticum: progress in diagnostics and research towards treatment – summary of the 2010 PXE International Research Meeting. *Am J Med Genet A.* 2011;155A:1517-1526.
92. Luo H, Faghankhani M, Cao Y, et al. Molecular genetics and modifier genes in pseudoxanthoma elasticum, a hereditable multisystem ectopic mineralization disorder. *J Invest Dermatol.* 2020;141(5):1148-1156.
93. Luft FC. Pseudoxanthoma elasticum revealed. *J Mol Med (Berl).* 2000;78:237-238.
94. Ghorbani AJ, Eichler C. Scurvy. *J Am Acad Dermatol.* 1994;30:881-883.
95. Levine M. New concepts in the biology and biochemistry of ascorbic acid. *N Engl J Med.* 1986;314:892-902.
96. Léger D. Scurvy: reemergence of nutritional deficiencies. *Can Fam Physician.* 2008;54:1403-1406.
97. Schuster S, Scarbourough H. Senile purpura. *Q J Med.* 1961;30:33-40.
98. Wong HY. Hypothesis: senile purpura is a prognostic feature in elderly patients. *Age Ageing.* 1988;17(6):422-424.
99. Jennette JC, Falk RJ, Andrassy K, et al. Nomenclature of systemic vasculitides. Proposal of an international consensus conference. *Arthritis Rheum.* 1994;37:187-192.
100. Koutkia P, Mylonakis E, Rounds S, Erickson A. Leukocytoclastic vasculitis: an update for the clinician. *Scand J Rheumatol.* 2001;30:315-322.
101. Stevens GL, Adelman HM, Wallach PM. Palpable purpura: an algorithmic approach. *Am Fam Physician.* 1995;52:1355-1362.

102. Wintrobe MM, Buell MV. Hyperproteinemia associated with multiple myeloma: with report of a case in which an extraordinary hyperproteinemia was associated with thrombosis of the retinal veins and symptoms suggesting Raynaud's disease. *Bull Johns Hopkins Hosp.* 1933;52:156-165.
103. Cohen SJ, Pittelkow MR, Su WP. Cutaneous manifestations of cryoglobulinemia: clinical and histopathologic study of seventy-two patients. *J Am Acad Dermatol.* 1991;25:21-27.
104. Waldenström J. Clinical methods for determination of hyperproteinemia and their practical value for diagnosis. *Nord Med.* 1943;20:2228-2295.
105. Senecal JL, Chartier S, Rothfield N. Hypergammaglobulinemic purpura in systemic autoimmune rheumatic diseases: predictive value of anti-Ro (SSA) and anti-La (SSB) antibodies and treatment with indomethacin and hydroxychloroquine. *J Rheumatol.* 1995;22:868-875.
106. Hewitt P, Davies S, Cohen H, Machin S. Therapy of Waldenström's benign hypergammaglobulinemia by regular plasmapheresis. *Acta Haematol.* 1984;71:345-349.
107. Venzor J, Lee WL, Huston DP. Urticarial vasculitis. *Clin Rev Allergy Immunol.* 2002;23:201-216.
108. Caksen H, Odabas D, Kosen M, et al. Report of eight infants with acute infantile hemorrhagic edema and review of the literature. *J Dermatol.* 2002;29:290-295.
109. Mills JA, Michel BA, Bloch DA, et al. The American College of Rheumatology 1990 criteria for the classification of Henoch-Schönlein purpura. *Arthritis Rheum.* 1990;33:1114-1121.
110. Patrignelli R, Sheikh SH, Shaw-Stiffel TA. Henoch-Schönlein purpura. A multisystem disease also seen in adults. *Postgrad Med.* 1995;97:123-134.
111. Saulsbury FT. Epidemiology of Henoch-Schönlein purpura. *Cleve Clin J Med.* 2002;69(suppl 2):SII87-SII89.
112. Van Hale HM, Gibson LE, Schroeter AL. Henoch-Schönlein vasculitis: direct immunofluorescence study of uninvolved skin. *J Am Acad Dermatol.* 1986;15:665-670.
113. Levy M, Broyer M, Arsan A, Levy-Bentolila D, Habib R. Anaphylactoid purpura nephritis in childhood: natural history and immunopathology. *Adv Nephrol Necker Hosp.* 1976;6:183-228.
114. Kaufmann RH, Herrmann WA, Meyer CJ, Daha MR, Van Es LA. Circulating IgA–immune complexes in Henoch-Schönlein purpura. A longitudinal study of their relationship to disease activity and vascular deposition of IgA. *Am J Med.* 1980;69:859-866.
115. Pillebout E, Thervet E, Hill G, Alberti C, Vanhille P, Nochy D. Henoch-Schönlein purpura in adults: outcome and prognostic factors. *J Am Soc Nephrol.* 2002;13:1271-1278.
116. Katz S, Borst M, Seekri I, Grosfeld JL. Surgical evaluation of Henoch–Schönlein purpura: experience with 110 children. *Arch Surg.* 1991;126:849-854.
117. Ha TS, Lee JS. Scrotal involvement in childhood Henoch-Schönlein purpura. *Acta Paediatr.* 2007;96:552-555.
118. Uppal SS, Hussain MA, A1-Raqum HA, et al. Henoch-Schönlein purpura in adults versus children/adolescents: a comparative study. *Clin Exp Rheumatol.* 2006;24(2 suppl 41):S26-S30.
119. Hetland LE, Susrud KS, Lindahl KH, Bygum A. Henoch-Schönlein purpura: a literature review. *Acta Derm Venereol.* 2017;97:1160-1166.
120. Shenoy M, Ognjanovic MV, Coulthard MG. Treating severe Henoch-Schönlein purpura and IgA nephritis with plasmapheresis alone. *Pediatr Nephrol.* 2007;22:1167-1171.
121. Cherqaoui B, Chausset A, Stephan JL, Merlin E. Intravenous immunoglobulins for severe gastrointestinal involvement in pediatric Henoch-Schonlein purpura: a French retrospective study. *Arch Pediatr.* 2016;23:584-590.
122. Gigli I, Rosen FS. Angioedema associated with complement abnormalities. In: Fitzpatrick TB, Eisen AZ, Wolff K, et al., eds. *Dermatology in General Medicine.* 4th ed. McGraw-Hill; 1993:1494-1500.
123. Kingston ME, Mackey D. Skin clues in the diagnosis of life-threatening infections. *Rev Infect Dis.* 1986;8:1-11.
124. Nielsen HE, Andersen EA, Anderson J, et al. Diagnostic assessment of haemorrhagic rash and fever. *Arch Dis Child.* 2001;85:160-165.
125. Harms M, Feldmann R, Saurat JH. Papular-purpuric "gloves and socks" syndrome. *J Am Acad Dermatol.* 1990;23:850-854.
126. Guibal F, Buffet P, Mouly F, Morel P, Rybojad M. Papular-purpuric gloves and socks syndrome with hepatitis B infection. *Lancet.* 1996;347:473.
127. McNeely M, Friedman J, Pope E. Generalized petechial eruption induced by parvovirus B19 infection. *J Am Acad Dermatol.* 2005;52:S109-S113.
128. Gentile GA, Lang JE. Tick-borne diseases. In: Auerbach PS, ed. *Wilderness Medicine.* 4th ed. Mosby; 2001:769-806.
129. Peters CJ, Zaki SR. Role of endothelium in viral hemorrhagic fevers. *Crit Care Med.* 2002;30(5 suppl):S268-S273.
130. Schittler HJ, Feldman H. Viral hemorrhagic fever—a vascular disease? *Thromb Haemost.* 2003;89:967-972.
131. Bray M. Pathogenesis of viral hemorrhagic fever. *Curr Opin Immunol.* 2005;17:399-400.
132. Borio L, Inglesby T, Peters CJ. Hemorrhagic fever viruses as biologic weapons. Medical and public health management. *JAMA.* 2002;287:2391-2405.
133. Smith SB, Arkin C. Cryofibrinogenemia: incidence, clinical correlations and a review of the literature. *Am J Clin Pathol.* 1972;58:524-530.
134. Moiseev S, Luqmani R, Novikov P, Shevtsova T. Cryofibrinogenaemia—a neglected disease. *Rheumatology.* 2017;56:1445-1451.
135. Klein AD, Kerdel FA. Purpura and recurrent ulcers on the lower extremities. Essential cryofibrinogenemia. *Arch Dermatol.* 1991;127:115.
136. Jantunen E, Soppi E, Neittaanmaki H, Lahtinen R. Essential cryofibrinogenaemia, leukocytoclastic vasculitis and chronic purpura. *J Intern Med.* 1993;234:331-333.
137. Falanga V, Kirsner RS, Eaglstein WH, Katz MH, Kerdel FA. Stanozolol in the treatment of leg ulcers due to cryofibrinogenemia. *Lancet.* 1991;338:347-348.
138. Falanga V, Fine MJ, Kapora WN. The cutaneous manifestations of cholesterol crystal embolization. *Arch Dermatol.* 1986;122:1194-1198.
139. Sherertz EF. Pigmented purpuric eruptions. *Semin Thromb Hemost.* 1984;10:190-195.
140. Ratnam KV, Su WP, Peters MS. Purpura simplex (inflammatory purpura without vasculitis): a clinicopathologic study of 174 cases. *J Am Acad Dermatol.* 1991;25:642-647.
141. Tristani-Firouzi P, Meadows KP, Vanderhooft S. Pigmented purpuric eruptions of childhood: a series of cases and review of the literature. *Pediatr Dermatol.* 2001;18:299-304.
142. Sardana K, Sarkar R, Sehgal VN. Pigmented purpuric dermatoses: an overview. *Int J Dermatol.* 2004;43:482-488.
143. Gardner FH, Diamond LK. Autoerythrocyte sensitization. A form of purpura producing painful bruises following autosensitization to red blood cells in certain women. *Blood.* 1955;10:675-690.
144. Ratnoff OD. The psychogenic purpuras: a review of autoerythrocyte sensitization, autosensitization to DNA, "hysterical" and factitial bleeding, and the religious stigmata. *Semin Hematol.* 1980;17(3):192-213.
145. Agle DP, Ratnoff OD. Purpura as a psychosomatic entity. *Archives Intern Med.* 1962;109:89-98.
146. Silny W, Marciniak A, Czarnecka-Operacz M, Zaba R, Schwartz RA. Gardner-Diamond syndrome. *Int J Dermatol.* 2010;49:1178-1181.
147. Ivanov OL, Lvov AN, Michenko AV, Künzel J, Mayser P, Gieler U. Autoerythrocyte sensitization syndrome (Gardner-Diamond syndrome): review of the literature. *J Eur Acad Dermatol Venereol.* 2009;23:499-504.

Chapter 52 ■ Thrombocytosis and Essential Thrombocythemia

TSEWANG TASHI • GEORGE M. RODGERS

INTRODUCTION

The normal reference interval for platelet counts in adults approximates 150,000 to 450,000/μL; patients with platelet counts higher than the upper limit of normal are said to have "thrombocytosis," which can be broadly classified as primary (clonal or essential), secondary (reactive), or inherited (Table 52.1). Primary thrombocytosis is also known as essential thrombocythemia (ET), which is an acquired clonal disorder, a part of classical Philadelphia chromosome–negative chronic myeloproliferative neoplasms (MPNs). Routine screening of healthy individuals has identified persons with asymptomatic thrombocytosis; some of these people will have ET.[1] In contrast, hospitalized patients with elevated platelet counts usually have reactive thrombocytosis.[2] At least 90% of all patients with thrombocytosis are reactive due to an underlying clinical disorder.[3] It is important to distinguish ET from reactive and inherited thrombocytosis because ET is an MPN with inherent risk of ischemic or bleeding complications, and long-term evolution to myelofibrosis or acute leukemia. Secondary thrombocytosis usually requires only treatment of their underlying medical condition, and in the case of inherited thrombocytosis, usually minimal or no treatment is required.

SECONDARY (REACTIVE) THROMBOCYTOSIS

Epidemiology and Pathophysiology

A retrospective Turkish survey of the incidence and etiology of thrombocytosis over a 5-year period demonstrated that of 124,340 patients who had platelet counts determined, 2000 patients (1.6%) had at least one platelet count ≥500 000/mL.[4] Reactive thrombocytosis was identified in 96.7% of these 2000 patients, with infection being the most common cause. Another survey found that tissue injury (surgery) was the most common cause of reactive thrombocytosis.[5]

Increased thrombopoiesis seen in infectious, inflammatory, or malignant disorders results from cytokines and other acute-phase response mediators active in these circumstances. Mediators that have been linked to reactive thrombocytosis include interleukin (IL)-6, interferon-γ (INF-γ), and thrombopoietin (TPO).[6,7] IL-6 has been shown to enhance thrombopoiesis by stimulating hepatic TPO production.[8] The hematologic effects of INF-γ include suppression of erythropoiesis and stimulation of macrophages to secrete inflammatory cytokines.

Table 52.1. Classification of Thrombocytosis

Primary (Clonal)	Secondary (Reactive)	Inherited
Essential thrombocythemia	Infection	THPO mutations
Other myeloid neoplasms:	Inflammation	MPL mutations
a) Polycythemia vera	Malignancy	GSN mutations
b) Chronic myeloid leukemia	Iron deficiency	
	Hemolytic anemia	
c) Myelofibrosis	Asplenia or hyposplenia	
d) Myelodysplasia		
e) MDS/MPN overlap syndrome	Recovery from thrombocytopenia	
	Tissue injury:	
	a) Surgery	
	b) Burns	

Abbreviations: GSN, gelsolin; MDS, myelodysplastic syndrome; MPL, thrombopoietin receptor gene; MPN, myeloproliferative neoplasm; THPO, thrombopoietin gene.
Gene mutation details are described in Hong WJ, Gotlib J. Hereditary erythrocytosis, thrombocytosis and neutrophilia. Best Pract Res Clin Haematol. 2014;27(2):95-106.

These cytokines lead to megakaryocytic growth and differentiation, resulting in enhanced thrombopoiesis.[9] TPO may act as an acute-phase protein in some, but not in all circumstances.[6] Thrombocytosis is a common finding in iron deficiency, whereas thrombocytopenia is also reported but rare.[10,11] An animal model of iron deficiency found that increased megakaryocyte differentiation was associated with reactive thrombocytosis[12] as the megakaryocytic/erythroid progenitors displayed lineage bias toward megakaryocytic lineage.[13] Some have suggested that the thrombocytosis in iron deficiency anemia in part can be attributed to the effects of increased erythropoietin (EPO) level resulting from anemia, as megakaryocytic progenitors also display EPO receptors.[14] However, the underlying pathophysiologic mechanism of thrombocytosis in iron deficiency still remains unclear but complex. Clinically, these patients will have microcytic anemia and elevated platelet counts, and can be confirmed with their low serum iron indices. Patients with solid tumors (e.g., lung and ovarian cancers) have a 30% to 40% incidence of thrombocytosis.[3,7] Extreme thrombocytosis may occur after splenectomy or in patients with hyposplenia or asplenia.[3,15]

Treatment

Although no trials have formally addressed the need for treating reactive thrombocytosis, the general recommendation is to identify and address the underlying cause, and not to treat the elevated platelet count in itself.[3] However, case reports have described thrombotic events in patients with reactive thrombocytosis, and studies have identified a thrombosis risk in hospitalized patients or cancer patients with reactive thrombocytosis.[16,17] However, in general, these patients have well-established cardiovascular risk factors, such as smoking, diabetes, older age, obesity, or they have venous thromboembolism (VTE) risk factors such as cancer. Therefore, in patients with cardiovascular risk factors, antiplatelet therapy can be considered. Hospitalized patients with reactive thrombocytosis should receive VTE prophylaxis, and primary therapy for all patients with reactive thrombocytosis should focus on treating the underlying disorder. A cohort study of critically ill patients found that reactive thrombocytosis was associated with a fivefold increased risk of VTE and a twofold increased risk of death.[18]

Inherited Thrombocytosis

Inherited thrombocytosis is suspected in patients with a life-long history of asymptomatic thrombocytosis, especially if other family members are also affected. The genetic mutations in inherited thrombocytosis are heterogeneous and may or may not involve mutations in the thrombopoietin gene (THPO) or its receptor (MPL).[3] At least five different mutations in THPO associated with increased TPO production and inherited thrombocytosis have been described in European and Japanese kindreds.[19,20] The TPO molecule in these patients is normal, and increased translation appears to explain the elevated levels of TPO.[19] At least four different MPL mutations have been linked to inherited thrombocytosis; affected kindreds are of European, African-American, Arabic, and Japanese ancestry.[19,20] Approximately 7% of African-Americans are heterozygous for the MPL-Baltimore mutation.[21] Thrombocytosis in patients with MPL mutations appears to result from either constitutive receptor activation or reduced receptor binding affinity for TPO. More recently, mutations in the JAK2 or gelsolin (GSN) genes have been reported.[20] In almost all cases, thrombocytosis was inherited as an autosomal dominant trait.

Clinical findings in patients with inherited thrombocytosis can be classified by whether the patients have THPO or MPL mutations. In general, those with THPO mutations have elevated TPO levels and mild splenomegaly, but a low incidence of vascular complications and low risk of evolution to acute leukemia and myelofibrosis although development of bone marrow disease was described in two family members with inherited thrombocytosis due to *THPO* mutations.[19,22] Some patients with *MPL* mutations and inherited thrombocytosis have been reported to experience thrombosis, splenomegaly, and myelofibrosis, but these complications have not been reported in African-American patients with MPL-Baltimore.[19]

Clonal Thrombocytosis Other Than Essential Thrombocythemia

Clonal or primary thrombocytosis includes not only ET (discussed later) but also is a prominent feature of the other MPNs and certain MDS. Patients with chronic myeloid leukemia (CML), polycythemia vera (PV), or myelofibrosis may all manifest elevated platelet counts. The diagnosis, clinical aspects, and management of these disorders are discussed in Chapters 81 to 85.

Clonal thrombocytosis is also seen in MDS although the frequency is lower than in MPNs. MDS/MPN with ringed sideroblasts and thrombocytosis (MDS/MPN-RS-T) is a rare entity recognized in 2016 World Health Organization (WHO) classification of myeloid neoplasms that have dysplastic features of MDS, but with marked thrombocytosis and hypercellular marrow as seen in MPNs.[23] MDS are discussed in Chapter 80.

DIFFERENTIAL DIAGNOSIS AND CLINICAL APPROACH TO THROMBOCYTOSIS

When evaluating a patient with thrombocytosis, the key consideration is to differentiate clonal hematological disorders, such as MPN or MDS from reactive thrombocytosis or inherited thrombocytosis and other disorders. Therefore, testing for *BCR-ABL* translocation, *JAK2*, *CALR*, and *MPL* mutations, and cytogenetic testing are important for diagnostic evaluation of primary hematological disorders. Patients with reactive thrombocytosis usually will have evidence of an underlying inflammatory, infectious, or a malignant disorder. However, patients with occult malignancy may initially present without obvious cancer symptoms. Postsplenectomy thrombocytosis will usually be obvious from their history as well as presence of a vestigial spleen or no splenic tissue on abdominal imaging. These patients will usually have Howell-Jolly bodies on the blood smear. Thrombocytosis in patients with iron deficiency anemia is usually evident from the microcytic anemia and low serum iron indices.

The WHO criteria for ET are discussed in the next section. These criteria provide no direct definitions of reactive thrombocytosis. Thus, the physician is left with practical clinical criteria to suggest reactive thrombocytosis if a patient does not have an obvious underlying disorder. Such criteria might include the presence of fever, an elevated C-reactive protein or erythrocyte sedimentation rate, a blood smear showing reactive or toxic changes in the leukocytes, the presence of iron deficiency, or the postsplenectomy state.

One approach to the evaluation of thrombocytosis is shown in *Figure 52.1*. Inherited thrombocytosis can be rapidly excluded if there is no life-long history of thrombocytosis and the family history is negative. Patients who may possibly have inherited thrombocytosis can be further evaluated with testing for *THPO* and *MPL* (and other) mutations. Because the majority of patients with thrombocytosis will have a reactive etiology, every effort should be made in trying to exclude secondary thrombocytosis before considering testing for MPNs, including ET.

ESSENTIAL THROMBOCYTHEMIA

Definition

ET is a clonal MPN characterized by excessive production of platelets due to an acquired somatic mutation in the hematopoietic stem cell and is intrinsically associated with risk of thrombotic and hemorrhagic complications, progression to myelofibrosis and albeit rarely, to secondary acute leukemia. This thrombocytosis is in many ways analogous to the erythrocytosis characteristic of the related disorder, PV. This "family resemblance" between what we now recognize as Philadelphia chromosome–negative MPN was initially pointed out by William Dameshek more than 60 years ago.[24]

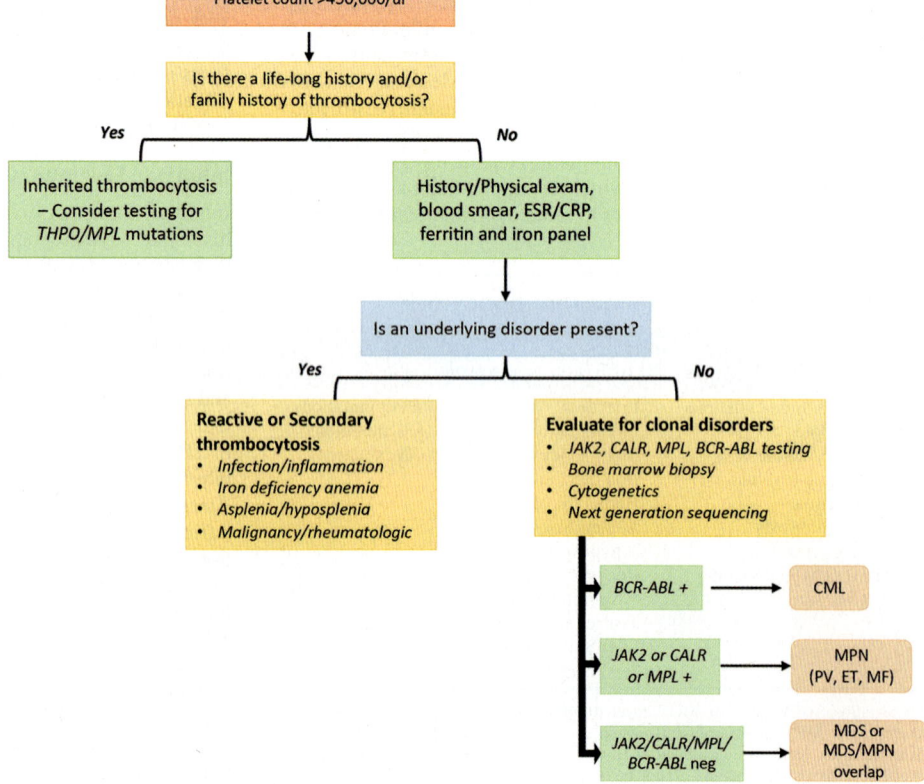

FIGURE 52.1 An approach to evaluating thrombocytosis. A life-long personal and family history of thrombocytosis would suggest inherited thrombocytosis. If that diagnosis is excluded, secondary etiologies should be next considered. If an underlying cause is identified and is treatable, thrombocytosis should resolve with appropriate therapy. If neither inherited nor secondary thrombocytosis is likely, testing for clonal thrombocytosis should be performed; this should include BCR-ABL, JAK2, CALR, and MPL testing. The appropriate tests include bone marrow evaluation and cytogenetics for myeloproliferative neoplasms and myelodysplasia. CALR, calreticulin; CML, chronic myeloid leukemia; CRP, C-reactive protein; ESR, erythrocyte sedimentation rate; ET, essential thrombocytosis; JAK2, Janus kinase 2; MDS, myelodysplastic syndrome; MF, myelofibrosis; MPL, thrombopoietin receptor gene; MPN, myeloproliferative neoplasm; PV, polycythemia vera; THPO, thrombopoietin gene.

Epidemiology

Estimated incidence rate of ET from large studies is reported to be about 1.5 per 100,000 population per year.[25,26] However, disease prevalence is usually much higher because of the chronic nature of the disease. Based on data from large health care plans in the United States between 2008 and 2010, prevalence has been reported to be about 38 to 57 cases per 100,000 population.[27]

The median age at diagnosis is in the mid-50s in large reported series, and unlike other MPNs, women have about twice the higher incidence rate than men.[26,27] ET in children is very uncommon and boys represent the majority of childhood cases.[28] Large population cohort studies have shown an increased risk of ET or other chronic MPNs in first-degree relatives of patients with a chronic MPN.[29] Risk for developing ET appears to be associated with environmental factors linked to other myeloid neoplasms, such as radon and gamma irradiation.[30,31]

Pathophysiology

The primary focus of pathophysiologic investigation in ET is on the role of cytokine signaling involving the TPO signaling pathway. *JAK2* is a cytoplasmic tyrosine kinase that is essential for TPO receptor signaling. Somatic gain-of-function point mutation in the exon 14 of *JAK2*, V617F causes an alteration in the autoinhibitory pseudokinase domain, leading to constitutive activation of the JAK/STAT signaling pathway, and is found in about 50% of the ET patients. In addition to TPO receptor signaling, JAK/STAT pathway is also involved in EPO, granulocyte-colony stimulating factor, and interferon receptor signaling. As such, *JAK2V617F* mutation can be commonly found in other myeloid neoplasms, and especially in PV, it can be detected in about 98% of the cases.[32]

Expression of *JAK2V617F* in hematopoietic progenitors in vitro and in murine models leads to an MPN phenotype resembling PV.[33] It has been proposed that increased *JAK2V617F* allele burden predisposes to thrombosis and identifies a population of patients with ET whose natural history more closely resembles PV.[34]

Somatic mutations in *CALR* gene were discovered in 2013 and are found in about 35% of ET and a similar proportion in MF, but not in PV. *CALR* gene encodes calreticulin protein—a chaperone protein in the endoplasmic reticulum—and mutations in the *CALR* genes are all either from deletions or insertions. There are number of different mutations described so far, but the two most frequently found are the 52 base-pair deletion, called type 1 variant and a 5 base-pair insertion, called type 2 variant. All these indels are located in exon 9 and cause frameshift mutation that results in a mutant protein with altered C-terminus that has impaired calcium binding. The mutant CALR protein is transported to the membrane and binds to the TPO receptor, activating the JAK/STAT signaling pathway.[35,36]

An acquired gain-of-function mutation of the TPO receptor gene—*MPL*—is found in about 3% to 5% of the ET patients, who lack *JAK2* or *CALR* mutations. Somatic *MPLW515L/K* mutation, located in the juxtamembrane domain, leads to constitutive activation of the TPO receptor complex, and is the most commonly observed, although there are several others that have been described.[37] Gain-of-function mutation in the transmembrane domain, *MPLS505N*, has been described in familial ET and is reported to have higher risk for thrombosis progression to myelofibrosis.[38]

Constitutive activation of JAK2/STAT signaling pathway is the common denominator in all the three driver mutations (*JAK2, CALR,* and *MPL*) in chronic MPN. In about 10% to 15% of ET, none of these three common driver mutations can be detected, and are termed as "triple-negative" ET. Rare cases of ET, as well as PV, harbor mutations in *LNK*—a negative regulator of JAK/STAT signaling pathway.[39] In some ET patients, mutations in epigenetic modifier genes such as ten-eleven translocation oncogene family member 2 (*TET2*), DNA methyl transferase 3α (*DNMT3A*), and enhancer of zeste homolog 2 (*EZH2*) may coexist with *JAK2/CALR/MPL* mutations.[35]

Clinical and Laboratory Features

Most patients with ET are asymptomatic at the time of presentation, although some may be diagnosed after a thrombotic event or in the course of evaluation of vasomotor symptoms such as dizziness and headache, which may reflect vascular occlusion. Erythromelalgia (burning dysesthesia in the fingers or toes relieved almost instantly by aspirin) is a characteristic symptom of myeloproliferative thrombocytosis, whether from ET or PV.[40] Distal ischemia ("blue toes syndrome") and cutaneous changes such as livedo reticularis or ulceration are occasionally found.[41,42]

Presenting blood counts and physical examination results from three series are shown in *Table 52.2*. Hemoglobin concentration is usually normal, and higher than normal hemoglobin concentration should raise suspicion for PV. White blood cell counts are typically normal, but leukocytosis >15 × 10^9/L may be found in 15% to 20% of patients.[43] The white blood cell differential is usually normal, but may show the basophilia, eosinophilia, or left-shift characteristic of myeloproliferative disorders. Splenomegaly, whether palpable or radiographic, is found in fewer than 25% of cases without transformation to myelofibrosis.

The characteristic bone marrow feature is a proliferation of large, mature-appearing megakaryocytes (*Figure 52.2*). Marrow cellularity is increased in approximately a third of cases, especially if *JAK2V617F* mutation is positive, but is otherwise normal.[44,46] The presence of significant reticulin deposition, dyserythropoiesis, or dysmyelopoiesis should raise suspicion for other diagnoses, such as myelofibrosis, MDS, or MDS/MPN overlap syndromes.

Patients with ET exhibit evidence of aspirin-reversible increased platelet activation in vivo (increased circulating levels of beta-thromboglobulin, platelet factor 4, and thrombomodulin and increased urinary thromboxane B_2 excretion) while paradoxically exhibiting defective platelet function in vitro, both by classic platelet aggregation and platelet function analyzer-100 studies.[47,48]

Some patients with ET having platelet counts >1000 × 10^9/L develop a bleeding diathesis due to an acquired type 2 von Willebrand syndrome that is reversed by platelet reduction.[47] Therefore, aspirin should be avoided in patients with extremely high platelet counts until a reasonable reduction in platelet count is achieved.

Diagnostic Criteria

For many years, the diagnosis of ET was based on the demonstration of significant sustained thrombocytosis (typically greater than 600 × 10^9/L) in the absence of a reactive etiology, but with the discovery of driver mutations and the demonstration that about 80% of ET patients have mutations in either *JAK2, CALR,* or *MPL* genes, the diagnostic accuracy of ET has significantly improved.

The 2016 WHO criteria for the diagnosis of ET are shown in *Table 52.3*.[23] This is a revised and updated version of the prior 2008 WHO criteria. The first criterion represents a reduction in the

Table 52.2. Clinical and Laboratory Features of Essential Thrombocythemia Patients From Three Series

	United States[43]	Spain[44]	Japan[45]
N	585[a]	92	381
Age, years	57	51	58
Female/male, %	66/34	65/35	55/45
White blood count, × 10^9/L	8.6	9.6	11.3
Hemoglobin, g/dL	13.9	14.4	13.6
Platelet count, × 10^9/L	1000	711	1066
Splenomegaly present, %	23	18	11

Median values from the US and Spanish series; mean values from Japanese series.
[a]Patients with leukemic transformation excluded.

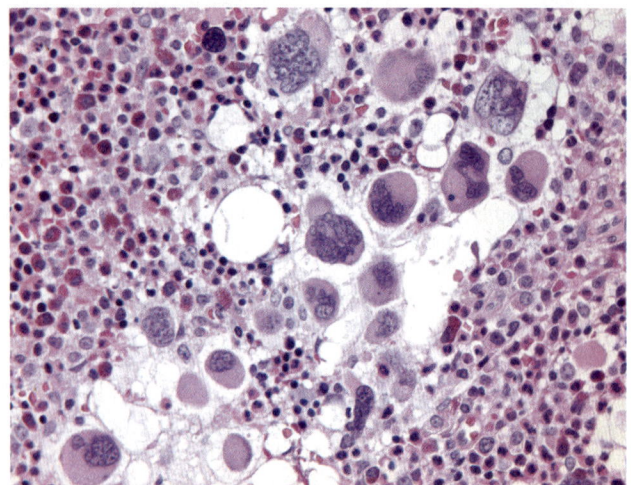

FIGURE 52.2 Characteristic megakaryocyte proliferation in a marrow specimen from an essential thrombocythemia patient.

threshold for thrombocytosis to 450×10^9/L, addressing the concerns that the higher threshold prevented the detection of early disease.[49,50] The second criterion requires demonstration of the characteristic bone marrow morphology of megakaryocytic hyperplasia and demonstrating very rare reticulin fibrosis (grade 1). This is an important criterion in order to differentiate ET from prefibrotic MF and holds therapeutic and prognostic implications.[51,52]

As discussed earlier in this chapter, a number of other myeloid neoplasms may be associated with thrombocytosis. This is particularly true when employing the lower platelet threshold of the revised WHO criteria. The third criterion requires exclusion of these disorders. PV is excluded by the absence of an elevated hematocrit or hemoglobin concentration with adequate iron stores demonstrated on a Prussian blue–stained marrow specimen or a normal serum ferritin: if iron stores are absent, a trial of iron replacement that does not elevate the hematocrit or hemoglobin above normal may be required. Primary myelofibrosis is excluded by the absence of excessive reticulin deposition on the marrow biopsy. CML is excluded by the absence of the *BCR-ABL* rearrangement. MDS and other myeloid neoplasms are excluded by absence of characteristic marrow abnormalities, such as dysplasia and ringed sideroblasts.

Table 52.3. 2016 WHO Diagnostic Criteria for Essential Thrombocythemia

Diagnosis requires meeting all four major criteria *or* meeting the first three major criteria and the minor criterion

Major Criteria
1. Platelet count ≥ 450×10^9/L
2. Bone marrow biopsy specimen showing proliferation mainly of the megakaryocyte lineage with increased numbers of enlarged mature megakaryocytes with hyperlobulated nuclei; no significant increase or left shift in neutrophil granulopoiesis or erythropoiesis; and very rarely minor (grade 1) increase in reticulin fibers
3. Not meeting WHO criteria for polycythemia vera, primary myelofibrosis, chronic myelogenous leukemia, myelodysplastic syndrome, or other myeloid neoplasms
4. Presence of *JAK2*, *CALR*, or *MPL* mutation.

Minor Criterion
Presence of a clonal marker or absence of evidence for reactive thrombocytosis

Abbreviations: *CALR*, calreticulin; *JAK2*, Janus kinase 2; *MPL*, thrombopoietin receptor gene; WHO, World Health Organization.
Reprinted from Arber DA, Orazi A, Hasserjian R, et al. The 2016 revision to the World Health Organization classification of myeloid neoplasms and acute leukemia. *Blood*. 2016;127(20):2391-2405. Copyright © 2016 American Society of Hematology. With permission.

The fourth criterion requires demonstration of mutations in one of the described "driver" genes for ET: *JAK2*, *CALR*, or *MPL*. *JAK2V617F* mutation is reported in 45% to 55% of adult patients with ET.[36] Alternate *JAK2* mutations have been reported in patients with PV lacking the *JAK2V617F* mutation: although similar findings have been reported in ET, they occur far less commonly.[53] *CALR* mutations occur in 30% to 35% of adult patients with ET.[35,36] It was initially reported that *CALR* and *JAK2V617F* mutations were mutually exclusive; although that is generally true, some rare exceptions have been reported.[54] *MPL* mutations, which can also be a cause of familial thrombocytosis, are seen in 3% to 4% of adult patients with ET.[55]

For the 15% to 20% of adult patients who lack mutations in either *JAK2*, *CALR*, or *MPL* (so called "triple-negative" ET), meeting the diagnostic criteria requires either demonstration of a different clonal marker or exclusion of a reactive process causing the thrombocytosis. The differential diagnosis of reactive thrombocytosis was discussed earlier in the chapter. Other additional nondriver mutations that have been reported in ET include additional sex combs–like 1, Casitas B-lineage lymphoma, *DNMT3A*, *EZH2*, isocitrate dehydrogenase 1 and 2, *LNK* (lymphocyte-specific adaptor protein), the TPO receptor/ligand *MPL* (myeloproliferative leukemia virus), *SF3B1* (splicing factor gene B1), nuclear factor 1, suppressor of zeste 2 homolog, and *TET2*.[32,55] These non–driver somatic mutations can be seen in range of other myeloid neoplasms and underscore the genetic complexity of the disease. In the related disorder PV, there are reports that the order of mutation acquisition may influence the clinical features. Patients who acquire *TET2* mutation prior to *JAK2* may attenuate the proliferative characteristic of *JAK2* mutation, while acquiring *JAK2* prior to *TET2* may present more as PV and also may be more responsive to *JAK2* inhibition therapies.[56]

Natural History and Prognosis

The median overall survival of patients with ET appears to exceed 22 years and does not significantly differ from that of the age-adjusted general population.[57] Reported risk factors for reduced overall survival include age >60 years, history of thrombosis, anemia, and leukocytosis >15×10^9/L.[43] The presence of additional non–driver somatic mutations has been associated with greater risk of progression to myelofibrosis and decreases overall survival, as these may indicate more clonal complexity.[32,55,58] A plurality (40%) of deaths is unrelated to ET; the next greatest contributor is thrombosis (26%). Solid tumors (14%) are the next most common cause of death, followed by leukemia, either de novo or postmyelofibrotic (8%) and myelofibrosis (4%).[57] Age, anemia, and platelet count >1000×10^9/L are reported risk factors for leukemic transformation.[43] *MPL* mutations may be associated with a higher fibrotic risk.[59] Compared to patients with PV, the 15-year cumulative risks of thrombosis (27% vs 17%), leukemia (7% vs 2%), and myelofibrosis (6% vs 4%) are lower in patients with ET.[57]

Studies have reported that *CALR*-mutated ET patients have a lower thrombotic risk than *JAK2V617F* or *MPL*-mutated patients.[60] However, this lower risk may reflect the association of *CALR* mutations with other predictors of decreased thrombotic risk, such as younger age and fewer previous thrombotic episodes.[55] In contrast, the *JAK2V617F* allele burden itself may or may not predict a greater thrombotic diathesis.[61] Among the different *CALR* variants, patients with *CALR* type 2 mutation can present with higher platelet count, lower risk of thrombosis, and overall indolent clinical course compared to patients with *CALR* type 1 mutation, which has a more myelofibrosis-type phenotype and higher risk of myelofibrotic transformation.[62]

Models to predict thrombotic risk for individual patients have traditionally been based on age >60 years and personal history of thrombosis. The International Prognostic Score for Essential Thrombocythemia-thrombosis (IPSET-thrombosis) added two additional factors: the presence of cardiovascular risk factors and *JAK2V617F* mutation status. The revised IPSET utilizes three factors—age > 60 years, presence of *JAK2V617F* mutation, and history of

Table 52.4. Risk Categories and Treatment Recommendations Based on Revised IPSET-Thrombosis[63]

Risk Category	Risk Factor	Treatment Recommendation
Very low	None	Observation or aspirin
Low	JAK2 V617F mutation	Aspirin only
Intermediate	Age > 60 years	Aspirin with or without cytoreduction
High	Thrombosis history or *both* JAK2 V617F mutation and age >60 years	Cytoreduction required Aspirin

Abbreviations: IPSET-thrombosis, International Prognostic Score for Essential Thrombocythemia-Thrombosis; JAK2, Janus kinase 2.

thrombosis—to designate four categories: very low risk and low, intermediate, and high risk[63] (see *Table 52.4*). It should be noted that even a markedly elevated platelet count by itself does not define advanced or high-risk disease.[64] However, cytoreduction may be needed in some cases with markedly high platelet count to mitigate bleeding risk from acquired von Willebrand syndrome.

TREATMENT

The goal of treatment in ET is the prevention of thrombotic events, the primary cause of morbidity and mortality.[57] Therefore, treatment strategy is based on thrombotic risk stratification. As a general guide, low-risk patients can be managed with low-dose aspirin or, under some circumstances, observation only. Cytoreduction of the platelet count is recommended for high-risk patients. Intermediate-risk patients may benefit from cytoreduction in some cases.

Aspirin

Aspirin therapy, usually at 100 mg/d or less, is generally well tolerated in patients with ET, with a low risk of bleeding.[65] Antiplatelet agents such as aspirin reduce the risk of venous thrombosis in patients with the JAK2V617F mutation, and reduce the risk of arterial thrombosis in patients with cardiovascular risk factors. Its benefits in other lower-risk patients are less.[66] Aspirin and antiplatelet agents should be avoided in patients with a history of bleeding. Although markedly elevated platelet counts are not a risk factor per se for aspirin-induced bleeding, acquired von Willebrand syndrome may be unmasked by aspirin in patients with platelet counts greater than $1000 \times 10^9/L$.[47] It is prudent to assess von Willebrand factor activity before initiating aspirin in such patients. The bleeding associated with acquired von Willebrand syndrome in ET can be resolved by reduction of the platelet count to a value approximating normal.[67]

Cytoreductive Therapy
Hydroxyurea

Hydroxyurea is the first-line cytoreductive agent in ET.[64,68] Some of the beneficial effects of hydroxyurea in ET and other myeloproliferative disorders may reflect reduction of leukocytosis and leukocyte–platelet interactions.[69] The extent to which hydroxyurea reduces JAK2V617F allele burden in patients with ET is disputed: most reports indicate it does not reduce allele burden in ET,[70,71] and one study reporting reduced allele burden in response to hydroxyurea noted that the effect was less in ET than in PV.[72] In a randomized study of PV patients, hydroxyurea was shown to decrease JAK2V617F allelic burden transiently in the first 2 years, but rebounded to baseline thereafter, compared to patients treated with pegylated interferon.[73] The risk of leukemic transformation with use of hydroxyurea has always been a concern, but so far there is no evidence to support this.[74]

Anagrelide

The platelet-reducing drug anagrelide has been a customary second choice for patients intolerant of, or unresponsive to, hydroxyurea.[68] Initial study comparing hydroxyurea and anagrelide for high-risk ET showed anagrelide was associated with cardiovascular, gastrointestinal, and neurological events, and although it reduced VTE, the anagrelide group had a higher rate of bleeding, arterial thromboembolism, and transformation to myelofibrosis.[75] However, later in the ANHYDRATE study published in 2013, anagrelide was shown to be noninferior to hydroxyurea, as there were no significant differences in the overall outcome.[76] However, anagrelide is not included as first-line therapy in the European LeukemiaNet guidelines for MPNs.[77] Response to anagrelide appears to be similar regardless of the driver mutations.[78,79] Unlike hydroxyurea, interferon, or busulfan, it does not affect leukocytosis or marrow cellular proliferation, and it can be used in combination with hydroxyurea.

Interferon

Administration of recombinant interferon can also be considered in patients refractory to hydroxyurea or to both hydroxyurea and anagrelide.[64,68] Pegylated formulations of interferon are much better tolerated with lesser side effects and weekly injections. High-risk pregnant women with ET can be successfully managed with interferon.[68] Aspirin should be considered for all pregnant women with ET in discussion with their obstetrician.[80] Several early phase clinical trials have reported that recombinant interferon can induce molecular response by reducing JAK2 allelic burden, and in some cases, reversion to polyclonal hematopoiesis.[81-83] Subsequent studies have shown long-term durable molecular responses when compared with hydroxyurea,[84] and thus interferon is the preferred first-line agent in younger patients.[68] However, although it is very effective and widely used in MPN, its use is still considered off-label in the United States, as the US Food and Drug Administration has not approved it for MPN. This may change in future as there are newer forms of pegylated interferon that are currently in clinical trials for MPN.

Other Agents/Modalities

Busulfan is an agent of established efficacy in myeloproliferative disorders such as ET,[64,68] however, its risk profile as an alkylating agent makes it less attractive than hydroxyurea, anagrelide, or interferon, particularly in younger patients. Apheresis can be utilized to obtain rapid reduction in the platelet count in emergencies associated with severe thrombocytosis such as bleeding with acquired von Willebrand syndrome or limb gangrene or in preparation for surgery, but its use should be accompanied by cytoreductive drugs.[67] Unlike in PV and in myelofibrosis where JAK2 inhibitors are approved, they have not yet been shown to be beneficial in ET.[85]

Post–Essential Thrombocythemia Myelofibrosis

Myelofibrosis may be a late complication of ET, with an incidence of approximately 1.6 per 1000 person-years of follow-up, and is the cause of death in approximately 4% of ET patients.[57] Myelofibrosis that develops as a progression from ET is termed as "post-ET myelofibrosis." Patients may develop transfusion-dependent anemia and/or thrombocytopenia and symptomatic splenomegaly. JAK2 inhibitors are first-line therapy in the management of myelofibrosis as outlined for primary myelofibrosis in Chapter 84.

References

1. Jensen MK, de Nully Brown P, Nielsen OJ, Hasselbalch HC. Incidence, clinical features and outcome of essential thrombocythaemia in a well defined geographical area. *Eur J Haematol.* 2000;65(2):132-139.
2. Buss DH, Cashell AW, O'Connor ML, Richards F,IInd, Case LD. Occurrence, etiology, and clinical significance of extreme thrombocytosis: a study of 280 cases. *Am J Med.* 1994;96(3):247-253.
3. Vannucchi AM, Barbui T. Thrombocytosis and thrombosis. *Hematology Am Soc Hematol Educ Program.* 2007:363-370.
4. Aydogan T, Kanbay M, Alici O, Kosar A. Incidence and etiology of thrombocytosis in an adult Turkish population. *Platelets.* 2006;17(5):328-331.

5. Griesshammer M, Bangerter M, Sauer T, Wennauer R, Bergmann L, Heimpel H. Aetiology and clinical significance of thrombocytosis: analysis of 732 patients with an elevated platelet count. *J Intern Med.* 1999;245(3):295-300.
6. Ceresa IF, Noris P, Ambaglio C, Pecci A, Balduni CL. Thrombopoietin is not uniquely responsible for thrombocytosis in inflammatory disorders. *Platelets.* 2007;18(8):579-582.
7. Stone RL, Nick AM, McNeish IA, et al. Paraneoplastic thrombocytosis in ovarian cancer. *N Engl J Med.* 2012;366(7):610-618.
8. Kaser A, Brandacher G, Steurer W, et al. Interleukin-6 stimulates thrombopoiesis through thrombopoietin: role in inflammatory thrombocytosis. *Blood.* 2001;98(9):2720-2725.
9. Morales-Mantilla DE, King KY. The role of interferon-gamma in hematopoietic stem cell development, htomeostasis, and disease. *Curr Stem Cell Rep.* 2018;4(3):264-271.
10. Dan K. Thrombocytosis in iron deficiency anemia. *Intern Med.* 2005;44(10):1025-1026.
11. Ibrahim R, Khan A, Raza S, et al. Triad of iron deficiency anemia, severe thrombocytopenia and menorrhagia-a case report and literature review. *Clin Med Insights Case Rep.* 2012;5:23-27.
12. Evstatiev R, Bukaty A, Jimenez K, et al. Iron deficiency alters megakaryopoiesis and platelet phenotype independent of thrombopoietin. *Am J Hematol.* 2014;89(5):524-529.
13. Xavier-Ferrucio J, Scanlon V, Li X, et al. Low iron promotes megakaryocytic commitment of megakaryocytic-erythroid progenitors in humans and mice. *Blood.* 2019;134(18):1547-1557.
14. Loo M, Beguin Y. The effect of recombinant human erythropoietin on platelet counts is strongly modulated by the adequacy of iron supply. *Blood.* 1999;93(10):3286-3293.
15. Imashuku S, Kudo N, Kubo K, Takahashi N, Tohyama K. Persistent thrombocytosis in elderly patients with rare hyposplenias that mimic essential thrombocythemia. *Int J Hematol.* 2012;95(6):702-705.
16. Zecchina G, Ghio P, Bosio S, Cravino M, Camaschella C, Scagliotti GV. Reactive thrombocytosis might contribute to chemotherapy-related thrombophilia in patients with lung cancer. *Clin Lung Cancer.* 2007;8(4):264-267.
17. Ghaffari S, Pourafkari L. Acute myocardial infarction in a patient with postsplenectomy thrombocytosis: a case report and review of literature. *Cardiol J.* 2010;17(1):79-82.
18. Ho KM, Yip CB, Duff O. Reactive thrombocytosis and risk of subsequent venous thromboembolism: a cohort study. *J Thromb Haemost.* 2012;10(9):1768-1774.
19. Teofili L, Larocca LM. Advances in understanding the pathogenesis of familial thrombocythaemia. *Br J Haematol.* 2011;152(6):701-712.
20. Hong WJ, Gotlib J. Hereditary erythrocytosis, thrombocytosis and neutrophilia. *Best Pract Res Clin Haematol.* 2014;27(2):95-106.
21. Moliterno AR, Williams DM, Gutierrez-Alamillo LI, Salvatori R, Ingersoll RG, Spivak JL. Mpl Baltimore: a thrombopoietin receptor polymorphism associated with thrombocytosis. *Proc Natl Acad Sci U S A.* 2004;101(31):11444-11447.
22. Posthuma HL, Skoda RC, Jacob FA, van der Maas AP, Valk PJ, Posthuma EF. Hereditary thrombocytosis not as innocent as thought? Development into acute leukemia and myelofibrosis. *Blood.* 2010;116(17):3375-3376.
23. Arber DA, Orazi A, Hasserjian R, et al. The 2016 revision to the World Health Organization classification of myeloid neoplasms and acute leukemia. *Blood.* 2016;127(20):2391-2405.
24. Dameshek W. Some speculations on the myeloproliferative syndromes. *Blood.* 1951;6(4):372-375.
25. Moulard O, Mehta J, Fryzek J, Olivares R, Iqbal U, Mesa RA. Epidemiology of myelofibrosis, essential thrombocythemia, and polycythemia vera in the European Union. *Eur J Haematol.* 2014;92(4):289-297.
26. Srour SA, Devesa SS, Morton LM, et al. Incidence and patient survival of myeloproliferative neoplasms and myelodysplastic/myeloproliferative neoplasms in the United States, 2001-12. *Br J Haematol.* 2016;174(3):382-396.
27. Mehta J, Wang H, Iqbal SU, Mesa R. Epidemiology of myeloproliferative neoplasms in the United States. *Leuk Lymphoma.* 2014;55(3):595-600.
28. Fu R, Liu D, Cao Z, et al. Distinct molecular abnormalities underlie unique clinical features of essential thrombocythemia in children. *Leukemia.* 2016;30(3):746-749.
29. Landgren O, Goldin LR, Kristinsson SY, Helgadottir EA, Samuelsson J, Bjorkholm M. Increased risks of polycythemia vera, essential thrombocythemia, and myelofibrosis among 24,577 first-degree relatives of 11,039 patients with myeloproliferative neoplasms in Sweden. *Blood.* 2008;112(6):2199-2204.
30. Mele A, Visani G, Pulsoni A, et al. Risk factors for essential thrombocythemia: a case-control study. Italian Leukemia Study Group. *Cancer.* 1996;77(10):2157-2161.
31. Falcetta R, Sacerdote C, Bazzan M, et al. Occupational and environmental risk factors for essential thrombocythemia: a case-control study. [Article in Italian]. *G Ital Med Lav Ergon.* 2003;25(suppl3):9-12.
32. Nangalia J, Green AR. Myeloproliferative neoplasms: from origins to outcomes. *Blood.* 2017;130(23):2475-2483.
33. Bumm TG, Elsea C, Corbin AS, et al. Characterization of murine JAK2V617F-positive myeloproliferative disease. *Cancer Res.* 2006;66(23):11156-11165.
34. Borowczyk M, Wojtaszewska M, Lewandowski K, et al. The JAK2 V617F mutational status and allele burden may be related with the risk of venous thromboembolic events in patients with Philadelphia-negative myeloproliferative neoplasms. *Thromb Res.* 2015;135(2):272-280.
35. Nangalia J, Massie CE, Baxter EJ, et al. Somatic CALR mutations in myeloproliferative neoplasms with nonmutated JAK2. *N Engl J Med.* 2013;369(25):2391-2405.
36. Klampfl T, Gisslinger H, Harutyunyan AS, et al. Somatic mutations of calreticulin in myeloproliferative neoplasms. *N Engl J Med.* 2013;369(25):2379-2390.
37. Pardanani AD, Levine RL, Lasho T, et al. MPL515 mutations in myeloproliferative and other myeloid disorders: a study of 1182 patients. *Blood.* 2006;108(10):3472-3476.
38. Teofili L, Giona F, Torti L, et al. Hereditary thrombocytosis caused by MPLSer505Asn is associated with a high thrombotic risk, splenomegaly and progression to bone marrow fibrosis. *Haematologica.* 2010;95(1):65-70.
39. McMullin MF, Cario H. LNK mutations and myeloproliferative disorders. *Am J Hematol.* 2016;91(2):248-251.
40. Michiels JJ, Berneman Z, Schroyens W, et al. Platelet-mediated erythromelalgic, cerebral, ocular and coronary microvascular ischemic and thrombotic manifestations in patients with essential thrombocythemia and polycythemia vera: a distinct aspirin-responsive and coumadin-resistant arterial thrombophilia. *Platelets.* 2006;17(8):528-544.
41. Gerry JL Jr, Persich D, Gumbart CH, Schramel RJ. Primary thrombocythemia: another cause of the "blue toe syndrome". *J La State Med Soc.* 1986;138(4):38-40.
42. Itin PH, Winkelmann RK. Cutaneous manifestations in patients with essential thrombocythemia. *J Am Acad Dermatol.* 1991;24(1):59-63.
43. Gangat N, Wolanskyj AP, McClure RF, et al. Risk stratification for survival and leukemic transformation in essential thrombocythemia: a single institutional study of 605 patients. *Leukemia.* 2007;21(2):270-276.
44. Kwon M, Osorio S, Munoz C, Sanchez JM, Buno I, Diez-Martin JL. Essential thrombocythemia in patients with platelet counts below 600x10(9)/L: applicability of the 2008 World Health Organization diagnostic criteria revision proposal. *Am J Hematol.* 2009;84(7):452-454.
45. Dan K, Yamada T, Kimura Y, et al. Clinical features of polycythemia vera and essential thrombocythemia in Japan: retrospective analysis of a nationwide survey by the Japanese Elderly Leukemia and Lymphoma Study Group. *Int J Hematol.* 2006;83(5):443-449.
46. Campbell PJ, Scott LM, Buck G, et al. Definition of subtypes of essential thrombocythaemia and relation to polycythaemia vera based on JAK2 V617F mutation status: a prospective study. *Lancet.* 2005;366(9501):1945-1953.
47. Michiels JJ, Berneman ZN, Schroyens W, Van Vliet HH. Pathophysiology and treatment of platelet-mediated microvascular disturbances, major thrombosis and bleeding complications in essential thrombocythaemia and polycythaemia vera. *Platelets.* 2004;15(2):67-84.
48. Tsantes AE, Dimoula A, Bonovas S, et al. The role of the Platelet Function Analyzer (PFA)-100 and platelet aggregometry in the differentiation of essential thrombocythemia from reactive thrombocytosis. *Thromb Res.* 2010;125(2):142-146.
49. Lengfelder E, Hochhaus A, Kronawitter U, et al. Should a platelet limit of 600 x 10(9)/l be used as a diagnostic criterion in essential thrombocythaemia? An analysis of the natural course including early stages. *Br J Haematol.* 1998;100(1):15-23.
50. Thiele J, Kvasnicka HM. A critical reappraisal of the WHO classification of the chronic myeloproliferative disorders. *Leuk Lymphoma.* 2006;47(3):381-396.
51. Gisslinger H, Jeryczynski G, Gisslinger B, et al. Clinical impact of bone marrow morphology for the diagnosis of essential thrombocythemia: comparison between the BCSH and the WHO criteria. *Leukemia.* 2016;30(5):1126-1132.
52. Thiele J, Kvasnicka HM, Mullauer L, Buxhofer-Ausch V, Gisslinger B, Gisslinger H. Essential thrombocythemia versus early primary myelofibrosis: a multicenter study to validate the WHO classification. *Blood.* 2011;117(21):5710-5718.
53. Milosevic Feenstra JD, Nivarthi H, Gisslinger H, et al. Whole-exome sequencing identifies novel MPL and JAK2 mutations in triple-negative myeloproliferative neoplasms. *Blood.* 2016;127(3):325-332.
54. Kang MG, Choi HW, Lee JH, et al. Coexistence of JAK2 and CALR mutations and their clinical implications in patients with essential thrombocythemia. *Oncotarget.* 2016;7(35):57036-57049.
55. Shammo JM, Stein BL. Mutations in MPNs: prognostic implications, window to biology, and impact on treatment decisions. *Hematology Am Soc Hematol Educ Program.* 2016;2016(1):552-560.
56. Ortmann CA, Kent DG, Nangalia J, et al. Effect of mutation order on myeloproliferative neoplasms. *N Engl J Med.* 2015;372(7):601-612.
57. Passamonti F, Rumi E, Pungolino E, et al. Life expectancy and prognostic factors for survival in patients with polycythemia vera and essential thrombocythemia. *Am J Med.* 2004;117(10):755-761.
58. Spivak JL. Myeloproliferative neoplasms. *N Engl J Med.* 2017;376(22):2168-2181.
59. Elala YC, Lasho TL, Gangat N, et al. Calreticulin variant stratified driver mutational status and prognosis in essential thrombocythemia. *Am J Hematol.* 2016;91(5):503-506.
60. Rotunno G, Mannarelli C, Guglielmelli P, et al. Impact of calreticulin mutations on clinical and hematological phenotype and outcome in essential thrombocythemia. *Blood.* 2014;123(10):1552-1555.
61. Larsen TS, Pallisgaard N, Moller MB, Hasselbalch HC. High prevalence of arterial thrombosis in JAK2 mutated essential thrombocythaemia: independence of the V617F allele burden. *Hematology.* 2008;13(2):71-76.
62. Pietra D, Rumi E, Ferretti VV, et al. Differential clinical effects of different mutation subtypes in CALR-mutant myeloproliferative neoplasms. *Leukemia.* 2016;30(2):431-438.
63. Haider M, Gangat N, Lasho T, et al. Validation of the revised International Prognostic Score of Thrombosis for Essential Thrombocythemia (IPSET-thrombosis) in 585 Mayo clinic patients. *Am J Hematol.* 2016;91(4):390-394.
64. Tefferi A, Barbui T. Polycythemia vera and essential thrombocythemia: 2017 update on diagnosis, risk-stratification, and management. *Am J Hematol.* 2017;92(1):94-108.
65. Finazzi G, Carobbio A, Thiele J, et al. Incidence and risk factors for bleeding in 1104 patients with essential thrombocythemia or prefibrotic myelofibrosis diagnosed according to the 2008 WHO criteria. *Leukemia.* 2012;26(4):716-719.

66. Alvarez-Larran A, Cervantes F, Pereira A, et al. Observation versus antiplatelet therapy as primary prophylaxis for thrombosis in low-risk essential thrombocythemia. *Blood*. 2010;116(8):1205-1210. quiz 387.
67. Elliott MA, Tefferi A. Pathogenesis and management of bleeding in essential thrombocythemia and polycythemia vera. *Curr Hematol Rep*. 2004;3(5):344-351.
68. Rumi E, Cazzola M. How I treat essential thrombocythemia. *Blood*. 2016;128(20):2403-2414.
69. Trelinski J, Tybura M, Smolewski P, Robak T, Chojnowski K. The influence of low-dose aspirin and hydroxyurea on platelet-leukocyte interactions in patients with essential thrombocythemia. *Blood Coagul Fibrinolysis*. 2009;20(8):646-651.
70. Antonioli E, Carobbio A, Pieri L, et al. Hydroxyurea does not appreciably reduce JAK2 V617F allele burden in patients with polycythemia vera or essential thrombocythemia. *Haematologica*. 2010;95(8):1435-1438.
71. Zalcberg IR, Ayres-Silva J, de Azevedo AM, Solza C, Daumas A, Bonamino M. Hydroxyurea dose impacts hematologic parameters in polycythemia vera and essential thrombocythemia but does not appreciably affect JAK2-V617F allele burden. *Haematologica*. 2011;96(3):e18-e20.
72. Besses C, Alvarez-Larran A, Martinez-Aviles L, et al. Modulation of JAK2 V617F allele burden dynamics by hydroxycarbamide in polycythaemia vera and essential thrombocythaemia patients. *Br J Haematol*. 2011;152(4):413-419.
73. Gisslinger H, Klade C, Georgiev P, et al. Ropeginterferon alfa-2b versus standard therapy for polycythaemia vera (PROUD-PV and CONTINUATION-PV): a randomised, non-inferiority, phase 3 trial and its extension study. *Lancet Haematol*. 2020;7(3):e196-e208.
74. Bjorkholm M, Derolf AR, Hultcrantz M, et al. Treatment-related risk factors for transformation to acute myeloid leukemia and myelodysplastic syndromes in myeloproliferative neoplasms. *J Clin Oncol*. 2011;29(17):2410-2415.
75. Harrison CN, Campbell PJ, Buck G, et al. Hydroxyurea compared with anagrelide in high-risk essential thrombocythemia. *N Engl J Med*. 2005;353(1):33-45.
76. Gisslinger H, Gotic M, Holowiecki J, et al. Anagrelide compared with hydroxyurea in WHO-classified essential thrombocythemia: the ANAHYDRET Study, a randomized controlled trial. *Blood*. 2013;121(10):1720-1728.
77. Barbui T, Tefferi A, Vannucchi AM, et al. Philadelphia chromosome-negative classical myeloproliferative neoplasms: revised management recommendations from European LeukemiaNet. *Leukemia*. 2018;32(5):1057-1069.
78. Cascavilla N, De Stefano V, Pane F, et al. Impact of JAK2(V617F) mutation status on treatment response to anagrelide in essential thrombocythemia: an observational, hypothesis-generating study. *Drug Des Devel Ther*. 2015;9:2687-2694.
79. Mela Osorio MJ, Ferrari L, Goette NP, et al. Long-term follow-up of essential thrombocythemia patients treated with anagrelide: subgroup analysis according to JAK2/CALR/MPL mutational status. *Eur J Haematol*. 2016;96(4):435-442.
80. Passamonti F, Rumi E, Randi ML, Morra E, Cazzola M. Aspirin in pregnant patients with essential thrombocythemia: a retrospective analysis of 129 pregnancies. *J Thromb Haemost*. 2010;8(2):411-413.
81. Kiladjian JJ, Cassinat B, Chevret S, et al. Pegylated interferon-alfa-2a induces complete hematologic and molecular responses with low toxicity in polycythemia vera. *Blood*. 2008;112(8):3065-3072.
82. Quintas-Cardama A, Kantarjian H, Manshouri T, et al. Pegylated interferon alfa-2a yields high rates of hematologic and molecular response in patients with advanced essential thrombocythemia and polycythemia vera. *J Clin Oncol*. 2009;27(32):5418-5424.
83. Swierczek S, Lima LT, Tashi T, Kim SJ, Gregg XT, Prchal JT. Presence of polyclonal hematopoiesis in females with Ph-negative myeloproliferative neoplasms. *Leukemia*. 2015;29(12):2432-2434.
84. Yacoub A, Mascarenhas J, Kosiorek H, et al. Pegylated interferon alfa-2a for polycythemia vera or essential thrombocythemia resistant or intolerant to hydroxyurea. *Blood*. 2019;134(18):1498-1509.
85. Harrison CN, Mead AJ, Panchal A, et al. Ruxolitinib vs best available therapy for ET intolerant or resistant to hydroxycarbamide. *Blood*. 2017;130(17):1889-1897.

Chapter 53 ■ Qualitative Disorders of Platelet Function

EMANUELA FALCINELLI • LOREDANA BURY • PAOLO GRESELE

INTRODUCTION

Platelets, discovered by Giulio Bizzozero in 1882,[1] are small, disc-shaped anucleate cells deriving from megakaryocytes that play a key role in the arrest of hemorrhage. When a vessel wound occurs, the formation of a hemostatic platelet plug is rapidly triggered as a finely regulated process that includes (1) the initial adhesion of platelets to subendothelial collagen fibrils, (2) the activation of adherent platelets, (3) the release of granular and metabolic products, (4) the recruitment of other platelets mediated by released soluble agonists, and (5) the interaction of activated platelet integrin $\alpha_{IIb}\beta_3$ with fibrinogen resulting in aggregation. In addition, when platelets get activated, negatively charged phospholipids move from the inner to the outer leaflet of the membrane bilayer providing the phospholipid surface for the optimal interaction between enzymes and cofactors of the coagulation system resulting in the formation of a fibrin clot.

In addition, clot retraction, effected by platelet actin-myosin fibers, contributes to draw the wound edges near and to stabilize the platelet clot.[2,3]

A defect altering any of these steps affects the formation or the effectiveness of the hemostatic plug and, consequently, leads to abnormal bleeding. Qualitative defects of platelet function, also defined inherited platelet function disorders (IPFDs), are characterized by mild to severe mucocutaneous bleeding, sometimes associated with reduced platelet number, and by a wide phenotypic and genotypic heterogeneity.

The exact prevalence of the different IPFDs is unknown, but estimates go from as low as 2/1,000,000[4] to more than 1/100.[5] A recent analysis of 125,748 exomes from the general population examining naturally occurring loss-of-function (LoF) variants in known platelet-associated genes estimated the probability of having a clinically relevant platelet-related LoF at 0.329%.[6]

The introduction of new laboratory tests, enhanced standardization of the established assays, and the ever growing diffusion of high-throughput gene sequencing techniques have led to great improvements in diagnosis and to the discovery of many novel forms (*Figure 53.1*).

DIAGNOSTIC APPROACH TO INHERITED PLATELET FUNCTION DISORDERS

The diagnostic approach to a patient with a bleeding disorder of suspected platelet origin should be based on clinical evaluation and a panel of laboratory tests of increasing complexity.[7-9]

A detailed personal and family history helps to establish whether there is an abnormal bleeding tendency and if the disorder may be hereditary or acquired. The hemorrhagic tendency may be of variable severity, with spontaneous mucocutaneous bleedings and hemorrhage after surgery, trauma, or delivery. Typical manifestations are epistaxis, oral cavity bleeding, especially during tooth brushing, and hemorrhage following dental extraction, menorrhagia, and skin bruising. Rare manifestations are muscle hematomas, central nervous system bleeds (reported in Glanzmann thrombasthenia [GT]), hematuria, gastrointestinal bleeding (hematemesis, melena, hematochezia), and ovulation bleeding.[8]

Some IPFDs show peculiar clinical features, such as the Quebec platelet disorder (QPD), which is associated with delayed bleeding typically starting 12 to 24 hours after surgery or trauma, or the Scott syndrome, which is associated with postoperative or posttrauma bleeding but rarely with spontaneous hemorrhage.

The use of a bleeding assessment tool is strongly encouraged to standardize the evaluation of bleeding severity, improve diagnostic accuracy and sensitivity, and possibly predict the future risk of bleeding.[10] The International Society on Thrombosis and Haemostasis (ISTH) Bleeding Assessment Tool (ISTH-BAT) is a clinical diagnostic instrument for mild/moderate bleeding disorders which has recently been validated for inherited platelet disorders (IPDs).[11] A study in a large cohort of patients with a well-defined IPD diagnosis showed that the bleeding score was higher in patients with IPFD compared with von Willebrand disease type 1, inherited thrombocytopenia (IT), and healthy controls (HCs) and that it allowed to differentiate IPFD from HC and potentially from IT.[11] Moreover, the ISTH-BAT has also been investigated for bleeding prediction in patients with IPD in a prospective study, confirming that this tool has a prognostic value for future bleeding incidence and may identify cases requiring more intensive prophylactic treatment.[12]

Besides bleeding history, associated organ involvement should also be sought, given that some inherited platelet disorders are part of a systemic syndrome. Drug-related or immunological causes of platelet dysfunction should be ruled out.[13]

Preliminary laboratory tests, including a full blood count, blood clotting screening (prothrombin time, partial thromboplastin time, fibrinogen), and von Willebrand factor (VWF) screening (VWF antigen, ristocetin cofactor activity, and factor VIII coagulant activity), should be performed before specific platelet function studies are started. A reduced platelet number, especially if mild, does not preclude further testing when there is clinical suspicion because several IPFD are associated with thrombocytopenia.[8] If the above screening tests exclude other bleeding disorders, laboratory investigations for possible IPFD should be undertaken.[10,13]

Initial tests should include an examination of a peripheral blood smear, light transmission aggregometry (LTA), the measurement of platelet granule release, and the evaluation of the main surface glycoproteins (GPs) by flow cytometry; all assays now available in the majority of the hemostasis laboratories.[9] A second set of laboratory tests, to be performed in patients in whom the first step has not yielded a diagnosis or has provided inconclusive results, should include LTA with an expanded range of agonists, flow cytometry with antibodies directed toward additional surface GPs, the measurement of granule contents, clot retraction, serum TxB_2 and transmission electron microscopy (TEM). Finally, the very special cases still evading diagnosis and for which a strong clinical suspicion persists may be studied with a series of additional, highly specialized, third step tests (*Figure 53.2*).[13]

The search for the causative variant by molecular biology, which previously played mainly a confirmatory role, is now increasingly used in the initial diagnosis of a suspected IPFD.[8,14]

Genotyping is recommended for conditions in which a genotype/phenotype correlation has been established and for those in which the phenotype, including platelet function testing, is not conclusive (*Figure 53.2*). However, genotyping is complex, cumbersome, still relatively expensive, and requires great expertise not only in molecular biology and bioinformatics but also in platelet function studies in order to assess the possible clinical relevance of the many missense variants that are usually detected.[8] Next-generation sequencing (NGS) has provided improved resolution for identifying variants associated with platelet disorders, proving to be an efficient method for discovering pathogenic variants in novel genes.[14,15] However, aggregations of high-quality exomes in the Exome Aggregation Consortium (ExAC) 22 and Genome Aggregation Database (gnomAD) have identified millions of naturally occurring exonic variants

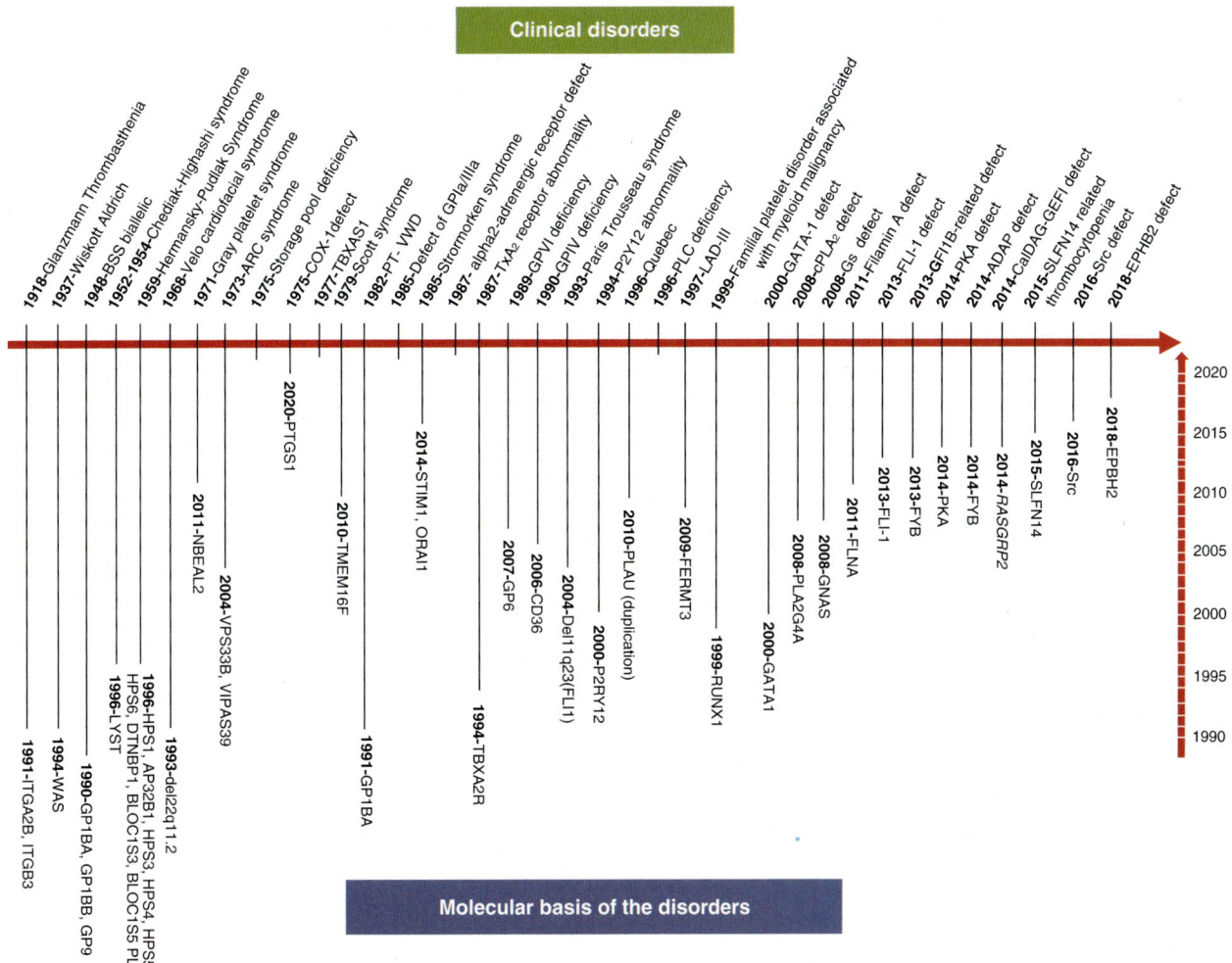

FIGURE 53.1 Timeline of IPFD discovery. ADAP, adhesion and degranulation-promoting adaptor protein; ARC, arthrogryposis, renal dysfunction, and cholestasis; CalDAG-GEFI, calcium and DAG-regulated guanine exchange factor-1; COX-1, cyclooxygenase-1; cPLA2, cytosolic phospholipase A2; EPHB2, Ephrin type B receptor 2; FLI-1, friend leukemia integration 1; GP, glycoprotein; HPS, Hermansky-Pudlak syndrome; LAD-III, leukocyte adhesion deficiency-III; PKA, protein kinase A; PLC, phospholipase C; PT-VWD, Platelet-type von Willebrand disease.

in a cross-section of the general population[6]; therefore, most of the new variants identified are classified as of uncertain pathogenicity. The Scientific and Standardization Committee on Genetics in Thrombosis and Haemostasis of the ISTH has thus developed an open-access gene variant submission interface aimed at curating variants for diagnostic-grade (TIER-1) genes and to improve variant classification.[16] Moreover, an up-to-date TIER1 gene-disease list for coagulation and platelet disorders, useful for clinical genetic testing for the design of gene panel tests, or for filtering whole exome or whole-genome sequencing data, has been developed.[17]

Based on the above considerations, although NGS-based methods are changing the approach to IPFDs diagnosis and in perspective may become the initial diagnostic technique, clinical and laboratory phenotypic characterization still remain crucial.

HEREDITARY DISORDERS OF PLATELET FUNCTION

IPFD are a very heterogeneous group of hemorrhagic diseases, and for several of them the causative molecular defect is unknown. They include at least 42 disorders caused by variants in 46 different genes. *Table 53.1* lists the main characteristics of the currently known IPFDs.

In this chapter they are classified according to the main function of the defective protein generated by the mutated gene or, when this is not known, the main structural or functional abnormality (*Table 53.2*).

Abnormalities of Adhesive Protein Receptors
Glanzmann Thrombasthenia

GT has been the first disorder of platelet function to be described clinically, and it was called by Eduard Glanzmann in 1918 hereditary hemorrhagic thrombasthenia. The cause of the disorder was identified in the absence of platelet surface glycoprotein (GP)IIb/IIIa only in the 1970s and the first causative gene variant only in 1991.[18,19]

GT is a rare autosomal recessive disorder characterized by the complete absence of platelet aggregation and defective clot retraction, with normal platelet number and volume. The prevalence of GT is estimated to be about 1/1,000,000, but it is higher in some populations in which consanguinity is frequent, like South Indian Hindus, Iraqi Jews, French Manouche gypsies, and Jordanian nomadic tribes. The molecular basis of the defect resides in quantitative and/or qualitative abnormalities of integrin $\alpha_{IIb}\beta_3$, or GPIIb/IIIa, the most abundant platelet surface receptor that binds fibrinogen (in addition to VWF, vitronectin, fibronectin, and thrombospondin).

GT is classified in types I, II and III based on the amount of residual $\alpha_{IIb}\beta_3$ expression and severity of the platelet function defect. Patients with type I express 0% to 5% of $\alpha_{IIb}\beta_3$ and have a profound defect of clot retraction; patients with type II express 10% to 20% $\alpha_{IIb}\beta_3$ and have an only moderately defective clot retraction; patients with type III, also called variant GT, express from 30% to 100% $\alpha_{IIb}\beta_3$ and show defective aggregation and a variable impairment of

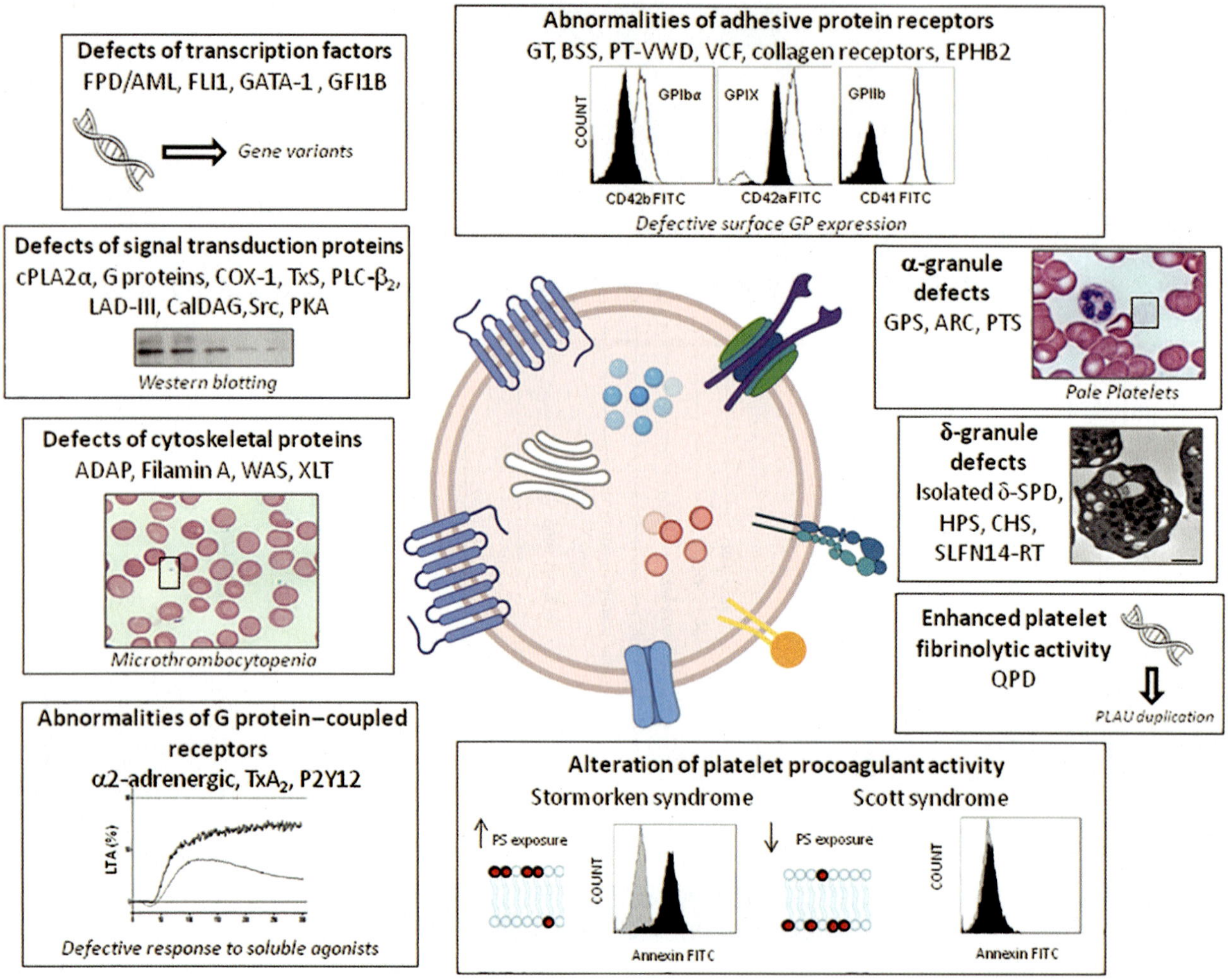

FIGURE 53.2 The figures show IPFDs according to the protein and/or platelet function element that is affected by the genetic anomaly and the most typical laboratory finding.

clot retraction. So far there is no evidence for a correlation between the intensity of bleeding manifestations and residual $\alpha_{IIb}\beta_3$ expression; therefore, there is no reliable test to predict the severity of the disease, which furthermore may differ considerably among the affected members of the same family. The expression of 50% of normal $\alpha_{IIb}\beta_3$ is sufficient to guarantee platelet aggregation, and thus heterozygous carriers are usually asymptomatic. Disease-causative variants affect the ITGA2B and ITGB3 genes, which are located close to each other at 17q21-23 and encode for the α_{IIb} and the β_3 subunits of the receptor, respectively. To date at least 149 different variants have been described, including deletions, insertions, and nonsense, frameshift, and missense variants. Most of them prevent $\alpha_{IIb}\beta_3$ subunit biosynthesis or the transport of pro-$\alpha_{IIb}\beta_3$ complexes from the endoplasmic reticulum to the Golgi apparatus and/or their translocation to the platelet surface. Rarer variants, causing type III GT, generate abnormal $\alpha_{IIb}\beta_3$ complexes that are nonfunctional, because they are unable either to bind its ligands (variants affecting the globular head)[20] or to transduce signals (variants affecting the cytoplasmic tail).

Gain-of-function variants that generate an $\alpha_{IIb}\beta_3$ complex constitutively activated, locked in a high affinity state able to spontaneously bind fibrinogen, are also associated with platelet dysfunction, mild macrothrombocytopenia, and hemorrhagic manifestations similar to classical recessive GT. In these forms, constitutive $\alpha_{IIb}\beta_3$ activation leads to receptor internalization and to altered cytoskeletal reorganization, which is the main effector of platelet dysfunction and macrothrombocytopenia.[21]

Bleeding manifestations of GT are moderate to severe, with purpura, epistaxis, gingival bleeding, and menorrhagia (which can be severe since menarche) as nearly constant features. Gastrointestinal bleeding and hematuria are less common, and hemarthroses and intracranial hemorrhage are relatively rare but may occur differently from most IPFD. Since bleeding manifestations are precocious, GT is usually diagnosed before 5 years of age and often soon after birth. Posttraumatic, postsurgical, and postpartum bleeding may be severe.[22,23] In spite of this, patients with GT are not protected from atherosclerosis or venous thromboembolism.[24,25]

Typical laboratory findings are the absence of platelet aggregation to all agonists but normal ristocetin-induced platelet agglutination, a prolonged bleeding time, normal platelet size and number, and impaired clot retraction. The diagnosis is confirmed by flow cytometry, with strikingly reduced or absent platelet surface CD41 (GPIIb) and CD61 (GPIIIa). Impaired platelet spreading on fibrinogen or collagen are also typical. In the rare cases with normal or only slightly reduced $\alpha_{IIb}\beta_3$ surface expression but a dysfunctional receptor, measurement of the binding of monoclonal antibody PAC-1, recognizing the active form of $\alpha_{IIb}\beta_3$ to stimulated platelets, is a clue to diagnosis.

Genetic testing is not mandatory, because the above described functional pattern is pathognomic, but it is required for prenatal diagnosis or for the diagnosis of autosomal dominant variant forms.

Bernard-Soulier Syndrome

Bernard-Soulier syndrome (BSS) was described clinically for the first time in 1948 and called hemorrhagiparous thrombocytic dystrophy.[26]

Table 53.1. Clinical and Laboratory Characteristics of the Congenital Disorders of Platelet Function

Disease	Syndromic Manifestations	Laboratory Findings
Abnormalities of Adhesive Protein Receptors		
Glanzmann thrombasthenia	-	• Absent platelet aggregation • Quantitative or qualitative defect of $\alpha_{IIb}\beta_3$ • Variants in *ITGA2B* or *ITGB3*
Bernard-Soulier syndrome	-	• Macrothrombocytopenia • Quantitative or qualitative defect of GPIb/IX/V • Absent or markedly reduced RIPA • Variants in *GP1BA* or *GP1BB* or *GP9*
Platelet-type VWD	-	• Mild macrothrombocytopenia • Loss of HMW-VWF multimers • Enhanced RIPA • Variants in *GP1BA*
22q11.2 Deletion syndrome	Heart disease, palate abnormalities, developmental delay, immune deficiency, facial dysmorphisms, vertebral anomalies, gastrointestinal abnormalities, deafness, renal anomalies, dental anomalies, learning disabilities, psychiatric disorders	• Macrothrombocytopenia • Quantitative or qualitative defect of GPIb/IX/V • Absent or markedly reduced RIPA • 22q11.2 deletion
Defect of $\alpha_2\beta_1$	-	• Absent platelet activation and aggregation by collagen • Decreased expression of $\alpha_2\beta_1$
Defect of GPVI	-	• Absent platelet activation and aggregation by collagen CRP and convulxin • Decreased expression of GPVI • Variants in *GP6*
Defect of GPIV	-	• Reduced expression of CD36 • Reduced adhesion of platelets to collagen under flow conditions • Variants in *CD36*
Abnormalities of G Protein–Coupled Receptors		
Defect of the α_2-adrenoreceptor	-	• Absent aggregation in response to adrenaline
Defect of the TxA$_2$ receptor (TP)	-	• Absent platelet aggregation by U46619 and arachidonic acid • Reduced secondary wave aggregation by ADP and adrenaline • Variants in *TBXA2R*
Defect of the ADP receptor (P2Y$_{12}$)	-	• Defective platelet aggregation in response to ADP • Defective inhibition of adenylyl cyclase by ADP • Variants in *P2RY12*
Defect of the PAR-1 receptor	-	• Decreased expression of PAR-1 • Impaired aggregation and secretion by PAR-1-activating peptide • Decreased procoagulant activity
Defects of Platelet Granules (Isolated/Syndromic)		
Isolated δ-storage pool deficiency	-	• Absence of δ-granules (TEM), decreased platelet nucleotide content, and increased ATP/ADP ratio (± decreased 5-HT content) • Absent secondary wave aggregation
Hermansky-Pudlak syndrome	• Oculocutaneous albinism, nystagmus and visual acuity loss • Pulmonary fibrosis, granulomatous colitis, or immunodeficiency depending on subtype	• Absence of δ-granules (TEM), decreased platelet nucleotide content, and increased ATP/ADP ratio (± decreased 5-HT content) • Absent secondary wave aggregation • Variants in *HPS1, AP32B1, HPS3, HPS4, HPS5, HPS6, DTNBP1, BLOC1S3, BLOC1S5 AP3B1,* or *PLDN*
Chediak-Higashi syndrome	• Oculocutaneous albinism • Recurrent infections • Severe immunological deficiency • Neurological problems	• Absence of δ-granules (TEM) or decrease in platelet nucleotide content and increased ATP/ADP ratio (± decreased 5-HT content) • Diminished secondary aggregation • Variants in *LYST*
SLFN14-related thrombocytopenia	-	• Thrombocytopenia • Reduction in δ-granules, impaired ATP secretion by ADP, collagen, and TRAP-6 • Variants in *SLFN14*
Autism with platelet dense granule defect	• Autism	• Decreased platelet ATP secretion • Reduction in δ-granules (TEM) • Variants in *NBEA*
Gray platelet syndrome (GPS)	• Bone marrow fibrosis (not always)	• Absence of α-granules • Reduced aggregation by thrombin or TRAP-6 • Increased vitamin B12 in plasma • Variants in *NBEAL2*

Table 53.1. Clinical and Laboratory Characteristics of the Congenital Disorders of Platelet Function (continued)

Disease	Syndromic Manifestations	Laboratory Findings
Arthrogryposis, renal dysfunction and cholestasis (ARC) syndrome	• Arthrogryposis, renal dysfunction, cholestasis, cerebral malformations, deafness, congenital heart disease, diabetes	• Macrothrombocytopenia • Absence of α-granules • Decreased P-selectin expression • Impaired aggregation by epinephrine, ADP, collagen, and arachidonic acid • Variants in *VPS33B* or *VIPAS39*
Paris-Trousseau syndrome	• Facial and skull dysmorphisms • Mental retardation • Congenital heart defects	• Macrothrombocytopenia • Giant α-granules • Impaired aggregation by epinephrine, ADP, collagen, and arachidonic acid • del11q23
α/δ-Storage pool deficiency	-	• Deficiency of α- and δ-granules
Signal Transduction Proteins Defects		
Gα$_{i1}$ deficiency	-	• Impaired aggregation by ADP and epinephrine • Absent inhibition of forskolin-stimulated cAMP increase by ADP, thrombin, or epinephrine • Diminished Gα$_{i1}$
Gα$_q$ deficiency	-	• Impaired aggregation and secretion by ADP, epinephrine, collagen, U46619, PAF • Defective TxA$_2$ production in response to ADP and thrombin • Defective Ca^{2+} mobilization in response to ADP and thrombin • Impaired GTPase activity • Diminished Gα$_q$ • Variants in *GNAQ* promoter
Gα$_s$ hyperfunction	-	• Enhanced cAMP generation upon stimulation • Sensitivity to inhibition by agents that elevate cAMP • Higher membrane-associated Gα$_s$ by Western blotting • Variants in *GNAS1*
Gα$_s$ hypofunction	-	• Reduced cAMP production after stimulation of Gs-coupled receptors • Impaired platelet shape change • Variants in *GNAS1*
Cytosolic phospholipase A$_2$α (cPLA$_2$α) defect	Bleeding from gastrointestinal ulcers	• Impaired aggregation and secretion by ADP and collagen (normal by arachidonic acid). • Reduction of urinary metabolites of PGE$_2$, PGD$_2$, PGI$_2$, and TxA$_2$ • Decreased serum TxB$_2$ • Decreased cPLA$_2$ • Variants in *PLA2G4A*
Cyclo-oxygenase-1 (COX-1) defect	-	• Impaired aggregation by ADP, collagen, epinephrine, and AA (normal by PGH$_2$). • Reduced platelet TXA$_2$ production in response to AA but normal in response to PGH$_2$ • Absence of COX-1 • Variants in *PTGS1*
Thromboxane synthase defect	Ghosal syndrome (increased bone density with predominant diaphyseal involvement, corticosteroid-sensitive anemia) (in some patients)	• Absent aggregation by AA, impaired by ADP and epinephrine • Decreased serum TxB$_2$ • Absence of thromboxane synthase by Western blotting • Variants in *TBXAS1*
Phospholipase C defect	-	• Impaired aggregation and Ca^{2+} mobilization by ADP, PAF, U46619, collagen, and thrombin • Decreased expression of PLC-β2 by Western blotting • Diminished formation of IP3 and DAG by thrombin and PAF
Leukocyte adhesion deficiency-III (LAD-III)	Predisposition to recurrent infections	• GT-like platelet phenotype • Leukocyte function defect • Variants in *FERMT3*
CalDAG-GEFI defect	-	• GT-like platelet phenotype • Variants in *RASGRP2*
Src defect	• Myelofibrosis • Bone defects	• Defect of platelet granules • Platelet cytoplasmic vacuoles • Variants in *SRC*
PKA defect	Macrothrombocytopenia	• Defective α$_{IIb}$β$_3$ activation, P-selectin exposure, and Ca^{2+} mobilization • Defective phosphorylation of filamin A • Variants in *PRKACG*

(Continued)

Table 53.1. Clinical and Laboratory Characteristics of the Congenital Disorders of Platelet Function *(continued)*

Disease	Syndromic Manifestations	Laboratory Findings
Defects of Transcription Factors		
Familial platelet disorder with associated myeloid malignancy (FPD/MM)	Increased risk of developing myeloid hematological malignancies	• Mild thrombocytopenia • Defective content and release of δ-granules • Variable reduction of α-granules • Impaired aggregation by epinephrine, ADP, and arachidonic acid • Presence of MYH10 in platelets • Variants in *RUNX1*
FLI1-related δ-granule defect	Alopecia, eczema, recurrent viral infections, psoriasis	• Mild thrombocytopenia • δ-Granules secretion defect • Presence of MYH10 in platelets • Variants in *FLI1*
GATA1 defect	Dyserythropoiesis, anemia, β-thalassemia, congenital erythropoietic porphyria	• Large platelets • Reduced number of α-granules • Reduced aggregation in response to collagen and ristocetin • Decreased expression of GPIbα • Variants in *GATA1*
GFI1B-related defect		• Reduction in α- and δ-granules • Variants in *GFI1B*
Defects of Cytoskeletal Proteins		
ADAP defect		• Microthrombocytopenia • Increased expression of P-selectin and PAC-1 • Reduced activation by ADP • Variants in *FYB*
Filamin A defects		• Macrothrombocytopenia • Impaired aggregation and secretion by collagen • Heterogeneous distribution of α-granules • Abnormal distribution of FLNa in platelets • Variants in *FLNA*
Wiskott-Aldrich syndrome/XLT	Eczema, immune dysfunction, enhanced susceptibility to infections, autoimmune diseases, malignancy (only in WAS)	• Microthrombocytopenia • δ-SPD • Reduction of GPIb, GPIa, GPIIb-IIIa • Impaired activation of GPIIb-IIIa • Impaired aggregation and expression of P-selectin • Variants in *WAS*
Defects of Membrane Phospholipids		
Scott syndrome	-	• Impaired platelet procoagulant activity • Variants in *TMEM16F*
Stormorken syndrome	Miosis, muscle weakness, dyslexia, ichthyosis, asplenia	• Increased platelet procoagulant activity • Variants in *STIM1* or *ORAI1*
Enhanced Platelet Fibrinolytic Activity		
Quebec platelet disorder	-	• Low levels of platelet factor V • Absent aggregation by epinephrine • Variants in *PLAU*
Unclassified		
Primary secretion defect	-	• Not well-defined platelet function abnormality always including defective platelet secretion • Normal granule content

It is characterized by mild thrombocytopenia, giant and dysfunctional platelets resulting in a severe bleeding tendency. The demonstration of defective platelet glycoprotein Ibα (GPIbα) as the causative alteration was given in the 1980s and contributed to identify GPIbα as a main effector of platelet adhesion.

BSS is a rare autosomal recessive disorder due to quantitative or qualitative defects of the GPIb/IX/V complex, a key adhesive protein platelet receptor formed by four subunits, GPIbα, GPIbβ, GPIX, and GPV, associated at a 2:4:2:1 ratio. GPIbα mediates the interaction of platelets with subendothelium-bound VWF during the early phases of primary hemostasis. BSS has an estimated incidence of 1/1,000,000 and is associated with a severe bleeding diathesis despite the mild thrombocytopenia (60×10^9/L platelets), while heterozygous carriers are asymptomatic and have a normal platelet count and function, but they show slightly enlarged platelets and mildly decreased platelet surface GPIb/IX/V expression. Indeed, here too 50% expression of the GPIb/IX/V complex is sufficient to guarantee normal adhesion.

Variants can be found in the GP1BA, GP1BB, and GP9 genes, coding for GPIbα, GPIbβ, and GPIX, while no defects in the GP5 gene, coding for the GPV subunit, have been reported. In the majority of patients, the receptor complex is absent or severely reduced; however, rare cases with normal receptor expression but a functional defect have been reported.

Defective platelet function is due to the impaired interaction of platelets with VWF, while macrothrombocytopenia derives from defective megakaryocyte membrane skeleton organization. In fact, GPIbα anchors the plasma membrane to the underlying skeleton, mainly composed of spectrin and filamin A, by a direct interaction

Table 53.2. Inherited Platelet Function Disorders: a Revised Classification

Abnormalities of Adhesive Protein Receptors
Glanzmann thrombasthenia ($\alpha_{IIb}\beta_3$)
Bernard-Soulier syndrome (GPIb/IX/V)
Platelet-type VWD (GPIb/IX/V)
22q11.2 Deletion syndrome (GPIb/IX/V)
Defects of collagen receptors ($\alpha_2\beta_1$, GPVI)
Defect of GPIV
Abnormalities of G Protein-Coupled Receptors
Defect of the α_2-adrenoreceptor
Defect of the TP receptor (TxA$_2$ receptor)
Defect of the P2 purinergic receptors
Defect of the PAR-1 receptor
Defects of Platelet Granules (Isolated/Syndromic)
δ-Granules
Isolated δ-storage pool deficiency
Hermansky-Pudlak syndrome
Chediak-Higashi syndrome
SLFN14-related thrombocytopenia
Autism with platelet dense granule defect
α-Granules
Gray platelet syndrome (GPS)
Arthrogryposis, renal dysfunction and cholestasis (ARC) syndrome
Paris-Trousseau syndrome
α/δ-Storage pool deficiency
Signal Transduction Proteins Defects
G proteins defects
Cytosolic phospholipase A$_2$α (cPLA$_2$α) defect
Cyclooxygenase-1 (COX-1) deficiency
Thromboxane synthase deficiency
Phospholipase C deficiency
Leukocyte adhesion deficiency-III (LAD-III)
CalDAG-GEFI defect
SRC defect
PKA defect
Defects of Transcription Factors
Familial platelet disorder with associated myeloid malignancy (FPD/MM)
FLI1-related δ-granule defect
GATA1 defect
GFI1B-related defect
Defects of Cytoskeletal Proteins
ADAP defect
Filamin A defects
Wiskott-Aldrich syndrome/XLT
Defects of Membrane Phospholipids
Scott syndrome
Stormorken syndrome
Enhanced Platelet Fibrinolytic Activity
Quebec platelet disorder
Unclassified
Primary secretion defect

of its cytoplasmic domain with filamin A. In patients with absent GPIbα this interaction is impaired leading to defective proplatelet formation.

Bleeding is usually severe, but its seriousness may differ between individuals. Hemorrhagic manifestations begin shortly after birth or in early childhood and include purpura, epistaxis, gingival bleeding, menorrhagia, and more rarely gastrointestinal bleeding, hematomas, or hematuria. Serious bleeding may result from surgery, trauma, or childbirth.[22,23]

Distinctive laboratory abnormalities are mild thrombocytopenia with giant platelets associated with absent aggregation to ristocetin but normal to all other agonists. Diagnosis is confirmed by reduced or absent platelet surface CD42a (GPIX) and CD42b (GPIbα) at flow cytometry. Genetic testing is not usually required, but it may be adopted for prenatal diagnosis. BSS is sometimes confused with immune thrombocytopenic purpura, but the simple measurement of platelet diameter on a blood film may be discriminating.[27]

Monoallelic BSS caused by variants in GP1BA and GP1BB is characterized by a mild, usually asymptomatic, macrothrombocytopenia.[28,29]

Platelet-Type von Willebrand Disease

Platelet-type von Willebrand disease (PT-VWD), or pseudo–von Willebrand disease, is a very rare autosomal dominant bleeding disorder due to gain-of-function variants in *GP1BA* conferring to platelet GPIbα-enhanced affinity for VWF and associated with mild thrombocytopenia with enhanced platelet volume and a variable hemorrhagic diathesis. The cause of bleeding and mild macrothrombocytopenia are poorly understood, and they are supposed to derive from the clearance from the circulation of high-molecular-weight VWF multimer-platelet complexes.

PT-VWD is probably an underdiagnosed bleeding disorder, with only 55 patients reported so far despite autosomal dominant inheritance, possibly due to its similarity to type 2B-VWD, a bleeding disorder in which gain-of-function variants of VWF cause increased affinity for GPIbα. A study in 110 patients initially diagnosed as type 2B-VWD showed that around 15% were actually PT-VWD.[30]

Seven variants of GPIbα causing PT-VWD have been described so far: five in the C-terminal disulfide loop of the VWF-binding domain (Gly233Val, Met239Val, Gly233Ser, Asp235Tyr, Trp246Leu), one in the macroglycopeptide (421-429del),[30] and one (p.Arg127Gln) in the leucine-rich repeat 5 (LRR-5). This last recently described mutation shows that gain-of-function variants occurring outside the GPIbα C-terminal disulfide loop may be pathogenic and may cause allosteric conformational changes in the C-terminal disulfide loop of GPIbα inducing a conformation with high affinity for VWF.[31]

In PT-VWD mucocutaneous bleeding is usually mild, with nosebleeds and hemorrhage after dental extractions or surgery; however, it may become serious during pregnancy or inflammatory conditions, probably due to the enhanced levels of VWF and the accelerated platelet clearance.[31-33]

Typical findings are a mild thrombocytopenia with increased platelet volume, platelet aggregates in the blood smear, prolonged bleeding time, normal or mildly reduced VWF:Ag, but low VWF activity with enhanced antigen/activity ratio, and reduced high-molecular-weight VWF multimers. Ristocetin-induced platelet agglutination is enhanced. A recent study unraveling the mechanism of platelet dysfunction in PT-VWD shows that platelets from a patient with PT-VWD carrying the Met239Val variant show the constitutive binding of VWF to GPIba which triggers phosphorylation of the platelet SFK Lyn that induces a negative-feedback loop downregulating platelet activation through phosphorylation of PECAM1.[33]

Recent consensus guidelines for the standardized diagnostic and management approach to PT-VWD[34] show that tests essential in the diagnostic workup are platelet count and size, ristocetin-induced platelet aggregation with mixing tests or cryoprecipitate challenge,[35] or genetic analysis.[8]

A flow cytometry mixing test has been shown to be feasible and more sensitive than platelet aggregation for differential diagnosis.[35]

22q11.2 Deletion Syndrome

The 22q11.2 deletion syndrome (22q11DS), also known as DiGeorge or velocardiofacial (VCF) syndrome, is an autosomal dominant genetic disease with an estimated prevalence of 1/2000 to 6000 live births and characterized by a broad phenotypic variability. The chromosomal aberration, which originates de novo in 90% of cases, causes congenital malformations associated in some cases with mild macrothrombocytopenia.

The chromosomal deletion involves the GP1BB gene, located at 22q11.2, and causes macrothrombocytopenia in 20% of patients with VCF syndrome, reduced expression of GPIb/IX/V, and impaired or absent platelet agglutination by ristocetin similar to BSS.

The clinical phenotype includes heart malformations; palatal abnormalities; mild facial dysmorphisms; vertebral, gastrointestinal, renal, and dental anomalies; immune deficiency; deafness; learning disabilities; and developmental delay of variable severity.

Diagnosis is suspected by the above-mentioned syndromic manifestations, and the identification of the 22q11.2 deletion, by fluorescence in situ hybridization or microarray, is conclusive.[36]

Defects of Collagen Receptors

Defects of GPVI and $\alpha_2\beta_1$ (GPIa/IIa) have been reported in only few patients with mucocutaneous bleeding, normal platelet count and morphology or mild macrothrombocytopenia, and typically absent aggregation in response to collagen, collagen-related peptide (CRP), and convulxin, associated with reduced platelet surface expression of the main collagen receptors, GPVI or $\alpha_2\beta_1$.

GPVI Defect

Defect of platelet GPVI is an autosomal recessive disorder caused by GP6 gene variants. Six patients have been described with a lifelong moderate to severe bleeding diathesis; normal platelet number and morphology; absent aggregation in response to collagen, convulxin, and CRP[37-39]; absent δ-granule secretion in response to collagen;[37] and reduced thrombus formation on a collagen surface under flow.[37-40] Flow cytometry and immunoblotting showed reduced levels of platelet GPVI.

$\alpha_2\beta_1$ Defect

The defect of $\alpha_2\beta_1$ is transmitted in an autosomal dominant manner. Two cases with a lifelong mild easy bruising history have been reported associated with reduced expression of $\alpha_2\beta_1$, impaired platelet adhesion to collagen under flow or static conditions, and defective platelet aggregation in response to fibrillar collagen.[41,42]

No gene variants have been identified so far after sequencing of the genes encoding for the two subunits of the receptor.

GPIV Defect

GPIV (CD36) defect is caused by homozygous or compound heterozygous variants of the CD36 gene and can be classified as type I, in which the receptor is absent in platelets and monocytes/macrophages, and type II, with GPIV defect only in platelets. GPIV defect is rather frequent in Japanese, Thai, and African populations (2%-3%) but rarer in Europeans and Americans (0.3%).[43]

This defect is not associated with hemorrhagic manifestations or platelet dysfunction, but in type I subjects isoantibodies against GPIV may develop during pregnancy or transfusion leading to neonatal alloimmune thrombocytopenia, refractoriness to HLA-matched platelet transfusions, or posttransfusion purpura.

Reduced expression of platelet CD36 at flow cytometry and sometimes reduced adhesion to collagen are found.[43]

Ephrin Type B Receptor 2 (EPHB2) Defect

The gene *EPHB2* encodes for a transmembrane tyrosine kinase receptor, which plays a role in platelet signaling causing aggregation and adhesion. Platelet-type bleeding disorder-22 (BDPLT22) is caused by homozygous mutations in the EPHB2 gene and is associated with impaired platelet aggregation. In two siblings with BDPLT22 born from consanguineous parents, Berrou et al[44] identified a homozygous missense mutation in the EPHB2 gene, which is located within the highly conserved intracellular tyrosine kinase motif, essential for the adenosine triphosphate–dependent kinase active site of EPHB2. Patients presented with spontaneous subcutaneous bleeding and excessive bleeding after minor injuries. Platelet counts were normal, but electron microscopy revealed abnormal platelet morphology, including an altered shape, large dimensions, and circulating large megakaryocyte fragments.[44] Platelets showed strongly impaired $\alpha_{IIb}\beta_3$ activation and aggregation in response to ADP and thrombin, decreased thrombus formation on collagen under flow, and defective granule secretion (dense and α-granules) and activation of integrin $\alpha_{IIb}\beta_3$. Response to ristocetin was normal, and platelets had normal levels of alpha and dense granules.[44]

Abnormalities of G Protein–Coupled Receptors

Soluble platelet agonists, such as ADP, TxA$_2$, and thrombin, act via G protein–coupled receptors (GPCRs), often synergistically, generating a positive-feedback loop that amplifies the initial signal to ensure rapid activation and recruitment of platelets to the growing platelet plug. Hereditary platelet function disorders associated with defects of several GPCRs have been described.

α_2-Adrenergic Receptor

Selective defect of epinephrine-induced aggregation associated with easy bruising and epistaxis and reduced expression of platelet α_2-adrenoceptors has been reported as a heritable trait.[45,46]

Impaired aggregation and secretion in response to epinephrine with normal response to other agonists, a mildly prolonged bleeding time, and decreased number of platelet α_2-adrenergic receptors are typical laboratory features of this disorder.[46]

However, it should be noted that aggregation to epinephrine is highly variable in normal individuals and that impaired or absent aggregation is a common finding,[3] possibly due to variations in α_2 adrenoreceptor number.[47] Thus, the causative role of deficient response to epinephrine for bleeding remains uncertain. A recent study assessing the spectrum of platelet function abnormalities in a cohort of individuals referred for bleeding manifestations concluded that defective aggregation to low doses of epinephrine (6 µM) is a common trait in subjects with inherited platelet disorders.[48]

Thromboxane A$_2$ Receptor

Defective TxA$_2$ (TP) receptor function is associated with impaired platelet aggregation to arachidonic acid (AA) and to stable TxA$_2$ analogs and with a mild bleeding tendency. An Arg60 to Leu variant in the first cytoplasmic loop of TP (R60L), leading to reduced coupling with its effector G proteins (G$_q$ and G$_{12/13}$) and with phospholipase C, was found in five unrelated Japanese patients.[49] The variant was inherited in an autosomal dominant way and was phenotypically expressed also in the heterozygous family members, suggesting a dominant negative effect.

Others heterozygous variants have been identified, some associated with reduced ligand binding (D304N, W29C, and V241G) but normal surface expression, others associated with defective surface expression of the receptor (c.167dupG and N42S).[50-54] Very recently a novel TBXA2R*c.908T>C mutation leading to a leucine to proline substitution at position 303 (p.L303P) was identified and shown as potentially pathogenic by prediction tools.[55]

The bleeding diathesis associated with these variants was of variable severity, with bleeding symptoms like menorrhagia and mucocutaneous bleeding in many affected subjects but no bleeding in patients heterozygous for the R60L and the D304N TxA2R substitution.

Normal platelet count and morphology, absent or severely impaired response to AA and TxA$_2$ analogues, reduced aggregation to collagen, and absent secondary wave to ADP and epinephrine, associated with defective granule secretion, are typical laboratory findings.

Defects in platelet cyclooxygenase (COX) or Tx-synthase may have laboratory results similar to the TxA$_2$ receptor defect but can be distinguished by the conserved aggregation response to TxA$_2$ analogues.

Platelet P2 Purinergic Receptors

Platelets express two GPCRs for ADP, the Gq-coupled receptor P2Y$_1$ and the Gi-coupled receptor P2Y$_{12}$. P2Y$_1$ triggers ADP-induced intracellular calcium mobilization and shape change and a weak, transient aggregation response, while the P2Y$_{12}$ receptor triggers adenylylcyclase inhibition and plays a major potentiating action of platelet activation induced by a wide range of agonists promoting the formation of stable platelet aggregates. Platelets also express a ligand-gated purinergic ion-channel receptor, P2X$_1$, activated by ATP, which amplifies the aggregation responses to low levels of collagen and thrombin. Case reports or case series of patients with a bleeding diathesis associated with defects of each of the platelet P2 receptors have been reported.

P2Y$_{12}$ Defect

P2Y$_{12}$ receptor (P2Y$_{12}$R) defect is an autosomal recessive disorder, with homozygous or compound heterozygous variants reported.

Most patients display a severe decrease of P2Y$_{12}$R usually due to frameshift variants of the P2RY12 gene resulting in the premature truncation of the protein with consequent impaired surface expression. Heterozygous individuals display an only mild abnormality of platelet function.

Other molecular defects are associated with normal surface expression of the P2Y$_{12}$ receptor, which is, however, dysfunctional, with defective ligand binding, compromised P2Y$_{12}$R recycling, and impaired P2Y$_{12}$R signaling.[56]

Common clinical findings are a lifelong mucocutaneous bleeding history, easy bruising, and excessive postoperative and posttraumatic bleeding. The severity of the bleeding diathesis is variable, with ISTH bleeding scores ranging from 8 to 13, while the bleeding score of heterozygous P2Y$_{12}$ defects is normal.[57]

Typical laboratory findings are a normal platelet count and morphology, mildly to severely prolonged bleeding time, absent or severely impaired platelet aggregation by high doses of ADP (>10 μM), and variably impaired aggregation to other agonists. Platelets have a normal granular content but impaired release. Heterozygous individuals may show reduced secondary wave aggregation to ADP. Absent adenylylcyclase inhibition by ADP, assessed by the measurement of cAMP or VASP phosphorylation after incubation with prostaglandin E1, confirms diagnosis.

Other P2 Receptors Defects

The case of a patient with a history of bleeding following surgery and impaired ADP-induced platelet aggregation was reported under abstract form in 1999.[58] The defect was associated with reduced platelet P2Y$_1$ mRNA (75% of normal), suggestive of deficient P2Y$_1$ gene transcription. ADP failed to elicit intraplatelet Ca^{2+} increase, but no further details have been published.

The same group described a patient with an in-frame deletion of three nucleotides in the P2X$_1$ gene, resulting in the expression of a nonfunctional P2X$_1$ channel.

The patient showed a severe bleeding diathesis associated with normal platelet count, size, and morphology and a selective impairment of ADP-induced platelet aggregation with normal response to TRAP, AA, and ristocetin.[59]

Protease-Activated Receptor 1

The thrombin receptors of human platelets, protease-activated receptor (PAR)-1 and -4, belong to the seven transmembrane domain receptors family.

So far, no defects of PAR receptors have been reported, suggesting that their absence is incompatible with life. Recently a loss-of-function polymorphism of the gene for PAR-1 in combination with a variant of P2Y$_{12}$ has been found in a patient suffering from chronic bleeding. This polymorphism was associated with decreased platelet surface expression of PAR-1, impaired aggregation and secretion in response to PAR-1-activating peptide, and decreased platelet procoagulant activity, suggesting that reduced PAR-1 contributed to the bleeding phenotype.[60]

Moreover, some patients with the gray platelet syndrome (GPS) show defective response to thrombin and to PAR1 and PAR4 activation peptides associated with reduced PAR-1 platelet expression. However, no variant of the PAR1 gene was identified in these patients.[61]

Abnormalities of Platelet Granules

Under the name of platelet storage pool disease (SPD) a heterogeneous group of disorders characterized by a decrease of platelet α- and/or δ-granules are grouped. Three subtypes of SPD can be identified: α-granules deficiency (α-SPD), δ-granules deficiency (δ-SPD), and combined α- and δ-granules deficiency (αδ-SPD).

Results of a recent global survey demonstrated that δ-granule disorders represent 9.3% of newly diagnosed inherited platelet defects.[9] This percentage may be underestimated because most patients with suspected IPFD do not undergo platelet granule content and release studies during diagnostic workup and because the molecular basis of isolated inherited SPD remains currently unknown.

δ-Storage Pool Disease

The term δ-storage pool disease (δ-SPD) defines a congenital structural abnormality of platelets characterized by a deficiency of δ-granules in megakaryocytes and platelets. δ-Granules are storage organelles for serotonin, calcium (which confers them electron density at electron microscopy), ADP and ATP (storage pool), and pyrophosphate and polyphosphate. ATP and ADP are also contained in a metabolic pool inside platelets, but with a markedly different ATP/ADP ratio as compared with granules (ADP prevails in the storage pool while ATP in the metabolic pool).

Autosomal recessive or autosomal dominant inheritance have been reported for δ-SPD, but neither the causative gene variant nor the defective platelet protein have been identified yet. The recent discovery of RUNX1 or FLI1 variants in some patients with platelet δ-granule defects as well as reduced δ-granule content of platelets from patients with SFLN14-RT (see below) suggest that δ-SPD may have a heterogeneous genetic basis.[62]

Patients with δ-SPD show a mild to moderate bleeding diathesis, with easy bruising, epistaxis, menorrhagia or, in the most severe forms, postsurgical bleeding complications and excessive postpartum hemorrhage.

Defects of δ-granules are characterized by normal primary aggregation to ADP and epinephrine but diminished or absent second-wave aggregation. Also aggregation in response to collagen is reduced. Agglutination by ristocetin and aggregation by AA are normal. A decrease of platelet ADP content with an increased ATP/ADP ratio, an impaired release of ATP upon activation, and reduced or absent δ-granules at whole-mount platelet TEM are diagnostic. A subtype of δ-SPD characterized by reduced platelet ADP but normal serotonin content associated with a deficiency of MRP4 (ABCC4), an ADP transporter, has been described.[63] Platelet count is normal, although a recent report documented mild thrombocytopenia in 20% to 40% of patients, and the bleeding time prolonged.

Deficiency of δ-granules in platelets associated with abnormalities of lysosome-related organelles in other cells give rise to syndromic phenotypes, such as the Hermansky-Pudlak or the Chediak-Higashi syndromes.

Hermansky-Pudlak Syndrome

Hermansky-Pudlak syndrome (HPS), so called after the two Czech pathologists who first described it, is an inherited multisystem disorder caused by a defect of lysosome-related subcellular organelles in various tissues, like δ-granules in platelets or melanosomes in melanocytes.

HPS is characterized by oculocutaneous albinism with nystagmus and visual acuity loss, bleeding diathesis and, in some cases, pulmonary fibrosis, granulomatous colitis, and immunodeficiency.

The prevalence of HPS is not well established, and less than 1000 cases have been described worldwide, but it seems to be particularly high in north Puerto Rico where up to 1 in 1800 people are affected.[64] Variants in 10 human genes, HPS1, AP3B1/HPS2, HPS3, HPS4, HPS5, HPS6, HPS-7/dysbindin, BLOC1S3, BLOC1S5, and PLDN, have been associated with HPS. Most proteins encoded by the HPS gene interact with one another in complexes called BLOCS (biogenesis of lysosome related organelle complexes) whose precise function is not well known but seems to be related to lysosome and late endosome biogenesis and transport, except AP3B1, which encodes for a subunit (β3A) of an ubiquitous cytosolic adaptor protein 3 complex (AP-3) that participates in vesicular transport.[65] Moreover, homozygous variants of the AP3D1 gene leading to destabilization of the AP3δ subunit of the AP3 complex cause a newly described severe neurologic disorder with immunodeficiency and albinism, which has been proposed to be classified as a novel type of Hermansky-Pudlak syndrome

(HPS-10).[66] Platelets from these patients were normal in number and size but showed a complete absence of δ-granules.[66,67]

HPS is an autosomal recessive disorder, and heterozygous carriers have no clinical manifestations. Bleeding diathesis is characterized by easy bruising, recurrent epistaxis, gingival bleeding, postpartum hemorrhage, colorectal bleeding, and prolonged bleeding after tooth extraction, circumcision, and surgery.

HPS diagnosis is established clinically by skin, eye, and sometimes hair hypopigmentation; strabismus; and/or nystagmus associated with absent or markedly reduced platelet δ-granule content at TEM. Prolonged bleeding time, absent secondary wave aggregation to ADP and epinephrine, and reduced aggregation to collagen are typical platelet function abnormalities. Molecular genetic testing confirms diagnosis and is important for prognostic evaluation.[68]

Chediak-Higashi Syndrome

Chediak-Higashi syndrome (CHS) is a rare autosomal recessive disorder affecting multiple organs and associated with a platelet δ-granule deficiency and oculocutaneous albinism. Affected subjects are also characterized by severe immunologic deficiency, with defective natural killer cell function, recurrent infections, and progressive neurological dysfunction with weakness, clumsiness, ataxia, sensory deficits, and walking impairment.

Approximately 85% of affected individuals develop hemophagocytic lymphohistiocytosis, in a phase defined "accelerated" characterized by multiorgan dysfunction, usually lethal unless allogeneic bone marrow transplantation is performed. However, about 10% to 15% of patients follow a less severe clinical course.

This disorder is rare, with less than 500 cases reported so far.

A hallmark of CHS is the presence of giant irregular lysosome-like organelles in the cytoplasm of various cells, such as leukocytes, fibroblasts, platelets, neutrophils, and melanocytes. CHS is due to variants in the lysosomal traffic regulator (LYST) gene, which encodes for a cytoplasmic protein with a not completely understood function supposed to be involved in the regulation of the fission of lysosomal fusion intermediates, giving rise to enlarged organelles. More than 60 different variants have been identified, all leading to a truncated LYST protein.[69,70] Frameshift and nonsense variants, particularly in exon 8, are the most common and are associated with severe forms while missense variants are usually associated with a milder phenotype.[71]

Bleeding diathesis and platelet function abnormalities are superimposable to those of δ-SPD.

Platelet δ-granules at TEM are reduced in number or are irregular and often enlarged.[72] Peroxidase-positive granules can be seen at immunocytochemistry in polymorphonuclear leukocytes, megakaryocytes, hepatocytes, renal tubular epithelial cells, and neurons.

Diagnosis is suspected by oculocutaneous albinism, neutropenia with recurrent infections, and platelet dysfunction and is confirmed by the identification of variants in the CHS gene.

Autism With Platelet Dense Granule Defect

Autism is a developmental disorder of the central nervous system characterized by impairment of social interaction and communication and associated with restricted repetitive and stereotyped behavior. It is generally assumed that in most cases autism has a polygenic cause, but the pathogenesis is still unknown. Neurobeachin (NBEA) has recently been identified as a candidate gene for autism in a patient with a de novo chromosomal translocation and in three patients with a monoallelic deletion. The exact function of NBEA, a multidomain scaffolding protein, is currently unknown but has been suggested to be involved in neuronal post-Golgi membrane traffic.[73]

Platelet function studies in nonsyndromic autistic spectrum disorder subjects with an NBEA heterozygous null allele showed increased platelet count, defective second-wave aggregation to epinephrine, decreased platelet ATP secretion,[74] and a reduced number of dense granules at TEM.[75] In one patient a lifelong bleeding tendency (ISTH BAT score 11) was described.[75]

SLFN14-Related Thrombocytopenia

Monoallelic variants in the schlafen 14 (SLFN14) gene has been identified by whole-exome sequencing as a novel cause of IT with platelet dysfunction. The function of the SLFN family proteins is poorly known, and they are supposed to play a role in cell-cycle regulation and cell proliferation and differentiation. SLFN14 and its mRNA have been detected in human and murine platelets and megakaryocytes,[76,77] but their role in platelet biogenesis or function is unknown.

Four different missense SLFN14 variants, resulting in substitutions within the ATPase-AAA-4 domain of the SLFN14 protein, have been identified in 10 patients belonging to 5 different families.[78]

Patients with SLFN14 variants have moderate thrombocytopenia with disproportionate mucocutaneous bleeding, experiencing severe bruising, prolonged bleeding from wounds and after dental surgery, and menorrhagia. Megakaryocyte differentiation is normal, but proplatelet formation is impaired, with short and barely branched protrusions.

Platelets display a reduced number of δ-granules and decreased ATP secretion in response to ADP, collagen, and TRAP-6.[76,79]

Gray Platelet Syndrome

GPS is a rare disease of platelets and megakaryocytes (MKs), first described by Raccuglia in 1971, also known as α-storage pool disease (α-SPD). It is characterized by mild to moderate thrombocytopenia, slightly enlarged platelets that show a unique ghost-like, gray appearance in May-Grünwald Giemsa-stained blood smears. Both autosomal recessive and autosomal dominant inheritance have been reported, implicating more than one gene in the etiology of the disease.

Approximately 60 cases from various countries have been reported, with a similar incidence in males and females.

The autosomal recessive form of GPS is associated with biallelic variants in NBEAL2 (neurobeachin-like 2 gene),[80,81] a gene encoding for a protein containing a BEACH domain with an unknown function supposed to be involved in vesicular trafficking.[82] Missense, nonsense, and frameshift variants as well as splice site alteration variants have been described, all causing essentially the same phenotype.

Platelet α-granule proteins are reduced, including PF4, βTG, VWF, fibrinogen, albumin, and IgG, while the expression of the α-granule membrane marker P-selectin varies, being reduced in some patients with GPS and normal in others, suggesting that α-granule membranes are normally formed in patients with GPS.[83]

Proteins leaking from MKs lead to bone marrow fibrosis.

The bleeding syndrome is mild to moderate, but trauma- and surgery-related severe hemorrhages have been reported. Patients with GPS exhibit a highly heterogeneous platelet dysfunction, with some showing minimally impaired aggregation and others clearly defective activation by thrombin and/or collagen. Surface GPs are normal but occasional patients with reduced GPVI expression have been reported.[84,85] Decreased expression of the platelet thrombin receptors, PAR-1 and PAR-4, may contribute to the impaired platelet response to thrombin.[85]

Increased vitamin B12 in plasma is a typical, although unexplained, finding in GPS.[86] Key diagnostic laboratory features are slightly enlarged platelets with the characteristic gray appearance, moderate thrombocytopenia, and reduced platelet α-granule proteins.

Recent studies extend the abnormalities associated with NBEAL2 mutations to immune cells: low leukocyte count, decreased neutrophil granulation, and impaired neutrophil extracellular trap formation represent prominent findings in patients with GPS, reflecting deranged innate immunity.[87] In addition, there is evidence of a deregulated adaptive immune response with frequent autoimmune involvement of different organs (Hashimoto thyroiditis, rheumatoid arthritis, and skin diseases, such as alopecia, discoid lupus erythematosus, and vitiligo) and a spectrum of autoantibodies (rheumatoid factor, perinuclear antineutrophil cytoplasmic, antithyroperoxidase, and antinuclear antibodies).[88]

Arthrogryposis, Renal Dysfunction, and Cholestasis Syndrome

The arthrogryposis, renal dysfunction and cholestasis (ARC) syndrome is a rare, autosomal recessive multisystem disorder characterized by neonatal cholestatic jaundice, renal tubular leak, hypotonia-related arthrogryposis, failure to thrive, and death within the first year of life, initially described by LutzRichner and Landolt in 1973. Additional features may be cerebral malformations, deafness, congenital heart disease, diabetes, and a bleeding tendency occurring in around half of patients.

ACR has been recently shown to derive from variants in the *VPS33B* (15q26.1) or *VIPAS39* (14q24.3) genes that encode for two ubiquitary protein-sorting proteins (VPS33B and VIPAR) involved in vesicle trafficking and fusion, required for platelet α-granule biogenesis.[89] VPS33B variants are detected in approximately 75% of the patients with a clinical diagnosis of ARC syndrome.

Platelets are large and show reduced α-granules. The defect involves proteins of granules and granular membranes, with P-selectin expression severely decreased.

Impaired platelet aggregation in response to epinephrine, ADP, collagen, and AA have been observed in ~25% of cases.[90]

Diagnosis relies on the identification of the typical severe, syndromic manifestations. Affected individuals usually do not survive their first year due to recurrent infections, severe dehydration, metabolic acidosis, and internal hemorrhages.

Paris-Trousseau-Jacobsen Syndrome

Jacobsen syndrome (JS) is a very rare disorder caused by a partial deletion of chromosome 11q23, initially described by the Danish geneticist Petrea Jacobsen in 1973 who reported a three-generation family in which several affected members had an unbalanced translocation involving chromosomes 11 and 21. Since Jacobsen's initial description, over 200 patients with the Jacobsen syndrome have been reported.[91] The disease is characterized by facial and skull dysmorphisms, with hypertelorism and eyelid ptosis, epicanthal folds, and small and low-set ears, and other abnormalities, including mental retardation and heart malformations.

Deletions of the long arm of chromosome 11q can range from 7 to 16 Mb, with the loss of multiple genes contributing to the overall clinical phenotype. When deletions include the FLI1 gene, coding for a member of the ETS family of transcription factors that transactivate several genes involved in megakaryocyte differentiation and maturation, they cause the Paris-Trousseau syndrome, a moderate to severe thrombocytopenia with giant α-granules in platelets. Approximately 90% of patients with JS have the Paris-Trousseau syndrome.[92-95]

Thrombocytopenia can be severe (10,000-30,000/μL), but it often clears up over the first few years of life, and associates with platelet dysfunction, which is instead usually persistent. The bleeding time is markedly prolonged. Both giant (approximately 85%) and normal platelets with giant α-granules (approximately 15%)[95] are found in peripheral blood. Abnormal granules fail to release their contents upon stimulation with thrombin. Moreover, an increased number of small megakaryocytes, with delayed maturation, are found in bone marrow.[93]

The bleeding phenotype is of variable severity and persists after platelet count normalization, implicating the intrinsic platelet function defect in its genesis.

Recently a homozygous c.970C>T FLI1 variant, mimicking the Paris-Trousseau thrombocytopenia but lacking the other features of the 11q23 deletion syndrome, was reported.[96] Affected individuals showed lifelong moderate to severe mucosal bleeding and moderate macrothrombocytopenia with large granules in 4% of circulating platelets. Light transmission aggregometry revealed absence of collagen-induced platelet aggregation, reduced aggregation to ADP and epinephrine, and normal aggregation to AA and ristocetin. Nonmuscle myosin heavy chain IIB (MYH10), absent from normal platelets, was found in patient platelets.[97]

Diagnosis is based on the syndromic features (mental retardation, facial dysmorphisms, and thrombocytopenia) and is confirmed by cytogenetic analysis.

α,δ-Storage Pool Deficiency

α,δ-SPD is a congenital bleeding disorder characterized by platelet α- and δ-granules deficiency. In 1979, Weiss et al first described α,δ-SPD in seven patients, and this was followed by a few reports of patients with a heterogeneous degree of α- and δ-granules defect.

Inheritance seems to be autosomal dominant, although sporadic recessive cases have been reported.

A more detailed study in four patients belonging to three generations of the same family showed a severe defect of both α- and δ-platelet granules and suggested that in this disorder platelet granules fuse with the open canalicular system and shed their contents to the outside in the absence of cell activation.[98]

Bleeding symptoms and platelet aggregation abnormalities are similar to those of δ-SPD. Measurement of platelet δ- and α-granule markers and/or TEM demonstration of α- and δ-granule platelet defect are required for diagnosis. Lysosomal content of platelets is normal.[98]

Defects of Signal Transduction Proteins

G-Protein Defects

Guanine nucleotide–binding proteins, also known as G proteins, belong to two distinct families: small G proteins and heterotrimeric G proteins. Small G proteins, part of the Ras superfamily of small GTPases, bind to GTP and GDP transmitting signals across the cell while heterotrimeric G proteins, composed of α, β, and γ subunits, transmit signals from the outside to the inside of cells. They are activated by GPCRs that in turn activate specific signal transduction pathways. They are classified in Gsα, Giα, Gq/$_{11}$α, and G$_{12/13}$α. Variants in the imprinted gene cluster GNAS1, encoding for Gsα, lead to Albright hereditary osteodystrophy, pseudohypoparathyroidism Ia (PHPIa), and pseudopseudohypoparathyroidism (PPHP), while methylation defects of GNAS1 lead to pseudohypoparathyroidism Ib (PHPIb). Patients with PHPIa and PPHP show short stature, round face, subcutaneous calcifications, mental retardation, obesity, and brachydactyly together with platelet Gsα hypofunction associated with a thrombotic phenotype. Indeed, activation of Gsα upregulates cAMP formation, which dampens platelet responsiveness, while platelets from patients with PHPIb show an only mild Gsα hypofunction, with decreased inhibition of platelet aggregation by Gsα stimulation with high concentrations of Gsα agonists. Finally, a congenital Gsα hyperfunction syndrome associated with enhanced trauma-related bleeding and a variable degree of mental retardation was described in some patients with a paternally inherited insertion in the extra-large stimulatory Gsα isoform (XLαs).[99]

A patient with decreased expression of Gqα, due to a variant in the Gqα promoter, showing mild bleeding and abnormal platelet aggregation and secretion in response to different agonists, has been reported.[100] Finally, one patient with strikingly reduced Gαi1 (25% of normal), a chronic bleeding diathesis and defective aggregation in response to ADP and epinephrine has been reported but no variant of the Gαi1 gene was found.[101]

Diagnosis of these rare defects requires complex biochemical studies to clarify the G protein involved. Western blotting may identify Gαq or Gαi1 defects, while the lack of Gsα may be highlighted functionally by Gsα agonists: no inhibition of platelet aggregation by PGI$_2$ or PGE$_1$ and hyperreactive platelets are features of Gsα hypofunction.[99]

Cytosolic Phospholipase A$_{2α}$ Defect

Cytosolic phospholipase A$_{2α}$ (cPLA$_{2α}$) hydrolyzes AA from membrane phospholipids, providing the substrate for the synthesis of eicosanoids, such as prostaglandins and leukotrienes. Four patients, belonging to three different families, with a cPLA$_{2α}$ defect have been described. Interestingly, all suffered gastrointestinal ulcer bleeding and two of them other bleeding manifestations, including menorrhagia. Platelet function in response to ADP and collagen was impaired while response to AA was normal. cPLA$_{2α}$ in platelets, measured by Western blotting, was reduced as well as thromboxane B$_2$ synthesis. One patient had a compound heterozygous variant of the gene coding for cPLA$_{2\alpha}$, PLA2G4A, while for the other patients no genetic analysis was performed.[102]

Differential diagnosis for the COX-1, thromboxane synthase, or TP-receptor defects is established by normal aggregation by AA and severely reduced serum thromboxane B$_2$, but genetic analysis is warranted for confirmation.

Cyclooxygenase-1 Defect

Cyclooxygenase-1 (COX-1) catalyzes the transformation of AA into prostaglandin endoperoxides (PGG$_2$ and PGH$_2$) and is coded by the PTGS1 gene. A familial bleeding disorder with epistaxis and easy bruising associated with platelet COX-1 defect has been reported in few cases, mostly with a dominant inheritance pattern.

Platelets show impaired aggregation to ADP, collagen, epinephrine, and AA and defective secretion, while response to the stable thromboxane A$_2$ analog U46619 and to PGH$_2$ are normal. Expression of COX-1 in platelet lysates may be severely defective (type 1) or normal but with functionally inactive enzyme (type 2).[103]

To date only a few cases with variants of PTGS1, the gene encoding for COX-1, have been reported. One patient with a severe bleeding diathesis carried the PTGS1 common single nucleotide variants (SNVs) c.22C>T (p.Arg8Trp) and c.50C>T (p.Pro17Leu) while another showed reduced TxA$_2$ synthesis associated with the heterozygous variants c.337C>T (p.Arg113Cys) and c.1003G>A (p.Val481Ile).[104]

Recently, the BRIDGE Consortium reported a pedigree with an autosomal recessive variant c.965G>C (p.Trp322Ser), which abrogated COX-1 expression resulting in an aspirin-like platelet dysfunction.[105]

Finally, a patient with a lifelong mild bleeding history associated with platelet dysfunction and a heterozygous PTGS1 variant c.428A>G (p.Asn143Ser) generating a dysfunctional hypoglycosylated COX-1, with an apparent dominant negative effect, was described.[106]

COX-1 deficiency may be suspected when defective aggregation in response to ADP, collagen, epinephrine, and AA with reduced TXA$_2$ production in response to AA but normal aggregation in response to U46619 and/or PGH2 are found. For the diagnosis of this disorder aspirin or nonsteroidal anti-inflammatory drugs intake must be carefully excluded and COX-1 defect should be confirmed by the reduced expression of COX-1 by Western blotting and confirmed by genetic analysis.

Thromboxane Synthase Defect

The TBXAS1 gene encodes for the member of the cytochrome P450 mono-oxygenases thromboxane synthase A1 (TxS), which converts prostaglandin H$_2$ to thromboxane A$_2$. Only two reports have described patients with a TxS defect: one girl with a severe bleeding tendency, defective platelet aggregation in response to ADP and epinephrine, absent aggregation in response to AA, and strikingly reduced serum thromboxane B$_2$, and one family with moderate bleeding, absent aggregation to AA but normal aggregation by TxA$_2$ analogues, reversible aggregation to ADP and epinephrine, and reduced thromboxane B$_2$ in serum. However, no variants in the TBXAS1 gene have been reported so far in patients with bleeding problems.[107,108] Variants in TBXAS1 have instead been found in families with the Ghosal hematodiaphyseal dysplasia syndrome (GHDD), a rare autosomal recessive disorder characterized by increased bone density with predominant diaphyseal involvement. Platelets from subjects with GHDD show defective AA-induced aggregation and P-selectin expression with normal response to U46619 and normal surface expression of platelet GPs. These patients do not show any bleeding symptoms.[109]

TxS defect may be suspected when platelet aggregation in response to ADP, epinephrine, and AA are defective together with a reduction of serum thromboxane B$_2$. TxS defect should be confirmed by Western blotting. Differential diagnosis between the COX-1 and the TxS defects can be made by testing platelet aggregation to PGH$_2$: in COX-1 defect, aggregation is normal, while in the case of TBXAS1 it is defective. U46619 instead triggers aggregation in both the COX-1 and TxS defects because the TP receptor is normally expressed and functional. Moreover, a redirection of AA metabolism toward PGE$_2$ and PGD$_2$, which are increased in stimulated platelets, occurs in platelets from patients with the TxS defect but not in those with a COX-1 defect.[110]

Phospholipase C-β$_2$ Defect

The stimulation of platelet receptors coupled to Gαq and Gα11 (e.g., P2Y$_{12}$ and TP) activates phospholipase C-β$_2$ (PLC-β$_2$), which catalyzes the hydrolysis of phosphatidylinositol 4,5-bisphosphate (PIP$_2$) with diacyl glycerol (DAG) and inositol 1,4,5-trisphosphate (IP$_3$) release. IP$_3$ binds to an IP$_3$ receptor on the endoplasmic reticulum, which serves as a Ca^{2+} channel, causing the release of Ca^{2+} from intracellular stores with consequent increase in the cytosol with activation of platelets. A unique platelet function defect characterized by platelet PLC-β$_2$ deficiency has been reported. The proposita and her son had impaired platelet aggregation, serotonin secretion, mobilization of cytoplasmic Ca^{2+}, and PLC-β$_2$ activation, assayed using ^{3}H-PIP$_2$ as substrate, in response to several agonists, including ADP, thrombin, platelet-activating factor (PAF), and U46619. Platelet PLC-β$_2$ was strikingly decreased compared with controls, and mRNA expression was strongly reduced.[111] However, the responsible gene variant was not identified.

Leukocyte Adhesion Deficiency-III

Leukocyte adhesion deficiency-III (LAD-III) is an autosomal recessive disorder characterized by a dysfunction of β$_1$, β$_2$, and β$_3$ integrin signaling in leukocytes and platelets but normal integrin expression. Patients with LAD-III have a predisposition to recurrent infections and a moderate to severe hemorrhagic diathesis with a platelet functional phenotype similar to that of Glanzmann thrombasthenia because α$_{IIb}$β$_3$ integrin activation is severely compromised. The disorder is caused by variants in the FERMT3 gene encoding for the hematopoietic line-specific integrin-activating cytoplasmic protein Kindlin-3. Kindlin-3 and Talin-1 are strictly involved in α$_{IIb}$β$_3$ activation, and also in the activation of other integrins, such as α$_2$β$_1$, the platelet receptor for collagen, and indeed adhesion to collagen under flow conditions is also impaired.[112] Less than 40 cases of LAD-III have been reported so far.[113]

CalDAG-GEFI Defect

Similarly to kindlin-3 CalDAG-GEFI (calcium- and DAG-regulated guanine exchange factor-1), a guanine nucleotide exchange factor for the small GTPase Rap1, plays a crucial role in α$_{IIb}$β$_3$ inside-out activation. Twenty-three subjects with mucocutaneous bleeding mainly consisting of severe epistaxis, ecchymosis, bleeding after tooth extraction, and in the female patient also severe menorrhagia, and chronic anemia have been described with a variant of RASGRP2, the gene coding for CalDAG-GEFI.[114-116]

Platelets from these individuals show reduced Rap1 and α$_{IIb}$β$_3$ activation. The platelet phenotype is similar to that of GT, with impaired aggregation to all agonists except ristocetin, defective α$_{IIb}$β$_3$ activation, impaired spreading on fibrinogen, and reduced adhesion to collagen under flow. Normal α$_{IIb}$β$_3$ expression differentiates this disorder from type I and II GT, while differential diagnosis from GT variants requires genetic analysis or the measurement of Rap-1b activation.

Src Defect

Eleven patients with a gain-of-function variant of the gene coding for the tyrosine kinase Src, commonly implicated in various types of tumors, have been described.[117-119] The variant was initially found by whole-genome sequencing analysis of patients enrolled in the BRIDGE-Bleeding and Platelet Disorders (BPD) study[117] and was shown to cause constitutive activation of Src. This variant is associated with thrombocytopenia, myelofibrosis, a severe bleeding diathesis (epistaxis, petechiae, easy bruising, menorrhagia, and severe bleeding after tooth extraction), and bone defects (edentulism and bone dysmorphisms). Platelets are deficient in granules and rich in vacuoles, similar to platelets of patients with the GPS, and megakaryocytes display a severe proplatelet formation defect.[117]

Protein Kinase A Defect

The gene PRKACG encodes for the γ isoform of the catalytic subunit of cAMP-dependent protein kinase A (PKA). PKA is activated by cAMP and phosphorylates proteins involved in platelet activation (e.g., RAP1b, Gα_{13}, IP$_3$, VASP), inhibiting them and thus maintaining circulating platelets in a resting state. Moreover, PKA phosphorylates filamin A inhibiting its proteolysis.

Recently, a missense variant of PRKACG was reported to be responsible for an autosomal recessive disorder characterized by severe thrombocytopenia with giant platelets and defective platelet $\alpha_{IIb}\beta_3$ activation and P-selectin expression in response to TRAP6 and Ca^{2+} mobilization in response to thrombin. Although PKA was normally expressed in platelets, phosphorylation of filamin A was almost absent and intracellular levels of cAMP were higher. Megakaryocyte proplatelet formation was defective, explaining thrombocytopenia.[120]

Transcription Factors Defects

Hematopoietic transcription factors (TFs) are proteins regulating the transcription of genes involved in hematopoiesis. TFs control hematopoietic lineage differentiation, megakaryopoiesis, and platelet production. Variants in hematopoietic TFs cause defects in platelet production and function. Variants of genes encoding for four different TFs have been linked to platelet function disorders, namely, RUNX1, FLI1, GATA1, and GFI1B, and a fifth, the variant of ETV6, to thrombocytopenia.

Familial Platelet Disorder With Associated Myeloid Malignancy

RUNX1 downregulates myeloid progenitors development and promotes lymphopoiesis and megakaryopoiesis. Numerous genes encoding for proteins involved in platelet structure and function are targets of RUNX1, such as the PF4 (platelet factor 4) and thrombopoietin receptor MPL genes.

Familial platelet disorder with associated myeloid malignancy (FPD/MM) is an autosomal dominant disorder caused by heterozygous variants in the Runt-related transcription factor 1 (RUNX1), also called CBFA2 or AML1. Acquired variants of *RUNX1*, mainly chromosomal translocations involving this gene, are common in myeloid malignancies. The inherited forms are instead rare, with about 70 patients described so far,[121] but their frequency may be underestimated because screening for the *RUNX1* variant is rarely performed. Causative variants include missense, nonsense, frameshift, insertion, deletion, and translocations disrupting the gene. Some act via haploinsufficiency while others generate proteins with a dominant-negative action.[122]

Patients with FPD/MM present mild thrombocytopenia and a platelet function defect associated with moderate/severe mucocutaneous bleeding. They have a significantly increased risk of developing myeloid hematologic malignancies, such as acute myelogenous leukemia, myelodysplastic syndromes, and myeloproliferative disorders and in rare cases acute lymphoblastic T-cell leukemia. The lifetime risk of developing one of these malignancies has been estimated to be as high as 35%, with a mean age of onset of 35 to 40 years.

A recent study has suggested that variants causing haploinsufficiency lead only to thrombocytopenia, whereas predisposition to hematological malignancies would occur when the mutated *RUNX1* allele causes a dominant negative effect. Myeloid malignancy develops when an additional somatic variant in the second *RUNX1* allele, or in other genes, occurs.[123]

Platelet count is moderately reduced with normal size. Platelets show reduced content and release of δ-granules, with variable decrease of α-granules. Platelet aggregation in response to epinephrine, ADP, and AA is defective. The presence in platelets of MYH10, a protein downregulated by RUNX1 and FLI1, is a surrogate marker for FLI1 and RUNX1 defects.[62] Detecting RUNX1 variants is important for the obvious prognostic implications and, although at the moment there are no preventive strategies to reduce leukemic transformation, diagnosis may allow to establish a medical monitoring program and to perform a preliminary screening for compatible bone marrow donors thus excluding carriers of *RUNX1* variants among family members as potential donors.

Friend Leukemia Integration 1 Defect

Friend leukemia integration 1 (FLI1) plays a major role in early and late megakaryopoiesis, regulating the expression of several megakaryocyte-specific proteins, such as GPIbα, GPIX, MPL, and PF4. The FLI1 gene is localized on chromosome 11q23.3–24, and the partial deletion of chromosome 11 in a region that includes *FLI1* results in the Jacobsen or Paris-Trousseau syndrome (described under "Paris-Trousseau syndrome"). Germline variants in FLI1 have been found in some families with normal platelet count or mild thrombocytopenia, a δ-granule secretion defect, excessive bleeding, alopecia, eczema, recurrent viral infections, and psoriasis.

Diagnosis of FLI1 defect is based on defective platelet δ-granules secretion, impaired aggregation in response to collagen and PAR-1 activating peptide, mild thrombocytopenia, and the presence of MYH10 in platelets.[62]

GATA-1 Defect

GATA-1 is a DNA-binding transcription factor that plays a critical role in the development of hematopoietic cells, including megakaryocytes. FOG (friend of GATA-1) interacts with the NF domain of GATA1 and cooperates with it to promote differentiation.

The GATA-1 defect is an X-linked disorder characterized by macrothrombocytopenia and platelet dysfunction of variable severity, sometimes associated with dyserythropoietic anemia, beta-thalassemia, or congenital erythropoietic porphyria. Patients show a severe hemorrhagic diathesis, with spontaneous bruising and excessive bleeding after minor cuts. Most of the variants of GATA-1 are found in the NF domain and cause decreased affinity of GATA-1 for FOG1. Females may have mild to moderate symptoms depending on the proportion of cells containing the mutated GATA1 allele on the active X chromosome.

Thrombocytopenia of variable severity, large platelets with a reduced number of α-granules, decreased expression of GPIbα, and reduced aggregation in response to collagen and ristocetin are typical of this defect. Conclusive diagnosis can be obtained only by the unraveling of a variant in *GATA1*.[124]

GFI1B-Related Defect

Heterozygous variants of the transcription factor gene *GFI1B*, which encodes for a nuclear zinc finger protein that binds DNA and functions as a transcriptional repressor (GFI1B growth factor independent 1B transcriptional repressor) implicated in megakaryopoiesis, have been reported to be associated with an autosomal dominant macrothrombocytopenia with deficiency of α-granules.[125,126] A nonsense variant introduces a premature stop codon that leads to the formation of a truncated protein lacking the DNA-binding domain with consequent inability to repress transcription. The truncated GFI1B exerts a dominant-negative action on the normal protein and causes abnormal megakaryocyte maturation and platelet biogenesis. Bleeding severity is variable with some affected individuals experiencing spontaneous bleeding while others only bleed after invasive procedures. Two recently reported cases suggest an association of α,δ-SPD with GFIB1 variants. Both patients had additional anomalies, like hypospadia, periventricular nodular heterotopia, syndactyly, or patent ductus arteriosus.[127]

Defects of Cytoskeletal Proteins
ADAP Defect

Two recent reports have described eight patients in two families with a new congenital, autosomal recessive microthrombocytopenia associated with a variant in the FYB gene.[128,129] The FYB gene encodes for the adhesion and degranulation-promoting adaptor protein (ADAP), a hematopoietic cell-specific protein expressed by platelets, T cells, natural killer cells, myeloid cells, and dendritic cells involved in platelet activation, cell motility and proliferation, actin polymerization, and integrin-mediated cell adhesion.

ADAP participates in inside-out activation of $\alpha_{IIb}\beta_3$ and in the binding of fibrinogen by the interaction with the integrin-regulatory adapters talin and kindlin-3,[130] and also in collagen-induced platelet activation through integrin $\alpha_2\beta_1$.[131]

A homozygous c.393G>A nonsense variant of the FYB gene has been found in five individuals of Arab Christian ancestry with microthrombocytopenia and bleeding tendency.[129]

The autosomal recessive bleeding phenotype included petechial rash and mild epistaxis. None of the patients had immune defects, infections, or growth abnormalities.

Laboratory investigations showed mild thrombocytopenia with reduced platelet volume, increased expression of P-selectin and PAC-1 on circulating platelets, but impaired activation upon stimulation and mildly reduced adhesion to fibrinogen and VWF.[129]

Filamin A Defects

Filamin A (FLNa) is a major component of the platelet cytoskeleton and plays a critical role in the attachment of GPIb/IX/V and GPIIb/IIIa to actin. Heterozygous variants in the FLNA gene cause a spectrum of rare X-linked developmental abnormalities, the most frequent of which is periventricular nodular heterotopia (FLNA-PVNH), a neuronal migration disorder characterized by nodules of neurons lining the brain ventricles instead of the normal cortex tissue.

Patients have a moderate bleeding phenotype, mild macrothrombocytopenia and impaired platelet aggregation and secretion triggered by GPVI.

Platelet anisocytosis, with both giant and normal platelets, abnormalities of α-granules, and absence of FLNa from a fraction (~20%) of the platelet population at fluorescence microscopy, addresses the diagnosis that needs to be confirmed by molecular genetic analysis.[132]

Wiskott-Aldrich Syndrome and X-Linked Thrombocytopenia

Wiskott-Aldrich syndrome (WAS) is a X-linked recessive disorder caused by hemizygous variants in the WAS gene (Xp11.4-p11.21) coding for the Wiskott-Aldrich syndrome protein (WASp), a protein expressed exclusively in hematopoietic cells, which has a major role in the reorganization of the actin cytoskeleton, signal transduction, and apoptosis. WAS is characterized by severe to moderate thrombocytopenia (5,000-150,000/μL) with very small platelets associated with eczema and immune dysfunction, enhanced susceptibility to infections and to the development of autoimmune disorders and lymphoid malignancy.[133,134]

A milder form of the disease, without immune deficiency and infections, is known as hereditary X-linked thrombocytopenia (XLT) and is characterized by moderate to severe thrombocytopenia with small-sized platelets and no other abnormalities except only occasionally transient eczema.

More than 160 WAS variants have been found, scattered throughout the gene, the most common being missense variants and small insertions followed by nonsense and splice site variants and insertions, which result in either the decreased expression or in the absence of WASp.

Variants completely suppressing WASp expression lead to the more severe, syndromic phenotype while missense variants resulting in reduced WASP most often are associated with the XLT phenotype. There are, however, exceptions to this rule, rendering it difficult to make a prognostic evaluation based only on the WAS gene variant.

Bleeding diathesis is mild/moderate. Bone marrow megakaryocyte number and morphology is normal, but there may be ineffective thrombocytopoiesis with premature proplatelet formation in the bone marrow and reduced platelet survival.

Physical examination, showing petechiae and eczema, the typical X-linked genetic transmission, and severe to moderate thrombocytopenia (ranging from 5000 to 50,000/μL) with clearly reduced platelet size are strong clues to diagnosis. Moreover, several platelet structural and functional abnormalities have been reported including δ-SPD; reduced GPIb, GPIa, and GPIIb/IIIa; impaired GPIIb/IIIa activation; impaired platelet aggregation; and defective expression of P-selectin in response to thrombin stimulation, with a preserved response to ADP.[134] Absent or decreased WAS protein in platelets and the detection of WAS gene variants allow conclusive diagnosis.

Abnormalities of Membrane Phospholipids
Scott Syndrome

In 1979, Weiss et al reported a patient with a history of moderate to severe bleeding and an impaired platelet procoagulant activity as the sole hemostatic abnormality. This extremely rare bleeding disorder has subsequently been referred to as Scott syndrome (after the first described patient, Mrs. M.A. Scott, 1939-1996). The disease is caused by a defect in the translocation of phosphatidylserine (PS) from the inner to the outer layer of the phospholipid platelet membrane, thus compromising blood clotting factor assembly on the platelet surface. This leads to decreased fibrin formation at sites of vascular injury with impaired hemostasis. PS translocation is mediated by Ca^{2+}-dependent phospholipid scramblases that transport phospholipids bidirectionally.

A similar defect in PS translocation has also been demonstrated in red blood cells and Epstein-Barr virus–transformed lymphocytes of patients with Scott syndrome.

To date, only six female patients have been reported.[135-139] This syndrome, transmitted as an autosomal recessive trait, is caused by loss of function variants of the TMEM16F gene encoding for the transmembrane protein 16F that acts as a Ca^{2+}-activated chloride channel and is required for the activation of phospholipid scramblases.[140,141]

Patients with Scott syndrome have a history of postoperative bleeding, trauma-related hematoma, or bleeding after tooth extraction but rarely spontaneous events, except for menorrhagia resulting in iron-deficiency anemia. Postpartum bleeding may be extremely severe.

Blood clotting factors and platelet count and structure are normal, and no abnormalities of platelet secretion, aggregation, granule content, or platelet adhesion have been detected. Scott platelets show an isolated defect of PS exposure upon activation, which can be detected by flow cytometry using high-affinity probes for phosphatidylserine (such as annexin V, lactadherin).[142] A reduced shedding of platelet microparticles (PMPs) after calcium ionophore stimulation has also been reported (~50% lower than in healthy subjects).[143]

Stormorken Syndrome

Stormorken syndrome, first described in 1985 by Stormorken et al in a Norwegian family, is defined as an inverse Scott syndrome because it is characterized by an enhanced externalization of phosphatidylserine, with resting platelets displaying full procoagulant activity. Its prevalence is estimated at <1/1,000,000, and near 20 patients belonging to unrelated families have been described.

Stormorken syndrome is characterized by a mild bleeding tendency, mild to moderate thrombocytopenia, and circulating platelets expressing PS on their surface and is associated with tubular aggregate myopathy (TAM), a rare form of myopathy with progressive loss of strength, cramps and muscle pain induced by exercise, and tubular aggregates in muscle fibers. Other manifestations include mild anemia, asplenia, miosis, headache, ichthyosis, impaired cognitive function, enophthalmos, hypotelorism, short stature, low body weight, and hypocalcemia.

Stormorken syndrome is caused by heterozygous gain-of-function variants of the gene STIM1, coding for the stromal interaction molecule 1 (STIM1),[144,145] the main Ca^{2+} sensor in the endoplasmic reticulum, and shows an autosomal dominant transmission pattern.

Store-operated calcium entry is regulated by the Ca^{2+} release-activated Ca^{2+} (CRAC) channel, composed of the pore-forming subunits ORAI1–3 and the Ca^{2+} sensors, STIM1 and STIM2. STIM1 is a single transmembrane-spanning protein that, in resting cells, exists as a dimer located in the membrane of the endoplasmic reticulum (ER). When the ER Ca^{2+} stores are empty, STIM1 molecules oligomerize, move to the plasma membrane, bind to ORAI1, and activate the CRAC channel allowing the entry of Ca^{2+} into the cell.

A variant in exon 7 of STIM1 (c.910C>T), resulting in a single amino acid substitution (p.R304W) in the C terminus of STIM1 and causing constitutive activation of CRAC channels and Ca^{2+} influx, is the cause of Stormorken syndrome. Recently, a novel c.252T>A (p.D84E) missense variant, affecting a highly conserved EF domain of STIM1, was found in a Portuguese patient with platelet features of Stormorken syndrome but without associated syndromic manifestations.[146] Moreover, gain-of-function heterozygous variants of ORAI1 resulting in hyperactivation of the CRAC channel have been found in patients with a mild form of Stormorken syndrome,[147,148] with TAM and miosis but without asplenia, bleeding diathesis, and thrombocytopenia.

Patients with Stormorken syndrome have mild to moderate thrombocytopenia with resting platelets expressing procoagulant activity and platelet surface PS and releasing spontaneously PMPs.[149] In addition, increased surface expression of CD63 and CD62P on circulating platelets but defective GPIIb/IIIa activation and reduced platelet aggregation and ATP secretion in response to collagen[144,149] with normal response to all other agonists and abnormal clot retraction are part of the picture. These observations suggest that platelets from patients with Stormorken syndrome are in a preactivated state, which may associate with impaired reactivity to stimuli and reduced platelet adhesion explaining the mild bleeding tendency.[144,150]

Enhanced Platelet Fibrinolytic Activity
Quebec Platelet Disorder

QPD is an autosomal dominant bleeding disorder due to a tandem duplication of the gene PLAU encoding for urokinase plasminogen activator, with consequent increased urokinase-type plasminogen activator (uPA) in platelet α-granules causing the degradation of granular proteins.[151] The structure of platelet α-granules is normal,[152] and systemic fibrinolysis as well as uPA levels in plasma and urine are normal.

Patients with QPD have been reported in Canada and the United States, and most of them have a common ancestry in a single family of French origin from the Canadian province of Quebec, where the prevalence of this disorder is 1:300,000.[153]

The increase of uPA in platelet α-granules leads to the local generation of plasmin that degrades α-granular proteins, for example, thrombospondin-1, von Willebrand factor, fibrinogen, and factor V. Degradation spares the α-granule membranes, and thus it does not involve platelet cytosolic proteins or δ-granules. Increased fibrinolytic activity of α-granules is the cause of bleeding, because platelet activation leads to the release of uPA with untimely clot lysis.

This disorder has peculiar clinical features, with moderate to severe bleeding starting late, typically 12 to 24 hours after surgery or trauma, and particularly sensitive to antifibrinolytic agents but not platelet transfusions.

The characteristic laboratory finding is a reduced level of platelet α-granule clotting factor V with normal plasma factor V. Many cases may go undiagnosed because there are no characteristic morphologic features or platelet function abnormalities, with only aggregation in response to epinephrine either absent or missing second wave.[154] Platelet count is normal or mildly reduced. Genetic testing for the duplication of PLAU is mandatory for diagnosis.[153]

Unclassified Abnormalities
Primary Secretion Defect

Any mild bleeding disorder associated with impaired platelet secretion but normal platelet granules content and normal AA metabolism has been defined as primary secretion defect (PSD). Bleeding tendency is usually mild to moderate, but asymptomatic patients have also been reported. The platelet function defect is heterogeneous with reduced secretion and, although not always, aggregation induced by several agonists.

Patients with PSD display abnormalities of platelet function that are similar to those of heterozygous carriers of the $P2Y_{12}$ receptor variant, suggesting that at least a fraction of patients labeled as PSD are indeed heterozygous $P2Y_{12}$ receptor defects.[155]

Studies in large series of patients with mild mucocutaneous bleeding suggested that PSD affects up to one-fifth of all patients, but no association between the degree of platelet dysfunction and bleeding severity was shown.[5,155]

The diagnosis of PSD is thus a generic definition of patients with a mild mucocutaneous bleeding disorder, normal blood coagulation, and a not well-defined platelet function abnormality always including defective platelet secretion, and it may be expected that with the expanding knowledge of the platelet function mechanisms and genes regulating platelet function, this group will progressively shrink and possibly disappear.

PROPHYLAXIS AND TREATMENT OF PLATELET FUNCTION DISORDERS

Despite progress in the diagnosis and understanding of IPFD, options for prophylaxis and treatment remain rather limited and not specific. Patient management is mainly focused on the prevention of bleeding after surgery or invasive procedures and on the control of major hemorrhagic events, while minor hemorrhages usually are disregarded, although they may be disturbing to patients.

General Prophylaxis Measures

Patients should be advised to avoid medications that interfere with platelet function (e.g., aspirin and nonsteroidal anti-inflammatory drugs), to perform regular dental hygiene, to avoid or limit intramuscular injections and, for the most serious forms, to avoid contact sports. Moreover, as these patients may require transfusions during their lifetime, they should be vaccinated against hepatitis A and B and should be typified for the human leukocyte antigen (HLA) in order to allow the transfusion of HLA-matched platelets in case of need to minimize the risk of alloimmunization. Patients affected by the most severe IPFD forms should carry an emergency health card with information about their disease, possible therapy, and drugs to be avoided. Correction of iron deficiency is often required, especially in children and young women, by cyclic iron therapy. For the most serious forms, prenatal diagnosis by genetic analysis of fetal cells and screening of potential sibling donors for disorders predisposing to acute leukemia should be considered.

Local Measures

Some types of localized bleeding, such as nose or gum bleeding, may be stopped by local measures such as electrocautery and nasal packing for epistaxis and mouthwashes with tranexamic acid or plugging with fibrin sealant or absorbable thrombin-soaked gelatin sponges for gingival bleeding. Compression, suturing, and application of gelatin sponges or gauzes soaked in tranexamic acid are useful for accidental or surgical wounds. Autologous platelet-rich clots have been used to accelerate wound healing in patients with type I GT.[156]

Desmopressin

Desmopressin (1-desamino-8-D-arginine vasopressin; DDAVP), a synthetic analogue of the antidiuretic hormone vasopressin, is an approved treatment for the prevention of bleeding in patients with mild hemophilia A and VWD because of its ability to transiently increase plasma levels of factor VIII and VWF. DDAVP is also useful in IPFDs, although the mechanism of its hemostatic effect in these disorders remains poorly understood, causing increased platelet adhesiveness, aggregation at high shear rate,[157] and procoagulant activity.[158] The drug should be used with caution in elderly patients, in those with a history of cardiovascular disease, and in infants. Moreover, it should be avoided in patients with PT-VWD because it might exacerbate thrombocytopenia due to release of HMW-VWF multimers and their binding to platelets with subsequent clearance from the circulation.[33] A meta-analysis showed that DDAVP may be a useful agent to reduce bleeding and transfusion for patients with platelet dysfunction or with a history of recent antiplatelet drug administration undergoing cardiac surgery.[159]

Antifibrinolytic Agents

Antifibrinolytic agents, such as ε-aminocaproic acid or tranexamic acid, are effective in arresting epistaxis, gingival bleeding, or menorrhagia and for the prevention of bleeding following minor surgery in IPFD, either as single drugs or in association with other treatments such as recombinant factor VIIa, DDAVP, or platelet transfusions. They can be administered intravenously or orally. Antifibrinolytic agents are considered contraindicated in hematuria for the risk of clot formation and occlusion of the urinary tract, but successful treatment of severe hematuria with no complications in patients with polycystic kidney has been reported,[160] and tranexamic acid is indicated in lower urinary tract bleedings.[161]

Activated Recombinant Factor VIIa

Recombinant activated factor VII (rFVIIa, NovoSeven, Novo Nordisk, Bagsvaerd, Denmark), originally developed for the treatment of hemophiliacs with inhibitor, is now used in several serious bleeding situations including in patients with severe IPFDs. In platelet disorders rFVIIa arrests bleeding by increasing thrombin generation, enhancing platelet adhesion to extracellular matrix, and restoring platelet procoagulant function.[162] In 2014, the US Food and Drug Administration approved rFVIIa for the treatment of severe bleeding and for perioperative management of patients with GT refractory to platelet transfusions.[163]

For other IPFDs, like BSS, PT-VWD, and δ-SPD, only case reports on the efficacy of rFVIIa are available. Severe adverse events associated with rFVIIa use, including myocardial infarction, ischemic stroke, and venous thromboembolism, have been reported.

Hormonal Treatment

Menarche may be associated with excessive bleeding, sometimes requiring blood transfusions, in patients with IPFD. Severe menometrorrhagia can be treated by intravenous high-dose conjugated estrogen for 24 to 48 hours followed by high doses of oral estrogen-progestins. Thereafter, combined oral contraceptives can be given for 2 to 3 months.[164,165]

Antifibrinolytic agents given orally on the first few days of menstruation are usually effective, but when they fail, long-term oral contraceptives should be given, especially when recurrent iron deficiency anemia develops.

Platelet Transfusions

Platelet transfusions have been used for many years; however, there is still debate about indications for platelet transfusion, frequency, and doses and prophylactic versus therapeutic use. Given the risks of allo- and Rh immunization, infection, and allergic reactions, platelet transfusions should be used in IPFD only when other agents have failed. HLA-matched platelets should be used to prevent HLA-alloimmunization, and when alloimmune antibodies develop, immunosuppression and/or plasmapheresis may be required to restore efficacy. Platelet transfusions can be used to arrest acute severe bleeding or in the preparation to surgery and should be continued after surgery until wound healing has occurred or for at least 2 days after hemorrhage arrest.[166] Platelet concentrates can be used to treat major spontaneous bleeding or for prophylaxis in patients with IPFDs at high bleeding risk who require invasive procedures. The Italian Society for Haemostasis and Thrombosis (SISET) guidelines on the management of bleeding and of invasive procedures in patients with platelet disorders suggested that concentrates from one apheresis unit, or 8 U of random-donor concentrates, can be used (at least $50\text{-}70 \times 10^8$ platelets/kg of body weight).[167]

Hematopoietic Stem Cell Transplantation and Gene Therapy

Hematopoietic stem cells (HSCs) can be derived from umbilical cord blood or from bone marrow of HLA-matched siblings or matched-unrelated or mismatched donors. HSC transplantation has been performed successfully in at least 23 patients with severe GT, but the largest study was conducted in patients with WAS. For 122 patients with WAS 5-year survival was 100% if transplanted from HLA-matched siblings and 90% for those transplanted from HLA-matched unrelated or from mismatched related donors.[168] Bone marrow transplantation from HLA-matched donors has also been used with success in BSS with severe hemorrhage and/or alloantibodies.[169] However, a careful evaluation of the risk-benefit ratio must be made before deciding on bone marrow transplantation.

Research on gene therapy for GT is ongoing: gene transfer in hematopoietic CD34+ cells using murine leukemia retroviral vectors, restoring GPIIb/IIIa expression, was successfully obtained in vitro[170] and in vivo in mice[171] with amelioration of platelet function. However, no attempts in humans have been performed so far. The feasibility of gene therapy for a platelet disorder in humans has been demonstrated in patients with WAS who showed sustained clinical benefit in 10 of 11 cases after infusion of gene-modified autologous HSCs, while one patient died of infection. Platelet counts and mean platelet volume increased in 6 of 11, but remained below normal; however, no patient experienced any major bleeding after gene therapy.[172-174]

Management of Delivery

Pregnancy is a matter of concern for patients with IPFDs because both the mother and the newborn are at risk of bleeding. Two large international collaborative studies have assessed the incidence of bleeding at delivery and pregnancy outcome in a large series of patients with well-defined IPDs and have shown that the risk of delivery-related bleeding is higher in IPDs than in healthy pregnant women and that severity of thrombocytopenia and previous bleeding history are predictive of postpartum hemorrhage (PPH). Bleeding rate was not different between vaginal deliveries and caesarean sections, and apparently it was not reduced by prophylactic platelet transfusions.[22,175] The highest incidence of PPH was observed in GT (50% of deliveries), and it was not prevented by prophylactic platelet transfusions: immunization against platelet antigens or inappropriate use of platelet concentrates are possible reasons for this failure.[175]

Delivery-related newborn bleedings are instead rare, although occasionally fatal cerebral hemorrhages have been reported. Case reports of delivery in patients with BSS, HPS, PT-VWD, and δ-SPD also suggest that maternal peripartum hemorrhage is not infrequent.[175]

Management of Surgery

Excessive bleeding at surgery is a feared complication in patients with IPFD; however, very few studies have evaluated the frequency of surgical bleeding in these conditions. Data from a large international study on the bleeding risk of surgery and invasive procedures in patients with IPDs, promoted by the Scientific Working Group on Thrombocytopenias and Platelet Function Disorders of the European Hematology Association, suggest that IPFDs are associated with a significant surgical bleeding risk (excessive bleeding in around 20% of all procedures), depending on diagnosis and type of surgery. A history of severe bleeding and a platelet count $<68 \times 10^9$/L are predictive of excessive bleeding at surgery. Prophylactic platelet transfusions, antifibrinolytic agents, desmopressin, or rFVIIa are empirically used.[166] Oral tranexamic acid can be employed for dental extractions, rFVIIa may be used for minor or major surgery, while HLA-matched platelets, alone or in association with rFVIIa, are recommended for major surgery.[23] The largest experience reported so far shows that both rFVIIa and platelets are effective in arresting or preventing bleeding associated with minor and major procedures in GT.[163]

MANAGEMENT OF THROMBOTIC RISK IN PATIENTS WITH IPFD

Despite their bleeding diathesis, patients with platelet disorders can develop transient or permanent prothrombotic conditions that necessitate prophylactic or therapeutic treatment. The thrombotic manifestations are often provoked by a transient risk factor such as surgery or a central venous catheter, which highlights the relevance of thromboprophylaxis.

Anticoagulation was reported for IPFD patients with GT, bBSS and MYH9-RT who developed VTE.[176] Long-term anticoagulation was mainly performed with vitamin K antagonists or low molecular weight heparin (LMWH), and anticoagulation related bleeding was rare.

The incidence of VTE in patients with IPD undergoing surgical procedures is unknown, and only little information on the use and safety of thromboprophylaxis in these patients is available. A recent study evaluating 210 surgical procedures carried out in 155 patients with well-defined forms of IPD showed that thromboprophylaxis was used only in 23.3% of procedures. The most frequently employed thromboprophylaxis was mechanical and appeared to be effective, with no patients developing thrombosis. LMWH use was low (10.5%), but it did not seem to influence the incidence of postsurgical bleeding. VTE incidence is low in these patients, with only two thromboembolic events registered, both occurring in patients who did not receive thromboprophylaxis.[24]

Although prophylactic anticoagulation should be considered if the thrombotic risk is high, caution is crucial and physicians should carefully assess bleeding events and thrombosis risks before and during anticoagulation. Recently a perioperative thromboprophylaxis guide in patients with IPD according to the *Caprini score*, a score that assesses the risk of surgery-associated VTE, has been proposed.[176] Briefly, the authors suggest mechanical prophylaxis when the thrombotic risk is only low or intermediate and prophylactic anticoagulation with LMWH when the VTE risk is high. In case of postsurgical excessive bleeding, LMWH should be postponed until effective hemostasis has been achieved.

References

1. de Gaetano G. Historical overview of the role of platelets in hemostasis and thrombosis. *Haematologica*. 2001;86:349-356.
2. Cohen I. The contractile system of blood platelets and its function. *Methods Achiev Exp Pathol*. 1979;9:40-86.
3. Lam WA, Chaudhuri O, Crow A, et al. Mechanics and contraction dynamics of single platelets and implications for clot stiffening. *Nat Mater*. 2011;10:61-66. doi: 10.1038/nmat2903
4. Israels SJ, Kahr WHA, Blanchette VS, Luban NLC, Rivard GE, Rand ML. Platelet disorders in children: a diagnostic approach. *Pediatr Blood Cancer*. 2011;56:975-983. doi:10.1002/pbc.22988
5. Quiroga T, Goycoolea M, Panes O, et al. High prevalence of bleeders of unknown cause among patients with inherited mucocutaneous bleeding. A prospective study of 280 patients and 299 controls. *Haematologica*. 2007;92:357-365. doi: 10.3324/haematol.10816
6. Oved JH, Lambert MP, Kowalska MA, Poncz M, Karczewski KJ. Population based frequency of naturally occurring loss-of-function variants in genes associated with platelet disorders. *J Thromb Haemost*. 2021;19:248-254. doi: 10.1111/jth.15113
7. Gresele P, Falcinelli E, Bury L. Inherited platelet function disorders. Diagnostic approach and management. *Hamostaseologie*. 2016;36:265-278. doi: 10.5482/HAMO-16-02-0002
8. Gresele P, Bury L, Falcinelli E. Inherited platelet function disorders: algorithms for phenotypic and genetic investigation. *Semin Thromb Hemost*. 2016;42:292-305. doi: 10.1055/s-0035-1570078
9. Gresele P, Harrison P, Bury L, et al. Diagnosis of suspected inherited platelet function disorders: results of a worldwide survey. *J Thromb Haemost*. 2014;12(9):1562-1569. doi:10.1111/jth.12650
10. Rodeghiero F, Pabinger I, Ragni M, et al. Fundamentals for a systematic approach to mild and moderate inherited bleeding disorders: an EHA consensus report. *Hemasphere*. 2019;3(4):e286. doi: 10.1097/HS9.0000000000000286
11. Gresele P, Orsini S, Noris P, et al. Validation of the ISTH/SSC bleeding assessment tool for inherited platelet disorders: a communication from the Platelet Physiology SSC. *J Thromb Haemost*. 2020;18(3):732-739. doi: 10.1111/jth.14683
12. Gresele P, Falcinelli E, Bury L, et al. The ISTH bleeding assessment tool as predictor of bleeding events in inherited platelet disorders: communication from the ISTH SSC Subcommittee on Platelet Physiology. *J Thromb Haemost*. 2021;19(5):1364-1371. doi: 10.1111/jth.15263
13. Gresele P. Subcommittee on platelet physiology of the international society on thrombosis and hemostasis. Diagnosis of inherited platelet function disorders: guidance from the SSC of the ISTH. *J Thromb Haemost*. 2015;13(2):314-322. doi: 10.1111/jth.12792
14. Simeoni I, Stephens JC, Hu F, et al. A high-throughput sequencing test for diagnosing inherited bleeding, thrombotic, and platelet disorders. *Blood*. 2016;127(23):2791-2803. doi: 10.1182/blood-2015-12-688267
15. Johnson B, Lowe GC, Futterer J, et al. Whole exome sequencing identifies genetic variants in inherited thrombocytopenia with secondary qualitative function defects. *Haematologica*. 2016;101(10):1170-1179. doi: 10.3324/haematol.2016.146316
16. Megy K, Downes K, Morel-Kopp MC, et al. GoldVariants, a resource for sharing rare genetic variants detected in bleeding, thrombotic, and platelet disorders: communication from the ISTH SSC Subcommittee on Genomics in Thrombosis and Hemostasis. *J Thromb Haemost*. 2021;19(10):2612-2617. doi: 10.1111/jth.15459
17. Megy K, Downes K, Simeoni I, et al. Curated disease-causing genes for bleeding, thrombotic, and platelet disorders: communication from the SSC of the ISTH. *J Thromb Haemost*. 2019;17(8):1253-1260. doi: 10.1111/jth.14479
18. Coller BS, Shattil SJ. The GPIIb/IIIa (integrin alphaIIbbeta3) odyssey: a technology-driven saga of a receptor with twists, turns, and even a bend. *Blood*. 2008;112(8):3011-3025. doi: 10.1182/blood-2008-06-077891
19. Newman PJ, Seligsohn U, Lyman S, Coller BS. The molecular genetic basis of Glanzmann thrombasthenia in the Iraqi-Jewish and Arab populations in Israel. *Proc Natl Acad Sci U S A*. 1991;88(8):3160-3164. doi:10.1073/pnas.88.8.3160
20. Nurden AT, Pillois X, Wilcox DA. Glanzmann thrombasthenia: state of the art and future directions. *Semin Thromb Hemost*. 2013;39(6):642-655. doi: 10.1055/s-0033-1353393
21. Bury L, Falcinelli E, Chiasserini D, Springer TA, Italiano JE, Gresele P. Cytoskeletal perturbation leads to platelet dysfunction and thrombocytopenia in variant forms of Glanzmann thrombasthenia. *Haematologica*. 2016;101(1):46-56. doi: 10.3324/haematol.2015.130849
22. Noris P, Schlegel N, Klersy C, et al. Analysis of 339 pregnancies in 181 women with 13 different forms of inherited thrombocytopenia. *Haematologica*. 2014;99(8):1387-1394. doi: 10.3324/haematol.2014.105924
23. Orsini S, Noris P, Bury L, et al. Bleeding risk of surgery and its prevention in patients with inherited platelet disorders. *Haematologica*. 2017;102(7):1192-1203. doi: 10.3324/haematol.2016.160754
24. Paciullo F, Bury L, Noris P, et al. Antithrombotic prophylaxis for surgery-associated venous thromboembolism risk in patients with inherited platelet disorders. The SPATA-DVT Study. *Haematologica*. 2020;105(7):1948-1956. doi:10.3324/haematol.2019.227876
25. Shpilberg O, Rabi I, Schiller K, et al. Patients with Glanzmann thrombasthenia lacking platelet glycoprotein alpha(IIb)beta(3) (GPIIb/IIIa) and alpha(v)beta(3) receptors are not protected from atherosclerosis. *Circulation*. 2002;105(9):1044-1048. doi:10.1161/hc0902.104676
26. Bernard J, Soulier JP. On a new variety of congenital thrombocytary hemoragiparous dystrophy. *Sem Hop*. 1948;24:3217-3223. Spec. No..
27. Noris P, Klersy C, Gresele P, et al. Platelet size for distinguishing between inherited thrombocytopenias and immune thrombocytopenia: a multicentric, real life study. *Br J Haematol*. 2013;162(1):112-119. doi: 10.1111/bjh.12349
28. Savoia A, Balduini CL, Savino M, et al. Autosomal dominant macrothrombocytopenia in Italy is most frequently a type of heterozygous Bernard-Soulier syndrome. *Blood*. 2001;97(5):1330-1335. doi: 10.1182/blood.v97.5.1330
29. Sivapalaratnam S, Westbury SK, Stephens JC, et al. Rare variants in GP1BB are responsible for autosomal dominant macrothrombocytopenia. *Blood*. 2017;129(4):520-524. doi: 10.1182/blood-2016-08-732248
30. Othman M, Kaur H, Favaloro EJ, et al. Platelet type von Willebrand disease and registry report: communication from the SSC of the ISTH. *J Thromb Haemost*. 2016;14(2):411-414. doi: 10.1111/jth.13204
31. Bury L, Falcinelli E, Kuchi Bhotla H, et al. A p.Arg127Gln variant in GPIbα LRR5 allosterically enhances affinity for VWF: a novel form of platelet-type VWD. *Blood Adv*. 2021;6(7):2236-2246. doi: 10.1182/bloodadvances.2021005463
32. Othman M, Kaur H, Emsley J. Platelet-type von Willebrand disease: new insights into the molecular pathophysiology of a unique platelet defect. *Semin Thromb Hemost*. 2013;39(6):663-673. doi: 10.1055/s-0033-1353442
33. Bury L, Falcinelli E, Mezzasoma AM, Guglielmini G, Momi S, Gresele P. Platelet dysfunction in platelet-type von Willebrand disease due to the constitutive triggering of the Lyn-PECAM1 inhibitory pathway. *Haematologica*. 2022;107:1643-1654. doi: 10.3324/haematol.2021.278776
34. Othman M, Gresele P. Guidance on the diagnosis and management of platelet-type von Willebrand disease: a communication from the Platelet Physiology Subcommittee of the ISTH. *J Thromb Haemost*. 2020;18(8):1855-1858. doi: 10.1111/jth.14827
35. Giannini S, Cecchetti L, Mezzasoma AM, Gresele P. Diagnosis of platelet-type von Willebrand disease by flow cytometry. *Haematologica*. 2010;95(6):1021-1024. doi: 10.3324/haematol.2009.015990
36. McDonald-McGinn DM, Sullivan KE, Marino B, et al. 22q11.2 deletion syndrome. *Nat Rev Dis Primers*. 2015;1:15071. doi: 10.1038/nrdp.2015.71
37. Hermans C, Wittevrongel C, Thys C, Smethurst PA, Van Geet C, Freson K. A compound heterozygous mutation in glycoprotein VI in a patient with a bleeding disorder. *J Thromb Haemost*. 2009;7(8):1356-1363. doi: 10.1111/j.1538-7836.2009.03520.x
38. Dumont B, Lasne D, Rothschild C, et al. Absence of collagen-induced platelet activation caused by compound heterozygous GPVI mutations. *Blood*. 2009;114(9):1900-1903. doi: 10.1182/blood-2009-03-213504
39. Matus V, Valenzuela G, Sáez CG, et al. An adenine insertion in exon 6 of human GP6 generates a truncated protein associated with a bleeding disorder in four Chilean families. *J Thromb Haemost*. 2013;11(9):1751-1759. doi: 10.1111/jth.12334
40. Jandrot-Perrus M, Hermans C, Mezzano D. Platelet glycoprotein VI genetic quantitative and qualitative defects. *Platelets*. 2019;30(6):708-713. doi: 10.1080/09537104.2019.1610166
41. Noris P, Guidetti GF, Conti V, et al. Autosomal dominant thrombocytopenias with reduced expression of glycoprotein Ia. *Thromb Haemost*. 2006;95(3):483-489. doi: 10.1160/TH05-06-0421
42. Nieuwenhuis HK, Akkerman JW, Houdijk WP, Sixma JJ. Human blood platelets showing no response to collagen fail to express surface glycoprotein Ia. *Nature*. 1985;318(6045):470-472. doi: 10.1038/318470a0
43. Yamamoto N, Ikeda H, Tandon NN, et al. A platelet membrane glycoprotein (GP) deficiency in healthy blood donors: naka- platelets lack detectable GPIV (CD36). *Blood*. 1990;76(9):1698-1703.
44. Berrou E, Soukaseum C, Favier R, et al. A mutation of the human EPHB2 gene leads to a major platelet functional defect. *Blood*. 2018;132(19):2067-2077. doi: 10.1182/blood-2018-04-845644
45. Tamponi G, Pannocchia A, Arduino C, et al. Congenital deficiency of alpha-2-adrenoceptors on human platelets: description of two cases. *Thromb Haemost*. 1987;58(4):1012-1016.
46. Rao AK, Willis J, Kowalska MA, Wachtfogel YT, Colman RW. Differential requirements for platelet aggregation and inhibition of adenylate cyclase by epinephrine. Studies of a familial platelet alpha 2-adrenergic receptor defect. *Blood*. 1988;71(2):494-501.
47. Lin TM, Lin JS, Tseng JY, Wu SY, Chen TY. Impaired responsiveness of platelets to epinephrine due to α2A adrenoreceptor deficiency in Male Chinese. *Platelets*. 2016;27(2):149-154. doi: 10.3109/09537104.2015.1049137
48. Hayward CPM, Pai M, Liu Y, et al. Diagnostic utility of light transmission platelet aggregometry: results from a prospective study of individuals referred for bleeding disorder assessments. *J Thromb Haemost*. 2009;7(4):676-684. doi: 10.1111/j.1538-7836.2009.03273.x

49. Hirata T, Kakizuka A, Ushikubi F, Fuse I, Okuma M, Narumiya S. Arg60 to Leu mutation of the human thromboxane A2 receptor in a dominantly inherited bleeding disorder. *J Clin Invest.* 1994;94(4):1662-1667. doi: 10.1172/JCI117510
50. Mumford AD, Dawood BB, Daly ME, et al. A novel thromboxane A2 receptor D304N variant that abrogates ligand binding in a patient with a bleeding diathesis. *Blood.* 2010;115(2):363-369. doi: 10.1182/blood-2009-08-236976
51. Flamm MH, Colace TV, Chatterjee MS, et al. Multiscale prediction of patient-specific platelet function under flow. *Blood.* 2012;120(1):190-198. doi: 10.1182/blood-2011-10-388140
52. Kamae T, Kiyomizu K, Nakazawa T, et al. Bleeding tendency and impaired platelet function in a patient carrying a heterozygous mutation in the thromboxane A2 receptor. *J Thromb Haemost.* 2011;9(5):1040-1048. doi: 10.1111/j.1538-7836.2011.04245.x
53. Nisar SP, Lordkipanidzé M, Jones ML, et al. A novel thromboxane A2 receptor N42S variant results in reduced surface expression and platelet dysfunction. *Thromb Haemost.* 2014;111(5):923-932. doi: 10.1160/TH13-08-0672
54. Mumford AD, Nisar S, Darnige L, et al. Platelet dysfunction associated with the novel Trp29Cys thromboxane A$_2$ receptor variant. *J Thromb Haemost.* 2013;11(3):547-554. doi: 10.1111/jth.12117
55. Bugert P, Fischer L, Althaus K, Knöfler R, Bakchoul T. Platelet dysfunction caused by a novel thromboxane A2 receptor mutation and congenital thrombocytopenia in a case of mild bleeding. *Platelets.* 2020;31(2):276-279. doi: 10.1080/09537104.2019.1652264
56. Cattaneo M. P2Y12 receptors: structure and function. *J Thromb Haemost.* 2015;13(suppl 1):S10-S16. doi: 10.1111/jth.12952
57. Cattaneo M. Molecular defects of the platelet P2 receptors. *Purinergic Signal.* 2011;7(3):333-339. doi:10.1007/s11302-011-9217-z
58. Oury C, Lenaerts T, Peerlink K. Congenital deficiency of the phospholipase C coupled platelet P2Y1 receptor leads to a mild bleeding disorder. *Thromb Haemost.* 1999;85(suppl):20.
59. Oury C, Toth-Zsamboki E, Van Geet C, et al. A natural dominant negative P2X1 receptor due to deletion of a single amino acid residue. *J Biol Chem.* 2000;275(30):22611-22614. doi: 10.1074/jbc.C000305200
60. Patel YM, Lordkipanidzé M, Lowe GC, et al. A novel mutation in the P2Y12 receptor and a function-reducing polymorphism in protease-activated receptor 1 in a patient with chronic bleeding. *J Thromb Haemost.* 2014;12(5):716-725. doi: 10.1111/jth.12539
61. De Candia E, Pecci A, Ciabattoni G, et al. Defective platelet responsiveness to thrombin and protease-activated receptors agonists in a novel case of gray platelet syndrome: correlation between the platelet defect and the alpha-granule content in the patient and four relatives. *J Thromb Haemost.* 2007;5(3):551-559. doi: 10.1111/j.1538-7836.2007.02329.x
62. Stockley J, Morgan NV, Bem D, et al. Enrichment of FLI1 and RUNX1 mutations in families with excessive bleeding and platelet dense granule secretion defects. *Blood.* 2013;122(25):4090-4093. doi: 10.1182/blood-2013-06-506873
63. Jedlitschky G, Cattaneo M, Lubenow LE, et al. Role of MRP4 (ABCC4) in platelet adenine nucleotide-storage: evidence from patients with delta-storage pool deficiencies. *Am J Pathol.* 2010;176(3):1097-1103. doi: 10.2353/ajpath.2010.090425
64. Sánchez-Guiu I, Torregrosa JM, Velasco F, et al. Hermansky-Pudlak syndrome. Overview of clinical and molecular features and case report of a new HPS-1 variant. *Hamostaseologie.* 2014;34(4):301-309. doi: 10.5482/HAMO-14-06-0024
65. Dell'Angelica EC, Shotelersuk V, Aguilar RC, Gahl WA, Bonifacino JS. Altered trafficking of lysosomal proteins in Hermansky-Pudlak syndrome due to mutations in the beta 3A subunit of the AP-3 adaptor. *Mol Cell.* 1999;3(1):11-21. doi: 10.1016/s1097-2765(00)80170-7
66. Ammann S, Schulz A, Krägeloh-Mann I, et al. Mutations in AP3D1 associated with immunodeficiency and seizures define a new type of Hermansky-Pudlak syndrome. *Blood.* 2016;127(8):997-1006. doi: 10.1182/blood-2015-09-671636
67. Mohammed M, Al-Hashmi N, Al-Rashdi S, et al. Biallelic mutations in AP3D1 cause Hermansky-Pudlak syndrome type 10 associated with immunodeficiency and seizure disorder. *Eur J Med Genet.* 2019;62(11):103583. doi: 10.1016/j.ejmg.2018.11.017
68. Velázquez-Díaz P, Nakajima E, Sorkhdini P, et al. Hermansky-Pudlak syndrome and lung disease: pathogenesis and therapeutics. *Front Pharmacol.* 2021;12:644671. doi: 10.3389/fphar.2021.644671
69. Certain S, Barrat F, Pastural E, et al. Protein truncation test of LYST reveals heterogenous mutations in patients with Chediak-Higashi syndrome. *Blood.* 2000;95(3):979-983.
70. Nagle DL, Karim MA, Woolf EA, et al. Identification and mutation analysis of the complete gene for Chediak-Higashi syndrome. *Nat Genet.* 1996;14(3):307-311. doi: 10.1038/ng1196-307
71. Karim MA, Suzuki K, Fukai K, et al. Apparent genotype-phenotype correlation in childhood, adolescent, and adult Chediak-Higashi syndrome. *Am J Med Genet.* 2002;108(1):16-22.
72. Huizing M, Helip-Wooley A, Westbroek W, Gunay-Aygun M, Gahl WA. Disorders of lysosome-related organelle biogenesis: clinical and molecular genetics. *Annu Rev Genomics Hum Genet.* 2008;9:359-386. doi: 10.1146/annurev.genom.9.081307.164303
73. Volders K, Nuytens K, Creemers JWM. The autism candidate gene neurobeachin encodes a scaffolding protein implicated in membrane trafficking and signaling. *Curr Mol Med.* 2011;11(3):204-217. doi: 10.2174/156652411795243432
74. Bijl N, Thys C, Wittevrongel C, et al. Platelet studies in autism spectrum disorder patients and first-degree relatives. *Mol Autism.* 2015;6:57. doi: 10.1186/s13229-015-0051-y
75. Leinøe E, Zetterberg E, Kinalis S, et al. Application of whole-exome sequencing to direct the specific functional testing and diagnosis of rare inherited bleeding disorders in patients from the Öresund Region, Scandinavia. *Br J Haematol.* 2017;179(2):308-322. doi: 10.1111/bjh.14863
76. Rowley JW, Oler AJ, Tolley ND, et al. Genome-wide RNA-seq analysis of human and mouse platelet transcriptomes. *Blood.* 2011;118(14):e101-e111. doi: 10.1182/blood-2011-03-339705
77. Fletcher SJ, Johnson B, Lowe GC, et al. SLFN14 mutations underlie thrombocytopenia with excessive bleeding and platelet secretion defects. *J Clin Invest.* 2015;125(9):3600-3605. doi:10.1172/JCI80347
78. Stapley RJ, Pisareva VP, Pisarev AV, Morgan NV. SLFN14 gene mutations associated with bleeding. *Platelets.* 2020;31(3):407-410. doi: 10.1080/09537104.2019.1648781
79. Marconi C, Di Buduo CA, Barozzi S, et al. SLFN14-related thrombocytopenia: identification within a large series of patients with inherited thrombocytopenia. *Thromb Haemost.* 2016;115(5):1076-1079. doi: 10.1160/TH15-11-0884
80. Albers CA, Cvejic A, Favier R, et al. Exome sequencing identifies NBEAL2 as the causative gene for gray platelet syndrome. *Nat Genet.* 2011;43(8):735-737. doi: 10.1038/ng.885
81. Gunay-Aygun M, Falik-Zaccai TC, Vilboux T, et al. NBEAL2 is mutated in gray platelet syndrome and is required for biogenesis of platelet α-granules. *Nat Genet.* 2011;43(8):732-734. doi: 10.1038/ng.883
82. Kahr WHA, Hinckley J, Li L, et al. Mutations in NBEAL2, encoding a BEACH protein, cause gray platelet syndrome. *Nat Genet.* 2011;43(8):738-740. doi: 10.1038/ng.884
83. Lages B, Sussman, Levine SP, Coletti D, Weiss HJ. Platelet alpha granule deficiency associated with decreased P-selectin and selective impairment of thrombin-induced activation in a new patient with gray platelet syndrome (alpha-storage pool deficiency). *J Lab Clin Med.* 1997;129(3):364-375. doi: 10.1016/s0022-2143(97)90185-2
84. Nurden AT, Nurden P. The gray platelet syndrome: clinical spectrum of the disease. *Blood Rev.* 2007;21(1):21-36. doi: 10.1016/j.blre.2005.12.003
85. Larocca LM, Heller PG, Podda G, et al. Megakaryocytic emperipolesis and platelet function abnormalities in five patients with gray platelet syndrome. *Platelets.* 2015;26(8):751-757. doi: 10.3109/09537104.2014.994093
86. Gunay-Aygun M, Zivony-Elboum Y, Gumruk F, et al. Gray platelet syndrome: natural history of a large patient cohort and locus assignment to chromosome 3p. *Blood.* 2010;116(23):4990-5001. doi: 10.1182/blood-2010-05-286534
87. Sims MC, Mayer L, Collins JH, et al. Novel manifestations of immune dysregulation and granule defects in gray platelet syndrome. *Blood.* 2020;136(17):1956-1967. doi: 10.1182/blood.2019004776
88. Glembotsky AC, De Luca G, Heller PG. A deep dive into the pathology of gray platelet syndrome: new insights on immune dysregulation. *J Blood Med.* 2021;12:719-732. doi: 10.2147/JBM.S270018
89. Gissen P, Johnson CA, Morgan NV, et al. Mutations in VPS33B, encoding a regulator of SNARE-dependent membrane fusion, cause arthrogryposis-renal dysfunction-cholestasis (ARC) syndrome. *Nat Genet.* 2004;36(4):400-404. doi: 10.1038/ng1325
90. Weyand AC, Lombel RM, Pipe SW, Shavit JA. The role of platelets and ε-aminocaproic acid in arthrogryposis, renal dysfunction, and cholestasis (ARC) syndrome associated hemorrhage. *Pediatr Blood Cancer.* 2016;63(3):561-563. doi: 10.1002/pbc.25814
91. Mattina T, Perrotta CS, Grossfeld P. Jacobsen syndrome. *Orphanet J Rare Dis.* 2009;4:9. doi: 10.1186/1750-1172-4-9
92. Breton-Gorius J, Favier R, Guichard J, et al. A new congenital dysmegakaryopoietic thrombocytopenia (Paris-Trousseau) associated with giant platelet alpha-granules and chromosome 11 deletion at 11q23. *Blood.* 1995;85(7):1805-1814.
93. Krishnamurti L, Neglia JP, Nagarajan R, et al. Paris-Trousseau syndrome platelets in a child with Jacobsen's syndrome. *Am J Hematol.* 2001;66(4):295-299. doi: 10.1002/ajh.1061
94. Favier R, Akshoomoff N, Mattson S, Grossfeld P. Jacobsen syndrome: advances in our knowledge of phenotype and genotype. *Am J Med Genet C Semin Med Genet.* 2015;169(3):239-250. doi: 10.1002/ajmg.c.31448
95. Favier R, Jondeau K, Boutard P, et al. Paris-Trousseau syndrome: clinical, hematological, molecular data of ten new cases. *Thromb Haemost.* 2003;90(5):893-897. doi: 10.1160/TH03-02-0120
96. Stevenson WS, Rabbolini DJ, Beutler L, et al. Paris-Trousseau thrombocytopenia is phenocopied by the autosomal recessive inheritance of a DNA-binding domain mutation in FLI1. *Blood.* 2015;126(17):2027-2030. doi: 10.1182/blood-2015-06-650887
97. Antony-Debré I, Bluteau D, Itzykson R, et al. MYH10 protein expression in platelets as a biomarker of RUNX1 and FLI1 alterations. *Blood.* 2012;120(13):2719-2722. doi: 10.1182/blood-2012-04-422352
98. White JG, Keel S, Reyes M, Burris SM. Alpha-delta platelet storage pool deficiency in three generations. *Platelets.* 2007;18(1):1-10. doi: 10.1080/09537100600800172
99. Freson K, Hoylaerts MF, Jaeken J, et al. Genetic variation of the extra-large stimulatory G protein alpha-subunit leads to Gs hyperfunction in platelets and is a risk factor for bleeding. *Thromb Haemost.* 2001;86(3):733-738.
100. Gabbeta J, Yang X, Kowalska MA, Sun L, Dhanasekaran N, Rao AK. Platelet signal transduction defect with Galpha subunit dysfunction and diminished Galphaq in a patient with abnormal platelet responses. *Proc Natl Acad Sci U S A.* 1997;94(16):8750-8755. doi: 10.1073/pnas.94.16.8750
101. Patel YM, Patel K, Rahman S, et al. Evidence for a role for Galphai1 in mediating weak agonist-induced platelet aggregation in human platelets: reduced Galphai1 expression and defective Gi signaling in the platelets of a patient with a chronic bleeding disorder. *Blood.* 2003;101(12):4828-4835. doi: 10.1182/blood-2002-10-3080
102. Faioni EM, Razzari C, Zulueta A, et al. Bleeding diathesis and gastro-duodenal ulcers in inherited cytosolic phospholipase-A2 alpha deficiency. *Thromb Haemost.* 2014;112(6):1182-1189. doi: 10.1160/TH14-04-0352

103. Dubé JN, Drouin J, Aminian M, Plant MH, Laneuville O. Characterization of a partial prostaglandin endoperoxide H synthase-1 deficiency in a patient with a bleeding disorder. *Br J Haematol.* 2001;113(4):878-885. doi: 10.1046/j.1365-2141.2001.02867.x
104. Palma-Barqueros V, Bohdan N, Revilla N, Vicente V, Bastida JM, Rivera J. PTGS1 gene variations associated with bleeding and platelet dysfunction. *Platelets.* 2021;32(5):710-716. doi: 10.1080/09537104.2020.1782370
105. Chan MV, Hayman MA, Sivapalaratnam S, et al. Identification of a homozygous recessive variant in PTGS1 resulting in a congenital aspirin-like defect in platelet function. *Haematologica.* 2021;106(5):1423-1432. doi: 10.3324/haematol.2019.235895
106. Palma-Barqueros V, Crescente M, de la Morena ME, et al. A novel genetic variant in PTGS1 affects N-glycosylation of cyclooxygenase-1 causing a dominant-negative effect on platelet function and bleeding diathesis. *Am J Hematol.* 2021;96(3):E83-E88. doi: 10.1002/ajh.26076
107. Mestel F, Oetliker O, Beck E, Felix R, Imbach P, Wagner HP. Severe bleeding associated with defective thromboxane synthetase. *Lancet.* 1980;1(8160):157. doi: 10.1016/s0140-6736(80)90642-x
108. Defreyn G, Machin SJ, Carreras LO, Dauden MV, Chamone DA, Vermylen J. Familial bleeding tendency with partial platelet thromboxane synthetase deficiency: reorientation of cyclic endoperoxide metabolism. *Br J Haematol.* 1981;49(1):29-41. doi: 10.1111/j.1365-2141.1981.tb07194.x
109. Geneviève D, Proulle V, Isidor B, et al. Thromboxane synthase mutations in an increased bone density disorder (Ghosal syndrome). *Nat Genet.* 2008;40(3):284-286. doi: 10.1038/ng.2007.66
110. Vezza R, Mezzasoma AM, Venditti G, Gresele P. Prostaglandin endoperoxides and thromboxane A2 activate the same receptor isoforms in human platelets. *Thromb Haemost.* 2002;87(1):114-121.
111. Lee SB, Rao AK, Lee KH, Yang X, Bae YS, Rhee SG. Decreased expression of phospholipase C-beta 2 isozyme in human platelets with impaired function. *Blood.* 1996;88(5):1684-1691.
112. van de Vijver E, De Cuyper IM, Gerrits AJ, et al. Defects in Glanzmann thrombasthenia and LAD-III (LAD-1/v) syndrome: the role of integrin β1 and β3 in platelet adhesion to collagen. *Blood.* 2012;119(2):583-586. doi: 10.1182/blood-2011-02-337188
113. Saultier P, Szepetowski S, Canault M, et al. Long-term management of leukocyte adhesion deficiency type III without hematopoietic stem cell transplantation. *Haematologica.* 2018;103(6):e264-e267. doi: 10.3324/haematol.2017.186304
114. Canault M, Ghalloussi D, Grosdidier C, et al. Human CalDAG-GEFI gene (RASGRP2) mutation affects platelet function and causes severe bleeding. *J Exp Med.* 2014;211(7):1349-1362. doi: 10.1084/jem.20130477
115. Lozano ML, Cook A, Bastida JM, et al. Novel mutations in RASGRP2, which encodes CalDAG-GEFI, abrogate Rap1 activation, causing platelet dysfunction. *Blood.* 2016;128(9):1282-1289. doi: 10.1182/blood-2015-11-683102
116. Palma-Barqueros V, Ruiz-Pividal J, Bohdan N, et al. RASGRP2 gene variations associated with platelet dysfunction and bleeding. *Platelets.* 2019;30(4):535-539. doi: 10.1080/09537104.2019.1585528
117. Turro E, Greene D, Wijgaerts A, et al. A dominant gain-of-function mutation in universal tyrosine kinase SRC causes thrombocytopenia, myelofibrosis, bleeding, and bone pathologies. *Sci Transl Med.* 2016;8(328):328ra30. doi: 10.1126/scitranslmed.aad7666
118. De Kock L, Thys C, Downes K, et al. De novo variant in tyrosine kinase SRC causes thrombocytopenia: case report of a second family. *Platelets.* 2019;30(7):931-934. doi: 10.1080/09537104.2019.1628197
119. Barozzi S, Di Buduo CA, Marconi C, et al. Pathogenetic and clinical study of a patient with thrombocytopenia due to the p.E527K gain-of-function variant of SRC. *Haematologica.* 2021;106(3):918-922. doi: 10.3324/haematol.2020.268516
120. Manchev VT, Hilpert M, Berrou E, et al. A new form of macrothrombocytopenia induced by a germ-line mutation in the PRKACG gene. *Blood.* 2014;124(16):2554-2563. doi:10.1182/blood-2014-01-551820
121. Galera P, Dulau-Florea A, Calvo KR. Inherited thrombocytopenia and platelet disorders with germline predisposition to myeloid neoplasia. *Int J Lab Hematol.* 2019;41(suppl 1):131-141. doi: 10.1111/ijlh.12999
122. Song WJ, Sullivan MG, Legare RD, et al. Haploinsufficiency of CBFA2 causes familial thrombocytopenia with propensity to develop acute myelogenous leukaemia. *Nat Genet.* 1999;23(2):166-175. doi: 10.1038/13793
123. Antony-Debré I, Manchev VT, Balayn N, et al. Level of RUNX1 activity is critical for leukemic predisposition but not for thrombocytopenia. *Blood.* 2015;125(6):930-940. doi: 10.1182/blood-2014-06-585513
124. Nichols KE, Crispino JD, Poncz M, et al. Familial dyserythropoietic anaemia and thrombocytopenia due to an inherited mutation in GATA1. *Nat Genet.* 2000;24(3):266-270. doi: 10.1038/73480
125. Monteferrario D, Bolar NA, Marneth AE, et al. A dominant-negative GFI1B mutation in the gray platelet syndrome. *N Engl J Med.* 2014;370(3):245-253. doi: 10.1056/NEJMoa1308130
126. Aminkeng F. GFI1B mutation causes autosomal dominant gray platelet syndrome. *Clin Genet.* 2014;85(6):534-535. doi: 10.1111/cge.12380
127. Ferreira CR, Chen D, Abraham SM, et al. Combined alpha-delta platelet storage pool deficiency is associated with mutations in GFI1B. *Mol Genet Metab.* 2017;120(3):288-294. doi: 10.1016/j.ymgme.2016.12.006
128. Hamamy H, Makrythanasis P, Al-Allawi N, Muhsin AA, Antonarakis SE. Recessive thrombocytopenia likely due to a homozygous pathogenic variant in the FYB gene: case report. *BMC Med Genet.* 2014;15:135. doi: 10.1186/s12881-014-0135-0
129. Levin C, Koren A, Pretorius E, et al. Deleterious mutation in the FYB gene is associated with congenital autosomal recessive small-platelet thrombocytopenia. *J Thromb Haemost.* 2015;13(7):1285-1292. doi: 10.1111/jth.12966
130. Kasirer-Friede A, Kang J, Kahner B, Ye F, Ginsberg MH, Shattil SJ. ADAP interactions with talin and kindlin promote platelet integrin αIIbβ3 activation and stable fibrinogen binding. *Blood.* 2014;123(20):3156-3165. doi: 10.1182/blood-2013-08-520627
131. Jarvis GE, Bihan D, Hamaia S, et al. A role for adhesion and degranulation-promoting adapter protein in collagen-induced platelet activation mediated via integrin α(2) β(1). *J Thromb Haemost.* 2012;10(2):268-277. doi: 10.1111/j.1538-7836.2011.04567.x
132. Berrou E, Adam F, Lebret M, et al. Heterogeneity of platelet functional alterations in patients with filamin A mutations. *Arterioscler Thromb Vasc Biol.* 2013;33(1):e11-e18. doi: 10.1161/ATVBAHA.112.300603
133. Buchbinder D, Nugent DJ, Fillipovich AH. Wiskott-Aldrich syndrome: diagnosis, current management, and emerging treatments. *Appl Clin Genet.* 2014;7:55-66. doi: 10.2147/TACG.S58444
134. Shcherbina A, Cooley J, Lutskiy MI, Benarafa C, Gilbert GE, Remold-O'Donnell E. WASP plays a novel role in regulating platelet responses dependent on alphaIIb-beta3 integrin outside-in signalling. *Br J Haematol.* 2010;148(3):416-427. doi: 10.1111/j.1365-2141.2009.07959.x
135. Toti F, Satta N, Fressinaud E, Meyer D, Freyssinet JM. Scott syndrome, characterized by impaired transmembrane migration of procoagulant phosphatidylserine and hemorrhagic complications, is an inherited disorder. *Blood.* 1996;87(4):1409-1415.
136. Munnix ICA, Harmsma M, Giddings JC, et al. Store-mediated calcium entry in the regulation of phosphatidylserine exposure in blood cells from Scott patients. *Thromb Haemost.* 2003;89(4):687-695.
137. Weiss HJ, Vicic WJ, Lages BA, Rogers J. Isolated deficiency of platelet procoagulant activity. *Am J Med.* 1979;67(2):206-213. doi: 10.1016/0002-9343(79)90392-9
138. Flores-Nascimento MC, Orsi FLA, Yokoyama AP, et al. Diagnosis of Scott syndrome in patient with bleeding disorder of unknown cause. *Blood Coagul Fibrinolysis.* 2012;23(1):75-77. doi: 10.1097/MBC.0b013e32834d0c81
139. Millington-Burgess SL, Harper MT. Gene of the issue: ANO6 and Scott syndrome. *Platelets.* 2020;31(7):964-967. doi: 10.1080/09537104.2019.1693039
140. Suzuki J, Umeda M, Sims PJ, Nagata S. Calcium-dependent phospholipid scrambling by TMEM16F. *Nature.* 2010;468(7325):834-838. doi: 10.1038/nature09583
141. Castoldi E, Collins PW, Williamson PL, Bevers EM. Compound heterozygosity for 2 novel TMEM16F mutations in a patient with Scott syndrome. *Blood.* 2011;117(16):4399-4400. doi: 10.1182/blood-2011-01-332502
142. Rubak P, Nissen PH, Kristensen SD, Hvas AM. Investigation of platelet function and platelet disorders using flow cytometry. *Platelets.* 2016;27(1):66-74. doi: 10.3109/09537104.2015.1032919
143. Zwaal RFA, Comfurius P, Bevers EM. Scott syndrome, a bleeding disorder caused by defective scrambling of membrane phospholipids. *Biochim Biophys Acta.* 2004;1636(2-3):119-128. doi: 10.1016/j.bbalip.2003.07.003
144. Misceo D, Holmgren A, Louch WE, et al. A dominant STIM1 mutation causes Stormorken syndrome. *Hum Mutat.* 2014;35(5):556-564. doi: 10.1002/humu.22544
145. Morin G, Bruechle NO, Singh AR, et al. Gain-of-Function mutation in STIM1 (P.R304W) is associated with Stormorken syndrome. *Hum Mutat.* 2014;35(10):1221-1232. doi: 10.1002/humu.22621
146. Noury JB, Böhm J, Peche GA, et al. Tubular aggregate myopathy with features of Stormorken disease due to a new STIM1 mutation. *Neuromuscul Disord.* 2017;27(1):78-82. doi: 10.1016/j.nmd.2016.10.006
147. Lacruz RS, Feske S. Diseases caused by mutations in ORAI1 and STIM1. *Ann N Y Acad Sci.* 2015;1356:45-79. doi: 10.1111/nyas.12938
148. Nesin V, Wiley G, Kousi M, et al. Activating mutations in STIM1 and ORAI1 cause overlapping syndromes of tubular myopathy and congenital miosis. *Proc Natl Acad Sci U S A.* 2014;111(11):4197-4202. doi: 10.1073/pnas.1312520111
149. Solum NO. Procoagulant expression in platelets and defects leading to clinical disorders. *Arterioscler Thromb Vasc Biol.* 1999;19(12):2841-2846. doi: 10.1161/01.atv.19.12.2841
150. Holme PA, Solum NO, Brosstad F, Egberg N, Lindahl TL. Stimulated Glanzmann's thrombasthenia platelets produced microvesicles. Microvesiculation correlates better to exposure of procoagulant surface than to activation of GPIIb-IIIa. *Thromb Haemost.* 1995;74(6):1533-1540.
151. Paterson AD, Rommens JM, Bharaj B, et al. Persons with Quebec platelet disorder have a tandem duplication of PLAU, the urokinase plasminogen activator gene. *Blood.* 2010;115(6):1264-1266. doi: 10.1182/blood-2009-07-233965
152. Kahr WH, Zheng S, Sheth PM, et al. Platelets from patients with the Quebec platelet disorder contain and secrete abnormal amounts of urokinase-type plasminogen activator. *Blood.* 2001;98(2):257-265. doi: 10.1182/blood.v98.2.257
153. Diamandis M, Paterson AD, Rommens JM, et al. Quebec platelet disorder is linked to the urokinase plasminogen activator gene (PLAU) and increases expression of the linked allele in megakaryocytes. *Blood.* 2009;113(7):1543-1546. doi: 10.1182/blood-2008-08-175216
154. Hayward CP, Rivard GE, Kane WH, et al. An autosomal dominant, qualitative platelet disorder associated with multimerin deficiency, abnormalities in platelet factor V, thrombospondin, von Willebrand factor, and fibrinogen and an epinephrine aggregation defect. *Blood.* 1996;87(12):4967-4978.
155. Lotta LA, Maino A, Tuana G, et al. Prevalence of disease and relationships between laboratory phenotype and bleeding severity in platelet primary secretion defects. *PLoS One.* 2013;8(4):e60396. doi: 10.1371/journal.pone.0060396
156. Nurden P, Youlouz-Marfak I, Siberchicot F, et al. Use of autologous platelet-rich clots for the prevention of local injury bleeding in patients with severe inherited mucocutaneous bleeding disorders. *Haemophilia.* 2011;17(4):620-624. doi: 10.1111/j.1365-2516.2010.02480.x
157. Cattaneo M, Pareti FI, Zighetti M, Lecchi A, Lombardi R, Mannucci PM. Platelet aggregation at high shear is impaired in patients with congenital defects of platelet secretion and is corrected by DDAVP: correlation with the bleeding time. *J Lab Clin Med.* 1995;125(4):540-547.

158. Colucci G, Stutz M, Rochat S, et al. The effect of desmopressin on platelet function: a selective enhancement of procoagulant COAT platelets in patients with primary platelet function defects. *Blood*. 2014;123(12):1905-1916. doi: 10.1182/blood-2013-04-497123
159. Desborough MJR, Oakland KA, Landoni G, et al. Desmopressin for treatment of platelet dysfunction and reversal of antiplatelet agents: a systematic review and meta-analysis of randomized controlled trials. *J Thromb Haemost*. 2017;15(2):263-272. doi: 10.1111/jth.13576
160. Vujkovac B, Sabovic M. A successful treatment of life-threatening bleeding from polycystic kidneys with antifibrinolytic agent tranexamic acid. *Blood Coagul Fibrinolysis*. 2006;17(7):589-591. doi: 10.1097/01.mbc.0000245293.41774.c8
161. Kumar S, Randhawa MS, Ganesamoni R, Singh SK. Tranexamic acid reduces blood loss during percutaneous nephrolithotomy: a prospective randomized controlled study. *J Urol*. 2013;189(5):1757-1761. doi: 10.1016/j.juro.2012.10.115
162. Lisman T, De Groot PG. Mechanism of action of recombinant factor VIIa. *J Thromb Haemost*. 2003;1(6):1138-1139. doi: 10.1046/j.1538-7836.2003.00225.x
163. Poon MC. The evidence for the use of recombinant human activated factor VII in the treatment of bleeding patients with quantitative and qualitative platelet disorders. *Transfus Med Rev*. 2007;21(3):223-236. doi: 10.1016/j.tmrv.2007.03.003
164. Franchini M, Lippi G, Guidi GC. The use of recombinant activated factor VII in platelet-associated bleeding. *Hematology*. 2008;13(1):41-45. doi: 10.1179/102453308X315816
165. Demers C, Derzko C, David M, Douglas J; Society of Obstetricians and Gynaecologists of Canada. Gynaecological and obstetric management of women with inherited bleeding disorders. *Int J Gynaecol Obstet*. 2006;95(1):75-87. doi: 10.1016/j.ijgo.2006.02.004
166. Seligsohn U. Treatment of inherited platelet disorders. *Haemophilia*. 2012;18(suppl 4):161-165. doi: 10.1111/j.1365-2516.2012.02842.x
167. Tosetto A, Balduini CL, Cattaneo M, et al. Management of bleeding and of invasive procedures in patients with platelet disorders and/or thrombocytopenia: guidelines of the Italian Society for Haemostasis and Thrombosis (SISET). *Thromb Res*. 2009;124(5):e13-e18. doi: 10.1016/j.thromres.2009.06.009
168. Moratto D, Giliani S, Bonfim C, et al. Long-term outcome and lineage-specific chimerism in 194 patients with Wiskott-Aldrich syndrome treated by hematopoietic cell transplantation in the period 1980-2009: an international collaborative study. *Blood*. 2011;118(6):1675-1684. doi: 10.1182/blood-2010-11-319376
169. Locatelli F, Rossi G, Balduini C. Hematopoietic stem-cell transplantation for the Bernard-Soulier syndrome. *Ann Intern Med*. 2003;138(1):79. doi: 10.7326/0003-4819-138-1-200301070-00028
170. Wilcox DA, White GC. Gene therapy for platelet disorders: studies with Glanzmann's thrombasthenia. *J Thromb Haemost*. 2003;1(11):2300-2311. doi: 10.1046/j.1538-7836.2003.00476.x
171. Fang J, Hodivala-Dilke K, Johnson BD, et al. Therapeutic expression of the platelet-specific integrin, αIIbβ3, in a murine model for Glanzmann thrombasthenia. *Blood*. 2005;106(8):2671-2679. doi: 10.1182/blood-2004-12-4619
172. Hacein-Bey Abina S, Gaspar HB, Blondeau J, et al. Outcomes following gene therapy in patients with severe Wiskott-Aldrich syndrome. *JAMA*. 2015;313(15):1550-1563. doi: 10.1001/jama.2015.3253
173. Aiuti A, Biasco L, Scaramuzza S, et al. Lentiviral hematopoietic stem cell gene therapy in patients with Wiskott-Aldrich syndrome. *Science*. 2013;341(6148):1233151. doi: 10.1126/science.1233151
174. Pala F, Morbach H, Castiello MC, et al. Lentiviral-mediated gene therapy restores B cell tolerance in Wiskott-Aldrich syndrome patients. *J Clin Invest*. 2015;125(10):3941-3951. doi: 10.1172/JCI82249
175. Civaschi E, Klersy C, Melazzini F, et al. Analysis of 65 pregnancies in 34 women with five different forms of inherited platelet function disorders. *Br J Haematol*. 2015;170(4):559-563. doi: 10.1111/bjh.13458
176. Zaninetti C, Thiele T. Anticoagulation in patients with platelet disorders. *Hamostaseologie*. 2021;41(2):112-119. doi: 10.1055/a-1344-7279

Section 3 ■ COAGULATION DISORDERS

Chapter 54 ■ Inherited Coagulation Disorders

MING Y. LIM • GEORGE M. RODGERS

INTRODUCTION

Inherited disorders of coagulation result from the deficiency or functional abnormality of one of the plasma proteins involved in providing normal coagulation.[1] If von Willebrand disease (vWD) is included, the inherited coagulation abnormalities (*Table 54.1*) are common; for example, vWD may affect up to 1% of the population. The other inherited coagulation disorders occur less often.

As the purpose of the coagulation cascade is to rapidly generate fibrin to form a clot, the clinical manifestation of any deficiency or functional abnormality in any coagulation protein will be similar, that is, clinical bleeding, with greater bleeding associated with more severe deficiency. Therefore, the manifestations and complications of clinical bleeding will be described in this chapter in the section on Hemophilia A. A review of treatment of hemophilia has been published.[2]

NOMENCLATURE

The international Roman numeral designations for these disorders are summarized in *Table 54.1*. Like abnormal hemoglobins, qualitatively abnormal fibrinogens are designated by the name of the city in which they were first discovered, as in *fibrinogen Paris*.

Table 54.1. Inherited Disorders of Coagulation

X-linked Recessive Traits
Hemophilia A (Factor VIII deficiency)
Hemophilia B (Factor IX deficiency)

Autosomal Recessive Traits
Factor XI deficiency
Prothrombin deficiency
Factor V deficiency
Factor VII deficiency
Factor X deficiency (i.e., Prower variant, Stuart variant, Friuli variant, others)
Afibrinogenemia
Hypofibrinogenemia
Factor XII deficiency
Factor XIII deficiency

Autosomal Dominant Traits
von Willebrand disease
Dysfibrinogenemias

Combined Abnormalities
Associated with factor VIII deficiency (i.e., factor V deficiency, hemophilia B, factor XI deficiency, factor VII deficiency, von Willebrand disease, dysfibrinogenemias, platelet dysfunction)
Involving vitamin K–dependent factors (i.e., factors II, VII, IX, and X; factors IX and XII; others)

Miscellaneous
Prekallikrein deficiency
High-molecular-weight kininogen deficiency
Deficiency of physiologic inhibitors (i.e., α_2-antiplasmin, abnormal α_1-antitrypsin [antithrombin Pittsburgh])

PRINCIPLES OF PATHOPHYSIOLOGY

With the exception of fibrinogen and prothrombin, the coagulation factors are trace proteins. Clinical laboratory measurements of their activity depend on bioassays, which detect both quantitative absence of a specific factor and a qualitative functional abnormality in a factor that is present in normal amounts. Further laboratory testing is required to determine the actual concentration of the protein, usually by enzyme-linked immunosorbent assay (ELISA) methodology. Thus, for example, in hemophilia A, the bioassay measures *factor VIII coagulant activity* (factor VIIIc) and refers to the functional property of the factor VIII molecule that corrects the coagulation defect of patients with hemophilia A. The amount of protein measures the amount of antigen by ELISA and is referred to as *factor VIIIAg* (*Table 54.2*). Many hemophilia treatment centers (HTCs) currently proceed to determine the genotype for individual persons with inherited coagulation disorders; such analysis is helpful to predict the severity of the clinical phenotype, to predict the risk of inhibitor development, and to aid in family counseling.

Most qualitative abnormalities in coagulation factors result in loss of function of the protein in the coagulation cascade. However, some mutations produce qualitative abnormalities that result in "gain of function." Such factors are called *abnormal* or *aberrant factors* to distinguish them. The most clearly defined disorders of this type are the dysfibrinogenemias, in which the abnormal fibrinogen typically is not completely nonfunctional, but may also inhibit the function of normal fibrinogen. Other disorders characterized by aberrant coagulation factors include the B_m variant of hemophilia B and some of the variants of prothrombin deficiency. Aberrant procoagulant proteins may also be synthesized in acquired deficiencies of the vitamin K–dependent factors (see Chapter 55). An example of a "gain-of-function" mutation

Table 54.2. Nomenclature for Factor VIII and von Willebrand Factor

Definition	International Nomenclature
Protein lacking or aberrant in hemophilia A	Factor VIII
Functional property of factor VIII that is deficient in hemophilia A and measured using coagulation assays	Factor VIIIc
Antigenic property of factor VIII that is measured by immunoassays in which homologous antibodies are used	Factor VIII$_{Ag}$
Protein required for normal platelet adhesion that is aberrant or deficient in von Willebrand disease	von Willebrand factor (vWF)
Antigenic property of vWF that is measured by immunoassays in which heterologous antibodies are used	vWF antigen (vWF$_{Ag}$)
Property of vWF required for platelet agglutination by ristocetin	Ristocetin cofactor activity (vWF:RCo)

This table is based on recommendations of the International Committee on Thrombosis and Haemostasis.
From Marder VJ, Mannucci PM, Firkin BG, Hoyer LW, Meyer D. Standard nomenclature for factor VIII and von Willebrand factor: a recommendation by the International Committee on Thrombosis and Haemostasis. *Thromb Haemost*. 1985;54:871-872; Mazurier C, Rodeghiero F. Recommended abbreviations for von Willebrand factor and its activities. *Thromb Haemost*. 2001;86:712.

for factor IX is factor IX Padua, in which a leucine was substituted for arginine at position 338 (R338L) and, despite a normal concentration of factor IX protein in plasma, the factor IX clotting activity was 8 times normal, resulting in clinically significant thrombosis.[3]

HEMOPHILIA A

Hemophilia A refers to the inherited coagulation disorder characterized by deficiency of function of the coagulation protein called factor VIII. Except for vWD, it is the most common inherited coagulation disorder, and is X-linked. Complete monographs have reviewed the early literature.[4] However, the bleeding disorder that occurred in males throughout the royal families of Europe because of a mutation that arose with Queen Victoria, long assumed to be the more common hemophilia A, turned out, after extensive medical forensic investigation, to be hemophilia B.[5]

Pathophysiology

The hemostatic abnormality in hemophilia A (factor VIII deficiency, classic hemophilia) is a deficiency or functional abnormality of the plasma protein factor VIII. It normally circulates in the plasma bound to a much larger molecule, von Willebrand factor (vWF). The half-life of factor VIII in the absence of vWF is much shorter, as seen in individuals with the vWF Normandy mutation, resulting in loss of the protein sequences for the binding interaction site between factor VIII and vWF, and causing low levels of factor VIII and clinical bleeding that appears similar to the bleeding seen in patients with hemophilia A. The production of vWF is coded by an autosomal gene, and this protein is qualitatively normal and is present in normal or increased amounts in patients with hemophilia A.[6] The function of the coagulation protein factor VIII is to serve (when activated) as a cofactor for the serine protease enzyme factor IX, and accelerate activation of factor X.

Incidence

Using a meta-analysis of registry data from Australia, Canada, France, Italy, New Zealand, and the United Kingdom, the prevalence for all severities of hemophilia A is estimated at 17.1 cases per 100 000 males.[7] In the United States, data from the US HTC network reported an average hemophilia A incidence of 1 case per 5617 live male births.[8]

Genetics

Hemophilia A is a classic example of an X-linked recessive trait. In such a disorder, the defective gene is located on the X chromosome[9]; the factor VIII gene maps to Xq28, on the distal end of the long arm of the X chromosome. In males who lack a normal allele, the defect is manifested by clinical hemophilia (*Figure 54.1*; generation I, number 1). The affected male does not transmit the disorder to his sons (generation II, numbers 4 and 5) because his Y chromosome is normal. However, all of his daughters are obligate carriers of the trait because they inherit his X chromosome (generation II, numbers 2 and 3). The female carrier transmits the disorder to half of her sons (generation III, numbers 6 and 7) and the carrier state to half of her daughters (generation III, numbers 8 and 9). Female carriers may or may not be affected clinically because of the presence of a normal allele from the mother. Because of lyonization of the X chromosome, if the normal factor VIII allele is inactivated more often by chance, then some of the female carriers may have clinical bleeding. The severity of their bleeding depends on their factor VIII activity level, and, rarely, a woman can have very low factor VIII activity and present with symptoms of moderate or even severe hemophilia.

The severity of bleeding varies in different kindreds, and closely depends on the particular genetic defect. As the same gene defect is present in the kindred, each of the affected males will have very similar clinical phenotypes.[10] Occasionally, however, the coinheritance of other genetic defects can influence the clinical symptoms of hemophilia A patients. An example is the coinheritance of the factor V Leiden mutation with hemophilia A. These patients have a milder clinical phenotype than expected for the same molecular defect in

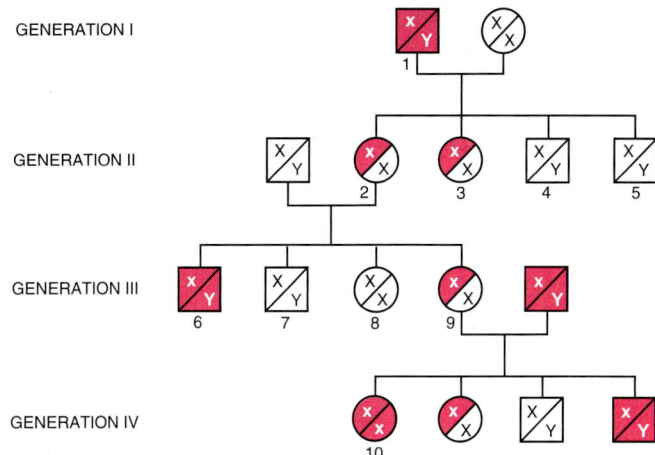

FIGURE 54.1 The inheritance of hemophilia A and hemophilia B. The pedigree is hypothetical. Squares indicate male; circles indicate female; fully shaded squares or circles indicate affected members; half-shaded circles indicate carriers. X, normal X chromosome; x, abnormal X chromosome; Y, normal Y chromosome.

factor VIII.[11] The coinheritance of the factor V Leiden mutation or other prothrombotic risk factors in children with severe hemophilia A may delay the first symptomatic bleeding event.[12]

Intriguing, and yet to be fully explained, is the fact that in over a third of families with hemophilia A, there is no evidence or history of abnormal bleeding in other members of the family.[13] This percentage is consistent with the Haldane hypothesis, which predicted that maintenance of a consistent frequency of a genetic disorder in the population would require that approximately one-third of cases result from spontaneous mutation. In other instances, neonatal deaths or the passage of the trait through a succession of female carriers may explain the negative family history. For practical purposes, therefore, a negative family history is of little value in excluding the possibility of hemophilia A. The large size of the factor VIII gene (186 kb), the presence of hot spots (e.g., CpG dinucleotides), and the fact that the X chromosome is unpaired in males may predispose for the factor VIII gene to undergo spontaneous mutation.[14,15]

Thousands of individuals with hemophilia worldwide have had their factor VIII genes analyzed; this genetic information is available through the Centers for Disease Control and Prevention Hemophilia Mutation Project (CHAMP and CHBMP), and includes mutations listed originally in the Hemophilia A Mutation, Structure, Test and Resource Site database.[16] In the United States, the *My Life Our Future* program enrolled over 6000 males with hemophilia A and provided hemophilia genotype analysis for these patients.[17]

The genetic defects of hemophilia A encompass deletions, insertions, and mutations throughout the factor VIII gene.[18] Point mutations involving CpG dinucleotides are especially common. Approximately 5% of patients with hemophilia A have large (>50 nucleotides) deletions in the factor VIII gene.[19]

Approximately 45% of severe hemophilia A cases result from a major inversion of a section of the tip of the long arm of the X chromosome, one breakpoint of which is situated within intron 22 of the factor VIII gene.[20] This common inversion is associated with severe hemophilia A, and a higher incidence of inhibitor formation. It is presumed that in the absence of homologous X chromosome pairing during male meiosis, an intrachromosomal recombination event occurs on the single X chromosome, resulting in this inversion. This event typically occurs in the father of the mother of a child with severe hemophilia A. Another common inversion (intron 1) accounts for 5% of patients with severe factor VIII deficiency.[21] Thus, two inversions of the factor VIII gene are seen in nearly one-half of all severely affected patients with hemophilia A. In contrast, point mutations are most likely found in patients with mild to moderate hemophilia A.[22] More than 98% of hemophilia A patients have mutations detected.[15,17] Approximately

2% of hemophilia A patients have no detectable mutations in the coding region of the factor VIII gene[23]; use of next generation sequencing identifies deep intronic mutations in these patients.[24]

There is a strong association between genetic mutations that lead to the absence of large portions of the factor VIII protein and the development of antibodies to therapeutic factor VIII infusions. These antibodies generally develop within the first 50 infusions of factor VIII, as expected when the immune system detects a protein to which it has not been exposed previously.

Variants

Hemophilia A with autosomal dominant transmission has been reported; however, it is important to distinguish these "variant hemophilia A patients" with negative X-linked transmission from patients with variant vWD (type 2N, vWD Normandy), an autosomal vWD subtype caused by defective factor VIII binding to vWF and with a clinical picture similar to hemophilia A.[25]

Carrier Detection

Despite the high rate of spontaneous de novo mutations in hemophilia A, detection of females who are carriers is important. When the family history of a patient suggests risk for being a carrier, then coagulation-based assays are performed, followed by DNA testing. The daughter of a man with hemophilia is an obligate carrier, irrespective of whether she has symptomatic bleeding or not. Similarly, if a female has two sons with hemophilia, then she is likely a carrier; if she has one son with hemophilia and a family history of hemophilia, then she is likely a carrier; but if she has one son with hemophilia and a negative family history, then the odds are approximately 67% that she is a carrier. It is most efficient and less expensive if the DNA of the relative with hemophilia is available to identify the specific genetic mutation in that kindred; then only that specific mutation is evaluated in the potential carrier.[26]

Coagulation-Based Assays

Coagulation-based assays are not useful in confirming or excluding the carrier state due to their limitations. The regularity with which the abnormal factor VIII gene is suppressed by the normal allele in female carriers of hemophilia varies because of the phenomenon of random X chromosome inactivation (the Lyon hypothesis). Thus, although the mean concentration of factor VIIIc in the plasma of heterozygous female carriers is ~50% of that in normal women,[10,27] observed values scatter widely around this mean and often overlap with those found in the normal population. This is a result, in part, of the large error of assay methods and the wide range of factor VIIIc levels in normal subjects.

Although the demonstration of low levels of factor VIIIc by means of the usual assay methods strongly suggests the presence of the carrier state, the converse statement cannot be made with equal certainty—that is, the presence of normal levels of factor VIIIc does not reliably exclude the carrier state.[28] Furthermore, pregnancy and hormonal medications may increase the levels of factor VIIIc in female carriers.[29] Normal women and carriers with blood type A, B, or AB have higher levels of factor VIIIc and vWFAg than those with blood type O.[30]

The use of immunoassays for vWF improves carrier detection in hemophilia A.[31] These methods allow measurement of levels of vWF, which are normal[32] or increased in carriers of the disorder, despite mild but variable deficiencies of factor VIIIc. Results obtained when a bioassay and an immunoassay are performed on the same sample, and the ratio of VIIIc to vWF is computed, differentiate between the carrier population and the normal population with minimal overlap. This ratio normally ranges from 0.74 to 2.20 and was found to be from 0.18 to 0.90 in obligatory carriers. The overall detection rate ranged from 72% to 94% in such obligatory carriers[33] and from 48% to 51% in women without hemophilic sons or fathers.[31] In the latter group (possible carriers), 50% would be predicted to be carriers. Abnormally low ratios of VIIIc:vWF (false positives) have been encountered in an occasional normal subject, which may be attributable to nonspecific variables such as stress.[33] Pregnancy and the use of oral contraceptives, blood type,[30] or contamination of plasma samples with thrombin[33] or other proteolytic enzymes may produce falsely high ratios (false negatives) in documented obligatory carriers.

DNA-Based Assays

Molecular analyses of the factor VIII gene identify mutations in over 98% of hemophilia A patients.[17] Based on the frequency of the intron 22 inversion, severe hemophilia A patients should be initially screened for this defect. Inversion-negative patients and those with mild or moderate hemophilia A should have systematic sequencing of the factor VIII promoter, exons, and splice junctions performed. The subject of genetic counseling in hemophilia has been reviewed.[34]

Hemophilia in the Female

Hemophilia has been well documented in females.[35] The most common form is that seen in a minority of heterozygous carriers, discussed previously, in whom X chromosome inactivation may occur at an unusually early stage of embryogenesis, resulting in unusually low levels of factor VIII. A second cause of female hemophilia is a mating between an affected male and a carrier female (*Figure 54.1*; generation IV, number 10).[36] One-half of the female offspring of such a match would inherit two abnormal X chromosomes, one from the father and one from the mother.

Clinical Manifestations of Hemophilia

Prior to effective replacement therapy, the life expectancy for a child born with severe hemophilia was less than 20 years. These boys would die from exsanguinating hemorrhage after a trivial traumatic injury, from spontaneous internal bleeding, or from spontaneous intracranial hemorrhage. It is dramatic that a boy born today with severe hemophilia A can expect to have a normal life expectancy.

The most characteristic bleeding manifestations in hemophilia are spontaneous bleeding in weight-bearing joints, leading to severe hemarthrosis. The frequency and severity of these joint bleeds are related to the functional activity level of factor VIII in plasma[37] (*Table 54.3*). Three categories of severity have been defined by a consensus committee on the basis of FVIII activity levels (*Table 54.3*).[38] Severe hemophilia (factor VIII level <1 IU/dL) is manifested clinically by repeated and severe hemarthroses, resulting almost invariably in crippling arthropathy in the absence of factor replacement therapy. Moderate hemophilia (factor VIII level of 1-5 IU/dL) is associated with less frequent and less severe hemarthroses but can result in serious orthopedic disability for those presenting with a severe phenotype. In mild hemophilia (factor VIII

Table 54.3. Prevalence and Severity of Hemophilia A and Hemophilia B in the United States

Factor VIII or IX Level (IU/dL)	Clinical Picture[a]	Percentage of Patients Seen at US HTC (%)[b]	
		Hemophilia A	Hemophilia B
<1	Severe, spontaneous bleeding	48	27
1-5	Moderate bleeding with minimal trauma or surgery	16	36
6-40	Mild bleeding with major trauma or surgery	34	35

[a]The criteria for classifying hemophilia severity are taken from White GC II, Rosendaal F, Aledort M, Lusher JM, Rothschild C, Ingerslev J; Factor VIII and Factor IX Subcommittee. Definitions in hemophilia. Recommendation of the scientific subcommittee on factor VIII and factor IX of the scientific and standardization committee of the International Society on Thrombosis and Haemostasis. *Thromb Haemost.* 2001;85:560.
[b]Numbers are from analyses of the 2016-2018 CDC Community Counts data of hemophilia patients who received care at United States hemophilia treatment centers (HTC) and are taken from Schieve LA, Byams VR, Dupervil B, et al. Evaluation of CDC's Hemophilia Surveillance Program — Universal Data Collection (1998-2011) and Community Counts (2011-2019), United States. *MMWR Surveill Summ.* 2020;69(5):1-18.

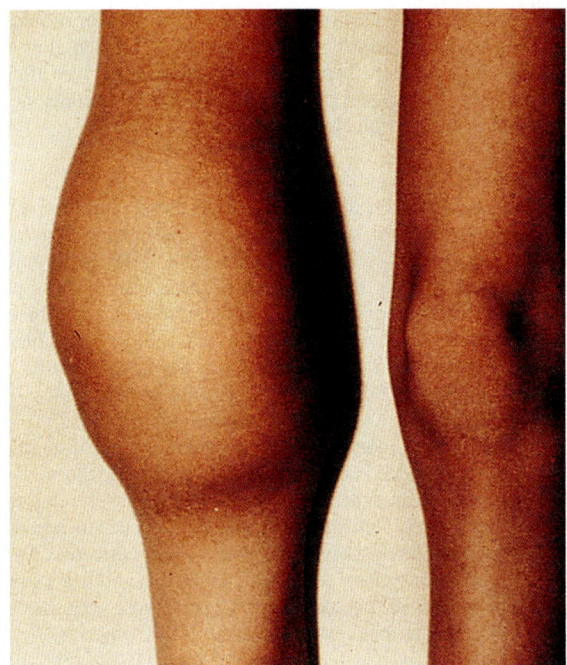

FIGURE 54.2 Hemophilic arthropathy. This figure illustrates the sequelae of recurrent joint bleeding.

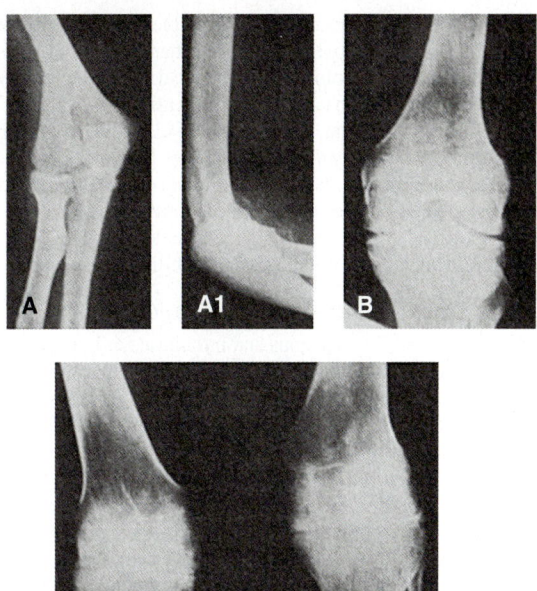

FIGURE 54.3 Elbow and knee joints in a patient with hemophilia A. Thickening of synovium with deposition of calcium is shown in (A) and (A1); increased intercondylar notch is shown in (B); increased density and decreased interarticular space are shown in (A-C); and lipping along the borders of the joint surfaces is shown in (C).

level of 6-40 IU/dL), hemarthroses and other spontaneous bleeding manifestations may be absent altogether, although serious bleeding may follow surgical procedures or traumatic injury.[39] As indicated in *Table 54.3*, most patients with hemophilia A have severe disease.

Hemarthrosis

Hemarthrosis is the most common manifestation of the inherited coagulation disorders (*Figure 54.2*). Joint bleeding and the consequent damage to weight-bearing joints remain the most common debilitating symptom in severe hemophilia.

Pathophysiology

Bleeding presumably originates from the synovial vessels and develops spontaneously or as the result of trivial trauma. Hemorrhage occurs in the joint cavity or in the diaphysis or epiphysis of the bone. In the acute stage, the synovial space is distended with blood. Muscular spasm further increases the intrasynovial pressure. Hemorrhage in the periarticular structures is a common complicating feature that occurs most often around small joints. In many patients, permanent joint damage, detectable by MRI, appears to occur after only one or two minor bleeds in a single joint.[40] An in vitro study demonstrated that interleukin-1β is the key cytokine mediating the destructive effects of blood on cartilage.[41]

The joint may regain normal function after the first few episodes of hemarthrosis. More often, however, the absorption of intra-articular blood is incomplete, and acute bleeding leads to chronic inflammation of the synovial membrane with the development of long-term damage to the joint. Sometimes, the joint remains swollen, tender, and painful for months, and in this setting may often suffer episodes of rebleeding. Such a joint is often termed a "target joint," and should be treated aggressively with physical therapy and appropriate factor replacement to interrupt the vicious cycle of inflammation, swollen synovium, and recurrent bleeding. Release of inflammatory cell cytokines and proteolytic enzymes mediates destruction of cartilage and bone.[41,42]

Acute hemarthroses almost invariably recur from time to time. With each recurrence, the synovium becomes progressively more thickened and vascular; folds and villi, which predispose to synovial injury during even minimal activity, may form. Proliferating synovium often fills and distends the joint, which remains swollen and enlarged in the absence of bleeding or pain (chronic proliferative synovitis).[43] Together with the weakening of the periarticular supporting structures, this process predisposes the joint to recurrent episodes of bleeding.

Repeated episodes of hemarthrosis, with the associated subchondral and synovial ischemia, result in progressive loss of hyaline cartilage, particularly at the margins of the joint. Through disuse, diffuse demineralization of the involved bones may also occur.

The terminal stage of hemarthrosis is called *chronic hemophilic arthropathy*.[44] It is manifested by fibrous or bony ankylosis of larger joints; complete destruction may take place in the smaller articulations because of the weaker joint structure and the thinner cortices of the smaller bones. Other permanent sequelae of hemarthrosis include atrophy and proliferation of bone, roughening of the articular surfaces with lipping and osteophyte formation, bone necrosis and cyst formation, stunted growth as the result of interference with the nutrition of the bone, and accelerated development and overgrowth of the epiphyses caused by excessive blood flow (*Figures 54.2* and *54.3*). Chronic hemophilic arthropathy is less common now because of widespread use of prophylactic replacement therapy. The challenges of chronic hemophilia arthropathy are reviewed here.[45]

Magnetic resonance imaging is superior to standard radiography for assessment of early arthropathy.[46] A scoring system for magnetic resonance joint evaluation has been reported[46] (*Table 54.4*).

Clinical Presentation

Most persons with severe hemophilia report a characteristic warm, tingling sensation before the onset of symptoms of joint bleeding and hemarthrosis; this is called the *aura*. The earliest definite symptom is pain, which in the acute form may be excruciating. Physical examination reveals muscle spasm and limited motion of the affected joint. If

Table 54.4. Scoring System for Hemophilic Arthropathy Using Magnetic Resonance Imaging

Score	Abnormalities on Imaging
0	None
I	Minimal hemosiderin
II	Large amount of hemosiderin and cartilaginous erosion
III	Cartilage destruction, bone erosion, subchondral cysts
IV	Osteoarthritis with or without ankylosis

therapy is not initiated immediately, typically within approximately 30 minutes, then the bleed may progress so that the joint is warm and grossly distended and discolored, but external evidence of bleeding may be minimal or absent in chronically damaged large joints because of thickening of the articular capsule. The weight-bearing joints are most commonly affected, and the knees are the joints most often severely affected. However, because of the success of total knee and total hip replacement surgeries, the ankles are the most commonly affected joints that lead to chronic problems that interfere with the quality of life for persons with severe hemophilia.

Subcutaneous and Intramuscular Hematomas

Large ecchymoses and subcutaneous and intramuscular hematomas were common in severe hemophilia A prior to the use of regular factor infusion therapy. With modern treatment protocols designed to keep plasma factor VIII levels above 1% of normal, and immediate home infusion when a bleeding episode occurs, the frequency of large soft-tissue bleeds has decreased dramatically. Such hemorrhages, when not treated promptly, characteristically spread within fascial spaces and dissect deeper structures (see Figure 46.2). When not treated promptly with factor infusion, the bleeding continues; and at the site of origin, the tissue is hard, indurated, raised, and purplish black. From this center, the hemorrhage extends in all directions, with each successive concentric extension less deeply colored. The point of origin of the hemorrhage may be absorbed entirely while the margin is still progressing. Intramuscular and subcutaneous hematomas may produce leukocytosis, fever, and severe pain in the absence of significant discoloration of the overlying skin.

Hematomas may produce serious consequences from the compression of vital structures. Bleeding in the tongue, throat, or neck may develop spontaneously and is especially dangerous because it may compromise the airway with surprising rapidity.[47] Gangrene may result from pressure on arteries; the development of compartment syndrome and, if not promptly treated, ischemic contractures are common sequelae of hemorrhage in the calves or forearms. Peripheral nerve lesions of varying severity are common complications of untreated hemorrhage in joints or muscles. Hemophilic cysts are discussed in the section Special Aspects of Treatment.

Psoas and Retroperitoneal Hematomas

Spontaneous hemorrhage in internal fascial spaces and muscles of the abdomen is common in severe hemophilia A, reflecting plasma factor levels less than 1% of normal. Bleeding in or around the iliopsoas muscle produces pain of progressively increasing severity and tenderness; when it occurs on the right side, it may closely simulate acute appendicitis. Femoral nerve involvement may be partial or complete, with the development of pain on the anterior surface of the thigh. The psoas sign is positive, and the hip is held in partial flexion. Paresthesias, partial or complete anesthesia, and, ultimately, weakness or paralysis of the thigh extensors with eventual muscular atrophy may ensue. Retroperitoneal hemorrhage and intraperitoneal hemorrhage are also common. Prompt factor infusion is critical to normalize coagulation and should be continued until the hematoma has resolved completely, as any residual hematoma is at higher risk for rebleeding and pseudocyst formation.

Gastrointestinal and Genitourinary Bleeding

Hemorrhage from the mouth, gums, lips, frenulum, and tongue is common and often serious. The eruption and shedding of deciduous teeth usually occur without abnormal bleeding, but may occasionally be accompanied by hemorrhage that lasts for days or weeks if not treated. Epistaxis occurs in many patients and may be of exsanguinating proportions.

Hematemesis, melena, or both are not uncommon. The source of the bleeding is usually the upper gastrointestinal tract. In most patients in whom bleeding is persistent or recurrent, it originates from a structural lesion, most commonly a peptic ulcer or gastritis. Hemorrhage may be accompanied by abdominal pain, distention, increased peristalsis, fever, and leukocytosis. Intramural bleeding in the intestinal wall may result in intussusception or obstruction.

Hematuria is more common than gastrointestinal bleeding, but it is less often the result of a demonstrable pathologic condition in the genitourinary tract. The bleeding may arise in the bladder or in one or both kidneys and may persist for days or weeks.[48] When clots form, ureteral colic may develop. Typically, the hematuria resolves after factor infusion, but if persistent, then a short course of prednisone may prove helpful to shorten the course of hematuria.[49]

Traumatic Bleeding

Patients with coagulation disorders seldom bleed abnormally from small cuts such as razor nicks, reflecting the normal function of platelets, as measured by platelet function tests. After larger injuries, however, hemorrhage out of proportion to the extent of the injury is characteristic. The bleeding reflects both increased acute bleeding rates beyond what is expected after the trauma, and persistent bleeding as slow continuous oozing occurs for days, weeks, or months. Such traumatic bleeding may be massive and life-threatening unless factor replacement therapy is provided by immediate factor infusion.

Delayed bleeding is common. Thus, although hemostasis after an injury or a minor surgical procedure may appear to be adequate, hemorrhage, often of sudden onset and serious proportions, may develop several hours or even days later. This phenomenon apparently occurs because the processes of primary hemostasis are only temporarily effective. Delayed bleeding may occur in patients with mild hemophilia and is a significant hazard after minor surgical procedures, particularly those performed on an outpatient basis, such as tooth extraction and tonsillectomy.

Other Clinical Aspects

Infants usually are asymptomatic because they are insulated from trauma.[50] However, trauma during birth or afterward may trigger life-threatening bleeding. Infants of women who are known carriers may be at risk during delivery, and instrumentation during vaginal delivery should be avoided. Currently, the usual standard of care is to allow normal vaginal delivery with backup Caesarean section available if any difficulties arise during birth. Typically, hematomas are seen first when children become active, and hemarthroses seldom develop until they begin to walk. Occasionally, evidence of the disorder is not seen until patients reach teenage years or young adult life. Spontaneous hemorrhage may be cyclic in nature. Hemorrhage from the umbilical cord or stump is unusual, but prolonged bleeding after circumcision is common and brought hemophilia to the attention of the ancient Hebrews. Spontaneous rupture of the spleen has been reported. Intracranial bleeding is discussed in the section Special Aspects of Treatment. The website of the National Hemophilia Foundation (www.hemophilia.org) contains useful information and links to more detailed information on this bleeding disorder.

Course and Prognosis

In recent years, the prognosis in severe hemophilia has improved dramatically.[51] With modern therapy using regular factor infusions to maintain adequate plasma factor concentrations to prevent nearly all spontaneous bleeding episodes, a person born with severe hemophilia A can expect to live an essentially normal life span. No other genetic disease has made such dramatic progress in the past 50 years. It is not yet clear whether hemophilia protects older hemophilia patients from thromboembolic disorders,[52] atherosclerosis,[53] or cardiovascular diseases.[53] Despite the lack of stringent prospective clinical studies for this emerging problem of aging patients with severe hemophilia and other medical problems, reviews of current practice and expert opinion on how to treat aging patients with severe hemophilia have been published.[54-56] A recent CDC database analysis identified liver failure from hepatitis C infection as the most common cause of death in men with severe hemophilia.[51]

Laboratory Diagnosis

The activity of the various coagulation factors is expressed in terms of units, defined as the activity present in 1 mL of fresh plasma from normal donors. The concentration of all coagulation factors in normal pooled plasma is thus 1 IU/mL or 100 IU/dL, or 100% activity. It should be noted that the activity levels in blood bank plasma are somewhat lower, approximately 80 IU/dL because of the dilution with anticoagulant.

The presence or absence of anemia or of signs of blood regeneration depends on the severity and frequency of bleeding, as in any individual patient. Neutrophilia may accompany severe hemorrhage, and the destruction of red blood cells in the hematoma may be reflected in elevated lactate dehydrogenase, aspartate aminotransferase, or bilirubin. As in other instances of posthemorrhagic anemia, the bone marrow reflects the response to blood loss.

Screening Tests of Hemostasis and Coagulation

The partial thromboplastin time (PTT) usually is prolonged in patients with hemophilia A (*Table 54.5*). The biochemical conditions for most laboratory assays of PTT are set so that the PTT is abnormal if the factor VIII level is <25% of normal; however, some PTT reagents are insensitive to mild factor VIII deficiency.[57] Therefore, in most situations, the abnormality of the PTT can be normalized by mixing the patient's plasma with normal plasma in a ratio of 1:1; and this test, called a mixing study, is routinely used to detect whether neutralizing factor VIII antibodies are present. The platelet count usually is normal, but may be elevated in the stress reaction to hemorrhage.

Factor VIIIc Assays

Assay of factor VIII is a simple technique, but requires trained and experienced technicians, as the results are sensitive to errors in laboratory technique, or to errors in proper handling of the blood specimen. Two-stage methods,[58] one-stage methods,[59] and micromethods[60] are suitable for diagnosis. The one-stage techniques are used most widely because they are simple to perform. Two-stage assays detect approximately 20% more factor VIII than do one-stage methods,[61] and they are less subject to variables[62] such as fluctuations attributable to contaminating traces of thrombin or other proteolytic enzymes.

The World Health Organization makes international standards, but many laboratories purchase commercial secondary standards that are calibrated to the international standard. Under most circumstances, a pool of citrated plasma carefully collected from normal subjects and frozen in individual laboratories also serves as an acceptable standard.

Chromogenic substrate assays or typical one-stage PTT assays using physiologic phospholipids are needed to quantitate factor VIII levels accurately in patients receiving B domain–deleted factor VIII.[63] Alternatively, a standard one-stage PTT assay using B domain–deleted factor VIII as the assay standard would be appropriate. The increasing use of modified (extended half-life) factor VIII products which may not be accurately measured by standard one-stage coagulation assays is a potential clinical problem.[64] The Scientific Subcommittee on Standards of the International Society of Thrombosis and Haemostasis is involved in defining appropriate standards for these new products. The appropriate choice of assays for laboratory measurement of FVIII replacement therapy for patients with hemophilia has been reviewed.[65]

Differential Diagnosis

The diagnosis of hemophilia A is seldom difficult, especially in the severely affected patient with repeated and often serious hemorrhagic manifestations, including such characteristic signs as hemarthrosis. Typically, the PTT is abnormal and leads to specific assays for clotting factor activity and mixing studies to rule out neutralizing inhibitors of coagulation activity. Hemarthrosis with significant orthopedic disability is rare in patients with coagulation disorders other than hemophilia A or B.

In patients with mild forms of the disorder, however, failure to recognize the existence of the disease or to make the correct diagnosis is more likely. Such patients rarely have a history of spontaneous bleeding, and the family history tends to be vague or negative. A history of abnormal bleeding after minor trauma may be difficult to establish because of variability in bleeding. Occasionally, mild hemophilia A may present with a normal PTT when the factor VIII activity assay result is greater than 25%; thus, a normal PTT may be misleading. It must be emphasized that individuals with mild hemophilia are still at risk for hazardous hemorrhage after trauma or during surgical procedures.[66] A survey of hemophilia carriers found that mild reduction in factor VIII or IX levels (41-60 IU/dL) was associated with excessive bleeding.[67] In the mildly affected patient, specific factor assays and occasionally genetic testing must be performed to confirm or exclude the diagnosis of hemophilia.

The results of screening tests (*Table 54.5*) usually are sufficient to exclude the possibility of acquired hemorrhagic disorders associated

Table 54.5. Laboratory Findings in Common Inherited Coagulation Disorders

Disorder	Partial Thromboplastin Time (PTT)	Prothrombin Time	Thrombin Time	Ancillary Tests
Hemophilia A	A	N	N	vWF antigen and activities are normal or increased; ratio of VIIIc:vWF is low.
Hemophilia B[a]	A	N[a]	N	–
von Willebrand disease[a,b]	A or N	N	N	vWF antigen and VIIIc are usually low; ratio of VIIIc:vWF is variable; ristocetin-induced platelet aggregation and ristocetin cofactor activity are usually diminished.
Afibrinogenemia	A	A	A	Platelet function may be abnormal.
Dysfibrinogenemia[a]	vA	vA	A[c,d]	Hypofibrinogenemia,[e] reptilase time is prolonged,[a] fibrin(o)gen degradation products levels are increased.[a]
Hypoprothrombinemia[a]	A	A	N	Two-stage assay is abnormal.[f]
Factor V deficiency	A	A	N	–
Factor VII deficiency[a]	N	A	N	Stypven (Russell viper venom) time is normal.
Factor X deficiency[a]	A	A	N	Stypven time is abnormal.
Factor XI deficiency	A	N	N	–
Factor XII deficiency	A	N	N	–
Factor XIII deficiency	N	N	N	Clot solubility tests are abnormal.

Certain PTT reagents may not detect mild deficiency of factors VIII, IX, and XI.
Abbreviations: A, abnormal; N, normal; v, variable; vWF, von Willebrand factor.
[a]Findings are significantly different in some variants.
[b]Coagulation abnormalities are caused by deficiency of factor VIIIc.
[c]Patient's plasma may inhibit normal coagulation.
[d]Abnormality may be corrected by increasing calcium concentration and may be magnified by diluting the thrombin solution.
[e]Abnormality varies depending on technique.
[f]Results of one-stage techniques may be uninterpretable.

with serious bleeding. Such disorders are seldom associated with a prolonged PTT and a normal prothrombin time (PT), a combination that strongly suggests an inherited disorder or an inhibitor. Among the inherited disorders characterized by this combination of findings (hemophilia A, hemophilia B, and deficiencies of factors XI, XII, prekallikrein, and high-molecular-weight kininogen [HMWK]), deficiency of the latter three factors can be readily excluded because their deficiency is not associated with excessive clinical bleeding. Factor XI deficiency in males may mimic mild hemophilia, and hemophilia B is clinically identical to hemophilia A. Both factor XI deficiency and hemophilia B must be distinguished from hemophilia A in the laboratory using specific factor activity assays. The best way to accomplish this goal in evaluating patients with an isolated prolonged PTT is by performing specific assays of these three factors in the order of their statistical frequency—that is, VIII, IX, and XI. A PTT mixing study should also be performed to exclude an inhibitor. A definitive diagnosis is of great importance because specific products are used to treat each of these disorders.

Severe vWD in males may be indistinguishable from mild hemophilia A. Confirmatory tests for vWD are needed to make this distinction. Patients with the uncommon type 2N vWD may also be clinically indistinguishable from patients with hemophilia A. This diagnosis is important to establish, because therapeutic infusions of recombinant factor VIII (r-FVIII) would be ineffective because of the shortened half-life of factor VIII resulting from the absence of effective binding to von Willebrand protein. An X-linked family history of bleeding supports a diagnosis of hemophilia A in these patients, and an autosomal recessive family history of bleeding supports a diagnosis of type 2N vWD. Statistically, one would expect a rare family that might carry both genetic disorders; clearly that situation may be problematic to resolve without additional genetic testing.

Intra-abdominal bleeding raises particularly serious diagnostic and therapeutic problems in the patient with hemophilia, even when the hemophilia condition has been accurately diagnosed. Thus, hemorrhage into the psoas, when on the right side, may simulate acute appendicitis so closely that, in the opinion of many experienced clinicians, there is no reliable clinical means to differentiate between the two diagnoses. A retroperitoneal hematoma may be mistaken for an appendiceal abscess. Intraperitoneal hemorrhage and bleeding into and around other viscera may simulate perforating peptic ulcer, bowel obstruction, or virtually any acute intra-abdominal condition. Computed tomography scanning and sonography may be particularly helpful in differentiating between intraabdominal conditions that require surgical intervention and retroperitoneal and psoas hemorrhages. In any case, early therapeutic infusion of factor VIII will prevent further bleeding and carries no additional risk for the individual with hemophilia. Therefore, when there is a question and further diagnostic tests are planned, factor VIII should be administered first and promptly before the diagnostic tests are performed.

HEMOPHILIA B

Hemophilia B was recognized as a separate disorder from hemophilia A in 1947.[68] Hemophilia B (Christmas disease, factor IX deficiency) was established as different from hemophilia A by Aggeler et al in 1952.[69,70] Hemophilia A is approximately 5 times more common than hemophilia B, with an estimated prevalence for all severities of hemophilia B at 3.8 cases per 100 000 males.[7] As expected, it appears that the severity of hemophilia B is a consequence of the plasma factor IX concentration, and that for any particular plasma concentration, the clinical severity is similar for hemophilia A and B. However, in contrast with hemophilia A, most of the genetic causes of hemophilia B are not large deletions or inversions; therefore, in many patients there is some antigenic protein, and often some low level of function of the mutated protein. Consequently, the clinical phenotype may be less severe. As with hemophilia A, hemophilia B is classified as severe, moderate, or mild based on the percentage of functional factor IX in coagulation activity assays. In addition, because of the presence of low levels of factor IX protein in more patients with hemophilia B, there are fewer persons with hemophilia B who develop neutralizing inhibitors (approximately 3% vs more than 25% in hemophilia A).

In a disorder called *hemophilia B Leyden*,[71] the clinical manifestations tend to diminish during puberty in association with a rise in the factor IX level from as low as 1 IU/dL in childhood to levels of 20 IU/dL or more in adult life. The genetic basis for factor IX Leyden is that mutations occur in the factor IX gene promoter region; this region contains an androgen response element that, with age, stimulates factor IX gene transcription and protein synthesis.[72]

Numerous factor IX mutations have been recognized.[15,73] Factor IX purified from the plasma of affected members of one kindred did not fragment normally when activated in vitro (hemophilia B Chapel Hill).[74] The molecular defect was found to be a substitution of histidine for arginine at position 145, a defect that inhibits cleavage by factor XIa.[74] Studies of factor IX obtained from another family revealed biochemical abnormalities identical to those characteristic of the descarboxy analog of this factor that is found in vitamin K deficiency or produced by coumarin drugs. Such molecules lack Ca^{2+}-binding sites and do not undergo conformational changes induced by Ca^{2+}.

Genetics

Hemophilia B is inherited as an X-linked recessive trait, but the locus on the X chromosome of the gene controlling factor IX production is remote from that involved with factor VIII biosynthesis.[75] Factor IX levels <10% have been documented in a few women, including some with chromosomal abnormalities.[76,77] An updated listing of mutations is available at www.factorix.org.[78] Unlike hemophilia A, the spontaneous mutation rate is low,[13] and most patients with hemophilia B have positive family histories.

Factor IX defects may be severe, moderate, or mild. Severe defects result from large gene deletions, nonsense mutations, and inversions; these defects are associated with absence of factor IX protein. Milder gene defects such as splice-site or missense mutations result in a dysfunctional protein with some residual activity. Missense mutations account for ~80% of mutations in severe hemophilia B patients.[15,78,79]

Detection of Carriers

Detection of heterozygous carriers of hemophilia B involves the same principles and limitations as described for hemophilia A. Carrier detection based on coagulation assay alone is slightly more reliable than is the case with hemophilia A.[80] In one series of 45 obligatory carriers, the mean factor IX level in the plasma was 33 IU/dL; 40 from the group had levels <50 IU/dL, and 10 had levels <25 IU/dL. As a consequence of these low levels of factor IX, abnormal bleeding symptoms are not uncommon in carriers of hemophilia B.

Results of immunoassays of factor IX and the ratio of factor IX–related antigen to coagulant factor IX levels in the carrier population overlap with the normal population to a considerable degree, particularly in the cross-reacting material (CRM)–positive variants.[81] The use of DNA probes[82] provides highly accurate methods for determining carrier status. Rapid carrier testing using allele-specific microarray methods has been described. This method permits detection of a majority of common factor IX mutations in a single assay.[83] Determination of carrier status is based on several factors, including pedigree analysis, factor IX assay results, and genotype.[84,85]

Clinical Features

Severely affected patients (those with factor IX activity levels <1 IU/dL) are less common than in hemophilia A (*Table 54.3*). Specific factor assays are necessary to distinguish between hemophilia A and hemophilia B. Mild factor IX deficiency should always be considered in the differential diagnosis of patients with coagulation-type bleeding and normal routine coagulation test results (PT, PTT).[86] Many PTT reagents do not detect mild factor IX deficiency (factor IX levels of 20%-30%).[57]

Laboratory Diagnosis

The laboratory diagnosis of hemophilia B involves the same approach and methods as those described for the recognition of hemophilia A

(*Table 54.5*). One-stage and two-stage assays for factor IX use the same principles as those discussed for factor VIIIc. Certain modified (extended half-life) factor IX products may not be accurately measured by standard one-stage coagulation assays, and chromogenic assays may be necessary for monitoring patients receiving these products.[65,87]

VON WILLEBRAND DISEASE

The historical confusion that has surrounded the pathogenesis of vWD is apparent from the many names that have been applied to this disorder. These designations include *angiohemophilia, vascular hemophilia, pseudohemophilia, constitutional thrombopathy,* and *idiopathic prolonged bleeding time*. von Willebrand first recognized the disorder in a 1926 study of the inhabitants of the Åland Islands.[88] Three cardinal manifestations of this bleeding disorder are mucocutaneous hemorrhage rather than hemarthrosis and deep-muscle bleeds; autosomal dominant inheritance, rather than sex-linked as seen in hemophilia A; and prolonged bleeding time. Evaluation of one large kindred revealed variable severity of bleeding symptoms, with some obligate heterozygote carriers being asymptomatic. von Willebrand thought that the hemostatic defect resulted from combined defects in platelet function and vascular endothelium. The discovery that plasma from normal volunteers or patients with hemophilia A corrected the hemostatic defect of vWD suggested that a plasma protein distinct from factor VIII caused vWD. In 1972, vWF was purified. Genetic variants were correlated with various vWF structural abnormalities, and demonstration of the heterogeneous nature of vWD was furthered by development of vWF multimer analysis by gel electrophoresis.[89] In its most common form (type 1), the disorder is characterized by mild mucocutaneous hemorrhage, which is attributable to deficiency of both vWF and factor VIIIc. The disorder is not homogeneous, however, in part because of the multiple physiologic functions played by vWF. The recognition of a number of variants, together with the demonstration of multiple genetic patterns, suggested that vWD is very heterogeneous. However, all forms of vWD can be traced to insufficient amounts of vWF or defective function of this protein. Recent reviews of this area have been published,[90,91] and a multidisciplinary guideline that included patient representatives on the diagnosis and management of vWD was recently published.[92,93]

Incidence

Epidemiologic studies indicate that vWD is the most common bleeding disorder, affecting about 1% of the population.[94] The high incidence of the disease is not limited to certain ethnic groups[94]; however, only a fraction of people come to medical attention because of bleeding symptoms. This may be because of either the relatively mild nature of the disease in many affected individuals or a lack of recognition by patients of excessive bleeding in response to either physiologic challenge (e.g., heavy menstrual bleeding) or trauma.

Nomenclature

The identification of numerous variants of vWD has led to a simplified classification of this disorder (*Table 54.6*). Quantitative defects are divided into partial deficiency (type 1) and severe deficiency with virtually complete absence of vWF (type 3). The qualitative defects (type 2) are divided into four categories according to the nature of the defect of vWF function. Type 2A refers to variants with impaired interaction between vWF and platelets, resulting from a deficiency of intermediate- and high-molecular-weight multimers of vWF. Type 2B refers to variants in which vWF exhibits increased affinity for its receptor, platelet GPIb. Paradoxically, bleeding in these patients develops as a result of clearance of larger vWF multimers and platelets from the circulation. Type 2M refers to variants with defective interaction between vWF and the platelet GPIb receptor that is not caused by a deficiency of high-molecular-weight multimers of vWF from plasma, but rather results from defects within the GPIb-binding domain of vWF. Finally, variants of vWD in which decreased affinity of vWF for factor VIII results in depressed plasma factor VIII levels are classified as type 2N.

Table 54.6. Revised Classification of von Willebrand Disease

Revised Type	Features
1	Partial deficiency of vWF
2	Qualitative vWF defects
2A	vWF variants with loss of high-molecular-weight multimers and decreased vWF-dependent platelet adhesion
2B	vWF variants with loss of high-molecular-weight multimers caused by increased affinity for platelet glycoprotein Ib
2M	vWF variants with decreased vWF-dependent platelet adhesion not associated with the loss of high-molecular-weight multimers
2N	vWF variants with decreased binding affinity for factor VIII
3	Severe deficiency of vWF

Abbreviation: vWF, von Willebrand factor.
Adapted from Sadler JE, Budde U, Eikenboom JC, et al. Update on the pathophysiology and classification of von Willebrand disease: a report of the Subcommittee on von Willebrand Factor. *J Thromb Haemost.* 2006;4(10):2103-2114. Copyright © 2006 International Society on Thrombosis and Haemostasis. With permission.

Thus, six major categories of vWD are defined, each having distinct pathophysiology.

Genetics

A gene on chromosome 12 codes for the synthesis of the vWF macromolecule. The genetic message is composed of 52 exons.[95,96] The vWF gene encodes for a protein with multiple copies of homologous motifs, including three "A," three "B," two "C," and four "D" motifs (see *Figure 54.4*). These motifs in turn encode protein domains that subserve the various functions of vWF. The A1 domain contains binding sites for platelet GPIb, ristocetin, and collagen, the A2 domain contains a protease-sensitive domain that may have a role in regulating vWF function, the A3 domain contains a second collagen-binding domain, the C1 domain has an RGD sequence capable of interacting with platelet glycoprotein IIb/IIIa, and the D′ and D3 domains contain a factor VIII–binding sequence.[97,98]

vWD appears to be inherited by multiple genetic mechanisms (*Table 54.7*). The most common form of the disorder (type 1 vWD) accounts for ~70% of all cases of vWD. Diagnostic criteria for type 1 vWD have been proposed, including a history of bleeding symptoms, a positive family history of bleeding symptoms, and bleeding that is attributable to quantitatively low vWF levels. Population screening suggests that the prevalence of vWD may be as high as 1% of the population, but only a minority of these patients subsequently present with clinically significant bleeding.[99] vWD is inherited as an incompletely dominant autosomal trait with variable penetrance, even among members within a single kindred. Because of variable penetrance and expression of vWD, only ~33% of children may be affected. *Figure 54.5* illustrates one of the original pedigrees described by von Willebrand.

Twin studies demonstrated that ~60% of the variation in vWF level and ~50% of the variation in factor VIII level is attributable to genetic factors.[100] Genetic loci outside of the vWF gene also contribute to variation of vWF level. Individuals with blood group O have vWF levels that are on average 30% lower than those of people with blood group A, B, or AB,[101] and it is likely that carbohydrate groups attached to vWF play a subtle role in clearance of vWF from plasma.[102] In addition, variation in expression of levels of other hemostatically active proteins, such as variation in the level of platelet adhesion receptors, may modulate the severity of symptoms conferred by vWF deficiency.[103] vWF levels are under hormonal and other controls, which further complicates disease expression. Variation in levels of as much as 20% has been reported with menstrual cycles, with levels lowest in the early follicular phase (before day 7 of the cycle); and levels increase with age, rising ~15% for each decade increase in

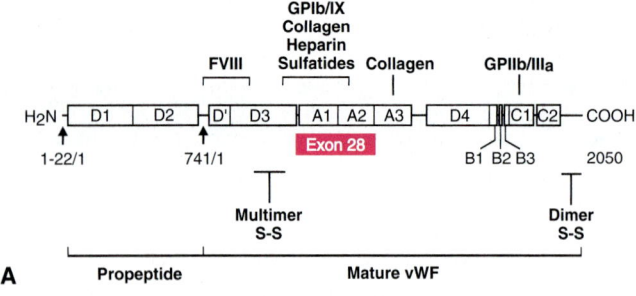
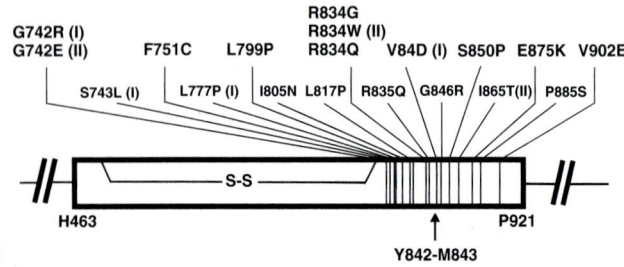
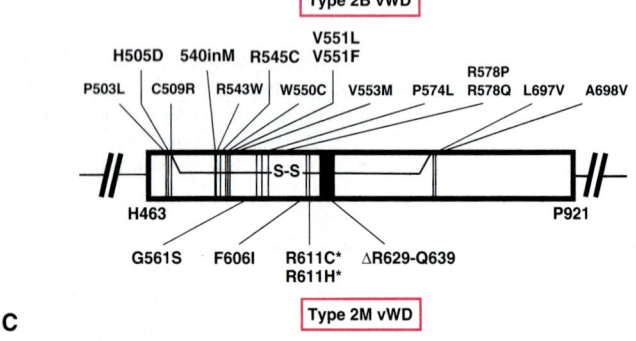

FIGURE 54.4 A, Structure and functional domains of von Willebrand factor (vWF). The open rectangles indicate domains of pre–pro-vWF. The first 22 amino acids of pre–pro-vWF are the signal sequence. The left arrow identifies the site of cleavage of the signal peptide, resulting in pre-vWF monomers. Pro-vWF monomers form dimers, and the vWF propeptide (vWAgII) is cleaved from mature vWF (right arrow indicates cleavage site). Dimer S–S and multimer S–S indicate locations of disulfide bonds that covalently link monomeric vWF into dimers and dimeric vWF into multimers, respectively. The red rectangle identifies exon 28, which encodes the A1 and A2 domains of mature vWF. Functional domains are identified above the open rectangles. The factor VIII binding site is located in the D′ and D3 domains in the amino-terminal 272 amino acids of mature vWF. The A domains of vWF contain the binding site for the platelet glycoprotein (GP) Ib/IX complex, as well as binding sites for heparin, collagen, and sulfatides. The GPIIb/IIIa complex binding site of activated platelets is located at the carboxy-terminal portion of the C1 domain and contains the Arg-Gly-Asp sequence. The numbers below the open rectangles indicate amino acid numbers: signal peptide, 22 amino acids; propeptide (vWAgII), 741 amino acids; mature vWF, 2050 amino acids. B, Mutations associated with type 2A von Willebrand disease (vWD). The open rectangle represents vWF exon 28 encoding domains A1 and A2. The arrow indicates the site of proteolysis seen in type 2A vWD. Mutations are identified using the single-letter code for amino acids. I and II identify group I and group II missense mutations that result in impaired synthesis of vWF or increased sensitivity to proteolysis in plasma, respectively. The disulfide bridge shown represents the boundary of the Cys 509-Cys 695 loop in the A1 domain. Type 2A vWD mutations associated with defective vWF multimerization are not shown in this figure; these latter mutations occur in the propeptide (vWAgII) D1 and D2 domains. C, Mutations associated with types 2B and 2M vWD. The large open rectangle represents exon 28, which encodes domains A1 and A2 of vWF. The mutations responsible for type 2B vWD are shown above the rectangle. Most type 2B mutations lie between residues 540 and 578 of mature vWF. The mutations responsible for type 2M vWD are shown below the rectangle. Asterisks identify mutations that reduce the platelet-dependent function of vWF and vWF multimeric size. Delta indicates deletion of an amino acid sequence. (Modified from the Symposium Proceedings of the National Hemophilia Foundation's 1995 Annual Meeting. Diagnosis and management of severe von Willebrand disease [types 2 and 3]. Kroner PA, Montgomery RR. The molecular basis of von Willebrand disease. *Baillieres Clin Haematol*. 1996:15-25.)

age.[104-106] As will be discussed later, the criteria for diagnosing quantitative vWD deficiency, and the specificity of historic bleeding, have courted controversy in what constitutes type 1 vWD and have led to the potential for the new diagnostic entity of "low vWF."[99,107]

Very low vWF levels in the range of 5 to 20 IU/dL tend to be highly inheritable and are frequently associated with "dominant negative"–acting mutations. Mutations in these patients with type 1 vWD appear to be different than those with type 3 disease, such that type 1 disease is not simply explained by being heterozygous for a type 3 allele. Genetic defects associated with these more severe type 1 phenotypes encode amino acid changes that in turn lead to defects in protein expression. Mechanisms responsible for decreased plasma vWF level include reduced secretion related to impaired intracellular transport of vWF subunits, increased clearance from the circulation, or accelerated catabolism as a result of increased susceptibility to degradation by ADAMTS13. Changes that were most likely to cause a "dominant negative" mechanism are often missense mutations that change the number of cysteine residues in the vWF protein. Although such changes probably affect vWF synthesis and trafficking in the cell, at least one common mutation (Tyr1584Cys) also results in enhanced degradation by ADAMTS13.[108,109] One non–cysteine-related mutation is seen in vWD Vicenza. In these patients, a mutation encoding for Arg1205His results in accelerated clearance of plasma vWF, with levels of vWF in the range of 15 IU/dL. With 1-deamino-8-D-arginine vasopressin (DDAVP) stimulation, timed plasma sampling revealed that the released vWF had a circulation half-life that was approximately one-sixth of normal.[110] Several other similar mutations have also been described.[111]

At higher levels of vWF, linkage of the vWF level to the vWF gene is found less often. The European type 1 vWF cohort study demonstrated this observation. Almost all families with vWF levels <30 IU/dL showed linkage to the vWF gene, but the proportion fell to only 51% with vWF levels >30 IU/dL.[108] These data were corroborated in a Canadian study.[109]

Complete absence of vWF is responsible for the most extreme form of vWD, and this is classified as type 3 vWD. As one might predict, a large variety of genetic abnormalities scattered throughout the vWF gene have been reported in families with type 3 vWD. These have included large gene deletions, small gene deletions, frameshift mutations, splice-site mutations, nonsense mutations, and point mutations.[112]

Type 2 vWD is characterized by the production of a qualitatively defective protein, and the genetics of these variant forms is more straightforward than that of type 1 vWD. In families affected by types 2B and 2M, as well as in the majority of families with type 2A vWD, inheritance is autosomal dominant. Rare cases of type 2A disease are transmitted in an autosomal recessive fashion, as are most cases of type 2N disease. vWF gene sequencing studies combined with vWF mutation-expression analysis have revealed that single missense point mutations underlie the majority of type 2 disorders. Type 3 vWD is also inherited as a recessive trait and occurs when both copies of the vWF gene are defective. In type 3 disease, gene abnormalities include large or partial gene deletions, disruption of orderly messenger RNA transcription (frameshift mutation, splice-site, or nonsense mutation), and missense mutation. For patients with recessively inherited vWD phenotypes (type 2N, type 3, or some rare type 2A), genetic analysis may reveal either homozygous or compound heterozygous gene

Table 54.7. Features of Common Variants of von Willebrand Disease

Features	Type 1	Type 2A	Type 2B	Type 3	Platelet Type
Inheritance	Autosomal dominant	Autosomal dominant	Autosomal dominant	Autosomal recessive	Autosomal dominant
Factor VIIIc in plasma	Normal or reduced	Normal or reduced	Normal or reduced	Markedly reduced	Normal or reduced
vWF antigen	Normal or reduced	Normal or reduced	Normal or reduced; increased affinity for platelets	Markedly reduced	Normal or reduced; increased affinity for platelets
Ristocetin cofactor activity	Normal or reduced	Reduced	Normal or reduced	Markedly reduced	Normal or reduced
vWF multimeric analysis	Normal (plasma and platelets)	Absence of large and intermediate-sized multimers in plasma	Absence of large multimers from plasma; normal in platelets	Small multimers or absent multimers in plasma and platelets	Reduction in large multimers caused by "consumption" by platelets
Ristocetin-induced platelet aggregation	Normal or diminished	Diminished	Increased aggregation at low ristocetin concentrations	Markedly diminished	Hyperaggregation with patient's platelets, normal plasma, and low concentration of ristocetin
vWF in platelets	Normal or reduced	Normal or absence of large and intermediate-sized multimers	Normal	Absent	Normal
Ancillary findings	DDAVP usually produces significant increase in plasma VIIIc and vWF	DDAVP produces rise in factor VIIIc, but functional vWF increase is variable and may be of short duration	Variable response to DDAVP, with intravascular platelet aggregation and thrombocytopenia in some cases; ristocetin-induced platelet aggregation enhanced in the presence of patient's plasma; cryoprecipitate does not aggregate platelets in vitro unless ristocetin is added	Response to DDAVP lacking; endothelial vWF absent	Transfusion of vWF or DDAVP may produce intravascular platelet aggregation and thrombocytopenia; cryoprecipitate produces in vitro platelet aggregation

Abbreviations: DDAVP, 1-deamino-8-D-arginine vasopressin; vWF, von Willebrand factor.

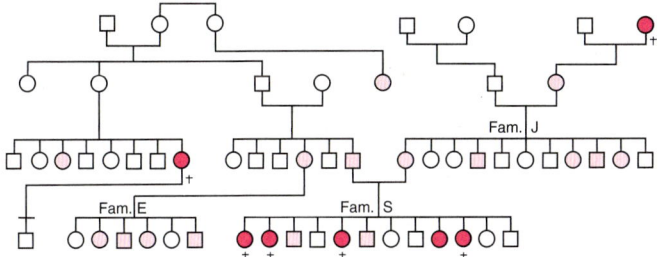

FIGURE 54.5 Pedigree of patients described by von Willebrand. Three families are emphasized: S, E, and J. Clinical details of bleeding events in these families have been reported. Open circles indicate female nonbleeders; open squares indicate male nonbleeders. Shaded circles and squares indicate female and male bleeders, respectively. Solid symbols indicate family members who experienced severe bleeding, and crosses indicate family members who experienced hemorrhagic deaths. (Modified from von Willebrand EA. Über hereditäre pseudohämophilie. *Acta Med Scand*. 1931;76(4-6):521-550. Copyright © 1931 Association for the Publication of the Journal of Internal Medicine. Reprinted by permission of John Wiley & Sons, Inc.)

abnormalities. Members of the International Society of Thrombosis and Hemostasis maintain a database of vWD mutations (www.vwf.group.shef.ac.uk).

Pathophysiology

The basic defect in vWD is a deficiency or abnormality of vWF function. vWF is synthesized in endothelial cells and megakaryocytes. The primary transcription product is 2813 amino acids in length and undergoes extensive further processing, including dimerization and polymerization, to form very-large-molecular-weight "multimers." Multimerization and intracellular trafficking of vWF through the endoplasmic reticulum and Golgi apparatus and into storage granules is directed by the vWF propeptide (vWFpp). vWFpp is cleaved off the "mature subunit" after multimer assembly. Large vWF multimers, which may exceed 20 million Da in size, are stored in endothelial cells in Weibel-Palade bodies and in platelet α-granules.

The majority of circulating vWF is present in plasma, with a concentration of ~10 μg/mL. The circulating half-life of plasma vWF is ~8 to 12 hours. Approximately 15% of circulating vWF is present intracellularly within platelets. Ultralarge multimers released from endothelial cells into the plasma are further degraded to smaller multimers through the activity of a "vWF cleaving protease."[98] The cDNA sequence identified this protein to be the 13th member of the ADAMTS family (a disintegrin-like and metalloproteinase with thrombospondin type 1 motifs, ADAMTS13).[113,114] vWF is cleaved between tyrosine 1605 and methionine 1606 located in the A2 domain. High shear stress and tethering of vWF by platelets most likely enhance exposure of the cleavage site.[115] The physiologic importance of enzymatic degradation of vWF after release is demonstrated clinically by the association of an inherited form of thrombotic microangiopathy (Upshaw-Schulman syndrome) with congenital absence of the protein because of defects of the ADAMTS13 gene,[113] and the observation of plasma deficiency of the protein with the presence of autoantibody in most patients with immune-mediated thrombotic thrombocytopenic purpura.[116] Endothelial cell stores of vWF can be released therapeutically with administration of desmopressin.[117]

vWF is required for normal platelet adhesion (see Chapter 19) and also acts as a carrier of factor VIII in the plasma. When vWF is deficient or aberrant, both factor VIII deficiency and abnormalities in the early steps of primary hemostasis result. vWD is thus manifested as a multifaceted hemostatic defect. Both abnormalities—factor VIII deficiency and abnormal primary hemostasis—give rise to characteristic and distinct laboratory abnormalities, and both defects contribute to the bleeding tendency.

Abnormalities of Primary Hemostasis

Convincing evidence exists that platelets, although intrinsically normal, do not adhere to the subendothelium normally in the setting of deficient or defective vWF. This abnormality is well demonstrated by methods that measure platelet adhesion to subendothelial surfaces under flow conditions (the Baumgartner technique). The physiologic stimulus for interaction of vWF with platelets is not completely defined, but tethering of vWF on exposed subendothelial cell matrix or shear stress may cause vWF to undergo conformational change. Results of experimental studies suggest that in the absence of vWF, platelet adhesion to collagen in a flowing stream of blood may be particularly deficient at high rates of shear, when only a short time is available for formation of a platelet-collagen bond.[118] Deficient platelet plug formation has been observed directly in experimental wounds.[119] In vitro, the interaction of vWF with the platelet GPIb receptor can be induced by the addition of the antibiotic ristocetin, by the snake venom protein botrocetin, or by subjecting platelets to high shear stress in the presence of vWF. For the effective support of platelet adhesion, vWF is multimerized into long chains (strings), which can exceed 2 μm in length. Plasma vWF demonstrates a spectrum of sizes; however, the longest vWF multimers are the most efficient at supporting platelet adhesion.

Abnormalities of Secondary Hemostasis

A second function of vWF is as a molecular chaperone for factor VIII, increasing the plasma half-life of factor VIII approximately fivefold.[120] This effect may occur through protection of factor VIII from activated protein C–mediated degradation.[121] Furthermore, the binding of vWF to the subendothelium at sites of vascular injury could serve to colocalize factor VIII, where it can participate in the regulation of hemostasis on the activated platelet membrane. Whereas vWF is synthesized in endothelial cells and megakaryocytes, factor VIII is synthesized primarily by hepatic endothelial cells.[122] When the drug desmopressin (DDAVP) is administered to normal subjects or to individuals with mild quantitative deficiency of vWF or factor VIII, levels of both molecules rise. Studies of hemophilia patients and patients with type 3 vWD on replacement therapies suggest that both vWF and factor VIII must be endogenously synthesized in order for there to be coordinated release after DDAVP.

Response to Transfusion

When blood products containing the vWF-factor VIII complex are infused in patients with severe hemophilia A, peak levels of factor VIIIc are present immediately after the infusion; this activity then declines rapidly, with an overall half-life of 8 to 10 hours. Twenty-four hours later, factor VIIIc activity is minimal. In most patients with vWD, the infusion of normal vWF-factor VIII complex produces an initial rise in factor VIIIc that is predicted from the preinfusion level and the amount of factor infused. This is followed by a sustained but variable rise in factor VIIIc activity that reaches a plateau about 24 hours later and may persist for 48 to 72 hours. This phenomenon is highly variable and irregular; in some patients, a rapid initial fall of factor VIIIc is followed by a secondary rise in activity. This disproportionate response to transfused factor VIII has been called the secondary transfusion response, a feature that is apparently unique to vWD. Various hypotheses have been advanced to explain the disproportionate response to transfusion described above. The leading hypothesis is that the infused vWF results in stimulation of increased factor VIII release into the plasma with the attachment of the newly released factor VIII onto infused vWF. A study of patients with vWD who received plasma infusion from patients with severe hemophilia A observed a sustained increase in factor VIII levels even though there was no factor VIII present in the infused plasma (Figure 54.6).

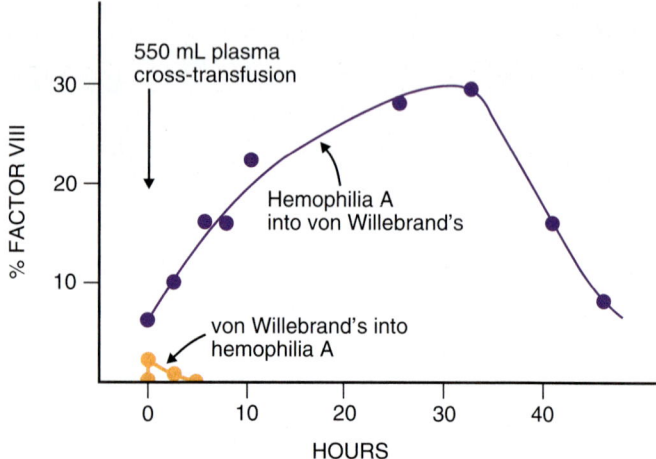

FIGURE 54.6 **The phenomenon of new factor VIII synthesis in patients with von Willebrand disease (vWD) who receive plasma transfusion.** Purple circles indicate changes in the plasma factor VIII levels of a patient with vWD after infusion of plasma from a patient with severe hemophilia A. A significant and sustained increase in the factor VIII levels of the recipient was observed even though no active factor VIII was present in the infused plasma. Orange circles indicate effects of infusing plasma from a patient with vWD to a patient with severe hemophilia A. The factor VIII level in the infused plasma was 15% of normal. Note the slight and transitory effects. (From Shulman NR, Cowan DH, Libre EP, et al. The physiologic basis for therapy of classic hemophilia (factor VIII deficiency) and related disorders. *Ann Intern Med.* 1967;67(4):856-882. Copyright © 1967 American College of Physicians. All Rights Reserved. Reprinted with the permission of American College of Physicians, Inc.)

Transfusions of blood products containing vWF shorten the bleeding time to a variable degree in patients with vWD. This corrective effect seldom persists for more than a few hours, even after massive transfusions that raise vWF to high levels. The correction of the bleeding time apparently requires the large molecular forms of vWF that are present in cryoprecipitate and select intermediate-purity factor VIII concentrates,[123] but that are completely absent from monoclonally purified or recombinant concentrates of factor VIII.[124]

Clinical Manifestations

The bleeding manifestations in vWD are heterogeneous but consistent with the dual roles of vWF in supporting both primary and secondary hemostasis. Thus, in the mild forms of vWD, the clinical picture is dominated by cutaneous and mucosal bleeding, which appears to be mainly the result of disordered primary hemostasis. In the most severe forms of the disorder, in which factor VIII levels are low, hemarthroses and dissecting intramuscular hematomas may develop. As in mild classic hemophilia, serious hemorrhage resulting from traumatic injuries or after surgical procedures is a significant hazard in severe vWD.

The bleeding manifestations in the usual patient with type 1 vWD are mild, however, and many patients are virtually asymptomatic. Easy bruising is common in vWD, but it is not specific. Mucosal bleeding is particularly common. Childhood epistaxis, a lifelong history of easy bruising, bleeding with dental extraction, heavy menstrual bleeding, or anemia attributed to excessive menstrual blood losses, or postpartum hemorrhage are all included in the spectrum of vWD symptomatology. Systemic bleeding disorders are often not considered in women with menorrhagia,[125] but clinical studies reveal that the prevalence of vWD is significant in individuals who present with this complaint.[126] Angiodysplasia of various vascular beds, particularly those in the gut, has been demonstrated in some patients with vWD and may be an important contributory factor in chronic gastrointestinal bleeding.[127] In type 1 vWD, symptoms usually become milder during pregnancy or with estrogen therapy, when the vWF and factor VIIIc levels rise significantly.[29] The disorder may also decrease in severity with advancing age. Bleeding manifestations tend to be more prominent in patients with more severe quantitative deficiency and in patients with qualitative (type 2) defects.

While eliciting the history of bleeding, one should bear in mind that women are often inaccurate assessors of whether their menstrual flow is normal or excessive. Retrospective studies of women with vWD show that abnormal bleeding can often be traced to menarche.[128] Family history also may provide important clues to a diagnosis. The physician should specifically seek a history of the response to hemostatic challenge, such as dental extraction, tonsillectomy, surgical procedures, menstruation, peripartum hemorrhage, and transfusion. The use of a standardized questionnaire with a scoring system has been recommended to identify subjects who should be screened for vWD.[129] Coexistent conditions or drug effects can strongly influence the severity of bleeding symptoms. Risk of hemorrhage may increase in patients with concomitant liver disease, uremia, gastrointestinal ulcer, or angiodysplasia. Excessive bleeding in response to challenge with aspirin may also point toward a bleeding disorder, but this history is not specific for vWD. Valproic acid use can result in lower vWF activity levels, as may hypothyroidism and valvular heart disease. Conversely, oral contraception frequently ameliorates menorrhagia. Of note, vWD patients have a reduced prevalence of arterial thrombosis.[130]

Laboratory Diagnosis

Criteria for the laboratory diagnosis of vWD are imperfect. Even with the more elaborate confirmatory tests now available, the diagnosis of this disorder may be difficult and may require repeated observations over a period of time. Both vWF and factor VIII are "acute-phase reactants," increasing with stress, trauma, estrogen therapy, or pregnancy, such that levels may fluctuate from time to time. Evaluation of a patient at a time remote from acute infection, pregnancy, or strenuous activity is preferable. However, pregnancy and acute-phase reaction are unlikely to obscure diagnosis in patients with more severe quantitative deficiency or qualitative defects.

Diagnosis of vWD is complicated, because of both the breadth of vWF functions and the spectrum of disorders that constitutes vWD. Consequently, a battery of studies should be considered to evaluate a patient conclusively for vWD. Screening tests such as bleeding time, Platelet Function Analyzer-100 (PFA-100), and PTT lack sensitivity; specific tests such as those for vWF antigen, vWF activity, and factor VIII level are preferred. Correlating the values of these various quantitative assays with each other, or obtaining qualitative tests such as vWF multimer analysis or low-dose ristocetin–induced platelet aggregation (RIPA), may provide important clues toward a diagnosis of type 2 vWD (Table 54.7).

Bleeding Time and Platelet Function Analyzer-100

The template bleeding time or the Ivy bleeding time may be useful in detecting the abnormality characteristic of vWD. However, the bleeding time may be normal in many patients with vWD.[126] Consequently, the bleeding time has little clinical utility in the diagnosis and management of patients with vWD, and is rarely performed nowadays.

The PFA-100 evaluates platelet adhesion and aggregation to collagen in a whole-blood assay under high shear conditions.[131,132] Citrate-anticoagulated whole blood is aspirated through an aperture in a collagen-coated membrane, and the device measures the time from first flow until flow ceases as the "closure time." PFA-100 closure times are sensitive to multiple factors, including vWF function, platelet count, platelet function, and hematocrit. Initial studies using the PFA-100 in patients with diagnosed vWD indicated that the assay was sensitive to most forms of vWD. However, when the closure time test was applied in clinical settings where patients were referred for evaluation of bleeding symptoms, the sensitivity of the PFA-100 for diagnosis of vWD ranged from 62% to 80%, with specificity ranging from 84% to 89%.[133] In addition, the closure time may remain normal in acquired vWD despite a very reduced plasma vWF level, because the platelet vWF level may remain normal. The PFA-100 closure time may also be normal in patients with type 2N vWD, in which the major defect is low factor VIII levels.

Partial Thromboplastin Time and Factor VIIIc Assay

Among the simple screening tests (Table 54.5), the PTT may be abnormal, reflecting reduced levels of factor VIIIc. Plasma levels of factor VIIIc vary greatly in this disorder and range from as low as 3 IU/dL in patients with type 3 vWD to normal levels in patients with mild type 1 vWD. Because factor VIIIc deficiency is often mild in patients with vWD, a diagnosis of vWD may be missed by the routine screening PTT. Consequently, a specific assay is required to reliably detect factor VIIIc deficiency in patients with vWD.

von Willebrand Factor Immunoassay

The immunoassay of vWF is a quantitative measure of vWF protein that is one of the most sensitive methods available for the diagnosis of vWD.[134] A variety of methods have been used, all of which depend on antibodies specific to vWF. The electroimmunodiffusion method of Laurell was initially widely used because it was simple to perform, but ELISA or automated assays using related methodologies have now largely replaced this technique. Average levels of vWF antigen (vWF:Ag) obtained by different laboratories will vary, but a level of ~45 to 50 IU/dL is the lower limit of normal reported by many laboratories. The ratio of factor VIII to vWF also varies by laboratory but normally ranges from ~0.7 to 2.2. Plasma levels of vWF:Ag are regulated to some extent by carbohydrate residues attached to the protein; ~25% lower vWF antigenic levels have been noted in patients with blood type O compared to patients with other blood types.[101] The contribution of blood group O is more marked in patients with mild quantitative vWF deficiency, where the low vWF level is less likely to be related to abnormalities of the vWF gene.[108,109] Whether these patients actually have vWD type I is subject to debate, and the role of blood group in the diagnosis of vWF deficiency remains to be resolved. Patients with type 2 vWD may have normal vWF:Ag levels, emphasizing the need to use more than just a vWF antigen assay to evaluate a patient for vWD.

von Willebrand Factor Functional Assays

vWF has multiple functions, and assays have been devised to specifically evaluate many of these. The function most often clinically assessed is its ability to interact with platelets. An assay that evaluates the ability of vWF to interact with collagen has also been proposed as a functional assay. The relevance of collagen-binding activity analysis is being increasingly demonstrated.[135] Finally, vWF binding of factor VIII can be assessed in special circumstances when questioning whether mild factor VIII deficiency is caused by failure of vWF chaperone function. vWF functional assay generally correlates well with vWF:Ag in patients with quantitative disorders of vWF. Observing a discrepancy between vWF function and vWF:Ag provides a useful clue for qualitative defects, provided that the testing laboratory uses the same control plasma for determining both assays.[136]

Ristocetin Cofactor Activity and Ristocetin-Induced Platelet Aggregation

The assay for ristocetin cofactor activity (vWF:RCo) is a quantitative technique for estimating the ability of vWF in patient plasma to bind target platelets that are specially prepared or preserved for use in the assay.[137] Ristocetin induces an activated conformation of vWF such that it will then bind platelets via the platelet GPIb receptor, mimicking the in vivo sequence of events that allows interaction between subendothelial tissue–bound vWF and platelets. Quantitation of vWF:RCo is held to be the single most sensitive and specific assay for vWD by multiple authorities.[138,139] vWF:RCo activity is adversely affected by loss of the larger-molecular-weight vWF multimers. The discrepancy between vWF:RCo and vWF:Ag that is observed in qualitative defects characterized by loss of both the intermediate- and higher-molecular-weight multimers (such as type 2A vWD) is thought to result from this. Ristocetin cofactor activity is also generally utilized to follow a vWD patient's response to therapeutic interventions. However, obtaining typical ristocetin cofactor activity is a time-consuming procedure, and assay standardization remains somewhat problematic. Automation of the vWF:RCo assay has resulted in a clinically more available, but less sensitive technique, which requires modification to detect levels below ~10 to 20 IU/dL. Simpler ELISA-based methods using monoclonal antibody to the GPIb-binding domain of vWF have been explored for estimating vWF activity.¹⁴⁰ Unfortunately, commercial functional epitope assays have not performed sufficiently well to allow them to replace vWF:RCo assay,¹⁴¹ and these assays do not measure the increased functionality of the larger vWF multimers directly. One advance in the area of improved vWF functional assays is the availability of the vWF:GPIbM assay which uses a mutant GPIb that does not require ristocetin to bind vWF, and has shown superior precision and sensitivity compared with the vWF:RCo assay.¹⁴²

RIPA is a distinct test from ristocetin cofactor activity. RIPA is a qualitative test that involves evaluating the rate or extent of agglutination of patient-derived platelet-rich plasma in response to the addition of the antibiotic ristocetin. The concentration of vWF and platelets present in the test plasma, as well as the amount of ristocetin added, affect RIPA. The assay is relatively insensitive to mild deficiency of vWF, but decreased aggregation response is observed in both more severe deficiency and in patients with Bernard-Soulier syndrome (in which platelets are missing the GPIb receptor). Titrating down the amount of ristocetin added in the assay may be of specific interest in defining variants of vWD in which there are "gain-of-function" mutations (type 2B and platelet-type [pseudo] vWD). These two conditions are characterized by increased sensitivity of patient vWF or platelets to the effect of ristocetin. However, insensitivity of patient samples to low-dose ristocetin aggregation is seen in occasional patients with type 2B vWD in whom there is marked reduction in the amount of high- and intermediate-molecular-weight multimers, and genetic analysis may be required to distinguish some cases of type 2B from type 2A vWD. In addition, low-dose ristocetin aggregation of patient-derived platelet-rich plasma cannot differentiate type 2B vWD from the rarer platelet-type (pseudo) vWD, and mixing studies using patient plasma and donor platelets have been devised to help make that distinction at the phenotypic level.¹⁴³

von Willebrand Collagen–Binding Activity

vWF contains collagen-binding sites in both the A1 and A3 domains of the vWF protein, and collagen-binding activity (vWF:CB) may be an important function that allows vWF to adhere to platelets at sites of vascular injury. Like ristocetin cofactor activity, vWF:CB is dependent on multimer size, with the larger multimers binding collagen more avidly. The assay is generally done in an ELISA format, in which type I and/or type III collagen is plated in microtiter wells, and the amount of vWF captured is assayed.¹⁴⁴ vWF:CB correlates well with vWF:Ag in normal individuals and those with quantitative deficiency of vWF, and discrepant results are indicative of vWD subtypes that are characterized by deficiency of larger vWF multimers.¹⁴⁴ One report suggests that vWF:CB assays may substitute for multimeric analysis assays.¹³⁵

Assay of von Willebrand Factor's Ability to Bind Factor VIII

Factor VIII binding by vWF (vWF:FVIIIB) can be measured in a few reference coagulation laboratories and is indicated for the evaluation of patients suspected of having factor VIII deficiency on the basis of defective vWF chaperone function (type 2N vWD).¹⁴⁵ In this ELISA format assay, ELISA plate wells are coated with antibody to vWF in order to capture vWF from patient plasma. After washing patient-derived factor VIII from the well, the ability of patient-derived vWF to capture r-FVIII is assessed using a chromogenic or immunoassay for factor VIII, and the quantity of patient-derived vWF:Ag in the well is quantified by the standard ELISA technique. The calculated ratio of captured r-FVIII to vWF:Ag is expected to be in the normal range when testing plasma from a patient with hemophilia A, whereas it will be abnormally low in the rare cases of type 2N vWD.¹⁴⁶

Multimeric Analysis of von Willebrand Factor

Normal vWF in plasma consists of a complex series of multimers, ranging in size from about 500 to 20,000 kDa. vWD initially diagnosed by abnormal assays for factor VIIIc, vWF antigen, or ristocetin cofactor activity should be further characterized by multimeric analysis. In this test, the spectrum of vWF molecular sizes of the patient's vWF is assessed by size-based separation of vWF multimers via agarose gel electrophoresis, and vWF multimers are imaged by immunologic methods coupled to autoradiography or other detection methods.¹⁴⁷ Multimer

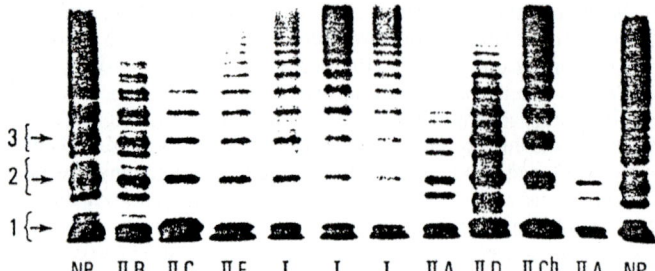

FIGURE 54.7 Multimeric composition of von Willebrand factor from normal plasma and that from types I, IIA, IIB, IIC, IID, and IIE von Willebrand disease (vWD), as well as from a type IIC heterozygote (IICh). Using the revised classification scheme, these types would correspond to 1, 2A, 2B, 2A, 2A, and 2A, respectively. The three brackets include the smallest normal oligomers, with arrows pointing to the central predominant band in each. In type 1 vWD, the relative concentration of large multimers varies. (Reprinted from Zimmerman TS, Ruggeri ZM. von Willebrand disease. *Hum Pathol.* 1987;18(2):140-152. Copyright © 1987 Elsevier. With permission.)

analysis is characterized as either "low-resolution" (which differentiates the largest multimer forms from the intermediate and smaller forms), or "high-resolution" (which resolves each multimer band into three to five satellite bands), which inform on the activity of ADAMTS13 on plasma vWF. Multimer analysis will confirm the presence of the entire spectrum of vWF multimers in normal individuals and those with type 1 vWD, and allows identification of the loss of intermediate- or high-molecular-weight multimers of vWF as is characteristic of the type 2A and type 2B qualitative defects.¹⁴⁷ Unfortunately, the distinction between type 2A and type 2B vWD is not always possible using multimer analysis alone, necessitating further testing. Multimeric analysis is a very labor-intensive test and is usually performed only in coagulation reference laboratories. The multimeric composition of plasma from normal subjects and patients with vWD is shown in *Figure 54.7*. This methodology has been reviewed.¹⁴⁸

von Willebrand Factor Propeptide Assay

After vWF is released from storage sites into the plasma, the vWFpp dissociates from vWF. vWF and the vWFpp are cleared independently and the ratio between vWFpp and vWF:Ag can be used to classify vWD subtypes.¹⁴⁹

Genetic Testing in von Willebrand Disease

Direct mutational analysis by vWF gene sequencing, allele-specific PCR, or restriction enzyme analysis is useful in confirming a diagnosis of type 2 variant vWD.¹⁵⁰ The functional domain structure of the vWF gene results in clustering of the various type 2 vWD defects in limited areas of the vWF sequence. vWF exon 28 encodes for the A1 loop of vWF responsible for the interaction of vWF with platelet GPIb, and vWD variants characterized by defects of this interaction (types 2B and 2M) are encoded by genetic mutations clustered in this exon.¹⁵¹ Exon 28 also encodes the A2 domain, which contains the ADAMTS13-sensitive bond tyrosine 1605–methionine 1606. Mutations that increase the susceptibility of this bond to cleavage by ADAMTS13 underlie a high fraction of type 2A vWD. Less commonly, type 2A vWD results from a defect of the multimerization process. The carboxy terminus of the vWF peptide (encoded by exons 51-52) is involved in initial vWF dimer formation in the rough endoplasmic reticulum. The vWFpp (encoded by exons 3-17) directs further multimerization via cross-linkage of the amino-terminal D′ and D3 of the mature vWF protein (encoded by exons 18-28). As one might expect, type 2A vWD on the basis of failure of multimerization has been attributed to genetic abnormalities in each of these regions of the genome. Mutations responsible for defective interaction of vWF with factor VIII (type 2N vWD) are predominantly clustered in exons 18 to 20, which encode for the factor VIII–binding domain of vWF; however, rare cases have been attributed to mutations in exons 24 and 25. An online database of defects found in vWD patients can be accessed at www.vwf.group.shef.ac.uk. *Figure 54.4* shows the location of these various genetic abnormalities schematically. Rapid, complete vWF gene sequencing has been reported.[152]

Genetics of Type 1 and Type 3 vWD

Mild to moderate quantitative deficiency of vWF characterizes patients with type 1 vWD, whereas virtual absence of vWF characterizes type 3 disease. Genetic analysis is not generally required to make these diagnoses, but may provide useful additional information concerning pathogenesis of a patient's condition, responsiveness to DDAVP, or risk for alloantibody formation. Distinct from type 2 vWD, genetic defects underlying quantitative vWF deficiency are distributed throughout the vWF gene, complicating evaluation. In addition, for families with patients who demonstrate normal multimer structure and higher vWF levels, the chances of finding linkage to the vWF gene are reduced,[108,109] and family members are usually asymptomatic.[99] Type 3 patients with large gene deletions are particularly prone to develop anti-vWF alloantibodies after treatment with vWF-containing concentrates.

Type 1 von Willebrand Disease and "Low von Willebrand Factor"

Patients with bleeding attributed to decreased production of qualitatively normal vWF are classified as having type 1 vWD. Most patients with vWD (70%-80%) fall into this category. The majority of patients have a mildly symptomatic disorder, but bleeding may increase with physical trauma, surgery, or during menstruation. vWF levels are low, with concordant reduction in vWF:Ag and vWF:RCo (and vWF:CB, if that is measured). Factor VIII levels are generally equal to or higher than vWF levels, and all vWF multimers should be present. The diagnosis of type 1 vWD may be simpler in an individual with mucosal bleeding symptoms, a strong family history of similar symptoms, and quantitative vWF level (vWF:Ag and/or vWF:RCo) <30 IU/dL. Although not required for a diagnosis of type 1 vWD, the probability of finding linkage of the phenotype to the vWF gene in such an individual would be high, such that both therapeutic choices and genetic counseling would be straightforward.

Unfortunately, many factors make the diagnosis of type 1 vWD difficult.[107] Mild bleeding symptoms are common in hemostatically normal people (see Chapter 46). In addition, the relative risk of bleeding for individuals with only modest reductions in vWF level appears to be minimal. Finally, because of the strong influence of blood group on vWF levels, there is a high prevalence of blood group O among individuals with mildly depressed vWF levels. These observations have led to the recent proposal of the concept of "low vWF."[99,107] The term "low vWF" could be applied to patients with vWF levels below the normal reference range but above some lower limit. Studies of families of patients with a diagnosis of type 1 vWD suggest that linkage to the vWF gene is less often seen when the vWF level rises above 30 IU/dL, suggesting that this might be a candidate for the lower limit of the "low vWF" category.[108,153] Two population-based studies have shown that "low vWF" causes increased bleeding.[154,155] These latter studies would suggest that abnormally low ristocetin cofactor activity, and not the presence of a mutation, should primarily be used to identify bleeders. Empiric therapy to raise vWF levels in patients with "low vWF" at times of hemostatic challenge would be reasonable for patients with a history of bleeding, but the genetic counseling issues would clearly be different.[107]

A recently published multidisciplinary guideline recommends that patients with abnormal bleeding and a vWF level of <0.50 IU/mL confirms the diagnosis of type 1 vWD.[92] This less restrictive diagnostic criteria was recommended to avoid missing the diagnosis and to ensure that management to treat bleeds was provided.[92]

Type 3 von Willebrand Disease

Type 3 vWD is the most severe form of vWD, because it results from complete failure of vWF synthesis. This bleeding disorder is generally diagnosed during infancy. Hematoma formation is common, epistaxis may be life threatening, and hemarthrosis may occur as a result of the low factor VIII levels. Plasma from patients with type 3 vWD contains virtually no detectable vWF, and vWF is not present in either platelets or endothelial cells. Factor VIII level is generally in the range of 1 to 10 IU/dL, similar to that seen in moderate to mild hemophilia A. Multimeric analysis of the little vWF present yields variable results, in some cases revealing only small multimers.[147] Type 3 vWD is rare, with an estimated frequency of 1 in a million people.[156] Genetic analysis reveals either homozygous or compound (double) heterozygous defects of the vWF gene, with gene deletions, frameshift mutations, missense mutations, or nonsense mutations. Careful laboratory evaluation of the parents of patients with type 3 disease may reveal mild quantitative deficiency of vWF. In a review of 117 obligate heterozygotes, the mean plasma vWF level was 45 IU/dL, with a range from 5 to 130 IU/dL.[107] Parents are frequently asymptomatic, consistent with the impression that type 3 disease is inherited as a recessive trait. Consanguinity is common in kindreds with this variant. In some patients with type 3 vWD, large gene deletions have been identified on one or both vWF alleles.[157] Such patients are at increased risk of developing inhibitory alloantibodies to vWF after transfusion therapy.[157]

Because these patients lack vWF in their endothelial cells and platelets, there is no rise in vWF level in response to DDAVP. For replacement therapy, these patients require vWF-containing concentrates. This is usually provided in the form of specific intermediate-purity factor VIII concentrates that have been documented to contain intact vWF.[117] Because these patients possess a normal *factor VIII* gene but are missing the vWF chaperone, posttransfusion factor VIII recovery and survival may be longer in a patient with type 3 vWD than in a patient with hemophilia A, owing to endogenous factor VIII production. Although life-threatening bleeds require immediate replacement of both vWF and factor VIII, replacement with vWF alone may be sufficient if therapy is begun 12 to 24 hours before elective surgery.[158]

Qualitative Defects of von Willebrand Factor

Several subsets of patients with vWD differ substantially from those with the common quantitative deficiency states (*Table 54.6*). Classified as type 2 variants, these qualitative defects of vWF are less common, but they may represent up to 20% to 25% of cases of vWD. Type 2 forms of vWD are suspected when the severity of the patient's symptoms seems in excess of the observed vWF and factor VIII levels, when there is discordant reduction between vWF antigen and vWF functional activity or factor VIII assay, or when there is concomitant vWF deficiency and thrombocytopenia. Discrimination between qualitatively normal and abnormal vWF can be difficult; however, when the ratio of vWF:RCo to vWF:Ag or vWF:CB to vWF:Ag is found to be <0.7, type 2 vWD should be considered.[92] The sensitivity and specificity of such ratio screening depend to a large extent on the expertise and precision of the laboratory performing the assays, but the predictive value of ratios decreases when the level of vWF antigen is <20 IU/dL. Examining the multimeric structure of patient vWF may provide further definition of the nature of the qualitative defect. If required, further information is provided by supplemental studies of vWF function, or via genetic analysis of the vWF gene (*Figure 54.4*).[89,147]

Type 2A von Willebrand Disease

vWD with defective interaction of vWF with platelets caused by deficiency of intermediate- and high-molecular-weight forms of vWF is classified as type 2A vWD. This form of the disorder is generally inherited as an autosomal dominant trait,[159] and it accounts for the majority of patients with type 2 defects. Levels of factor VIIIc and vWF:Ag in the plasma may be normal or reduced. The vWF activity as assayed by either vWF:RCo or vWF:CB is significantly lower than vWF:Ag because of the absence of the larger multimers (which are more potent in their ability to interact with platelet GPIb and collagen). Analysis of vWF multimers reveals a relative reduction in intermediate- and high-molecular-weight species. Protein studies followed by genetic analysis of the basis of type 2A vWD revealed multiple mechanisms for the generation of this disorder.[160,161] In some patients, there is failure to synthesize full-length multimers. Mutations associated with impaired vWF multimerization have been localized to the vWFpp, the region of the mature vWF protein associated with the amino terminus area of multimer formation, and the carboxy terminus region that is involved in initial dimer formation. The spectrum of multimers released into the plasma after DDAVP administration would not be expected to improve significantly in these patients whose defects prevent normal multimer assembly.

A second group of type 2A patients has been described in whom there is excessive catabolism of fully multimerized vWF after vWF is released into the plasma. These patients demonstrate mutations in exon 28, encoding the A1 and A2 regions of vWF. These mutations allow increased proteolysis of multimerized vWF by ADAMTS13. Again, high-resolution multimer gel studies may be informative by demonstrating increased "satellite" band intensity, which accumulates as a result of excessive ADAMTS13 activity. Because intracellular vWF is protected from cleavage by ADAMTS13, these patients may demonstrate very transient improvement in both vWF activity and multimer spectrum after DDAVP administration.

Inheritance of type 2A vWD is generally autosomal dominant, with the majority of cases caused by mutations clustered in the region of exon 28, which encodes the vWF A2 homologous repeat (*Figure 54.4*). Rare recessive forms of type 2A vWD have been reported with some multimerization defects. Because of the underlying structural abnormality of the vWF produced in these patients, neither stress nor pregnancy significantly increases the functional amount of vWF protein in the plasma.

Type 2B von Willebrand Disease

Type 2B vWD is a paradoxical bleeding disorder, characterized by increased interaction of patient vWF with platelets which is demonstrated in vitro in the presence of low doses of ristocetin. Increased in vivo interaction of the larger multimers of type 2B vWF with platelets is thought to result from mutations that either allow increased access of platelets to the A1 loop of vWF or that stabilize that interaction. This may in turn allow increased generation of vWF-platelet complexes, which are subsequently cleared from circulation, resulting in thrombocytopenia.

This bleeding disorder is characterized by deficient vWF function attributable to mild reduction in vWF:Ag, a somewhat more marked deficiency of vWF:RCo activity (and vWF:CB, if measured). Multimeric analysis reveals a deficiency of the highest-molecular-weight vWF multimers. Measurements of factor VIIIc are variable. Many patients with the type 2B variant have mild persistent thrombocytopenia.[162] The platelet count may fall further during physiologic stresses, pregnancy, in association with surgical procedures, or after the administration of DDAVP.[163]

Additional laboratory evaluation is required to support a diagnosis of type 2B vWD. In most cases, multimeric analysis reveals the absence of higher-molecular-weight forms of plasma vWF, but distinction of type 2B from type 2A vWD is not possible by multimeric analysis alone. To show the distinct "gain in function" in type 2B disease, RIPA studies are done to reveal enhanced interaction of patient vWF and platelets with low doses of the drug. Finally, to differentiate the more common type 2B vWD from the rare platelet-type (pseudo) vWD, one should prove that the defect resides in vWF. This is done either through performing mixing studies of patient plasma with donor platelets[143] or by analysis of the patient's vWF gene.

Type 2B vWD is inherited as an autosomal dominant trait. A small cluster of mutations within the portion of vWF exon 28 that encodes the vWF A1 domain that interacts with platelet GPIb accounts for all the cases of type 2B vWD that have been reported (*Figure 54.4*).

Evaluation of a large number of patients with type 2B vWD mutations revealed diversity in laboratory findings.[164] Not all patients had reduced vWF:RCo activity or abnormal multimeric analysis, and not all patients had thrombocytopenia.[164] Type 2B patients with normal multimers did not develop thrombocytopenia.

Type 2M von Willebrand Disease

The type 2M vWD variant is defined by diminished platelet-dependent vWF function that is not attributed to deficiency of vWF multimers. Thus, these patients have an initial laboratory profile that in many ways is similar to that of patients with type 2A vWD, revealing variable deficiency of vWF:Ag but disproportionately decreased interaction of vWF with platelets in the presence of ristocetin as measured by the vWF:RCo assay. Factor VIII level is proportionate to vWF:Ag, and the platelet counts are normal. What differentiates type 2M vWD from the type 2A patients is that the vWF multimeric analysis is normal (and, if measured, the vWF:CB is usually similar to vWF:Ag). Type 2M vWD is inherited as an autosomal dominant trait, and, when investigated, mutations have been found in the region of exon 28 that encodes the A1 domain of vWF. Unlike the type 2B mutations, 2M mutations cause impairment of the binding of vWF to the GPIb receptor and have been shown to be localized to an alternative area in the A1 domain (*Figure 54.4*).[151]

One case classified as a type 2M defect was described in which the vWF interaction with collagen was defective. In that case, a mutation in the A3 domain that contributes to the interaction of vWF with collagen was found.[165]

Type 2N von Willebrand Disease

Mutations affecting the association of vWF with factor VIII can result in "autosomal hemophilia" in which factor VIII levels are significantly reduced relative to vWF. Affected patients have factor VIII levels in the range of 5 to 30 IU/dL, attributed to mutations at the factor VIII–binding site near the amino terminus of the vWF subunit.[166] Indeed, genetic studies indicate that the majority of mutations underlying type 2N vWD involve vWF exons 18, 19, and 20, which encode the bulk of the factor VIII–binding domain of vWF. The other functions of vWF in patients with type 2N vWD are qualitatively normal, and thus, vWF laboratory parameters (vWF:Ag, ristocetin cofactor activity, etc) are usually normal (unless there is coinheritance of type 1 vWD). This variant was originally named vWD Normandy but has been renamed type 2N vWD in the revised classification. The factor VIII–binding defect in these patients is inherited in an autosomal recessive manner, and thus affected patients must inherit 2N alleles from each of their two parents, or inherit type 1 vWD from one parent while inheriting a 2N allele from the other. Patients with factor VIII deficiency and a bleeding disorder that is not clearly transmitted as an X-linked disorder or who demonstrate an unexpectedly short in vivo survival of infused factor VIII should be evaluated for type 2N vWD.[167] Diagnosis requires performance of an assay that assesses the interaction of factor VIII with vWF,[145,146] or genetic studies of the vWF gene. A survey of almost 400 unrelated patients with either hemophilia A or type 1 vWD indicated a prevalence of type 2N vWD in these patient populations of 3% and 1.5%, respectively.[168] Consideration of this diagnosis is important because both therapy and genetic counseling are distinct from that of mild hemophilia A.

Platelet-Type (Pseudo) von Willebrand Disease

Platelet-type (pseudo) vWD resembles type 2B vWD in most respects, except that the basis for platelet-type vWD is a structural defect in platelet GPIb[169] rather than a defect of vWF (thus platelet-type [pseudo] vWD is a form of platelet dysfunction). However, as with type 2B vWD, a genetic defect results in increased interaction between GPIb and vWF. Phenotypically, platelet-type (pseudo) vWD is manifested by mild thrombocytopenia, a prolonged bleeding time, and variable deficiency of plasma vWF and factor VIIIc. The reductions in plasma vWF and factor VIIIc may be a result of the attachment of these proteins to platelets that are subsequently removed from the circulation. This "consumption" of vWF and platelets results in preferential loss of high-molecular-weight multimers from patient plasma.[169] In vitro platelet aggregation studies reveal platelet agglutination at unusually low concentrations of ristocetin. Spontaneous intravascular platelet clumping may also occur. Platelet-type (pseudo) vWF is inherited as an autosomal dominant trait in most families.[169,170]

Distinction of platelet-type vWD from type 2B vWD is based on showing that the enhanced interaction of platelets with vWF is either platelet based or resides in the plasma phase (type 2B vWD).[171] This can sometimes be demonstrated through low-dose ristocetin–based agglutination assays using mixtures of normal donor and patient samples, or genetic analysis can be used. To date, all cases of platelet-type vWD have been traced to genetic variations of platelet GPIbα and are available at the PT-VWD Registry (www.pt-vwd.com). These include missense mutations that alter the amino acid sequence from Gly233 to Met 239. This region of the protein adopts a β-sheet conformation after interaction with vWF, and these mutations may function to stabilize this conformation.[172] In addition, a 27-bp gene deletion that encodes for deletion of proline 421 through serine 429 has been shown to underlie platelet-type vWD in one kindred. Thus, genetic analysis of the GPIbα gene could confirm a diagnosis of platelet-type vWD in cases in which phenotypic studies were unsuccessful. A consensus recommendation for the standardized diagnostic and management of platelet-type (pseudo) VWD is available.[173]

CLINICAL DISORDERS OF THE FIBRINOGEN MOLECULE

The clinical disorders of fibrinogen are complex, and depending on the types of mutation, patients may present with bleeding or with thrombotic symptoms, or both. These disorders can be divided based on whether the defect is predominantly a quantitative or qualitative abnormality of the fibrinogen molecule.[174] Quantitative abnormalities are disorders associated with the complete absence of fibrinogen (afibrinogenemia) or with low levels of fibrinogen (hypofibrinogenemia). Qualitative abnormalities are disorders resulting from synthesis of an abnormal fibrinogen molecule (dysfibrinogenemia) with altered functional properties. An illustrated overview of fibrinogen and fibrin summarizes the history, biochemistry, genetics, and clinical relevance of the fibrinogen molecule.[175]

Fibrinogen is a 340-kDa plasma protein that circulates at a concentration of 1.5 to 3.5 mg/mL. It is a symmetric disulfide-linked dimer with a central E domain linked via "coiled coil" peptide chains to outer D domains.[176] Each half-molecule consists of a set of three different peptide chains, termed Aα, Bβ, and γ, which are linked at their amino termini by disulfide bonds to form the E domain. The D domains are formed by disulfide linkages near the carboxy termini of the peptides. Fibrinogen is synthesized in hepatocytes[177] by coordinated expression of three separate genes on chromosome 4.[178] The rate-limiting step in fibrinogen synthesis is transcription of the Bβ gene. Fibrinogen is an acute-phase reactant, and levels may rise considerably with inflammation. The circulation half-life of plasma fibrinogen is ~4 days. Fibrinogen participates in multiple physiologic processes, including fibrin clot formation mediated by the enzymatic activities of thrombin and factor XIIIa, and cohesion of activated platelets through interaction with the GPIIb/IIIa receptor. Fibrinogen also acts as a plasma carrier for factor XIII.

The congenital disorders of fibrinogen associated with afibrinogenemia and hypofibrinogenemia are reviewed in the next section, followed by a discussion of the dysfibrinogenemias. Afibrinogenemia is a very uncommon condition. The first case was described in 1920,[179] and at least 300 cases have been reported since then (see database at isth.org). Congenital hypofibrinogenemia was first reported in 1935,[180] and at least 40 cases have been reported in the literature. However, it is likely that many of the cases of hypofibrinogenemia were actually cases of dysfibrinogenemia with a reduced level of circulating clottable fibrinogen. Congenital disorders of fibrinogen are rare, and, in practice, most commonly observed disorders are acquired as a result of liver disease or consumptive processes.

Pathogenesis of Quantitative Fibrinogen Disorders

In congenital afibrinogenemia and hypofibrinogenemia, defects in synthesis, secretion, or intracellular processing of the final gene product result in deficiency of plasma fibrinogen.[181] When newly synthesized fibrinogen is not secreted, the protein may accumulate in the rough endoplasmic reticulum of hepatocytes or other cells, resulting in amyloid-like accumulations.[182] In both afibrinogenemia and hypofibrinogenemia, the fibrinolytic system and other coagulation pathways are completely normal. Similarly, there is no evidence of blood coagulation activation, which could cause consumption, or degradation of the fibrinogen molecule. The fibrinogen gene locus is located on chromosome 4; it contains three distinct genes that encode for the Aα, Bβ, and γ peptide chains that compose the fibrinogen molecule.[183] The inheritance pattern of afibrinogenemia is autosomal recessive in nature,[180] and many reported cases are the result of consanguineous relationships between asymptomatic parents with symptomatic homozygote offspring. The molecular basis for quantitative fibrinogen disorders has been reviewed.[184] Genetic defects are scattered throughout the three fibrinogen genes that code for the three polypeptide chains—Aα, Bβ, and γ. Multiple genetic defects have been reported, including deletions, point mutations, missense mutations, and uniparental isodisomy.[184] Deletion of an 11-kb region of the fibrinogen α gene appears to be a recurrent finding in unrelated families with afibrinogenemia from both Europe and the United States.[185]

Afibrinogenemia

Inherited afibrinogenemia is a rare autosomal recessive disorder, with an estimated frequency of 1 in a million individuals.[185] It is somewhat of an anomaly that patients who are afibrinogenemic have little hemorrhage, despite the fact that their blood cannot clot normally. This may in part be due to the presence of functional vWF, which allows platelet adhesion and aggregation, with the formation of loose thrombi even in the absence of fibrinogen.[186] A similar phenotype was described for afibrinogenemic mice created by gene-targeted knockout.[187] In patients with afibrinogenemia, life-threatening hemorrhages do occur, but in many situations the bleeding is not as severe as is seen in hemophilia. The diagnosis is often made early in infancy, when prolonged umbilical stump bleeding occurs.[188] A major cause of death is intracranial hemorrhage during infancy or childhood.[189] The clinical manifestations include mucosal membrane bleeding, such as epistaxis, menorrhagia, or gastrointestinal hemorrhage. A review of the cases entered into the North American Rare Bleeding Disorder Registry indicated that most bleeding events were triggered by trauma, with only 20% to 30% occurring spontaneously.[190]

Increased incidence of first-trimester abortion, placental abruption, and postpartum hemorrhage has been observed in patients with afibrinogenemia.[191] Fetuses of female afibrinogenemic patients rarely reach full term unless replacement therapy is given.[192] Replacement therapy for patients with afibrinogenemia is available,[193] although there may be some concern with increased risk of thrombosis during therapy. Patients with congenital hypofibrinogenemia do not typically have any spontaneous bleeding unless the fibrinogen level is <50 mg/dL. These patients may actually have hypodysfibrinogenemia, which is discussed in a later section of this chapter.

Laboratory Diagnosis

Screening coagulation tests from afibrinogenemic and hypofibrinogenemic patients typically show a marked prolongation of all tests where the endpoint is the appearance of fibrin clot, as severe fibrinogen deficiency renders plasma nonclottable. These tests include the PT, PTT, thrombin clotting time, and reptilase time. These test abnormalities, when caused by functional deficiency of clottable fibrinogen, are usually corrected when patient plasma is mixed with normal plasma.[194] A diagnosis of afibrinogenemia depends on the specific finding of undetectable fibrinogen antigen in the plasma of these patients. Platelet fibrinogen is also absent. Mild thrombocytopenia has been reported in some afibrinogenemic patients, but typically the platelet count is usually not lower than 100,000/μL.[195] Afibrinogenemic patients who undergo hypersensitivity reaction skin testing do not typically show an induration response to allergens. They show only erythema because the later phases of the hypersensitivity reaction depend on the deposition of subcutaneous fibrin.[196] Laboratory recommendations for the diagnosis of congenital fibrinogen disorders by the ISTH have been published.[174]

Differential Diagnosis and Therapy of Afibrinogenemia

Congenital quantitative defects in fibrinogen must be carefully distinguished from acquired quantitative defects in the fibrinogen molecule, which are often seen in the setting of liver disease or disseminated intravascular coagulation. Acquired hypofibrinogenemia has been reported after therapy with L-asparaginase, which impairs hepatic synthesis of fibrinogen,[197] and in patients with aplastic anemia treated with antithymocyte globulin and corticosteroids.[198] In the absence of purified fibrinogen concentrates, cryoprecipitate administration is used for replacement therapy for patients with severe afibrinogenemia. Prophylactic therapy is recommended for pregnant patients, or patients with a history of central nervous system (CNS) hemorrhage.[188] Replacement therapy is indicated for any episode of acute active bleeding and preoperatively. Fibrinogen levels between 50 and 100 mg/dL are usually adequate for normal hemostasis.[188] Levels >100 mg/dL are recommended for maintenance during pregnancy, based on empiric clinical observations.[188] Weekly infusions are recommended, but one should be aware that fibrinogen requirements may rise significantly around the time of parturition, and that levels as high as 150 mg/mL may be helpful to avert abruption.[199] Each bag of cryoprecipitate contains ~250 mg of fibrinogen, and one bag of cryoprecipitate typically raises plasma fibrinogen levels of an adult by ~10 mg/dL; thus, 5 to 10 bags of cryoprecipitate are usually sufficient in the average adult patient. Because the fractional catabolic rate of fibrinogen is 25% per day, acute-care patients should receive one-third of their loading dose daily for as long as fibrinogen support is desired.[193] There are plasma concentrates of fibrinogen now available that may provide advantages over the use of cryoprecipitate.[200] Measurement of plasma fibrinogen levels after infusion is recommended to confirm that a patient has obtained the desired therapeutic effect. The complications of replacement therapy in afibrinogenemia include allergic reactions, development of antifibrinogen antibodies, and anaphylaxis.[201] Thromboembolic complications following cryoprecipitate infusions include deep venous thrombosis and pulmonary emboli; the risk of these complications may be increased when an inhibitor of fibrinolysis or oral contraceptive therapy is also administered.[202] Low-molecular-weight heparin in combination with fibrinogen replacement has been used to avoid these thromboembolic complications.[203] Antifibrinolytics alone may be sufficient to prevent bleeding from mucosal sites, but caution should be exercised in patients with a personal or family history of thrombosis. Treatment of rare bleeding disorders, including afibrinogenemia, has been reviewed.[204]

Dysfibrinogenemia

The first reported case of dysfibrinogenemia mediated by a qualitatively abnormal fibrinogen molecule occurred in 1965, and since that time, >300 families have been reported with this disorder. The molecular genetic basis of fibrinogen dysfunction has been fairly well established in many families that have been studied. There is an intriguing report of an increased association of dysfibrinogenemia with chronic thromboembolic pulmonary hypertension.[205]

Molecular Basis of Dysfibrinogenemia

The reported abnormalities in the fibrinogen molecule include defects in each of the major steps of fibrin formation and stabilization. The conversion of fibrinogen to an insoluble fibrin clot requires that the molecule first be cleaved by thrombin between arginine 16 and glycine 17 of the Aα chain to release fibrinopeptide A, and between arginine 14 and valine 15 of the Bβ chain to release fibrinopeptide B. This produces a fibrin monomer capable of undergoing the second step, fibrin polymerization. Once these molecules polymerize, they are stabilized by the action of factor XIIIa. Fibrinogen also supports the hemostatic process through interaction with platelets during platelet cohesion (aggregation). Finally, during the process of wound healing and tissue remodeling, the fibrin clot undergoes fibrinolysis by concerted activities of plasminogen and plasminogen activators. Fibrinogen dysfunction may affect any of these various steps of fibrin clot formation, platelet interaction, or lysis. It is therefore expected that the dysfibrinogenemias can be associated with abnormal clinical bleeding, thrombotic tendency, disorders of wound healing, or no clinically apparent disease. Domain location of a mutation does not necessarily predict the associated disease phenotype. Defects of fibrinopeptide release have been associated with both hemorrhagic and thrombotic complications. Similarly, disruption of D-D interactions has been associated with both bleeding and thrombosis. Patients who have heterozygous dysfibrinogenemia typically have ~50% of normal fibrinogen levels, which should be adequate for hemostasis. Clottable fibrinogen protein measurements may not be a reliable indicator of plasma fibrinogen concentration, because functionally abnormal molecules are not always incorporated into the clot. An abnormal fibrinogen may inhibit the conversion of normal fibrinogen to fibrin, so the tendency for many of these patients to bleed is higher than one would suspect. Hypodysfibrinogenemia occurs when an abnormality of the fibrinogen molecule results in decreased secretion or increased clearance of the protein. More than 50 cases have been reported with hypodysfibrinogenemia.[206] Autosomal amyloidosis has been attributed to genetic disorders of fibrinogen, as well as to genetic disorders of several other proteins (including transthyretin, gelsolin, apolipoprotein A, and lysozyme). Hereditary renal amyloid disease has been associated with genetic defects of the Aα chain, and renal amyloid has recurred in renal transplants. Hepatic amyloid disease has also been attributed to abnormalities of fibrinogen.[207]

Dysfibrinogenemia is typically inherited as an autosomal dominant trait with high levels of penetrance. Most of these patients are heterozygotes, but a few homozygotes and some rare compound heterozygotes have been reported in the literature. Approximately 40% of dysfibrinogenemic patients are asymptomatic, and 45% to 50% have a bleeding disorder.[208] The remaining 10% to 15% have either a thrombotic disorder (venous or arterial) or both bleeding and thrombotic tendencies. The bleeding associated with dysfibrinogenemia is generally mild and includes soft-tissue hemorrhage, easy bruising, and menorrhagia. Although intraoperative and postoperative bleeding has been reported, most bleeding is not life threatening.

There are only a few families in which a thrombotic tendency can be unambiguously associated with dysfibrinogenemia, and criteria for making this association have been proposed. These criteria include a demonstrated molecular defect, thrombosis at an early age or in multiple family members, presence of no other predisposing factor for thrombosis, strong association between the fibrinogen defect and thrombus complications within a family, and association of the same molecular defect with thrombosis in another, unrelated kindred.[209] The true prevalence of thrombosis among patients with dysfibrinogenemia is unknown. Studies indicate a distinct thrombotic tendency in individuals with dysfibrinogenemia related to defects in the α-C domain of the Aα chain of fibrinogen, especially if new cysteine residues are encoded that can become disulfide linked to albumin. In contrast, dysfibrinogenemic patients with defective cross-linking experience primarily defective wound healing.

Laboratory Diagnosis of Dysfibrinogenemia

The thrombin clotting time remains a sensitive screening test for dysfibrinogenemias,[194] and the PT appears to be more sensitive than the PTT to the effects of dysfibrinogenemia. In some cases, clot formation may be absent. Reptilase is a snake venom enzyme that differs from thrombin in that it cleaves only fibrinopeptide A of fibrinogen. The reptilase time is often more prolonged than the thrombin clotting time, especially in patients who have defective fibrinopeptide A release. Some dysfibrinogenemias exhibit a very short thrombin clotting time, and these patients may have thrombotic complications. The fibrinogen concentration can be either low or normal in these patients. Most patients with dysfibrinogenemia have a significant discrepancy between the level of clottable fibrinogen and that detected by immunologic methods. Criteria for diagnosing dysfibrinogens using ratios of immunologic and functional fibrinogen assays have been reported.[210] Laboratory testing for fibrinogen abnormalities has been reviewed.[174] Recommendations also include genotyping to confirm the diagnosis and facilitate family screening.

The diagnosis of inherited dysfibrinogenemia must be distinguished from hypofibrinogenemia, which is either acquired or congenital in nature. Acquired dysfibrinogenemia occurs typically in the setting of severe liver disease,[211] and the suspicion can be readily investigated by evaluation of liver function tests. Acquired dysfibrinogenemias are also associated with malignancies that produce an abnormal fibrinogen molecule, such as some hepatomas (see Chapter 55), multiple myeloma,[212] as well as autoimmune disorders. An algorithm has been proposed for the orderly evaluation of patients in whom dysfibrinogenemia is a consideration.[194]

Acquired inhibitors to fibrin formation that interfere with fibrinogen-to-fibrin conversion may also be confused with dysfibrinogenemia. These acquired inhibitors include heparin-like molecules, elevated levels of fibrin split products, and antibodies at concentrations such as may occur in macroglobulinemia, multiple myeloma, or other disorders that interfere with fibrin polymerization.[213] Acquired antibodies against the fibrinogen molecule are quite rare but have been reported in association with a variety of diseases.[214]

Therapy

The majority of patients with dysfibrinogenemia do not require any specific therapy. Any bleeding complications that develop can be managed with transfusion of either plasma or cryoprecipitate. The role of the newer fibrinogen concentrates in treating patients with dysfibrinogenemia has not been clarified through appropriate clinical trials yet. Antifibrinolytic drugs have been used in some patients but should be especially avoided in patients who have thrombotic tendencies. Patients who have repeated venous thrombotic episodes may actually require long-term antithrombotic therapy. In women with dysfibrinogenemia, recurrent miscarriages may be prevented using prophylactic cryoprecipitate, and successful pregnancy outcomes in such cases have been reported.[188]

FACTOR XIII DEFICIENCY

The initial hemostatic plug is not sufficient to prevent blood loss unless it is stabilized by the action of plasma factor XIII (fibrin-stabilizing factor). A complex set of reactions among thrombin, fibrin, and plasma factor XIII is necessary for clot stabilization (see Chapter 20). Factor XIIIa transforms the unstable, noncovalently associated fibrin clot to a stable covalently cross-linked set of fibrin fibers that are mechanically stronger, more rigid, and more elastic. A cross-linked fibrin clot is more resistant to mechanical as well as enzymatic degradation by plasmin than uncross-linked fibrin because α_2-plasmin inhibitor is also cross-linked to fibrin to inhibit plasmin activity. Factor XIIIa is a transglutaminase that catalyzes the formation of intermolecular γ-glutamyl-ϵ-lysyl covalent (isopeptide) bonds between the γ chains and α chains of fibrin strands within the clot. In addition, several other plasma and extracellular matrix proteins are linked to the fibrin clot through the action of factor XIII. Cross-linking of thrombin-activatable fibrinolysis inhibitor into fibrin clots further increases the resistance of the clot to plasmin degradation.[215] Cross-linkage of fibrin to adhesive proteins such as vWF, fibronectin, thrombospondin, and vitronectin may improve adhesion to vessel walls and may play a role in cell migration during angiogenesis and wound healing.

Pathogenesis

In 1944, Robbins postulated that deficiency of fibrin-stabilizing factor, which later became known as factor XIII, would produce a serious bleeding disorder.[216] However, it was not until the first case of factor XIII deficiency was described in 1960 that the severe nature of this bleeding disorder was recognized.[217] Over 200 cases of congenital factor XIII deficiency have been reported in the literature.[218] It is estimated that ~1 person in every 1 million to 5 million people has factor XIII deficiency. The disorder is inherited as an autosomal recessive trait.[188,219]

The factor XIII molecule is present in both plasma and in blood platelets and monocytes. The plasma concentration of factor XIII is 14 to 28 µg/mL. Approximately half of that concentration circulates within blood platelets. Tissue-based factor XIII resides in monocyte/macrophages. Structurally, platelet and monocyte factor XIII consists of only A dimers present within the cytoplasm of both platelets and megakaryocytes. The plasma factor XIII molecular complex is a heterotetramer, containing two of each of the A and B subunits. The A subunit mediates factor XIII function, containing an activation peptide, calcium-binding site, and enzymatic domain with an active site sulfhydryl residue that is characteristic of this class of enzymes.[220] The B subunit appears to promote stabilization of the A subunit in plasma and may play an important role in regulating both the localization of the A subunit to the fibrin clot and thrombin-dependent activation of the protein. Two distinct forms of factor XIII deficiency have been described, based on whether the A and B subunits are absent or present.[215] In type I deficiency, there is absence of the B subunit, with resultant decreased concentration of the A subunit in plasma, but platelet A subunit content is maintained. In type II deficiency, the A subunit is absent and the B subunit is present.

Molecular Genetics

Since the protein was initially described in human serum in 1944, both the A and B subunits have been purified, and cDNA sequence and gene structure have been established.[215] The A subunit is encoded on chromosome 6, containing 15 exons and spanning a region of 160 kb. A common genetic polymorphism of the A subunit has been described that results in Val34 replacement by Leu just three amino acid residues from the site of cleavage of the activation peptide. This polymorphism may influence factor XIII activation and has been investigated in reference to risk for myocardial infarction.[221] The B subunit is encoded by chromosome 1.[222] Because the mode of inheritance of factor XIII deficiency is autosomal recessive in nature, only homozygotes or compound heterozygotes are clinically symptomatic. The homozygotes reported in the literature are often children of consanguineous marriages.[223]

Factor XIII deficiency is more frequently attributed to mutation of the gene encoding the A subunit, confirming the functional importance of this subunit. To date, over 70 mutations have been described.[218] The majority of defects observed are "point mutations" resulting in stop codons, missense errors, or frameshifts and small deletions. Factor XIII B chain deficiency is a very rare autosomal recessive disorder, with very few reported cases in the literature.[224] Only ~5 mutations have been reported in the B chain gene.[218]

Clinical Aspects

Clinically affected factor XIII–deficient patients typically have plasma levels that are <1% of normal,[215] with bleeding attributed to accelerated fibrin clot degradation. The bleeding phenotype in patients with inherited factor XIII deficiency is unusually severe. Abnormal bleeding manifests shortly after birth, when bleeding from the healthy umbilical cord remnant occurs.[225] This has been a prominent feature, reported in up to 80% of cases,[223] but this complication was observed in only 22% of the 34 cases reported to the North American Rare Bleeding Disorders Registry.[190] Umbilical stump bleeding is an uncommon presentation for other congenital bleeding disorders. Rebleeding at circumcision is also common. Other bleeding manifestations in these patients include soft-tissue hemorrhage, hemarthrosis, hematomas, and the development of large pseudocysts.[225] The most life-threatening complication of factor XIII deficiency is spontaneous intracranial hemorrhage. Intracranial hemorrhage is more prevalent in factor XIII deficiency than in other inherited bleeding disorders. Approximately 25% of factor XIII–deficient patients experience intracranial hemorrhage.[226] Bleeding is usually spontaneous, and prevention of intracranial hemorrhage forms the basis for the recommendation of prophylactic therapy of factor XIII–deficient patients. Surgery in these patients is often complicated by abnormal wound healing and excessive postoperative bleeding, which can occur either immediately or later. Poor wound healing is reported in ~20% of patients with factor XIII deficiency. The affected males in some families also have oligospermia, resulting in infertility. Furthermore, infertility in affected females results from spontaneous abortions. Females with this deficiency cannot carry a pregnancy to term unless plasma factor XIII levels are maintained at levels that prevent bleeding.[227] The manifestations of factor XIII deficiency vary greatly among patients and may not necessarily present as bleeding symptoms. The protean biologic activities of factor XIII have been summarized.[228]

Differential Diagnosis

Congenital or acquired factor XIII deficiency must be considered when a patient has a major bleeding disorder and all of the initial screening laboratory tests are normal, including PT, PTT, and platelet count. Bleeding can occur spontaneously or after major surgery. It remains imperative in the adult to exclude both inherited and acquired factor XIII deficiency, because patients can develop antibodies to factor XIII that interfere with fibrin stabilization. Specific antibodies to factor XIII were reported in patients taking isoniazid, phenytoin, procainamide, penicillin, and valproic acid.[215] Factor XIII antibodies also occur in association with autoimmune disease, in patients with monoclonal gammopathy, or as an idiopathic occurrence. Acquired factor XIII deficiency has been reported in Henoch-Schönlein purpura, liver disease, Crohn disease, and ulcerative colitis.[215]

Laboratory Diagnosis

The PT and PTT assays are normal (*Table 54.5*). The solubility of a fibrin clot in 5 M urea or 1% monochloroacetic acid (clot stability assay) is the most useful screening test for factor XIII deficiency. In these conditions, clots formed in the absence of factor XIII activity dissolve within 60 minutes.[215] In contrast, normal clots covalently modified by factor XIIIa remain insoluble for at least 24 hours. This is a qualitative assay, and as little as 5% of the normal factor XIII activity level can render a clot insoluble in urea. Unfortunately, clot stability testing is not well standardized. If clot solubility is found, a mixing study with normal plasma is recommended to exclude factor XIII inhibitor. Deficiency of α_2-antiplasmin may also cause a bleeding disorder with normal coagulation screening studies and increased urea clot solubility; a specific assay for α_2-antiplasmin should be considered to exclude this possibility. Quantitative measurements of factor XIII activity can also be done, and these tests are useful to confirm factor XIII deficiency that is suspected based on an abnormal qualitative clot solubility assay. Specialized laboratories may measure either ammonia production (an end product of the factor XIIIa reaction) or the incorporation of fluorescent or radioactive amines (such as dansyl-cadaverine) into proteins such as casein. Quantitative factor XIII activity assays perform better than clot solubility assays in detecting factor XIII deficiency; however, some quantitative activity assays overestimate low factor XIII levels.[229]

PROTHROMBIN DEFICIENCY

Inherited prothrombin deficiency is an exceedingly rare, autosomal recessive bleeding disorder, with a frequency of 1 in ~2 million.[230,231] To date, <50 mutations have been identified from <100 reported cases (isth.org database). As with some of the other factor deficiencies, the frequency of prothrombin deficiency is greater in countries where consanguineous marriages occur. Phenotypically, prothrombin deficiency is classified as either *hypoprothrombinemia* (type I), distinguished by reduced prothrombin activity and reduced prothrombin antigen, or *dysprothrombinemia* (type II), distinguished by reduced prothrombin activity but normal prothrombin antigen.

Pathophysiology

By convention, these mutant prothrombins have been named according to the proband's origin, for example, prothrombin Cardeza.[231] The prevalence of prothrombin deficiency in Puerto Ricans led to the recent description of several unrelated families of Puerto Rican ancestry having a common mutation, prothrombin Puerto Rico I, with characteristics of both hypoprothrombinemia and dysprothrombinemia.[232] Dysprothrombins with amino acid substitutions at or near the factor Xa cleavage sites inhibit activation to thrombin.[233] Amino acid substitutions elsewhere in prothrombin can affect the function determined by that region, including the catalytic domain (Quick II),[234] Molise, Perijé, and fibrinogen binding (Quick I).[235]

Clinical Features

Epistaxis, menorrhagia, and posttraumatic bleeding are the most common complaints. Hemarthroses and muscle hematomas have also been reported.[230] The extent of prothrombin deficiency does not necessarily correlate with clinical bleeding. Although hemostasis can be maintained by prothrombin levels >25% of normal, significant bleeding is usually seen when prothrombin levels are <2% of normal.[236] Of the severe prothrombin deficiency patients reported to the Rare Bleeding Disorders Registry, 20% experienced intracranial bleeding.[190] Prothrombin-deficient heterozygotes have 40% to 60% of normal prothrombin activity; compound heterozygotes and homozygotes usually have >10% of normal prothrombin activity.[237] As of yet, no human cases of total prothrombin deficiency have been reported. Based on studies with knockout mice, such a complete deficiency is thought to be incompatible with life, leading to a loss of vascular integrity, arrested development, and tissue necrosis, ultimately resulting in embryonic or neonatal lethality.[238] This effect is thought to result from a developmental activity of thrombin on yolk sac vasculature. The genetic elimination of prothrombin in an adult mouse model was also not compatible with survival.[239]

Laboratory Diagnosis

A summary of laboratory findings in prothrombin deficiency is included in *Table 54.5*. Prothrombin deficiency is associated with normal thrombin times but prolonged PT and aPTT, which can be corrected in mixing studies. Specific factor assays for prothrombin are used in diagnosis. Acquired prothrombin deficiency, caused by either vitamin K deficiency or an antiprothrombin antibody associated with antiphospholipid antibodies, should be considered before making the diagnosis of inherited prothrombin deficiency. Fresh-frozen plasma (FFP) and prothrombin complex concentrates (PCCs) are used to treat prothrombin deficiency,[204] as outlined later, in *Table 54.8*.

FACTOR V DEFICIENCY

Inherited factor V deficiency, also known as *labile factor deficiency*, *proaccelerin deficiency*, and *parahemophilia*, is a rare autosomal recessive bleeding disorder first described by Owren,[240] with an estimated frequency of 1 in 1 million. To date, there are over 200 reported cases,[241,242] and a database at isth.org lists >120 factor V mutations. As with some of the other factor deficiencies, the frequency of factor V deficiency is greater in countries where consanguineous marriages occur. This subject has been recently reviewed.[243]

Pathophysiology

The majority of factor V deficiencies result from a failure to either synthesize or secrete factor V. The mutants responsible for these deficiencies are CRM negative (type I); CRM-positive factor V mutations (type II) have also been detected.[244] The CRM-negative form is a product of missense, nonsense, insertion, or deletion mutations and is characterized by a true deficiency of factor V, with a strong correlation between functional assays and immunoassays. Factor V New Brunswick, a CRM-positive form, is caused by a missense mutation and is characterized by antigenically competent factor V with reduced activity, most likely because of reduced stability of factor Va.[245]

By convention, many of these mutant factor Vs have been named according to the proband's origin, for example, factor V Stanford[246] and factor V Ogden.[247] Factor V Quebec is associated with a moderate reduction in plasma factor V levels and a severe reduction in platelet factor V, but also other α-granule proteins, including multimerin (a factor V carrier molecule within platelets), and is thus more properly considered a platelet disorder.[248] Approximately 20% of the circulating pool of factor V is contained within platelets. This platelet pool of factor V and low levels of tissue factor pathway inhibitor seen in factor V–deficient patients may explain the milder bleeding phenotype in this bleeding disorder.[242,243]

Clinical Features

Epistaxis, menorrhagia, and posttraumatic bleeding are the most common complaints. Trauma-induced hemarthroses and muscle hematomas have also been reported.[242] Gastrointestinal or CNS bleeding is observed very rarely. Hemostasis can be maintained by factor V levels >10% to 20% of normal, but moderately severe bleeding is usually seen when factor V levels are <10% of normal. Factor V–deficient heterozygotes have 40% to 60% of normal factor V activity; compound heterozygotes and homozygotes usually have <10% of normal factor

Table 54.8. Replacement Therapy in Inherited Coagulation Disorders

Disorder	Therapeutic Product	Loading Dose	Maintenance Dose
von Willebrand disease	Humate-P[a]	40-60 IU/kg	40-50 IU/kg every 12-24 h for up to 7 d
	Wilate[a]	40-60 IU/kg	20-40 IU/kg every 12-24 h for up to 7 d
	Vonvendi[a]	50-80 IU/kg	40-60 IU/kg every 8-24 h for up to 7 d
	Cryoprecipitate[b]	Not required	1 bag/10 kg daily
Fibrinogen deficiency	Cryoprecipitate	1-2 bags/10 kg	1 bag/10 kg every other d
	Purified fibrinogen	50-100 mg/kg	20 mg/kg every other d
Prothrombin deficiency	Fresh-frozen plasma[c]	15 mL/kg	5-10 mL/kg daily
Dysprothrombinemia	Purified prothrombin complex[d]	20 IU/kg	10 IU/kg daily
Factor V deficiency	Fresh-frozen plasma	20 mL/kg	10 mL/kg every 12-24 h
Factor VII deficiency	Recombinant factor VIIa	15-30 mcg/kg	15-30 mcg/kg every 4-6 hours until hemostasis is achieved
	Fresh-frozen plasma[c]	20 mL/kg	5 mL/kg every 6-24 h
	Purified prothrombin complex[d]	30 IU/kg	10-20 IU/kg every 6-24 h
Factor X deficiency	Plasma-derived factor X	25 IU/kg	25 IU/kg daily
	Fresh-frozen plasma[c]	15-20 mL/kg	5-10 mL/kg daily
	Purified prothrombin complex[d]	15 IU/kg	10 IU/kg daily
Factor XI deficiency	Fresh-frozen plasma[c]	15-20 mL/kg	5 mL/kg every 12-24 h
Factor XIII deficiency	Plasma or recombinant factor XIII	35-40 IU/kg	35-40 IU/kg monthly
	Fresh-frozen plasma	5 mL/kg every 1-2 wk	Not usually required

The replacement therapy regimens suggested in this table are for major bleeding or surgical prophylaxis. Patients with minor bleeding may require lower dosages of these replacement products. Confirmation of hemostatic levels of the appropriate coagulation factor being replaced should be done, with dosage adjustments performed as needed.
[a]Labeled in ristocetin cofactor units. Alphanate and Wilate can also be used to treat von Willebrand disease, Vonvendi therapy may require initial therapy with factor VIII.
[b]Recommended only if purified factor replacement therapy is not available.
[c]Plasma after removal of cryoprecipitate is satisfactory.
[d]Prothrombin complex concentrates are thrombogenic and should be used only for major bleeding or major surgery. Antifibrinolytic drugs (ε-aminocaproic acid, tranexamic acid) should not be used in conjunction with prothrombin complex concentrates.

V activity. Bleeding symptoms may correlate better with platelet factor V content rather than the plasma factor V level.[248]

A genetic model of factor V deficiency utilizing factor V–knockout mice underscores the importance of factor V in not only hemostasis but development, as fetal loss in utero is markedly increased.[249] Based on these knockout-mouse studies, complete factor V deficiency is apparently incompatible with life, but <0.1% of normal factor V activity is sufficient to rescue completely deficient mice.[250] As of yet, no human cases of total factor V deficiency have been reported, and even patients with a homozygous or compound heterozygous factor V deficiency usually have some residual factor V activity.

Laboratory Diagnosis

A summary of laboratory findings in factor V deficiency is included in *Table 54.5*. Factor V deficiency is associated with normal thrombin times but prolonged PT and aPTT, which can be corrected in mixing studies. A PT–based factor V assay or an ELISA can be used to verify quantitative reductions in factor V. Acquired factor V deficiency, caused by liver disease, disseminated intravascular coagulation, or antibodies to factor V, should be excluded before making the diagnosis of inherited factor V deficiency. Upon confirmation of factor V deficiency, however, a specific assay for factor VIII should also be performed to rule out the rare combined factor V/factor VIII deficiency,[251] the treatment of which entails a different replacement therapy. Currently, FFP or platelet transfusion is used to treat factor V deficiency, as outlined later, in *Table 54.8*.

FACTOR VII DEFICIENCY

Factor VII deficiency was first described in 1951 by Alexander et al under the name *serum prothrombin conversion accelerator deficiency*. Approximately 200 cases of true factor VII deficiency have been reported, and the population prevalence is estimated to be 1 in 500,000,[252] making it the most common of the "rare bleeding disorders." Also known as *stable factor* or *proconvertin deficiency*, the condition is inherited as an autosomal recessive trait that produces severe deficiency in the homozygote and mild deficiency, usually without clinical manifestations, in the heterozygote. As in other rare bleeding disorders, it is more common in cultures where consanguineous marriage is practiced.

Pathophysiology

Factor VII is secreted as a single-chain proenzyme glycoprotein of ~50 kDa by hepatocytes. Factor VII has the shortest plasma half-life of all coagulation factors (~5 hours), and its plasma concentration is very low, ~500 ng/mL.[253] Factor VIIa is detectable in trace amounts in normal plasma,[254] and sensitive assays indicate that <1% of circulating factor VII is in the activated form.[254] Tissue factor increases the rate of activation of factor VII significantly, and current theory is that coagulation is initiated in the presence of tissue factor that is exposed at sites of vascular injury or contributed by blood monocytes.[255]

In a mouse knockout model in which factor VII is completely lacking, fatal hemorrhage occurs perinatally.[256] In humans, factor VII deficiency occurs as a recessive trait resulting from homozygous or compound heterozygous mutations. Many mutations of the factor VII gene have been reported, with >200 mutations listed in a database at isth.org. Most reported genetic defects are single-base substitutions, including missense, splice-site, and nonsense mutations. Most mutations affect only a few patients, but one mutation (Ala242Val) was detected in 23 "apparently" unrelated Jews in Israel.[257] The association of Dubin-Johnson syndrome with factor VII deficiency[258] may simply reflect a high consanguinity rate. Combined deficiency of factor VII along with the other vitamin K–dependent coagulation proteins or as a deficiency with a single other coagulation protein has been reported in rare families (see section Miscellaneous Inherited Coagulation Disorders).

Clinical Features

Only severe factor VII deficiency is associated with hemorrhagic symptoms, and heterozygous carriers are usually asymptomatic. Factor VII levels do not completely correlate with the severity of symptoms, and this may in part reflect heterogeneity in the molecular basis of factor VII deficiency or the tissue factor–containing reagents used to quantify the factor VII activity level in patients.[259] However, patients with levels of >10 to 15 IU/dL rarely manifest bleeding.[260] Patients with levels between 5 and 10 IU/dL tend to have milder symptoms, such as epistaxis, gingival bleeding, or genitourinary and gastrointestinal bleeding. Patients with levels <1 IU/dL may have symptoms similar to patients with hemophilia A or hemophilia B, with spontaneous joint and deep-muscle bleeding, but some patients with factor VII levels of <1 IU/dL have been asymptomatic.[252] Bleeding in the CNS is particularly common, being observed in 15% to 60% of patients with factor VII levels <2 IU/dL.[261] CNS bleeds often present during the neonatal period, and the risk of recurrence is high enough that prophylaxis with factor replacement therapy should be considered in patients who present with this complication.[262] The severity of bleeding after trauma or surgical procedures varies to a surprising degree in this disorder, with oral and urogenital cavity procedures being particularly troublesome, possibly reflecting the high local fibrinolytic activity in these regions of the body. Prior clinical bleeding symptoms are an important prognostic factor predicting surgical bleeding complications in patients with factor VII deficiency.

Some reports indicate that patients with factor VII deficiency may also be more prone to various thromboembolic manifestations.[263] The explanation for this phenomenon is unknown, but thrombophilic markers have been observed in most of these cases.[264]

Laboratory Diagnosis

In factor VII deficiency, normal results are obtained with coagulation tests that bypass the extrinsic pathway of coagulation and factor VII (*Table 54.5*), that is, the PTT, thrombin time, and, if tested, the Stypven (Russell viper venom) time. Thus, a diagnosis of factor VII deficiency is suspected in a patient with a lifelong history of bleeding when there is an isolated prolonged PT and normal PTT. The PT will correct on 1:1 mixing of patient plasma with normal plasma, but a diagnosis of factor VII deficiency requires a specific factor VII assay for confirmation. The use of human recombinant thromboplastin in the PT assay is recommended, as results with this reagent better predict bleeding risk.[252] A factor VII mutation (factor VII Padua) has been described in African-American patients who are asymptomatic; this defect results in low factor VII activity levels when rabbit brain thromboplastin is used, but normal factor VII activity when human thromboplastin is used.[265] Confirmation of low factor VII antigen level can be obtained by ELISA. Levels of factor VII in heterozygous carriers overlap the normal range. Before making a diagnosis of factor VII deficiency, one should exclude causes for acquired abnormalities such as vitamin K deficiency, liver disease, or warfarin therapy. Also, rare conditions such as combined deficiency of all vitamin K–dependent factors, and combined factor VII and factor X deficiency should be considered. Autoantibody directed to factor VII occurs, but few case reports have been published.

Treatment of factor VII deficiency with recombinant human factor VIIa, plasma, or PCCs is discussed later in this chapter. Although the necessity for correcting factor VII deficiency has been questioned,[266] patients who have factor VII deficiency and a history of excessive clinical bleeding should be given replacement therapy before surgery. Numerous clinical reviews confirm that the patient's clinical bleeding history is the best predictive parameter of bleeding risk.[252,267] Patients with factor VII deficiency who have factor VII levels >10% when assayed using human thromboplastin reagents have minimal bleeding symptoms.

FACTOR X DEFICIENCY

Inherited factor X deficiency, first described in the Prower[268] and Stuart[269] kindreds, is a rare autosomal recessive bleeding disorder with an estimated frequency of 1 in 1 million.[204,270] Factor X deficiency represents ~10% of all rare bleeding disorders. Over 100 mutations have been identified,[270] with the majority being missense mutations.[271] As with some of the other factor deficiencies, the frequency of factor X deficiency is greater in countries where consanguineous marriages occur. Phenotypically, factor X deficiency is classified as either type I, distinguished by reduced factor X activity and reduced factor X antigen, or type II, distinguished by reduced factor X activity but normal factor X antigen.

Pathophysiology

The CRM-negative form is a product of missense, insertion, or deletion mutations, and is characterized by a true deficiency of factor X, with a strong correlation between functional assays and immunoassays. The CRM-reduced and -positive forms are products of missense mutations and are characterized by low to normal levels of antigenically competent factor X but with disproportionately reduced factor X activity. Deletion mutations result in premature termination and thus the loss of the factor X catalytic domain, whereas missense mutations may affect not only the catalytic domain, but phospholipid binding, activation, secretion, or even synthesis of factor X. By convention, these mutant factor Xs have been named according to the proband's origin, for example, factor X San Antonio I[272] and factor X Friuli.[273]

Clinical Features

The symptoms of factor X deficiency tend to be the most severe of the inherited coagulation deficiencies.[270] Epistaxis, menorrhagia, and posttraumatic bleeding are common complaints, and hemarthroses and hematomas have been reported in two-thirds of factor X–deficient patients. Umbilical stump, gastrointestinal, and CNS bleeding are also frequently observed. Heterozygotes generally appear asymptomatic, as hemostasis can be maintained by factor X levels >10% of normal. However, compound heterozygotes and homozygotes with factor X levels <1% of normal suffer from severe bleeding. Experiments utilizing factor X–knockout mice resulted in either neonatal death or postnatal death, caused by intraabdominal or intracranial bleeding.[274]

Laboratory Diagnosis

A summary of laboratory findings in factor X deficiency is included in *Table 54.5*. Factor X deficiency is associated with normal thrombin times but prolonged PT, aPTT, and often Stypven (Russell viper venom) time, particularly among the CRM-negative variants. Unfortunately, factor X–deficient variants have been described with isolated prolonged PT or aPTT values.[275,276] Upon ruling out other inherited bleeding disorders, a factor X–specific assay can be used to verify factor X deficiency. Acquired factor X deficiency, caused by liver disease, warfarin therapy, amyloidosis,[277] or antibodies to factor X, should be excluded before making the diagnosis of inherited factor X deficiency. Currently, FFP, PCCs and a plasma-derived factor X concentrate (Coagadex) are used to treat factor X deficiency, as outlined in *Table 54.8*.

FACTOR XI DEFICIENCY

Factor XI deficiency (plasma thromboplastin antecedent deficiency) was first recognized by Rosenthal et al in 1953[278] and was called *hemophilia C*. Factor XI deficiency is transmitted as an incompletely recessive autosomal trait manifested either as a major defect in homozygous patients with factor XI levels <20 IU/dL or as a minor defect in heterozygous patients with levels ranging from 30 to 65 IU/dL.[279] The incidence of this disorder varies widely, with estimates of frequency in the general population being 1 in 1 million persons. A particularly high frequency of the disorder exists in people of Jewish extraction,[279-281] with an estimated gene frequency of 5% to 11% in Ashkenazi Jews.[282] Up to 0.3% of this population is homozygous for factor XI deficiency.[282]

Factor XI deficiency has been reported to result from three major types of mutations: type I mutations result in disruption of splicing; type II mutations result in a stop codon and nonfunctional molecule; and type III mutations result in amino acid substitutions and a dysfunctional molecule.[283] Patients with type II mutations have the greatest bleeding tendency.[284] Type II and III mutations are most common in Ashkenazi Jews.

A more recent classification scheme for factor XI–deficient cases that are CRM-negative includes three mechanistic categories: (1) mutations that reduce or prevent polypeptide synthesis, (2) mutations resulting in polypeptides that fail to form intracellular dimers, and (3) mutations resulting in polypeptides that form dimers that are not secreted.[285] Mechanism (3) may account for some kindreds with apparent autosomal dominant factor XI deficiency.[286] In general, most factor XI mutations result in decreased factor XI protein proportionate to factor XI clotting activity. Over 200 factor XI mutations have been reported[287,288] (database at isth.org).

Clinical Features

The clinical manifestations of factor XI deficiency are extremely variable and generally milder than those of hemophilia A or B.[280,287,289] As a rule, spontaneous bleeding is rare, and hemorrhage usually occurs only after trauma or a surgical procedure. The extent of factor XI deficiency may not correlate with bleeding.[280,287,289] Hemarthrosis is uncommon, but delayed bleeding is a particularly treacherous feature in some patients,[290] especially for surgical procedures involving tissues rich in fibrinolytic activity.[188] Mild factor XI deficiency may be associated with Noonan syndrome[291] and Gaucher disease.[292] Hemorrhagic manifestations may be absent in certain patients,[293] especially in those with type I mutations. Approximately one-half of heterozygous factor XI–deficient patients have a bleeding tendency.[294] Factor XI deficiency should be considered in female patients with menorrhagia.[295] In one study of women with menorrhagia, the prevalence of factor XI deficiency was 4%.[125]

Laboratory Diagnosis and Treatment

In the homozygous form of factor XI deficiency,[296] the PTT is prolonged. In most of these patients, factor XI levels in the plasma are in the range of 3 to 15 IU/dL. In people with the mild form of the disorder, the PTT often is normal because most PTT reagents are insensitive to mild factor XI deficiency.[57,188] Abnormalities in the plasma of such mildly affected patients may be removed by freezing. Specific factor assays are used to diagnose factor XI deficiency. The thrombin time is normal. Factor XI deficiency has also been reported in combination with inherited factor IX deficiency (type VI familial multiple factor deficiency).[297] Treatment of factor XI deficiency with plasma is summarized in *Table 54.8*. The management of factor XI deficiency in pregnancy has been reviewed.[298]

FACTOR XII DEFICIENCY

Factor XII deficiency was discovered by Ratnoff and Colopy during routine preoperative coagulation studies on John Hageman, an adult who had no evidence or history of abnormal bleeding.[299,300] The disorder, subsequently named *Hageman factor deficiency*, is inherited as an autosomal recessive trait. Factor XII deficiency has been identified in 1.5% to 3.0% of a healthy blood donor population.[301]

Pathophysiology

The plasma of most patients with factor XII deficiency does not contain material that reacts with antibodies to this factor. Radioimmunoassays with heterologous antibodies have demonstrated antigenic material identical to normal factor XII in only 2 of 42[302] separate kindreds. One large study of 31 factor XII–deficient kindreds identified most mutations in the serine protease domain.[303]

Clinical Features

Factor XII deficiency usually is not associated with hemorrhagic manifestations.[299,304] It is noteworthy that myocardial infarction and thrombophlebitis have been observed in patients with severe factor XII deficiency,[305] and that Hageman died of thromboembolic complications.[306] It was originally thought that factor XII deficiency might actually predispose to thrombosis, possibly as the result of deficient activation of fibrinolysis.[307] However, surveys indicate that factor XII deficiency is not associated with an excessive risk of thrombosis[52,308,309]; thrombotic events in factor XII–deficient patients may be explained by the presence of other prothrombotic gene defects in these patients.[310]

In vitro experiments suggest that factor XII has a central role in the initiation of the intrinsic pathway of coagulation and mediates a variety of other processes such as fibrinolysis, complement activation, inflammation, and chemotaxis.[311]

The discrepancy between in vitro evidence of grossly abnormal blood coagulation and the absence of hemorrhagic manifestations in factor XII deficiency poses a fundamental question regarding the role of the intrinsic coagulation pathway in hemostasis and the significance of laboratory measurements of coagulation. Alternative mechanisms for initiation of coagulation are discussed in Chapters 20 and 56.

Results of an animal model of arterial thrombosis have raised the question of whether factor XII has a role in thrombosis.[312] When factor XII–deficient mice were exposed to arterial vascular injury, defective platelet-rich thrombosis was observed, a defect that was corrected by administration of exogenous factor XII.[312] Results from a mouse stroke model indicate that factor XII deficiency protects affected mice from ischemic brain injury.[313] Although a large body of clinical evidence suggests that factor XII is not important for hemostasis, the animal model data suggest that factor XII is important for pathologic (arterial) thrombosis, perhaps by factor XII$_a$–mediated factor XI activation.[314] A summary of data supporting a role for factor XII (and other contact activation pathway proteins) in thrombosis risk has been published.[315]

Laboratory Diagnosis

Factor XII–deficient patients typically present with a negative history of clinical bleeding and an isolated, prolonged PTT that corrects with mixing with normal plasma. Normal levels of factor XII range from 50 to 150 IU/dL. Laboratory demonstration of the heterozygous state is difficult. The mean level of factor XII in the plasma of carriers is ~50% of normal, but observed values are distributed in a bimodal manner, an observation interpreted as suggesting the presence of multiple abnormal alleles.

PREKALLIKREIN DEFICIENCY

An additional abnormality of the intrinsic pathway of coagulation was defined and named *Fletcher factor deficiency* by Hathaway in 1965.[316] In 1972, Wuepper et al established that Fletcher factor was identical to plasma prekallikrein, a protein that had been studied for many years in terms of its role in inflammation.[317] The convergence of these two avenues of research demonstrated that prekallikrein, in addition to its role in inflammation and chemotaxis, is essential for the optimal activation and fragmentation of factor XII in the early steps of coagulation.

Pathophysiology and Genetics

Prekallikrein deficiency is inherited as an autosomal recessive trait.[318] Over 100 cases have been reported.[318] Heterozygotes with ~50% of normal plasma levels of prekallikrein can be identified. The prevalence of severe prekallikrein deficiency is ~1:150,000; in Africans the prevalence is ~1:5000.[318] Severe deficiency is associated with mutations in KLKB1, but other mutations have been reported.[318]

Clinical Features

Prekallikrein deficiency, like factor XII deficiency, is not associated with abnormal bleeding. Studies of affected patients revealed variable deficiencies in stress-induced fibrinolysis, chemotaxis, immediate and delayed inflammatory responses, and responses to preformed permeability–enhancing activity.[319] These abnormalities are not associated with any apparent deleterious effects. Most patients with prekallikrein deficiency are of African ancestry.[318] Prekallikrein deficiency is not associated with an excessive risk of either bleeding or thrombosis[52]; however, as with factor XII deficiency, prekallikrein-deficient mice are protected from arterial thrombosis.[314]

Laboratory Diagnosis

Prekallikrein deficiency is associated with a moderate prolongation of the PTT. The PT and thrombin time are normal. The disorder is characterized by abnormally slow contact activation. Thus, the PTT may be normalized by prolonged incubation (10-15 minutes) of plasma with particulate activators.[320] This phenomenon appears to result from autoactivation of factor XII.[320] Specific assays for prekallikrein are based on traditional coagulation techniques and chromogenic substrate assays.

HIGH-MOLECULAR-WEIGHT KININOGEN DEFICIENCY

A unique inherited coagulation abnormality associated with deficiencies of kinin formation and fibrinolysis was described in three unrelated kindreds in 1975. The disorder received the names of the affected families (Fitzgerald trait,[321] Williams trait,[322] Flaujeac trait, and Fujiwara trait)[323] and has subsequently been found to be the result of deficiency of HMWK. Patients with this disorder are asymptomatic. HMWK functions in its nonactivated form as a cofactor, binding prekallikrein, and factor XI to anionic surfaces, accelerating their activation by surface-bound factor XIIa (see Chapter 20).

Pathophysiology

Deficiency of HMWK appears to be inherited as an autosomal recessive trait. Mildly affected heterozygotes have been identified in some families. Detailed biochemical studies of five kindreds revealed considerable heterogeneity.[322,323] Thus, HMWK levels in the plasma ranged from nil[321] to 50 IU/dL.[322] With the exception of the Fitzgerald kindred, associated deficiencies in low-molecular-weight kininogen have been demonstrated in all families. Variable deficiency of prekallikrein also was present in the Williams, Fitzgerald, and Fujiwara kindreds; prekallikrein levels were normal in the Flaujeac kindred. The absence of the stabilizing effects of HMWK may lead to accelerated degradation and deficiency of prekallikrein in this disorder.[324] However, as discussed earlier with deficiency of either factor XII or prekallikrein, deficiency of HMWK is also associated with arterial thrombosis protection.[314] HMWK deficiency is not associated with excessive clinical bleeding or thrombosis. There is limited information on the genetic basis for HMWK deficiency.[325-327]

Laboratory Diagnosis

Deficiency of HMWK is manifested by an isolated, prolonged PTT. The PTT assay results are abnormal irrespective of whether particulate or soluble contact activators are used, and values are not normalized by prolonged incubation of the plasma with particulate activators.

MISCELLANEOUS INHERITED COAGULATION DISORDERS

Combined Defects

Of unusual interest are reports concerning the presence of combined deficiencies of two or more coagulation factors. Deficiency of factors V and VIII and combined deficiency of various vitamin K–dependent factors appear to be the most common combined deficiency disorders.[328] Several other combined coagulation defects have been described (*Table 54.1*).

Deficiency of Factors V and VIII

Combined deficiency of factors V and VIII, reported in <200 patients, is inherited as an autosomal recessive trait.[329] This combined defect manifests clinically with mild mucosal and cutaneous bleeding. Severe posttraumatic and postsurgical bleeding is common (e.g., after tooth extractions).[329] Hemarthrosis is rare. Laboratory findings in homozygous patients include a prolonged PTT and PT and levels of factor VIIIc and Vc that average 15 IU/dL. Levels of factor VIIIAg (VIIIcAg) and VAg are low and are proportional to those obtained by coagulation measurements.[330]

Linkage analysis of combined factor V and VIII deficiency to chromosome 18q excluded all known hemostasis proteins, suggesting that the basis for the disease is a defect affecting a process common to the biosynthesis of factors V and VIII. Indeed, subsequent studies by two groups identified the genetic basis for most patients with the disorder as mutations in the endoplasmic reticulum–Golgi intermediate compartment protein 53 (also known as lectin mannose–binding type 1 [LMAN1]). Other patients with this combined defect have mutations in another protein termed multiple coagulation factor deficiency-2 (MCFD2).[331-333] LMAN1 and MCFD2 form a complex that acts as a receptor (chaperone) or cargo receptor for transport of several secreted proteins, including factors V and VIII.[332,334] This rare bleeding disorder has been reviewed.[335]

Combined Deficiency of Factors II, VII, IX, and X

Combined deficiency of factors II, VII, IX, and X is an autosomal recessive coagulation disorder that has been identified in only a small number of patients.[190,328,336] In addition to low levels of the vitamin K–dependent factors, skeletal abnormalities may also be seen, resulting from effects on bone Gla proteins.[337] Levels of the vitamin K–dependent proteins range from <12% to 50% of normal; thus, clinical bleeding manifestations may vary widely. Both the PT and PTT are prolonged. Measurement of serum warfarin levels may be necessary to exclude surreptitious anticoagulant use. Mutations in the γ-glutamyl carboxylase gene have been identified in a few patients with this disorder,[338-340] and another group has identified a second gene locus (vitamin K epoxide reductase complex, subunit 1) causing this defect.[341] Some patients have clinical improvement and correction of the coagulopathy with vitamin K therapy.[336-339]

ABNORMALITIES OF PROTEASE INHIBITORS

Rare abnormalities of three plasma antiproteases, which are associated with bleeding, are described in this section. Other, more numerous abnormalities of the components of the antiprotease system and the fibrinolytic enzyme system that may be associated with thrombosis are discussed in Chapter 56.

α2-Antiplasmin Deficiency

Severe bleeding, including hemarthrosis, was associated with deficiency of α_2-antiplasmin in several kindreds.[342-345] This disorder appears to be inherited as an autosomal recessive trait, in which heterozygotes have detectable deficiencies of this antiprotease but only mild bleeding. A report published in 2008 identified 15 cases; seven cases had genetic abnormalities defined.[346] Most cases had mutations in exon 10, which is the location of the active site, and the plasminogen-binding site.[346] Modifications of α_2-antiplasmin may occur in vivo to regulate its activity.[347]

Bleeding presumably is the result of premature lysis of hemostatically important fibrin plugs caused by unregulated plasmin activity. The laboratory findings are variable. Hypofibrinogenemia and increased clot solubility in urea have been reported. Fibrinogen degradation product levels and platelet counts were normal in most cases.[345] When assayed qualitatively by fluorometric or photochromogenic techniques, α_2-antiplasmin levels usually are <10 IU/dL. Treatment of bleeding episodes with tranexamic acid and other antifibrinolytic agents may be helpful. α_2-Antiplasmin deficiency should be considered as a cause of bleeding in patients with unknown bleeding disorders.[348,349]

Plasminogen Activator Inhibitor-1 Deficiency

Deficiency of plasminogen activator inhibitor (PAI)-1 is associated with a moderate bleeding disorder.[350] Fewer than 40 patients have been reported.[349] One study investigated a large kindred with multiple family members who were homozygous for this disorder.[351] Homozygous, but not heterozygous, patients exhibited clinical bleeding.[351] The null gene mutation responsible for PAI-1 deficiency was identified in this kindred.[351] Another case was described; the phenotype was severe hemorrhage and prolonged wound healing.[352] PAI-1 deficiency is also associated with miscarriage and preterm birth.[349] The basis of the bleeding is similar to that described for α_2-antiplasmin deficiency: excessive plasmin activity, caused in this case by excessive activation of plasminogen. Laboratory screening studies are typically normal, but the euglobulin clot lysis time is shortened. It is recommended that measurement of PAI-1 antigen and activity in both serum and plasma be done to screen for PAI-1 deficiency.[351] The in vitro activities and clinical relevance of PAI-1 have been reviewed.[353]

α_1-Antitrypsin Pittsburgh

A lifelong hemorrhagic diathesis in a 14-year-old boy was associated with a unique qualitatively abnormal form of α_1-antitrypsin (antithrombin III Pittsburgh).[354] This disorder is the result of the substitution of a single amino acid (arginine for methionine at position 358 in the α_1-antitrypsin molecule).[354] This site corresponds to the P1 residue or "bait" amino acid of the molecule, and the substitution produced a mutation of α_1-antitrypsin, a weak antiprotease with little affinity for thrombin, into a potent antithrombin that impaired blood coagulation to a significant degree. The mutant molecule also is a potent inhibitor of factor XIa, factor XIIf, and kallikrein, a property lacking in the normal molecule.[355] The plasma concentration of the abnormal molecule increased after trauma, possibly as the result of an acute-phase response. The patient ultimately died of bleeding. Additional patients with this disorder have been identified to date.[356]

Tissue Factor Deficiency

One case of heterozygous tissue factor deficiency was described.[357] The patient had a bleeding disorder with normal routine coagulation tests; the disorder was identified by screening thrombosis patients using whole genome sequencing.

TREATMENT OF INHERITED COAGULATION DISORDERS

The principal treatment for the inherited coagulation disorders is replacement therapy—that is, the intravenous administration of the required factor in the form of blood products derived from normal people or animals, or recombinant coagulation proteins. Estrogens may be useful in treating female patients with vWD.[358] Topical hemostatics (thrombin) may be temporarily effective in small injuries or nosebleeds, and certain other treatments such as DDAVP and inhibitors of fibrinolysis are useful adjunctive therapy under specific circumstances such as dental surgery.[359] Additionally, novel therapeutics are being used to treat hemophilic patients, including small interfering RNAs, bispecific antibodies, and gene therapy.[360-362]

Replacement Therapy

The objective of replacement therapy is to obtain a concentration of the required factor at the bleeding site such that coagulation may become hemostatically effective. The pharmacokinetic (PK) properties of the various coagulation factors (Table 54.9) and clinical assessment of the severity of the hemorrhagic risk are important considerations in determining appropriate doses and duration for therapy. Replacement products are dosed on the basis of actual body weight (Tables 54.8 and 54.10) or plasma volume. This latter method may be more precise in patients who do not have a normal plasma volume because of bleeding. In one such method, blood volume is considered to be 7% of body weight; plasma volume is then calculated using the patient's hematocrit. Next, the therapeutic objective is assessed (e.g., the desired incremental increase in factor VIII level). For example, if a patient with severe hemophilia A (<1% factor VIII) has a plasma volume of 3000 mL and requires major surgery, the target factor VIII level should be 100% of normal. Infusion of 3000 IU of factor VIII would result in a calculated peak factor VIII level of 1 IU/mL (100% of normal). Peak factor levels should be monitored to determine whether the expected response was achieved, and then further dosage adjustments can be calculated if necessary. Subsequent doses are scheduled according to the predicted half-life of the factor, with laboratory tests to verify actual levels when appropriate. Case reports and clinical experience detailing management of hemophilia A during surgery have been published.[2,363-365]

Table 54.9. Biodynamic Properties of Coagulation Factors of Concern in Replacement Therapy

Disorder	Hemostatic Level (IU/dL)[a]		Biologic Half-Life (h)
	[b]	[c]	
Hemophilia A (factor VIII deficiency)	25-30		12
Hemophilia B (factor IX deficiency)	20-60		20-24
Fibrinogen deficiency	100 mg/dL	>100 mg/dL	77-106
Prothrombin deficiency	40-50		72-96
Factor V deficiency	10-30	12	15-36
Factor VII deficiency	10-20	25	4-7
Factor X deficiency	10-40	56	32-48
Factor XI deficiency	20-30	26	40-80
Factor XIII deficiency	10	31	280
von Willebrand disease	20-50		20-40

[a]Patients undergoing major surgery or experiencing major bleeding should receive dosages to achieve higher factor levels; for example, patients with hemophilia A should have replacement such that factor VIII levels approach 100% of normal. For patients with factor XIII deficiency and major trauma, plasma factor XIII levels of at least 30% should be achieved.
[b]Data in this column are taken from Teruya J, Ramsey G. Blood components for hemostasis. Lab Med. 2001;32:31-35.
[c]Data in this column are taken from Peyvandi F, Palla R, Menegatti M, et al; European Network of Rare Bleeding Disorders Group. Coagulation factor activity and clinical bleeding severity in rare bleeding disorders: results from the European Network of Rare Bleeding Disorders. J Thromb Haemost. 2012;10:615-621.

Hemostatic Levels

The *hemostatic level* may be defined as the lowest plasma concentration of a given coagulation factor that is required for normal hemostasis (Table 54.9). This value was determined by purely empiric means—that is, by measurement of the blood levels of the deficient factor at which bleeding appeared to stop in patients with one of the inherited coagulation disorders during the course of replacement therapy. Such estimates obviously may be inaccurate. In patients with hemophilia A, the hemostatic level of factor VIIIc is ~25 to 30 IU/dL; in those with hemophilia B, values range from 20 to 60 IU/dL. However, for patients with major trauma or those undergoing surgery, higher plasma levels of these coagulation proteins should be achieved (i.e., 100% for factors VIII or IX; 25%-50% for factor XIII).

In Vivo Recovery and Survival of Infused Coagulation Factors

When a coagulation factor is infused intravenously in a recipient who is deficient in that factor, the levels present in the circulation after intravascular mixing usually are significantly lower than those that would be expected from mere dilution in the recipient's plasma. That this initial in vivo recovery of infused coagulation factors (Table 54.9) is <100% presumably is the result of loss of these proteins from the intravascular space. The adsorption of coagulation factors by platelets and various cell and vascular surfaces may also be involved. The initial recovery of infused coagulation factors is difficult to quantify and ranges from nearly 100% for factor XI to as low as 30% for factor IX. Typically, because the range of in vivo recovery in a population is so variable, clinicians will determine the in vivo recovery for each individual by laboratory testing of blood samples drawn 10 to 20 minutes (peak level) after the therapeutic infusion.

Table 54.10. Replacement Therapy in Hemophilia A and Hemophilia B

Disorder	Therapeutic Product	Minor Bleeding (i.e., Uncomplicated Hemarthroses; Hematomas in Noncritical Areas; Hematuria; Dressing Changes[a]; Arthrocentesis[a]; Removal of Sutures and Drains[a])		Major Bleeding (Hematomas in Critical Locations; Traumatic Injuries; Multiple Tooth Extractions; Major Surgical Procedures)	
		Loading Dose	Maintenance Dose	Loading Dose	Maintenance Dose
Hemophilia A (factor VIII deficiency)	Purified factor VIII[b]	Not required	10-15 IU/kg every 12 h for 2-4 d	50 IU/kg	30-40 IU/kg every 12 h
	Cryoprecipitate[c]	Not required	1.25-1.75 bags/10 kg every 12 h for 1-3 d	3.5 bags/10 kg	1.75 bags/10 kg every 8 h for 1-2 d; every 12 h thereafter
Hemophilia B (factor IX deficiency)	Purified factor IX[b,d]	20-30 IU/kg	15 IU/kg every 24 h for 2-4 d	80-100 IU/kg	30-50 IU/kg every 24 h
	Prothrombin complex[b,c]	20-30 IU/kg	15 IU/kg every 24 h for 2-4 d	40-60 IU/kg	20-25 IU/kg every 24 h

Because weight-based calculations may not correctly predict plasma volumes in bleeding patients, confirmation of the hemostatic level of the coagulation factor being replaced should always be performed for patients with major bleeding indications, with appropriate dosage adjustments performed based on these results.
[a]Single dose of 15 IU/kg or equivalent amounts of concentrated product usually are sufficient.
[b]Initial in vivo recovery of active factor varies somewhat depending on preparation.
[c]Recommended only if purified factor replacement therapy is not available. Antifibrinolytic therapy should not be used with prothrombin complex concentrates.
[d]Certain recombinant factor IX products may require higher doses.

The biologic half-life and the hemostatic level for the factor of concern are the main determinants of the frequency of administration and the size of the maintenance dose of therapeutic product. For example, ~80% of factor VIII infused is initially recovered in the circulation; its initial (diffusion) and subsequent (biologic) half-lives are ~6 and 12 hours, respectively.[366] Thus, in the treatment of patients with hemophilia A, doses are administered every 8 to 12 hours. In patients with hemophilia B, the initial recovery of factor IX is 50% or less; its initial and subsequent half-lives are ~3 and 24 hours, respectively.[367] Hence, larger doses of factor IX are required initially, but dosing is usually once a day to maintain adequate hemostasis. After a large loading dose or after several courses of therapeutic product have been administered, the survival curves of infused coagulation factors become nearly monophasic, presumably because extravascular spaces and the other mechanisms that remove infused coagulation factors from the circulation are saturated. New extended half-life factor VIII and IX products are available. Half-life extension results from pegylation, glycopegylation, albumin fusion, or Fc fusion technologies.[368,369]

Products

Before 1960, plasma was the only agent generally available for the treatment of the inherited coagulation disorders. The life expectancy of a boy born in 1960 with severe hemophilia A was approximately 20 years, and now the life expectancy is essentially normal with modern therapeutic products and the comprehensive care of HTCs.[370] Tables 54.10-54.13 summarize therapeutic choices available to treat certain inherited bleeding disorders.

Plasma

Although most current replacement therapies of coagulation factor deficiencies involve sterile purified concentrates, recombinant proteins, or nonfactor products, plasma therapy is still important in treating some deficient states such as factor XI deficiency. FFP is usually preferred for therapeutic purposes. For factor VIII and fibrinogen deficiencies, and vWD, the appropriate coagulation factors are concentrated in cryoprecipitate. Both the rate of administration and the total dose of plasma administered are limited by the possibility of acute or chronic circulatory overload. The volume expansion resulting from even moderate doses of plasma also limits the blood levels of the missing coagulation factor that can be attained. As a consequence, therapy with plasma alone can be expected to increase the levels of a deficient factor no more than 20 IU/dL above baseline values. When plasma is the only therapeutic agent available, plasmapheresis may be of adjunctive value.[371] Sterile solvent-detergent–treated plasma preparations are available, but activity of certain coagulation proteases and inhibitors in these products is not equivalent to that of FFP.[372,373] A British guideline for the use of FFP and cryoprecipitate has been published.[374]

Table 54.11. Plasma-Derived Factor VIII and IX Products

Factor VIII products licensed to treat hemophilia A Alphanate Hemofil M Koate-DVI
Factor VIII/vWF products licensed to treat vWD Alphanate Humate-P Wilate
Factor IX products licensed to treat hemophilia B AlphaNine SD

Products listed are licensed to treat hemophilia or vWD in the United States.
Abbreviation: vWD, von Willebrand disease.

Table 54.12. Recombinant Factor VIII and IX Products

Standard half-life factor VIII products	Extended half-life factor VIII products
Advate Afstyla Kovaltry Novoeight Nuwiq Recombinate Xyntha	Adynovate Eloctate Jivi Esperoct
Standard half-life factor IX products	Extended half-life factor IX products
BeneFIX Ixinity Rixubis	Alprolix Idelvion Rebinyn

Table 54.13. Comparison of Miscellaneous Antihemophilic Agents

Agent	Manufacturer/Site	Labeled Uses
Factor VIIa, recombinant (Novoseven RT, recombinant)	Novo Nordisk A/S Denmark	• Surgical prophylaxis and treatment of bleeding in patients with hemophilia A with inhibitors to factor VIII • Surgical prophylaxis and treatment of bleeding in patients with hemophilia B with inhibitors to factor IX • Surgical prophylaxis and treatment of bleeding in patients with acquired hemophilia • Surgical prophylaxis and treatment of bleeding in patients with congenital factor VII deficiency
Factor VIIa, recombinant (Sevenfact)	Hema Biologics, USA	• Treatment and control of bleeding episodes in adults and adolescents with hemophilia A or B with inhibitors
Factor X, human (Coagadex, human plasma derived)	Bio Products Laboratory, UK	• Control of bleeding episodes and perioperative management of factor X deficiency
Factor XIII, human (Corifact, human plasma derived)	CSL Behring, GmbH Germany	• Routine prophylaxis in patients with congenital factor XIII deficiency
Factor XIII, human (Tretten, human recombinant)	Novo Nordisk, Denmark	• Prophylaxis of bleeding in patients with inherited factor XIII A-subunit deficiency
Anti-inhibitor coagulant complex (Feiba NF, human plasma derived)	Baxter Healthcare Corporation, USA	• Surgical prophylaxis and treatment of bleeding in patients with hemophilia A and hemophilia B with inhibitors to factor VIII or factor IX
Fibrinogen, human (RiaSTAP, human plasma derived)	CSL Behring, GmbH, Germany	• Acute bleeding episodes in patients with afibrinogenemia or hypofibrinogenemia
Fibrinogen, human Fibryga, human plasma derived	Octapharma, Austria	• Treatment of acute bleeding episodes in adults and adolescents with congenital fibrinogen deficiency, including afibrinogenemia and hypofibrinogenemia

Purified or Concentrated Coagulation Factors

Cryoprecipitate

A major advance in the therapy of hemophilia A was the demonstration by Pool et al that cold insoluble material obtained from plasma contains high concentrations of factor VIII and fibrinogen.[375] Cryoprecipitate, which for many years was discarded during clarification of plasma, is prepared by slowly thawing rapidly frozen plasma at 2 °C to 4 °C, then harvesting the precipitate by centrifugation. Cryoprecipitate prepared from 200 mL of fresh plasma (1 U) contains 50 to 120 U of factor VIII, ~250 mg of fibrinogen, and therapeutically useful amounts of factor XIII and vWF that is rich in high-molecular-weight multimers.

Purified Factor VIII

Among the many methods developed to purify factor VIII, several are suitable for the large-scale production of concentrates of the human protein for therapeutic use, and sufficiently robust to attain in vivo factor VIIIc levels as high as 100 IU/dL in hemophilic patients without significant expansion of the plasma volume.

Nearly all individuals with severe or moderate hemophilia require frequent therapeutic intravenous infusions and therefore, as the concentrated factor products became available in the late 1970s, most patients learned how to administer these infusions themselves at home.

Unfortunately, before the mid-1980s, the risk of viral transmission accompanied the use of these concentrated preparations, because they were prepared from large plasma pools and specific virucidal treatment was not used. The risk of virus transmission has been greatly diminished by serologic testing of the plasma for viruses and by sterilization of the concentrate by solvent-detergent treatment and/or heat sterilization.[376] High-potency preparations of factor VIII can be obtained by affinity chromatography using monoclonal antibodies. The initial (first-generation) r-FVIII products contain human albumin. Second-generation products eliminated albumin, but human and/or animal protein components are utilized in the manufacturing process. Third-generation products have removed all exogenous human and animal proteins from the manufacturing process. Recombinant products with extended half-life for factors VIII and IX are now available.[368,377]

Although modern production methods have reduced the risk of transmitting lipid-enveloped viruses (e.g., human immunodeficiency virus [HIV] and hepatitis B and C), transmission of non–lipid-enveloped viruses, such as hepatitis A and parvovirus B19, has been reported with sterilized plasma–derived products.[378,379] *Tables 54.11* and *54.12* summarize information on currently available products used to treat hemophilia A and hemophilia B.

Prothrombin Complex Concentrates, Factor IX, and Factor VII (VIIa)

Concentrates of vitamin K–dependent coagulation factors may contain small but significant amounts of activated coagulation factors that may be thrombogenic when administered in large doses or for extended periods of time. The thrombogenicity of such concentrates varies from preparation to preparation and from lot to lot and has been variously attributed to thrombin, factor VIIa, factor Xa, factor IXa,[380,381] and coagulant phospholipids.[382] Attention has been directed to the serious and even fatal thromboembolic complications of these products, including disseminated intravascular coagulation.[380,383] Such complications are particularly common in infants and in patients with liver disease,[384] as discussed in Chapter 55. The availability of monoclonally purified and recombinant factor IX products has led to decreased use of PCCs in the treatment of hemophilia B.[385,386] PCCs are now used primarily to treat patients with inhibitors to factor VIII, a condition in which the presence of thrombogenic proteins is clinically useful.[387,388] PCCs are also useful in treating deficiencies of prothrombin and factors VII and X, and for reversal of warfarin anticoagulation.[389]

When treating hemophilia B with replacement factor IX products, it should be noted that factor IX distributes to both intravascular and extravascular compartments. Consequently, loading doses required to achieve 100% of the normal plasma factor IX level are usually 1.5 to 2 times greater than those calculated from the patient's plasma volume. Thus, when purified factor IX products are used, twice the calculated amount of factor IX should be given for the initial dose. However, PCCs are thrombogenic, and when these products are used to treat patients with hemophilia B, the dosage should be reduced below that given when the purified products are used.

Recombinant factor VIIa is being used primarily for treatment of bleeding episodes in patients with hemophilia with inhibitors,[390] but also in patients with bleeding resulting from refractory thrombocytopenia, platelet dysfunction, factor VII deficiency (discussed in the section Factor VII Deficiency), or severe liver disease (discussed in Chapter 55).

Detailed summaries of prior, current, and future coagulation factor products have been published.[391,392] Nonfactor therapies to treat hemophilia A and B are an emerging area of interest. Three such products include emicizumab, a bispecific antibody factor VIII mimetic that is highly effective in treating hemophilia A patients with inhibitors; fitusiran, a small inhibitory RNA that induces antithrombin deficiency; and concizumab, a monoclonal antibody to tissue factor pathway inhibitor.[360,361,393,394]

Emicizumab, originally developed to treat hemophilia A patients with inhibitors, is also indicated to treat noninhibitor hemophilia A patients, with either weekly, biweekly, or monthly subcutaneous dosing. If it is necessary to monitor factor VIII levels in patients receiving emicizumab, chromogenic factor VIII assays are required.

Adjunctive Therapies

A congener of vasopressin, DDAVP, was originally developed for the treatment of diabetes insipidus. Its extrarenal actions stimulate vascular endothelial cells to release several proteins, including vWF in amounts sufficient to raise the plasma levels of this protein and associated factor VIII 2 to 5 times (*Figure 54.8*).[395] This effect is therapeutically useful in most patients with type 1 vWD[396] and in some patients with mild hemophilia A,[397] and it is particularly useful because the biohazards of blood products are avoided. Excellent responses were obtained in the prevention of bleeding after minor surgical procedures, such as tooth extractions, and in some major surgical procedures.[398,399] It has been noted that young boys with mild to moderate hemophilia A have a lower response rate to DDAVP; the response rate of these patients improves later in life, and nonresponder children are candidates for retesting when they are older.[400]

The vWF released in response to DDAVP is rich in high-molecular-weight multimers[401] that increase adhesion and spreading of platelets at injury sites. This effect may explain the therapeutic efficacy of the drug in several disorders of platelet function, including uremia.[402]

DDAVP also induces the release of endothelial cell–derived plasminogen activators and has produced exaggerated fibrinolytic phenomena in several rare cases. For this reason, it is sometimes given with ε-aminocaproic acid (EACA) or other fibrinolytic enzyme inhibitors. Compared to vasopressin, DDAVP is markedly less potent as a pressor agent, but does retain significant antidiuretic activity. Neither effect has proved to be a major problem in its therapeutic use, but most experienced clinicians use caution when treating patients with hypertension or congestive heart failure. Reports of hyponatremia and seizures in children less than 2 years of age have led to cautious use of DDAVP in this population. Serum sodium should be monitored in adults who receive more than three or four sequential doses of DDAVP because of the side effect of hyponatremia, and in these patients water restriction is advised. DDAVP should not be administered more than once a day, and repeated doses of DDAVP may produce progressively diminishing amounts of vWF (tachyphylaxis), presumably because of exhaustion of stored vWF.[403] DDAVP is available in a formulation for parenteral use or by a nasal spray.[397,404] DDAVP should be used cautiously in older patients with vascular disease because of the potential risk of drug-induced thrombosis.[404,405] Limitations of DDAVP in the pediatric population have been summarized.[406]

Inhibitors of fibrinolysis, such as EACA or tranexamic acid, may diminish bleeding from mucosal membranes where the concentrations of fibrinolytic enzymes are high, in patients with inherited coagulation disorders: for example, with bleeding in the mouth, tongue, tonsils, and pharynx, and with bleeding associated with operative dental procedures.[407] These drugs act to protect labile hemostatic plugs from fibrinolytic degradation. The use of EACA alone has been effective in the treatment of patients with mild hemophilia A (plasma levels of factor VIII >5 IU/dL)[408] and those with other mild inherited coagulation disorders such as vWD or factor XI deficiency. Some clinicians have used EACA as an adjunct to single dose[409] or various other factor replacement regimens. EACA can be administered in oral doses (pills or syrup) of 6 g every 6 hours to adults and 100 mg/kg every 6 hours to children, for 3 to 4 days after tooth extraction. Doses of as little as 1 g every 6 hours may be as effective in most adult patients. The drug can be given intravenously (1 g/h) for patients who cannot swallow. Hematuria or abnormal renal function is a contraindication to the use of this drug because of the hazard of intrarenal or ureteral obstruction by blood clots.[410] EACA also should not be given to patients with disseminated intravascular coagulation or active hepatitis, or to patients receiving PCCs, although an EACA mouthwash can be used with these latter drugs.[407,411] Tranexamic acid is also available; the recommended adult dosage is two 650 mg tablets orally 3 times daily. These drugs may be teratogenic and should be used with caution in pregnant women.

MAJOR AND MINOR BLEEDING

General treatment guidelines for patients, including newborns with hemophilia and other bleeding disorders, have been published.[411,412] Additional detailed guidelines are available on the National Hemophilia Foundation's website, www.hemophilia.org, under Medical and Scientific Advisory Council recommendations.

For purposes of replacement therapy, the various bleeding manifestations commonly encountered in the inherited coagulation disorders are often divided subjectively into major and minor bleeding. Manifestations falling into the minor category include bleeding associated with uncomplicated hemarthrosis, symptomatic hematomas in noncritical areas, and minor traumatic injuries, as well as such therapeutic procedures as minor dental procedures, arthrocentesis, and dressing changes. Small cuts and scratches, removal of stitches or drains, superficial ecchymoses, and small hematomas may require no replacement therapy.

Major bleeding is by definition life threatening and includes hematomas in critical locations and bleeding resulting from traumatic injuries, particularly those in which external blood loss is significant. Major bleeding occurs in surgical procedures, including tonsillectomy

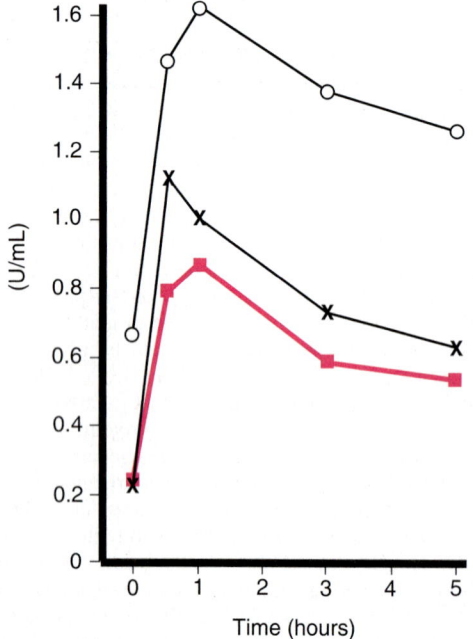

FIGURE 54.8 **The response to desmopressin infusion (0.3 μg/kg body weight) in a hemophilic patient.** Open circles indicate von Willebrand factor antigen; solid boxes indicate factor VIIIc activity; and crosses indicate factor VIIIc antigen. (From de la Fuente B, Kasper CK, Rickles FR, et al. Response of patients with mild and moderate hemophilia A and von Willebrand's disease to treatment with desmopressin. *Ann Intern Med.* 1985;103(1):6-14. Copyright © 1985 American College of Physicians. All Rights Reserved. Reprinted with the permission of American College of Physicians, Inc.)

and the extraction of molar teeth. In the treatment of major bleeding, general guidelines recommend that the in vivo levels of the missing factor should be maintained above 60% to 80% to provide effective hemostasis until bleeding has stopped and appropriate healing has occurred so that there is no risk of rebleeding. In bleeding of a particularly critical nature, such as intracranial hemorrhage, or for the prevention of excessive bleeding during neurosurgery, factor levels should be maintained at 100% of normal.

Hemophilia A Minor Bleeding

DDAVP is effective in the treatment of minor bleeding manifestations in individuals with hemophilia A with baseline factor VIIIc levels >5 IU/dL, if patients have been previously demonstrated to respond to DDAVP with therapeutic levels of factor VIIIc after administration of DDAVP.[398,399] Side effects of DDAVP are more prominent if the total dose exceeds 24 μg. Administration of DDAVP produces significant increases in factor VIIIc and vWF.[413] Repeated doses of DDAVP at approximately daily intervals may produce useful increments of factor VIII in many patients. At least 24 hours should elapse before repeat administration of the drug in order for the endothelial cell stores of vWF to be replenished. Patients should be tested before surgery for their response to DDAVP by documenting adequate hemostatic levels of factor VIII levels 30 to 60 minutes after treatment, to ensure that the drug will be effective in appropriate responders. Only small amounts of factor VIII are produced by DDAVP in persons with severe hemophilia, and the use of this drug in patients with factor VIII levels <5 IU/dL is seldom useful and therefore is not recommended, even for minor bleeding manifestations. EACA (6 g orally every 6 hours) or tranexamic acid (25 mg/kg orally every 6-8 hours) has been administered together with DDAVP in an attempt to minimize fibrinolysis.[407,408] For maximal effectiveness, antifibrinolytic drugs should be started prior to surgical procedures.

Although effective in minor bleeding, plasma or cryoprecipitate is not currently recommended for use in the treatment of patients with hemophilia A. Factor VIII concentrates are widely available and are the most useful therapeutic products. The regimens summarized in *Table 54.10* illustrate one approach to treating hemophilia A. For some minor bleeding manifestations, treatment for a minimum of 3 days is required, but in most cases, a single dose of 10 to 15 IU/kg of factor VIII is usually sufficient.[414] In the treatment of minor bleeding, loading doses are not required, and laboratory monitoring of in vivo factor VIII levels is unnecessary. The minor bleeding treatment regimens summarized in *Table 54.10* typically result in peak factor VIII levels of ~30%. Occasionally, if the minor bleeding episode is not treated promptly and bleeding is prolonged, then a hematoma may form, and often, additional doses of factor products at higher doses are needed to prevent continued bleeding around the hematoma and potential pseudocyst formation. It is generally recommended in such cases of delayed treatment that full (100%) doses be administered to maintain adequate hemostatic levels until the hematoma is completely resolved.

Hemophilia A Major Bleeding

To treat major bleeding in patients with hemophilia A, sufficient factor VIII must be given often enough to ensure that the blood level does not fall to <30 to 50 IU/dL for any length of time. Most experienced clinicians target trough levels of more than 50% IU/dL until bleeding has stopped and substantial healing has taken place. Maintenance doses usually are administered every 8 to 12 hours. Regimens of continuous infusion of factor VIII are being used with increasing frequency during hospitalization, and have been shown to save total factor use by as much as 30%.[415-417] The administration of 2 IU/kg/h of factor VIII produces a mean factor VIIIc level in the plasma of ~50 IU/dL and appears to be more cost-effective than twice-daily intravenous bolus treatments.[418] However, in a recent study of adult hemophilia patients undergoing major orthopedic surgery, the total dose of factor per kg body weight received in the postoperative period was similar with continuous infusion and bolus infusion, with comparable safety and efficacy.[419] Even so, continuous infusion has the advantage of maintaining a consistent, therapeutic factor level. It is important to note that the treatment of postsurgical or major traumatic hemorrhage in patients with mild hemophilia A requires nearly as much therapeutic product as is needed for the severely affected patient. Many experts recommend treatment for 10 to 14 days after major surgical procedures, whereas others administer the full doses indicated in *Table 54.10* for 10 days and continue half-doses for longer periods as healing continues and the patient is undergoing increasingly active physical therapy, especially after major orthopedic surgeries.

Determination in the laboratory of the in vivo levels of factor VIIIc is recommended during the treatment of patients with major hemorrhage. The use of the PTT to guide factor VIII replacement therapy is not recommended, because the results of these tests may be normal at levels of factor VIII that do not provide adequate hemostasis.[57] Clinicians should be aware that some of the new hemophilia products available or under development may not be reliably assayed by standard coagulation laboratory assays and may require chromogenic factor assay measurement.[65]

von Willebrand Disease

Fortunately, in many patients with vWD, bleeding manifestations are mild, and replacement therapy is seldom required. Unlike the situation in hemophilia, in which there is a close correlation between factor levels and clinical outcome, treatment decisions are more complicated in vWD because it is unclear which measurement (vWF, factor VIII, or platelet function) correlates best with the severity of bleeding or clinical outcome. Many experts recommend following vWF:RCo and factor VIII levels,[420] but little information exists about the level of vWF:RCo that is critical for control of mucosal bleeding or the prevention of surgical bleeding. Bleeding times may not normalize, but a normal bleeding time is not required for a satisfactory response, and monitoring of bleeding time is not recommended.[117] Therapeutic goals include resolution of active bleeding and prevention of excessive bleeding in response to invasive procedures or trauma. Unlike the situation with hemophilia A or B, chronic prophylaxis therapy is rarely required, but should be considered in patients with severe vWD who have recurrent menorrhagia, gastrointestinal, or joint hemorrhage.

The spectrum of therapeutic interventions in vWD includes desmopressin (DDAVP), concentrate infusion, and adjunctive therapy with medications that modulate bleeding symptoms by affecting either menstrual pattern or fibrinolysis. Dosing recommendations in vWD are empiric. In the case of a patient with major surgery or trauma, one recommendation is that clinicians attempt to bring the vWF (and factor VIII) level to near 100 IU/dL, and maintain it >40 to 50 IU/dL for the first 3 to 5 days, after which one recommended goal is to maintain the factor VIII level at >40 IU/dL for a total of 7 to 10 days or until healing is completed.[117] In surgical settings, monitoring of factor levels seems prudent, but monitoring of the bleeding time is discouraged, as surgeries have been done successfully in patients with type 3 vWD in the face of only partial correction of bleeding time.[117]

DDAVP is the mainstay of treatment for patients with mild forms of type 1 vWD.[117] The dosage, route of administration, and contraindications described under the discussion of hemophilia A also apply to the use of the drug in vWD. vWF and factor VIII levels generally increase by twofold to fourfold over baseline. Because responsiveness to therapy between patients is variable, a test dose given at the time of diagnosis or before elective surgery is advised. Obtaining both vWF:RCo and factor VIII levels 1 hour after DDAVP administration is recommended in order to confirm a patient's responsiveness. It may also be informative to obtain a second sample 4 hours after DDAVP to confirm that vWF has the expected 8- to 10-hour half-life after release.[110] Concerns regarding tachyphylaxis, hyponatremia, and rare thrombotic complications are similar to those when treating patients with hemophilia A. Note that whereas patients with type 1 vWD are likely to have a satisfactory response, patients with non–type 1 vWD respond poorly or unpredictably to DDAVP. Type 3 patients have essentially no endogenous vWF synthesis, and are DDAVP-nonresponsive. In one large series of patients with type 2B vWD, the platelet count fell from an average of 86,000 to 60,000/μL after administration of this drug.[164] Because thrombocytopenia may worsen after administration of DDAVP to patients with type 2B vWD and the platelet-type form of the disorder, patients with these variants should not be treated routinely with DDAVP. However, some authors report good-responder type 2B vWD patients who received DDAVP.[421] Response in type 2A vWD is variable and may be of shorter duration than in type 1 patients, because of increased vWF proteolysis. Similarly, factor VIII levels may rise in response to DDAVP in patients with type 2N vWD, but because of the deficient factor VIII–stabilizing activity of vWF in this variant, levels of factor VIII then fall at an accelerated rate.[422] Because of interindividual variability, a documented therapeutic response to DDAVP should be obtained before surgical prophylaxis with the drug, to ensure adequate hemostasis postoperatively. It is recommended that this DDAVP trial be performed at the time of diagnosis of vWD.

Transfusion therapy with plasma-derived products is the current therapy of choice in DDAVP-unresponsive patients who require factor support or those with major bleeding or surgery. In order to treat both the factor VIII deficiency and the defect in primary hemostasis seen in patients with severe vWD, it is necessary to give a product with factor VIII activity that also contains high-molecular-weight multimers of vWF. The concentrations of vWF and factor VIII in FFP are insufficient for appropriate therapy. Cryoprecipitate contains ~80 to 100 U per bag, 5 to 10 times the concentration of these factors compared to plasma. Cryoprecipitate has a small residual risk of viral transmission and is not currently suited for virus-inactivation therapy; consequently, pathogen-inactivated, intermediate-purity factor VIII concentrates with demonstrated preservation of vWF multimers are the preferred replacement product. At the time of this writing, three commercial plasma-derived products are licensed in the United States for this indication (Humate-P, known as Haemate-P in Europe; Wilate; and Alphanate SD/HT) (*Table 54.12*). A Canadian multicenter study confirmed "excellent" or "good" outcomes in 97% of patients treated with Humate-P, with a median recovery of 1.23 IU/kg per IU/kg infused.[423] Similarly, Alphanate was shown to ultimately control all bleeding episodes in one large multicenter trial.[424] Alphanate is currently not licensed for treatment of type 3 vWD; it is labeled only in factor VIII units, but vWF:RCo has been reported to be ~50% lower than the labeled factor VIII content.[424] A PK clinical trial compared Wilate vs Humate-P and found similar PK parameters for the two products; however, Wilate achieved a 1:1 ratio for vWF:factor VIII, suggesting simpler dosing of Wilate.[425] A recombinant vWF product is now available (vonicog alfa).[426] Coadministration of an initial dose of r-FVIII appears to be required when the recombinant vWF product is used. Very-high-purity plasma-derived factor VIII concentrates and r-FVIII concentrates are essentially devoid of vWF, and they should not be used to treat vWD, unless used in conjunction with recombinant vWF.[426]

Suggested doses and target factor levels for treatment of vWD patients have been published.[90,427,428] Recommended doses in ristocetin cofactor units are similar to factor VIII doses, because both have similar in vivo recovery (~2 IU/dL rise in plasma concentration for each IU/kg of factor administered). Monitoring response to therapy with both factor VIII and vWF:RCo is appropriate. Although vWF levels can be expected to fall between doses of vWF-containing concentrate, which has a half-life of 8 to 10 hours, factor VIII levels may continue to rise in response to the patient's endogenous factor VIII production. Avoidance of unusually high factor VIII levels is suggested in order to minimize venous thrombotic risk.[429]

Platelets are estimated to contain ~15% of the total body vWF. Some authors suggest using platelet transfusion in patients with severe vWD who exhibit bleeding despite plasma factor VIII concentrate therapy.[117] Thrombocytopenia may be exacerbated by the administration of normal exogenous vWF in platelet-type (pseudo) vWD,[430] but not in type 2B vWD. Patients with platelet-type vWD should receive platelet transfusions for significant bleeding or surgery.

Adjunctive therapy for vWD patients with menorrhagia usually takes the form of oral contraception or other hormonal intervention.[117] Antifibrinolytic therapy and DDAVP have also found a role in control of menorrhagia[407,431] and oral bleeding. Doses of DDAVP administered every 24 hours for up to 3 days, or EACA up to 5 g 3 times per day, or tranexamic acid, may be useful in control of menorrhagia, but toxicity profiles should also be considered. Failure of medical therapy may lead to surgical approaches, such as endometrial resection or even hysterectomy.

Pregnancy is a special situation for patients with vWD. vWF levels generally improve in patients with type 1 vWD as pregnancy proceeds, but improvement is less likely in type 2A vWD, and thrombocytopenia may actually worsen in patients with type 2B and platelet-type (pseudo) vWD variants. Current information indicates that the patient's factor VIIIc at delivery predicts the risk of bleeding, with a factor VIII level less than 50% of normal at term being associated with excessive bleeding.[432] If sufficient factor VIII levels are achieved, aggressive surgical hemostasis and efficient uterine contraction should prevent peripartum bleeding. Thus, factor levels should be determined before delivery. If sufficient factor VIII levels are not achieved before delivery and the patient is known to respond to DDAVP, this drug can be given to the mother immediately postpartum, although electrolytes and urine output need to be closely monitored due to the side effects of DDAVP causing fluid retention. If the patient does not respond to DDAVP, then vWF/factor VIII concentrate should be administered peripartum. Although endogenous vWF levels rise during pregnancy in patients with type 1 vWD, the vWF levels fall quickly after parturition,[433] and patients should be advised to report late bleeding. DDAVP or replacement therapy may be useful to prevent late bleeding in patients with vWD.

Alloantibodies to vWF develop in a minority of patients with type 3 vWD after replacement therapy.[434] The risk appears to be highest in patients with large gene deletions. Administration of vWF-containing concentrates to these allosensitized patients has been associated with anaphylactic reactions. Alternative therapies that have been successful include high-dose r-FVIII or recombinant factor VIIa.[434]

Hemophilia B Treatment

Most of the guidelines for replacement therapy of patients with hemophilia A apply to the treatment of those with hemophilia B (*Table 54.10*). Because of the low initial in vivo recovery and the rapid initial disappearance of factor IX from the circulation, higher initial doses are recommended, even for the treatment of minor bleeding. In patients with hemophilia B, purified factor IX concentrates or recombinant factor IX products (summarized in *Tables 54.11* and *54.12*) are recommended for the treatment of major or minor hemorrhage because of the thrombotic potential of PCCs.[380,383]

An unusual complication of hemophilia B therapy is anaphylaxis. These patients typically have severe factor IX deficiency with complete gene deletions.[435,436] These patients may require bypass therapy with PCCs or recombinant factor VIIa, although there are reports of successful desensitization with factor IX products.[437]

Gene Therapy for Hemophilia

Gene therapy for the inherited bleeding disorders is now promising, after many years of frustrating failures. A major success was published involving patients with severe factor IX deficiency.[438] Ten of ten subjects with severe hemophilia B were treated with adeno-associated viral vector carrying a variant factor IX gene (factor IX Padua), and had factor IX levels of ~30%. This trial had ~9 years of follow-up. Similar success has been reported in patients with severe hemophilia A who received an adeno-associated viral vector encoding a B-domain-deleted human factor VIII gene.[439] A major focus of gene therapy research is to develop a gene delivery system that is efficient, safe, nonimmunogenic, and provides long-term gene expression.[362] Issues of concern related to hemophilia gene therapy include the presence of pre-existing antibodies to vectors, potential liver toxicity and requirement for immunosuppression, factor levels achieved, duration of response, long-term safety, and costs.[362]

Factor VII Deficiency

Unlike in patients with severe hemophilia A or B, bleeding in a patient with factor VII deficiency undergoing surgery is variable, so multiple issues should be considered in the perioperative care of factor VII–deficient patients,[440-442] including the individual patient's prior experiences and symptomatology: patients with a history of hemarthrosis or CNS hemorrhage are at a higher risk for bleeding complications. The oral and urogenital tracts are areas of high local fibrinolytic activity. Patients with factor VII levels <3 IU/dL are at high risk for bleeding, whereas patients with levels of 15 to 25 IU/dL are less likely to develop bleeding complications associated with surgery. Finally, one should consider the logistics of therapy, because factor VII has a short half-life, possibly as short as 3.5 hours. Volume overload is likely, as plasma is commonly used as a source for factor replacement.

Traditionally, FFP, PCCs, or plasma-derived factor VII concentrate has been used for factor VII replacement therapy, and more recently, recombinant human activated factor VIIa (rFVIIa) has been the recommended product.[443-447] In general, doses of between 15 and 30 μg/kg of rFVIIa are administered at intervals of 4 to 6 hours. The half-life of recombinant factor VIIa is between 2.5 and 3 hours, and the roles of continuous factor infusion and laboratory monitoring remain to be defined in treating factor VII–deficient patients. Antibody to factor VII has developed in response to therapy in some individuals with congenital factor VII deficiency.[448] The risk of thrombosis should be considered when rFVIIa is being used, especially when treating a condition that itself is associated with thrombosis, such as orthopedic surgery.

Although the half-life of factor VII is short, rFVIIa infusions have been successful in chronic infusion prophylaxis programs to prevent spontaneous CNS and joint bleeding. Factor VIIa was administered every other day or twice weekly, suggesting that an additional mechanism of action independent of the short plasma half-life was operative in these cases.

Although it is no longer the "product of choice," plasma can be used for replacement therapy for factor VII in emergency situations when other products are not available. For patients treated with plasma, a loading dose of 15 to 20 mL/kg, followed by 4 to 6 mL/kg every 6 hours for 7 to 10 days, has been recommended. Plasma exchange therapy has been used in some patients to avoid volume overload. PCCs have been used, but carry some thrombotic risk, which may be associated with the generation of unnecessarily high levels of other activated vitamin K–dependent coagulation proteins.[449] This is especially a problem with extended PCC use or use of PCCs in the setting of liver disease. PCCs are not generally labeled with their factor IX content, but the factor VII content is usually available from the manufacturer. Recovery studies indicate that an administered factor VII dose of 1 IU/kg will raise the patient's plasma factor level by ~2 IU/dL. If available, the use of purified factor VII concentrate might decrease the thrombotic risk associated with the use of less-specific PCCs. A heat-treated intermediate-purity factor VII concentrate (manufactured by Immuno A.G.) had been used for treatment of acute bleeds, perioperative prophylaxis, and for prevention of recurrent CNS hemorrhage. Factor VII levels rose ~2.33 IU/dL for each IU/kg infused, and the factor VII half-life was ~6 hours. For replacement therapy in a surgical setting, factor-level monitoring is recommended, to ensure that perioperative factor levels are >25 IU/dL.

Factor XIII Deficiency Treatment

Therapy for congenital factor XIII deficiency is based on the principle that only a small quantity of factor XIII must be present in human plasma to promote normal hemostasis.[450] The long half-life of factor XIII (estimated as being between 9 and 19 days in the literature)[451] makes prophylactic therapy both practical and highly advisable given the high frequency of intracranial hemorrhage.[252] This long half-life may not be present in some situations in newborn infants with severe FXIII deficiency.[452] FFP and factor concentrates have been used successfully to prevent factor XIII–associated bleeding, and these remain possible treatment options. Pasteurized factor XIII concentrate that contained only the A subunit prepared from human placenta has been replaced by plasma-derived preparations that contain both A and B subunits.[453] A plasma-derived factor XIII preparation is available (Corifact, *Table 54.13*) to treat congenital factor XIII deficiency. Recommended dosing is 40 IU/kg every 4 weeks with dose adjustments based on achieving a trough level of 5% to 20%. Two other preparations that have been used therapeutically are Fibrogammin-P, which is licensed in several countries (but not the United States or Canada), and a factor XIII preparation from Bio Products Laboratory that has been used in the United Kingdom. A recombinant factor XIII concentrate composed of the A subunit is also available.[454] Tretten (*Table 54.13*) is the drug name. It is strongly recommended that all patients with severe factor XIII deficiency be placed on lifelong prophylaxis in order to prevent the devastating complication of intracranial hemorrhage. Prophylactic therapy of affected patients undergoing surgery may actually require more intensive replacement therapy. If concentrates are unavailable, patients can be given either FFP or cryoprecipitate.[455] A typical plasma dose is 10 to 20 mL/kg body weight, every 4 to 6 weeks. Cryoprecipitate at a dose of 1 bag per 10 to 20 kg of body weight every 3 to 4 weeks is an alternative therapy that has the advantage of requiring transfusion of a smaller volume. It is recommended that factor XIII levels be kept between 25% and 50% of normal to achieve normal hemostasis following major trauma in these patients; doses of concentrate recommended are 35 IU/kg preoperatively, followed by 10 IU/kg/d for 5 more days. Affected patients with a history of spontaneous abortions can complete a normal pregnancy when they are managed with prophylactic FFP or factor XIII concentrates. Factor XIII levels fall during pregnancy, and replacement therapy is recommended every 21 days.[456] Monitoring of factor XIII trough levels may also be helpful. Formation of antibody inhibitors to factor XIII after replacement therapy appears to be rare. A review of the Rare Bleeding Disorders Registry indicated that a minimal factor XIII level of 15% should be a target for prophylaxis.[457]

Treatment Considerations for Miscellaneous Disorders

Therapeutic regimens recommended for the treatment of patients with any of the less common inherited coagulation disorders are summarized in *Table 54.8*.

The management of major bleeding caused by deficiencies of prothrombin and factor X has been facilitated by the availability of PCCs. The majority of these plasma-derived products contain three factors (prothrombin, factor IX, and factor X), but four-factor concentrates are also available. Factor IX content has generally been used to label the potency of these concentrates, but factor content of the other vitamin K–dependent factors relative to the factor IX content is often available, either in published reports or from the manufacturer. The currently available PCC products are subjected to virus attenuation steps to inactivate hepatitis B, hepatitis C, and HIV. However, the thrombogenicity of these products remains a concern,[380,383] and concomitant use of antifibrinolytics may increase that risk. In the absence of a specific factor concentrate, plasma transfusion may also be used to replace vitamin K–dependent coagulation factors.

There are few data on which to base recommendations on treating the rare bleeding disorders. It is estimated that 1 IU/kg of infused PCC will raise the prothrombin level by 1 IU/dL. Relatively low levels of prothrombin are required for normal hemostasis, and target values of 40 to 50 IU/dL are recommended for surgery. The half-life of prothrombin is ~72 hours, so infrequent postoperative infusions, every 2 to 3 days, is reasonable.[458] Guidelines for the treatment of factor X deficiency vary. The biologic half-life of factor X is 20 to 40 hours. Calculation of the factor X dose is based on the empiric observation that for each 1 IU/kg infused, factor X levels rise ~1.5 IU/kg. Factor X levels varying from 5 IU/dL to as high as 40 IU/dL have been recommended for surgery; however, levels >20 IU/dL were suggested by the United Kingdom Haemophilia Centre Doctors' Organisation.[188] Monitoring of the factor level achieved is prudent. A plasma-derived, factor X concentrate is now available (Coagadex) to treat factor X deficiency.[459]

There are currently no factor V concentrates, so patients with factor V deficiency who require replacement therapy are treated with plasma. The United Kingdom Haemophilia Centre Doctors' Organisation recommends target levels >15 IU/dL, whereas others have suggested levels of 25 to 30 IU/dL.[188] The half-life of plasma factor V is reported to be 12 to 36 hours. In the United States, some blood collection organizations are moving away from production of FFP toward production of plasma that is separated and frozen within 24 hours after collection (FP-24). Although factor V has been called "labile factor," levels of factor V in FP-24 are only modestly reduced compared to those in FFP.[460] In addition, factor V appears to be relatively stable in "thawed plasma" held up to 5 days in transfusion service refrigerators at 0 °C to 4 °C. Loading plasma doses of 20 mL/kg are often given, followed by maintenance infusions of 3 to 6 mL/kg every 12 hours. Cryoprecipitate does not contain sufficient factor V to be used as an alternative to plasma. Finally, in the setting of acquired factor V autoantibody, platelet transfusion has been used successfully. Similarly, platelet transfusion might hold some promise in the treatment of a patient with congenital factor V with alloantibody[188]; platelet transfusion appears to also be effective in patients with inherited factor V deficiency.[461]

Patients with factor XI deficiency usually respond well to FFP. A solvent-detergent plasma preparation has been developed and may be the desired therapy not only for factor XI deficiency, but for other factor deficiencies for which sterile concentrates are not available. Unfortunately, some of the factor XI concentrates were shown to be thrombogenic in early clinical studies,[188] and their clinical utility may be limited by this toxicity.

Cryoprecipitate is used in replacement therapy for afibrinogenemia, hypofibrinogenemia, and dysfibrinogenemia. Two sterile fibrinogen concentrates RiaSTAP and Fibryga are available. Treatment of rare bleeding disorders has been reviewed.[204]

SPECIAL ASPECTS OF TREATMENT

Hemarthrosis

All patients with hemarthrosis should receive adequate replacement therapy in order to prevent the development of permanent disability because of repeated bleeding in a joint. Pain usually is relieved promptly and is a reliable index of the therapeutic response. Supportive therapy follows the acronym of RICE: rest through immobilization, ice to cool the inflammation and reduce the swelling, compression to reduce the swelling and bleeding, and elevation to reduce the swelling. The administration of analgesics that do not interfere with platelet function is appropriate to relieve the pain of bleeding in the joint.

Arthrocentesis usually is unnecessary if therapeutic infusion is accomplished early, but it may be of significant benefit when the joint is severely distended or when resolution of the hemarthrosis is delayed despite adequate replacement therapy.[462] Large volumes of blood seldom can be aspirated, but even a small volume may relieve symptoms. If arthrocentesis is performed, it should be done immediately after the administration of a therapeutic dose of factor.

Early physiotherapy aimed at restoring the full range of motion of the affected joint should be instituted as soon as the acute stage of hemarthrosis has resolved. More energetic physiotherapeutic techniques should be carried out only in conjunction with an adequate course of replacement therapy. Various orthopedic devices (orthotics), such as braces and removable bivalve plaster casts, which provide additional support for chronically injured joints, have proved useful in reducing the frequency of recurrent hemarthrosis, particularly in the knee and ankle joints.[463] Anti-inflammatory drugs such as salsalate (Disalcid) or choline magnesium trisalicylate (Trilisate) or the newer cyclooxygenase-2 inhibitors (Celebrex) may be useful in patients with bleeding disorders, because these drugs have anti-inflammatory activity but do not impair platelet function.[464]

Regular infusions of factor concentrates may prevent or significantly delay progression of hemophilic arthropathy. A randomized clinical trial in boys demonstrated the markedly better results of a prophylaxis program vs episodic treatment on long-term joint function.[40] This study demonstrated a significant reduction in joint damage and other bleeding episodes in the prophylaxis group.

A second clinical trial looked at whether late prophylaxis would be effective in reversing arthropathy. Although late prophylaxis reduced joint bleeding and improved quality of life, there was no improvement in arthropathy.[465] Thus, optimal treatment of hemophilic arthropathy relies on early initiation of early prophylaxis to prevent this complication.

Prophylaxis therapy is regarded as optimal treatment for patients with severe hemophilia. One report compared two prophylaxis regimens for hemophilia A—standard prophylaxis (20-40 IU/kg every other day) vs PK-tailored prophylaxis (20-80 IU/kg every third day). Annualized bleeding rates, factor consumption, and adverse events were similar.[466] Adherence to prophylaxis should be easier with increasing use of extended half-life products and use of nonfactor products. Improved clinical outcomes should also be seen with these therapies.

Reconstructive surgical procedures are available to improve the function of chronically damaged joints.[45,467,468] Favorable results have been reported with total knee arthroplasty in several series.[468] Long-term follow-up (>5 years) indicates adequately functioning prostheses and persistent pain relief in most patients. Synovectomy is effective in reducing the frequency of hemarthrosis that cannot be controlled by replacement therapy.[469] Radioisotopic synovectomy is also effective therapy for hemophilic arthropathy.[470] A review of the literature on radioisotopic synovectomy indicates that ~80% of patients benefit from the procedure,[471] but an updated safety review identified two patients who subsequently developed acute lymphocytic leukemia.[472] Although not statistically significant, this report raised a safety question about radioisotopic synovectomy. A subsequent case-control study found no increase in prevalence of malignancy in patients with bleeding disorders who had undergone RS, which may help to address safety concerns.[473]

Hemophilic Cysts

Hemophilic cysts are very rare with modern treatment, but once were a serious complication that developed in patients with severe hemophilia A or B who had recurrent bleeding with inadequate treatment. Also known as *hemophilic pseudotumors*, such cysts are gradually expanding blood-filled loculations that apparently originate from hemorrhages into confined subperiosteal, tendinous, or fascial spaces. The osmotic pressure created by breakdown products of blood in such confined spaces may produce further influx of fluid; this, together with recurrent bleeding, explains the progressive increase in the size of the cyst and its ability to erode contiguous structures. Such cysts most commonly develop in the thigh and may destroy bone as well as the soft tissues as they increase in size. Hemophilic cysts are readily prevented, but difficult to treat. Although long-term replacement therapy combined with x-ray treatment has been successful in a few cases,[474] hemophilic pseudocysts may require radical surgical procedures such as extensive resections or amputations. Surgical and nonsurgical approaches to manage pseudotumors have been reported and reviewed.[475,476]

Intracranial Bleeding

Despite the widespread use of prophylaxis programs, hemorrhage, including intracranial hemorrhage, remains a leading cause of death among persons with hemophilia. After the neonatal period, intracranial hemorrhage affects 3% to 10% of hemophilia patients not receiving prophylaxis.[477] An estimate of the incidence of intracranial hemorrhage placed the risk at 1 in 200 per year, proportional to the time spent with factor levels below 1 IU/dL.[477] A systematic review reported that in persons of all ages with hemophilia, the pooled intracranial hemorrhage incidence and mortality rates were 2.3 (95% CI 1.2-4.8) and 0.8 (95% CI 0.5-1.2) per 1000 person-years, respectively.[478] Approximately 50% of cases are associated with head injury[479]; the etiology is not apparent in 38% of cases (spontaneous cases).[480] Bleeding may be subdural, epidural, or intracerebral. Subarachnoid bleeding occurs least commonly, but it carries the best prognosis. Hemorrhage also may develop in the spinal cord or spinal meninges. In cases associated with head trauma, the presence of a lucid interval and the absence of localizing neurologic signs at the time of presentation are commonly seen.[480]

Significant head injury must be treated early and intensively in patients with inherited coagulation disorders. Those with hemophilia

A and B should immediately receive sufficient factor product to raise the plasma level of deficient factor to 100 IU/dL. Samples for essential coagulation studies should be drawn before administration of replacement therapy, but treatment should not be delayed while waiting for results of these studies. Radiologic procedures, such as computed tomography scanning, should be performed after the therapeutic product is administered. If it is performed expertly, lumbar puncture usually can be carried out without serious risk, but many clinicians prefer to wait until replacement therapy has been given. In one series, replacement therapy given within 6 hours of head injury prevented any intracranial bleeding.[481]

In cases involving major cranial trauma, if neurologic signs or symptoms develop, or if intracranial bleeding is confirmed radiologically or otherwise, the administration of factor VIII or factor IX concentrates should continue on a schedule in doses sufficient to keep the nadir levels of the deficient factor >50 IU/dL. Treatment should be maintained for 10 to 14 days.[480] Before the widespread use of factor VIII concentrates, the mortality rate after intracranial bleeding was greater than 70%.[479] For treatment of patients who have suffered from an episode of spontaneous intracranial hemorrhage, most experts recommend prophylaxis therapy so that the factor level rarely is below 1 IU/dL, as the risk of recurrence is significantly higher in such patients. It is expected that the morbidity and mortality of intracranial bleeding will be reduced further with increased use of the extended half-life factor products and nonfactor products now in clinical use.

Viral Transmission From Past Factor Concentrates: HIV and Hepatitis C

Acquired immunodeficiency syndrome (AIDS) was first recognized in 1978 and was found to be transmitted in blood products in the early 1980s,[482] infecting approximately 70% of persons with severe hemophilia using factor concentrates prior to 1984. HIV transmission through factor concentrate was reduced to zero after 1985, through the inclusion of virucidal steps in the manufacturing process, the institution of stringent donor testing, and the availability of recombinant products. Improvements in therapy for HIV have allowed many persons with hemophilia to become long-term survivors, although there remain many seropositive patients who have not progressed to AIDS.

In the United States mortality survey of hemophilia A patients between 1995 and 1998, liver disease was listed as a cause of death in 15% of patients.[483] It is estimated that approximately 90% of persons with severe hemophilia who used factor concentrates prior to 1984 were infected by the hepatitis C virus transmitted in the factor concentrate.[484] Nearly 20% of these individuals were able to eradicate the virus, thus becoming hepatitis C antibody positive, but hepatitis C virus negative. However, for other patients, the hepatitis C virus has progressed inexorably with many dying from chronic liver disease. A prospective study of US hemophilia patients found that 66% of the hepatitis C–infected hemophilia patients also had HIV infection,[484] and that coinfection was associated with a fivefold to fourfold increase in end-stage liver disease. Modern manufacturing methods render factor concentrates free of hepatitis C virus and other lipid-enveloped viruses. No hepatitis C viral transmission has been connected with factor concentrates since 1986. Patients who are seronegative for the hepatitis A and B viruses should receive immunizations for these viruses. However, standard solvent-detergent–inactivated products may still transmit non–lipid-enveloped viruses such as parvovirus,[485] hepatitis A,[486] and other viruses.[487] An unresolved issue is the transmission potential of the agent that causes Creutzfeldt-Jakob disease, but the manufacturers of plasma-derived factor concentrates have taken steps to reduce the risk of transmitting this agent also.[488]

Antibodies to Coagulation Factors

A major problem with current therapeutic products in hemophilia A is the development of neutralizing antibodies (inhibitors) to factor VIII. This complication is less common in patients with hemophilia B and other inherited coagulation disorders. Such antibodies may seriously complicate the treatment of these patients (see Chapter 55).

Home Treatment Programs

In general, current recommended therapy of hemophilia is replacement therapy or prophylaxis treatment to prevent any spontaneous bleeding episodes, rather than treating bleeding episodes after they occur, termed "on demand." A prospective randomized clinical trial demonstrated that joint damage is minimized if treatment is begun immediately after the onset of symptoms.[40] Such programs have resulted in decreased bleeding episodes and improved preservation of joint function.[489,490] Typical prophylactic regimens with standard half-life products are 25 to 40 IU/kg of factor VIII 3 times per week for hemophilia A, and 25 to 40 IU/kg of factor IX twice per week for hemophilia B. Such therapy usually maintains the trough factor level at or above 1% of normal. In older hemophilia patients with significant joint arthropathy, higher doses often are needed, whereas in younger patients with essentially normal joints, lower factor doses are sufficient. A 30-year follow-up report confirmed the efficacy of prophylaxis.[491] An economic analysis of prophylaxis found that although higher costs were associated with prophylaxis programs, the approach was justified on medical grounds.[492] It is recommended that patients begin prophylaxis soon after the first joint bleed.[493]

References

1. Ratnoff OD. The molecular basis of hereditary clotting disorders. *Prog Hemost Thromb.* 1972;1:39-74.
2. Peyvandi F, Garagiola I, Young G. The past and future of haemophilia: diagnosis, treatments, and its complications. *Lancet.* 2016;388:187-197.
3. Simioni P, Tormene D, Tognin G, et al. X-linked thrombophilia with a mutant factor IX (factor IX Padua). *N Engl J Med.* 2009;361:1671-1675.
4. Ingram GI. The history of haemophilia. *J Clin Pathol.* 1976;29:469-479.
5. Rogaev EI, Grigorenko AP, Faskhutdinova G, Kittler EL, Moliaka YK. Genotype analysis identifies the cause of the "royal disease". *Science.* 2009;326:817.
6. Hoyer LW. Immunologic properties of antihemophilic factor. *Prog Hematol.* 1973;8:191-221.
7. Iorio A, Stonebraker JS, Chambost H, et al. Data and demographics committee of the World federation of hemophilia. Establishing the prevalence and prevalence at birth of hemophilia in males: a meta-analytic approach using national registries. *Ann Intern Med.* 2019;171(8):540-546.
8. Soucie JM, Miller CH, Dupervil B, Le B, Buckner TW. Occurrence rates of haemophilia among males in the United States based on surveillance conducted in specialized haemophilia treatment centres. *Haemophilia.* 2020;26(3):487-493.
9. Graham JB. Genetic control of factor VIII. *Lancet.* 1980;1:340-342.
10. Pitney WR, Arnold BJ. Plasma antihaemophilic factor (AHF) concentrations in families of patients with haemorrhagic states. *Br J Haematol.* 1959;5:184-193.
11. Nichols WC, Amano K, Cacheris PM, et al. Moderation of hemophilia A phenotype by the factor V R506Q mutation. *Blood.* 1996;88:1183-1187.
12. Escuriola Ettingshausen C, Halimeh S, Kurnik K, et al. Symptomatic onset of severe hemophilia A in childhood is dependent on the presence of prothrombotic risk factors. *Thromb Haemost.* 2001;85:218-220.
13. Barrai I, Cann HM, Cavalli-Sforza LL, De Nicola P. The effect of parental age on rates of mutation for hemophilia and evidence for differing mutation rates for hemophilia A and B. *Am J Hum Genet.* 1968;20:175-196.
14. Lawn RM. The molecular genetics of hemophilia: blood clotting factors VIII and IX. *Cell.* 1985;42:405-406.
15. Miller CH, Benson J, Ellingsen D, et al. F8 and F9 mutations in US haemophilia patients: correlation with history of inhibitor and race/ethnicity. *Haemophilia.* 2012;18:375-382.
16. Centers for Disease Control and Prevention. *CDC Hemophilia Mutation Project (CHAMP & CHBMP).* Accessed August 27, 2021. https://www.cdc.gov/ncbddd/hemophilia/champs.html
17. Johnsen JM, Fletcher SN, Dove A, et al. Results of genetic analysis of 11,341 participants enrolled in the My Life, Our Future (MLOF) hemophilia genotyping initiative. *J Thromb Haemost.* 2022;20:2022-2034.
18. Antonarakis SE, Kazazian HH, Tuddenham EG. Molecular etiology of factor VIII deficiency in hemophilia A. *Hum Mutat.* 1995;5:1-22.
19. Antonarakis SE, Kazazian HH, Gitschier J, Hutter P, de Moerloose P, Morris MA. Molecular etiology of factor VIII deficiency in hemophilia A. *Adv Exp Med Biol.* 1995;386:19-34.
20. Antonarakis SE, Rossiter JP, Young M, et al. Factor VIII gene inversions in severe hemophilia A: results of an international consortium study. *Blood.* 1995;86:2206-2212.
21. Bagnall RD, Waseem N, Green PM, Giannelli F. Recurrent inversion breaking intron 1 of the factor VIII gene is a frequent cause of severe hemophilia A. *Blood.* 2002;99:168-174.
22. Amano K, Sarkar R, Pemberton S, Kemball-Cook G, Kazazian HH Jr, Kaufman RJ. The molecular basis for cross-reacting material-positive hemophilia A due to missense mutations within the A2-domain of factor VIII. *Blood.* 1998;91:538-548.
23. Klopp N, Oldenburg J, Uen C, Schneppenheim R, Graw J. 11 Hemophilia A patients without mutations in the factor VIII encoding gene. *Thromb Haemost.* 2002;88:357-360.

24. Pezeshkpoor B, Zimmer N, Marquardt N, et al. Deep intronic "mutations" cause hemophilia A: application of next generation sequencing in patients without detectable mutation in F8 cDNA. *J Thromb Haemost*. 2013;11(9):1679-1687.
25. Nishino M, Girma JP, Rothschild C, Fressinaud E, Meyer D. New variant of von Willebrand disease with defective binding to factor VIII. *Blood*. 1989;74:1591-1599.
26. Balak DM, Gouw SC, Plug I, et al. Prenatal diagnosis for haemophilia: a nationwide survey among female carriers in the Netherlands. *Haemophilia*. 2012;18:584-592.
27. Mulder E, Mochtar IA, Van Creveld, Cardozo EB. Factor-8 activity in carriers of haemophilia A. *Br J Haematol*. 1965;11:206-209.
28. Rapaport SI, Patch MJ, Casey JE. The antihemophilic globulin in plasma; content of freshly frozen single-donor plasma units prepared by the Los Angeles Red Cross Blood Center. *Calif Med*. 1960;93:208-210.
29. Bennett B, Ratnoff OD. Changes in antihemophilic factor (AHF, factor 8) procoagulant activity and AHF-like antigen in normal pregnancy, and following exercise and pneumoencephalography. *J Lab Clin Med*. 1972;80:256-263.
30. Blann AD, Daly RJ, Amiral J. The influence of age, gender and ABO blood group on soluble endothelial cell markers and adhesion molecules. *Br J Haematol*. 1996;92:498-500.
31. Ratnoff OD, Jones PK. The laboratory diagnosis of the carrier state for classic hemophilia. *Ann Intern Med*. 1977;86:521-528.
32. Seligsohn U, Zivelin A, Perez C, Modan M. Detection of haemophilia A carriers by replicate factor VIII activity and factor VIII antigenicity determinations. *Br J Haematol*. 1979;42:433-439.
33. Göbel U, von Kries R, Jürgens H, von Voss H. Problems in the detection of carriers of hemophilia A: the influence of stress and thrombin. *Blut*. 1978;37:37-41.
34. Miller R. Counselling about diagnosis and inheritance of genetic bleeding disorders: haemophilia A and B. *Haemophilia*. 1999;5:77-83.
35. Gilchrist GS, Hammond D, Melnyk J. Hemophilia A in a phenotypically normal female with XX-XO mosaicism. *N Engl J Med*. 1965;273:1402-1406.
36. Merskey C. The occurrence of haemophilia in the human female. *Q J Med*. 1951;20:299-312.
37. Mannucci PM, Tuddenham EG. The hemophilias—from royal genes to gene therapy. *N Engl J Med*. 2001;344:1773-1779.
38. White GC II, Rosendaal F, Aledort LM, et al. Definitions in hemophilia. Recommendation of the scientific subcommittee on factor VIII and factor IX of the scientific and standardization committee of the International Society on Thrombosis and Haemostasis. *Thromb Haemost*. 2001;85:560.
39. Graham JB, McLendon WW, Brinkhous KM. Mild hemophilia; allelic form of the disease. *Am J Med Sci*. 1953;225:46-53.
40. Manco-Johnson MJ, Abshire TC, Shapiro AD, et al. Prophylaxis versus episodic treatment to prevent joint disease in boys with severe hemophilia. *N Engl J Med*. 2007;357:535-544.
41. van Vulpen LF, Schutgens RE, Coeleveld K, et al. IL-1β, in contrast to TNFα, is pivotal in blood-induced cartilage damage and is a potential target for therapy. *Blood*. 2015;126:2239-2246.
42. Roosendaal G, Vianen ME, Wenting MJ, et al. Iron deposits and catabolic properties of synovial tissue from patients with haemophilia. *J Bone Joint Surg Br*. 1998;80:540-545.
43. Gilbert MS. Musculoskeletal manifestations of hemophilia. *Mt Sinai J Med*. 1977;44:339-358.
44. Arnold WD, Hilgartner MW. Hemophilic arthropathy. Current concepts of pathogenesis and management. *J Bone Joint Surg Am*. 1977;59:287-305.
45. Gualtierotti R, Solimeno LP, Peyvandi F. Hemophilic arthropathy: current knowledge and future perspectives. *J Thromb Haemost*. 2021;19(9):2112-2121.
46. Soler R, López-Fernβndez F, Rodríguez E, Marini M. Hemophilic arthropathy. A scoring system for magnetic resonance imaging. *Eur Radiol*. 2002;12:836-843.
47. Leatherdale RA. Respiratory obstruction in haemophilic patients. *Br Med J*. 1960;1:1316-1320.
48. Prentice CR, Lindsay RM, Barr RD, et al. Renal complications in haemophilia and Christmas disease. *Q J Med*. 1971;40:47-61.
49. Abildgaard CF, Simone JV, Schulman I. Steroid treatment of hemophilic hematuria. *J Pediatr*. 1965;66:117-119.
50. Baehner RL, Strauss HS. Hemophilia in the first year of life. *N Engl J Med*. 1966;275:524-528.
51. Mazepa MA, Monahan PE, Baker JR, Riske BK, Soucie JM; US Hemophilia Treatment Center Network. Men with severe hemophilia in the United States: birth cohort analysis of a large national database. *Blood*. 2016;127(24):3073-3081.
52. Goodnough LT, Saito H, Ratnoff OD. Thrombosis or myocardial infarction in congenital clotting factor abnormalities and chronic thrombocytopenias: a report of 21 patients and a review of 50 previously reported cases. *Medicine (Baltimore)*. 1983;62:248-255.
53. Sood SL, Cheng D, Ragni M, et al. A cross-sectional analysis of cardiovascular disease in the hemophilia population. *Blood Adv*. 2018;2(11):1325-1333.
54. Shapiro S, Makris M. Haemophilia and ageing. *Br J Haematol*. 2019;184(5):712-720.
55. Franchini M, Mannucci PM. Management of hemophilia in older patients. *Drugs Aging*. 2017;34(12):881-889.
56. Fogarty PF, Olin JW, Kessler CM, Konkle BA, Aledort LM. An algorithmic approach to peripheral artery disease in hemophilia: extrapolation of management principles from noncoagulopathic patients. *Blood Coagul Fibrinolysis*. 2012;23:23-29.
57. Martin BA, Branch DW, Rodgers GM. The preparation of a sensitive partial thromboplastin reagent from bovine brain. *Blood Coagul Fibrinolysis*. 1992;3:287-294.
58. Kekwick RA, Walton PL. An assay for antihaemophilic factor (factor VIII) with some considerations affecting the establishment of a standard reference preparation. *Br J Haematol*. 1964;10:299-313.
59. Margolis J. An improved procedure for accurate assays of factor VIII. *Pathology*. 1979;11:149-159.
60. Vermylen C, Verstraete M. A simple method for the assay of factor 8, using 20 microlitres of capillary blood. *Br J Haematol*. 1968;14:241-245.
61. Kirkwood TB, Barrowcliffe TW. Discrepancy between one-stage and two-stage assay of factor VIII:C. *Br J Haematol*. 1978;40:333-338.
62. Blombäck M, Kjellman H, Allain JP, Hedner U, Schimpf K, Wiechel B. On the unreliability of one-stage factor VIII:C clotting assays after infusion of factor VIII concentrates. *Scand J Clin Lab Invest*. 1987;47:561-566.
63. Mikaelsson M, Oswaldsson U, Sandberg H. Influence of phospholipids on the assessment of factor VIII activity. *Haemophilia*. 1998;4:646-650.
64. Sommer JM, Moore N, McGuffie-Valentine B, et al. Comparative field study evaluating the activity of recombinant factor VIII Fc fusion protein in plasma samples at clinical haemostasis laboratories. *Haemophilia*. 2014;20:294-300.
65. Gray E, Kitchen S, Bowyer A, et al. Laboratory measurement of factor replacement therapies in the treatment of congenital haemophilia: a United Kingdom Haemophilia Centre Doctors' Organisation guideline. *Haemophilia*. 2020;26(1):6-16.
66. Richards M, Lavigne Lissalde G, Combescure C, et al. Neonatal bleeding in haemophilia: a European Cohort Study. *Br J Haematol*. 2012;156:374-382.
67. Plug I, Mauser-Bunschoten EP, Bröcker-Vriends AH, et al. Bleeding in carriers of hemophilia. *Blood*. 2006;108:52-56.
68. Pavlovsky A. Contribution to the pathogenesis of hemophilia. *Blood*. 1947;2:185-191.
69. Aggeler PM, White SG, Glendening MB, Page EW, Leake TB, Bates G. Plasma thromboplastin component (PTC) deficiency; a new disease resembling hemophilia. *Proc Soc Exp Biol Med*. 1952;79:692-694.
70. Aggeler PM, Spaet TH, Emery BB. Purification of plasma thromboplastin factor B (plasma thromboplastin component) and its identification as a beta2 globulin. *Science*. 1954;119:806.
71. Veltkamp JJ, Meilof J, Remmelts HG, van der Vlerk D, Loeliger EA. Another genetic variant of haemophilia B: haemophilia B Leyden. *Scand J Haematol*. 1970;7:82-90.
72. Crossley M, Ludwig M, Stowell KM, De Vos P, Olek K, Brownlee GG. Recovery from hemophilia B Leyden: an androgen-responsive element in the factor IX promoter. *Science*. 1992;257:377-379.
73. Payne AB, Bean CJ, Hooper WC, Miller CH. Utility of multiplex ligation-dependent probe amplification (MLPA) for hemophilia mutation screening. *J Thromb Haemost*. 2012;10(9):1951-1954.
74. Noyes CM, Griffith MJ, Roberts HR, Lundblad RL. Identification of the molecular defect in factor IX Chapel Hill: substitution of histidine for arginine at position 145. *Proc Natl Acad Sci U S A*. 1983;80:4200-4202.
75. Davies SH, Gavin J, Goldsmith KL, et al. The linkage relations of hemophilia A and hemophilia B (Christmas disease) to the Xg blood group system. *Am J Hum Genet*. 1963;15:481-492.
76. Bithell TC, Pizarro A, MacDiarmid WD. Variant of factor IX deficiency in female with 45, X Turner's syndrome. *Blood*. 1970;36:169-179.
77. Nisen P, Stamberg J, Ehrenpreis R, et al. The molecular basis of severe hemophilia B in a girl. *N Engl J Med*. 1986;315:1139-1142.
78. Rallapalli PM, Kemball-Cook G, Tuddenham EG, Gomez K, Perkins SJ. An interactive mutation database for human coagulation factor IX provides novel insights into the phenotypes and genetics of hemophilia B. *J Thromb Haemost*. 2013;11:1329-1340.
79. Hamasaki-Katagiri N, Salari R, Simhadri VL, et al. Analysis of F9 point mutations and their correlation to severity of haemophilia B disease. *Haemophilia*. 2012;18(6):933-940.
80. Didisheim P, Vandervoort RL. Detection of carriers for factor IX (PTC) deficiency. *Blood*. 1962;20:150-155.
81. Orstavik KH, Veltkamp JJ, Bertina RM, Hermans J. Detection of carriers of haemophilia B. *Br J Haematol*. 1979;42:293-301.
82. Poon MC, Chui PH, Patterson M, Starozik DM, Dimnik LS, Hoar DI. Hemophilia B (Christmas disease) variants and carrier detection analyzed by DNA probes. *J Clin Invest*. 1987;79:1204-1209.
83. Chan K, Sasanakul W, Mellars G, et al. Detection of known haemophilia B mutations and carrier testing by microarray. *Thromb Haemost*. 2005;94:872-878.
84. Peyvandi F, Jayandharan G, Chandy M, et al. Genetic diagnosis of haemophilia and other inherited bleeding disorders. *Haemophilia*. 2006;12(suppl 3):82-89.
85. Ljung R, Tedgard U. Genetic counseling of hemophilia carriers. *Semin Thromb Hemost*. 2003;29:31-36.
86. Aggeler PM, Hoag MS, Wallerstein RO, Whissell D. The mild hemophilias. Occult deficiencies of AHF, PTC and PTA frequently responsible for unexpected surgical bleeding. *Am J Med*. 1961;30:84-94.
87. Sommer JM, Buyue Y, Bardan S, et al. Comparative field study: impact of laboratory assay variability on the assessment of recombinant factor IX Fc fusion protein (rFIXFc) activity. *Thromb Haemost*. 2014;112:932-940.
88. Nyman D, Eriksson AW, Blomback M, Frants RR, Wahlberg P. Recent investigations of the first bleeder family in Åland (Finland) described by von Willebrand. *Thromb Haemost*. 1981;45:73-76.
89. Federici AB, Mannucci PM. Advances in the genetics and treatment of von Willebrand disease. *Curr Opin Pediatr*. 2002;14:23-33.
90. Laffan MA, Lester W, O'Donnell JS, et al. The diagnosis and management of von Willebrand disease: a United Kingdom Haemophilia Centre Doctors Organization guideline approved by the British Committee for Standards in Haematology. *Br J Haematol*. 2014;167:453-465.
91. Weyand AC, Flood VH. Von Willebrand disease: current status of diagnosis and management. *Hematol Oncol Clin North Am*. 2021;35(6):1085-1101.
92. James PD, Connell NT, Ameer B, et al. ASH ISTH NHF WFH 2021 guidelines on the diagnosis of von Willebrand disease. *Blood Adv*. 2021;5(1):280-300.

93. Connell NT, Flood VH, Brignardello-Petersen R, et al. ASH ISTH NHF WFH 2021 guidelines on the management of von Willebrand disease. *Blood Adv*. 2021;5(1):301-325.
94. Werner EJ, Broxson EH, Tucker EL, Giroux DS, Shults J, Abshire TC. Prevalence of von Willebrand disease in children: a multiethnic study. *J Pediatr*. 1993;123:893-898.
95. Ginsberg D, Handin RI, Bonthron DT, et al. Human von Willebrand factor (vWF): isolation of complementary DNA (cDNA) clones and chromosomal localization. *Science*. 1985;228:1401-1406.
96. Sadler JE, Shelton-Inloes BB, Sorace JM, Harlan JM, Titani K, Davie EW. Cloning and characterization of two cDNAs coding for human von Willebrand factor. *Proc Natl Acad Sci U S A*. 1985;82:6394-6398.
97. Jenkins PV, Pasi KJ, Perkins SJ. Molecular modeling of ligand and mutation sites of the type A domains of human von Willebrand factor and their relevance to von Willebrand's disease. *Blood*. 1998;91:2032-2044.
98. Furlan M, Robles R, Lammle B. Partial purification and characterization of a protease from human plasma cleaving von Willebrand factor to fragments produced by in vivo proteolysis. *Blood*. 1996;87:4223-4234.
99. Sadler JE. New concepts in von Willebrand disease. *Annu Rev Med*. 2005;56:173-191.
100. Orstavik KH, Magnus P, Reisner H, Berg K, Graham JB, Nance W. Factor VIII and factor IX in a twin population. Evidence for a major effect of ABO locus on factor VIII level. *Am J Hum Genet*. 1985;37:89-101.
101. Gill JC, Endres-Brooks J, Bauer PJ, Marks WJ Jr, Montgomery RR. The effect of ABO blood group on the diagnosis of von Willebrand disease. *Blood*. 1987;69:1691-1695.
102. Gallinaro L, Cattini MG, Sztukowska M, et al. A shorter von Willebrand factor survival in O blood group subjects explains how ABO determinants influence plasma von Willebrand factor. *Blood*. 2008;111:3540-3545.
103. Di Paola J, Federici AB, Mannucci PM, et al. Low platelet $\alpha_2 2\beta_2 1$ levels in type I von Willebrand disease correlate with impaired platelet function in a high shear stress system. *Blood*. 1999;93:3578-3582.
104. Kadir RA, Economides DL, Sabin CA, Owens D, Lee CA. Variations in coagulation factors in women: effects of age, ethnicity, menstrual cycle and combined oral contraceptive. *Thromb Haemost*. 1999;82:1456-1461.
105. Abou-Ismail MY, Ogunbayo GO, Secic M, Kouides PA. Outgrowing the laboratory diagnosis of type 1 von Willebrand disease: a two decade study. *Am J Hematol*. 2018;93(2):232-237.
106. Biguzzi E, Siboni SM, le Cessie S, et al. Increasing levels of von Willebrand factor and factor VIII with age in patients affected by von Willebrand disease. *J Thromb Haemost*. 2021;19(1):96-106.
107. Sadler JE. Von Willebrand disease type 1: a diagnosis in search of a disease. *Blood*. 2003;101:2089-2093.
108. Goodeve A, Eikenboom J, Castaman G, et al. Phenotype and genotype of a cohort of families historically diagnosed with type 1 von Willebrand disease in the European study, Molecular and Clinical Markers for the Diagnosis and Management of Type I von Willebrand Disease (MCMDM–1VWD). *Blood*. 2007;109:112-121.
109. James PD, Notley C, Hegadorn C, et al. The mutational spectrum of type 1 von Willebrand disease: results from a Canadian cohort study. *Blood*. 2007;109:145-154.
110. Casonato A, Pontara E, Sartorello F, et al. Reduced von Willebrand factor survival in type Vicenza von Willebrand disease. *Blood*. 2002;99:180-184.
111. Haberichter SL, Balistreri M, Christopherson P, et al. Assay of the von Willebrand factor (VWF) propeptide to identify patients with type 1 von Willebrand disease with decreased VWF survival. *Blood*. 2006;108:3344-3351.
112. Baronciani L, Cozzi G, Canciani MT, et al. Molecular characterization of a multiethnic group of 21 patients with type 3 von Willebrand disease. *Thromb Haemost*. 2000;84:536-540.
113. Levy GG, Nichols WC, Lian EC, et al. Mutations in a member of the ADAMTS gene family cause thrombotic thrombocytopenic purpura. *Nature*. 2001;413:488-494.
114. Zheng X, Chung D, Takayama TK, Majerus EM, Sadler JE, Fujikawa K. Structure of von Willebrand factor-cleaving protease (ADAMTS13), a metalloprotease involved in thrombotic thrombocytopenic purpura. *J Biol Chem*. 2001;276:41059-41063.
115. Dong JF, Moake JL, Nolasco L, et al. ADAMTS13 metalloprotease rapidly cleaves newly secreted ultralarge von Willebrand factor multimers on the endothelial surface under flowing conditions. *Blood*. 2002;100:4033-4039.
116. Lammle B, Kremer Hovinga JA, Alberio L. Thrombotic thrombocytopenic purpura. *J Thromb Haemost*. 2005;3:1663-1675.
117. Mannucci PM. Treatment of von Willebrand's disease. *N Engl J Med*. 2004;351:683-694.
118. Baumgartner HR, Tschopp TB, Meyer D. Shear rate dependent inhibition of platelet adhesion and aggregation on collagenous surfaces by antibodies to human factor VIII/von Willebrand factor. *Br J Haematol*. 1980;44:127-139.
119. Hovig T, Stormorken H. Ultrastructural studies on the platelet plug formation in bleeding time wounds from normal individuals and patients with von Willebrand's disease. *Acta Pathol Microbiol Scand Suppl*. 1974;(suppl 248):105-122.
120. Brinkhous KM, Sandberg H, Garris JB, et al. Purified human factor VIII procoagulant protein: comparative hemostatic response after infusions into hemophilic and von Willebrand disease dogs. *Proc Natl Acad Sci U S A*. 1985;82:8752-8756.
121. Koedam JA, Meijers JC, Sixma JJ, Bouma BN. Inactivation of human factor VIII by activated protein C. Cofactor activity of protein S and protective effect of von Willebrand factor. *J Clin Invest*. 1988;82:1236-1243.
122. Everett LA, Cleuren AC, Khoriaty RN, Ginsburg D. Murine coagulation factor VIII is synthesized in endothelial cells. *Blood*. 2014;123:3697-3705.
123. Agrawal YP, Dzik W. The vWF content of factor VIII concentrates. *Transfusion*. 2001;41:153-154.
124. Weinstein M, Deykin D. Comparison of factor VIII-related von Willebrand factor proteins prepared from human cryoprecipitate and factor VIII concentrate. *Blood*. 1979;53:1095-1105.
125. Dilley A, Drews C, Lally C, Austin H, Barnhart E, Evatt B. A survey of gynecologists concerning menorrhagia: perceptions of bleeding disorders as a possible cause. *J Womens Health Gend Based Med*. 2002;11:39-44.
126. Kadir RA, Economides DL, Sabin CA, Owens D, Lee CA. Frequency of inherited bleeding disorders in women with menorrhagia. *Lancet*. 1998;351:485-489.
127. Franchini M, Mannucci PM. Gastrointestinal angiodysplasia and bleeding in von Willebrand disease. *Thromb Haemost*. 2014;112:427-431.
128. Ragni MV, Bontempo FA, Hassett AC. von Willebrand disease and bleeding in women. *Haemophilia*. 1999;5:313-317.
129. Rodeghiero F, Castaman G, Tosetto A, et al. The discriminant power of bleeding history for the diagnosis of type 1 von Willebrand disease: an international, multicenter study. *J Thromb Haemost*. 2005;3:2619-2626.
130. Sanders YV, Eikenboom J, de Wee EM, et al. Reduced prevalence of arterial thrombosis in von Willebrand disease. *J Thromb Haemost*. 2013;11:845-854.
131. Fressinaud E, Veyradier A, Truchaud F, et al. Screening for von Willebrand disease with a new analyzer using high shear stress: a study of 60 cases. *Blood*. 1998;91:1325-1331.
132. Kundu SK, Heilmann EJ, Sio R, Garcia C, Davidson RM, Ostgaard RA. Description of an in-vitro platelet function analyzer—PFA-100. *Semin Thromb Hemost*. 1995;21(suppl 2):106-112.
133. Quiroga T, Goycoolea M, Munoz B, et al. Template bleeding time and PFA-100 have low sensitivity to screen patients with hereditary mucocutaneous hemorrhages: comparative study in 148 patients. *J Thromb Haemost*. 2004;2:892-898.
134. Sultan Y, Simeon J, Maisonneuve P, Caen JP. Immunologic studies in von Willebrand's disease: alteration of factor VIII/von Willebrand protein after transfusion with plasma concentrates in patients with von Willebrand's disease. *Thromb Haemost*. 1976;35:110-119.
135. Flood VH, Gill JC, Friedman KD, et al. Collagen binding provides a sensitive screen for variant von Willebrand disease. *Clin Chem*. 2013;59:684-691.
136. Federici AB, Canciani MT, Forza I, Cozzi G. Ristocetin cofactor and collagen binding activities normalized to antigen levels for a rapid diagnosis of type 2 von Willebrand disease: single center comparison of four different assays. *Thromb Haemost*. 2000;84:1127-1128.
137. Brinkhous KM, Read MS. Preservation of platelet receptors for platelet aggregating factor/von Willebrand factor by air drying, freezing, or lyophilization: a new stable platelet preparation for von Willebrand factor assays. *Thromb Res*. 1978;13:591-597.
138. Rodeghiero F, Castaman G, Tosetto A. von Willebrand factor antigen is less sensitive than ristocetin-cofactor for the diagnosis of type I von Willebrand disease: results based on an epidemiological investigation. *Thromb Haemost*. 1990;64:349-352.
139. Favaloro EJ, Smith J, Petinos P, Hertzberg M, Koutts J. Laboratory testing for von Willebrand's disease: an assessment of current diagnostic practice and efficacy by means of a multi-laboratory survey. RCPA Quality Assurance Program (QAP) in Haematology Haemostasis Scientific Advisory Panel. *Thromb Haemost*. 1999;82:1276-1282.
140. Goodall AH, Jarvis J, Chand S, et al. An immunoradiometric assay for human factor VIII/von Willebrand factor (VIII:VWF) using a monoclonal antibody that defines a functional epitope. *Br J Haematol*. 1985;59:565-577.
141. Sharma R, Flood VH. Advances in the diagnosis and treatment of von Willebrand disease. *Blood*. 2017;130:2386-2391.
142. Patzke J, Budde U, Huber A, et al. Performance evaluation and multicentre study of a von Willebrand factor activity assay based on GPIb binding in the absence of ristocetin. *Blood Coagul Fibrinolysis*. 2014;25:860-870.
143. Scott JP, Montgomery RR. The rapid differentiation of type IIb von Willebrand's disease from platelet-type (pseudo-) von Willebrand's disease by the "neutral" monoclonal antibody binding assay. *Am J Clin Pathol*. 1991;96:723-728.
144. Favaloro EJ. Collagen binding assay for von Willebrand factor (VWF:CBA): detection of von Willebrand disease and discrimination of von Willebrand disease subtypes, depends on collagen source. *Thromb Haemost*. 2000;83:127-135.
145. Casonato A, Pontara E, Zerbinati P, Zucchetto A, Girolami A. The evaluation of factor VIII binding activity of von Willebrand factor by means of an ELISA method: significance and practical implications. *Am J Clin Pathol*. 1998;109:347-352.
146. Kroner PA, Foster PA, Fahs SA, Montgomery RR. The defective interaction between von Willebrand factor and factor VIII in a patient with type 1 von Willebrand disease is caused by substitution of Arg19 and His54 in mature von Willebrand factor. *Blood*. 1996;87:1013-1021.
147. Zimmerman TS, Ruggeri ZM. von Willebrand disease. *Hum Pathol*. 1987;18:140-152.
148. Ledford-Kraemer MR. Analysis of von Willebrand factor structure by multimer analysis. *Am J Hematol*. 2010;85:510-514.
149. Sanders YV, Groeneveld D, Meijer K, et al. von Willebrand factor propeptide and the phenotypic classification of von Willebrand disease. *Blood*. 2015;125:3006-3013.
150. Hambleton J. Diagnosis and incidence of inherited von Willebrand disease. *Curr Opin Hematol*. 2001;8:306-311.
151. Hillery CA, Mancuso DJ, Evan Sadler J, et al. Type 2M von Willebrand disease: F606I and I662F mutations in the glycoprotein Ib binding domain selectively impair ristocetin- but not botrocetin-mediated binding of von Willebrand factor to platelets. *Blood*. 1998;91:1572-1581.
152. Corrales I, Ramírez L, Altisent C, Parra R, Vidal F. Rapid molecular diagnosis of von Willebrand disease by direct sequencing. Detection of 12 novel putative mutations in VWF gene. *Thromb Haemost*. 2009;101:570-576.
153. James PD, Paterson AD, Notley C, et al. Genetic linkage and association analysis in type 1 von Willebrand disease: results from the Canadian type 1 VWD study. *J Thromb Haemost*. 2006;4:783-792.
154. Gudmundsdottir BR, Marder VJ, Onundarson PT. Risk of excessive bleeding associated with marginally low von Willebrand factor and mild platelet dysfunction. *J Thromb Haemost*. 2007;5:274-281.

155. Lethagen S, Hillarp A, Ekholm C, Mattson E, Halldén C, Friberg B. Distribution of von Willebrand factor levels in young women with and without bleeding symptoms: influence of ABO blood group and promoter haplotypes. *Thromb Haemost.* 2008;99:1013-1018.
156. Mannucci PM, Bloom AL, Larrieu MJ, Nilsson IM, West RR. Atherosclerosis and von Willebrand factor. I. Prevalence of severe von Willebrand's disease in Western Europe and Israel. *Br J Haematol.* 1984;57:163-169.
157. Mancuso DJ, Tuley EA, Castillo R, de Bosch N, Mannucci PM, Sadler JE. Characterization of partial gene deletions in type III von Willebrand disease with alloantibody inhibitors. *Thromb Haemost.* 1994;72:180-185.
158. Borel-Derlon A, Federici AB, Roussel-Robert V, et al. Treatment of severe von Willebrand disease with a high-purity von Willebrand factor concentrate (Wilfactin): a prospective study of 50 patients. *J Thromb Haemost.* 2007;5:1115-1124.
159. Hill FG, Enayat MS, George AJ. Investigation including VIIIR: AG multimeric analysis of a large kindred with type IIa von Willebrand's disease showing a dominant inheritance and similar gene expression in four generations. *Thromb Haemost.* 1983;50:735-739.
160. Berkowitz SD, Dent J, Roberts J, et al. Epitope mapping of the von Willebrand factor subunit distinguishes fragments present in normal and type IIA von Willebrand disease from those generated by plasmin. *J Clin Invest.* 1987;79:524-531.
161. Gralnick HR, Williams SB, McKeown LP, et al. In vitro correction of abnormal multimeric structure of von Willebrand factor in type IIa von Willebrand disease. *Proc Natl Acad Sci U S A.* 1985;82:5968-5972.
162. Kyrle PA, Niessner H, Dent J, et al. IIB von Willebrand disease: pathogenetic and therapeutic studies. *Br J Haematol.* 1988;69:55-59.
163. Holmberg L, Nilsson IM, Borge L, Gunnarsson M, Sjörin E. Platelet aggregation induced by 1-desamino-8-D-arginine vasopressin (DDAVP) in type IIB von Willebrand disease. *N Engl J Med.* 1983;309:816-821.
164. Federici AB, Mannucci PM, Castaman G, et al. Clinical and molecular predictors of thrombocytopenia and risk of bleeding in patients with von Willebrand disease type 2B: a cohort study of 67 patients. *Blood.* 2009;113:526-534.
165. Ribba AS, Loisel I, Lavergne JM, et al. Ser968Thr mutation within the A3 domain of von Willebrand factor (VWF) in two related patients leads to a defective binding of VWF to collagen. *Thromb Haemost.* 2001;86:848-854.
166. Foster PA, Fulcher CA, Marti T, Titani K, Zimmerman TS. A major factor VIII binding domain resides within the amino-terminal 272 amino acid residues of von Willebrand factor. *J Biol Chem.* 1987;262:8443-8446.
167. Mazurier C. von Willebrand disease masquerading as hemophilia A. *Thromb Haemost.* 1992;67:391-396.
168. Schneppenheim R, Budde U, Krey S, et al. Results of a screening for von Willebrand disease type 2N in patients with suspected haemophilia A or von Willebrand disease type 1. *Thromb Haemost.* 1996;76:598-602.
169. Miller JL, Castella A. Platelet-type von Willebrand's disease: characterization of a new bleeding disorder. *Blood.* 1982;60:790-794.
170. Bryckaert MC, Pietu G, Ruan C, et al. Abnormality of glycoprotein Ib in two cases of "pseudo"-von Willebrand disease. *J Lab Clin Med.* 1985;106:393-400.
171. Favaloro EJ, Patterson D, Denholm A, et al. Differential identification of a rare form of platelet-type (pseudo-) von Willebrand disease (VWD) from type 2B VWD using a simplified ristocetin-induced-platelet-agglutination mixing assay and confirmed by genetic analysis. *Br J Haematol.* 2007;139:623-626.
172. Huizinga EG, Tsuji S, Romijn RA, et al. Structures of glycoprotein Ibα and its complex with von Willebrand factor A1 domain. *Science.* 2002;297:1176-1179.
173. Othman M, Gresele P. Guidance on the diagnosis and management of platelet-type von Willebrand disease: a communication from the Platelet Physiology Subcommittee of the ISTH. *J Thromb Haemost.* 2020;18:1855-1858.
174. Casini A, Undas A, Palla R, et al. Diagnosis and classification of congenital fibrinogen disorders: communication from the SSC of the ISTH. *J Thromb Haemost.* 2018;16:1887-1890.
175. Pieters M, Wolberg AS. Fibrinogen and fibrin: an illustrated review. *Res Pract Thromb Haemost.* 2019;3:161-172.
176. Mosesson MW. Fibrinogen and fibrin structure and functions. *J Thromb Haemost.* 2005;3:1894-1904.
177. Fuller GM, Nickerson JM, Adams MA. Translational and cotranslational events in fibrinogen synthesis. *Ann N Y Acad Sci.* 1983;408:440-448.
178. Chung DW, Rixon MW, Que BG, Davie EW. Cloning of fibrinogen genes and their cDNA. *Ann N Y Acad Sci.* 1983;408:449-456.
179. De Silva CC, Thanabalasundaram RS. Congenital afibrinogenemia. *Br Med J.* 1951;2:86-88.
180. de Moerloose P, Neerman-Arbez M. Congenital fibrinogen disorders. *Semin Thromb Hemost.* 2009;35:356-366.
181. Uzan G, Courtois G, Besmond C, et al. Analysis of fibrinogen genes in patients with congenital afibrinogenemia. *Biochem Biophys Res Commun.* 1984;120:376-383.
182. Callea F, Tortura O, Kojima T, et al. Hypofibrinogenemia and fibrinogen storage disease. In: Mosesson MW, Amrani DL, Siebenlist KR, DiOrio JP, eds. *Fibrinogen 3: Biochemistry, Biological Functions, Gene Regulation, and Expression.* Elsevier Science; 1988:247-250.
183. Kant JA, Fornace AJ Jr, Saxe D, Simon MI, McBride OW, Crabtree GR. Evolution and organization of the fibrinogen locus on chromosome 4: gene duplication accompanied by transposition and inversion. *Proc Natl Acad Sci U S A.* 1985;82:2344-2348.
184. Asselta R, Duga S, Tenchini ML. The molecular basis of quantitative fibrinogen disorders. *J Thromb Haemost.* 2006;4:2115-2129.
185. Neerman-Arbez M. The molecular basis of inherited afibrinogenaemia. *Thromb Haemost.* 2001;86:154-163.
186. Ni H, Denis CV, Subbarao S, et al. Persistence of platelet thrombus formation in arterioles of mice lacking both von Willebrand factor and fibrinogen. *J Clin Invest.* 2000;106:385-392.
187. Suh TT, Holmbäck K, Jensen NJ, et al. Resolution of spontaneous bleeding events but failure of pregnancy in fibrinogen-deficient mice. *Genes Dev.* 1995;9:2020-2033.
188. Bolton-Maggs PH, Perry DJ, Chalmers EA, et al. The rare coagulation disorders—review with guidelines for management from the United Kingdom Haemophilia Centre Doctors' Organisation. *Haemophilia.* 2004;10:593-628.
189. Fried K, Kaufman S. Congenital afibrinogenemia in 10 offspring of uncle-niece marriages. *Clin Genet.* 1980;17:223-227.
190. Acharya SS, Coughlin A, Dimichele DM. Rare Bleeding Disorder Registry: deficiencies of factors II, V, VII, X, XIII, fibrinogen and dysfibrinogenemias. *J Thromb Haemost.* 2004;2:248-256.
191. Goodwin TM. Congenital hypofibrinogenemia in pregnancy. *Obstet Gynecol Surv.* 1989;44:157-161.
192. Mensah PK, Oppenheimer C, Watson C, Pavord S. Congenital afibrinogenaemia in pregnancy. *Haemophilia.* 2011;17:167-168.
193. Bornikova L, Peyvandi F, Allen G, Bernstein J, Manco-Johnson MJ. Fibrinogen replacement therapy for congenital fibrinogen deficiency. *J Thromb Haemost.* 2011;9:1687-1704.
194. Cunningham MT, Brandt JT, Laposata M, Olson JD. Laboratory diagnosis of dysfibrinogenemia. *Arch Pathol Lab Med.* 2002;126:499-505.
195. Yamagata S, Mori K, Kayaba T, Hiratsuka I, Kitamura T. A case of congenital afibrinogenemia and review of reported cases in Japan. *Tohoku J Exp Med.* 1968;96:15-35.
196. Colvin RB, Mosesson MW, Dvorak HF. Delayed-type hypersensitivity skin reactions in congenital afibrinogenemia lack fibrin deposition and induration. *J Clin Invest.* 1979;63:1302-1306.
197. Ramsay NK, Coccia PF, Krivit W, Nesbit ME, Edson JR. The effect of L-asparaginase of plasma coagulation factors in acute lymphoblastic leukemia. *Cancer.* 1977;40:1398-1401.
198. Fischer M, Lechner K, Hinterberger W, et al. Deficiency of fibrinogen and factor VII following treatment of severe aplastic anaemia with anti-thymocyte globulin and high-dose methylprednisolone. *Scand J Haematol.* 1985;34:312-316.
199. Frenkel E, Duksin C, Herman A, Sherman DJ. Congenital hypofibrinogenemia in pregnancy: report of two cases and review of the literature. *Obstet Gynecol Surv.* 2004;59:775-779.
200. Manco-Johnson MJ, Dimichele D, Castaman G, et al. Pharmacokinetics and safety of fibrinogen concentrate. *J Thromb Haemost.* 2009;7:2064-2069.
201. De Vries A, Rosenberg T, Kochwa S, Boss JH. Precipitating antifibrinogen antibody appearing after fibrinogen infusions in a patient with congenital afibrinogenemia. *Am J Med.* 1961;30:486-494.
202. Ruiz-Saez A. Thrombosis in rare bleeding disorders. *Hematology.* 2012;17(suppl 1):S156-S158.
203. Calenda E, Borg JY, Peillon C, et al. Perioperative management of a patient with congenital hypofibrinogenemia. *Anesthesiology.* 1989;71:622-623.
204. Menegatti M, Peyvandi F. Treatment of rare factor deficiencies other than hemophilia. *Blood.* 2019;133:415-424.
205. Morris TA, Marsh JJ, Chiles PG, et al. High prevalence of dysfibrinogenemia among patients with chronic thromboembolic pulmonary hypertension. *Blood.* 2009;114:1929-1936.
206. Casini A, Brungs T, Lavenu-Bombled C, et al. Genetics, diagnosis and clinical features of congenital hypodysfibrinogenemia: a systematic literature review and report of a novel mutation. *J Thromb Haemost.* 2017;15:876-888.
207. Benson MD. Amyloidosis. In: Scriver CR, Beaudet A, Sly WS, Valle D, eds. *The Metabolic Basis of Inherited Disease.* 7th ed. McGraw-Hill; 1995:4159-4191.
208. Francis RB Jr. Clinical disorders of fibrinolysis: a critical review. *Blut.* 1989;59:1-14.
209. Mosesson MW. Dysfibrinogenemia and thrombosis. *Semin Thromb Hemost.* 1999;25:311-319.
210. Rodgers GM, Garr SB. Comparison of functional and antigenic fibrinogen values from a normal population. *Thromb Res.* 1992;68:207-210.
211. Pluta A, Gutkowski K, Hartleb M. Coagulopathy in liver diseases. *Adv Med Sci.* 2010;55:16-21.
212. Post GR, James L, Alapat D, Guillory V, Cottler-Fox M, Nakagawa M. A case of acquired dysfibrinogenemia in multiple myeloma treated with therapeutic plasma exchange. *Transfus Apher Sci.* 2013;48:35-38.
213. Galanakis DK, Ginzler EM, Fikrig SM. Monoclonal IgG anticoagulants delaying fibrin aggregation in two patients with systemic lupus erythematosus (SLE). *Blood.* 1978;52:1037-1046.
214. Marciniak E, Greenwood MF. Acquired coagulation inhibitor delaying fibrinopeptide release. *Blood.* 1979;53:81-92.
215. Greenberg CS, Sane DC, Lai TS. Factor XIII and fibrin stabilization. In: Colman RW, Marder VJ, Clowes AW, et al, eds. *Hemostasis and Thrombosis: Basic Principles and Clinical Practice.* Lippincott Williams & Wilkins; 2006:317-334.
216. Robbins KC. A study on the conversion of fibrinogen to fibrin. *Am J Physiol.* 1944;142:581-588.
217. Duckert F, Jung E, Shmerling DH. A hitherto undescribed congenital haemorrhagic diathesis probably due to fibrin stabilizing factor deficiency. *Thromb Diath Haemorrh.* 1960;5:179-186.
218. Kohler HP, Ichinose A, Seitz R, et al. Diagnosis and classification of factor XIII deficiencies. *J Thromb Haemost.* 2011;9:1404-1406.
219. Dorgalaleh A, Rashidpanah J. Blood coagulation factor XIII and factor XIII deficiency. *Blood Rev.* 2016;30:461-475.
220. Takagi T, Doolittle RF. Amino acid sequence studies on factor XIII and the peptide released during its activation by thrombin. *Biochemistry.* 1974;13:750-756.
221. Kohler HP, Strickland MH, Ossei-Gerning N, Carter A, Mikkola H, Grant PJ. Association of a common polymorphism in the factor XIII gene with myocardial infarction. *Thromb Haemost.* 1998;79:8-13.
222. Webb GC, Coggan M, Ichinose A, Board PG. Localization of the coagulation factor XIII B subunit gene (F13B) to chromosome bands 1q31-32.1 and restriction fragment length polymorphism at the locus. *Hum Genet.* 1989;81:157-160.

223. Kitchens CS, Newcomb TF. Factor XIII. *Medicine (Baltimore)*. 1979;58:413-429.
224. Greenberg DL, Davie EW. Blood coagulation factors: their complementary DNAs, genes, and expression. In: Colman RW, Hirsh J, Marder VJ, et al, eds. *Hemostasis and Thrombosis: Basic Principles and Clinical Practice*. 4th ed. Lippincott Williams & Wilkins; 2001:21-57.
225. Britten AF. Congenital deficiency of factor XIII (fibrin-stabilizing factor): report of a case and review of the literature. *Am J Med*. 1967;43:751-761.
226. Duckert F. Documentation of the plasma factor XIII deficiency in man. *Ann N Y Acad Sci*. 1972;202:190-199.
227. Ikkala E. Transfusion therapy in congenital deficiencies of plasma factor XIII. *Ann N Y Acad Sci*. 1972;202:200-203.
228. Mitchell JL, Mutch NJ. Let's cross-link: diverse functions of the promiscuous cellular transglutaminase factor XIII-A. *J Thromb Haemost*. 2019;17:19-30.
229. Hsu P, Zantek ND, Meijer P, et al. Factor XIII Assays and associated problems for laboratory diagnosis of factor XIII deficiency: an analysis of International Proficiency testing results. *Semin Thromb Hemost*. 2014;40:232-238.
230. Lancellotti S, Basso M, De Cristofaro R. Congenital prothrombin deficiency: an update. *Semin Thromb Hemost*. 2013;39:596-606.
231. Shapiro SS, Martinez J, Holburn RR. Congenital dysprothrombinemia: an inherited structural disorder of human prothrombin. *J Clin Invest*. 1969;48:2251-2259.
232. Lefkowitz JB, Weller A, Nuss R, Santiago-Borrero PJ, Brown DL, Ortiz IR. A common mutation, Arg457→Gln, links prothrombin deficiencies in the Puerto Rican population. *J Thromb Haemost*. 2003;1:2381-2388.
233. Rabiet MJ, Furie BC, Furie B. Molecular defect of prothrombin Barcelona. Substitution of cysteine for arginine at residue 273. *J Biol Chem*. 1986;261:15045-15048.
234. Henriksen RA, Mann KG. Substitution of valine for glycine-558 in the congenital dysthrombin thrombin Quick II alters primary substrate specificity. *Biochemistry*. 1989;28:2078-2082.
235. Henriksen RA, Mann KG. Identification of the primary structural defect in the dysthrombin thrombin Quick I: substitution of cysteine for arginine-382. *Biochemistry*. 1988;27:9160-9165.
236. Shapiro SS, McCord S. Prothrombin. *Prog Hemost Thromb*. 1978;4:177-209.
237. Girolami A, Scarano L, Saggiorato G, Girolami B, Bertomoro A, Marchiori A. Congenital deficiencies and abnormalities of prothrombin. *Blood Coagul Fibrinolysis*. 1998;9:557-569.
238. Xue J, Wu Q, Westfield LA, et al. Incomplete embryonic lethality and fatal neonatal hemorrhage caused by prothrombin deficiency in mice. *Proc Natl Acad Sci U S A*. 1998;95:7603-7607.
239. Mullins ES, Kombrinck KW, Talmage KE, et al. Genetic elimination of prothrombin in adult mice is not compatible with survival and results in spontaneous hemorrhagic events in both heart and brain. *Blood*. 2009;113:696-704.
240. Owren PA. The coagulation of blood: investigations on a new clotting factor. *Acta Med Scand*. 1947;194:1-327.
241. Vos HL. An online database of mutations and polymorphisms in and around the coagulation factor V gene. *J Thromb Haemost*. 2007;5:185-188.
242. Duckers C, Simioni P, Rosing J, Castoldi E. Advances in understanding the bleeding diathesis in factor V deficiency. *Br J Haematol*. 2009;146:17-26.
243. Tabibian S, Shiravand Y, Shams M, et al. A comprehensive overview of coagulation factor V and congenital factor V deficiency. *Semin Thromb Haemost*. 2019;45:523-543.
244. Chiu HC, Whitaker E, Colman RW. Heterogeneity of human factor V deficiency: evidence for the existence of antigen-positive variants. *J Clin Invest*. 1983;72:493-503.
245. Steen M, Miteva M, Villoutreix BO, Yamazaki T, Dahlbäck B. Factor V New Brunswick: Ala221Val associated with FV deficiency reproduced in vitro and functionally characterized. *Blood*. 2003;102:1316-1322.
246. Zehnder JL, Hiraki DD, Jones CD, Gross N, Grumet FC. Familial coagulation factor V deficiency caused by a novel 4 base pair insertion in the factor V gene: factor V Stanford. *Thromb Haemost*. 1999;82:1097-1099.
247. Kling SJ, Griffee M, Flanders MM, Rodgers GM. Factor V deficiency caused by a novel missense mutation, Ile417Thr, in the A2 domain. *J Thromb Haemost*. 2006;4:481-483.
248. Tracy PB, Giles AR, Mann KG, Eide LL, Hoogendoorn H, Rivard GE. Factor V (Quebec): a bleeding diathesis associated with a qualitative platelet factor V deficiency. *J Clin Invest*. 1984;74:1221-1228.
249. Cui J, O'Shea KS, Purkayastha A, Saunders TL, Ginsburg D. Fatal haemorrhage and incomplete block to embryogenesis in mice lacking coagulation factor V. *Nature*. 1996;384:66-68.
250. Yang TL, Cui J, Taylor JM, Yang A, Gruber SB, Ginsburg D. Rescue of fatal neonatal hemorrhage in factor V deficient mice by low level transgene expression. *Thromb Haemost*. 2000;83:70-77.
251. Fischer RR, Giddings JC, Roisenberg I. Hereditary combined deficiency of clotting factors V and VIII with involvement of von Willebrand factor. *Clin Lab Haematol*. 1988;10:53-62.
252. de Moerloose P, Schved JF, Nugent D. Rare coagulation disorders: fibrinogen, factor VII and factor XIII. *Haemophilia*. 2016;22(suppl 5):61-65.
253. Fair DS. Quantitation of factor VII in the plasma of normal and warfarin-treated individuals by radioimmunoassay. *Blood*. 1983;62:784-791.
254. Morrissey JH, Macik BG, Neuenschwander PF, Comp PC. Quantitation of activated factor VII levels in plasma using a tissue factor mutant selectively deficient in promoting factor VII activation. *Blood*. 1993;81:734-744.
255. Edgington TS, Dickinson CD, Ruf W. The structural basis of function of the TF. VIIa complex in the cellular initiation of coagulation. *Thromb Haemost*. 1997;78:401-405.
256. Rosen ED, Chan JC, Idusogie E, et al. Mice lacking factor VII develop normally but suffer fatal perinatal bleeding. *Nature*. 1997;390:290-294.
257. Tamary H, Fromovich Y, Shalmon L, et al. Ala244Val is a common, probably ancient mutation causing factor VII deficiency in Moroccan and Iranian Jews. *Thromb Haemost*. 1996;76:283-291.
258. Marder VJ, Shulman NR. Clinical aspects of congenital factor VII deficiency. *Am J Med*. 1964;37:182-194.
259. Roberts HR, Escobar MA. Inherited disorders of prothrombin conversion. In: Colman RW, Marder VJ, Clowes AW, et al, eds. *Hemostasis and Thrombosis: Basic Principles and Clinical Practice*. Lippincott Williams & Wilkins; 2006:923-937
260. Triplett DA, Brandt JT, Batard MA, Dixon JL, Fair DS. Hereditary factor VII deficiency: heterogeneity defined by combined functional and immunochemical analysis. *Blood*. 1985;66:1284-1287.
261. Ragni MV, Lewis JH, Spero JA, Hasiba U. Factor VII deficiency. *Am J Hematol*. 1981;10:79-88.
262. Cohen LJ, McWilliams NB, Neuberg R, et al. Prophylaxis and therapy with factor VII concentrate (human) immuno, vapor heated in patients with congenital factor VII deficiency: a summary of case reports. *Am J Hematol*. 1995;50:269-276.
263. Perry DJ. Factor VII deficiency. *Br J Haematol*. 2002;118:689-700.
264. Girolami A, Tezza F, Scandellari R, Vettore S, Girolami B. Associated prothrombotic conditions are probably responsible for the occurrence of thrombosis in almost all patients with congenital FVII deficiency. Critical review of the literature. *J Thromb Thrombolysis*. 2010;30:172-178.
265. Pollak ES, Russell TT, Ptashkin B, Smith-Whitley K, Camire RM, Bauer KA. Asymptomatic factor VII deficiency in African Americans. *Am J Clin Pathol*. 2006;126:128-132.
266. Yorke AJ, Mant MJ. Factor VII deficiency and surgery: is preoperative replacement therapy necessary? *J Am Med Assoc*. 1977;238:424-425.
267. Giansily-Blaizot M, Schved JF. Potential predictors of bleeding risk in inherited factor VII deficiency. Clinical, biological and molecular criteria. *Thromb Haemost*. 2005;94:901-906.
268. Telfer TP, Denson KW, Wright DR. A "new" coagulation defect. *Br J Haematol*. 1956;2:308-316.
269. Hougie C, Barrow EM, Graham JB. Stuart clotting defect. I. Segregation of an hereditary hemorrhagic state from the heterogeneous group heretofore called stable factor (SPCA, proconvertin, factor VII) deficiency. *J Clin Invest*. 1957;36:485-496.
270. Menegatti M, Peyvandi F. Factor X deficiency. *Semin Thromb Hemost*. 2009;35:407-415.
271. Peyvandi F, Menegatti M, Santagostino E, et al. Gene mutations and three-dimensional structural analysis in 13 families with severe factor X deficiency. *Br J Haematol*. 2002;117:685-692.
272. Reddy SV, Zhou ZQ, Rao KJ, et al. Molecular characterization of human factor X san Antonio. *Blood*. 1989;74:1486-1490.
273. James HL, Girolami A, Fair DS. Molecular defect in coagulation factor XFriuli results from a substitution of serine for proline at position 343. *Blood*. 1991;77:317-323.
274. Dewerchin M, Liang Z, Moons L, et al. Blood coagulation factor X deficiency causes partial embryonic lethality and fatal neonatal bleeding in mice. *Thromb Haemost*. 2000;83:185-190.
275. Bertina RM, Alderkamp GJH, DeNooy E. A variant of factor X that is defective only in extrinsic coagulation. *Thromb Haemost*. 1981;46:88.
276. Parkin JD, Madaras F, Sweet B, Castaldi PA. A further inherited variant of coagulation factor X. *Aust N Z J Med*. 1974;4:561-564.
277. Greipp PR, Kyle RA, Bowie EJ. Factor-X deficiency in amyloidosis: a critical review. *Am J Hematol*. 1981;11:443-450.
278. Rosenthal RL, Dreskin OH, Rosenthal N. New hemophilia-like disease caused by deficiency of a third plasma thromboplastin factor. *Proc Soc Exp Biol Med*. 1953;82:171-174.
279. Rapaport SI, Proctor RR, Patch MJ, Yettra M. The mode of inheritance of PTA deficiency: evidence for the existence of major PTA deficiency and minor PTA deficiency. *Blood*. 1961;18:149-165.
280. Gomez K, Bolton-Maggs P. Factor XI deficiency. *Haemophilia*. 2008;14:1183-1189.
281. Seligsohn U, Modan M. Definition of the population at risk of bleeding due to factor XI deficiency in Ashkenazi Jews and the value of activated partial thromboplastin time in its detection. *Isr J Med Sci*. 1981;17:413-415.
282. Seligsohn U. High gene frequency of factor XI (PTA) deficiency in Ashkenazi Jews. *Blood*. 1978;51:1223-1228.
283. Asakai R, Chung DW, Ratnoff OD, Davie EW. Factor XI (plasma thromboplastin antecedent) deficiency in Ashkenazi Jews is a bleeding disorder that can result from three types of point mutations. *Proc Natl Acad Sci U S A*. 1989;86:7667-7671.
284. Asakai R, Chung DW, Davie EW, Seligsohn U. Factor XI deficiency in Ashkenazi Jews in Israel. *N Engl J Med*. 1991;325:153-158.
285. Kravtsov DV, Monahan PE, Gailani D. A classification system for cross-reactive material-negative factor XI deficiency. *Blood*. 2005;105:4671-4673.
286. Kravtsov DV, Wu W, Meijers JC, et al. Dominant factor XI deficiency caused by mutations in the factor XI catalytic domain. *Blood*. 2004;104:128-134.
287. Bolton-Maggs PH. Factor XI deficiency and its management. *Haemophilia*. 2000;6(suppl 1):100-109.
288. Duga S, Salomon O. Congenital factor XI deficiency: an update. *Semin Thromb Hemost*. 2013;39:621-631.
289. Seligsohn U. Factor XI deficiency. *Thromb Haemost*. 1993;70:68-71.
290. Rosenthal RL, Dreskin OH, Rosenthal N. Plasma thromboplastin antecedent (PTA) deficiency: clinical, coagulation, therapeutic and hereditary aspects of a new hemophilia-like disease. *Blood*. 1955;10:120-131.
291. Kitchens CS, Alexander JA. Partial deficiency of coagulation factor XI as a newly recognized feature of Noonan syndrome. *J Pediatr*. 1983;102:224-227.
292. Berrebi A, Malnick SD, Vorst EJ, Stein D. High incidence of factor XI deficiency in Gaucher's disease. *Am J Hematol*. 1992;40:153.

293. Edson JR, White JG, Krivit W. The enigma of severe factor XI deficiency without hemorrhagic symptoms. Distinction from Hageman factor and "Fletcher factor" deficiency; family study; and problems of diagnosis. *Thromb Diath Haemorrh.* 1967;18:342-348.
294. Bolton-Maggs PH, Patterson DA, Wensley RT, Tuddenham EG. Definition of the bleeding tendency in factor XI-deficient kindreds: a clinical and laboratory study. *Thromb Haemost.* 1995;73:194-202.
295. Kadir RA, Economides DL, Lee CA. Factor XI deficiency in women. *Am J Hematol.* 1999;60:48-54.
296. De Vries SI, Braat-van Straaten MA. Haemorrhagic diathesis as the result of severe deficiency of plasma thromboplastin antecedent (PTA, factor XI). *Thromb Diath Haemorrh.* 1964;11:167-186.
297. Soff GA, Levin J, Bell WR. Familial multiple coagulation factor deficiencies. II. Combined factor VIII, IX, and XI deficiency and combined factor IX and XI deficiency: two previously uncharacterized familial multiple factor deficiency syndromes. *Semin Thromb Hemost.* 1981;7:149-169.
298. Wheeler AP, Hemingway C, Gailani D. The clinical management of factor XI deficiency in pregnant women. *Expert Rev Hematol.* 2020;13:719-729.
299. Ratnoff OD, Colopy JE. A familial hemorrhagic trait associated with a deficiency of a clot-promoting fraction of plasma. *J Clin Invest.* 1955;34:602-613.
300. Ratnoff OD, Rosenblum JM. Role of Hageman factor in the initiation of clotting by glass; evidence that glass frees Hageman factor from inhibition. *Am J Med.* 1958;25:160-168.
301. Halbmayer WM, Haushofer A, Schon R, et al. The prevalence of moderate and severe FXII (Hageman factor) deficiency among the normal population: evaluation of the incidence of FXII deficiency among 300 healthy blood donors. *Thromb Haemost.* 1994;71:68-72.
302. Saito H, Scott JG, Movat HZ, Scialla SJ. Molecular heterogeneity of Hageman trait (factor XII deficiency): evidence that two of 49 subjects are cross-reacting material positive (CRM+). *J Lab Clin Med.* 1979;94:256-265.
303. Schloesser M, Zeerleder S, Lutze G, et al. Mutations in the human factor XII gene. *Blood.* 1997;90:3967-3977.
304. Wachtfogel YT, De La Cadena RA, Colman RW. Structural biology, cellular interactions and pathophysiology of the contact system. *Thromb Res.* 1993;72:1-21.
305. Glueck HI, Roehill W Jr. Myocardial infarction in a patient with a Hageman (factor XII) defect. *Ann Intern Med.* 1966;64:390-396.
306. Ratnoff OD, Busse RJ, Sheon RP. The demise of John hageman. *N Engl J Med.* 1968;279:760-761.
307. Lodi S, Isa L, Pollini E, Bravo AF, Scalvini A. Defective intrinsic fibrinolytic activity in a patient with severe factor XII-deficiency and myocardial infarction. *Scand J Haematol.* 1984;33:80-82.
308. Koster T, Rosendaal FR, Briet E, Vandenbroucke JP. John Hageman's factor and deep-vein thrombosis: Leiden thrombophilia study. *Br J Haematol.* 1994;87:422-424.
309. Zeerleder S, Schloesser M, Redondo M, et al. Reevaluation of the incidence of thromboembolic complications in congenital factor XII deficiency: a study on 73 subjects from 14 Swiss families. *Thromb Haemost.* 1999;82:1240-1246.
310. Girolami A, Randi ML, Gavasso S, Lombardi AM, Spiezia F. The occasional venous thromboses seen in patients with severe (homozygous) FXII deficiency are probably due to associated risk factors: a study of prevalence in 21 patients and review of the literature. *J Thromb Thrombolysis.* 2004;17:139-143.
311. Schmaier AH, Stavrou EX. Factor XII- What's important but not commonly thought about. *Res Pract Thromb Haemost.* 2019;3:599-606.
312. Renne T, Pozgajova M, Gruner S, et al. Defective thrombus formation in mice lacking coagulation factor XII. *J Exp Med.* 2005;202:271-281.
313. Kleinschnitz C, Stoll G, Bendszus M, et al. Targeting coagulation factor XII provides protection from pathological thrombosis in cerebral ischemia without interfering with hemostasis. *J Exp Med.* 2006;203:513-518.
314. Cheng Q, Tucker EI, Pine MS, et al. A role for factor XIIa-mediated factor XI activation in thrombus formation in vivo. *Blood.* 2010;116:3981-3989.
315. Schmaier AH. Antithrombotic potential of the contact activation pathway. *Curr Opin Hematol.* 2016;23:445-452.
316. Hathaway WE, Belhasen LP, Hathaway HS. Evidence for a new plasma thromboplastin factor. I. Case report, coagulation studies and physiochemical properties. *Blood.* 1965;26:521-532.
317. Wuepper KD. Prekallikrein deficiency in man. *J Exp Med.* 1973;138:1345-1355.
318. Barco S, Sollfrank S, Trinchero A, et al. Severe plasma prekallikrein deficiency: clinical characteristics, novel KLKB1 mutations, and estimated prevalence. *J Thromb Haemost.* 2020;18:1598-1617.
319. Weiss AS, Gallin JI, Kaplan AP. Fletcher factor deficiency: a diminished rate of Hageman factor activation caused by absence of prekallikrein with abnormalities of coagulation, fibrinolysis, chemotactic activity, and kinin generation. *J Clin Invest.* 1974;53:622-633.
320. Asmis LM, Sulzer I, Furlan M, Lammle B. Prekallikrein deficiency. The characteristic normalization of the severely prolonged aPTT following increased preincubation time is due to autoactivation of factor XII. *Thromb Res.* 2002;105:463-470.
321. Saito H, Ratnoff OD, Waldman R, Abraham JP. Fitzgerald trait. *J Clin Invest.* 1975;55:1082-1089.
322. Colman RW, Bagdasarian A, Talamo RC, et al. Williams trait. Human kininogen deficiency with diminished levels of plasminogen proactivator and prekallikrein associated with abnormalities of the Hageman factor-dependent pathways. *J Clin Invest.* 1975;56:1650-1662.
323. Oh-Ishi S, Ueno A, Uchida Y, et al. Abnormalities in the contact activation through factor-XII in Fujiwara trait: a deficiency in both high and low-molecular-weight kininogens with low-level of prekallikrein. *Tohoku J Exp Med.* 1981;133:67-80.
324. Donaldson VH, Kleniewski J, Saito H, Sayed JK. Prekallikrein deficiency in a kindred with kininogen deficiency and Fitzgerald trait clotting defect: evidence that high-molecular-weight kininogen and prekallikrein exist as a complex in normal human plasma. *J Clin Invest.* 1977;60:571-583.
325. Hayashi H, Ishimaru F, Fujita T, Tsurumi N, Tsuda T, Kimura I. Molecular genetic survey of five Japanese families with high-molecular-weight kininogen deficiency. *Blood.* 1990;75:1296-1304.
326. Cheung PP, Kunapuhi SP, Scott CF, Wachtfogel YT, Colman RW. Genetic basis of total kininogen deficiency in Williams' trait. *J Biol Chem.* 1993;268:23361-23365.
327. Krijanovski Y, Proulle V, Mahdi F, Dreyfus M, Müller-Esterl W, Schmaier AH. Characterization of molecular defects of Fitzgerald trait and another novel high-molecular-weight kininogen-deficient patient: insights into structural requirements for kininogen expression. *Blood.* 2003;101:4430-4436.
328. Zhang B, Ginsburg D. Familial multiple coagulation factor deficiencies: new biologic insight from rare genetic bleeding disorders. *J Thromb Haemost.* 2004;2:1564-1572.
329. Peyvandi F, Tuddenham EG, Akhtari AM, Lak M, Mannucci PM. Bleeding symptoms in 27 Iranian patients with the combined deficiency of factor V and factor VIII. *Br J Haematol.* 1998;100:773-776.
330. Seligsohn U, Zivelin A, Zwang E. Combined factor V and factor VIII deficiency among non-Ashkenazi Jews. *N Engl J Med.* 1982;307:1191-1195.
331. Nichols WC, Seligsohn U, Zivelin A, et al. Mutations in the ER-Golgi intermediate compartment protein ERGIC-53 cause combined deficiency of coagulation factors V and VIII. *Cell.* 1998;93:61-70.
332. Zhang B, McGee B, Yamaoka JS, et al. Combined deficiency of factor V and factor VIII is due to mutations in either *LMAN1* or *MCFD2*. *Blood.* 2006;107:1903-1907.
333. Mohanty D, Ghosh K, Shetty S, Spreafico M, Garagiola I, Peyvandi F. Mutations in the *MCFD2* gene and a novel mutation in the *LMAN1* gene in Indian families with combined deficiency of factor V and VIII. *Am J Hematol.* 2005;79:262-266.
334. Zheng C, Liu HH, Yuan S, Zhou J, Zhang B. Molecular basis of LMAN1 in coordinating LMAN1-MCFD2 cargo receptor formation and ER-to-Golgi transport of FV/FVIII. *Blood.* 2010;116:5698-5706.
335. Zheng C, Zhang B. Combined deficiency of coagulation factors V and VIII: an update. *Semin Thromb Hemost.* 2013;39:613-620.
336. Napolitano M, Mariani G, Lapecorella M. Hereditary combined deficiency of the vitamin K-dependent clotting factors. *Orphanet J Rare Dis.* 2010;5:21.
337. Goldsmith GH Jr, Pence RE, Ratnoff OD, Adelstein DJ, Furie B. Studies on a family with combined functional deficiencies of vitamin K-dependent coagulation factors. *J Clin Invest.* 1982;69:1253-1260.
338. Brenner B, Sanchez-Vega B, Wu SM, Lanir N, Stafford DW, Solera J. A missense mutation in γ-glutamyl carboxylase gene causes combined deficiency of all vitamin K-dependent blood coagulation factors. *Blood.* 1998;92:4554-4559.
339. Spronk HM, Farah RA, Buchanan GR, Vermeer C, Soute BA. Novel mutation in the γ-glutamyl carboxylase gene resulting in congenital combined deficiency of all vitamin K-dependent blood coagulation factors. *Blood.* 2000;96:3650-3652.
340. Darghouth D, Hallgren KW, Shtofman RL, et al. Compound heterozygosity of novel missense mutations in the gamma-glutamyl-carboxylase gene causes hereditary combined vitamin K-dependent coagulation factor deficiency. *Blood.* 2006;108:1925-1931.
341. Rost S, Fregin A, Ivaskevicius V, et al. Mutations in *VKORC1* cause warfarin resistance and multiple coagulation factor deficiency type 2. *Nature.* 2004;427:537-541.
342. Aoki N, Saito H, Kamiya T, Koie K, Sakata Y, Kobakura M. Congenital deficiency of α_2-plasmin inhibitor associated with severe hemorrhagic tendency. *J Clin Invest.* 1979;63:877-884.
343. Aoki N, Sakata Y, Matsuda M, Tateno K. Fibrinolytic states in a patient with congenital deficiency of α_2-plasmin inhibitor. *Blood.* 1980;55:483-488.
344. Collen D. α_2-Antiplasmin inhibitor deficiency. *Lancet.* 1979;1:1039-1040.
345. Favier R, Aoki N, de Moerloose P. Congenital $\alpha_2$2-plasmin inhibitor deficiencies: a review. *Br J Haematol.* 2001;114:4-10.
346. Maino A, Garagiola I, Artoni A, Al-Humood S, Peyvandi F. A novel mutation of alpha2-plasmin inhibitor gene causes an inherited deficiency and a bleeding tendency. *Haemophilia.* 2008;14:166.
347. Abdul S, Leebeek FW, Rijken DC, Uitte de Willige S. Natural heterogeneity of α2-antiplasmin: functional and clinical consequences. *Blood.* 2016;127:538-545.
348. Mehic D, Pabinger I, Ay C, Gebhart J. Fibrinolysis and bleeding of unknown cause. *Res Pract Thromb Haemost.* 2021;5:e12511.
349. Saes JL, Schols SEM, Van Heerde WL, Nijziel MR. Hemorrhagic disorders of fibrinolysis: a clinical review. *J Thromb Haemost.* 2018;16:1498-1509.
350. Lee MH, Vosburgh E, Anderson K, McDonagh J. Deficiency of plasma plasminogen activator inhibitor 1 results in hyperfibrinolytic bleeding. *Blood.* 1993;81:2357-2362.
351. Fay WP, Parker AC, Condrey LR, Shapiro AD. Human plasminogen activator inhibitor-1 (PAI-1) deficiency: characterization of a large kindred with a null mutation in the PAI-1 gene. *Blood.* 1997;90:204-208.
352. Iwaki T, Tanaka A, Miyawaki Y, et al. Life-threatening hemorrhage and prolonged wound healing are remarkable phenotypes manifested by complete plasminogen activator inhibitor-1 deficiency in humans. *J Thromb Haemost.* 2011;9:1200-1206.
353. Horrevoets AJ. Plasminogen activator inhibitor 1 (PAI-1): in vitro activities and clinical relevance. *Br J Haematol.* 2004;125:12-23.
354. Owen MC, Brennan SO, Lewis JH, Carrell RW. Mutation of antitrypsin to antithrombin: α-1-antitrypsin Pittsburgh (358 Met leads to Arg), a fatal bleeding disorder. *N Engl J Med.* 1983;309:694-698.
355. Scott CF, Carrell RW, Glaser CB, Kueppers F, Lewis JH, Colman RW. Alpha-1-antitrypsin Pittsburgh: a potent inhibitor of human plasma factor XI_a, kallikrein, and factor XII_f. *J Clin Invest.* 1986;77:631-634.
356. Henneuse A, Suchon P, Chambost H, Morange PE, Frere C, Alessi MC. α_1-Antitrypsin Pittsburgh and plasmin-mediated proteolysis. *J Thromb Haemost.* 2016;14:2023-2026.

357. Schulman S, El-Darzi E, Florido MH, et al. A coagulation defect arising from heterozygous premature termination of tissue factor. *J Clin Invest.* 2020;130:5302-5312.
358. Alperin JB. Estrogens and surgery in women with von Willebrand's disease. *Am J Med.* 1982;73:367-371.
359. Green D, Smith NJ. Hemophilia. Current concepts in management. *Med Clin North Am.* 1972;56:105-117.
360. Shima M, Hanabusa H, Taki M, et al. Factor VIII-mimetic function of humanized bispecific antibody in hemophilia A. *N Engl J Med.* 2016;374:2044-2053.
361. Sehgal A, Barros S, Ivanciu L, et al. An RNAi therapeutic targeting antithrombin to rebalance the coagulation system and promote hemostasis in hemophilia. *Nat Med.* 2015;21:492-497.
362. Batty P, Lillicrap D. Hemophilia gene therapy: Approaching the first licensed product. *Hemasphere.* 2021;5(3):e540.
363. Fogarty PF, Kouides P. How we manage prostate biopsy and prostate cancer therapy in men with haemophilia. *Haemophilia.* 2012;18:e88-e90.
364. Ljung RC, Knobe K. How to manage invasive procedures in children with haemophilia. *Br J Haematol.* 2012;157:519-528.
365. Aryal KR, Wiseman D, Siriwardena AK, Bolton-Maggs PH, Hay CR, Hill J. General surgery in patients with a bleeding diathesis: how we do it. *World J Surg.* 2011;35:2603-2610.
366. Abildgaard CF, Cornet JA, Fort E, Schulman I. The in vivo longevity of antihaemophilic factor (factor VIII). *Br J Haematol.* 1964;10:225-237.
367. Smith KJ, Thompson AR. Labeled factor IX kinetics in patients with hemophilia-B. *Blood.* 1981;58:625-629.
368. Peyvandi F, Garragiola I, Biguzzi E. Advances in the treatment of bleeding disorders. *J Thromb Haemost.* 2016;14:2095-2106.
369. Santagostino E, Negrier C, Klamroth R, et al. Safety and pharmacokinetics of a novel recombinant fusion protein linking coagulation factor IX with albumin (rIX-FP) in hemophilia B patients. *Blood.* 2012;120(12):2405-2411.
370. Soucie JM, Nuss R, Evatt B, et al. Mortality among males with hemophilia: relations with source of medical care. The Hemophilia Surveillance System Project Investigators. *Blood.* 2000;96:437-442.
371. Perkins HA. Plasmapheresis of the patient as a method for achieving effective levels of plasma coagulation factors using fresh frozen plasma. *Transfusion.* 1966;6:293-301.
372. Keller MK, Krebs M, Spies C, et al. Clotting factor activity in thawed OctaplasLG during storage at 2-6 degree C for 6 days from a quality assurance point of view. *Transfu Apher Sci.* 2012;46:129-136.
373. Leebeek FW, Schipperus MR, van Vliet HH. Coagulation factor levels in solvent/detergent-treated plasma. *Transfusion.* 1999;39:1150-1151.
374. O'Shaughnessy DF, Atterbury C, Bolton-Maggs P, et al. Guidelines for the use of fresh-frozen plasma, cryoprecipitate and cryosupernatant. *Br J Haematol.* 2004;126:11-28.
375. Pool JG, Shannon AE. Production of high-potency concentrates of antihemophilic globulin in a closed-bag system. *N Engl J Med.* 1965;273:1443-1447.
376. Brettler DB, Levine PH. Factor concentrates for treatment of hemophilia: which one to choose? *Blood.* 1989;73:2067-2073.
377. Laffan M. New products for the treatment of haemophilia. *Br J Haematol.* 2016;172:23-31.
378. Ragni MV, Koch WC, Jordan JA. Parvovirus B19 infection in patients with hemophilia. *Transfusion.* 1996;36:238-241.
379. Gaboulaud V, Parquet A, Tahiri C, et al. Prevalence of IgG antibodies to human parvovirus B19 in haemophilia children treated with recombinant factor (F) VIII only or with at least one plasma-derived FVIII or FIX concentrate: results from the French haemophilia cohort. *Br J Haematol.* 2002;116:383-389.
380. White GC II, Roberts HR, Kingdon HS, Lundblad RL. Prothrombin complex concentrates: potentially thrombogenic materials and clues to the mechanism of thrombosis in vivo. *Blood.* 1977;49:159-170.
381. Hultin MB. Activated clotting factors in factor IX concentrates. *Blood.* 1979;54:1028-1038.
382. Giles AR, Nesheim ME, Hoogendoorn H, Tracy PB, Mann KG. The coagulant-active phospholipid content is a major determinant of in vivo thrombogenicity of prothrombin complex (factor IX) concentrates in rabbits. *Blood.* 1982;59:401-407.
383. Campbell EW, Neff S, Bowdler AJ. Therapy with factor IX concentrate resulting in DIC and thromboembolic phenomena. *Transfusion.* 1979;18:94-97.
384. Blatt PM, Lundblad RL, Kingdon HS, McLean G, Roberts HR. Thrombogenic materials in prothrombin complex concentrates. *Ann Intern Med.* 1974;81:766-770.
385. Shapiro AD, Ragni MV, Lusher JM, et al. Safety and efficacy of monoclonal antibody purified factor IX concentrate in previously untreated patients with hemophilia B. *Thromb Haemost.* 1996;75:30-35.
386. Mannucci PM, Bauer KA, Gringeri A, et al. Thrombin generation is not increased in the blood of hemophilia B patients after the infusion of a purified factor IX concentrate. *Blood.* 1990;76:2540-2545.
387. Lusher JM, Shapiro SS, Palascak JE, Rao AV, Levine PH, Blatt PM. Efficacy of prothrombin-complex concentrates in hemophiliacs with antibodies to factor VIII: a multicenter therapeutic trial. *N Engl J Med.* 1980;303:421-425.
388. Teitel J, Berntorp E, Dolan G, et al. A consensus statement on clinical trials of bypassing agent prophylaxis in inhibitor patients. *Haemophilia.* 2011;17:516-521.
389. Rodgers GM. Prothrombin complex concentrates in emergency bleeding disorders. *Am J Hematol.* 2012;87:898-902.
390. Glazer S, Hedner U, Falch JF. Clinical update on the use of recombinant factor VII. *Adv Exp Med Biol.* 1995;386:163-174.
391. Tomeo F, Mariz S, Brunetta AL, et al. Haemophilia, state of the art and new therapeutic opportunities, a regulatory perspective. *Br J Clin Pharmacol.* 2021;87(11):4183-4196.
392. Mancuso ME, Mahlangu JN, Pipe SW. The changing treatment landscape in hemophilia: from standard half-life clotting factor concentrates to gene editing. *Lancet.* 2021;397(10274):630-640.
393. Oldenburg J, Mahlangu JN, Kim B, et al. Emicizumab prophylaxis in hemophilia A with inhibitors. *N Engl J Med.* 2017;377:809-818.
394. Mahlangu JN. Progress in the development of anti-tissue factor pathway inhibitors for haemophilia management. *Front Med (Lausanne).* 2021;8:670526.
395. Cash JD, Gader AM, da Costa J. Proceedings: the release of plasminogen activator and factor VIII to lysine vasopressin, arginine vasopressin, I-desamino-8-d-arginine vasopressin, angiotensin and oxytocin in man. *Br J Haematol.* 1974;27:363-364.
396. Theiss W, Schmidt G. DDAVP in von Willebrand's disease: repeated administration and the behaviour of the bleeding time. *Thromb Res.* 1978;13:1119-1123.
397. Mannucci PM. Desmopressin (DDAVP) in the treatment of bleeding disorders: the first 20 years. *Blood.* 1997;90:2515-2521.
398. Warrier AI, Lusher JM. DDAVP: a useful alternative to blood components in moderate hemophilia A and von Willebrand disease. *J Pediatr.* 1983;102:228-233.
399. de la Fuente B, Kasper CK, Rickles FR, Hoyer LW. Response of patients with mild and moderate hemophilia A and von Willebrand's disease to treatment with desmopressin. *Ann Intern Med.* 1985;103:6-14.
400. Revel-Vilk S, Blanchette VS, Sparling C, Stain AM, Carcao MD. DDAVP challenge tests in boys with mild/moderate haemophilia A. *Br J Haematol.* 2002;117:947-951.
401. Ruggeri ZM, Mannucci PM, Lombardi R, Federici AB, Zimmerman TS. Multimeric composition of factor VIII/von Willebrand factor following administration of DDAVP: implications for pathophysiology and therapy of von Willebrand's disease subtypes. *Blood.* 1982;59:1272-1278.
402. Kobrinsky NL, Israels ED, Gerrard JM, et al. Shortening of bleeding time by 1-deamino-8-D-arginine vasopressin in various bleeding disorders. *Lancet.* 1984;1:1145-1148.
403. Dunn AL, Powers JR, Ribeiro MJ, Rickles FR, Abshire TC. Adverse events during use of intranasal desmopressin acetate for haemophilia A and von Willebrand disease: a case report and review of 40 patients. *Haemophilia.* 2000;6:11-14.
404. Mannucci PM. Desmopressin: a nontransfusional form of treatment for congenital and acquired bleeding disorders. *Blood.* 1988;72:1449-1455.
405. Bond L, Bevan D. Myocardial infarction in a patient with hemophilia treated with DDAVP. *N Engl J Med.* 1988;318:121.
406. Sutor AH. DDAVP is not a panacea for children with bleeding disorders. *Br J Haematol.* 2000;108:217-227.
407. Mannucci PM. Hemostatic drugs. *N Engl J Med.* 1998;339:245-253.
408. Kasper CK, Dietrich SL. Comprehensive management of haemophilia. *Clin Haematol.* 1985;14:489-512.
409. Evans BE, Aledort LM. Hemophilia and dental treatment. *J Am Dent Assoc.* 1978;96:827-834.
410. Stark SN, White JG, Lange RL Jr, Krivit W. Epsilon amino caproic acid therapy as a cause of intrarenal obstruction in haematuria of haemophiliacs. *Scand J Haematol.* 1965;2:99-107.
411. Kasper CK. Hereditary plasma clotting factor disorders and their management. *Haemophilia.* 2000;6(suppl 1):13-27.
412. Moorehead PC, Chan AKC, Lemyre B, et al. A practical guide to the management of the fetus and newborn with hemophilia. *Clin Appl Thromb Hemost.* 2018;24(9 suppl):29S-41S.
413. Köhler M, Hellstern P, Miyashita C, von Blohn G, Wenzel E. Comparative study of intranasal, subcutaneous and intravenous administration of desamino-D-arginine vasopressin (DDAVP). *Thromb Haemost.* 1986;55:108-111.
414. Ashenhurst JB, Langehannig PL, Seeler RA. Early treatment of bleeding episodes with 10 U/kg of factor VIII. *Blood.* 1977;50:181-182.
415. Bona RD, Weinstein RA, Weisman SJ, Bartolomeo A, Rickles FR. The use of continuous infusion of factor concentrates in the treatment of hemophilia. *Am J Hematol.* 1989;32:8-13.
416. Batorova A, Martinowitz U. Intermittent injections vs. continuous infusion of factor VIII in haemophilia patients undergoing major surgery. *Br J Haematol.* 2000;110:715-720.
417. Takedani H. Continuous infusion during total joint arthroplasty in Japanese haemophilia A patients: comparison study among two recombinants and one plasma-derived factor VIII. *Haemophilia.* 2010;16:740-746.
418. Hathaway WE, Christian MJ, Clarke SL, Hasiba U. Comparison of continuous and intermittent factor VIII concentrate therapy in hemophilia A. *Am J Hematol.* 1984;17:85-88.
419. Pabinger I, Mamonov V, Windyga J, et al. Results of a randomized phase III/IV trial comparing intermittent bolus versus continuous infusion of antihaemophilic factor (recombinant) in adults with severe or moderately severe haemophilia A undergoing major orthopaedic surgery. *Haemophilia.* 2021;27(3):e331-e339.
420. Lusher JM. Clinical guidelines for treating von Willebrand disease patients who are not candidates for DDAVP—a survey of European physicians. *Haemophilia.* 1998;4(suppl 3):11-14.
421. Fowler WE, Berkowitz LR, Roberts HR. DDAVP for type IIB von Willebrand disease. *Blood.* 1989;74:1859-1860.
422. Mazurier C, Gaucher C, Jorieux S, Goudemand M. Biological effect of desmopressin in eight patients with type 2N ("Normandy") von Willebrand disease. Collaborative Group. *Br J Haematol.* 1994;88:849-854.
423. Lillicrap D, Poon MC, Walker I, et al. Efficacy and safety of the factor VIII/von Willebrand factor concentrate, Haemate-P/Humate-P: ristocetin cofactor unit dosing in patients with von Willebrand disease. *Thromb Haemost.* 2002;87:224-230.
424. Mannucci PM, Chediak J, Hanna W, et al. Treatment of von Willebrand disease with a high-purity factor VIII/von Willebrand factor concentrate: a prospective, multicenter study. *Blood.* 2002;99:450-456.
425. Kessler CM, Friedman K, Schwartz BA, et al. The pharmacokinetic diversity of two von Willebrand factor (VWF)/factor VIII (FVIII) concentrates in subjects with congenital von Willebrand disease. Results from a prospective, randomised crossover study. *Thromb Haemost.* 2011;106:279-288.

426. Gill JC, Castaman G, Windyga J, et al. Hemostatic efficacy, safety, and pharmacokinetics of a recombinant von Willebrand factor in severe von Willebrand disease. *Blood.* 2015;126:2038-2046.
427. Thompson AR, Gill JC, Ewenstein BM, et al. Successful treatment for patients with von Willebrand disease undergoing urgent surgery using factor VIII/VWF concentrate (Humate-P). *Haemophilia.* 2004;10:42-51.
428. Leebeek FWG, Eikenboom JCJ. von Willebrand's disease. *N Engl J Med.* 2016;375:2067-2080.
429. Makris M, Colvin B, Gupta V, Shields ML, Smith MP. Venous thrombosis following the use of intermediate purity FVIII concentrate to treat patients with von Willebrand disease. *Thromb Haemost.* 2002;88:387-388.
430. Miller JL, Kupinski JM, Castella A, Ruggeri ZM. von Willebrand factor binds to platelets and induces aggregation in platelet-type but not type IIB von Willebrand disease. *J Clin Invest.* 1983;72:1532-1542.
431. Kouides PA. Current understanding of von Willebrand's disease in women—some answers, more questions. *Haemophilia.* 2006;12(suppl 3):143-151.
432. Conti M, Mari D, Conti E, Muggiasca ML, Mannucci PM. Pregnancy in women with different types of von Willebrand disease. *Obstet Gynecol.* 1986;68:282-285.
433. James AH, Konkle BA, Kouides P, et al. Postpartum von Willebrand factor levels in women with and without von Willebrand disease and implications for prophylaxis. *Haemophilia.* 2015;21:81-87.
434. James PD, Lillicrap D, Mannucci PM. Alloantibodies in von Willebrand disease. *Blood.* 2013;122:636-640.
435. Thorland EC, Drost JB, Lusher JM, et al. Anaphylactic response to factor IX replacement therapy in haemophilia B patients: complete gene deletions confer the highest risk. *Haemophilia.* 1999;5:101-105.
436. Jadhav M, Warrier I. Anaphylaxis in patients with hemophilia. *Semin Thromb Hemost.* 2000;26:205-208.
437. Clough AM, Gilreath JA, McPherson JP, et al. Design and implementation of a recombinant factor IX Fc fusion protein desensitization protocol. *J Thromb Haemost.* 2017;23:e227-e230.
438. George LA, Sullivan SK, Giermasz A, et al. Hemophilia B gene therapy with a high-specific-activity factor IX variant. *N Engl J Med.* 2017;377:2215-2227.
439. Pasi KJ, Rangarajan S, Mitchell N, et al. Multiyear follow-up of AAV5-hFVIII-SQ gene therapy for hemophilia A. *N Engl J Med.* 2020;382(1):29-40.
440. Livnat T, Shenkman B, Spectre G, et al. Recombinant factor VIIa treatment for asymptomatic factor VII deficient patients going through major surgery. *Blood Coagul Fibrinolysis.* 2012;23:379-387.
441. Benlakhal F, Mura T, Schved JF, et al. A retrospective analysis of 157 surgical procedures performed without replacement therapy in 83 unrelated factor VII-deficient patients. *J Thromb Haemost.* 2011;9:1149-1156.
442. Giansily-Blaizot M, Biron-Andreani C, Aguilar-Martinez P, et al. Inherited factor VII deficiency and surgery: clinical data are the best criteria to predict the risk of bleeding. *Br J Haematol.* 2002;117:172-175.
443. Mariani G, Konkle BA, Ingerslev J. Congenital factor VII deficiency: therapy with recombinant activated factor VII—a critical appraisal. *Haemophilia.* 2006;12:19-27.
444. Mariani G, Herrmann FH, Bernardi F, Schved JF, Auerswald G, Ingerslev J. Clinical manifestations, management, and molecular genetics in congenital factor VII deficiency: the International Registry on Congenital Factor VII Deficiency (IRF7). *Blood.* 2000;96:374.
445. Mariani G, Herrmann FH, Dolce A, et al. Clinical phenotypes and factor VII genotype in congenital factor VII deficiency. *Thromb Haemost.* 2005;93:481-487.
446. Mariani G, Dolce A, Batorova A, et al. Recombinant, activated factor VII for surgery in factor VII deficiency: a prospective evaluation—the surgical STER. *Br J Haematol.* 2011;152:340-346.
447. Mariani G, Dolce A, Napolitano M, et al. Invasive procedures and minor surgery in factor VII deficiency. *Haemophilia.* 2012;18:e63-e65.
448. Ingerslev J, Christiansen K, Sorensen B. Inhibitor to factor VII in severe factor VII deficiency: detection and course of the inhibitory response. *J Thromb Haemost.* 2005;3:799-800.
449. Wilde JT. Evidence for the use of activated prothrombin complex concentrates (aPCCs) in the treatment of patients with haemophilia and inhibitors. *Pathophysiol Haemost Thromb.* 2002;32(suppl 1):9-12.
450. Ichinose A. Factor XIII is a key molecule at the intersection of coagulation and fibrinolysis as well as inflammation and infection control. *Int J Hematol.* 2012;95:362-370.
451. Lovejoy AE, Reynolds TC, Visich JE, et al. Safety and pharmacokinetics of recombinant factor XIII-A2 administration in patients with congenital factor XIII deficiency. *Blood.* 2006;108:57-62.
452. Fujii N, Souri M, Ichinose A. A short half-life of the administered factor XIII (FXIII) concentrates after the first replacement therapy in a newborn with severe congenital FXIII deficiency. *Thromb Haemost.* 2012;107:592-594.
453. Gootenberg JE. Factor concentrates for the treatment of factor XIII deficiency. *Curr Opin Hematol.* 1998;5:372-375.
454. Inbal A, Oldenburg J, Carcao M, Rosholm A, Tehranchi R, Nugent D. Recombinant factor XIII: a safe and novel treatment for congenital factor XIII deficiency. *Blood.* 2012;119:5111-5117.
455. Greenberg LH, Schiffman S, Wong YS. Factor XIII deficiency. Treatment with monthly plasma infusions. *J Am Med Assoc.* 1969;209:264-265.
456. Rodeghiero F, Castaman GC, Di Bona E, Ruggeri M, Dini E. Successful pregnancy in a woman with congenital factor XIII deficiency treated with substitutive therapy. Report of a second case. *Blut.* 1987;55:45-48.
457. Menegatti M, Palla R, Boscarino M, et al. Minimal factor XIII activity level to prevent major spontaneous bleeds. *J Thromb Haemost.* 2017;15:1728-1736.
458. Meeks SL, Abshire TC. Abnormalities of prothrombin: a review of the pathophysiology, diagnosis, and treatment. *Haemophilia.* 2008;14:1159-1163.
459. Escobar MA, Auerswald G, Austin S, Huang JN, Norton M, Millar CM. Experience of a new high-purity factor X concentrate in subjects with hereditary factor X deficiency undergoing surgery. *Haemophilia.* 2016;22:713-720.
460. Cardigan R, Lawrie AS, Mackie IJ, Williamson LM. The quality of fresh-frozen plasma produced from whole blood stored at 4 degrees C overnight. *Transfusion.* 2005;45:1342-1348.
461. Gavva C, Yates SG, Rambally S, Sarode R. Transfusion management of factor V deficiency: three case reports and review of the literature. *Transfusion.* 2016;56:1745-1749.
462. Ingram GI, Mathews JA, Bennett AE. A controlled trial of joint aspiration in acute haemophilic haemarthrosis. *Br J Haematol.* 1972;23:649-654.
463. Querol F, Aznar JA, Haya S, Cid A. Orthoses in haemophilia. *Haemophilia.* 2002;8:407-412.
464. Rattray B, Nugent DJ, Young G. Celecoxib in the treatment of haemophilic synovitis, target joints, and pain in adults and children with haemophilia. *Haemophilia.* 2006;12:514-517.
465. Manco-Johnson MJ, Lundin B, Funk S, et al. Effect of late prophylaxis in hemophilia on joint bleeds: a randomized trial. *J Thromb Haemost.* 2017;15:2115-2124.
466. Valentino LA, Mamonov V, Hellmann A, et al. A randomized comparison of two prophylaxis regimens and a paired comparison of on-demand and prophylaxis treatments in hemophilia A management. *J Thromb Haemost.* 2012;10:359-367.
467. Rana NA, Shapiro GR, Green D. Long-term follow-up of prosthetic joint replacement in hemophilia. *Am J Hematol.* 1986;23:329-337.
468. Wang K, Street A, Dowrick A, Liew S. Clinical outcomes and patient satisfaction following total joint replacement in haemophilia—23-year experience in knees, hips and elbows. *Haemophilia.* 2012;18:86-93.
469. McCollough NC III, Enis JE, Lovitt J, Lian EC, Niemann KN, Loughlin EC Jr. Synovectomy or total replacement of the knee in hemophilia. *J Bone Joint Surg Am.* 1979;61:69-75.
470. Molho P, Verrier P, Stieltjes N, et al. A retrospective study on chemical and radioactive synovectomy in severe haemophilia patients with recurrent haemarthrosis. *Haemophilia.* 1999;5:115-123.
471. Dunn AL, Busch MT, Wyly JB, Abshire TC. Radionuclide synovectomy for hemophilic arthropathy: a comprehensive review of safety and efficacy and recommendation for a standardized treatment protocol. *Thromb Haemost.* 2002;87:383-393.
472. Dunn AL, Manco-Johnson M, Busch MT, Balark KL, Abshire TC. Leukemia and P32 radionuclide synovectomy for hemophilic arthropathy. *J Thromb Haemost.* 2005;3:1541-1542.
473. Lim MY, Cheng D, Aschman D, et al. Radionuclide synovectomy in patients with bleeding disorders: a review of malignancy and myeloproliferative neoplasms from the ATHNdataset. *Haemophilia.* 2017;23:e160-e162.
474. Hilgartner MW, Arnold WD. Hemophilic pseudotumor treated with replacement therapy and radiation. Report of a case. *J Bone Joint Surg Am.* 1975;57:1145-1146.
475. Rodriguez-Merchan EC. Haemophilic cysts (pseudotumours). *Haemophilia.* 2002;8:393-401.
476. Lim MY, Nielsen B, Ma A, Key NS. Clinical features and management of haemophilic pseudotumours: a single US centre experience over a 30-year period. *Haemophilia.* 2014;20(1):e58-e62.
477. Ljung RC. Intracranial haemorrhage in haemophilia A and B. *Br J Haematol.* 2008;140:378-384.
478. Zwagemaker AF, Gouw SC, Jansen JJ, et al. Incidence and mortality rates of intracranial hemorrhage in hemophilia: a systematic review and meta-analysis. *Blood.* 2021;138(26):2853-2873. doi:10.1182/blood.2021011849
479. Silverstein A. Intracranial bleeding in hemophilia. *Arch Neurol.* 1960;3:141-157.
480. Eyster ME, Gill FM, Blatt PM, Hilgartner MW, Ballard JO, Kinney TR. Central nervous system bleeding in hemophiliacs. *Blood.* 1978;51:1179-1188.
481. Andes WA, Wulff K, Smith WB. Head trauma in hemophilia. A prospective study. *Arch Intern Med.* 1984;144:1981-1983.
482. Curran JW, Lawrence DN, Jaffe H, et al. Acquired immunodeficiency syndrome (AIDS) associated with transfusions. *N Engl J Med.* 1984;310:69-75.
483. Chorba TL, Holman RC, Clarke MJ, Evatt BL. Effects of HIV infection on age and cause of death for persons with hemophilia A in the United States. *Am J Hematol.* 2001;66:229-240.
484. Goedert JJ, Eyster ME, Lederman MM, et al. End-stage liver disease in persons with hemophilia and transfusion-associated infections. *Blood.* 2002;100:1584-1589.
485. Lefrere JJ, Mariotti M, Thauvin M. B19 parvovirus DNA in solvent/detergent-treated anti-haemophilia concentrates. *Lancet.* 1994;343:211-212.
486. Mannucci PM, Gdovin S, Gringeri A, et al. Transmission of hepatitis A to patients with hemophilia by factor VIII concentrates treated with organic solvent and detergent to inactivate viruses. The Italian Collaborative Group. *Ann Intern Med.* 1994;120:1-7.
487. Giangrande PL. Hepatitis in haemophilia. *Br J Haematol.* 1998;103:1-9.
488. Cardone F, Simoneau S, Arzel A, et al. Comparison of nanofiltration efficacy in reducing infectivity of centrifuged versus ultracentrifuged 263K scrapie-infected brain homogenates in "spiked" albumin solutions. *Transfusion.* 2012;52:953-962.
489. Helske T, Ikkala E, Myllylä G, Nevanlinna HR, Rasi V. Joint involvement in patients with severe haemophilia A in 1957-59 and 1978-79. *Br J Haematol.* 1982;51:643-647.
490. Nilsson IM, Berntorp E, Löfqvist T, Pettersson H. Twenty-five years' experience of prophylactic treatment in severe haemophilia A and B. *J Intern Med.* 1992;232:25-32.
491. Löfqvist T, Nilsson IM, Berntorp E, Pettersson H. Haemophilia prophylaxis in young patients—a long-term follow-up. *J Intern Med.* 1997;241:395-400.
492. Bohn RL, Avorn J, Glynn RJ, Choodnovskiy I, Haschemeyer R, Aledort LM. Prophylactic use of factor VIII: an economic evaluation. *Thromb Haemost.* 1998;79:932-937.
493. Fischer K, van der Bom JG, Mauser-Bunschoten EP, et al. The effects of postponing prophylactic treatment on long-term outcome in patients with severe hemophilia. *Blood.* 2002;99:2337-2341.

Chapter 55 ■ Acquired Coagulation Disorders

GEORGE M. RODGERS • MING Y. LIM

INTRODUCTION

Acquired coagulopathies can complicate many medical disorders (*Table 55.1*). Unlike inherited bleeding disorders in which deficiency or abnormality of a single factor is characteristic, the acquired forms are usually associated with compound hemostatic defects that can cause multiple coagulation abnormalities, often complicated by thrombocytopenia, deficient platelet function, and abnormal inhibitors of coagulation. As a result, the severity of bleeding often correlates poorly with the results of laboratory tests in these patients, and replacement therapy may be ineffective. With some notable exceptions, however, bleeding is usually less severe than in the inherited forms, and the clinical picture is often complicated by signs and symptoms of the underlying disease.

DEFICIENCIES OF VITAMIN K–DEPENDENT FACTORS

Vitamin K is required for hepatic synthesis of prothrombin; factors VII, IX, and X; and proteins C and S (see Chapter 20 and *Figure 55.1*).[1] When vitamin K stores are deficient or abnormal, hypofunctional analogs of these factors are synthesized, which inhibit normal coagulation. These descarboxy analogs do not bind to cellular phospholipid surfaces or participate in cell-associated coagulation reactions.[2] This may occur in disorders in which intake or absorption of vitamin K is deficient and in disorders that impair the biosynthetic capacity of the liver (*Figure 55.1*). A similar coagulation abnormality may be produced by vitamin K antagonist anticoagulant drugs such as coumarin and indanediones, which antagonize the action of vitamin K (see Chapter 56).

Vitamin K Deficiency Bleeding in Infancy

Vitamin K deficiency bleeding (VKDB) in infancy, which was historically termed hemorrhagic disease of the newborn, was formerly a major cause of bleeding.[3] This disorder is now uncommon because of the routine administration of vitamin K at birth; however, it may be encountered in economically deprived populations or when vitamin K prophylaxis is refused.[4]

Pathophysiology

The normal newborn has a moderate deficiency of the vitamin K–dependent coagulation factors, which decrease further during the first 2 to 5 days of life, rise again when the infant is 7 to 14 days old, and attain normal adult levels by about 6 months (see also Table 46.6). This relative deficiency at birth and gradual increase toward adult levels presumably arises from intrinsic liver immaturity because neither of these physiologic phenomena is affected by vitamin K administration. Conversely, prophylactic vitamin K at birth prevents the nadir at age 2 to 5 days, and which may also reoccur thereafter, arising from transitory physiologic deficiency of this vitamin. Impairment of uptake of vitamin K from the intestine or of hepatic synthetic capacity predisposes to VKDB. This may occur in (1) prematurity (vitamin K–dependent factors at birth are approximately proportional to gestational age and birth weight); (2) placental transfer of maternal medications that impair vitamin K activity, including certain anticonvulsants and antibiotics; (3) inadequate dietary intake; (4) delayed gut colonization by bacteria; (5) various obstetric and perinatal complications; (6) possibly maternal deficiency of vitamin K; and (7) bowel or hepatobiliary disease, particularly cholestasis. The causes of deficient intake of vitamin K often overlap with delayed colonization of the gut by bacteria, including delayed feeding, breastfeeding, vomiting, severe diarrhea, and antibiotics, including those present in maternal milk. Human milk and colostrum are poor sources of vitamin K.[5]

Clinical Features and Laboratory Diagnosis

Bleeding in classic VKDB is severe, with melena, large cephalohematomas, and bleeding from the umbilical stump and after circumcision. Generalized ecchymoses (often without petechiae), intracranial bleeding, and large intramuscular hemorrhages may also develop.

VKDB may be classified as idiopathic (no cause other than breast-feeding) or secondary (malabsorption of vitamin K, liver disease, and drugs). VKDB can also be classified in terms of age of onset: early (onset < 24 hours of age), classic (onset usually between 3 and 5 days), and late (onset on or after 8 days). Early VKDB is uncommon and usually results from placental transfer of maternal drugs that antagonize vitamin K in the newborn. Late VKDB occurs almost exclusively in breast-fed infants, particularly those who may also have hepatobiliary disease.

Laboratory diagnosis is relatively simple (*Table 55.2*), provided coagulation test results are compared to age-matched expected physiologic reference ranges, potentially additionally modified for gestational age (see Table 46.6). In VKDB, the prothrombin time (PT) always is prolonged. The partial thromboplastin time (PTT) is also prolonged. Factors V and VIII, as well as fibrinogen, are normal. In

Table 55.1. Acquired Coagulation Disorders

Deficiencies of vitamin K–dependent coagulation factors
Vitamin K deficiency bleeding in infancy (hemorrhagic disease of the newborn)
Biliary obstruction (gallstone, strictures, fistulas)
Malabsorption of vitamin K (sprue, idiopathic steatorrhea, celiac disease, ulcerative colitis, regional enteritis, gastrocolic fistulas, *Ascaris* infestation)
Nutritional deficiency
Drugs
1. Pharmacologic antagonists of vitamin K (coumarins, indandiones, rodenticides) 2. Those that alter gut flora (broad-spectrum antibiotics, sulfonamides) 3. Miscellaneous (cholestyramine)
Liver disease (see *Table 55.3*)
Accelerated destruction of coagulation factors
Disseminated intravascular coagulation (see *Table 55.4*)
Fibrinolysis (liver disease, thrombolytic agents, tumors, after surgery)
Inhibitors of coagulation
Specific inhibitors (antibodies) (see *Table 55.6*)
Antiphospholipid-protein antibodies (see *Table 55.7*)
Miscellaneous (antithrombins, paraproteinemias)
Miscellaneous
After massive transfusion
After extracorporeal circulation
Drugs (antibiotics, antineoplastic agents, others)
Other disorders (polycythemia vera, congenital heart disease, amyloidosis, nephrotic syndrome, Sheehan syndrome, Gaucher disease, leukemia, others)

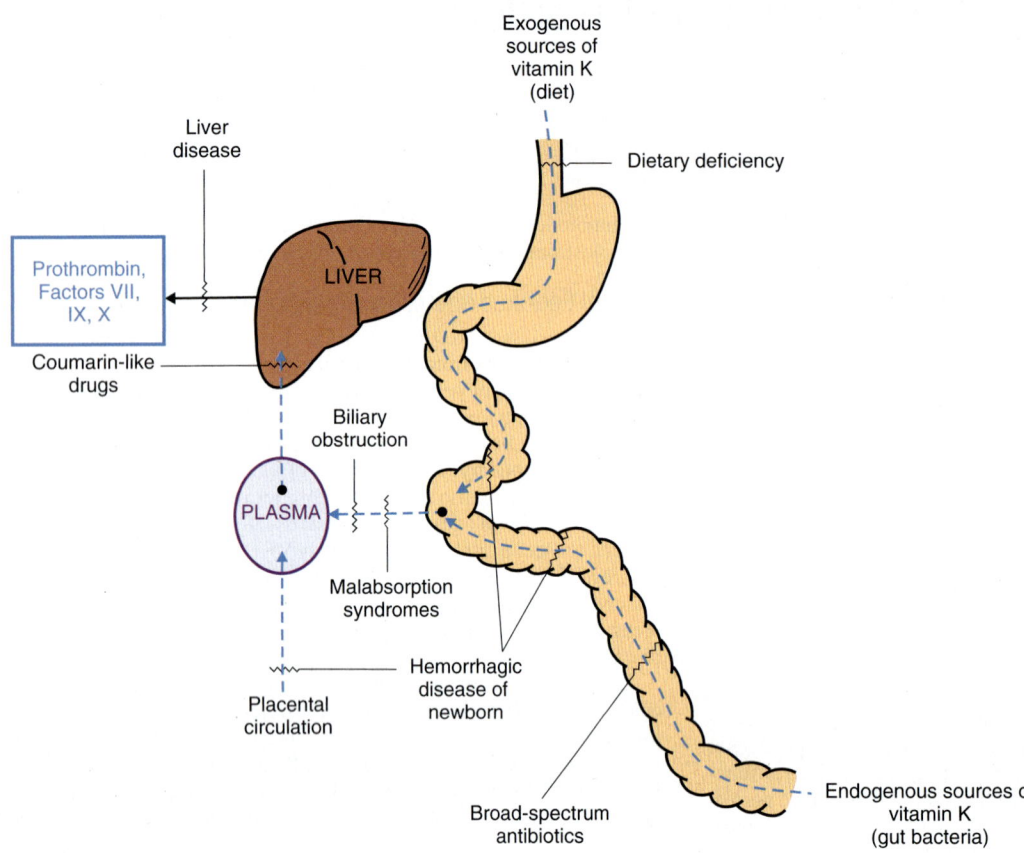

FIGURE 55.1 Etiologies of vitamin K deficiency. Sources of vitamin K include the diet and gut bacterial synthesis. Processes leading to vitamin K deficiency are indicated with a solid line ending in a squiggle.

clinical practice, the triad of a prolonged PT value, a normal fibrinogen level, and a normal platelet count defines the diagnosis, as well as a prompt response within hours to vitamin K. In specific settings, such as possible nonaccidental injury, confirmatory tests such as enzyme immunoassay of uncarboxylated prothrombin (protein induced by vitamin K absence or antagonism-II) may occasionally be appropriate. If performed, specific factor assays reveal functional deficiencies of prothrombin; factors VII, IX, and X; and proteins C and S in conjunction with normal antigenic levels of these vitamin K–dependent factors by immunoassay.

The clinician should not assume that bleeding in the neonate is invariably the result of vitamin K deficiency. The differential diagnosis includes virtually all causes of bleeding, particularly thrombocytopenia (see Chapter 47) and disseminated intravascular coagulation (DIC).[6] Inherited coagulation disorders (see Chapter 54) may produce serious hemorrhage in the neonatal period, but significant prolongation of the PT is not found in the most common forms, for example, hemophilia A and hemophilia B. Umbilical bleeding and hemorrhage after circumcision are relatively less common in the inherited coagulation disorders than in VKDB.

Treatment

Approaches to prophylaxis and treatment vary between different countries; the clinician should consult local guidelines.[7] An American Academy of Pediatrics consensus report summarized recommendations for vitamin K therapy for prevention of early and late VKDB.[8] Vitamin K_1 (0.5-1.0 mg given intramuscularly) is dramatically effective in the treatment of VKDB[9]; the 0.5-mg dose appears to be more than adequate.[10] The PT usually shortens within 6 hours, and levels of vitamin K–dependent factors seen in normal neonates are usually attained within 24 hours of administration. Larger (2 mg) or repeated (every 4-8 hours) doses of vitamin K_1 may be required to counteract the effects of coumarin drugs in infants. In premature infants, the response is often incomplete. The administration of large doses of vitamin K may produce hemolysis, hyperbilirubinemia, and even kernicterus in the neonate. These complications appear to be associated more commonly with the synthetic derivatives than with vitamin K_1, but even the latter may be dangerous in large doses.

In severe cases of VKDB, the transfusion of plasma may be helpful. Concentrates of vitamin K–dependent coagulation factors are effective but have led to thrombosis and intravascular coagulation in some infants, particularly in premature infants. This has been attributed to immaturity of hepatic clearance and to physiologic deficiency of antithrombin.

VKDB is primarily a disease of breast-fed infants[11]; accordingly, VKDB can be prevented by the administration of vitamin K to the mother before delivery. Most authorities, however, recommend administering vitamin K_1 to the infant. Further prophylactic administration of vitamin K_1 may be given to infants 1 to 5 months of age, especially those who are breast-fed or who have a disorder that may impair vitamin K absorption. The usual dosage in such older infants is 50 to 100 µg daily or 1 mg monthly.

Other Causes of Vitamin K Deficiency

Both intrahepatic and extrahepatic biliary tract obstruction commonly produce vitamin K deficiency because of the absence of bile salts in the gut. Complete obstruction may lead to severe coagulation abnormalities and bleeding within 2 to 4 weeks. Before the discovery of vitamin K, this was a major obstacle to surgical procedures on the biliary tract.

Most malabsorption syndromes and various other chronic gastrointestinal disorders may also give rise to vitamin K deficiency. Such disorders include celiac disease, sprue, gastrocolic fistulas, ulcerative colitis, regional enteritis, extensive gut resections, and protracted diarrhea of any cause, *Ascaris* infestations, and cystic fibrosis.[12] Nevertheless, because vitamin K is normally available from two

Table 55.2. Laboratory Findings in Acquired Coagulation Disorders

	Vitamin K Deficiency Bleeding in Infancy	Severe Liver Disease	Disseminated Intravascular Coagulation	Primary Fibrinolysis	Antibodies to Factor VIII	Inhibitors of Lupus Type
Screening Tests						
Platelet count[a]	N	vD	D	uN	N	V[a]
Prothrombin time[b]	I	I	I	vI	N	V[a]
Partial thromboplastin time[b]	I	I	V	vI	I	I
Thrombin time[b]	vI	uI	I	I	N	N
Erythrocyte morphology[a]	Macrocytes	Target cells and macrocytes	Schistocytes and microspherocytes	uN	uN[a]	uN[a]
Specific Assays						
Fibrinogen	N	vD	D	vD	N	N
Prothrombin[b]	D	D	V	uN	N	vD[c]
Factor V	N	uD	uD	vD	N	N[c]
Factor VII[b]	D	D	V	uN	N	N[c]
Factor VIIIc	N	uI	uD[c]	vD	D	N[c]
von Willebrand factor	N	uI	vI	V	N	N
Factor IX[b]	D	D	V[c]	uN	N	N[c]
Factor X[b]	D	D	vD	uN	N	N[c]
Factor XI[b]	vD	vD	uN	uN[c]	N	N[c]
Factor XIII[d]	uN	vD	uD	vD	N	N
Tests for Fibrinolysis and FDP						
FDP	uN	uI	I	I	N	N[e]
Plasminogen[b]	vD	vD	D	D	N	N
α₂-Antiplasmin	uN	vD	V	vD	N	N
Plasmin	N	vI	uI	uI	N	N
D-Dimer	uN	uN	I	uN	N	N[e]
Miscellaneous Tests						
Antithrombin	N	vD	vD	uN	N	N
Protein C	D	D	V	uN	N	uN
Protein S	D	D	V	uN	N	V

[a]May reveal effects of acute bleeding or abnormality characteristic of underlying disease.
[b]Results may differ from adult norms in normal neonates.
[c]One-stage assays may yield aberrant results.
[d]Hypofibrinogenemia may alter results.
[e]The presence of immunoglobulin M rheumatoid factors in certain patients may lead to a false-positive result in latex agglutination assays.
Abbreviations: D, decreased; FDP, fibrin(ogen) degradation products; I, increased; N, normal; u, usually; v, variably; V, variable.

independent sources (*Figure 55.1*), neither nutritional deficiency nor gut sterilization alone produces significant coagulation abnormalities.

In normal adults, the daily oral intake of vitamin K must be reduced to 20 μg or less for several weeks to produce significant hypoprothrombinemia. Nevertheless, vitamin K deficiency can occur in hospitalized patients with poor oral food intake, especially if they are also taking antibiotics.[13] Coagulation abnormalities can arise rapidly in such patients and may be confused with DIC or may present with serious, unexpected postoperative hemorrhage. Antimicrobial agents presumably impair vitamin K production by inhibiting the synthesis of menadiones by gut bacteria, but they may also directly affect carboxylation reactions.[14,15] Vitamin K deficiency may also result from cholestyramine,[16] which binds bile salts, or mineral oil and other cathartics when used for protracted periods. Vitamin E may antagonize the metabolic action of vitamin K and potentiate the action of coumarins. When taken in large doses, this vitamin may prolong the PT.[17] Antibiotic therapy, poor diet, or any of the aforementioned disorders may predispose patients to coumarin toxicity (see Chapter 56).[18] Large doses of aspirin, as given to treat rheumatoid disorders or in amounts associated with overdosage of the drug, may also induce vitamin K deficiency.[19]

Treatment

In adults, the parenteral administration of 10 mg of vitamin K_1 abolishes coagulation abnormalities within 12 to 24 hours if they are the consequence of a deficiency of this vitamin. Failure of vitamin K to normalize the PT is evidence for the presence of a complicating process, such as liver disease or DIC, or super-warfarin ingestion.[20] The synthetic vitamin K_3 (menadiones) may be absorbed in the absence of bile salts and in various malabsorption syndromes. However, these congeners of vitamin K have a more transient effect than the natural forms of this vitamin and offer minimal therapeutic advantage in the usual case. Replacement therapy with fresh-frozen plasma or prothrombin complex concentrates (PCCs) is effective in the treatment of emergent vitamin K deficiency.[21]

Intravenous (IV) administration of vitamin K may produce hemolytic anemia in patients with inherited deficiencies of various red cell enzymes and may be associated with a risk of anaphylaxis.[22]

Table 55.3. Abnormalities of Hemostasis and Coagulation in Liver Disease

Deficient biosynthesis
Of fibrinogen; prothrombin; coagulation factors V,[25] VII, IX, X, XI, XII, and XIII; prekallikrein; high–molecular-weight kininogen
Of antiplasmins, antithrombin, proteins C and S
Aberrant biosynthesis
Of abnormal fibrinogen,[26,27] factor V
Of abnormal inhibitory analogs of prothrombin, factors VII, IX, and X
Deficient clearance
Of hemostatic "products" (e.g., fibrin monomers, fibrin[ogen] degradation products, platelet factor-3)
Of activated coagulation factors (IXa, Xa, XIa)
Of plasminogen activators
Accelerated destruction of coagulation factors
Disseminated intravascular coagulation[28-30]
Abnormal fibrinolysis[31]
Thrombocytopenia
Hypersplenism (portal hypertension)
Folic acid deficiency
Chronic ethanol intoxication
Disseminated intravascular coagulation
Platelet dysfunction
Acute and chronic ethanol intoxication
Effects of products of fibrinogen degradation[32]
Uremia
Miscellaneous
Inhibition of coagulation by products of fibrinogen degradation[33]
Loss or consumption of coagulation factors in ascitic fluid[34]

Malnourished patients receiving broad-spectrum antibiotic therapy should receive vitamin K prophylactically, 5 mg twice weekly, orally, or subcutaneously.[23]

Commercially available rodenticides (super-warfarins) that exhibit long-acting vitamin K antagonism have been associated with significant bleeding disorders when these compounds have been ingested by humans.[20] These drugs are chemically distinct from warfarin, are 100 times more potent than warfarin, and can induce vitamin K deficiency lasting for months. In 1995 alone, more than 13000 people were exposed to these agents and treated.[24] Initial treatment of these patients may require up to 100 mg of vitamin K daily to normalize vitamin K metabolism.[24]

LIVER DISEASE

Severe hepatic disease affects virtually every hemostatic function (Table 55.3)[35] as the result of failure of both the biosynthetic and clearance functions of the liver. The pathophysiology of these abnormalities is multifactorial, including thrombocytopenia (see Chapter 47), platelet dysfunction (see Chapter 53), abnormal coagulation factors, intravascular coagulation and fibrinolysis, and the effects of products of fibrinogen catabolism on hemostasis (see section, Pathophysiology).

Pathophysiology

Thrombocytopenia

Significant liver disease is associated with portal hypertension. The associated splenomegaly is associated with splenic sequestration of platelets, contributing to thrombocytopenia. The liver is also the major site of production of thrombopoietin, the principal humoral factor involved in megakaryocyte maturation, and platelet formation (see Chapter 17). Although there has been some controversy, relative deficiency of thrombopoietin can occur in liver disease.[36] This may, along with decreased expression of the thrombopoietin receptor, c-Mpl,[37] contribute to thrombocytopenia. Additionally, increased thrombopoietin degradation by platelets sequestered in the spleen may also contribute to thrombocytopenia.[38]

Deficient or Aberrant Synthesis of Coagulation Factors

In patients with liver disease, all coagulation factors, except factor VIII, may be deficient as a consequence of synthetic failure in the hepatic cells. Failure of biosynthesis of coagulation factors loosely correlates with the severity of hypoalbuminemia. Deficiencies of prothrombin; factors VII, IX, and X; and proteins C and S result mainly from impaired synthesis. For example, factor VII expression in liver biopsies from patients with liver disease decreases as the severity of hepatic dysfunction increases.[39] Impaired carboxylation of precursors may contribute to the defect. Superimposed vitamin K deficiency may result from a poor diet or malabsorption caused by insufficient production of bile salts or by exocrine pancreatic insufficiency.[40] The failure of these coagulation abnormalities to respond to vitamin K administration provides good evidence of hepatic cell dysfunction.

Factors V, XI, and XIII are synthesized by the liver, but are not vitamin K dependent[25]; all of these factors may be deficient in patients with severe liver disease. Plasma levels of factor XII, prekallikrein (Fletcher factor), and high–molecular-weight kininogen (Fitzgerald factor) may be low in association with liver disease. Deficiencies of these latter three factors do not contribute to a bleeding diathesis.

Hypofibrinogenemia may rarely result from deficient hepatic biosynthesis[25] or may be the consequence of fibrinogenolysis or DIC, as discussed subsequently. In many patients with liver disease, prolongation of the thrombin time can be significant in the absence of hypofibrinogenemia or increased levels of fibrin(ogen) degradation products (FDPs).[26] This apparently is the result of a qualitatively abnormal fibrinogen that is synthesized by the diseased hepatic cell. Such acquired dysfibrinogenemia has been reported in most forms of liver disease, ranging from mild acute hepatitis to acute hepatic necrosis and cirrhosis.[41] Fibrin monomer polymerization is delayed, and the abnormal fibrinogen molecule acts as an antithrombin.[26] This dysfibrinogen may have an abnormally high content of sialic acids[42] and may produce a structurally defective fibrin clot.[27] Acquired dysfibrinogenemia, abnormal inhibitors of fibrinolysis, and the presence within the plasma of descarboxy analogs of prothrombin have been reported in patients with hepatocellular carcinoma.[43]

Fibrinogenolysis and Fibrinolysis

Endogenous plasminogen activators are normally removed from the circulation by the liver. In patients with severe liver disease, however, they may circulate for an abnormally long time and lead to the chronic or intermittent activation of the fibrinolytic enzyme system.[31] This process may be a contributory factor in the pathogenesis of hypofibrinogenemia in patients with liver disease. It also leads to the production of large amounts of FDP, which persist in the circulation for abnormally long periods because of deficient hepatic clearance, and may impair blood coagulation and platelet function.[32] Such proteolytic activity may also produce a shift in the mean molecular weight of circulating fibrinogen from the normal species to a less reactive species of lower molecular weight, thereby contributing to the "antithrombins of liver disease."[33]

The incidence of hyperfibrinolysis was surveyed in patients with cirrhotic and noncirrhotic liver disorders.[44] Hyperfibrinolysis, as measured by a shortened euglobulin clot lysis time, was present in approximately 30% of cirrhotic patients but not present in noncirrhotic patients.[44] The role of thrombin-activatable fibrinolysis inhibitor (TAFI) deficiency in liver disease in contributing to hyperfibrinolysis has been studied. TAFI levels are reduced in liver disease, with lower levels seen in more severe liver disease.[45] However, there was no association of low TAFI levels with hyperfibrinolysis, even in cirrhotic patients suggesting a corresponding profibrinolytic reduction. This suggests that uncompensated hyperfibrinolysis is not common in liver disease, even in cirrhosis.

Intravascular Coagulation

Severe liver disease theoretically predisposes individuals to the development of DIC because of deficient hepatic clearance of activated coagulation factors and other coagulant substances. The in vivo turnover rates of prothrombin,[46] fibrinogen,[47] plasminogen,[46] and antithrombin are often accelerated in patients with cirrhosis. Plasma levels of fibrinopeptide A are elevated in most patients with cirrhosis.[48] All of these abnormalities may be normalized in some cases by the administration of heparin.[49] It has been hypothesized that accelerated catabolism of coagulation factors in these disorders is the result of DIC. The nature of the initiating process is unclear, but one suggestion is that DIC is activated by hypoperfusion of the congested portal bed. Indirect evidence suggests that in severe liver disease, activators of coagulation, possibly endotoxin, may originate in the gut.

Low-grade DIC or localized intravascular coagulation indeed may occur in association with severe liver disease, but overt DIC is responsible only rarely for bleeding in the absence of other etiologic factors that trigger this process, for instance, sepsis, shock, and cancer.[28,29] This conclusion is supported by findings in patients with stable cirrhosis that demonstrated no increased levels of markers of activation of coagulation, such as prothrombin fragment 1 + 2 and thrombin-antithrombin complex.[30]

Evidence for accelerated fibrinogen turnover in ascitic fluid suggests that the loss or consumption of coagulation factors in peritoneal fluid may be a contributory factor in the coagulopathy of chronic liver failure. Shunting of ascitic fluid into the venous circulation by means of LeVeen shunts consistently produces coagulation abnormalities consistent with DIC in cirrhotic patients.[50] Although this phenomenon is usually attributed to intravascular coagulation, evidence shows that it may result, in part, from the presence of plasminogen activators and active plasmin[34] or collagen in peritoneal fluid.

A transitory coagulation disorder that resembles intravascular coagulation with active fibrinolysis has been documented during liver transplantation procedures. Coagulation abnormalities disappear promptly if the graft is successful. The complex coagulopathy seen with liver transplantation has been reviewed.[51]

Prothrombotic Changes

The individual contribution of specific changes to the increased risk of thrombosis seen in patients with liver disease is uncertain. However, plasma levels of protein C, antithrombin, antiplasmin, and plasminogen are subnormal. Plasma levels of factor VIIIc are usually elevated in both parenchymal and cholestatic liver disease.[52] This arises not from increased transcriptional activity of factor VIII in the liver but instead likely results from decreased clearance associated with increased liver synthesis of von Willebrand factor (vWF) and decreased levels of lipoprotein receptor–related protein, both of which regulate clearance of plasma factor VIII levels.[52] Patients with acute liver failure who had higher vWF levels and lower ADAMTS13 levels had worse clinical outcomes.[53]

Clinical Manifestations

Despite the increased risk of bleeding that has been conceptually linked to these numerous abnormalities of individual hemostatic parameters in severe liver disease, many patients do not bleed abnormally. Clinically, overall coagulation function in liver disease within an individual patient is often functionally rebalanced because of parallel reductions in both procoagulant and anticoagulant factors,[54] albeit with an increased vulnerability to tilt toward either bleeding or thrombosis.[55] Additional clinical stimuli can disrupt this new tenuous equilibrium, with increased tendency to bleeding or thrombosis or both.

Gastrointestinal hemorrhage is the most common bleeding manifestation, but it almost always originates from a local lesion, such as esophageal varices, peptic ulcer, or gastritis. The degree to which specific coagulation abnormalities contribute to such bleeding is uncertain. In one large series, gastrointestinal bleeding was not significantly more severe or protracted in patients with coagulation abnormalities than in those without them.[56] Moderate generalized bleeding manifestations, such as recurrent ecchymoses and epistaxis, are not uncommon, and severe generalized bleeding may complicate surgical procedures, including biopsies, tooth extractions, and other minor procedures. Standard coagulation tests, such as the PT, do not measure major in vivo regulators of coagulation such as thrombomodulin and do not adequately reflect hemostasis in these patients.[35,54]

Portal vein thrombosis has been increasingly appreciated in liver disease. Therapy with closely monitored anticoagulation is considered in acute thrombosis, especially when patients are symptomatic with abdominal pain. Anticoagulation is usually not given if the diagnosis is radiologically uncertain, or if there are no symptoms, or with chronic thrombus. Owing to the risks of bleeding, including from varices, anticoagulation is usually limited to 3 months of therapy.[55] In patients listed for liver transplantation, long-term anticoagulation may be considered to prevent rethrombosis due to the impact of portal vein thrombosis on mortality in the posttransplant setting.[57]

Laboratory Diagnosis

The laboratory findings in liver disease vary with the cause and severity of the underlying disorder and range from a slight prolongation of the PT in anicteric hepatitis to the findings summarized in *Table 55.2*, which are seen in severe decompensated cirrhosis. The PT is a calculation factor in both Child-Pugh and Model for End-Stage Liver Disease scores of the severity of liver disease. In cirrhosis, coagulation abnormalities correlate with the presence of portal hypertension and may be minimal in inactive cirrhosis; thrombocytopenia alone is common in association with portal hypertension. Acute fibrinogenolysis is significantly more common in patients with cirrhosis[44] than in those with acute hepatocellular disease, such as hepatitis, although elevations of FDP are consistently found in people with chronic aggressive hepatitis.[41] Coagulation abnormalities are seldom marked in biliary cirrhosis, and some patients with this disorder have abnormally high levels of prothrombin and factors VII and X. Hemostatic abnormalities of any sort are rare in metastatic liver disease. In severe acute liver failure, the PT value has prognostic value, potentially indicative of the need for liver transplantation.[58]

Although screening tests of coagulation are almost invariably performed before liver biopsy, they lack predictive value in anticipating or preventing hemorrhage after this and other minor surgical procedures.[35,54,59] Similarly, the bleeding time test is of little clinical use in predicting bleeding.[60] Many physicians use the international normalized ratio (INR) as a substitute coagulation test for the PT.[61] When measured with a sensitive thromboplastin, the INR can quantitate vitamin K deficiency due to liver disease, but results should not be interpreted as in patients receiving warfarin.[61]

Treatment

Not all patients with the coagulopathy of liver disease require hemostatic correction before procedures such as liver biopsy. A retrospective study looked at the PT ratio (patient PT/mean of reference range PT) and degree of thrombocytopenia to determine the necessity of plasma and platelet transfusion.[62] In patients with platelet counts of 50,000/μL or greater, there was no increased bleeding with liver biopsy compared with patients with normal platelet counts. With regard to elevated PT values, if the PT ratio was <1.5, no increased bleeding was observed.[62] A British guidelines committee on the use of plasma products suggests that "patients with liver disease and a PT more than 4 seconds longer than control are unlikely to benefit from FFP."[63] This recommendation is based on expert opinion. Therefore, many patients with moderate thrombocytopenia and liver disease coagulopathy do not need routine hemostatic correction with blood products. However, additional diagnoses of concern may include intercurrent infection or kidney insufficiency. Patients with a diagnosis of malignancy may have a higher bleeding risk, possibly due to chronic DIC and elevated FDP levels.[62]

Elevated FDP levels may be a significant hemostasis risk factor in liver disease. High levels of FDP may impair platelet function and fibrin monomer polymerization. The thrombin time can screen for the latter defect. A prolonged thrombin time in a patient with a normal functional fibrinogen level and high FDP levels, who is not receiving heparin, may constitute a significant bleeding risk, especially in the setting of moderate thrombocytopenia.

Vitamin K_1, in a dose of 10 mg, produces some improvement in the coagulation abnormalities in approximately 30% of patients, usually those with milder liver disease, but the PT often becomes prolonged again after an initially favorable response. Patients with severe liver disease have minimal response to vitamin K therapy.[64]

Replacement therapy with fresh-frozen plasma is indicated only in the presence of serious bleeding or before surgical procedures, and its effect is often disappointing in patients with liver disease. The reasons for this may include the short in vivo half-life of factor VII, hypervolemia, the loss of transfused factors into ascitic fluid, and the fact that the in vivo recovery of transfused factor IX is significantly lower than that of other factors, even in the absence of liver disease. Older concentrates of vitamin K–dependent coagulation factors (PCC) have been used in the replacement therapy of bleeding in patients with liver disease with variable success but, in several cases, have led to thromboembolic complications and DIC.[65] Thrombosis presumably develops because such concentrates contain trace amounts of activated coagulation factors, particularly factors IXa and Xa,[65] that normally are not cleared from the circulation by the diseased liver and because of antithrombin deficiency, which is commonly present. Newer PCCs also contain proteins C and S in addition to the procoagulant vitamin K–dependent factors. These products have not been well studied in liver disease coagulopathy, but appear to be effective in reversing warfarin coagulopathy.[66] Fresh-frozen plasma is one option, but the effects of even maximum doses (20-30 mL/kg of body weight) are often transitory. Cryoprecipitate is useful to maintain fibrinogen levels over 100 mg/dL. A controlled trial found that 1-desamino-8-D-arginine vasopressin (DDAVP) is not helpful in management of variceal bleeding in cirrhotic patients.[67]

The most current concept of hemostasis in liver disease is that cirrhosis is a prothrombotic condition. Epidemiologic data[68] and laboratory data[69] support this concept. American Gastroenterological Association guidelines recommend not correcting thrombocytopenia and coagulopathy before low-risk procedures (paracentesis, endoscopy) and using the newer four-factor PCCs instead of plasma for high-risk procedures.[70]

Recombinant factor VIIa (rVIIa) is a potential therapy for liver disease patients with significant clinical coagulopathy. However, the drug is not indicated for use in variceal bleeding, partial hepatectomy, or liver transplantation.[71] Disadvantages of rVIIa include its high cost and risk of DIC and thromboembolic complications.

Correction of thrombocytopenia may be difficult in patients with severe liver disease. There is often only a transitory increase in platelet number and function. In the absence of rigorous prospective data, there is no consensus on the appropriate threshold values for prophylactic platelet transfusions, but these can be considered with platelet counts below 50,000/μL.[72] Two thrombopoietin-mimetic agents are approved to treat thrombocytopenia associated with liver disease—avatrombopag and lusutrombopag.[70] For patients requiring liver biopsy who are deemed high risk from a hemostasis perspective, various anatomical or surgical approaches, such as transjugular access, may be considered.[73]

DISSEMINATED INTRAVASCULAR COAGULATION

The syndrome of DIC (defibrination syndrome and consumption coagulopathy) has been one of the most intensively studied subjects in hematology. This large body of information has been summarized in many detailed reviews and monographs.[74,75] A consensus definition of DIC has been proposed: "DIC is an acquired syndrome characterized by the intravascular activation of coagulation with loss of localization arising from different causes. It can originate from and cause damage to the microvasculature, which, if sufficiently severe, can produce organ dysfunction."[76]

Table 55.4. Etiologies of Disseminated Intravascular Coagulation

Obstetric complications
Abruptio placentae, septic abortion and chorioamnionitis, amniotic fluid embolism, intrauterine fetal death, miscellaneous (degenerating hydatidiform moles and leiomyomas, postpartum hemolytic-uremic syndrome, abdominal pregnancy, tetracycline-induced hepatorenal failure, fetomaternal blood passage).
Infections
Viral (herpes, rubella, smallpox, acute hepatitis, Reye syndrome, cytomegalic inclusion disease, various epidemic hemorrhagic fevers, others)
Rickettsial (Rocky Mountain spotted fever, others)
Bacterial (meningococcemia, septicemia, particularly that due to gram-negative organisms, many others)
Mycotic (histoplasmosis, aspergillosis)
Protozoal (malaria, kala-azar, trypanosomiasis)
Neoplasms
Carcinomas[77] (prostate, pancreas, breast, lung, ovary, many others)
Miscellaneous (metastatic carcinoid, rhabdomyosarcoma, neuroblastoma, others)
Disorders of the hematopoietic system
Acute leukemia (promyelocytic,[78] other types)
Intravascular hemolysis (transfusion of incompatible blood, paroxysmal nocturnal hemoglobinuria, freshwater submersion)
Histiocytic medullary reticulosis
Vascular disorders
Malformation (giant hemangiomas [Kasabach-Merritt syndrome],[79] aneurysms, coarctations of the aorta and other large vessels, Takayasu aortitis, large prosthetic arterial grafts, cyanotic congenital cardiac lesions)
Collagen vascular disorders
Hypoxia and hypoperfusion, myocardial infarction, cardiac arrest, various forms of shock, hypothermia
Massive tissue injury
Large traumatic injuries and burns, extensive surgical intervention, extracorporeal circulation, fat embolism
Miscellaneous
Acute iron toxicity, head trauma, snakebite,[80] anaphylaxis, concentrates of vitamin K–dependent coagulation factors,[65] heatstroke, allograft rejection, graft-vs-host disease, severe respiratory distress syndrome, diabetic acidosis, status epilepticus, acute pancreatitis, homozygous deficiency of protein C

Etiology and Incidence

DIC has been well documented in association with the disorders summarized in *Table 55.4*. Several retrospective studies suggest that DIC remains a relatively uncommon entity, but in one large general hospital, its overall incidence was 1 in 1000 admissions.[81] The most prevalent etiologic factor was infection,[81] but in another study, more than 50% of cases were obstetric patients.[82] A Japanese study found that in a hospital population, 45% of DIC cases were associated with malignancy.[83] In many of the disorders listed in *Table 55.4*, DIC develops only in an occasional case. Thus, it is rare in heatstroke, autoimmune disorders, and hemolytic anemias. DIC is present in most cases of venomous snakebite, which is probably one of the most common causes of the disorder worldwide.

Pathophysiology

Mechanisms by Which Disseminated Intravascular Coagulation is Initiated

The pathophysiology of DIC is complex. The mechanisms that trigger or activate DIC act on processes that are involved in normal

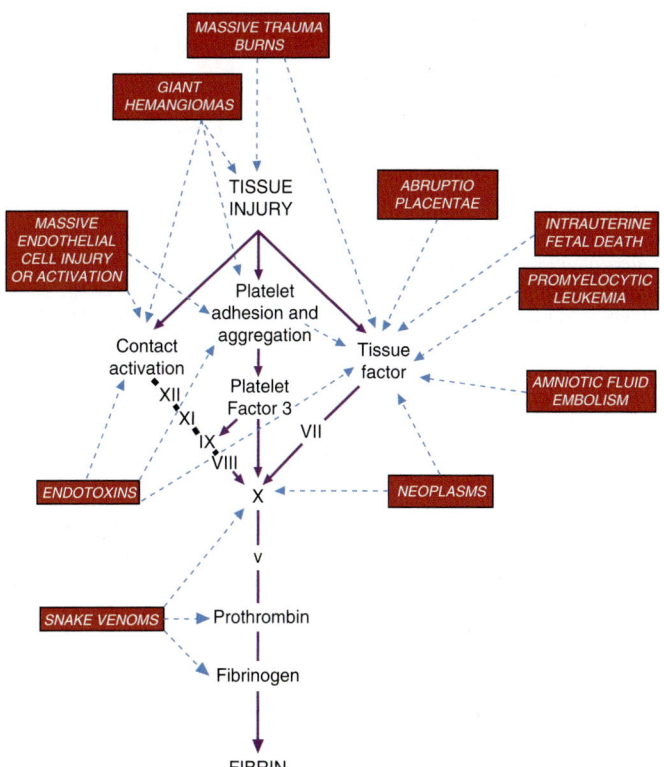

FIGURE 55.2 Initiating mechanisms of disseminated intravascular coagulation (DIC). The solid arrows indicate normal hemostatic pathways, and dotted arrows indicate pathways by which certain disorders associated with DIC initiate or promote the coagulopathy of DIC. Initiation of coagulation by expression of tissue factor activity is probably the most important mechanism triggering DIC.

hemostasis, including platelet adhesion and aggregation, contact-activated (intrinsic), and tissue factor–activated (extrinsic) pathways of coagulation (*Figure 55.2*). These drivers have in common the capacity, in terms of either the magnitude or the duration of the activating stimulus, to exceed normal compensatory processes. Thrombin is persistently generated, and fibrin is formed in the circulating blood. Fibrinogen, various other coagulation factors, and platelets are consumed. The fibrinolytic mechanism is initially activated, and large amounts of FDP are produced, which further impair hemostatic function. Subsequently, fibrinolysis is inhibited. Bleeding, shock, and vascular occlusion commonly supervene and produce profound alterations in the function of various organ systems. Normal compensatory processes may become impaired, creating a self-perpetuating vicious cycle. The ultimate outcome is determined by a dynamic interplay between the various pathologic processes and compensatory mechanisms, in other words, fibrin deposition vs fibrinolysis; depletion vs repletion of coagulation factors and platelets; and production vs clearance of fibrin, FDPs, and other products of coagulation (*Figure 55.3*). Different etiologies of DIC may have differing phenotypes; for example, patients with acute promyelocytic leukemia may exhibit primarily hemorrhage due to hyperfibrinolysis, whereas patients with disorders associated with hypofibrinolysis may experience thrombosis and organ dysfunction.

Tissue Factor

The exposure of procoagulant tissue extracts to blood is a major contributory factor in most forms of DIC and is of major pathogenetic importance in cases associated with abruptio placentae, intrauterine fetal death, acute promyelocytic leukemia, amniotic fluid embolism, massive trauma, and various neoplasms.[84] The active component of such extracts is tissue factor (thromboplastin), which interacts with factor VIIa to activate the extrinsic pathway of coagulation.

DIC can be associated with a variety of pregnancy complications.[77] In abruptio placentae,[85] decidual fragments, serum-containing activated coagulation factors, and other substances from the placental site enter the intervillous "maternal lake" and, hence, the venous circulation. This process is initiated by rupture of the basal decidual plate. In amniotic fluid embolism, relatively weak thromboplastins that increase in potency with gestational age and large amounts of particulate matter enter the circulation suddenly. In intrauterine fetal death, thromboplastic substances from the dead fetus are slowly but continuously absorbed, producing a picture of chronic but progressive DIC.

In neoplasms, tumor microemboli and tumor "vesicles"[86] are thought to enter the circulation and act as thromboplastins.[84,87] Tumor cell surface expression of tissue factor has been demonstrated.[88] Some neoplasms may secrete a factor X activator.[89]

DIC in association with acute leukemia presumably results from the formation or release of tissue factor by leukemic cells.[90] Additionally, leukocyte enzymes such as elastase may contribute to DIC and fibrin(ogen)olysis by proteolysis of coagulation zymogens and fibrinogen.[91] Malignant promyelocytes, as seen in promyelocytic leukemia, express high levels of annexin II, a phospholipid-binding protein, and receptor for plasminogen and tissue plasminogen activator.[92] This overexpression of annexin II results in enhanced plasmin production and increased fibrinolytic activity.[92] The granules of various "blast" forms contain tissue factor, with the promyelocyte containing particularly high concentrations.[90]

In DIC associated with massive trauma,[93] major surgical procedures, or large burns, damaged tissue expressing tissue factor activity presumably is a major initiating factor. In such cases, additional abnormalities and complications are important contributory factors, such as "hypercoagulability," azotemia, shock, intravascular hemolysis, massive transfusions of stored blood, septicemia, and hypoxia. Cerebral trauma of sufficient magnitude to produce significant brain destruction induces a brief episode of DIC, which, although transitory, may be significant in that it may perpetuate cerebral bleeding.[94]

Vascular Endothelium

In addition to monocytes or macrophages, vascular endothelium can be induced to express tissue factor activity in the setting of experimental DIC.[95] Endothelium can also be downregulated in terms of anticoagulant properties (e.g., thrombomodulin activity and fibrinolysis) by stimuli relevant in the pathogenesis of DIC (see Chapter 21). This altered endothelium is referred to as *activated*; properties of activated endothelium include conversion of the normally anticoagulant phenotype to a procoagulant phenotype, expression of adhesion molecules, production of inflammatory mediators, and production of vasoactive agents.[96] Many of these pathologic events are amplified by endothelial cell protease–activated receptors (PARs) (see Chapter 21). Vascular endothelium may also promote coagulation by formation of thrombogenic microparticles, which express anionic phospholipid. Microparticles in DIC may also originate from platelets or granulocytes.[97]

Thrombin generation caused by activation of factor XII in DIC appears to be less important than that initiated by tissue factor.[98] Contact activation, instead, appears critical in mediating DIC-associated hypotension.[99]

Role of Cytokines

Although there are numerous etiologies for DIC (*Table 55.4*), a common pathway for activation of coagulation by these disorders is cytokine release.[75] Important mediators include endotoxin, interleukin-1 (IL-1), IL-6, IL-8, platelet-activating factor, and tumor necrosis factor (TNF). TNF and IL-1 both increase monocyte and endothelial cell tissue factor activity and inhibit protein C activation. Elevated levels of IL-8 correlate with sepsis mortality and DIC.[100]

Infections

DIC often accompanies septicemia as a result of bacteria that possess potent endotoxins. This correlation has led to the intensive study of the effects of endotoxin on the hemostatic mechanism. Purified endotoxin produces several effects that may lead to DIC, namely, activation of factor XII,[101] platelet aggregation, inhibition of fibrinolysis, leukocyte aggregation, direct endothelial injury,[102] cellular induction of tissue factor activity,[103] and impairment of compensatory clearance functions.

Shock, Hypoperfusion, and Hypoxemia

Hypoperfusion, even of normal vessels, acidosis, and hypoxemia produce hypercoagulability and favor intravascular platelet aggregation. Furthermore, splanchnic hypoperfusion impairs reticuloendothelial and hepatic clearance functions and is present in virtually all forms of shock. Shock may also impair hepatic synthesis of coagulation factors and thus contribute to the coagulation defect in DIC. Activated neutrophils may generate oxygen radicals and proteases to alter vascular permeability. Vascular injury may also occur with ischemia/reperfusion that elicits inflammatory responses.

DIC in association with giant hemangiomas (Kasabach-Merritt syndrome)[104] or with aneurysms of the aorta or other large vessels[105] has been attributed to hypoperfusion and stasis in local vascular beds.

Miscellaneous Activating Stimuli

Snake venoms contain enzymes that may trigger coagulation in unique ways. Venom extracts may produce defibrination without affecting other coagulation factors, such as ancrod, an enzyme purified from the venom of the Malayan pit viper (*Calloselasma rhodostoma*). Other venoms contain thrombin-like enzymes or substances that specifically activate factor X or prothrombin.[106] Crude venoms also contain substances that act as thromboplastins and produce intravascular red cell hemolysis and massive vascular damage.[107] An inventory of the biochemical properties of snake venoms and their constituent enzymes has been summarized elsewhere.[108]

Consumption of Coagulation Factors and Impaired Anticoagulant Pathways

Generalizations based on the consumption of coagulation factors during in vitro coagulation are not always consistent with laboratory findings in patients with DIC. Plasma levels of factors that are normally consumed, such as fibrinogen, prothrombin, and factors V and XIII, are often reduced in severe DIC, but factors that normally are not consumed may also be deficient, such as factors VII, IX, and X. Significant hypoprothrombinemia reflects either massive and protracted activation of coagulation or complicating factors, because in animals, severe depletion of platelets, fibrinogen, and factors V and VIII results from activation of only 10% of plasma prothrombin.[109]

Antithrombin is the principal inhibitor of thrombin and activated factor X; low levels of antithrombin in DIC result from consumption because of persistent neutralization of thrombin, degradation by elastase released from activated neutrophils, and decreased hepatic synthesis. Other natural anticoagulant pathways—the protein C pathway and tissue factor pathway inhibitor—are also diminished in DIC.[110] Proinflammatory cytokines (TNF and IL-1) downregulate endothelial cell thrombomodulin activity, resulting in decreased levels of activated protein C (APC). Low levels of APC not only fail to inhibit activation of coagulation (by inactivating factors Va and VIIIa) but also contribute to failure to downregulate inflammation. Additionally, the endothelial protein C receptor is downregulated in DIC, further reducing activity of the protein C pathway.[111] Thus, impairment of the protein C pathway in DIC contributes to the procoagulant and inflammatory phenotype seen in the disorder.

The numerous and diverse defense processes that are mediated by factor XIIa are activated in DIC, including the complement system and the kallikrein system. It has been suggested that the hypotensive effects of bradykinin may explain the conspicuous presence of hypotension in patients with DIC triggered by activation of factor XII,[112] for example, that associated with endotoxemia.

Consumption of Platelets

In DIC, the platelet count is often depressed out of proportion to the severity of coagulation abnormalities. Thrombocytopenia may result from processes other than the consumption of platelets in thrombotic lesions. These processes include adhesion to denuded or damaged endothelial cell surfaces and intravascular aggregation with subsequent sequestration, which may be caused by endotoxin, antigen-antibody complexes, thrombin, particulate matter, and, possibly, fibrin-FDP complexes.

All of these agents initiate the platelet release reaction, which may produce a population of partially activated platelets that are depleted of storage nucleotides (acquired storage pool disease). Partially activated platelets may contribute to impairment of clearance functions. Epinephrine and serotonin are released from the platelets and may reach extremely high concentrations in hypoperfused vascular beds. This process may produce sustained constriction of the afferent renal arteriole and may predispose to cortical necrosis. Serotonin may also produce pulmonary and cerebral hypoperfusion.

A mouse model of DIC investigated the role of PARs in mediating the endothelial cell and platelet response to activation of coagulation. In this model of endotoxemia, activation of coagulation occurred, but knockout of PARs failed to improve survival or thrombocytopenia. Although this model may not extrapolate to human DIC, it suggests that PARs may not mediate the DIC response and that thrombocytopenia in DIC may result from mechanisms other than thrombin activation.[113]

Intravascular Fibrin Formation

The formation of fibrin, in the form of small strands and "microclots," is the immediate result of DIC; the ultimate consequence of this process is determined by a balance between the rate of fibrin formation and the rate of its clearance from the circulation or lysis by the fibrinolytic enzyme system.

Erythrocytes are injured mechanically during passage through fibrin networks in the microcirculation. Such microangiopathic hemolysis leads to the production of schistocytes and microspherocytes. It should be noted that red cell fragmentation is not seen in all patients with DIC.[114]

Fibrinolysis

Fibrinolysis is present in virtually every patient with DIC, but it generally plays a homeostatic rather than a pathologic role. In the setting of DIC, this "secondary fibrinolysis" is an appropriate response to persistent thrombin generation. Fibrinolysis may be activated by several mechanisms. The major endogenous source of plasminogen activators is in the vascular endothelium of the microcirculation, and in DIC, such activators, especially tissue plasminogen activator, are released as a result of thrombin formation and fibrin deposition on endothelial surfaces, endothelial injury, or hypoxia. Many of the thromboplastic substances that initiate DIC, such as tumor tissues and extracts of leukemic cells, also contain plasminogen activators. The release of plasminogen activators from platelets and leukocytes may also be significant. Finally, factor XIIa activates plasminogen by interacting with normal proactivators and the kinin system.

Fibrinolysis must be distinguished clearly from the process of fibrinogenolysis, in which fibrinogen and other coagulation factors are proteolytically destroyed in the circulation. Fibrinogenolysis may be an inappropriate response in DIC associated with amniotic fluid embolism, heatstroke, and, rarely, carcinoma. It is uncommon in other forms of DIC; when present, it is usually transitory and overshadowed by marked fibrinolysis. Disorders in which fibrinogenolysis arises in the absence of DIC (primary fibrinolysis) are discussed elsewhere in this chapter.

Following the initial enhanced fibrinolytic response to DIC, suppression of fibrinolysis occurs as a result of elevated levels of plasminogen activator inhibitor-1; this inhibition of fibrinolysis was associated with a poorer clinical outcome.[115] Increased thrombin generation seen in DIC would activate TAFI and exacerbate thrombosis and organ dysfunction.[116]

Fibrin(ogen) Degradation Products

The stepwise process by which fibrin is degraded proteolytically and the biologic effects of the various products of the process (FDPs) are discussed in Chapter 20. These protein fragments act as antithrombins,[33] inhibit fibrin polymerization, produce a structurally defective fibrin polymer,[117] and may impair platelet[32] and reticuloendothelial clearance functions. The presence of large amounts of FDP in the circulation is a major factor in the production of hemorrhage in many patients with DIC.

The infusion of large amounts of FDP (fragment D) into rabbits produces changes that resemble the posttraumatic respiratory distress syndrome in humans.[118] This observation suggests that large amounts of FDP may directly damage the pulmonary vasculature, leading to respiratory distress syndrome, which has been reported in association with DIC and the use of thrombolytic agents.[119]

In DIC, a large amount of fibrin remains in a soluble state as a consequence of the formation of complexes between fibrin monomers, various FDPs, and fibrinogen. This solubility has been regarded as a final defense against vascular occlusion. In vitro, the complexes dissociate in the presence of alcohol or protamine sulfate to form gels or precipitates of various types (paracoagulation).

Impairment of Clearance Mechanisms

The numerous processes that normally remove procoagulant material from the circulation are of the utmost importance in DIC because of the presence of massive amounts of both activators and products of coagulation. Most of the products of intravascular coagulation (prothrombinase, platelet factor-3 activity, and various types of FDPs and complexes thereof),[120] as well as various initiators of the process (tissue fragments, endotoxin, antigen-antibody complexes, tissue factor, and red cell stroma), are removed from the circulation by the reticuloendothelial system (*Figure 55.3*). The Kupffer cells of the liver[121] and splenic macrophages are of particular importance. In certain forms of DIC, large amounts of relatively inert particulate matter (e.g., amniotic fluid embolism) place an additional burden on the reticuloendothelial system. The hepatic cells are of primary importance in the clearance of activated coagulation factors, such as factors IXa, Xa,[122] and XIa.

Chronic or "Compensated" Disseminated Intravascular Coagulation

Certain forms of DIC result from a weak or intermittent activating stimulus. In such patients, destruction and production of coagulation factors and platelets are balanced (*Figure 55.3*). The pathophysiology of such chronic, subacute, or "compensated" DIC is fundamentally the same as that in the acute case. Nevertheless, the distinction is valuable because the clinical picture and laboratory findings in the chronic form are quite variable and may be diagnostically confusing.

Chronic DIC has been described in many patients with intrauterine fetal death or giant hemangiomas (Kasabach–Merritt syndrome) and in many cases of adenocarcinoma.[84] Other etiologic factors that may produce chronic DIC include various forms of vasculitis, acute leukemia, aneurysms, hemangiomatous transformation of the spleen, and renal allograft rejection.

In cancer patients, a virtually continuous spectrum of clinical and laboratory features has been described; these range from recurrent venous thrombosis or arterial embolism[84] with high levels of platelets and coagulation factors to acute DIC with severe

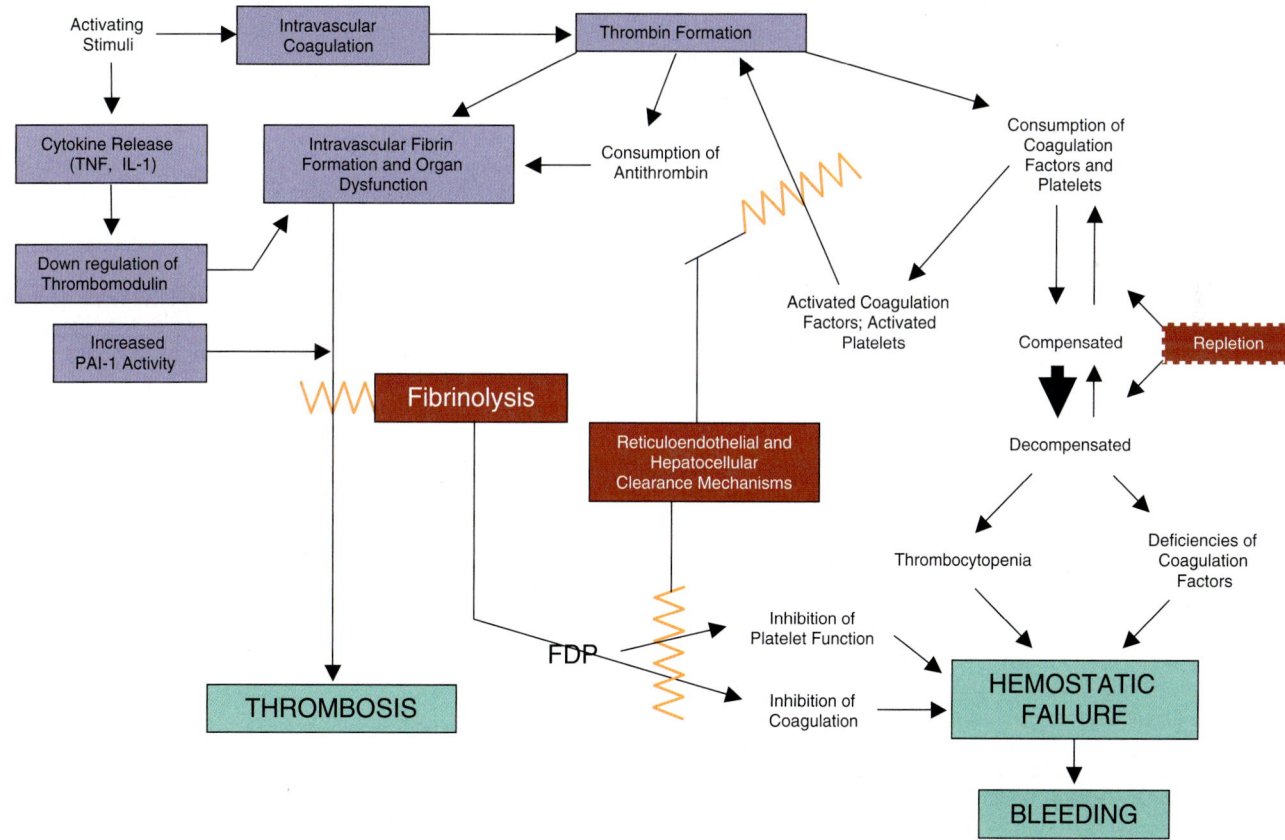

FIGURE 55.3 Pathophysiology of disseminated intravascular coagulation (DIC). The critical event in DIC is the generation of thrombin in an unregulated fashion. The clinical consequences of thrombin production depend on the rate of thrombin formation as well as underlying host factors (marrow reserve of platelet production, liver function). Patients with adequate compensatory responses (ability to compensate for platelet or coagulation factor production, fibrinolysis, intact clearance mechanisms) may have minimal symptoms, whereas other patients with defective compensatory responses may bleed or thrombose or both. Increased levels of cytokines occur (TNF and IL-1) that contribute to the proinflammatory state by downregulating fibrinolysis and thrombomodulin activity, leading to enhancement of intravascular fibrin formation and organ dysfunction. Major compensatory factors that influence clinical events are indicated in colored blocks. The zig-zag line indicates interruption of an adverse clinical event by a compensatory factor. FDP, fibrin(ogen) degradation product; IL-I, interleukin-1; PAI-1, plasminogen activator inhibitor-1; TNF, tumor necrosis factor.

hemorrhage.[84] The clinical and experimental evidence is incontrovertible that pregnancy, the best-studied form of hypercoagulability, is associated with an increased propensity for the development of DIC.[123] Indeed, even normal pregnancy has been suggested as a form of low-grade "physiologic" DIC,[123] which, at term, becomes overt for a short time.

Clinical Features

The major clinical features of DIC are bleeding, often of serious magnitude and abrupt onset; a variable element of shock that is often out of proportion to apparent blood loss; and symptoms of hypoperfusion of various vascular beds. Acute renal failure is common, and thromboembolic manifestations are often noted.[110,124] Any of these features or signs and symptoms of the underlying disorder may predominate in a given case.

Evidence of major organ dysfunction is a common finding in patients with DIC, most often including signs, symptoms, and laboratory evidence of abnormal pulmonary, renal, hepatic, and central nervous system function. Although virtually all of these manifestations have been attributed to the underlying DIC, the clinical manifestations that have been described were usually the result of the underlying disorder. For example, one study observed that patients with DIC due to aortic aneurysm had laboratory features of DIC but minimal clinical manifestations. Patients with DIC due to obstetric disorders all had bleeding, but only 20% had organ dysfunction. In contrast, of patients with DIC due to sepsis, only 15% had bleeding, but 76% had organ failure.[83] These results suggest that marked heterogeneity exists in clinical manifestations of DIC and that the etiology of DIC is a major predictor of clinical events.[83]

In this section, the clinical manifestations and diagnosis of DIC are discussed in general terms. Various specific clinical features and details regarding treatment of the most common forms follow in a separate section.

Acute Disseminated Intravascular Coagulation

Bleeding manifestations of virtually every kind have been described, and they may evolve rapidly in the patient with acute DIC. Generalized ecchymoses, petechiae, and bleeding from previously intact venipuncture sites or around indwelling IV needles or catheters are noted in many patients. Large, spreading, hemorrhagic skin lesions are often superimposed on familiar exanthems in patients with rickettsial and viral infections. "Geographic" acral cyanosis is a prominent feature in some patients. Large, sharply demarcated ecchymotic areas may result from thrombotic occlusion of dermal vessels and may progress to skin infarction. Such infarcts are particularly common in patients with purpura fulminans and are also seen in coumarin-induced skin necrosis and inherited homozygous deficiency of protein C (see Chapter 56). In patients with meningococcemia, cutaneous hemorrhage may be striking. Bleeding from apparently normal gingivae, epistaxis, gastrointestinal bleeding, pulmonary hemorrhage, and hematuria are common. In patients who develop DIC after surgical procedures, alarming hemorrhage may develop around drains and tracheostomies.

Chronic Disseminated Intravascular Coagulation

Superficial but extensive ecchymoses of the extremities, often without petechiae, may develop intermittently or may persist. Recurrent episodes of epistaxis or more serious internal mucosal bleeding may punctuate the course. Trousseau sign (recurrent migratory thrombophlebitis in association with cancer) in most instances is a manifestation of chronic DIC. More serious hemorrhagic manifestations may develop because the underlying disease progresses or may arise with dramatic suddenness after surgical procedures such as a prostatectomy. In some patients, evidence of vascular obstruction (e.g., impairment of renal function, confusion, transitory neurologic syndromes, or repeated episodes of cerebral thrombosis) may develop with minimal bleeding.

Laboratory Diagnosis

The laboratory findings in DIC are summarized in Table 55.2. Contrary to what is commonly assumed, they may be quite variable. The plasma fibrinogen level, PTT, PT, platelet count, and estimates of FDP or D-dimer are the cornerstones on which the diagnosis of DIC is based. These simple tests should always be performed first. Additional information may confirm, but seldom refutes, the diagnosis of DIC if typical abnormalities are demonstrated by these tests. Laboratory data may change with remarkable rapidity in DIC based on disease progression or therapy.

Laboratory data must be interpreted with caution. Levels of platelets and various coagulation factors, fibrinogen, and factor VIII, in particular, may be elevated in many of the conditions associated with DIC, including pregnancy. Thus, a fibrinogen level of 200 mg/dL, although within the normal range determined in healthy subjects, may represent a significant decrease in a patient whose baseline level was 800 mg/dL owing to acute-phase changes.

The best test for diagnosing DIC is the D-dimer assay.[125] The semiquantitative method is sensitive,[126] and D-dimer values >2000 ng/mL have been reported to be consistent with DIC.[127] More sensitive, quantitative D-dimer assays are now available; one study reported that a sensitive D-dimer assay result <8.2 μg/mL optimized sensitivity and negative predictive value in patients with DIC.[128]

Basic Blood Examinations

In patients with DIC, routine hematologic tests may reveal evidence of acute bleeding, accelerated red cell destruction, or signs of the underlying disease. Examination of the blood smear reveals schistocytes in approximately 50% of cases,[82,114] but the degree of schistocytosis bears no necessary correlation with other facets of the disorder. More subtle evidence of intravascular hemolysis is often found, such as increased serum levels of lactate dehydrogenase and diminished haptoglobin levels.

Coagulation Defect

The PTT, PT, and thrombin time are prolonged in most patients with acute DIC. Early in the course of the disorder and in chronic DIC, the PTT may be normal or even shorter than normal, which may be the result of the procoagulant effects of activated coagulation factors or elevated factor VIII levels.

Occasionally, one can follow the process of DIC from its inception, and specific assays for various coagulation factors obtained at the time of diagnosis reveal a variable and rapidly changing picture. The plasma levels of fibrinogen and of factors V and XIII are usually significantly depressed; fibrinogen and factor V are the most consistently affected.[129] The level of factor X may be lower than that of other "stable" factors (factors VII, IX, and XI), which are usually present in normal amounts.[129]

The levels of factors VIII, IX, and XI as determined by one-stage assays may fluctuate widely as the result of the presence of activated factors, such as thrombin and factor Xa.[130] This problem is minimized in two-stage assays.[129] Levels of factor VIIIc are often normal or increased, particularly when assayed by two-stage techniques.[131] The thrombin time may be prolonged out of proportion to the reduction in the fibrinogen level, because of elevated FDP levels.

Tests for Fibrinolysis: Fibrin Monomers, Fibrin(ogen) Degradation Products, and D-Dimer

In most patients with DIC, FDP levels as determined by quantitative methods are 25-μg fibrinogen "equivalents"/mL or higher.[129] All methods are most sensitive to large or "early" FDPs. These fragments, particularly fragment X, retain thrombin-binding sites or may form a complex with fibrinogen and consequently be removed during the preparation of serum for FDP tests. This phenomenon or the presence of only small FDPs may explain the normal levels of FDPs in some patients with otherwise typical DIC. Fibrinopeptide A and certain fibrinogen fragments that are formed by the lysis of cross-linked fibrin, such as the DD-dimer and the DD-dimer-E complex, can be demonstrated using special techniques. These latter FDPs provide direct evidence of the action of thrombin on fibrinogen and provide a means of differentiating fibrin degradation products from fibrinogen degradation products.[132]

The simplicity, specificity, and sensitivity of the D-dimer test have led many laboratories to replace less sensitive or less convenient tests for DIC with the D-dimer test. Because false-positive results may be seen with FDP latex agglutination tests in patients with dysfibrinogenemia, the D-dimer test may be more specific in diagnosing DIC, especially in distinguishing the coagulopathy of liver disease from DIC.[29,126,133] False-positive D-dimer latex agglutination tests may occur in patients with elevated levels of immunoglobulin M (IgM) (rheumatoid factor).

"Paracoagulation" techniques are simple to perform, but they are less specific than tests for FDPs. Results of protamine gelation tests are usually positive,[134] but abnormal results are obtained in numerous other disorders, including many that are commonly associated with DIC.

Other Laboratory Findings

Plasma levels of fibrinopeptide A[135] are a sensitive indicator of DIC and may be abnormal even in patients with normal levels of FDP. Levels of antithrombin,[136] α_2-antiplasmin, and proteins C and S may be diminished in some cases. In a primate model of gram-negative sepsis, a number of molecular markers of coagulation were investigated for their use in monitoring DIC.[137] Markers such as soluble thrombomodulin and soluble fibrin monomer are useful in assessing the status of microvascular injury.

The clinical role of these assays in diagnosing or managing DIC patients at this time is uncertain. The best test for diagnosis and monitoring DIC appears to be a sensitive D-dimer assay. The International Society on Thrombosis and Haemostasis (ISTH) has proposed clinical and laboratory criteria to better define the spectrum of DIC cases.[138]

Differential Diagnosis

The syndrome of DIC is seldom difficult to recognize. Problems arise when the diagnosis simply is not considered or in chronic forms, or when the underlying coagulation disorder may be masked by features of the basic disease or by thromboembolic complications.[139]

Two disorders, however, produce laboratory abnormalities that resemble DIC: severe liver disease, which is common, and primary fibrinogenolysis or "pathologic" fibrinolysis, which is rare (Table 55.2). In patients with primary fibrinogenolysis, the following conditions may be evident: hypofibrinogenemia; increased levels of FDP; abnormalities of the PTT, PT, and thrombin time; and deficiencies of factors V and VIIIc. However, the platelet count is usually normal, the D-dimer level should be normal or only minimally elevated, and protamine sulfate tests should be negative. Hypoprothrombinemia and deficiencies of stable coagulation factors VII, IX, X, and XI are rare. Thus, routine coagulation tests should be able to distinguish DIC from primary fibrinogenolysis.

In patients with liver disease, coagulation abnormalities and thrombocytopenia may originate from many pathologic processes (Table 55.3). Chronic or intermittent fibrinogenolysis with high levels of FDP is common, particularly in patients with cirrhosis. In such patients, the exclusion of the diagnosis of DIC may be difficult. Factor VIIIc levels are usually elevated when liver disease is severe, and the levels of factors VII and IX typically are low. A helpful test in discriminating between the coagulopathy of liver disease and DIC is the D-dimer test, the results of which should be abnormal in DIC but normal in liver disease (unless additional disorders coexist).[29,133]

DIC, particularly that associated with carcinoma, may be confused with various microangiopathic hemolytic anemias, such as thrombotic thrombocytopenic purpura and hemolytic-uremic syndrome; in these disorders, the clinical picture may resemble that of DIC in many respects. High levels of FDP may be encountered in patients with microangiopathic hemolytic anemias, but significant coagulation abnormalities are not commonly present. Many other disorders may produce slight-to-moderate elevations of FDP, including, pulmonary embolism and chronic renal disease with uremia.

Treatment

DIC is always the end result of a serious underlying disorder. Although the patient may benefit greatly from the replacement of depleted coagulation factors and platelets, correction of the syndrome depends on prompt and energetic treatment of the primary disorder. This—not the therapeutic measures described in this section—remains the cornerstone of therapy.

Anticoagulants

Heparin is a specific activator of the physiologic antithrombin system and thereby inhibits a number of proteolytic enzymes, including factors IXa and Xa and thrombin (see Chapter 56). In view of the complexity of DIC, inhibition of coagulation alters only one facet, albeit a fundamental one, of the pathophysiologic cycle. Appreciation of the role of anticoagulation and inflammatory pathways has led to consideration of novel therapies, including replacement of anticoagulant proteins such as antithrombin, APC, and soluble thrombomodulin.[110]

In patients with chronic DIC, the results of heparin therapy are usually favorable and may be dramatic. In most patients, heparin would not be expected to alter ultimate mortality because of the nature of the underlying diseases; however, this drug typically does reduce the severity of bleeding and thromboembolic manifestations and produces parallel improvement in the abnormalities of laboratory test values. Elevated levels of D-dimer and FDPs drop rapidly, and accelerated fibrinolysis, if present, disappears after the administration of heparin, often before the coagulation defect has been alleviated. The response of the platelet count to heparin therapy for DIC is slow and often erratic.

In patients with acute DIC, particularly that associated with sepsis, the results of heparin therapy have been less encouraging.[140] Most clinicians are reluctant to use heparin in patients with acute DIC. Because baseline PTT values are usually prolonged in acute DIC, heparin levels may be required to monitor therapy (see Chapter 56).

Replacement Therapy With Platelets and Coagulation Factors

The major aim of replacement therapy with blood products in DIC is to replenish fibrinogen. This goal is best accomplished by the administration of cryoprecipitate, each unit of which contains approximately 250 mg of fibrinogen.[141] The amount of cryoprecipitate given should be sufficient to elevate the plasma fibrinogen level to at least 100 to 150 mg/dL. As a general guide, 3 g of fibrinogen can be expected to raise the plasma level of an adult patient approximately 100 mg/dL. Fibrinogen administration probably should be restricted to the occasional patient with hypofibrinogenemia and significant bleeding, in whom DIC is self-limited. Two fibrinogen concentrates are available for bleeding episodes related to congenital deficiency (RiaSTAP and Fibryga); they are not labeled in the United States for use in DIC.

Patients with DIC, bleeding, and platelet counts <50,000/µL should be considered for platelet transfusion. Owing to the acquired storage pool defect seen with DIC, as well as FDP inhibition of platelet function, DIC patients may require a higher platelet count for adequate hemostasis than patients with thrombocytopenia in the absence of platelet dysfunction.

The availability of purified, sterile antithrombin concentrates has led to its investigation in treating DIC. As seen in most studies,[142] although antithrombin concentrates can normalize plasma levels of this protein in patients with DIC and improve hemostasis parameters, consistent clinical benefit in terms of survival is not evident. A large clinical trial demonstrated that high-dose antithrombin therapy in patients with sepsis had no effect on mortality.[143] A posthoc analysis of this clinical trial indicated that high-dose antithrombin therapy may be effective in improving survival in the subset of patients with severe sepsis and high risk of death, especially if concomitant heparin treatment is avoided.[144]

Other Therapeutic Measures

Treatment of shock should be immediate and vigorous in all patients with DIC. Packed erythrocytes should be given promptly if indicated. The indiscriminate use of ε-aminocaproic acid (EACA) and other antifibrinolytic drugs should be discouraged. Because of the potential risks, fibrinolytic enzyme inhibitors should be administered only to carefully selected patients, that is, those in whom DIC has resulted from a transitory stimulus or has been arrested by heparin administration and in whom fibrinogenolysis or inappropriate fibrinolysis, hypofibrinogenemia, and adequate renal function have been clearly documented. The therapeutic use of EACA in fibrinogenolysis and appropriate dosage schedules are discussed elsewhere in this chapter.

Specific Features of Various Forms of Disseminated Intravascular Coagulation

Obstetric Disorders

Abruptio Placentae

DIC complicates abruptio placentae in approximately 10% of cases[145] in which fetal compromise occurs. Shock develops rapidly, but vaginal bleeding may be minimal or absent for a time and bears little relationship to the extent of abruption. Brisk external hemorrhage may originate from episiotomies and lacerations, and large amounts of blood may be concealed behind the placenta and within the wall of the uterus.

Hemorrhage is the major factor leading to shock and renal complications in abruptio placentae, and the most essential therapeutic measures are the vigorous treatment of blood loss and the prompt evacuation of the uterus. Extensive replacement therapy seldom is required. Often, fibrinogen replacement is given if immediate surgical treatment is necessary. Fibrinogen replacement may be most useful in patients with fetal death requiring cesarean delivery. If the coagulation defect and thrombocytopenia are severe or persist for an unusually long time, the administration of platelets, fibrinogen in the form of cryoprecipitate, and fresh-frozen plasma[146] may reduce hemorrhage. Most obstetricians do not administer heparin because it may increase bleeding and because rapid spontaneous remission of DIC is usual when the uterus is evacuated.

Intrauterine Fetal Death

In the event of intrauterine fetal death, definite laboratory abnormalities are not seen until the dead fetus has been retained for ≥5 weeks[145]; plasma levels of FDPs then begin to rise, and the platelet count and fibrinogen level gradually decline. Bleeding may be inconspicuous, but a progressive loss of renal function is not uncommon. In most women in whom delivery of the dead fetus is induced promptly according to usual obstetric practice, bleeding is not serious, even in the presence of low-grade DIC. Operative intervention is dangerous when hypofibrinogenemia is severe, and such patients should receive heparin until safe fibrinogen levels are restored.[147]

Amniotic Fluid Embolism

In women who survive amniotic fluid embolism (mortality rate of up to 80% in early studies), DIC with severe hemorrhage may develop within 1 to 2 hours.[148] More recent surveys indicate a mortality rate of 20% to 30%. Hypoxia and other sequelae of pulmonary vascular obstruction dominate the clinical picture and usually determine the outcome. The release of serotonin and other vasoactive substances from platelets may contribute to the profound pulmonary vasoconstriction.

The International Society of Thrombosis and Haemostasis has published recommendations on the diagnosis and management of obstetrical DIC.[149]

Disseminated Intravascular Coagulation in Neonates and Infants

Several disorders unique to the neonate and infant may be associated with DIC (Table 55.2).[150] The transplacental passage of thromboplastins or other procoagulant substances has been the apparent cause of DIC in neonates born of mothers affected with DIC owing to abruptio placentae, eclampsia, or septicemia. Asphyxia may be a common precipitating factor for DIC in these disorders. Bacterial infection and generalized viral infections (e.g., herpes simplex, cytomegalic inclusion disease, and rubella), acidosis, and hypoxia are more common causes of DIC in infants than in adults. DIC secondary to giant hemangiomas and purpura fulminans has been reported in neonates.

Management of septic DIC in the neonate should emphasize treatment of underlying infection. A controlled study that compared treatment with heparin, extensive replacement therapy with blood products, and supportive care only revealed no significant differences in outcome for the three groups.[151] A more recent study confirms that clinical trials in neonatal sepsis have not identified a beneficial therapy.[152]

In many patients, no additional measures other than treating infection and shock (if present) are required. No evidence has been cited that heparin has diminished mortality. A Cochrane database review of the effects of recombinant APC in neonates with sepsis concluded that there were insufficient data to support the use of the drug in the pediatric setting,[153] similar to that seen in the adult setting.[154]

Purpura Fulminans

The hemorrhagic manifestations of purpura fulminans develop several days after an acute infection; these are most commonly scarlet fever or various viral respiratory diseases. Purpura fulminans is most common in children but is also well documented in adults. The most common manifestations are symmetric ecchymoses of the lower extremities and buttocks, sharply circumscribed infarcts of the skin and genitalia, and gangrene of the extremities that often involves the digits symmetrically.[155] These ecchymotic lesions often become necrotic, ultimately forming blood-filled bullae. Petechiae are rare. Fever and prostration are seen, but visceral lesions, including renal involvement, are relatively uncommon.

The mortality rate associated with purpura fulminans ranges from 18%[156] to 40% to 70%.[157] Heparin in therapeutic doses has often proved therapeutically effective, and it has been suggested that poor results obtained previously with this anticoagulant reflect late treatment of moribund patients. In patients with purpura fulminans, relapses are particularly common after cessation of heparin therapy,[156] and the administration of this anticoagulant, possibly in reduced doses, should be continued for 2 to 3 weeks. The subject of purpura fulminans diagnosis and treatment has been reviewed.[158] Evidence that purpura fulminans may be a manifestation of homozygous protein C deficiency is discussed in Chapter 56. Unlike drotrecogin alfa (recombinant APC), which was voluntarily withdrawn from use in severe sepsis,[153] protein C concentrate from human plasma is indicated in severe congenital protein C deficiency for the prevention and treatment of venous thrombosis and purpura fulminans.

Neoplastic Disorders

Carcinoma

In patients with DIC associated with carcinoma, the clinical picture is quite variable and often consists of a combination of bleeding and thromboembolic phenomena, including arterial embolism.[84,87,88] The association of chronic DIC, thromboembolism, and cancer is often called *Trousseau syndrome.*[84] Laboratory findings are variable. Evidence of chronic DIC, hypercoagulability, or acute DIC may be found. In a study of more than 1000 patients with solid tumors, 7% were diagnosed with DIC using standard coagulation tests (platelet count, fibrinogen, D-dimer, and FDPs).[159] Risk factors associated with the occurrence of DIC included older age, male gender, advanced disease, breast cancer, and necrosis of the tumor specimen.[159]

Analysis of a large database of Medicare patients with cancer identified tissue-specific differences in thrombotic risks among cancers.[160] Those cancers with a high risk of thrombosis included uterine, brain, leukemia, ovary, and pancreas (twofold or greater risk), whereas prostate, liver, head or neck, bladder, and breast cancer had less than a onefold risk (compared to noncancer patients).[160]

DIC in association with carcinoma resolves with effective treatment of the underlying tumor. Heparin or low–molecular-weight heparin (LMWH) in therapeutic doses has proved effective in controlling the hemorrhagic and thromboembolic symptoms.[84,87,161] However, a Cochrane review of the effects of heparin on cancer patient survival found no effect on mortality at 12 and 24 months.[162]

A significant minority of patients with cancer and thrombosis will experience recurrent thrombosis with warfarin[84] and will benefit from long-term heparin or LMWH.[163] Clinical trial data indicate that three oral factor X_a inhibitors (rivaroxaban, apixaban, and edoxaban) are also safe and effective to treat cancer-associated thrombosis.[164] In the case of DIC associated with prostate cancer, adjunctive therapy with ketoconazole[165] or antiandrogens[166] has been useful. The spectrum of mechanisms of thrombosis in Trousseau syndrome has been reviewed.[167]

Acute Promyelocytic Leukemia

DIC has been reported in association with all forms of acute leukemia, but it is most common in the "hypergranular" promyelocytic variety (APL),[168] in which it may occur in 60% to 100% of cases. The cause of the coagulopathy is multifactorial: tissue factor is present in the granules of the abnormal promyelocytes[90] as well as leukocyte proteases, including elastase.[78] Enhanced fibrinolysis also results from increased promyelocyte expression of annexin II, a receptor for plasminogen and tissue plasminogen activator.[92] The clinical picture is usually one of chronic progressive DIC with a significant fibrinolytic component that may antedate the other manifestations of the disease. Acute fulminant DIC may develop spontaneously or may be triggered by the administration of chemotherapeutic agents, which cause the release of thromboplastic contents of the promyelocytes.

In some patients with acute leukemia, accelerated fibrinolysis is a conspicuous finding. In one study, depletion of α_2-antiplasmin developed during induction of chemotherapy, a finding that was more predictive of bleeding complications than traditional indices of DIC, such as levels of fibrinogen, antithrombin, and plasminogen.[169] This study suggests that unregulated fibrinolysis, by destroying functional hemostatic plugs and depleting fibrinogen, may be more important than DIC in some cases.

Current protocols for APL combine ATRA with either arsenic trioxide or chemotherapy. The use of antifibrinolytic agents concurrently with ATRA should be avoided.[170] Replacement therapy for hypofibrinogenemia and thrombocytopenia may still be required. ATRA is more effective than chemotherapy alone in improving the coagulopathy; however, aberrant cytokine expression may temporarily persist in some patients, regardless of therapeutic approach, leading to hypercoagulability.[171]

Kasabach-Merritt Syndrome (Giant Hemangiomas)

The severity and incidence of DIC tends to parallel the size of the vascular tumors in the Kasabach-Merritt syndrome.[172] Platelet consumption, activation of coagulation, and microangiopathic red cell destruction take place mainly within the hemangioma ("sequestered" or localized intravascular coagulation), but laboratory evidence of DIC in the general circulation is usually clear-cut.[104,172] Recurrent bleeding from the surface of the tumor is the major hemorrhagic manifestation; in the presence of DIC, this bleeding may be intractable. Periodic swelling of the lesions is often observed. This phenomenon may be a consequence of intermittent obstruction of blood outflow from the hemangioma and may provoke serious hemorrhage. Surgical removal of the tumors has ultimately been required in most patients.[104,172] Interferon-α has been successful in some patients; this cytokine probably acts as an antiproliferative/antiangiogenic agent.[172] Antifibrinolytic therapy has been reported to be useful in controlling the coagulopathy.[79] Data indicate that sirolimus, a drug that targets a signaling pathway of lymphangiogenesis, is useful in these patients.[173]

For patients with aneurysms associated with DIC, LMWH has been reported to be useful in resolving the coagulopathy.[174]

The Coagulopathy of COVID-19 Infection

As of December 2022, the pandemic caused by the SARS-Cov-2 (COVID-19) virus has resulted in over 600,000,000 cases and almost 7 million deaths worldwide (data from the Johns Hopkins Coronavirus Resource Center). Two striking features of this infection are its coagulopathy[175] and thrombosis risk.[176] An elevated D-dimer is a prominent feature of the COVID-19 coagulopathy, affecting ~50% of hospitalized patients, with higher levels (>2 μg/mL) correlating with mortality.[177] Although elevated D-dimer levels in COVID-19 infection suggest DIC, other clinical features of the disorder are not consistent with DIC.[177] For example, thrombocytopenia in COVID-19 infection is usually mild and hypofibrinogenemia is uncommon. Additionally, levels of antithrombin, protein C, and protein S are usually preserved,[178] which would limit thrombin generation and suppress D-dimer increases. Clinical features of COVID-19 infection are mostly thrombotic [venous thrombosis incidence ~ 20%][176] instead of hemorrhagic. Indeed, some aspects of COVID-19 infection more resemble a thrombotic microangiopathy, with endothelial cell infection and platelet mircothrombosis, especially in the lungs.[177]

A major clinical question regarding COVID-19 patient management is optimal thrombosis prophylaxis. At this time, a consensus panel of the American Society of Hematology[179] recommends prophylactic intensity anticoagulation. Randomized trials are investigating whether higher intensity anticoagulation is more effective.

Hemolytic Transfusion Reactions

DIC is present in many patients with hemolytic transfusion reactions. Severe, acute hemolytic transfusion events are triggered by antigen-antibody reactions that initiate complement activation and activation of coagulation. These reactions are usually a result of ABO incompatibility. These patients may experience not only DIC but also shock and renal failure. Primary therapy is directed to control of hypotension and restoration of renal blood flow. Fluid, diuretics, and dopamine may be useful therapies.

Snakebite

DIC associated with snakebite differs from the usual form of the syndrome in several respects. Hemorrhage may be relatively inconspicuous,[80] even in the presence of incoagulable blood. When present, it is mainly the result of a vascular toxin. Platelets are often spared, although the venom of the timber rattlesnake (*Crotalus horridus horridus*) contains a unique serine protease that acts as a potent platelet activator.[180] The specific coagulopathy seen in individual patients in large part depends on venom constituents present in the particular snake species.

The treatment of snakebite involves the administration of specific antivenom and intensive supportive care. Heparin therapy has proved marginally effective at best.[181] In general, it is not indicated when specific antivenom is available. Cryoprecipitate should be given to maintain the fibrinogen level over 100 mg/dL.

Pathology

The fatality rate associated with DIC is up to 60%.[182] In many cases, death is attributed to bleeding or thrombosis. Mortality increases with age, underlying comorbidities, the number of clinical manifestations, and the severity of laboratory abnormalities.

The deposition of fibrin in small vessels represents the ultimate result of DIC. In many patients, fibrin can be formed and lysed without significant vascular occlusion. Indeed, at autopsy, fibrin thrombi in some subjects were absent or were demonstrated only with special stains or by electron microscopy. This may result from postmortem lysis or from deposition of thin films of fibrin on the vast endothelial surface and on the erythrocytes. The localization of fibrin thrombi varies somewhat with the cause of DIC. The kidney is the single most common site of fibrin thrombi. Renal lesions range from patchy tubular necrosis to massive bilateral cortical necrosis and have been attributed to a sieving effect of the renal microvasculature. Nonthrombotic endocarditis and pulmonary hyaline membranes have been found in many patients,[84,183] especially those with cancer.

Emerging Therapies for Disseminated Intravascular Coagulation

The recognition of pathogenic mechanisms critical in initiation or progression of DIC has led to investigation of new therapeutic agents in animal models of DIC and clinical trials in humans. High-dose antithrombin replacement therapy had no effect on mortality in patients with severe sepsis.[143] The role of protein C in ameliorating the mortality of sepsis has also been demonstrated; neutralization of protein C activity in an animal model exacerbated the lethal response,[184] and infusion of protein C[185] prevented the lethal response in humans with meningococcemia. An initial clinical trial with recombinant soluble thrombomodulin in patients with sepsis and DIC was positive, but a follow-up trial was negative.[186] Anticoagulant strategies used in clinical trials in the management of DIC associated with sepsis have been reviewed.[187]

PRIMARY FIBRINOLYSIS (FIBRINOGENOLYSIS)

Fibrinolysis is an appropriate response to thrombosis and necessary in the re-establishment of blood flow. This localized response, termed *physiologic fibrinolysis*, is discussed in Chapter 20. The term *pathologic fibrinolysis* has been used indiscriminately to refer to any situation in which in vitro evidence of fibrinolysis was associated with bleeding. In retrospect, it seems probable that fibrinolysis in many cases was secondary to DIC and that in others it represented an essentially physiologic response to anoxia, shock, or stress. In isolated primary fibrinogenolysis, on the other hand, the proteolytic destruction of fibrinogen and other proteins occurs in the general circulation, and severe bleeding may develop. The pathophysiology of fibrinogenolysis may represent a disproportionate or "inappropriate" response to underlying DIC or may result from a defective fibrinolytic mechanism that may be inherited or acquired.

Etiology

Fibrinogenolysis may complicate various disorders, among which severe liver disease is the most common. Fibrinogenolysis is a predominant laboratory feature in several patients with disseminated neoplasms,[188,189] especially urogenital neoplasms.[190] The mechanism for enhanced fibrinolysis in these patients is probably increased tumor cell secretion of plasminogen activators, such as urokinase.[188] Enhanced fibrinolysis has also been associated with cardiac bypass surgery[191] and aortic clamping during vascular surgery.[192] Inherited deficiency of plasminogen activator inhibitor type-1[193] or α_2-plasmin inhibitor[194] also results in hyperfibrinolysis and a bleeding tendency.

Pathophysiology

Fibrinogenolysis is a consequence of the generation of plasmin within the general circulation (plasminemia). Potent plasmin inhibitors (antiplasmins) normally neutralize free plasmin rapidly (see Chapter 20); the result is that the proteolytic effects of this enzyme normally are restricted to fibrin. Fibrinogenolysis occurs only when the neutralizing capacity of the antiplasmins is exceeded.

The proteolytic action of plasmin is nonspecific. In addition to fibrin and fibrinogen, this enzyme may degrade factor VIIIc, factor XIII, other coagulation factors, and a wide variety of other plasma proteins, such as complement and various hormones. Free plasmin may also activate bradykinin, a phenomenon that may underlie the marked hypotension present in some patients with fibrinogenolysis. Thus, *pathologic proteolysis* is an appropriate synonym for *fibrinogenolysis*.

Fibrinogenolysis is activated by mechanisms that are remarkably similar to those that initiate DIC. Therefore, tumor tissue contains plasminogen activators in addition to tissue factor.[188] The secretion of these activators into the circulation may rapidly activate most of the circulating plasminogen.

Hypoxia and hypoperfusion may lead to plasminogen activation and, occasionally, to fibrinogenolysis. However, in many of these patients, bleeding is minimal; when present, it cannot be clearly related to the presence of fibrinogenolysis. In these patients, fibrinogenolysis probably is a nonspecific, essentially physiologic response. Fibrinogenolysis may also result from therapy with thrombolytic agents, as discussed in Chapter 56.

Clinical Features and Laboratory Diagnosis

The clinical picture in most reported cases of fibrinogenolysis is similar to that of DIC. The usual laboratory findings are summarized in *Table 55.2* and are discussed in an earlier section of this chapter. Hypofibrinogenemia may be seen. The PTT, PT, and thrombin time may be prolonged because of the anticoagulant effects of FDPs. Among the coagulation factors, factors V and VIIIc are the most sensitive to the proteolytic action of plasmin; factor XIII is also deficient in some patients. The plasma levels of other factors (e.g., factors VII and IX), including some that are degraded by plasmin in vitro, are usually normal in patients with fibrinogenolysis. Depletion of plasminogen and α_2-antiplasmin and the presence of PAP complexes in the plasma may also be demonstrated in many patients with fibrinogenolysis and in those with DIC and active fibrinolysis.[195]

The standard FDP test does not discriminate between fibrinogen degradation products and fibrin degradation products. Measurements of fibrinopeptide A and the D-dimer, which is a specific indication of degraded cross-linked fibrin, yield normal results in fibrinogenolysis. Thus, patients with hypofibrinogenemia, prolonged PT and PTT values, elevated FDP levels, and a normal D-dimer may have primary fibrinogenolysis. In the absence of intravascular coagulation, paracoagulable complexes containing fibrin monomers do not form in plasma; thus, plasma protamine gelation tests are negative in fibrinogenolysis. Assays for plasminogen and for the various inhibitors of the fibrinolytic enzyme system may reveal a pattern of depletion. In addition to normal results for D-dimer, patients with fibrinogenolysis have normal platelet counts or mild thrombocytopenia with bleeding out of proportion to the reduction in platelet count.

Treatment

Antifibrinolytic agents would seem therapeutically desirable in the treatment of fibrinogenolysis; however, these drugs are hazardous in the presence of DIC. EACA and tranexamic acid are specific and potent inhibitors of fibrinolysis and fibrinogenolysis.[196] The clinical effectiveness of these drugs is dramatic in carefully selected patients.[197] For severe bleeding, EACA should be administered IV with a 5 g loading dose, followed by 1 g/h.[198] The drug can also be given orally. The total EACA dosage should not exceed 30 g in a 24-hour period.[198] Tranexamic acid is a newer antifibrinolytic agent that, like EACA, possesses the ability to bind to the lysine-binding sites of plasminogen, thereby preventing plasmin that is generated from binding to fibrin. The oral dosage of tranexamic acid is 25 mg/kg, three or four times daily. The IV dosage is 10 mg/kg given three or four times daily.

Because antifibrinolytic agents are potentially dangerous drugs in the presence of DIC,[199] the diagnosis of DIC should be excluded in these patients using a specific test, such as D-dimer, before administering these agents. Patients with DIC and a substantial secondary fibrinolytic component should be considered for heparin therapy before administration of antifibrinolytics.[190]

Patients with hormone-refractory prostate cancer and fibrinogenolysis have been reported to benefit from docetaxel, with resolution of bleeding symptoms and laboratory evidence of hyperfibrinolysis.[200] A literature review of hyperfibrinolysis in solid tumor patients identified 21 case reports[201]; 76% of cases were metastatic prostate cancer.

PATHOLOGIC INHIBITORS OF COAGULATION

Circulating anticoagulants are pathologic endogenous inhibitors that can act at any stage in the process of coagulation.[202] Most are antibodies that act as specific inhibitors, inactivating a single coagulation protein. The clinical and laboratory manifestations resemble the corresponding inherited coagulation disorders in many respects. Antibody disorders with wider effects on the coagulation system are sometimes seen, especially in the antiphospholipid-protein antibody (APA) disorders. Other inhibitors of coagulation often have heparin-like activities and are much less common.

Antibodies to Factor VIII

Factor VIII is the most common target of monospecific-acquired anticoagulant antibodies. Conditions that are associated with monospecific factor VIII antibodies are outlined in Table 55.5. Factor VIII inhibitors are termed alloantibodies when they appear in treated hemophilia patients and autoantibodies when they appear in nonhemophilia patients.

Alloantibodies in Hemophilia A

Frequency of Inhibitors

A systematic review of prospective studies found that the cumulative risk of inhibitor development was as high as 39%.[203] However, many patients have only transient inhibitors; the aforementioned systematic review reported an overall prevalence of inhibitors in unselected hemophiliac populations of 5% to 7%.[203] Those at high risk of development of inhibitors include patients with severe hemophilia A with large deletions, nonsense mutations, and intron 22 inversions,[204] or patients with mild or moderate hemophilia A whose factor VIII missense mutation in the A2 domain or near the junction of the C1-C2 domains results in an abnormal factor VIII molecule.[205] Other factors affecting the risk of inhibitor development include the patient's human leukocyte antigen (HLA) class II haplotype, African American ancestry,[206] periods of intensive therapy,[207] and early use of factor VIII at the time of a major bleed or surgery.[208] Additional reports have confirmed these conclusions in patients with mild-to-moderate hemophilia.[209,210] Whether the type of factor VIII product (plasma-derived vs recombinant) is a risk factor for inhibitor development remains controversial. A prospective cohort study of previously untreated hemophilia A patients observed that both plasma-derived and recombinant factor VIII products conferred similar risk of inhibitor development,[211] whereas a randomized trial, Survey of Inhibitors in Plasma-Product Exposed Toddlers, assessing the incidence of inhibitors in previously untreated hemophilia A patients receiving plasma-derived vs recombinant products found that recombinant factor VIII products were associated with nearly twice the rate of inhibitor development as plasma-derived products.[212] At this time, the World Federation of Hemophilia does not express a preference for product type.[213] Patient age at initiation of therapy may also be an independent risk factor for inhibitor development. Patients beginning therapy before 6 months of age had three times the rate of inhibitors than patients beginning therapy after 1 year of age,[214] but a subsequent study showed no association between inhibitor development and age at first FVIII exposure.[215] A UK epidemiology study reported that there is a bimodal distribution of factor VIII antibodies in hemophilia A patients, with peaks in early childhood and >60 years of age.[216]

Induced Antibody Titer

It is recognized, particularly in previously treated hemophilia A patients, that up to 30% of inhibitors are subclinical, occur relatively early (median of 10 days) after product exposure, are of low titer, are transient, and often resolve even with continuing product exposure.[217] Hemophiliacs with inhibitors can be categorized as either strong or weak responders to administered factor VIII. Once an antibody has developed in a hemophiliac, further administered factor VIII may act as an inducing antigen. Additionally, it has been appreciated that certain recombinant factor VIII products, depending on the manufacturing process, may be immunogenic in hemophilia A patients.[218]

Autoantibodies to Factor VIII in the Nonhemophilic Patient

It is estimated that acquired factor VIII autoantibodies are seen in one to two persons per million population annually.[219] Neutralizing immunoglobulin G (IgG) autoantibodies to factor VIII can arise spontaneously in association with various autoimmune and chronic inflammatory diseases, such as systemic lupus erythematosus (SLE), rheumatoid arthritis, and ulcerative colitis.[220] Antibodies to factor VIII can develop in the puerperium,[219] usually appearing at term or within several months after parturition in association with a first pregnancy. The antibody may disappear spontaneously in postpartum patients after 12 to 18 months. Reappearance during subsequent pregnancy seems to be very unusual, and in those patients who have persistent antibodies, remission can occur during a subsequent pregnancy.[221] Acquired hemophilia may also be seen in association with hematologic malignancies and solid tumors[222,223]; certain medications such as penicillin, sulfa antibiotics, chlorpromazine, and phenytoin; and dermatologic conditions such as psoriasis and pemphigus vulgaris. Most often, acquired factor VIII antibodies are idiopathic, particularly in older persons without apparent underlying disease.[219,220]

Pathophysiology of Development of Antibodies to Factor VIII

The genetic and immunologic aspects of induction of anti–factor VIII alloantibodies in hemophilia patients have been extensively reviewed.[224,225] Although inhibitor development is more common in more severely affected patients, inhibitors are also seen in mild hemophilic patients.[226] Specific associations between factor VIII genotype and HLA class II phenotype have been made,[227] but the associations are weak. Genetic influences on inhibitor development are postulated to be additive and polygenic.[227] A high frequency (70%) of inhibitor development is seen in patients with either large, multidomain deletions or nonsense mutations in the factor VIII A3 domain.[228] However, the presence of inhibitors is not consistent, even in a given family with similar factor VIII mutations, suggesting that other factors contribute to induction of factor VIII antibodies.

Another hypothesis as to how inhibitors to factor VIII might occur is that these antibodies arise from the expansion of pre-existing natural factor VIII clones that possess neutralizing properties[229]; such antibodies have been identified from the IgG fraction of plasma from normal people.[229] Clonal expansion of anti–factor VIII antibodies may be modulated by the presence of anti-idiotypic antibodies.[230]

Table 55.5. Conditions Associated With Monospecific Factor VIII Antibodies

Alloantibodies in hemophilia A
Autoantibodies in nonhemophilic patients
Autoimmune disease
Systemic lupus erythematosus
Rheumatoid arthritis
Inflammatory bowel disease
Dermatologic conditions
Psoriasis
Pemphigus vulgaris
Pregnancy (peripartum)
Malignancy
Lymphoproliferative disorders
Plasma cell dyscrasias
Medications: penicillin, sulfa antibiotics, chloramphenicol, phenytoin
Idiopathic

In nonhemophilic patients, the development of autoantibodies to factor VIII is thought to occur due to a breakdown in immune tolerance (IT) that is modulated by a combination of genetic and environmental factors.[219]

Characteristics of Factor VIII Inhibitory Antibodies

The majority of antibodies to factor VIII are IgG inhibitors that appear to be specific for the coagulant subunit of the factor VIII complex (VIIIc).[231] Common epitopes for allo- and autoantibodies include those in the A2 domain or the C2 domain or both. Typically, hemophilic alloantibodies recognize both domains,[232] whereas autoantibodies recognize the C2 domain more frequently than the A2 domain. Circulating factor VIII immune complexes have been identified in plasma from patients with acquired hemophilia A with autoantibodies.[233] IgA or IgM inhibitors are rare, as are antibodies that inhibit both VIIIc and vWF. Antibodies to factor VIII are disproportionately often of the IgG4 subclass and do not fix complement.

Antibodies inactivate factor VIII in a time- and temperature-dependent process,[234] the kinetics and stoichiometry of which are variable. Two types of antibody inhibition are described[235]: type I inhibitors completely inhibit factor VIII activity following second-order kinetics (linear time course of inactivation); these antibodies are seen in hemophilia patients.[236] Type II inhibitors have complex kinetics and do not completely inhibit factor VIII activity; these are autoantibodies seen in nonhemophilic patients.[237] The type II inhibition phenomenon may produce aberrations in the assay system and may explain certain puzzling laboratory features in atypical cases, such as detectable factor VIII clotting activity in a patient with a high-titer inhibitor.

Laboratory Evaluation

Simple mixing techniques based on the PTT usually suggest the presence of an inhibitor. Factor VIII levels are usually undetectable in severely affected hemophilia patients with alloantibodies, but may be detectable in patients with autoantibodies. Specific tests for antibodies involve the demonstration of progressive and time-dependent inactivation of factor VIII in vitro by the plasma or serum of the patient. Methods for detecting low-titer inhibitors and for quantifying the levels of antibody have been devised,[238] and standardized inhibitor units (the Bethesda unit in the United States[239] and the New Oxford unit in Britain)[240] have been defined. In the Bethesda assay, in vitro tests are performed at 37 °C using 2-hour incubation mixtures of various dilutions of patient plasma with normal plasma. The inhibitor titer is the reciprocal of the dilution of inhibitor plasma that neutralizes 50% of normal factor VIII activity. Because the Bethesda assay may underestimate the inhibitor titer in acquired hemophilia, it is recommended that the titer should be calculated from the lowest dilution that results in 50% residual factor VIII activity after the incubation period. The New Oxford method measures residual activity at 37 °C after a 4-hour incubation. A Bethesda unit is generally equivalent to 1.21 Oxford units. The standard Bethesda assay does not control pH, permitting variable low-level inactivation of factor VIII by nonimmunologic mechanisms. The Nijmegen modification controls pH, thus improving classification of positive and negative samples.[239] The Nijmegen modification of the Bethesda assay has been endorsed by the ISTH.[241] Although an inhibitor unit does not imply that any specific number of factor VIII units infused into the patient will neutralize any specific number of inhibitor units, the titer provides a general estimate of the initial likelihood of response to infusion of factor VIII products.

Clinical Manifestations

The bleeding manifestations resulting from antibodies to factor VIII are often similar to those seen in severe hemophilia A.[219] However, prolonged or unexpectedly severe hemorrhage may occur after comparatively trivial trauma, postoperatively, or postpartum. Soft-tissue or muscle hematomas, hematuria, and spontaneous and intractable epistaxis seem relatively more common; hemarthrosis is relatively less common in acquired hemophilia than in congenital hemophilia A. Figure 55.4 illustrates soft-tissue hematomas occurring in a nonhemophilic patient with an acquired inhibitor to factor VIII. When antibodies arise in patients with mild hemophilia A, bleeding typical of severe deficiency may develop; more significantly, the bleeding may be refractory to replacement therapy. This condition may have serious consequences, and fatal events are seen in 10% to 20% of clinically symptomatic patients.[219,242] Antibodies to factor VIII arising during pregnancy may cross the placenta.

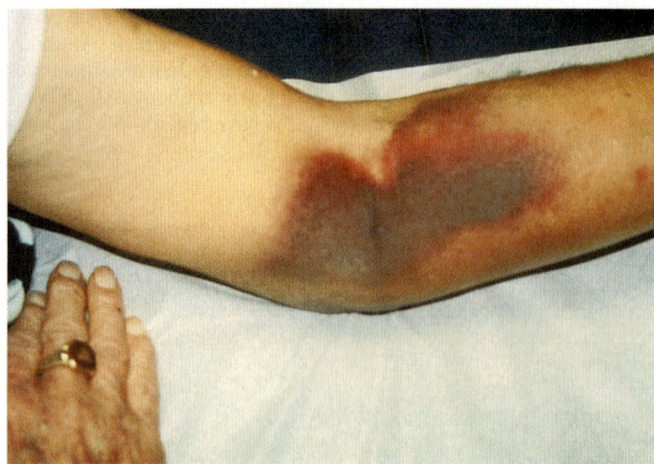

FIGURE 55.4 Soft-tissue hemorrhage in a 76-year-old man with a high-titer factor VIII inhibitor. This patient has a history of ischemic cardiomyopathy and diabetes and developed spontaneous extremity bruising as shown. The antihuman factor VIII antibody titer was 10 Bethesda units. (Courtesy of Alan Grosset.)

Treatment

The treatment of bleeding in patients with antibodies to factor VIII presents several challenges.[243] No adequate randomized trials have been conducted to evaluate different forms of therapy or to investigate the timing and sequence of their application; therefore, practical treatment decisions are based on expert consensus with estimates of benefits and risks deduced from retrospective literature review and consideration of each patient's circumstances and comorbidities. A consensus group from the United Kingdom has published guidelines on treatment of inhibitors in patients with hemophilia,[244] and an international panel has summarized treatment recommendations for acquired hemophilia.[245] An algorithm that has some general applicability is shown in Figure 55.5. As a first step, basic clinical information should be obtained, including whether the inhibitor arose in the setting of hemophilia or is acquired, the severity of bleeding, anticipated surgical procedures, inhibitor titer and persistence, prior inhibitor response and relation in time to previous factor infusions, possible triggering events such as recent medication exposure or pregnancy, and the presence of other diseases. For example, the mere presence of an inhibitor may in itself not warrant immediate therapy because many inhibitors are present in low titer and are often transient. Spontaneous remissions may occur in a significant number of patients, particularly if the inhibitor develops during the puerperium.[221] At the other end of the spectrum, an unfortunate clinical scenario might involve significant spontaneous clinical hemorrhage, a persistent high-titer inhibitor, and incidental comorbidities such as cardiac, hepatic, or renal insufficiency. Principles of management include stopping bleeding using bypass therapy, eradication of the inhibitor with immunosuppression, and recognizing and treating any underlying disorder that may have triggered autoantibodies to factor VIII.

The inhibitor titer and its prior response to factor VIII infusion is of particular use in guiding therapeutic decisions (Figure 55.5). In patients with low-titer inhibitors who do not have any clinical bleeding and for whom no surgical procedures are foreseen, the most reasonable approach may be to monitor the abnormal laboratory finding. For patients with minor bleeding who have residual factor VIII activity >5% of normal with low inhibitor titers, recombinant

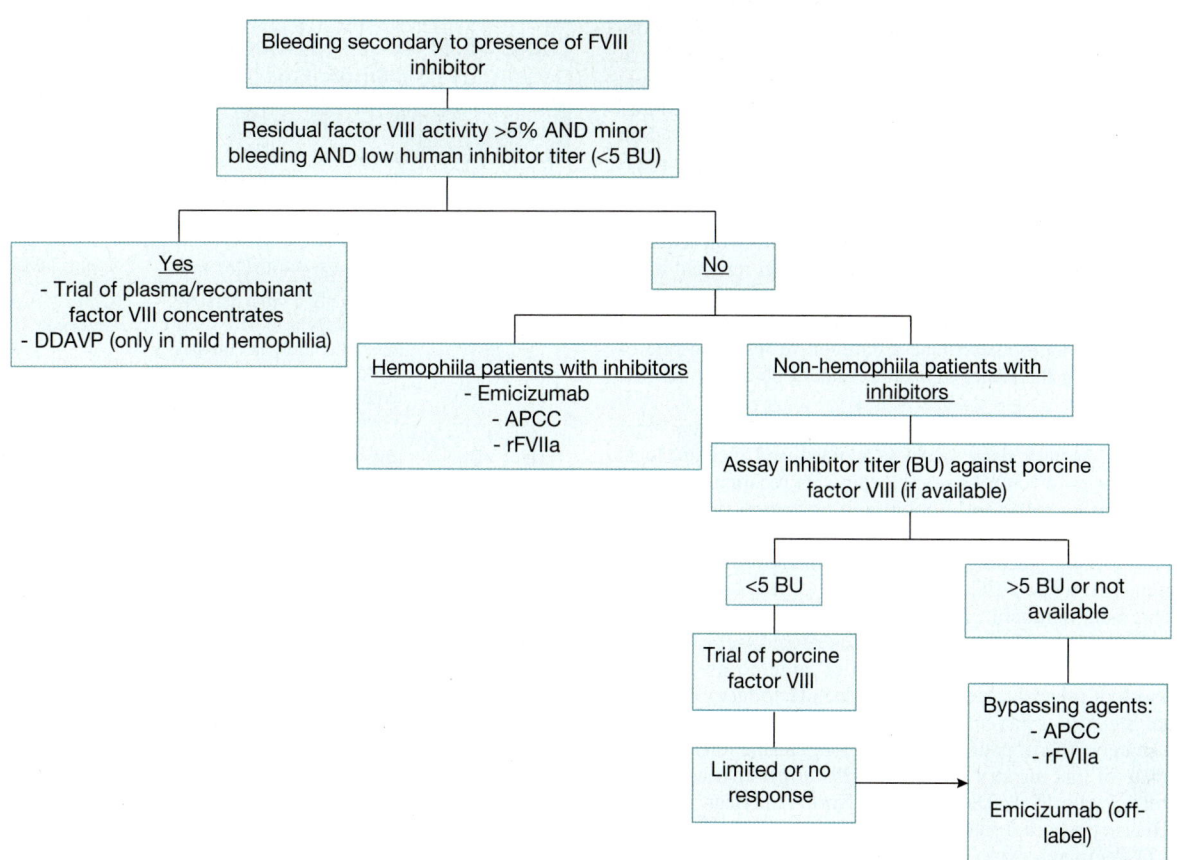

FIGURE 55.5 A strategy for management of factor VIII inhibitors in hemophilic and nonhemophilic patients. Key decisions are based on antihuman and antiporcine factor VIII inhibitor titers. Multiple options for patients not responding to human or porcine factor VIII are available. The underlined options are preferred. Emicizumab is a new treatment option for these patients. Immunosuppression options include rituximab, steroids, and cytotoxic drugs. APCC, activated prothrombin complex concentrate; BU, Bethesda units; DDAVP, 1-desamino-8-D-arginine vasopressin. (Information in this figure is from the literature, including Morrison AE, Ludlam CA. Acquired hemophilia and its management. *Br J Haematol.* 1995;89:231-236.)

or plasma-derived human factor VIII concentrates could be considered only if bypassing agents or recombinant porcine factor VIII are unavailable.[245] As a rule, replacement therapy with factor VIII in the usual doses is ineffective. If clinical bleeding mandates active therapy, patients with a low Bethesda inhibitor titer (<5 U/mL), particularly if they are known to be low responders, may respond to high purity or recombinant human factor VIII given as a large initial 150 U/kg bolus followed by a continuous infusion of 1000 U/h. The therapeutic response to human factor VIII should be clinically assessed; factor VIII levels and repeat assays of inhibitor titer response may be helpful. Desmopressin could be considered in patients with mild hemophilia and a low-titer inhibitor[244] but is of limited utility and no longer recommended for acquired hemophilia.[219,245]

In patients with high-titer inhibitors (>5 Bethesda U/mL) or a history of an anamnestic response, or routinely in medical centers that prefer to reduce the uncertain risk of inducing an increased inhibitor titer, bypassing agents including APCCs (factor VIII inhibitor–bypassing activity, FEIBA) and rVIIa are usually first-line treatments.[244,245] Therapy with human factor VIII is seldom successful in patients with high-titer antibodies. A typical dose for FEIBA during the acute bleed setting is 50 to 75 U/kg every 8 to 12 hours.[219] FEIBA has been successfully used as a prophylaxis therapy for hemophilia patients with inhibitors at a dose of 85 U/kg three times per week.[246]

rVIIa is another treatment option for inhibitor patients.[247] This drug was originally thought to exert activity by binding to tissue factor at sites of vascular injury to initiate coagulation. More recent data indicate that at the pharmacologic concentrations of factor VIIa achieved during rVIIa therapy, there may be platelet-dependent, tissue factor–independent mechanisms to mediate hemostasis.[248] The standard dose of rVIIa is 90 μg/kg every 2 hours for serious bleeding or 90 μg/kg every 3 hours for mild-to-moderate bleeding. Recent trial data indicate that a single rVIIa dose of 270 μg/kg is an effective home treatment for hemarthroses in hemophilia patients with inhibitors.[249] rVIIa can also be used in the prophylaxis setting for hemophilia patients with inhibitors at a dose of 90 to 270 μg/kg daily.[250] Continuous infusion of rVIIa is also effective, targeting factor VII levels to 30 to 40 U/mL. Both rVIIa and FEIBA therapy are associated with potential thrombotic complications; a comparative evaluation of the thrombotic event rate of rVIIa vs FEIBA revealed that rVIIa was associated with approximately three-fold more thrombotic events than APCC.[251]

There is no consensus as to the best therapeutic approach between these two options. A Cochrane systematic review found that the efficacy and safety of FEIBA vs rVIIa were similar in hemophilia A patients with inhibitors.[252] A European registry reported the efficacy and safety of FEIBA vs rVIIa in treating bleeding events in acquired hemophilia and concluded that efficacy between the two products was similar.[253] Typically, if one agent is not successful in stopping bleeding, the other agent should be used.[254] For patients refractory to both drugs used as single agents, sequential therapy with FEIBA and rVIIa has been reported.[255]

Another therapeutic option in acquired hemophilia is recombinant porcine factor VIII which is approved for use in the United States, Canada, and Europe.[256] Obtaining an antiporcine antibody titer is useful, but as a rule of thumb, the initial antiporcine titer is often 5% to 10% of the antihuman titer. However, the antiporcine titer may rapidly rise after administration of porcine factor VIII, resulting in decrease treatment efficacy. International consensus groups recommend porcine factor VIII an as appropriate first-line treatment option.[245]

Immunosuppressive therapies are not indicated when inhibitors arise in patients with congenital hemophilia A, but they are effective in the setting of nonhemophilic patients.[245] Numerous treatment options exist.[245,254] Corticosteroids alone (e.g., prednisone in doses of 1.0 mg/kg/d) produced improvement in 58% of patients, whereas combination of cyclophosphamide (1-2 mg/kg/d) with prednisone achieved remission in 80% of patients in one European registry.[253]

Rituximab, a monoclonal antibody to the CD20 antigen on B cells, has been reported to be effective in case series of patients with acquired factor VIII antibodies.[257,258] Cyclosporine A has been reported to be useful in patients failing first-line eradication therapy.[259] A literature review[260] of the efficacy of intravenous Ig (IVIg) in the treatment of acquired factor VIII antibodies found a cumulative response rate of only 12%, suggesting that other modalities should be attempted first for these patients.

In addition, procedures or medications (antiplatelet drugs) that would increase hemostatic risks should be avoided, and ancillary local therapeutic measures to control minor bleeding are recommended and may in themselves be sufficient. Antifibrinolytic therapy, such as the administration of EACA or tranexamic acid, may be helpful, especially for oral or nasal bleeding; however, this therapy should not be used in conjunction with APCCs or rVIIa.

In patients with hemophilia A who have developed alloantibodies to factor VIII, infused factor VIII provokes a rapid increase in the antibody titer. However, the administration of large doses of factor VIII for periods of months to years may produce IT to factor VIII. An international registry of patients treated with this approach reported that approximately 70% of patients achieved long-lasting tolerance.[261] A 1997 update of this registry found that 52% of patients were successfully treated with IT.[262] Data from the North American Immune Tolerance Registry reported an overall success rate of 70%.[263]

Several IT regimens exist. The International Immune Tolerance Study compared high-dose (200 U/kg daily) vs low-dose (50 U/kg daily) factor VIII. Both dosage regimens were equivalent in terms of inducing tolerance; however, the low-dose regimen was associated with more bleeding.[264] The use of factor VIII products that contain vWF may be more effective in IT induction.[265] The addition of immunosuppressive agents to standard IT has had varying success.[266,267] The topic of IT induction in hemophilia A and B patients has been reviewed.[268] The cost-effectiveness of IT therapy has been demonstrated.[269]

In the past 5 years, several emerging therapies have been developed, including substitutive and rebalancing therapies, to treat hemophilia A patients with FVIII inhibitors. The first substitutive therapy is emicizumab, a humanized bispecific, monoclonal antibody that mimics the cofactor function of activated FVIII. In clinical studies, the use of emicizumab in hemophilia A patients with FVIII inhibitors resulted in substantial improvements in health-related outcomes including reduction in number of bleeding events, missed workdays, and days of hospitalization.[270,271] Globally, emicizumab is approved for routine prophylaxis in hemophilia A patients with FVIII inhibitors in over 100 countries. Rebalancing therapies targeting tissue factor pathway inhibitor, antithrombin, and APC are currently undergoing clinical trials. These innovative approaches and their nuances have been reviewed.[272]

Monospecific Antibodies to Other Coagulation Factors

Table 55.6 summarizes certain conditions associated with antibodies to other coagulation factors.

Factor IX

Inhibitors of factor IX have been demonstrated in approximately 5% of patients with hemophilia B[273] and rarely in previously normal persons (acquired hemophilia).[274] Hemophilia B patients who acquire antibodies to factor IX often have deletion or nonsense mutations.[275] One series of eight hemophilia B inhibitor patients found that antibodies typically were IgG1 and IgG4 and that the antibodies targeted the Gla domain and protease domain epitopes of factor IX.[276] rVIIa[277] or IT therapy[263] has been used to treat these patients, although IT for hemophilia B inhibitor patients may be less effective than that for hemophilia A inhibitor patients.[278] Patients with antibodies to factor IX may experience anaphylaxis when treated with factor IX–containing products[278]; rVIIa may be an option for this patient group, or a desensitization protocol may be effective.[279] A British consensus group has published guidelines on treating factor IX inhibitor patients,[244] and an international registry of factor IX inhibitor patients has been established.[280] The rebalancing therapies targeting tissue factor pathway inhibitor and antithrombin may be a promising therapy for factor IX inhibitor patients.[272]

Factor V

Inhibitors of factor V[281] have developed spontaneously in previously normal older persons after administration of antibiotics, mainly beta-lactams,[282] and after surgical procedures. More rarely, factor V inhibitors have been associated with malignancies, autoimmune conditions such as bullous pemphigoid, and COVID-19 infections.[282,283] These antibodies are usually of IgG isotype. It is a rare entity with

Table 55.6. Acquired Disorders Associated With Deficiency of a Single Coagulation Factor

Deficient Factor	Specific Inhibitors[a]	Other Disorders
Fibrinogen	Hereditary afibrinogenemia; lupus erythematosus; liver disease	—
Prothrombin	Previously normal persons	Lupus inhibitors
Factor V	Previously normal persons; often associated with streptomycin; rarely in inherited factor V deficiency; postoperative patients who received bovine thrombin	Chronic myelocytic leukemia
Factor VII	Bronchogenic carcinoma, acquired immunodeficiency syndrome	Aplastic anemia, liposarcoma
Factor VIII (VIIIc)	Hemophilia A; puerperium; inflammatory disorders; drug reactions; in the absence of underlying disease	—
von Willebrand factor	Previously normal persons; lymphoproliferative disorders; rarely in von Willebrand disease; thrombocytosis	Wilms tumor
Factor IX	Hemophilia B; rarely in previously normal persons	Nephrotic syndrome; Sheehan syndrome; Gaucher disease
Factor X	—	Amyloidosis; upper respiratory infection; other associations
Factor XI	Lupus erythematosus; rarely in inherited factor XI deficiency and chronic lymphocytic leukemia; previously normal persons	—
Factor XII	Lupus erythematosus, rarely	Nephrotic syndrome; chronic myelocytic leukemia
Factor XIII	Previously normal persons, often associated with isoniazid; rarely in inherited factor XIII deficiency; other associations	Acute and chronic leukemia; Crohn disease

[a]Evidence suggests that these inhibitors are antibodies. In patients with inherited deficiencies of the various factors, their development is usually related to transfusion of blood or blood products.

an estimated incidence of <0.5 per million person-years.[284,285] Alloantibodies to factor V may occur in factor V–deficient patients who receive blood products.[286]

Previously, an iatrogenic coagulopathy had been identified: the occurrence of antibodies to thrombin and factor V in patients treated with bovine thrombin during surgery.[286,287] Bovine thrombin contains small amounts of bovine factor V that can elicit a potent immune response. In a large surgical series of patients exposed to bovine thrombin, more than 95% of patients developed antibodies to bovine thrombin or factor V, and 50% of these patients had antibodies cross-reacting to human coagulation proteins.[288] No increased risk for adverse outcomes was observed in those with elevated antibody levels to bovine or human coagulation proteins after surgery.[288] A review of the literature found that one-third of bovine thrombin–induced factor V inhibitor patients developed bleeding.[287] This iatrogenic condition led to bovine thrombin falling out of favor, especially with the development of human recombinant thrombin.[289]

In contrast to bovine thrombin–induced factor V inhibitors, spontaneous factor V inhibitors have significant bleeding; 72% in one literature review of reported cases with 17% of these cases resulting in death.[287] Another literature review identified a bleeding mortality rate of 12% in patients with factor V antibodies not because of exposure to bovine factor V or noninherited-acquired factor V antibodies.[285] Treatment of these bleeding episodes typically involves platelet transfusion or fresh frozen plasma. In several patients with severe hemorrhage, platelet transfusions were therapeutically more effective than plasma.[285,290,291] This clinical benefit of platelet transfusions likely relates to platelet α-granule content of factor V which is released at sites of bleeding to improve local hemostasis. Plasmapheresis,[292] immunosuppression, and IVIgG[293] have been reported to be effective in resolving antibodies to factor V. In some cases, these antibodies resolve spontaneously.

A small number of patients have been described with thrombosis symptoms associated with factor V antibodies. These patients may or may not[294] have coexisting antiphospholipid (aPL) antibodies.

von Willebrand Factor

Acquired von Willebrand disease (vWD) has been reported in association with a variety of disorders, primarily including patients with lymphoproliferative disorders, myeloproliferative disorders, solid tumors, autoimmune disease, aortic stenosis, and artificial heart devices. An international registry identified lymphoproliferative and myeloproliferative disease as accounting for more than 60% of acquired vWD.[295] A literature review concluded that most cases of acquired vWD result from an antibody that recognizes high-molecular-weight multimers of vWF and mediates subsequent antigen-antibody clearance.[296] Another mechanism for the development of this disorder includes adsorption of vWF by tumor cells[297] or platelets. Acquired vWD has also been reported in patients with aortic stenosis[298] and in patients with ventricular-assist devices and artificial hearts.[299,300] In these cardiac conditions, vWF is subjected to shear stress and proteolysis.[300] Ristocetin cofactor activity is usually decreased, whereas factor VIII activity may be normal.[296] In most patients, the hemostatic abnormalities disappear when the underlying disorder is treated.[301] For patients with acquired vWD associated with monoclonal gammopathy of uncertain significance, a scoping review of 75 published cases found that the overall clinical success rates for hemostatic control using DDAVP, vWF concentrates, and IVIg were 43.8%, 33.3%, and 85.4%, respectively.[302] Other strategies including myeloma-directed therapies, plasma exchange, rFVIIa, and antifibrinolytics were also helpful, whereas immunosuppressive agents including corticosteroids and rituximab were largely ineffective.[302]

Acquired vWD may also be associated with angiodysplasia and gastrointestinal bleeding.[303] Loss of vWF may be linked to increased ADAMTS13 activity and enhanced angiogenesis (see Chapter 21).[304]

Factor XIII

Inhibitors of factor XIII have been described after transfusions in patients with inherited deficiency of this proenzyme and in previously normal persons.[305] Many of the latter group had received isoniazid,[306] and it was suggested that this drug may alter factor XIII in such a manner that it becomes antigenic.[307] These inhibitors may recognize the zymogen, impair the activation of factor XIII by thrombin, or be directed against the cross-linking sites of fibrin, or to the B-subunit.[308,309] A summary of 93 factor XIII inhibitor patients found that approximately 50% of cases were idiopathic, and the remainder were associated with autoimmune disorder and malignancy.[310] Therapeutic options include factor XIII replacement therapy (plasma and cryoprecipitate), rVIIa, as well as inhibitor eradication options (steroids, cyclophosphamide, rituximab, etc).[309] A factor XIII concentrate, fibrogammin, if available, may also be useful.[310] A survey of hemophilia treatment centers reported that approximately 38% of inherited factor XIII–deficient patients developed antibodies as a treatment complication[311]; these patients may require bypassing agents to treat bleeding.

Fibrinogen and Prothrombin

A precipitating antibody to fibrinogen has been demonstrated after transfusions in patients with hereditary afibrinogenemia.[312] Acquired hypofibrinogenemia is usually seen in acute DIC. Dysfibrinogenemia may occur in patients with liver disease or hepatoma, or in plasma cell disorders (discussed in the section "Deficient or Aberrant Synthesis of Coagulation Factors"). Antibodies to prothrombin have also been reported.[313] Acquired hypoprothrombinemia usually occurs in the setting of the lupus anticoagulant (LA) when patients have antibodies to prothrombin that clear prothrombin activity from blood.[314]

Factor XI

A survey of prevalence of acquired inhibitors to factor XI in patients with inherited factor XI deficiency found that approximately 5% of patients with severe deficiency developed antibodies after plasma therapy.[315] Of those factor XI–deficient patients homozygous for a null allele, one-third developed antibodies.[315] A combination of low-dose rVIIa and tranexamic acid was reported to be safe and effective for such patients requiring surgery.[316] Specific inhibitors of factor XI have been described primarily in association with autoimmune disease.[317,318]

Factor X

Acquired factor X deficiency has been frequently reported in amyloidosis (see section, Acquired Deficiencies of Single Coagulation Factors). However, antibodies to factor X are very uncommon. A literature review identified 34 cases of acquired factor X deficiency not associated with vitamin K deficiency or amyloidosis, with most cases associated with a preceding viral illness.[319] Yet in these 34 cases, inhibitors to factor X were only established in 9 cases.[319] The coagulopathy resolved in all cases.[319] Treatment modalities include using PCCs,[320] IVIg, steroids, or plasma exchange.[319,321]

Factor VII

Antibodies to factor VII are rare, with fewer than 20 cases reported in the English literature.[322] They have been associated with lung cancer[323] and human immunodeficiency virus infection[324] and with no apparent disorder.[325,326] Immunosuppression has been used successfully in anecdotal case reports of autoantibodies to factor VII.[327]

Tissue Factor

Antibodies to tissue factor are very uncommon, with one group reporting two patients who developed anti–tissue factor antibodies after liver surgery.[328] Similar to patients who acquire antithrombin and anti–factor V antibodies after use of topical bovine thrombin,[286,290] the patients who developed anti–tissue factor antibodies were both treated with a topical hemostatic agent prepared from bovine tissue that contained tissue factor. The antibodies to bovine tissue factor did not cause clinical bleeding, but did prolong PT values.[328]

Antiphospholipid-Protein Antibodies: Lupus Anticoagulants and Anticardiolipin Antibodies

Historical Considerations and Nomenclature

The two best-known clinical types of APAs are traditionally called LA and anticardiolipin (aCL) antibodies. These antibodies are associated in some patients, but not in others, with clinical illness[329-331] of varying severity. Individual patients may manifest arterial or venous thromboembolic disease, recurrent pregnancy loss, thrombocytopenia or other cytopenias, and neurologic and skin abnormalities. The clinical importance, particularly of the LA or higher titer aCL antibodies, has been increasingly recognized; these antibodies or their functional consequences are found in approximately 10% of patients with venous thromboembolic events.[332,333] Bleeding is quite uncommon, and when present, it is usually the result of severe thrombocytopenia, platelet dysfunction, hypoprothrombinemia, or the effects of an underlying disease. On the other hand, thrombosis and its many manifestations are common.

Synonyms for LA and aCL antibodies include aPL antibodies, APAs, and autoantibodies to phospholipid-binding plasma proteins.[334] The associated clinical manifestations including thrombosis are variously called the LA syndrome, antiphospholipid syndrome (APS), or antiphospholipid-protein syndrome. APS without a known well-defined autoimmune disease is termed primary APS (PAPS). A few patients with APA develop an acute, severe, multiple organ APS illness. These patients are designated as having catastrophic APS (CAPS).

The existence of these antibodies was first detected more than 60 years ago when it became apparent that approximately 15% of patients with active SLE have a false-positive venereal disease research laboratory (VDRL) test.[335] The VDRL test assesses antibody reactivity to "reagin" (antigen), an acidic-phospholipid complex that is chemically extracted from bovine heart tissue. Reagin consists of a mixture of lecithin, cholesterol, and cardiolipin. A nonspecific antibody reaction to reagin is also seen less often in other autoimmune disorders and in some apparently healthy patients. Other laboratory assays discussed in this section identified a family of antibodies that were initially thought to have direct specificity to various phospholipids, although it is now known that the antibodies recognize phospholipid-protein complexes. The proteins often serve a critical cofactor role,[336] and the antibodies collectively are thus most accurately called APAs.[337]

Coagulation assays are sensitive to some of these antibodies. Plasma samples from some patients with SLE, often those with the abnormal VDRL tests, show an in vitro inhibitor effect in several coagulation assays. This association gave rise to the term LA.[338] Most often, a prolonged PTT result that is not corrected on mixing with normal plasma is observed; other phospholipid-dependent assays, including the modified Stypven time (dilute Russell viper venom time [DRVVT]), are also affected. Despite persistent clinical use, it is now known that most patients with an LA phenomenon do not have SLE. Moreover, clinical thrombosis is much more often seen than is bleeding with APS antibodies. Patients with SLE occasionally have inhibitors to other hemostatic factors,[339] but these inhibitors are not considered LAs.

In addition to the biologically false-positive VDRL results and the paradoxic in vitro LA effect, laboratory studies found a third phenomenon, initially detected by radioimmunoassay: antibodies to cardiolipin.[340] In aCL antibody assay systems, serum Igs bind to various anionic phospholipid-protein complexes, most commonly to cardiolipin in a coated microwell enzyme-linked immunosorbent assay (ELISA). The sensitivity and specificity of this assay are substantially higher than those of the VDRL. A phospholipid-binding protein, β_2-glycoprotein I ($\beta_2$gpI), has been identified,[341] and antibodies to this antigen can also be demonstrated in patients with APS.[342] Thus, the most useful assays to evaluate patients for aPL antibodies include the LA, aCL antibodies, and antibodies to $\beta_2$gpI.

Epitope Specificity

In these disorders, the antibodies were initially thought to react with anionic phospholipids directly, but the presence of specific plasma proteins associated with phospholipids is now known to be of great importance.[343] In the case of LAs, the seemingly paradoxic discordance between laboratory screening test results and clinical symptoms is frequently the consequence of antibodies that bind to a complex of phospholipid-bound prothrombin.[314,344] This antibody binding impairs the function of the standard prothrombin-binding synthetic anionic phospholipids[345] that are used routinely in the laboratory to replace platelets in phospholipid-dependent coagulation assays, such as the PTT. Other more natural phospholipids, or platelets themselves, are less affected by this phenomenon and are used in some assays as correction factors in mixing studies.

In the case of aCL antibodies, especially in autoimmune and drug-induced aCL, $\beta_2$gpI[346] serves as a mandatory protein cofactor.[341] Patient-derived antibodies directed against $\beta_2$gpI that have LA activity have also been reported.[347] $\beta_2$gpI is a 57-kDa plasma protein with an uncertain physiologic role, but it is often considered a noncomplement member of the complement-control family of proteins, with structural similarity to complement factor H. One study reported that $\beta_2$gpI inhibited complement activation at the level of C3.[348] $\beta_2$gpI has a number of anticoagulant activities,[349] but inherited deficiency of $\beta_2$gpI has no thrombophilic association. The antibodies in these settings are often of the IgG isotype, are relatively persistent and high in titer, are associated with an LA phenomenon in approximately 60% of patients, and are clearly associated with the clinical syndromes discussed subsequently. IgM and IgA antibodies occur less often. aCL antibodies are not directed primarily against cardiolipin itself, but against epitopes formed after $\beta_2$gpI binds to anionic phospholipid membranes or anionic synthetic surfaces. One study observed that pathogenic antibodies targeted an epitope in domain 1 of $\beta_2$gpI and that these antibodies had LA activity.[350] $\beta_2$gpI may also mediate aCL binding to endothelial cell membranes.[351] Other proteins have been occasionally implicated as possible obligatory cofactors, including annexin A5,[352] annexin A2,[353] factor Xa, protein C, protein S, and vimentin. Anti-$\beta_2$gpI antibodies have been reported to induce acquired resistance to APC.[354]

It was previously thought that APA recognized neoepitopes of the above phospholipid-binding proteins expressed on cell surface binding. Another hypothesis is that the true antibody target is an appropriate density ("clustering") of proteins bound to phospholipid surfaces, which is necessary for antibody recognition.[355] For example, based on in vitro data, it has been proposed that $\beta_2$gpI acts as an antigen in vivo only when the antigen ($\beta_2$gpI) clusters on membrane surfaces such as endothelium. When clustering occurs, this increased antigenic density allows antibody recognition to occur, leading to antibody binding and endothelial cell activation and potentially triggering cellular events resulting in thrombosis.[356] *Figure 55.6* illustrates how this phenomenon might occur. Additional studies found that $\beta_2$gpI undergoes a conformational change (circular to "fishhook") upon cell binding to anionic phospholipids, leading to clustering[357] and antibody binding.[358] Involvement of the MyD88 signal transduction pathway in antibody-mediated endothelial cell activation has been described,[359] and others have reported involvement of the p38 mitogen–activated protein kinase pathway.[360] Receptors that have been described that could possibly mediate the APA response include a toll-like receptor on the endothelium.[331] A recent report identified endothelial cells as the major target for anti-$\beta_2$gpI antibodies and characterized the signaling pathway involving the apolipoprotein E receptor 2.[361]

In other settings, particularly those related to infection, the aCL antibodies are often of IgM isotype, are often of low titer and relatively transitory, and have no identified cofactor protein.[336] Although $\beta_2$gpI is an absolute protein cofactor requirement for aCL activity in autoimmune settings, it may, in contrast, be inhibitory in the infection-related circumstance. The clinical association of IgM antibodies with thrombophilia is less strong,[362] particularly thrombosis occurring after drug administration,[363] although exceptions to this generalization have been noted.[364]

Another key question related to the pathogenesis of APS is, how are aPL antibodies generated? One potential explanation is that oxidation of $\beta_2$gpI increases its immunogenicity, and patients with APS have increased amounts of oxidized $\beta_2$gpI.[365]

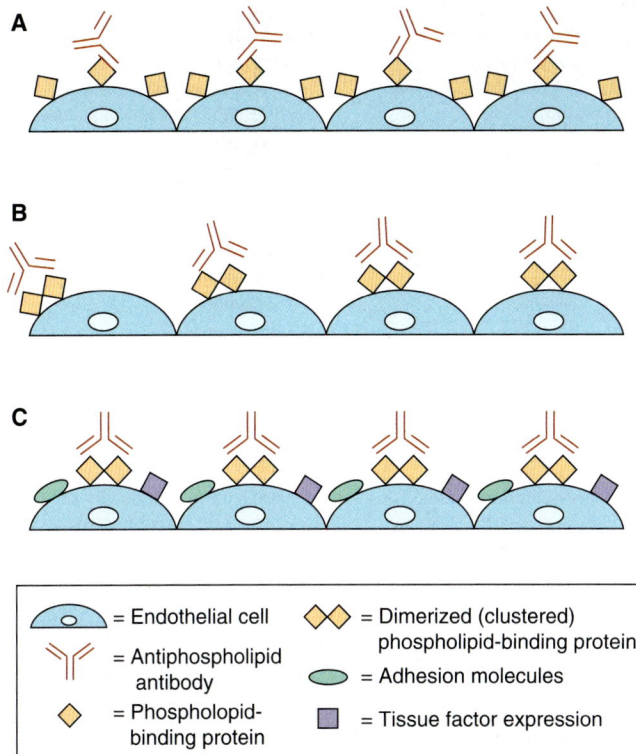

FIGURE 55.6 A proposed mechanism by which antiphospholipid antibodies induce endothelial cell activation and thrombosis. A, Endothelial cells express a phospholipid-binding protein (e.g., $\beta_2$gpI). In the absence of high antigenic density ("clustering"), antibody binding is inefficient. B, Endothelial cells display dimerized ("clustered") antigen, which allows for efficient antibody binding, resulting in endothelial cell activation and promotion of thrombosis (C).

Mechanism of Thrombosis

Potential mechanisms to explain how aPL induces thrombosis[331,332] include (1) endothelial cell activation, (2) oxidant-mediated vascular injury, (3) interference with the function of phospholipid-binding proteins in regulating coagulation, (4) platelet activation, and (5) complement activation. In the first hypothesis, aPL antibodies directly bind to endothelium to upregulate expression of adhesion molecules and cytokine secretion. In the second hypothesis, autoantibodies to oxidized low-density lipoprotein occur with aCL antibodies, and aCL antibodies recognize oxidized phospholipids and phospholipid-binding proteins.[366] In the third hypothesis, aPL antibodies may interfere with the anticoagulant functions of protein C or annexin V or enhance procoagulant activity.[329,352,353] In the fourth hypothesis, complement activation by aPL antibodies leads to neutrophil expression of tissue factor.[367] Additional pathogenic mechanisms for APS have been reviewed.[368]

Immunologic studies lend strong support for a direct pathophysiologic role of these antibodies in the clinically observed thrombotic syndromes.[369] In animal models using standardized vessel injury to induce thrombosis, either passively conferred APA[370] or active induction of antibody with APA or $\beta_2$gpI[371] resulted in thrombosis; this suggested that APAs are not merely epiphenomena of thrombi arising for other reasons but, in some cases, play a direct role in initiation, propagation, or maintenance of thrombosis. Immunization of mice or rabbits with $\beta_2$gpI produces two populations of antibodies: one with specificity for $\beta_2$gpI alone without binding to phospholipids and the other with specificities for both cardiolipin and $\beta_2$gpI.[372] This dual specificity of antibodies is also seen with those aPLs that are present in patients with autoimmune diseases.

The concept of hexagonal-phase configuration has been popularized. This configuration is thought to arise in vivo in response to membrane damage.[373] Normally, polar heads of phospholipids exist on the external surface, whereas in the hexagonal phase, lipid cylinders exist with internal aqueous channels formed by polar head groups.[374] LA and aCL may represent antibodies generated in response to these neoantigens. APAs have been generated in mice immunized with hexagonal-phase phospholipid[375]; these antibodies reacted with cardiolipin and possessed functional LA activity.

The precise cause of thrombosis in APS is uncertain and is likely multifactorial.[368] Presumably, APAs act by interfering with coagulation,[330] possibly involving dysfunction or apoptosis[376] of endothelial cells, platelets, and coagulation proteins, and affect pregnancy outcome by interfering with embryo implantation and fetal development.[329]

Specific mechanisms of thrombosis that have been implicated include inhibition of APC,[330] acquired free protein S deficiency, platelet activation, and abnormalities in the antigenic levels or activity of endothelium-derived hemostatic factors, including inhibition of prostacyclin secretion, fibrinolysis, nitric oxide synthesis, or disruption of annexin A5 or A2.[368] High-avidity anti–protein C antibodies have been postulated as a marker for recurrent venous or arterial thrombosis despite therapeutic anticoagulation.[377] The thrombogenicity of APAs may also result from their interference with endothelial cell phospholipids required for antithrombin and proteins C and S anticoagulant activity, and increased endothelial cell expression of the following procoagulants: tissue factor, vWF, platelet-activating factor, and plasminogen activator inhibitor type-1.[329-331,333,368,378,379] Tissue factor was identified as a mediator of complement-induced APS fetal loss in a mouse model.[366,380]

Epidemiology and Clinical Associations

Young, apparently healthy control subjects are reported to have a prevalence of 1% to 5% of aPL antibodies.[381] In patients with systemic lupus, aPL occurs in 12% to 34%. After prolonged follow-up, APS may develop in more than 50% of patients with systemic lupus.[329]

LA and aCL antibodies have been reported in a variety of clinical disorders, including SLE and other autoimmune and connective tissue diseases and in disorders that are unrelated to SLE (Table 55.7). The presence of phospholipid-binding antibodies could in some cases be an epiphenomenon. In other cases, APAs may be of profound direct etiologic relevance. In general terms, although there are individual patient exceptions, clinical symptoms are seen less often with aCL than with LA, particularly when APAs are associated with infection or medication, are of low titer, and are of IgM isotype.

Interpretation of estimates of APA frequency must consider the sensitivity of the diverse assay systems that have been used by investigators. Different LA assay systems have been tested with plasma samples from a rigorously defined group of patients with the antiphospholipid-protein syndrome, confirming the importance of variables such as the concentration and composition of phospholipids used in the assay,[382] phospholipid reagent conformation,[374] and so forth.

In a large series of internal medicine patients, 7% were APA positive, and 2% fulfilled the criteria of antiphospholipid-antibody syndrome.[383] The most commonly associated diseases were cancer and chronic or acute alcoholic intoxication. In another study, elevations of APA were found in approximately 20% of an unselected autopsy population, 10% of age- and sex-matched controls, and 2% of healthy normal subjects.[384]

Inhibitors of the lupus type were originally recognized in association with SLE. The prevalence of LA in patients with SLE strongly depends on the type of LA assay system used; three standard PTT reagents detected LA in only 10% of SLE patients.[385] A modified PTT with a reduced concentration of phospholipid detected LA activity in approximately 50% of SLE patients.[385,386] The kaolin clotting time, a test similar to the PTT, detected LA in 70% of patients with SLE.[387] LA activity was associated with higher mortality in SLE patients[388] and in patients without SLE.[389] APAs have been seen in other connective tissue disorders, including rheumatoid arthritis and Behçet syndrome.

APAs are present in many patients with malignancy.[390] APAs have been associated with monoclonal gammopathy of undetermined

Table 55.7. Clinical Diagnoses Associated With Antiphospholipid-Protein Antibodies

Primary antiphospholipid-protein antibody syndrome
Autoimmune disorder with no apparent cause
Secondary autoimmune disorders
Systemic lupus erythematosus; other autoimmune and connective tissue diseases; drug induced: procainamide, hydralazine, quinidine, phenothiazines, penicillin
Malignancies
Leukemia, lymphoproliferative and plasmacytic disorders, solid tumors, essential thrombocytosis
Infections
Viral, bacterial, protozoal, fungal
Neurologic disorders
Liver disease
Valvular heart disease
Peripheral arterial disease
Chronic renal failure
Sickle cell disease
Ethylenediaminetetraacetic acid–dependent pseudothrombocytopenia

Table 55.8. Criteria for Diagnosis of the APS

Clinical Event	Laboratory Abnormality
Venous thrombosis	Positive lupus anticoagulant test (according to guideline in *Table 55.11*)
Or	Or
Arterial thrombosis	Positive anticardiolipin antibody test (moderate-titer or high-titer IgG or IgM antibodies)
Or	Or
	Positive $\beta_2$gpI antibody test (titer >99th percentile, IgG or IgM antibodies)
	And
Small-vessel thrombosis	Laboratory abnormality should persist for two or more occasions at least 12 wk apart
Or	
Complications of pregnancy	
One or more unexplained deaths of normal fetuses at or after 10 wk of gestation with normal fetal morphology	
One or more premature births of normal neonates before 34 wk of gestation	
Three or more unexplained consecutive spontaneous abortions before 10 wk of gestation, excluding anatomic, hormonal, and chromosomal abnormalities	

A diagnosis of definite APS requires the presence of at least one clinical event and at least one laboratory abnormality.
Abbreviations: APS, antiphospholipid syndrome; Ig, immunoglobulin.
Criteria reprinted from Miyakis S, Lockshin MD, Atsumi T, et al. International consensus statement on an update of the classification criteria for definite antiphospholipid syndrome (APS). *J Thromb Haemost.* 2006;4(2):295-306. Copyright © 2006 International Society on Thrombosis and Haemostasis. With permission.

significance and Waldenström macroglobulinemia. APAs have been identified in liver disease, the prevalence increasing significantly as the liver disease progresses; APA positivity was as high as 80% in patients with alcoholic hepatitis or cirrhosis.[391] The antibodies have been found in many infections, including hepatitis C,[392] infection with human immunodeficiency virus,[393] human T-cell lymphotrophic virus-1–associated tropical spastic paraparesis, Q fever, and malaria.[394] Children with viral infections often acquire a transient LA effect. Perhaps as a result of the structural changes in the red cell membrane with increased hexagonal-phase content, APAs are common in sickle cell disease.[395] Patients with transient ischemic attacks and cardiac valve lesions had a high incidence of APAs.[384] APAs have been seen in a variety of unrelated neurologic disorders.[396] Patients with essential thrombocytosis have an increased prevalence of APA and increased risk of thrombosis.[397]

Several medications are associated with APA, most often, phenothiazines such as chlorpromazine,[363] procainamide,[398] quinine and quinidine,[399] hydralazine, and penicillin.[400] APAs were common in patients with ethylenediaminetetraacetic acid–dependent pseudothrombocytopenia.[401] aCL antibodies can occur in both active and quiescent Crohn disease, usually without concomitant LA expression,[402] but their role in the thrombotic complications that can occur in the active phase of this disease is uncertain.

APA positivity is a common finding in patients with idiopathic thrombocytopenic purpura,[403] with either LA or elevated aCL antibodies in almost one half of patients. Moreover, APA levels were not influenced by immunosuppressive therapy with steroids and are not related to the activity of idiopathic thrombocytopenic purpura.

aCL antibodies and, less often, LA are seen in apparently healthy people,[381,404] especially in the elderly.[405] In studies of normal blood donors, 5% to 10% have aCL antibodies, often present transiently and in relatively low titer without a concomitant LA effect; these donors do not have an increased risk of developing thrombosis.[406] An inherited predisposition to the development of lupus inhibitors was suggested by their presence in familial studies.[407] Further investigations have suggested associations with certain HLA types.[408,409]

Clinical Manifestations

Although LAs are immunologically distinct from aCL antibodies, clinical manifestations associated with each antibody appear to be similar. Clinical experience suggests that venous thrombosis is more likely associated with the LA, and arterial thrombosis is more likely associated with high-titer aCL antibodies. However, a literature meta-analysis found that the LA was a stronger risk factor for all thrombosis.[410]

The antiphospholipid-antibody syndrome is characterized by the clinical events of pregnancy morbidity or thromboembolic disease (arterial, venous, or small vessel) or both (*Table 55.8*).[411] These clinical features are most highly associated with aPL antibodies in prospective studies.[411] Older definitions included immune thrombocytopenia as a clinical event, but the newer classification omits thrombocytopenia. A wide variety of clinical features may be seen with APA.[330,331,411-414] However, many patients with APA are asymptomatic. A proportion of asymptomatic patients develop SLE[415] or other disorders.[416] The diverse clinical manifestations of APA are listed in *Table 55.9*.

Arterial and Venous Thromboembolic Disease

The most common clinical presentation of patients with LA or aCL antibodies or both is arterial or venous thromboembolism,[330,417,418] affecting up to 70% of patients in some series but averaging approximately 30% to 40% of patients in most studies.[386,418,419] The most common site is extremity deep vein thrombosis, but occasionally, unusual sites are involved, such as the axillary, retinal, and hepatic veins and cerebral venous sinus thrombosis. Cerebral thrombosis, often heralded by repeated transient ischemic attacks, is a common arterial lesion.[330,420] Mesenteric artery occlusion, adrenal infarction, gastrointestinal ischemia or ulceration, and subclavian thrombosis with "pulseless" disease have also been described. Multiple cerebral infarcts with dementia in addition to coronary occlusions have occurred in unusually young age groups.[421] A paradoxic syndrome of cerebral infarction with concurrent severe thrombocytopenia and

Table 55.9. Clinical Manifestations of Antiphospholipid Antibodies

Asymptomatic

Arterial and venous thromboembolism

Avascular osteonecrosis

Hematologic

Cytopenias: thrombocytopenia, autoimmune hemolytic anemia, leukopenia

Coagulopathy: platelet dysfunction, prothrombin deficiency, lupus anticoagulant

Neurologic

Acute ischemia (cerebrovascular accident, transient ischemic attack, encephalopathy); severe migraine; multiple infarct dementia; cognitive dysfunction; seizures

Dermatologic

Livedo reticularis; acrocyanosis (distal cutaneous ischemia, ulceration, gangrene); widespread cutaneous necrosis; pyoderma gangrenosum–like skin lesions; anetoderma

Cardiopulmonary

Marantic endocarditis; myocardial ischemia and infarction; intracardiac thrombotic mass; peripheral arterial disease; thromboembolic; and non-thrombotic pulmonary hypertension

Obstetric

Recurrent spontaneous abortion; intrauterine growth restriction; pre-eclampsia; chorea gravidarum; low Apgar scores; prematurity

Catastrophic antiphospholipid syndrome

---

bleeding has been reported in several cases.[420] Antibodies to $\beta_2$gpI are highly associated with venous thrombosis,[422] and in other studies, assays for the LA correlated best with thrombosis, compared with assays for other APAs.[410,423] Another unusual ischemic syndrome associated with APA is avascular osteonecrosis.[424]

Thrombocytopenia

Moderate immune thrombocytopenia is noted in approximately 50% of patients with lupus inhibitors, but in many cases, it apparently is the result of the underlying disorder.[425] Immune thrombocytopenia is no longer considered a clinical criterion for diagnosis of APS.[411] When bleeding occurs in patients with aPLs,[426] this is generally attributed to coexistent thrombocytopenia, platelet dysfunction,[427] prothrombin deficiency,[428] or other underlying coagulopathies. Other cytopenias may be associated with APA, including autoimmune hemolytic anemia and leukopenia.

Neurologic Syndromes

Various neurologic disorders have been linked with APA, including dementia, migraines, chorea, seizures, transverse myelopathy, Guillain-Barré syndrome, mononeuritis multiplex, transient global amnesia, and myasthenia gravis. Many of these disorders are not associated with ischemia or thrombosis, and the pathologic relationship of these disorders with APA is uncertain. A consensus statement on stroke and APS proposed criteria to determine the likelihood that APA is associated with ischemic stroke.[429] A literature survey determined that the presence of APA in patients with ischemic stroke did not predict recurrence of stroke or differential response to treatment and that routine screening for APA in these patients was not warranted.[430] A recent review summarized neurological manifestations of APS.[431]

Dermatologic Disorders

A variety of ischemic-dermatologic syndromes have been associated with aCL antibodies, including livedo reticularis, acrocyanosis (distal cutaneous ischemia, ulceration, and gangrene), widespread cutaneous necrosis, and pyoderma gangrenosum–like skin lesions.[411,432] Livedo reticularis is more prevalent among APS patients with systemic lupus, and in females.[411]

Cardiac Disorders

A high incidence of APA is seen in patients with peripheral arterial disease who experience an associated increased risk of early graft thrombosis.[433] This may justify routine testing for APA before reconstructive vascular surgery, with consideration of perioperative antiplatelet agents or anticoagulation. Some reports have noted the presence of APA in survivors of myocardial infarction.[434] A variety of valvular heart lesions is associated with APS.[411] The consensus group recommends that patients with biopsy-proven myocardial small-vessel thrombosis or those with intracardiac thrombi be considered for meeting criteria for APS. Coronary artery disease also fulfills the APS thrombosis criterion.[411]

Pulmonary Disorders

Ischemic and thrombotic pulmonary disease is linked to APA, including pulmonary embolism, pulmonary hypertension, intra-alveolar pulmonary hemorrhage, and adult respiratory distress syndrome.[435,436] The latter syndrome has been reported in patients with CAPS.[436]

Obstetric Aspects

APAs are associated with obstetric complications,[329,411,437,438] including intrauterine growth restriction, pre-eclampsia, chorea gravidarum, and, primarily, recurrent spontaneous fetal loss (RSFL). Pregnancy losses in women with aPLs are often caused by fetal death despite normal fetal karyotypes. Spontaneous fetal loss is perhaps most common in the first trimester, but paradoxically, early first-trimester pregnancy losses are relatively less common than in other patients with recurrent fetal loss.[439] The international consensus statement listed obstetric criteria for diagnosis of APA: (1) one or more unexplained deaths of a morphologically normal fetus at or beyond the 10th week of gestation (with normal fetal morphology); (2) one or more premature births of a morphologically normal neonate before the 34th week of gestation because of pre-eclampsia, eclampsia, or placental insufficiency; or (3) three or more unexplained consecutive spontaneous abortions before the 10th week of pregnancy (with maternal anatomic or hormonal abnormalities, and paternal and maternal chromosomal causes excluded).[411]

There is a significantly increased incidence of elevated APA in women with a history of two or more miscarriages in the first trimester of pregnancy.[440] Women with a history of RSFL should be tested for both LA and aCL antibodies.[441] Repeat testing is important because only 66% of LA-positive, 37% of IgG aCL-positive, and 36% of IgM aCL-positive women had a positive test result on repeat evaluation. Laboratory screening for LA is confounded in pregnancy because altered coagulation factor concentrations in normal pregnancy may change the observed normal range of coagulation tests, including the PTT. In two studies, the DRVVT was the most frequently positive test for the LA in this population. Rigorous adherence to diagnostic criteria is particularly appropriate in pregnancy because treatment may require potentially hazardous antithrombotic therapy. Elevated maternal serum levels of α-fetoprotein[442] or human chorionic gonadotrophin[443] are common in women with aPLs and are significantly associated with fetal loss. Maternal APA testing may be appropriate if prenatal screening reveals an elevated human chorionic gonadotropin level, and ultrasonography demonstrates an otherwise normal singleton gestation.

It is generally considered not appropriate to screen for APA in asymptomatic pregnancies without a history of RSFL.[444] APAs were identified at the first prenatal visit in almost 25% of healthy pregnant women.[445] LA appears to be much rarer than aCL antibodies in pregnancy.[446] It appears that women with isolated IgM aCL or with low levels of IgG aCL are a distinct group that is not at risk for APA-related complications beyond the risk conferred by their medical histories.[447]

Although the mechanism by which APA causes recurrent pregnancy loss has not been fully explained, these antibodies may induce intervillous thrombosis and intravillous infarctions, resulting in poor placental perfusion, and have been shown to affect cytotrophoblast tissue in vitro. The thrombotic phenomenon may be mediated by aPL antibodies interfering with trophoblastic annexin V.[330,448]

The role of inflammation and the complement pathway in APS-associated pregnancy complications was reported.[449] Anticoagulants that prevented complement activation (unfractionated or LMWH) were successful in preventing pregnancy loss in an animal model of APS; anticoagulants that did not inhibit complement activation (fondaparinux and hirudin) did not prevent pregnancy loss. These data suggest that the beneficial effects of anticoagulants in APS-associated pregnancy loss result from inhibition of complement activation.[449]

Seronegative Antiphospholipid-Antibody Syndrome

While the consensus criteria define a homogeneous group with APS, patients with clinical manifestations highly suggestive of APS, but who have repeatedly negative conventional antibodies may be classified as having seronegative APS (SNAPS). Various "noncriteria" antibodies can be identified in about one-third of these patients.[450] A recent review summarized noncriteria clinical manifestations and laboratory tests.[451]

Catastrophic Antiphospholipid-Antibody Syndrome

Some patients with APA develop an acute, severe, multiorgan illness[329,331,436,452] characterized by diffuse small-vessel ischemia and occlusion with extensive tissue damage, including myocardial infarction, limb ischemia, DIC, and a high mortality rate of 50%.[453] The patients present with a dramatic illness, often without an obvious precipitating event, that prompts consideration of a wide differential diagnosis, including severe lupus vasculitis, thrombotic thrombocytopenic purpura, or severe DIC. The syndrome is defined by clinical involvement of at least three different organ systems with histologic evidence of thrombosis.[453] Typically, small-vessel thrombotic lesions occur, with common sites of involvement including the kidney, lung, central nervous system, heart, and skin.[452,453] In a larger series of CAPS patients, nearly one-half of the cases had systemic lupus, and 40% had PAPS.[454] Precipitating factors for development of CAPS included infections, trauma/procedures, cancer, and subtherapeutic anticoagulation.[454] LA activity and, particularly, high aCL antibody titers are usually present. Central nervous system symptoms and hypertension are common, and leukocytosis and a significantly elevated sedimentation rate are often also present. The clinical manifestations of this syndrome can include all the symptoms and signs indicated in Table 55.9. Effective therapies include therapeutic anticoagulation, steroids, IVIg, plasma exchange, and cyclophosphamide.[453] A literature review of rituximab use in CAPS found encouraging results.[455] A summary of CAPS registry cases reported that anticoagulation with steroids ± plasma exchange/IVIg was associated with at least a 70% success rate.[456] Based on these data, a consensus group recommended this combination therapy as first-line treatment for CAPS.[457] Eculizumab has been found to be effective in some patients with refractory CAPS.[452] A recent study found that patients with CAPS had high rates of rare germline variants in complement regulatory genes similar to that of patients with atypical hemolytic uremic syndrome.[458] The implications of complement in the pathophysiology of thrombosis in CAPS have been summarized.[459]

Laboratory Diagnosis of Antiphospholipid-Protein Antibodies

LA and high-titer aCL antibodies have similar clinical implications, although studies suggest a higher thrombotic risk in patients with the LA.[410,423] In patients with SLE, the LA is the best predictor for both venous and arterial thrombosis. The laboratory should perform both fibrin-based coagulation assays to detect LA and solid-phase ELISA assays for aCL and $\beta_2$gpI antibodies in patients suspected of having APA.

A considerable array of phospholipid-responsive laboratory tests, such as the PTT, dilute PTT, kaolin clotting time, and DRVVT, may serve to screen for the LA.[336] LA may be defined as an immunoglobulin (IgG, IgM, IgA, or a mixture) that interferes with one or more of these in vitro, phospholipid-dependent coagulation tests. A more recent definition of the LA would be antibodies to $\beta_2$gpI or to prothrombin that prolong phospholipid-dependent coagulation assays. Coagulation tests that are phospholipid independent are not affected by LA. Unless concurrent additional factor deficiencies are present, the standard PT is usually normal because of the large amount of phospholipids in this reagent. No individual test seems to have a universal detection rate; this observation may reflect LA subtypes with distinct activities or the requirement of various cofactors. Consequently, it is recommended to perform at least two independent assays for the LA.[411,460] A simplified algorithm approach for diagnosis of the LA has been described that uses two assays, the DRVVT and a hexagonal-phase assay.[461] Comparative studies suggest that activated PTT reagents with reduced levels or different types of phospholipids are more sensitive than routine PTT reagents.[336,462] Platelet-poor plasma should be used in these screening assays, particularly if fresh-frozen plasma samples are to be tested.[463] Two LA guidelines have reviewed these issues.[464,465] Table 55.10 indicates some of the clinical and laboratory differences between specific anticoagulant antibodies to particular factors, such as factor VIII and LA. Other nonspecific anticoagulants are uncommon but include the heparin-like anticoagulants discussed in the section "Other Acquired Coagulation Disorders." Confirmatory tests for LA based on activated PTT or DRVVT include abnormal mixing studies with normal plasma and correction with mixing using phospholipids, such as lysed washed platelets (platelet neutralization procedure), or with added hexagonal-phase phospholipids.[466]

The ideal test to identify the LA is controversial; some investigators reported the kaolin clotting time to be the most sensitive test.[462,467] On the other hand, some DRVVT assays are more able to identify LA associated with thrombosis.[468] A subgroup of patients with unexplained thrombosis with antibodies to phosphatidylethanolamine as the only abnormal APA test has been identified.[469] Optimal detection of the LA requires more than one of the phospholipid-dependent assays described earlier.[411,464,470] This latter suggestion is supported by reports that different phospholipid-dependent coagulation tests detect different populations of LA antibodies.[471] Table 55.11 summarizes the recommendations of an ISTH consensus group on laboratory diagnosis of LA.[411]

Several clinical points are worth stating. The search for LA or aCL antibodies should not be abandoned even if normal plasma in a mixing study corrects the test patient plasma, particularly in a human immunodeficiency virus–positive population.[472] It is sometimes important for the clinician to discern the possible effect that heparin in the test patient plasma can have on the confirmatory laboratory assay; satisfactory correction procedures should be resistant to heparin, and many commercial LA reagents have heparin neutralizers. LA testing is usually feasible in patients being treated with vitamin K antagonists.

Direct oral anticoagulants are associated with false-positive LA results, particularly with many DRVVT testing systems.[473,474] When feasible, LA testing should be avoided while using these agents. However, clinical practicalities may require testing at the medication's trough level, together with careful adjudication of any positive result. Apixaban appears to have a lesser incidence of false-positive LA tests.[474] Argatroban has also been associated with false-positive LA results.

aPLs may also be detected by ELISA[411] or by radioimmunoassay. Commercial ELISA systems are reasonably well standardized. The aCL antibody assay used to improve sensitivity and specificity has undergone several modifications. Using anti-$\beta_2$gpI–dependent assay systems is useful to discriminate between transiently positive aCL antibodies that are associated with infection, which characteristically do not have a $\beta_2$gpI cofactor requirement, and those aCL antibodies associated with an increased risk of thrombosis.[475] IgA aCL antibodies should not be considered a laboratory criterion for diagnosis of APS.

Definitional standardization of the criteria for clinical and laboratory APA has been published.[329,411] For the diagnosis of APS, in addition to a clinical event (e.g., at least one venous, arterial, or

Table 55.10. Comparison of Factor VIII Antibodies and Antiphospholipid-Protein Antibodies

Clinical Event or Laboratory Test	Factor VIII Antibodies	Antiphospholipid-Protein Antibodies
Bleeding	Often severe	Uncommon
Thrombosis	Rare	Common
Obstetric complications (abortion and intrauterine fetal death)	Rare	Common
Prothrombin time	Normal	May be prolonged
Thrombin time	Normal	Occasionally prolonged
Thrombocytopenia	Rare	Common
Inhibitory effect in plasma mixtures	Usually time dependent	Often is instantaneous; occasionally, mixing studies show time-dependent inhibition
Prothrombin level	Normal	Occasionally deficient
Factor VIII level	Deficient; one-stage assay curve is aberrant with low-affinity antibodies	Normal when assayed in a dilute system; all one-stage assay curves are aberrant
Anticardiolipin and $\beta_2$gpI antibodies	Rare	Common
Phospholipid or platelet correction of abnormal assay result	No	Usually

Abbreviations: $\beta_2$gpI, β_2-glycoprotein I; Ig, immunoglobulin.

Table 55.11. Laboratory Diagnosis of Lupus Anticoagulant: International Society on Thrombosis and Haemostasis Criteria

- Prolongation of at least two phospholipid-dependent coagulation tests with the use of platelet-poor plasma (e.g., the activated partial thromboplastin time, dilute prothrombin time, dilute Russell viper venom time, kaolin clotting time). The DRVVT should be the first test considered.
- Failure to correct the prolonged coagulation time by mixing patient and normal plasma.
- Confirmation of lupus anticoagulant by demonstrating correction of the prolonged coagulation time by addition of excess phospholipids or freeze-thawed platelets.
- Exclusion of alternative coagulopathies using specific assays (e.g., factor VIII antibodies).

Abbreviation: DRVVT, dilute Russell viper venom time.
Diagnostic criteria from Levine JS, Branch DW, Rauch J. The antiphospholipid syndrome. *N Engl J Med.* 2002;346:752-763; Brandt JT, Triplett DA, Alving B, Scharrer I. Criteria for the diagnosis of lupus anticoagulants: an update. On behalf of the Subcommittee on Lupus Anticoagulant/Antiphospholipid Antibody of the Scientific and Standardisation Committee of the ISTH. *Thromb Haemost.* 1995;74:1185-1190. Additional laboratory details and patient selection criteria are discussed in Devreese KMJ, de Groot PG, de Laat B, et al. Guidance from the Scientific and Standardization Committee for lupus anticoagulant/antiphospholipid antibodies of the International Society on Thrombosis and Haemostasis: Update of the guidelines for lupus anticoagulant detection and interpretation. *J Thromb Haemost.* 2020;18(11):2828-2839.

small-vessel thrombosis, pregnancy morbidity/mortality), positive laboratory tests for LA, aCL, or $\beta_2$gpI antibodies (in medium or high titer) should be found on two occasions at least 12 weeks apart (*Table 55.8*). It is recommended that aCL antibodies be measured by a standardized ELISA for $\beta_2$gpI–dependent antibodies.[329,411] Although consensus criteria require persistence of the laboratory abnormality for at least 12 weeks, in clinical practice, a functional definition taking into account the number of clinical manifestations and the titer of aCL antibodies or positivity for the LA on even a single occasion may help categorize patients as having definite, probable, or doubtful APS and may direct immediate treatment options. A "triple positive" profile (positive results for all three assays: LA, aCL antibodies, and $\beta_2$gpI antibodies) has been identified as a strong independent risk factor for thrombosis.[476] A 2018 update of ISTH recommendations on APS laboratory testing confirms previous recommendations and does not recommend additional APA tests.[477]

Even if the patient is asymptomatic, lupus inhibitors should always be identified correctly when discovered, despite the costly, time-consuming laboratory study required. If the cause for a prolonged PTT is not identified, the necessity for definitive laboratory evaluation almost invariably arises again, often in the context of an emergency. This may result in the unnecessary use of blood products and a delay of required surgical procedures.

Primary Prevention

Depending on the clinical symptoms, patients with APA may need no treatment or may need anticoagulant and/or immunosuppressive therapy. Although spontaneous remissions are uncommon and aCL antibodies and LA can be associated with life-threatening thromboembolic events, only 10% to 15% of asymptomatic patients with APA develop these complications. Based on the uncertainty of predicting when thrombotic events might occur in non-SLE patients with aCL or LA positivity, as well as the risks of anticoagulation, neither aspirin alone nor the combination of aspirin with low-dose warfarin is routine in the primary prevention setting, with the possible exception of use in individuals with additional thrombotic risk factors,[478] or as a short-term intervention when additional thrombophilic hazards such as immobilization or surgery are anticipated. Conversely, with SLE and a positive LA or persistent medium-high aCL levels, aspirin is recommended.[478]

Hydroxychloroquine, an immunosuppressive agent used to treat patients with SLE, decreases thrombosis risk in SLE patients,[479] perhaps by interfering with aPL antibody binding to phospholipid.[480] Although well tolerated, its utility in patients without SLE has not been confirmed.

Thrombosis Treatment

Patients with significant thrombotic events (e.g., deep vein thrombosis, arterial ischemia, or fetal loss) are appropriate candidates for antithrombotic therapy. Two randomized trials investigated the optimal intensity of warfarin therapy in APS patients.[481,482] Both studies found that high-intensity warfarin (INR 3.1-4.0 or 4.5) was not superior to standard-intensity warfarin (INR 2.0-3.0).[481,482] Long-term treatment with oral anticoagulation therapy is advised because of the high rate of recurrence even if the venous or arterial occlusion occurred many years previously.[483,484] Patients receiving oral anticoagulants had no recurrence over 8 years, whereas patients in whom anticoagulant drugs had been discontinued had a 50% probability of a recurrent venous thromboembolic episode after 2 years and an almost 80% probability of recurrence after 8 years.[485] This strategy is supported by a study that found that APS patients with thrombosis benefited from prolonged oral anticoagulation because persistent elevation of aCL levels predicted an increased risk of thrombosis recurrence and death.[486] This mortality signal has been confirmed in a more recent study.[389] Many investigators follow this approach,[330] unless all laboratory evidence of LA and aCL in patients in whom high titers were initially detected or in whom a thrombotic risk was attributed to APA has been continually absent for at least 6 months; no other thrombophilic risk is present; and close surveillance is feasible. An alternative treatment strategy in APS patients is to consider single-positivity test results for $\beta_2$gpI or aCL antibodies as a lesser risk for recurrent thrombosis, and perhaps less intense or shorter duration treatment periods.[330]

APS patients with ischemic stroke can receive either aspirin or low-intensity warfarin (INR 2.0-3.0).[487] For noncerebral arterial thrombosis, combined therapy with low-intensity warfarin (INR 2.0-3.0) plus aspirin (81 mg) is recommended.[487]

Numerous case series[488] and two prospective trials[489,490] indicate that warfarin is preferable to direct-acting oral anticoagulants in treating APS thrombosis. Given these data, the latest 2021 American College of Chest Physicians (CHEST) guidelines suggest the use of warfarin over direct-acting oral anticoagulants in patients with confirmed APS being managed with anticoagulant.[491] Occasionally, maintenance therapy with enoxaparin[333] or fondaparinux may be required.

Patients with the uncommon LA hypoprothrombinemia syndrome who either have bleeding or need surgery may benefit from steroid therapy or IVIgG.[492]

Patients with the LA and acute thrombosis pose difficulty in terms of monitoring heparin anticoagulation. The usually prolonged PTT value seen with the LA renders this test unreliable. These patients can be monitored using heparin assays, which are available by automated methodology (see Chapter 56). Alternatively, patients can be treated using a LMWH, without the necessity for laboratory monitoring (see Chapter 56).

In those patients with an LA and hypoprothrombinemia, or an LA that affects the PT, the use of the INR to monitor anticoagulation has been questioned. These patients may require monitoring with a test that is insensitive to the LA, such as a prothrombin-proconvertin assay or a chromogenic factor X assay.[493]

Corticosteroid use often diminishes or abolishes the coagulation abnormalities and immune thrombocytopenia of APA syndrome within a short time. However, for most patients, the role of steroids, other immunosuppressive agents, or aspirin is uncertain. Although immunosuppression with cyclophosphamide in pulse form is effective in reducing elevated antibody levels, there is often a rapid rebound to pretreatment levels shortly after discontinuation of the therapy. Consequently, additional therapies with aspirin or steroids or more aggressive immunosuppression are not used unless recurrent thrombotic or ischemic events are seen despite optimal warfarin therapy. High-dose corticosteroid therapy has equivocal efficacy and considerable toxicity and is reserved for treatment of underlying comorbid conditions such as active lupus and not for the laboratory phenomena of the antiphospholipid-antibody syndrome itself.

In patients with CAPS who experience multisystem involvement, intensive treatment with corticosteroids, immunosuppression, IVIg, plasmapheresis, or eculizumab (for refractory cases) may be useful.[333,452,455] In one literature analysis of CAPS therapy, the highest response to therapy occurred in patients treated with anticoagulation and steroids (64%).[454] Immune thrombocytopenia and autoimmune hemolytic anemia in patients with APA are treated similarly as in patients without APA.

Obstetric Treatment

Because the risk of pregnancy loss in women with APS and prior pregnancy loss may exceed 60%, a history of recurrent fetal loss is an indication for treatment during pregnancy. Several randomized studies have provided information about useful treatment strategies in pregnancy-associated APS.[329,494] IVIg is of no benefit in these patients, and heparin may be more effective than aspirin. A meta-analysis recommends that a combination of unfractionated heparin (5000 U subcutaneously twice daily) and low-dose aspirin be used.[494] A recent systematic review found a small increase in live births and a small reduction in preeclampsia in women taking heparins, with or without aspirin.[495] For dosing, consensus guidelines recommend "prophylactic or intermediate-dose unfractionated heparin or prophylactic LMWH combined with low-dose aspirin (75-100 mg/d)."[496] For women with APS and prior thrombosis, aspirin and therapeutic LMWH are recommended.[331]

Transfusion-Associated Coagulation Abnormalities

The administration of blood products in a volume >1.5 times the patient's estimated blood volume or replacement of total blood volume in <24 hours constitutes massive blood transfusion.[497] Traditional resuscitation efforts were initiated with large volumes of crystalloid and packed red cell transfusions; a new paradigm is termed "damage control resuscitation" which includes administration of tranexamic acid for cases of uncontrolled hemorrhage, use of a massive transfusion protocol with fixed blood product ratios, avoidance of large volume crystalloid use, and usage of permissive hypotension.[498-500] Some protocols include using blood viscoelastic hemostasis assays, such as thromboelastography (TEG) and rotational thromboelastometry (ROTEM).[501] On the other hand, literature reviews on the clinical utility of TEG and ROTEM monitoring demonstrate insufficient data to recommend their routine use.[502] This remains an area of active research.

The importance of core body temperature on hemostasis parameters has been demonstrated; at a temperature of 33 °C, platelet function is impaired. Below 33 °C, both coagulation factor activity and platelet function are reduced.[503]

Bleeding Associated With Extracorporeal Circulation

Defective hemostasis with cardiopulmonary bypass is associated with multiple contributory causes, including hemodilution of coagulation factors, inadequate neutralization of heparin, acquired platelet dysfunction, and thrombocytopenia. These latter two defects are further discussed in Chapter 53. In general, extracorporeal-circulation–induced hemostatic defects may be ascribed to activation of platelets and coagulation proteins by artificial surfaces.

Platelet dysfunction (acquired storage pool defect) is considered the major hemostatic insult induced by bypass.[504] Although DDAVP was shown to reduce bleeding and transfusion requirements in these patients in earlier studies, subsequent trials indicated no benefit from DDAVP.[505] Aprotinin should not be used in this setting.[506] A practical approach to this group of patients has been summarized.[507]

Drug-Induced Coagulation Abnormalities

Broad-spectrum antibiotics, such as the β-lactam antibiotics, may induce a coagulopathy by inhibition of vitamin K synthesis by gut bacteria and direct inhibition of essential carboxylation reactions.[14] A number of antibiotics may also inhibit platelet function (see Chapter 53).

L-Asparaginase produces hypofibrinogenemia and deficiency of other coagulation factors.[508] Hematin produces a complex coagulopathy.[509] Valproic acid therapy has been associated with acquired vWD.[510]

Acquired Deficiencies of Single Coagulation Factors

An uncommon phenomenon is the development of deficiency of a single coagulation factor during the course of an acquired disorder. Isolated deficiency of factor X is well documented in patients with primary amyloidosis and amyloidosis associated with multiple myeloma.[511] Factor X levels in these patients do not rise even after massive replacement therapy, and studies using ^{125}I-labeled factor X suggest that this proenzyme is bound to subendothelial amyloid fibrils in blood vessels.[512] Splenectomy abolished the factor X deficiency and produced complete remission of bleeding in several cases,[513] presumably because of extensive amyloid infiltration in the splenic vasculature. Chemotherapy with melphalan and prednisone was associated with resolution of factor X deficiency in amyloidosis.[514] High-dose chemotherapy with stem cell transplantation is also effective therapy.[515] A detailed literature review of acquired factor X deficiency has been published.[319]

Hypoprothrombinemia has been reported as an isolated finding,[516] most commonly in association with LAs, as discussed previously. Deficiencies of prothrombin, factors IX and XII, plasminogen, and antithrombin have been reported in some patients with the nephrotic syndrome,[517-521] presumably as the result of massive protein loss in the urine. Isolated deficiency of factor IX in several patients with Gaucher disease has also been documented.[522]

Acquired factor VII deficiency has been reported with aplastic anemia[523] and liposarcoma.[524]

Factor XIII deficiency has been associated with chronic myeloid leukemia and with various forms of acute leukemia.[525] Factor XIII deficiency has also been associated with inflammatory bowel disease,[526] and isoniazid-induced antibodies to factor XIII have been reported.[305,306,527] Factor V deficiency has been reported in chronic myeloid leukemia and in celiac disease. Acquired vWD was discussed earlier in the section "von Willebrand Factor."

Other Acquired Coagulation Disorders

Heparin-like anticoagulants have been reported in patients with hematologic malignancies (e.g., plasma cell dyscrasias[528] or leukemias[529,530] or solid tumors).[531] A prolonged thrombin time and normal reptilase clotting time are typically seen in these patients. Significant clinical bleeding may occur with heparin-like anticoagulants; a titrated protamine sulfate infusion may be helpful in these patients.

Malignancy may also be associated with other inhibitors of coagulation, including FDPs and paraproteins, dysfibrinogenemias, and specific antibodies to coagulation factors (discussed earlier). A monoclonal antithrombin antibody associated with bleeding has been reported in a patient with myeloma.[532]

References

1. Doolittle RF. Some important milestones in the field of blood clotting. *J Innate Immun*. 2016;8:23-29.
2. Furie B, Furie BC. Molecular basis of vitamin K-dependent gamma-carboxylation. *Blood*. 1990;75:1753-1762.
3. Sutor AH, von Kries R, Cornelissen EA, McNinch AW, Andrew M. Vitamin K deficiency bleeding (VKDB) in infancy. ISTH pediatric/perinatal subcommittee. International society on thrombosis and haemostasis. *Thromb Haemost*. 1999;81:456-461.
4. Mihatsch WA, Braegger C, Bronsky J, et al. ESPGHAN Committee on Nutrition. Prevention of vitamin K deficiency bleeding in newborn infants: a position paper by the ESPGHAN committee on nutrition. *J Pediatr Gastroenterol Nutr*. 2016;63:123-129.
5. Shearer MJ. Vitamin K deficiency bleeding (VKDB) in early infancy. *Blood Rev*. 2009;23:49-59.
6. Hathaway WE. The bleeding newborn. *Semin Hematol*. 1975;12:175-188.
7. Accessed December 1, 2022. https://www.ncbi.nlm.nih.gov/pubmedhealth/PMH0078451/pdf/PubMedHealth_PMH0078451.pdf
8. American Academy of Pediatrics Committee on Fetus and Newborn. Controversies concerning vitamin K and the newborn. *Pediatrics*. 2003;112(pt 1):191-192.
9. Zipursky A. Prevention of vitamin K deficiency bleeding in newborns. *Br J Haematol*. 1999;104:430-437.
10. Costakos DT, Greer FR, Love LA, Dahlen LR, Suttie JW. Vitamin K prophylaxis for premature infants: 1 mg versus 0.5 mg. *Am J Perinatol*. 2003;20:485-490.
11. Greer FR. Are breast-fed infants vitamin K deficient? *Adv Exp Med Biol*. 2001;501:391-395.
12. Jagannath VA, Thaker V, Chang AB, Price AI. Vitamin K supplementation for cystic fibrosis. *Cochrane Database Syst Rev*. 2020;6(6):CD008482.
13. Mercer KW, Gail Macik B, Williams ME. Hematologic disorders in critically ill patients. *Semin Respir Crit Care Med*. 2006;27:286-296.
14. Allison PM, Mummah-Schendel LL, Kindberg CG, Harms CS, Bang NU, Suttie JW. Effects of a vitamin K-deficient diet and antibiotics in normal human volunteers. *J Lab Clin Med*. 1987;110:180-188.
15. Brown RB, Klar J, Lemeshow S, Teres D, Pastides H, Sands M. Enhanced bleeding with cefoxitin or moxalactam. Statistical analysis within a defined population of 1493 patients. *Arch Intern Med*. 1986;146:2159-2164.
16. Vroonhof K, van Rijn HJ, van Hattum J. Vitamin K deficiency and bleeding after long-term use of cholestyramine. *Neth J Med*. 2003;61:19-21.
17. Corrigan JJ Jr, Marcus FI. Coagulopathy associated with vitamin E ingestion. *J Am Med Assoc*. 1974;230:1300-1301.
18. Holbrook AM, Pereira JA, Labiris R, et al. Systematic overview of warfarin and its drug and food interactions. *Arch Intern Med*. 2005;165:1095-1106.
19. Goldsweig HG, Kapusta M, Schwartz J. Bleeding, salicylates, and prolonged prothrombin time: three case reports and a review of the literature. *J Rheumatol*. 1976;3:37-42.
20. Spahr JE, Maul JS, Rodgers GM. Superwarfarin poisoning: a report of two cases and review of the literature. *Am J Hematol*. 2007;82:656-660.
21. Rodgers GM. Prothrombin complex concentrates in emergency bleeding disorders. *Am J Hematol*. 2012;87:898-902.
22. de la Rubia J, Grau E, Montserrat I, Zuazu I, Payá A. Anaphylactic shock and vitamin K1. *Ann Intern Med*. 1989;110:943.
23. Alperin JB. Coagulopathy caused by vitamin K deficiency in critically ill, hospitalized patients. *J Am Med Assoc*. 1987;258:1916-1619.
24. Schulman S, Furie B. How I treat poisoning with vitamin K antagonists. *Blood*. 2015;125:438-442.
25. Losowsky MS, Simmons AV, Miloszewski K. Coagulation abnormalities in liver disease. *Postgrad Med*. 1973;53:147-152.
26. Palascak JE, Martinez J. Dysfibrinogenemia associated with liver disease. *J Clin Invest*. 1977;60:89-95.
27. Soria J, Soria C, Ryckewaert JJ, Samama M, Thomson JM, Poller L. Study of acquired dysfibrinogenaemia in liver disease. *Thromb Res*. 1980;19:29-41.
28. Bloom AL. Intravascular coagulation and the liver. *Br J Haematol*. 1975;30:1-7.
29. VanDeWater L, Carr JM, Aronson D, McDonagh J. Analysis of elevated fibrin (ogen) degradation product levels in patients with liver disease. *Blood*. 1986;67:1468-1473.
30. Ben-Ari Z, Osman E, Hutton RA, Burroughs AK. Disseminated intravascular coagulation in liver cirrhosis: fact or fiction? *Am J Gastroenterol*. 1999;94:2977-2982.
31. Fletcher AP, Biederman O, Moore D. Abnormal plasminogen-plasmin system activity (fibrinolysis) in patients with hepatic cirrhosis: its cause and consequences. *J Clin Invest*. 1964;43:681-695.
32. Ballard HS, Marcus AJ. Platelet aggregation in portal cirrhosis. *Arch Intern Med*. 1976;136:316-319.
33. Fletcher AP, Alkjaersig N, Sherry S. Pathogenesis of the coagulation defect developing during pathological plasma proteolytic ("fibrinolytic") states. I. The significance of fibrinogen proteolysis and circulating fibrinogen breakdown products. *J Clin Invest*. 1962;41:896-916.
34. Henderson JM, Stein SF, Kutner M, Wiles MB, Ansley JD, Rudman D. Analysis of twenty-three plasma proteins in ascites. The depletion of fibrinogen and plasminogen. *Ann Surg*. 1980;192:738-742.
35. Tripodi A, Mannucci PM. The coagulopathy of chronic liver disease. *N Engl J Med*. 2011;365:147-156.
36. Peck-Radosavljevic M. Thrombocytopenia in chronic liver disease. *Liver Int*. 2017;37:778-793.
37. Ishikawa T, Ichida T, Sugahara S, et al. Thrombopoietin receptor (c-Mpl) is constitutively expressed on platelets of patients with liver cirrhosis, and correlates with its disease progression. *Hepatol Res*. 2002;23:115-121.
38. Rios R, Sangro B, Herrero I, Quiroga J, Prieto J. The role of thrombopoietin in the thrombocytopenia of patients with liver cirrhosis. *Am J Gastroenterol*. 2005;100:1311-1316.
39. Rodríguez-Iñigo E, Bartolomé J, Quiroga JA, et al. Expression of factor VII in the liver of patients with liver disease: correlations with the disease severity and impairment in the hemostasis. *Blood Coagul Fibrinolysis*. 2001;12:193-199.
40. Yanofsky RA, Jackson VG, Lilly JR, Stellin G, Klingensmith WC III, Hathaway WE. The multiple coagulopathies of biliary atresia. *Am J Hematol*. 1984;16:171-180.
41. Ruggiero G, De Biasi R, Attanasio S, Bile G, Giusti G. Hemostatic abnormalities in chronic aggressive hepatitis and liver cirrhosis. *Acta Hepatogastroenterol (Stuttg)*. 1975;22:221-228.
42. Martinez J, Palascak JE, Kwasniak D. Abnormal sialic acid content of the dysfibrinogenemia associated with liver disease. *J Clin Invest*. 1978;61:535-538.
43. Liebman HA, Furie BC, Tong MJ, et al. Des-gamma-carboxy (abnormal) prothrombin as a serum marker of primary hepatocellular carcinoma. *N Engl J Med*. 1984;310:1427-1431.
44. Hu KQ, Yu AS, Tiyyagura L, Redeker AG, Reynolds TB. Hyperfibrinolytic activity in hospitalized cirrhotic patients in a referral liver unit. *Am J Gastroenterol*. 2001;96:1581-1586.
45. Lisman T, Leebeek FW, Mosnier LO, et al. Thrombin-activatable fibrinolysis inhibitor deficiency in cirrhosis is not associated with increased plasma fibrinolysis. *Gastroenterology*. 2001;121:131-139.
46. Collen D, Rouvier J, Chamone DA, Verstraete M. Turnover of radiolabeled plasminogen and prothrombin in cirrhosis of the liver. *Eur J Clin Invest*. 1978;8:185-188.
47. Tytgat GN, Collen D, Verstraete M. Metabolism of fibrinogen in cirrhosis of the liver. *J Clin Invest*. 1971;50:1690-1701.
48. Coccheri S, Mannucci PM, Palareti G, Gervasoni W, Poggi M, Viganò S. Significance of plasma fibrinopeptide A and high molecular weight fibrinogen in patients with liver cirrhosis. *Br J Haematol*. 1982;52:503-509.
49. Cordova C, Musca A, Violi F, Alessandri C, Vezza E. Improvement of some blood coagulation factors in cirrhotic patients treated with low doses of heparin. *Scand J Haematol*. 1982;29:235-240.
50. Stein SF, Fulenwider JT, Ansley JD, et al. Accelerated fibrinogen and platelet destruction after peritoneovenous shunting. *Arch Intern Med*. 1981;141:1149-1151.
51. Ozier Y, Steib A, Ickx B, et al. Haemostatic disorders during liver transplantation. *Eur J Anaesthesiol*. 2001;18:208-218.
52. Hollestelle MJ, Geerteen HGM, Straatsburg IH, van Gulik TM, van Mourik JA. Factor VIII expression in liver disease. *Thromb Haemost*. 2004;91:267-275.
53. Driever EG, Stravitz RT, Zhang J, et al. vWF/ASAMTS13 imbalance, but not global coagulation or fibrinolysis, is associated with outcome and bleeding in acute liver failure. *Hepatology*. 2021;73:1882-1891.
54. Lisman T, Porte RJ. Rebalanced hemostasis in patients with liver disease: evidence and clinical consequences. *Blood*. 2010;116:878-885.
55. Ribic C, Crowther M. Thrombosis and anticoagulation in the setting of renal or liver disease. *Hematology Am Soc Hematol Educ Program*. 2016;2016:188-195.
56. Chalmers TC, Bigelow FS, Desforges JF. The effects of massive gastrointestinal hemorrhage on hemostasis. II. Coagulation factors. *J Lab Clin Med*. 1954;43:511-517.
57. Zanetto A, Rodriguez-Kastro KI, Germani G, et al. Mortality in liver transplant recipients with portal vein thrombosis - an updated meta-analysis. *Transpl Int*. 2018;31:1318-1329.
58. O'Grady JG, Alexander GJ, Hayllar KM, Williams R. Early indicators of prognosis in fulminant hepatic failure. *Gastroenterology*. 1989;97:439-445.
59. Mannucci PM. Abnormal hemostasis tests and bleeding in chronic liver disease: are they related? No. *J Thromb Haemost*. 2006;4:721-723.
60. McGill DB. Predicting hemorrhage after liver biopsy. *Dig Dis Sci*. 1981;26:385-387.
61. Deitcher SR. Interpretation of the international normalised ratio in patients with liver disease. *Lancet*. 2002;359:47-48.

62. McVay PA, Toy PT. Lack of increased bleeding after liver biopsy in patients with mild hemostatic abnormalities. *Am J Clin Pathol.* 1990;94:747-753.
63. O'Shaughnessy DF, Atterbury C, Bolton Maggs P, et al; British Committee for Standards in Haematology, Blood Transfusion Task Force. Guidelines for the use of fresh-frozen plasma, cryoprecipitate and cryosupernatant. *Br J Haematol.* 2004;126:11-28.
64. Saja MF, Abdo AA, Sanai FM, Shaikh SA, Gader AG. The coagulopathy of liver disease; does vitamin K help? *Blood Coagul Fibrinolysis.* 2013;24:10-17.
65. Blatt PM, Lundblad RL, Kingdon HS, McLean G, Roberts HR. Thrombogenic materials in prothrombin complex concentrates. *Ann Intern Med.* 1974;81:766-770.
66. Scott LJ. Prothrombin complex concentrate (Beriplex P/N). *Drugs.* 2009;69:1977-1984.
67. De Franchis R, Arcidiacono PG, Carpinelli L, et al. Randomized controlled trial of desmopressin plus terlipressin vs. terlipressin alone for the treatment of acute variceal hemorrhage in cirrhotic patients: a multicenter, double-blind study. New Italian Endoscopic Club. *Hepatology.* 1993;18:1102-1107.
68. Sogaard KK, Horvath-Puho E, Gronbaek H, et al. Risk of venous thromboembolism in patients with liver disease: a nationwide population-based case-control study. *Am J Gastroenterol.* 2009;104:96-101.
69. Tripodi A, Primignani M, Chantarangkul V, et al. An imbalance of pro-vs-anticoagulation factors in plasma from patients with cirrhosis. *Gastroenterology.* 2009;137:2105-2111.
70. O'Leary JG, Greenberg CS, Patton HM, Caldwell SH. AGA clinical practice update: coagulation in cirrhosis. *Gastroenterology.* 2019;157:34-43.
71. Lisman T, Porte RJ. Recombinant factor VIIa to treat severe bleeding in patients with liver disease: pitfalls and possibilities. *J Hepatol.* 2011;55:950-951.
72. Hayashi H, Beppu T, Shirabe K, Maehara Y, Baba H. Management of thrombocytopenia due to liver cirrhosis: a review. *World J Gastroenterol.* 2014;20:2595-2605.
73. Dohan A, Guerrache Y, Boudiaf M, Gavini JP, Kaci R, Soyer P. Transjugular liver biopsy: indications, technique and results. *Diagn Interv Imaging.* 2014;95:11-15.
74. Levi M, Toh CH, Thachil J, Watson HG. Guidelines for the diagnosis and management of disseminated intravascular coagulation. British Committee for Standards in Haematology. *Br J Haematol.* 2009;145:24-33.
75. Levi M, van der Poll T. A short contemporary history of disseminated intravascular coagulation. *Semin Thromb Hemost.* 2014;40:874-880.
76. Taylor FB, Toh CH, Hoots K, Wada H, Levi M; Scientific Subcommittee on Disseminated Intravascular Coagulation (DIC) of the International Society on Thrombosis and Haemostasis (ISTH). Towards a definition, clinical and laboratory criteria and a scoring system for disseminated intravascular coagulation. *Thromb Haemost.* 2001;86:1327-1330.
77. Erez O, Mastrolia SA, Thachil J. Disseminated intravascular coagulation in pregnancy: insights in pathophysiology, diagnosis, and management. *Am J Obstet Gynecol.* 2015;213:452-463.
78. Tallman MS, Kwaan HC. Reassessing the hemostatic disorder associated with acute promyelocytic leukemia. *Blood.* 1992;79:543-553.
79. Warrell RP Jr, Kempin SJ. Treatment of severe coagulopathy in the Kasabach-Merritt syndrome with aminocaproic acid and cryoprecipitate. *N Engl J Med.* 1985;313:309-312.
80. Hasiba U, Rosenbach LM, Rockwell D, Lewis JH. DIC-like syndrome after envenomation by the snake, *Crotalus horridus* horridus. *N Engl J Med.* 1975;292:505-507.
81. Siegal T, Seligsohn U, Aghai E, Modan M. Clinical and laboratory aspects of disseminated intravascular coagulation (DIC): a study of 118 cases. *Thromb Haemost.* 1978;39:122-134.
82. Jacobson RJ, Jackson DP. Erythrocyte fragmentation in defibrination syndromes. *Ann Intern Med.* 1974;81:207-209.
83. Okajima K, Sakamoto Y, Uchiba M. Heterogeneity in the incidence and clinical manifestations of disseminated intravascular coagulation: a study of 204 cases. *Am J Hematol.* 2000;65:215-222.
84. Sack GH Jr, Levin J, Bell WR. Trousseau's syndrome and other manifestations of chronic disseminated coagulopathy in patients with neoplasms: clinical, pathophysiologic, and therapeutic features. *Medicine (Baltimore).* 1977;56:1-37.
85. Sutton DM, Hauser R, Kulapongs P, Bachmann F. Intravascular coagulation in abruptio placentae. *Am J Obstet Gynecol.* 1971;109:604-614.
86. Dvorak HF, Van DeWater L, Bitzer AM, et al. Procoagulant activity associated with plasma membrane vesicles shed by cultured tumor cells. *Cancer Res.* 1983;43:4434-4442.
87. Rickles FR, Edwards RL. Activation of blood coagulation in cancer: Trousseau's syndrome revisited. *Blood.* 1983;62:14-31.
88. Callander N, Rapaport SI. Trousseau's syndrome. *West J Med.* 1993;158:364-371.
89. Gordon SG, Cross BA. A factor X-activating cysteine protease from malignant tissue. *J Clin Invest.* 1981;67:1665-1671.
90. Gralnick HR, Abrell E. Studies of the procoagulant and fibrinolytic activity of promyelocytes in acute promyelocytic leukaemia. *Br J Haematol.* 1973;24:89-99.
91. Plow EF. Leukocyte elastase release during blood coagulation. A potential mechanism for activation of the alternative fibrinolytic pathway. *J Clin Invest.* 1982;69:564-572.
92. Menell JS, Cesarman GM, Jacovina AT, McLaughlin MA, Lev EA, Hajjar KA. Annexin II and bleeding in acute promyelocytic leukemia. *N Engl J Med.* 1999;340:994-1004.
93. McKay DG. Trauma and disseminated intravascular coagulation. *J Trauma.* 1969;9:646-660.
94. Goodnight SH, Kenoyer G, Rapaport SI, Patch MJ, Lee JA, Kurze T. Defibrination after brain-tissue destruction: a serious complication of head injury. *N Engl J Med.* 1974;290:1043-1047.
95. Drake TA, Cheng J, Chang A, Taylor FB Jr. Expression of tissue factor, thrombomodulin, and E-selectin in baboons with lethal *Escherichia coli* sepsis. *Am J Pathol.* 1993;142:1458-1470.
96. Hack CE, Zeerleder S. The endothelium in sepsis: source of and a target for inflammation. *Crit Care Med.* 2001;29:S21-S27.
97. Nieuwland R, Berckmans RJ, McGregor S, et al. Cellular origin and procoagulant properties of microparticles in meningococcal sepsis. *Blood.* 2000;95:930-935.
98. Pixley RA, De La Cadena R, Page JD, et al. The contact system contributes to hypotension but not disseminated intravascular coagulation in lethal bacteremia. In vivo use of a monoclonal anti-factor XII antibody to block contact activation in baboons. *J Clin Invest.* 1993;91:61-68.
99. Schapira M, Ramus MA, Waeber B, et al. Protection by recombinant α 1-anti-trypsin Ala357 Arg358 against arterial hypotension induced by factor XII fragment. *J Clin Invest.* 1987;80:582-585.
100. Damas P, Canivet JL, de Groot D, et al. Sepsis and serum cytokine concentrations. *Crit Care Med.* 1997;25:405-412.
101. Mason JW, Colman RW. The role of Hageman factor in disseminated intravascular coagulation induced by septicemia, neoplasia, or liver disease. *Thromb Diath Haemorrh.* 1971;26:325-331.
102. McGrath JM, Stewart GJ. The effects of endotoxin on vascular endothelium. *J Exp Med.* 1969;129:833-848.
103. Colucci M, Balconi G, Lorenzet R, et al. Cultured human endothelial cells generate tissue factor in response to endotoxin. *J Clin Invest.* 1983;71:1893-1896.
104. Hillman RS, Phillips LL. Clotting-fibrinolysis in a cavernous hemangioma. *Am J Dis Child.* 1967;113:649-653.
105. Bieger R, Vreeken J, Stibbe J, Loeliger EA. Arterial aneurysm as a cause of consumption coagulopathy. *N Engl J Med.* 1971;285:152-154.
106. Kornalik F, Blombäck B. Prothrombin activation induced by Ecarin—a prothrombin converting enzyme from *Echis carinatus* venom. *Thromb Res.* 1975;6:57-63.
107. Gold BS, Dart RC, Barish RA. Bites of venomous snakes. *N Engl J Med.* 2002;347:347-356.
108. Swenson S, Markland FS Jr. Snake venom fibrin(ogen)olytic enzymes. *Toxicon.* 2005;45:1021-1039.
109. Rapaport SI, Hjort PF, Patch MJ, Jeremic M. Consumption of serum factors and prothrombin during intravascular clotting in rabbits. *Scand J Haematol.* 1966;3:59-75.
110. Levi M, Scully M. How I treat disseminated intravascular coagulation. *Blood.* 2018;131:845-854.
111. Taylor FB Jr, Stearns-Kurosawa DJ, Kurosaw S, et al. The endothelial cell protein C receptor aids in host defense against *Escherichia coli* sepsis. *Blood.* 2000;95:1680-1686.
112. Mason JW, Kleeberg U, Dolan P, Colman RW. Plasma kallikrein and Hageman factor in gram-negative bacteremia. *Ann Intern Med.* 1970;73:545-551.
113. Camerer E, Cornelissen I, Kataoka H, Duong DN, Zheng YW, Coughlin SR. Roles of protease-activated receptors in a mouse model of endotoxemia. *Blood.* 2006;107:3912-3921.
114. Visudhiphan S, Piankijagum A, Sathayapraseart P, Mitrchai N. Erythrocyte fragmentation in disseminated intravascular coagulation and other diseases. *N Engl J Med.* 1983;309:113.
115. Mesters RM, Flörke N, Ostermann H, Kienast J. Increase of plasminogen activator inhibitor levels predicts outcome of leukocytopenic patients with sepsis. *Thromb Haemost.* 1996;75:902-907.
116. Nesheim M, Wang W, Boffa M, Nagashima M, Morser J, Bajzar L. Thrombin, thrombomodulin and TAFI in the molecular link between coagulation and fibrinolysis. *Thromb Haemost.* 1997;78:386-391.
117. Bang NU, Fletcher AP, Alkjaersig N, Sherry S. Pathogenesis of the coagulation defect developing during pathological plasma proteolytic ("fibrinolytic") states. III. Demonstration of abnormal clot structure by electron microscopy. *J Clin Invest.* 1962;41:935-948.
118. Rinaldo JE, Rogers RM. Adult respiratory-distress syndrome: changing concepts of lung injury and repair. *N Engl J Med.* 1982;306:900-909.
119. Martin TR, Sandblom RL, Johnson RJ. Adult respiratory distress syndrome following thrombolytic therapy for pulmonary embolism. *Chest.* 1983;83:151-153.
120. Sherman LA, Lee J, Jacobson A. Quantitation of the reticuloendothelial system clearance of soluble fibrin. *Br J Haematol.* 1977;37:231-238.
121. Oka K, Shimamura K, Nakazawa M, Tsunoda R, Kojima M. The role of Kupffer's cells in disseminated intravascular coagulation. A morphologic study in thrombin-infused rabbits. *Arch Pathol Lab Med.* 1983;107:570-576.
122. Deykin D, Cochios F, DeCamp G, Lopez A. Hepatic removal of activated factor X by the perfused rabbit liver. *Am J Physiol.* 1968;214:414-419.
123. Letsky EA. Disseminated intravascular coagulation. *Best Pract Res Clin Obstet Gynaecol.* 2001;15:623-644.
124. Deykin D. The clinical challenge of disseminated intravascular coagulation. *N Engl J Med.* 1970;283:636-644.
125. Johnson ED, Schell JC, Rodgers GM. The D-dimer assay. *Am J Hematol.* 2019;94:833-839.
126. Greenberg CS, Devine DV, McCrae KM. Measurement of plasma fibrin D-dimer levels with the use of a monoclonal antibody coupled to latex beads. *Am J Clin Pathol.* 1987;87:94-100.
127. Calverley DC, Liebman HA. Disseminated intravascular coagulation. In: Hoffman R, Benz EJ, Shattil SJ, eds. *Hematology: Basic Principles and Practice.* 3rd ed. Churchill Livingstone; 2000:1983-1995.
128. Lehman CM, Wilson LW, Rodgers GM. Analytic validation and clinical evaluation of the STA LIATEST immunoturbidimetric D-dimer assay for the diagnosis of disseminated intravascular coagulation. *Am J Clin Pathol.* 2004;122:178-184.
129. Merskey C, Johnson AJ, Kleiner GJ, Wohl H. The defibrination syndrome: clinical features and laboratory diagnosis. *Br J Haematol.* 1967;13:528-549.

130. Niemetz J, Nossel HL. Activated coagulation factors: in-vivo and in-vitro studies. *Br J Haematol.* 1969;16:337-351.
131. Giles AR, Nesheim ME, Mann KG. Studies of factors V and VIII:C in an animal model of disseminated intravascular coagulation. *J Clin Invest.* 1984;74:2219-2225.
132. Whitaker AN, Rowe EA, Masci PP, Gaffney PJ. Identification of D dimer-E complex in disseminated intravascular coagulation. *Thromb Res.* 1980;18:453-459.
133. Carr JM, McKinney M, McDonagh J. Diagnosis of disseminated intravascular coagulation. Role of D-dimer. *Am J Clin Pathol.* 1989;91:280-287.
134. Niewiarowski S, Gurewich V. Laboratory identification of intravascular coagulation. The serial dilution protamine sulfate test for the detection of fibrin monomer and fibrin degradation products. *J Lab Clin Med.* 1971;77:665-676.
135. Nossel HL. Radioimmunoassay of fibrinopeptides in relation to intravascular coagulation and thrombosis. *N Engl J Med.* 1976;295:428-432.
136. Tanaka H, Kobayashi N, Maekawa T. Studies on production of antithrombin III with special reference to endotoxin-induced DIC in dogs. *Thromb Haemost.* 1986;56:137-143.
137. Wada H, Yamamuro M, Inoue A, et al. Comparison of the responses of global tests of coagulation with molecular markers of neutrophil, endothelial, and hemostatic system perturbation in the baboon model of *E. coli* sepsis-toward a distinction between uncompensated overt DIC and compensated non-overt DIC. *Thromb Haemost.* 2001;86:1489-1494.
138. Toh CH, Hoots WK; SSC on Disseminated Intravascular Coagulation of the ISTH. The scoring system of the Scientific and Standardisation Committee on Disseminated Intravascular Coagulation of the International Society on Thrombosis and Haemostasis: a 5-year overview. *J Thromb Haemost.* 2007;5:604-606.
139. Kim HS, Suzuki M, Lie JT, Titus JL. Clinically unsuspected disseminated intravascular coagulation (DIC): an autopsy survey. *Am J Clin Pathol.* 1976;66:31-39.
140. Iba T, Levy JH, Warkentin TE, et al. Diagnosis and management of sepsis-induced coagulopathy and disseminated intravascular coagulation. *J Thromb Haemost.* 2019;17:1989-1994.
141. Ness PM, Perkins HA. Cryoprecipitate as a reliable source of fibrinogen replacement. *J Am Med Assoc.* 1979;241:1690-1691.
142. Lechner K, Kyrle PA. Antithrombin III concentrates–are they clinically useful? *Thromb Haemost.* 1995;73:340-348.
143. Warren BL, Eid A, Singer P, et al; KyberSept Trial Study Group. Caring for the critically ill patient. High-dose antithrombin III in severe sepsis: a randomized controlled trial. *J Am Med Assoc.* 2001;286:1869-1878.
144. Wiedermann CJ, Hoffmann JN, Juers M, KyberSept Investigators. High-dose antithrombin III in the treatment of severe sepsis in patients with a high risk of death: efficacy and safety. *Crit Care Med.* 2006;34:285-292.
145. Montagnana M, Franchi M, Danese E, Gotsch F, Guidi GC. Disseminated intravascular coagulation in obstetric and gynecologic disorders. *Semin Thromb Hemost.* 2010;36:404-418.
146. Cunningham FG, Nelson DB. Disseminated intravascular coagulation syndromes in obstetrics. *Obstet Gynecol.* 2015;126:999-1011.
147. Strauss JH, Ballard JO, Chamlian D. Consumption coagulopathy associated with intrauterine fetal death: the role of heparin therapy. *Int J Gynaecol Obstet.* 1978;16:225-227.
148. Society for Maternal-Fetal Medicine (SMFM); Pacheco LD, Saade G, Hankins GD, Clark SL. Amniotic fluid embolism: diagnosis and management. *Am J Obstet Gynecol.* 2016;215:B16-B24.
149. Rabinovich A, Abdul-Kadir R, Thachil J, et al. DIC in obstetrics: diagnostic score, highlights in management, and international registry-communication from the DIC and Women's Health SSCs of the International Society of Thrombosis and Haemostasis. *J Thromb Haemost.* 2019;17:1562-1566.
150. Rajaqopal R, Thachil J, Monagle P. Disseminated intravascular coagulation in paediatrics. *Arch Dis Child.* 2017;102:187-193.
151. Gross SJ, Filston HC, Anderson JC. Controlled study of treatment for disseminated intravascular coagulation in the neonate. *J Pediatr.* 1982;100:445-448.
152. Kreuz W, Veldmann A, Fischer D, Schlösser M, Volk WR, Ettingshausen CE. Neonatal sepsis: a challenge in hemostaseology. *Semin Thromb Hemost.* 1999;25:531-535.
153. Martí-Carvajal AJ, Solà I, Gluud C, Lathyris D, Cardona AF. Human recombinant protein C for severe sepsis and septic shock in adult and paediatric patients. *Cochrane Database Syst Rev.* 2012;12(12):CD004388.
154. Ranieri VM, Thompson BT, Barie PS, et al. Drotrecogin alfa (activated) in adults with septic shock. *N Engl J Med.* 2012;366(22):2055-2064.
155. Dudgeon DL, Kellogg DR, Gilchrist GS, Woolley MM. Purpura fulminans. *Arch Surg.* 1971;103:351-358.
156. Spicer TE, Rau JM. Purpura fulminans. *Am J Med.* 1976;61:566-571.
157. Gamper G, Oschatz E, Herkner H, et al. Sepsis-associated purpura fulminans in adults. *Wien Klin Wochenschr.* 2001;113:107-112.
158. Chalmers E, Cooper P, Forman K, et al. Purpura fulminans: recognition, diagnosis and management. *Arch Dis Child.* 2011;96:1066-1071.
159. Sallah S, Wan JY, Nguyen NP, Hanrahan LR, Sigounas G. Disseminated intravascular coagulation in solid tumors: clinical and pathologic study. *Thromb Haemost.* 2001;86:828-833.
160. Thodiyil PA, Kakkar AK. Variation in relative risk of venous thromboembolism in different cancers. *Thromb Haemost.* 2002;87:1076-1077.
161. Walsh-McMonagle D, Green D. Low-molecular-weight heparin in the management of Trousseau's syndrome. *Cancer.* 1997;80:649-655.
162. Akl EA, Kahale LA, Hakoum MB, et al. Parenteral anticoagulation in ambulatory patients with cancer. *Cochrane Database Syst Rev.* 2017;9(9):CD006652.
163. Lee AY, Levine MN, Baker RI, et al; Randomized Comparison of Low-Molecular-Weight Heparin Versus Oral Anticoagulant Therapy for the Prevention of Recurrent Venous Thromboembolism in Patients With Cancer (CLOT) Investigators. Low-molecular-weight heparin versus a coumarin for the prevention of recurrent venous thromboembolism in patients with cancer. *N Engl J Med.* 2003;349:146-153.
164. Ng S, Carrier M. Prevention and treatment of cancer-associated thrombosis. *Curr Oncol.* 2020;27:275-278.
165. Litt MR, Bell WR, Lepor HA. Disseminated intravascular coagulation in prostatic carcinoma reversed by ketoconazole. *J Am Med Assoc.* 1987;258:1361-1362.
166. Martinez JF, Tabernero Redondo MD, Alberca Silva I, Lopez-Borrasca A. Disseminated intravascular coagulation in prostatic carcinoma reversed by antiandrogenic therapy. *J Am Med Assoc.* 1988;260:2507.
167. Varki A. Trousseau's syndrome: multiple definitions and multiple mechanisms. *Blood.* 2007;110:1723-1729.
168. Sultan C, Heilmann-Gouault M, Tulliez M. Relationship between blast-cell morphology and occurrence of a syndrome of disseminated intravascular coagulation. *Br J Haematol.* 1973;24:255-259.
169. Schwartz BS, Williams EC, Conlan MG, Mosher DF. Epsilon-aminocaproic acid in the treatment of patients with acute promyelocytic leukemia and acquired α-2-plasmin inhibitor deficiency. *Ann Intern Med.* 1986;105:873-877.
170. Brown JE, Olujohungbe A, Chang J, et al. All-trans retinoic acid (ATRA) and tranexamic acid: a potentially fatal combination in acute promyelocytic leukaemia. *Br J Haematol.* 2000;110:1010-1012.
171. Tallman MS, Lafebvre P, Baine RM, et al. Effects of all-trans retinoic acid or chemotherapy on the molecular regulation of systemic blood coagulation and fibrinolysis in patients with acute promyelocytic leukemia. *J Thromb Haemost.* 2004;2:1341-1350.
172. Hall GW. Kasabach-Merritt syndrome: pathogenesis and management. *Br J Haematol.* 2001;112:851-862.
173. O'Rafferty C, O'Regan G, Irvine AD, Smith OP. Recent advances in the pathobiology and management of Kasabach-Merritt phenomenon. *Br J Haematol.* 2015;171:38-51.
174. Cummins D, Segal H, Hunt BJ, et al. Chronic disseminated intravascular coagulation after surgery for abdominal aortic aneurysm: clinical and haemostatic response to dalteparin. *Br J Haematol.* 2001;113:658-660.
175. Connors JM, Levy JH. COVID19 and its implications for thrombosis and anticoagulation. *Blood.* 2020;135:2033-2040.
176. Nopp S, Moik F, Jilma B, et al. Risk of venous thromboembolism in patients with COVID-19: a systematic review and meta-analysis. *Res Pract Thromb Haemost.* 2020;4(7):1178-1191.
177. Levi M, Iba T. COVID-19 coagulopathy: is it disseminated intravascular coagulation? *Int Emerg Med.* 2021;16(2):309-312.
178. Goshua G, Pine AB, Meizlish ML, et al. Endotheliopathy in COVID-19-associated coagulopathy: evidence from a single-centre, cross-sectional study. *Lancet Haematol.* 2020;7(8):e575-e582.
179. Cuker A, Tseng EK, Nieuwlaat R, et al. American Society of Hematology 2021 guidelines on the use of anticoagulation for thromboprophylaxis in patients with COVID-19. *Blood Adv.* 2021;5(3):872-888.
180. Schmaier AH, Claypool W, Colman RW. Crotalocytin: recognition and purification of a timber rattlesnake platelet aggregating protein. *Blood.* 1980;56:1013-1019.
181. Warrell DA, Pope HM, Prentice CR. Disseminated intravascular coagulation caused by the carpet viper (*Echis carinatus*): trial of heparin. *Br J Haematol.* 1976;33:335-342.
182. Spero JA, Lewis JH, Hasiba U. Disseminated intravascular coagulation. Findings in 346 patients. *Thromb Haemost.* 1980;43:28-33.
183. Kim HS, Suzuki M, Lie JT, Titus JL. Nonbacterial thrombotic endocarditis (NBTE) and disseminated intravascular coagulation (DIC): autopsy study of 36 patients. *Arch Pathol Lab Med.* 1977;101:65-68.
184. Taylor FB Jr, Chang A, Esmon CT, D'Angelo A, Vigano-D'Angelo S, Blick KE. Protein C prevents the coagulopathic and lethal effects of *Escherichia coli* infusion in the baboon. *J Clin Invest.* 1987;79:918-925.
185. White B, Livingstone W, Murphy C, Hodgson A, Rafferty M, Smith OP. An open-label study of the role of adjuvant hemostatic support with protein C replacement therapy in purpura fulminans-associated meningococcemia. *Blood.* 2000;96:3719-3724.
186. Vincent J, Francois B, Zabolotskikh I, et al. Effect of a recombinant human soluble thrombomodulin on mortality in patients with sepsis-associated coagulopathy: the SCARLET randomized clinical trial. *J Am Med Assoc.* 2019;321(20):1993-2002.
187. Thachil J. Managing sepsis-associated coagulopathy remains an enigma. *J Thromb Haemost.* 2019;17:1586-1589.
188. Bennett B, Croll AM, Robbie LA, Herriot R. Tumour cell u-PA as a cause of fibrinolytic bleeding in metastatic disease. *Br J Haematol.* 1997;99:570-574.
189. Bell WR. The fibrinolytic system in neoplasia. *Semin Thromb Hemost.* 1996;22:459-478.
190. Taylor RN, Lacey CG, Shuman MA. Adenocarcinoma of Skene's duct associated with a systemic coagulopathy. *Gynecol Oncol.* 1985;22:250-256.
191. Kevy SV, Glickman RM, Bernhard WF, Diamond LK, Gross RE. The pathogenesis and control of the hemorrhagic defect in open heart surgery. *Surg Gynecol Obstet.* 1966;123:313-318.
192. Illig KA, Green RM, Ouriel K, et al. Primary fibrinolysis during supraceliac aortic clamping. *J Vasc Surg.* 1997;25:244-251, discussion 252-254.
193. Lee MH, Vosburgh E, Anderson K, McDonagh J. Deficiency of plasma plasminogen activator inhibitor 1 results in hyperfibrinolytic bleeding. *Blood.* 1993;81:2357-2362.

194. Aoki N, Saito H, Kamiya T, Koie K, Sakata Y, Kobakura. Congenital deficiency of alpha 2-plasmin inhibitor associated with severe hemorrhagic tendency. *J Clin Invest*. 1979;63:877-884.
195. Booth NA, Bennett B. Plasmin-α 2-antiplasmin complexes in bleeding disorders characterized by primary or secondary fibrinolysis. *Br J Haematol*. 1984;56:545-556.
196. Bachmann F. Disorders of fibrinolysis and use of antifibrinolytic agents. In: Beutler E, Lichtman MA, Coller BS, et al, eds. *Williams Hematology*. 6th ed. McGraw-Hill; 2001:1829-1840.
197. Nilsson IM, Andersson L, Bjorkman SE. Epsilon-aminocaproic acid (ε-ACA) as a therapeutic agent based on 5 years' clinical experience. *Acta Med Scand Suppl*. 1966;448:1-46.
198. Accessed December 1, 2022. https://www.pdr.net-Amicar-aminocaproic-acid-1954
199. Naeye RL. Thrombotic state after a hemorrhagic diathesis, a possible complication of therapy with epsilon-aminocaproic acid. *Blood*. 1962;19:694-701.
200. Sallah S, Gagnon GA. Reversion of primary hyperfibrinogenolysis in patients with hormone-refractory prostate cancer using docetaxel. *Cancer Invest*. 2000;18:191-196.
201. Winther-Larsen A, Sandfeld-Paulsen B, Hvas AM. Hyperfibrinolysis in patients with solid malignant neoplasms: a systematic review. *Semin Thromb Hemost*. 2021;47(5):581-588.
202. Franchini M, Castaman G, Coppola A, et al. Acquired inhibitors of clotting factors: AICE recommendations for diagnosis and management. *Blood Transfus*. 2015;13:498-513.
203. Wight J, Paisley S. The epidemiology of inhibitors in haemophilia A: a systematic review. *Haemophilia*. 2003;9:418-435.
204. Schwaab R, Brackmann HH, Meyer C, et al. Haemophilia A: mutation type determines risk of inhibitor formation. *Thromb Haemost*. 1995;74(6):1402-1406.
205. Eckhardt CL, van Velzen AS, Peters M, et al. Factor VIII gene (F8) mutation and risk of inhibitor development in nonsevere hemophilia A. *Blood*. 2013;122(11):1954-1962.
206. Viel KR, Ameri A, Abshire TC, et al. Inhibitors of factor VIII in black patients with hemophilia. *N Engl J Med*. 2009;360:1618-1627.
207. Gouw SC, van den Berg HM, le Cessis S, van der Bom JG. Treatment characteristics and the risk of inhibitor development: a multicenter cohort study among previously untreated patients with severe hemophilia A. *J Thromb Haemost*. 2007;5:1383-1390.
208. Ragni MV. FVIII, CD4, and liaisons dangereuses. *Blood*. 2011;117:6060-6061.
209. Abdi A, Eckhardt CL, van Velzen AS, et al. Treatment-related risk factors for inhibitor development in non-severe hemophilia A after 50 cumulative exposure days: a case-control study. *J Thromb Haemost*. 2021;19(9):2171-2181.
210. van Velzen AS, Eckhardt CL, Peters M, et al. Intensity of factor VIII treatment and the development of inhibitors in non-severe hemophilia A patients: results of the INSIGHT case-control study. *J Thromb Haemost*. 2017;15(7):1422-1429.
211. Gouw SC, van der Bom JG, Ljung R, et al; PedNet and RODIN Study Group. Factor VIII products and inhibitor development in severe hemophilia A. *N Engl J Med*. 2013;368:231-239.
212. Peyvandi F, Mannucci PM, Garagiola I, et al. A randomized trial of factor VIII and neutralizing antibodies in hemophilia A. *N Engl J Med*. 2016;374:2054-2064.
213. Srivastava A, Santagostino E, Dougall A, et al. WFH guidelines for the management of hemophilia. 3rd edition. *Haemophilia*. 2020;26(suppl 6):1-158.
214. Lorenzo JI, López A, Altisent C, Aznar JA. Incidence of factor VIII inhibitors in severe haemophilia: the importance of patient age. *Br J Haematol*. 2001;113:600-603.
215. Maclean PS, Richards M, Williams M, et al. Treatment related factors and inhibitor development in children with severe haemophilia A. *Haemophilia*. 2011;17(2):282-287.
216. Hay CR, Palmer B, Chalmers E, et al; United Kingdom Haemophilia Centre Doctors' Organisation (UKHCDO). Incidence of factor VIII inhibitors throughout life in severe hemophilia A in the United Kingdom. *Blood*. 2011;118:6367-6370.
217. Iorio A, Barbara AM, Makris M, et al. Natural history and clinical characteristics of inhibitors in previously treated haemophilia A patients: a case series. *Haemophilia*. 2017;23(2):255-263.
218. Volkers P, Hanschmann KM, Calvez T, et al. Recombinant factor VIII products and inhibitor development in previously untreated patients with severe haemophilia A: combined analysis of three studies. *Haemophilia*. 2019;25(3):398-407.
219. Kruse-Jarres R, Kempton CL, Baudo F, et al. Acquired hemophilia A: updated review of evidence and treatment guidance. *Am J Hematol*. 2017;92(7):695-705.
220. Green D, Lechner K. A survey of 215 non-hemophilic patients with inhibitors to factor VIII. *Thromb Haemost*. 1981;45:200-203.
221. Solymoss S. Postpartum acquired factor VIII inhibitors: results of a survey. *Am J Hematol*. 1998;59:1-4.
222. Hauser I, Lechner K. Solid tumors and factor VIII antibodies. *Thromb Haemost*. 1999;82:1005-1007.
223. Sallah S, Nguyen NP, Abdallah JM, Hanrahan LR. Acquired hemophilia in patients with hematologic malignancies. *Arch Pathol Lab Med*. 2000;124:730-734.
224. Cormier M, Batty P, Tarrant J, Lillicrap D. Advances in knowledge of inhibitor formation in severe haemophilia A. *Br J Haematol*. 2020;189:39-53.
225. Scott DW, Pratt KP. Factor VIII: perspectives on immunogenicity and tolerogenic strategies. *Front Immunol*. 2020;10:3078.
226. Franchini M, Salvagno GL, Lippi G. Inhibitors in mild/moderate haemophilia: an update. *Thromb Haemost*. 2006;96:113-118.
227. Frommel D, Allain JP. Genetic predisposition to develop factor VIII antibody in classic hemophilia. *Clin Immunol Immunopathol*. 1977;8:34-38.
228. Tuddenham EG, McVey JH. The genetic basis of inhibitor development in haemophilia A. *Haemophilia*. 1998;4:543-545.
229. Moreau A, Lacroix-Desmazes S, Stieltjes N, et al. Antibodies to the FVIII light chain that neutralize FVIII procoagulant activity are present in plasma of nonresponder patients with severe hemophilia A and in normal polyclonal human IgG. *Blood*. 2000;95:3435-3441.
230. Sultan Y, Kazatchkine MD, Maisonneuve P, Nydegger UE. Anti-idiotypic suppression of autoantibodies to factor VIII (antihaemophilic factor) by high-dose intravenous gammaglobulin. *Lancet*. 1984;2:765-768.
231. Allain JP, Gaillandre A, Frommel D. Acquired haemophilia: functional study of antibodies to factor VIII. *Thromb Haemost*. 1981;45:285-289.
232. Prescott R, Nakai H, Saenko EL, et al. The inhibitor antibody response is more complex in hemophilia A patients than in most nonhemophiliacs with factor VIII autoantibodies. Recombinate and Kogenate Study Groups. *Blood*. 1997;89:3663-3671.
233. Nogami K, Shima M, Giddings JC, et al. Circulating factor VIII immune complexes in patients with type 2 acquired hemophilia A and protection from activated protein C-mediated proteolysis. *Blood*. 2001;97:669-677.
234. Pool JG, Miller RG. Assay of the immune inhibitor in classic haemophilia: application of virus-antibody reaction kinetics. *Br J Haematol*. 1972;22:517-528.
235. Gawryl MS, Hoyer LW. Inactivation of factor VIII coagulant activity by two different types of human antibodies. *Blood*. 1982;60:1103-1109.
236. Biggs R, Austen DE, Denson KW, Rizza CR, Borrett R. The mode of action of antibodies which destroy factor VIII. I. Antibodies which have second-order concentration graphs. *Br J Haematol*. 1972;23:125-135.
237. Biggs R, Austen DE, Denson KW, Borrett R, Rizza CR. The mode of action of antibodies which destroy factor VIII. II. Antibodies which give complex concentration graphs. *Br J Haematol*. 1972;23:137-155.
238. Kasper CK, Aledort LM, Counts RB. Proceedings: a more uniform measurement of factor VIII inhibitors. *Thromb Diath Haemorrh*. 1975;34:869-872.
239. Verbruggen B, Novakova I, Wessels H, Boezeman J, van den Berg M, Mauser-Bunschoten E. The Nijmegen modification of the Bethesda assay for factor VIII: C inhibitors: improved specificity and reliability. *Thromb Haemost*. 1995;73:247-251.
240. Rizza CR, Biggs R. The treatment of patients who have factor-VIII antibodies. *Br J Haematol*. 1973;24:65-82.
241. Giles AR, Verbruggen B, Rivard GE, Teitel J, Walker I. A detailed comparison of the performance of the standard versus the Nijmegen modification of the Bethesda assay in detecting factor VIII: C inhibitors in the haemophilia A population of Canada. Association of Hemophilia Centre Directors of Canada. Factor VIII/IX Subcommittee of Scientific and Standardization Committee of International Society on Thrombosis and Haemostasis. *Thromb Haemost*. 1998;79:872-875.
242. Lottenberg R, Kentro TB, Kitchens CS. Acquired hemophilia. A natural history study of 16 patients with factor VIII inhibitors receiving little or no therapy. *Arch Intern Med*. 1987;147:1077-1081.
243. Aledort LM, White GC. Challenges in the treatment of haemophilia with inhibitors. *Haemophilia*. 1999;5(suppl 3):1-51.
244. Collins PW, Chalmers E, Hart DP, et al. Diagnosis and treatment of factor VIII and IX inhibitors in congenital haemophilia: (4th edition). UK Haemophilia Centre Doctors Organization. *Br J Haematol*. 2013;160(2):153-170.
245. Tiede A, Collins P, Knoebl P, et al. International recommendations on the diagnosis and treatment of acquired hemophilia A. *Haematologica*. 2020;105(7):1791-1801.
246. Leissinger C, Gringeri A, Antmen B, et al. Anti-inhibitor coagulant complex prophylaxis in hemophilia with inhibitors. *N Engl J Med*. 2011;365:1684-1692.
247. Hay CR, Negrier C, Ludlam CA. The treatment of bleeding in acquired haemophilia with recombinant factor VIIa: a multicentre study. *Thromb Haemost*. 1997;78:1463-1467.
248. Monroe DM, Hoffman M, Oliver JA, Roberts HR. A possible mechanism of action of activated factor VII independent of tissue factor. *Blood Coagul Fibrinolysis*. 1998;9(suppl 1):S15-S20.
249. Key NS, Aledort LM, Beardsley D, et al. Home treatment of mild to moderate bleeding episodes using recombinant factor VIIa (Novoseven) in haemophiliacs with inhibitors. *Thromb Haemost*. 1998;80:912-918.
250. Konkle BA, Ebbesen LS, Erhardtsen E, et al. Randomized, prospective clinical trial of recombinant factor VIIa for secondary prophylaxis in hemophilia patients with inhibitors. *J Thromb Haemost*. 2007;5(9):1904-1913.
251. Aledort LM. Comparative thrombotic event incidence after infusion of recombinant factor VII$_a$ versus factor VIII inhibitor bypass activity. *J Thromb Haemost*. 2004;2:1700-1708.
252. Matino D, Makris M, Dwan K, D'Amico R, Iorio A. Recombinant factor VIIa concentrate versus plasma-derived concentrates for treating acute bleeding episodes in people with haemophilia and inhibitors. *Cochrane Database Syst Rev*. 2015;2015(12):CD004449.
253. Baudo F, Collins P, Huth-Kuhne A, et al; EACH2 Registry Contributors. Management of bleeding in acquired hemophilia A: results from the European Acquired Haemophilia (EACH2) Registry. *Blood*. 2012;120:39-46.
254. Sborov DW, Rodgers GM. How I manage patients with acquired hemophilia A. *Br J Haematol*. 2013;161:157-165.
255. Ingerslev J, Sørensen B. Parallel use of by-passing agents in haemophilia with inhibitors: a critical review. *Br J Haematol*. 2011;155:256-262.
256. Kruse-Jarres R, St-Louis J, Greist A, et al. Efficacy and safety of OB-1, an antihaemophilia factor VIII (recombinant), porcine sequence, in subjects with acquired haemophilic A. *Haemophilia*. 2015;21:162-170.
257. Wiestner A, Cho HJ, Asch AS, et al. Rituximab in the treatment of acquired factor VIII inhibitors. *Blood*. 2002;100:3426-3428.
258. Onitilo AA, Skorupa A, Lal A, et al. Rituximab in the treatment of acquired factor VIII inhibitors. *Thromb Haemost*. 2006;96:84-87.
259. Brox AG, Laryea H, Pelletier M. Successful treatment of acquired factor VIII inhibitors with cyclosporin. *Am J Hematol*. 1998;57:87-88.

260. Crenier L, Ducobu J, des Grottes JM, Cerny J, Delaunoit C, Capel P. Low response to high-dose intravenous immunoglobulin in the treatment of acquired factor VIII inhibitor. *Br J Haematol.* 1996;95:750-753.
261. Mariani G, Ghirardini A, Bellocco R. Immune tolerance in hemophilia–principal results from the International Registry. Report of the factor VIII and IX Subcommittee. *Thromb Haemost.* 1994;72:155-158.
262. Mariani G, Kroner B. International immune tolerance registry, 1997 update. *Vox Sang.* 1999;77(suppl 1):25-27.
263. DiMichele DM, Kroner BL. The North American Immune Tolerance Registry: practices, outcomes, outcome predictors. *Thromb Haemost.* 2002;87:52-57.
264. Hay CR, DiMichele DM; International Immune Tolerance Study. The principal results of the International Immune Tolerance Study: a randomized dose comparison. *Blood.* 2012;119:1335-1344.
265. Ettingshausen CE, Kreuz W. Role of von Willebrand factor in immune tolerance induction. *Blood Coagul Fibrinolysis.* 2005;16(suppl 1):S27-S31.
266. Nilsson IM, Berntorp E, Zettervall O. Induction of immune tolerance in patients with hemophilia and antibodies to factor VIII by combined treatment with intravenous IgG, cyclophosphamide, and factor VIII. *N Engl J Med.* 1988;318:947-950.
267. Leissinger C, Josephson CD, Granger S, et al. Rituximab for treatment of inhibitors in haemophilia A. A Phase II study. *Thromb Haemost.* 2014;112(3):445-458.
268. DiMichele DM. Immune tolerance in haemophilia: the long journey to the fork in the road. *Br J Haematol.* 2012;159:123-134.
269. Colowick AB, Bohn RL, Avorn J, Ewenstein BM. Immune tolerance induction in hemophilia patients with inhibitors: costly can be cheaper. *Blood.* 2000;96:1698-1702.
270. Oldenburg J, Mahlangu JN, Kim B, et al. Emicizumab prophylaxis in hemophilia A with inhibitors. *N Engl J Med.* 2017;377:809-818.
271. Oldenburg J, Mahlangu JN, Bujan W, et al. The effect of emicizumab prophylaxis on health-related outcomes in persons with haemophilia A with inhibitors: HAVEN 1 Study. *Haemophilia.* 2019;25(1):33-44.
272. Croteau SE, Wang M, Wheeler AP. Clinical trials update: innovations in hemophilia therapy. *Am J Hematol.* 2021;96:128-144.
273. Ljung RC. Gene mutations and inhibitor formation in patients with hemophilia B. *Acta Haematol.* 1995;94(suppl 1):49-52.
274. Largo R, Sigg P, von Felten A, Straub PW. Acquired factor-IX inhibitor in a non-haemophilic patient with autoimmune disease. *Br J Haematol.* 1974;26:129-140.
275. Ljung R, Petrini P, Tengborn L, Sjörin E. Haemophilia B mutations in Sweden: a population-based study of mutational heterogeneity. *Br J Haematol.* 2001;113:81-86.
276. Christophe OD, Lenting PJ, Cherel G, et al. Functional mapping of antifactor IX inhibitors developed in patients with severe hemophilia B. *Blood.* 2001;98:1416-1423.
277. Ekert H, Brewin T, Boey W, Davey P, Tilden D. Cost-utility analysis of recombinant factor VIIa (NovoSeven) in six children with long-standing inhibitors to factor VIII or IX. *Haemophilia.* 2001;7:279-285.
278. Lusher JM. Inhibitor antibodies to factor VIII and factor IX: management. *Semin Thromb Hemost.* 2000;26:179-188.
279. Clough AM, Gilreath JA, McPherson JP, Link NC, Rodgers GM, Nance D. Implementation of a recombinant factor IX Fc fusion protein extended-infusion desensitization protocol. *Haemophilia.* 2017;23:e227-e230.
280. Chitlur M, Warrier I, Rajpurkar M, Lusher JM. Inhibitors in factor IX deficiency a report of the ISTH-SSC international FIX inhibitor registry (1997-2006). *Haemophilia.* 2009;15:1027-1031.
281. Feinstein DI. Acquired inhibitors of factor V. *Thromb Haemost.* 1978;39:663-674.
282. Goulenok T, Vasco C, Faille D, et al. Acquired factor V inhibitor: a nation-wide study of 38 patients. *Br J Haematol.* 2021;192:892-899.
283. Bennett J, Cunningham MT, Howard C, Hoffmann M, Plapp FV. Acquired factor V inhibitor in the setting of coronavirus disease 2019 infection. *Blood Coagul Fibrinolysis.* 2021;32(4):294-297.
284. Favaloro EJ, Bonar R, Duncan E, et al. Identification of factor inhibitors by diagnostic haemostasis laboratories: a large multi-centre evaluation. *Thromb Haemost.* 2006;96(1):73-78.
285. Ang AL, Kuperan P, Ng CH, Ng HJ. Acquired factor V inhibitor. A problem-based systematic review. *Thromb Haemost.* 2009;101:852-859.
286. Ortel TL. Clinical and laboratory manifestations of anti-factor V antibodies. *J Lab Clin Med.* 1999;133:326-334.
287. Streiff MB, Ness PM. Acquired factor V inhibitors: a needless iatrogenic complication of bovine thrombin exposure. *Transfusion.* 2002;42:18-26.
288. Ortel TL, Mercer MC, Thames EH, Moore KD, Lawson JH. Immunologic impact and clinical outcomes after surgical exposure to bovine thrombin. *Ann Surg.* 2001;233:88-96.
289. Diesen DL, Lawson JH. Bovine thrombin: history, use, and risk in the surgical patient. *Vascular.* 2008 Mar-Apr;16(suppl 1):S29-S36.
290. Ness P, Creer M, Rodgers GM, et al; Recognition, Evaluation and Treatment of Acquired Coagulopathy Consensus (RETACC) Panel. Building an immune-mediated coagulopathy consensus: early recognition and evaluation to enhance post-surgical patient safety. *Patient Saf Surg.* 2009;3:8.
291. Chediak J, Ashenhurst JB, Garlick I, Desser RK. Successful management of bleeding in a patient with factor V inhibitor by platelet transfusions. *Blood.* 1980;56:835-841.
292. Grace CS, Wolf P. Proceedings: a high titre circulating inhibitor of human factor V. Clinical, biochemical and immunological features and its treatment by plasmapheresis. *Thromb Diath Haemorrh.* 1975;34:322.
293. DeRaucourt E, Barbier C, Sinda P, Dib M, Peltier JY, Ternisien C. High-dose intravenous immunoglobulin treatment in two patients with acquired factor V inhibitors. *Am J Hematol.* 2003;74:187-190.
294. Kalafatis M, Simioni P, Tormene D, Beck DO, Luni S, Girolami A. Isolation and characterization of an antifactor V antibody causing activated protein C resistance from a patient with severe thrombotic manifestations. *Blood.* 2002;99:3985-3992.
295. Federici AB, Rand JH, Bucciarelli P, et al; Subcommittee on von Willebrand Factor. Acquired von Willebrand syndrome: data from an international registry. *Thromb Haemost.* 2000;84:345-349.
296. Rinder MR, Richard RE, Rinder HM. Acquired von Willebrand's disease: a concise review. *Am J Hematol.* 1997;54:139-145.
297. Veyradier A, Jenkins CS, Fressinaud E, Meyer D. Acquired von Willebrand syndrome: from pathophysiology to management. *Thromb Haemost.* 2000;84:175-182.
298. Vincentelli A, Susen S, Le Tourneau T, et al. Acquired von Willebrand syndrome in aortic stenosis. *N Engl J Med.* 2003;349:343-349.
299. Heilmann C, Geisen U, Beyersdorf F, et al. Acquired von Willebrand syndrome in patients with ventricular assist device or total artificial heart. *Thromb Haemost.* 2010;103:962-967.
300. Nascimbene A, Neelamegham S, Frazier OH, Moake JL, Dong JF. Acquired von Willebrand syndrome associated with left ventricular assist device. *Blood.* 2016;127:3133-3141.
301. Tiede A, Rand JH, Budde U, Ganser A, Federici AB. How I treat the acquired von Willebrand syndrome. *Blood.* 2011;117:6777-6785.
302. Abou-Ismail MY, Rodgers GM, Bray PF, Lim MY. Acquired von Willebrand syndrome in monoclonal gammopathy—a scoping review on hemostatic management. *Res Pract Thromb Haemost.* 2021;5(2):356-365.
303. Franchini M, Mannucci PM. Von Willebrand disease-associated angiodysplasia: a few answers, still many questions. *Br J Haematol.* 2013;161:177-182.
304. Randi AM. Endothelial dysfunction in von Willebrand disease: angiogenesis and angiodysplasia. *Thromb Res.* 2016;141(suppl 2):S55-S58.
305. Lorand L, Jacobsen A, Bruner-Lorand J. A pathological inhibitor of fibrin cross-linking. *J Clin Invest.* 1968;47:268-273.
306. Lewis JH, Szeto IL, Ellis LD, Bayer WL. An acquired inhibitor to coagulation factor XIII. *Johns Hopkins Med J.* 1967;120:401-407.
307. Lorand L, Maldonado N, Fradera J, Atencio AC, Robertson B, Urayama T. Haemorrhagic syndrome of autoimmune origin with a specific inhibitor against fibrin stabilizing factor (factor XIII). *Br J Haematol.* 1972;23:17-27.
308. Ajzner E, Schlammadinger A, Kerényi A, et al. Severe bleeding complications caused by an autoantibody against the B subunit of plasma factor XIII: a novel form of acquired factor XIII deficiency. *Blood.* 2009;113:723-725.
309. Luo YY, Zhang GS. Acquired factor XIII inhibitor: clinical features, treatment, fibrin structure and epitope determination. *Haemophilia.* 2011;17:393-398.
310. Ichinose A. Autoimmune acquired factor XIII deficiency due to anti-factor XIII/13 antibodies. A summary of 93 patients. *Blood Rev.* 2017;31:37-45.
311. Acharya SS, Coughlin A, DiMichele DM. Rare Bleeding Disorder Registry: deficiencies of factors II, V, VII, X, XIII, fibrinogen and dysfibrinogenemias. *J Thromb Haemost.* 2003;2:248-256.
312. DeVries A, Rosenberg T, Kochwa S, Boss JH. Precipitating antifibrinogen antibody appearing after fibrinogen infusions in a patient with congenital afibrinogenemia. *Am J Med.* 1961;30:486-494.
313. Scully MF, Ellis V, Kakkar VV, Savidge GF, Williams YF, Sterndale H. An acquired coagulation inhibitor to factor II. *Br J Haematol.* 1982;50:655-664.
314. Bajaj SP, Rapaport SI, Fierer DS, Herbst KD, Schwartz DB. A mechanism for the hypoprothrombinemia of the acquired hypoprothrombinemia-lupus anticoagulant syndrome. *Blood.* 1983;61:684-692.
315. Salomon O, Zivelin A, Livnat T, et al. Prevalence, causes, and characterization of factor XI inhibitors in patients with inherited factor XI deficiency. *Blood.* 2003;101:4783-4788.
316. Livnat T, Tamarin I, Mor Y, et al. Recombinant activated factor VII and tranexamic acid are haemostatically effective during major surgery in factor XI-deficient patients with inhibitor antibodies. *Thromb Haemost.* 2009;102:487-492.
317. Reece EA, Clyne LP, Romero R, Hobbins JC. Spontaneous factor XI inhibitors. Seven additional cases and a review of the literature. *Arch Intern Med.* 1984;144:525-529.
318. Bortoli R, Monticielo OA, Chakr RM, et al. Acquired factor XI inhibitor in systemic lupus erythematosus—case report and literature review. *Semin Arthritis Rheum.* 2009;39:61-65.
319. Lee G, Duan-Porter W, Metjian A. Acquired, non-amloid related factor X deficiency: review of the literature. *Haemophilia.* 2012;18:655-663.
320. Henson K, Files JC, Morrison FS. Transient acquired factor X deficiency: report of the use of activated clotting concentrate to control a life-threatening hemorrhage. *Am J Med.* 1989;87:583-585.
321. Hsia CC, Keeney M, Bosco AA, Xenocostas A. Treatment of acquired factor X inhibitor by plasma exchange with concomitant intravenous immunoglobulin and corticosteroids. *Am J Hematol.* 2008;83:318-320.
322. Aguilar C, Lucia JF, Hernandez P. A case of an inhibitor autoantibody to coagulation factor VII. *Haemophilia.* 2003;9:119-120.
323. Campbell E, Sanal S, Mattson J, et al. Factor VII inhibitor. *Am J Med.* 1980;68:962-964.
324. Ndimbie OK, Raman B, Saeed SM. Lupus anticoagulant associated with specific inhibition of factor VII in a patient with AIDS. *Am J Clin Pathol.* 1989;91:491-493.
325. Delmer A, Horellou MH, Andreu G, et al. Life-threatening intracranial bleeding associated with the presence of an antifactor VII autoantibody. *Blood.* 1989;74:229-232.
326. Alqarni NS, Algairaigri AH. A neonate with acquired factor VII deficiency successfully managed with immunomodulatory therapy. *Int J Pediatr Adolesc Med.* 2021;8(3):195-197.

327. Okajima K, Ishii M. Life-threatening bleeding in a case of autoantibody-induced factor VII deficiency. *Int J Hematol.* 1999;69:129-132.
328. Tsuda H, Higashi S, Iwanaga S, Kubota T, Morita T, Yanaga K. Development of antitissue factor antibodies in patients after liver surgery. *Blood.* 1993;82:96-102.
329. Levine JS, Branch DW, Rauch J. The antiphospholipid syndrome. *N Engl J Med.* 2002;346:752-763.
330. Ruiz-Irastorza G, Crowther M, Branch W, Khamashta MA. Antiphospholipid syndrome. *Lancet.* 2010;376:1498-1509.
331. Chaturvedi S, McCrae KR. Diagnosis and management of the antiphospholipid syndrome. *Blood Rev.* 2017;31:406-417.
332. Doig RG, O'Malley CJ, Dauer R, McGrath KM. An evaluation of 200 consecutive patients with spontaneous or recurrent thrombosis for primary hypercoagulable states. *Am J Clin Pathol.* 1994;102:797-801.
333. Garcia D, Erkan D. Diagnosis and management of the antiphospholipid syndrome. *N Engl J Med.* 2018;378:2010-2021.
334. Roubey RA. Autoantibodies to phospholipid-binding plasma proteins: a new view of lupus anticoagulants and other "antiphospholipid" autoantibodies. *Blood.* 1994;84:2854-2867.
335. Moore JE, Lutz WB. The natural history of systemic erythematosus: an approach to its study through chronic biologic false-positive reactors. *J Chron Dis.* 1955;1:297-316.
336. Triplett DA. Antiphospholipid-protein antibodies: laboratory detection and clinical relevance. *Thromb Res.* 1995;78:1-31.
337. Vermylen J, Arnout J. Is the antiphospholipid syndrome caused by antibodies directed against physiologically relevant phospholipid-protein complexes? *J Lab Clin Med.* 1992;120:10-12.
338. Mueller JF, Ratnoff O, Heinle RW. Observations on the characteristics of an unusual circulating anticoagulant. *J Lab Clin Med.* 1951;38:254-261.
339. Simone JV, Cornet JA, Abildgaard CF. Acquired von Willebrand's syndrome in systemic lupus erythematosus. *Blood.* 1968;31:806-812.
340. Harris EN, Gharavi AE, Boey ML, et al. Anticardiolipin antibodies: detection by radioimmunoassay and association with thrombosis in systemic lupus erythematosus. *Lancet.* 1983;2:1211-1214.
341. McNeil HP, Simpson RJ, Chesterman CN, Krilis SA. Anti-phospholipid antibodies are directed against a complex antigen that includes a lipid-binding inhibitor of coagulation: beta 2-glycoprotein I (apolipoprotein H). *Proc Natl Acad Sci U S A.* 1990;87:4120-4124.
342. Gomez-Pacheco L, Villa AR, Drenkard C, Cabiedes J, Cabral AR, Alarcón-Segovia D. Serum anti-beta2-glycoprotein-I and anticardiolipin antibodies during thrombosis in systemic lupus erythematosus patients. *Am J Med.* 1999;106:417-423.
343. Roubey RA. Antigenic specificities of "antiphospholipid" autoantibodies. *Springer Semin Immunopathol*; 1994;16:211-222.
344. Bevers EM, Galli M, Barbui T, Comfurius P, Zwaal RF. Lupus anticoagulant IgG's (LA) are not directed to phospholipids only, but to a complex of lipid-bound human prothrombin. *Thromb Haemost.* 1991;66:629-632.
345. Simmelink MJ, Horbach DA, Derksen RH, et al. Complexes of anti-prothrombin antibodies and prothrombin cause lupus anticoagulant activity by competing with the binding of clotting factors for catalytic phospholipid surfaces. *Br J Haematol.* 2001;113:621-629.
346. Kandiah DA, Krilis SA. Beta 2-glycoprotein I. *Lupus.* 1994;3:207-212.
347. Dienava-Verdoold I, Boon-Spijker MG, de Groot PG, et al. Patient-derived monoclonal antibodies directed towards beta2 glycoprotein-1 display lupus anticoagulant activity. *J Thromb Haemost.* 2011;9:738-747.
348. Gropp K, Weber N, Reuter M, et al. β$_2$-glycoprotein I, the major target in antiphospholipid syndrome, is a special human complement regulator. *Blood.* 2011;118:2774-2783.
349. Nimpf J, Wurm H, Kostner GM. Beta 2-glycoprotein-I (apo-H) inhibits the release reaction of human platelets during ADP-induced aggregation. *Atherosclerosis.* 1987;63:109-114.
350. de Laat HB, Derksen RH, Urbanus RT, Roest M, de Groot PG. β$_2$-glycoprotein I–dependent lupus anticoagulant highly correlates with thrombosis in the antiphospholipid syndrome. *Blood.* 2004;104:3598-3602.
351. Le Tonqueze M, Salozhin K, Dueymes M, et al. Role of beta 2-glycoprotein I in the antiphospholipid antibody binding to endothelial cells. *Lupus.* 1995;4:179-186.
352. Rand JH, Wa XX, Lapinski R, et al. Detection of antibody-mediated reduction of annexin A5 anticoagulant activity in plasmas of patients with the antiphospholipid syndrome. *Blood.* 2004;104:2783-2790.
353. Cesarman-Maus G, Ríos-Luna NP, Deora AB, et al. Autoantibodies against the fibrinolytic receptor, annexin 2, in antiphospholipid syndrome. *Blood.* 2006;107:4375-4382.
354. Galli M, Ruggeri L, Barbui T. Differential effects of anti-beta 2-glycoprotein I and antiprothrombin antibodies on the anticoagulant activity of activated protein C. *Blood.* 1998;91:1999-2004.
355. Sheng Y, Kandiah DA, Krilis SA. Anti-beta 2-glycoprotein I autoantibodies from patients with the "antiphospholipid" syndrome bind to beta 2-glycoprotein I with low affinity: dimerization of beta 2-glycoprotein I induces a significant increase in anti-beta 2-glycoprotein I antibody affinity. *J Immunol.* 1998;161:2038-2043.
356. Triplett DA, Asherson RA. Pathophysiology of the catastrophic antiphospholipid syndrome (CAPS). *Am J Hematol.* 2000;65:154-159.
357. Gamsjaeger R, Johs A, Gries A, et al. Membrane binding of beta2-glycoprotein I can be described by a two-state reaction model: an atomic force microscopy and surface plasmon resonance study. *Biochem J.* 2005;389:665-673.
358. Agar C, van Os GM, Mörgelin M, et al. Beta2-glycoprotein I can exist in 2 conformations: implications for our understanding of the antiphospholipid syndrome. *Blood.* 2010;116:1336-1343.
359. Raschi E, Testoni C, Bosisio D, et al. Role of the MyD88 transduction signaling pathway in endothelial activation by antiphospholipid antibodies. *Blood.* 2003;101:3495-3500.
360. Vega-Ostertag M, Casper K, Swerlick R, Ferrara D, Harris EN, Pierangeli SS. Involvement of p38 MAPK in the up-regulation of tissue factor on endothelial cells by antiphospholipid antibodies. *Arthritis Rheum.* 2005;52:1545-1554.
361. Sacharidou A, Chambliss KL, Ulrich V, et al. Antiphospholipid antibodies induce thrombosis by PP2A activation via apoER2-Dab2-SHC1 complex formation in endothelium. *Blood.* 2018;131:2097-2110.
362. Pierangeli SS, Goldsmith GH, Krnic S, Harris EN. Differences in functional activity of anticardiolipin antibodies from patients with syphilis and those with antiphospholipid syndrome. *Infect Immun.* 1994;62:4081-4084.
363. Canoso RT, Sise HS. Chlorpromazine-induced lupus anticoagulant and associated immunologic abnormalities. *Am J Hematol.* 1982;13:121-129.
364. Triplett DA, Brandt JT, Musgrave KA, Orr CA. The relationship between lupus anticoagulants and antibodies to phospholipid. *J Am Med Assoc.* 1988;259:550-554.
365. Passam FH, Giannakopoulos B, Mirarabshahi P, Krilis SA. Molecular pathophysiology of the antiphospholipid syndrome: the role of oxidative posttranslational modification of beta 2 glycoprotein I. *J Thromb Haemost.* 2011;9(suppl 1):275-282.
366. Hörkkö S, Miller E, Dudl E, et al. Antiphospholipid antibodies are directed against epitopes of oxidized phospholipids. Recognition of cardiolipin by monoclonal antibodies to epitopes of oxidized low density lipoprotein. *J Clin Invest.* 1996;98:815-825.
367. Redecha P, Tilley R, Tencati M, et al. Tissue factor: a link between C5a and neutrophil activation in antiphospholipid antibody induced fetal injury. *Blood.* 2007;110:2423-2431.
368. Giannakopoulos B, Krilis SA. The pathogenesis of the antiphosholipid syndrome. *N Engl J Med.* 2013;368:1033-1044.
369. Pierangeli SS, Barker JH, Stikovac D, et al. Effect of human IgG antiphospholipid antibodies on an in vivo thrombosis model in mice. *Thromb Haemost.* 1994;71:670-674.
370. Pierangeli SS, Liu XW, Barker JH, Anderson G, Harris EN. Induction of thrombosis in a mouse model by IgG, IgM and IgA immunoglobulins from patients with the antiphospholipid syndrome. *Thromb Haemost.* 1995;74:1361-1367.
371. Yodfat O, Blank M, Krause I, Shoenfeld Y. The pathogenic role of anti-phosphatidylserine antibodies: active immunization with the antibodies leads to the induction of antiphospholipid syndrome. *Clin Immunol Immunopathol.* 1996;78:14-20.
372. Gharavi AE, Sammaritano LR, Bovastro JL Jr, Wilson WA. Specificities and characteristics of beta 2 glycoprotein I-induced antiphospholipid antibodies. *J Lab Clin Med.* 1995;125:775-778.
373. Casciola-Rosen L, Rosen A, Petri M, Schlissel M. Surface blebs on apoptotic cells are sites of enhanced procoagulant activity: implications for coagulation events and antigenic spread in systemic lupus erythematosus. *Proc Natl Acad Sci U S A.* 1996;93:1624-1629.
374. Rauch J, Tannenbaum M, Tannenbaum H, et al. Human hybridoma lupus anticoagulants distinguish between lamellar and hexagonal phase lipid systems. *J Biol Chem.* 1986;261:9672-9677.
375. Aguilar L, Ortega-Pierres G, Campos B, et al. Phospholipid membranes form specific nonbilayer molecular arrangements that are antigenic. *J Biol Chem.* 1999;274(36):25193-25196.
376. Bordron A, Dueymes M, Levy Y, et al. The binding of some human antiendothelial cell antibodies induces endothelial cell apoptosis. *J Clin Invest.* 1998;101:2029-2035.
377. Arachchillage DR, Efthymiou M, Mackie IJ, Lawrie AS, Machin SJ, Cohen H. Anti-protein C antibodies are associated with resistance to endogenous protein C activation and a severe thrombotic phenotype in antiphospholipid syndrome. *J Thromb Haemost.* 2014;12:1801-1809.
378. Esmon NL, Smirnov MD, Esmon CT. Thrombogenic mechanisms of antiphospholipid antibodies. *Thromb Haemost.* 1997;78:79-82.
379. López-Pedrera C., Buendía P, Aguirre MA, Velasco F, Cuadrado MJ. Antiphospholipid syndrome and tissue factor: a thrombotic couple. *Lupus.* 2006;15:161-166.
380. Redecha P, Franzke CW, Ruf W, Mackman N, Girardi G. Neutrophil activation by the tissue factor/Factor VIIa/PAR2 axis mediates fetal death in a mouse model of antiphospholipid syndrome. *J Clin Invest.* 2008;118:3453-3461.
381. Petri M. Epidemiology of the antiphospholipid antibody syndrome. *J Autoimmun.* 2000;15:145-151.
382. Kelsey PR, Stevenson KJ, Poller L. The diagnosis of lupus anticoagulants by the activated partial thromboplastin time–the central role of phosphatidyl serine. *Thromb Haemost.* 1984;52:172-175.
383. Schved JF, Dupuy-Fons C, Biron C, Quéré I, Janbon C. A prospective epidemiological study on the occurrence of antiphospholipid antibody: the Montpellier Antiphospholipid (MAP) Study. *Haemostasis.* 1994;24:175-182.
384. Ford SE, Kennedy L, Ford PM. Clinicopathologic correlations of antiphospholipid antibodies. An autopsy study. *Arch Pathol Lab Med.* 1994;118:491-495.
385. Feinstein DI, Francis RB. The lupus anticoagulant and anticardiolipin antibodies. In: Wallace DJ, Hahn BH, eds. *Dubois' Lupus Erythematosus.* 4th ed. Lea & Febiger; 1993:246-253.
386. Boey ML, Colaco CB, Gharavi AE, Elkon KB, Loizou S, Hughes GR. Thrombosis in systemic lupus erythematosus: striking association with the presence of circulating lupus anticoagulant. *Br Med J.* 1983;287:1021-1023.
387. Exner T, Rickard KA, Kronenberg H. A sensitive test demonstrating lupus anticoagulant and its behavioural patterns. *Br J Haematol.* 1978;40:143-151.

388. Jouhikainen T, Stephansson E, Leirisalo-Repo M. Lupus anticoagulant as a prognostic marker in systemic lupus erythematosus. *Br J Rheumatol*. 1993;32:568-573.
389. Gebhart J, Posch F, Koder S, et al. Increased mortality in patients with the lupus anticoagulant: the vienna lupus anticoagulant and thrombosis study (LATS). *Blood*. 2015;125:3477-3483.
390. Stasi R, Stipa E, Masi M, et al. Antiphospholipid antibodies: prevalence, clinical significance and correlation to cytokine levels in acute myeloid leukemia and non-Hodgkin's lymphoma. *Thromb Haemost*. 1993;70:568-572.
391. Chedid A, Chadalawada KR, Morgan TR, et al. Phospholipid antibodies in alcoholic liver disease. *Hepatology*. 1994;20:1465-1471.
392. Prieto J, Yuste JR, Beloqui O, et al. Anticardiolipin antibodies in chronic hepatitis C: implication of hepatitis C virus as the cause of the antiphospholipid syndrome. *Hepatology*. 1996;23:199-204.
393. Bloom EJ, Abrams DI, Rodgers G. Lupus anticoagulant in the acquired immunodeficiency syndrome. *J Am Med Assoc*. 1986;256:491-493.
394. Facer CA, Agiostratidou G. High levels of anti-phospholipid antibodies in uncomplicated and severe Plasmodium falciparum and in P. vivax malaria. *Clin Exp Immunol*. 1994;95:304-309.
395. Kucuk O, Gilman-Sachs A, Beaman K, Lis LJ, Westerman MP. Antiphospholipid antibodies in sickle cell disease. *Am J Hematol*. 1993;42:380-383.
396. Levine SR, Welch KM. The spectrum of neurologic disease associated with antiphospholipid antibodies. Lupus anticoagulants and anticardiolipin antibodies. *Arch Neurol*. 1987;44:876-883.
397. Harrison CN, Donohoe S, Carr P, Dave M, Mackie I, Machin SJ. Patients with essential thrombocythaemia have an increased prevalence of antiphospholipid antibodies which may be associated with thrombosis. *Thromb Haemost*. 2002;87:802-807.
398. Bell WR, Boss GR, Wolfson JS. Circulating anticoagulant in the procainamide-induced lupus syndrome. *Arch Intern Med*. 1977;137:1471-1473.
399. Bird MR, O'Neill AI, Buchanan RR, Ibrahim KM, Des Parkin J. Lupus anticoagulant in the elderly may be associated with both quinine and quinidine usage. *Pathology*. 1995;27:136-139.
400. Orris DJ, Lewis JH, Spero JA, Hasiba U. Blocking coagulation inhibitors in children taking penicillin. *J Pediatr*. 1980;97:426-429.
401. Bizzaro N, Brandalise M. EDTA-dependent pseudothrombocytopenia. Association with antiplatelet and antiphospholipid antibodies. *Am J Clin Pathol*. 1995;103:103-107.
402. Chamouard P, Grunebaum L, Wiesel ML, et al. Prevalence and significance of anticardiolipin antibodies in Crohn's disease. *Dig Dis Sci*. 1994;39:1501-1504.
403. Stasi R, Stipa E, Masi M, et al. Prevalence and clinical significance of elevated antiphospholipid antibodies in patients with idiopathic thrombocytopenic purpura. *Blood*. 1994;84:4203-4208.
404. Shi W, Krilis SA, Chong BH, Gordon S, Chesterman CN. Prevalence of lupus anticoagulant and anticardiolipin antibodies in a healthy population. *Aust N Z J Med*. 1990;20:231-236.
405. Manoussakis MN, Tzioufas AG, Silis MP, Pange PJ, Goudevenos J, Moutsopoulos HM. High prevalence of anti-cardiolipin and other autoantibodies in a healthy elderly population. *Clin Exp Immunol*. 1987;69:557-565.
406. Vila P, Hernández MC, López-Fernández MF, Batlle J. Prevalence, follow-up and clinical significance of the anticardiolipin antibodies in normal subjects. *Thromb Haemost*. 1994;72:209-213.
407. Goldberg SN, Conti-Kelly AM, Greco TP. A family study of anticardiolipin antibodies and associated clinical conditions. *Am J Med*. 1995;99:473-479.
408. Camps MT, Cuadrado MJ, Ocón P, et al. Association between HLA class II antigens and primary antiphospholipid syndrome from the south of Spain. *Lupus*. 1995;4:51-55.
409. Colucci AT, Di Lorenzo G, Ingrassia A, et al. Blood antiphospholipid antibody levels are influenced by age, sex and HLA-B8,DR3 phenotype. *Exp Clin Immunogenet*. 1992;9:72-79.
410. Galli M, Luciani D, Bertolini G, Barbui T. Lupus anticoagulants are stronger risk factors for thrombosis than anticardiolipin antibodies in the antiphospholipid syndrome: a systematic review of the literature. *Blood*. 2003;101:1827-1832.
411. Miyakis S, Lockshin MD, Atsumi T, et al. International consensus statement on an update of the classification criteria for definite antiphospholipid syndrome (APS). *J Thromb Haemost*. 2006;4:295-306.
412. Morgan M, Downs K, Chesterman CN, Biggs JC. Clinical analysis of 125 patients with the lupus anticoagulant. *Aust N Z J Med*. 1993;23:151-156.
413. Cervera R, Asherson RA, Lie JT. Clinicopathologic correlations of the antiphospholipid syndrome. *Semin Arthritis Rheum*. 1995;24:262-272.
414. Triplett DA. Protean clinical presentation of antiphospholipid-protein antibodies (APA). *Thromb Haemost*. 1995;74:329-337.
415. Derksen RH, Gmelig-Meijling FH, de Groot PG. Primary antiphospholipid syndrome evolving into systemic lupus erythematosus. *Lupus*. 1996;5:77-80.
416. Silver RM, Draper ML, Scott JR, Lyon JL, Reading J, Branch DW. Clinical consequences of antiphospholipid antibodies: an historic cohort study. *Obstet Gynecol*. 1994;83:372-377.
417. Bowie EWJ, Thompson JH Jr, Pascuzzi CA, Owen CA Jr. Thrombosis in systemic lupus erythematosus despite circulating anticoagulants. *J Lab Clin Med*. 1963;62:416-430.
418. Gastineau DA, Kazmier FJ, Nichols WL, Bowie EJ. Lupus anticoagulant: an analysis of the clinical and laboratory features of 219 cases. *Am J Hematol*. 1985;19:265-275.
419. Mueh JR, Herbst KD, Rapaport SI. Thrombosis in patients with the lupus anticoagulant. *Ann Intern Med*. 1980;92:156-159.
420. Coull BM, Levine SR, Brey RL. The role of antiphospholipid antibodies in stroke. *Neurol Clin*. 1992;10:125-143.
421. Levine SR, Brey RL, Sawaya KL, et al. Recurrent stroke and thrombo-occlusive events in the antiphospholipid syndrome. *Ann Neurol*. 1995;38:119-124.
422. Sanmarco M, Soler C, Christides C, et al. Prevalence and clinical significance of IgG isotype anti-beta 2-glycoprotein I antibodies in antiphospholipid syndrome: a comparative study with anticardiolipin antibodies. *J Lab Clin Med*. 1997;129:499-506.
423. Horbach DA, van Oort E, Donders RC, Derksen RH, de Groot PG. Lupus anticoagulant is the strongest risk factor for both venous and arterial thrombosis in patients with systemic lupus erythematosus. Comparison between different assays for the detection of antiphospholipid antibodies. *Thromb Haemost*. 1996;76:916-924.
424. Asherson RA, Liote F, Page B, et al. Avascular necrosis of bone and antiphospholipid antibodies in systemic lupus erythematosus. *J Rheumatol*. 1993;20:284-288.
425. Galli M, Finazzi G, Barbui T. Thrombocytopenia in the antiphospholipid syndrome. *Br J Haematol*. 1996;93:1-5.
426. Ordi J, Vilardel M, Oristrell J, et al. Bleeding in patients with lupus anticoagulant. *Lancet*. 1984;2:868-869.
427. Dorsch CA, Meyerhoff J. Mechanisms of abnormal platelet aggregation in systemic lupus erythematosus. *Arthritis Rheum*. 1982;25:966-973.
428. Natelson EA, Cyprus GS, Hettig RA. Absent factor II in systemic lupus erythematosus. Immunologic studies and response to corticosteroid therapy. *Arthritis Rheum*. 1976;19:79-82.
429. Brey RL, Chapman J, Levine SR, et al. Stroke and the antiphospholipid syndrome: consensus meeting Taormina 2002. *Lupus*. 2003;12:508-513.
430. Levine SR, Brey RL, Tilley BC, et al. Antiphospholipid antibodies and subsequent thrombo-occlusive events in patients with ischemic stroke. *J Am Med Assoc*. 2004;291:576-584.
431. Leal Rato M, Bandeira M, Romão VC, Aguiar de Sousa D. Neurologic manifestations of the antiphospholipid syndrome - an update. *Curr Neurol Neurosci Rep*. 2021;21(8):41.
432. Alegre VA, Gastineau DA, Winkelmann RK. Skin lesions associated with circulating lupus anticoagulant. *Br J Dermatol*. 1989;120:419-429.
433. Fligelstone LJ, Cachia PG, Ralis H, et al. Lupus anticoagulant in patients with peripheral vascular disease: a prospective study. *Eur J Vasc Endovasc Surg*. 1995;9:277-283.
434. Hamsten A, Norberg R, Bjorkholm M, de Faire U, Holm G. Antibodies to cardiolipin in young survivors of myocardial infarction: an association with recurrent cardiovascular events. *Lancet*. 1986;1:113-116.
435. Asherson RA, Mackworth-Young CG, Boey ML, et al. Pulmonary hypertension in systemic lupus erythematosus. *Br Med J*. 1983;287:1024-1025.
436. Asherson RA. The catastrophic antiphospholipid syndrome. *J Rheumatol*. 1992;19:508-512.
437. Branch DW, Scott JR, Kochenour NK, Hershgold E. Obstetric complications associated with the lupus anticoagulant. *N Engl J Med*. 1985;313:1322-1326.
438. Shapiro GA. Antiphospholipid syndrome in obstetrics and gynecology. *Semin Thromb Hemost*. 1994;20:64-70.
439. Oshiro BT, Silver RM, Scott JR, Yu H, Branch DW. Antiphospholipid antibodies and fetal death. *Obstet Gynecol*. 1996;87:489-493.
440. MacLean MA, Cumming GP, McCall F, Walker ID, Walker JJ. The prevalence of lupus anticoagulant and anticardiolipin antibodies in women with a history of first trimester miscarriages. *Br J Obstet Gynaecol*. 1994;101:103-106.
441. Rai RS, Regan L, Clifford K, et al. Antiphospholipid antibodies and beta 2-glycoprotein-I in 500 women with recurrent miscarriage: results of a comprehensive screening approach. *Hum Reprod*. 1995;10:2001-2005.
442. Silver RM, Draper ML, Byrne JL, Ashwood EA, Lyon JL, Branch DW. Unexplained elevations of maternal serum alpha-fetoprotein in women with antiphospholipid antibodies: a harbinger of fetal death. *Obstet Gynecol*. 1994;83:150-155.
443. Clark F, Dickinson JE, Walters BN, Marshall LR, O'Leary PC. Elevated mid-trimester hCG and maternal lupus anticoagulant. *Prenat Diagn*. 1995;15:1035-1039.
444. Harris EN, Spinnato JA. Should anticardiolipin tests be performed in otherwise healthy pregnant women? *Am J Obstet Gynecol*. 1991;165:1272-1277.
445. Lynch A, Marlar R, Murphy J, et al. Antiphospholipid antibodies in predicting adverse pregnancy outcome. A prospective study. *Ann Intern Med*. 1994;120:470-475.
446. Rix P, Stentoft J, Aunsholt NA, et al. Lupus anticoagulant and anticardiolipin antibodies in an obstetric population. *Acta Obstet Gynecol Scand*. 1992;71:605-609.
447. Silver RM, Porter TF, van Leeuween I, Jeng G, Scott JR, Branch DW. Anticardiolipin antibodies: clinical consequences of "low titers". *Obstet Gynecol*. 1996;87:494-500.
448. Rand JH, Wu XX, Andree HA, et al. Pregnancy loss in the antiphospholipid-antibody syndrome—a possible thrombogenic mechanism. *N Engl J Med*. 1997;337:154-160.
449. Girardi G, Redecha P, Salmon JE. Heparin prevents antiphospholipid antibody-induced fetal loss by inhibiting complement activation. *Nat Med*. 2004;10:1222-1226.
450. Cervera R, Conti F, Doria A, Iaccarino L, Valesini G. Does seronegative antiphospholipid syndrome really exist? *Autoimmun Rev*. 2012;11:581-584.
451. Sciascia S, Amigo MC, Roccatello D, Khamashta M. Diagnosing antiphospholipid syndrome: "extra-criteria" manifestations and technical advances. *Nat Rev Rheumatol*. 2017;13:548-560.
452. Rodriguez-Pinto I, Espinosa G, Cervera R. Catastrophic antiphospholipid syndrome: the current management approach. *Best Pract Res Clin Rheumatol*. 2016;30:239-249.
453. Asherson RA, Cervera R, Piette JC, et al. Catastrophic antiphospholipid syndrome. Clinical and laboratory features of 50 patients. *Medicine (Baltimore)*. 1998;77:195-207.

454. Asherson RA, Cervera R, Piette JC, et al. Catastrophic antiphospholipid syndrome: clues to the pathogenesis from a series of 80 patients. *Medicine (Baltimore)*. 2001;80:355-377.
455. Erre GL, Pardini S, Faedda R, Passiu G. Effect of rituximab on clinical and laboratory features of antiphospholipid syndrome: a case report and a review of literature. *Lupus*. 2008;17:50-55.
456. Cervera R, CAPS Registry Project Group. Catastrophic antiphospholipid syndrome (CAPS): update from the "CAPS Registry". *Lupus*. 2010;19:412-418.
457. Legault K, Schunemann H, Hillis C, et al. McMaster RARE-Bestpractices clinical practice guideline on diagnosis and management of the catastrophic antiphospholipid syndrome. *J Thromb Haemost*. 2018;16:1656-1664.
458. Chaturvedi S, Braunstein EM, Yuan X, et al. Complement activity and complement regulatory gene mutations are associated with thrombosis in APS and CAPS. *Blood*. 2020;135(4):239-251.
459. Chaturvedi S, Braunstein EM, Brodsky RA. Antiphospholipid syndrome: complement activation, complement gene mutations, and therapeutic implications. *J Thromb Haemost*. 2021;19(3):607-616.
460. Wisloff F, Jacobsen EM, Liestol S. Laboratory diagnosis of the antiphospholipid syndrome. *Thromb Res*. 2003;108:263-271.
461. Zhang L, Whitis JG, Embry MB, Hollensead SC. A simplified algorithm for the laboratory detection of lupus anticoagulants. *Am J Clin Pathol*. 2005;124:894-901.
462. Martin BA, Branch DW, Rodgers GM. Sensitivity of the activated partial thromboplastin time, the dilute Russell's viper venom time, and the kaolin clotting time for the detection of the lupus anticoagulant: a direct comparison using plasma dilutions. *Blood Coagul Fibrinolysis*. 1996;7:31-38.
463. Brien WF, Schaus MR, Cooper KE, O'Keefe BT, Inwood M. Lupus anticoagulant testing: effect of the platelet count on the activated partial thromboplastin time. *Br J Biomed Sci*. 1993;50:114-116.
464. Pengo V, Tripodi A, Reber G, et al. Subcommittee on lupus anticoagulant/antiphospholipid antibody of the scientific and standardisation committee of the international society on thrombosis and haemostasis. Update of the guidelines for lupus anticoagulant detection. *J Thromb Haemost*. 2009;7:1737-1740.
465. Keeling D, Mackie I, Moore GW, et al. Guidelines on the investigation and management of antiphospolipid syndrome. *Br J Haematol*. 2012;157:47-58.
466. Rauch J, Tannenbaum M, Janoff AS. Distinguishing plasma lupus anticoagulants from anti-factor antibodies using hexagonal (II) phase phospholipids. *Thromb Haemost*. 1989;62:892-896.
467. Lo SC, Oldmeadow MJ, Howard MA, Firkin BG. Comparison of laboratory tests used for identification of the lupus anticoagulant. *Am J Hematol*. 1989;30:213-220.
468. Galli M, Dlott J, Norbis F, et al. Lupus anticoagulants and thrombosis: clinical association of different coagulation and immunologic tests. *Thromb Haemost*. 2000;84:1012-1016.
469. Sanmarco M, Alessi MC, Harle JR, et al. Antibodies to phosphatidyl-ethanolamine as the only antiphospholipid antibodies found in patients with unexplained thromboses. *Thromb Haemost*. 2001;85:800-805.
470. Brandt JT, Triplett DA, Alving B, Scharrer I. Criteria for the diagnosis of lupus anticoagulants: an update. On behalf of the subcommittee on lupus anticoagulant/antiphospholipid antibody of the scientific and standardisation committee of the ISTH. *Thromb Haemost*. 1995;74:1185-1190.
471. Kandiah DA, Krillis SA. Heterogeneity of lupus anticoagulant (LA) antibodies: LA activity in dilute Russell's Viper Venom Time and dilute Kaolin Clotting Time detect different populations of antibodies in patients with the "antiphospholipid" syndrome. *Thromb Haemost*. 1998;80:250-257.
472. Clyne LP, Yen Y, Kriz NS, Breitenstein MG. The lupus anticoagulant. High incidence of "negative" mixing studies in a human immunodeficiency virus-positive population. *Arch Pathol Lab Med*. 1993;117:595-601.
473. Moore GW. Recent guidelines and recommendations for laboratory detection of lupus anticoagulants. *Semin Thromb Haemost*. 2014;40:163-171.
474. Hoxha A, Banzato A, Ruffatti A, Pengo V. Detection of lupus anticoagulant in the era of direct oral anticoagulants. *Autoimmun Rev*. 2017;16:173-178.
475. McNally T, Purdy G, Mackie IJ, Machin SJ, Isenberg DA. The use of an anti-beta 2-glycoprotein-I assay for discrimination between anticardiolipin antibodies associated with infection and increased risk of thrombosis. *Br J Haematol*. 1995;91:471-473.
476. Pengo V, Biasiolo A, Pegoraro C, Cucchini U, Noventa F, Iliceto S. Antibody profiles for the diagnosis of antiphospholipid syndrome. *Thromb Haemost*. 2005;93:1147-1152.
477. Devreese KMJ, Ortel TL, Pengo V, et al. Laboratory criteria for antiphospholipid syndrome: communication from the SSC of the ISTH. *J Thromb Haemost*. 2018;16:809-813.
478. Lim W. Prevention of thrombosis in antiphospholipid syndrome. *Hematology Am Soc Hematol Educ Program*. 2016;2016:707-713.
479. Petri M. Thrombosis and systemic lupus erythematosus: the Hopkins Lupus Cohort perspective. *Scand J Rheumatol*. 1996;25:191-193.
480. Rand JH, Wu XX, Quinn AS, Chen PP, Hathcock JJ, Taatjes DJ. Hydroxychloroquine directly reduces the binding of antiphospholipid antibody-β2-glycoprotein I complexes to phospholipid bilayers. *Blood*. 2008;112:1687-1695.
481. Crowther MA, Ginsberg JS, Julian J, et al. A comparison of two intensities of warfarin for the prevention of recurrent thrombosis in patients with the antiphospholipid antibody syndrome. *N Engl J Med*. 2003;349:1133-1138.
482. Finazzi G, Marchioli R, Brancaccio V, et al. A randomized clinical trial of high-intensity warfarin vs conventional antithrombotic therapy for the prevention of recurrent thrombosis in patients with the antiphospholipid syndrome (WAPS). *J Thromb Haemost*. 2005;3:848-853.
483. Ordi-Ros J, Perez-Peman P, Monasterio J. Clinical and therapeutic aspects associated to phospholipid binding antibodies (lupus anticoagulant and anticardiolipin antibodies). *Haemostasis*. 1994;24:165-174.
484. Khamashta MA, Hughes GR. Antiphospholipid antibodies and antiphospholipid syndrome. *Curr Opin Rheumatol*. 1995;7:389-394.
485. Derksen RH, de Groot PG, Kater L, Nieuwenhuis HK. Patients with antiphospholipid antibodies and venous thrombosis should receive long term anticoagulant treatment. *Ann Rheum Dis*. 1993;52:689-692.
486. Schulman S, Svenungsson E, Granqvist S. Anticardiolipin antibodies predict early recurrence of thromboembolism and death among patients with venous thromboembolism following anticoagulant therapy. Duration of Anticoagulation Study Group. *Am J Med*. 1998;104:332-338.
487. Crowther MA, Wisloff F. Evidence based treatment of the antiphospholipid syndrome II. Optimal anticoagulant therapy for thrombosis. *Thromb Res*. 2005;115:3-8.
488. Dufrost V, Risse J, Zuily S, Wahl D. Direct oral anticoagulants use in antiphospholipid syndrome: are these drugs an effective and safe alternative to warfarin? A systematic review of the literature. *Curr Rheumatol Rep*. 2016;18:74.
489. Cohen H, Hunt BJ, Efthymiou M, et al; RAPS trial investigators, et al. Rivaroxaban versus warfarin to treat patients with thrombotic antiphospholipid syndrome, with or without systemic lupus erythematosus (RAPS): a randomized, controlled, open label phase 2/3, non-inferiority trial. *Lancet Haematol*. 2016;3:e426-e436.
490. Pengo V, Denas G, Zoppellaro G, et al. Rivaroxaban vs warfarin in high-risk patients with antiphospholipid syndrome. *Blood*. 2018;132(13):1365-1371.
491. Stevens SM, Woller SC, Baumann Kreuziger L, et al. Antithrombotic therapy for VTE disease: second update of the CHEST guideline and expert panel report - executive summary. *Chest*. 2021;160(6):e545-e608.
492. Pernod G, Arvieux J, Carpentier PH, Mossuz P, Bosson JL, Polack B. Successful treatment of lupus anticoagulant-hypoprothrombinemia syndrome using intravenous immunoglobulins. *Thromb Haemost*. 1997;78:969-970.
493. Moll S, Ortel TL. Monitoring warfarin therapy in patients with lupus anticoagulants. *Ann Intern Med*. 1997;127:177-185.
494. Empson M, Lassere M, Craig J, Scott J. Prevention of recurrent miscarriage for women with antiphospholipid antibody or lupus anticoagulant. *Cochrane Database Syst Rev*. 2005;(2):CD002859.
495. Guerby P, Fillion A, O'Connor S, Bujold E. Heparin for preventing adverse obstetrical outcomes in pregnant women with antiphospholipid syndrome, a systematic review and meta-analysis. *J Gynecol Obstet Hum Reprod*. 2021;50(2):101974.
496. Bates SM, Greer IA, Middeldorp S, Veenstra DL, Prabulos AM, Vandvik PO. VTE, thrombophilia, antithrombotic therapy, and pregnancy: antithrombotic therapy and prevention of thrombosis, 9th ed. American College of Chest Physicians Evidence-Based Clinical Practice Guidelines. *Chest*. 2012;141(suppl 2):e691S-e736S.
497. Donaldson MD, Seaman MJ, Park GR. Massive blood transfusion. *Br J Anaesth*. 1992;69:621-630.
498. Young PP, Cotton BA, Goodnough LT. Massive transfusion protocols for patients with substantial hemorrhage. *Transfus Med Rev*. 2011;25:293-303.
499. Cherkas D. Traumatic hemorrhagic shock: advances in fluid management. *Emerg Med Pract*. 2011;13:1-19.
500. Hunt BJ. Bleeding and coagulopathies in critical care. *N Engl J Med*. 2014;370:847-859.
501. Johansson PI, Stensballe J, Oliveri R, Wade CE, Ostrowski SR, Holcomb JB. How I treat patients with massive hemorrhage. *Blood*. 2014;124:3052-3058.
502. Hunt H, Stanworth S, Curry N, et al. Thromboelastography (TEG) and rotational thromboelastometry (ROTEM) for trauma induced coagulopathy in adult trauma patients with bleeding. *Cochrane Database Syst Rev*. 2015;2:CD010438.
503. Wolberg AS, Meng ZH, Monroe DM, Hoffman M. A systematic evaluation of the effect of temperature on coagulation enzyme activity and platelet function. *J Trauma*. 2004;56:1221-1228.
504. Woodman RC, Harker LA. Bleeding complications associated with cardiopulmonary bypass. *Blood*. 1990;76:1680-1697.
505. de Prost O, Barbier-Boehm G, Hazebroucq J, et al. Desmopressin has no beneficial effect on excessive postoperative bleeding or blood product requirements associated with cardiopulmonary bypass. *Thromb Haemost*. 1992;68:106-110.
506. Schneeweiss S, Seeger JD, Landon J, Walker AM. Aprotinin during coronary-artery bypass grafting and risk of death. *N Engl J Med*. 2008;358:771-783.
507. Davidson S. State of the art—how I manage coagulopathy in cardiac surgery patients. *Br J Haematol*. 2014;164:779-789.
508. Ramsay NK, Coccia PF, Krivit W, Nesbit ME, Edson JR. The effect of l-asparaginase on plasma coagulation factors in acute lymphoblastic leukemia. *Cancer*. 1977;40:1398-1401.
509. Glueck R, Green D, Cohen I, Ts'ao CH. Hematin: unique effects of hemostasis. *Blood*. 1983;61:243-249.
510. Kreuz W, Linde R, Funk M, et al. Valproate therapy induces von Willebrand disease type I. *Epilepsia*. 1992;33:178-184.
511. Thompson CA, Kyle R, Gertz M, Heit J, Pruthi R, Pardanani A. Systemic AL amyloidosis with acquired factor X deficiency: a study of perioperative bleeding risk and treatment outcomes in 60 patients. *Am J Hematol*. 2010;85:171-173.
512. Furie B, Voo L, McAdam KP, Furie BC. Mechanism of factor X deficiency in systemic amyloidosis. *N Engl J Med*. 1981;304:827-830.
513. Rosenstein ED, Itzkowitz SH, Penziner AS, Cohen JI, Mornaghi RA. Resolution of factor X deficiency in primary amyloidosis following splenectomy. *Arch Intern Med*. 1983;143:597-599.
514. Camoriano JK, Greipp PR, Bayer GK, Bowie EJ. Resolution of acquired factor X deficiency and amyloidosis with melphalan and prednisone therapy. *N Engl J Med*. 1987;316:1133-1135.

515. Choufani EB, Sanchorawala V, Ernst T, et al. Acquired factor X deficiency in patients with amyloid light-chain amyloidosis: incidence, bleeding manifestations, and response to high-dose chemotherapy. *Blood*. 2001;97:1885-1887.
516. Karpatkin S, Ingram GIC, Graham JB. Severe isolated prothrombin deficiency: an acquired state with complete recovery. *Thromb Diath Haemorrh*. 1962;8:221-234.
517. Vaziri ND, Toohey J, Paule P, et al. Urinary excretion and deficiency of prothrombin in nephrotic syndrome. *Am J Med*. 1984;77:433-436.
518. Natelson EA, Lynch EC, Hettig RA, Alfrey CP Jr. Acquired factor IX deficiency in the nephrotic syndrome. *Ann Intern Med*. 1970;73:373-378.
519. Thompson AR. Factor XII and other hemostatic protein abnormalities in nephrotic syndrome patients. *Thromb Haemost*. 1982;48:27-32.
520. Kauffmann RH, Veltkamp JJ, Van Tilburg NH, Van Es LA. Acquired antithrombin III deficiency and thrombosis in the nephrotic syndrome. *Am J Med*. 1978;65:607-613.
521. Panicucci F, Sagripanti A, Vispi M, et al. Comprehensive study of haemostasis in nephrotic syndrome. *Nephron*. 1983;33:9-13.
522. Boklan BF, Sawitsky A. Factor IX deficiency in Gaucher disease. An in vitro phenomenon. *Arch Intern Med*. 1976;136:489-492.
523. Weisdorf D, Hasegawa D, Fair DS. Acquired factor VII deficiency associated with aplastic anaemia: correction with bone marrow transplantation. *Br J Haematol*. 1989;71:409-413.
524. de Raucourt E, Dumont MD, Tourani JM, Hubsch JP, Riquet M, Fischer AM. Acquired factor VII deficiency associated with pleural liposarcoma. *Blood Coagul Fibrinolysis*. 1994;5:833-836.
525. Rasche H, Dietrich M, Gaus W, Schleyer M. Factor XIII-activity and fibrin subunit structure in acute leukemia. *Biomedicine*. 1974;21:61-66.
526. Oshitani N, Kitano A, Hara J, et al. Deficiency of blood coagulation factor XIII in Crohn's disease. *Am J Gastroenterol*. 1995;90:1116-1118.
527. Nijenhuis AVM, van Bergeijk L, Huijgens PC, Zweegman S. Acquired factor XIII deficiency due to an inhibitor: a case report and review of the literature. *Haematologica*. 2004;89:ECR14.
528. Khoory MS, Nesheim ME, Bowie EJ, Mann KG. Circulating heparan sulfate proteoglycan anticoagulant from a patient with a plasma cell disorder. *J Clin Invest*. 1980;65:666-674.
529. Bussel JB, Steinherz PG, Miller DR, Hilgartner MW. A heparin-like anticoagulant in an 8-month-old boy with acute monoblastic leukemia. *Am J Hematol*. 1984;16:83-90.
530. Llamas P, Outeiriño J, Espinoza J, Santos AB, Román A, Tomás JF. Report of three cases of circulating heparin-like anticoagulants. *Am J Hematol*. 2001;67:256-258.
531. Rodgers GM, Corash L. Acquired heparinlike anticoagulant in a patient with metastatic breast carcinoma. *West J Med*. 1985;143:672-675.
532. Colwell NS, Tollefsen DM, Blinder MA. Identification of a monoclonal thrombin inhibitor associated with multiple myeloma and a severe bleeding disorder. *Br J Haematol*. 1997;97:219-226.

Section 4 ■ THROMBOSIS

Chapter 56 ■ Thrombosis and Antithrombotic Therapy
STACY A. JOHNSON • GEORGE M. RODGERS

INTRODUCTION

The term *thrombosis* refers to the formation, from the constituents of the blood, of a mass within the venous or arterial vasculature of a living animal. Hemostatic thromboses, namely, self-limited and localized thromboses that prevent excessive blood loss, represent the body's natural and desired response to acute vascular injury. Pathologic thromboses, such as deep venous thrombosis (DVT), pulmonary embolism (PE), coronary arterial thrombosis leading to myocardial infarction (MI), and cerebrovascular thrombotic occlusion, represent the body's undesired response to acute and chronic perturbations of the vasculature or blood or both. The terms *coagulated blood* and *clot* are not synonymous with thrombosis and refer to the formation of a solid mass of blood components outside the vascular tree. Examples of clots include soft tissue, body cavity (e.g., peritoneal), and visceral hematomas. Coagulated blood best describes clots formed ex vivo.

Thrombosis of the veins and arteries, together with complicating embolic phenomena, is perhaps the most important cause of sickness and death in the developed countries of the world at the present time. Deaths from MI and thrombotic stroke consistently represent the major causes of death in the United States, numbering >700,000 people annually (almost 25% of all deaths) in a recent report.[1] Venous thromboembolic disease is the third most common cardiovascular disease, after atherosclerotic heart disease and stroke. It has been estimated that between 500,000 and 2 million venous thromboembolic events (VTEs), including calf vein thrombosis, proximal DVT (e.g., lower extremity and pelvic veins), and PE, occur annually in the United States alone.[2] A committee of the International Society on Thrombosis and Haemostasis (ISTH) reported that VTE was a major contributor to global disease burden with incidence rates of VTE ranging between 0.75 and 2.69 per 1000 people.[3]

In this chapter, the pathophysiology of arterial and venous thrombosis and mechanisms of action of antithrombotic pharmacologic agents, including antiplatelet drugs, anticoagulants, and fibrinolytic agents, are summarized and discussed. Inherited conditions that predispose an individual to thrombosis, also termed *hypercoagulable states*, and the management of venous thromboembolic disease are also covered. The management of arterial thrombotic events is beyond the scope of this chapter, and the reader is referred to several review articles.[4-6]

PHYSIOLOGY AND PATHOPHYSIOLOGY OF THROMBOSIS

The human hemostatic system consists of multiple independent, yet integrally related, cellular and protein components that function to maintain blood fluidity under normal conditions and promote localized, temporary thrombus (hemostatic thrombus) formation at the sites of vascular injury. An abnormal hemostatic system can result in pathologic bleeding or vascular thrombosis or both.

The hemostatic system is composed of six major components: platelets, vascular endothelium, procoagulant plasma protein "factors," natural anticoagulant proteins, fibrinolytic proteins, and antifibrinolytic proteins. Each of these six hemostatic components must be present in fully functional form, in adequate quantity, and at the proper location to prevent excessive blood loss after vascular trauma and, at the same time, to prevent pathologic thrombosis. The hemostatic system is highly regulated and maintains a delicate balance between a prohemorrhagic state and a prothrombotic state. Any significant acquired or congenital imbalance in the hemostatic "scales" can lead to a pathologic outcome.

Normal hemostasis in response to vascular injury can be divided into two major processes of equal importance, known as primary hemostasis and secondary hemostasis. *Primary hemostasis* comprises the reactions needed to form a platelet plug at a site of vascular damage, whereas *secondary hemostasis* comprises a series of reactions (coagulation cascade) needed to generate cross-linked fibrin required to stabilize the platelet plug and form a durable thrombus. Despite separation of hemostasis into these two phases, experimental models of thrombosis suggest that platelet aggregation and fibrin formation occur simultaneously.[7] Natural anticoagulants (antithrombin [AT] and activated protein C [APC]) function to confine thrombus formation to the sites of vascular injury and limit thrombus size to prevent vessel occlusion and flow interruption in the affected vessel. The activity of AT is greatly enhanced by endothelial cell heparan sulfate and pharmacologic heparins. The function of APC is enhanced by its cofactor, protein S. Physiologic fibrinolysis is initiated by endothelial cell–derived tissue-type plasminogen activator (t-PA), which converts plasminogen to plasmin. Plasmin can degrade cross-linked fibrin, limit thrombus size, and help dissolve a thrombus once the vascular injury has been repaired. The fibrinolytic system is regulated and localized by antiplasmin and PA inhibitor (PAI)-1. Details of the hemostatic mechanisms and endothelial cell regulation of hemostasis are given in Chapters 20 and 21.

Specific alterations in the quantitative and qualitative status of any hemostatic cellular or protein element can lead to pathologic thrombosis. A marked increase in the platelet count (thrombocytosis) and accentuated platelet aggregation ("sticky platelet syndrome") are associated with thromboembolic events. Elevated levels of procoagulant factors, such as fibrinogen and factors VIII, IX, XI, and VII, as well as resistance to inactivation of factor Va by APC are recognized risk factors for vascular disease and thrombosis. Deficiency of a natural anticoagulant protein, such as protein C, protein S, or AT, is associated with venous thromboembolic disease. Abnormalities in fibrinolysis, such as excess plasma levels of the fibrinolytic inhibitor PAI-1, have been linked to arterial thrombosis. It is the net balance between the participating and, at times, opposing groups of proteins and not the level of any individual factor that is most critical to hemostatic regulation.

VIRCHOW TRIAD

In the mid-19th century (1854), a German pathologist, Rudolph Virchow postulated that vascular obstruction was precipitated by, and thrombosis resulted from, three interrelated factors: (a) "decreased blood flow" (stasis of blood flow), (b) "inflammation of near or near the blood vessels" (vascular endothelial injury), and (c) "intrinsic alterations in the nature of the blood itself" (hypercoagulability).[8] Many students of coagulation medicine, though, do not realize that Virchow actually recognized his "triad" as being the result of vascular occlusion, not necessarily as the original precipitant of vascular thrombosis. Nonetheless, the vascular, rheologic, and hematologic aspects of thrombosis, known as the Virchow triad, remain relevant and instructive today (*Figure 56.1*).

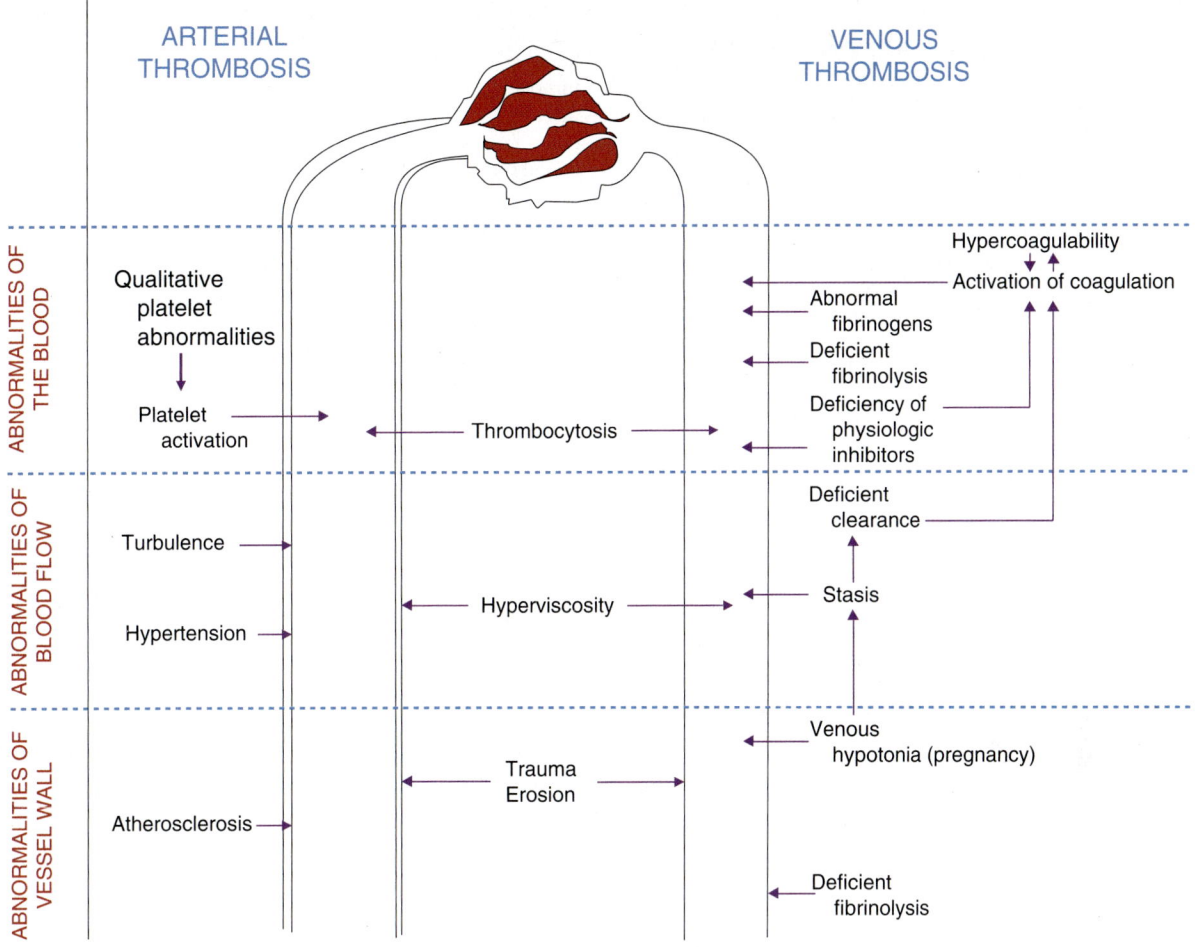

FIGURE 56.1 Pathophysiology of thrombosis. Factors implicated in the pathogenesis of arterial thrombosis (left) and venous thrombosis (right) are depicted. Examples of disorders leading to platelet activation and arterial thrombosis include atherosclerosis, the myeloproliferative disorders, heparin-associated thrombocytopenia/thrombosis syndrome, thrombotic thrombocytopenic purpura, and certain platelet polymorphisms. Examples of disorders leading to venous thrombosis in the category of deficiency of physiologic inhibitors include the inherited disorders, factor V Leiden, protein C and protein S deficiencies, and antithrombin deficiency. Many patients with thrombosis may have more than one of the risk factors listed. Estrogen therapy is a risk factor for venous thrombosis; its use is associated with activation of coagulation.

Abnormalities of Blood Flow

Arterial thrombosis initially occurs under conditions of rapid blood flow (high shear stress), a condition in which von Willebrand factor (vWF) is critical for platelet adhesion.[9] Arterial thrombi are usually composed of tightly coherent masses of platelets, which contain small amounts of fibrin and a few erythrocytes and leukocytes. These thrombi are the classic "white thrombi," which resemble, in many respects, normal hemostatic plugs. As arterial thrombi enlarge, progressive or intermittent deposition of new layers of platelets and fibrin produces the characteristic lines of Zahn; partial or complete obstruction of blood flow may produce a "tail" of "red thrombus." The most serious consequences of arterial thrombosis are vascular occlusion with resultant ischemia and infarction of tissue and distal thrombus embolization.

Hypertension, turbulent blood flow at arterial branch points and at the sites of focal atherosclerosis, and hyperviscosity may be the contributory factors in certain forms of arterial thrombosis. The causes of plasma hyperviscosity that can precipitate thrombosis and exacerbate ischemia include acute myeloid leukemia, myeloproliferative syndromes such as polycythemia rubra vera, cryoglobulinemia, and the plasma cell dyscrasias, including multiple myeloma and Waldenström macroglobulinemia. Immunoglobulin (Ig) paraproteins produced by plasma cell dyscrasias can increase viscosity and promote red blood cell agglutination.

Venous thrombosis typically develops under conditions of slow blood flow (low shear stress) and is augmented by further retardation and stagnation of flow caused by the developing thrombus itself. Right-sided heart failure, preexistent venous thrombosis, extrinsic vascular compression by tumor, and chronic venous insufficiency all promote venous stasis, blood pooling, and a concentration of procoagulant factors.[10] The anatomic structure of venous valves results in retrograde eddy currents, which produce pockets of stasis even in normal veins.[11] The venous arcades in the soleus muscles of the calves may represent another site of physiologic venous stasis. These structures may enlarge and lose vascular tone with aging.[12] These facts may partially explain why DVT most commonly occurs in the valve cusps and veins of the pelvis and lower extremities, and why older age is an important risk factor for venous thrombosis.[13]

Venous thrombi are composed of large amounts of fibrin containing numerous erythrocytes. In these loose, friable masses (the red thrombi), the platelets and leukocytes are enmeshed in a random manner. Venous thrombi resemble blood clots formed in vitro, and they usually produce significant obstruction to blood flow from the outset, but their most serious consequence is embolization. Blood flow obstruction secondary to venous thrombosis itself promotes the further formation of thrombus. Although traditional teaching holds that risk factors for arterial and venous thrombotic diseases are distinct, newer epidemiologic data suggest that common risk factors exist for both disorders and that appropriate management of thrombosis patients should address secondary prevention of both arterial and venous thrombosis.[14] The pathogenesis of both venous and arterial thrombosis has been reviewed.[15]

Vascular Injury

Permanent and transient vascular injuries play major roles in the development of arterial thrombosis. Intraluminal vascular endothelial cell injury, atherosclerotic plaque rupture, hyperhomocysteinemia, arterial outflow obstruction, aneurysm formation, and vessel dissection are among the recognized risk factors for arterial thrombosis.[16] Arterial thrombosis usually begins with platelet adhesion to an abnormal vascular endothelial surface or exposed subendothelial constituent, such as collagen. The adherent platelets become activated, leading to the release of α- and dense-granule contents.[15] Platelet-dense granules (dense bodies) release adenosine diphosphate (ADP), adenosine triphosphate (ATP), calcium, and serotonin into the surrounding milieu, resulting in the recruitment and activation of additional platelets.[16] This release reaction and platelet synthesis of thromboxane A_2 (TXA_2) and other agonists induce the aggregation of more platelets and enlargement of the temporary platelet plug. In addition to the recruitment of additional platelets, the original nidus of adherent platelets provides a phospholipid surface rich in phosphatidylserine to support and concentrate the generation of thrombin and fibrin necessary to reinforce and stabilize the platelet plug.

New insights into arterial thrombus formation have been gleaned from experiments using confocal and wide-field microscopy to image real-time thrombus formation in arterioles of the live mouse cremaster muscle.[17] Thrombosis is precipitated by laser-induced endothelial injury. These experiments demonstrated that the initiation of blood coagulation in vivo involves the initial accumulation of tissue factor (TF) on the upstream and thrombus–vessel wall interface of the developing thrombus. The TF is biologically active and is associated with intrathrombus fibrin generation. TF density is highest at the thrombus–vessel wall interface and is eventually observed throughout the thrombus. Leukocyte rolling is noted approximately 2 minutes after endothelial cell injury and correlates with P-selectin expression on the outer aspect of the thrombus. Minimal TF and fibrin are detected in platelet thrombi formed in mice lacking P-selectin or the P-selectin glycoprotein ligand 1.

In venous thrombosis, the luminal surface of the vessel wall is usually histologically normal, and factors extrinsic to the vessel appear to have a major pathophysiologic role.[18] Exceptions to this generalization are direct venous trauma, extrinsic venous compression, and vascular endothelial cell injury resulting from the toxic effect of cancer chemotherapy and elevated levels of homocysteine. A generalized reduction in venous tone may be an important pathophysiologic factor in venous thrombosis in pregnant women and in women taking oral contraceptives.[19] One study indicates that human platelets express TF pre-mRNA and, when activated, splice this message into mature mRNA that is expressed.[20] These results suggest that both platelets and the vessel wall may contribute to the initiation of thrombosis. Additional mechanisms may contribute to a prothrombotic state, including upregulation of stress-response genes, endothelial cell activation, formation of neutrophil extracellular traps, and activation of the intrinsic coagulation pathway.[21]

Abnormalities of the Blood: Hypercoagulability

The term *hypercoagulable state* and its synonym *thrombophilia* refer to any inherited or acquired abnormality of the hemostatic system that places an individual at increased risk for venous thrombosis or arterial thrombosis (or both). Blood from patients with active thrombosis or with a hypercoagulable state may clot at an abnormally rapid rate in vitro.[22] The concept of hypercoagulability has gained widespread acceptance, and it is generally appreciated that these hemostatic changes are important in the pathogenesis of thrombosis; however, whether testing for these disorders may be helpful in patient management is uncertain.[23,24]

Platelet Abnormalities

Although platelets may be incorporated into any thrombus, they appear to be pathogenetically most important in arterial thrombosis. Increased platelet turnover (shortened platelet survival and compensated platelet destruction) occurs in vascular disease and thrombosis, including arterial and venous thrombosis, coronary artery disease, vasculitis, hyperhomocysteinemia, and valvular heart disease.[25-27] Increased platelet turnover can also be seen in patients with risk factors for vascular disease, including those who use tobacco and those with hyperlipidemia.[28,29] Increased platelet turnover and activation can reflect thromboembolic disease and also probably contribute to an exacerbation of thrombotic events.

Vascular endothelium possesses multiple antiplatelet properties that may be important in preventing platelet adhesion, promoting vasodilation, and inhibiting platelet aggregation.[30-32] However, interruption of endothelial cell prostacyclin synthesis by aspirin does not result in a net thrombotic tendency. The potential role of hyperactive platelets in patients with thrombosis, as well as the use of platelet function testing in this setting, is somewhat controversial.

Because of the importance of vWF in mediating platelet adhesion to subendothelium, the role of vWF in human vascular disease has been a topic of investigation. An association between elevated plasma vWF levels and recurrent MI has been demonstrated, and vWF antigen is an independent predictor of coronary artery disease.[33]

Platelet polymorphisms have been evaluated as risk factors for arterial thrombosis. These include polymorphisms for glycoprotein (GP) IIIa (Pl^{A2}), GPIa (807 T allele), and GPIbα.[34] The Pl^{A2} polymorphism is linked with coronary artery disease; Pl^{A2}-positive platelets exhibit a lower threshold for activation and also have variable aspirin sensitivity.[34]

Coagulation Abnormalities

Coagulation disorders that can contribute to hypercoagulability can be divided into three risk factor categories: transient, inherited, and acquired.[35] *Transient risk factors* represent well-defined, temporary clinical circumstances that are associated with increased thrombosis risk both while they are present and for a short period after they have resolved. Examples include surgery, prolonged immobilization, oral contraceptive pill (OCP) use, hormone replacement therapy (HRT), pregnancy, cancer chemotherapy, and heparin-induced thrombocytopenia (HIT). *Inherited risk factors* represent genetic mutations and polymorphisms that result in deficiency of a natural anticoagulant (e.g., protein C, protein S, or AT), procoagulant factor accumulation (e.g., prothrombin G20210A), or coagulation factor resistance to inactivation by a natural anticoagulant (i.e., factor V G1691A, also known as factor V Leiden). These conditions are characterized by a disruption in the normally highly regulated coagulation mechanism, resulting in greater thrombin generation and an increased risk of clinical thrombosis. *Acquired risk factors* result from either medical conditions or nonfamilial hematologic abnormalities that interfere with normal hemostasis or blood rheology. Examples include cancer, inflammatory bowel disease, nephrotic syndrome, vasculitis, antiphospholipid antibodies, myeloproliferative syndromes, paroxysmal nocturnal hemoglobinuria, and hyperviscosity syndromes. These acquired risk factors are distinct from transient risk factors by the fact that they represent alterations in hemostatic homeostasis as a result of disease or, for the most part, nonreversible processes. In contrast, transient risk factors result from either a therapeutic intervention or an adverse reaction to such an intervention. Hyperhomocysteinemia and increased factor VIII functional activity are examples of thrombosis risk factors that can be acquired in nature or have a genetic predisposition.[36,37] Age defies categorization but remains the single most predictable risk factor for thrombosis. The estimated baseline annual age-associated risk of VTE is 1 in 10,000 people aged <40 years, increasing to 1 in 100 people aged >75 years.[38]

A large number of reports have implicated elevated levels of various coagulation proteins (fibrinogen and factors V, VII, VIII, X, and XI) in thrombosis patients. However, detailed analyses of these reports suggest that for most of these coagulation proteins, their link to thrombophilia is uncertain, and testing for these analytes is not recommended.[39] Abnormal fibrinolysis has been linked to arterial vascular disease. Low fibrinolytic activity (measured by dilute clot lysis) was a significant determinant of coronary artery disease in the Northwick Park Heart Study, and elevated PAI-1 activity was associated with major ischemic events in other studies.[40,41]

ACTIVATION OF COAGULATION

The mechanisms leading to activation of coagulation in patients with thrombosis have been proposed. TF is thought to be the primary initiator of in vivo coagulation.[42,43] In the absence of TF expression, endothelial cells actively maintain thromboresistance. TF may be expressed in trace amounts during various physiologic processes, such as during normal parturition and after even minimal trauma, including minor head injuries. Immunologic injury of endothelium may lead to the exposure of TF. Antibodies formed to exogenous heparin may bind to heparan sulfate on the endothelium, resulting in cell injury, the expression of TF, and the initiation of coagulation.[44] In a similar manner, endothelial cells may be induced to express TF by interleukin-1, homocysteine, tumor necrosis factor, and endotoxin.[45-48] TF antigen expression by endothelium has been demonstrated in pathologic primate and human tissues.[49-51] Activation of coagulation may also occur on monocytes, and platelets can be activated to mediate factor Xa–catalyzed prothrombin conversion to thrombin.[52,53] Deficient hepatic clearance of activated coagulation factors may represent an important thrombogenic factor in premature infants and in patients with liver disease, especially after administration of prothrombin complex concentrates (PCCs) that contain trace amounts of activated vitamin K–dependent coagulation factors.

Various other mechanisms may be responsible for low-grade in vivo coagulation under certain conditions. Certain tumor cells can promote thrombin generation directly by producing TF, expressing the coagulation factor X activator known as *cancer procoagulant*, or displaying surface sialic acid residues that can support nonenzymatic factor X activation.[54,55] Tumor cells can also promote thrombin generation indirectly by eliciting TF expression by monocytes and endothelial cells. Tumor-associated coagulation cascade activation can result in the generation of thrombin that can promote angiogenesis by signaling through protease-activated receptors.

A laboratory picture similar to that described in the hypercoagulable state may also be seen in patients with chronic disseminated intravascular coagulation (DIC).[56] In such patients, the prothrombin time (PT) and the activated partial thromboplastin time (aPTT) may be shortened because of the presence of traces of thrombin or other activated coagulation factors. High levels of factor V and factor VIII-activity may reflect the presence of thrombin-activated forms of these factors in the circulation. Pregnancy, which can be regarded as a hypercoagulable state, has also been described as a physiologic form of chronic DIC by some clinicians.[57] Pregnancy increases the risk of venous thromboembolism (VTE) approximately five-fold among the general population, and female patients who have experienced prior venous thrombosis have a three-fold risk of venous thrombosis during pregnancy.[58] The use of estrogen-containing oral contraceptives and estrogen HRT is clearly associated with an increased risk of VTE.[59] A prospective study of these patients indicates that estrogens induce activation of coagulation as well as reduction in levels of natural anticoagulants, such as AT and protein S.[60] However, many patients who experience VTE while taking oral contraceptives have a common inherited thrombotic disorder, APC resistance (APC-R), or prothrombin G20210A.[61] Another report indicated that oral contraceptives induced "acquired APC-R" in women.[62] The relative risk of VTE in postmenopausal women using estrogen replacement is 2.14, and the risk is highest during the first year of use.[63] Whether transdermal estrogen products are safer than oral estrogens is uncertain.[64] A literature review of reports of progestin-only contraceptives found that patients using an oral progestin or a progestin-only intrauterine device experienced no excess risk of VTE while depot administration of progestin more than doubled VTE risk.[65] Testosterone therapy in males is associated with a two-fold increased risk of VTE.[66] *Table 56.1* summarizes acquired etiologies that predispose to thrombosis.

Table 56.1. Acquired Disorders Predisposing to Thrombosis

Vascular Disorders
Atherosclerosis
Diabetes
Vasculitis
Prosthetic materials (grafts, valves, indwelling vascular catheters)
Abnormal Rheology
Stasis (immobilization, surgery, congestive heart failure)
Hyperviscosity (polycythemia vera, Waldenström macroglobulinemia, acute leukemia, sickle cell disease)
Other Disorders Associated With Hypercoagulability
Cancer (Trousseau syndrome)
Cancer chemotherapeutic agents, thalidomide, bevacizumab
Oral contraceptives, estrogen therapy, selective estrogen-receptor modulators
Pregnancy
Testosterone therapy
Infusion of prothrombin complex concentrates and recombinant factor VIIa
Nephrotic syndrome
Myeloproliferative disorders
Paroxysmal nocturnal hemoglobinuria
Inflammatory bowel disease
Thrombotic thrombocytopenic purpura
Disseminated intravascular coagulation
Antiphospholipid antibody syndrome
Heparin-induced thrombocytopenia/thrombosis
Human immunodeficiency virus infection

INHERITED THROMBOTIC DISORDERS

Several monographs and reviews have covered the topic of inherited thrombotic disorders in detail.[18,35,67-69] *Table 56.2* summarizes the prevalence of selected inherited and acquired hypercoagulable states in different populations. Many patients who experience thrombosis are found to have a combination of defects, for example, APC-R plus the use of oral contraceptive agents,[61] or a combination of inherited defects.[35] Although people with inherited hypercoagulable states are at a greater risk for developing a thrombotic event than those without such disorders, not all people with a well-defined hypercoagulable state develop an overt thrombosis. Testing for an inherited hypercoagulable state is likely to uncover an abnormality in >60% of patients presenting with idiopathic (i.e., spontaneous or unprovoked) venous thrombosis.[68] Although the remaining 30% to 40% have unremarkable test results, this does not imply a true absence of a hypercoagulable state. Some of these individuals may have an acquired condition such as cancer or antiphospholipid antibodies, whereas others may have a disorder or genetic defect that has not yet been discovered or characterized.

Antithrombin Deficiency

AT, formally known as *AT-III*, deficiency was first described by Egeberg in 1965.[70] AT, a serine protease inhibitor, regulates coagulation by inactivating thrombin and other procoagulant enzymes, including factors Xa, IXa, XIa, and XIIa. As are most inherited thrombotic disorders, AT deficiency is inherited as an autosomal dominant disorder.[71,72] A blood bank survey reported that 1 in 600 people has AT

Table 56.2. Prevalence of Selected Inherited and Acquired Hypercoagulable States in Different Patient Populations

Hypercoagulable State	General Population (%)	Patients With First Venous Thromboembolism (%)	Thrombophilic Families (%)
Factor V Leiden	3-7[a]	20	50
Prothrombin G20210A	1-3	6	18
Protein C deficiency	0.2-0.4	3	6-8
Protein S deficiency	N/A	1-2	3-13
Antithrombin deficiency	0.02	1	4-8
Mild hyperhomocysteinemia	5-10	10-25	N/A
Elevated factor VIII	11	25	N/A
Lupus anticoagulant	0-3	5-15	N/A
Elevated anticardiolipin antibodies	2-7	14	N/A

Abbreviation: N/A, not available or unknown.
[a]Prevalence as high as 15% in northern Europe.

deficiency.[73] The interactions of unfractionated heparin (UFH) and low-molecular-weight heparin (LMWH) with AT are discussed in section "Heparin." In addition to its anticoagulant function, AT also possesses anti-inflammatory and antibacterial activities.[74]

Pathophysiology and Genetics

Patients with AT deficiency may have either type I (quantitative deficiency) or type II (qualitative abnormality) disease. Type I AT-deficient patients usually have concordant reductions in AT measured by both immunologic and functional assays. Type II AT-deficient patients have reduced functional AT activity associated with normal amounts of AT protein. Plasma concentrations of the thrombin activation peptide, prothrombin fragment 1 + 2, are elevated in patients with AT deficiency, indicating persistent activation of coagulation as a result of deficient neutralization of factor Xa in these patients.[75]

The genetic basis for type I AT deficiency is either deletion of a gene segment or the occurrence of point mutations or deletions, resulting in a nonsense mutation and an incomplete protein. The genetic basis for type II AT deficiency is the occurrence of point mutations that do not impair synthesis of the protein, but that result in a dysfunctional protease inhibitor. A database of AT mutations is located at https://www.imperial.ac.uk/immunology-inflammation/research/haematology/haemostasis-and-thrombosis/database. In general, mutant AT molecules exhibit deficient heparin binding or deficient protease inhibition or both. Abnormalities in glycosylation of AT[76] and transient AT deficiency[77] have been described.

Clinical Aspects

AT deficiency is manifested primarily by recurrent VTE.[70,71] Almost every vein site has been reported to be involved with thrombosis in AT-deficient patients, including unusual sites such as mesenteric vessels. Thrombosis may occur in the absence of precipitating factors or may result from events, such as pregnancy, estrogen use, trauma, or surgery. AT deficiency may result in heparin resistance manifesting as a normal to minimally increased aPTT in patients receiving large doses of heparin.[78] In family-based studies, venous thrombosis occurred in 85% of AT-deficient relatives before 55 years of age.[78] The estimated increased lifetime relative risk of venous thrombosis has been reported to be up to 40-fold.[79] Early studies reported pregnancy-related venous thrombosis rates as high as 70% for AT-deficient women.[80] Most AT-deficient patients are heterozygotes and possess ~50% of normal activity levels. Although homozygotes have been reported in consanguineous kindreds, in general, homozygous type I AT deficiency is believed to be fatal in utero[81] (*Table 56.3*).

Laboratory Diagnosis

The results of the PT and aPTT are normal in AT-deficient patients. A variety of commercial assays is available to measure AT levels, including functional and immunologic assays. Functional assays are preferable because they detect both type I and type II patients. One report found that 2% of patients with AT deficiency had type II disease.[82] Functional assays for AT measure heparin cofactor activity using a

Table 56.3. Clinical Presentations of Venous Thromboembolism That May Suggest Certain Hypercoagulable States

Venous Thromboembolism Presentation	Hypercoagulable State
Cerebral vein thrombosis in women using oral contraceptives	Prothrombin G20210A mutation
Cerebral vein thrombosis in general	Paroxysmal nocturnal hemoglobinuria, essential thrombocythemia, antiphospholipid antibodies, antithrombin deficiency, PT G20210A mutation
Intra-abdominal vein thrombosis (inferior vena cava, renal vein, portal vein, mesenteric and hepatic veins)	Antiphospholipid antibodies, paroxysmal nocturnal hemoglobinuria, myeloproliferative syndromes, cancer, antithrombin deficiency
Warfarin skin necrosis	Protein C and protein S deficiencies
Unexplained recurrent fetal loss	Antiphospholipid antibodies; factor V Leiden
Recurrent superficial thrombophlebitis	Factor V Leiden, polycythemia vera, protein C, protein S, or antithrombin deficiency
Migratory superficial thrombophlebitis (Trousseau syndrome)	Adenocarcinoma (particularly of the gastrointestinal tract)
Neonatal purpura fulminans	Homozygous protein C or protein S deficiency

Abbreviation: PT, prothrombin.

chromogenic substrate method to quantitate thrombin or factor Xa neutralization.[83]

Immunologic assays for AT use Laurell rocket immunoelectrophoresis, microlatex particle-mediated immunoassay, radial immunodiffusion, or enzyme-linked immunosorbent assay (ELISA) methods.[84] Ideally, patients should be evaluated for AT deficiency at a time when they are not receiving therapeutic heparin or oral anticoagulants because heparin depresses AT levels, whereas long-term warfarin therapy increases plasma AT levels in some patients.[71,85] Laboratory testing recommendations for AT deficiency have been summarized.[86]

Treatment

Some AT-deficient patients may experience heparin resistance, requiring the administration of AT by using virally inactivated, plasma-derived concentrates, or fresh-frozen plasma. Supplemental AT may make it easier to achieve therapeutic anticoagulation with heparin in these patients.[87] Patients with recurrent thrombosis should receive long-term warfarin therapy at a dosage to maintain an international normalized ratio (INR) value of 2.0 to 3.0 (discussed in section "Warfarin"). Patients with a single thrombotic event should receive at least 3 to 6 months of warfarin therapy and, because of an increased recurrence rate, should be considered for long-term therapy beyond 6 months. Patients with massive venous thrombosis or PE may be candidates for thrombolytic therapy. AT-deficient patients who become pregnant or who will undergo general surgery should be considered for anticoagulant prophylaxis, including AT concentrate administration.[87,88] Most asymptomatic patients should not be treated, but should be prophylaxed during high-risk situations. The avoidance of estrogens should be considered in AT-deficient patients who are not therapeutically anticoagulated.

Acquired Antithrombin Deficiency

AT deficiency is also associated with numerous disorders, including DIC, liver disease, nephrotic syndrome, and preeclampsia, and is seen in patients taking oral contraceptive agents and during pregnancy.[89-92] Although logic suggests that correction of AT deficiency might be clinically useful in disorders such as DIC or liver disease, there are no conclusive data supporting AT replacement therapy outside the setting of prophylaxis of high-risk patients, such as AT-deficient pregnant patients.[93]

Heparin Cofactor II Deficiency

Heparin cofactor II (HCII) is another heparin-dependent thrombin inhibitor differing from AT in that a glycosaminoglycan other than heparin, dermatan sulfate, catalyzes this inhibitor of coagulation.[94] HCII deficiency is inherited as an autosomal dominant trait. Although there have been anecdotal studies of thrombosis associated with HCII-deficient kindreds, a larger study has concluded that HCII deficiency by itself is not an inherited risk factor for thrombosis.[95]

Protein C Deficiency

Protein C is a vitamin K–dependent plasma protein that, when activated by the thrombin-thrombomodulin complex to APC, inactivates factors Va and VIIIa to inhibit coagulation.[96] APC also possesses profibrinolytic activity that results from neutralization of PAI-3 activity.[97] Inherited deficiency of protein C and its association with thrombosis were first described by Griffin and coworkers in 1981.[98] Protein C deficiency was believed to be inherited in an autosomal dominant pattern with incomplete penetrance. More recent studies have suggested that protein C deficiency may be an autosomal recessive disorder and that coinheritance of another defect (particularly factor V Leiden) results in a high degree of penetrance that appears as the dominant inheritance in double heterozygous carriers.[99,100]

Pathophysiology and Genetics

As with AT deficiency, patients with protein C deficiency may have type I (quantitative deficiency) or type II (qualitative abnormality) disease. Most patients are heterozygotes with ~50% of normal protein C levels. A hypercoagulable state can be demonstrated in nonanticoagulated protein C–deficient patients using activation peptide (fragment 1 + 2) assays.[101]

In type I protein C deficiency, more than half of the gene mutations identified are missense mutations. Point mutations affecting protein function appear to be common in patients with type II protein C deficiency. At least 195 different gene abnormalities have been associated with both types of protein C deficiency.[102] Despite the clear association of protein C deficiency with thrombosis in large epidemiologic studies, there are also definitive data indicating that many protein C–deficient patients are asymptomatic.[99,103] For example, one report found that heterozygous protein C deficiency occurred in approximately 1 in 250 subjects, whereas a large Scottish study estimated the prevalence to be approximately 1 in 500.[104,105] No patient in either study had a history of symptomatic venous thrombosis. These findings indicate that additional risk factors—acquired or genetic or both—are necessary to provoke thrombosis in heterozygous protein C–deficient patients. Indeed, in one study, up to 20% of symptomatic protein C–deficient patients also had APC-R, supporting the concept that many patients with recurrent thrombosis have more than one risk factor.[100]

Clinical Aspects

Three clinical syndromes are associated with protein C deficiency: VTE in heterozygous adults, neonatal purpura fulminans in homozygous newborns, and warfarin-induced skin necrosis in certain heterozygous adults. The predominant clinical symptom of protein C–deficient patients is recurrent VTE, although arterial thrombotic events, including stroke, have been reported.[105,106] As mentioned previously, many patients are found to have risk factors other than inherited protein C deficiency on investigation, such as APC-R, the use of oral contraceptive agents, and pregnancy. Protein C deficiency has also been linked to fetal loss.[107]

Neonatal purpura fulminans is seen in homozygous newborns of heterozygous parents. These children develop DIC at birth, associated with extensive venous thrombosis or arterial thrombosis (or both) and very low levels of protein C (<5% of normal).[108] Warfarin-induced skin necrosis is an unusual syndrome seen in certain patients with heterozygote protein C deficiency.[109] Most patients who develop this syndrome have received large doses of warfarin in the absence of concomitant overlapping therapeutic parenteral anticoagulation. The basis for this syndrome is that warfarin therapy, especially in large loading doses, reduces protein C levels more rapidly than the vitamin K–dependent procoagulant factors, leading to exacerbation of the basal hypercoagulable state and thrombosis.

In family-based studies, venous thrombosis occurred in 50% of protein C–deficient relatives of affected probands before 40 years of age.[110] The estimated increased lifetime relative risk of venous thrombosis has been reported to be up to 31-fold.[78] As stated earlier, other studies did not detect an increased thrombosis risk in carriers of protein C deficiency. Differences in risk between family- and population-based studies can be in part explained by greater difficulty in obtaining reliable population-based estimates because of the overall low prevalence of this and other natural anticoagulant deficiencies. In studies of unselected patients with venous thrombosis, the odds ratio (OR) of having protein C deficiency is increased six- to nine-fold compared to controls.[35,103,110,111] An annual absolute risk of venous thrombosis of 4.3% has been reported in women carriers of a natural anticoagulant deficiency, such as protein C deficiency, who also use OCPs.[112]

Laboratory Diagnosis

Patients with heterozygous protein C deficiency have normal PT and aPTT values, whereas patients with homozygous protein C deficiency have abnormal coagulation tests consistent with DIC. Because both type I and type II disorders may occur, functional assays are suggested to optimize identification of affected patients. Some investigators prefer the clot endpoint-based assay because it measures complete function of the protein C molecule, including those patients with abnormal protein C molecules who possess normal activity by a chromogenic substrate assay. However, therapeutic heparin levels affect the clot-based assay. The College of American Pathologists' Consensus

Conference on Thrombophilia recommends the use of the chromogenic substrate assay.[113] One report indicated that measurement of the ratio of protein C to protein S antigen was useful in identifying carriers of protein C deficiency.[114]

Protein C levels can also be measured by immunologic methods, including Laurell rocket immunoelectrophoresis and ELISA. However, immunologic assays may not detect type II patients and may overestimate protein C levels in warfarin-treated patients. Immunologic assays may be more useful in evaluating patients with homozygous deficiency and DIC.

Age-related changes occur with protein C levels.[115] Consequently, it is important to consider this when testing younger patients (<30 years); otherwise, normal subjects may be misclassified as protein C deficient.

A common problem faced by laboratories is measuring protein C levels in patients taking oral anticoagulants. Many clinicians forget that protein C is a vitamin K–dependent molecule and that otherwise hemostatically normal people taking warfarin may have low protein C levels. Griffin and coworkers suggested that protein C data be normalized against the level of another vitamin K–dependent protein to distinguish inherited protein C–deficient patients from normal subjects taking warfarin.[98] One author reported that using a ratio between protein C and prothrombin optimally categorized patients.[116] However, for this method to be useful, patients must be stably anticoagulated for at least 2 weeks, and the laboratory must obtain plasma samples and reference ranges from patients taking warfarin for reasons other than recurrent thrombosis. The consensus conference did not recommend assaying protein C levels in patients on oral anticoagulants.[113] Laboratory test recommendations for protein C deficiency by the ISTH have been reviewed.[117]

Treatment

Many patients with protein C deficiency are asymptomatic, especially those identified in screening studies. Asymptomatic patients should not be treated but should be considered for prophylaxis when they experience high-risk procedures, such as surgery. Symptomatic protein C–deficient patients should be anticoagulated with heparin and then considered for long-term secondary prophylaxis with warfarin at an INR of 2.0 to 3.0. Those patients with a single thrombotic event should receive at least 3 to 6 months of warfarin. Patients with more than one thrombotic event, patients with a single life-threatening thromboembolic event, and those with a significant family history of thrombosis should be considered for long-term anticoagulation. Patients with massive thrombosis or PE may be candidates for thrombolytic therapy.

Infants with neonatal purpura fulminans should be treated with protein C replacement therapy. Protocols using a purified protein C concentrate or PCCs have been described.[118] The use of the purified concentrate normalizes activation of coagulation in these homozygous patients. The protein C product is called Ceprotin.[119]

Acquired Protein C Deficiency

Because protein C is a vitamin K–dependent protein, any disorder associated with vitamin K deficiency may result in protein C deficiency, including warfarin use, liver disease, and malnutrition.[120] Protein C levels are also reduced in DIC, presumably reflecting thrombin activation of the zymogen and consumption of APC.[121] Protein C levels may also be reduced in renal disease, especially the nephrotic syndrome.[122] Protein C levels are not generally reduced with acute VTE.[123]

Protein S Deficiency

Protein S is a vitamin K–dependent plasma protein that facilitates the anticoagulant activity of APC. Protein S deficiency in association with inherited thrombotic disease was first described by two groups in 1984.[124,125] As with AT and protein C deficiencies, protein S deficiency is inherited as an autosomal dominant trait. Many patients with a previous diagnosis of protein S deficiency actually have APC-R.[126] This diagnostic error results from interference in the functional protein S assay of patients with the inherited disorder, APC-R, and misclassification of patients. These patients have a "pseudo" protein S deficiency, often display a type II deficiency pattern, and have protein S activity levels that correlate with the APC ratio. Based on these reports and the high incidence of APC-R in the general population, the true importance of protein S deficiency in inherited thrombosis is uncertain.[126] A population-based, case-control study found that low protein S levels rarely identified subjects at risk for VTE and that protein S testing should not be done on unselected VTE patients.[127]

Pathophysiology and Genetics

As described for AT and protein C deficiencies, patients with protein S deficiency may have quantitative or qualitative disorders. Under normal circumstances, protein S exists in plasma in two forms: bound to C4b-binding protein (60% of total protein S) and free (40% of total). Because only free protein S has APC cofactor activity, a revised classification system has been proposed for protein S deficiency.[128] Type I protein S deficiency is a quantitative disorder in which protein S functional activity, total antigen, and free antigen levels are equally reduced to ~50% of normal. Type IIa protein S deficiency is a deficiency of free protein S with preserved normal levels of total protein S. In type IIb protein S deficiency, the levels of both total and free protein S antigen are normal. A listing of protein S gene mutations and polymorphisms can be found at www.ISTH.org.

As with protein C deficiency, many patients with protein S deficiency and thrombosis have additional risk factors. In one study, among patients with protein S deficiency, ~40% also had APC-R; of family members with thrombosis, 72% had both defects, whereas <20% of patients with single defects experienced thrombosis.[129]

Clinical Aspects

Like AT and protein C–deficient patients, most patients with protein S deficiency and thrombosis have experienced VTE.[124,125] However, unlike most other inherited thrombotic disorders, up to 25% of patients with protein S deficiency may experience arterial thrombosis, including stroke.[106,130] As mentioned previously, many patients with protein S deficiency and thrombosis have other risk factors, including APC-R, estrogen use, or pregnancy.[129] Neonatal purpura fulminans, fetal loss, and warfarin-induced skin necrosis have also been associated with protein S deficiency.[107,131]

Laboratory Diagnosis

Patients with heterozygous protein S deficiency have normal PT and aPTT values. The laboratory diagnosis of protein S deficiency is complicated by four factors: the levels of C4b-binding protein, the coexistence of APC-R in certain patients, elevated factor VIII activity levels, and warfarin therapy. C4b-binding protein is an acute-phase reactant protein S–binding protein, often elevated in thromboembolism, resulting in reduced free protein S levels from the patient's true baseline. Consequently, measurement of protein S levels in patients with acute thrombosis may yield misleading results. Similarly, false-positive results may be seen when functional protein S assays are performed on patients who have APC-R or factor VIII activity levels ≥250%.[129] Patients should not be assumed to have protein S deficiency (diagnosed by functional assay) until APC-R has been excluded. Lastly, because protein S is a vitamin K–dependent protein, warfarin therapy and vitamin K deficiency pose the same difficulty as described for patients evaluated for protein C deficiency. Protein S levels may also be decreased in the setting of pregnancy but are not necessarily associated with thrombotic events.

Both functional and immunologic assays are commercially available to quantitate plasma protein S levels. Functional assays may be PT- or aPTT based, measuring inhibition of factor Va by APC.[132] These assays have the advantage of measuring free protein S activity. Immunologic assays to measure either total (free plus C4b-binding protein bound) or free protein S levels are available.[133,134] Immunologic assays may be useful in evaluating patients who have coexisting APC-R. Total protein S levels are measured using Laurell rocket immunoelectrophoresis or ELISA. In the interpretation of immunologic assays, one should consider the report that the mean plasma level of protein S antigen in males is higher than that in females.[134]

Treatment

Asymptomatic patients should not be treated but should be considered for prophylaxis when they experience high-risk procedures, such as surgery. Symptomatic protein S–deficient patients should be anticoagulated as described for protein C–deficient patients.

Protein Z Deficiency

Protein Z is a vitamin K–dependent plasma protein that serves as a cofactor for activated factor X inhibition by the protein Z–dependent protease inhibitor.[135] Reduced circulating levels of protein Z have been implicated in thrombosis.[136] Protein Z deficiency has also been linked to early and late fetal demise and intrauterine growth restriction.[136] Protein Z deficiency has also been found in the setting of acute coronary syndromes, whereas a deficiency state and the presence of a series of protein Z variants that modulate protein Z plasma levels have been associated with stroke.[136,137] However, a more recent literature review found no association of protein Z deficiency and stroke.[138]

Activated Protein C Resistance (Factor V Leiden)

Before 1993, most patients with idiopathic venous thrombosis evaluated for inherited thrombosis were not given a diagnosis because AT, protein C, and protein S deficiencies together were found in <20% of patients. In 1993, Dahlback and colleagues in Sweden postulated that certain patients with recurrent thrombosis might have additional abnormalities of the protein C pathway, resulting in a hypercoagulable state.[139] They found that addition of APC to plasma obtained from patients with recurrent thrombosis did not prolong the aPTT to the same degree as that seen when APC was added to normal plasma.[139] These patients did not have any previously recognized inherited thrombotic disorder. The term *APC resistance* was used for these patients. Other investigators then used the aPTT-based APC screening test to examine other populations for this phenotype. APC-R was found in 20% to 60% of patients with recurrent thrombosis.[140-142] Like other inherited thrombotic disorders, APC-R was inherited in an autosomal dominant manner.

Pathophysiology and Genetics

APC inactivates factor Va in an orderly and sequential series of cleavages, first at Arg506 and then at Arg306 and Arg679.[143,144] Although the affected factor V cleavage site in APC-R is not directly responsible for complete inactivation of factor Va, APC cleavage at this site is necessary for subsequent proteolytic events. This "partial resistance" is explained by the fact that cleavage of factor Va by APC at Arg306 continues to occur, albeit at a slower rate.[145] In fact, factor V Arg506Gln (factor V Leiden) is inactivated 10 times more slowly than normal factor Va. This provides a pathophysiologic explanation for why factor V Leiden, although common, is a relatively weak risk factor for VTE. Because factor Va functions as a cofactor in the conversion of prothrombin to thrombin, the mutation results in greater amounts of factor Va being available for coagulation reactions, "shifting" the hemostatic balance toward greater thrombin generation.

APC-R caused by factor V Leiden is the most common inherited predisposition to hypercoagulability in Caucasian populations of northern European background. Factor V Leiden follows a geographic and an ethnic distribution: the mutation occurs most frequently in northern and western Europe but is rare in the Asian and African continents as well as in ethnic groups of Asian descent, such as Inuit Eskimos, Amerindians, Australian Aborigines, and Polynesians.[146] In the United States, factor V Leiden is most commonly seen in Caucasians (6.0%), with lower prevalences in Hispanics (2.2%), African and Native Americans (1.2%), and Asian Americans (0.45%).[147]

Factor V Leiden accounts for 92% of cases of APC-R, with the remaining 8% of cases resulting from pregnancy, oral contraceptive use, cancer, selected antiphospholipid antibodies, plasma glucosylceramide deficiency,[148] and other factor V point mutations. Therefore, the terms *factor V Leiden* and *APC-R* should not be considered synonymous; in fact, APC-R is an independent risk factor for VTE even in the absence of factor V Leiden.[149] It is estimated that the mutation arose in a single Caucasian ancestor some 21,000 to 34,000 years ago, well after the evolutionary separation of non-Africans from Africans (~100,000 years ago) and of Caucasoid (white Caucasians) from Mongoloid (Asians) subpopulations (~60,000 years ago).[150]

Clinical Aspects

Heterozygous carriers of factor V Leiden have a 2- to 10-fold increased lifetime relative risk of developing VTE.[112,140,151] This risk is further increased in combination with pregnancy (9-fold), OCP use (36-fold), and HRT (13- to 16-fold).[152-154] VTE is the most common clinical symptom of APC-R in patients who experience thrombosis. In general, there is a notable lack of association of APC-R with arterial thrombosis.[155] Another clinical association with APC-R is recurrent miscarriage, with one study reporting that 20% of patients with second-trimester pregnancy loss have APC-R.[107,156] Factor V Leiden does not appear to be a cause of recurrent pregnancy loss occurring late in the first trimester.[156] Neonatal purpura fulminans has been reported in a patient with factor V Leiden who did not have protein C or protein S deficiency.[157] The factor V Leiden mutation has also been identified in children who experience thrombosis.[158] However, this mutation does not appear to play a major role in the hypercoagulability of cancer.[159] There are conflicting data on the role of factor V Leiden heterozygosity as an independent risk factor for VTE recurrence.[160,161]

Homozygous carriers of the factor V Leiden mutation are estimated to have an 80-fold increased lifetime relative risk of VTE.[155] A more recent estimate, derived from a pooled analysis of a larger population, has confirmed an increased risk of VTE but of lower magnitude (10-fold).[151] The discrepancy is likely caused by the very low prevalence of factor V Leiden homozygosity found in the healthy controls from the general population. Most homozygous carriers present with VTE before 40 years of age, but some can live thrombosis free until the sixth or seventh decade of life or even remain asymptomatic for life.[162] The majority of VTE is situational, and women appear more likely to develop VTE than men, suggesting an important role of OCP use and pregnancy in triggering thrombosis.[162,163] Based on data from the first prospective Duration of Anticoagulation trial, the risk of VTE recurrence is significantly increased in homozygous factor V Leiden carriers (36.4% at 48 months) compared to heterozygous carriers (16.1%) and controls (12.4%).[164]

Laboratory Diagnosis

The intense interest in this common inherited thrombotic disorder has focused substantial attention on laboratory methods for its diagnosis. Laboratory aspects of its discovery have been reviewed by Dahlback.[165] The disorder can be evaluated by coagulation assays that have as their basis inhibition of factor Va by APC and prolongation of the clotting time. Typically, APC is added to patient plasma, and a clotting assay is performed (usually the PTT), with results expressed as the following ratio:

$$\frac{\text{Patient PTT} + \text{APC}}{\text{Patient PTT}}$$

Reference ranges are established for normal patients with and without addition of APC. Affected patients with mutant factor V have clotting times prolonged to a lesser extent (lower ratio) than normals. Alternatively, a DNA test can be done to look specifically for the Arg506Gln mutation; this highly conserved point mutation is present in most patients with APC-R.

With properly collected plasma samples, the APC-R clotting test can correctly classify nearly 100% of patients, when normalized to a control plasma pool.[166] Predilution of the patient sample with factor V–deficient plasma has improved the performance characteristics of most currently available commercial assays.[167] Samples from patients with baseline abnormal coagulation studies (e.g., anticoagulant therapy, lupus anticoagulants, and liver disease) yield uninterpretable results. A TF-dependent factor V assay has been described that is useful in patients taking oral anticoagulants or with the lupus anticoagulant.[168] Consensus recommendations on methodologies to assay for factor V Leiden and APC-R have been presented.[169,170] Although factor V Leiden is the most common cause of APC-R, other factor V mutations have been described, resulting in milder or more severe APC-R and thrombotic phenotypes.[171]

Treatment

Therapy of VTE in patients with APC-R is similar to that described for patients without an identified hypercoagulable state. Long-term secondary prophylaxis is not necessary for heterozygotes unless they experience more than one thrombotic event or experience life-threatening thromboembolism. Asymptomatic patients with APC-R should not be treated, but female patients with this disorder should be informed about the additional thrombotic risk associated with oral contraceptive use, pregnancy, and HRT.[62] Prophylaxis for high-risk situations, such as surgery, should be given. Homozygotes who experience VTE should be considered for long-term anticoagulation.

Prothrombin Mutations

The prothrombin G20210A mutation is the second most common inherited predisposition to hypercoagulability. Heterozygous prothrombin G20210A has been found in 18% of probands of thrombophilic families, 6% of unselected patients with DVT, and 2% of normal Caucasian individuals.[35,172]

Additionally, a single-point mutation of the prothrombin gene at position 20,209 has been reported in four unrelated patients, two of whom had a history of VTE and one of whom had a history of stroke.[173] Although the clinical significance of the prothrombin C20209T mutation is unknown, it may be underrecognized because it is not detected by the polymerase chain reaction/digestion assay commonly used for prothrombin gene mutation testing. Interestingly, all four reported individuals with prothrombin C20209T were African Americans.

Pathophysiology and Genetics

Prothrombin G20210A is a single-point mutation (G-to-A substitution at nucleotide 20,210) in the 3′ untranslated region of the prothrombin gene.[172] This autosomal dominant mutation results in elevated concentrations of plasma prothrombin.[172] In fact, the VTE risk increases as the plasma prothrombin level increases, with levels >115 IU/dL leading to a 2.1-fold increased relative risk of VTE.[172] The G20210A mutation leads to a "gain of function" of the prothrombin gene, perhaps by resulting in an altered polyadenylation pattern in mutant prothrombin mRNA.[174] An in vitro study of thrombin generation found that increasing prothrombin levels to 150% of normal resulted in enhanced thrombin activity.[175]

The mutation appears to follow a geographic and ethnic distribution, with the highest prevalence occurring, unlike factor V Leiden, in Caucasians from southern Europe (3%).[176] This prevalence is nearly twice that observed in northern Europe (1.7%).[176] Similar to factor V Leiden, the prothrombin G20210A mutation is also found in the Middle East and Indian regions, but it is virtually absent in individuals of Asian and African backgrounds.[176] These distributions provide support to the estimate that both mutations (factor V Leiden and prothrombin G20210A) originated relatively recently in the European founding population, after the evolutionary divergences of subpopulations.

Clinical Aspects

Heterozygous prothrombin G20210A is associated with a 2- to 6-fold increased lifetime relative risk of VTE.[35,172,177] The risk appears to be further increased in combination with pregnancy (15-fold) and OCP use (16-fold).[152,178] The relative risk of cerebral vein thrombosis is increased 10-fold in women with this mutation who are not on OCPs, as opposed to 150-fold in OCP users.[179] Homozygosity for prothrombin G20210A has an estimated population prevalence of 0.014%, and homozygous carriers appear to have greater predisposition to develop early (before 40 years of age) idiopathic recurrent VTE than heterozygotes.[172,180] Three prospective studies, which each included 28 to 52 patients, found no increased risk of recurrent VTE in heterozygous prothrombin G20210A carriers.[164,181,182] A large case-control study of >14,000 men revealed no increased risk of stroke or MI associated with this abnormal prothrombin gene.[183]

Laboratory Diagnosis

The prothrombin G20210A and C20209T mutations can only be reliably and routinely identified using molecular biologic techniques. Measurements of functional prothrombin activity do not sufficiently differentiate between carriers and noncarriers of these gene mutations. Genetic testing can be performed accurately despite concomitant treatment with any form of anticoagulation.

Treatment

Treatment paradigms for patients with prothrombin G20210A heterozygosity parallel those for patients with heterozygous factor V Leiden. Patients with concomitant prothrombin G20210A heterozygosity and factor V Leiden heterozygosity should be considered for long-term anticoagulation following a first thrombotic event.

Hyperhomocysteinemia

Homocysteine is a sulfhydryl amino acid formed during the conversion of methionine to cysteine. Hyperhomocysteinemia results when homocysteine metabolism is abnormal. Hyperhomocysteinemia has been identified as an independent risk factor for stroke, MI, peripheral arterial disease, and venous thrombotic disease.[184-186] Even mild-to-moderate hyperhomocysteinemia is a significant risk factor for vascular disease. However, lowering homocysteine levels with vitamin therapy has not resulted in improved outcomes in vascular disease and thrombosis.[187]

Pathophysiology and Genetics

The amino acid homocysteine is normally metabolized via the transsulfuration pathway by the enzyme cystathionine β-synthase (CBS), which requires vitamin B_6 as cofactor, and via the remethylation pathway by the enzymes methylenetetrahydrofolate reductase (MTHFR), which is folate dependent, and methionine synthase, which requires vitamin B_{12} as cofactor.[36] Inherited severe hyperhomocysteinemia (plasma level >100 μmol/L), as seen in classic homocystinuria, may result from homozygous MTHFR and CBS deficiencies and, more rarely, from inherited errors of cobalamin metabolism.[36] Inherited mild-to-moderate hyperhomocysteinemia (plasma level >15-100 μmol/L) may result from heterozygous MTHFR and CBS deficiencies, but most commonly results from the thermolabile variant of MTHFR (tlMTHFR) that is encoded by the *C677T* gene polymorphism.[36]

Acquired hyperhomocysteinemia may be caused by folate deficiency, vitamin B_6 or vitamin B_{12} deficiency, renal insufficiency, hypothyroidism, type 2 diabetes mellitus, pernicious anemia, inflammatory bowel disease, advanced age, climacteric state, carcinoma (particularly involving breast, ovaries, or pancreas), and acute lymphoblastic leukemia, as well as methotrexate, theophylline, and phenytoin therapy.[36]

The precise mechanisms underlying the thrombogenicity of homocysteine remain unclear. Several diverse mechanisms have been proposed, including endothelial cell desquamation, low-density lipoprotein (LDL) oxidation, promotion of monocyte adhesion to endothelium, and factor V activation and promotion of thrombin generation.[36,188] Homocysteine also enhances platelet aggregation and adhesiveness as well as turnover, presumably as a result of endothelial cell injury.[189] One study found that moderate hyperhomocysteinemia does not impair the activation of protein C by thrombin and the inactivation of factor Va by APC.[190]

Severe homocysteinemia usually results from homozygous CBS deficiency. The incidence of this disorder is ~1 in 335,000 live births. Classic symptoms for homozygous patients include premature vascular disease and thrombosis, mental retardation, ectopic lens, and skeletal abnormalities.[191] Heterozygous homocysteinemia has been recognized as a disease entity; this disorder may affect 0.3% to 1.0% of the general population.[191]

Clinical Aspects

Heterozygous carriers of the tlMTHFR mutation have normal plasma homocysteine levels unless folate levels are reduced.[192] More important, the majority of case-control studies have not demonstrated an increased VTE risk in homozygous carriers of the tlMTHFR, and the majority of individuals with hyperhomocysteinemia do not have the tlMTHFR polymorphism. Thus, characterization of the tlMTHFR polymorphism is not useful to determine an individual's VTE risk. VTE risk is most closely related to elevated fasting plasma homocysteine levels, regardless of etiology. Hyperhomocysteinemia (plasma level >18.5 μmol/L) has been associated with a 2- to 4-fold increased VTE risk.[193,194]

The majority of reports linking hyperhomocysteinemia to thrombosis have focused on venous thromboembolic disease. Kottke-Marchant et al compared 23 patients with documented arterial peripheral thrombosis to age- and sex-matched controls.[195] Elevated homocysteine levels (>13 μmol/L) conferred an OR of 7.8 for thrombosis. Elevated homocysteine levels were found in 73% of cases vs 28% of controls. Only smoking and homocysteine level were independent risk factors for arterial thrombosis.

Laboratory Diagnosis

The initial step in the evaluation of the patient with suspected hyperhomocysteinemia involves measurement of fasting total plasma homocysteine (the sum of nonprotein bound and protein bound).[36] Many laboratories report homocysteine values in reference to published "normal" ranges such as 5 to 15 μmol/L, but, ideally, a local, laboratory-specific normal range should always be established. Testing 2 to 8 hours after an oral methionine load (100 mg/kg) increases the sensitivity of detecting occult vitamin B_6 deficiency and obligate heterozygotes for CBS deficiency,[196] but methionine loading is not routinely recommended.[197] Vitamin B_{12} and folate deficiency do not affect postmethionine-loading homocysteine values. In patients found to have elevated levels of homocysteine, testing for vitamin B_{12} deficiency is advocated to avoid missing subclinical deficiency before beginning oral folic acid therapy. Methodologies to measure homocysteine levels have been reviewed.[198]

Treatment

Folic acid supplementation is the mainstay of effective hyperhomocysteinemia therapy.[36] A meta-analysis of 1114 patients enrolled in 12 randomized studies of vitamin supplementation to lower homocysteine levels demonstrated a 25% reduction in homocysteine levels, with similar effects across a dosage range from 0.5 to 5.0 mg daily.[199] The usual recommended dose is 0.4 to 1.0 mg daily. Because patients with subclinical vitamin B_{12} deficiency may be prone to developing peripheral neuropathy if they receive folic acid supplementation alone, additional treatment with 0.5 mg/d of oral vitamin B_{12} has been advocated. In the same meta-analysis, an additional 7% reduction of homocysteine levels was noted with vitamin B_{12} supplementation.[199] Vitamin B_{12} administration results in normalization of homocysteine levels in B_{12}-deficient individuals. Vitamin B_6 supplementation did not appear to have any effect on homocysteine levels. Betaine, a nutritional supplement derived from beets, functions as an alternative methyl donor in the remethylation of homocysteine to methionine. Betaine has been used in individuals with homocystinuria and may facilitate homocysteine reduction in individuals who are not responsive to folate and vitamin B_6.[200]

Thrombotic events in hyperhomocysteinemic patients should be treated as described for other inherited disorders. An additional treatment strategy is to lower plasma homocysteine levels, with the hope of alleviating a risk factor for recurrent thrombosis. However, results of the Heart Outcomes Prevention Evaluation 2 (HOPE-2) trial and Norwegian Vitamin (NORVIT) trial do not support the utility of homocysteine lowering in patients with arterial disease.[201,202] In NORVIT trial, folic acid and vitamin B_{12}, with or without vitamin B_6, did not reduce risk for the composite endpoint of MI, stroke, or death from coronary artery disease in patients with an index MI.[202] Secondary analysis of the HOPE-2 trial regarding effects of vitamin therapy on VTE risk found that there was no significant risk reduction in VTE with vitamin therapy.[203] These trials yielding negative results with vitamin therapy raise questions about the utility of testing and treating homocysteinemia.

Increased Factor VIII Activity

Elevated levels of certain procoagulant coagulation factors, in addition to deficiencies of natural anticoagulant proteins, are risk factors for VTE. Factor VIII levels >1.5 IU/mL (150%) are associated with a 3- and 6-fold greater relative risk of VTE compared to levels <1.5 IU/mL (150%) and <1.0 IU/mL (100%), respectively.[204] VTE risk is increased 11-fold with levels >200%, but it does not appear to be accentuated by concomitant OCP use.[205] Elevated activity levels of factor VIII associated with VTE risk seem to be persistent and not solely attributable to acute-phase response.[206] Transiently elevated factor VIII levels associated with acute-phase response, though, may in part explain the hypercoagulability associated with inflammatory disorders, such as inflammatory bowel disease and cancer. Individuals with plasma factor VIII activity >234% (above the 90th percentile cutoff point for the study population) have a 6.7-fold increased relative risk of recurrent VTE compared to those with activity levels <120%.[37]

Because factor VIII is indeed an acute-phase reactant and its levels can be affected by many factors, including blood type and vWF concentration, determination of the true meaning of an elevated factor VIII level in an individual patient with VTE is challenging. In the study by Koster et al, in which blood samples for factor VIII activity were obtained a minimum of 6 months after the VTE, it was impossible to distinguish completely between inherited elevation and postthrombotic transient elevation of factor VIII.[204] More recent studies support the concept that elevated factor VIII levels are a significant risk factor in asymptomatic individuals for both arterial and venous thrombosis.[207] The College of American Pathologists' consensus conference recommendations are not to routinely measure factor VIII levels in patients with venous thrombosis or arterial thrombosis (Table 56.4).[208]

Increased Levels of Factors IX, X, XI, and XIII

The Longitudinal Investigation of Thromboembolism Etiology study investigated the possible role of elevated factors IX, X, XI, and XIII in VTE risk[209] and found that of these coagulation proteins, only elevated factor XI levels were associated with VTE risk. Elevated factor XI levels have also been linked to stroke and coronary disease.[210]

Impaired Endogenous Fibrinolysis

The endogenous fibrinolytic system is composed of plasminogen, PAs, and antifibrinolytic-regulatory proteins. Intravascular plasminogen is converted to the active fibrinolytic enzyme plasmin primarily by t-PA derived from vascular endothelial cells and by urokinase-type PA (u-PA) from leukocytes. The principal physiologic inhibitor of t-PA is PAI-1, whereas plasmin itself is inactivated by circulating and thrombus-bound α_2-antiplasmin and, to a lesser extent, α_2-macroglobulin. Decreased endogenous fibrinolytic activity as a result of qualitative and quantitative abnormalities of plasminogen, an inadequate release of t-PA in response to vascular injury, and excessive production of PAI-1, such as is found in inflammatory and malignant diseases, can result in impaired endogenous fibrinolysis and accumulation of pathologic thrombus.[211]

Abnormal fibrinolysis was previously thought to account for a large proportion of patients with inherited thrombosis. However, the discovery of APC-R as a common inherited disorder and a literature review that concluded that a causal relationship between abnormal fibrinolysis and inherited thrombosis had not been clearly demonstrated diminished enthusiasm for routinely evaluating patients with recurrent thrombosis for abnormal fibrinolysis.[212] However, newer data from the Leiden Thrombophilia study indicate that reduced plasma fibrinolytic potential is a risk factor for venous thrombosis,[213] and another group identified an elevated level of thrombin-activatable fibrinolysis inhibitor as a risk factor for recurrent venous thrombosis.[214] Additionally,

Table 56.4. Summary of the College of American Pathologists Recommendations on Laboratory Testing for Inherited Thrombosis

Thrombotic Disorder	Who Should Be Tested?	Test Method(s)	Comments
FVL	First VTE at age <50 y Recurrent VTE First unprovoked VTE First VTE, unusual site First VTE, positive family history First VTE related to pregnancy or hormonal therapy Unexplained second- or third-trimester pregnancy loss	APC-R assay using factor V–deficient plasma *or* DNA-based assay	Patients with relatives who are known to have FVL should be tested directly with DNA-based assays. Patients with positive APC-R assays should have confirmatory DNA tests.
Prothrombin gene mutation	As above	DNA-based assay	Prothrombin activity assays should not be used.
Homocysteinemia	Arterial vascular disease; controversial for VTE	High-performance liquid chromatography or immunoassays	Genotyping for methylenetetrahydrofolate reductase mutations is not recommended. Fasting may not be necessary. Proper sample processing is necessary. Testing in VTE patients may be appropriate to identify and treat affected patients with vitamins.
PC deficiency	Infants with neonatal purpura fulminans; VTE patient from a family with known PC deficiency Asymptomatic female from a known PC-deficient family before hormonal therapy	Chromogenic substrate assays preferred Functional assays are useful Immunologic assays are discouraged	Avoid testing during acute thrombosis or anticoagulant therapy. Exclude causes of acquired PC deficiency. Consider age-dependent reference ranges.
PS deficiency	Patient with VTE from a family with known PS deficiency	Functional assay *or* immunoassay for free PS Total PS antigen assays not recommended	Abnormal functional assay results should be confirmed with an immunoassay for free PS. Exclude acquired causes of PS deficiency. Avoid testing during acute thrombosis, anticoagulant therapy, and pregnancy. Consider age- and gender-dependent reference ranges.
AT deficiency	Patient with VTE from a family with known AT deficiency Asymptomatic female from a known AT-deficient family before hormonal therapy	Chromogenic substrate assays preferred AT antigen assays not recommended	Exclude acquired causes of AT deficiency. Avoid testing during acute thrombosis or anticoagulant therapy.
Elevated factor VIII levels	Controversial	Factor VIII activity assay	Test 6 mo after thrombosis. Avoid anticoagulant therapy.
Dysfibrinogenemia	Not recommended		
Heparin cofactor II	Not recommended		
Factor XIII polymorphisms	Not recommended		
Plasminogen activator inhibitor 1	Not recommended		
Plasminogen deficiency	Test in non-DVT patients with ligneous conjunctivitis		

Abbreviations: APC-R, activated protein C resistance; AT, antithrombin; DVT, deep venous thrombosis; FVL, factor V Leiden; PC, protein C; PS, protein S; VTE, venous thromboembolism.
From College of American Pathologists. Consensus Conference XXXVI: diagnostic issues in thrombophilia. *Arch Pathol Lab Med.* 2001;126:1277-1433.

elevated levels of α_2-antiplasmin are linked to increased risk of MI,[215] and elevated levels of PAI-1 are associated with venous thrombosis.[216]

Plasminogen Deficiency

Quantitative and qualitative abnormalities of plasminogen have been reported in patients with recurrent venous thrombosis.[217,218] Quantitative deficiency is inherited as an autosomal dominant disorder, whereas qualitative plasminogen defects (dysplasminogenemia) are usually inherited as autosomal recessive disorders. Dysplasminogenemia is more common in Japanese subjects, and a single mutation accounts for >90% of cases in this population.[219] However, two reports have suggested that quantitative plasminogen deficiency[220] and dysplasminogenemia[221] may not be risk factors for thrombosis, and a large series of 50 patients with quantitative plasminogen deficiency found the major clinical manifestation to be ligneous conjunctivitis; venous thrombosis was not observed.[222] The College of American Pathologists' Consensus Conference on Thrombophilia does not recommend routine assay for plasminogen deficiency in thrombophilia patients.[223]

Tissue Plasminogen Activator Deficiency

Defective synthesis or release of t-PA from the vessel wall represents a potential mechanism for thrombosis. Plasma t-PA activity is unstable, and for accurate assays, citrated plasma samples must be immediately acidified and red blood cells removed.[224,225] Addition of a platelet activation inhibitor to the blood collection tube may help reduce the release of platelet-derived PAI-1, which can interfere with t-PA activity quantification. A plasminogen-chromogenic substrate assay is used to measure t-PA activity; t-PA antigen can be measured by ELISA using citrated plasma. The College of American Pathologists' Consensus Conference on Thrombophilia does not recommend routine assay for t-PA deficiency in thrombophilia patients.[223]

Increased Plasminogen Activator Inhibitor 1 Levels

Increased levels of PAI-1 have been associated with venous thrombosis or arterial thrombosis. Plasma PAI-1 activity is measured in citrated plasma using a back-titration method with single-chain t-PA.[226] Because blood fibrinolytic activity exhibits a diurnal rhythm (decreased fibrinolysis in the morning as a result of peak PAI-1 levels; increased fibrinolysis in the evening as a result of low PAI-1 levels), plasma samples should be obtained at standardized times, such as between 8:00 and 9:00 AM.[227] In addition, because fibrinolytic component levels can be affected by acute-phase changes, patients should not be evaluated for abnormal fibrinolysis until 2 to 3 months after an acute thrombotic event.

Elevated levels of PAI-1 effectively reduce t-PA activity levels, thereby inducing impaired fibrinolysis that may ultimately lead to thrombosis. Theoretically, markedly elevated levels of PAI-1 might also impair attempts at pharmacologic thrombolysis in the setting of acute arterial and venous thrombosis.[228] Defects in endogenous fibrinolytic capacity have also been found in young patients with unexplained arterial thromboembolism. Deficient t-PA release was found in 45% of such patients, and elevated levels of PAI-1 were found in 59%.[229] Similar defects have been detected in individuals with recurrent venous thrombosis.[216] It has been noted that patients who have undergone major surgical procedures might experience a transient "fibrinolytic shutdown" as a result of elevated PAI-1 levels as part of an acute-phase response.[230]

Avoidance of obesity and associated insulin resistance, correction of hypertriglyceridemia, cessation of smoking, and exercise may improve the innate fibrinolytic status.[231,232] Treatment of hypertension with angiotensin-converting enzyme inhibitors or angiotensin II receptor antagonists has been associated with significantly reduced PAI-1 production.[233,234] The lipid-lowering agent gemfibrozil has also been shown to decrease the PAI-1 synthesis rate.[235] Modest alcohol consumption and hormone replacement treatment in postmenopausal women also seem to be beneficial.[236,237]

Dysfibrinogenemia

The clinical and biochemical aspects of dysfibrinogens are reviewed in Chapter 54. In general, dysfibrinogens associated with thrombosis have as their molecular defect generation of an abnormal fibrin that is resistant to fibrinolysis. Dysfibrinogenemia as a cause of inherited thrombosis is uncommon.

Certain patients with dysfibrinogenemia may have a prolonged PT; more typically, these patients are detected by prolonged thrombin and reptilase times, suggesting a defect in the conversion of fibrinogen to fibrin.[238] Confirmation of a dysfibrinogen can be done by simultaneous measurement of functional and immunologic fibrinogen levels. Typically, immunologic levels are found to be higher than levels measured by functional assay. Published data for the healthy population indicate that for fresh plasma samples, the ratio of immunologic to functional fibrinogen ranges from 1.12 to 1.65; ratios >1.65 are suggestive of dysfibrinogenemia.[239]

Another potentially useful test to evaluate patients for dysfibrinogenemia is the fibrinogen lysis time. This test requires partial purification of the patient's fibrinogen, followed by clotting and lysis in a standardized assay.[240] Dysfibrinogens may also result in a false-positive test for fibrin(ogen)-degradation products (FDPs) as assayed by latex agglutination because residual fibrinogen remains in serum after clotting and is detected by the antibody-coated latex beads. An algorithm for the laboratory diagnosis of dysfibrinogenemia has been reported.[241]

Thrombomodulin Deficiency

Thrombomodulin complexed with thrombin is required to activate protein C. In theory, thrombomodulin deficiency should result in hypercoagulability. A number of mutations in the thrombomodulin gene have been identified in patients with venous thrombosis and their families.[242] Routine laboratory testing for this disorder is not yet available, but an Italian study of thrombosis patients indicated that thrombomodulin deficiency is not a common cause of thrombosis.[243] Thrombomodulin gene mutations have been linked to MI.[244] In the prospective Atherosclerosis Risk in Communities study, soluble thrombomodulin levels had a graded inverse association with, and were a good predictor of, coronary artery disease.[245]

Lipoprotein(a)

Lipoprotein(a) (Lp[a]) is a lipoprotein moiety similar to LDL cholesterol in core lipid composition, and it has apolipoprotein (apo) B-100 as a surface apolipoprotein. In addition, Lp(a) has a unique glycoprotein, apo(a), which is bound to apoB-100. Apo(a) is structurally similar to plasminogen but lacks fibrinolytic activity.[246] Lp(a) has both atherogenic and thrombogenic properties. Its thrombogenic effect is derived from stimulation of PAI-1 synthesis, promotion of intercellular adhesion molecule-1 expression by vascular endothelium, inhibition of both plasminogen and t-PA binding to fibrin, inhibition of plasminogen activation by t-PA, and competition with plasminogen for binding sites on endothelial cells and fibrin.[247] The cumulative effect is impaired activation of plasminogen to plasmin at the vessel wall, inhibition of fibrinolysis, and increased risk for thrombosis.

Measurement of Lp(a) should be considered mainly in individuals with atherosclerosis in the absence of classic risk factors, rapidly progressive atherosclerotic lesions despite aggressive risk factor modification, and individuals with acute arterial thrombosis.[248,249] Because it is an acute-phase reactant, an elevated Lp(a) level must be carefully interpreted if drawn shortly after surgery, acute thrombosis, or acute coronary syndromes.[250]

Tissue Factor Pathway Inhibitor

Tissue factor pathway inhibitor (TFPI) is a major anticoagulant, present in plasma, and associated with vascular endothelium. TFPI binds to and neutralizes the TF–factor VIIa complex to inhibit activation of factor X. Low levels of TFPI are a weak risk factor for a first venous thrombosis as well as recurrent VTE events.[251,252] Studies have also linked TFPI deficiency to arterial thrombosis.[253]

Combined Defects

Compound heterozygosity for two different natural anticoagulant deficiencies is extremely rare because of the low prevalence of each individual defect. Double heterozygosity for factor V Leiden and a natural anticoagulant deficiency has been described in some families.[100,254] In families with both factor V Leiden and protein C deficiency, 73% of compound heterozygotes reported a history of VTE, compared with 31% and 13% of relatives with protein C deficiency only and factor V Leiden only, respectively.[100] In families with factor V Leiden and AT deficiency, 92% of double heterozygous carriers had a history of VTE, as opposed to 57% and 20% of individuals with AT deficiency only and factor V Leiden only, respectively.[254] Combined heterozygosity for both the factor V Leiden and prothrombin G20210A mutations, which is estimated to occur in 1 in 1000 persons, does appear to be associated with an increased relative risk of both first and recurrent VTE.[255] The frequency of recurrent VTE was 16% for carriers of factor V Leiden, 20% for carriers of PT G20210A, and 36% for carriers of both mutations.[255]

The prevalence of factor V Leiden carriership in combination with acquired hypercoagulable states has also been studied. Factor V Leiden appears to increase the risk of VTE in patients with antiphospholipid antibodies but is not a prerequisite for the development of VTE in those patients.[256] The interaction between factor V Leiden and hyperhomocysteinemia has been a matter of interest since the observation, not corroborated by further studies, that factor V Leiden appeared to be a prerequisite for VTE in individuals from families with classic homocystinuria.[257] In the large Physicians' Health study, the concomitant presence of both conditions did appear to be synergistic.[258]

Inherited Risk Factors in Childhood Venous Thrombosis

Many of the common inherited thrombotic disorders described in adult patients have been linked to pediatric thrombosis. A prospective European study identified a single genetic risk factor in 54% of pediatric thrombosis patients.[259] Common defects identified were factor V Leiden (32%), protein C deficiency (9%), protein S deficiency (6%), prothrombin gene mutation (4%), and AT deficiency (3%).[259] In most patients, thrombosis is precipitated by superimposed nongenetic risk factors that included central venous catheters, cancer, sepsis, immobility, surgery, trauma, or the use of oral contraceptives.[260] For neonatal patients with thrombosis, the most significant factor associated with thrombosis is the presence of a central venous catheter.[261] In children with recurrent thrombosis, the factor V Leiden mutation is present in most patients.[262] Homozygous deficiencies of protein C or protein S are causal in neonatal purpura fulminans.[108,131] When pediatric patients are evaluated for protein C, protein S, or AT deficiency, pediatric reference ranges are mandatory because age-related changes occur in the levels of these proteins.[263]

A consensus panel of the ISTH has recommended that pediatric patients with thrombosis be routinely tested for both inherited and acquired disorders in a comprehensive manner.[264] However, many of the suggested tests are not recommended by the College of American Pathologists' consensus panel, and there are no data to indicate that patients with a genetic predisposition to thrombosis—children or adults—should be treated differently[265,266] from those without risk factors (discussed in the following section). A large study investigated the association of perinatal stroke with thrombophilia, and concluded that thrombophilia testing was not useful or indicated for these patients.[267] The American College of Chest Physicians (ACCP) Guidelines on Antithrombotic Therapy has pediatric recommendations.[268]

Perspective on Laboratory Testing for Inherited Thrombotic Disorders

Increased availability of hypercoagulable-state test "panels" and enhanced ability to identify an abnormality in tested patients have prompted widespread testing of thrombosis patients. Testing for acquired and inherited hypercoagulable states uncovers an abnormality in >50% of patients presenting with an initial VTE but may have minimal actual impact on management in most of these patients.[23,24,266,267,269,270] Such laboratory screening should be reserved for patients for whom the results of individual tests significantly affect the choice of anticoagulant agent, intensity of anticoagulant therapy, therapeutic monitoring, family screening, family planning, prognosis determination, and, most of all, duration of antithrombotic therapy. Testing "just to know" is neither cost-effective nor clinically appropriate.

Patients should be considered for evaluation of these disorders if they are young (<45 years of age) with recurrent thrombosis, or if they have had a single idiopathic thrombotic event and have a positive family history.[68] This recommendation is based on the fact that, with the exception of hyperhomocysteinemia and qualitative abnormalities of plasminogen, inherited thrombotic disorders, especially the five most common (APC-R, prothrombin G20210A, protein C deficiency, protein S deficiency, and AT deficiency) are autosomal dominant disorders, and most patients with these disorders (but not all)[271] have supportive family histories. Patients without a family history of thrombosis should be evaluated for common acquired etiologies for thrombosis, including malignancy, myeloproliferative disorders, paroxysmal nocturnal hemoglobinuria, and antiphospholipid antibodies.[68] Because thrombosis may induce an acute-phase response that may affect functional coagulation assays, testing is ideally done when the patient has fully recovered from the acute event and is not receiving anticoagulants. Functional assays are preferred over immunologic assays so that both type I and type II disorders can be detected. An important exception to this recommendation is APC-R, which can be screened for using a DNA test that is not affected by acute-phase responses or anticoagulant therapy. Diagnosis of protein C or protein S deficiency in patients already anticoagulated with warfarin can be facilitated by parental testing, testing symptomatic family members who are not receiving anticoagulation, referral to a reference laboratory that has standardized assays for these natural anticoagulants in anticoagulated patients, or temporary cessation of warfarin therapy (minimum of 3-4 weeks).[68] Patients with arterial thrombosis should be considered for testing for hyperhomocysteinemia, Lp(a), and, possibly, protein S deficiency and antiphospholipid antibodies.[4]

In addition to a positive family history of thrombosis, other clinical features may suggest inherited thrombosis, including recurrent spontaneous thromboses, thrombosis in unusual sites (mesenteric vein), thrombosis at an early age, heparin resistance (suggestive of AT deficiency), warfarin-induced skin necrosis and neonatal purpura fulminans (suggestive of protein C or protein S deficiency), and thrombosis occurring with estrogen therapy or pregnancy (suggestive of APC-R or prothrombin G20210A). The presence of these clinical events may justify laboratory evaluation of these patients. Even in situations in which the relative risk of thrombosis and recurrent thrombosis is increased, the absolute risk for a particular patient may not warrant the risks of chronic anticoagulation. Thus, one should always assess the pretest use of hypercoagulable-state testing before embarking on an expensive investigation.

A more fundamental question is whether routine laboratory testing for inherited thrombotic disorders will change treatment (intensity or duration of anticoagulation). This is a controversial subject because the available data do not support the contention that patients with an inherited thrombotic disorder should be managed differently from patients without such a disorder.[23,269,270] One study found that thrombophilia testing at a major urban medical center was overutilized and that a majority of tests were ordered at suboptimal times.[272]

There are three thrombotic risk factors that may influence treatment strategy: the presence of antiphospholipid antibodies (discussed in Chapter 55), AT deficiency, and (perhaps) hyperhomocysteinemia. Patients with antiphospholipid antibodies may require a longer duration of oral anticoagulation, and some patients with hyperhomocysteinemia may respond to vitamin therapy to resolve this thrombosis risk factor, although clinical trial data have not demonstrated a benefit of lowering homocysteine levels.[202,203] Patients identified as having AT deficiency may benefit from this diagnosis because availability of AT concentrates may optimize their management. *Table 56.4* summarizes the clinical laboratory testing recommendations of the College of American Pathologists' Consensus Conference on Thrombophilia.

Laboratory Testing for the Prethrombotic State

Levels of FDPs, including cross-linked FDPs (D-dimer), are usually increased in the presence of acute VTE. The absence of an elevated level of D-dimer in patients undergoing an evaluation for acute DVT or PE has an excellent negative predictive value for thrombosis.[273] D-dimer measured 3 months after oral anticoagulation for DVT treatment was discontinued has been shown to have a negative predictive value of 95.6% for VTE recurrence.[274] It has also been shown that baseline elevations of D-dimer are strongly and positively related to the occurrence of future venous thrombosis.[275] Plasma levels of fibrinopeptide A can be increased in venous thrombosis patients, but this assay has the disadvantage of requiring rigorous attention to specimen collection to avoid an activated plasma sample. The activation peptide generated when prothrombin is cleaved to form thrombin, prothrombin fragment 1 + 2, is a sensitive measure of thrombin formation.[276] In patients with COVID-19 infection, the prothrombin fragment 1 + 2 is a better predictor of thrombosis than D-dimer.[277] Other markers of activation of coagulation include thrombin-AT complex and plasmin-antiplasmin complex.

Combining results of a sensitive D-dimer assay with clinical criteria optimizes exclusion of VTE[278,279] or risk of recurrent VTE.[280-282] *Figure 56.2* depicts one strategy algorithm to incorporate D-dimer testing in thrombosis evaluation. Some investigators recommend using age-adjusted D-dimer cutoff values.[283]

ANTITHROMBOTIC THERAPY

Arterial and venous thrombotic events combined, including acute coronary syndromes, stroke, peripheral arterial thrombosis, DVT, and PE, are likely responsible for more morbidity and mortality than any other condition in the developed world.[3]

Cardiovascular disease was reported to be the underlying cause of death in ~25% of all deaths in the United States in 2018.[1] Every year, 750,000 new strokes occur in the United States, of which 85% are ischemic in nature.[284] Because approximately one-third of these patients die as a direct or an indirect result of their cerebrovascular thrombosis–related occlusion, stroke is the third leading cause of

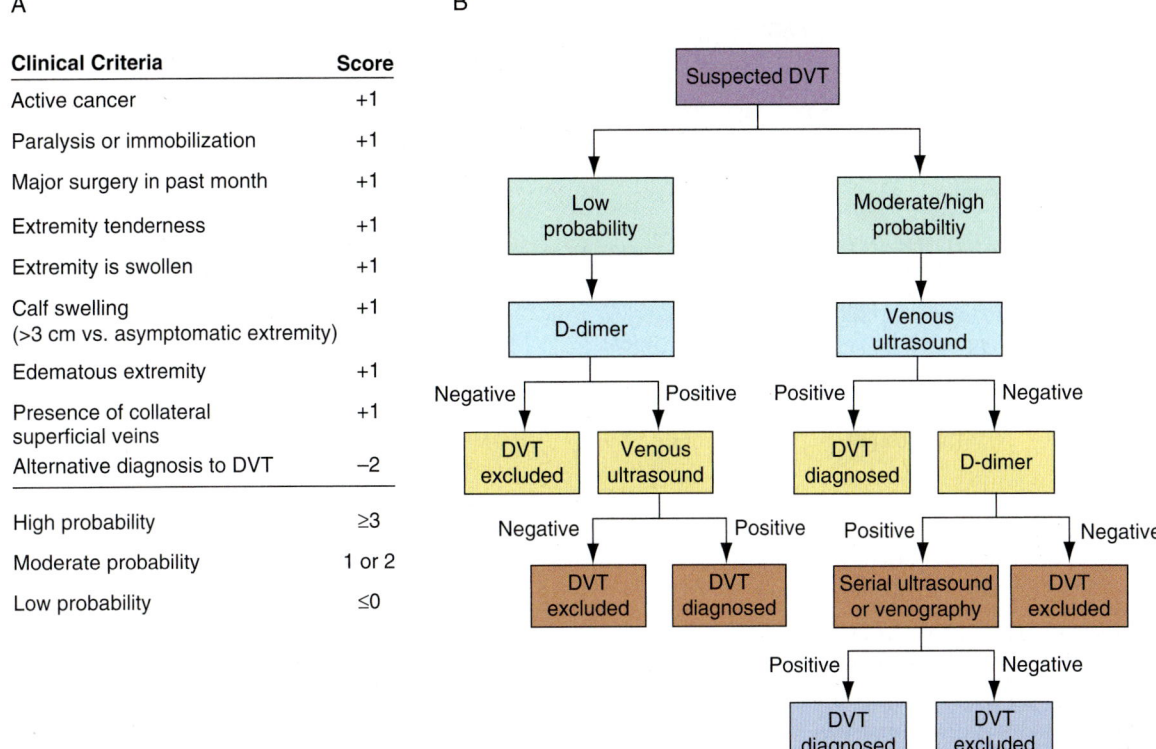

FIGURE 56.2 Algorithm for excluding deep venous thrombosis (DVT) using clinical criteria, D-dimer testing, and venous ultrasound. A, Based on clinical criteria fulfilled by the patient, the cumulative score is tallied. High probability is a score ≥3, moderate probability is 1 or 2, and low probability is ≤0. B, The probability score is used with D-dimer assay and ultrasound to determine which patients may be excluded from DVT testing. (A, Adapted from Wells PS, Anderson DR, Bormanis J, et al. Value of assessment of pretest probability of deep-vein thrombosis in clinical management. *Lancet.* 1997;350(9094):1795-1798. Copyright © 1997 Elsevier. With permission.; B, Adapted from Hirsh J, Lee AY. How we diagnose and treat deep vein thrombosis. *Blood.* 2002;99(9):3102-3110. Copyright © 2002 American Society of Hematology. With permission.)

death in this country. In addition, stroke is the leading cause of serious long-term disability in the United States, with roughly 5 million total stroke survivors. Acute limb ischemia secondary to peripheral arterial thrombosis and thromboembolism involving native and prosthetic vessels is a relatively uncommon but ominous form of vascular accident. National databases suggest a rate of 16 events annually per 100,000 population.[285] In a manner similar to coronary artery thrombosis, acute peripheral arterial thrombosis typically develops at the sites of preexisting peripheral atherosclerotic occlusive disease (PAOD). PAOD has been diagnosed in as many as 17% of men and 20% of women aged >55 years and is highly predictive for the coexistence of coronary and cerebral vascular disease. It has been estimated that PAOD progresses to critical limb ischemia in 15% to 20% of patients.[286]

Acute VTE, including DVT and PE, is a common, potentially life-threatening, often preventable vascular condition associated with trauma, major surgery, advanced congestive heart failure, pregnancy, HRT, malignancy, and inherited hypercoagulability. Proximal lower extremity DVT can result in venous limb gangrene (phlegmasia cerulea dolens), chronic stasis changes related to the postthrombotic syndrome (PTS), and symptomatic PE. PE in its most severe presentation can result in pulmonary hypertension, right-sided heart failure, cardiopulmonary collapse, and death.

A common feature of the management of all thromboembolic vascular diseases is the use of antithrombotic agents. Antithrombotic agents, including antiplatelet drugs, anticoagulants, and thrombolytic agents, are used to prevent thrombotic events, prevent or mitigate the complications of thrombotic events, and restore vascular patency to prevent loss of tissue, organ, and limb function, as well as life. Based on the pathologic basis of thrombosis involving different vascular beds, drugs that inhibit platelet activation and aggregation play a primary role in arterial disease management, whereas drugs that inhibit thrombin and fibrin generation play a primary role in venous disease management. The following sections describe the pharmacodynamics, pharmacokinetics, and clinical uses of select antithrombotic agents.

Antiplatelet Drugs

Given the important role of platelets in mediating arterial thrombosis and the significant morbidity and mortality of arterial thrombotic disorders, the safety and efficacy of antiplatelet drugs have been evaluated in numerous primary and secondary prevention trials. A 1988 meta-analysis indicated that antiplatelet treatment reduced overall mortality from vascular disease by 15% and nonfatal vascular events by 30%.[287] A 2002 update on this subject supports the original observation of the efficacy of antiplatelet therapy.[288] The ACCP 2012 consensus conference summarized the status of clinical trials with aspirin and other antiplatelet drugs.[289]

Numerous potential targets exist for antiplatelet therapy (*Figure 56.3*). Platelet cyclooxygenase (COX-1) is the target of acetylation and irreversible inactivation by aspirin.[290,291] ADP-induced platelet aggregation can be selectively inhibited by the thienopyridines, ticlopidine, clopidogrel, prasugrel, and by ticagrelor, a member of the cyclopentyltriazolopyrimidine class of drugs.[289,291] Dipyridamole alters platelet function, in part, by inhibition of cyclic nucleotide phosphodiesterase to increase platelet cyclic adenosine monophosphate levels.[289] Other potential targets for antiplatelet therapy include the platelet membrane receptor, GPIb, mediator of platelet adhesion, and inhibitors to thrombin, the most potent stimulus to platelet activation.[289,291] Interference with fibrinogen-mediated platelet aggregation by anti-GPIIb-IIIa antibodies and peptides is well established.[289]

Aspirin

Aspirin (acetylsalicylic acid) is the prototypical antiplatelet drug, exerting its antithrombotic action by irreversibly inactivating (by acetylation) the COX activity of platelet prostaglandin H synthase 1 (COX-1) and prostaglandin H synthase 2 (COX-2).[292] This COX

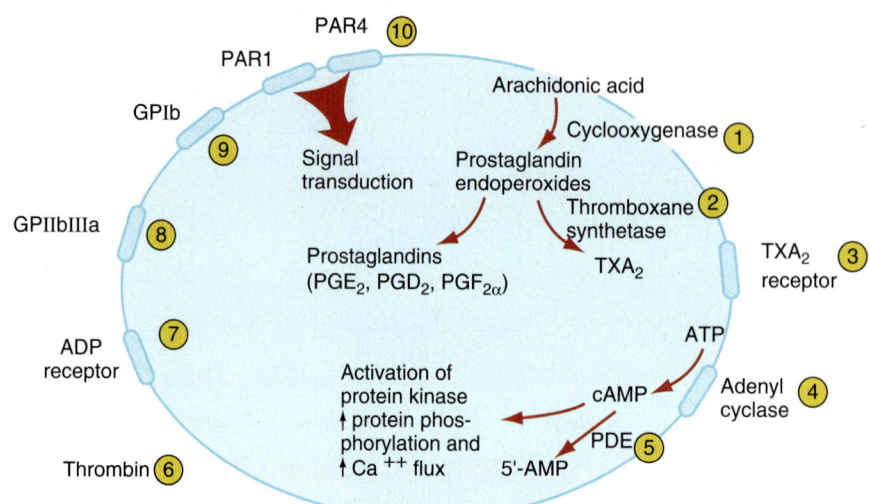

FIGURE 56.3 Targets for antiplatelet agents. This diagram summarizes certain aspects of platelet function relevant to antiplatelet therapy. Platelet metabolic pathways, membrane receptors, and enzymes are depicted with specific therapeutic targets enumerated. Four target categories for antiplatelet drugs are the arachidonic acid pathway, which regulates production of prostaglandins (PGs) and thromboxanes; the cyclic adenosine monophosphate (cAMP) mechanism, which modulates important metabolic events; platelet membrane glycoproteins (GPs), which act as receptors for platelet agonists; and thrombin, a key stimulus to platelet activation. Specific targets for antiplatelet therapies include the following: (1) Cyclooxygenase is the target of acetylation and irreversible inactivation by aspirin, as well as reversible inactivation by the nonsteroidal anti-inflammatory agents; (2) inhibitors to thromboxane synthetase prevent generation of thromboxane A2 (TXA_2); (3) an example of a TXA_2 receptor antagonist is BM 531; (4) infusion of prostaglandin E_1 (PGE_1) or stable analogs of prostacyclin (Iloprost) increases platelet concentrations of cAMP via stimulation of adenylate cyclase; (5) dipyridamole increases platelet cAMP concentrations by inhibition of cyclic nucleotide phosphodiesterase (PDE), and cilostazol inhibits PDE3 to increase platelet cGMP concentrations; (6) because thrombin is the most potent stimulus to platelet activation, inhibitors of thrombin (heparin, argatroban, and bivalirudin) are important agents in preventing platelet-dependent thrombosis; (7) ticlopidine, clopidogrel, prasugrel, and ticagrelor inhibit platelet activation by inhibition of adenosine diphosphate (ADP)-induced aggregation; (8) monoclonal antibodies or peptides directed against the GPIIb-IIIa complex inhibit fibrinogen binding to platelets and subsequent platelet aggregation; (9) inhibitors to the von Willebrand factor receptor (GPIb) are being developed to prevent platelet adhesion; and (10) inhibitors to protease-activated receptors 1 and 4 (PAR1 and 4) such as vorapaxar antagonize thrombin activation of platelets. ATP, adenosine triphosphate. (Reproduced and modified from Greenberg PL, Negrin R, Rodgers GM. Hematologic disorders. In: Melmon KL, Morrelli HF, Hoffman BB, et al, eds. *Clinical Pharmacology: Basic Principles in Therapeutics*. 3rd ed. McGraw-Hill; 1992:524-599.)

inhibition leads to the prevention of TXA_2 synthesis and impairment of platelet secretion and aggregation.[293] A variety of nonsteroidal anti-inflammatory drugs can inhibit TXA_2-dependent platelet function via competitive reversible inhibition of COX-1. A lesser degree of COX-1 inhibition may explain why long-term use of nonaspirin nonsteroidal anti-inflammatory drugs is not protective against first MIs in postmenopausal women.[294] Aspirin is the least expensive, most widely studied, and most widely used antiplatelet drug.

Aspirin (when not enteric coated) is rapidly absorbed from the upper gastrointestinal tract; plasma salicylate concentrations peak within 1 hour of ingestion. The effects of aspirin on platelet function occur within 1 hour and last for the duration of the affected platelets' life span (~1 week). The toxicity of aspirin is dose related, explaining why clinical studies have focused on finding the lowest effective antithrombotic dose of the drug. Toxicities include gastrointestinal discomfort and blood loss, and the risk of systemic bleeding. Clinical trials suggest that aspirin doses as low as 75 or 30 mg/d are antithrombotic.[289]

In addition to reducing aspirin toxicity, lower aspirin doses inhibit vascular endothelial cell prostacyclin production to a lesser extent because inhibition of endothelial cell COX is of shorter duration and requires higher aspirin doses than does platelet COX inhibition.[295] The inhibitory effects of chronic low-dose aspirin administration are cumulative.[296] However, even when taken chronically in large doses, aspirin is not believed to be thrombogenic.[297]

The 2012 ACCP consensus conference statement on antiplatelet therapy indicates that aspirin has been convincingly demonstrated in over 100 randomized trials to be effective in treatment of thrombotic disorders, such as stable and unstable angina, acute MI, transient ischemic attack and incomplete stroke, stroke after carotid artery surgery, atrial fibrillation (low risk), and prosthetic heart valves (in combination with warfarin).[289] The minimum effective aspirin dose for these indications is 75 to 325 mg/d. Aspirin has also been shown to reduce mortality post–coronary artery bypass surgery.[298]

Although early clinical trials suggested that aspirin was effective for primary prevention of cardiovascular events, more recent trials showed little or no clinical benefit of aspirin for this indication, and some trials suggested harm from aspirin use.[299]

Data from the Clopidogrel for High Atherothrombotic Risk and Ischemic Stabilization, Management, and Avoidance (CHARISMA) trial highlight aspirin's preeminent antiplatelet role in cardioprevention.[300] CHARISMA assessed whether adding clopidogrel (75 mg/d) to aspirin therapy (75-162 mg/d) provided any benefit over aspirin monotherapy in preventing MI, stroke, or death from cardiovascular disease. The study showed that the addition of clopidogrel to aspirin did not result in a significant lowering of risk of the primary composite endpoint. In addition, the rate of severe bleeding was 1.7% and 1.3% for the clopidogrel-plus-aspirin and aspirin-only groups, respectively. Clopidogrel in addition to aspirin did reduce the relative risk of a recurrent MI, stroke, or cardiovascular death by 12.5% in the subgroup of patients with established atherothrombotic disease. The subgroup of patients with multiple risk factors, but no clearly established vascular disease did not benefit from the addition of clopidogrel and actually had nonstatistically significant increases in cardiovascular events and bleeding. Clopidogrel plus aspirin remains an approved and standard therapy in conjunction with coronary artery stenting.

Aspirin may modify the natural history of intermittent claudication from lower extremity arteriosclerosis. Because these patients are at high risk for future cardiovascular and cerebrovascular atherothrombotic events, lifelong aspirin therapy is recommended.[4] Similar therapy is advisable after peripheral arterial bypass surgery and carotid endarterectomy.

The Pulmonary Embolism Prevention trial was a large-scale, double-blind, multicenter study of 13,356 patients undergoing surgery for hip fracture and an additional 4088 patients undergoing elective knee or hip arthroplasty.[301] Patients were assigned to a regimen of 160 mg of aspirin or placebo once daily for 5 weeks, with the first dose given before surgery. Other forms of prophylaxis were allowed, and 40% of patients received UFH or LMWH in addition to the aspirin. The study demonstrated that aspirin reduced the incidence of fatal PE (58% risk reduction) and symptomatic nonfatal DVT or PE (36% risk reduction) in patients with hip fracture.[301] Although beneficial when compared to placebo, aspirin cannot be recommended as first-line VTE prophylaxis in hip fracture patients because the benefit of aspirin is less effective than anticoagulants.[302] The potential role of aspirin in treating VTE has been resurrected by the results of a VTE treatment trial that demonstrated that aspirin therapy, begun after 6 to 18 months of oral anticoagulant treatment, reduced VTE recurrence by ~40% compared to placebo.[303] Aspirin, used as prophylaxis for VTE recurrence, would have the advantage of being an active drug to also prevent arterial thrombosis.[304]

The concept of "aspirin resistance" has been popularized. This term refers to persistent platelet activation that occurs in patients treated with aspirin who experience treatment failure. There are numerous reasons for aspirin resistance[305]; current recommendations are to not test routinely for aspirin resistance and to not change therapy based on such test results.[306] One literature review concluded that the most common cause for aspirin resistance was noncompliance.[307] Routine laboratory monitoring for aspirin resistance is not recommended.[308] The etiologies of aspirin resistance have been summarized.[309]

The bleeding risk of continuing antiplatelet therapy at the time of surgery was explored in a literature meta-analysis in which the impact of aspirin, clopidogrel, and dual antiplatelet therapy was studied in noncardiac surgery patients.[310] Continued antiplatelet therapy resulted in minimal bleeding risk; thus it may not be necessary to discontinue these drugs prior to noncardiac surgery.[310]

Thienopyridines

Ticlopidine and clopidogrel are structurally related compounds that selectively inhibit ADP-induced platelet aggregation and likely ADP-mediated amplification of the platelet response to other agonists.[311] A lack of in vitro platelet aggregation inhibition suggests that in vivo hepatic transformation to an active metabolite is necessary for an antiplatelet effect. Both agents were initially used as aspirin substitutes in aspirin-intolerant patients. Enthusiasm for ticlopidine has been dampened by associated hematologic complications, including neutropenia, thrombocytopenia, aplastic anemia, and thrombotic thrombocytopenic purpura.[312,313]

Clopidogrel, an irreversible inhibitor of the P2Y12 ADP receptor, is rapidly absorbed and extensively metabolized. The plasma half-life of the main systemic metabolite, SR 26334, is roughly 8 hours.[314] Platelet function returns to normal approximately 7 days after the last dose of clopidogrel. The Clopidogrel vs Aspirin in Patients at Risk of Ischemic Events trial compared clopidogrel to aspirin in patients who had experienced a recent stroke or a recent MI and in those presenting with symptomatic peripheral arterial disease.[315] The annual ischemic event rate for aspirin was 5.83% compared to 5.32% for clopidogrel. The majority of the difference in efficacy occurred in the patients who entered the trial because of symptomatic peripheral arterial disease, with a 23.8% relative risk reduction.[315] The Clopidogrel in Unstable Angina to Prevent Recurrent Events trial has demonstrated an advantage of clopidogrel plus aspirin over aspirin alone in patients with acute coronary syndromes.[316] Clopidogrel, like ticlopidine, can rarely precipitate thrombotic thrombocytopenic purpura.[317]

Despite the current standard antiplatelet regimen of aspirin and clopidogrel (with or without GPIIb/IIIa inhibitors) in percutaneous coronary intervention (PCI) patients, peri- and postprocedural ischemic events continue to occur.[318] Prasugrel, a newer potent thienopyridine P2Y12 receptor antagonist, can achieve more rapid and higher levels of inhibition of ADP-induced platelet aggregation than clopidogrel.[319] However, although a major clinical trial with prasugrel found that it did not reduce overall mortality, it did increase major bleeding.[318]

Ticagrelor, an antiplatelet agent of the cyclopentyltriazolopyrimidine class, reversibly inhibits the P2Y12 ADP receptor in platelets.[289] An international trial that compared clopidogrel vs ticagrelor in patients with an acute coronary syndrome found that although the overall trial results demonstrated that ticagrelor was the superior drug, the results for US patients showed the opposite, with clopidogrel associated with better outcomes. Major bleeding rates between the two drugs were similar.[318] Perioperative management of patients on antiplatelet therapy has been reviewed.[320]

The use of dual antiplatelet therapy (ASA plus either clopidogrel, prasugrel, or ticagrelor) is commonplace, but there is no agreement as to which drug to combine with ASA. A recent British guideline summarizes the data for specific acute coronary syndrome situations.[321]

Vorapaxar is an analog of himbacine that inhibits PAR-1 to prevent thrombin-induced platelet aggregation.[291] The drug is approved to reduce the risk of MI, stroke, cardiovascular death, and revascularization in patients with a previous MI and in patients with peripheral vascular disease. As with the other antiplatelet agents, vorapaxar is associated with a bleeding risk.[322]

Integrin $\alpha_{IIb}\beta_3$ (Glycoprotein IIb/IIIa) Receptor Antagonists

Because of the multitude of pathways that lead to platelet aggregation, it is not surprising that the clinical efficacy of the antiplatelet agents described earlier is only partial. Even combination therapy with clopidogrel and aspirin, resulting in partial inhibition of TXA_2- and ADP-mediated platelet aggregation, leaves platelets susceptible to agonists, such as thrombin and collagen. Because expression of functionally active GPIIb/IIIa on platelet surfaces is the final common pathway of platelet aggregation regardless of initial stimulus, it is logical to target this glycoprotein receptor with antiplatelet agents for maximal platelet inhibition.

GPIIb/IIIa is a member of the integrin family of receptors. These receptors recognize the amino acid sequence arginine-glycine-aspartate (Arg-Gly-Asp [RGD]), which represents the cell attachment regulation sequence present in certain adhesive proteins, such as fibrinogen.[323] Inhibitors of fibrinogen binding to GPIIb/IIIa, called the *disintegrins*, include a chimeric monoclonal antibody against the receptor, naturally occurring RGD sequence-containing peptides from snake (pit viper) venoms, synthetic RGD peptides, synthetic Lys-Gly-Asp (KGD) peptides, peptidomimetics, and nonpeptide RGD mimetics.[323-325]

Three parenteral GPIIb/IIIa inhibitors have been extensively studied, primarily in the settings of PCI, unstable angina, and non–Q-wave MI: abciximab, eptifibatide, and tirofiban.[325] Abciximab (c7E3 Fab) is a chimeric Fab fragment of human and murine protein that binds to GPIIb/IIIa. Abciximab is unique among the GPIIb/IIIa antagonists because it also blocks the $\alpha_v\beta_3$ receptor.[326] Eptifibatide is a synthetic cyclic heptapeptide with a KGD sequence that is more specific for GPIIb/IIIa than the RGD sequence. Tirofiban is a synthetic peptidomimetic based on the RGD sequence. Oral GPIIb/IIIa inhibitors have been generally unsuccessful. Current and emerging antiplatelet therapies have been reviewed.[289,291,322]

Anticoagulant Drugs

Anticoagulant drugs are ubiquitous in medical and surgical practice. Anticoagulants are used to prevent and treat thrombosis. Traditionally, short-term anticoagulation is provided in the form of an intravenous infusion or subcutaneous injection, whereas more chronic anticoagulation is facilitated using oral agents. The narrow-spectrum (single protein target) oral anticoagulants referred to as direct oral anticoagulants (DOACs) (e.g., dabigatran, rivaroxaban, apixaban, and edoxaban) have largely replaced broad-spectrum anticoagulants (e.g., heparin and warfarin) for VTE and atrial fibrillation management.[327]

Heparin

Heparin is a naturally occurring, highly sulfated glycosaminoglycan that is normally present in human tissues (*Figure 56.4*). Commercial UFH is obtained from either bovine lung or porcine intestinal mucosa and consists of a heterogeneous mixture of polysaccharides

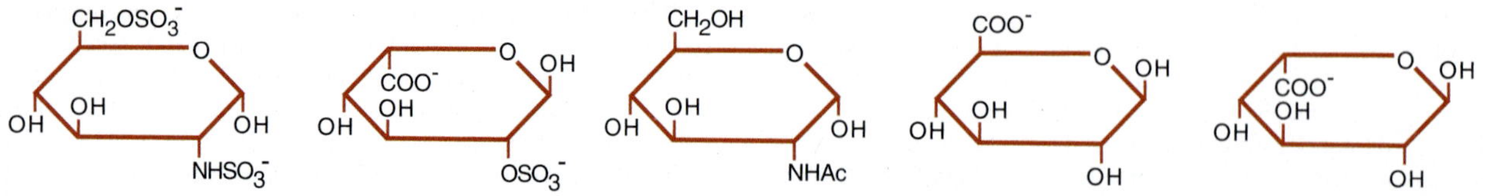

FIGURE 56.4 Structure of the common active saccharide moieties found in commercial unfractionated heparin. These polymeric structures are termed *glycosaminoglycans*. From left to right, the saccharide structures are 2-deoxy-2-sulfamino-α-d-glucose-6-sulfate, α-l-iduronic acid-2-sulfate, 2-acetamido-2-deoxy-α-d-glucose, β-d-glucuronic acid, and α-l-iduronic acid. (Reproduced with permission from Greenberg PL, Negrin R, Rodgers GM. Hematologic disorders. In: Melmon KL, Morrelli HF, Hoffman BB, et al, eds. *Clinical Pharmacology: Basic Principles in Therapeutics*. 3rd ed. McGraw-Hill; 1992:524-599. Copyright © 1992 by McGraw-Hill Inc. All rights reserved.)

(glycosaminoglycans) with molecular weights ranging from 4000 to 30,000 Da, with a mean molecular weight of approximately 15,000 Da (approximately 45 saccharide units). UFH molecules with anticoagulant activity constitute approximately one-third by weight of commercial heparin products.[328] Heparin structure consists of alternating residues of uronic acid and glucosamine that are variably sulfated.[329] Sulfation is a major determinant of the anticoagulant activity of a given heparin preparation; the heparin molecules with anticoagulant activity exhibit high-affinity binding to AT.

UFH molecules contain a randomly distributed unique pentasaccharide sequence that binds to AT. Once bound to UFH, the natural anticoagulant effect of AT is potentiated, resulting in the accelerated binding and inactivation of serine proteases in general, and particularly factor Xa and thrombin.[330,331] The inhibition of these factors affects the common pathway of coagulation, resulting in decreased formation of thrombin and fibrin.

Heparin's interaction with AT is thought to occur as follows and is depicted in *Figure 56.5*. A ternary complex with heparin, thrombin, and AT first occurs; this association permits inactivation of thrombin by the active-site inhibitor domain of AT. Lastly, heparin dissociates from the AT-thrombin complex to subsequently catalyze additional AT-mediated reactions.[332] A pentasaccharide series interacts only with the AT-binding sequence and promotes factor Xa inhibition substantially but has minimal effect on thrombin inhibition.[333] In this case, only the conformational change induced by the pentasaccharide is necessary for factor Xa inhibition to occur. Oligosaccharides of greater length (at least 18 residues) are necessary for enhancement of thrombin inhibition by AT. It is likely that in this latter case, a ternary complex of AT, thrombin, and heparin forms to mediate protease inhibition.[334] In vitro experiments suggest that UFH exerts its major anticoagulant effect by promoting AT suppression of thrombin-dependent amplification reactions.[335]

In addition to its anticoagulant activity, heparin possesses other unrelated biologic effects.[336] Heparin hydrolyzes triglycerides from chylomicrons and very LDLs by the release of endothelial cell lipoprotein lipase into the blood.[337] Heparin can also activate platelets, suppress cell-mediated immunity, and affect metabolism of aldosterone and thyroxine. Heparin is active when given parenterally, either intravenously or subcutaneously. Because of its highly charged nature and inability to cross biologic membranes alone, oral use of heparin has historically been viewed as impossible.

The half-life of heparin varies with the dosage given, with the half-life increasing with increasing dosage.[338] A 100-U/kg intravenous dose is cleared with a half-life of ~1 hour. The clearance of heparin is also affected by the extent of thromboembolism, with extensive thrombosis decreasing heparin half-life.[339] Heparin is cleared by the reticuloendothelial system and metabolized by the liver, and metabolic products are excreted in the urine. The anticoagulant effect of heparin is also altered by its nonspecific binding to plasma proteins and cells.[340] Given these numerous variables affecting the plasma half-life of heparin, therapeutic use of this drug requires close laboratory monitoring to achieve a therapeutic effect and regulation of heparin activity within a targeted range to optimize safety and efficacy. When using intravenous heparin, the use of established nomogram-guided therapy is preferred.[341] *Table 56.5* illustrates an example of a weight-based nomogram for using UFH. This assumes that the hospital laboratory has calibrated the aPTT values such that an aPTT range from 1.5 to 2.5 times the mean laboratory control aPTT is equivalent to plasma heparin levels of 0.3 to 0.7 U/mL, as measured by anti–factor Xa activity.[341]

Pharmacologic reversal of UFH anticoagulant activity can be achieved with protamine sulfate. Protamine is a positively charged moiety derived from salmon sperm that can interact with the negatively charged UFH to form a stable complex that lacks anticoagulant activity. One milligram of protamine can inactivate ~100 U of UFH. Protamine, in excess, can promote an anticoagulant state. Because of clinically meaningful risks of bradycardia, hypotension, and anaphylaxis, protamine has typically been reserved for cases of life-threatening bleeding or UFH overdose, and reversal of anticoagulation following cardiopulmonary bypass or major vascular surgery.[341,342]

An additional challenge to the use of heparin is the development of heparin resistance. "True" heparin resistance manifests as inadequate

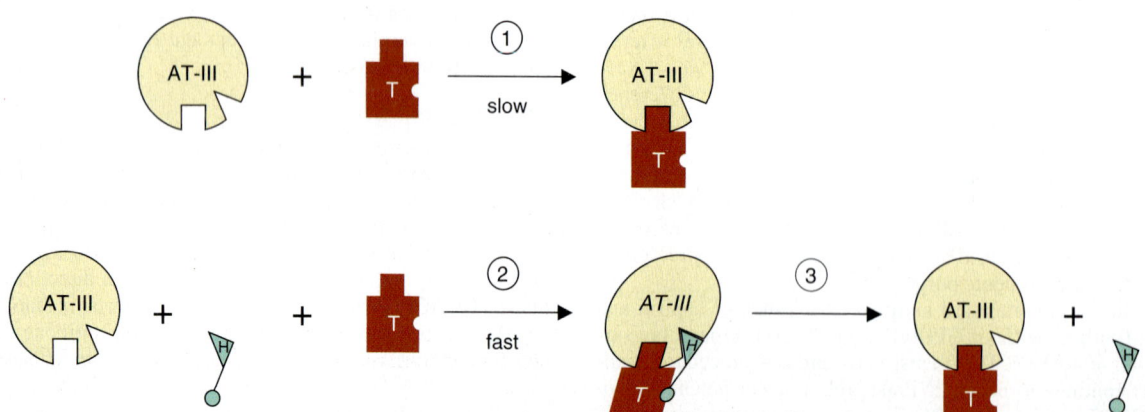

FIGURE 56.5 Inhibition of thrombin activity by the heparin (H)-antithrombin (AT) mechanism. Reaction *1* indicates that in the absence of heparin catalysis, AT can irreversibly inactivate thrombin (T), albeit in an inefficient manner. In the presence of H, a conformation change occurs in the AT molecule, and heparin also acts as a template to bind both AT and T, promoting rapid inactivation of coagulation (reaction 2). In reaction 3, heparin is released from the AT-T complex and is available to catalyze subsequent reactions. Inhibition of factor Xa by AT-H does not require binding of heparin to the factor Xa molecule.

Table 56.5. Weight-Based Nomogram of UFH in Treatment of Venous Thromboembolism

Initial UFH bolus	80 U/kg
Initial UFH infusion rate	18 U/kg/h
Check aPTT after 6 h of IV infusion; modify infusion rate as follows:	
If aPTT <1.2 × control, repeat bolus (80 U/kg) and increase infusion rate by	4 U/kg/h
If aPTT is 1.2-1.5 × control, repeat bolus (40 U/kg) and increase infusion rate by	2 U/kg/h
If aPTT is 1.5-2.3 × control, no change	—
If aPTT is 2.3-3.0 × control, decrease infusion rate by	2 U/kg/h
If aPTT >3 × control, hold infusion for 1 h, then decrease infusion by	3 U/kg/h

Abbreviations: aPTT, activated partial thromboplastin time; IV, intravenous; UFH, unfractionated heparin.
Data from Raschke RA, Reilly BM, Guidry JR, Fontana JR, Srinivas S. The weight-based heparin dosing nomogram compared with a "standard care" nomogram: a randomized, controlled trial. *Ann Intern Med.* 1993;119:874-881.

anticoagulant and antithrombotic responses from what would otherwise be perceived as an adequate weight-based dose. Some have deemed a requirement of >35,000 U of heparin per 24-hour period, regardless of patient weight, to reflect this form of heparin resistance.[343] With true heparin resistance, both a measurement of anticoagulant activity such as the aPTT and a measurement of antithrombotic activity such as the anti–factor Xa activity assay demonstrate inadequate degrees of heparin activity. True heparin resistance most likely results from the nonspecific binding of heparin to mononuclear white blood cells, vascular endothelial cells, and acute-phase proteins, such as histidine-rich glycoprotein, vitronectin, and PF4, resulting in an inadequate quantity of free or AT-bound heparin.[341] Another potential cause of heparin resistance is acquired AT deficiency that can be seen in patients with the nephrotic syndrome, liver disease, malnutrition, DIC, or malignancy.[342,343]

Patients can also manifest an "apparent" heparin resistance characterized by dissociation between the aPTT and heparin assays.[344] In these patients, the aPTT may be normal or near normal, whereas the anti–factor Xa activity assay reveals an appropriate target heparin activity level between 0.3 and 0.7 U/mL. Simply escalating the dose of heparin to achieve the desired aPTT without checking a heparin assay may result in a pronounced bleeding risk. Dissociation between the aPTT and heparin concentration likely reflects elevated levels of factor VIII or fibrinogen that can shorten the in vitro aPTT without affecting the antithrombotic actions of the drug.

Low-Molecular-Weight Heparins

LMWH is derived from the enzymatic or chemical cleavage of UFH to produce a mixture of low-molecular-weight glycosaminoglycan molecules with a mean molecular weight of ~5000 Da (~15 saccharide units).[340] For example, enoxaparin sodium is produced by benzylation followed by alkaline hydrolysis, dalteparin sodium is produced by controlled nitrous acid depolymerization, and tinzaparin sodium is produced by enzymatic digestion with heparinase. LMWH binds AT via the same pentasaccharide sequence as UFH.[340] However, because of the predominance of molecules <18 saccharide units in length, LMWH has limited antithrombin (IIa) activity compared to its anti–factor Xa activity. Whereas UFH has an anti–factor Xa to anti-IIa activity ratio of 1:1, LMWHs have reported ratios of 1.9:1 to 4.1:1.[340] Because of limited thrombin inhibition, LMWH therapy cannot be monitored using the aPTT. Other differences between LMWH preparations include the degree of TF pathway inhibitor release, sulfation, and stimulated vWF release.[345-347]

At low doses, subcutaneous LMWH has 90% bioavailability compared to 30% for UFH. LMWHs have limited nonspecific binding to plasma proteins, platelets, endothelial cells, and macrophages compared to UFH, as well as a predictable clearance and a longer half-life that facilitates once- or twice-daily administration.[340,348] Unlike UFH, the half-life of LMWH is not dose dependent.[340] These characteristics make LMWH preferred in settings that may normally result in heparin resistance. These advantages of LMWH allow these drugs to be given subcutaneously, once or twice daily and without the need for routine laboratory monitoring.[340] Similar to UFH, absolute contraindications for LMWH include active bleeding, HIT, or a history of HIT, and known sensitivity to LMWH, UFH, or pork products.

LMWHs have substantial renal clearance; therefore, multiday therapeutic use of LMWH in patients with significant renal insufficiency (creatinine clearance [CrCl] < 30 mL/min) should be avoided.[23] In the setting of less severe renal insufficiency, LMWH should be used with caution and with a reduced dosing frequency. The anti–factor Xa activity assay is used to guide LMWH dose adjustment in patients with renal insufficiency and extremes of body weight.[349] Approximately 60% of LMWH anticoagulant activity can be reversed after the administration of protamine sulfate.[350] Novel agents are under development that appear more effective for LMWH reversal.[351,352] Table 56.6 summarizes the LMWH products available in the United States and their properties and U.S. Food and Drug Administration (FDA)-approved indications.

Heparinoids

Heparinoids are low-molecular-weight glycosaminoglycans that are not derived from heparin. Heparinoids include dermatan sulfate and danaparoid sodium. Dermatan sulfate and low-molecular-weight dermatan sulfate act as anticoagulants by activating HCII.[353,354] Danaparoid sodium is a glycosaminoglycan mixture derived from porcine intestinal mucosa and composed of heparan sulfate (84%), dermatan sulfate (12%), and chondroitin sulfate (4%).[355] Danaparoid has an anti–factor Xa activity to anti-IIa activity ratio of greater than 22:1 (compared to a 1:1 ratio for heparin), which explains why it is minimally neutralized by protamine sulfate.[341]

The largest collection of clinical experience with danaparoid is in the setting of HIT. Danaparoid may cross-react with 10% to 50% of HIT sera, but in vivo cross-reactivity, although reported, has not been commonly observed.[356] Danaparoid has a relatively long half-life of ~24 hours, which may make its use less desirable in patients at high risk for developing bleeding or those likely to need surgery. Significant experience exists with the administration of danaparoid by both intravenous and subcutaneous routes. Danaparoid anticoagulation is monitored using an anti–factor Xa activity chromogenic assay calibrated with danaparoid standards. The target therapeutic anti–factor Xa activity is 0.5 to 0.8 U/mL. Danaparoid's potential for cross-reactivity and the longer half-life make it less desirable than a direct thrombin inhibitor (DTI) for the treatment of patients with HIT.[341]

Pentasaccharides

Because factor Xa is situated at the start of the common pathway of coagulation and upstream of thrombin in the cascade, it is an attractive target for anticoagulants. By not directly inhibiting thrombin activity, factor Xa inhibitors might allow small amounts of thrombin to be generated, facilitating hemostasis and theoretically leading to a more favorable bleeding risk profile. Fondaparinux is an FDA-approved synthetic pentasaccharide (molecular weight, 1728 Da) that causes selective indirect (i.e., AT-mediated) inhibition of factor Xa.[341] Fondaparinux is administered subcutaneously, has a half-life of ~17 hours, and does not require therapeutic monitoring. Fondaparinux elimination is prolonged in patients with renal impairment. The reduction in clearance increases as the CrCl decreases. Elimination is also prolonged in patients aged >75 years and in those weighing <50 kg. Fondaparinux has been used with success to treat HIT[357] and is approved for the prevention and treatment of VTE.

Idraparinux and idrabiotaparinux are long-acting hypermethylated synthetic pentasaccharides with half-lives up to 130 hours designed to allow once-weekly subcutaneous dosing.[358] Based on disappointing clinical trial results the manufacturer halted further development of both compounds.[359,360]

Table 56.6. Low-Molecular-Weight Heparin and Polysaccharide Products Available in the United States

Low-Molecular-Weight Heparin	Approved Indications	FDA-Approved Dosage Regimen
Dalteparin (Fragmin)	DVT/PE prophylaxis for abdominal surgery	2500 U SC daily, starting 1-2 h before surgery and continued 5-10 d postoperatively.
		High-risk patients (e.g., malignancy): 5000 U SC daily, starting the evening before surgery and continued for 5-10 d postoperatively. Or, give 2500 U SC 1-2 h before surgery, then 2500 U SC 12 h later, and 5000 U SC daily for 5-10 d postoperatively.
	DVT/PE prophylaxis for hip replacement surgery	Preoperative start, evening before surgery: 5000 U SC daily, starting 10-14 h before surgery. The usual duration is 5-10 d postoperatively, although 14 d has been studied. Allow 24 h between doses.
		Preoperative start, day of surgery: 2500 U SC within 2 h before surgery, then 2500 U SC 4-8 h after surgery, and 5000 U SC daily postoperatively. The usual duration is 5-10 d postoperatively, although 14 d has been studied. Allow at least 6 h between the first postoperative dose and the next postoperative dose.
		Postoperative start: 2500 U SC 4-8 h after surgery, then 5000 U SC daily. The usual duration is 5-10 d postoperatively, although 14 d has been studied. Allow at least 6 h between the first postoperative dose and the next postoperative dose.
	DVT/PE prophylaxis in medical patients with severely restricted mobility due to acute illness	5000 U SC daily for 12-14 d.
	Prophylaxis of ischemic complications of non–Q-wave myocardial infarction in patients on concurrent aspirin therapy	120 U/kg SC every 12 h for 5-8 d, given concurrently with aspirin 75-165 mg/d PO. Do not exceed 10,000 U/dose. Continue until patient is clinically stabilized.
	Prophylaxis of ischemic complications of unstable angina in patients on concurrent aspirin therapy	120 U/kg SC every 12 h for 5-8 d, given concurrently with aspirin 75-165 mg/d PO. Do not exceed 10,000 U/dose. Continue until patient is clinically stabilized.
	Extended treatment of DVT/PE in cancer patients	200 U/kg SC daily (max. 18,000 U) for 1 mo, then 150 U/kg SC daily (max. 18,000 U) for 5 mo
Enoxaparin (Lovenox)	DVT/PE prophylaxis for abdominal surgery	40 mg SC daily, starting 2 h before surgery. The usual duration is 7-10 d postoperatively, although 12 d has been studied.
	DVT/PE prophylaxis for hip replacement surgery	30 mg SC every 12 h, starting 12-24 h after surgery. The usual duration is 7-10 d postoperatively, although 14 d has been studied.
		An alternative regimen is 40 mg SC daily, starting 9-15 h before surgery and continued for 3 wk.
	DVT/PE prophylaxis for knee replacement surgery	30 mg SC every 12 h, starting 12-24 h after surgery. The usual duration is 7-10 d postoperatively, although 14 d has been studied.
	DVT/PE prophylaxis in medical patients with severely restricted mobility due to acute illness	40 mg SC daily. The usual duration is 6-11 d, although 14 d has been studied.
	Treatment of DVT with or without PE (inpatient therapy) in patients starting on warfarin sodium	1 mg/kg SC every 12 h, or 1.5 mg/kg SC daily (at the same time each day). Start warfarin when appropriate (usually within 72 h of starting enoxaparin). Continue enoxaparin for at least 5 d, until INR is therapeutic; usually an additional 7 d is needed, although up to 17 d may be required.
	Treatment of DVT without PE (outpatient therapy) in patients starting on warfarin sodium	1 mg/kg SC every 12 h. Start warfarin when appropriate (usually within 72 h of starting enoxaparin). Continue enoxaparin for at least 5 d, until INR is therapeutic; usually an additional 7 d is needed, although up to 17 d may be required.
	Prophylaxis of ischemic complications of non–Q-wave myocardial infarction in patients on concurrent aspirin therapy	1 mg/kg SC every 12 h given concurrently with aspirin 100-325 mg/d PO. The usual duration is 2-8 d, although up to 12.5 d has been studied.
	Prophylaxis of ischemic complications of unstable angina in patients on concurrent aspirin therapy	1 mg/kg SC every 12 h given concurrently with aspirin 100-325 mg/d PO. The usual duration is 2-8 d, although up to 12.5 d has been studied.
Fondaparinux (Arixtra)	DVT/PE prophylaxis following abdominal surgery	2.5 mg SC daily, starting 6-8 h after surgery. The usual duration is 5-9 d, although up to 10 d has been studied.
	DVT/PE prophylaxis following hip replacement surgery	2.5 mg SC daily, starting 6-8 h after surgery. The usual duration is 5-9 d, although up to 11 d has been studied.
	DVT/PE prophylaxis following hip fracture surgery	2.5 mg SC daily, starting 6-8 h after surgery. The usual duration is 5-9 d, although up to 11 d has been studied.
	DVT/PE prophylaxis following knee replacement surgery	2.5 mg SC daily, starting 6-8 h after surgery. The usual duration is 5-9 d, although up to 11 d has been studied.
	Treatment of DVT and PE in patients starting on warfarin sodium	5 mg SC daily for patients <50 kg, 7.5 mg SC daily for patients 50-100 kg, or 10 mg SC daily for patients >100 kg. Start warfarin when appropriate (usually within 72 h of starting fondaparinux). Continue fondaparinux for at least 5 d, until INR is therapeutic; the usual duration is 5-9 d, although up to 26 d has been studied.

Abbreviations: DVT, deep venous thrombosis; INR, international normalized ratio; IV, intravenous; PE, pulmonary embolism; PO, orally; SC, subcutaneously.
Data from *Arixtra (fondaparinux sodium injection)*. Package Insert. GlaxoSmithKline; 2005; *Lovenox (enoxaparin sodium injection)*. Package Insert. Sanofi-Aventis U.S. LLC; 2006; *Fragmin (dalteparin sodium injection)*. Package Insert. Pfizer Inc; 2008.

Parenteral Direct Thrombin Inhibitors

The parenteral DTIs have been studied for use in patients with acute coronary events, but are most widely utilized in patients with HIT. In these patients, elimination of all heparin exposure is an essential treatment strategy. This includes discontinuing heparin intravenous catheter flushes, prophylactic subcutaneous heparin or LMWH, and heparin-coated indwelling catheters. Yet, despite heparin discontinuation and platelet count recovery, patients with isolated, serologically confirmed HIT have up to a 50% risk of developing a confirmed thrombotic event during the 30-day period after heparin cessation.[361] The persistent prothrombotic tendency associated with HIT and the patient's original indication for heparin therapy warrant the use of an alternative anticoagulant agent, such as DTIs or DOACs, after heparin cessation (Table 56.7).

Hirudins

Hirudin, a polypeptide originally isolated from the salivary glands of the medicinal leech, directly inhibits thrombin. Two recombinant forms of hirudin have been developed, lepirudin and desirudin. Lepirudin differs from native hirudin in that it lacks sulfation on the tyrosine at position 63 and has a leucine at position 1 rather than isoleucine.[362] Lepirudin is a potent DTI that lacks any structural homology with heparin, does not cross-react with heparin, has a short half-life (~80 minutes), is able to inactivate clot-bound thrombin, and can be monitored using the ubiquitous aPTT assay or the less readily available ecarin clotting time.[363] The major challenges of lepirudin treatment are the lack of an antidote, the extreme care needed when treating patients with even mild renal insufficiency, and immunogenicity. Lepirudin received FDA approval in 1998 for the treatment of HIT with thrombosis. Subsequently, the manufacturer discontinued production and marketing in 2012 unrelated to safety concerns. Desirudin, another recombinant form or hirudin that was approved for VTE prevention after elective hip replacement surgery in the United States, has similarly been discontinued.

Argatroban

Argatroban is a synthetic, small-molecule, L-arginine derivative that is FDA approved for prophylaxis and treatment of thrombosis in patients with HIT. Argatroban is a rapid and reversible DTI, in contrast to lepirudin, which is an irreversible thrombin inhibitor. Argatroban can inhibit both free and fibrin-associated thrombin. Argatroban exerts its antithrombotic effects by inhibiting thrombin-mediated reactions, including fibrin formation; activation of coagulation factors V, VIII, and XIII; activation of the natural anticoagulant protein C; and platelet activation.[364] Like lepirudin, argatroban does not cross-react with heparin. Argatroban is metabolized by the liver with biliary excretion and has a half-life of approximately 40 minutes. Renal excretion has also been documented; however, renal impairment has been shown to have little adverse effect on drug clearance and half-life. Unlike lepirudin, argatroban does not require dose adjustment in the setting of renal insufficiency.[365] Dose reduction is required in patients with significant hepatic dysfunction.[366,367]

Argatroban is administered as a weight-based intravenous infusion. The recommended initial infusion rate is 2 μg/kg/min in patients with normal hepatic function. The initial rate should be reduced to 0.5 μg/kg/min in patients with significant hepatic dysfunction. Critical illness with multiorgan dysfunction, severe anasarca, and postcardiac surgery may warrant initial dose reduction between 0.5 and 1.2 μg/kg/min.[368] Regular aPTT monitoring and dose adjustments are recommended to target an aPTT of 1.5 to 3.0 times the baseline value. Therapy may also be monitored by whole-blood ACT or the ecarin clotting time. Argatroban prolongs the PT as well as the aPTT. This PT prolongation makes determination of an accurate INR during conversion to oral warfarin therapy a challenge.[369] Holding the infusion for 4 to 6 hours before INR determination is prudent. Argatroban has been shown to provide adequate anticoagulation with minimal bleeding risk while enabling procedural success in HIT patients undergoing PCI. Patients were given a 250 to 350 μg/kg bolus of argatroban followed by 10 to 25 μg/kg/min infusion titrated to achieve an ACT of 250 to 450 seconds.[370] Argatroban use during cardiopulmonary bypass has been less successful and is not recommended.[371,372]

Bivalirudin

Bivalirudin is a semisynthetic, bivalent DTI consisting of a dodecapeptide analog of the carboxy-terminus of hirudin.[373] The short half-life of bivalirudin (~25 minutes) may enhance its safety profile. Bivalirudin use in patients presenting with acute coronary syndrome increased after clinical trials demonstrated similar efficacy to heparin with GPIIb/IIIa inhibition and an improved safety profile.[374,375] Follow-up studies suggest the bleeding reduction from bivalirudin use is largely attributable to arterial access location and increased bleeding with GPIIb/IIIa coadministration with UFH.[376] Direct comparison of bivalirudin with UFH for primary PCI demonstrated similar bleeding rates and reduced ischemic events with UFH use.[377] Bivalirudin use for PCI has subsequently declined.[376]

Bivalirudin has also been evaluated for the management of patients with HIT, especially those requiring cardiac surgery. The recommended dose of bivalirudin is a bolus of 0.75 mg/kg, followed by an infusion of 1.75 mg/kg/h for the duration of the procedure.[341] This dose should be reduced in patients with moderate-to-severe renal impairment and those requiring hemodialysis.[378]

Table 56.7. Comparison of Parenteral Direct Thrombin Inhibitors

Drug Profile	Lepirudin (Refludan)[a]	Argatroban (Argatroban)	Bivalirudin (Angiomax)
Derivative	Recombinant hirudin	L-Arginine derivative	Synthetic hirudin-based peptide
Action	Direct thrombin inhibitor	Direct thrombin inhibitor	Direct thrombin inhibitor
Clearance	Renal	Hepatic	Renal
Administration	IV (or SC)	IV	IV or SC
Half-life	1.5 h	40 min	25 min
Monitoring	aPTT	aPTT	aPTT or ACT
Heparin cross-reactivity	None	None	None
Effect on international normalized ratio	Yes	Yes	Yes
Approved for heparin-induced thrombocytopenia	Yes	Yes	Yes
Immunogenic	Yes	No	Unknown

Abbreviations: ACT, activated clotting time; aPTT, activated partial thromboplastin time; IV, intravenous; SC, subcutaneous.
[a]No longer available in the United States.

Warfarin

In the 1920s, cattle developed a bleeding disorder when they were fed spoiled sweet clover. Campbell and Link later identified the active agent as bishydroxycoumarin (dicoumarol).[379] Drugs that inhibit the biosynthesis of the vitamin K–dependent coagulation proteins are derived from either 4-hydroxycoumarin or 1,3-indanedione. Although the indanediones are used in Europe, a coumarin derivative, warfarin, is the major formulation used in the United States. Warfarin inhibits γ-carboxylation of select glutamic acid residues in the N-terminus of prothrombin and factors VII, IX, and X, as well as the vitamin K–dependent natural anticoagulants, protein C and protein S.[380] Warfarin inhibits the two enzymes critical for the generation of reduced vitamin K, namely, vitamin K epoxide reductase and vitamin K reductase.[381,382] Reduced vitamin K is necessary for catalyzing γ-carboxylation of glutamic acid residues. Inhibition of γ-carboxylation by warfarin leads to synthesis of incomplete, hypofunctional coagulation proteins that are unable to bind to cellular surfaces to mediate coagulation reactions. The effect of warfarin on vitamin K–dependent procoagulant protein production is depicted in *Figure 56.6*. Details of vitamin K metabolism are presented in Chapter 20.

Commercially available warfarin is a racemic mixture of levorotatory and dextrorotatory forms of the drug. The half-life of warfarin in blood is ~36 hours.[383] Laboratory monitoring of warfarin therapy is best done using functional coagulation tests, such as the PT. Plasma warfarin levels are most useful in evaluating the unusual patient who does not respond to standard warfarin dosages or in whom malabsorption, noncompliance, or inherited drug resistance is an issue.[382,384]

Because factor X and prothrombin have half-lives >2 days, reduction of all vitamin K–dependent coagulation proteins into the therapeutic range (TTR [time in therapeutic range]) (~20% of normal) requires 4 to 5 days of therapy.[385] This is the basis for the "parenteral anticoagulant overlap" period of 5 days during which patients receive therapeutic parenteral anticoagulant while waiting to achieve the therapeutic effects of warfarin.[386]

Warfarin dosage is influenced by numerous variables, including the patient's age, body mass, dietary stores of vitamin K, liver function, coexisting medical disorders, concurrent medications,[387] and the presence or absence of cytochrome P-450 complex (CYP2C9) and vitamin K epoxide reductase complex subunit 1 (VKORC1) single-nucleotide polymorphisms that affect coumarin metabolism or sensitivity.[388-390] Patients with liver disease, malnutrition, or other factors associated with sensitivity to warfarin should receive lower warfarin dosages. The most common adverse interaction of warfarin use occurs in a patient with marginal dietary vitamin K intake (postoperative state) who is given a broad-spectrum antibiotic, reducing enteric bacterial synthesis of vitamin K, resulting in increased sensitivity to warfarin.[382] Starting warfarin therapy the same day as parenteral anticoagulation has many advantages, including earlier hospital discharge on adequate oral anticoagulation and potential reduction in the incidence of HIT.[391] The metabolism of warfarin may be affected by other drugs metabolized by the cytochrome P-450 enzyme complex, drugs that displace albumin-bound warfarin into the circulation, drugs that impair gastrointestinal absorption, and many antibiotics that alter the natural flora of the colon (an endogenous source of vitamin K)[382,387] (*Table 56.8*).

Table 56.8. Drugs and Medical Conditions Affecting Warfarin Potency

Potentiators	Antagonists
Drugs	**Drugs**
Acetaminophen	Adrenal corticosteroids
Anabolic steroids	Barbiturates
Broad-spectrum antibiotics	Carbamazepine
Chloral hydrate	Chlordiazepoxide
Cimetidine	Cholestyramine
Clofibrate	Efavirenz
Disulfiram	Griseofulvin
Fluconazole	Nafcillin
Indomethacin	Rifampin
Influenza vaccine	Sucralfate
Lovastatin	Trazodone
Metronidazole	**Medical Conditions**
Omeprazole	Excess dietary vitamin K
Phenylbutazone	Inherited resistance to warfarin
Phenytoin	Hypothyroidism
Propranolol	Nephrotic syndrome
Protease inhibitors (except ritonavir)	
Quinine/quinidine	
Salicylates	
Tamoxifen	
Thyroid drugs	
Trimethoprim/sulfamethoxazole	
Medical Conditions	
Older age	
Liver disease	
Biliary disease	
Malabsorption	
Congestive heart failure	
Fever	
Hyperthyroidism	
Malnutrition	
Vitamin K deficiency	
Cancer	

Data from the *Physicians' Desk Reference*. Thomson Healthcare; 2003; Hirsh J, Dalen JE, Anderson DR, et al. Oral anticoagulants: mechanism of action, clinical effectiveness, and optimal therapeutic range. *Chest*. 2001;119(1 suppl):8S-21S.

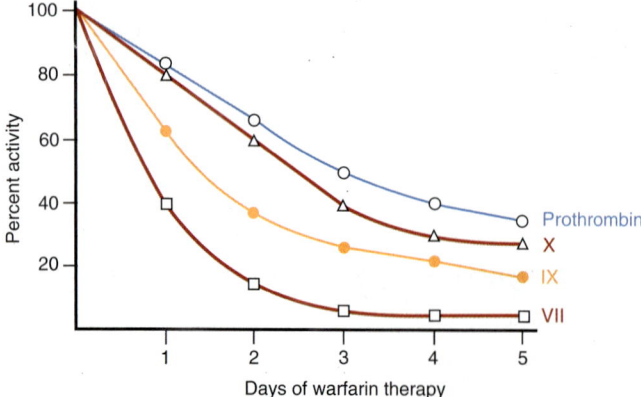

FIGURE 56.6 **Effects of standard warfarin therapy on the plasma vitamin K–dependent procoagulant coagulation proteins.** Administration of 5 to 10 mg daily of warfarin results in inhibition of synthesis of functional vitamin K–dependent proteins. The coagulant activity of these proteins in plasma declines as a function of their half-life. Half-lives of factors VII, IX, and X and prothrombin are 6, 24, 40, and 60 hours, respectively. Although 1 to 2 days of warfarin prolongs the prothrombin time assay (because of the rapid decrease in factor VII concentration), therapeutic anticoagulation requires at least 4 to 5 days. (Data from O'Reilly RA. The pharmacodynamics of the oral anticoagulant drugs. *Prog Hemost Thromb*. 1974;2:175-213; reproduced with permission from Greenberg PL, Negrin R, Rodgers GM. Hematologic disorders. In: Melmon KL, Morrelli HF, Hoffman BB, et al, eds. *Clinical Pharmacology: Basic Principles in Therapeutics*. 3rd ed. McGraw-Hill; 1992:524-599. Copyright © 1992 by McGraw-Hill Inc. All rights reserved.)

Certain genotypes for CYP2C9 and VKORC1 have a significant effect on the pharmacokinetic and pharmacodynamic response to warfarin dosing, respectively. Although there is a clear gene-dose relationship, the routine use of genotype-guided warfarin dosing does not improve clinical outcomes.[392] Genotype-guided warfarin dosing does not increase the TTR compared to validated clinical dosing algorithms for warfarin initiation and maintenance.[392]

Certain patients may require very large doses of warfarin (>50 mg/d) to achieve therapeutic anticoagulation; the term *warfarin resistance* has been applied.[384] Patients who are difficult to anticoagulate with warfarin, either because they exhibit warfarin resistance or because they are very sensitive to the drug and cannot be safely regulated, should be switched to a DOAC unless a contraindication exists (e.g., mechanical heart valve).

Laboratory Monitoring of Warfarin Therapy

The PT assay is used to monitor warfarin therapy because this assay measures three vitamin K–dependent coagulation proteins: factors VII, X, and prothrombin. The PT is particularly sensitive to factor VII deficiency; with a half-life of 4 to 6 hours, the factor VII level may drop rapidly after only 1 day of warfarin therapy and prolong the PT value. However, because the other vitamin K–dependent proteins have longer half-lives, therapeutic anticoagulation takes 4 to 5 days. There is no advantage to giving larger loading doses of warfarin (e.g., >10 mg); this regimen only results in a more rapid drop in factor VII levels, delay in attainment of a stable PT, a precipitous fall in protein C levels, and predisposition to warfarin-induced skin necrosis.[383,393,394]

To understand warfarin monitoring, it is important to appreciate the concept of the INR, a method that standardizes PT assays.[382,395] An international reference thromboplastin preparation has been adopted by the World Health Organization (WHO). Each new commercial thromboplastin is calibrated against the primary WHO reference preparation. These results are used to calculate the relative sensitivity of the unknown preparation compared with the WHO standard (international sensitivity index [ISI]). The method to determine the ISI for a particular thromboplastin is depicted in *Figure 56.7*. By adjusting for the ISI of a particular thromboplastin, an INR, defined as the PT ratio (measured PT/mean normal PT) that would have been obtained if the WHO standard thromboplastin had been used, can be determined. The INR is calculated using the following formula: $INR = (PT\ ratio)^{ISI}$ (*Figure 56.8*).

Moderate-intensity warfarin therapy (INR, 2.0-3.0) is recommended for all indications except prosthetic mechanical heart valves, for which higher intensity warfarin therapy (INR, 2.5-3.5) is suggested.[396] Low-intensity warfarin therapy (INR, 1.5-1.9) is less effective than moderate-intensity warfarin for the prevention of recurrent VTE and has a similar bleeding risk.[397] Higher intensity warfarin therapy, for indications other than prosthetic mechanical heart valves, is generally associated with increased bleeding risk without meaningful reductions in thromboembolism rates.[398,399]

POC INR devices have been developed, allowing patient self-testing (PST) and patient self-management (PSM) of warfarin. These devices use a fingerstick sample of whole blood to measure clotting time, estimating the INR. Device manufacturers calculate conversion formulas to estimate the INR by comparing POC results against thromboplastin assays calibrated against the WHO reference preparation.[382] The lack of a universally accepted POC device calibration method has led to discordance between POC and laboratory INR results, especially as the INR increases above 3.5 to 4.0.[400] Although discrepancies between POC and laboratory INR results may lead to different warfarin dosing recommendations, the effect on clinical outcomes remains uncertain. Despite these limitations, PST and PSM offer greater convenience and are associated with improved TTR and reductions in thromboembolic events and deaths, without an increase in major bleeding among select patients.[401]

Adverse Effects of Warfarin Therapy

Bleeding. A direct relationship exists between the risk of bleeding and the intensity of anticoagulation, with patients receiving higher intensity (INR >3.0) therapy having a fivefold greater risk of bleeding.[398] Other major factors contributing to bleeding include coexisting conditions, such as structural gastrointestinal lesions, hypertension, renal disease, and cerebrovascular disease.[402,403] Investigation of patients who experience visceral bleeding while on warfarin therapy often results in identification of structural disease.[404] Highest bleeding rates occur early in the course of warfarin therapy and in patients with cerebrovascular disease.[402,405] For patients given moderate-intensity warfarin therapy for prophylaxis of VTE, the risk of major bleeding is <1% annually.[397] Antiplatelet medications or other drugs

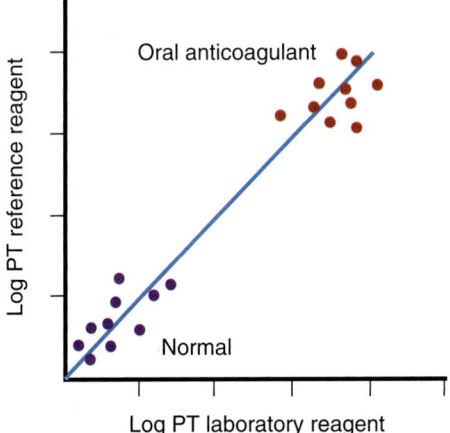

FIGURE 56.7 Method for determination of an international sensitivity index (ISI) value for a laboratory thromboplastin preparation. Log prothrombin time (PT) values are determined using a reference thromboplastin reagent and the commercial laboratory thromboplastin reagent on patients receiving stable (2 weeks) oral anticoagulant therapy and a group of normal, untreated volunteers. The best-fit line is determined, and the slope of this line multiplied by the ISI of the reference thromboplastin reagent is the ISI value for the commercial thromboplastin reagent. (From Rodgers GM. Laboratory monitoring of anticoagulant and fibrinolytic therapy. In: Kjeldsberg C, McKenna R, Perkins S, et al, eds. *Practical Diagnosis of Hematologic Disorders*. 2nd ed. ASCP Press; 1995:745-755. Copyright © 1995 by American Society for Clinical Pathologists.)

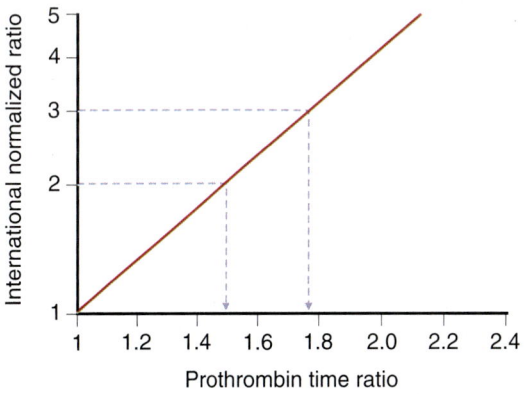

FIGURE 56.8 Relationship between a patient's prothrombin time (PT) ratio on warfarin therapy and the corresponding international normalized ratio (INR) value. The slope of the line represents the international sensitivity index (ISI) value of the particular thromboplastin preparation used in the laboratory PT assay. In this example, for moderate-intensity warfarin therapy (INR 2.0-3.0), a PT ratio between 1.50 and 1.75 would be required. Thromboplastins with higher ISI values would have slopes greater than that shown and would be less sensitive reagents for the PT assay, whereas thromboplastins with lower ISI values would have slopes less than that shown (more sensitive reagents). (Reproduced with permission from Greenberg PL, Negrin R, Rodgers GM. Hematologic disorders. In: Melmon KL, Morrelli HF, Hoffman BB, et al, eds. *Clinical Pharmacology: Basic Principles in Therapeutics*. 3rd ed. McGraw-Hill; 1992:524-599. Copyright © 1992 by McGraw-Hill Inc. All rights reserved.)

that potentiate warfarin activity are important contributors to bleeding (Table 56.8).

Treatment strategy of bleeding in patients receiving warfarin depends on several factors: the duration of expected warfarin therapy, the severity of bleeding, and the extent of INR elevation. Patients with minor bleeding (bruising and microscopic hematuria) and an INR of <6.0 can have warfarin withheld until the INR approaches the desired INR target. Warfarin can then be resumed at a lower maintenance dosage. If patients have visceral bleeding that is not immediately life threatening, their coagulopathy can be reversed with vitamin K, 2.5 to 10 mg, intravenously or orally. Patients with severe life-threatening bleeding should be reversed with a PCC or recombinant factor VII a, in addition to parenterally administered vitamin K. Fresh-frozen plasma (4-5 U) can be used if PCCs and recombinant factor VII are unavailable. If the INR is <10 and no clinical bleeding exists, several warfarin doses should be held and the INR reassessed; the routine administration of vitamin K in these patients does not lead to improved outcomes and is not recommended.[382,406] For an INR >10 in patients without bleeding, oral vitamin K can be given (2-10 mg) and repeated at 12- to 24-hour intervals, depending on posttreatment INR values and the patient's clinical condition. Failure of vitamin K to correct the coagulopathy suggests that another process is present, such as liver disease or DIC. The management of warfarin overdosage and reversal has been reviewed.[382]

Patients who ingest rodenticides that contain long-acting vitamin K antagonists (VKAs) ("superwarfarins") may require massive daily doses (≥100 mg) of vitamin K to correct the coagulopathy, for periods of weeks to months (see Chapter 55).

Most patients on long-term warfarin therapy who require temporary interruption for procedures or elective surgery do not require bridging therapy with a parenteral anticoagulant during the periprocedural interruption (i.e., when warfarin is discontinued 4-5 days before surgery). The observed risk of thromboembolism is <1% in the periprocedural period. Bridging anticoagulation does not significantly reduce thromboembolic events and is associated with a 3- to 10-fold increase in major and clinically relevant bleeding periprocedurally.[407-409] Patients at high risk for thromboembolism (e.g., mechanical mitral valve, acute VTE within 4 weeks) warrant an individualized risk-benefit assessment to determine the need for bridging because these patients have not been well studied (Table 56.9). Postoperatively, LMWH or UFH can be used to achieve anticoagulation overlap until reinitiation of therapeutic warfarin has been achieved. Following a major surgical procedure, the use of therapeutically dosed parenteral anticoagulants should be avoided in the first 48 to 72 hours postoperatively owing to the high risk of bleeding.[410]

Nonhemorrhagic adverse effects of warfarin therapy include alopecia, gastrointestinal discomfort, rash, liver dysfunction, and calciphylaxis.[393] A warfarin embryopathy can occur when pregnant mothers receive warfarin during the first trimester. A bone matrix protein, osteocalcin, is vitamin K dependent, and in the presence of vitamin K deficiency induced by warfarin, osteocalcin is synthesized in a nonfunctional manner, resulting in fetal bone malformations.[411] Additional fetal abnormalities have been noted when warfarin is used during pregnancy. Because of these fetal risks, warfarin use during pregnancy should be avoided.[412] Similar to warfarin embryopathy, the reduction of osteocalcin and other γ-carboxyglutamic acid (Gla) containing proteins has been implicated as a precipitant for calciphylaxis in patients with chronic kidney disease and normal renal function.[413,414] Warfarin should be halted in patients with suspected or biopsy-confirmed calciphylaxis, followed by vitamin K administration and initiation of another anticoagulant (e.g., UFH, LMWH, or DOAC).

Warfarin-Induced Skin Necrosis. Skin necrosis is an unusual but devastating complication of warfarin therapy, occurring within the first week of initiating therapy. Affected patients have usually received large loading doses of warfarin, perhaps in the absence of heparin coadministration. The basis for this complication is thought to be a warfarin-induced rapid reduction in protein C levels in patients with a preexisting protein C deficiency that results in a hypercoagulable state and thrombosis. Not all heterozygous protein C–deficient patients receiving warfarin experience this complication, and not all patients with this complication have inherited protein C deficiency.

Clinically, the skin lesions begin on certain subcutaneous areas of the body (breasts, abdomen, and thighs) as erythematous patches.[415] Lesions progress to blebs followed by demarcated skin necrosis. Skin biopsy reveals generalized thrombosis of dermal and subcutaneous vessels. This complication may require amputation or reconstructive surgery or both. The use of standard maintenance doses of warfarin (5-10 mg/d) beginning after patients are therapeutically anticoagulated with heparin may avoid this complication. Patients who experience warfarin-induced skin necrosis should be heparinized, warfarin should be discontinued, and vitamin K should be administered promptly. Patients experiencing this complication should be screened for protein C deficiency. A few cases of warfarin-induced skin necrosis have been reported in protein S–deficient patients.[416] A literature review of warfarin-induced skin necrosis found that warfarin therapy could be reinstituted in affected patients; smaller initial doses of warfarin and heparin coadministration until the INR is >2 were recommended.[417]

Direct Oral Anticoagulants. VKAs (e.g., warfarin, acenocoumarol, phenprocoumon, and fluindione) were the mainstay of oral anticoagulation therapy until the development of several narrow-spectrum anticoagulants, collectively referred to DOACs. Warfarin and other VKAs have substantial limitations, including inter- and intrapatient dosing variability, drug-drug and dietary interactions, and a narrow therapeutic index. These limitations necessitate routine laboratory monitoring and dose adjustment that may be burdensome for patients and healthcare systems. Since their introduction, DOACs have been demonstrated to be a safe and effective form of anticoagulation with notable benefits including: predictable pharmacology; few drug-drug

Table 56.9. General Approach to Periprocedural Anticoagulation for Patients on Long-Term Warfarin Therapy

Thromboembolic Risk Group	Indication for Anticoagulation		
	Mechanical Heart Valve	Atrial Fibrillation	Venous Thromboembolism (VTE)
High Management strategy: consider bridging	• Mechanical mitral valve • Older generation (e.g., ball-in-cage) • Prior stroke with anticoagulation interruption • Mechanical aortic valve with risk factors (e.g., atrial fibrillation, ejection fraction <35%)	• $CHADS_2$[a] score ≥5 • CHA_2DS_2VASc[b] score ≥7 • Recent stroke or systemic embolism within 3 mo • Prior stroke during transient anticoagulation interruption	• VTE within prior 6 wk • Severe thrombophilia (e.g., antiphospholipid syndrome, protein C deficiency) • Recurrent VTE during transient anticoagulation interruption
Low Management strategy: no bridging	• Any patient not meeting high-risk criteria		

[a]$CHADS_2$ stroke score is calculated by adding 1 point for each of congestive heart failure, hypertension, age ≥75 years, diabetes mellitus, and 2 points for prior stroke or transient ischemic attack.
[b]CHA_2DS_2VASc score is calculated by adding 1 point for congestive heart failure, hypertension, age 65 to 74 years, diabetes mellitus, vascular disease, female sex, and 2 points for age ≥75 years or prior stroke/transient ischemic attack.

Table 56.10. Pharmacology of Direct Oral Anticoagulants

	Dabigatran (Pradaxa)	Rivaroxaban (Xarelto)	Apixaban (Eliquis)	Edoxaban (Savaysa)
Target	**Thrombin** (binds reversibly)	**Factor Xa** (binds reversibly)	**Factor Xa** (binds reversibly)	**Factor Xa** (binds reversibly)
Dosage form	Capsule	Tablet	Tablet	Tablet
Bioavailability	6%	60%-80%	50%-85%	62%
Time to peak	1-2 h	2-4 h	1-3 h	1-2 h
Metabolism	Conjugation; no CYP involvement	Oxidation (via CYP3A4 + CYP2J2) + hydrolysis	Oxidation (via CYP3A4) + conjugation	Biliary and renal excretion; minimal CYP involvement
Drug interactions	Strong P-GP inducers and inhibitors	Strong P-GP and CYP3A4 inducers and inhibitors	Strong P-GP and CYP3A4 inducers and inhibitors	Strong P-GP inducers and inhibitors
Renal excretion	80%	35%	25%	50%
Half-life	14-17 h	5-13 h	12 h	10-14 h
Dosing frequency, major trials	BID	QD	BID	QD

Abbreviations: BID, twice daily; CYP, cytochrome P-450; P-GP, P-glycoprotein; QD, daily.

or dietary interactions; and they do not require frequent laboratory monitoring. The oral DTI dabigatran etexilate and the oral factor Xa inhibitors (e.g., rivaroxaban, apixaban, and edoxaban) have several FDA-approved indications. *Table 56.10* summarizes the properties of the DOACs available for clinical use.

Dabigatran Etexilate

Dabigatran etexilate is an oral prodrug that is rapidly converted by serum esterases to dabigatran, a potent univalent DTI. Oral bioavailability is ~3% to 7% and uptake is reduced by proton-pump inhibitors and delayed with food. However, these pharmacokinetic alterations are not believed to be clinically significant or require dose adjustment. Peak dabigatran serum levels occur ~2 hours after an oral dose; dabigatran is primarily eliminated by renal clearance (~80%), and has a half-life of ~12 to 17 hours.[418] Although a reduced dose (75 mg) is available for use in the United States for patients with a CrCl between 15 and 30 mL/min, solely based upon drug kinetic modeling, the safety and efficacy outcomes of this dose are unknown.[419] Dabigatran etexilate use is contraindicated in patients with a creatinine clearance <15 mL/min or on hemodialysis.[418] Strong P-glycoprotein (P-GP) inhibitors (e.g., dronedarone and ketoconazole) and inducers (e.g., rifampin and St. John's wort) affect serum levels. In patients with moderate renal impairment (CrCl 30-50 mL/min), coadministration of P-GP inhibitors may necessitate a dose adjustment (refer to prescribing information).[418]

The predictable dose-response makes routine laboratory monitoring unnecessary. However, if laboratory assessment of the anticoagulant activity is required (e.g., need for urgent surgery or management of bleeding), a normal aPTT, thrombin time, or ecarin clotting time implies that little drug activity is present. Conversely, the INR is insensitive to the presence of dabigatran and is not a useful measure of anticoagulant activity.[420] *Table 56.11* suggests a management approach for patients requiring periprocedural interruption.

Dabigatran is approved for the prevention of stroke and systemic embolism in patients with nonvalvular atrial fibrillation, acute VTE treatment, and the prevention of VTE in patients undergoing elective total hip arthroplasty. In patients with nonvalvular atrial fibrillation, dabigatran 150 mg twice daily was more effective than warfarin for the prevention of stroke and systemic embolism, with similar bleeding risks. Conversely, a lower dabigatran dose (110 mg twice daily) demonstrated similar thromboembolic event rates and a reduced bleeding risk compared to warfarin.[421] Dabigatran appears to be

Table 56.11. Periprocedural Management of Direct Oral Anticoagulants

Preprocedure	Half-Life (Range) h	Low Bleeding Risk Procedures (Average of 2-3 Drug Half-Lives Separate Last Dose and Surgery)	Moderate-to-High Bleeding Risk (Average of 5 Drug Half-Lives Separate Last Dose and Surgery)
Dabigatran			
CrCl >50	14 h (11-24)	Skip 2 doses (1 d)	Skip 4 doses (2 d)
CrCl 30-50	18 h (13-23)	Skip 4 doses (2 d)	Skip 6-8 doses (3-4 d)
CrCl <30	27 h (22-35)	Skip 4-10 doses (2-5 d)	Skip >10 doses (>5 d)
Rivaroxaban			
CrCl >50	8 h	Skip 1 dose (1 d)	Skip 2 doses (2 d)
CrCl <50	9-10 h	Skip 2 doses (2 d)	Skip 3-4 doses (3-4 d)
Apixaban			
	12 h	Skip 2 doses (1 d)	Skip 4 doses (2 d)
Edoxaban			
	12 h (10-14)	Skip 1 dose (1 d)	Skip 4 doses (2 d)
Postprocedure	Delay reinitiation until hemostasis is certain (24-72 h) and no epidural catheter is present		

Abbreviation: CrCl, creatinine clearance (mL/min).

superior to warfarin among patients who have a low TTR (e.g., <55%), whereas the benefits are less certain in those with well-controlled warfarin (e.g., TTR >70%).[422] Among patients with acute VTE, dabigatran 150 mg twice daily was as effective as warfarin and demonstrated a similar safety profile.[423] Notably, when dabigatran is chosen for acute VTE treatment, at least 5 days of parenteral anticoagulation (e.g., UFH or LMWH) administration is required prior to the initiation of oral dabigatran.[418] When assessed for VTE prophylaxis following total knee arthroplasty, dabigatran was less effective than enoxaparin.[424] Following total hip arthroplasty, dabigatran appears more effective than enoxaparin 40 mg once daily for VTE prophylaxis, although dabigatran was not directly compared to the usual North American dosing regimen of enoxaparin 30 mg twice daily.[425] Dabigatran is not an effective thromboprophylactic agent in patients with prosthetic mechanical heart valves[426]; clinical guidelines recommend against its use in this population.[427]

Rivaroxaban

Rivaroxaban is a reversible, orally administered, direct factor Xa inhibitor that binds to and inactivates both fluid-phase factor Xa and factor Xa associated with the prothrombinase complex. Rivaroxaban has a bioavailability of ~80%, with peak levels achieved 2 to 3 hours after oral administration. The drug is metabolized in part by both CYP3A4-dependent and CYP3A4-independent pathways, and has an elimination half-life of ~5 to 9 hours in young healthy patients, prolonging to ~11 to 13 hours in elderly patients.[428] The kidneys eliminate approximately 35% of active drug as well as inactive metabolites. Potent combined P-GP and CYP3A4 inhibitors (e.g., ketoconazole, itraconazole, lopinavir/ritonavir, ritonavir, indinavir/ritonavir, and conivaptan) and inducers (e.g., carbamazepine, phenytoin, rifampin, St. John's wort) should be avoided in patients on rivaroxaban because they can significantly increase or decrease plasma drug concentrations, respectively. Dose reduction is recommended for patients with nonvalvular atrial fibrillation and moderate renal impairment (CrCl ≤50 mL/min) or end-stage renal disease on hemodialysis.[428]

The predictable pharmacology of rivaroxaban eliminates the need for routine laboratory monitoring of its anticoagulant effect. Baseline assessment of renal function is prudent to guide dose reduction when initiating therapy. In patients with chronic kidney disease or those at risk of acutely worsening renal function (e.g., patients treated with diuretics), periodic assessment of renal function is recommended.[429] Detection of anticoagulant activity may be desirable to guide clinical management in patients requiring urgent surgery or those with serious life-threatening bleeding (e.g., intracranial hemorrhage). This is best achieved through rivaroxaban-calibrated anti–factor Xa activity assays, although commercial assays are not widely available. LMWH-calibrated anti–factor Xa activity assays appear to correlate with rivaroxaban concentrations up to 500 ng/mL.[430] Most PT and aPTT assays are capable of detecting the anticoagulant activity of rivaroxaban at trough and peak levels, although assay sensitivity varies significantly between reagents, and some assays are insensitive to low levels of rivaroxaban.[431] Therefore, the PT and aPTT assays should not be used in scenarios where the presence of low levels of rivaroxaban would alter clinical management.

Rivaroxaban is approved for stroke and systemic embolism prophylaxis in patients with nonvalvular atrial fibrillation, acute VTE treatment, VTE prophylaxis following total hip or knee arthroplasty, and secondary prophylaxis in coronary artery disease and peripheral arterial disease.[428] Patients with mechanical heart valves should not receive rivaroxaban for thromboembolism prophylaxis.[427] Similarly, after transcatheter aortic-valve replacement (TAVR) rivaroxaban is associated with higher rates of thromboembolism and bleeding compared to antiplatelet agents in patients without an established indication for anticoagulation.[432]

Apixaban

Apixaban is a reversible, orally administered, direct factor Xa inhibitor that binds to and inactivates both fluid-phase and clot-bound factor Xa. Its oral bioavailability is ~50%, achieves peak levels 3 to 4 hours after an oral dose, has an elimination half-life of ~12 hours, and is mainly metabolized via CYP3A4. Renal excretion accounts for ~25% of drug clearance.[433] Similar to rivaroxaban, coadministration with potent inhibitors or inducers of CYP3A4 should be avoided.[433] When prescribed for nonvalvular atrial fibrillation, dose reduction is recommended when two or more of the following risk factors are present: age ≥80 years, weight ≤60 kg, or serum creatinine ≥1.5 mg/dL.[433]

Apixaban is FDA approved for use in patients with end-stage renal disease requiring hemodialysis.[433] Notably this approval was based on a small, open-label, single-dose pharmacokinetic study.[434] Several observational studies suggest apixaban use in patients with advanced kidney disease (e.g., CrCl <15) or requiring dialysis may be associated with improved clinical outcomes compared to warfarin, although high-quality studies are needed to confirm these results.[435-437]

As with rivaroxaban, the pharmacology of apixaban is predictable, and routine laboratory monitoring is unnecessary. In patients with nonvalvular atrial fibrillation, similar recommendations apply for initial and periodic assessment of renal function to guide dose reduction.[429] The anticoagulant activity measured via LMWH-calibrated anti–factor Xa activity assays appears to correlate linearly with apixaban serum concentrations.[430] PT assays demonstrate modest correlation to apixaban concentration, whereas aPTT assays are insensitive and unacceptable for apixaban detection.[430]

Apixaban is approved for the prevention of stroke and systemic embolism in patients with nonvalvular atrial fibrillation, acute VTE treatment, and the prevention of VTE in patients undergoing elective total hip or knee arthroplasty.[433] In patients with nonvalvular atrial fibrillation, apixaban is more effective and safer than warfarin.[438] Apixaban for acute VTE treatment is as effective as warfarin, associated with less bleeding, and does not require an initial course of parenteral anticoagulation.[439] After completing at least 6 months of VTE treatment, extended VTE prophylaxis with reduced dose apixaban (2.5 mg twice daily) appears to be safe and effective.[440] In patients undergoing total hip or knee arthroplasty, apixaban for VTE prophylaxis was more effective than enoxaparin (40 mg daily), with similar bleeding risk.[441,442] Compared to the North American dosing regimen of enoxaparin (30 mg twice daily) for total knee arthroplasty, apixaban was inferior.[443] Apixaban should not be used for thromboembolism prophylaxis in patients with mechanical heart valves.[427] Among patients undergoing TAVR, apixaban was not superior to antiplatelet therapy in patients without an indication for oral anticoagulation; whereas in patients with an indication for anticoagulation, apixaban use is favored over VKAs.[444]

Edoxaban

Edoxaban shares similar characteristics with rivaroxaban and apixaban. It is a reversible, orally administered, direct factor Xa inhibitor. Edoxaban has an oral bioavailability of ~62%, achieves peak levels 1 to 2 hours after an oral dose, has an elimination half-life of 10 to 14 hours, and is minimally metabolized via CYP3A4. Renal excretion accounts for ~50% of drug clearance with the remainder cleared through biliary and intestinal excretion.[445] Use with P-GP inducers (e.g., rifampin) should be avoided, whereas no dose adjustments are recommended for P-GP inhibitors.[445] Readers are referred to the prescribing information for specific dose adjustments depending on renal function, weight, and indication.[445]

Similar to other oral factor Xa inhibitors, edoxaban exerts a modest effect on PT and aPTT assays with a high degree of variability between reagents.[446] Anti–factor Xa activity assays calibrated for LMWH correlate linearly with edoxaban concentrations; commercial edoxaban calibrators are unavailable.[447]

Edoxaban is approved for the prevention of stroke and systemic embolism prophylaxis in patients with nonvalvular atrial fibrillation and acute VTE treatment. Details of edoxaban clinical trials will not be reviewed here, although two observations are noteworthy. First, edoxaban is less effective than warfarin for the prevention of stroke in patients with normal renal function. Hence, edoxaban should not be prescribed to patients with atrial fibrillation and a CrCl >95 mL/min.[445] Next, acute VTE treatment necessitates a 5- to 10-day course of parenteral anticoagulation prior to initiation of oral edoxaban, limiting the convenience compared to other oral factor Xa inhibitor regimens.[448]

Reversal of Direct Oral Anticoagulants

DOAC-associated major bleeding is defined as life-threatening, bleeding into a critical space or organ (e.g., intracranial, epidural, intraocular), or uncontrolled bleeding despite supportive measures. Administration of a reversal agent is suggested when DOAC-associated major bleeding is present, or when a DOAC-treated patient requires an invasive procedure that cannot be safely delayed performed in the presence of anticoagulation. Administration of a targeted reversal agent is suggested when available.[449] Targeted reversal of dabigatran is accomplished by idarucizumab, a monoclonal antibody fragment that rapidly and completely reverses the anticoagulant effect of dabigatran within minutes.[450] When idarucizumab is unavailable, activated PCC 50 units/kg is suggested. Andexanet-alfa is suggested for the targeted reversal of oral factor Xa inhibitors (e.g., rivaroxaban, apixaban). The dose of andexanet-alfa varies depending on the target agent to be reversed (rivaroxaban vs apixaban) and the time elapsed from the last dose. When andexanet-alfa is unavailable, four-factor PCC 2000 units is suggested instead.[449]

Special Populations

DOACs are simple, effective, and reliable forms of anticoagulation for most patients. However, special populations exist where DOACs may be ineffective or hazardous, relative to warfarin. Future studies should aim to clarify areas of clinical uncertainty.

Extremes of body weight may require DOAC dose adjustment. Dose reduction of apixaban and edoxaban is recommended in patients with a low body mass (<60 kg), depending on indication and other factors.[433,445] In morbidly obese patients (>120 kg or body mass index >40 kg/m^2), DOACs were previously discouraged unless drug-specific peak and trough levels were within expected ranges.[451] However, these concerns do not appear to be clinically significant based on meta-analyses of observational studies suggesting similar efficacy to warfarin, and possibly a lower risk of major bleeding in morbidly obese patients.[452,453]

DOACs should be used with caution, or avoided altogether, due to unpredictable bioavailability and/or clearance in patients with cirrhosis or intestinal malabsorption (e.g., gastric bypass surgery or small intestinal inflammatory bowel disease). Poorly adherent patients may benefit from warfarin use in place of a DOAC because of its longer duration of action and adherence reinforced through frequent monitoring. Lastly, in patients with triple positive antiphospholipid syndrome or surgically implanted devices requiring anticoagulation (e.g., left ventricular assist device or mechanical valve replacement), DOACs should be avoided.[454,455]

Thrombolytic Agents

The major reaction of the fibrinolytic system involves the conversion by plasminogen activators (PAs) of the inactive proenzyme, plasminogen, into the active enzyme, plasmin. Plasmin degrades fibrinogen, fibrin monomers, and cross-linked fibrin (as found in thrombi); fragments are collectively referred to as FDPs. These plasmin-mediated reactions generate many species of FDPs such as fragment X from fibrinogenolysis, and cross-linked FDPs such as (DD)E- and D-dimer from cross-linked fibrin.[456,457] Knowledge of these reactions is necessary to appreciate the mechanisms of action and limitations of commercial PAs.

A common feature of the management of all thromboembolic diseases is the desire to restore vascular patency in a timely manner to prevent loss of tissue, organ, or limb function, as well as life. Acute arterial thrombosis warrants an attempt at immediate thrombolysis, whereas venous thrombosis only warrants such intervention in extreme cases. Recognition of the importance of the endogenous fibrinolytic system in limiting the size of hemostatic thrombi, clearing hemostatic thrombi after vascular repair, and preventing pathologic thrombosis have resulted in the development of pharmacologic fibrinolytic (thrombolytic) agents to facilitate rapid restoration of vascular patency. Most thrombolytic agents are recombinant forms of physiologic PAs. The commercially available PAs differ with regard to plasma half-life, fibrin selectivity, primary clinical usage, infusion strategy, and immunogenicity. Currently available and investigational PAs and their key characteristics are summarized in *Table 56.12*.

Most thrombolytic agents are fashioned after endogenous t-PA or urokinase. Traditional thrombolytic drugs include bacteria-derived streptokinase (SK), anisoylated plasminogen SK activator complex, urokinase (two-chain u-PA), and recombinant t-PA (rt-PA). Newer molecules have been and are being developed to improve upon the traditional agents. Major goals of new thrombolytic agent development include increasing fibrin specificity, theoretically to reduce bleeding complications, prolonging initial plasma half-life to facilitate single- or double-bolus administration, reducing sensitivity to inactivation by PAI-1, and improving production efficiency. New thrombolytic agents include mutants of PAs, chimeric PAs, conjugates of PAs with monoclonal antibodies, and novel PAs from animal or bacterial origin.

Table 56.12. Properties of Currently Available and Investigational Thrombolytic Agents

Thrombolytic Agent	Molecular Weight (Da)	Plasma Half-Life (min)	Key Properties
Streptokinase	47,000	20 (drug) 90 (lytic effect)	Complexes with plasminogen to achieve activity
Anisoylated plasminogen streptokinase activator complex	131,000	40-90	Streptokinase and plasminogen complex
Urokinase	34,000/54,000	15	Direct plasminogen activator derived from fetal kidney cells
Recombinant urokinase	54,000	7	Recombinant high-molecular-weight urokinase
Recombinant prourokinase	49,000	7	Active after conversion to urokinase
Alteplase	65,000	4-8	A recombinant t-PA
Reteplase (recombinant plasminogen activator)	39,000	15	Truncated t-PA with an extended half-life
Tenecteplase	65,000	20 (initial) 90-130 (terminal)	A modified t-PA with an extended half-life, enhanced plasminogen activator inhibitor 1 resistance, and greater fibrin specificity
Desmoteplase (rDSPAα1)	52,000	2.8 h	Highly fibrin specific and lacking in neurotoxic effects of alteplase
Plasmin	85,000	—	Catheter-directed therapy

Abbreviation: t-PA, tissue-type plasminogen activator.

Non-PA thrombolytic agents that can degrade fibrin and/or fibrinogen directly (e.g., microplasmin, alfimeprase, and ancrod) are also under investigation.[458]

Streptokinase

SK is obtained from cultures of β-hemolytic streptococci. By itself, SK has no PA activity, but after combining with plasminogen, a complex is formed that is capable of activating other plasminogen molecules to plasmin.[459] Purified SK has a molecular weight of 47,000 Da. SK was the first clinically used thrombolytic agent. It is not fibrin selective in that its therapeutic use results in systemic fibrin(ogen)olysis and what is termed the *lytic state* from proteolysis of fibrinogen, factors V and VIII, and other plasma proteins.[459] Platelet function may also be perturbed because plasmin can proteolyze key platelet membrane receptors.[460] Generation of FDPs also contributes to the significant hemostatic defect of thrombolytic therapy. Although the lytic state predisposes patients to bleeding, the benefit of decreased blood viscosity that results from the lytic state may be clinically important. The half-life of SK is ~20 minutes. Because SK is a bacterial protein, it is antigenic, and allergic reactions occur in ~6% of patients. Anaphylaxis during SK use occurs in ~0.1% of patients.[461] Patients exposed to SK or those with previous streptococcal infections may acquire long-lasting antistreptococcal antibody levels sufficient to neutralize the activity of SK.[462] Therefore, all patients receiving SK should be monitored to ensure attainment of the lytic state. This can be done with the thrombin time assay. SK has been used primarily to treat VTE and MI. Although it is no longer commercially available in the United States, it remains the sole thrombolytic agent on the WHO's list of essential medicines.[463]

Urokinase-Type Plasminogen Activator

In the past, u-PA was obtained from human fetal kidney cell cultures. It is currently produced using nonhuman mammalian tissue cultures. Its molecular weight is 34,000 Da. u-PA is not fibrin selective, and this drug also produces a lytic state. The half-life of u-PA is ~15 minutes. u-PA is used to treat VTE, MI, and thrombolysis of clotted catheters. Urokinase is no longer commercially available.

Tissue-Type Plasminogen Activator

Currently, t-PA (alteplase) is produced by recombinant technology as a two-chain species, with a molecular weight of ~65,000 Da.[464,465] In vitro, t-PA is fibrin specific because of its high affinity for fibrin with which it forms a ternary complex with plasminogen. However, with t-PA dosage regimens currently being used, the lytic state is produced in vivo.[466] Consequently, bleeding complications with t-PA are similar to those with SK or u-PA.[467] The half-life of t-PA (~5 minutes) is much shorter than that of SK or u-PA. t-PA is used to treat acute massive PE, acute MI, acute ischemic stroke (within 4.5 hours of stroke onset), and central venous catheter occlusion.[467–473] Laboratory monitoring of t-PA therapy is usually not recommended.

Tissue-Type Plasminogen Activator Variants

r-PA (reteplase) is a nonglycosylated deletion mutant of wild-type human t-PA composed of only the kringle 2 and the protease domains of the parent molecule. Lack of the finger domain imparts lower fibrin-binding affinity.[474] Lack of glycosylation, a finger domain, and an epidermal growth factor domain extend the half-life to ~15 minutes. The longer half-life allows for a double-bolus administration 30 minutes apart, in the setting of acute MI. Reteplase is no longer available in the United States.

Tenecteplase (TNK) is a recombinant form of t-PA with two-point mutations in kringle 1 and a tetra-alanine substitution in the protease domain. These mutations render TNK more fibrin specific than t-PA, and extend the half-life to ~20 minutes. TNK is administered as a single, weight-based bolus for the treatment of acute MI and PE.[475,476]

Lanoteplase (nPA) is another recombinant form of t-PA that lacks the fibronectin fingerlike and epidermal growth factor domains, thus prolonging the half-life to ~37 minutes.[477] nPA is less fibrin specific relative to t-PA. When administered as a single weight-based bolus for acute MI, the safety and efficacy of nPA appear comparable to those of t-PA.[477]

Other Plasminogen Activators

Recombinant glycosylated prourokinase (single-chain u-PA) has a greater stability than recombinant nonglycosylated prourokinase and has been evaluated for catheter-directed, intra-arterial treatment of stroke.[478] Staphylokinase is produced by *Staphylococcus aureus*. It appears to have substantial thrombolytic activity, but it may also be immunogenic.[479] Vampire bat (*Desmodus rotundus*) salivary PA (rDSPAα1, desmoteplase) possesses >72% primary structure homology to human t-PA but lacks a kringle 2 domain,[480] which may impart greater fibrin specificity. Finally, although not a PA, plasmin therapy has been investigated in arterial vascular disease.[458]

Thrombolytic Therapy–Associated Bleeding

Bleeding is the most common complication associated with thrombolytic therapy, regardless of the agent. The bleeding stems from plasmin's inability to distinguish between hemostatic and pathologic thrombi. This complication can range from minor bleeding at an intravenous infusion site to life-threatening hemorrhage.[481] Symptomatic intracranial hemorrhage is a relatively uncommon but serious complication of thrombolytic therapy occurring in ~2% to 6% of patients.[470,482]

The factors that increase the risk for bleeding during thrombolytic therapy are not fully understood. Several demographic, physiologic, and clinical factors are associated with an increased risk of bleeding, including age >75 years, female sex, low body mass (e.g., <65 kg), systolic blood pressure >160 mm Hg, diastolic blood pressure >100 mm Hg, recent or active bleeding, recent surgery or trauma, prior intracranial hemorrhage, structural intracranial disease, recent ischemic stroke, anticoagulation, and traumatic cardiopulmonary resuscitation.[470,483] It is also possible that the dose administered and intrinsic properties of the thrombolytic agent also contribute to bleeding complications.[484]

Thrombolytic Fibrin Specificity and Hemorrhagic Risk

Thrombolytic agents can be characterized along a variety of dimensions, but one that is often mentioned is fibrin specificity.[485] The ability of a thrombolytic agent (PA) to distinguish between plasminogen in the general circulation and plasminogen bound to fibrin surfaces dictates its fibrin specificity. Activation of fibrin-bound plasminogen results in the generation of fibrin-bound plasmin that is protected from inactivation by α_2-antiplasmin. Bound plasmin generates soluble FDPs; circulating plasmin degrades fibrinogen into FDPs. Fibrin specificity differs from fibrin affinity, which is a measure of how avidly a given agent binds to fibrin, but not its specificity for this molecule.[485] At present, there is little evidence to support the view that differences in fibrin affinity among PAs are significantly correlated with either the efficacy or the safety of these preparations.[486] High fibrin specificity is thought to be associated with lower risk for hemorrhagic complications in patients undergoing thrombolytic therapy because of the belief that plasmin generated on the fibrin surface of a thrombus restricts its activity only to that surface. This view is not universally supported by available data from large-scale clinical trials.

A relationship between high fibrin specificity and reduced bleeding risk has been demonstrated.[476] The results of the Assessment of the Safety and Efficacy of a New Thrombolytic-2 trial, which included 16,949 patients with acute MI, showed that the use of the highly fibrin-specific thrombolytic agent TNK, compared with alteplase, was associated with a significantly lower risk for major noncerebral bleeding.[486] This lower rate of bleeding complications was correlated with a significant reduction in the need for blood transfusions. Intracranial bleeding rates were comparable with the two agents.

Results from other large-scale studies support the opposing view that high fibrin specificity may actually be associated with increased risk for intracranial bleeding. For example, the Global Utilization of Streptokinase and Tissue Plasminogen Activator for Occluded

Coronary Arteries trial showed that the risk of intracranial bleeding was slightly higher in patients who received alteplase compared to SK.[487] Findings from another large-scale comparison of SK with alteplase for acute MI showed a significantly higher risk of stroke in patients who received alteplase, the more fibrin-specific agent.[476] Additionally, the hemorrhagic stroke risk was increased nearly 1.5-fold with alteplase relative to SK use.

There are several potential explanations for the association between high fibrin specificity and increased intracranial bleeding. These include the inability of fibrin-specific agents to distinguish between pathologic thrombi and hemostatic thrombi, and the possibility that treatment with fibrin-specific agents resulted in greater degradation of hemostatic fibrinogen and other circulating coagulation factors. Fibrin-specific therapy may result in increased production and accumulation of fragment X, enhancing the bleeding risk.[488] Lastly, instead of fibrin specificity or affinity, observed differences in intracranial bleeding may be attributable to different PA doses used in clinical trials.[489]

VENOUS THROMBOEMBOLIC DISEASE

VTE, encompassing both DVT and PE, is a common disease that carries a substantial risk of morbidity and mortality, is associated with high health care costs, and for many patients can be prevented. The age- and sex-adjusted annual incidence of VTE is estimated to be ~1.17 per 1000 persons.[490] Applying this figure to current population estimates, as many as 900,000 VTE cases occur annually in the United States alone. This number may underestimate the actual incidence because up to 50% of DVT and PE are asymptomatic or undetected.[2]

The major clinical consequences of extremity DVT include the PTS, which manifests as chronic swelling, stasis dermatitis, stasis ulceration, and venous claudication: all secondary to venous insufficiency, and PE. Major clinical consequences of PE include acute lung infarction, chronic dyspnea, chronic thromboembolic pulmonary hypertension, and death. DVT restricted to the calf veins uncommonly results in clinically important PE and is rarely associated with a fatal outcome. In contrast, inadequately treated DVT involving the popliteal or more proximal leg veins is associated with a 20% to 50% risk of clinically relevant recurrence and is strongly associated with both symptomatic and fatal PE.[491,492] In untreated patients, death from PE occurs most frequently within 24 to 48 hours of initial presentation. All-cause mortality rates in treated patients with PE are as high as 11% at 2 weeks and 17% at 3 months.[2] Even small PE in patients with emphysema, cardiac disease, or lung involvement with malignancy may result in death. Any VTE in a patient with a contraindication to anticoagulation presents a therapeutic challenge and greater likelihood of adverse outcome.

Management of Venous Thromboembolism

The treatment of patients with VTE traditionally consists of an initial treatment phase (first 5-7 days) wherein a therapeutically dosed parenteral anticoagulant (e.g., heparin or LMWH) and simultaneous initiation of long-term therapy (e.g., VKA), followed by a long-term treatment phase (from 5-7 days to 3 months) where the parenteral anticoagulant is discontinued and VKA therapy is continued, followed by an extended treatment phase (3 months to indefinite) where there is a decision to continue treatment or not.[493-495] The introduction of DOACs into the clinical landscape has greatly simplified VTE treatment, where some regimens eliminate the need for parenteral anticoagulation.[438,496,497]

Initial Treatment of Venous Thromboembolism

The mainstay of pharmacologic therapy for VTE is anticoagulation. A delay in achieving therapeutic anticoagulant intensity may negatively impact a patient's long-term VTE recurrence rate.[495,498] DOACs have largely replaced VKAs for VTE treatment based on the predictable pharmacology, fixed dosing regimens, few drug-drug and drug-food interactions, lack of obligatory lab monitoring, and generally favorable safety profile.[499] Two DOACs (rivaroxaban and apixaban) were compared to standard VTE treatment regimens (e.g., LMWH and warfarin) utilizing a novel approach to initial VTE therapy, the omission of parenteral anticoagulation. The EINSTEIN trial's high dose of rivaroxaban (15 mg twice daily) was administered for the first 21 days of VTE therapy, in place of parenteral anticoagulation, followed by rivaroxaban 20 mg daily.[500,501] Similarly, in the AMPLIFY trial, a high dose of apixaban (10 mg twice daily) was used for the first 7 days, followed by apixaban 5 mg twice daily.[440] This convenient approach proved safe and effective for these two agents, and appears to increase patient satisfaction.[502] Monotherapy has not been studied with other available DOACs. Dabigatran and edoxaban both require an initial 5- to 10-day course of parenteral anticoagulation for VTE treatment.[423,448] In patients who are ineligible for DOAC-based VTE treatment, VKA-based therapy should be used unless a contraindication exists. VKAs have a delayed onset of action; therefore a rapid-onset parenteral anticoagulant (e.g., heparin) must be initiated in patients with acute VTE during VKA initiation.[503] As long as warfarin is dosed to a therapeutic level, overlap therapy with heparins can be minimized to 5 days.[328,504,505]

UFH is the preferred initial parenteral anticoagulant for a minority of patients with an acute VTE, such as those with end-stage renal disease or recent major bleeding. When UFH is used, weight-based dosing (80 U/kg bolus followed by 18 U/kg/h infusion) with subsequent dose adjustments based on a standardized nomogram (Table 56.5) facilitates achieving a target aPTT.[506] The use of a published nomogram expedites the achievement of target intensity anticoagulation. Adjusted-dose subcutaneous UFH, intermittent intravenous UFH boluses, and fixed dose subcutaneous heparin have also been used effectively in the treatment of VTE.[493,507,508] The therapeutic intensity of UFH is monitored using either the aPTT or anti–factor Xa activity assays. An aPTT therapeutic range that correlates with an anti–factor Xa activity level of 0.3 to 0.7 U/mL is preferred.[343] The aPTT or anti–factor Xa activity should be checked every 6 hours until they surpass the lower limit of the therapeutic range.

When a heparin-based anticoagulant is chosen for the initial treatment of VTE, weight-based subcutaneous LMWH is recommended over UFH for most patients.[485] Numerous comparative trials and meta-analyses have demonstrated that LMWH is more effective and safer than adjusted-dose UFH for the initial treatment of VTE.[509] Thrombotic complications occurred less often (OR 0.70; 95% CI, 0.57-0.85), thrombus size was reduced (OR 0.69; 95% CI, 0.59-0.81), major bleeding was lower (OR 0.58; 95% CI, 0.40-0.83), and fewer patients died (OR 0.77; 95% CI, 0.63-0.93) when treated with LMWH compared to UFH.[509] Enoxaparin sodium can be dosed at 1.0 mg/kg body weight every 12 hours or 1.5 mg/kg once daily, although VTE treatment guidelines prefer the higher dose utilized with twice-daily administration.[485,510] Tinzaparin is dosed at 175 U/kg once daily.[485] Dalteparin is dosed at 200 U/kg once daily, with clinical practice guidelines suggesting against dose cap (i.e., 18,000 U) in obese patients.[511] Fondaparinux is an effective and safe alternative to LMWH and is also recommended over UFH for initial VTE treatment.[485,510]

When VKA-based treatment is selected, efficient initial dosing of VKA therapy in patients with VTE minimizes excessive duration (i.e., beyond 5-7 days) of potentially costly parenteral anticoagulants and may shorten hospitalizations. The use of standardized warfarin initiation dosing nomograms has been shown to be efficient and safe.[396,510,512] In two separate studies of predominantly inpatients, dosing nomograms using a 5-mg initial dose was compared to 10 mg and shown to be effective in achieving a therapeutic INR within 5 days with less risk of excessive anticoagulation.[396,510] Among outpatients, a 10-mg initial VKA dose nomogram had a greater percentage of patients achieving a therapeutic INR by day 5 with no difference in excessive anticoagulation or adverse events compared to a lower initial dose.[512] Lower initial doses (e.g., 5 mg or less) may be most appropriate for those patients who are elderly, have low body weight, are on interacting medications, or have poor nutrition.

Historically, the initial treatment of VTE was confined to the inpatient setting; however, several clinical trials have demonstrated outpatient DVT treatment is safe, effective, and less costly.[513-515] Initial

DVT treatment is recommended to occur in the outpatient setting, assuming the home environment is suitable, the patient has adequate caregiver support and the ability to return to the hospital promptly, comorbidities are stable, and symptoms are controlled.[485] The approach to patients presenting with acute PE should be more cautious. Unlike patients with acute DVT, patients with acute PE represent a heterogeneous risk group with 3-month mortality rates ranging from 1.4% to 17.4%.[2,516] Carefully selected, low-risk patients can be safely managed in the outpatient setting.[517,518] Utilizing a validated risk-stratification tool such as the PE severity index, combined with an assessment of the patient's comorbid illnesses and social support system, is recommended to identify low-risk patients eligible for outpatient PE therapy.[485,517]

Initial Treatment Considerations in Special Populations With Venous Thromboembolism

In occasional patients with thrombosis, the aPTT assay may not be a reliable method to monitor UFH therapy, for example, patients with the lupus anticoagulant and a prolonged baseline aPTT. In these patients, an alternative strategy for monitoring UFH is to use an anti–factor Xa activity assay. In this scenario, the targeted therapeutic range is 0.3 to 0.7 U/mL. Alternatively, these patients could receive LMWH or fondaparinux, with the dosage determined solely by body weight without laboratory monitoring of the anticoagulant activity.[511] Patients with marked elevation in factor VIII or fibrinogen levels may also be more reliably anticoagulated using LMWH.[346,348]

Obese patients are underrepresented in VTE treatment trials and that has led to uncertainty about optimal LMWH dosing in these patients.[23,351] Studies evaluating drug activity with the use of anti–factor Xa activity levels suggest that the pharmacodynamics of LMWHs in obese patients (weighing up to 190 kg) are similar to nonobese patients.[351,519,520] Consequently, weight-based dosing (using total body weight) in obese patients without dose capping and without anti–factor Xa activity monitoring is suggested.[343,351,511] However, owing to limited published experience, anti–factor Xa activity monitoring with subsequent dose adjustment should be considered in patients at extreme weights, such as those over 190 kg in whom LMWH is used.[351]

Renal insufficiency (CrCl <30 mL/min) is associated with worse outcomes, including fatal bleeding, in patients with VTE.[521] LMWHs have a significant degree of renal clearance, and drug accumulation occurs in patients with a CrCl <30 mL/min.[343] Unadjusted LMWH therapy is associated with more bleeding (OR 2.25, 95% CI 1.19-4.27) in patients with CrCl <30 mL/min compared to those without renal impairment.[522] Because of potentially worse outcomes with LMWHs in patients with significant renal impairment, weight-based adjusted-dose UFH is recommended over LMWH for VTE treatment in these patients.[23,343,351] DOAC-based monotherapy with apixaban may be a reasonable VTE treatment strategy in patients with severe renal insufficiency (i.e., CrCl <15 or requiring hemodialysis), although prospective studies are needed to validate this approach.[436]

Extended Treatment of Venous Thromboembolism

The optimal duration of anticoagulation should be determined for each patient. Patients with a provoked VTE attributable to a reversible or transient risk factor, such as recent surgery, immobilization, trauma, or pregnancy, should be anticoagulated for ~3 months as long as the provoking risk factor has resolved.[328] Patients with unprovoked VTE or ongoing major risk factors, such as malignancy or triple-positive antiphospholipid antibody syndrome, require indefinite therapy as long as the bleeding risk does not outweigh the benefit of anticoagulant therapy.[328,523] In general, patients with an unprovoked VTE have a risk of recurrence of ~10% to 15% during the first year after stopping anticoagulation. This risk remains elevated with a ~5% to 7.5% annual risk of recurrence thereafter.[485] Continuation of anticoagulation beyond 3 months (e.g., 6 or 12 months) reduces this risk as long as the patient remains on anticoagulation, but the heightened long-term recurrence risk remains unchanged once anticoagulation is discontinued. For these reasons, guidelines recommend extended therapy (i.e., beyond initial 3 months) for patients with unprovoked VTE as long as the bleeding risk is not high.[328]

D-dimer has been proposed as a method to differentiate between patients whose anticoagulation can be safely discontinued and those who require indefinite anticoagulation for unprovoked VTE. Early studies demonstrated an increased risk of VTE recurrence among patients who had a persistently elevated D-dimer after stopping anticoagulation, compared to those with a normal D-dimer.[282,524] Follow-up studies in patients with unprovoked VTE (treated for at least 3 months) and two negative D-dimers (one prior to stopping anticoagulation and another 1 month after stopping anticoagulation) failed to consistently identify patients with a risk of VTE recurrence sufficiently low enough to recommend stopping anticoagulation.[282] Men appeared to have a higher risk of recurrence compared to women, despite similarly normal D-dimer results.[282] Based on the available evidence, D-dimer does not appear to be a reliable enough method to guide safe anticoagulation discontinuation for patients with an unprovoked VTE.

Guidelines for the duration of anticoagulant therapy are suggested in Table 56.13.

The intensity of oral anticoagulation has been the subject of controversy for patients assigned to extended VTE treatment, with aims to minimize the risks of bleeding and VTE recurrence. Following an initial course of full-dose DOAC therapy, dose-reduced DOAC therapy appears to be as effective as full-dose therapy, while also having a lower risk of major bleeding.[525] For VKA-based therapy, a consensus group concluded that low-intensity oral anticoagulation (INR 1.5-2.0) was less effective and no safer than standard intensity therapy (INR 2.0-3.0).[526]

All patients prescribed warfarin should be educated to maintain a stable diet. Patients are encouraged to consume a constant intake of dietary vitamin K, avoiding large variations in their diet. Because of the numerous drug-drug interactions that exist between warfarin and other drugs (Table 56.8), patients should be instructed to inform their physician of the addition or withdrawal of any medication during warfarin therapy. In addition, patients should be encouraged to avoid over-the-counter vitamin supplements or herbal preparations containing vitamin K or vitamin K analogs and those known to influence warfarin (e.g., ginkgo biloba).

The risk of anticoagulation-related bleeding should be explained to all patients. It is strongly recommended that patients avoid high-risk activities, such as contact sports, and the use of appropriate protective equipment (e.g., bicycle helmets) should be emphasized. Patients should be instructed to seek medical attention for severe bleeding or bleeding that is not controlled after 10 to 15 minutes of continuous compression. Patients should be instructed to wear a medical identification bracelet or necklace, and carry a wallet card, that identifies their use of an anticoagulant. Patient education is best provided by specialists that focus on anticoagulation management. Studies suggest that anticoagulation management services offer better control of VKA-based anticoagulation.[527] In carefully selected patients treated with

Table 56.13. Duration of Anticoagulation in Venous Thromboembolic Disease

Disease	Duration
Provoked DVT or PE (transient/reversible risk factors)	3 mo
Initial unprovoked DVT or PE	3 mo (high bleeding risk) Indefinite (low-to-moderate bleeding risk)
Recurrent unprovoked DVT or PE	Indefinite
DVT with ongoing risk factors[a]	Long-term/indefinite
Calf vein DVT	3 mo

Abbreviations: DVT, deep venous thrombosis; PE, pulmonary embolism.
[a]For example, malignancy, triple-positive antiphospholipid antibody syndrome, high-risk thrombophilia.

VKAs, PST and PSM may reduce thromboembolic events and mortality, without an increase in major bleeding.[528,529] Whether PST and PSM are cost-effective strategies for warfarin management remains undetermined.[401]

In select cases, LMWH may be used in lieu of oral anticoagulants for extended treatment. Because of its teratogenic effects, warfarin therapy is contraindicated in pregnancy, so long-term heparin or LMWH is prudent for pregnant patients; LMWH is preferred in pregnancy because osteopenia occurs less often with LMWH than with UFH.[530] The safety of DOACs during pregnancy remains unclear and should generally be avoided.[531] Patients with variable oral intake, episodic vomiting, malabsorption, and difficulty in regulating INR may be better served by extended LMWH therapy. Additionally, in patients who experience a recurrent VTE while on VKA or DOAC therapy, LMWH should be initiated and continued for at least 1 month in place of the non-LMWH agent.[328,532] A few patients may even experience a recurrent VTE while receiving therapeutic doses of LMWH, a situation that warrants escalation of the LMWH dose by ~25% to 33%.[328,532]

Patients with cancer are more likely to develop VTE compared to patients without cancer, and experience higher rates of major bleeding and VTE recurrence during anticoagulation therapy; findings that are not explained by anticoagulant intensity.[533] Several clinical trials have compared dose-adjusted VKA therapy to LMWH for extended treatment of VTE, demonstrating significant reductions in recurrent VTE without an increased risk of bleeding.[534,535] A meta-analysis of seven randomized controlled trials concluded that LMWH significantly reduces the risk of recurrent VTE (hazard ratio 0.47; 95% CI, 0.32-0.71), without significant differences in mortality or bleeding.[536] DOAC therapy for cancer-associated VTE is at least as effective as LMWH.[537,538] Major bleeding and clinically relevant nonmajor bleeding may be increased with rivaroxaban and edoxaban, whereas apixaban does not appear to be associated with increased major bleeding.[537] Based on these findings, extended therapy with LMWH or a DOAC is recommended over VKA therapy in patients with cancer-associated VTE.[539]

Isolated Distal Deep Venous Thrombosis of the Leg

Many clinicians perceive an isolated distal DVT of the leg (i.e., DVT involving only calf veins) is of limited clinical significance. This misunderstanding and underappreciation of the potential morbidity and mortality associated with isolated distal DVT have resulted in a lack of clear consensus on the optimal management strategy of this condition. Isolated distal DVT may account for as few as 6.2% of all symptomatic acute DVT and as many as 43.0% of all acute VTE.[540] Although distal DVT and proximal DVT may be considered separate conditions at their outset, ~15% of distal DVT propagate into the proximal veins within 2 to 3 weeks wherein a risk of embolism ensues.[328,541,542] Such proximal extension renders what was initially a distal DVT just as dangerous as a proximal DVT.

The primary goal of proximal DVT treatment is the prevention of DVT recurrence and PE, whereas the goals of distal DVT treatment are to treat severe symptoms and to prevent proximal extension. Current treatment approaches for isolated distal DVT are to implement either anticoagulant therapy or serial duplex ultrasound surveillance. Surveillance typically consists of repeat ultrasound imaging at 1 and 2 weeks (or sooner if concerning symptoms) after the initial ultrasound study, the usual time frame for proximal extension. Limitations of serial imaging include cost, compliance, and inconvenience associated with multiple return visits. Anticoagulant therapy confers similar limitations of cost and inconvenience and introduces the risk of bleeding. Anticoagulation is suggested for patients with a low bleeding risk who have severe symptoms or risk factors for proximal extension (thrombus length >5 cm, involves multiple calf veins, thrombus is close to proximal veins, and ongoing underlying risk factors, such as immobility or cancer, history of VTE).[328] When anticoagulant therapy is initiated for isolated distal DVT of the leg, the approach and intensity should be the same as that for proximal DVT. The recommended treatment duration is 3 months, irrespective of the presence or absence of provoking factors.[328] Consideration should also be given to individual patient preferences. Some patients may wish to avoid anticoagulant therapy because of the associated bleeding risk, opting for serial imaging, whereas others may opt for anticoagulant therapy because of unacceptable fear of thrombus extension during the surveillance period.

Isolated Subsegmental Pulmonary Embolism

The introduction of multidetector computed tomography (CT) scanners in 1998 has been associated with an increase in the PE detection rate.[543] In spite of a near doubling of the PE incidence (62.1-112.3 per 100,000 US adults), the number of PE-related deaths remained unchanged (12.3-11.9 per 100,000), whereas the case fatality rate decreased by approximately one-third (12.1%-7.8%).[543,544] These findings imply that more clinically insignificant PE is being detected because the effectiveness of anticoagulant therapy has not changed. In fact, the small pulmonary artery filling defects noted on CT imaging may represent false-positive findings instead of true PE[545]; or they may represent a normal physiologic process wherein the lungs capture small thrombi, preventing more serious systemic embolization, previously unidentified by less sensitive imaging techniques (e.g., nuclear medicine ventilation-perfusion scan).[543]

Clinical practice guidelines suggest withholding anticoagulation is reasonable in patients with good cardiopulmonary reserve, without ongoing VTE risk factors (e.g., active cancer, prior VTE), and provided that DVT has been excluded with bilateral lower extremity duplex ultrasounds. Upper extremity evaluation is also necessary if a central venous catheter is present.[328] However, these recommendations were based on observational studies with conflicting risk estimates.[546-548] More recently, a well-designed randomized trial reported the risk of recurrent VTE was higher than anticipated (3.1%) during the 90-day follow-up period.[549] This observation may impact anticoagulation strategies for isolated subsegmental PE in future guidelines.

Advanced Therapies for Venous Thromboembolism
Vena Caval Filter

Patients with an acute VTE and active bleeding or a contraindication to anticoagulation may require placement of an inferior vena cava (IVC) filter.[550] Relative contraindications to anticoagulation are listed in *Table 56.14*. It is important to note that active bleeding may be a treatable and transient contraindication to anticoagulation. Recurrent VTE while on therapeutic anticoagulation is no longer considered an indication for IVC filter placement.[550] Addressing factors associated with anticoagulation failure (e.g., nonadherence, poor TTR, underdosing) is important prior to IVC filter placement. In patients with IVC filters placed because of bleeding, appropriate anticoagulation should begin after the bleeding source has been adequately treated or sufficient time has elapsed to allow healing at the bleeding site (e.g., peptic ulcer). An IVC filter should not be viewed as an equivalent substitute to anticoagulation in the setting of acute VTE and is certainly not an "insurance policy" against subsequent PE. In fact, IVC filter placement does not further reduce the risk of recurrent PE when combined with anticoagulation therapy.[551]

Table 56.14. Relative Contraindications to Anticoagulation Therapy

Bacterial endocarditis
Recent organ biopsy or noncompressible arterial intervention site
Recent gastrointestinal or genitourinary bleeding (<10 d)
Thrombocytopenia or marked anemia
History of a bleeding disorder
History of spontaneous intracranial, spinal, or ocular bleeding
Recent (<2 wk) history of major surgery, stroke, or trauma
Hepatic insufficiency

Their use has been associated with an increased risk of recurrent DVT, reduced PE, little to no difference in overall mortality, and low rates of filter retrieval.[552-555] Placement and subsequent removal of a temporary (or retrievable) IVC filter once the contraindication to anticoagulation has passed is ideal because severe complications, such as IVC occlusion, visceral perforation, and myocardial perforation, from filter embolization have been reported.[556-558] Guidelines regarding appropriate use of IVC filters have been published.[550]

Catheter-Directed Thrombolysis of Deep Venous Thrombosis

Catheter-directed thrombolytic therapy is usually reserved for patients with extensive DVT involving the IVC or iliac veins and for patients who have signs and symptoms of actual or impending phlegmasia cerulea dolens.[559-564] An initial venogram is performed via a distal vessel, usually a popliteal or foot vein, to delineate fully the extent of the DVT. Placement of a vascular access sheath is best accomplished via the popliteal vein, typically using ultrasound guidance to assure nontraumatic, single-puncture catheter placement. A multiple side hole or ultrasound-assisted catheter is advanced and embedded within the thrombus.[565] Thrombolytic agent is infused through this catheter. At a minimum, low-dose heparin (500 U/h) should be infused through the sheath to prevent sheath thrombosis. Periodic surveillance with venography should be performed to assess resolution of the DVT. As lysis is achieved, the infusion catheter may require repositioning to maintain infusion within the thrombus.[560]

Thrombolytic therapy for DVT carries the same contraindications as for thrombolysis of PE. Active bleeding is an absolute contraindication to the procedure; relative contraindications include those for any anticoagulant. In addition, a history of contrast allergy or renal insufficiency is a relative contraindication to the procedure. The major complication associated with the use of thrombolytic agents is bleeding, with access site bleeding occurring most often. Bleeding in the popliteal space may be particularly significant because the popliteal vein is poorly compressible. Additional complications, such as intracranial bleeding, are also seen with DVT thrombolysis. PE, potentially fatal, has been reported in patients undergoing DVT thrombolytic therapy, leading some proceduralists to place an IVC filter prior to catheter-directed thrombolysis.[550]

After the completion of thrombolytic therapy, patients should be anticoagulated with an appropriate parenteral agent (UFH, LMWH, or DTI) and converted to warfarin or a DOAC in the usual manner. Patients who have a contraindication to pharmacologic thrombolysis may be able to derive some benefit from mechanical thrombectomy performed at the time of venography/intervention. However, mechanical thrombectomy should not be attempted in patients with a contraindication to anticoagulation because any benefit from suction thrombectomy would likely be lost without maintenance of therapeutic anticoagulation.

The purported benefits of DVT thrombolysis include the ability to subsequently diagnose and treat any underlying venous stenosis, venous compression (as in May-Thurner syndrome), or venous webs that may be discovered after thrombolysis.[561,562] The use of angioplasty or stent placement or both may improve outcomes in these patients.[563] The combined use of localized pharmacomechanical intervention has been suggested to reduce subsequent PTS occurrence but increased overall bleeding.[566,567] These findings are important because the primary goal of catheter-based interventions for the management of DVT is to reduce the subsequent occurrence of PTS, which develops in ~20% to 50% of patients with symptomatic DVT.[568] Pain, swelling, edema, pigmentation changes, and skin ulcers may occur. PTS results from damage to venous valves by thrombotic material, leading to valvular incompetence and venous reflux.[568] The management of PTS involves the administration of high-quality anticoagulation for acute DVT treatment and secondary prophylaxis. The use of graduated elastic compression stockings does not prevent PTS, but may alleviate associated symptoms.[568] The role of catheter-directed thrombolysis for the treatment of proximal DVT (i.e., ileofemoral) and prevention of PTS remains controversial. Results from the Acute Venous Thrombosis: Thrombus Removal with Adjunctive Catheter-Directed Thrombolysis (ATTRACT) trial, a randomized trial of pharmacomechanical catheter-directed thrombolysis vs anticoagulation alone, resulted in a higher risk of bleeding and did not significantly lower the risk of PTS after 24 months of follow-up.[569] Current guidelines do not recommend the routine use of thrombolytic therapy.[328,526]

Thrombolysis for Pulmonary Embolism

The majority of patients with symptomatic PE should be treated solely with anticoagulation. Select patients with PE may benefit from thrombolytic therapy to actively degrade the thrombus obstructing the pulmonary vasculature. When compared to anticoagulation alone, thrombolytic therapy results in more rapid thrombus lysis, early improvement in pulmonary blood flow, and improvement of right ventricular function.[570] Systemic thrombolytic therapy has also been demonstrated to improve survival in patients with high-risk or massive PE and is recommended in these patients.[328,571,572] However, these improvements in cardiopulmonary function have not resulted in decreased mortality in patients without significant hemodynamic compromise. Among patients with intermediate-risk PE, defined as right ventricular dysfunction identified on imaging (echocardiogram or CT pulmonary angiography) combined with myocardial injury (elevated troponin), thrombolytic therapy did not reduce early (within 7 days) or late mortality (within 30 days).[475] Furthermore, long-term mortality, residual dyspnea, and right ventricular dysfunction were not reduced after a median follow-up of 38 months.[573] The routine use of thrombolytic therapy is not recommended for patients with intermediate- or low-risk PE, unless they have a low risk of bleeding and develop signs of significant hypotension (systolic blood pressure <90 mm Hg) or clinical instability after initial presentation.[328,526,571]

Catheter-assisted thrombolysis is an alternative method for the treatment of high-risk PE and is particularly useful in patients with a high bleeding risk. Catheter-based therapy facilitates the delivery of a high concentration of the thrombolytic agent directly into the obstructing thrombus, and can be combined with thrombus aspiration or mechanical thrombus fragmentation.[571] This approach uses a lower total dose of the thrombolytic agent and achieves hemodynamic improvements similar to systemic thrombolysis, without a high risk of bleeding.[574,575]

Thrombolytic therapy is contraindicated in patients with active bleeding, prior intracranial hemorrhage, recent ischemic stroke (within 3 months), recent brain or spinal surgery, recent traumatic brain injury or cranial fracture, and known bleeding diathesis.[571] Other relative contraindications include recent organ biopsy or arterial puncture in a noncompressible site, recent traumatic cardiopulmonary resuscitation, uncontrolled hypertension, pregnancy, recent surgery, pericarditis, advanced age (>75 years), recent bleeding episode, and current anticoagulation use (e.g., warfarin or DOAC). For all patients, the potential benefits of lysis must be weighed heavily against the potential risks of bleeding.

Major hemorrhage rates have varied between 4% and 22% in studies at the currently recommended doses. Intracranial hemorrhage rates vary between 1% and 3%, approximately one-half of which are fatal.[571,576] Heparin generally should not be administered concomitantly with thrombolytic agents. An aPTT should be determined at the completion of the lysis; if the aPTT is ≤2.5 times the control, then heparin infusion should be started/resumed. If the aPTT is >2.5 times the control, the aPTT should be repeated every 4 hours; once it decreases into an acceptable range, the heparin infusion may be initiated. If a complication of therapy occurs, the lytic agent and any other anticoagulants should be held. Fresh-frozen plasma or PCCs and cryoprecipitate may be used to replete fibrinogen and clotting factors. Consideration should be given to the use of antifibrinolytic agents to reverse excessive fibrinolysis.[577]

PREVENTION OF VENOUS THROMBOEMBOLIC DISEASE

If clinicians focused more on VTE prophylaxis, much less time would be needed to emphasize methods for VTE diagnosis and treatment. Fatal PE is considered to be one of the most common preventable causes of hospital death.[578] Because the clinical diagnosis of VTE is unreliable and serial surveillance of all high-risk patients is expensive, widespread use of anticoagulants (or other prophylactic measures) has been recommended and is the subject of comprehensive practice guidelines by multiple professional societies.[302,579-581]

Optimal delivery of thromboprophylaxis requires an assessment of risk vs benefit, and this is particularly relevant to medically ill patients wherein the absolute risk of clinically relevant VTE may be less than in patients undergoing major surgical procedures. There is an abundance of literature supporting the benefits of thromboprophylaxis in surgical patients, but the absolute clinical impact in nonsurgical patients is less certain. This is highlighted in a meta-analysis of medically ill patients; those who received pharmacologic prophylaxis had reduced incidence of symptomatic PE (number needed to treat 306), but increased bleeding events (number needed to harm 296 for major bleeding), and no reduction in total mortality.[582] Risk assessment, however, is imperfect and can be viewed as group risk (e.g., all orthopedic patients) or individualized risk (e.g., based upon individual patient characteristics). *Figure 56.9* illustrates several VTE risk assessment models that have been validated.[583-585] It is important to note that not all patients at risk develop a thrombosis, and not all thromboses result in symptoms, morbidity, or death. The benefit of pharmacologic thromboprophylaxis must always be weighed against the bleeding risk. Patients at high risk of bleeding should still receive prophylaxis in the form of an intermittent pneumatic compression device or thromboembolism-deterrence stockings or both. Furthermore, prophylaxis strategies must consider whether a patient has a history of HIT. *Figure 56.10* illustrates a general approach to thromboprophylaxis, and *Table 56.14* lists relative contraindications to anticoagulant therapy.

The duration of thromboprophylaxis has also received attention. In general, extended prophylaxis (i.e., up to 4 weeks) has been suggested for patients undergoing elective hip arthroplasty, hip fracture repair, and high-risk abdominal-pelvic cancer surgery. Extending prophylaxis in medically ill patients after hospitalization, however, has not been shown to be effective and is associated with increased bleeding.[586,587] In contrast, routine thromboprophylaxis is recommended for selected high-risk ambulatory patients with cancer (Khorana score ≥2)[588] and those receiving thalidomide- or lenalidomide-based treatment for multiple myeloma.[539]

HEPARIN-INDUCED THROMBOCYTOPENIA

Although bleeding is the most common adverse event associated with heparin and LMWH therapy, HIT, also known as the *white clot syndrome*, is recognized as a potentially severe, albeit paradoxic, immune-mediated complication of heparin therapy.[589,590] HIT is a "clinical-pathologic" syndrome, meaning that the diagnosis is based on compatible clinical features as well as laboratory assay results positive for heparin-dependent antibodies. In vivo platelet activation results in the release of platelet factor-4 (PF4), a tetrameric platelet α-granule constituent, into blood where it may also bind to the external platelet surface. Heparin is a chain of negatively charged oligosaccharides that can bind to positively charged PF4 tetramers, resulting in heparin-PF4 complex formation that is immunogenic under certain circumstances.[591] Binding of IgG to the heparin-PF4 complex forms an immune complex that triggers cross-linking of the platelet FcγIIa receptor, an event that leads to platelet activation and formation of thrombogenic microparticles.[592] The end result is the development of thrombocytopenia in the setting of a profound hypercoagulable state.

HIT typically develops between 5 and 14 days after the commencement of heparin therapy and produces a variable but often moderate degree of thrombocytopenia wherein nadir platelet counts are typically in the range of 60,000/μL and the development of severe thrombocytopenia (<20,000/μL) is unusual.[589] A platelet count fall that begins before day 5 of heparin is unlikely to represent HIT except in patients with a recent (within 3 months) heparin exposure.[593] These patients may experience an abrupt onset of thrombocytopenia on reexposure to heparin as a result of acute platelet activation caused by preformed, circulating HIT-associated antibodies. In contrast, delayed-onset HIT represents a clinical challenge because patients may develop thrombocytopenia with or without thrombosis, days to weeks after heparin cessation.[594]

The incidence of HIT varies between different patient populations and the type of heparin administered. Patients exposed to bovine lung–derived UFH have been reported to have a 3- to 4-fold increased risk of developing HIT compared to those exposed to porcine intestine–derived UFH, with HIT occurring in up to 3% to 5% of patients exposed to unfractionated porcine intestine–derived heparin.[595] UFH induces pathogenic HIT antibodies up to 10 times more often

All Hospitalized[a]		Medical[b]	
Risk Factor	Points	Risk Factor	Points
Cancer	3	Prior VTE	3
Prior VTE	3	Thrombophilia	2
Thrombophilia	3	LE paralysis	2
Major surgery	2	Cancer	2
Age >75 y	1	Immobility 7+ days	1
Obesity	1	ICU/CCU	1
Bed rest	1	Age >60 y	1
Hormones	1		
High risk = 4+ points		High risk = 4+ points	

Nonorthopedic Surgical Patients[c]
5 points each: Joint replacement surgery, hip/pelvic/leg fracture, stroke, multiple trauma, SCI
3 points each: Age >75, history of VTE, family history of thrombosis, HIT, thrombophilia
2 points each: Age 60–74, cancer, major surgery, laparoscopic or arthroscopic surgery, CVC, bed rest >72 h, immobilizing cast
1 point each: Age 41-60, minor surgery, IBD, edema, BMI > 25, sepsis, serious lung disease, medical patient on bed rest, CHF, AMI, varicose veins, OCP/ERT, pregnant/postpartum
High risk = 8+ points
Low risk = 0–1+ points

- High risk = >4% Symptomatic VTE rate
- Greater # RF = Greater RAM sensitivity

FIGURE 56.9 Individualized venous thromboembolism risk assessment models (RAMs). Individualized risk assessment for venous thromboembolism using validated RAMs may optimize patient selection and subsequent net benefit of thromboprophylaxis for acutely ill hospitalized patients or those undergoing major surgical intervention. In general, RAMs have a good positive predictive value in identifying high-risk patients, but may be relatively less useful in identifying lower risk patients. AMI, acute myocardial infarction; BMI, body mass index; CHF, congestive heart failure; CVC, central venous catheter; HIT, heparin-induced thrombocytopenia; IBD, inflammatory bowel disease; ICU/CCU, intensive care unit/critical care unit; LE, lower extremity; OCP/ERT, oral contraceptives/estrogen replacement therapy; SCI, spinal cord injury; VTE, venous thromboembolism. (Adapted from [a]Kucher N, Koo S, Quiroz R, et al. Electronic alerts to prevent venous thromboembolism among hospitalized patients. *N Engl J Med.* 2005;352:969-977; [b]Spyropoulos AC, Anderson FA Jr, Fitzgerald G, et al. Predictive and associative models to identify hospitalized medical patients at risk for VTE. *Chest.* 2011;140:706-714; [c]Bahl V, Hu HM, Henke PK, Wakefield TW, Campbell DA Jr, Caprini JA. A validation study of a retrospective venous thromboembolism scoring method. *Ann Surg.* 2010;251:344-350.)

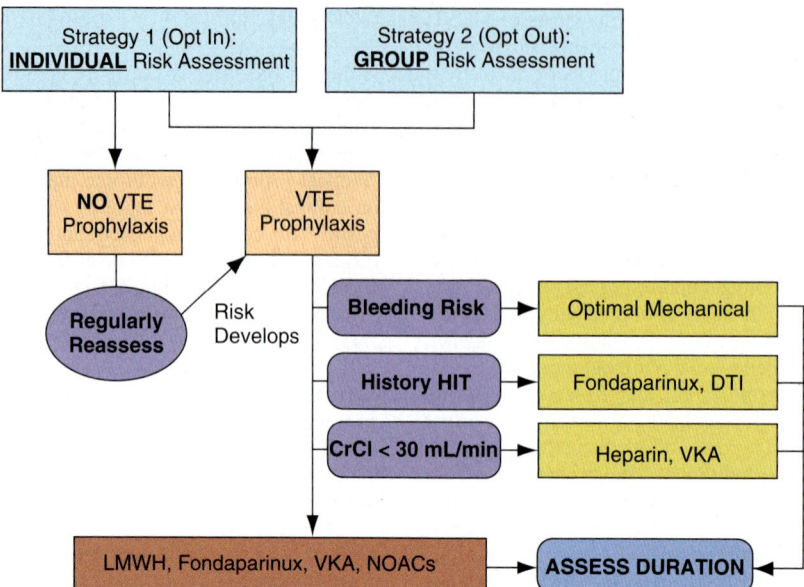

FIGURE 56.10 **A general approach to venous thromboembolism (VTE) prophylaxis in hospitalized patients.** Some form of VTE risk assessment should be performed in patients admitted to the hospital to identify those patients who are most likely to benefit from thromboprophylaxis. Risk assessment can be either individualized or considering at-risk patient groups (e.g., orthopedic surgery patients). Once risk has been identified, the choice of prophylactic strategy should be based upon the patient's bleeding risk, history of heparin-induced thrombocytopenia, renal function, duration of therapy, and cost. CrCl, creatinine clearance; DTI, direct thrombin inhibitor; HIT, heparin-induced thrombocytopenia; LMWH, low-molecular-weight heparin; NOACs, novel oral anticoagulants; VKA, vitamin K antagonist.

than LMWH.[595,596] Warkentin et al evaluated the incidence of HIT in 665 patients randomized to receive subcutaneous UFH or LMWH for venous thromboprophylaxis after elective hip surgery. HIT was diagnosed in 2.7% (9/332) of patients given UFH vs 0% (0/333) of those given LMWH. HIT with thrombosis developed in 88.9% (8/9) of the patients who developed HIT, compared with a thrombosis rate of 17.8% (117/656) in patients without HIT.[597] Patients undergoing cardiac surgery who receive UFH have a higher incidence of pathogenic HIT antibodies (2.5%) compared to medical (<1%) or obstetric (<0.1%) patients. HIT also appears to develop more often in women.[593,595]

The most feared complication of HIT is thrombosis, which occurs in one-third to one-half of patients diagnosed with HIT.[598] The thrombotic tendency associated with HIT can last for at least 30 days, and HIT with thrombosis may develop well after the discontinuation of heparin and platelet count recovery. Venous thrombosis is more common than arterial thrombosis in HIT patients, especially in those who receive UFH for postoperative VTE prophylaxis.[599,600] Extremity DVT is the most frequently encountered venous thrombotic complication in HIT patients followed in frequency by PE and cerebral sinus thrombosis. Most HIT-associated arterial thromboses involve the extremities, although stroke, MI, and renal artery thrombosis related to heparin infusions have been described. HIT with thrombosis after coronary artery bypass grafting may present as bypass graft occlusion, left atrial thrombus formation, valvular thrombosis, or PE.[601] Acute graft occlusion secondary to HIT has been described in vascular surgery patients even after platelet count normalization. It is reasonable to assume that patients with preexisting vascular lesions, intravascular catheters, sepsis, or postoperative venous stasis are particularly susceptible to the thrombotic complications of HIT.

Other clinical manifestations of HIT include heparin-induced skin lesions, heparin "resistance," and adrenal vein thrombosis leading to hemorrhagic infarction.[602,603] Heparin-induced skin lesions have been observed in ~10% to 20% of patients who generate HIT-IgG in response to subcutaneous UFH injections. The skin lesions develop at heparin injection sites with an appearance ranging from painful red plaques to overt skin necrosis reminiscent of warfarin-induced skin necrosis. Thrombocytopenia may not develop in the majority of patients with heparin-induced skin lesions, but those who do develop skin lesions and thrombocytopenia appear to be at extremely high risk for arterial thrombosis. The thrombocytopenia that develops in HIT is not typically associated with hemorrhagic events, and platelet transfusion is associated with an increased risk of arterial thrombosis and mortality.[604]

HIT is primarily a clinical diagnosis and must be strongly suspected in any patient who develops thrombocytopenia while receiving heparin in any dose or by any route of administration. Whereas HIT is usually associated with a platelet count below the lower limits of normal (150,000/μL in most laboratories), the extent of thrombocytopenia is quite variable, and the diagnosis should be considered if the platelet count falls below 50% of the baseline value (even if still within the normal range) after the fifth day of heparin treatment.[598] Similarly, a 30% to 50% decrease in baseline platelet count combined with any form of thrombosis in a patient receiving heparin should be attributed to HIT until proven otherwise. Thrombotic events occurring or progressing during therapeutic intensity heparin therapy, even if the platelet count is normal, may also constitute a HIT variant.[605-607] An autoimmune variant of HIT has also been described wherein anti-PF4-polyanion antibodies activate platelets in the absence of heparin.[608]

Limitations of laboratory assays for HIT (discussed below) have led to the development of a clinical scoring system to determine the pretest probability of HIT to rapidly identify patients with a probable diagnosis. The "4T's" scoring system (*Table 56.15*) uses easily available clinical information (platelet count nadir, timing of thrombocytopenia, the presence or absence of thrombosis, and alternative explanations for thrombocytopenia) to classify patients into high (score of 6-8), intermediate (score of 4-5), or low (score of ≤3) probability of HIT.[609] Several systematic reviews indicate this scoring system has a high negative predictive value.[610-612] Consequently, a low pretest score is useful in ruling out a HIT diagnosis.[598] A meta-analysis of clinical trials using the 4T's scoring system reported the negative predictive value of a low 4T score was 99.8%, whereas the positive predictive value for patients with an intermediate-to-high 4T score ranged from 22% to 63%.[610]

In vitro diagnostic assays for HIT are either immunoassays or functional assays. Immunoassays detect the presence of heparin-PF4 antibodies using ELISA methodology. HIT ELISAs have high sensitivity, but poor specificity for the diagnosis.[613] Early generation

Table 56.15. The 4T's Clinical Prediction Score for the Diagnosis of Heparin-Induced Thrombocytopenia

4T's	Score = 2 Points	Score = 1 Point	Score = 0 Points
Thrombocytopenia	Platelet count fall >50% and platelet count nadir ≥20,000 and no surgery within preceding 3 d	Platelet count fall 30%-50% or platelet count nadir 10-19,000 Or Platelet count fall >50% but surgery within preceding 3 d	Platelet count fall <30% Or Platelet count nadir <10,000
Timing of platelet count fall	Onset of fall 5-10 d after heparin start Or Platelet count fall ≤1 d after heparin start with prior heparin exposure within 30 d	Uncertain as to time course but likely platelet count fall 5-10 d after heparin start Or Platelet count fall after day 10 of heparin start Or Platelet count fall within 1 d after heparin start with prior heparin exposure in past 31-100 d	Platelet count fall ≤4 d after heparin start and no heparin exposure in past 100 d
Thrombosis (or other clinical events)	Confirmed new thrombosis Or Skin necrosis at injection site Or Acute systemic reaction to IV UFH Or Adrenal hemorrhage	Recurrent VTE in a patient receiving therapeutic anticoagulation Or Suspected thrombosis Or Erythematous skin lesions at heparin injection sites	Thrombosis not suspected
Other cause for thrombocytopenia	No alternative explanation for platelet decline	Possible other cause	Probable/definite (DIC, sepsis, drug-induced, surgery within 3 d, etc)

Each 4T's parameter is evaluated and scored; patients with scores ≤3 points are at low risk for HIT. Those with scores of 4 to 5 points are at intermediate risk, and patients with scores of 6 to 8 points are at high risk of HIT.
Abbreviations: DIC, disseminated intravascular coagulation; UFH, unfractionated heparin; VTE, venous thromboembolism.
Adapted from Warkentin TE, Linkins LA. Non-necrotizing heparin-induced skin lesions and the 4T's score. *J Thromb Haemost.* 2010;8(7):1483-1485. Copyright © 2010 International Society on Thrombosis and Haemostasis. With permission.

ELISAs detected IgG, IgM, and IgA antibodies, though only IgG antibodies are pathogenic in this disorder, which resulted in a high rate of false-positive tests and unnecessary parenteral DTI therapy.[614] In addition, not all antibodies to the heparin-PF4 complex will induce platelet activation. The improved reliability of commercially available IgG-specific ELISAs is useful to consider the "positivity" of the result. ELISA optical density (OD) results near the upper limit of the normal range (typically ~0.4 OD units) are less likely to be associated with clinical HIT than a much higher positive result (≥2.0 OD units).[598,615]

Functional assays detect platelet aggregation or platelet activation after exposure to suspected HIT serum and heparin. Functional assays include the platelet aggregation test, the heparin-induced platelet aggregation test, heparin-induced platelet release of ATP detected by lumi-aggregometry, the ^{14}C-serotonin release assay (^{14}C-SRA), heparin-induced platelet microparticle formation detected by flow cytometry, and enzyme immunoassay detection of platelet serotonin release. Traditionally, the ^{14}C-SRA has been considered the "gold standard" for HIT diagnostic confirmation. However, most studies evaluating the diagnostic use of the available functional assays and immunoassays, including studies of ^{14}C-SRA, used a clinical diagnosis of HIT as the true "gold standard." The SRA is tedious to perform, has a lengthy turnaround time, and is offered by few laboratories.[613] Patients should first be assessed clinically (*Table 56.15*) using the 4T's scoring system to determine their likelihood of having HIT. Those patients with a low pretest likelihood for HIT usually do not require further testing or alternative anticoagulation, unless the 4T score is difficult to assess because of missing information (e.g., platelet count). Conversely, patients with an intermediate or high pretest probability for HIT and an ongoing need for anticoagulation should receive a nonheparin anticoagulant while further testing is performed.[598] A negative immunoassay result effectively rules out HIT, and heparin can be restarted. Patients with an intermediate pretest probability and a positive immunoassay result should undergo confirmatory testing with a functional assay to definitively diagnose HIT. Patients with a high pretest probability should be managed similar to those with intermediate probability, with a confirmatory functional assay performed, especially if the immunoassay is only weakly positive (e.g., OD 0.4-1.0). A strongly positive immunoassay (e.g., OD > 2.0) may obviate the need for confirmatory testing in high pretest probability patients.[598] *Figure 56.11* suggests an initial diagnostic and management approach to HIT.

The initial treatment of HIT with or without thrombosis is to discontinue all exposure to heparin or LMWHs (including heparin-coated catheters) and immediately begin a nonheparin anticoagulant such as argatroban, bivalirudin, danaparoid, fondaparinux, or a DOAC. In patients with life- or limb-threatening thrombosis, the efficacy of DOAC therapy is uncertain and DTI therapy may be preferable.[598] Parenteral DTIs are continued as monotherapy until normalization of the platelet count, followed by a transition to an oral anticoagulant. Warfarin may be desired for long-term therapy, but should never be initiated in the absence of a nonheparin anticoagulant as it is reported to be a major factor contributing to limb amputation from progression of otherwise unremarkable DVTs to phlegmasia cerulea dolens in patients with HIT.[616] The combination of HIT-associated hypercoagulability and warfarin-induced protein C deficiency may result in a profound procoagulant state leading to venous limb gangrene. Vitamin K should be administered to patients on warfarin therapy when alternative anticoagulation is started, thereby reversing any procoagulant effect of protein C deficiency.[598] After the platelet count normalizes, warfarin can be initiated. Warfarin therapy requires overlap with a DTI for at least 5 days, and until a therapeutic INR (2.0-3.0) is achieved on warfarin alone. DOACs may be preferable to warfarin in clinically stable patients with platelet recovery given their generally favorable bleeding risk.[598]

In isolated HIT (i.e., without thrombosis) anticoagulation should be continued at least until the platelet count normalizes (≥150 × 10^9/L), with some experts recommending up to 4 weeks of therapeutic anticoagulation.[372,598] HIT with thrombosis requires therapeutically dosed anticoagulation for at least 3 months.[372,598]

Patients should be informed that they should not be exposed to heparin again, although protocols are available in which short-term exposure can be safely done in patients who require temporary heparin exposure (e.g., cardiopulmonary bypass).[598]

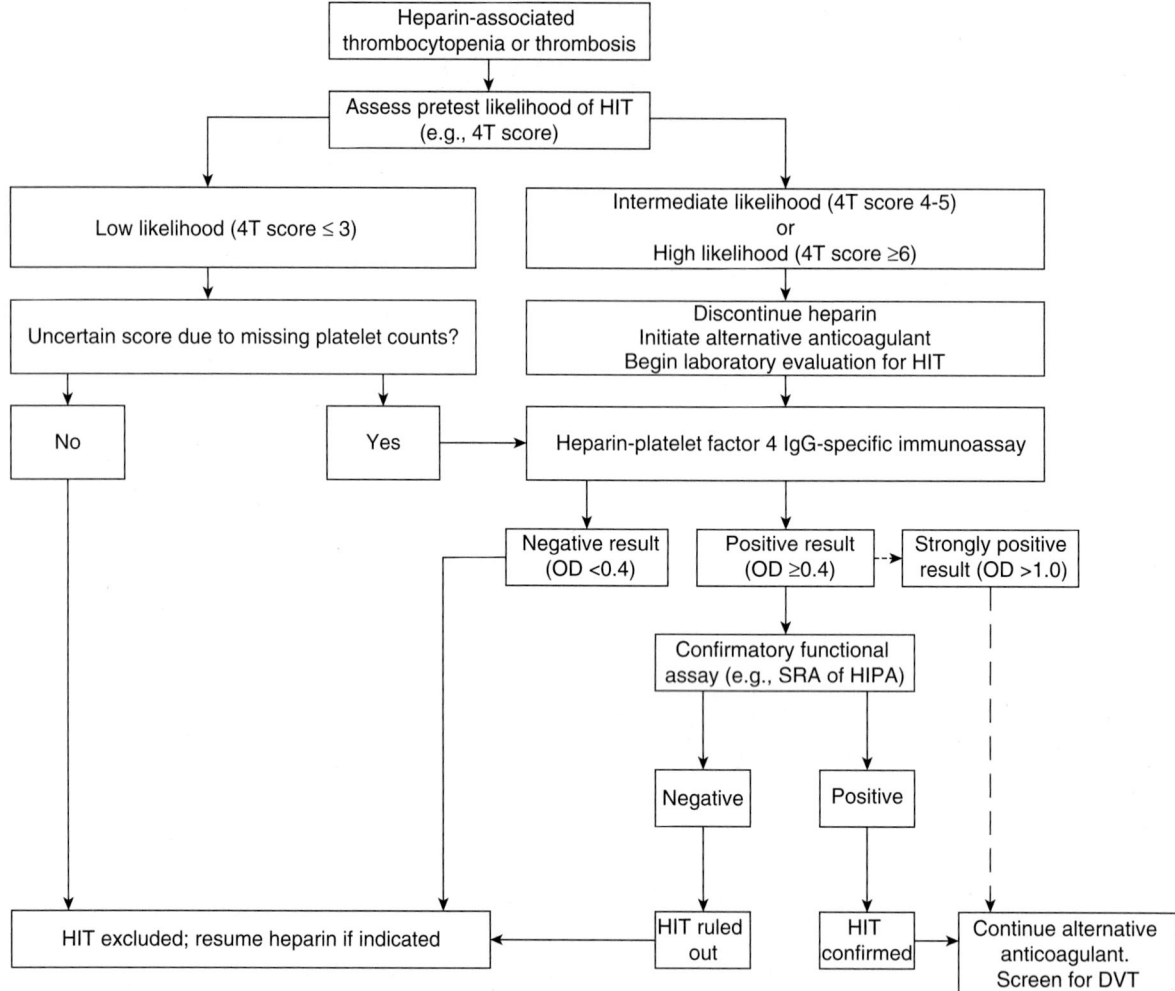

FIGURE 56.11 Initial management of patients with suspected heparin-induced thrombocytopenia (HIT). Patients with suspected HIT should be approached in a rapid and evidence-based manner, wherein a pretest probability assessment is completed (e.g., using the 4T's scoring system, *Table 56.15*) and application of an immunoassay test, in particular to those patients at intermediate-to-high pretest probability. While awaiting immunoassay test results, implementation of an alternative anticoagulant (e.g., direct thrombin inhibitor) is recommended. Patients with positive immunoassay results should undergo additional testing with a functional platelet activation assay, such as the serotonin release assay (SRA). DVT, deep venous thrombosis; HIPA, heparin-induced platelet aggregation; OD, optical density. (Adapted from Greinacher A. Clinical practice. Heparin-induced thrombocytopenia. *N Engl J Med*. 2015;373(3):252-261.)

Considering the complexity of HIT diagnosis and treatment, HIT prevention must be emphasized. Patients receiving UFH should have platelet count monitoring at baseline and at least every third day between day 5 and day 14 of heparin exposure.[598] Appropriate medical record documentation and patient education may help avert heparin reexposure in patients with a history of HIT. Reexposure to heparin in patients with past HIT should be delayed at least 3 months, kept to a minimum duration to provide succinct anamnesis, and avoided whenever possible. DOACs and fondaparinux are preferable to LMWH and UFH for the treatment and prevention of thromboembolic disease in patients with a known history of HIT.[598] For those patients with acute or subacute HIT who require urgent cardiac surgery or PCI, the use of bivalirudin is recommended, and in rare circumstances plasma exchange to remove circulating HIT antibodies.[598]

References

1. Murphy SL, Xu J, Kochanek KD, Arias E, Tejada-Vera B. Deaths: final data for 2018. *Natl Vital Stat Rep*. 2021;69(13):1-83.
2. Goldhaber SZ, Visani L, De Rosa M. Acute pulmonary embolism: clinical outcomes in the International Cooperative Pulmonary Embolism Registry (ICOPER). *Lancet*. 1999;353(9162):1386-1389.
3. ISTH Steering Committee for World Thrombosis Day. Thrombosis: a major contributor to the global disease burden. *J Thromb Haemost*. 2014;12(10):1580-1590.
4. Alonso-Coello P, Bellmunt S, McGorrian C, et al. Antithrombotic therapy in peripheral artery disease: antithrombotic therapy and prevention of thrombosis, 9th ed. American College of Chest Physicians Evidence-Based Clinical Practice Guidelines. *Chest*. 2012;141(2 suppl):e669S-e690S.
5. Lansberg MG, O'Donnell MJ, Khatri P, et al. Antithrombotic and thrombolytic therapy for ischemic stroke: antithrombotic therapy and prevention of thrombosis, 9th ed. American College of Chest Physicians Evidence-Based Clinical Practice Guidelines. *Chest*. 2012;141(2 suppl):e601S-e636S.
6. Rodriguez F, Harrington RA. Management of antithrombotic therapy after acute coronary syndromes. *N Engl J Med*. 2021;384(5):452-460.
7. Furie B. Pathogenesis of thrombosis. *Hematology Am Soc Hematol Educ Program*. 2009;2009:255-258.
8. Virchow R. *Gesammelte Abhandlungen zur Wissenschaftlichen Medicin*. Science History Publications; 1856.
9. Badimon L, Badimon JJ, Galvez A, Chesebro JH, Fuster V. Influence of arterial damage and wall shear rate on platelet deposition. Ex vivo study in a swine model. *Arteriosclerosis*. 1986;6(3):312-320.
10. Thomas DP. Overview of venous thrombogenesis. *Semin Thromb Hemost*. 1988;14(1):1-8.
11. Strandness DE Jr, Ward K, Krugmire R Jr. The present status of acute deep venous thrombosis. *Surg Gynecol Obstet*. 1977;145(3):433-445.
12. Nicolaides AN, Kakkar VV, Renney JT. Soleal sinuses and stasis. *Br J Surg*. 1971;58(4):307.
13. van Langevelde K, Sramek A, Rosendaal FR. The effect of aging on venous valves. *Arterioscler Thromb Vasc Biol*. 2010;30(10):2075-2080.
14. Lowe GD. Common risk factors for both arterial and venous thrombosis. *Br J Haematol*. 2008;140(5):488-495.
15. Turpie AG, Esmon C. Venous and arterial thrombosis–pathogenesis and the rationale for anticoagulation. *Thromb Haemost*. 2011;105(4):586-596.
16. Ross R. The pathogenesis of atherosclerosis: a perspective for the 1990s. *Nature*. 1993;362(6423):801-809.

17. Falati S, Gross P, Merrill-Skoloff G, Furie BC, Furie B. Real-time in vivo imaging of platelets, tissue factor and fibrin during arterial thrombus formation in the mouse. *Nat Med.* 2002;8(10):1175-1181.
18. Preston RJS, O'Sullivan JM, O'Donnell JS. Advances in understanding the molecular mechanisms of venous thrombosis. *Br J Haematol.* 2019;186(1):13-23.
19. Goodrich SM, Wood JE. Peripheral venous distensibility and velocity of venous blood flow during pregnancy or during oral contraceptive therapy. *Am J Obstet Gynecol.* 1964;90:740-744.
20. Schwertz H, Tolley ND, Foulks JM, et al. Signal-dependent splicing of tissue factor pre-mRNA modulates the thrombogenicity of human platelets. *J Exp Med.* 2006;203(11):2433-2440.
21. Reitsma PH, Versteeg HH, Middeldorp S. Mechanistic view of risk factors for venous thrombosis. *Arterioscler Thromb Vasc Biol.* 2012;32(3):563-568.
22. Hirsh J. Hypercoagulability. *Semin Hematol.* 1977;14(4):409-425.
23. Rondina MT, Pendleton RC, Wheeler M, Rodgers GM. The treatment of venous thromboembolism in special populations. *Thromb Res.* 2007;119(4):391-402.
24. Coppens M, Reijnders JH, Middeldorp S, Doggen CJ, Rosendaal FR. Testing for inherited thrombophilia does not reduce the recurrence of venous thrombosis. *J Thromb Haemost.* 2008;6(9):1474-1477.
25. Harker LA, Slichter SJ. Arterial and venous thromboembolism: kinetic characterization and evaluation of therapy. *Thromb Diath Haemorrh.* 1974;31(2):188-203.
26. Abrahamsen AF, Eika C, Godal HC, Lorentsen E. Effect of acetylsalicylic acid and dipyridamole on platelet survival and aggregation in patients with atherosclerosis obliterans. *Scand J Haematol.* 1974;13(4):241-245.
27. Steele P, Weily H, Davies H, Ppppas G, Genton E. Platelet survival time following aortic valve replacement. *Circulation.* 1975;51(2):358-362.
28. Miller GJ, Bauer KA, Cooper JA, Rosenberg RD. Activation of the coagulant pathway in cigarette smokers. *Thromb Haemost.* 1998;79(3):549-553.
29. Harker LA, Hazzard W. Platelet kinetic studies in patients with hyperlipoproteinemia: effects of clofibrate therapy. *Circulation.* 1979;60(3):492-496.
30. Moncada S. Prostacyclin and arterial wall biology. *Arteriosclerosis.* 1982;2(3):193-207.
31. Radomski MW, Palmer RM, Moncada S. Endogenous nitric oxide inhibits human platelet adhesion to vascular endothelium. *Lancet.* 1987;2(8567):1057-1058.
32. Marcus AJ, Broekman MJ, Drosopoulos JH, et al. The endothelial cell ecto-ADPase responsible for inhibition of platelet function is CD39. *J Clin Invest.* 1997;99(6):1351-1360.
33. Thompson SG, Kienast J, Pyke SD, Haverkate F, van de Loo JC. Hemostatic factors and the risk of myocardial infarction or sudden death in patients with angina pectoris. European Concerted Action on Thrombosis and Disabilities Angina Pectoris Study Group. *N Engl J Med.* 1995;332(10):635-641.
34. Williams MS, Bray PF. Genetics of arterial prothrombotic risk states. *Exp Biol Med (Maywood).* 2001;226(5):409-419.
35. Rosendaal FR. Venous thrombosis: a multicausal disease. *Lancet.* 1999;353(9159):1167-1173.
36. Welch GN, Loscalzo J. Homocysteine and atherothrombosis. *N Engl J Med.* 1998;338(15):1042-1050.
37. Kyrle PA, Minar E, Hirschl M, et al. High plasma levels of factor VIII and the risk of recurrent venous thromboembolism. *N Engl J Med.* 2000;343(7):457-462.
38. Oger E. Incidence of venous thromboembolism: a community-based study in western France. EPI-GETBP study group. Groupe d'Etude de la Thrombose de Bretagne Occidentale. *Thromb Haemost.* 2000;83(5):657-660.
39. Franchini M, Martinelli I, Mannucci PM. Uncertain thrombophilia markers. *Thromb Haemost.* 2016;115(1):25-30.
40. Meade TW, Ruddock V, Stirling Y, Chakrabarti R, Miller GJ. Fibrinolytic activity, clotting factors, and long-term incidence of ischaemic heart disease in the Northwick Park Heart Study. *Lancet.* 1993;342(8879):1076-1079.
41. Cortellaro M, Cofrancesco E, Boschetti C, et al. Increased fibrin turnover and high PAI-1 activity as predictors of ischemic events in atherosclerotic patients. A case-control study. The PLAT Group. *Arterioscler Thromb.* 1993;13(10):1412-1417.
42. Nemerson Y. Tissue factor and hemostasis. *Blood.* 1988;71(1):1-8.
43. Steffel J, Luscher TF, Tanner FC. Tissue factor in cardiovascular diseases: molecular mechanisms and clinical implications. *Circulation.* 2006;113(5):722-731.
44. Visentin GP, Ford SE, Scott JP, Aster RH. Antibodies from patients with heparin-induced thrombocytopenia/thrombosis are specific for platelet factor 4 complexed with heparin or bound to endothelial cells. *J Clin Invest.* 1994;93(1):81-88.
45. Bevilacqua MP, Pober JS, Majeau GR, Cotran RS, Gimbrone MA Jr. Interleukin 1 (IL-1) induces biosynthesis and cell surface expression of procoagulant activity in human vascular endothelial cells. *J Exp Med.* 1984;160(2):618-623.
46. Fryer RH, Wilson BD, Gubler DB, Fitzgerald LA, Rodgers GM. Homocysteine, a risk factor for premature vascular disease and thrombosis, induces tissue factor activity in endothelial cells. *Arterioscler Thromb.* 1993;13(9):1327-1333.
47. Nawroth PP, Stern DM. Modulation of endothelial cell hemostatic properties by tumor necrosis factor. *J Exp Med.* 1986;163(3):740-745.
48. Colucci M, Balconi G, Lorenzet R, et al. Cultured human endothelial cells generate tissue factor in response to endotoxin. *J Clin Invest.* 1983;71(6):1893-1896.
49. Courtney MA, Haidaris PJ, Marder VJ, Sporn LA. Tissue factor mRNA expression in the endothelium of an intact umbilical vein. *Blood.* 1996;87(1):174-179.
50. Drake TA, Cheng J, Chang A, Taylor FB Jr. Expression of tissue factor, thrombomodulin, and E-selectin in baboons with lethal Escherichia coli sepsis. *Am J Pathol.* 1993;142(5):1458-1470.
51. Speiser W, Kapiotis S, Kopp CW, et al. Effect of intradermal tumor necrosis factor-alpha-induced inflammation on coagulation factors in dermal vessel endothelium. An in vivo study of human skin biopsies. *Thromb Haemost.* 2001;85(2):362-367.
52. Edwards RL, Rickles FR, Bobrove AM. Mononuclear cell tissue factor: cell of origin and requirements for activation. *Blood.* 1979;54(2):359-370.
53. Miletich JP, Jackson CM, Majerus PW. Properties of the factor Xa binding site on human platelets. *J Biol Chem.* 1978;253(19):6908-6916.
54. Callander N, Rapaport SI. Trousseau's syndrome. *West J Med.* 1993;158(4):364-371.
55. Gordon SG, Cross BA. A factor X-activating cysteine protease from malignant tissue. *J Clin Invest.* 1981;67(6):1665-1671.
56. Taylor FB Jr, Kinasewitz GT. The diagnosis and management of disseminated intravascular coagulation. *Curr Hematol Rep.* 2002;1(1):34-40.
57. Weiner CP, Kwaan H, Hauck WW, Duboe FJ, Paul M, Wallemark CB. Fibrin generation in normal pregnancy. *Obstet Gynecol.* 1984;64(1):46-48.
58. Pabinger I, Grafenhofer H, Kyrle PA, et al. Temporary increase in the risk for recurrence during pregnancy in women with a history of venous thromboembolism. *Blood.* 2002;100(3):1060-1062.
59. van Hylckama Vlieg A, Middeldorp S. Hormone therapies and venous thromboembolism: where are we now? *J Thromb Haemost.* 2011;9(2):257-266.
60. Quehenberger P, Loner U, Kapiotis S, et al. Increased levels of activated factor VII and decreased plasma protein S activity and circulating thrombomodulin during use of oral contraceptives. *Thromb Haemost.* 1996;76(5):729-734.
61. Vandenbroucke JP, Koster T, Briet E, Reitsma PH, Bertina RM, Rosendaal FR. Increased risk of venous thrombosis in oral-contraceptive users who are carriers of factor V Leiden mutation. *Lancet.* 1994;344(8935):1453-1457.
62. Rosing J, Tans G, Nicolaes GA, et al. Oral contraceptives and venous thrombosis: different sensitivities to activated protein C in women using second- and third-generation oral contraceptives. *Br J Haematol.* 1997;97(1):233-238.
63. Miller J, Chan BK, Nelson HD. Postmenopausal estrogen replacement and risk for venous thromboembolism: a systematic review and meta-analysis for the U.S. Preventive Services Task Force. *Ann Intern Med.* 2002;136(9):680-690.
64. Abou-Ismail MY, Citla Sridhar D, Nayak L. Estrogen and thrombosis: a bench to bedside review. *Thromb Res.* 2020;192:40-51.
65. Mantha S, Karp R, Raghavan V, Terrin N, Bauer KA, Zwicker JI. Assessing the risk of venous thromboembolic events in women taking progestin-only contraception: a meta-analysis. *Br Med J.* 2012;345:e4944.
66. Walker RF, Zakai NA, MacLehose RF, et al. Association of Testosterone therapy with risk of venous thromboembolism among men with and without hypogonadism. *JAMA Intern Med.* 2020;180(2):190-197.
67. Khor B, Van Cott EM. Laboratory evaluation of hypercoagulability. *Clin Lab Med.* 2009;29(2):339-366.
68. Robetorye RS, Rodgers GM. Update on selected inherited venous thrombotic disorders. *Am J Hematol.* 2001;68(4):256-268.
69. Varga EA, Kujovich JL. Management of inherited thrombophilia: guide for genetics professionals. *Clin Genet.* 2012;81(1):7-17.
70. Egeberg O. Inherited antithrombin deficiency causing thrombophilia. *Thromb Diath Haemorrh.* 1965;13:516-530.
71. Cosgriff TM, Bishop DT, Hershgold EJ, et al. Familial antithrombin III deficiency: its natural history, genetics, diagnosis and treatment. *Medicine (Baltimore).* 1983;62(4):209-220.
72. Marciniak E, Farley CH, DeSimone PA. Familial thrombosis due to antithrombin 3 deficiency. *Blood.* 1974;43(2):219-231.
73. Tait RC, Walker ID, Perry DJ, et al. Prevalence of antithrombin deficiency in the healthy population. *Br J Haematol.* 1994;87(1):106-112.
74. Rezaie AR, Giri H. Antithrombin: an anticoagulant, anti-inflammatory and antibacterial serpin. *J Thromb Haemost.* 2020;18(3):528-533.
75. Bauer KA, Rosenberg RD. The pathophysiology of the prethrombotic state in humans: insights gained from studies using markers of hemostatic system activation. *Blood.* 1987;70(2):343-350.
76. de la Morena-Barrio ME, Martinez-Martinez I, de Cos C, et al. Hypoglycosylation is a common finding in antithrombin deficiency in the absence of a SERPINC1 gene defect. *J Thromb Haemost.* 2016;14(8):1549-1560.
77. Navarro-Fernandez J, de la Morena-Barrio ME, Padilla J, et al. Antithrombin Dublin (p.Val30Glu): a relatively common variant with moderate thrombosis risk of causing transient antithrombin deficiency. *Thromb Haemost.* 2016;116(1):146-154.
78. Hirsh J, Piovella F, Pini M. Congenital antithrombin III deficiency. Incidence and clinical features. *Am J Med.* 1989;87(3B):34S-38S.
79. Patnaik MM, Moll S. Inherited antithrombin deficiency: a review. *Haemophilia.* 2008;14(6):1229-1239.
80. Toglia MR, Weg JG. Venous thromboembolism during pregnancy. *N Engl J Med.* 1996;335(2):108-114.
81. Boyer C, Wolf M, Vedrenne J, Meyer D, Larrieu MJ. Homozygous variant of antithrombin III: AT III Fontainebleau. *Thromb Haemost.* 1986;56(1):18-22.
82. Harper PL, Luddington RJ, Daly M, et al. The incidence of dysfunctional antithrombin variants: four cases in 210 patients with thromboembolic disease. *Br J Haematol.* 1991;77(3):360-364.
83. Holmes EW, Fareed J, Bermes EW Jr. Automation of plasma antithrombin III assays. *Clin Chem.* 1981;27(6):816-818.
84. Buller HR, ten Cate JW. Acquired antithrombin III deficiency: laboratory diagnosis, incidence, clinical implications, and treatment with antithrombin III concentrate. *Am J Med.* 1989;87(3B):44S-48S.
85. Marciniak E, Gockerman JP. Heparin-induced decrease in circulating antithrombin-III. *Lancet.* 1977;2(8038):581-584.
86. Van Cott EM, Orlando C, Moore GW, et al. Recommendations for clinical laboratory testing for antithrombin deficiency; Communication from the SSC of the ISTH. *J Thromb Haemost.* 2020;18(1):17-22.
87. Rodgers GM. Role of antithrombin concentrate in treatment of hereditary antithrombin deficiency. An update. *Thromb Haemost.* 2009;101(5):806-812.
88. Brandt P. Observations during the treatment of antithrombin-III deficient women with heparin and antithrombin concentrate during pregnancy, parturition, and abortion. *Thromb Res.* 1981;22(1-2):15-24.

89. Damus PS, Wallace GA. Immunologic measurement of antithrombin III-heparin cofactor and alpha2 macroglobulin in disseminated intravascular coagulation and hepatic failure coagulopathy. *Thromb Res.* 1975;6(1):27-38.
90. Kauffmann RH, Veltkamp JJ, Van Tilburg NH, Van Es LA. Acquired antithrombin III deficiency and thrombosis in the nephrotic syndrome. *Am J Med.* 1978;65(4):607-613.
91. Friedman KD, Borok Z, Owen J. Heparin cofactor activity and antithrombin III antigen levels in preeclampsia. *Thromb Res.* 1986;43(4):409-416.
92. Ball AP, McKee PA. Fibrin formation and dissolution in women receiving oral contraceptive drugs. *J Lab Clin Med.* 1977;89(4):751-762.
93. Lechner K, Kyrle PA. Antithrombin III concentrates–are they clinically useful? *Thromb Haemost.* 1995;73(3):340-348.
94. Tollefsen DM, Pestka CA, Monafo WJ. Activation of heparin cofactor II by dermatan sulfate. *J Biol Chem.* 1983;258(11):6713-6716.
95. Bertina RM, van der Linden IK, Engesser L, Muller HP, Brommer EJ. Hereditary heparin cofactor II deficiency and the risk of development of thrombosis. *Thromb Haemost.* 1987;57(2):196-200.
96. Esmon CT. The roles of protein C and thrombomodulin in the regulation of blood coagulation. *J Biol Chem.* 1989;264(9):4743-4746.
97. Esmon CT. The regulation of natural anticoagulant pathways. *Science.* 1987;235(4794):1348-1352.
98. Griffin JH, Evatt B, Zimmerman TS, Kleiss AJ, Wideman C. Deficiency of protein C in congenital thrombotic disease. *J Clin Invest.* 1981;68(5):1370-1373.
99. Miletich J, Sherman L, Broze G Jr. Absence of thrombosis in subjects with heterozygous protein C deficiency. *N Engl J Med.* 1987;317(16):991-996.
100. Koeleman BP, Reitsma PH, Allaart CF, Bertina RM. Activated protein C resistance as an additional risk factor for thrombosis in protein C-deficient families. *Blood.* 1994;84(4):1031-1035.
101. Bauer KA, Broekmans AW, Bertina RM, et al. Hemostatic enzyme generation in the blood of patients with hereditary protein C deficiency. *Blood.* 1988;71(5):1418-1426.
102. D'Ursi P, Marino F, Caprera A, Milanesi L, Faioni EM, Rovida E. ProCMD: a database and 3D web resource for protein C mutants. *BMC Bioinformatics.* 2007;8(suppl 1):S11.
103. Koster T, Rosendaal FR, Briet E, et al. Protein C deficiency in a controlled series of unselected outpatients: an infrequent but clear risk factor for venous thrombosis (Leiden Thrombophilia Study). *Blood.* 1995;85(10):2756-2761.
104. Tait RC, Walker ID, Reitsma PH, et al. Prevalence of protein C deficiency in the healthy population. *Thromb Haemost.* 1995;73(1):87-93.
105. Bovill EG, Bauer KA, Dickerman JD, Callas P, West B. The clinical spectrum of heterozygous protein C deficiency in a large New England kindred. *Blood.* 1989;73(3):712-717.
106. Mahmoodi BK, Brouwer JL, Veeger NJ, van der Meer J. Hereditary deficiency of protein C or protein S confers increased risk of arterial thromboembolic events at a young age: results from a large family cohort study. *Circulation.* 2008;118(16):1659-1667.
107. Preston FE, Rosendaal FR, Walker ID, et al. Increased fetal loss in women with heritable thrombophilia. *Lancet.* 1996;348(9032):913-916.
108. Marlar RA, Montgomery RR, Broekmans AW. Report on the diagnosis and treatment of homozygous protein C deficiency. Report of the working party on homozygous protein C deficiency of the ICTH-subcommittee on protein C and protein S. *Thromb Haemost.* 1989;61(3):529-531.
109. McGehee WG, Klotz TA, Epstein DJ, Rapaport SI. Coumarin necrosis associated with hereditary protein C deficiency. *Ann Intern Med.* 1984;101(1):59-60.
110. Allaart CF, Poort SR, Rosendaal FR, Reitsma PH, Bertina RM, Briet E. Increased risk of venous thrombosis in carriers of hereditary protein C deficiency defect. *Lancet.* 1993;341(8838):134-138.
111. van der Meer FJ, Koster T, Vandenbroucke JP, Briet E, Rosendaal FR. The leiden thrombophilia study (LETS). *Thromb Haemost.* 1997;78(1):631-635.
112. Simioni P, Sanson BJ, Prandoni P, et al. Incidence of venous thromboembolism in families with inherited thrombophilia. *Thromb Haemost.* 1999;81(2):198-202.
113. Kottke-Marchant K, Comp P. Laboratory issues in diagnosing abnormalities of protein C, thrombomodulin, and endothelial cell protein C receptor. *Arch Pathol Lab Med.* 2002;126(11):1337-1348.
114. Libourel EJ, Meinardi JR, de Kam PJ, et al. Protein C/S ratio, an accurate and simple tool to identify carriers of a protein C gene mutation. *Br J Haematol.* 2002;118(2):615-618.
115. Tait RC, Walker ID, Islam SI, et al. Age related changes in protein C activity in healthy adult males. *Thromb Haemost.* 1991;65(3):326-327.
116. Pabinger I, Kyrle PA, Speiser W, Stoffels U, Jung M, Lechner K. Diagnosis of protein C deficiency in patients on oral anticoagulant treatment: comparison of three different functional protein C assays. *Thromb Haemost.* 1990;63(3):407-412.
117. Cooper PC, Pavlova A, Moore GW, Hickey KP, Marlar RA. Recommendations for clinical laboratory testing for protein C deficiency, for the subcommittee on plasma coagulation inhibitors of the ISTH. *J Thromb Haemost.* 2020;18(2):271-277.
118. Dreyfus M, Magny JF, Bridey F, et al. Treatment of homozygous protein C deficiency and neonatal purpura fulminans with a purified protein C concentrate. *N Engl J Med.* 1991;325(22):1565-1568.
119. Conard J, Bauer KA, Gruber A, et al. Normalization of markers of coagulation activation with a purified protein C concentrate in adults with homozygous protein C deficiency. *Blood.* 1993;82(4):1159-1164.
120. Vigano D'Angelo S, Comp PC, Esmon CT, D'Angelo A. Relationship between protein C antigen and anticoagulant activity during oral anticoagulation and in selected disease states. *J Clin Invest.* 1986;77(2):416-425.
121. Griffin JH, Mosher DF, Zimmerman TS, Kleiss AJ. Protein C, an antithrombotic protein, is reduced in hospitalized patients with intravascular coagulation. *Blood.* 1982;60(1):261-264.
122. Sorensen PJ, Knudsen F, Nielsen AH, Dyerberg J. Protein C activity in renal disease. *Thromb Res.* 1985;38(3):243-249.
123. Kovacs MJ, Kovacs J, Anderson J, Rodger MA, Mackinnon K, Wells PS. Protein C and protein S levels can be accurately determined within 24 hours of diagnosis of acute venous thromboembolism. *Clin Lab Haematol.* 2006;28(1):9-13.
124. Comp PC, Esmon CT. Recurrent venous thromboembolism in patients with a partial deficiency of protein S. *N Engl J Med.* 1984;311(24):1525-1528.
125. Schwarz HP, Fischer M, Hopmeier P, Batard MA, Griffin JH. Plasma protein S deficiency in familial thrombotic disease. *Blood.* 1984;64(6):1297-1300.
126. Cooper PC, Hampton KK, Makris M, Abuzenadah A, Paul B, Preston FE. Further evidence that activated protein C resistance can be misdiagnosed as inherited functional protein S deficiency. *Br J Haematol.* 1994;88(1):201-203.
127. Pintao MC, Ribeiro DD, Bezemer ID, et al. Protein S levels and the risk of venous thrombosis: results from the MEGA case-control study. *Blood.* 2013;122(18):3210-3219.
128. Comp PC. Measurement of the natural anticoagulant protein S. How and when. *Am J Clin Pathol.* 1990;94(2):242-243.
129. Zoller B, Berntsdotter A, Garcia de Frutos P, Dahlback B. Resistance to activated protein C as an additional genetic risk factor in hereditary deficiency of protein S. *Blood.* 1995;85(12):3518-3523.
130. Sie P, Boneu B, Bierme R, Wiesel ML, Grunebaum L, Cazenave JP. Arterial thrombosis and protein S deficiency. *Thromb Haemost.* 1989;62(3):1040.
131. Mahasandana C, Suvatte V, Chuansumrit A, et al. Homozygous protein S deficiency in an infant with purpura fulminans. *J Pediatr.* 1990;117(5):750-753.
132. Boyer-Neumann C, Bertina RM, Tripodi A, et al. Comparison of functional assays for protein S: European collaborative study of patients with congenital and acquired deficiency. *Thromb Haemost.* 1993;70(6):946-950.
133. Hubbard AR, Wong MY. A collaborative study on the measurement of protein S antigen in plasma. *Thromb Haemost.* 1992;68(2):115-118.
134. Edson JR, Vogt JM, Huesman DA. Laboratory diagnosis of inherited protein S deficiency. *Am J Clin Pathol.* 1990;94(2):176-186.
135. Broze GJ Jr. Protein Z-dependent regulation of coagulation. *Thromb Haemost.* 2001;86(1):8-13.
136. Sofi F, Cesari F, Abbate R, Gensini GF, Broze G Jr, Fedi S. A meta-analysis of potential risks of low levels of protein Z for diseases related to vascular thrombosis. *Thromb Haemost.* 2010;103(4):749-756.
137. Vasse M, Guegan-Massardier E, Borg JY, Woimant F, Soria C. Frequency of protein Z deficiency in patients with ischaemic stroke. *Lancet.* 2001;357(9260):933-934.
138. Slomka A, Kowalewski M, Zekanowska E, Suwalski P, Lorusso R, Eikelboom JW. Plasma levels of protein Z in ischemic stroke: a systematic review and meta-analysis. *Thromb Haemost.* 2020;120(5):815-822.
139. Dahlback B, Carlsson M, Svensson PJ. Familial thrombophilia due to a previously unrecognized mechanism characterized by poor anticoagulant response to activated protein C: prediction of a cofactor to activated protein C. *Proc Natl Acad Sci U S A.* 1993;90(3):1004-1008.
140. Koster T, Rosendaal FR, de Ronde H, Briet E, Vandenbroucke JP, Bertina RM. Venous thrombosis due to poor anticoagulant response to activated protein C: Leiden Thrombophilia Study. *Lancet.* 1993;342(8886-8887):1503-1506.
141. Svensson PJ, Dahlback B. Resistance to activated protein C as a basis for venous thrombosis. *N Engl J Med.* 1994;330(8):517-522.
142. Griffin JH, Evatt B, Wideman C, Fernandez JA. Anticoagulant protein C pathway defective in majority of thrombophilic patients. *Blood.* 1993;82(7):1989-1993.
143. Bertina RM, Koeleman BP, Koster T, et al. Mutation in blood coagulation factor V associated with resistance to activated protein C. *Nature.* 1994;369(6475):64-67.
144. Kalafatis M, Haley PE, Lu D, Bertina RM, Long GL, Mann KG. Proteolytic events that regulate factor V activity in whole plasma from normal and activated protein C (APC)-resistant individuals during clotting: an insight into the APC-resistance assay. *Blood.* 1996;87(11):4695-4707.
145. Heeb MJ, Kojima Y, Greengard JS, Griffin JH. Activated protein C resistance: molecular mechanisms based on studies using purified Gln506-factor V. *Blood.* 1995;85(12):3405-3411.
146. De Stefano V, Chiusolo P, Paciaroni K, Leone G. Epidemiology of factor V Leiden: clinical implications. *Semin Thromb Hemost.* 1998;24(4):367-379.
147. Ridker PM, Miletich JP, Hennekens CH, Buring JE. Ethnic distribution of factor V Leiden in 4047 men and women. Implications for venous thromboembolism screening. *J Am Med Assoc.* 1997;277(16):1305-1307.
148. Castoldi E, Rosing J. APC resistance: biological basis and acquired influences. *J Thromb Haemost.* 2010;8(3):445-453.
149. Rodeghiero F, Tosetto A. Activated protein C resistance and factor V Leiden mutation are independent risk factors for venous thromboembolism. *Ann Intern Med.* 1999;130(8):643-650.
150. Zivelin A, Griffin JH, Xu X, et al. A single genetic origin for a common caucasian risk factor for venous thrombosis. *Blood.* 1997;89(2):397-402.
151. Middeldorp S, Henkens CM, Koopman MM, et al. The incidence of venous thromboembolism in family members of patients with factor V Leiden mutation and venous thrombosis. *Ann Intern Med.* 1998;128(1):15-20.
152. Gerhardt A, Scharf RE, Beckmann MW, et al. Prothrombin and factor V mutations in women with a history of thrombosis during pregnancy and the puerperium. *N Engl J Med.* 2000;342(6):374-380.
153. Rosendaal FR, Vessey M, Rumley A, et al. Hormonal replacement therapy, prothrombotic mutations and the risk of venous thrombosis. *Br J Haematol.* 2002;116(4):851-854.
154. Herrington DM, Vittinghoff E, Howard TD, et al. Factor V Leiden, hormone replacement therapy, and risk of venous thromboembolic events in women with coronary disease. *Arterioscler Thromb Vasc Biol.* 2002;22(6):1012-1017.

155. Ridker PM, Hennekens CH, Lindpaintner K, Stampfer MJ, Eisenberg PR, Miletich JP. Mutation in the gene coding for coagulation factor V and the risk of myocardial infarction, stroke, and venous thrombosis in apparently healthy men. *N Engl J Med*. 1995;332(14):912-917.
156. Kutteh WH, Park VM, Deitcher SR. Hypercoagulable state mutation analysis in white patients with early first-trimester recurrent pregnancy loss. *Fertil Steril*. 1999;71(6):1048-1053.
157. Pipe SW, Schmaier AH, Nichols WC, Ginsburg D, Bozynski ME, Castle VP. Neonatal purpura fulminans in association with factor V R506Q mutation. *J Pediatr*. 1996;128(5 pt 1):706-709.
158. Gurgey A, Mesci L, Renda Y, Olcay L, Kocak N, Erdem G. Factor V Q 506 mutation in children with thrombosis. *Am J Hematol*. 1996;53(1):37-39.
159. Otterson GA, Monahan BP, Harold N, Steinberg SM, Frame JN, Kaye FJ. Clinical significance of the FV: Q506 mutation in unselected oncology patients. *Am J Med*. 1996;101(4):406-412.
160. Ridker PM, Miletich JP, Stampfer MJ, Goldhaber SZ, Lindpaintner K, Hennekens CH. Factor V Leiden and risks of recurrent idiopathic venous thromboembolism. *Circulation*. 1995;92(10):2800-2802.
161. Simioni P, Prandoni P, Lensing AW, et al. The risk of recurrent venous thromboembolism in patients with an Arg506-->Gln mutation in the gene for factor V (factor V Leiden). *N Engl J Med*. 1997;336(6):399-403.
162. Emmerich J, Alhenc-Gelas M, Aillaud MF, et al. Clinical features in 36 patients homozygous for the ARG 506-->GLN factor V mutation. *Thromb Haemost*. 1997;77(4):620-623.
163. Rintelen C, Mannhalter C, Ireland H, et al. Oral contraceptives enhance the risk of clinical manifestation of venous thrombosis at a young age in females homozygous for factor V Leiden. *Br J Haematol*. 1996;93(2):487-490.
164. Lindmarker P, Schulman S, Sten-Linder M, Wiman B, Egberg N, Johnsson H. The risk of recurrent venous thromboembolism in carriers and non-carriers of the G1691A allele in the coagulation factor V gene and the G20210A allele in the prothrombin gene. DURAC Trial Study Group. Duration of anticoagulation. *Thromb Haemost*. 1999;81(5):684-689.
165. Dahlback B. The discovery of activated protein C resistance. *J Thromb Haemost*. 2003;1(1):3-9.
166. de Ronde H, Bertina RM. Laboratory diagnosis of APC-resistance: a critical evaluation of the test and the development of diagnostic criteria. *Thromb Haemost*. 1994;72(6):880-886.
167. Jorquera JI, Montoro JM, Fernandez MA, Aznar JA, Aznar J. Modified test for activated protein C resistance. *Lancet*. 1994;344(8930):1162-1163.
168. Le DT, Griffin JH, Greengard JS, Mujumdar V, Rapaport SI. Use of a generally applicable tissue factor–dependent factor V assay to detect activated protein C-resistant factor Va in patients receiving warfarin and in patients with a lupus anticoagulant. *Blood*. 1995;85(7):1704-1711.
169. Press RD, Bauer KA, Kujovich JL, Heit JA. Clinical utility of factor V Leiden (R506Q) testing for the diagnosis and management of thromboembolic disorders. *Arch Pathol Lab Med*. 2002;126(11):1304-1318.
170. Johnson NV, Khor B, Van Cott EM. Advances in laboratory testing for thrombophilia. *Am J Hematol*. 2012;87(suppl 1):S108-S112.
171. Nogami K, Shinozawa K, Ogiwara K, et al. Novel FV mutation (W1920R, FVNara) associated with serious deep vein thrombosis and more potent APC resistance relative to FVLeiden. *Blood*. 2014;123(15):2420-2428.
172. Poort SR, Rosendaal FR, Reitsma PH, Bertina RM. A common genetic variation in the 3'-untranslated region of the prothrombin gene is associated with elevated plasma prothrombin levels and an increase in venous thrombosis. *Blood*. 1996;88(10):3698-3703.
173. Warshawsky I, Hren C, Sercia L, et al. Detection of a novel point mutation of the prothrombin gene at position 20209. *Diagn Mol Pathol*. 2002;11(3):152-156.
174. Pollak ES, Lam HS, Russell JE. The G20210A mutation does not affect the stability of prothrombin mRNA in vivo. *Blood*. 2002;100(1):359-362.
175. Butenas S, van't Veer C, Mann KG. "Normal" thrombin generation. *Blood*. 1999;94(7):2169-2178.
176. Rosendaal FR, Doggen CJ, Zivelin A, et al. Geographic distribution of the 20210 G to A prothrombin variant. *Thromb Haemost*. 1998;79(4):706-708.
177. Margaglione M, Brancaccio V, Giuliani N, et al. Increased risk for venous thrombosis in carriers of the prothrombin G-->A20210 gene variant. *Ann Intern Med*. 1998;129(2):89-93.
178. Martinelli I, Taioli E, Bucciarelli P, Akhavan S, Mannucci PM. Interaction between the G20210A mutation of the prothrombin gene and oral contraceptive use in deep vein thrombosis. *Arterioscler Thromb Vasc Biol*. 1999;19(3):700-703.
179. Martinelli I, Sacchi E, Landi G, Taioli E, Duca F, Mannucci PM. High risk of cerebral-vein thrombosis in carriers of a prothrombin-gene mutation and in users of oral contraceptives. *N Engl J Med*. 1998;338(25):1793-1797.
180. Kyrle PA, Mannhalter C, Beguin S, et al. Clinical studies and thrombin generation in patients homozygous or heterozygous for the G20210A mutation in the prothrombin gene. *Arterioscler Thromb Vasc Biol*. 1998;18(8):1287-1291.
181. De Stefano V, Martinelli I, Mannucci PM, et al. The risk of recurrent venous thromboembolism among heterozygous carriers of the G20210A prothrombin gene mutation. *Br J Haematol*. 2001;113(3):630-635.
182. Eichinger S, Minar E, Hirschl M, et al. The risk of early recurrent venous thromboembolism after oral anticoagulant therapy in patients with the G20210A transition in the prothrombin gene. *Thromb Haemost*. 1999;81(1):14-17.
183. Ridker PM, Hennekens CH, Miletich JP. G20210A mutation in prothrombin gene and risk of myocardial infarction, stroke, and venous thrombosis in a large cohort of US men. *Circulation*. 1999;99(8):999-1004.
184. Clarke R, Daly L, Robinson K, et al. Hyperhomocysteinemia: an independent risk factor for vascular disease. *N Engl J Med*. 1991;324(17):1149-1155.
185. Stampfer MJ, Malinow MR, Willett WC, et al. A prospective study of plasma homocyst(e)ine and risk of myocardial infarction in US physicians. *J Am Med Assoc*. 1992;268(7):877-881.
186. Molgaard J, Malinow MR, Lassvik C, Holm AC, Upson B, Olsson AG. Hyperhomocyst(e)inaemia: an independent risk factor for intermittent claudication. *J Intern Med*. 1992;231(3):273-279.
187. Study of the Effectiveness of Additional Reductions in Cholesterol and Homocysteine Collaborative Group; Armitage JM, Bowman L, et al. Effects of homocysteine-lowering with folic acid plus vitamin B12 vs placebo on mortality and major morbidity in myocardial infarction survivors: a randomized trial. *J Am Med Assoc*. 2010;303(24):2486-2494.
188. Rees MM, Rodgers GM. Homocysteinemia: association of a metabolic disorder with vascular disease and thrombosis. *Thromb Res*. 1993;71(5):337-359.
189. Harker LA, Slichter SJ, Scott CR, Ross R. Homocystinemia. Vascular injury and arterial thrombosis. *N Engl J Med*. 1974;291(11):537-543.
190. Lentz SR, Piegors DJ, Fernandez JA, et al. Effect of hyperhomocysteinemia on protein C activation and activity. *Blood*. 2002;100(6):2108-2112.
191. Mudd SH, Levy HL, Skovby F. Disorders of transsulfuration. In: Scriver CR, Beaudet AL, Sly WS, Valle D, eds. *The Metabolic Basis of Inherited Disease*. 6th ed. McGraw-Hill; 1989:693-734.
192. Hanson NQ, Aras O, Yang F, Tsai MY. C677T and A1298C polymorphisms of the methylenetetrahydrofolate reductase gene: incidence and effect of combined genotypes on plasma fasting and post-methionine load homocysteine in vascular disease. *Clin Chem*. 2001;47(4):661-666.
193. den Heijer M, Koster T, Blom HJ, et al. Hyperhomocysteinemia as a risk factor for deep-vein thrombosis. *N Engl J Med*. 1996;334(12):759-762.
194. Simioni P, Prandoni P, Burlina A, et al. Hyperhomocysteinemia and deep-vein thrombosis. A case-control study. *Thromb Haemost*. 1996;76(6):883-886.
195. Kottke-Marchant K, Green R, Jacobsen DW, et al. High plasma homocysteine: a risk factor for arterial and venous thrombosis in patients with normal coagulation profiles. *Clin Appl Thromb Hemost*. 1997;3(4):239-244.
196. Van Cott EM, Laposata M. Laboratory evaluation of hypercoagulable states. *Hematol Oncol Clin North Am*. 1998;12(6):1141-1166.
197. Key NS, McGlennen RC. Hyperhomocyst(e)inemia and Thrombophilia. *Arch Pathol Lab Med*. 2002;126(11):1367-1375.
198. Ueland PM, Refsum H, Stabler SP, Malinow MR, Andersson A, Allen RH. Total homocysteine in plasma or serum: methods and clinical applications. *Clin Chem*. 1993;39(9):1764-1779.
199. Homocysteine Lowering Trialists' Collaboration. Lowering blood homocysteine with folic acid based supplements: meta-analysis of randomised trials. Homocysteine Lowering Trialists' Collaboration. *Br Med J* 1998;316(7135):894-898.
200. Wilcken DE, Wilcken B, Dudman NP, Tyrrell PA. Homocystinuria–the effects of betaine in the treatment of patients not responsive to pyridoxine. *N Engl J Med*. 1983;309(8):448-453.
201. Lonn E, Yusuf S, Arnold MJ, et al. Homocysteine lowering with folic acid and B vitamins in vascular disease. *N Engl J Med*. 2006;354(15):1567-1577.
202. Bonaa KH, Njolstad I, Ueland PM, et al. Homocysteine lowering and cardiovascular events after acute myocardial infarction. *N Engl J Med*. 2006;354(15):1578-1588.
203. Ray JG, Kearon C, Yi Q, Sheridan P, Lonn E. Heart Outcomes Prevention Evaluation I. Homocysteine-lowering therapy and risk for venous thromboembolism: a randomized trial. *Ann Intern Med*. 2007;146(11):761-767.
204. Koster T, Blann AD, Briet E, Vandenbroucke JP, Rosendaal FR. Role of clotting factor VIII in effect of von Willebrand factor on occurrence of deep-vein thrombosis. *Lancet*. 1995;345(8943):152-155.
205. Bloemenkamp KW, Helmerhorst FM, Rosendaal FR, Vandenbroucke JP. Venous thrombosis, oral contraceptives and high factor VIII levels. *Thromb Haemost*. 1999;82(3):1024-1027.
206. O'Donnell J, Mumford AD, Manning RA, Laffan M. Elevation of FVIII: C in venous thromboembolism is persistent and independent of the acute phase response. *Thromb Haemost*. 2000;83(1):10-13.
207. Bank I, van de Poel MH, Coppens M, et al. Absolute annual incidences of first events of venous thromboembolism and arterial vascular events in individuals with elevated FVIII:c. A prospective family cohort study. *Thromb Haemost*. 2007;98(5):1040-1044.
208. Chandler WL, Rodgers GM, Sprouse JT, Thompson AR. Elevated hemostatic factor levels as potential risk factors for thrombosis. *Arch Pathol Lab Med*. 2002;126(11):1405-1414.
209. Cushman M, O'Meara ES, Folsom AR, Heckbert SR. Coagulation factors IX through XIII and the risk of future venous thrombosis: the Longitudinal Investigation of Thromboembolism Etiology. *Blood*. 2009;114(14):2878-2883.
210. Yang DT, Flanders MM, Kim H, Rodgers GM. Elevated factor XI activity levels are associated with an increased odds ratio for cerebrovascular events. *Am J Clin Pathol*. 2006;126(3):411-415.
211. Hong JJ, Kwaan HC. Hereditary defects in fibrinolysis associated with thrombosis. *Semin Thromb Hemost*. 1999;25(3):321-331.
212. Prins MH, Hirsh J. A critical review of the evidence supporting a relationship between impaired fibrinolytic activity and venous thromboembolism. *Arch Intern Med*. 1991;151(9):1721-1731.
213. Lisman T, de Groot PG, Meijers JC, Rosendaal FR. Reduced plasma fibrinolytic potential is a risk factor for venous thrombosis. *Blood*. 2005;105(3):1102-1105.
214. Eichinger S, Schonauer V, Weltermann A, et al. Thrombin-activatable fibrinolysis inhibitor and the risk for recurrent venous thromboembolism. *Blood*. 2004;103(10):3773-3776.
215. Meltzer ME, Doggen CJ, de Groot PG, Rosendaal FR, Lisman T. Plasma levels of fibrinolytic proteins and the risk of myocardial infarction in men. *Blood*. 2010;116(4):529-536.

216. Meltzer ME, Lisman T, de Groot PG, et al. Venous thrombosis risk associated with plasma hypofibrinolysis is explained by elevated plasma levels of TAFI and PAI-1. *Blood*. 2010;116(1):113-121.
217. Aoki N, Moroi M, Sakata Y, Yoshida N, Matsuda M. Abnormal plasminogen. A hereditary molecular abnormality found in a patient with recurrent thrombosis. *J Clin Invest*. 1978;61(5):1186-1195.
218. Dolan G, Greaves M, Cooper P, Preston FE. Thrombovascular disease and familial plasminogen deficiency: a report of three kindreds. *Br J Haematol*. 1988;70(4):417-421.
219. Tsutsumi S, Saito T, Sakata T, Mlyata T, Ichinose A. Genetic diagnosis of dysplasminogenemia: detection of an Ala601-Thr mutation in 118 out of 125 families and identification of a new Asp676-Asn mutation. *Thromb Haemost*. 1996;76(2):135-138.
220. Shigekiyo T, Uno Y, Tomonari A, et al. Type I congenital plasminogen deficiency is not a risk factor for thrombosis. *Thromb Haemost*. 1992;67(2):189-192.
221. Schuster V, Hugle B, Tefs K. Plasminogen deficiency. *J Thromb Haemost*. 2007;5(12):2315-2322.
222. Tefs K, Gueorguieva M, Klammt J, et al. Molecular and clinical spectrum of type I plasminogen deficiency: a series of 50 patients. *Blood*. 2006;108(9):3021-3026.
223. Brandt JT. Plasminogen and tissue-type plasminogen activator deficiency as risk factors for thromboembolic disease. *Arch Pathol Lab Med*. 2002;126(11):1376-1381.
224. Chandler WL, Trimble SL, Loo SC, Mornin D. Effect of PAI-1 levels on the molar concentrations of active tissue plasminogen activator (t-PA) and t-PA/PAI-1 complex in plasma. *Blood*. 1990;76(5):930-937.
225. Chandler WL, Schmer G, Stratton JR. Optimum conditions for the stabilization and measurement of tissue plasminogen activator activity in human plasma. *J Lab Clin Med*. 1989;113(3):362-371.
226. Chandler WL, Loo SC, Nguyen SV, Schmer G, Stratton JR. Standardization of methods for measuring plasminogen activator inhibitor activity in human plasma. *Clin Chem*. 1989;35(5):787-793.
227. Angleton P, Chandler WL, Schmer G. Diurnal variation of tissue-type plasminogen activator and its rapid inhibitor (PAI-1). *Circulation*. 1989;79(1):101-106.
228. Stringer HA, van Swieten P, Heijnen HF, Sixma JJ, Pannekoek H. Plasminogen activator inhibitor-1 released from activated platelets plays a key role in thrombolysis resistance. Studies with thrombi generated in the Chandler loop. *Arterioscler Thromb*. 1994;14(9):1452-1458.
229. Juhan-Vague I, Valadier J, Alessi MC, et al. Deficient t-PA release and elevated PA inhibitor levels in patients with spontaneous or recurrent deep venous thrombosis. *Thromb Haemost*. 1987;57(1):67-72.
230. D'Angelo A, Kluft C, Verheijen JH, Rijken DC, Mozzi E, Mannucci PM. Fibrinolytic shut-down after surgery: impairment of the balance between tissue-type plasminogen activator and its specific inhibitor. *Eur J Clin Invest*. 1985;15(6):308-312.
231. Hamsten A, Wiman B, de Faire U, Blomback M. Increased plasma levels of a rapid inhibitor of tissue plasminogen activator in young survivors of myocardial infarction. *N Engl J Med*. 1985;313(25):1557-1563.
232. Meade TW, Chakrabarti R, Haines AP, North WR, Stirling Y. Characteristics affecting fibrinolytic activity and plasma fibrinogen concentrations. *Br Med J*. 1979;1(6157):153-156.
233. Vaughan DE, Rouleau JL, Ridker PM, Arnold JM, Menapace FJ, Pfeffer MA. Effects of ramipril on plasma fibrinolytic balance in patients with acute anterior myocardial infarction. HEART Study Investigators. *Circulation*. 1997;96(2):442-447.
234. Pahor M, Franse LV, Deitcher SR, et al. Fosinopril versus amlodipine comparative treatments study: a randomized trial to assess effects on plasminogen activator inhibitor-1. *Circulation*. 2002;105(4):457-461.
235. Fujii S, Sobel BE. Direct effects of gemfibrozil on the fibrinolytic system. Diminution of synthesis of plasminogen activator inhibitor type 1. *Circulation*. 1992;85(5):1888-1893.
236. Gebara OC, Mittleman MA, Sutherland P, et al. Association between increased estrogen status and increased fibrinolytic potential in the Framingham Offspring Study. *Circulation*. 1995;91(7):1952-1958.
237. Ridker PM, Vaughan DE, Stampfer MJ, Glynn RJ, Hennekens CH. Association of moderate alcohol consumption and plasma concentration of endogenous tissue-type plasminogen activator. *J Am Med Assoc*. 1994;272(12):929-933.
238. Bithell TC. Hereditary dysfibrinogenemia. *Clin Chem*. 1985;31(4):509-516.
239. Rodgers GM, Garr SB. Comparison of functional and antigenic fibrinogen values from a normal population. *Thromb Res*. 1992;68(3):207-210.
240. Carrell N, Gabriel DA, Blatt PM, Carr ME, McDonagh J. Hereditary dysfibrinogenemia in a patient with thrombotic disease. *Blood*. 1983;62(2):439-447.
241. Cunningham MT, Brandt JT, Laposata M, Olson JD. Laboratory diagnosis of dysfibrinogenemia. *Arch Pathol Lab Med*. 2002;126(4):499-505.
242. Kunz G, Ohlin AK, Adami A, Zoller B, Svensson P, Lane DA. Naturally occurring mutations in the thrombomodulin gene leading to impaired expression and function. *Blood*. 2002;99(10):3646-3653.
243. Faioni EM, Franchi F, Castaman G, Biguzzi E, Rodeghiero F. Mutations in the thrombomodulin gene are rare in patients with severe thrombophilia. *Br J Haematol*. 2002;118(2):595-599.
244. Ireland H, Kunz G, Kyriakoulis K, Stubbs PJ, Lane DA. Thrombomodulin gene mutations associated with myocardial infarction. *Circulation*. 1997;96(1):15-18.
245. Salomaa V, Matei C, Aleksic N, et al. Soluble thrombomodulin as a predictor of incident coronary heart disease and symptomless carotid artery atherosclerosis in the Atherosclerosis Risk in Communities (ARIC) Study: a case-cohort study. *Lancet*. 1999;353(9166):1729-1734.
246. Scanu AM. Structural and functional polymorphism of lipoprotein(a): biological and clinical implications. *Clin Chem*. 1995;41(1):170-172.
247. Kullo IJ, Gau GT, Tajik AJ. Novel risk factors for atherosclerosis. *Mayo Clin Proc*. 2000;75(4):369-380.
248. Miles LA, Plow EF. Lp(a): an interloper into the fibrinolytic system? *Thromb Haemost*. 1990;63(3):331-335.
249. Scanu AM. Lipoprotein(a). A genetic risk factor for premature coronary heart disease. *J Am Med Assoc*. 1992;267(24):3326-3329.
250. Maeda S, Abe A, Seishima M, Makino K, Noma A, Kawade M. Transient changes of serum lipoprotein(a) as an acute phase protein. *Atherosclerosis*. 1989;78(2-3):145-150.
251. Dahm A, Van Hylckama Vlieg A, Bendz B, Rosendaal F, Bertina RM, Sandset PM. Low levels of tissue factor pathway inhibitor (TFPI) increase the risk of venous thrombosis. *Blood*. 2003;101(11):4387-4392.
252. Hoke M, Kyrle PA, Minar E, et al. Tissue factor pathway inhibitor and the risk of recurrent venous thromboembolism. *Thromb Haemost*. 2005;94(4):787-790.
253. Winckers K, Siegerink B, Duckers C, et al. Increased tissue factor pathway inhibitor activity is associated with myocardial infarction in young women: results from the RATIO study. *J Thromb Haemost*. 2011;9(11):2243-2250.
254. van Boven HH, Reitsma PH, Rosendaal FR, et al. Factor V Leiden (FV R506Q) in families with inherited antithrombin deficiency. *Thromb Haemost*. 1996;75(3):417-421.
255. Margaglione M, D'Andrea G, Colaizzo D, et al. Coexistence of factor V Leiden and Factor II A20210 mutations and recurrent venous thromboembolism. *Thromb Haemost*. 1999;82(6):1583-1587.
256. Dizon-Townson D, Hutchison C, Silver R, Branch DW, Ward K. The factor V Leiden mutation which predisposes to thrombosis is not common in patients with antiphospholipid syndrome. *Thromb Haemost*. 1995;74(4):1029-1031.
257. Mandel H, Brenner B, Berant M, et al. Coexistence of hereditary homocystinuria and factor V Leiden–effect on thrombosis. *N Engl J Med*. 1996;334(12):763-768.
258. Ridker PM, Hennekens CH, Selhub J, Miletich JP, Malinow MR, Stampfer MJ. Interrelation of hyperhomocyst(e)inemia, factor V Leiden, and risk of future venous thromboembolism. *Circulation*. 1997;95(7):1777-1782.
259. Junker R, Koch HG, Auberger K, Munchow N, Ehrenforth S, Nowak-Gottl U. Prothrombin G20210A gene mutation and further prothrombotic risk factors in childhood thrombophilia. *Arterioscler Thromb Vasc Biol*. 1999;19(10):2568-2572.
260. Sifontes MT, Nuss R, Hunger SP, Waters J, Jacobson LJ, Manco-Johnson M. Activated protein C resistance and the factor V Leiden mutation in children with thrombosis. *Am J Hematol*. 1998;57(1):29-32.
261. Chalmers EA. Neonatal thrombosis. *J Clin Pathol*. 2000;53(6):419-423.
262. Nowak-Gottl U, Junker R, Kreuz W, et al. Risk of recurrent venous thrombosis in children with combined prothrombotic risk factors. *Blood*. 2001;97(4):858-862.
263. Flanders MM, Phansalkar AR, Crist RA, Roberts WL, Rodgers GM. Pediatric reference intervals for uncommon bleeding and thrombotic disorders. *J Pediatr*. 2006;149(2):275-277.
264. Manco-Johnson MJ, Grabowski EF, Hellgreen M, et al. Laboratory testing for thrombophilia in pediatric patients. On behalf of the subcommittee for perinatal and pediatric thrombosis of the scientific and standardization committee of the International Society of Thrombosis and Haemostasis (ISTH). *Thromb Haemost*. 2002;88(1):155-156.
265. Tormene D, Simioni P, Prandoni P, et al. The incidence of venous thromboembolism in thrombophilic children: a prospective cohort study. *Blood*. 2002;100(7):2403-2405.
266. Raffini L, Thornburg C. Testing children for inherited thrombophilia: more questions than answers. *Br J Haematol*. 2009;147(3):277-288.
267. Curtis C, Mineyko A, Massicotte P, et al. Thrombophilia risk is not increased in children after perinatal stroke. *Blood*. 2017;129(20):2793-2800.
268. Monagle P, Chan AKC, Goldenberg NA, et al. Antithrombotic therapy in neonates and children: antithrombotic therapy and prevention of thrombosis, 9th ed. American College of Chest Physicians Evidence-Based Clinical Practice Guidelines. *Chest*. 2012;141(2 suppl):e737S-e801S.
269. Schafer AI. Hypercoagulable states: molecular genetics to clinical practice. *Lancet*. 1994;344(8939-8940):1739-1742.
270. Bauer KA. The thrombophilias: well-defined risk factors with uncertain therapeutic implications. *Ann Intern Med*. 2001;135(5):367-373.
271. van Sluis GL, Sohne M, El Kheir DY, Tanck MW, Gerdes VE, Buller HR. Family history and inherited thrombophilia. *J Thromb Haemost*. 2006;4(10):2182-2187.
272. Somma J, Sussman II, Rand JH. An evaluation of thrombophilia screening in an urban tertiary care medical center: a "real world" experience. *Am J Clin Pathol*. 2006;126(1):120-127.
273. Turkstra F, van Beek EJ, ten Cate JW, Buller HR. Reliable rapid blood test for the exclusion of venous thromboembolism in symptomatic outpatients. *Thromb Haemost*. 1996;76(1):9-11.
274. Palareti G, Legnani C, Cosmi B, Guazzaloca G, Pancani C, Coccheri S. Risk of venous thromboembolism recurrence: high negative predictive value of D-dimer performed after oral anticoagulation is stopped. *Thromb Haemost*. 2002;87(1):7-12.
275. Cushman M, Folsom AR, Wang L, et al. Fibrin fragment D-dimer and the risk of future venous thrombosis. *Blood*. 2003;101(4):1243-1248.
276. Teitel JM, Bauer KA, Lau HK, Rosenberg RD. Studies of the prothrombin activation pathway utilizing radioimmunoassays for the F2/F1 + 2 fragment and thrombin–antithrombin complex. *Blood*. 1982;59(5):1086-1097.
277. Al-Samkari H, Song F, Van Cott EM, Kuter DJ, Rosovsky R. Evaluation of the prothrombin fragment 1.2 in patients with coronavirus disease 2019 (COVID-19). *Am J Hematol*. 2020;95(12):1479-1485.
278. Kearon C, Ginsberg JS, Douketis J, et al. Management of suspected deep venous thrombosis in outpatients by using clinical assessment and D-dimer testing. *Ann Intern Med*. 2001;135(2):108-111.
279. Douma RA, Tan M, Schutgens RE, et al. Using an age-dependent D-dimer cut-off value increases the number of older patients in whom deep vein thrombosis can be safely excluded. *Haematologica*. 2012;97(10):1507-1513.

280. Palareti G, Cosmi B, Legnani C, et al. D-dimer testing to determine the duration of anticoagulation therapy. *N Engl J Med.* 2006;355(17):1780-1789.
281. Ageno W, Cosmi B, Ghirarduzzi A, et al. The negative predictive value of D-dimer on the risk of recurrent venous thromboembolism in patients with multiple previous events: a prospective cohort study (the PROLONG PLUS study). *Am J Hematol.* 2012;87(7):713-715.
282. Kearon C, Spencer FA, O'Keeffe D, et al. D-dimer testing to select patients with a first unprovoked venous thromboembolism who can stop anticoagulant therapy: a cohort study. *Ann Intern Med.* 2015;162(1):27-34.
283. Goodwin AJ, Higgins RA, Moser KA, et al. Issues surrounding age-adjusted d-dimer cutoffs that practicing physicians need to know when evaluating patients with suspected pulmonary embolism. *Ann Intern Med.* 2017;166(5):361-363.
284. Furlan AJ, Fisher M. Devices, drugs, and the Food and Drug Administration: increasing implications for ischemic stroke. *Stroke.* 2005;36(2):398-399.
285. Davies B, Braithwaite BD, Birch PA, Poskitt KR, Heather BP, Earnshaw JJ. Acute leg ischaemia in Gloucestershire. *Br J Surg.* 1997;84(4):504-508.
286. Ouriel K. Peripheral arterial disease. *Lancet.* 2001;358(9289):1257-1264.
287. Antiplatelet Trialists' Collaboration. Secondary prevention of vascular disease by prolonged antiplatelet treatment. *Br Med J* 1988;296(6618):320-331.
288. Antithrombotic Trialists' Collaboration. Collaborative meta-analysis of randomised trials of antiplatelet therapy for prevention of death, myocardial infarction, and stroke in high risk patients. *Br Med J.* 2002;324(7329):71-86.
289. Eikelboom JW, Hirsh J, Spencer FA, Baglin TP, Weitz JI. Antiplatelet drugs: antithrombotic therapy and prevention of thrombosis, 9th ed. American College of Chest Physicians Evidence-Based Clinical Practice Guidelines. *Chest.* 2012;141(2 suppl):e89S-e119S.
290. De Meyer SF, Vanhoorelbeke K, Broos K. Salles, II, Deckmyn H. Antiplatelet drugs. *Br J Haematol.* 2008;142(4):515-528.
291. Michelson AD. Advances in antiplatelet therapy. *Hematology Am Soc Hematol Educ Program.* 2011;2011:62-69.
292. Roth GJ, Majerus PW. The mechanism of the effect of aspirin on human platelets. I. Acetylation of a particulate fraction protein. *J Clin Invest.* 1975;56(3):624-632.
293. Catella-Lawson F, Reilly MP, Kapoor SC, et al. Cyclooxygenase inhibitors and the antiplatelet effects of aspirin. *N Engl J Med.* 2001;345(25):1809-1817.
294. Garcia Rodriguez LA, Varas C, Patrono C. Differential effects of aspirin and non-aspirin nonsteroidal antiinflammatory drugs in the primary prevention of myocardial infarction in postmenopausal women. *Epidemiology.* 2000;11(4):382-387.
295. Masotti G, Galanti G, Poggesi L, Abbate R, Neri Serneri GG. Differential inhibition of prostacyclin production and platelet aggregation by aspirin. *Lancet.* 1979;2(8154):1213-1217.
296. Patrignani P, Filabozzi P, Patrono C. Selective cumulative inhibition of platelet thromboxane production by low-dose aspirin in healthy subjects. *J Clin Invest.* 1982;69(6):1366-1372.
297. Hirsh J. The optimal antithrombotic dose of aspirin. *Arch Intern Med.* 1985;145(9):1582-1583.
298. Mangano DT; Multicenter Study of Perioperative Ischemia Research G. Aspirin and mortality from coronary bypass surgery. *N Engl J Med.* 2002;347(17):1309-1317.
299. Raber I, McCarthy CP, Vaduganathan M, et al. The rise and fall of aspirin in the primary prevention of cardiovascular disease. *Lancet.* 2019;393(10186):2155-2167.
300. Bhatt DL, Fox KA, Hacke W, et al. Clopidogrel and aspirin versus aspirin alone for the prevention of atherothrombotic events. *N Engl J Med.* 2006;354(16):1706-1717.
301. Prevention of pulmonary embolism and deep vein thrombosis with low dose aspirin: pulmonary Embolism Prevention (PEP) trial. *Lancet.* 2000;355(9212):1295-1302.
302. Falck-Ytter Y, Francis CW, Johanson NA, et al. Prevention of VTE in orthopedic surgery patients: antithrombotic therapy and prevention of thrombosis, 9th ed. American College of Chest Physicians Evidence-Based Clinical Practice Guidelines. *Chest.* 2012;141(2 suppl):e278S-e325S.
303. Becattini C, Agnelli G, Schenone A, et al. Aspirin for preventing the recurrence of venous thromboembolism. *N Engl J Med.* 2012;366(21):1959-1967.
304. Warkentin TE. Aspirin for dual prevention of venous and arterial thrombosis. *N Engl J Med.* 2012;367(21):2039-2041.
305. Sanderson S, Emery J, Baglin T, Kinmonth AL. Narrative review: aspirin resistance and its clinical implications. *Ann Intern Med.* 2005;142(5):370-380.
306. Michelson AD, Cattaneo M, Eikelboom JW, et al. Aspirin resistance: position paper of the working group on aspirin resistance. *J Thromb Haemost.* 2005;3(6):1309-1311.
307. Dalen JE. Aspirin resistance: is it real? Is it clinically significant? *Am J Med.* 2007;120(1):1-4.
308. Smock KJ, Rodgers GM. Laboratory evaluation of aspirin responsiveness. *Am J Hematol.* 2010;85(5):358-360.
309. Du G, Lin Q, Wang J. A brief review on the mechanisms of aspirin resistance. *Int J Cardiol.* 2016;220:21-26.
310. Columbo JA, Lambour AJ, Sundling RA, et al. A meta-analysis of the impact of aspirin, clopidogrel, and dual antiplatelet therapy on bleeding complications in non-cardiac surgery. *Ann Surg.* 2018;267(1):1-10.
311. Quinn MJ, Fitzgerald DJ. Ticlopidine and clopidogrel. *Circulation.* 1999;100(15):1667-1672.
312. Gent M, Blakely JA, Easton JD, et al. The Canadian American Ticlopidine Study (CATS) in thromboembolic stroke. *Lancet.* 1989;1(8649):1215-1220.
313. Chen DK, Kim JS, Sutton DM. Thrombotic thrombocytopenic purpura associated with ticlopidine use: a report of 3 cases and review of the literature. *Arch Intern Med.* 1999;159(3):311-314.
314. Herbert JMFD, Vallee E, Kieffer G, et al. Clopidogrel, A novel antiplatelet and antithrombotic agent. *Cardiovasc Drug Rev.* 1993;11(2):180-198.
315. Caprie Steering Committee. A randomised, blinded, trial of clopidogrel versus aspirin in patients at risk of ischaemic events (CAPRIE). CAPRIE Steering Committee. *Lancet.* 1996;348(9038):1329-1339.
316. Mehta SR, Yusuf S, Peters RJ, et al. Effects of pretreatment with clopidogrel and aspirin followed by long-term therapy in patients undergoing percutaneous coronary intervention: the PCI-CURE study. *Lancet.* 2001;358(9281):527-533.
317. Bennett CL, Connors JM, Carwile JM, et al. Thrombotic thrombocytopenic purpura associated with clopidogrel. *N Engl J Med.* 2000;342(24):1773-1777.
318. Gurbel PA, Myat A, Kubica J, Tantry US. State of the art: oral antiplatelet therapy. *JRSM Cardiovasc Dis.* 2016;5:2048004016652514.
319. Wiviott SD, Antman EM, Winters KJ, et al. Randomized comparison of prasugrel (CS-747, LY640315), a novel thienopyridine P2Y12 antagonist, with clopidogrel in percutaneous coronary intervention: results of the Joint Utilization of Medications to Block Platelets Optimally (JUMBO)-TIMI 26 trial. *Circulation.* 2005;111(25):3366-3373.
320. Ortel TL. Perioperative management of patients on chronic antithrombotic therapy. *Blood.* 2012;120(24):4699-4705.
321. National Guideline Centre. *Evidence Review for Dual Antiplatelet Therapy: Acute Coronary Syndromes. Evidence Review A.* National Institute for Health and Care Excellence; 2020.
322. Tscharre M, Michelson AD, Gremmel T. Novel antiplatelet agents in cardiovascular disease. *J Cardiovasc Pharmacol Ther.* 2020;25(3):191-200.
323. Hynes RO. Integrins: versatility, modulation, and signaling in cell adhesion. *Cell.* 1992;69(1):11-25.
324. Dennis MS, Henzel WJ, Pitti RM, et al. Platelet glycoprotein IIb-IIIa protein antagonists from snake venoms: evidence for a family of platelet-aggregation inhibitors. *Proc Natl Acad Sci U S A.* 1990;87(7):2471-2475.
325. Topol EJ, Byzova TV, Plow EF. Platelet GPIIb-IIIa blockers. *Lancet.* 1999;353(9148):227-231.
326. Coller BS. Binding of abciximab to alpha V beta 3 and activated alpha M beta 2 receptors: with a review of platelet-leukocyte interactions. *Thromb Haemost.* 1999;82(2):326-336.
327. Barnes GD, Lucas E, Alexander GC, Goldberger ZD. National trends in ambulatory oral anticoagulant use. *Am J Med.* 2015;128(12):1300.e1302-1305.e1302.
328. Kearon C, Akl EA, Ornelas J, et al. Antithrombotic therapy for VTE disease: CHEST guideline and expert panel report. *Chest.* 2016;149(2):315-352.
329. McLean J. The thromboplastic action of cephalin. *Am J Physiol.* 1916;41:250-257.
330. Lam LH, Silbert JE, Rosenberg RD. The separation of active and inactive forms of heparin. *Biochem Biophys Res Commun.* 1976;69(2):570-577.
331. Rosenberg RD, Edelberg JM, Zhang L. *The heparin/antithrombin system: a natural anticoagulant mechanism. Hemostasis and Thrombosis: Basic Principles and Clinical Practice.* 4th ed. Lippincott Williams & Wilkins; 2001:711-732.
332. Bjork I, Jackson CM, Jornvall H, Lavine KK, Nordling K, Salsgiver WJ. The active site of antithrombin. Release of the same proteolytically cleaved form of the inhibitor from complexes with factor IXa, factor Xa, and thrombin. *J Biol Chem.* 1982;257(5):2406-2411.
333. Choay J, Petitou M, Lormeau JC, Sinay P, Casu B, Gatti G. Structure-activity relationship in heparin: a synthetic pentasaccharide with high affinity for antithrombin III and eliciting high anti-factor Xa activity. *Biochem Biophys Res Commun.* 1983;116(2):492-499.
334. Olson ST, Bjork I. Predominant contribution of surface approximation to the mechanism of heparin acceleration of the antithrombin-thrombin reaction. Elucidation from salt concentration effects. *J Biol Chem.* 1991;266(10):6353-6364.
335. Olson ST, Bjork I, Sheffer R, Craig PA, Shore JD, Choay J. Role of the antithrombin-binding pentasaccharide in heparin acceleration of antithrombin-proteinase reactions. Resolution of the antithrombin conformational change contribution to heparin rate enhancement. *J Biol Chem.* 1992;267(18):12528-12538.
336. Danielsson A, Raub E, Lindahl U, Bjork I. Role of ternary complexes, in which heparin binds both antithrombin and proteinase, in the acceleration of the reactions between antithrombin and thrombin or factor Xa. *J Biol Chem.* 1986;261(33):15467-15473.
337. Ofosu FA, Hirsh J, Esmon CT, et al. Unfractionated heparin inhibits thrombin-catalysed amplification reactions of coagulation more efficiently than those catalysed by factor Xa. *Biochem J.* 1989;257(1):143-150.
338. Bengtsson-Olivecrona G, Olivecrona T. Binding of active and inactive forms of lipoprotein lipase to heparin. Effects of pH. *Biochem J.* 1985;226(2):409-413.
339. Paliwal R, Paliwal SR, Agrawal GP, Vyas SP. Recent advances in search of oral heparin therapeutics. *Med Res Rev.* 2012;32(2):388-409.
340. Nyman D, Thurnherr N, Duckert F. Heparin dosage in extracorporeal circulation and its neutralization. *Thromb Diath Haemorrh.* 1975;33(1):102-104.
341. Hirsh J, van Aken WG, Gallus AS, Dollery CT, Cade JF, Yung WL. Heparin kinetics in venous thrombosis and pulmonary embolism. *Circulation.* 1976;53(4):691-695.
342. Hirsh J, Warkentin TE, Shaughnessy SG, et al. Heparin and low-molecular-weight heparin: mechanisms of action, pharmacokinetics, dosing, monitoring, efficacy, and safety. *Chest.* 2001;119(1 suppl):64S-94S.
343. Garcia DA, Baglin TP, Weitz JI, Samama MM. Parenteral anticoagulants: antithrombotic therapy and prevention of thrombosis, 9th ed. American College of Chest Physicians Evidence-Based Clinical Practice Guidelines. *Chest.* 2012;141(2 suppl):e24S-e43S.
344. Maclean PS, Tait RC. Hereditary and acquired antithrombin deficiency: epidemiology, pathogenesis and treatment options. *Drugs.* 2007;67(10):1429-1440.
345. Newhall KA, Saunders EC, Larson RJ, Stone DH, Goodney PP. Use of protamine for anticoagulation during carotid endarterectomy: a meta-analysis. *JAMA Surg.* 2016;151(3):247-255.
346. Levine MN, Hirsh J, Gent M, et al. A randomized trial comparing activated thromboplastin time with heparin assay in patients with acute venous thromboembolism requiring large daily doses of heparin. *Arch Intern Med.* 1994;154(1):49-56.
347. Nader HB, Walenga JM, Berkowitz SD, Ofosu F, Hoppensteadt DA, Cella G. Preclinical differentiation of low molecular weight heparins. *Semin Thromb Hemost.* 1999;25(suppl 3):63-72.

348. Casu B, Torri G. Structural characterization of low molecular weight heparins. *Semin Thromb Hemost.* 1999;25(suppl 3):17-25.
349. Montalescot G, Collet JP, Lison L, et al. Effects of various anticoagulant treatments on von Willebrand factor release in unstable angina. *J Am Coll Cardiol.* 2000;36(1):110-114.
350. Palm M, Mattsson C. Pharmacokinetics of heparin and low molecular weight heparin fragment (Fragmin) in rabbits with impaired renal or metabolic clearance. *Thromb Haemost.* 1987;58(3):932-935.
351. Nutescu EA, Spinler SA, Wittkowsky A, Dager WE. Low-molecular-weight heparins in renal impairment and obesity: available evidence and clinical practice recommendations across medical and surgical settings. *Ann Pharmacother.* 2009;43(6):1064-1083.
352. Wolzt M, Weltermann A, Nieszpaur-Los M, et al. Studies on the neutralizing effects of protamine on unfractionated and low molecular weight heparin (Fragmin) at the site of activation of the coagulation system in man. *Thromb Haemost.* 1995;73(3):439-443.
353. Lu G, DeGuzman FR, Hollenbach SJ, et al. A specific antidote for reversal of anticoagulation by direct and indirect inhibitors of coagulation factor Xa. *Nat Med.* 2013;19(4):446-451.
354. Ansell JE, Laulicht BE, Bakhru SH, Hoffman M, Steiner SS, Costin JC. Ciraparantag safely and completely reverses the anticoagulant effects of low molecular weight heparin. *Thromb Res.* 2016;146:113-118.
355. Tollefsen DM. Insight into the mechanism of action of heparin cofactor II. *Thromb Haemost.* 1995;74(5):1209-1214.
356. Miglioli M, Pironi L, Ruggeri E, et al. Bioavailability of Desmin, a low molecular weight dermatan sulfate, after subcutaneous administration to healthy volunteers. *Int J Clin Lab Res.* 1997;27(3):195-198.
357. Kang M, Alahmadi M, Sawh S, Kovacs MJ, Lazo-Langner A. Fondaparinux for the treatment of suspected heparin-induced thrombocytopenia: a propensity score-matched study. *Blood.* 2015;125(6):924-929.
358. Herbert JM, Herault JP, Bernat A, et al. Biochemical and pharmacological properties of SANORG 34006, a potent and long-acting synthetic pentasaccharide. *Blood.* 1998;91(11):4197-4205.
359. Paty I, Trellu M, Destors JM, Cortez P, Boelle E, Sanderink G. Reversibility of the anti-FXa activity of idrabiotaparinux (biotinylated idraparinux) by intravenous avidin infusion. *J Thromb Haemost.* 2010;8(4):722-729.
360. Hagemeyer CE, Tomic I, Jaminet P, et al. Fibrin-targeted direct factor Xa inhibition: construction and characterization of a recombinant factor Xa inhibitor composed of an anti-fibrin single-chain antibody and tick anticoagulant peptide. *Thromb Haemost.* 2004;92(1):47-53.
361. van Gogh I, Buller HR, Cohen AT, et al. Idraparinux versus standard therapy for venous thromboembolic disease. *N Engl J Med.* 2007;357(11):1094-1104.
362. Warkentin TE, Kelton JG. A 14-year study of heparin-induced thrombocytopenia. *Am J Med.* 1996;101(5):502-507.
363. Markwardt F. The development of hirudin as an antithrombotic drug. *Thromb Res.* 1994;74(1):1-23.
364. Hursting MJ, Alford KL, Becker JC, et al. Novastan (brand of argatroban): a small-molecule, direct thrombin inhibitor. *Semin Thromb Hemost.* 1997;23(6):503-516.
365. Guzzi LM, McCollum DA, Hursting MJ. Effect of renal function on argatroban therapy in heparin-induced thrombocytopenia. *J Thromb Thrombolysis.* 2006;22(3):169-176.
366. Levine RL, Hursting MJ, McCollum D. Argatroban therapy in heparin-induced thrombocytopenia with hepatic dysfunction. *Chest.* 2006;129(5):1167-1175.
367. Yarbrough PM, Varedi A, Walker A, Rondina MT. Argatroban dose reductions for suspected heparin-induced thrombocytopenia complicated by child-pugh class C liver disease. *Ann Pharmacother.* 2012;46(11):e30.
368. Schiele F, Vuillemenot A, Kramarz P, et al. Use of recombinant hirudin as antithrombotic treatment in patients with heparin-induced thrombocytopenia. *Am J Hematol.* 1995;50(1):20-25.
369. Harder S, Graff J, Klinkhardt U, et al. Transition from argatroban to oral anticoagulation with phenprocoumon or acenocoumarol: effects on prothrombin time, activated partial thromboplastin time, and Ecarin Clotting Time. *Thromb Haemost.* 2004;91(6):1137-1145.
370. Rossig L, Genth-Zotz S, Rau M, et al. Argatroban for elective percutaneous coronary intervention: the ARG-E04 multi-center study. *Int J Cardiol.* 2011;148(2):214-219.
371. Follis F, Filippone G, Montalbano G, et al. Argatroban as a substitute of heparin during cardiopulmonary bypass: a safe alternative? *Interact Cardiovasc Thorac Surg.* 2010;10(4):592-596.
372. Linkins LA, Dans AL, Moores LK, et al. Treatment and prevention of heparin-induced thrombocytopenia: antithrombotic therapy and prevention of thrombosis, 9th ed. American College of Chest Physicians Evidence-Based Clinical Practice Guidelines. *Chest.* 2012;141(2 suppl):e495S-e530S.
373. Maraganore JM, Bourdon P, Jablonski J, Ramachandran KL, Fenton JW II. Design and characterization of hirulogs: a novel class of bivalent peptide inhibitors of thrombin. *Biochemistry.* 1990;29(30):7095-7101.
374. Lincoff AM, Bittl JA, Kleiman NS, et al. Comparison of bivalirudin versus heparin during percutaneous coronary intervention (the randomized evaluation of PCI linking angiomax to reduced clinical events [REPLACE]-1 trial). *Am J Cardiol.* 2004;93(9):1092-1096.
375. Lincoff AM, Bittl JA, Harrington RA, et al. Bivalirudin and provisional glycoprotein IIb/IIIa blockade compared with heparin and planned glycoprotein IIb/IIIa blockade during percutaneous coronary intervention: REPLACE-2 randomized trial. *J Am Med Assoc.* 2003;289(7):853-863.
376. Secemsky EA, Kirtane A, Bangalore S, et al. Use and effectiveness of bivalirudin versus unfractionated heparin for percutaneous coronary intervention among patients with ST-segment elevation myocardial infarction in the United States. *JACC Cardiovasc Interv.* 2016;9(23):2376-2386.
377. Shahzad A, Kemp I, Mars C, et al. Unfractioned heparin versus bivalirudin in primary percutaneous coronary intervention (HEAT-PPCI): an open-label, single centre, randomised controlled trial. *Lancet.* 2014;384(9957):1849-1858.
378. Tsu LV, Dager WE. Bivalirudin dosing adjustments for reduced renal function with or without hemodialysis in the management of heparin-induced thrombocytopenia. *Ann Pharmacother.* 2011;45(10):1185-1192.
379. Campbell HA, Link KP. Studies on the hemorrhagic sweet clover disease: IV. The isolation and crystallization of the hemorrhagic agent. *J Biol Chem.* 1941;138:21-33.
380. Furie B, Furie BC. Molecular basis of vitamin K-dependent gamma-carboxylation. *Blood.* 1990;75(9):1753-1762.
381. Fasco MJ, Principe LM, Walsh WA, Friedman PA. Warfarin inhibition of vitamin K 2,3-epoxide reductase in rat liver microsomes. *Biochemistry.* 1983;22(24):5655-5660.
382. Ageno W, Gallus AS, Wittkowsky A, Crowther M, Hylek EM, Palareti G. Oral anticoagulant therapy: antithrombotic therapy and prevention of thrombosis, 9th ed. American College of Chest Physicians Evidence-Based Clinical Practice Guidelines. *Chest.* 2012;141(2 suppl):e44S-e88S.
383. O'Reilly RA. The pharmacodynamics of the oral anticoagulant drugs. *Prog Hemost Thromb* 1974;2:175-213.
384. O'Reilly RA, Aggeler PM, Hoag MS, Leong LS, Kropatkin ML. Hereditary transmission of exceptional resistance to coumarin anticoagulant drugs. The first reported kindred. *N Engl J Med.* 1964;271:809-815.
385. Zivelin A, Rao LV, Rapaport SI. Mechanism of the anticoagulant effect of warfarin as evaluated in rabbits by selective depression of individual procoagulant vitamin K-dependent clotting factors. *J Clin Invest.* 1993;92(5):2131-2140.
386. Choueiri T, Deitcher SR. Why shouldn't we use warfarin alone to treat acute venous thrombosis? *Cleve Clin J Med.* 2002;69(7):546-548.
387. Holbrook AM, Pereira JA, Labiris R, et al. Systematic overview of warfarin and its drug and food interactions. *Arch Intern Med.* 2005;165(10):1095-1106.
388. Wells PS, Holbrook AM, Crowther NR, Hirsh J. Interactions of warfarin with drugs and food. *Ann Intern Med.* 1994;121(9):676-683.
389. Deitcher SR. Interpretation of the international normalised ratio in patients with liver disease. *Lancet.* 2002;359(9300):47-48.
390. International Warfarin Pharmacogenetics Consortium; Klein TE, Altman RB, et al. Estimation of the warfarin dose with clinical and pharmacogenetic data. *N Engl J Med.* 2009;360(8):753-764.
391. Deitcher SR. Heparin-induced thrombocytopenia: pathogenesis, management, and prevention. *Formulary.* 2001;36(1):26-41.
392. Kimmel SE, French B, Kasner SE, et al. A pharmacogenetic versus a clinical algorithm for warfarin dosing. *N Engl J Med.* 2013;369(24):2283-2293.
393. Hirsh J. Oral anticoagulant drugs. *N Engl J Med.* 1991;324(26):1865-1875.
394. Harrison L, Johnston M, Massicotte MP, Crowther M, Moffat K, Hirsh J. Comparison of 5-mg and 10-mg loading doses in initiation of warfarin therapy. *Ann Intern Med.* 1997;126(2):133-136.
395. Hirsh J, Poller L. The international normalized ratio. A guide to understanding and correcting its problems. *Arch Intern Med.* 1994;154(3):282-288.
396. Guyatt GH, Akl EA, Crowther M, et al. Executive summary: antithrombotic therapy and prevention of thrombosis, 9th ed. American College of Chest Physicians Evidence-Based Clinical Practice Guidelines. *Chest.* 2012;141(2 suppl):7S-47S.
397. Kearon C, Ginsberg JS, Kovacs MJ, et al. Comparison of low-intensity warfarin therapy with conventional-intensity warfarin therapy for long-term prevention of recurrent venous thromboembolism. *N Engl J Med.* 2003;349(7):631-639.
398. Hull R, Hirsh J, Jay R, et al. Different intensities of oral anticoagulant therapy in the treatment of proximal-vein thrombosis. *N Engl J Med.* 1982;307(27):1676-1681.
399. Crowther MA, Ginsberg JS, Julian J, et al. A comparison of two intensities of warfarin for the prevention of recurrent thrombosis in patients with the antiphospholipid antibody syndrome. *N Engl J Med.* 2003;349(12):1133-1138.
400. Ryan F, O'Shea S, Byrne S. The reliability of point-of-care prothrombin time testing. A comparison of CoaguChek S and XS INR measurements with hospital laboratory monitoring. *Int J Lab Hematol.* 2010;32(1 pt 1):e26-e33.
401. Bloomfield HE, Krause A, Greer N, et al. Meta-analysis: effect of patient self-testing and self-management of long-term anticoagulation on major clinical outcomes. *Ann Intern Med.* 2011;154(7):472-482.
402. Levine MN, Raskob G, Beyth RJ, Kearon C, Schulman S. Hemorrhagic complications of anticoagulant treatment: the seventh ACCP conference on antithrombotic and thrombolytic therapy. *Chest.* 2004;126(3 suppl):287S-310S.
403. Beyth RJ, Quinn LM, Landefeld CS. Prospective evaluation of an index for predicting the risk of major bleeding in outpatients treated with warfarin. *Am J Med.* 1998;105(2):91-99.
404. Landefeld CS, Rosenblatt MW, Goldman L. Bleeding in outpatients treated with warfarin: relation to the prothrombin time and important remediable lesions. *Am J Med.* 1989;87(2):153-159.
405. Fang MC, Go AS, Hylek EM, et al. Age and the risk of warfarin-associated hemorrhage: the anticoagulation and risk factors in atrial fibrillation study. *J Am Geriatr Soc.* 2006;54(8):1231-1236.
406. Crowther MA, Ageno W, Garcia D, et al. Oral vitamin K versus placebo to correct excessive anticoagulation in patients receiving warfarin: a randomized trial. *Ann Intern Med.* 2009;150(5):293-300.
407. Clark NP, Witt DM, Davies LE, et al. Bleeding, recurrent venous thromboembolism, and mortality risks during warfarin interruption for invasive procedures. *JAMA Intern Med.* 2015;175(7):1163-1168.
408. Daniels PR, McBane RD, Litin SC, et al. Peri-procedural anticoagulation management of mechanical prosthetic heart valve patients. *Thromb Res.* 2009;124(3):300-305.
409. Douketis JD, Spyropoulos AC, Kaatz S, et al. Perioperative bridging anticoagulation in patients with atrial fibrillation. *N Engl J Med.* 2015;373(9):823-833.

410. Strebel N, Prins M, Agnelli G, Buller HR. Preoperative or postoperative start of prophylaxis for venous thromboembolism with low-molecular-weight heparin in elective hip surgery? *Arch Intern Med.* 2002;162(13):1451-1456.
411. Hall JG, Pauli RM, Wilson KM. Maternal and fetal sequelae of anticoagulation during pregnancy. *Am J Med.* 1980;68(1):122-140.
412. Ginsberg JS, Hirsh J, Turner DC, Levine MN, Burrows R. Risks to the fetus of anticoagulant therapy during pregnancy. *Thromb Haemost.* 1989;61(2):197-203.
413. Saifan C, Saad M, El-Charabaty E, El-Sayegh S. Warfarin-induced calciphylaxis: a case report and review of literature. *Int J Gen Med.* 2013;6:665-669.
414. Nigwekar SU, Kroshinsky D, Nazarian RM, et al. Calciphylaxis: risk factors, diagnosis, and treatment. *Am J Kidney Dis.* 2015;66(1):133-146.
415. Faraci PA, Deterling RA Jr, Stein AM, Rheinlander HF, Cleveland RJ. Warfarin induced necrosis of the skin. *Surg Gynecol Obstet.* 1978;146(5):695-700.
416. Grimaudo V, Gueissaz F, Hauert J, Sarraj A, Kruithof EK, Bachmann F. Necrosis of skin induced by coumarin in a patient deficient in protein S. *Br Med J.* 1989;298(6668):233-234.
417. Jillella AP, Lutcher CL. Reinstituting warfarin in patients who develop warfarin skin necrosis. *Am J Hematol.* 1996;52(2):117-119.
418. Boerhinger Ingelheim Pharmaceuticals, Inc. *Pradaxa (Dabigatran Etexilate) Prescribing Information.* 2022. Accessed January 26, 2022. https://docs.boehringer-ingelheim.com/Prescribing%20Information/PIs/Pradaxa/Pradaxa.pdf
419. Kooiman J, van der Hulle T, Maas H, et al. Pharmacokinetics and pharmacodynamics of dabigatran 75 mg b.i.d. in patients with severe chronic kidney disease. *J Am Coll Cardiol.* 2016;67(20):2442-2444.
420. Crowther MA, Warkentin TE. Managing bleeding in anticoagulated patients with a focus on novel therapeutic agents. *J Thromb Haemost.* 2009;7(suppl 1):107-110.
421. Connolly SJ, Ezekowitz MD, Yusuf S, et al. Dabigatran versus warfarin in patients with atrial fibrillation. *N Engl J Med.* 2009;361(12):1139-1151.
422. Wallentin L, Yusuf S, Ezekowitz MD, et al. Efficacy and safety of dabigatran compared with warfarin at different levels of international normalised ratio control for stroke prevention in atrial fibrillation: an analysis of the RE-LY trial. *Lancet.* 2010;376(9745):975-983.
423. Schulman S, Kearon C, Kakkar AK, et al. Dabigatran versus warfarin in the treatment of acute venous thromboembolism. *N Engl J Med.* 2009;361(24):2342-2352.
424. Ginsberg JS, Davidson BL, Comp PC, et al. Oral thrombin inhibitor dabigatran etexilate vs North American enoxaparin regimen for prevention of venous thromboembolism after knee arthroplasty surgery. *J Arthroplasty.* 2009;24(1):1-9.
425. Eriksson BI, Dahl OE, Huo MH, et al. Oral dabigatran versus enoxaparin for thromboprophylaxis after primary total hip arthroplasty (RE-NOVATE II*). A randomised, double-blind, non-inferiority trial. *Thromb Haemost.* 2011;105(4):721-729.
426. Eikelboom JW, Connolly SJ, Brueckmann M, et al. Dabigatran versus warfarin in patients with mechanical heart valves. *N Engl J Med.* 2013;369(13):1206-1214.
427. Nishimura RA, Otto CM, Bonow RO, et al. 2014 AHA/ACC guideline for the management of patients with valvular heart disease. Executive summary: a report of the American College of Cardiology/American Heart Association Task Force on Practice Guidelines. *J Am Coll Cardiol.* 2014;63(22):2438-2488.
428. Janssen Pharmaceuticals, Inc. *Xarelto (Rivaroxaban) Prescribing Information.* Published 2021. Accessed January 2022. https://www.janssenlabels.com/package-insert/product-monograph/prescribing-information/XARELTO-pi.pdf
429. Kirchhof P, Benussi S, Kotecha D, et al. 2016 ESC Guidelines for the management of atrial fibrillation developed in collaboration with EACTS. *Eur Heart J.* 2016;37(38):2893-2962.
430. Cuker A, Siegal DM, Crowther MA, Garcia DA. Laboratory measurement of the anticoagulant activity of the non-vitamin K oral anticoagulants. *J Am Coll Cardiol.* 2014;64(11):1128-1139.
431. Samama MM, Martinoli JL, LeFlem L, et al. Assessment of laboratory assays to measure rivaroxaban–an oral, direct factor Xa inhibitor. *Thromb Haemost.* 2010;103(4):815-825.
432. Dangas GD, Tijssen JGP, Wohrle J, et al. A controlled trial of rivaroxaban after transcatheter aortic-valve replacement. *N Engl J Med.* 2020;382(2):120-129.
433. *Eliquis (Apixaban) Prescribing Information.* Bristol-Myers Squibb Company; Published 2021. Accessed January 2022. https://packageinserts.bms.com/pi/pi_eliquis.pdf
434. Wang X, Tirucherai G, Marbury TC, et al. Pharmacokinetics, pharmacodynamics, and safety of apixaban in subjects with end-stage renal disease on hemodialysis. *J Clin Pharmacol.* 2016;56(5):628-636.
435. Siontis KC, Zhang X, Eckard A, et al. Outcomes associated with apixaban use in patients with end-stage kidney disease and atrial fibrillation in the United States. *Circulation.* 2018;138(15):1519-1529.
436. Schafer JH, Casey AL, Dupre KA, Staubes BA. Safety and efficacy of apixaban versus warfarin in patients with advanced chronic kidney disease. *Ann Pharmacother.* 2018;52(11):1078-1084.
437. Makani A, Saba S, Jain SK, et al. Safety and efficacy of direct oral anticoagulants versus warfarin in patients with chronic kidney disease and atrial fibrillation. *Am J Cardiol.* 2020;125(2):210-214.
438. Granger CB, Alexander JH, McMurray JJ, et al. Apixaban versus warfarin in patients with atrial fibrillation. *N Engl J Med.* 2011;365(11):981-992.
439. Agnelli G, Buller HR, Cohen A, et al. Oral apixaban for the treatment of acute venous thromboembolism. *N Engl J Med.* 2013;369(9):799-808.
440. Agnelli G, Buller HR, Cohen A, et al. Apixaban for extended treatment of venous thromboembolism. *N Engl J Med.* 2013;368(8):699-708.
441. Lassen MR, Raskob GE, Gallus A, et al. Apixaban versus enoxaparin for thromboprophylaxis after knee replacement (ADVANCE-2): a randomised double-blind trial. *Lancet.* 2010;375(9717):807-815.
442. Lassen MR, Gallus A, Raskob GE, et al. Apixaban versus enoxaparin for thromboprophylaxis after hip replacement. *N Engl J Med.* 2010;363(26):2487-2498.
443. Lassen MR, Raskob GE, Gallus A, Pineo G, Chen D, Portman RJ. Apixaban or enoxaparin for thromboprophylaxis after knee replacement. *N Engl J Med.* 2009;361(6):594-604.
444. Collet JP. *ATLANTIS: Apixaban Not Superior to Standard of Care After TAVR*; Published 2021. Accessed January 5, 2022. https://www.acc.org/latest-in-cardiology/articles/2021/05/12/18/51/sat-9am-atlantis-acc-2021
445. *Savaysa (Edoxaban) Prescribing Information.* Daiichi Sankyo, Inc; Published 2020. Accessed January 2022. https://daiichisankyo.us/prescribing-information-portlet/getPIContent?productName=Savaysa&inline=true
446. Wolzt M, Samama MM, Kapiotis S, Ogata K, Mendell J, Kunitada S. Effect of edoxaban on markers of coagulation in venous and shed blood compared with fondaparinux. *Thromb Haemost.* 2011;105(6):1080-1090.
447. Samuelson BT, Cuker A. Measurement and reversal of the direct oral anticoagulants. *Blood Rev.* 2017;31(1):77-84.
448. Hokusai VTEI, Buller HR, Decousus H, et al. Edoxaban versus warfarin for the treatment of symptomatic venous thromboembolism. *N Engl J Med.* 2013;369(15):1406-1415.
449. Cuker A, Burnett A, Triller D, et al. Reversal of direct oral anticoagulants: guidance from the anticoagulation forum. *Am J Hematol.* 2019;94(6):697-709.
450. Pollack CV Jr, Reilly PA, Eikelboom J, et al. Idarucizumab for dabigatran reversal. *N Engl J Med.* 2015;373(6):511-520.
451. Martin K, Beyer-Westendorf J, Davidson BL, Huisman MV, Sandset PM, Moll S. Use of the direct oral anticoagulants in obese patients: guidance from the SSC of the ISTH. *J Thromb Haemost.* 2016;14(6):1308-1313.
452. Mai V, Marceau-Ferron E, Bertoletti L, et al. Direct oral anticoagulants in the treatment of acute venous thromboembolism in patients with obesity: a systematic review with meta-analysis. *Pharmacol Res.* 2021;163:105317.
453. Elshafei MN, Mohamed MFH, El-Bardissy A, et al. Comparative effectiveness and safety of direct oral anticoagulants compared to warfarin in morbidly obese patients with acute venous thromboembolism: systematic review and a meta-analysis. *J Thromb Thrombolysis.* 2021;51(2):388-396.
454. Otto CM, Nishimura RA, Bonow RO, et al. 2020 ACC/AHA guideline for the management of patients with valvular heart disease: a report of the American College of Cardiology/American Heart Association Joint Committee on clinical practice guidelines. *Circulation.* 2021;143(5):e72-e227.
455. Tektonidou MG, Andreoli L, Limper M, et al. EULAR recommendations for the management of antiphospholipid syndrome in adults. *Ann Rheum Dis.* 2019;78(10):1296-1304.
456. Collen D, Lijnen HR. Molecular basis of fibrinolysis, as relevant for thrombolytic therapy. *Thromb Haemost.* 1995;74(1):167-171.
457. Eisenberg PR, Sobel BE, Jaffe AS. Characterization in vivo of the fibrin specificity of activators of the fibrinolytic system. *Circulation.* 1988;78(3):592-597.
458. Marder VJ, Novokhatny V. Direct fibrinolytic agents: biochemical attributes, preclinical foundation and clinical potential. *J Thromb Haemost.* 2010;8(3):433-444.
459. Marder VJ, Bell WR. *Fibrinolytic therapy. Hemostasis and Thrombosis: Basic Principles and Clinical Practice.* 2nd ed. JB Lippincott; 1987.
460. Stricker RB, Wong D, Shiu DT, Reyes PT, Shuman MA. Activation of plasminogen by tissue plasminogen activator on normal and thrombasthenic platelets: effects on surface proteins and platelet aggregation. *Blood.* 1986;68(1):275-280.
461. Sharma GV, Cella G, Parisi AF, Sasahara AA. Thrombolytic therapy. *N Engl J Med.* 1982;306(21):1268-1276.
462. Squire IB, Lawley W, Fletcher S, et al. Humoral and cellular immune responses up to 7.5 years after administration of streptokinase for acute myocardial infarction. *Eur Heart J.* 1999;20(17):1245-1252.
463. *WHO Model Lists of Essential Medicines.* World Health Organization (WHO). Published 2021. Accessed January 2022. https://www.who.int/publications/i/item/WHO-MHP-HPS-EML-2021.02
464. Bell WR. Present-day thrombolytic therapy: therapeutic agents–pharmacokinetics and pharmacodynamics. *Rev Cardiovasc Med.* 2002;3(suppl 2):S34-S44.
465. Pennica D, Holmes WE, Kohr WJ, et al. Cloning and expression of human tissue-type plasminogen activator cDNA in E. coli. *Nature.* 1983;301(5897):214-221.
466. Collen D, Bounameaux H, De Cock F, Lijnen HR, Verstraete M. Analysis of coagulation and fibrinolysis during intravenous infusion of recombinant human tissue-type plasminogen activator in patients with acute myocardial infarction. *Circulation.* 1986;73(3):511-517.
467. Goldhaber SZ, Vaughan DE, Markis JE, et al. Acute pulmonary embolism treated with tissue plasminogen activator. *Lancet.* 1986;2(8512):886-889.
468. Rapaport E. Thrombolytic agents in acute myocardial infarction. *N Engl J Med.* 1989;320(13):861-864.
469. Neuhaus KL, Feuerer W, Jeep-Tebbe S, Niederer W, Vogt A, Tebbe U. Improved thrombolysis with a modified dose regimen of recombinant tissue-type plasminogen activator. *J Am Coll Cardiol.* 1989;14(6):1566-1569.
470. National Institute of Neurological D, Stroke rt PASSG. Tissue plasminogen activator for acute ischemic stroke. *N Engl J Med.* 1995;333(24):1581-1587.
471. Deitcher SR, Fesen MR, Kiproff PM, et al. Safety and efficacy of alteplase for restoring function in occluded central venous catheters: results of the cardiovascular thrombolytic to open occluded lines trial. *J Clin Oncol.* 2002;20(1):317-324.
472. Hacke W, Kaste M, Bluhmki E, et al. Thrombolysis with alteplase 3 to 4.5 hours after acute ischemic stroke. *N Engl J Med.* 2008;359(13):1317-1329.
473. Jauch EC, Saver JL, Adams HP Jr, et al. Guidelines for the early management of patients with acute ischemic stroke: a guideline for healthcare professionals from the American Heart Association/American Stroke Association. *Stroke.* 2013;44(3):870-947.
474. Kohnert U, Rudolph R, Verheijen JH, et al. Biochemical properties of the kringle 2 and protease domains are maintained in the refolded t-PA deletion variant BM 06.022. *Protein Eng.* 1992;5(1):93-100.

475. Meyer G, Vicaut E, Danays T, et al. Fibrinolysis for patients with intermediate-risk pulmonary embolism. *N Engl J Med*. 2014;370(15):1402-1411.
476. Van De Werf F, Adgey J, Ardissino D, et al. Single-bolus tenecteplase compared with front-loaded alteplase in acute myocardial infarction: the ASSENT-2 double-blind randomised trial. *Lancet*. 1999;354(9180):716-722.
477. InTime-II Investigators. Intravenous NPA for the treatment of infarcting myocardium early; InTIME-II, a double-blind comparison of single-bolus lanoteplase vs accelerated alteplase for the treatment of patients with acute myocardial infarction. *Eur Heart J*. 2000;21(24):2005-2013.
478. Furlan A, Higashida R, Wechsler L, et al. Intra-arterial prourokinase for acute ischemic stroke. The PROACT II study: a randomized controlled trial. Prolyse in Acute Cerebral Thromboembolism. *J Am Med Assoc*. 1999;282(21):2003-2011.
479. Verstraete M. Third-generation thrombolytic drugs. *Am J Med*. 2000;109(1):52-58.
480. Liberatore GT, Samson A, Bladin C, Schleuning WD, Medcalf RL. Vampire bat salivary plasminogen activator (desmoteplase): a unique fibrinolytic enzyme that does not promote neurodegeneration. *Stroke*. 2003;34(2):537-543.
481. Berkowitz SD, Granger CB, Pieper KS, et al. Incidence and predictors of bleeding after contemporary thrombolytic therapy for myocardial infarction. The Global Utilization of Streptokinase and Tissue Plasminogen Activator for Occluded Coronary Arteries (GUSTO) I Investigators. *Circulation*. 1997;95(11):2508-2516.
482. Wahlgren N, Ahmed N, Davalos A, et al. Thrombolysis with alteplase 3-4.5 h after acute ischaemic stroke (SITS-ISTR): an observational study. *Lancet*. 2008;372(9646):1303-1309.
483. Brass LM, Lichtman JH, Wang Y, Gurwitz JH, Radford MJ, Krumholz HM. Intracranial hemorrhage associated with thrombolytic therapy for elderly patients with acute myocardial infarction: results from the Cooperative Cardiovascular Project. *Stroke*. 2000;31(8):1802-1811.
484. Kearon C, Akl EA, Comerota AJ, et al. Antithrombotic therapy for VTE disease: antithrombotic therapy and prevention of thrombosis, 9th ed. American College of Chest Physicians Evidence-Based Clinical Practice Guidelines. *Chest*. 2012;141(2 suppl):e419S-e496S.
485. Wang C, Zhai Z, Yang Y, et al. Efficacy and safety of low dose recombinant tissue-type plasminogen activator for the treatment of acute pulmonary thromboembolism: a randomized, multicenter, controlled trial. *Chest*. 2010;137(2):254-262.
486. Ouriel K. Comparison of safety and efficacy of the various thrombolytic agents. *Rev Cardiovasc Med*. 2002;3(suppl 2):S17-S24.
487. Lijnen HR, Collen D. Remaining perspectives of mutant and chimeric plasminogen activators. *Ann N Y Acad Sci*. 1992;667:357-364.
488. Gore JM, Granger CB, Simoons ML, et al. Stroke after thrombolysis. Mortality and functional outcomes in the GUSTO-I trial. Global use of strategies to open occluded coronary arteries. *Circulation*. 1995;92(10):2811-2818.
489. Maggioni AP, Franzosi MG, Santoro E, White H, Van de Werf F, Tognoni G. The risk of stroke in patients with acute myocardial infarction after thrombolytic and antithrombotic treatment. Gruppo Italiano per lo Studio della Sopravvivenza nell'Infarto Miocardico II (GISSI-2), and the International Study Group. *N Engl J Med*. 1992;327(1):1-6.
490. Deitcher SR, Jaff MR. Pharmacologic and clinical characteristics of thrombolytic agents. *Rev Cardiovasc Med*. 2002;3(suppl 2):S25-S33.
491. Huang X, MacIsaac R, Thompson JL, et al. Tenecteplase versus alteplase in stroke thrombolysis: an individual patient data meta-analysis of randomized controlled trials. *Int J Stroke*. 2016;11(5):534-543.
492. Silverstein MD, Heit JA, Mohr DN, Petterson TM, O'Fallon WM, Melton LJ III. Trends in the incidence of deep vein thrombosis and pulmonary embolism: a 25-year population-based study. *Arch Intern Med*. 1998;158(6):585-593.
493. Hull RD, Raskob GE, Hirsh J, et al. Continuous intravenous heparin compared with intermittent subcutaneous heparin in the initial treatment of proximal-vein thrombosis. *N Engl J Med*. 1986;315(18):1109-1114.
494. Prandoni P, Lensing AW, Cogo A, et al. The long-term clinical course of acute deep venous thrombosis. *Ann Intern Med*. 1996;125(1):1-7.
495. Trust; CDEaR, Trust; CCDEaR, Forum; EV, Forum; IST, Angiology; IUo, Phlebologie UId. Prevention and treatment of venous thromboembolism. International Consensus Statement (guidelines according to scientific evidence). *Int Angiol*. 2006;25(2):101-161.
496. Investigators E, Bauersachs R, Berkowitz SD, et al. Oral rivaroxaban for symptomatic venous thromboembolism. *N Engl J Med*. 2010;363(26):2499-2510.
497. Investigators E-P, Buller HR, Prins MH, et al. Oral rivaroxaban for the treatment of symptomatic pulmonary embolism. *N Engl J Med*. 2012;366(14):1287-1297.
498. Snow V, Qaseem A, Barry P, et al. Management of venous thromboembolism: a clinical practice guideline from the American College of Physicians and the American Academy of Family Physicians. *Ann Intern Med*. 2007;146(3):204-210.
499. Lutsey PL, Walker RF, MacLehose RF, Alonso A, Adam TJ, Zakai NA. Direct oral anticoagulants and warfarin for venous thromboembolism treatment: trends from 2012 to 2017. *Res Pract Thromb Haemost*. 2019;3(4):668-673.
500. Bauersachs R, Berkowitz SD, Brenner B, et al. Oral rivaroxaban for symptomatic venous thromboembolism. *N Engl J Med*. 2010;363(26):2499-2510.
501. Buller HR, Prins MH, Lensin AW, et al. Oral rivaroxaban for the treatment of symptomatic pulmonary embolism. *N Engl J Med*. 2012;366(14):1287-1297.
502. Prins MH, Bamber L, Cano SJ, et al. Patient-reported treatment satisfaction with oral rivaroxaban versus standard therapy in the treatment of pulmonary embolism; results from the EINSTEIN PE trial. *Thromb Res*. 2015;135(2):281-288.
503. Brandjes DP, Heijboer H, Buller HR, de Rijk M, Jagt H, ten Cate JW. Acenocoumarol and heparin compared with acenocoumarol alone in the initial treatment of proximal-vein thrombosis. *N Engl J Med*. 1992;327(21):1485-1489.
504. Gallus A, Jackaman J, Tillett J, Mills W, Wycherley A. Safety and efficacy of warfarin started early after submassive venous thrombosis or pulmonary embolism. *Lancet*. 1986;2(8519):1293-1296.
505. Hull RD, Raskob GE, Rosenbloom D, et al. Heparin for 5 days as compared with 10 days in the initial treatment of proximal venous thrombosis. *N Engl J Med*. 1990;322(18):1260-1264.
506. Raschke RA, Reilly BM, Guidry JR, Fontana JR, Srinivas S. The weight-based heparin dosing nomogram compared with a "standard care" nomogram. A randomized controlled trial. *Ann Intern Med*. 1993;119(9):874-881.
507. Prandoni P, Carnovali M, Marchiori A, Galilei I. Subcutaneous adjusted-dose unfractionated heparin vs fixed-dose low-molecular-weight heparin in the initial treatment of venous thromboembolism. *Arch Intern Med*. 2004;164(10):1077-1083.
508. Kearon C, Ginsberg JS, Julian JA, et al. Comparison of fixed-dose weight-adjusted unfractionated heparin and low-molecular-weight heparin for acute treatment of venous thromboembolism. *J Am Med Assoc*. 2006;296(8):935-942.
509. Erkens PM, Prins MH. Fixed dose subcutaneous low molecular weight heparins versus adjusted dose unfractionated heparin for venous thromboembolism. *Cochrane Database Syst Rev*. 2010;(9):CD001100.
510. Merli G, Spiro TE, Olsson CG, et al. Subcutaneous enoxaparin once or twice daily compared with intravenous unfractionated heparin for treatment of venous thromboembolic disease. *Ann Intern Med*. 2001;134(3):191-202.
511. Witt DM, Nieuwlaat R, Clark NP, et al. American Society of Hematology 2018 guidelines for management of venous thromboembolism: optimal management of anticoagulation therapy. *Blood Adv*. 2018;2(22):3257-3291.
512. Buller HR, Davidson BL, Decousus H, et al. Fondaparinux or enoxaparin for the initial treatment of symptomatic deep venous thrombosis: a randomized trial. *Ann Intern Med*. 2004;140(11):867-873.
513. Koopman MM, Prandoni P, Piovella F, et al. Treatment of venous thrombosis with intravenous unfractionated heparin administered in the hospital as compared with subcutaneous low-molecular-weight heparin administered at home. The Tasman Study Group. *N Engl J Med*. 1996;334(11):682-687.
514. Levine M, Gent M, Hirsh J, et al. A comparison of low-molecular-weight heparin administered primarily at home with unfractionated heparin administered in the hospital for proximal deep-vein thrombosis. *N Engl J Med*. 1996;334(11):677-681.
515. O'Brien B, Levine M, Willan A, et al. Economic evaluation of outpatient treatment with low-molecular-weight heparin for proximal vein thrombosis. *Arch Intern Med*. 1999;159(19):2298-2304.
516. Douketis JD, Kearon C, Bates S, Duku EK, Ginsberg JS. Risk of fatal pulmonary embolism in patients with treated venous thromboembolism. *J Am Med Assoc*. 1998;279(6):458-462.
517. Aujesky D, Roy PM, Verschuren F, et al. Outpatient versus inpatient treatment for patients with acute pulmonary embolism: an international, open-label, randomised, non-inferiority trial. *Lancet*. 2011;378(9785):41-48.
518. Otero R, Uresandi F, Jimenez D, et al. Home treatment in pulmonary embolism. *Thromb Res*. 2010;126(1):e1-e5.
519. Bazinet A, Almanric K, Brunet C, et al. Dosage of enoxaparin among obese and renal impairment patients. *Thromb Res*. 2005;116(1):41-50.
520. Hainer JW, Barrett JS, Assaid CA, et al. Dosing in heavy-weight/obese patients with the LMWH, tinzaparin: a pharmacodynamic study. *Thromb Haemost*. 2002;87(5):817-823.
521. Wilson SJ, Wilbur K, Burton E, Anderson DR. Effect of patient weight on the anticoagulant response to adjusted therapeutic dosage of low-molecular- weight heparin for the treatment of venous thromboembolism. *Haemostasis*. 2001;31(1):42-48.
522. Falga C, Capdevila JA, Soler S, et al. Clinical outcome of patients with venous thromboembolism and renal insufficiency. Findings from the RIETE registry. *Thromb Haemost*. 2007;98(4):771-776.
523. Lim W, Dentali F, Eikelboom JW, Crowther MA. Meta-analysis: low-molecular-weight heparin and bleeding in patients with severe renal insufficiency. *Ann Intern Med*. 2006;144(9):673-684.
524. Douketis J, Tosetto A, Marcucci M, et al. Patient-level meta-analysis: effect of measurement timing, threshold, and patient age on ability of D-dimer testing to assess recurrence risk after unprovoked venous thromboembolism. *Ann Intern Med*. 2010;153(8):523-531.
525. Vasanthamohan L, Boonyawat K, Chai-Adisaksopha C, Crowther M. Reduced-dose direct oral anticoagulants in the extended treatment of venous thromboembolism: a systematic review and meta-analysis. *J Thromb Haemost*. 2018;16(7):1288-1295.
526. Ortel TL, Neumann I, Ageno W, et al. American Society of Hematology 2020 guidelines for management of venous thromboembolism: treatment of deep vein thrombosis and pulmonary embolism. *Blood Adv*. 2020;4(19):4693-4738.
527. van Walraven C, Jennings A, Oake N, Fergusson D, Forster AJ. Effect of study setting on anticoagulation control: a systematic review and metaregression. *Chest*. 2006;129(5):1155-1166.
528. Gardiner C, Williams K, Longair I, Mackie IJ, Machin SJ, Cohen H. A randomised control trial of patient self-management of oral anticoagulation compared with patient self-testing. *Br J Haematol*. 2006;132(5):598-603.
529. Matchar DB, Jacobson A, Dolor R, et al. Effect of home testing of international normalized ratio on clinical events. *N Engl J Med*. 2010;363(17):1608-1620.
530. Ginsberg JS, Kowalchuk G, Hirsh J, et al. Heparin effect on bone density. *Thromb Haemost*. 1990;64(2):286-289.
531. Beyer-Westendorf J, Tittl L, Bistervels I, et al. Safety of direct oral anticoagulant exposure during pregnancy: a retrospective cohort study. *Lancet Haematol*. 2020;7(12):e884-e891.
532. Lai N, Jones AE, Johnson SA, Witt DM. Anticoagulant therapy management of venous thromboembolism recurrence occurring during anticoagulant therapy: a descriptive study. *J Thromb Thrombolysis*. 2021;52(2):414-418.
533. Prandoni P, Lensing AW, Piccioli A, et al. Recurrent venous thromboembolism and bleeding complications during anticoagulant treatment in patients with cancer and venous thrombosis. *Blood*. 2002;100(10):3484-3488.

534. Lee AY, Levine MN, Baker RI, et al. Low-molecular-weight heparin versus a coumarin for the prevention of recurrent venous thromboembolism in patients with cancer. *N Engl J Med*. 2003;349(2):146-153.
535. Hull RD, Pineo GF, Brant RF, et al. Long-term low-molecular-weight heparin versus usual care in proximal-vein thrombosis patients with cancer. *Am J Med*. 2006;119(12):1062-1072.
536. Akl EA, Kahale L, Barba M, et al. Anticoagulation for the long-term treatment of venous thromboembolism in patients with cancer. *Cochrane Database Syst Rev*. 2014;(7):CD006650.
537. Agnelli G, Becattini C, Meyer G, et al. Apixaban for the treatment of venous thromboembolism associated with cancer. *N Engl J Med*. 2020;382(17):1599-1607.
538. Li A, Garcia DA, Lyman GH, Carrier M. Direct oral anticoagulant (DOAC) versus low-molecular-weight heparin (LMWH) for treatment of cancer associated thrombosis (CAT): a systematic review and meta-analysis. *Thromb Res*. 2019;173:158-163.
539. Key NS, Khorana AA, Kuderer NM, et al. Venous thromboembolism prophylaxis and treatment in patients with cancer: ASCO clinical practice guideline update. *J Clin Oncol*. 2020;38(5):496-520.
540. Schulman S, Rhedin AS, Lindmarker P, et al. A comparison of six weeks with six months of oral anticoagulant therapy after a first episode of venous thromboembolism. Duration of Anticoagulation Trial Study Group. *N Engl J Med*. 1995;332(25):1661-1665.
541. Masuda EM, Kistner RL, Musikasinthorn C, Liquido F, Geling O, He Q. The controversy of managing calf vein thrombosis. *J Vasc Surg*. 2012;55(2):550-561.
542. Hughes MJ, Stein PD, Matta F. Silent pulmonary embolism in patients with distal deep venous thrombosis: systematic review. *Thromb Res*. 2014;134(6):1182-1185.
543. Wiener RS, Schwartz LM, Woloshin S. Time trends in pulmonary embolism in the United States: evidence of overdiagnosis. *Arch Intern Med*. 2011;171(9):831-837.
544. Burge AJ, Freeman KD, Klapper PJ, Haramati LB. Increased diagnosis of pulmonary embolism without a corresponding decline in mortality during the CT era. *Clin Radiol*. 2008;63(4):381-386.
545. Donato AA, Khoche S, Santora J, Wagner B. Clinical outcomes in patients with isolated subsegmental pulmonary emboli diagnosed by multidetector CT pulmonary angiography. *Thromb Res*. 2010;126(4):e266-e270.
546. Carrier M, Righini M, Le Gal G. Symptomatic subsegmental pulmonary embolism: what is the next step?. *J Thromb Haemost*. 2012;10(8):1486-1490.
547. Stein PD, Goodman LR, Hull RD, Dalen JE, Matta F. Diagnosis and management of isolated subsegmental pulmonary embolism: review and assessment of the options. *Clin Appl Thromb Hemost*. 2012;18(1):20-26.
548. den Exter PL, van Es J, Klok FA, et al. Risk profile and clinical outcome of symptomatic subsegmental acute pulmonary embolism. *Blood*. 2013;122(7):1144-1149, quiz 1329.
549. Le Gal G, Kovacs MJ, Bertoletti L, et al. Risk for recurrent venous thromboembolism in patients with subsegmental pulmonary embolism managed without anticoagulation: a multicenter prospective cohort study. *Ann Intern Med*. 2022;175(1):29-35.
550. Kaufman JA, Barnes GD, Chaer RA, et al. Society of interventional radiology clinical practice guideline for inferior vena cava filters in the treatment of patients with venous thromboembolic disease: developed in collaboration with the American College of Cardiology, American College of Chest Physicians, American College of Surgeons Committee on Trauma, American Heart Association, Society for Vascular Surgery, and Society for Vascular Medicine. *J Vasc Interv Radiol*. 2020;31(10):1529-1544.
551. Mismetti P, Laporte S, Pellerin O, et al. Effect of a retrievable inferior vena cava filter plus anticoagulation vs anticoagulation alone on risk of recurrent pulmonary embolism: a randomized clinical trial. *J Am Med Assoc*. 2015;313(16):1627-1635.
552. Decousus H, Leizorovicz A, Parent F, et al. A clinical trial of vena caval filters in the prevention of pulmonary embolism in patients with proximal deep-vein thrombosis. Prevention du Risque d'Embolie Pulmonaire par Interruption Cave Study Group. *N Engl J Med*. 1998;338(7):409-415.
553. Prepic Study Group. Eight-year follow-up of patients with permanent vena cava filters in the prevention of pulmonary embolism: the PREPIC (Prevention du Risque d'Embolie Pulmonaire par Interruption Cave) randomized study. *Circulation*. 2005;112(3):416-422.
554. Haut ER, Garcia LJ, Shihab HM, et al. The effectiveness of prophylactic inferior vena cava filters in trauma patients: a systematic review and meta-analysis. *JAMA Surg*. 2014;149(2):194-202.
555. Sarosiek S, Crowther M, Sloan JM. Indications, complications, and management of inferior vena cava filters: the experience in 952 patients at an academic hospital with a level I trauma center. *JAMA Intern Med*. 2013;173(7):513-517.
556. Williams ZB, Organ NM, Deane S. Inferior vena caval filter strut perforation causing intramural duodenal haematoma. *J Surg Case Rep*. 2016;2016(11).
557. Ollila T, Naeem S, Poppas A, McKendall G, Ehsan A. Embolization of inferior vena cava filter tyne and right ventricular perforation: a cardiac missile. *Ann Thorac Surg*. 2016;102(6):e515-e516.
558. Zhou D, Spain J, Moon E, McLennan G, Sands MJ, Wang W. Retrospective review of 120 celect inferior vena cava filter retrievals: experience at a single institution. *J Vasc Interv Radiol*. 2012;23(12):1557-1563.
559. Mewissen MW, Seabrook GR, Meissner MH, Cynamon J, Labropoulos N, Haughton SH. Catheter-directed thrombolysis for lower extremity deep venous thrombosis: report of a national multicenter registry. *Radiology*. 1999;211(1):39-49.
560. Patel NH, Stookey KR, Ketcham DB, Cragg AH. Endovascular management of acute extensive iliofemoral deep venous thrombosis caused by May-Thurner syndrome. *J Vasc Interv Radiol*. 2000;11(10):1297-1302.
561. O'Sullivan GJ, Semba CP, Bittner CA, et al. Endovascular management of iliac vein compression (May-Thurner) syndrome. *J Vasc Interv Radiol*. 2000;11(7):823-836.
562. AbuRahma AF, Perkins SE, Wulu JT, Ng HK. Iliofemoral deep vein thrombosis: conventional therapy versus lysis and percutaneous transluminal angioplasty and stenting. *Ann Surg*. 2001;233(6):752-760.
563. Schweizer J, Kirch W, Koch R, et al. Short- and long-term results after thrombolytic treatment of deep venous thrombosis. *J Am Coll Cardiol*. 2000;36(4):1336-1343.
564. Comerota AJ, Throm RC, Mathias SD, Haughton S, Mewissen M. Catheter-directed thrombolysis for iliofemoral deep venous thrombosis improves health-related quality of life. *J Vasc Surg*. 2000;32(1):130-137.
565. Grommes J, Strijkers R, Greiner A, Mahnken AH, Wittens CH. Safety and feasibility of ultrasound-accelerated catheter-directed thrombolysis in deep vein thrombosis. *Eur J Vasc Endovasc Surg*. 2011;41(4):526-532.
566. Enden T, Haig Y, Klow NE, et al. Long-term outcome after additional catheter-directed thrombolysis versus standard treatment for acute iliofemoral deep vein thrombosis (the CaVenT study): a randomised controlled trial. *Lancet*. 2012;379(9810):31-38.
567. Sharifi M, Bay C, Mehdipour M, Sharifi J, Investigators T. Thrombus obliteration by rapid percutaneous endovenous intervention in deep venous occlusion (TORPEDO) trial: midterm results. *J Endovasc Ther*. 2012;19(2):273-280.
568. Kahn SR, Galanaud JP, Vedantham S, Ginsberg JS. Guidance for the prevention and treatment of the post-thrombotic syndrome. *J Thromb Thrombolysis*. 2016;41(1):144-153.
569. Vedantham S, Goldhaber SZ, Julian JA, et al. Pharmacomechanical catheter-directed thrombolysis for deep-vein thrombosis. *N Engl J Med*. 2017;377(23):2240-2252.
570. Konstantinides S, Tiede N, Geibel A, Olschewski M, Just H, Kasper W. Comparison of alteplase versus heparin for resolution of major pulmonary embolism. *Am J Cardiol*. 1998;82(8):966-970.
571. Konstantinides SV, Meyer G, Becattini C, et al. 2019 ESC Guidelines for the diagnosis and management of acute pulmonary embolism developed in collaboration with the European Respiratory Society (ERS). *Eur Heart J*. 2020;41(4):543-603.
572. Giri J, Sista AK, Weinberg I, et al. Interventional therapies for acute pulmonary embolism. Current status and principles for the development of novel evidence: a scientific statement from the American Heart Association. *Circulation*. 2019;140(20):e774-e801.
573. Konstantinides SV, Vicaut E, Danays T, et al. Impact of thrombolytic therapy on the long-term outcome of intermediate-risk pulmonary embolism. *J Am Coll Cardiol*. 2017;69(12):1536-1544.
574. Kucher N, Boekstegers P, Muller OJ, et al. Randomized, controlled trial of ultrasound-assisted catheter-directed thrombolysis for acute intermediate-risk pulmonary embolism. *Circulation*. 2014;129(4):479-486.
575. Kuo WT, Banerjee A, Kim PS, et al. Pulmonary embolism response to fragmentation, embolectomy, and catheter thrombolysis (PERFECT): initial results from a prospective multicenter registry. *Chest*. 2015;148(3):667-673.
576. Kanter DS, Mikkola KM, Patel SR, Parker JA, Goldhaber SZ. Thrombolytic therapy for pulmonary embolism. Frequency of intracranial hemorrhage and associated risk factors. *Chest*. 1997;111(5):1241-1245.
577. Makris M, Van Veen JJ, Tait CR, Mumford AD, Laffan M, British Committee for Standards in H. Guideline on the management of bleeding in patients on antithrombotic agents. *Br J Haematol*. 2013;160(1):35-46.
578. Marynard G. *Preventing Hospital-Associated Venous Thromboembolism: A Guide for Effective Quality Improvement*. Agency for Healthcare Research and Quality; Published 2016. Accessed January, 2022. https://www.ahrq.gov/sites/default/files/publications/files/vteguide.pdf
579. Guyatt GH, Eikelboom JW, Gould MK, et al. Approach to outcome measurement in the prevention of thrombosis in surgical and medical patients: antithrombotic therapy and prevention of thrombosis, 9th ed. American College of Chest Physicians Evidence-Based Clinical Practice Guidelines. *Chest*. 2012;141(2 suppl):e185S-e194S.
580. Kahn SR, Lim W, Dunn AS, et al. Prevention of VTE in nonsurgical patients: antithrombotic therapy and prevention of thrombosis, 9th ed. American College of Chest Physicians Evidence-Based Clinical Practice Guidelines. *Chest*. 2012;141(2 suppl):e195S-e226S.
581. Gould MK, Garcia DA, Wren SM, et al. Prevention of VTE in nonorthopedic surgical patients: antithrombotic therapy and prevention of thrombosis, 9th ed. American College of Chest Physicians Evidence-Based Clinical Practice Guidelines. *Chest*. 2012;141(2 suppl):e227S-e277S.
582. Lederle FA, Zylla D, MacDonald R, Wilt TJ. Venous thromboembolism prophylaxis in hospitalized medical patients and those with stroke: a background review for an American College of Physicians Clinical Practice Guideline. *Ann Intern Med*. 2011;155(9):602-615.
583. Kucher N, Koo S, Quiroz R, et al. Electronic alerts to prevent venous thromboembolism among hospitalized patients. *N Engl J Med*. 2005;352(10):969-977.
584. Spyropoulos AC, Anderson FA Jr, FitzGerald G, et al. Predictive and associative models to identify hospitalized medical patients at risk for VTE. *Chest*. 2011;140(3):706-714.
585. Bahl V, Hu HM, Henke PK, Wakefield TW, Campbell DA Jr, Caprini JA. A validation study of a retrospective venous thromboembolism risk scoring method. *Ann Surg*. 2010;251(2):344-350.
586. Hull RD, Schellong SM, Tapson VF, et al. Extended-duration venous thromboembolism prophylaxis in acutely ill medical patients with recently reduced mobility: a randomized trial. *Ann Intern Med*. 2010;153(1):8-18.
587. Goldhaber SZ, Leizorovicz A, Kakkar AK, et al. Apixaban versus enoxaparin for thromboprophylaxis in medically ill patients. *N Engl J Med*. 2011;365(23):2167-2177.
588. Khorana AA, Kuderer NM, Culakova E, Lyman GH, Francis CW. Development and validation of a predictive model for chemotherapy-associated thrombosis. *Blood*. 2008;111(10):4902-4907.
589. Greinacher A. CLINICAL PRACTICE. Heparin-induced thrombocytopenia. *N Engl J Med*. 2015;373(3):252-261.

590. Warkentin TE, Greinacher A. Management of heparin-induced thrombocytopenia. *Curr Opin Hematol.* 2016;23(5):462-470.
591. Amiral J, Bridey F, Dreyfus M, et al. Platelet factor 4 complexed to heparin is the target for antibodies generated in heparin-induced thrombocytopenia. *Thromb Haemost.* 1992;68(1):95-96.
592. Warkentin TE, Hayward CP, Boshkov LK, et al. Sera from patients with heparin-induced thrombocytopenia generate platelet-derived microparticles with procoagulant activity: an explanation for the thrombotic complications of heparin-induced thrombocytopenia. *Blood.* 1994;84(11):3691-3699.
593. Warkentin TE, Sheppard JA, Sigouin CS, Kohlmann T, Eichler P, Greinacher A. Gender imbalance and risk factor interactions in heparin-induced thrombocytopenia. *Blood.* 2006;108(9):2937-2941.
594. Warkentin TE, Kelton JG. Delayed-onset heparin-induced thrombocytopenia and thrombosis. *Ann Intern Med.* 2001;135(7):502-506.
595. Bell WR, Royall RM. Heparin-associated thrombocytopenia: a comparison of three heparin preparations. *N Engl J Med.* 1980;303(16):902-907.
596. Martel N, Lee J, Wells PS. Risk for heparin-induced thrombocytopenia with unfractionated and low-molecular-weight heparin thromboprophylaxis: a meta-analysis. *Blood.* 2005;106(8):2710-2715.
597. Warkentin TE, Levine MN, Hirsh J, et al. Heparin-induced thrombocytopenia in patients treated with low-molecular-weight heparin or unfractionated heparin. *N Engl J Med.* 1995;332(20):1330-1335.
598. Cuker A, Arepally GM, Chong BH, et al. American Society of Hematology 2018 guidelines for management of venous thromboembolism: heparin-induced thrombocytopenia. *Blood Adv.* 2018;2(22):3360-3392.
599. Warkentin TE, Kelton JG. Heparin-induced thrombocytopenia. *Prog Hemost Thromb.* 1991;10:1-34.
600. Hunter JB, Lonsdale RJ, Wenham PW, Frostick SP. Heparin induced thrombosis: an important complication of heparin prophylaxis for thromboembolic disease in surgery. *Br Med J.* 1993;307(6895):53-55.
601. Singer RL, Mannion JD, Bauer TL, Armenti FR, Edie RN. Complications from heparin-induced thrombocytopenia in patients undergoing cardiopulmonary bypass. *Chest.* 1993;104(5):1436-1440.
602. Warkentin TE. Heparin-induced skin lesions. *Br J Haematol.* 1996;92(2):494-497.
603. Ansell J, Deykin D. Heparin-induced thrombocytopenia and recurrent thromboembolism. *Am J Hematol.* 1980;8(3):325-332.
604. Goel R, Ness PM, Takemoto CM, Krishnamurti L, King KE, Tobian AA. Platelet transfusions in platelet consumptive disorders are associated with arterial thrombosis and in-hospital mortality. *Blood.* 2015;125(9):1470-1476.
605. Klement D, Rammos S, Kries Rv, Kirschke W, Kniemeyer HW, Greinacher A. Heparin as a cause of thrombus progression. Heparin-associated thrombocytopenia is an important differential diagnosis in paediatric patients even with normal platelet counts. *Eur J Pediatr.* 1996;155(1):11-14.
606. Hach-Wunderle V, Kainer K, Salzmann G, Muller-Berghaus G, Potzsch B. Heparin-related thrombosis despite normal platelet counts in vascular surgery. *Am J Surg.* 1997;173(2):117-119.
607. Calaitges JG, Liem TK, Spadone D, Nichols WK, Silver D. The role of heparin-associated antiplatelet antibodies in the outcome of arterial reconstruction. *J Vasc Surg.* 1999;29(5):779-785, discussion 785-776.
608. Greinacher A, Selleng K, Warkentin TE. Autoimmune heparin-induced thrombocytopenia. *J Thromb Haemost.* 2017;15(11):2099-2114.
609. Lo GK, Juhl D, Warkentin TE, Sigouin CS, Eichler P, Greinacher A. Evaluation of pretest clinical score (4 T's) for the diagnosis of heparin-induced thrombocytopenia in two clinical settings. *J Thromb Haemost.* 2006;4(4):759-765.
610. Cuker A, Gimotty PA, Crowther MA, Warkentin TE. Predictive value of the 4Ts scoring system for heparin-induced thrombocytopenia: a systematic review and meta-analysis. *Blood.* 2012;120(20):4160-4167.
611. Nagler M, Bachmann LM, ten Cate H, ten Cate-Hoek A. Diagnostic value of immunoassays for heparin-induced thrombocytopenia: a systematic review and meta-analysis. *Blood.* 2016;127(5):546-557.
612. Sun L, Gimotty PA, Lakshmanan S, Cuker A. Diagnostic accuracy of rapid immunoassays for heparin-induced thrombocytopenia. A systematic review and meta-analysis. *Thromb Haemost.* 2016;115(5):1044-1055.
613. Warkentin TE. How I diagnose and manage HIT. *Hematology Am Soc Hematol Educ Program.* 2011;2011:143-149.
614. Sylvester KW, Fanikos J, Anger KE, et al. Impact of an immunoglobulin G-specific enzyme-linked immunosorbent assay on the management of heparin-induced thrombocytopenia. *Pharmacotherapy.* 2013;33(11):1191-1198.
615. Bakchoul T, Giptner A, Najaoui A, Bein G, Santoso S, Sachs UJ. Prospective evaluation of PF4/heparin immunoassays for the diagnosis of heparin-induced thrombocytopenia. *J Thromb Haemost.* 2009;7(8):1260-1265.
616. Warkentin TE. Heparin-induced thrombocytopenia: IgG-mediated platelet activation, platelet microparticle generation, and altered procoagulant/anticoagulant balance in the pathogenesis of thrombosis and venous limb gangrene complicating heparin-induced thrombocytopenia. *Transfus Med Rev.* 1996;10(4):249-258.

Part 6

DISORDERS OF LEUKOCYTES, IMMUNODEFICIENCY, AND THE SPLEEN

Chapter 57 ■ Diagnostic Approach to Tissue Examination and Testing

AARON C. SHAVER • ADAM C. SEEGMILLER

In the diagnosis and monitoring of hematologic disorders, one of the most indispensable steps in many cases is the examination of tissue, whether peripheral blood, bone marrow, body fluid, or lymphoid tissue. Just as with any other test performed on a patient, the success of tissue examination depends on proper attention to preanalytic characteristics, followed by careful choice of the appropriate analytic modalities to be pursued. Careful collaboration is necessary between the hematologist caring for the patient and the pathologists and laboratorians involved in the analysis.

This chapter begins by listing the considerations involved in morphologic examination of different tissue types of concern to the hematologist. Next, the categories of ancillary testing are reviewed, along with their strengths and weaknesses, as well as the situations in which they can complement or even replace morphologic review. A range of strategies for the assessment of various tissues in the different clinical settings is provided. Finally, these topics are brought together in a discussion of systems for ordering and coordinating testing, with the goal of minimizing inappropriate testing and maximizing patient care quality. Some of these topics will be treated more fully in other sections, but the goal of this chapter is to consider the diagnostic approach as a coordinated system, rather than as individual modalities.

TISSUE-BASED APPROACH

When considering the proper approach to acquiring tissue for examination and considering ancillary testing to pursue, the tissue of origin is of paramount importance. Peripheral blood material collected for examination will be subject to a different set of testing than material acquired via forceps during endoscopy, for example. This section considers in turn the most common tissues of interest to hematologists and discusses the advantages and limitations of each tissue, as well as issues to be considered in the preanalytic phase of testing: how best to acquire the tissue, what ancillary testing may be ordered, and what follow-up testing may be required.

Peripheral Blood

Routine examination of peripheral blood is one of the most commonly performed tests in most hospitals, with complete blood count (CBC) indices representing one of the most common laboratory tests performed. More extensive morphologic review of peripheral blood smears beyond enumeration and measurement of cellular elements (cell counts, hemoglobin levels, etc.) is somewhat more uncommon, particularly in larger hospitals where testing volume and requirements for reasonable turnaround times preclude actual visual examination of peripheral blood smears in all but a small percentage of cases. Most clinical hematology laboratories have a set of defined criteria by which peripheral smears are triaged for more intensive examination, with only samples demonstrating some significant abnormality destined for microscopic visual review by a medical technologist or pathologist. With this in mind, the practicing hematologist should be alert for patients in whom the clinical setting suggests a need for microscopic review, either by the hematologist themselves or by the hematology laboratorians, and should communicate this need to the laboratory.

In those samples that undergo microscopic review, the ubiquitous standard is the peripheral blood smear stained with Wright-Giemsa or related stains. A peripheral smear is produced by placing a drop of blood on a glass slide, and then smearing it across the slide by drawing another slide across the top. Performed properly, this creates a gradient of cell density across the smear such that the cell types in the peripheral blood (red cells, white cells, and platelets) are properly preserved for morphologic interpretation without artifact. The leading "feathered" edge of the smear often preserves large objects, if present, such as clumps of platelets, infectious organisms, or abnormal cellular elements such as large lymphocytes or megakaryocyte fragments.

Indications for peripheral blood examination occur naturally to the hematologist, since many of the indications for hematology consultation arise from clinically measurable abnormalities in peripheral blood elements. Examination of the peripheral blood plays an important role in the differential diagnosis of a variety of cytoses and cytopenias, as will be discussed in a subsequent section. Abnormal circulating populations, such as leukemic blasts or the circulating component of a lymphoma, are often first recognized in a peripheral blood smear. In the case of patients for whom myelodysplasia is in the differential diagnosis, the peripheral blood smear is an important tool for the assessment of morphologic dysplasia, particularly for the myeloid elements (neutrophils). In the case of certain infectious organisms, predominantly intracellular organisms such as *Plasmodium*, *Ehrlichia*, *Babesia*, and others but more rarely extracellular parasites such as filarial worms, morphologic examination of the peripheral smear is still the mainstay of diagnosis.

Consideration of possible pre-analytic complications is important in every clinical test, and peripheral blood examination is no exception. Collection in tubes with improper anticoagulation,[1] or improper treatment during storage and transport,[2] can lead to complications like clotting and cellular lysis that can skew CBC cell counts and create morphologic artifacts. Patient characteristics create important considerations; a sample from a few-day old infant will often have markedly left-shifted erythroid and myeloid maturation, with circulating immature granulocytes and nucleated red cells a common sight in ill infants at levels that would be sure signs of a hematologic malignancy in an adult. A patient undergoing or recovering from cytotoxic chemotherapy might have so few circulating granulocytes that assessment for morphologic abnormality or infectious organisms is impracticable. Finally, certain clinical conditions of interest to the hematologist are simply unlikely to manifest themselves directly in the peripheral blood. The malignant cells of Hodgkin lymphoma, for example, do not circulate and the only signs of Hodgkin disease in the peripheral blood are likely to be a non-specific, cytokine-driven neutrophilia.[3]

Beyond morphologic examination, peripheral blood provides a key substrate for performing a wide range of ancillary testing, the details of which will be elaborated in subsequent sections. Peripheral blood is an optimal material for flow cytometry, with utility in a wide range of clinical conditions both for diagnosis and in monitoring. Fluorescent in situ hybridization (FISH) can also easily be performed on peripheral blood samples, as can molecular genetic techniques.

Bone Marrow

Examination of bone marrow material is an important and necessary step for many of the differential diagnoses that will confront the hematologist. Bone marrow examination can be used to determine the etiology of a variety of cytopenias and cytoses, with the capacity to assess for disease processes including neoplasia, infection, autoimmunity, and idiopathic conditions. For proper examination of the bone marrow, both solid bone marrow core biopsy and semiliquid bone marrow aspirate specimens are necessary (Table 57.1). Proper technique during the marrow sampling process is necessary to prevent artifact which can limit the interpretation of the specimen (see below).[4]

The semiliquid aspirate material is typically smeared onto slides and stained with Wright-Giemsa or similar stains. Like a peripheral blood smear, this technique allows for optimal examination of the morphology of individual cells, where features such as chromatin quality, cytoplasmic color and granularity, and general cell size and shape can be accurately and reproducibly assessed. The aspirate is particularly important for assessment of the myeloid and erythroid lineages; examination of megakaryocytes is also important in the aspirate, but the core biopsy also presents a good opportunity for examination of that lineage. An important quality measure for examination of aspirate smears is the presence of bone marrow particles.[5] These relatively intact fragments of bone marrow material are difficult to assess directly on an aspirate smear, since the material in the particles may be too thick to be well visualized even after smearing, but the presence of particles indicates that the material being examined is truly bone marrow aspirate and not hemodilute (i.e., contaminated by peripheral blood leaking into the marrow space during the biopsy procedure). When particles are present in the aspirate, the material immediately surrounding them will be enriched for bone marrow elements that are well spread out and amenable to individual cytomorphologic examination, and this is the area in which morphologic review will best be concentrated. In addition to their presence or absence, the condition of the bone marrow particles permits correlation with the cellularity of the aspirate smear to determine the quality of the aspirate. In a patient with a paucicellular aspirate smear, it may not be clear whether the patient's marrow material is truly hypocellular or the material is artifactually dilute. The presence of hypocellular marrow particles may reinforce the conclusion of true marrow hypocellularity, while the absence of particles may argue for hemodilution. A final advantage to the presence of bone marrow particles is that they can contribute a sense of geographic distribution to the aspirate material. Rather than a homogeneous fluid without spatial organization, such as in peripheral blood, aspirate with particles will often have cells clustered around their particles of origin. This may help with assessment of heterogeneously distributed marrow elements, with local aggregation of cells such as lymphocytes, plasma cells, or blasts leading to recognition of abnormalities that an overall measure like manual differential counts might not reflect.

Samples with adequate bone marrow particles can save any particles left over after creating smears and process the leftover particles through a tissue processor, resulting in paraffin-embedded aspirate material that can be examined in methods similar to a bone marrow core biopsy (see below). This collection of material is referred to as a particle preparation or particle block, and has many of the advantages of the core biopsy, including long-term archival and availability for special staining and some ancillary testing. Finally, liquid aspirate material may be processed and frozen for specimen banking purposes, providing an important source of viable, unfixed material for future clinical or research studies.

Some patients will not yield an adequate bone marrow aspiration sample regardless of proper biopsy technique. As would be expected, poor aspirate materials are often obtained from patients with extensive marrow fibrosis or from patients whose marrows are extensively replaced with neoplastic populations (either primary or metastatic) that are tightly packed or extensively necrotizing. Poor aspirates may also be seen in patients who have undergone repeat marrow biopsies in the same location or who have other reasons for extensive bony remodeling or osteosclerosis at the site of biopsy. In patients such as these, appropriate triage of the core biopsy specimen presents an opportunity to at least potentially retain the cytomorphologic and ancillary testing advantages of the aspirate smear. Touch preparations of the core biopsy are simple to perform and do not consume potentially scarce diagnostic material. In this technique, the fresh core biopsy specimen is repeatedly pressed against a glass slide or coverslip, depositing individual cells onto the slip. This process is less efficient than aspirate smears, but can result in a significant number of cells being left behind, particularly in patients who have marrows packed with cells, but less so in marrows that are fibrotic. The touch preparations can be stained for morphologic examination, or saved unstained and potentially used for molecular genetics studies, although this may be limited by total cellularity. If touch preparations are inadequate, or if viable cells are required for techniques such as flow cytometry or karyotyping, then an additional core biopsy can be obtained and, instead of being saved in formalin and processed for tissue examination, can be stored in tissue culture medium and mechanically disaggregated in order to recover viable cells. Similar to touch preparations, this technique of core disaggregation is most effective in patients with densely cellular packed marrows and less effective in fibrotic ones.

Bone marrow core biopsy specimens serve a complementary function to the aspirate. The core biopsy is just what it sounds—a long core of bone marrow material, resembling a thick pencil lead in size and shape, containing both fragments of the cancellous bony support structure of the marrow as well as the intervening hematopoietic elements. The core biopsy is preserved in formalin or other fixate, typically subjected to chemical decalcification to permit clean sectioning of the bone during slide preparation, and then processed for histologic examination. The most important advantage of the bone marrow core biopsy is that it preserves the bone marrow elements in situ without the disruption and loss of geographic context that comes from aspiration. Examination of the core biopsy under the microscope permits assessment of cellularity (proportion of marrow space taken up by hematopoietic elements rather than adipocytes), as well as assessment of heterogeneous patterns of distribution that may not be fully apparent in the aspirate smear.[6] Clustering or aggregation of lymphocytes, plasma cells, or blasts plays an important role in the assessment for neoplastic

Table 57.1. Bone Marrow Aspirate and Core Biopsy

	Bone Marrow Aspirate	Core Biopsy
Morphologic features	High-power cytomorphology	Low-power architecture
Morphologic dysplasia	Can assess all three lineages	Best for assessing megakaryocytic lineage
Architectural organization	Somewhat preserved, especially near intact particles	Preserved intact
Immunophenotypic examination	Flow cytometry, or IHC on particle preparation	IHC
Ancillary studies	Viable cells, can be submitted for wide range of testing	Formalin-fixed, paraffin-embedded tissue; often decalcified, which limits testing options
Long-term storage	Frozen as liquid aspirate, or paraffin-embedded as particle preparation	Paraffin-embedded
Potential artifacts limiting interpretation	Hemodilution because of packed or fibrotic marrow or poor aspiration technique	Aspiration artifact because of poor technique; fragmentation or lack of subcortical space

Abbreviation: IHC, immunohistochemistry.

disease. The core biopsy is the most important sample to examine in diseases known to have heterogeneous distributions in the marrow, especially those such as follicular lymphoma or Hodgkin lymphoma that, by the nature of their infiltrate, are less likely to be seen in the aspirate material, or in rarer disease processes such as hepatosplenic T-cell lymphoma, where the pattern of the lymphocytic involvement is an important clue to involvement of the marrow. Other subtler factors, such as the pattern of myelo- and erythropoiesis and the localization of immature progenitor cells, can be relevant to assessment of disease such as myelodysplastic syndrome.[7] Additionally, while megakaryocyte morphology can be examined in the aspirate, they may be better represented in the biopsy specimen, where the large size of the cells permits easy examination. Smaller cells in the erythroid, myeloid, and lymphoid lineages are more difficult to assess cytomorphologically in the core biopsy specimen and are best evaluated in the aspirate and peripheral blood smears.

Because of their fixation in formalin and preservation in paraffin, bone marrow core biopsy specimens can be preserved for decades, available for further clinical or research studies. The paraffin-embedded material can be evaluated by immunohistochemical (IHC) staining to evaluate cellular immunophenotypes in the context of morphology, or special staining for microorganisms or other processes such as fibrosis or amyloid deposition in appropriate cases. The treatment necessary to decalcify the bony fragments in a core biopsy renders the specimen inappropriate for some ancillary testing, but some techniques are robust to this process and can continue to be used.[8,9] It is important to note that particle preparations (discussed above) are typically not decalcified but are otherwise preserved in a manner similar to core biopsies, and thus serve an important role as archival material suitable for a broad range of testing.

For the reasons described above, the optimal bone marrow biopsy will include both semiliquid aspirate and solid core biopsy material. Some considerations are necessary in order to ensure high-quality material for both samples. First of all, appropriate technique in inserting the bone marrow needle is necessary; biopsies performed at the wrong angle relative to the direction of the pelvic brim will result in a biopsy consisting primarily of the periosteum, cartilage, and cortical bone. Once the needle has been inserted at the proper angle, the needle needs to be inserted to the appropriate depth. Shallow biopsies tend to produce aspirates that are largely hemodilute, and core specimens from such biopsies may be markedly hypocellular, particularly in older patients due to the age-related phenomenon where the hematopoietic elements tend to be concentrated in the central portions of the marrow, while the peripheral portions become largely fatty.[10] In addition to older patients, biopsies in post–stem cell transplant patients must be sufficiently long, as there is often significant marrow heterogeneity posttransplant. Finally, once the sample has been aspirated, the needle must be reseated before the core biopsy is obtained; failure to reseat the needle will result in a core sample with extensive hemorrhagic aspiration artifact.

Lymph Nodes

Examination of material from lymph nodes or lymphoid organs is a major part of the workup for unexplained lymphadenopathy. More so than either peripheral blood or bone marrow, acquisition of lymph node material for examination can proceed by multiple pathways, ranging from less to more invasive (Table 57.2). As a general rule, the more invasive the procedure, the more potentially informative the tissue examination will be, and there are some diagnoses (Hodgkin lymphoma or morphologic transformation of non-Hodgkin lymphoma, for example) that are very difficult to render on smaller samples. However, unless the diagnosis is known or strongly suspected a priori, less-invasive procedures may still have a chance of rendering a diagnosis, thus making unnecessary further procedures that might carry some risk to the patient.

Fine needle aspiration (FNA) is the least invasive of the tissue acquisition modalities available. For superficial palpable nodes, FNA can be performed without anesthesia in the clinic setting and with very little risk to the patient, making it a flexible and desirable approach. For deeper lesions, FNA can still be performed endoscopically or percutaneous with image guidance. The tissue obtained from FNA consists of individual, disaggregated cells which are viable and intact, meaning they can be used for techniques like flow cytometry or conventional karyotyping. Morphologic examination of FNA material is similar to bone marrow aspirate: cells are either smeared on glass slides and stained, or collected into a tissue block and embedded in paraffin. The decision on how to triage FNA tissue for morphologic review depends on some of the same considerations encountered with bone marrow material: individual cell cytomorphology is best assessed by smear, but immunophenotyping via IHC staining can only be done on a cell block. Low-power geographic assessment is not generally possible in FNA specimens, due to the disaggregated nature of the specimen, and requires more significant interventions (see below).

FNA is well suited for the diagnosis of processes that involve homogenous populations of readily identifiable cells, such as chronic lymphocytic leukemia/small lymphocytic lymphoma (CLL/SLL) or Burkitt lymphoma. In contrast, FNA is unlikely to yield satisfactory results in neoplasms with rare malignant cells, like Hodgkin lymphoma, or in disease processes that are unlikely to give adequate FNA results due to properties like fibrosis, as is commonly encountered in primary mediastinal B-cell lymphoma. In patients for whom these diseases are very high on the pretest differential diagnosis, it may be advisable to proceed directly to one of the more invasive techniques described below; although the risk to the patient of FNA is low, the hematologist can avoid wasting the patient's time and resources by skipping a test that may be predicted to be of low diagnostic yield.

Lymph node core biopsy is another diagnostic modality that is of relatively low risk to the patient and has some advantages over FNA in terms of its diagnostic yield. Core biopsy is particularly

Table 57.2. Methods for Lymph Node Examination

	Fine Needle Aspiration	Core Biopsy	Excisional Biopsy
Architectural organization	Disrupted	Locally intact, loss of large-scale heterogeneity	Intact, including large-scale heterogeneity
Morphological features	High-power cytomorphology	Low-power architecture limited by size of biopsy	Low-power architecture
Invasiveness of procedure	Minimally invasive, office or bedside	Minor procedure, percutaneous or endoscopic	Surgical procedure
Limitations	Unsuitable for cases with rare malignant cells or architectural features limiting aspiration (fibrosis, necrosis)	Unsuitable for cases needing examination of large-scale heterogeneity or very rare malignant cells	May not be easily obtainable depending on anatomic location (retroperitoneum, mediastinum, etc.)
Best suited for	Homogeneous populations of immunophenotypically aberrant cells	Homogeneous or mixed populations of aberrant cells, or with striking architectural patterns	Rare malignant cells or diagnostic features depending on low-power architectural distortion

appropriate for biopsy of deep or relatively inaccessible lesions that are not easily amenable to surgical resection. In cases such as these, core biopsies can be obtained endoscopically or percutaneously without exposing the patient to significant procedures. A core biopsy can be obtained during the same procedure as FNA material, combining the strengths of these two modalities in a way similar to the combination of bone marrow aspirate and core biopsy. For more superficial nodes, surgical excision may be relatively simple and of much higher potential diagnostic yield than core biopsy, and may be preferred in these situations.

The core biopsy specimen provides many of the advantages of FNA, including a reasonable number of viable cells suitable for morphologic examination or ancillary testing. While FNA samples are disaggregated and best used for high-power cytomorphologic review of individual cells, core biopsy specimens permit examination, at least to some degree, of low-power architecture, including the organization of the lymphoid material and examination of potentially abnormal cells in their appropriate histologic context. With a core biopsy specimen, hints of the overall architecture of the node can be appreciated, if not fully examined as in an excisional specimen. The presence or absence of normal lymphoid follicles can be noted, as well as other morphologic cues that may indicate the presence of reactive or paraneoplastic processes. Because the core biopsy does not depend on disaggregated cells, a wider range of neoplastic processes can be assessed, including metastatic nonhematologic malignancies like carcinoma or small round blue cell tumors. Hematolymphoid processes that are not suitable for FNA, such as Hodgkin lymphoma, can often be appreciated in core biopsy specimens, although care must be taken to exclude other elements of the differential diagnosis in these cases.

Core biopsy specimens still have limitations, and definitive diagnosis of certain processes can be difficult without additional tissue. In these cases, excisional biopsy is the technique most likely to provide a definitive diagnosis. Although it is a surgical procedure and thus more complicated to schedule and perform, an excisional biopsy provides the best context for diagnosing the abnormality, both in terms of low-power architecture and high-power cytomorphology. Patterns of architectural distortion that can be difficult to appreciate on a core biopsy specimen may be obvious with an excisional biopsy, and rare populations of cells, either in diseases like Hodgkin lymphoma or in cases of focal metastasis in epithelial malignancies, have the highest chance of being found in an excisional specimen. Appropriate tissue triage at the time of biopsy will allow additional studies to be done, including high-power cytomorphology (via touch preparations), ancillary studies like flow cytometry (via preservation of viable tissue), or other studies such as microbial culture that might be indicated by the clinical presentation.

With these considerations and trade-offs in mind, planning an approach for diagnosis in a patient with lymphadenopathy requires careful assessment of the clinical and radiographic context. If the suspicion for a disease such as a small B-cell lymphoma is high, then FNA is likely to be of high value, particularly if adequate material is collected for flow cytometry. In patients with a high likelihood of a disease such as Hodgkin lymphoma, or nonneoplastic conditions such as inflammatory lymphadenitis, then FNA or even core biopsy is likely to be of little use and may cause a delay in diagnosis. On the other hand, for patients with lymphadenopathy in relatively inaccessible areas such as the mediastinum or retroperitoneum, FNA and core biopsy may be the only realistic methods for obtaining a sample, and exertion should be made on the part of the hematologist and pathologist to at least refine the differential, if not provide a definitive diagnosis, to avoid invasive procedures.

Body Fluid

Assessment of body fluids such as cerebrospinal fluid (CSF), pleural or peritoneal effusions, or bronchoalveolar lavage is a relatively specialized topic, where the approach depends largely on the particular body fluid and the clinical presentation. One property all of these specimens have in common is that they are typically assessed by techniques similar to those used in workup of an FNA specimen: stained smears for cytomorphology, collected tissue fragments for tissue embedding into a cell block, and collection of viable material for ancillary testing such as culture, flow cytometry, or genetic studies. In contrast to an adequate FNA specimen, body fluids will often be relatively paucicellular, particularly those from small-volume or relatively sterile sites, making some of these techniques—such as cell block or flow cytometry—of limited utility.

CSF is one of the most commonly encountered body fluids in hematology. In patients with known prior central nervous system (CNS) involvement by their hematolymphoid malignancy, or in patients whose disease process is known to have a high rate of CNS involvement, such as B lymphoblastic leukemia, repeat CSF examinations will be part of standard care.[11] Another common presentation is in a patient newly presenting with a CNS lesion where lymphoma or other hematologic malignancy is in the clinical or radiographic differential diagnosis. Although CSF sampling requires lumbar puncture (LP), this is certainly a less-invasive procedure than direct biopsy of CNS tissue, and thus diagnostic LP is an important first step in the workup of such a patient. Morphologically abnormal circulating cells in the CSF can lead to a diagnosis in the absence of neurosurgical biopsy, and the diagnosis can be confirmed by flow cytometry or genetic studies on the CSF when appropriate.

Although CSF examination can be of great diagnostic utility when definitively abnormal cells are present, it is important to note that CSF examination is a specific but not sensitive technique for diagnosis of CNS disease. In other words, the absence of abnormal cells in a CSF sample from a patient with a CNS lesion provides very little negative predictive value about the nature of the lesion, even in patients with diffuse disease or whose lesion appears radiographically to communicate with the CSF.[12] Flow cytometry, often thought of as a more sensitive modality than morphologic examination, is not well suited to relatively paucicellular specimens like CSF, and has been shown to add very little diagnostic utility in cases with no other evidence of disease.[13]

Other types of body fluids also present diagnostic challenges, particularly in cases with very few cells available for analysis. One extreme example is vitreous fluid, which is rarely encountered but is of prime diagnostic importance in a small set of cases. For patients in whom intraocular lymphoma is suspected, examination of aspirated vitreous fluid is the only available diagnostic modality short of enucleation. However, the diagnostic material is available only in small volumes, and to make matters worse, the patients are often pretreated with high-dose steroids, potentially preserving the patient's sight but killing a majority of the neoplastic cells, reducing even further the number of cells available to make a diagnosis. In these cases, proper tissue triage is of utmost importance, and preference may be shown for specialized genetic testing over more general but less clinically sensitive techniques like morphologic review.[14]

Nonlymphoid Tissue

Lymphomas can often involve extranodal sites, and leukemias can present with soft-tissue deposits outside the typical hematopoietic tissues. Examination of these tissues may be required in order to render a primary diagnosis or to stage an already diagnosed patient. In some respects, strategies for assessment of these tissues are similar to those described above for lymphoid tissues. Diagnostic modality may be constrained by anatomic location (endoscopy for gastrointestinal [GI] lesions, for example) or may be amenable to more generous biopsy (such as skin lesions). While many of the same ancillary modalities are available for nonlymphoid tissues, important consideration must be made by the coordinating hematologist to issues of specimen triage. Specialists in areas such as GI or GU endoscopy may be less used to the particular requirements of hematologic tissue triage (fresh material for flow cytometry, for example), and a careful plan needs to be laid out for apportioning of biopsy tissue before the procedure in order not to waste scant material.

CONSIDERATIONS FOR ANCILLARY TESTING

Part of choosing a plan for how to sample tissue for examination includes choosing what, if any, ancillary testing needs to be performed. Making this choice requires an understanding of what questions need to be answered in a particular clinical setting. The major modalities of ancillary testing—with some of the most frequently performed including immunohistochemistry, flow cytometry, conventional karyotype, FISH, and a wide range of molecular genetic studies—all answer different and sometimes overlapping questions, and thus should be ordered accordingly. This section will review the most common types of ancillary testing, their strengths and weaknesses, and special considerations related to tissue acquisition and suitability for testing.

Immunophenotype

The set of markers displayed on the surface or interior of a cell is referred to as that cell's immunophenotype. Immunophenotyping can serve as a useful adjunct to morphologic review, especially for tumors that lack a pathognomonic morphologic appearance, because carefully chosen markers can give clues as to the cell's lineage in a way that may assist in diagnosis. For example, distinction between T and B lymphocytes cannot be done by morphology, but is easily performed by referring to immunophenotypic markers, such as CD3 or CD19. In addition to making diagnostic assessments about cell lineage, immunophenotyping can provide prognostic information (such as the Ki67 proliferative index in mantle cell lymphoma)[15] or serve as a guide for administering targeted therapeutics (such as CD20 and rituximab).

Immunophenotyping is generally performed by allowing the cells to interact with targeted antibodies specific to the markers of interest. The specific techniques differ in how the binding of these antibodies is assayed. Immunohistochemistry (IHC) is a technique in which the specific antibodies are conjugated to a developer molecule, whose presence is assayed by a secondary reaction subsequent to the antibody binding step. This secondary reaction results in a color change (usually brown or red) in the area where the antibody bound. Thus, the pattern of brown coloration on an IHC slide indicates where the molecule of interest is distributed in the tissue. A similar technique called in situ hybridization uses DNA/RNA base recognition and hydrogen bonding rather than antibody specificity to localize the developer molecule, and thus can be used to assay the distribution of nucleic acids rather than proteins. Flow cytometry is another technique that employs antibody-specific binding and differs from IHC in that it uses fluorophore-tagged antibodies with disaggregated cells in suspension, rather than developer-tagged antibodies with fixed cells in tissue blocks.

With two separate and complementary techniques for performing immunophenotyping, it is important to understand the strengths and weaknesses of each (*Table 57.3*). IHC has two primary strengths, one related to the types of tissue it can be performed on and one related to how it can assist in diagnosis. First, IHC can be performed on formalin-fixed, paraffin-embedded material and thus can be performed on archival material. This permits older cases to be re-examined, either for diagnostic reasons or for research, either as new clinical questions arise or as new markers become available. This is of particular benefit in occasions where only small samples are available, such as endoscopic biopsy, where triaging tissue to separate storage conditions may be difficult, or the need to perform immunophenotyping may not have become apparent until the procedure was already performed. In these cases, IHC can be performed on the same tissue used for morphologic examination. The second primary benefit is that, since IHC is performed on tissue in situ in the same sections used for morphologic examination, direct correlates can be drawn between immunophenotypic patterns and morphology. In cases with rare abnormal cells, or with geographically distinct areas of abnormality, the IHC pattern can be directly mapped onto morphology.

Although IHC has many strengths and is a ubiquitous part of the diagnostic toolkit, it does have some weaknesses that make alternative methods of immunophenotyping important. Where IHC uses one

Table 57.3. Methods of Immunophenotyping

	Flow Cytometry	Immunohistochemistry
Number of markers assayed per test	Many (up to 8-12 in most clinical laboratories)	One (rarely two)
Range of detectable intensity	Wide	Narrow
Type of data obtained	Quantitative	Qualitative
Turnaround time	Rapid (<1 h)	Slower (hours)
Sample required	Intact, disaggregated cells	Frozen tissue or formalin-fixed, paraffin-embedded tissue
Correlation with morphologic findings	Indirect	Direct
Best suited for	Viable samples of discohesive cells where multiple markers must be examined per cell, and correlation with morphology is not essential	Paraffin-embedded samples or populations not suited to disaggregation; few markers per cell; relatively rare populations of morphologically abnormal cells

antibody at a time, and multiple sections must be examined to assay multiple markers, flow cytometry uses panels of different specific antibodies, each tagged with a separate fluorophore, to investigate multiple markers in the same population of cells at the same time. This allows flow cytometry to overcome one of IHC's major drawbacks, which is that trying to analyze a complex immunophenotype (positive for one marker, but negative for two others, for example) requires shifting back and forth between multiple IHC-stained slides in order to get a picture of the overall pattern. With flow cytometry, a single analysis can provide a complex immunophenotype for a single population of cells with great reliability. IHC also suffers from the method in which its results are read out: because it results in colored stain on a slide, only areas with significant color reaction to be seen in the microscope can be read as positive, and the results are semiquantitative at best (faint, dark, variable, etc.). Flow cytometry, in contrast, has a wider range of sensitivity and can detect levels of positivity that are clinically relevant but too low to be apparent by IHC. In addition, the results of flow cytometry are fully quantitative and can be used (with proper calibration) to make reliable relative comparisons between populations staining with different intensity. Another benefit of flow cytometry is related to turnaround time, or how rapidly the test can be performed and interpreted. IHC requires fixation and processing of the tissue, as well as incubation of the antibody and the developing reaction. In all, this process can take several hours and typically has a 12- to 24-hour turnaround time in many clinical laboratories. Flow cytometry, on the other hand, can be performed rapidly, and results can be reported in less than an hour from acquisition of the material in the laboratory. This makes flow cytometry particularly useful in the diagnosis of newly arising and clinically acute conditions such as acute leukemia.

Flow cytometry, in turn, has weaknesses and limitations that explain the wide utility of IHC in clinical diagnostics. The primary issue lies in sample requirements: flow cytometry requires individual cells in suspension. This means that previously fixed tissue is not suitable, since the fixation prevents the cells from being effectively dissociated from each other. Epithelial tissues or ones with a great deal of fibrosis or other connective tissue are also less amenable to flow cytometry, since the abundant cell-cell connections in tissues such as these make the recovery individual cells much less efficient. For a sample that can be triaged at the time of acquisition, sample can be stored unfixed for flow cytometry or other testing, but this cannot be done retrospectively, unless a portion of the sample was stored unfixed and frozen for other purposes. As noted above, IHC can be performed on fixed tissue stored in paraffin for any length of time, and is well suited to retrospective analysis. The need for disaggregated cells in flow cytometry leads to another major drawback for the technique: loss of the geographic context that can be so important to interpretation of IHC. If a small population of abnormal cells is detected by flow cytometry, then only indirect evidence or intuition can permit identification of that population with rare abnormal cells seen by morphologic examination.

Newer cytometry modalities, such as mass cytometry[16] or spectral flow cytometry,[17] amplify many of the benefits and overcome some of the limitations of more traditional modalities like flow cytometry. Mass cytometry, which uses antibodies labeled with heavy metals of varying atomic weights and analyzes the antibody-bound phenotype via mass spectroscopy rather than laser-induced fluorescence, has the same need for disaggregated cells in suspension as traditional flow cytometry. However, the much large number of available heavy metals for tagging allows for higher parameter analysis when combined with the reduced need to perform postanalytic "compensation," which is the mathematical adjustment necessary in traditional flow cytometry to account for overlap or spillover of the spectra of different tagged antibodies. Spectral flow cytometry is similar to classical flow cytometry in its methods for sample setup but uses a different method for analyzing the fluorescence patterns in order to avoid the need for compensation.

Their overlapping strengths and weaknesses make it clear why both IHC and flow cytometry are used frequently in the examination of tissue for hematologic disorders. Some particular diagnoses are more suitable to one modality or the other: IHC rather than flow for Hodgkin lymphoma, for example, or flow cytometry for the assessment of small B-cell clonality. In some cases, both IHC and flow cytometry may need to be performed in the same specimen; for example, if flow cytometry detects an abnormal population, then IHC for a subset of the same markers can be used to verify that the abnormal immunophenotype maps onto a particular set of cells seen by morphologic examination.

Cytogenetics

Analysis of chromosome structure for large-scale genetic abnormalities is referred to as cytogenetics. This technique plays an important role in the diagnosis and evaluation of many hematologic neoplasms, due to the high frequency of chromosome scale abnormalities in this set of diseases. Gain or loss of entire chromosomes or portions of chromosomes, known as aneuploidy, is frequently seen in a wide range of diseases, and can be of major prognostic significance. Reciprocal translocation—exchange of two portions of chromosomes at the site of a double DNA strand break—is another frequent culprit in hematologic disease, and its detection is central to diagnosis, prognosis, and in some cases choice of therapy for many diseases. For this reason, cytogenetic analysis has one of the longest histories of any ancillary diagnostic technique, and multiple approaches are available. Three of the most common will be discussed here: conventional karyotyping, FISH, and comparative genomic hybridization (CGH) (Table 57.4).

Conventional karyotyping is the oldest of these techniques and is still widely used. This technique relies on stimulating viable cells to go through the cell cycle in ex vivo culture, and then arresting the cells at mitotic metaphase via treatment with compounds such as colchicine. Cells arrested at metaphase will have their chromatin condensed into individual chromatids, which can then be Giemsa stained and analyzed under the microscope. The staining results in complex banding patterns on the chromosomes, associated with packed versus unpacked DNA, and these banding patterns can be used to identify individual chromosomes and assess for abnormalities. This technique is well suited for detection of aneuploidy, since the presence or absence of individual arms or whole chromosomes is readily apparent by this analysis. In the hands of properly trained experts, somewhat more subtle abnormalities, such as translocations or smaller scale interstitial deletions or amplifications, can also be detected. Additionally, because conventional karyotyping proceeds by examining every chromosome in a cell in an unbiased fashion, a broad range of possible abnormalities, including potentially unexpected ones, can be detected, rather than needing an a priori idea of what to look for. This makes conventional karyotyping very useful in disease processes such as myelodysplasia, where a broad range of possible abnormalities may occur, and where the range of abnormalities may evolve over time.

While it is a very powerful technique, conventional karyotyping does come with its own set of limitations. Because of the effort involved in performing a complete karyotype for every cell examined, the number of cells assayed in each test is relatively low, usually around 20, which necessarily limits the clinical sensitivity of the test. The lower limit of resolution, or the smallest possible abnormalities than can be detected, varies to some degree since it depends on the banding pattern of the chromosome, but is on the order of several megabases, meaning that a wide range of clinically relevant genetic abnormalities are undetectable by this test. Because evaluation of a karyotype requires a refined understanding of the normal chromosome banding patterns, highly trained technologists and cytogeneticists are necessary to interpret the results. Finally, the requirement for viable cells that can be grown in culture limits both the methods for sample acquisition, since fresh, viable cells are necessary, and the types of cells that can be analyzed, since some cell types are less amenable to growth and replication in culture than others, although specialized culture regimens can help overcome some of these limitations.[18]

FISH overcomes some of the obstacles presented by conventional karyotyping. This method for cytogenetic analysis depends on matching long, sequence-specific DNA probes labeled with many copies of the same fluorophore to regions of interest in the target cells' genome. By examining these cells under the microscope, patterns of fluorescence can be observed that correspond to the distribution of that target sequence in the genome. The presence of additional areas of fluorescence in a cell indicates amplification of a particular genetic element, for example, either by intrachromosomal amplification or by additional copies of the chromosome bearing the genetic region. Combinations of probes using different fluorophores can be used to detect translocations, by detecting when fluorescent signals for genetic regions that should be far apart come together, or vice versa. Because the probes are targeted to specific DNA elements based on their sequence, the results from FISH are relatively specific. Compared to conventional karyotyping, the assay is relatively easily to interpret, since it requires enumerating areas of fluorescence rather than interpreting banding patterns, and thus a larger number of cells can be assayed: usually 200 to 500 in most clinical testing. The increased reliability of the results and the higher number of cells assayed increases the clinical sensitivity of the test, making it more useful for evaluating

Table 57.4. Methods of Cytogenetic Analysis

	Conventional Karyotype	FISH	CGH
Types of changes detected	Untargeted	Targeted	Untargeted
Number of cells assayed	Few (~20)	Many (~200)	Pooled sample
Lower limit of resolution	~5-10 Mb	~100-500 kb	~100 kb
Sample required	Viable cells, stimulated in culture	Viable or fixed cells	Viable or fixed cells
Types of abnormalities detected	Gains, losses, or balanced translocations	Gains, losses, or translocations, depending on primer design	Gains or losses only

Abbreviations: CGH, comparative genomic hybridization; FISH, fluorescence in situ hybridization.

low levels of disease. The targeted nature of the probes also makes the technique more sensitive at evaluating smaller abnormalities; the resolution of FISH is on the order of hundreds of kilobases, which is several times more precise than the megabase-level resolution of conventional karyotyping. A final advantage of FISH is that it can be performed on fixed tissue, allowing it to be performed retrospectively on archived material, or performed in cases where viable cells are not easy to obtain or stimulate in culture.

Drawbacks to FISH are primarily related to the targeted nature of the technique. Because FISH analysis depends on evaluating the fluorescence pattern for a particular targeted probe, any cytogenetic changes at sites not involving the probe will remain undetected. In order to evaluate many genetic regions, multiple probes must be used, which rapidly increases the complexity of the test and its expense. This makes FISH an inefficient technique for monitoring changes across a wide range of locations throughout the genome, particularly if the changes are large enough to be readily detectable by conventional karyotyping. Additionally, without appropriate context, the changes seen by FISH can be difficult to interpret; for example, an extra copy of a probe might indicate an additional copy of the chromosome that carries that element, or it could indicate a chromosomal rearrangement involving that sequence, or it could indicate amplification of that sequence within a single chromosome.

One of the newest techniques in cytogenetic karyotyping is CGH. This method combines many of the advantages of conventional karyotyping and of FISH to create a powerful technique for detecting copy number abnormalities in chromosomes with high resolution. In array CGH, the form in which it is most often used clinically, the target genome is fluorescently labeled and hybridized to an array of genetic elements from a standard reference genome. The degree of fluorescence at each element on the array gives a measure of the copy number of the genome at the site of that array element, and reading the fluorescence across every member of the array provides a map of where chromosomal or subchromosomal gains or losses are located. The resolution of array CGH is determined by the number of elements that are used in the array, and can be decreased to the order of tens or hundreds of kilobases. Since array CGH requires only target DNA, it can be performed on preserved tissue, and since the hybridization array can cover sites across the entire genome, it does not suffer from the "tunnel vision" complications of FISH.

While it is a very powerful technique, array CGH does have some limitations. The most prominent one for hematologic applications is its inability to detect balanced chromosomal abnormalities such as reciprocal translocations. Because it relies on detecting copy number variations, chromosome changes like translocations that result in abnormal chromosomes with no gain or less of chromosome material will be effectively invisible to CGH. Since balanced translocations are some of the most important abnormalities to detect in hematologic malignancies, this is a significant issue that means that FISH and conventional cytogenetics continue to have a major role in diagnostics. Another, somewhat paradoxical, limitation that CGH shares with next-generation sequencing (NGS) (see below) is that it can detect so many previously undescribed abnormalities that many of the abnormalities detected in patient samples cannot be placed in a relevant clinical context. Since some copy number variations are benign or incidental, the mere presence of an abnormality at this level of resolution is not sufficient to indicate that it is associated with a neoplastic process.[19] This level of ambiguity about what appear to be abnormal results can be difficult for both physicians and patients to deal with, and can lead to overdiagnosis if proper caution is not exercised.

Molecular Genetics

While cytogenetic analysis is suited for identifying chromosomal level abnormalities, the level of resolution of even the more sensitive modern techniques such as array CGH is at the level of kilobases. Thus, cytogenetic techniques are not useful for detecting point mutations, small insertions or deletions, and other fine-scale genetic abnormalities. For these purposes, a variety of molecular genetic techniques have been developed and rapidly incorporated into testing algorithms.

This method of testing represents the fastest growing area in diagnostic science, both in hematology and in other areas such as solid tumor oncology. There is a proliferation of techniques that vary in important details but that can be collected into a few major groups, which are described in more detail here. The major groups include amplification-based techniques, Sanger sequencing, and NGS (Table 57.5).

Amplification-based assays use polymerase chain reaction (PCR) or related techniques to amplify target areas of either DNA or RNA. These target areas can then be examined by a range of secondary techniques, including size estimation, hybridization, copy number estimation, or sequencing to determine more about the genetic sequence of interest. Most of these assays use sequence-specific DNA primers to define the target area of interest. Depending on the design of the primers and the specifics of the technique, the mere presence or absence of the amplified target at the end of the experiment can indicate whether the target sequence is present in the sample being assayed. Other experimental setups, for example those using real-time PCR, are quantitative and can be used in serial monitoring of a patient over time to track response using a sequence of clinical interest. Still others can detect small insertions or deletions by measuring the size of the amplified target and comparing it to a normal standard. Either DNA or RNA can be used as the substrate for testing depending on the methodology, although care must be taken with RNA-based assays due to the greater danger of RNA degradation.

Because the sequence-specific nature of these amplification-based assays leads to a targeted set of questions being addressed, and because the experimental conditions can be standardized to provide reliability and reproducibility, these tests are well suited to use in the regulated setting of a clinical laboratory. The well-established nature of many of these procedures, and the presence of reliable and in some cases highly automated instruments for performing the test and measuring the results, means that many of these tests are widely available and can be performed in a wide range of clinical labs. Since the samples depend only on DNA, most of these tests can be performed on fixed tissue. The power of amplification allows very low-level abnormalities to be detected with a strong signal, meaning that these types of techniques can be very clinically sensitive, and are appropriate for use in following very low levels of disease, such as in minimal residual disease analysis in acute leukemia.[20]

Much as is the case with FISH and other targeted techniques, the targeted nature of amplification-based techniques creates weaknesses as well as strengths. The "tunnel vision" problem arises again: if there are abnormalities outside the area of DNA that is amplified, they will never be detected by these targeted techniques. Thus, these assays are best used for analysis of hotspots, areas of the genome where abnormalities are frequently detected at the same site. Many of the most common hematologic malignancies have mutational hotspots of proven prognostic or diagnostic utility, and targeted molecular tests are very useful for those regions. However, nonhotspot mutations are also

Table 57.5. Methods for Molecular Genetic Analysis

	Amplification-Based	Sequencing
Method of sample analysis	Fragment size, sequence hybridization, copy number quantification	Direct evaluation of nucleotide sequence
Sequence specificity	Specificity determined by sequence-specific primers	Nonspecific (whole genome or whole exome) or specific (targeted panels)
Analytic sensitivity	Highly sensitive	Determined by the capacity of sequence platform, typically less sensitive than amplification-based
Volume of data produced	Limited to the specific targets of the assay	Very high volume

quite common and are of increasingly recognized importance in the era of NGS (see below), and are not amenable to efficient investigation by the types of techniques described so far. The other major limitation of amplification-based techniques lies in their dependence on specific sequences as targets for amplification. If these amplification targets are absent or significantly altered, due to extensive mutation, large deletions, or translocations, then the amplification assay will fail.

Sequencing-based techniques can perform many of the tasks in which amplification-based techniques are lacking. When coupled with high-throughput techniques and modern analysis software, sequencing can become efficient enough that it even replaces older amplification-based techniques for many tasks, although amplification-based approach still provides superior or at least equivalent analytical sensitivity in most cases, along with relative simplicity in test setup and interpretation. As the name implies, sequencing techniques involve isolating and sequencing stretches of DNA or RNA, giving a direct impression of the target sequence rather than the more indirect appreciation provided by some of the amplification-based techniques. Older sequencing approaches primarily employed the Sanger technique, named after the originator, which used fluorescently or radiologically tagged terminating nucleotides to create an array of differently sized fragments, where the size and label of each fragment corresponded to the identity of the base at that site.[21] This technique is time tested and relatively straightforward to interpret, but does not scale well in a high-throughput setting. Modern techniques for sequencing, collectively termed NGS, are designed to be easily scalable for high-throughput analysis; although the specifics vary between techniques, generally each round of sequencing is performed simultaneously on a large number of individual samples corresponding to individual sequence fragments. Thus, scaling up the technique only requires being able to assay more samples at one time.

Sequencing, particularly in its high-throughput modern NGS incarnation, markedly reduces the "tunnel vision" problem of older amplification-based techniques. Although many of the NGS techniques in clinical use do use some sort of sequence-specific selection to focus their sequencing efforts, the number of targets that can be selected is high enough that large numbers of genes can be sequenced across all of their coding and relevant noncoding sequence. This allows clinically important but nonhotspot genes, such as TP53 in hematologic neoplasms,[22] to be easily assayed. Using this strategy, disease-specific panels of tens to hundreds of genes are assayed with NGS techniques, providing a compromise between the expense and complexity of whole-genome or whole-exome sequencing and the need for larger amounts of data as more clinically relevant genetic associations are uncovered. Additionally, marrying the high bandwidth of NGS with a relatively small number of target genes allows more coverage of each gene target, resulting in an analytic sensitivity significantly better than Sanger sequencing, although usually not approaching the levels seen in amplification-based techniques such as allele-specific PCR. At the same time, whole-exome sequencing, often combined with RNA-based assays designed to detect fusion signals resulting from chromosomal rearrangement, is in increasing use in clinical NGS testing.[23,24]

The shortcomings of NGS are related to the complexity of the testing and data analysis and the sheer volume of data produced. Analytical pipelines, the informatics processes employed in screening raw NGS data and transforming it into a clinically relevant list of genetic abnormalities, are still as much of an art as a science, and different centers employ different and dissimilar techniques. This can make comparing sequencing results from different centers or different technologies difficult. Similar to array CGH (described above), NGS can result in such large amounts of data that it is difficult to sift the clinically relevant results away from the neutral variants or the population polymorphisms. Even genetic lesions that have been proven to be associated with specific diseases may be difficult to associate with a particular prognostic or therapeutic role, as even well-powered research studies can fail to identify specific associations between disease phenotype and some genetic abnormalities. Although the associations between genetic lesions and disease behavior will presumably grow clearer as more data are acquired, the increasing number of genes proven to be disease-associated and the unfortunate reality of gene-gene interactions means that the problem of assigning clinical relevance is a combinatorial one, with statistical power requirements swiftly outpacing the size of even the largest clinical studies.

IMPORTANCE OF THE CLINICAL SETTING

Putting together an understanding of the limitations imposed by the type of tissue to be examined and the opportunities provided by the variety of ancillary tests that are available, the final decision for how to approach testing in a particular patient depends on the clinical setting. The approach to testing is different for a new diagnosis of an unknown disease than it is for confirmation of successful treatment of a known and previously diagnosed process. This section will consider several common clinical scenarios and discuss the approach to choosing ancillary testing.

Uncertain New Diagnosis

In a patient whose clinical presentation results in a broad differential diagnosis with no clear favorite, the approach to testing is fraught with potential difficulties. Although the temptation is to order a large number of tests to cover a wide range of possibilities, such an approach may be wasteful of resources and raises the specter of having to deal with false positives or negatives. Since no testing modality is absolutely sensitive and specific, care must be taken to maximize the pretest probability of success. Ordering testing in cases where the pretest probability of positivity is relatively low markedly reduces the positive predictive value of the test, and thus markedly increases the likelihood of acquiring a false positive. This is especially true for assays designed to be screening tests with relatively permissive cutoffs for positivity, which are meant to be followed up by more rigorous confirmatory testing but which may cause stress and confusion to the patient who has received an initial positive screening result before the confirmatory testing is performed.

As is usual in building and refining complicated differential diagnoses, attention should be focused first on the most likely and the most clinically acute diagnostic possibilities, with other less likely or less dangerous diagnoses explored in a triaged manner. An example of a case where specific testing would be indicated early in the workup would be bone marrow biopsy and flow cytometry for lymphoblastic leukemia in a child with unexplained cytopenias, due to the acuity and frequency of that diagnosis as an explanation for pediatric pancytopenia.

Confirming a Likely Diagnosis

With a patient for whom there is a single most likely diagnosis, the goal of testing is to choose the single most appropriate test or set of tests without wasting resources or potentially getting a false positive or negative that muddies the diagnostic waters. To take the example of a patient with leukocytosis, if all of the clinical and morphologic evidence strongly supported a diagnosis of chronic myeloid leukemia (CML), then the question would be how best to evaluate for that disease. Multiple testing modalities—conventional karyotyping, FISH, translocation-specific PCR—are available for this disease. While the natural inclination might be to choose all of them, this is often not the best course. In the simplest case, if all of the tests come back positive, then extraneous resources have been spent to confirm a diagnosis that could have been arrived at more efficiently. In a more complicated case, perhaps one or more of these tests come back negative—perhaps because of a sample processing error, or perhaps because of limitations of the test (a nonstandard translocation was present and not picked up by the PCR, for example). This situation creates ambiguity in the testing results, which can cause confusion for the patient or physicians and can result in a delay in diagnosis.

For these reasons, care should be taken in this clinical situation to choose testing carefully based on cost and test performance characteristics. In the CML example discussed above, FISH has been established as the most clinically sensitive method for detecting the diagnostic *BCR::ABL1* translocation. Conventional karyotyping retains the ability to detect other secondary cytogenetic abnormalities, and PCR would be able to more reliably detect a smaller population of disease, but neither of these advantages are relevant in the diagnosis of florid de novo disease, and their increased likelihood of returning negative results for non–standard, cryptic translocations argues against using them in this setting.

Monitoring Disease

A situation encountered far more frequently in hematology than in solid-tissue oncology is repeat testing of the same patient to monitor his or her disease process over time. The relative ease of access to materials like peripheral blood or even bone marrow means that patients are frequently resampled multiple times over the course of their therapy and even for years afterward for monitoring of remission. In this setting, testing is ordered with the goal of monitoring levels of disease and being alert for disease evolution. Here, there is generally more information about what abnormalities were present at diagnosis, and specific tests can be chosen to follow the patient based on what was initially present, as well as abnormalities generally known to arise during disease evolution. For these situations, analytical sensitivity—the ability to detect low levels of disease in a sample—is more important than clinical sensitivity—the ability to detect disease in a population of patients, since presumably the test has been proven to work on the patient at diagnosis. Tests with high analytical sensitivity, such as flow cytometry or PCR, are favored in these settings. On the other hand, there is also a role for nontargeted testing such a conventional karyotyping in certain situations, such as when disease evolution or potential development of secondary therapy–related disease is suspected.

SYSTEMS FOR ORDERING AND COORDINATING TESTING

As the number and complexity of diagnostic tests increases, their value to clinical care becomes more apparent, but simultaneously the appropriate utilization of these tests becomes a more significant concern.[25] Definitions of appropriate testing differ, but in general, the primary consideration is whether the result of an ordered test is likely to inform patient care. In the context of hematology, this can be distilled into four clinical questions:

1. Does the result help make or help rule out a specific diagnosis?
2. Does the result provide information about patient prognosis?
3. Does the result inform therapy?
4. Can the result be used to track patient response to therapy?

If a clinician can affirmatively answer one or more of these questions, the test is likely to be appropriate. It is important to note, however, that the answers to these questions may change depending upon the clinical phase of a patient's care. For example, at initial diagnosis, it may be important to test broadly in an attempt to account for all potential abnormalities that could define diagnosis, subclassification, prognosis, and therapy. However, subsequent testing to measure disease response to therapy may be narrower, focusing on only those abnormalities present at diagnosis that can help assess for persistent disease. In this situation, understanding analytic sensitivity is also important, as one would want to use the testing modality with the greatest ability to detect residual disease at low levels. It may be useful to test broadly again at relapse, as there may be clonal evolution that impacts the therapeutic approach.

Inappropriate utilization falls into two major categories: overutilization, which means ordering tests when they are not indicated, and underutilization, which is failing to order a test that is indicated. A number of studies have demonstrated that both of these forms of inappropriate utilization of laboratory tests are a consistent problem in the practice of medicine.[26-30] This is true of hematology as well: a study of cytogenetic and molecular tests performed on bone marrow biopsies indicated more than 35% overutilization, and indicated that underutilization is also a problem.[31]

Inappropriate utilization has a number of consequences.[32] First, it consumes resources unnecessarily, both financial resources related to testing costs and the resource of patient blood.[33] Second, it affects test performance. When tests are ordered unnecessarily, they generally have a low pretest probably for abnormal results, which reduces the positive predictive value, increasing the risk of false-positive results. Third, when tests are underutilized, important information about diagnosis, classification, prognosis, and therapy may be absent, resulting in insufficient information to optimally care for patients.

Approaches to Test Ordering Improvement

A number of practices have been developed to effectively ensure that tests are ordered appropriately and to decrease overutilization.[34] A few of these are listed below.

Testing Guidelines

Clinical practice guidelines are statements, generally developed by specialty organizations, that outline the parameters of accepted good practice in a particular specialty. In some cases, these include recommendations on which diagnostic tests are appropriate to evaluate particular diseases. In general, these are evidence based and generated by consensus of experts in the field.

For example, the National Comprehensive Cancer Network, which is an alliance of leading cancer centers, publishes consensus guidelines (available at www.nccn.org), which make recommendations on the prevention, diagnosis, treatment, and support of patients with cancer. In hematology, these include guidelines on acute lymphoblastic and myeloid leukemias, CLL/SLL, chronic myeloid leukemia, hairy cell leukemia, Hodgkin and non-Hodgkin lymphomas, plasma cell neoplasms, myelodysplastic syndrome, and myeloproliferative neoplasms.

Clinical practice guidelines are also produced by professional organizations, such as the American Society of Hematology, American Society of Clinical Oncology, the British Society for Haematology, and the European Society for Medical Oncology, among others. Similarly, professional pathology organizations, such as the College of American Pathologists, have guidelines for testing and reporting in particular diseases and for specific types of specimens.

Recently, a consortium of professional societies has taken a different approach to guidelines. The "Choosing Wisely" campaign has produced lists of diagnostic tests, procedures, and interventions that should not be performed in particular circumstances.[35] Lists including items relevant to clinical hematology have been produced by a number of national and international organizations (see www.choosingwisely.org).[36-39] Application of these guidelines has been shown to reduce unnecessary testing.[40-42]

Automated Decision Support

The implementation of electronic medical records and computerized physician order entry systems has facilitated the implementation of clinical guidelines and standardization of best practices. Many of these systems allow intervention at the point of order entry to guide physicians to best test ordering practices. These interventions come in different forms with varying degrees of restriction.

At one end are so-called best practice alerts. These are messages that appear at the time of order entry giving information and/or suggestions about function and utility of a test to the ordering physician without restricting the order. At the other end are "hard stop" restrictions that block a test order, either restricting it completely or limiting it to particular providers or particular groups of patients. In the middle are restrictions that can be termed "soft stops," which require the ordering provider to input additional information about the patient or the test before allowing it to be ordered.

Studies show that computerized decision support tools can be effective in changing test ordering behavior.[43,44] However, the more restrictive approaches appear to more effective.[45]

Diagnostic Management Teams

Diagnostic management teams (DMTs) are collaborations between clinicians, pathologists, and laboratorians, the focus of which is creation and implementation of processes and guidelines that ensure proper ordering and interpretation of laboratory testing.[31] DMTs have been applied to many areas of laboratory testing, but one of the best examples is in hematologic malignancies, specifically the genetic and molecular testing performed on bone marrow biopsies.

In this model, clinical hematologists and hematopathologists worked together to establish standard ordering protocols (SOPs) defining what tests are appropriate. These are evidence based and specific to the patient's diagnosis and clinical and testing history. The SOPs are applied by the pathologist at the time that the biopsy is viewed, delaying testing decisions until maximum information is known. The SOPs are adaptable and are regularly reviewed and updated as new evidence emerges, as clinical practice changes, and as new therapies and tests are implemented.

Implementation of the hematologic malignancies DMT at one institution resulted in significant reduction in both under- and over-utilization of tests with two predicted results: decreased costs and increase in positive tests.[31] Periodic iterative refinement of the SOPs led to further improvements.[46]

Institutional Formulary Committees

Implementation of any of these measures works best when done under the aegis of institutional leadership. In some institutions, this has been accomplished by the creation of laboratory formulary or utilization management committees.[47-49] These function similar to pharmacy formulary or blood product utilization committees in that they collect data, set institutional policies and guidelines, approve new tests, and provide enforcement. When systematically studied, these organizations appear to have positive effects on test utilization.

References

1. Payne BA, Pierre RV. Pseudothrombocytopenia: a laboratory artifact with potentially serious consequences. *Mayo Clin Proc*. 1984;59(2):123-125.
2. Bond MM, Richards-Kortum RR. drop-to-Drop variation in the cellular components of fingerprick blood. *Am J Clin Pathol*. 2015;144(6):885-894. doi:10.1309/AJCP1L7DKMPCHPEH
3. Swerdlow SH, Campo E, Harris NL, et al. *WHO Classification of Tumours of Haematopoietic and Lymphoid Tissues*. World Health Organization; 2017.
4. Malempati S, Joshi S, Lai S, Braner DAV, Tegtmeyer K. Bone marrow aspiration and biopsy. *N Engl J Med*. 2009;361(15):e28. doi:10.1056/NEJMvcm0804634
5. Fadem RS, Berlin I, Yalow R. Comparisons between bone marrow differentials prepared from particles and from random samples of aspirate and determinations of the dilution of aspirate with peripheral blood utilizing radioactive phosphorous (P32). *Blood*. 1951;6:160-174.
6. Schmidt B, Kremer M, Götze K, et al. Bone marrow involvement in follicular lymphoma: comparison of histology and flow cytometry as staging procedures. *Leuk Lymphoma*. 2006;47(9):1857-1862. doi:10.1080/10428190600709127
7. Mangi MH, Salisbury JR, Mufti GJ. Abnormal localization of immature precursors (ALIP) in the bone marrow of myelodysplastic syndromes: current state of knowledge and future directions. *Leuk Res*. 1991;15(7):627-639.
8. Singh VM, Salunga RC, Huang VJ, et al. Analysis of the effect of various decalcification agents on the quantity and quality of nucleic acid (DNA and RNA) recovered from bone biopsies. *Ann Diagn Pathol*. 2013;17(4):322-326. doi:10.1016/j.anndiagpath.2013.02.001
9. Schrijver WAME, van der Groep P, Hoefnagel LD, et al. Influence of decalcification procedures on immunohistochemistry and molecular pathology in breast cancer. *Mod Pathol*. 2016;29(12):1460-1470. doi:10.1038/modpathol.2016.116
10. Ricci C, Cova M, Kang YS, et al. Normal age-related patterns of cellular and fatty bone marrow distribution in the axial skeleton: MR imaging study. *Radiology*. 1990;177(1):83-88. doi:10.1148/radiology.177.1.2399343
11. Sison EAR, Silverman LB. CNS prophylaxis in pediatric acute lymphoblastic leukemia. *Hematology*. 2014;2014(1):198-201. doi:10.1182/asheducation-2014.1.198
12. Glantz MJ, Cole BF, Glantz LK, et al. Cerebrospinal fluid cytology in patients with cancer: minimizing false-negative results. *Cancer*. 1998;82(4):733-739.
13. Kovach AE, DeLelys ME, Kelliher AS, et al. Diagnostic utility of cerebrospinal fluid flow cytometry in patients with and without prior hematologic malignancy. *Am J Hematol*. 2014;89(10):978-984. doi:10.1002/ajh.23806
14. Bonzheim I, Giese S, Deuter C, et al. High frequency of MYD88 mutations in vitreoretinal B-cell lymphoma: a valuable tool to improve diagnostic yield of vitreous aspirates. *Blood*. 2015;126(1):76-79. doi:10.1182/blood-2015-01-620518
15. Katzenberger T, Petzoldt C, Höller S, et al. The Ki67 proliferation index is a quantitative indicator of clinical risk in mantle cell lymphoma. *Blood*. 2006;107(8):3407. doi:10.1182/blood-2005-10-4079
16. Spitzer MH, Nolan GP. Mass cytometry: single cells, many features. *Cell*. 2016;165(4):780-791. doi:10.1016/j.cell.2016.04.019
17. Nolan JP, Condello D. Spectral flow cytometry. *Curr Protoc Cytom*. 2013;63(1):1.27.1-1.27.13. doi:10.1002/0471142956.cy0127s63
18. Heerema NA, Byrd JC, Dal Cin PS, et al. Stimulation of chronic lymphocytic leukemia cells with CpG oligodeoxynucleotide gives consistent karyotypic results among laboratories: a CLL Research Consortium (CRC) Study. *Cancer Genet Cytogenet*. 2010;203(2):134-140. doi:10.1016/j.cancergencyto.2010.07.128
19. Whitby H, Tsalenko A, Aston E, et al. Benign copy number changes in clinical cytogenetic diagnostics by array CGH. *Cytogenet Genome Res*. 2008;123(1-4):94-101. doi:10.1159/000184696
20. van Dongen JJM, van der Velden VHJ, Bruggemann M, Orfao A. Minimal residual disease diagnostics in acute lymphoblastic leukemia: need for sensitive, fast, and standardized technologies. *Blood*. 2015;125(26):3996-4009. doi:10.1182/blood-2015-03-580027
21. Sanger F, Coulson AR. A rapid method for determining sequences in DNA by primed synthesis with DNA polymerase. *J Mol Biol*. 1975;94(3):441-448.
22. Xu P, Liu X, Ouyang J, Chen B. TP53 mutation predicts the poor prognosis of non-Hodgkin lymphomas: evidence from a meta-analysis. *PLoS One*. 2017;12(4):e0174809. doi:10.1371/journal.pone.0174809
23. Beaubier N, Bontrager M, Huether R, et al. Integrated genomic profiling expands clinical options for patients with cancer. *Nat Biotechnol*. 2019;37(11):1351-1360. doi:10.1038/s41587-019-0259-z
24. He J, Abdel-Wahab O, Nahas MK, et al. Integrated genomic DNA/RNA profiling of hematologic malignancies in the clinical setting. *Blood*. 2016;127(24):3004-3014. doi:10.1182/blood-2015-08-664649
25. Hallworth MJ, Epner PL, Ebert C, et al. Current evidence and future perspectives on the effective practice of patient-centered laboratory medicine. *Clin Chem*. 2015;61(4):589-599. doi:10.1373/clinchem.2014.232629
26. Bates DW, Boyle DL, Rittenberg E, et al. What proportion of common diagnostic tests appear redundant? *Am J Med*. 1998;104(4):361-368.
27. Castellví-Boada JM, Castells-Oliveres X. Appropriateness of physicians' requests of laboratory examinations in primary health care: an over- and under-utilisation study. *Clin Chem Lab Med*. 1999;37(1):65-69. doi:10.1515/CCLM.1999.010
28. Rehmani R, Amanullah S. Analysis of blood tests in the emergency department of a tertiary care hospital. *Postgrad Med*. 1999;75(889):662-666.
29. Zhi M, Ding EL, Theisen-Toupal J, Whelan J, Arnaout R. The landscape of inappropriate laboratory testing: a 15-year meta-analysis. *PLoS One*. 2013;8(11):e78962. doi:10.1371/journal.pone.0078962
30. Leaf DE, Srivastava A, Zeng X, et al. Excessive diagnostic testing in acute kidney injury. *BMC Nephrol*. 2016;17:9. doi:10.1186/s12882-016-0224-8
31. Seegmiller AC, Kim AS, Mosse CA, et al. Optimizing personalized bone marrow testing using an evidence-based, interdisciplinary team approach. *Am J Clin Pathol*. 2013;140(5):643-650. doi:10.1309/AJCP8CKE9NEINQFL
32. Epner PL, Gans JE, Graber ML. When diagnostic testing leads to harm: a new outcomes-based approach for laboratory medicine. *BMJ Qual Saf*. 2013;22(suppl 2):ii6-ii10. doi:10.1136/bmjqs-2012-001621
33. Shander A, Corwin HL. A narrative review on hospital-acquired anemia: keeping blood where it belongs. *Transfus Med Rev*. 2020;34(3):195-199. doi:10.1016/j.tmrv.2020.03.003
34. Rubinstein M, Hirsch R, Bandyopadhyay K, et al. Effectiveness of practices to support appropriate laboratory test utilization. *Am J Clin Pathol*. 2018;149(3):197-221. doi:10.1093/ajcp/aqx147
35. Cassel CK. Choosing wisely. *JAMA*. 2012;307(17):1801. doi:10.1001/jama.2012.476
36. Hicks LK, Bering H, Carson KR, et al. The ASH Choosing Wisely® campaign: five hematologic tests and treatments to question. *Blood*. 2013;122(24):3879-3883. doi:10.1182/blood-2013-07-518423
37. Hicks LK, Bering H, Carson KR, et al. Five hematologic tests and treatments to question. *Blood*. 2014;124(24):3524-3528. doi:10.1182/blood-2014-09-599399
38. Bhella S, Majhail NS, Betcher J, et al. Choosing wisely BMT: American society for blood and marrow transplantation and Canadian blood and marrow transplant group's list of 5 tests and treatments to question in blood and marrow transplantation. *Biol Blood Marrow Transplant*. 2018;24(5):909-913. doi:10.1016/j.bbmt.2018.01.017
39. O'Brien SH, Badawy SM, Rotz SJ, et al. The ASH-ASPHO Choosing Wisely Campaign: 5 hematologic tests and treatments to question. *Blood Adv*. 2022;6(2):679-685. doi:10.1182/bloodadvances.2020003635
40. Erard Y, del Giorno R, Zasa A, et al. A multi-level strategy for a long lasting reduction in unnecessary laboratory testing: a multicenter before and after study in a teaching hospital network. *Int J Clin Pract*. 2019;73(3):e13286. doi:10.1111/ijcp.13286
41. Ruka M, Moore H, O'Keeffe D. Inherited thrombophilia testing in a large tertiary hospital in New Zealand: implementation of a choosing wisely protocol to reduce unnecessary testing and costs. *N Z Med J*. 2020;133(1512):45-58.
42. Cliff BQ, Avancena ALv, Hirth RA, Lee SYD. The impact of choosing wisely interventions on low-value medical services: a systematic review. *Milbank Q*. 2021;99(4):1024-1058. doi:10.1111/1468-0009.12531
43. van Wijk MA, van der Lei J, Mosseveld M, Bohnen AM, van Bemmel JH. Assessment of decision support for blood test ordering in primary care. A randomized trial. *Ann Intern Med*. 2001;134(4):274-281.
44. Poley MJ, Edelenbos KI, Mosseveld M, et al. Cost consequences of implementing an electronic decision support system for ordering laboratory tests in primary care: evidence from a controlled prospective study in The Netherlands. *Clinical Chem*. 2007;53(2):213-219. doi:10.1373/clinchem.2006.073908
45. Roshanov PS, Fernandes N, Wilczynski JM, et al. Features of effective computerised clinical decision support systems: meta-regression of 162 randomised trials. *BMJ (Clinical research ed)*. 2013;346:f657.
46. Seegmiller AC, Kim AS, Mosse CA, et al. Data-driven iterative refinement of bone marrow testing protocols leads to progressive improvement in cytogenetic and molecular test utilization. *Am J Clin Pathol*. 2016;146(5):585-593. doi:10.1093/ajcp/aqw180
47. Kim JY, Dzik WH, Dighe AS, Lewandrowski KB. Utilization management in a large urban academic medical center: a 10-year experience. *Am J Clin Pathol*. 2011;135(1):108-118. doi:10.1309/AJCP4GS7KSBDBACF
48. Warren JS. Laboratory test utilization program: structure and impact in a large academic medical center. *Am J Clin Pathol*. 2013;139(3):289-297. doi:10.1309/AJCP4G6UAUXCFTQF
49. Zhang YV, Smoller BR, Levy PC. Laboratory formulary: a model for high-value evidence-based medicine. *Clin Chem*. 2017;63(7):1299-1300. doi:10.1373/clinchem.2016.270819

Chapter 58 ■ Neutropenia

NATHALIE JAVIDI-SHARIFI • NANCY BERLINER

INTRODUCTION

The normal range for the peripheral white blood count (WBC) is between 4.5×10^9 and $10.0 \times 10^9/L$, with a mean of $7.5 \times 10^9/L$. The total WBC includes neutrophils and lymphocytes, as well as smaller numbers of monocytes, basophils, and eosinophils. Leukopenia, a depressed WBC, may reflect either neutropenia or lymphopenia. Neutrophils constitute about 60% of the peripheral WBC, and, therefore, the reduction of WBC number most commonly reflects a decreased absolute neutrophil count (ANC). Neutropenia can occur as a secondary manifestation of an underlying disease or exposure or it may reflect primary hematologic disease. This chapter focuses on the primary and secondary causes of neutropenia.

NORMAL NEUTROPHIL KINETICS

The circulating neutrophil pool represents only ~5% of the body's total neutrophil number. It is therefore a fairly distant reflection of the dynamics of neutrophil maturation within the bone marrow.[1] Neutrophils arise in the bone marrow from a multipotent progenitor cell that also gives rise to all other formed elements of the blood. Maturation of neutrophil precursors occurs over 6 to 10 days. The majority of mature neutrophils constitute a storage pool that remains in the bone marrow poised for release as needed. The proliferating pool and storage pool together make up about 95% of the total granulocyte mass. Of the remaining 5% of neutrophils that enter the peripheral circulation, about 60% are a "marginating pool" that adheres to the vascular endothelium. These marginated neutrophils are easily mobilized into the circulation in response to stress. Circulating neutrophils survive for only 6 to 24 hours; when mobilized to sites of infection or inflammation, they can migrate into tissues where they survive for 1 to 4 days. Neutropenia can occur upon disruption of any of these processes: it may reflect decreased marrow production, increased margination (especially in the setting of splenomegaly and sequestration by the spleen), or peripheral immune destruction of mature cells.

DEFINITION AND CLASSIFICATION OF NEUTROPENIA

Neutropenia is defined by a decreased ANC, calculated by multiplying the total WBC by the percentage of neutrophils and bands noted on the differential cell count. What constitutes a low ANC differs by age, sex, genetic variability, and other factors; the normal range for the ANC for a given population, then, is defined as the mean ANC for that population ±2 SD.[2,3] In general, however, an ANC less than $1.5 \times 10^9/L$ is considered neutropenic in most patient populations. Neutropenia can be further classified as mild, moderate, or severe based on the degree of ANC depression: an ANC of 1.0 to $1.5 \times 10^9/L$ is considered mild, 0.5 to $1.0 \times 10^9/L$ is considered moderate, and less than $0.5 \times 10^9/L$ is considered severe. Although this classification is useful in predicting the risk of severe bacterial infection, other features may modify the risk. The risk of infection may be modified by the neutrophil storage pool.[4] Risk may also be modified by the cause of neutropenia. For instance, chemotherapy-induced neutropenia is associated with a much greater risk of serious infection than chronic immune or nonimmune neutropenia. The risk of infection is also a function of both the degree and duration of neutropenia.[5]

DIFFERENTIAL DIAGNOSIS

The differential diagnosis of neutropenia includes pseudoneutropenia, primary or congenital neutropenias (*Table 58.1*), and acquired neutropenias (*Table 58.2*). Global marrow defects such as aplastic anemia, leukemia, myelodysplasia, or myeloproliferative disorders can also cause neutropenia and are discussed in other chapters. Here we outline and discuss the causes of isolated neutropenia.

Pseudoneutropenia

Neutropenia may be the result of laboratory or clerical error, an artifact due to prolonged processing time of a peripheral blood specimen, the consequence of neutrophil clumping due to the presence of a paraprotein or certain anticoagulants, or as a result of marginalization of the circulating neutrophil pool.[6,7] In each of these situations, the ANC is not actually low and these patients are not at increased risk of infection. Manual examination of the peripheral blood smear and repeated measurements can help differentiate these causes of pseudoneutropenia from true neutropenia.

Primary Causes of Neutropenia
Duffy Null Phenotype

An ANC of less than $1.5 \times 10^9/L$ can result from homozygosity of a single-nucleotide polymorphism (SNP) in the promoter region of the Duffy antigen receptor for chemokines gene (*DARC*). Homozygosity at this SNP results in a red blood cell membrane antigen phenotype termed Duffy null. The Duffy null phenotype is found in 1% of those with European or Asian ancestry but is very common in individuals from sub-Saharan Africa (80%-100%) and the Arabian Peninsula (50%-70%).[8-11] The Duffy antigen is the receptor for *Plasmodium vivax*, and therefore the Duffy-negative phenotype is protective against malaria and selected for in areas of the world where malaria is endemic.[12] This physiologic genetic variance was formerly described as benign ethnic neutropenia; however, the term Duffy-negative phenotype is a more accurate description and avoids the suggestion that ethnicity alone is causal or that this common variant is abnormal.[13] There is also an autosomal dominantly inherited condition called *benign familial neutropenia* characterized by neutrophil counts in the 0.8 to $1.4 \times 10^9/L$ range, for which the responsible gene is not known.

Duffy-negative phenotype and benign familial neutropenias are not associated with an increased risk of infection.[14,15] Bone marrow biopsies have normal cellularity, but a reduction in mature granulocytes and neutrophil kinetic studies reveals a reduced myeloid precursor pool in the marrow, reduced mitotic pool size, and reduced concentration of colony-forming unit culture consistent with the faulty release of mature neutrophils from the bone marrow.[16,17]

Nonfamilial Chronic Benign and Idiopathic Chronic Severe Neutropenia

Nonfamilial chronic benign neutropenia is a condition defined by neutropenia in the absence of a familial pattern and without an increased risk of infection. There is often a compensatory monocytosis and eosinophilia, and bone marrow biopsies show hypercellularity and myeloid hyperplasia with maturation arrest at the band stage of myeloid ontogeny. Neutrophil counts do rise, however, under conditions of stress such as infection or exogenous epinephrine or corticosteroid administration, perhaps explaining the absence of risk for infection.[18] Some cases are associated with the presence of autoantibodies pointing toward an immune mechanism in the pathophysiology of this condition.[19,20] Other cases seem to be the result of abnormal phagocytosis of normal marrow neutrophils by macrophages or the result of T-cell- and cytokine-mediated suppression of granulopoiesis in the bone marrow.[21,22] Included in this diagnosis is chronic benign granulocytopenia of infancy and childhood, which typically resolves spontaneously around age 4.[18] Although neutrophil counts do rise in

Table 58.1. Differential Diagnosis and Features of Congenital Neutropenia

Syndrome	Inheritance Pattern	Gene (Frequency)	Clinical Features
Normal neutrophil count for Duffy-negative phenotype	Unknown	DARC SNPs (unknown frequency)	African-American, Yemenite and Falasha Jews, African Bedouins; mild and clinically insignificant neutropenia
Benign familial neutropenia	AD	Unknown	Mild and clinically insignificant neutropenia
Severe congenital neutropenia	AR, AD, X-linked	Unknown (~40%), HAX1 (~0%-2%), G6PC3 (~4%), ELANE (~55%), WASP (~2%)	Severe (ANC < 500), chronic neutropenia; increased risk of severe infection and MDS/AML; responsive to G-CSF
Cyclic neutropenia	AD	ELANE (100%)	Severe (ANC <200) neutropenia for 3-5 d every 21 d; increased risk of infection during nadir; responsive to G-CSF; no increased risk of MDS/AML; sporadic forms a/w diseases such as LGL
Shwachman-Diamond syndrome	AR	SBDS (100%)	ANC 200-800 at infancy; progresses to marrow failure; pancreatic dysfunction, skeletal abnormalities, and developmental retardation; increased risk of MDS/AML; responsive to G-CSF and SCT
Fanconi anemia	AR, X-linked	FANCA[a]-SLX4	Marrow failure; short stature with upper limb abnormalities; café-au-lait spots; increased risk of malignancies; neutropenia is responsive to G-CSF and RIC SCT
Dyskeratosis congenital	X-linked, AD, AR	DKC1 (~80%), TERC (0%-20%), TERT (0%-20%), Misc (0%-20%)	Marrow failure; nail dystrophy; leukoplakia; skin pigmentation abnormalities; pulmonary and liver fibrosis; osteoporosis; premature graying of the hair; increased risk of MDS/AML; and other malignancies
Glycogen storage disease Ib	AR	SLC37A4 (100%)	Hepatomegaly; metabolic crises; neutropenia
Myelokathexis	AD	CXCR4 (100%)	Neutropenia due to marrow retention; can be part of the WHIM syndrome; responsive to G-CSF and the CXCR4 antagonist plerixafor
Chediak-Higashi syndrome	AR	LYST (100%)	Oculocutaneous albinism; platelet dysfunction; neurologic disease; neutropenia; risk of HLH
Griscelli syndrome II	AR	RAB27A (100%)	Oculocutaneous albinism; neutropenia
Hermansky-Pudlak syndrome II	AR	AP3B1 (100%)	Oculocutaneous albinism; platelet dysfunction; pulmonary fibrosis; neutropenia
Cartilage-hair hypoplasia	AR	RMRP (100%)	Moderate-severe neutropenia; short-limb dwarfism; fine hair; defects in cellular immunity

Abbreviations: AD, autosomal dominant; ANC, absolute neutrophil count; AR, autosomal recessive; a/w, associated with; G-CSF, granulocyte colony–stimulating factor; HLH, hemophagocytic lymphohistiocytosis; LGL, large granular lymphocytosis; MDS/AML, myelodysplastic syndrome/acute myelogenous leukemia; Misc, miscellaneous; RIC, reduced intensity conditioning; SCT, stem cell transplantation; SNPs, single-nucleotide polymorphisms; WHIM syndrome, warts, hypogammaglobulinemia, immunodeficiency, myelokathexis syndrome.
[a]Indicates the most commonly mutated complementation group in Fanconi anemia.

response to granulocyte colony-stimulating factor (G-CSF) administration, G-CSF therapy is not recommended given the relatively benign clinical course associated with this condition.[23,24]

Idiopathic chronic severe neutropenia is distinguished from this benign condition in that it typically affects patients in their late childhood or as adults and has a more severe clinical course with increased risk and number of infections.[25] There is evidence of myeloid hypoplasia, maturation arrest, or abnormal myeloid morphology on bone marrow biopsy; the form associated with severe myeloid hypoplasia is called *chronic hypoplastic neutropenia*.[26,27] To diagnose patients with idiopathic chronic severe neutropenia, other causes of neutropenia must be ruled out, including autoimmune etiologies. The pathogenesis of this form of severe neutropenia is completely unknown. Despite ANCs that may be in the 0.1 to 2.5×10^9/L range, these patients have a remarkably benign course, although some have recurrent infections requiring chronic cytokine support with G-CSF.

A large body of literature has focused on chronic neutropenia in Greece. The incidence of neutropenia on the island of Crete is quite high. This should be distinguished from chronic severe neutropenia, in that nearly all these patients have an ANC in the 0.8 to 1.4×10^9/L range, and rarely if ever have ANC of $<0.5 \times 10^9$/L. There is evidence that these patients may have a cytokine-mediated, inflammatory component to their illness.[22] It is unknown whether these patients have an increased prevalence of the DARC polymorphism associated with neutropenia.

Severe Congenital Neutropenia

Severe congenital neutropenia (SCN) is a disorder of severe neutropenia first described in 1956 by Rolf Kostmann. He postulated that this was the first described congenital disorder of neutrophil number, presenting as an autosomal recessive disorder in neonates and infants with neutrophil counts <500 cells/μL associated with recurrent bacterial infections, most commonly due to *Staphylococcus aureus*, *Escherichia coli*, and *Pseudomonas aeruginosa*.[28,29] His original report described this syndrome in nine families from a remote region in northern Sweden where consanguinity was common, explaining the increased incidence of this rare autosomal recessive syndrome.[28] The syndrome was named infantile genetic agranulocytosis, which later was renamed SCN or Kostmann syndrome. Afflicted children suffer from infections that can occur as early as the first months of life and often include omphalitis and perirectal abscesses; otitis media, pneumonia, gingivitis, and urinary tract infections are also common. The diagnosis is usually apparent within the first 3 months of life. Death may occur as a result of septicemia, peritonitis, and enteritis, with fatal infections common in infancy and early childhood. All patients have severe neutropenia with an ANC $<0.5 \times 10^9$/L, but often $<0.2 \times 10^9$/L, and there is often an increase in other myeloid cell lines including monocytes and eosinophils. SCN was previously hypothesized to be the result of a deficiency in G-CSF or its receptor, but further studies have demonstrated that G-CSF production is not impaired in patients with SCN. Granulocyte colony–stimulating factor receptor (G-CSFR)

Table 58.2. Differential Diagnosis and Features of Acquired Neutropenias

Cause	Mechanism	Management
Infection		
Viral	Redistribution; decreased production; immune destruction	Supportive care; treatment of the underlying infection; G-CSF or WBC transfusions reserved for protracted or severe cases; IVIg may be useful for immune- or complement-mediated neutrophil destruction
Atypical organisms	Redistribution; decreased production; immune- and complement-mediated destruction; direct marrow suppression	
Sepsis	Consumption of the marrow neutrophil reserve; increased margination	
Drug-Induced		
Penicillin, PTU, gold	Immune-mediated destruction via hapten-induced antibody formation and complement fixation or the formation of circulating immune complexes	Supportive care; removal of the offending agent; G-CSF reserved for protracted or severe cases
Valproic acid, carbamazepine, β-lactams	Dose-dependent inhibition of CFU-GM resulting in marrow suppression	
Immune-Mediated		
Systemic/autoimmune disease	Pan-reactive antibodies against neutrophils and neutrophil precursors	Supportive care; treatment of the underlying condition; G-CSF as needed
LGL/Felty syndrome	Antineutrophil antibodies and immune complex–mediated neutrophil destruction; increased neutrophil adhesion to the endothelium; FAS-mediated apoptosis of neutrophils; impaired myelopoiesis; splenic destruction	Supportive care; immunosuppression with methotrexate, cyclosporine, cyclophosphamide, and/or rituximab; G-CSF as needed
Neonatal alloimmune neutropenia	Maternal IgG antibodies to paternally inherited neutrophil antigens	Self-limited; supportive care with antibiotics as needed; plasma exchange, IVIg, maternal neutrophils for life-threatening infections
Autoimmune neutropenia of infancy and childhood	Antibody-mediated neutrophil destruction, usually against a specific neutrophil antigen	
Primary autoimmune neutropenia of adults	Cellular and humoral immune mediated; associated with thymoma	Supportive care; G-CSF therapy to prevent recurrent or severe infection
Pure white cell aplasia	C5a and complement activation leading to increased adhesion and aggregation within pulmonary vessels; splenic sequestration	Thymectomy; adjuvant cyclophosphamide, steroids, cyclosporine, IVIg, and/or SCT
Neutrophil margination/hypersplenism		
Nutritional deficiency (B_{12}, folate, copper)	Ineffective myelopoiesis and maturation arrest	Vitamin and mineral replacement

Abbreviations: CFU-GM, colony-forming unit granulocyte macrophages; G-CSF, granulocyte colony–stimulating factor; IgG, immunoglobulin class G; IVIg, intravenous immunoglobulin; LGL, large granular lymphocytosis; PTU, propylthiouracil; SCT, stem cell transplantation; WBC, white blood cell.

---

number and function are normal in patients with SCN, and the administration of G-CSF results in correction of neutropenia and improved clinical outcomes.[30-34] Kostmann's early studies suggested that intramedullary apoptosis of myeloid precursors was a prominent feature of SCN, and more recent studies have confirmed that accelerated apoptosis is a central defect of this disorder, suggesting that G-CSF functions to correct the phenotype in part through its activity as an antiapoptotic agent.[35-38]

Since the initial description in 1956, SCN has come to be recognized as a syndrome resulting from a heterogeneous mix of genetic mutations with different patterns of inheritance. SCN can follow autosomal dominant, autosomal recessive, and X-linked patterns of inheritance and has been shown to be associated with mutations in a variety of genes including those for neutrophil elastase (*ELANE*), *HAX-1*, *WAS* (*WASP*), *GFI1*, Shwachman-Bodian-Diamond syndrome (*SBDS*), and *G6PC3*.[39-43] Neutrophil elastase (ELANE) is a serine protease that is synthesized predominantly at the promyelocyte stage of neutrophil maturation and stored in primary granules. It has been hypothesized that *ELANE* mutations lead to cytoplasmic accumulation of defective protein, subsequently triggering apoptosis. Evidence supports activation of the unfolded protein response as the driver of apoptosis in ELANE-associated SCN.[44,45] SCN due to *ELANE* mutations is inherited in an autosomal dominant manner. It was the first SCN gene to be identified and is responsible for the majority of cases of SCN. It is not the mutation found in the original Swedish cohort described by Kostmann, however, which is an autosomal recessive disorder that results from mutations in *HAX-1*.[46] "Kostmann syndrome" now refers only to SCN with mutant *HAX-1*.[42] HAX-1 is a mitochondrial protein with weak homology to BCL-2 and its absence results in mitochondrial-dependent apoptosis. WASP regulates actin polymerization in hematopoietic cells. Absolute deficiency in this protein resulting from gene-inactivating mutations results in the Wiskott-Aldrich syndrome, characterized by thrombocytopenia, small platelets, sinopulmonary infections, and eczema. *WASP* mutations resulting in hypomorphic alleles, however, may lead to X-linked thrombocytopenia and neutropenia.[41,43] *GFI1* encodes a transcription factor, growth factor independent-1, that regulates the expression of genes involved in granulopoiesis, *SBDS* gene encodes a gene involved in ribosomal RNA regulation and is responsible for Shwachman-Diamond syndrome (SDS) (which is discussed in a later section), and *G6PC3* encodes the catalytic subunit 3 of glucose-6-phosphatase. Mutations in each of these three genes have been associated with SCN.[47-49] The gene(s) responsible for approximately 40% of SCN, however, remain unknown.[41]

Although G-CSFR signaling is intact in the vast majority of patients with SCN, rare cases have been described in which SCN arises from a congenital abnormality in the G-CSFR. Not surprisingly, these patients are marked by resistance to therapy with G-CSF.[50-53] The most important observation to emerge from the studies of the G-CSFR in SCN, however, is the finding of frequent somatic mutations in the G-CSFR arising in patients with SCN on cytokine therapy. When searching for potential constitutional mutations in the G-CSFR that might cause SCN, investigators identified a somatic missense mutation that appeared to be associated with transformation to myelodysplastic syndrome (MDS) and acute myelogenous leukemia (AML).[50] This mutation introduces a stop codon leading to truncation of the distal intracellular domain of the receptor. The distal portion of the receptor is known to be the site of JAK-STAT activation and maturation signaling.[50] Some investigators have postulated that the mutation causes proliferation at the expense of maturation, explaining why patients with this mutation have a higher risk of MDS/AML.[54] It has clearly been demonstrated that the mutation shifts the dose-response curve for G-CSF, rendering the cells hyperproliferative, and permitting clonal dominance of the mutant clone in the setting of G-CSF therapy. Whether the mutation actually blocks differentiation or merely predisposes to further genetic events by virtue of increasing cell proliferation remains controversial. Regardless, these G-CSFR mutations have been found to confer resistance to apoptosis and enhance cell survival in patients with SCN.[55]

In general, patients with SCN have an increased risk of developing MDS and AML at a rate of ~2% to 8% per year.[56-58] In patients who do develop MDS and/or AML, there appears to be a sequential gain of mutations that were not present in the subpopulation of progenitor cells in the early SCN phase such that over two-thirds of patients with SCN who develop MDS or leukemia have a G-CSF receptor mutation (*CSF3R*). Transformation is also associated with acquisition of other genetic changes, including mutations associated with MDS/AML such as *RUNX1* and *ASXL1*.[59] Increasing mutations in the *G-CSF* receptor gene point toward a role for aberrant G-CSFR signaling in leukemogenesis.[59,60] The role of G-CSF in causing or promoting these mutations remains unknown and a subject of considerable controversy.

G-CSF has revolutionized the treatment and management of SCN. Before the development of G-CSF as a clinical agent, SCN was almost uniformly fatal, with death from infection occurring in infancy or early childhood. Patients were treated with corticosteroids, testosterone, splenectomy, vitamin B_6, and lithium, all of which were largely ineffective.[61-64] The use of G-CSF for this disease began in the 1980s and has prevented infection in the vast majority of patients (80%-90%), although some patients require higher doses.[58,65] The resultant increased life expectancy of these patients has coincided with an increased incidence of MDS and AML. This has led some to posit that G-CSF therapy facilitates the transformation to these malignant diseases, whereas others contend that prolonged survival allows for the emergence of a predisposition to MDS/AML as part of the natural history of this disease. The potential role of G-CSF in the development of MDS/AML in SCN is discussed later on in this chapter. Chronic G-CSF therapy in this disease has led to other complications, including osteoporosis, vasculitis, splenomegaly, hepatomegaly, and glomerulonephritis.[58,65]

Cyclic Neutropenia

Cyclic neutropenia (CN) is a periodic disorder characterized by neutropenia (ANC $\leq 0.2 \times 10^9$/L) occurring at approximately 21-day intervals, although one-quarter of patients may have cycles as short as 12 days or as long as 36 days.[66-68] Nadirs of the ANC last 3 to 5 days and may be associated with recurrent fevers, aphthous ulcers, and infections of the skin, upper respiratory tract, and ears. The severity of infection reflects the severity and duration of neutropenia.[69] Fatal infections are uncommon, however, owing to the relatively brief period of neutropenia that is the hallmark of this disease, and as a result patients enjoy favorable overall survivals. With time, the cyclic nature of the disorder becomes less prominent, however, and patients can look more like patients with chronic neutropenia.[70] It was first described in 1910 in an infant with recurrent episodes of fever, stomatitis, skin infections, and neutropenia.[71] Diagnosis of CN can be demonstrated by documenting intermittent neutropenia via blood counts every 2 to 3 weeks over a course of 6 weeks, but can now be confirmed by the detection of a pathogenic mutation in the setting of a suggestive pattern of WBC fluctuation. CN is inherited as an autosomal dominant disorder, although it may arise sporadically. CN can also be acquired in association with systemic diseases such as large granular lymphocytosis.[72,73] Virtually 100% of patients with congenital CN also have point mutations in the gene for neutrophil elastase (*ELANE*).[74] These mutations are largely distinct from those associated with SCN, although both syndromes have been seen arising from the same mutation within the same pedigree.[75,76] Levels of secretory leukocyte protease inhibitor (SLPI) in myeloid cells are diminished in SCN but not CN patients, and normal levels of SLPI in patients with CN may protect them from the unfolded protein response induced by *ELANE* mutations.[77]

Serial measurements of other hematopoietic cells in patients with CN reveal a periodicity to the numbers of platelets, reticulocytes, monocytes, and eosinophils as well, and the condition is sometimes referred to as *cyclic hematopoiesis*.[78] As opposed to the depression seen in the neutrophil count, these other cells are often increased in number on or around periods of neutropenia.[79] Bone marrow biopsies done during times of neutropenia and times of normal neutrophil counts reveal an absence of neutrophils and neutrophil precursors immediately preceding the period of neutropenia, whereas neutrophil precursors increase in number before recovery of peripheral neutrophil counts.[80] The periodicity of the cell counts is thought to be the result of variations in the rate of release of mature cells from the marrow. Although knock-in mice fail to reproduce the phenotype of either SCN or CN, a dog model of CN has provided insight into its pathogenesis.[81] In gray collie dogs, the disease can be transmitted to unaffected animals following bone marrow transplantation from an affected animal and can be cured following transplantation from an unaffected animal.[82] In humans, a patient with acute lymphoblastic leukemia treated with a stem cell transplant from a sibling donor with this disorder developed the disease.[83] These observations and experiments support the notion that this disease is the result of an intrinsic stem cell regulatory defect, possibly related to accelerated apoptosis.[84] A comparison of bone marrow biopsies from patients with CN and SCN and normal subjects revealed that there were no differences in the frequency of CD34, KIT, and G-CSFR expression on marrow precursor cells between patients with CN and normal subjects.[85] Differences emerged, however, in response to hematopoietic growth factors with impaired granulopoiesis in both $CD34^+/KIT^+/G\text{-}CSFR^+$ and $CD34^+/KIT^+/G\text{-}CSFR^-$ cells in patients with CN; in SCN, impaired granulopoiesis was observed only in the former.

Despite the impairment of granulopoiesis observed in response to hematopoietic growth factors, this disease is successfully treated with G-CSF and is not associated with an increased risk of leukemic transformation.[58,70,86] G-CSF therapy does not prevent the cyclic depressions in neutrophil counts, but does decrease the duration of neutropenia. Granulocyte-macrophage colony-stimulating factor (GM-CSF) therapy, on the other hand, has been noted to prevent the cycles but not to increase the neutrophil numbers to the same extent as seen with G-CSF.[87] G-CSF remains the treatment of choice for this disease when therapy is required. Lower doses of G-CSF are needed for the treatment of CN than for SCN, with a median dose of 2.5 μg/kg/d in one cohort.[66] G-CSF is safe and well tolerated, although patients may develop a gradual asymptomatic splenic enlargement.[70] The acquired, adult-onset forms of CN associated with systemic diseases are treated differently and are often successfully managed with immunosuppression including daily or alternate-daily corticosteroids or cyclosporine.[88,89] These therapies are not successful in the congenital forms of this disease.[66,69]

Congenital Immune Defects With Associated Neutropenia

Patients with inherited immunodeficiencies of humoral and/or cellular immunity are at risk of developing neutropenia. The infectious consequences in such patients are magnified because of the coexisting immune defects. Diseases involving immunoglobulin (Ig) production, including X-linked agammaglobulinemia, hyper-IgM syndrome, dysgammaglobulinemia type I, isolated IgA deficiency, and familial forms of hypogammaglobulinemia have all been associated with periodic neutropenia, and in some are thought to be related to the production of autoantibodies.[90-94] These patients should be treated with intravenous immunoglobulin (IVIg), which may correct both immune defects, with growth factors reserved for patients who do not respond to Ig replacement.[95] Likewise, neutropenia has been associated with defects in cellular immunity; one familial syndrome was described in 1976 in which patients manifested severe neutropenia coincident with decreased antibody production in response to tetanus and poliomyelitis vaccines with resultant infectious complications.[96] Finally, reticular dysgenesis is a rare immunodeficiency marked by severe neutropenia, lymphopenia, agammaglobulinemia, and absent cellular immunity believed to be due to an inherent defect in hematopoietic stem cells committed to myeloid and lymphoid development.[97,98] Mutations in adenylate kinase isozyme 2 are thought to be responsible for this disorder.[99,100] It is not responsive to G-CSF, but can be cured with stem cell transplantation.[101-103]

Other Congenital Syndromes With Associated Neutropenia

Neutropenia is an important feature of several other congenital disorders (see also Chapter 38). These include SDS, Fanconi anemia (FA), dyskeratosis congenita (DKC), glycogen storage disease Ib, myelokathexis, Chediak-Higashi syndrome (CHS), Griscelli syndrome type II (GS2), Hermansky-Pudlak syndrome II (HPSII), and cartilage-hair hypoplasia.

SDS usually presents with neutropenia in infancy and subsequently progresses to marrow failure. It is also associated with pancreatic dysfunction and skeletal abnormalities.[104] It was initially described in 1964 and is also associated with anemia, thrombocytopenia, developmental and mental retardation, diarrhea, weight loss, failure to thrive, eczema, recurrent otitis media and pneumonia, and neutrophil motility defects.[105-107] SDS is an autosomal recessive disease caused by mutations in the *SBDS* gene on chromosome 7q, which is involved in the regulation of ribosomal RNA processing.[48] Neutropenia, in the range of 0.2 to 0.8×10^9/L, appears to be the result of myeloid hypoplasia.[108] The mechanism of neutropenia is unknown, but neutrophils from affected patients appear to have increased ubiquitin-proteasome–rich cytoplasmic structures.[109] Patients with SDS are predisposed to the development of MDS/AML, with myelodysplasia or clonal cytogenetic abnormalities (usually monosomy 7) present in up to one-third of patients. The risk of severe hematologic complications is greatest in patients with cytopenias and symptoms before 3 months of age.[110,111] Before the use of G-CSF for this disease, mortality reached 25% and was the result of infection, marrow failure, and/or malignancy.[112] The use of G-CSF, at an average dose of 4.3 μg/kg/d, corrects the neutropenia and decreases the risk and mortality from infection.[113] As seen in SCN, however, the use of G-CSF and improvements in survival have also been associated with increased risk of MDS and AML and it is unclear if this is due to G-CSF or the natural history of the disease; the risk of MDS/AML is similar to that seen in SCN in the International Registry, but was slightly lower than this in the French Registry.[114] Stem cell transplantation can be curative, but is associated with increased transplant-related morbidity and mortality and thus requires careful consideration and consultation with experienced transplant centers.[115-118] The successful use of reduced intensity conditioning transplantation for this disease may make transplant a more widely available option for these patients.[119]

FA is the most common cause of congenital aplastic anemia. It can be inherited in an autosomal recessive or X-linked manner and is due to mutations in genes involved in DNA repair. Marrow failure develops somewhat later than in other congenital marrow syndromes (median age 7 years), presumably because marrow failure occurs secondary to acquired mutations in the setting of defective DNA repair.[120-122] Multiple genes have been found to be mutated in FA and 15 complementation groups have been identified (*FANCA-SLX4 I* [*FA-P*]), with *FANCA* being the most common.[123] In addition to marrow dysfunction, up to two-thirds of patients with FA have a constellation of other abnormalities, including short stature with upper limb anomalies, and hyperpigmented, café-au-lait spots. Patients with FA are at increased risk for malignancies, especially MDS/AML and squamous cell carcinomas.[124] The diagnosis of FA is established by demonstrating chromosomal fragility following exposure to diepoxybutane or mitomycin C; subsequent gene analysis can then identify mutations in one of the genes involved in the DNA repair complex.[125] Stem cell transplantation can treat the hematologic manifestations of the disease, but carries a high risk of morbidity and mortality due to the effects of conditioning on these patients with impaired DNA repair; consequently, reduced intensity conditioning regimens are necessary.[126-130] Other therapies for the hematologic manifestations of this disease include androgens, which may be effective in half of the patients with FA, and growth factors such as G-CSF at doses starting at 5 μg/kg/d.[131,132]

DKC is a rare multiorgan syndrome associated with neutropenia and/or aplastic anemia; patients may also have other abnormalities, including nail dystrophy, leukoplakia, and abnormal skin pigmentation.[133-135] Additional clinical manifestations include premature graying of the hair, idiopathic pulmonary fibrosis, cancer predisposition (including AML and solid tumors including squamous cell carcinomas), osteoporosis, and cirrhosis.[136] The majority of cases involve mutations in the *DKC1* gene on chromosome Xq28, but DKC can also be due to genetic mutations that are inherited in an autosomal dominant or recessive manner such as mutations in *TERT* and *TERC*.[137,138] The *DKC1* gene encodes dyskerin, a protein that is involved in RNA function and telomere maintenance. *TERT* and *TERC* are the genes for the reverse transcriptase portion of telomerase and the telomerase RNA component, respectively, and, as is *DKC1*, are crucial for maintenance of telomere length. Clinical manifestations reflect progressive telomere shortening and are therefore not present at birth; clinical symptoms typically do not present until the second decade of life. The severity and penetrance of some variants of DKC are unpredictable. However, inasmuch as offspring of affected individuals will inherit shortened telomeres, this is a syndrome that can manifest anticipation, with earlier and more severe symptoms occurring in consecutive generations. Telomere length in three different lymphocyte subsets can be measured to screen for this disease; patients with DKC have telomere lengths less than the first percentile for age in all three cell lines.[139] Genetic testing for known mutations can be helpful, but does not rule out the disease because a subset of patients lack identifiable mutations. G-CSF or GM-CSF is effective in improving neutrophil counts in patients with DKC, and allogeneic stem cell transplantation, with reduced intensity conditioning given the sensitivity to genotoxic agents, is effective in treating the hematologic manifestations of this disease.[134,140-142] DKC affects other organ systems, however, which will not improve following stem cell transplantation, and pulmonary disease and solid tumors remain a major source of morbidity and mortality following stem cell transplantation.

Glycogen storage disease Ib is an autosomal recessive disorder caused by mutations in the gene for glucose-6-phosphatase translocase. This leads to hepatomegaly and a metabolic disorder related to intracellular accumulation of polysaccharide. It is also associated with defects in the neutrophil respiratory burst that increase apoptosis of circulating neutrophils and lead to neutropenia.[143,144] Patients typically present at 6 months of age with hepatomegaly, hypoglycemia, and lactic acidosis.[145] Neutropenia presents within the first year of life in the majority of patients, and although it is usually intermittent, it has no faithful periodicity or cycle.[146] Diagnosis is made by looking for the most common genetic mutations; but if none are identified, liver biopsy to confirm excess glycogen stores and steatosis without prominent fibrosis is recommended. A strict carbohydrate-restricted diet is necessary to control the disease, and G-CSF can be used to treat the neutropenia.[147,148] Liver transplantation has been used to correct many complications of this disease, but neutropenia persists.[149] Neutropenia has also been reported in other metabolic disorders, including propionic academia, methylmalonic academia, and isovaleric academia.[150-152]

Myelokathexis is a rare syndrome in which mature neutrophils are retained in the bone marrow, leading to a decreased peripheral ANC.[153] The retained neutrophils display an abnormal morphology with cytoplasmic vacuolization, pyknotic nuclei, nuclear hypersegmentation, and thin nuclear strands connecting nuclear lobes.[154] There is also evidence that neutrophils undergo accelerated apoptosis in affected patients, resulting in a shortened peripheral lifespan. Evidence suggests that this is a cell-intrinsic defect, because neutrophil survival is also reduced following injection into unaffected volunteers.[154,155] Accelerated apoptosis may be due to decreased expression of Bcl-x, an inhibitor of apoptosis. The storage pool of mature neutrophils is not reduced, and neutrophil counts rise in response to infection in patients with myelokathexis, making the risk of overwhelming infectious complications low. There is a female predominance in this disease, and most patients are diagnosed in infancy.[156] The combination of myelokathexis with hypogammaglobulinemia and warts is termed *WHIM syndrome* (warts, hypogammaglobulinemia, immunodeficiency, myelokathexis),[157] which is caused by heterozygous mutations in the gene for the chemokine receptor *CXCR4*.[158] These mutations cause hyperreactivity of CXCR4, leading to retention of neutrophils in the marrow. These patients respond to growth factor therapy with G-CSF or GM-CSF, which downregulate the expression of CXCR4.[159,160] The CXCR4 antagonist, plerixafor, has been given to nine patients with the WHIM syndrome with resultant transient normalization of WBC counts.[161-163]

Congenital disorders of vesicular trafficking are also associated with neutropenia. These include CHS, GS2, and HPSII.[164] These diseases are also associated with disorders of other granulated cells, leading to oculocutaneous albinism (from disrupted melanin granules), bleeding (from abnormal platelet secretory granules), and neurologic disease (from abnormal trafficking and release of neuronal granules). All of these diseases can enter a terminal phase of hemophagocytic syndrome, often in the setting of Epstein-Barr virus (EBV) infection. In all cases, this is postulated to occur because of abnormal secretion of perforin-containing granules into the immunologic synapse, impairing natural killer cell–mediated killing. CHS is an autosomal recessive disorder caused by mutations in the *LYST* gene (lysosomal trafficking regulatory gene) and is associated with characteristic neutrophils containing giant granules.[164-166] Three-quarters of patients with CHS develop moderate to severe neutropenia, thought to be the result of increased destruction of peripheral neutrophils and decreased marrow release of neutrophils.[165,167] Infectious risk is increased above that expected for the ANC because of concomitant humoral and cellular immune defects in this disease.[168,169] GS2 is also an autosomal recessive disorder due to mutations in a small GTPase *RAB27A*, which is part of the protein complex necessary for granule release.[170,171] HPSII is due to defects in *AP3B1*, which encodes a part of a protein transport complex that mediates sorting of lysosomal proteins.[172] Defects in *AP3B1* lead to widespread functional impairment of cells carrying secretory granules. As for many of the syndromes and diseases noted earlier, stem cell transplantation can cure the hematologic manifestations of these diseases and may be necessary to control the hemophagocytosis associated with CHS and GS2, but does not treat the other systemic findings.[173,174] Otherwise, growth factor support and antibiotics provide supportive care, and steroids, splenectomy, IVIg, and chemotherapy have been used to manage the accelerated phase of CHS.[175,176]

Lastly, cartilage-hair hypoplasia is a rare syndrome associated with moderate to severe neutropenia, as well as short-limb dwarfism, fine hair, and defects in cellular immunity.[177] It is inherited in an autosomal recessive manner and has increased prevalence in the Amish and Finnish populations.[178,179] It is caused by mutations in the *RMRP* gene on chromosome 9, which has an unknown function but is a noncoding RNA essential for early murine development.[180,181] As in other syndromes with combined neutropenia and cellular immune defects, infectious risk is additive. G-CSF is effective and stem cell transplantation can cure the hematologic and immunologic manifestations of this disease.[182,183]

Secondary Causes of Neutropenia
Postinfectious Neutropenia

Several viral infections have been shown to cause a transient neutropenia, including varicella, measles, rubella, hepatitis A and B, EBV, influenza, parvovirus, and cytomegalovirus. Neutropenia typically corresponds to the period of peak viremia during the first 1 to 2 days of clinical symptoms. Neutropenia usually resolves within 3 to 7 days. Neutropenia results from a combination of decreased production and immune destruction of neutrophils; in addition, some viral infections increase neutrophil adherence to the vasculature, causing increased margination.[184,185] Because neutropenia is short lived, it rarely results in bacterial superinfection regardless of its severity. However, the neutropenia associated with hepatitis B and EBV infections can be more prolonged and thus more dangerous. Human immunodeficiency virus infection is commonly associated with neutropenia that arises from a combination of decreased marrow production of neutrophils and peripheral immune destruction.[186] As with EBV and hepatitis B infection, this neutropenia may be protracted as a result of direct viral infection of hematopoietic precursor cells or as a result of antineutrophil antibodies. Moderate neutropenia can also be seen in association with atypical bacterial infections, including those caused by *Mycobacterium tuberculosis*, ehrlichiosis, rickettsia, tularemia, and brucellosis. This may be related to by direct bone marrow suppression of myelopoiesis by toxins released by the pathogenic organisms, decreased neutrophil production as a result of infection-mediated decrease in growth factor production, and complement-mediated peripheral neutrophil destruction. Neutropenia is fairly common in the setting of overwhelming sepsis and reflects consumption of marrow reserves of neutrophils. This is usually seen at the extremes of life, in infants, and in the elderly, in which patients typically have decreased marrow reserves.[187] Management of patients with infection-related neutropenia requires good supportive care with treatment of the underlying infection. G-CSF or WBC transfusions are reserved for protracted and severe cases.[188,189] IVIg may be effective for neutropenia that results from autoimmune or complement-mediated destruction as a result of the underlying infection.[190]

Drug-Induced Neutropenia and Neutropenia Due to Marrow Injury

Although accurate estimates of the incidence of drug-induced neutropenia are not readily available, a 10-year Swedish experience, a 5-year Dutch experience, a 22-year Spanish experience, and the International Aplastic Anemia and Agranulocytosis Study demonstrate an annual incidence of severe drug-induced neutropenia of 1.0 to 3.4 cases per million population per year.[191-193] Multiple drugs have been implicated in neutropenia and agranulocytosis, both in predictable and idiosyncratic patterns. Antineoplastic, antiviral, and immunosuppressive agents all cause an expected dose-dependent decrease in neutrophils, often accompanied by general marrow suppression. Common drugs known to cause neutropenia that is more idiosyncratic include clozapine, the thionamides, and sulfasalazine. Most drugs cause direct dose-dependent marrow suppression and others incite immune-mediated destruction; these mechanisms may not be mutually exclusive.[194-197] Immune-mediated destruction may occur by one of two mechanisms: the drug may act as a hapten and induce antibody formation and complement fixation, or the drug can cause the formation of circulating immune complexes that bind to neutrophils. The former is the mechanism associated with penicillin, propylthiouracil, and gold and the latter is associated with quinine administration. Marrow suppression, on the other hand, is the result of dose-dependent inhibition of colony-forming unit granulocyte macrophages and can be seen with valproic acid, carbamazepine, and β-lactam antibiotics. Finally, drugs can cause damage to the marrow microenvironment and myeloid precursors; certain patients with specific genetic polymorphisms or other medical problems may be at increased risk for drug-induced neutropenia by this mechanism.[198-200]

Drug-induced neutropenia typically occurs after 1 to 2 weeks of exposure to the drug, although it may occur after a longer period of exposure. Recovery usually begins within days of stopping the drug, but this pattern is highly variable depending on the mechanism of neutropenia. For example, immune-mediated neutropenia may be immediate, occurring within hours of administration of the drug especially if there has been a previous exposure and prior antibody production, whereas drugs that cause direct marrow suppression or toxicity follow the abovementioned paradigm.[201] Some patients may present with agranulocytosis, fever, and possibly sepsis; in these patients, mortality may be significant. Neutrophil recovery is often preceded by the appearance of monocytes and immature neutrophil forms. Although marrow examination is rarely necessary, one can roughly predict the duration of neutropenia from the cellularity of the marrow, because patients with hypercellular marrows or marrows with abundant metamyelocytes and later forms tend to have more rapid reconstitution following discontinuation of the offending medication. Management is similar to that for postinfectious neutropenia with supportive care and removal of the offending agent, although growth factor support is recommended for patients presenting with agranulocytosis.[202]

Radiation can also result in acute or chronic marrow failure. Exposure to radiation is also a risk factor for AML/MDS. These diseases are discussed in greater detail in Chapters 76 and 80, respectively. Likewise, metastatic carcinoma to the bone can also cause marrow failure because the marrow becomes increasingly occupied by the metastatic cells.

Immune Neutropenia

As discussed previously, infection and drugs can cause immune-mediated neutrophil destruction. However, primary immune neutropenia can occur in the absence of other inciting events or can also arise in association with an underlying systemic autoimmune disease. Antineutrophil antibodies are implicated in mediating neutrophil destruction either by destruction in the spleen or by intravascular complement-mediated neutrophil lysis. A number of neutrophil-specific antigens have been identified in patients with a history of autoimmune neutropenia, including human neutrophil antigen (HNA)-1, an isoform of the Fcγ IIIB receptor, and HNA-4 and HNA-5, which are CD11b and CD11a, respectively.[203,204] The clinical presentation is variable, and depends on whether the antineutrophil antibodies react primarily with mature neutrophils or with myeloid progenitor cells, whether the antibodies are primary or secondary to an underlying condition, and whether the antibody is of restricted or nonrestricted clonality.[205,206] Some patients may have an absence of only mature neutrophils, whereas others may be missing all or some myeloid forms. In primary immune neutropenia, antibodies are more likely to be directed against a neutrophil-specific antigen, whereas secondary conditions are commonly associated with pan-reactive antibodies. Similarly, antibodies that are produced as a result of an exposure to a foreign antigen are more likely to be polyclonal and short lived, whereas those due to the loss of suppression of a clone of cells producing an autoantibody are associated with a more protracted and severe course of neutropenia. Bone marrow biopsy findings will depend on the stage in neutrophil maturation against which the antibodies are directed; but in most cases, the marrow is hyper- or normocellular with a "maturation arrest" that reflects destruction of later stage cells.

Hyperthyroidism, Wegener granulomatosis, rheumatoid arthritis (RA), systemic lupus erythematosus (SLE), chronic hepatitis and other systemic infections, and malignancy are autoimmune and systemic disorders associated with antineutrophil antibodies. In many of these diseases, especially SLE, neutropenia is often mild and reflects the activity of the underlying disease. It rarely requires treatment outside of treatment of the underlying disease.[207]

Felty syndrome and large granular lymphocytic (LGL) leukemia can also cause immune-mediated neutrophil destruction, and may be associated with profound neutropenia and increased infections. LGL is a syndrome of autoimmune neutropenia in association with marrow infiltration by clonal large granular lymphocytes.[208] These lymphocytes are cytotoxic T cells with the following immunophenotype: CD3⁻, CD8⁻, CD16⁻, and CD57⁺. LGL can occur sporadically or in association with systemic autoimmune diseases, especially RA.[209] LGL is closely related to Felty syndrome, a syndrome associated with splenomegaly and neutropenia in the setting of RA.[210] Ninety percent of patients with Felty syndrome and LGL associated with RA are human leukocyte antigen (HLA)-DR4⁺, leading many investigators to postulate that the two syndromes are in a spectrum of the same disease.[211] The pathophysiology of neutropenia is complex, including both antibody-mediated and cell-mediated destruction, immune complexes, and increased FAS-mediated apoptosis.[212-216] The neutropenia is responsive to G-CSF, which is usually utilized until the primary disease can be treated.[217] Treatment options for LGL and Felty syndrome include immunosuppressive therapies including methotrexate, cyclosporine, cyclophosphamide, and, most recently, rituximab for Felty syndrome.[218-222]

Neonatal neutropenia, or neonatal alloimmune neutropenia, is caused by transplacental passage of maternal IgG antibodies against paternal neutrophil antigens, resulting in neutropenia in a manner similar to anemia in Rh hemolytic disease. During gestation, the mother is sensitized to unique fetal neutrophil antigens and produces IgG antibodies against these antigens that can cross the placenta. These antigens will be shared with the father and so will be reactive against the father's neutrophils, thus facilitating the diagnosis. Neutropenia typically resolves within 2 months, and appropriate antibiotics will usually be sufficient to support the patient. In the event of severe or life-threatening infection, plasma exchange, IVIg, and transfusion of maternal neutrophils have all been used.[223]

Autoimmune neutropenia of infancy and childhood, termed *primary immune neutropenia*, occurs in children ages 6 months to 10 years and is the most frequent primary immune neutropenia.[224] Infections tend to be mild and include otitis media, gastroenteritis, and/or cellulitis. Resolution of neutropenia occurs in over 95% of patients by age 2.[225] Primary autoimmune neutropenia in adults is rare and tends to be more chronic. However, even adults tend to have a mild clinical course.

Lastly, pure white cell aplasia is a rare disease associated with severe pyogenic infections and is associated with a thymoma in over two-thirds of cases.[226] It has also occurred following ibuprofen therapy.[227] There is a complete absence of myeloid precursors on bone marrow examination. It is immune mediated, but removal of the thymoma in thymoma-associated cases may not be sufficient for remission. Adjuvant therapy with cytoxan, steroids, cyclosporine, IVIg, and even stem cell transplantation may be needed.[228-230]

Neutropenia Due to Increased Margination and Hypersplenism

Complement activation increases margination of neutrophils and can suppress the peripheral ANC.[231] This has been seen in patients suffering from burns and transfusion reactions and as a result of exposure to artificial membranes used in dialysis, cardiopulmonary bypass, apheresis, and extracorporeal membrane oxygenation.[232-234] Neutropenia in the setting of transfusion is due to an anamnestic response to foreign antigens on neutrophils in a prior transfused blood product. Complement activation may also lead to direct neutrophil destruction, as in the case of paroxysmal nocturnal hemoglobinuria. Splenomegaly with hypersplenism can also reduce the neutrophil count.[235]

Neutropenia Due to Nutritional Deficiency

Neutropenia is part of the clinical spectrum of megaloblastic anemia arising from deficiency of vitamin B_{12}, folate, and copper.[236,237] These diseases typically cause pancytopenia because of disordered maturation of all cell lines.

CLINICAL PRESENTATION AND DIAGNOSTIC APPROACH TO NEUTROPENIA

One of the first definitions of the syndrome of neutropenia and infection was in 1922 by Werner Schultz who described the findings of sore throat, prostration, and neutropenia in a cohort of middle-aged women and called this entity agranulocytosis.[238] This fulminant form of neutropenia has sometimes been referred to as Schultz disease.[239] The description highlights that the first evidence of neutropenia is often the development of infection, and that severe neutropenia is associated with a risk for spontaneous infection. Although the lower level of the normal ANC is 1500 cells/μL, patients rarely develop infectious complications of neutropenia until their ANC falls below 500 cells/μL, and, in fact, patients with chronic neutropenia rarely develop fever unless their ANC is below 200 cells/μL. Common sites of infection include the oral cavity and mucous membranes including mouth ulcers, pharyngeal inflammation, and periodontitis, the skin with rashes, cellulitis, abscesses, and poor wound healing, the perirectal and anal areas, and the respiratory tract. Endogenous flora are the primary pathogens. It should be remembered that most of the signs and symptoms of infection are generated by neutrophils. Consequently, patients with neutropenia may have minimal signs and symptoms of infection, with minimal inflammatory infiltrates. Fever is the most informative sign in patients with neutropenia and should be evaluated emergently, because in the setting of profound neutropenia, patients may rapidly develop fatal sepsis. A presentation of neutropenia should prompt a careful evaluation for signs and symptoms of infection with cultures and antibiotic administration when indicated.

In children presenting for the first time with neutropenia, growth and development should be documented (*Figure 58.1*). Attention should be paid to the skin, bones/appendages, and nails as abnormalities in these may point toward one of the congenital neutropenia syndromes. Family history of recurrent infections and sudden death may be helpful in this regard. If congenital neutropenia is suspected, appropriate genetic testing should be obtained. In adults previously known to have a normal ANC who present with profound neutropenia (agranulocytosis) and an otherwise normal complete blood count, the diagnosis is almost invariably drug-induced neutropenia. These patients usually present with an acute febrile episode. A thorough history of drug and toxin exposure should be obtained and all potential offending agents discontinued. For patients of all ages, the perineum and perirectal area should be examined, in addition to a complete physical examination. The peripheral blood smear should be examined and tests for vitamin B_{12} and folate levels obtained. Older tests included hydrocortisone stimulation tests (for marrow myeloid reserve), the epinephrine challenge test (for estimation of the size of the marginated neutrophil pool), and the Rebuck skin window (which evaluates neutrophil margination into tissues), but these are rarely used today.[240-242] Bone marrow examination is not required unless there are other features to suggest an alternative diagnosis.

In patients presenting with unexplained neutropenia in the absence of a well-documented normal ANC in the past, evaluation depends on the severity of the neutropenia (*Figure 58.2*). There is little information to be gained from an extensive evaluation of healthy subjects with no history of infections and ANC of 1.2 to 1.5×10^9 cells/L that has been present for many years. In individuals of appropriate ancestry, the diagnosis of constitutional neutropenia obviates the need for further evaluation. Even in patients who do not have a clear Duffy-negative phenotype or familial neutropenia, studies to rule out marrow pathology in the absence of clinical sequelae or evidence of continued decrease in the blood counts are unlikely to be informative.

In patients with severe neutropenia of indeterminate duration, the pace and extent of diagnosis should be determined by the clinical presentation. In patients in whom cycling is suspected, genetic testing for *ELANE* mutations and peripheral blood flow cytometry and T-cell receptor rearrangement studies to assess for LGL should be obtained. In the cases of a selective severe chronic neutropenia, even in the absence of a history of infection or drug/toxin exposure or an evident B_{12} or folate deficiency, a single bone marrow examination is recommended to assess for myelodysplasia. If marrow morphology is unremarkable and cytogenetics are normal, repeated bone marrow examination is not recommended unless there is a significant change in the peripheral blood counts that suggests a new intervening diagnosis. Bone marrow biopsy should be performed in all patients with bi- or tricytopenias to evaluate the adequacy of hematopoietic marrow pools, the relative maturation of these pools, and the morphology of these pools for clues as to the etiology of the cytopenias.

MANAGEMENT OF NEUTROPENIA

Decisions regarding the treatment of neutropenia depend primarily on the presence or absence of fever. Neutropenia with fever should be treated as a medical emergency, with the goal of evaluating patients and initiating antibiotics within 30 to 60 minutes. The administration of empiric broad-spectrum antibiotics to patients with febrile neutropenia has been demonstrated to improve survival.[243,244] Third- or fourth-generation cephalosporins as single agents have become the standard initial empiric therapy, replacing previous combinations that emphasized double coverage for pseudomonal species.[245] In patients with indwelling lines, the addition of vancomycin may be considered, and patients at increased risk for fungal infection or who remain febrile despite 3 to 5 days of antibiotics should receive antifungal agents.[246]

For patients with mild neutropenia and infections, outpatient antibiotic therapy may be warranted and is based on the clinical judgment of the treating physician. The cause of neutropenia is important in determining further therapies: transient neutropenia due to a drug, infection, or chemotherapy administration may require no further therapy. G-CSF can be used for high-risk patients with pneumonia, hypotension, and/or fungemia, whereas neutropenia due to autoantibodies, an underlying systemic disease, or a congenital syndrome may require preventative approaches including immunologic therapies such as corticosteroids, IVIg, and/or plasmapheresis, treatment of the underlying disease, G-CSF therapy, or possibly a hematopoietic stem cell

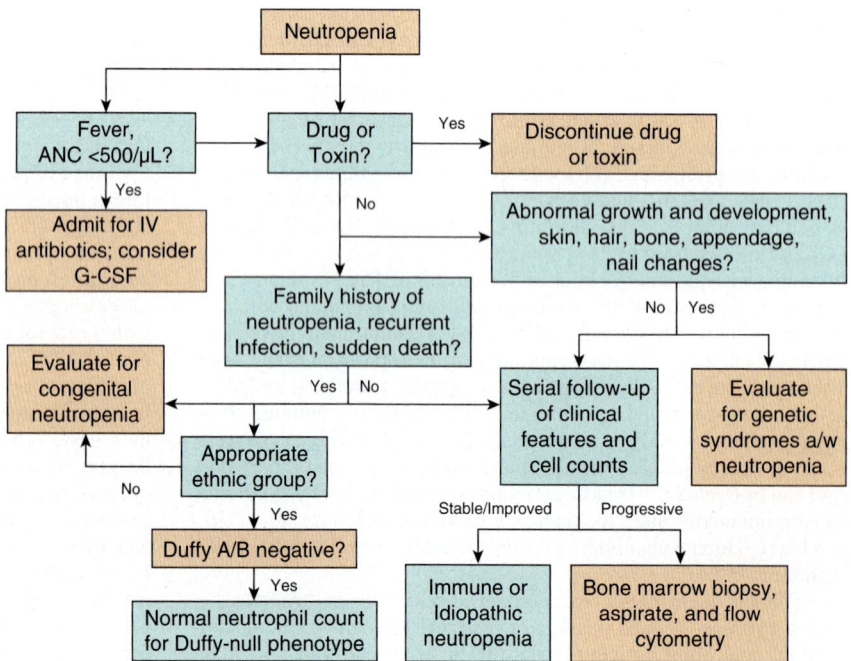

FIGURE 58.1 Diagnostic approach to neutropenia in the infant. a/w, associated with; ANC, absolute neutrophil count; G-CSF, granulocyte colony-stimulating factor; IV, intravenous.

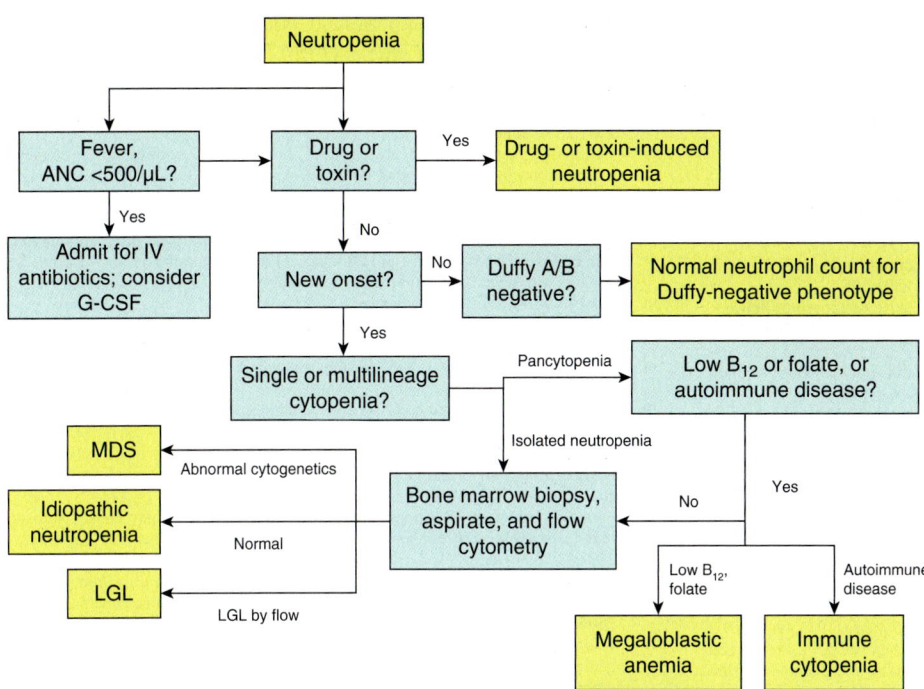

FIGURE 58.2 Diagnostic approach to neutropenia in the adult. ANC, absolute neutrophil count; G-CSF, granulocyte colony–stimulating factor; IV, intravenous; LGL, large granular lymphocytosis; MDS, myelodysplastic syndrome.

transplant. For cases of severe life-threatening infection that is unresponsive to antibiotics, granulocyte transfusion may be warranted.[247]

In patients with neutropenia who have not had a history of infection, treatment is rarely necessary. Patients should be educated about simple approaches to preventing infection, including skin and mouth care, good oral and dental hygiene, avoidance of rectal trauma by rectal thermometers and prevention of constipation with stool softeners, proper cleaning, and topical antibiotic application to all skin abrasions. Patients with profound neutropenia not on G-CSF should be instructed to notify a physician as soon as they develop a fever. It is advisable that they also be supplied with prophylactic antibiotics such as trimethoprim-sulfamethoxazole or ciprofloxacin to take in the event there is a delay in seeking medical attention. It should be emphasized, however, that use of these agents is for emergencies only and should not be used in place of seeking appropriate medical evaluation and care.

Patients with SCN require lifelong G-CSF therapy. The use of G-CSF has extended the life expectancy for these patients from 2 to 3 years to adulthood.[58] Some patients with CN also require G-CSF, but can often restrict treatment to low daily doses of G-CSF or cyclical administration during the period around the nadir of the ANC. Dose requirements vary depending on G-CSF response.[58,70,86] As previously mentioned, with improved survival of patients with SCN, a significant risk of MDS/AML has emerged.[55-57] The risk of MDS/AML appears to be associated with higher doses of G-CSF, but whether this is a reflection of the underlying disease phenotype or whether transformation is enhanced or accelerated by G-CSF itself is unknown.[54,55,59,60]

Other congenital syndromes associated with neutropenia, such as SDS, FA, and DKC, respond to doses of G-CSF similar to those used in SCN. These patients are also at increased risk of MDS and/or AML, but again it is not clear if this is due to the G-CSF or the underlying disease.[113,132,135] Patients with idiopathic neutropenia and CN, as well as neutropenia associated with glycogen storage Ib, and myelokathexis, however, do not develop MDS or AML, despite therapy with G-CSF.[70,86,148,159] One could argue, though, that this may be a dose-dependent phenomenon because patients with SCN, SDS, FA, and DKC require higher doses of G-CSF than do those with idiopathic neutropenia and CN. Long-term use of G-CSF or GM-CSF has been associated with osteoporosis and organomegaly.

Severe drug-induced neutropenia/agranulocytosis requires the permanent discontinuation of the causative agent. However, agents that cause dose-related marrow suppression and mild neutropenia can be continued if necessary, provided the neutropenia is not progressive or severe. Patients with agranulocytosis frequently present with life-threatening infections. They should be admitted to the hospital for broad-spectrum antibiotics. G-CSF speeds the recovery of the ANC and, given the morbidity and mortality associated with this syndrome, is recommended.

Immune neutropenia related to SLE or other systemic autoimmune disease rarely needs direct treatment, and ANC usually responds to decreased disease activity with therapy directed at the underlying rheumatologic disorder. Patients with LGL respond well to low-dose immunosuppression with cyclophosphamide or methotrexate.

Finally, stem cell transplantation can be useful to reverse the hematologic effects and neutropenia associated with a number of the congenital neutropenia and bone marrow failure syndromes such as SDS, FA, DKC, and cartilage-hair hypoplasia. The risk of transplant in many of these patients is greater than that seen in transplantation for hematologic malignancies due to the nature of the underlying genetic disorder. Furthermore, many of these disorders are associated with disease of other organs, including pulmonary fibrosis, or a risk of solid tumors. Transplantation does nothing to prevent these manifestations of the underlying disease and should be considered before undertaking the procedure.

G-CSF Biosimilars

A biosimilar product is a biological product that is approved following demonstration that it is highly similar to an FDA-approved (US Food and Drug Administration) biological product, known as a reference product. It has no clinically meaningful differences from the reference product in terms of safety and effectiveness. Zarxio (filgrastim-sndz) was the first biosimilar for filgrastim and the reference product Neupogen to gain FDA approval in the United States in 2015. A second filgrastim biosimilar, Nivestym (filgrastim-aafi), was approved in 2018. Granix (tbo-filgrastim) entered the US market in 2013. Although Granix's structure, formulation, and mechanism do not differ significantly from Neupogen's, Granix was reviewed prior to the adoption of the biosimilar approval pathway. Additionally, the reference product for long-acting filgrastim, Neulasta (pegfilgrastim), currently has four biosimilars on the US market. They include Udenyca, Fulphila, Ziextenzo, and Nyvepria.

ACKNOWLEDGMENT

We would like to gratefully acknowledge the contributions of Caron A. Jacobson, MD, to this chapter.

References

1. von Vietinghoff S, Ley K. Homeostatic regulation of blood neutrophil counts. *J Immunol*. 2008;181(8):5183-5188.
2. Weetman RM, Boxer LA. Childhood neutropenia. *Pediatr Clin North Am*. 1980;27(2):361-376.
3. Reed WW, Diehl LF. Leukopenia, neutropenia, and reduced hemoglobin levels in healthy American blacks. *Arch Intern Med*. 1991;151(3):501-505.
4. Bodey GP, Buckley M, Sathe YS, Freireich EJ. Quantitative relationships between circulating leukocytes and infection in patients with leukemia. *Ann Intern Med*. 1966;64:328-340.
5. Alario AJ, O'Shea JS. Risk of infectious complications in well-appearing children with transient neutropenia. *Am J Dis Child*. 1989;143(8):973-976.
6. Galifi M, Schinella M, Nicoli M, Lippi G. Instrumental reports and effect of anticoagulants in a case of neutrophil agglutination in vitro. *Haematologica*. 1993;78(6):364-370.
7. Joyce RA, Boggs DR, Hasiba U, Srodes CH. Marginal neutrophil pool size in normal subjects and neutropenic patients as measured by epinephrine infusion. *J Lab Clin Med*. 1976;88(4):614-620.
8. Djaldetti M, Joshua H, Kalderon M, et al. Familial leukopenia-neutropenia in Yemenite Jews. *Bull Res Counc Isr*. 1961;9E:24-28.
9. Shaper AG, Lewis P. Genetic neutropenia in people of African origin. *Lancet*. 1971;2(7732):1021-1023.
10. Jacobs P. Familial benign chronic neutropenia [letter]. *S Afr Med J*. 1975;49(17):692.
11. Denic S, Showqi S, Klein C, Takala M, Nagelkerke N, Agarwal MM. Prevalence, phenotype and inheritance of benign neutropenia in Arabs. *BMC Blood Disord*. 2009;9:3.
12. Reich D, Nalls MA, Kao WH, et al. Reduced neutrophil count in people of African descent is due to a regulatory variant in the Duffy antigen receptor for chemokines gene. *PLoS Genet*. 2009;5(1):e1000360.
13. Merz L, Achebe M. When non-Whiteness becomes a condition. *Blood*. 2021;137(1):13-15.
14. Stabholz A, Soskolne V, Machtei E, Or R, Soskolne WA. Effect of benign familial neutropenia on the periodontium of Yemenite Jews. *J Periodontol*. 1990;61(1):51-54.
15. Shoenfeld Y, Alkan ML, Asaly A, Carmeli Y, Katz M. Benign familial leukopenia and neutropenia in different ethnic groups. *Eur J Haematol*. 1988;41(3):273-277.
16. Mintz U, Sachs L. Normal granulocyte colony-forming cells in the bone marrow of Yemenite Jews with genetic neutropenia. *Blood*. 1973;41(6):745-751.
17. Joyce RA, Boggs DR, Chervenick PA. Neutrophil kinetics in hereditary and congenital neutropenias. *N Engl J Med*. 1976;295(25):1385-1390.
18. Jonsson OG, Buchanan GR. Chronic neutropenia during childhood. A 13-year experience in a single institution. *Am J Dis Child*. 1991;145(2):232-235.
19. Komiyama A, Ishiguro A, Kubo T, et al. Increases in neutrophil counts by purified human urinary colony-stimulating factor in chronic neutropenia of childhood. *Blood*. 1988;71(1):41-45.
20. Sabbe LJ, Claas FH, Langerak J, et al. Group-specific auto-immune antibodies directed to granulocytes as a cause of chronic benign neutropenia in infants. *Acta Haematol*. 1982;68(1):20-27.
21. Parmley RT, Crist WM, Ragab AH, Boxer LA, Malluh A, Findley H. Phagocytosis of neutrophils by marrow macrophages in childhood chronic benign neutropenia. *J Pediatr*. 1981;98(2):207-212.
22. Papadaki HA, Pontikoglou C. Pathophysiologic mechanisms, clinical features and treatment of idiopathic neutropenia. *Expert Rev Hematol*. 2008;1(2):217-229.
23. Jakubowski AA, Souza L, Kelly F, et al. Effects of human granulocyte colony-stimulating factor in a patient with idiopathic neutropenia. *N Engl J Med*. 1989;320(1):38-42.
24. Sonoda Y, Yashige H, Fujii H, Maekawa T, Abe T. Treatment of idiopathic neutropenia in the elderly with recombinant human granulocyte colony-stimulating factor. *Acta Haematol*. 1991;85(3):146-152.
25. Kyle RA. Natural history of chronic idiopathic neutropenia. *N Engl J Med*. 1980;302(16):908-909.
26. Lipton A. Chronic idiopathic neutropenia. Treatment with corticosteroids and mercaptopurine. *Arch Intern Med*. 1969;123(6):694-700.
27. Spaet TH, Dameshek W. Chronic hypoplastic neutropenia. *Am J Med*. 1952;13(1):35-45.
28. Kostman R. Infantile genetic agranulocytosis. A review with presentation of ten new cases. *Acta Paediatr Scand*. 1975;64(3):362-368.
29. Kostmann R. Infantile genetic agranulocytosis. *Acta Paediatr Scand*. 1956;45(suppl 105):1-78.
30. Pietsch T, Buhrer C, Mempel K, et al. Blood mononuclear cells from patients with severe congenital neutropenia are capable of producing granulocyte colony-stimulating factor. *Blood*. 1991;77(6):1234-1237.
31. Kyas U, Pietsch T, Welte K. Expression of receptors for granulocyte colony-stimulating factor on neutrophils from patients with severe congenital neutropenia and cyclic neutropenia. *Blood*. 1992;79(5):1144-1147.
32. Guba SC, Sartor CA, Hutchinson R, Boxer LA, Emerson SG. Granulocyte colony-stimulating factor (G-CSF) production and G-CSF receptor structure in patients with congenital neutropenia. *Blood*. 1994;83(6):1486-1492.
33. Welte K, Zeidler C, Reiter A, et al. Differential effects of granulocyte-macrophage colony-stimulating factor and granulocyte colony-stimulating factor in children with severe congenital neutropenia. *Blood*. 1990;75(5):1056-1063.
34. Mempel K, Pietsch T, Menzel T, Zeidler C, Welte K. Increased serum levels of granulocyte colony-stimulating factor in patients with severe congenital neutropenia. *Blood*. 1991;77(9):1919-1922.
35. Dale DC, Liles WC, Garwicz D, Aprikyan AG. Clinical implications of mutations of neutrophil elastase in congenital and cyclic neutropenia. *J Pediatr Hematol Oncol*. 2001;23(4):208-210.
36. Carlsson G, Aprikyan AA, Tehranchi R, et al. Kostmann syndrome: severe congenital neutropenia associated with defective expression of Bcl-2, constitutive mitochondrial release of cytochrome c, and excessive apoptosis of myeloid progenitor cells. *Blood*. 2004;103(9):3355-3361.
37. Nakamura K, Kobayashi M, Konishi N, et al. Abnormalities of primitive myeloid progenitor cells expressing granulocyte colony-stimulating factor receptor in patients with severe congenital neutropenia. *Blood*. 2000;96(13):4366-4369.
38. Konishi N, Kobayashi M, Miyagawa S, Sato T, Katoh O, Ueda K. Defective proliferation of primitive myeloid progenitor cells in patients with severe congenital neutropenia. *Blood*. 1999;94(12):4077-4083.
39. Welte K, Zeidler C, Dale DC. Severe congenital neutropenia. *Semin Hematol*. 2006;43(3):189-195.
40. Dale DC, Person RE, Bolyard AA, et al. Mutations in the gene encoding neutrophil elastase in congenital and cyclic neutropenia. *Blood*. 2000;96(7):2317-2322.
41. Xia J, Bolyard AA, Rodger E, et al. Prevalence of mutations in ELANE, GFI1, HAX1, SBDS, WAS and G6PC3 in patients with severe congenital neutropenia. *Br J Haematol*. 2009;147(4):535-542.
42. Klein C, Grudzien M, Appaswamy G, et al. HAX1 deficiency causes autosomal recessive severe congenital neutropenia (Kostmann disease). *Nat Genet*. 2007;39(1):86-92.
43. Ancliff PJ, Blundell MP, Cory GO, et al. Two novel activating mutations in the Wiskott-Aldrich syndrome protein result in congenital neutropenia. *Blood*. 2006;108(7):2182-2189.
44. Kollner I, Sodeik B, Schreek S, et al. Mutations in neutrophil elastase causing congenital neutropenia lead to cytoplasmic protein accumulation and induction of the unfolded protein response. *Blood*. 2006;108(2):493-500.
45. Grenda DS, Murakami M, Ghatak J, et al. Mutations of the ELA2 gene found in patients with severe congenital neutropenia induce the unfolded protein response and cellular apoptosis. *Blood*. 2007;110(13):4179-4187.
46. Carlsson G, Aprikyan AA, Ericson KG, et al. Neutrophil elastase and granulocyte colony-stimulating factor receptor mutation analyses and leukemia evolution in severe congenital neutropenia patients belonging to the original Kostmann family in northern Sweden. *Haematologica*. 2006;91(5):589-595.
47. Zarebski A, Velu CS, Baktula AM, et al. Mutations in growth factor independent-1 associated with human neutropenia block murine granulopoiesis through colony stimulating factor-1. *Immunity*. 2008;28(3):370-380.
48. Boocock GR, Morrison JA, Popovic M, et al. Mutations in SBDS are associated with Shwachman-Diamond syndrome. *Nat Genet*. 2003;33(1):97-101.
49. Boztug K, Appaswamy G, Ashikov A, et al. A syndrome with congenital neutropenia and mutations in G6PC3. *N Engl J Med*. 2009;360(1):32-43.
50. Dong F, Hoefsloot LH, Schelen AM, et al. Identification of a nonsense mutation in the granulocyte-colony-stimulating factor receptor in severe congenital neutropenia. *Proc Natl Acad Sci U S A*. 1994;91(10):4480-4484.
51. Ward AC, van Aesch YM, Gits J, et al. Novel point mutation in the extracellular domain of the granulocyte colony-stimulating factor (G-CSF) receptor in a case of severe congenital neutropenia hyporesponsive to G-CSF treatment. *J Exp Med*. 1999;190(4):497-507.
52. Sinha S, Zhu QS, Romero G, Corey SJ. Deletional mutation of the external domain of the human granulocyte colony-stimulating factor receptor in a patient with severe chronic neutropenia refractory to granulocyte colony-stimulating factor. *J Pediatr Hematol Oncol*. 2003;25(10):791-796.
53. Druhan LJ, Ai J, Massullo P, Kindwall-Keller T, Ranalli MA, Avalos BR. Novel mechanism of G-CSF refractoriness in patients with severe congenital neutropenia. *Blood*. 2005;105(2):584-591.
54. Dong F, Brynes RK, Tidow N, Welte K, Lowenberg B, Touw IP. Mutations in the gene for the granulocyte colony-stimulating-factor receptor in patients with acute myeloid leukemia preceded by severe congenital neutropenia. *N Engl J Med*. 1995;333(8):487-493.
55. Hunter MG, Avalos BR. Granulocyte colony-stimulating factor receptor mutations in severe congenital neutropenia transforming to acute myelogenous leukemia confer resistance to apoptosis and enhance cell survival. *Blood*. 2000;95(6):2132-2137.
56. Freedman MH, Alter BP. Risk of myelodysplastic syndrome and acute myeloid leukemia in congenital neutropenias. *Semin Hematol*. 2002;39(2):128-133.
57. Dale DC, Cottle TE, Fier CJ, et al. Severe chronic neutropenia: treatment and follow-up of patients in the severe chronic neutropenia international registry. *Am J Hematol*. 2003;72(2):82-93.
58. Rosenberg PS, Alter BP, Bolyard AA, et al. The incidence of leukemia and mortality from sepsis in patients with severe congenital neutropenia receiving long-term G-CSF therapy. *Blood*. 2006;107(12):4628-4635.
59. Beekman R, Valkhorf MG, Sanders MA, et al. Sequential gain of mutations in severe congenital neutropenia progressing to acute myeloid leukemia. *Blood*. 2012;119(22):5071-5077.
60. Tschan CA, Pilz C, Zeidler C, Welte K, Germeshausen M. Time course of increasing numbers of mutations in the granulocyte colony-stimulating factor receptor gene in a patient with congenital neutropenia who developed leukemia. *Blood*. 2001;97(6):1882-1884.
61. Gilman PA, Jackson DP, Guild HG. Congenital agranulocytosis: prolonged survival and terminal acute leukemia. *Blood*. 1970;36(5):576-585.
62. Lang JE, Cutting HO. Infantile genetic agranulocytosis. *Pediatrics*. 1965;35:596-600.
63. Beard ME, Newmark P, Smith ME, Franklin AW. Infantile genetic agranulocytosis associated with changes in serum vitamin B_{12} binding proteins. *Acta Paediatr Scand*. 1972;61(5):526-532.

64. Wriedt K, Kauder E, Mauer AM. Defective myelopoiesis in congenital neutropenia. *N Engl J Med.* 1970;283(20):1072-1077.
65. Dale DC, Bolyard AA, Schwinzer BG, et al. The severe chronic neutropenia international registry: 10-year follow-up report. *Support Cancer Ther.* 2006;3(4):220-231.
66. Dale DC, Bolyard AA, Aprikyan A. Cyclic neutropenia. *Semin Hematol.* 2002;39(2):89-94.
67. Haurie C, Dale DC, Mackey MC. Cyclical neutropenia and other periodic hematological disorders: a review of mechanisms and mathematical models. *Blood.* 1998;92(8):2629-2640.
68. Lange RD. Cyclic hematopoiesis: human cyclic neutropenia. *Exp Hematol.* 1983;11(6):435-451.
69. Wright DG, Dale DC, Fauci AS, Wolff SM. Human cyclic neutropenia: clinical review and long-term follow-up of patients. *Medicine (Baltimore).* 1981;60(1):1-13.
70. Dale DC, Bolyard AA, Hammond WP. Cyclic neutropenia: natural history and effects of long-term treatment with recombinant human granulocyte colony-stimulating factor. *Cancer Invest.* 1993;11(2):219-223.
71. Leale M. Recurrent furunculosis in an infant showing an unusual blood picture. *JAMA.* 1910;54:1854-1855.
72. Morley AA, Carew JP, Baikie AG. Familial cyclical neutropenia. *Br J Haematol.* 1967;13(5):719-738.
73. Loughran TP, Jr, Clark EA, Price TH, Hammond WP. Adult-onset cyclic neutropenia is associated with increased large granular lymphocytes. *Blood.* 1986;68(5):1082-1087.
74. Horwitz M, Benson KF, Person RE, Aprikyan AG, Dale DC. Mutations in ELA2, encoding neutrophil elastase, define a 21-day biological clock in cyclic haematopoiesis. *Nat Genet.* 1999;23(4):433-436.
75. Berliner N, Horwitz M, Loughran TP, Jr. Congenital and acquired neutropenia. *Hematology Am Soc Hematol Educ Program.* 2004;15:63-79.
76. Newburger PE, Pindyck TN, Zhu Z, et al. Cyclic neutropenia and severe congenital neutropenia in patients with a shared ELANE mutation and paternal haplotype: evidence for phenotype determination by modifying genes. *Pediatr Blood Cancer.* 2010;55(2):314-317.
77. Nustede R, Klimiankou M, Klimenkova O, et al. ELANE mutant-specific activation of different UPR pathways in congenital neutropenia. *Br J Haematol.* 2016;172:219-227.
78. Guerry DT, Dale DC, Omine M, Perry S, Wolff SM. Periodic hematopoiesis in human cyclic neutropenia. *J Clin Invest.* 1973;52(12):3220-3230.
79. Engelhard D, Landreth KS, Kapoor N, et al. Cycling of peripheral blood and marrow lymphocytes in cyclic neutropenia. *Proc Natl Acad Sci U S A.* 1983;80(18):5734-5738.
80. Quesenberry PJ. Cyclic hematopoiesis: disorders of primitive hematopoietic stem cells. *Exp Hematol.* 1983;11(8):687-700.
81. Lund JE, Padgett GA, Ott RL. Cyclic neutropenia in grey collie dogs. *Blood.* 1967;29(4):452-461.
82. Dale DC, Graw RG, Jr. Transplantation of allogenic bone marrow in canine cyclic neutropenia. *Science.* 1974;183(4120):83-84.
83. Krance RA, Spruce WE, Forman SJ, et al. Human cyclic neutropenia transferred by allogeneic bone marrow grafting. *Blood.* 1982;60(6):1263-1266.
84. Aprikyan AA, Liles WC, Rodger E, Jonas M, Chi EY, Dale DC. Impaired survival of bone marrow hematopoietic progenitor cells in cyclic neutropenia. *Blood.* 2001;97(1):147-153.
85. Sera Y, Kawaguchi H, Nakamura K, et al. A comparison of the defective granulopoiesis in childhood cyclic neutropenia and in severe congenital neutropenia. *Haematologica.* 2005;90(8):1032-1041.
86. Hammond WP, Price TH, Souza LM, Dale DC. Treatment of cyclic neutropenia with granulocyte colony-stimulating factor. *N Engl J Med.* 1989;320(20):1306-1311.
87. Wright DG, Kenney RF, Oette DH, LaRussa VF, Boxer LA, Malech HL. Contrasting effects of recombinant human granulocyte-macrophage colony-stimulating factor (CSF) and granulocyte CSF treatment on the cycling of blood elements in childhood-onset cyclic neutropenia. *Blood.* 1994;84(4):1257-1267.
88. Wright DG, Fauci AS, Dale DC, Wolff SM. Correction of human cyclic neutropenia with prednisolone. *N Engl J Med.* 1978;298(6):295-300.
89. Selleri C, Catalano L, Alfinito F, De Rosa G, Vaglio S, Rotoli B. Cyclosporin A in adult-onset cyclic neutropenia. *Br J Haematol.* 1988;68(1):137-138.
90. Winkelstein JA, Marino MC, Lederman HM, et al. X-linked agammaglobulinemia: report on a United States registry of 201 patients. *Medicine (Baltimore).* 2006;85(4):193-202.
91. Rosen FS, Janeway CA. Diagnosis and treatment of antibody deficiency syndromes. *Postgrad Med.* 1968;43(5):188-194.
92. Kozlowski C, Evans DI. Neutropenia associated with X-linked agammaglobulinaemia. *J Clin Pathol.* 1991;44(5):388-390.
93. Ng RP, Prankerd TA. Ig A deficiency and neutropenia. *Br Med J.* 1976;1(6009):563.
94. Lonsdale D, Deodhar SD, Mercer RD. Familial granulocytopenia and associated immunoglobulin abnormality. Report of three cases in young brothers. *J Pediatr.* 1967;71(6):790-801.
95. Rieger CH, Moohr JW, Rothberg RM. Correction of neutropenia associated with dysgammaglobulinemia. *Pediatrics.* 1974;54(4):508-511.
96. Bjorksten B, Lundmark KM. Recurrent bacterial infections in four siblings with neutropenia, eosinophilia, hyperimmunoglobulinemia A, and defective neutrophil chemotaxis. *J Infect Dis.* 1976;133(1):63-71.
97. de VO, Seynhaeve V. Reticular dysgenesia. *Lancet.* 1959;2(7112):1123-1125.
98. Roper M, Parmley RT, Crist WM, Kelly DR, Cooper MD. Severe congenital leukopenia (reticular dysgenesis). Immunologic and morphologic characterizations of leukocytes. *Am J Dis Child.* 1985;139(8):832-835.
99. Pannicke U, Honig M, Hess I, et al. Reticular dysgenesis (aleukocytosis) is caused by mutations in the gene encoding mitochondrial adenylate kinase 2. *Nat Genet.* 2009;41:101-105.
100. Lagresle-Peyrou C, Six EM, Picard C, et al. Human adenylate kinase 2 deficiency causes a profound hematopoietic defect associated with sensorineural deafness. *Nat Genet.* 2009;41:106-111.
101. Levinsky RJ, Tiedeman K. Successful bone-marrow transplantation for reticular dysgenesis. *Lancet.* 1983;1(8326, pt 1):671-672.
102. Bertrand Y, Muller SM, Casanova JL, Morgan G, Fischer A, Friedrich W. Reticular dysgenesis: HLA non-identical bone marrow transplants in a series of 10 patients. *Bone Marrow Transplant.* 2002;29(9):759-762.
103. Bujan W, Ferster A, Azzi N, Devalck C, Leriche A, Sariban E. Use of recombinant human granulocyte colony stimulating factor in reticular dysgenesis. *Br J Haematol.* 1992;81(1):128-130.
104. Shwachman H, Diamond LK, Oski FA, Khaw KT. The syndrome of pancreatic insufficiency and bone marrow dysfunction. *J Pediatr.* 1964;65:645-663.
105. Shimamura A. Shwachman-Diamond syndrome. *Semin Hematol.* 2006;43(3):178-188.
106. Hall GW, Dale P, Dodge JA. Shwachman-Diamond syndrome: UK perspective. *Arch Dis Child.* 2006;91(6):521-524.
107. Aggett PJ, Harries JT, Harvey BA, Soothill JF. An inherited defect of neutrophil mobility in Shwachman syndrome. *J Pediatr.* 1979;94(3):391-394.
108. Saunders EF, Gall G, Freedman MH. Granulopoiesis in Shwachman's syndrome (pancreatic insufficiency and bone marrow dysfunction). *Pediatrics.* 1979;64(4):515-519.
109. Necchi V, Minelli A, Sommi P, et al. Ubiquitin-proteasome-rich cytoplasmic structures in neutrophils of patients with Shwachman-Diamond syndrome. *Haematologica.* 2012;97(7):1057-1063.
110. Ginzberg H, Shin J, Ellis L, et al. Shwachman syndrome: phenotypic manifestations of sibling sets and isolated cases in a large patient cohort are similar. *J Pediatr.* 1999;135(1):81-88.
111. Donadieu J, Fenneteau O, Beaupain B, et al. Classification and risk factors of hematological complications in a French national cohort of 102 patients with Shwachman-Diamond syndrome. *Haematologica.* 2012;97(9):1312-1319.
112. Woods WG, Roloff JS, Lukens JN, Krivit W. The occurrence of leukemia in patients with the Shwachman syndrome. *J Pediatr.* 1981;99(3):425-428.
113. Ventura A, Dragovich D, Luxardo P, Zanazzo G. Human granulocyte colony-stimulating factor (rHuG-CSF) for treatment of neutropenia in Shwachman syndrome. *Haematologica.* 1995;80(3):227-229.
114. Donadieu J, Leblanc T, Bader Meunier B, et al. Analysis of risk factors for myelodysplasias, leukemias and death from infection among patients with congenital neutropenia. Experience of the French severe chronic neutropenia study group. *Haematologica.* 2005;90(1):45-53.
115. Donadieu J, Michel G, Merlin E, et al. Hematopoietic stem cell transplantation for Shwachman-Diamond syndrome: experience of the French neutropenia registry. *Bone Marrow Transplant.* 2005;36(9):787-792.
116. Cesaro S, Oneto R, Messina C, et al. Haematopoietic stem cell transplantation for Shwachman-Diamond disease: a study from the European Group for blood and marrow transplantation. *Br J Haematol.* 2005;131(2):231-236.
117. Okcu F, Roberts WM, Chan KW. Bone marrow transplantation in Shwachman-Diamond syndrome: report of two cases and review of the literature. *Bone Marrow Transplant.* 1998;21(8):849-851.
118. Hsu JW, Vogelsang G, Jones RJ, Brodsky RA. Bone marrow transplantation in Shwachman-Diamond syndrome. *Bone Marrow Transplant.* 2002;30(4):255-258.
119. Bhatla D, Davies SM, Shenoy S, et al. Reduced-intensity conditioning is effective and safe for transplantation of patients with Shwachman-Diamond syndrome. *Bone Marrow Transplant.* 2008;42(3):159-165.
120. Taniguchi T, D'Andrea AD. Molecular pathogenesis of Fanconi anemia: recent progress. *Blood.* 2006;107(11):4223-4233.
121. Wang W. Emergence of a DNA-damage response network consisting of Fanconi anaemia and BRCA proteins. *Nat Rev Genet.* 2007;8(10):735-748.
122. Giampietro PF, Adler-Brecher B, Verlander PC, Pavlakis SG, Davis JG, Auerbach AD. The need for more accurate and timely diagnosis in Fanconi anemia: a report from the International Fanconi Anemia Registry. *Pediatrics.* 1993;91(6):1116-1120.
123. Fanconi anaemia/Breast cancer consortium. Positional cloning of the Fanconi anaemia group A gene. *Nat Genet.* 1996;14(3):324-328.
124. Kutler DI, Singh B, Satagopan J, et al. A 20-year perspective on the international Fanconi anemia registry (IFAR). *Blood.* 2003;101(4):1249-1256.
125. Seyschab H, Friedl R, Sun Y, et al. Comparative evaluation of diepoxybutane sensitivity and cell cycle blockage in the diagnosis of Fanconi anemia. *Blood.* 1995;85(8):2233-2237.
126. Gluckman E, Auerbach AD, Horowitz MM, et al. Bone marrow transplantation for Fanconi anemia. *Blood.* 1995;86(7):2856-2862.
127. Socie G, Devergie A, Girinski T, et al. Transplantation for Fanconi's anaemia: long-term follow-up of fifty patients transplanted from a sibling donor after low-dose cyclophosphamide and thoraco-abdominal irradiation for conditioning. *Br J Haematol.* 1998;103(1):249-255.
128. Guardiola P, Pasquini R, Dokal I, et al. Outcome of 69 allogeneic stem cell transplantations for Fanconi anemia using HLA-matched unrelated donors: a study on behalf of the European Group for Blood and Marrow Transplantation. *Blood.* 2000;95(2):422-429.
129. Pasquini R, Carreras J, Pasquini MC, et al. HLA-matched sibling hematopoietic stem cell transplantation for Fanconi anemia: comparison of irradiation and non-irradiation containing conditioning regimens. *Biol Blood Marrow Transplant.* 2008;14(10):1141-1147.

130. Torjemane L, Ladeb S, Ben Othman T, Abdelkefi A, Lakhal A, Ben Abdeladhim A. Bone marrow transplantation from matched related donors for patients with Fanconi anemia using low-dose busulfan and cyclophosphamide as conditioning. *Pediatr Blood Cancer*. 2006;46(4):496-500.
131. Shahidi NT, Diamond LK. Testosterone-induced remission in aplastic anemia of both acquired and congenital types. Further observations in 24 cases. *N Engl J Med*. 1961;264:953-967.
132. Rackoff WR, Orazi A, Robinson CA, et al. Prolonged administration of granulocyte colony-stimulating factor (filgrastim) to patients with Fanconi anemia: a pilot study. *Blood*. 1996;88(5):1588-1593.
133. Trowbridge AA, Sirinavin C, Linman JW. Dyskeratosis congenita: hematologic evaluation of a sibship and review of the literature. *Am J Hematol*. 1977;3:143-152.
134. Sirinavin C, Trowbridge AA. Dyskeratosis congenita: clinical features and genetic aspects. Report of a family and review of the literature. *J Med Genet*. 1975;12(4):339-354.
135. Putterman C, Safadi R, Zlotogora J, Banura R, Eldor A. Treatment of the hematological manifestations of dyskeratosis congenita. *Ann Hematol*. 1993;66(4):209-212.
136. Armanios MY, Chen JJ, Cogan JD, et al. Telomerase mutations in families with idiopathic pulmonary fibrosis. *N Engl J Med*. 2007;356(13):1317-1326.
137. Mitchell JR, Wood E, Collins K. A telomerase component is defective in the human disease dyskeratosis congenita. *Nature*. 1999;402(6761):551-555.
138. Yamaguchi H, Calado RT, Ly H, et al. Mutations in TERT, the gene for telomerase reverse transcriptase, in aplastic anemia. *N Engl J Med*. 2005;352(14):1413-1424.
139. Alter BP, Baerlocher GM, Savage SA, et al. Very short telomere length by flow fluorescence in situ hybridization identifies patients with dyskeratosis congenita. *Blood*. 2007;110(5):1439-1447.
140. Russo CL, Glader BE, Israel RJ, Galasso F. Treatment of neutropenia associated with dyskeratosis congenita with granulocyte-macrophage colony-stimulating factor. *Lancet*. 1990;336(8717):751-752.
141. Mahmoud HK, Schaefer UW, Schmidt CG, Becher R, Gotz GF, Richter HJ. Marrow transplantation for pancytopenia in dyskeratosis congenita. *Blut*. 1985;51(1):57-60.
142. Langston AA, Sanders JE, Deeg HJ, et al. Allogeneic marrow transplantation for aplastic anaemia associated with dyskeratosis congenita. *Br J Haematol*. 1996;92(3):758-765.
143. Melis D, Fulceri R, Parenti G, et al. Genotype/phenotype correlation in glycogen storage disease type 1b: a multicentre study and review of the literature. *Eur J Pediatr*. 2005;164(8):501-508.
144. Gerin I, Veiga-da-Cunha M, Achouri Y, Collet JF, Van Schaftingen E. Sequence of a putative glucose 6-phosphate translocase, mutated in glycogen storage disease type Ib. *FEBS Lett*. 1997;419(2-3):235-238.
145. Rake JP, Visser G, Labrune P, Leonard JV, Ullrich K, Smit GP. Glycogen storage disease type I: diagnosis, management, clinical course and outcome. Results of the European Study on Glycogen Storage Disease Type I (ESGSD I). *Eur J Pediatr*. 2002;161(suppl 1):S20-S34.
146. Visser G, Rake JP, Fernandes J, et al. Neutropenia, neutrophil dysfunction, and inflammatory bowel disease in glycogen storage disease type Ib: results of the European Study on Glycogen Storage Disease type I. *J Pediatr*. 2000;137(2):187-191.
147. Visser G, Rake JP, Labrune P, et al. Consensus guidelines for management of glycogen storage disease type 1b—European Study on Glycogen Storage Disease Type 1. *Eur J Pediatr*. 2002;161(suppl 1):S120-S123.
148. Schroten H, Roesler J, Breidenbach T, et al. Granulocyte and granulocyte-macrophage colony-stimulating factors for treatment of neutropenia in glycogen storage disease type Ib. *J Pediatr*. 1991;119(5):748-754.
149. Matern D, Starzl TE, Arnaout W, et al. Liver transplantation for glycogen storage disease types I, III, and IV. *Eur J Pediatr*. 1999;158(suppl 2):S43-S48.
150. Childs B, Nyhan WL. Further observations of a patient with hyperglycinemia. *Pediatrics*. 1964;33:403-412.
151. Matsui SM, Mahoney MJ, Rosenberg LE. The natural history of the inherited methylmalonic acidemias. *N Engl J Med*. 1983;308(15):857-861.
152. Sidbury JB, Jr, Smith EK, Harlan W. An inborn error of short-chain fatty acid metabolism. The odor-of-sweaty-feet syndrome. *J Pediatr*. 1967;70(1):8-15.
153. Mamlok RJ, Juneja HS, Elder FF, Haggard ME, Schmalstieg FC, Goldman AS. Neutropenia and defective chemotaxis associated with binuclear, tetraploid myeloid-monocytic leukocytes. *J Pediatr*. 1987;111(4):555-558.
154. Zuelzer WW. "Myelokathexis"—a new form of chronic granulocytopenia. Report of a case. *N Engl J Med*. 1964;270:699-704.
155. Aprikyan AA, Liles WC, Park JR, Jonas M, Chi EY, Dale DC. Myelokathexis, a congenital disorder of severe neutropenia characterized by accelerated apoptosis and defective expression of bcl-x in neutrophil precursors. *Blood*. 2000;95(1):320-327.
156. Hord JD, Whitlock JA, Gay JC, Lukens JN. Clinical features of myelokathexis and treatment with hematopoietic cytokines: a case report of two patients and review of the literature. *J Pediatr Hematol Oncol*. 1997;19(5):443-448.
157. Gorlin RJ, Gelb B, Diaz GA, Lofsness KG, Pittelkow MR, Fenyk JR, Jr. WHIM syndrome, an autosomal dominant disorder: clinical, hematological, and molecular studies. *Am J Med Genet*. 2000;91(5):368-376.
158. Hernandez PA, Gorlin RJ, Lukens JN, et al. Mutations in the chemokine receptor gene CXCR4 are associated with WHIM syndrome, a combined immunodeficiency disease. *Nat Genet*. 2003;34(1):70-74.
159. Weston B, Axtell RA, Todd RF, III, et al. Clinical and biologic effects of granulocyte colony stimulating factor in the treatment of myelokathexis. *J Pediatr*. 1991;118(2):229-234.
160. Wetzler M, Talpaz M, Kellagher MJ, Gutterman JU, Kurzrock R. Myelokathexis: normalization of neutrophil counts and morphology by GM-CSF. *JAMA*. 1992;267(16):2179-2180.
161. McDermott DH, Liu Q, Ulrick J, et al. The CXCR4 antagonist plerixafor corrects panleukopenia in patients with WHIM syndrome. *Blood*. 2011;118(18):4957-4962.
162. Dale DC, Bolyard AA, Kelley ML, et al. The CXCR4 antagonist plerixafor is a potential therapy for myelokathexis, WHIM syndrome. *Blood*. 2011;118(18):4963-4966.
163. McDermott DH, Liu Q, Velez L, et al. A phase 1 clinical trial of long-term, low-dose treatment of WHIM syndrome with the CXCR4 antagonist plerixafor. *Blood*. 2014;123:2308-2316.
164. Huizing M, Anikster Y, Gahl WA. Hermansky-Pudlak syndrome and Chediak-Higashi syndrome: disorders of vesicle formation and trafficking. *Thromb Haemost*. 2001;86(1):233-245.
165. Blume RS, Wolff SM. The Chediak-Higashi syndrome: studies in four patients and a review of the literature. *Medicine (Baltimore)*. 1972;51(4):247-280.
166. Certain S, Barrat F, Pastural E, et al. Protein truncation test of LYST reveals heterogenous mutations in patients with Chediak-Higashi syndrome. *Blood*. 2000;95(3):979-983.
167. Blume RS, Bennett JM, Yankee RA, Wolff SM. Defective granulocyte regulation in the Chediak-Higashi syndrome. *N Engl J Med*. 1968;279(19):1009-1015.
168. Root RK, Rosenthal AS, Balestra DJ. Abnormal bactericidal, metabolic, and lysosomal functions of Chediak-Higashi syndrome leukocytes. *J Clin Invest*. 1972;51(3):649-665.
169. Merino F, Amesty C, Henle W, Layrisse Z, Bianco N, Ramirez-Duque P. Chediak-Higashi syndrome: immunological responses to Epstein-Barr virus studies in gene heterozygotes. *Clin Immunol*. 1986;6(3):242-248.
170. Menasche G, Pastural E, Feldmann J, et al. Mutations in RAB27A cause Griscelli syndrome associated with haemophagocytic syndrome. *Nat Genet*. 2000;25(2):173-176.
171. Kurowska M, Goudin N, Nehme NT, et al. Terminal transport of lytic granules to the immune synapse is mediated by the kinesin-1/Slp3/Rab27a complex. *Blood*. 2012;119(17):3879-3889.
172. Di Pietro SM, Dell'Angelica EC. The cell biology of Hermansky-Pudlak syndrome: recent advances. *Traffic*. 2005;6(7):525-533.
173. Eapen M, DeLaat CA, Baker KS, et al. Hematopoietic cell transplantation for Chediak-Higashi syndrome. *Bone Marrow Transplant*. 2007;39(7):411-415.
174. Pachlopnik Schmid J, Moshous D, Boddaert N, et al. Hematopoietic stem cell transplantation in Griscelli syndrome type 2: a single-center report on 10 patients. *Blood*. 2009;114(1):211-218.
175. Aslan Y, Erduran E, Gedik Y, Mocan H, Yildiran A. The role of high dose methylprednisolone and splenectomy in the accelerated phase of Chediak-Higashi syndrome. *Acta Haematol*. 1996;96(2):105-107.
176. Ayas M, Al-Ghonaium A. In patients with Chediak-Higashi syndrome undergoing allogeneic SCT, does adding etoposide to the conditioning regimen improve the outcome? *Bone Marrow Transplant*. 2007;40(6):603.
177. Lux SE, Johnston RB, Jr, August CS, et al. Chronic neutropenia and abnormal cellular immunity in cartilage-hair hypoplasia. *N Engl J Med*. 1970;282(5):231-236.
178. McKusick VA, Eldridge R, Hostetler JA, Ruangwit U, Egeland JA. Dwarfism in the Amish. II. Cartilage-hair hypoplasia. *Bull Johns Hopkins Hosp*. 1965;116:285-326.
179. Makitie O, Kaitila I. Cartilage-hair hypoplasia—clinical manifestations in 108 Finnish patients. *Eur J Pediatr*. 1993;152(3):211-217.
180. Hermanns P, Tran A, Munivez E, et al. RMRP mutations in cartilage-hair hypoplasia. *Am J Med Genet A*. 2006;140(19):2121-2130.
181. Rosenbluh J, Nijhawan D, Chen Z, Wong KK, Masutomi K, Hahn WC. RMRP is a non-coding RNA essential for early murine development. *PLoS One*. 2011;6(10):e26270.
182. O'Reilly RJ, Brochstein J, Dinsmore R, Kirkpatrick D. Marrow transplantation for congenital disorders. *Semin Hematol*. 1984;21(3):188-221.
183. Ammann RA, Duppenthaler A, Bux J, Aebi C. Granulocyte colony-stimulating factor-responsive chronic neutropenia in cartilage-hair hypoplasia. *J Pediatr Hematol Oncol*. 2004;26(6):379-381.
184. MacGregor RR, Friedman HM, Macarak EJ, Kefalides NA. Virus infection of endothelial cells increases granulocyte adherence. *J Clin Invest*. 1980;65(6):1469-1477.
185. Schooley RT, Densen P, Harmon D, et al. Antineutrophil antibodies in infectious mononucleosis. *Am J Med*. 1984;76(1):85-90.
186. Zon LI, Groopman JE. Hematologic manifestations of the human immune deficiency virus (HIV). *Semin Hematol*. 1988;25(3):208-218.
187. Christensen RD, Rothstein G. Exhaustion of mature marrow neutrophils in neonates with sepsis. *J Pediatr*. 1980;96(2):316-318.
188. Cairo MS. Review of G-CSF and GM-CSF. Effects on neonatal neutrophil kinetics. *Am J Pediatr Hematol Oncol*. 1989;11(2):238-244.
189. Cairo MS. Granulocyte transfusions in neonates with presumed sepsis. *Pediatrics*. 1987;80(5):738-740.
190. Cairo MS, Worcester CC, Rucker RW, et al. Randomized trial of granulocyte transfusions versus intravenous immune globulin therapy for neonatal neutropenia and sepsis. *J Pediatr*. 1992;120(2 pt 1):281-285.
191. Bottiger LE, Furhoff AK, Holmberg L. Drug-induced blood dyscrasias. A ten-year material from the Swedish Adverse Drug Reaction Committee. *Acta Med Scand*. 1979;205(6):457-461.
192. van der Klauw MM, Goudsmit R, Halie MR, et al. A population-based case-cohort study of drug-associated agranulocytosis. *Arch Intern Med*. 1999;159(4):369-374.
193. Ibanez L, Vidal X, Ballarin E, Laporte JR. Population-based drug-induced agranulocytosis. *Arch Intern Med*. 2005;165(8):869-874.
194. Salama A, Schutz B, Kiefel V, Breithaupt H, Mueller-Eckhardt C. Immune-mediated agranulocytosis related to drugs and their metabolites: mode of sensitization and heterogeneity of antibodies. *Br J Haematol*. 1989;72(2):127-132.
195. Eisner EV, Carr RM, MacKinney AR. Quinidine-induced agranulocytosis. *JAMA*. 1977;238(8):884-886.
196. Neftel KA, Hauser SP, Muller MR. Inhibition of granulopoiesis in vivo and in vitro by beta-lactam antibiotics. *J Infect Dis*. 1985;152(1):90-98.

197. Irvine AE, French A, Daly A, Ranaghan L, Morris TC. Drug-induced neutropenia due to direct effects on CFU-C-ten years of culture experience. *Eur J Haematol.* 1994;52(1):21-27.
198. Hodinka L, Geher P, Meretey K, Gyodi EK, Petranyi GG, Bozsoky S. Levamisole-induced neutropenia and agranulocytosis: association with HLA B27 leukocyte agglutinating and lymphocytotoxic antibodies. *Int Arch Allergy Appl Immunol.* 1981;65(4):460-464.
199. Duchin KL, Singhvi SM, Willard DA, Migdalof BH, McKinstry DN. Captopril kinetics. *Clin Pharmacol Ther.* 1982;31(4):452-458.
200. Pisciotta AV, Kaldahl J. Studies on agranulocytosis. IV. Effects of chlorpromazine on nucleic acid synthesis of bone marrow cells in vitro. *Blood.* 1962;20:364-376.
201. Pisciotta AV. Immune and toxic mechanisms in drug-induced agranulocytosis. *Semin Hematol.* 1973;10(4):279-310.
202. Muroi K, Ito M, Sasaki R, Suda T, Sakamoto S, Miura Y. Treatment of drug-induced agranulocytosis with granulocyte-colony stimulating factor. *Lancet.* 1989;2(8653):55.
203. Stroncek D, Bux J. Is it time to standardize granulocyte alloantigen nomenclature? *Transfusion.* 2002;42(4):393-395.
204. Lalezari P, Jiang AF, Yegen L, Santorineou M. Chronic autoimmune neutropenia due to anti-NA2 antibody. *N Engl J Med.* 1975;293(15):744-747.
205. Harmon DC, Weitzman SA, Stossel TP. The severity of immune neutropenia correlates with the maturational specificity of antineutrophil antibodies. *Br J Haematol.* 1984;58(2):209-215.
206. Bruin MC, von dem Borne AE, Tamminga RY, Kleijer M, Buddelmeijer L, de Haas M. Neutrophil antibody specificity in different types of childhood autoimmune neutropenia. *Blood.* 1999;94(5):1797-1802.
207. Starkebaum G. Chronic neutropenia associated with autoimmune disease. *Semin Hematol.* 2002;39(2):121-127.
208. Loughran TP, Jr, Kadin ME, Starkebaum G, et al. Leukemia of large granular lymphocytes: association with clonal chromosomal abnormalities and autoimmune neutropenia, thrombocytopenia, and hemolytic anemia. *Ann Intern Med.* 1985;102(2):169-175.
209. Saway PA, Prasthofer EF, Barton JC. Prevalence of granular lymphocyte proliferation in patients with rheumatoid arthritis and neutropenia. *Am J Med.* 1989;86(3):303-307.
210. Felty AR. Chronic arthritis in the adult, associated with splenomegaly and neutropenia. *Johns Hopkins Med J.* 1924;35:16.
211. Sokol L, Loughran TP, Jr. Large granular lymphocyte leukemia. *Curr Hematol Malig Rep.* 2007;2(4):278-282.
212. Campion G, Maddison PJ, Goulding N, et al. The Felty syndrome: a case-matched study of clinical manifestations and outcome, serologic features, and immunogenetic associations. *Medicine (Baltimore).* 1990;69(2):69-80.
213. Breedveld FC, Lafeber GJ, de Vries E, van Krieken JH, Cats A. Immune complexes and the pathogenesis of neutropenia in Felty's syndrome. *Ann Rheum Dis.* 1986;45(8):696-702.
214. Liu JH, Wei S, Lamy T, et al. Chronic neutropenia mediated by fas ligand. *Blood.* 2000;95(10):3219-3222.
215. Papadaki HA, Eliopoulos AG, Kosteas T, et al. Impaired granulocytopoiesis in patients with chronic idiopathic neutropenia is associated with increased apoptosis of bone marrow myeloid progenitor cells. *Blood.* 2003;101(7):2591-2600.
216. Vincent PC, Levi JA, Macqueen A. The mechanism of neutropenia in Felty's syndrome. *Br J Haematol.* 1974;27(3):463-475.
217. Choi MF, Mant MJ, Turner AR, Akabutu JJ, Aaron SL. Successful reversal of neutropenia in Felty's syndrome with recombinant granulocyte colony stimulating factor. *Br J Haematol.* 1994;86(3):663-664.
218. Loughran TP, Jr, Kidd PG, Starkebaum G. Treatment of large granular lymphocyte leukemia with oral low-dose methotrexate. *Blood.* 1994;84(7):2164-2170.
219. Rashba EJ, Rowe JM, Packman CH. Treatment of the neutropenia of Felty syndrome. *Blood Rev.* 1996;10(3):177-184.
220. Burks EJ, Loughran TP, Jr. Perspectives in the treatment of LGL leukemia. *Leuk Res.* 2005;29(2):123-125.
221. Narvaez J, Domingo-Domenech E, Gomez-Vaquero C, et al. Biological agents in the management of Felty's syndrome: a systematic review. *Semin Arthritis Rheum.* 2012;41(5):658-668.
222. Lamy T, Loughran TP, Jr. How I treat LGL leukemia. *Blood.* 2011;117(10):2764-2774.
223. Lalezari P, Nussbaum M, Gelman S, Spaet TH. Neonatal neutropenia due to maternal isoimmunization. *Blood.* 1960;15:236-243.
224. Bux J, Behrens G, Jaeger G, Welte K. Diagnosis and clinical course of autoimmune neutropenia in infancy: analysis of 240 cases. *Blood.* 1998;91(1):181-186.
225. Bruin M, Dassen A, Pajkrt D, Buddelmeyer L, Kuijpers T, de Haas M. Primary autoimmune neutropenia in children: a study of neutrophil antibodies and clinical course. *Vox Sang.* 2005;88(1):52-59.
226. Levitt LJ, Ries CA, Greenberg PL. Pure white-cell aplasia. Antibody-mediated autoimmune inhibition of granulopoiesis. *N Engl J Med.* 1983;308(19):1141-1146.
227. Mamus SW, Burton JD, Groat JD, Schulte DA, Lobell M, Zanjani ED. Ibuprofen-associated pure white-cell aplasia, *N Engl J Med*, 1986, 314(10):624-625.
228. Barbui T, Bassan R, Viero P, Minetti B, Comotti B, Buelli M. Pure white cell aplasia treated by high dose intravenous immunoglobulin. *Br J Haematol.* 1984;58(3):554-555.
229. Chakupurakal G, Murrin RJ, Neilson JR. Prolonged remission of pure white cell aplasia (PWCA), in a patient with CLL, induced by rituximab and maintained by continuous oral cyclosporin. *Eur J Haematol.* 2007;79(3):271-273.
230. Passweg JR, Rabusin M, Musso M, et al. Haematopoetic stem cell transplantation for refractory autoimmune cytopenia. *Br J Haematol.* 2004;125(6):749-755.
231. Sacks T, Moldow CF, Craddock PR, Bowers TK, Jacob HS. Oxygen radicals mediate endothelial cell damage by complement-stimulated granulocytes. An in vitro model of immune vascular damage. *J Clin Invest.* 1978;61(5):1161-1167.
232. Craddock PR, Fehr J, Dalmasso AP, Brighan KL, Jacob HS. Hemodialysis leukopenia. Pulmonary vascular leukostasis resulting from complement activation by dialyzer cellophane membranes. *J Clin Invest.* 1977;59(5):879-888.
233. Boogaerts MA, Roelant C, Goossens W, Verwilghen RL. Complement activation and adult respiratory distress syndrome during intermittent flow apheresis procedures. *Transfusion.* 1986;26(1):82-87.
234. Sirchia G, Rebulla P, Mascaretti L, et al. The clinical importance of leukocyte depletion in regular erythrocyte transfusions. *Vox Sang.* 1986;51(suppl 1):2-8.
235. Amorosi EL. Hypersplenism. *Semin Hematol.* 1965;2:249-285.
236. Dunlap WM, James GW, III, Hume DM. Anemia and neutropenia caused by copper deficiency. *Ann Intern Med.* 1974;80(4):470-476.
237. Drenick EJ, Alvarez LC. Neutropenia in prolonged fasting. *Am J Clin Nutr.* 1971;24(7):859-863.
238. Schultz W. Uber eigenartige Halserkrankungen. *Dtsch Med Wochenschr.* 1922;48:1495.
239. Hartl W. Drug allergic agranulocytosis (Schultz's disease). *Semin Hematol.* 1965;2(4):313-337.
240. Senn H, Holland JF, Banerjee T. Kinetic and comparative studies on localized leukocyte mobilization in normal man. *J Lab Clin Med.* 1969;74(5):742-756.
241. Athens JW, Haab OP, Raab SO, et al. Leukokinetic studies. IV. The total blood, circulating and marginal granulocyte pools and the granulocyte turnover rate in normal subjects. *J Clin Invest.* 1961;40:989-995.
242. Rebuck JW, Crowley JH. A method of studying leukocytic functions in vivo. *Ann N Y Acad Sci.* 1955;59(5):757-805.
243. Schimpff S, Satterlee W, Young VM, Serpick A. Empiric therapy with carbenicillin and gentamicin for febrile patients with cancer and granulocytopenia. *N Engl J Med.* 1971;284(19):1061-1065.
244. Calandra T, Klastersky J, Gaya H, Glauser MP, Meunier F, Zinner SH. The EORTC International Antimicrobial Therapy Cooperative Group. Ceftazidime combined with a short or long course of amikacin for empirical therapy of gram-negative bacteremia in cancer patients with granulocytopenia. *N Engl J Med.* 1987;317(27):1692-1698.
245. Pizzo PA, Hathorn JW, Hiemenz J, et al. A randomized trial comparing ceftazidime alone with combination antibiotic therapy in cancer patients with fever and neutropenia. *N Engl J Med.* 1986;315(9):552-558.
246. Vancomycin added to empirical combination antibiotic therapy for fever in granulocytopenic cancer patients. European Organization for Research and Treatment of Cancer (EORTC) international antimicrobial therapy cooperative group and the national cancer institute of Canada-Clinical trials group. *J Infect Dis.* 1991;163(5):951-958.
247. Bishton M, Chopra R. The role of granulocyte transfusions in neutropenic patients. *Br J Haematol.* 2004;127(5):501-508.

Chapter 59 ■ Qualitative Disorders of Leukocytes

LAURA C. MICHAELIS

INTRODUCTION

The disorders considered here are generally rare and typically congenital. The consequence of each abnormality is an impairment of host defense due to failure of the neutrophil to conduct normal bactericidal activities—including leukocyte adhesion and rolling, chemotaxis, phagocytosis, or oxidative killing. The conditions may reflect a general metabolic defect, the major manifestation of which may be serious in other organs of the body as well. Some of these conditions may have morphologic abnormalities detectable on the peripheral smear and may therefore come to the attention of the hematologist or hematopathologist. Others may be diagnosed due to patient or family history and/or abnormalities in complete blood count.

The normal function of the leukocyte is reviewed, in depth, in Chapter 7. The fundamental activity of the leukocyte is to search out and engage bacterial and fungal pathogens.[1] When micro-organisms invade a tissue, a variety of vasoactive and chemotactic mediators are released by the involved tissue, including interleukin (IL)-1, endotoxin, and tumor necrosis factor-alpha (TNF-α). These mediators upregulate adhesion molecules on local endothelial cells and provide a chemotactic gradient to attract leukocytes. The leukocytes express integrins and carbohydrate moieties that then initiate attachment, rolling, and margination. In the area of inflammation, the leukocytes ingest and kill the invading organisms and may act as effector cells, releasing cytokines that modify both neutrophils and other immunologic participants. Given the complexity of this infection-fighting process, it should be apparent that defects in one of more of the activities may result in pathologic states.

In this chapter we will review the qualitative disorders of leukocytes and divide the defects by activity: those that impair (1) adhesion and margination, (2) chemotaxis, (3) phagocytosis, and (4) oxidative killing[2] (Figure 59.1). This division is somewhat arbitrary and simplistic, of course, as there is overlap in the impacts of the pathologies. This chapter will end with a description of some of the morphologic aberrancies that may be seen in leukocytes, but which are not linked to significant diminishment in activity.

FUNCTIONAL NEUTROPHIL DISORDERS

Defects Affecting Adhesion And/Or Margination

Leukocyte adhesion deficiencies are primary immunodeficiencies which result, generally, in impaired rolling and adhesion as well as disruption of normal macrophage activity at the site of infection. As such, these rare conditions impair the inflammatory response and lead to increased morbidity and mortality from infection[3] (Table 59.1).

Leukocyte Adhesion Deficiency Type I

Leukocyte adhesion deficiency type I (LADI) is a rare, often fatal, autosomal recessive disorder of leukocyte function. It is the most common of the leukocyte adhesion deficiency syndromes; hundreds of cases have been reported. It usually is detected in infancy or early childhood as a result of frequent bacterial (and sometimes viral) infections or delayed umbilical cord separation, and high neutrophil counts.[4] Infections are recurrent, often life threatening or fatal, and usually involve the skin and subcutaneous tissues, middle ear, and oropharynx, including abscesses caused by *Staphylococcus aureus* or gram-negative enteric organisms. Periodontal disease may be severe.

Neutrophils are present in the blood in increased numbers (even between infections) and appear normal. However, they too fail to migrate to the sites of infection in normal numbers, and pus is not formed. When studied in vitro, neutrophils exhibit defects in motility, phagocytosis, granule secretion, and particle-stimulated respiratory burst activity. Humoral (immunoglobulins and complement) and cellular immunity (skin tests and lymphocyte stimulation tests) otherwise appear normal, although T-cell function may be impaired.[5] Interesting, novel work has demonstrated that some manifestations of the condition are a microbe-induced hyperinflammatory response.[6]

The disorder results from mutations in *ITGB2* gene, which encodes CD18, the common chain of the β₂ integrin family.[7] Mutations in the *ITGB2* gene lead to absent, reduced, or aberrant CD18 expression and therefore reduction in the β₂ integrins essential to adhesion. In LADI, mutations in the common CD18 chain disrupt the formation of leukocyte glycoprotein complexes and result in the inability of the cells to

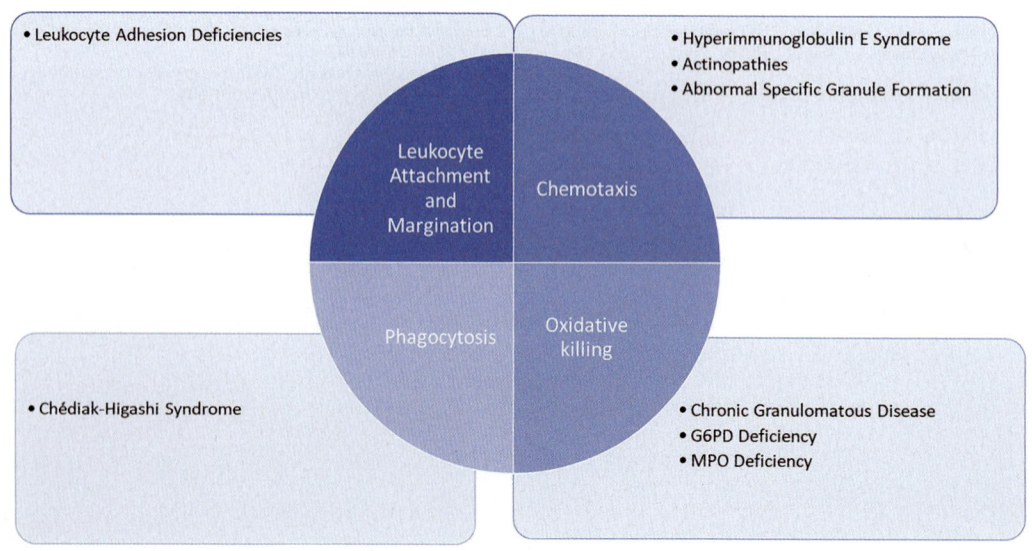

FIGURE 59.1 Select qualitative disorders of leukocytes.

Table 59.1. Characteristics of Leukocyte Adhesion Deficiencies[3]

	Mutation	Gene Location	Clinical Phenotype
LADI	ITGB2 (integrin ß2, CD18)	21q22.3	Granulocytosis common. Presenting symptoms can include omphalitis, absence of pus formation. Life-threatening, recurrent bacterial and fungal infections. Typically, infections are of the skin and mucosal surfaces.
LADII	SLC35C1 or FUCT1	11p11.2	Granulocytosis common, with a somewhat milder clinical course than LADI. May be accompanied by short stature and impaired post–natal weight gain and microcephaly.
LADIII	FERMT3	11q13.1	Similar nonpurulent infections, severe Glanzmann thrombasthenia–like bleeding disorder.

Adapted with permission from van de Vijver E, van den Berg TK, Kuijpers TW. Leukocyte adhesion deficiencies. *Hematol Oncol Clin North Am.* 2013;27:101-116, viii.

interact with intercellular adhesion molecule-1 proteins on endothelial cells; the consequence is severely defective neutrophil adhesion and migration of leukocytes. They therefore are not present at the site of infection to be consumed by the local macrophages.[8] The condition is diagnosed by flow cytometry, which will demonstrate the absence of CD11b/CD18 on peripheral blood leukocytes or by genetic analysis. Severe disease is typically characterized by <2% of CD18-expressing neutrophils. Less severe phenotypes are associated with levels of CD18-expressing neutrophils of 2% to 30%, although these individuals still suffer from a shortened life expectancy.[9]

As described in Chapter 7, the CD11/CD18 family consists of three heterodimeric proteins, each composed of a noncovalently associated α (α_L, α_M, or α_X) and β (β_2) chain (Tables 7.7 and 59.2). Translocation of α- and β-chains to the cell surface requires assembly of the αβ heterodimer. Mutations in the β_2-chain prevent normal assembly of the αβ heterodimer and subsequent translocation to the surface. CD11/CD18-deficient neutrophils roll normally on endothelial cells but do not adhere or migrate with chemotactic stimulation. The severity of clinical manifestations correlated directly with the degree of glycoprotein deficiency.[9,10] Multiple mutations in CD18 have been identified.[9,11,12]

It has long been known that severe periodontitis accompanies this disorder thought to be due to impaired neutrophil surveillance of periodontal tissue.[8] However, recent research identified a dysregulated IL-23/IL-17 inflammatory axis as the critical mediator of the associated periodontal destruction.[13] With the absence of migratory capacity of the leukocytes in this disease, macrophages do not ingest the leukocytes and subsequently IL-23 production is unchecked.[6] This results in excess IL-17 production from T cells in the extravascular space at the site of inflammation and infection. The elegant description of this aberrant inflammatory axis in LADI patients prompted some investigators to attempt therapy with ustekinumab, a monoclonal antibody against IL-23 and IL-12 that impedes downstream production of IL-17. The administration of this agent to a patient with chronic oral disease and a severe sacral wound led to a resolution of these conditions. The reader is referred to the primary report for a review of this patient's case and a video description of the clinical rationale for this intervention.[6]

Treatment for LADI may be conservative in patients with a mild-to-moderate phenotype, including antibiotics for infections; however, even in those with partial expression of LADI, morbidity may arise from periodontal disease, bacterial infections, or delayed healing. Although encouraging, the utility of ustekinumab requires additional study to determine safety and efficacy, particularly in patients with more severe disease who might experience adverse effects from prolonged additional immune suppression. An ongoing clinical trial is investigating this option in patients (NCT03366142). Gene therapy is also currently under investigation. Allogeneic hematopoietic stem cell transplant is curative for this disease and currently recommended.[14] A retrospective review of transplant for this indication was published in 2021.[15] Researchers from the European Society for Blood and Marrow Transplantation identified all transplants for leukocyte adhesion disorders that were performed between 2007 and 2017. A total of 69 patients were transplanted for LADI. The 3-year overall survival (OS) rate was 84% for LADI patients.

Table 59.2. Leukocyte β_2 Integrins

Neutrophil Integrin	Expression	Ligand
$\alpha_L\beta_2$ LFA-1, CD11a/CD18	All leukocytes	ICAM-1 (CD54)
		ICAM-2 (CD102)
		ICAM-3 (CD50)
$\alpha_M\beta_2$ HMac-1, CD11b/CD18	Monocytes, neutrophils, some natural killer cells	ICAM-1, iC3b, fibrinogen, factor X
$\alpha_X\beta_2$ p150,95, CD11c/CD18	Monocytes, neutrophils	iC3b, fibrinogen

Leukocyte Adhesion Deficiency Type II

Additional forms of adhesion deficiencies have been described. Leukocyte adhesion deficiency type II is an exceedingly rare variant which results from mutations in the membrane transporter for fucose. Distinct clinical and genetic results include disorders in intellectual development, short stature, characteristic facial appearance, the Bombay (hh) blood phenotype, and recurrent bacterial infections, including pneumonia, otitis media, periodontitis, and localized cellulitis without the accumulation of pus, in association with an elevated white count.[16-18] In this variant of disease, phagocytosis has been described as normal, but motility and homotypic aggregation are defective. Surface CD18 expression is typically normal.

As described in Chapter 7, cell surface selectins, including CD62E (E-selectin), CD62P (P-selectin), and CD62L (L-selectin), and their ligands (carbohydrates whose structures appear to be related to sialyl-Lex [CD15s]) play an important role in neutrophil adhesion. LADII neutrophils have been found to lack CD15s expression and did not bind IL-1β–stimulated endothelial cells (which express E-selectin). The critical structure of CD15s is NeuAc α2 → 3 Gal β1 → 4, [Fuc α1 → 3] GlcNAc and the Bombay phenotype is a deficiency of Fuc α1 → 2 Gal linkages, which serve as the core of the A, B, and O blood groups.[19]

Because these patients had deficiencies of several fucosylated carbohydrates, the syntheses of which depend on different fucosyltransferase genes, a general defect in fucose metabolism was postulated.[17,20] This syndrome has since been termed *congenital disorder of glycosylation*, type IIc, and is a member of a group of disorders characterized by defects in processing protein-bound glycans. In some of these patients, mutations in *SLC35C1*, a GDP-fucose transporter, have been described.[18,21] LADII neutrophils do not roll well on endothelial cells and do not adhere under shear stress.[22] However, under static conditions, LADII neutrophils can adhere and migrate. Few cases have been described, and these may represent different biochemical defects. Oral fucose supplementation may be useful in some patients.[23,24] Bone marrow transplantation might be considered in some cases.

Leukocyte Adhesion Deficiency Type III

Leukocyte adhesion deficiency type III (LADIII), a third form of LAD, has also been described.[3,25] (Some refer to this as LADI/variant.) This condition results from defects in integrin activation following stimulation of G protein–coupled chemokine receptors. LADIII follows an autosomal recessive pattern and is associated with recurrent infections, leukocytosis, and a bleeding tendency similar to Glanzmann thrombasthenia. Patients experience recurrent, nonpurulent infections and may also demonstrate an osteopetrosis-like bone defect. LADIII results from mutations of *FERMT3*, or *KIND3*, which codes for kindlin-3, a protein that associates with β-integrins.[26,27] These mutations interfere with β-integrin activation in both leukocytes and platelets.[28] As described in Chapter 65, integrin activation follows binding of talins to NPxY sites on the cytoplasmic domains of β-integrin. Talins also tether integrins to the actin cytoskeleton. Kindlins, like talins, can bind NPxY sites and NxxY sites.[29] Because kindlin-3 is also expressed in other hematopoietic cells, including platelets, LADIII also has platelet dysfunction with associated hemostatic defects.[30]

Diagnosis is established in the right clinical condition with genetic confirmation of mutations in *FERMT3*. Like LADI, there is a substantially shortened lifespan for affected individuals with a mortality rate of over 75% by 2 years of age.[15] Allogeneic stem cell transplant may be curative, and in their 2021 retrospective review, European transplant researchers documented a 3-year OS rate of 75%.[15]

Defects Impacting Chemotaxis

Several rare conditions can result in defects of chemotaxis—the process by which neutrophils move through a gradient of chemotactic agents and are drawn to site of infection.

Autosomal Dominant Hyperimmunoglobulin E Syndrome (Job Syndrome)

Hyperimmunoglobulin E syndrome (HIES) may occur sporadically, but most information has been gleaned from study of the most common form, which is an autosomal dominant condition characterized by impaired chemotaxis with generally preserved phagocytic function.[31-33] Autosomal dominant hyperimmunoglobulin E syndrome (AD-HIES) arises from a defect in the signal transducer and activator of transcription 3 (*STAT3*) gene. The most commonly reported mutations are dominant-negative missense variants in the Src homology 2 and DNA-binding domain regions of *STAT3*.[34-36] While AD-HIES is recognized as the prototype condition, several other genetically characterized immunodeficiency disorders have been identified over the past decade, including autosomal recessive mutations in the *DOCK8*, *ZNF431*, and *PGM3* gene as well as mutations that result in alterations in the *CARD11* gene.[37-40]

These clinical conditions are typically associated with eczema, a significantly elevated IgE level, and recurrent skin and pulmonary infections. The skin and lung infections are typically caused by staphylococcal infections. The phenotype is due to the downstream consequences of *STAT3* mutations and subsequent impairment of T-helper cell type 17 (Th17) activity and function. Generally, the STAT3 mutations cause increased production of immunoglobulin E by B lymphocytes. As IL-6 plays an essential role in the genesis of Th17 cells, the lack of this cytokine leads to a deficiency of Th17 cells in Job syndrome. The absence of CD4 + Th17 cells diminishes the defense against infections, mainly bacteria and extracellular fungi.

The original reports of what was dubbed Job syndrome were in two unrelated girls with red hair and fair skin who suffered from repeated staphylococcal cold abscesses, sinusitis, eczema, and pulmonary disease. The affliction was likened to the biblical story of Job. As originally described, the leukocytes of these patients were capable of normal phagocytosis, bacterial killing, nitroblue tetrazolium (NBT) reduction, and iodine fixation, unlike those of patients with chronic granulomatous disease (CGD).[41,42] However, hyperimmunoglobulinemia E and defective chemotaxis were demonstrated. The defects in chemotaxis appeared to be independent of fluctuations in serum IgG. It has since been shown that this disorder is seen in both sexes and in patients of varied racial backgrounds and hair colors.[43-45] The common features are increased susceptibility to bacterial and candida infections (usually evident in the first 6 weeks of life), chronic dermatitis, and hyperimmunoglobulinemia E.[46] HIES is now recognized as a multisystem disease, characterized not only by the features described above, but also by retained primary dentition, unusual facial phenotype, bone fragility, and hyperextensible joints.[40,47] The signs and symptoms may be quite variable.[48,49]

Individuals with these conditions are typically not neutropenic (although cytopenias may occur in those with variants other than AD-HIES). Their neutrophils can perform phagocytosis. But in approximately 80% of patients there are chemotactic defects. Inflammation is minimal, which causes the resulting "cold," that is, noninflamed abscesses.[35,50] Patients' serum IgE levels are significantly elevated, especially in childhood (i.e., >2000 IU/mL). The defect in chemotaxis appears to be unrelated to IgE level, however,[8] and is rather due to alterations in both proinflammatory and anti-inflammatory cytokines.[51] Defective Th17 cell production of IL-17 may be responsible for the impairment of neutrophil chemotaxis and proliferation, and pulmonary and tracheal epithelial cells are dependent on IL-117 for cell killing and antifungal responses. There may also be secondary effects on interferon-gamma (IFN-γ) secretion.

Genetic diagnosis has allowed more patients to be identified and the complete clinical repertoire of the disease is now being realized. Fungal, viral, and bacterial infections are common. A risk for lymphoma is higher in these patients. Survivors with *DOCK8* mutations have developed T-cell lymphomas and squamous cell carcinoma of the skin in early adulthood.[52] Management should be with a specialist in immune deficiency disorders. Prophylactic treatment with dicloxacillin or trimethoprim-sulfamethoxazole may be helpful in managing afflicted patients. The role of IFN-γ is unclear[53] and there is currently study of antibody therapy, although this is only investigational. The clinical course of *DOCK8*-deficient HIES appears to be more severe than that of autosomal dominant HIES. Hematopoietic cell transplantation (HCT), especially if done early in life, might be lifesaving.[54]

Actinopathies and "Lazy-Leukocyte Syndrome"

Genetic disorders effecting neutrophil actin function (actinopathies) may also cause chemotactic impairment, and syndromes have been described with a phenotype of recurrent bacterial infections, and defects in chemotaxis, adhesion, and phagocytosis have also been described.[55-57] In conditions like these, single-gene defects result in impaired cytoskeletal function at the cellular level and can be differentiated from leukocyte adhesion deficiencies based on the characteristic LAD findings of neutrophilia and lack of pus formation.[55] The conditions that fall into this category may lead to infection or may have syndromic features other than infection. As summarized in a recent review, they include the "Lazy-Leukocyte Syndrome" or a related mutation in WDR1 with an alternative clinical phenotype that has also been reported.[55,58-60]

Additional actinopathies include, for example, Wiskott-Aldrich syndrome (WAS),[61] X-linked neutropenia caused by gain-of-function mutation in the cdc42-binding site of the WAS gene,[61] WAS interacting protein deficiency, DOCK8 deficiency,[62] RASGRP1 deficiency, CORONIN-1A deficiency, DOCK2 deficiency, Rac2 deficiency (see below), beta-actin deficiency, and ARPC1B deficiency.[55,61,62]

A recent report[63] has illustrated at least one of the genetic underpinnings of an actin dysfunction syndrome which had been dubbed the "Lazy-leukocyte syndrome." Initially reported more than in the 1970s,[64-66] this condition was characterized by recurrent infections, stomatitis, neutropenia, abnormal neutrophil random (chemokinesis) and directed (chemotaxis) migration, and defective neutrophil mobilization.[66] Actin activity and function remains essential for supporting the formation of lamellipodia; however, disassembly of actin is also critical for neutrophil movement. Actin-depolymerizing protein (ADP) (also called cofilin) has been identified as critical for helping actin break down and be severed, and notably, ADP/cofilin is partially dependent on actin-interacting protein-1 for potentiation and efficacy.

In a high-profile study published recently, researchers were able to identify biallelic mutations in *WDR1* affecting distinct antiparallel b-strands of actin-interacting protein-1 in four children from three different families.[59] All of the children had a similar clinical phenotype of recurrent infections, mild neutropenia, and stomatitis. The new primary immune deficiency which arises from WDR1 mutation affects neutrophil motility, morphology, and function.[67]

In other conditions, the leukocytes appear to have actin that does not polymerize well and had lower levels of F-actin in both the resting state and after stimulation. Subsequent studies after the death of the index case found that one, but not both, parent was heterozygous for LAD1. Most patients with LAD1 do not have abnormal actin polymerization. Cases of patients with this syndrome and overexpression of 47- and 89-kDa proteins (NAD 47/89) were also described.[56,57,68] A more recent case was described with overexpression of leufactin—an F-actin–binding protein that regulates microfilaments—and NAD with serious infections. Leufactin was shown to be the 47-kDa protein overexpressed in NAD 47/89.[68,69] Overexpression of leufactin, also known as lymphocyte-specific protein-1, can create the morphologic and motility abnormalities seen in leufactin-overexpressing neutrophils.[69,70]

Rac2 GTPase Mutation

A defect of neutrophil adhesion, oxidase activation, degranulation, and chemotaxis in response to chemoattractants has been reported in one patient who had a double negative mutation in Rac2 GTPase.[71,72] This patient had leukocytosis with a deficiency of pus at sites of infection, exhibiting a phenotype similar to that of Rac2 knockout mice.[73-75]

Localized Juvenile Periodontitis

Localized juvenile periodontitis is an adolescent disease characterized by alveolar bone loss, most prominently of the incisors and first molars and severe periodontal infections.[76,77] Interestingly, these patients do not have demonstrable problems with extraoral infections. Abnormal neutrophil chemotaxis to f-met-leu-phe (FMLP) and C5a in these patients has been reported, and a similar chemotactic defect was also observed in siblings of patients before developing clinical disease.[78,79] Neutrophils from patients with localized juvenile periodontitis have been reported to generate the lipoxin LXA4, which might function as an immunomodulatory in the pathogenesis of periodontitis. The mechanism of this abnormality has not been defined.

CARD9 Deficiency

Autosomal recessive defects in *CARD9* (caspase recruitment domain–containing protein 9) have been described in several kindreds.[80-82] Common clinical manifestations include fungal infections such as meningoencephalitis caused by *Candida*, disseminated *Exophiala* and *Phialophora* infections, and deep dermatophytoses.[83] CARD9 functions as an adaptor protein in the immune-signaling cascades downstream of C-type lectin receptor and toll-like receptors in myeloid cells.[84] The mechanisms by which CARD9 deficiency leads to invasive fungal infections are still not completely understood. However, recruitment of neutrophils to the site of candida infection, including the central nervous system (CNS) is impaired in CARD9-deficient patients and animals.[85]

Abnormal Specific (Secondary) Granule Formation

A syndrome of recurrent staphylococcal skin and sinus infections associated with abnormal chemotaxis, impaired staphylococcal killing, and morphologic abnormalities in the neutrophils was described in a 14-year-old boy.[86] No other family members were affected. The patient's polymorphonuclear neutrophils exhibited bilobed nuclei with unevenly distributed chromatin, drumstick-like nuclear projections, and nearly absent cytoplasmic granules that stained with peroxidase but not with alkaline phosphatase. Electron microscopy revealed primary granules, but specific granules were small and reduced in number. These neutrophils were capable of phagocytosis, generated H_2O_2, reduced NBT dye, and killed *Candida*, but staphylococcal killing was impaired.

Since the original report, multiple cases of specific granule deficiency (SGD) have been identified with both sexes affected.[87,88] SGD neutrophils exhibit decreased chemotaxis and bacterial killing in vitro and decreased migration into skin windows in vivo, and they fail to upregulate CD11/CD18, laminin, or FMLP receptors after activation.[2,89] These neutrophils are significantly deficient in many important microbicidal granule proteins, including lactoferrin and the defensins. However, oxygen radical generation is apparently normal. Myeloperoxidase (MPO)-positive primary granules are present, but the specific secondary granules appeared to be absent in Wright-stained blood smears and were decreased in number and small when viewed with electron microscopy. The specific granule constituents lactoferrin and B_{12}-binding protein are reduced or absent.

Lactoferrin deficiency in patients with SGD is tissue specific (ie, confined to myeloid cells, whereas lactoferrin is secreted normally in nasal secretions) and is secondary to a deficiency of RNA transcripts.[90] Because morphologic changes have been described in the primary granule and because other granule proteins, such as primary granule defensin and "tertiary" granule gelatinase, are also deficient in SGD neutrophils, it was suggested that the basic defect in SGD is one of the regulations of production of these proteins.[91] Thus, this disorder may be one of the incomplete granule syntheses rather than a true SGD.[92]

SGD neutrophils demonstrate relatively severe chemotactic defects, resulting from significantly fewer or absent intracellular leukocyte adhesion molecules—molecules which would normally mobilize to the cell surface in response to inflammation. Patients with this condition present with challenging infections due to bacteria or fungi, normally involving the skin and lungs.[2]

CCATT/enhancer-binding protein epsilon (C/EBPE) is an important regulator of neutrophil secondary granule genes, and mutations in the C/EBPE gene have been found in patients with SGD.[93,94] Neutrophils from Cebpe-deficient mice have functional defects very similar to those of patients with SGD,[93,95,96] and these mice have defects in eosinophil and macrophage function as well.[97,98] Monocyte/macrophage abnormalities have also been noted in a patient with SGD.[99] One case of SGD has been reported with no mutation in the C/EBPE gene.[100]

Defects Affecting Phagocytosis and Degranulation

Appropriate microbial killing requires that following phagocytosis, neutrophil granules can release proteases, enzymes, and antibacterial proteins into the lumen of the phagosome. Among the more common conditions that impair this process are complement deficiencies and primary B-cell deficiencies.[2] Congenital neutrophil abnormalities that result in failure of proper bacterial ingestion or degranulation are very uncommon but critical for the hematologist to recognize. Among the most well known is Chédiak-Higashi syndrome (CHS), which was actually initially described by neither of the individuals included in the name, but rather a Cuban physician—Antonio Beguez-Cesar—who noted atypical enlarged granules within leukocytes in an affected patient.[101]

Chédiak-Higashi Syndrome

This rare syndrome is an autosomal recessive disorder with a worldwide incidence estimated at less than one in a million cases. It is characterized by partial ocular and cutaneous albinism, increased susceptibility to pyogenic infections, the presence of large lysosome-like organelles in most granule-containing cells, and a bleeding tendency. Among other consequences, the defects from granulopoeisis result in delayed and incomplete degranulation. The abnormal granules are most readily seen in blood and marrow leukocytes, especially granulocytes (*Figure 59.2*) and in melanocytes.

In the first families that were reported with this anomaly, the mothers noted that some of their children exhibited pale hair (*Figure 59.3*) and photophobia. Indeed, the symptoms of CHS may be apparent during early infancy. Affected children may have photosensitivity and/or nystagmus. Because these children often had infections and adenopathy and died at an early age, the children born subsequently who were similarly affected were brought to medical attention in the hope of avoiding a fatal outcome.[102] It was then that the large, peroxidase-positive granules were noted in their blood and marrow granulocytes. Nevertheless, without definitive treatment, most patients die in infancy or early childhood; only a few survive into early adult life.[103]

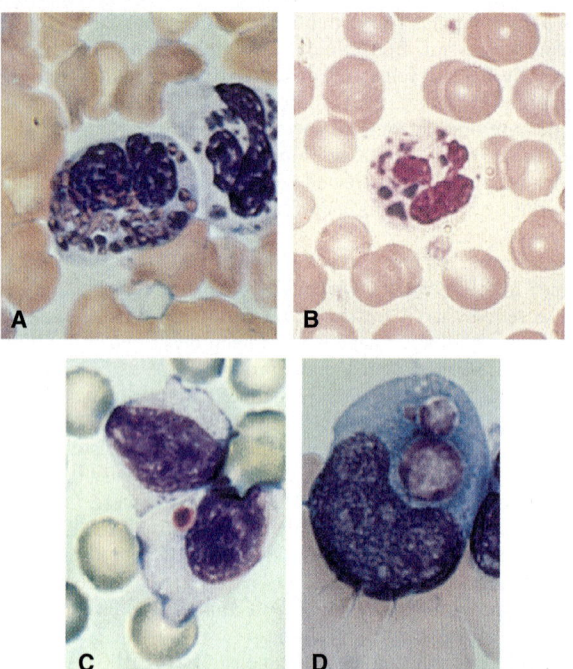

FIGURE 59.2 Inclusion bodies in Chédiak-Steinbrink-Higashi anomaly. A and B, Neutrophils. C, A lymphocyte. D, A monocytoid cell.

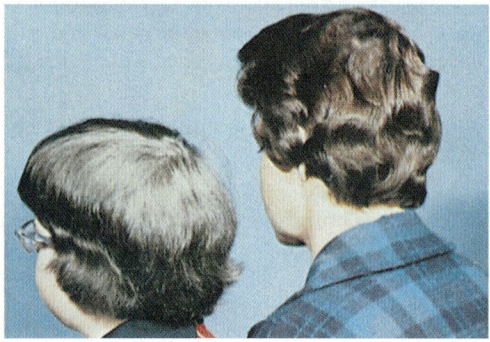

FIGURE 59.3 The characteristic silver-gray hair of a child (left) with Chédiak-Steinbrink-Higashi anomaly contrasted with that of her mother. (Courtesy of Dr Dorothy Windhorst, National Institutes of Health.)

During the 30 years after the first description of CHS, 59 cases were reported. The similar disorder in animals is of use in investigations of the pathogenic defect and is of significant economic impact in mink, in that affected animals inbred for their unusual color, seldom survive more than a year, and exhibit increased susceptibility to a slow viral infection that produces hepatitis and a myeloma-like illness (Aleutian mink disease).

Etiology and Pathogenesis

The pathology of CHS lies in the aberrations resulting from impaired organellar protein trafficking and subsequent defective fusion of vesicles and failure to transport lysosomes.[104] Researchers discovered the responsible gene initially in mice (who were beige in color) and then the human homologue was cloned. The mouse gene and the defective human gene, called CHS1/LYST at 1q42.1-2, are part of the BEACH (Beige and Chediak-Higashi) family of vesicle trafficking regulatory proteins.[104,105] The majority of reported mutations are nonsense or null mutations, which lead to an absent CHS/LYST protein; however, since the genetics of the disease have been discovered, some individuals with a less severe phenotype have been described and this may be due to missense mutations or genotypes with residual function preserved.[106-108] The protein produced by the CHS1/LYST gene is, normally, widely expressed in cytosol and critical for membrane fusion and fission by regulating the size and trafficking of lysosomes.

The manifestations of this disorder appear to result from abnormal intracellular protein transport, resulting in abnormal granule fusion with larger, fewer-than-normal, and perhaps defective granules being formed in most granule-containing cells throughout the body. The giant azurophilic granules do not release their contents in response to bacterial or viral infection.[109] Chemotaxis is also defective for the neutrophils of patients with CHS.[110] The cytotoxic granules of T lymphocytes are aberrant as well, with limited mobility, and the mutations in LYST appear to impact the trafficking of effectors involved in exocytosis required for the terminal maturation of perforin-containing vesicles into secretory cytotoxic granules.[111]

The resulting abnormalities can be found in the hematopoietic tissues, hair, ocular pigment, skin, adrenal glands, pituitary gland, gastrointestinal organs, peripheral nerves, and elsewhere.[112-114]

In neutrophils, the anomalously large, peroxidase-positive granules seen by light microscopy[115,116] have been shown by electron microscopy to be abnormal primary (azurophilic) granules, the contents of which remain pleomorphic, the normal granule crystalloid structure not being formed.[113,117] Characterization of the abnormal granules by means of immunofluorescence microscopy demonstrated that they were formed by the progressive aggregation and fusion of azurophilic granules.[118,119]

In a subsequent electron microscopic study, investigators demonstrated the presence of two types of giant peroxidase-positive granules in CHS neutrophils: large, round, or oval granules with homogeneous internal structure similar to normal azurophilic granules and irregular granules much larger than those of the first type. Because basophils and eosinophils from patients with CHS do not contain type 2 granules, and because type 2 granules are less common in promyelocytes, myelocytes, and young neutrophils in the bone marrow than in blood neutrophils, the authors suggested that normal primary (azurophil) granules are formed, but progressive granule fusion occurs during maturation, especially in the blood. In this process, granules and bits of cytoplasm are trapped within the fused granules.[120] Also noted is an increased tendency to autophagic vacuole formation in Chédiak-Higashi neutrophils, perhaps because of increased permeability and leakage of injurious materials from the massive granules.[114] A secretory defect appears to prevent granule release in CHS T cells.[121] Abnormal granules have been observed less often in erythroid cells, whereas in megakaryocytes and platelets, the granules appear normal by light microscopy. By electron microscopy, however, a decrease in dense bodies was seen, and decreased serotonin, adenosine triphosphate, and adenosine diphosphate levels were noted.[113]

Similar large granules containing a glycolipid have been observed in the Schwann cells of peripheral nerves, in neurons in the CNS, in renal tubular cells, and in the vascular endothelium and fibroblasts.[114,122-124] In addition, giant pigment granules have been demonstrated in melanosomes and in hair strands. In the several different tissues affected, the consistent feature is that the histochemical reactions of the large abnormal granules are those usually seen in normal granules of that cell line; no qualitative alteration in granule enzyme content is noted, but some decrease in granule enzymes and an increase in cytoplasmic enzyme content have been described.[122,125] The effects of the abnormality in different tissues depend on granule function in that tissue. Thus, the large but fewer melanin granules produce pigment dilution, which explains the peculiar hair color, partial albinism, photophobia, and nystagmus.

The abnormal large granules in neutrophils lead to increased susceptibility to infection. Patients experience frequent *S. aureus* infections, among others. Infection occurs despite an above-normal rate of phagocytosis and a normal post–phagocytic metabolic burst (H_2O_2 production).[126] Apparently, the intracellular destruction of some bacteria by Chédiak-Higashi leukocytes is delayed because the postphagocytic delivery of lysosomal enzymes into phagosomes is inefficient and incomplete. A similar defect in granule extrusion has been noted in the renal tubule.[127,128] There are two different models that have been presented to explain the dysregulation of lysosomal size. A summary of these is provided in a recent review: one model suggests that

LYST is required for lysosomal fusion to occur; the other model suggests that LYST may contribute to lysosomal membrane fission events instead of fusion.[101]

Chédiak-Higashi neutrophils from humans lack cathepsin G and elastase[129] and have reduced C3bi receptor expression.[130] Because measurements of elastase and cathepsin G were normal in the bone marrow of beige mice, the primary lesion was thought not to be a gene defect but rather is likely a disorder of protein processing, protein synthesis, or granule assembly. Studies have also shown that lysosomes function as calcium-regulated secretory compartments and may play an important role in membrane resealing. Lysosomal exocytosis triggered by membrane wounding is defective in human CHS and beige mouse fibroblasts, and this defect may be central to the CHS phenotype.[131]

Inheritance
The disorder is inherited as an autosomal recessive trait. Male and female subjects are affected at about equal numbers. A high proportion of marriages producing affected children have been consanguineous. Some heterozygotes may be identifiable by the presence of granulation in some of their lymphocytes.[132,133] There does not appear to be a higher risk for any particular ethnic or racial group. There are less than 500 cases of the disease on record.[109]

Clinical Features and Course
The partial albinism (more properly, pigment dilutional defect), silvery hair, and photophobia are usually noted early in infancy. The poor resistance to respiratory and cutaneous infection, especially by *Staphylococcus* and other gram-positive organisms, soon becomes evident. Four patients studied for more than a year experienced 29 episodes of fever and pyogenic infection.[134] Increased bleeding with abnormal platelet function has also been recognized, although not as impactful as patients with Hermansky-Pudlak syndrome. Many of the afflicted children develop potentially fatal infections during infancy or early childhood. In others, the disease remains quiescent until, in more than 85% of patients, it changes to an *accelerated* phase that is characterized by lymphadenopathy, hepatosplenomegaly, neuropathy, anemia, neutropenia, and, less often, thrombocytopenia.[135,136] During this phase, infiltration of the tissues by mononuclear cells is widespread, and the accelerated phase is now considered akin to the disorder *hemophagocytic lymphohistiocytosis* (HLH),[101,109] which has a high mortality associated with it.

Neurologic manifestations come in two forms: developmental delay with learning difficulties at an early age and degenerative disorders, which worsen with age and may include progressive reflex disorders, signs of cerebellar dysfunction, neuronopathy, weakness, spasticity and a Parkinson-like syndrome. Brain imaging is typically unrevealing.[101,109]

Laboratory Findings
The characteristic microscopic findings are the large, often multiple, peroxidase-positive lysosomal granules in the granulocytes of the blood and bone marrow and the large melanosomes in the hair. Less common are granules in the lymphocytes. Abnormal platelet aggregation can be demonstrated regularly. During the early phases of the disease, blood counts yield normal values, but as the disease progresses, anemia, neutropenia, and thrombocytopenia often develop.

Management
Infections require aggressive antimicrobial therapy. Once the diagnosis is established, prevention of infections is key with prophylactic antibacterial and antiviral agents. Accelerated phase is managed with immune suppression, much like in HLH. HCT is the treatment of choice and corrects the immunologic and hematologic manifestation of the disease. However, it does not alter the neurologic deterioration.[137-139] Given outcomes, transplant should be considered prior to the development of an accelerated phase. Bone marrow transplant corrects the immune and bleeding abnormalities and prevents the development of the accelerated phase. Bleeding can be managed with desmopressin or platelet transfusions, if necessary. Genetic counseling, recommendations to limit sun exposure, and standard screening for cancers are advisable.

Disorders of Bacterial Killing and Respiratory Burst
Chronic Granulomatous Disease
CGD is a genetically heterogeneous, rare, clinical syndrome caused by mutations in one of five genes coding for subunits of the neutrophil nicotinamide dinucleotide phosphate (NADPH) oxidase and resulting in recurrent, life-threatening bacterial and fungal infections and granuloma formation.[140] The incidence of this condition is approximately 1/200,000 live births in the United States, although it may be more common in the Israeli Arab population.[141] Recent reviews have been published.[140,142-144]

Normally, phagocytosis is followed by fusion of lysosomes with the phagocytic vacuole, discharge of lysosomal enzymes into the phagosome, and a burst of post–phagocytic metabolic activity. These events are usually accompanied by bacterial death and digestion (see Chapter 7). The NADH oxidase is a multicomponent enzyme with both membrane-bound and cytosolic subunits. This enzyme is critical to neutrophil anti-infective activities as it transfers electrons to molecular oxygen resulting in superoxide anion and hydrogen peroxide and the subsequent reactive metabolites.

Early studies of CGD cited a deficiency of NADPH oxidase or an abnormality in its activation as the underlying cause of this syndrome. Activation of the NADPH oxidase requires functional protein kinases, lipid-mobilizing enzymes, and factors that activate the Rac GTPase; thus, the CGD phenotype may arise from a variety of mutational defects. The finding that iodination of bacteria in the phagosome appears to be one mode of bacterial killing, and that this process is defective in CGD leukocytes and can be partially repaired by the insertion of an oxidase into the phagosome, either carried on oxidase-coated polystyrene particles or as part of the ingested bacteria,[145-147] provided strong evidence incriminating defective generation of H_2O_2, superoxide, or related ions as the pathogenic defect in this disorder.[148,149] Although most studies have focused on neutrophils, eosinophils, monocytes, macrophages, and neutrophils fail to generate superoxide, hydrogen peroxide, and other oxygen radicals after particle phagocytosis (or other stimulation), and thus have decreased microbicidal activity.[140,141] The impaired superoxide production leads to recurrent bacterial and fungal infections, most commonly at epithelial surfaces. The platelets appear normal.

CGD was first noted in male children with a history, beginning in early childhood, of recurrent suppurative infections caused by organisms of low-grade pathogenicity, including fungi, or by staphylococci. The eczematoid, granulomatous, and sometimes purulent skin infections recur repeatedly and clear slowly. Associated adenopathy develops and may persist. Pulmonary and other infections (e.g., osteomyelitis) also are common, and progressive granulomatous disease of the lungs, liver, and other sites develops. Hepatosplenomegaly is common, and biopsy reveals necrotizing granulomas, often with associated purulent inflammation. Although rare, CGD has assumed great importance as a prototype of defects in leukocyte bactericidal capacity.[142,143]

History and Molecular Genetics
CGD was first described from 1954 to 1957 as affecting only men.[150] By 1970, more than 90 cases were reported. X-linked inheritance was established, and female heterozygotes were identifiable by the presence of defective leukocyte bactericidal capacity intermediate in degree between that of affected patients and that of normal individuals.[151] Measurements of postphagocytic release of $(^{14})CO_2$ from glucose-1-$(^{14})C$ or reduction of NBT dye were used to detect the defect. By means of the NBT dye test, female carriers were found to have a mixed population of neutrophils, approximately one-half being NBT negative and one-half being NBT positive. The defect is most commonly transmitted on an X chromosome, and the degree of deficit in female subjects varies according to random X chromosome inactivation. Consequently, one may expect to find an occasional female

carrier with clinical disease as severe as that in male patients.[151,152] In the late 1960s and 1970s, an autosomal recessive form of CGD was described.[146,147] It is clinically identical to the X-linked forms, with the exception that the parents of affected children usually have normal neutrophil function.

NADPH oxidase is a multi–protein enzyme complex comprised of five subunits. Mutations in genes encoding each of the subunits have been found in CGD. The most common (two-thirds) of these are in the *CYBB* gene, on the X chromosome, encoding for gp91phox (also called NOX2). The second most common (~25%) are autosomal recessive mutations in *NCF1*, with the corresponding protein subunit being p47phox. Less common mutations in the remaining subunits have also been described.[142] All the mutations result in loss of function and near complete loss of NADPH oxidase enzymatic activity, although some retain minor function that might explain milder phenotypes. Rare variants have also been found such as missense mutations in X-linked *CYBB* that cause selective reduction of NADPH oxidase activity in macrophages but not in neutrophils.[153] An alteration in the B-cell compartment in patients with CGD has also been reported.[154] It appears that CGD is associated with a reduction in the peripheral blood memory B-cell compartment, suggesting a role for NADPH in memory B-cell formation.

Clinical and Laboratory Features

Recurrent infections are the hallmark clinical feature of CGD. Infections usually begin in early childhood, most commonly affecting the lungs, skin, lymph nodes, bones, and the gastrointestinal tract, including liver abscesses. Organisms typically implicated are *Staphylococci, Burkholderia, Nocardia, Serratia,* and *Salmonella* species.[155] In areas where *Bacillus Calmette-Guérin* vaccination is practiced, disseminated infections with this mycobacterium strain are encountered. Fungal infections, particularly *Aspergillus* pneumonia, are also common. Many of these bacterial species are catalase producers, and it is thought that catalase-positive bacteria generate much lower levels of endogenous H_2O_2, which is insufficient for CGD phagocytes to utilize in generating hypochlorous (HOCL) acid. Chronic and recurrent infections lead to lymph node enlargements, hepatomegaly, and granulomas. However, some of the granulomas may be unrelated to infections such as the granulomatous enterocolitis. Chronic inflammation in the gastrointestinal and urinary tracts can result in obstruction. The underlying pathophysiology of chronic inflammation in CGD is not completely understood, but might involve dysregulation of inflammatory cytokine pathways that depend on reactive oxygen species production. Other noninfectious complications of CGD include HLH, discoid lupus, and microvascular liver disease.

The classic method for diagnosing CGD is the post–phagocytic, intraphagosomal reduction of almost colorless NBT dye to blue-black formazan. When tests are properly standardized with respect to time of incubation of leukocytes with the dye-tagged zymosan particles, affected patients and most carriers are readily recognized. When the reaction to this test is negative in suspected carriers, the reaction to the quantitative dye reduction test usually is positive. However, currently, the preferred method is flow cytometry–based detection of the conversion of the nonfluorescent dye dihydrorhodamine (DHR) to its oxidized form that emits green fluorescence.[156] The sensitivity and quantitative nature of this test make it more reliable and also allow for detection of residual oxidase activity that can be important in prognosis.[157]

There is considerable heterogeneity in the severity of the clinical course of patients with CGD. There is a distinct correlation between the severity of the disease and the specific gene defect, with *NCF1* (p47phox) mutations associated with less severe disease. This is partly explained by the residual activity of NADPH oxidase in patients with *NCF1* mutations.

Treatment

Without treatment, this disease usually runs a progressive downhill course because of repeated infections and granuloma formation. The average life expectancy was reported to be 5 to 7 years in 1968. In 2008, one-half of patients were projected to survive into the fourth decade.[158,159]

Treatment of infections with appropriate antibiotics and surgical procedures remains the cornerstone of management.[140,144] Prolonged use of antimicrobial therapy may be required even for commonplace infections. Voriconazole or posaconazole may be empirically used if mold infection is suspected, and reports have been published on the use of granulocyte transfusions, although this may complicate future allogeneic stem cell transplantation.[160] The overall incidence and severity of infections decreases in the second decade of life, but the overall increased risk of infections is lifelong. Prophylactic use of antibiotics, including trimethoprim-sulfamethoxazole and itraconazole with or without IFN-γ, is generally recommended.[155,161]

In some patients with CGD, the administration of IFN-γ has induced partial correction of cytochrome b content and restored phagocyte bactericidal capacity toward normal, and reports have suggested that IFN-γ increases the ability of CGD neutrophils to kill *Aspergillus* and decreases the number of serious infections in patients with CGD.[162,163] The exact mechanism by which IFN-γ exerts its beneficial effect in CGD is unclear and may include other effects in addition to augmentation of the respiratory burst.[164] Inflammatory complications are treated with systemic corticosteroids. Allogeneic HCT is the only cure for CGD, although aggressive research on gene therapy is advancing.[140] High-risk patients include those with severe infection or autoinflammation. Since levels of residual superoxide production have correlated well with OS, HSCT has been recommended in patients with X-linked or autosomal recessive CGD if a matched donor is identified, and if no residual oxidase activity or if severe disease complications develop.[165]

CGD was one of the first diseases to be treated with gene therapy. Early studies resulted in successful correction of NADPH oxidase deficiency and resolution of infections. However, the retrovirus used in gene delivery resulted in activation of neighboring oncogenes, eventually inducing leukemia.[166] More recently, studies on lentiviral-based gene therapy have been conducted.[167]

CGD Variants and Additional Conditions Associated With Defective Respiratory Burst

Because the clinical picture of CGD results from delayed killing of catalase-positive bacteria, enzymatic defects in the bactericidal system other than decreased NADPH oxidase may produce an almost identical picture. Multiple examples are in the literature of such biochemical variants exist. For example, in a brother and sister with the clinical picture of CGD, after phagocytosis of latex particles by their neutrophils, all oxidative metabolic reactions were absent. If the latex particles were opsonized with immunoglobulin, however, post–phagocytic oxidative changes were stimulated dramatically.[168] Another patient was reported in whom no oxidative changes (measured by chemiluminescence) occurred after phagocytosis of a variety of opsonized particles (latex, bacteria, or zymosan), but normal chemiluminescent responses occurred when the neutrophils were stimulated with soluble agents (concanavalin A and phorbol myristate acetate).[169] These patients appear to have a defect in signal transduction and activation of the oxidase system rather than in the oxidase enzyme(s). Another patient with clinically mild, X-linked CGD exhibited normal membrane depolarization (and therefore presumably normal activation), but NADPH oxidase apparently had a low affinity for NADPH and thus produced low but measurable amounts of superoxide.[170]

Lipochrome Histiocytosis

A clinical variant, lipochrome histiocytosis, was described in three sisters with rheumatoid arthritis, hyperglobulinemia, splenomegaly, pulmonary infiltrates, and increased susceptibility to infection.[171,172] No granulomas were found in tissue biopsies, but lipochrome pigmentation in large macrophages was present throughout the tissues. Studies of blood leukocyte function in two of the sisters revealed impaired postphagocytic respiration, NBT reduction, and hexose monophosphate shunt activity identical to that seen in patients with CGD.

Glucose-6-Phosphate Dehydrogenase Deficiency

NADPH is the major substrate for the respiratory burst oxidase. A bactericidal defect similar to CGD has been described in a patient with a complete deficiency of G6PD, an enzyme important in the generation of NADPH.[173] Apparently, almost complete absence of G6PD activity is necessary to interfere with bacterial killing because no difference from normal could be detected in cells with 25% activity or greater.[174]

Glutathione Peroxidase Deficiency

Two unrelated 9- and 13-year-old girls presented a clinical picture similar to that of CGD and with decreased bactericidal capacity.[175] The findings in these girls differed from those in men with CGD only in that no heterozygotes were detected in their families and their clinical course was somewhat milder. These patients were reported before the nature of the NADPH oxidase was known, and it was suggested that the CGD phenotype was due to glutathione peroxidase deficiency, resulting in inhibition of the oxidase by accumulated peroxides. A subsequent study, however, suggested that glutathione peroxidase activity was normal in these patients and that both had mutations in the NADPH oxidase.[176] Thus, there is no firm evidence that glutathione peroxidase deficiency is a cause of the CGD phenotype.

Glutathione Synthetase or Reductase Deficiency

Reduced glutathione (GSH) plays an important role in protecting neutrophils (including the NADPH oxidase system) from reactive metabolites, including H_2O_2. Because GSH levels are generated by both direct synthesis via glutathione synthetase (GSS) and the reduction of oxidized glutathione by glutathione reductase, deficiencies of these enzymes might be expected to result in defective neutrophil function. GSS deficiency is an autosomal recessive disorder and three groups of affected patients are recognized: mildly affected, moderately affected, and severely affected.[177]

As initially described, the neutrophils of a normally growing infant with a relatively benign history of recurrent otitis and repeated episodes of neutropenia were found to have 5% of normal GSS activity and 10% to 20% of normal glutathione content. The cells ingested particles and metabolized 1-(^{14}C) glucose normally, but after phagocytosis, excess peroxide accumulated and impaired iodination and killing of bacteria were demonstrable. Electron microscopic examination showed damage to the microtubules and membranes of the neutrophils.[178,179] Neutrophil dysfunction resulting from a deficiency of glutathione reductase has also been reported.[180]

Patients with glutathione reductase deficiency or GSS deficiency have heterogeneous outcomes—with some having no symptoms, others with an isolated hemolytic anemia, and those with moderate or severe disease having episodes of metabolic acidosis or even progressive nervous system dysfunction in addition to hemolysis and increased susceptibility to infection. Sodium bicarbonate and high doses of vitamin C and vitamin E may be useful in patients with severe GSS deficiency.[175]

Catalase Deficiency

The neutrophil is protected from products of the NADPH oxidase not only by glutathione but also by superoxide dismutase, which generates H_2O_2 from superoxide, and by catalase, which converts H_2O_2 to H_2O and O_2. A deficiency in neutrophil catalase has been reported in which the surface of the neutrophil was more susceptible to damage by H_2O_2 than normal.[181] These patients do not appear to have severe complications with infections.

Immunodeficiency States and Neutrophil Dysfunction

Neutrophil dysfunction also occurs in a variety of immunodeficiency states. Defects in any of the steps of oxidase assembly and activation could result in decreased superoxide production. In the primary immunodeficiency state, IL-1R–associated kinase 4 deficiency, there was decreased phosphorylation of p47phox and decreased translocation to the membrane of p47phox, p67phos, and other oxidase components with associated decreased oxidase activity.[182]

In NF-κB essential modulator (NEMO) deficiency, NEMO-deficient cells had similar but less prominent changes, although p47phox translocation was normal.[182] With Bruton tyrosine kinase (BTK) deficiency (also known as X-linked agammaglobulinemia), the picture is less clear. In patients with X-linked agammaglobulinemia, there is both a deficiency of the kinase BTK and neutropenia.[183] Studies suggest that in humans, BTK-deficient neutrophils produce excessive NADPH oxidase activity after various stimuli and that this was associated with increased apoptosis. It appears that the NADPH oxidase complex is partially assembled in resting BTK-deficient human neutrophils, making them ready for activation, that is, human BTK-deficient neutrophils are in a primed state. This is in contrast to studies of BTK-deficient mouse neutrophils where impaired NADPH oxidase activity was found. The model is that in humans BTK functions as a cytosolic component that inhibits translocation of NADPH oxidase components to the membrane and subsequent interactions with other NADPH components. Patients receiving the BTK-inhibitor ibrutinib for the treatment of chronic lymphocytic leukemia or other lymphoid malignancies are at significant risk for fungal infections, in particular, invasive aspergillosis.[184,185]

Myeloperoxidase Deficiency

The autosomal recessive inherited deficiency of MPO was initially described in 1954.[186] A 49-year-old man, one of his two sisters, and all four sons exhibited decreased MPO activity; no increased frequency of infections accompanied this defect. In two other families, apparently similarly affected, no increase in infection was noted.[187] Since that time, with the development of flow cytometry and automated differential cell-counting techniques, however, MPO deficiency has been commonly detected (~1 in 2000 subjects) during routine hematologic evaluation of patients admitted to the hospital. It is now known to be the most common inherited disorder of phagocytes with a complete deficiency occurring in 1 in 4000 individuals.[188,189] This disorder is now known to be autosomal recessive with mutations localized in the *MPO* gene on chromosome 17q23.[186] While impaired microbial killing has been documented, deficiency is not typically associated with clinical symptoms.

Most studies of MPO-deficient neutrophils reveal that bacteria and fungi are phagocytized normally, and ingestion is followed by a vigorous respiratory burst. Bactericidal killing, however, is somewhat delayed, reaching normal levels only after 1 to 3 hours. Findings of these studies and the rarity of clinical infections in MPO-deficient individuals support the concept of MPO-independent microbicidal mechanisms.[187,190] In contrast, although ingested normally, several *Candida* species and *Aspergillus* are killed poorly, if at all, and some MPO-deficient patients, including one of the first reported cases, suffered from disseminated fungal infection. MPO-deficient mice also have impaired defense against *Candida* and have also been noted to have increased atherogenesis.[189,191] In spite of these abnormalities, the majority of the patients are asymptomatic and only a small percentage suffer from *Candida* infections.[192-195] It is possible that co-occurrence of other defects are responsible for these rare infectious events and not just MPO deficiency. It should also be noted that complete MPO deficiency can be misdiagnosed as CGD because of reduced oxidation of the DHR dye.[195]

MPO deficiency also occurs as an acquired defect in a variety of situations (eg, pregnancy, lead intoxication, Hodgkin lymphoma, and activated coagulation),[190] but it is encountered most commonly in association with acute myeloblastic leukemia (up to 48% of patients), myeloproliferative states (20%-60% in chronic myelogenous leukemia, 32% in myelofibrosis), and myelodysplastic syndromes (25%). In many of these conditions, only some of the circulating myeloid cells are deficient, presumably those produced by the abnormal clone.[190]

Cystic Fibrosis

As described, an important mechanism of bacterial killing by neutrophils involves the production of HOCl acid from H_2O_2 and chloride. Cystic fibrosis (CF) is caused by mutations in the gene encoding the cystic fibrosis transmembrane conductance regulator (CFTR), a cyclic adenosine monophosphate–regulated chloride channel. CFTR is present in neutrophil secretory vesicles and phagolysosomes. Although CF neutrophils produce extracellular HOCl normally, they have impaired chlorination and killing of phagocytosed bacteria because of defective HOCl production in phagolysosomes.[195,196]

Papillon-Lefèvre Syndrome
Papillon-Lefèvre syndrome, characterized by juvenile periodontitis leading to tooth loss and hyperkeratosis palmoplantaris, is an uncommon autosomal recessive disorder.[197,198] One patient with this syndrome was found to have a mutation in *CTSC* that inactivates dipeptidyl peptidase 1 (or cathepsin C). This enzyme removes two N-terminal amino acids that block the active site of neutrophil proteases.[198,199] This patient's neutrophils lacked the primary granule enzymes elastase, cathepsin G, proteinase 3, and neutrophil serine protease 4, but did not have frequent or severe infections. However, ~25% of these patients do suffer from frequent infection.[200]

Acquired Conditions of Impaired Bacterial Killing
Desensitization
After previous exposure to a stimulus, neutrophils react less to subsequent stimulation by the same stimulus. This phenomenon has been termed *desensitization*.[201] In some cases, the desensitization appears specific to the original stimulus, but in other cases, desensitization to different stimuli is also observed (cross-desensitization). Such desensitization has been observed in patients undergoing hemodialysis, in which exposure of blood to a cuprophane dialyzer membrane results in the generation of C5a, which causes a transient neutropenia due to pulmonary leukostasis, as described in Chapter 7. Although C5a generation persists throughout dialysis, the neutropenia is transient.[202-204] In contrast to neutrophils obtained at the start of dialysis, neutrophils obtained after 2 hours of dialysis (after the leukostasis has resolved) do not aggregate in response to plasma leaving the dialyzer membrane, demonstrating desensitization in vivo. A patient with cytomegalovirus infection and serum-induced granulocyte aggregation (presumably due to C5a) did not experience neutropenia during dialysis; and his neutrophils did not aggregate in response to serum leaving the dialyzer, in contrast to control cells, also demonstrating in vivo desensitization.[204] It is likely that neutrophil desensitization may also occur in other pathologic states, including infection, trauma, and multiorgan failure syndrome, and may contribute to neutrophil dysfunction, although the clinical significance of this phenomenon is unclear.

Viral Infection
Neutrophil dysfunction has been reported to occur in response to influenza A exposure. Both influenza A virus and its purified hemagglutinin activate neutrophils, and neutrophil responses to other stimuli are depressed after preexposure to influenza A and parainfluenza.[204,205] Neutrophils from patients with human immunodeficiency virus (HIV) infection also may exhibit abnormal function. In one study, neutrophils from patients with early HIV infection had enhanced superoxide production in response to bacterial products. Another study found evidence for neutrophil activation in patients with HIV infection as manifested by increased CD11b expression, decreased CD62L expression, increased H_2O_2 production, and increased actin polymerization.[206,207] Interestingly, H_2O_2 production, in response to FMLP after TNF and IL-8 priming, was decreased, and CD62L downregulation in response to FMLP was less complete; these abnormalities correlated with the clinical stage of disease. Whether these abnormalities are a direct effect of the HIV virus, a manifestation of desensitization as described in the previous section, or the result of another mechanism is unclear. These observations suggest that neutrophil dysfunction may occur in response to other viral infections as well, although the clinical significance of such a phenomenon is unclear.

Hyperalimentation Hypophosphatemia
In the past, the use of hyperalimentation without adequate phosphate occasionally resulted in hypophosphatemia that was associated with neutrophil dysfunction, including impaired chemotaxis.[208] The exact mechanism of this defect is unclear, and this syndrome is now rarely encountered, although evidence suggests that the impairment of phagocytosis seen in phosphate depletion may result from an increase in intracellular calcium.[209]

Hyperglycemia
Abnormalities have been observed in several neutrophil functions in patients with poorly controlled diabetes, including phagocytosis, chemotaxis, adhesion, and the oxidative burst.[210,211] Improvement in glucose control is associated with an improvement in neutrophil function. Improvement in neutrophil function can occur after incubation with insulin for as little as 15 minutes.[212] In patients with non–insulin-dependent diabetes, neutrophil dysfunction is associated with an increased intracellular calcium that returns to normal in association with normalization of phagocytic function when glucose control is improved.[210]

Neutrophil Dysregulation in the Systemic Inflammatory Response Syndrome
Although this chapter has primarily addressed disorders resulting in decreased neutrophil function, neutrophil activity may also be increased. For example, one study reported increased neutrophil functional activity in patients with severe acute pancreatitis.[213] There are accumulating data that one of the reasons for the high levels of morbidity associated with infection with the novel Coronavirus (SARS-CoV-2) was the uncontrolled formation of neutrophil extracellular traps and their by-products.[214,215] The reader is referred to a number of reviews on this phenomenon, which is, at this writing, a subject of investigation.[216-218]

FREQUENCY OF IDENTIFIABLE QUALITATIVE NEUTROPHIL DISORDERS

Most patients suspected of having a defect in neutrophil function do not have a well-defined abnormality. In one study of 100 patients referred for evaluation of a suspected neutrophil abnormality, only 4 were identified as a described syndrome. Some degree of impaired chemotaxis or superoxide production was found in 53 of 100 patients, but no abnormality was found in 41 of 100.[219]

MORPHOLOGIC CHANGES IN PHAGOCYTIC LEUKOCYTES

The hematologist should also be aware of conditions where there are clearly apparent morphologic morphologic changes in the neutrophil, but where there is little-to-no systemic impact on the leukocyte function. In the remainder of this chapter, we will summarize several of these findings, as they may be faced in clinical practice.

Pelger-Huët Anomaly
Pelger-Huët anomaly is a benign anomaly of leukocytes and is inherited as a non–sex-linked, dominant trait. It is characterized by distinctive shapes of the nuclei of leukocytes, a reduced number of nuclear segments (best seen in the neutrophils), and coarseness of the chromatin of the nuclei of neutrophils, lymphocytes, and monocytes. The nuclei appear rod like, dumbbell shaped, peanut shaped, and spectacle like ("pince-nez") with smooth, round, or oval individual lobes, contrasted with the irregular lobes seen in normal neutrophils.[220] The incidence of this disorder in different studies has ranged from as high as 1 in 1000 persons to 1 in 4000, 6000, or even 10,000.[221] The practical importance of identifying the Pelger-Huët anomaly lies in distinguishing this defect from the shift to the left that occurs in association with infection.

The discovery of this anomaly in rabbits led to breeding experiments and the production of homozygotes. In rabbits, the homozygous form was often lethal, with most animals dying in utero; some survivors suffered skeletal malformations. In human homozygotes, the cytoplasm of the neutrophils appeared mature, but the nuclei were round or oval in all the neutrophils, in contrast to the fewer than 40% single-lobed neutrophils present in heterozygotes (*Table 59.3*). In the

Table 59.3. Distribution of Nuclear Lobes in Neutrophils of Normal Persons and in Those With Pelger-Huët Anomaly

	Cases Examined	Number of Lobes[a]				
		1	2	3	4	5
Normals[b]	50	2.8 ±2.8	22.0 ±6.3	54.3 ±5.3	18.1 ±6.9	2.8 ±2.1
Pelger-Huët heterozygotes[b]	34	31.3 ±9.2	63.8 ±9.5	4.9 ±3.7	0.3 —	0 —
Pelger-Huët Homozygotes	2	100.0	—	—	—	—

[a]Mean and variance.
[b]Modified from Davidson WM, Lawler SD, Ackerly AG. The Pelger-Huët anomaly: investigation of family "A". *Ann Hum Genet*. 1954;19(1):1. Reprinted by permission of John Wiley & Sons, Inc.

homozygotes, the eosinophils, basophils, and megakaryocytes also were characterized by dense nuclear chromatin and rounded nuclear lobes; these individuals had fewer nuclear lobes than normal subjects. Examination of the bone marrow revealed normal morphologic features in myeloid precursors through the myelocyte stage, and electron microscopy revealed persistence of nucleoli in the otherwise mature neutrophils that contained single oval nuclei. This finding was interpreted as indicating some retardation of nuclear maturation because no cytochemical defects were noted in the cytoplasm. Pelger-Huët syndrome is now known to be due to mutations in the lamin B receptor gene, a gene important in maintaining nuclear structure.[221-225]

Pelger–Huët cells appear to be normal functionally, are able to phagocytize and kill microorganisms, and survive normally in the circulation.[226,227] The Pelger-Huët heterozygote is recognized by finding (1) 69% to 93% of the neutrophils to be of the bilobed, pince-nez type; (2) few cells with three lobes (usually <10%); and (3) rare or no cells with four lobes (*Table 59.1*). In normal blood smears, no more than 27% of the cells are bilobed, and significant numbers of cells have three or more lobes. The presence of similar abnormalities in the blood smear in other family members also is helpful in establishing the diagnosis. In heterozygotes, mature neutrophils with round or oval nuclei of the type that is characteristic of the homozygous state may increase after stress such as the injection of colchicine.

Pseudo– or Acquired Pelger-Huët Anomaly

Cells with morphologic changes, such as those just described, have been observed occasionally in association with myxedema, acute enteritis, agranulocytosis, multiple myeloma, malaria, leukemoid reactions secondary to metastases to the bone marrow, drug sensitivity, or chronic lymphocytic leukemia.[228-230] More commonly, pseudo–Pelger-Huët cells (*Figure 59.4*)[22] are seen in patients with myeloid leukemia, either acute or chronic or in those with myelodysplastic syndrome or who are being treated for such.[231-234]

Alder-Reilly Anomaly

Alder-Reilly anomaly, inherited as a recessive trait, apparently does not interfere with leukocyte function.[235] It is characterized by the presence of larger-than-normal azurophil and basophil granules (Alder-Reilly bodies), which may be easily confused with granulations due to toxic states (*Figure 59.5*). These granules stain dark lilac with Wright-Giemsa stains and are seen in patients with various types of bone and cartilage abnormalities. They are most common, however, in association with mucopolysaccharidoses such as Hurler syndrome, Hunter syndrome, and Maroteaux-Lamy polydystrophic syndrome.[236-238]

Similar inclusions may be seen in blood lymphocytes (Gasser cells) and monocytes.[239] The lymphocyte inclusions stain dark red or purple with May-Grünwald Giemsa stain and metachromatically with toluidine blue; normal azurophilic granules do not stain at all. Such lymphocyte granules are found in all types of mucopolysaccharidoses except Morquio syndrome, but they are most common in the Hurler, Hunter, Sanfilippo, and Maroteaux-Lamy syndromes. They tend to

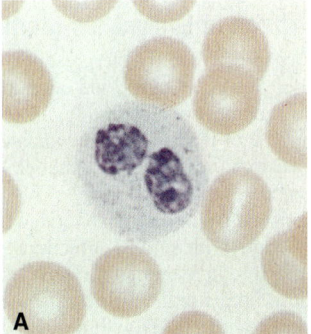
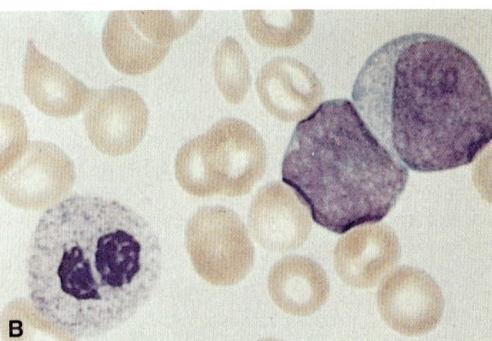

FIGURE 59.4 A, Pseudo–Pelger-Huët cells. B, From a patient with acute myeloblastic leukemia.

occur in clusters rather than diffusely throughout the cytoplasm, are surrounded by vacuoles, and are shaped like a dot or a comma. In one series of 19 patients, 8% to 50% of the lymphocytes contained the inclusions, and their presence was thought to be of diagnostic significance.

The type of inclusion seen is not diagnostic of a particular type of mucopolysaccharidosis, and the frequency of the inclusions is not correlated with clinical severity.[240] The basic defect in this group of diseases lies in the incomplete degradation of the protein-carbohydrate complexes known as *glycosaminoglycans* (*GAGs*), and the different forms of mucopolysaccharidosis involve different enzymatic deficiencies. The accumulation of partially degraded GAG within lysosomes has been demonstrated by electron microscopy; the degradation of the protein core of the GAG appears to proceed normally, but catabolism of the carbohydrate side chains is impaired.[236]

May-Hegglin Anomaly

The May-Hegglin anomaly is a rare, dominantly inherited disorder characterized by large (2-5 μm), well-defined, basophilic, and pyroninophilic inclusions in granulocytes (neutrophils, eosinophils, basophils, monocytes) and accompanied by variable thrombocytopenia and giant platelets containing few granules.[241] For the most part, affected family members have not been ill, but occasionally abnormal bleeding has occurred.[242,243] The granulocyte inclusions are similar to Döhle bodies in appearance, but they often are larger, are more round and discrete, and may be present in a large percentage of the cells.

Mutations in *MYH9*, the gene encoding NMMHC-A, have been found in this syndrome.[244] NMMHC-A is a nonmuscle myosin heavy chain that is part of a family of genes coding for proteins that form part of the actin-myosin force generating complexes. Mutations in *MYH9* are inherited in an autosomal dominant manner, but depending on the mutation generate a spectrum of clinical findings manifest as several syndromes because of variable expressivity of the clinical features.[245] These clinical syndromes include May-Hegglin anomaly, Sebastian syndrome, Fechtner syndrome, and Epstein syndrome and are characterized by giant platelets, leukocyte inclusions, and variable thrombocytopenia, in addition to problems with hearing, vision, or renal function.[245]

Familial Vacuolization of Leukocytes (Jordan Anomaly)

Jordan anomaly is characterized by the presence of vacuoles in the cytoplasm of granulocytes, monocytes, and occasionally lymphocytes and plasma cells. In members of one family, all of the blood neutrophils and more than 70% of the monocytes contained 3 to 10 vacuoles ranging in size from 2 to 5 µm; fewer and smaller vacuoles were seen in eosinophils, basophils, and lymphocytes. This type of vacuolization must be distinguished from that characterized by fat-staining vacuoles occurring in people with serious infections, toxic hepatitis, or diabetic ketoacidosis. Jordan's anomaly is now recognized as a feature of familial neutral lipid storage disorders (NLSDs). Mutations in PNPLA2 are associated with NLSD with myopathy, while Chanarin-Dorfman syndrome, an NLSD with ichthyosis, is caused by mutations in ABHD5.[246-248]

Other Inclusions in Leukocytes

In an infant with congenital bile duct atresia, amorphous, round to oval bodies stained green or gray-green with Romanowsky stains in 3% to 13% of the blood neutrophils and in 1% to 5% of the monocytes.[249] Similar inclusions were present in all stages of myeloid cells in the bone marrow but not in lymphocytes or plasma cells. Electron microscopic analysis showed that the inclusions were not enclosed in a phagocytic vesicle.

In the blood monocytes of patients with the Hermansky-Pudlak syndrome,[250] a rare familial disorder characterized by albinism, mild bleeding related to platelet dysfunction, accumulation of ceroid-like pigment in marrow macrophages, and deficiency of the tetraspan protein CD63 in platelets,[86] lipopigment bodies, as well as another type of inclusion, were demonstrated.

Hereditary Giant Neutrophilia

Neutrophils with a diameter of ~17 µm (as compared with a normal diameter of about 13 µm) are rare in blood smears from normal people (1 in 20,000 neutrophils or less). They may be seen with greater frequency in patients who are ill, but even then the number rarely exceeds 0.2% unless a disease involving leukocyte production is present or a reaction to a cytotoxic drug occurs. A family with giant neutrophils in healthy members of three generations has been reported. Over several years, the propositus had an average of 1.6% giant neutrophils in the blood. The large neutrophils appeared to be nearly double the normal cell volume and contained from 6 to 10 nuclear lobes. Therefore, it was suggested that the cells may have been tetraploid. This anomaly appeared to be transmitted as an autosomal dominant trait.[251]

Hereditary Hypersegmentation of Neutrophil Nuclei

Several families have been described whose members had a hereditary (autosomal dominant) increase in the number of neutrophil nuclear segments (*Figure 59.6*).[252] The proportion of neutrophils containing five lobes or more exceeded 10% in most heterozygotes and was >14% in several suspected homozygotes, as compared with no more than 10% in normal controls. The bone marrow findings suggested a tendency toward nuclear indentation in early myeloid forms (eosinophils and basophils as well as neutrophils). The normal size of these neutrophils was thought to provide evidence against tetraploidy, but in one study of five female family members, the mean number of nuclear drumsticks appeared to be increased above normal.[253] The chief significance of this anomaly is in its differentiation from other causes of hypersegmentation such as folate or vitamin B_{12} deficiency.

Hypersegmentation of Eosinophils and Negative Staining for Peroxidase and Phospholipids

Hypersegmentation of eosinophils can be inherited as an autosomal recessive trait, and the abnormality is characterized by a lack of sudanophilia and peroxidase activity in all of the eosinophils, whereas these histochemical reactions remain positive in the neutrophils and monocytes.[254,255] In addition, the number of eosinophilic granules per cell appears to be reduced, and some hypersegmentation of the eosinophil nucleus may occur. No disease accompanies the disorder. This has been most commonly reported in people of Jewish (predominantly Yemenite) extraction, although members of other races have not been studied adequately.

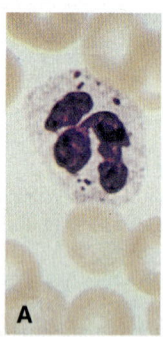

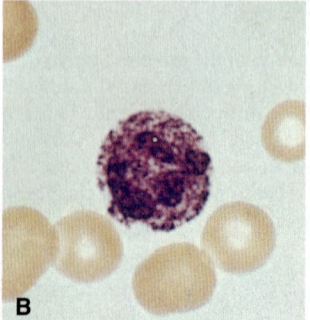 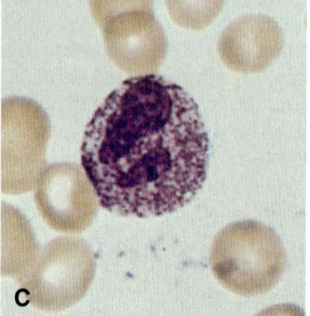

FIGURE 59.5 Neutrophils with Alder-Reilly bodies (A) compared with neutrophils exhibiting toxic granulation (B and C).

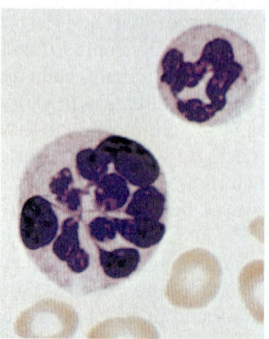

FIGURE 59.6 Hypersegmented neutrophil.

CONCLUSION

In this chapter, we have attempted to catalog the most commonly encountered and scientifically interesting of the qualitative disorders of leukocytes. While many are of historical interest, they retain importance as we learn more and more about the molecular structure of neutrophils and of how their phenotype is influenced by both genetic and epigenetic phenomenon. The reader is referred to several websites, listed below, that should allow for additional information on hematologic ramifications of primary immune deficiency.

WEBSITE RESOURCES

www.jmfworld.com/
https://www.niaid.nih.gov/diseases-conditions/primary-immune-deficiency-diseases-pidds
http://primaryimmune.org/

ACKNOWLEDGMENTS

The author acknowledges the tremendous contributions of Dr. Ashish Kumar and Dr. Keith M. Skubitz. Their previous edition of this chapter served as the basis for the present revision.

References

1. Boxer LA, Blackwood RA. Leukocyte disorders: quantitative and qualitative disorders of the neutrophil, Part 1. *Pediatr Rev.* 1996;17:19-28.
2. Dinauer MC. Neutrophil defects and diagnosis disorders of neutrophil function: an overview. *Methods Mol Biol.* 2020;2087:11-29.
3. van de Vijver E, van den Berg TK, Kuijpers TW. Leukocyte adhesion deficiencies. *Hematol Oncol Clin North Am.* 2013;27:101-116. viii.
4. Todd RF, III, Freyer DR. The CD11/CD18 leukocyte glycoprotein deficiency. *Hematol Oncol Clin North Am.* 1988;2:13-31.
5. Etzioni A. Leukocyte adhesion deficiencies: molecular basis, clinical findings, and therapeutic options. *Adv Exp Med Biol.* 2007;601:51-60.
6. Moutsopoulos NM, Zerbe CS, Wild T, et al. Interleukin-12 and interleukin-23 blockade in leukocyte adhesion deficiency type 1. *N Engl J Med.* 2017;376:1141-1146.
7. Crowley CA, Curnutte JT, Rosin RE, et al. An inherited abnormality of neutrophil adhesion. Its genetic transmission and its association with a missing protein. *N Engl J Med.* 1980;302:1163-1168.
8. Dinauer MC. Inflammatory consequences of inherited disorders affecting neutrophil function. *Blood.* 2019;133:2130-2139.
9. Almarza Novoa E, Kasbekar S, Thrasher AJ, et al. Leukocyte adhesion deficiency-I: a comprehensive review of all published cases. *J Allergy Clin Immunol Pract.* 2018;6:1418-1420.e10.
10. Anderson DC, Schmalsteig FC, Finegold MJ, et al. The severe and moderate phenotypes of heritable Mac-1, LFA-1 deficiency: their quantitative definition and relation to leukocyte dysfunction and clinical features. *J Infect Dis.* 1985;152:668-689.
11. Harlan JM. Leukocyte adhesion deficiency syndrome: insights into the molecular basis of leukocyte emigration. *Clin Immunol Immunopathol.* 1993;67:S16-S24.
12. Wright AH, Douglass WA, Taylor GM, et al. Molecular characterization of leukocyte adhesion deficiency in six patients. *Eur J Immunol.* 1995;25:717-722.
13. Moutsopoulos NM, Konkel J, Sarmadi M, et al. Defective neutrophil recruitment in leukocyte adhesion deficiency type I disease causes local IL-17-driven inflammatory bone loss. *Sci Transl Med.* 2014;6:229ra40.
14. Qasim W, Cavazzana-Calvo M, Davies EG, et al. Allogeneic hematopoietic stem-cell transplantation for leukocyte adhesion deficiency. *Pediatrics.* 2009;123:836-840.
15. Bakhtiar S, Salzmann-Manrique E, Blok HJ, et al. Allogeneic hematopoietic stem cell transplantation in leukocyte adhesion deficiency type I and III. *Blood Adv.* 2021;5:262-273.
16. Gazit Y, Mory A, Etzioni A, et al. Leukocyte adhesion deficiency type II: long-term follow-up and review of the literature. *J Clin Immunol.* 2010;30:308-313.
17. Etzioni A, Frydman M, Pollack S, et al. Brief report: recurrent severe infections caused by a novel leukocyte adhesion deficiency. *N Engl J Med.* 1992;327:1789-1792.
18. Lubke T, Marquardt T, von Figura K, et al. A new type of carbohydrate-deficient glycoprotein syndrome due to a decreased import of GDP-fucose into the golgi. *J Biol Chem.* 1999;274:25986-25989.
19. Le Pendu J, Cartron JP, Lemieux RU, et al. The presence of at least two different H-blood-group-related beta-D-gal alpha-2-L-fucosyltransferases in human serum and the genetics of blood group H substances. *Am J Hum Genet.* 1985;37:749-760.
20. Karsan A, Cornejo CJ, Winn RK, et al. Leukocyte Adhesion Deficiency Type II is a generalized defect of de novo GDP-fucose biosynthesis. Endothelial cell fucosylation is not required for neutrophil rolling on human nonlymphoid endothelium. *J Clin Invest.* 1998;101:2438-2445.
21. Luhn K, Wild MK, Eckhardt M, et al. The gene defective in leukocyte adhesion deficiency II encodes a putative GDP-fucose transporter. *Nat Genet.* 2001;28:69-72.
22. von Andrian UH, Berger EM, Ramezani L, et al. In vivo behavior of neutrophils from two patients with distinct inherited leukocyte adhesion deficiency syndromes. *J Clin Invest.* 1993;91:2893-2897.
23. Etzioni A, Tonetti M. Leukocyte adhesion deficiency II-from A to almost Z. *Immunol Rev.* 2000;178:138-147.
24. Etzioni A, Tonetti M. Fucose supplementation in leukocyte adhesion deficiency type II. *Blood.* 2000;95:3641-3643.
25. Alon R, Etzioni A. LAD-III, a novel group of leukocyte integrin activation deficiencies. *Trends Immunol.* 2003;24:561-566.
26. McDowall A, Svensson L, Stanley P, et al. Two mutations in the KINDLIN3 gene of a new leukocyte adhesion deficiency III patient reveal distinct effects on leukocyte function in vitro. *Blood.* 2010;115:4834-4842.
27. Svensson L, Howarth K, McDowall A, et al. Leukocyte adhesion deficiency-III is caused by mutations in KINDLIN3 affecting integrin activation. *Nat Med.* 2009;15:306-312.
28. Kuijpers TW, van de Vijver E, Weterman MA, et al. LAD-1/variant syndrome is caused by mutations in FERMT3. *Blood.* 2009;113:4740-4746.
29. Borregaard N. Neutrophils, from marrow to microbes. *Immunity.* 2010;33:657-670.
30. Hogg N, Patzak I, Willenbrock F. The insider's guide to leukocyte integrin signalling and function. *Nat Rev Immunol.* 2011;11:416-426.
31. Minegishi Y, Saito M, Tsuchiya S, et al. Dominant-negative mutations in the DNA-binding domain of STAT3 cause hyper-IgE syndrome. *Nature.* 2007;448:1058-1062.
32. Holland SM, DeLeo FR, Elloumi HZ, et al. STAT3 mutations in the hyper-IgE syndrome. *N Engl J Med.* 2007;357:1608-1619.
33. Minegishi Y, Karasuyama H. Hyperimmunoglobulin E syndrome and tyrosine kinase 2 deficiency. *Curr Opin Allergy Clin Immunol.* 2007;7:506-509.
34. Woellner C, Gertz EM, Schäffer AA, et al. Mutations in STAT3 and diagnostic guidelines for hyper-IgE syndrome. *J Allergy Clin Immunol.* 2010;125:424-432.e8.
35. Mogensen TH. STAT3 and the Hyper-IgE syndrome: clinical presentation, genetic origin, pathogenesis, novel findings and remaining uncertainties. *JAK-STAT.* 2013;2:e23435.
36. Kumánovics A, Wittwer CT, Pryor RJ, et al. Rapid molecular analysis of the STAT3 gene in Job syndrome of hyper-IgE and recurrent infectious diseases. *J Mol Diagn.* 2010;12:213-219.
37. Zhang Q, Davis JC, Lamborn IT, et al. Combined immunodeficiency associated with DOCK8 mutations. *N Engl J Med.* 2009;361:2046-2055.
38. Hsu AP, Davis J, Puck JM, et al. STAT3 hyper IgE syndrome. In: Adam MP, Mirzaa GM, Pagon RA, et al, eds. *GeneReviews((R))*. 1993.
39. Al-Shaikhly T, Ochs HD. Hyper IgE syndromes: clinical and molecular characteristics. *Immunol Cell Biol.* 2019;97:368-379.
40. Gharehzadehshirazi A, Amini A, Rezaei N. Hyper IgE syndromes: a clinical approach. *Clin Immunol.* 2022;237:108988.
41. Davis SD, Schaller J, Wedgwood RJ. Job's Syndrome. Recurrent, "cold," staphylococcal abscesses. *Lancet.* 1966;1:1013-1015.
42. White LR, Iannetta A, Kaplan EL, et al. Leucocytes in Job's syndrome. *Lancet.* 1969;1:630.
43. Leung DY, Geha RS. Clinical and immunologic aspects of the hyperimmunoglobulin E syndrome. *Hematol Oncol Clin North Am.* 1988;2:81-100.
44. Schopfer K, Baerlocher K, Price P, et al. Staphylococcal IgE antibodies, hyperimmunoglobulinemia E and *Staphylococcus aureus* infections. *N Engl J Med.* 1979;300:835-838.
45. Sillaber C, Valent P. New insights into the pathogenesis of the hyperimmunoglobulinaemia E syndrome. *Eur J Clin Invest.* 2005;35:667-668.
46. Grimbacher B, Holland SM, Puck JM. Hyper-IgE syndromes. *Immunol Rev.* 2005;203:244-250.
47. Grimbacher B, Schäffer AA, Holland SM, et al. Genetic linkage of hyper-IgE syndrome to chromosome 4. *Am J Hum Genet.* 1999;65:735-744.
48. Chandesris MO, Melki I, Natividad A, et al. Autosomal dominant STAT3 deficiency and hyper-IgE syndrome: molecular, cellular, and clinical features from a French national survey. *Medicine (Baltimore).* 2012;91:e1-e19.
49. Hsu AP, Sowerwine KJ, Lawrence MG, et al. Intermediate phenotypes in patients with autosomal dominant hyper-IgE syndrome caused by somatic mosaicism. *J Allergy Clin Immunol.* 2013;131:1586-1593.
50. Van Scoy RE, Hill HR, Ritts RE, et al. Familial neutrophil chemotaxis defect, recurrent bacterial infections, mucocutaneous candidiasis, and hyperimmunoglobulinemia E. *Ann Intern Med.* 1975;82:766-771.
51. Mandola AB, Levy J, Nahum A, et al. Neutrophil functions in immunodeficiency due to DOCK8 deficiency. *Immunol Invest.* 2019;48:431-439.
52. Su HC, Jing H, Zhang Q. DOCK8 deficiency. *Ann N Y Acad Sci.* 2011;1246:26-33.
53. Jeppson JD, Jaffe HS, Hill HR. Use of recombinant human interferon gamma to enhance neutrophil chemotactic responses in Job syndrome of hyperimmunoglobulinemia E and recurrent infections. *J Pediatr.* 1991;118:383-387.
54. Aydin SE, Kilic SS, Aytekin C, et al. DOCK8 deficiency: clinical and immunological phenotype and treatment options - a review of 136 patients. *J Clin Immunol.* 2015;35:189-198.
55. Etzioni A, Ochs HD. Lazy leukocyte syndrome—an enigma finally solved? *J Clin Immunol.* 2020;40:9-12.
56. Coates TD, Torkildson JC, Torres M, et al. An inherited defect of neutrophil motility and microfilamentous cytoskeleton associated with abnormalities in 47-Kd and 89-Kd proteins. *Blood.* 1991;78:1338-1346.
57. Southwick FS, Howard TH, Holbrook T, et al. The relationship between CR3 deficiency and neutrophil actin assembly. *Blood.* 1989;73:1973-1979.
58. Pfajfer L, Mair NK, Jiménez-Heredia R, et al. Mutations affecting the actin regulator WD repeat–containing protein 1 lead to aberrant lymphoid immunity. *J Allergy Clin Immunol.* 2018;142:1589-1604.e11.
59. Kuhns DB, Fink DL, Choi U, et al. Cytoskeletal abnormalities and neutrophil dysfunction in WDR1 deficiency. Blood. *J Am Soc Hematol.* 2016;128:2135-2143.

60. Standing AS, Malinova D, Hong Y, et al. Autoinflammatory periodic fever, immunodeficiency, and thrombocytopenia (PFIT) caused by mutation in actin-regulatory gene WDR1. *J Exp Med.* 2017;214:59-71.
61. Janssen E, Geha RS. Primary immunodeficiencies caused by mutations in actin regulatory proteins. *Immunol Rev.* 2019;287:121-134.
62. Tangye SG, Bucciol G, Casas-Martin J, et al. Human inborn errors of the actin cytoskeleton affecting immunity: way beyond WAS and WIP. *Immunol Cell Biol.* 2019;97:389-402.
63. Kuhns DB, Fink DL, Choi U, et al. Cytoskeletal abnormalities and neutrophil dysfunction in WDR1 deficiency. *Blood.* 2016;128:2135-2143.
64. Miller ME, Oski FA, Harris MB. Lazy-leucocyte syndrome. A new disorder of neutrophil function. *Lancet.* 1971;1:665-669.
65. Goldman JM, Foroozanfar N, Gazzard BG, et al. Lazy leukocyte syndrome. *J R Soc Med.* 1984;77:140-141.
66. Pinkerton PH, Robinson JB, Senn JS. Lazy leucocyte syndrome—disorder of the granulocyte membrane? *J Clin Pathol.* 1978;31:300-308.
67. Southwick FS. The lazy leukocyte syndrome revisited. *Blood.* 2016;128:2112-2113.
68. Howard T, Li Y, Torres M, et al. The 47-kD protein increased in neutrophil actin dysfunction with 47- and 89-kD protein abnormalities is lymphocyte-specific protein. *Blood.* 1994;83:231-241.
69. Howard TH, Hartwig J, Cunningham C. Lymphocyte-specific protein 1 expression in eukaryotic cells reproduces the morphologic and motile abnormality of NAD 47/89 neutrophils. *Blood.* 1998;91:4786-4795.
70. Li Y, Guerrero A, Howard TH. The actin-binding protein, lymphocyte-specific protein 1, is expressed in human leukocytes and human myeloid and lymphoid cell lines. *J Immunol.* 1995;155:3563-3569.
71. Ambruso DR, Knall C, Abell AN, et al. Human neutrophil immunodeficiency syndrome is associated with an inhibitory Rac2 mutation. *Proc Natl Acad Sci U S A.* 2000;97:4654-4659.
72. Williams DA, Tao W, Yang F, et al. Dominant negative mutation of the hematopoietic-specific Rho GTPase, Rac2, is associated with a human phagocyte immunodeficiency. *Blood.* 2000;96:1646-1654.
73. Kim C, Dinauer MC. Rac2 is an essential regulator of neutrophil nicotinamide adenine dinucleotide phosphate oxidase activation in response to specific signaling pathways. *J Immunol.* 2001;166:1223-1232.
74. Ming W, Li S, Billadeau DD, et al. The Rac effector p67phox regulates phagocyte NADPH oxidase by stimulating Vav1 guanine nucleotide exchange activity. *Mol Cell Biol.* 2007;27:312-323.
75. Roberts AW, Kim C, Zhen L, et al. Deficiency of the hematopoietic cell-specific Rho family GTPase Rac2 is characterized by abnormalities in neutrophil function and host defense. *Immunity.* 1999;10:183-196.
76. Genco RJ, Van Dyke TE, Levine MJ, et al. 1985 Kreshover lecture. Molecular factors influencing neutrophil defects in periodontal disease. *J Dent Res.* 1986;65:1379-1391.
77. Van Dyke TE, Levine MJ, Genco RJ. Neutrophil function and oral disease. *J Oral Pathol.* 1985;14:95-120.
78. Van Dyke TE, Levine MJ, Tabak LA, et al. Reduced chemotactic peptide binding in juvenile periodontitis: a model for neutrophil function. *Biochem Biophys Res Commun.* 1981;100:1278-1284.
79. Kantarci A, Oyaizu K, Van Dyke TE. Neutrophil-mediated tissue injury in periodontal disease pathogenesis: findings from localized aggressive periodontitis. *J Periodontol.* 2003;74:66-75.
80. Glocker E-O, Hennigs A, Nabavi M, et al. A homozygous CARD9 mutation in a family with susceptibility to fungal infections. *N Engl J Med.* 2009;361:1727-1735.
81. Drewniak A, Gazendam RP, Tool AT, et al. Invasive fungal infection and impaired neutrophil killing in human CARD9 deficiency. *Blood.* 2013;121:2385-2392.
82. Lanternier F, Pathan S, Vincent QB, et al. Deep dermatophytosis and inherited CARD9 deficiency. *N Engl J Med.* 2013;369:1704-1714.
83. Drummond RA, Franco LM, Lionakis MS. Human CARD9: a critical molecule of fungal immune surveillance. *Front Immunol.* 2018;9:1836.
84. de Diego RP, Sánchez-Ramón S, López-Collazo E, et al. Genetic errors of the human caspase recruitment domain–B-cell lymphoma 10–mucosa-associated lymphoid tissue lymphoma-translocation gene 1 (CBM) complex: molecular, immunologic, and clinical heterogeneity. *J Allergy Clin Immunol.* 2015;136:1139-1149.
85. Drummond RA, Lionakis MS. Mechanistic insights into the role of C-type lectin receptor/CARD9 signaling in human antifungal immunity. *Front Cell Infect Microbiol.* 2016;6:39.
86. Nishibori M, Cham B, McNicol A, et al. The protein CD63 is in platelet dense granules, is deficient in a patient with Hermansky-Pudlak syndrome, and appears identical to granulophysin. *J Clin Invest.* 1993;91:1775-1782.
87. Schim van der Loeff I, Sprenkeler EGG, Tool ATJ, et al. Defective neutrophil development and specific granule deficiency caused by a homozygous splice-site mutation in SMARCD2. *J Allergy Clin Immunol.* 2021;147:2381-2385.e2.
88. Yucel E, Karakus IS, Krolo A, et al. Novel frameshift autosomal recessive loss-of-function mutation in SMARCD2 encoding a chromatin remodeling factor mediates granulopoiesis. *J Clin Immunol.* 2021;41:59-65.
89. Boxer LA, Smolen JE. Neutrophil granule constituents and their release in health and disease. *Hematol Oncol Clin North Am.* 1988;2:101-134.
90. Gallin JI. Neutrophil specific granule deficiency. *Annu Rev Med.* 1985;36:263-274.
91. Lomax KJ, Gallin JI, Rotrosen D, et al. Selective defect in myeloid cell lactoferrin gene expression in neutrophil specific granule deficiency. *J Clin Invest.* 1989;83:514-519.
92. Parmley RT, Gilbert CS, Boxer LA. Abnormal peroxidase-positive granules in "specific granule" deficiency. *Blood.* 1989;73:838-844.
93. Gombart AF, Koeffler HP. Neutrophil specific granule deficiency and mutations in the gene encoding transcription factor C/EBP(epsilon). *Curr Opin Hematol.* 2002;9:36-42.
94. Lekstrom-Himes JA, Dorman SE, Kopar P, et al. Neutrophil-specific granule deficiency results from a novel mutation with loss of function of the transcription factor CCAAT/enhancer binding protein epsilon. *J Exp Med.* 1999;189:1847-1852.
95. Gombart AF, Shiohara M, Kwok SH, et al. Neutrophil-specific granule deficiency: homozygous recessive inheritance of a frameshift mutation in the gene encoding transcription factor CCAAT/enhancer binding protein—epsilon. *Blood.* 2001;97:2561-2567.
96. Yamanaka R, Barlow C, Lekstrom-Himes J, et al. Impaired granulopoiesis, myelodysplasia, and early lethality in CCAAT/enhancer binding protein epsilon-deficient mice. *Proc Natl Acad Sci U S A.* 1997;94:13187-13192.
97. Gombart AF, Krug U, O'Kelly J, et al. Aberrant expression of neutrophil and macrophage-related genes in a murine model for human neutrophil-specific granule deficiency. *J Leukoc Biol.* 2005;78:1153-1165.
98. Shiohara M, Gombart AF, Sekiguchi Y, et al. Phenotypic and functional alterations of peripheral blood monocytes in neutrophil-specific granule deficiency. *J Leukoc Biol.* 2004;75:190-197.
99. Chumakov AM, Grillier I, Chumakova E, et al. Cloning of the novel human myeloid-cell-specific C/EBP-epsilon transcription factor. *Mol Cell Biol.* 1997;17:1375-1386.
100. Wynn RF, Sood M, Theilgaard-Mönch K, et al. Intractable diarrhoea of infancy caused by neutrophil specific granule deficiency and cured by stem cell transplantation. *Gut.* 2006;55:292-293.
101. Sharma P, Nicoli ER, Serra-Vinardell J, et al. Chediak-Higashi syndrome: a review of the past, present, and future. *Drug Discov Today Dis Model.* 2020;31:31-36.
102. Bell TG, Meyers KM, Prieur DJ, et al. Decreased nucleotide and serotonin storage associated with defective function in Chediak-Higashi syndrome cattle and human platelets. *Blood.* 1976;48:175-184.
103. Toro C, Nicoli ER, Malicdan MC, Adams DR, Introne WJ. Chediak-Higashi syndrome. In: Adam MP, Everman DB, Mirzaa GM, et al., eds. *GeneReviews®* [Internet]. University of Washington, Seattle; 1993-2022. PMID: 20301751.
104. Barbosa MD, Nguyen QA, Tchernev VT, et al. Identification of the homologous beige and Chediak-Higashi syndrome genes. *Nature.* 1996;382:262-265.
105. Nagle DL, Karim MA, Woolf EA, et al. Identification and mutation analysis of the complete gene for Chediak-Higashi syndrome. *Nat Genet.* 1996;14:307-311.
106. Introne W, Boissy RE, Gahl WA. Clinical, molecular, and cell biological aspects of Chediak-Higashi syndrome. *Mol Genet Metabol.* 1999;68:283-303.
107. Introne WJ, Westbroek W, Groden CA, et al. Neurologic involvement in patients with atypical Chediak-Higashi disease. *Neurology.* 2017;88:e57-e65.
108. Karim MA, Suzuki K, Fukai K, et al. Apparent genotype–phenotype correlation in childhood, adolescent, and adult Chediak-Higashi syndrome. *Am J Med Genet.* 2002;108:16-22.
109. Kaplan J, De Domenico I, Ward DM. Chediak-Higashi syndrome. *Curr Opin Hematol.* 2008;15:22-29.
110. Clark RA, Kimball HR. Defective granulocyte chemotaxis in the Chediak-Higashi syndrome. *J Clin Invest.* 1971;50:2645-2652.
111. Sepulveda FE, Burgess A, Heiligenstein X, et al. LYST controls the biogenesis of the endosomal compartment required for secretory lysosome function. *Traffic.* 2015;16:191-203.
112. Barak Y, Nir E. Chediak-Higashi syndrome. *Am J Pediatr Hematol Oncol.* 1987;9:42-55.
113. Davis WC, Douglas SD. Defective granule formation and function in the Chediak-Higashi syndrome in man and animals. *Semin Hematol.* 1972;9:431-450.
114. White JG. The Chediak-Higashi syndrome: cytoplasmic sequestration in circulating leukocytes. *Blood.* 1967;29:435-451.
115. Chediak MM. New leukocyte anomaly of constitutional and familial character. *Rev Hematol.* 1952;7:362-367.
116. Sato A. Chédiak and Higashi's disease: probable identity of a new leucocytal anomaly (Chédiak) and congenital gigantism of peroxidase granules (Higashi). *Tohoku J Exp Med.* 1955;61:201-210.
117. Efrati P, Danon D. Electron-microscopical study of bone marrow cells in a case of Chediak-Higashi-Steinbrinck syndrome. *Br J Haematol.* 1968;15:173-176.
118. Kjeldsen L, Calafat J, Borregaard N. Giant granules of neutrophils in Chediak-Higashi syndrome are derived from azurophil granules but not from specific and gelatinase granules. *J Leukoc Biol.* 1998;64:72-77.
119. Rausch PG, Pryzwansky KB, Spitznagel JK. Immunocytochemical identification of azurophilic and specific granule markers in the giant granules of Chediak-Higashi neutrophils. *N Engl J Med.* 1978;298:693-698.
120. White JG, Krumwiede M. Normal-sized primary lysosomes are present in Chediak-Higashi syndrome neutrophils. *Pediatr Res.* 1987;22:208-215.
121. Baetz K, Isaaz S, Griffiths GM. Loss of cytotoxic T lymphocyte function in Chediak-Higashi syndrome arises from a secretory defect that prevents lytic granule exocytosis. *J Immunol.* 1995;154:6122-6131.
122. Windhorst DB, Zelickson AS, Good RA. Chediak-Higashi syndrome: hereditary gigantism of cytoplasmic organelles. *Science.* 1966;151:81-83.
123. Blume RS, Wolff SM. The Chediak-Higashi syndrome: studies in four patients and a review of the literature. *Medicine (Baltimore).* 1972;51:247-280.
124. Burkhardt JK, Wiebel FA, Hester S, et al. The giant organelles in beige and Chediak-Higashi fibroblasts are derived from late endosomes and mature lysosomes. *J Exp Med.* 1993;178:1845-1856.
125. Kimball HR, Ford GH, Wolff SM. Lysosomal enzymes in normal and Chediak-Higashi blood leukocytes. *J Lab Clin Med.* 1975;86:616-630.
126. Root RK, Rosenthal AS, Balestra DJ. Abnormal bactericidal, metabolic, and lysosomal functions of Chediak-Higashi Syndrome leukocytes. *J Clin Invest.* 1972;51:649-665.
127. Stossel TP, Root RK, Vaughan M. Phagocytosis in chronic granulomatous disease and the Chediak–Higashi syndrome. *N Engl J Med.* 1972;286:120-123.
128. Brandt EJ, Elliott RW, Swank RT. Defective lysosomal enzyme secretion in kidneys of Chediak-Higashi (beige) mice. *J Cell Biol.* 1975;67:774-788.

129. Ganz T, Metcalf JA, Gallin JI, et al. Microbicidal/cytotoxic proteins of neutrophils are deficient in two disorders: Chediak-Higashi syndrome and "specific" granule deficiency. *J Clin Invest.* 1988;82:552-556.
130. Cairo MS, Vandeven C, Toy C, et al. Fluorescent cytometric analysis of polymorphonuclear leukocytes in Chediak-Higashi syndrome: diminished C3bi receptor expression (OKM1) with normal granular cell density. *Pediatr Res.* 1988;24:673-676.
131. Huynh C, Roth D, Ward DM, et al. Defective lysosomal exocytosis and plasma membrane repair in Chediak-Higashi/beige cells. *Proc Natl Acad Sci U S A.* 2004;101:16795-16800.
132. Douglas SD, Blume RS, Wolff SM. Fine structural studies of leukocytes from patients and heterozygotes with the Chediak-Higashi syndrome. *Blood.* 1969;33:527-540.
133. Moran TJ, Estevez JM. Chediak-Higashi disease. Morphologic studies of a patient and her family. *Arch Pathol.* 1969;88:329-339.
134. Wolff SM. The Chediak-Higashi syndrome: studies of host defenses. *Ann Intern Med.* 1972;76:293-306.
135. Blume RS, Bennett JM, Yankee RA, et al. Defective granulocyte regulation in the Chediak-Higashi syndrome. *N Engl J Med.* 1968;279:1009-1015.
136. Rubin CM, Burke BA, McKenna RW, et al. The accelerated phase of Chediak-Higashi syndrome. An expression of the virus-associated hemophagocytic syndrome? *Cancer.* 1985;56:524-530.
137. Ward DM, Shiflett SL, Kaplan J. Chediak-Higashi syndrome: a clinical and molecular view of a rare lysosomal storage disorder. *Curr Mol Med.* 2002;2:469-477.
138. Tardieu M, Lacroix C, Neven B, et al. Progressive neurologic dysfunctions 20 years after allogeneic bone marrow transplantation for Chediak-Higashi syndrome. *Blood.* 2005;106:40-42.
139. Eapen M, DeLaat CA, Baker KS, et al. Hematopoietic cell transplantation for Chediak-Higashi syndrome. *Bone Marrow Transplant.* 2007;39:411-415.
140. Yu HH, Yang YH, Chiang BL. Chronic granulomatous disease: a comprehensive review. *Clin Rev Allergy Immunol.* 2021;61:101-113.
141. Rider NL, Jameson MB, Creech CB. Chronic granulomatous disease: epidemiology, pathophysiology, and genetic basis of disease. *J Pediatric Infect Dis Soc.* 2018;7:S2-S5.
142. Dinauer MC. Primary immune deficiencies with defects in neutrophil function. *Hematology Am Soc Hematol Educ Program.* 2016;2016:43-50.
143. Dinauer MC. Disorders of neutrophil function: an overview. *Methods Mol Biol.* 2014;1124:501-515.
144. Wolach B, Gavrieli R, de Boer M, et al. Chronic granulomatous disease: clinical, functional, molecular, and genetic studies. The Israeli experience with 84 patients. *Am J Hematol.* 2017;92:28-36.
145. Baehner RL, Nathan DG, Karnovsky ML. Correction of metabolic deficiencies in the leukocytes of patients with chronic granulomatous disease. *J Clin Invest.* 1970;49:865-870.
146. Johnston RB, Jr, Baehner RL. Improvement of leukocyte bactericidal activity in chronic granulomatous disease. *Blood.* 1970;35:350-355.
147. Klebanoff SJ, White LR. Iodination defect in the leukocytes of a patient with chronic granulomatous disease of childhood. *N Engl J Med.* 1969;280:460-466.
148. Curnutte JT, Whitten DM, Babior BM. Defective superoxide production by granulocytes from patients with chronic granulomatous disease. *N Engl J Med.* 1974;290:593-597.
149. Fridovich I. Editorial: superoxide radical and the bactericidal action of phagocytes. *N Engl J Med.* 1974;290:624-625.
150. Berendes H, Bridges RA, Good RA. A fatal granulomatosus of childhood: the clinical study of a new syndrome. *Minn Med.* 1957;40:309-312.
151. Windhorst DB, Page AR, Holmes B, et al. The pattern of genetic transmission of the leukocyte defect in fatal granulomatous disease of childhood. *J Clin Invest.* 1968;47:1026-1034.
152. Dupree E, Smith CW, MacDougall NL, et al. Undetected carrier state in chronic granulomatous disease. *J Pediatr.* 1972;81:770-774.
153. Bustamante J, Arias AA, Vogt G, et al. Germline CYBB mutations that selectively affect macrophages in kindreds with X-linked predisposition to tuberculous mycobacterial disease. *Nat Immunol.* 2011;12:213-221.
154. Bleesing JJ, Souto-Carneiro MM, Savage WJ, et al. Patients with chronic granulomatous disease have a reduced peripheral blood memory B cell compartment. *J Immunol.* 2006;176:7096-7103.
155. Marciano BE, Spalding C, Fitzgerald A, et al. Common severe infections in chronic granulomatous disease. *Clin Infect Dis.* 2015;60:1176-1183.
156. Vowells SJ, Sekhsaria S, Malech HL, et al. Flow cytometric analysis of the granulocyte respiratory burst: a comparison study of fluorescent probes. *J Immunol Methods.* 1995;178:89-97.
157. Kuhns DB, Alvord WG, Heller T, et al. Residual NADPH oxidase and survival in chronic granulomatous disease. *N Engl J Med.* 2010;363:2600-2610.
158. Martire B, Rondelli R, Soresina A, et al. Clinical features, long-term follow-up and outcome of a large cohort of patients with chronic granulomatous disease: an Italian multicenter study. *Clin Immunol.* 2008;126:155-164.
159. Arnold DE, Heimall JR. A review of chronic granulomatous disease. *Adv Ther.* 2017;34:2543-2557.
160. Bielorai B, Toren A, Wolach B, et al. Successful treatment of invasive aspergillosis in chronic granulomatous disease by granulocyte transfusions followed by peripheral blood stem cell transplantation. *Bone Marrow Transplant.* 2000;26:1025-1028.
161. Slack MA, Thomsen IP. Prevention of infectious complications in patients with chronic granulomatous disease. *J Pediatric Infect Dis Soc.* 2018;7:S25-S30.
162. Gallin JI, Farber JM, Holland SM, et al. Interferon-gamma in the management of infectious diseases. *Ann Intern Med.* 1995;123:216-224.
163. A controlled trial of interferon gamma to prevent infection in chronic granulomatous disease. *N Engl J Med.* 1991;324:509-516.
164. Rex JH, Bennett JE, Gallin JI, et al. In vivo interferon-gamma therapy augments the in vitro ability of chronic granulomatous disease neutrophils to damage Aspergillus hyphae. *J Infect Dis.* 1991;163:849-852.
165. Åhlin A, Fasth A. Chronic granulomatous disease–conventional treatment vs. hematopoietic stem cell transplantation: an update. *Curr Opin Hematol.* 2015;22:41-45.
166. Ott MG, Schmidt M, Schwarzwaelder K, et al. Correction of X-linked chronic granulomatous disease by gene therapy, augmented by insertional activation of MDS1-EVI1, PRDM16 or SETBP1. *Nat Med.* 2006;12:401-409.
167. Kohn DB, Booth C, Kang EM, et al. Lentiviral gene therapy for X-linked chronic granulomatous disease. *Nat Med.* 2020;26:200-206.
168. Weening RS, Roos D, Weemaes CM, et al. Defective initiation of the metabolic stimulation in phagocytizing granulocytes: a new congenital defect. *J Lab Clin Med.* 1976;88:757-768.
169. Harvath L, Andersen BR. Defective initiation of oxidative metabolism in polymorphonuclear leukocytes. *N Engl J Med.* 1979;300:1130-1135.
170. Lew PD, Southwick FS, Stossel TP, et al. A variant of chronic granulomatous disease: deficient oxidative metabolism due to a low-affinity NADPH oxidase. *N Engl J Med.* 1981;305:1329-1333.
171. Ford DK, Price GE, Culling CF, et al. Familial lipochrome pigmentation of histiocytes with hyperglobulinemia, pulmonary infiltration, splenomegaly, arthritis and susceptibility to infection. *Am J Med.* 1962;33:478-489.
172. Rodey GE, Park BH, Ford DK, et al. Defective bactericidal activity of peripheral blood leukocytes in lipochrome histiocytosis. *Am J Med.* 1970;49:322-327.
173. Cooper MR, DeChatelet LR, McCall CE, et al. Complete deficiency of leukocyte glucose-6-phosphate dehydrogenase with defective bactericidal activity. *J Clin Invest.* 1972;51:769-778.
174. Cooper MR, Dechatelet L, Mccall C, et al. Leucocyte g.-6-pD deficiency. *Lancet.* 1970;296:110.
175. Holmes B, Park BH, Malawista SE, et al. Chronic granulomatous disease in females. *N Engl J Med.* 1970;283:217-221.
176. Newburger PE, Malawista SE, Dinauer MC, et al. Chronic granulomatous disease and glutathione peroxidase deficiency, revisited. *Blood.* 1994;84(11):3861-3869.
177. Njålsson R. Glutathione synthetase deficiency. *Cell Mol Life Sci.* 2005;62:1938-1945.
178. Boxer LA, Oliver JM, Spielberg SP, et al. Protection of granulocytes by vitamin E in glutathione synthetase deficiency. *N Engl J Med.* 1979;301:901-905.
179. Spielberg SP, Boxer LA, Oliver JM, et al. Oxidative damage to neutrophils in glutathione synthetase deficiency. *Br J Haematol.* 1979;42:215-223.
180. Roos D, Weening RS, Voetman AA, et al. Protection of phagocytic leukocytes by endogenous glutathione: studies in a family with glutathione reductase deficiency. *Blood.* 1979;53:851-866.
181. Roos D, Weening RS, Wyss SR, et al. Protection of human neutrophils by endogenous catalase: studies with cells from catalase-deficient individuals. *J Clin Invest.* 1980;65:1515-1522.
182. Singh A, Zarember KA, Kuhns DB, et al. Impaired priming and activation of the neutrophil NADPH oxidase in patients with IRAK4 or NEMO deficiency. *J Immunol.* 2009;182:6410-6417.
183. Honda F, Kano H, Kanegane H, et al. The kinase Btk negatively regulates the production of reactive oxygen species and stimulation-induced apoptosis in human neutrophils. *Nat Immunol.* 2012;13:369-378.
184. Ghez D, Calleja A, Protin C, et al. Early-onset invasive aspergillosis and other fungal infections in patients treated with ibrutinib. *Blood.* 2018;131:1955-1959.
185. Blez D, Blaize M, Soussain C, et al. Ibrutinib induces multiple functional defects in the neutrophil response against Aspergillus fumigatus. *Haematologica.* 2020;105:478-489.
186. Ren R, Fedoriw Y, Willis M. The molecular pathophysiology, differential diagnosis, and treatment of MPO deficiency. *J Clinic Experiment Pathol.* 2012;2:109. doi:10.4172/2161-0681.1000109.
187. Lehrer RI, Cline MJ. Leukocyte myeloperoxidase deficiency and disseminated candidiasis: the role of myeloperoxidase in resistance to Candida infection. *J Clin Invest.* 1969;48:1478-1488.
188. Klebanoff SJ, Kettle AJ, Rosen H, et al. Myeloperoxidase: a front-line defender against phagocytosed microorganisms. *J Leukoc Biol.* 2013;93:185-198.
189. Parry MF, Root RK, Metcalf JA, et al. Myeloperoxidase deficiency: prevalence and clinical significance. *Ann Intern Med.* 1981;95:293-301.
190. Nauseef WM. Myeloperoxidase deficiency. *Hematol/Oncol Clin.* 1988;2:135-158.
191. Suzuki K, Muso E, Nauseef WM. Contribution of peroxidases in host-defense, diseases and cellular functions. *Jpn J Infect Dis.* 2004;57:S1-S2.
192. Hansson M, Olsson I, Nauseef WM. Biosynthesis, processing, and sorting of human myeloperoxidase. *Arch Biochem Biophys.* 2006;445:214-224.
193. Nauseef WM. Lessons from MPO deficiency about functionally important structural features. *Jpn J Infect Dis.* 2004;57:S4-S5.
194. Tobler A, Selsted ME, Miller CW, et al. Evidence for a pretranslational defect in hereditary and acquired myeloperoxidase deficiency. *Blood.* 1989;73(7):1980-1986.
195. Milligan KL, Mann D, Rump A, et al. Complete myeloperoxidase deficiency: beware the "false-positive" dihydrorhodamine oxidation. *J Pediatr.* 2016;176:204-206.
196. Biswas L, Götz F. Molecular mechanisms of Staphylococcus and Pseudomonas interactions in cystic fibrosis. *Front Cell Infect Microbiol.* 2021;11:824042.
197. Giannetti L, Apponi R, Dello Diago AM, et al. Papillon-Lefèvre syndrome: oral aspects and treatment. *Dermatol Ther.* 2020;33:e13336.
198. Sørensen OE, Clemmensen SN, Dahl SL, et al. Papillon-Lefevre syndrome patient reveals species-dependent requirements for neutrophil defenses. *J Clin Invest.* 2014;124:4539-4548.
199. Nauseef WM. Proteases, neutrophils, and periodontitis: the NET effect. *J Clin Investig.* 2014;124:4237-4239.

200. Noack B, Görgens H, Schacher B, et al. Functional Cathepsin C mutations cause different Papillon–Lefévre syndrome phenotypes. *J Clin Periodontol.* 2008;35:311-316.
201. O'Flaherty J, Kreutzer D, Showell H, et al. Selective neutrophil desensitization to chemotactic factors. *J Cell Biol.* 1979;80:564-572.
202. Craddock PR, Fehr J, Dalmasso A, et al. Hemodialysis leukopenia. Pulmonary vascular leukostasis resulting from complement activation by dialyzer cellophane membranes. *J Clin Invest.* 1977;59:879-888.
203. Craddock P, Hammerschmidt D, White J, et al. Complement (C5-a)-induced granulocyte aggregation in vitro. A possible mechanism of complement-mediated leukostasis and leukopenia. *J Clin Invest.* 1977;60:260-264.
204. Skubitz KM, Craddock PR. Reversal of hemodialysis granulocytopenia and pulmonary leukostasis: a clinical manifestation of selective down-regulation of granulocyte responses to C5a desArg. *J Clin Investig.* 1981;67:1383-1391.
205. Cassidy L, Lyles D, Abramson J. Depression of polymorphonuclear leukocyte functions by purified influenza virus hemagglutinin and sialic acid-binding lectins. *J Immunol.* 1989;142:4401-4406.
206. Bandres J, Trial J, Musher D, et al. Increased phagocytosis and generation of reactive oxygen products by neutrophils and monocytes of men with stage 1 human immunodeficiency virus infection. *JID (J Infect Dis).* 1993;168:75-83.
207. Elbim C, Prevot M, Bouscarat F, et al. Polymorphonuclear neutrophils from human immunodeficiency virus-infected patients show enhanced activation, diminished fMLP-induced L-selectin shedding, and an impaired oxidative burst after cytokine priming. *Blood.* 1994;84(8):2759-2766.
208. Craddock P, Yawata Y, VanSanten L, et al. Acquired phagocyte dysfunction: a complication of the hypophosphatemia of parenteral hyperalimentation. *N Engl J Med.* 1974;290:1403-1407.
209. Kiersztejn M, Chervu I, Smogorzewski M, et al. On the mechanisms of impaired phagocytosis in phosphate depletion. *J Am Soc Nephrol.* 1992;2:1484-1489.
210. Alexiewicz JM, Kumar D, Smogorzewski M, et al. Polymorphonuclear leukocytes in non-insulin-dependent diabetes mellitus: abnormalities in metabolism and function. *Ann Intern Med.* 1995;123:919-924.
211. Andersen B, Goldsmith GH, Spagnuolo PJ. Neutrophil adhesive dysfunction in diabetes mellitus: the role of cellular and plasma factors. *J Lab Clin Med.* 1988;111:267-274.
212. Repine JE, Clawson C, Goetz FC. Bactericidal function of neutrophils from patients with acute bacterial infections and from diabetics. *JID (J Infect Dis).* 1980;142:869-875.
213. Simms HH, D'amico R. Polymorphonuclear leukocyte dysregulation during the systemic inflammatory response syndrome. *Blood.* 1994;83(5):1398-1407.
214. Thierry Alain R, Roch B. SARS-CoV2 may evade innate immune response, causing uncontrolled neutrophil extracellular traps formation and multi-organ failure. *Clin Sci.* 2020;134:1295-1300.
215. McMichael T, Currie D, Clark S, et al. Epidemiology of Covid-19 in a long-term care facility in King County, Washington: *N Engl J Med.* 2020;382(21):2005-2011.
216. Taylor Erin B. Casting a wide NET: an update on uncontrolled NETosis in response to COVID-19 infection. *Clin Sci.* 2022;136:1047-1052.
217. Loyer C, Lapostolle A, Urbina T, et al. Impairment of neutrophil functions and homeostasis in COVID-19 patients: association with disease severity. *Crit Care.* 2022;26:155.
218. Zhu Y, Chen X, Liu X. NETosis and neutrophil extracellular traps in COVID-19: immunothrombosis and beyond. *Front Immunol.* 2022;13:838011.
219. Ottonello L, Dapino P, Pastorino G, et al. Neutrophil dysfunction and increased susceptibility to infection. *Eur J Clin Invest.* 1995;25:687-692.
220. Klein A, Hussar AE, Bornstein S. Pelger–huët anomaly of the leukocytes. *N Engl J Med.* 1955;253:1057-1062.
221. Colella R, Hollensead SC. Understanding and recognizing the Pelger-Huët anomaly. *Am J Clin Pathol.* 2012;137:358-366.
222. Speeckaert MM, Verhelst C, Koch A, et al. Pelger-Huët anomaly: a critical review of the literature. *Acta Haematol.* 2009;121:202-206.
223. Best S, Salvati F, Kallo J, et al. Lamin B receptor (LBR) mutations in Pelger-Huet anomaly. *Blood.* 2002;100:924.
224. Cohen TV, Klarmann KD, Sakchaisri K, et al. The lamin B receptor under transcriptional control of C/EBPε is required for morphological but not functional maturation of neutrophils. *Hum Mol Genet.* 2008;17:2921-2933.
225. Hoffmann K, Dreger CK, Olins AL, et al. Mutations in the gene encoding the lamin B receptor produce an altered nuclear morphology in granulocytes (Pelger-Huët anomaly). *Nat Genet.* 2002;31:410-414.
226. Skendzel LP, Hoffman GC. The Pelger anomaly of leukocytes: forty-one cases in seven families. *Am J Clin Pathol.* 1962;37:294-301.
227. Rosse WF, Gurney CW. The Pelger-Huët anomaly in three families and its use in determining the disappearance of transfused neutrophils from the peripheral blood. *Blood.* 1959;14:170-186.
228. Shanbrom E, Tanaka KR. Acquired Pelger-Huet granulocytes in severe myxedema. *Acta Haematol.* 1962;27:289-293.
229. Kaplan JM, Barrett O, Jr. Reversible pseudo-Pelger anomaly related to sulfisoxazole therapy. *N Engl J Med.* 1967;277:421-422.
230. Dusse LM, Moreira AM, Vieira LM, et al. Acquired Pelger-Huët: what does it really mean? *Clin Chim Acta.* 2010;411:1587-1590.
231. Robier C, Knaus G, Egger M. Acquired Pelger-Huet anomaly in two patients with chronic lymphocytic leukemia treated with venetoclax. *Clin Chem Lab Med.* 2021;59:e395-e397.
232. Kaur J, Catovsky D, Valdimarsson H, et al. Familial acute myeloid leukaemia with acquired Pelger-Huet anomaly and aneuploidy of C group. *Br Med J.* 1972;4:327-331.
233. Dorr AD, Moloney WC. Acquired pseudo-Pelger anomaly of granulocytic leukocytes. *N Engl J Med.* 1959;261:742-746.
234. Shanbrom E, Collins Z, Miller S. "Acquired" Pelger-Huet cells in blood dyscrasias. *Am J Med Sci.* 1960;240:732-738.
235. Jordans GH. Hereditary granulation anomaly of the leucocytes (Alder). *Acta Med Scand.* 1947;129:348-351.
236. Groover RV, Burke EC, Gordon H, et al. The genetic mucopolysaccharidoses. *Semin Hematol.* 1972;9:371-402.
237. Leal AF, Nieto WG, Candelo E, et al. Hematological findings in lysosomal storage disorders: a perspective from the medical laboratory. *Ejifcc.* 2022;33:28-42.
238. Jain R, Khurana U, Bhan BD, et al. Mucopolysaccharidosis: a case report highlighting hematological aspects of the disease. *J Lab Physicians.* 2019;11:97-99.
239. Mittwoch U. Abnormal lymphocytes in gargoylism. *Br J Haematol.* 1959;5:365-368.
240. Matsaniotis N, Kattamis C, Lehmann H, et al. Urinary excretion of acid mucopolysaccharide in sibs with Morquio's syndrome and Reilly's granules in leucocytes. *Arch Dis Child.* 1967;42:652-653.
241. Buchanan JG, Pearce L, Wetherley-Mein G. The may-hegglin anomaly; a family report and chromosome study. *Br J Haematol.* 1964;10:508-512.
242. Untanu RV, Vajpayee N. *May Hegglin anomaly, StatPearls.* StatPearls Publishing; 2022. Copyright © 2022, StatPearls Publishing LLC.
243. Lusher JM, Schneider J, Mizukami I, et al. The May-Hegglin anomaly: platelet function, ultrastructure and chromosome studies. *Blood.* 1968;32:950-961.
244. Seri M, Pecci A, Di Bari F, et al. MYH9-related disease: may-Hegglin anomaly, Sebastian syndrome, Fechtner syndrome, and Epstein syndrome are not distinct entities but represent a variable expression of a single illness. *Medicine (Baltimore).* 2003;82:203-215.
245. Dong F, Li S, Pujol-Moix N, et al. Genotype-phenotype correlation in MYH9-related thrombocytopenia. *Br J Haematol.* 2005;130:620-627.
246. Jordans GH. The familial occurrence of fat containing vacuoles in the leukocytes diagnosed in two brothers suffering from dystrophia musculorum progressiva (ERB). *Acta Med Scand.* 1953;145:419-423.
247. Fischer J, Lefèvre C, Morava E, et al. The gene encoding adipose triglyceride lipase (PNPLA2) is mutated in neutral lipid storage disease with myopathy. *Nat Genet.* 2007;39:28-30.
248. Lefèvre C, Jobard F, Caux F, et al. Mutations in CGI-58, the gene encoding a new protein of the esterase/lipase/thioesterase subfamily, in Chanarin-Dorfman syndrome. *Am J Hum Genet.* 2001;69:1002-1012.
249. Smith H. Unidentified inclusions in haemopoietic cells, congenital atresia of the bile ducts and livedo reticularis in an infant: a new syndrome. *Br J Haematol.* 1967;13:695-705.
250. White JG, Witkop CJ, Jr, Gerritsen SM. The Hermansky-Pudlak syndrome: inclusions in circulating leucocytes. *Br J Haematol.* 1973;24:761-765.
251. Davidson WM, Milner RDG, Lawler SD, et al. Giant neutrophil leucocytes: an inherited anomaly. *Br J Haematol.* 1960;6:339-343.
252. Undritz E. A new family with hereditary-constitutional hypersegmentation of neutrophil nuclei. *Schweiz Med Wochenschr.* 1958;88:1000-1001.
253. Lueers T. The numerical count of sex-specific nuclear drumsticks in hereditary-constitutional hypersegmentation of neutrophil nucleus of Undriz. *Schweiz Med Wochenschr.* 1960;90:246-248.
254. Joshua H, Spitzer A, Presentey B. The incidence of peroxidase and phospholipid deficiency in eosinophilic granulocytes among various Jewish groups in Israel. *Am J Hum Genet.* 1970;22:574-578.
255. Presentey BZ. A new anomaly of eosinophilic granulocytes. *Tech Bull Registry Med Tech.* 1968;38:131-134.

Chapter 60 ■ Lysosomal Abnormalities of the Monocyte-Macrophage System: Gaucher and Niemann-Pick Diseases

MARGARET M. MCGOVERN • ROBERT J. DESNICK

INTRODUCTION

Abnormalities of the monocyte-macrophage system include certain inherited lysosomal storage diseases that result from specific defects that impair lysosomal function. Most of these disorders are caused by the deficiency of a particular hydrolytic enzyme, but others are due to impaired receptors, transporters, or deficiencies of crucial cofactors or protective proteins. Prevalent among these disorders are the sphingolipidoses, which are a unique family of diverse diseases related by their molecular pathology. Here, the clinical, biochemical, and genetic features of two of these disorders are presented: Niemann-Pick types A and B disease, caused by defects in the acid sphingomyelinase (*SMPD1*) gene, and Gaucher disease, caused by defects in the acid α-glucosidase (*GBA*) gene. In each of these autosomal recessive disorders, mutations in the gene that encodes the lysosomal enzyme result in a defective enzyme that is unable to perform its normal function as a hydrolase. The deficiency of these lysosomal hydrolases results in abnormal metabolism of the enzyme's specific sphingolipid substrate, and the substrate accumulates in the cells of the monocyte-macrophage system, causing the clinical manifestations. For example, in Gaucher disease and Niemann-Pick types A and B diseases, anemia, thrombocytopenia, leukopenia, and/or hepatosplenomegaly can be the presenting symptoms. Thus, these disorders are frequently diagnosed by the hematologist and must be included in the differential diagnosis for patients with monocyte-macrophage involvement.

PATHOPHYSIOLOGY OF THE LYSOSOMAL STORAGE DISEASES

The underlying defect in the inherited lipidoses is the accumulation of metabolites, including glycolipids and sphingomyelin. The glycosphingolipids, which are present in the membranes of many cell types, are formed by the addition of various carbohydrates to a ceramide backbone (*Figure 60.1*). The fatty acid portion of ceramide consists primarily of stearic acid (C_{18}) in the brain, whereas in nonneural tissues it is somewhat longer (C_{20}-C_{24}). Each sphingolipid is characterized by the nature of the compound that is esterified to the first carbon of the ceramide molecule. For example, the addition of hexoses and *N*-acetylneuraminic acid to ceramide forms the gangliosides, which are found in brain, whereas the neutral glycolipids are found more ubiquitously in cell membranes. The blood group antigens are also glycosphingolipids. In the lysosomal storage diseases, these lipid compounds vary in amount in different cell types, so their rate and amount of accumulation because of a specific lysosomal enzyme defect will vary, leading to their cell-related manifestations (*Figure 60.2*). *Tables 60.1* and *60.2* outline the biochemical and phenotypic characteristics and the molecular basis of the lysosomal storage diseases, respectively.

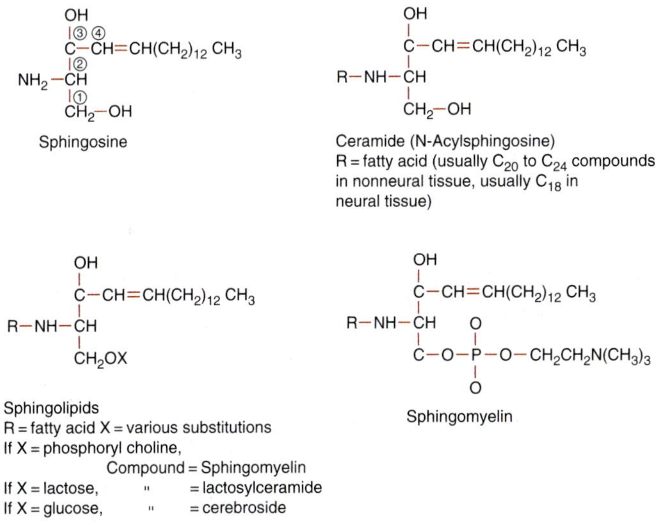

GAUCHER DISEASE

Definition and History

Gaucher disease is a lipid storage disease characterized by the deposition of glucocerebroside in cells of the macrophage-monocyte system. It was first described by Gaucher in 1882, and the storage of glucocerebroside was first recognized by Epstein in 1924. The metabolic defect, which is the deficiency of the lysosomal hydrolase acid β-glucosidase, or β-glucocerebrosidase, was identified by Brady et al.[1] There are three clinical subtypes, which are delineated by the absence or presence and progression of neurologic involvement: type 1 or the nonneuronopathic form; type 2, the infantile-onset, acute neuronopathic form; and type 3, the juvenile-onset neuronopathic form.[2] All three subtypes are inherited as autosomal recessive traits. Type 1 disease is the most common lysosomal storage disease and one of the most prevalent genetic disorders among Ashkenazi Jewish individuals, with an incidence of about 1 in 1000 and a carrier frequency of about 1 in 15.[3]

Etiology and Pathogenesis

All three subtypes of Gaucher disease result from the deficient activity of the lysosomal hydrolase, acid β-glucosidase (*Table 60.1*). The major acid β-glucosidase gene mutations that cause Gaucher disease among Ashkenazi Jewish patients have been identified (*Table 60.2*). Genotype/phenotype correlations have been made for the different subtypes and provide insight into the molecular basis for the remarkable clinical variation in Gaucher disease. Presumably, the amount of residual enzymatic activity determines disease subtype and severity. For example, the mutations that cause the severe type 2 (infantile) disease express little, if any, enzymatic activity in vitro, whereas type 1 patients who are homozygous for the milder N370S mutation tend to have a later onset and a milder course than patients with one N370S allele and another mutant allele. However, the wide variability in clinical presentation among Gaucher disease patients cannot be fully explained by the underlying acid β-glucosidase mutations, and presumably other "modifier" genes can influence disease severity.

Pathology

The pathologic hallmark in Gaucher disease is the presence of Gaucher cells in the macrophage-monocyte system, particularly in the bone marrow. These cells, which are 20 to 100 μm in diameter, have a characteristic wrinkled paper appearance resulting from intracytoplasmic substrate deposition. These cells stain strongly positive with periodic acid-Schiff reagent, and their presence in bone marrow and/or other tissues suggests the diagnosis (*Figure 60.3*). The accumulated

FIGURE 60.1 Formulas of some of the sphingolipids.

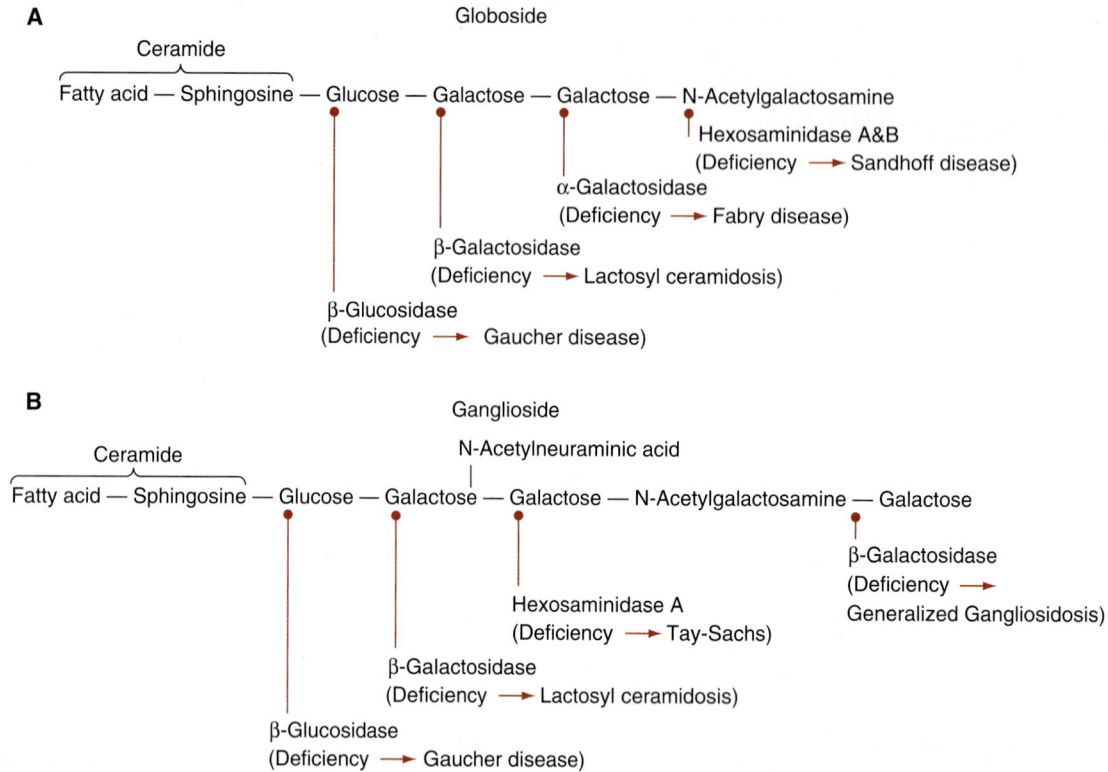

FIGURE 60.2 Schematic structures of globoside (A) and ganglioside (B) to show the site of action of several catabolic enzymes, which result in one of the storage diseases when defective.

Table 60.1. Biochemical and Phenotypic Characteristics of Gaucher and Niemann-Pick Diseases

Disease	Enzyme Deficiency	Substance Accumulated	Site	Complications
Gaucher Disease				
Type 1	Acid β-glucosidase	Primarily glucosylceramide	Macrophage-monocyte system	Infiltration of bone marrow, progressive hepatosplenomegaly, skeletal complications
Type 2	Acid β-glucosidase	Primarily glucosylceramide	Macrophage-monocyte system, CNS	Infiltration of bone marrow, progressive hepatosplenomegaly, skeletal complications, neurodegeneration
Type 3	Acid β-glucosidase	Primarily glucosylceramide	Macrophage-monocyte system, CNS	Progressive neurodegeneration
Niemann-Pick Disease				
Type A	Acid sphingomyelinase	Sphingomyelin	Monocyte-macrophage system, CNS	Hepatosplenomegaly, progressive neurodegeneration
Type B	Acid sphingomyelinase	Sphingomyelin	Monocyte-macrophage system	Progressive hepatosplenomegaly, infiltrative lung disease
Type C	Abnormal cholesterol transport	Primarily cholesterol	Most cells, especially liver, CNS	Hepatosplenomegaly, progressive neurodegeneration

Abbreviation: CNS, central nervous system.

glycosphingolipid, glucosylceramide, is derived primarily from the phagocytosis and degradation of senescent leukocytes and, to a lesser extent, erythrocyte membranes. Glucosylceramide storage results in organomegaly and pulmonary infiltration. Neuronal cell loss in patients with types 2 and 3 disease presumably results from the neural accumulation of the cytotoxic glycosphingolipid, glucosphingosine, due to the severe deficiency of acid β-glucosidase activity. Glucosylceramide accumulation in the bone marrow, liver, spleen, lungs, and kidney leads to pancytopenia, massive hepatosplenomegaly, diffuse infiltrative pulmonary disease, and nephropathy or glomerulonephritis. The progressive infiltration of Gaucher cells in the bone marrow causes thinning of the cortex, pathologic fractures, bone pain, bony infarcts, and osteopenia, particularly in type 1 disease. Central nervous system (CNS) involvement occurs only in patients with types 2 and 3 disease.

Clinical Manifestations
Type 1 Disease

There is a broad spectrum of clinical expression among type 1 disease patients, in part because of the combination of different mutant alleles. Onset of clinical manifestations occurs from early childhood to late adulthood, with more symptomatic patients presenting in childhood

Table 60.2. Molecular Basis of Gaucher and Niemann-Pick Diseases

Disease	Chromosome Assignment	Molecular Characteristics	Comments
Gaucher disease	1q21	cDNA, functional and pseudogenomic sequences, >200 mutant alleles known	Four mutations (N370S, L444P, 84insG, IVS2$^+$1) account for 90 to >95% of mutant alleles in Ashkenazi Jewish patients
Niemann-Pick disease			
Types A and B	11p15.1 to p15.4	cDNA, entire genomic sequence, >70 mutant alleles known	Four mutations account for >95% of mutant alleles in Ashkenazi Jewish patients with type A disease
Type C	18q11-q12 region	cDNA, entire genomic sequence, >100 mutant alleles known	More than 100 mutations in NPC1 gene

Abbreviation: cDNA, complementary DNA.

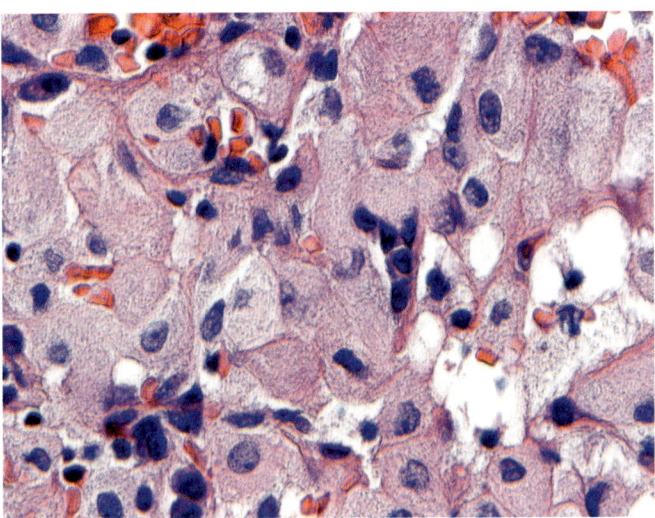

FIGURE 60.3 Splenic histopathology in Gaucher disease. There are sheets of histiocytes with bland nuclei and abundant pink cytoplasm with a fine "tissue paper" appearance.

or adolescence. At presentation, patients may have easy bruisability resulting from thrombocytopenia, chronic fatigue secondary to anemia, hepatomegaly with or without elevated liver function tests, splenomegaly, and bone pain or pathologic fractures. Occasionally patients present with pulmonary involvement. Patients who are diagnosed in the first 5 years of life are frequently non-Jewish and typically have a more malignant disease course. Those with milder disease are discovered later in life during evaluations for hematologic or skeletal problems or are found to have splenomegaly on routine examinations. In symptomatic patients, splenomegaly is progressive and can become massive. Clinically apparent bony involvement can present as bone pain or pathologic fractures. Most patients have radiologic evidence of skeletal involvement, including an "Erlenmeyer flask" deformity of the distal femur, which is an early skeletal change. In patients with symptomatic bone disease, lytic lesions can develop in the long bones, ribs, and pelvis, and osteosclerosis may be evident at an early age. Bone crises with severe pain and swelling can occur. Bleeding secondary to thrombocytopenia may manifest as epistaxis and bruising and is frequently overlooked until other symptoms become apparent. Children with massive splenomegaly are short of stature because of the energy expenditure required by the enlarged organ.

Type 2 Disease

Infants with the rare and panethnic type 2 subtype have a rapid neurodegenerative course with extensive visceral involvement and death within the first 2 years of life. The disease presents in infants with increased tone, strabismus, and organomegaly. Failure to thrive and stridor resulting from laryngospasm are typical. The progressive psychomotor degeneration leads to death, usually due to respiratory compromise.

Type 3 Disease

Patients with type 3 Gaucher disease typically present in infancy or childhood. In addition to the organomegaly and bony involvement, neurologic involvement is present. There is a high frequency of type 3 disease in Sweden (1 in 50,000), which has been traced to a common founder in the 17th century. Type 3 has been further classified as type 3a or 3b based on the extent of neurologic involvement and whether there is progressive myotonia and dementia (type 3a) or isolated supranuclear gaze palsy (type 3b).

Diagnosis

Gaucher disease should be considered in the differential diagnosis of patients who present with unexplained organomegaly, easy bruisability, and/or bone pain.[4] In the past, bone marrow examination revealing the presence of Gaucher cells was used for diagnosis. Today, all suspect diagnoses should be confirmed by demonstrating deficient acid β-glucosidase activity in isolated leukocytes. For genotype/phenotype correlations, the specific acid β-glucosidase gene mutation should be determined, particularly in Ashkenazi Jewish patients. Carrier identification can be achieved by enzymatic assay, although in the Ashkenazi this can be best achieved by targeted sequencing analysis of the common founder mutations. Testing should be offered to all family members, keeping in mind that heterogeneity even among members of the same kindred can be significant and that asymptomatic affected individuals may be diagnosed during such testing. Prenatal diagnosis is available by determining the parent's specific mutations in chorionic villi or cultured amniotic fluid cells.

Treatment

Enzyme replacement with recombinant acid β-glucosidase (imiglucerase [Cerezyme, Genzyme Corporation, Cambridge, MA] or velaglucerase alfa [Vpriv, Shire HGT, Lexington, MA]) is the standard of care for the treatment of patients with type 1 disease. Clinical trials have demonstrated that most extraskeletal symptoms are reversed within 12 to 36 months by a dose of 60 U/kg administered by intravenous infusion every other week. Initial higher doses may be indicated in patients with severe disease (type 3) at the time of diagnosis and in those with rapid progression or significant comorbidities.[5] Early treatment may be efficacious in normalizing linear growth and bone morphology in affected children. Experience during the last 20 years has proven enzyme replacement therapy (ERT) to be safe and effective in preventing the complications of type 1 disease. However, enzyme replacement does not alter the neurologic progression of patients with Gaucher disease types 2 and 3. It has been used as a palliative measure in type 3 patients with severe visceral involvement. Alternative treatments rely on orally administered glucosylceramide synthase inhibitors including miglustat (Zavesca, Actelion), although its efficacy on hematological parameters is not as effective as ERT.

A second and more effective substrate inhibitor, eliglustat (Cerdelga, Sanofi Genzyme), received marketing approval in 2015. In clinical studies it had demonstrated significant efficacy versus placebo and was not inferior to imiglucerase making this an alternative first-line treatment for patients with type 1 disease.

NIEMANN-PICK DISEASE

Definition

Niemann-Pick disease (NPD) types A and B are lipid storage disorders that result from the deficiency of the lysosomal enzyme, acid sphingomyelinase, and the subsequent accumulation of its substrate, sphingomyelin.[6] The original description of NPD referred to what is now known as type A NPD, which is a fatal neurodegenerative disorder of infancy characterized by failure to thrive, hepatosplenomegaly, and a rapidly progressive neurodegenerative course that leads to death by the age of 2 or 3 years. Type B NPD has a wide phenotypic spectrum that can include neurologic manifestations, but typically does not.[6-8] Type C NPD is a neurodegenerative disorder that results from defective intracellular cholesterol transport and accumulation of unesterified cholesterol in lysosomes.[7,8] Previously, a type D disease was identified in patients from Nova Scotia; however, these patients actually have type C disease. All the subtypes are inherited as autosomal recessive traits and display variable clinical features.

Etiology and Pathogenesis

Types A and B NPD result from the deficient activity of the lysosomal hydrolase, acid sphingomyelinase (Table 60.1). In type C NPD, the genetic defect involves the defective transport of cholesterol from the lysosome to the cytosol. Two different genes causing the altered cholesterol transport in type C disease have been identified (*NPC1* and *NPC2*), permitting more precise diagnosis, carrier detection, and prenatal diagnosis in affected families. Only types A and B are discussed here; for type C, see Patterson et al and Vanier.[7,8]

Pathology

Types A and B Niemann-Pick Disease

The pathologic hallmark in types A and B NPD is the histochemically characteristic lipid-laden foam cell, often referred to as the "Niemann-Pick cell." These cells, which can be readily distinguished from Gaucher cells by their histologic and histochemical characteristics, are not pathognomonic for NPD, because histologically similar cells are found in patients with Wolman disease, cholesterol ester storage disease, lipoprotein lipase deficiency, and in some patients with GM_1 gangliosidosis, type 2 (Figure 60.4). Sphingomyelin is the major lipid that accumulates in the cells and tissues of patients with types A and B NPD. In most normal tissues, sphingomyelin constitutes from 5% to 20% of the total cellular phospholipid content; however, in patients with types A and B NPD, the sphingomyelin levels may be elevated up to 50-fold, constituting ~70% of the total phospholipid fraction. Lysosomal sphingomyelin accumulation in the liver, kidney, and lungs has been documented with organs from types A and B NPD patients containing about the same amount of sphingomyelin, with the notable finding of significant sphingomyelin and psychosphingosine in the CNS of type A NPD patients. In general, patients with type A disease have <5% of normal acid sphingomyelinase activity when assayed in cultured fibroblasts and/or lymphocytes, whereas cells from type B patients typically have >5% of normal activity, which presumably prevents the development of the neurologic symptoms.

Clinical Manifestations

Types A and B Niemann-Pick Disease

The clinical presentation and course of type A NPD is relatively uniform and is characterized by a normal appearance at birth. Hepatosplenomegaly and psychomotor retardation are evident by 6 months of life, followed by rapid neurodegeneration and death by 3 years. The loss of motor function and the deterioration of intellectual capabilities are progressive. In later stages, spasticity and rigidity are evident, with affected infants experiencing complete loss of contact with their environment.

In contrast to the stereotyped type A phenotype, the clinical presentation and course of patients with type B disease are more variable. Most patients are diagnosed in infancy or childhood, when enlargement of the liver and/or spleen is detected during a routine physical examination. At diagnosis, type B patients also have evidence of mild pulmonary involvement, usually detected as a diffuse reticular or finely nodular infiltration on the chest roentgenogram. In most patients, hepatosplenomegaly is particularly prominent in childhood, but with increasing linear growth, the abdominal protuberance decreases and becomes less conspicuous. In mildly affected patients, the splenomegaly may not be noted until adulthood, and there may be minimal disease manifestations. In most type B patients, decreased pulmonary diffusion resulting from alveolar infiltration becomes evident in childhood and progresses with age. Severely affected individuals may experience significant pulmonary compromise by age 15 to 20 years. Such patients have low pO_2 values and dyspnea on exertion. Life-threatening bronchopneumonias may occur, and cor pulmonale has been described. Severely affected patients also may have liver involvement leading to life-threatening cirrhosis, portal hypertension, and ascites. Clinically significant pancytopenia resulting from secondary hypersplenism may necessitate partial or total splenectomy, although removal of the spleen can exacerbate the pulmonary disease.

Cholesterol abnormalities characterized by low high-density lipoprotein cholesterol and increased total cholesterol are found in most patients and can be associated with early atherosclerotic changes. Some type B patients have neurologic involvement, which can include cerebellar signs and nystagmus, extrapyramidal involvement, mental retardation, and psychiatric disorders. As in other lysosomal storage diseases, it is evident that neurologic manifestations in acid sphingomyelinase deficiency (ASMD) may occur along a continuum among patients. Nevertheless, there is a distinctive, fatal neurodegenerative form (NPD-A), characterized by a brief period of normal development followed by a severe neurodegenerative course and death in early childhood.

Patients with NPD type C disease often have prolonged neonatal jaundice, appear normal for 1 to 2 years, and then experience a slowly progressive and variable neurodegenerative course. Their hepatosplenomegaly is less severe than that in patients with type A or B disease, and they may survive into adulthood.

Diagnosis

Type A NPD patients are diagnosed in the first year of life with failure to thrive, organomegaly, and severe psychomotor retardation. In type B NPD patients, splenomegaly is usually noted early in childhood; however, in very mildly affected patients, the enlargement may be subtle and detection may be delayed until adolescence or

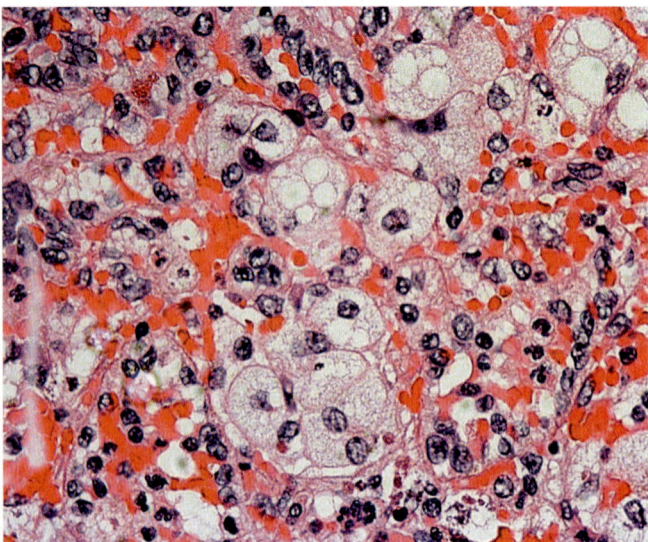

FIGURE 60.4 Splenic histology in Niemann-Pick disease type B. Aggregates of histiocytes are present with distinct vacuoles. Although some large vacuoles are seen, most are small. (Image provided by Professor Attilio Orazi, Department of Pathology, Indiana University.)

adulthood. The presence of the characteristic Niemann-Pick cells in the bone marrow supports the diagnosis. However, patients with type C disease also have extensive infiltration of these cells in the bone marrow. Thus, all suspect cases should be evaluated enzymatically for type B or by mutation analysis for both types to confirm the clinical diagnosis by measuring the acid sphingomyelinase activity in peripheral leukocytes or cultured fibroblasts and/or lymphoblasts. Patients with type A or B disease will have markedly decreased levels of enzymatic activity (1%-10% of normal), patients with type C disease may have slightly decreased sphingomyelinase activities (50%-75% of normal), and patients with Gaucher disease and other storage disorders presenting with hepatosplenomegaly and/or neurologic involvement will have normal or near-normal acid sphingomyelinase levels. Type C NPD can be documented biochemically by demonstrating the cholesterol transport defect in cultured fibroblasts by filipin staining or by determining the specific mutations in the *NPC1* or *NPC2* genes.

The enzymatic identification of type A and B carriers is problematic. However, in families in which the specific molecular lesion has been identified, family members can be accurately tested for heterozygote status by DNA analysis. Prenatal diagnosis of types A and B disease may be made reliably by measuring the acid sphingomyelinase activity in cultured amniocytes or chorionic villi. In families in which the specific gene mutations are known, the prenatal diagnosis can be made by DNA analysis of fetal cells. Historically, the diagnosis of Niemann-Pick type C relied on the demonstration of the cholesterol transport defect in cultured fibroblasts by filipin staining but is now made by genetic testing of the NPC1 and NPC2 genes and the measurement of oxidative cholesterol metabolites.

Treatment

Orthotopic liver transplantation in an infant with type A disease and amniotic cell transplantation in several type B patients have been attempted, with little or no success. Bone marrow transplantation of type B patients has reduced the spleen and liver volumes, the sphingomyelin content of the liver, the number of Niemann-Pick cells in the marrow, and the radiologic infiltration of the lungs. However, no long-term information is available, as these patients often lose their engraftment or have significant morbidity and mortality in the posttransplant period. To date, lung transplantation has not been reported in any severely compromised type B patient. A 26-week phase 1b study of ERT with olipudase alpha in adult patients with NPD B established initial proof of concept in this patient group.[9] A phase 1/2 pediatric trial (ASCEND-Peds/NCT02292654) in children with chronic ASMD also demonstrated that ERT was generally well tolerated with improvements in disease pathology, and a phase 1/2 clinical trial in pediatric patients and a randomized phase 2/3 trial in adults (ASCEND) with ASMD documented improvement in lung function and spleen size.

Clinical trials of miglustat (Actelion, Basel, Switzerland) also have been performed and the drug has been approved in Europe for the treatment of type C disease. Treatment of type A disease is limited by the severe neurologic involvement.

Web Sites

www.gaucherdisease.com
www.nnpdf.org
www.ninds.nih.gov/health_and_medical/disorders/niemann.doc.htm

References

1. Brady RO, Kanfer JN, Bradley RM, Shapiro D. Demonstration of a deficiency of glucocerebroside-cleaving enzyme in Gaucher's disease. *J Clin Invest.* 1966;45:1112-1115.
2. Grabowski GA, Petsko GA, Kolodny EH. Gaucher disease. In: Valle D, Beaudet AL, Vogelstein B, et al., eds. *The Online Metabolic and Molecular Bases of Inherited Disease-OMMBID.* McGraw-Hill; 2014:Chapter 186www.ommbid.com.
3. McGovern MM, Avetisyan R, Sanson BJ, Lidove O. Disease manifestations and burden of illness in patients with acid sphingomyelinase deficiency (ASMD) Orphanet. *J Rare Dis.* 2017;12:41.
4. Charrow J, Esplin JA, Gribble TJ, et al. Gaucher disease: recommendations on diagnosis, evaluation, and monitoring. *Arch Intern Med.* 1998;158:1754-1760.
5. Mistry PK, Cappellini MD, Lukina E, et al. A reappraisal of Gaucher disease-diagnosis and disease management algorithms. *Am J Hematol.* 2011;86:110-115.
6. Schuchman EH, Desnick RJ. Niemann-Pick disease types A and B: acid sphingomyelinase deficiencies. In: Valle D, Beaudet AL, Vogelstein B, et al., eds. *The Online Metabolic and Molecular Bases of Inherited Disease-OMMBID.* McGraw-Hill; 2014:Chapter 144http://ommbid.mhmedical.com/content.aspx?bookid=971&sectionid=62632315.
7. Patterson M, Vanier MT, Suzuki K, et al. Niemann-Pick disease type C: a lipid trafficking disorder. In: Valle D, Beaudet AL, Vogelstein B, et al., eds. *The Online Metabolic and Molecular Bases of Inherited Disease-OMMBID.* McGraw-Hill; 2010:Chapter 145www.ommbid.com.
8. Vanier MT. Niemann-Pick disease type C. *Orphanet J Rare Dis.* 2010;5:16.
9. Wasserstein MP, Diaz GA, Lachmann RH, et al. Olipudase alfa for treatment of acid sphingomyelinase deficiency (ASMD): safety and efficacy in adults treated for 30 months. *J Inherit Metab Dis.* 2018;41:829-838.

Chapter 61 ■ Langerhans Cell Histiocytosis

AMIT RAJARAM • MICHAEL M. HENRY

INTRODUCTION

Langerhans cell histiocytosis (LCH) is a disorder characterized by clonal proliferation of cells in the mononuclear phagocyte system. Since the first case was described more than a century ago,[1] LCH has often been a source of confusion, perhaps best demonstrated by the several labels given to the disorder during the past 100 years. Since 1985, *Langerhans cell histiocytosis* has been the preferred term,[2,3] replacing *histiocytosis X*, coined in 1953.[4] The *X* demonstrated the lack of knowledge about the etiology and pathophysiology of LCH, and about how the different clinical syndromes were related. The term *histiocytosis X* did serve to bind the syndromes, which included Hand-Schüller-Christian syndrome, Letterer-Siwe disease, eosinophilic granuloma, Hashimoto-Pritzker syndrome,[5] self-healing histiocytosis,[6] and pure cutaneous histiocytosis,[7] into one clinical entity. The term *Langerhans cell histiocytosis* reflects the central role of the Langerhans cell in these diseases. LCH also distinguishes these disorders from other histiocytic syndromes, which include primary and secondary hemophagocytic lymphohistiocytosis, Rosai-Dorfman disease, and neoplastic disorders such as acute monocytic leukemia, malignant histiocytosis, and true histiocytic lymphoma.[2] This chapter focuses on LCH.

HISTORY

The history of LCH in the medical literature begins with a suspicious case described by Hippocrates in 400 to 450 BC of a patient with a "nonfatal" disease associated with painful skull lesions.[8] In 1865, Smith was the first to describe a patient with "impetiginous" lesions in the skin and lytic lesions in the skull.[9] Although there is no empirical evidence to confirm the diagnosis, it is quite possible that the impetiginous lesions represented cutaneous manifestations of LCH. In 1868, Langerhans described "epidermal, nonpigmentary, dendritic cells" in the skin of patients who were likely affected by LCH.[10] Shortly thereafter, in 1893, Hand described a child with polyuria and exophthalmos, which at the time was attributed to tuberculosis.[11] In 1915, Schüller[12] and in 1920, Christian[13] independently described patients with similar skull defects, exophthalmos, and diabetes insipidus (DI). The clinical triad of defects in membranous bone, exophthalmos, and polyuria in children, which became known as *Hand-Schüller-Christian disease*,[14] was described in 1921 in a review by Hand.[15] Hand described the first six reported cases, including those of Christian, Schüller, and his own first case reported in 1893.[1] All six patients had hepatosplenomegaly, lymphadenopathy, and bone lesions. However, not all patients had exophthalmos and polyuria. Attempts to link the disorder to xanthoma tuberosum, lipid storage disease, and the xanthomatoses proved unsuccessful; and to this day, no evidence exists that a specific biochemical defect is responsible for the condition. The foamy, or xanthoma, cell came to be regarded as a pathognomonic feature of the syndrome.[16]

A different syndrome, consisting of fever, localized bone tumors, hepatosplenomegaly, coagulopathy, anemia, and hyperplasia of non–lipid-storing macrophages and adenopathy in a young infant who died, was described by Letterer in 1924.[17] In 1933, Siwe described a 16-month-old girl who died after a similar 3-month illness characterized by fever, hepatosplenomegaly, lymphadenopathy, neutrophilia, and a destructive lesion in her fibula.[18] At autopsy, massive infiltrates of large cells resembling histiocytes were found. Siwe reviewed five other cases from the literature (including that of Letterer) and concluded that they constituted a single clinical entity.[18]

In 1940, two groups of investigators described a syndrome in which a characteristic feature was infiltration of bone by eosinophilic granulomas.[19,20] In 1941 to 1942, Green and Farber described a series of patients with eosinophilic granulomas of bone, which usually healed promptly after irradiation or curettage.[21,22] They noted that these cases shared pathologic features like those of the Letterer-Siwe and Hand-Schüller-Christian syndromes. In 1953, because of the similarity of the histiocytes observed in these three disorders, Lichtenstein combined them into a single entity called *histiocytosis X* to indicate their unknown cause.[4] The recognition that these three disorders were related was an important contribution to our understanding of LCH. In 1973, Nezelof showed that "histiocytosis X" was the result of a proliferation of abnormal Langerhans cells.[23] The term *LCH*, proposed in 1985, reflects an improved understanding of these disorders.[2,24] *Figure 61.1* represents a summary of these discoveries.

Despite our understanding of the central role played by the Langerhans cells in LCH, little is known about the etiology of LCH.

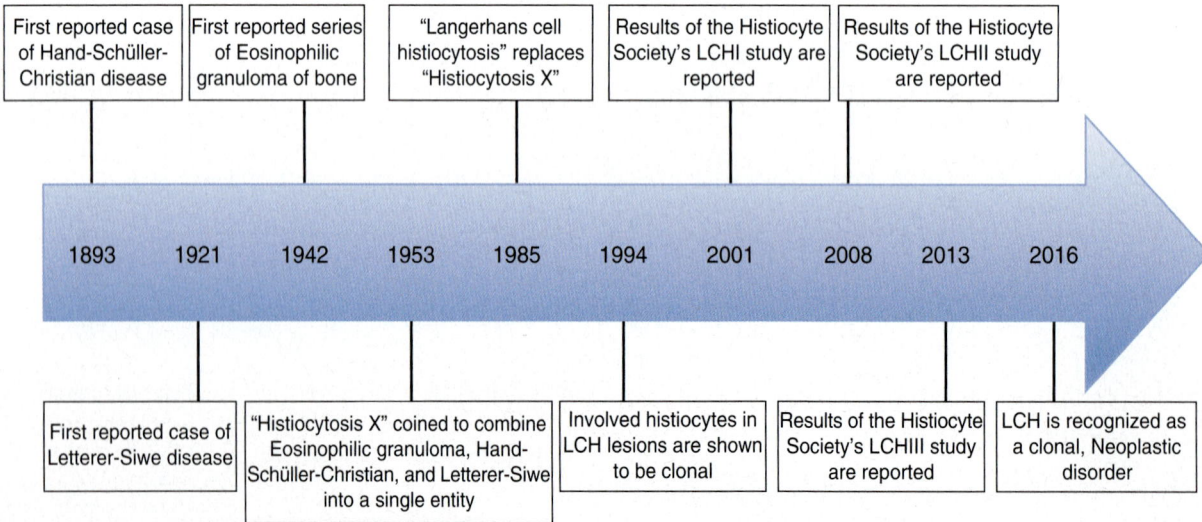

FIGURE 61.1 Historical timeline demonstrating the major discoveries regarding the pathogenesis and treatment of Langerhans cell histiocytosis (LCH).

Although clinical features of LCH were first recognized over a century ago, the pathogenesis remains uncertain. In 1994, two separate groups detected clonality of the involved histiocytes from LCH lesions.[25,26] Clonality was demonstrated in LCH cells from unifocal lesions as well as disseminated disease. It is now recognized that genetic mutations leading to aberrant cell-signaling pathways are important in the pathophysiology of LCH, and these findings have led to the redefinition of LCH as a neoplasm.[27]

EPIDEMIOLOGY

The annual childhood incidence of LCH has been estimated to be ~4 to 9 cases per million.[28-30] The discrepancy between epidemiologic studies is likely due to variation in reporting and data collection. Across studies, there is consistently a slight predominance of cases in men.[29-31] LCH occurs less frequently in adults, with an incidence of 1 to 2 cases per million per year.[32] The disease is more common and tends to be more severe in younger children. For children under 1 year of age, the annual incidence is 9.9 cases per million.[33] A majority of multisystem LCH occurs before 5 years of age.[28,34,35] In an exploratory case-control study comparing 177 children with LCH to children with cancer and community controls,[31] LCH was associated with a family history of benign tumors and was less strongly associated with feeding problems during infancy. Other factors associated with LCH in this study were maternal urinary tract infections during pregnancy and blood transfusions during infancy. Factors not associated with LCH were the typical childhood viral infections and medication use. In a case-control study of 459 children with LCH, which compared risk factors in children with LCH to those in both community and cancer controls,[36] LCH was associated with neonatal infections, solvent exposure, and thyroid disease in the proband or the family. Childhood immunizations appeared to be protective. Reports of seasonal variation in incidence are conflicting.[28,29] Familial clustering of LCH has been observed, suggesting that a genetic predisposition may exist.[37] The concordance rates between dizygotic and monozygotic twins are 33% and 80%, respectively. In addition, patients with LCH may have a predisposition to cancer and vice versa. Links with both solid tumors and leukemia have been documented.[38] Several cases of LCH developing in patients with acute lymphoblastic and acute myelogenous leukemia have been reported.[39-42] Patients with LCH have genetic instability and increased chromosomal breakage, which also suggests a genetic predisposition to malignancy.[43-45]

PATHOLOGY AND PATHOPHYSIOLOGY

The basic histologic lesion in LCH is granulomatous, with lesions containing histiocytes, mature eosinophils, and lymphocytes.[46] Other cells present may include giant cells, neutrophils, and plasma cells. Initially, lesions are proliferative and dominated by histiocytes, some of which are Langerhans cells. Although mitotic figures may be occasionally identified, the histiocytes are not neoplastic by histologic criteria. As lesions progress, necrosis may develop, and the number of eosinophils and phagocytic cells containing cellular debris increases. Ultimately, xanthomatous changes and fibrosis may occur; and late in the course of disease, Langerhans cells may no longer be demonstrable. Multinucleated giant cells occasionally are prominent, especially in bone and lymph nodes. These histologic findings do not correlate with the extent or aggressiveness of disease.[24]

The Langerhans cell is the sine qua non of the diagnostic lesion. Langerhans cells are dendritic antigen-presenting cells that are normally found in skin and other organs, and they are classified as dendritic cells because of their capacity to form long cytoplasmic extensions, through which they establish intimate contact with other cells. The presence of fascin, a highly selective marker of dendritic cells, on the surface of Langerhans cells confirms their derivation from dendritic cells.[47] Langerhans cells are found primarily in normal epidermis, but also are evident in lymph nodes and spleen. A hematopoietic progenitor of Langerhans cells has been identified in normal bone marrow.[47] In the skin, Langerhans cells form a trap for external contact antigens and are involved in delayed hypersensitivity. Despite low phagocytic activity, they fix antigens for presentation to other cells, especially T lymphocytes.[48]

Although its demonstration is essential for diagnosis, the Langerhans cell may constitute no more than a small proportion of histiocytes within lesions. Viewed by light microscopy, these cells appear as large mononuclear cells with few cytoplasmic vacuoles and little or no phagocytic material.[49] The nuclei are irregularly shaped and contain a fine chromatin pattern. Electron microscopic or immunohistochemical studies may be required to identify Langerhans cells with confidence. The former method demonstrates structures known as *Birbeck granules* (Langerhans bodies, X granules),[50,51] rod-shaped organelles with a central striation, and occasional terminal vesicular dilation, giving them a tennis racket appearance. Birbeck granules are thought to be produced by invagination of the cell membrane, and their function is not known. The other feature that conclusively establishes the diagnosis of LCH is the demonstration of either CD1a antigen or CD207 (langerin) on the surface of LCH cells by immunohistochemical staining.[49,52] Langerin is a cell-surface receptor that induces the formation of Birbeck granules.[53] Langerin expression recently has been recognized as a sensitive and relatively specific marker in establishing the diagnosis of LCH. Other distinctive features of Langerhans cells that can be demonstrated with immunohistochemical techniques include the expression of S-100 protein,[49] Ia-like antigen,[54] and CD101.[55]

The intralesional histiocytes of LCH were previously thought to be like normal Langerhans cells found in skin. It is now recognized, however, that pathologic Langerhans cells or LCH cells are a less-differentiated and more-activated type of dendritic cell.[56] CD1a-positive LCH cells from bone lesions express CD14 and CD68, which are monocyte antigens that are not expressed in, or are expressed at low levels in, normal skin Langerhans cells.[57] A relatively recent study demonstrated a gene expression profile of intralesional LCH cells that was distinct from that of normal skin Langerhans cells.[58] LCH cells also express the immature dendritic cell marker CCR6 in the absence of CCR7, which is expressed on mature dendritic cells.[59] LCH cells exhibit a degree of migration capability, which is absent in mature dendritic cells. LCH cells can be induced to differentiate in the presence of CD40 ligand in vitro.[57] Because CD40 ligand is abundant in LCH lesions, however, the reason for maturational arrest is unclear.[60] Abnormal cellular adhesion molecules in LCH cells, suggested by the presence of CD2, CD11a, CD11b, and CD11d, may contribute to the migration of Langerhans cells into LCH lesions, as well as their abnormal persistence and proliferation.[61] Compared to normal Langerhans cells, LCH cells are defective in their alloantigen-presenting activity.[62]

The focal accumulation of Langerhans cells, macrophages, lymphocytes, and eosinophils suggests that LCH is immunologically mediated. This reasoning is supported by both histologic abnormalities of the thymus and disturbances of immunoregulation in patients with active disease.[63] Thymic abnormalities were noted by Letterer in his initial description of the disorder, later known as Letterer-Siwe disease.[17] Abnormalities noted on pre–therapy thymic biopsy samples and postmortem materials include dysmorphic changes, dysplasia, and nonspecific involution.[64-66] In patients with LCH, the number of normal thymocytes (expressing CD6) and late differentiating suppressor lymphocytes (expressing CD8) is decreased.[67] These abnormalities are noted even when the disease is limited in its distribution.

Recognition of the possible pathogenic significance of thymic abnormalities prompted several studies of T lymphocytes in the blood. The demonstration of decreased numbers of H_2 receptors on blood lymphocytes suggests loss of T-suppressor cells.[68] This loss was confirmed by quantitation of T-cell subsets in patients with active disease. Both the relative and absolute numbers of suppressor T lymphocytes (CD8+ cells) are decreased, resulting in an increased T4-to-T8 lymphocyte ratio. Suppressor cell activity, as measured by the concanavalin A and indomethacin stimulation assays, also is poor.[68] That T-suppressor cell deficiency may be causally related to a functionally abnormal thymus is suggested by the normalization of T4-to-T8 ratios with thymic extract.[66] Moreover, the apparent ability of crude thymic extract to reverse disease activity in some patients suggests that the T-cell abnormalities may be of primary pathogenic significance.[66]

Although less consistent, other abnormalities in immune regulation also have been described, including hypergammaglobulinemia,[69] deficiency in antibody-dependent monocyte-mediated cytotoxicity,[70] and abnormal in vitro response to mitogens and antigens.[64] However, most investigators note normal mitogen-induced responses and normal delayed hypersensitivity.[71] Several cytokines also are increased in LCH.[72,73] Cytokines serve as mediators of inflammation, regulators of lymphocyte growth and differentiation, and activators of specialized effector cells. In tissue culture, Langerhans cells purified from bony LCH lesions secrete interleukin (IL)-1 and prostaglandin E_2, both of which induce bone resorption in vitro.[74] These lesions also secrete angiotensin-converting enzyme, transforming growth factor-β_1 and IL-2.[75] These mediators are probably responsible for the osteolytic lesions that are a prominent clinical feature of LCH. Other cytokines that have been demonstrated to be increased in the serum of LCH patients include granulocyte-macrophage colony-stimulating factor (GM-CSF), IL-3, IL-8, IL-10, and tumor necrosis factor-α (TNF-α).[76] These cytokines are related to local activation of T lymphocytes and other inflammatory leukocytes. In addition, GM-CSF receptors are expressed by Langerhans cells.[77] GM-CSF induces Langerhans cell proliferation and activation in vitro, and serum levels of GM-CSF have been correlated with the extent of disease.[77]

The link between proliferation of Langerhans cells and immune dysfunction has not entirely been elucidated. One suggestion is that the disorder results from a physiologically appropriate response of the Langerhans cell to an external antigen or neoantigen, possibly infectious in origin. The lack of seasonal variation or geographic clustering, however, argues against an infectious basis. In addition, no direct evidence for a viral etiology (viral particles or nuclear material) in LCH lesions has been demonstrated.[78,79] Alternatively, LCH may result from an appropriate response of the Langerhans cell to abnormal signals from other cells in the immune system, perhaps from T lymphocytes. In either event, deficiency of T-suppressor cells may disrupt the mechanism for termination of immune responses. Failure of this homeostatic mechanism could result in unrestrained macrophage proliferation. Indeed, patients with interferon-γ deficiency present with findings that mimic LCH.[80]

Whether LCH is primarily a reactive or neoplastic process has long been debated. The predominant theory has been that LCH is a reactive process to an unknown stimulus.[81] In 1994, however, two groups showed that the lesional cells are clonal.[25,26] Clonality occurred in patients with all forms of LCH, including acute disseminated LCH and unifocal LCH, and in those with intermediate forms of the disease. T cells within LCH lesions are polyclonal.[25] Interestingly, LCH occurs in some individuals with malignant disorders.[38] Most cases of malignancy occur after treatment for LCH, although acute lymphoblastic leukemia in particular may precede the diagnosis of LCH.[41,42] The presence of chromosomal instability and mutational events reported in a few studies support a neoplastic process.[43,44] However, at least some cases of pulmonary LCH are not clonal.[82] Moreover, the immature phenotype of LCH cells appears dependent on the microenvironment, suggesting a reactive process.

In addition to the finding of clonality, recent insights into genetic mutations implicated in altered cell-signaling pathways that give rise to LCH have strengthened the notion that LCH is a neoplasm and not just a reactive disorder.[27,83-94] Indeed, LCH is included in the World Health Organization's classification of mature lymphoid, histiocytic, and dendritic neoplasms.[94] The current understanding of altered molecular mechanisms in the pathogenesis of LCH involves activation of *ERK* via somatic mutations in upstream proteins, including *B-RAF*, *MEK*, *K-RAS*, and *MAPK* in ~60% to 85% of patients with LCH.[27,85,87-89,91,92,95-97] Dysregulation of the *AKT* pathway, a protein kinase that has a role in cell survival, also has been implicated in the development of LCH proliferation.[98] The potential to therapeutically target these aberrant molecular pathways has led to an exciting new frontier for drug development.[83,84,90,91,97,99-101]

CLINICAL FEATURES

LCH presents along a continuum of illness, ranging from indolent to explosive disease. In some patients, pathologic lesions are solitary, whereas in others they are widely disseminated. Moreover, the distribution of lesions in each patient may vary considerably over time. Although LCH can occur at any age, it occurs with greatest frequency in infants and children. The median age at diagnosis for all disease variants is 3 to 6 years.[29,30] The acute disseminated form of the disease characteristically occurs in younger children and almost all cases occur before the age of 5.[28] Children younger than 1 year of age often present with multiple-organ involvement.[33,102] The more indolent forms of LCH occur primarily in older children and young adults.[103] Approximately 70% of cases of LCH in children involve a single-organ system, with bone being the most common site.[28-30,33] *Table 61.1* shows the distribution of involved sites by age at diagnosis of LCH. The most commonly involved organ in adults is the bone, often accompanied by an adjacent soft-tissue mass.[104] Other organs that are involved less often in adults include the lungs and pituitary gland. In adults, multisystem disease, including liver, lymph node, and bone marrow involvement, is extremely rare.[32]

The traditional classification of clinical variants was based on patterns of organ involvement.[14] Eosinophilic granuloma was used to describe a syndrome characterized by single- or multiple-bone lesions in the absence of visceral involvement.[19] When granulomas involved the liver, spleen, lymph nodes, skin, central nervous system (CNS), or bone marrow, as well as bones, the disorder was called *Letterer-Siwe disease*.[17,18] The triad of multiple-bone lesions, exophthalmos (resulting from retro-orbital granulomas), and DI (the result of hypothalamic or pituitary involvement) constituted *Hand-Schüller-Christian disease*.[15] The separation of eosinophilic granuloma of bone from syndromes characterized by visceral dissemination proved to be useful from a prognostic standpoint, but the distinction between Letterer-Siwe disease and Hand-Schüller-Christian disease was often subtle and clinically irrelevant. The current classification of LCH is based on the number of organ systems involved and the number of sites involved within an organ system.[34,105] The main classifications of disease are "nonrisk organ" and "risk organ." "Non–risk organ" disease comprises single-system, single-site disease (usually in bone) and single-system, multiple-site disease (usually in bone). "Risk organ" disease refers to multisystem involvement, particularly in the liver, spleen, or bone marrow. Pulmonary involvement was originally considered to be a risk organ; but based on several analyses, this association has fallen out of favor,[106-108] and pulmonary involvement is not included in the definition of "risk organ" involvement in the current LCH-IV clinical trial that is being conducted by the Histiocyte Society. The presence and degree of organ dysfunction are important distinctions in those with multisystem disease.[105]

Bone is the most commonly involved organ in LCH, with the skull being the most commonly involved site in both children and adults.[109,110] Unifocal LCH of the bone is the most common form of the disease.[16,111] Multifocal bone involvement may or may not be associated with visceral disease. Characteristically, patients note mild discomfort at the site of bone involvement. Skull lesions are often painless, however, and are found only because of a soft-tissue exophytic mass over the bony defect. In young children, multifocal lesions of the skull are often associated with other head and neck manifestations. Gingival swelling and inflammation, usually associated with cervical adenopathy, may be the first manifestations of disease. Premature eruption or loss of teeth and breakdown of the lower alveolar ridge result from involvement of the mandible.[112] Mandibular lesions may be palpable and painful, giving rise to facial swelling.[113] The maxilla and upper gingival ridge are involved less often. Involvement of the petrus ridge of the temporal bone and mastoid is common, predisposing to chronic otitis media. Vertebral lesions pose special problems because of the risk of injury to the spinal cord. Vertebral collapse gives rise to vertebral plana (*Figure 61.2*), which can lead to failed diagnostic biopsy attempts because of lack of diagnostic tissue in unifocal cases.[114] Extension of granulomas into the spinal space may compress

Table 61.1. Systems Affected on Diagnosis of Langerhans Cell Histiocytosis by Age

Age Group	Number	Multisystem Disease (%)	Percentage of Cases With Each System Affected on Diagnosis						
			Bone	Skin	Soft Tissue	Lymph Nodes	Liver/ Spleen	Lung	Ear	Other
<1	25	64	32	76	24	24	28	16	36	8
1-4	52	71	69	35	27	21	17	31	13	4
5-14	24	17	100	0	8	8	0	0	4	0
0-14	101	56	67	37	22	19	16	20	17	4
P value[a]		<0.001	<0.001	<0.001	0.19	0.32	0.02	0.003	0.01	0.54

[a]P value for proportion of cases with involvement of each system varying by age group.
From Alston RD, Tatevossian RG, McNally RJ, Kelsey A, Birch JM, Eden TO. Incidence and survival of childhood Langerhans cell histiocytosis in Northwest England from 1954 to 1998. *Pediatr Blood Cancer.* 2007;48:555-560. Copyright © 2006 Wiley-Liss, Inc. Reprinted by permission of John Wiley & Sons, Inc.

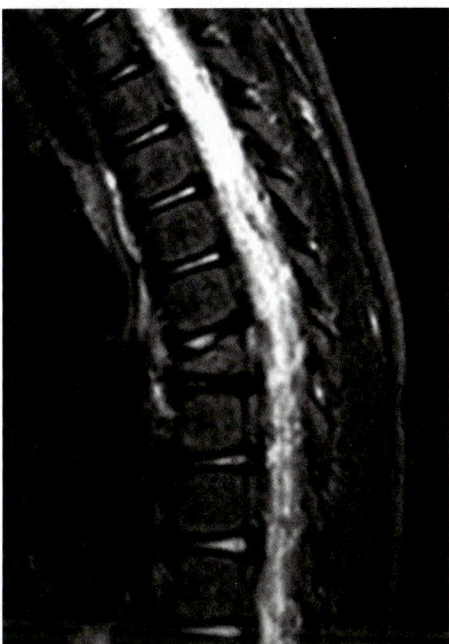

FIGURE 61.2 Sagittal magnetic resonance image of the thoracic spine showing collapse of the T8 vertebral body, more prominent in the anterior aspect, in a patient with reactivation of Langerhans cell histiocytosis.

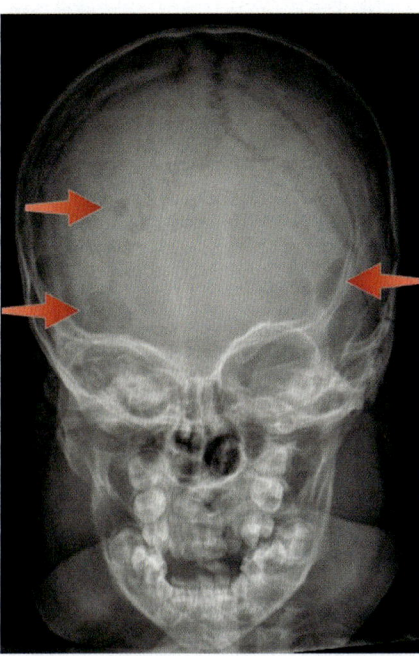

FIGURE 61.3 Skull radiograph showing active osteolytic lesions (arrows) in a patient with disseminated Langerhans cell histiocytosis. Note absence of reactive sclerosis.

the spinal cord, causing permanent neurologic damage. Recurrent bony lesions in children, particularly those involving the craniofacial region, are often associated with DI.[115,116]

Radiographically, skeletal lesions are characterized by sharply demarcated rarefactions of the medullary portions of bone, producing a "punched out" appearance (*Figure 61.3*).[110,111] Reactive sclerosis in surrounding uninvolved bone is unusual at diagnosis, but when present, signifies that healing has begun. As healing occurs, the sharp endosteal margins become less distinct, and sclerosis is often seen. Both tables of the skull characteristically are involved, the outer table more so than the inner table. Erosion of mandibular bone around unerupted teeth gives them the appearance of floating in space. Skeletal lesions are well delineated with conventional radiography, computed tomography (CT), and magnetic resonance imaging (MRI).[117,118] The relative benefit of radionuclide bone scintigraphy, on the other hand, is controversial.[119-121] Radionuclide bone scans often are falsely negative for skull lesions, but may be more sensitive in identifying lesions in the ribs, spine, and pelvis.[122,123] Positron emission tomography (PET) may have greater specificity in identifying active osseous lesions, and its clinical utility in LCH is likely superior to other imaging modalities.[124,125] Indeed, PET/CT is the preferred imaging modality at most large institutions to monitor the response to therapy.

Skin involvement occurs in about one-third of patients overall.[28,33] While skin manifestations are seen in only 10% of patients with single-system disease, it is a much more common feature of acute disseminated histiocytosis.[111,126] Even in those with skin-only disease, the rate of progression to multisystem disease is 30% to 40%.[127] The skin lesions are typically vesiculopustular and may have a hemorrhagic crust. They are similar in appearance to those of seborrheic dermatitis. A diagnosis of LCH is often suspected after a seborrheic rash fails to respond to treatment. The rash has a predilection for the scalp, postauricular areas, and diaper area (*Figure 61.4*). The back, axillae, and intertriginous areas also may be involved.[126] With advanced stages of the disease, the entire integument may be affected. Breakdown of severely affected areas is common, and concurrent thrombocytopenia imparts a hemorrhagic component to the rash.

A rash indistinguishable from that seen in acute disseminated histiocytosis may occur as a congenital, self-limited phenomenon not associated with skeletal or visceral disease. This form of histiocytosis has been called *congenital self-healing histiocytosis* or *Hashimoto-Pritzker syndrome.*[5,128] The lesions are present at birth or appear within the first 2 or 3 weeks of life. The lesions are most numerous over the scalp and face, and they also may extend over the trunk and proximal extremities. Mucous membranes are spared. Langerhans

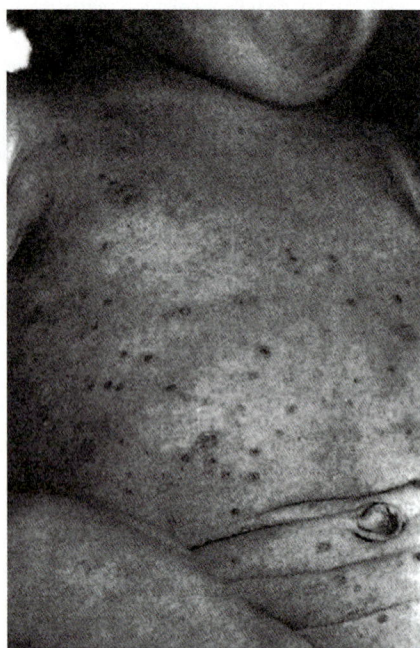

FIGURE 61.4 Erythematous maculopapular rash in a baby boy with disseminated Langerhans cell histiocytosis. (Reprinted from Esterly NB, Maurer HS, Gonzalez-Crussi F. Histiocytosis X: a seven year experience at a children's hospital. *J Am Acad Dermatol*. 1985;13:481-496. Copyright © 1985 Elsevier. With permission.)

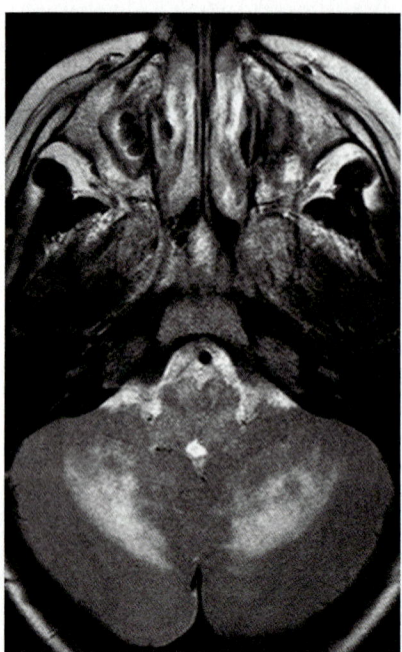

FIGURE 61.5 Axial magnetic resonance imaging scan showing diffuse bilateral signal abnormality in the cerebellum in a patient with neurodegenerative Langerhans cell histiocytosis.

cells present in biopsy material have the same immunophenotypic characteristics as those in the other variants of histiocytosis, although they contain fewer Birbeck granules.[128] The lesions typically undergo spontaneous regression, with complete healing by the time the patient is 3 to 4 months of age. The prognosis is generally excellent without therapy, although occasionally isolated cutaneous LCH in infants can progress to multisystem disease.[129] A study[130] of patients with skin-limited LCH revealed that the 3-year overall survival was 100%. In the same study, patients with multisystem disease and cutaneous manifestations had a 3-year progression rate of 77% compared with 30% in patients with just cutaneous disease. Periodic testing of peripheral blood for cell-free DNA harboring the *BRAF V600E* mutation may be helpful in identifying extracutaneous dissemination of LCH, provided that the skin lesions demonstrate the *BRAF V600E* mutation.[130]

CNS involvement is increasingly appreciated as a problem in LCH.[131,132] CNS involvement occurs by contiguous spread of skull lesions into brain substance or by granulomatous infiltration of deep brain structures. CNS disease can be classified as either focal mass lesions or lesions associated with progressive neurodegeneration. LCH demonstrates a predilection for the hypothalamic nuclei[133] and cerebellum,[134,135] although focal lesions may occur in the temporal lobe, occipital lobe, and spinal cord. In addition to brain parenchymal lesions, CNS disease can also present as masses in the meninges and choroid plexus.[132] Rarely, CNS lesions are found in patients who have no other evidence of histiocytosis. Neurologic signs and symptoms include ataxia, nystagmus, dysmetria, seizures, dysphagia, cranial nerve deficits, and spastic paraparesis.[136] DI resulting from infiltration of the hypothalamus or pituitary stalk is common[137] and is the most common initial finding of CNS LCH.[138] Mass lesions are satisfactorily visualized by CT or MRI, whereas infiltrative lesions within the hypothalamus and elsewhere often are of similar density to adjacent brain tissue and produce little or no mass effect. Some of these lesions may be seen with MRI.[131] CNS involvement may leave survivors with permanent sequelae.[116,131]

Neurodegenerative disease is the next most common CNS consequence of LCH after DI.[139] The typical MRI findings are diffuse, symmetrical signal changes of variable intensity in the basal ganglia or cerebellum (*Figure 61.5*).[140-142] PET/CT scans can show either increased or decreased fluorodeoxyglucose (18F) uptake.[143-145]

Patients with LCH-associated neurodegenerative disease demonstrate variable manifestations of disease. Some patients have no neurologic signs or symptoms, whereas others may have significant neurologic deficits. Clinical signs may include tremor, ataxia, spasticity, dysarthria, and behavioral or psychiatric problems. Some may also develop cerebellar syndrome with spastic tetraparesis, pseudobulbar palsy, and cognitive deterioration.[116,137,139,146-150] The time course of disease progression is variable, but neurologic deterioration may be severe and devastating. Histologic evaluation of neurodegenerative lesions shows a T-cell–mediated inflammatory process with tissue degeneration and, importantly, absence of CD1a-positive cells, in contrast to CNS mass lesions.[151] There is no known effective treatment for neurodegeneration, but intravenous immunoglobulin (IVIG) has been demonstrated to be a promising therapy to halt disease progression in some patients.[152] Systemic chemotherapy has been shown to stabilize disease progression and CNS function.[147,153,154]

Of the endocrinopathies associated with LCH, DI is the most common.[155] LCH is a common cause of DI in both adults and children.[156] DI is caused by infiltration of the hypothalamus, pituitary stalk, or posterior pituitary gland by Langerhans cells. The prevalence of DI in large series of patients ranges from 10% to 50%.[6,11,115,138,155-158] In a study of 1741 children with LCH, the cumulative risk of DI was 20% at 15 years from diagnosis.[115] DI is more common in patients with multisystem disease and in those with proptosis.[138] Patients with multiple craniofacial bone lesions are also at increased risk.[115] DI is not typically a complication of unifocal bone disease not involving the skull. Characteristically, the onset of DI occurs after the diagnosis of LCH is made, but symptoms of DI can occur at or preceding the diagnosis of LCH in one-third of patients.[116] However, LCH should be considered in the differential diagnosis in patients who present with central DI.[156,159-161] In such cases, a thickened pituitary stalk seen on MRI may be the only radiographic manifestation (*Figure 61.6*).[159] For most children, symptoms occur within 2 years of diagnosis and rarely, if ever, after 4 to 5 years.[138,162] Although most affected patients have complete absence of antidiuretic hormone, partial deficiency may be present. Progression from partial to complete DI may occur. Once complete DI has developed, it cannot be reversed, except as described in a few anecdotal case reports.[163,164] Whether systemic chemotherapy for LCH may prevent the development of DI is unclear. However, more rapid response to therapy and shorter disease duration correspond to a

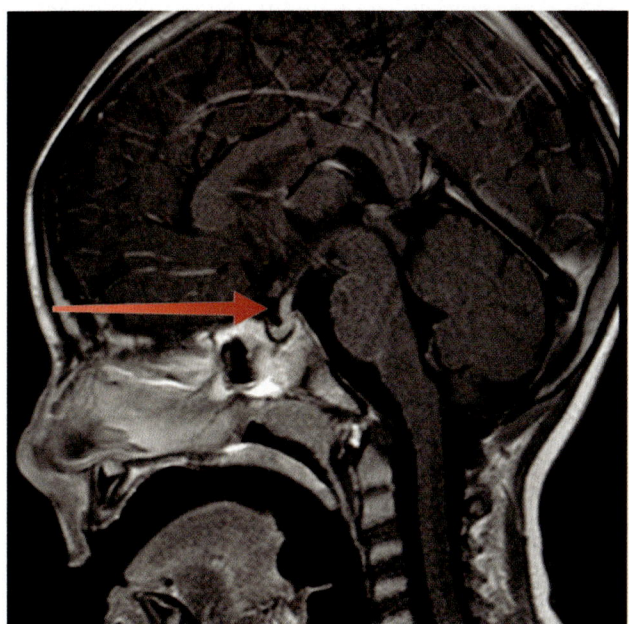

FIGURE 61.6 Sagittal magnetic resonance imaging scan showing thickened pituitary stalk (arrow).

decreased incidence of DI.[115] Reactivation of disease after complete resolution is associated with an increased risk of DI.[115]

Growth retardation resulting from growth hormone (GH) deficiency is another complication of LCH.[155,156] GH deficiency occurs in approximately 10% of patients with LCH overall and up to 60% of patients with LCH-associated DI.[116,165] Loss of GH, along with deficiency of other anterior pituitary hormones, is usually due to involvement of the hypothalamus or anterior pituitary gland by Langerhans cells.[165] GH replacement has been shown to be safe and effective in children with LCH and GH deficiency.[166]

Thyroid involvement by histiocytosis gives rise to goiter and may lead to hypothyroidism.[157] Obstruction of the upper airway by diffuse enlargement of the thyroid gland has been described.[167] Most children with thyroid involvement have DI and other evidence of disseminated disease.[155] Treatment of choice for isolated LCH involvement of the thyroid is surgical resection since there is no evidence that chemotherapy or radiation therapy provides a therapeutic benefit.[168]

Enlargement of the liver, often associated with abnormal liver function, is observed in many children with the disseminated form of LCH.[169-171] In some patients, liver involvement leads to portal cirrhosis or intrahepatic cholestasis.[169] Tissue from liver biopsies obtained from children with hepatomegaly infrequently shows the infiltrates of Langerhans cells, eosinophils, and lymphocytes that are hallmarks of the disease in other organs. Instead, subtle changes in the portal triads are observed, including triaditis, bile duct proliferation, and fibrosis.[170] Patients with triaditis alone at diagnosis are less likely to have abnormal liver function or progressive liver disease than those with fibrohistiocytic or cirrhotic changes. Persistent abnormality of liver function is a well-recognized adverse prognostic indicator.[172]

Involvement of the lymph nodes and spleen is often a feature of disseminated disease.[34] Lymph nodes may be involved because of contiguous bone or skin disease or because of widespread histiocytic dissemination. Splenomegaly is caused by portal hypertension or involvement of the spleen by large numbers of histiocytes. Curiously, Birbeck granules are rarely seen in otherwise characteristic Langerhans cells in the spleen and liver.[46,51]

Although not common, the lungs may be involved with disseminated histiocytosis.[173] As with other forms of disseminated disease, lung involvement occurs primarily in infants and young children. In contrast, primary pulmonary histiocytosis is principally a disease of young and middle-aged adults,[174-177] although it occasionally does occur in children. Smoking is often associated with pulmonary LCH.[178,179] Affected patients do not have apparent multisystem disease at diagnosis; but with further evaluation, some patients have asymptomatic bone lesions,[180] and as many as 10% subsequently develop DI.[181] Signs and symptoms of pulmonary involvement may be subtle or may include growth failure or weight loss, dyspnea, tachypnea, and hemoptysis. Recurrent pneumothoraces occur in as many as 20% to 25% of cases.[182] Lung involvement is characterized radiographically by diffuse micronodular densities with cyst formation, sometimes giving rise to a picture of "honeycomb lung." Lesions are usually prominent in the perihilar regions and the upper lung fields. Costophrenic angles are usually spared, and enlargement of hilar nodes is unusual. Permanent pulmonary sequelae often occur,[183] and reactivation in the lungs may be associated with smoking.[178]

Bone marrow involvement by Langerhans cells has been described most often in infants with disseminated disease.[34,35,184] This condition is characterized by anemia, neutropenia, and thrombocytopenia, occurring singly or together. Erythrophagocytosis may rarely be a factor in the pathogenesis of anemia.[185] Because bone marrow and splenic involvement often occur together, splenic sequestration of blood cells may further exaggerate the cytopenia of bone marrow involvement.

DIAGNOSIS

The clinical and radiographic features of LCH are distinctive enough to suggest the diagnosis in most patients. However, the diagnosis must be made pathologically; and for a definitive diagnosis, the presence of langerin and/or CD1a on the surface of LCH cells must be demonstrated.[186]

Assessment of the extent of disease is critical. To help standardize the workup and management of patients with LCH, the Histiocyte Society has published guidelines on how to evaluate and follow up patients.[187] A thorough physical examination is necessary to evaluate for hepatomegaly, splenomegaly, lymphadenopathy, and any bone or soft-tissue masses. Bony lesions may be diagnosed by either bone scan or skeletal survey. Each modality has been shown to discover lesions missed by the other, and radionucleotide bone scan may miss osteolytic lesions that do not have any osteoblastic characteristics. This is particularly true for skull lesions.[122,123] Other required studies include a chest radiograph, complete blood count, assessment of liver function (including gamma-glutamyl transferase due to higher incidence of portal triad infiltration), and determination of renal concentrating ability. A bone marrow examination is required if cytopenias exist, and a chest CT scan may be necessary if signs and symptoms suggest pulmonary involvement.[188] Newer imaging modalities, including PET scans, may be useful in LCH, but they require additional study.[125,144,189]

Several staging or scoring systems have been proposed as having prognostic and therapeutic relevance. Most cite age (younger than 2 years being a liability), extent of disease, and involved organ function as the most important prognostic variables.[34,35,190] An important distinction made by the Histiocyte Society and proved to be highly prognostic is whether "risk" organs are involved. "Risk" organ involvement is defined as at least two cytopenias (with or without documented bone marrow involvement), or involvement of LCH in the spleen or liver. The lungs were thought to be a "risk" organ in the past, but new analyses have suggested that pulmonary involvement is a less-prognostic factor than originally thought.[106-108] The presence of "CNS-risk" lesions (those involving the craniofacial bones, particularly those around the eyes, ears, and oral cavity)[115] results in a higher risk of developing DI. The LCH Study Group of the Histiocyte Society recognizes three distinct groups of patients: those with single-system LCH, those with multisystem LCH (with or without "risk" organ involvement), and those with "CNS-risk" lesions that were described previously.

PROGNOSIS

For most patients with LCH, the prognosis is excellent. Although the disease course of LCH may wax and wane over the years, most patients improve over time. Patients with multisystem disease may

Table 61.2. Outcome Data

Group	No Reactivation or Progression	Progression	Reactivation	Death	4-Year Event-Free Survival (%)
Single bone (n = 48)	46	0	2	0	89.7
Multiple bone (n = 40)	26	1	13	0	58.1
Multiple organ					
All (n = 34)	10	7	17	7	24
Age < 1 y (n = 19)	5	6	8	7	22

From Jubran RF, Marachelian A, Dorey F, et al. Predictors of outcome in children with Langerhans cell histiocytosis. *Pediatr Blood Cancer*. 2005;45(1):37-42. Copyright © 2005 Wiley-Liss, Inc. Reprinted by permission of John Wiley & Sons, Inc.

experience fulminant organ failure, which can be fatal. Outcomes by single-bone, multiple-bone, and multiple-organ involvement are shown in *Table 61.2*.

Many patients with unifocal bone disease experience complete resolution of lesions with or without treatment. Progression of bone erosion and recurrences at new sites are the exception rather than the rule.[191] In a study of 48 patients with single-bone involvement, the recurrence rate was 8% and no deaths were reported.[102] In contrast, disease that is multifocal at the time of diagnosis is often characterized by one or more recurrences after disease control.[102,109] Patients with multiple-bone lesions, particularly those with skull involvement, have a much higher incidence of disease reactivation than those with single-bone lesions.[102] In addition, most patients with multiple-site involvement will experience disease recurrence. In one large series, 72% of patients with multisystem disease who initially responded to treatment experienced recurrent LCH from 2 months to more than 5 years after cessation of therapy, and most recurrences were in previously uninvolved sites.[103] Young children, especially those younger than 2 years of age at diagnosis, are at higher risk for multiple relapses. However, in most patients, the disease appears to burn out eventually.[192,193] *BRAF-V600E* mutations also have been linked to increase the risk multiple relapse.[3]

Despite the favorable prognosis for most patients, mortality from disease progression can occur. Approximately one-third of adults with pulmonary LCH die of the disease.[177] The highest incidence of mortality, however, is seen in children with multiple "risk" organ involvement at the time of diagnosis, although the outcome of these patients has significantly improved in the past several years thanks to advances in the understanding of disease pathophysiology and markedly improved treatments.[81,116,193,194] After disease resolution, LCH survivors may be left with permanent complications, including DI, pulmonary difficulties, neurologic complications, orthopedic abnormalities, neuropsychological impairment, dental problems, chronic otitis, or hearing impairment.[81,116,193] Patients with one or more reactivations after initial therapy are more likely to have long-term sequelae from LCH.[195]

MANAGEMENT AND TREATMENT

Management is dictated by the likely natural history of the disease based on the location and extent of lesions and by the presence of specific organ involvement and/or dysfunction. Given that LCH tends to improve with time, most patients do not require treatment aimed at ablating the disease. In most patients, disease manifestations are reversed with therapy that is far less intensive than that used for other neoplastic disease. As noted previously, however, multiple courses of treatment may be required for recurrences. Unfortunately, DI is not ameliorated by chemotherapy. Although some authors describe reversal of DI with low-dose chemotherapy[163] or radiotherapy directed to the hypothalamus-pituitary region soon after the onset of symptoms,[196] the consensus is that radiotherapy, like chemotherapy, is typically without benefit in this situation.[157,197]

Treatment decisions should be based on the number of systems involved and on whether a particular lesion is likely to result in disability. Children with single-system disease, particularly if they have a solitary lesion of bone (e.g., eosinophilic granuloma of bone), may require no therapy other than curettage,[191] although there is ongoing debate as to whether this approach is superior to systemic treatment.[111,198] Many patients have aggressive disease, however, warranting treatment with multiagent chemotherapy.[100,199-201] In addition, multiple courses of treatment may be required for disease recurrences.[201-208] Rarely, aggressive approaches, such as bone marrow transplantation, are required for relapsed or refractory disease.[202,205,206,209]

Because unifocal bone disease is associated with a uniformly excellent prognosis,[111] therapy with potential late effects should be avoided. The surgical procedure required for diagnostic purposes often is definitively therapeutic as well.[210] Lesions other than those for which curettage is performed for diagnostic purposes often heal spontaneously.[211] Lesions in weight-bearing sites, such as the neck of the femur, may require curettage and autologous bone grafting. Direct steroid injection into the lesion has been used,[212] but the benefit of this treatment has never been proved in a randomized manner. Radiation therapy has been used with anecdotal success.[213,214] As a single modality, however, it is not adequate to prevent recurrence in most cases, and its use should be limited to clinical instances that require immediate mass decompression.[197,215] In addition, radiation therapy can have significant short- and long-term sequelae that do not justify its use in most cases.[213]

Isolated histiocytosis of the skin in infants usually regresses spontaneously and does not require systemic therapy.[6,128,216] Skin lesions in older children or adults may respond at least temporarily to phototherapy[217] topical therapies, such as imiquimod,[218] nitrogen mustard,[219] methotrexate,[220] and α-interferon.[221] Various systemic therapies have anecdotal success with skin lesions as well.[222] For refractory, cutaneous disease, radiation therapy has shown some efficacy.[223] *BRAF* inhibitors, such as vemurafenib and dabrafenib, and *MEK* inhibitors, such as trametinib, have shown promising results against lesions positive for the *BRAF-V600E* mutation.[224-227] Patients with cutaneous-only LCH need to be monitored for progression to systemic disease. Periodic radiographic imaging and testing of peripheral blood for the presence of *BRAF V600E* are suggested as the most effective methods to monitor these patients.[130]

Systemic therapy is required for multisystem disease and for single-system disease in which multiple bones are involved. Approximately 50% of patients requiring systemic therapy respond to corticosteroids alone.[228] Because of the toxicity of corticosteroids when used for more than brief periods, however, other chemotherapeutic agents are now the mainstay of management and are used in combination with lower cumulative doses of corticosteroids. Vinblastine, vincristine, 6-mercaptopurine, methotrexate, alkylating agents, anthracyclines, and etoposide, singly or in combinations, are effective in controlling LCH.[190] Patients with liver or bone marrow dysfunction as well as those at high risk for adverse CNS outcomes are best treated with combination chemotherapy. In a clinical trial in which patients were stratified by risk, treatment included induction chemotherapy with vinblastine, etoposide, and prednisone followed by maintenance chemotherapy with etoposide, vinblastine, prednisone, 6-mercaptopurine, and methotrexate.[172] Two-thirds of those patients with organ dysfunction achieved a complete remission, as did approximately 90% of those with either multisite bony disease or soft-tissue disease without organ dysfunction.

The Histiocyte Society has conducted several multinational randomized clinical trials in LCH.[105,229,230] In the first international trial (LCH I),[105] 143 patients were randomized to receive 24 weeks of vinblastine (6 mg/m² intravenously weekly) or etoposide (150 mg/m²/d intravenously for 3 days, every 3 weeks). All patients received 3 days of methylprednisolone. Both of those monotherapies had similar outcomes. Owing to the risk of secondary leukemias with etoposide, subsequent studies have been based on the vinblastine arm. One robust finding in this study was that the response at 6 weeks was strongly prognostic, regardless of initial treatment. However, LCH I did not produce superior results compared to studies from the German/Austrian group, DAL-HX 83 and DAL-HX 90.[231] Survival was similar, but the DAL-HX studies had superior reactivation rates and reactivation rate intervals and fewer permanent disabilities.[172,231]

The Histiocyte Society's LCH II trial demonstrated that intensified treatment increased early response in patients younger than 2 years with multisystem disease and risk organ involvement.[229] The study showed that the addition of etoposide to a regimen of vinblastine, prednisone, and daily 6-mercaptopurine reduced the risk of mortality for these patients. The LCH III trial evaluated the effect of adding methotrexate to the combination of vinblastine and prednisone for patients with "risk" organ involvement while treating all "risk" organ patients for 12 months, compared to the 6-month treatment regimens in LCH I and LCH II. This trial also evaluated therapy prolongation to 12 months for patients with "nonrisk" organs compared with 6 months of treatment. The study found that although the addition of methotrexate did not improve outcomes in patients at higher risk, therapy prolongation to 12 months produced a better outcome compared with historical controls. Patients without "risk" organ involvement who received 12 months of treatment also had improved outcomes compared with patients who received 6 months of treatment.[230] The current LCH IV trial is an all-encompassing study with seven treatment strata that is investigating optimal therapies and outcomes for single-site disease, multisite disease, low-risk recurrent disease, high-risk recurrent disease, bone marrow transplantation, neurodegeneration, and observation only (no treatment) in LCH.

Agents that have been evaluated for relapsed/refractory LCH include cladribine (2-chlorodeoxyadenosine).[208,232-236] In a phase 2 study, cladribine showed benefit in patients with reactivation of disease in nonrisk organs,[208] but cladribine proved no more beneficial than standard therapy for patients with multisystem disease and risk organ involvement. Cladribine monotherapy also has the benefit of a more favorable side effect profile compared to other agents, with the common effects of immunosuppression and bone marrow suppression with prolonged courses of therapy.[237] The combination of cladribine with other agents such as cytarabine or etoposide may be more effective for relapsed or refractory multisystem LCH involvement, but these agents carry the risk of more pronounced bone marrow suppression and hematologic toxicity.[203,204] Other agents that have shown promise in small patient series include clofarabine,[207,238,239] bisphosphonates,[240,241] indomethacin,[242,243] hydroxyurea,[244] and etanercept.[245] In a prospective, multicenter, phase II trial, clofarabine was found to be tolerated well and had an 82% 1-year PFS/OS. In the same trial, clofarabine was found to be efficacious in non-LCH histiocytosis.[246] Indomethacin inhibits the cyclooxygenase (COX) pathway, which may allow this drug to target LCH cells selectively because they strongly express COX-2.[247] Etanercept inhibits TNF-α, which is highly expressed in Langerhans cells, lymphocytes, and macrophages of LCH lesions, and promotes proliferation of Langerhans cells.[57,248] Finally, BRAF/MEK inhibitors, such as vemurafenib, dabrafenib, or trametinib, have been used as effective salvage therapy for refractory LCH, but they are usually unsuccessful in eradicating the disease without more intensive therapy.[226]

Treatment of LCH with CNS involvement is quite variable depending on whether mass lesions are present or if LCH-associated neurodegeneration has occurred.[249] In general, CNS mass lesions are treated per the current standards based on LCH III, which call for curettage of isolated lesions and corticosteroids and vinblastine and prednisone for multifocal lesions.[230] Patients who have "CNS-risk" bone lesions (sinuses, skull base, and orbit), parenchymal lesions, and pituitary lesions require systemic chemotherapy.[146,250] Neurodegeneration in LCH has no defined treatment plan and most of the therapies associated with it are aimed at halting progression of the disease. IVIG has immunomodulatory effects[251] and has been shown in multiple case reports to prevent further advancement of neurodegenerative symptoms.[252,253] Systemic chemotherapy also has efficacy in treating neurodegeneration. Cladribine has shown activity against CNS mass lesions,[143] but has not been studied extensively in neurodegeneration in LCH. Cytarabine is also a reasonable agent, as it has the ability to cross the blood-brain barrier and accumulate in the CSF.[254] Case reports have anecdotally noted improvement in neurodegenerative symptoms with IV cytarabine.[255,256] IVIG and cytarabine are being investigated as possible treatments for neurodegeneration and/or CNS LCH in the ongoing LCH IV clinical trial.

Several patients with recurrent, progressive LCH that is refractory to conventional therapy have benefited from allogeneic hematopoietic stem cell transplantation (HSCT).[202,205,206,257-261] Toxicity from HSCT in these patients has been an issue, however, with high rates of transplant-related mortality. A few patients have undergone HSCT with reduced-intensity conditioning with decreased transplant-related morbidity and mortality.[259] The most effective conditioning regimens and appropriate timing of HSCT are yet to be determined.

References

1. Hand A. General tuberculosis. *Trans Pathol Soc Phila*. 1893;16:282.
2. Writing group of the histiocyte society. Histiocytosis syndromes in children. *Lancet*. 1987;1:208-209.
3. Chu A, Favara BE, Ladisch S, Nezelof C, Prichard J. Report and recommendations of the workshop on the childhood histiocytoses: concepts and controversies. *Med Pediatr Oncol*. 1986;14:116-117.
4. Lichtenstein L. Histiocytosis X; integration of eosinophilic granuloma of bone, Letterer-Siwe disease, and Schuller-Christian disease as related manifestations of a single nosologic entity. *AMA Arch Pathol*. 1953;56:84-102.
5. Hashimoto K, Pritzker MS. Electron microscopic study of reticulohistiocytoma. An unusual case of congenital, self-healing reticulohistiocytosis. *Arch Dermatol*. 1973;107:263-270.
6. Hashimoto K, Griffin D, Kohsbaki M. Self-healing reticulohistiocytosis: a clinical, histologic, and ultrastructural study of the fourth case in the literature. *Cancer*. 1982;49:331-337.
7. Wolfson SL, Botero F, Hurwitz S, Pearson HA. "Pure" cutaneous histiocytosis-X. *Cancer*. 1981;48:2236-2238.
8. Donadieu J, Prichard J. Langerhans cell histiocytosis—400 BC? *Med Pediatr Oncol*. 1999;33:520.
9. Coppes-Zantinga A, Egeler RM. The Langerhans cell histiocytosis X files revealed. *Br J Haematol*. 2002;116:3-9.
10. Lampert F. Langerhans cell histiocytosis. Historical perspectives. *Hematol Oncol Clin North Am*. 1998;12:213-219.
11. Hand A. Polyuria and tuberculosis. *Arch Pediatr*. 1893;10:673-675.
12. Schüller A. Uber eigenartige schadeldefekte im jugendalter. *Fortschritte Auf der Gebiete Röntgenstrahlen*. 1915;23:12-18.
13. Christian HA. Defects in membranous bones, exophthalmos, and diabetes insipidus: an unusual syndrome of dyspituitarism. *Med Clin North Am*. 1920;3:849-871.
14. Komp DM. Historical perspectives of Langerhans cell histiocytosis. *Hematol Oncol Clin North Am*. 1987;1:9-21.
15. Hand A. Defects of membranous bones, exophthalmos and polyuria in childhood. *Am J Med Sci*. 1921;162:509-515.
16. Lieberman PH, Jones CR, Dargeon HW, Begg CF. A reappraisal of eosinophilic granuloma of bone, Hand-Schuller-Christian syndrome and Letterer-Siwe syndrome. *Medicine (Baltimore)*. 1969;48:375-400.
17. Letterer E. Aleukamische Retikulose (ein Beitrag zu den proliferativen Erkrankungen des Reticuloendothelialapparates). *Frankfurter Zeitchritte Pathol*. 1924;30:377-394.
18. Siwe SA. Die Reitiiculoendotheliose—ein neues Krankheitsbild unter den Hepatosplenomegalien. *Z Kinderheilk*. 1933;55:212-247.
19. Lichtenstein L, Jeffe HL. Eosinophilic granuloma of bone: with report of a case. *Am J Pathol*. 1940;16:595-604.3.
20. Otani S, Ehrlich JC. Solitary granuloma of bone: simulating primary neoplasm. *Am J Pathol*. 1940;16:479-490.7.
21. Farber S. The nature of solitary or eosinophilic granuloma of bone. *Am J Pathol*. 1941;17:625-629.
22. Green WT FS. "Eosinophilic or solitary granuloma" of bone. *J Bone Joint Surg Am*. 1942;24(3):499-526.
23. Nezelof C, Basset F, Rousseau MF. Histiocytosis X histogenetic arguments for a Langerhans cell origin. *Biomedicine*. 1973;18:365-371.
24. Risdall RJ, Dehner LP, Duray P, Kobrinsky N, Robinson L, Nesbit ME. Histiocytosis X (Langerhans' cell histiocytosis). Prognostic role of histopathology. *Arch Pathol Lab Med*. 1983;107:59-63.
25. Willman CL, Busque L, Griffith BB, et al. Langerhans'-cell histiocytosis (histiocytosis X): a clonal proliferative disease. *N Engl J Med*. 1994;331:154-160.

26. Yu RC, Chu AC, Chu C, Buluwela L. Clonal proliferation of Langerhans cells in Langerhans cell histiocytosis. *Lancet.* 1994;343:767-768.
27. Egeler RM, Katewa S, Leenen PJM, et al. Langerhans cell histiocytosis is a neoplasm and consequently its recurrence is a relapse: in memory of Bob Arceci. *Pediatr Blood Cancer.* 2016;63:1704-1712.
28. Guyot-Goubin A, Donadieu J, Barkaoui M, Bellec S, Thomas C, Clavel J. Descriptive epidemiology of childhood Langerhans cell histiocytosis in France, 2000-2004. *Pediatr Blood Cancer.* 2008;51:71-75.
29. Salotti JA, Nanduri V, Pearce MS, Parker L, Lynn R, Windebank KP. Incidence and clinical features of Langerhans cell histiocytosis in the UK and Ireland. *Arch Dis Child.* 2009;94:376-380.
30. Stalemark H, Laurencikas E, Karis J, Gavhed D, Fadeel B, Henter JI. Incidence of Langerhans cell histiocytosis in children: a population-based study. *Pediatr Blood Cancer.* 2008;51:76-81.
31. Hamre M, Hedberg J, Buckley J, et al. Langerhans cell histiocytosis: an exploratory epidemiologic study of 177 cases. *Med Pediatr Oncol.* 1997;28:92-97.
32. Baumgartner I, von Hochstetter A, Baumert B, Luetolf U, Follath F. Langerhans'-cell histiocytosis in adults. *Med Pediatr Oncol.* 1997;28:9-14.
33. Alston RD, Tatevossian RG, McNally RJQ, Kelsey A, Birch JM, Eden TOB. Incidence and survival of childhood Langerhans cell histiocytosis in Northwest England from 1954 to 1998. *Pediatr Blood Cancer.* 2007;48:555-560.
34. Komp DM, Herson J, Starling KA, Vietti TJ, Hvizdala E. A staging system for histiocytosis X: a southwest oncology group study. *Cancer.* 1981;47:798-800.
35. Nezelof C, Frileux-Herbet F, Cronier-Sachot J. Disseminated histiocytosis X: analysis of prognostic factors based on a retrospective study of 50 cases. *Cancer.* 1979;44:1824-1838.
36. Bhatia S, Nesbit ME, Egeler M, Buckley JD, Mertens A, Robison LL. Epidemiologic study of Langerhans cell histiocytosis in children. *J Pediatr.* 1997;130:774-784.
37. Arico M, Nichols K, Whitlock JA, et al. Familial clustering of Langerhans cell histiocytosis. *Br J Haematol.* 1999;107:883-888.
38. Egeler RM, Neglia JP, Aricò M, et al. The relation of Langerhans cell histiocytosis to acute leukemia, lymphomas, and other solid tumors. The LCH-Malignancy Study Group of the Histiocyte Society. *Hematol Oncol Clin North Am.* 1998;12:369-378.
39. Chiles LR, Christian MM, McCoy DK, Hawkins HK, Yen AH, Raimer SS. Langerhans cell histiocytosis in a child while in remission for acute lymphocytic leukemia. *J Am Acad Dermatol.* 2001;45:S233-S234.
40. Kager L, Heise A, Minkov M, et al. Occurrence of acute nonlymphoblastic leukemia in two girls after treatment of recurrent, disseminated Langerhans cell histiocytosis. *Pediatr Hematol Oncol.* 1999;16:251-256.
41. Raj A, Bendon R, Moriarty T, Suarez C, Bertolone S. Langerhans cell histiocytosis following childhood acute lymphoblastic leukemia. *Am J Hematol.* 2001;68:284-286.
42. Trebo MM, Attarbaschi A, Mann G, Minkov M, Kornmüller R, Gadner H. Histiocytosis following T-acute lymphoblastic leukemia: a BFM study. *Leuk Lymphoma.* 2005;46:1735-1741.
43. Betts DR, Leibundgut K, Feldges A, Plüss H, Niggli F. Cytogenetic abnormalities in Langerhans cell histiocytosis. *Br J Cancer.* 1998;77:552-555.
44. Murakami I, Gogusev J, Fournet JC, Glorion C, Jaubert F. Detection of molecular cytogenetic aberrations in langerhans cell histiocytosis of bone. *Hum Pathol.* 2002;33:555-560.
45. Scappaticci S, Danesino C, Rossi E, et al. Cytogenetic abnormalities in PHA-stimulated lymphocytes from patients with Langerhans cell histiocytosis. *Br J Haematol.* 2000;111:258-262.
46. Favara BE, Jaffe R. The histopathology of Langerhans cell histiocytosis. *Br J Cancer Suppl.* 1994;23:S17-S23.
47. Reid CD, Fryer P, Clifford C, Kirk A, Tikerpae J, Knight S. Identification of hematopoietic progenitors of macrophages and dendritic Langerhans cells (DL-CFU) in human bone marrow and peripheral blood. *Blood.* 1990;76:1139-1149.
48. Choi KL, Sauder DN. The role of Langerhans cells and keratinocytes in epidermal immunity. *J Leukoc Biol.* 1986;39:343-358.
49. Favara BE, McCarthy RC, Mierau GW. Histiocytosis X. *Hum Pathol.* 1983;14:663-676.
50. Birbeck M, Breathnach A, Everall J. An electron microscope study of basal melanocytes and high-level clear cells (langerhans cells) in vitiligo. *J Invest Dermatol.* 1961;37:51-64.
51. Mierau GW, Favara BE, Brenman JM. Electron microscopy in histiocytosis X. *Ultrastruct Pathol.* 1982;3:137-142.
52. Lau SK, Chu PG, Weiss LM. Immunohistochemical expression of Langerin in Langerhans cell histiocytosis and non-Langerhans cell histiocytic disorders. *Am J Surg Pathol.* 2008;32:615-619.
53. Valladeau J, Ravel O, Dezutter-Dambuyant C, et al. Langerin, a novel C-type lectin specific to langerhans cells, is an endocytic receptor that induces the formation of Birbeck granules. *Immunity.* 2000;12:71-81.
54. Rowden G. Expression of Ia antigens on Langerhans cells in mice, Guinea pigs, and man. *J Invest Dermatol.* 1980;75:22-31.
55. Bouloc A, Boulland ML, Geissmann F, et al. CD101 expression by Langerhans cell histiocytosis cells. *Histopathology.* 2000;36:229-232.
56. Chu T, Jaffe R. The normal Langerhans cell and the LCH cell. *Br J Cancer Suppl.* 1994;23:S4-S10.
57. Geissmann F, Lepelletier Y, Fraitag S, et al. Differentiation of Langerhans cells in Langerhans cell histiocytosis. *Blood.* 2001;97:1241-1248.
58. Allen CE, Li L, Peters TL, et al. Cell-specific gene expression in Langerhans cell histiocytosis lesions reveals a distinct profile compared with epidermal Langerhans cells. *J Immunol.* 2010;184:4557-4567.
59. Annels NE, da Costa CET, Prins FA, Willemze R, Hogendoorn PCW, Egeler RM. Aberrant chemokine receptor expression and chemokine production by Langerhans cells underlies the pathogenesis of Langerhans cell histiocytosis. *J Exp Med.* 2003;197:1385-1390.
60. Egeler RM, Favara BE, Laman JD, Claassen E. Abundant expression of CD40 and CD40-ligand (CD154) in paediatric Langerhans cell histiocytosis lesions. *Eur J Cancer.* 2000;36:2105-2110.
61. de Graaf JH, Tamminga RY, Kamps WA, Timens W. Expression of cellular adhesion molecules in Langerhans cell histiocytosis and normal Langerhans cells. *Am J Pathol.* 1995;147:1161-1171.
62. Yu RC, Alaibac M, Chu AC. Functional defect in cells involved in Langerhans cell histiocytosis. *Arch Dermatol Res.* 1995;287:627-631.
63. Leikin SL. Immunobiology of histiocytosis-X. *Hematol Oncol Clin North Am.* 1987;1:49-61.
64. Nesbit ME, Jr, O'Leary M, Dehner LP, Ramsay NK. The immune system and the histiocytosis syndromes. *Am J Pediatr Hematol Oncol.* 1981;3:141-149.
65. Newton WA, Jr, Hamoudi AB, Shannon BT. Role of the thymus in histiocytosis-X. *Hematol Oncol Clin North Am.* 1987;1:63-74.
66. Osband ME, Lipton JM, Lavin P, et al. Histiocytosis-X. *N Engl J Med.* 1981;304:146-153.
67. Bove KE, Hurtubise P, Wong KY. Thymus in untreated systemic histiocytosis X. *Pediatr Pathol.* 1985;4:99-115.
68. Shannon BT, Newton WA. Suppressor-cell dysfunction in children with histiocytosis-X. *J Clin Immunol.* 1986;6:510-518.
69. Lahey ME, Heyn R, Ladisch S, et al. Hypergammaglobulinemia in histiocytosis X. *J Pediatr.* 1985;107:572-574.
70. Kragballe K, Zachariae H, Herlin T, Jensen J. Histiocytosis X: an immune deficiency disease? Studies on antibody-dependent monocyte-mediated cytotoxicity. *Br J Dermatol.* 1981;105:13-18.
71. Leikin S, Puruganan G, Frankel A, Steerman R, Chandra R. Immunologic parameters in histiocytosis-X. *Cancer.* 1973;32:796-802.
72. Ishii R, Morimoto A, Ikushima S, et al. High serum values of soluble CD154, IL-2 receptor, RANKL and osteoprotegerin in Langerhans cell histiocytosis. *Pediatr Blood Cancer.* 2006;47:194-199.
73. Kannourakis G, Abbas A. The role of cytokines in the pathogenesis of Langerhans cell histiocytosis. *Br J Cancer Suppl.* 1994;23:S37-S40.
74. Arenzana-Seisdedos F, Barbey S, Virelizier JL, Kornprobst M, Nezelof C. Histiocytosis X. Purified (T6+) cells from bone granuloma produce interleukin 1 and prostaglandin E2 in culture. *J Clin Invest.* 1986;77:326-329.
75. Brown RE. Angiotensin-converting enzyme, transforming growth factor beta(1), and interleukin 11 in the osteolytic lesions of Langerhans cell histiocytosis. *Arch Pathol Lab Med.* 2000;124:1287-1290.
76. Andersson By U, Tani E, Andersson U, Henter JI. Tumor necrosis factor, interleukin 11, and leukemia inhibitory factor produced by Langerhans cells in Langerhans cell histiocytosis. *J Pediatr Hematol Oncol.* 2004;26:706-711.
77. Emile JF, Fraitag S, Andry P, Leborgne M, Lellouch-Tubiana A, Brousse N. Expression of GM-CSF receptor by Langerhans' cell histiocytosis cells. *Virchows Arch.* 1995;427:125-129.
78. McClain K, Jin H, Gresik V, Favara B. Langerhans cell histiocytosis: lack of a viral etiology. *Am J Hematol.* 1994;47:16-20.
79. Mierau GW, Wills EJ, Steele PO. Ultrastructural studies in Langerhans cell histiocytosis: a search for evidence of viral etiology. *Pediatr Pathol.* 1994;14:895-904.
80. Edgar JD, Smyth AE, Pritchard J, et al. Interferon-gamma receptor deficiency mimicking Langerhans' cell histiocytosis. *J Pediatr.* 2001;139:600-603.
81. Komp DM. Langerhans cell histiocytosis. *N Engl J Med.* 1987;316:747-748.
82. Yousem SA, Colby TV, Chen YY, Chen WG, Weiss LM. Pulmonary Langerhans' cell histiocytosis: molecular analysis of clonality. *Am J Surg Pathol.* 2001;25:630-636.
83. Abla O, Weitzman S. Treatment of Langerhans cell histiocytosis: role of BRAF/MAPK inhibition. *Hematology Am Soc Hematol Educ Program.* 2015;2015:565-570.
84. Allen CE, Parsons DW. Biological and clinical significance of somatic mutations in Langerhans cell histiocytosis and related histiocytic neoplastic disorders. *Hematology Am Soc Hematol Educ Program.* 2015;2015:559-564.
85. Berres ML, Lim KPH, Peters T, et al. BRAF-V600E expression in precursor versus differentiated dendritic cells defines clinically distinct LCH risk groups. *J Exp Med.* 2014;211:669-683.
86. Berres ML, Merad M, Allen CE. Progress in understanding the pathogenesis of Langerhans cell histiocytosis: back to Histiocytosis X? *Br J Haematol.* 2015;169:3-13.
87. Chakraborty R, Hampton OA, Shen X, et al. Mutually exclusive recurrent somatic mutations in MAP2K1 and BRAF support a central role for ERK activation in LCH pathogenesis. *Blood.* 2014;124:3007-3015.
88. Emile JF, Abla O, Fraitag S, et al. Revised classification of histiocytoses and neoplasms of the macrophage-dendritic cell lineages. *Blood.* 2016;127:2672-2681.
89. Gatalica Z, Bilalovic N, Palazzo JP, et al. Disseminated histiocytoses biomarkers beyond BRAFV600E: frequent expression of PD-L1. *Oncotarget.* 2015;6:19819-19825.
90. Heritier S, Jehanne M, Leverger G, et al. Vemurafenib use in an infant for high-risk langerhans cell histiocytosis. *JAMA Oncol.* 2015;1:836-838.
91. Hutter C, Minkov M. Insights into the pathogenesis of Langerhans cell histiocytosis: the development of targeted therapies. *ImmunoTargets Ther.* 2016;5:81-91.
92. Nelson DS, Halteren A, Quispel WT, et al. MAP2K1 and MAP3K1 mutations in Langerhans cell histiocytosis. *Genes Chromosomes Cancer.* 2015;54:361-368.
93. Rollins BJ. Genomic alterations in langerhans cell histiocytosis. *Hematol Oncol Clin North Am.* 2015;29:839-851.
94. Swerdlow SH, Campo E, Pileri SA, et al. The 2016 revision of the World Health Organization classification of lymphoid neoplasms. *Blood.* 2016;127:2375-2390.
95. Badalian-Very G, Vergilio JA, Degar BA, et al. Recurrent BRAF mutations in Langerhans cell histiocytosis. *Blood.* 2010;116:1919-1923.

96. Chakraborty R, Burke TM, Hampton OA, et al. Alternative genetic mechanisms of BRAF activation in Langerhans cell histiocytosis. *Blood.* 2016;128:2533-2537.
97. Heritier S, Emile JF, Barkaoui MA, et al. BRAF mutation correlates with high-risk langerhans cell histiocytosis and increased resistance to first-line therapy. *J Clin Oncol.* 2016;34:3023-3030.
98. Brown RE. Brief communication: morphoproteomic analysis of osteolytic Langerhans cell histiocytosis with therapeutic implications. *Ann Clin Lab Sci.* 2005;35:131-136.
99. Arceci RJ, Allen CE, Dunkel IJ, et al. A phase IIa study of afuresertib, an oral pan-AKT inhibitor, in patients with Langerhans cell histiocytosis. *Pediatr Blood Cancer.* 2017;64(5). doi:10.1002/pbc.26325.
100. Arico M. Langerhans cell histiocytosis in children: from the bench to bedside for an updated therapy. *Br J Haematol.* 2016;173:663-670.
101. Zinn DJ, Chakraborty R, Allen CE. Langerhans cell histiocytosis: emerging insights and clinical implications. *Oncology (Williston Park).* 2016;30:122-132. 139.
102. Jubran RF, Marachelian A, Dorey F, Malogolowkin M. Predictors of outcome in children with Langerhans cell histiocytosis. *Pediatr Blood Cancer.* 2005;45:37-42.
103. Matus-Ridley M, Raney RB, Thawerani H, Meadows AT. Histiocytosis X in children: patterns of disease and results of treatment. *Med Pediatr Oncol.* 1983;11:99-105.
104. Islinger RB, Kuklo TR, Owens BD, et al. Langerhans' cell histiocytosis in patients older than 21 years. *Clin Orthop Relat Res.* 2000;379:231-235.
105. Gadner H, Grois N, Arico M, et al. A randomized trial of treatment for multisystem Langerhans' cell histiocytosis. *J Pediatr.* 2001;138:728-734.
106. Braier J, Latella A, Balancini B, et al. Outcome in children with pulmonary Langerhans cell Histiocytosis. *Pediatr Blood Cancer.* 2004;43:765-769.
107. Odame I, Li P, Lau L, et al. Pulmonary Langerhans cell histiocytosis: a variable disease in childhood. *Pediatr Blood Cancer.* 2006;47:889-893.
108. Ronceray L, Pötschger U, Janka G, Gadner H, Minkov M. Pulmonary involvement in pediatric-onset multisystem Langerhans cell histiocytosis: effect on course and outcome. *J Pediatr.* 2012;161:129-133.e1-3.
109. Howarth DM, Gilchrist GS, Mullan BP, et al. Langerhans cell histiocytosis: diagnosis, natural history, management, and outcome. *Cancer.* 1999;85:2278-2290.
110. Kilpatrick SE, Wenger DE, Gilchrist GS, Shives TC, Wollan PC, Unni KK. Langerhans' cell histiocytosis (histiocytosis X) of bone. A clinicopathologic analysis of 263 pediatric and adult cases. *Cancer.* 1995;76:2471-2484.
111. Titgemeyer C, Grois N, Minkov M, Flucher-Wolfram B, Gatterer-Menz I, Gadner H. Pattern and course of single-system disease in Langerhans cell histiocytosis data from the DAL-HX 83- and 90-study. *Med Pediatr Oncol.* 2001;37:108-114.
112. Hartman KS. Histiocytosis X: a review of 114 cases with oral involvement. *Oral Surg Oral Med Oral Pathol.* 1980;49:38-54.
113. Smith RJ, Evans JN. Head and neck manifestations of histiocytosis-X. *Laryngoscope.* 1984;94:395-399.
114. Yeom JS, Lee CK, Shin HY, Lee CS, Han CS, Chang H. Langerhans' cell histiocytosis of the spine. Analysis of twenty-three cases. *Spine.* 1999;24:1740-1749.
115. Grois N, Pötschger U, Prosch H, et al. Risk factors for diabetes insipidus in langerhans cell histiocytosis. *Pediatr Blood Cancer.* 2006;46:228-233.
116. Haupt R, Nanduri V, Calevo MG, et al. Permanent consequences in langerhans cell histiocytosis patients: a pilot study from the histiocyte society-late effects study group. *Pediatr Blood Cancer.* 2004;42:438-444.
117. Azouz EM, Saigal G, Rodriguez MM, Podda A. Langerhans' cell histiocytosis: pathology, imaging and treatment of skeletal involvement. *Pediatr Radiol.* 2005;35:103-115.
118. Moore JB, Kulkarni R, Crutcher DC, Bhimani S. MRI in multifocal eosinophilic granuloma: staging disease and monitoring response to therapy. *Am J Pediatr Hematol Oncol.* 1989;11:174-177.
119. Crone-Munzebrock W, Brassow F. A comparison of radiographic and bone scan findings in histiocytosis X. *Skeletal Radiol.* 1983;9:170-173.
120. Parker BR, Pinckney L, Etcubanas E. Relative efficacy of radiographic and radionuclide bone surveys in the detection of the skeletal lesions of histiocytosis X. *Radiology.* 1980;134:377-380.
121. Siddiqui AR, Tashjian JH, Lazarus K, Wellman HN, Baehner RL. Nuclear medicine studies in evaluation of skeletal lesions in children with histiocytosis X. *Radiology.* 1981;140:787-789.
122. Dogan AS, Conway JJ, Miller JH, Grier D, Bhattathiry MM, Mitchell CS. Detection of bone lesions in Langerhans cell histiocytosis: complementary roles of scintigraphy and conventional radiography. *J Pediatr Hematol Oncol.* 1996;18:51-58.
123. Van Nieuwenhuyse JP, Clapuyt P, Malghem J, et al. Radiographic skeletal survey and radionuclide bone scan in Langerhans cell histiocytosis of bone. *Pediatr Radiol.* 1996;26:734-738.
124. Binkovitz LA, Olshefski RS, Adler BH. Coincidence FDG-PET in the evaluation of Langerhans' cell histiocytosis: preliminary findings. *Pediatr Radiol.* 2003;33:598-602.
125. Phillips M, Allen C, Gerson P, McClain K. Comparison of FDG-PET scans to conventional radiography and bone scans in management of Langerhans cell histiocytosis. *Pediatr Blood Cancer.* 2009;52:97-101.
126. Winkelmann RK. The skin in histiocytosis X. *Mayo Clin Proc.* 1969;44:535-548.
127. Lau L, Krafchik B, Trebo MM, Weitzman S. Cutaneous Langerhans cell histiocytosis in children under one year. *Pediatr Blood Cancer.* 2006;46:66-71.
128. Kanitakis J, Zambruno G, Schmitt D, Cambazard F, Jacquemier D, Thivolet J. Congenital self-healing histiocytosis (Hashimoto-Pritzker). An ultrastructural and immunohistochemical study. *Cancer.* 1988;61:508-516.
129. Kapur P, Erickson C, Rakheja D, Carder KR, Hoang MP. Congenital self-healing reticulohistiocytosis (Hashimoto-Pritzker disease): ten-year experience at Dallas Children's Medical Center. *J Am Acad Dermatol.* 2007;56:290-294.
130. Simko SJ, Garmezy B, Abhyankar H, et al. Differentiating skin-limited and multisystem Langerhans cell histiocytosis. *J Pediatr.* 2014;165:990-996.
131. Barthez MA, Araujo E, Donadieu J. Langerhans cell histiocytosis and the central nervous system in childhood: evolution and prognostic factors. Results of a collaborative study. *J Child Neurol.* 2000;15:150-156.
132. Grois N, Fahrner B, Arceci RJ, et al. Central nervous system disease in Langerhans cell histiocytosis. *J Pediatr* 2010;156:873-881.e1.
133. Rothman JG, Snyder PJ, Utiger RD. Hypothalamic endocrinopathy in Hand-Schuller-Christian disease. *Ann Intern Med.* 1978;88:512-513.
134. Grois N, Barkovich AJ, Rosenau W, Ablin AR. Central nervous system disease associated with Langerhans' cell histiocytosis. *Am J Pediatr Hematol Oncol.* 1993;15:245-254.
135. Shuper A, Stark B, Yaniv Y, et al. Cerebellar involvement in Langerhans' cell histiocytosis: a progressive neuropsychiatric disease. *J Child Neurol.* 2000;15:824-826.
136. Whitsett SF, Kneppers K, Coppes MJ, Egeler RM. Neuropsychologic deficits in children with Langerhans cell histiocytosis. *Med Pediatr Oncol.* 1999;33:486-492.
137. Mittheisz E, Seidl R, Prayer D, et al. Central nervous system-related permanent consequences in patients with Langerhans cell histiocytosis. *Pediatr Blood Cancer.* 2007;48:50-56.
138. Dunger DB, Broadbent V, Yeoman E, et al. The frequency and natural history of diabetes insipidus in children with Langerhans-cell histiocytosis. *N Engl J Med.* 1989;321:1157-1162.
139. Wnorowski M, Prosch H, Prayer D, Janssen G, Gadner H, Grois N. Pattern and course of neurodegeneration in Langerhans cell histiocytosis. *J Pediatr.* 2008;153:127-132.
140. Martin-Duverneuil N, Idbaih A, Hoang-Xuan K, et al. MRI features of neurodegenerative Langerhans cell histiocytosis. *Eur Radiol.* 2006;16:2074-2082.
141. Prayer D, Grois N, Prosch H, Gadner H, Barkovich AJ. MR imaging presentation of intracranial disease associated with Langerhans cell histiocytosis. *AJNR Am J Neuroradiol.* 2004;25:880-891.
142. Prosch H, Grois N, Wnorowski M, Steiner M, Prayer D. Long-term MR imaging course of neurodegenerative Langerhans cell histiocytosis. *AJNR Am J Neuroradiol.* 2007;28:1022-1028.
143. Buchler T, Cervinek L, Belohlavek O, et al. Langerhans cell histiocytosis with central nervous system involvement: follow-up by FDG-PET during treatment with cladribine. *Pediatr Blood Cancer.* 2005;44:286-288.
144. Calming U, Bemstrand C, Mosskin M, Elander SS, Ingvar M, Henter JI. Brain 18-FDG PET scan in central nervous system langerhans cell histiocytosis. *J Pediatr.* 2002;141:435-440.
145. Ribeiro MJ, Idbaih A, Thomas C, et al. 18F-FDG PET in neurodegenerative Langerhans cell histiocytosis: results and potential interest for an early diagnosis of the disease. *J Neurol.* 2008;255:575-580.
146. Grois N, Tsunematsu Y, Barkovich AJ, et al. Central nervous system disease in Langerhans cell histiocytosis. *Br J Cancer Suppl.* 1994;23:S24-S28.
147. Imashuku S, Ishida S, Koike K, et al. Cerebellar ataxia in pediatric patients with Langerhans cell histiocytosis. *J Pediatr Hematol Oncol.* 2004;26:735-739.
148. Nanduri VR, Lillywhite L, Chapman C, Parry L, Pritchard J, Vargha-Khadem F. Cognitive outcome of long-term survivors of multisystem langerhans cell histiocytosis: a single-institution, cross-sectional study. *J Clin Oncol.* 2003;21:2961-2967.
149. Porto L, Schöning S, Hattingen E, Sörensen J, Jurcoane A, Lehrnbecher T. Central nervous system imaging in childhood Langerhans cell histiocytosis—a reference center analysis. *Radiol Oncol.* 2015;49:242-249.
150. Van't Hooft I, Gavhed D, Laurencikas E, Henter JI. Neuropsychological sequelae in patients with neurodegenerative Langerhans cell histiocytosis. *Pediatr Blood Cancer.* 2008;51:669-674.
151. Grois N, Prayer D, Prosch H, Lassmann H; CNS LCH Co-operative Group. Neuropathology of CNS disease in Langerhans cell histiocytosis. *Brain.* 2005;128:829-838.
152. Gavhed D, Laurencikas E, Åkefeldt SO, Henter JI. Fifteen years of treatment with intravenous immunoglobulin in central nervous system Langerhans cell histiocytosis. *Acta Paediatr.* 2011;100:e36-e39.
153. Allen CE, Flores R, Rauch R, et al. Neurodegenerative central nervous system Langerhans cell histiocytosis and coincident hydrocephalus treated with vincristine/cytosine arabinoside. *Pediatr Blood Cancer.* 2010;54:416-423.
154. Sieni E, Barba C, Mortilla M, et al. Early diagnosis and monitoring of neurodegenerative langerhans cell histiocytosis. *PLoS One.* 2015;10:e0131635.
155. Nanduri VR, Bareille P, Pritchard J, Stanhope R. Growth and endocrine disorders in multisystem Langerhans' cell histiocytosis. *Clin Endocrinol.* 2000;53:509-515.
156. Maghnie M, Cosi G, Genovese E, et al. Central diabetes insipidus in children and young adults. *N Engl J Med.* 2000;343:998-1007.
157. Braunstein GD, Kohler PO. Endocrine manifestations of histiocytosis. *Am J Pediatr Hematol Oncol.* 1981;3:67-75.
158. Grois N, Flucher-Wolfram B, Heitger A, Mostbeck GH, Hofmann J, Gadner H. Diabetes insipidus in langerhans cell histiocytosi: results from the DAL-HX 83 study. *Med Pediatr Oncol.* 1995;24:248-256.
159. Leger J, Velasquez A, Garel C, Hassan M, Czernichow P. Thickened pituitary stalk on magnetic resonance imaging in children with central diabetes insipidus. *J Clin Endocrinol Metab.* 1999;84:1954-1960.
160. Marchand I, Barkaoui MA, Garel C, Polak M, Donadieu J. Central diabetes insipidus as the inaugural manifestation of Langerhans cell histiocytosis: natural history and medical evaluation of 26 children and adolescents. *J Clin Endocrinol Metab.* 2011;96:E1352-E1360.
161. Prosch H, Grois N, Prayer D, et al. Central diabetes insipidus as presenting symptom of Langerhans cell histiocytosis. *Pediatr Blood Cancer.* 2004;43:594-599.
162. Helbock H, Krivit W, Nesbit ME, Jr. Patterns of anti-diuretic function in diabetes insipidus caused by histiocytosis X. *J Lab Clin Med.* 1971;78:194-202.

163. Abla O, Palmert MR. Reversal of LCH-related diabetes insipidus and reappearance of posterior pituitary bright spot with low-dose chemotherapy. *Pediatr Blood Cancer.* 2012;59:201-202.
164. Ottaviano F, Finlay JL. Diabetes insipidus and Langerhans cell histiocytosis: a case report of reversibility with 2-chlorodeoxyadenosine. *J Pediatr Hematol Oncol.* 2003;25:575-577.
165. Dean HJ, Bishop A, Winter JS. Growth hormone deficiency in patients with histiocytosis X. *J Pediatr.* 1986;109:615-618.
166. Howell SJ, Wilton P, Shalet SM. Growth hormone replacement in patients with Langerhan's cell histiocytosis. *Arch Dis Child.* 1998;78:469-473.
167. Lahey ME, Rallison ML, Hilding DA, Ater J. Involvement of the thyroid in histiocytosis X. *Am J Pediatr Hematol Oncol.* 1986;8:257-259.
168. Patten DK, Wani Z, Tolley N. Solitary langerhans histiocytosis of the thyroid gland: a case report and literature review. *Head and Neck Pathology.* 2012;6:279-289.
169. Braier J, Ciocca M, Latella A, de Davila MG, Drajer M, Inventarza O. Cholestasis, sclerosing cholangitis, and liver transplantation in Langerhans cell Histiocytosis. *Med Pediatr Oncol.* 2002;38:178-182.
170. Heyn RM, Hamoudi A, Newton WA, Jr. Pretreatment liver biopsy in 20 children with histiocytosis X: a clinicopathologic correlation. *Med Pediatr Oncol.* 1990;18:110-118.
171. Leblanc A, Hadchouel M, Jehan P, Odièvre M, Alagille D. Obstructive jaundice in children with histiocytosis X. *Gastroenterology.* 1981;80:134-139.
172. Gadner H, Heitger A, Grois N, Gatterer-Menz I, Ladisch S. Treatment strategy for disseminated Langerhans cell histiocytosis. DAL HX-83 Study Group. *Med Pediatr Oncol.* 1994;23:72-80.
173. Carlson RA, Hattery RR, O'Connell EJ, Fontana RS. Pulmonary involvement by histiocytosis X in the pediatric age group. *Mayo Clin Proc.* 1976;51:542-547.
174. Basset F, Corrin B, Spencer H, et al. Pulmonary histiocytosis X. *Am Rev Respir Dis.* 1978;118:811-820.
175. Friedman PJ, Liebow AA, Sokoloff J. Eosinophilic granuloma of lung. Clinical aspects of primary histiocytosis in the adult. *Medicine (Baltimore).* 1981;60:385-396.
176. Marcy TW, Reynolds HY. Pulmonary histiocytosis X. *Lung.* 1985;163:129-150.
177. Vassallo R, Ryu JH, Schroeder DR, Decker PA, Limper AH. Clinical outcomes of pulmonary Langerhans'-cell histiocytosis in adults. *N Engl J Med.* 2002;346:484-490.
178. Bernstrand C, Cederlund K, Ashtröm L, Henter JI. Smoking preceded pulmonary involvement in adults with pulmonary Langerhans cell histiocytosis diagnosed in childhood. *Acta Paediatr.* 2000;89:1389-1392.
179. Watanabe R, Tatsumi K, Hashimoto S, Tamakoshi A, Kuriyama T, The Respiratory Failure Research Group of Japan. Clinico-epidemiological features of pulmonary histiocytosis X. *Intern Med.* 2001;40:998-1003.
180. Nondahl SR, Finlay JL, Farrell PM, Warner TF, Hong R. A case report and literature review of "primary" pulmonary histiocytosis X of childhood. *Med Pediatr Oncol.* 1986;14:57-62.
181. Lewis JG. Eosinophilic granuloma and its variants with special reference to lung involvement. A report of 12 patients. *Q J Med.* 1964;33:337-359.
182. Roland AS, Merdinger WF, Froeb HF. Recurrent spontaneous pneumothorax; a clue to the diagnosis of histiocytosis X. *N Engl J Med.* 1964;270:73-77.
183. Bernstrand C, Cederlund K, Sandstedt B, et al. Pulmonary abnormalities at long-term follow-up of patients with Langerhans cell histiocytosis. *Med Pediatr Oncol.* 2001;36:459-468.
184. Berry DH, Gresik MV, Humphrey GB, et al. Natural history of histiocytosis X: a pediatric oncology group study. *Med Pediatr Oncol.* 1986;14:1-5.
185. Favara BE, Jaffe R, Egeler RM. Macrophage activation and hemophagocytic syndrome in langerhans cell histiocytosis: report of 30 cases. *Pediatr Dev Pathol.* 2002;5:130-140.
186. Jaffe RW, Weiss LM, Facchetti F. Tumors derived from Langerhans cells. In: Swerdlow SH, Campo E, Harris NL, et al., eds. *WHO Classification of Tumors of Hematopoietic and Lymphoid Tissues.* IARC Press; 2008:358-360.
187. Haupt R, Minkov M, Astigarraga I, et al. Langerhans cell histiocytosis (LCH): guidelines for diagnosis, clinical work-up, and treatment for patients till the age of 18 years. *Pediatr Blood Cancer.* 2013;60:175-184.
188. Al-Trabolsi HA, Alshehri M, Al-Shomrani A, Shabanah M, Al-Barki AA. "Primary" pulmonary Langerhans cell histiocytosis in a two-year-old child: case report and literature review. *J Pediatr Hematol Oncol.* 2006;28:79-81.
189. Lastoria S, Montella L, Catalano L, Rotoli B, Muto P, Palmieri G. Functional imaging of Langerhans cell histiocytosis by (111)In-DTPA-D-Phe(1)-octreotide scintigraphy. *Cancer.* 2002;94:633-640.
190. Minkov M. Multisystem Langerhans cell histiocytosis in children: current treatment and future directions. *Paediatr Drugs.* 2011;13:75-86.
191. Berry DH, Gresik M, Maybee D, Marcus R. Histiocytosis X in bone only. *Med Pediatr Oncol.* 1990;18:292-294.
192. Bernstrand C, Sandstedt B, Åhström L, Henter JI. Long-term follow-up of Langerhans cell histiocytosis: 39 years' experience at a single centre. *Acta Paediatr.* 2007;94:1073-1084.
193. Willis B, Ablin A, Weinberg V, Zoger S, Wara WM, Matthay KK. Disease course and late sequelae of Langerhans' cell histiocytosis: 25-year experience at the University of California, San Francisco. *J Clin Oncol.* 1996;14:2073-2082.
194. Rigaud C, Barkaoui MA, Thomas C, et al. Langerhans cell histiocytosis: therapeutic strategy and outcome in a 30-year nationwide cohort of 1478 patients under 18 years of age. *Br J Haematol.* 2016;174:887-898.
195. Pollono D, Rey G, Latella A, Rosso D, Chantada G, Braier J. Reactivation and risk of sequelae in Langerhans cell histiocytosis. *Pediatr Blood Cancer.* 2007;48:696-699.
196. Cassady JR. Current role of radiation therapy in the management of histiocytosis-X. *Hematol Oncol Clin North Am.* 1987;1:123-129.
197. Selch MT, Parker RG. Radiation therapy in the management of Langerhans cell histiocytosis. *Med Pediatr Oncol.* 1990;18:97-102.
198. Chellapandian D, Shaikh F, van den Bos C, et al. Management and outcome of patients with langerhans cell histiocytosis and single-bone CNS-risk lesions: a multi-institutional retrospective study. *Pediatr Blood Cancer.* 2015;62:2162-2166.
199. Allen CE, Ladisch S, McClain KL. How I treat Langerhans cell histiocytosis. *Blood.* 2015;126:26-35.
200. Arico M, Astigarraga I, Braier J, et al. Lack of bone lesions at diagnosis is associated with inferior outcome in multisystem langerhans cell histiocytosis of childhood. *Br J Haematol.* 2015;169:241-248.
201. Uppuluri R, Ramachandrakurup S, Subburaj D, Bakane A, Raj R. Excellent remission rates with limited toxicity in relapsed/refractory Langerhans cell histiocytosis with pulse dexamethasone and lenalidomide in children. *Pediatr Blood Cancer.* 2017;64:110-112.
202. Akkari V, Donadieu J, Piguet C, et al. Hematopoietic stem cell transplantation in patients with severe Langerhans cell histiocytosis and hematological dysfunction: experience of the French Langerhans Cell Study Group. *Bone Marrow Transplant.* 2003;31:1097-1103.
203. Bernard F, Thomas C, Bertrand Y, et al. Multi-centre pilot study of 2-chlorodeoxyadenosine and cytosine arabinoside combined chemotherapy in refractory Langerhans cell histiocytosis with haematological dysfunction. *Eur J Cancer.* 2005;41:2682-2689.
204. Donadieu J, Bernard F, van Noesel M, et al. Cladribine and cytarabine in refractory multisystem Langerhans cell histiocytosis: results of an international phase 2 study. *Blood.* 2015;126:1415-1423.
205. Kinugawa N, Imashuku S, Hirota Y, et al. Hematopoietic stem cell transplantation (HSCT) for Langerhans cell histiocytosis (LCH) in Japan. *Bone Marrow Transplant.* 1999;24:935-938.
206. Nagarajan R, Neglia J, Ramsay N, Baker KS. Successful treatment of refractory Langerhans cell histiocytosis with unrelated cord blood transplantation. *J Pediatr Hematol Oncol.* 2001;23:629-632.
207. Rodriguez-Galindo C, Jeng M, Khuu P, McCarville MB, Jeha S. Clofarabine in refractory Langerhans cell histiocytosis. *Pediatr Blood Cancer.* 2008;51:703-706.
208. Stine KC, Saylors RL, Williams LL, Becton DL. 2-Chlorodeoxyadenosine (2-CDA) for the treatment of refractory or recurrent Langerhans cell histiocytosis (LCH) in pediatric patients. *Med Pediatr Oncol.* 1997;29:288-292.
209. Veys PA, Nanduri V, Baker KS, et al. Haematopoietic stem cell transplantation for refractory Langerhans cell histiocytosis: outcome by intensity of conditioning. *Br J Haematol.* 2015;169:711-718.
210. Rivera JC, Wylie E, Dell'Orfano S, et al. Approaches to treatment of unifocal langerhans cell histiocytosis: is biopsy alone enough? *J Pediatr Orthop.* 2014;34:820-824.
211. Womer RB, Raney RB, Jr, D'Angio GJ. Healing rates of treated and untreated bone lesions in histiocytosis X. *Pediatrics.* 1985;76:286-288.
212. Cohen M, Zornoza J, Cangir A, Murray JA, Wallace S. Direct injection of methylprednisolone sodium succinate in the treatment of solitary eosinophilic granuloma of bone: a report of 9 cases. *Radiology.* 1980;136:289-293.
213. Kotecha R, Venkatramani R, Jubran RF, Arkader A, Olch AJ, Wong K. Clinical outcomes of radiation therapy in the management of Langerhans cell histiocytosis. *Am J Clin Oncol.* 2014;37:592-596.
214. Kriz J, Eich HT, Bruns F, et al. Radiotherapy in langerhans cell histiocytosis - a rare indication in a rare disease. *Radiat Oncol.* 2013;8:233.
215. Gramatovici R, D'Angio GJ. Radiation therapy in soft-tissue lesions in histiocytosis X (Langerhans' cell histiocytosis). *Med Pediatr Oncol.* 1988;16:259-262.
216. Larralde M, Rositto A, Giardelli M, Gatti CF, Munoz AS. Congenital self-healing histiocytosis (Hashimoto-Pritzker). *Int J Dermatol.* 1999;38:693-696.
217. Iwatsuki K, Tsugiki M, Yoshizawa N, Takigawa M, Yamada M, Shamoto M. The effect of phototherapies on cutaneous lesions of histiocytosis X in the elderly. *Cancer.* 1986;57:1931-1936.
218. Dodd E, Hook K. Topical imiquimod for the treatment of childhood cutaneous langerhans cell histiocytosis. *Pediatr Dermatol.* 2016;33:e184-e185.
219. Lindahl LM, Fenger-Gron M, Iversen L. Topical nitrogen mustard therapy in patients with Langerhans cell histiocytosis. *Br J Dermatol.* 2012;166:642-645.
220. Steen AE, Steen KH, Bauer R, Bieber T. Successful treatment of cutaneous Langerhans cell histiocytosis with low-dose methotrexate. *Br J Dermatol.* 2001;145:137-140.
221. Chang SE, Koh GJ, Choi JH, et al. Widespread skin-limited adult Langerhans cell histiocytosis: long-term follow-up with good response to interferon alpha. *Clin Exp Dermatol.* 2002;27:135-137.
222. McClain KL. Drug therapy for the treatment of Langerhans cell histiocytosis. *Expert Opin Pharmacother.* 2005;6:2435-2441.
223. Girschikofsky M, Arico M, Castillo D, et al. Management of adult patients with Langerhans cell histiocytosis: recommendations from an expert panel on behalf of Euro-Histio-Net. *Orphanet J Rare Dis.* 2013;8:72.
224. Charles J, Beani JC, Fiandrino G, Busser B. Major response to vemurafenib in patient with severe cutaneous Langerhans cell histiocytosis harboring BRAF V600E mutation. *J Am Acad Dermatol.* 2014;71:e97-e99.
225. Hazim AZ, Ruan GJ, Ravindran A, et al. Efficacy of BRAF-inhibitor therapy in BRAF(V600E)-mutated adult langerhans cell histiocytosis. *Oncol.* 2020;25:1001-1004.
226. Kolenová A, Schwentner R, Jug G, et al. Targeted inhibition of the MAPK pathway: emerging salvage option for progressive life-threatening multisystem LCH. *Blood Advances.* 2017;1:352-356.
227. Yang Y, Wang D, Li N, et al. Improvement in pituitary imaging after targeted therapy in three children with BRAF-mutated langerhans cell histiocytosis with pituitary involvement. *OncoTargets Ther.* 2020;13:12357-12363.

228. Lahey ME. Histiocytosis X: comparison of three treatment regimens. *J Pediatr.* 1975;87:179-183.
229. Gadner H, Grois N, Pötschger U, et al. Improved outcome in multisystem Langerhans cell histiocytosis is associated with therapy intensification. *Blood.* 2008;111:2556-2562.
230. Gadner H, Minkov M, Grois N, et al. Therapy prolongation improves outcome in multisystem Langerhans cell histiocytosis. *Blood.* 2013;121:5006-5014.
231. Minkov M, Grois N, Heitger A, Pötschger U, Westermeier T, Gadner H. Treatment of multisystem Langerhans cell histiocytosis. Results of the DAL-HX 83 and DAL-HX 90 studies. DAL-HX Study Group. *Klin Pädiatr.* 2000;212:139-144.
232. Grau J, Ribera JM, Indiano JM, et al. Resultados del tratamiento con 2-clorodesoxiadenosina en la histiocitosis de células de langerhans resistente o en recaída. Estudio de 9 pacientes. *Med Clínica.* 2001;116:339-342.
233. Rodriguez-Galindo C, Kelly P, Jeng M, Presbury GG, Rieman M, Wang W. Treatment of children with Langerhans cell histiocytosis with 2-chlorodeoxyadenosine. *Am J Hematol.* 2002;69:179-184.
234. Watts J, Files B. Langerhans cell histiocytosis: central nervous system involvement treated successfully with 2-chlorodeoxyadenosine. *Pediatr Hematol Oncol.* 2001;18:199-204.
235. Weitzman S, Braier J, Donadieu J, et al. 2'-Chlorodeoxyadenosine (2-CdA) as salvage therapy for Langerhans cell histiocytosis (LCH). results of the LCH-S-98 protocol of the Histiocyte Society. *Pediatr Blood Cancer.* 2009;53:1271-1276.
236. Weitzman S, Wayne AS, Arceci R, Lipton JM, Whitlock JA. Nucleoside analogues in the therapy of Langerhans cell histiocytosis: a survey of members of the histiocyte society and review of the literature. *Med Pediatr Oncol.* 1999;33:476-481.
237. Barkaoui MA, Queheille E, Aladjidi N, et al. Long-term follow-up of children with risk organ-negative Langerhans cell histiocytosis after 2-chlorodeoxyadenosine treatment. *Br J Haematol.* 2020;191:825-834.
238. Abraham A, Alsultan A, Jeng M, Rodriguez-Galindo C, Campbell PK. Clofarabine salvage therapy for refractory high-risk langerhans cell histiocytosis. *Pediatr Blood Cancer.* 2013;60:E19-E22.
239. Simko SJ, Tran HD, Jones J, et al. Clofarabine salvage therapy in refractory multifocal histiocytic disorders, including Langerhans cell histiocytosis, juvenile xanthogranuloma and Rosai-Dorfman disease. *Pediatr Blood Cancer.* 2014;61:479-487.
240. Arzoo K, Sadeghi S, Pullarkat V. Pamidronate for bone pain from osteolytic lesions in Langerhans'-cell histiocytosis. *N Engl J Med.* 2001;345:225.
241. Farran RP, Zaretski E, Egeler RM. Treatment of Langerhans cell histiocytosis with pamidronate. *J Pediatr Hematol Oncol.* 2001;23:54-56.
242. Braier J, Rosso D, Pollono D, et al. Symptomatic bone langerhans cell histiocytosis treated at diagnosis or after reactivation with indomethacin alone. *J Pediatr Hematol Oncol.* 2014;36:e280-e284.
243. Munn SE, Olliver L, Broadbent V, Pritchard J. Use of indomethacin in Langerhans cell histiocytosis. *Med Pediatr Oncol.* 1999;32:247-249.
244. Zinn DJ, Grimes AB, Lin H, Eckstein O, Allen CE, McClain KL. Hydroxyurea: a new old therapy for Langerhans cell histiocytosis. *Blood.* 2016;128:2462-2465.
245. Henter JI, Karlén J, Calming U, Bernstrand C, Andersson U, Fadeel B. Successful treatment of Langerhans'-cell histiocytosis with etanercept. *N Engl J Med.* 2001;345:1577-1578.
246. Degar B, et al. *Clofarabine for relapsed/refractory LCH and non-LCH histiocytosis. 36th Annual Meeting of the Histiocyte Society*; 2020. Virtual Meeting: Pediatric Blood and Cancer.
247. Henry M, Dickman P. *The expression of COX-2 in langerhans cell histiocytosis. The 27th Meeting of the Histiocyte Society.* Vienna, Austria; 2011.
248. Egeler RM, Favara BE, van Meurs M, Laman JD, Claassen E. Differential in situ cytokine profiles of Langerhans-like cells and T cells in Langerhans cell histiocytosis: abundant expression of cytokines relevant to disease and treatment. *Blood.* 1999;94:4195-4201.
249. Yeh EA, Greenberg J, Abla O, et al. Evaluation and treatment of Langerhans cell histiocytosis patients with central nervous system abnormalities: current views and new vistas. *Pediatr Blood Cancer.* 2018;65.
250. Grois N, Prayer D, Prosch H, Minkov M, Pötschger U, Gadner H. Course and clinical impact of magnetic resonance imaging findings in diabetes insipidus associated with Langerhans cell histiocytosis. *Pediatr Blood Cancer.* 2004;43:59-65.
251. Misra N, Bayry J, Ephrem A, et al. Intravenous immunoglobulin in neurological disorders: a mechanistic perspective. *J Neurol.* 2005;252(suppl 1):I1-I6.
252. Imashuku S, Fujita N, Shioda Y, et al. Follow-up of pediatric patients treated by IVIG for Langerhans cell histiocytosis (LCH)-related neurodegenerative CNS disease. *Int J Hematol.* 2015;101:191-197.
253. Imashuku S, Okazaki N, Nakayama M, et al. Treatment of neurodegenerative CNS disease in Langerhans cell histiocytosis with a combination of intravenous immunoglobulin and chemotherapy. *Pediatr Blood Cancer.* 2008;50:308-311.
254. Damon L, Plunkett W, Linker C. Plasma and cerebrospinal fluid pharmacokinetics of 1-beta-D-arabinofuranosylcytosine and 1-beta-D-arabinofuranosyluracil following the repeated intravenous administration of high- and intermediate-dose 1-beta-D-arabinofuranosylcytosine. *Cancer Res.* 1991;51:4141-4145.
255. Egeler RM, de Kraker J, Voute PA. Cytosine-arabinoside, vincristine, and prednisolone in the treatment of children with disseminated Langerhans cell histiocytosis with organ dysfunction: experience at a single institution. *Med Pediatr Oncol.* 1993;21:265-270.
256. Ehrhardt MJ, Karst J, Donohoue PA, et al. Recognition and treatment of concurrent active and neurodegenerative langerhans cell histiocytosis: a case report. *J Pediatr Hematol Oncol.* 2015;37:e37-e40.
257. Greinix HT, Storb R, Sanders JE, Petersen FB. Marrow transplantation for treatment of multisystem progressive Langerhans cell histiocytosis. *Bone Marrow Transplant.* 1992;10:39-44.
258. Hale GA, Bowman LC, Woodard JP, et al. Allogeneic bone marrow transplantation for children with histiocytic disorders: use of TBI and omission of etoposide in the conditioning regimen. *Bone Marrow Transplant.* 2003;31:981-986.
259. Steiner M, Matthes-Martin S, Attarbaschi A, et al. Improved outcome of treatment-resistant high-risk Langerhans cell histiocytosis after allogeneic stem cell transplantation with reduced-intensity conditioning. *Bone Marrow Transplant.* 2005;36:215-225.
260. Stoll M, Freund M, Schmid H, et al. Allogeneic bone marrow transplantation for Langerhans' cell histiocytosis. *Cancer.* 1990;66:284-288.
261. Suminoe A, Matsuzaki A, Hattori H, Ishii S, Hara T. Unrelated cord blood transplantation for an infant with chemotherapy-resistant progressive Langerhans cell histiocytosis. *J Pediatr Hematol Oncol.* 2001;23:633-636.

Chapter 62 ■ Pathology of Langerhans Cell Histiocytosis and Other Histiocytic Proliferations

ANDREW L. FELDMAN

INTRODUCTION

Langerhans cell histiocytosis (LCH) and other tumors of histiocytes, dendritic cells, and associated immune accessory cells are rare neoplasms arising from cells involved in antigen presentation and related immune functions.[1] Dendritic cells are myeloid-derived antigen-presenting cells that express human leukocyte antigen (HLA) class II and play a role in activating naïve T cells.[2] Langerhans cells are specialized dendritic cells that occur mostly in the skin and are involved in antigen trafficking to lymph nodes, where they present antigen to T cells. Interdigitating dendritic cells (IDCs) reside mostly in the lymph nodes and perform a similar function.[3] Plasmacytoid dendritic cells produce interferon-α and play a role in immune tolerance.[4] Follicular dendritic cells (FDCs), despite their name, are of stromal cell origin[5]; tumors derived from them are addressed here because of their immune accessory function, playing a critical role in the formation and organization of lymphoid follicles. Histiocytes are noncirculating cells that represent the tissue equivalent of monocytes, including macrophages.[6] Table 62.1 summarizes the main tumors derived from these cell types along with recurrent genetic abnormalities, particularly in the mitogen-activated protein kinase (MAPK) and phosphatidylinositol 3-kinase pathways, that shed light on their molecular pathogenesis and form the basis for existing or potential therapies.[7]

LANGERHANS CELL HISTIOCYTOSIS AND LANGERHANS CELL SARCOMA

LCH is a neoplastic proliferation of Langerhans cells that occurs particularly in children, although there is a wide age range. LCH is most common in Caucasians; males are affected more than females (3.7:1). Most cases presenting in the lung are associated with smoking.[8] The disease may affect one anatomic site, one system with multiple sites, or multiple systems.[9] Single-site LCH commonly involves bone, especially skull, and typically presents as a lytic bone lesion with cortical erosion. Other sites include the skin, lung, and lymph node. Multifocal lesions with single-system involvement also usually affect the bone, particularly in children; cranial involvement may lead to diabetes insipidus. Multisystem disease typically affects infants and involves the bone, skin, liver, spleen, and bone marrow. Marrow involvement may be associated with cytopenias at presentation.

Like normal Langerhans cells, the neoplastic cells in LCH are typically oval and often have folded or grooved ("coffee-bean") nuclei with minimal atypia (Figure 62.1A). The background often contains eosinophils and may also have non-Langerhans histiocytes (including multinucleated giant cells), small lymphocytes, and neutrophils. In lymph nodes, there often is a sinusoidal pattern of involvement; in spleen, the red pulp is involved. LCH of the liver preferentially involves the intrahepatic biliary tree and may lead to sclerosing cholangitis. Bone marrow involvement may be associated with fibrosis. Ultrastructurally, the neoplastic cells have tennis racket-shaped, cytoplasmic Birbeck granules. By immunohistochemistry (IHC), they express S100, CD1a (Figure 62.1B), langerin, cyclin D1,[10] CD4, CD45, CD68, HLA-DR, and often PD-L1.[11] They typically lack markers of monocytes/macrophages (e.g., CD14, CD163, and OCT2) and FDCs (e.g., CD21 and CD35).

LCH is a clonal disorder, except some pulmonary cases in adults.[12] Immunoglobulin or T-cell receptor gene rearrangements have been reported in up to 30% of cases[13]; occasional cases are clonally related to underlying lymphoid neoplasms, likely via transdifferentiation.[14,15] BRAF V600E mutations are present in about 50% and can be detected by IHC; about 25% of cases have MAP2K1 mutations, usually

Table 62.1. Summary of Features of Langerhans Cell Histiocytosis and Other Histiocytic Disorders

Disease	Group(s)[a]	Cell of Origin	Typical Phenotype	Genetics
Langerhans cell histiocytosis; Langerhans cell sarcoma	L,M	Langerhans cell	CD1a, CD68, cyclin D1, S100, langerin	BRAF alterations (V600E, other abnormalities); mutations in MAP2K1, ARAF, KRAS
Follicular dendritic cell sarcoma	n/i	Follicular dendritic cell	CD21, CD23, CD35, clusterin	Loss-of-function alterations of NFKBIA, CYLD, CDKN2A, RB1; BRAF V600E; gains of 9p24
Interdigitating dendritic cell sarcoma	M	Interdigitating dendritic cell	S100	BRAF V600E (frequency unknown), other MAPK gene mutations
Blastic plasmacytoid dendritic cell neoplasm	n/i	Plasmacytoid dendritic cell	CD4, CD56, CD123, CD303, TCL1A	Complex karyotypes; CDKN2A deletions; mutations in TET2 (most common), NPM1, NRAS, ATM, and other RAS-family genes
Histiocytic sarcoma	M	Histiocyte	CD68, CD163	Mutations in BRAF (V600E and others), HRAS, and KMT2D
Disseminated juvenile xanthogranuloma; Erdheim-Chester disease	L,C	Histiocyte	CD14, CD68, CD163, factor XIIIa	BRAF V600E (most common); mutations in PIK3CA, NRAS, KRAS, MAP2K1
Rosai-Dorfman disease	R,C	Histiocyte	CD68, CD163, cyclin D1, OCT2, S100	Some cases reactive; others with mutations in KRAS, NRAS, ARAF, MAP2K1
ALK-positive histiocytosis	n/i	Histiocyte	CD68, CD163, S100 (variable), ALK	ALK fusions (usually KIF5B-ALK)
Hemophagocytic lymphohistiocytosis	H	Histiocyte (activated)	CD68, CD163	Reactive; primary and some secondary cases associated with germline mutations (see text)

[a]Based on the Histiocyte Society classification.[1] ALK, anaplastic lymphoma kinase; C, cutaneous/mucocutaneous group; H, hemophagocytic/macrophage activation group; L, Langerhans group; M, malignant group; n/i, not included; R, Rosai-Dorman group.

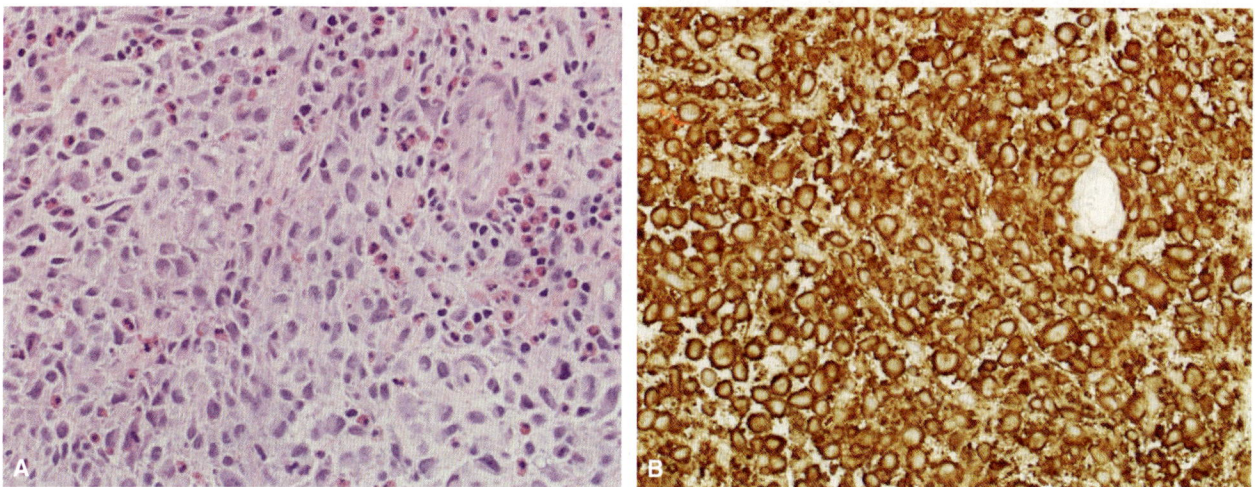

FIGURE 62.1 Langerhans cell histiocytosis. A, Hematoxylin and eosin (H&E) stain. The cells are oval with some showing folded or grooved nuclei. There are numerous eosinophils in the background. B, CD1a stain. The neoplastic cells show strong and uniform membranous staining.

exclusive of *BRAF* mutations.[16] Other mutations include *MAP3K1*, *ARAF*, or non-V600E *BRAF* variants.[16,17] The clinical course is related primarily to stage of disease at presentation, with excellent outcomes in patients with unifocal disease and high mortality rates in infants with refractory multisystem disease.

Langerhans cell sarcoma (LCS) is a rare tumor with malignant cytology and a Langerhans cell phenotype. It typically presents in adults with multiorgan involvement, including the skin, soft tissue, lymph node, lung, liver, spleen, and bone. The neoplastic cells show marked nuclear pleomorphism and prominent nucleoli (*Figure 62.2A*). Occasional nuclear grooves may aid in diagnosis. Background inflammatory cells, including eosinophils, are less frequent than in LCH. The phenotype is similar to that of LCH, including expression of S100, CD1a, and langerin (*Figure 62.2B*), although staining for individual markers is more variable than in LCH. *BRAF* V600E and *KRAS* mutations have been reported.[18] The clinical behavior of LCS is aggressive, and prognosis is poor.

FOLLICULAR DENDRITIC CELL SARCOMA

FDC sarcoma is a rare neoplasm of FDCs that predominantly affects adults without a sex predisposition. It sometimes arises in association with Castleman disease. Patients typically present with a large, localized, slow-growing mass, often at extranodal sites such as tonsil, soft tissue, gastrointestinal tract, and lung. Systemic symptoms are rare. Nodal presentation also occurs, particularly in the neck. Metastasis to the lung, liver, and lymph nodes may be seen; some patients develop paraneoplastic pemphigus.

FDC sarcomas are composed of oval to spindled cells arranged in a fascicular, whorled, or storiform pattern (*Figure 62.3A*). The nuclei are elongated and often bland, but cases with more nuclear pleomorphism may be seen. Multinucleate cells occur commonly. There often is a background of scattered small lymphocytes. Tumor cells express one or more FDC markers, including CD21 (*Figure 62.3B*), CD23, and CD35. CXCL13, clusterin, podoplanin, and epidermal growth factor receptor are often expressed but are less specific. Epithelial membrane antigen, smooth muscle actin, S100, CD68, and occasionally CD30 may be expressed.[7] CD1a, cytokeratins, and myeloid markers are typically absent. *Terminal deoxynucleotidyl transferase (*TdT)–positive T cells may be present in the background.[19]

FDC sarcomas may have clonal immunoglobulin gene rearrangements.[20] Karyotypes typically are complex. Recurrent genetic alterations include loss-of-function events in genes negatively regulating nuclear factor-κB (*CYLD*, *NFKBIA*, *SOCS3*, *TNFAIP3*, *TRAF3*) and the cell cycle (*CDKN2A*, *RB1*, *TP53*), and 9p24 copy number gains involving *MYC*, *CCND2*, and 9p24; MAPK gene mutations are typically absent.[18,21] FDC sarcoma usually is treated surgically with good outcomes in the absence of metastasis. Adverse prognostic factors include tumor size ≥6 cm, necrosis, high mitotic rate, and atypia.

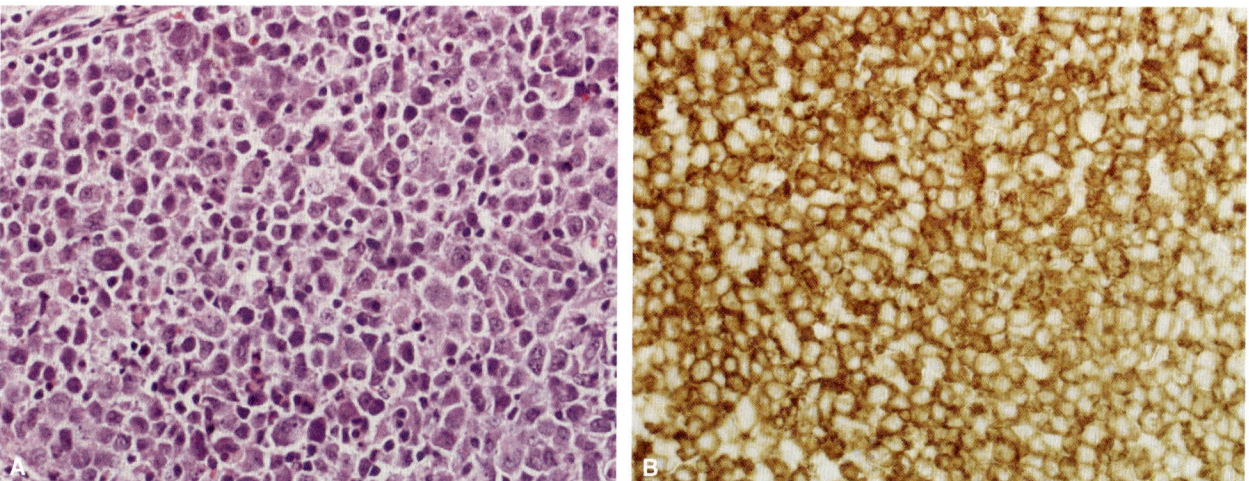

FIGURE 62.2 Langerhans cell sarcoma. A, H&E stain. The cells show significant nuclear pleomorphism. B, CD1a stain. The neoplastic cells show strong and uniform membranous staining.

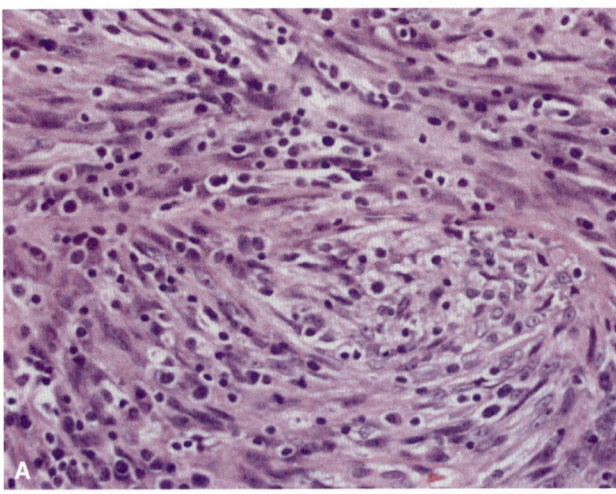 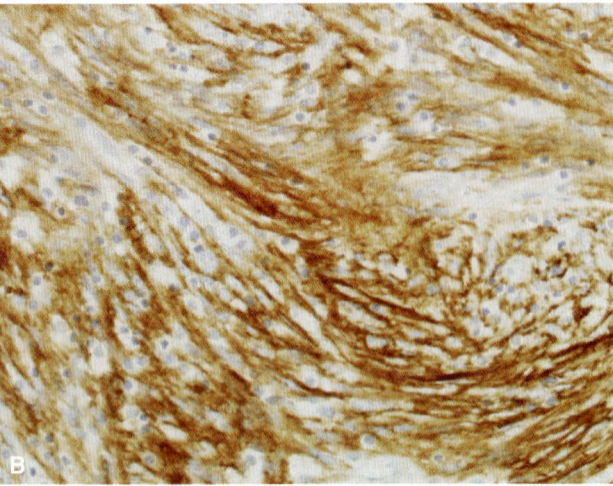

FIGURE 62.3 Follicular dendritic cell sarcoma. A, H&E stain. The neoplastic cells are spindled and show whorl formation. There are scattered small lymphocytes in the background. B, CD21 stain. The neoplastic cells show strong staining.

A variant of FDC sarcoma, inflammatory pseudotumor-like follicular/fibroblastic dendritic cell sarcoma, primarily involves the liver and/or spleen of young women. The tumors harbor Epstein-Barr virus (EBV) and show more variable FDC marker expression than FDC sarcomas. Recurrent genetic alterations have not been reported.[22] The clinical course typically is indolent but may be marked by multiple intra-abdominal recurrences.

INTERDIGITATING DENDRITIC CELL SARCOMA AND OTHER DENDRITIC CELL SARCOMAS

IDC sarcoma is a rare neoplasm that typically occurs in adults with a slight male predominance and affects lymph nodes as an asymptomatic mass or occasionally widespread lymphadenopathy. Skin and soft-tissue involvement or hepatosplenomegaly may be present.

Lymph node biopsy shows paracortical expansion, often sparing residual follicles. The neoplastic cells are oval to spindled with variable atypia and are arranged in a fascicular, whorled, or storiform pattern (*Figure 62.4*). Multinucleate cells may be present. The background often contains abundant reactive lymphocytes. Ultrastructural examination shows interdigitating processes. The tumor cells express S100 and vimentin but are negative for CD1a, langerin, myeloperoxidase, CD30, CD34, keratins, and FDC markers, which is important since FDC sarcomas may be indistinguishable morphologically. Staining for CD45, CD68, and lysozyme is variable. The background lymphocytes are mostly T cells.

Indeterminate dendritic cell tumors are spindle cell neoplasms with a phenotype similar to indeterminate cells, which may represent Langerhans cell precursors.[23] They typically present in the skin, although nodal or splenic presentation has been reported. The tumors involve the dermis and contain cells resembling Langerhans cells. Eosinophils are less frequent than in LCH. The cells express S100 and CD1a but not langerin. They may express CD4, CD45, CD68, or lysozyme, but lack FDC markers and CD163. Fibroblastic reticular cell tumors are very rare. They have been reported in the lymph nodes, spleen, and soft tissue and are composed of spindled cells similar to those seen in FDC or IDC sarcomas. They variably express smooth muscle actin, desmin, cytokeratins, and CD68.

IDC sarcomas and other dendritic cell tumors may have immunoglobulin gene rearrangements,[20] occasionally associated with underlying B-cell lymphomas.[24,25] *BRAF* V600E and other MAPK gene mutations have been reported.[18,26] IDC sarcomas usually are clinically aggressive; the clinical behavior of other dendritic cell neoplasms varies widely.

BLASTIC PLASMACYTOID DENDRITIC CELL NEOPLASM

Blastic plasmacytoid dendritic cell neoplasm (BPDCN) is a rare, aggressive tumor of plasmacytoid dendritic cell precursors typically occurring in older adults with a male predominance. Some cases are associated with or evolve into chronic myelomonocytic leukemia or other myeloid neoplasms.[27] BPDCN involves the skin, bone marrow, and peripheral blood, although other sites may be affected. Initial diagnosis most frequently is made on biopsy of skin lesions, which tend to be isolated, often purple nodules. Occasional patients present with localized papules, while others present with widespread skin involvement. Regional lymphadenopathy may be present. The diagnosis may be established on peripheral blood or bone marrow examination in patients without cutaneous manifestations. Cytopenias may be present.

The tumor cells in BPDCN are medium-sized blasts with dispersed chromatin and scant cytoplasm (*Figure 62.5*). Skin biopsy shows marked infiltration of the dermis extending into subcutaneous fat but sparing the epidermis and adnexa. In lymph nodes, the follicles tend to be spared. Bone marrow findings vary from interstitial infiltration to near total replacement by tumor. The neoplastic cells express CD4, CD56, CD123, CD303, TCL1A, and cytoplasmic CD68. CD2, CD5, CD7, CD33, and TdT are variably expressed. Some cases, particularly

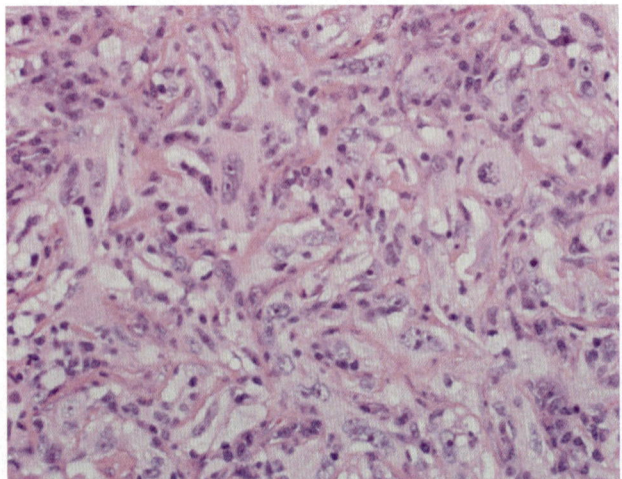

FIGURE 62.4 Interdigitating dendritic cell sarcoma, H&E stain. The neoplastic cells have oval nuclei and abundant cytoplasm and are arranged in a storiform pattern.

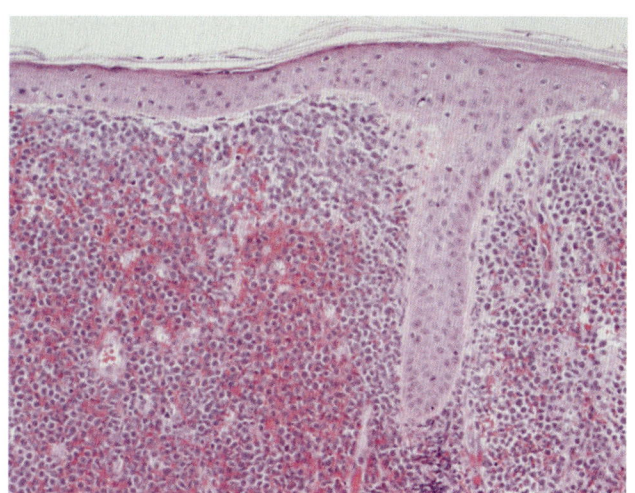

FIGURE 62.5 Blastic plasmacytoid dendritic cell neoplasm, H&E stain. Skin biopsy shows extensive dermal infiltrate of medium-sized cells with dispersed chromatin, with sparing of the epidermis.

in children, express S100. CD13, CD16, lysozyme, and myeloperoxidase are absent. Blastic neoplasms without sufficient phenotypic features for a diagnosis of BPDCN are best classified as acute leukemia of ambiguous lineage.

BPDCNs have complex karyotypes, with recurrent abnormalities of 5q, 6q, 9, 12p, 13q, and 15q.[28] *CDKN2A* deletions are common. Recurrent mutations are seen in *KRAS*, *NRAS*, *TET2*, *ASXL1*, *SUZ12*, *ARID1A*, and other epigenetic modifiers.[29] Transcription factor 4 has been identified as a master transcriptional regulator, suggesting potential therapeutic targets.[30] BPDCNs are clinically aggressive, with frequent relapse despite initial response to chemotherapy. Adverse prognostic factors include older age, extensive marrow or blood involvement, TdT negativity, CD303 positivity, *CDKN2A/B* mutations, and mutations in genes involved in DNA methylation.

HISTIOCYTIC SARCOMA

Histiocytic sarcoma (HS) is a rare malignancy of mature tissue histiocytes and must be distinguished from tissue-based manifestations of acute monocytic leukemia. It predominantly affects adults with a possible male predominance. Most present with a solitary extranodal mass, especially in the skin, soft tissue, or gastrointestinal tract (sometimes causing obstruction). Lymph nodes may be involved, and systemic symptoms are common. Widespread disease at presentation has been referred to as malignant histiocytosis.

The tumor cells in HS typically are large with pleomorphic nuclei and abundant, eosinophilic cytoplasm (*Figure 62.6A*). Multinucleated cells are common; spindled cells also may be seen. Some cells may show hemophagocytosis. The growth pattern usually is diffuse but may be sinusoidal in lymph nodes. The background contains reactive immune cells, including small lymphocytes, plasma cells, neutrophils, and eosinophils, which are sometimes so numerous that identification of the tumor cells is difficult. Most cases express CD45, CD68, CD163 (*Figure 62.6B*), and lysozyme. They are negative for CD1a, langerin, and FDC markers. S100 may be partially expressed.

Some HS have immunoglobulin gene rearrangements,[20] which may be related to underlying B-cell neoplasms.[24,25,31] Mutations of *BRAF* (V600E and others, as well as *BRAF* fusions), *HRAS*, *KRAS*, *NRAS*, and *MAP2K1* have been reported.[18] Most cases are clinically aggressive and have poor responses to therapy. Clinical stage is the best characterized prognostic factor.

DISSEMINATED JUVENILE XANTHOGRANULOMA AND ERDHEIM-CHESTER DISEASE

Disseminated juvenile xanthogranuloma (JXG) and Erdheim-Chester disease (ECD) are related but distinct mature histiocytic neoplasms.[1,32] Disseminated JXG is a disease of childhood and is not believed to arise from solitary dermal JXG. It is associated with type 1 neurofibromatosis and increased risk of juvenile myelomonocytic leukemia.[33] Skin, soft tissue, mucosal surfaces, the central nervous system, eye, liver, lung, lymph node, and bone marrow are commonly involved sites. Eye lesions may lead to glaucoma; central nervous system involvement may cause diabetes insipidus or neuropsychiatric symptoms. Some patients develop a macrophage activation syndrome, which can be fatal.

The neoplastic cells of JXG are small, oval cells with xanthomatous change; Touton-like giant cells may be seen. There is a background of mixed inflammatory cells. The tumor cells are positive for CD14, CD68, CD163, factor XIIIa, and vimentin. Partial S100 may be present. CD1a and langerin are absent. *BRAF* V600E and *MAPK1* mutations may occur occasionally, but genetics are poorly understood.[17,34] Though considered benign, severe consequences can result from local mass effect (particularly in the CNS) or macrophage activation syndrome.

ECD is related to JXG but has differing clinical and genetic features. It is rare, typically affects adults, and has a male predominance. Nearly any anatomic site can be affected, but the skeletal system is usually involved; the cardiovascular and central nervous systems are

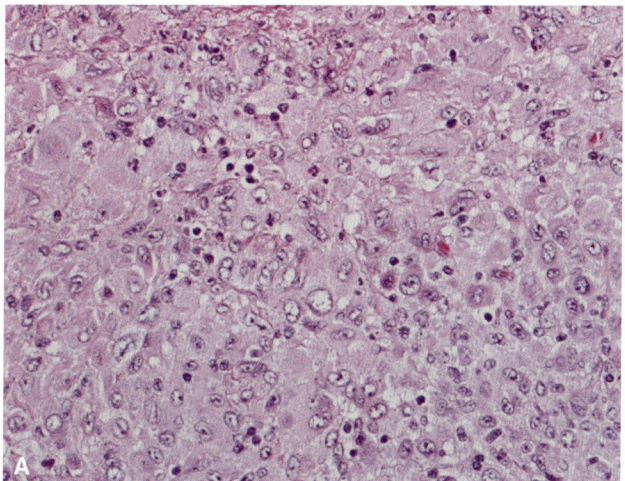
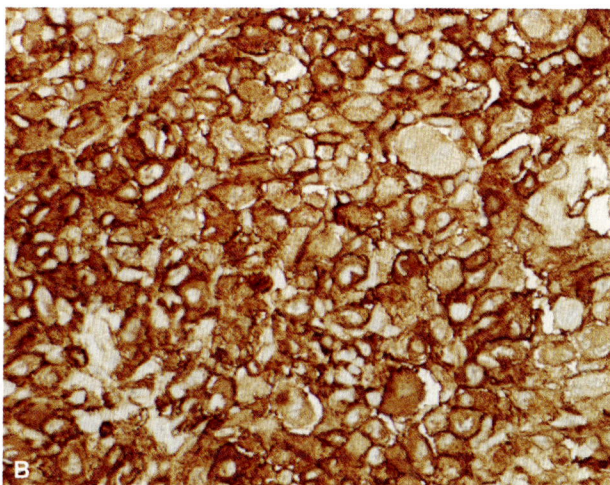

FIGURE 62.6 Histiocytic sarcoma. A, H&E stain. The neoplastic cells are large and have pleomorphic nuclei and abundant eosinophilic cytoplasm. B, CD163 stain. The neoplastic cells show strong and uniform staining.

other common sites. Skin involvement often presents as xanthelasma around the eyes. ECD may coexist with LCH in the same or different lesions.[1] The cytological features are similar to those of JXG. Fibrosis often is present. The phenotype also is similar to that of JXG, with expression of CD14, CD68, CD163, factor XIIIa, and vimentin.

BRAF V600E is present in over 50% of cases of ECD and recurrent mutations in *PIK3CA*, *NRAS*, *KRAS*, and *MAP2K1* also have been reported.[17,35] ECD is a chronic disease; outcomes are related principally to the sites and extent of disease. Interferon-α or BRAF inhibitors have shown therapeutic efficacy.

ROSAI-DORFMAN DISEASE

Rosai-Dorfman disease (RDD), or sinus histiocytosis with massive lymphadenopathy, is a rare histiocytic proliferation. The median age is 20 years; males are affected slightly more than females. The etiology is unknown, though relationships with viral infections, autoimmune lymphoproliferative syndrome, lupus, and IgG4-related diseases have been suggested. Most patients present with massive cervical lymphadenopathy, often with a variety of systemic symptoms and laboratory abnormalities.[36] Extranodal involvement occurs in one-third of patients, including skin and soft tissue, bone, central nervous system, and the upper respiratory tract.

The lymph nodes of RDD show sinusoidal accumulation of large histiocytes with one or multiple nuclei and prominent nucleoli; emperipolesis, with intact lymphocytes and plasma cells in the cytoplasm, is a characteristic though nonspecific feature (*Figure 62.7*). The cells express CD4, CD14, CD33, CD68, CD163, cyclin D1,[37] OCT2,[38] and S100, which facilitate visualizing the emperipolesis.

While some cases of RDD have been found to be polyclonal, suggesting a reactive process, occasional cases are neoplastic; MAPK gene mutations, including *KRAS*, *NRAS*, *ARAF*, and *MAP2K1*, occur but at a lower frequency than in LCH, JXG, and ECD.[17] The clinical course is generally indolent and self-limited; most cases resolve in 3 to 9 months, though prolonged disease episodes may occur. The main treatment is surgical.

ANAPLASTIC LYMPHOMA KINASE–POSITIVE HISTIOCYTOSIS

Anaplastic lymphoma kinase (ALK)–positive histiocytosis has been reported since 2008[39]; recently, the clinicopathologic features have become more fully understood and it has been proposed as a distinct entity.[40] Clinical presentations have been grouped into infants (Group 1A) or older patients (Group 1B) with multisystem disease and patients

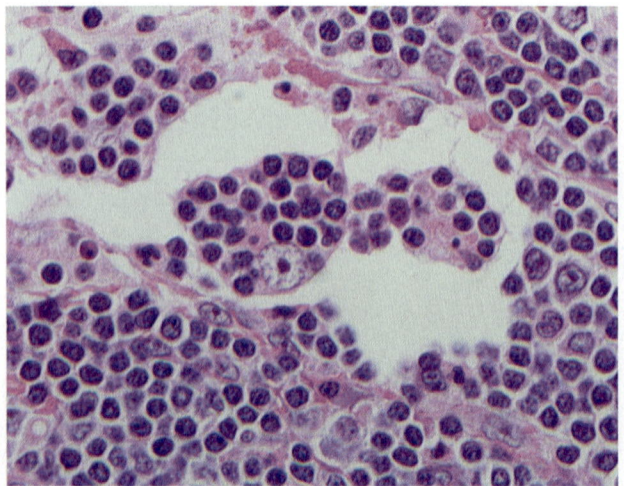

FIGURE 62.7 Rosai-Dorfman disease, H&E stain. A large histiocyte within a sinusoid shows a single nucleus with a central nucleolus, and multiple intact intracytoplasmic lymphocytes (emperipolesis).

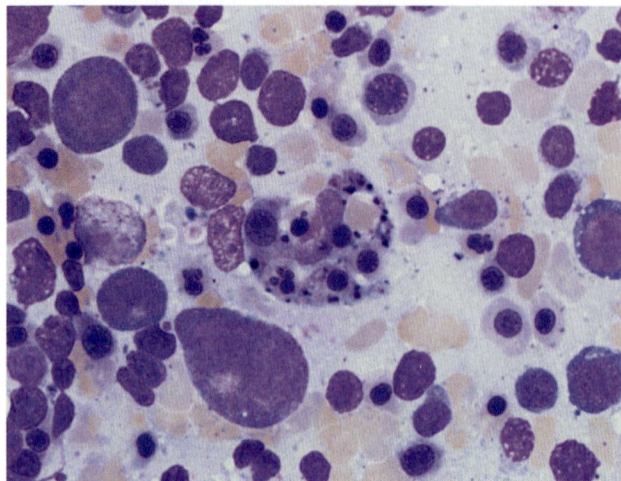

FIGURE 62.8 Hemophagocytic lymphohistiocytosis, Wright-Giemsa stain. A histiocyte from a bone marrow aspirate smear shows marked hemophagocytosis.

with single-system disease (Group 2). Neurologic involvement is seen in about half of patients, particularly in Groups 1B and 2.

Histologically, ALK-positive histiocytosis shows xanthogranulomatous features in about 1/3 of cases; the remaining cases are more monomorphic with a variety of cytological appearances including cases with spindled or epithelioid cells, which may mimic mesenchymal neoplasms or reactive processes.[40-42] ALK-positive histiocytosis shares immunophenotypic features with other histiocytic neoplasms but expresses ALK. It typically expresses CD68 and CD163 with variable S100 and lacks expression of CD1a, langerin, and BRAF-V600E.[41] Most cases bear *KIF5B-ALK* fusions, which typically show a cytoplasmic staining pattern with dot-like Golgi accentuation by ALK IHC; occasionally, *ALK* rearrangements with non-*KIF5B* partner genes are seen.[40,41] ALK inhibitors have shown durable responses.[40]

HEMOPHAGOCYTIC LYMPHOHISTIOCYTOSIS

Hemophagocytic lymphohistiocytosis (HLH) comprises a spectrum of disorders with extensive hemophagocytosis, classified into primary and secondary types.[1,17] Both are characterized by immune activation and cytokine dysregulation accompanied by cytopenias, systemic symptoms, and accumulation of macrophages at various tissue sites with hepatosplenomegaly. Primary HLH is a disease of children with a known familial history in about half of cases. Secondary HLH has a wide age range, though children are predominantly affected, and typically is triggered by infection, autoimmune disease, or underlying malignancy.

HLH manifests as an accumulation of benign histiocytes showing hemophagocytosis, particularly of red blood cells and neutrophils (*Figure 62.8*). The reticuloendothelial system is extensively affected, as well as other sites such as the central nervous system. The bone marrow is commonly affected; however, hemophagocytosis may be absent early in the disease course, and high clinical suspicion should prompt further evaluation such as liver biopsy. The hemophagocytic cells show expression of histiocytic markers such as CD68 and CD163.

HLH is a reactive condition. Familial cases have been associated with germline alterations in a variety of genes, including *PRF1*, *UNC13D*, *STX11*, *STXBP2*, *LYST*, *RAB27A*, *AP3B1*, *SH2D1A*, and *XIAP*.[1] The functional consequence of the mutation is associated with age of presentation and clinical severity.[17] Children with primary immunodeficiency syndromes may develop HLH in the setting of immune challenge such as EBV infection; these cases are not considered true primary HLH. While primary HLH was previously nearly uniformly fatal, improved survival rates are being seen with immunosuppression, cytotoxic therapy, and/or transplantation.

References

1. Emile JF, Abla O, Fraitag S, et al. Revised classification of histiocytoses and neoplasms of the macrophage-dendritic cell lineages. *Blood.* 2016;127(22):2672-2681.
2. Banchereau J, Briere F, Caux C, et al. Immunobiology of dendritic cells. *Annu Rev Immunol.* 2000;18:767-811.
3. Geissmann F, Dieu-Nosjean MC, Dezutter C, et al. Accumulation of immature Langerhans cells in human lymph nodes draining chronically inflamed skin. *J Exp Med.* 2002;196(4):417-430.
4. Geissmann F, Manz MG, Jung S, Sieweke MH, Merad M, Ley K. Development of monocytes, macrophages, and dendritic cells. *Science.* 2010;327(5966):656-661.
5. Munoz-Fernandez R, Blanco FJ, Frecha C, et al. Follicular dendritic cells are related to bone marrow stromal cell progenitors and to myofibroblasts. *J Immunol.* 2006;177(1):280-289.
6. Gordon S. The macrophage: past, present and future. *Eur J Immunol.* 2007;37(suppl 1):S9-S17.
7. Facchetti F, Pileri SA, Lorenzi L, et al. Histiocytic and dendritic cell neoplasms: what have we learnt by studying 67 cases. *Virchows Arch.* 2017;471(4):467-489.
8. Roden AC, Yi ES. Pulmonary langerhans cell histiocytosis: an update from the pathologists' perspective. *Arch Pathol Lab Med.* 2016;140(3):230-240.
9. Lieberman PH, Jones CR, Steinman RM, et al. Langerhans cell (eosinophilic) granulomatosis. A clinicopathologic study encompassing 50 years. *Am J Surg Pathol.* 1996;20(5):519-552.
10. Shanmugam V, Craig JW, Hornick JL, Morgan EA, Pinkus GS, Pozdnyakova O. Cyclin D1 is expressed in neoplastic cells of langerhans cell histiocytosis but not reactive langerhans cell proliferations. *Am J Surg Pathol.* 2017;41(10):1390-1396.
11. Gatalica Z, Bilalovic N, Palazzo JP, et al. Disseminated histiocytoses biomarkers beyond BRAFV600E: frequent expression of PD-L1. *Oncotarget.* 2015;6(23):19819-19825.
12. Willman CL, Busque L, Griffith BB, et al. Langerhans'-cell histiocytosis (histiocytosis X)—a clonal proliferative disease. *N Engl J Med.* 1994;331(3):154-160.
13. Chen W, Wang J, Wang E, et al. Detection of clonal lymphoid receptor gene rearrangements in langerhans cell histiocytosis. *Am J Surg Pathol.* 2010;34(7):1049-1057.
14. Feldman AL, Berthold F, Arceci R, et al. Clonal relationship between precursor T-lymphoblastic leukaemia/lymphoma and Langerhans-cell histiocytosis. *Lancet Oncol.* 2005;6(6):435-437.
15. West DS, Dogan A, Quint PS, et al. Clonally related follicular lymphomas and langerhans cell neoplasms: expanding the spectrum of transdifferentiation. *Am J Surg Pathol.* 2013;37(7):978-986.
16. Chakraborty R, Burke TM, Hampton OA, et al. Alternative genetic mechanisms of BRAF activation in Langerhans cell histiocytosis. *Blood.* 2016;128(21):2533-2537.
17. McClain KL, Bigenwald C, Collin M, et al. Histiocytic disorders. *Nat Rev Dis Prim.* 2021;7(1):73.
18. Massoth LR, Hung YP, Ferry JA, et al. Histiocytic and dendritic cell sarcomas of hematopoietic origin share targetable genomic alterations distinct from follicular dendritic cell sarcoma. *Oncologist.* 2021;26(7):e1263-e1272.
19. Ohgami RS, Zhao S, Ohgami JK, et al. TdT+ T-lymphoblastic populations are increased in Castleman disease, in Castleman disease in association with follicular dendritic cell tumors, and in angioimmunoblastic T-cell lymphoma. *Am J Surg Pathol.* 2012;36(11):1619-1628.
20. Chen W, Lau SK, Fong D, et al. High frequency of clonal immunoglobulin receptor gene rearrangements in sporadic histiocytic/dendritic cell sarcomas. *Am J Surg Pathol.* 2009;33(6):863-873.
21. Facchetti F, Simbeni M, Lorenzi L. Follicular dendritic cell sarcoma. *Pathologica.* 2021;113(5):316-329.
22. Bruehl FK, Azzato E, Durkin L, Farkas DH, Hsi ED, Ondrejka SL. Inflammatory pseudotumor-like follicular/fibroblastic dendritic cell sarcomas of the spleen are EBV-associated and lack other commonly identifiable molecular alterations. *Int J Surg Pathol.* 2021;29(4):443-446.
23. Dalia S, Shao H, Sagatys E, Cualing H, Sokol L. Dendritic cell and histiocytic neoplasms: biology, diagnosis, and treatment. *Cancer Control.* 2014;21(4):290-300.
24. Feldman AL, Arber DA, Pittaluga S, et al. Clonally related follicular lymphomas and histiocytic/dendritic cell sarcomas: evidence for transdifferentiation of the follicular lymphoma clone. *Blood.* 2008;111(12):5433-5439.
25. Shao H, Xi L, Raffeld M, et al. Clonally related histiocytic/dendritic cell sarcoma and chronic lymphocytic leukemia/small lymphocytic lymphoma: a study of seven cases. *Mod Pathol.* 2011;24(11):1421-1432.
26. O'Malley DP, Agrawal R, Grimm KE, et al. Evidence of BRAF V600E in indeterminate cell tumor and interdigitating dendritic cell sarcoma. *Ann Diagn Pathol.* 2015;19(3):113-116.
27. Khoury JD, Medeiros LJ, Manning JT, Sulak LE, Bueso-Ramos C, Jones D. CD56(+) TdT(+) blastic natural killer cell tumor of the skin: a primitive systemic malignancy related to myelomonocytic leukemia. *Cancer.* 2002;94(9):2401-2408.
28. Leroux D, Mugneret F, Callanan M, et al. CD4(+), CD56(+) DC2 acute leukemia is characterized by recurrent clonal chromosomal changes affecting 6 major targets: a study of 21 cases by the Groupe Francais de Cytogenetique Hematologique. *Blood.* 2002;99(11):4154-4159.
29. Sapienza MR, Abate F, Melle F, et al. Blastic plasmacytoid dendritic cell neoplasm: genomics mark epigenetic dysregulation as a primary therapeutic target. *Haematologica.* 2019;104(4):729-737.
30. Ceribelli M, Hou ZE, Kelly PN, et al. A druggable TCF4- and BRD4-dependent transcriptional network sustains malignancy in blastic plasmacytoid dendritic cell neoplasm. *Cancer Cell.* 2016;30(5):764-778.
31. Feldman AL, Minniti C, Santi M, Downing JR, Raffeld M, Jaffe ES. Histiocytic sarcoma after acute lymphoblastic leukaemia: a common clonal origin. *Lancet Oncol.* 2004;5(4):248-250.
32. Swerdlow S, Campo E, Harris N, et al., eds. *WHO Classification of Tumours of Haematopoietic and Lymphoid Tissues.* Revised 4th ed. International Agency for Research on Cancer; 2017. Bosman F, Jaffe E, Lakhani S, Ohgaki H, eds. World Health Organization Classification of Tumours.
33. Zvulunov A, Barak Y, Metzker A. Juvenile xanthogranuloma, neurofibromatosis, and juvenile chronic myelogenous leukemia. World statistical analysis. *Arch Dermatol.* 1995;131(8):904-908.
34. Chakraborty R, Hampton OA, Abhyankar H, et al. Activating MAPK1 (ERK2) mutation in an aggressive case of disseminated juvenile xanthogranuloma. *Oncotarget.* 2017;8(28):46065-46070.
35. Haroun F, Millado K, Tabbara I. Erdheim-chester disease: comprehensive review of molecular profiling and therapeutic advances. *Anticancer Res.* 2017;37(6):2777-2783.
36. Foucar E, Rosai J, Dorfman R. Sinus histiocytosis with massive lymphadenopathy (Rosai-Dorfman disease): review of the entity. *Semin Diagn Pathol.* 1990;7(1):19-73.
37. Baraban E, Sadigh S, Rosenbaum J, et al. Cyclin D1 expression and novel mutational findings in Rosai-Dorfman disease. *Br J Haematol.* 2019;186(6):837-844.
38. Ravindran A, Goyal G, Go RS, Rech KL, Mayo Clinic Histiocytosis Working G. Rosai-dorfman disease displays a unique monocyte-macrophage phenotype characterized by expression of OCT2. *Am J Surg Pathol.* 2021;45(1):35-44.
39. Chan JK, Lamant L, Algar E, et al. ALK+ histiocytosis: a novel type of systemic histiocytic proliferative disorder of early infancy. *Blood.* 2008;112(7):2965-2968.
40. Kemps PG, Picarsic J, Durham BH, et al. ALK-positive histiocytosis: a new clinicopathologic spectrum highlighting neurologic involvement and responses to ALK inhibition. *Blood.* 2022;139(2):256-280.
41. Chang KTE, Tay AZE, Kuick CH, et al. ALK-positive histiocytosis: an expanded clinicopathologic spectrum and frequent presence of KIF5B-ALK fusion. *Mod Pathol.* 2019;32(5):598-608.
42. Kashima J, Yoshida M, Jimbo K, et al. ALK-positive histiocytosis of the breast: a clinicopathologic study highlighting spindle cell histology. *Am J Surg Pathol.* 2021;45(3):347-355.

Chapter 63 ■ Infectious Mononucleosis and Other Epstein-Barr Virus–Related Disorders

LAURA F. WALSH • RICHARD F. AMBINDER

INTRODUCTION

Epstein-Barr virus (EBV) infects more than 90% of the world's adult population. Most primary infection is asymptomatic, but particularly in adolescents and young adults primary infection is associated with infectious mononucleosis (IM). The virus is also associated with other disorders including hemophagocytic lymphohistiocytosis (HLH) and multiple sclerosis (MS); B-, T-, and natural killer (NK)-cell lymphoproliferative disorders; and a variety of other malignancies including nasopharyngeal carcinoma and gastric carcinoma. This chapter reviews the biology of the virus and the hematologic diseases associated with EBV infection.

HISTORICAL BACKGROUND

EBV was first identified in 1964 by electron microscopy that revealed herpesvirus-like particles in cell cultures from biopsies of endemic Burkitt lymphoma (BL), a rapidly growing lymphoma initially identified in children from equatorial Africa.[1] In 1967, it was reported that EBV would immortalize cultured B lymphocytes in vitro.[2,3] Shortly thereafter, when a laboratory technician lacking EBV-neutralizing antibodies contracted IM and EBV antibody titers and heterophile titers turned positive, the relationship between primary EBV infection and IM was discovered.[4,5] The syndrome of IM had been recognized decades earlier.[6] It was characterized by enlarged tonsils, sore throat, and increased numbers of mononuclear cells.[7-10] Serum antibodies against antigens on sheep red blood cells were recognized as characteristic of IM ("heterophile antibodies").[11] Subsequently, EBV DNA was identified in nasopharyngeal carcinoma, posttransplant lymphoproliferative disease (PTLD), Hodgkin lymphoma (HL), peripheral T-cell lymphoma, and a variety of other malignancies.[12-16] More recently, evidence has emerged that EBV infection is likely etiologic in most cases of MS.[17]

VIRAL BIOLOGY/LYMPHOCYTE IMMORTALIZATION/ VIRAL GENE EXPRESSION

EBV is a gammaherpesvirus.[18] Virions contain linear double-stranded DNA of ~173,000 bp. It encodes ~100 proteins. Infection is mainly transmitted through saliva.[19,20] B cells in the oral mucosa become infected (Figure 63.1). Viral entry into lymphocytes is mediated by several viral glycoproteins interacting with cell surface receptors that lead to fusion of the viral envelope with the cell membrane.[21] The envelope glycoprotein gp350 binds to either CD21 (complement receptor type 2) or CD35 (complement receptor type 1) which leads to endocytosis of the virion. Following endocytosis, the viral capsid moves to the nucleus, where the linear EBV genome circularizes to form a nuclear plasmid or episome.[22,23] Latent infection is established in some of the infected cells, that is, virion production ceases but expression of latency genes continues. Viral gene expression drives the proliferation of these cells. The progeny cells also harbor viral episomes. The result is that cells harboring viral genomes spread through the B-cell compartment (blood, lymph nodes, spleen, and bone marrow).[24,25] In the normal host, immune responses are established that control infection. However, latently infected cells harboring viral genomes will persist for life in a small subset of resting memory B cells. These cells elude immune surveillance in part because of restricted viral gene expression. Occasional activation of lytic viral replication leads to lifelong intermittent viral shedding in saliva.

In vitro infection of B lymphocytes results in immortalization such that the infected cells grow indefinitely as lymphoblastoid cell lines. The immortalized B cells are tumorigenic in immunodeficient mice. The process of immortalization has been studied extensively. Nine viral proteins are expressed in these cell lines: Epstein-Barr nuclear antigen 1 (EBNA1), EBNA2, EBNA3A, EBNA3B, EBNA3C, EBNA leader protein, latency membrane protein 1 (LMP1), latency membrane protein 2A (LMP2A), and latency membrane protein 2B.[26,27] Not all of the latency proteins expressed in immortalized cells are required for the process of immortalization. Among those that are required are EBNA1, a protein important in the replication and maintenance of the viral episome; EBNA2, a transcription factor that activates Notch pathway signaling; and LMP1, a constitutively active member of the tumor necrosis factor receptor superfamily.[28,29] Although lymphocyte immortalization has been studied as a model for lymphomagenesis, some caution is required insofar as most EBV-associated lymphomas show much more restricted patterns of viral gene expression.

Although not required for lymphocyte immortalization, other EBV genes expressed in immortalized lymphocytes may also play a role in EBV-driven lymphomagenesis. These include EBER1 and EBER2, two RNA polymerase 3 transcripts that may be important for regulating apoptotic pathways and are secreted in exosomes.[30,31] The virus also encodes 44 mature microRNAs that may function in cell transformation and proliferation.[32] Viral gene expression may also perturb normal lymphocyte biology. Thus, LMP1 expression upregulates activation-induced (cytidine) deaminase expression, which facilitates somatic hypermutation and immunoglobulin class switching.[33] LMP1 expression may also be important in the conversion of naïve B cells to postgerminal center memory B cells. LMP2A allows B cells that lack normal immunoglobulin expression to escape regulatory checkpoints and survive.[34]

In latency, there is no virion production. Viral genomes are replicated in tandem with the cell cycle. The only viral protein required for viral genome replication in latency is EBNA1. Several different patterns of EBV latency gene expression are recognized as illustrated in Figure 63.2. In latency 1, EBNA1 is the only viral protein expressed. This is the pattern of viral gene expression associated with BL and primary effusion lymphoma (PEL). In latency 2, EBNA1, LMP1, and LMP2 (A or B) are expressed. This is the pattern associated with HL, some PTLDs, EBV-associated NK/T-cell lymphoma, and some AIDS diffuse large B-cell lymphoma (DLBCL). In latency 3, all of the EBNAs and all of the LMPs are expressed. This is the pattern associated with some PTLDs and some AIDS lymphomas, particularly primary central nervous system (CNS) lymphomas. More recently, latency 0 has been recognized in resting memory B cells that harbor EBV episomes. These cells which lack any viral protein expression are thus completely shielded from CD4 and CD8 T-cell immune surveillance.

Transition to lytic replication results when transcription of EBV immediate early proteins ZTA or RTA triggers a cascade of viral gene expression that results in synthesis of viral enzymes involved in nucleic acid metabolism and synthesis as well as of viral proteins that will form the viral capsid. Complete viral replication results in the lysis and death of the host cell and release of virions. Antiviral agents such as acyclovir and ganciclovir inhibit the viral DNA polymerase and block lytic replication. In contrast, these agents have no impact on replication of the viral genome in latency.

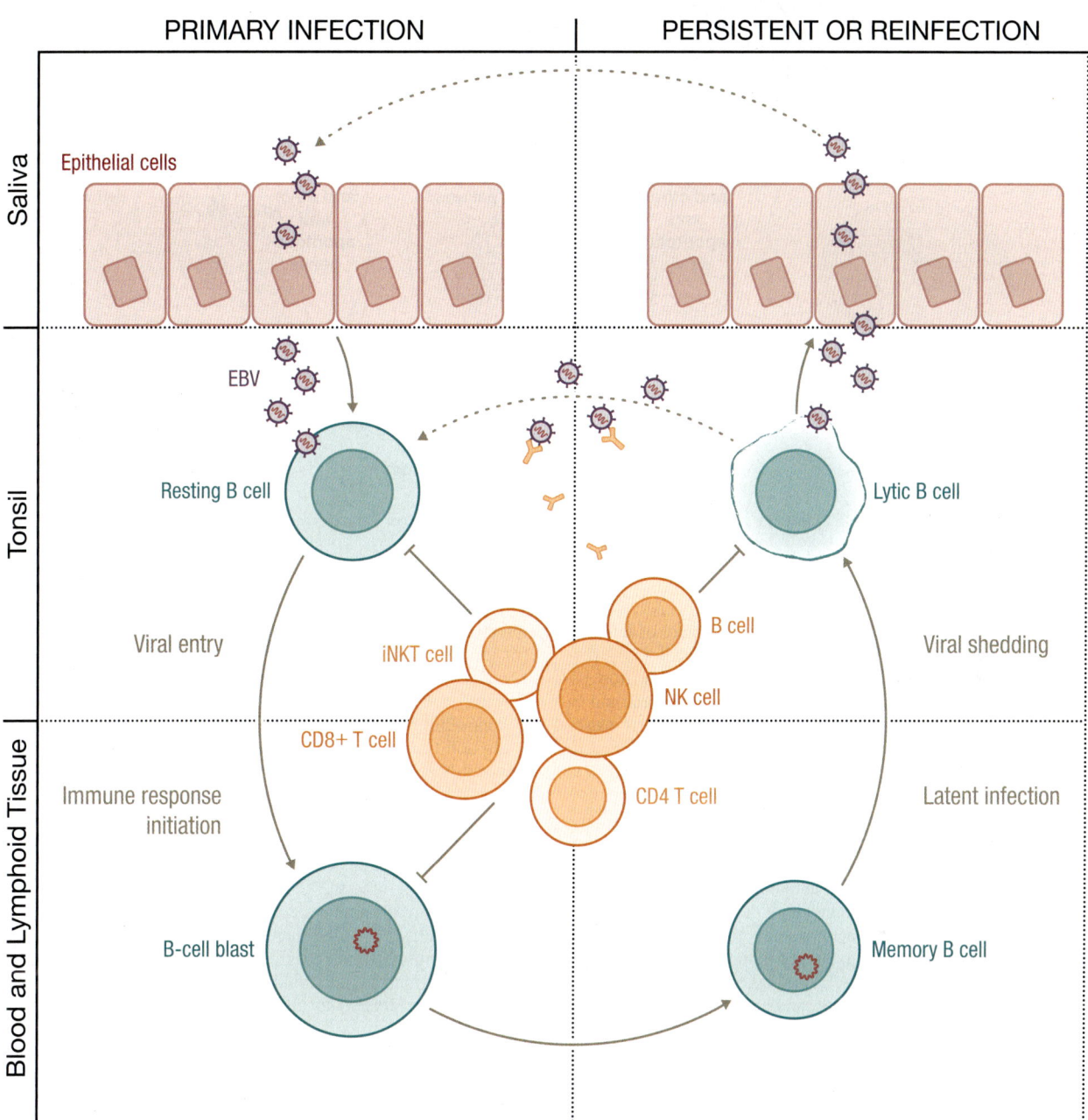

FIGURE 63.1 Schematic depicting Epstein-Barr virus (EBV) infection and the antiviral immune response. EBV infects resting B cells just under the surface of the oropharyngeal epithelium. Following virus entry into B cells, a series of events takes place, including delivery of linear viral DNA into the nucleus, formation of a circular episome, and expression of the full complement of viral proteins, leading to B-cell activation and proliferation. Subsequently, the genes that drive B-cell proliferation are shut off, and the virus assumes a state of latency within memory B cells, where only a limited array of viral proteins is expressed. Memory B cells circulating through oropharyngeal lymphoid tissues occasionally initiate viral replication, leading to release of lytic virus that may directly reinfect additional resting B cells or be released into the saliva, only to start the infectious cycle again (represented by dashed arrows). All but latently infected resting memory B cells are susceptible to attack by components of the host immune system, including CD8+ and CD4+ T cells, NK cells, and perhaps invariant NKT cells. NK, natural killer; NKT, natural killer T. Adapted from Cohen JI. Epstein-Barr virus infection. *N Engl J Med.* 2000;343(7):481-492; Odumade OA, Hogquist KA, Balfour HH Progress and problems in understanding and managing primary Epstein-Barr virus infections. *Clin Microbiol Rev.* 2011; 24(1):193-209. Joshua Stokes from The Department of Biomedical Communication at St. Jude Children's Research Hospital (SJCRH) provided assistance in drafting this figure.

IMMUNE RESPONSE TO EPSTEIN-BARR VIRUS INFECTION

In healthy individuals, NK cells are thought to play an important role in controlling the virus early in infection. With time, there is a brisk cellular and humoral immune response that constrains the outgrowth of EBV-infected B cells. Cytotoxic T lymphocytes (CTLs) reactive to EBV lytic proteins account for up to 50% of the large atypical lymphocytes visible in the blood of individuals with acute IM.[1,35-37] The marked expansion of CTL is accompanied by an increase in serum levels of proinflammatory and immunoregulatory cytokines, such as interferon-γ, tumor necrosis factor-α, interleukin (IL)-6, IL-10, and transforming growth factor-β, which further enhance and direct the antiviral immune response.[37,38] These T-helper cells secrete cytokines, facilitate generation of T-cell–dependent antibody responses, and sometimes exhibit cytotoxic activity.[38] Despite the vigorous EBV-specific T-cell response, virus-infected B cells are never completely eradicated. Accordingly, approximately 1 in 10,000 to 100,000 memory B cells remain infected

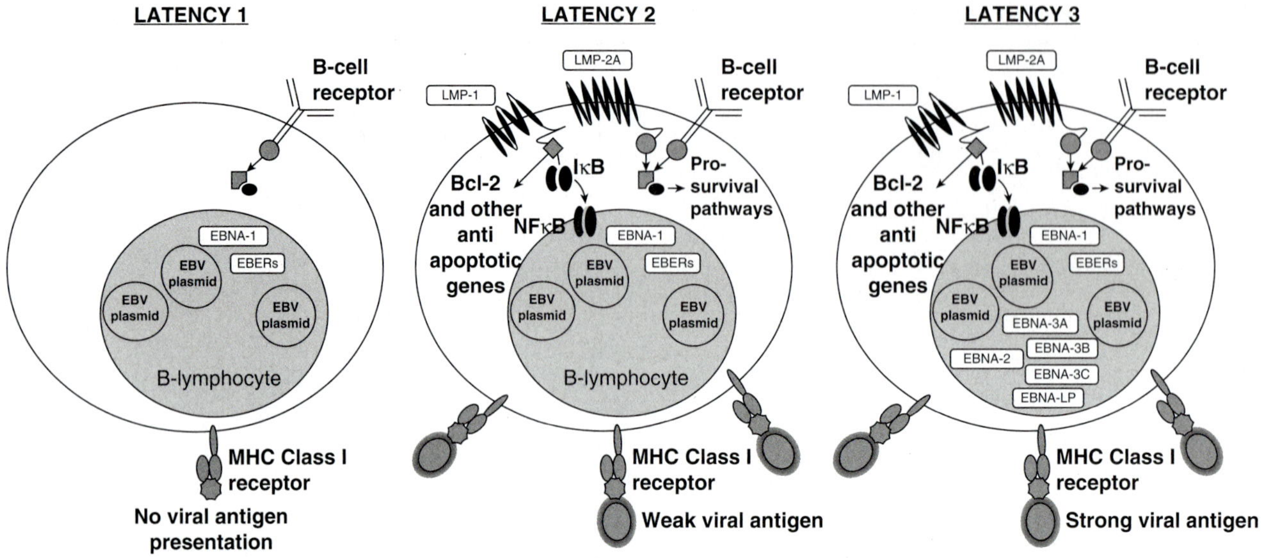

FIGURE 63.2 Epstein-Barr virus (EBV) latency gene patterns. Three gene expression patterns are illustrated and EBV-associated lymphomas in which these patterns of viral gene expression are seen. Note that viral gene expression in PTLD and AIDS lymphomas is variable. LMP, latency membrane protein; MHC, major histocompatibility complex, NFκB, nuclear factor kappa B; PTLD, posttransplant lymphoproliferative disease

throughout the life of the host.[23] It is likely from this pool of infected memory B cells that the virus periodically reactivates leading to intermittent viral shedding that occurs throughout the lifetime of the host.

The humoral response to EBV has been well characterized, and in healthy individuals, the detection of EBV-specific antibodies is a useful method to diagnose acute or prior EBV infection as illustrated in Figure 63.3.[39,40] However, measurement of EBV-specific antibodies is less useful in immunocompromised individuals. Virtually, all healthy individuals will develop antibodies to EBV viral capsid antigen (VCA). These antibodies are the earliest to appear following primary infection and include immunoglobulin M (IgM) and, later, IgG.[40] IgG anti-VCA antibodies peak 2 to 3 weeks after IgM antibodies and persist for life.[41] Subsequently, about 60% to 80% of individuals develop an IgG response to the EBV early antigen (EA) that peaks at 3 to 4 weeks following infection.[39] In approximately 20% to 30% of individuals, these anti-EA IgG responses are retained for years.[42] Antibodies against EBNA1 are the last to emerge. These antibodies appear weeks to months following infection, with titers rising slowly over 1 to 2 years and then persisting for life. In young children, anti-VCA and anti-EA antibodies may be lower in quantity, and it may take longer for anti-EBNA antibodies to emerge.[43] The possible importance of antibodies against EBV antigens in controlling viral infection remains poorly understood.

In addition to the production of EBV-specific antibodies, EBV-infected B cells produce a wide array of other antibodies that are not directed against the virus. Some of these represent autoantibodies and can cause disease. These include cold-reactive anti-I antibodies; Donath-Landsteiner antibodies; antibodies against smooth muscle, thyroid, and stomach[44]; antinuclear antibodies[45,46]; and rheumatoid factors[47] among others.[48,49] In 1932, Paul and Bunnell demonstrated that sera from IM patients contained antibodies reactive with sheep red blood cells.[11,50] Subsequently, these antibodies were termed "heterophile" antibodies in recognition of the fact that they interact with epitopes to which an individual has never been exposed. Because these antibodies are present in most individuals who have been recently

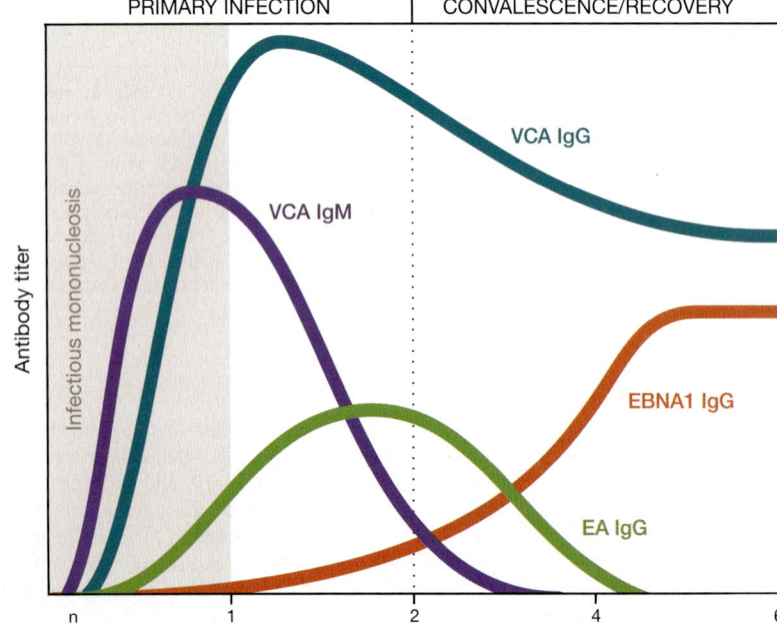

FIGURE 63.3 Schematic depicting development of the humoral response to Epstein-Barr virus (EBV). The humoral response to EBV develops over a period of several weeks following primary infection and begins with the production of IgM and IgG antibodies reactive with the viral capsid antigen (VCA). This is followed by an IgG response to the early antigen (EA) and last to EBNA1. Owing to the highly predictable nature of the humoral response, assessment of antibody titers can greatly aid in the diagnosis and staging of EBV infection in immunocompetent individuals. Ig, immunoglobulin. Joshua Stokes from The Department of Biomedical Communication at SJCRH provided assistance in drafting this figure.

infected with EBV, their presence has become a standard tool in establishing the diagnosis of acute EBV infection.

INFECTIOUS MONONUCLEOSIS

Epidemiology

Serologic studies have established that IM is associated with primary infection in adolescents and young adults.[1] The populations of seroconverters that have been best studied are college students. The most detailed studies come from the University of Minnesota where 74% experienced IM, with a median duration of illness of 18 days. Deep kissing is the major risk factor for IM in adolescents and young adults and thus IM is commonly referred to as the "kissing disease."[51,52] Other modes of exposure to saliva include premastication and shared food or eating utensils. Infection may be transmitted by breast feeding, organ transplantation, and transfusion of blood or hematopoietic cells.[53] Screening and leukoreduction of blood products reduce, but do not eliminate, the risk of transfusion-associated EBV transmission.[54]

Clinical Features

The presentation of IM varies at least in part as a function of patient age.[55] Most newly infected children are asymptomatic, whereas adolescents and adults present with the classic clinical triad of fever, pharyngitis, and adenopathy.[56] Development of symptoms occurs after an incubation period of four to 7 weeks.[57]

Pharyngitis varies in intensity, but rarely, massive tonsillar and pharyngeal edema can cause severe pharyngeal obstruction. The presence of white tonsillar exudates helps to distinguish IM from bacterial tonsillitis. Anorexia is also seen, with intensity and duration linked to severity of pharyngitis. Fatigue, malaise, and myalgia may also occur and be accompanied by fever, sweating, and chills. Most symptoms develop over the first 1 to 2 weeks and then subside after 2 to 4 weeks, with approximately 20% of patients reporting persistent sore throat at 4 weeks.[57] Lymphadenopathy usually appears during the first week of illness and slowly resolves thereafter. Cervical node enlargement is almost always present, and palpable axillary and inguinal nodes are common. Radiographically detectable hilar adenopathy is rare (<1%).[58] The spleen is palpable in half to three-fourths of patients, but massive splenomegaly is rare.[59] Ultrasound studies show that splenomegaly appears within 2 weeks of symptom onset and resolves within 4 to 6 weeks.[60] Hepatomegaly is detected in 15% to 25% of patients and may be associated with tenderness.[59] Headaches, photophobia, ocular myalgia, edema, conjunctivitis, dry eyes, keratitis, uveitis, choroiditis, retinitis, papillitis, and ophthalmoplegia are all described.[61] Drug rashes are common, especially with ampicillin.[62,63]

Laboratory Findings

Most patients with IM have slightly or moderately increased total white blood cell counts in the range of 10.0 to 20.0×10^9 cells/L.[64] Atypical lymphocytes account for >20% of total lymphocytes. These cells vary in size and shape and possess a nucleus that may be oval, kidney shaped, or lobulated (Figure 63.4). Leukopenia has been observed and may manifest as lymphopenia or granulocytopenia. Mild thrombocytopenia is common. Severe neutropenia and/or thrombocytopenia are concerning and may be signs of EBV-induced HLH.

Subclinical hepatitis as evident by elevated levels of alanine aminotransferase is seen in about 75% of patients, and in 5% to 10%, overt hepatitis with tender hepatomegaly and jaundice can occur. About one-third of patients have mild-to-moderate elevations of serum bilirubin values; levels above 8 mg/dL (135 μmol/L) are rare.[64,65] Occasionally, proteinuria or hematuria is present, but renal function is usually normal. When lumbar puncture has been performed, the cerebrospinal fluid pressure may be elevated; pleocytosis and increased levels of protein are often noted. The glucose content is normal. In a few patients, heterophile antibodies have been demonstrated in the cerebrospinal fluid.[66]

IM, without development of heterophile antibodies, also occurs in children but is less well studied. IM also occurs in adults over the age of 40 but is mainly the focus of case reports or small series.[67-69] In these reports which undoubtedly present a skewed picture, protracted fever, jaundice, pleural effusion, and Guillain-Barré syndrome often dominate the clinical picture.

Histologic Findings

The main histologic feature observed in tissues from patients with IM is expansion of the reticuloendothelial system, especially within the lymph nodes and spleen. Given the marked accumulation and activation of lymphocytes, it may be difficult to distinguish between malignant

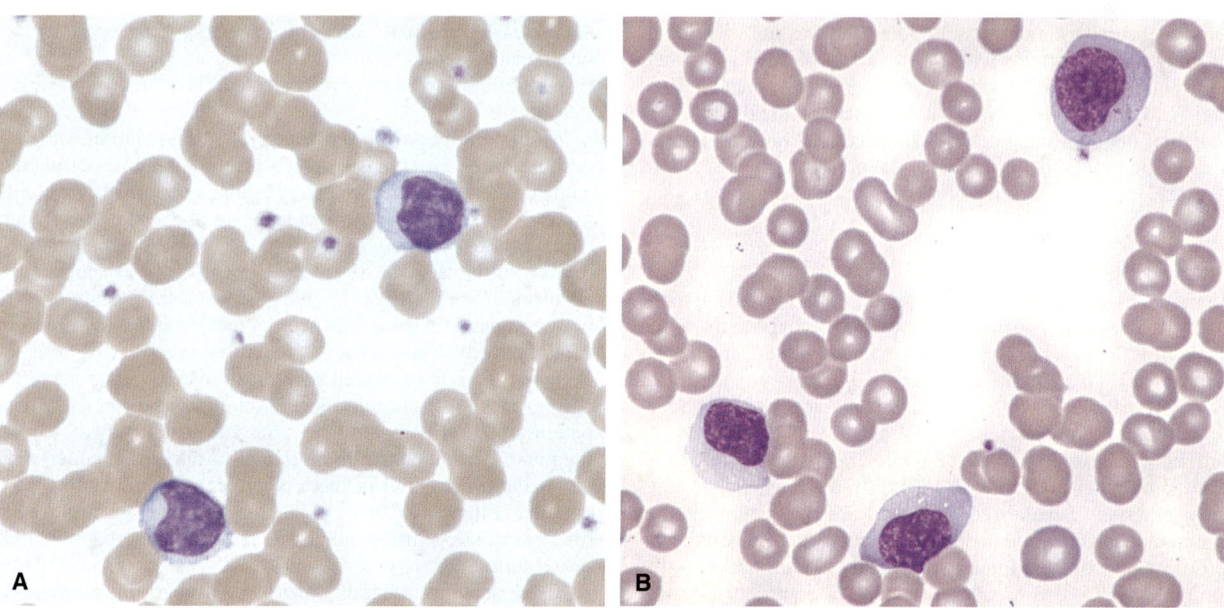

FIGURE 63.4 **Photomicrographs of normal human peripheral blood lymphocytes and the atypical lymphocytes seen in infectious mononucleosis (IM).** A, Normal peripheral blood lymphocytes. B, Atypical lymphocytes observed in the blood of an individual with IM. These cells may vary in size and shape but are generally larger than normal lymphocytes, have round to oval or indented nuclei with dense chromatin and distinct nucleoli, and increased amounts of cytoplasm that may contain granules or vacuoles. Photomicrographs are shown at ×100 magnification. Photomicrographs provided by Tina Motroni from the Department of Pathology at SJCRH.

lymphoma and nonmalignant lymphoproliferation, especially in those with underlying immunodeficiency. The lymph node architecture is generally intact, but may be distorted. Other morphologic features mimicking lymphoma include extensive immunoblastic proliferation with significant cellular atypia. Clonality studies are sometimes helpful in distinguishing IM from malignant disease. Germinal centers (GCs) are usually identifiable, but follicular prominence is diminished, probably because of the irregular and vaguely defined borders that result from the lymphocytic and reticuloendothelial hyperplasia of paracortical structures and, to a lesser extent, the medullary cords. This intense proliferative activity within the paracortical areas is in keeping with the characterization of atypical lymphocytes as T cells. The spleen is striking for infiltration of its fibromuscular structures by mononuclear cells.[70] The capsule and trabeculae are often thin and invaded by proliferating lymphocytes, which may explain the occurrence of splenic rupture. The bone marrow may exhibit hyperplasia of erythroid, myeloid, and megakaryocytic elements.[71,72]

Diagnosis

The presence of typical clinical features, atypical lymphocytosis, and a positive heterophile antibody test is usually sufficient to establish a diagnosis of IM.[1] Heterophile antibodies can usually be identified using the "Monospot" assay, which detects antibody-mediated agglutination of sheep red blood cell. That said, heterophile antibodies are not specific for IM and may not develop in all cases. In particular, heterophile antibodies are less sensitive and specific in young children and should not be used in children under 4 years old.[73] EBV-specific antibody tests may also be used to diagnose and stage infection. During acute infection, one generally observes high titers of anti-VCA IgM and IgG, high titers of anti-EA antibodies, and the absence of anti-EBNA1 antibodies. In contrast, a prior infection is diagnosed based on disappearance of anti-VCA IgM and appearance of anti-EBNA1 IgG.[39,40]

Molecular diagnostic techniques are also available for the identification of EBV. These tests are particularly useful for immunocompromised patients who may not mount a normal humoral response and for patients who have received intravenous Ig infusions, both of which make serologic testing challenging. Polymerase chain reaction (PCR)–mediated detection of EBV DNA in peripheral blood (PB) mononuclear cells, plasma, or whole blood provides evidence of an EBV infection. In a hospital-based study, detection of EBV in plasma was more specific for EBV-associated disease than EBV in mononuclear cells.[74] The copy number of EBV detected was not of value in distinguishing among patients with IM, a variety of EBV-associated tumors, or patients with illness that was not EBV associated. Thus, it appears that EBV may reactivate with a variety of stresses and that EBV detection may not indicate any causative relationship between the virus and the illness that has brought the patient to medical attention. EBV detection in the plasma of patients in intensive care is quite frequent.[75]

Differential Diagnosis

The differential diagnosis of IM, characterized by pharyngitis, lymphadenopathy, and malaise, includes streptococcal pharyngitis, acute cytomegalovirus (CMV), primary HIV, *Toxoplasma gondii*, and human herpesvirus 6 (HHV6).[76] Acute CMV and *T. gondii* share additional features with IM including splenomegaly, hepatomegaly, lymphocytosis, and atypical lymphocytosis. CMV and toxoplasmosis can be distinguished with serology. Acute HIV infection is more likely to be accompanied by mucocutaneous lesions, rash, diarrhea, weight loss, nausea, and emesis.[77] Generalized lymph node enlargement, including the postauricular and occipital nodes, is characteristic of rubella.[78]

The differential of pharyngitis specifically, which accounts for 6% of outpatient visits, is broader and includes respiratory viruses (rhinovirus, coronavirus, influenza virus adenovirus, parainfluenza virus), CMV, herpes simplex virus, coxsackievirus A, HIV, HHV6, bacteria (Group A streptococci, Group C and Group G streptococci, *Arcanobacterium haemolyticum*, *Corynebacterium diphtheriae*, *Neisseria gonorrhoeae*, *Mycoplasma pneumoniae*), and *T. gondii*.

Group A beta-hemolytic streptococcal infection is the most common bacterial cause of pharyngitis; it is important to distinguish this from IM because the former warrants antibiotic treatment to prevent sequelae. Patients suspected of having pharyngitis as part of IM may be screened for Group A streptococci by using swabs with rapid antigen tests or culture. IM and Group A pharyngitis may co-occur together; however, the incidence of co-occurrence is unclear.[76] Therefore, a positive strep test does not rule out the presence of a concomitant EBV infection. Drug fever and serum sickness–like reactions may also suggest IM because they are also characterized by fever, jaundice, lymph node enlargement, and the presence of atypical lymphocytes.[78]

The PB lymphocytosis in IM mimics that observed with both malignant and benign diseases related to infections or drugs. Malignant causes of monoclonal peripheral lymphocytosis include chronic lymphocytic leukemia, hairy cell leukemia, splenic marginal zone lymphoma, lymphoplasmacytic lymphoma, follicular lymphoma, mantle cell lymphoma, adult T-cell leukemia or lymphoma, and Sézary syndrome. Although the leukocytes of patients with IM appear abnormal, few contain nucleoli (a common feature of leukemia or lymphoma cells), and patients with IM only rarely develop severe thrombocytopenia and/or anemia. The bone marrow examination can be used to differentiate IM from acute leukemia or other hematologic processes. In IM, the bone marrow morphology is generally normal, whereas in leukemia, there will be infiltration with lymphoblasts, and in HLH, there may be an excessive number of activated macrophages with evidence of hemophagocytosis. CMV and EBV are the most common infectious causes of peripheral lymphocytosis. Other infectious causes include primary HIV infection, coxsackie A and B6 viruses, echovirus, adenovirus, HHV6, rubella, virus, varicella, human T lymphotropic virus-1, hepatitis viruses. Non–viral infectious causes include *T. gondii* and *Bordetella pertussis*.[79]

Complications

A variety of problems can arise during IM; however, severe or even fatal complications are present in ≤1% of patients.[1] Hematologic complications are among the most common, observed in 25% to 50% of IM cases.[76] This includes hemolytic anemia (3%), neutropenia (50%-80%), thrombocytopenia (25%-50%), and rarely, aplastic anemia, thrombotic thrombocytopenic purpura or hemolytic-uremic syndrome, and disseminated intravascular coagulation.[76,80]

Hemolytic anemia should be suspected in patients with IM with jaundice. Direct antiglobulin testing should be obtained to confirm the diagnosis. In around 70% of patients, titers of cold agglutinins are increased,[81] usually with anti-I specificity.[82] Occasionally, hemolysis is attributed to Donath-Landsteiner antibodies,[83,84] and in some cases, no antibodies are ever detected. Treatment is typically with steroids.[85,86]

Severe thrombocytopenia generally attributed to increased platelet destruction by an enlarged spleen or production of antiplatelet antibodies. When bone marrow examination is performed, myeloid hyperplasia is usually seen with increased numbers of promyelocytes, but depletion of more mature neutrophils.[87] Neutropenia occurs in 50% to 80% of cases, with severe neutropenia (<1000 neutrophils/mm^3) occurring in <3% of cases. While profound suppression of the marrow is rare, aplastic anemia has been noted.[88] Generally, it is related to EBV-induced HLH.

One of the most feared complications is splenic rupture.[80] The diagnosis of a ruptured spleen should be entertained whenever a patient with IM has pain below the left costal margin, especially if the pain is accompanied by radiation to the left shoulder and supraclavicular area, or when there is evidence of impending peripheral vascular collapse. Other signs include peritoneal irritation, abdominal tenderness, and shifting dullness if massive intra-abdominal bleeding has occurred.[89,90]

Complications affecting other organ systems including neurologic manifestations such as headache,[80] encephalitis, meningitis, cranial nerve palsies, and mononeuropathies may occur in up to 7% of patients.[91] Cardiac complications involve myocarditis/pericarditis,[92] mediastinitis,[93] and cardiac tamponade.[94] The most serious respiratory complication is acute airway obstruction, which usually results from extreme hyperplasia of the tonsils and pharyngeal lymphatic tissue. Interstitial pneumonia and pleuritis are rare pulmonary complications. Asymptomatic elevations in transaminases occur in 50% to 80% of cases.[80] Hepatic necrosis or liver failure is rarely seen, usually in patients with EBV–associated hemophagocytic lymphohistiocytosis (EBV-HLH) or underlying immunodeficiency.[95]

Treatment

Most patients experiencing uncomplicated acute IM require only supportive care. Acetaminophen and nonsteroidal anti-inflammatory agents may be used for fever, pharyngitis, and malaise. Nonsteroidal anti-inflammatory drugs should be avoided in cases with severe hepatitis. Aspirin should be avoided because it interferes with platelet function and increases the risk of bleeding in thrombocytopenic patients. Concern with splenic rupture has led some to recommend that contact sports be avoided for 3 weeks.[96]

Corticosteroids, which have anti-inflammatory and lympholytic properties, are best reserved for severe complications of IM; for example, they are appropriate in cases of severe airway obstruction, carditis, lymphoid interstitial pneumonitis, and cerebral involvement. With regards to mild cases of IM, the cumulative results of several small, controlled clinical trials suggest that corticosteroids hasten resolution of fever and pharyngitis in patients with uncomplicated IM, but do not provide significant benefits in reducing lymphadenopathy or hepatosplenomegaly.[97] Another study showed early improvement in sore throat with corticosteroids, but the effects were not sustained at follow-up visits.[98] Systematic reviews have concluded that there is insufficient evidence of clinical benefit to routinely recommend corticosteroid treatment.[99]

Several antiviral agents, such as acyclovir, valacyclovir, ganciclovir, zidovudine, foscarnet, and the interferons have been shown to inhibit the replication of EBV in vitro.[100] Only the linear form of the genome, not the latent circular form, is susceptible to inhibition. The efficacy of acyclovir in the therapy of uncomplicated IM has been assessed in several controlled trials.[101-103] In general, acyclovir reduces viral shedding during the time of therapy, but viral shedding resumes when therapy is discontinued. Clinical trials have documented few clinical benefits as measured by duration of illness and sore throat, weight loss, or the absence from school or work, even when acyclovir was given in combination with steroids. A small randomized study of 20 college students found that subjects receiving valacyclovir had less oropharyngeal shedding and a reduction in symptom severity [16]. PB EBV copy numbers were similar between groups. A separate study treated healthy subjects with valacyclovir or no antiviral therapy for 1 year and periodically measured the levels of EBV DNA. Subjects receiving valacyclovir had reduced levels of EBV-infected B cells.[104]

OTHER EPSTEIN-BARR VIRUS–RELATED HEMATOLOGIC DISEASES

In addition to IM, EBV infection has been linked to a wide spectrum of nonmalignant and malignant diseases. Although association has been demonstrated, the mechanisms underlying disease pathogenesis remain poorly understood for many of these disorders.

Chronic Active Epstein-Barr Virus Infection

Chronic active EBV infection (CAEBV) is a rare disorder in which EBV-infected T cells and NK cells cause systemic inflammation and the development of neoplasms.[105] In 2016, the World Health Organization, based on research supporting clonal evolution of infected T and NK cells, defined CAEBV as an EBV-T/NK-lymphoproliferative disorder.[105,106] The criteria for diagnosis of CAEBV are (1) sustained or recurrent IM-like symptoms persisting for more than 3 months; (2) an elevated EBV genome load in the PB or a tissue lesion; (3) EBV infection of T or NK cells in the affected tissues or the PB; and (4) exclusion of other possible diagnoses including primary EBV infection (IM), autoimmune diseases, congenital immunodeficiencies, HIV, and other immunodeficiencies.[105] Clinically, CAEBV is characterized by systemic inflammation and neoplastic disease. This manifests as recurrent IM-like symptoms, including fever, lymphadenopathy, and splenomegaly, liver dysfunction, thrombocytopenia, and anemia, and occurs most commonly in patients who develop IM as older children or young adults.[107-109] Infected T and NK cells may invade the vasculature causing vasculitis leading to vascular aneurysms, ischemic organ damage, and uveitis. CAEBV may progress to HLH and chemotherapy-resistant lymphoma if clonal expansion occurs.[105] Life-threatening complications include HLH (21%), coronary artery aneurysm (21%), hepatic failure (18%), malignant lymphoma (16%), and interstitial pneumonia (12%).[109] Most deaths are caused by HLH or lymphoma, which may be of T-cell, B-cell, or NK-cell phenotype.

Two skin conditions, severe mosquito bite allergy (sMBA) and hydroa vacciniforme (HV), are also characterized by EBV-infected T and NK cells. In contrast to CAEBV, symptoms and inflammation are confined to the skin. sMBA presents with hypersensitivity to mosquito bites and patients develop high fevers, ulcers, necrosis, and scarring after the bite. HV presents with recurrent eruptions of vesicles in sun-exposed areas and may resemble herpetic lesions. These conditions are rare and their pathogenesis and relation to CAEBV are poorly understood.[105,110]

In CAEBV, high levels of EBV DNA are found in $CD4^+$ T cells and NK cells, but not in B cells, as is seen in typical EBV infection.[111] The EBV genome in CAEBV patients has also been found to contain unique intragenic deletions also seen in other EBV neoplastic disorders such as DLBCL and extranodal NK/T-cell lymphoma; notably, these deletions are not seen in IM or posttransplant lymphoproliferative disorders.[112,113] This suggests that the presence of certain genomic deletions may drive the development of CAEBV after initial infection with EBV. The deletions studied to date are thought to reactivate the viral lytic cycle while also downregulating viral production and cell lysis, thus driving lymphomagenesis. CAEBV is thought to occur more commonly in patients from Asia and South America, but is also seen in North American and European populations. In some CAEBV patients as well as their parents, CTL and NK-cell activity are reduced, suggesting a heritable cellular defect. It has been suggested that gain-of-function mutations in DDX3X may be driver mutations that lead to lymphoma or leukemia.[105] Biallelic inactivating mutations in the gene encoding perforin have been described.[114] CAEBV clinically overlaps with EBV-HLH.

The only curative therapy for CAEBV is allogeneic hematopoietic stem cell transplant.[115] A variety of cytotoxic and antiviral agents may be used to temporize the disease until the patient is ready for transplant.[107,115] HLH-directed immunochemotherapy (eg, etoposide, corticosteroids, and cyclosporin A) has been used to control symptoms and treat hemophagocytic manifestations,[108] whereas lymphomas have been treated with standard non-Hodgkin lymphoma (NHL) therapy.[108] Adoptive T-cell therapies have been tried with limited success.[107]

Epstein-Barr Virus–Associated Hemophagocytic Lymphohistiocytosis

EBV-associated HLH is an aggressive life-threatening syndrome of excessive immune activation that can occur in patients with genetic defects associated with dysregulation of the immune response (familial HLH) or arise in patients with infection or malignancy (nonfamilial or secondary HLH).[116] Diagnosis and treatment of HLH are considered in other chapters. For the purposes of this chapter, we note EBV-HLH is recognized in the context of HLH with elevated EBV as assessed by PCR in the blood or by Epstein-Barr virus (EBV)-encoded small RNAs in situ hybridization that identifies EBV-infected lymphocytes in the marrow. Primary EBV infection may serve as a trigger of familial HLH or immunodeficiency syndromes such as X-linked lymphoproliferative (XLP) disease or in patients without inherited predisposition. Finally EBV-associated lymphoproliferative disorders and lymphomas, particularly T/NK cell can be associated with HLH. Whereas in healthy seropositives, EBV in the blood is found almost exclusively in B cells, in many patients with EBV-HLH, viral DNA is detected in T or NK cells. Thus, while some have advocated rituximab for EBV-HLH in addition to other therapies, there is neither consensus nor randomized data that this is useful.[117] Similarly, although acyclovir or valacyclovir are widely used in this setting, there is little if any evidence that they improve outcome. At a first approximation, treatment for EBV-HLH is not virus specific.[78]

EPSTEIN-BARR VIRUS–ASSOCIATED LYMPHOMA

EBV is seen in association with approximately 1% of the worldwide burden of human cancer, including lymphoid, epithelial, and mesenchymal malignancies.[1] In what follows, we address the lymphoid malignancies. Before discussing these tumors, it is worth noting how a relationship with a tumor type is established. Because many tumor types harbor predominantly latent EBV with very limited viral protein expression, the standard approach to virus detection in lymphoma tissues is EBER in situ hybridization. EBER1 and EBER2 are small non–coding RNA polymerase 3 transcripts that are expressed at very high levels in most latently infected cells and thus ideal targets for in situ hybridization.[118] Originally detected by autoradiography, the abundance of the target made it ideal for immunohistochemistry, and assay for EBER expression has become a standard pathologic tool. In HL which has a latency 2 pattern of viral gene expression, the results of EBER in situ hybridization and immunohistochemistry for LMP1 are comparable, whereas only EBER in situ hybridization will detect tumors with more restricted patterns of viral expression such as in BL.[119]

Burkitt Lymphoma

Endemic BL occurs in children in areas where malaria is holoendemic including equatorial Africa and Papua New Guinea, the disease characteristically arises as a rapidly enlarging jaw or abdominal mass, and is almost uniformly associated with EBV.[120] It is among the most common childhood tumors (~5/100,000) in endemic areas, and more common in boys than in girls. Outside these regions, the clinical presentation and EBV association of BL is distinct. Sporadic BL is much less common (~0.1/100,000), has a much broader age distribution, only rarely presents as a jaw mass, and is variably EBV associated. Outside the endemic regions, less than 30% of cases are EBV associated.[121] Among people living with HIV in the United States, the incidence of BL is almost as high as in the regions where BL is endemic in Africa (~3/100,000).[122] It is not yet clear what the impact of HIV infection is on the incidence of endemic BL.[123]

Whether endemic, sporadic, or HIV associated, the pattern of viral gene expression appears to be consistent: EBNA1 is the only viral protein consistently expressed.[123] A small percentage of tumor cells show evidence of lytic infection. Tumor cell lines are readily established in the laboratory. Chromosomal translocations that bring the c-myc gene under the control of the immunoglobulin heavy or less commonly immunoglobulin light chain loci c-myc are found in BL independent of the association with EBV, although differences in precise chromosomal breakpoints have been reported. EBV-associated BL has fewer driver mutations affecting cell survival pathways.[124]

Key aspects of the pathogenesis of EBV-associated BL and its cofactors malaria and HIV are not understood.[123] Evidence has been presented that malaria may increase EBV DNA copy number in blood. Malaria may alter the risk or the impact of primary EBV infection in very young children, blunt EBV-specific cytotoxic T-cell responses, activate toll-like receptors, and increase double-strand breaks and translocations. EBV gene expression, especially noncoding RNAs, may confer resistance to apoptosis in the genetically unstable infected lymphocytes. And while it is tempting to attribute the increased incidence of BL in people with HIV to global immunocompromise, the evidence points to a more complex relationship. In contrast to other EBV-associated non-HLs, its incidence has not fallen with the introduction of effective antiretroviral therapy (ART) and in contrast to some other EBV-associated lymphomas in people living with HIV, absolute CD4 T-cell counts are typically greater than 200. And finally, many AIDS BLs, perhaps most, are not EBV associated. Thus, malaria and HIV are both identified as cofactors that increase the risk of BL many fold, but the details of pathogenesis remain largely speculative.

Hodgkin Lymphoma

EBV is detected in the tumor cells of HL in 20% to 100% of cases.[125] When virus is detected in tumor cells, it is usually detected at presentation and relapse and at all sites of tumor involvement. Factors associated with the presence of EBV in tumor cells include histologic subtype (mixed cellularity HL is most commonly EBV positive), male gender, very young or very old age, Hispanic ethnicity primary or acquired immunocompromise (HIV, PTLD, or iatrogenic immunosuppression), and history of symptomatic IM.[126-130]

The pattern of viral gene expression in HL is latency 2 (EBNA1, LMP1, LMP2A), but it is distinctive with regard to the very high-level expression of LMP1 and LMP2A (in comparison with nasopharyngeal carcinoma, another tumor with latency 2 expression).[131] These viral proteins activate signaling pathways that may be important in the pathogenesis of the tumor.[132] Crippling immunoglobulin gene mutations are more commonly seen in the tumor cells of EBV-positive HL cases vs EBV-negative cases. Noting that LMP2A mimics immunoglobulin receptor signaling and that in mouse models, deletion of surface Ig-negative cells in the GC can be inhibited by LMP2A, it has been speculated that LMP2A expression protects the tumor cells in HL from deletion. LMP1 leads to activation of the nuclear factor kappa B (NFκB) pathway and also promotes cell survival. In EBV-negative cases, biallelic-inactivating mutations in *TNFAIP3* (a negative regulator of NFκB) are common.[133] Thus, the paths to EBV-associated and EBV-negative HL may be different.

Tumor cells in HL that are EBV associated express major histocompatibility complex class 1, while those that are EBV-negative do not.[131,134] Taken together with the observation that CD8+ CTLs can consistently be isolated from the PB of patients with EBV(+) HL[135] suggests that the tumor cells in EBV-associated HL are somehow protected from cytotoxic T-cell surveillance. Amplification of the programmed death-ligand 1/2 locus which is characteristic of EBV-associated and EBV-negative HL is presumed to play a role in insulating the tumor cells from cytotoxic killing.

Posttransplant Lymphoproliferative Disease

The increased frequency of lymphoma in the posttransplant period led to the recognition of PTLD. The original cases were EBV associated but EBV-negative PTLD are now recognized. Lymphoproliferative disease or lymphoma arises weeks to decades after solid organ transplantation (SOT) or hematopoietic cell transplantation (HCT). EBV-associated PTLD predominates in the first year. In contrast, PTLD occurring many years after transplantation is rarely EBV associated. Changes in pharmacologic immunosuppression have lowered the incidence of EBV-associated PTLD.

The incidence of PTLD varies as a function of the organ or tissue transplanted, the immunosuppressive regimen used, and prior exposure to EBV infection.[136] The highest incidences of PTLD occurred in the setting of T-cell depleted HCT, in cardiac transplant recipients treated with OKT3 (an antibody targeting CD3), or in seronegative recipients of gut transplants. PTLDs are heterogeneous in histology and clinical presentation. EBV-associated PTLD may be polyclonal or clonal. Although most commonly of B-cell lineage, they may also be of T/NK lineage. In HCT recipients, the tumors are typically derived from donor B cells, whereas in SOT recipients, the tumors are typically derived from host B cells. The EBV-associated lymphoproliferative lesions may present as nondestructive lesions (plasmacytic hyperplasia, IM, or florid follicular hyperplasia), polymorphic lesions, or monomorphic lesions that most commonly resemble diffuse large B-cell lymphoma, BL, plasma cell myeloma, peripheral T-cell lymphoma, or classic HL.[137] They are commonly extranodal and often associated with B symptoms. Gastrointestinal tract and CNS involvement are common. Although many different lymphomas may occur in the posttransplant setting, a subset of these tumors arising in the most profoundly immunocompromised are almost unique insofar as they show a latency 3 pattern of expression.

Successful treatment of PTLD necessitates controlling the B-cell proliferation and facilitating the development of an appropriate cytotoxic T-cell (EBV-CTL) response. Surgery, radiotherapy, or the combination is sometimes effective in curing localized disease. The use of antiviral agents, such as acyclovir or ganciclovir, and/or intravenous Ig may reduce risk insofar as they lower viral replication and thereby limit the number of infected B cells; however, their efficacy remains unproven and there is little reason to believe that established PTLD ever responds to these interventions. Therapy of EBV-associated B-cell tumors commonly involves B-cell targeted therapies such as rituximab, often augmented with cytotoxic chemotherapy. In some instances, reduction or change in immunosuppressive regimens alone may be adequate to induce remission. Adoptive cellular immunotherapy is sometimes effective.[138]

Natural Killer/T-Cell Lymphoma

Extranodal NK/T-cell lymphoma; nasal type, formerly known as lethal midline granuloma; and aggressive NK-cell leukemia are more common in Asia and Central and South America, but occur worldwide.[139] EBV is detected by in situ hybridization. These lymphomas occur primarily in the nose and upper airway (80%), less commonly in the skin, gastrointestinal tract, and testes; and rarely as a fulminant leukemia. Quantification of plasma EBV is a prognostic factor and can be used for monitoring response to therapy.

HV-like lymphoma is another EBV-driven lymphoproliferative disorder that occurs mainly in Central and South America and Asia. The illness generally affects children and is characterized by skin lesions on the face and other sun-exposed areas. Some patients have hypersensitivity to mosquito bites. They can have either a T-cell or NK phenotype and can progress to a systemic peripheral T-cell lymphoma that is relatively chemoresistant.[140]

Epstein-Barr Virus in People Living With HIV

The clinical spectrum of lymphoma in HIV includes DLBCL, primary CNS lymphoma, plasmablastic lymphoma, HL, and PEL.[141,142] In association with HIV, EBV is detected in approximately 40% DLBCL, 90% of plasmablastic lymphoma, virtually all primary CNS lymphomas, and approximately 90% of HL.[143] PEL merits special comment. It occurs almost exclusively in AIDS patients recipients, is virtually always Kaposi's sarcoma-associated herpesvirus associated, and usually EBV associated as well, that is, most tumor cells are dually infected.[144] How the viruses interact in the pathogenesis of PEL is not understood.

Also poorly understood are the very different associations of absolute CD4 T-cell counts with these EBV-associated lymphomas. Low absolute CD4 T-cell counts are a risk factor for lymphoma and other HIV-associated diseases. Among people living with HIV, primary CNS lymphoma occurs almost exclusively in people with very low absolute CD4 T-cell counts, while HL occurs almost exclusively in people with preserved CD4 T-cell counts. Following the introduction of ART, there has been an increase in CD4 T cells in the HIV population, a marked decrease in primary CNS lymphoma, and lesser decrease in systemic diffuse large B-cell lymphoma; however, the incidence of HL seemingly remains unchanged.[145,146] Thus, while the role of HIV in the development of primary CNS lymphoma may be global immunosuppression, the role in the pathogenesis of HL is likely more complex.

Other EBV-Associated Lymphomas and Lymphoid Lesions

There are a variety of other EBV-associated lymphoid lesions worthy of comment.[147] EBV mucocutaneous ulcer is an entity characterized by a well-circumscribed ulcer, most commonly in the oropharyngeal mucosa, characterized by a mixed inflammatory background and a variable number of EBV-positive, CD30-positive cells which may be indistinguishable from the tumor cells of HL. A rim of CD3-positive small lymphocytes usually demarcates the base of the lesion. These lesions are seen in elderly or immunocompromised patients. Spontaneous regression is common. Lymphomatoid granulomatosis is a rare disorder that usually occurs in the lungs, CNS, skin, kidney, or liver. It is an angiocentric and angiodestructive B-cell disorder. EBV is almost always associated. The clinical course is highly variable with some patients having asymptomatic indolent disease, whereas others have very aggressive disease. Treatment usually follows a lymphoma paradigm. These patients are also treated with an aggressive lymphoma paradigm.[148] DLBCL associated with chronic inflammation typically arises in body cavities. Originally identified as pyothorax-associated lymphoma, it was first described in Japanese patients treated for pulmonary tuberculosis with artificial pneumothorax (in the preantibiotic era). It may also arise in the setting of chronic osteomyelitis, metallic implants, and skin ulcers or in association with hematomas or thrombi. There is typically more than 10 years between the inciting event and the diagnosis of lymphoma. Lesions associated with hematomas or thrombi (so called "fibrin-associated") are typically more indolent and often treated with surgical excision alone. Angioimmunoblastic T-cell lymphoma is a malignancy of mature T-follicular helper cells that typically presents with lymphadenopathy, fever, skin rash, and polyclonal hypergammaglobulinemia.[149] Biopsies typically show scattered EBER-positive B cells distinct from the malignant T cells that are EBER negative. EBER-positive B-cell lymphomas sometimes arise in association with angioimmunoblastic T-cell lymphoma.

EBV–ASSOCIATED DISORDERS IN PRIMARY IMMUNODEFICIENCY

Many primary immunodeficiency diseases (PIDDs) are linked to increased risk of lymphoma. These are typically disorders of T-cell number or function or of innate immunity. In many of these PIDDs, lymphoproliferative disease is variably associated with EBV, while in others, the association is consistent. EBV lymphoma may present as the first manifestation of these disorders.

XLP1 is a rare immunodeficiency in which primary EBV infection is often fulminant leading to HLH or lymphoma. It affects approximately 1 out of every million male individuals.[150] A distinctive feature is the increased susceptibility of affected boys to EBV but not other childhood infections. Three phenotypes are common and include (1) fatal infectious mononucleosis (referred to here as EBV-HLH), (2) malignant manifestation, and (3) dysgammaglobulinemia. Less common manifestations include vasculitis, pulmonary lymphomatoid granulomatosis, and aplastic anemia.[151] Some XLP patients with evidence of current or prior EBV infection never develop EBV-HLH.[150] Allogeneic-HSCT is the only curative approach.[152,153] Dysgammaglobulinemia affects approximately 50% of affected boys.[152,154] Most boys manifesting this phenotype demonstrate global decreases of serum Ig levels; however, some have increased IgM or IgA or both, as well as variable deficiencies in IgG1 and IgG3 subclasses.[155] Although hypogammaglobulinemia often occurs after EBV infection, some XLP patients develop hypogammaglobulinemia without prior evidence of EBV infection. Immunoglobulin replacement therapy is standard for such patients. NHL develops in approximately 25% of XLP patients.[150] Most are of B-cell phenotype and are characterized by Burkitt or diffuse large cell histology. The role of EBV in the lymphoma development in XLP is unclear because ~50% of boys with lymphoma have no evidence of prior EBV infection, and EBV is detectable in only 25% of tumor specimens. Although chemotherapy may induce remissions, the risk of relapse or other fatal complications is very high.[153] The disease is the result of a mutation in SH2D1A, a gene which encodes a small cytoplasmic adaptor protein known as signaling lymphocyte activation molecule (SLAM)-associated protein (SAP).[156-158] SAP is an SH2 domain–containing adaptor molecule that regulates intracellular signaling downstream of the SLAM family of receptors expressed on hematopoietic cells. Studies of SAP-deficient cells have revealed critical roles for this protein in the promotion of stable interactions between T and B cells, which are required for the recognition and killing of B cells by CD8$^+$ CTL and the induction of B-cell–dependent humoral responses by CD4$^+$ follicular T-helper cells.[37,159] Collectively, defects in these processes are proposed to underlie the inability of T and NK cells to recognize and eradicate EBV-infected cells. The diagnosis of XLP1 can be strongly suspected based on reduced or lack of SAP protein expression by flow cytometric assessment of PB lymphocytes and confirmed by identification of inactivating mutations in SH2D1A. Historically, XLP was considered highly lethal, with 75% of patients dying by 10 years of age. However, improved recognition and earlier interventions have led to a current survival rate of 71.4%.[154] The role for preemptive HSCT prior to the development of XLP1 manifestations remains a matter of debate; however, it is important to recognize that outcomes are significantly better for those who undergo allo-HSCT prior to developing EBV-HLH.[152]

In 2006, a second X-linked disorder associated with EBV-HLH was described.[160,161] In addition to HLH, these patients may develop inflammatory bowel disease, hypogammaglobulinemia, cytopenias, and a variety of other autoinflammatory conditions. In contrast to XLP, they do not develop lymphoma. The similarity in EBV sensitivity between patients with SAP and XIAP deficiency initially led to the naming of this condition as XLP2. Over time, however, as the differences came to be better appreciated, XIAP has come to be the preferred term. Diagnosis of XIAP deficiency is often suspected based on reduced or lack of XIAP expression by flow cytometry. The gold standard is the identification of an *XIAP* inactivating mutation.[162] Reduced intensity allogeneic HSCT is a standard curative approach.

ITK encodes the IL-2–inducible T-cell kinase, a nonreceptor tyrosine kinase expressed by hematopoietic cells that is involved in proximal T-cell receptor (TCR) signaling via its regulation of phospholipase C-γ phosphorylation.[37] Biallelic-inactivating mutations in *ITK* cause an interesting autosomal-recessive primary immunodeficiency disorder associated with the development of EBV-positive HL. The disorder was originally identified in two female siblings from a consanguineous family who developed EBV-HLH–like symptoms with progression to HL.[163] Including this original report, 11 patients from 8 unrelated families have been identified, 21 of whom presented with EBV viremia and lymphoproliferation that often progressed to HL.[37] Patients also exhibited CD4+ T-cell lymphopenia, reduced invariant NK T (iNKT) cells, and progressive hypogammaglobulinemia. Although most of the patients responded favorably to HL-directed chemotherapy, many experienced a relapse. Of the 13 reported cases, only 5 (42%) were alive at the time of reporting, with 2 having received allo-HSCT. Collectively, these reports suggest that genetic defects that impair ITK function are an important cause of HL, especially when it occurs in young children and in the setting of EBV infection. Although the mechanisms underlying the sensitivity to EBV and development of HL remain to be determined, it is possible that ITK deficiency leads to disease by compromising TCR activation, which is further compounded by a reduction of iNKT cells.

CONCLUSION

EBV is a ubiquitous virus that leads to lifelong infection. Primary infection may be asymptomatic or associated with the syndrome of IM. It is associated with a variety of B-, T- and NK-cell neoplasms. Some are associated with particular infectious cofactors such as African BL with malaria, or a variety of B-cell lymphomas with HIV. Others are associated with genetic disorders, immunosuppression, or chronic inflammation. Some like BL are rapidly fatal if untreated, and others like mucocutaneous ulcer are indolent and may require only observation. Although there is a growing role for adoptive cellular immunotherapy that targets EBV antigens, most EBV-associated diseases are not yet treated with virus specific therapies. In this regard, it should be noted that standard antiviral therapies have little if any role in the management of either primary EBV infection or the treatment of EBV-associated malignancies.

ACKNOWLEDGMENTS

The authors thank Troy Messick and Kim Nichols for providing the prior version of this chapter for editing and updating.

References

1. Dunmire SK, Verghese PS, Balfour HH. Primary Epstein-Barr virus infection. *J Clin Virol*. 2018;102:84-92.
2. Henle W, Diehl V, Kohn G, Zur Hausen H, Henle G. Herpes-type virus and chromosome marker in normal leukocytes after growth with irradiated Burkitt cells. *Science*. 1967;157:1064-1065.
3. Pope J. Establishment of cell lines from peripheral leucocytes in infectious mononucleosis. *Nature*. 1967;216:810-811.
4. Henle G, Henle W, Diehl V. Relation of Burkitt's tumor-associated herpes-type virus to infectious mononucleosis. *Proc Natl Acad Sci U S A*. 1968;59:94.
5. De-Thé G. Epidemiology of Epstein–Barr virus and associated diseases in man. *The herpesviruses*. 1982;1:25-103.
6. Evans AS. The history of infectious mononucleosis. *Am J Med Sci*. 1974;267:189-195.
7. Türk W. Septische Erkrankungen bei Verkümmerung des granulozytensystems. *Wien Klin Wochenschr*. 1907;20:157.
8. Sprunt TP, Evans FA. Mononuclear leucocytosis in reaction to acute infections ("infectious mononucleosis"). *Bull Johns Hopkins Hosp*. 1920;31:410-417.
9. Downey H, McKinlay C. Acute lymphadenosis compared with acute lymphatic leukemia. *Arch Intern Med*. 1923;32:82-112.
10. Baldridge C, Rohner F, Hansmann G. Glandular fever (infectious mononucleosis). *Arch Intern Med*. 1926;38:413-448.
11. Paul JR, Bunnell W. The presence of heterophile antibodies in infectious mononucleosis. *Rev Infect Dis*. 1982;4(5):1062-1068.
12. Hausen HZ, Schulte-Holthausen H, KLEIN G, et al. Epstein–Barr virus in Burkitt's lymphoma and nasopharyngeal carcinoma: EBV DNA in biopsies of Burkitt tumours and anaplastic carcinomas of the nasopharynx. *Nature*. 1970;228:1056-1058.
13. Wolf H, Hausen HZ, Becker V. EB viral genomes in epithelial nasopharyngeal carcinoma cells. *Nat New Biol*. 1973;244:245-247.
14. Nagington J, Gray J. Cyclosporin A immunosuppression, Epstein-Barr antibody, and lymphoma. *Lancet*. 1980;315:536-537.
15. Weiss LM, Strickler JG, Warnke R, Purtilo D, Sklar J. Epstein-Barr viral DNA in tissues of Hodgkin's disease. *Am J Pathol*. 1987;129:86.
16. Jones JF, Shurin S, Abramowsky C, et al. T-cell lymphomas containing Epstein–Barr viral DNA in patients with chronic Epstein–Barr virus infections. *N Engl J Med*. 1988;318:733-741.
17. Bjornevik K, Cortese M, Healy BC, et al. Longitudinal analysis reveals high prevalence of Epstein-Barr virus associated with multiple sclerosis. *Science*. 2022;375:296-301.
18. Farrell PJ. Epstein–Barr virus strain variation. *Epstein Barr Virus*. 2015;1:45-69.
19. Young LS, Yap LF, Murray PG. Epstein–Barr virus: more than 50 years old and still providing surprises. *Nat Rev Cancer*. 2016;16:789.
20. Thorley-Lawson DA, Hawkins JB, Tracy SI, Shapiro M. The pathogenesis of Epstein-Barr virus persistent infection. *Curr Opin Virol*. 2013;3:227-232.
21. Smith NA, Coleman CB, Gewurz BE, Rochford R. CD21 (Complement Receptor 2) is the receptor for Epstein-Barr virus entry into T cells. *J Virol*. 2020;94:00428-20.
22. Longnecker RM, Kieff E, Cohen JI. *Epstein-barr Virus, Fields Virology*. 6th ed. Wolters Kluwer Health Adis (ESP); 2013.
23. Thorley-Lawson DA. EBV persistence—introducing the virus. *Epstein Barr Virus*. 2015;1:151-209.
24. Minamitani T, Ma Y, Zhou H, et al. Mouse model of Epstein–Barr virus LMP1-and LMP2A-driven germinal center B-cell lymphoproliferative disease. *Proc Natl Acad Sci USA*. 2017;114:4751-4756.
25. Wirtz T, Weber T, Kracker S, Sommermann T, Rajewsky K, Yasuda T. Mouse model for acute Epstein–Barr virus infection. *Proc Natl Acad Sci USA*. 2016;113:13821-13826.
26. Kang M-S, Kieff E. Epstein–Barr virus latent genes. *Exp Mol Med*. 2015;47:e131.
27. Frappier L. Ebna1. *Epstein Barr Virus*. 2015;2:3-34.
28. Fish K, Longnecker R. EBV germinates lymphoma from the germinal center in a battle with T and NK cells. *Proc Natl Acad Sci USA*. 2017;114:4571-4573.
29. Kanda T. *EBV-encoded latent genes. Human Herpesviruses*. Springer; 2018:377-394.
30. Iwakiri D. Multifunctional non-coding Epstein–Barr virus encoded RNAs (EBERs) contribute to viral pathogenesis. *Virus Res*. 2016;212:30-38.
31. Canitano A, Venturi G, Borghi M, Ammendolia MG, Fais S. Exosomes released in vitro from Epstein–Barr virus (EBV)-infected cells contain EBV-encoded latent phase mRNAs. *Cancer Lett*. 2013;337:193-199.
32. Vereide DT, Seto E, Chiu Y-F, et al. Epstein–Barr virus maintains lymphomas via its miRNAs. *Oncogene*. 2014;33:1258-1264.
33. Epeldegui M, Hung Yee P, McQuay A, Ambinder Richard F, Martínez-Maza O. Infection of human B cells with Epstein-Barr virus results in the expression of somatic hypermutation-inducing molecules and in the accrual of oncogene mutations. *Mol Immunol*. 2007;44:934-942.
34. Rovedo M, Longnecker R. Epstein-Barr virus latent membrane protein 2A preferentially signals through the Src family kinase Lyn. *J Virol*. 2008;82:8520-8528.
35. Callan M, Tan L, Annels N, et al. Direct visualization of antigen-specific CD8+ T cells during the primary immune response to Epstein-Barr virus in vivo. *J Exp Med*. 1998;187:1395-1402.
36. Cohen JI. Epstein–Barr virus infection. *N Engl J Med*. 2000;343:481-492.
37. Tangye SG, Palendira U, Edwards ES. Human immunity against EBV—lessons from the clinic. *J Exp Med*. 2017;214:269-283.
38. Long HM, Chagoury OL, Leese AM, et al. MHC II tetramers visualize human CD4+ T cell responses to Epstein–Barr virus infection and demonstrate atypical kinetics of the nuclear antigen EBNA1 response. *J Exp Med*. 2013;210:933-949.
39. Henle W, Henle GE, Horwitz CA. Epstein-barr virus specific diagnostic tests in infectious mononucleosis. *Hum Pathol*. 1974;5:551-565.
40. Evans AS, Neiderman JC, Cenabre LC, West B, Richards VA. A prospective evaluation of heterophile and Epstein-Barr virus-specific IgM antibody tests in clinical and subclinical infectious mononucleosis: specificity and sensitivity of the tests and persistence of antibody. *J Infect Dis*. 1975;132:546-554.
41. Nikoskelainen J, Neel E, Stevens DA. Epstein-Barr virus-specific serum immunoglobulin A as an acute-phase antibody in infectious mononucleosis. *J Clin Microbiol*. 1979;10:75-79.

42. De Paschale M, Clerici P. Serological diagnosis of Epstein-Barr virus infection: problems and solutions. *World J Virol.* 2012;1:31.
43. Durbin WA, Sullivan JL. Epstein-Barr virus infection. *Pediatr Rev.* 1994;15:63-68.
44. Garzelli C, Taub F, Scharff J, Prabhakar B, Ginsberg-Fellner F, Notkins A. Epstein-Barr virus-transformed lymphocytes produce monoclonal autoantibodies that react with antigens in multiple organs. *J Virol.* 1984;52:722-725.
45. Elling P, Faber V. Antinuclear antibodies in infectious mononucleosis. *Lancet.* 1968;291:918-919.
46. Kaplan ME. Cryoglobulinemia in infectious mononucleosis: quantitation and characterization of the cryoproteins. *J Lab Clin Med.* 1968;71:754-765.
47. Capra JD, Winchester RJ, Kunkel HG. Cold-reactive rheumatoid factors in infectious mononucleosis and other diseases. *Arthritis Rheum.* 1969;12:67-73.
48. Grubb R. The Gm system. Anti-Gm's: characteristics in rheumatoid arthritis; experimental induction without resort to allotype; frequent occurrence in mononucleosis. *Scand J Rheumatol.* 1988;17:227-232.
49. Misra R, Venables P, Plater-Zyberk C, Watkins P, Maini R. Anti-cardiolipin antibodies in infectious mononucleosis react with the membrane of activated lymphocytes. *Clin Exp Immunol.* 1989;75:35.
50. Kano K, Milgrom F. Heterophile antigens and antibodies in medicine. *Curr Top Microbiol Immunol.* 1977;77:43-69.
51. Hoagland RJ. The transmission of infectious mononucleosis. *Am J Med Sci.* 1955;229:262-272.
52. Grimm JM, Schmeling DO, Dunmire SK, et al. Prospective studies of infectious mononucleosis in university students. *Clin Trans Immunol.* 2016;5:e94.
53. Daud II, Coleman CB, Smith NA, et al. Breast milk as a potential source of epstein-Barr virus transmission among infants living in a malaria-endemic region of Kenya. *J Infect Dis.* 2015;212:1735-1742.
54. Trottier H, Buteau C, Robitaille N, et al. Transfusion-related Epstein-Barr virus infection among stem cell transplant recipients: a retrospective cohort study in children. *Transfusion.* 2012;52:2653-2663.
55. Rostgaard K, Balfour HH, Jr, Jarrett R, et al. Primary Epstein-Barr virus infection with and without infectious mononucleosis. *PLoS One.* 2019;14:e0226436.
56. Fugl A, Andersen CL. Epstein-Barr virus and its association with disease - a review of relevance to general practice. *BMC Fam Pract.* 2019;20:62.
57. Lennon P, Crotty M, Fenton JE. Infectious mononucleosis. *BMJ.* 2015;350:h1825.
58. Rosenthal T, Hertz M. Mediastinal lymphadenopathy in infectious mononucleosis: report of two cases. *JAMA.* 1975;233:1300-1301.
59. Kilpatrick ZM. Structural and functional abnormalities of liver in infectious mononucleosis. *Arch Intern Med.* 1966;117:47-53.
60. Hosey RG, Kriss V, Uhl TL, DiFiori J, Hecht S, Wen DY. Ultrasonographic evaluation of splenic enlargement in athletes with acute infectious mononucleosis. *Br J Sports Med.* 2008;42:974-977.
61. Matoba AY. Ocular disease associated with Epstein-Barr virus infection. *Surv Ophthalmol.* 1990;35:145-150.
62. Brown GL, Kanwar B. Drug rashes in glandular fever. *Lancet.* 1967;290:1418.
63. McKenzie H, Parratt D, White R. IgM and IgG antibody levels to ampicillin in patients with infectious mononucleosis. *Clin Exp Immunol.* 1976;26:214.
64. Wright DH. *Burkitt's lymphoma and infectious mononucleosis. The Immunopathology of Lymphoreticular Neoplasms.* Springer; 1978:391-424.
65. Fuhrman SA, Gill R, Horwitz CA, et al. Marked hyperbilirubinemia in infectious mononucleosis: analysis of laboratory data in seven patients. *Arch Intern Med.* 1987;147:850-853.
66. Freedman MJ, Odland LT, Cleve EA. Infectious mononucleosis with diffuse involvement of nervous system: report of a case. *AMA Arch Neurol Psychiatry.* 1953;69:49-54.
67. Young L, Rowe M. Epstein-Barr virus, lymphomas and Hodgkin's disease. *Semin Cancer Biol.* 1992;3(5):273-284.
68. Carter J, Edson R, Kennedy C. Infectious mononucleosis in the older patient. *Mayo Clin Proc.* 1978;53(3):146-150.
69. Schmader KE, van der Horst CM, Klotman ME. Epstein-Barr virus and the elderly host. *Rev Infect Dis.* 1989;11:64-73.
70. Prange E, Trautmann JC, Kreipe H, Radzun HJ, Parwaresch MR. Detection of Epstein-Barr virus in lymphoid tissues of patients with infectious mononucleosis by in situ hybridization. *J Pathol.* 1992;166:113-119.
71. Boyd J, Reid D. Bone marrow in nine cases of clinical glandular fever and a review of the literature. *J Clin Pathol.* 1968;21:683-690.
72. Martin M. Atypical infectious mononucleosis with bone marrow granulomas and pancytopenia. *Br Med J.* 1977;2:300.
73. Marshall-Andon T, Heinz P. How to use... the Monospot and other heterophile antibody tests. *Arch Dis Child Educ Pract.* 2017;102:188-193.
74. Kanakry JA, Hegde AM, Durand CM, et al. The clinical significance of EBV DNA in the plasma and peripheral blood mononuclear cells of patients with or without EBV diseases. *Blood.* 2016;127:2007-2017.
75. Coşkun O, Yazici E, Şahiner F, et al. Cytomegalovirus and Epstein–Barr virus reactivation in the intensive care unit. *Med Klin Intensivmed Notfallmed.* 2017;112:239-245.
76. Luzuriaga K, Sullivan JL. Infectious mononucleosis. *N Engl J Med.* 2010;362:1993-2000.
77. Ebell MH. Epstein-Barr virus infectious mononucleosis. *Am Fam Physician.* 2004;70:1279-1287.
78. Greiner T, Gross T. *Atypical Immune Lymphoproliferations. Hematology: Basic Principles and Practice.* 3rd ed. WB Saunders; 2000.
79. Mims MP. Lymphocytosis, lymphocytopenia, hypergammaglobulinemia, and hypogammaglobulinemia. *Hematology.* 2018:682-690.
80. Jenson HB. Acute complications of Epstein-Barr virus infectious mononucleosis. *Curr Opin Pediatr.* 2000;12:263-268.
81. Mahoney DH, Fernbach DJ. *The hematologic response. Infectious Mononucleosis.* Springer; 1989:80-88.
82. Hossaini AA. Anti-i in infectious mononucleosis. *Am J Clin Pathol.* 1970;53:198-203.
83. Uzokwe C, Gwynn A, Gorst D, Adamson A. Infectious mononucleosis complicated by haemolytic anaemia due to the Donath Landsteiner antibody and by severe neutropenia. *Clin Lab Haematol.* 1993;15:137-140.
84. Wishart M, Davey M. Infectious mononucleosis complicated by acute haemolytic anaemia with a positive Donath-Landsteiner reaction. *J Clin Pathol.* 1973;26:332-334.
85. Akin M, Kuuml K, Gozkeser E, Erdoan F. Direct antiglobulin test (Coombs) positive autoimmune hemolytic anemia induced by Epstein-Barr virus infectious mononucleosis in two children. *J Infect Dis Immun.* 2011;3:14-16.
86. Garefalakis K, Tsiodra P, Charalampopoulos A. Acute hemolytic anemia following infectious mononucleosis. *Eur J Intern Med.* 2007;18:260.
87. Stevens D, Everett E, Boxer L, Landefeld R. Infectious mononucleosis with severe neutropenia and opsonic antineutrophil activity. *South Med J.* 1979;72:519-521.
88. Baranski B, Armstrong G, Truman JT, Quinnan GV, Jr, Straus SE, Young NS. Epstein-Barr virus in the bone marrow of patients with aplastic anemia. *Ann Intern Med.* 1988;109:695-704.
89. Aldrete JS. *Spontaneous Rupture of the Spleen in Patients with Infectious Mononucleosis.* Elsevier; 1992:910-912.
90. Farley DR, Zietlow SP, Bannon MP, Farnell MB. *Spontaneous Rupture of the Spleen Due to Infectious Mononucleosis.* Elsevier; 1992:846-853.
91. Connelly KP, DeWitt LD. Neurologic complications of infectious mononucleosis. *Pediatr Neurol.* 1994;10:181-184.
92. Sabbatani S, Manfredi R, Ortolani P, Trapani FF, Viale P. Myopericarditis during a primary Epstein-Barr virus infection in an otherwise healthy young adult. An unusual and insidious complication. Case report and a 60-year literature review. *Infezioni Med Le.* 2012;20:75-81.
93. Lloyd T, Tran VK. Acute mediastinitis as a complication of Epstein-Barr virus. *Can J Emerg Med.* 2016;18:149-151.
94. Ho KM, Mitchell SC. An unusual presentation of cardiac tamponade associated with Epstein-Barr virus infection. *BMJ Case Rep.* 2015;2015:bcr2015209659.
95. Markin RS, Linder J, Zuerlein K, et al. Hepatitis in fatal infectious mononucleosis. *Gastroenterology.* 1987;93:1210-1217.
96. Putukian M, O'Connor FG, Stricker P, et al. Mononucleosis and athletic participation: an evidence-based subject review. *Clin J Sport Med.* 2008;18:309-315.
97. McGowan JE, Chesney PJ, Crossley KB, LaForce FM. Guidelines for the use of systemic glucocorticosteroids in the management of selected infections. *J Infect Dis.* 1992;165:1-13.
98. Roy M, Bailey B, Amre DK, Girodias JB, Bussieres JF, Gaudreault P. Dexamethasone for the treatment of sore throat in children with suspected infectious mononucleosis: a randomized, double-blind, placebo-controlled, clinical trial. *Arch Pediatr Adolesc Med.* 2004;158:250-254.
99. Candy B, Hotopf M. Steroids for symptom control in infectious mononucleosis. *Cochrane Database Syst Rev.* 2006;(3):CD004402. doi:10.1002/14651858.CD004402.pub2.
100. Straus SE. Epstein-Barr virus and human herpes virus type 6. In: Galasso GJ, Whitley RJ, Merigan TC, eds. *Antiviral Agents and Viral Diseases of Man.* Raven Press; 1990:647-668.
101. Andersson J, Sköldenberg B, Henle W, et al. Acyclovir treatment in infectious mononucleosis: a clinical and virological study. *Infection.* 1987;15:S14-S20.
102. Tynell E, Aurelius E, Brandell A, et al. Acyclovir and prednisolone treatment of acute infectious mononucleosis: a multicenter, double-blind, placebo-controlled study. *J Infect Dis.* 1996;174:324-331.
103. van der Horst C, Joncas J, Ahronheim G, et al. Lack of effect of peroral acyclovir for the treatment of acute infectious mononucleosis. *J Infect Dis.* 1991;164:788-792.
104. Hoshino Y, Katano H, Zou P, et al. Long-term administration of valacyclovir reduces the number of Epstein-Barr virus (EBV)-infected B cells but not the number of EBV DNA copies per B cell in healthy volunteers. *J Virol.* 2009;83:11857-11861.
105. Arai A. Advances in the study of chronic active Epstein-Barr virus infection: clinical features under the 2016 WHO classification and mechanisms of development. *Front Pediatr.* 2019;7:14.
106. Swerdlow SH, Campo E, Pileri SA, et al. The 2016 revision of the World Health Organization classification of lymphoid neoplasms. *Blood.* 2016;127:2375-2390. J Am Soc Hematol.
107. Cohen JI. Optimal treatment for chronic active Epstein-Barr virus disease. *Pediatr Transplant.* 2009;13:393.
108. Okano M, Kawa K, Kimura H, et al. Proposed guidelines for diagnosing chronic active Epstein-Barr virus infection. *Am J Hematol.* 2005;80:64-69.
109. Kimura H, Hoshino Y, Kanegane H, et al. Clinical and virologic characteristics of chronic active Epstein-Barr virus infection. *Blood.* 2001;98:280-286.
110. Kimura H, Ito Y, Kawabe S, et al. EBV-associated T/NK–cell lymphoproliferative diseases in nonimmunocompromised hosts: prospective analysis of 108 cases. *Blood.* 2012;119:673-686.
111. Cohen JI. Primary immunodeficiencies associated with EBV disease. *Curr Top Microbiol Immunol.* 2015;390:241-265.
112. Okuno Y, Murata T, Sato Y, et al. Defective Epstein–Barr virus in chronic active infection and haematological malignancy. *Nat Microbiol.* 2019;4:404-413.
113. Venturini C, Houldcroft CJ, Lazareva A, et al. Epstein–Barr virus (EBV) deletions as biomarkers of response to treatment of chronic active EBV. *Br J Haematol.* 2021;195:249-255.
114. Katano H, Ali MA, Patera AC, et al. Chronic active Epstein-Barr virus infection associated with mutations in perforin that impair its maturation. *Blood.* 2004;103:1244-1252.

115. Bollard CM, Cohen JI. How I treat T-cell chronic active Epstein-Barr virus disease. *Blood.* 2018;131:2899-2905.
116. El-Mallawany NK, Curry CV, Allen CE. Haemophagocytic lymphohistiocytosis and Epstein–Barr virus: a complex relationship with diverse origins, expression and outcomes. *Br J Haematol.* 2022;196:31-44.
117. Chellapandian D, Das R, Zelley K, et al. Treatment of Epstein Barr virus-induced haemophagocytic lymphohistiocytosis with rituximab-containing chemo-immunotherapeutic regimens. *Br J Haematol.* 2013;162:376-382.
118. Wu TC, Mann RB, Charache P, et al. Detection of EBV gene expression in Reed-Sternberg cells of Hodgkin's disease. *Int J Cancer.* 1990;46:801-804.
119. Glaser Sally L, Gulley Margaret L, Borowitz Michael J, et al. Inter- and intra-observer reliability of Epstein-Barr virus detection in Hodgkin lymphoma using histochemical procedures. *Leuk Lymphoma.* 2004;45:489-497.
120. Peprah S, Ogwang MD, Kerchan P, et al. Risk factors for Burkitt lymphoma in East African children and minors: a case–control study in malaria-endemic regions in Uganda, Tanzania and Kenya. *Int J Cancer.* 2020;146:953-969.
121. Hämmerl L, Colombet M, Rochford R, Ogwang DM, Parkin DM. The burden of Burkitt lymphoma in Africa. *Infect Agents Cancer.* 2019;14:1-6.
122. Mbulaiteye SM, Anderson WF, Bhatia K, Rosenberg PS, Linet MS, Devesa SS. Trimodal age-specific incidence patterns for Burkitt lymphoma in the United States, 1973-2005. *Int J Cancer.* 2010;126:1732-1739.
123. Shannon-Lowe C, Rickinson A. The global landscape of EBV-associated tumors. *Front Oncol.* 2019;9:713.
124. Grande BM, Gerhard DS, Jiang A, et al. Genome-wide discovery of somatic coding and noncoding mutations in pediatric endemic and sporadic Burkitt lymphoma. *Blood.* 2019;133:1313-1324.
125. Kanakry JA, Li H, Gellert LL, et al. Plasma Epstein-Barr virus DNA predicts outcome in advanced Hodgkin lymphoma: correlative analysis from a large North American cooperative group trial. *Blood.* 2013;121:3547-3553.
126. Glaser SL, Lin RJ, Stewart SL, et al. Epstein-Barr virus-associated Hodgkin's disease: epidemiologic characteristics in international data. *Int J Cancer.* 1997;70:375-382.
127. Glaser SL, Clarke CA, Gulley ML, et al. Population-based patterns of human immunodeficiency virus-related Hodgkin lymphoma in the greater san francisco bay area, 1988-1998. *Cancer.* 2003;98:300-309.
128. Ambinder RF, Browning PJ, Lorenzana I, et al. Epstein-Barr virus and childhood Hodgkin's disease in Honduras and the United States. *Blood.* 1993;81:462-467.
129. Hjalgrim H, Jarrett RF. Epidemiology of Hodgkin lymphoma. In: Engert A, Younes A, eds. *Hodgkin Lymphoma: A Comprehensive Overview*. Springer International Publishing; 2020:3-23, doi:10.1007/978-3-030-32482-7_1
130. Connors JM, Cozen W, Steidl C, et al. Hodgkin lymphoma. *Nat Rev Dis Prim.* 2020;6:1-25.
131. Murray PG, Constandinou CM, Crocker J, Young LS, Ambinder RF. Analysis of major histocompatibility complex class I, TAP expression, and LMP2 epitope sequence in Epstein-Barr virus-positive Hodgkin's disease. *Blood.* 1998;92:2477-2483.
132. Cen O, Longnecker R. Latent membrane protein 2 (LMP2). *Curr Top Microbiol Immunol.* 2015;391:151-180.
133. Schmitz R, Hansmann M-L, Bohle V, et al. TNFAIP3 (A20) is a tumor suppressor gene in Hodgkin lymphoma and primary mediastinal B cell lymphoma. *J Exp Med.* 2009;206:981-989.
134. Cader FZ, Schackmann RCJ, Hu X, et al. Mass cytometry of Hodgkin lymphoma reveals a CD4(+) regulatory T-cell-rich and exhausted T-effector microenvironment. *Blood.* 2018;132:825-836.
135. Sing AP, Ambinder RF, Hong DJ, et al. Isolation of Epstein-Barr virus (EBV)-specific cytotoxic T lymphocytes that lyse Reed-Sternberg cells: implications for immune-mediated therapy of EBV+ Hodgkin's disease. *Blood.* 1997;89:1978-1986.
136. Lindsay J, Othman J, Heldman MR, Slavin MA. Epstein-Barr virus posttransplant lymphoproliferative disorder: update on management and outcomes. *Curr Opin Infect Dis.* 2021;34:635-645.
137. Swerdlow SH, Campo E, Harris NL, et al. *WHO Classification of Tumours of Haematopoietic and Lymphoid Tissues*. Vol 2. International agency for research on cancer; 2008.
138. Heslop HE, Sharma S, Rooney CM. Adoptive T-cell therapy for epstein-Barr virus-related lymphomas. *J Clin Oncol.* 2021;39:514-524.
139. Tse E, Kwong YL. The diagnosis and management of NK/T-cell lymphomas. *J Hematol Oncol.* 2017;10:1-13.
140. Quintanilla-Martinez L, Ridaura C, Nagl F, et al. Hydroa vacciniforme-like lymphoma: a chronic EBV+ lymphoproliferative disorder with risk to develop a systemic lymphoma. *Blood.* 2013;122:3101-3110. J Am Soc Hematol.
141. McClain K. Epstein-Barr virus and HIV-AIDS-associated diseases. *Biomed Pharmacother.* 2001;55:348-352.
142. Bibas M, Antinori A. EBV and HIV-related lymphoma. *Mediterr J Hematol Infect Dis.* 2009;1(2):e2009032.
143. MacMahon E, Charache P, Glass D, et al. Epstein-Barr virus in AIDS-related primary central nervous system lymphoma. *Lancet.* 1991;338:969-973.
144. Cesarman E, Chang Y, Moore PS, Said JW, Knowles DM. Kaposi's sarcoma-associated herpesvirus-like DNA sequences in AIDS-related body-cavity-based lymphomas. *N Engl J Med.* 1995;332:1186-1191.
145. Matthews GV, Bower M, Mandalia S, Powles T, Nelson MR, Gazzard BG. Changes in acquired immunodeficiency syndrome-related lymphoma since the introduction of highly active antiretroviral therapy. *Blood.* 2000;96:2730-2734.
146. Besson C, Goubar A, Gabarre J, et al. Changes in AIDS-related lymphoma since the era of highly active antiretroviral therapy. *Blood.* 2001;98:2339-2344. J Am Soc Hematol.
147. Rezk SA, Weiss LM. EBV–Associated lymphoproliferative disorders: update in classification. *Surg Pathol Clin.* 2019;12:745-770.
148. Noy A, Lensing SY, Moore PC, et al. Plasmablastic lymphoma is treatable in the HAART era. A 10 year retrospective by the AIDS Malignancy Consortium. *Leuk Lymphoma.* 2016;57:1731-1734.
149. Yabe M, Dogan A, Horwitz SM, Moskowitz AJ. Angioimmunoblastic T-cell lymphoma. In: Querfeld C, Zain J, Rosen S, eds. *T-Cell and NK-Cell Lymphomas*. Cancer Treatment and Research. Vol 176. Springer, Cham; 2019. https://doi.org/10.1007/978-3-319-99716-2_5.
150. Seemayer TA, Gross TG, Egeler RM, et al. X-linked lymphoproliferative disease: twenty-five years after the discovery. *Pediatr Res.* 1995;38:471-478.
151. Talaat KR, Rothman JA, Cohen JI, et al. Lymphocytic vasculitis involving the central nervous system occurs in patients with X-linked lymphoproliferative disease in the absence of Epstein-Barr virus infection. *Pediatr Blood Cancer.* 2009;53:1120-1123.
152. Booth C, Gilmour KC, Veys P, et al. X-linked lymphoproliferative disease due to SAP/SH2D1A deficiency: a multicenter study on the manifestations, management and outcome of the disease. *Blood.* 2011;117:53-62.
153. Lankester A, Visser L, Hartwig N, et al. Allogeneic stem cell transplantation in X-linked lymphoproliferative disease: two cases in one family and review of the literature. *Bone Marrow Transplant.* 2005;36:99-105.
154. Sumegi J, Huang D, Lanyi A, et al. Correlation of mutations of the SH2D1A gene and Epstein-Barr virus infection with clinical phenotype and outcome in X-linked lymphoproliferative disease. *Blood.* 2000;96:3118-3125.
155. Grierson HL, Skare J, Hawk J, Pauza M, Purtilo DT. Immunoglobulin class and subclass deficiencies prior to Epstein-Barr virus infection in males with X-linked lymphoproliferative disease. *Am J Med Genet.* 1991;40:294-297.
156. Coffey AJ, Brooksbank RA, Brandau O, et al. Host response to EBV infection in X-linked lymphoproliferative disease results from mutations in an SH2-domain encoding gene. *Nat Genet.* 1998;20:129-135.
157. Nichols KE, Harkin DP, Levitz S, et al. Inactivating mutations in an SH2 domain-encoding gene in X-linked lymphoproliferative syndrome. *Proc Natl Acad Sci USA.* 1998;95:13765-13770.
158. Sayos J, Wu C, Morra M, et al. The X-linked lymphoproliferative-disease gene product SAP regulates signals induced through the co-receptor SLAM. *Nature.* 1998;395:462-469.
159. Cohen JI. Primary immunodeficiencies associated with EBV disease. *Epstein Barr Virus.* 2015;1:241-265.
160. Rigaud S, Fondaneche MC, Lambert N, et al. XIAP deficiency in humans causes an X-linked lymphoproliferative syndrome. *Nature.* 2006;444:110-114.
161. Mudde ACA, Booth C, Marsh RA. Evolution of our understanding of XIAP deficiency. *Front Pediatr.* 2021;9:557.
162. Gifford CE, Weingartner E, Villanueva J, et al. Clinical flow cytometric screening of SAP and XIAP expression accurately identifies patients with SH2D1A and XIAP/BIRC4 mutations. *Cytometry B Clin Cytometry.* 2014;86:263-271.
163. Huck K, Feyen O, Niehues T, et al. Girls homozygous for an IL-2-inducible T cell kinase mutation that leads to protein deficiency develop fatal EBV-associated lymphoproliferation. *J Clin Invest.* 2009;119:1350-1358.

Chapter 64 ■ Primary Immunodeficiency Diseases

TROY R. TORGERSON

INTRODUCTION

Primary immunodeficiency disorders (PIDDs) were traditionally described in patients with unusually severe, persistent, or atypical infections. These disorders were initially characterized clinically (for example, agammaglobulinemia, severe combined immunodeficiency [SCID]), then cellularly (for example, absence of B cells in X-linked agammaglobulinemia [XLA]), and then genetically (e.g., *BTK* gene mutations as the cause of XLA). Now, mutations in more than 450 different genes have been associated with immune-related diseases that have clinical presentations ranging from traditional PIDDs with severe or unusual infections to primary immune regulatory disorders in which patients present with few infections but have severe, early-onset autoimmunity or inflammatory disease.[1] This wealth of genetic information has led to an understanding that PIDDs originally described based on clinical features can be caused by defects in many different genes. For example, defects in more than 20 genes have now been associated with a clinical phenotype of SCID.[1] Recent studies have also demonstrated that acquired (somatic) mutations may cause immune-related diseases indistinguishable from those that occur when the mutation is present from birth (germline).[2]

Discoveries in patients with immune-related diseases have markedly extended our understanding of the role of numerous molecules and functional pathways in immune system function and homeostasis. Identification of the genetic cause of disease in a growing number of patients with immune-related diseases has also created opportunities to utilize targeted therapies to treat patients, which has improved outcomes and quality of life.

MAJOR COMPARTMENTS OF THE IMMUNE SYSTEM

A simple, four-compartment framework is useful for thinking about immune-related diseases including immunodeficiencies and immune dysregulation disorders. In this model, the four major compartments of the immune system are complement, phagocytes, B cells and antibodies, and T cells (*Figure 64.1*). The complement and phagocyte compartments, along with skin and epithelial barriers, make up most of the "innate" portion of the immune system, while the B-cell and T-cell compartments make up most of the "adaptive" portion of the immune system. Many immunodeficiency disorders are caused by a defect in only one compartment of the immune system, while others are "combined" immunodeficiencies with defects in multiple compartments. In general, defects in each compartment of the immune system are associated with susceptibilities to certain types of infections or predisposition to particular forms of autoimmunity or inflammatory disease, which are discussed below in context.

COMPLEMENT

The complement system consists of a family of proteins that are present in the plasma and extracellular fluid that become activated in various ways upon encountering pathogens. Activation of early complement components initiates a cascade of protein cleavage and activation events that ultimately lead to formation of the membrane attack complex (MAC) consisting of complement proteins C5, 6, 7, 8, and 9 (*Figure 64.2*). Regulatory proteins including C1 esterase inhibitor, factor H, factor I, MCP (membrane cofactor protein), and CD59 control complement activation, thereby preventing inappropriate complement fixation. The complement cascade can be activated via three major mechanisms: (1) the *Classical Pathway*, which is initiated by antigen/antibody complexes; (2) the *Alternative Pathway*, which is initiated when the active fragment (C3b) of spontaneously hydrolyzed C3 covalently binds to pathogens; and (3) the *Lectin Pathway*, which is initiated by carbohydrate moieties present in bacterial membranes.

Complement deficiencies make up a relatively small proportion (~2%) of all primary immune deficiencies.[3] Defective activation of the entire complement cascade can be caused by the absence or dysfunction of only 1 of more than 20 different complement proteins. The proteins most often affected are C2, C3, and C4.[4]

Clinical Presentation

Patients with mutations that affect activation of the three complement pathways typically present with invasive infections with encapsulated organisms. *Streptococcus pneumoniae* and *Haemophilus influenzae*

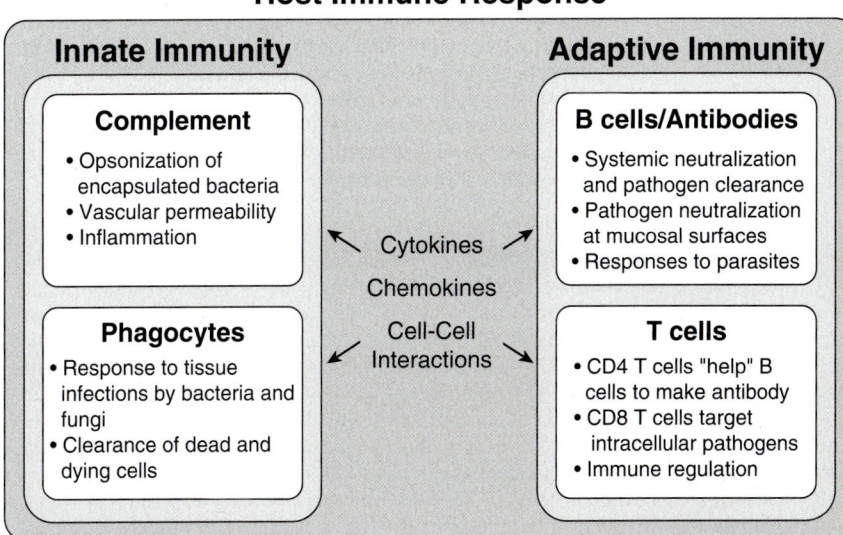

FIGURE 64.1 Compartments of the immune system.

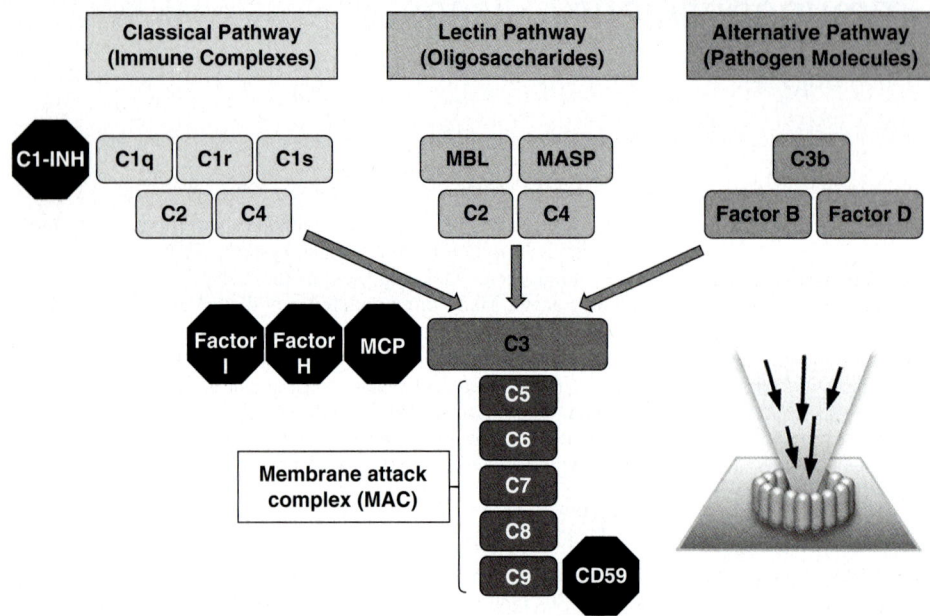

FIGURE 64.2 Complement activation.

are particularly problematic in the setting of early classical pathway (C1-C4) defects, reflecting the importance of the classical pathway for opsonization of carbohydrate-coated organisms. Invasive infections with *Neisseria* species are more common among patients with defects in MAC proteins (C5-C9). Patients with early classical pathway defects (C1-C4) are also at high risk for developing systemic lupus erythematosus (SLE) or glomerulonephritis reflective of the important role that early classical pathway proteins also play in opsonizing fragments of our own dead and dying cells for clearance.[4]

Patients with defects in complement regulatory proteins have fewer problems with infections but instead have problems related to dysregulated activation of complement proteins. C1 esterase inhibitor deficiency causes hereditary angioedema (HAE) in which allergic or mechanical stimuli can trigger massive, localized, severe attacks of edema that can be life-threatening if they involve the airway. Patients with defects in factor I, factor H, or MCP are at risk of developing atypical hemolytic uremic syndrome and age-related macular degeneration.[5,6]

Specific Disorders
C2 Deficiency
C2 deficiency is the most common complement component deficiency associated with susceptibility to infections, occurring in approximately 1 of 20,000 people. As indicated above, patients with early complement cascade defects (C1-C4) are susceptible to invasive infections with encapsulated organisms, *S. pneumoniae* being a particularly fulminant pathogen in these patients. The infectious susceptibility is compounded by functional antibody deficiency in some patients. In addition, patients with C1, C2, or C4 deficiency are at high risk of developing autoimmunity (lupus or glomerulonephritis). In the case of homozygous C2 deficiency, approximately 50% of patients develop lupus or glomerulonephritis.[4]

C1 Esterase Inhibitor Deficiency
C1 esterase inhibitor deficiency causes HAE. Unlike many of the other early complement component deficiencies, absence of C1 esterase inhibitor does not lead to increased risk for infection. C1 esterase inhibitor does regulate the C1 complex, but importantly, it also regulates the activity of kallikrein, blocking its ability to act on factor XII and kininogen. Consequently, minor irritants cause unabated production of bradykinin and other mediators of vascular permeability, leading to rapid swelling of the soft tissues (angioedema), severe abdominal pain, and at times, acute obstruction of the airway.

Effective treatments are now available for HAE including purified C1 esterase inhibitor, a kallikrein inhibitor, and a bradykinin B2 receptor antagonist.[7,8] Because of the expense of these agents, they are often administered at the beginning of an attack to abort symptoms rather than prophylactically to prevent the onset of an attack. In addition to genetic deficiency, C1 inhibitor deficiency can also be acquired in the setting of complement consumption (e.g., in neoplastic disorders like B-cell lymphomas) or due to a functionally neutralizing autoantibody targeting C1 esterase inhibitor as seen occasionally in monoclonal gammopathies or other autoimmune diseases.[9]

Diagnosis
Screening for complement deficiency should be performed in patients with recurrent episodes of bacteremia, bacterial meningitis, or disseminated gonorrhea. Since more than 30% of patients with recurrent *Neisseria* infections have complement deficiency, it is imperative that prompt testing of the complement system be done in these individuals. The CH50 test functionally screens the activity of the entire classical pathway; therefore it is a good, plasma-based screen for the most common complement deficiencies. If an alternative pathway defect is suspected however, an analogous test (the AH50), can be performed. For the CH50 to give accurate results, the blood specimen needs to be handled carefully since complement is heat labile. In general, it is recommended that any abnormal CH50 test should be repeated to confirm a complement deficiency. The CH50 is typically very low or absent in patients with a true complement component deficiency. A CH50 that is only moderately low is often seen in situations where the specimen was handled incorrectly or in patients with autoimmune disease such as lupus or mixed connective tissue disease. Once an abnormal CH50 test is confirmed, specialized testing to identify the specific complement component that is absent can be performed.

Treatment
Patients with complement deficiency are susceptible to fulminant sepsis and other deep-seated infections caused by encapsulated organisms. For this reason, patients should be given a letter or laminated card to carry at all times with contact information for their primary care physician and clinical immunologist and a message indicating that they have a complement deficiency and there should be no delay in giving parenteral antibiotics should they be ill. For patients who live at a distance from skilled medical care, consideration should be given to providing a dose of parenteral antibiotic such as ceftriaxone that can be administered by the patient or a family member when they become ill, prior to a lengthy trip to the hospital. The efficacy of chronic

prophylactic antibiotics to prevent infection in patients with complement deficiency is not well studied and remains a significant question in this group of disorders. In addition to preparing for and treating infections, patients should also be regularly screened for autoimmunity by history, physical exam (i.e., blood pressure monitoring), and laboratory testing including BUN (blood urea nitrogen), creatinine, and urinalysis to monitor for signs of glomerulonephritis.

PHAGOCYTES

One of the major roles of phagocytic cells (neutrophils, monocytes, macrophages, and dendritic cells) is to continuously survey the body for signs of infection. If an infection occurs, phagocytes migrate toward the site where they begin to ingest both opsonized and nonopsonized pathogens and debris. The ingested material is processed, and fragments of digested proteins are loaded into class II MHC (major histocompatibility complex) molecules that are presented at the cell surface where they can be recognized by cells of the adaptive immune system. Phagocytes that ingest pathogens and debris can either remain at the site of infection or migrate back to local draining lymph nodes to present antigen. Phagocytic disorders typically fall into one of three classes: (1) a lack of phagocytes (e.g., congenital neutropenia); (2) defective phagocyte migration (e.g., leukocyte adhesion deficiency, WHIM syndrome, etc.); (3) inability of phagocytes to process or degrade organisms that have been ingested (e.g., chronic granulomatous disease).[10]

Clinical Presentation

Because of the role that phagocytes play in controlling bacterial and fungal pathogens, patients with phagocytic defects often present with infections and abscesses of skin, deep tissues, and organs caused by bacteria and fungi. Symptoms can include boils and/or cellulitis with or without pus, lymphadenitis, pneumonia, delayed shedding of the umbilical cord, hepatic abscesses, gastrointestinal disorders, gingivitis, and unexplained fever, malaise and fatigue. The onset of symptoms of phagocytic cell disorders is typically in infancy or early childhood.

Specific Disorders
Congenital Neutropenia and Severe Congenital Neutropenia

The congenital neutropenias are described in more detail elsewhere (see Chapter 58), so will be covered only briefly here. Mutations in more than 25 different genes have now been associated with congenital neutropenia with a subset of these associated with the most severe forms of the disease. Autosomal dominant mutations in the neutrophil elastase gene, *ELANE*, are the most commonly identified genetic defect in congenital neutropenia, accounting for up to 45% of cases.[11] The range of severities reported for *ELANE*-associated congenital neutropenia can vary from cyclic neutropenia to severe congenital neutropenia (SCN). Some genetic disorders of congenital neutropenia are associated with broader syndromic features (e.g., G6PC3 deficiency, Shwachman-Diamond syndrome) as well.

In all cases, clinical management involves a heightened suspicion for infections and aggressive treatment if these arise. Treatment of acute infections may require antibiotics combined with granulocyte colony-stimulating factor (G-CSF) to increase neutrophil counts. Despite there being little evidence supporting the use of prophylactic antibiotics specifically in SCN, extrapolation from data in leukemic patients with neutropenia suggests a benefit; therefore they are used in most patients. Prophylactic, long-term therapy with G-CSF is typically utilized only in those patients who have recurrent, severe bacterial infections despite antibiotic prophylaxis or in patients with fungal infections. Bone marrow transplantation is effective in SCN although there is little to no reported experience in some of the genetic disorders that are rarer.

Leukocyte Adhesion Deficiency

Leukocyte adhesion deficiency (LAD) is caused by the absence of functional adhesion receptors that are required for the migration of phagocytes from the circulation into the tissues. The characteristic clinical features of LAD include recurrent skin and soft-tissue infections that often lead to development of deep ulcers despite there being highly elevated peripheral blood leukocyte counts. Interestingly, the inability of leukocytes to migrate to these sites of infection leads to an absence of pus in the lesions, which can be a useful diagnostic clue. Wound healing is also compromised, and patients typically have marked gingivostomatitis. Three forms of LAD have been described: *LAD-I*, the most common form of LAD, is caused by mutations in the *ITGB2* gene encoding the β2-integrin CD18. Mutations cause an absence of the CD11/CD18 integrin complex on the surface of leukocytes, which can be readily discerned by flow cytometry. *LAD-II* is caused by mutations in the *SLC35C1* gene encoding the GDP-fucose transporter. These mutations cause defective expression of sialyl Lewis X (sLe^X), a fucose-containing ligand on neutrophils. sLe^X is the ligand for E- and P-selectins, which are expressed on the surface of cytokine-activated endothelial cells and allow neutrophil rolling. As a result of the fucose defect, all patients with LAD-II also have the rare Bombay blood group, which is a useful diagnostic test for suspected LAD-II. *LAD-III* is caused by mutations in the *FERMT3* gene that encodes kindlin-3, a co-activator that is required for activation and function of β1-, β2-, and β3-integrins. Absence of functional kindlin-3 leads to dysfunction of CD18 and causes a LAD phenotype (see LAD-I above). In addition, patients with LAD-III also have a Glanzmann-type bleeding disorder resulting from dysfunctional integrin-mediated aggregation of platelets.[12,13]

Patients with LAD-I and LAD-III typically present in childhood and often have a severe course with early mortality, whereas patients with LAD-II are often milder and may live into adulthood. Treatment of LAD can be more complicated than some of the other phagocytic disorders because in addition to aggressively treating infections with antibiotics, active soft-tissue infections may require recurrent donor white cell infusions of functional neutrophils to clear the infection. Since the primary defects of LAD are intrinsic to hematopoietic cells, bone marrow transplantation can be curative.[14,15]

WHIM Syndrome

WHIM syndrome (Warts, Hypogammaglobulinemia, recurrent bacterial Infections, and Myelokathexis [retention of neutrophils in the bone marrow]) is caused by autosomal dominant mutations in CXCR4, the receptor for the chemokine CXCL12 (stromal cell–derived factor 1). Patients with WHIM typically present in childhood with recurrent bacterial otitis media, sinusitis, bronchitis, pneumonia, and cellulitis. The bacterial susceptibility is a result of the combination of hypogammaglobulinemia and neutropenia. In addition to bacterial infections, patients with WHIM have a particular susceptibility to papillomavirus infections, which can be severe and lead to early malignancy. The mechanisms that underlie the viral susceptibility are not entirely understood but are thought to possibly be intrinsic to the epithelial cells. In the hematopoietic system, CXCL12 causes homing of cells to the bone marrow and controls release of these cells from the marrow. Neutrophils and lymphocytes from patients with WHIM have an increased chemotactic response to CXCL12, suggesting that the neutropenia and lymphopenia observed in WHIM are the result of inappropriate cell retention in the marrow.[16] Treatment with G-CSF or granulocyte macrophage-colony stimulating factor can normalize the neutrophil counts although these often cause significant bone pain at the doses required to mitigate the neutropenia.[17,18] Recent studies using the CXCR4 antagonist plerixafor in adults with WHIM syndrome have shown promise for improving neutrophil counts by mobilizing neutrophils from the bone marrow.[19,20] Antibiotics and immunoglobulin replacement can significantly reduce the risk of bacterial infections. There is very little reported experience regarding bone marrow transplantation for WHIM although anecdotal evidence suggests that it may correct the neutropenia and hypogammaglobulinemia but may not alter the papillomavirus susceptibility.[21,22]

Chronic Granulomatous Disease

Chronic granulomatous disease (CGD) is the most frequently diagnosed phagocytic cell immune defect. The most common form is

X-linked recessive, caused by mutations in the *CYBB* gene and accounting for approximately two-thirds of all CGD cases. The remaining forms, caused by mutations in the *CYBA*, *NCF1*, *NCF2*, or *NCF4* genes, are all autosomal recessive. All mutations affect the formation or function of the NADPH oxidase complex, on neutrophil phagolysosomes. The NADPH oxidase is required to generate a burst of reactive oxygen species in response to phagocytosis of pathogens. Reactive oxygen species activate proteases in the phagolysosomes that destroy ingested bacteria. In CGD, the oxidative burst cannot be generated, leading to defective processing of ingested organisms and an inability to appropriately eliminate bacterial and fungal pathogens. Catalase-positive organisms including *Staphylococcus* species, *Aspergillus* species, *Burkholderia cepacia*, *Serratia marcescens*, and others are the most common pathogens. The most common types of infection at presentation are pneumonia, lymphadenitis, cellulitis, and hepatic abscesses (particularly with *Aspergillus* sp.). The most common cause of premature death is *Aspergillus* infection.[23,24] In addition to the infectious susceptibilities of CGD, a substantial percentage of patients struggle with inflammatory complications that are common to this disorder including an inflammatory colitis that occurs in approximately 40%, hepatic dysfunction, gingivitis, and others.[25]

Treatment of CGD revolves around aggressive management of acute infections followed by prophylaxis against future infections using a combination of daily antibiotic (typically trimethoprim-sulfamethoxazole), daily antifungal (typically itraconazole), and thrice-weekly interferon-γ (IFN-γ) injections. This combination has dramatically improved outcomes in CGD; however, despite appropriate use of this regimen, some patients ultimately have increasing symptoms that lead to a decline in survival beginning in the late-teens or early twenties. The prospects for long-term survival appear to be correlated with the amount of residual oxidative burst activity that can be generated by a particular patient's phagocytes.[26] This has led to a renewed interest in bone marrow transplantation for CGD, which has been quite successful in the modern era, likely due to improved antimicrobials and transplant conditioning regimens with reduced toxicity. Many now recommend that for patients who have mutations that severely impact oxidative burst activity, bone marrow transplant should be considered preemptively, early in life before patients develop comorbidities.[27]

Diagnosis

Assessment of patients for a possible phagocytic disorder requires that both the number and the function of phagocytes be evaluated. Numbers are easily evaluated using a complete blood count with differential. If there is a concern for cyclic neutropenia, neutrophil counts may need to be evaluated three times weekly for three to 4 weeks to identify the nadir.[28] Functional testing includes evaluation of CD11/CD18 integrin expression on myeloid cells by flow cytometry if the patient has symptoms suggestive of LAD. In cases of suspected CGD, evaluation of neutrophil oxidative burst function is essential. Traditionally this was done using nitrobluetetrazoleum but is now performed using dihydrorhodamine (DHR), a reagent that permeates neutrophils and fluoresces in response to a normal neutrophil oxidative burst. Fluorescence is measured by flow cytometry. The DHR test is sensitive enough to differentiate most cases of X-linked CGD from autosomal recessive CGD, making it a particularly useful clinical assay.[29,30]

Treatment

As noted above, management of phagocytic disorders revolves around having a heightened suspicion for infections, aggressively treating acute infections using antibiotics and G-CSF as necessary, and developing a prophylaxis regimen that is both effective and reasonable from a patient standpoint. At times, patients continue to have recurrent or severe infections despite these efforts and require more definitive therapy. As indicated above, hematopoietic cell transplantation (HCT) has been shown to be effective in many, but not all, phagocytic disorders. Gene therapy has been moderately successful in X-linked CGD, but some patients experienced inflammatory complications after treatment and at this point is still considered experimental.[31,32] Gene therapy for other neutrophil disorders including LAD-1 has largely been unsuccessful.

B CELLS/ANTIBODIES

B cells play an important role in the immune system as antigen-presenting cells and producers of key cytokines, but their predominant role is to make antibodies (immunoglobulins) in response to antigen challenge (pathogens, vaccines, etc.). The absence of functional antibodies causes susceptibility to bacterial and viral infections. Antibody deficiency can occur in one of three different ways: (1) hypogammaglobulinemia or low levels of one or more immunoglobulin classes (IgG, IgA, IgM, or IgE) occurring because of decreased antibody production, often associated with a specific genetic defect; (2) hypogammaglobulinemia caused by excessive antibody loss, typically through the kidneys as proteinuria or through the gut as protein-losing enteropathy; (3) functional antibody deficiency, in which immunoglobulin levels are normal but the Ig lacks the quality required to bind and opsonize pathogens.

Clinical Presentation

Patients who lack sufficient levels of functional antibody typically develop recurrent bacterial sinopulmonary infections (sinusitis, otitis media, bronchitis, and pneumonia). In addition, patients may develop bowel infections caused by microorganisms such as *Giardia* or *Cryptosporidium* that are often only modestly pathogenic to normal individuals. In addition to these symptoms, patients with certain antibody-deficiency disorders have characteristic clinical features that can provide clues to the specific diagnosis. These are covered below.

Specific Disorders
X-Linked Agammaglobulinemia

XLA is caused by mutations in the Bruton tyrosine kinase (*BTK*) gene. BTK is a member of the Tec family of cytoplasmic tyrosine kinases and is required for the maturation of B-cell precursors in the bone marrow. Mutations in BTK therefore cause an arrest of B-cell development at the Pre-B-cell stage leading to virtually absent B cells in the peripheral blood. Mutations that only partially interfere with the enzymatic function of BTK have also been described and are associated with milder forms of the disease that only have defects in generation of specific antibody responses.[33]

XLA is typically suspected in male patients with recurrent bacterial sinopulmonary infections and <2% circulating CD19$^+$ B cells. Other infections that may occur in patients with XLA prior to the initiation of IgG replacement therapy include skin infections (furunculosis, pyoderma, and cellulitis) and sepsis. The diagnosis can be confirmed either by identifying a mutation in the *BTK* gene or by demonstrating absence of the BTK protein in monocytes or platelets. A positive family history suggestive of an X-linked recessive mode of inheritance increases the suspicion for XLA. It is uncommon for patients with XLA to develop symptoms in the first months of life because newborns are protected from most infections by transplacentally acquired maternal IgG. There are few distinguishing physical features of XLA that can provide clues to the diagnosis, but absence of visible tonsils or adenoids (by x-ray or CT scan) is a useful clue.

In addition to the common sinopulmonary pathogens, patients with XLA are also susceptible to infections by particular opportunistic organisms that are rarer and fastidious, which can cause unusual clinical syndromes. For example, non–*Helicobacter pylori Helicobacter* species (*cinaedi*, *canis*, *bilis*, etc.) can cause a syndrome of dermatomyositis and cellulitis that presents with cutaneous ulcerations, particularly on the lower legs.[34] The organisms can sometimes be recovered from the blood, but they are fastidious and difficult to culture using usual methods. The ability to culture the organisms and evaluate their antibiotic sensitivity is crucial in most cases since they are frequently antibiotic resistant. A combination of antibiotics is often needed to effectively clear the infection.[35] Similarly, *Mycoplasma* species, including *Mycoplasma hominis,* can cause lung, abdominal, or bone infections that are difficult to eradicate and *Ureaplasma urealyticum* infections are a rare cause of arthritis, urethritis, and pneumonia.[36]

Prior to the widespread use of IgG supplementation in XLA, opportunistic viral infections, particularly with viruses that require an extracellular phase, were especially problematic. For example, echovirus encephalitis was estimated to be the cause of death in ~10% of boys with XLA in the 1970s, but that number has fallen dramatically with aggressive use of IgG supplementation. There continue to be rare cases of echovirus encephalitis in patients with XLA, even in those on adequate IgG replacement therapy, but these are thought to be caused by viral strains for which there may not be high antibody titers in the particular IgG preparation being used.[37,38] Similarly, a mink astrovirus strain was identified by deep sequencing from the brain of an XLA patient who developed a neurodegenerative disorder as a teen. Interestingly, he had lived next to a mink farm as a child but was started on immunosuppression early in his teens for inflammatory bowel disease, which may have allowed the virus to escape control.[39] Lastly, infections with vaccine-strain poliovirus were pathogenic in undiagnosed patients with XLA who were immunized with the live-viral vaccine after transplacentally acquired maternal antibody had waned. The shift from live attenuated to killed poliovirus for immunization has essentially eliminated new cases.

Hyperimmunoglobulin M Syndromes

Under normal circumstances, binding of antigen to cell-surface IgM on naïve B cells induces B-cell activation. The antigen, bound to surface IgM on the B cell, is ingested, proteolytically digested, and antigenic peptide fragments are displayed on the B-cell surface in MHC class II molecules. Antigen-specific T cells then engage the B cell via MHC II/TCR interactions. Once engaged, the activated helper T cell (Th) provides additional co-stimulatory signals to the B cell that are critical to promote immunoglobulin class-switching from IgM to IgG, IgA, and IgE. The most important of these co-stimulatory signals comes via the interaction of CD40 ligand on activated T cells with CD40 on B cells. Additional co-stimulatory signals come from ICOS on activated T cells and ICOS ligand (B7-H2) on B cells. Activation of the B cell through CD40 and cytokines that are secreted by the helper T cell cause it to undergo class-switch recombination (CSR) during which the μ-heavy chain gene segment within the immunoglobulin gene is replaced by either a γ, α, or ε gene segment. This is accomplished by nicking and double-strand breakage of the DNA in the immunoglobulin heavy-chain locus, which requires a series of enzymatic steps that involve activation-induced cytidine deaminase (AID), uracil DNA glycosylase (UNG), and others. Genetic defects that affect CD40 ligand (CD40L), CD40, AID, or UNG can therefore prevent CSR thus thwarting the B cell's ability to make significant amounts of any antibody isotype besides IgM.

The overwhelming majority of patients with hyper-IgM syndrome have the X-linked form caused by X-linked recessive mutations in CD40 ligand (CD40L/CD154), which is encoded by the *CD40LG* gene on the X-chromosome.[40] CD40L and its receptor CD40 are members of the tumor necrosis factor superfamily of ligands and receptors. In lymphocytes, CD40L is expressed only on activated T cells but is also expressed on platelets where its role is unknown. Affected boys may present with recurrent bacterial sinopulmonary infections caused by low IgG, IgA, and IgE, while IgM is normal or elevated. In addition to the usual bacterial pathogens, patients with CD40L mutations also demonstrate unique susceptibilities to fungal infections, particularly *Pneumocystis jirovecii* that causes pneumonia, and to a protozoan, *Cryptosporidium parvum* that causes bowel infections. B lymphocytes are present, and T-cell numbers are generally normal. In almost all cases, the diagnosis can be made by using flow cytometry to evaluate the expression and function of the CD40L protein on activated T cells. Expression is evaluated using antibodies specific to the CD40L protein and the function is evaluated by measuring the binding of a CD40-Ig heavy chain fusion protein to the expressed CD40L. Gene sequencing can be performed to identify a specific mutation.

The susceptibility to *Pneumocystis* and possibly other fungal pathogens has been somewhat of a puzzle because patients do not have other signs of a significant cellular immune defect such as severe or recurrent viral infections. Interestingly, the susceptibility to *P. jirovecii* pneumonia (PJP) appears to wane in most patients by the age of 5. PJP can be readily prevented by prophylactic trimethoprim-sulfamethoxazole administration and active disease is amenable to treatment using higher doses of the same drug. Recent data have suggested that the fungal susceptibility in CD40L deficiency may be a result of defective CD40L signaling to dendritic cells and monocytes that express CD40.[41]

C. parvum bowel infections are more difficult to diagnose and manage in patients with CD40L deficiency. *C. parvum* may cause abdominal pain, bloating, diarrhea, malabsorption, and weight loss. It may require multiple stool samples to identify the oocysts and occasionally, the diagnosis can only be made on endoscopically obtained biopsy specimens. *C. parvum* infections can result in chronic inflammation of the gut and biliary tree, which seems a likely contributor to the high incidence of bile duct cancers seen in these patients.[42,43]

Treatment involves the use of IgG replacement therapy combined with prophylactic antibiotics for prevention of PJP at least until the age of 5. The role of bone marrow transplantation for CD40L deficiency is still being evaluated. Even though numerous patients have undergone successful bone marrow transplantation, the role of bone marrow transplantation remains somewhat controversial although concerns about the poor prognosis of patients who develop hepatobiliary disease are considered to balance the risks of transplantation.[44,45]

Autosomal recessive mutations in CD40, AID, and UNG can also cause a hyper-IgM phenotype. CD40 deficiency is phenotypically like CD40 ligand deficiency, but AID and UNG deficiency tend to be milder. Patients with AID or UNG deficiency typically live into adulthood and do not demonstrate the same susceptibility to PJP and *C. parvum* bowel infections. Patients with mutations in AID deficiency do however have a significant propensity to develop autoimmunity affecting various organ systems. Patients are typically treated with IgG replacement therapy and antibiotics for acute infections. There are no reports of bone marrow transplantation for AID or UNG deficiency.

Common Variable Immunodeficiency Syndromes

Common variable immunodeficiency (CVID) is a heterogeneous disorder that is likely caused by a variety of molecular mechanisms that ultimately lead to a similar clinical phenotype. This has been borne out by recent studies demonstrating that causative genetic defects in more than 15 genes can be identified in 25% to 30% of patients with CVID.[46,47] In an effort to standardize the diagnosis of CVID, the European Society of Immunodeficiencies (ESID) has proposed diagnostic criteria that include the following: (1) plasma IgG levels that are less than 2 standard deviations below the mean for age combined with a "marked decrease" in either IgM or IgA; (2) age of onset of immunodeficiency >2 years; (3) absent isohemagglutinins or poor responses to vaccines; (4) defined causes of hypogammaglobulinemia have been excluded.[48]

The peak age of onset of CVID is in the second or third decade of life and 50% to 60% of patients have a clinical phenotype consisting almost exclusively of increased bacterial sinopulmonary infections. With IgG supplementation, this group of patients has a relatively benign course with long-term survival that is not unlike the normal population. The other 30% to 40% of patients have a complicated disease course with autoimmunity or lymphoproliferative disease that can involve the hematopoietic system, lungs, lymph nodes, liver, and bowel. The long-term outcome of this population is significantly worse, approaching only 40% survival over 40 years.[49]

Among the more clinically impactful disorders that occur in CVID patients with inflammatory disease is granulomatous, lymphoproliferative, interstitial lung disease that affects approximately 30% to 40% of patients.[50] This typically presents with decreasing lung function manifested by cough, decreased exercise tolerance, and sometimes hypoxemia. Typical findings on chest CT scan include diffuse nodules within the lung, opacities that have a "ground glass" appearance, bronchial wall thickening, and bronchiectasis. Lung biopsy generally demonstrates a lymphocytic interstitial pneumonitis with noncaseating granulomas and a follicular bronchiolitis with lymphoid aggregates of both B and T cells. This pattern is sometimes mistaken for sarcoidosis. Over time, this inflammatory process in the lungs causes destruction of alveoli and will contribute to development of bronchiectasis. There continues to be some debate among providers about whether this process should be treated if the patient is not demonstrating pulmonary compromise.[51] If unchecked, there is evidence that irreversible damage and fibrosis may develop. Studies using a combination of anti-CD20 monoclonal antibody (rituximab) therapy and azathioprine have led to functional improvement in a significant percentage of treated patients.[52,53]

In addition to pulmonary symptoms, gastrointestinal complaints are common in CVID, affecting 20% to 30% of patients.[54,55] Patients who develop disease demonstrate a hypertrophic lymphoproliferation of Peyer patches that causes a nodular lymphoid hyperplasia in the bowel. This is associated with abdominal discomfort, diarrhea, malabsorption, and weight loss and can cause significant morbidity. A variety of approaches have been taken to treat this process, but none have offered particularly dramatic results although nonabsorbable steroid preparations have shown some benefit with minimal side effects. Nodular regenerative hyperplasia of the liver is a more troubling complication observed in 5% to 10% of patients. It often presents with increased transaminases and can cause severe hepatic dysfunction with development of hepatosplenomegaly and ascites.[56] Recent studies have hypothesized that this may be related to increased permeability of the gut mucosa leading to increased circulating lipopolysaccharides and bacterial products.[57]

B-cell numbers are normal in the majority of CVID patients, but there are some that have B-cell lymphopenia. In patients with normal B-cell numbers, B-cell maturation, memory development, and immunoglobulin class-switching are often abnormal and can be assessed by detailed flow-cytometry-based immunophenotyping of B cells. Varying classification schemes have been proposed to subtype patients according to their B-cell phenotype and these subsets have been correlated with differences in risk for autoimmunity, etc. In addition to the humoral immune deficiency, some patients with CVID have impaired T-cell function with decreased CD4 or CD8 T-cell numbers as well as abnormal T-cell proliferative responses to mitogens and antigens in vitro. To differentiate these patients with features of a combined immunodeficiency from the more typical CVID, some have proposed that they be termed late-onset combined immunodeficiency.[58,59]

Selective Immunoglobulin a Deficiency

Two isoforms of IgA are made predominantly at mucosal surfaces where they play a critical role in neutralizing pathogens and maintaining mucosal integrity. Subjects >4 years of age with serum IgA levels consistently <7 mg/dL but normal IgG and IgM levels are considered to have selective IgA deficiency (SIgAD). SIgAD can be difficult to diagnose in childhood because adult blood levels of IgA (50-200 mg/dL) are not usually attained until 12 years of age or older. The molecular mechanisms by which this occurs are largely unknown. Interestingly, despite low IgA, the frequency of cell-surface IgA-positive B cells is normal in many patients with SIgAD. Up to 20% of IgA-deficient subjects have reduced levels of at least one IgG subclass as well—mostly IgG_2.

Selective IgA deficiency is the most common immune deficiency with an incidence as high as 1 in 300 in blood bank studies. The majority (>50%) of patients with selective IgA-deficiency have no apparent symptoms that can be directly linked to their immune defect. In the patients who do have symptoms, they are typically more suggestive of immune dysregulation and autoimmunity (allergy, arthritis, diarrhea, celiac disease, etc.) than immune deficiency (sinusitis, otitis media, bronchitis, and pneumonia). In patients who are truly IgA deficient, sensitization to IgA itself can be a problem, leading to anaphylactic reactions during infusions of blood products including IVIg, red blood cells, platelets, etc. Complete deficiency of IgA is, however, quite uncommon and risks for infusion-related anaphylaxis can often be managed by pretreatment with benadryl, acetaminophen, and steroids.[60]

Transient Hypogammaglobulinemia

Maternal IgG is actively transported across the placenta from mother to infant. The rate of transfer increases in the last month of pregnancy. Premature infants will therefore have low IgG levels, but term newborns have IgG concentrations virtually equal to their mother's. Since the half-life of IgG is approximately 21 days, the level of maternal IgG falls as the infant grows and IgG is catabolized. For most term infants, the IgG level in blood reaches a nadir between 200 and 400 mg/dL, typically between 3 and 4 months of age. As the infant's own immune system matures and begins to generate more IgG of its own, the immunoglobulin levels begin to rise again. There are however children whose IgG levels dip below 200 mg/dL and may remain low for a prolonged period before they begin to rise into the normal range again. Despite this, the response to protein antigen vaccines is often normal. This phenomenon is termed *transient hypogammaglobulinemia of infancy (THI)* and immunoglobulin levels typically return to normal by 2 to 6 years of age. There are almost no data about the mechanism by which THI occurs although it has been suggested that it may be the result of delayed B-cell maturation. This has however not been borne out by B-cell immunophenotyping studies.[61] The true incidence of THI is unknown because immunoglobulin levels are usually only requested if patients are having symptoms (ie, recurrent infections). There is no consensus on how to manage THI although most would agree that if patients are having frequent infections, they might require IgG supplementation until their own IgG levels normalize. One approach has been to immunize affected infants with killed vaccines and to start supplemental IgG therapy on those that make no significant antibody response. Infants who do respond to immunization with a protective specific antibody titer are usually safe with symptomatic management or with prophylactic antibiotics alone.

Diagnosis

The diagnosis of antibody deficiency needs to evaluate both the quantity and the quality of the antibody response. Quantity is easily evaluated by measuring quantitative immunoglobulin levels (IgG, IgM, IgA, and IgE) in the blood and comparing these to the age-appropriate normal ranges. Evaluating the quality of the antibody response can be done by measuring specific antibody titers to vaccines the patient has received. Generally, responses to both protein antigens (tetanus, diphtheria, hepatitis B, etc.) and carbohydrate antigens (23-valent unconjugated Pneumovax) need to be assessed to confirm normal antibody responses. Patients who respond appropriately to protein antigens but do not respond to carbohydrate antigens may have *specific antibody deficiency* and may require additional workup. Guidelines regarding the interpretation and use of diagnostic vaccination have been published.[62]

In addition to evaluating antibody quantity and quality, it is essential to determine whether patients have normal B-cell numbers by evaluating lymphocyte subsets. The use of more detailed B-cell immunophenotyping to evaluate B-cell development, absence of $CD27^+$ memory B cells, and the ability of memory B cells to undergo immunoglobulin class-switching have been utilized as prognostic biomarkers and have become commonplace in many clinics.[63,64]

Flow cytometry testing to assess the expression of specific proteins that are defective in B cell and antibody deficiency disorders including BTK, CD40 ligand, CD40, ICOS, CD27, BAFF receptor, etc. can be performed in specialty laboratories and offer the ability to rapidly obtain a molecular diagnosis. This is typically supplemented by sequencing of specific genes.

Treatment
Immunoglobulin Replacement

In patients with antibody deficiency, replacement of IgG is critical to maintain health and prevent long-term complications associated with recurrent infections. Immunoglobulin replacement therapy has been found to be effective when administered intravenously (IVIg), subcutaneously (SCIg), or intramuscularly (IMIg) and there are currently FDA-approved products that support administration via any of these routes. That said, because of significant discomfort associated with IMIg administration, this route is typically not preferred by patients. Most are maintained on either IVIg or SCIg depending on preference and provider recommendations related to each patient's clinical need. Because the half-life of IgG in the circulation is ~21 days under normal circumstances, IVIg is typically administered every 3 to 4 weeks providing high peak levels followed by a decline over the ensuing weeks to a trough prior to the next infusion. In contrast, SCIg is typically administered 1 to 2 times per week in smaller doses providing a more "steady-state" level of IgG in the circulation. IgG products are prepared from pooled plasma collected from thousands of healthy donors and therefore they contain a broad range of antibodies. A reasonable starting dose of either IVIg or SCIg is 400 to 500 mg/kg/mo. This can be divided into the number of doses required to administer the necessary monthly volume (IgG preparations range in concentration from 5 g/100 cc [5%] to 20 g/100 cc [20%]). In most patients, a trough IgG level of 600 mg/dL in the blood is a reasonable initial target, but the dose should then be adjusted to achieve a trough IgG level that prevents both acute infections and development of progressive lung disease. There is evidence that at least for bacterial pneumonia, higher IgG trough levels are directly correlated with a decreased risk of infection.[65] Supplemental IgG is generally very effective at preventing lower respiratory tract infections (bronchitis and pneumonia), but the response of upper tract disease (particularly sinusitis) is more variable. Some patients have persistent sinus symptoms that can be a significant clinical problem despite IgG therapy. In these patients, the addition of prophylactic antibiotics or increasing the frequency or dose of IgG infusions may be beneficial.

Side effects with IVIg therapy are relatively common, occurring in as many as 25% of treated patients.[66] Side effects include headaches, nausea, vomiting, chills, fatigue, fever, rash, and aseptic meningitis. These can often be managed by changing the IgG product, pretreating with benadryl, acetaminophen, and steroids (0.5-1 mg/kg) prior to infusion, or slowing the rate of infusion. Patients who have persistent symptoms despite these measures can often tolerate subcutaneous IgG supplementation (SCIg).

Prophylactic Antibiotics

It is increasingly recognized that in many patients with antibody deficiency, replacement of IgG (even to normal levels) may not prevent all clinically significant infections. The addition of prophylactic antibiotics has been used as an adjunct to IgG therapy to try and improve control of infections and decrease morbidity. Since many patients with antibody deficiency have evidence of bronchiectasis and chronic lung disease, some providers, extrapolating from lung transplant and cystic fibrosis literature, have utilized thrice weekly macrolide antibiotics as a prophylactic regimen in an attempt to prevent progression of lung pathology. A recent prospective, double-blind, placebo controlled trial of low-dose azithromycin in primary antibody deficiency patients demonstrated a decrease in infectious exacerbations, a reduction in the need for additional antibiotic courses, and decreased hospitalizations in the antibiotic treated group.[67] Other antibiotic prophylaxis regimens have not yet undergone a similar rigor of testing in clinical trials so cannot be directly compared for efficacy, but existing data suggest potential benefit.

T CELLS

Disorders characterized by the absence of T cells were described more than 60 years ago, but identification of several new genetic defects has expanded this group of disorders substantially. Some of these are characterized by significant, generalized T-cell lymphopenia, while others are characterized by the absence of specialized subsets of T cells.

Clinical Presentation

In general, absence of T cells causes susceptibility to unusual or severe infections caused by viruses including cytomegalovirus (CMV), Epstein-Barr virus (EBV), and adenoviruses; fungal infections caused by organisms such as *P. jirovecii* that commonly causes pneumonias in this group of patients; and mycobacteria such as Bacille Calmette-Guérin (BCG) in areas of the world where this is used. In addition, patients with T-cell deficiencies frequently have symptoms of autoimmunity including diarrhea (secondary to autoimmune enteropathy), cytopenias (autoimmune hemolytic anemia and idiopathic thrombocytopenic purpura), and hepatitis.

Specific Disorders
22q11 Deletion Syndrome (DiGeorge Syndrome)

Deletions within the 22q11.2 region of the long arm of chromosome 22 have been associated with various clinical syndromes including DiGeorge syndrome (DGS), velocardiofacial syndrome, conotruncal anomaly face syndrome, CATCH22 syndrome, and others. DiGeorge syndrome is the name most associated with immune deficiency so will be the focus of this discussion. While DGS is a complex syndrome that has been associated with a wide array of symptoms, the diagnostic criteria proposed by the ESID are relatively straightforward. These propose that a diagnosis of DGS should be strongly considered in patients who have <500 CD3+ T cells/mm^3 and any two of the following three characteristics: (1) conotruncal cardiac defect (truncus arteriosus, tetralogy of Fallot, interrupted aortic arch, or aberrant right subclavian); (2) hypocalcemia requiring therapy for >3 weeks; (3) deletion of chromosome 22q11.2. This chromosomal deletion syndrome occurs in approximately 1 in 4000 to 5000 births and causes haploinsufficiency of the genes encompassed in the deletion that can extend to include as much as 3 Mb of the chromosome.[68,69]

The characteristic T-cell lymphopenia of DGS is thought to arise primarily from the absence of adequate thymic tissue and at times, the diagnosis is suspected when the cardiac surgeon correcting a congenital heart defect finds little or no thymic tissue in the mediastinum. Most affected infants have low, but not absent T cells and absolute counts tend to improve over the first year of life. Both CD4+ and CD8+ T cells are low; however, CD8+ T-cell numbers tend to be more affected in most patients. Despite low T-cell counts, most patients do not have significant problems with recurrent or severe viral or fungal infections. Some patients may have recurrent candidiasis. Bacterial infections of the upper respiratory tract including otitis media and sinusitis do occur but may be related more to anatomical issues associated with the facial anomalies than to the immunodeficiency per se. Rare patients have severe T-cell lymphopenia with essentially no T cells and are termed "complete" DiGeorge. These patients may have a clinical phenotype like SCID.[68,69]

Other prominent clinical features include hypocalcemia that can be severe and persistent due to parathyroid hypoplasia; dysmorphic facial features that include small low-set ears, hypertelorism, and micrognathia; renal anomalies including horseshoe kidney and a duplicated collecting system; and developmental delay including problems with speech acquisition, learning disabilities, and behavioral problems. Patients with DGS have also been found to have an increased incidence of autoimmunity including cytopenias (particularly affecting red cells and platelets), juvenile idiopathic arthritis, and thyroiditis.

In symptomatic patients, the diagnosis of DGS is typically made by confirming a deletion within the 22q11.2 region by fluorescence in situ hybridization or by quantitative polymerase chain reaction for deletion of the *TBX1* gene that lies within the deletion.[70] In approximately 10% of patients, deletion of this region cannot be detected despite the presence of the classic clinical features.

Treatment of DiGeorge initially involves supportive care that may include cardiac support and calcium supplementation. In patients with severe T-cell lymphopenia or evidence of decreased T-cell function, prophylaxis against PJP pneumonia and IgG supplementation may be required. Blood for these patients should be irradiated to prevent the risk of graft-versus-host disease (GvHD). For those patients with the severe, "complete" form of the syndrome, grafting of allogeneic thymus slices into the thigh muscle has proven to be successful in recovering the T-cell lymphopenia, improving T-cell responses to mitogens, and correcting the infectious susceptibility.[71,72] HCT has been utilized in a handful of patients with mixed results. In general, HCT restores

T-cell counts and protects patients against further infection, but in the absence of a thymus, the T-cell graft likely consists of long-lived committed lymphoid progenitor T cells and not of cells derived from donor bone marrow stem cells. As a result, there is concern that the T-cell grafts may senesce over time, once again leaving the patient lymphopenic and susceptible to infection.

Severe Combined Immune Deficiency

Made famous by *The Boy in the Plastic Bubble*, a 1976 made-for-TV movie starring John Travolta, SCID is among the most severe immunodeficiencies. It is now known that this category of diseases is made up of a variety of related disorders caused by mutations in more than 20 different genes. The commonality between all forms of SCID is deficiency of one or more subsets of T cells. Depending on the genetic defect, patients may also lack B cells and/or natural killer (NK) cells. This has led to the useful convention of defining cases of SCID by their cellular phenotype (ie, $T^{neg}B^+NK^+$, $T^{neg}B^+NK^{neg}$, $T^{neg}B^{neg}NK^+$, $T^{neg}B^{neg}NK^{neg}$, etc.). The cellular phenotype suggests which underlying genetic defect may cause the disease (*Table 64.1*).[1] Because of the absence of functional T cells, patients with SCID typically come to medical attention because of severe or chronic viral infections, fungal infections, or autoimmunity. In the overwhelming majority of SCID cases, this leads to death in infancy or early childhood if patients don't undergo curative treatment such as HCT or gene therapy. Unfortunately, infections create complications for HCT or gene therapy and substantially decrease the likelihood of survival. This led to the addition of SCID to newborn screening panels performed on dried blood spot cards after birth universally in the United States and increasingly in other countries. This has led to the recognition that the incidence of SCID is approximately 1 in 40,000 live births in the United States, more than double initial estimates.[73,74]

Table 64.1. Molecular Defects Associated With Specific Cellular Phenotypes in SCID

Cellular Phenotype	Gene	Inheritance	Other Features
$T^{neg}B^{neg}NK^{neg}$			
• Adenosine deaminase deficiency	*ADA1*	AR	Costochondral abnormalities, neonatal hepatitis
• Purine nucleotide phosphorylase deficiency	PNP	AR	Progressive neurologic problems
• Reticular dysgenesis	AK2	AR	Also has deficiency of myeloid lineage cells, sensorineural deafness
$T^{neg}B^{neg}NK^+$			
• RAG1 deficiency	RAG1	AR	
• RAG2 deficiency	RAG2	AR	
• Artemis deficiency	DCLRE1C	AR	Radiosensitivity
• DNA-PKcs deficiency	PRKDC	AR	Radiosensitivity
• DNA ligase IV deficiency	LIG4	AR	Radiosensitivity, microcephaly, growth retardation
• Cernunnos/XLF deficiency	NHEJ1	AR	Radiosensitivity, microcephaly, growth retardation
$T^{neg}B^+NK^{neg}$			
• Common γ chain deficiency	IL2RG	XL	
• JAK3 deficiency	JAK3	AR	
• CD45	PTPRC	AR	Some NK cells may be present
$T^{neg}B^+NK^+$			
• IL-7 receptor-α (CD127) deficiency	IL7RA	AR	
• DiGeorge syndrome	22q11.2 del	AD	Hypoparathyroidism, cardiac defects, dysmorphic facies
• CHARGE syndrome	CHD7	AD	Multiple anomalies make up the clinical complex of CHARGE syndrome
• CD3δ deficiency	CD3D	AR	
• CD3ε deficiency	CD3E	AR	
• CD3γ deficiency	CD3G	AR	
• CD3ζ deficiency	CD3Z	AR	
• LCK deficiency	LCK	AR	
• Coronin-1A deficiency	CORO1A	AR	Lymphadenopathy
$T^+B^+NK^+$			
• MHC II deficiency	CIITA	AR	CD4+ T cells are typically decreased but not absent
	RFXANK	AR	
	RFX5	AR	
	RFXAP	AR	
• ORAI1 deficiency	ORAI1	AR	Myopathy, calcium flux defect in B and T cells, poor lymphocyte proliferation
• STIM1 deficiency	STIM1	AR	Myopathy, calcium flux defect in B and T cells, poor lymphocyte proliferation

Modified from Van Horebeek L, Dubois B, Goris A. Somatic variants: new kids on the block in human immunogenetics. *Trends Genet.* 2019;35(12):935-947.
Abbreviations: AD, autosomal dominant; AR, autosomal recessive; SCID, severe combined immunodeficiency; XL, X-linked recessive.

SCID Caused by Defective Cytokine Signaling in T Cells
T cells are highly dependent on interleukin (IL)-2 and IL-7 for growth, survival, activation, and differentiation. Defects in molecules that disrupt IL-2 or IL-7 signaling lead to T-cell deficiency.

X-Linked Severe Combined Immunodeficiency
X-linked SCID is the most common type of SCID, accounting for ~40% of all cases. It occurs because of mutations in the *IL2RG* gene, encoding the common γ receptor chain (γc) utilized by cytokine receptors for IL-2, IL-4, IL-7, IL-9, IL-15, and IL-21. In the absence of a functional γc chain, cells are unable to respond to these cytokines. Since IL-2 and IL-7 are key growth factors for T cells, and IL-15 is the key growth factor for NK cells, patients with X-SCID lack T and NK cells but usually have normal numbers of circulating B cells. The ability to make antibodies is nevertheless severely impaired due to the lack of T-cell help.

If not identified by newborn screening, infants with X-SCID typically present with severe infections. PJP is common and often accompanied by severe viral infections with CMV, EBV, respiratory syncytial virus, rotavirus, metapneumovirus, and others. Adenovirus is particularly lethal in SCID, causing not only pneumonitis but also a severe, fulminant hepatitis. In countries where BCG is still used for vaccination, SCID patients often develop severe, systemic BCG-osis. Other symptoms frequently associated with X-SCID include diarrhea, failure to thrive, and candidiasis. The physical exam and associated studies offer few clues to the diagnosis of X-SCID other than a paucity of palpable lymph nodes and absence of a thymic shadow on chest x-ray.

Flow cytometry can be used to evaluate tyrosine phosphorylation of the STAT3 transcription factor in response to IL-21 stimulation and can provide rapid functional assessment of whether a patient may have an IL2RG or JAK3 defect. Under normal circumstances, IL-21 stimulation of B cells causes rapid tyrosine phosphorylation of STAT3 that is absent in patients with IL2RG or JAK3 deficiency. The diagnosis is ultimately confirmed by sequencing of the *IL2RG* gene.

HCT using a variety of pretransplant conditioning regimens has been the mainstay of therapy for X-SCID. Some have strongly advocated the use of T-cell-depleted grafts from a haploidentical parent because they are readily available, but some patients transplanted using that approach have failed to obtain significant donor chimerism in the B-cell compartment, so have remained dependent on IgG supplementation posttransplant.[75,76] X-SCID was also the first disorder successfully treated by gene therapy. Unfortunately, the retroviral gene therapy vector used to deliver the normal copy of the *IL2RG* gene had an unknown propensity to integrate within the T-cell oncogene *LMO2*, causing T-cell leukemias in a subset of treated patients.[77,78] Newer generation lentiviral gene therapy vectors have thus far avoided this complication while demonstrating excellent immune reconstitution.[79]

JAK3-Deficient SCID
JAK3 is the tyrosine kinase immediately downstream of the common gamma chain (γc). It transduces signals from cytokine receptors to the STAT5 transcription factor and to other intracellular signaling molecules. As a result, patients with pathogenic JAK3 mutations have a $T^{neg}B^+NK^{neg}$ cellular phenotype and a clinical presentation like that observed in γc-deficiency (see X-SCID above). Approximately one-third of patients have milder mutations that cause hypomorphic JAK3 function, allowing them to develop some T cells but these are typically dysfunctional.[80] Sequencing of the *JAK3* gene is required to confirm a diagnosis.

Interleukin-7 Receptor–Deficient SCID
Defects in the α-chain of the IL-7 receptor gene, *IL7RA*, cause SCID with a $T^{neg}B^+NK^+$ phenotype since IL-7 is only required for growth and homeostatic expansion of T cells.

SCID Caused by Defective T-Cell Receptor Structure, Function, or Activation
T-cell survival and activation is dependent on expression of a functional T-cell receptor (TCR) at the cell surface, the ability of that TCR to bind to MHC molecules expressing antigenic peptide, and the capacity of the TCR to initiate an appropriate activation signal into the cells.

CD3 Component and CD45-Deficient SCID
CD3γ, δ, ε, and ζ chains are essential subunits of the TCR complex. The TCR, including CD3 subunits, assembles in the endoplasmic reticulum and Golgi complex before trafficking to the cell surface. If any of the receptor subunits are absent (including any of the CD3 chains), most of the receptors are recycled, never making it to the outer cell membrane. Consequently, cells are unable to receive essential TCR stimulation as they traffic through the thymus and die by "neglect." Patients with CD3 subunit deficiencies therefore typically have a $T^{neg}B^+NK^+$ phenotype. Since the number of T-cell precursors entering the thymus is normal however, the CD3 defects are unusual among SCID disorders in that the size of the thymus is generally normal. Defects in all 4 CD3 chains have been identified, but CD3γ deficiency is often the mildest with only moderate T-cell lymphopenia and recurrent pneumonia and otitis.[81]

Zap-70 (Kinase) and CD45 (Phosphatase)-Deficient SCID
Zap-70 is a tyrosine kinase that is downstream of CD3 in the TCR signaling pathway. Absence of functional enzyme results in a characteristic SCID phenotype with decreased CD4$^+$ T cells but virtually absent CD8$^+$ T cells. Immunoglobulin levels are often decreased and antibody responses to vaccination are typically absent because of the lack of effective T-cell help. CD4$^+$ T cells that are present do not respond to antigen or mitogen stimulation that utilizes the TCR but they do proliferate and make cytokines in response to phorbol and ionomycin stimulation, which mimics TCR stimulation by activating kinases and calcium flux through downstream mechanisms.[82] Bone marrow transplantation is effective in this disorder.

CD45 is a transmembrane tyrosine phosphatase present on most white blood cells. It regulates intracellular Src-family tyrosine kinases that are important for TCR function and activation. Autosomal recessive mutations of CD45 lead to T-cell deficiency and a SCID phenotype in affected infants.[83,84]

Defects in Antigen Presentation by MHC I or MHC II
The class I MHC complex is expressed by virtually all nucleated cells in the body and presents peptide antigens derived from intracellular proteins. Proteolytically derived peptides are bound to the MHC I complex as it is generated and trafficked through the endoplasmic reticulum. Peptides generated in the cytosol are transported into the inner lumen of the endoplasmic reticulum by the peptide transporters TAP1 and TAP2 where they bind to newly generated MHC I complexes, stabilizing them for transport to the cell membrane. Mutations in either of these, or of tapasin to which they bind, prevent antigenic peptides from being transported into the endoplasmic reticulum; therefore expression of MHC I complexes on the cell surface is markedly decreased. Since CD8$^+$ T cells require MHC-I antigen presentation to activate the TCR, CD8$^+$ T-cell and NK-cell counts are frequently (but not uniformly) decreased in these patients. Other cell subsets are typically normal. Heterogeneity in the phenotype may reflect differences in the underlying mutation and in the gene affected. MHC I deficiency is typically associated with recurrent viral infections, and recurrent sinusitis and bronchitis. Some patients may survive into the third decade. Since MHC I is expressed on virtually all nucleated cells in the body, the role of HCT in MHC I deficiency is unclear. The diagnosis is usually confirmed by a combination of genetic testing and flow cytometry to demonstrate an absence of MHC I on cells.[85]

The class II MHC complex is expressed only by cells considered to be professional antigen-presenting cells (phagocytes and B cells). The reason for this is that MHC II generally presents peptide antigens derived from material ingested (phagocytosed) from outside the cell. Defects that interfere with the assembly or cell-surface expression of the class II MHC–peptide complex prevent effective antigen recognition by CD4$^+$ T cells, resulting in a SCID syndrome characterized by CD4+ T-cell lymphopenia but normal CD8+ T-cell numbers. Patients typically present in infancy with chronic diarrhea, failure to thrive, and occasionally with autoimmune cytopenias. Some patients can have a mild disease course and can live well into adulthood with only supportive care, while others with the same mutation may have a more severe phenotype. Bone marrow transplantation for MHC II deficiency has been challenging with reported survival rates of approximately 50%. In addition, there is a high rate of severe GvHD, possibly because thymic epithelial cells that play a role in positive and negative T-cell selection are not replaced by HCT and still do not express MHC II.[86] MHC II deficiency can result from defects in one of four DNA-binding proteins that regulate transcription of the MHC class II gene (*CIITA*, *RFXANK*, *RFX5*, and *RFXAP*). Founder mutations (particularly in RFXANK) are most common in the Mediterranean and have led to most affected patients having some familial ties to this geographical region. A rapid preliminary diagnosis can be made by evaluating MHC II complex expression on peripheral blood cells by flow cytometry. A definitive molecular diagnosis can then be confirmed by genetic testing to identify mutations in one of the four causative genes. Since mutations in either MHC I or MHC II lead to problems with development and function of only a subset of T cells, total T-cell numbers are usually decreased but not absent. As a result, patients may be missed by SCID newborn screening.[87]

SCID Caused by Defects in DNA Recombination (DNA Double-Strand Breakage and Repair)

Rearrangement of the V, D, J, and constant regions of TCR gene and the B-cell immunoglobulin gene requires that double-stranded breaks be made in the DNA and that these breaks then be repaired after removal of intervening chromosomal fragments. The recombinase activating genes *RAG1* and *RAG2* are expressed in T and B cells and play an essential role in creating the necessary double-stranded DNA breaks in the TCR and immunoglobulin loci. A large complex of proteins including Artemis (DCLRE1C), DNA-PKcs, Cernunnos/XLF (XRCC4-like factor), and DNA Ligase IV (LIG4) then play a role in repair of the DNA double-stranded breaks needed to create the final, recombined TCR or Ig locus. Since productive rearrangement of the TCR or Ig locus is a necessary developmental step during T- and B-cell maturation, complete failure in one of these processes results in lymphopenia, with few if any T or B cells in the blood, while generation of NK cells is generally unaffected. Because radiation induces double-stranded breaks in DNA, cells from patients with mutations in any of the proteins involved in DNA repair (Artemis, DNA-PKcs, Cernunnos, Ligase IV) demonstrate decreased survival in vitro after radiation exposure (radiation-sensitivity). This can be a valuable diagnostic clue in making a diagnosis.

Patients who have null mutations of any of these proteins have a clear $T^{neg}B^{neg}NK^+$ cell phenotype. There are however many mutations, particularly missense mutations or small in-frame deletions, that allow expression of a partially functional protein that can occasionally productively recombine a TCR or Ig gene locus. The cell in which this occurs is then able to pass the developmental block and proliferate to fill the lymphopenic void that is otherwise present in SCID. These forms of SCID are termed "leaky" because they allow a small number of T (and occasionally B) cells to "leak" past the developmental block. Omenn syndrome, originally described in leaky RAG1 or RAG2 mutants, is a clinical phenotype that results from this leaky form of SCID. Affected infants typically develop a desquamative erythroderma after birth that is associated with the presence of oligoclonal, activated T cells in the skin, hepatosplenomegaly, lymphadenopathy, eosinophilia, and elevated IgE. Some develop autoimmune enteropathy and cytopenias. Affected patients are typically treated with T-cell-directed immunosuppression such as cyclosporine or FK506, followed by bone marrow transplantation. Leaky forms of SCID have now been described in several SCID-associated molecular defects including RAG1, RAG2, Artemis, Ligase IV, IL7RA, IL2RG, RMRP, and others.[88,89]

SCID Caused by Metabolic Defects

Adenosine Deaminase and Purine Nucleotide Phosphorylase-Deficient SCID

In the 1970s, adenosine deaminase (ADA) deficiency became the first molecularly defined immunodeficiency with the discovery that patients with SCID lacked the enzymatic activity of ADA in peripheral blood. ADA catalyzes the conversion of adenosine triphosphate (ATP), guanosine triphosphate (GTP), and their deoxy counterparts to adenosine diphosphate (ADP) and guanosine diphosphate (GDP). When enzyme activity is impaired or absent, intracellular levels of deoxy-ATP (dATP) rise to interfere with ribonucleotide reductase, such that DNA synthesis and repair are slowed and lymphocyte apoptosis is increased. Purine nucleotide phosphorylase (PNP) works further down this same metabolic pathway to convert deoxyinosine to hypoxanthine. Mutations interfering with this function cause deoxy-GTP accumulation and the inhibition of ribonucleotide reductase and DNA synthesis. In both cases, affected infants typically have a $T^{neg}B^{neg}NK^{neg/low}$ cellular phenotype due to the toxic nature of the accumulated metabolites on lymphocyte maturation and development. Patients typically present with severe or recurrent viral infections or recurrent sinopulmonary infections in the first year of life.

Both syndromes are associated with other, nonimmune symptoms including skeletal abnormalities and osseochondrous dysplasia in ADA deficiency and neurologic deficits, developmental delay, and spasticity, in PNP deficiency. In both cases, the diagnosis can be made by detecting high levels of the toxic metabolites that build up in the peripheral blood in the absence of enzymatic activity. Sequencing of the *ADA* or *PNP* genes can be done to confirm the diagnosis. ADA deficiency accounts for 20% or more of autosomal recessive SCID cases.

Aside from bone marrow transplantation, ADA-deficient infants can be treated with recombinant, PEGylated ADA, which is injected intramuscularly once per week. Treatment efficacy is gauged by measuring plasma ADA activity and red cell deoxyATP levels. Enzyme treatment has the advantage of speed of response coupled with safety.[90,91] The treatment is very expensive and some patients exhibit decreasing efficacy over time. Hematopoietic stem cell transplant (HSCT) is effective in ADA deficiency but less so in PNP deficiency as it does not correct the neurologic deficits. Gene therapy for ADA deficiency has been highly successful and unlike X-linked SCID, there have been no reported cases of leukemia.[92,93]

Treatment of Severe Combined Immunodeficiency Syndromes

SCID was uniformly lethal in the first years of life until Good and colleagues successfully reconstituted an affected infant with a transplant of sibling bone marrow.[94] Experience in subsequent years has shown that patients with B-cell-positive SCID (IL2RG, JAK3, IL7RA, etc.) readily reconstitute their T-cell deficiency but may not develop significant B-cell chimerism. The reasons for this are not entirely understood, but various hypotheses have been put forward. From a practical standpoint, a lack of donor B-cell engraftment may lead to a chronic need for IgG replacement therapy even after transplant since patients may not be able to mount sufficient antibody responses. Patients with B-cell-negative SCID are more likely to have successful donor engraftment of both T- and B-cell lineages and more likely to recover full humoral immune function.

One of the most significant challenges in the treatment of SCID is that in the absence of a family history, most patients come to attention because of infections. These are most commonly PJP and severe viral infections (see above). PJP can be treated but may lead to lung damage, whereas the viral infections may or may not be controllable.[95] In addition, many SCID infants have significant diarrhea and weight loss by the time they reach a transplant center. Together, these complications increase the risk of adverse outcomes during transplantation for SCID and have been the major impetus for adding SCID to state newborn screening panels. Initial management prior to transplant involves aggressive supportive care, antimicrobials to treat any intercurrent infections (bacterial, viral, and fungal), antimicrobial prophylaxis to prevent future infections, and IgG replacement therapy.

There is significant debate about the best pretransplant conditioning regimen for patients with SCID to balance safety and efficacy. In general, those patients that have a matched sibling donor receive no conditioning prior to receiving unmanipulated bone marrow. For other patients, a variety of conditioning regimens ranging from no conditioning to fully myeloablative regimens have been tried. Similarly, a range of manipulated and unmanipulated stem cell sources have been tried including matched, mismatched, or haploidentical bone marrow or peripheral blood stem cells or cord blood. Lastly, a variety of prophylactic immunosuppressive regimens have been used in the early posttransplant period to limit GvHD and prevent graft rejection. Each option has advantages and disadvantages, which has led to a spectrum of transplant regimens that has been attempted for SCID. A number of ongoing studies assess which regimens offer the best outcomes and lowest risk.[76,96-98]

OTHER COMPLEX OR COMBINED IMMUNODEFICIENCY DISORDERS

Wiskott-Aldrich Syndrome

Wiskott-Aldrich syndrome (WAS) is unique among immunodeficiency disorders because affected patients have both an infectious susceptibility and a bleeding disorder. The bleeding problems stem from the platelets being small (mean platelet volume < 5fL), dysfunctional, and few in number (usually platelet counts < 70,000/μL). Patients with WAS typically present in infancy with bloody diarrhea and/or bruising, recurrent upper respiratory tract infections, and eczema. The incidence of hematopoietic malignancies is high. IgE levels are often elevated. Serum IgG levels and T-cell counts are often normal in infancy but often decrease over time. Responses to vaccination, particularly with carbohydrate antigens such as Pneumovax are often abnormal.[99]

WAS is caused by mutations in the *WAS* gene located on the short arm of the X chromosome. Inheritance is X-linked recessive. There is a distinct genotype/phenotype correlation of mutations in WAS: mutations that destroy WAS protein (WASp) expression lead to the full syndrome of immunodeficiency and platelet dysfunction. Mutations that allow expression of a mutant WASp are typically associated with a milder X-linked thrombocytopenia (XLT) phenotype in which the platelet dysfunction persists but the immunodeficiency is very mild. Point mutations in the CDC42 binding domain of the WASp lead to a third phenotype of X-linked neutropenia that is generally not accompanied by bleeding abnormalities.[100]

The WASp is expressed primarily in lymphoid and myeloid cells where it functions to nucleate actin polymerization in the cell. Patients with WAS therefore have problems with directed migration of neutrophils and with clustering and signaling through T-cell and B-cell antigen receptors (this causes decreased signaling into the cell and abnormal proliferative responses).[101,102] A diagnosis of WAS can be confirmed by demonstrating the absence of WASp in cells by flow cytometry or western blotting, or by identifying a mutation in the *WAS* gene.

Treatment of WAS initially involves supportive care including treatment of any acute infections and management of any bleeding episodes. In general, repeated platelet transfusions are avoided because of the concern that patients will become sensitized to a wide array of HLA types, which may increase the risk of graft rejection during subsequent HSCT. Splenectomy can increase platelet counts; however, it also increases the risk that patients may die of sepsis with encapsulated organisms so there continues to be significant controversy surrounding the role of splenectomy in WAS. Patients with the full WAS phenotype should be evaluated for HSCT with matched related or unrelated donor bone marrow or cord blood.[103,104] Haploidentical transplants in WAS have proven to be complicated. The role of HCT in XLT remains controversial.[105] Some have advocated that the benefits for curing the bleeding problems are worth the risk if a matched sibling donor is available. Gene therapy has been successful in a small number of patients with WAS but like the X-SCID gene therapy trials, some treated patients developed T-cell leukemias because of integration of the viral gene therapy vector near an oncogene.[106]

Radiation Sensitive Disorders: Ataxia Telangiectasia and Nijmegen Breakage Syndrome

Ataxia telangiectasia (AT) is disorder associated with progressive neurologic decline, immunodeficiency, and propensity to malignancy. It is caused by autosomal recessive mutations in the *ATM* gene that encodes a serine/threonine kinase that acts together with the NBS1 protein as one of the major sensors of double-stranded DNA breaks in the cell. ATM phosphorylates key proteins involved in activation of the DNA damage repair checkpoint, leads to cell-cycle arrest, and then double-stranded DNA break repair. In the absence of functional ATM or NBS1, cells have a marked sensitivity to ionizing radiation. Since rearrangement of the TCR gene and the immunoglobulin gene loci also require double-stranded DNA break repair, these processes may be affected as well.

Patients with AT usually present in early childhood (most commonly between 2 and 5 years of age) with cerebellar ataxia that progresses to unsteady gait and over time, to choreoathetosis. Telangiectasias (small tufts of dilated blood vessels under the surface of the skin or mucus membranes) typically develop first on the conjunctivae and later are seen on the nose, ears, and shoulders. They can be an important diagnostic clue in a child with progressive ataxia. Most patients have immunoglobulin deficiency of varying degrees and can develop sinopulmonary symptoms and sepsis. The progressive neurodegeneration can compromise coughing, so it is hard to determine whether respiratory infections occur because of the immunodeficiency or the motor defects. Most affected individuals have elevated serum α-fetoprotein levels, which can be useful diagnostically. Malignancies are an important complication because of the DNA-repair defect. Acute T-cell leukemias are common and often have chromosomal translocations that affect the TCR gene loci. B-cell lymphomas also occur and are usually associated with 11q22 to 23 chromosomal deletions. There is also an increase in the frequency of epithelial tumors in both homozygotes and ATM mutation carriers. Affected patients usually die in the second or third decade of life.

Other DNA repair defects that cause varying degrees of ataxia and/or mild mental retardation include an ataxia-like syndrome caused my mutations in *MRE11* and Nijmegen breakage syndrome (NBS), caused by mutations in *NBS1*. In addition to an immunodeficiency like that observed in AT, patients with NBS have marked microcephaly, mild developmental delay/mental retardation, and a strong propensity to develop lymphomas. Another DNA repair defect, Bloom syndrome, caused by mutations in the DNA helicase RECQL3, results in excess sister chromatid exchanges; it is associated principally with lymphomas and cancer. Multiple primary tumors occurring at an early age are common. Reduced growth in childhood results in a proportional dwarfism that, with cutaneous telangiectasias, is a useful physical sign. Inheritance is autosomal recessive, and most common within Ashkenazi Jewish populations where there is a founder mutation. Chronic lung disease occurs and may be related to the low levels of IgA and IgM.[107]

Cartilage-Hair Hypoplasia

Cartilage-hair hypoplasia (CHH) is a complex disorder characterized by skeletal dysplasia with short limbs (metaphyseal chondrodysplasia), sparse hypoplastic hair, gastrointestinal problems, and a variable immunodeficiency. CHH is caused by mutations in the *RMRP* gene, which encodes the 267 base-pair RNA component of the RNase MRP complex that plays a role in processing of precursor ribosomal RNA. The mechanism by which autosomal recessive mutations in *RMRP* cause the clinical features of CHH is unknown. The largest populations of CHH patients have been identified among the Old Order Amish and Finnish populations. Virtually all patients with CHH have some degree of immunodeficiency that can range from a mild humoral defect with decreased vaccine responses to a SCID-like phenotype associated with progressive lymphopenia and severe infections with bacteria, viruses, and fungi. A leaky-SCID phenotype has also been described in RMRP deficiency. The diagnosis of CHH can be made based on the clinical phenotype and confirmed by sequencing of the *RMRP* gene. The immunologic features of CHH can be corrected by HSCT but the other features persist.[108,109]

Mammalian Susceptibility to Mycobacterial Disease

Under normal circumstances, intracellular pathogens like mycobacteria induce production of IL-12 and IL-23, which play a role in driving maturation of naïve T cells into activated T helper type I (Th1) cells that produce IFN-γ. IFN-γ then acts on a variety of cells including phagocytes (neutrophils, monocytes, and dendritic cells) to activate a program of IFN-inducible genes. Multiple molecules in this signaling pathway have been found to be defective in patients with intact cellular immunity who have invasive, nontuberculous mycobacterial infections. Mutations in genes encoding the IL-12 p40 subunit (*IL12B*), the IL-12 receptor β1 chain (*IL12RB1*), the TYK2 tyrosine kinase (*TYK2*) that associates with the IL-12 receptor and phosphorylates the STAT4 transcription factor, the IFN-γ receptor subunits (*IFNGR1* and *IFNGR2*), and the STAT1 transcription factor that is activated in response to IFN-γ (*STAT1*) are associated with an unusual susceptibility to mycobacterial infections. Mutations in this pathway are also associated with other infections including invasive salmonellosis and severe viral infections (*STAT1*). In addition to these gene defects, patients with invasive mycobacterial disease have now been identified with neutralizing autoantibodies to IFN-γ. Together these discoveries demonstrate a major role for the IL-12/IL-23/IFN-γ axis in normal human immunity to mycobacterias. For patients with the milder, autosomal dominant IFN-γ receptor defects, IL-12 p40 defects, IL-12 receptor defects, and TYK2 defects, antimicrobial therapy and IFN-γ treatment are often sufficient to treat invasive mycobacterial infections and to prevent future infections. For patients with the more severe, autosomal recessive IFN-γ receptor defects, IFN-γ supplementation provides no benefit and HSCT is warranted.[110]

Toll-Like Receptors and Innate Signaling Pathway Defects

The Toll-like receptors are a family of at least 10 pattern recognition receptors that are expressed in varying combinations on a broad array of immune and nonimmune cells. They recognize particular types (patterns) of molecules derived from pathogens (e.g., bacterial lipopolysaccharide, flagellin, mannan, CpG dinucleotides, viral dsDNA). Triggering of Toll-like receptors activates intracellular signaling pathways, many of which converge on a common pathway utilizing the IRAK proteins and MyD88, which in turn activate the IκB kinase complex (NEMO/IκKα/IκKβ), ultimately leading to phosphorylation and degradation of IκBα and activation of the NF-κB transcription factor complex.

Loss-of-function mutations in TLR signaling pathways are associated with major infectious susceptibilities: Mutations in *IRAK4* and *MyD88* have been identified in patients with susceptibility to invasive pyogenic bacterial infections, particularly *S. pneumoniae*, *Staphylococcus aureus*, and *Pseudomonas aeruginosa*. Interestingly, patients with IRAK4 or MyD88 deficiency tend to have problems with invasive pyogenic bacterial infections in childhood but these subside over time, assumed to be the result of adaptive immune response covering the innate defect. Mutations in *TLR3*, *TRIF*, *TRAF3*, and *UNC-93B* have been identified in patients with susceptibility to herpes simplex virus encephalitis and recently described defects in TLR7 lead to susceptibility to severe SARS-CoV-2 infection.[111,112] Defects in NEMO and IκBα also cause susceptibility to infections with pyogenic bacteria and mycobacteria and are associated with an anhidrotic ectodermal dysplasia phenotype.

Gain-of-function (GOF) mutations in TLRs 7 and 8 have also been recently described and both lead to immune dysregulation, autoimmunity, and autoinflammation. In the case of TLR7, GOF mutations cause SLE, whereas GOF mutations in TLR8 lead to autoinflammation, bone marrow failure, and resulting neutropenia.[113,114]

Chronic Mucocutaneous Candidiasis Syndromes

Chronic mucocutaneous candidiasis (CMC) is a clinical syndrome associated with chronic and recurrent candidal infections of mucosae, particularly oral and vaginal, together with nail-bed infections but generally without systemic infection. CMC can occur in isolation or as part of a broader clinical syndrome such as in APECED (Autoimmune PolyEndocrinopathy, Candidiasis, Ectodermal Dystrophy). Recent discoveries have determined that in almost all cases, CMC is associated with abnormalities in development of Th17 effector T cells or with the production of, or responses to the cytokine IL-17. These include autosomal recessive mutations in IL-17F or the IL-17 receptor α-subunit, dominant loss-of-function mutations in STAT3, and dominant GOF mutations in STAT1.[115]

CMC associated with APECED was originally thought to be the result of autoantibodies to type-1 IFNs, IL-17, and IL-22, but recent evidence suggests that defective mucosal barrier immunity characterized by increased IFN-γ may be a greater contributor.[116,117] APECED is caused by mutations in AIRE1, a nuclear protein that regulates the expression of self-antigens by thymic medullary epithelial cells where it plays a role in T-cell selection and maturation. Other features of this disorder include interstitial lung disease, endocrinopathies (hypoparathyroidism, adrenal insufficiency, and diabetes), alopecia areata, nail dystrophy, and vitiligo.[118]

IMMUNE REGULATORY DISORDERS

There are a growing number of genetic immune disorders characterized primarily by severe early-onset autoimmunity or inflammatory disease. These highlight a variety of important mechanisms utilized by the immune system to maintain homeostasis. When these are absent or dysfunctional, immune dysregulation ensues.

Immune Dysregulation, Polyendocrinopathy, Enteropathy, X-Linked

Immune dysregulation, polyendocrinopathy, enteropathy, X-linked (IPEX) is a syndrome of regulatory T-cell deficiency. Natural regulatory T cells comprise a subset of CD4+ T cells that regulate immune responses and play a critical role in peripheral immune tolerance. IPEX is caused by mutations in the *FOXP3* gene located on the X chromosome that encodes a key transcription factor that is required for the generation of functional regulatory T cells (Treg). In the absence of FOXP3, patients present with severe, early-onset, systemic autoimmunity that is the result of having decreased Treg cell function. Almost all patients with IPEX present with enteropathy within the first 6 months of life. The enteropathy is typically characterized by profuse watery diarrhea (often nonbloody) and villus atrophy. Most patients have an eczematous dermatitis that typically begins in the first months of life. 60% to 70% of patients also develop an early-onset endocrinopathy that is almost exclusively either thyroiditis or type 1 diabetes. The most consistent laboratory abnormality among patients is a significantly elevated serum IgE level. In addition to these characteristic clinical and lab features, patients also have a high incidence of other severe autoimmune disorders including hemolytic anemia, thrombocytopenia, neutropenia, hepatitis, renal disease, and others.

Recognition of the clinical features of IPEX is the first step in diagnosing this disorder. Sequencing of the *FOXP3* gene remains the gold standard for making a diagnosis although sequencing needs to encompass noncoding areas of the gene including the upstream noncoding exon and the polyadenylation signal sequence in order to cover all regions in which pathogenic mutations have been identified.[119] Patients have varying degrees of FOXP3+ Treg deficiency due to the fact that mutant FOXP3 may not support normal Treg development.

Initial therapy for IPEX typically consists of aggressive supportive care (parenteral nutrition, insulin, thyroid hormone, etc.) combined with T-cell-directed immune suppression using agents such as tacrolimus, cyclosporine, or rapamycin. HCT is currently the only curative therapy for IPEX. Survival has been reported to be approximately 70%.[119,120]

Susceptibility to Hemophagocytic Lymphohistiocytosis and Severe EBV Infection

Several defects affecting intracellular trafficking of vesicles and granules are associated with susceptibility to hemophagocytic lymphohistiocytosis (HLH). This group includes some phenotypes that are quite distinctive including Chédiak-Higashi (CHS) and Griscelli (GS) syndromes, which are both associated with a partial oculocutaneous albinism. Patients with CHS have pyogenic infections and periodontitis: their neutrophils have reduced chemotaxis and contain giant inclusion bodies (lysosomes). Patients with GS also have neurologic defects ranging from developmental delay to fatal neurodegeneration. Their neutrophils are dysfunctional, but they lack the giant granules of CHS. In vitro tests show low NK cell and cytotoxic cell function. CHS, GS, and X-linked lymphoproliferative syndrome (XLP) share susceptibility for HLH—an accelerated inflammatory process that in the case of XLP, may be triggered by EBV. The genes responsible for these syndromes include *LYST*, *RAB27A*, *SH2D1A*, and *XIAP*, respectively. Defects associated with decreased perforin expression or unloading of lytic lysosomes containing perforin at the cell surface of NK and CD8+ cytotoxic T cells (*PRF1*, *UNC13D*, *STX11*, *STXBP2*) also lead to familial forms of HLH.[121,122]

Autoimmune Lymphoproliferative Syndrome

The clinical phenotype of autoimmune lymphoproliferative syndrome (ALPS) is typically characterized by massive lymphadenopathy and splenomegaly. Patients also have problems with recurrent episodes of autoimmune hemolytic anemia and thrombocytopenia. The defects that have been identified in patients with this group of disorders are all associated with abnormalities in lymphocyte apoptosis. These include *FAS* (CD95), Fas ligand (*FASL*), *FADD*, Caspase 10 (*CASP10*), *NRAS*, and *KRAS*. Peripheral blood T- and B-cell counts are generally normal, but in many cases, there is an increased percentage of αβ-TCR+ double-negative T cells that lack expression of both CD4 and CD8. A predisposition to developing lymphoid malignancies has been described in ALPS but is thought to be primarily in those patients that have mutations in the death domain of FAS. In addition to elevated double-negative T cells, patients with ALPS frequently have elevated levels of soluble FAS ligand, IL-10, and vitamin-B_{12} in the blood, which can be valuable diagnostically in patients with suspected ALPS. Patients with mutations in Caspase 8 (*CASP8*) were previously classified as ALPS but are now considered to be a unique syndrome that may have lymphadenopathy and splenomegaly, but recurrent respiratory tract infections and mucocutaneous herpesvirus infections are prominent, both unusual features in ALPS.[123,124]

A variety of immunosuppressive therapies have been tried to control the recurrent autoimmune cytopenias, lymphadenopathy, and severe splenomegaly characteristic of ALPS. Most of these, including splenectomy, were only modestly successful but rapamycin has shown dramatic therapeutic benefit, often causing rapid shrinkage of lymph nodes and spleen.[125,126]

BASIC LABORATORY WORKUP FOR IMMUNE DEFICIENCY

A basic laboratory workup to screen for significant defects in each of the four major compartments of the immune system can be done by most practitioners prior to making a referral to a Clinical Immunologist for further, detailed evaluation (*Figure 64.3*). In simple terms, this workup should include evaluation of numbers and function for each of the four immune system compartments. A recommended workup using this approach is outlined in *Figure 64.4*.

Complement	Phagocytes	B cells/Antibodies	T cells
• Invasive infections with encapsulated bacteria (*S. pneumoniae*, *H. influenzae*, etc.) (C1-C4) • Recurrent, invasive *Neisseria* infections (MAC) • Hereditary angioedema (C1 inhibitor) • Autoimmunity (lupus, glomerulonephritis) (C1-C4) • Familial hemolytic uremic syndrome (HUS) (factor I, factor H, MCP)	• Skin and soft-tissue abscesses, boils, and lymphadenitis • Infections with catalase+ organisms (*S. aureus*, *Serratia*, *Aspergillus*, etc.) • Poor wound healing (LAD) • Chronic gingivitis and periodontal disease (LAD) • Mucosal ulcerations, colitis • Delayed separation of the umbilical cord/omphalitis	• Recurrent bacterial sinopulmonary infections • Unexplained bronchiectasis • Chronic or recurrent gastroenteritis (*Giardia*, *Cryptosporidium*, enterovirus, etc.) • Echovirus encephalomyelitis (BTK)	• *Pneumocystis jirovecii* pneumonia (SCID) • Recurrent, severe, or unusual viral infections (CMV, EBV, adenovirus, papillomavirus, etc.) (SCID) • Invasive fungal or mycobacterial infections (SCID) • GvHD (rash, abnormal LFTs, chronic diarrhea) (SCID) • Failure to thrive • Early-onset autoimmunity (FOXP3, SCID)

FIGURE 64.3 **Common presentations associated with defects in each of the four major immune compartments.** Unless indicated, clinical presentations apply to most disorders in this group. BTK, Bruton tyrosine kinase; CMV, cytomegalovirus; EBV, Epstein-Barr virus; GvHD, graft-vs-host disease; LAD, leukocyte adhesion deficiency; LFTs, liver function tests; MAC, membrane attack complex; MCP, membrane cofactor protein; SCID, severe combined immunodeficiency.

Complement	Phagocytes	B cells/Antibodies	T cells
Numbers: • Plasma levels of specific complement components (C1 esterase inhibitor, C2, C3, C4, etc.) **Function:** • CH50—functional test for classical pathway • AH50—functional test for alternative pathway	**Numbers:** • CBC with differential to evaluate neutrophil counts **Function:** • Neutrophil oxidative burst using dihydrorhodamine 123 (DHR) or nitrobluetetrazoleum (NBT) • Expression of the CD11b/CD18 integrin on leukocytes	**Numbers:** • CBC with differential to evaluate lymphocyte counts • Lymphocyte subsets to evaluate T, B, and NK cell counts **Function:** • Vaccine titers: protein antigens (tetanus titers, diphtheria titers, etc.) • Vaccine titers: carbohydrate antigens (Pneumococcal titers)	**Numbers:** • CBC with differential to evaluate lymphocyte counts • Lymphocyte subsets to evaluate T, B, and NK cell counts **Function:** • T cell proliferation to mitogens/antigens • Vaccine titers: protein antigens (tetanus titers, diphtheria titers, etc.)

FIGURE 64.4 **Suggested lab tests for basic evaluation of each compartment of the immune system.** The lab evaluation for immunodeficiency should be individualized to each patient's clinical presentation. CBC, complete blood count.

Useful Web Sites

www.primaryimmune.org
www.info4pi.org
www.nlm.nih.gov/medlineplus/immunesystemanddisorders.html
www.genome.gov/13014325

References

1. Tangye SG, Al-Herz W, Bousfiha A, et al. Human inborn errors of immunity: 2019 update on the classification from the international union of immunological societies expert committee. *J Clin Immunol*. 2020;40(1):24-64.
2. Van Horebeek L, Dubois B, Goris A. Somatic variants: new Kids on the block in human immunogenetics. *Trends Genet*. 2019;35(12):935-947.
3. Errante PR, Franco JL, Espinosa-Rosales FJ, Sorensen R, Condino-Neto A. Advances in primary immunodeficiency diseases in Latin America: epidemiology, research, and perspectives. *Ann N Y Acad Sci*. 2012;1250:62-72.
4. Frank MM, Sullivan KE. Chapter 42: complement deficiencies. In: Sullivan KE, Stiehm ER, eds. *Stiehm's Immune Deficiencies*. 2nd ed. Academic Press; 2020:919-947.
5. Santacroce R, D'Andrea G, Maffione AB, Margaglione M, d'Apolito M. The genetics of hereditary angioedema: a review. *J Clin Med*. 2021;10(9):2023.
6. Schramm EC, Java A, Liszewski MK, Atkinson JP. Complement deficiencies associated with atypical hemolytic uremic syndrome. In: MacKay I, Rose N, Eds. *Encyclopedia of Medical Immunology*. Springers; 2016. https://doi.org/10.1007/978-1-4614-9209-2_5-1.
7. Craig TJ. Recent advances in hereditary angioedema self-administration treatment: summary of an international hereditary angioedema expert meeting. *Int Arch Allergy Immunol*. 2013;161(suppl 1)26-27.
8. Zafra H. Hereditary angioedema: a review. *Wis Med J*. 2022;121(1):48-53.
9. Cicardi M, Zingale LC, Pappalardo E, Folcioni A, Agostoni A. Autoantibodies and lymphoproliferative diseases in acquired C1-inhibitor deficiencies. *Medicine*. 2003;82(4):274-281.
10. Rosenzweig SD, Holland SM. Phagocyte immunodeficiencies and their infections. *J Allergy Clin Immunol*. 2004;113(4):620-626.
11. Skokowa J, Dale DC, Touw IP, Zeidler C, Welte K. Severe congenital neutropenias. *Nat Rev Dis Primers*. 2017;3:17032.
12. Almarza Novoa E, Kasbekar S, Thrasher AJ, et al. Leukocyte adhesion deficiency-I: a comprehensive review of all published cases. *J Allergy Clin Immunol Pract*. 2018;6(4):1418-1420.e10.
13. Kambli PM, Bargir UA, Yadav RM, et al. Clinical and genetic spectrum of a large cohort of patients with leukocyte adhesion deficiency type 1 and 3: a multicentric study from India. *Front Immunol*. 2020;11:612703.
14. Qasim W, Cavazzana-Calvo M, Davies EG, et al. Allogeneic hematopoietic stem-cell transplantation for leukocyte adhesion deficiency. *Pediatrics*. 2009;123(3):836-840.
15. Bakhtiar S, Salzmann-Manrique E, Blok HJ, et al. Allogeneic hematopoietic stem cell transplantation in leukocyte adhesion deficiency type I and III. *Blood Adv*. 2021;5(1):262-273.
16. Balabanian K, Lagane B, Pablos JL, et al. WHIM syndromes with different genetic anomalies are accounted for by impaired CXCR4 desensitization to CXCL12. *Blood*. 2005;105(6):2449-2457.
17. Lanini LLS, Prader S, Siler U, Reichenbach J. Modern management of phagocyte defects. *Pediatr Allergy Immunol*. 2017;28(2):124-134.
18. Dotta L, Tassone L, Badolato R. Clinical and genetic features of warts, hypogammaglobulinemia, infections and Myelokathexis (WHIM) syndrome. *Curr Mol Med*. 2011;11(4):317-325.
19. McDermott DH, Liu Q, Ulrick J, et al. The CXCR4 antagonist plerixafor corrects panleukopenia in patients with WHIM syndrome. *Blood*. 2011;118(18):4957-4962.
20. McDermott DH, Pastrana DV, Calvo KR, et al. Plerixafor for the treatment of WHIM syndrome. *N Engl J Med*. 2019;380(2):163-170.
21. Kriván G, Erdos M, Kallay K, et al. Successful umbilical cord blood stem cell transplantation in a child with WHIM syndrome. *Eur J Haematol*. 2010;84(3):274-275.
22. Kawahara Y, Oh Y, Kato T, Zaha K, Morimoto A. Transient marked increase of γδ T cells in WHIM syndrome after successful HSCT. *J Clin Immunol*. 2018;38(5):553-555.
23. Segal BH, Leto TL, Gallin JI, Malech HL, Holland SM. Genetic, biochemical, and clinical features of chronic granulomatous disease. *Medicine*. 2000;79(3):170-200.
24. Marciano BE, Spalding C, Fitzgerald A, et al. Common severe infections in chronic granulomatous disease. *Clin Infect Dis*. 2015;60(8):1176-1183.
25. Marciano BE, Rosenzweig SD, Kleiner DE, et al. Gastrointestinal involvement in chronic granulomatous disease. *Pediatrics*. 2004;114(2):462-468.
26. Kuhns DB, Alvord WG, Heller T, et al. Residual NADPH oxidase and survival in chronic granulomatous disease. *N Engl J Med*. 2010;363(27):2600-2610.
27. Chiesa R, Wang J, Blok HJ, et al. Hematopoietic cell transplantation in chronic granulomatous disease: a study of 712 children and adults. *Blood*. 2020;136(10):1201-1211.
28. Walkovich K, Boxer LA. How to approach neutropenia in childhood. *Pediatr Rev*. 2013;34(4):173-184.
29. Jirapongsananuruk O, Malech HL, Kuhns DB, et al. Diagnostic paradigm for evaluation of male patients with chronic granulomatous disease, based on the dihydrorhodamine 123 assay. *J Allergy Clin Immunol*. 2003;111(2):374-379.
30. Vowells SJ, Sekhsaria S, Malech HL, Shalit M, Fleisher TA. Flow cytometric analysis of the granulocyte respiratory burst: a comparison study of fluorescent probes. *J Immunol Methods*. 1995;178(1):89-97.
31. Kang HJ, Bartholomae CC, Paruzynski A, et al. Retroviral gene therapy for X-linked chronic granulomatous disease: results from phase I/II trial. *Mol Ther*. 2011;19(11):2092-2101.
32. Kohn DB, Booth C, Kang EM, et al. Lentiviral gene therapy for X-linked chronic granulomatous disease. *Nat Med*. 2020;26(2):200-206.
33. Vihinen M, Mattsson PT, Smith CI. Bruton tyrosine kinase BTK in X-linked agammaglobulinemia XLA. *Front Biosci*. 2000;5:d917-d928.
34. Romo-Gonzalez C, Bustamante-Ogando JC, Yamazaki-Nakashimada MA, et al. Infections with enterohepatic non-H. pylori Helicobacter species in X-linked agammaglobulinemia: clinical cases and review of the literature. *Front Cell Infect Microbiol*. 2021;11:807136.
35. Turvey SE, Leo SH, Boos A, et al. Successful approach to treatment of Helicobacter bilis infection in X-linked agammaglobulinemia. *J Clin Immunol*. 2012;32(6):1404-1408.
36. Kainulainen L, Nikoskelainen J, Vuorinen T, Tevola K, Liippo K, Ruuskanen O. Viruses and bacteria in bronchial samples from patients with primary hypogammaglobulinemia. *Am J Respir Crit Care Med*. 1999;159(4 pt 1):1199-1204.
37. Misbah SA, Spickett GP, Ryba PC, et al. Chronic enteroviral meningoencephalitis in agammaglobulinemia: case report and literature review. *J Clin Immunol*. 1992;12(4):266-270.
38. Bearden D, Collett M, Quan PL, Costa-Carvalho BT, Sullivan KE. Enteroviruses in X-linked agammaglobulinemia: update on epidemiology and therapy. *J Allergy Clin Immunol Pract*. 2016;4(6):1059-1065.
39. Quan PL, Wagner TA, Briese T, et al. Astrovirus encephalitis in boy with X-linked agammaglobulinemia. *Emerg Infect Dis*. 2010;16(6):918-925.
40. Lee W-I, Torgerson TR, Schumacher MJ, Yel L, Zhu Q, Ochs HD. Molecular analysis of a large cohort of patients with the hyper immunoglobulin M (IgM) syndrome. *Blood*. 2005;105(5):1881-1890.
41. Cabral-Marques O, Schimke LF, Pereira PVS, et al. Expanding the clinical and genetic spectrum of human CD40L deficiency: the occurrence of paracoccidioidomycosis and other unusual infections in Brazilian patients. *J Clin Immunol*. 2012;32(2):212-220.
42. Hayward AR, Levy J, Facchetti F, et al. Cholangiopathy and tumors of the pancreas, liver, and biliary tree in boys with X-linked immunodeficiency with hyper-IgM. *J Immunol*. 1997;158(2):977-983.
43. Bucciol G, Nicholas SK, Calvo PL, et al. Combined liver and hematopoietic stem cell transplantation in patients with X-linked hyper-IgM syndrome. *J Allergy Clin Immunol*. 2019;143(5):1952-1956.e6.
44. Carruthers V-A, Lum SH, Flood T, Slatter MA, Gennery AR. Hematopoietic cell transplant for CD40 ligand deficiency—comparing busulfan versus treosulfan. *J Clin Immunol*. 2022;42(3):703-705.
45. Ferrua F, Galimberti S, Courteille V, et al. Hematopoietic stem cell transplantation for CD40 ligand deficiency: results from an EBMT/ESID-IEWP-SCETIDE-PIDTC study. *J Allergy Clin Immunol*. 2019;143(6):2238-2253.
46. Maffucci P, Filion CA, Boisson B, et al. Genetic diagnosis using whole exome sequencing in common variable immunodeficiency. *Front Immunol*. 2016;7:220.
47. Christiansen M, Offersen R, Jensen JMB, Petersen MS, Larsen CS, Mogensen TH. Identification of novel genetic variants in CVID patients with autoimmunity, autoinflammation, or malignancy. *Front Immunol*. 2019;10:3022.
48. Ameratunga R, Woon S-T, Gillis D, Koopmans W, Steele R. New diagnostic criteria for CVID. *Expert Rev Clin Immunol*. 2014;10(2):183-186.
49. Resnick ES, Moshier EL, Godbold JH, Cunningham-Rundles C. Morbidity and mortality in common variable immune deficiency over 4 decades. *Blood*. 2012;119(7):1650-1657.
50. Somogyi V, Eichinger M, Lasitschka F, Kappes J, Kreuter M. Interstitial lung disease in CVID (GLILD): clinical presentation and comparison to CVID without ILD. *Rare ILD/DPLD*. 2019;54:PA1409. doi:10.1183/13993003.congress-2019.pa1409
51. van de Ven AAJM, Alfaro TM, Robinson A, et al. Managing granulomatous-lymphocytic interstitial lung disease in common variable immunodeficiency disorders: e-GLILDnet international clinicians survey. *Front Immunol*. 2020;11:606333.
52. Chase NM, Verbsky JW, Hintermeyer MK, et al. Use of combination chemotherapy for treatment of granulomatous and lymphocytic interstitial lung disease (GLILD) in patients with common variable immunodeficiency (CVID). *J Clin Immunol*. 2013;33(1):30-39.
53. Verbsky JW, Hintermeyer MK, Simpson PM, et al. Rituximab and antimetabolite treatment of granulomatous and lymphocytic interstitial lung disease in common variable immunodeficiency. *J Allergy Clin Immunol*. 2021;147(2):704-712.e17.
54. Jørgensen SF, Reims HM, Frydenlund D, et al. A cross-sectional study of the prevalence of gastrointestinal symptoms and pathology in patients with common variable immunodeficiency. *Am J Gastroenterol*. 2016;111(10):1467-1475.
55. Pikkarainen S, Martelius T, Ristimaki A, Siitonen S, Seppanen MRJ, Farkkila M. A high prevalence of gastrointestinal manifestations in common variable immunodeficiency. *Am J Gastroenterol*. 2019;114(4):648-655.
56. Ward C, Lucas M, Piris J, Collier J, Chapel H. Abnormal liver function in common variable immunodeficiency disorders due to nodular regenerative hyperplasia. *Clin Exp Immunol*. 2008;153(3):331-337.
57. Ho HE, Radigan L, Bongers G, El-Shamy A, Cunningham-Rundles C. Circulating bioactive bacterial DNA is associated with immune activation and complications in common variable immunodeficiency. *JCI Insight*. 2021;6(19):e144777.
58. López-Granados E. Late-onset combined immunodeficiencies (LOCID). In: D'Elios MM, Rizzi M, eds. *Humoral Primary Immunodeficiencies*. Springer International Publishing; 2019:57-66.
59. Malphettes M, Gerard L, Carmagnat M, et al. Late-onset combined immune deficiency: a subset of common variable immunodeficiency with severe T cell defect. *Clin Infect Dis*. 2009;49(9):1329-1338.
60. Lilic D, Sewell WAC. IgA deficiency: what we should—or should not—be doing. *J Clin Pathol*. 2001;54(5):337-338.

61. Bukowska-Strakova K, Kowalczyk D, Baran J, Siedlar M, Kobylarz K, Zembala M. The B-cell compartment in the peripheral blood of children with different types of primary humoral immunodeficiency. *Pediatr Res*. 2009;66(1):28-34.
62. Orange JS, Ballow M, Stiehm ER, et al. Use and interpretation of diagnostic vaccination in primary immunodeficiency: a working group report of the basic and clinical immunology interest section of the American academy of allergy, asthma & immunology. *J Allergy Clin Immunol*. 2012;130(3 suppl):S1-S24.
63. Yazdani R, Seify R, Ganjalikhani-Hakemi M, et al. Comparison of various classifications for patients with common variable immunodeficiency (CVID) using measurement of B-cell subsets. *Allergol Immunopathol*. 2017;45(2):183-192.
64. Carsetti R, Rosado MM, Donnanno S, et al. The loss of IgM memory B cells correlates with clinical disease in common variable immunodeficiency. *J Allergy Clin Immunol*. 2005;115(2):412-417.
65. Orange JS, Grossman WJ, Navickis RJ, Wilkes MM. Impact of trough IgG on pneumonia incidence in primary immunodeficiency: a meta-analysis of clinical studies. *Clin Immunol*. 2010;137(1):21-30.
66. Pierce LR, Jain N. Risks associated with the use of intravenous immunoglobulin. *Transfus Med Rev*. 2003;17(4):241-251.
67. Milito C, Pulvirenti F, Cinetto F, et al. Double-blind, placebo-controlled, randomized trial on low-dose azithromycin prophylaxis in patients with primary antibody deficiencies. *J Allergy Clin Immunol*. 2019;144(2):584-593.e7.
68. McDonald-McGinn DM, Sullivan KE. Chromosome 22q11.2 deletion syndrome (DiGeorge syndrome/velocardiofacial syndrome). *Medicine*. 2011;90:1-18.
69. Bassett AS, McDonald-McGinn DM, Devriendt K, et al. Practical guidelines for managing patients with 22q11.2 deletion syndrome. *J Pediatr*. 2011;159(2):332-339.e1.
70. Tomita-Mitchell A, Mahnke DK, Larson JM, et al. Multiplexed quantitative real-time PCR to detect 22q11.2 deletion in patients with congenital heart disease. *Physiol Genomics*. 2010;42A(1):52-60.
71. Davies EG, Cheung M, Gilmour K, et al. Thymus transplantation for complete DiGeorge syndrome: European experience. *J Allergy Clin Immunol*. 2017;140(6):1660-1670.e16.
72. Markert ML, Gupton SE, McCarthy EA. Experience with cultured thymus tissue in 105 children. *J Allergy Clin Immunol*. 2022;149(2):747-757.
73. Currier R, Puck JM. SCID newborn screening: what we've learned. *J Allergy Clin Immunol*. 2021;147(2):417-426.
74. Puck JM, Gennery AR. Establishing newborn screening for SCID in the USA; experience in California. *Int J Neonatal Screen*. 2021;7(4):72.
75. Buckley RH, Win CM, Moser BK, Parrott RE, Sajaroff E, Sarzotti-Kelsoe M. Post-transplantation B cell function in different molecular types of SCID. *J Clin Immunol*. 2013;33(1):96-110.
76. Heimall J, Logan BR, Cowan MJ, et al. Immune reconstitution and survival of 100 SCID patients post-hematopoietic cell transplant: a PIDTC natural history study. *Blood*. 2017;130(25):2718-2727.
77. Hacein-Bey-Abina S, Von Kalle C, Schmidt M, et al. LMO2-associated clonal T cell proliferation in two patients after gene therapy for SCID-X1. *Science*. 2003;302(5644):415-419.
78. Yamada K, Tsukahara T, Yoshino K, et al. Identification of a high incidence region for retroviral vector integration near exon 1 of the LMO2 locus. *Retrovirology*. 2009;6:79.
79. Mamcarz E, Zhou S, Lockey T, et al. Lentiviral gene therapy combined with low-dose busulfan in infants with SCID-X1. *N Engl J Med*. 2019;380(16):1525-1534.
80. O'Shea JJ, Husa M, Li D, et al. Jak3 and the pathogenesis of severe combined immunodeficiency. *Mol Immunol*. 2004;41:727-737.
81. Fischer A, de Saint Basile G, Le Deist F. CD3 deficiencies. *Curr Opin Allergy Clin Immunol*. 2005;5(6):491-495.
82. Turul T, Tezcan I, Artac H, et al. Clinical heterogeneity can hamper the diagnosis of patients with ZAP70 deficiency. *Eur J Pediatr*. 2009;168(1):87-93.
83. Tchilian EZ, Wallace DL, Wells RS, Flower DR, Morgan G, Beverley PC. A deletion in the gene encoding the CD45 antigen in a patient with SCID. *J Immunol*. 2001;166(2):1308-1313.
84. Sullivan KEA. Deletion in the gene encoding the CD45 antigen in a patient with SCID. *Pediatrics*. 2002;110:467.
85. Reith W, Mach B. The bare lymphocyte syndrome and the regulation of MHC expression. *Annu Rev Immunol*. 2001;19:331-373.
86. Kallen ME, Pullarkat ST. Type II bare lymphocyte syndrome: role of peripheral blood flow cytometry and utility of stem cell transplant in treatment. *J Pediatr Hematol Oncol*. 2015;37(4):e245-e249.
87. Kuo CY, Chase J, Garcia Lloret M, et al. Newborn screening for severe combined immunodeficiency does not identify bare lymphocyte syndrome. *J Allergy Clin Immunol*. 2013;131(6):1693-1695.
88. Rigoni R, Fontana E, Dobbs K, et al. Cutaneous barrier leakage and gut inflammation drive skin disease in Omenn syndrome. *J Allergy Clin Immunol*. 2020;146(5):1165-1179.e11.
89. Villa A. Omenn Syndrome: inflammation and autoimmunity. *J Transl Med*. 2011;9:I5.
90. Booth C, Gaspar HB. Pegademase bovine (PEG-ADA) for the treatment of infants and children with severe combined immunodeficiency (SCID). *Biologics*. 2009;3:349-358.
91. Kohn DB, Gaspar HB. How we manage adenosine deaminase-deficient severe combined immune deficiency (ADA SCID). *J Clin Immunol*. 2017;37(4):351-356.
92. Ferrua F, Aiuti A. Twenty-five years of gene therapy for ADA-SCID: from Bubble babies to an approved drug. *Hum Gene Ther*. 2017;28(11):972-981.
93. Kohn DB, Booth C, Shaw KL, et al. Autologous ex vivo lentiviral gene therapy for adenosine deaminase deficiency. *N Engl J Med*. 2021;384(21):2002-2013.
94. Gatti RA, Meuwissen HJ, Allen HD, Hong R, Good RA. Immunological reconstitution of sex-linked lymphopenic immunological deficiency. *Lancet*. 1968;2(7583):1366-1369.
95. Dorsey MJ, Wright NAM, Chaimowitz NS, et al. Infections in infants with SCID: isolation, infection screening, and prophylaxis in PIDTC centers. *J Clin Immunol*. 2021;41(1):38-50.
96. Haddad E, Logan BR, Griffith LM, et al. Genotype, phenotype and T cell counts at one year predict survival and long term immune reconstitution after transplantation in severe combined immune deficiency (SCID)—the primary immune deficiency treatment consortium (PIDTC). *Biol Blood Marrow Transplant*. 2017;23:S133-S134.
97. Heimall J, Logan BR, Cowan MJ, et al. Poor T cell reconstitution at 100 Days after T cell-replete hematopoietic cell transplantation (HCT) for SCID is associated with later risk of death or need for 2nd transplant in the 6901 prospective study of the pidtc. *Biol Blood Marrow Transplant*. 2016;22:S101-S102.
98. Eissa H, Thakar MS, Shah AJ, et al. A primary immune deficiency treatment consortium (PIDTC) study of chronic and late onset medical complications after initial hematopoietic cell transplantation (HCT) for severe combined immunodeficiency disease (SCID). *Transplantation and Cellular Therapy*. 2022;28:S339-S340.
99. Hosahalli Vasanna S, Pereda MA, Dalal J. Clinical features, cancer biology, transplant approach and other integrated management strategies for wiskott-aldrich syndrome. *J Multidiscip Healthc*. 2021;14:3497-3512.
100. Jin Y, Mazza C, Christie JR, et al. Mutations of the Wiskott-Aldrich Syndrome Protein (WASP): hotspots, effect on transcription, and translation and phenotype/genotype correlation. *Blood*. 2004;104(13):4010-4019.
101. Sun J, Zhong X, Fu X, et al. The actin regulators involved in the function and related diseases of lymphocytes. *Front Immunol*. 2022;13:799309.
102. Dupré L, Boztug K, Pfajfer L. Actin dynamics at the T cell synapse as revealed by immune-related actinopathies. *Front Cell Dev Biol*. 2021;9:665519.
103. Albert MH, Slatter MA, Gennery AR, et al. Hematopoietic stem cell transplantation for wiskott-aldrich syndrome: an EBMT inborn errors working party analysis. *Blood*. 2022;139(13):2066-2079.
104. Burroughs LM, Petrovic A, Brazauskas R, et al. Excellent outcomes following hematopoietic cell transplantation for Wiskott-Aldrich syndrome: a PIDTC report. *Blood*. 2020;135(23):2094-2105.
105. Albert MH, Bittner TC, Nonoyama S, et al. X-linked thrombocytopenia (XLT) due to WAS mutations: clinical characteristics, long-term outcome and treatment options. *Blood*. 2010;115(16):3231-3238.
106. Braun CJ, Boztug K, Paruzynski A, et al. Gene therapy for wiskott-aldrich syndrome—long-term efficacy and genotoxicity. *Sci Transl Med*. 2014;6(227):227ra33.
107. Arora H, Chacon AH, Choudhary S, et al. Bloom syndrome. *Int J Dermatol*. 2014;53(7):798-802.
108. Vakkilainen S, Taskinen M, Mäkitie O. Immunodeficiency in cartilage-hair hypoplasia: pathogenesis, clinical course and management. *Scand J Immunol*. 2020;92(4):e12913.
109. Ridanpää M, van Eenennaam H, Pelin K, et al. Mutations in the RNA component of RNase MRP cause a pleiotropic human disease, cartilage-hair hypoplasia. *Cell*. 2001;104(2):195-203.
110. Roesler J, Horwitz ME, Picard C, et al. Hematopoietic stem cell transplantation for complete IFN-γ receptor 1 deficiency: a multi-institutional survey. *J Pediatr*. 2004;145(6):806-812.
111. Asano T, Boisson B, Onodi F, et al. X-linked recessive TLR7 deficiency in ~1% of men under 60 years old with life-threatening COVID-19. *Sci Immunol*. 2021;6(62):eabl4348.
112. Maglione PJ, Simchoni N, Cunningham-Rundles C. Toll-like receptor signaling in primary immune deficiencies. *Ann N Y Acad Sci*. 2015;1356:1-21.
113. Brown GJ, Canete PF, Wang H, et al. TLR7 gain-of-function genetic variation causes human lupus. *Nature*. 2022;605(7909):349-356. doi:10.1038/s41586-022-04642-z
114. Aluri J, Bach A, Kaviany S, et al. Immunodeficiency and bone marrow failure with mosaic and germline TLR8 gain-of-function. *Blood*. 2021;137(18):2450-2462. doi:10.1182/blood.2020009620
115. Li J, Casanova JL, Puel A. Mucocutaneous IL-17 immunity in mice and humans: host defense vs. excessive inflammation. *Mucosal Immunol*. 2018;11(3):581-589.
116. Puel A, Döffinger R, Natividad A, et al. Autoantibodies against IL-17A, IL-17F, and IL-22 in patients with chronic mucocutaneous candidiasis and autoimmune polyendocrine syndrome type I. *J Exp Med*. 2010;207(2):291-297.
117. Break TJ, Oikonomou V, Dutzan N, et al. Response to Comments on "Aberrant type 1 immunity drives susceptibility to mucosal fungal infections". *Science*. 2021;373(6561):eabi8835.
118. Ferre EMN, Rose SR, Rosenzweig SD, et al. Redefined clinical features and diagnostic criteria in autoimmune polyendocrinopathy-candidiasis-ectodermal dystrophy. *JCI Insight*. 2016;1(13):e88782.
119. Gambineri E, Ciullini Mannurita S, Hagin D, et al. Clinical, immunological, and molecular heterogeneity of 173 patients with the phenotype of immune dysregulation, polyendocrinopathy, enteropathy, X-linked (IPEX) syndrome. *Front Immunol*. 2018;9:2411.
120. Barzaghi F, Amaya Hernandez LC, Neven B, et al. Long-term follow-up of IPEX syndrome patients after different therapeutic strategies: an international multicenter retrospective study. *J Allergy Clin Immunol*. 2018;141(3):1036-1049.e5.
121. Degar B. Familial hemophagocytic lymphohistiocytosis. *Hematol Oncol Clin North Am*. 2015;29(5):903-913.
122. Janka GE, Aricò M. Clinical features, diagnosis and therapy of familial haemophagocytic lymphohistiocytosis. *Acta Paediatr*. 2021;110(10):2723-2728.

123. Oliveira JB, Gupta S. Disorders of apoptosis: mechanisms for autoimmunity in primary immunodeficiency diseases. *J Clin Immunol*. 2008;28(suppl 1):S20-S28.
124. Oliveira JB, Bleesing JJ, Dianzani U, et al. Revised diagnostic criteria and classification for the autoimmune lymphoproliferative syndrome (ALPS): report from the 2009 NIH International Workshop. *Blood*. 2010;116(14):e35-e40.
125. Klemann C, Esquivel M, Magerus-Chatinet A, et al. Evolution of disease activity and biomarkers on and off rapamycin in 28 patients with autoimmune lymphoproliferative syndrome. *Haematologica*. 2017;102(2):e52-e56.
126. Rao VK. Approaches to managing autoimmune cytopenias in novel immunological disorders with genetic underpinnings like autoimmune lymphoproliferative syndrome. *Front Pediatr*. 2015;3:65.

Chapter 65 ■ Human Immunodeficiency Virus Infection

ARIELA NOY • ROY M. GULICK

HUMAN IMMUNODEFICIENCY VIRUS INFECTION AND ACQUIRED IMMUNODEFICIENCY SYNDROME

Human immunodeficiency virus (HIV) infection is a true pandemic, an infection that affects individuals in every country of the world.[1] A diagnosis of acquired immunodeficiency syndrome (AIDS) is made when a person with HIV infection progresses to develop severe immunodeficiency as demonstrated by a CD4 lymphocyte count of less than 200/μL or the development of specific AIDS-associated diseases.[2] The first cases of AIDS were described over 40 years ago in 1981 in five young gay men in Los Angeles.[3] Since the beginning of the HIV pandemic, an estimated 70 million people worldwide acquired HIV infection and over half of them died.[1] Currently, an estimated 38 million people are living with HIV infection, more than two-thirds of whom are living in sub-Saharan Africa. An estimated 1.2 million people currently live with HIV infection in the United States with a prevalence of 0.4%; about 14% are not aware of their diagnosis.[4] The development of effective antiretroviral treatment in 1996 changed the natural history and clinical course of HIV infection dramatically, with remarkable decreases in HIV-associated illnesses and deaths.[5] In parallel, many of the hematologic complications of HIV infection happen less commonly today. Cytopenias caused by HIV disease or its treatment occurred frequently in the past, but now are uncommon. Coagulation abnormalities occur occasionally. Hematologic malignancies remain an important challenge, even in the setting of effective HIV treatment. This chapter discusses HIV infection and the diagnosis and management of associated hematologic complications. A complete discussion of antiretroviral therapy (ART) and opportunistic diseases can be found elsewhere.[6,7]

Background

HIV-1 was discovered by two independent groups in 1983 to 1984.[8] A related virus, HIV-2, was discovered in 1986, but remains localized to residents and immigrants from Western Africa and countries with historical ties to Western African countries.[9] HIV is transmitted most commonly worldwide by sexual contact and also by intravenous drug use, transfusion of infected blood or blood products, and perinatally from an infected mother to her child.[10] HIV may be transmitted by infected blood, blood products, bloody fluids, or genital secretions, but not by saliva, sweat, urine, other nonbloody fluids, or feces. In the absence of HIV treatment, the time from initial HIV infection to the development of severe immunodeficiency and AIDS is approximately 10 years.[11] The US Centers for Disease Control and Prevention (CDC) define AIDS in individuals who are HIV-1 antibody positive with a CD4 cell count <200/μL (regardless of symptoms) or who have one of 25 AIDS-defining illnesses, including opportunistic infections (OIs) and malignancies.[2] Effective ART suppresses viremia and, thereby, changes the natural history of the disease, preventing HIV disease progression and prolonging survival.

Pathophysiology

HIV-1 is a retrovirus with a genome that contains the structural genes *gag*, *pol*, and *env* that code for viral core proteins that control viral replication (e.g., HIV reverse transcriptase, HIV integrase, and HIV protease), as well as the envelope glycoproteins, gp160, 120, and 41.[12] Additional regulatory genes, *rev* and *tat*, code for viral-specific proteins that control viral transcription and processing of viral messenger RNA. Other viral genes mediate infectivity and interactions with the host cell (*nef*, *vif*, *vpr*, *vpu*).

HIV entry is the first step in HIV-1 infection and consists of three substeps: CD4 receptor binding, chemokine receptor binding (to the CCR5 and/or CXCR4 receptor), and membrane fusion.[13] In the first substep, the viral outer membrane glycoprotein, gp120, binds to the CD4 receptor on the surface of the target cell. Cells that express CD4 receptors include the CD4 lymphocyte, macrophages, and dendritic cells. Following binding of gp120 to the CD4 receptor, gp120 undergoes a conformational change that allows binding to a second coreceptor, the chemokine receptor, either CCR5 or CXCR4.[14] Individuals who lack the gene that codes for the CCR5 receptor are relatively resistant to HIV infection; individuals who are heterozygotes for this gene demonstrate a slower progression of HIV disease.[15] Following binding to the coreceptor, gp120 undergoes a second conformational change that allows a second HIV membrane glycoprotein, gp41, to bind and attach to the cell surface and then allows the viral membrane to fuse with the host cell membrane.

After HIV entry, the contents of the viral particle, including viral RNA and viral proteins, are extruded into the cytoplasm of the target cell. Viral RNA is transcribed to complementary viral DNA by the viral-specific enzyme HIV reverse transcriptase. The viral DNA forms a double-stranded complex that migrates to the nucleus of the cell, where the viral-specific enzyme HIV integrase inserts the viral DNA randomly into the host cell genome. An HIV-infected CD4 lymphocyte may enter a latency period that can extend to 70 years, constituting a long-lived viral reservoir.[16] The latently infected cell may be activated, and then genomic DNA along with incorporated viral DNA is transcribed to viral RNA that is translated to viral proteins, including *gag* and *pol* gene products that assemble with viral RNA at the surface of the cell and then bud off into new viral particles. Post budding, precursor viral proteins are cleaved by another viral-specific enzyme, HIV protease, in a step that is required for viral maturation and infectiousness.[17] A single latently infected cell can produce hundreds to thousands of virions. When enough viral particles have budded off from an infected cell, the membrane becomes compromised and cell death occurs.

The characteristic decrease in CD4 lymphocytes over the course of untreated HIV disease occurs from a combination of increased apoptosis and decreased lymphopoiesis, although this is not completely understood.[18] An estimated one in a million resting CD4 lymphocytes are latently infected in an HIV-infected individual with controlled infection on ART.[19] Although the relative number of latently infected CD4 cells is small, apoptosis may occur in uninfected CD4 cells. Untreated HIV infection also was recognized early on to be associated with immune activation, CD8 cell dysfunction, B-cell dysfunction, and impaired antibody production and general immune dysregulation.[20,21]

Diagnosis

The US Preventive Services Task Force recommends routine HIV screening for all individuals aged 15 to 65, *not* based on risk, and for younger adolescents and older adults who are at increased risk of infection, as a "grade A" recommendation.[22] Standard HIV testing starts with a combination immunoassay that detects antibodies to both HIV-1 and HIV-2 as well as HIV-1 p24 antigen.[23] Reactive specimens are then tested with a second immunoassay that differentiates HIV-1 from HIV-2. The Western blot test is no longer used routinely as a confirmatory test. False-negative HIV antibody tests can occur because of the window period (now about 3 weeks), that is, the time between viral infection and the development of a detectable antibody response.

Rapid tests detect HIV antibodies in blood or oral fluids, and results are available within 20 minutes or less. Although the rapid test is very specific (>99%), with a high positive predictive value (≥90%), a positive rapid test must be confirmed with an immunoblot test.[24] Some rapid tests are now Clinical Laboratory Improvement Amendments-waived and may be performed in nonhealthcare settings (e.g., street fairs, mobile vans, or even self-administered at home), allowing more widespread testing.

HIV can be detected directly by the viral p24 antigen or HIV RNA, and this reduces the window period to 10 to 14 days: p24 antigen testing was added to the HIV antibody test, in the next-generation test, to detect HIV infections earlier, including acute infection.[25] Nucleic acid–based testing has been used both in individual cases and in blood bank screening programs.[26] Using these newer tests along with pretransfusion screening, the risk of acquiring HIV infection through a blood transfusion in the United States is less than 1 per 2.8 million units transfused.[27]

Clinical Features of HIV-1 Infection

Acute HIV infection can present as a nonspecific illness characterized by fever, oral ulcers, and maculopapular rash; however, at least 70% of newly infected individuals may be completely asymptomatic.[28] The clinical illness will subside over several weeks, and then the patient enters an asymptomatic phase, often with nonspecific generalized lymphadenopathy, which may last years as the CD4 lymphocyte count gradually declines over time. HIV-related diseases occurring at higher CD4 counts (>300 cells/µL) include those caused by more aggressive pathogens (e.g., tuberculosis, herpes zoster, and pneumococcal pneumonia) as well as Kaposi sarcoma (KS). As the CD4 cell count declines below 300/µL, other HIV-related illnesses also occur, including oral hairy leukoplakia, oral thrush, and seborrheic dermatitis. As the CD4 cell count declines below 200/µL, profound immunodeficiency occurs, the case definition of AIDS is met, and AIDS-defining illnesses may occur, including *Pneumocystis jiroveci* (formerly *carinii*) pneumonia, central nervous system (CNS) toxoplasmosis, and cryptococcal meningitis. Multiple opportunistic illnesses can occur simultaneously in a single patient.

Hematologic disorders such as leukopenia, anemia, immune and thrombotic thrombocytopenia, bone marrow failure, coagulation disorders including thrombosis, and malignancies all occurred commonly in HIV-infected individuals.[29,30] Some of these complications were caused by viremia and immune dysregulation, and others by toxicity from HIV therapies.[31] With the development of effective ART, hematologic disorders and HIV-associated malignancies have decreased markedly,[32] and currently, ART-related hematologic toxicities are rare.

Treatment

In the 1980s and early 1990s, the average life expectancy of a patient with AIDS was less than 1 year. Today, it is estimated that an individual diagnosed with HIV infection and appropriately managed with antiretroviral treatment will have an average life expectancy similar to that of the general population.[33] ART changes the natural history of HIV infection by inhibiting viral replication. Currently, there are 33 U.S. Food and Drug Administration–approved unique drugs for the treatment of HIV infection; combination regimens with two, three or more drugs are standard treatment. Current US HIV treatment guidelines recommend starting ART in all HIV-infected individuals, regardless of symptoms, HIV viral load, or CD4 cell count.[6] The life cycle of the virus and the specific sites targeted by ART are shown in *Figure 65.1*.

The oldest mechanistic classes of drugs are the HIV reverse transcriptase inhibitors of two kinds, the nucleoside analogs and the nonnucleoside analogs. The nucleoside analogs mimic the structures of the four DNA bases and when bound to the active site and incorporated into the elongating viral DNA, result in chain termination: adenosine analogs, didanosine (ddI) and tenofovir (two formulations, TAF, tenofovir alafenamide, and TDF, tenofovir disoproxil fumarate)); cytosine analogs, emtricitabine (FTC), lamivudine (3TC), zalcitabine (ddC); guanine analog, abacavir (ABC); and thymidine analogs, stavudine (d4T) and zidovudine (ZDV, formerly known as AZT, azidothymidine). The nonnucleoside analogs also inhibit the HIV reverse transcriptase enzyme but do so by binding a site remote to the active site and include delavirdine, doravirine, efavirenz, etravirine, nevirapine, and rilpivirine (RPV).

In the mid-1990s, the third antiretroviral drug class was approved, the HIV protease inhibitors, that target a step late in the viral life cycle. Following budding of the viral particles from the infected cell, viral precursor proteins must be chemically cleaved by the viral-specific

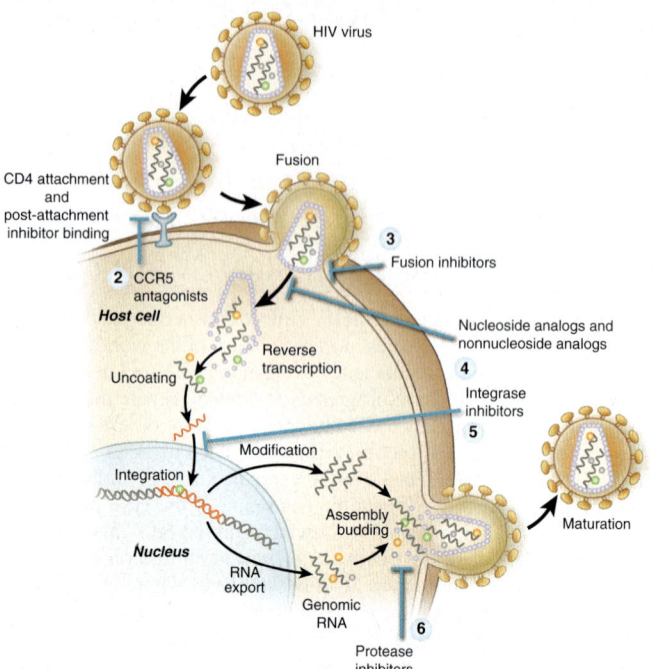

FIGURE 65.1 The human immunodeficiency virus (HIV) life cycle, deciphered with the help of genomic analyses, is unusually complex in its details, but all viruses undergo the same basic steps to infect cells and reproduce. Points at which antiretrovirals act are marked.

enzyme, HIV protease. These compounds were the most potent known against HIV and when used in combination regimens resulted in suppression of HIV RNA levels and dramatic decreases in morbidity and mortality.[5] Each of the 10 approved protease inhibitors binds in the active site of the protease and blocks this cleavage: amprenavir and its prodrug fosamprenavir, atazanavir, darunavir (DRV), indinavir (IDV), lopinavir, nelfinavir (NFV), ritonavir (RTV), saquinavir, and tipranavir.

The newer mechanistic classes of approved HIV drugs are four different kinds of HIV entry inhibitors and the HIV integrase inhibitors. The approved CD4 attachment inhibitor is fostemsavir, a small molecule that binds to HIV gp120. The approved CD4 postattachment inhibitor is ibalizumab, a monoclonal antibody that targets the CD4 receptor. The approved chemokine receptor antagonist is maraviroc that binds to the host cell CCR5 receptor and prevents viral binding. The approved HIV fusion inhibitor is a small peptide, enfuvirtide (T-20), that targets the viral glycoprotein gp41 and prevents fusion of the viral and cellular membranes; as a peptide, it requires twice-daily subcutaneous dosing and is used uncommonly. Bictegravir (BIC), cabotegravir (CAB), dolutegravir (DTG), elvitegravir, and raltegravir inhibit the viral-specific enzyme HIV integrase that inserts the viral DNA into the host cell DNA. HIV integrase inhibitor–based regimens are potent and well tolerated and have emerged as the treatment of choice for HIV/AIDS. CAB and the nonnucleoside RPV constitute the first approved monthly (or bimonthly) all-injectable antiretroviral regimen that is effective in maintaining suppressed viral load levels.

Current treatment guidelines recommend the following two- or three-drug combination antiretroviral regimens for most people with HIV on the basis of potency, tolerability, and convenience[6]: (1) TAF/emtricitabine/BIC (coformulated as one pill, taken once daily); (2) abacavir/lamivudine/DTG (coformulated as one pill, taken once daily); (3) tenofovir (TAF or TDF)/(emtricitabine or lamivudine) (coformulated) + DTG (two or three pills taken once daily); and (4) DTG/lamivudine (coformulated as one pill, taken once daily). The goal of current HIV treatment is maximal virologic suppression; current virologic suppression rates on initial therapy regimens approach or even exceed 90%. CD4 cell counts typically increase 100/µL over baseline in the first weeks or months following initiation of therapy and then continue to increase at a slower rate.[34] The reconstituted CD4 cells generally are of the memory type (CD45RO$^+$ or CD34RA$^+$), with naïve cells increasing more slowly; thymic function also improves. Immune reconstitution may result in IRIS, the immune-related inflammatory syndrome usually managed symptomatically.[35] Appropriate increases in CD4 cell counts allow discontinuation of opportunistic maintenance therapy and prophylaxes. Specific immune-based therapies, including interleukin (IL)-2, have failed to demonstrate additional clinical benefits and are not recommended currently.[6,36]

An HIV-infected individual who is stable taking ART will typically see the treating physician every 3 to 6 months to check for side effects and monitor the HIV RNA. A CD4 cell count also is obtained at baseline and every 3 to 6 months until the level returns to 300 to 500/μL for at least 2 years, and then it is checked annually; when the CD4 cell count increases to >500/μL for at least 2 years, checking the count is considered optional.[6] In the case of virologic failure, drug resistance testing is performed and a new regimen selected on the basis of treatment history, drug resistance testing results, and available drug options. The goal is to construct a regimen with two fully active drugs, including a drug with a high barrier to resistance (e.g. BIC, DTG, or DRV), and this will result in resuppression of HIV RNA in the majority of patients. HIV therapy currently is lifelong. Treatment interruptions are associated with clinical events[6] and should be avoided. Virologic suppression also reduces the risk of sexual transmission >95%.[37] HIV prevention with postexposure and preexposure prophylaxis are effective strategies to administer antiretroviral drugs to at-risk, uninfected individuals to avoid establishment of HIV infection with exposure.[34]

Several ongoing challenges remain in the management of HIV disease. Life-long adherence to ART poses challenges that newer long-acting formulations may address. Despite potent suppression of virologic replication, some patients experience ongoing inflammation and immune activation, and this has been linked to nontraditional HIV illnesses such as cardiac, hepatic, renal, and neurologic diseases, and non-AIDS malignancies. In addition, despite dramatic improvements in life expectancy, cure of HIV disease remains elusive. The first patient considered cured of HIV infection is the unique case of a man with HIV disease controlled on ART who developed acute myelogenous leukemia and underwent a bone marrow transplant from a donor with a deletion in the gene coding for the CCR5 receptor.[38] Cure, defined either as chronic suppression of HIV without ART, or complete eradication of HIV, remains challenging because of the long-lived latently infected CD4 cell reservoir; much current research is focused on this goal.[39]

HEMATOLOGIC COMPLICATIONS OF HIV INFECTION

Anemia

Anemia is the most frequent cytopenia observed in HIV-1 infection. Striking anemia with transfusion dependence was common early in the epidemic when high doses of ZDV were in use, but severe depression of hemoglobin levels are now rarely observed, except in patients with advanced disease.[40] In several large multicenter studies, persistent anemia was associated with shorter survival, independent of the degree of immunosuppression.[41,42]

As in other persons, anemia occurs because of one of three major factors: either ineffective hematopoiesis; blood loss caused by involvement of the intestines by infection such as cytomegalovirus (CMV) or KS; or red blood cell destruction.

Red blood cell production can be affected by HIV itself because of cytokines that interfere with hematopoiesis,[43-45] highly active ART, and medications used to treat HIV-associated infections (Table 65.1, including high-dose trimethoprim-sulfamethoxazole for *P. jiroveci* pneumonia and ganciclovir for CMV), HIV-associated cancers such as lymphomatous infiltration of the marrow, low erythropoietin, or HIV-associated hypogonadism.[46]

Table 65.1. Hematologic Toxicities of Antiretroviral Drugs

Medication	Type of Activity	Hematologic Toxicity
Zidovudine	Nucleoside analogs, antiretroviral	Anemia, neutropenia (dose dependent)
Stavudine	Nucleoside analogs, antiretroviral	Anemia, neutropenia (dose dependent)
Ganciclovir	Cytomegalovirus infection	Leukopenia, thrombocytopenia
Trimethoprim/ sulfamethoxazole	Antibiotic, *Pneumocystis* pneumonia	Dose-related neutropenia, anemia; methemoglobinemia, especially in persons with G6PD deficiency
Primaquine	Antibiotic, *Pneumocystis* pneumonia	Rare agranulocytosis, thrombocytopenia; methemoglobinemia, especially in G6PD deficiency
Pentamidine	*Pneumocystis* pneumonia	Infrequent anemia, leukopenia, thrombocytopenia
Sulfadiazine	Toxoplasmosis	Leukopenia in 40%; thrombocytopenia in 12%
Clindamycin/ pyrimethamine	Toxoplasmosis	Cytopenias in 31%
Amphotericin B	Antifungal, cryptococcal meningitis	Anemia

Abbreviation: G6PD, glucose-6-phosphate dehydrogenase.

The Effect of Antiretroviral Therapy on Anemia

Nucleoside analogs other than ZDV are not associated with anemia. ZDV is commonly associated with marrow toxicity, particularly with long-term administration. Use of lower ZDV doses in combination with other nonmyelosuppressive antiviral drugs (such as the protease inhibitors or other nucleoside analogs) has significantly decreased the frequency of anemia, although patients with advanced disease on doses of ZDV of <500 mg/d still demonstrate significantly decreased hemoglobin levels when compared to similarly immunosuppressed HIV-infected patients not taking the drug.[47] Although the mechanism responsible for ZDV-associated anemia, inhibition of thymidine kinase, and DNA chain termination should theoretically also affect cells of other lineages, neutropenia is a less frequent toxicity and thrombocytopenia is very uncommon. In contradistinction to ZDV, protease inhibitors, such as IDV, RTV, and NFV, alone or in combination with ZDV or other nucleoside analogs, have little or no effect on hematopoiesis.[31,48] It is important to note that ART itself improves anemia, as shown in a single center retrospective series in the ART era. ART was associated with hemoglobin levels >140 g/L in 42% of patients, irrespective of use of ZDV as part of ART regimen, compared with 31% of patients who did not use ART.[49]

Treatable causes of anemia include nutritional/vitamin deficiency, gastrointestinal losses, parvovirus B19 infection,[50,51] HIV-related kidney disease, and low erythropoietin levels independent of normal renal function. In HIV infection, erythropoietin levels are low in some patients, in part because tumor necrosis factor-α (TNF-α) acts to block erythropoietin release in response to low hemoglobin levels.[52] Patients with low erythropoietin levels respond better to its administration than do patients with normal or elevated levels of the hormone. In one meta-analysis, patients with erythropoietin levels below 500 IU/L demonstrated significant increases in hemoglobin levels, decreases in transfusion requirements, and improvement in quality of life, whereas replacement was ineffective in patients with high erythropoietin levels.[53]

Some patients with HIV infection have significant anemia, requiring frequent transfusion. Clinical and experimental evidence suggests transfusion may be associated with substantial morbidity in

HIV-infected patients. In one study, transfused patients with advanced disease had an increased incidence of CMV infection and death.[54] Laboratory data suggest transfusion may be associated with HIV viral activation. Allogeneic lymphocytes present in transfused blood components activate viral production by HIV-infected lymphocytes in vitro.[55] When quantitative polymerase chain reaction (PCR) was used to measure circulating HIV, viral load was increased in HIV-infected patents 5 days after transfusion.[56] However, when leuko-depleted blood components were used, no significant differences in viremia or infectious complications occurred.[57]

Red Blood Cell Destruction

Red blood cells can be destroyed in the setting of HIV infection through a variety of mechanisms. This includes autoimmune disease,[58] hemophagocytic syndrome, disseminated intravascular coagulation typically seen with infection or cancer, sulfa use in the setting of glucose-6-phosphate dehydrogenase deficiency, or thrombotic thrombocytopenic purpura (TTP) (see "Thrombotic Thrombocytopenia Purpura"). Drugs can also cause hemolysis.

Parvovirus is a rare but treatable cause of anemia. Parvovirus affects erythroid lineage cells. This is a self-limited infection in immunocompetent patients but is serious in patients who cannot clear the infection or who have other hemolytic problems. For parvovirus infection, commercial immune globulin infusion (400 mg/kg/d for 5-10 days or 1 g/kg/d for 2 days) is almost always associated with marked improvement in hemoglobin levels with resolution of anemia.[51,59] Maintenance intravenous immune globulin (IVIG) at doses of 0.4 g/kg/d every 4 weeks following the initial IVIG treatment dose can prevent relapse in patients with low CD4 cell counts (e.g., <100 cells/μL).[60]

Thrombocytopenia

Thrombocytopenia occurs in the setting of HIV infection because of decreased production, increased destruction, or splenic sequestration secondary to other causes such as lymphoma or hepatitis C. Although mild- to moderate thrombocytopenia is common in patients with HIV, it is rarely associated with bleeding. Thrombocytopenia is generally associated with decreased platelet survival, except in patients with advanced disease where bone marrow failure is more prominent.[61] OIs, splenomegaly, and fever all decrease platelet survival.

Idiopathic thrombocytopenia (ITP) is a feature of HIV infection and is a diagnosis of exclusion. Notably, patients can present in advance of other symptoms of HIV. Consequently, HIV should be ruled out in new cases of ITP. CD4$^+$ lymphocyte counts in reported series of patients with HIV-ITP have averaged between 300 and 600 cells/μL.

Although platelet-associated antibodies increase in prevalence with HIV disease progression, it is not clear if they play a major role in most patients. Technical difficulties in detecting platelet-associated antibody have led to a very high false-positive rate.[62] Furthermore, for any condition (including sepsis and TTP) associated with platelet injury, antibody can be detected on the platelet surface. Specific platelet-associated antibody has nonetheless been carefully characterized in a limited number of patients. One study demonstrated that platelet-associated immune complexes are made up of antiplatelet integrin, glycoprotein IIIa (β), antibody (Ab), and its anti-idiotype blocking Ab.[63] Some of the antibodies also bound epitopes with homology to HIV-1 proteins *nef*, *gag*, *env*, and *pol*, suggesting molecular mimicry. The presence of this Ab was associated with thrombocytopenia and produced thrombocytopenia when infused into mice.[64] The associated platelet fragmentation was due to generation of the membrane-damaging peroxide and other reactive oxygen species. Antibodies to a cleavage product of talin, which can be generated by platelet activation or exposure to HIV-1 protease, have also been characterized. These may result from an immune response to talin-H, a neoantigen that may have been created by platelet fragmentation.[65]

Defective megakaryocytopoiesis may also contribute to thrombocytopenia, particularly in patients with advanced disease. Megakaryocytes can be infected with certain strains of HIV, some of which can be cytopathic for the megakaryocytes.[66] In addition, megakaryocytes arising from HIV-1–infected CD34$^+$ progenitor cells are defective in their ability to produce platelets.[67]

Treatment

Generally, patients with modest thrombocytopenia (platelet count > 50×10^9/L) require no treatment. For others with clinically significant thrombocytopenia, short-term steroids produce rapid responses in 60% to 80% of patients. However, steroids are immunosuppressive and are associated with long-term infectious complications and can accelerate the development of KS. HIV-specific ART will result in improvements of platelet counts in most patients. Although most of the original work was done with ZDV, other antiretrovirals are effective. Both antiretroviral agents and steroids improve thrombocytopenia by increasing platelet production, without significantly affecting platelet survival.[68,69] Splenectomy will increase platelet counts in those not responding to ART and does not appear to accelerate the underlying HIV disease.[70] Intravenous immune globulin also is effective but its high cost, limited availability, and short duration of action make this a less attractive treatment. Anti-Rh immune globulin has the advantages of wide availability and cheaper cost but is also limited by its short duration of action[71] and is associated with a mild hemolysis that can be clinically problematic in patients with preexisting anemia, requiring transfusion prior to administration of anti-Rh immune globulin. Vincristine is effective when given monthly, although its administration is complicated by neuropathy. IL-11, a cytokine that promotes megakaryocyte maturation, is licensed for treatment of chemotherapy-related thrombocytopenia, but no studies have reported efficacy in HIV-infected patients. Three newer treatments for ITP in the general population include the anti–B-cell antibody rituximab, effective in approximately 60% of patients, and the thrombopoietin mimetics, romiplostim and eltrombopag, each associated with a 60% to 85% response.[72,73] Remarkably, these drugs have not been systematically studied in HIV-associated ITP. Romiplostim increased platelet counts in five patients, but two patients succumbed to thromboembolic complications.[74]

Neutropenia

Mild neutropenia is relatively common in patients with HIV infection. Although generally not of clinical significance, a deficiency in the bone marrow reserve may become clinically apparent when administration of cytotoxic chemotherapy or other marrow-suppressive drugs becomes necessary. In fact, cytotoxic chemotherapy generally requires prophylactic use of hematopoietic growth factors. Antineutrophil antibodies can frequently be seen,[62] but their presence does not correlate with the degree of neutropenia. Progenitor cell numbers are generally normal except in patients with advanced disease when they are modestly decreased.[75]

Treatment

Neutropenic (absolute neutrophil count, $<1.0 \times 10^9$/L) HIV-positive patients may experience increased frequency of significant bacterial infections. In a case-controlled study, Tumbarello et al[76] compared the neutrophil counts of groups of HIV-infected patients with and without bacteremia. An absolute neutrophil count of $<1.0 \times 10^9$/L as present in 38% of bacteremic patients was compared with 19% of asymptomatic patients. A matched cohort study[77] found the frequency of bacteremia increased in neutropenic patients to 12.60 events per 100 patient months compared with 0.87 events per 100 patient months in the nonneutropenia controls. In another study of 1645 patients with an absolute neutrophil count of $<0.5 \times 10^9$/L, the risk of gram-negative infection increased eightfold.[78]

Recombinant growth factors can reduce the incidence of infection and number of hospitalizations. Granulocyte colony–stimulating factor (G-CSF) enhances the proliferation and differentiation of neutrophils and improves neutrophil function, whereas granulocyte-macrophage colony–stimulating factor (GM-CSF) stimulates the proliferation and differentiation of a variety of myeloid progenitor cells and inhibits migration of neutrophils, enhancing the function of mature neutrophils and macrophages.[71,79] G-CSF is the most widely used hematopoietic growth factor in HIV-infected patients, has fewer side effects, and increases the neutrophil count more rapidly. Although GM-CSF has been associated with an increase in HIV-1 replication in vitro, no consistent observation of acceleration of disease progression or increase in p24 antigen levels in patients receiving the drug has been demonstrated. G-CSF is primarily used to increase the tolerance of patients undergoing chemotherapy.

HIV-infected patients can also have a number of defects in neutrophil function. These include reduced L-selectin shedding and decreased H_2O_2 production[80] as well as defects in leukocyte migration, chemotaxis, and chemiluminescence during phagocytosis. These defects were more prominent in patients with advanced disease.[81] G-CSF and GM-CSF both improve leukocyte function in vitro. These cytokines demonstrate potential benefits in animal models of immunosuppression. In a murine model of *P. jiroveci* pneumonia, $CD4^+$-depleted immunosuppressed mice that received G-CSF after experiential pulmonary infection with *P. jiroveci* demonstrated improved survival when compared with control mice receiving placebo. Similar benefits were demonstrated using mouse models of disseminated *Mycobacterium avium* infection, systemic candidiasis, and streptococcal pneumonia.[82] No clinical study using either G-CSF or GM-CSF to enhance leukocyte function has been performed.

Lymphopenia

Increases in both CD4 and CD8 cell death and impairment in function are the sine qua non of HIV infection. IL-2 partially corrects the impaired lymphocyte proliferation and cytotoxicity seen in HIV infection in vitro. It can also partially block the enhanced tendency of lymphocytes obtained from HIV-infected patients to undergo programmed cell death (apoptosis).[38] In phase I trials of IL-2 in HIV-infected patients, it increased CD4 cell number and improved lymphocyte function.[83] The development of a long-acting polyethylene glycol–modified IL-2, which increases the half-life by 10- to 15-fold, allows for intermittent administration of the drug. Administration of doses of 1 to 5 million U/m^2, two to three times weekly, resulted in modest but sustained increases in CD4 counts and improvement in natural killer activity in a patient with CD4 counts >400 cells/µL[84] in 3 to 6 months. Fever, rash, and capillary leak are the most common toxicities.[85] More recently, administration of very high doses of IL-2 (7.5 million IU twice daily to patients with early HIV infection) resulted in substantial increases in CD4 counts, compared with those seen in the group administered lower doses (1.5 million IU twice daily).[86] Of greater importance is the suggestion that intermittent administration of IL-2 in combination with ART may lead to reduction in $CD4^+$ T-lymphocyte cells that contain replication-competent HIV.[87] None of these approaches is currently standard of care.

Thrombotic Thrombocytopenic Purpura

TTP is more common among patients with HIV infection. HIV-1 infection has been reported to account for up to 30% of TTP/hemolytic-uremic syndrome.[88] The risk of microangiopathy has declined significantly after institution of ART, although the reasons for this are unclear.[89] Although no controlled studies comparing HIV-related TTP with classic TTP have been conducted, HIV-related TTP is generally thought to be associated with a milder course and a better response to therapy than classic TTP.[90]

A number of different possible pathophysiologic mechanisms have been proposed. HIV can infect endothelial cells, and viral p24 antigen has been detected by immunochemical stain in splenic endothelial cells, spinal cord specimens, and bone marrow microvascular endothelial cells.[91] Whether infection results in vascular dysfunction has not been clearly demonstrated. TNF-α and IL-1β, two cytokines that are increased in HIV infection, could potentially lead to increases in endothelial expression of certain adhesion molecules, such as vascular cell adhesion molecule-1, intercellular adhesion molecule, and E-selectin, promoting localization of inflammatory cells to the endothelium with transmigration of lymphocytes through the endothelial wall. CMV, a virus that appeared to be associated with TTP in one large AIDS Clinical Treatment Group drug study, increases procoagulant activity in cultures of endothelial cells, potentially by binding and activating coagulation factor X/Xa.[92] Endothelial cells from small vessels undergo apoptosis when exposed to plasma from patients with TTP.[92-94] Recently, severe ADAMTS13 (a disintegrin-like and metalloprotease with thrombospondin type 1 repeats) deficiency has been reported in TTP unassociated with HIV.[95]

Treatment

Although the treatment of choice of TTP is plasmapheresis or plasma exchange, successes with antiplatelet agents, vincristine, splenectomy, and plasma infusion have been reported.[96] In one study of HIV-TTP, most patients undergoing plasma exchange in addition to other therapies achieved a complete response.[90] Patients with advanced HIV disease and OIs who present with thrombotic microangiopathy tend to respond to simple plasma infusion, whereas patients with less progressive HIV disease tend to behave like those with idiopathic TTP, requiring plasma exchange rather than simple plasma infusion.[97]

Plasma exchange is currently recommended to replace 35 to 40 mL/kg per exchange using the lactate dehydrogenase (LDH) values and platelet counts to follow the course of the disease. A platelet count above $50 \times 10^9/L$ and a normalized LDH are general aims of effective therapy. Platelets should not be transfused, because doing so may lead to thrombotic events.

Pathophysiology of Bone Marrow Suppression in HIV Infection

Diverse factors responsible for impaired hematopoiesis in HIV infection include suppression of the bone marrow by the virus or by viral proteins, immune dysregulation, actual infection of the bone marrow progenitor cells by HIV, and alteration of stromal cell elements. A number of studies demonstrate that CD34 cells have both HIV receptors necessary for infection (i.e., CD4 and the chemokine receptors CXCR4 or CCR5).[98] Chemokines are cytokines that induce chemotaxis. CD4 expression, as well as CXCR4 and CCR5 coreceptor expression, increases with maturation of the CD34 cell, and the expression of each correlates with potential infectability.[99] In addition, CXCR5 may be upregulated by a number of different cytokines. Although it is clear that the CD34 cell can be infected by HIV under a number of conditions, it appears that bone marrow progenitor cells do not represent a significant reservoir of infection.[100] In one study, HIV was detected in CD34 cells in only 14% of HIV-infected patients recruited in the United States and in 36% of HIV-infected persons in Zaire.[101] When found, CD34 infection was present in those patients with far-advanced disease. Many investigators could not detect HIV infection in any stem cells.[102,103] In another study, purified $CD34^+$ cells were infected in vitro and cultured on allogeneic stroma for extended periods of time.[104] A highly sensitive PCR failed to detect HIV-1 in the most primitive long-term colony-initiating cells (i.e., the secondary colonies generated from clonogenic cells harvested from stroma). Thus, it appears that although some committed progenitor cells can be infected with HIV-1 under some circumstances, the most immature stem cells appear not to be susceptible to HIV-1 infection.

The effects of HIV-1 on colony formation have been studied, either using bone marrow cells derived from HIV-1–infected patients[102,105] or after in vitro infection of hematopoietic cells from bone marrow of normal donors.[67,102] Results have been surprisingly divergent. Although the growth potential of committed bone marrow progenitor cells in methylcellulose cultures after challenge with HIV-1 appears to be diminished, normal growth frequently has also been reported.[102] Similar disparity exists in the results of studies performed with patient bone marrow. Such differences may be related to techniques in assaying colony growth (total bone marrow vs purified $CD34^+$ cells), culture conditions (use of specific cytokines or growth factors), or patient selection. In some reports, inhibition of colony formation by virus was observed only in cultures of total bone marrow cells and not with isolated $CD34^+$ cells.[45] Of interest is one report of abnormal progenitor cell function in HIV-negative infants born to infected mothers,[106] implying that direct infection was not necessary for marrow suppression.

Marrow stromal function has been examined in patients with HIV infection. Stromal cells from some HIV-1–infected patients may be infected by the virus, demonstrating the importance of stromal infection in causing dysregulation of hematopoiesis. In one study,[107] decreased colony formation has been observed when stroma infected in vitro was used to support growth of normal uninfected bone marrow progenitor cells. In another study, stroma obtained from HIV-infected patients supported growth of normal CD34+ cells equally as well as stroma obtained from normal uninfected controls.[75]

Although the stem cell compartment appears to be relatively well preserved early in the disease, in patients with low CD4 counts and history of OIs, long-term colony-initiating cell numbers are modestly reduced.[75] However, the long-term colony-initiating cell numbers were far better preserved in this population than in patients with aplastic anemia with similar blood counts, implying that OIs; pharmacotherapy with antiparasitic, antimicrobial, antiviral, or cytotoxic agents; vitamin deficiencies; or poorly understood virally mediated immunomodulatory changes were the major contributors to bone marrow failure in patients with advanced HIV disease.

Inconsistencies in the results of experiments attempting to demonstrate the role of direct infection of HIV-1 on hematopoiesis have stimulated further search for pathophysiologic mechanisms of bone marrow suppression. Several cytokines released during the course of HIV-1 infection are potent inhibitors of hematopoiesis. Not only native virus and productive infection[45,108] but also viral products, such as gp120, gp160, and viral *tat* proteins, induce the secretion of an array of cytokines, including TNF-α, lymphotoxin-β (TNF-β), and IL-6.[109] Perhaps the most prominent cytokine implicated in an array of pathophysiologic reactions in AIDS is TNF-α (or cachexin).[110,111] In addition to its effect on body metabolism and the immune system, TNF-α has inhibitory effects on hematopoiesis.[112] High levels of interferon-γ (IFN-γ) were not only associated with a poor prognosis in HIV-1 infection, but also correlated with the degree of anemia.[113] Although disordered cytokine production by both lymphoid tissue and bone marrow clearly occurs in HIV-1 infection, it is difficult to determine its ultimate role in suppression of hematopoiesis. Many inhibitory cytokines are produced in greatest quantities early in the course of HIV-1 infection when marrow suppression is least, and their levels decline as the disease progresses (when marrow suppression becomes most marked). In addition, increased levels of stimulatory cytokines have been observed in HIV-1 infection, and many cytokines never reach significant levels in the circulation. Local production of growth factors in bone marrow may be more important than systemically secreted factors. In support of this hypothesis, one study of genetically engineered stromal cells, designed to produce low levels of IFN-γ constitutively, showed significant suppression of normal hematopoietic colony growth on IFN-γ stroma, which could only be replicated by addition of large amounts of exogenous IFN-γ to marrow grown on normal stroma.

Apoptosis of hematopoietic progenitor cells through the Fas-L/Fas-R pathway is a mechanism by which activated T cells can kill virus-infected cells.[114] It is likely that Fas-L and other cytokine products of activated T cells contribute to the hematopoietic inhibition seen in HIV-1 infection. Increased levels of Fas-L have been reported in patients with AIDS, and triggering of Fas-R on hematopoietic cells results in apoptosis.

Bone Marrow Examination in HIV-1 Infection

The majority of bone marrow samples from HIV-1–infected patients will exhibit morphologic abnormalities, but most are nonspecific except in OI, in which the bone marrow examination provides valuable diagnostic information. Therefore, the bone marrow examination rarely yields substantial clinical information except in the diagnosis of concurrent *M. avium-intracellulare*, tuberculosis, or fungal infection or as part of staging for malignancy.[115]

The histopathologic findings in the bone marrow of HIV-1–infected patients are varied. In one large study of 216 bone marrow examinations performed in 178 HIV-1–infected patients for evaluation of cytopenia, 69% of patients exhibited hypercellular marrow, 69% showed myelodysplastic changes, and 20% showed significant fibrosis; only 5% of the biopsies were hypocellular. Granulomas were found in 13% and lymphoid aggregates in 36% (but in other studies, in up to 50%) of specimens. Higher numbers of plasma cells and elevated numbers of eosinophils were also present, especially in conjunction with increased reticulum. Hyperplasia involving the granulocytic and erythrocytic lineages has been most commonly reported; the myeloid-to-erythroid ratio has varied from 2:1 to 5:1.[116]

Morphologic changes tend to be more pronounced in more immunosuppressed patients and increase in frequency as disease progresses. All lineages can be involved. Megaloblastic changes and ringed sideroblasts are frequent. Using the morphologic criteria established for primary myelodysplastic syndromes, dysplasia involving at least one lineage was diagnosed in 69% of patients. Dysplastic changes increase with disease progression. However, in one study, the numbers of erythroid precursors and the morphology of megakaryocytes clearly differentiated patients with AIDS from those with myelodysplastic syndrome.[117] The cumulative effects of drug toxicities, direct HIV-1 infection of marrow cells, and dysregulated cytokine production may be responsible for the morphologic changes that occur late in AIDS. However, the dysplastic changes in an individual lineage and specific cytopenias are not correlated.

Coagulation Abnormalities

A number of retrospective epidemiologic studies[118-124] found the incidence of thrombosis in HIV-infected patients was increased 2- to 10-fold over what would be expected in a healthy control population of the same age. However, except for isolated cases of protein S deficiency, no study has compared these patients to equally sick uninfected patients whose immobility, lymphedema, and hypoalbuminemia predispose them to hypercoagulability. Patients with HIV are more likely to develop antiphospholipid antibodies such as lupus anticoagulant (found in 1% of patients)[125] and antiphosphatidylcholine and anticardiolipin autoantibodies (found in about 50% of patients with HIV infection)[126,127]; however, many of these studies were performed before ART became the standard of care. Apart from diagnostic problems related to a falsely elevated partial prothrombin time, these antibodies do not appear to be associated with an increased frequency of thrombosis, as they are in uninfected patients.[128,129]

Increased levels of complement-binding protein 4, which attaches to protein S and renders the protein inactive, can be detected in as many as 27% to 73% of patients. These patients demonstrate decreased functional protein S when a functional assay is used to measure activity. The risk of thrombosis in these patients is substantially increased. No clear guidelines are available for treatment or other protein-S–deficient patients, but most hematologists recommend anticoagulation for an undefined period of time for those with a history of unprovoked thrombosis.

AIDS-RELATED MALIGNANCIES

Cancer is the leading cause of death for HIV-1–infected persons on ART. Twenty-five to 40% of HIV-positive patients will develop a malignancy.[32,33,130-135] Although KS, aggressive B-cell lymphomas, and cervical cancer are said to be AIDS defining when occurring in the setting of HIV infection and occur more frequently in HIV infection, death from non–AIDS-defining cancers is more common. The development of malignancies is related to a number of factors, including immunosuppression and concurrent infections with other viruses such as human herpes virus 8 (HHV8) and Epstein-Barr virus (EBV), or the human papillomavirus, which foster malignant transformation. These viruses carry oncogenic proteins and cytokines that contribute to malignant pathogenesis. Additionally, HIV infection reduces the ability to clear the viral infection. The Strategies for Management of Antiretroviral Therapy study demonstrated that ART interruptions in so-called drug conservation strategies increase the risk of cancer sixfold.[136] That being said, the prevalence of ART use leads to a striking change in the epidemiology with KS and non-Hodgkin lymphoma (NHL) generally now occurring at higher CD4 counts and lower HIV viral loads without an increased cancer risk on a per patient basis. In fact, in recent years, KS is more frequently encountered after ART initiation.[137]

Although the incidence of KS and certain lymphomas has decreased after ART was introduced, the frequency of other tumors such as cervical cancer has undergone little change. CNS lymphoma, although once accounting for 18% of AIDS-related lymphomas, is now extremely rare. Several new drugs and therapies have been developed for KS and AIDS-related lymphomas, and these treatments, plus the development of ART, have contributed to improvements in morbidity and mortality. Given the introduction of ART and our increased ability to treat infections effectively, the life span of patients with HIV has increased, eventually leading to substantial increases in individuals living with HIV-1.[33] One analysis projected a median life expectancy of 75 years assuming a high rate of HIV diagnosis (median CD4 cell count at diagnosis, 432 cells/μL), and 71.5 years with a low diagnosis rate (diagnosis only when symptomatic, median CD4 cell count 140/μL). Cumulative risks of death by 5 and 10 years after infection were 2.3% and 5.2%, respectively.[138] This makes treating malignancies more attractive than in the pre-ART era. Although these malignancies also occur in the HIV-uninfected population, their presentation, as well as their appropriate treatment, is quite different in the HIV-infected patient.

AIDS-RELATED LYMPHOMA

The remainder of this chapter will concentrate on the hematologic malignancies associated with HIV, specifically NHL and Hodgkin lymphoma (HL), which occur with increased frequency in patients infected with HIV. Original estimates were a 25- to 150-fold increase compared to the general population.[139-141] More recently, the risk is estimated as 4% to 10% lifetime with a 11- to 17-fold increase dependent on the subtype of lymphoma.[142]

Recent studies also demonstrate the duration and depth of the CD4 nadir and the duration of viremia increase the incidence of NHL. Decreased immune surveillance, B-cell dysregulation,[143] and, in certain subtypes, infections with HHV8 and EBV are also involved in the pathophysiology of the disorder.

A number of changes have occurred in the HIV-related lymphomas since widespread institution of ART. The overall incidence of HIV-associated lymphomas has declined for NHL, and survival has increased (*Figure 65.2*).[144] This decrease has primarily affected lymphomas occurring at low CD4 counts, whereas NHL occurring at higher CD4 counts has been relatively unaffected.[145]

AIDS-defining lymphoma subtypes as designated by the CDC include Burkitt lymphoma, diffuse large B-cell lymphoma (DLBCL) and its variants, and primary CNS lymphoma (*Figure 65.3*). These are grouped in *Table 65.2* with subtypes noted, although the World Health Organization classification does not specifically address HIV-associated lymphoma. Current estimates are that 4% to 5% of all NHL deaths are related to HIV, including higher contributions in the HIV-specific subtypes: 7% of DLBCL, 33% of Burkitt, and 18% of primary CNS lymphoma.[144] Of note, these subtypes differ in their clinical presentations, in their underlying pathogenesis, and in their response to therapy. The majority of HIV-related lymphomas are of B-cell origin. T-cell lymphomas are rare, as are primary effusion lymphomas (PELs), which lack B-, T-, and hematopoietic cell markers.

The frequency of NHL increases with the degree of immunosuppression, particularly for CNS lymphoma. Thus, CNS lymphoma is rarely seen in developed countries where ART is available, except in socioeconomic sectors where standard of care HIV therapy is not ubiquitous. In addition, patients with poorer virologic control on ART suffer a significantly higher incidence of lymphoma and worse outcomes following therapy.[146]

Some studies have suggested genetic factors play a role in the development of NHL. One study demonstrated HIV-infected patients who are heterozygous for the CCR5D32 deletion are less likely to develop lymphoma, whereas those with stromal-cell–derived factor-1 mutations are more likely to develop lymphoma.[147]

For patients receiving combination chemotherapy, the optimal timing of ART with combination chemotherapy is controversial. Currently, oncologists generally continue antiretrovirals during chemotherapy, as drug-drug interactions and increased toxicities can be eliminated with a judicious selection of ART. Drug discontinuation has been challenged by six randomized studies in infections showing immune reconstitution occurring within the first month of ART, leading to a decrease in infection mortality.[148] This suggests that ART discontinuation or deferment of initiation after a concurrent HIV and lymphoma diagnosis could be detrimental. Nonetheless, in a retrospective Italian study comparing toxicities between patients receiving CHOP (cyclophosphamide, doxorubicin, vincristine, and prednisone) plus ART versus CHOP or a comparable regimen without ART, the group receiving ART experienced greater neurotoxicity and anemia but a decreased frequency of infection.[149] The differences in favor of ART may have been due to improvements in supportive care gained during the 1990s. Moreover, with an expansion of the panoply of ART medications, it is now possible to avoid specific ART components to minimize drug-drug interaction. A retrospective analysis of a prospective study suggested more rapid immune reconstitution with concurrent rather than delayed ART.[150] However, no controlled clinical trial has yet been performed to assess the contribution of continuing ART

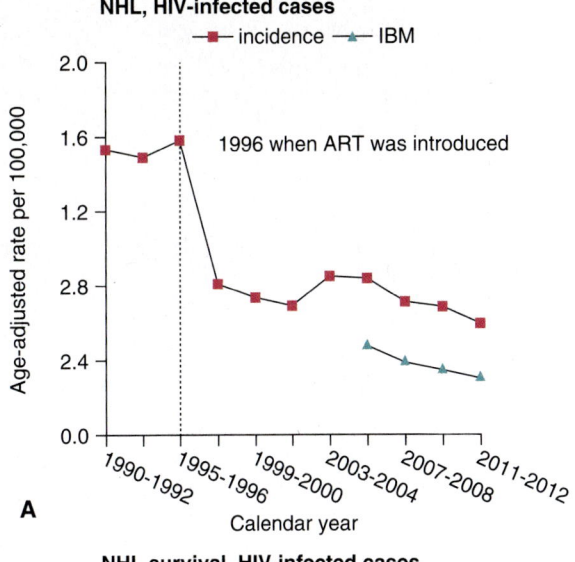

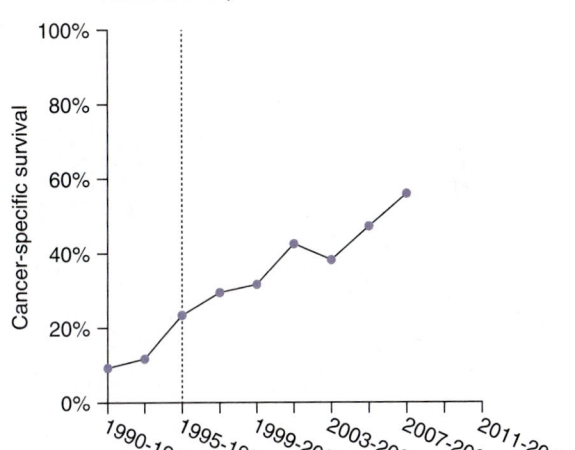

FIGURE 65.2 A, Non-Hodgkin lymphoma (NHL) incidence and incidence-based mortality (IBM) for HIV patients following the introduction of antiretroviral therapy (ART) in the United States. B, Improving 5-year survival according to year of NHL diagnosis for HIV patients, based on the Survival, Epidemiology, and End Results (SEER) database. (Adapted from Howlader N, Shiels MS, Mariotto AB, et al. Contributions of HIV to non-Hodgkin mortality trends in the United States. *Cancer Epidemiol Biomarkers Prev.* 2016;25:1289-1296. Copyright © 2016 American Association for Cancer Research. With permission from AACR.)

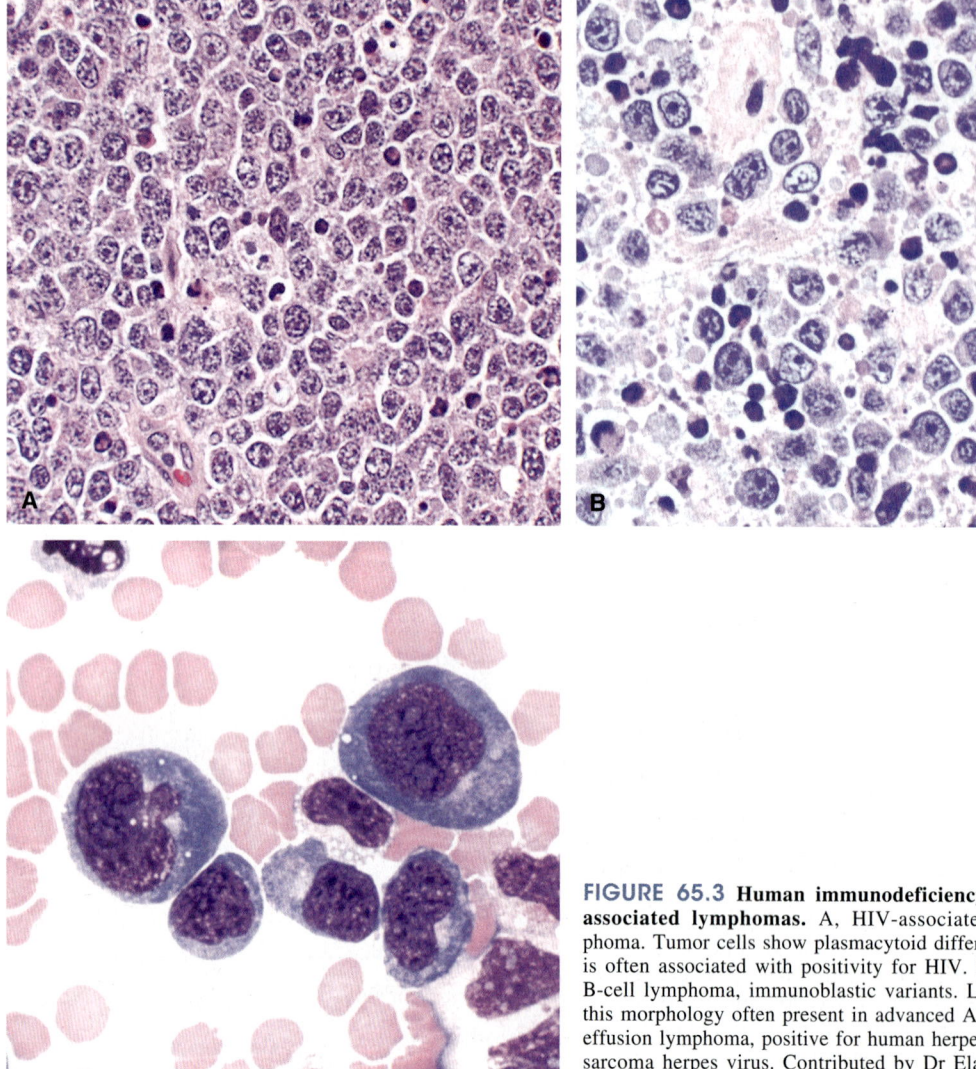

FIGURE 65.3 Human immunodeficiency virus (HIV)–associated lymphomas. A, HIV-associated Burkitt lymphoma. Tumor cells show plasmacytoid differentiation, which is often associated with positivity for HIV. B, Diffuse large B-cell lymphoma, immunoblastic variants. Lymphomas with this morphology often present in advanced AIDS. C, Primary effusion lymphoma, positive for human herpes virus 8/Kaposi sarcoma herpes virus. Contributed by Dr Elaine Jaffe, Chief Hematopathology Section and Acting Chief Laboratory of Pathology, National Cancer Institute.

therapy to improvement in viral replication and lymphoma control. It is unlikely that such a study will be conducted.

The role of viruses in the pathophysiology of HIV-related lymphomas is dependent on subtype.[151] For example, CNS lymphomas are virtually always associated with EBV infection, and PEL is associated with HHV8 infection. EBV encodes for a number of cytokines promoting cell growth. AIDS-Burkitt is variably associated with EBV, but also contains activating mutations in the *cMYC* proto-oncogene, frequent inactivation of p53, as well as point mutations in *BCL-6*. One study showed that loss of EBV-specific CD8+ T cells in subjects progressing to EBV-related NHL correlated with loss of CD4+ T cells and that these cells were better preserved in equally immunocompromised patients not developing lymphoma.[152] In patients on ART, coinfection with hepatitis B and C also appears to increase the risk of NHL.[153] Beyond coviruses, HIV itself may have direct pathogenic effects by secreting proteins into the microenvironment, promoting lymphogenesis.[154,155]

Patients with HIV-NHL frequently present with advanced stage III or IV disease. The majority will present with a rapidly growing mass or the development of systemic B symptoms (i.e., fever, night sweats, and unexplained weight loss). The clinical presentation is dependent on the site of involvement. Extranodal involvement including the bone marrow (25%-40%), gastrointestinal tract (26%), and CNS (17%-32%) is common. Leptomeningeal disease may be present and detected by flow cytometry only at a higher frequency than the immunocompetent population, where it is rare, with a surprising 22% among 51 newly diagnosed patients in one study in which 11 (22%) were detected by flow cytometry and only 1 by cytology.[156] Involvement of the small bowel and rectum is also prevalent, particularly in those with large cell histology. An AIDS-related lymphoma score consists of three components: age-adjusted International Prognostic Index, number of involved extranodal sites, and an HIV score that incorporates baseline CD4 count, HIV viral load, and prior history of AIDS.[157]

Clinical Manifestations
Therapy

Prior to ART, patients with lymphoma were more debilitated and experienced significant toxicity associated with chemotherapy. Multiple trials focused on reduced-intensity chemotherapy, which generally resulted in shorter remission durations. Treatment of HIV lymphoma has changed radically after the institution of ART, and remission has been anecdotally reported after institution of ART alone. However, this is not the standard of care, and most trials now focus on more intensive therapy.

The French Italian Cooperative Group tailored treatment to the level of preexisting immunosuppression, examining low- vs high-dose therapy in patients with moderate and severe immunosuppression.

Table 65.2. Classification of Human Immunodeficiency Virus–Associated Lymphomas

Primary central nervous system lymphoma
Diffuse large B-cell lymphoma (DLBCL)
Centroblastic
Immunoblastic ± plasmacytoid
Burkitt lymphoma (BL) ± plasmacytoid
Unclassifiable lymphoma with features intermediate between BL and DLBCL
Plasmablastic lymphoma
Oral cavity type
Other site
Primary effusion lymphoma
Classic variant in the absence of other masses
Solid variant ± serous effusions
Multicentric Castleman disease–associated large cell lymphoma
Hodgkin lymphoma
Other rare histologies including
Polymorphic B-cell lymphoma (posttransplant lymphoproliferative disorder-like) and peripheral T-cell lymphomas

Patients with CD4 counts over 200 cells/μL received a dose-intensified regimen of ACVB (doxorubicin, cyclophosphamide, vindesine, bleomycin, methylprednisolone, methotrexate) versus standard CHOP because of evidence from previous trials of NHL unrelated to HIV showing that patients receiving an intensified regimen had more durable remissions.[158] Both groups of HIV-infected patients in this trial had comparable responses, but toxicity was better in the CHOP arm. Patients with one adverse prognostic factor were randomly assigned to CHOP or dose-reduced CHOP. High-risk patients were treated with dose-reduced CHOP or vincristine plus prednisone. In the intermediate-risk group, standard-dose CHOP was superior to dose-reduced CHOP, but overall survival remained similar in the two groups. This risk-adapted approach has not been adapted universally because of the results of other trials.

Although alternative infusional regimens like cyclophosphamide, doxorubicin, and etoposide (CDE)[159,160] have been studied, EPOCH (etoposide, prednisone vincristine, cyclophosphamide, and doxorubicin-cyclophosphamide dose adjusted to CD4 count) has emerged as the predominant approach because it produced responses of 79% in a preliminary study.[161] Antiviral therapy was suspended during treatment in this protocol, for fear of concurrent toxicities, leading to transient increases in viral load and decreases in CD4 counts. A multicenter trial by the AIDS malignancy consortium investigated EPOCH with concurrent versus sequential rituximab and found the CR rate to be higher in the concurrent arm.[162] The vast majority of patients remained on ART during treatment, challenging the earlier assertion that ART must be suspended as also discussed above. Overall, the more intensive regimens may have increased efficacy in AIDS-NHL based on pooled analysis, but not studied in a random assignment trial.[163] Phase II studies have suggested some patients can receive fewer cycles of treatment.[164,165] Additionally, patients with myc-driven tumors may have a more adverse prognosis.[166]

Anti-CD20 monoclonal antibody (rituximab) has become a ubiquitous component of B-cell NHL in the general population. Preliminary studies show that it can be added to chemotherapy without evidence of added toxicity.[167] Rituximab administered with CDE and concomitant ART has yielded 2-year survival rate of 80%.[168] However, a randomized phase III study of CHOP with or without rituximab failed to demonstrate any added benefit of rituximab and suggested increased toxicity in those with a CD4 count less than 50 cells/μL.[169] In contrast, another study, rituximab adjunction to CHOP produced a complete response rate of 77% and a 2-year survival rate of 75% in patients with AIDS-related NHL, without increasing the risk of life-threatening infections.[170] The current standard of care is to use rituximab with attention to infection, including hematopoietic growth factors and antibiotic prophylaxis in those at highest risk.

Primary Central Nervous System Lymphoma

Primary CNS NHL typically affects the most immunocompromised with $CD4^+$ lymphocyte counts less than 50 cells/μL and is now rarely seen in patients receiving ART. Most are diffuse large B-cell lymphomas and are multifocal.[171] Confusion, memory loss, lethargy, and focal neurologic findings are the most frequent presenting symptoms and signs. The response to therapy in patients with primary CNS lymphoma has been very disappointing. Palliation with steroids and whole-brain radiation (3000-5400 Gy) has response rates of 75%, and treatment with high-dose methotrexate has reportedly given similar results, but the response duration is short with a median survival of 2 to 4 months regardless of CD4 count. A pilot study using only antivirals and immunomodulation was very promising with two of five patients treated remaining in complete remission at 28 and 52 months, respectively, but closed early because of low accrual.[172] HIV patients have been excluded from trials of chemotherapy with upfront autologous stem cell transplant which has become an accepted approach in those without HIV.[173]

Primary Effusion Lymphoma

PEL comprises approximately 1% to 5% of AIDS-related lymphoma cases. Clinically, the disease is characterized by malignant effusions with the absence of nodal disease. Diagnosis is made by pericardiocentesis, thoracentesis, or paracentesis with cytologic examination of the fluid and immunohistochemical evaluation. PEL cells have pleomorphic morphology and lack expression of B-cell–associated genes, including surface immunoglobulin, although immunoglobulin gene rearrangements are usually positive, indicating a clonal B-cell origin. The gene expression profile of PEL cells suggests plasmablastic derivation.[174] The malignant clone is almost always found to be infected with HHV8, whereas concurrent infection with EBV is frequent. PEL may extend into tissues underlying the serous cavities, including the omentum, lymph nodes, mediastinum, and lung. In one study of 277 NHL patients, PEL was diagnosed in 11 patients (4%). Patients treated with doxorubicin, vincristine, and prednisone achieved a complete response rate of 42%. However, median survival time was only 6 months.[175] The decision to undergo therapy should be based on the functional status of the patient, the degree of immunosuppression, and the likelihood that the quality of life would be improved. A report of antiviral therapy alone leading to sustained remission has been documented.[176] As with other lymphomas, outcome may be better in the ART era.[177]

Burkitt Lymphoma

Burkitt lymphoma is highly overrepresented in patients living with HIV. Before the era of ART, treatments were curtailed from fears of prolonged and profound neutropenia associated with the intensive therapies that had become standard in the general population. One small retrospective[178] and one small prospective study[179] initially challenged the prevailing dogma and found that intensive therapies such as cyclophosphamide, vincristine, doxorubicin, methotrexate, ifosfamide, etoposide, cytarabine or hyper-cyclophosphamide, vincristine, doxorubicin, dexamethasone with methotrexate and high-dose cytarabine could be safely given with ART with success rates of 80% to 90%. More recent publications have also suggested the same.[180] AIDS Malignancy Consortium 048 demonstrated efficacy and less toxicity by adding rituximab and modifying dose and schedules of CODOX-M/IVAC.[181] The National Cancer Institute reported favorable results with less toxicity than the intensive regimens with dose-adjusted R-EPOCH for both HIV and non-HIV patients with Burkitt lymphoma[182] and expanded this to a multicenter trial showing equal results in the 25% with HIV compared to the remainder of the 113 patient trial.[183]

Plasmablastic Lymphoma

Plasmablastic lymphoma is a very rare CD20-negative variant of HIV-associated NHL.[183] It was originally described as almost exclusively associated with HIV and nearly always fatal in the pre-ART era.[184] The sine qua non of stage I disease is a mass in the jaw, but disseminated disease, including numerous bone lesions, is common. Retrospective studies suggested curability in the ART era in both HIV-positive and HIV-negative patients.[185,186] Optimal management will be difficult to define because of the rarity of the disease; however, 17 patients were accrued to a wider DLBCL REPOCH study and enjoyed a 75% 2-year event-free survival.[166]

Hodgkin Lymphoma

Although HL is not considered an AIDS-defining illness, a marked increase is seen in HIV. Moreover, although the risk of NHL has decreased with better therapy, the incidence of HL among patients with HIV infection has increased.[187] Unlike HL in HIV-uninfected patients, B symptoms are often present; mixed cellularity HL is the predominant pathologic subtype of disease; and advanced, extranodal disease is expected in the majority. One study showed 70% to 90% of patients present with B symptoms, and 74% to 96% of patients have advanced disease (stage III or IV) at the time of diagnosis with frequent involvement of extranodal sites (60%), including bone marrow, liver, and spleen involvement. Unlike those not infected with HIV, noncontiguous spread of disease is common and mediastinal involvement is far less. Bone marrow involvement occurs in 40% to 50% of patients and may be their first indication of the disease. Another characteristic distinguishing the HIV-associated HL from that not associated with HIV is the predominance of Reed-Sternberg cell–rich cases. AIDS-HL, like AIDS-NHL, is characterized by a high frequency of EBV infection when compared to HL in the HIV-negative population. The pathologic role of EBV in HL is evidenced by the Reed-Sternberg cell expression of EBV-transforming protein.

Treatment

Prior to ART, response to standard chemotherapy ABVD (doxorubicin, bleomycin, vinblastine, and dacarbazine), and median overall survival of 1.5 years was lower than that of patients without HIV infection. Similar to NHL, recent studies in the ART era show outcomes comparable to the general population with 2-year overall and progression-free survival of 94% and 89%, respectively.[188] A US intergroup study (S0816) showed similar results in a small cohort.[189] The novel and highly potent brentuximab vedotin, an anti-CD30 antibody conjugated to an antitubulin drug, is approved for relapsed and refractory non-HIV Hodgkin and proved superior in combination with AVD as first-line therapy compared to ABVD for advanced stage HL in the general population. A phase II study of brentuximab vedotin in combination with AVD in an AIDS Malignancy Consortium of untreated advanced stage HIV-HL showed comparable efficacy and toxicity to the general population.[190]

Transplantation for Hodgkin Lymphoma and Non-Hodgkin Lymphoma

Myeloablative autologous transplants have been performed in patients with both NHL and HL. The City of Hope reported the first prospective study of 12 patients with NHL beyond first complete remission.[191] OIs were seen in three patients; transient increases in viral load were seen in seven (related to ART noncompliance). Three patients died, including two with relapsed lymphoma, but all others were alive at 18.5 months. Another study included eight patients with relapsed or resistant lymphoma, four with HL and four with NHL. Seven of eight continued ART during transplant, and seven engrafted successfully. Although six of seven patients engrafted, only four patients went into complete remission.[192] Another pilot of 16 patients with relapsed and refractory lymphoma reported 6 of 16 alive at a median of 8 months after second-line therapy, high-dose conditioning, and autologous stem cell support.[193] The European Cooperative Study Group on AIDS and Tumors reported the largest study and the only one enrolling patients before second-line therapy with 27 of 50 going on to autologous transplant and a median overall survival of 33 in all 50 eligible patients.[194] In addition, two retrospective case control studies have suggested no difference in outcome between HIV-positive and HIV-negative patients undergoing autologous transplant for the same indications.[195,196] The AIDS Malignancy Consortium and Bone Marrow Clinical Trials Network have demonstrated multicenter feasibility and recommend autologous transplant as a standard therapy for relapsed, chemosensitive HIV-related lymphoma.[197] Finally, gene therapy pilot studies are ongoing to test the feasibility of engineered hematopoietic stem cell HIV resistance at the time of transplant for malignancy.[198]

Nonmyeloablative allogeneic transplantation has been used in patients with refractory disease and has produced short-term remissions (12 months), but was associated with little toxicity and few OIs.[199] A case has been reported of simultaneous treatment of acute myelogenous leukemia and eradication of HIV infection using a donor with homozygous CCR5 deletion, a receptor necessary for HIV infection.[200] However, the rarity of this deletion makes this approach unique. The AIDS Malignancy Consortium and Bone Marrow Clinical Trials Network have recently reported an allogeneic transplant pilot study of 19 HIV-infected patients with a wide variety of hematologic malignancies.[201] Transplant-related mortality at 100 days was zero and full chimerism was achieved resulting in HIV viral suppression.

CONCLUSION

Patients with HIV infections are living longer and having a better quality of life than ever before. Life expectancy is now similar to that of the general population. Treatment of HIV-infected patients with ART has altered the natural history of HIV infection by decreasing the frequency of OIs and altering the expected frequency of hematologic complications and AIDS-related malignancies. Cytopenias, particularly anemia, are more common in advanced stages of HIV and result both from bone marrow failure and peripheral destruction. With the development and application of ART, both AIDS-defining and non–AIDS-defining malignancies represent an ever-increasing cause of death in this population. Lymphomas are highly prevalent among HIV-infected patients, although CNS lymphoma is now very rare on ART. Intensive curative therapies are now the norm except in patients with advanced AIDS. In the future, different strategies directed toward controlling the underlying inciting viral infections associated with malignancy (EBV, HHV8) and focusing on immune reconstitution in addition to standard chemotherapy may improve response rates and survival.

ACKNOWLEDGMENTS

Elaine M. Sloand and Jerome P. Groopman coauthored a previous version of this chapter in the 12th edition.

References

1. *UNAIDS Data 2020*. Accessed June 9, 2021. http://www.unaids.org/en/resources/documents/2020/unaids-data
2. Centers for Disease Control (CDC). 1993 revised classification system for HIV infection and expanded surveillance case definition for AIDS among adolescents and adults. *MMWR Recomm Rep (Morb Mortal Wkly Rep)*. 1992;41(RR-17):1-19.
3. Centers for Disease Control (CDC). *Pneumocystis* pneumonia—Los Angeles. *MMWR Morb Mortal Wkly Rep*. 1981;30:250-252.
4. Centers for Disease Control and Prevention (CDC). *Estimated HIV Incidence and Prevalence in the United States, 2014-2018*. HIV Surveillance Supplemental Report 2020;25(No. 1)http://www.cdc.gov/hiv/library/reports/hiv-surveillance.html. 2020. Accessed June 9, 2021.
5. Palella FJ, Jr, Delaney KM, Moorman AC, et al. Declining morbidity and mortality among patients with advanced human immunodeficiency virus infection. HIV Outpatient Study Investigators. *N Engl J Med*. 1998;338:853-860.
6. Panel on Antiretroviral Guidelines for Adults and Adolescents. *Guidelines for the Use of Antiretroviral Agents in Adults and Adolescents with HIV*. Department of Health and Human Services. Accessed June 9, 2021. https://clinicalinfo.hiv.gov/sites/default/files/inline-files/AdultandAdolescentGL.pdf
7. Panel on Guidelines for the Prevention and Treatment of Opportunistic Infections in Adults and Adolescents with HIV. *Guidelines for the Prevention and Treatment of Opportunistic Infections in HIV-infected Adults and Adolescents: Recommendations from the Centers for Disease Control and Prevention, the National Institutes of Health, and the HIV Medicine Association of the Infectious Diseases Society of America*. Accessed June 9, 2021. https://clinicalinfo.hiv.gov/sites/default/files/inline-files/adult_oi.pdf

8. Gallo RC, Montagnier L. The discovery of HIV as the cause of AIDS. *N Engl J Med.* 2003;349:2283-2285.
9. Clavel F, Guetard D, Brun-Vezinet F, et al. Isolation of a new human retrovirus from West African patients with AIDS. *Science.* 1986;233:343-346.
10. Patel P, Borkowf CB, Brooks JT, Lasry A, Lansky A, Mermin J. Estimating per-act HIV transmission risk: a systematic review. *AIDS.* 2014;28:1509-1519.
11. Grossman Z, Meier-Schellersheim M, Paul WE, Picker LJ. Pathogenesis of HIV infection: what the virus spares is as important as what it destroys. *Nat Med.* 2006;12(3):289-295.
12. Engelman A, Cherepanov P. The structural biology of HIV-1: mechanistic and therapeutic insights. *Nat Rev Microbiol.* 2012;10:279-290.
13. Chen B. Molecular mechanism of HIV-1 entry. *Trends Microbiol.* 2019;27:878-891.
14. Schuitemaker H, van 't Wout AB, Lusso P. Clinical significance of HIV-1 coreceptor usage. *J Transl Med.* 2011;9:S5.
15. Marmor M, Sheppard HW, Donnell D, et al. Homozygous and heterozygous CCR5-Delta32 genotypes are associated with resistance to HIV infection. *J Acquir Immune Defic Syndr.* 2001;27:472-481.
16. Cohn LB, Chomont N, Deeks SG. The biology of the HIV-1 latent reservoir and implications for cure strategies. *Cell Host Microbe.* 2020;27:519-530.
17. Kohl NE, Emini EA, Schleif WA, et al. Active human immunodeficiency virus protease is required for viral infectivity. *Proc Natl Acad Sci U S A.* 1988;85:4686-4690.
18. Doitsh G, Greene WC. Dissecting how CD4 T cells are lost during HIV infection. *Cell Host Microbe.* 2016;19:280-291.
19. Dufour C, Gantner P, Fromentin R, Chomont N. The multifaceted nature of HIV latency. *J Clin Invest.* 2020;130:3381-3390.
20. Martínez-Maza O, Crabb E, Mitsuyasu RT, Fahey JL, Giorgi JV. Infection with the human immunodeficiency virus (HIV) is associated with an in vivo increase in B lymphocyte activation and immaturity. *J Immunol.* 1987;138:3720-3724.
21. Margolick JB, Volkman DJ, Folks TM, Fauci AS. Amplification of HTLV-III/LAV infection by antigen-induced activation of T cells and direct suppression by virus of lymphocyte blastogenic responses. *J Immunol.* 1987;138:1719-1723.
22. US Preventive Services Task Force; Owens DK, Davidson KW, Krist AH, et al. Screening for HIV infection: US Preventive Services Task Force recommendation statement. *JAMA.* 2019;321:2326-2336.
23. Centers for Disease Control (CDC). National HIV testing day and new testing recommendations. *MMWR Morb Mortal Wkly Rep.* 2014;63:537.
24. Wesolowski LG, MacKellar DA, Facente SN, et al. Post-marketing surveillance of OraQuick whole blood and oral fluid rapid HIV testing. *AIDS.* 2006;20:1661-1666.
25. Weber B, Fall EH, Berger A, Doerr HW. Reduction of diagnostic window by new fourth-generation human immunodeficiency virus screening assays. *J Clin Microbiol.* 1998;36:2235-2239.
26. Pilcher CD, Fiscus SA, Nguyen TQ, et al. Detection of acute infections during HIV testing in North Carolina. *N Engl J Med.* 2005;352:1873-1883.
27. Grebe E, Busch MP, Notari EP, et al. HIV incidence in US first-time blood donors and transfusion risk with a 12-month deferral for men who have sex with men. *Blood.* 2020;136:1359-1367.
28. Robb ML, Eller LA, Kibuuka H, et al. Prospective study of acute HIV-1 infection in adults in East Africa and Thailand. *N Engl J Med.* 2016;374:2120-2130.
29. Doweiko JP. Hematologic aspects of HIV infection. *AIDS.* 1993;7:753-757.
30. Mitsuyasu R. Oncological complications of human immunodeficiency virus disease and hematological consequences of their treatment. *Clin Infect Dis.* 1999;29:35-43.
31. Pluda JM, Mitsuya H, Yarchoan R. Hematologic effects of AIDS therapies. *Hematol Oncol Clin North Am.* 1991;5:229-248.
32. Bower M, Palmieri C, Dhillon T. AIDS-related malignancies: changing epidemiology and the impact of highly active antiretroviral therapy. *Curr Opin Infect Dis.* 2006;19:14-19.
33. Lohse N, Obel N. Update of survival for persons with HIV infection in Denmark. *Ann Intern Med.* 2016;165:749-750.
34. Saag MS, Gandhi RT, Hoy JF, et al. Antiretroviral drugs for treatment and prevention of HIV infection in adults: 2020 recommendations of the international antiviral society-USA panel. *JAMA.* 2020;324:1651-1669.
35. Müller M, Wandel S, Colebunders R, et al. Immune reconstitution inflammatory syndrome in patients starting antiretroviral therapy for HIV infection: a systematic review and meta-analysis. *Lancet Infect Dis.* 2010;10:251-261.
36. INSIGHT-ESPRIT Study Group, SILCAAT Scientific Committee; Abrams D, Lévy Y, Losso MH, et al. Interleukin-2 therapy in patients with HIV infection. *N Engl J Med.* 2009;361:1548-1559.
37. Cohen MS, Chen YQ, McCauley M, et al. Antiretroviral therapy for the prevention of HIV-1 transmission. *N Engl J Med.* 2016;375:830-839.
38. Hütter G, Nowak D, Mossner M, et al. Long-term control of HIV by CCR5 Delta32/Delta32 stem-cell transplantation. *N Engl J Med.* 2009;360(7):692-698.
39. Cillo AR, Mellors JW. Which therapeutic strategy will achieve a cure for HIV-1? *Curr Opin Virol.* 2016;18:14-19.
40. Murphy EL, Collier AC, Kalish LA, et al. Highly active antiretroviral therapy decreases mortality and morbidity in patients with advanced HIV disease. *Ann Intern Med.* 2001;135:17-26.
41. Sullivan PS, Hanson DL, Chu SY, et al. Epidemiology of anemia in human immunodeficiency virus (HIV)-infected persons: results from the multistate adult and adolescent spectrum of HIV disease surveillance project. *Blood.* 1998;91:301-308.
42. Saah AJ, Munoz A, Kuo V, et al. Predictors of the risk of development of acquired immunodeficiency syndrome within 24 months among gay men seropositive for human immunodeficiency virus type 1: a report from the Multicenter AIDS Cohort Study. *Am J Epidemiol.* 1992;135:1147-1155.
43. Zauli G, Re MC, Visani G, et al. Evidence for a human immunodeficiency virus type-1 mediated suppression of uninfected hematopoietic (CD34+) cells in AIDS patients. *J Infect Dis.* 1992;166:710-716.
44. Zauli G, Davis BR, Re MC, Visani G, Furlini G, LaPlaca M. Tat protein stimulates production of transforming growth factor-β 1 by bone marrow macrophages: a potential mechanism for human immunodeficiency virus-1–induced hematopoietic suppression. *Blood.* 1992;80:3036.
45. Maciejewski JP, Weichold FF, Young NS. HIV-1 suppression of hematopoiesis in vitro mediated by envelope glycoprotein and TNF-α. *J Immunol.* 1994;153:4303-4310.
46. Dobs AS. Androgen therapy in AIDS wasting. *Baillieres Clin Endocrinol Metab.* 1998;12(3):379-390.
47. Koch MA, Volberding PA, Lagakos SW, et al. Toxic effects of zidovudine in asymptomatic human immunodeficiency virus-infected individuals with CD4+ cell counts of 0.50×10^9/L or less. Detailed and updated results from protocol 019 of the AIDS Clinical Trials Group. *Arch Intern Med.* 1992;152:2286-2292.
48. Sandstrom EG, Kaplan JC. Antiviral therapy in AIDS. Clinical pharmacological properties and therapeutic experience to date. *Drugs.* 1987;34:372-390.
49. Moore RD, Forney D. Anemia in HIV-infected patients receiving highly active antiretroviral therapy. *J Acquir Immune Defic Syndr.* 2002;29(1):54-57.
50. Abkowitz JL, Brown KE, Wood RW, et al. Clinical relevance of parvovirus B19 as a cause of anemia in patients with human immunodeficiency virus infection. *J Infect Dis.* 1997;176:269-273.
51. Frickhofen N, Abkowitz JL, Safford M, et al. Persistent B19 parvovirus infection in patients infected with human immunodeficiency virus type 1 (HIV-1): a treatable cause of anemia in AIDS. *Ann Intern Med.* 1990;113:926-933.
52. Kreuzer KA, Rockstroh JK, Jelkmann W, Theisen A, Spengler U, Sauerbruch T. Inadequate erythropoietin response to anaemia in HIV patients: relationship to serum levels of tumour necrosis factor-alpha, interleukin-6 and their soluble receptors. *Br J Haematol.* 1997;96:235-239.
53. Henry DH, Beall GN, Benson CA, et al. Recombinant human erythropoietin in the treatment of anemia associated with human immunodeficiency virus (HIV) infection and zidovudine therapy. Overview of four clinical trials. *Ann Intern Med.* 1992;117:739-748.
54. Sloand E, Kumar P, Klein HG, Merritt S, Sacher R. Transfusion of blood components to persons infected with human immunodeficiency virus type 1: relationship to opportunistic infection. *Transfusion.* 1994;34:48-53.
55. Busch MP, Lee TH, Heitman J. Allogeneic leukocytes but not therapeutic blood elements induce reactivation and dissemination of latent human immunodeficiency virus type 1 infection: implications for transfusion support of infected patients. *Blood.* 1992;80:2128-2135.
56. Mudido PM, Georges D, Dorazio D, et al. Human immunodeficiency virus type 1 activation after blood transfusion. *Transfusion.* 1996;36:860-865.
57. Ariga H, Lee TH, Laycock ME, et al; Viral Activation Transfusion Study. Residual WBC subsets in filtered prestorage RBCs. *Transfusion.* 2003;43:98-106.
58. McGinniss MH, Macher AM, Rook AH, Alter HJ. Red cell autoantibodies in patients with acquired immune deficiency syndrome. *Transfusion.* 1986;26(5):405.
59. Fuller A, Moaven L, Spelman D, et al. Parvovirus B19 in HIV infection: a treatable cause of anemia. *Pathology.* 1996;28:277-280.
60. Koduri PR. Parvovirus B19-related anemia in HIV-infected patients. *AIDS Patient Care STDS.* 2000;14(1):7.
61. Savona S, Nardi MA, Lennette ET, Karpatkin S. Thrombocytopenic purpura in narcotics addicts. *Ann Intern Med.* 1985;102:737-741.
62. Klaassen RJ, Mulder JW, Vlekke AB, et al. Autoantibodies against peripheral blood cells appear early in HIV infection and their prevalence increases with disease progression. *Clin Exp Immunol.* 1990;81:11-17.
63. Li Z, Nardi MA, Karpatkin S. Role of molecular mimicry to HIV-1 peptides in HIV-1-related immunologic thrombocytopenia. *Blood.* 2005;106:572-576.
64. Nardi M, Feinmark SJ, Hu L, Li Z, Karpatkin S. Complement-independent Ab-induced peroxide lysis of platelets requires 12-lipoxygenase and a platelet NADPH oxidase pathway. *J Clin Invest.* 2004;113:973-980.
65. Koefoed K, Ditzel HJ. Identification of talin head domain as an immunodominant epitope of the antiplatelet antibody response in patients with HIV-1-associated thrombocytopenia. *Blood.* 2004;104:4054-4062.
66. Kunzi MS, Groopman JE. Identification of a novel human immunodeficiency virus strain cytopathic to megakaryocytic cells. *Blood.* 1993;81:3336-3342.
67. Zauli G, Re MC, Davis B, et al. Impaired in vitro growth of purified (CD34+) hematopoietic progenitors in human immunodeficiency virus-1 seropositive thrombocytopenic individuals. *Blood.* 1992;79:2680-2687.
68. Gernsheimer T, Stratton J, Ballem PJ, Slichter SJ. Mechanisms of response to treatment in autoimmune thrombocytopenic purpura. *N Engl J Med.* 1989;320:974-980.
69. Ballem PJ, Belzberg A, Devine DV, et al. Kinetic studies of the mechanism of thrombocytopenia in patients with human immunodeficiency virus infection. *N Engl J Med.* 1992;327:1779-1784.
70. Barbui T, Cortelazzo S, Minetti B, Galli M, Buelli M. Does splenectomy enhance risk of AIDS in HIV-positive patients with chronic thrombocytopenia? *Lancet.* 1987;2:342-343.
71. Oksenhendler E, Bierling P, Brossard Y, et al. Anti-RH immunoglobulin therapy for human immunodeficiency virus-related immune thrombocytopenic purpura. *Blood.* 1988;71:1499-1502.
72. Ahmad HN, Ball C, Height SE, Rees DC. Rituximab in chronic, recurrent HIV-associated immune thrombocytopenic purpura. *Br J Haematol.* 2004;127:607-608.
73. Arnold DM, Nazi I, Kelton JG. New treatments for idiopathic thrombocytopenic purpura: rethinking old hypotheses. *Expert Opin Investig Drugs.* 2009;18(6):805-819.
74. Kowalczyk M, Rubinstein PG, Aboulafia DM. Initial experience with the use of thrombopoetin receptor agonists in patients with refractory HIV-associated immune thrombocytopenic purpura: a case series. *J Int Assoc Provid AIDS Care.* 2015;14(3):211-216. doi:10.1177/2325957414557266

75. Sloand EM, Young NS, Sato T, et al. Secondary colony formation after long-term bone marrow culture using peripheral blood and bone marrow of HIV-infected patients. *AIDS.* 1997;11:1547-1553.
76. Tumbarello M, Tacconelli E, Caponera S, Cauda R, Ortona L. The impact of bacteraemia on HIV infection. Nine years experience in a large Italian university hospital. *J Infect.* 1995;31:123-131.
77. Keiser P, Higgs E, Smith J. Neutropenia is associated with bacteremia in patients infected with the human immunodeficiency virus. *Am J Med Sci.* 1996;312:118-122.
78. Mathews WC, Caperna J, Toerner JG, Barber RE, Morgenstern H. Neutropenia is a risk factor for gram-negative bacillus bacteremia in human immunodeficiency virus-infected patients: results of a nested case-control study. *Am J Epidemiol.* 1998;148:1175-1183.
79. Pui CH, Boyett JM, Hughes WT, et al. Human granulocyte colony-stimulating factor after induction chemotherapy in children with acute lymphoblastic leukemia. *N Engl J Med.* 1997;336:1781-1787.
80. Elbim C, Prevot MH, Bouscarat F, et al. Impairment of polymorphonuclear neutrophil function in HIV-infected patients. *J Cardiovasc Pharmacol.* 1995;25(suppl 2):S66-S70.
81. Flo RW, Naess A, Nilsen A, Harthug S, Solberg CO. A longitudinal study of phagocyte function in HIV-infected patients. *AIDS.* 1994;8:771-777.
82. Coffey MJ, Phare SM, George S, Peters-Golden M, Kazanjian PH. Granulocyte colony-stimulating factor administration to HIV-infected subjects augments reduced leukotriene synthesis and anticryptococcal activity in neutrophils. *J Clin Invest.* 1998;102:663-670.
83. Kovacs JA, Vogel S, Albert JM, et al. Controlled trial of interleukin-2 infusions in patients infected with the human immunodeficiency virus. *N Engl J Med.* 1996;335:1350-1356.
84. Levy Y, Capitant C, Houhou S, et al. Comparison of subcutaneous and intravenous interleukin-2 in asymptomatic HIV-1 infection: a randomised controlled trial. ANRS 048 study group. *Lancet.* 1999;353:1923-1929.
85. Wood R, Montoya JG, Kundu SK, Schwartz DH, Merigan TC. Safety and efficacy of polyethylene glycol-modified interleukin-2 and zidovudine in human immunodeficiency virus type 1 infection: a phase I/II study. *J Infect Dis.* 1993;167:519-525.
86. Davey RT, Jr, Chaitt DG, Albert JM, et al. A randomized trial of high-versus low-dose subcutaneous interleukin-2 outpatient therapy for early human immunodeficiency virus type 1 infection. *J Infect Dis.* 1999;179:849-858.
87. Chun TW, Fauci AS. Latent reservoirs of HIV-obstacles to the eradication of virus. *Proc Natl Acad Sci U S A.* 1999;96:10958-10961.
88. Leaf AN, Laubenstein LJ, Raphael B, Hochster H, Baez L, Karpatkin S. Thrombotic thrombocytopenic purpura associated with human immunodeficiency virus type 1 (HIV-1) infection. *Ann Intern Med.* 1988;109:194-197.
89. Gervasoni C, Ridolfo AL, Vaccarezza M, et al. Thrombotic microangiopathy in patients with acquired immunodeficiency syndrome before and during the era of introduction of highly active antiretroviral therapy. *Clin Infect Dis.* 2002;35:1534-1540.
90. Bell WR, Chulay JD, Feinberg JE. Manifestations resembling thrombotic microangiopathy in patients with advanced human immunodeficiency virus (HIV) disease in a cytomegalovirus prophylaxis trial (ACTG 204). *Medicine (Baltimore).* 1997;76:369-380.
91. Del AA, Martinez MA, Pena JM, et al. Thrombotic thrombocytopenic purpura associated with human immunodeficiency virus infection: demonstration of p24 antigen in endothelial cells. *Clin Infect Dis.* 1993;17:360-363.
92. Laurence J, Mitra D, Steiner M, Staiano-Coico L, Jaffe E. Plasma from patients with idiopathic and human immunodeficiency virus-associated thrombotic thrombocytopenic purpura induces apoptosis in microvascular endothelial cells. *Blood.* 1996;87:3245-3254.
93. Mitra D, Kim J, MacLow C, Karsan A, Laurence J. Role of caspases 1 and 3 and Bcl-2-related molecules in endothelial cell apoptosis associated with thrombotic microangiopathies. *Am J Hematol.* 1998;59:279-287.
94. Laurence J, Mitra D. Apoptosis of microvascular endothelial cells in the pathophysiology of thrombotic thrombocytopenic purpura/sporadic hemolytic uremic syndrome. *Semin Hematol.* 1997;34:98-105.
95. Vesely SK, George JN, Lammle B, et al. ADAMTS13 activity in thrombotic thrombocytopenic purpura-hemolytic uremic syndrome: relation to presenting features and clinical outcomes in a prospective cohort of 142 patients. *Blood.* 2003;102:60-68.
96. Eldor A. Thrombotic thrombocytopenic purpura: diagnosis, pathogenesis and modern therapy. *Baillieres Clin Haematol.* 1998;11:475-495.
97. Warner NC, Vaughan LB, Wenzel RP. Human immunodeficiency virus associated thrombotic thrombocytopenic purpura, a clinical conundrum. *J Clin Apher.* 2017;32(6):567-570.
98. Ruiz ME, Cicala C, Arthos J, et al. Peripheral Blood-derived CD34+ progenitor cells: CXC chemokine receptor 4 and CC chemokine receptor 5 expression and infection by HIV. *J Immunol.* 1998;161:4169-4176.
99. Chelucci C, Casella I, Federico M, et al. Lineage-specific expression of human immunodeficiency virus (HIV) receptor/coreceptors in differentiating hematopoietic precursors: correlation with susceptibility to T- and M-tropic HIV and chemokine-mediated HIV resistance. *Blood.* 1999;94:1590-1600.
100. Kitano K, Abboud CN, Ryan DH, Quan SG, Baldwin GC, Golde DW. Macrophage-active colony-stimulating factors enhance human immunodeficiency virus type 1 infection in bone marrow stem cells. *Blood.* 1991;77:1699-1705.
101. Stanley SK, Kessler SW, Justement JS, et al. CD34+ bone marrow cells are infected with HIV in a subset of seropositive individuals. *J Immunol.* 1992;149:689-697.
102. Molina JM, Scadden DT, Sakaguchi M, Fuller B, Woon A, Groopman JE. Lack of evidence for infection of or effect on growth of hematopoietic progenitor cells after in vivo or in vitro exposure to human immunodeficiency virus. *Blood.* 1990;76:2476-2482.
103. Neal TF, Holland HK, Baum CM, et al. CD34+ progenitor cells from asymptomatic patients are not a major reservoir for human immunodeficiency virus-1. *Blood.* 1995;86:1749-1756.
104. Weichold FF, Zella D, Barabitskaja O, et al. Neither human immunodeficiency virus-1 (HIV-1) nor HIV-2 infects most-primitive human hematopoietic stem cells as assessed in long-term bone marrow cultures. *Blood.* 1998;91:907-915.
105. Louache F, Henri A, Bettaieb A, et al. Role of human immunodeficiency virus replication in defective in vitro growth of hematopoietic progenitors. *Blood.* 1992;80:2991-2999.
106. Nielsen SD, Jeppesen DL, Kolte L, et al. Impaired progenitor cell function in HIV-negative infants of HIV-positive mothers results in decreased thymic output and low CD4 counts. *Blood.* 2001;98:398-404.
107. Rieckmann P, Poli G, Fox CH, Kehrl JH, Fauci AS. Recombinant gp120 specifically enhances tumor necrosis factor-alpha production and Ig secretion in B lymphocytes from HIV-infected individuals but not from seronegative donors. *J Immunol.* 1991;147:2922-2927.
108. Voth R, Rossol S, Klein K, et al. Differential gene expression of IFN-alpha and tumor necrosis factor-alpha in peripheral Blood mononuclear cells from patients with AIDS related complex and AIDS. *J Immunol.* 1990;144:970-975.
109. Clouse KA, Cosentino LM, Weih KA, et al. The HIV-1 gp120 envelope protein has the intrinsic capacity to stimulate monokine secretion. *J Immunol.* 1991;147:2892-2901.
110. Lau AS, Williams BR. The role of interferon and tumor necrosis factor in the pathogenesis of AIDS. *J Exp Pathol.* 1990;5:111-122.
111. Odeh M. The role of tumour necrosis factor-alpha in the pathogenesis of complicated falciparum malaria. *Cytokine.* 2001;14:11-18.
112. Selleri C, Sato T, Anderson S, Young NS, Maciejewski JP. Interferon-gamma and tumor necrosis factor-alpha suppress both early and late stages of hematopoiesis and induce programmed cell death. *J Cell Physiol.* 1995;165:538-546.
113. Fuchs D, Reibnegger G, Werner ER, Vinazzer H, Wachter H. Low haemoglobin in haemophilia children is associated with chronic immune activation. *Acta Haematol.* 1991;85:62-65.
114. Kagi D, Vignaux F, Ledermann B, et al. Fas and perforin pathways as major mechanisms of T cell-mediated cytotoxicity. *Science.* 1994;265:528-530.
115. Karcher DS, Frost AR. The bone marrow in human immunodeficiency virus (HIV)-related disease. Morphology and clinical correlation. *Am J Clin Pathol.* 1991;95:245-252.
116. Zon LI, Arkin C, Groopman JE. Haematologic mainifestations of the human immune deficiency virus (HIV). *Br J Haematol.* 1987;66:251-256.
117. Thiele J, Titius BR, Quitmann H, et al. Megakaryocytopoiesis in bone marrow biopsies of patients with acquired immunodeficiency syndrome (AIDS). An immunohistochemical and morphometric evaluation with special emphasis on myelodysplastic features and precursor cells. *Pathol Res Pract.* 1992;188:722-728.
118. Sullivan PS, Dworkin MS, Jones JL, Hooper WC. Epidemiology of thrombosis in HIV-infected individuals. The adult/adolescent spectrum of HIV disease project. *AIDS.* 2000;14:321-324.
119. Saber AA, Aboolian A, LaRaja RD, Baron H, Hanna K. HIV/AIDS and the risk of deep vein thrombosis: a study of 45 patients with lower extremity involvement. *Am Surg.* 2001;67:645-647.
120. Saif MW, Bona R, Greenberg B. AIDS and thrombosis: retrospective study of 131 HIV-infected patients. *AIDS Patient Care STDS.* 2001;15:311-320.
121. Jacobson MC, Dezube BJ, Aboulafia DM. Thrombotic complications in patients infected with HIV in the era of highly active antiretroviral therapy: a case series. *Clin Infect Dis.* 2004;39:1214-1222.
122. Majluf-Cruz A, Silva-Estrada M, Sanchez-Barboza R, et al. Venous thrombosis among patients with AIDS. *Clin Appl Thromb Hemost.* 2004;10:19-25.
123. Fultz SL, McGinnis KA, Skanderson M, Ragni MV, Justice AC. Association of venous thromboembolism with human immunodeficiency virus and mortality in veterans. *Am J Med.* 2004;116:420-423.
124. Klein SK, Slim EJ, de Kruif MD, et al. Is chronic HIV infection associated with venous thrombotic disease? A systematic review. *Neth J Med.* 2005;63:129-136.
125. Abuaf N, Laperche S, Rajoely B, et al. Autoantibodies to phospholipids and to the coagulation proteins in AIDS. *Thromb Haemost.* 1997;77:856-861.
126. De Larranaga GF, Forastiero RR, Carreras LO, Alonso BS. Different types of antiphospholipid antibodies in AIDS: a comparison with syphilis and the antiphospholipid syndrome. *Thromb Res.* 1999;96:19-25.
127. Weiss L, You JF, Giral P, Alhenc-Gelas M, Senger D, Kazatchkine MD. Anti-cardiolipin antibodies are associated with anti-endothelial cell antibodies but not with anti-beta 2 glycoprotein I antibodies in HIV infection. *Clin Immunol Immunopathol.* 1995;77:69-74.
128. Falco M, Sorrenti A, Priori R, et al. Anti-cardiolipin antibodies in HIV infection are true antiphospholipids not associated with antiphospholipid syndrome. *Ann Ital Med Int.* 1993;8:171-174.
129. Hassell KL, Kressin DC, Neumann A, Ellison R, Marlar RA. Correlation of anti-phospholipid antibodies and protein S deficiency with thrombosis in HIV-infected men. *Blood Coagul Fibrinolysis.* 1994;5:455-462.
130. Shiels MS, Pfeiffer RM, Gail MH, et al. Cancer burden in the HIV-infected population in the United States. *J Natl Cancer Inst.* 2011;103:753-762.
131. Patel P, Hanson DL, Sullivan PS; Adult and Adolescent Spectrum of Disease Project and HIV Outpatient Study Investigators, et al. Incidence of types of cancer among HIV-infected persons compared with the general population in the United States, 1992-2003. *Ann Intern Med.* 2008;148:728-736.
132. Shiels MS, Pfeiffer RM, Hall HI, et al. Proportions of Kaposi sarcoma, selected non-Hodgkin lymphomas, and cervical cancer in the United States occurring in persons with AIDS, 1980-2007. *JAMA.* 2011;305:1450-1459.
133. D'Souza G, Wiley DJ, Li X, et al. Incidence and epidemiology of anal cancer in the multicenter AIDS cohort study. *J Acquir Immune Defic Syndr.* 2008;48:491-499.

134. Puoti M, Bruno R, Soriano V, et al; HIV HCC Cooperative Italian-Spanish Group. Hepatocellular carcinoma in HIV-infected patients: epidemiological features, clinical presentation and outcome. *AIDS*. 2004;18:2285.
135. Seaberg EC, Wiley D, Martinez-Maza O, et al; Multicenter AIDS Cohort Study (MACS). Cancer incidence in the multicenter AIDS cohort study before and during the HAART era: 1984 to 2007. *Cancer*. 2010;116:5507-5516.
136. Simard EP, Pfeiffer RM, Engels EA. Spectrum of cancer risk late after AIDS onset in the United States. *Arch Intern Med*. 2010;170:1337-1345.
137. Silverberg MJ, Neuhaus J, Bower M, et al. Risk of cancers during interrupted antiretroviral therapy in the SMART study. *AIDS*. 2007;21:1957-1963.
138. Yanik EL, Achenbach CJ, Gopal S, et al. Changes in clinical context for Kaposi's sarcoma and non-Hodgkin lymphoma among people with HIV infection in the United States. *J Clin Oncol*. 2016;34:3276-3283.
139. Nakagawa F, Lodwick RK, Smith CJ, et al. Projected life expectancy of people with HIV according to timing of diagnosis. *AIDS*. 2012;26:335-343.
140. Zoufaly A, Stellbrink HJ, Heiden MA; ClinSurv Study Group, et al. Cumulative HIV viremia during highly active antiretroviral therapy is a strong predictor of AIDS-related lymphoma. *J Infect Dis*. 2009;200(1):79-87.
141. Bower M, Fisher M, Hill T; UK CHIC Steering Committee, et al. CD4 counts and the risk of systemic non-Hodgkin's lymphoma in individuals with HIV in the UK. *Haematologica*. 2009;94:875-880.
142. Lewden C, Bouteloup V, De Wit S; The Collaboration of Observational HIV Epidemiological Research Europe (COHERE) in EuroCoord, et al. All-cause mortality in treated HIV-infected adults with CD4 ≥500/mm^3 compared with the general population: evidence from a large European observational cohort collaboration. *Int J Epidemiol*. 2012;41:433-445.
143. Silverberg MJ, Lau B, Achenbach CJ; North American AIDS Cohort Collaboration on Research and Design of the International Epidemiologic Databases to Evaluate AIDS, et al. Cumulative incidence of cancer among persons with HIV in North America: a cohort study. *Ann Intern Med*. 2015;163:507-518.
144. Howlader N, Shiels MS, Mariotto AB, Engels EA. Contributions of HIV to non-Hodgkin mortality trends in the United States. *Cancer Epidemiol Biomarkers Prev*. 2016;25:1289-1296.
145. Landgren O, Goedert J, Rabkin CS, et al. Circulating serum free light chains as predictive markers of AIDS-related lymphoma. *J Clin Oncol*. 2010;5:773-779.
146. Wolf T, Brodt HR, Fichtlscherer S, et al. Changing incidence and prognostic factors of survival in AIDS-related non-Hodgkin's lymphoma in the era of highly active antiretroviral therapy (HAART). *Leuk Lymphoma*. 2005;46:207-215.
147. Rabkin CS, Yang Q, Goedert JJ, Nguyen G, Mitsuya H, Sei S. Chemokine and chemokine receptor gene variants and risk of non-Hodgkin's lymphoma in human immunodeficiency virus-1-infected individuals. *Blood*. 1999;93:1838-1842.
148. Lawn SD, Török ME, Wood R. Optimum time to start antiretroviral therapy during HIV-associated opportunistic infections. *Curr Opin Infect Dis*. 2011;24:34-42.
149. Tirelli U, Bernardi D. Impact of HAART on the clinical management of AIDS-related cancers. *Eur J Cancer*. 2001;37:1320-1324.
150. Tan CRC, Barta SK, Lee J, Rudek MA, Sparano JA, Noy A. Combination antiretroviral therapy accelerates immune recovery in patients with HIV-related lymphoma treated with EPOCH: a comparison within one prospective trial AMC034. *Leuk Lymphoma*. 2018;59(8):1851-1860. doi:10.1080/10428194.2017.1403597
151. Carbone A, Cesarman E, Spina M, Gloghini A, Schultz TF. HIV-associated lymphomas and gamma-herpesviruses. *Blood*. 2009;113:1213-1224.
152. Piriou E, van Dort K, Nanlohy NM, van Oers MH, Miedema F, van Baarle D. Loss of EBNA1-specific memory CD4+ and CD8+ T cells in HIV-infected patients progressing to AIDS-related non-Hodgkin lymphoma. *Blood*. 2005;106:3166-3174.
153. Wang Q, De Luca A, Smith C, Zangerle R; Hepatitis coinfection and non-Hodgkin lymphoma project team for the Collaboration of Observational HIV Epidemiological Research Europe (COHERE) in EuroCoord, et al. Chronic hepatitis B and C virus infection and risk for non-Hodgkin lymphoma in HIV-infected patients: a cohort study. *Ann Intern Med*. 2017;166:9-17.
154. Martorelli D, Muraro E, Mastorci K, et al. A natural HIV p17 protein variant up-regulates the LMP-1 EBV oncoprotein and promotes the growth of EBV-infected B-lymphocytes: implications for EBV-driven lymphomagenesis in the HIV setting. *Int J Cancer*. 2015;137:1374-1385.
155. Dolcetti R, Giagulli C, He W, et al. Role of HIV-1 matrix protein p17 variants in lymphoma pathogenesis. *Proc Natl Acad Sci U S A*. 2015;112:14331-14336.
156. Hegde U, Filie A, Little RF, et al. High incidence of occult leptomeningeal disease detected by flow cytometry in newly diagnosed aggressive B-cell lymphomas at risk for central nervous system involvement: the role of flow cytometry versus cytology. *Blood*. 2005;105:496-502.
157. Barta SK, Xue X, Wang D, et al. A new prognostic score for AIDS-related lymphomas in the rituximab-era. *Haematologica*. 2014;99:1731-1737.
158. Gisselbrecht C, Oksenhendler E, Tirelli U, et al. Human immunodeficiency virus-related lymphoma treatment with intensive combination chemotherapy. French-Italian Cooperative Group. *Am J Med*. 1993;95:188-196.
159. Sparano JA, Wiernik PH, Strack M, et al. Infusional cyclophosphamide, doxorubicin and etoposide in HIV-related non-Hodgkin's lymphoma: a follow-up report of a highly active regimen. *Leuk Lymphoma*. 1994;14:263-271.
160. Sparano JA, Weller E, Nazeer T, et al. Phase 2 trial of infusional cyclophosphamide, doxorubicin, and etoposide in patients with poor-prognosis, intermediate-grade non-Hodgkin lymphoma: an Eastern Cooperative Oncology Group trial (E3493). *Blood*. 2002;100:1634-1640.
161. Little RF, Pittaluga S, Grant N, et al. Highly effective treatment of acquired immunodeficiency syndrome-related lymphoma with dose-adjusted EPOCH: impact of antiretroviral therapy suspension and tumor biology. *Blood*. 2003;101:4653-4659.
162. Sparano JA, Lee JY, Kaplan LD; AIDS Malignancy Consortium, et al. Rituximab plus concurrent infusional EPOCH chemotherapy is highly effective in HIV-associated B-cell non-Hodgkin lymphoma. *Blood*. 2010;115(15):3008-3016.
163. Barta SK, Xue X, Wang D, et al. Treatment factors affecting outcomes in HIV-associated non-Hodgkin lymphomas: a pooled analysis of 1546 patients. *Blood*. 2013;122:3251-3262.
164. Dunleavy K, Little RF, Pittaluga S, et al. The role of tumor histogenesis, FDG-PET, and short-course EPOCH with dose-dense rituximab (SC-EPOCH-RR) in HIV-associated diffuse large B-cell lymphoma. *Blood*. 2010;115(15):3017-3024. doi:10.1182/blood-2009-11-253039
165. Sparano JA, Lee JY, Kaplan LD, et al. Response-adapted therapy with infusional EPOCH chemotherapy plus rituximab in HIV-associated, B-cell non-Hodgkin's lymphoma. *Haematologica*. 2021;106(3):730-735. doi:10.3324/haematol.2019.243386
166. Ramos JC, Sparano JA, Chadburn A, et al. Impact of Myc in HIV-associated non-Hodgkin lymphomas treated with EPOCH and outcomes with vorinostat (AMC-075 trial). *Blood*. 2020;136(11):1284-1297. doi:10.1182/blood.2019003959
167. Spina M, Tirelli U. Rituximab for HIV-associated lymphoma: weighing the benefits and risks. *Curr Opin Oncol*. 2005;17:462-465.
168. Tirelli U, Spina M, Jaeger U, et al. Infusional CDE with rituximab for the treatment of human immunodeficiency virus-associated non-Hodgkin's lymphoma: preliminary results of a phase I/II study. *Recent Results Cancer Res*. 2002;159:149-153.
169. Kaplan LD, Lee JY, Ambinder RF, et al. Rituximab does not improve clinical outcome in a randomized phase 3 trial of CHOP with or without rituximab in patients with HIV-associated non-Hodgkin lymphoma: AIDS-Malignancies Consortium Trial 010. *Blood*. 2005;106:1538-1543.
170. Boue F, Gabarre J, Gisselbrecht C, et al. Phase II trial of CHOP plus rituximab in patients with HIV-associated non-Hodgkin's lymphoma. *J Clin Oncol*. 2006;24:4123-4128.
171. Navarro WH, Kaplan LD. AIDS-related lymphoproliferative disease. *Blood*. 2006;107:13-20.
172. Aboulafia DM, Ratner L, Miles SA, Harrington WJ, Jr; AIDS Associated Malignancies Clinical Trials Consortium. Antiviral and immunomodulatory treatment for AIDS-related primary central nervous system lymphoma: AIDS Malignancies Consortium pilot study 019. *Clin Lymphoma Myeloma*. 2006;6(5):399-402.
173. Omuro A, Correa DD, DeAngelis LM, et al. R-MPV followed by high-dose chemotherapy with TBC and autologous stem-cell transplant for newly diagnosed primary CNS lymphoma. *Blood*. 2015;125(9):1403-1410. doi:10.1182/blood-2014-10-604561
174. Klein U, Gloghini A, Gaidano G, et al. Gene expression profile analysis of AIDS-related primary effusion lymphoma (PEL) suggests a plasmablastic derivation and identifies PEL-specific transcripts. *Blood*. 2003;101:4115-4121.
175. Simonelli C, Spina M, Cinelli R, et al. Clinical features and outcome of primary effusion lymphoma in HIV-infected patients: a single-institution study. *J Clin Oncol*. 2003;21:3948-3954.
176. Ghosh SK, Wood C, Boise LH, et al. Potentiation of TRAIL-induced apoptosis in primary effusion lymphoma through azidothymidine-mediated inhibition of NF-kappa B. *Blood*. 2003;101(6):2321-2327.
177. Guillet S, Gérard L, Meignin V, et al. Classic and extracavitary primary effusion lymphoma in 51 HIV-infected patients from a single institution. *Am J Hematol*. 2016;91(2):233-237.
178. Wang ES, Straus DJ, Teruya-Feldstein J, et al. Intensive chemotherapy with cyclophosphamide, doxorubicin, high-dose methotrexate/ifosfamide, etoposide, and high-dose cytarabine (CODOX-M/IVAC) for human immunodeficiency virus-associated Burkitt lymphoma. *Cancer*. 2003;98:1196-1205.
179. Cortes J, Thomas D, Rios A, et al. Hyperfractionated cyclophosphamide, vincristine, doxorubicin, and dexamethasone and highly active antiretroviral therapy for patients with acquired immunodeficiency syndrome-related Burkitt lymphoma/leukemia. *Cancer*. 2002;94:1492-1499.
180. Rodrigo JA, Hicks LK, Cheung MC, et al. HIV-associated Burkitt lymphoma: good efficacy and tolerance of intensive chemotherapy including CODOX-M/IVAC with or without rituximab in the HAART era. *Adv Hematol*. 2012;2012:735392.
181. Noy A, Lee JY, Cesarman E, et al. AMC 048: modified CODOX-M/IVAC-rituximab is safe and effective for HIV-associated Burkitt lymphoma. *Blood*. 2015;126(2):160-166.
182. Dunleavy K, Pittaluga S, Shovlin M, et al. Low-intensity therapy in adults with Burkitt's lymphoma. *N Engl J Med*. 2013;369:1915-1925.
183. Roschewski M, Dunleavy K, Abramson JS, et al. Multicenter study of risk-adapted therapy with dose-adjusted EPOCH-R in adults with untreated Burkitt lymphoma. *J Clin Oncol*. 2020;38(22):2519-2529. doi:10.1200/JCO.20.00303
184. Delecluse HJ, Anagnostopoulos I, Dallenbach F, et al. Plasmablastic lymphomas of the oral cavity: a new entity associated with the human immunodeficiency virus infection. *Blood*. 1997;89(4):1413-1420.
185. Teruya-Feldstein J, Chiao E, Filippa DA, et al. CD20-negative large-cell lymphoma with plasmablastic features: a clinically heterogenous spectrum in both HIV-positive and-negative patients. *Ann Oncol*. 2004;15(11):1673-1679.
186. Noy A, Lensing SY, Moore PC, et al. Plasmablastic lymphoma is treatable in the HAART era. A 10 year retrospective by the AIDS Malignancy Consortium. *Leuk Lymphoma*. 2016;57:1731-1734.
187. Biggar RJ, Jaffe ES, Goedert JJ, et al. Hodgkin lymphoma and immunodeficiency in persons with HIV/AIDS. *Blood*. 2006;108:3786-3791.
188. Besson C, Lancar R, Prevot S, et al. High risk features contrast with favorable outcomes in HIV-associated Hodgkin lymphoma in the modern cART era, ANRS CO16 LYMPHOVIR cohort. *Clin Infect Dis*. 2015;61:1469-1475.
189. Danilov AV, Li H, Press OW, et al. Feasibility of interim positron emission tomography (PET)-adapted therapy in HIV-positive patients with advanced Hodgkin lymphoma (HL): a sub-analysis of SWOG S0816 phase 2 trial. *Leuk Lymphoma*. 2017;58:461-465.

190. Rubinstein PG, Moore P, Henry DH, Ratner L, Sharon E, Noy A. AMC-085: a pilot trial of AVD and brentuximab vedotin in the upfront treatment of stage II-IV HIV-associated Hodgkin lymphoma. A Trial of the AIDS Malignancy Consortium. *Blood*. 2015;126:1526.
191. Krishnan A, Molina A, Zaia J, et al. Durable remissions with autologous stem cell transplantation for high-risk HIV-associated lymphomas. *Blood*. 2005;105:874-878.
192. Gabarre J, Azar N, Autran B, Katlama C, Leblond V. High-dose therapy and autologous haematopoietic stem-cell transplantation for HIV-1-associated lymphoma. *Lancet*. 2000;355:1071-1072.
193. Re A, Cattaneo C, Michieli M, et al. High-dose therapy and autologous peripheral-blood stem-cell transplantation as salvage treatment for HIV-associated lymphoma in patients receiving highly active antiretroviral therapy. *J Clin Oncol*. 2003;21:4423-4427.
194. Re A, Michieli M, Casari S, et al. High-dose therapy and autologous peripheral blood stem cell transplantation as salvage treatment for AIDS-related lymphoma: long-term results of the Italian Cooperative Group on AIDS and Tumors (GICAT) study with analysis of prognostic factors. *Blood*. 2009;114:1306-1313.
195. Balsalobre P, Díez-Martín JL, Re A, et al. Autologous stem-cell transplantation in patients with HIV-related lymphoma. *J Clin Oncol*. 2009;27:2192-2198.
196. Krishnan A, Palmer JM, Zaia JA, Tsai N, Alvarnas J, Forman SJ. HIV status does not affect the outcome of autologous stem cell transplantation (ASCT) for non-Hodgkin lymphoma (NHL). *Biol Blood Marrow Transplant*. 2010;16:1302-1308.
197. Alvarnas JC, Rademacher JL, Wang Y. Autologous hematopoietic cell transplantation for HIV-related lymphoma: results of the (BMT CTN) 0803/(AMC) 071 trial. *Blood*. 2016;128:1050-1058.
198. DiGiusto DL, Krishnan A, Li L, et al. RNA-based gene therapy for HIV with lentiviral vector–modified CD34+ cells in patients undergoing transplantation for AIDS-related lymphoma. *Sci Transl Med*. 2010;2:36ra43.
199. Kang EM, De WM, Malech H, et al. Nonmyeloablative conditioning followed by transplantation of genetically modified HLA-matched peripheral Blood progenitor cells for hematologic malignancies in patients with acquired immunodeficiency syndrome. *Blood*. 2002;99:698-701.
200. Knops E, Kobbe G, Kaiser R, et al. Treatment of HIV and acute myeloid leukemia by allogeneic CCR5-d32 blood stem cell transplantation [abstract]. *J Clin Virol*. 2016;82:S86.
201. Ambinder RF, Wu J, Logan B, et al. Allogeneic hematopoietic cell transplant for HIV patients with hematologic malignancies: the BMT CTN-0903/AMC-080 trial. *Biol Blood Marrow Transplant*. 2019;25(11):2160-2166. doi:10.1016/j.bbmt.2019.06.033

Chapter 66 ▪ Disorders of the Spleen

WILLIAM C. CHAPMAN JR • WILLIAM C. CHAPMAN

INTRODUCTION

The spleen is a small, maroon, sponge-like organ found in the left upper abdominal quadrant.[1] Although there is no mention of the spleen in the Bible, it receives considerable attention in the Talmud and post-Talmudic literature. Classically identified as the seat of laughter, there has been much debate over whether the spleen is truly necessary.[2] It is said that Galen called it an "organ full of mystery" as early as the 2nd century AD. Although we have come to understand much about the structure and function of the spleen since those times, much of what intrigued Galen still remains a mystery today. The spleen has been classified into different organ systems including the circulatory, hematopoietic, mononuclear phagocyte, and lymphatic systems. However, it is probably most accurate to describe the spleen as a clearinghouse for circulating cellular elements—a place where multiple organ systems converge in both structure and function.

DEVELOPMENT AND ANATOMY

The spleen is derived from embryonic mesoderm. The developing organ first becomes apparent during the fifth week of gestation as mesodermal cells coalesce between the leaflets of the dorsal mesogastrium, posterior to the developing stomach. While the origin of the splenic progenitor mesenchymal tissue remains debated, current evidence points to the pancreatic bud as its initial site of proliferation. Around week 5 of gestation, the splenic mesenchyme separates from the pancreatic bud and migrates into the left upper quadrant.[3] As development continues, independent lobules enveloped by mesogastrium become evident. In time, they fuse to form a multilobulated mass that eventually differentiates into a well-formed organ by late fetal life.[4] Occasionally, a stray lobule may fail to fuse with the others, develop independently, and give rise to an accessory spleen, a functioning mass of splenic tissue set apart from the body of the organ proper. The mesogastrium enveloping the lobules eventually gives rise to the organ's capsule and trabecular skeleton, and the posterior and anterior attachments give rise to the primary supporting structures: the splenorenal and gastrosplenic ligaments, respectively.[5] The colonization of the cellular elements of the spleen occurs first with the erythroid and myeloid progenitors, followed by the first hematopoietic stem cells. Finally, lymphoid-tissue-inducer cells are observed and provide the necessary local cellular signals to trigger the unique architecture of the splenic cellular elements. This development is highly similar to that of lymph nodes.

Gross Anatomy

Grossly, the spleen may appear in a variety of shapes. It may be wedge shaped (44%), tetrahedral (42%), or triangular (14%), depending on its relationships with the stomach, left kidney, pancreas, and colon. The average adult spleen measures 13 to 15 cm in length, 8 to 10 cm in width, and 4 cm in thickness, with a weight up to 250 g and a corresponding blood volume of ~300 mL. However, the size of the spleen varies with age, immunologic status, and nutritional status.[1]

The nonperfused organ appears purplish in color with a solid, sponge-like texture throughout. It is covered by a fibrous connective tissue capsule that is 1.5 mm thick and composed of collagen and elastin fibers.[1] This capsule surrounds all but the hilum of the spleen.[5] Continuous with the capsule, involutions penetrate the body of the organ to form trabeculae, the fibrous supporting skeleton of the spleen. Finally, a serosal membrane, derived from peritoneum, covers the organ externally and adheres to the capsule. This mesothelial membrane covers the entire organ except at its hilum and the reflections of its primary supporting ligaments.[1]

In the majority of people, the spleen is divided into the superior lobe and the inferior lobe, but further division into subsegmental lobes can be seen. Avascular planes separate each lobe, which are defined by discrete, non–anastomosing circulatory pathways.[1,4]

Location and Relationships

The spleen is located in the left upper quadrant of the abdominal cavity, posteriorly, at the level of the ninth to eleventh thoracic vertebrae. The superior, or diaphragmatic, surface of the organ is convex in shape, smooth, and abuts the left hemidiaphragm superiorly, whereas the inferior, or visceral, surface is somewhat triangular and is intimately associated with the splenic flexure of the colon, greater curve of the stomach, and tail of the pancreas.[1,5]

The medial portion of the spleen is concave and divided by a longitudinal ridge into a gastric surface anteriorly and a renal surface posteriorly. The gastric surface contains the hilum of the organ and relates to the fundus of the stomach and the tail of the pancreas. The tail of the pancreas lies in close approximation to the splenic hilum, contributing to the risk of pancreatic injury in patients undergoing splenectomy.[6] The renal surface borders the superolateral surface of the left kidney and left adrenal gland. *Figure 66.1* shows the gross appearance of the spleen as well as its relationship to the adjacent pancreatic tail and branch vessels of the splenic artery.

The spleen is supported by a number of suspensory ligaments: the splenorenal posteriorly, the gastrosplenic anteromedially, the splenophrenic superiorly, and the splenocolic inferiorly.[1] The splenorenal and gastrosplenic ligaments provide the majority of support to the organ and are considered primary. The splenorenal ligament supports the organ posteriorly and serves as a conduit for the organ's neurovascular bundle, whereas the gastrosplenic ligament stabilizes the spleen anteromedially to the greater curvature of the stomach and contains the short gastric and gastroepiploic vessels. The other ligaments of the spleen play a secondary role in the support of the organ and are generally avascular.[1,5,6] However, in certain pathologic states, such as portal hypertension, significant collateral circulation through these planes may occur.

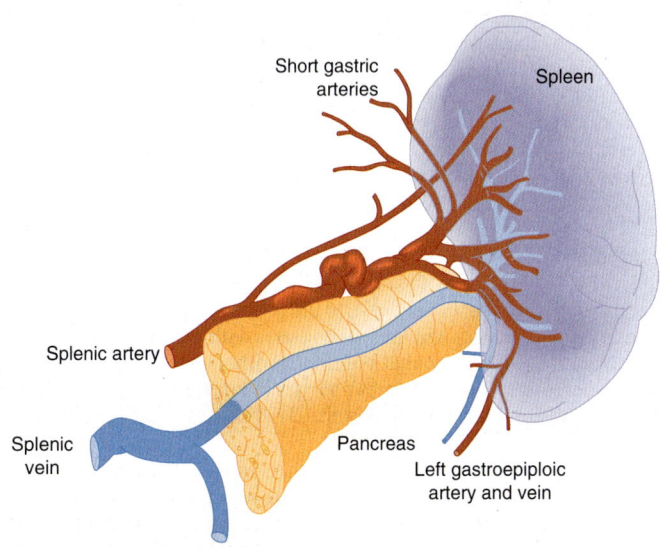

FIGURE 66.1 Illustration of the spleen and relationship to the adjacent pancreatic tail and branch vessels of the splenic artery and vein. (Redrawn and modified from Cameron JL, ed. *Atlas of Surgery*. Mosby, Inc; 1994. Copyright © 1994 Elsevier. With permission.)

Vascular Supply

The spleen is a highly perfused organ. Although it represents only ~0.2% of the total body weight, it receives >5% of the total cardiac output.[7] The main blood supply to the spleen is through the highly variable splenic artery, which delivers 250 to 300 mL of arterial blood per minute. It arises as a branch of the aorta's celiac trunk in the midline and follows a tortuous course to the left, enveloped within the splenorenal ligament, to supply the organ.[1]

The splenic artery is a highly unpredictable vessel that displays variations in course and dimension. In 95% of the population, it travels along the upper border of the pancreas, but it may also travel in front of, within, or behind the pancreatic tissue. Along its tortuous course, the splenic artery gives rise to the left gastroepiploic artery and the short gastric arteries, both of which run within the gastrosplenic ligament. At its terminal end, the splenic artery branches into a number of smaller arteries, or segmental branches, before penetrating the hilum of the organ. Two dominant patterns of splenic artery branching are referred to as magistral (30% of the population) and distributed (70% of all-comers); while the magistral pattern is organized and results in polar and terminal branching at the hilum, distributed patterns result in irregular branches arising further from the root of the organ.[6] These smaller arteries are also highly variable but are most often four in number and include the superior polar, superior middle, inferior middle, and inferior polar splenic arteries. The segmental branches penetrate the organ by traveling within the trabeculae (sheaths of fibrous connective tissue derived from the involution of the spleen's fibrous capsule) and ramify within the body of the organ. Additional sources of arterial blood to the spleen include direct tributaries and collateral circulation provided by branches of the pancreatic and short gastric arteries.[1,5]

Venous drainage is facilitated primarily by the splenic vein. It is formed by the coalescence of the segmental splenic veins, as they leave the hilum of the organ, and the left gastroepiploic vein. Occasionally, short gastric veins may also participate. The splenic vein courses toward the midline along the superior border of the pancreas, where it joins the superior mesenteric vein to form the portal vein. Along the way, the splenic vein receives venous tributaries from the pancreas and, in 60% of cases, also receives the inferior mesenteric vein.[1,5]

Lymphatics

The spleen, which is considered by many to be a lymphatic organ, has no afferent lymphatics, yet a significant amount of lymph fluid is expressed by the organ and drains via efferent vessels that form around the arterioles. The lymphatics travel with the neurovascular bundle through the trabeculae, exiting at the hilum.[4] In turn, the lymphatic fluid is directed toward the nodes of the splenic hilum, the splenic artery, and the pancreas (the pancreatico-splenic nodes), eventually terminating at the nodes of the celiac axis.[5]

Innervation

The spleen is innervated by fibers of the sympathetic nervous system which originate at the level of T-6 to T-8 and travel with the greater thoracic splanchnic nerve to the celiac ganglion.[8] From there, they pass to the organ via the arterial tree, with resulting vasomotor function.[1] It is believed that, similar to other mammals, the autonomic nervous system regulates changes in spleen volume, resulting in the expulsion of stored red blood cells during times of physiologic stress.[9,10]

Of interest are studies that relate the sympathetic innervation of the spleen to the immune system.[11] These studies suggest that catecholaminergic terminals penetrate the lymphocytic white pulp of the spleen, and that the innervation is plastic and able to be remodeled depending on the host's current immune state.[12] While the direct mechanism for sympathetic communication with lymphocytes remains unclear, increasing evidence suggests that these hard-wired connections may mediate a number of immunomodulatory effects including stress-induced immunosuppression.[13,14]

Benign Anatomic Variants

Accessory Spleen

An accessory spleen is a functioning lobule of splenic tissue set apart from the body of the spleen proper. It is an anatomic variant present in 10% to 30% of the general population and appears to be found with greater frequency in patients with hematologic disorders. *Figure 66.2* shows a typical example of an accessory spleen.

These supernumerary organs arise during embryologic development when an encapsulated lobule of precursor cells fails to fuse with others forming the spleen proper; they are solitary in ~88% but can be multiple in 10% of cases.[15] In the majority of cases, accessory spleens receive their blood supply from a tributary of the splenic artery and are found most often near the hilum of the organ or within one of the primary supporting ligaments. However, they may be found within secondary supporting ligaments or within the greater omentum or even in as remote a location as the pelvis of the female or the scrotum of the male.[16] They may be mistaken for malignancy on imaging studies, such as computed tomography (CT) or endoscopic ultrasound.

Because accessory spleens perform the same functions as the spleen proper, they are subject to the same pathologic conditions that affect the parent organ. Therefore, they may enlarge after splenectomy, causing a relapse of the disease process for which the spleen was removed. The presence of an unrecognized accessory spleen can account for failure of certain surgical procedures such as splenectomy for immune thrombocytopenic purpura (ITP).[8,9,17,18] In patients who continue to have thrombocytopenia after splenectomy, a search for a missed accessory spleen should be considered. Diagnosis may be made using abdominal sonography, CT, magnetic resonance imaging, nuclear scintigraphy, or Doppler sonography.[19]

Splenosis

In addition to accessory spleen, extrasplenic tissue may occur via traumatic autotransplantation in the form of splenosis—the migration and subsequent proliferation of dislodged splenic tissue. While most commonly occurring in the abdomen, splenosis may also be found in the pelvis, the thorax, of even the subcutaneous tissue of the trunk.[20-22] Histologic examination of ectopic splenic tissue reveals the same elements of the parent organ: white pulp, red pulp, and marginal zones. It follows, therefore, that such tissue should preserve at least some

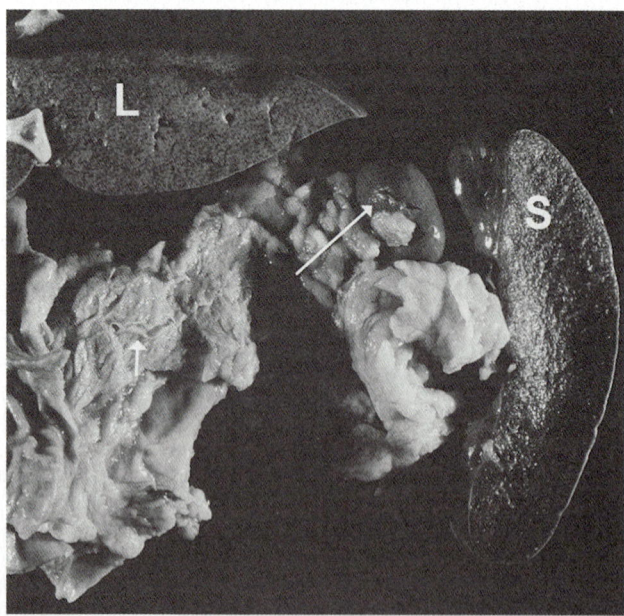

FIGURE 66.2 Autopsy photograph demonstrating accessory spleen (large arrow) and its relationship to the splenic hilum, pancreas (small arrow), and adjacent liver. L, liver; S, spleen. (Photograph provided by Hedi Wingard, MD, Department of Pathology, Vanderbilt University Medical Center.)

splenic function. Indeed, it has been observed that postsplenectomy patients with splenosis do retain the ability to clear erythrocytes of Howell-Jolly inclusion bodies.[21,23] However, it has not been demonstrated that this provides sufficient protection from post–splenectomy infectious complications, and the practice of splenic tissue reimplantation after splenectomy is obsolete.[24]

Wandering Spleen

Wandering, or ectopic, spleen refers to migration of the spleen from its normal location in the left upper quadrant. With an incidence of <0.5% in splenectomy series, the major complication of an ectopic spleen is torsion, either acutely or chronically. Signs and symptoms include vague or chronic abdominal discomfort and a tender abdominal mass; CT assessment of viability and degree of ischemia on exploration typically determines definitive treatment with either splenectomy or splenopexy.[25]

Microscopic Anatomy

Splenic tissue is supported by a scaffold of trabeculae, a dense, fibrous connective-tissue skeleton that gives rise to an intrasplenic meshwork of collagen fibers. Vascular elements enter the spleen at the hilum, branch through the trabeculae, and penetrate the body of the organ to supply the microcirculation.[1] As the arterial elements enter the parenchyma, they become surrounded by an aggregate of lymphoid tissue, which follows vessels in a sheath-like distribution. Aggregates of lymphoid tissue are collectively called the white pulp. White pulp may be arranged in this coaxial fashion, or it may appear as isolated follicles within the parenchyma of the organ. The balance of splenic tissue beneath the capsule is known as the red pulp. It is composed of vascular, circulatory, and mononuclear phagocytic elements. Additionally, an intermediate region can be observed at the junction between the white and red pulp; it is known as the marginal zone. Nerves and lymphatics follow the distribution of the larger vessels throughout the body of the organ.[1]

White Pulp

The white pulp structure resembles that of a lymph node, with organized T-cell and B-cell compartments surrounding branching arterial vessels. The organization of the cellular elements within the white pulp is created and maintained by local chemokine gradients specific to T- and B-cells.[4,9] White pulp may be observed in one of two arrangements: a periarteriolar lymphatic sheath (PALS) or a lymphoid follicle. The PALS is a collection of T lymphocytes that surrounds intraparenchymal arterioles and follows these vessels in a coaxial fashion for several millimeters throughout their terminal distribution. Within the PALS, T-cells interact with dendritic cells and passing B-cells. The lymphoid follicles are spherical collections of B-lymphocytes. These follicles are usually distributed along the length of the PALS in an eccentric fashion and house-activated B-cells undergoing clonal expansion.[7]

Red Pulp

The red pulp represents approximately three-fourths of the splenic volume and is composed primarily of vascular elements surrounded by a fibrocellular reticulum that contains mononuclear phagocytic cell lines and circulating elements of blood in transit.[1] The chief vascular component of the red pulp is the splenic sinus, a preliminary venous element whose structure is unique to this organ. The sinus is composed of an incomplete lining of elongated endothelial cells surrounded by a highly fenestrated basement membrane. The structure is supported externally by reticulin fibers wrapped in a transverse fashion. These stress fibers also have actin- and myosin-like filaments that regulate the porosity of the sinus. The unique architecture of the splenic sinus has been compared to the structure of a wooden barrel, with the elongated endothelial cells resembling the wooden staves and the external reticulin fibers representing the metal hoops.[4]

The splenic sinuses permeate the surrounding fibrocellular reticulum that supports them. Two-dimensional histologic observation reveals an intervening reticulum arranged in cords called splenic cords or cords of Billroth.[1] These cords actually are a three-dimensional meshwork of densely packed elements (fibroblasts, collagen fibers, and cells of the mononuclear phagocytic lines). Terminal arterioles and capillaries deliver circulating blood to this meshwork that percolates through the cord toward the sinuses. Thus, circulating elements of blood in transit are also packed within the cords: erythrocytes, platelets, macrophages, lymphocytes, plasma cells, and granulocytes.[1,4,7]

Marginal Zone

The marginal zone is a transitional region between the white and red pulp and contains both lymphocytic and mononuclear phagocytic elements. Within this transitional zone, three distinct regions can be identified. Moving from white to red pulp are the marginal sinus, the marginal zone proper, and the perimarginal cavernous sinus plexus.[4]

The marginal sinus is a vascular sinus that surrounds the white pulp and is a region where arterioles terminate into an anastomosing complex of vascular spaces. External to the marginal sinus is the marginal zone. This transitional region contains elements of both white and red pulp and is where much of the circulating blood is presented to lymphocytic and mononuclear phagocytic cells.[4] *Figure 66.3* illustrates a schematic view of the microcirculation within the spleen.

Many different cell types reside in the marginal zone. The structural foundation is a framework of reticular fibroblasts which is continuous with the reticular fibroblasts of the red pulp and the cells lining the marginal sinus. The marginal zone macrophage, metallophilic macrophage, and B-cell are the key cell types in this transitional zone. The marginal zone B-cell is a specialized subset of B-cells that differ phenotypically and functionally from follicular B-cells and are considered a bridge between the innate and adaptive immune systems.[10] Interactions between these cells are key in the marginal zone's organization and integrity. Many transient cells pass through this area as they circulate into the red pulp and back into the blood stream. Diapedesis of lymphocytes and dendritic cells occurs through a barrier cell layer from the marginal sinus into the white pulp; however, the exact mechanism of this localization remains unknown.[10,26]

Microvasculature

As the splenic artery approaches the body of the organ, it divides into a series of branches, the proper splenic arteries. On average, four proper splenic arteries then enter the organ at the hilum and branch into trabecular arteries, so named because they run within the framework of the fibrous connective tissue skeleton, the trabeculae. Trabecular arteries leave the fibrous trabeculae and penetrate the parenchyma by branching into central arteries that immediately become surrounded by a cuff of white pulp, the PALS.[4,7]

As the central arteries pass through the white pulp, they give off lateral branches at right angles, most of which terminate in and supply the marginal sinuses, and others that terminate within the marginal zone or red

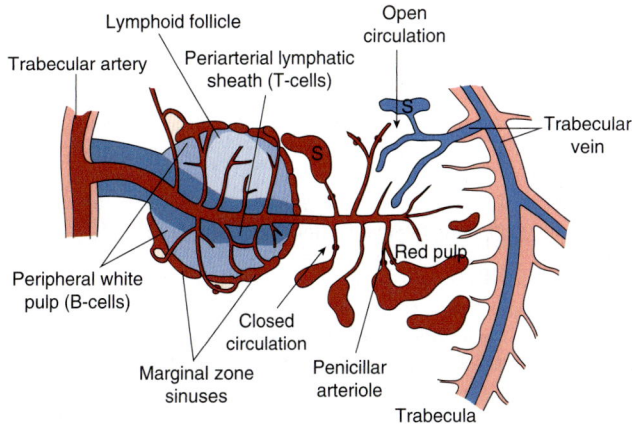

FIGURE 66.3 Schematic illustration of the microcirculation of the spleen. S, splenic sinus. (Redrawn and modified from Greep RO, ed. *The Spleen*. McGraw-Hill; 1966.)

pulp.[7] The right angle by which these lateral tributaries branch off from the central artery is thought to mediate a plasma-skimming effect that functions to hemoconcentrate the blood with a greater number of cellular elements.[27] This skimming effect may also help regulate plasma volume.

Central arteries continue from the white pulp sheath through the marginal zone and eventually terminate in the red pulp, giving off additional lateral branches along the way that are known as penicillar arterioles.[1] The penicillar arterioles, which are named for their resemblance to *Penicillium* molds, terminate in one of three fashions. They may circle back and supply the marginal sinus; they may terminate in the red pulp, supplying the splenic cords; and a minority may terminate directly into the venous sinuses for direct venous return. Eventually, the central artery itself terminates within the red pulp.[27]

Circulating elements of splenic blood flow begin their return to the venous system by first entering the splenic sinuses. Flow may enter the sinuses directly from arterial connections in a closed circulatory fashion. Alternatively, plasma and blood cells may reach the sinuses only after percolating through the reticulum of the parenchyma in an open circulatory fashion. Eventually, the venous sinuses coalesce and drain into trabecular veins that give rise to the segmental veins and, finally, the splenic vein.[27]

The exact details of splenic microcirculation remain elusive despite much research since its first description in 1901. The currently accepted models that describe the flow of blood through the vessels of the spleen discuss this in terms of the pathway, or route, and kinetics, or speed of flow. Closed circulation implies that blood passes directly from artery to capillary to vein. In terms of the spleen, blood traveling along a closed circulatory path follows the terminal arterioles to capillaries and, eventually, into the venous sinuses. Indeed, such direct connections have been observed.[27] The term "open circulation" implies that cells and plasma circulate outside of endothelium-lined vascular channels. As it pertains to the spleen, circulating blood may follow one of two open pathways. Passing through the endothelium-lined marginal sinus, blood traverses the white pulp and drains into the open-ended sinuses of the perimarginal cavernous sinus plexus. Or, it may leave penicillar arterioles that terminate in stroma of the red pulp, traverse the splenic cords, and re-enter the venous sinuses through their fenestrations.[7,27,28]

Another model for discussing splenic microcirculation describes it in terms of kinetics or speed of flow.[1,27] Accordingly, intrasplenic circulation may be fast, intermediate, or slow, traversing the organ in seconds, minutes, or hours.[1] Fast flow, which accounts for approximately 90% of total flow, follows the open circulation of the marginal zone and, to a lesser extent, the closed circulation of direct arterial, capillary, and sinus connections. Intermediate flow composes approximately 9% of splenic circulation and facilitates red blood cell processing, known as pitting and culling. Finally, around 1% of splenic flow is comprised of a slow-moving pool of reticulocytes thought to be undergoing final maturation.[7]

SPLENIC FUNCTION

The functions of the spleen are best understood in terms of its unique structure. Composed of several different tissue types, it functions as a unique lymphoid organ where elements of the circulatory, reticuloendothelial, and immune systems interact. Thus, it is ideally suited to play a critical role in the surveillance, filtration, and storage of circulating blood. Additionally, the spleen may have a number of other responsibilities, including hematopoiesis, hemoglobin degradation and iron recovery, and plasma volume regulation.

Circulating Blood Filtration

One of the primary functions of the spleen is to filter blood. Elements removed from circulation by the spleen include aging or abnormal red blood cells, erythrocyte inclusions, and foreign particulate matter.[4]

Culling

Culling, or the removal of aging or abnormal red blood cells by the spleen, occurs within the cords of Billroth by three likely mechanisms. First, cells bound for destruction become trapped within the reticulum meshwork and, as their splenic transit time increases, undergo phagocytosis by resident macrophages. Second, as erythrocytes age, they lose significant amounts of cytoplasmic membrane. Senescent cells therefore lack the deformability necessary to negotiate the meshwork and ultimately become trapped. Morphologically abnormal red blood cells, such as in congenital disorders like sickle cell anemia and hereditary spherocytosis, are also destroyed by this process. Third, self-directed antibodies bind to aging red blood cells with increasing frequency. Once opsonized with antibody, senescent cells are easily trapped by cordal macrophages and destroyed.[4,7,29]

Pitting

In addition to culling, the spleen also cleanses intraerythrocyte inclusions from circulating red blood cells. The ability of the spleen to clear these inclusions while maintaining the integrity of the red blood cell itself is known as pitting and is an exclusive function of splenic tissue.

Undesirable intracellular elements removed by the spleen include circulating particulate matter, Heinz bodies (denatured hemoglobin), Howell-Jolly bodies (nuclear remnants), and Pappenheimer bodies (iron granules). Pitting occurs as cells within the cords attempt to re-enter the circulation through the splenic sinuses. To do this, they must pass through slit-like fenestrations of the sinus endothelium. As this occurs, the deformable portion of the cell bends to negotiate the opening, whereas the inclusion, which is nondeformable, is unable to pass through the narrow passage; thus, it is left behind to be phagocytized by resident macrophages. The passage of red blood cells through the slits is mediated by active changes within the sinus endothelial cell stress fibers. These cells have been shown to have cytoskeletons that include the contractile protein components actin and myosin.[4,29] *Figure 66.4* is a schematic representation of the process of pitting.

As expected, asplenic and hyposplenic patients lose their ability to clear damaged red blood cells and intraerythrocyte inclusion bodies from the circulation. These patients display peripheral blood smears with an abnormal variety of erythrocytes, many with intracellular inclusions. In fact, determining the percentage of pitted erythrocytes is a well-established method of assessing splenic function.[29]

Clearance of Particulate Matter

Another important filtering function of the spleen is its ability to remove particulate matter from the circulation. As blood travels through the meshwork of the cords, foreign particles are exposed to splenic macrophages that clear them by phagocytosis.[30]

Immune Function

Because the spleen is composed of lymphocytic tissue, circulatory elements, and mononuclear phagocytic cell lines, it is ideally suited to modulate both nonspecific as well as specific immune function. The nonspecific immune functions of the spleen include the clearance of pathogens, the clearance of opsonized erythrocytes and platelets, and the production of complement. The ability of the spleen to clear blood-borne microorganisms and debris combined with its highly organized lymphoid compartment makes the spleen the most important organ for antibacterial and antifungal immune reactivity.[7,30]

The spleen plays a significant role in the removal of blood-borne pathogens from the circulation. Once coated with complement, bacteria and viruses become circulating immune complexes.[30] Although the liver clears some of these complexes, many others are delivered to the spleen and eliminated by marginal zone cells expressing specific receptors including pattern-recognition receptors, C-type lectin SIGNR1, and type 1 scavenger receptor MARCO.[31] Marginal zone metallophilic macrophages also function to concentrate pathogens in the spleen, leading to their opsonization, and produce high levels of interferon-α and interferon-β after viral exposure. Marginal zone B-cells are specialized to detect circulating pathogens, after which they rapidly differentiate into immunoglobulin (Ig) M producing plasma cells or antigen presenting cells capable of $CD4^+$ T-cell activation. The contribution of the spleen to this process is supported by the fact that asplenic patients display a higher level of circulating immune complexes than do spleen-competent subjects.[26]

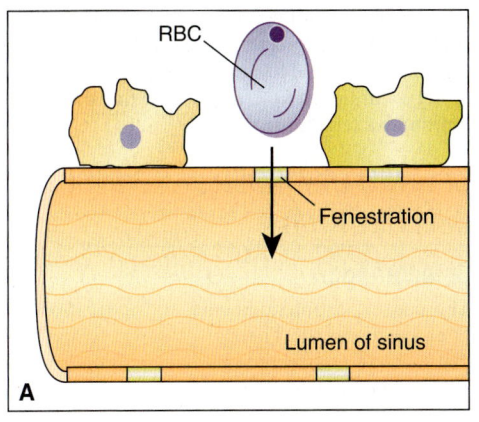
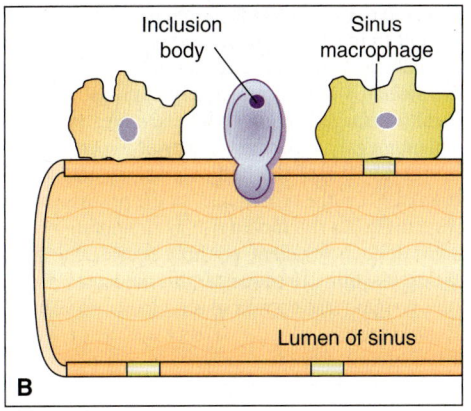
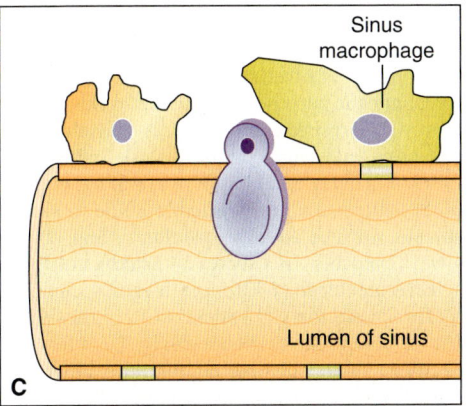
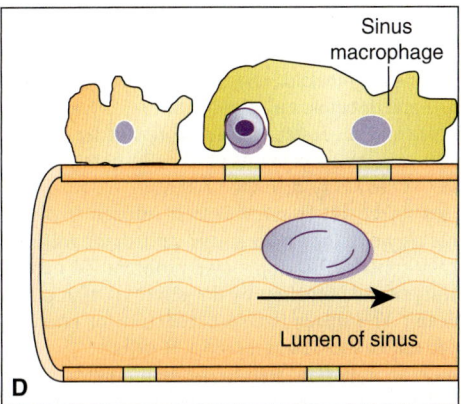

FIGURE 66.4 **Schematic representation of process of pitting by the spleen.** This process is believed to be responsible for removal of undesirable elements from circulation, including particulate matter, Heinz bodies (denatured hemoglobin), Howell-Jolly bodies (nuclear remnants), and Pappenheimer bodies (iron granules). A, Red blood cell (RBC) flows from open circulation and approaches fenestration of sinus. B, RBC begins to enter sinus through fenestration; note inclusion body within RBC. C, RBC transverses sinus; membrane-bound inclusion body lags behind. Sinus macrophage begins to approach inclusion body. D, RBC within sinus returns to venous circulation. Inclusion body succumbs to sinus macrophage. (Modified from Weintraub LR. Splenectomy: who, when, and why? *Hosp Pract.* 1994;29(6):27-34. Reprinted by permission of Taylor & Francis Ltd. http://www.tandfonline.com)

The ability of the spleen to clear encapsulated bacteria is especially significant. Because these organisms have the ability to evade antibody and complement binding, their clearance depends on prolonged contact between pathogen and macrophage. It is well recognized that asplenic or hyposplenic patients are prone to a syndrome of fulminant septicemia, most often involving encapsulated bacteria (see section Overwhelming Postsplenectomy Infection).[29]

The spleen also plays a major role in the removal of opsonized erythrocytes and platelets from the circulation. In certain pathologic states, such as autoimmune hemolytic anemia or ITP, circulating elements become opsonized with IgG antibody. The resulting cell-antibody complexes enter the spleen and encounter Fc receptor-laden macrophages in the marginal zone, where they are destroyed.[4]

Several proteins and glycoproteins of the complement system are synthesized by mononuclear phagocytic cells in the spleen, namely properdin and tuftsin. Properdin is an opsonin that plays a critical role in the alternative pathway and has been detected in spleen monocytes. Tuftsin stimulates interleukin-1 production and binds to granulocytes to initiate phagocytosis.[4] Although these elements are also produced by extrasplenic tissues, the spleen's significant contribution is demonstrated by the lower concentrations found in the circulation of asplenic or hyposplenic patients. Patients who have lost their spleens also display a decreased concentration of C3 and factor B.[32]

Specific Immune Response

The spleen is also uniquely suited to play a coordinating role in the specific arm of the immune response. Because white pulp and vascular elements lie adjacent to each other, this may serve as an interface between the lymphocytic populations of T- and B-cells and the elements of circulating blood.

As circulating blood enters the spleen, 90% of it passes through the marginal sinuses and surrounding zones. Here, foreign antigens inoculate the lymphocytic tissue of the PALS and follicles, stimulating them to respond. After antigen-specific differentiation in the white pulp follicles, plasmablasts migrate to the bridging channels of the marginal zone within the red pulp.[33] The anatomic localization of the plasmablasts in the spleen resembles that found in lymph nodes. Antibodies produced at this location rapidly enter the circulation.

The spleen also plays an important role in the induction of cell-mediated immunity. Once activated, antigen-presenting cells enter the white pulp, resulting in the activation of T-cells. Activated T-cells then localize to the periphery of the B-cell follicles where costimulatory signals are exchanged, resulting in B-cell isotype switching in the follicle. These activated B-cells then either migrate to the marginal zone or remain in the germinal center. Although these functions also occur within lymph nodes, white pulp uniquely collects antigen from the blood and is therefore maximally positioned to respond to blood-borne pathogens. Nodal tissue, on the other hand, relies on lymph for antigen presentation.[34,35]

Cellular Reservoir Function

The ability of the spleen to function as a reservoir for circulating blood elements has been the subject of much study. Platelet sequestration by the spleen is well documented.[36] Newer evidence supports the spleen as a primary site of production and a reservoir for white blood cells as well.[4]

The spleen is considered a reservoir for platelets because it can sequester large quantities of thrombocytes and, in turn, release them on demand. In nonpathologic states, the spleen sequesters ~30% of the body's platelets and can release them into the circulation in response to certain stimuli. For example, in response to an increase in circulating catecholamines, the spleen releases significant numbers of sequestered leukocytes and thrombocytes into the circulation.[37]

This function of the spleen is most dramatically demonstrated by the fact that pathologically enlarged spleens sequester greater quantities of platelets. In splenomegaly secondary to portal hypertension, the organ can sequester up to 90% of the body's reserves and result in severe thrombocytopenia.[38] On the other hand, in the postoperative period after splenectomy, there is a significant rise in circulating platelet counts. Sometimes this effect is transient, possibly because the liver compensates by increasing its ability to sequester thrombocytes.[36]

The spleen also stores a significant portion of red blood cell volume during times of inactivity, reducing blood viscosity and heart workload.[39] Increases in the hematocrit after exercise reproducibly occur secondary to release of erythrocytes from the spleen. Splenic volume and the retention of erythrocytes in the splenic sinuses is thought to be mediated through the contractility of the stress fibers supporting the splenic sinuses.[4] The mechanism of splenic volume change likely involves both direct innervation by autonomic fibers as well as the hormonal effects of catecholamines.[13] α-Adrenergic blockade abolishes the responses of the spleen to norepinephrine and direct neural stimulation.[11]

The ability to produce and sequester various groups of leukocytes allows the spleen to act as a mediator between the different arms of the immune response.[14] One study has shown that as blood enters the spleen, lymphocytes selectively migrate to their respective zones: T-cells to the lymphatic tissue of the PALS and B-cells to the follicles and red pulp. Mitogen-stimulated B-lymphocyte proliferation can be upregulated in the setting of inflammation by the serotonin-rich platelets located in the spleen.[4] The spleen is also a reservoir for granulocytes, readily mobilized under stress, and memory B-cells.

The spleen also plays an important role in the coordination of the cellular innate immune response. Large numbers of innate immune cells including undifferentiated myeloid cells reside in the spleen and greatly outnumber those found in active circulation. These myeloid cells cluster in the cords of the subcapsular red pulp and can be released in response to injury, inflammation, and sepsis to regulate the host's immune response.[40] Interestingly, this population of undifferentiated myeloid cells has been implicated as an important mediator of tumor-induced immune suppression. In cancer patients, these cells have been termed myeloid-derived suppressor cells and are upregulated in the spleen and peripheral circulation. The degree of this upregulation correlates to the disease stage.[41]

Erythropoietic Function

The spleen produces red blood cells during fetal development and during certain pathologic states. During the fifth month of fetal development, it is a major source of red blood cell production, after which it loses this ability. Pathologic states associated with splenic hematopoiesis include myeloid metaplasia. However, the production of cells by the spleen under these abnormal conditions results not from the reactivation of fetal stem cells but from displaced bone marrow cells that take up residence in the confines of the organ.[12]

Iron Metabolism

As red blood cells are destroyed within the splenic cords, their contents are degraded in the phagolysosome of sinusoid macrophages. The hemoglobin is recycled into heme and sent to the bone marrow for use in the manufacture of new erythrocytes or stored as ferritin. Large complexes of ferritin form into hemosiderin, both of which can be mobilized into the circulation during times of iron deficiency.[42] The spleen's storage ability of iron is clearly demonstrated by the fact that asplenic patients display lower serum iron levels for a considerable amount of time after splenectomy.[29]

The spleen also scavenges hemoglobin released from intravascular destruction of erythrocytes. Intravascular hemoglobin is rapidly bound by haptoglobin, which is removed in the spleen through a receptor-mediated endocytosis directed by CD163, a hemoglobin-specific receptor on the surface of macrophages.[43]

The ability to scavenge for iron also plays an important antibacterial role. Iron is a necessary nutrient for many bacterial pathogens that secrete siderophores to compete for iron in host serum and tissues. Specialized macrophages in the red pulp of the spleen can be stimulated by these bacteria through toll-like receptors resulting in the secretion of lipocalin-2, a molecule that complexes with siderophores, limiting bacterial growth.[44]

SPLENIC DISORDERS AND INDICATIONS FOR SPLENECTOMY

Splenomegaly

The causes of splenomegaly and indications for splenectomy can often be confusing. There are many potential causes of splenomegaly that must be considered in any patient undergoing evaluation with an unknown diagnosis. Patients without a known cause of splenomegaly should rarely undergo splenectomy, and then only after a thorough workup has been completed to assess the likely etiology of this finding.

Splenomegaly is often secondary to another condition, not a primary pathologic state. The spleen rarely harbors a primary malignancy not apparent at other sites. The temptation to perform a splenectomy for diagnostic purposes early in the workup of the stable patient should be strongly resisted. It is unlikely to yield a diagnosis, and, in some situations, may entail significant risk to the patient with no benefit (as in splenomegaly resulting from portal hypertension).

Splenic size is not a reliable guide to splenic function; palpable spleens are not always pathologic, and abnormal spleens are not always palpable. In a survey of healthy college athletes, over 7% had spleens greater than 13 cm in length, technically meeting size criteria for splenectomy.[45] Patients with cirrhosis and portal hypertension almost always have splenomegaly. Therefore, consideration for splenectomy should involve additional evaluation of abnormal splenic function and the responsible etiology.[46]

Chauffard introduced the concept of hypersplenism in 1907, although the exact clinical definition remains confusing in practice.[47] The criteria for this diagnosis generally include four features: cytopenia with anemia, thrombocytopenia, leukopenia, or some combination; compensatory bone marrow hyperplasia; splenomegaly; and improvement or resolution in these findings after splenectomy. Given the nonspecific nature of this diagnosis and uncertainties regarding its therapeutic implications, it is used less often today.

Perhaps a more useful guide in the assessment of splenomegaly is to consider the mechanisms responsible for the splenic enlargement. The causes of splenomegaly are classically divided into six major categories, listed in *Table 66.1*.[48] The likely mechanisms for resulting cytopenias in specific disease states are shown in *Table 66.2*. Interestingly, the degree of splenomegaly does not appear to correlate with the magnitude of cytopenia. Overall, splenectomy is rarely recommended for treatment of otherwise undifferentiated splenomegaly.

Immune Thrombocytopenic Purpura

ITP is an acquired, isolated thrombocytopenia in which circulating antiplatelet antibodies bind to platelets, triggering clearance by phagocytic cells (see Chapter 48).[49] The humoral cause of the disease was established in 1951, when a hematologist-in-training infused himself with the plasma from a patient with ITP and developed thrombocytopenia and platelet destruction. Today, between 40% and 80% of patients with ITP have identified autoantibodies to platelet-specific glycoproteins, including GPIIb/IIIa and GPIb/IX.[50] In addition, dendritic cells with upregulated costimulatory molecules appear to play a major role in the pathophysiology of the disease through the enhancement of B-cell and T-cell responses to platelets.[51] The spleen likely has a dual role in this disease by both producing IgG and providing the location for removal of platelets from the circulatory system.

ITP most commonly presents in women in their 20s and 30s, often presenting with bleeding after minor trauma. There are typically few additional physical findings, and importantly, the spleen is frequently normal in size. The primary laboratory abnormality is thrombocytopenia with platelet counts typically under 50×10^9/L. Peripheral smear reveals immature platelets, and bone marrow evaluation reveals elevated numbers of megakaryocytes. ITP in childhood often follows a

Table 66.1. Classification of Splenomegaly by Mechanism

Mechanism	Causative Disease Examples
Immune response work hypertrophy	Subacute bacterial endocarditis Infectious mononucleosis Felty syndrome
Red blood cell destruction work hypertrophy	Spherocytosis Thalassemia major Early sickle cell anemia
Congestive (venous outflow obstruction)	Cirrhosis and portal hypertension Splenic vein thrombosis
Infiltrative	Niemann-Pick disease Amyloidosis Gaucher disease
Neoplastic	Lymphoma Polycythemia vera Angiosarcoma Metastatic carcinoma
Miscellaneous	Trauma Splenic cysts Iron deficiency anemia

Data from Kasper DL. Lymphadenopathy and splenomegaly. In: *Harrison's Manual of Medicine*. 19th ed. McGraw-Hill Education Medical; 2016; Eichner ER, Whitfield CL. Splenomegaly. An algorithmic approach to diagnosis. *JAMA*. 1981;246:2858-2861; Poulose BK, Holtzman MD. The spleen. In: Townsend CM, ed. *Sabiston Textbook of Surgery*. 20th ed. WB Saunders; 2017;1556-1571.

Table 66.2. Etiology of Splenomegaly and Cytopenia in Selected Disease States

Disease Condition	Probable Mechanism
Portal hypertension	Increased pooling of blood cells
Hairy cell leukemia	Retention of hairy cells in splenic pulp
Felty syndrome	Immune system work hypertrophy
Thalassemia major	Reticuloendothelial system work hypertrophy
Gaucher disease	Increased pooling and flow–induced dilutional anemia
Myelofibrosis	Extramedullary hematopoiesis

Data from Kasper DL. Lymphadenopathy and Splenomegaly. In: *Harrison's Manual of Medicine*. 19th ed. McGraw-Hill Education Medical; 2016; Eichner ER, Whitfield CL. Splenomegaly. An algorithmic approach to diagnosis. *JAMA*. 1981;246:2858-2861; Poulose BK, Holtzman MD. The spleen. In: Townsend CM, ed. *Sabiston Textbook of Surgery*. 20th ed. WB Saunders; 2017;1556-1571.

viral illness and frequently resolves spontaneously within 6 months to 1 year.[52] Compared to adults, children with ITP experience severe, extracranial bleeding complications more frequently (20.2% vs 9.6%, $P < .01$) but have lesser intracranial hemorrhage (0.4% vs 1.4%, $P < .01$).[53]

First-line treatment of patients with ITP and symptomatic bleeding or platelet counts $<30 \times 10^9$/L is with corticosteroids, with the goal of achieving and maintaining a hemostatic platelet count.[54] Typical regimens include daily oral prednisone or pulses of high-dose dexamethasone. While optimal dosing regimens have been debated for over 50 years, a recent randomized trial by Wei and colleagues demonstrated increased incidence of initial response in a shorter time course with fewer treatment-related complications in patients treated with dexamethasone.[55] However, recent work has highlighted the burden of heavy corticosteroid usage; almost 95% of patients treated for ITP with steroids report adverse events, and over 30% require dose reductions of therapy cessation due to complications.[56] In thrombocytopenic crises and overt bleeding, a rapid increase in platelet count may be achieved with IVIg (1 g/kg) or anti-D (for Rh-positive patients) infusions followed by platelet transfusion and steroid administration.[57]

Almost all patients with ITP will progress to second-line treatment as remission with corticosteroids is infrequently durable and the long-term side effects are unacceptable. Options for patients who fail steroid treatment include rituximab, TPO-receptor agonists, or splenectomy.[17,57-59]

Splenectomy remains an effective treatment of ITP. In a systematic review evaluating the efficacy of splenectomy in patients with ITP over 58 years of age, complete remission was achieved in 66% of patients, partial response in 22%, and recurrence was uncommon.[18] Splenectomy can usually be performed electively unless patients have active, ongoing bleeding. However, the use of splenectomy for ITP has declined from 50% to 60% to between 20% and 25% in recent series, due largely to medical management improvements and concerns over post–splenectomy operative and infectious complications.[60] Since circulating platelets function normally and destruction by the spleen is rapid, preoperative platelet transfusions are usually unnecessary and ineffective.[61]

Rituximab or TPO-receptor agonists are also effective second-line therapies for ITP or those patients who fail splenectomy. Although normal platelet counts ($>150 \times 10^9$/L) were achieved in 44% of patients and a partial response was seen in 63% ($>30 \times 10^9$/L) with administration of rituximab, median duration of response was only 10.5 months. While the early use of rituximab in ITP was associated with significant toxicity and mortality rates, recent series demonstrate serious adverse event rates of less than 2% and mortality less than 1%. TPO-receptor agonists effectively achieve durable increases in platelet counts, but require continuous treatment. Platelet counts respond in approximately 80% of patients, including those who have failed splenectomy and rituximab.[62-65]

Importantly, postsplenectomy failures should also prompt a search for accessory spleens. Accessory spleens have been reported in 10% to 30% of patients with ITP.[8,9] Technetium sulfa-colloid scanning or I^{111}-labeled scanning is useful to demonstrate accessory splenic tissue and areas of platelet sequestration.[19,36]

Thrombotic Thrombocytopenic Purpura

Thrombotic thrombocytopenic purpura (TTP) is characterized by thrombocytopenia, microangiopathic hemolytic anemia, neurologic abnormalities, renal failure, and fever and generally occurs in young and middle-aged women (see Chapter 49). Associated with genetic mutations in the *ADAMTS13* gene, the von Willebrand factor–cleaving protease, or acquired autoantibody inhibitors after therapy with ticlopidine or clopidogrel, TTP is likely to be the result of the abnormal platelet-aggregating agent in the circulation. Studies indicate that this agent is von Willebrand factor, which is found in excess in patients with TTP. Platelet aggregation leads to microvascular thrombi, typically in the brain, heart, spleen, kidneys, pancreas, and adrenals. Nearly 90% of adults with *ADAMTS13* deficiency will respond to daily plasma exchange with plasmapheresis and transfusion of fresh-frozen plasma. Patients with acquired autoantibodies can be treated with high-dose glucocorticoids, rituximab, or splenectomy. Monoclonal antibody therapy, most frequently with rituximab, has become a mainstay of therapy due to durability of response and overall safety profile of the medication.[66] Eculizumab, a complement-inhibiting anti-C5 monoclonal antibody, has been used in refractory cases.[67] Surgical treatment is considered in patients who have frequent relapses of TTP and may prolong the disease-free interval.[68,69]

Hereditary Anemias

Hereditary spherocytosis is inherited as an autosomal dominant disease in which the red blood cell membrane includes a defective protein, spectrin (see Chapter 29). The spleen destroys the resulting defective, spherical red blood cells, resulting in an anemia and significant reticulocytosis. Peripheral smears demonstrate spherocytes, and these patients have a negative Coombs test. Elective splenectomy will correct the anemia. Ideally, splenectomy is performed after the age of 5 or 6 years to minimize the potential risks of postsplenectomy sepsis. Because of the rapid red blood cell turnover, these patients often develop calcium bilirubinate gallstones, and consideration should be given to concomitant cholecystectomy at the time of splenectomy if they are present.[9]

Sickle cell anemia is an autosomal recessive condition that also results in defective red blood cells (see Chapter 34). Because of the frequency of sludging and thrombosis in small vessels, these patients more often develop infarcts in the spleen, which over time results in autosplenectomy. In rare patients, however, splenectomy may be indicated for acute splenic sequestration crisis, hypersplenism, massive splenic infarction, and splenic abscess.[70,71] Unlike hereditary spherocytosis, splenectomy has little effect on anemia related to the sickle cell condition.

Thalassemia major is an autosomal dominant condition in which abnormal hemoglobin forms protein precipitates in the red blood cell, recognized as Heinz bodies on a peripheral smear (see Chapter 35). These patients can develop significant splenomegaly with resulting cytopenia. In this condition, splenectomy can lessen the need for transfusion but is rarely indicated in the primary treatment of the disease.[72]

Malignant Tumors of the Spleen

Malignant diseases affecting the spleen can be divided into lymphoproliferative disorders, myeloproliferative disorders, metastatic lesions, and primary splenic neoplasms. Most metastatic lesions usually reflect vastly disseminated disease secondary to hematogenous spread. Melanoma, breast, lung, renal, and ovarian lesions are the main sources. Solitary metastasis to the spleen is rare, though improvement in radiographic imaging in recent years has increased its incidence.[73]

Primary tumors of the spleen are exceedingly rare (Chapter 67). They include hemangiosarcoma, hemangiopericytoma, plasmacytomas, and malignant fibrous histiocytomas. All of these conditions may present with splenomegaly and are uniformly treated with splenectomy.[74,75]

Lymphoma

Lymphoma is a common tumor leading to splenomegaly or a splenic mass, although the spleen is rarely the primary site (see Chapters 89 and 90). Non-Hodgkin lymphoma, including splenic marginal zone lymphoma, can present with massive splenomegaly. Although splenectomy has been shown to be a therapeutic treatment of hypersplenism by increasing blood counts, it has not improved long-term survival among patients with lymphoma.[76]

Hodgkin Lymphoma

Hodgkin lymphoma, described by Thomas Hodgkin in 1832, is a highly curable malignant lymphoma characterized by typical multinucleated giant cells (Reed-Sternberg) and predictable stepwise progression from one lymph node basin to another (see Chapters 94 and 95). Histologic subtypes fall into five categories: lymphocyte-rich classical, lymphocyte predominant, nodular sclerosing, mixed cellularity, and lymphocyte depleted. Most patients initially present with asymptomatic peripheral lymphadenopathy, most often in the cervical region (60%-80%). Other nodal regions, including the mediastinal, axillary, inguinal, and retroperitoneal regions, are less often involved at initial presentation. The presence of B symptoms, including fever, weight loss >10%, and night sweats, is noted. Extralymphatic and splenic involvement is used to stage patients. Below the diaphragm, the first nodal tissue involved is the spleen, with 35% of stage I or II patients having occult splenic disease.[77]

Historically, staging laparotomy was used in patients with Hodgkin lymphoma suspected of harboring subdiaphragmatic disease. In this procedure, lymph nodes were sampled from the para-aortic, paracaval, and iliac regions, and liver biopsies were performed along with splenectomy. With the enhanced accuracy of CT for staging purposes, utilization of positron emission tomography scanning to assess treatment response, the increased effectiveness of medical treatments, and inherent surgical risks, the performance of surgical staging has essentially been eliminated.[77]

Leukemia

In chronic lymphocytic leukemia (Chapter 91) and less often in chronic myelogenous leukemia (Chapter 82), massive splenomegaly may be treated by splenectomy to palliate significant symptoms from the mass effect of the enlarged spleen. Likewise, patients with refractory cytopenia unresponsive to conventional medical measures (i.e., corticosteroids, immunosuppression) may undergo splenectomy. The decision to operate must be made with caution, because these patients often are immunosuppressed and malnourished and have higher operative mortality and morbidity risk.[78]

Hairy cell leukemia (Chapter 92) can lead to infiltrative splenomegaly and pancytopenia, which may limit cytotoxic chemotherapy. With the introduction of effective medical therapies, the indications for splenectomy are now limited to palliative responses to end-stage issues such as spontaneous splenic rupture and severe thrombocytopenia with bleeding.[79]

Myelofibrosis

Myelofibrosis describes a group of disorders characterized by acquired mutations that target the hematopoietic stem cells and induce dysregulation of cellular signaling, clonal proliferation, and abnormal cytokine signaling (see Chapter 84). Prominent bone marrow fibrosis and disruption of normal hematopoiesis result in, and can be associated with, enlargement of the liver and spleen as a result of extramedullary hematopoiesis.[80] Massive splenomegaly may lead to pancytopenia, portal hypertension, early satiety, and pain; splenectomy remains a viable treatment when significantly symptomatic. Within 12 months of operation, approximately 50% of patients are rendered transfusion independent, and most experience resolution of mechanical symptoms.[81] Caution must be taken with splenectomy in patients with myelofibrosis, though, as the procedure carries a perioperative mortality rate around 10% and a morbidity rate of approximately 25% with a relatively modest median survival of 1.5 years.[81]

Splenic Cysts

Cystic lesions of the spleen are rare and represent a challenge for physicians to diagnose and treat. The number of asymptomatic cysts incidentally diagnosed continues to rise because of increased utilization of high-resolution abdominal imaging including CT, ultrasound, and magnetic resonance.[82]

Splenic cysts are categorized based on the presence or absence of an epithelial lining. Primary cysts, those with an epithelial lining, can be further subdivided into parasitic or nonparasitic. Secondary cysts, or pseudocysts, lack an epithelium and are believed to result from trauma in the majority of cases (*Figure 66.5*).[83,84]

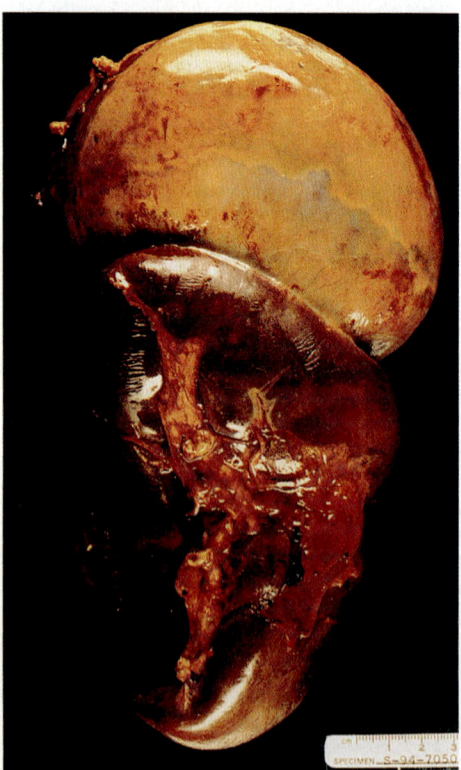

FIGURE 66.5 Large symptomatic splenic pseudocyst developing after blunt trauma to the spleen.

Chapter 66: Disorders of the Spleen

therapy with mebendazole, an effective antiparasitic therapy, is an alternative. Treatment of a single or few cysts can be managed sequentially with medical treatment, chemical sterilization (cetrimide 0.1%), cyst evacuation, and partial splenectomy.[85] Where resection is necessitated by contraindications to medical therapy or refractory infections, total splenectomy remains the standard of care; however, partial splenectomy is a potential option in select cases.[85,86]

Nonparasitic primary cysts, usually congenital, are divided into endodermoid, dermoid, or epidermoid cysts. Epidermoid cysts are the most common congenital cysts (~90%) and present most often in children and young adults. They are derived from inclusions of splenic surface epithelial lining into the splenic parenchyma during development or from an accelerated secretion of lining cells from an unknown cause.[87] Dermoid cysts are exceedingly rare; they contain all three embryonic germ layers and make up the remainder of nonparasitic congenital cysts. Endodermoid cysts are not true cysts, but rather cystic vascular lesions composed of several ectatic vessels best described as lymphangioma or hemangioma (*Figure 66.6*). These benign tumors are most often incidentally discovered with imaging or laparotomy for an alternative purpose. Typically, follow-up imaging adequately demonstrates the benign nature of these masses. Rarely, however, the patient may develop significant splenomegaly and cytopenia with these cysts, requiring diagnostic or symptomatic splenectomy.[83]

The spleen is one of the most frequently injured organs by abdominal trauma. Although 75% of nonparasitic splenic cysts are posttraumatic, 30% of patients cannot recall the inciting event.[84] Pseudocysts may contain a mixture of blood and necrotic debris, as they commonly form after intraparenchymal or subcapsular hematomas organize and degenerate (*Figure 66.7*). Certain pancreatic lesions may also invade the adjacent splenic tissue, rarely masquerading as a secondary splenic cyst.

Splenic cysts are often asymptomatic (70%) but may present with vague abdominal pain. The pain can be constant or intermittent, left-sided or epigastric, and occasionally radiates to the left shoulder. Radiologic examination with ultrasound, CT, or magnetic resonance imaging can characterize the cyst and provide insight into anatomic relationships. Prior to any invasive procedure, determination of parasitic antibody titers is of great importance to rule out parasitic infection. Ultrasound-guided percutaneous cyst aspiration may be useful for obtaining definitive diagnosis, decreasing the size of the cyst, and excluding communicating pancreatic origin.

The majority of patients with splenic cysts are asymptomatic and do not require specific treatment. However, for cysts greater than 5 cm or causing significant symptoms, surgical intervention is often offered. Although percutaneous drainage and alcohol ablation is often successful in initially reducing the size of the cyst, the procedure is plagued with a high incidence of recurrence.[88,89] For single, unilocular superficial cysts, laparoscopic marsupialization or fenestration with splenic preservation should be undertaken. Deep cysts, or those located at either splenic pole, can be resected with partial splenectomy,

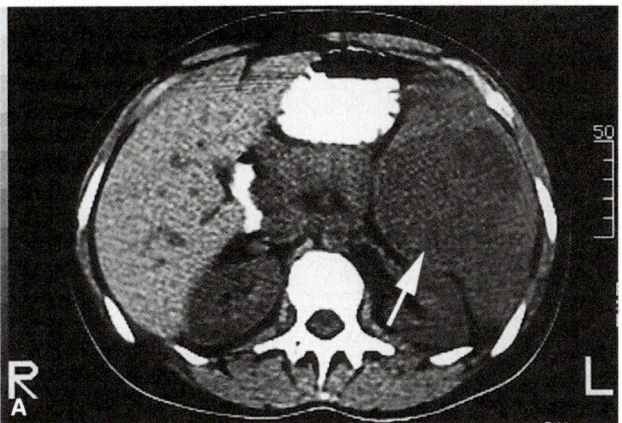
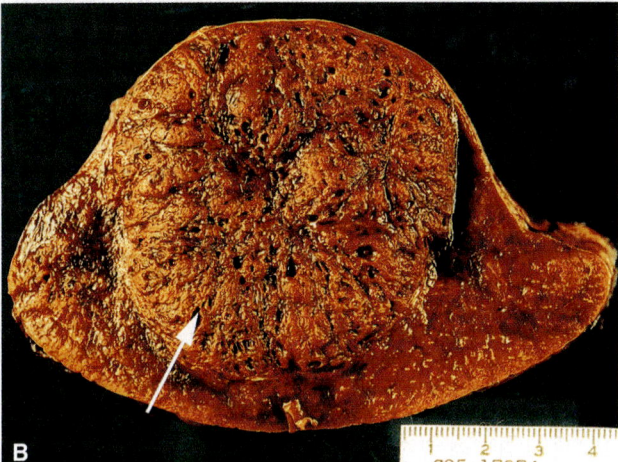

FIGURE 66.6 Computed tomographic scan (A) and gross photograph (B) of the spleen in a 35-year-old woman with marked splenomegaly from splenic hemangioma. The arrow demonstrates central hemangioma with surrounding uninvolved splenic parenchyma. This benign tumor had caused significant thrombocytopenia, resulting in spontaneous bleeding before splenectomy.

Primary, parasitic cysts are most often multilocular, associated with hepatic cysts, and occur most commonly after infection with *Echinococcus granulosus*. They make up the majority of splenic cysts worldwide and are endemic in South America and the Mediterranean. Parasitic cysts, however, are rare among Western nations. Surgery must be undertaken carefully, as rupture can result in anaphylactic shock or disseminated scolexal infection. In the presence of large numbers of cysts, surgical treatment is contraindicated and medical

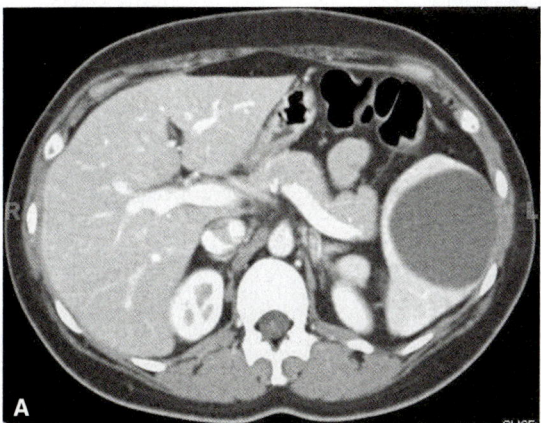
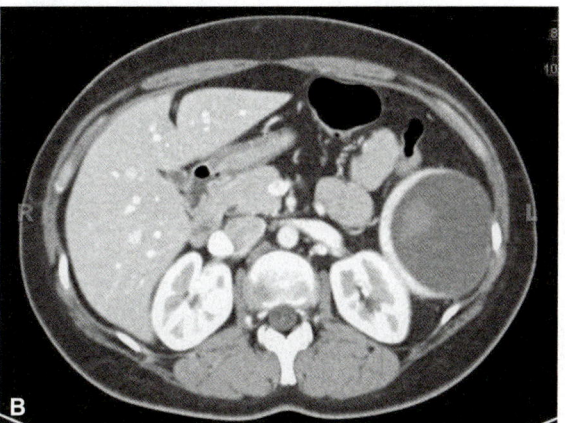

FIGURE 66.7 A, Computed tomography (CT) of a 43-year-old woman who was scanned after developing left upper quadrant pain. She had no history of trauma. CT showed a splenic pseudocyst. B, After aspiration, some blood is seen in the cyst lumen. The cyst rapidly reaccumulated, and the patient subsequently had a successful laparoscopic cyst deroofing.

which provides immunologic protection and improved outcomes when compared to splenic autotransplantation.[90] Complete splenectomy is indicated in cases of giant cysts surrounded by splenic parenchyma or multilocular cysts.[9,84,87]

Splenic Abscess

Splenic abscesses may occur primarily, usually from a hematogenous source, or from secondary infection. Typical sources of hematogenous seeding include distant infection or intravenous drug abuse. Immunocompromised states or splenic infarction, as in patients with sickle cell disease, predisposes to primary abscess formation. Specific symptoms suggesting splenic abscess are rare, although left upper quadrant tenderness may be present in patients with significant abscess cavities along with more classic symptoms of recurrent fevers and idiopathic leukocytosis. Abdominal CT with contrast is the most helpful imaging modality, often demonstrating low-density lesions that may contain gas and present peripheral enhancement.[89] The majority of cases can be successfully treated with image-guided percutaneous drainage. Multilocular abscesses with thick septations or necrotic debris generally require surgery, although percutaneous catheter drainage may successfully temporize significant infections as a bridge to surgery.[88,89] Antimicrobial therapy is based on aspirate culture data, with *Staphylococcus* and *Streptococcus* species being common pathogens.

Felty Syndrome

Felty syndrome, a triad of rheumatoid arthritis, neutropenia, and splenomegaly, is found in <1% of patients with rheumatoid arthritis (see Chapter 58). Clinically, patients present with severe joint destruction and other systemic manifestations such as leg ulcers, rheumatoid nodules, vasculitis, lymphadenopathy, and hepatomegaly. Antibody-coated neutrophils are cleared from the circulation in the spleen, and neutropenia can develop. Recurrent bacterial infections, a major source of morbidity, are owing to the decreased granulopoiesis, increased peripheral destruction of neutrophils, and defects in neutrophil function. Methotrexate or other disease-modifying antirheumatic drugs (DMARDs) are the first-line treatment for Felty syndrome with granulocytopenia. If DMARD treatment is unsuccessful, low-dose granulocyte colony-stimulating factor may prove therapeutic. Splenectomy is indicated only in treatment-resistant cases in which splenomegaly is present; splenectomy is contraindicated in patients with large granular lymphocyte expansion, as the procedure has no effect and may actually cause deterioration.[91-93]

Table 66.3. AAST Grades of Splenic Injury (1994 Revision)

Grade 1	Minor subcapsular tear 1 cm or subcapsular hematoma <10% SA
Grade 2	Capsular tear not involving trabecular vessels, <3 cm or subcapsular hematoma between 10% and 50% SA
Grade 3	Laceration >3 cm parenchymal depth involving trabecular vessels or subcapsular hematoma >50% S, or expanding or ruptured hematoma
Grade 4	Laceration involving the hilum with >25% devascularization of the spleen or intraparenchymal hemorrhage with active bleeding
Grade 5	Completely shattered spleen

Abbreviations: AAST, American Association for the Surgery of Trauma; SA, surface area.

Abdominal Trauma and Splenic Injury

Splenic preservation is the main goal of the modern management of blunt traumatic splenic injuries. Nonoperative management is successful in more than 90% of patients.[94] The degree of splenic injury is measured using contrast-enhanced CT scans and graded according to the American Association for the Surgery of Trauma criteria (*Table 66.3*). Most injuries of grade 3 or less are successfully managed nonoperatively, whereas the presence of a high-grade injury (grade 4 or 5) or a contrast blush predicts the need for intervention (*Figure 66.8*).[95] The primary requirement for nonoperative management is hemodynamic stability, and therefore, close monitoring is required in all cases. A continued transfusion requirement and hypotension in the face of adequate resuscitation are indications for urgent intervention. A meta-analysis of 24,615 patients demonstrated that 12% of patients failed conservative management, ultimately requiring intervention. It also suggested that failure of conservative management in older patients may be associated with increased mortality.[96,97]

Options for operative intervention consist primarily of open splenectomy, with splenic repair and partial splenectomy utilized rarely. In addition to splenectomy, splenic artery embolization has become an integral adjunct in the management of high-grade splenic injuries and in patients with active contrast extravasation. With adequate patient selection, angioembolization has decreased the failure rate of nonoperative management to 4% in some recent series.[95,98]

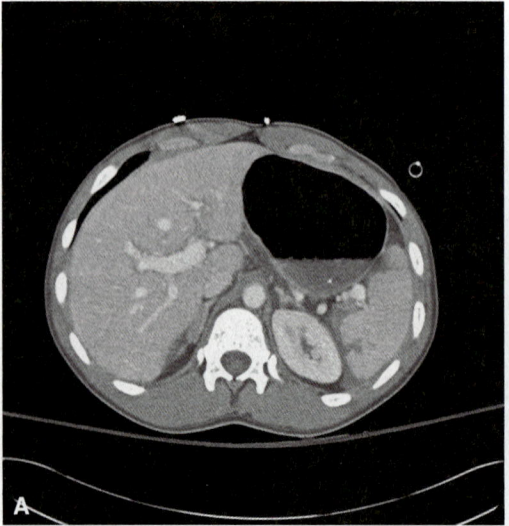 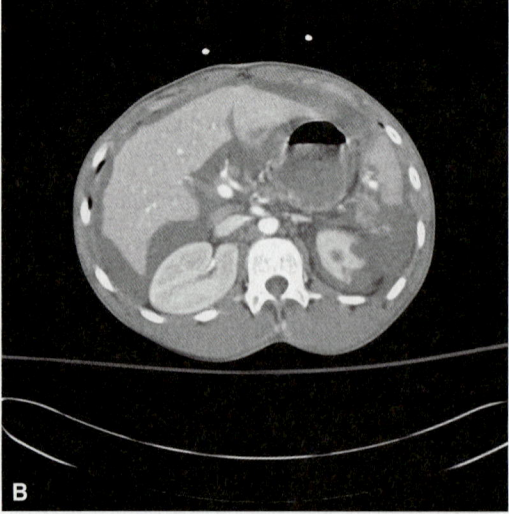

FIGURE 66.8 A, Contrast-enhanced computed tomography (CT) showing a grade 1 splenic laceration in the inferior pole, with associated hemoperitoneum; the patient was successfully managed conservatively. B, Contrast-enhanced CT showing a grade 5 splenic laceration with evidence of active extravasation and perisplenic hematoma. This patient required urgent splenectomy.

Delayed Splenic Rupture

Delayed splenic rupture has been reported in patients experiencing blunt abdominal trauma, a setting in which patients develop splenic hemorrhage >7 days after their original injury.[99] These patients usually have an initial splenic contusion that continues to slowly enlarge and, at some later date, results in disruption of the splenic capsule. This is an exceedingly uncommon occurrence, especially with the introduction of high-resolution CT. But, it should be considered in any patient who develops significant left upper quadrant pain, distention, and signs of bleeding or shock after an episode of trauma.[100] The treatment is urgent intervention with angiography or splenectomy, depending on the patient's clinical picture.

Spontaneous Splenic Rupture

Spontaneous rupture of the spleen is extremely rare and for unknown reasons occurs predominantly in males. Predisposing conditions include splenic infarctions, coagulation disorders, thrombocytopenia, portal hypertension, vasculitis, venous thrombosis in the spleen and focal splenic lesions, lymphoma, and leukemia. Spontaneous rupture is most often secondary to a neoplastic etiology. Overall mortality with rupture is about 12% with splenomegaly, advanced age (>40 years), and a neoplastic etiology predicting an increased risk of death.[101]

These patients usually develop acute left upper quadrant pain that may be associated with referred pain in the left shoulder. Initially, this may be contained beneath the splenic capsule as a subcapsular hematoma, but if intraperitoneal rupture occurs, patients may present with acute severe pain and hypovolemic shock. Ultrasonography or CT scanning confirms the diagnosis with intraperitoneal fluid (blood) and subcapsular hematoma. Urgent or emergent splenectomy is definitive treatment for these patients. Splenic conservation may be a viable option depending on degree of instability and injury grade.

SPLENECTOMY: SURGICAL TECHNIQUE

Open Splenectomy

Historically, splenectomy has been performed via a midline or left subcostal incision, depending on the surgeon's preference and the degree of splenomegaly. In patients with massive splenomegaly (>2000 g), a midline incision may be preferred to allow adequate mobilization and delivery of the spleen into the operative field.

In the setting of significant splenomegaly, initial ligation of the splenic artery near its origin prior to dissection of the organ may be advantageous. This maneuver decreases splenic distention and limits bleeding should a capsular tear occur. To achieve this, the surgeon first divides the avascular gastrohepatic ligament above the pancreas and isolates the splenic artery near its point of origin on the celiac axis. The vessel can then be suture ligated between clamps or stapled. Care must be taken to avoid injury to the adjacent pancreas. If the artery is not readily accessible, this step may be omitted to avoid pancreatic injury.

Next, the ligamentous attachments to the spleen must be divided. The avascular phrenosplenic and splenocolic attachments may be divided with sharp dissection. The gastrosplenic ligament (and short gastric vessels) must then be suture ligated or taken with hemostatic electrosurgical instruments; significant bleeding may occur if not dissected in hemostatic fashion. Finally, the vessels of the splenic hilum are individually ligated, taking care during this portion of the procedure to avoid injury to the tail of the pancreas. Closed suction drainage of the splenic bed is performed only in cases of suspected pancreatic injury; evacuation of pancreatic fluid reduces incidence of abscess formation and creates a controlled pancreatic fistula that will usually seal with observation alone. Finally, a careful search of the abdomen is made for accessory spleens, which are most often found in the splenic hilum or in the mesentery of the intestine.

Partial splenectomy is not indicated in the setting of marked splenomegaly but may be an option for patients with splenic pseudocysts that simply require unroofing. Patients with limited splenic trauma may be candidates for splenorrhaphy or subtotal splenectomy.

Minimally Invasive Splenectomy

Since laparoscopic splenectomy was first described in 1991 by Delaitre et al, minimally invasive approaches have become the standard for elective operative treatment of many benign and malignant diseases of the spleen.[8,9,102] Numerous studies have demonstrated the advantages of the laparoscopic approach compared to open splenectomy, including decreased blood loss, shorter hospital stays, accelerated recovery, and decreased convalescence; recent adoption of surgical robotic platforms has also demonstrated capability for minimally invasive splenectomy.[103] Over the past decade, the indications for minimally invasive splenectomy have gradually expanded and now include ITP, hereditary spherocytosis, hemolytic anemia, TTP, leukemias, splenic myelofibrosis, sickle cell disease, lymphomas, myelodysplastic syndrome, multiple myeloma, and accessory splenectomy.

Massive splenomegaly is no longer an absolute contraindication for a minimally invasive approach. Superior outcomes over open splenectomy in patients with massive spleens, including decreased blood loss, reduced transfusion requirement, fewer reoperations for bleeding, and an average reduction in hospital stay by 8 days, have been shown. Decreased blood loss and opioid usage continue to be the great advantages of minimally invasive splenectomy in patients who are coagulopathic and at risk for massive hemorrhage.[104,105] The decision to perform laparoscopic splenectomy in a patient with splenomegaly is a multifactorial decision that depends on the underlying disease process, comorbidities, and surgeon experience. The effect of the surgeon's learning curve has been clearly demonstrated in laparoscopic splenectomy, with the average conversion rate depending on experience and ranging from 1.2% to 15%.[104] Though less explored to date, robotic surgical platforms also demonstrate improved outcomes later in a surgeon's learning curve.

The operative approach for laparoscopic splenectomy continues to evolve with the introduction of new surgical technology. After induction of general anesthesia, a nasogastric tube and Foley catheter are inserted to decompress the stomach and bladder, respectively. The patient is moved into the right lateral decubitus position, and three or four working ports are placed for the introduction of the laparoscopic instruments, including an angled laparoscope. The lateral port is most often placed at the level of the 11th rib tip, the medial port in midline, and the middle port halfway between the two, approximately 4 cm below the inferior tip of the spleen. In patients with a supramassive spleen (>22 cm in craniocaudal length or 19 cm in width), the addition of a hand port has been shown to greatly reduce operative time without increasing length of stay or convalescence. This approach allows the insertion of the surgeon's nondominant hand into the abdominal cavity while maintaining pneumoperitoneum. Positioning is slightly altered by placing the patient's side at a 45° angle. After accessing the abdomen, a careful inspection of the abdomen is carried out to identify other disease or the presence of accessory spleens, focused on the hilum, omentum, and lesser sac.[105]

The dissection then proceeds in five stages: division of the short gastric vessels, division of the splenocolic ligament, ligation of the inferior polar vessels, hilar control, and division of the phrenic attachments of the spleen. Much of the dissection may be carried out with harmonic shears, and the hilar structures are ligated and divided with an endoscopic stapling device. The spleen is then placed in an extraction bag, morcellated in situ, and the fragments removed. Generally, robotic splenectomy proceeds in similar fashion with minor adjustments in accordance with system requirements.

COMPLICATIONS OF SPLENECTOMY

The perioperative complication rate for laparoscopic splenectomy is approximately 10%.[106] The most common complications of splenectomy include bleeding, injury to the adjacent pancreas with resulting pancreatitis, and pancreatic pseudocyst, abscess, or fistula formation. These patients can also develop injury to the adjacent stomach or splenic flexure of the colon if care is not taken in dividing the ligamentous attachments to these structures.

Postoperative thrombocytosis can occur, and low-dose aspirin should be considered if the platelet count is >1000 × 10⁹/L to minimize the risks of thrombosis or embolism. The thrombocytosis is usually transient, with return of platelet counts to normal ranges by 2 years after splenectomy.

Thrombosis of the portal venous system is a unique and potentially life-threatening semiacute complication after splenectomy via any approach. These patients are particularly at risk owing to the propensity for clot formation in the remnant splenic vein to propagate into the portal vein. Although this complication was once believed to be rare, improvements in radiologic techniques have demonstrated portal venous thrombosis much more frequently than previously thought, with a number of cases occurring asymptomatically. The reported incidence of portal venous thrombosis varies greatly within the literature. Initial retrospective reviews demonstrated incidences between 5% and 15%. When prospectively analyzed, however, 19% to 55% of patients developed portal venous thrombosis. Of these, 33% to 66% remained asymptomatic. Patients with larger-diameter splenic veins and those operated on for hematologic malignancy were found to be at highest risk for thrombosis.[107-109]

When symptomatic, portal venous thrombosis most often presents between 2 and 22 days postoperatively with nonspecific complaints including decreased appetite, vague abdominal pain, nausea, and malaise. Abdominal pain is a rare sign that is present most typically in cases of severe vascular congestion. Fever and leukocytosis are common. Risk factors highly associated with portal venous thrombosis include splenomegaly, hematologic malignancy, and thrombocytosis. Normal D-dimer levels have a 98% negative predictive value. Contrast-enhanced CT scanning is the preferred method of evaluation as it can assess the portal circulation as well as other common etiologies of abdominal pain.[109,110]

Once the diagnosis of portal venous thrombosis is made, systemic anticoagulation should be started immediately. With prompt anticoagulation, recanalization can occur rapidly in over 90% of patients. Although treatment with thrombolytics and antiplatelet agents has been reported, indications for routine use are yet to be determined.[109,111]

Infection Risk Postsplenectomy

Infectious complications occur after splenectomy in both the early and late postoperative periods. The rate of early postoperative infections is particularly high when multiple other procedures are performed (e.g., after complex injuries in the setting of polytrauma).[112] The complication of overwhelming postsplenectomy infection (OPSI) has received significant attention. In addition to OPSI, postsplenectomy patients are at risk for multiple and recurrent episodes of severe infection requiring hospitalization.[113]

Overwhelming Postsplenectomy Infection

One of the most important developments affecting the surgical treatment of the spleen has been the recognition of life-long increased risk of severe infection and sepsis after splenectomy. In 1969, Diamond described a case of post–splenectomy fulminant bacteremia leading to rapid death and popularized the term OPSI.[114]

Pathophysiology

While staphylococci and enteric Gram-negative bacilli are often implicated in early postoperative infections, the most common organisms isolated in cases of true OPSI are encapsulated bacteria. *Streptococcus pneumonia* is the most common (incidence of 50%-90%), followed by *Neisseria meningitidis, Escherichia coli, Haemophilus influenzae,* and *Staphylococcus aureus*.[115] Infections occur at rates that range from 7% to 12%.[116]

The special susceptibility of the asplenic patient to encapsulated organisms is likely owing to compromised humoral immunity. After splenectomy, the subset of IgM memory B cells that respond to bacterial polysaccharide antigen is severely depleted. These particular B-cells, having developed specific antibody production in response to a specific antigen, are responsible for immediate antibody generation upon re-exposure to encapsulated organisms. Responsible for the immediate, T-cell–independent immune response, these B-cells require a functional spleen for their generation and survival.[117] Studies confirm that bacteria-specific IgM production in asplenic patients is both delayed and diminished.[118]

In addition to delayed antibody production, asplenic patients also maintain lower circulating levels of plasma factors necessary to activate complement in the absence of antibody such as properdin, tuftsin, C3, and factor B.[119] Tuftsin is a tetrapeptide that stimulates bacterial phagocytosis by binding to specific receptors on granulocytes, monocytes, macrophages, and natural killer cells. Properdin, also produced by the spleen, plays a crucial role in propagating complement activation in the absence of antibody by driving conversion of C3 to C3b through the stabilization of C3 convertase.

There is also evidence that splenectomy results in defects of cellular immunity. After splenectomy, multiple cohorts of patients have demonstrated a significant reduction in the percentage of CD4⁺ T-cells, specifically in the CD45RA⁺ subset. This change lasts for years after splenectomy and portends impaired primary immune responsiveness.[120]

Incidence

OPSI is most common in the very young, in patients with underlying malignancies or other medical conditions, and within the first 2 years after splenectomy (although it has been reported 20-40 years after surgery). The precise incidence of OPSI is controversial, but is estimated to be around 0.23% per year; published estimates vary widely secondary to different disease definition, duration of follow-up, age stratification, indication for splenectomy, and age.[113,115,116,119,121,122] OPSI is greatest in the very young and diminishes with age: 15.7% in infants, 10.4% in children <5 years old, 4.4% in children <16 years old, and 0.9% in adults. Although the incidence in adults is similar to that of the general population, mortality from sepsis is increased 58-fold in the asplenic population, with a fatality rate between 50% and 90%. Underlying pathology, like youth, also imparts an increased risk of OPSI with the highest risk associated with underlying immune disorders and Hodgkin lymphoma.[113,115,116,119,121]

Clinical Course

OPSI usually presents with fever and brief upper respiratory tract infection and pursues a rapid course with evolution to sepsis, shock, disseminated intravascular coagulation, and multiorgan failure within hours. All asplenic patients with fever should be evaluated for possible OPSI. Key to successful treatment is prompt administration of broad-spectrum intravenous antibiotics. A complete septic workup, including routine laboratory tests, appropriate imaging, and microbiology cultures, should be performed, but never delay the initiation of antibiotics. In fully developed OPSI, mortality rates of 50% to 90% have been reported; 80% of deaths occur within 48 hours.[113,115] Therefore, rapid recognition and treatment initiation are crucial.

Prevention of Overwhelming Postsplenectomy Infection

The guidelines for the prevention of OPSI center around vaccination, antibiotic prophylaxis, patient education, and splenic preservation strategies.[123] Vaccines against meningococcus, *Haemophilus*, and pneumococcus are generally recommended. For patients undergoing elective splenectomy, vaccination should be performed at least 2 weeks before surgery to maximize antibody development against T-cell–dependent immunogens. In emergent cases, patients should be vaccinated 14 days after their surgery.[116,123]

In adults, the Centers for Disease Control and Prevention currently recommends pneumococcal, meningococcal, and *Haemophilus* vaccination schedules of varying complexity. For pneumococcus, patients should receive the 13-valent vaccine initially, with follow-up administration of the 23-valent vaccine 8 weeks and 5 years after initial administration. The recommended meningococcal vaccination regimen includes two initial doses of the quadrivalent conjugate vaccine followed by the serogroup B vaccine; no redosing is recommended. And for *Haemophilus*, a single administration of the conjugate vaccine is recommended only in adults who have not been previously immunized.[124]

Children less than 5 years old, in addition to aggressive immunization, also require antibiotic prophylaxis after splenectomy. Initial vaccination is provided with the *H. influenzae* vaccine, meningococcal vaccine, and 7-valent pneumococcal conjugate vaccine. If not previously immunized against pneumococcus, an additional dose of the 7-valent vaccine is recommended no less than 6 to 8 weeks after the first dose, with a final 23-valent vaccine booster 3 to 5 years later. Daily antibiotic prophylaxis with penicillin V potassium (125 mg twice a day until 3 years of age and 250 mg twice a day thereafter) is recommended for all children under the age of 5 years. If no invasive pneumococcal infections are experienced, prophylaxis may be discontinued after the age of 5 years after appropriate immunizations have been obtained.[125,126]

One of the most important, and most overlooked, aspects of prevention is patient education. Up to 50% of asplenic patients are unaware of their increased risk of serious infection, and 30% to 40% do not recall being vaccinated.[115] Few are provided with antibiotics to take empirically at the onset of fever, and one-half would not spontaneously tell an uninformed emergency department doctor about their splenectomies.[116] Asplenic patients should be extensively counseled about their health risks, the need for reimmunization, and the importance of informing future caregivers of their condition.

Autotransplantation of Splenic Tissue

Extrasplenic tissue may emerge secondary to traumatic autotransplantation, known as splenosis. Although this tissue appears as normal spleen, with white pulp, red pulp, and marginal zones, extrasplenic tissue is insufficient to recapitulate the host immune response and is not a recommended practice for patients undergoing splenectomy.[20,24]

References

1. Standring S. *Gray's Anatomy: The Anatomical Basis of Clinical Practice.* 41st ed. Elsevier Limited; 2016.
2. McClusky DA, IIIrd, Skandalakis LJ, Colborn GL, Skandalakis JE. Tribute to a triad: history of splenic anatomy, physiology, and surgery—part 1. *World J Surg.* 1999;23:311-325.
3. Burn SF, Boot MJ, de Angelis C, et al. The dynamics of spleen morphogenesis. *Dev Biol.* 2008;318:303-311.
4. Mebius RE, Kraal G. Structure and function of the spleen. *Nat Rev Immunol.* 2005;5:606-616.
5. Skandalakis LJ, Skandalakis JE, Skandalakis PN. *Surgical Anatomy and Technique: A Pocket Manual.* 3rd ed. Springer; 2009.
6. Courtney MT, Townsend CM, Beauchamp RD, Evers BM, Mattox KL. *Sabiston Textbook of Surgery: The Biological Basis of Modern Surgical Practice.* 20th ed. Elsevier; 2016.
7. Cesta MF. Normal structure, function, and histology of the spleen. *Toxicol Pathol.* 2006;34:455-465.
8. Duperier T, Brody F, Felsher J, Walsh RM, Rosen M, Ponsky J. Predictive factors for successful laparoscopic splenectomy in patients with immune thrombocytopenic purpura. *Arch Surg.* 2004;139:61-66. discussion 6.
9. Rosen M, Brody F, Walsh RM, Tarnoff M, Malm J, Ponsky J. Outcome of laparoscopic splenectomy based on hematologic indication. *Surg Endosc.* 2002;16:272-279.
10. Nolte MA, Arens R, Kraus M, et al. B cells are crucial for both development and maintenance of the splenic marginal zone. *J Immunol.* 2004;172:3620-3627.
11. Nance DM, Sanders VM. Autonomic innervation and regulation of the immune system (1987-2007). *Brain Behav Immun.* 2007;21:736-745.
12. Rosas-Ballina M, Tracey KJ. The neurology of the immune system: neural reflexes regulate immunity. *Neuron.* 2009;64:28-32.
13. Verlinden TJM, van Dijk P, Hikspoors J, Herrler A, Lamers WH, Köhler SE. Innervation of the human spleen: a complete hilum-embedding approach. *Brain Behav Immun.* 2019;77:92-100.
14. Murray K, Godinez DR, Brust-Mascher I, Miller EN, Gareau MG, Reardon C. Neuroanatomy of the spleen: mapping the relationship between sympathetic neurons and lymphocytes. *PLoS One.* 2017;12:e0182416.
15. Varga I, Galfiova P, Adamkov M, et al. Congenital anomalies of the spleen from an embryological point of view. *Med Sci Monit.* 2009;15:RA269-RA276.
16. Cowles RA, Lazar EL. Symptomatic pelvic accessory spleen. *Am J Surg.* 2007;194:225-226.
17. George JN. Sequence of treatments for adults with primary immune thrombocytopenia. *Am J Hematol.* 2012;87(suppl 1):S12-S15.
18. Kojouri K, Vesely SK, Terrell DR, George JN. Splenectomy for adult patients with idiopathic thrombocytopenic purpura: a systematic review to assess long-term platelet count responses, prediction of response, and surgical complications. *Blood.* 2004;104:2623-2634.
19. Phom H, Kumar A, Tripathi M, et al. Comparative evaluation of Tc-99m-heat-denatured RBC and Tc-99m-anti-D IgG opsonized RBC spleen planar and SPECT scintigraphy in the detection of accessory spleen in postsplenectomy patients with chronic idiopathic thrombocytopenic purpura. *Clin Nucl Med.* 2004;29:403-409.
20. Fremont RD, Rice TW. Splenosis: a review. *South Med J.* 2007;100:589-593.
21. Bramos A, Stengle J. Chest wall subcutaneous splenosis after remote trauma. *Surgery.* 2016;159:1689-1690.
22. Chang NJ, Yeh JT, Lin YT, Lin CH. Subcutaneous splenosis in gunshot outlet: case report. *J Trauma.* 2009;66:E55-E56.
23. Yeh CJ, Chuang WY, Kuo TT. Unusual subcutaneous splenosis occurring in a gunshot wound scar: pathology and immunohistochemical identification. *Pathol Int.* 2006;56:336-339.
24. Connell NT, Brunner AM, Kerr CA, Schiffman FJ. Splenosis and sepsis: the born-again spleen provides poor protection. *Virulence.* 2011;2:4-11.
25. Chauhan NS, Kumar S. Torsion of a wandering spleen presenting as acute abdomen. *Pol J Radiol.* 2016;81:110-113.
26. Lopes-Carvalho T, Kearney JF. Development and selection of marginal zone B cells. *Immunol Rev.* 2004;197:192-205.
27. Steiniger B, Bette M, Schwarzbach H. The open microcirculation in human spleens: a three-dimensional approach. *J Histochem Cytochem.* 2011;59:639-648.
28. Steiniger BS. Human spleen microanatomy: why mice do not suffice. *Immunology.* 2015;145:334-346.
29. Lammers AJ, de Porto AP, Bennink RJ, et al. Hyposplenism: comparison of different methods for determining splenic function. *Am J Hematol.* 2012;87:484-489.
30. Borges da Silva H, Fonseca R, Pereira RM, Cassado AA, Álvarez JM, D'Império Lima MR. Splenic macrophage subsets and their function during blood-borne infections. *Front Immunol.* 2015;6:480.
31. Gordon S. Pattern recognition receptors: doubling up for the innate immune response. *Cell.* 2002;111:927-930.
32. Ge Y, Gao H, Kong XT. Immunoglobulins and complement in splenectomised and autotransplanted subjects. *Ann Med.* 1989;21:265-267.
33. Sze DM, Toellner KM, Garcia de Vinuesa C, Taylor DR, MacLennan IC. Intrinsic constraint on plasmablast growth and extrinsic limits of plasma cell survival. *J Exp Med.* 2000;192:813-821.
34. Gretz JE, Norbury CC, Anderson AO, Proudfoot AE, Shaw S. Lymph-borne chemokines and other low molecular weight molecules reach high endothelial venules via specialized conduits while a functional barrier limits access to the lymphocyte microenvironments in lymph node cortex. *J Exp Med.* 2000;192:1425-1440.
35. Nolte MA, Belien JA, Schadee-Eestermans I, et al. A conduit system distributes chemokines and small blood-borne molecules through the splenic white pulp. *J Exp Med.* 2003;198:505-512.
36. Navez J, Hubert C, Gigot JF, et al. Does the site of platelet sequestration predict the response to splenectomy in adult patients with immune thrombocytopenic purpura? *Platelets.* 2015;26:573-576.
37. Ajmo CT, Jr, Vernon DO, Collier L, et al. The spleen contributes to stroke-induced neurodegeneration. *J Neurosci Res.* 2008;86:2227-2234.
38. Sarpatwari A, Provan D, Erqou S, Sobnack R, David Tai FW, Newland AC. Autologous 111 In-labelled platelet sequestration studies in patients with primary immune thrombocytopenia (ITP) prior to splenectomy: a report from the United Kingdom ITP Registry. *Br J Haematol.* 2010;151:477-487.
39. Stewart IB, McKenzie DC. The human spleen during physiological stress. *Sports Med.* 2002;32:361-369.
40. Swirski FK, Nahrendorf M, Etzrodt M, et al. Identification of splenic reservoir monocytes and their deployment to inflammatory sites. *Science.* 2009;325:612-616.
41. Gabrilovich DI, Ostrand-Rosenberg S, Bronte V. Coordinated regulation of myeloid cells by tumours. *Nat Rev Immunol.* 2012;12:253-268.
42. Knutson M, Wessling-Resnick M. Iron metabolism in the reticuloendothelial system. *Crit Rev Biochem Mol Biol.* 2003;38:61-88.
43. Kristiansen M, Graversen JH, Jacobsen C, et al. Identification of the haemoglobin scavenger receptor. *Nature.* 2001;409:198-201.
44. Flo TH, Smith KD, Sato S, et al. Lipocalin 2 mediates an innate immune response to bacterial infection by sequestrating iron. *Nature.* 2004;432:917-921.
45. Hosey RG, Mattacola CG, Kriss V, Armsey T, Quarles JD, Jagger J. Ultrasound assessment of spleen size in collegiate athletes. *Br J Sports Med.* 2006;40:251-254. discussion -4.
46. Motykova G, Steensma DP. Why does my patient have lymphadenopathy or splenomegaly? *Hematol Oncol Clin North Am.* 2012;26:395-408. ix.
47. Lv Y, Lau WY, Li Y, et al. Hypersplenism: history and current status. *Exp Ther Med.* 2016;12:2377-2382.
48. Kasper DL. *Harrison's Manual of Medicine.* 19th ed. McGraw Hill Education Medical; 2016.
49. van Leeuwen EF, van der Ven JT, Engelfriet CP, von dem Borne AE. Specificity of autoantibodies in autoimmune thrombocytopenia. *Blood.* 1982;59:23-26.
50. Feng R, Liu X, Zhao Y, et al. GPIIb/IIIa autoantibody predicts better rituximab response in ITP. *Br J Haematol.* 2018;182:305-307.
51. Semple JW. Infections, antigen-presenting cells, T cells, and immune tolerance: their role in the pathogenesis of immune thrombocytopenia. *Hematol Oncol Clin North Am.* 2009;23:1177-1192.
52. Cines DB, Bussel JB, Liebman HA, Prak Luning ET. The ITP syndrome: pathogenic and clinical diversity. *Blood.* 2009;113:6511-6521.
53. Neunert C, Noroozi N, Norman G, et al. Severe bleeding events in adults and children with primary immune thrombocytopenia: a systematic review. *J Thromb Haemost.* 2015;13:457-464.
54. Mazzucconi MG, Fazi P, Bernasconi S, et al; Party GIMEdAGTW. Therapy with high-dose dexamethasone (HD-DXM) in previously untreated patients affected by idiopathic thrombocytopenic purpura: a GIMEMA experience. *Blood.* 2007;109:1401-1407.
55. Wei Y, Ji XB, Wang YW, et al. High-dose dexamethasone vs prednisone for treatment of adult immune thrombocytopenia: a prospective multicenter randomized trial. *Blood.* 2016;127:296-302. quiz 70.
56. Cuker A, Liebman HA. Corticosteroid overuse in adults with immune thrombocytopenia: cause for concern. *Res Pract Thromb Haemost.* 2021;5:e12592.
57. Neunert C, Lim W, Crowther M, et al. The American Society of Hematology 2011 evidence-based practice guideline for immune thrombocytopenia. *Blood.* 2011;117:4190-4207.

58. Provan D, Stasi R, Newland AC, et al. International consensus report on the investigation and management of primary immune thrombocytopenia. *Blood.* 2010;115:168-186.
59. Audia S, Mahévas M, Nivet M, Ouandji S, Ciudad M, Bonnotte B. Immune thrombocytopenia: recent advances in pathogenesis and treatments. *Hemasphere.* 2021;5:e574.
60. Rodeghiero F, Ruggeri M. Is splenectomy still the gold standard for the treatment of chronic ITP? *Am J Hematol.* 2008;83:91.
61. Chaturvedi S, Arnold DM, McCrae KR. Splenectomy for immune thrombocytopenia: down but not out. *Blood.* 2018;131:1172-1182.
62. Arnold DM, Dentali F, Crowther MA, et al. Systematic review: efficacy and safety of rituximab for adults with idiopathic thrombocytopenic purpura. *Ann Intern Med.* 2007;146:25-33.
63. Bennett CM, Rogers ZR, Kinnamon DD, et al. Prospective phase 1/2 study of rituximab in childhood and adolescent chronic immune thrombocytopenic purpura. *Blood.* 2006;107:2639-2642.
64. Godeau B, Porcher R, Fain O, et al. Rituximab efficacy and safety in adult splenectomy candidates with chronic immune thrombocytopenic purpura: results of a prospective multicenter phase 2 study. *Blood.* 2008;112:999-1004.
65. Tran H, Brighton T, Grigg A, et al. A multi-centre, single-arm, open-label study evaluating the safety and efficacy of fixed dose rituximab in patients with refractory, relapsed or chronic idiopathic thrombocytopenic purpura (R-ITP1000 study). *Br J Haematol.* 2014;167:243-251.
66. Page EE, Kremer Hovinga JA, Terrell DR, Vesely SK, George JN. Rituximab reduces risk for relapse in patients with thrombotic thrombocytopenic purpura. *Blood.* 2016;127:3092-3094.
67. Chapin J, Weksler B, Magro C, Laurence J. Eculizumab in the treatment of refractory idiopathic thrombotic thrombocytopenic purpura. *Br J Haematol.* 2012;157:772-774.
68. Zipfel PF, Heinen S, Skerka C. Thrombotic microangiopathies: new insights and new challenges. *Curr Opin Nephrol Hypertens.* 2010;19:372-378.
69. Joly BS, Coppo P, Veyradier A. Thrombotic thrombocytopenic purpura. *Blood.* 2017;129:2836-2846.
70. Al-Salem AH. Splenic complications of sickle cell anemia and the role of splenectomy. *ISRN Hematol.* 2011;2011:864257.
71. Naymagon L, Pendurti G, Billett HH. Acute splenic sequestration crisis in adult sickle cell disease: a report of 16 cases. *Hemoglobin.* 2015;39:375-379.
72. Crowther M. *Evidence-based Hematology.* Wiley-Blackwell; 2008.
73. Comperat E, Bardier-Dupas A, Camparo P, Capron F, Charlotte F. Splenic metastases: clinicopathologic presentation, differential diagnosis, and pathogenesis. *Arch Pathol Lab Med.* 2007;131:965-969.
74. Batouli A, Fairbrother SW, Silverman JF, et al. Primary splenic angiosarcoma: clinical and imaging manifestations of this rare aggressive neoplasm. *Curr Probl Diagn Radiol.* 2016;45:284-287.
75. Suzuki K, Nakazato T, Mihara A, Sanada Y, Kakimoto T. Primary splenic angiosarcoma mimicking splenic lymphoma. *Intern Med.* 2010;49:203-204.
76. Fallah J, Olszewski AJ. Diagnostic and therapeutic splenectomy for splenic lymphomas: analysis of the National Cancer Data Base. *Hematology.* 2019;24:378-386.
77. Hoppe RT, Advani RH, Ai WZ, et al. Hodgkin lymphoma. *J Natl Compr Canc Netw.* 2011;9:1020-1058.
78. Hodgson K, Ferrer G, Pereira A, Moreno C, Montserrat E. Autoimmune cytopenia in chronic lymphocytic leukaemia: diagnosis and treatment. *Br J Haematol.* 2011;154:14-22.
79. Kreitman RJ. Hairy cell leukemia: present and future directions. *Leuk Lymphoma.* 2019;60:2869-2879.
80. Mesa RA, Nagorney DS, Schwager S, Allred J, Tefferi A. Palliative goals, patient selection, and perioperative platelet management: outcomes and lessons from 3 decades of splenectomy for myelofibrosis with myeloid metaplasia at the Mayo Clinic. *Cancer.* 2006;107:361-370.
81. Tefferi A. Primary myelofibrosis: 2021 update on diagnosis, risk-stratification and management. *Am J Hematol.* 2021;96:145-162.
82. Ingle SB, Hinge Ingle CR, Patrike S. Epithelial cysts of the spleen: a minireview. *World J Gastroenterol.* 2014;20:13899-13903.
83. Hansen MB, Moller AC. Splenic cysts. *Surg Laparosc Endosc Percutaneous Tech.* 2004;14:316-322.
84. Morgenstern L. Nonparasitic splenic cysts: pathogenesis, classification, and treatment. *J Am Coll Surg.* 2002;194:306-314.
85. Sharma A. Splenectomy or partial splenectomy should be preferred treatment for large splenic hydatid cysts. *Am J Trop Med Hyg.* 2016;94:1436.
86. Arikanoglu Z, Taskesen F, Gumus H, et al. Selecting a surgical modality to treat a splenic hydatid cyst: total splenectomy or spleen-saving surgery? *J Gastrointest Surg.* 2012;16:1189-1193.
87. Cowles RA, Yahanda AM. Epidermoid cyst of the spleen. *Am J Surg.* 2000;180:227.
88. Singh AK, Shankar S, Gervais DA, Hahn PF, Mueller PR. Image-guided percutaneous splenic interventions. *Radiographics.* 2012;32:523-534.
89. Thanos L, Dailiana T, Papaioannou G, Nikita A, Koutrouvelis H, Kelekis DA. Percutaneous CT-guided drainage of splenic abscess. *AJR Am J Roentgenol.* 2002;179:629-632.
90. Chen J, Yu S, Xu L. Laparoscopic partial splenectomy: a safe and feasible treatment for splenic benign lesions. *Surg Laparosc Endosc Percutaneous Tech.* 2018;28:287-290.
91. Balint GP, Balint PV. Felty's syndrome. *Best Pract Res Clin Rheumatol.* 2004;18:631-645.
92. Rashba EJ, Rowe JM, Packman CH. Treatment of the neutropenia of Felty syndrome. *Blood Rev.* 1996;10:177-184.
93. Liatsos GD, Tsironi I, Vassilopoulos D, Dourakis S. Severe pancytopenia and splenomegaly associated with Felty's syndrome, both fully responsive solely to corticosteroids. *Clin Case Rep.* 2018;6:509-512.
94. Stassen NA, Bhullar I, Cheng JD, et al. Selective nonoperative management of blunt splenic injury: an Eastern Association for the Surgery of Trauma practice management guideline. *J Trauma Acute Care Surg.* 2012;73:S294-S300.
95. Bhullar IS, Frykberg ER, Siragusa D, et al. Selective angiographic embolization of blunt splenic traumatic injuries in adults decreases failure rate of nonoperative management. *J Trauma Acute Care Surg.* 2012;72:1127-1134.
96. Bhangu A, Nepogodiev D, Lal N, Bowley DM. Meta-analysis of predictive factors and outcomes for failure of non-operative management of blunt splenic trauma. *Injury.* 2012;43:1337-1346.
97. McIntyre LK, Schiff M, Jurkovich GJ. Failure of nonoperative management of splenic injuries: causes and consequences. *Arch Surg.* 2005;140:563-568. discussion 8-9.
98. O'Connor SC, Doud AN, Sieren LM, Miller PR, Zeller KA. The spleen not taken: differences in management and outcomes of blunt splenic injuries in teenagers cared for by adult and pediatric trauma teams in a single institution. *J Trauma Acute Care Surg.* 2017;83:368-372.
99. Clancy AA, Tiruta C, Ashman D, Ball CG, Kirkpatrick AW. The song remains the same although the instruments are changing: complications following selective non-operative management of blunt spleen trauma – a retrospective review of patients at a level I trauma centre from 1996 to 2007. *J Trauma Manag Outcomes.* 2012;6:4.
100. Gorg C, Colle J, Gorg K, Prinz H, Zugmaier G. Spontaneous rupture of the spleen: ultrasound patterns, diagnosis and follow-up. *Br J Radiol.* 2003;76:704-711.
101. Renzulli P, Hostettler A, Schoepfer AM, Gloor B, Candinas D. Systematic review of atraumatic splenic rupture. *Br J Surg.* 2009;96:1114-1121.
102. Delaitre B, Maignien B. Splenectomy by the laparoscopic approach. Report of a case. [Article in French]. *Presse Med.* 1991;20:2263.
103. Shelby R, Kulaylat AN, Villella A, Michalsky MP, Diefenbach KA, Aldrink JH. A comparison of robotic-assisted splenectomy and laparoscopic splenectomy for children with hematologic disorders. *J Pediatr Surg.* 2021;56:1047-1050.
104. Grahn SW, Alvarez J,IIIrd, Kirkwood K. Trends in laparoscopic splenectomy for massive splenomegaly. *Arch Surg.* 2006;141:755-761. discussion 61-2.
105. Kercher KW, Matthews BD, Walsh RM, Sing RF, Backus CL, Heniford BT. Laparoscopic splenectomy for massive splenomegaly. *Am J Surg.* 2002;183:192-196.
106. Tessier DJ, Pierce RA, Brunt LM, et al. Laparoscopic splenectomy for splenic masses. *Surg Endosc.* 2008;22:2062-2066.
107. Winslow ER, Brunt LM, Drebin JA, Soper NJ, Klingensmith ME. Portal vein thrombosis after splenectomy. *Am J Surg.* 2002;184:631-635. discussion 5-6.
108. Danno K, Ikeda M, Sekimoto M, et al. Diameter of splenic vein is a risk factor for portal or splenic vein thrombosis after laparoscopic splenectomy. *Surgery.* 2009;145:457-464. discussion 65-66.
109. James AW, Rabl C, Westphalen AC, Fogarty PF, Posselt AM, Campos GM. Portomesenteric venous thrombosis after laparoscopic surgery: a systematic literature review. *Arch Surg.* 2009;144:520-526.
110. Ikeda M, Sekimoto M, Takiguchi S, et al. High incidence of thrombosis of the portal venous system after laparoscopic splenectomy: a prospective study with contrast-enhanced CT scan. *Ann Surg.* 2005;241:208-216.
111. Stamou KM, Toutouzas KG, Kekis PB, et al. Prospective study of the incidence and risk factors of postsplenectomy thrombosis of the portal, mesenteric, and splenic veins. *Arch Surg.* 2006;141:663-669.
112. Demetriades D, Scalea TM, Degiannis E, et al. Blunt splenic trauma: splenectomy increases early infectious complications – a prospective multicenter study. *J Trauma Acute Care Surg.* 2012;72:229-234.
113. Kyaw MH, Holmes EM, Toolis F, et al. Evaluation of severe infection and survival after splenectomy. *Am J Med.* 2006;119:276 e1-e7.
114. Diamond LK. Splenectomy in childhood and the hazard of overwhelming infection. *Pediatrics.* 1969;43:886-889.
115. Sumaraju V, Smith LG, Smith SM. Infectious complications in asplenic hosts. *Infect Dis Clin North Am.* 2001;15:551-565. x.
116. Moffett SL. Overwhelming postsplenectomy infection: managing patients at risk. *JAAPA.* 2009;22:3645-3649.
117. Kruetzmann S, Rosado MM, Weber H, et al. Human immunoglobulin M memory B cells controlling Streptococcus pneumoniae infections are generated in the spleen. *J Exp Med.* 2003;197:939-945.
118. Tracy ET, Haas KM, Gentry T, et al. Partial splenectomy but not total splenectomy preserves immunoglobulin M memory B cells in mice. *J Pediatr Surg.* 2011;46:1706-1710.
119. Ram S, Lewis LA, Rice PA. Infections of people with complement deficiencies and patients who have undergone splenectomy. *Clin Microbiol Rev.* 2010;23:740-780.
120. Karakantza M, Theodorou GL, Mouzaki A, Theodori E, Vagianos C, Maniatis A. In vitro study of the long-term effects of post-traumatic splenectomy on cellular immunity. *Scand J Immunol.* 2004;59:209-219.
121. Price VE, Blanchette VS, Ford-Jones EL. The prevention and management of infections in children with asplenia or hyposplenia. *Infect Dis Clin North Am.* 2007;21:697-710. viii-ix.
122. Davidson RN, Wall RA. Prevention and management of infections in patients without a spleen. *Clin Microbiol Infect.* 2001;7:657-660.
123. Davies JM, Lewis MP, Wimperis J, et al. Review of guidelines for the prevention and treatment of infection in patients with an absent or dysfunctional spleen: prepared on behalf of the British Committee for Standards in Haematology by a working party of the Haemato-Oncology task force. *Br J Haematol.* 2011;155:308-317.
124. Prevention CfDCa. *Adult Immunization Schedule by Medical and Other Indications.* 2017. https://www.cdc.gov/vaccines/schedules/hcp/imz/adult-conditions.html
125. Howdieshell TR, Heffernan D, Dipiro JT; Therapeutic Agents Committee of the Surgical Infection S. Surgical infection society guidelines for vaccination after traumatic injury. *Surg Infect (Larchmt).* 2006;7:275-303.
126. Bayrhuber M, Anka N, Camp J, Glattacker M, Farin E, Rieg S. Prevention of postsplenectomy sepsis in patients with asplenia - a study protocol of a controlled trial. *BMC Infect Dis.* 2020;20:41.

Chapter 67 ■ Tumors of the Spleen

DANIEL A. ARBER

INTRODUCTION

A variety of tumors and tumorous proliferations may involve the spleen, and there are several that are unique to this organ. This chapter focuses on the unique proliferations as well as other neoplastic causes of splenomegaly. Splenomegaly, however, is not restricted to neoplastic causes and may occur with secondary hypersplenism, which may be secondary to autoimmune or paraneoplastic causes, infectious processes, and passive congestion due to other non–neoplastic medical disorders.

PATTERNS OF TUMOROUS SPLEEN PROLIFERATIONS

Although splenomegaly is often present with splenic neoplasia, some tumors and tumorous proliferations may be found incidentally in normal-sized spleens during radiologic staging or in spleens removed owing to traumatic rupture or incidentally removed during other surgical procedures. The pattern of splenic infiltration may be helpful in the differential diagnosis of splenic tumors, and the gross disease patterns tend to mimic histologic patterns (*Figure 67.1* and *Table 67.1*).[1] The most common disease patterns are diffuse, miliary, and nodular disease. Diffuse disease generally results in splenomegaly with complete infiltration of the splenic parenchyma. This often imparts a glassy and homogeneous red appearance to the cut surface of the spleen. This is usually due to obliteration of the normal splenic white pulp by a cellular proliferation of the red pulp. This disease pattern has traditionally been attributed to leukemic infiltration, T-cell lymphomas, and histiocytic tumors. Many of the red pulp proliferations previously considered to be histiocytic, however, have now been shown to represent T-cell neoplasms. The miliary pattern shows small, punctate tan or white areas throughout the cut surface of the spleen. These usually represent expansion of the splenic white pulp, the normal B-cell compartment of the spleen. However, a similar gross appearance may occur with granulomatous infections. The white pulp expansion pattern most commonly occurs in florid reactive hyperplasia and with low-grade B-cell lymphomas. The nodular disease pattern is characterized by one or more distinct tumor nodules in the spleen that may be identified incidentally on imaging studies. These nodules are usually firm and tan or white in cases of large cell lymphoma, Hodgkin disease, or metastatic tumors and are bloody with a beefy red appearance in vascular proliferations. Cystic lesions of the spleen may also show a nodular pattern of involvement.

CYSTS AND ABSCESSES

Cysts of the spleen are found in <1% of splenectomy specimens.[2] They occur most commonly in men in the third decade of life. They are usually asymptomatic; however, they may cause a splenic mass and be associated with abdominal pain. Splenic cysts may be essentially any size but are on average 10 cm in diameter, and some are associated with elevations of serum carcinogenic antigen 19-9[3] that may cause clinical concern for a malignant neoplasm. Splenic cysts may be designated as primary or secondary, also considered true and false cysts, respectively. Both types are usually unilocular, but some small primary cysts are multilocular. Primary cysts are reported to represent approximately 20% of all splenic cysts, but small primary cysts of the spleen are probably underrepresented in older studies, and more extensive evaluation of nonparasitic cysts shows that the vast majority are true cysts.[4,5] Primary cysts have a firm, rough, and trabecular cyst wall that shows fibrosis and an epithelial lining on histologic examination (*Figure 67.2*). The lining may be of mesothelial or squamous epithelium, with the latter probably representing a metaplastic change. The epithelial lining of primary cysts may be patchy, with denuded

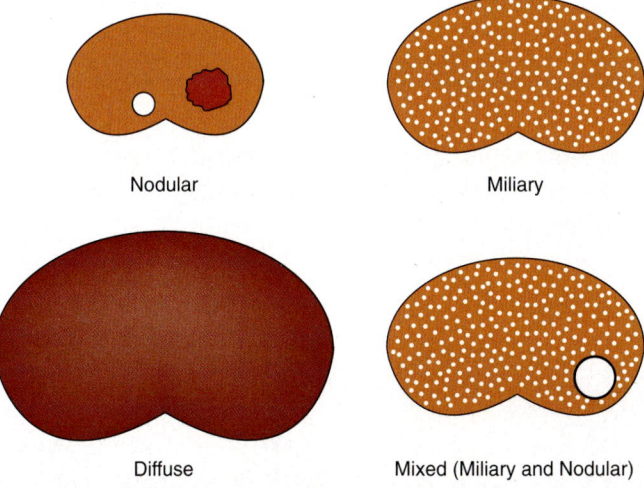

FIGURE 67.1 Gross patterns of splenic tumor involvement. Nodular tumor infiltrates may form solid firm masses or may be hemorrhagic masses. The miliary pattern shows small punctate white foci that usually correspond to expansions of the white pulp. The diffuse pattern shown is usually associated with massive splenomegaly and corresponds to a red pulp expansion. Mixed patterns may be seen when the spleen is involved by more than one process or when a low-grade lymphoma transforms to high-grade disease.

Table 67.1. Patterns of Splenic Tumor Involvement

Diffuse (Predominantly Red Pulp) Disease	Miliary (Predominantly White Pulp) Disease	Predominantly Nodular Disease
Peliosis	Marked white pulp hyperplasia	Cysts
Hemangiomatosis	Chronic lymphocytic leukemia/small lymphocytic lymphoma	Abscess
Lymphangiomatosis		Inflammatory pseudotumor-like follicular/fibroblastic dendritic cell sarcoma
Acute leukemias		
Hairy cell leukemia		
Hairy cell leukemia variant		
Diffuse red pulp small B-cell lymphoma	Prolymphocytic leukemia	Hamartoma
Chronic myeloproliferative neoplasms	Most follicular lymphomas	Hemangioma
	Mantle cell lymphoma	Sclerosing angiomatoid nodular transformation
Lymphoblastic lymphoma	Splenic marginal zone lymphoma	Littoral cell angioma
Hepatosplenic T-cell lymphoma	Lymphoplasmacytic lymphoma[a]	Epithelioid hemangioendothelioma
Large granular lymphocytosis	Early involvement by large B-cell lymphoma	Angiosarcoma
Lymphoplasmacytic lymphoma[a]		Metastatic tumors
		Most large B-cell lymphomas
		Hodgkin lymphoma

[a]More than one pattern may occur with some diseases.

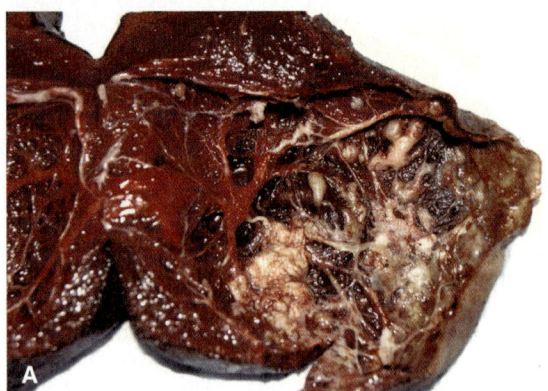 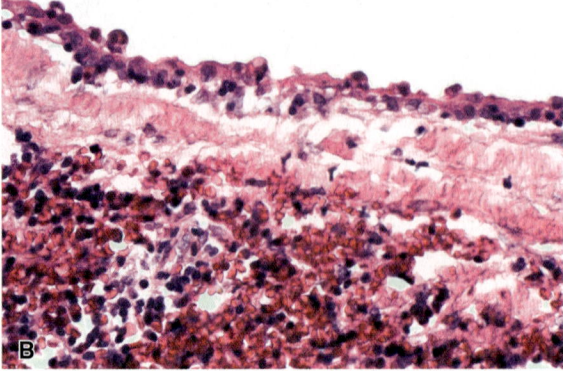

FIGURE 67.2 Primary cysts. A, Primary cyst of the spleen showing a trabeculated inner surface on gross examination. B, The cyst showing an epithelial lining on histologic sections, a feature that is definitional of a primary cyst.

areas present that may simulate a secondary cyst. Primary cysts can be further subdivided into parasitic and nonparasitic types. Primary parasitic cysts related to echinococcal infection (hydatid cysts) are common worldwide, but are uncommon in Western countries. Parasitic cysts are readily identified by the presence of parasite scolices in the cyst contents. Nonparasitic primary cysts appear to arise from congenital inclusions of capsular mesothelium. Small multilocular primary cysts of the spleen occurring at the splenic capsule have in the past been mistaken for lymphangiomas.[6] Primary cysts are usually treated with splenectomy, and partial resection by laparoscopic methods often leads to recurrence.[7]

Secondary cysts are reportedly more common, representing approximately 80% of splenic cysts in most studies, but more detailed evaluation can confirm many of these as having a focal epithelial lining, and thus, they are really primary.[3] The true secondary cysts are often associated with a history of abdominal trauma and are probably acquired after hematoma or infection. The cysts are unilocular and usually have a smooth lining. They differ histologically from primary cysts by the complete absence of an epithelial lining and are thus unlikely to recur even if only partially resected. The cyst wall may contain hemosiderin or calcification.

Some secondary cysts of the spleen may represent resolved abscesses. Multiple small splenic abscesses usually do not develop associated fibrosis with resolution, but larger abscesses are often single and develop a wall of surrounding fibrosis virtually identical to that seen in secondary cysts. Although relatively uncommon, splenic abscesses are most often associated with sepsis or endocarditis. They may also occur following abdominal trauma, including splenic rupture, by contiguous spread of infection from other organs, or in association with functional asplenia in sickle cell anemia.[8] Most splenic abscesses are due to polymicrobial infection, but common organisms include *Streptococcus, Staphylococcus, Escherichia coli,* and *Salmonella.*[9]

Partial splenectomy has been used successfully in the treatment of nonparasitic splenic cysts.[10]

VASCULAR PROLIFERATIONS

Vascular tumors are the most common tumors of the spleen.[11] Vascular proliferations may be diffuse or may form a tumor mass. Peliosis is a rare, diffuse vascular proliferation that is usually an incidental finding occurring in adults.[12] It may be associated with hepatic peliosis and may occur with anabolic steroid use, in association with malignancies, and following solid organ transplantation, as well as in patients with hepatic cirrhosis, tuberculosis, and aplastic anemia. Peliosis results in dilated vascular spaces, usually 1 mm or less in diameter, that involve the entire splenic parenchyma (*Figure 67.3*). Splenic peliosis appears to be associated with an increased risk of splenic rupture.[13]

Hemangiomas are benign tumors that are also usually asymptomatic, but may cause splenomegaly, abdominal pain, and hypersplenism.[2,14-16]

Most hemangiomas are localized and form single or multiple tumor nodules that contain cystic blood-filled spaces grossly. These spaces are lined by endothelial cells, and papillary projections may occur in areas with thrombi. The tumor nodules are usually surrounded by fibrosis and may show calcification. Plain abdominal radiographs, computed tomographic scans, and sonograms are nonspecific, but all show discrete solid and cystic masses, often with evidence of calcification.[17] Diffuse hemangiomatosis of the spleen is less common, is often associated with systemic hemangiomatosis, results in massive splenomegaly, and may be associated with coagulopathies.[18] Diffuse hemangiomatosis differs from peliosis by the presence of intervening fibrosis in hemangiomatosis, which is not a feature of peliosis.

Localized lymphangiomas of the spleen may be difficult to distinguish from hemangiomas or primary cysts, but usually contain proteinaceous fluid rather than the blood of a hemangioma.[2,14,19] Diffuse lymphangiomatosis may be localized to the spleen, but is usually a systemic process and most commonly occurs in children and young adults with massive splenomegaly.[19,20] The splenic parenchyma is replaced by multiple cysts, up to 3 cm in diameter, imparting a spongy appearance (*Figure 67.4*). The cysts are filled with thick pink to brown fluid. Large localized lymphangiomas and lymphangiomatosis of the spleen may be treated with splenectomy.[19]

Although hemangiomas and lymphangiomas of the spleen are similar to those of other sites, there are two unique vascular proliferations of the spleen. Littoral cell angioma is a tumor presumably derived from the normal splenic lining cell, also known as the littoral cell.[15,21,22] These tumors may occur at any age and usually cause mild-to-moderate

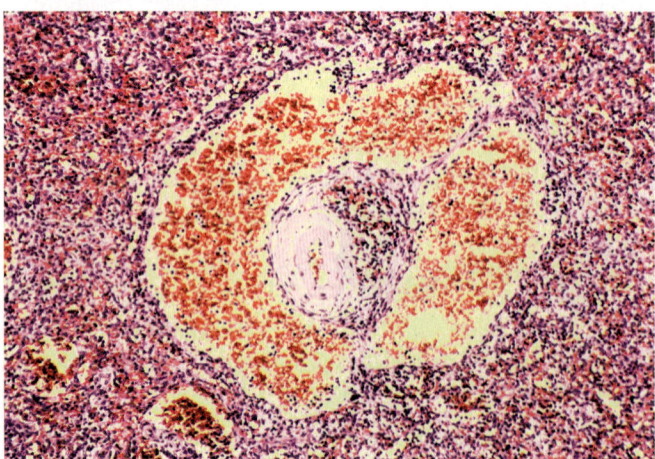

FIGURE 67.3 Splenic peliosis. Peliosis of the spleen shows expanded small vessels that diffusely involve the spleen without forming a nodular mass and without intervening fibrosis.

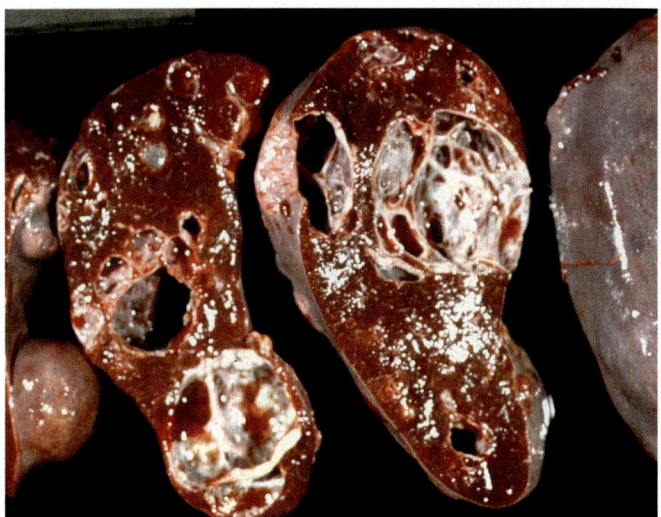

FIGURE 67.4 Lymphangiomatosis. Cut surface of a spleen. Multiple, variably sized cysts are present.

splenomegaly. Many tumors, however, are found incidentally. An association with visceral malignancies is reported.[22] The tumor forms multiple spongy dark red nodules that can measure up to 9 cm in diameter (*Figure 67.5*). Histologically, these tumors differ from hemangiomas in that the vascular spaces are lined by plump cells with nuclear enlargement and often show papillary areas and lining cells sloughing into the vascular spaces. The lining cells of littoral cell angioma have a unique immunophenotype, expressing vascular, histiocytic, and dendritic-associated markers such as CD31, VEGFR-2, ERG, LMO2, CD68, CD163, and CD21. The basilar layer of the lining cells shows unusual expression of langerin.[23] In contrast to hemangiomas and normal sinus-lining cells, the lining cells of littoral cell angioma do not express CD34 or CD8. Most cases of littoral cell angioma are treated with splenectomy without recurrence, but there are reports of late abdominal and liver metastases.[24,25] Those cases showed solid foci of clear cells and probably represent littoral cell hemangioendotheliomas.

Sclerosing angiomatoid nodular transformation (SANT) is the other vascular proliferation unique to the spleen.[26-28] The vast majority of cases of SANT occur in adults, usually presenting as an incidental mass, and less commonly with splenomegaly or abdominal pain. It usually forms a single fibrotic nodule that contains vascular spaces, including slitlike spaces, fibrosis with spindled cells, and splenic sinus-lining cells without nuclear atypia, mitotic figures, or necrosis. Cases of this type have been interpreted in the past as epithelioid and spindled hemangioendotheliomas or as inflammatory pseudotumors, but they have not recurred or metastasized after splenectomy. SANT is now felt to be a reactive fibrous entrapment of altered red pulp, presumably following some form of splenic injury, rather than a true neoplasm. Some reports have described an increase in immunoglobulin G4–positive plasma cells in SANT,[27] but they are not generally believed to be part of the spectrum of IgG4-related disease.

Angiosarcoma of the spleen occurs most commonly in adults and is usually associated with splenomegaly, abdominal pain, and cytopenias.[15,29] Splenic rupture is common in these patients. Because most angiosarcomas involving the spleen are high-grade sarcomas with dissemination, it is often difficult to determine whether the splenic tumor is primary or secondary. The tumor forms an infiltrating mass that may have areas of cystic hemorrhage. The histologic appearance may be varied; however, angiosarcomas characteristically show cytologic atypia, high mitotic activity, and necrosis. Many cases may be difficult to differentiate from other high-grade sarcomas, and immunohistochemical detection of vascular antigen expression, such as CD31, CD34, and von Willebrand factor, is necessary to diagnose such cases. High-grade angiosarcomas involving the spleen have a generally poor prognosis, with most patients dying of disease within 1 year of diagnosis; however, rare cares with long-term survival following splenectomy have been reported.

Low-grade angiosarcomas, also known as epithelioid hemangioendotheliomas, are much less common than high-grade tumors.[30,31] These are reported to occur in both children and adults, but some of the adult cases have features similar to those more recently described for SANT. Patients usually present with anemia and may have hypersplenism or hyposplenism. These tumors are better circumscribed than high-grade angiosarcomas with more bland epithelioid cells, vascular spaces, and prominent fibrosis. They also usually lack necrosis. The cells may show intracellular lumina and will express vascular-associated antigens. These tumors may be incidental findings, are usually localized to the spleen, and do not tend to recur after splenectomy.

LYMPHOID PROLIFERATIONS

Essentially, any lymphoproliferative disorder may involve the spleen, and splenic involvement may be the first evidence of disease. Despite this, most lymphoid proliferations involving the spleen are disseminated at the time of splenic involvement and are accompanied by lymphadenopathy.[32,33] Two types of splenic lymphoma, however, are unique to the spleen and present with splenomegaly without lymphadenopathy.

Splenic marginal zone lymphoma was originally described as a splenic lymphoma with features that mimicked hairy cell leukemia.[34] Although sharing some morphologic and immunophenotypic features, splenic marginal zone lymphoma appears to be distinct from both nodal and extranodal (nonsplenic) marginal zone lymphomas.[35,36] It is the most common lymphoma type in patients with so-called splenic lymphoma with circulating villous lymphocytes.[37-40] Splenic marginal zone lymphoma most commonly occurs in elderly patients with massive splenomegaly (*Figure 67.6*).[33,41-43] Although splenic hilar lymph

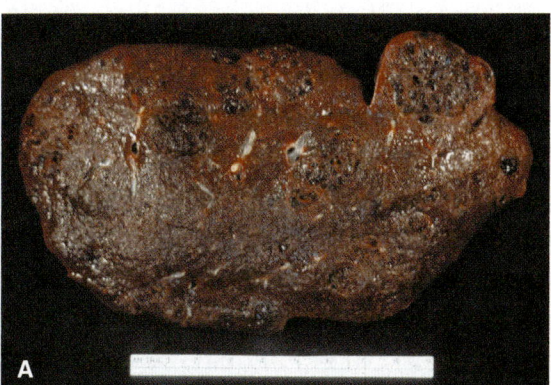
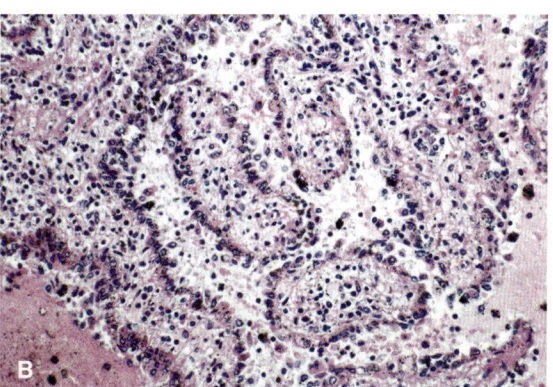

FIGURE 67.5 Littoral cell angioma. A, Multinodular hemorrhagic lesions of the spleen in littoral cell angioma. B, Microscopically, there are papillary vascular spaces with plump-lining cells and histiocytes.

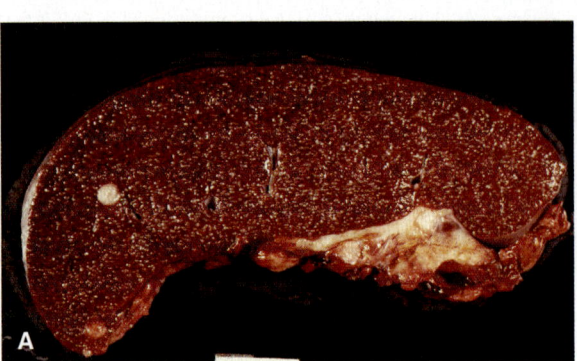
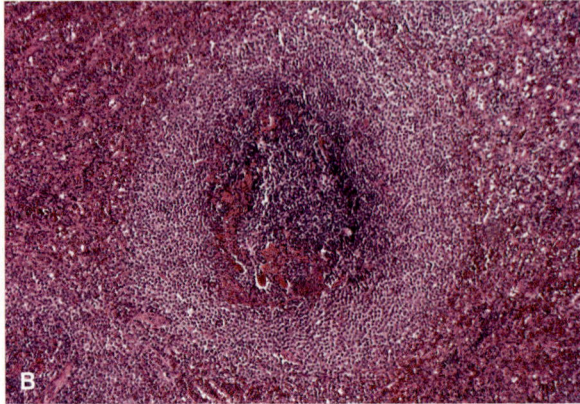

FIGURE 67.6 Splenic marginal zone lymphoma and metastatic carcinoma. A, Gross appearance of the miliary pattern of splenic involvement by splenic marginal zone lymphoma. Note the white, larger mucoid lesion at the left, which represents metastatic papillary serous ovarian carcinoma resulting in a mixed disease pattern of infiltration. B, The splenic marginal zone lymphoma showing a biphasic cellular composition of the white pulp with small round cells in the center and larger lymphocytes with more cytoplasm in the outer marginal zones. Similar cells with clear cytoplasm are also present in the adjacent red pulp.

nodes are often involved by disease, other adenopathy is not usually present. Patients frequently have a lymphocytosis. The abnormal lymphoid cells may vary in appearance, but some cases have circulating lymphocytes with villous cytoplasmic projections that differ from hairy cell leukemia lymphocytes by having only unipolar or bipolar projections as opposed to the more uniform villous projections of hairy cell leukemia. The spleen is uniformly enlarged without a distinct mass. The white pulp is massively expanded by a biphasic population of small lymphocytes that may cause a gross miliary pattern of the spleen parenchyma. The central white pulp lymphocytes are small with scant cytoplasm and are surrounded by a bandlike proliferation of more irregular small lymphocytes with abundant clear to pink cytoplasm on histologic sections. These cells are CD20+ B cells that express BCL2, but do not express CD10, or CD43. A subset of cases may express CD5. The pattern of infiltration is distinct from hairy cell leukemia, hairy cell variant and splenic diffuse red pulp small B-cell lymphoma, which cause a diffuse red pulp infiltrate, and splenic marginal zone lymphoma does not usually demonstrate tartrate-resistant acid phosphatase (TRAP) positivity or expression of annexin A1, CD25, or CD103 of hairy cell leukemia.

Although peripheral blood and bone marrow involvement by splenic marginal zone lymphoma is common,[44] most cases are indolent and do well with splenectomy with or without chemotherapy.[41,45] In a series of 60 patients, all treated with splenectomy and almost half receiving chemotherapy, the overall survival was 103 months with a range of 2 to 164 months. The subset of more aggressive cases tended to show involvement of bone marrow and nonhematopoietic sites.[45] Other features reported to be associated with more aggressive disease include increased numbers of large lymphoma cells, p53 overexpression, and loss of chromosomal regions 7q and 17p.[45-48] A large series of 309 patients found a 76% 5-year cause-specific survival, with factors associated with worse survival on multivariant analysis being hemoglobin <12 g/dL, lactate dehydrogenase levels greater than normal, and albumin levels <3.5 g/dL.[49] More recently, patients have shown excellent responses to rituximab alone or with chemotherapy without splenectomy,[50] but mutations of *NOTCH2* and *TP53* are associated with worse outcome.[51] Rare cases have recurred in lymph nodes with transformation to diffuse large B-cell lymphoma,[52] and one report described cases with transformation to micronodular T-cell–rich large B-cell lymphoma.[53] Cases of splenic marginal zone lymphoma with hepatitis C virus infection and mixed cryoglobulinemia are reported to have regressed with hepatitis C antiviral therapy.[54,55] Most cases, however, occur in the absence of hepatitis C infection, and rituximab with or without chemotherapy appears to have major activity in these patients.[56] Splenic red pulp small B-cell lymphoma and hairy cell leukemia variant share some similarities with splenic marginal zone lymphoma and both remain as provisional entities in the 2016 World Health Organization classification.[57,58] They differ from splenic marginal zone lymphoma by being primarily red pulp small B-cell proliferations. All are CD5 and CD10 negative B-cell proliferations. Hairy cell leukemia variant is typically composed of cells similar to prolymphocytes with prominent nucleoli, but these cells also show cytoplasmic projections suggestive of hairy cells. Despite the morphologic similarity to hairy cell leukemia, hairy cell leukemia variant does not usually express CD25 or annexin A1, markers typically expressed in hairy cell leukemia. It is important to distinguish hairy cell leukemia variant from splenic marginal zone lymphoma because hairy cell leukemia variant is a more aggressive disease.[59]

Hepatosplenic T-cell lymphoma is the other lymphoma type unique to the spleen. It also presents with massive splenomegaly as well as hepatomegaly and usually with bone marrow disease.[60-63] This lymphoma most commonly occurs in young adults with a male predominance. Patients present with fever, weight loss, and jaundice in addition to hepatosplenomegaly and may have pancytopenia and circulating lymphoma cells in the peripheral blood. Rare cases have occurred after solid organ transplantation,[64,65] and cases associated with inflammatory bowel disease and rheumatoid arthritis have been reported. These latter cases may occur in older patients and may be associated with immunomodulator and tumor necrosis factor-α inhibitor therapies,[66] but this remains controversial.[67] This tumor was originally described as erythrophagocytic Tγ lymphoma[68] and has also been referred to as hepatosplenic γδ T-cell lymphoma. The lymphoma diffusely expands the spleen without a discrete mass, and medium-sized cells with irregular nuclear contours and abundant cytoplasm infiltrate the splenic red pulp (*Figure 67.7*), often with loss of the splenic white

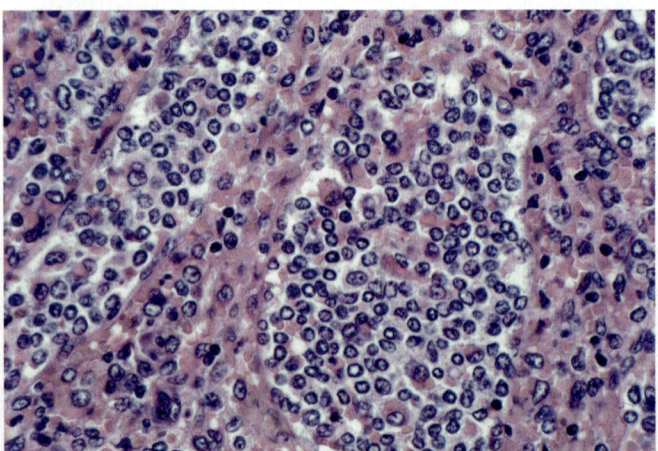

FIGURE 67.7 Hepatosplenic T-cell lymphoma. Medium-sized lymphoma cells are infiltrating the splenic red cords and sinuses of the red pulp.

pulp. The liver involvement is sinusoidal rather than forming a tumor mass. Hemophagocytosis may also be present, and some cases in the past may have been interpreted as malignant histiocytosis. The cells express T-cell–associated markers, such as CD2, CD3, CD5, CD7, and CD43, but may show aberrant loss of one or more of these markers. The cells also usually express CD16, CD56, and TIA-1, but do not show other features of natural killer cells. The cells are negative for Epstein-Barr virus (EBV), granzyme B, and perforin. Most cases are neoplasms of γδ T cells, which do not express CD4, CD8, or T-cell receptor β-chains. However, some cases are αβ T-cell neoplasms, and there appears to be little significance to subdividing this lymphoma by T-cell type[63]; cases with both immunophenotypes show the characteristic combined cytogenetic abnormalities of isochromosome 7q and trisomy 8.[69] Hepatosplenic T-cell lymphoma is an aggressive disease that may show initial improvement following splenectomy and/or chemotherapy, but usually behaves aggressively with a median survival of 8 months (range 0-42 months) reported in one study. Patients with longer survival have received a variety of combination chemotherapy and hematopoietic cell transplantation approaches.[63,70]

Secondary involvement of the spleen by lymphoproliferative disorders is also common.[33] Hairy cell leukemia is one that frequently presents with splenomegaly without lymphadenopathy. The patients are usually elderly, with pancytopenia that includes monocytopenia. Peripheral blood and bone marrow are virtually always involved to some degree, although blood involvement may be minimal. The spleen is enlarged by a diffuse or red pulp infiltrate of small lymphocytes. The white pulp is decreased or absent, and dilated blood-filled spaces, often termed red blood cell "lakes," are common in the red pulp. The blood, bone marrow, and splenic lymphocytes are monotypic B cells that lack CD5 and express CD11c, CD25, annexin A1, CD103, and BRAF V600E mutant protein, as well as being positive by cytochemistry or immunohistochemistry for TRAP. A subset of cases shows expression of CD10 or lacks expression of CD11c, CD25, or CD103.[71] In the past, TRAP cytochemistry was considered the gold standard for diagnosis of hairy cell leukemia, but it has been largely replaced by immunophenotypic evaluation. The blood changes of circulating lymphocytes with villous cytoplasmic projections may be difficult to distinguish from splenic lymphoma with villous lymphocytes, usually secondary to splenic marginal zone lymphoma. However, the pattern of the splenic infiltration between the two diseases differs, with a red pulp or diffuse pattern in hairy cell leukemia and a predominantly white pulp expansion in splenic marginal zone lymphoma.

Other lymphomas of small B lymphocytes may secondarily involve the spleen resulting in splenomegaly and include chronic lymphocytic leukemia/small lymphocytic lymphoma, lymphoplasmacytic lymphoma, mantle cell lymphoma, and follicular lymphoma. With the exception of a subset of cases of lymphoplasmacytic lymphoma, these disorders all infiltrate and expand the splenic white pulp. The majority of large B-cell lymphomas and virtually all cases of Hodgkin lymphoma involving the spleen form distinct tumor nodules with adjacent uninvolved splenic tissue. A subset of large B-cell lymphomas and lymphoplasmacytic lymphomas will primarily involve the splenic red pulp and before immunophenotyping may mimic other disorders, including leukemic infiltrates in the case of red pulp large B-cell lymphoma and, possibly, hairy cell leukemia in the case of red pulp lymphoplasmacytic lymphoma. T-cell lymphomas and the rare histiocytic tumors typically enlarge the spleen by expanding the splenic red pulp in a diffuse manner.

ACUTE LEUKEMIA AND MYELOPROLIFERATIVE NEOPLASMS

In acute leukemia, splenomegaly may be caused by an increase in either lymphoblasts or myeloblasts in the red pulp. This is rarely an isolated finding and does not usually create diagnostic difficulty. Myeloproliferative neoplasms characteristically cause splenomegaly, and in some cases, this enlargement is massive. Primary myelofibrosis most commonly causes massive splenomegaly, usually over

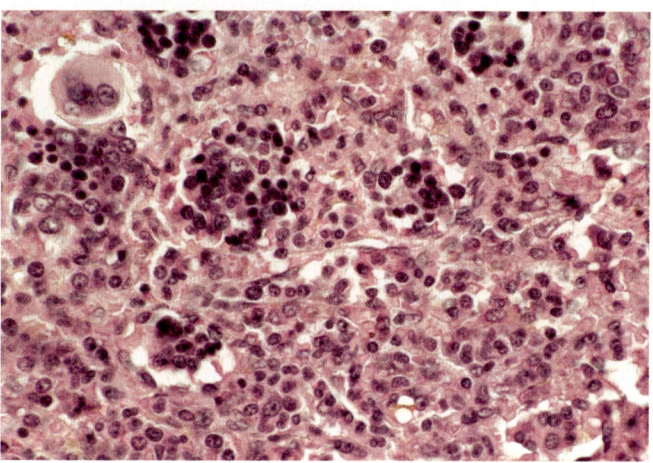

FIGURE 67.8 Chronic myeloid leukemia involving the spleen. The red pulp is expanded by aggregates of erythroid and myeloid precursors admixed with scattered megakaryocytes.

1000 g.[72,73] The splenomegaly may be associated with a wasting syndrome that is improved with splenectomy. Splenectomy in this disorder, however, is associated with an increased risk for blast transformation.[73] The cause of splenomegaly in most myeloproliferative neoplasms is expansion of the splenic red pulp by abnormal hematopoiesis. The red pulp cords and sinuses are filled with varying numbers of nucleated red blood cells, maturing granulocytes, and atypical megakaryocytes (*Figure 67.8*). There may be other causes of noticeable splenomegaly in patients with myeloproliferative neoplasms. A rapidly enlarging spleen may signal accelerated phase or blast transformation. Detection of increased numbers of CD34+ immature cells in the red pulp may be a useful clue to such transformation. In essential thrombocythemia, the spleen may be enlarged because of increased numbers of platelet-filled macrophages in the red pulp. In the early phase of polycythemia vera, massive congestion by red blood cells may be the cause of splenomegaly.[74]

OTHER TUMOROUS PROLIFERATIONS

Splenic hamartomas are also known as splenomas or spleen-in-spleen syndrome and are benign splenic proliferations.[75-77] They may occur at any age and are usually incidental findings, although up to 30% of patients have cytopenias due to hypersplenism. They form single or multiple, sometimes scarring masses of the splenic parenchyma. They are grossly bulging masses when the spleen is cut (*Figure 67.9*), but are more indistinct on histologic sections because these proliferations represent a reduplication of splenic red pulp tissue with normal splenic sinus-lining cells and a lack of normal white pulp. They are also associated with fibrosis, which may include bizarre stromal cells, but these proliferations have no malignant potential. It is not clear whether splenic hamartomas are actually neoplasms or represent an unusual reparative process.

Inflammatory pseudotumor-like follicular/fibroblastic dendritic cell sarcoma (also known as EBV-positive inflammatory follicular dendritic cell tumor), previously known as inflammatory pseudotumor of the spleen and liver, is distinct from inflammatory pseudotumors or inflammatory myofibroblastic tumors of other sites.[78] In the spleen, these tumors occur more commonly in adult women who may present with symptoms that may include fever, weight loss, malaise, anemia, leukocytosis, thrombocytosis, polyclonal hypergammaglobulinemia, and an elevation of the erythrocyte sedimentation rate.[79-81] Infectious disease evaluations are usually negative. The splenic mass is usually solitary and may be up to 12 cm in diameter. The tumor is a dense nodule containing a mixed inflammatory infiltrate and fibrosis. The spindled fibrotic cells of this unique tumor contain evidence of clonal EBV, and the infected spindled cells in some cases express the follicular dendritic cell marker CD21. Some

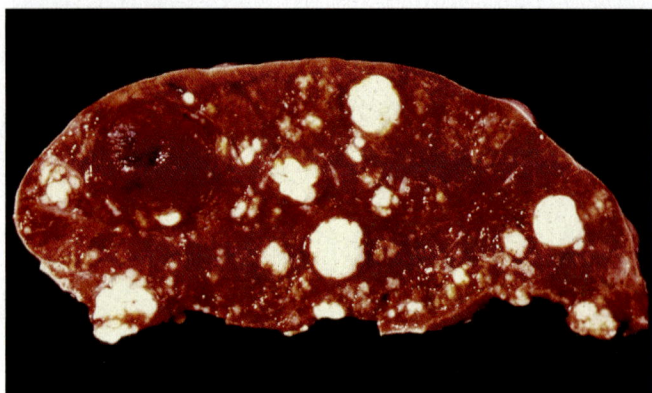

FIGURE 67.9 Splenic hamartoma and splenic involvement by classic Hodgkin lymphoma. The hamartoma represents a bulging red mass to the left, whereas the Hodgkin lymphoma forms multiple firm white nodules throughout the spleen. Hamartomas are often incidental findings in spleens removed for other reasons.

hepatic cases have recurred, but splenic cases treated with splenectomy have not. Although now considered as an unusual type of follicular dendritic cell tumor,[82] other follicular dendritic cell tumors are not associated with the EBV.

Primary sarcomas, other than angiosarcoma, and carcinomas of the spleen are extremely uncommon. Reported cases of sarcoma include malignant fibrous histiocytoma, fibrosarcoma, leiomyosarcoma, rhabdomyosarcoma, histiocytic sarcoma, interdigitating dendritic cell sarcoma, and fibroblastic reticular cell tumor.[3,83-88] Primary carcinomas reported include squamous cell carcinoma arising in a cyst, mucinous cystadenocarcinoma and carcinosarcoma both possibly arising from peritoneal surface epithelium, and primary transitional cell carcinoma.[89-92] Although still rare, carcinoma of the spleen from metastasis or direct tumor extension is more common than primary disease. One-third of metastatic tumors are only identified on microscopic examination,[93] so the frequency of splenic involvement may be underestimated by imaging studies. Lung, gastric, ovarian, and breast carcinoma primaries are the most common to involve the spleen, and splenectomy may be performed for solitary splenic metastases.[94,95]

References

1. Arber DA. Spleen. In: Goldblum JRLL, McKenney JK, Myers JL, eds. *Rosai and Ackerman's Surgical Pathology*. 11th ed. Elsevier; 2018.
2. McClure RD, Altemeier WA. Cysts of the spleen. *Ann Surg*. 1942;116(1):98-102.
3. Matsui T, Matsubayashi H, Sugiura T, et al. A splenic epithelial cyst: increased size, exacerbation of symptoms, and elevated levels of serum carcinogenic antigen 19-9 after 6-year follow-up. *Intern Med*. 2016;55(18):2629-2634.
4. Vajda P, Kereskai L, Czauderna P, et al. Re-evaluation of histological findings of nonparasitic splenic cysts. *Eur J Gastroenterol Hepatol*. 2012;24(3):316-319.
5. Pang WB, Zhang TC, Chen YJ, Zhang JZ. Space-occupying benign lesions in spleen: experiences in a single institute. *Pediatr Surg Int*. 2009;25(1):31-35.
6. Arber DA, Strickler JG, Weiss LM. Splenic mesothelial cysts mimicking lymphangiomas. *Am J Surg Pathol*. 1997;21(3):334-338.
7. Ganti AL, Sardi A, Gordon J. Laparoscopic treatment of large true cysts of the liver and spleen is ineffective. *Am Surg*. 2002;68(11):1012-1017.
8. Al-Salem AH, Qaisaruddin S, Jam'a AA, Al-Kalaf J, El-Bashier AM. Splenic abscess and sickle cell disease. *Am J Hematol*. 1998;58:100-104.
9. Brook I, Frazier EH. Microbiology of liver and spleen abscesses. *J Med Microbiol*. 1998;47(12):1075-1080.
10. Szczepanik AB, Meissner AJ. Partial splenectomy in the management of nonparasitic splenic cysts. *World J Surg*. 2009;33(4):852-856.
11. Sangiorgio VFI, Arber DA. Vascular neoplasms and non-neoplastic vascular lesions of the spleen. *Semin Diagn Pathol*. 2021;38(2):154-158.
12. Tsokos M, Puschel K. Isolated peliosis of the spleen: report of 2 autopsy cases. *Am J Forensic Med Pathol*. 2004;25(3):251-254.
13. Kohr RM, Haendiges M, Taube RR. Peliosis of the spleen: a rare cause of spontaneous splenic rupture with surgical implications. *Am Surg*. 1993;59(3):197-199.
14. Morgenstern L, Rosenberg J, Geller SA. Tumors of the spleen. *World J Surg*. 1985;9:468-476.
15. Arber DA, Strickler JG, Chen YY, Weiss LM. Splenic vascular tumors: a histologic, immunophenotypic, and virologic study. *Am J Surg Pathol*. 1997;21(7):827-835.
16. Willcox TM, Speer RW, Schlinkert RT, Sarr MG. Hemangioma of the spleen: presentation, diagnosis, and management. *J Gastrointest Surg*. 2000;4(6):611-613.
17. Abbott RM, Levy AD, Aguilera NS, Gorospe L, Thompson WM. From the archives of the AFIP: primary vascular neoplasms of the spleen – radiologic-pathologic correlation. *Radiographics*. 2004;24(4):1137-1163.
18. Shiran A, Naschitz JE, Yeshurun D, Misselevitch I, Boss JH. Diffuse hemangiomatosis of the spleen: splenic hemangiomatosis presenting with giant splenomegaly, anemia, and thrombocytopenia. *Am J Gastroenterol*. 1990;85:1515-1517.
19. Morgenstern L, Bello JM, Fisher BL, Verham RP. The clinical spectrum of lymphangiomas and lymphangiomatosis of the spleen. *Am Surg*. 1992;58:599-604.
20. Marymont JV, Knight PJ. Splenic lymphangiomatosis: a rare cause of splenomegaly. *J Pediatr Surg*. 1987;22(5):461-462.
21. Falk S, Stutte HJ, Frizzera G. Littoral cell angioma. A novel splenic vascular lesion demonstrating histiocytic differentiation. *Am J Surg Pathol*. 1991;15(11):1023-1033.
22. Peckova K, Michal M, Hadravsky L, et al. Littoral cell angioma of the spleen: a study of 25 cases with confirmation of frequent association with visceral malignancies. *Histopathology*. 2016;69(5):762-774.
23. Selove W, Picarsic J, Swerdlow SH. Langerin staining identifies most littoral cell angiomas but not most other splenic angiomatous lesions. *Hum Pathol*. 2019;83:43-49.
24. Ben Izhak O, Bejar J, Ben Eliezer S, Vlodavsky E. Splenic littoral cell haemangioendothelioma: a new low-grade variant of malignant littoral cell tumour. *Histopathology*. 2001;39(5):469-475.
25. Fernandez S, Cook GW, Arber DA. Metastasizing splenic littoral cell hemangioendothelioma. *Am J Surg Pathol*. 2006;30(8):1036-1040.
26. Martel M, Cheuk W, Lombardi L, Lifschitz-Mercer B, Chan JK, Rosai J. Sclerosing angiomatoid nodular transformation (SANT): report of 25 cases of a distinctive benign splenic lesion. *Am J Surg Pathol*. 2004;28(10):1268-1279.
27. Kuo TT, Chen TC, Lee LY. Sclerosing angiomatoid nodular transformation of the spleen (SANT): clinicopathological study of 10 cases with or without abdominal disseminated calcifying fibrous tumors, and the presence of a significant number of IgG4+ plasma cells. *Pathol Int*. 2009;59(12):844-850.
28. Chang KC, Lee JC, Wang YC, et al. Polyclonality in sclerosing angiomatoid nodular transformation of the spleen. *Am J Surg Pathol*. 2016;40(10):1343-1351.
29. Falk S, Krishnan J, Meis JM. Primary angiosarcoma of the spleen. A clinicopathologic study of 40 cases. *Am J Surg Pathol*. 1993;17(10):959-970.
30. Suster S. Epithelioid and spindle-cell hemangioendothelioma of the spleen. Report of a distinctive splenic vascular neoplasm of childhood. *Am J Surg Pathol*. 1992;16(8):785-792.
31. Kaw YT, Duwaji MS, Kinsley RE, Esparza AR. Hemangioendothelioma of the spleen. *Arch Pathol Lab Med*. 1992;116:1079-1082.
32. Falk S, Stutte HJ. Primary malignant lymphomas of the spleen. A morphologic and immunohistochemical analysis of 17 cases. *Cancer*. 1990;66:2612-2619.
33. Arber DA, Rappaport H, Weiss LM. Non-Hodgkin's lymphoproliferative disorders involving the spleen. *Mod Pathol*. 1997;10(1):18-32.
34. Neiman RS, Sullivan AL, Jaffe R. Malignant lymphoma simulating leukemic reticuloendotheliosis. A clinicopathologic study of ten cases. *Cancer*. 1979;43:329-342.
35. Sol Mateo M, Mollejo M, Villuendas R, et al. Analysis of the frequency of microsatellite instability and p53 gene mutation in splenic marginal zone and MALT lymphomas. *J Clin Pathol*. 1998;51:262-267.
36. Bonfiglio F, Bruscaggin A, Guidetti F, et al. Genetic and phenotypic attributes of splenic marginal zone lymphoma. *Blood*. 2022;139(5):732-747.
37. Melo JV, Hegde U, Parreira A, Thompson I, Lampert IA, Catovsky D. Splenic B cell lymphoma with circulating villous lymphocytes: differential diagnosis of B cell leukaemias with large spleens. *J Clin Pathol*. 1987;40:642-651.
38. Mulligan SP, Matutes E, Dearden C, Catovsky D. Splenic lymphoma with villous lymphocytes: natural history and response to theraepy in 50 cases. *Br J Haematol*. 1991;78:206-209.
39. Troussard X, Valensi F, Duchayne E, et al. Splenic lymphoma with villous lymphocytes: clinical presentation, biology and prognostic factors in a series of 100 patients. *Br J Haematol*. 1996;93:731-736.
40. Isaacson PG, Matutes E, Burke M, Catovsky D. The histopathology of splenic lymphoma with villous lymphocytes. *Blood*. 1994;84(11):3828-3834.
41. Schmid C, Kirkham N, Diss T, Isaacson PG. Splenic marginal zone cell lymphoma. *Am J Surg Pathol*. 1992;16(5):455-466.
42. Mollejo M, Men rguez J, Lloret E, et al. Splenic marginal zone lymphoma: a distinctive type of low-grade B-cell lymphoma - a clinicopathological study of 13 cases. *Am J Surg Pathol*. 1995;19(10):1146-1157.
43. Hammer RD, Glick AD, Greer JP, Collins RD, Cousar JB. Splenic marginal zone lymphoma. A distinct B-cell neoplasm. *Am J Surg Pathol*. 1996;20(5):613-626.
44. Arber DA, George TI. Bone marrow biopsy involvement by non-Hodgkin's lymphoma: frequency of lymphoma types, patterns, blood involvement, and discordance with other sites in 450 specimens. *Am J Surg Pathol*. 2005;29(12):1549-1557.
45. Chacon JI, Mollejo M, Munoz E, et al. Splenic marginal zone lymphoma: clinical characteristics and prognostic factors in a series of 60 patients. *Blood*. 2002;100(5):1648-1654.
46. Lloret E, Mollejo M, Mateo MS, et al. Splenic marginal zone lymphoma with increased number of blasts: an aggressive variant? *Hum Pathol*. 1999;30(10):1153-1160.
47. Hernandez JM, Garcia JL, Gutierrez NC, et al. Novel genomic imbalances in B-cell splenic marginal zone lymphomas revealed by comparative genomic hybridization and cytogenetics. *J Pathol*. 2001;158(5):1843-1850.
48. Algara P, Mateo MS, Sanchez-Beato M, et al. Analysis of the IgV(H) somatic mutations in splenic marginal zone lymphoma defines a group of unmutated cases with frequent 7q deletion and adverse clinical course. *Blood*. 2002;99(4):1299-1304.
49. Arcaini L, Lazzarino M, Colombo N, et al. Splenic marginal zone lymphoma: a prognostic model for clinical use. *Blood*. 2006;107(12):4643-4649.

50. Bennett M, Schechter GP. Treatment of splenic marginal zone lymphoma: splenectomy versus rituximab. *Semin Hematol.* 2010;47(2):143-147.
51. Parry M, Rose-Zerilli MJ, Ljungstrom V, et al. Genetics and prognostication in splenic marginal zone lymphoma: revelations from deep sequencing. *Clin Cancer Res.* 2015;21(18):4174-4183.
52. Camacho FI, Mollejo M, Mateo MS, et al. Progression to large B-cell lymphoma in splenic marginal zone lymphoma - a description of a series of 12 cases. *Am J Surg Pathol.* 2001;25(10):1268-1276.
53. Wang SA, Olson N, Zukerberg L, Harris NL. Splenic marginal zone lymphoma with micronodular T-cell rich B-cell lymphoma. *Am J Surg Pathol.* 2006;30(1):128-132.
54. Hermine O, Lefrere F, Bronowicki JP, et al. Regression of splenic lymphoma with villous lymphocytes after treatment of hepatitis C virus infection. *N Engl J Med.* 2002;347(2):89-94.
55. Saadoun D, Suarez F, Lefrere F, et al. Splenic lymphoma with villous lymphocytes, associated with type II cryoglobulinemia and HCV infection: a new entity? *Blood.* 2005;105(1):74-76.
56. Tsimberidou AM, Catovsky D, Schlette E, et al. Outcomes in patients with splenic marginal zone lymphoma and marginal zone lymphoma treated with rituximab with or without chemotherapy or chemotherapy alone. *Cancer.* 2006;107(1):125-135.
57. Mollejo M, Algara P, Mateo MS, et al. Splenic small B-cell lymphoma with predominant red pulp involvement: a diffuse variant of splenic marginal zone lymphoma? *Histopathology.* 2002;40(1):22-30.
58. Matutes E, Wotherspoon A, Catovsky D. The variant form of hairy-cell leukaemia. *Best Pract Res Clin Haematol.* 2003;16(1):41-56.
59. Hockley SL, Else M, Morilla A, et al. The prognostic impact of clinical and molecular features in hairy cell leukaemia variant and splenic marginal zone lymphoma. *Br J Haematol.* 2012;158(3):347-354.
60. Gaulard P, Bourquelot P, Kanavaros P, et al. Expression of the alpha/beta and gamma/delta T-cell receptors in 57 cases of peripheral T-cell lymphomas. Identification of a subset of γ/δ T-cell lymphomas. *Am J Pathol.* 1990;137(3):617-628.
61. Cooke CB, Krenacs L, Stetler-Stevenson M, et al. Hepatosplenic T-cell lymphoma: a distinct clinicopathologic entity of cytotoxic γδ T-cell origin. *Blood.* 1996;88(11):4265-4274.
62. Salhany KE, Feldman M, Kahn MJ, et al. Hepatosplenic γδ T-cell lymphoma: ultrastructural, immunophenotypic, and functional evidence for cytotoxic T lymphocyte differentiation. *Hum Pathol.* 1997;28(6):674-685.
63. Macon WR, Levy NB, Kurtin PJ, et al. Hepatosplenic alpha beta T-cell lymphomas - a report of 14 cases and comparison with hepatosplenic gamma delta T-cell lymphomas. *Am J Surg Pathol.* 2001;25(3):285-296.
64. Ross CW, Schnitzer B, Sheldon S, Braun DK, Hanson CA. Gamma/delta T-cell prostransplantation lymphoproliferative disorder primarily in the spleen. *Am J Clin Pathol.* 1994;102:310-315.
65. Kraus MD, Crawford DF, Kaleem Z, Shenoy S, MacArthur CA, Longtine JA. T γ/δ hepatosplenic lymphoma in a heart transplant patient after and Epstein-Barr positive lymphoproliferative disorder. A case report. *Cancer.* 1998;82:983-992.
66. Parakkal D, Sifuentes H, Semer R, Ehrenpreis ED. Hepatosplenic T-cell lymphoma in patients receiving TNF-alpha inhibitor therapy: expanding the groups at risk. *Eur J Gastroenterol Hepatol.* 2011;23(12):1150-1156.
67. Mercer LK, Regierer AC, Mariette X, et al. Spectrum of lymphomas across different drug treatment groups in rheumatoid arthritis: a European registries collaborative project. *Ann Rheum Dis.* 2017;76(12):2025-2030.
68. Kadin ME, Kamoun M, Lamberg J. Erythrophagocytic Tγ lymphoma. A clinicopathologic entity resembling malignant histiocytosis. *N Engl J Med.* 1981;304(11):648-653.
69. Jonveaux P, Daniel MT, Martel V, Maarek O, Berger R. Isochromosome 7q and trisomy 8 are consistent primary, non-random chromosomal abnormalities associated with hepatosplenic T gamma/delta lymphoma. *Leukemia.* 1996;10:1453-1455.
70. Weidmann E. Hepatosplenic T cell lymphoma. A review on 45 cases since the first report describing the disease as a distinct lymphoma entity in 1990. *Leukemia.* 2000;14(6):991-997.
71. Chen YH, Tallman MS, Goolsby C, Peterson L. Immunophenotypic variations in hairy cell leukemia. *Am J Clin Pathol.* 2006;125(2):251-259.
72. Falk S, Mix D, Stutte HJ. The spleen in osteomyelofibrosis. A morphologic and immunohistochemical study of 30 cases. *Virchows Arch A Pathol Anat Histopathol.* 1990;416:437-442.
73. Theile J, Klein H, Falk S, Bertsch HP, Fischer R, Stutte HJ. Splenic megakaryocytopoiesis in primary (idiopathic) osteomyelofibrosis. An immunohistochemical and morphometric study with comparison of corresponding bone marrow features. *ActaHaematol.* 1992;87:176-180.
74. Wolf BC, Banks PM, Mann RB, Neiman RS. Splenic hematopoiesis in polycythemia vera. A morphologic and immunohistochemical study. *Am J Clin Pathol.* 1988;89:69-75.
75. Falk S, Stutte HJ. Hamartomas of the spleen: a study of 20 biopsy cases. *Histopathology.* 1989;14:603-612.
76. Cheuk W, Lee AK, Arora N, Ben Arie Y, Chan JK. Splenic hamartoma with bizarre stromal cells. *Am J Surg Pathol.* 2005;29(1):109-114.
77. Sangiorgio VFI, Arber DA. Non-hematopoietic neoplastic and pseudoneoplastic lesions of the spleen. *Semin Diagn Pathol.* 2021;38(2):159-164.
78. Arber DA, Kamel OW, van de Rijn M, et al. Frequent presence of the Epstein-Barr virus in inflammatory pseudotumor. *Hum Pathol.* 1995;26(10):1093-1098.
79. Cotelingam JD, Jaffe ES. Inflammatory pseudotumor of the spleen. *Am J Surg Pathol.* 1984;8(5):375-380.
80. Selves J, Meggetto F, Brousset P, et al. Inflammatory pseudotumor of the liver. Evidence for follicular dendritic reticulum cell proliferation associated with clonal Epstein-Barr virus. *Am J Surg Pathol.* 1996;20(6):747-753.
81. Neuhauser TS, Derringer GA, Thompson LD, et al. Splenic inflammatory myofibroblastic tumor (inflammatory pseudotumor): a clinicopathologic and immunophenotypic study of 12 cases. *ArchPathol Lab Med.* 2001;125(3):379-385.
82. Cheuk W, Chan JK, Shek TW, et al. Inflammatory pseudotumor-like follicular dendritic cell tumor: a distinctive low-grade malignant intra-abdominal neoplasm with consistent Epstein-Barr virus association. *Am J Surg Pathol.* 2001;25(6):721-731.
83. Wick MR, Smith SL, Scheithauer BW, Beart RW, Jr. Primary nonlymphoreticular malignant neoplasms of the spleen. *Am J Surg Pathol.* 1982;6(3):229-242.
84. Feakins RM, Norton AJ. Rhabdomyosarcoma of the spleen. *Histopathology.* 1996;29:577-579.
85. Martel M, Sarli D, Colecchia M, et al. Fibroblastic reticular cell tumor of the spleen: report of a case and review of the entity. *Hum Pathol.* 2003;34(9):954-957.
86. Audouin J, Vercelli-Retta J, le Tourneau A, et al. Primary histiocytic sarcoma of the spleen associated with erythrophagocytic histiocytosis. *Pathol Res Pract.* 2003;199(2):107-112.
87. Kawachi K, Nakatani Y, Inayama Y, Kawano N, Toda N, Misugi K. Interdigitating dendritic cell sarcoma of the spleen: report of a case with a review of the literature. *Am J Surg Pathol.* 2002;26(4):530-537.
88. Colovic N, Cemerikic-Martinovic V, Colovic R, Zogovic S. Primary malignant fibrous histiocytoma of the spleen and liver. *MedOncol.* 2001;18(4):293-297.
89. Elit L, Aylward B. Splenic cyst carcinoma presenting in pregnancy. *Am J Hematol.* 1989;32:57-60.
90. Morinaga S, Ohyama R, Koizumi J. Low-grade mucinous cystadenocarcinoma in the spleen. *Am J Surg Pathol.* 1992;16(9):903-908.
91. Westra WH, Anderson BO, Klimstra DS. Carcinosarcoma of the spleen. An extragenital malignant mixed müllerian tumor? *Am J Surg Pathol.* 1994;18(3):309-315.
92. Naik S, Kapoor S, Sharma S, Sewkani A, Juneja M, Varshney S. Primary transitional cell carcinoma of spleen. *Indian J Gastroenterol.* 2006;25(4):215.
93. Marymont JH, Gross S. Patterns of metastatic cancer in the spleen. *Am J Clin Pathol.* 1963;40(1):58-66.
94. Klein B, Stein M, Kuten A, et al. Splenomegaly and solitary spleen metastasis in solid tumors. *Cancer.* 1987;60(1):100-102.
95. Lam KY, Tang V. Metastatic tumors to the spleen: a 25-year clinicopathologic study. *Arch Pathol Lab Med.* 2000;124(4):526-530.

Part 7

HEMATOLOGIC MALIGNANCIES

Section 1 ■ GENERAL ASPECTS

Chapter 68 ■ Hematopoietic Neoplasms: Principles of Pathologic Diagnosis

DANIEL A. ARBER

INTRODUCTION

The hematopoietic neoplasms consist of acute and chronic leukemias, Hodgkin and non-Hodgkin lymphomas, plasma cell tumors, and the rare histiocytic and dendritic neoplasms. Each of these disease categories is now recognized to represent various heterogeneous disease groups that include a large number of distinct biologic entities.[1-4] In view of the great advances in targeted therapies and molecular genetic discoveries made in the area of hematopoietic tumors, the number of distinct entities will continue to grow. Although the diagnosis and classification of these tumors were originally based primarily on morphologic features, sometimes supplemented by cytochemical studies,[5-9] diagnosis of hematopoietic tumors now requires a complex battery of specialized tools that almost always include immunophenotyping and frequently require cytogenetic and molecular genetic studies. Despite these advances, morphologic evaluation remains the cornerstone of the pathologic diagnosis for most diseases. Morphologic evaluation allows for cost-effective tissue processing and triaging for appropriate ancillary tests, which becomes increasingly important as the number of molecular genetic tests grows in this area.

PREOPERATIVE CONSIDERATIONS

Special considerations are often needed prior to sampling of tissue that is suspected to contain a hematopoietic neoplasm.[10-14] The testing that will be needed depends on the clinical differential diagnosis as well as the initial pathologic impression of the sample. Guidelines have been recently published for the evaluation of patients suspected of having acute leukemia[15] and lymphoid neoplasms.[16] If the correct specimen types for ancillary tests are not saved prior to the initial pathologic review, the tissue may not be sufficient for these additional tests. Therefore, the hematologist, pathologist, or surgeon performing the procedure should have a clear understanding of the specimen requirements for the various tests that might be needed to confirm or rule out all suspected diseases. This often requires direct communication with the surgical pathologist or hematopathologist who will ultimately receive the sample prior to obtaining tissue. Submission of fresh tissue on saline-soaked gauze is ideal for tissue samples; however, this may not be feasible if the sample is taken at night or in a clinic that is physically separate from where the sample is processed. Even in the latter setting, the sample may be couriered to a remote location quickly so that the tissue can be correctly triaged. If the sample has not been centrally processed, the physician performing the procedure must be aware of how to collect samples that are adequate for immunophenotyping studies, molecular and cytogenetic studies, and possible cultures. This problem is even more complicated when reference laboratories are used for different types of testing, an increasingly common practice, resulting in the need to split what may be very small samples prior to sending them out for these studies.

Ideally, the entire fresh sample is submitted to the pathology department within minutes of removal. There it may be received by a resident, technician, pathology assistant, or pathologist. No matter who receives the specimen, the clinical indication for the biopsy and any special clinical concerns or testing requirements need to be clearly communicated. For tissues removed to rule out lymphoma, specimens should be sampled in the fresh state. One protocol for lymph node sampling is provided in *Figure 68.1*[10] and discussed in more detail in what follows. Hematologists and pathologists should work together to establish a suitable protocol for their institution. Special needs should be communicated to the pathologist before obtaining the sample, to ensure that the supporting testing areas, such as cytogenetics or microbiology, are prepared to receive the sample or to make arrangements to send samples quickly to the appropriate reference laboratory. It is worth noting that surgical pathologists receive lymph node specimens for a variety of indications, most of which do not require special processing and are simply formalin fixed. Without adequate clinical information and communication alerting them to the possibility of lymphoma or another hematopoietic tumor, tissue may not be sent for flow cytometry or cytogenetic studies or saved for possible molecular genetic studies. Because the differential diagnosis of malignant lymphoma often includes infectious etiologies, the need for cultures or other infectious disease testing requiring fresh tissue or other special tissue preparation must also be communicated. Similarly, if a suspicion of acute leukemia is not conveyed to the pathologist, adequate material may not be saved for appropriate molecular genetic studies that may be triggered by features identified during the course of the pathologic evaluation of the disease. With appropriate clinical information, the pathologist may bank frozen cells or prepare a nondecalcified clot section of the marrow specimen for possible future studies.

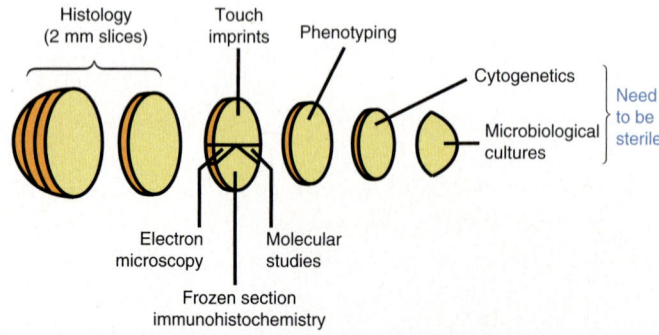

FIGURE 68.1 Schematic of protocol for processing lymph node biopsies from patients suspected of having lymphoid malignancies.

SPECIMEN PROCESSING

Triaging Protocols

How a sample for a suspected hematologic disorder is triaged often depends on the specimen type and the approach developed by the institution. Peripheral blood, bone marrow aspirate, and fine-needle aspirate samples are often triaged at the bedside by the physician collecting the sample. In this setting, the treating physician often orders flow cytometry immunophenotyping, cytogenetics, molecular genetics, and even cultures on samples collected in different tubes. Because the diagnosis of most disorders is still based in large part on morphologic features, it is advisable to use the initial bone marrow aspirate material for fresh smears, prepared at the bedside, or to make touch preparations for morphology in all cases with inadequate aspirate material (see Chapter 1). Subsequent aspirations may be more hemodiluted but are usually still suitable for ancillary studies. Some institutions, however, have moved to having bone marrow testing triaged after receipt in the laboratory based on protocols developed between treating physicians and pathologists. This approach is sure to result in more timely and cost-effective testing.[17,18] In contrast to marrow specimens, the triaging of tissue biopsy specimens is historically performed after the sample is submitted to the laboratory, as mentioned previously and illustrated in Figure 68.1.[10,11] If lymphoma is suspected, sections of fresh material should be fixed for morphologic evaluation. If enough tissue is obtained, a portion of fresh tissue may also be sent for flow cytometry and possibly for cytogenetics or cultures. Additional material may be frozen for future molecular genetic studies. The exact tests performed, however, will depend on the clinical indication for the biopsy and communication between the pathologist and the treating hematologist, but most lymphoma-associated genetic testing, especially fluorescence in situ hybridization (FISH) testing, can now be performed on formalin-fixed, paraffin-embedded tissue.

Tissue Fixation and Processing

Proper specimen fixation and processing are essential for morphologic evaluation as well as for the optimal performance of ancillary studies.[12-14] If lymphoma is suspected, thin sections of fresh material should be fixed for morphologic evaluation. In the past, special fixatives containing heavy metals such as mercuric chloride were used to improve cell morphology, but these fixatives are less commonly used today because of difficulties in disposing of the mercury. Such fixatives also disrupt nucleic acids, making molecular studies often impossible. More routine formalin fixation will usually provide appropriate sections, as long as the tissue is fixed adequately; usually this means overnight fixation of thin sections in fresh neutral buffered formalin. Formalin-fixed tissue is satisfactory for many DNA-based molecular assays, but some tests cannot be performed on fixed tissue. Tissue that is frozen should be stored at the lowest possible temperature (preferably −70 to −80 °C) and not in defrostable freezers.

Bone marrow aspirate specimens should be sent fresh after collection with minimal anticoagulant. Bone marrow biopsies should also be submitted fresh or in fixative if delivery to the laboratory may be delayed. Again, heavy metal fixatives are less commonly available today, and formalin or Bouin fixation is more frequently used. Bone marrow biopsies also must undergo decalcification, which may degrade some antigens and may reduce the ability to perform some assays. Decalcification in ethylenediaminetetraacetic acid is considered the most gentle for antigen preservation,[18] but some methods take several days to obtain adequate decalcification; hence, this method is not routinely performed in many laboratories.

SAMPLING METHODS AND THEIR LIMITATIONS

Open Biopsy

The ideal specimen for pathologic evaluation is a large portion of tissue, received fresh and taken from an open biopsy. Such samples allow the maximum amount of tissue for morphologic analysis and ancillary studies. However, the increasing use of less-invasive procedures requires different approaches for different specimen types.

Peripheral Blood

Peripheral blood is often the easiest sample to obtain for an initial evaluation for a hematologic malignancy. Analysis of blood may allow for a diagnosis of leukemia or even peripheral blood involvement by lymphoma, although the absence of neoplastic cells in blood cannot exclude disease elsewhere. Limitations to blood analysis include the inability to classify blast proliferations with <20% circulating blasts and the lack of architecture needed for classification of some lymphomas involving blood. Despite these limitations, when blood is involved by a hematopoietic tumor, morphologic, immunophenotypic, and molecular genetic studies of blood may be of value in some patients. However, if a bone marrow is to be performed, duplication of testing on both blood and marrow is usually unnecessary.

Bone Marrow Aspirate and Biopsy

Evaluation of marrow material will often provide much more information than peripheral blood alone in terms of classifying leukemic processes and determining the marrow blast percentage. In addition, some acute leukemias with monocytic features will have an increase in marrow blasts but show maturation of neoplastic cells in blood that may mimic chronic myelomonocytic leukemia; therefore, bone marrow assessment is essential in that setting. Both aspirate and biopsy materials provide critical information. Some diseases, such as lymphomas and metastatic tumors, may focally involve the marrow and are often associated with fibrosis, both factors that may make them undetectable on aspirate smears alone. When such focal disease processes are suspected, biopsies from more than one site will produce a higher yield for disease detection.[19]

Fine-Needle Aspirate and Core Biopsy

Fine-needle aspiration has become a common evaluation tool for solid tumors and even lymphoma because it is a relatively noninvasive procedure. The technique is ideal for evaluation of the relapse of disease but is now often used for initial patient evaluation. Although fine-needle aspiration coupled with flow cytometry immunophenotyping is ideal for the diagnosis of many low-grade lymphomas,[20,21] it has significant limitations because of the inability to determine architectural features of the lymphoma, to grade some lymphomas properly, and to identify focal disease or transformation. The addition of needle biopsies with or without aspiration and immunophenotyping overcomes some of these limitations, but a significant number of cases will need to go on to open biopsy for diagnosis and/or classification. Because of these limitations, excisional biopsy of easily accessible lymph nodes, when available, is preferred over lymph node aspiration or needle biopsy as an initial diagnostic procedure.

Laparoscopic Biopsy

Laparoscopic biopsies and other more invasive biopsy techniques often obtain more tissue than core biopsies but often fragment the specimen, especially with laparoscopic splenectomy specimens.[22] Despite this, the fragments are usually large enough to determine the architectural pattern of the lymphoid infiltrate.

IMMUNOPHENOTYPING

Immunophenotyping is now essential in the diagnosis and classification of most hematopoietic tumors. It is necessary to distinguish precursor B- from precursor T-cell acute lymphoblastic leukemia/lymphoma (ALL) and early T-cell precursor from usual type T-ALL, to detect aberrant immunophenotypes in both lymphoid and myeloid leukemias and to determine B-cell clonality and disease-associated aberrancies in malignant lymphomas. Flow cytometry and immunohistochemistry are the primary methods currently used, and they have different advantages in the evaluation of these diseases.

Flow Cytometry

Flow cytometry is ideal for tumors involving blood and bone marrow because the cells are already in a cell suspension, a necessary factor for this analytic technique. This method, however, is also ideal for nonsclerotic lymph node specimens, in which a cell suspension can often be made easily. The method requires the processing of unfixed tissue, either fresh or in transport media. As described in Chapter 2, flow cytometry is ideal for evaluating surface antigen expression on cell suspensions and allows for the evaluation of multiple antigens on a given cell. This method is most helpful for acute leukemias and lymphomas of small B cells in which aberrant antigen expression in combinations is common on the neoplastic cells.[23,24] Detection of nuclear and cytoplasmic antigens, such as cyclin D1 and BCL2, is more difficult with this methodology.

Immunohistochemistry

Immunohistochemistry can be performed on fixed, paraffin-embedded tissue and allows for morphologic correlation with antigen expression. This is most useful in tumors with only scattered tumor cells, such as Hodgkin lymphoma, which is usually not detectable by flow cytometry methods currently used. Paraffin section immunohistochemistry also allows for detection of cytoplasmic and nuclear antigens that do not routinely work well by flow cytometry and enable fairly complete immunophenotyping of disorders that do not have fresh tissue available,[25] although the number of markers detectable by this method is still less than those that can be assessed by flow cytometry immunophenotyping.

GENETIC TESTING

Genetic analysis has become increasingly important in the diagnosis, classification, and prognosis assessment of hematopoietic tumors (see Chapters 4, 73, and 89). These techniques are described in more detail in those chapters; however, it is important to understand the general utility of the various assays that are currently available. Gene array analysis has contributed greatly to our understanding of a variety of hematopoietic tumors in recent years, but it is not used as a diagnostic tool in most laboratories and is being largely supplanted by sequencing methods in the research setting. Karyotype analysis is still the best overall screening method for most tumors and detects most gross chromosomal abnormalities, including translocations, deletions, and aneuploidy. This method has the advantage of overall screening of all chromosomes, compared to the more targeted detection of abnormalities with the other molecular genetic methods, and should be performed on all suspected acute leukemias or myeloproliferative neoplasms. The submission of samples for karyotype analysis in cases of suspected malignant lymphoma shows more institutional variability.

Many important genetic abnormalities, however, are cryptic at the karyotype level of detection, and these include some translocations, such as the t(12;21)(p13.2;q22.1) and internal amplification of chromosome 21 in pediatric ALL; B- and T-cell antigen-receptor rearrangements of malignant lymphomas; and gene mutations, such as those seen in many acute myeloid leukemias. Karyotype analysis is also difficult on slow-growing tumors, such as low-grade lymphomas, plasma cell myeloma, and chronic lymphocytic leukemia, and will not work on fixed tissues. Therefore, a variety of other techniques are also commonly used to evaluate the molecular genetic changes of these tumors. Although Southern blot analysis has traditionally been considered the gold standard for the detection of gene rearrangements, the need for large amounts of fresh or frozen tumor tissue, the complexity of the assay, and the relatively long turnaround time of this assay have resulted in the abandonment of this method as a clinical test. FISH is a commonly used technique that can be performed on metaphases or intact cell nuclei, and this method is ideal for the detection of translocations, deletions, and trisomies. FISH panels to detect common, disease-specific abnormalities with prognostic significance are now routine assays performed at diagnosis for cases of suspected chronic lymphocytic lymphoma and plasma cell myeloma and are becoming more common for other neoplasms. The various polymerase chain reaction (PCR) methods are rapid means of detecting translocations and gene rearrangements and can detect lower tumor volumes than FISH methods. Quantitative PCR assays are used to determine levels of minimal residual disease, for example, in patients being treated for chronic myeloid leukemia. Other in situ hybridization methods are useful to localize infectious agents, in particular the Epstein-Barr virus, in specific cell types, and the PCR method is often used in the diagnosis of classical Hodgkin lymphoma and nasal natural killer/T-cell lymphoma. The introduction of next-generation sequencing (NGS) platforms into clinical laboratories has increased the number of genetic targets for a given case, and NGS panels are now commonly performed for acute leukemia.[15] Therefore, a variety of molecular diagnostic tools are now available to supplement karyotype analysis in the evaluation of hematopoietic tumors.

OTHER ANCILLARY METHODS

While new molecular genetic technology has become available for diagnostic use, other more traditional ancillary techniques are actually becoming less common in the routine diagnosis of hematopoietic tumors. Specifically, electron microscopy is rarely used and has been largely supplanted by immunophenotypic methods. Similarly, the diagnostic utility of many histochemical and cytochemical assays has also diminished. Although the proper classification of some of the acute myeloid leukemias in the "not otherwise specified" group of the World Health Organization (WHO) classification still has cytochemical criteria, it is now generally recognized that subgroups of acute myeloid leukemia defined solely by these methods have little clinical relevance.[26]

THE DIAGNOSTIC REPORT

The diagnostic report for hematopoietic tumors should ideally summarize all diagnostic material and testing from a sample.[15,27,28] This would include a combination of peripheral blood, marrow aspirate, and marrow biopsy for bone marrow samples. The morphologic review should be performed and interpreted in combination with immunophenotyping and cytogenetic and molecular genetic studies. The report should state the relevant clinical information and indication for biopsy/aspiration. In addition, the report should clearly define the methodology used for any special studies (e.g., flow cytometry vs immunohistochemistry; PCR vs FISH); the antibodies studied, along with the results; a summary of the interpretation of each special study; and a final interpretation of the significance of all of the assays performed. The final diagnosis should clearly identify the site from which the specimen was obtained and should, when possible, provide a diagnosis using the most current classification of hematopoietic tumors. At the time of writing this chapter, the 2016 (revised 4th edition) WHO classification was the standard and that classification is used throughout the text of this edition. However, in 2022 a 5th edition of the WHO and a clinical advisory committee meeting driven International Consensus Classification (ICC) sponsored by the Society for Hematopathology and the European Association for Haematopathology are being developed. The ICC classification[3,4] is summarized in *Tables 68.1* to *68.8*. Comprehensive reports are more complicated to produce but are necessary to classify most hematopoietic neoplasms properly. This approach may require amending initial interpretations, based on morphology and immunophenotyping, to provide the complete assessment, including cytogenetic and molecular genetic results.

The pathologic diagnosis of hematopoietic tumors now requires a broad approach that involves very close interactions between hematologists and pathologists as well as interactions with a variety of laboratories. Excellent communication between the physician performing the diagnostic procedure and the laboratories is needed to ensure that the specimen is handled in the most efficient manner and to obtain the most accurate and rapid diagnosis for the patient.

Table 68.1. International Consensus Classification of Mature B-Cell Neoplasms

Chronic lymphocytic leukemia (CLL)/small lymphocytic lymphoma
- *Monoclonal B-cell lymphocytosis*
  - CLL type
  - Non-CLL type

B-cell prolymphocytic leukemia

Splenic marginal zone lymphoma

Hairy cell leukemia

Splenic B-cell lymphoma/leukemia, unclassifiable
- *Splenic diffuse red pulp small B-cell lymphoma*
- *Hairy cell leukemia variant*

Lymphoplasmacytic lymphoma
- Waldenström macroglobulinemia

IgM monoclonal gammopathy of undetermined significance (MGUS)
- IgM MGUS, plasma cell type[a]
- IgM MGUS, NOS[a]

Primary cold agglutinin disease[a]

Heavy chain diseases

Mu heavy chain disease

Gamma heavy chain disease

Alpha heavy chain disease

Plasma cell neoplasms

Non-IgM monoclonal gammopathy of undetermined significance

Multiple myeloma (Plasma cell myeloma)[a]
- Multiple myeloma not otherwise specified (NOS)
- Multiple myeloma with recurrent genetic abnormality
  - Multiple myeloma with *CCND* family translocation
  - Multiple myeloma with *MAF* family translocation
  - Multiple myeloma with *NSD2* translocation
  - Multiple myeloma with hyperdiploidy Solitary plasmacytoma of bone

Extraosseous plasmacytoma

Monoclonal immunoglobulin deposition diseases

Immunoglobulin light chain amyloidosis (AL)[a]

Localized AL amyloidosis[a]

Light chain and heavy chain deposition disease

Extranodal marginal zone lymphoma of mucosa–associated lymphoid tissue (MALT lymphoma)

Primary cutaneous marginal zone lymphoproliferative disorder[a]

Nodal marginal zone lymphoma

Pediatric nodal marginal zone lymphoma

Follicular lymphoma

In situ follicular neoplasia

Duodenal-type follicular lymphoma

BCL2-R negative, CD23-positive follicle center lymphoma

Primary cutaneous follicle center lymphoma

Pediatric-type follicular lymphoma

Testicular follicular lymphoma[a]

Large B-cell lymphoma with IRF4 rearrangement[a]

Mantle cell lymphoma

In situ mantle cell neoplasia

Leukemic non–nodal mantle cell lymphoma

Diffuse large B-cell lymphoma (DLBCL), NOS
- Germinal center B-cell subtype
- Activated B-cell subtype

Table 68.1. International Consensus Classification of Mature B-Cell Neoplasms (Continued)

Large B-cell lymphoma with 11q aberration[a]
Nodular lymphocyte predominant B-cell lymphoma[a]
T cell/histiocyte-rich large B-cell lymphoma
Primary DLBCL of the central nervous system
Primary DLBCL of the testis[a]
Primary cutaneous DLBCL, leg type
Intravascular large B-cell lymphoma
HHV-8 and Epstein-Barr virus (EBV)-negative primary effusion-based lymphoma[a]
EBV-positive mucocutaneous ulcer[a]
EBV-positive DLBCL, NOS
DLBCL associated with chronic inflammation Fibrin-associated DLBCL
Lymphomatoid granulomatosis
EBV-positive polymorphic B-cell lymphoproliferative disorder, NOS[a]
ALK-positive large B-cell lymphoma
Plasmablastic lymphoma
HHV8-associated lymphoproliferative disorders
Multicentric Castleman disease
HHV8-positive germinotropic lymphoproliferative disorder
HHV8-positive DLBCL, NOS
Primary effusion lymphoma
Burkitt lymphoma
High-grade B-cell lymphoma, with *MYC* and *BCL2* rearrangements[a]
High-grade B-cell lymphoma with MYC and BCL6 rearrangements[a]
High-grade B-cell lymphoma, NOS
Primary mediastinal large B-cell lymphoma
Mediastinal gray zone lymphoma[a]

[a]Changes from the 2016 WHO classification.
Italics: Provisional tumor entities.

Table 68.2. International Consensus Classification of Classic Hodgkin Lymphoma

Nodular Sclerosis Classic Hodgkin Lymphoma
Lymphocyte-rich classic Hodgkin lymphoma
Mixed cellularity classic Hodgkin lymphoma
Lymphocyte–depleted classic Hodgkin lymphoma

Table 68.3. International Consensus Classification of Mature T- and NK-cell Neoplasms

T-cell prolymphocytic leukemia
T-cell large granular lymphocytic leukemia
Chronic lymphoproliferative disorder of natural killer (NK) cells
Adult T-cell leukemia/lymphoma
Epstein-Barr virus (EBV)-positive T/NK lymphoproliferative disorder (LPD) of childhood[a]
Hydroa vacciniforme LPD
Classic
Systemic
Severe mosquito bite allergy
Chronic active EBV disease, systemic (T and NK-cell phenotype)
Systemic EBV-positive T-cell lymphoma of childhood
Extranodal NK/T-cell lymphoma, nasal type
Aggressive NK cell leukemia

(Continued)

Table 68.3. International Consensus Classification of Mature T- and NK-cell Neoplasms (Continued)

Primary nodal EBV-positive T/NK-cell lymphoma[a]
Enteropathy-associated T-cell lymphoma
Type II refractory celiac disease[a]
Monomorphic epitheliotropic intestinal T-cell lymphoma
Intestinal T-cell lymphoma, not otherwise specified (NOS)
Indolent clonal T-cell lymphoproliferative disorder of the gastrointestinal tract[a]
Indolent NK cell lymphoproliferative disorder of the gastrointestinal tract[a]
Hepatosplenic T-cell lymphoma
Mycosis fungoides
Sézary syndrome
Primary cutaneous CD30-positive T-cell lymphoproliferative disorders
Lymphomatoid papulosis
Primary cutaneous anaplastic large cell lymphoma
Primary cutaneous small/medium CD4-positive T-cell lymphoproliferative disorder
Subcutaneous panniculitis–like T-cell lymphoma
Primary cutaneous gamma-delta T-cell lymphoma
Primary cutaneous acral CD8-positive T-cell lymphoproliferative disorder[a]
Primary cutaneous CD8-positive aggressive epidermotropic cytotoxic T-cell lymphoma
Peripheral T-cell lymphoma, NOS
Follicular helper T-cell lymphoma[a]
Follicular helper T-cell lymphoma, angioimmunoblastic type (angioimmunoblastic T-cell lymphoma)
Follicular helper T-cell lymphoma, follicular type
Follicular helper T-cell lymphoma, NOS
Anaplastic large cell lymphoma, ALK-positive
Anaplastic large cell lymphoma, ALK-negative
Breast implant-associated anaplastic large cell lymphoma

[a]Changes from the 2016 WHO classification.
Italics: Provisional tumor entities.

Table 68.4. International Consensus Classification of Immunodeficiency-Associated Lymphoproliferative Disorders

Post-transplant Lymphoproliferative Disorders (PTLDs)
Plasmacytic hyperplasia PTLD
Infectious mononucleosis PTLD
Florid follicular hyperplasia PTLD
Polymorphic PTLD
Monomorphic PTLD (B- and T/natural killer (NK)-cell types)[a]
Classic Hodgkin lymphoma PTLD[a]
Other iatrogenic immunodeficiency associated lymphoproliferative disorders

[a]These lesions are classified according to the lymphoma to which they correspond.

Table 68.5. International Consensus Classification of Histiocytic and Dendritic Cell Neoplasms

Histiocytic Sarcoma
Langerhans cell histiocytosis
Langerhans cell sarcoma
Indeterminate dendritic cell histiocytosis[a]
Interdigitating dendritic cell sarcoma[a]
ALK-positive histiocytosis[a]
Disseminated juvenile xanthogranuloma
Erdheim/Chester disease
Rosai-Dorfman-Destombes disease[a]
Follicular dendritic cell sarcoma
Fibroblastic reticular cell sarcoma[a]
Epstein-Barr virus (EBV)–positive inflammatory follicular dendritic cell/fibroblastic reticular cell tumor[a]

[a]Changes from the 2016 WHO classification.

Table 68.6. International Consensus Classification of Myeloid Neoplasms and Acute Leukemias

Myeloproliferative Neoplasms
Chronic myeloid leukemia
Polycythemia vera
Essential thrombocythemia
Primary myelofibrosis
Early/prefibrotic primary myelofibrosis
Overt primary myelofibrosis
Chronic neutrophilic leukemia
Chronic eosinophilic leukemia, not otherwise specified (NOS)
Myeloproliferative neoplasm, unclassifiable
Myeloid/lymphoid neoplasms with eosinophilia and tyrosine kinase gene fusions
Myeloid/lymphoid neoplasm with *PDGFRA* rearrangement
Myeloid/lymphoid neoplasm with *PDGFRB* rearrangement
Myeloid/lymphoid neoplasm with *FGFR1* rearrangement
Myeloid/lymphoid neoplasm with *JAK2* rearrangement
Myeloid/lymphoid neoplasm with *FLT3* rearrangement
Myeloid/lymphoid neoplasm with *ETV6::ABL1*
Mastocytosis
Cutaneous mastocytosis
Urticaria pigmentosa/maculopapular cutaneous mastocytosis
Diffuse cutaneous mastocytosis
Mastocytoma of skin
Systemic mastocytosis
Indolent systemic mastocytosis
Smoldering systemic mastocytosis
Aggressive systemic mastocytosis
Mast cell leukemia
Systemic mastocytosis with an associated myeloid neoplasm
Mast cell sarcoma
Myelodysplastic/myeloproliferative neoplasms
Chronic myelomonocytic leukemia
Clonal cytopenia with monocytosis of undetermined significance
Clonal monocytosis of undetermined significance

(Continued)

Table 68.6. International Consensus Classification of Myeloid Neoplasms and Acute Leukemias (Continued)

Atypical chronic myeloid leukemia
Myelodysplastic/myeloproliferative neoplasm with thrombocytosis and *SF3B1* mutation
Myelodysplastic/myeloproliferative neoplasm with ring sideroblasts and thrombocytosis, NOS
Myelodysplastic/myeloproliferative neoplasm, unclassifiable
Pre-malignant clonal cytopenias and myelodysplastic syndromes
Clonal cytopenia of undetermined significance
Myelodysplastic syndrome with mutated *SF3B1*
Myelodysplastic syndrome with del(5q)
Myelodysplastic syndrome with mutated *TP53*
Myelodysplastic syndrome, not otherwise specified (MDS, NOS)
MDS, NOS without dysplasia
MDS, NOS with single lineage dysplasia
MDS, NOS with multilineage dysplasia
Myelodysplastic syndrome with excess blasts
Myelodysplastic syndrome/acute myeloid leukemia (MDS/AML)
MDS/AML with mutated *TP53*
MDS/AML with myelodysplasia–related gene mutations
MDS/AML with myelodysplasia–related cytogenetic abnormalities
MDS/AML, not otherwise specified
Pediatric and/or germline mutation-associated disorders
Juvenile myelomonocytic leukemia
Juvenile myelomonocytic leukemia-like neoplasms
Noonan syndrome-associated myeloproliferative disorder
Refractory cytopenia of childhood
Hematologic neoplasms with germline predisposition
Acute myeloid leukemias (Table 68.7)
Myeloid proliferations associated with Down syndrome
Blastic plasmacytoid dendritic cell neoplasm
Acute leukemia of ambiguous lineage
Acute undifferentiated leukemia
Mixed phenotype acute leukemia (MPAL) with t(9;22) (q34.1;q11.2); *BCR::ABL1*
MPAL, with t(v;11q23.3); *KMT2A* rearranged
MPAL, B/myeloid, NOS
MPAL, T/myeloid, NOS
B-lymphoblastic leukemia/lymphoma (Table 68.8)
T-lymphoblastic leukemia/lymphoma (Tables 68.8)

Table 68.7. International Consensus Classification of Acute Myeloid Leukemia (AML)

Acute promyelocytic leukemia (APL) with t(15;17)(q24.1;q21.2)/*PML::RARA*
APL with other *RARA* rearrangements
AML with t(8;21) (q22;q22.1)/*RUNX1::RUNX1T1*
AML with inv(16) (p13.1q22) or t(16;16) (p13.1;q22)/*CBFB::MYH11*
AML with t(9;11) (p21.3;q23.3)/*MLLT3::KMT2A*
AML with other *KMT2A* rearrangements
AML with t(6;9) (p22.3;q34.1)/*DEK::NUP214*
AML with inv(3) (q21.3q26.2) or t(3;3) (q21.3;q26.2)/*GATA2; MECOM(EVI1)*

Table 68.7. International Consensus Classification of Acute Myeloid Leukemia (AML) (Continued)

AML with other *MECOM* rearrangements
AML with other rare recurring translocations
AML with t(9;22) (q34.1;q11.2)/*BCR::ABL1*[b]
AML with mutated *NPM1*
AML with in-frame bZIP *CEBPA* mutations
AML with mutated *TP53*[a]
AML with myelodysplasia-related gene mutations[a]
Defined by mutations in *ASXL1, BCOR, EZH2, RUNX1, SF3B1, SRSF2, STAG2, U2AF1,* or *ZRSR2*
AML with myelodysplasia–related cytogenetic abnormalities[a]
Defined by detecting a complex karyotype (≥3 unrelated clonal chromosomal abnormalities in the absence of other class-defining recurring genetic abnormalities), del(5q)/t(5q)/add(5q), -7/del(7q), +8, del(12p)/t(12p)/add(12p), i(17q), -17/add(17p) or del(17p), del(20q), and/or idic(X) (q13) clonal abnormalities
AML not otherwise specified (NOS)[a]
Myeloid sarcoma

All AML categories other than myeloid sarcoma require at least 10% bone marrow or peripheral.
[a]Bone marrow or peripheral blood blast count of >20% required. Cases with 10% to 19% bone marrow or peripheral blood blast counts will now be designated as MDS/AML.
[b]The category of MDS/AML will not be used for AML with *BCR::ABL1* due to its overlap with progression of chronic myeloid leukemia, *BCR:ABL1*-positive.

Table 68.8. International Consensus Classification of Lymphoblastic Leukemia/Lymphoma

B-lymphoblastic Leukemia/lymphoma (B-ALL)

B-lymphoblastic leukemia/lymphoma with recurrent genetic abnormalities
  B-lymphoblastic leukemia/lymphoma with t(9;22) (q34.1;q11.2)/*BCR::ABL1*
    with lymphoid only involvement
    with multilineage involvement
  B-lymphoblastic leukemia/lymphoma with t(v;11q23.3)/*KMT2A* rearranged
  B-lymphoblastic leukemia/lymphoma with t(12;21) (p13.2;q22.1)/*ETV6::RUNX1*
  B-lymphoblastic leukemia/lymphoma, low hypodiploid
  B-lymphoblastic leukemia/lymphoma, near haploid
  B-lymphoblastic leukemia/lymphoma with t(5;14) (q31.1;q32.3)/*IL3::*IGH
  B-lymphoblastic leukemia/lymphoma with t(1;19) (q23.3;p13.3)/*TCF3::PBX1*
  B-lymphoblastic leukemia/lymphoma, *BCR::ABL1*–like, ABL1 class rearranged
  B-lymphoblastic leukemia/lymphoma, *BCR::ABL1*–like, JAK-STAT activated
  B-lymphoblastic leukemia/lymphoma, *BCR::ABL1*–like, not otherwise specified (NOS)
  B-lymphoblastic leukemia/lymphoma with iAMP21
  B-lymphoblastic leukemia/lymphoma with *MYC* rearrangement
  B-lymphoblastic leukemia/lymphoma with *DUX4* rearrangement
  B-lymphoblastic leukemia/lymphoma with *MEF2D* rearrangement
  B-lymphoblastic leukemia/lymphoma with *ZNF384(362)* rearrangement
  B-lymphoblastic leukemia/lymphoma with *NUTM1* rearrangement
  B-lymphoblastic leukemia/lymphoma with *HLF* rearrangement
  B-lymphoblastic leukemia/lymphoma with *UBTF::ATXN7L3/PAN3,CDX2* ("CDX2/UBTF")
  B-lymphoblastic leukemia/lymphoma with mutated *IKZF1* N159Y
  B-lymphoblastic leukemia/lymphoma with mutated *PAX5* P80 R
  B-lymphoblastic leukemia/lymphoma, ETV6::RUNX1-like
  B-lymphoblastic leukemia/lymphoma, with PAX5 alteration
  B-lymphoblastic leukemia/lymphoma, with mutated ZEB2 (p.H1038 R)/IGH::CEBPE
  B-lymphoblastic leukemia/lymphoma, ZNF384 rearranged-like
  B-lymphoblastic leukemia/lymphoma, KMT2A rearranged-like
B-lymphoblastic leukemia/lymphoma, NOS

T-lymphoblastic leukemia/lymphoma

Early T-cell precursor lymphoblastic leukemia/lymphoma with *BCL11B* rearrangement

Early T-cell precursor lymphoblastic leukemia/lymphoma, NOS

T-lymphoblastic leukemia/lymphoma, NOS

Natural killer (NK) cell lymphoblastic leukemia/lymphoma

Italics: Provisional tumor entities.

References

1. Arber DA, Orazi A, Hasserjian R, et al. The 2016 revision to the World Health Organization classification of myeloid neoplasms and acute leukemia. *Blood.* 2016;127(20):2391-2405.
2. Swerdlow SH, Campo E, Pileri SA, et al. The 2016 revision of the World Health Organization classification of lymphoid neoplasms. *Blood.* 2016;127(20):2375-2390.
3. Arber DA, Orazi A, Hasserjian RP, et al. The International Consensus classification of myeloid neoplasms and acute leukemias: integrating morphological, clinical, and genomic data. *Blood.* 2022;140(11):1200-1228.
4. Campo E, Jaffe ES, Cook JA, et al. The International Consensus classificaiton of mature lymphoid neoplasms: a report from the clinical advisory committee. *Blood.* 2022;140(11):1229-1253.
5. Bennett JM, Catovsky D, Daniel MT, et al. Proposals for the classification of the acute leukemias. *Br J Haematol.* 1976;33:451-458.
6. Bennett JM, Catovsky D, Daniel MT, et al. Proposed revised criteria for the classification of acute myeloid leukemia. A report of the French-American-British Cooperative Group. *Ann Intern Med.* 1985;103(4):626-629.
7. Bennett JM, Catovsky D, Daniel MT, et al. Proposals for the classification of the myelodysplastic syndromes. *Br J Haematol.* 1982;51:189-199.
8. Rappaport H. *Tumors of the Hematopoietic System.* Armed Forces Institute of Pathology; 1966:1-442.
9. National Cancer Institute sponsored study of classifications of non-Hodgkin's lymphomas: summary and description of a working formulation for clinical usage. The Non-Hodgkin's Lymphoma Pathologic Classification Project. *Cancer.* 1982;49(10):2112-2135.
10. Collins RD. Lymph node examination. What is an adequate workup? *ArchPathol Lab Med.* 1985;109(9):797-799.
11. Cousar JB. Surgical pathology examination of lymph nodes. Practice survey by American Society of Clinical Pathologists. *Am J Clin Pathol.* 1995;104(2):126-132.
12. Foucar K. Procurement and indications for bone marrow examination. In: Foucar K, Reichard K, Czuchlewski D, eds. *Bone Marrow Pathology.* 3rd ed. ASCP Press; 2010:52-65.
13. Prakash SBPM. Technical factors in the preparation and evaluation of lymph node biopsies. In: Orazi A, Weiss LM, Foucar K, Knowles DM, eds. *Knowles' Neoplastic Hematopathology.* 3rd ed. Wolters Kluwer; 2014:286-292.
14. Nguyen PL. Collection, processing, and examination of bone marrow specimens. In: Jaffe ES, Arber DA, Campo E, Harris NL, Quintanilla-Martinez L, eds. *Hematopathology.* 2nd ed. Elsevier; 2017:29-40.
15. Arber DA, Borowitz MJ, Cessna M, et al. Initial diagnostic workup of acute leukemia: guideline from the college of American pathologists and the American society of hematology. *Arch Pathol Lab Med.* 2017;141(10):1342-1393.
16. Kroft SH, Sever CE, Bagg A, et al. Laboratory workup of lymphoma in adults: guideline from the American society for clinical pathology and the college of American pathologists. *Arch Pathol Lab Med.* 2021;145(3):269-290.
17. Seegmiller AC, Kim AS, Mosse CA, et al. Optimizing personalized bone marrow testing using an evidence-based, interdisciplinary team approach. *Am J Clin Pathol.* 2013;140(5):643-650.
18. Arber JM, Weiss LM, Chang KL, Battifora H, Arber DA. The effect of decalcification on in situ hybridization. *Mod Pathol.* 1997;10(10):1009-1014.
19. Wang J, Weiss LM, Chang KL, et al. Diagnostic utility of bilateral bone marrow examination: significance of morphologic and ancillary technique study in malignant. *Cancer.* 2002;94(5):1522-1531.
20. Zeppa P, Marino G, Troncone G, et al. Fine-needle cytology and flow cytometry immunophenotyping and subclassification of non-Hodgkin lymphoma: a critical review of 307 cases with technical suggestions. *Cancer.* 2004;102(1):55-65.
21. Laane E, Tani E, Bjorklund E, et al. Flow cytometric immunophenotyping including Bcl-2 detection on fine needle aspirates in the diagnosis of reactive lymphadenopathy and non-Hodgkin's lymphoma. *Cytometry B Clin Cytom.* 2005;64(1):34-42.
22. Bernard T, Rhodes M, Turner GE, Wimperis JZ, Deane AM. Laparoscopic splenectomy: single-centre experience of a district general hospital. *Br J Haematol.* 1999;106(4):1065-1067.
23. Davis BH, Holden JT, Bene MC, et al. 2006 Bethesda International Consensus recommendations on the flow cytometric immunophenotypic analysis of hematolymphoid neoplasia: medical indications. *Cytometry B Clin Cytom.* 2007;72(suppl 1):S5-S13.
24. Wood BL, Arroz M, Barnett D, et al. 2006 Bethesda International Consensus recommendations on the immunophenotypic analysis of hematolymphoid neoplasia by flow cytometry: optimal reagents and reporting for the flow cytometric diagnosis of hematopoietic neoplasia. *Cytometry B Clin Cytom.* 2007;72(suppl 1):S14-S22.
25. Pittaluga S, Barry TS, Raffeld M. Immunohistochemistry for the hematopathology laboratory. In: Jaffe ES, Arber DA, Campo E, Harris NL, Quintanilla-Martinez L, eds. *Hematopathology.* 2nd ed. Elsevier; 2017:41-52.
26. Walter RB, Othus M, Burnett AK, et al. Significance of FAB subclassification of "acute myeloid leukemia, NOS" in the 2008 WHO classification: analysis of 5848 newly diagnosed patients. *Blood.* 2013;121(13):2424-2431.
27. Mohanty SK, Piccoli AL, Devine LJ, et al. Synoptic tool for reporting of hematological and lymphoid neoplasms based on World Health Organization classification and College of American Pathologists checklist. *BMC Cancer.* 2007;7:144.
28. Ohgami RS, Arber DA. Challenges in consolidated reporting of hematopoietic neoplasms. *Surg Pathol Clin.* 2013;6(4):795-806.

Chapter 69 ■ Principles of Targeted Therapies for Hematologic Malignancies

NITIN JAIN • SHILPA PAUL • NAVEEN PEMMARAJU • VARSHA GANDHI

INTRODUCTION

Cancer management has undergone significant evolution with increasing use of targeted therapies for treatment of hematologic malignancies in the last decade. Such approaches "target" a specific disease pathway. These may include a surface protein such as CD20, CD19, and others with monoclonal antibodies or intracellular signaling transduction inhibitors such as inhibitors of ABL, BTK, IDH2, and others. For several hematologic malignancies, targeted therapies are being combined with chemotherapy. In some diseases such as chronic lymphocytic leukemia (CLL), targeted therapies have largely supplanted chemotherapy.

To optimally treat patients with blood cancer, clinicians should understand the principles of targeted therapies as well as the pharmacology of the drugs they are administering. Recently approved targeted therapies and immunotherapy agents have expanded management options and improved survival for patients with selected blood cancers. It is also important for clinicians to recognize common toxicities with targeted therapies, which most often are unique to a particular class of drug. In this chapter, we summarize targeted therapies for several hematologic malignancies. Details about their role in the clinical management of a particular entity are included in disease-focused chapters.

GENERAL PRINCIPLES OF TARGETED THERAPIES

As mentioned previously, targeted therapies address a specific disease pathway or marker. This may include a surface receptor or an intracellular protein. With chemotherapy, there is typically a need to assess maximal-tolerated doses (MTDs) during phase 1 trials as generally there is a dose-response relationship (and therefore need to administer to the highest possible dose of chemotherapy to maximize therapy benefit). With targeted therapies, one might not need to dose patients at MTD as the biological effect (and thereby therapeutic effect) can be seen at a lower dose, sometimes called optimal biological dose.

Adverse events of targeted therapies can result from either on-target or off-target effects. On-target toxicity refers to a toxic effect as a result of inhibition of the intended target; for example, PD1 inhibition causes immune activation leading to immunological toxicities; navitoclax, a BCL2/BCL-xL inhibitor, causes thrombocytopenia due to dependency of platelets to BCL-xl. Off-target toxicity refers to toxicities resulting from additional targets, beyond the intended target, being affected by the drug. For example, ibrutinib, a BTK inhibitor, inhibits several additional kinases, other than BTK, which are postulated to lead to ibrutinib-associated adverse events such as atrial fibrillation, diarrhea, and skin rash. Specific toxicities may also result from the toxin "payload" of antibody-drug conjugates (ADCs). Inotuzumab ozogamicin is a CD22-targeted ADC with calicheamicin as toxin. Calicheamicin can lead to liver toxicity.

Another important aspect of targeted therapy for cancer is recognition of tumor heterogeneity. Tumor heterogeneity can occur within the same patient (intrapatient) or between different patients (interpatient). As targeted therapies are directed against a specific disease-specific process, it is important to assess how frequent the target is present within the tumor of a particular patient. For example, CD19-targeted therapy is unlikely to be active if the tumor is CD19 negative. An individual patient's tumor may have multiple clones, each expressing a different set of tumor targets. This is now becoming a common scenario with the introduction of next-generation sequencing and other methodologies to assess tumor cells.

Understanding the resistance mechanisms to targeted therapies is an important area of research and can help direct the next line of therapy. Resistance to ABL1 tyrosine kinase inhibitors (TKIs) is commonly associated with mutations in the ABL1 kinase domain, and the type of mutation present can help with selection of the subsequent TKI. Similarly, acquisition of BTK mutation in a patient with CLL on ibrutinib therapy is associated with ibrutinib resistance.

Several of the targeted therapies are metabolized by CYP3A4 pathway, and it is important to assess for drug-drug interactions when prescribing targeted therapies, especially oral targeted therapies. For example, the dose of venetoclax should be reduced when given in combination with azole antifungal therapy due to drug-drug interaction, which increases venetoclax blood levels.

Although pharmacokinetic (PK) and pharmacodynamic markers are routinely assessed for targeted therapies in clinical trials, for most targeted therapies, these have limited utility in routine clinical care, largely due to lack of clear response relationship and lack of validated laboratory assays.

A comprehensive review of the pharmacology of all targeted therapy agents is beyond the scope of this chapter. This section focuses on those agents that are US Food and Drug Administration (FDA) approved and commonly used in the therapy of hematologic malignancies. Important information necessary for the optimal use of these drugs requires knowledge of their (a) mechanism of action; (b) pharmacology, including bioavailability, routes of elimination, and important drug interactions; and (c) toxicities.

MONOCLONAL ANTIBODIES AND IMMUNE ANTIBODY-DRUG CONJUGATES

Monoclonal antibodies were among the first targeted therapies for hematologic malignancies with the introduction of anti-CD20 monoclonal antibody rituximab in the 1990s and more recently a second-generation anti-CD20 monoclonal antibody obinutuzumab.[1,2] *Figure 69.1* shows several approved monoclonal antibodies and ADCs with their respective cell surface target. A review of these targets (*Table 69.1*) is provided below.

CD22

The CD22 cell surface marker is overexpressed in majority of patients with B-cell acute lymphoblastic leukemia (B-ALL) and therefore is a potential target for pharmacological intervention. Inotuzumab ozogamicin is an ADC with an anti-CD22 humanized antibody that is conjugated with the toxin calicheamicin (the same toxin as in the anti-CD33-ADC gemtuzumab ozogamicin). In a phase 2 clinical trial, inotuzumab demonstrated clinical activity as a monotherapy in relapsed/refractory (R/R) B-ALL.[3] This was followed by phase 3 trial, which reported improved outcomes with inotuzumab compared with standard chemotherapy in R/R B-ALL.[4] The most notable safety signal with inotuzumab is risk of veno-occlusive disease (VOD) of the liver due to toxin calicheamicin; this is especially important for patients undergoing allogeneic stem cell transplant after receiving inotuzumab. Ongoing trials are exploring inotuzumab with chemotherapy and other targeted therapies, both in R/R and in frontline B-ALL.

Moxetumomab pasudotox is another ADC that targets CD22. The toxin is a modified bacterial toxin (pseudomonas based). The drug is approved for treatment of patients with R/R hairy cell leukemia. Notably, for this agent that most common adverse event that led to drug discontinuation was hemolytic uremic syndrome.[5,6]

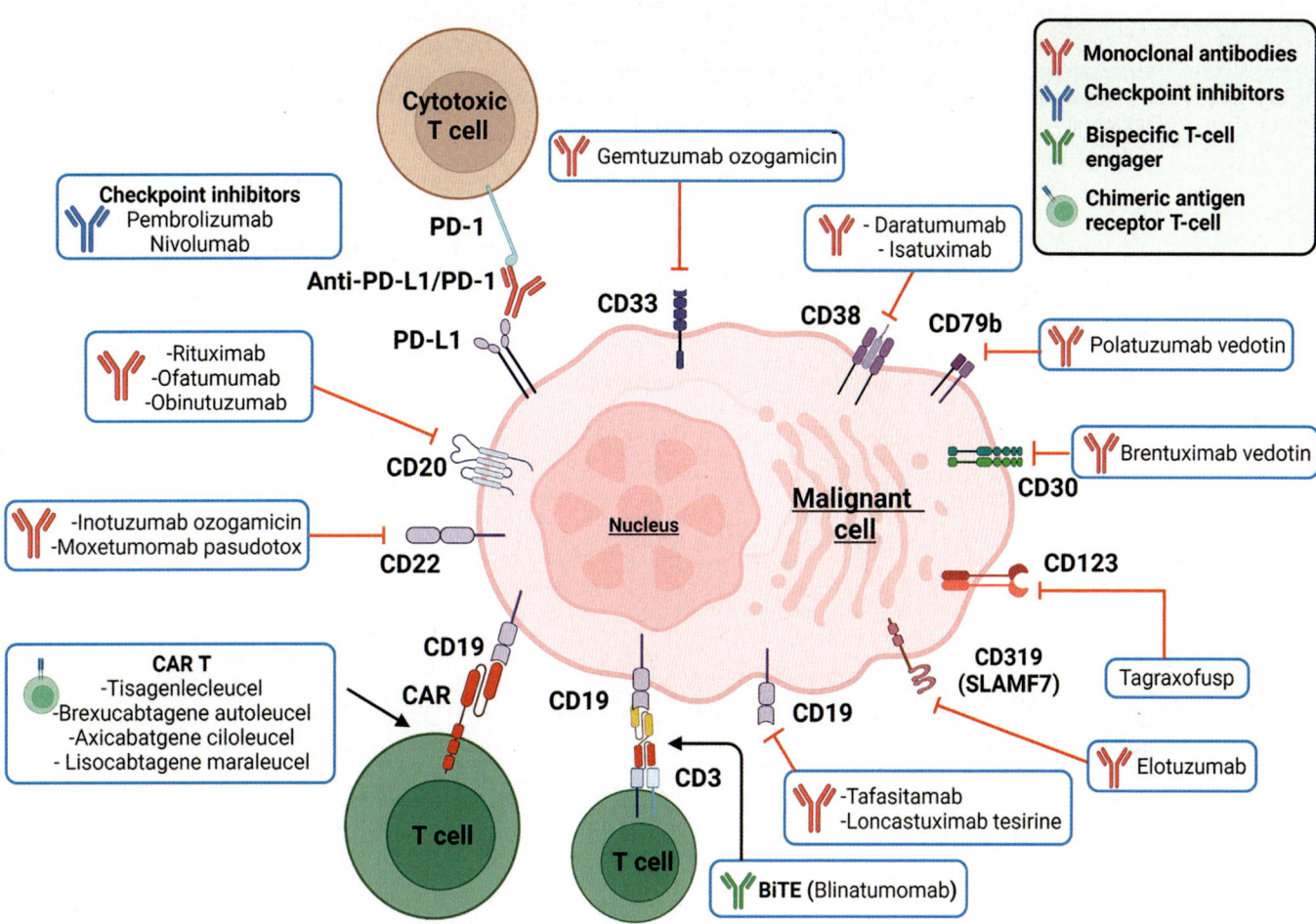

FIGURE 69.1 Therapeutic targeting of cell surface targets. (Figure made on BioRender.com.)

CD30

Brentuximab vedotin is an ADC directed against CD30 and conjugated to the toxin monomethyl auristatin E (MMAE). In the phase I study, brentuximab as monotherapy demonstrated durable clinical responses and tumor regression in the majority of patients with R/R CD30+ lymphomas.[7] Brentuximab has also been combined with frontline doxorubicin, vinblastine, and dacarbazine (AVD) chemotherapy for Hodgkin lymphoma.[8] Additional studies have combined brentuximab with other novel agents such as PD1 checkpoint inhibition.[9] An important side effect of brentuximab is peripheral neuropathy due to MMAE toxin.

CD52

Alemtuzumab targets CD52, which is a surface antigen present on both T and B cells, NK cells, and various other hematopoietic cells. An older drug that has been available for decades, alemtuzumab has been used for treatment of a variety of diseases including, but not limited to, CLL, multiple sclerosis, aplastic anemia, and T-cell large granular lymphocyte/T-cell prolymphocytic leukemia (T-PLL). The mechanism of action includes CD52+ site attachment binding leading to antibody-dependent cellular lysis of cancer cells. Notably, alemtuzumab is associated with an increased risk of opportunistic infections, especially *Pneumocystis jirovecii* pneumonia and cytomegalovirus, prolonged myelosuppression, and infusion-related events. Interestingly, alemtuzumab has been even incorporated into lymphodepletion conditioning regimens in some of the allogeneic chimeric antigen receptor T (CAR T) programs with the goal of enhanced host T-cell suppression to allow for improved CAR T persistence.

CD79b

Polatuzumab vedotin is an ADC that targets CD79b. It was approved by the FDA in 2019, in combination with rituximab and bendamustine (P + BR) for treatment of adult patients with R/R diffuse large B-cell lymphoma (DLBCL) after two or more prior lines of treatment.[10] Most common toxicities of P + BR included cytopenias, fatigue, peripheral neuropathy, and diarrhea. Polatuzumab has also been investigated in frontline DLBCL in combination with modified R-CHOP (Pola-R-CHP) versus standard RCHOP, and improved outcomes have been reported.[11]

CD33

Gemtuzumab ozogamicin is an ADC that consists of an anti-CD33 monoclonal antibody conjugated to the cytotoxin agent calicheamicin via covalent linker. Gemtuzumab originally received FDA accelerated approval in the year 2000, but it subsequently was voluntarily withdrawn in 2010 as it was not able to demonstrate confirmatory results.[12] With additional analysis, including final efficacy results from the phase 3 ALFA-0701 clinical trial, which demonstrated that addition of gemtuzumab to intensive chemotherapy did have improved clinical benefit for patients with acute myeloid leukemia (AML), the drug ultimately gained full FDA approval in 2017. Importantly, the most notable toxicity is "black-box warning" for hepatotoxicity and VOD/sinusoidal obstructive syndrome of the liver.[13]

CD123

Targeting CD123, also known as IL3Rα, has been of therapeutic interest in the leukemia field.[14] Pharmacological development targeting CD123 has included a variety of approaches, including monoclonal antibodies, CAR T, and ADCs. The first approved targeted agent specifically against CD123, indicated for treatment of patients with blastic plasmacytoid dendritic cell neoplasm (BPDCN), is a novel agent tagraxofusp, which consists of a truncated diphtheria toxin conjugated with recombinant human IL-3.[15] The most notable toxicity observed is capillary leak syndrome, which can be managed with

Table 69.1. Selected Approved Monoclonal Antibodies in Hematologic Malignancies

Target	Drug Name	Toxin	Indication	Main Adverse Events
CD19	Tafasitamab	–	DLBCL	Myelosuppression
	Loncastuximab tesirine	Pyrrolobenzodiazepine (PBD) dimer	DLBCL	Myelosuppression, Pleural effusion, edema, rash
CD20	Rituximab	–	Multiple disease indications	Infusion reaction
	Ofatumumab	–	CLL	Infusion reaction
	Obinutuzumab	–	CLL, follicular lymphoma	Infusion reaction, myelosuppression
CD22	Moxetumomab pasudotox	Pseudomonas exotoxin	Hairy cell leukemia	Capillary leak syndrome, hemolytic uremic syndrome
	Inotuzumab ozogamicin	Calicheamicin	B-cell acute lymphoblastic leukemia	Hepatotoxicity including hepatic veno-occlusive disease, thrombocytopenia
CD30	Brentuximab vedotin	Monomethyl auristatin E (MMAE)	Hodgkin lymphoma, Anaplastic large cell lymphoma	Peripheral neuropathy
CD33	Gemtuzumab ozogamicin	Calicheamicin	Acute myeloid leukemia	Hepatotoxicity including hepatic veno-occlusive disease, thrombocytopenia
CD38	Daratumumab	–	Multiple myeloma	Infusion reaction
	Isatuximab	–	Multiple myeloma	Infusion reaction
CD52	Alemtuzumab	–	CLL	Infusion reaction, opportunistic infections
CD79b	Polatuzumab vedotin	MMAE	DLBCL	Peripheral neuropathy
CD123	Tagraxofusp	Diphtheria toxin	BPDCN	Capillary leak syndrome, hepatotoxicity
SLAMF7	Elotuzumab	–	Multiple myeloma	Infusion reaction, hepatotoxicity
BCMA	Belantamab mafodotin	Monomethyl auristatin F (MMAF)	Multiple myeloma	Corneal toxicity, thrombocytopenia
CCR4	Mogamulizumab	–	Mycosis fungoides	Skin toxicity, infusion reaction

specific preventative/mitigation clinical measures.[16] Tagraxofusp was FDA approved (12 μg/kg/dose, 5 days intravenously [IV] per cycle) for patients with BPDCN. Ongoing trials are investigating tagraxofusp in combination with other active therapies for patients with BPDCN as well as for patients with AML.

B-cell Maturation Antigen

Targeting of B-cell maturation antigen (BCMA) is a recent area of growing clinical interest. This is present on mature B lymphocytes and overexpressed in multiple myeloma (MM), and there are now three approved drugs targeting BCMA in the MM field with other agents in active development in a variety of approaches and platforms.[17] Two of the approvals are CAR T directed against BCMA: idecabtagene vicleucel ("ide-cel") and ciltacabtagene autoleucel ("cita-cel") have reported promising results, with expected toxicities of cytokine release syndrome (CRS) and neurotoxicity to be aware of as with all CAR T constructs. Both are approved for patients with relapsed/refractory MM. In addition, there is a BCMA-targeted ADC, known as belantamab, which is now approved for patients with R/R MM who have had at least four prior therapies. The most notable toxicity for belantamab is ocular toxicity, which requires close monitoring.[18]

CD38

CD38 is a glycoprotein marker that is overexpressed on the surface of MM cells, therefore making it an attractive therapeutic target. Daratumumab is a monoclonal antibody specifically targeting CD38, approved for both frontline and R/R MM. Major toxicities include infusion-related reactions and a known interference phenomenon with red blood cell antigen screening/cross-matching and cytopenias.[19] Isatuximab is another CD38-targeting IV monoclonal antibody approved for patients with MM. Similar to daratumumab, this agent requires close monitoring for infusion-related reactions and cytopenias.[20]

SLAMF7

SLAMF7 (Signaling-lymphocytic activation-molecule), or CD319, is a surface marker found on plasma cells and MM cells. The drug elotuzumab was the first-in-class approved targeting agent in this field. It is approved in combination with lenalidomide plus dexamethasone for patients with R/R MM. Patients should be closely monitored for infusion-related reactions and cytopenias.[21]

PD-1

Targeting of the immune checkpoint axis in cancer cells has been a long quest by multiple researchers for decades and have transformed the cancer care for multiple malignancies, especially solid tumors. Nivolumab and pembrolizumab are anti-PD-1 monoclonal antibodies and are approved for patients with Hodgkin lymphoma.[22] Patients should be closely monitored for autoimmune "-itis" syndromes (such as colitis and thyroiditis).

BISPECIFIC T-CELL ENGAGERS

Blinatumomab is a bispecific T-cell engager (BiTE) composed of two single-chain antibodies, one engaging CD3 on cytotoxic T cells and the other targeting CD19 on B cells.[23] Blinatumomab mediates a bivalent binding of CD3 and CD19 cells leading to a catalytic synapse activating T cells. This causes an upregulation of expression of adhesion molecules, perforin-mediated direct cell killing of B cells, release of concomitant inflammatory cytokines, and T-cell proliferation.[23] CD19 on B cells is an ideal target for therapeutic development due to its high expression on malignant B cells in several lymphoid malignancies, including B-ALL.

Blinatumomab has a short terminal half-life of approximately 2 hours requiring administration as a continuous intravenous infusion (CIVI). T-cell expansion after blinatumomab is largely driven by expansion of effector memory CD8+ and CD4+ T cells.[24] Blinatumomab was approved by the FDA in 2014 for B-ALL. Currently, it has two approved indications: 1) positive minimal residual disease (MRD+) in B-ALL; 2) R/R B-ALL. In the R/R setting, for patients ≥45 kg, blinatumomab is administered as a CIVI at 9 μg/d on days 1 to 7, followed by 28 μg/d on days 8 to 28 during the first 6-week cycle. During cycles 2 to 5, it is administered as 28 μg/d continuously for 28 days. Dexamethasone 20 mg is given as a premedication prior to starting each cycle, on day of dose escalation, and any time there is a dose interruption for ≥4 hours. In patients (≥45 kg) with MRD+ disease, the dose is 28 μg/d CIVI on days 1 to 28 of cycles 1 to 4, without a lead-in phase due to the low burden of disease and decreased risk for CRS.

Blinatumomab reported superior progression-free survival (PFS) and overall survival (OS) compared with standard chemotherapy in R/R B-ALL in a phase 3 trial leading to FDA approval in R/R B-ALL.[25] Owing to its promising activity in the R/R setting, blinatumomab is currently being combined with chemoimmunotherapy in the frontline setting with an aim to induce deeper and more sustainable remissions. Blinatumomab in combination with BCR-ABL1 TKIs is currently being explored in several trials for Ph+ ALL.

The two most common adverse effects of blinatumomab are CRS and neurotoxicity. These are due to T-cell activation that up regulates cytokines and other inflammatory markers. CRS mainly occurs during the first cycle as its incidence is proportional to disease burden. CRS symptoms include fever, hypotension, tachycardia, nausea/vomiting, and hypoxia. Management is based on severity of the CRS; for grade 1, continue infusion with close monitoring, whereas grade 4 requires discontinuing the infusion, use of systemic steroids, and other supportive measures. Neurotoxicity with blinatumomab may include aphasia, tremors, confusion, ataxia, headaches, or seizures. Neurotoxicity can occur at any time, but the incidence is higher in the first cycle. Infusion should be held and dexamethasone administered for seizures and G3-4 neurotoxicity. Myelosuppression can occur but is less common compared with conventional cytotoxic chemotherapy.

SIGNAL TRANSDUCTION INHIBITORS

Since the identification of the first oncogene[26] and associated protein kinase activity,[27] there have been attempts to block the oncogenic signaling for treatment of cancer. The signaling event that initiates at the apex involves a multitude of proteins in an orderly and logical path. In this section we systematically describe small molecules that have been utilized in hematologic oncology to block signals that have been identified as oncogenic emanating either from an oncoprotein or downstream of that protein. The majority of these oncogenic signals are involved in cell proliferation, cell survival, initiation and activation of transcription or translation, and motility of cells.

Most of these signal transduction inhibitors directly or indirectly target protein kinases. Early studies identified epidermal growth factor receptor tyrosine kinase or HER-2/neu oncogene inhibition as beneficial in solid tumors.[28-30] For hematological malignancies, the breakthrough occurred when Bcr-abl kinase was targeted by imatinib. *Figure 69.2* provides details of many signal transduction inhibitors and other relevant therapeutic targets.

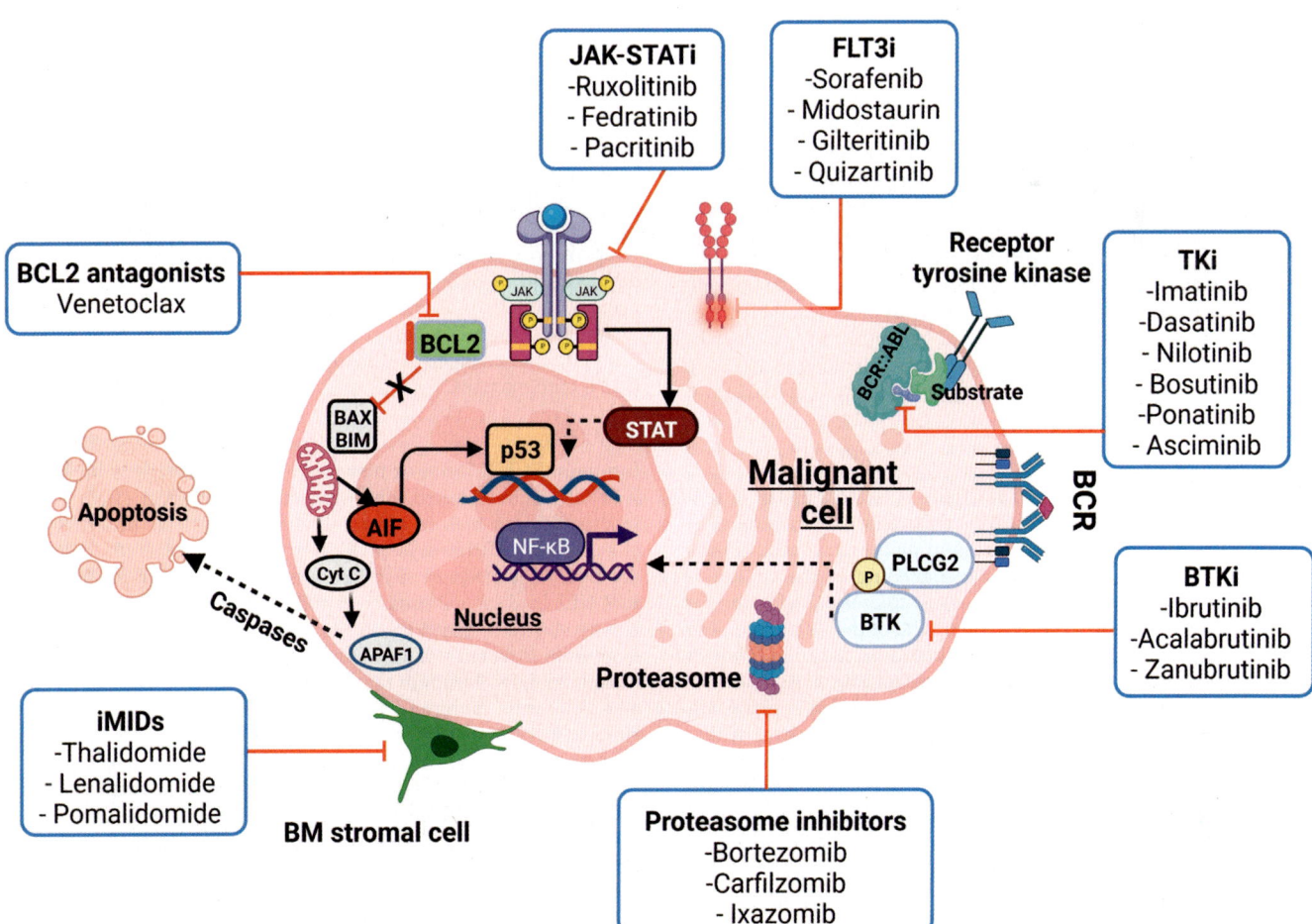

FIGURE 69.2 Therapeutic targeting of intracellular signaling pathways. (Figure made on BioRender.com.)

ABL Kinase Inhibitors

One of the major transformative events that occurred in hematologic oncology was the discovery of imatinib, which targets Bcr-abl kinase. This was the beginning of a new era in hematology for the development and testing of a plethora of kinase inhibitors that are now established approved agents.

The common thread for all ABL kinase inhibitors is Philadelphia (Ph) chromosome, which results from the reciprocal translocation between chromosome 9 and 22.[31] *ABL* is located on chromosome 9 while *BCR* is present on chromosome 22. The *ABL* gene encodes Abl tyrosine kinase, which is disrupted when these genes are fused. *BCR-ABL* is on the 22q– chromosome (the Ph chromosome); this encodes a 210-kd protein in patients with chronic myelogenous leukemia (CML) and Ph+ acute lymphoblastic leukemia (Ph+ ALL) with constitutively active Abl-tyrosine kinase.[32,33] Downstream events from the Bcr-Abl include multiple intracellular signaling pathways that increase cell proliferation, genomic instability due to inhibition of DNA repair processes, and increased motility. Defined structure of the protein and identification that this is a solo driver for the disease were the primary impetus to create unique chemical candidates that can occupy this protein and block its activity. While the first molecule was imatinib, this research area is highly proliferative with several drugs (imatinib, dasatinib, nilotinib, bosutinib, ponatinib, asciminib) tested and approved. Clinical activity of imatinib validated the pathogenetic role of BCR-ABL tyrosine kinase. This was the genesis of kinase-targeted small molecule signal transduction inhibitors (STIs) or TKIs.

Imatinib

Originally known as STI571 or CGP571488, imatinib was tested initially in cells harboring the Bcr-Abl fusion gene and protein. Drug-inhibited cellular proliferation and was selective for cells with this mutation.[34] This was validated in a phase 1 dose-escalation clinical trial for patients with CML where complete hematologic responses were observed in majority of the patients. Importantly, off-target effects were minimal and hence the drug was well tolerated.[35] Responses, albeit not that impressive, in advanced blast crisis disease further elucidated the importance of this fusion gene in the pathogenesis of CML in blast crisis.[36] Long-term follow-up study with imatinib further indicated that responses were durable and deepened with continuous dosing. Randomized trials further substantiated early trial data.[37] The approved dose of imatinib for chronic phase CML is 400 mg orally once daily. Continuous and long-term use of imatinib was required, and this is where development of resistance was observed, which was due to multiple BCR-ABL kinase domain mutations.[38-40] One mechanism of kinase domain mutation was decreased binding of the drug where scientists focused on dose increases and other approaches to increase efficacy.[41-43]

Dasatinib

Despite the enormous success of imatinib, it became apparent that a subset of patients treated with CML in the chronic phase develop resistance to imatinib. Since reduced drug binding was the primary mechanism of resistance through understanding of the crystallographic structure of the protein, a focus was to create conformation-specific drugs that bind to the ATP-binding site of the Abl kinase. The first in this series was BMS-354825, now known as dasatinib,[39] which showed objective responses in imatinib-resistant Ph+ leukemias.[44,45] Complete cytogenetic responses were higher in patients with CML treated with dasatinib in contrast to imatinib-treated disease with a faster rate of achievement of molecular responses compared with imatinib.[46,47] Dasatinib can cause pleural/pericardial effusions and pulmonary hypertension. The approved dose of dasatinib for chronic-phase CML is 100 mg orally once daily.

Nilotinib

Similar to dasatinib, nilotinib was discovered and designed to overcome Bcr-Abl point mutation–mediated resistance. AMN107, now known as nilotinib, is a selective inhibitor of native and mutant Bcr-Abl.[48] The drug was effective in patients with Ph+ disease that was either imatinib resistance or intolerant.[49] Nilotinib was compared with imatinib in a randomized trial and found to be superior to imatinib for achievement of molecular responses and improvement in the time to progression to the accelerated or blast phase.[50] Both dasatinib and nilotinib can work against several imatinib-resistant ABL1 kinase domain mutations but are not effective on T315I-mutant CML.

Bosutinib

Bosutinib, SKI-606, is a dual Src/Abl kinase inhibitor that showed potent activity against multiple mutant Bcr-Abl kinases and in cell lines harboring imatinib-resistant Bcr-Abl and in patients with imatinib-resistant disease.[51,52] Randomized trial compared bosutinib with imatinib and noted improved responses with bosutinib.[53] Gastrointestinal (GI) toxicity and transaminase elevations are common with bosutinib.

Ponatinib

Ponatinib (previously called AP24534) was the first Abl kinase inhibitor that in model systems was able to target T315I-mutated Bcr-Abl along with many other Bcr-Abl mutants in cellular and biochemical assays.[54] The drug was evaluated for patients with Ph+ leukemia with T315I Bcr-Abl-mutant disease and in those with resistance to other Bcr-Abl TKIs.[55]

The judicious use of TKIs to tackle CML disease serves as a model for drug design, development, and testing in the clinical setting of targeted agents, their challenges, and overcoming those limitations.

BTK Inhibitors

The B-cell antigen receptor (BCR) is critical for the development and maturation of B cells.[56] BCR signaling is initiated after an antigen-specific immunoglobulin binds to the receptor. Upon this ligation, the complex recruits multiple kinases and adaptor molecules that stimulate a nexus of signaling cascades. Active BTK phosphorylates immediate molecule phospholipase Cγ2 (PLCG2) accompanied by Ca^{2+} mobilization. Stimulation of this pathway ultimately leads to activation of NF-κB and MAP kinase pathways, which in turn results in increased proliferation, survival, and migration of B cells. The role of BCR activation has been recently recognized as a key driver of B-cell malignancies, including CLL, DLBCL, and mantle cell lymphoma (MCL).[57,58] This understanding provided impetus for the development of BCR pathway inhibitors, and PI3K, AKT, and BTK became attractive targets to design clinical candidate drugs. What imatinib did to the CML space, ibrutinib did in the B-cell malignancies field and changed the therapeutic landscape of CLL and other B-cell malignancies.

Ibrutinib

Ibrutinib, PCI-32765, is a first-in-class oral irreversible inhibitor of BTK and demonstrated inhibition of the biological effect of BTK inactivation on mature B-cell function as well as progression of B-cell disease.[59] It binds covalently to the cysteine 481 residue of the BTK. The efficacy of ibrutinib was seen in early-phase trials in R/R CLL and later in treatment-naïve CLL.[60-63] Randomized studies demonstrated that PFS and in some studies OS were prolonged in ibrutinib-treated patients compared with chemoimmunotherapy-treated patients. Ibrutinib represented a significant clinical advance, and as a result, the drug has been incorporated into treatment algorithms as a primary option for many B-cell malignancies.[64] Yet, there are some limitations that include a low CR rate, resistance development due to *BTK* and other BCR pathway (*PLCG2*) mutations,[65-68] the risk of off-target toxic effects, and need for long-term use and associated high cost. These constraints have led to development of more selective agents and/or in combining ibrutinib with other agents. Major adverse events with ibrutinib include atrial fibrillation, which can occur in 5% to 15% of patients; increased bleeding risk; and hypertension.[69]

Acalabrutinib

Ibrutinib investigations clearly suggested the need for a more selective BTK inhibitor. Acalabrutinib is a second-generation BTK inhibitor and is more selective than ibrutinib.[70] In whole cell evaluations, biological activities of both drugs were similar in CLL cells but different in normal T cells, which were more affected by ibrutinib.[71,72] Clinically, the drug showed impressive activity in patients with CLL in phase I trials,[73] MCL,[74] and Waldenström macroglobulinemia.[75] Comparison with ibrutinib in a randomized trial in CLL demonstrated noninferior PFS and fewer cardiovascular adverse events.[76] Comparison of twice daily (BID) vs once daily dosing suggested BID as a preferred schedule for this drug.[77]

Zanubrutinib

Success of ibrutinib provided two key points of information: BTK is an actionable target and is a driver in many B-cell malignancies and ibrutinib has many off-target effects. Zanubrutinib (BGB-3111), another irreversible BTK inhibitor for the treatment of B-cell malignancies, was designed to have favorable characteristics for binding to the target and PK properties. Preclinical investigations demonstrated pleiotropic actions and activity of this drug in cell lines and murine MCL models.[78] The drug has been investigated for CLL and several other B-cell malignancies.[79-81] Similar to acalabrutinib, zanubrutinib was shown to be better tolerated compared with ibrutinib in patients with R/R CLL.

A common thread among all these three inhibitors is that they all bind covalently to the C481 residue in the kinase domain. Hence, mutations in this site would result in resistance to any of these three drugs. This issue has led to the design of new agents that bind to different pockets of the enzyme and reversibly inhibit the enzyme.

PI3K Inhibitors

The phosphatidylinositol 3-kinases (PI3Ks) have regulatory and catalytic subunits that must work in concert for their activities.[82] In contrast to other kinases that phosphorylate proteins, PI3Ks are atypical kinases that phosphorylate lipid; the regulatory subunits of PI3Ks facilitate membrane localization, receptor binding, and activation, whereas the catalytic subunits phosphorylate phosphatidylinositol-4,5-bisphosphate (PIP2) to yield the lipid-based second messenger phosphatidylinositol-3,4,5-triphosphate (PIP3). The PI3K pathway regulates a multitude of cellular processes, such as proliferation, survival, migration, and glucose metabolism through downstream signaling cascades AKT, PDK1, and mTOR[83-85] and is highly deregulated in many human cancers.[82,86]

Class I PI3K is composed of four enzymes characterized by four catalytic subunits: p110α, -β, -δ or -γ. While p110α and p110β are ubiquitously expressed, p110δ and p110γ are predominantly expressed in hematopoietic cells and are involved in the regulation of immune function.[87-89] Several studies have reported overexpression of PI3Kδ in B-cell malignancies through multiple mechanisms,[90,91] and this observation provided a rationale to create isoform-specific inhibitors for B-cell malignancies.

Idelalisib

Idelalisib (CAL-101 or GS-563117) is a potent inhibitor of PI3Kdelta and in preclinical studies showed biological activity in B-cell malignancies[92,93] through inhibition of translational machinery.[94] This was the first-in-class PI3Kδ-specific inhibitor that was tested clinically[95,96] and FDA approved. Although not recognized during clinical trials in patients with relapsed/refractory disease, immune toxicities became apparent during clinical trials in R/R disease and at a higher incidence in treatment-naïve patients.[97-100] Expression of other isoforms and the MAPK pathway are associated with development of resistance.[101]

Duvelisib

Success and limitations of idelalisib or inhibition of only one isoform, that is, PI3K-delta, spurred an interest in inhibiting the PI3K gamma isoform.[102] A dual inhibitor of both delta and gamma, IPI-145, now duvelisib,[103] inhibited the PI3K/AKT/S6 pathway1[104] and metabolism[105] and induced apoptosis. Similar to idelalisib, duvelisib also lowered Mcl-1 protein levels, which resulted in sensitization of cells to venetoclax.[106] Activity was demonstrated in a phase 1 trial,[107] and a phase 2 trial showed meaningful response rates with similar toxicity profile to idelalisib.[108] In the phase 3 registration trial, duvelisib demonstrated significant improvement in PFS compared with those achieved with ofatumumab.[109] In 2018, duvelisib was approved for patients with R/R CLL.

Copanlisib

It was identified during idelalisib clinical trials that activation of PI3K alpha isoform may limit activities of idelalisib.[110] This spurred an interest in pan-class I PI3K inhibitors. Screening and structure-activity relationship identified BAY80-6946 or copanlisib as a clinical candidate for pan-PI3K inhibitor.[111] In fact, simultaneous inhibition of alpha and delta in preclinical studies in lymphomas showed regression of tumors using copanlisib.[112] In a phase II trial for R/R non-Hodgkin lymphoma, objective responses along with complete remissions were observed with transient hyperglycemia.[113,114] Because this drug inhibits all PI3K isoforms, its use in solid tumors is actively being pursued.

JAK Inhibitors

In contrast to other signaling pathways that were identified through the respective oncogenes that activate them, the Janus kinase/signal transducers and activators of transcription (JAK/STAT) pathway was discovered from the signaling response to interferons.[115] These are cytoplasmic protein kinases and have four variants: JAK1, JAK2, JAK3, and TYK2. Their importance became evident when it was recognized that this pathway is stimulated via a plethora of cytokines, growth factors, and interferons. The initial event after ligand binding is the phosphorylation of tyrosine residues in the receptor mediated by JAKs. They then phosphorylate cytoplasmic STATs, which activates other signaling.[116,117] Depending on the stimulus, cross talk with different partners and interactions occur,[118-120] including the MAPK cascade or the PI3K/AKT/mTOR triad and downstream signaling.[121] Like other signal transduction pathways, JAK activation also results in proliferation, migration, differentiation, and survival of cells. These kinases play a significant role in hematopoiesis, and this pathway is activated in many malignancies such as Ph-negative myeloproliferative neoplasms (MPNs),[122-126] T-cell leukemia/lymphoma,[127,128] "Ph-like" ALL,[129] and T-PLL.[130] Consequently, several JAKi are approved or being investigated for patients with MPNs, while others are approved for autoimmune and inflammatory diseases.[131,132]

Ruxolitinib

Ruxolitinib, previously known as INCB018424, is an oral, selective, and potent inhibitor of both JAK1 and JAK2 (IC50 for both <4 nM). Ruxolitinib inhibited cytokine-induced activation of JAK/STAT signaling, as well as activity of V617F mutant JAK2. This was recapitulated in vivo in an animal model driven by JAK2V617F.[133] The most prevalent, gain-of-function V617F mutation in JAK2 in MPNs ("driver mutation") served as the impetus to test JAKi in these disorders. Ruxolitinib was the first JAKi approved for myelofibrosis[134,135] and later for polycythemia vera[136,137] and provides marked symptom and quality-of-life benefits to patients, ameliorates splenomegaly and associated symptoms, and prolongs survival in patients with higher-risk myelofibrosis. Newer studies indicate potential utility in T-cell lymphomas.[138] In general, ruxolitinib is well tolerated and hematological toxicities is the primary adverse event; opportunistic infections and nonmelanoma skin cancer may occur. Mechanisms of resistance have not been well defined, but one might be the "persistence" phenomenon of transactivation of JAK2 due to heterodimerization with other JAK family members.[139]

Fedratinib

Fedratinib, formerly TG101348, is a JAK2 and FLT3 inhibitor.[140] Uniquely, this drug binds to the kinase domain both at the

ATP-binding site as well as the peptide-substrate binding site. This dual binding may provide fewer opportunities for development of resistance.[141] This drug is approved for patients with myelofibrosis. It has been tested in previously ruxolitinib-treated, as well as JAKi-naïve patients.[142-144] GI toxicities are frequent with fedratinib, besides anemia and thrombocytopenia. The drug carries a black box warning for Wernicke encephalopathy, although the mechanisms remain poorly understood.

Pacritinib

Pacritinib, formerly SB1518, is a JAK2, FLT3, and IRAK1 inhibitor approved for the treatment of patients with myelofibrosis and severe thrombocytopenia. The unique attribute of this agent is its relative lack of myelosuppression. Pacritinib has, thus, been studied in (both JAKi-naïve and JAKi-exposed) patients with myelofibrosis without regard to baseline thrombocytopenia.[145-147] It is the only drug specifically approved for patients with platelets $<50 \times 10^9$/L, where data are lacking for both ruxolitinib and fedratinib, providing spleen and symptom benefits in this difficult group of patients while maintaining blood counts.

FLT3 Inhibitors

Among the genetic alterations in AML, mutations in the FMS-like tyrosine kinase (FLT3) gene have been identified as one of the most common lesion.[148] Albeit at a lower rate, FLT3 mutations are also present in patients with ALL[149] and MDS.[148] The human FLT3 gene, cloned by two groups,[150,151] encodes a membrane-bound 993-amino-acid-long receptor tyrosine kinase. This receptor tyrosine kinase is activated by FLT3 ligand, which is secreted by many hematopoietic cells, which leads to phosphorylation of the tyrosine-kinase domain thereby activating the signal transduction cascade. Wild-type FLT3 is critical in proliferation, differentiation, and apoptosis of normal hematopoietic cells. Two types of mutations in FLT3 gene have been identified: internal tandem duplication (ITD)[152-155] and point mutation in the tyrosine kinase domain (TKD).[155-157] The most common change is at 835 codon with a substitution of aspartic acid to tyrosine (D835Y). Other point mutations have been more recently reported especially in the setting of resistance to FLT3 inhibitors. In addition, other mutations have been identified around codon 835 location. Mutated FLT3 is independent of ligand and hence constitutively active.[158,159] In AML, ITD is more prevalent than TKD mutations and is linked to poor prognosis and clinical outcomes. Success of Bcr-abl kinase targeting in CML and prevalence of FLT3 mutations in acute leukemias garnered interest in designing, developing, and testing FLT3 inhibitors (FLT3is). Several FLT3is have been tested in preclinical and clinical settings.[160]

Midostaurin

Midostaurin, previously known as PKC412, was FDA approved in 2017. Chemically, it is 4′-N-benzoylstaurosporin. The drug inhibits Flt3 kinase, and inhibitory plasma levels were achieved to inhibit this kinase,[161] yet unlike ABL kinase inhibitors, midostaurin or other FLT3is had limited monotherapy activity.[162-167] Addition to chemotherapy led to improved outcomes with midostaurin.[168,169] GI, hematological, and skin toxicities were at higher prevalence in the arm containing midostaurin. Although mechanisms of resistance are not clearly identified, development of additional and diverse mutations have also been indicated.[170]

Gilteritinib

Unlike midostaurin, gilteritinib is more selective with inhibition of FLT3 and AXL[171]; the latter is expressed in AML[172] and considered to be responsible for prevention of FLT3i resistance development.[173,174] Pharmacodynamic-driven trials of this drug showed a dose-dependent increase in plasma levels along with an inhibitory effect on FLT3 phosphorylation.[175] Even as a single agent, this inhibitor resulted in a 40% overall response rate. In phase 3 trial, gilteritinib was evaluated against salvage chemotherapy in R/R AML.[176] Compared with the chemotherapy arm, the gilteritinib arm resulted in higher rates of overall response with longer survival, thus establishing single agent activity of FLT3 inhibition strategy.

IDH1/2 Inhibitors

Isocitrate dehydrogenase (IDH) 1 and 2 share similar structures and are key enzymes involved in cellular metabolism. In oncology, initial discoveries identified mutations in these enzymes in gliomas and glioblastomas.[177,178] Although they were at a much lower rate than in solid tumors, sequencing of the AML genome identified IDH1/2 mutations.[179,180] In parallel it was discovered that IDH1/2 mutations result in the production of 2-hydroxyglutarate (2-HG) from alpha-ketoglutarate,[181] which acts as an oncometabolite and is a culprit for the development and/or progression of cancer. In addition to being involved in metabolism, IDH1/2 enzymes are involved in the cellular redox state, hypermethylation and epigenetic regulation,[182] and DNA repair[183,184] and they interconnect epigenetics to cellular signaling.[185] Mutations in these enzymes induce BCL-2 dependence in AML.[186] Involvement of these enzymes in multiple cancers was an impetus for the identification and design of molecules that target these proteins.

Ivosidenib and Enasidenib

Ivosidenib inhibits IDH1 enzyme while enasidenib inhibits IDH2 enzyme, and both these drugs were FDA approved for treatment of AML.[187-190] These inhibitors prevent the formation of 2-HG, which promotes differentiation of myeloid blasts. Several mechanisms of resistance have been identified including trans-cis dimer-interface mutations,[191] clonal heterogeneity,[192] and co-occurring mutations.[193] Combinations of these inhibitors with azacytidine, chemotherapy, or venetoclax are being pursued to circumvent resistance mechanisms.[194-196]

PROTEASOME INHIBITORS

Bortezomib and ixazomib, reversibly, and carfilzomib, irreversibly, inhibit the proteasome, a large enzyme complex that breaks down proteins that have been selected for degradation.[197] The proteasome inhibitors inhibit the degradation of proteins involved in regulation of cell proliferation and survival. It deregulates signaling molecules that are critical to the interaction of tumor cells with the bone marrow microenvironment, leading to growth inhibition and apoptosis. Several intracellular molecules important in apoptosis, including NF-κB, JNK, Bcl-2, p53, and gp130, are modulated by proteasome degradation. Unlike bortezomib and carfilzomib, ixazomib is an orally available proteasome inhibitor. The primary mechanism of bortezomib clearance is oxidative metabolism via the cytochrome P450 enzyme system; no dosage adjustment is necessary for renal impairment. Carfilzomib is primarily metabolized via peptidase cleavage and epoxide hydrolysis with minimal metabolism through cytochrome P450 enzymes; no dosage adjustment is necessary for preexisting renal impairment. Ixazomib is primarily metabolized via multiple CYP enzymes and non-CYP proteins; dose reduction is required for severe renal impairment. The most frequent toxicities associated with proteasome inhibitors treatment include herpes zoster reactivation, myelosuppression (neutropenia/thrombocytopenia), and peripheral neuropathy. The peripheral neuropathy caused from bortezomib is a sensory neuropathy affecting the hands and feet in a "stocking and glove" distribution and is frequently painful. The incidence and severity are higher with bortezomib than with carfilzomib and ixazomib. The risk of peripheral neuropathy with bortezomib is lower with less frequent schedule (weekly vs more frequently) and with subcutaneous route rather than IV administration. For patients who develop neuropathy, treatment discontinuation or dose modification leads to improvement/resolution of symptoms in majority of patients within 3 months; for some patients' neuropathy can persist for longer duration. Carfilzomib can be associated with cardiovascular side effects, including hypertension, heart failure, and arrhythmias. Herpes zoster reactivation has been observed with the proteasome inhibitors, and therefore, patients receiving proteasome inhibitors should receive herpes simplex virus prophylaxis.

IMMUNOMODULATORY DRUGS

Thalidomide, lenalidomide, and pomalidomide are immunomodulatory drugs (IMiDs) with a wide range of potential antineoplastic actions, particularly against multiple myeloma.[198] Pomalidomide and lenalidomide were developed after thalidomide and are more potent with fewer side effects. These IMiDs activate T cells and stimulate endogenous cytokine release, including IL-2, and IFN-α production. They inhibit TNF-α synthesis and block the activation of NF-κB. The specific mechanism of antineoplastic immunomodulation of these three agents remains uncertain, although they have been shown to interact with the ubiquitin E3 ligase cereblon, leading to degradation of Ikaros transcription factors. Because thalidomide is mainly hydrolyzed and passively excreted, its clearance is not expected to be altered in patients with impaired liver or renal function. Lenalidomide is excreted in its unchanged form via the kidneys and has a reduced clearance in the setting of renal impairment; dose adjustments are needed for patients with renal dysfunction. Pomalidomide is metabolized extensively by the liver, and therefore, dose adjustment is not necessary for mild to moderate renal dysfunction; dose adjustment is required for patients with hepatic impairment.

Thalidomide is a potent teratogen. Use of thalidomide as a sedative in the late 1950s resulted in birth defects in >10,000 infants. Birth defects included absent or hypoplastic limbs, ear or eye deformities, and heart defects. Thalidomide administration to pregnant women is absolutely contraindicated. Women of childbearing age must have a negative pregnancy test before starting IMiDs and use appropriate birth control measures. Common IMiDs toxicities include neuropathy, somnolence, and myelosuppression. The toxicity profile of IMiDs increases when given in combination with drugs such as corticosteroids. Clinical features are tingling or painful distal paresthesias affecting primarily the feet but sometimes the hands. There is increased risk of venous and arterial thrombosis, with higher risk in older patients and in combination with steroids. Constipation develops a few days after starting treatment in >50% of patients receiving IMiDs. Another common IMiDs toxicity is reversible myelosuppression (neutropenia and thrombocytopenia). An increased risk of development of second malignancies has been reported with IMiDs.

CHIMERIC ANTIGEN RECEPTOR T-CELL THERAPY

CAR T cell therapy represents a major advance for the field of hematologic malignancies and are currently approved for R/R B-ALL, non-Hodgkin lymphoma (NHL), and MM. Approved CAR T are autologous products derived from the patient's own T cells that have undergone ex vivo transduction to introduce the CAR molecule. CD19-directed CAR T are approved for B-ALL and NHL, including MCL, whereas BCMA-directed CAR T are approved for MM (Table 69.2). A detailed description of the CAR T, their toxicities, and role in the management of a particular disease are provided in disease-specific chapters.

OTHER NOVEL AGENTS

BCL2 Inhibition

Venetoclax is a small molecule oral B-cell lymphoma-2 homology 3 (BH3) mimetic. It selectively inhibits the B-cell lymphoma 2 (BCL2) protein. BCL2 is upregulated in many hematologic malignancies, particularly in CLL and AML. Once venetoclax binds to the BH3-binding groove of BCL2 within the tumor cell, it displaces BIM and other proapoptotic BH3 proteins enabling them to activate BAX and BAK. Activation of BAX/BAK leads to their oligomerization, mitochondrial outer membrane permeabilization, and activation of caspases leading to apoptosis.

Venetoclax has a mean terminal half-life of approximately 14 to 18 hours with different doses. It peaks 5 to 8 hours after administration with a low-fat meal. It is hepatically metabolized, mainly via cytochrome P450 (CYP3A) enzymes, and excreted primarily through feces. Based on PK studies, venetoclax doses of 20 to 1200 mg once daily given with low- and high-fat meals increased venetoclax exposure by almost 4-fold compared with a fasting state. Venetoclax should be administered within 30 minutes of a meal regardless of the fat content. Since venetoclax is predominately metabolized through CYP3A, appropriate dose modification with concomitant moderate and strong CY3A4 inhibitors that increase its serum concentration by reducing metabolism is imperative to prevent toxicities. In general, venetoclax dose should be reduced by 50% with moderate CYP3A4 inhibitors and by at least 75% with strong CYP3A4 inhibitors.

Venetoclax has two approved indications: (1) newly diagnosed AML in adults ≥75 years of age or with comorbidities precluding them from receiving intensive chemotherapy and (2) CLL. CLL is very sensitive to venetoclax therapy due to its high BCL-2 expression, which increases the risk of tumor lysis syndrome (TLS) upon treatment initiation. Therefore, a 5-week dose ramp-up is recommended with a weekly dose increase (20-50-100-200-400 mg) until maximum dose of 400 mg is established. In AML, venetoclax 400 mg is combined with hypomethylating agents and 600 mg is given with low-dose cytarabine. To reduce the risk of TLS in AML, starting therapy with white blood cell of <10 K is preferred along with a 3-day dose ramp-up. Duration of venetoclax is based on the chosen combination regimen as well as patient- and disease-related factors. Modifications are often necessary after induction based on time to hematologic recovery and tolerability.

The main adverse effects of venetoclax are TLS, cytopenias, and GI toxicity (nausea/vomiting/diarrhea). Risk of TLS is higher in CLL than in AML, due to higher BCL2 expression, but close monitoring of TLS labs and prophylaxis with a uric acid–lowering agent and hydration should be administered. Dose ramp-up, as stated earlier, is also necessary to reduce the risk of TLS. In CLL, patients are risk stratified to low, intermediate, and high for TLS based on their absolute lymphocyte count and lymph node size. The main difference in management based on risk stratification is that low-risk patients and moderate risk with good renal function can be treated in the outpatient setting while those with moderate risk with poor renal function and high-risk should be admitted for at least 24 to 48 hours for close monitoring upon treatment initiation and dose ramp-up. Management of cytopenias includes dose interruption or dose adjustment, empiric prophylactic antimicrobials, and/or administration of granulocyte colony-stimulating factor.

The main mechanism of resistance of venetoclax is upregulation of MCL-1, BCL-xL, and AKT phosphorylation and decreased expression of BAX, PTEN, and BIM. In patients with CLL, BCL2 mutations have been described at the time of venetoclax resistance. Increased knowledge of these resistance mechanisms has prompted development of several investigational agents to help overcome resistance. In addition, patients with AML who harbor adverse cytogenetics such as *TP53* and *FLT3* mutations were identified to have lower duration of response.

Table 69.2. Selected Approved CAR-T Therapies in Hematologic Malignancies

Target	Drug Name	Costimulatory Domain	Indication
CD19	Tisagenlecleucel	4-1BB	B-ALL (pediatric) DLBCL, FL
	Axicabtagene ciloleucel	CD28	DLBCL, FL
	Brexucabtagene autoleucel	CD28	B-ALL (adult) Mantle cell lymphoma
	Lisocabtagene maraleucel	4-1BB	DLBCL
BCMA	Idecabtagene vicleucel	4-1BB	Multiple myeloma
	Ciltacabtagene autoleucel	4-1BB	Multiple myeloma

Asparaginase

Asparaginase is an endogenous enzyme that hydrolyses L-asparagine to ammonia and L-aspartic acid and glutamine to glutamic acid.[199] Asparagine is an amino acid needed for protein synthesis and cell growth. Hence, insufficient levels of asparagine promote the cell to activate apoptotic mechanisms. Lymphoblastic leukemia cells are unable to make asparagine due to low levels of asparaginase synthetase intracellularly; thus, they are dependent on extracellular asparagine for survival. Therapeutic asparaginase depletes asparagine promoting cell death through apoptosis.

Asparaginase is derived from two bacterial species, *Escherichia coli* and *Erwinia carotovora*. *E. coli* asparaginase; pegaspargase, a pegylated form of the native product; and calaspargase pegol, pegylated with the addition of succinimidyl carbamate, come from *E. coli*, and asparaginase *Erwinia chrysanthemi* comes from *E. carotovora*. The three available and FDA-approved formulations for treatment of ALL are pegaspargase, *Erwinia* asparaginase, and calaspargase pegol.

Although all three kill leukemic cells equivalently, their PK profiles differ. Pegaspargase can be administered through IV or intramuscularly, but the latter route of administration is less common. Duration of asparagine depletion is longer, due to it being pegylated, at 2 to 4 weeks with IV. The duration of asparagine depletion with *Erwinia* asparaginase is shorter at 48 to 72 hours. Calaspargase pegol, only available as an IV, has the longest half-life of approximately 16 days. Owing to the differences in their PK, these products are not easily interchangeable as their dose and, most importantly, dosing schedules differ.

Asparaginase is a key component of ALL treatment, particularly in children. The dose and frequency of each agent differs due to their unique PK profile. The most clinically utilized product is pegaspargase. Pediatric and young adults receive higher doses than older adults because of better tolerance. The dose also differs depending on the protocol and combination regimen utilized. Calaspargase has the same dose as pegaspargase but is administered every 21 days.

Erwinia asparaginase may be substituted for an *E. coli* product like pegaspargase in case of intolerance, but its dose and frequency differ significantly from those of the other products. There are no dose adjustments required for renal or hepatic impairment, although all three agents can cause hepatotoxicity, so caution is advised in patients with hepatic disease. Aside from the PK differences, there can also be interpatient variability.

There are numerous trials establishing the efficacy and safety of each product, mostly as part of a combination regimen, in treatment of ALL. The CALGB 10403 trial in adolescent and young adults (AYAs) was a large prospective trial demonstrating efficacy and safety of utilizing a pediatric inspired regimen, which includes pegaspargase.[200] A higher incidence of asparaginase-related toxicity such as hepatic and thrombotic complications was noted in the AYA group.

Adverse effects of asparaginase differ by age. Adults tend to have higher rates of hyperglycemia, hyperbilirubinemia, pancreatitis, elevated liver enzymes, and hypofibrinogenemia. Therapeutic drug monitoring of asparaginase levels can help evaluate effectiveness in real time and improve outcomes.[201] Hypersensitivity reactions can also occur with all formulations and may be mild to moderate such as flushing, chill, hypotension, and fever or severe, causing chest pain, bronchospasm, or anaphylaxis. If symptoms developed on an *E. coli*–derived product then *Erwinia* should be used and vice versa because all *E. coli*–derived products have cross-resistance. Premedications can help reduce allergic reactions.

Glasdegib

The hedgehog (Hh) signaling pathway is an important regulator in stem cells, cell differentiation and proliferation. Some cancers overexpress the hedgehog pathway. Glasdegib is a Hh inhibitor that binds to Smoothened protein, a transmembrane protein important in hedgehog signal transduction, and inhibits its translocation thereby halting downstream activation of the Hh pathway.[202] In AML, glasdegib is thought to sensitize leukemic cells to cytotoxic chemotherapy by promoting quiescent leukemic stem cells to differentiate.

Glasdegib is a major substrate of CYP3A4 and mainly metabolized by CYP3A4 and to lesser extent by CYP2C8 and UGT1A9. Therefore, strong, or moderate, inhibitors or inducers of CYP3A4 can either increase or decrease glasdegib serum concentration, respectively. Glasdegib is currently approved in combination with low-dose cytarabine in patients ≥75 years of age or with comorbidities who have a diagnosis of AML.[203] The most common and unique adverse effects of glasdegib are elevated liver enzymes including bilirubin, musculoskeletal pain, muscle spasm, electrolyte disturbances, specifically hyponatremia, and hypomagnesemia.

Selinexor

Selinexor is an oral first-in-class, reversible, selective inhibitor of nuclear export for growth regulators, tumor suppressor proteins, and oncogenic proteins that covalently binds to exportin 1 (XPO1).[204] Selinexor inhibits XPO1, which halts loading and export of cargo, causing accumulation of tumor suppressor protein in the nucleus thereby reducing oncoprotein messenger RNA translation and inhibiting NF-κB that leads to cell cycle arrest and apoptosis.

Selinexor is an oral agent approved in adults with R/R DLBCL and MM.[205,206] Selinexor can cause hematologic toxicities, especially when combined with other therapies. Prophylactic antimicrobials and growth factor support may be necessary. Selinexor has a moderate to high emetogenicity requiring antiemetic prophylaxis. It can cause diarrhea, nausea, vomiting, constipation, and anorexia. Hyponatremia is common. Selinexor can also lead to neurologic toxicities such as dizziness, confusion, delirium, or cognitive impairment possibly due to its ability to cross the blood-brain barrier.

All-*trans* Retinoic Acid

Acute promyelocytic leukemia (PML) is characterized by chromosome translocation t(15;17) (q22;q21), which causes a reciprocal translocation in the gene encoding for PML and retinoic acid receptor-alpha (RAR*a*) creating a fusion protein called *PML-RARa*. The oncoprotein *PML-RARa* causes a maturation block of promyelocytes preventing their differentiation along the myeloid lineage. All-*trans* retinoic acid (ATRA), also known as tretinoin, is a retinoid, which is a derivative of vitamin A, important for cell growth and development. ATRA binds to the *RARa* moiety of the *PML-RARAa* oncoprotein allowing for differentiation of the promyelocyte to neutrophils.

ATRA is well absorbed and reaches peak plasma levels in 1 to 2 hours. It is hepatically metabolized through the CYP enzymes with its primary metabolite being 4-oxo-all *trans*-retinoic acid. The dose of ATRA is 45 mg/m^2/d orally divided in two doses, rounded to the nearest 10 mg, given until achievement of complete remission during induction. During consolidation, it is given at the same dose but only on days 1 to 14 of a 28-day cycle. It is commonly combined with arsenic trioxide as the frontline treatment of APL.[207] ATRA can cause differentiation syndrome, hepatotoxicity, and pseudomotor cerebri. Differentiation syndrome, a potentially fatal complication, is manifested by dyspnea, pleural effusion and/or pericardial effusion, pulmonary infiltrates, unexplained fever, hypotension, acute renal failure, or weigh gain. The median time of onset is typically 7 to 12 days after treatment initiation. Treatment with ATRA should be initiated inpatient during induction with close monitoring of labs and vitals. If differentiation syndrome occurs, dexamethasone should be administered. In addition, supportive care measures such as diuretics for volume overload should be used. Pseudomotor cerebri is a rare but a serious side effect for which the symptoms include headache, visual disturbance, tinnitus, papilledema, and nausea/vomiting. Symptoms can often be managed with acetazolamide.

Arsenic Trioxide

Arsenic trioxide (ATO) mechanism of action is not well elucidated, but it causes morphologic changes and DNA fragmentation leading to apoptosis of leukemic cell and degrades and damages the fusion oncoprotein PML/RAR*a*. ATO, once in solution, is immediately hydrolyzed to arsenous acid (AA), which is the most active form. AA is mainly excreted through the urine; patients with severe renal dysfunction receiving ATO have demonstrated higher exposure to AA and its metabolites, and therefore, ATO should be avoided or used with caution in patients with severe renal dysfunction. Several studies have demonstrated the efficacy of ATO in combination with ATRA for treatment of APL. Differentiation syndrome, QT prolongation, nausea/vomiting, rash, hepatotoxicity, and hematologic toxicity are some of the more common toxicities with ATO.

Crizotinib

Translocation of anaplastic lymphoma kinase (ALK) creates an oncogenic fusion protein that dysregulates and activates ALK expression and signaling causing cell proliferation and survival. Crizotinib is a first-generation ALK inhibitor preventing its phosphorylation and signal transduction. Crizotinib is indicated in R/R ALK-positive anaplastic large cell lymphoma (ALCL) in both pediatric and young adult patients and in metastatic ALK-positive or ROS1-positive non–small cell lung cancer. Dose adjustments are necessary for renal impairment (CrCl <30 mL/min) and for moderate to severe hepatic impairment. Concomitant CYPA4 inhibitors and inducers should be avoided. ALK is a driver mutation in ALCL. Although ALK-positive ALCL responds to chemotherapy, relapses occur. Crizotinib reported high rates of ORR in patients with R/R ALCL. Crizotinib can cause ocular, cardiac, pulmonary, hepatic, and GI toxicities.

Tazemetostat

Tazemetostat is an oral, selective, first-in-class potent inhibitor of EZH2. EZH2 is an epigenetic regulator, the catalytic subunit of PRC2, that mediates gene repression. *EZH2* aberrations or mutations enhance oncogenic transformation and histone methylation and cause dependency to EZH2 activity promoting tumor progression. Tazemetostat is hepatically metabolized via CYP3A to inactive metabolites in the form EPZ006931 and EPZ-6930. It is approved for R/R follicular lymphoma at 800 mg twice daily continuously until disease progression or unacceptable toxicity. Most common side effects are cytopenia, mainly thrombocytopenia, and GI symptoms.

NOVEL EMERGING TARGETS IN CLINICAL TRIALS

There are several agents in clinical trials targeting novel therapeutic pathways. Many ongoing trials are exploring these agents as single agent or in combination with either chemotherapy or other targeted therapies.

CD20 Bispecific Antibodies

Several CD20 bispecific antibodies are in clinical development. These antibodies are similar in concept to blinatumomab, a CD19-targeting bispecific antibody, but they target a different surface protein, namely, CD20. These drugs target CD20 on the surface of tumor cells and CD3 on the surface of T cells. This leads to T-cell activation and, thereby, tumor cell killing. Several of these antibodies are in clinical trials including mosunetuzumab, odronextamab, glofitamab, and epcoritamab.[208] Some of these antibodies are given IV; for others subcutaneous formulation is being developed for ease of administration. Encouraging single-agent activity has been reported in clinical trials in patients with relapsed/refractory NHL, and several of these agents are being combined with chemoimmunotherapy. Important adverse events are secondary to T-cell activation, which include CRS and neurological toxicity.

BCL-xL Inhibitors

The expression of BCL-2 family proteins, perturbed in multiple types of leukemias and solid tumors, is associated with disease progression and with resistance to chemotherapy. Venetoclax, described in a previous section of this chapter, is a small-molecule BH3 mimetic that selectively binds BCL-2. BCL-xL is expressed in several hematologic malignancies and is associated with chemotherapy resistance and with venetoclax resistance. Navitoclax is a dual BCL2/BCL-xL, which was limited in its use due to on-target off-tumor effect on mature platelets, which are dependent on BCL-xL for survival.[209] Initial studies in CLL reported clinical activity of navitoclax, but with dose-dependent thrombocytopenia.[210] More recently, navitoclax has been explored in combination with venetoclax and chemotherapy with relapsed/refractory ALL,[211] and in combination with ruxolitinib in patients with myelofibrosis.[212] Additional BCL-xL and dual BCL2/BCL-xL inhibitors are in clinical development.

MCL1 Inhibitors

MCL1 is a member of the BCL-2 family antiapoptotic proteins. Given the clinical success of venetoclax, a selective BCL-2 inhibitor, and the role of MCL1 overexpression in venetoclax refractory leukemias, there are several selective MCL1 inhibitors in clinical development. Only limited clinical data are available so far, and some of the trials have been put on hold due to on-target off-tumor cardiac toxicity.[213]

Several other novel targets including but not limited to proteolysis-targeting chimera (PROTAC),[214] inhibitor of apoptosis proteins (IAPs),[215] cyclin-dependent kinase inhibitors,[216] bromodomain inhibitors,[217] and other targets are in clinical development.

FUTURE OF TARGETED THERAPY

Additional genes, signaling pathway molecules, and posttranslational events important in the development and growth of hematologic cancers will continue to be discovered, as will potential new pathways for therapy. A number of clinical trials are ongoing exploring these novel targets in different hematologic malignancies (http://www.clinicaltrials.gov). Overall, there is increasing shift from chemotherapy to targeted therapies in majority of hematologic malignancies; this is especially true for diseases such as CML, CLL, and APL where chemotherapy has been largely replaced by targeted therapies. For other disease subsets, an increasing number of targeted therapies, either as monotherapy or in combination, are being developed, and it is likely that we will rely more and more on targeted therapies than chemotherapy in future.

References

1. McLaughlin P, Grillo-Lopez AJ, Link BK, et al. Rituximab chimeric anti-CD20 monoclonal antibody therapy for relapsed indolent lymphoma: half of patients respond to a four-dose treatment program. *J Clin Oncol*. 1998;16(8):2825-2833.
2. Mossner E, Brunker P, Moser S, et al. Increasing the efficacy of CD20 antibody therapy through the engineering of a new type II anti-CD20 antibody with enhanced direct and immune effector cell-mediated B-cell cytotoxicity. *Blood*. 2010;115(22):4393-4402.
3. Kantarjian H, Thomas D, Jorgensen J, et al. Inotuzumab ozogamicin, an anti-CD22-calecheamicin conjugate, for refractory and relapsed acute lymphocytic leukaemia: a phase 2 study. *Lancet Oncol*. 2012;13(4):403-411.
4. Kantarjian HM, DeAngelo DJ, Stelljes M, et al. Inotuzumab ozogamicin versus standard therapy for acute lymphoblastic leukemia. *N Engl J Med*. 2016;375(8):740-753.
5. Kreitman RJ, Dearden C, Zinzani PL, et al. Moxetumomab pasudotox in relapsed/refractory hairy cell leukemia. *Leukemia*. 2018;32(8):1768-1777.
6. Kreitman RJ, Pastan I. Antibody fusion proteins: anti-CD22 recombinant immunotoxin moxetumomab pasudotox. *Clin Cancer Res*. 2011;17(20):6398-6405.
7. Younes A, Bartlett NL, Leonard JP, et al. Brentuximab vedotin (SGN-35) for relapsed CD30-positive lymphomas. *N Engl J Med*. 2010;363(19):1812-1821.
8. Connors JM, Radford JA. Brentuximab vedotin for stage III or IV Hodgkin's lymphoma. *N Engl J Med*. 2018;378(16):1560-1561.
9. Herrera AF, Moskowitz AJ, Bartlett NL, et al. Interim results of brentuximab vedotin in combination with nivolumab in patients with relapsed or refractory Hodgkin lymphoma. *Blood*. 2018;131(11):1183-1194.
10. Sehn LH, Herrera AF, Flowers CR, et al. Polatuzumab vedotin in relapsed or refractory diffuse large B-cell lymphoma. *J Clin Oncol*. 2020;38(2):155-165.
11. Tilly H, Morschhauser F, Sehn LH, et al. Polatuzumab vedotin in previously untreated diffuse large B-cell lymphoma. *N Engl J Med*. 2022;386(4):351-363.
12. Ravandi F, Estey EH, Appelbaum FR, et al. Gemtuzumab ozogamicin: time to resurrect? *J Clin Oncol*. 2012;30(32):3921-3923.
13. Lambert J, Pautas C, Terre C, et al. Gemtuzumab ozogamicin for de novo acute myeloid leukemia: final efficacy and safety updates from the open-label, phase III ALFA-0701 trial. *Haematologica*. 2019;104(1):113-119.
14. Jordan CT, Upchurch D, Szilvassy SJ, et al. The interleukin-3 receptor alpha chain is a unique marker for human acute myelogenous leukemia stem cells. *Leukemia*. 2000;14(10):1777-1784.
15. Frankel AE, Woo JH, Ahn C, et al. Activity of SL-401, a targeted therapy directed to interleukin-3 receptor, in blastic plasmacytoid dendritic cell neoplasm patients. *Blood*. 2014;124(3):385-392.

16. Pemmaraju N, Lane AA, Sweet KL, et al. Tagraxofusp in blastic plasmacytoid dendritic-cell neoplasm. *N Engl J Med.* 2019;380(17):1628-1637.
17. Shah N, Chari A, Scott E, Mezzi K, Usmani SZ. B-cell maturation antigen (BCMA) in multiple myeloma: rationale for targeting and current therapeutic approaches. *Leukemia.* 2020;34(4):985-1005.
18. Abeykoon JP, Vaxman J, Patel SV, et al. Impact of belantamab mafodotin-induced ocular toxicity on outcomes of patients with advanced multiple myeloma. *Br J Haematol.* 2022;199(1):95-99.
19. Facon T, Kumar S, Plesner T, et al. Daratumumab plus lenalidomide and dexamethasone for untreated myeloma. *N Engl J Med.* 2019;380(22):2104-2115.
20. Attal M, Richardson PG, Rajkumar SV, et al. Isatuximab plus pomalidomide and low-dose dexamethasone versus pomalidomide and low-dose dexamethasone in patients with relapsed and refractory multiple myeloma (ICARIA-MM): a randomised, multicentre, open-label, phase 3 study. *Lancet.* 2019;394(10214):2096-2107.
21. Lonial S, Dimopoulos M, Palumbo A, et al. Elotuzumab therapy for relapsed or refractory multiple myeloma. *N Engl J Med.* 2015;373(7):621-631.
22. Ansell SM, Lesokhin AM, Borrello I, et al. PD-1 blockade with nivolumab in relapsed or refractory Hodgkin's lymphoma. *N Engl J Med.* 2015;372(4):311-319.
23. Nagorsen D, Kufer P, Baeuerle PA, Bargou R. Blinatumomab: a historical perspective. *Pharmacol Ther.* 2012;136(3):334-342.
24. Bargou R, Leo E, Zugmaier G, et al. Tumor regression in cancer patients by very low doses of a T cell-engaging antibody. *Science.* 2008;321(5891):974-977.
25. Kantarjian H, Stein A, Gokbuget N, et al. Blinatumomab versus chemotherapy for advanced acute lymphoblastic leukemia. *N Engl J Med.* 2017;376(9):836-847.
26. Beemon K, Hunter T. In vitro translation yields a possible Rous sarcoma virus src gene product. *Proc Natl Acad Sci U S A.* 1977;74(8):3302-3306.
27. Collett MS, Erikson RL. Protein kinase activity associated with the avian sarcoma virus src gene product. *Proc Natl Acad Sci U S A.* 1978;75:2021-2024.
28. Slamon DJ, Godolphin W, Jones LA, et al. Studies of the HER-2/neu proto-oncogene in human breast and ovarian cancer. *Science.* 1989;244(4905):707-712.
29. Ullrich A, Schlessinger J. Signal transduction by receptors with tyrosine kinase activity. *Cell.* 1990;61(2):203-212.
30. Schlessinger J. Cell signaling by receptor tyrosine kinases. *Cell.* 2000;103(2):211-225.
31. Rowley JD. Letter: a new consistent chromosomal abnormality in chronic myelogenous leukaemia identified by quinacrine fluorescence and Giemsa staining. *Nature.* 1973;243(5405):290-293.
32. Heisterkamp N, Stephenson JR, Groffen J, et al. Localization of the c-abl oncogene adjacent to a translocation break point in chronic myelocytic leukaemia. *Nature.* 1983;306(5940):239-242.
33. Bartram CR, de Klein A, Hagemeijer A, et al. Translocation of c-abl oncogene correlates with the presence of a Philadelphia chromosome in chronic myelocytic leukaemia. *Nature.* 1983;306(5940):277-280.
34. Druker BJ, Tamura S, Buchdunger E, et al. Effects of a selective inhibitor of the Abl tyrosine kinase on the growth of Bcr-Abl positive cells. *Nat Med.* 1996;2(5):561-566.
35. Druker BJ, Talpaz M, Resta DJ, et al. Efficacy and safety of a specific inhibitor of the BCR-ABL tyrosine kinase in chronic myeloid leukemia. *N Engl J Med.* 2001;344(14):1031-1037.
36. Druker BJ, Sawyers CL, Kantarjian H, et al. Activity of a specific inhibitor of the BCR-ABL tyrosine kinase in the blast crisis of chronic myeloid leukemia and acute lymphoblastic leukemia with the Philadelphia chromosome. *N Engl J Med.* 2001;344(14):1038-1042.
37. O'Brien SG, Guilhot F, Larson RA, et al. Imatinib compared with interferon and low-dose cytarabine for newly diagnosed chronic-phase chronic myeloid leukemia. *N Engl J Med.* 2003;348(11):994-1004.
38. Shah NP, Nicoll JM, Nagar B, et al. Multiple BCR-ABL kinase domain mutations confer polyclonal resistance to the tyrosine kinase inhibitor imatinib (STI571) in chronic phase and blast crisis chronic myeloid leukemia. *Cancer Cell.* 2002;2:117-125.
39. Shah NP, Tran C, Lee FY, Chen P, Norris D, Sawyers CL. Overriding imatinib resistance with a novel ABL kinase inhibitor. *Science.* 2004;305(5682):399-401.
40. Braun TP, Eide CA, Druker BJ. Response and resistance to BCR-ABL1-targeted therapies. *Cancer Cell.* 2020;37(4):530-542.
41. Larson RA, Druker BJ, Guilhot F, et al. Imatinib pharmacokinetics and its correlation with response and safety in chronic-phase chronic myeloid leukemia: a subanalysis of the IRIS study. *Blood.* 2008;111:4022-4028.
42. Hehlmann R, Lauseker M, Jung-Munkwitz S, et al. Tolerability-adapted imatinib 800 mg/d versus 400 mg/d versus 400 mg/d plus interferon-α in newly diagnosed chronic myeloid leukemia. *J Clin Oncol.* 2011;29(12):1634-1642.
43. Marin D, Bazeos A, Mahon FX, et al. Adherence is the critical factor for achieving molecular responses in patients with chronic myeloid leukemia who achieve complete cytogenetic responses on imatinib. *J Clin Oncol.* 2010;28(14):2381-2388.
44. Talpaz M, Shah NP, Kantarjian H, et al. Dasatinib in imatinib-resistant Philadelphia chromosome-positive leukemias. *N Engl J Med.* 2006;354(24):2531-2541.
45. Hochhaus A, Kantarjian HM, Baccarani M, et al. Dasatinib induces notable hematologic and cytogenetic responses in chronic-phase chronic myeloid leukemia after failure of imatinib therapy. *Blood.* 2007;109(6):2303-2309.
46. Cortes JE, Jones D, O'Brien S, et al. Results of dasatinib therapy in patients with early chronic-phase chronic myeloid leukemia. *J Clin Oncol.* 2010;28(3):398-404.
47. Kantarjian H, Shah NP, Hochhaus A, et al. Dasatinib versus imatinib in newly diagnosed chronic-phase chronic myeloid leukemia. *N Engl J Med.* 2010;362(24):2260-2270.
48. Weisberg E, Manley PW, Breitenstein W, et al. Characterization of AMN107, a selective inhibitor of native and mutant Bcr-Abl. *Cancer Cell.* 2005;7(2):129-141.
49. Kantarjian HM, Giles F, Gattermann N, et al. Nilotinib (formerly AMN107), a highly selective BCR-ABL tyrosine kinase inhibitor, is effective in patients with Philadelphia chromosome-positive chronic myelogenous leukemia in chronic phase following imatinib resistance and intolerance. *Blood.* 2007;110(10):3540-3546.
50. Saglio G, Kim DW, Issaragrisil S, et al. Nilotinib versus imatinib for newly diagnosed chronic myeloid leukemia. *N Engl J Med.* 2010;362(24):2251-2259.
51. Puttini M, Coluccia AML, Boschelli F, et al. In vitro and in vivo activity of SKI-606, a novel Src-Abl inhibitor, against imatinib-resistant Bcr-Abl+ neoplastic cells. *Cancer Res.* 2006;66(23):11314-11322.
52. Cortes JE, Kantarjian HM, Brümmendorf TH, et al. Safety and efficacy of bosutinib (SKI-606) in chronic phase Philadelphia chromosome-positive chronic myeloid leukemia patients with resistance or intolerance to imatinib. *Blood.* 2011;118(17):4567-4576.
53. Cortes JE, Gambacorti-Passerini C, Deininger MW, et al. Bosutinib versus imatinib for newly diagnosed chronic myeloid leukemia: results from the randomized BFORE trial. *J Clin Oncol.* 2018;36(3):231-237.
54. O'Hare T, Shakespeare WC, Zhu X, et al. AP24534, a pan-BCR-ABL inhibitor for chronic myeloid leukemia, potently inhibits the T315I mutant and overcomes mutation-based resistance. *Cancer Cell.* 2009;16(5):401-412.
55. Cortes JE, Kim DW, Pinilla-Ibarz J, et al. A phase 2 trial of ponatinib in Philadelphia chromosome-positive leukemias. *N Engl J Med.* 2013;369(19):1783-1796.
56. Stevenson FK, Krysov S, Davies AJ, Steele AJ, Packham G. B-cell receptor signaling in chronic lymphocytic leukemia. *Blood.* 2011;118(16):4313-4320.
57. Burger JA. Treatment of chronic lymphocytic leukemia. *N Engl J Med.* 2020;383(5):460-473.
58. Stevenson FK, Forconi F, Kipps TJ. Exploring the pathways to chronic lymphocytic leukemia. *Blood.* 2021;138(10):827-835.
59. Honigberg LA, Smith AM, Sirisawad M, et al. The Bruton tyrosine kinase inhibitor PCI-32765 blocks B-cell activation and is efficacious in models of autoimmune disease and B-cell malignancy. *Proc Natl Acad Sci U S A.* 2010;107(29):13075-13080.
60. Advani RH, Buggy JJ, Sharman JP, et al. Bruton tyrosine kinase inhibitor ibrutinib (PCI-32765) has significant activity in patients with relapsed/refractory B-cell malignancies. *J Clin Oncol.* 2013;31(1):88-94.
61. Byrd JC, Furman RR, Coutre SE, et al. Targeting BTK with ibrutinib in relapsed chronic lymphocytic leukemia. *N Engl J Med.* 2013;369(1):32-42.
62. Burger JA, Tedeschi A, Barr PM, et al. Ibrutinib as initial therapy for patients with chronic lymphocytic leukemia. *N Engl J Med.* 2015;373(25):2425-2437.
63. Byrd JC, Brown JR, O'Brien S, et al. Ibrutinib versus ofatumumab in previously treated chronic lymphoid leukemia. *N Engl J Med.* 2014;371(3):213-223.
64. Timofeeva N, Gandhi V. Ibrutinib combinations in CLL therapy: scientific rationale and clinical results. *Blood Cancer J.* 2021;11(4):79.
65. Burger JA, Landau DA, Taylor-Weiner A, et al. Clonal evolution in patients with chronic lymphocytic leukaemia developing resistance to BTK inhibition. *Nat Commun.* 2016;7:11589.
66. Furman RR, Cheng S, Lu P, et al. Ibrutinib resistance in chronic lymphocytic leukemia. *N Engl J Med.* 2014;370(24):2352-2354.
67. Liu TM, Woyach JA, Zhong Y, et al. Hypermorphic mutation of phospholipase C, γ2 acquired in ibrutinib-resistant CLL confers BTK independency upon B-cell receptor activation. *Blood.* 2015;126(1):61-68.
68. Woyach JA, Ruppert AS, Guinn D, et al. BTK(C481S)-Mediated resistance to ibrutinib in chronic lymphocytic leukemia. *J Clin Oncol.* 2017;35(13):1437-1443.
69. Christensen BW, Zaha VG, Awan FT. Cardiotoxicity of BTK inhibitors: ibrutinib and beyond. *Expet Rev Hematol.* 2022;15(4):321-331.
70. Herman SEM, Montraveta A, Niemann CU, et al. The Bruton tyrosine kinase (BTK) inhibitor acalabrutinib demonstrates potent on-target effects and efficacy in two mouse models of chronic lymphocytic leukemia. *Clin Cancer Res.* 2017;23(11):2831-2841.
71. Patel V, Balakrishnan K, Bibikova E, et al. Comparison of acalabrutinib, A selective Bruton tyrosine kinase inhibitor, with ibrutinib in chronic lymphocytic leukemia cells. *Clin Cancer Res.* 2017;23(14):3734-3743.
72. Patel VK, Lamothe B, Ayres ML, et al. Pharmacodynamics and proteomic analysis of acalabrutinib therapy: similarity of on-target effects to ibrutinib and rationale for combination therapy. *Leukemia.* 2018;32(4):920-930.
73. Byrd JC, Harrington B, O'Brien S, et al. Acalabrutinib (ACP-196) in relapsed chronic lymphocytic leukemia. *N Engl J Med.* 2016;374(4):323-332.
74. Wang M, Rule S, Zinzani PL, et al. Acalabrutinib in relapsed or refractory mantle cell lymphoma (ACE-LY-004): a single-arm, multicentre, phase 2 trial. *Lancet.* 2018;391(10121):659-667.
75. Owen RG, McCarthy H, Rule S, et al. Acalabrutinib monotherapy in patients with Waldenström macroglobulinemia: a single-arm, multicentre, phase 2 study. *Lancet Haematol.* 2020;7:e112-e121.
76. Byrd JC, Hillmen P, Ghia P, et al. Acalabrutinib versus ibrutinib in previously treated chronic lymphocytic leukemia: results of the first randomized phase III trial. *J Clin Oncol.* 2021;39(31):3441-3452.
77. Sun C, Nierman P, Kendall EK, et al. Clinical and biological implications of target occupancy in CLL treated with the BTK inhibitor acalabrutinib. *Blood.* 2020;136(1):93-105.
78. Li CJ, Jiang C, Liu Y, et al. Pleiotropic action of novel Bruton's tyrosine kinase inhibitor BGB-3111 in mantle cell lymphoma. *Mol Cancer Ther.* 2019;18(2):267-277.
79. Tam C, Grigg AP, Opat S, et al. The BTK inhibitor, Bgb-3111, is safe, tolerable, and highly active in patients with relapsed/refractory B-cell malignancies: initial report of a phase 1 first-in-human trial. *Blood.* 2015;126:832.
80. Tam CS, Opat S, Simpson D, et al. Zanubrutinib for the treatment of relapsed or refractory mantle cell lymphoma. *Blood Adv.* 2021;5(12):2577-2585.
81. Tam CS, Trotman J, Opat S, et al. Phase 1 study of the selective BTK inhibitor zanubrutinib in B-cell malignancies and safety and efficacy evaluation in CLL. *Blood.* 2019;134(11):851-859.

82. Vanhaesebroeck B, Stephens L, Hawkins P. PI3K signalling: the path to discovery and understanding. *Nat Rev Mol Cell Biol.* 2012;13(3):195-203.
83. Manning BD, Cantley LC. AKT/PKB signaling: navigating downstream. *Cell.* 2007;129(7):1261-1274.
84. Alessi DR, James SR, Downes CP, et al. Characterization of a 3-phosphoinositide-dependent protein kinase which phosphorylates and activates protein kinase Balpha. *Curr Biol.* 1997;7(4):261-269.
85. Sarbassov DD, Guertin DA, Ali SM, Sabatini DM. Phosphorylation and regulation of Akt/PKB by the rictor-mTOR complex. *Science.* 2005;307(5712):1098-1101.
86. Fruman DA, Rommel C. PI3K and cancer: lessons, challenges and opportunities. *Nat Rev Drug Discov.* 2014;13(2):140-156.
87. Okkenhaug K. Signaling by the phosphoinositide 3-kinase family in immune cells. *Annu Rev Immunol.* 2013;31:675-704.
88. Vanhaesebroeck B, Welham MJ, Kotani K, et al. P110delta, a novel phosphoinositide 3-kinase in leukocytes. *Proc Natl Acad Sci U S A.* 1997;94(9):4330-4335.
89. Chantry D, Vojtek A, Kashishian A, et al. p110delta, a novel phosphatidylinositol 3-kinase catalytic subunit that associates with p85 and is expressed predominantly in leukocytes. *J Biol Chem.* 1997;272(31):19236-19241.
90. Tzenaki N, Papakonstanti EA. p110δ PI3 kinase pathway: emerging roles in cancer. *Front Oncol.* 2013;3:40.
91. Pauls SD, Lafarge ST, Landego I, Zhang T, Marshall AJ. The phosphoinositide 3-kinase signaling pathway in normal and malignant B cells: activation mechanisms, regulation and impact on cellular functions. *Front Immunol.* 2012;3:224.
92. Meadows SA, Vega F, Kashishian A, et al. PI3Kδ inhibitor, GS-1101 (CAL-101), attenuates pathway signaling, induces apoptosis, and overcomes signals from the microenvironment in cellular models of Hodgkin lymphoma. *Blood.* 2012;119(8):1897-1900.
93. Herman SEM, Gordon AL, Wagner AJ, et al. Phosphatidylinositol 3-kinase-δ inhibitor CAL-101 shows promising preclinical activity in chronic lymphocytic leukemia by antagonizing intrinsic and extrinsic cellular survival signals. *Blood.* 2010;116(12):2078-2088.
94. Yang Q, Chen LS, Ha MJ, Do KA, Neelapu SS, Gandhi V. Idelalisib impacts cell growth through inhibiting translation-regulatory mechanisms in mantle cell lymphoma. *Clin Cancer Res.* 2017;23(1):181-192.
95. Gopal AK, Kahl BS, de Vos S, et al. PI3Kδ inhibition by idelalisib in patients with relapsed indolent lymphoma. *N Engl J Med.* 2014;370(11):1008-1018.
96. Furman RR, Sharman JP, Coutre SE, et al. Idelalisib and rituximab in relapsed chronic lymphocytic leukemia. *N Engl J Med.* 2014;370(11):997-1007.
97. Lampson BL, Kasar SN, Matos TR, et al. Idelalisib given front-line for treatment of chronic lymphocytic leukemia causes frequent immune-mediated hepatotoxicity. *Blood.* 2016;128(2):195-203.
98. Coutré SE, Barrientos JC, Brown JR, et al. Management of adverse events associated with idelalisib treatment: expert panel opinion. *Leuk Lymphoma.* 2015;56(10):2779-2786.
99. Jones JA, Robak T, Brown JR, et al. Efficacy and safety of idelalisib in combination with ofatumumab for previously treated chronic lymphocytic leukaemia: an open-label, randomised phase 3 trial. *Lancet Haematol.* 2017;4:e114-e126.
100. Zelenetz AD, Barrientos JC, Brown JR, et al. Idelalisib or placebo in combination with bendamustine and rituximab in patients with relapsed or refractory chronic lymphocytic leukaemia: interim results from a phase 3, randomised, double-blind, placebo-controlled trial. *Lancet Oncol.* 2017;18(3):297-311.
101. Murali I, Kasar S, Naeem A, et al. Activation of the MAPK pathway mediates resistance to PI3K inhibitors in chronic lymphocytic leukemia. *Blood.* 2021;138(1):44-56.
102. Rommel C, Camps M, Ji H. PI3K delta and PI3K gamma: partners in crime in inflammation in rheumatoid arthritis and beyond? *Nat Rev Immunol.* 2007;7(3):191-201.
103. Winkler DG, Faia KL, DiNitto JP, et al. PI3K-δ and PI3K-γ inhibition by IPI-145 abrogates immune responses and suppresses activity in autoimmune and inflammatory disease models. *Chem Biol.* 2013;20(11):1364-1374.
104. Balakrishnan K, Peluso M, Fu M, et al. The phosphoinositide-3-kinase (PI3K)-delta and gamma inhibitor, IPI-145 (Duvelisib), overcomes signals from the PI3K/AKT/S6 pathway and promotes apoptosis in CLL. *Leukemia.* 2015;29(9):1811-1822.
105. Vangapandu HV, Havranek O, Ayres ML, et al. B-Cell receptor signaling regulates metabolism in chronic lymphocytic leukemia. *Mol Cancer Res.* 2017;15(12):1692-1703.
106. Patel VM, Balakrishnan K, Douglas M, et al. Duvelisib treatment is associated with altered expression of apoptotic regulators that helps in sensitization of chronic lymphocytic leukemia cells to venetoclax (ABT-199). *Leukemia.* 2017;31(9):1872-1881.
107. Horwitz SM, Koch R, Porcu P, et al. Activity of the PI3K-δ, γ inhibitor duvelisib in a phase 1 trial and preclinical models of T-cell lymphoma. *Blood.* 2018;131(8):888-898.
108. Flinn IW, Miller CB, Ardeshna KM, et al. DYNAMO: a phase II study of duvelisib (IPI-145) in patients with refractory indolent non-Hodgkin lymphoma. *J Clin Oncol.* 2019;37(11):912-922.
109. Flinn IW, Hillmen P, Montillo M, et al. The phase 3 DUO trial: duvelisib vs ofatumumab in relapsed and refractory CLL/SLL. *Blood.* 2018;132(23):2446-2455.
110. Iyengar S, Clear A, Bödör C, et al. P110α-mediated constitutive PI3K signaling limits the efficacy of p110δ-selective inhibition in mantle cell lymphoma, particularly with multiple relapse. *Blood.* 2013;121(12):2274-2284.
111. Scott WJ, Hentemann MF, Rowley RB, et al. Discovery and SAR of novel 2,3-dihydroimidazo[1, 2-c]quinazoline PI3K inhibitors: identification of copanlisib (BAY 80-6946). *ChemMedChem.* 2016;11(14):1517-1530.
112. Paul J, Soujon M, Wengner AM, et al. Simultaneous inhibition of PI3Kδ and PI3Kα induces ABC-DLBCL regression by blocking BCR-dependent and -independent activation of NF-κB and AKT. *Cancer Cell.* 2017;31(1):64-78.
113. Dreyling M, Santoro A, Mollica L, et al. Phosphatidylinositol 3-kinase inhibition by copanlisib in relapsed or refractory indolent lymphoma. *J Clin Oncol.* 2017;35:3898-3905.
114. Patnaik A, Appleman LJ, Tolcher AW, et al. First-in-human phase I study of copanlisib (BAY 80-6946), an intravenous pan-class I phosphatidylinositol 3-kinase inhibitor, in patients with advanced solid tumors and non-Hodgkin's lymphomas. *Ann Oncol.* 2016;27(10):1928-1940.
115. Darnell JE Jr, Kerr IM, Stark GR. Jak-STAT pathways and transcriptional activation in response to IFNs and other extracellular signaling proteins. *Science.* 1994;264(5164):1415-1421.
116. Ihle JN, Witthuhn BA, Quelle FW, Yamamoto K, Silvennoinen O. Signaling through the hematopoietic cytokine receptors. *Annu Rev Immunol.* 1995;13:369-398.
117. Ihle JN, Witthuhn BA, Quelle FW, et al. Signaling by the cytokine receptor superfamily: JAKs and STATs. *Trends Biochem Sci.* 1994;19(5):222-227.
118. Heinrich PC, Behrmann I, Haan S, Hermanns HM, Müller-Newen G, Schaper F. Principles of interleukin (IL)-6-type cytokine signalling and its regulation. *Biochem J.* 2003;374(Pt 1):1-20.
119. Rane SG, Reddy EP. Janus kinases: components of multiple signaling pathways. *Oncogene.* 2000;19(49):5662-5679.
120. Shuai K. Modulation of STAT signaling by STAT-interacting proteins. *Oncogene.* 2000;19(21):2638-2644.
121. Foster FM, Traer CJ, Abraham SM, Fry MJ. The phosphoinositide (PI) 3-kinase family. *J Cell Sci.* 2003;116(pt 15):3037-3040.
122. Baxter EJ, Scott LM, Campbell PJ, et al. Acquired mutation of the tyrosine kinase JAK2 in human myeloproliferative disorders. *Lancet.* 2005;365(9464):1054-1061.
123. Kralovics R, Passamonti F, Buser AS, et al. A gain-of-function mutation of JAK2 in myeloproliferative disorders. *N Engl J Med.* 2005;352(17):1779-1790.
124. James C, Ugo V, Le Couédic JP, et al. A unique clonal JAK2 mutation leading to constitutive signalling causes polycythaemia vera. *Nature.* 2005;434(7037):1144-1148.
125. Levine RL, Wadleigh M, Cools J, et al. Activating mutation in the tyrosine kinase JAK2 in polycythemia vera, essential thrombocythemia, and myeloid metaplasia with myelofibrosis. *Cancer Cell.* 2005;7(4):387-397.
126. Scott LM, Tong W, Levine RL, et al. JAK2 exon 12 mutations in polycythemia vera and idiopathic erythrocytosis. *N Engl J Med.* 2007;356(5):459-468.
127. Elliott NE, Cleveland SM, Grann V, Janik J, Waldmann TA, Davé UP. FERM domain mutations induce gain of function in JAK3 in adult T-cell leukemia/lymphoma. *Blood.* 2011;118(14):3911-3921.
128. Manso R, Sánchez-Beato M, González-Rincón J, et al. Mutations in the JAK/STAT pathway genes and activation of the pathway, a relevant finding in nodal Peripheral T-cell lymphoma. *Br J Haematol.* 2018;183(3):497-501.
129. Mullighan CG, Zhang J, Harvey RC, et al. JAK mutations in high-risk childhood acute lymphoblastic leukemia. *Proc Natl Acad Sci U S A.* 2009;106(23):9414-9418.
130. Wahnschaffe L, Braun T, Timonen S, et al. JAK/STAT-Activating genomic alterations are a Hallmark of T-PLL. *Cancers.* 2019;11(12):1833.
131. Schwartz DM, Kanno Y, Villarino A, Ward M, Gadina M, O'Shea JJ. JAK inhibition as a therapeutic strategy for immune and inflammatory diseases. *Nat Rev Drug Discov.* 2017;17(1):78-62.
132. Papp K, Gordon K, Thaçi D, et al. Phase 2 trial of selective tyrosine kinase 2 inhibition in psoriasis. *N Engl J Med.* 2018;379(14):1313-1321.
133. Quintás-Cardama A, Vaddi K, Liu P, et al. Preclinical characterization of the selective JAK1/2 inhibitor INCB018424: therapeutic implications for the treatment of myeloproliferative neoplasms. *Blood.* 2010;115(15):3109-3117.
134. Verstovsek S, Mesa RA, Gotlib J, et al. A double-blind, placebo-controlled trial of ruxolitinib for myelofibrosis. *N Engl J Med.* 2012;366(9):799-807.
135. Harrison C, Kiladjian JJ, Al-Ali HK, et al. JAK inhibition with ruxolitinib versus best available therapy for myelofibrosis. *N Engl J Med.* 2012;366(9):787-798.
136. Vannucchi AM, Kiladjian JJ, Griesshammer M, et al. Ruxolitinib versus standard therapy for the treatment of polycythemia vera. *N Engl J Med.* 2015;372(17):1670-1671.
137. Passamonti F, Griesshammer M, Palandri F, et al. Ruxolitinib for the treatment of inadequately controlled polycythaemia vera without splenomegaly (RESPONSE-2): a randomised, open-label, phase 3b study. *Lancet Oncol.* 2017;18(1):88-99.
138. Moskowitz AJ, Ghione P, Jacobsen E, et al. A phase 2 biomarker-driven study of ruxolitinib demonstrates effectiveness of JAK/STAT targeting in T-cell lymphomas. *Blood.* 2021;138(26):2828-2837.
139. Koppikar P, Bhagwat N, Kilpivaara O, et al. Heterodimeric JAK–STAT activation as a mechanism of persistence to JAK2 inhibitor therapy. *Nature.* 2012;489(7414):155-159.
140. Wernig G, Kharas MG, Okabe R, et al. Efficacy of TG101348, a selective JAK2 inhibitor, in treatment of a murine model of JAK2V617F-induced polycythemia vera. *Cancer Cell.* 2008;13(4):311-320.
141. Kesarwani M, Huber E, Kincaid Z, et al. Targeting substrate-site in Jak2 kinase prevents emergence of genetic resistance. *Sci Rep.* 2015;5:14538.
142. Pardanani A, Harrison C, Cortes JE, et al. Safety and efficacy of fedratinib in patients with primary or secondary myelofibrosis: a randomized clinical trial. *JAMA Oncol.* 2015;1(5):643-651.
143. Harrison CN, Schaap N, Vannucchi AM, et al. Janus kinase-2 inhibitor fedratinib in patients with myelofibrosis previously treated with ruxolitinib (JAKARTA-2): a single-arm, open-label, non-randomised, phase 2, multicentre study. *Lancet Haematol.* 2017;4(7):e317-e324.
144. Harrison CN, Schaap N, Vannucchi AM, et al. Fedratinib in patients with myelofibrosis previously treated with ruxolitinib: an updated analysis of the JAKARTA2 study using stringent criteria for ruxolitinib failure. *Am J Hematol.* 2020;95(6):594-603.
145. Mesa RA, Vannucchi AM, Mead A, et al. Pacritinib versus best available therapy for the treatment of myelofibrosis irrespective of baseline cytopenias (PERSIST-1): an international, randomised, phase 3 trial. *Lancet Haematol.* 2017;4(5):e225-e236.

146. Mascarenhas J, Hoffman R, Talpaz M, et al. Pacritinib vs best available therapy, including ruxolitinib, in patients with myelofibrosis: a randomized clinical trial. *JAMA Oncol.* 2018;4(5):652-659.
147. Gerds AT, Savona MR, Scott BL, et al. Determining the recommended dose of pacritinib: results from the PAC203 dose-finding trial in advanced myelofibrosis. *Blood Adv.* 2020;4(22):5825-5835.
148. Stirewalt DL, Radich JP. The role of FLT3 in haematopoietic malignancies. *Nat Rev Cancer.* 2003;3(9):650-665.
149. Xu F, Taki T, Yang HW, et al. Tandem duplication of the FLT3 gene is found in acute lymphoblastic leukaemia as well as acute myeloid leukaemia but not in myelodysplastic syndrome or juvenile chronic myelogenous leukaemia in children. *Br J Haematol.* 1999;105(1):155-162.
150. Rosnet O, Schiff C, Pébusque MJ, et al. Human FLT3/FLK2 gene: cDNA cloning and expression in hematopoietic cells. *Blood.* 1993;82(4):1110-1119.
151. Small D, Levenstein M, Kim E, et al. STK-1, the human homolog of Flk-2/Flt-3, is selectively expressed in CD34+ human bone marrow cells and is involved in the proliferation of early progenitor/stem cells. *Proc Natl Acad Sci U S A.* 1994;91(2):459-463.
152. Nakao M, Yokota S, Iwai T, et al. Internal tandem duplication of the flt3 gene found in acute myeloid leukemia. *Leukemia.* 1996;10(12):1911-1918.
153. Meshinchi S, Woods WG, Stirewalt DL, et al. Prevalence and prognostic significance of Flt3 internal tandem duplication in pediatric acute myeloid leukemia. *Blood.* 2001;97(1):89-94.
154. Schnittger S, Schoch C, Dugas M, et al. Analysis of FLT3 length mutations in 1003 patients with acute myeloid leukemia: correlation to cytogenetics, FAB subtype, and prognosis in the AMLCG study and usefulness as a marker for the detection of minimal residual disease. *Blood.* 2002;100(1):59-66.
155. Thiede C, Steudel C, Mohr B, et al. Analysis of FLT3-activating mutations in 979 patients with acute myelogenous leukemia: association with FAB subtypes and identification of subgroups with poor prognosis. *Blood.* 2002;99(12):4326-4335.
156. Yamamoto Y, Kiyoi H, Nakano Y, et al. Activating mutation of D835 within the activation loop of FLT3 in human hematologic malignancies. *Blood.* 2001;97(8):2434-2439.
157. Abu-Duhier FM, Goodeve AC, Wilson GA, Care RS, Peake IR, Reilly JT. Identification of novel FLT-3 Asp835 mutations in adult acute myeloid leukaemia. *Br J Haematol.* 2001;113(4):983-988.
158. Kiyoi H, Towatari M, Yokota S, et al. Internal tandem duplication of the FLT3 gene is a novel modality of elongation mutation which causes constitutive activation of the product. *Leukemia.* 1998;12(9):1333-1337.
159. Hayakawa F, Towatari M, Kiyoi H, et al. Tandem-duplicated Flt3 constitutively activates STAT5 and MAP kinase and introduces autonomous cell growth in IL-3-dependent cell lines. *Oncogene.* 2000;19(5):624-631.
160. Weisberg E, Meng C, Case AE, et al. Comparison of effects of midostaurin, crenolanib, quizartinib, gilteritinib, sorafenib and BLU-285 on oncogenic mutants of KIT, CBL and FLT3 in haematological malignancies. *Br J Haematol.* 2019;187(4):488-501.
161. Propper DJ, McDonald AC, Man A, et al. Phase I and pharmacokinetic study of PKC412, an inhibitor of protein kinase C. *J Clin Oncol.* 2001;19(5):1485-1492.
162. Kindler T, Lipka DB, Fischer T. FLT3 as a therapeutic target in AML: still challenging after all these years. *Blood.* 2010;116(24):5089-5102.
163. Weisberg E, Boulton C, Kelly LM, et al. Inhibition of mutant FLT3 receptors in leukemia cells by the small molecule tyrosine kinase inhibitor PKC412. *Cancer Cell.* 2002;1(5):433-443.
164. Knapper S, Burnett AK, Littlewood T, et al. A phase 2 trial of the FLT3 inhibitor lestaurtinib (CEP701) as first-line treatment for older patients with acute myeloid leukemia not considered fit for intensive chemotherapy. *Blood.* 2006;108(10):3262-3270.
165. Stone RM, DeAngelo DJ, Klimek V, et al. Patients with acute myeloid leukemia and an activating mutation in FLT3 respond to a small-molecule FLT3 tyrosine kinase inhibitor, PKC412. *Blood.* 2005;105(1):54-60.
166. Smith BD, Levis M, Beran M, et al. Single-agent CEP-701, a novel FLT3 inhibitor, shows biologic and clinical activity in patients with relapsed or refractory acute myeloid leukemia. *Blood.* 2004;103(10):3669-3676.
167. Cortes JE, Kantarjian H, Foran JM, et al. Phase I study of quizartinib administered daily to patients with relapsed or refractory acute myeloid leukemia irrespective of FMS-like tyrosine kinase 3-internal tandem duplication status. *J Clin Oncol.* 2013;31(29):3681-3687.
168. Stone RM, Fischer T, Paquette R, et al. Phase IB study of the FLT3 kinase inhibitor midostaurin with chemotherapy in younger newly diagnosed adult patients with acute myeloid leukemia. *Leukemia.* 2012;26(9):2061-2068.
169. Stone RM, Mandrekar SJ, Sanford BL, et al. Midostaurin plus chemotherapy for acute myeloid leukemia with a FLT3 mutation. *N Engl J Med.* 2017;377(5):454-464.
170. Alvarado Y, Kantarjian HM, Luthra R, et al. Treatment with FLT3 inhibitor in patients with FLT3-mutated acute myeloid leukemia is associated with development of secondary FLT3-tyrosine kinase domain mutations. *Cancer.* 2014;120(14):2142-2149.
171. Lee LY, Hernandez D, Rajkhowa T, et al. Preclinical studies of gilteritinib, a next-generation FLT3 inhibitor. *Blood.* 2017;129(2):257-260.
172. Neubauer A, Fiebeler A, Graham DK, et al. Expression of axl, a transforming receptor tyrosine kinase, in normal and malignant hematopoiesis. *Blood.* 1994;84(6):1931-1941.
173. Park IK, Mishra A, Chandler J, Whitman SP, Marcucci G, Caligiuri MA. Inhibition of the receptor tyrosine kinase Axl impedes activation of the FLT3 internal tandem duplication in human acute myeloid leukemia: implications for Axl as a potential therapeutic target. *Blood.* 2013;121(11):2064-2073.
174. Park IK, Mundy-Bosse B, Whitman SP, et al. Receptor tyrosine kinase Axl is required for resistance of leukemic cells to FLT3-targeted therapy in acute myeloid leukemia. *Leukemia.* 2015;29(12):2382-2389.
175. Perl AE, Altman JK, Cortes J, et al. Selective inhibition of FLT3 by gilteritinib in relapsed or refractory acute myeloid leukaemia: a multicentre, first-in-human, open-label, phase 1-2 study. *Lancet Oncol.* 2017;18(8):1061-1075.
176. Perl AE, Martinelli G, Cortes JE, et al. Gilteritinib or chemotherapy for relapsed or refractory FLT3-mutated AML. *N Engl J Med.* 2019;381(18):1728-1740.
177. Parsons DW, Jones S, Zhang X, et al. An integrated genomic analysis of human glioblastoma multiforme. *Science.* 2008;321(5897):1807-1812.
178. Yan H, Parsons DW, Jin G, et al. IDH1 and IDH2 mutations in gliomas. *N Engl J Med.* 2009;360(8):765-773.
179. Mardis ER, Ding L, Dooling DJ, et al. Recurring mutations found by sequencing an acute myeloid leukemia genome. *N Engl J Med.* 2009;361(11):1058-1066.
180. Figueroa ME, Abdel-Wahab O, Lu C, et al. Leukemic IDH1 and IDH2 mutations result in a hypermethylation phenotype, disrupt TET2 function, and impair hematopoietic differentiation. *Cancer Cell.* 2010;18(6):553-567.
181. Dang L, White DW, Gross S, et al. Cancer-associated IDH1 mutations produce 2-hydroxyglutarate. *Nature.* 2009;462(7274):739-744.
182. Sasaki M, Knobbe CB, Munger JC, et al. IDH1(R132H) mutation increases murine haematopoietic progenitors and alters epigenetics. *Nature.* 2012;488(7413):656-659.
183. Molenaar RJ, Thota S, Nagata Y, et al. Clinical and biological implications of ancestral and non-ancestral IDH1 and IDH2 mutations in myeloid neoplasms. *Leukemia.* 2015;29(11):2134-2142.
184. Molenaar RJ, Maciejewski JP, Wilmink JW, van Noorden CJF. Wild-type and mutated IDH1/2 enzymes and therapy responses. *Oncogene.* 2018;37(15):1949-1960.
185. M Gagné L, Boulay K, Topisirovic I, Huot MÉ, Mallette FA. Oncogenic activities of IDH1/2 mutations: from epigenetics to cellular signaling. *Trends Cell Biol.* 2017;27(10):738-752.
186. Chan SM, Thomas D, Corces-Zimmerman MR, et al. Isocitrate dehydrogenase 1 and 2 mutations induce BCL-2 dependence in acute myeloid leukemia. *Nat Med.* 2015;21:178-184.
187. Stein EM, DiNardo CD, Pollyea DA, et al. Enasidenib in mutant IDH2 relapsed or refractory acute myeloid leukemia. *Blood.* 2017;130(6):722-731.
188. Stein EM, DiNardo CD, Fathi AT, et al. Molecular remission and response patterns in patients with mutant-IDH2 acute myeloid leukemia treated with enasidenib. *Blood.* 2019;133(7):676-687.
189. DiNardo CD, Stein EM, de Botton S, et al. Durable remissions with ivosidenib in IDH1-mutated relapsed or refractory AML. *N Engl J Med.* 2018;378(25):2386-2398.
190. Roboz GJ, DiNardo CD, Stein EM, et al. Ivosidenib induces deep durable remissions in patients with newly diagnosed IDH1-mutant acute myeloid leukemia. *Blood.* 2020;135(7):463-471.
191. Intlekofer AM, Shih AH, Wang B, et al. Acquired resistance to IDH inhibition through trans or cis dimer-interface mutations. *Nature.* 2018;559(7712):125-129.
192. Quek L, David MD, Kennedy A, et al. Clonal heterogeneity of acute myeloid leukemia treated with the IDH2 inhibitor enasidenib. *Nat Med.* 2018;24(8):1167-1177.
193. Wang F, Morita K, DiNardo CD, et al. Leukemia stemness and co-occurring mutations drive resistance to IDH inhibitors in acute myeloid leukemia. *Nat Commun.* 2021;12(1):2607.
194. DiNardo CD, Schuh AC, Stein EM, et al. Enasidenib plus azacitidine versus azacitidine alone in patients with newly diagnosed, mutant-IDH2 acute myeloid leukaemia (AG221-AML-005): a single-arm, phase 1b and randomised, phase 2 trial. *Lancet Oncol.* 2021;22(11):1597-1608.
195. DiNardo CD, Stein AS, Stein EM, et al. Mutant isocitrate dehydrogenase 1 inhibitor ivosidenib in combination with azacitidine for newly diagnosed acute myeloid leukemia. *J Clin Oncol.* 2021;39:57-65.
196. Stein EM, DiNardo CD, Fathi AT, et al. Ivosidenib or enasidenib combined with intensive chemotherapy in patients with newly diagnosed AML: a phase 1 study. *Blood.* 2021;137(13):1792-1803.
197. Manasanch EE, Orlowski RZ. Proteasome inhibitors in cancer therapy. *Nat Rev Clin Oncol.* 2017;14(7):417-433.
198. Kumar SK, Rajkumar V, Kyle RA, et al. Multiple myeloma. *Nat Rev Dis Primers.* 2017;3:17046.
199. Muller HJ, Boos J. Use of L-asparaginase in childhood ALL. *Crit Rev Oncol Hematol.* 1998;28(2):97-113.
200. Stock W, Luger SM, Advani AS, et al. A pediatric regimen for older adolescents and young adults with acute lymphoblastic leukemia: results of CALGB 10403. *Blood.* 2019;133(14):1548-1559.
201. van der Sluis IM, Vrooman LM, Pieters R, et al. Consensus expert recommendations for identification and management of asparaginase hypersensitivity and silent inactivation. *Haematologica.* 2016;101(3):279-285.
202. Queiroz KCS, Ruela-de-Sousa RR, Fuhler GM, et al. Hedgehog signaling maintains chemoresistance in myeloid leukemic cells. *Oncogene.* 2010;29(48):6314-6322.
203. Cortes JE, Heidel FH, Hellmann A, et al. Randomized comparison of low dose cytarabine with or without glasdegib in patients with newly diagnosed acute myeloid leukemia or high-risk myelodysplastic syndrome. *Leukemia.* 2019;33(2):379-389.
204. Etchin J, Sun Q, Kentsis A, et al. Antileukemic activity of nuclear export inhibitors that spare normal hematopoietic cells. *Leukemia.* 2013;27(1):66-74.
205. Kalakonda N, Maerevoet M, Cavallo F, et al. Selinexor in patients with relapsed or refractory diffuse large B-cell lymphoma (SADAL): a single-arm, multinational, multicentre, open-label, phase 2 trial. *Lancet Haematol.* 2020;7:e511-e522.
206. Chari A, Vogl DT, Gavriatopoulou M, et al. Oral selinexor-dexamethasone for triple-class refractory multiple myeloma. *N Engl J Med.* 2019;381(8):727-738.
207. Lo-Coco F, Avvisati G, Vignetti M, et al. Retinoic acid and arsenic trioxide for acute promyelocytic leukemia. *N Engl J Med.* 2013;369(2):111-121.
208. Karmali R. Relapsed disease: off-the-shelf immunotherapies vs customized engineered products. *Hematology Am Soc Hematol Educ Program.* 2021;2021(1):164-173.

209. Mason KD, Carpinelli MR, Fletcher JI, et al. Programmed anuclear cell death delimits platelet life span. *Cell*. 2007;128(6):1173-1186.
210. Roberts AW, Seymour JF, Brown JR, et al. Substantial susceptibility of chronic lymphocytic leukemia to BCL2 inhibition: results of a phase I study of navitoclax in patients with relapsed or refractory disease. *J Clin Oncol*. 2012;30(5):488-496.
211. Pullarkat VA, Lacayo NJ, Jabbour E, et al. Venetoclax and navitoclax in combination with chemotherapy in patients with relapsed or refractory acute lymphoblastic leukemia and lymphoblastic lymphoma. *Cancer Discov*. 2021;11(6):1440-1453.
212. Harrison CN, Garcia JS, Somervaille TCP, et al. Addition of navitoclax to ongoing ruxolitinib therapy for patients with myelofibrosis with progression or suboptimal response: phase II safety and efficacy. *J Clin Oncol*. 2022;40(15):1671-1680.
213. Roberts AW, Wei AH, Huang DCS. BCL2 and MCL1 inhibitors for hematologic malignancies. *Blood*. 2021;138(13):1120-1136.
214. Bekes M, Langley DR, Crews CM. PROTAC targeted protein degraders: the past is prologue. *Nat Rev Drug Discov*. 2022;21(3):181-200.
215. Cetraro P, Plaza-Diaz J, MacKenzie A, Abadia-Molina F. A review of the current impact of inhibitors of apoptosis proteins and their repression in cancer. *Cancers (Basel)*. 2022;14(7):1671.
216. Zhang M, Zhang L, Hei R, et al. CDK inhibitors in cancer therapy, an overview of recent development. *Am J Cancer Res*. 2021;11(5):1913-1935.
217. Schwalm MP, Knapp S. BET bromodomain inhibitors. *Curr Opin Chem Biol*. 2022;68:102148.

Chapter 70 ■ Infectious Complications in Hematologic Malignancies

MARKUS PLATE • ALEXANDER DRELICK • MICHAEL J. SATLIN

INTRODUCTION

Patients with hematologic neoplasms are at significant risk for infectious complications from both their underlying malignancy and its treatment. Infections are one of the most common complications in this population and cause substantial morbidity and mortality. The risk of infection is related to broad deficits in both innate and acquired immunity.

Deficits in Host Defense Mechanisms

Patients with hematologic malignancies may have global or specific immune abnormalities preceding the diagnosis and treatment. Characteristic infections seen with certain functional immune deficiencies, such as impaired phagocytosis or antibody production, are highlighted in *Table 70.1*.[1] Lymphoid disorders with impaired T and B-cell function predispose to intracellular and encapsulated bacterial infections, respectively. Associated chronic comorbidities also contribute to infection risk and influence management decisions. Understanding the immunosuppression associated with each disease and associated therapies allows for an individualized assessment of infectious risk, which can lead to the optimal design of infection prevention strategies for each patient.

Neutrophil Defects

Neutrophils are produced in the bone marrow under the influence of an array of cytokines and play a critical role in the innate immune response, mediating antimicrobial and inflammatory responses.[2] They are the most abundant phagocytes and are essential to host defense, placing considerable demand on the marrow for their constitutive production. The life span and production of neutrophils are adaptive to the physiologic needs of pathologic conditions such as inflammation or infection.[3] In the setting of chemotherapy-induced neutropenia, the absence of neutrophils combines with damage to the integrity of the gastrointestinal mucosal barrier to create a high-risk setting for translocation of gut bacteria into the bloodstream.[4]

Neutropenia is defined quantitatively as a decrease in the peripheral blood neutrophil count below 1.5×10^9/L. The risk of bacterial and fungal infection begins to increase when the absolute neutrophil count (ANC) decreases to less than 1×10^9/L.[5] The two most important risk factors for infection are severity and duration of neutropenia, with neutrophil counts $<0.1 \times 10^9$/L and neutropenia duration of >1 week greatly increasing the risk of serious infections.[5] Localizing signs and symptoms suggesting infection are often absent in the setting of severe neutropenia due to the lack or blunting of the normal inflammatory response generated by granulocytes.[6] Fever may be the sole manifestation of a life-threatening infection.

Neutropenia is often present at the time of diagnosis of acute leukemia and is universally seen following induction therapy. The myeloblasts and lymphoblasts of acute leukemia are of no functional benefit to the patient against infection. In the myeloproliferative neoplasms, neutropenia may coincide with the development of blast crisis or evolution to myelofibrosis. Mild neutropenia may be found in patients with multiple myeloma or lymphoma but is less frequent in the absence of treatment or advanced disease. The neutropenia of other disorders such as hairy cell leukemia may be secondary to marrow invasion, splenomegaly with sequestration, or both. Profound neutropenia and its complications may be the initial clue in the diagnosis of T cell large granular lymphocytic leukemia.[7]

Myelodysplastic syndrome (MDS) is characterized by ineffective hematopoiesis and cytopenias. Infections are a leading cause of morbidity and mortality in patients with MDS[8]; however, with improved supportive care, infectious complications are no longer the primary cause of death in these patients.[9] Morphologically, normal neutrophils may still possess numerous functional defects. In some patients with MDS, impaired neutrophil mobilization, adhesion, and chemotaxis are combined with deficits in enzyme generation and phagocytic capabilities.[9] The neutrophils in patients with untreated chronic myeloid leukemia are partially defective in phagocytosis, oxygen consumption, and bactericidal capacity, with decreased concentrations of lactoferrin, elastase, collagenase, and peroxidase.[10]

Defects in Humoral Immunity

The humoral immune system responds to antigens with activation of B cells and generation of the antibody response. Impairment of this process is a major cause of frequent and severe infections in patients with hematologic malignancies, particular those caused by encapsulated bacteria (e.g., pneumococcus, *Haemophilus influenzae*, and *Neisseria meningitidis*) and respiratory viruses.[11,12] Diminished immunoglobulin synthesis is observed in many patients with chronic lymphocytic leukemia (CLL), multiple myeloma, and some B cell non-Hodgkin lymphomas.[13,14] Plasma cell dyscrasias including multiple myeloma may have relative or functional hypogammaglobulinemia despite normal or elevated total immunoglobulin levels. Prior splenectomy or functional asplenia due to tumor infiltration also results in impaired antibody responses and can result in fulminant presentations of infections caused by encapsulated organisms.[15] Vaccinations are of paramount importance in asplenic patients to mitigate this risk.[16] Functional hyposplenism has also been demonstrated in patients following allogeneic hematopoietic cell transplantation (HCT).[17]

Anti-CD20 therapies that are commonly used in the treatment of lymphoid malignancies, such as rituximab, deplete peripheral blood B cells, which impairs responses to vaccines.[18] However, these therapies usually do not significantly reduce the levels of existing antibodies because most antigen-specific immunoglobulins are produced by plasma cells that do not express CD20.[19] Although one would expect Bruton tyrosine kinase inhibitors (e.g., ibrutinib) to impair humoral immunity because they inhibit B-cell signaling, it is challenging to distinguish their effects from those caused by underlying lymphoid malignancies.[20]

Defects in Cellular Immunity

T lymphocytes, macrophages, and natural killer cells recognize and combat intracellular pathogens through cell-mediated immunity. T lymphocytes are activated by antigen-presenting cells, such as dendritic cells, macrophages, and B lymphocytes, which present foreign antigens to the T-cell receptor.[21] Cytotoxic CD8$^+$ T cells directly attack and lyse host cells that express foreign antigens. Helper CD4$^+$ T cells stimulate the proliferation of B cells and the production of immunoglobulins. Defects in cell-mediated immunity characterized by impaired T_H1 CD4$^+$ T lymphocytes and/or macrophage function result in increased risk of infections with intracellular bacteria, fungi, parasites, and viruses.

Impaired cellular immunity is influenced by the underlying hematologic disorder and stage, as well as the agents employed in treatment. For example, patients with advanced-stage CLL frequently have both quantitative and qualitative abnormalities of T cells and NK cells.[13] Depressed cellular immunity is not a primary feature of acute leukemias, but is a well-recognized complication of maintenance therapy for acute lymphoblastic leukemia (ALL), with prolonged deficits observed after completion of treatment.[22] In contrast, while the humoral immune response recovers slowly, the cellular immune response rebounds relatively quickly after treatment for acute myeloid leukemia (AML).[23]

Approach to Infection in the Neutropenic Host

The initial approach to and assessment of the neutropenic patient with a hematologic malignancy is critical. The initial evaluation should focus on assessing the patient's severity of illness and identifying potential sites and causative organisms of infection. Careful histories and physical examinations must be performed with special attention to the most common sites of infection: skin, oropharynx, nares, sinuses, lungs, gastrointestinal tract (including perianal area), soft tissues, and indwelling catheters. Although neutropenic patients are usually able to produce a fever in the presence of an infection, other physical exam findings related to infection may be absent.[6] For example, in patients with severe neutropenia, pharyngitis is less likely to present with exudates and pneumonia may lack the common manifestations of cough, productive sputum, and consolidation on exam.

Fever and Neutropenia

Fever and neutropenia is defined as a single oral temperature of 38.3 °C or a temperature of 38 °C sustained over a 1-hour period.[4] Patients with fever and neutropenia resulting from chemotherapy frequently do not have microbiologically documented infections. For example, in a study of 2142 patients with fever and neutropenia, 499 (23%) had documented bacteremia.[34] Gram-positive bacteremias (57% of total episodes) were more common than Gram-negative bacteremias (34%) and polymicrobial bacteremias (10%). Other studies have confirmed these findings and Gram-positive bacteria consistently cause the majority of bloodstream infections in neutropenic patients.[35] However, mortality rates of neutropenic patients with Gram-negative bacteremia are greater than those with Gram-positive bacteremia (18% vs 5%).[34] Despite immediate antimicrobial therapy for fever and neutropenia, 30-day mortality rates remain as high.[36] Although anaerobes are prominent members of gastrointestinal flora, they are uncommon causes of bacteremia in patients with fever and neutropenia.[36]

Initial risk assessment in fever and neutropenia helps stratify the severity of illness and estimate the risk of complications. Stratification may influence the selection of empirical antimicrobial therapy (oral vs intravenous administration), venue of treatment (inpatient vs outpatient), and duration of prescribed treatment. The most commonly used tool to differentiate patients with febrile neutropenia into low vs high risk for complications is the Multinational Association for Supportive Care in Cancer index (MASCC, see Table 70.2).[37] Independent factors found to be predictive of lower risk for complications include the following: (1) burden of illness characterized by low or moderate symptoms, (2) absence of hypotension, (3) absence of chronic obstructive

Table 70.1. Immune Deficits and Examples of Associated Infections

Defect	Infections
Neutropenia	Gram-negative bacteria 　*Escherichia coli* 　*Klebsiella pneumoniae* 　*Pseudomonas aeruginosa* Gram-positive bacteria 　Viridans group streptococci 　*Staphylococcus aureus* 　Coagulase-negative staphylococci 　Enterococci Fungi 　*Candida* spp. 　*Aspergillus* spp. 　Mucorales
Humoral immunity	Encapsulated organisms 　*Streptococcus pneumoniae* 　*Haemophilus influenzae* 　*Neisseria meningitidis* Respiratory viral infections (e.g., influenza)
Cellular immunity	Intracellular bacteria 　*Listeria monocytogenes* 　*Salmonella* Mycobacteria 　*Legionella* spp. 　*Nocardia* spp. Viruses 　Herpes simplex virus 　Varicella-zoster virus 　Cytomegalovirus 　Respiratory viral infections (e.g., influenza) Fungi 　*Pneumocystis jirovecii* 　*Cryptococcus neoformans* 　*Coccidioides immitis* 　*Histoplasma capsulatum* Parasites 　*Toxoplasma gondii* 　*Strongyloides stercoralis*

Numerous therapies for hematologic malignancies impair cell-mediated immunity. Purine analogs such as fludarabine cause quantitative and qualitative T-cell abnormalities and are associated with opportunistic infections caused by organisms such as *Listeria monocytogenes*, *Pneumocystis*, and herpesviruses, particularly when combined with corticosteroids.[24,25] Newer agents for hematologic malignancies, such as idelalisib and ibrutinib, are also associated with cell-mediated immune impairment and increased risk of opportunistic infections.[26,27] Alemtuzumab, an anti-CD52 monoclonal antibody, causes a profound and long-lasting depletion of B-cell and T-cell lymphocytes, natural killer cells, and monocytes, which predisposes to viral, bacterial, and fungal infections.[28]

Host Genetic Factors in Immunity

Inherited global deficiencies in host immunity, such as X-linked agammaglobulinemia, severe combined immunodeficiency, and complement pathway deficiencies, are well described with their accompanying predilection for characteristic infections.[29-31] However, less well-known host factors such as genetic variants in the innate immune system also appear to have a distinct influence on the course of infections in cancer patients. For example, polymorphisms associated with decreased levels of mannose-binding lectin were associated with a doubling of the duration of febrile neutropenia in pediatric cancer patients compared to wildtype.[32,33] The growing fields of bioinformatics and personalized medicine may have a future role in prognostic and management decisions in the treatment of the patient with a hematologic disorder.

Table 70.2. The MASCC Risk-Index Score: Determining the Risk of Serious Complications in Febrile Neutropenia

Category	Weight[a]
Burden of illness: no or mild symptoms	5
No hypotension	5
No chronic obstructive pulmonary disease	4
Solid tumor or no previous invasive fungal infection	4
No dehydration	3
Burden of illness: moderate symptoms	3
Outpatient status	3
Age <60 y	2

Abbreviation: MASCC, Multinational Association of Supportive Care in Cancer.
[a]Low risk: score ≥ 21; High risk: score < 21.
Reprinted with permission from Klastersky J, Paesmans M, Rubenstein EB, et al. The multinational association for supportive care in cancer risk index: a multinational scoring system for identifying low-risk febrile neutropenic cancer patients. *J Clin Oncol*. 2000;18(16):3038-3051. Copyright © 2000 by American Society of Clinical Oncology.

pulmonary disease, (4) presence of solid tumor or absence of previous fungal infection in patients with hematologic malignancies, (6) outpatient status, (7) absence of dehydration, and (8) age less than 60 years. These variables assessed at fever onset were assigned an integer weight, and a risk-index score consisting of the sum of these integers was derived. In a prospective evaluation, a score of 21 or greater identified patients at low risk for complications with a positive predictive value of 91%, specificity of 68%, and sensitivity of 71%.[37] In general, most experts consider high-risk patients to be those with anticipated prolonged (>7 days duration) and profound neutropenia (ANC < 0.1×10^9/L), significant medical comorbid conditions, or who are clinically unstable (e.g., hypotension, pneumonia, new abdominal pain, or neurologic changes).[4] High-risk patients warrant inpatient therapy with intravenous antibiotics. Low-risk patients, including those with anticipated brief (<7 days duration) neutropenic periods and few comorbidities, are candidates for empirical oral therapy with close outpatient follow-up.

The initial evaluation of neutropenic fever should include a focused history, physical examination with attention to occasionally overlooked areas such as the perineum and venous catheter sites. Laboratory investigations should include a complete blood count with differential, serum chemistry, including hepatic and renal assessment, and at least two sets of blood cultures. Preferably, a set of blood cultures should be collected simultaneously from lumens of existing central venous catheters (CVCs), if present, and from a peripheral venipuncture site.[4] Other investigations should be directed by signs and symptoms. For example, urine should be obtained for urinalysis and culture if signs or symptoms of a urinary tract infection are present, and stool should be sent for *Clostridioides difficile* testing if diarrhea is present. In patients with signs or symptoms of a respiratory tract infection, such as cough, a nasopharyngeal swab should be collected and analyzed for respiratory viruses and a chest radiograph should be obtained. Sputum samples should be obtained for Gram stain and culture if a productive cough is present. Skin lesions should be aspirated and/or biopsied, where feasible and appropriate, with specimens sent for direct staining, culture, and/or cytological/pathological testing. Additional radiographic tests, such as computed tomography (CT) scans of the sinuses, chest, and abdomen as well as examination of cerebrospinal fluid may be necessary in selected patients. Noninfectious causes of fever, such as drug reactions, mucositis, or graft-vs-host disease (GVHD) should also be considered.

Initial Antimicrobial Therapy

Fever and neutropenia represents an emergent clinical situation because insidious infections may progress rapidly to shock and multiorgan system failure. The goal of initial empirical antibacterial therapy is to prevent serious morbidity and mortality due to bacterial pathogens until further culture results are available. In the 1960s, prior to the routine initiation of empirical antibacterial therapy for fever and neutropenia, one-half of neutropenic patients infected with *Pseudomonas aeruginosa* died within 72 hours.[38] In the early 1970s, the empiric use of broad-spectrum antibacterial agents with activity against *P. aeruginosa* and other Gram-negative bacteria at the onset of fever led to dramatic decreases in mortality. The immediate initiation of antibacterial therapy with a spectrum of activity that includes Gram-negatives, including *P. aeruginosa*, has become a cornerstone of the treatment of fever and neutropenia.[39] The initial antimicrobial selection should be based on the risk status of the patient (low vs high), localizing signs or symptoms, and the epidemiologic and antimicrobial resistance patterns of the treating facility.[4] Evidence-based guidelines from the Infectious Diseases Society of America (IDSA), American Society of Clinical Oncology (ASCO), and European Society for Medical Oncology (ESMO) are available for guidance on antimicrobial therapy for neutropenic patients with fever.[4,40,41] Our recommendations are summarized in *Figure 70.1* and outlined below.

Lower Risk Patients With Fever and Neutropenia

Outpatient management with close monitoring and follow-up may be appropriate for patients with MASCC scores >21 who are at lower risk for complications. Expert panels support the use of outpatient oral antibiotic therapy in carefully selected lower risk patients with neutropenic fever.[4,40,41] An oral fluoroquinolone with amoxicillin-clavulanate is recommended for adult patients, but clindamycin may be substituted for amoxicillin-clavulanate in patients with penicillin allergies.[40] Fluoroquinolones retain an important role in the outpatient management of febrile neutropenia as they are the only class of oral antimicrobial agents with activity against *P. aeruginosa*. However, their use is not appropriate for patients who develop fever and neutropenia while receiving fluoroquinolone prophylaxis. The IDSA/ASCO guidelines recommend observing patients who are treated as an outpatient for fever and neutropenia for ≥4 hours before having them return home.[40] These patients require frequent follow-up and assessment to ensure rapid identification of any worsening of their clinical status that would require hospitalization.

Initial Treatment for High-Risk Patients

Broad-spectrum antibacterial therapy should be administered as soon as possible after collection of blood cultures and no later than 1 hour after presentation with fever and neutropenia.[40] One study identified that 28-day mortality increased by 18% for every hour there was a delay in antibacterial therapy after the onset of fever

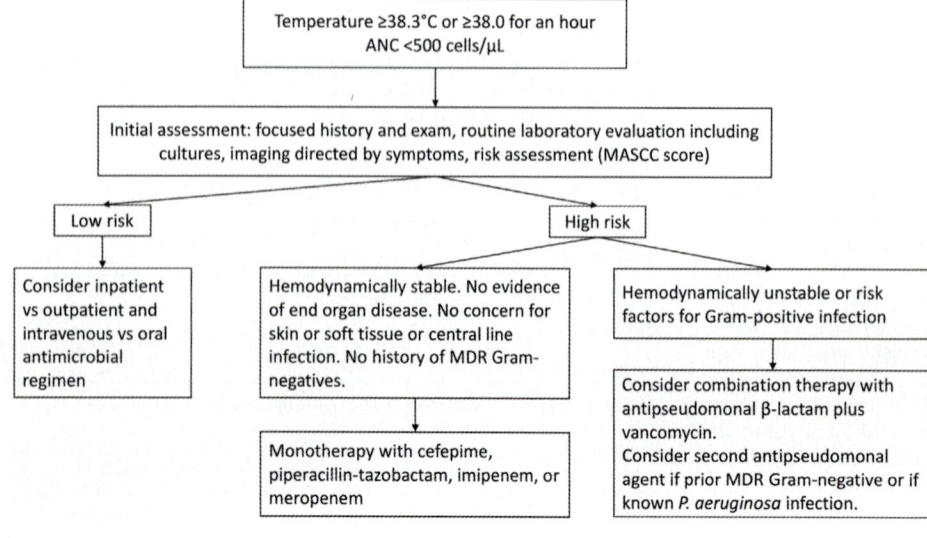

FIGURE 70.1 Empiric approach to fever and neutropenia. ANC, absolute neutrophil count; MASCC, Multinational Association for Supportive Care in Cancer.

and neutropenia.[42] The goal of empirical therapy is to cover the pathogens most likely to cause life-threatening infections in neutropenic patients, including Enterobacterales (e.g., *Escherichia coli, Klebsiella pneumoniae*), *P. aeruginosa,* and streptococci.[37] Concerns of treatment failure promoted the historical practice of double coverage for *P. aeruginosa* with combinations of β-lactams and aminoglycosides as initial empirical therapy.[43] Multiple randomized trials have since demonstrated comparable outcomes between anti–pseudomonal β-lactam monotherapy and combination therapy for initial treatment of fever and neutropenia.[44-49] The efficacy of monotherapy was confirmed by a Cochrane database review of randomized trials that also noted increased toxicity in the combination therapy arms of these trials, primarily as a result of antimicrobial-related nephrotoxicity.[50]

Recommended initial empirical antimicrobial therapies for fever and neutropenia in a high-risk patient include cefepime, piperacillin-tazobactam, imipenem-cilastatin, or meropenem.[4,41,51] Ceftazidime is also a potential option, but its diminished activity against Gram-positive bacteria may limit its use as a routine therapy for fever and neutropenia.[52,53] A recent meta-analysis identified decreased treatment success and greater need for therapy modification when ceftazidime was used as initial therapy.[54] Carbapenems are often reserved for second-line use, but may be appropriate empirical therapies in centers with a high prevalence of extended-spectrum-β-lactamase (ESBL)–producing organisms or in patients known to be colonized with these organisms.[4,55,56] Fluoroquinolones are generally not recommended as initial empirical therapy in high-risk neutropenic cancer patients, especially if the patient previously received fluoroquinolone prophylaxis.[4,50] The choice of initial empirical therapy for fever and neutropenia should take into account the local antimicrobial susceptibility patterns of the institution and may be optimized by an integrated antimicrobial stewardship program.[57]

Combination Therapy

Randomized trials have not demonstrated a benefit to the routine addition of a glycopeptide (e.g., vancomycin) for broad-spectrum Gram-positive coverage in the initial management of fever and neutropenia.[58,59] Furthermore, the addition of a glycopeptide leads to increased nephrotoxicity.[59] Thus, glycopeptides and other broad-spectrum Gram-positive agents should not be routinely used for fever and neutropenia. However, the empirical addition of vancomycin or another glycopeptide should be considered in certain situations, such as hemodynamic instability, suspected infection of a venous catheter, skin or soft tissue infection, or history of colonization with methicillin-resistant *Staphylococcus aureus* (MRSA).[4,51] Although treatment with a single anti–pseudomonal β-lactam agent is the recommended approach for most patients with fever and neutropenia, the addition of a second Gram-negative agent, such as an aminoglycoside or fluoroquinolone, may be appropriate in patients who have previously been infected or colonized with Gram-negative bacteria that are resistant to standard anti–pseudomonal β-lactam agents.[4]

Penicillin-Allergic Patients

Patients with hematologic malignancies who have reported β-lactam allergies have worse clinical outcomes because they rely on second-line antibacterial agents.[60] Thus, a detailed patient history is necessary to distinguish IgE-mediated immediate allergic reactions (e.g., bronchospasm, hives) or serious delayed reactions (e.g., Stevens-Johnson syndrome) from side effects, drug intolerance, or non–immediate allergic reactions. Most penicillin-allergic patients who do not have documented anaphylactic or serious delayed reactions tolerate antipseudomonal cephalosporins and carbapenems, and thus, these agents remain appropriate empirical therapies for fever and neutropenia in this setting.[4,61] For patients with anaphylaxis or serious delayed reactions from penicillins, vancomycin, and aztreonam are recommended for empirical treatment of fever and neutropenia.[4,51] The rationale for adding vancomycin to aztreonam is because aztreonam has no activity against Gram-positive bacteria. Clindamycin plus a fluoroquinolone is another potential option for patients who did not receive fluoroquinolone prophylaxis.

Modification of Initial Empirical Therapy

Modifications of the initial antimicrobial regimen are recommended based on clinical and/or microbiologic data. The addition of vancomycin is reasonable for patients who are found to have bacterial infections due to Gram-positive cocci while awaiting organism identification and antimicrobial susceptibility testing results. The addition of linezolid or daptomycin may be considered in patients known to be colonized with vancomycin-resistant enterococci (VRE) who develop infections due to Gram-positive cocci in pairs or chains, with the caveat that daptomycin is not effective for pneumonia because it is inactivated by pulmonary surfactant.[62] Given that *P. aeruginosa* can be resistant to first-line β-lactam therapies for fever and neutropenia and that it causes infections with high-mortality rates if effective treatment is delayed,[38] the addition of a second antipseudomonal agent (e.g., aminoglycoside or fluoroquinolone) is reasonable for a neutropenic patient found to have a *P. aeruginosa* infection while awaiting antimicrobial susceptibility testing results.[63]

Neutropenic patients who have persistent fever despite the addition of appropriate antimicrobial therapies warrant continued clinical assessment. The median time to defervescence in neutropenic patients with hematologic malignancies and HCT recipients who are successfully treated is 5 days, compared to 2 days in patients with solid tumors.[64,65] Thus, the initial antimicrobial therapy typically does not need to be modified in patients who have persistent fever for 2 to 4 days despite antibacterial therapy, but who are clinically stable. In a randomized trial of neutropenic patients with persistent fever for 48 to 60 hours after the initiation of piperacillin-tazobactam monotherapy, the addition of intravenous vancomycin did not lead to improved clinical outcomes compared to placebo.[66] In contrast, neutropenic patients who clinically decompensate warrant a broadening of their antibacterial coverage to cover resistant pathogens.[4]

The standard approach to duration of empirical therapy has been to continue until neutrophil recovery (ANC > 0.5×10^9/L).[4] However, increasing awareness and concern over the rising prevalence of resistant organisms has led to efforts to decrease antimicrobial exposure when safely permissible. A recent randomized trial suggests that continuing empirical antibacterial therapy until neutrophil recovery may not always be necessary.[67] This trial enrolled 157 adult patients with hematologic malignancies and HCT recipients who developed high-risk fever and neutropenia without a clinical or microbiologic diagnosis of infection. Subjects were randomized to stop empirical therapy once afebrile for 72 hours and clinically stable regardless of the neutrophil count or to continue empirical therapy until neutrophil recovery. Those who stopped empirical therapy received fewer days of antibiotic therapy and did not have increased risk of recurrent fever, infection, or adverse events. This early de-escalation approach is advocated by the 2011 European Conference on Infections in Leukemia.[68] However, others, including the National Comprehensive Cancer Network (NCCN) and IDSA, recommend continuing empirical treatment until neutrophil recovery (ANC > 0.5×10^9/L) with the option to de-escalate to fluoroquinolone prophylaxis in select cases.[4,69] Regardless of the preferred clinical guidelines, individual assessment of each case in clinical context is key, and reevaluation of the antimicrobial regimen with additional clinical and microbiologic data throughout the course is required to tailor the treatment (*Figure 70.2*). In cases where a specific infectious organism or site is identified, the antibiotic regimen should be narrowed as able with susceptibility results, and the duration of therapy should be determined by the specific syndrome and/or documented pathogen.

Historical autopsy series found high rates of invasive fungal infections (IFIs) diagnosed postmortem among patients with hematologic malignancies and HCT recipients, with *Candida* spp. and *Aspergillus* spp. being the most common etiologies.[70] The risk of IFI correlates strongly with the duration of neutropenia, increasing significantly after 1 week of severe neutropenia.[5] Persistent fever despite antibacterial therapy is often the first sign of IFI, and thus patients who

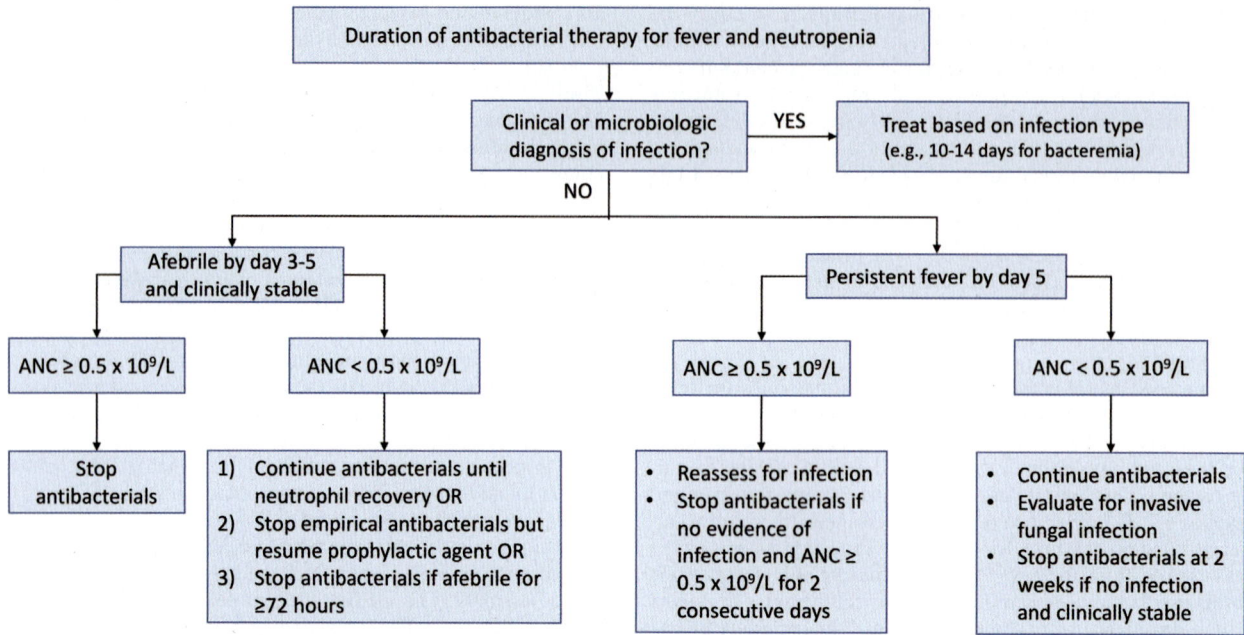

FIGURE 70.2 Duration of antimicrobial therapy and common modifications. ANC, absolute neutrophil count.

have received broad-spectrum antibacterial therapy for 4 to 7 days with persistent fever and who have had neutropenia for greater than 1 week should be evaluated for the presence of IFI.[4] This work-up may include blood tests for (1→3)-β-D-glucan and *Aspergillus* galactomannan, CT imaging of the chest and sinuses, and attempts to isolate fungal specimens on culture or tissue through biopsy, bronchoscopy with bronchoalveolar lavage (BAL), or aspiration of involved areas.

While these investigations are being performed, empirical antifungal therapy may be considered. The choice of antifungal agent for empirical antifungal therapy should reflect the most likely fungal pathogens, taking into account the use of antifungal prophylaxis and toxicities of antifungal therapies. Although amphotericin B deoxycholate was the initial antifungal agent used for empirical antifungal therapy in patients with prolonged fever and neutropenia,[71] voriconazole, echinocandins, and lipid formulations of amphotericin B are now preferred agents based on their efficacy and favorable toxicity profiles.[72-74]

An alternate approach to empirical antifungal therapy is to pursue a preemptive approach, where the decision to initiate antifungal therapy incorporates radiographic findings (CT imaging of the sinuses and chest) and laboratory data (*Aspergillus* galactomannan antigen or (1→3)-β-D-glucan assay) to determine the likelihood of invasive disease. In a preemptive approach, antifungal therapy may be withheld in patients who do not have radiographic or laboratory data suggestive of an IFI. In a randomized clinical trial of high-risk, febrile, neutropenic patients, a preemptive approach to antifungal therapy was noninferior to an empirical approach for the primary outcome of mortality but was associated with an increased risk of proven or probable IFI (9.1% vs 2.7%).[75] The preemptive approach did not decrease nephrotoxicity compared to the empirical approach but did decrease costs of antifungal therapy. The IDSA supports both preemptive and empirical approaches to antifungal therapy, with an emphasis on individualized treatment.[4]

Other Therapies: Colony-Stimulating Factors

Myeloid colony-stimulating factors (CSFs, also known as hematopoietic growth factors) are recommended as primary prophylaxis to decrease the duration of neutropenia and associated complications when the risk of fever and neutropenia is ≥20% (*Figure 70.3*).[4,41,76] Several meta-analyses of randomized trials have demonstrated that use of CSFs in high-risk patients decreases the risk of fever and infections during neutropenia; however, no mortality benefit from the prophylactic use of CSFs has been demonstrated.[77-80] Use of CSFs as secondary prophylaxis for subsequent chemotherapy cycles in patients who had an episode of fever and neutropenia in a prior cycle is controversial. There is no role for initiating CSFs in afebrile patients who have already developed severe neutropenia. In a randomized, placebo-controlled trial, the use of CSFs in this setting did not decrease the risk of hospitalization, antibiotic use, or infection, although it decreased the duration of neutropenia by 2 days.[81] Widespread therapeutic use of CSFs in all cases of fever and neutropenia is not recommended, but CSFs may be considered in certain situations. A meta-analysis of 14 randomized trials did not identify a statistically significant decrease in overall mortality or infection-related mortality with the use of CSFs and antibiotics compared to antibiotics alone in patients with fever and neutropenia.[82] Therapeutic CSF was associated with decreased duration of hospitalization and antibiotic use, and faster recovery from fever, but was also associated with a higher incidence of bone or joint pain or flu-like symptoms. Although neither the IDSA nor ASCO recommends routine use of CSFs for the treatment of fever and neutropenia, the ASCO recommends consideration of CSFs in patients who are at high risk of infection-associated complications or who have prognostic factors predictive of poor clinical outcomes, such as expected prolonged and profound neutropenia, advanced age, uncontrolled primary disease, pneumonia, hypotension and sepsis, or IFI.[4,76]

Other Therapies: Granulocyte Transfusions

Although the infusion of granulocytes in the neutropenic patient with an infection has a clear biologic rationale and the technical capabilities have been available for more than half a century, the role for granulocyte transfusions in clinical practice remains unclear. A recent review of available literature found low-grade evidence that prophylactic use may decrease the rates of bacteremia and fungemia with dose-dependent results.[83] The RING (Resolving Infection in Neutropenia with Granulocytes) trial attempted to answer this question in patients with established infections through a multicenter randomized trial, but it failed to demonstrate a benefit in the primary outcome of survival and microbial response.[84] The trial was hindered in statistical power due to limited subject accrual. Enthusiasm for the potential benefit of granulocytes in neutropenic patients for the prevention and treatment of infections remains, but there are insufficient data for their use outside of a clinical trial.

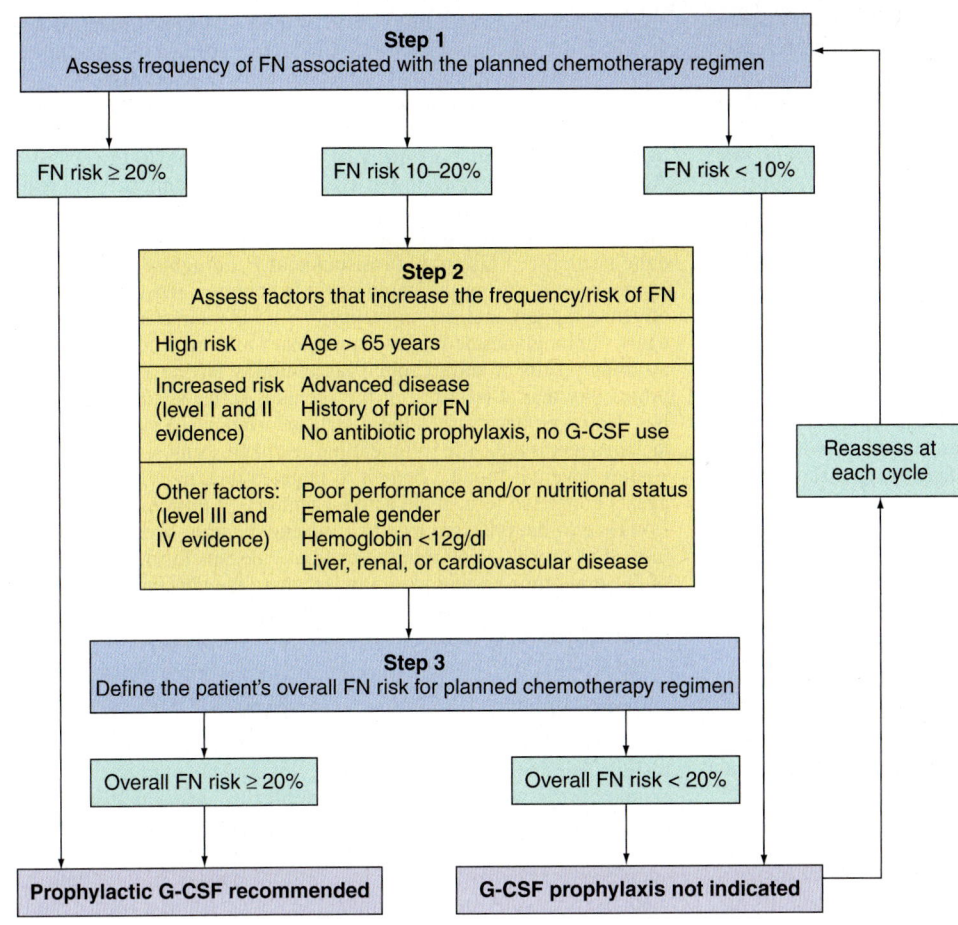

FIGURE 70.3 Algorithm for use of prophylactic G-CSF. FN, febrile neutropenia; G-CSF, granulocyte colony–stimulating factor. (With permission from Aapro MS, Bohlius J, Cameron DA, et al. 2010 update of EPRTC guidelines for the use of granulocyte colony-stimulating factor to reduce the incidence of chemotherapy-induced febrile neutropenia in adult patients with lymphoproliferative disorders and solid tumors. (Reprinted from Aapro MS, Bohlius J, Cameron DA, et al. 2010 update of EORTC guidelines for the use of granulocyte-colony stimulating factor to reduce the incidence of chemotherapy-induced febrile neutropenia in adult patients with lymphoproliferative disorders and solid tumors. *Eur J Cancer.* 2011;47(1):8-32. Copyright © 2010 Elsevier. With permission.)

SPECIFIC INFECTIOUS SYNDROMES, PATHOGENS, AND TREATMENTS

The spectrum of clinical presentations in hematology patients with infections is broad. Patients may have objective findings suggesting the source of infection (e.g., cellulitis, pulmonary infiltrates), but microbiologic confirmation is found in less than half of cases.[4] The course may be insidious with fever as the sole manifestation of bacteremia, or patients may present with septic shock and multisystem organ failure. Cancer is both a risk factor and adverse prognostic marker for the development and outcome of sepsis.[85] Given the wide differential diagnosis of infection in patients with hematologic malignancies, including bacterial, fungal, and viral pathogens, there is a low threshold for pursuing a work-up to establish a microbiologic diagnosis in these patients.

Bloodstream Infections

At least two sets of blood cultures should be obtained in all hematology patients with fever and suspected infection. If a CVC is present, one set should be collected simultaneously from each catheter lumen and one from a peripheral venipuncture site.[4] If no central device is present, two separate peripheral venipuncture sites are recommended. For several decades, the incidence of Gram-positive bacteremia has increased and now accounts for the majority of bacteremias in neutropenic patients.[34] However, recent trends indicate a potential shift in the epidemiologic patterns, with Gram-negative organisms becoming increasingly common in some centers around the world.[35] More alarming than the shift in etiology of bacteremia in cancer patients is the rising prevalence of antimicrobial resistance among the bacterial pathogens.[36,86]

Gram-Positive Bacteremia

S. aureus is the most virulent of the *Staphylococcus* spp., but coagulase-negative staphylococci are the most common cause of bacteremia in patients with hematologic malignancies.[34] The increased use of indwelling CVCs may be responsible for the increased incidence of infections due to common Gram-positive skin flora like coagulase-negative staphylococci.[87] *S. aureus* bacteremia in patients with hematologic malignancies is associated with 15% to 25% 30-day mortality.[34,88] The increased virulence of *S. aureus* should prompt the clinician to proceed with careful evaluation for endovascular infection and metastatic complications when this organism is the cause of bacteremia. The percentage of *S. aureus* isolates that are methicillin resistant varies geographically. Among *S. aureus* central line–associated bloodstream infections from cancer patients reported to the Centers for Disease Control and Prevention (CDC) in 2009 to 2012, 46% were methicillin resistant.[89] Anti–staphylococcal β-lactams, such as cefazolin, oxacillin, or nafcillin, are treatments of choice for methicillin-susceptible *S. aureus* bacteremia.[90] In a cohort study where 20% of patients had a hematologic malignancy, infection-related mortality was more than threefold lower with anti–staphylococcal β-lactam therapy compared to vancomycin therapy.[91]

Vancomycin remains the most widely used agent for MRSA bacteremia. The use of vancomycin for MRSA bacteremia in patients with hematologic malignancies requires therapeutic drug monitoring to optimize efficacy and minimize toxicity. Prior recommendations were to measure trough concentrations and adjust the dosage to achieve trough concentrations of 15 to 20 μg/mL.[92] However, experts now recommend measuring vancomycin area under the curve concentrations over 24 hours (AUC) and using AUC/minimum inhibitory concentration ratios (AUC/MIC) to guide vancomycin therapy for MRSA infections in hospitals where this type of monitoring is available.[93] Daptomycin is an alternative to vancomycin for MRSA bacteremia and was associated with similar outcomes compared to vancomycin-based therapy in a randomized trial.[94] Linezolid has in vitro activity against MRSA and yielded similar outcomes to vancomycin in a randomized trial of patients with suspected MRSA infections.[95] However, most patients in this trial had skin and soft-tissue infection or pneumonia; few had a bloodstream infection. Furthermore, linezolid is bacteriostatic and has accompanying risks of thrombocytopenia, delayed neutrophil recovery, and serotonin syndrome when used with selective serotonin reuptake inhibitors.[96-98] Thus, linezolid is not considered a first-line therapy for MRSA bacteremia. Other agents with oral formulations, such as clindamycin, doxycycline, and trimethoprim-sulfamethoxazole (TMP-SMX), have in vitro activity against MRSA but are not recommended for the treatment of MRSA bacteremia. Consultation with an infectious diseases specialist about antimicrobial management, diagnostic evaluation for endocarditis and other complications, and duration of treatment is recommended for S. aureus bacteremia because this consultation is consistently associated with decreased mortality with these infections.[99,100]

Viridans group streptococci are the next most common causes of Gram-positive bacteremia in patients with hematologic malignancies and are particularly common pathogens in patients with severe chemotherapy-induced mucositis.[4,34] Viridans group streptococcal infections have been associated with a shock syndrome characterized by hypotension, rash, and adult respiratory distress syndrome in neutropenic patients.[101,102] Agents recommended for fever and neutropenia by IDSA (cefepime, piperacillin-tazobactam, and carbapenems) generally have activity against viridans group streptococci, although resistance to these β-lactam agents has been increasingly reported.[103] Thus, the use of vancomycin may be considered in septic neutropenic patients with bacteremia due to viridans group streptococci while awaiting antimicrobial susceptibility testing results.

Enterococcus spp. are the third most common Gram-positive pathogens isolated among cancer patients, with Enterococcus faecalis and Enterococcus faecium accounting for the majority of cases.[90] Although often considered less virulent than Staphylococcus and Streptococcus spp., enterococcal infections are associated with high mortality rates among hematology patients.[104,105] VRE are increasingly common pathogens in this population and these organisms are typically also resistant to β-lactam agents. Thus, VRE bacteremia typically requires treatment with daptomycin or linezolid. If daptomycin is used for the treatment of VRE bacteremia, dosages of 8 to 12 mg/kg/d are recommended.[106] Common predisposing risk factors for VRE in hematology cohorts include nosocomial acquisition, prior antibiotic exposure, prolonged neutropenia, and stem cell transplantation.[107]

Gram-Negative Bacteremia

Surveillance studies indicate the number of infections attributed to Gram-negative pathogens is patients with hematologic malignancies is increasing.[35] Gram-negative bacteremia in neutropenic patients with cancer is associated with increased mortality compared to Gram-positive bacteremia. Unfortunately, the resurgence of infections with Gram-negative organisms has also been associated with drug-resistant strains, including multidrug-resistant P. aeruginosa, ESBL-producing and carbapenem-resistant Enterobacterales (CRE), and Stenotrophomonas maltophilia.[36,86] Enterobacterales, specifically E. coli and K. pneumoniae, are the most common causes of Gram-negative bacteremia.[34] These infections are typically from translocation of gut bacteria into the bloodstream in the setting of chemotherapy-induced neutropenia.[4,56,108] Depending on the geographic location, 17% to 37% of Enterobacterales bloodstream isolates in patients with hematologic malignancies produce ESBL enzymes that hydrolyze many β-lactam antibiotics.[55,109,110] Neutropenic patients with bacteremia due to ESBL-producing Enterobacterales (ESBL-E) have increased mortality compared to those with bacteremia due to Enterobacterales that do not produce ESBLs. Carbapenems are the treatments of choice for ESBL-E bacteremia in neutropenic patients because they are associated with decreased mortality compared to alternative therapies like piperacillin-tazobactam and cefepime.[111,112] CRE bacteremia in patients with hematologic malignancies was associated with nearly 50% mortality when the only available therapies were polymyxins, tigecycline, and aminoglycosides.[113-115] However, novel β-lactam/β-lactamase inhibitors, such as ceftazidime-avibactam, meropenem-vaborbactam, imipenem-relebactam, are now available that are highly effective against many CRE.[116] Use of these agents has been associated with decreased mortality with CRE infections and they should be utilized with consultation from infectious diseases specialists.[117-119]

P. aeruginosa does not cause Gram-negative bacteremia as frequently as E. coli in patients with hematologic malignancies, but P. aeruginosa bacteremia is associated with a higher mortality rate.[34,120] Additionally, P. aeruginosa bacteremia in neutropenic patients may manifest with ecthyma gangrenosum, where the bacteria invades the arteries and veins of the dermis and epidermis and causes ischemic necrosis.[121] Given that resistance of P. aeruginosa to first-line agents used for fever and neutropenia is common and that delays of effective therapy increase mortality,[38,63,122] the addition of a second agent (aminoglycoside or fluoroquinolone) may be considered while awaiting results of antimicrobial susceptibility testing to increase the probability that at least one of the agents is active against the organism. However, once susceptibility data are available, a single active β-lactam agent is typically sufficient for treatment, as most observational studies have not found a benefit to targeted therapy with two active agents compared to a single active agent.[123-125] Prolonging the infusion time of the β-lactam by administering the drug over 2 to 4 hours instead of over 30 to 60 minutes may provide benefit in the treatment of P. aeruginosa bacteremia by maintaining the concentration of the antibiotic above the MIC for a longer duration of the dosing interval. Clinical data supporting this approach are primarily from observational studies[126,127]; data from randomized trials are mixed.[128,129]

Catheter-Related Bloodstream Infection

CVCs are frequently necessary for the treatment of hematologic malignancies because they provide access for safe administration of chemotherapy, for routine laboratory evaluation, and for outpatient use of intravenous medications. However, they also serve as a source for bloodstream infections.[130] The risk of infectious complications varies among catheter types and increases with the number of CVC manipulations. Surgically implanted tunneled venous catheters and central venous ports generally have a lower risk of infection than nontunneled catheters. Other preventive measures, such as patient and staff education about catheter management and proper hand hygiene, are important and effective interventions. Staff and patient awareness of the issue of infectious risk and implementation of preventive protocols have been shown to reduce catheter-related bloodstream infections (CRBSIs).[131] Given that many bloodstream infections in patients with hematologic malignancies who have chemotherapy-induced neutropenia and mucositis are from gut translocation of bacteria and not an infection of the CVC, a new surveillance definition of mucosal barrier injury laboratory-confirmed bloodstream infections (MBI-LCBIs) was introduced.[132] A retrospective analysis of oncology, hematology, and transplant units at a large academic center found that 71% of CRBSIs met MBI-LCBI criteria.[133] The removal of MBI-LCBIs from the CRBSI category allows for accurate recognition of areas in which central line management changes are most needed.[134]

When cultures are obtained from indwelling catheters and peripheral venipuncture sites simultaneously, differential time to positivity of blood cultures obtained from the central line at least 120 minutes before a positive peripheral blood culture has been prospectively validated as a sensitive and specific test for establishing the presence of CRBSI.[135,136] Once confirmed, management of CRBSIs is tailored to the clinical scenario and specific organism isolated. In addition to antimicrobial therapy, removal of the catheter is recommended for patients with CRBSIs caused by S. aureus, P. aeruginosa, fungi, and mycobacteria, but catheter removal may not always be necessary for CRBSIs caused by coagulase-negative staphylococci and Enterobacterales.[4] In addition, catheter removal is recommended for CRBSIs associated with tunnel infection, mediport pocket site infection, septic thrombosis, endocarditis, sepsis with hemodynamic instability, and persistently bacteremic patients. In scenarios where catheter removal is not pursued, antibiotic lock therapy may serve as an adjunct to systemic antibiotic therapy. Antibiotic lock therapy refers to the instillation of a concentrated antibiotic solution in the catheter lumen with the goal of achieving a concentration of the antibiotic that is high enough to kill bacteria within the biofilm of the catheter.[137] Most cases of CRBSIs in immunocompromised patients require a 10 to 14 days of antimicrobial therapy after documentation of clearance of the infection with negative cultures.[4] Cases involving attempts to salvage the catheter, deep tissue infections, or other more complex scenarios may require longer durations of therapy.

Candidemia

The vast majority of fungemias in patients with hematologic malignancies are caused by *Candida* spp. The identification of *Candida* in a blood culture warrants prompt initiation of antifungal therapy, as the mortality rates with candidemia in patients with hematologic malignancies are approximately 40%.[138,139] Risk factors for candidemia in patients with hematologic malignancies include neutropenia, receipt of glucocorticoids, broad-spectrum antibiotics, and total parenteral nutrition, and use of a CVC.[139-141] In part due to the widespread use of fluconazole prophylaxis, candidemia is more frequently caused by species other than *Candida albicans* in patients with hematologic malignancies, such as *Candida krusei* and *Candida glabrata*.[138,140] *Candida parapsilosis* is a common cause of catheter-related candidemia.[140]

Echinocandins (e.g., caspofungin, micafungin, anidulafungin) are generally recommended for initial therapy of candidemia in patients with hematologic malignancies.[142] In a randomized, double-blind trial of 245 patients with candidemia, 76% of patients randomized to an echinocandin (anidulafungin) had successful treatment, compared to only 60% of those randomized to fluconazole ($P = .02$).[143] The benefit of echinocandin therapy in this trial even occurred in patients infected with *C. albicans*, even though *C. albicans* is typically susceptible to fluconazole.[144] Echinocandin therapy was also found to be associated with decreased mortality in a meta-analysis of seven randomized trials of patients with candidemia and invasive candidiasis.[145] Transition from an echinocandin to fluconazole is reasonable only after the patient has achieved clinical stability, blood cultures have cleared, and the bloodstream isolate has demonstrated susceptibility to fluconazole.[142]

Patients with candidemia who have CVCs should generally have their catheters removed as soon as possible if the source of infection is thought to be the catheter and it can be safely removed.[142] Although no randomized trials have assessed the efficacy of catheter removal for candidemia, observational studies and secondary analyses of aggregated data from trials comparing antifungal therapies suggest improved mortality with early catheter removal.[145-147] The role of catheter removal is less clear in patients with hematologic malignancies who have chemotherapy-induced neutropenia, where the gastrointestinal tract is a more likely source of the candidemia than the CVC.[142,148] Furthermore, the risks of catheter removal and replacement are greater in neutropenic and thrombocytopenic patients. In addition to consideration of catheter removal, patients with candidemia should undergo evaluation for metastatic sites of infection, including chorioretinitis and endophthalmitis and liver and spleen abscesses.[142] IDSA recommends a dilated ophthalmological examination for all patients with candidemia to screen for chorioretinitis and endophthalmitis.[142] For patients who are neutropenic, it is recommended to delay this exam until recovery from neutropenia because ocular findings may be obscured during neutropenia. In contrast, the American Academy of Ophthalmology favors routine ophthalmologic examination only in patients with candidemia who have ocular symptoms or cannot report symptoms.[149] *Candida* chorioretinitis and endophthalmitis is typically treated with at least 4 to 6 weeks of antifungal therapy, usually fluconazole, with the final duration depending on resolution of the lesions by repeated ophthalmological exams. In certain situations, an intravitreal injection of antifungal therapy or vitrectomy may be necessary.

Pulmonary Infections

Infection is the most common cause of pulmonary infiltrates in patients with hematologic malignancies and pneumonia is a leading cause of morbidity and mortality in this population.[150-152] However, the differential diagnosis for pulmonary findings in these patients is broad, including a large number of infectious and noninfectious complications (*Table 70.3*).[152,153] Noninfectious pulmonary syndromes such as transfusion-related acute lung injury and diffuse alveolar hemorrhage may mimic infection with fever, hypoxia, and alveolar opacities. New targeted agents for hematologic malignancies may simultaneously predispose to idiosyncratic reactions such as pneumonitis and opportunistic infections.[27,154,155] Profound neutropenia may

Table 70.3. Differential Diagnosis of Pulmonary Infiltrates in Patients With Hematologic Malignancies

Category	Etiology	Implicated Organism, Agents, or Clinical Setting
Infectious	Bacterial	Community-acquired organisms: *Streptococcus pneumoniae*, *Haemophilus influenzae*, *Moraxella catarrhalis*, *Mycoplasma pneumoniae*, *Legionella* spp., *Chlamydia* spp.
		Hospital or healthcare-associated or opportunistic organisms: *Staphylococcus aureus*, *Pseudomonas aeruginosa*, *Klebsiella* spp., *Enterobacter* spp., *Serratia marcescens*, *Stenotrophomonas maltophilia*, *Nocardia* spp.
	Fungal	*Aspergillus* spp., Mucorales, *Pneumocystis jirovecii*, *Cryptococcus* spp., *Histoplasma capsulatum*, *Coccidioides* spp.
	Viral	SARS-CoV-2, influenza, respiratory syncytial virus, parainfluenza virus, human metapneumovirus, rhinovirus, cytomegalovirus, herpes simplex virus
	Parasites	*Toxoplasma gondii*, *Strongyloides stercoralis*
Noninfectious	Pulmonary embolism	Westermark sign, Hampton hump
	Radiation pneumonitis	Anthracyclines, gemcitabine, carboplatin, cyclophosphamide
	Drug toxicity	Methotrexate, bleomycin, cyclophosphamide, sirolimus, cytarabine, dasatinib, ibrutinib, idelalisib
	Pulmonary edema	Congestive heart failure, volume overload
	Transfusion related	Transfusion-related acute lung injury, transfusion associated circulatory overload
	Hemorrhage	Diffuse alveolar hemorrhage
	Leukostasis	Acute leukemia (blasts > 50×10^9/L)
	Hematopoietic cell transplant related	Idiopathic pneumonia syndrome, organizing pneumonia, engraftment syndrome, pulmonary graft-vs-host disease, pulmonary alveolar proteinosis
	Differentiation syndrome	Acute promyelocytic leukemia with all-trans retinoic acid or arsenic trioxide therapy
	Cytokine release syndrome	Bispecific antibodies for leukemia or chimeric antigen receptor T cell therapy

Abbreviation: SARS-CoV-2, severe acute respiratory syndrome coronavirus 2.

blunt the inflammatory response and typical findings such as productive sputum, consolidation, or radiographic opacities may be absent on initial presentation.[6] As with other infections, pulmonary infections in the immunocompromised patient may progress rapidly with life-threatening complications. Prompt recognition, empirical treatment, and judicious pursuit of an accurate microbiologic diagnosis are critical for appropriate management.[156-160] Many patients with concern for infection warrant admission and evaluation in the inpatient setting to expedite the diagnostic work-up and to provide supportive care and appropriate empirical therapies.

Diagnostic Evaluation

In addition to blood cultures, patients with suspected pulmonary infection and a productive cough should have sputum obtained for Gram stain and culture. Use of induced sputum samples with hypertonic saline or other inhaled agents is not routinely recommended in patients with hematologic malignancies. Induced sputum has only been shown to be beneficial in the diagnosis of pneumonia due to *Pneumocystis jirovecii* and mycobacteria, and even for these infections the benefit has primarily been observed in HIV-infected patients.[161-163] The diagnostic workup for pneumonia is guided by the clinical presentation and risk for invasive or atypical infectious pathogens. Polymerase chain reaction (PCR) testing of nasopharyngeal swab samples for common respiratory viral and atypical bacterial pathogens permits rapid identification of these infections with a high degree of sensitivity.[164] Use of PCR assays for respiratory viruses may be particularly helpful during seasonal cycles of respiratory illnesses or local outbreaks, with the caveat that molecular detection of viral pathogens in hematology patients with upper respiratory tract symptoms is common, and positive tests may represent colonization or be associated with bacterial coinfection.[165,166] The serum β-D-glucan assay is a useful tool to screen for fungal pneumonia due to *Aspergillus* and *P. jirovecii*. The sensitivity is modest for invasive aspergillosis (IA) but is very high for *P. jirovecii* pneumonia (PJP), where a negative test makes PJP very unlikely.[167-170] The serum *Aspergillus* galactomannan assay is another valuable test to detect IA, with a sensitivity and specificity of approximately 70% and 90%, respectively, in patients with hematologic malignancies.[171] Urinary antigen tests for *Legionella pneumophila* serotype 1, which causes the majority of *Legionella* infections, and *S. pneumoniae* are also useful diagnostic tools, with each assay having approximately 70% sensitivity for detection of *Legionella* and pneumococcal pneumonia, respectively.[172,173]

CT of the chest has an important diagnostic role in patients with hematologic malignancies and should be considered in patients with normal chest roentgenograms when there is high clinical suspicion for pulmonary disease. In a high-risk patient with fever who also has cough, pleurisy, or hypoxia, obtaining CT imaging of the chest has been shown to alter management and may allow for earlier identification of opportunistic infections.[160,174,175] Patients with a normal plain chest film who remain febrile after 48 hours of empirical antimicrobial therapy may have abnormal chest CT imaging in up to 50% of cases.[175] Even for patients with abnormal chest X-rays, CT imaging can provide additional resolution to better inform the differential diagnosis of the pulmonary infiltrates and decisions on potential diagnostic procedures.

Appropriate use of systemic therapies is best tailored when the diagnosis is known. In the case of pulmonary infections, invasive procedures for a microbiologic or tissue diagnosis are often warranted. Inherent risks of complications related to the procedure (e.g., bleeding, pneumothorax) should be weighed against the potential benefit of increasing the probability of obtaining an accurate diagnosis. Diagnostic procedures include bronchoscopy and BAL with or without a transbronchial biopsy, percutaneous needle biopsy, video-assisted thoracoscopic biopsy, or open lung biopsy. The optimal procedure depends partially on the nature and location of the pulmonary lesions, with diffuse lesions better sampled by BAL and/or transbronchial biopsy and discrete peripheral nodules better sampled by percutaneous needle or surgical biopsy. A systematic review comparing open lung biopsy to BAL found that both procedures reached a diagnosis in a similar proportion of cases overall.[157] However, open lung biopsy was more likely to identify a noninfectious cause and bronchoscopy with BAL was more likely to identify an infectious cause. The complication rate and procedure-related mortality of lung biopsy were significantly higher than the bronchoscopic approach. There may be a tendency to delay diagnostic procedures in hematology patients due to clinical instability, thrombocytopenia, or the general desire to avoid invasive measures, but earlier bronchoscopy within the first 4 days of clinical presentation has been shown to have a higher diagnostic yield and improve outcomes in HCT recipients.[158] In a study of febrile patients with hematologic malignancies and pulmonary infiltrates, bronchoscopy with BAL yielded a causative pathogen in 118 (48%) out of 246 BAL samples.[176] BAL samples should be tested for a variety of pathogens depending on the clinical scenario, including viral, protozoal, fungal, and mycobacterial, as well as the traditional Gram stain and bacterial culture. *Aspergillus* galactomannan antigen testing on BAL samples increases the diagnostic yield and is discussed in the section on Aspergillosis.

Aspergillosis

Aspergillus spp. are ubiquitous in the environment, but the development of invasive disease is infrequent and typically only occurs in immunocompromised patients. Despite advances in the diagnosis and the management of IA, it remains a leading cause of infectious death among hematology patients.[177] Prolonged neutropenia and use of high doses of corticosteroids are major risk factors for IA. European registries have demonstrated that as many as 13% of patients with acute leukemia and 6% of allogeneic HCT recipients develop IA.[178,179] Development of acute or chronic GVHD (cGVHD) following HCT increases the risk in transplant patients even after the recovery from neutropenia.[180] The lungs are the most common site of invasive disease (*Figure 70.4*), but the classic triad of pleuritic chest pain, hemoptysis, and fever is often absent. Symptoms or radiographic findings may be absent or nonspecific. Definitive diagnosis of invasive disease by detecting invading fungal hyphae on tissue biopsy or a positive culture from a sterile site is often challenging. Thus, guidelines for the diagnosis of "probable" IA may be applied, which incorporate host factors,

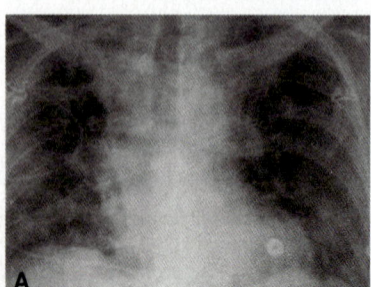
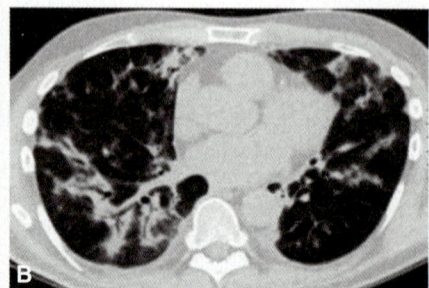
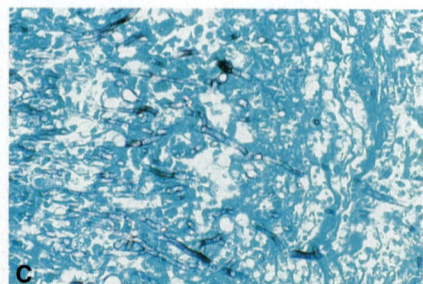

FIGURE 70.4 A, Plain chest radiograph and B, Chest CT in a hematopoietic cell transplant recipient who developed a pneumonia approximately 2 years after initial diagnosis of acute myeloid leukemia. C, Photomicrograph of characteristic 45-degree branching of the septate hyphal form of *Aspergillus*. Gomori methenamine silver stain ×400. (Photomicrograph courtesy of Margie Scott, MD.)

radiographic findings, and mycological evidence, including a positive *Aspergillus* galactomannan test.[181] Chest CT imaging in the evaluation of neutropenic fever, especially after failure to defervesce with antimicrobial therapy, should be considered to evaluate for the possibility of invasive fungal pneumonia, and implementation of this practice leads to earlier diagnosis of invasive pulmonary aspergillosis.[182,183] Radiographic findings may include the classic well-circumscribed pulmonary nodule, with or without a "halo" of ground-glass attenuation representing angioinvasion, but the radiographic presentations of invasive pulmonary aspergillosis are variable.[184,185] With treatment, nodules may progress to a cavitary lesion known as an "air crescent" sign that appears with recovery of the granulocyte count.[185] Cultures have only modest sensitivity for diagnosing aspergillosis and require days to yield a result, and invasive tissue sampling may be challenging to obtain because of thrombocytopenia.[186] Disseminated disease may involve the skin, brain, eyes, heart, or other vital structures and is associated with a poor prognosis.[187]

Early diagnosis of aspergillosis improves outcomes.[187] The challenge of establishing a histopathologic diagnosis has led to increasing use of the serum markers β-D-glucan and galactomannan antigen to establish a diagnosis.[181] A positive β-D-glucan assay may also occur with other IFIs, including candidiasis and PJP, and false-positive results may occur with receipt of hemodialysis, intravenous immunoglobulin (IVIG), or albumin.[188] The galactomannan antigen is more specific for aspergillosis, but the assay may cross-react with other mycoses such as histoplasmosis or *Fusarium* infection, and the sensitivity is decreased by concurrent use of mold-active antifungal therapy.[189,190] Galactomannan results are reported as an optical density (OD) and a cutoff value of 0.5 OD in a meta-analysis resulted in assay sensitivity of 82% and specificity of 81%, with reduced sensitivity in nonneutropenic patients.[191] As a positive galactomannan result may precede clinical or radiographic changes by several days, serial galactomannan testing may be considered as a screening tool in high-risk patients who are not receiving antimold prophylaxis.[192] Although these serum assays are helpful initial screening tests, a bronchoscopy with BAL is often indicated to evaluate for invasive pulmonary aspergillosis. BAL samples should initially be stained with calcofluor white with 10% potassium hydroxide to directly detect fungal hyphae, followed by fungal culture.[193] *Aspergillus* spp. are often visible in culture after 1 to 3 days of incubation and inspection of spore-bearing structures can provide identification to the species level. Galactomannan testing can also be performed on BAL samples, where it has a higher sensitivity for the diagnosis of pulmonary aspergillosis compared to galactomannan testing of serum samples.[194,195] Lung biopsy specimens can also be examined for hyphal forms using Gomori methenamine silver or periodic acid-Schiff staining. *Aspergillus* spp. present as narrow septate hyaline hyphae with acute angle branching in tissue specimens. Molecular diagnostics, including PCR assays, are emerging diagnostic tools, but are not currently in routine use.[181,196] Ongoing prospective evaluations are underway with hopes that newer molecular diagnostics will allow for accurate, timely, and noninvasive diagnosis of pulmonary aspergillosis in high-risk patients.

Voriconazole, posaconazole, and isavuconazole are first-line therapies for IA. Voriconazole is recommended in IDSA guidelines based on extensive clinical experience and its improved responses and survival compared to amphotericin B deoxycholate in a randomized trial.[197,198] Posaconazole and isavuconazole have been shown to be effective and better tolerated than voriconazole in randomized trials.[199,200] Some experts recommend adding an echinocandin to triazole therapy based on a trend toward improved survival with this combination compared to monotherapy in a randomized trial.[201] Antifungal therapy should be continued for a minimum of 6 to 12 weeks, and continued until radiographic abnormalities have stabilized and signs of active infection have resolved.[197] Therapeutic drug monitoring is recommended for voriconazole and posaconazole.[181,202] Whenever possible, the degree of immunosuppression should be decreased as an adjunct to antifungal therapy.[181] Surgery may have a role in patients with a solitary lung lesion, or in patients with recurrent hemoptysis or invasion into the chest wall or pleural space.

Pneumocystis

P. jirovecii, formerly *Pneumocystis carinii*, is now classified taxonomically as a fungus rather than a protozoon and is a prototypical cause of opportunistic infection in the immunocompromised host.[203,204] Risk factors for PJP include glucocorticoid use,[205,206] maintenance therapy for ALL,[204] allogeneic HCT,[207] and use of alkylating agents such as temozolomide,[208] the purine analog fludarabine,[24] monoclonal antibodies rituximab and alemtuzumab,[209,210] and the targeted agents idelalisib and ibrutinib.[26,155] The most common symptoms include fever, dyspnea, and cough.[211] Compared with HIV-infected patients, patients with hematologic malignancies may have a more fulminant presentation, with increased need for intensive care and mechanical ventilation, and increased mortality.[212] The predominant radiographic pattern is bilateral interstitial infiltrates and hypoxia is frequently present.[211] Lactate dehydrogenase may be elevated with PJP, but this finding has less clinical utility among patients with hematologic malignancies.[169] Serum β-D-glucan is almost always elevated in patients with PJP, but may also be elevated in other fungal infections such as candidiasis and aspergillosis.[169] A normal serum β-D-glucan indicates that PJP is unlikely in hematology and transplant patients.[169,170] *Pneumocystis* cannot be grown in culture in the microbiology laboratory, and the diagnosis is traditionally made by staining and microscopy of induced sputum or BAL fluid.[213] Immunofluorescent stains with monoclonal antibodies can visualize both trophic forms and cysts and have increased yield compared to standard stains that only detect trophic forms.[214] The sensitivity of staining and microscopy to diagnose PJP is lower in patients with hematologic malignancies than in HIV-infected patients because of reduced organism burden.[162,215] PCR assays are also available for use on sputum and BAL samples that have greater sensitivity than staining and microscopy, but may also detect patients colonized with *P. jirovecii*.[215,216] Thus, these molecular assays should only be used in patients with a high clinical suspicion of PJP.

TMP-SMX is the treatment of choice for PJP based on its superior efficacy compared to other agents in randomized trials of HIV-infected patients.[217,218] TMP-SMX is typically administered for 21 days at dosage of 15 to 20 mg/kg/d (based on the trimethoprim component),[219] although lower dosages of TMP-SMX may yield similar effectiveness with less toxicity.[220] The combination of clindamycin plus primaquine and intravenous pentamidine are second-line treatments for severe PJP,[217,221,222] and patients should be evaluated for glucose-6-phosphate dehydrogenase deficiency prior to using primaquine.[223] In adults with HIV and moderate or severe PJP (hypoxia, increased alveolar-arterial oxygen gradient, or decreased arterial partial pressure of oxygen), adjunctive corticosteroids reduce the inflammatory response and improve outcomes.[224-226] Supportive data for corticosteroids in patients with hematologic malignancies are less clear,[227-229] but their use may be considered in hypoxic patients, particularly given the more fulminant course in this population. Prophylaxis against PJP is discussed later in this chapter.

Mucormycosis

Mucorales, such as *Rhizopus*, *Mucor*, and *Rhizomucor*, are increasingly common causes of IFI in patients with hematologic malignancies and HCT recipients.[230,231] Voriconazole does not have activity against the Mucorales and use of voriconazole prophylaxis is a risk factor for invasive mucormycosis.[232] In contrast to patients with diabetes, who typically have rhino-orbital-cerebral infection, pulmonary infection is the most common manifestation in patients with hematologic malignancies and HCT recipients.[231] Mucormycosis is rapidly progressive, resulting in parenchymal infarction and potentially disseminated disease. Imaging may reveal nodules, consolidation, pleural effusions, and/or a "reverse halo" sign.[233] The diagnosis of mucormycosis typically relies on identification of compatible hyphae in tissue on histopathology and/or isolating the organism in culture.[234] Treatment of mucormycosis involves antifungal therapy, typically with lipid formulations of amphotericin B, combined with surgical debridement and reduction of immunosuppression, where feasible.[235]

Other Fungal and Atypical Organisms

The endemic dimorphic fungi *Blastomyces, Coccidioides,* and *Histoplasma* have regional distributions and can cause primary infections or reactivation disease in previously exposed patients.[236] Although the primary route of infection is respiratory, these endemic mycoses can disseminate to involve virtually any organ in immunocompromised patients with hematologic malignancies.[237] The clinical manifestations may be protean, and diagnosis can be difficult and delayed. These pathogens should be included in the differential diagnosis for any immunocompromised patient with pulmonary infiltrates.[160] Serum and urine antigen testing has improved the ability to diagnose disseminated disease in immunocompromised patients.[238] Urine antigen testing is also available for *L. pneumophila*, a potential etiology of pneumonia in immunocompromised patients that has a high mortality rate in cancer patients.[172,239] The partially acid-fast bacterial pathogen *Nocardia* and the endemic fungus *Cryptococcus* may cause cavitary lung lesions in the immunocompromised patient with potential for central nervous system dissemination.[240,241]

Coronavirus Disease 2019 (COVID-19)

Emerging in December 2019 and being declared a pandemic in March 2020, COVID-19 has affected nearly every aspect of care for patients with hematologic malignancies. Patients with hematologic malignancies have an increased risk of mortality from COVID-19 compared to the general patient population and compared to patients with solid tumors.[242,243] Diagnostic testing by reverse transcription-PCR or rapid antigen testing for severe acute respiratory syndrome coronavirus 2 (SARS-CoV-2) should be performed for any hematology patient with new symptoms of a respiratory tract infection and/or fever. Testing may also be indicated in asymptomatic patients prior to chemotherapy or transplantation.[244]

Given their high risk of developing severe COVID-19, treatment with either an antiviral agent or a monoclonal antibody should be initiated as soon as the diagnosis is established in patients with hematologic malignancies. Nirmatrelvir-ritonavir is a combination of oral protease inhibitors that decreased the risk of progression to severe COVID-19 by 89% compared to placebo when administered early in the course of infection.[245] A thorough review of medications for possible drug interactions is essential prior to prescribing nirmatrelvir-ritonavir, because it is a potent inhibitor of CYP3A enzymes.[246] Early treatment with remdesivir, an inhibitor of viral replication, is also effective in preventing progression to severe disease, but its use in outpatients is limited by the need for 3 days of an intravenous infusion.[247] Molnupiravir is a nucleoside analog that inhibits SARS-CoV-2 replication, but is considered a second-line therapy because of limited efficacy.[248] Monoclonal antibodies are effective in preventing severe COVID-19, but require either subcutaneous or intravenous administration and the optimal therapies are subject to change depending on the SARS-CoV-2 variant that is circulating.[249-251]

Corticosteroids decrease mortality in patients who are hospitalized for COVID-19 and are hypoxic.[252-254] In the largest randomized trial to demonstrate a mortality benefit, 6 mg of daily dexamethasone was used for up to 10 days.[252] Janus kinase inhibitors (e.g., baricitinib) or interleukin-6 pathway inhibitors (e.g., tocilizumab) may provide additional benefit when combined with corticosteroids in patients who have rapidly progressive respiratory failure and elevated inflammatory markers.[255-257]

Remdesivir has not been shown to decrease mortality in patients hospitalized with COVID-19.[258] However, given that it shortens the time to clinical recovery,[259] it should be considered in patients with hematologic malignancies who are hospitalized, particularly given that these immunocompromised patients have prolonged viral replication.[260] Given the high rate of thromboembolic complications among hospitalized patients with COVID-19,[261] pharmacologic prophylaxis against venous thromboembolism should be considered in patients without thrombocytopenia or contraindications.[262] Patients with hematologic malignancies may have prolonged viral shedding and therefore may require prolonged isolation in healthcare settings.[263]

Given the poor outcomes associated with COVID-19 in patients with hematologic malignancies, vaccination to lower the risk of infection and severe disease is critical. COVID-19 vaccinations are generally safe in patients with cancer, including HCT recipients,[264] with similar risks of adverse events compared to patients without cancer.[265] None of the available COVID-19 vaccines contain infectious virus. However, the effectiveness of COVID-19 vaccines is lower in patients with hematologic malignancies than in patients with solid tumors or in the general population.[266] Humoral immunologic responses to COVID-19 vaccines are impaired in patients receiving active treatment for hematologic malignancies, particularly B cell-targeted therapies.[267,268] Given these diminished immunologic responses, three doses of an mRNA vaccine are considered a primary vaccination series in patients with hematologic malignancies. The addition of a third dose of mRNA vaccine in this population was shown to increase the likelihood of obtaining SARS-CoV-2 neutralizing antibodies, even against the omicron variant.[269] Additionally, given the waning immunity provided by COVID-19 vaccines and the decreased efficacy against certain variants,[269] a booster (or fourth) dose is recommended at least 3 months after completion of the primary three-dose series.[270] Due to the suboptimal protection provided by COVID-19 vaccines in patients with hematologic malignancies, use of the long-lasting monoclonal antibody tixagevimab-cilgavimab should be considered in addition to vaccination.[271] Given the rapidly changing information related to COVID-19, providers should frequently review the latest recommendations from the CDC.

Pneumonia Due to Viral Pathogens Other Than COVID-19

Primary infection with viral pathogens is a frequent cause of fever and respiratory symptoms in patients with hematologic malignancies.[165] The morbidity and associated complications of respiratory viral infections are greater in patients with hematologic malignancies than in the general population.[272] Influenza, respiratory syncytial virus (RSV), and human metapneumovirus (hMPV) are seasonal viruses that have the highest incidence in winter months, whereas parainfluenza viruses have the highest incidence in the spring and summer.[272] Rhinovirus is the most common respiratory viral infection in patients with hematologic malignancies and HCT recipients and may be present throughout the year.[273,274]

Advances in diagnostic testing now permit rapid identification of the most common viral pathogens by PCR.[275] Detecting the etiology of a respiratory viral infection other than COVID-19 in patients with hematologic malignancies has important infection control and treatment implications. Hematology patients with influenza benefit from treatment with a neuraminidase inhibitor such as oseltamivir even if they begin treatment more than 2 days after the onset of symptoms.[276,277] Baloxavir is another potential treatment option for influenza, but is not a first-line agent in immunocompromised patients because its use has been associated with the emergence of resistance.[278] Ribavirin therapy for upper respiratory tract infections due to RSV has been associated with decreased risk of progression to pneumonia and death in HCT recipients,[279,280] and recent data suggest that oral ribavirin therapy is safe and as effective as aerosolized ribavirin.[281] Most studies have not shown a benefit to adding IVIG or the monoclonal antibody palivizumab to ribavirin for RSV infections.[282,283] In contrast to influenza and RSV, treatment of respiratory infections caused by parainfluenza virus, hMPV, rhinovirus, and seasonal coronaviruses is largely supportive, with a focus on reducing immunosuppression where feasible.[284] Most observational studies have not identified a benefit to administering IVIG for these infections, although its role warrants additional investigation.[285,286] Secondary infections with bacteria and fungi are common after viral respiratory tract infections in patients with hematologic malignancies and HCT recipients, and thus vigilance is warranted to detect and treat these coinfections.[287,288]

Cytomegalovirus

CMV pneumonia is a major cause of infectious morbidity and mortality among allogeneic HCT recipients.[289] The most important risk factor for CMV disease after allogeneic HCT is recipient CMV seropositivity.[290-292] Other risk factors include GVHD, T-cell depletion, use of haploidentical, cord blood, or mismatched donor grafts, lymphopenia, older age, and use of high doses of corticosteroids. The incidence of CMV disease in the first 3 months after transplant has been reduced from 20% to 30% to less than 5% because of the widespread use of preemptive and prophylactic antiviral strategies.[292,293] The preemptive approach involves serial testing of blood or plasma for CMV DNA by PCR and initiating antiviral therapy (usually valganciclovir or ganciclovir) upon detection of CMV reactivation.[290,293,294] The rationale for this approach is that asymptomatic CMV viremia typically precedes the onset of CMV disease, particularly CMV pneumonia, by 1 to 2 weeks.[294] Widespread adoption of this approach has now made CMV gastrointestinal tract disease more common than CMV pneumonia, likely because there is a weaker correlation between CMV viremia and gastrointestinal disease.[295,296] The prophylactic approach is beginning to be used more due to the availability of letermovir, an antiviral agent with activity against CMV that does not cause myelosuppression like ganciclovir. In a randomized trial of CMV-seropositive allogeneic HCT recipients, patients randomized to letermovir were less likely to develop CMV infection and had lower 24-week mortality than those randomized to placebo.[297]

CMV pneumonia typically presents radiographically as bilateral symmetric interstitial infiltrates[298] (*Figure 70.5*). The definitive diagnosis of CMV pneumonia frequently requires a biopsy of infected lung to identify CMV inclusion bodies and/or CMV viral antigens in lung histopathology. Given that lung biopsies may be challenging to perform in HCT recipients, particularly those with thrombocytopenia, CMV PCR is frequently performed on BAL samples to establish the diagnosis.[299] A negative result rules out CMV pneumonia, but a positive result should be interpreted in context with the clinical picture. Higher quantities of viral DNA detected by PCR correlate with an increased likelihood of CMV pneumonia, as opposed to nonspecific shedding of virus into the respiratory tract.[299] Ganciclovir and foscarnet are first-line treatment options for CMV pneumonia, with the choice of agent depending on patient characteristics that impact toxicity risk, such as graft function and underlying kidney disease.[300] It is unclear whether the addition of immunoglobulin to these antiviral agents improves outcomes.[301] Maribavir is a potential treatment option for CMV infection that is resistant or refractory to ganciclovir and/or foscarnet,[302] but data supporting its use for CMV pneumonia are limited.

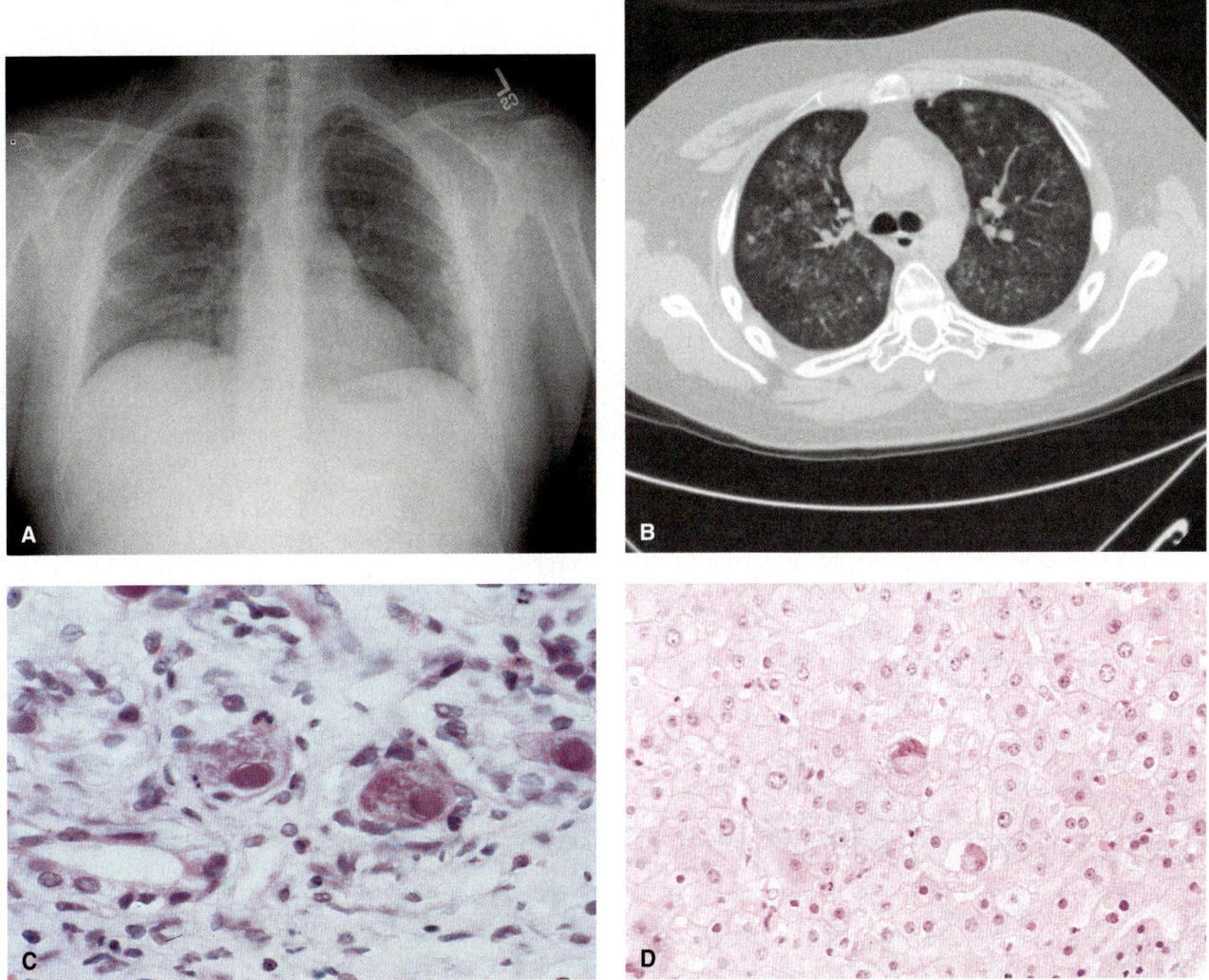

FIGURE 70.5 **The spectrum of cytomegalovirus (CMV) disease in the abnormal human host.** A, Chest radiograph demonstrating diffuse interstitial infiltrates in a patient 60 days after cord blood transplant. B, Chest CT showing bilateral fine nodular infiltrates. C, CMV inclusion disease of the colon. Typical infected cells show cellular ballooning with dense primary nuclear inclusions surrounded by a thin, cleared rim; secondary inclusions appear as cytoplasmic granules after the nucleus has filled with virions. D, CMV hepatitis demonstrated on liver biopsy. Viral cytopathic effect may be difficult to establish, but rare viral inclusions with surrounding parenchymal changes are diagnostic of CMV. Hematoxylin and eosin stain ×400. (Courtesy of Margie Scott, MD.)

Sinus Infections

Patients with hematologic disorders are at risk for the same spectrum of rhinosinusitis issues as the immunocompetent host, with the added potential complication of acute invasive fungal rhinosinusitis.[303] Risk factors for invasive fungal rhinosinusitis in patients with hematologic malignancies include prolonged neutropenia, allogeneic HCT, use of corticosteroids, and diabetes.[304,305] It is characterized by hyphae invasion of blood vessels resulting in tissue infarction and is most commonly associated with *Aspergillus, Fusarium,* and Mucorales. Clinical manifestations include fever, sinus pain, headache, rhinorrhea, epistaxis, and/or cranial nerve deficits. Early involvement of an otolaryngologist for endoscopic evaluation and possible biopsy is critical for timely diagnosis and definitive treatment.[306] CT imaging may suggest acute sinusitis but is insufficient to distinguish between bacterial and fungal etiologies.[307] The diagnosis is made by histologic demonstration of invasive hyphae on tissue biopsy. Empirical therapy typically consists of lipid formulations of amphotericin B. Mucorales can often be ruled out by inspection of lung histopathology and therapy can be transitioned to voriconazole if the characteristics of the hyphae are not compatible with mucormycosis. Antifungal therapy alone is often insufficient, and surgical debridement is usually required.[197,308]

Abdominal Infections

Receipt of chemotherapy that causes prolonged neutropenia and disruption of the mucosal barrier of the gastrointestinal tract predisposes patients with hematologic malignancies to develop neutropenic enterocolitis. Commonly referred to as typhlitis, this term implies inflammation of the cecal region, but any portion of the small or large intestine may be involved.[309] Gram-positive, Gram-negative, and anaerobic (e.g., *Clostridium septicum*) bacteria, as well as *Candida* spp., are implicated in the pathogenesis of neutropenic enterocolitis, and polymicrobial bloodstream infections are common in this setting.[310] Fever and abdominal pain in patients with prolonged neutropenia and recent chemotherapy should alert the clinician to the possibility of typhlitis and lead to evaluation with CT imaging.[311] Bowel wall thickening is universally present, but other radiographic findings may include mesenteric stranding, pneumatosis intestinalis, or perforation.[312] In addition to obtaining a CT scan, blood cultures and tests for *Clostridioides* (formerly *Clostridium*) *difficile* should be performed. Bowel rest, intravenous fluids, blood product support, broad-spectrum antimicrobials, and consideration of nasogastric tube placement for suction are the primary supportive interventions for patients with neutropenic enterocolitis.[311] Antimicrobial therapy should target Gram-negative enteric bacteria, *P. aeruginosa*, and anaerobes, with piperacillin-tazobactam, carbapenems, and cefepime plus metronidazole all being reasonable empirical choices. Empirical antifungal therapy should be added in patients who have persistent fever despite antibacterial therapy. Early consultation with a general surgeon is recommended, as severe cases with obstruction, perforation, or hemorrhage may require operative intervention.[309]

C. difficile infection is also a common cause of fever, abdominal pain, and diarrhea in patients with hematologic malignancies. Watery diarrhea (≥3 loose stools in 24 hours) is the most common manifestation, but *C. difficile* may also cause fulminant colitis, toxic megacolon, and multiorgan system failure.[313] Prior antimicrobial use is a major risk factor for *C. difficile* colitis, with clindamycin, fluoroquinolones, cephalosporins, and β-lactams being the most commonly implicated agents.[314] Diagnostic tests for *C. difficile* either detect the gene that encodes for toxin B by PCR or detect the toxin itself from stool samples.[315] The diagnosis of *C. difficile* infection requires clinical correlation because asymptomatic carriage is common among hospitalized patients, particularly patients with hematologic malignancies and HCT recipients.[316,317] Therefore, *C. difficile* testing should not be performed on formed stool samples or in patients who develop diarrhea after receiving laxatives.[318]

Guidelines now recommend fidaxomicin as the preferred treatment for *C. difficile* infection, with oral vancomycin as an acceptable alternative.[319,320] Fidaxomicin has a more limited spectrum of activity against commensal flora compared to vancomycin and its use is associated with a lower risk of recurrent disease.[321,322] Fidaxomicin does not disrupt the gastrointestinal microbiome like oral vancomycin does,[323] and this feature may be particularly important in allogeneic HCT recipients, where gut dysbiosis has been associated with posttransplant mortality.[324] Fulminant *C. difficile* disease with hypotension, shock, or toxic megacolon should be treated with high-dose vancomycin by mouth or nasogastric tube and intravenous metronidazole, with the addition of rectal vancomycin if an ileus is present.[319] Abdominal imaging should also be considered in such patients to evaluate for complications such as toxic megacolon or bowel perforation that may necessitate surgical consultation. Bezlotoxumab is a monoclonal antibody that binds to toxin B of *C. difficile* and is administered as a single intravenous infusion.[325] It use is recommended as an adjunct to antibacterial therapy in patients who have had a recurrence of *C. difficile* within the previous 6 months.[319] For patients with multiple recurrences who do not respond to appropriate therapies, fecal microbiota transplantation may be considered with careful screening of donor specimens to prevent transmission of potentially harmful pathogens.[319,326] Strict adherence to contact precautions with gowns, gloves, and handwashing with soap and water is critical for hospitalized patients with *C. difficile* to prevent nosocomial transmission.[318] *C. difficile* spores have been identified on almost every object tested in patient rooms and are resistant to alcohol-based hand sanitizing solutions.[327,328]

Skin and Soft-Tissue Infections

Skin infections in the neutropenic patient may lack the characteristic features of redness, pain, warmth, and swelling.[6] Noninfectious causes of skin lesions include Sweet syndrome, erythema multiforme, vasculitis, and leukemia cutis, all of which may be difficult to differentiate from infection. Intravenous catheter and bone marrow biopsy sites should be carefully examined. The perineum should also be closely inspected to evaluate for perirectal infections, but digital rectal examinations are avoided in the neutropenic patient.[4,329] Biopsies should be considered for cutaneous findings of unclear etiology to establish a diagnosis, a practice that was demonstrated to change management in up to one-half of cases in pediatric patients.[330] Patients with undifferentiated febrile syndromes and concern for skin and soft-tissue infection should be treated empirically with vancomycin or an agent with a similar spectrum of activity against *Staphylococcus* and *Streptococcus* spp.[4] Ecthyma gangrenosum is a rapidly progressive deep ulcerative lesion that often becomes necrotic because of perivascular bacterial invasion.[121] It is most commonly observed in immunocompromised patients with *P. aeruginosa* bacteremia and sepsis, but similar-appearing lesions may occur with IFIs,[331,332] highlighting the importance of biopsy for definitive diagnosis and management. Cultures taken directly from the skin are less useful for establishing a microbiologic diagnosis. When viral pathogens are suspected (e.g., herpes simplex virus [HSV]), the base of the vesicle should be tested with culture, direct fluorescent antibody tests, or PCR.[69]

Central Nervous System

As with other infectious/inflammatory conditions in the immunocompromised patient, typical symptoms may be absent with a CNS infection. The diagnosis of CNS infections is typically made through imaging and cerebrospinal fluid analysis. Patients with hematologic malignancies who have impaired humoral immunity and allogeneic HCT recipients are at increased risk of meningitis due to *Streptococcus pneumoniae* and other encapsulated bacteria.[333,334] Hematology patients with pronounced cell-mediated immune impairment may be at increased risk of developing meningitis due to cryptococcus or *Listeria monocytogenes*.[335,336] Cryptococcal meningitis may have a subacute presentation with subtle symptoms and is diagnosed by performing cryptococcal antigen testing on cerebrospinal fluid.[337,338] Tuberculosis meningitis is a rare complication in patients with hematologic malignancies.[339]

Viral encephalitis is more common in patients with hematologic malignancies than in the in the general population.[340] HSV and varicella-zoster virus (VZV) are the most common causes of viral

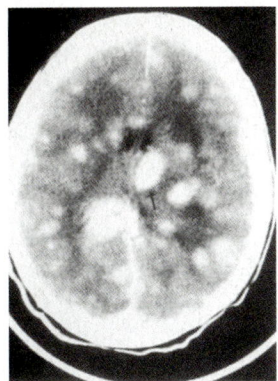 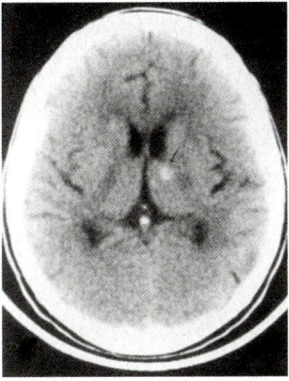

FIGURE 70.6 Central nervous system toxoplasmosis. Magnetic resonance imaging of the brain before (A) and after (B) therapy with pyrimethamine and sulfadiazine.

encephalitis and are important to rapidly diagnose because they can be effectively treated with prompt initiation of antiviral therapy.[341,342] Human herpesvirus 6 (HHV-6) is an important cause of viral encephalitis in allogeneic HCT recipients, typically occurring within 6 weeks after transplantation.[343] Ganciclovir or foscarnet are considered the treatments of choice for HHV-6 encephalitis.[344] Given that these etiologies of viral encephalitis are treatable, rapid diagnosis is critical. Thus, a lumbar puncture should be considered in patients with altered mental status or focal neurologic deficits without an obvious explanation, and the cerebrospinal fluid should be tested by PCR for these viral pathogens. Multiplexed PCR assays are now available that rapidly detect herpes viruses and other infections etiologies of meningitis and encephalitis.[345] In addition to herpes viruses, enterovirus and arboviruses such as West Nile Virus can cause viral encephalitis in patients with hematologic malignancies.[346,347]

Molds such as *Aspergillus* spp., Mucorales, *Fusarium* spp., and *Scedosporium* spp. are capable of causing CNS infections in patients who are neutropenic or recipients of glucocorticoids or allogeneic HCT.[348] These infections typically manifest as brain abscesses and may arise from direct extension from paranasal sinuses, eye, or middle ear or from hematogenous dissemination. Although a definitive diagnosis requires a brain biopsy, given that this is a highly invasive procedure, the diagnosis is often made by identifying invasive mold infections at other body sites. *Toxoplasmosis gondii* may present with pneumonitis, encephalitis, or disseminated disease with a predilection for CNS involvement (*Figure 70.6*). Allogeneic HCT recipients who are seropositive for *T. gondii* are at highest risk of developing this infection.[349] Some centers screen blood samples of seropositive allogeneic HCT recipients for *T. gondii* DNA and initiate preemptive therapy when reactivation is detected.[350]

Progressive multifocal leukoencephalopathy (PML) due to polyomavirus John Cunningham virus reactivation is typically seen only in the setting of profound immunosuppression, such as after allogeneic HCT or with the use of purine analogs, alkylating agents, rituximab, or brentuximab.[351,352] Clinical manifestations of PML include altered mental status, motor deficits, ataxia, and visual disturbance, and imaging typically reveals white matter lesions without mass effect.[353] PML is typically diagnosed by imaging findings and cerebrospinal fluid testing for JC virus by PCR. There are no specific antiviral therapies for PML and the mortality rate in patients with hematologic malignancies is high.[354] Treatment primarily consists of withdrawing immunosuppressive therapies. Small case series suggest a potential role for immune checkpoint inhibitors in PML therapy,[355] but further investigations are needed prior to routine use of these agents.

HEMATOPOIETIC CELL TRANSPLANTATION

HCT recipients have a unique set of infectious disease risks above and beyond that attributable to prolonged cytopenias and the underlying hematologic disorder. The indication for the transplant, conditioning regimen, type of graft, immunosuppressive regimen, and complications (e.g., GVHD) are all factors in the overall risk for infectious complications after HCT.[289] The pattern of immunosuppression and associated complications and opportunistic infections are variable for each patient, but a general timeline is provided in *Figure 70.7*.

Pre-Engraftment Period

Prior to engraftment, the major risk factors for infection are neutropenia and breakdown of protective barriers (e.g., gastrointestinal mucositis, central access devices). The most common pathogens are bacteria and fungi, similar to the pathogens encountered in neutropenic patients with hematologic malignancies who have not received a transplant.[289] Bloodstream infections, intra-abdominal infections (neutropenic enterocolitis and *C. difficile* colitis), pneumonia, and catheter-related infections are the most common infections prior to engraftment. Engraftment syndrome can occur around the time of neutrophil recovery and typically manifests as fever and rash with a negative infectious work-up, frequently with diarrhea and pulmonary infiltrates.[356] Engraftment syndrome may masquerade as pulmonary infection (peri-engraftment respiratory distress syndrome) and may be more common following autologous HCT.[357] Hemorrhagic cystitis in the pre-engraftment period is usually related to the conditioning regimen rather than BK virus infection.[358]

Early Postengraftment

The second defined period of risk is after engraftment until approximately 3 months after the transplant. Progressive recovery of cellular immunity in this phase is accompanied with reduced infection risk, and this occurs much more quickly following autologous than allogeneic HCT. Pneumonia is a major cause of infectious morbidity and mortality in the early postengraftment period in allogeneic HCT recipients, with invasive fungal pneumonia leading to a particularly high mortality.[359] Acute GVHD and CMV disease are the major risk factors for IFIs after allogeneic HCT.[360] The high mortality associated with invasive fungal disease necessitates an early and aggressive approach to diagnosis with CT imaging, serum antigen testing, and BAL with galactomannan antigen testing to reach a diagnosis. Antifungal prophylaxis is indicated in HCT recipients and regimens are discussed later in this chapter. Empirical therapy should be initiated early, while the diagnostic algorithm is underway when the clinical picture is consistent with possible IFI.[197] Diffuse pulmonary infiltrates are more commonly associated with respiratory viral pathogens, PJP, or CMV than with molds. However, the incidence of PJP and CMV pneumonia during the early postengraftment period has decreased significantly with widespread use of PJP prophylaxis and preemptive therapy for CMV.[295,361] Gastrointestinal GVHD is a common cause of diarrhea during the early postengraftment period but is clinically indistinguishable from and may coexist with common enteric pathogens including CMV, adenovirus, norovirus, enteropathogenic *E. coli*, and *C. difficile*.[362,363] In addition to testing of stool for enteric pathogens, endoscopy with biopsy is often necessary to distinguish GVHD from colitis due to CMV or adenovirus. This is particularly important because the treatment of GVHD requires the addition of immunosuppressive agents,[364] whereas the treatment of CMV or adenovirus colitis includes decreasing immunosuppression.[365]

GVHD is also one of the most common causes of hepatic abnormalities (usually detected by routine labs) in the first 3 months after transplant, but the differential diagnosis is broad and includes infectious etiologies such as viruses and disseminated candidiasis with hepatosplenic involvement.[366] Hepatic sinusoidal obstruction syndrome (veno-occlusive disease) typically presents within the first month after transplant.[367] Reactivation of hepatitis B virus (HBV) can occur in patients with serologic evidence of past infection who are not administered antiviral prophylaxis posttransplant.[368] BK polyomavirus and adenovirus infections are most commonly implicated in the development of postengraftment hemorrhagic cystitis.[369-371] The risk of BK virus–associated hemorrhagic cystitis increases with the use of myeloablative regimens, grafts that are HLA donor mismatched or

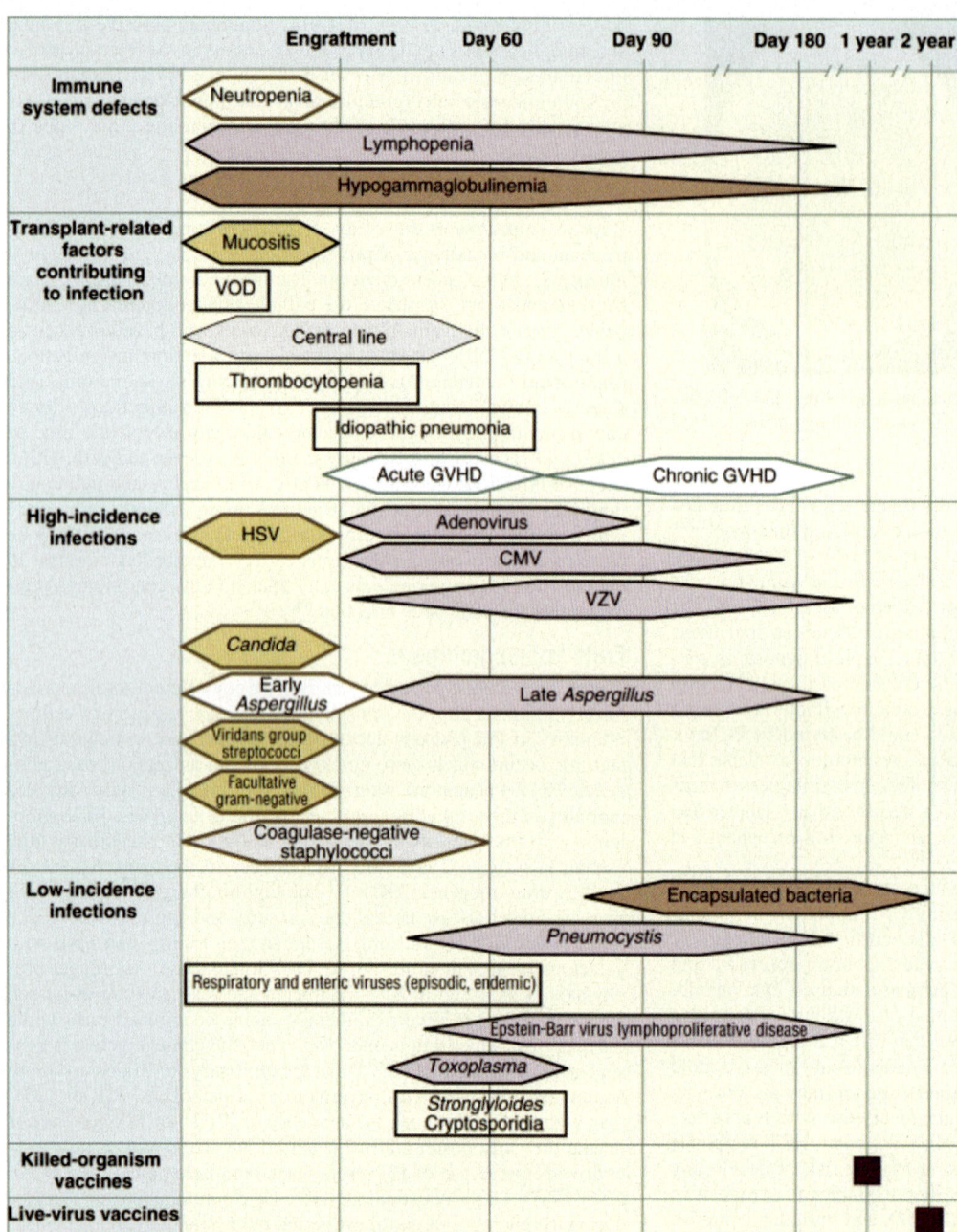

FIGURE 70.7 Phases of predictable immune suppression and timing of common opportunistic infections among allogeneic hematopoietic cell transplant recipients. CMV, cytomegalovirus; GVHD, graft-vs-host disease; HSV, herpes simplex virus; VOD, veno-occlusive disease; VZV, varicella-zoster virus. (Reprinted from Freifeld AG, Kaul DR. Infection in the patient with cancer. In: Niederhuber JE, Armitage JO, Doroshow JH et al, eds. *Abeloff's Clinical Oncology*. 5th ed. Churchill Livingstone; 2014:562-580.e5. Copyright © 2014 Elsevier. With permission.)

from haploidentical donors or umbilical cord blood,[372,373] and alemtuzumab as part of the conditioning regimen.[374]

Reactivation of latent herpes viruses is most common during the early postengraftment period. The incidence of HSV and VZV reactivation has been reduced by antiviral (e.g., acyclovir) prophylaxis.[375,376] Preemptive and prophylaxis strategies have also decreased the risk of CMV disease, as outlined earlier in this chapter. Epstein-Barr virus (EBV) reactivation is common after engraftment in allogeneic HCT recipients, particularly those who received T-cell depleted transplants, and may lead to posttransplant lymphoproliferative disorders (PTLDs).[377] HHV-6 reactivation is very common early after engraftment in allogeneic HCT recipients, but only a small minority of these patients will progress to develop HHV-6 encephalitis. Confusion, altered mental status, memory disturbance, or other neurologic findings early after engraftment should raise concern for the possibility of HHV-6 encephalitis. Reactivation of adenovirus or primary infection can also occur after engraftment, with clinical manifestations ranging from asymptomatic viremia to disseminated disease with multiorgan system involvement.[378] Treatment of adenovirus infection after HCT consists of antiviral therapy with cidofovir and adenovirus-specific T-cell therapy, where available, but mortality rates with disseminated disease are high.[379,380]

Toxoplasmosis most commonly presents within the first 3 months after allogeneic HCT.[350] It can present as brain abscesses, pneumonitis, or as disseminated disease and the diagnosis is typically made by histologic confirmation of biopsied tissue or PCR testing. Risk factors for posttransplant toxoplasmosis include prior exposure based on pretransplant seropositivity, T-cell depletion, and lack of prophylaxis with TMP-SMX.[381] Another parasitic infection to consider in HCT recipients is *Strongyloides stercoralis*. Immunocompromised HCT recipients with prior *S. stercoralis* infection can develop hyperinfection and life-threatening disseminated disease in the setting of immunosuppression.[382] HCT candidates who are from endemic areas should be screened for serologic evidence of infection and empirically treated with ivermectin prior to their transplant in the setting of a positive test result or unexplained eosinophilia.

Late Postengraftment

The late postengraftment period has no exact endpoint and may extend up to 6 to 12 months after autologous transplant and up to 1 to 2 years after allogeneic transplant, during which B- and T-cell immunity continues to recover.[383] Use of rituximab or glucocorticoids may delay recovery of B- and T-cell subsets, respectively. cGVHD, CMV serostatus (donor-negative, recipient-positive), and use of radiation with conditioning are risk factors for the development of late bacterial, fungal, and viral infections. Infectious complications account for a majority of the long-term mortality seen after HCT.[384] Encapsulated organisms such as pneumococcus are common pathogens in the last postengraftment period, causing respiratory, bloodstream, or CNS infections.[385] The presence of cGVHD increases the risk of developing late IFIs.[207,383] Allogeneic HCT recipients are also at risk of developing EBV-related PTLD in the late postengraftment phase, particularly in patients whose graft has been T-cell depleted.[386] Late onset of VZV infection is common in both autologous and allogeneic HCT recipients, often coinciding with discontinuation of antiviral prophylaxis. In one study, VZV was the most common late postengraftment infection.[384] In addition to opportunistic infections, HCT recipients are also vulnerable to developing severe manifestations of common causes of community-acquired infections.

PREVENTION OF INFECTION

Infection Prevention Practices

Effective infection control measures can reduce the exposure of patients with hematologic malignancies and HCT recipients to nosocomial pathogens. Transmission of pathogens from one patient to another is directly linked to the healthcare worker's hands and is reduced with the use of soap and water or alcohol-based sanitizers.[387] Standard (universal) precautions to prevent transmission of nosocomial pathogens include hand hygiene and use of appropriate personal protective equipment (e.g., gloves, surgical masks or eye protection, gowns) during procedures that are likely to generate splashes of body fluid, secretions, or cause soiling of clothing.[388] For patients infected with SARS-CoV-2, use of properly fitted N95 respirators may further decrease the risk of viral transmission compared to the use of surgical masks.[389] Daily bathing of patients with chlorhexidine-impregnated washcloths may further reduce the risk of hospital-acquired infections.[390]

For allogeneic HCT patients, the American Society for Transplantation and Cellular Therapy (ASTCT) recommends using single-occupancy patient rooms, high efficiency particulate air filters, directed airflow, positive air pressure rooms, and self-closing doors to minimize exposure of at-risk patients to other nosocomial pathogens or environmental molds or spores.[383] Patient rooms on transplant units should be cleaned daily, with a focus on preventing the accumulation of dust. Plants and flowers should not be allowed on transplant units to reduce exposure to molds and bacteria. In addition, if constructions or renovations are performed, intensive strategies should be implemented to minimize the amount of fungal spores in patient rooms. Excavations adjacent to a hospital have been linked to increased rates of IFIs,[391] and hospital construction guidelines recommend sealed windows in transplant units to limit external exposures.[383] Frequently used among hospitalized hematology patients, the "neutropenic diet" limits intake of raw food (e.g., fruits, vegetables), some soft cheeses, and certain animal products.[392] However, data to support the efficacy of this diet are limited. Pediatric patients randomized to the neutropenic diet or the FDA Safe Food Guideline handout (for one cycle of chemotherapy) saw no difference between the two dietary strategies for infection prevention.[393]

Prophylaxis to Reduce Infection Risks

Antibacterial

Patients who develop prolonged chemotherapy-induced neutropenia are at high risk of bacterial infections,[5] and strategies are needed to prevent these infections (*Table 70.4*). A randomized trial of 760 adult patients who were expected to have chemotherapy-induced neutropenia for >7 days found that levofloxacin decreased the risk of fever and neutropenia, bacteremia, and microbiologically documented infections compared to placebo.[400] Another randomized trial in patients with solid tumors and lymphoma identified lower rates of febrile episodes and hospitalization with levofloxacin compared to placebo.[401] Although neither randomized trial demonstrated a statistically significant mortality benefit, a systematic review found that antibacterial prophylaxis significantly reduced all-cause mortality by 34%.[402] These benefits must be balanced against the potential for adverse effects of fluoroquinolones and the potential for selecting for infections due to viridans group streptococci and ESBL-E.[56,403,404] Based on these considerations, ASCO, IDSA, NCCN, and ASTCT all recommend consideration of fluoroquinolone prophylaxis during neutropenia for patients who are expected to have prolonged chemotherapy-induced neutropenia, including most patients being treated for MDS or AML and patients receiving HCT with myeloablative conditioning regimens.[40,69,394] Allogeneic HCT recipients with cGVHD are at high risk of developing serious infections due to encapsulated bacteria, with pneumococcus being the most common pathogen.[405] In addition to pneumococcal vaccination, antibacterial prophylaxis with penicillin has been recommended in such patients to prevent pneumococcal infections.[383]

Antifungal

Prior to routine antifungal prophylaxis (*Table 70.4*), patients with hematologic malignancies and HCT recipients with prolonged fever and neutropenia frequently had IFIs diagnosed postmortem.[406] *Candida* spp. were the most common etiologies of IFI,[406] frequently causing catheter-related infections or bloodstream infections after translocation from the gastrointestinal tract in neutropenic patients.[407] In a randomized, placebo-controlled trial, fluconazole was shown to decrease the risk of invasive candidiasis and any IFI when administered during neutropenia in both autologous and allogeneic HCT recipients.[408] In a subsequent randomized placebo-controlled trial in mostly allogeneic HCT recipients, fluconazole was administered for 75 days after transplant and was found to not only decrease the risk of invasive candidiasis and IFI, but also decrease mortality.[409,410] Based on these trials, plus an additional trial in patients with acute leukemia,[411] fluconazole prophylaxis became the standard of care in HCT recipients and patients with acute leukemia. However, with adoption of fluconazole prophylaxis, which does not prevent mold infections, IA replaced invasive candidiasis as the most common IFI in HCT recipients.[412] Two subsequent randomized placebo-controlled trials of the mold-active antifungal agent posaconazole were conducted in patient populations at high risk of IA. The first trial was conducted in patients with AML and MDS who were receiving induction chemotherapy and found that posaconazole decreased the risk of IFI and increased survival compared to fluconazole or itraconazole.[395] Posaconazole is now the recommended prophylactic antifungal agent in this population.[69] The second trial was conducted in allogeneic HCT recipients with GVHD who were being treated with corticosteroids and found that posaconazole decreased the risk of IFI compared to fluconazole.[397] Although posaconazole is now recommended in allogeneic HCT recipients at high risk of IA,[396] such as patients receiving corticosteroids for GVHD, mold-active prophylaxis may not be necessary in all patients receiving an allogeneic HCT. A randomized trial of voriconazole vs fluconazole prophylaxis for 100 days after allogeneic HCT did not identify significant differences in IFI or survival in the setting of a structured fungal screening program using serial serum galactomannan tests.[413] Thus, fluconazole is a recommended prophylactic agent in allogeneic HCT recipients at low risk of IA.[69,396] Adverse reactions of the mold active azoles include hallucinations, liver function test abnormalities, QTc prolongation, and drug interactions via CYP3A4 inhibition, which require close drug monitoring of concomitant immunosuppressive therapies. Isavuconazole has activity against *Aspergillus* and *Mucorales* spp. with a favorable side effect profile, but data on prophylaxis are limited.[414] The echinocandins

Table 70.4. Prophylaxis of Infections in Hematopoietic Stem Cell Transplant Recipients and Hematologic Cancer Patients

Prophylaxis	Indication	Agent[a]	Duration/Comments
Bacteria			
Antibacterial prophylaxis[40,394]	Patients who are expected to be neutropenic for ≥7 d	Levofloxacin (cefpodoxime may be used for those allergic or intolerant of fluoroquinolones)	Start when ANC < 1×10^9/L and continue until resolution of neutropenia
Pneumococcal prophylaxis[383]	Allogeneic HCT recipients with chronic GVHD	Penicillin is the drug of choice. Alternatives include second-generation cephalosporins, macrolides, TMP-SMX, and fluoroquinolones.	Pneumococcal vaccination is also recommended.
Fungi			
Antifungal prophylaxis	Induction therapy for AML or MDS[69,395]	Posaconazole is the drug of choice if high risk for aspergillosis. Alternatives include voriconazole or an echinocandin (may choose to use fluconazole prophylaxis if risk of aspergillosis is low)	Begin with initiation of chemotherapy and continue until resolution of neutropenia. Azoles are cytochrome P-450 enzyme inhibitors and can decrease the metabolism of some chemotherapeutic agents and immunosuppressive medications.
	ALL[69]	Fluconazole[b] or an echinocandin.	Continue prophylaxis for duration of neutropenia.
	Autologous HCT recipients[69,396]	Fluconazole[b] or echinocandin	Continue prophylaxis for duration of neutropenia.
	Allogeneic HCT recipients: Low risk[69,396]	Fluconazole[b] or echinocandin	Continue prophylaxis through day 75 after transplant
	Allogeneic HCT recipients: High risk[c,396,397]	Posaconazole is the drug of choice. Alternatives include voriconazole or an echinocandin.	Continue prophylaxis through day 75 after transplant and beyond if ongoing risk factors such as GVHD
Pneumocystis jirovecii prophylaxis[40,383]	ALL, allogeneic HCT recipients, patients receiving alemtuzumab, fludarabine, corticosteroids (≥20 mg of prednisone equivalent for ≥1 mo) with other immunosuppression, or temozolomide with radiation therapy	TMP-SMX is drug of choice. Alternatives include dapsone, atovaquone, or inhaled pentamidine.	In allogeneic HCT, continue for at least 6 months and longer if remain on immunosuppressive therapy. In patients treated with alemtuzumab, continue prophylaxis for 2 mo. after the last dose or until the CD4 count is >200 cells/mm^3.
Viruses			
Prophylaxis for HSV[40,383]	HSV-seropositive HCT recipients or patients with acute leukemia receiving induction chemotherapy. Patients treated with alemtuzumab	Acyclovir or valacyclovir	Continue prophylaxis until engraftment and resolution of mucositis or through day 30. In patients treated with alemtuzumab, continue prophylaxis for 2 mo. after the last dose or until the CD4 count is >200 cells/mm^3.
Prophylaxis for VZV[69,383,398]	HCT recipients	Acyclovir or valacyclovir	Continue for 1 year after allogeneic HCT and for 6-12 mo after autologous HCT. Extend longer if remain on immunosuppressive therapy.
Prophylaxis and preemptive therapy for CMV[69,290,297]	Primary prophylaxis for allogeneic HCT recipients who are CMV-seropositive. Screening for viremia with preemptive therapy for: 1. Allogeneic HCT recipients who are CMV-seronegative, but whose donor(s) are CMV-seropositive 2. Autologous HCT recipients receiving a CD34-enriched autograft 3. Patients treated with alemtuzumab	Prophylaxis: Letermovir (surveillance for CMV viremia should still be performed despite use of prophylaxis) Preemptive therapy for detection of asymptomatic CMV viremia: Oral valganciclovir or intravenous ganciclovir. Foscarnet is an alternative. Continue therapy for at least 2 wk and until CMV viral load in blood undetectable.	Continue letermovir for primary prophylaxis for at least 100 d. CMV surveillance: 1. Allogeneic HCT recipients: once per week from the time of transplant until at least day 100. Patients who receive letermovir prophylaxis, have CMV infection, GVHD requiring high-dose prednisone, lymphopenia (<100 lymphocytes/mm^3), or lack CMV-specific T-cell immunity require prolonged surveillance after day 100. 2. Recipients of CD34-enriched autologous grafts: day 30 to day 100 and until the CD4$^+$ count is >100 cells/mm^3. 3. Alemtuzumab recipients: time of initiation until at least 2 mo after completion of therapy and until the CD4 count is >100 cells/mm^3.
Prophylaxis against HBV reactivation[399]	All patients receiving systemic anticancer therapy should be tested for HBV surface antigen (HBsAg), core antibody (anti-HBc), and antibody to surface antigen. Patients have chronic infection if HBsAg-positive and prior infection if HBsAg-negative and anti-HBc-positive.	Chronic HBV: Entecavir or tenofovir Prior HBV: Entecavir of tenofovir if receive anti-CD20 monoclonal antibodies or HCT Prior HBV: other therapies: HBsAg and ALT testing every 3 mo	Continue prophylaxis for a minimum of 12 mo after completion of therapy. HBV DNA should be measured at baseline and followed every 6 mo during antiviral therapy.

Abbreviations: ALL, acute lymphoblastic leukemia; AML, acute myeloid leukemia; ANC, absolute neutrophil count; CMV, cytomegalovirus; DS, double strength; GVHD, graft-vs-host disease; HBV, hepatitis B virus; HCT, hematopoietic cell transplant; HSV, herpes simplex virus; MDS, myelodysplastic syndrome; PCR, polymerase chain reaction; TMP-SMX, trimethoprim-sulfamethoxazole; VZV, varicella-zoster virus.

Adapted from the NCCN Clinical Practice Guidelines in Oncology. Prevention and Treatment of Cancer-Related Infection. NCCN. Version 1.2018 and the clinical practice guideline for the use of antimicrobial agents in neutropenic patients with cancer: 2011 update by the Infectious Diseases Society of America (IDSA).

[a]Recommended dosages of prophylactic oral agents in adults, assuming normal kidney function: acyclovir: 400 mg three times daily or 800 mg twice daily; atovaquone: 1500 mg daily; cefpodoxime: 200 mg twice daily; dapsone: 100 mg daily; letermovir: 480 mg daily (240 mg if also receiving cyclosporine); levofloxacin: 500 mg daily; posaconazole: 300 mg daily (after loading dose of 300 mg twice daily for 1 day); TMP-SMX: 1 double strength tablet (TMP 160 mg + SMX 800) daily or 3 days per week; valacyclovir: 500 mg twice daily; valganciclovir: 900 mg twice daily (induction) or 900 mg daily (maintenance).

[b]Fluconazole is effective as prophylaxis against candidiasis, but not against mold infections. If prophylactic fluconazole is used in patients with prolonged neutropenia, a strategy of empirical modification to a mold-active drug in patients with persistent fever despite antibacterial therapy should be considered.

[c]Allogeneic HCT recipients who are at high risk of invasive aspergillosis include patients with a pretransplant history of invasive aspergillosis, use of a graft from an HLA-mismatched, haploidentical, or cord blood donor, prior prolonged neutropenia, GVHD, and receipt of corticosteroid therapy (>1 mg/kg/d prednisone equivalent).

are administered intravenously and can be used as an alternative for antifungal prophylaxis when azole-related toxicities are of concern. They have broad activity against *Candida* spp. but are only fungistatic against *Aspergillus* spp., and do not have activity against most other molds.[415]

The efficacy of TMP-SMX for the prevention of PJP was established more than 4 decades ago.[416] Patients receiving induction and maintenance therapy for ALL,[204] allogeneic HCT,[207] alemtuzumab,[210] or high-dose glucocorticoids (at least 20 mg of prednisone daily for 4 weeks or greater) are at highest risk for PJP.[205] Prophylaxis is recommended for the duration of therapy for ALL, for at least 6 months following allogeneic HCT, and for at least 2 months following the last dose of alemtuzumab,[69] but the patient profile at risk for PJP is continually evolving and there are increased reports of opportunistic infections with targeted therapies.[27,155,209] For patients intolerant or allergic to TMP-SMX, dapsone may be used after screening for G6PD deficiency.[417] Atovaquone and inhaled pentamidine are additional options for PJP prophylaxis.

Antiviral

The risk of reactivation of herpes viruses correlates with the degree of suppression of cellular immunity and is particularly common after allogeneic HCT.[418] However, HSV reactivation is also common in seropositive patients during induction therapy for acute leukemia.[419] Acyclovir prophylaxis was shown to be effective in reducing HSV reactivation in seropositive patients in a randomized trial,[420] and IDSA/ASCO guidelines support the use of prophylactic acyclovir (or valacyclovir) during induction chemotherapy for acute leukemia[40] (Table 70.4). Acyclovir prophylaxis was also shown to be effective in seropositive HCT recipients,[421] and acyclovir or valacyclovir prophylaxis is also recommended in seropositive autologous and allogenic HCT recipients.[40,383] VZV reactivation is also common after HCT.[422] Acyclovir prophylaxis for 1 year after allogeneic HCT was found to decrease the risk of VZV infection by 84% compared to placebo in a randomized trial.[398] Extended acyclovir or valacyclovir prophylaxis for up to 1 year is now recommended in HCT recipients, with consideration of extending the prophylaxis for allogeneic HCT recipients who remain on immunosuppressive therapy.[69,383] Alemtuzumab causes significant and prolonged T-cell suppression requiring antiviral prophylaxis for several months following completion of therapy.[423] VZV reactivation is less common outside of the transplant setting, and prophylaxis is usually not required. An exception is the increased risk of herpes zoster in patients with multiple myeloma who are treated with proteasome inhibitors, specifically bortezomib.[424,425] Acyclovir prophylaxis decreases the risk of shingles in patients with multiple myeloma who are treated with bortezomib.[426] Similar increases in the risk of VZV infection have been observed in trials of other proteasome inhibitors (carfilzomib and ixazomib),[427] and thus, acyclovir or valacyclovir prophylaxis is indicated to prevent VZV infection in patients who receive any proteasome inhibitor.

CMV reactivation is common after allogeneic HCT with the greatest risk in CMV-seropositive recipients.[293] Letermovir prophylaxis is recommended for CMV-seropositive allogeneic HCT recipients.[290] Letermovir is well tolerated and in a randomized trial it reduced CMV infection and all-cause mortality at week 24 posttransplant.[297] It can be given orally and has widely replaced valganciclovir for primary CMV prophylaxis. However, it has no HSV or VZV activity, requiring it to be coadministered with acyclovir or valacyclovir.[428] Serial surveillance for CMV reactivation with preemptive therapy for reactivation is an alternate strategy and typically used for CMV-seronegative recipients who receive CMV-seropositive grafts. CMV prophylaxis is not typically warranted in autologous HCT recipients or other patients with hematologic malignancies.

HBV persists in the body despite viral clearance and serologic recovery. Previously infected patients can reactivate the virus when receiving immunosuppressive therapies, and this can lead to fulminant hepatitis and even death.[429] Patients initiating therapies for hematologic malignancies should be screened for chronic or past infection with HBV by evaluating for HBV surface antigen (HBsAg) and for core (anti-HBc) and surface antigen antibodies.[399] Those found to have chronic infection (HBsAg-positive) should begin treatment with entecavir or tenofovir for at least 1 year after completion of their anticancer therapy.[399,430] These antivirals are preferred to lamivudine because they have a higher barrier to resistance.[431] For patients found to have past infection (HBsAg-negative, anti-HBC-positive), the need for antiviral prophylaxis to prevent reactivation depends on the therapies used for their malignancy.[399] Antiviral prophylaxis is recommended for patients receiving anti-CD20 antibody therapy (e.g., rituximab) and patients undergoing HCT. Other patients with past infection should be followed carefully to detect HBV reactivation during treatment for their malignancy, including HBsAg and ALT testing every 3 months, with subsequent HBV DNA testing if these tests suggest reactivation. Antiviral therapy would then be indicated if the patient becomes HBsAg-positive or develops significant viremia.

Immunization

Immunizations are an important part of a comprehensive strategy to decrease the risks of infection in immunocompromised hosts. Depending on the immune status of the patient, patients with hematologic malignancies may be less likely to mount a protective immune response to vaccines compared to immunocompetent patients.[432] Furthermore, live vaccines (e.g., measles-mumps-rubella vaccine) are generally avoided in patients receiving ongoing immunosuppressive therapies.[383,432] SARS-CoV-2 vaccines were previously discussed in this chapter. Patients with hematologic malignancies and their household contacts should receive annual influenza vaccination with an inactivated vaccine.[69,432] Immune responses may be low in patients receiving intensive chemotherapy or those who have received anti-CD20 therapies in the previous 6 months, and individualized decision-making is necessary in regard to the timing of influenza vaccine in such patients.[432] New pneumococcal conjugate vaccines (PCVs) that cover additional serotypes compared to prior versions became available in 2021, including a 20-valent vaccine (PCV20) and a 15-valent vaccine (PCV15).[433] Updated recommendations in patients with hematologic malignancies are to administer one dose of PCV20 or one dose of PCV15 followed by a dose of the 23-valent polysaccharide vaccine (PPSV23) 1 year later. A shorter time interval (≥8 weeks) between the PCV15 and PPSV23 vaccines is indicated in high-risk patients. There are no current recommendations to administer the new conjugate vaccine to those who previously received the 13-valent vaccine (PCV13). The live attenuated VZV vaccine has now been replaced by a recombinant VZV vaccine that is more effective and safer in immunocompromised hosts because it is not a live virus vaccine.[434,435] In a randomized trial in patients with hematologic malignancies, this recombinant VZV vaccine yielded robust and persistent humoral and cell-mediated immune responses and resulted in an 87% reduction in the incidence of herpes zoster infection compared to placebo.[436] Local adverse effects such as pain and erythema at the injection site were common with the vaccine, but no serious safety concerns were identified. Two doses of the recombinant VZV vaccine are now recommended in all immunocompromised adults who have a history of prior varicella infection or vaccination, not just those >50 years old.[437]

HCT recipients have unique immunization considerations because they may enter the transplant with protective antibody responses toward organisms against which they were previously vaccinated but lose this protection after their transplant.[438-440] Thus, they should be reimmunized against these pathogens once they are likely to mount an immune response. It is generally recommended that HCT recipients initiate vaccination series against tetanus, diphtheria, and pertussis, poliovirus, *H. influenzae* type B, and HBV 6 to 12 months after their transplant.[383,432] PCV13, PCV15, or PCV20 may be administered as a three-dose series at 1-month intervals starting 3 to 6 months after transplant, followed by a dose of PPSV23 for those who received the PCV13 or PCV15 vaccine series at 12 months in patients without GVHD. Two doses of the recombinant VZV vaccine are recommended in autologous HCT recipients starting at 50 to 70 days after the transplant. This regimen was found to decrease the incidence of herpes zoster by 68% compared to placebo and decrease other zoster-associated complications, such as postherpetic neuralgia.[435]

SUMMARY

The prognosis of patients with hematologic malignancies has markedly improved following the understanding of molecular pathogenesis and the development of novel therapies. Part of the progress, however, can be attributed to better infectious diseases supportive care, with improved strategies to prevent, diagnose, and treat infectious complications. Appropriate management to deliver the optimal patient care frequently requires consultation from infectious diseases, pulmonary/critical care, gastroenterology, surgery, radiology, and pharmacists. This chapter provides an overview of some of the most common infectious complications encountered in hematologic neoplasms. For further guidance on these increasingly nuanced issues, the reader is directed to the following societal guidelines for review.

WEBSITE RESOURCES

National Comprehensive Cancer Network (NCCN) Guidelines for Supportive Care: www.nccn.org
American Society of Clinical Oncology (ASCO) Supportive Care and Treatment Related Issues: www.asco.org
European Society for Medical Oncology (ESMO) Management of Febrile Neutropaenia: www.esmo.org
Infectious Diseases Society of America (IDSA) Fever and Neutropenia in Adults with Cancer: www.idsociety.org

References

1. Donnelly JP, Blijlevens NMA, van der Velden WJ. Infections in the immunocompromised host: general principles. In: Bennett JE, Dolin R, Blaser MJ, eds. *Mandell, Douglas, and Bennett's Principles and Practice of Infectious Diseases*. Updated Edition. Elsevier; 2015:3384.e4-3394.e4.
2. Witko-Sarsat V, Rieu P, Descamps-Latscha B, Lesavre P, Halbwachs-Mecarelli L. Neutrophils: molecules, functions and pathophysiological aspects. *Lab Invest*. 2000;80(5):617.
3. Silvestre-Roig C, Hidalgo A, Soehnlein O. Neutrophil heterogeneity: implications for homeostasis and pathogenesis. *Blood*. 2016;127(18):2173-2181.
4. Freifeld AG, Bow EJ, Sepkowitz KA, et al. Clinical practice guideline for the use of antimicrobial agents in neutropenic patients with cancer: 2010 update by the Infectious Diseases Society of America. *Clin Infect Dis*. 2011;52(4):e56-e93.
5. Bodey GP, Buckley M, Sathe YS, Freireich EJ. Quantitative relationships between circulating leukocytes and infection in patients with acute leukemia. *Ann Intern Med*. 1966;64(2):328-340.
6. Sickles EA, Greene WH, Wiernik PH. Clinical presentation of infection in granulocytopenic patients. *Arch Intern Med*. 1975;135(5):715-719.
7. Zhang D, Loughran TP. Large granular lymphocytic leukemia: molecular pathogenesis, clinical manifestations, and treatment. *Hematology Am Soc Hematol Educ Program*. 2012;2012(1):652-659.
8. Pomeroy C, Oken MM, Rydell RE, Filice GA. Infection in the myelodysplastic syndromes. *Am J Med*. 1991;90(3):338-344.
9. Boogaerts MA, Nelissen V, Roelant C, Goossens W. Blood neutrophil function in primary myelodysplastic syndromes. *Br J Haematol*. 1983;55(2):217-227.
10. Olofsson T, Odeberg H, Olsson I. Granulocyte function in chronic granulocytic leukemia. II. Bactericidal capacity, phagocytic rate, oxygen consumption, and granule protein composition in isolated granulocytes. *Blood*. 1976;48(4):581-593.
11. Oksenhendler E, Gérard L, Fieschi C, et al. Infections in 252 patients with common variable immunodeficiency. *Clin Infect Dis*. 2008;46(10):1547-1554.
12. Kainulainen L, Vuorinen T, Rantakokko-Jalava K, Osterback R, Ruuskanen O. Recurrent and persistent respiratory tract viral infections in patients with primary hypogammaglobulinemia. *J Allergy Clin Immunol*. 2010;126(1):120-126.
13. Ravandi F, O'Brien S. Immune defects in patients with chronic lymphocytic leukemia. *Cancer Immunol Immunother*. 2006;55(2):197-209.
14. Pratt G, Goodyear O, Moss P. Immunodeficiency and immunotherapy in multiple myeloma. *Br J Haematol*. 2007;138(5):563-579.
15. Di Sabatino A, Carsetti R, Corazza GR. Post-splenectomy and hyposplenic states. *Lancet*. 2011;378(9785):86-97.
16. Theilacker C, Ludewig K, Serr A, et al. Overwhelming postsplenectomy infection: a prospective multicenter cohort study. *Clin Infect Dis*. 2016;62(7):871-878.
17. Cuthbert RJ, Iqbal A, Gates A, Toghill PJ, Russell NH. Functional hyposplenism following allogeneic bone marrow transplantation. *J Clin Pathol*. 1995;48(3):257-259.
18. Pescovitz MD, Torgerson TR, Ochs HD, et al. Effect of rituximab on human in vivo antibody immune responses. *J Allergy Clin Immunol*. 2011;128(6):1295-1302.e5.
19. Rao A, Kelly M, Musselman M, et al. Safety, efficacy, and immune reconstitution after rituximab therapy in pediatric patients with chronic or refractory hematologic autoimmune cytopenias. *Pediatr Blood Cancer*. 2008;50(4):822-825.
20. Reinwald M, Silva JT, Mueller NJ, et al. ESCMID Study Group for Infections in Compromised Hosts (ESGICH) Consensus Document on the safety of targeted and biological therapies: an infectious diseases perspective (Intracellular signaling pathways – tyrosine kinase and mTOR inhibitors). *Clin Microbiol Infect*. 2018;24(suppl 2):S53-S70.
21. Heath WR, Carbone FR. Dendritic cell subsets in primary and secondary T cell responses at body surfaces. *Nat Immunol*. 2009;10(12):1237-1244.
22. Perkins JL, Harris A, Pozos TC. Immune dysfunction after completion of childhood leukemia therapy. *J Pediatr Hematol Oncol*. 2017;39(1):1-5.
23. Goswami M, Prince G, Biancotto A, et al. Impaired B cell immunity in acute myeloid leukemia patients after chemotherapy. *J Transl Med*. 2017;15(1):155.
24. Anaissie EJ, Kontoyiannis DP, O'Brien S, et al. Infections in patients with chronic lymphocytic leukemia treated with fludarabine. *Ann Intern Med*. 1998;129(7):559-566.
25. Morrison VA, Rai KR, Peterson BL, et al. Impact of therapy with chlorambucil, fludarabine, or fludarabine plus chlorambucil on infections in patients with chronic lymphocytic leukemia: Intergroup Study Cancer and Leukemia Group B 9011. *J Clin Oncol*. 2011;19(16):3611-3621.
26. Jones JA, Robak T, Brown JR, et al. Efficacy and safety of idelalisib in combination with ofatumumab for previously treated chronic lymphocytic leukaemia: an open-label, randomised phase 3 trial. *Lancet Haematol*. 2017;4(3):e114-e126.
27. Tillman BF, Pauff JM, Satyanarayana G, Talbott M, Warner JL. Systematic review of infectious events with the BTK inhibitor ibrutinib in the treatment of haematologic malignancies. *Eur J Haematol*. 2018;100(4):325-334.
28. Lundin J, Porwit-MacDonald A, Rossmann ED, et al. Cellular immune reconstitution after subcutaneous alemtuzumab (anti-CD52 monoclonal antibody, CAMPATH-1H) treatment as first-line therapy for B-cell chronic lymphocytic leukaemia. *Leukemia*. 2004;18(3):484-490.
29. Shillitoe B, Gennery A. X-Linked Agammaglobulinaemia: outcomes in the modern era. *Clin Immunol*. 2017;183:54-62.
30. Shearer WT, Dunn E, Notarangelo LD, et al. Establishing diagnostic criteria for severe combined immunodeficiency disease (SCID), leaky SCID, and Omenn syndrome: the Primary Immune Deficiency Treatment Consortium experience. *J Allergy Clin Immunol*. 2014;133(4):1092-1098.
31. Kuijpers TW, Nguyen M, Hopman CT, et al. Complement factor 7 gene mutations in relation to meningococcal infection and clinical recurrence of meningococcal disease. *Mol Immunol*. 2010;47(4):671-677.
32. Neth O, Hann I, Turner MW, Klein NJ. Deficiency of mannose-binding lectin and burden of infection in children with malignancy: a prospective study. *Lancet*. 2001;358(9282):614-618.
33. Dommett R, Chisholm J, Turner M, Bajaj-Elliott M, Klein NJ. Mannose-binding lectin genotype influences frequency and duration of infectious complications in children with malignancy. *J Pediatr Hematol Oncol*. 2013;35(1):69-75.
34. Klastersky J, Ameye L, Maertens J, et al. Bacteraemia in febrile neutropenic cancer patients. *Int J Antimicrob Agents*. 2007;30(suppl 1):S51-S59.
35. Mikulska M, Viscoli C, Orasch C, et al. Aetiology and resistance in bacteraemias among adult and paediatric haematology and cancer patients. *J Infect*. 2014;68(4):321-331.
36. Gudiol C, Bodro M, Simonetti A, et al. Changing aetiology, clinical features, antimicrobial resistance, and outcomes of bloodstream infection in neutropenic cancer patients. *Clin Microbiol Infect*. 2013;19(5):474-479.
37. Klastersky J, Paesmans M, Rubenstein EB, et al. The multinational association for supportive care in cancer risk index: a multinational scoring system for identifying low-risk febrile neutropenic cancer patients. *J Clin Oncol*. 2000;18(16):3038-3051.
38. Schimpff SC, Greene WH, Young VM, Wiernik PH. *Pseudomonas* septicemia: incidence, epidemiology, prevention and therapy in patients with advanced cancer. *Eur J Cancer*. 1973;9(6):449-455.
39. Pizzo PA. Management of fever in patients with cancer and treatment-induced neutropenia. *N Engl J Med*. 1993;328(18):1323-1332.
40. Taplitz RA, Kennedy EB, Bow EJ, et al. Outpatient management of fever and neutropenia in adults treated for malignancy: American Society of Clinical Oncology and Infectious Diseases Society of America Clinical Practice Guideline update. *J Clin Oncol*. 2018;36(14):1443-1453.
41. Klastersky J, de Naurois J, Rolston K, et al. Management of febrile neutropenia: ESMO clinical practice guidelines. *Ann Oncol*. 2016;27(suppl 5):v111-v118.
42. Rosa RG, Goldani LZ. Cohort study of the impact of time to antibiotic administration on mortality in patients with febrile neutropenia. *Antimicrob Agents Chemother*. 2014;58(7):3799-3803.
43. Klastersky J, Daneau D, Henri A, Cappel R, Hensgens C. Antibiotic combinations of gram-negative infections in patients with cancer. *Eur J Cancer*. 1973;9(6):407-415.
44. Pizzo PA, Hathorn JW, Hiemenz J, et al. A randomized trial comparing ceftazidime alone with combination antibiotic therapy in cancer patients with fever and neutropenia. *N Engl J Med*. 1986;315(9):552-558.
45. Leyland MJ, Bayston KF, Cohen J, et al. A comparative study of imipenem versus piperacillin plus gentamicin in the initial management of febrile neutropenic patients with haematological malignancies. *J Antimicrob Chemother*. 1992;30(6):843-854.
46. De Pauw BE, Deresinski SC, Feld R, Lane-Allman EF, Donnelly JP. Ceftazidime compared with piperacillin and tobramycin for the empiric treatment of fever in neutropenic patients with cancer. A multicenter randomized trial. The Intercontinental Antimicrobial Study Group. *Ann Intern Med*. 1994;120(10):834-844.
47. Cometta A, Calandra T, Gaya H, et al. Monotherapy with meropenem versus combination therapy with ceftazidime plus amikacin as empiric therapy for fever in granulocytopenic patients with cancer. The International Antimicrobial Therapy Cooperative Group of the European Organization for Research and Treatment of Cancer and the Gruppo Italiano Malattie Ematologiche Maligne dell'Adulto infection program. *Antimicrob Agents Chemother*. 1996;40(5):1108-1115.

48. Del Favero A, Menichetti F, Martino P, et al. A multicenter, double-blind, placebo-controlled trial comparing piperacillin-tazobactam with and without amikacin as empiric therapy for febrile neutropenia. *Clin Infect Dis*. 2001;33(8):1295-1301.
49. Furno P, Bucaneve G, Del Favero A. Monotherapy or aminoglycoside-containing combinations for empirical antibiotic treatment of febrile neutropenic patients: a meta-analysis. *Lancet Infect Dis*. 2002;2(4):231-242.
50. Paul M, Dickstein Y, Schlesinger A, et al. Beta-lactam versus beta-lactam-aminoglycoside combination therapy in cancer patients with neutropenia. *Cochrane Database Syst Rev*. 2013;6:CD003038.
51. Heinz WJ, Buchheidt D, Christopeit M, et al. Diagnosis and empirical treatment of fever of unknown origin (FUO) in adult neutropenic patients: guidelines of the Infectious Diseases Working Party (AGIHO) of the German Society of Hematology and Medical Oncology (DGHO). *Ann Hematol*. 2017;96(11):1775-1792.
52. Fritsche TR, Sader HS, Jones RN. Comparative activity and spectrum of broad-spectrum beta-lactams (cefepime, ceftazidime, ceftriaxone, piperacillin/tazobactam) tested against 12,295 staphylococci and streptococci—report from the SENTRY antimicrobial surveillance program (North America: 2001-2002). *Diagn Microbiol Infect Dis*. 2003;47(2):435-440.
53. Jones RN, Sader HS, Fritsche TR, Pottumarthy S. Comparisons of parenteral broad-spectrum cephalosporins tested against bacterial isolates from pediatric patients: report from the SENTRY Antimicrobial Surveillance Program (1998-2004). *Diagn Microbiol Infect Dis*. 2007;57(1):109-116.
54. Horita N, Shibata Y, Watanabe H, Namkoong H, Kaneko T. Comparison of antipseudomonal β-lactams for febrile neutropenia empiric therapy: systematic review and network meta-analysis. *Clin Microbiol Infect*. 2017;23(10):723-729.
55. Kang CI, Chung DR, Ko KS, Peck KR, Song JH; Korean Network for Study of Infectious Diseases. Risk factors for infection and treatment outcome of extended-spectrum-β-lactamase-producing *Escherichia coli* and *Klebsiella pneumoniae* in patients with hematologic malignancy. *Ann Hematol*. 2021;91(1):115-121.
56. Satlin MJ, Chavda KD, Baker TM, et al. Colonization with levofloxacin-resistant extended-spectrum-β-lactamase-producing Enterobacteriaceae and risk of bacteremia in hematopoietic stem cell transplant recipients. *Clin Infect Dis*. 2018;67(11):1720-1728.
57. Gyssens IC, Kern WV, Livermore DM. ECIL-4, a joint venture of EBMT, EORTC, ICHS and ESGICH of ESCMID. The role of antibiotic stewardship in limiting antibacterial resistance among hematology patients. *Haematologica*. 2013;98(12):1821-1825.
58. Beyar-Katz O, Dickstein Y, Borok S, Vidal L, Leibovici L, Paul M. Empirical antibiotics targeting gram-positive bacteria for the treatment of febrile neutropenic patients with cancer. *Cochrane Database Syst Rev*. 2017;6(6):CD003914.
59. Vardakas KZ, Samonis G, Chrysanthopoulou A, Bliziotis IA, Falagas ME. Role of glycopeptides as part of initial empirical treatment of febrile neutropenic patients: a meta-analysis of randomised controlled trials. *Lancet Infect Dis*. 2005;5(7):431-439.
60. Huang KHG, Cluzet V, Hamilton K, Fadugba O. The impact of reported beta-lactam allergy in hospitalized patients with hematologic malignancies requiring antibiotics. *Clin Infect Dis*. 2018;67(1):27-33.
61. Kula B, Djordjevic G, Robinson JL. A systematic review: can one prescribe carbapenems to patients with IgE-mediated allergy to penicillins or cephalosporins? *Clin Infect Dis*. 2014;59(8):1113-1122.
62. Silverman JA, Mortin LI, Vanpraagh ADG, Li T, Adler J. Inhibition of daptomycin by pulmonary surfactant: *in vitro* modeling and clinical impact. *J Infect Dis*. 2005;191(12):2149-2152.
63. Micek ST, Lloyd AE, Ritchie DJ, Reichley RM, Fraser VJ, Kollef MH. *Pseudomonas aeruginosa* bloodstream infection: importance of appropriate initial antimicrobial treatment. *Antimicrob Agents Chemother*. 2005;49(4):1306-1311.
64. Bow EJ, Rotstein C, Noskin GA, et al. A randomized, open-label, multicenter comparative study of the efficacy and safety of piperacillin-tazobactam and cefepime for the empirical treatment of febrile neutropenic episodes in patients with hematologic malignancies. *Clin Infect Dis*. 2006;43(4):447-459.
65. Elting LS, Lu C, Escalanate CP, et al. Outcomes and cost of outpatient or inpatient management of 712 patients with febrile neutropenia. *J Clin Oncol*. 2008;26(4):606-611.
66. Cometta A, Kern WV, De Bock R, et al. Vancomycin versus placebo for treating persistent fever in patients with neutropenic cancer receiving piperacillin-tazobactam monotherapy. *Clin Infect Dis*. 2003;37(3):382-389.
67. Aguilar-Guisado M, Espigado I, Martín-Peña A, et al. Optimisation of empirical antimicrobial therapy in patients with haematological malignancies and febrile neutropenia (How Long study): an open-label, randomised, controlled phase 4 trial. *Lancet Haematol*. 2017;4(12):e573-e583.
68. Averbuch D, Orasch C, Cordonnier C, et al. European guidelines for empirical antibacterial therapy for febrile neutropenic patients in the era of growing resistance: summary of the 2011 4th European Conference on Infections in Leukemia. *Haematologica*. 2013;98(12):1826-1835.
69. Baden LR, Swaminathan S, Angarone M, et al. Prevention and treatment of cancer-related infections, version 2.2016, NCCN Clinical Practice Guidelines in Oncology. *J Natl Compr Canc Netw*. 2016;14(7):882-913.
70. Bodey G, Bueltmann B, Duguid W, et al. Fungal infections in cancer patients: an international autopsy survey. *Eur J Clin Microbiol Infect Dis*. 1992;11(2):99-109.
71. Pizzo PA, Robichaud KJ, Gill FA, Witebsky FG. Empiric antibiotic and antifungal therapy for cancer patients with prolonged fever and granulocytopenia. *Am J Med*. 1982;72(1):101-111.
72. Walsh TJ, Pappas P, Winston DJ, et al. Voriconazole compared with liposomal amphotericin B for empirical antifungal therapy in patients with neutropenia and persistent fever. *N Engl J Med*. 2002;346(4):225-234.
73. Walsh TJ, Teppler H, Donowitz GR, et al. Caspofungin versus liposomal amphotericin B for empirical antifungal therapy in patients with persistent fever and neutropenia. *N Engl J Med*. 2004;351(14):1391-1402.
74. Walsh TJ, Finberg RW, Arndt C, et al. Liposomal amphotericin B for empirical therapy in patients with persistent fever and neutropenia. National Institute of Allergy and Infectious Diseases Mycoses Study Group. *N Engl J Med*. 1999;340(10):764-771.
75. Cordonnier C, Pautas C, Maury S, et al. Empirical versus preemptive antifungal therapy for high-risk, febrile, neutropenic patients: a randomized, controlled trial. *Clin Infect Dis*. 2009;48(8):1042-1051.
76. Smith TJ, Bohlke K, Lyman GH, et al. Recommendations for the use of WBC growth factors: American Society of clinical oncology clinical practice guideline update. *J Clin Oncol*. 2015;33(28):3199-3212.
77. Kuderer NM, Dale DC, Crawford J, Lyman GH. Impact of primary prophylaxis with granulocyte colony-stimulating factor on febrile neutropenia and mortality in adult cancer patients receiving chemotherapy: a systematic review. *J Clin Oncol*. 2007;25(21):3158-3167.
78. Sung L, Nathan PC, Alibhai SM, Tomlinson GA, Beyene J. Meta-analysis: effect of prophylactic hematopoietic colony-stimulating factors on mortality and outcomes of infection. *Ann Intern Med*. 2007;147(6):400-411.
79. Bohlius J, Herbst C, Reiser M, Schwarzer G, Engert A. Granulopoiesis-stimulating factors to prevent adverse effects in the treatment of malignant lymphoma. *Cochrane Database Syst Rev*. 2008;2008(4):CD003189.
80. Wang L, Baser O, Kutikova L, Page JH, Barron R. The impact of primary prophylaxis with granulocyte colony-stimulating factors on febrile neutropenia during chemotherapy: a systematic review and meta-analysis of randomized controlled trials. *Support Care Cancer*. 2015;23(11):3131-3140.
81. Hartmann LC, Tschetter LK, Habermann TM, et al. Granulocyte colony-stimulating factor in severe chemotherapy-induced afebrile neutropenia. *N Engl J Med*. 1997;336(25):1776-1780.
82. Mhaskar R, Clark OA, Lyman G, et al. Colony-stimulating factors for chemotherapy-induced febrile neutropenia. *Cochrane Database Syst Rev*. 2014;10:CD003039.
83. Estcourt LJ, Stanworth S, Doree C, et al. Granulocyte transfusions for preventing infections in people with neutropenia or neutrophil dysfunction. *Cochrane Database Syst Rev*. 2015;6:CD005341.
84. Price TH, Boeckh M, Harrison RW, et al. Efficacy of transfusion with granulocytes from G-CSF/dexamethasone-treated donors in neutropenic patients with infection. *Blood*. 2015;126(18):2153-2161.
85. Danai PA, Moss M, Mannino DM, Martin GS. The epidemiology of sepsis in patients with malignancy. *Chest*. 2006;129(6):1432-1440.
86. Baker TM, Satlin MJ. The growing threat of multidrug-resistant Gram-negative infections in patients with hematologic malignancies. *Leuk Lymphoma*. 2016;57(10):2245-2258.
87. Raad I, Chaftari AM. Advances in prevention and management of central line-associated bloodstream infections in patients with cancer. *Clin Infect Dis*. 2014;59(suppl 5):S340-S343.
88. Ryu BH, Lee SC, Kim M, et al. Impact of neutropenia on the clinical outcomes of *Staphylococcus aureus* bacteremia in patients with hematologic malignancies: a 10-year experience in a tertiary care hospital. *Eur J Clin Microbiol Infect Dis*. 2020;39(5):937-943.
89. See I, Freifeld AG, Magill SS. Causative organisms and associated antimicrobial resistance in healthcare-associated, central line-associated bloodstream infections form oncology settings, 2009-2012. *Clin Infect Dis*. 2016;62(10):1203-1209.
90. Holland T, Fowler VG, Shelburne SA. Invasive gram-positive bacterial infection in cancer patients. *Clin Infect Dis*. 2014;59(suppl 5):S331-S334.
91. Kim SH, Kim KH, Kim HB, et al. Outcome of vancomycin treatment in patients with methicillin-susceptible *Staphylococcus aureus* bacteremia. *Antimicrob Agents Chemother*. 2008;52(1):192-197.
92. Rybak MJ, Lomaestro BM, Rotschafer JC, et al. Vancomycin therapeutic guidelines: a summary of consensus recommendations from the Infectious Diseases Society of America, the American Society of Health-System Pharmacists, and the Society of Infectious Diseases Pharmacists. *Clin Infect Dis*. 2009;49(3):325-327.
93. Rybak MJ, Le J, Lodise TP, et al. Therapeutic monitoring of vancomycin for serious methicillin-resistant *Staphylococcus aureus* infections: a revised consensus guideline and review by the American Society of Health-System Pharmacists, the Infectious Diseases Society of America, the Pediatric Infectious Diseases Society, and the Society of Infectious Diseases Pharmacists. *Clin Infect Dis*. 2020;71(6):1361-1364.
94. Fowler VG, Jr, Boucher HW, Corey GR, et al. Daptomycin versus standard therapy for bacteremia and endocarditis caused by *Staphylococcus aureus*. *N Engl J Med*. 2006;355(7):653-665.
95. Stevens DL, Herr D, Lampiris H, Hunt JL, Batts DH, Hafkin B. Linezolid versus daptomycin for the treatment of methicillin-resistant *Staphylococcus aureus* infections. *Clin Infect Dis*. 2002;34(11):1481-1490.
96. Attassi K, Hershberger E, Alam R, Zervos MJ. Thrombocytopenia associated with linezolid therapy. *Clin Infect Dis*. 2002;34(5):695-698.
97. Jaksic B, Martinelli G, Perez-Oteyza J, Hartman CS, Leonard LB, Tack KJ. Efficacy and safety of linezolid compared with vancomycin in a randomized, double-blind study of febrile neutropenic patients with cancer. *Clin Infect Dis*. 2006;42(5):597-607.
98. Lawrence KR, Adra M, Gillman PK. Serotonin toxicity associated with the use of linezolid: a review of postmarketing data. *Clin Infect Dis*. 2006;42(11):1578-1583.
99. Goto M, Schweizer ML, Vaughan-Sarrazin MS, et al. Association of evidence-based care processes with mortality in *Staphylococcus aureus* bacteremia at Veterans Health Administration Hospitals, 2003-2014. *JAMA Intern Med*. 2017;177(10):1489-1497.

100. Bai AD, Showler A, Burry L, et al. Impact of infectious disease consultation on quality of care, mortality, and length of stay in *Staphylococcus aureus* bacteremia: results from a large multicenter cohort study. *Clin Infect Dis.* 2015;60(10):1451-1461.
101. Kern W, Kurrle E, Schmeiser T. Streptococcal bacteremia in adult patients with leukemia undergoing aggressive chemotherapy. A review of 55 cases. *Infection.* 1990;18(3):138-145.
102. Elting LS, Bodey GP, Keefe BH. Septicemia and shock syndrome due to viridans streptococci: a case-control study of predisposing factors. *Clin Infect Dis.* 1992;14(6):1201-1207.
103. Shelburne SA, IIIrd, Lasky RE, Sahasrabhojane P, Tarrand JT, Rolston KVI. Development and validation of a clinical model to predict the presence of β-lactam resistance in viridans group streptococci causing bacteremia in neutropenic cancer patients. *Clin Infect Dis.* 2014;59(2):223-230.
104. Vydra J, Shanley RM, George I, et al. Enterococcal bacteremia is associated with increased risk of mortality in recipients of allogeneic hematopoietic stem cell transplantation. *Clin Infect Dis.* 2012;55(6):764-770.
105. Satlin MJ, Soave R, Racanelli AC, et al. The emergence of vancomycin-resistant enterococcal bacteremia in hematopoietic stem cell transplant recipients. *Leuk Lymphoma.* 2014;55(12):2858-2865.
106. Satlin MJ, Nicolau DP, Humphries RM, et al. Development of daptomycin susceptibility breakpoints for *Enterococcus faecium* and revision of the breakpoints for other enterococcal species by the Clinical and Laboratory Standards Institute. *Clin Infect Dis.* 2020;70(6):1240-1246.
107. Gudiol C, Ayats J, Camoez M, et al. Increase in bloodstream infection due to vancomycin-susceptible *Enterococcus faecium* in cancer patients: risk factors, molecular epidemiology and outcomes. *PLoS One.* 2013;8(9):e74734.
108. Satlin MJ, Chen L, Douglass C, et al. Colonization with fluoroquinolone-resistant Enterobacterales decreases the effectiveness of fluoroquinolone prophylaxis in hematopoietic cell transplant recipients. *Clin Infect Dis.* 2021;73(7):1257-1265.
109. Gudiol C, Calatayud L, Garcia-Vidal C, et al. Bacteremia due to extended-spectrum beta-lactamase-producing *Escherichia coli* (ESBL-EC) in cancer patients: clinical features, risk factors, molecular epidemiology and outcome. *J Antimicrob Chemother.* 2010;65(2):333-341.
110. Cornejo-Juárez P, Pérez-Jiménez C, Silva-Sánchez J, et al. Molecular analysis and risk factors for *Escherichia coli* producing extended-spectrum β-lactamase bloodstream infection in hematologic malignancies. *PLoS One.* 2012;7(4):e35780.
111. Harris PNA, Tambyah PA, Lye DC, et al. Effect of piperacillin-tazobactam vs meropenem on 30-day mortality for patients with *E. coli* or *Klebsiella pneumoniae* bloodstream infection and ceftriaxone resistance: a randomized clinical trial. *JAMA.* 2018;320(10):984-994.
112. Lee NY, Lee CC, Huang WH, Tsui KC, Hsueh PR, Ko WC. Cefepime therapy for monomicrobial bacteremia caused by cefepime-susceptible extended-spectrum beta-lactamase-producing Enterobacteriaceae: MIC matters. *Clin Infect Dis.* 2013;56(4):488-495.
113. Trecarichi EM, Pagano L, Martino B, et al. Bloodstream infections caused by *Klebsiella pneumoniae* in onco-hematological patients: clinical impact of carbapenem resistance in a multicenter prospective survey. *Am J Hematol.* 2016;91(11):1076-1081.
114. Satlin MJ, Cohen N, Ma KC, et al. Bacteremia due to carbapenem-resistant Enterobacteriaceae in neutropenic patients with hematologic malignancies. *J Infect.* 2016;73(4):336-345.
115. Girmenia C, Rossolini GM, Piciocchi A, et al. Infections by carbapenem-resistant *Klebsiella pneumoniae* in SCT recipients: a nationwide retrospective survey from Italy. *Bone Marrow Transplant.* 2015;50(2):282-288.
116. Tamma PD, Aitken SL, Bonomo RA, Mathers AJ, van Duin D, Clancy CJ. Infectious Diseases Society of America guidance on the treatment of extended-spectrum β-lactamase producing Enterobacterales (ESBL-E), carbapenem-resistant Enterobacterales (CRE), and *Pseudomonas aeruginosa* with difficult-to-treat resistance (DTR-*P. aeruginosa*). *Clin Infect Dis.* 2021;72(7):e169-e183.
117. Van Duin D, Lok JJ, Earley M, et al. Colistin versus ceftazidime-avibactam in the treatment of infections due to carbapenem-resistant Enterobacteriaceae. *Clin Infect Dis.* 2018;66(2):163-171.
118. Wunderink RG, Giamarellos-Bourboulis EJ, Rahav G, et al. Effect and safety of meropenem-vaborbactam versus best-available therapy in patients with carbapenem-resistant Enterobacteriaceae infections: the TANGO II randomized clinical trial. *Infect Dis Ther.* 2018;7(4):439-455.
119. Motsch J, Murta de Oliveira C, Stus V, et al. RESTORE-IMI 1: a multicenter, randomized, double-blind trial comparing efficacy and safety of imipenem/relebactam vs colistin plus imipenem in patients with imipenem-nonsusceptible bacterial infections. *Clin Infect Dis.* 2020;70(9):1799-1808.
120. Trecarichi EM, Pagano L, Candoni A, et al. Current epidemiology and antimicrobial resistance data for bacterial bloodstream infections in patients with hematologic malignancies: an Italian multicentre prospective survey. *Clin Microbiol Infect.* 2015;21(4):337-343.
121. Greene SL, Su WP, Muller SA. Ecthyma gangrenosum: report of clinical, histopathologic, and bacteriologic aspects of eight cases. *J Am Acad Dermatol.* 1984;11(5, pt 1):781-787.
122. Sader HS, Flamm RK, Carvalhaes CG, Castanheira M. Antimicrobial susceptibility of *Pseudomonas aeruginosa* to ceftazidime-avibactam, ceftolozane-tazobactam, piperacillin-tazobactam, and meropenem stratified by U.S. census divisions: results from the 2017 INFORM Program. *Antimicrob Agents Chemother.* 2018;62(12):e01 5877-18.
123. Babich T, Naucler P, Valik JK, et al. Combination versus monotherapy as definitive treatment for *Pseudomonas aeruginosa* bacteremia: a multicentre retrospective observational cohort study. *J Antimicrob Chemother.* 2021;76(8):2172-2181.
124. Peña C, Suarez C, Ocampo-Sosa A, et al. Effect of adequate single-drug vs combination antimicrobial therapy on mortality in *Pseudomonas aeruginosa* bloodstream infections: a post hoc analysis of a prospective cohort. *Clin Infect Dis.* 2013;57(2):208-216.
125. Chamot E, El Amari EB, Rohner P, Van Delden C. Effectiveness of combination antimicrobial therapy for *Pseudomonas aeruginosa* bacteremia. *Antimicrob Agents Chemother.* 2013;47(9):2756-2764.
126. Lodise TP, Jr, Lomaestro B, Drusano GL. Piperacillin-tazobactam for *Pseudomonas aeruginosa* infection: clinical implications of an extended-infusion strategy. *Clin Infect Dis.* 2007;44(3):357-363.
127. Bauer KA, West JE, O'Brien JM, Goff DA. Extended-infusion cefepime reduces mortality in patients with *Pseudomonas aeruginosa* infections. *Antimicrob Agents Chemother.* 2013;57(7):2907-2912.
128. Dulhunty JM, Roberts JA, Davis JS, et al. A multicenter randomized trial of continuous versus intermittent β-lactam infusion in severe sepsis. *Am J Respir Crit Care Med.* 2015;192(11):1298-1305.
129. Abdul-Aziz MH, Sulaiman H, Mat-Nor MB, et al. Beta-lactam infusion in severe sepsis (BLISS): a prospective, two-centre, open-labelled randomised controlled trial of continuous versus intermittent beta-lactam infusion in critically ill patients with severe sepsis. *Intensive Care Med.* 2016;42(10):1535-1545.
130. Maki DG, Kluger DM, Crnich CJ. The risk of bloodstream infection in adults with different intravascular devices: a systematic review of 200 published prospective studies. *Mayo Clin Proc.* 2006;81(9):1159-1171.
131. Pronovost P, Needham D, Berenholtz S, et al. An intervention to decrease catheter-related bloodstream infections in the ICU. *N Engl J Med.* 2006;355(26):2725-2732.
132. See I, Iwamoto M, Allen-Bridson K, et al. Mucosal barrier injury laboratory-confirmed bloodstream infection: results from a field test of a new National Healthcare Safety Network definition. *Infect Control Hosp Epidemiol.* 2013;34(8):769-776.
133. Metzger KE, Rucker Y, Callaghan M, et al. The burden of mucosal barrier injury laboratory-confirmed bloodstream infection among hematology, oncology, and stem cell transplant patients. *Infect Control Hosp Epidemiol.* 2015;36(2):119-124.
134. See I, Soe MM, Epstein L, et al. Impact of removing mucosal barrier injury laboratory-confirmed bloodstream infections from central line-associated bloodstream infection rates in the National Healthcare Safety Network, 2014. *Am J Infect Control.* 2017;45(3):321-323.
135. Blot F, Nitenberg G, Chachaty E, et al. Diagnosis of catheter-related bacteraemia: a prospective comparison of the time to positivity of hub-blood versus peripheral-blood cultures. *Lancet.* 1999;354(9184):1071-1077.
136. Raad I, Hanna HA, Alakech B, et al. Differential time to positivity: a useful method for diagnosing catheter-related bloodstream infections. *Ann Intern Med.* 2004;140(1):18-25.
137. Mermel LA, Allon M, Bouza E, et al. Clinical practice guidelines for the diagnosis and management of intravascular catheter-related infection: 2009 update by the Infectious Diseases Society of America. *Clin Infect Dis.* 2009;49(1):1-45.
138. Cornely OA, Gachot B, Akan H, et al. Epidemiology and outcome of fungemia in a cancer cohort of the Infectious Diseases Group (IDG) of the European Organization for Research and Treatment of Cancer (EORTC 65031). *Clin Infect Dis.* 2015;61(3):324-331.
139. Kullberg BJ, Arendrup MC. Invasive candidiasis. *N Engl J Med.* 2015;373(15):1445-1456.
140. Hachem R, Hanna H, Kontoyiannis D, Jiang Y, Raad I. The changing epidemiology of invasive candidiasis: *Candida glabrata* and *Candida krusei* as the leading causes of candidemia in hematologic malignancy. *Cancer.* 2008;112(11):2493-2499.
141. Pagano L, Antinori A, Ammassari A, et al. Retrospective study of candidemia in patients with hematological malignancies. Clinical features, risk factors and outcome of 76 episodes. *Eur J Haematol.* 1999;63(2):77-85.
142. Pappas PG, Kauffman CA, Andes DR, et al. Clinical practice guideline for the management of candidiasis: 2016 update by the Infectious Diseases Society of America. *Clin Infect Dis.* 2016;62(4):e1-e50.
143. Reboli AC, Rotstein C, Pappas PG, et al. Anidulafungin versus fluconazole for invasive candidiasis. *N Engl J Med.* 2007;356(24):2472-2482.
144. Pfaller MA, Moet GJ, Messer SA, Jones RN, Castanheira M. *Candida* bloodstream infections: comparison of species distributions and antifungal resistance patterns in community-onset and nosocomial isolates in the SENTRY Antimicrobial Surveillance Program, 2008-2009. *Antimicrob Agents Chemother.* 2011;55(2):561-566.
145. Andes DR, Safdar N, Baddley JW, et al. Impact of treatment strategy on outcomes in patients with candidemia and other forms of invasive candidiasis: a patient-level quantitative review of randomized trials. *Clin Infect Dis.* 2012;54(8):1110-1122.
146. Kollef M, Micek S, Hampton N, Doherty JA, Kumar A. Septic shock attributed to *Candida* infection: importance of empiric therapy and source control. *Clin Infect Dis.* 2012;54(12):1739-1746.
147. Labelle AJ, Micek ST, Roubinian N, Kollef MH. Treatment-related risk factors for hospital mortality in *Candida* bloodstream infections. *Crit Care Med.* 2008;36(11):2967-2972.
148. Nucci M, Anaissie E. Revisiting the source of candidemia: skin or gut? *Clin Infect Dis.* 2001;33(12):1959-1967.
149. Breazzano MP, Bond JB, IIIrd, Bearelly S, et al. American Academy of Ophthalmology recommendations on screening for endogenous *Candida* endophthalmitis. *Ophthalmology.* 2022;129(1):73-76.
150. Kuderer NM, Dale DC, Crawford J, Cosler LE, Lyman GH. Mortality, morbidity, and cost associated with febrile neutropenia in adult cancer patients. *Cancer.* 2006;106(10):2258-2266.
151. Rosenow EC. Diffuse pulmonary infiltrates in the immunocompromised host. *Clin Chest Med.* 1990;11(1):55-64.

152. Collin BA, Ramphal R. Pneumonia in the compromised host including cancer patients and transplant patients. *Infect Dis Clin North Am.* 1998;12(3):781-805. xi.
153. Escuissato DL, Warszawiak D, Marchiori E. Differential diagnosis of diffuse alveolar haemorrhage in immunocompromised patients. *Curr Opin Infect Dis.* 2015;28(4):337-342.
154. Barr PM, Saylors GB, Spurgeon SE, et al. Phase 2 study of idelalisib and entospletinib: pneumonitis limits combination therapy in relapsed refractory CLL and NHL. *Blood.* 2016;127(20):2411-2415.
155. Ahn IE, Jerussi T, Farooqui M, et al. Atypical *Pneumocystis jirovecii* pneumonia in previously untreated patients with CLL on single-agent ibrutinib. *Blood.* 2016;128(15):1940-1943.
156. Evans SE, Ost DE. Pneumonia in the neutropenic cancer patient. *Curr Opin Pulm Med.* 2015;21(3):260-271.
157. Chellapandian D, Lehrnbecher T, Phillips B, et al. Bronchoalveolar lavage and lung biopsy in patients with cancer and hematopoietic stem-cell transplantation recipients: a systematic review and meta-analysis. *J Clin Oncol.* 2015;33(5):501-509.
158. Shannon VR, Andersson BS, Lei X, Champlin RE, Kontoyiannis DP. Utility of early versus late fiberoptic bronchoscopy in the evaluation of new pulmonary infiltrates following hematopoietic stem cell transplantation. *Bone Marrow Transplant.* 2010;45(4):647-655.
159. Brownback KR, Thomas LA, Simpson SQ. Role of bronchoalveolar lavage in the diagnosis of pulmonary infiltrates in immunocompromised patients. *Curr Opin Infect Dis.* 2014;27(4):322-328.
160. Maschmeyer G, Donnelly JP. How to manage lung infiltrates in adults suffering from haematological malignancies outside allogeneic haematopoietic stem cell transplantation. *Br J Haematol.* 2016;173(2):179-189.
161. Fishman JA, Roth RS, Zanzot E, Enos EJ, Ferraro MJ. Use of induced sputum specimens for microbiologic diagnosis of infections due to organisms other than *Pneumocystis carinii. J Clin Microbiol.* 1994;32(1):131-134.
162. Limper AH, Offord KP, Smith TF, Martin WJ. *Pneumocystis carinii* pneumonia. Differences in lung parasite number and inflammation in patients with and without AIDS. *Am Rev Respir Dis.* 1989;140(5):1204-1209.
163. Pagano L, Fianchi L, Mele L, et al. *Pneumocystis carinii* pneumonia in patients with malignant haematological diseases: 10 years' experience of infection in GIMEMA centres. *Br J Haematol.* 2002;117(2):379-386.
164. Leber A, Everhart K, Daly J, et al. Multicenter evaluation of BioFire FilmArray Respiratory Panel 2 for detection of viruses and bacteria in nasopharyngeal swab samples. *J Clin Microbiol.* 2018;56(6):e01945-17.
165. Martino R, Rámila E, Rabella N, et al. Respiratory virus infections in adults with hematologic malignancies: a prospective study. *Clin Infect Dis.* 2003;36(1):1-8.
166. Jacobs SE, Lamson DM, Soave R, et al. Clinical and molecular epidemiology of human rhinovirus infections in patients with hematologic malignancy. *J Clin Virol.* 2015;71:51-58.
167. Karageorgopoulos DE, Vouloumanou EK, Ntziora F, Michalopoulos A, Rafailidis PI, Falagas ME. β-D-glucan assay for the diagnosis of invasive fungal infections: a meta-analysis. *Clin Infect Dis.* 2011;52(6):750-770.
168. Lamoth F, Cruciani M, Castagnola E, et al. β-glucan antigenemia assay for the diagnosis of invasive fungal infections in patients with hematologic malignancies: a systematic review and meta-analysis of cohort studies from the Third European Conference on Infections in Leukemia (ECIL-3). *Clin Infect Dis.* 2012;54(5):633-643.
169. Alanio A, Hauser PM, Lagrou K, et al. ECIL guidelines for the diagnosis of *Pneumocystis jirovecii* pneumonia in patients with haematological malignancies and SCT recipients. *J Antimicrob Chemother.* 2016;71(9):2386-2396.
170. Del Corpo O, Butler-Laporte G, Sheppard D, et al. Diagnostic accuracy of serum (1-3)-β-D-glucan for *Pneumocystis jirovecii* pneumonia: a systemic review and meta-analysis. *Clin Microbiol Infect.* 2020;26(9):1137-1143.
171. Pfeiffer CD, Fine JP, Safdar N. Diagnosis of invasive aspergillosis using a galactomannan assay: a meta-analysis. *Clin Infect Dis.* 2006;42(10):1417-1427.
172. Shimada T, Noguchi Y, Jackson JL, et al. Systematic review and metaanalysis: urinary antigen tests for Legionellosis. *Chest.* 2009;136(6):1576-1585.
173. Gutiérrez F, Masiá M, Rodríguez JC, et al. Evaluation of the immunochromatographic Binax NOW assay for detection of *Streptococcus pneumoniae* urinary antigen in a prospective study of community-acquired pneumonia in Spain. *Clin Infect Dis.* 2003;36(3):286-292.
174. Barloon TJ, Galvin JR, Mori M, Stanford W, Gingrich RD. High-resolution ultrafast chest CT in the clinical management of febrile bone marrow transplant patients with normal or nonspecific chest roentgenograms. *Chest.* 1991;99(4):928-933.
175. Heussel CP, Kauczor HU, Heussel GE, et al. Pneumonia in febrile neutropenic patients and in bone marrow and blood stem-cell transplant recipients: use of high-resolution computed tomography. *J Clin Oncol.* 1999;17(3):796-805.
176. Hummel M, Rudert S, Hof H, Hehlmann R, Buchheidt D. Diagnostic yield of bronchoscopy with bronchoalveolar lavage in febrile patients with hematologic malignancies and pulmonary infiltrates. *Ann Hematol.* 2008;87(4):291-297.
177. Segal BH. Aspergillosis. *N Engl J Med.* 2009;360(18):1870-1884.
178. Pagano L, Caira M, Picardi M, et al. Invasive aspergillosis in patients with acute leukemia: update on morbidity and mortality—SEIFEM-C Report. *Clin Infect Dis.* 2007;44(11):1524-1525.
179. Pagano L, Caira M, Nosari A, et al. Fungal infections in recipients of hematopoietic stem cell transplants: results of the SEIFEM B-2004 study—Sorveglianza Epidemiologica Infezioni Fungine Nelle Emopatie Maligne. *Clin Infect Dis.* 2007;45(9):1161-1170.
180. Harrison N, Mitterbauer M, Tobudic S, et al. Incidence and characteristics of invasive fungal diseases in allogeneic hematopoietic stem cell transplant recipients: a retrospective cohort study. *BMC Infect Dis.* 2015;15:584.
181. Donnelly JP, Chen SC, Kauffman CA, et al. Revision and update of the consensus definitions of invasive fungal disease from the European Organization for Research and Treatment of Cancer and the Mycoses Study Group Education and Research Consortium. *Clin Infect Dis.* 2020;71(6):1367-1376.
182. Caillot D, Casasnovas O, Bernard A, et al. Improved management of invasive pulmonary aspergillosis in neutropenic patients using early thoracic computed tomographic scan and surgery. *J Clin Oncol.* 1997;15(1):139-147.
183. Hauggaard A, Ellis M, Ekelund L. Early chest radiography and CT in the diagnosis, management and outcome of invasive pulmonary aspergillosis. *Acta Radiol. 1987.* 2002;43(3):292-298.
184. Horger M, Hebart H, Einsele H, et al. Initial CT manifestations of invasive pulmonary aspergillosis in 45 non-HIV immunocompromised patients: association with patient outcome? *Eur J Radiol.* 2005;55(3):437-444.
185. Greene RE, Schlamm HT, Oestmann J-W, et al. Imaging findings in acute invasive pulmonary aspergillosis: clinical significance of the halo sign. *Clin Infect Dis.* 2007;44(3):373-379.
186. Cuenca-Estrella M, Bassetti M, Lass-Flörl C, et al. Detection and investigation of invasive mould disease. *J Antimicrob Chemother.* 2011;66(suppl 1):i15-i24.
187. Upton A, Kirby KA, Carpenter P, Boeckh M, Marr KA. Invasive aspergillosis following hematopoietic cell transplantation: outcomes and prognostic factors associated with mortality. *Clin Infect Dis.* 2007;44(4):531-540.
188. Marty FM, Koo S. Role of (1→3)-beta-D-glucan in the diagnosis of invasive aspergillosis. *Med Mycol.* 2009;47(suppl 1):S233-S240.
189. Miceli MH, Maertens J. Role of non-culture-based tests, with an emphasis on galactomannan testing for the diagnosis of invasive aspergillosis. *Semin Respir Crit Care Med.* 2015;36(5):650-661.
190. Marr KA, Laverdiere M, Gugel A, Leisenring W. Antifungal therapy decreases sensitivity of the *Aspergillus* galactomannan enzyme immunoassay. *Clin Infect Dis.* 2005;40(12):1762-1769.
191. Leeflang MM, Debets-Ossenkopp YJ, Wang J, et al. Galactomannan detection for invasive aspergillosis in immunocompromised patients. *Cochrane Database Syst Rev.* 2015;12:CD007394.
192. Maertens J, Verhaegen J, Lagrou K, Van Eldere J, Boogaerts M. Screening for circulating galactomannan as a noninvasive diagnostic tool for invasive aspergillosis in prolonged neutropenic patients and stem cell transplantation recipients: a prospective validation. *Blood.* 2001;97(6):1604-1610.
193. Gray LD, Roberts GD. Laboratory diagnosis of systemic fungal diseases. *Infect Dis Clin North Am.* 1988;2(4):779-803.
194. D'Haese J, Theunissen K, Vermeulen E, et al. Detection of galactomannan in bronchoalveolar lavage fluid samples of patients at risk for invasive pulmonary aspergillosis: analytical and clinical validity. *J Clin Microbiol.* 2012;50(4):1258-1263.
195. Maertens J, Maertens V, Theunissen K, et al. Bronchoalveolar lavage fluid galactomannan for the diagnosis of invasive pulmonary aspergillosis in patients with hematologic diseases. *Clin Infect Dis.* 2009;49(11):1688-1693.
196. Arvanitis M, Ziakas PD, Zacharioudakis IM, Zervou FN, Caliendo AM, Mylonakis E. PCR in diagnosis of invasive aspergillosis: a meta-analysis of diagnostic performance. *J Clin Microbiol.* 2014;52(10):3731-3742.
197. Patterson TF, Thompson GR, Denning DW, et al. Practice guidelines for the diagnosis and management of aspergillosis: 2016 update by the Infectious Diseases Society of America. *Clin Infect Dis.* 2016;63(4):e1-e60.
198. Hebrecht R, Denning DW, Patterson TF, et al. Voriconazole versus amphotericin B for primary therapy of invasive aspergillosis. *N Engl J Med.* 2002;347(6):408-415.
199. Maertens JA, Raad II, Marr KA, et al. Isavuconazole versus voriconazole for primary treatment of invasive mould disease caused by *Aspergillus* and other filamentous fungi (SECURE): a phase 3, randomised-controlled, non-inferiority trial. *Lancet.* 2016;387(10020):760-769.
200. Maertens JA, Rahav G, Lee DG, et al. Posaconazole versus voriconazole for primary treatment of invasive aspergillosis: a phase 3, randomised, controlled, non-inferiority trial. *Lancet.* 2021;397(10273):499-509.
201. Marr KA, Schlamm HT, Hebrecht R, et al. Combination antifungal therapy for invasive aspergillosis: a randomized trial. *Ann Intern Med.* 2015;162(2):81-89.
202. Pascual A, Calandra T, Bolay S, Buclin T, Bille J, Marchetti O. Voriconazole therapeutic drug monitoring in patients with invasive mycoses improves efficacy and safety outcomes. *Clin Infect Dis.* 2008;46(2):201-211.
203. Edman JC, Kovacs JA, Masur H, et al. Ribosomal RNA sequence shows *Pneumocystis carinii* to be a member of the fungi. *Nature.* 1988;334(6182):519-522.
204. Hughes WT, Feldman S, Aur RJ, et al. Intensity of immunosuppressive therapy and the incidence of *Pneumocystis carinii* pneumonitis. *Cancer.* 1975;36(6):2004-2009.
205. Yale SH, Limper AH. *Pneumocystis carinii* pneumonia in patients without acquired immunodeficiency syndrome: associated illness and prior corticosteroid therapy. *Mayo Clin Proc.* 1996;71(1):5-13.
206. Sepkowitz KA, Brown AE, Telzak EE, Gottlieb S, Armstrong D. *Pneumocystis carinii* pneumonia among patients without AIDS at a cancer hospital. *JAMA.* 1992;267(6):832-837.
207. De Castro N, Neuville S, Sarfati C, et al. Occurrence of *Pneumocystis jirovecii* pneumonia after allogeneic stem cell transplantation: a 6-year retrospective study. *Bone Marrow Transplant.* 2005;36(10):879-883.
208. Schwarzberg AB, Stover EH, Sengupta T, et al. Selective lymphopenia and opportunistic infections in neuroendocrine tumor patients receiving temozolomide. *Cancer Invest.* 2007;25(4):249-255.
209. Martin-Garrido I, Carmona EM, Specks U, Limper AH. Pneumocystis pneumonia in patients treated with rituximab. *Chest.* 2013;144(1):258-265.
210. Rai KR, Freter CE, Mercier RJ, et al. Alemtuzumab in previously treated chronic lymphocytic leukemia patients who also had received fludarabine. *J Clin Oncol.* 2002;20(18):3891-3897.

211. Bollée G, Sarfati C, Thiéry G, et al. Clinical picture of *Pneumocystis jirovecii* pneumonia in cancer patients. *Chest.* 2007;132(4):1305-1310.
212. Nüesch R, Bellini C, Zimmerli W. *Pneumocystis carinii* pneumonia in human immunodeficiency virus (HIV)-positive and HIV-negative immunocompromised patients. *Clin Infect Dis.* 1999;29(6):1519-1523.
213. Thomas CF, Limper AH. Pneumocystis pneumonia. *N Engl J Med.* 2004;350(24):2487-2498.
214. Kovacs JA, Ng VL, Masur H, et al. Diagnosis of *Pneumocystis carinii* pneumonia: improved detection in sputum with use of monoclonal antibodies. *N Engl J Med.* 1988;318(10):589-593.
215. Azoulay É, Bergeron A, Chevret S, et al. Polymerase chain reaction for diagnosing pneumocystis pneumonia in non-HIV immunocompromised patients with pulmonary infiltrates. *Chest.* 2009;135(3):655-661.
216. Robert-Gangneux F, Belaz S, Revest M, et al. Diagnosis of *Pneumocystis jirovecii* pneumonia in immunocompromised patients by real-time PCR: a 4-year prospective study. *J Clin Microbiol.* 2014;52(9):3370-3376.
217. Sattler FR, Cowan R, Nielsen DM, Ruskin J. Trimethoprim-sulfamethoxazole compared with pentamidine for treatment of *Pneumocystis carinii* pneumonia in the acquired immunodeficiency syndrome. A prospective, noncrossover study. *Ann Intern Med.* 1988;109(4):280-287.
218. Hughes W, Leoung G, Kramer F, et al. Comparison of atovaquone (566C80) with trimethoprim-sulfamethoxazole to treat *Pneumocystis carinii* pneumonia in patients with AIDS. *N Engl J Med.* 1993;328(21):1521-1527.
219. Limper AH, Knox KS, Sarosi GA, et al. An official American Thoracic Society statement: treatment of fungal infections in adult pulmonary and critical care patients. *Am J Respir Crit Care Med.* 2011;183(1):96-128.
220. Butler-Laporte G, Smyth E, Amar-Zifkin A, Cheng MP, McDonald EG, Lee TC. Low-dose TMP-SMX in the treatment of *Pneumocystis jirovecii* pneumonia: a systematic review and meta-analysis. *Open Forum Infect Dis.* 2020;7(5):ofaa112.
221. Smego RA, Jr, Nagar S, Maloba B, Popara M. A meta-analysis of salvage therapy for *Pneumocystis carinii* pneumonia. *Arch Intern Med.* 2001;161(12):1529-1533.
222. Hughes WT, Feldman S, Chaudhary SC, Ossi MJ, Cox F, Sanyal SK. Comparison of pentamidine isethionate and trimethoprim-sulfamethoxazole in the treatment of *Pneumocystis carinii* pneumonia. *J Pediatr.* 1978;92(2):285-291.
223. Watson J, Taylor WR, Menard D, Kheng S, White NJ. Modelling primaquine-induced haemolysis in G6PD deficiency. *Elife.* 2017;6:e23061.
224. Montaner JS, Lawson LM, Levitt N, Belzberg A, Schechter MT, Ruedy J. Corticosteroids prevent early deterioration in patients with moderately severe *Pneumocystis carinii* pneumonia and the acquired immunodeficiency syndrome (AIDS). *Ann Intern Med.* 1990;113(1):14-20.
225. Bozzette SA, Sattler FR, Chiu J, et al. A controlled trial of early adjunctive treatment with corticosteroids for *Pneumocystis carinii* pneumonia in the acquired immunodeficiency syndrome. California Collaborative Treatment Group. *N Engl J Med.* 1990;323(21):1451-1457.
226. Gagnon S, Boota AM, Fischl MA, Baier H, Kirksey OW, La Voie L. Corticosteroids as adjunctive therapy for severe *Pneumocystis carinii* pneumonia in the acquired immunodeficiency syndrome. A double-blind, placebo-controlled trial. *N Engl J Med.* 1990;323(21):1444-1450.
227. Pareja JG, Garland R, Koziel H. Use of adjunctive corticosteroids in severe adult non-HIV *Pneumocystis carinii* pneumonia. *Chest.* 1998;113(5):1215-1224.
228. Delclaux C, Zahar JR, Amraoui G, et al. Corticosteroids as adjunctive therapy for severe *Pneumocystis carinii* pneumonia in non-human immunodeficiency virus-infected patients: retrospective study of 31 patients. *Clin Infect Dis.* 1999;29(3):670-672.
229. Wieruszewski PM, Barreto JN, Frazee E, et al. Early corticosteroids for *Pneumocystis* pneumonia in adults without HIV are not associated with better outcome. *Chest.* 2018;154(3):636-644.
230. Petrikkos G, Skiada A, Lortholary O, Roilides E, Walsh TJ, Kontoyiannis DP. Epidemiology and clinical manifestations of mucormycosis. *Clin Infect Dis.* 2012;54(suppl 1):S23-S34.
231. Roden MM, Zaoutis TE, Buchanan WL, et al. Epidemiology and outcome of zygomycosis: a review of 929 reported cases. *Clin Infect Dis.* 2005;41(5):634-653.
232. Kontoyiannis DP, Lionakis MS, Lewis RE, et al. Zygomycosis in a tertiary-care center in the era of *Aspergillus*-active antifungal therapy: a case-control observational study of 27 recent cases. *J Infect Dis.* 2005;191(8):1350-1360.
233. Georgiadou SP, Sipsas NV, Marom EM, Kontoyiannis DP. The diagnostic value of halo and reversed halo signs for invasive mold infections in compromised hosts. *Clin Infect Dis.* 2011;52(9):1144-1155.
234. Walsh TJ, Gamaletsou MN, McGinnis MR, Hayden RT, Kontoyiannis DP. Early clinical and laboratory diagnosis of invasive pulmonary, extrapulmonary, and disseminated mucormycosis (zygomycosis). *Clin Infect Dis.* 2012;54(suppl 1):S55-S60.
235. Cornely OA, Alastruey-Izquierdo A, Arenz D, et al. Global guideline for the diagnosis and management of mucormycosis: an initiative of the European Confederation of Medical Mycology in cooperation with the Mycoses Study Group Education and Research Consortium. *Lancet Infect Dis.* 2019;19(12):e405-e421.
236. Kauffman CA, Freifeld AG, Andes DR, et al. Endemic fungal infections in solid organ and hematopoietic cell transplant recipients enrolled in the Transplant-Associated Infection Surveillance Network (TRANSNET). *Transpl Infect Dis.* 2014;16(2):213-224.
237. Kauffman CA. Endemic mycoses in patients with hematologic malignancies. *Semin Respir Infect.* 2002;17(2):106-112.
238. Hage CA, Ribes JA, Wengenack NL, et al. A multicenter evaluation of tests for diagnosis of histoplasmosis. *Clin Infect Dis.* 2011;53(5):448-454.
239. Jacobson KL, Miceli MH, Tarrand JJ, Kontoyiannis DP. Legionella pneumonia in cancer patients. *Medicine.* 2008;87(3):152-159.
240. Schmalzle SA, Buchwald UK, Gilliam BL, Riedel DJ. *Cryptococcus neoformans* infection in malignancy. *Mycoses.* 2016;59(9):542-552.
241. Cattaneo C, Antoniazzi F, Caira M, et al. *Nocardia* spp infections among hematological patients: results of a retrospective multicenter study. *Int J Infect Dis.* 2013;17(8):e610-e614.
242. Chavez-MacGregor M, Lei X, Zhao H, Scheet P, Giordano SH. Evaluation of COVID-19 mortality and adverse outcomes in US patients with or without cancer. *JAMA Oncol.* 2022;8(1):69-78.
243. Lee LYW, Cazier JB, Starkey T, et al. COVID-19 prevalence and mortality in patients with cancer and the effect of primary tumour subtype and patient demographics: a prospective cohort study. *Lancet Oncol.* 2020;21(10):1309-1316.
244. Ljungman P, Mikulska M, de la Camara R, et al. The challenge of COVID-19 and hematopoietic cell transplantation; EBMT recommendations for management of hematopoietic cell transplant recipients, their donors, and patients undergoing CAR T-cell therapy. *Bone Marrow Transplant.* 2020;55(11):2071-2076.
245. Hammond J, Leister-Tebbe H, Gardner A, et al. Oral nirmatrelvir for high-risk, nonhospitalized adults with Covid-19. *N Engl J Med.* 2022;386(15):1397-1408.
246. Marzolini C, Kuritzkes DR, Marra F, et al. Prescribing nirmatrelvir-ritonavir: how to recognize and manage drug-drug interactions. *Ann Intern Med.* Published online 2022.
247. Gottlieb RL, Vaca CE, Paredes R, et al. Early remdesivir to prevent progression to severe Covid-19 in outpatients. *N Engl J Med.* 2022;386(4):305-315.
248. Bernal AJ, Gomes da Silva MM, Musungaie DB, et al. Molnupiravir for oral treatment of Covid-19 in nonhospitalized patients. *N Engl J Med.* 2022;386(6):509-520.
249. Gupta A, Gonzalez-Rojas Y, Juarez E, et al. Early treatment for Covid-19 with SARS-CoV-2 neutralizing antibody sotrovimab. *N Engl J Med.* 2021;385(21):1941-1950.
250. O'Brien MP, Forleo-Neto E, Musser BJ, et al. Subcutaneous REGEN-COV antibody combination to prevent Covid-19. *N Engl J Med.* 2021;385(13):1184-1195.
251. Dougan M, Nirula A, Azizad M, et al. Bamlanivimab plus etesevimab in mild or moderate Covid-19. *N Engl J Med.* 2021;385(15):1382-1392.
252. RECOVERY Collaborative Group; Horby P, Lim WS, Emberson JR, et al. Dexamethasone in hospitalized patients with Covid-19. *N Engl J Med.* 2021;384(8):693-704.
253. Angus DC, Derde L, Al-Beidh F, et al. Effect of hydrocortisone on mortality and organ support in patients with severe COVID-19: the REMAP-CAP COVID-19 Corticosteroid Domain Randomized Clinical Trial. *JAMA.* 2020;324(13):1317-1329.
254. WHO Rapid Evidence Appraisal for COVID-19 Therapies (REACT) Working Group; Sterne JAC, Murthy S, Diaz JV, et al. Association between administration of systemic corticosteroids and mortality among critically ill patients with COVID-19: a meta-analysis. *JAMA.* 2020;324(13):1330-1341.
255. WHO Solidarity Trial Consortium; Pan H, Peto R, Henao-Restrepo AM, et al. Repurposed antiviral drugs for Covid-19—Interim WHO Solidarity trial results. *N Engl J Med.* 2021;384(6):497-511.
256. Marconi VC, Ramanan AV, de Bono S, et al. Efficacy and safety of baricitinib for the treatment of hospitalized adults with COVID-19 (COV-BARRIER): a randomised, double-blind, parallel-group, placebo-controlled phase 3 trial. *Lancet Respir Med.* 2021;9(12):1407-1418.
257. RECOVERY Collaborative Group. Tocilizumab in patients admitted to the hospital with COVID-19 (RECOVERY): a randomised, controlled, open-label, platform trial. *Lancet.* 2021;397(10285):1637-1645.
258. Investigators REMAP-CAP; Gordon AC, Mouncey PR, Al-Beidh F, et al. Interleukin-6 receptor antagonists in critically ill patients with Covid-19. *N Engl J Med.* 2021;384(16):1491-1502.
259. Beigel JH, Tomashek KM, Dodd LE, et al. Remdesivir for the treatment of Covid-19—final report. *N Engl J Med.* 2020;383(19):1813-1826.
260. Lee CY, Shah MK, Hoyos D, et al. Prolonged SARS-CoV-2 infection in patients with lymphoid malignancies. *Cancer Discov.* 2022;12(1):62-73.
261. Bilaloglu S, Aphinyanaphongs Y, Jones S, Iturrate E, Hochman J, Berger JS. Thrombosis in hospitalized patients with COVID-19 in a New York City health system. *JAMA.* 2020;324(8):799-801.
262. REMAP-CAP Investigators; ACTIV-4a Investigators; ATTACC Investigators; Goligher EC, Bradbury CA, McVerry BJ, et al. Therapeutic anticoagulation with heparin in critically ill patients with Covid-19. *N Engl J Med.* 2021;385(9):777-789.
263. Aydillo T, Gonzalez-Reiche AS, Aslam S, et al. Shedding of viable SARS-CoV-2 after immunosuppressive therapy for cancer. *N Engl J Med.* 2020;383(26):2586-2588.
264. Piñana JL, López-Corral L, Martino R, et al. SARS-CoV-2-reactive antibody detection after SARS-CoV-2 vaccination in hematopoietic stem cell transplant recipients: prospective survey from the Spanish Hematopoietic Stem Cell Transplantation and Cell Therapy Group. *Am J Hematol.* 2022;97(1):30-42.
265. Shulman RM, Weinberg DS, Ross EA, et al. Adverse events reported by patients with cancer after administration of a 2-dose mRNA COVID-19 vaccine. *J Natl Compr Cancer Netw.* 2022;20(2):160-166.
266. Wu JT, La J, Branch-Elliman W, et al. Association of COVID-19 vaccination with SARS-CoV-2 infection in patients with cancer: a US nationwide Veterans Affairs study. *JAMA Oncol.* 2022;8(2):281-286.
267. Mair MJ, Berger JM, Berghoff AS, et al. Humoral immune response in hematooncological patients and health care workers who received SARS-CoV-2 vaccinations. *JAMA Oncol.* 2022;8(1):106-113.
268. Jurgens EM, Ketas TJ, Zhao Z, et al. Serologic response to mRNA COVID-19 vaccination in lymphoma patients. *Am J Hematol.* 2021;96(11):e410-e413.
269. Fendler A, Shepherd STC, Au L, et al. Omicron neutralizing antibodies after third COVID-19 vaccine dose in patients with cancer. *Lancet.* 2022;399(10328):905-907.
270. Centers for Disease Control and Prevention. *COVID-19 Vaccines for Moderately or Severely Immunocompromised People.* 2022. Accessed April 27, 2022.
271. Levin MJ, Ustianowski A, De Wit S, et al. Intramuscular AZD7442 (tixagevimab-cilgavimab) for prevention of Covid-19. *N Engl J Med.* 2022;386(23):2188-2200.

272. Fontana L, Strasfeld L. Respiratory virus infections of the stem cell transplant recipient and the hematologic malignancy patient. *Infect Dis Clin North Am*. 2019;33(2):523-544.
273. Jacobs SE, Soave R, Shore TB, et al. Human rhinovirus infections of the lower respiratory tract in hematopoietic stem cell transplant recipients. *Transpl Infect Dis*. 2013;15(5):474-486.
274. Eichenberger EM, Soave R, Zappetti D, et al. Incidence, significance, and persistence of human coronavirus infection in hematopoietic stem cell transplant recipients. *Bone Marrow Transplant*. 2019;54(7):1058-1066.
275. Hammond SP, Gagne LS, Stock SR, et al. Respiratory virus detection in immunocompromised patients with FilmArray respiratory panel compared to conventional methods. *J Clin Microbiol*. 2012;50(10):3216-3221.
276. Choi SM, Boudreault AA, Xie H, Englund JA, Corey L, Boeckh M. Differences in clinical outcomes after 2009 influenza A/H1N1 and seasonal influenza among hematopoietic cell transplant recipients. *Blood*. 2011;117(19):5050-5056.
277. Chemaly RF, Torres HA, Aguilera EA, et al. Neuraminidase inhibitors improve outcome of patients with leukemia and influenza: an observational study. *Clin Infect Dis*. 2007;44(7):964-967.
278. Hayden FG, Sugaya N, Hirotsu N, et al. Baloxavir marboxil for uncomplicated influenza in adults and adolescents. *N Engl J Med*. 2018;379(10):913-923.
279. Shah DP, Ghantoji SS, Shah JN, et al. Impact of aerosolized ribavirin on mortality in 280 allogeneic haematopoietic stem cell transplant recipients with respiratory syncytial virus infections. *J Antimicrob Chemother*. 2013;68(8):1872-1880.
280. Waghmare A, Campbell AP, Xie H, et al. Respiratory syncytial virus lower respiratory disease in hematopoietic cell transplant recipients: viral RNA detection in blood, antiviral treatment, and clinical outcomes. *Clin Infect Dis*. 2013;57(12):1731-1741.
281. Foolad F, Aitken SL, Shigle TL, et al. Oral versus aerosolized ribavirin for the treatment of respiratory syncytial virus infections in hematopoietic cell transplant recipients. *Clin Infect Dis*. 2019;68(10):1614-1649.
282. Seo S, Campbell AP, Xie H, et al. Outcome of respiratory syncytial virus lower respiratory tract disease in hematopoietic cell transplant recipients receiving aerosolized ribavirin: significance of stem cell source and oxygen requirement. *Biol Blood Marrow Transplant*. 2013;19(4):589-596.
283. Sicre de Fontbrune F, Robin M, Porcher R, et al. Palivizumab treatment of respiratory syncytial virus infection after allogeneic hematopoietic stem cell transplantation. *Clin Infect Dis*. 2007;45(8):1019-1024.
284. Waghmare A, Englund JA, Boeckh M. How I treat respiratory viral infections in the setting of intensive chemotherapy or hematopoietic cell transplantation. *Blood*. 2016;127(22):2682-2692.
285. Seo S, Xie H, Campbell AP, et al. Parainfluenza virus lower respiratory tract disease after hematopoietic cell transplant: viral detection in the lung predicts outcome. *Clin Infect Dis*. 2014;58(10):1357-1368.
286. Akhmedov M, Wais V, Sala E, et al. Respiratory syncytial virus and human metapneumovirus after allogeneic hematopoietic stem cell transplantation: impact of the immunodeficiency scoring index, viral load, and ribavirin treatment on the outcomes. *Transpl Infect Dis*. 2020;22(4):e13276.
287. Piñana JL, Gómez MD, Montoro J, et al. Incidence, risk factors, and outcome of pulmonary invasive fungal disease after respiratory virus infection in allogeneic hematopoietic stem cell transplantation recipients. *Transpl Infect Dis*. 2019;21(5):e13158.
288. Piñana JL, Gómez MD, Pérez A, et al. Community-acquired respiratory virus lower respiratory tract disease in allogeneic stem cell transplantation recipient: risk factors and mortality from pulmonary virus-bacterial mixed infections. *Transpl Infect Dis*. 2018;20(4):e12926.
289. Wingard JR, Hsu J, Hiemenz JW. Hematopoietic stem cell transplantation: an overview of infection risks and epidemiology. *Infect Dis Clin North Am*. 2010;24(2):257-272.
290. Hakki M, Aitken SL, Danziger-Isakov L, et al. American Society for transplantation and cellular therapy Series: #3-Prevention of cytomegalovirus infection and disease after hematopoietic cell transplantation. *Transplant Cell Ther*. 2021;27(9):707-719.
291. George B, Pati N, Gilroy N, et al. Pre-transplant cytomegalovirus (CMV) serostatus remains the most important determinant of CMV reactivation after allogeneic hematopoietic stem cell transplantation in the era of surveillance and preemptive therapy. *Transpl Infect Dis*. 2010;12(4):322-329.
292. Boeckh M, Nichols WG. The impact of cytomegalovirus serostatus of donor and recipient before hematopoietic stem cell transplantation in the era of antiviral prophylaxis and preemptive therapy. *Blood*. 2004;103(6):2003-2008.
293. Boeckh M, Nichols WG, Papanicolaou G, et al. Cytomegalovirus in hematopoietic stem cell transplant recipients: current status, known challenges, and future strategies. *Biol Blood Marrow Transplant*. 2003;9(9):543-558.
294. Einsele H, Ehninger G, Hebart H, et al. Polymerase chain reaction monitoring reduces the incidence of cytomegalovirus disease and the duration and side effects of antiviral therapy after bone marrow transplantation. *Blood*. 1995;86(7):2815-2820.
295. Travi G, Pergam SA. Cytomegalovirus pneumonia in hematopoietic stem cell recipients. *J Intensive Care Med*. 2014;29(4):200-212.
296. Green ML, Leisenring W, Stachel D, et al. Efficacy of a viral load-based, risk-adapted, preemptive treatment strategy for prevention of cytomegalovirus disease after hematopoietic cell transplantation. *Biol Blood Marrow Transplant*. 2012;18(11):1687-1699.
297. Marty FM, Ljungman P, Chemaly RF, et al. Letermovir prophylaxis for cytomegalovirus in hematopoietic-cell transplantation. *N Engl J Med*. 2017;377(25):2433-2444.
298. Ljungman P. CMV infections after hematopoietic stem cell transplantation. *Bone Marrow Transplant*. 2008;42(suppl 1):S70-S72.
299. Boeckh M, Stevens-Ayers T, Travi G, et al. Cytomegalovirus (CMV) DNA quantitation in bronchoalveolar lavage fluid from hematopoietic stem cell transplant recipients with CMV pneumonia. *J Infect Dis*. 2017;215(10):1514-1522.
300. Yong MK, Shigle TL, Kim YJ, Carpenter PA, Chemaly RF, Papanicolaou GA. American Society for Transplantation and Cellular Therapy Series: #4—cytomegalovirus treatment and management of resistant or refractory infections after hematopoietic cell transplantation. *Transplant Cell Ther*. 2021;27(12):957-967.
301. Erard V, Guthrie K, Seo S, et al. Reduced mortality of cytomegalovirus pneumonia after hematopoietic cell transplantation due to antiviral therapy and changes in transplantation practices. *Clin Infect Dis*. 2015;61(1):31-39.
302. Avery RK, Alain S, Alexander BD, et al. Maribavir for refractory cytomegalovirus infections with or without resistance post-transplant: results from a phase 3 randomized clinical trial. *Clin Infect Dis*. Published online 2021.
303. Chakrabarti A, Denning DW, Ferguson BJ, et al. Fungal rhinosinusitis: a categorization and definitional schema addressing current controversies. *Laryngoscope*. 2009;119(9):1809-1818.
304. Drakos PE, Nagler A, Or R, et al. Invasive fungal sinusitis in patients undergoing bone marrow transplantation. *Bone Marrow Transplant*. 1993;12(3):203-208.
305. deShazo RD, Chapin K, Swain RE. Fungal sinusitis. *N Engl J Med*. 1997;337(4):254-259.
306. DelGaudio JM, Clemson LA. An early detection protocol for invasive fungal sinusitis in neutropenic patients successfully reduces extent of disease at presentation and long term morbidity. *Laryngoscope*. 2009;119(1):180-183.
307. DelGaudio JM, Swain RE, Kingdom TT, Muller S, Hudgins PA. Computed tomographic findings in patients with invasive fungal sinusitis. *Arch Otolaryngol Head Neck Surg*. 2003;129(2):236-240.
308. Gillespie MB, O'Malley BW. An algorithmic approach to the diagnosis and management of invasive fungal rhinosinusitis in the immunocompromised patient. *Otolaryngol Clin North Am*. 2000;33(2):323-334.
309. Urbach DR, Rotstein OD. Typhlitis. *Can J Surg*. 1999;42(6):415-419.
310. Rolston KVI, Bodey GP, Safdar A. Polymicrobial infection in patients with cancer: an underappreciated and underreported entity. *Clin Infect Dis*. 2007;45(2):228-233.
311. Nesher L, Rolston KV. Neutropenic enterocolitis, a growing concern in the era of widespread use of aggressive chemotherapy. *Clin Infect Dis*. 2013;56(5):711-717.
312. Kirkpatrick ID, Greenberg HM. Gastrointestinal complications in the neutropenic patient: characterization and differentiation with abdominal CT. *Radiology*. 2003;226(3):668-674.
313. Bagdasarian N, Rao K, Malani PN. Diagnosis and treatment of *Clostridium difficile* in adults: a systematic review. *JAMA*. 2015;313(4):398-408.
314. Deshpande A, Pasupuleti V, Thota P, et al. Community-associated *Clostridium difficile* infection and antibiotics: a meta-analysis. *J Antimicrob Chemother*. 2013;68(9):1951-1961.
315. McDonald LC, Gerding DN, Johnson S, et al. Clinical practice guidelines for *Clostridium difficile* infection in adults and children: 2017 update by the Infectious Diseases Society of America (IDSA) and Society for Healthcare Epidemiology of America (SHEA). *Clin Infect Dis*. 2018;66(7):e1-e48.
316. Ford CD, Lopansri BK, Webb BJ, et al. *Clostridioides difficile* colonization and infection in patients with newly diagnosed acute leukemia: incidence, risk factors, and patient outcomes. *Am J Infect Control*. 2019;47(4):394-399.
317. Jain T, Croswell C, Urday-Cornejo V, et al. *Clostridium difficile* colonization in hematopoietic stem cell transplant recipients: a prospective study of the epidemiology and outcomes involving toxigenic and nontoxigenic strains. *Biol Blood Marrow Transplant*. 2016;22(1):157-163.
318. Leffler DA, Lamont JT. *Clostridium difficile* infection. *N Engl J Med*. 2015;372(16):1539-1548.
319. Johnson S, Lavergne V, Skinner AM, et al. Clinical practice guideline by the Infectious Diseases Society of America (IDSA) and Society for Healthcare Epidemiology of America (SHEA): 2021 focused update guidelines on management of *Clostridioides difficile* infection in adults. *Clin Infect Dis*. 2021;73(5):e10 29-e1044.
320. Alonso CD, Maron G, Kamboj M, et al. American Society for Transplantation and Cellular Therapy Series: #5-Management of *Clostridioides difficile* infection in hematopoietic cell transplant recipients. *Transplant Cell Ther*. 2022;28(5):225-232.
321. Louie TJ, Miller MA, Mullane KM, et al. Fidaxomicin versus vancomycin for *Clostridium difficile* infection. *N Engl J Med*. 2011;364(5):422-431.
322. Cornely OA, Crook DW, Esposito R, et al. Fidaxomicin versus vancomycin for infection with *Clostridium difficile* in Europe, Canada, and the USA: a double-blind, non-inferiority, randomised controlled trial. *Lancet Infect Dis*. 2012;12(4):281-289.
323. Louie TJ, Cannon K, Byrne B, et al. Fidaxomicin preserves the intestinal microbiome during and after treatment of *Clostridium difficile* infection (CDI) and reduces both toxin reexpression and recurrence of CDI. *Clin Infect Dis*. 2012;55(suppl 2):S132-S142.
324. Peled JU, Gomes ALC, Devlin SM, et al. Microbiota as predictor of mortality in allogeneic hematopoietic-cell transplantation. *N Engl J Med*. 2020;382(9):822-834.
325. Wilcox MH, Gerding DN, Poxton IR, et al. Bezlotoxumab for prevention of recurrent *Clostridium difficile* infection. *N Engl J Med*. 2017;376(4):305-317.
326. DeFilipp Z, Bloom PP, Soto MT, et al. Drug-resistant *E. coli* bacteremia transmitted by fecal microbiota transplant. *N Engl J Med*. 2019;381(21):2043-2050.
327. Otter JA, Yezli S, French GL. The role played by contaminated surfaces in the transmission of nosocomial pathogens. *Infect Control Hosp Epidemiol*. 2011;32(7):687-699.
328. Jabbar U, Leischner J, Kasper D, et al. Effectiveness of alcohol-based hand rubs for removal of *Clostridium difficile* spores from hands. *Infect Control Hosp Epidemiol*. 2010;31(6):565-570.
329. Barnes SG, Sattler FR, Ballard JO. Perirectal infections in acute leukemia. Improved survival after incision and debridement. *Ann Intern Med*. 1984;100(4):515-518.
330. Allen U, Smith CR, Prober CG. The value of skin biopsies in febrile, neutropenic, immunocompromised children. *Am J Dis Child*. 1986;140(5):459-461.

331. Fine JD, Miller JA, Harrist TJ, Haynes HA. Cutaneous lesions in disseminated candidiasis mimicking ecthyma gangrenosum. *Am J Med*. 1981;70(5):1133-1135.
332. Prins C, Chavaz P, Tamm K, Hauser C. Ecthyma gangrenosum-like lesions: a sign of disseminated Fusarium infection in the neutropenic patient. *Clin Exp Dermatol*. 1995;20(5):428-430.
333. Garcia Garrido HM, Knol MJ, Heijmans J, et al. Invasive pneumococcal disease among adults with hematological and solid organ malignancies: a population-based cohort study. *Int J Infect Dis*. 2021;106:237-245.
334. van Veen KEB, Brouwer MC, van der Ende A, van de Beek D. Bacterial meningitis in hematopoietic stem cell transplant recipients: a population-based prospective study. *Bone Marrow Transplant*. 2016;51(11):1490-1495.
335. Nematollahi S, Dioverti-Prono. Cryptococcal infection in haematologic malignancies and haematopoietic stem cell transplantation. *Mycoses*. 2020;63(10):1033-1046.
336. Mylonakis E, Hohmann EL, Calderwood SB. Central nervous system infection with *Listeria monocytogenes*. 33 years' experience at a general hospital and review of 776 episodes from the literature. *Medicine (Baltimore)*. 1998;77(5):313-336.
337. Pappas PG, Perfect JR, Cloud GA, et al. Cryptococcosis in human immunodeficiency virus-negative patients in the era of effective azole therapy. *Clin Infect Dis*. 2001;33(5):690-699.
338. Tanner DC, Weinstein MP, Fedorciw B, Joho KL, Thorpe JJ, Reller L. Comparison of commercial kits for detection of cryptococcal antigen. *J Clin Microbiol*. 1994;32(7):1680-1684.
339. Yang J, Moon S, Kwon M, Huh K, Jung CW. A case of tuberculosis meningitis after allogeneic hematopoietic stem cell transplantation for relapsed acute myeloid leukemia. *Transpl Infect Dis*. 2021;23(2):e13482.
340. Saylor D, Thakur K, Venkatesan A. Acute encephalitis in the immunocompromised individual. *Curr Opin Infect Dis*. 2015;28(4):330-336.
341. Mailles A, Stahl JP. Steering Committee and Investigators Group. Infectious encephalitis in France in 2007: a national prospective study. *Clin Infect Dis*. 2009;49(12):1838-1847.
342. Whitley RJ, Alford CA, Hirsch MS, et al. Vidarabine versus acyclovir therapy in herpes simplex encephalitis. *N Engl J Med*. 1986;314(3):144-149.
343. Ogata M, Satou T, Kadota J, et al. Human herpesvirus 6 (HHV-6) reactivation and HHV-6 encephalitis after allogeneic hematopoietic cell transplantation: a multicenter, prospective study. *Clin Infect Dis*. 2013;57(5):671-681.
344. Tunkel AR, Glaser CA, Bloch KC, et al. The management of encephalitis: clinical practice guidelines by the Infectious Diseases Society of America. *Clin Infect Dis*. 2008;47(3):303-327.
345. Leber AL, Everhart K, Balada-Llasat JM, et al. Multicenter evaluation of BioFire FilmArray Meningitis/Encephalitis Panel for detection of bacteria, viruses, and yeast in cerebrospinal fluid specimens. *J Clin Microbiol*. 2016;54(9):2251-2261.
346. Shaheen N, Mussai F. Enteroviral encephalitis in a child with CNS relapse of Burkitt leukemia treated with rituximab. *J Pediatr Hematol Oncol*. 2019;41(1):e27-e29.
347. Brenner W, Storch G, Buller R, Vij R, Devine S, DiPersio J. West Nile Virus encephalopathy in an allogeneic stem cell transplant recipient: use of quantitative PCR for diagnosis and assessment of viral clearance. *Bone Marrow Transplant*. 2005;36(4):369-370.
348. McCarthy M, Rosengart A, Schuetz AN, Kontoyiannis DP, Walsh TJ. Mold infections of the central nervous system. *N Engl J Med*. 2014;371(2):150-160.
349. Robert-Gangneux F, Meroni V, Dupont D, et al. Toxoplasmosis in transplant recipients, Europe, 2010-2014. *Emerg Infect Dis*. 2018;24(8):1497-1504.
350. Isa F, Saito K, Huang YT, et al. Implementation of molecular surveillance after a cluster of fatal toxoplasmosis at 2 neighboring transplant centers. *Clin Infect Dis*. 2016;63(4):565-568.
351. Carson KR, Evens AM, Richey EA, et al. Progressive multifocal leukoencephalopathy after rituximab therapy in HIV-negative patients: a report of 57 cases from the Research on Adverse Drug Events and Reports project. *Blood*. 2009;113(20):4834-4840.
352. Carson KR, Newsome SD, Kim EJ, et al. Progressive multifocal leukoencephalopathy associated with brentuximab vedotin therapy: a report of 5 cases from the Southern Network on Adverse Reactions (SONAR) project. *Cancer*. 2014;120(16):2464-2471.
353. Berger JR, Aksamit AJ, Clifford DB, et al. PML diagnostic criteria: consensus statement from the AAN Neuroinfectious Disease Section. *Neurology*. 2013;80(15):1430-1438.
354. Anand P, Hotan GC, Vogel A, Venna N, Mateen FJ. Progressive multifocal leukoencephalopathy: a 25-year retrospective cohort study. *Neurol Neuroimmunol Neuroinflamm*. 2019;6(6):e618.
355. Cortese I, Muranski P, Enose-Akahata Y, et al. Pembrolizumab treatment for progressive multifocal leukoencephalopathy. *N Engl J Med*. 2019;380(17):1597-1605.
356. Maiolino A, Biasoli I, Lima J, Portugal AC, Pulcheri W, Nucci M. Engraftment syndrome following autologous hematopoietic stem cell transplantation: definition of diagnostic criteria. *Bone Marrow Transplant*. 2003;31(5):393-397.
357. Afessa B, Abdulai RM, Kremers WK, et al. Risk factors and outcome of pulmonary complications after autologous hematopoietic stem cell transplant. *Chest*. 2012;141(2):442-450.
358. Zaia J, Baden L, Boeckh MJ, et al. Viral disease prevention after hematopoietic cell transplantation. *Bone Marrow Transplant*. 2009;44(8):471-482.
359. Baddley JW, Andes DR, Marr KA, et al. Factors associated with mortality in transplant patients with invasive aspergillosis. *Clin Infect Dis*. 2010;50(12):1559-1567.
360. Fukuda T, Boeckh M, Carter RA, et al. Risks and outcomes of invasive fungal infections in recipients of allogeneic hematopoietic stem cell transplants after nonmyeloablative conditioning. *Blood*. 2003;102(3):827-833.
361. Williams KM, Ahn KW, Chen M, et al. The incidence, mortality and timing of *Pneumocystis jirovecii* pneumonia after hematopoietic cell transplantation: a CIBMTR analysis. *Bone Marrow Transplant*. 2016;51(4):573-580.
362. Van Kraaij MG, Dekker AW, Verdonck LF, et al. Infectious gastro-enteritis: an uncommon cause of diarrhoea in adult allogeneic and autologous stem cell transplant recipients. *Bone Marrow Transplant*. 2000;26(3):299-303.
363. Rogers WS, Westblade LF, Soave R, et al. Impact of a multiplexed polymerase chain reaction panel on identifying diarrheal pathogens in hematopoietic cell transplant recipients. *Clin Infect Dis*. 2020;71(7):1693-1700.
364. Martin P, Rizzo JD, Wingard JR, et al. First- and second-line systemic treatment of acute graft-versus-host disease: recommendations of the American Society of Blood and Marrow Transplantation. *Biol Blood Marrow Transplant*. 2012;18(8):1150-1163.
365. El Chaer F, Shah DP, Chemaly RF. How I treat resistant cytomegalovirus infection in hematopoietic cell transplantation recipients. *Blood*. 2016;128(23):2624-2636.
366. Matsukuma KE, Wei D, Sun K, Ramsamooj R, Chen M. Diagnosis and differential diagnosis of hepatic graft versus host disease (GVHD). *J Gastrointest Oncol*. 2016;7(suppl 1):S21-S31.
367. McDonald GB. Hepatobiliary complications of hematopoietic cell transplantation, 40 years on. *Hepatology*. 2010;51(4):1450-1460.
368. Murt A, Elverdi T, Eskazan AE, et al. Hepatitis B reactivation in hematopoietic stem cell transplanted patients: 20 years of experience of a single center from a middle endemic country. *Ann Hematol*. 2020;99(11):2671-2677.
369. Erard V, Storer B, Corey L, et al. BK virus infection in hematopoietic stem cell transplant recipients: frequency, risk factors, and association with postengraftment hemorrhagic cystitis. *Clin Infect Dis*. 2004;39(12):1861-1865.
370. La Rosa AM, Champlin RE, Mirza N, et al. Adenovirus infections in adult recipients of blood and marrow transplants. *Clin Infect Dis*. 2001;32(6):871-876.
371. Gorczynska E, Turkiewicz D, Rybka K, et al. Incidence, clinical outcome, and management of virus-induced hemorrhagic cystitis in children and adolescents after allogeneic hematopoietic cell transplantation. *Biol Blood Marrow Transplant*. 2005;11(10):797-804.
372. Dalianis T, Ljungman P. Full myeloablative conditioning and an unrelated HLA mismatched donor increase the risk for BK virus-positive hemorrhagic cystitis in allogeneic hematopoietic stem cell transplanted patients. *Anticancer Res*. 2011;31(3):939-944.
373. Silva Lde P, Patah PA, Saliba RM, et al. Hemorrhagic cystitis after allogeneic hematopoietic stem cell transplants is the complex result of BK virus infection, preparative regimen intensity and donor type. *Haematologica*. 2010;95(7):1183-1190.
374. Park SH, Choi SM, Lee DG, et al. Infectious complications associated with alemtuzumab use for allogeneic hematopoietic stem cell transplantation: comparison with anti-thymocyte globulin. *Transpl Infect Dis*. 2009;11(5):413-423.
375. Gluckman E, Lotsberg J, Devergie A, et al. Prophylaxis of herpes infections after bone-marrow transplantation by oral acyclovir. *Lancet*. 1983;2(8352):706-708.
376. Erard V, Guthrie KA, Varley C, et al. One-year acyclovir prophylaxis for preventing varicella-zoster virus disease after hematopoietic cell transplantation: no evidence of rebound varicella-zoster virus disease after drug discontinuation. *Blood*. 2007;110(8):3071-3077.
377. van Esser JW, van der Holt B, Meijer E, et al. Epstein-Barr virus (EBV) reactivation is a frequent event after allogeneic stem cell transplantation (SCT) and quantitatively predicts EBV-lymphoproliferative disease following T-cell-depleted SCT. *Blood*. 2001;98(4):972-978.
378. Chaekal OK, Soave R, Chen Z, et al. Adenovirus viremia after *in vivo* T-cell depleted allo-transplant in adults: low lymphocyte counts are associated with uncontrolled viremia and fatal outcomes. *Leuk Lymphoma*. 2022;63(2):435-442.
379. Lindemans CA, Leen AM, Boelens JJ. How I treat adenovirus in hematopoietic stem cell transplant recipients. *Blood*. 2010;116(25):5476-5485.
380. Lee YJ, Huang YT, Kim SJ, et al. Adenovirus viremia in adult CD34(+) selected hematopoietic cell transplant recipients: low incidence and high clinical impact. *Biol Blood Marrow Transplant*. 2016;22(1):174-178.
381. Derouin F, Pelloux H; ESCMID Study Group on Clinical Parasitology. Prevention of toxoplasmosis in transplant patients. *Clin Microbiol Infect*. 2008;14(12):1089-1101.
382. Wirk B, Wingard JR. *Strongyloides stercoralis* hyperinfection in hematopoietic stem cell transplantation. *Transpl Infect Dis*. 2009;11(2):143-148.
383. Tomblyn M, Chiller T, Einsele H, et al. Guidelines for preventing infectious complications among hematopoietic cell transplantation recipients: a global perspective. *Biol Blood Marrow Transplant*. 2009;15(10):1143-1238.
384. Robin M, Porcher R, De Castro Araujo R, et al. Risk factors for late infections after allogeneic hematopoietic stem cell transplantation from a matched related donor. *Biol Blood Marrow Transplant*. 2007;13(11):1304-1312.
385. Youssef S, Rodriguez G, Rolston KV, et al. *Streptococcus pneumoniae* infections in 47 hematopoietic stem cell transplantation recipients: clinical characteristics of infections and vaccine-breakthrough infections, 1989-2005. *Medicine*. 2007;86(2):69-77.
386. Gündüz M, Özen M, Sahin U, et al. Subsequent malignancies after allogeneic hematopoietic stem cell transplantation. *Clin Transplant*. 2017;31(7). doi:10.1111/ctr.12987
387. Pittet D, Allegranzi B, Sax H, et al. Evidence-based model for hand transmission during patient care and the role of improved practices. *Lancet Infect Dis*. 2006;6(10):641-652.
388. Siegel JD, Rhinehart E, Jackson M, Chiarello L; Health care infection control practices Advisory Committee. 2007 Guideline for Isolation Precautions: Preventing transmission of infectious agents in the health care setting. *Am J Infect Control*. 2007;35(10 suppl 2):S65-S164.
389. Sims MD, Maine GN, Childers KL, et al. Coronavirus disease 2019 (COVID-19) seropositivity and asymptomatic rates in healthcare workers are associated with job function and masking. *Clin Infect Dis*. 2021;73(suppl 2):S154-S162.
390. Climo MW, Yokoe DS, Warren DK, et al. Effect of daily chlorhexidine bathing on hospital-acquired infection. *N Engl J Med*. 2013;368(6):533-542.

391. Pokala HR, Leonard D, Cox J, et al. Association of hospital construction with the development of healthcare associated environmental mold infections (HAEMI) in pediatric patients with leukemia. *Pediatr Blood Cancer*. 2014;61(2):276-280.
392. Pizzo PA, Purvis DS, Waters C. Microbiological evaluation of food items. For patients undergoing gastrointestinal decontamination and protected isolation. *J Am Diet Assoc*. 1982;81(3):272-279.
393. Moody KM, Baker RA, Santizo RO, et al. A randomized trial of the effectiveness of the neutropenic diet versus food safety guidelines on infection rate in pediatric oncology patients. *Pediatr Blood Cancer*. 2018;65(1). doi:10.1002/pbc.26711
394. Satlin MJ, Weissman SJ, Carpenter PA, Seo SK, Shelburne SA. American Society of Transplantation and Cellular Therapy Series, 1: Enterobacterales infection prevention and management after hematopoietic cell transplantation. *Transplant Cell Ther*. 2021;27(2):108-114.
395. Cornely OA, Maertens J, Winston DJ, et al. Posaconazole vs. fluconazole or itraconazole prophylaxis in patients with neutropenia. *N Engl J Med*. 2007;356(4):348-359.
396. Dadwal SS, Hohl TM, Fisher CE, et al. American Society of Transplantation and Cellular Therapy Series, 2: management and prevention of aspergillosis in hematopoietic cell transplantation recipients. *Transplant Cell Ther*. 2021;27(3):201-211.
397. Ullmann AJ, Lipton JH, Vesole DH, et al. Posaconazole or fluconazole for prophylaxis in severe graft-versus-host disease. *N Engl J Med*. 2007;356(4):335-347.
398. Boeckh M, Kim HW, Flowers MED, Meyers JD, Bowden RA. Long-term acyclovir for prevention of varicella zoster virus disease after allogeneic hematopoietic cell transplantation—a randomized double-blind placebo-controlled study. *Blood*. 2006;107(5):1800-1805.
399. Hwang JP, Feld JJ, Hammond SP, et al. Hepatitis B virus screening and management for patients with cancer prior to therapy: ASCO provisional clinical opinion update. *J Clin Oncol*. 2020;38(31):3698-3715.
400. Bucaneve G, Micozzi A, Menichetti F, et al. Levofloxacin to prevent bacterial infection in patients with cancer and neutropenia. *N Engl J Med*. 2005;353(10):977-987.
401. Cullen M, Steven N, Billingham L, et al. Antibacterial prophylaxis after chemotherapy for solid tumors and lymphomas. *N Engl J Med*. 2005;353(10):988-998.
402. Gafter-Gvili A, Fraser A, Paul M, et al. Antibiotic prophylaxis for bacterial infections in afebrile neutropenic patients following chemotherapy. *Cochrane Database Syst Rev*. 2012;1:CD004386.
403. Mehlhorn AJ, Brown DA. Safety concerns with fluoroquinolones. *Ann Pharamcother*. 2007;41(11):1859-1866.
404. Razonable RR, Litzow MR, Khaliq Y, et al. Bacteremia due to viridans group streptococci with diminished susceptibility to levofloxacin among neutropenic patients receiving levofloxacin prophylaxis. *Clin Infect Dis*. 2002;34(11):1469-1474.
405. Engelhard D, Cordonnier C, Shaw PJ, et al. Early and late invasive pneumococcal infection following stem cell transplantation: a European Bone Marrow Transplantation survey. *Br J Haematol*. 2002;117(2):444-450.
406. Cho SY, Choi HY. Opportunistic fungal infection among cancer patients. A ten-year autopsy study. *Am J Clin Pathol*. 1979;72(4):617-621.
407. Marr KA. Fungal infections in hematopoietic stem cell transplant recipients. *Med Mycol*. 2008;46:293-302.
408. Goodman JL, Winston DJ, Greenfield RA, et al. A controlled trial of fluconazole to prevent fungal infections in patients undergoing bone marrow transplantation. *N Engl J Med*. 1992;326(13):845-851.
409. Slavin MA, Osborne B, Adams R, et al. Efficacy and safety of fluconazole prophylaxis for fungal infections after marrow transplantation—a prospective, randomized, double-blind study. *J Infect Dis*. 1995;171(6):1545-1552.
410. Marr KA, Seidel K, Slavin MA, et al. Prolonged fluconazole prophylaxis is associated with persistent protection against candidiasis-related death in allogeneic marrow transplant recipients: long-term follow-up of a randomized, placebo-controlled trial. *Blood*. 2000;96(6):2055-2061.
411. Winston DJ, Chandrasekar PH, Lazarus HM, et al. Fluconazole prophylaxis of fungal infections in patients with acute leukemia. Results of a randomized, placebo-controlled, double-blind multicenter trial. *Ann Intern Med*. 1993;118(7):495-503.
412. Kontoyiannis DP, Marr KA, Park BJ, et al. Prospective surveillance for invasive fungal infections in hematopoietic stem cell transplant recipients, 2001-2006: overview of the Transplant-Associated Infection Surveillance Network (TRANSNET) Database. *Clin Infect Dis*. 2010;50(8):1091-1100.
413. Wingard JR, Carter SL, Walsh TJ, et al. Randomized, double-blind trial of fluconazole versus voriconazole for prevention of invasive fungal infection after allogeneic hematopoietic cell transplantation. *Blood*. 2010;116(24):5111-5118.
414. Bogler Y, Stern A, Su Y, et al. Efficacy and safety of isavuconazole compared with voriconazole as primary antifungal prophylaxis in allogeneic hematopoietic cell transplant recipients. *Med Mycol*. 2021;59(10):970-979.
415. Patil A, Majumdar S. Echinocandins in antifungal pharmacotherapy. *J Pharm Pharmacol*. 2017;69(12):1635-1660.
416. Hughes WT, Kuhn S, Chaudhary S, et al. Successful chemoprophylaxis for *Pneumocystis carinii* pneumonitis. *N Engl J Med*. 1977;297(26):1419-1426.
417. Cooley L, Dendle C, Wolf J, et al. Consensus guidelines for diagnosis, prophylaxis and management of *Pneumocystis jirovecii* pneumonia in patients with haematological and solid malignancies, 2014. *Intern Med J*. 2014;44(12b):1350-1363.
418. van Kraaij MGJ, Verdonck LF, Rozenberg-Arska M, Dekker AW. Early infections in adults undergoing matched related and matched unrelated/mismatched donor stem cell transplantation: a comparison of incidence. *Bone Marrow Transplant*. 2022;30(5):303-309.
419. Lam MT, Pazin GJ, Armstrong JA, Ho M. Herpes simplex infection in acute myelogenous leukemia and other hematologic malignancies: a prospective study. *Cancer*. 1981;48(10):2168-2171.
420. Saral R, Ambinder RF, Burns WH, et al. Acyclovir prophylaxis against herpes simplex virus infection in patients with leukemia. A randomized, double-blind, placebo-controlled study. *Ann Intern Med*. 1983;99(6):773-776.
421. Saral R, Burns WH, Laskin OL, Santos GW, Lietman PS. Acyclovir prophylaxis of herpes-simplex-virus infections. *N Engl J Med*. 1981;305(2):63-67.
422. Han CS, Miller W, Haake R, Weisdorf D. Varicella zoster infection after bone marrow transplantation: incidence, risk factors and complications. *Bone Marrow Transplant*. 1994;13(3):277-283.
423. Mikulska M, Lanini S, Guidol C, et al. ESCMID Study Group for Infections in Compromised Hosts (ESGICH) Consensus Document on the safety of targeted and biological therapies: an infectious diseases perspective (Agents targeting lymphoid cells surface antigens [I]—CD19, CD20, and CD52. *Clin Microbiol Infect*. 2018;24(suppl 2):S71-S82.
424. Richardson PG, Sonneveld P, Schuster MW, et al. Bortezomib or high-dose dexamethasone for relapsed multiple myeloma. *N Engl J Med*. 2005;352(24):2487-2498.
425. San Miguel JF, Schlag R, Khuageva NK, et al. Bortezomib plus melphalan and prednisone for initial treatment of multiple myeloma. *N Engl J Med*. 2008;359(9):906-917.
426. Minarik J, Pika T, Bacovsky J, Langova K, Scudla V. Low-dose acyclovir prophylaxis for bortezomib-induced herpes zoster in multiple myeloma patients. *Br J Haematol*. 2012;159(1):111-113.
427. Dimopoulos MA, Gay F, Schjesvold F, et al. Oral ixazomib maintenance following autologous stem cell transplantation (TOURMALINE-MM3): a double-blind, randomised, placebo-controlled phase 3 trial. *Lancet*. 2019;393(10168):253-264.
428. Chen K, Cheng MP, Hammond SP, Einsele H, Marty FM. Antiviral prophylaxis for cytomegalovirus infection in allogeneic hematopoietic cell transplantation. *Blood Adv*. 2018;2(16):2159-2175.
429. Gupta S, Govindarajan S, Fong TL, Redeker AG. Spontaneous reactivation in chronic hepatitis B: patterns and natural history. *J Clin Gastroenterol*. 1990;12(5):562-568.
430. Terrault NA, Lok ASF, McMahon BJ, et al. Update on prevention, diagnosis, and treatment of chronic hepatitis B: AASLD 2018 hepatitis B guidance. *Hepatology*. 2018;67(4):1560-1599.
431. Huang H, Li X, Zhu J, et al. Entecavir vs lamivudine for prevention of hepatitis B virus reactivation among patients with untreated diffuse large B-cell lymphoma receiving R-CHOP chemotherapy: a randomized clinical trial. *JAMA*. 2014;312(23):2521-2530.
432. Rubin LG, Levin MJ, Ljungman P, et al. 2013 IDSA clinical practice guideline for vaccination of the immunocompromised host. *Clin Infect Dis*. 2014;58(3):e44-e100.
433. Kobayashi M, Farrar JL, Gierke R, et al. Use of 15-valent pneumococcal conjugate vaccine and 20-valent pneumococcal conjugate vaccine among U.S. adults: updated recommendations of the Advisory Committee on Immunization Practices – United States, 2022. *MMWR Morb Mortal Wkly Rep*. 2022;71(4):109-117.
434. Lal H, Cunningham AL, Godeaux O, et al. Efficacy of an adjuvanted herpes zoster subunit vaccine in older adults. *N Engl J Med*. 2015;372(22):2087-2096.
435. Bastidas A, de la Serna J, El Idrissi M, et al. Effect of recombinant zoster vaccine on incidence of herpes zoster after autologous stem cell transplantation: a randomized clinical trial. *JAMA*. 2019;322(2):123-133.
436. Dagnew AF, Ilhan O, Lee WS, et al. Immunogenicity and safety of the adjuvanted recombinant zoster vaccine in adults with haematological malignancies: a phase 3, randomised clinical trial and post-hoc efficacy analysis. *Lancet Infect Dis*. 2019;19(9):988-1000.
437. Anderson TC, Masters NB, Guo A, et al. Use of recombinant zoster vaccine in immunocompromised adults aged ≥19 years: recommendations of the Advisory Committee on Immunization Practices—United States, 2022. *MMWR Morb Mortal Wkly Rep*. 2022;71(3):80-84.
438. Ljungman P, Wiklund-Hammarsten M, Duraj V, et al. Response to tetanus toxoid immunization after allogeneic bone marrow transplantation. *J Infect Dis*. 1990;162(2):496-500.
439. Nordøy T, Husebekk A, Aaberge IS, et al. Humoral immunity to viral and bacterial antigens in lymphoma patients 4-10 years after high-dose therapy with ABMT. Serological responses to revaccinations according to EBMT guidelines. *Bone Marrow Transplant*. 2001;28(7):681-687.
440. Ljungman P, Duraj V, Magnius L. Response to immunization against polio after allogeneic marrow transplantation. *Bone Marrow Transplant*. 1991;7(2):89-93.

Chapter 71 ■ Immunotherapy

TRISHA R. BERGER • MARCELA V. MAUS

HISTORICAL PERSPECTIVE

There probably is no field in medicine that has provided as much hope, or as much disappointment, as the field of tumor immunology. A major relationship between the immune system and the oversight of neoplasms was postulated in the early part of the last century by Paul Ehrlich.[1] This theory envisioned that, in long-lived animals, inheritable genetic changes in somatic cells must be common, and some proportion of these changes must represent steps toward malignant transformation. It was considered an evolutionary necessity, therefore, that some mechanisms exist for eliminating or inactivating such potentially dangerous mutant cells. This mechanism was thought to be immunologic. The theory of immunosurveillance was restated in the 1950s by Lewis Thomas, then popularized and championed by Sir Macfarlane Burnet (Figure 71.1).[2] Supported by these powerful figures in medicine, the theory of immunosurveillance was so inherently appealing that it was often accepted uncritically, and evidence to the contrary often overlooked.[3] For instance, although patients or animals who are immunosuppressed tend to have an increased incidence of tumors, these tumors are disproportionately of lymphoid origin or associated with an oncogenic virus. The development of common epithelial neoplasms (with the exception of certain skin cancers) in these patients occurs with much less impressive frequency.[4]

The most obvious evolutionary necessity of the immune system was to survey a variety of infections, especially viral infections. Early evidence seemed to indicate that immunity played a significant role in eradicating virally induced tumors.[4,5] On the other hand, it appeared to play a less significant, or less effective, role in prevention of tumors induced by physical or chemical carcinogens.[6,7] Experimentation in the early part of the 20th century demonstrated that spontaneously arising tumors in outbred animals could occasionally be transplanted from one animal to another of the same species and propagated in that manner. Attempts to immunize against transplantable tumors soon followed. Animals injected with a small number of tumor cells were often able to eliminate those tumor cells; that is, there appeared to be a threshold number of tumor cells required for tumor propagation. Animals that had eliminated a sublethal inoculum of tumor cells were often able to withstand inoculation with a large number of tumor cells that would have been lethal in a naive animal. Furthermore, preexposure to normal tissue of the donor often rendered the recipient resistant to challenge with a lethal number of tumor cells.[8] These experiments brought into question the idea of tumor-specific antigens and ultimately led to the discovery of major histocompatibility complex (MHC) genes and their products.[9,10]

Modern tumor immunology finds its roots in the classic experiments of Prehn and Main.[11] These investigators demonstrated, in genetically identical mice, that previous exposure to a chemically induced sarcoma rendered animals resistant to challenge with the same tumor, but that these animals would accept normal, nonneoplastic tissues transplanted from the tumor donor animal. Similarly, prior exposure to normal tissues from the donor animal did not render the recipient animal resistant to tumor challenge. These experiments revived the notion that tumor-specific (transplantation) antigens did exist. Subsequent experiments demonstrated that protection afforded by prior exposure to tumor cells was tumor specific.[5] Thus, the host response to transplanted tumors behaved like an adaptive immune response, demonstrating memory and specificity.

Tumor immunity could be passively conveyed from one animal to another by transfer of lymphoid cells.[12] The relevant cells for protection were shown to be T lymphocytes.[13] Thus, it should have been clear to workers in the field that the relevant tumor antigens were those that could be recognized by T lymphocytes. However, as this work was beginning, there was little understanding of how T lymphocytes recognized antigens or how those antigens were processed and presented to the T lymphocyte by antigen-presenting cells (APCs) or the tumor target cells. Much time and effort were expended in search of membrane structures or tumor cell products that would distinguish the tumor from all others. Particularly after the description of monoclonal antibody (mAb) technology,[14] a fervent search was undertaken to define structures on tumor cells that would be tumor specific and potential targets for therapeutic intervention. Although many cell surface structures were defined, and the contribution to the understanding

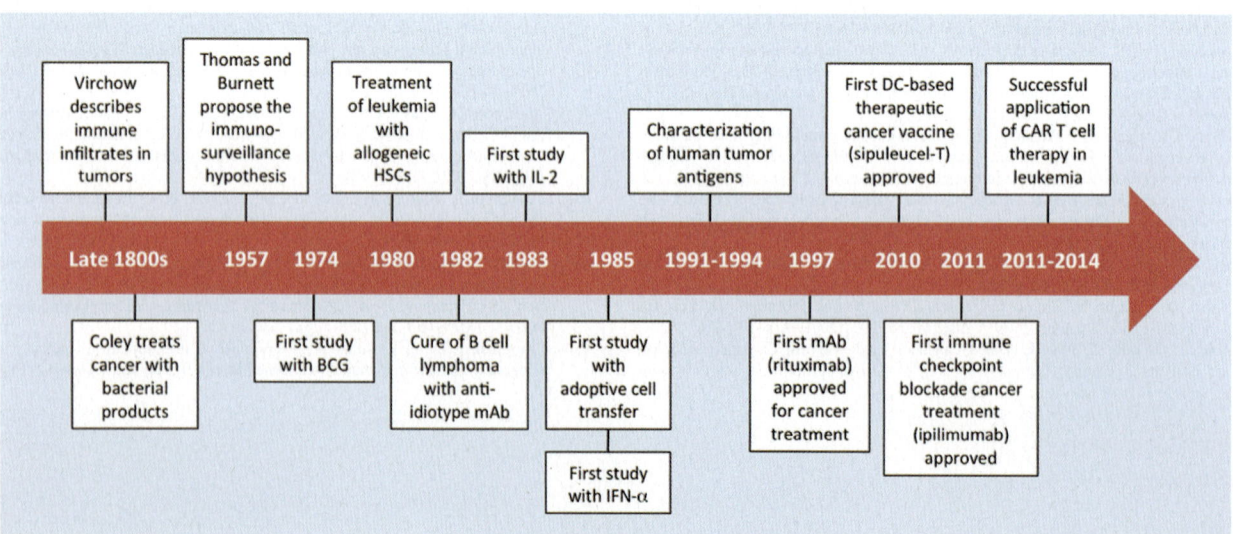

FIGURE 71.1 Timeline of major advances in cancer immunology and immunotherapy. Important basic immunologic studies of cancer and key clinical studies are shown. BCG, Bacillus Calmette-Guérin; CAR, chimeric antigen receptor; DC, dendritic cell; HSCs, hematopoietic stem cells; IFN-α, interferon-α; IL-2, interleukin-2; mAb, monoclonal antibody.

of biology cannot be overstated, this adventure produced only a single truly specific tumor antigen, the idiotype (Id) of clonally distributed immunoglobulin present on certain lymphomas.

Only during the past 2 decades has convincing evidence for an effect of immunosurveillance been produced.[15,16] This evidence relies, in great measure, on the availability of genetically manipulated animal systems. Thus, a variety of knockout mice with defects in components of immune activation or effector function develop, at high frequency, spontaneous tumors or tumors after carcinogen exposure.[15,16]

The concept that the immune system can recognize and possibly eliminate tumors has led to a variety of immunotherapies. Immunologic treatment of cancer has been attempted for over a century with sometimes surprising but not sustainable results. For example, William B. Coley, a surgeon in New York City, treated patients with live or killed bacteria called Coley toxins, which brought about partial or complete tumor regression in some patients.[17] Although appealing, Coley's approach was unpredictable and was eventually abandoned. Since these early attempts, new insights into the immune system and the immune response against cancer have renewed excitement in developing immunotherapies for cancer. Hematologic malignancies have been at the forefront of the effective application of cancer immunotherapies (*Figure 71.1*).[18]

INNATE IMMUNITY AGAINST TUMORS

The innate immune system is a widespread and evolutionarily ancient form of host defense against infection. In recent years, there has been an explosion of information regarding innate immunity, including its role in host defense and its regulation of inflammation and adaptive immunity.[19,20] The innate immune system is made up of many cells, including dendritic cells (DCs), macrophages, mast cells, neutrophils, eosinophils, innate lymphocytes such as natural killer (NK) cells, and innate-like lymphocytes such as natural killer T (NKT) cells and mucosal γδ T cells. Each of these cell types has been implicated in immune responses against tumors.

Phagocytic Cells

Many cells of the innate immune system, including neutrophils, macrophages, and DCs, bear receptors that detect "danger"[21] in the form of pathogen-associated molecular patterns (PAMPs). Examples of PAMPs include bacterial lipopolysaccharide, lipoprotein, peptidoglycan, and lipoteichoic acids; bacterial CpG DNA; and viral RNA and DNA. These PAMPs are recognized by a variety of pattern recognition receptors (PRRs) expressed by cells of the innate immune system.[22] The innate immune system is said to distinguish "infectious nonself" from "noninfectious self." The PRRs of the innate immune system are encoded in the germline. Unlike genes of the T-cell antigen receptor and the immunoglobulins, these genes do not undergo rearrangement. They are fixed and detect critical microbial components. Engagement of PRRs with PAMPs can result in pathogen uptake and/or cellular activation.[22] One important group of PRRs is the family of evolutionary conserved toll-like receptors (TLRs), which are critically important for innate immune cell activation. Thirteen TLRs, each with specificity for a different PAMP, have been described in mammals. Other PRR families include the nucleotide-binding domain leucine-rich repeats (NLR) receptors and the caspase recruitment domain-containing helicases.

Neutrophils and macrophages typically exert little antitumor activity, unless these cells are activated by bacteria, their products, or cytokines produced by tumor-specific T cells.[23,24] Recent studies have suggested that dying tumor cells or damaged tissues can release damage-associated molecular patterns (DAMPs) that can interact with PRRs and thus serve as danger signals.[25] NLR receptors such as NLR family pyrin domain–containing 3, which form large cytoplasmic signaling complexes called inflammasomes, are thought to play a critical role in detecting DAMPs and might regulate the development of tumors either positively or negatively.[26,27] Macrophages can kill tumor cells using the same mechanisms utilized for killing of microorganisms. These mechanisms include phagocytosis and release of cytotoxic molecules, such as reactive oxygen intermediates and nitric oxide. Activated macrophages also produce a variety of cytokines. Among these cytokines, tumor necrosis factor (TNF)-α plays a major role in the tumoricidal effects of macrophages in vitro.[28]

Another important role of phagocytes in tumor immunity is to present tumor antigens to T lymphocytes. DCs (and other APCs such as macrophages) can phagocytose tumor cells and present tumor antigens in the context of MHC molecules and costimulatory signals to T lymphocytes.[29]

Natural Killer Cells

It has been recognized for a long time that NK cells kill MHC class I–deficient tumor cells in vivo and in vitro.[30] However, the identity and characterization of receptors mediating NK activation proved elusive for many years. Activation of NK cells is now understood to be dependent on the balance of activating and inhibitory signals emanating from activating and inhibitory receptors on the NK cell surface.[31] These receptors fall into two major structural classes, those of the immunoglobulin superfamily (killer cell immunoglobulin-like receptors [KIRs] and leukocyte Immunoglobulin-like receptors [LIRs]) and those of the C-type lectin-like family (NKG2D, CD94/NKG2A, and Ly49). Most inhibitory receptors (e.g., CD94/NKG2A, KIR, and Ly49) recognize classic or nonclassic MHC molecules. An activating receptor on NK cells, NKG2D (also called KLRK1), has now been shown to recognize a variety of stress-induced MHC class I–like molecules (e.g., Rae-1, H60, and MICA/B). Of note, activated CD8+ T cells and mucosal γδ T cells also express NKG2D. Another activation receptor on NK cells is FcγRIII, which can target NK cells to immunoglobulin G (IgG) antibody–coated tumor cells and induce antibody-dependent cell-mediated cytotoxicity.

NK cells can also discriminate between different allelic variants of MHC molecules.[32] This phenomenon was originally identified in the context of the hybrid resistance transplant model in mice, where parental bone marrow grafts were rejected by a subset of host F1 NK cells. When faced with mismatched allogeneic targets, a subset of donor NK cells can sense the missing expression of self-human leukocyte antigen (HLA) class I alleles and mediate alloreactions. These alloreactive NK cells can improve engraftment and control the relapse of acute myeloid leukemia (AML) in mismatched hematopoietic transplants.[32]

Natural Killer T Cells

NKT cells are a subset of T lymphocytes that share receptor structures and functions with the NK cell lineage.[33] Prototypical NKT cells, often referred to as invariant NKT (iNKT) cells, express a semi-invariant T-cell receptor (TCR), which is specific for glycolipid antigens presented by the MHC class I–like protein CD1d. Although NKT cells express an antigen-specific receptor that is generated by somatic DNA rearrangement, these cells belong to the innate rather than the adaptive arm of the immune system.[34] The invariant TCR expressed by NKT cells recognizes a limited set of self- and foreign antigens and, therefore, bears similarity to the PRRs expressed by cells of the innate immune system. Further, NKT cells have a natural, activated phenotype and are unable to generate classic memory responses against their cognate glycolipid antigens.

Mice that are deficient in NKT cells have increased susceptibility to methylcholanthrene (MCA)-induced sarcomas, indicating that these cells contribute to natural immunity against tumors.[35] NKT cells in mice and humans respond to the marine sponge-derived glycosphingolipid α-galactosylceramide (α-GalCer), which has potent antimetastatic activities in mice.[35] α-GalCer and related NKT cell antigens are being explored as potential cancer immunotherapies.

Mucosal γδ T Cells

T cells expressing the γδ TCR are enriched in mucosal tissues, such as the mucosa of the gut and skin.[36] These mucosal γδ T cells have a highly restricted TCR repertoire, suggesting specificity for a limited set of antigens selectively expressed in their respective epithelial compartments. Like NKT cells, mucosal γδ T cells can be classified as being at the interface between innate and adaptive immunity.[34] Epidermal and intestinal γδ T cells express NKG2D and become activated when NKG2D binds to stress-induced MHC class I–related molecules.

γδ T cells play a crucial role in immunosurveillance against malignant epidermal cells. The incidence of cutaneous malignancies after treatment with a combination of initiator and promoter carcinogens was substantially increased in mice lacking the TCR δ-chain.[37] Activation of γδ T cells required both NKG2D and the γδ TCR, suggesting that engagement of NKG2D with its ligand(s) synergizes with signals received through the autoreactive γδ TCR.

ADAPTIVE IMMUNITY AGAINST TUMORS

The adaptive immune system is composed of B and T cells that express diverse antigen-specific receptors, immunoglobulins, and TCRs, respectively. Diversity of these receptors is generated by somatic DNA rearrangement, in a process referred to as variable-diversity-joining recombination.[38] Currently, there is little evidence that adaptive immunity plays a major role in natural immunity against tumors (with the exception of tumors induced by viruses). Although mice lacking T lymphocytes have increased susceptibility to the development of MCA-induced sarcomas, this might be largely due to the lack of iNKT cells and/or γδ T cells.[16] Nevertheless, it is clear that tumors can induce adaptive immune responses (*Figure 71.2*), which can be exploited for the development of cancer immunotherapies.

Antibodies and B Cells

The role of B cells in regulating tumor immunity remains poorly understood. In some tumor models, B cells appear to be important for priming of T-cell responses and tumor resistance, whereas in other models, B cells have an inhibitory effect on the generation of cytotoxic T-lymphocyte (CTL) responses and tumor rejection.[39] Nevertheless, it is clear that tumor-bearing hosts can produce antibodies against a variety of tumor antigens.[16] However, strong humoral responses rarely correlate with tumor resistance. Nevertheless, antibodies can be utilized for immunotherapy of cancer, in particular tumors of hematopoietic origin. Antibodies may kill tumor cells by activating complement and promoting phagocytosis by macrophages. Alternatively, antibody-coated tumor cells may be killed by antibody-dependent cell-mediated cytotoxicity, in which Fc receptor–bearing NK cells, macrophages, or neutrophils mediate the killing. In addition, in certain cases, antibodies may directly interfere with the growth of tumor cells, as illustrated by the beneficial effects of anti-HER-2/neu antibodies against breast cancer, which likely involves downregulation of the HER-2/neu growth factor receptor.[40]

T Lymphocytes

Classic studies with transplantable tumors have demonstrated a critical role of T lymphocytes in tumor immunity.[11] CTLs play a particularly important role in tumor rejection because these cells can directly lyse malignant cells that display tumor antigens in association with MHC class I molecules.[41] The importance of CD4+ T cells in tumor immunity is less clear. CD4+ T cells may secrete cytokines that promote the development of CD8+ T-cell responses, increase the sensitivity of tumor targets to CTL lysis by inducing MHC class I expression, and activate macrophages. Because of their critical role for the development of tumor immunotherapies, we briefly describe the mechanisms that lead to the induction of T-cell responses to tumors.

Antigen Processing and Presentation

T lymphocytes recognize peptide antigens in the context of MHC molecules, which are derived from two distinct pathways.[42] Peptides representing proteins sampled from the extracellular world are generally presented in the context of MHC class II proteins, whereas peptides resulting from intracellular synthesis of proteins are presented in the peptide groove of the MHC class I proteins (*Figure 71.3*).[43]

Peptides located in MHC class II molecules are derived from proteins that have been consumed by APCs[44] (*Figure 71.3A*). The proteins are taken up by phagocytosis, receptor-mediated endocytosis, or pinocytosis. Once internalized, the antigens are located in endosomes, which fuse with lysosomes.[44] There, disulfide bonds in proteins are first reduced by the enzyme interferon-γ (IFN-γ)–inducible lysosomal thiol reductase, and the resulting products are cleaved to peptides by proteases, predominantly cathepsins. The endosome fuses with an exocytic vesicle budding from the Golgi apparatus that contains newly made MHC class II molecules associated with invariant chain, which plays a critical role in the assembly, intracellular transport, and function of MHC class II molecules.[45] In addition, a chaperone, HLA-DM, facilitates binding of MHC class II with antigenic peptide.[45] Fusion of the endosome with the plasma membrane ultimately displays the MHC class II molecule-peptide complexes on the cell surface.

Peptides are prepared for presentation on class I molecules in a different manner (*Figure 71.3B*). These peptides are derived from intracellular protein synthesis.[46] After protein synthesis, proteins introduced into the cytoplasm may become the target of the proteasome, a cytoplasmic organelle whose major function is the degradation of proteins tagged for turnover by the addition of ubiquitin. During conditions of IFN-γ production such as infection, several proteasome subunits (LMP-2,

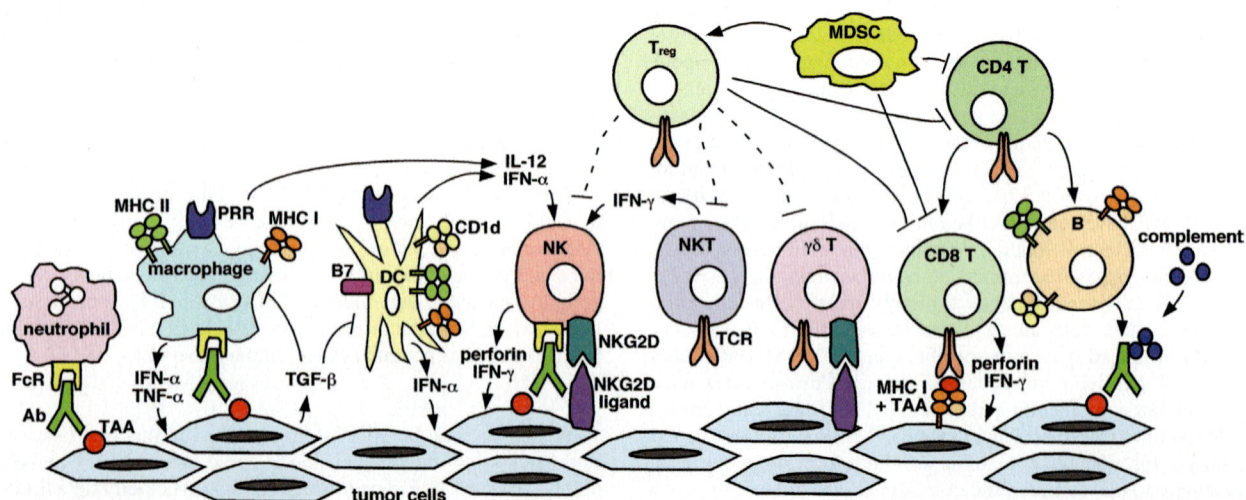

FIGURE 71.2 Immune responses against tumors. A variety of cells and soluble factors of innate and adaptive immunity can participate in immune responses against tumors. Examples of mechanisms that can suppress immune responses against tumors (i.e., production of TGF-β by tumor cells and induction of T_{reg}) are also depicted. Ab, antibody; FcR, Fc receptor; IFN, interferon; MDSC, myeloid-derived suppressor cell; MHC, major histocompatibility complex; NK, natural killer; NKT, natural killer T; PRR, pattern recognition receptor; TAA, tumor-associated antigen; TCR, T-cell receptor; TGF, transforming growth factor; TNF, tumor necrosis factor; T_{reg}, regulatory T cell.

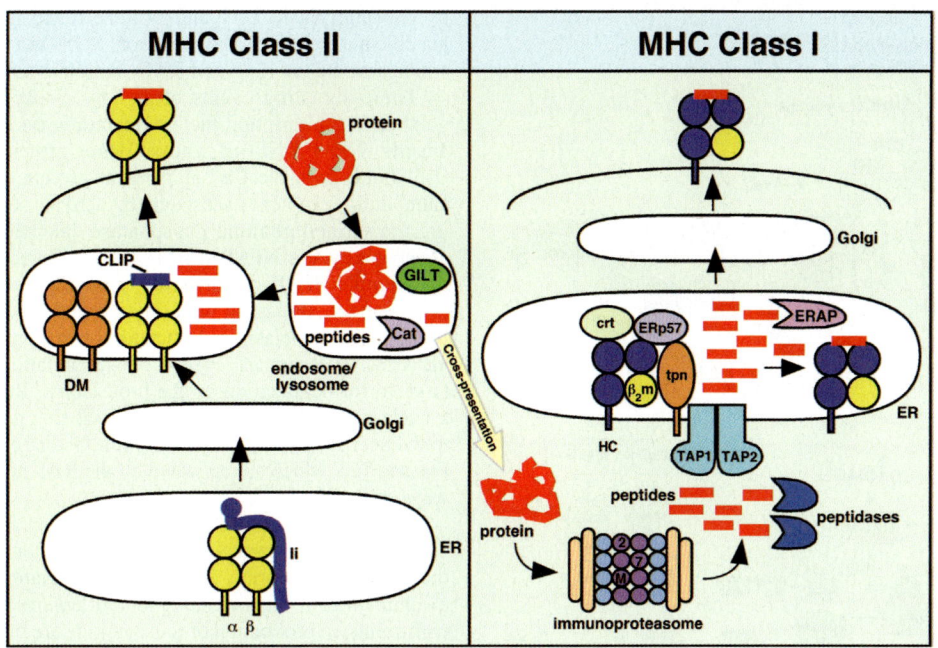

FIGURE 71.3 Presentation of peptides by major histocompatibility complex (MHC) molecules. A, MHC class II–restricted antigen processing and presentation to CD4 T cells. Exogenous protein antigens are taken up by APCs, disulfide bonds are reduced by the interferon (IFN)-γ–inducible lysosomal thiol reductase (GILT), and the proteins are then degraded in endosomal/lysosomal compartments by cathepsins (Cat). MHC class II α and β are synthesized in the endoplasmic reticulum (ER) and associated there with the MHC class II–associated invariant chain (Ii). The class II/Ii complexes then egress to endosomal compartments, where Ii is degraded by cathepsins, until only its class II–associated invariant chain (CLIP) region remains bound by class II. CLIP is then removed from class II by the human leukocyte antigen (HLA)-DM peptide exchange factor. Finally, class II is loaded with peptide and delivered to the cell surface for presentation to class II–restricted CD4 T cells. B, MHC class I–restricted antigen processing and presentation to CD8 T cells. Cytosolic proteins, derived from endogenously synthesized proteins or from cross-presented antigens (as indicated by the arrow), are degraded by immunoproteasomes that contain the interferon IFN-γ–inducible subunits LMP-2 (2), LMP-7 (7), and MECL-1 (M). Some of the resulting peptides are further processed in the cytoplasm by peptidases and then transported to the lumen of the ER by the transporter of antigen processing (TAP). Some of the peptides undergo further processing in the ER by ER-associated aminopeptidases (ERAPs). Peptide-receptive MHC class I heavy-chain (HC)/β$_2$-microglobulin (β$_2$m) heterodimers in the ER associate with a variety of chaperones, including calreticulin (crt), ERp57, and tapasin (tpn). After binding with peptides, class I molecules undergo a conformational change, permitting their egress to the cell surface for presentation to class I–restricted CD8 T cells.

LMP-7, and MECL-1) become upregulated and are incorporated into newly assembled proteasomes.[46] These peptides are then transported into the lumen of the endoplasmic reticulum (ER) by the transporter associated with antigen processing (TAP) proteins. Within the ER, peptides may be further trimmed by ER-resident aminopeptidases (i.e., ERAP1 and ERAP2). Within the ER, empty MHC class I molecules are associated with a variety of chaperones, including calnexin, calreticulin, ERp57, and tapasin. Tapasin is a transmembrane protein that tethers empty class I molecules in the ER to TAP.[46] The assembled MHC class I–peptide complex transits the Golgi apparatus, proceeds in a vesicle to the cell surface, and is displayed on the cell surface after fusion of the vesicle membrane with the plasma membrane.

There has been interest in the mechanisms whereby tumor cells initiate CD8+ T-cell responses. Few tumors are derived from professional APCs and, therefore, do not effectively prime naive CD8+ T cells. It has now been established that tumor cells can be processed and presented by host APCs, particularly DCs, in a process that is referred to as cross-presentation (*Figure 71.3*).[47] Tumor antigens are then processed inside the APCs, and peptides derived from these antigens are displayed on MHC class I molecules for recognition by CD8+ T cells. These APCs also express MHC class II molecules and can prime naive CD4+ T cells, which may be important for the generation of effective CD8+ memory responses. Once tumor antigen–specific CTLs are generated, they can kill tumor cells without the requirement for costimulation. While the precise mechanisms of cross-presentation remain poorly understood, the concept of cross-presentation has important applications in the development of tumor vaccines.[47]

T-Lymphocyte Activation

The goal of antigen processing and presentation is the activation of appropriate T lymphocytes to proliferate, produce cytokines, and promote an immunologic reaction or become cytotoxic cells. Although the interaction of the T-cell antigen receptor with antigen-MHC provides specificity of the response and initiates the crucial events of activation, the interactions are few and have low affinity.[48] The interaction between T lymphocytes and APCs or target cells is initially stabilized by a number of nonspecific receptor-counterreceptor interactions, leading to the development of an immunologic synapse with its central supramolecular activation cluster.[49] Chief among these interactions is the coupling of CD2 on the T lymphocyte with lymphocyte function antigen-3 on the APC. Also involved is the interaction of the lymphocyte function antigen-1 molecule with intercellular adhesion molecule-1 and intercellular adhesion molecule-2. Once the cells have been apposed, the specific interaction of the T-cell antigen receptor and the antigen-MHC can occur. It now appears that the T cell proceeds toward activation only if certain threshold numbers of TCR–MHC/antigen interactions occur.[50]

The signal transduction pathways that result in T-cell activation have been extensively reviewed,[51] and we will focus here on the most salient features (*Figure 71.4*). Ligation of the TCR with an agonist peptide/MHC complex results in phosphorylation of the cytoplasmic portions of the CD3 and ζ components of the TCR. The cytoplasmic domains of CD3 and ζ contain several conserved peptide sequences called immunoreceptor tyrosine-based activation motifs (ITAMs) that are targets for intracellular protein tyrosine kinases that catalyze the phosphorylation of tyrosine residues in various protein substrates. The tyrosine kinase lck interacts with the cytoplasmic domains of CD4 and CD8, and the tyrosine kinase fyn interacts with the TCR-CD3 complex. Binding of the TCR with peptide/MHC complexes results in receptor clustering, bringing CD4/CD8 and lck in closeness, proximity of the ITAMs within the CD3 and ζ-chains. Lck and fyn subsequently phosphorylate tyrosine residues within the ITAMs, which

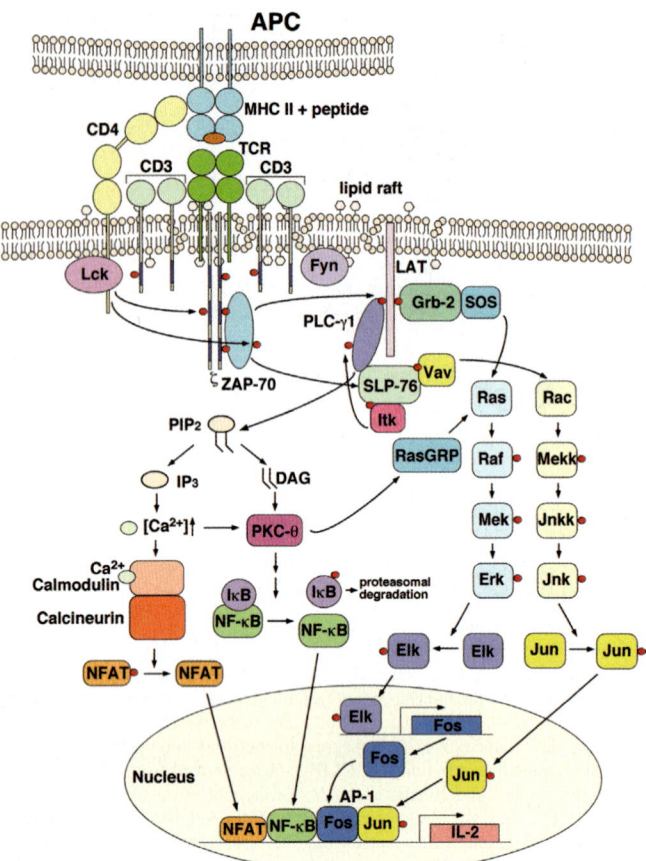

FIGURE 71.4 Overview of signal transduction events involved in T-lymphocyte activation. Interaction of the T-cell receptor (TCR) and coreceptors with major histocompatibility complex (MHC)–peptide complexes on antigen-presenting cells (APCs) results in multiple signaling events that lead to the activation of several transcription factors that stimulate expression of numerous genes (e.g., the interleukin-2 [*IL-2*] gene). Note that the precise interactions between different adaptor proteins that participate in proximal TCR signaling events remain incompletely understood. AP, activated protein; DAG, diacylglycerol; Elk, Ets-like transcription factor; Erk, extracellular signal–regulated kinase; Grb, growth factor receptor–bound protein; IκB, inhibitor of κB; IP_3, inositol triphosphate; Itk, interleukin-2–inducible tyrosine kinase; Jnk, Jun N-terminal kinase; Jnkk, Jnk kinase; LAT, linker of activated T cells; Lck, lymphocyte-specific protein tyrosine kinase; Mek, Mapk/Erk kinase; Mekk, Mapk/Erk kinase; NF, nuclear factor; NFAT, nuclear factor of activated T cells; PIP_2, phosphatidylinositol biphosphate; PKC, protein kinase; PLC, phospholipase C; RasGRP, Ras guanyl nucleotide–releasing protein; SLP-76, SH2 domain–containing leukocyte protein, 76-kDa; SOS, son of sevenless; ZAP-70, ζ-associated protein kinase, 70-kDa.

become docking sites for the ζ-associated protein, ZAP-70, a member of the syk family of protein tyrosine kinases. The bound ZAP-70 then becomes a substrate for lck, and phosphorylation of ZAP-70 results in its activation. Activated ZAP-70 phosphorylates several scaffolding proteins, including linker of activated T cells (LAT) and SLP-76 (adaptor protein involved in signaling through the T-cell antigen receptor complex), which, when phosphorylated, serve as docking sites for other proteins that, in turn, activate multiple signaling pathways. One of these signaling pathways involves changes in inositol lipid metabolism. Phospholipase Cγ1 (PLCγ1) becomes tyrosine phosphorylated and activated as it associates with LAT. Activation of PLCγ1 leads to the hydrolysis of a minor membrane lipid, phosphatidylinositol biphosphate, to yield inositol triphosphate (IP_3) and diacylglycerol (DAG). Each of these products activates downstream events. IP_3 induces a rapid increase in free Ca^{2+} by release from membrane-sequestered Ca^{2+} stores, whereas DAG and Ca^{2+} activate protein kinase C (PKC) θ. T-cell activation also results in the activation of the RAS and RAC signaling pathways. Adapter proteins that are activated by phosphorylated LAT and SLP-76 result in the activation of the guanine nucleotide exchange factors SOS (son of sevenless) and VAV, which activate the RAS and RAC signaling pathways, respectively.

These signaling events ultimately result in the activation of a number of transcription factors, including nuclear factor of activated T cells (NFAT), NF-κB, and activator protein 1 (AP-1). Cytosolic Ca^{2+} binds with the Ca^{2+}-dependent protein calmodulin, and Ca^{2+}-calmodulin complexes subsequently activate several enzymes, including the serine/threonine phosphatase calcineurin. Calcineurin then dephosphorylates NFAT, which uncovers a nuclear localization signal that permits NFAT to translocate to the nucleus. Activation of NF-κB is dependent, at least in part, on activated PKCθ. NF-κB is normally found in the cytoplasm in association with a protein called inhibitor of κB (IκB). TCR signals result in phosphorylation of IκB, which is then targeted for degradation by the proteasome. Release of IκB uncovers a nuclear translocation signal in NF-κB that permits its translocation to the nucleus. AP-1 is a transcription factor composed of the proteins Fos and Jun, which are activated by the RAS and RAC signaling pathways, respectively.

The net result of this extremely complex activation system is the expression of new proteins, the acquisition of functional capacity, or the ability to proliferate. T-lymphocyte activation is best understood as a culmination of events leading to interleukin (IL)-2 production.[51] The constraints on production of this cytokine are more rigorous than those relevant for production of other gene products (such as IL-2 receptor α-chain and transcription factors). The promoter of the *IL-2* gene is made up of a number of binding sites for transcription factors, including two NFAT sites, an NF-κB site, and an AP-1 site.[51] The combination of production of IL-2 receptor α-chain and IL-2 provides an adequate stimulus for the T lymphocyte to successfully proliferate, giving rise to the antigen-specific clonal expansion of lymphocytes characteristic of immunologic responses. However, there are extraordinary controls against inappropriate activation of T lymphocytes. In addition to a first signal delivered via the T-cell antigen receptor complex, full activation of T cells also requires a second signal.[52] The best characterized origin of these second signals is the interaction of CD28 on the T-lymphocyte surface with its cognate ligands CD80 (B7-1) and CD86 (B7-2) on the APC, the most potent of which is the DC. Failure to receive a second signal can lead the T lymphocyte to undergo anergy or apoptosis. Activation of T cells is also regulated by a variety of negative signals, referred to as immune checkpoints, including inhibitory receptors of the CD28 family such as CTL-associated protein 4 (CTLA-4), which interacts with CD80 and CD86, and programmed death 1 (PD-1), which interacts with PD-1 ligands, PD-L1 and PD-L2.[52]

TUMOR-ASSOCIATED ANTIGENS

Tumor antigens are like all other antigens of adaptive immunity. That is, with few exceptions, they are peptides that are presented to T lymphocytes in the cleft of an MHC-encoded protein.[41] The nature of peptide antigens responsible for immune responses to tumors has been described in a classic set of experiments that did not make assumptions regarding the nature of the antigenic peptides.[41] Most tumor-specific antigenic peptides discovered thus far have been derived from proteins not usually expressed in any normal adult tissues (with the exception of testis and ovary), such as P1A and MAGE-1, or they represent differentiation antigens characteristic of the cellular lineage of the tumor, such as tyrosinase, gp100, and MART1/Aa in melanoma.[53]

Early definition of tumor antigens focused on MHC class I–restricted peptides.[41] This seemed to be the obvious approach because most tumors express MHC class I structures, but few express MHC class II molecules. Also, the point of immunotherapy was to eliminate tumors—a job for cytolytic cells (i.e., for $CD8^+$ cytotoxic lymphocytes that recognize antigen in the context of MHC class I molecules). Early clinical immunization trials[54] demonstrated the feasibility and the potential efficacy of immunotherapy with peptides recognized by $CD8^+$ T cells. However, immune responses were, in general, weak and short-lived. At the same time that the trials were being conducted, there was a growing realization of the importance of $CD4^+$ T cells in the immune response against tumors.[55] It is likely that incorporation of both MHC class I– and class II–restricted epitopes in tumor vaccines will be required to generate potent antitumor responses.

While this direct approach to tumor antigen recognition has proceeded, other investigators have asked whether certain appealing target proteins could be immunogenic. In particular, molecules involved in the process of malignant transformation provide attractive targets for therapeutic intervention. Because loss variants of tumor cells bearing these oncogenic proteins would presumably be nonmalignant, an immunologic assault on these proteins might be particularly effective. Evidence has been provided that immune responses to both mutated and overexpressed oncogenic proteins can occur in patients with malignancy or can be elicited in animals. Target oncogenic proteins include mutated RAS, HER-2/Neu, BCR-ABL, PML-RARα, and mutated p53. TCRs specific to mutated oncogenic proteins have been analyzed in patients receiving adoptive T cell therapy (ACT), where tumor-infiltrating lymphocytes (TILs) are expanded ex vivo and reinjected. In one case of a successful response to ACT, the TILs were made up of four TCRs specific to the KRAS-G12D mutation and were restricted by HLA-C, which bound mutant KRAS peptides presented by the TCR but not WT.[56] This type of TCR identification provides important metrics for developing ACTs that will recognize oncogenic proteins.

Since these early studies, advances in genomics, proteomics, bioinformatics, and immunologic approaches have facilitated the identification of tumor neoantigens.[57] For example, such approaches were employed to identify personal tumor-specific neoantigens in chronic lymphocytic leukemia (CLL).[58] A new approach to identify neoantigen-specific TCRs involves coculturing patient TIL with autologous APCs that are transduced with tandem minigenes or pulsed with peptides. The TILs then undergo single-cell RNA sequencing analysis to identify TCR sequences in cells expressing high levels of IFN-g and IL-2.[59] These TCR sequences can then transduced into T cells and used for ACT.

TUMOR-HOST INTERACTIONS: BEYOND IMMUNOSURVEILLANCE

While the immune system can protect against the development of tumors, interactions between developing tumors and the host are complex. Tumors often develop means to evade immune responses, and tumors that develop in immunocompetent hosts are often more immunogenic than those that develop in immunodeficient hosts. Finally, it is now also well recognized that the immune system can play both tumor-suppressing and tumor-promoting roles.

Immune Evasion by Tumors

Many tumors have devised ways to evade immune responses.[16] First, tumors may lose expression of the antigens that were recognized by antibodies or CTLs. Second, many tumors downregulate expression of MHC class I molecules, rendering these cells resistant to lysis by CTLs. Third, tumors may fail to induce effective CTL responses because of the absence of costimulatory molecules and/or resistance to uptake by APCs and cross-presentation. Instead of inducing an effective immune response, some tumors may actively promote tolerance induction, by inducing anergy, exhaustion, or deletion of tumor antigen–specific T cells. This might involve the generation of tumor antigen–specific regulatory T cells (T_{regs}), induction of inhibitory costimulatory molecules such as CTLA-4 and PD-1 on tumor antigen–specific T cells, induction of tumor-associated macrophages that suppress T-cell effector functions, and/or expansion of myeloid-derived suppressor cells, a heterogeneous group of myeloid progenitor cells and immature myeloid cells that can inhibit lymphocyte function. Fourth, tumor cells may actively suppress immune responses by secretion of suppressive cytokines such as transforming growth factor β (TGF-β) or by expression of the Fas ligand, which may engage with Fas on lymphocytes to induce apoptosis. Fifth, the tumor microenvironment, most notably the tumor stroma, may be critical in preventing immunologic destruction of tumor cells by effectively generating an immune privileged site. Much progress has been made in devising approaches to overcome immune evasion mechanisms, as exemplified by the success of inhibitors targeting the CTLA-4 and PD-1 immune checkpoints in cancer immunotherapy (see Checkpoint Blockade).

Immune Sculpting of Tumors

In 2001, an important study showed that the immune system not only can protect against the development of tumors but also can influence the quality of tumors—that is, the immune system of the host in which a tumor develops influences the immunogenicity of the tumor.[60] These investigators showed that RAG2-deficient mice not only develop MCA-induced tumors at higher frequency but that a substantial portion of these tumors was spontaneously rejected upon transplantation in syngeneic immunocompetent mice. In sharp contrast, tumors derived from immunocompetent mice usually grew progressively in immunodeficient mice. Thus, these findings demonstrated that the immune system not only protects the host from tumor formation but also sculpts the immunogenicity of the tumors, in a process that is now referred to as cancer immunoediting.[16,61,62] Cancer immunoediting has been posited to proceed through three sequential stages: (1) an elimination phase where the immune system recognizes and destroys tumors before they become clinically apparent; (2) an equilibrium phase where tumor cells that escaped the elimination phase are continuously destroyed, with emergence of resistant tumor cell variants because of immune pressure; and (3) an escape phase where tumor cells that have successfully evaded immune responses progressively grow. The cancer immunoediting hypothesis represents an extension or modern version of the immunosurveillance hypothesis.

Tumor-Promoting Immune Responses

Discussion of tumor-host interactions would not be complete without at least a mention of the tumor-promoting role of the immune system.[63] Many environmental factors, including chronic infections, tobacco smoke, and inhaled pollutants, as well as dietary factors and obesity, are associated with a low-level chronic inflammation and represent risk factors for cancer development. Chronic inflammation can contribute to tumor genesis at all stages, by generating nontoxic stress during the initiation of cancer, inducing cellular proliferation to promote cancer development, and enhancing angiogenesis and tumor invasion to promote cancer progression.[63]

Approaches to Immunotherapy

Immunotherapy is the use of the immune system or its components to target and eradicate tumors. Improved understanding of the progressive mutations occurring in a single cell, recognition of tumor-associated antigens (TAAs) by the T cells, and elimination of numerous tumors by immunoediting have resulted in the development of a new class of drugs called immunotherapeutics, which exploit the delicate relationship between the immune system and carcinogenesis. The discovery that cancer cells use to escape mechanisms to avoid immune control has led to the development of drugs able to overcome this cancer escape route. CTLA-4, PD-1, and PD-L1 allow immunologic escape by cancer cells and are the targets for the class of drugs known collectively as the "checkpoint inhibitors." They suppress T-cell activity in different ways: CTLA-4 regulates T-cell activity at an early stage, whereas PD-1 regulates later effector T-cell activity within tissue and tumors. Checkpoint inhibitors have demonstrated significant effectiveness against a broadening range of cancers. However, expanding their applicability would require better understanding of the complex interaction between cancer and the immune system and clinical trials that combine therapies to target multiple events in the cancer-immunity cycle.

Antibody Approaches

The most common form of immunotherapy employed in the treatment of cancer is passive immunotherapy, which involves the administration of manufactured antibodies that target a particular antigen (*Table 71.1*). mAbs have emerged as a potent and effective molecularly targeted

Table 71.1. Personalized Active Immunotherapy vs Passive Immunotherapy

Personalized Active Immunotherapy	Passive Immunotherapy
Tumor-specific	Not tumor-specific
Stimulates host immune response	Does not stimulate host immune response
Induces immunologic memory	Temporary antitumor effect
May produce long-term immunity	Requires retreatment
Induces both the cellular and humoral arms of the immune system	Induces the humoral arm of the immune system only (ADCC, CDC)
Requires patient tumor sample for production	Does not require patient tumor sample

Abbreviations: ADCC, antibody-dependent cellular cytotoxicity; CDC, complement-dependent cytotoxicity.

therapy for human cancer and can be used either alone or in combination with chemotherapy.[64,65] Therapeutic mAbs, such as rituximab and brentuximab, are examples of a passive approach. Several lymphoma antigens have been successfully targeted. Examples include CD20 and CD22, which are present on cells of B-cell lineage and targeted with rituximab and inotuzumab, respectively, and CD30, which is present in Hodgkin lymphoma (HL) cells and targeted with brentuximab vedotin.[66-68]

Unconjugated Antibodies

Unaltered antibodies have been used since the earliest trials of mAb therapy in humans.[69,70] In early trials, success was limited by the absence of suitable tumor cell surface targets, antigenicity of first-generation (murine) mAbs in humans, modulation of the target structure from the tumor cell surface, and poor recruitment of immune effector mechanisms.[71,72] However, enthusiasm for this approach was rekindled by the enormous success of genetically engineered, chimeric, or fully humanized versions of mAbs, most notably rituximab for lymphoid malignancies and trastuzumab in breast cancer.[71] Rituximab was the first chimeric mAb with humanized framework and Fc regions to be widely used in clinical trials, particularly in lymphoma. It targets CD20, a pan–B-cell antigen that is present on pre–B cells and mature B cells, but not on terminally differentiated plasma cells. The function of CD20 remains poorly understood.[73] Some thoughts are that it is been implicated in B-cell activation, regulation of B-cell growth, and regulation of transmembrane calcium flux.[67,74,75] The pattern with which rituximab engages CD20 triggers apoptosis through complement system activation and antibody-dependent cellular cytotoxicity (ADCC).[67,74,75]

Rituximab was first approved for use as monotherapy in patients with low-grade or follicular CD20+ non-Hodgkin lymphoma (NHL) in 1997.[76] The pivotal trial involved 166 patients with relapsed or chemotherapy-resistant disease who received 4 weekly infusions of rituximab at 375 mg/m^2. Tumor response occurred in 48% of patients with a median duration of response of 11.8 months.[76] Several subsequent trials also demonstrated the efficacy of rituximab in relapsed, refractory low-grade NHL where patients were treated for either 4 or 8 weekly infusions and had overall response rates of 38% to 47% and 57%, respectively.[77]

Rituximab has also been used with success in patients with more aggressive lymphomas.[78,79] The addition of rituximab to cyclophosphamide, hydroxyl-daunomycin, oncovin (vincristine), and prednisone (CHOP) chemotherapy × 6 cycles in 33 previously untreated patients with advanced aggressive B-cell NHL produced an ORR of 94% and a CR rate of 61%. The 5-year survival rate was 88% (95% confidence interval [CI]: 72-97), and the 5-year PFS was 82% (95% CI: 64-93). The Groupe d'Etude des Lymphomes de l'Adulte compared eight cycles of rituximab-CHOP (RCHOP) (202 patients) with CHOP (197 patients) in elderly patients (age 60-80) with diffuse B-cell lymphoma.[80] RCHOP produced superior CR rate (76% vs 63% [P = .005]). The median PFS was 1.2 years (95% CI: 0.9-1.8) with CHOP compared to 4.8 years (95% CI: 2.7-7.6) for RCHOP. The 10-year PFS was 36.5% with RCHOP compared with 20% with CHOP alone, and the 10-year overall survival (OS) was 43.5% compared with 27.6%, respectively (95% CI: 36.4-5.4).[79]

Maintenance rituximab has also been found to prolong event-free survival (EFS) and response duration in follicular lymphoma.[81] In a randomized phase III study,[82,83] rituximab maintenance regimen provided significant PFS but not OS at 3-year[82,83] and 4-year follow-up assessments in both previously treated and untreated patients with follicular NHL.[82,84] In mantle cell lymphoma (MCL), the use of maintenance therapy with rituximab after RCHOP significantly improved survival (4-year OS 87% vs 63%, P = .005) compared with INF-α.[85] Biosimilar versions of rituximab are now available for many settings.

Possible mechanism of action of rituximab includes initiation of complement-mediated cell lysis, induction of ADCC, and signaling via CD20 leading to programmed cell death and/or sensitization to cytotoxic drugs. Pretreatment lymphoma cells from 29 patients were examined by flow cytometry for expression of complement inhibitors CD46, CD55, and CD59.[86] Expression of these cell surface inhibitors of complement activation was not predictive of outcome to rituximab therapy. There is evidence that induction of ADCC plays an important role in rituximab's antilymphoma effects. A rituximab-like antibody for which an IgG4γ framework was substituted for the IgG1 framework of rituximab was incapable of producing B-cell depletion in primates.[87] Rituximab was relatively ineffective in eliminating Raji B-cell implants in FcRγ$^{-/-}$/nu/nu knockout mice compared to nu/nu mice.[88,89] These mice lacked the activating receptor for Fc portions of antibodies, a critical component of the antibody-dependent cell-mediated cytotoxicity mechanism.

In patients, response to rituximab has been shown to be associated with homozygosity for the high-affinity allotype of the FcγRIIIa receptor.[90] Evidence also exists that rituximab signaling or interference with normal signaling via CD20 may directly induce apoptosis or sensitize cells to the deleterious effects of chemotherapeutic agents.[91] A direct, growth inhibitory effect of rituximab, with accompanying apoptosis, on cell lines cultured in the absence of complement was demonstrated.[92] Anti–CD20-associated apoptosis has been associated with upregulation of the proapoptotic protein, BAX,[93] and downregulation of antiapoptotic protein BCL-2 through inactivation of signal transducer and activator of transcription 3 (STAT3).[94] Downregulation of STAT3 appears to be a result of downregulation of an IL-10 autocrine pathway.[95] These changes and/or others may be responsible for increased sensitivity to chemotherapeutic agents.[96]

Human antichimeric antibodies have been described in patients treated with mAbs and can occasionally be associated with infusion reactions.[97-99] The most common adverse reactions associated with mAbs such as rituximab were a constellation of acute infusion-related events, including chills, fever, headache, rhinitis, pruritus, vasodilation, asthenia, and angioedema. This syndrome can progress to hypotension, urticaria, bronchospasm, and, very rarely, death. The risk is particularly great in patients with high-circulating white blood cell counts and large tumor burden.[99,100] Other toxicities were, in general, mild and infrequent.[101] Neutropenia and thrombocytopenia were unusual.[99] Circulating B cells were depleted and remained low until recovery at a median of 12 months. Although this trial did not report increased infections or hypogammaglobulinemia, subsequent studies, particularly those that involved rituximab maintenance, had increased pneumonia and sinusitis. Long-term use of rituximab can also result in reactivation of serious viral infections, including hepatitis B and polyomavirus JC.[102]

In the wake of the success of rituximab, a number of other antilymphoma mAbs have been studied in clinical trials.[103] Alemtuzumab is a humanized IgG1κ mAb directed against CD52, which is expressed on normal and malignant lymphocytes of B- and T-cell lineage, NK cells, monocytes, and macrophages. Alemtuzumab is indicated for the treatment of B-cell CLL in patients who have been treated with alkylating agents and who have failed fludarabine therapy based on a phase II trial of 93 patients.[104] Alemtuzumab is the most effective agent for T-prolymphocytic leukemia[105,106] and is used in preparative regimens as part of pretransplant conditioning.[107] The most common AEs were infusion related. Rigors occurred in 90% of patients (grade 3 in 14%), fever in 85% of patients (grade 3 or 4 in 20%), nausea in 53% of patients, and vomiting in 38% of patients. Infusion-associated side effects declined with subsequent infusions. A total of 55% of patients developed an infection during the study half of which were serious (grade 3 or 4). Opportunistic infections occurred in 12% of patients. Infusion-related events appear to result from ligation of CD16 on NK cells and were termed *cytokine storm*—release of IL-6, TNF-α, and INF-γ.[108] Prolonged immunosuppression after use of alemtuzumab can result in opportunistic infections.[99,109,110] Treatment schemas now include the routine use of prophylaxis with both antibiotics and antivirals. The widespread nature of the CD52 target (B cells, T cells, APC, and NK cells) probably contributed to the efficacy of this drug to induce immunosuppression. However, the severe immunosuppression, challenges with manufacturing and procurement, has greatly limited the utility of this drug in clinical practice.

To improve the immunogenicity and efficacy (e.g., of rituximab) and also limit toxicities (e.g., alemtuzumab), the paradigm has shifted toward CD20 targeting and away from CD52. There has been the development of novel anti-CD20 mAbs with enhanced antitumor activity resulting from increased complement-dependent cytotoxicity (CDC) and/or ADCC and increased Fc-binding affinity for the low-affinity variants of the FcγRIIIa receptor (CD16) on immune effector cells. These newer mAbs are classified into two groups, type I and type II. Type I are similar to rituximab and include ofatumumab, veltuzumab, and ocrelizumab.[111-113] They all localize into lipid rafts causing more CDC, induce ADCC, antibody-dependent cell-mediated phagocytosis but have a relatively lower propensity to cause cell death by apoptosis.[113] Ofatumumab, a fully human anti-CD20 IgG1 mAb, specifically recognizes an epitope encompassing both the small and large extracellular loops of the CD20 molecule and is more effective than rituximab at CDC induction and killing target cells. Veltuzumab (IMMU-106, hA20), a humanized anti-CD20 mAb with complementarity-determining regions similar to rituximab, has enhanced binding avidities and a stronger effect on CDC compared to rituximab. Ocrelizumab is another humanized mAb with the potential for enhanced efficacy in lymphoid malignancies compared to rituximab because of increased binding affinity for the low-affinity variants of the FcγRIIIa receptor.

The type II mAB in clinical use is obinutuzumab, a fully humanized mAbs with Fc specifically engineered to increase its binding affinity for the FcγRIIIa receptor. In CLL, obinutuzumab-chlorambucil had a higher CR rate (20.7% vs 7.0%) and a superior PFS than rituximab-chlorambucil.[114] Infusion-related reactions and neutropenia were more common with obinutuzumab, but infections were not increased. Other type II mAbs include AME-133v (ocaratumumab)[115] and PRO131921[116] (Table 71.2), both with enhanced affinity for the FcγRIIIa receptor and an enhanced ADCC activity compared to rituximab.[117]

Several other mAbs have been used in the treatment of lymphoma in the clinical trial setting.[103,118] Epratuzumab is a humanized IgG1 mAb directed against the CD22 antigen, a pan–B-cell antigen with distribution similar to that of CD20. Epratuzumab has a favorable safety profile. 88.2% of follicular lymphoma patients responded in a phase II trial and 60% remained in remission at the 3-year mark posttreatment.[119] The combination of epratuzumab (360 mg/m^2 intravenously [IV]) with RCHOP in 107 patients with untreated showed similar toxicity to standard RCHOP.[120] By intention to treat analysis, at a median follow-up of 43 months, the EFS and OS at 3 years in all 107 patients were 70% and 80%, respectively.[120]

Milatuzumab (hLL1, IMMU-115; Immunomedics) is a fully humanized mAb specific for CD74, a cell surface–expressed epitope of the HLA class II–associated invariant chain. CD74 plays an important role as an accessory signaling molecule and survival receptor in the maturation and proliferation of B cells by activating the PI3K/Akt and the NF-κB pathways.[121] Milatuzumab demonstrated antiproliferative activity that appears to be higher in malignant compared to nonmalignant cells. In clinical trials, milatuzumab had limited single-agent activity as described in a phase I study in multiple myeloma where no objective responses were seen but stabilization of disease noted.[122]

Table 71.2. Anti-CD20 Monoclonal Antibodies (mAbs) Approved or Potentially Useful for Lymphoid Malignancies

mAb	Company	Antibody Characteristics	ADCC	CDC	Direct Effects	Comparison With Rituximab
Rituximab (Rituxan, MabThera)	Hoffman La Roche	Type I, first-generation mouse/human chimeric IgG1	++	++	+	
Ofatumumab (Arzerra, HuMax-CD20)	GlaxoSmithKline plc/Genmab A/S	Type I, first-generation, human IgG1	++	++++	+	Binding to different CD20 epitope; more effective at CDC
Veltuzumab (IMMU-106, hA20)	Immunomedics Inc	Type I, second-generation, humanized IgG1	++	++	+	Slower off-rate, enhanced binding avidity, a superior CDC
Ocrelizumab	Genentech Inc/Biogen Idec Inc/Chugai Pharmaceutical Co Ltd/Roche Holding Ag	Type I, second-generation, Humanized fusion IgG1	+++	+/−	+	Binding to different CD20 epitope, enhanced ADCC, reduced CDC, enhanced affinity for FcγRIIIa RIIIa
PRO131921	Genentech, Inc	Type I, third-generation, humanized fusion IgG1	+++	+++	+	Improved binding to FcγRIIIa, better ADCC, superior antitumor efficacy
Ocaratuzumab (AME-133 v)	Lilly	Type I, third-generation, humanized fusion IgG1	+++	++	++	Enhanced affinity for FcγRIIIa, superior ADCC
Obinutuzumab (Gazyva, GA-101)	Glycart Biotechnology AG, Genentech, F Hoffmann-La Roche Ltd	Type II, third-generation, humanized IgG1	++++	−	++++	Superior ADCC and direct cell killing

+, indicates low cytotoxicity; ++, indicates intermediate cytotoxicity; +++, indicates high cytotoxicity; ++++, indicates very high cytotoxicity; +/−, indicates very low cytotoxicity; −, indicates lack of cytotoxicity; ?, indicates cytotoxicity unknown.
Abbreviations: ADCC, antibody-dependent cellular cytotoxicity; CDC, complement-dependent cytotoxicity; IgG, immunoglobulin G; SMIP, small modular immunopharmaceutical.

In another study, milatuzumab was combined with veltuzumab in 35 patients with refractory NHL. Treatment consisted of veltuzumab 200 mg/m² weekly combined with escalating doses of milatuzumab at 8, 16, and 20 mg/kg weekly for 4 weeks. ORR was 24%; median duration of response was 12 months. Responses were observed at all dose levels and in 50% of patient's refractory to rituximab. The investigators concluded that combination therapy with veltuzumab and milatuzumab demonstrated activity in a population of heavily pretreated patients with relapsed or refractory indolent NHL.[123]

Mogamulizumab (KW-0761) is humanized antichemokine receptor-4 (CCR4) mAb, which enhances ADCC, and is effective in mature T-cell neoplasms. In a phase II trial of 26 patients with relapsed CCR4-positive adult T-cell leukemia (ATL), the ORR was 50%, including 31% CR.[124] In a phase I/II study of 41 pretreated cutaneous T-cell lymphoma (CTCL) patients, there was no dose-limiting toxicity, and the dose in the phase II part was 1.0 mg/kg weekly for 4 weeks followed by every 2 weeks until progression.[125] The majority of AEs were grade 1/2: nausea (31.0%), chills (23.8%), headache (21.4%), and infusion-related reaction (21.4%). The ORR rate was 36.8%: 47.1% in Sézary syndrome and 28.6% in mycosis fungoides. Mogamulizumab was first approved for treatment of relapsed ATL in Japan in March 2012 and had a better PFS that vorinostat in a phase III trial of previously treated CTCL.[126]

In multiple myeloma, the cell surface glycoprotein CS1 (CD2 subset 1, CRACC, SLAMF7, and CD319) is highly expressed on myeloma cells, and there is restricted expression in normal tissues. Preclinical studies using a SCID-hu mouse model showed that elotuzumab (formerly known as HuLuc63; EMPLICITI), a humanized mAb targeting CS1, could induce patient-derived myeloma cell killing within the bone marrow microenvironment. It was also shown that the *CS1* gene and cell surface protein expression persisted on myeloma patient-derived plasma cells collected after bortezomib administration. In vitro bortezomib pretreatment of myeloma targets significantly enhanced elotuzumab-mediated ADCC, both for OPM2 myeloma cells using NK cells or peripheral blood mononuclear cells from healthy donors and for primary myeloma cells using autologous NK effector cells. In an OPM2 myeloma xenograft model, elotuzumab in combination with bortezomib exhibited significantly enhanced in vivo antitumor activity. In a phase I trial for relapsed/refractory myeloma,[127] elotuzumab was given at a dose of 2.5, 5.0, 10, or 20 mg/kg IV as well as bortezomib (1.3 mg/m² IV) on days 1 and 11 and days 1, 4, 8, and 11, respectively, in 21-day cycles using a 3 + 3 dose-escalation design. Maximum tolerated dose (MTD) was not reached up to the maximum planned dose of 20 mg/kg. The most frequent grades 3 to 4 AEs were lymphopenia (25%) and fatigue (14%). An objective response was observed in 13 (48%) of 27 evaluable patients and in 2 (67%) of 3 patients refractory to bortezomib. Median TTP was 9.46 months.[128,129]

In a randomized phase III clinical trial (ELOQUENT-2), the schema was lenalidomide and dexamethasone ± elotuzumab; 321 patients were assigned to the elotuzumab group and 325 to the lenalidomide dexamethasone alone (control group). Median PFS in the elotuzumab group was 19.4 months compared to 14.9 months in the control group (hazard ratio for progression or death in the elotuzumab group, 0.70; 95% CI: 0.57-0.85; $P < .001$). The ORR in the elotuzumab group was 79% vs 66% in the control group ($P < .001$). The trial concluded that elotuzumab added to the benefit from lenalidomide and dexamethasone with a 30% reduction in the risk of disease progression or death.[128,129]

Daratumumab (DARZALEX), a humanized antibody that targets CD38, was tested in the phase III setting in combination with other drugs in the treatment of relapsed, refractory multiple myeloma.[130] A total of 498 patients received bortezomib (1.3 mg/m² of body-surface area) and dexamethasone (20 mg) alone (control group) or in combination with daratumumab (16 mg/kg of body weight). The 12-month PFS was 60.7% in the daratumumab group vs 26.9% in the control group. The ORR was higher in the daratumumab group than in the control group (82.9% vs 63.2%, $P < .001$), as were the rates of very good partial response or better (59.2% vs 29.1%, $P < .001$) and complete response or better (19.2% vs 9.0%, $P = .001$). Three of the most common grade 3 or 4 AEs reported in the daratumumab group and the control group were thrombocytopenia (45.3% and 32.9%, respectively), anemia (14.4% and 16.0%, respectively), and neutropenia (12.8% and 4.2%, respectively). Infusion-related reactions with daratumumab treatment occurred in 45.3% of the patients in the daratumumab group. Most of the reactions (98.2%) occurred during the first infusion. Among patients with relapsed or refractory multiple myeloma, daratumumab added to the benefit from bortezomib and dexamethasone and resulted in significantly longer PFS. Daratumumab was approved as a monotherapy for multiple myeloma patients who had at least three prior lines of therapy in 2015 and in combination with lenalidomide or bortezomib and dexamethasone as a second-line therapy 1 year later. In 2019, it was approved for combination with bortezomib, thalidomide, and dexamethasone as a first-line therapy and is now considered the standard of care for multiple myeloma. One precaution when using daratumumab is that it can block the CD38 antigen, making it undetectable by flow cytometry, which is commonly used to evaluate plasma cell clonality to diagnose multiple myeloma and assess response to therapy.[131]

Anti-Idiotype Therapy

The search for tumor-specific antigens that can be targeted involved a laborious process of immunization and hybridization that revealed the Id of clonally distributed antibody expressed on the surface of certain B-cell lymphomas. The Id then serves as an antigen for antibody production, because it represents a unique protein structure, and an immunologic response to Id leads to tumor protection.[132] Anti-Id strategies have been explored in the clinic with some successes, but several interesting problems were noted in early studies: the interfering effect of circulating Id, the development of human antimouse antibody, and the emergence of Id-negative tumor cell variants.[133,134] Another limitation to further development along the lines of Id is the success of mAbs, either alone or in combination with other agents, in the treatment of lymphoma.

Radioimmunotherapy

The use of immunoglobulin-radionuclide conjugates in cancer treatment represents appropriation of a classic guided-missile strategy. In theory, the antibody homes to its antigenic target and delivers a cytotoxic assault on the cell to which it attaches. Unlike traditional external beam radiation that issues pulses of high-dose radiation, radioimmunotherapy (RIT) emits low-dose rate continuous and exponentially decreasing radiation. Radionuclides do not have to be internalized. They deliver radiation over distances of 1 to 5 mm, and cause limited collateral damage to normal tissues. The principles of radiation physics underlying RIT have been reviewed by Press and Rasey.[135] The most commonly used isotopes for RIT have been iodine 131 (I-131) and yttrium 90 (Y-90). They induce cell death primarily through emission of β particles, resulting in DNA strand breaks.

Several reviews have addressed the utility and evolution of this field.[136,137] The two products that have been tested in lymphoma are Y-90 ibritumomab-tiuxetan (Zevalin) and I-131 tositumomab (Bexxar) though only one (Zevalin) is now available for clinical use. They both target the CD20 antigen of B lymphocytes and have been administered after infusion of unconjugated anti-CD20 antibodies—rituximab in the case of Zevalin and tositumomab in the case of Bexxar. Both have used nuclear medicine imaging as a preparatory step to administration, but it is no longer required for Y-90 ibritumomab. Both have been studied most extensively in indolent lymphoma and have been approved for treatment of patients with relapsed or refractory follicular, including rituximab refractory, or transformed B (CD20⁺) NHL.

The approval for ibritumomab-tiuxetan rested primarily on two clinical studies.[138,139] The first was a randomized controlled comparison of the effectiveness of Y-90 ibritumomab-tiuxetan to that of rituximab in patients with relapsed or refractory, follicular, or transformed B-cell NHL.[138] The study involved 143 patients; 73 randomized to Y-90 ibritumomab-tiuxetan (single administration) and 70 randomized to rituximab (weekly × 4). Y-90 ibritumomab-tiuxetan produced a statistically superior response rate of 80% vs 56% ($P = .002$). The number of durable responders at 6 months favored Y-90 ibritumomab-tiuxetan–treated patients, but the significance of the observation was lost at 9 and 12 months. Median TTP was 11.2 months for patients treated with Y-90 ibritumomab-tiuxetan and 10.1 months for patients treated with rituximab ($P = .173$). The second was a phase II clinical trial of 57 patients who had failed to respond to rituximab or had a TTP of ≤6 months.[139] These patients had a median of four prior therapies, and 74% had bulky tumors (greatest diameter ≥5 cm). In this patient population, Y-90 ibritumomab-tiuxetan produced a response rate of 74% and CR rate of 15%. The median TTP was estimated at 6.8 months. Grade 4 neutropenia occurred in 35% of patients, grade 4 thrombocytopenia in 9% of patients, and grade 4 anemia in 4% of patients.

The pivotal study for I-131 tositumomab enrolled 60 patients with refractory or transformed low-grade NHL.[140] A statistically significant improvement in the primary endpoint was achieved with a longer duration of response (>30 days difference) after I-131 tositumomab therapy (74% vs 26%) of patients after their last qualifying chemotherapy (LQC) ($P < .001$). Improvements in secondary efficacy endpoints after I-131 tositumomab compared to those after LQC were also achieved: overall response (65% vs 28%; $P < .001$), duration of response (6.5 vs 3.4 months; $P < .001$), and CR (20% vs 3%; $P < .001$). Nine of 12 CR patients treated with Bexxar remained in CR with ongoing responses from 32 to 47 months.

The efficacy of I-131 tositumomab was also evaluated in patients who had progressed after rituximab.[141] Twenty-four patients had a longer (at least 30 days) duration of response after I-131 tositumomab than after rituximab; five patients had a longer duration of response after rituximab than after I-131 tositumomab; nine patients had equivalent durations of response; and two patients were censored ($P < .001$). A total of 14 patients (35%) had a TTP of 12 months or longer. The median PFS was 10.4 months (95% CI: 5.7-8.6) for all patients and 24.5 months for confirmed responders (95% CI: 16.8 to not reached). Median PFS for 15 confirmed CR patients was not reached with an estimated 3 years PFS of 73%. Prior response to rituximab did not significantly affect the confirmed OR rate, duration of response, or median PFS.

Retreatment with tositumomab and I-131 tositumomab has also been found possible in patients with progressive disease after treatment with I-131 tositumomab, who were able to receive subsequent therapy, including cytotoxic chemotherapy and stem cell transplantation.[142] In patients with prior response, I-131 tositumomab can produce second responses that can be durable.[143,144] Radioiodinated tositumomab and Y-90 ibritumomab-tiuxetan have been used at myeloablative doses with stem cell rescue in patients with relapsed B-cell lymphomas.[135,145-148] Twenty-one patients received therapeutic infusions of radioiodinated tositumomab (345-785 mCi) as a single agent followed by reinfusion of autologous hematopoietic stem cells.[145] All patients engrafted, and 18 responded with 16 achieving a CR. With a median follow-up of 2 years, a 2-year PFS was estimated at 62%, with OS estimated at 93%. Press et al subsequently combined radioiodinated tositumomab with chemotherapy and autologous stem cell transfusion in a series of patients with relapsed B-cell lymphomas.[146] Fifty-two patients received the planned RIT followed by etoposide, 60 mg/kg, and cyclophosphamide, 100 mg/kg (CY/VP16) prior to stem cell infusion at 2 years, the Kaplan-Meier estimates of OS and PFS for all treated patients were 83% and 68%, respectively, and were considered superior to results previously observed in patients who had undergone external beam total-body radiation with CY/VP16 preparation for transplantation in the same institution. In a trial of 31 patients with CD20+ NHL treated with high-dose Y-90 ibritumomab-tiuxetan in combination with CY/VP16 followed by autologous hematopoietic cell transplantation (HCT), the 2-year estimated OS and PFS rates were 92% and 78%, respectively.[147]

The use of RIT has also been investigated in the allogeneic HCT setting.[149-154] RIT with β-emitters has been successfully used for further dose intensification of myeloablative conditioning regimens for HCT. In two relapsed patients with NHL, Y-90 ibritumomab-tiuxetan was given as part of the conditioning for an HLA-matched donor transplant, and engraftment was rapid.[151] A "pretargeting" RIT method of slow distribution of the antibody has been explored in hematologic malignancies.[153,154] A phase II clinical trial of Y-90 ibritumomab-tiuxetan and reduced-intensity conditioning (RIC) HCT in 18 patients with high-risk relapsed/refractory aggressive NHL using related donors was done.[155] The conditioning regimen consisted of rituximab 250 mg (days −21 and −14), Y-90 ibritumomab IV (0.4 m Ci/kg, day −14), fludarabine 30 mg/m² IV (days −3 and −2) plus melphalan 70 mg/m² IV (days −3 and −2), or 1 dose of melphalan and thiotepa 5 mg/kg (day −8). Y-90-ibritumomab infusions were well tolerated, and nonrelapse mortality at 1 year was 28%. The 4-year OS and PFS were both 44.4% with a median follow-up of 46 (range, 39-55) months. Similar reports showed that Y-90 ibritumomab-tiuxetan can be safely added to RIC for allogeneic HCT and have led to the recommendation for a phase III clinical trial to clarify the contribution of RIT to RIC allogeneic HCT.[152]

Immunotoxins and Fusion Toxins

This category of treatment requires a targeting moiety (to identify and home to target) and a cytolytic moiety (usually a toxin) that is delivered to the target cell targets tumors through. The targeting moiety most often used are antibodies, lymphokines, growth factors, and so on, that specifically bind receptors on the surfaces of target tumor cells. Attached to the targeting moiety is the cytolytic moiety, which is usually a toxin, derived from plants or bacteria, and works by inhibiting protein synthesis. They kill either resting or dividing cells and require fewer than 10 molecules in the cytosol to be effective.[156,157] Toxins of this type tested in phase I trials include ricin A-chain, blocked ricin, saporin, pokeweed antiviral protein, *Pseudomonas* exotoxin A, and diphtheria toxin. Recently, calicheamicin, a highly potent antitumor antibiotic that cleaves double-stranded DNA at specific sequences,[158] has been successfully targeted to leukemia cells.[159]

A number of factors influence the efficacy of immunotoxins. These include the binding affinity of the ligand for its target and the target density on the tumor cell surface.[160] The epitope to which binding occurs can affect the potency of the immunotoxin.[161] Membrane-proximal epitopes appear to confer greater efficacy. Immunotoxin binding must lead to internalization of the target structure and the attached immunotoxin.[162] Once internalized, the toxin moiety must translocate to the cytoplasm to be effective. This process is aided by certain translocation sequences in the toxin. The need for translocation signals provides the rationale for using blocked ricin toxin; targeting via the binding subunit is eliminated, but translocation signals are preserved.[163] The site of translocation may vary for different toxins. Increasing lysosomal pH protects cells from *Pseudomonas* exotoxin and diphtheria toxin but increases sensitivity to ricin,[164,165] suggesting that ricin may undergo translocation in the Golgi apparatus. Finally, these toxins affect protein synthesis by ADP-ribosylating elongation factor 2[166] in the case of diphtheria toxin and *Pseudomonas* toxin, or by alteration of the 60S ribosomal subunit in the case of ricin.[167]

A number of phase I clinical trials using ricin-based, anti–pan-B-cell antibody immunotoxins have been reported in B-cell lymphoma.[168-172] These trials demonstrated that therapeutic doses of immunotoxins can be delivered with tolerable and reversible side effects. Toxicities include systemic symptoms of fever, nausea, vomiting, headache, and muscle aches; evidence of hepatocyte damage with transaminase elevations; and significant problems with capillary leak syndrome.[173] Again recognized were the problems of human anti–mouse antibody formation and rapid clearance of immunotoxin in the presence of circulating antigenemia.[170] Sporadic responses were seen in these trials, with response rates perhaps approaching 25% and CRs approaching 10%. There were hints that targeting via CD22 might be more useful than targeting via CD19.[170,174] Some experts have suggested that addressing the immunogenicity is an important step in advancing these therapies.[72,157,170]

Studies of recombinant immunotoxin containing anti-CD22 variable domain (Fv) fused to a truncated *Pseudomonas* exotoxin have produced CRs in patients with hairy-cell leukemia (HCL).[171] Of 16 patients with relapse refractory disease, 13 responded, and 11 had CRs.

Common side effects included transient elevations of liver enzymes and hypoalbuminemia. Median follow-up was 16 months, during which 3 of the 11 complete responders relapsed and were retreated with the immunotoxin. Two of the three patients developed hemolytic-uremic syndrome. Moxetumomab pasudotox is an improved, more active form of a predecessor recombinant immunotoxin and is up to 50-fold more active on lymphoma and leukemia cell lines. However, treatment remained complicated by a relatively high rate of development of hemolytic-uremic syndrome. Several phase I trials were done showing efficacy in acute lymphoblastic leukemia (ALL) but also a high prevalence of hemolytic-uremic syndrome and other toxicities, which has limited clinical development.[171,175-177]

Gemtuzumab ozogamicin (GO), also known as Mylotarg, is an immunotoxin composed of a recombinant human IgG4κ mAb conjugated with a cytotoxic antitumor antibiotic, calicheamicin,[178] and was previously approved for the treatment of elderly patients with CD33-positive AML in first relapse. The antibody is directed against the CD33 antigen found on the surface of leukemic blasts and normal immature cells of myelomonocytic lineage, but not on hematopoietic stem cells. CD33 is a sialic acid–dependent adhesion molecule. In a phase I dose-escalation trial, treatment with GO resulted in elimination of leukemic cells from peripheral blood and bone marrow in 8 of 40 patients.[179] The basis for approval of the drug was the experience in 142 patients participating in one of three similar trials designed to examine the efficacy and safety of GO in patients in first relapse of AML.[159] The median duration of first remission was 11.1 months, and median OS 5.9 months. Median relapse-free survival (RFS) for responders was 6.8 months. In all, 15% of patients experienced grade 3 or 4 bleeding events, and 11 patients died during the treatment period of causes other than disease progression. GO was withdrawn from the U.S. market in 2010 owing to lack of clinical benefit in subsequent trials, but it remained available in Japan and for selected investigator-initiated research.

However, on September 1, 2017, the U.S. Food and Drug Administration (FDA) once again approved GO to be marketed in the United States based on the results of clinical trials that suggested improved outcomes. In the phase III Alfa-0701 trial, 280 adults with new diagnosis of AML were randomized to receive 5 doses of IV GO (3 mg/m^2 on days 1, 4, and 7 during induction and day 1 of each of the two consolidation chemotherapy courses). The primary outcome was EFS and that was achieved in 40.8% in the GO group compared to 17.1% in the control group (hazard ratio 0.58, 95% CI: 0.43-0.78; $P = .0003$).[180] In another trial in 237 older patients (age >60) randomized to GO vs best supportive care (BSC), the median OS was 4.9 months (95% CI: 4.2-6.8 months) in the GO group and 3.6 months (95% CI: 2.6-4.2 months) in the BSC group (hazard ratio, 0.69; 95% CI: 0.53-0.90; $P = .005$); the 1-year OS rate was 24.3% with GO and 9.7% with BSC. The OS benefit with GO was consistent across most subgroups.[181]

Inotuzumab ozogamicin is a similar immunotoxin-linking calicheamicin to an IgG4 antibody against the B-cell marker CD22 and has been in trials for B-cell acute lymphoblastic leukemia (B-ALL) and B-cell lymphoma.[182-184] In a phase III trial of 326 adults with relapsed or refractory Philadelphia chromosome negative (Ph−) ALL randomized to inotuzumab vs standard therapy, CR was significantly higher in the inotuzumab ozogamicin group than standard therapy group (80.7% vs 29.4%, $P < .001$). More patients in the inotuzumab group were minimal residual disease (MRD) negative (78.4% vs 28.1%, $P < .001$). Median PFS was significantly longer in the inotuzumab group (5 vs 1.8 months; hazard ratio, 0.45; 97.5% CI: 0.34-0.61).[182-184] On August 17, 2017, the FDA approved inotuzumab ozogamicin (BESPONSA; Wyeth Pharmaceuticals Inc, a subsidiary of Pfizer Inc) for the treatment of adults with relapsed or refractory B-ALL.

Neoplasms bearing the high-affinity IL-2 receptor have been approached with a genetically engineered, bacterially expressed IL-2-diphtheria toxin fusion protein, denileukin diftitox.[185] Denileukin diftitox (ONTAK) was approved in 1998 for the treatment of patients with relapsed CTCL, but it was taken off the market in 2014 owing to side effects and problems in manufacturing.[186] The basis of approval was a trial conducted in 73 patients with refractory disease.[187] Patients were randomized to either a low dose (9 μg/kg/d) or high dose (18 μg/kg/d) of the fusion toxin for 5 consecutive days in 21-day cycles for up to eight cycles. Seventy-one patients received denileukin diftitox, and the responses were similar between the 2 doses with an ORR of 30% and a CR of 10%. AEs included flulike symptoms, acute infusion-related events, vascular leak syndrome, elevated transaminase levels, and hypoalbuminemia. Although approximately one-half of patients had antibodies against diphtheria toxin at baseline and almost all patients had antibodies after treatment, these did not appear to affect treatment outcome.[187]

A new formulation of denileukin diftitox, E7777, with improved purity and a larger amount of active protein monomer species is under evaluation (NCT01871727). Resimmune, a second-generation recombinant immunotoxin (composed of a catalytic and translocation domains of diphtheria toxin fused to two single-chain antibody fragments reactive with the extracellular domain of $CD3_\varepsilon$, which is expressed on skin-tropic T cells), had a 36% ORR (16% CR) in 25 patients with CTCL.[188] Capillary leak syndrome occurred in 40% of patients with 7% grade 4/5. Reactivation of cytomegalovirus or Epstein-Barr virus (EBV) was seen in 23% and transaminitis in 20%.

An anti-CD30 antibody, brentuximab vedotin, an antibody-drug conjugate composed of the anti-CD30 chimeric IgG1 mAb cAC10 and the potent antimicrotubule drug monomethyl auristatin E connected by a protease-cleavable linker, is increasingly being used in hematologic malignancies.[189] Several trials have shown durable antitumor activity with a manageable safety profile in patients with relapsed/refractory HL,[190,191] systemic anaplastic large-cell lymphoma (ALCL), or primary cutaneous CD30-positive lymphoproliferative disorders.[191] Treatment with single-agent brentuximab vedotin resulted in objective response rates and CR rates of 75% and 34%, respectively, in relapsed or refractory HL and of 86% and 57%, respectively, in relapsed or refractory systemic ALCL patients.[191] Peripheral sensory neuropathy and neutropenia were observed with brentuximab vedotin but were generally grades 1 and 2 in severity and manageable. In July 2011, brentuximab vedotin was approved in the United States for the treatment of HL after failure of autologous HCT or after failure of at least two prior multiagent chemotherapy regimens in HCT-ineligible candidates and for the treatment of systemic ALCL after failure of at least one prior multiagent chemotherapy regimen. Brentuximab vedotin given as consolidation after an autologous HCT for HL has been shown to improve PFS over placebo.[192] It was also approved for treatment of previously treated mycosis fungoides in 2017 following a phase III trial, showing an improved response vs methotrexate or bexarotene.[193] Brentuximab vedotin has also been more recently approved in combination with chemotherapy for advanced stage HL and CD30-positive T cell lymphoma. Details of these data are presented in other disease-specific chapters.

Bispecific Antibodies

Bispecific antibodies are antibody constructions that recognize a TAA with one arm and recognize and activate an immune effector cell structure with the other arm.[194-196] In theory, approximation of a tumor cell with an activated immune effector could result in tumor cell recognition and immune-mediated elimination. These bispecific antibodies can be obtained either by chemical heteroconjugation or by fusion of two hybridomas of desired specificity to yield a tetradoma. With either approach, chromatographic or other separation techniques are required to isolate the desired product.

Strategies using antibodies to activate phagocytic cells, NK cells, and T lymphocytes have been examined. Recognizing the need for costimulation in T-cell response, investigators have used a combination of bispecific antibodies, anti-CD3 × anti-TAA, and anti-CD28 × anti-TAA, with interesting results.[194]

Blinatumomab (BLINCYTO), a novel class of T-cell engaging bispecific single-chain antibody (BiTE antibodies), engages T cells for redirected lysis of CD19-positive target cells.[197] CD19 is expressed on cells of B-cell lineage, including malignancies. In a phase I trial of blinatumomab in NHL patients, doses as low as 0.005 mg/m^2/d led to elimination of target cells in blood, whereas partial and complete tumor regressions were observed at a dose level of 0.015 mg. All seven patients treated at a dose level of 0.06 mg experienced a tumor regression.[198] In another phase I/II study of B-lineage ALL patients with persistent or relapsed MRD, 76 patients were enrolled in a 3 + 3 design with the objective to determine AEs, MTD pharmacokinetics, pharmacodynamics, and ORR of continuous IV infusion blinatumomab in patients with relapsed/refractory NHL. Blinatumomab was administered over 4 or 8 weeks at seven different dose levels (0.5-90 μg/m²/d). Neurologic events were dose limiting, and 60 μg/m²/d was established as the MTD. Thirty-four additional patients were recruited to evaluate antilymphoma activity and strategies for mitigating neurologic events at a prespecified MTD. Grade 3 neurologic events occurred in 22% of patients (no grade 4/5). Among patients treated at 60 μg/m²/d (target dose; n = 35), the ORR was 69% across NHL subtypes and 55% for diffuse large B-cell lymphoma (DLBCL) (n = 11); median response duration was 404 days (95% CI: 207-1129 days). The authors concluded that treating NHL with blinatumomab was feasible with an MTD of 60 μg/m²/d and that blinatumomab single agent showed antilymphoma activity.

A phase II study of blinatumomab patients with B-lineage ALL, with persistent or relapsed MRD, resulted in an 80% MRD response rate. After a median follow-up of 33 months, the RFS of the whole evaluable study cohort of 20 patients was 61%, whereas 9 patients who received allogeneic HCT after blinatumomab treatment had a hematologic RFS rate of 65% (Kaplan-Meier estimate). Among patients who were Ph−, four of six MRD responders with no further therapy after blinatumomab were in ongoing hematologic and molecular remission. Thus, blinatumomab may have a role in inducing long-lasting CRs in B-lineage ALL patients with persistent or recurrent MRD.[199]

Bispecific antibodies have been used in the treatment of patients with refractory HL.[200,201] In an initial phase I/II trial,[200] 15 patients were treated with an NK cell–activating bispecific mAb directed against the Fcγ receptor III (CD16 antigen) and the Hodgkin-associated CD30 antigen. The antibody was administered every 3 to 4 days × 4. Dose-limiting toxicity was not encountered up to and including the highest dose administered which was 64 mg/m². Side effects were unusual, but included fever, pain in involved lymph nodes, and maculopapular rash. Of 15 patients, 9 developed a human anti–mouse antibody response that resulted in allergic reactions in 4 patients who were retreated. Duration of one CR was 16 months, and partial responses endured for a median of 3 months. These results prompted a second trial to investigate the effects of different administration schedules and the concomitant administration of cytokines on the effectiveness of the bispecific antibody.[202] Sixteen patients were treated with 25 mg of the construct four times, either as a continuous infusion for 4 days or a 1-hour infusion every other day. Patients who exhibited response were retreated at 4-week intervals, if possible. Patients with stable disease received retreatment after administration of IL-2 and granulocyte-macrophage colony-stimulating factor. Four patients responded to the treatment (three PRs and one CR). Durations of response were from 5 to 9 months.

In a single-arm phase II trial reported by Topp et al, 36 adult patients with relapsed or refractory B-precursor ALL were treated with blinatumomab in cycles of 4-week continuous infusion followed by a 2-week treatment-free interval. The primary endpoint was CR or CR with partial hematologic recovery (CRh), and secondary endpoints included MRD response, rate of allogeneic HCT realization, RFS, OS, and incidence of AEs. Twenty-five patients (69%) achieved a CR or CRh, with 88% of the responders achieving an MRD response. Median OS was 9.8 months (95% CI: 8.5-14.9), and median RFS was 7.6 months (95% CI: 4.5-9.5). Thirteen responders (52%) underwent HCT after achieving a CR or CRh. The most frequent AE during treatment was pyrexia (grade 1 or 2, 75%; grade 3, 6%). Treatment was interrupted in six patients with nervous system or psychiatric toxicity and in two with cytokine release syndrome (CRS). The authors concluded that blinatumomab is effective in the treatment of adult patients with relapsed or refractory ALL. In a subsequent multicenter single-arm, open-label phase II study in 189 adult patients with Ph−, primary refractory or relapsed refractory disease including relapse within 12 months after allogeneic HCT, blinatumomab was given as a continuous IV infusion 9 μg/d × 7 day and 28 μg/d thereafter × 4 weeks every 6 weeks for up to five cycles. The primary endpoint was CR or CRh of peripheral blood counts within the first two cycles. Analysis was by intention to treat. After two cycles, 81 patients (43%; 95% CI: 36-50) had achieved a CR or CRh. 32 patients (40%) underwent subsequent allogeneic HCT. The most frequent grade 3 or worse AEs were febrile neutropenia (25%). Three patients (2%) had grade 3 CRS. Grade 3 or 4 neurologic events occurred in 20 (11%) and 4 (2%) patients, respectively. The authors concluded that single-agent blinatumomab showed antileukemia activity in adult patients with relapsed or refractory B-precursor ALL characterized by negative prognostic factors. More recently a number of anti-CD20/CD3 bispecific antibodies (including mosunetuzumab, epcoritamab, glofitamab, and odronextamab) have shown clinical activity (including complete responses) in a variety of B cell malignancies including relapsed follicular lymphoma, MCL, and DLBCL. Toxicities include CRS, although they are largely able to be administered on an outpatient basis. Several of these agents are moving through the regulatory review process for approval, and combination studies are underway.

Bispecific antibody immunotherapy has also shown activity in the treatment of solid tumors.[203,204] This approach as an immunotherapeutic strategy is also being explored in overcoming drug resistance cell lines in B-cell malignancies,[205] as well as the allogeneic HCT setting, to enhance the graft-vs-tumor (GVT) effect, while minimizing graft-vs-host disease (GVHD).[206] Relatively minor results have not given rise to large-scale trials. Gupta et al in a preclinical study showed that two bispecific HexAbs (IgG-[Fab]4 constructed from veltuzumab [anti-CD20 IgG] and milatuzumab [anti-CD74 IgG]) show enhanced cytotoxicity in MCL and other lymphoma/leukemia cell lines, as well as patient tumor samples without a cross-linking Ab, compared with their parental mAb counterparts, alone or in combination. They may thus constitute a new class of therapeutic Abs by invoking the juxtaposition and engagement of two independent targets on a cancer cell.[207] A trifunctional bispecific antibody, FBTA05, demonstrated efficacy in preclinical studies,[208] including improved cytotoxicity of CLL patient cells ex vivo compared to alemtuzumab and rituximab,[209] and has been used as compassionate care in children with relapsed or refractory mature B cell NHL, Burkitt leukemia, or pre–B acute lymphoblastic leukemia.[210] It is designed to target human CD20 and human CD3, simultaneously binding B cells and T cells by its variable regions and recruiting FcγR-positive accessory immune cells by its intact Fc region. Of the 10 children treated with FBTA05, 9 had a clinical response with 3 SD, 1 PR, and 5 CR.[210] These unique approaches appear to further improve the antineoplastic efficacy of mAbs in hematologic malignancies.

Cytokines

Interferons

The IFNs constitute a family of cytokines that were initially recognized by their abilities to interfere with viral replication and cause tumor regression.[141,211,212] Two major classes of IFNs exist: type I, consisting primarily of IFN-α and IFN-β; and type II, consisting of IFN-γ. Type I IFNs are produced by many cell types. Type II IFN is produced by T lymphocytes. Signaling in this system involves the Janus kinase (JAK) family and the STATs.[213] Transmission of IFN-specific signals results in induction of a number of genes, including several transcription factors, MHC class I and class II (primarily in response to IFN-γ) molecules, and a number of proteins that are responsible for the antiviral activity of the IFNs, including the (2-5′) oligoadenylate synthase-nuclease system.[214] The most successful applications of these substances have been in chronic myelogenous leukemia (CML), HCL, and polycythemia vera.

In chronic-phase CML, IFN-α treatment resulted in complete cytogenetic responses in 25% of patients.[215-220] Side effects included flulike symptoms, fatigue, weight loss, neurotoxicity, depression, and insomnia. Other less common side effects include cardiac arrhythmias, congestive heart failure, hemolytic anemia, thrombocytopenia, rheumatologic disorders, hypothyroidism, and nephrotic syndrome. IFN is no longer used as first line in CML owing to the success of tyrosine kinase inhibitors. In a trial of 1106 patients randomized to imatinib or IFN-α plus low-dose cytarabine, after 18-month follow-up, more patients in the imatinib arm achieved complete cytogenetic response 76.2% vs 14.5% ($P < .001$). Based on this as well as other trials, the role of IFN in CML is now only of historical significance.[221-223]

In HCL, IFN-α became the first effective, nonsurgical treatment; splenectomy was the first treatment approach. A number of approaches demonstrated that approximately 75% of treated patients achieved a complete or partial response.[224,225] Median durations of response were 12 to 24 months, but virtually all patients eventually relapsed. Although IFN-α is an active agent in HCL, the nucleoside agents cladribine and deoxycoformycin have proven to be more effective in inducing sustained clinical CRs and have become the treatment of choice in most patients with the disease.

IFN-α has been used in the treatment of NHL as a single agent,[72] but it has little utility in the era of immunotherapy and novel agents; there was a suggestion that IFN might reduce the rate of transformation to higher grade lymphoma.[226]

IFN-α was part of the treatment of multiple myeloma before the development of novel agents.[227-229] When used in combination with chemotherapy, IFN-α appeared to add some benefit but the pattern was inconsistent. The randomized trial of 256 patients[228,230] showed improved disease-free survival of 17.8 vs 8.2 months for the control group and OS of 50.6 vs 34.4 months. However, in a large cooperative group trial,[229] no benefit was seen to IFN-α maintenance therapy, and a meta-analysis of 24 randomized studies involving more than 4000 subjects indicated that IFN-α improved RFS to a moderate degree and OS to a marginal degree in multiple myeloma. Furthermore, its usefulness has been questioned in melphalan-prednisone–treated patients,[231] in patients receiving high-dose steroids,[232] and in the elderly.[233]

Historically, recombinant IFN-γ1b was used to enhance the immune system in high-risk cancer patients treated with granulocyte transfusions, as well as to treat fungal infections in the allogeneic HCT setting.[234] Type I IFN (human lymphoblastoid interferon, IFN-α2b, and IFN-β) has been shown to enhance antileukemic cytotoxicity of γδ T cells in in vitro models.[235] IFN-α is effective in polycythemia vera, particularly in the young or pregnant patient.[236]

Interleukin-2

IL-2 was first recognized as a growth factor for T lymphocytes.[237,238] Its discovery allowed the cloning and long-term propagation of antigen-specific T-cell clones.[239,240] In addition, it was determined that IL-2 treatment led to gain of function, particularly increased cytotoxicity in T lymphocytes[241] and NK cells.[242] IL-2 binds specifically to receptors (IL-2R) on target cell surfaces.[243,244]

Early experience with IL-2 used increasing doses, seeking optimal effect. However, at high IV dose ($>10^{-8}$ M peak concentration, attempting to saturate intermediate-affinity IL-2R on target cells), IL-2 produced significant, life-threatening toxicities that have limited its use.[245] These side effects included fever and chills initially followed by a constellation of problems resulting from a capillary leak syndrome, including hypotension requiring pressor support in a majority of patients, significant weight gain, respiratory distress occasionally requiring intubation, oliguria, renal dysfunction, and death in approximately 1% of patients. Additional side effects included nausea, emesis, diarrhea, cardiac arrhythmia, liver dysfunction, mental status changes, anemia, and thrombocytopenia.

Investigators found that the administration of daily subcutaneous low-dose IL-2 in patients with active chronic GVHD rapidly induced preferential and sustained T_{reg} expansion, reversed advanced manifestations of chronic GVHD, and permitted a substantial reduction in the glucocorticoid dose.[246,247] Conversely, basiliximab and daclizumab, two IL-2 receptor antagonists (IL-2RAs) that bind to the α-subunit of the IL-2R (CD25), found predominantly on the surface of activated cytotoxic T cells, induced proliferation and provided selected immunosuppression, prevented GVHD efficiently, and contributed to a favorable outcome following unrelated donor HCT.[248]

Cellular Approaches

Graft-vs-Leukemia Effect

Multiple mechanisms of immune-mediated antileukemia effects in humans have been proposed, but most are T-cell mediated, though only part of the effect correlates with clinical GVHD, and highly suggestive of a graft-vs-leukemia (GVL) effect occurring in an allogeneic setting. Similar mechanism of action has been postulated to occur in an autologous setting and underlies the quest for autologous vaccines that can potentially induce a GVT effect.[249] Other pertinent clinical observations supporting a potent role for the GVL effect include (1) increased leukemia relapse risk in recipients of transplants from genetically identical twins compared to allotransplant recipients[250]; (2) decreased leukemia relapse risk in allotransplant recipients with GVHD compared to those without GVHD[251]; (3) increased leukemia relapse risk in recipients of T-cell–depleted allotransplants compared to T-cell–replete allotransplants (even when adjusted for GVHD); (4) antileukemia effects of stopping posttransplant immune suppression or infusing donor immune cells (referred to as donor leukocyte infusion [DLI]). Such approaches attempt to maximize the GVT effect conferred by donor T cells. Yet, responses are variable and acute GVHD is a major cause of treatment failure.

The potency of GVT effect differs among neoplasms, and the molecular and cellular mechanisms that underlie GVL effect are now better understood.[252-257] Antigens implicated in these processes have been described. While MHC differences have long been implicated in GVHD pathogenesis, the role played by minor histocompatibility antigen expression in GVHD and the GVL effect is now better understood[253-255,257] (*Figure 71.5*). Immune responses against tumor-specific antigens, such as the neoantigens expressed from the *BCR/ABL* fusion in CML, *PML/RαRα* fusion in acute promyelocytic leukemia, and *p53* oncoprotein in ovarian cancer, have been explored for association with clinical outcomes.[258-260]

The immunologic effectors of GVHD and GVL, principally the T lymphocytes, play a pivotal role in these reactions, and their removal results in a marked decrease in GVHD and marked increases in relapse frequencies.[261] There is a role for NK cells in mediating the GVL effect.[261,262] Preclinical studies in mice and humans have shown that different combinations of activating and inhibitory receptors on NK cells can reduce GVHD, promote engraftment, and provide superior GVT responses.[261-264] The use of KIR-ligand incompatibility produces a potent GVL effect in patients with AML at high risk of relapse.[262] Also, CD4+ T lymphocytes may be particularly important in the GVL effect.[263,265] Allografts selectively depleted of CD8+ T lymphocytes (CD4+ T lymphocytes preserved) demonstrated a low incidence of GVHD yet a preserved GVL effect similar to that seen with unfractionated HCT in patients with CML. Development of MHC-tetramer technology has provided a means to visualize antigen-specific T-cell responses.[266] In an early application of this approach, Mutis et al[267] showed that the frequencies of T cells specific for the HY and HA-1 minor histocompatibility antigens correlated with the severity of GVHD. Other strategies investigated over the past few years to enhance the GVL effect and reduce GVHD include a reduction in the total number of T lymphocytes used in transplantation,[268] delayed transfusion of donor lymphocytes,[264] depletion of CD8+ T-lymphocytes, ablation of thymidine kinase gene–transfected donor T lymphocytes with ganciclovir administration in case of GVHD,[269,270] incorporation of a safety switch, such as inducible caspase 9, to rapidly deplete transferred T cells,[271] administration of IL-2 and use of IL-2RAs, functional depletion of antihost lymphocytes without depletion of antimyeloid lymphocytes,[269,270,272] and ex vivo generation of leukemia-specific T lymphocytes,[273] or chimeric antigen receptor (CAR) T cells (discussed further below).[274]

Nonmyeloablative HCT or mini-allografting[275,276] has been used in augmenting the GVT effect. These low-dose regimens are designed, not to eradicate host hematopoiesis, but to allow induction of the GVL effect as the primary treatment mechanism. Early experience using such approach was described by Shimoni et al.[275,276] The investigators at the Center for International Blood and Marrow Transplant Research

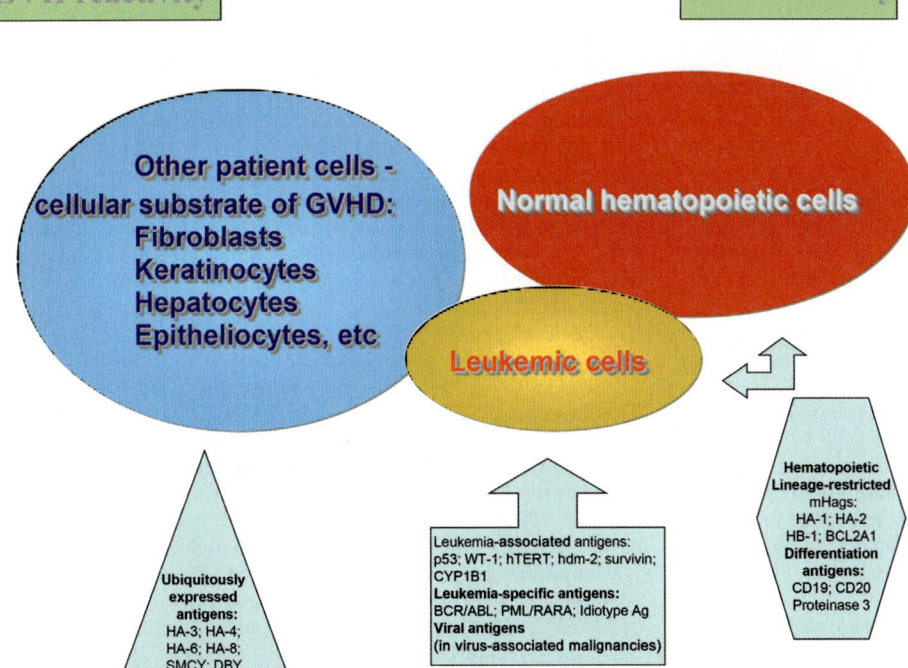

FIGURE 71.5 Antigenic basis of graft-vs-leukemia (GVL) and graft-vs-host (GVH) immune responses. GVL reactivity is mediated by immune responses specific to antigens with expression restricted to leukemic cells (leukemia-specific and certain viral antigens) and patient hematopoietic cells (hematopoietic lineage–restricted minor histocompatibility antigens, hematopoietic differentiation antigens). Reactivity to leukemia-associated antigens contributes to GVL mostly, although these antigens are expressed at low levels in normal tissues. Ubiquitously expressed antigens are a substrate of GVHD. Ag, antigen; GVHD, graft-vs-host disease; mHags, minor histocompatibility antigens. (Adapted from Ivanov R, Hagenbeek A, Ebeling S. Towards immunogene therapy of hematological malignancies. *Exp Hematol*. 2006;34(3):251-263. Copyright © 2006 International Society for Experimental Hematology. With permission.)

have determined that in the setting of HCT using myeloablative conditioning, GVHD had an adverse effect on transplant-related mortality with early modest augmentation of GVHD-associated GVL. While following RIC, GVL may be important in limiting both early and late leukemia recurrence.[277]

Donor Lymphocyte Infusions

Allogeneic HCT is a curative treatment modality for patients with malignant hematologic diseases. Relapse, however, remains one of the leading causes of treatment failure and typically portends a very poor prognosis. Strategies to induce a remission after relapse include withdrawal of immunosuppression medications and/or use of DLI. The goal is to optimize the GVL effect rendered by donor T cells, though responses are variable and acute GVHD is a major cause of treatment failure. The optimal timing and dose application of DLI in various hematologic malignancies following HCT are still being explored. Initial doses of 1×10^6 to 1×10^7 CD3$^+$/kg have been suggested in sibling and matched unrelated donor allogeneic HCT[278-280]; however, the starting dose for mismatched donors remains a matter of debate. There is a lack of consensus on the time interval between DLI infusions and the guidelines are institution-specfic; however, an 8-week interval is generally accepted, with the initial dose after 3 months following HCT. In a retrospective analysis, the European Bone Marrow Transplantation Acute Leukemia Working Party analyzed the data of 399 patients with AML in the first hematologic relapse after hematopoietic stem cell transplantation whose treatment did ($n = 171$) or did not ($n = 228$) include DLI. After a median follow-up of 27 to 40 months, respectively, estimated survival at 2 years was about 21% for patients who received DLI and 9% for patients who did not receive DLI. Improved outcome was associated with younger age (>37 years; $P = .008$), relapse occurring more than 5 months after HCT ($P < .0001$), and use of DLI ($P = .04$). Among DLI recipients, a lower tumor burden at relapse (>35% of bone marrow blasts; $P = .006$), female sex ($P = .02$), favorable cytogenetics ($P = .004$), and remission at time of DLI ($P < .0001$) were predictive for survival in a multivariate analysis. Two-year survival was 56% if the DLI was performed in remission or with favorable karyotype, compared to 15% if the DLI was given in aplasia or with active disease.[281] Anecdotal reports of responses have been generated in multiple myeloma, CLL, Fanconi anemia, and polycythemia rubra vera.[282] When applied to patients with ALL, HL, and NHL, few responses have been observed.[283]

DLIs have been used either alone or in combination with chemotherapy[284] or hypomethylating agents such as decitabine or 5-azacitidine.[285-288] In retrospective studies, patients with AML or myelodysplastic syndrome (MDS) treated with DLI plus chemotherapy achieved better outcomes compared to patients who received chemotherapy alone.[281,289,290] Treatment with chemotherapy plus DLI resulted in higher ORR compared to hypomethylating agent or DLI (68% vs 33%, $P = .07$). The use of prophylactic DLI to augment GVL effect is being explored in patients at high risk of relapse such as those with mixed chimerism[291,292] or any evidence of MRD,[291,293] following HCT for myeloid malignancies. However, the timing, dosing, and patient selection need further investigation. Studies so far have shown that early DLI in AML or MDS is feasible, although variably effective.[294]

DLIs are not without complications. The two most worrisome are GVHD and pancytopenia occurring within a few weeks after infusion.[295] Predictors of GVHD following DLI were T-lymphocyte depletion in the original transplant marrow and concomitant IFN-α usage. The GVHD induced by DLI appears to respond more readily to immunosuppressive measures than does the GVHD seen with transplantation. Predictors of myelosuppression include frank hematologic relapse and T-lymphocyte depletion.[283,296,297] Various forms of adoptive immunotherapy are being explored to reduce the incidence of acute GVHD associated with DLIs. Such approaches have included escalating doses of T cells, CD8$^+$-depleted DLI, antigen-specific CTLs, and NK cells.[298-300]

Cytokine-induced killer cells (CIK cells) are cytotoxic effector T cells, which are readily expandable and express in addition to the T-cell marker, CD3$^+$ markers typically associated with NK cells such as CD56$^+$ and NKG2D. CIK cells are generated by the in vitro culture of peripheral blood lymphocytes with IFN-γ, IL-2, and anti-CD3. T-cell expansion and activation occurs resulting in cytolytic cells, which recognize targets through NKG2D.[301] NKG2D is an activating receptor expressed on all NK cells and also serves as a T-cell costimulatory molecule that augments cytotoxic and proliferative responses of T cells upon encountering antigen.[302,303] CIK cell–mediated cytotoxicity is MHC unrestricted, and TCR independent as target killing occurs through NKG2D-mediated recognition. In preclinical studies, CIK cells have shown potent activity against several tumor cell lines and with a markedly reduced capacity of inducing GVHD in murine models.[301,304]

The results of a phase I feasibility study in which escalating doses of CIK cells derived from HLA-matched sibling donors were administered to recipients with hematologic malignancies who relapsed after allogeneic HCT showed significant GVL effect with minimal GVHD.[305] Significant cytotoxicity was demonstrated in vitro against a panel of human tumor cell lines. The study of included 18 patients, median age of 53 years (range 20-69), received CIK cell infusions based on $CD3^+$ cells/kg at escalating doses of 1×10^7 ($n = 4$), 5×10^7 ($n = 6$), and 1×10^8 ($n = 8$). The median expansion of $CD3^+$ cells was 12-fold (range 4- to 91-fold). $CD3^+CD56^+$ cells represented a median of 11% (range 4%-44%) of the harvested cells with a median 31-fold (range, 7- to 515-fold) expansion. Median $CD3^+CD314^+$ expression was 53% (range, 32%-78%) of harvested cells. Acute GVHD, grades I to II, were seen in two patients, and one patient has limited chronic GVHD. After a median follow-up of 20 months (range 1-69 months) from CIK infusion, the median OS was 28 months, and median EFS was 4 months. All deaths were caused by relapsed disease; however, five patients had longer remissions after infusion of CIK cells than from allogeneic transplantation.

Adoptive Cellular Immunotherapy

Allogeneic HCT is a potentially curative therapy for a variety of diseases, including hematologic malignancies,[306] solid tumors,[307] and other nonmalignant disorders.[308] Early and late complications after HCT include immunologic complications, such as GVHD, graft failure, disease relapse, and infections.[309] Successful outcome following HCT depends on numerous variables, such as the type of disease, age of the patient, disease status at HCT, and therapies used. In malignant disorders, GVT effects or recognition of cancer cells by donor T cells is the primary objective sought with this therapy. Unfortunately, GVHD and GVT are tightly associated, and the pathways of one can lead to the other. Therefore, novel methods of augmenting the GVT and complications after HCT are needed. Adoptive immunotherapeutic approaches including CTLs, γδ T cells, CIK cells, NK cells, and T_{regs} are being developed for use in patients with hematologic malignancies.

Lymphocyte-Activated Killer Cells

Rosenberg et al pioneered the development and use of lymphocyte-activated killer cells (LAK cells) plus IL-2.[310,311] LAK cells were derived from resting, autochthonous, peripheral blood mononuclear cells by culture ex vivo in high concentrations of IL-2. After culture, these cells were capable of lysing fresh tumor cells in an MHC-nonrestricted manner.[312] They were subsequently administered to patients with malignant tumors along with high-dose IL-2. LAK cells appear to be derived from the NK subset of human lymphocytes because they bore NK markers CD16 and CD56 and usually lacked CD3.[313,314] Initial reports with LAK plus IL-2 in patients suggested a significant response rate in NHL, but more emphasis was given to solid tumors, particularly renal cell carcinoma, melanoma, and lung cancer.[315-317] Studies showed that LAK cells' therapeutic effect was limited because they did not home to the site of tumor involvement on a consistent basis. Furthermore, there does not seem to be an advantage for the administration of LAK plus IL-2 over administration of IL-2 alone.[315]

Tumor-Infiltrating Lymphocytes

A search for more potent killer cells resulted in the description of TILs.[318] These cells could be isolated and grown from single-cell suspensions of tumor specimens in IL-2 in a complicated production process that can take up to 3 weeks or more.[319-321] They have the phenotype of classic cytotoxic T cells and kill tumor cells in an MHC-restricted manner. In animal studies, TILs are approximately 50 to 100 times more potent killers than are LAK cells. TILs also more efficiently home to and accumulate in tumor deposits.[322,323] Pilot trials[311,324] have demonstrated a response rate of 35% to 72% in patients with melanoma.[325,326] Longer telomeres of the infused cells, the number of $CD8^+CD27^+$ cells infused, and the persistence of the infused cells in the circulation at 1 month were associated with ORR.[326]

The TILs process uses specific properties of the immune system to target a malignant lesion. Some of these include the specificity of immune response to target tumor antigens without toxicity to the host, and persistence of the TILs long enough to eradicate the tumor. The enthusiasm for TIL treatments waned over time due to the rather modest response rates, the extremely labor-intensive nature of these treatments, and the serious toxicity of systemically administered IL-2.[327-332] However, there has recently been a resurgence of interest in TIL, following strong efficacy data in patients with melanoma and nonsmall cell lung cancer,[333,334] and TIL are now undergoing commercial development.

Viral Antigen–Specific T Cells

The success of adoptively transferred, virally specific, ex vivo expanded T lymphocytes for control of cytomegalovirus infection in patients after allogeneic HCT[335-337] suggests that, if appropriate tumor cell antigens can be found and exploited, this form of therapy may become a useful modality in the treatment of hematologic malignancies.[338-340] EBV has served as a target for >80% of posttransplant lymphoproliferative disorder (PTLD), 30% to 50% of HL, and a variety of EBV + NHL. The advantages of using autologous or allogeneic cytotoxic T cells that target viral antigens are the minimal toxicity, their long-term presence, lack of need for chemotherapy, and the relatively low cost compared to other therapies, particularly CAR T cells (see below).

In patients who were at risk for PTLD following T-depleted allogeneic HCT, EBV-specific CTLs from donors prevented the development of PTLD in all 101 patients receiving them for prophylaxis and achieved a sustained CR in 11 of 13 patients who developed PTLD.[341] Utilizing a bank of frozen EBV-specific CTLs from multiple donors for primarily solid-organ transplant patients ($n = 33$) who developed PTLD resulted in a 64% response at 5 weeks and 52% response (42% CR) at 6 months.[342]

Autologous T cells directed at EBV latent membrane protein (LMP)-2 or LMP-1 and LMP-2 antigens in high-risk patients with EBV^+ HL and NHL led to sustained remissions in 28 of 29 patients when given as adjuvant therapy and an 82% EFS at 2 years; and 13 responses (11 CR) in 21 patients with relapsed/resistant disease at the time of infusion.[343] In order to bypass TGF-β inhibition of immune responses against cancer, these tumor-specific T cells were further modified to be TGF-β resistant and were infused into eight patients with refractory EBV^+ HL; there were 3 responses in 7 evaluable patients with 2 sustained CRs beyond 4 years.[344]

Chimeric Antigen Receptors

The CAR construct: This consists of a protein structure that has an extracellular binding domain, typically derived from linking the variable chains of monoclonal antibodies into a single-chain variable fragment (scFv), that can bind specific antigen, and transmembrane and intracellular signaling domains that serve to activate the T cell through downstream signaling. The end result is the mounting of a robust T cell response that is directed to the target antigen in a non–MHC-restricted manner.[345,346] Several experiments in the 1980s and 1990s paved the way for the development of the essential components of the CAR construct.[345-349] The way the CAR protein structure is made is through the insertion of a single strand of DNA into the mature T lymphocyte using a γ retrovirus or lentivirus vector. Additional gene-transfer technologies, including transposon technologies, are also in clinical development.[350] The DNA fragment consists of the extracellular binder domain essential for antigen recognition, CD3 portion that affects the intracellular signaling cascade, and costimulatory domains (CD28 or 4-1BB) that allow the T cell to receive its costimulatory signal independent of the APC (*Figure 71.6*).[349,351,352] Although most CARs in clinical use a binder domain derived from a murine mAb, it is also possible to use humanized antibodies, camelid-derived single-domain

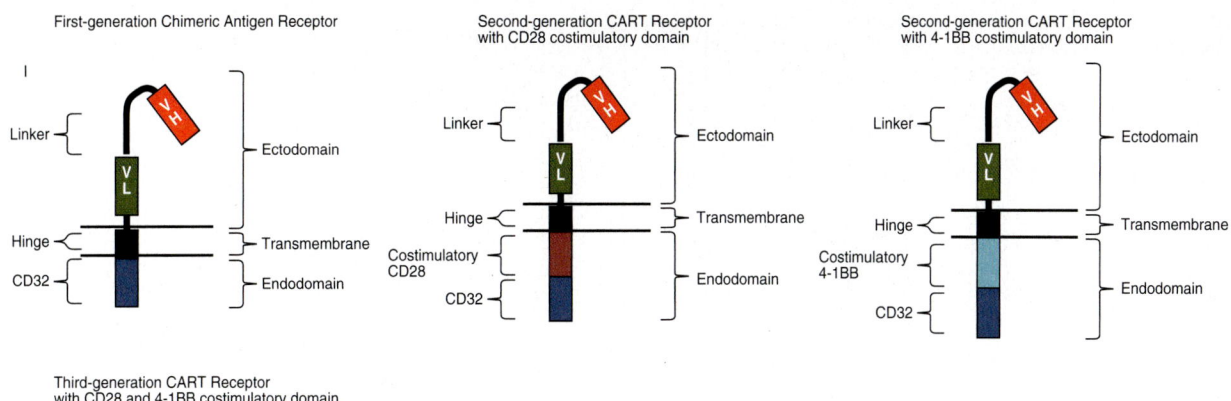
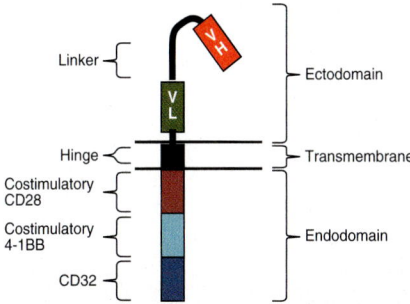

FIGURE 71.6 Schematic depiction of components of first-, second-, and third-generation chimeric antigen receptor (CAR) T receptors. First-generation CARs lacked the costimulatory domains and were of limited efficacy. Second-generation CARs have a single costimulatory domain, most commonly CD28 or the 4-1BB, which resulted in enhanced efficacy. Third-generation CARs have both the CD28 and 4-1BB costimulatory domains, or combinations of other costimulatory domains, and are still being developed.

antibodies, synthetic molecules such as ankyrins or darpins, or the natural ligands to receptors of interest.[353]

Early clinical data: The very first CARs were able to bind to the specified target but were unable to multiply and persist sufficiently to mount an effective immune response to the target because they lacked the costimulatory signal that would have been received through interaction with the APC (CD28 on the T cell and CD80/CD86 on the APC).[349,354] In order to overcome this problem, researchers included either CD28 or 4-1BB intracellular signaling domains into the CAR construct such that the T cell that was activated by the CAR construct will automatically be self-sufficient in the costimulatory signal necessary to mount a sustained immune response independent of the APC. These so-called second-generation CARs were able to mount an adequate immune response that was sufficiently robust, and they persisted sufficiently to ensure that meaningful response rates and a successfully eradicated the defined target, including malignant cells (*Table 71.3*). There are a number of other costimulatory domains that have been incorporated into CARs and tested, including CD27, OX40, DAP12, ICOS, MYD88-CD40, etc, but these have not yet entered the mainstream clinical development.[353]

Clinical trials using CAR T therapy: Several case series and nonrandomized clinical trials have been completed using CAR T therapy. The earliest trials were single institution phase I studies conducted entirely in academic medical centers. Though with small sample size, valuable insights were gained in efficacy and safety. Importantly, researchers also began to understand how to better predict for and manage toxicities that came with CAR therapy. Carefully constructed multicenter single-arm phase II clinical trials have now become the basis for the approval of several CAR T products in patients with relapsed or refractory lymphoid hematologic malignancies, including ALL, large cell lymphomas, follicular lymphoma, MCL, and multiple myeloma.

Chronic Lymphocytic Leukemia

Some of the earliest human experiments using CAR therapy were done in patients with relapsed/refractory CLL.[356,360,364] A phase I trial reported by Brentjens et al included a cohort of eight CLL patients with bulky and rapidly progressive/refractory disease and majority of whom had adverse-risk cytogenetics.[365] The first three patients had no lymphodepleting chemotherapy prior to infusion and were thought not to have responded owing to this limitation. Other patients treated had cyclophosphamide lymphodepleting chemotherapy prior to CAR T cells.[365] Three of the four patients achieved stabilization of disease ranging from 2 to 6 months. No patient achieved CR.[365] In another early phase trial reported by Porter et al,[364] 14 patients with CLL were treated with the CD19-4-1BB CAR T cells using lentiviral vector for the gene transfer mechanism. All received lymphodepleting chemotherapy, and median PFS was 7 months, median OS was 29 months, and 18 months PFS was 26.8%.[364] The first two subjects treated on this trial recently met a significant milestone of being in complete remission for over 10 years,[366] which has now been equated with "cure" in this previously uncurable disease. However, a dose-finding phase II study of this CAR T cell product, which was since named CTL019 and then tisagenlecleucel (tisa-cel), reported a complete remission rate of 33% in patients with CLL,[367] and the clinical development in this disease was paused.

Acute Lymphoblastic Leukemia

CAR T cellular immunotherapy has proven beneficial in ALL.[355,357,358,365,368,369] Davila et al reported on 16 patients with relapsed or refractory ALL treated with the second-generation CARs using CD19 to 28z construct that used murine gamma-retroviral vector for gene-transfer. All patients received lymphodepleting chemotherapy consisting of cyclophosphamide.[355] CR was noted in 88% patients, and median time to CR was 24.5 days. Seventy-five percent had no detectable MRD. CRS was observed in all patients, but the symptoms were generally reversible.[355] Lee et al also reported a single-arm phase I trial in 21 children and young adults with relapse refractory ALL, including eight who had relapsed after allogeneic hematopoietic stem cell transplant (HSCT). They were treated with the CD19 to 28 construct,[357] and all received lymphodepleting chemotherapy with fludarabine and cyclophosphamide. The results showed

Table 71.3. Early Clinical Trials in CD19 CART

First Author	Disease	Site	N	Phase	CAR Design	Median Age	Prep	Dose	CR (%)	CRS	Notes
Davila[355]	ALL	MSKCC	18	1	19-28	50	Cy 1.5-3.0 g/m²	3×10^6	88	Grade 0-2 56% Grade 3-4 44%	75% MRD negative, 44% bridged to allo-HCT
Maude[356]	ALL	UPENN	30	1	19-4-1BB	14	Physician choice	$1\text{-}10 \times 10^6$	90	Grade 0-2 73% Grade 3-4 27%	98% MRD negative, 10% bridged to allo-HCT, 67% EFS at 6 mo
Lee[357]	ALL	NCI	21	1	19-28	N/A	Flu 25 mg/m² D-5 to D-2 Cy 900 mg/m² D-2	1×10^6 or 3×10^6	70	Grade 0-2 76% Grade 3-4 28.4%	60% MRD negative, 48% bridged to allo-HCT, 51.6 EFS at 9.7 mo
Brentjens[358]	CLL	MSKCC	8	1	19-28	65.5	Cy 1.5-3 g/m²	$0.4\text{-}3.0 \times 10^7$	0	50% grade ≥3	38% PR/SD in CLL patients
Kochenderfer[359]	CLL PMBCL DLBCL SMZL	NCI	15	1	19-28	56	Cy 60-120 mg/kg	$1\text{-}5 \times 10^6$	53	80% grade ≥3	27% PR
Porter[360]	CLL	UPENN	14	1	19-4-1BB	66	21% FluCy 36% PenCy 43% Ben	$0.4\text{-}11 \times 10^8$	29	50% grade ≥3	57% ORR, 29% MRD negative
Neelapu[361]	DLBCL	21 US and 1 Israel study centers	101	2	19-28	58	Flu 30 mg/m² Cy 500 mg/m² D-5 to D-2	2×10^6	54	13% grade ≥3	82% ORR, 52% OS at 18 mo
Maude[362]	ALL	25 study sites in 11 countries across North America, Europe, Asia, and Australia	75	1-2a	19-4-1BB	11	Flu 30 mg/m² for 4 d Cy 500 mg/m² for 2 d	0.03×10^8 to 2.6×10^8 cells	60	46% grade ≥3	81% ORR, 50% EFS, 76% OS at 12 mo
Abramson[363]	LBCL	14 cancer centers in the US	269	2	19-4-1BB 1:1 CD4:CD8	63	Flu 30 mg/m² Cy 300 mg/m² for 3 d	$50\text{-}100 \times 10^6$	54	42% any grade 2% grade ≥3	73% ORR, 44% PFS 58% OS at 12 mo

Abbreviations: ALL, acute lymphoblastic leukemia; allo-HCT, allogeneic hematopoietic cell transplant; Ben, bendamustine; CLL, chronic lymphocytic leukemia; CAR, chimeric antigen receptor; CR, complete response; CRS, cytokine-release syndrome; Cy, cyclophosphamide; D, day; DLBCL, diffuse large B-cell lymphoma; EFS, event-free survival; Flu, fludarabine; MRD, minimal residual disease; MSKCC, Memorial Sloan-Kettering Cancer Center; NA, not available; NCI, National Cancer Institute; Pen, pentostatin; PFS, progression-free survival; PMBCL, primary mediastinal B-cell lymphoma; PR, partial response; SD, stable disease; SMZL, splenic marginal zone lymphoma; UPENN, University of Pennsylvania.

66.7% CR rate at 1 month of therapy, and 60% MRD-negative rate with additional follow-up. OS at a median follow-up of 10 months was 51.6% at 9.7 months.[357] CRS was noted in 76% of patients, most were grades 1 to 2 and not life-threatening.[357] In another trial, Maude reported on 30 children and adult patients with relapse refractory ALL, including 18 post–allogeneic HSCT relapses.[356] They were treated with the CD19-4-1BB CAR construct (CTL019). All patients received lymphodepleting chemotherapy at the discretion of the treating physician. The CR rate was 90%, 88% achieved MRD-negative status, and the median time to CR was 1 month. Follow-up was relatively short, but 78% OS and 76% EFS at 6 months was noted. All patients experienced CRS in varying degrees. The CARs in this study persisted for up to 6 months.[356] A phase 2 study of tisa-cel (named ELIANA) in 75 patients with relapsed or refractory ALL demonstrated an ORR of 81%, and 50% EFS and 76% OS at 12 months.[362] In August 2017, the FDA approved Kymriah (tisagenlecleucel) for pediatric and young adult patients (<26 years) with relapsed/refractory ALL. CD22 CAR T cells have induced remissions in B-ALL that was resistant to CD-19-targeted CAR immunotherapy, and bispecific (CD19 and CD22) CAR T cells are under investigation.[370]

Diffuse Large B-Cell Lymphoma

CAR T therapy has been applied in the treatment of patients with relapsed or refractory DLBCL. Nine patients with DLBCL were included in the 15 with advanced B-cell malignancies who received CD19 to 28z CAR T cells as reported by Kochenderfer et al.[359] All patients received cyclophosphamide and fludarabine lymphodepleting chemotherapy prior to CAR T infusion. Of the 15-patient cohort, 4 (53.3%) achieved CR and 4 (26.7%) PR. Four of the seven patients with DLBCL who were evaluable achieved CR. In another study of 28 patients with B-cell lymphomas, CR occurred in 6 of 14 patients with DLBCL (43%; 95% CI: 18-71). At a median follow-up of 28.6 months, 86% of responders remained without relapse suggesting durability.[371] This CAR-T product was then further developed and named axicabtagene ciloleucel. ZUMA-1 was a multiinstitutional trial of axicabtagene ciloleucel in which 101 (91%) of 111 patients with refractory aggressive B-cell NHL received CAR T and had an ORR of 82% (54% CR, 28% PR)[361,372]; at a median follow-up of 15.4 months, 42% of patients were in response, and 40% remained in CR. In October 2017, the FDA approved Yescarta (axicabtagene ciloleucel, also known as Axi-cel) for patients with certain types of DLBCL who were refractory or had relapsed after at least two other treatments.

Since then, axi-cel has been further developed and approved in several other indications: the ZUMA-5 study in follicular lymphoma showed an ORR of 92% and CR of 76% in 146 patients treated with axi-cel, with a 12-month PFS and OS of 92.9% and 73.9%.[373] A second CAR T cell product that used the same molecular design as axi-cel but had slight changes to the method of the manufacturing process for the T cell culture (named brexucabtagene autoleucel or brexu-cel) was tested and developed separately in mantle cell lymphoma (MCL) and in adults with ALL. The ZUMA-2 study was a single-arm Phase II study in 74 patients with relapsed or refractory MCL, which demonstrated an ORR of 85% and CR of 59%. At 12 months, there was 61% PFS and 83% OS.[374] This pivotal trial led to approval of brexu-cel for MCL in July 2020. The ZUMA-3 study was a single-arm Phase II study of brexu-cel in adults with relapsed or refractory ALL, and demonstrated complete remission or complete remission with incomplete hematological recovery in 39 of 55 treated patients (71%; 95% CI: 57-82), with 31(56%) patients reaching complete remission at a median follow-up of 16.4 months (range 13.8-19.6).[375] Brexu-cel became approved for this indication in April 2021. Notably, the lymphodepleting regimen for brexu-cel varies by disease indication. MCL patients receive 500 mg/m^2 cyclophosphamide and 30 mg/m^2 fludarabine IV on the fifth, fourth, and third days before infusion, whereas ALL patients receive 25 mg/m^2 fludarabine administered IV over 30 minutes on the fourth, third, and second days prior to infusion and 900 mg/m^2 cyclophosphamide administered IV over 60 minutes on the second day prior to infusion.

Lisocabtagene maraleucel (liso-cel) is another CD19-targeting CAR T cell product that has recently been approved by the FDA for the treatment of large B cell lymphomas. Liso-cel uses the same design as tisa-cel (CD19 scFV with a 4-1BB costimulatory domain) but with a CD28 hinge and transmembrane domain. Additionally, the CD4 and CD8 transduced T cells are isolated and infused at a 1:1 ratio. The TRANSCEND study demonstrated an objective response in 186 of 256 evaluable patients (73%; 95% CI:66.8-78.0) and a complete response in 136 (53%; CI: 46.8-59.4) patients.[363] This study led to the approval of lis-cel for relapsed or refractory large B cell lymphoma in February 2021. It has also demonstrated promising results in CLL and small lymphocytic lymphoma (SLL),[376] and the phase II portion of the study is ongoing.

Axi-cel, liso-cel, and tisa-cel have been compared to the standard of care for relapsed or refractory large B-cell lymphoma (chemotherapy followed by autologous stem cell transplantation) as second-line treatments in phase 3 studies. In the ZUMA-7 trial, there was an 83% response rate in the axi-cel group compared to 50% in the standard-care group (with 65% complete response vs 32%), and a median EFS of 8.3 months compared to 2.0 month at the median follow-up of 24.9 months.[377] In the TRANSFORM study, there was a complete response rate of 66% in the liso-cel treated group compared to 39% in the standard care group, a median EFS of 10.1 vs 2.3 months, and a median PFS of 14.8 vs 5.7 months.[378] Of the 91 patients treated with standard-care, 50 crossed over to receive liso-cel treatment. Both of these studies demonstrated significant outcome improvements with CAR T cells as the second-line therapy compared to the standard of care. Given these results, CAR T cell therapy is now being considered for second-line therapy (in patients with progression within 1 year of initial therapy) rather than waiting for end-stage disease. The exception to these results was the BELINDA trial, where tisa-cel did not demonstrate improved outcomes compared to the standard of care for second-line therapy. Both groups had median EFS of 3.0 months and responses occurred in 46.3% of the tisa-cel group compared to 42.5% in the standard-care group.[379] However, the percent of patient with high-grade lymphomas was higher in the tisa-cel group, as was the percentage with an international prognostic index score of 2 or higher. Therefore, additional studies of tisa-cel as a second-line therapy are needed to determine if certain patients may benefit from this approach.

Multiple Myeloma

Garfall reported the case of a patient with multiple myeloma who had relapsed after myeloablative chemotherapy with melphalan and autologous HCT. The patient was treated with CAR T cells targeting CD19 (tisagenlecleucel) and achieved complete response and without measurable serum or urine monoclonal protein 12 months after treatment. The author noted that the remission occurred despite no known expression of CD19 in myeloma cells.[380] Subsequent to this finding, CARs targeting the B-cell maturation antigen (BCMA) have been developed and are being tested in the clinical trial setting.[381] One BCMA-targeting CAR product has been approved by the FDA to treat patients with relapsed or refractory multiple myeloma. In a phase 2 trial name KarMMa, idecabtagene vicleucel (ide-cel, also called bb2121) demonstrated a 73% response rate, with 33% complete response or better, at a median follow-up of 13.3 months and an 8.8-month media PFS,[382] leading to its approval in March 2021. Another CAR product, ciltacabtagene autoleucel (cilta-cel, previously known as JNJ-4528) was designated as a breakthrough therapy by the FDA and is expected to be approved in early 2022. Results from its phase 1b/2 clinical trial CARTITUDE-1 demonstrated an overall response rate of 97% (95% CI: 91.2-99.4), with 67% complete stringent response, a 12-month PFS of 77% (95% CI: 66.0-84.3), and an OS of 89% (80.2-93.5).[383] Both CAR T cell products contain 41BB and CD3Z intracellular signaling domains, but they vary in their BCMA antigen binding domains; ide-cel contains a mouse scFv specific to BCMA while cilta-cel has two camelid Vhh domains. Additional CAR products targeting new antigens in multiple myeloma are rapidly developing and in clinical trials, including CD38, CD138, immunoglobulin κ light chain, SLAMF7, and others.[384]

Donor Lymphocyte CARs

Relapses do occur after allogeneic treatment of B-cell malignancies and pose a challenge to treatment because patients are often not in a position to receive cytotoxic chemotherapy, or have already received multiple lines pretransplant, meaning that the relapse disease has become relatively chemotherapy refractory. Several investigators have reported on the ability of CAR T cells from a donor to induce remissions in the posttransplant setting.[274,385,386] Kochenderfer reported a study that consisted of 10 patients with refractory CD19-positive malignancy after allogeneic HCT and standard of care DLIs.[274] A single dose of allogeneic anti–CD19-CAR T cells was given, and three of the ten patients had regression of disease including two with CLL and one with MCL. None of the patients treated developed GVHD. Toxicities of CAR therapy included transient hypotension and fever. They concluded that the CAR T cells can cause regression of B-cell malignancies that are resistant to standard care of DLIs without causing GVHD. Brudno also reported on a study of 20 patients with relapse refractory CD19-positive malignancies after allogeneic HCT.[385] They were treated with CART cells obtained from each recipient's allogeneic HCT donor. No lymphodepleting chemotherapy was given. Of the 20 patients treated, 8 developed objective responses (6 CR and 2 PR). Four of the five ALL patients treated achieved MRD-negative CR. No patient treated developed GVHD. Toxicities of the treatment included fever, tachycardia, and hypotension. They concluded that allogeneic CAR T cells have a role in the treatment of B-cell malignancies that progress after allogeneic HCT.[385]

"Off-the-Shelf" CAR Immune Cells

Though CAR T cells have been successful in patients, they are costly and time consuming to manufacture and can be difficult to produce if the patient was heavily pretreated. An attractive alternative is using healthy donor cells to make "off the self" CAR T cells that would be readily available. However, using allogeneic cells can lead to GVHD as well as rejection from the host. A number of methods have been explored to prevent this, including using umbilical cord blood or induced pluripotent stem cells to make the cells and having a bank from donors with varying HLA haplotypes, using donor-derived T cells in stem cell transplant recipients, selecting for virus-specific T cells, using non-ab T cells, or gene-editing the cells to remove the TCR.[387] One promising approach is to electroporate transcription activator-like effector nucleases specific to the T cell receptor constant a chain (TRAC) and CD52 into CD19-CAR T cells (named UCART19). This method results in TRAC and CD52 knockout CAR T cells that do not induce GVHD and can avoid allogeneic rejection through depletion of the host T cells with a CD52-specific mAb, alemtuzumab. In two phase 1 clinical trials, UCART19 manufactured from donor-derived T cells demonstrated for the first time the feasibility of using allogeneic CAR T cells in patients with relapsed or refractory B-cell ALL. In patients treated with alemtuzumab, UCART19 cells expanded and had antileukemic activity.[388]

Another approach avoids using ab T cells and instead uses NK cells to express the CAR, which when engaged will activate the NK cell's natural killing mechanisms.[389] One of the challenges with this approach is that CAR NK cells have limited persistence. This has been addressed by additionally engineering these cells to express IL-2 or IL-15 to enhance proliferation. Cord blood–derived NK cells expressing a CD19CAR, IL-15, and an iCasp9 safety switch resulted in 8 (73%) responses, including 7 complete remissions, in 11 patients with relapsed or refractory CD19-positive cancers.[390] CAR NK cells targeting other tumor antigens (including in solid tumors) and using other engineering strategies to improve their function are rapidly being developed and proceeding to clinical trials.[391]

Side Effects of CAR T Therapy

The use of CAR therapy is associated with specific side effects that occur owing to the nature of the immune response that the CARs induce. These side effects can be classified into CRS, neurologic events, and B-cell aplasia in the case of CD19-directed CARs.

Cytokine Release Syndrome

CRS is an immune-mediated condition that occurs as the infused CAR T cells expand and engage the antigen to which they have been targeted (*Table 71.4*). It consists of bulk T-cell activation, secretion of large amounts of proinflammatory cytokines, and the recruitment of other cells of the immune system, including macrophages.[355,357,364]

Table 71.4. Cytokine-Release Syndrome Grading System and Management

Grade	Toxicity	Therapy
Grade 1	Fever[a] ≥38.0 °C with no hypotension or hypoxia	Supportive medications
Grade 2	Fever ≥38.0 °C with hypotension not requiring vasopressors and/or[b] hypoxia requiring low-flow nasal cannula[c] or blow-by	In adults, tocilizumab may be considered. In pediatric patients with prolonged grade 2 CRS or intolerance to fever, tocilizumab may be administered. In elderly patients or patients with extensive comorbidities, tocilizumab should be considered earlier in the course of CRS.
Grade 3	Fever ≥38.0 °C with hypotension requiring a vasopressor with or without vasopressin and/or hypoxia requiring high-flow nasal cannula, face mask, non-rebreather mask, or venturi mask	In pediatric patients, tocilizumab should be administered. In both adults and children, if CRS does not improve after 1 dose of tocilizumab, then steroids should be administered with a second dose of tocilizumab.
Grade 4	Fever ≥38.0 °C with hypotension requiring multiple vasopressors (excluding vasopressin) and/or hypoxia requiring positive pressure (e.g., CPAP, BiPAP, intubation, and mechanical ventilation)	If CRS does not improve after 2 doses of tocilizumab (and steroids), third-line agents, including anakinra, siltuximab, and high-dose methylprednisolone, should be considered. If CRS does not improve after tocilizumab and steroids, infections should be considered again in the differential diagnosis and managed appropriately. If steroids are used in the management of CRS, a rapid taper should be used once symptoms begin to improve.

Organ toxicities associated with CRS may be graded according to CTCAE v5.0 but they do not influence CRS grading.
Abbreviations: BiPAP, bilevel positive airway pressure; CPAP, continuous positive airway pressure; CRS, cytokine release syndrome; CTCAE, Common Terminology Criteria for Adverse Events.
[a]Fever is defined as temperature 38 °C not attributable to any other cause. In patients who have CRS then receive antipyretic or anticytokine therapy such as tocilizumab or steroids, fever is no longer required to grade subsequent CRS severity. In this case, CRS grading is driven by hypotension and/or hypoxia.
[b]CRS grade is determined by the more severe event: hypotension or hypoxia not attributable to any other cause. For example, a patient with temperature of 39.5 °C, hypotension requiring 1 vasopressor, and hypoxia requiring low-flow nasal cannula is classified as grade 3 CRS.
[c]Low-flow nasal cannula is defined as oxygen delivered at ≤6 L/min. Low flow also includes blow-by oxygen delivery, sometimes used in pediatrics. High-flow nasal cannula is defined as oxygen delivered at >6 L/min.
Adapted from Lee DW, Santomasso BD, Locke FL, et al. ASTCT consensus grading for cytokine release syndrome and neurologic toxicity associated with immune effector cells. *Biol Blood Marrow Transplant*. 2019;25(4):625-638 and Maus MV, Alexander S, Bishop MR, et al. Society for Immunotherapy of Cancer (SITC) clinical practice guideline on immune effector cell-related adverse events. *J Immuother Cancer*. 2020;8(2):e001511.

CRS spans the spectrum from mild to life-threatening, and many but not all patients experience some form of this toxicity. The syndrome typically begins within 1 to 5 days of CAR T-cell infusion with fevers (often high grade >40 °C) that may or may not respond to antipyretics.[357,365,368,392] Proinflammatory cytokines that are upregulated include IL-2, IFN-γ, TNF, and IL-6.[357,365,368] Studies suggest a correlation between CRS and tumor burden, and CRS frequency and timing also vary with disease indication and type of CAR T product. In addition to fevers, patients could also experience respiratory distress, hypotension, and neurologic events.[357,365,368] Patients require close management (i.e., hospitalization) in order to prevent end-organ damage and mortality. This may involve vasopressors and intubation with mechanical ventilation and hemodialysis.[357,365,368]

In the study by Lee et al,[357] CRS occurred in 76% of patients. Most were grades 1 to 2 and did not appear to be life-threatening. The rate of severe CRS (grades 3 and 4) was 14.3% each. In the study by Davila et al,[355] all patients developed CRS, and 25% had grade 4. All recovered with supportive care and pharmacologic intervention. Maude et al[356] also reported that CRS occurred in all patients, and 27% had grades 3 to 4. Conservative management for mild cases and medical interventions are designed for more severe cases. Corticosteroids and/or tocilizumab are used in the more severe CRS. Tocilizumab is a mAb that binds the IL-6R, and it has been used successfully to ameliorate the severity of CRS.[369] Le et al performed a retrospective analysis of patients receiving tocilizumab to manage CRS resulting from treatment with tisa-cel or axi-cel during their prospective clinical trials. Of the 45 patients treated with tocilizumab following severe or life-threatening CRS after tisa-cel, 31 (69%) achieved a response as defined by resolution of CRS within 14 days of the first dose, requiring no more than 2 doses, or if no other drugs or corticosteroids were used for treatment. In the cohort of patients receiving axi-cel, 53% of the 15 patients treated with tocilizumab following CRS responded.[393] This study led to the FDA approval of tocilizumab for CRS that occurs with CAR T cell therapy. This approval occurred simultaneously with the approval of tisa-cel for patients up to 25 years old with relapsed or refractory B cell ALL. It was the first approval of CAR T cell therapy for pediatric ALL.

Neurologic Events

CAR T-cell–induced neurologic events occur in 28% to 43% (Table 71.5). Symptoms are reversible in most patients, but fatalities have been described. The mechanism is unclear but of interest is the fact that CAR T cell does migrate into the central nervous system (CNS) and is detected in the cerebrospinal fluid even in patients without detectable CNS disease.[355-357] It manifests as a spectrum of neurologic symptoms including tremors and various degrees of encephalopathy including aphasia, confusion, somnolence seizures, and fatal cerebral edema.[355-357,394] It is suspected that neurologic events are a separate process from the CRS, though the two seem to be related. Recently, a group of investigators developed a set of clinical tools and a uniform grading system to facilitate communication around the description of both CRS and neurotoxicity.[393] Because the neurotoxicity observed with CD19 CAR T cells has also been observed with other T cell engaging therapies, notably blinatumomab bispecific antibodies and CAR T cells directed to BCMA in multiple myeloma, the term "immune-effector cell–associated neurotoxicity syndrome," or ICANS, was coined. The clinical tool to describe the syndrome was termed an "ICE" score, and consists of an abbreviated mini-mental status exam (Table 71.5). Conservative medical management has been successful in patients with mild symptoms, whereas those with more severe symptoms require high doses of corticosteroids with the aim to decrease vasogenic edema; specific management strategies depend in part on the indication and the CAR T cell product, but there have also been consensus guidelines developed to guide clinicians.[395] Tocilizumab given in the prophylactic or treatment setting for CRS does not appear to prevent or ameliorate the neurologic toxicity.

B-Cell Aplasia

B-cell aplasia is an on-target off-tumor response that is seen in the setting of CAR T therapy when the CARs are directed to CD19.[364,396] All patients achieving a CR have some duration of B-cell aplasia.[3][55-357,364,396] In the study by Porter, patients developed prolonged B-cell aplasia that required IV IgG repletion on a periodic basis.[364] The B-cell aplasia lasted up to 4 years in certain individuals.[364] CAR T cells targeting other antigens such as BCMA do not lead to B cell aplasia but may lead to hypogammaglobulinemia due to plasma-cell targeting.

Mechanisms of Resistance to CAR T Cells

Despite the success of CAR T cell hematologic malignancies, many patients still relapse following CAR T cell therapy and CAR T cells have yet to be approved for solid tumors due to a lack of efficacy. Several mechanisms of resistance to CAR therapy have been identified, including downregulation of the targeted antigen by the tumor cells and outgrowth of antigen-negative clones, difficulty identifying target antigens that are uniformly expressed by the tumor and not by normal cells, poor expansion or persistence of the CAR T cells, suppression of the infused cells by the tumor microenvironment, or rejection of the CAR T cells if patients develop immunity to the nonhuman parts of the CAR. One of the main focuses of CAR T cell research is how to improve their function and prevent resistance from occurring. A number of strategies to further engineer CAR T cells or use combination therapies to combat these mechanisms are currently being explored in the lab and in the clinic.[397]

Future Directions

The CAR process has led to improved efficacy in selected relapsed malignancies and appears superior to chemotherapy alone. Although CAR T therapy has been used as a bridge to allogeneic transplant for some patients with B-ALL, responses have been sustained in some patients with ALL and other hematologic neoplasms, including CLL and other lymphomas. Owing to the success of CAR T cells, efforts are underway to extend this benefit to other malignancies, including HL (targeting CD30), cervical cancer and others that involve HPV (targeting E6 and E7), and colorectal cancer. The complex logistics, intensity of clinical care required, and high cost of CAR T will need to be addressed for this therapy to become more widely available for patients.

Placenta-Derived NK Cells

NK cells are involved in immune recognition of cancer and are closely involved in targeting malignant cells for destruction. Researchers have long been interested in developing NK cells to target malignant cells including AML, and some progress has been made in recent years. NK cell activity can be downregulated by T_{regs}; therefore, lymphodepleting chemotherapy is essential for the type of enhanced NK cell function that is required for cytotoxicity. Bachanova et al reported that NK cellular activity increased to 27% (up from 10%) when a more immunosuppressive therapy was given to the host because more immunosuppression leads to decreased T_{reg} function.[398] There are several clinical trials evaluating the role of placenta-derived NK cells in identifying malignant cells in relapse refractory AML.[398,399]

Checkpoint Blockade

The PD-1 pathway is a checkpoint to limit T-cell–mediated immune responses, and inhibitors of PD-1, its ligands, and CTLA-4, a protein that downregulates the immune system, have led to a major breakthrough in solid tumors, particularly melanoma, lung cancer, and renal cell cancer; are active in HL; and are under evaluation in a number of hematologic malignancies.[400] In classic HL, alterations of chromosome 9p24.1 are a recurrent genetic abnormality that amplifies the expression of PD-1 ligands, PD-L1 and PD-L2, and augments the JAK-STAT pathway that further promotes PD-L1 production. EBV, common in HL, also leads to PD-L1 expression, which, in turn, contributes to viral persistence.

Phase I trials evaluating the role of two PD-1 inhibitors, nivolumab and pembrolizumab, in hematologic cancers led to phase II trials in HL. In a study using nivolumab for 23 patients with relapsed, refractory HL, including 78% who had a prior autologous HCT and 78% who

Table 71.5. Neurologic Toxicity Grading and Management Guidance

Neurologic Event	Therapy	
	Concurrent CRS	No Concurrent CRS
Grade 1		
ICE score 7-9 Depressed level of consciousness[a]—awakens spontaneously Seizure—n/a Motor findings—n/a Elevated ICP/cerebral edema—n/a	Because of the possibility that tocilizumab may worsen neurotoxicity, the management of neurotoxicity may take precedence over the management of low-grade CRS • e.g., in the case of a patient with concomitant grade 1 CRS (fever) and grade 2 ICANS, steroids should be given. • This does not apply to higher-grade CRS.	Based on the expected neurotoxicities seen with different CAR T cell therapies, the management of ICANS should be risk-adjusted based on product-specific and patient-specific characteristics. • Patients with CNS involvement of their disease may need earlier intervention for ICANS. • Patients with history of inflammatory neurological conditions or current CNS disease involvement should be referred for additional neurological consultation prior to initiating CAR T cell therapy.
Grade 2		
ICE score 3-6 Depressed level of consciousness[a]—awakens to voice Seizure—n/a Motor findings—n/a Elevated ICP/cerebral edema—n/a	• After being treated with 4-1BB CAR T cell products, such as tisagenlecleucel, steroids may be considered. • After being treated with CD28 costimulated CAR T cell products such as axicabtagene ciloleucel and brexucabtagen autoleucel, steroids should be used to mitigate the duration and severity of ICANS • If steroids are used in the management of ICANS, at least 2 doses should be given and a fast taper should be used once there is improvement	
Grade 3		
ICE score 0-2[b] Depressed level of consciousness[a]—awakens only to tactile stimulus Seizure—any clinical seizure focal or generalized that resolves rapidly or nonconvulsive seizures on EEG that resolve with intervention Motor findings—n/a Elevated ICP/cerebral edema—focal/local edema on neuroimaging[c]	• Steroids are recommended • To manage seizures in patients treated with CAR T cell therapies, levetiracetam is recommended • There is insufficient evidence to recommend prophylactic antiseizure medications to all patients undergoing CAR T cell therapies. However, in patients deemed to be at high risk of developing neurotoxicity based on history, disease characteristics, or the product being administered, prophylactic levetiracetam may be considered	
Grade 4		
ICE score 0[b] (patient is unarousable) Depressed level of consciousness[a]—patient is unarousable or requires vigorous or repetitive tactile stimuli to arouse; stupor or coma Seizure—Life-threatening prolonged seizure (>5 min), repetitive clinical or electrical seizures without return to baseline in between Motor findings[d]—Deep focal motor weakness such as hemiparesis or paraparesis Elevated ICP/cerebral edema—Diffuse cerebral edema on neuroimaging, decerebrate or decorticate posturing, cranial nerve VI palsy, papilledema, or Cushing triad	• Steroids are recommended • For brain imaging in patients deemed high risk, MRI is preferred. If a patient is too unstable to transport, or fast-brain MRI is unavailable for pediatric patients (thus necessitating sedation), CT imaging may be used • If cerebral edema is suspected based on clinical signs and symptoms, patients should be immediately referred to intensive care where rapid imaging and management of intracranial hypertension should be performed	

ICANS grade is determined by the most severe event not attributable to any other cause.
Abbreviations: ASTCT, American Society for Transplantation and Cellular Therapy; CRS, cytokine release syndrome; CTCAE, Common Terminology Criteria for Adverse Events; EEG, electroencephalogram; ICANS, immune effector cell–associated neurotoxicity syndrome; ICE, effector cell–associated encephalopathy; ICP, intracranial pressure; n/a, not applicable.
[a]Attributable to no other cause (e.g., no sedating medication).
[b]A patient with an ICE score of 0 may be classified as grade 3 ICANS if awake with global aphasia, but a patient with an ICE score of 0 may be classified as grade 4 ICANS if unarousable.
[c]Intracranial hemorrhage with or without associated edema is not considered a neurotoxicity feature and is excluded from ICANS grading. It may be graded according to CTCAE V.5.0.
[d]Tremors and myoclonus associated with immune effector cell therapies may be graded according to CTCAE V.5.0, but they do not influence ICANS grading.
From Maus MV, Alexander S, Bishop MR, et al. Society for Immunotherapy of Cancer (SITC) clinical practice guideline on immune effector cell-related adverse events. *J Immuother Cancer*. 2020;8(2):e001511, with permission from BMJ Publishing Group Ltd. Adapted from Lee DW, Santomasso BD, Locke FL, et al. ASTCT consensus grading for cytokine release syndrome and neurologic toxicity associated with immune effector cells. *Biol Blood Marrow Transplant*. 2019;25(4):625-638. Copyright © 2018 American Society for Blood and Marrow Transplantation. With permission.

had received brentuximab vedotin, the ORR was 87% (17% CR and 70% PR), and the PFS at 6 months was 86%.[401] In a study using pembrolizumab for 31 patients with relapsed/refractory HL, all of whom had failed brentuximab vedotin, the ORR was 65% (16% CR and 48% PR), and the PFS was 69% at 6 months and 46% at 13 months.[402] Grade 3 and 4 toxicities were less than 20% in both trials and included immunologic events, such as colitis, pneumonitis, thyroiditis, and transaminitis. Pembrolizumab (Keytruda) was approved by the FDA in March 2017 for refractory HL or after three or more lines of therapy; and nivolumab (Opdivo) was approved in April 2017 for refractory HL after failing an autologous HCT. Ongoing trials are evaluating the use of immune checkpoint inhibitors as part of initial therapy with HL (primarily in combination with chemotherapy).

PD-1 inhibitors have not uniformly been as successful in NHL, but early trials have identified specific types that have high-response rates. In a phase I trial of 81 patients with relapsed/refractory B-cell NHL, the ORR with nivolumab was 28% with the highest response rates in follicular lymphoma and DLBCL at 40% and 36%, respectively, but only one patient had a sustained response beyond 6 months.[403] Subtypes of DLBCL with high-response rates to PD-1 inhibitors often have a high expression of PD-1 and its ligands and include large B-cell lymphoma of the mediastinum that also has a similar genetic profile with HL, primary CNS lymphoma, and primary testicular lymphoma.[404] Peripheral T-cell lymphomas that respond to PD-1 blockade include mycosis fungoides and nasal NKT cell lymphoma, an EBV-related neoplasm.[405,406]

Ipilimumab, a mAb that inhibits CTLA-4, is under investigation in hematologic malignancies as a single agent and in combination with other therapies. In a phase I trial of 18 patients with NHL, the ORR was only 11%, but there were two prolonged responses, a CR in DLBCL lasting 2.5 years and a PR in follicular lymphoma maintained for 1.5 years.[407] Ipilimumab appears to have higher responses in relapses after allogeneic HCT for a variety of hematologic cancers, including AML and lymphomas, by restoring donor-mediated GVT effect. In a phase I/Ib study of 28 patients, 6 (21%) had adverse immune events, and 4 (14%) had worsening GVHD preventing additional ipilimumab therapy.[408] Of 22 patients who received a dose of 10 mg/kg, 13 (59%) had a reduction in tumor burden, and 7 (32%) had an objective response (5 CR and 2 PR); the 1-year OS was 49% with a median follow-up of 15 months.

CONCLUSION

Immunotherapy is ushering in a paradigm shift in oncology with hematologic malignancies being among the most susceptible to immune targeting.[409] Many of the therapies are active by themselves, but it is probable that combinations will yield better results than single agents. Ongoing trials are evaluating checkpoint inhibitors with mAbs or chemotherapy and are screening for biomarkers that are associated with response. It is possible that CAR T cells that target both CD19 and CD22 could yield higher responses than those that target either alone by preventing an escape mechanism of antigen shifting by the malignant cell. Immunotherapy will continue to be investigated in transplantation, including studies to decrease relapse following autologous HCT and to augment the GVT effect with allogeneic HCT.

WEB SITES

http://www.anticancer.net/
http://www.cancerresearch.org/

ACKNOWLEDGMENTS

This chapter represents an edited and updated version of the chapter on "Immunotherapy" included in the 14th edition of this book. We, therefore, gratefully acknowledge the authors of the original chapter, Olalekan O. Oluwole, Adetola A. Kassim, and Luc Van Kaer for their important contributions.

References

1. Ehrlich P. Uebr den jetzigne stand der karzinomforschung. *Ned Tijdschr Geneeskd.* 1909;5:273-290.
2. Burnet FM. The concept of immunological surveillance. *Prog Exp Tumor Res.* 1970;13:1-27.
3. Moller G, Moller E. The concept of immunological surveillance against neoplasia. *Transplant Rev.* 1976;28:3-16.
4. Penn I. Tumors of the immunocompromised patient. *Annu Rev Med.* 1988;39:63-73.
5. Old LJ, Boyse EA. Antigens of tumors and leukemias induced by viruses. *Fed Proc.* 1965;24(5):1009-1017.
6. Groopman JE. Neoplasms in the acquired immune deficiency syndrome: the multidisciplinary approach to treatment. *Semin Oncol.* 1987;14(2 suppl 3):1-6.
7. Stutman O. Tumor development after 3-methylcholanthrene in immunologically deficient athymic-nude mice. *Science.* 1974;183(4124):534-536.
8. Woglom W. Immunity to transplantable tumors. *Cancer Res.* 1929;4:129-214.
9. Gorer PA. Some recent work on tumor immunity. *Adv Cancer Res.* 1956;4:149-186.
10. Snell GD. Studies in histocompatibility. *Science.* 1981;213(4504):172-178.
11. Prehn RT, Main JM. Immunity to methylcholanthrene-induced sarcomas. *J Natl Cancer Inst.* 1957;18(6):769-778.
12. Mitchison NA. Passive transfer of transplantation immunity. *Proc R Soc Lond B Biol Sci.* 1954;142(906):72-87.
13. Rouse BT, Rollinghoff M, Warner NL. Anti-theta serum-induced supression of the cellular transfer of tumour-specific immunity to a syngeneic plasma cell tumour. *Nat New Biol.* 1972;238(82):116-117.
14. Kohler G, Milstein C. Continuous cultures of fused cells secreting antibody of pre-defined specificity. *Nature.* 1975;256(5517):495-497.
15. Smyth MJ, Godfrey DI, Trapani JA. A fresh look at tumor immunosurveillance and immunotherapy. *Nat Immunol.* 2001;2(4):293-299.
16. Vesely MD, Kershaw MH, Schreiber RD, Smyth MJ. Natural innate and adaptive immunity to cancer. *Annu Rev Immunol.* 2011;29:235-271.
17. Coley WB. The treatment of malignant tumors by repeated inoculations of erysipelas. With a report of ten original cases. 1893. *Clin Orthop Relat Res.* 1991;262:3-11.
18. Bachireddy P, Burkhardt UE, Rajasagi M, Wu CJ. Haematological malignancies: at the forefront of immunotherapeutic innovation. *Nat Rev Cancer.* 2015;15(4):201-215.
19. Fearon DT, Locksley RM. The instructive role of innate immunity in the acquired immune response. *Science.* 1996;272(5258):50-53.
20. Janeway CA Jr, Medzhitov R. Innate immune recognition. *Annu Rev Immunol.* 2002;20:197-216.
21. Matzinger P. The danger model: a renewed sense of self. *Science.* 2002;296(5566):301-305.
22. Akira S, Uematsu S, Takeuchi O. Pathogen recognition and innate immunity. *Cell.* 2006;124(4):783-801.
23. Hibbs JB Jr, Lambert LH Jr, Remington JS. Possible role of macrophage mediated nonspecific cytotoxicity in tumour resistance. *Nat New Biol.* 1972;235(54):48-50.
24. Lichtenstein A. Granulocytes as possible effectors of tumor immunity. *Immunol Allergy Clin North Am.* 1990;10:731-746.
25. Sims GP, Rowe DC, Rietdijk ST, Herbst R, Coyle AJ. HMGB1 and RAGE in inflammation and cancer. *Annu Rev Immunol.* 2010;28:367-388.
26. Allen IC, TeKippe EM, Woodford RM, et al. The NLRP3 inflammasome functions as a negative regulator of tumorigenesis during colitis-associated cancer. *J Exp Med.* 2010;207(5):1045-1056.
27. Chow MT, Moller A, Smyth MJ. Inflammation and immune surveillance in cancer. *Semin Cancer Biol.* 2012;22(1):23-32.
28. Carswell EA, Old LJ, Kassel RL, Green S, Fiore N, Williamson B. An endotoxin-induced serum factor that causes necrosis of tumors. *Proc Natl Acad Sci U S A.* 1975;72(9):3666-3670.
29. Banchereau J, Palucka AK. Dendritic cells as therapeutic vaccines against cancer. *Nat Rev Immunol.* 2005;5(4):296-306.
30. Ljunggren HG, Karre K. In search of the "missing self": MHC molecules and NK cell recognition. *Immunol Today.* 1990;11(7):237-244.
31. Lanier LL. Up on the tightrope: natural killer cell activation and inhibition. *Nat Immunol.* 2008;9(5):495-502.
32. Ruggeri L, Mancusi A, Capanni M, Martelli MF, Velardi A. Exploitation of alloreactive NK cells in adoptive immunotherapy of cancer. *Curr Opin Immunol.* 2005;17(2):211-217.
33. Van Kaer L, Parekh VV, Wu L. Invariant natural killer T cells: bridging innate and adaptive immunity. *Cell Tissue Res.* 2011;343(1):43-55.
34. Bendelac A, Bonneville M, Kearney JF. Autoreactivity by design: innate B and T lymphocytes. *Nat Rev Immunol.* 2001;1(3):177-186.
35. Smyth MJ, Crowe NY, Hayakawa Y, Takeda K, Yagita H, Godfrey DI. NKT cells - conductors of tumor immunity? *Curr Opin Immunol.* 2002;14(2):165-171.
36. Hayday AC. γδ Cells: a right time and a right place for a conserved third way of protection. *Annu Rev Immunol.* 2000;18:975-1026.
37. Girardi M, Oppenheim DE, Steele CR, et al. Regulation of cutaneous malignancy by gammadelta T cells. *Science.* 2001;294(5542):605-609.
38. Tonegawa S. Somatic generation of antibody diversity. *Nature.* 1983;302(5909):575-581.
39. Qin Z, Richter G, Schuler T, Ibe S, Cao X, Blankenstein T. B cells inhibit induction of T cell-dependent tumor immunity. *Nat Med.* 1998;4(5):627-630.
40. Slamon DJ, Leyland-Jones B, Shak S, et al. Use of chemotherapy plus a monoclonal antibody against HER2 for metastatic breast cancer that overexpresses HER2. *N Engl J Med.* 2001;344(11):783-792.
41. Boon T, Cerottini JC, Van den Eynde B, van der Bruggen P, Van Pel A. Tumor antigens recognized by T lymphocytes. *Annu Rev Immunol.* 1994;12:337-365.
42. Germain RN. MHC-dependent antigen processing and peptide presentation: providing ligands for T lymphocyte activation. *Cell.* 1994;76(2):287-299.
43. Engelhard VH. Structure of peptides associated with class I and class II MHC molecules. *Annu Rev Immunol.* 1994;12:181-207.
44. Wolf PR, Ploegh HL. How MHC class II molecules acquire peptide cargo: biosynthesis and trafficking through the endocytic pathway. *Annu Rev Cell Dev Biol.* 1995;11:267-306.
45. Van Kaer L. Accessory proteins that control the assembly of MHC molecules with peptides. *Immunol Res.* 2001;23(2-3):205-214.
46. Van Kaer L. Major histocompatibility complex class I-restricted antigen processing and presentation. *Tissue Antigens.* 2002;60(1):1-9.
47. Segura E, Amigorena S. Cross-presentation in mouse and human dendritic cells. *Adv Immunol.* 2015;127:1-31.
48. Fremont DH, Rees WA, Kozono H. Biophysical studies of T-cell receptors and their ligands. *Curr Opin Immunol.* 1996;8(1):93-100.
49. Dustin ML, Depoil D. New insights into the T cell synapse from single molecule techniques. *Nat Rev Immunol.* 2011;11(10):672-684.
50. Viola A, Lanzavecchia A. T cell activation determined by T cell receptor number and tunable thresholds. *Science.* 1996;273(5271):104-106.
51. Smith-Garvin JE, Koretzky GA, Jordan MS. T cell activation. *Annu Rev Immunol.* 2009;27:591-619.
52. Greenwald RJ, Freeman GJ, Sharpe AH. The B7 family revisited. *Annu Rev Immunol.* 2005;23:515-548.
53. Pardoll DM. Tumour antigens. A new look for the 1990s. *Nature.* 1994;369(6479):357.
54. Rosenberg SA, Yang JC, Schwartzentruber DJ, et al. Immunologic and therapeutic evaluation of a synthetic peptide vaccine for the treatment of patients with metastatic melanoma. *Nat Med.* 1998;4(3):321-327.
55. Toes RE, Ossendorp F, Offringa R, Melief CJ. CD4 T cells and their role in antitumor immune responses. *J Exp Med.* 1999;189(5):753-756.

56. Sim MJW, Lu J, Spencer M, et al. High-affinity oligoclonal TCRs define effective adoptive T cell therapy targeting mutant KRAS-G12D. *Proc Natl Acad Sci USA*. 2020;117(23):12826-12835.
57. Gubin MM, Artyomov MN, Mardis ER, Schreiber RD. Tumor neoantigens: building a framework for personalized cancer immunotherapy. *J Clin Invest*. 2015;125(9):3413-3421.
58. Rajasagi M, Shukla SA, Fritsch EF, et al. Systematic identification of personal tumor-specific neoantigens in chronic lymphocytic leukemia. *Blood*. 2014;124(3):453-462.
59. Lu Y, Zheng Z, Robbins P, et al. An efficient single-cell RNA-seq approach to identify neoantigen-specific T cell receptors. *Mol Ther*. 2018;26(2):379-389.
60. Shankaran V, Ikeda H, Bruce AT, et al. IFNgamma and lymphocytes prevent primary tumour development and shape tumour immunogenicity. *Nature*. 2001;410(6832):1107-1111.
61. Dunn GP, Old LJ, Schreiber RD. The immunobiology of cancer immunosurveillance and immunoediting. *Immunity*. 2004;21(2):137-148.
62. Mittal D, Gubin MM, Schreiber RD, Smyth MJ. New insights into cancer immunoediting and its three component phases—elimination, equilibrium and escape. *Curr Opin Immunol*. 2014;27:16-25.
63. Grivennikov SI, Greten FR, Karin M. Immunity, inflammation, and cancer. *Cell*. 2010;140(6):883-899.
64. Adams GP, Weiner LM. Monoclonal antibody therapy of cancer. *Nat Biotechnol*. 2005;23(9):1147-1157.
65. Finn OJ. Cancer immunology. *N Engl J Med*. 2008;358(25):2704-2715.
66. Domagala A, Kurpisz M. CD52 antigen—a review. *Med Sci Monit*. 2001;7(2):325-331.
67. Tedder TF, Engel P. CD20: a regulator of cell-cycle progression of B lymphocytes. *Immunol Today*. 1994;15(9):450-454.
68. Tedder TF, Tuscano J, Sato S, Kehrl JH. CD22, a B lymphocyte-specific adhesion molecule that regulates antigen receptor signaling. *Annu Rev Immunol*. 1997;15:481-504.
69. Miller RA, Levy R. Response of cutaneous T cell lymphoma to therapy with hybridoma monoclonal antibody. *Lancet*. 1981;2(8240):226-230.
70. Nadler LM, Stashenko P, Hardy R, et al. Serotherapy of a patient with a monoclonal antibody directed against a human lymphoma-associated antigen. *Cancer Res*. 1980;40(9):3147-3154.
71. Glennie MJ, Johnson PW. Clinical trials of antibody therapy. *Immunol Today*. 2000;21(8):403-410.
72. Longo DL. Immunotherapy for non-Hodgkin's lymphoma. *Curr Opin Oncol*. 1996;8(5):353-359.
73. Riley JK, Sliwkowski MX. CD20: a gene in search of a function. *Semin Oncol*. 2000;27(6 suppl 12):17-24.
74. Grillo-Lopez AJ. Rituximab: an insider's historical perspective. *Semin Oncol*. 2000;27(6 suppl 12):9-16.
75. Grillo-Lopez AJ, White CA, Varns C, et al. Overview of the clinical development of rituximab: first monoclonal antibody approved for the treatment of lymphoma. *Semin Oncol*. 1999;26(5 suppl 14):66-73.
76. McLaughlin P, Grillo-Lopez AJ, Link BK, et al. Rituximab chimeric anti-CD20 monoclonal antibody therapy for relapsed indolent lymphoma: half of patients respond to a four-dose treatment program. *J Clin Oncol*. 1998;16(8):2825-2833.
77. Salles G, Barret M, Foà R, et al. Rituximab in B-cell hematologic malignancies: a review of 20 years of clinical experience. *Adv Ther*. 2017;34(2):2232-2273.
78. Vose JM, Link BK, Grossbard ML, et al. Phase II study of rituximab in combination with chop chemotherapy in patients with previously untreated, aggressive non-Hodgkin's lymphoma. *J Clin Oncol*. 2001;19(2):389-397.
79. Coiffier B, Thieblemont C, Van Den Neste E, et al. Long-term outcome of patients in the LNH-98.5 trial, the first randomized study comparing rituximab-CHOP to standard CHOP chemotherapy in DLBCL patients: a study by the Groupe d'Etudes des Lymphomes de l'Adulte. *Blood*. 2010;116(12):2040-2045.
80. Coiffier B, Lepage E, Briere J, et al. CHOP chemotherapy plus rituximab compared with CHOP alone in elderly patients with diffuse large-B-cell lymphoma. *N Engl J Med*. 2002;346(4):235-242.
81. Ghielmini M, Schmitz SF, Cogliatti SB, et al. Prolonged treatment with rituximab in patients with follicular lymphoma significantly increases event-free survival and response duration compared with the standard weekly × 4 schedule. *Blood*. 2004;103(12):4416-4423.
82. Hochster H, Weller E, Gascoyne RD, et al. Maintenance rituximab after cyclophosphamide, vincristine, and prednisone prolongs progression-free survival in advanced indolent lymphoma: results of the randomized phase III ECOG1496 Study. *J Clin Oncol*. 2009;27(10):1607-1614.
83. Van Oers MH, Hagenbeek A, Van Glabbeke M, Teodorovic I. Chimeric anti-CD20 monoclonal antibody (Mabthera) in remission induction and maintenance treatment of relapsed follicular non-Hodgkin's lymphoma: a phase III randomized clinical trial—Intergroup Collaborative Study. *Ann Hematol*. 2002;81(10):553-557.
84. Sohn BS, Kim SM, Yoon DH, et al. The comparison between CHOP and R-CHOP in primary gastric diffuse large B cell lymphoma. *Ann Hematol*. 2012;91(11):1731-1739.
85. Kluin-Nelemans HC, Hoster E, Hermine O, et al. Treatment of older patients with mantle-cell lymphoma. *N Engl J Med*. 2012;367(6):520-531.
86. Weng WK, Levy R. Expression of complement inhibitors CD46, CD55, and CD59 on tumor cells does not predict clinical outcome after rituximab treatment in follicular non-Hodgkin lymphoma. *Blood*. 2001;98(5):1352-1357.
87. Reff ME, Carner K, Chambers KS, et al. Depletion of B cells in vivo by a chimeric mouse human monoclonal antibody to CD20. *Blood*. 1994;83(2):435-445.
88. Clynes RA, Towers TL, Presta LG, Ravetch JV. Inhibitory Fc receptors modulate in vivo cytotoxicity against tumor targets. *Nat Med*. 2000;6(4):443-446.
89. Stavenhagen JB, Gorlatov S, Tuaillon N, et al. Fc optimization of therapeutic antibodies enhances their ability to kill tumor cells in vitro and controls tumor expansion in vivo via low-affinity activating Fcγ receptors. *Cancer Res*. 2007;67(18):8882-8890.
90. Cartron G, Dacheux L, Salles G, et al. Therapeutic activity of humanized anti-CD20 monoclonal antibody and polymorphism in IgG Fc receptor FcγRIIIa gene. *Blood*. 2002;99(3):754-758.
91. Wilson WH. Chemotherapy sensitization by rituximab: experimental and clinical evidence. *Semin Oncol*. 2000;27(6 suppl 12):30-36.
92. Shan D, Ledbetter JA, Press OW. Apoptosis of malignant human B cells by ligation of CD20 with monoclonal antibodies. *Blood*. 1998;91(5):1644-1652.
93. Mathas S, Rickers A, Bommert K, Dorken B, Mapara MY. Anti-CD20- and B-cell receptor-mediated apoptosis: evidence for shared intracellular signaling pathways. *Cancer Res*. 2000;60(24):7170-7176.
94. Alas S, Bonavida B. Rituximab inactivates signal transducer and activation of transcription 3 (STAT3) activity in B-non-Hodgkin's lymphoma through inhibition of the interleukin 10 autocrine/paracrine loop and results in down-regulation of Bcl-2 and sensitization to cytotoxic drugs. *Cancer Res*. 2001;61(13):5137-5144.
95. Alas S, Emmanouilides C, Bonavida B. Inhibition of interleukin 10 by rituximab results in down-regulation of bcl-2 and sensitization of B-cell non-Hodgkin's lymphoma to apoptosis. *Clin Cancer Res*. 2001;7(3):709-723.
96. Alas S, Bonavida B, Emmanouilides C. Potentiation of fludarabine cytotoxicity on non-Hodgkin's lymphoma by pentoxifylline and rituximab. *Anticancer Res*. 2000;20(5a):2961-2966.
97. Afif W, Loftus EV Jr, Faubion WA, et al. Clinical utility of measuring infliximab and human anti-chimeric antibody concentrations in patients with inflammatory bowel disease. *Am J Gastroenterol*. 2010;105(5):1133-1139.
98. Miele E, Markowitz JE, Mamula P, Baldassano RN. Human antichimeric antibody in children and young adults with inflammatory bowel disease receiving infliximab. *J Pediatr Gastroenterol Nutr*. 2004;38(5):502-508.
99. Keating MJ, Dritselis A, Yasothan U, Kirkpatrick P. Ofatumumab. *Nat Rev Drug Discov*. 2010;9(2):101-102.
100. Byrd JC, Waselenko JK, Maneatis TJ, et al. Rituximab therapy in hematologic malignancy patients with circulating blood tumor cells: association with increased infusion-related side effects and rapid blood tumor clearance. *J Clin Oncol*. 1999;17(3):791-795.
101. Kunkel L, Wong A, Maneatis T, et al. Optimizing the use of rituximab for treatment of B-cell non-Hodgkin's lymphoma: a benefit-risk update. *Semin Oncol*. 2000;27(6 suppl 12):53-61.
102. Gea-Banacloche JC. Rituximab-associated infections. *Semin Hematol*. 2010;47(2):187-198.
103. Press OW, Leonard JP, Coiffier B, Levy R, Timmerman J. Immunotherapy of non-Hodgkin's lymphomas. *Hematol Am Soc Hematol Educ Program*. 2001;2001:221-240.
104. Keating MJ, Flinn I, Jain V, et al. Therapeutic role of alemtuzumab (Campath-1H) in patients who have failed fludarabine: results of a large international study. *Blood*. 2002;99(10):3554-3561.
105. Dearden CE, Matutes E, Cazin B, et al. High remission rate in T-cell prolymphocytic leukemia with CAMPATH-1H. *Blood*. 2001;98(6):1721-1726.
106. Damlaj M, Sulai NH, Oliveira JL, et al. Impact of alemtuzumab therapy and route of administration in T-prolymphocytic leukemia: a single-center experience. *Clin Lymphoma Myeloma Leuk*. 2015;15(11):699-704.
107. Kennedy-Nasser AA, Bollard CM, Myers GD, et al. Comparable outcome of alternative donor and matched sibling donor hematopoietic stem cell transplant for children with acute lymphoblastic leukemia in first or second remission using alemtuzumab in a myeloablative conditioning regimen. *Biol Blood Marrow Transplant*. 2008;14(11):1245-1252.
108. Wing MG, Moreau T, Greenwood J, et al. Mechanism of first-dose cytokine-release syndrome by CAMPATH 1-H: involvement of CD16 (FcγRIII) and CD11a/CD18 (LFA-1) on NK cells. *J Clin Invest*. 1996;98(12):2819-2826.
109. O'Brien SM, Keating MJ, Mocarski ES. Updated guidelines on the management of cytomegalovirus reactivation in patients with chronic lymphocytic leukemia treated with alemtuzumab. *Clin Lymphoma Myeloma*. 2006;7(2):125-130.
110. Robak T. Alemtuzumab in the treatment of chronic lymphocytic leukemia. *BioDrugs*. 2005;19(1):9-22.
111. Edelmann J, Gribben JG. Obinutuzumab for the treatment of indolent lymphoma. *Future Oncol*. 2016;12(15):1769-1781.
112. Gagez AL, Cartron G. Obinutuzumab: a new class of anti-CD20 monoclonal antibody. *Curr Opin Oncol*. 2014;26(5):484-491.
113. Illidge T, Klein C, Sehn LH, Davies A, Salles G, Cartron G. Obinutuzumab in hematologic malignancies: lessons learned to date. *Cancer Treat Rev*. 2015;41(9):784-792.
114. Goede V, Fischer K, Busch R, et al. Obinutuzumab plus chlorambucil in patients with CLL and coexisting conditions. *N Engl J Med*. 2014;370(12):1101-1110.
115. Cheney CM, Stephens DM, Mo X, et al. Ocaratuzumab, an Fc-engineered antibody demonstrates enhanced antibody-dependent cell-mediated cytotoxicity in chronic lymphocytic leukemia. *MAbs*. 2014;6(3):749-755.
116. Casulo C, Vose JM, Ho WY, et al. A phase I study of PRO131921, a novel anti-CD20 monoclonal antibody in patients with relapsed/refractory CD20+ indolent NHL: correlation between clinical responses and AUC pharmacokinetics. *Clin Immunol*. 2014;154(1):37-46.
117. Robak T, Robak E. New anti-CD20 monoclonal antibodies for the treatment of B-cell lymphoid malignancies. *BioDrugs*. 2011;25(1):13-25.
118. Leonard JP, Link BK. Immunotherapy of non-Hodgkin's lymphoma with hLL2 (epratuzumab, an anti-CD22 monoclonal antibody) and Hu1D10 (apolizumab). *Semin Oncol*. 2002;29(1 suppl 2):81-86.
119. Grant BW, Jung SH, Johnson JL, et al. A phase 2 trial of extended induction epratuzumab and rituximab for previously untreated follicular lymphoma: CALGB 50701. *Cancer*. 2013;119(21):3797-3804.

120. Micallef IN, Maurer MJ, Wiseman GA, et al. Epratuzumab with rituximab, cyclophosphamide, doxorubicin, vincristine, and prednisone chemotherapy in patients with previously untreated diffuse large B-cell lymphoma. *Blood.* 2011;118(15):4053-4061.
121. Stein R, Mattes MJ, Cardillo TM, et al. CD74: a new candidate target for the immunotherapy of B-cell neoplasms. *Clin Cancer Res.* 2007;13(18 pt 2):5556s-5563s.
122. Kaufman JL, Niesvizky R, Stadtmauer EA, et al. Phase I, multicentre, dose-escalation trial of monotherapy with milatuzumab (humanized anti-CD74 monoclonal antibody) in relapsed or refractory multiple myeloma. *Br J Haematol.* 2013;163(4):478-486.
123. Christian BA, Poi M, Jones JA, et al. The combination of milatuzumab, a humanized anti-CD74 antibody, and veltuzumab, a humanized anti-CD20 antibody, demonstrates activity in patients with relapsed and refractory B-cell non-Hodgkin lymphoma. *Br J Haematol.* 2015;169(5):701-710.
124. Ishida T, Joh T, Uike N, et al. Defucosylated anti-CCR4 monoclonal antibody (KW-0761) for relapsed adult T-cell leukemia-lymphoma: a multicenter phase II study. *J Clin Oncol.* 2012;30(8):837-842.
125. Duvic M, Pinter-Brown LC, Foss FM, et al. Phase 1/2 study of mogamulizumab, a defucosylated anti-CCR4 antibody, in previously treated patients with cutaneous T-cell lymphoma. *Blood.* 2015;125(12):1883-1889.
126. Kim YH, Bagot M, Pinter-Brown L. Anti-CCR4 monoclonal antibody, mogamulizumab, demonstrates significant improvement in PFS compared to vorinostat in patients with previously treated cutaneous T-cell lymphoma (CTCL): results from the phase III MAVORIC study [abstract]. *Blood.* 2017;130:817.
127. van Rhee F, Szmania SM, Dillon M, et al. Combinatorial efficacy of anti-CS1 monoclonal antibody elotuzumab (HuLuc63) and bortezomib against multiple myeloma. *Mol Cancer Ther.* 2009;8(9):2616-2624.
128. Lonial S, Dimopoulos M, Palumbo A, et al. Elotuzumab therapy for relapsed or refractory multiple myeloma. *N Engl J Med.* 2015;373(7):621-631.
129. Lonial S, Kaufman J, Reece D, Mateos MV, Laubach J, Richardson P. Update on elotuzumab, a novel anti-SLAMF7 monoclonal antibody for the treatment of multiple myeloma. *Expert Opin Biol Ther.* 2016;16(10):1291-1301.
130. Palumbo A, Chanan-Khan A, Weisel K, et al. Daratumumab, bortezomib, and dexamethasone for multiple myeloma. *N Engl J Med.* 2016;375(8):754-766.
131. Perincheri S, Torres R, Tormey CA, Smith BR, Rinder HM, Siddon AJ. Daratumumab interferes with flow cytometric evaluation of multiple myeloma. *Blood.* 2016;128(22):5630.
132. Lynch RG, Graff RJ, Sirisinha S, Simms ES, Eisen HN. Myeloma proteins as tumor-specific transplantation antigens. *Proc Natl Acad Sci U S A.* 1972;69(6):1540-1544.
133. Meeker T, Lowder J, Cleary ML, et al. Emergence of idiotype variants during treatment of B-cell lymphoma with anti-idiotype antibodies. *N Engl J Med.* 1985;312(26):1658-1665.
134. Levy S, Mendel E, Kon S, Avnur Z, Levy R. Mutational hot spots in Ig V region genes of human follicular lymphomas. *J Exp Med.* 1988;168(2):475-489.
135. Press OW, Rasey J. Principles of radioimmunotherapy for hematologists and oncologists. *Semin Oncol.* 2000;27(6 suppl 12):62-73.
136. Stevens PL, Oluwole O, Reddy N. Advances and application of radioimmunotherapy in non-Hodgkin lymphoma. *Am J Blood Res.* 2012;2(2):86-97.
137. Illidge T, Morschhauser F. Radioimmunotherapy in follicular lymphoma. *Best Pract Res Clin Haematol.* 2011;24(2):279-293.
138. Witzig TE, Gordon LI, Cabanillas F, et al. Randomized controlled trial of yttrium-90-labeled ibritumomab tiuxetan radioimmunotherapy versus rituximab immunotherapy for patients with relapsed or refractory low-grade, follicular, or transformed B-cell non-Hodgkin's lymphoma. *J Clin Oncol.* 2002;20(10):2453-2463.
139. Witzig TE, Flinn IW, Gordon LI, et al. Treatment with ibritumomab tiuxetan radioimmunotherapy in patients with rituximab-refractory follicular non-Hodgkin's lymphoma. *J Clin Oncol.* 2002;20(15):3262-3269.
140. Kaminski MS, Zelenetz AD, Press OW, et al. Pivotal study of iodine I 131 tositumomab for chemotherapy-refractory low-grade or transformed low-grade B-cell non-Hodgkin's lymphomas. *J Clin Oncol.* 2001;19(19):3918-3928.
141. Horning SJ, Younes A, Jain V, et al. Efficacy and safety of tositumomab and iodine-131 tositumomab (Bexxar) in B-cell lymphoma, progressive after rituximab. *J Clin Oncol.* 2005;23(4):712-719.
142. Dosik AD, Coleman M, Kostakoglu L, et al. Subsequent therapy can be administered after tositumomab and iodine I-131 tositumomab for non-Hodgkin lymphoma. *Cancer.* 2006;106(3):616-622.
143. Kaminski MS, Radford JA, Gregory SA, et al. Re-treatment with I-131 tositumomab in patients with non-Hodgkin's lymphoma who had previously responded to I-131 tositumomab. *J Clin Oncol.* 2005;23(31):7985-7993.
144. Gopal AK, Rajendran JG, Gooley TA, et al. High-dose [131I]tositumomab (anti-CD20) radioimmunotherapy and autologous hematopoietic stem-cell transplantation for adults > or = 60 years old with relapsed or refractory B-cell lymphoma. *J Clin Oncol.* 2007;25(11):1396-1402.
145. Press OW, Eary JF, Appelbaum FR, et al. Phase II trial of 131I-B1 (anti-CD20) antibody therapy with autologous stem cell transplantation for relapsed B cell lymphomas. *Lancet.* 1995;346(8971):336-340.
146. Press OW, Eary JF, Gooley T, et al. A phase I/II trial of iodine-131-tositumomab (anti-CD20), etoposide, cyclophosphamide, and autologous stem cell transplantation for relapsed B-cell lymphomas. *Blood.* 2000;96(9):2934-2942.
147. Nademanee A, Forman S, Molina A, et al. A phase 1/2 study of high-dose yttrium-90-ibritumomab tiuxetan in combination with high-dose etoposide and cyclophosphamide followed by autologous stem cell transplantation in patients with poor-risk or relapsed non-Hodgkin lymphoma. *Blood.* 2005;106(8):2896-2902.
148. Alcindor T, Witzig TE. Radioimmunotherapy with yttrium-90 ibritumomab tiuxetan for patients with relapsed CD20+ B-cell non-Hodgkin's lymphoma. *Curr Treat Options Oncol.* 2002;3(4):275-282.
149. Gopal AK, Pagel JM, Rajendran JG, et al. Improving the efficacy of reduced intensity allogeneic transplantation for lymphoma using radioimmunotherapy. *Biol Blood Marrow Transplant.* 2006;12(7):697-702.
150. Bethge WA, Wilbur DS, Sandmaier BM. Radioimmunotherapy as non-myeloablative conditioning for allogeneic marrow transplantation. *Leuk Lymphoma.* 2006;47(7):1205-1214.
151. Fietz T, Uharek L, Gentilini C, et al. Allogeneic hematopoietic cell transplantation following conditioning with 90Y-ibritumomab-tiuxetan. *Leuk Lymphoma.* 2006;47(1):59-63.
152. Bouabdallah K, Furst S, Asselineau J, et al. 90Y-ibritumomab tiuxetan, fludarabine, busulfan and antithymocyte globulin reduced-intensity allogeneic transplant conditioning for patients with advanced and high-risk B-cell lymphomas. *Ann Oncol.* 2015;26(1):193-198.
153. Lin Y, Pagel JM, Axworthy D, Pantelias A, Hedin N, Press OW. A genetically engineered anti-CD45 single-chain antibody-streptavidin fusion protein for pretargeted radioimmunotherapy of hematologic malignancies. *Cancer Res.* 2006;66(7):3884-3892.
154. Pagel JM, Matthews DC, Kenoyer A, et al. Pretargeted radioimmunotherapy using anti-CD45 monoclonal antibodies to deliver radiation to murine hematolymphoid tissues and human myeloid leukemia. *Cancer Res.* 2009;69(1):185-192.
155. Cabrero M, Martin G, Briones J, et al. Phase II study of Yttrium-90-Ibritumomab Tiuxetan as part of reduced-intensity conditioning (with Melphalan, Fludarabine +/− Thiotepa) for allogeneic transplantation in relapsed or refractory aggressive B cell lymphoma: a GELTAMO trial. *Biol Blood Marrow Transplant.* 2017;23(1):53-59.
156. Ghetie MA, Vitetta ES. Recent developments in immunotoxin therapy. *Curr Opin Immunol.* 1994;6(5):707-714.
157. Kreitman RJ. Immunotoxins in cancer therapy. *Curr Opin Immunol.* 1999;11(5):570-578.
158. Zein N, Poncin M, Nilakantan R, Ellestad GA. Calicheamicin gamma 1I and DNA: molecular recognition process responsible for site-specificity. *Science.* 1989;244(4905):697-699.
159. Sievers EL, Larson RA, Stadtmauer EA, et al. Efficacy and safety of gemtuzumab ozogamicin in patients with CD33-positive acute myeloid leukemia in first relapse. *J Clin Oncol.* 2001;19(13):3244-3254.
160. Vallera DA. Immunotoxins: will their clinical promise be fulfilled? *Blood.* 1994;83(2):309-317.
161. May RD, Finkelman FD, Wheeler HT, Uhr JW, Vitetta ES. Evaluation of ricin A chain-containing immunotoxins directed against different epitopes on the delta-chain of cell surface-associated IgD on murine B cells. *J Immunol.* 1990;144(9):3637-3642.
162. Olsnes S, Sandvig K, Petersen OW, van Deurs B. Immunotoxins--entry into cells and mechanisms of action. *Immunol Today.* 1989;10(9):291-295.
163. Lambert JM, McIntyre G, Gauthier MN, et al. The galactose-binding sites of the cytotoxic lectin ricin can be chemically blocked in high yield with reactive ligands prepared by chemical modification of glycopeptides containing triantennary N-linked oligosaccharides. *Biochemistry.* 1991;30(13):3234-3247.
164. Casellas P, Bourrie BJ, Gros P, Jansen FK. Kinetics of cytotoxicity induced by immunotoxins. Enhancement by lysosomotropic amines and carboxylic ionophores. *J Biol Chem.* 1984;259(15):9359-9364.
165. Ramakrishnan S, Houston LL. Inhibition of human acute lymphoblastic leukemia cells by immunotoxins: potentiation by chloroquine. *Science.* 1984;223(4631):58-61.
166. Pappenheimer AM Jr. Diphtheria toxin. *Ann Rev Biochem.* 1977;46:69-94.
167. Endo Y, Mitsui K, Motizuki M, Tsurugi K. The mechanism of action of ricin and related toxic lectins on eukaryotic ribosomes. The site and the characteristics of the modification in 28 S ribosomal RNA caused by the toxins. *J Biol Chem.* 1987;262(12):5908-5912.
168. Grossbard ML, Fidias P. Prospects for immunotoxin therapy of non-Hodgkin's lymphoma. *Clin Immunol Immunopathol.* 1995;76(2):107-114.
169. Multani PS, O'Day S, Nadler LM, Grossbard ML. Phase II clinical trial of bolus infusion anti-B4 blocked ricin immunoconjugate in patients with relapsed B-cell non-Hodgkin's lymphoma. *Clin Cancer Res.* 1998;4(11):2599-2604.
170. Kreitman RJ, Stetler-Stevenson M, Margulies I, et al. Phase II trial of recombinant immunotoxin RFB4(dsFv)-PE38 (BL22) in patients with hairy cell leukemia. *J Clin Oncol.* 2009;27(18):2983-2990.
171. Kreitman RJ, Wilson WH, Bergeron K, et al. Efficacy of the anti-CD22 recombinant immunotoxin BL22 in chemotherapy-resistant hairy-cell leukemia. *N Engl J Med.* 2001;345(4):241-247.
172. Wayne AS, Kreitman RJ, Findley HW, et al. Anti-CD22 immunotoxin RFB4(dsFv)-PE38 (BL22) for CD22-positive hematologic malignancies of childhood: preclinical studies and phase I clinical trial. *Clin Cancer Res.* 2010;16(6):1894-1903.
173. Soler-Rodriguez AM, Ghetie MA, Oppenheimer-Marks N, Uhr JW, Vitetta ES. Ricin A-chain and ricin A-chain immunotoxins rapidly damage human endothelial cells: implications for vascular leak syndrome. *Exp Cell Res.* 1993;206(2):227-234.
174. Senderowicz AM, Vitetta E, Headlee D, et al. Complete sustained response of a refractory, post-transplantation, large B-cell lymphoma to an anti-CD22 immunotoxin. *Ann Intern Med.* 1997;126(11):882-885.
175. Kinjyo I, Matlawska-Wasowska K, Chen X, et al. Characterization of the anti-CD22 targeted therapy, moxetumomab pasudotox, for B-cell precursor acute lymphoblastic leukemia. *Pediatr Blood Cancer.* 2017;64(11):e26604.
176. Short NJ, Kantarjian H, Jabbour E, et al. A phase I study of moxetumomab pasudotox in adults with relapsed or refractory B-cell acute lymphoblastic leukaemia. *Br J Haematol.* 2018;182(3):442-444.
177. Wayne AS, Shah NN, Bhojwani D, et al. Phase 1 study of the anti-CD22 immunotoxin moxetumomab pasudotox for childhood acute lymphoblastic leukemia. *Blood.* 2017;130(14):1620-1627.

178. Hamann PR, Hinman LM, Hollander I, et al. Gemtuzumab ozogamicin, a potent and selective anti-CD33 antibody-calicheamicin conjugate for treatment of acute myeloid leukemia. *Bioconjug Chem*. 2002;13(1):47-58.
179. Sievers EL, Appelbaum FR, Spielberger RT, et al. Selective ablation of acute myeloid leukemia using antibody-targeted chemotherapy: a phase I study of an anti-CD33 calicheamicin immunoconjugate. *Blood*. 1999;93(11):3678-3684.
180. Castaigne S, Pautas C, Terre C, et al. Effect of gemtuzumab ozogamicin on survival of adult patients with de-novo acute myeloid leukaemia (ALFA-0701): a randomised, open-label, phase 3 study. *Lancet*. 2012;379(9825):1508-1516.
181. Amadori S, Suciu S, Selleslag D, et al. Gemtuzumab ozogamicin versus best supportive care in older patients with newly diagnosed acute myeloid leukemia unsuitable for intensive chemotherapy: results of the randomized phase III EORTC-GIMEMA AML-19 trial. *J Clin Oncol*. 2016;34(9):972-979.
182. Ricart AD. Antibody-drug conjugates of calicheamicin derivative: gemtuzumab ozogamicin and inotuzumab ozogamicin. *Clin Cancer Res*. 2011;17(20):6417-6427.
183. Kantarjian HM, DeAngelo DJ, Stelljes M, et al. Inotuzumab ozogamicin versus standard therapy for acute lymphoblastic leukemia. *N Engl J Med*. 2016;375(8):740-753.
184. Shor B, Gerber HP, Sapra P. Preclinical and clinical development of inotuzumab-ozogamicin in hematological malignancies. *Mol Immunol*. 2015;67(2 pt A):107-116.
185. Kreitman RJ, Pastan I. Recombinant single-chain immunotoxins against T and B cell leukemias. *Leuk Lymphoma*. 1994;13(1-2):1-10.
186. Apisarnthanarax N, Talpur R, Duvic M. Treatment of cutaneous T cell lymphoma: current status and future directions. *Am J Clin Dermatol*. 2002;3(3):193-215.
187. Olsen E, Duvic M, Frankel A, et al. Pivotal phase III trial of two dose levels of denileukin diftitox for the treatment of cutaneous T-cell lymphoma. *J Clin Oncol*. 2001;19(2):376-388.
188. Frankel AE, Woo JH, Ahn C, et al. Resimmune, an anti-CD3epsilon recombinant immunotoxin, induces durable remissions in patients with cutaneous T-cell lymphoma. *Haematologica*. 2015;100(6):794-800.
189. Gualberto A. Brentuximab Vedotin (SGN-35), an antibody-drug conjugate for the treatment of CD30-positive malignancies. *Expert Opin Investig Drugs*. 2012;21(2):205-216.
190. Younes A, Gopal AK, Smith SE, et al. Results of a pivotal phase II study of brentuximab vedotin for patients with relapsed or refractory Hodgkin's lymphoma. *J Clin Oncol*. 2012;30(18):2183-2189.
191. Fanale MA, Forero-Torres A, Rosenblatt JD, et al. A phase I weekly dosing study of brentuximab vedotin in patients with relapsed/refractory CD30-positive hematologic malignancies. *Clin Cancer Res*. 2012;18(1):248-255.
192. Moskowitz CH, Nademanee A, Masszi T, et al. Brentuximab vedotin as consolidation therapy after autologous stem-cell transplantation in patients with Hodgkin's lymphoma at risk of relapse or progression (AETHERA): a randomised, double-blind, placebo-controlled, phase 3 trial. *Lancet*. 2015;385(9980):1853-1862.
193. Prince HM, Kim YH, Horwitz SM, et al. Brentuximab vedotin or physician's choice in CD30-positive cutaneous T-cell lymphoma (ALCANZA): an international, open-label, randomised, phase 3, multicentre trial. *Lancet*. 2017;390(10094):555-566.
194. Renner C, Pfreundschuh M. Tumor therapy by immune recruitment with bispecific antibodies. *Immunol Rev*. 1995;145:179-209.
195. van Spriel AB, van Ojik HH, van De Winkel JG. Immunotherapeutic perspective for bispecific antibodies. *Immunol Today*. 2000;21(8):391-397.
196. Weiner GJ, Hillstrom JR. Bispecific anti-idiotype/anti-CD3 antibody therapy of murine B cell lymphoma. *J Immunol*. 1991;147(11):4035-4044.
197. Loffler A, Kufer P, Lutterbuse R, et al. A recombinant bispecific single-chain antibody, CD19 × CD3, induces rapid and high lymphoma-directed cytotoxicity by unstimulated T lymphocytes. *Blood*. 2000;95(6):2098-2103.
198. Bargou R, Leo E, Zugmaier G, et al. Tumor regression in cancer patients by very low doses of a T cell-engaging antibody. *Science*. 2008;321(5891):974-977.
199. Topp MS, Gokbuget N, Zugmaier G, et al. Long-term follow-up of hematologic relapse-free survival in a phase 2 study of blinatumomab in patients with MRD in B-lineage ALL. *Blood*. 2012;120(26):5185-5187.
200. Hartmann F, Renner C, Jung W, et al. Treatment of refractory Hodgkin's disease with an anti-CD16/CD30 bispecific antibody. *Blood*. 1997;89(6):2042-2047.
201. Koon HB, Junghans RP. Anti-CD30 antibody-based therapy. *Curr Opin Oncol*. 2000;12(6):588-593.
202. Hartmann F, Renner C, Jung W, et al. Anti-CD16/CD30 bispecific antibody treatment for Hodgkin's disease: role of infusion schedule and costimulation with cytokines. *Clin Cancer Res*. 2001;7(7):1873-1881.
203. Booy EP, Johar D, Maddika S, et al. Monoclonal and bispecific antibodies as novel therapeutics. *Arch Immunol Ther Exp*. 2006;54(2):85-101.
204. Pishvaian M, Morse MA, McDevitt J, et al. Phase 1 dose escalation study of MEDI-565, a bispecific T-cell engager that targets human carcinoembryonic antigen, in patients with advanced gastrointestinal adenocarcinomas. *Clin Colorectal Cancer*. 2016;15(4):345-351.
205. Gall JM, Davol PA, Grabert RC, Deaver M, Lum LG. T cells armed with anti-CD3 × anti-CD20 bispecific antibody enhance killing of CD20+ malignant B cells and bypass complement-mediated rituximab resistance in vitro. *Exp Hematol*. 2005;33(4):452-459.
206. Morecki S, Lindhofer H, Yacovlev E, Gelfand Y, Slavin S. Use of trifunctional bispecific antibodies to prevent graft versus host disease induced by allogeneic lymphocytes. *Blood*. 2006;107(4):1564-1569.
207. Gupta P, Goldenberg DM, Rossi EA, et al. Dual-targeting immunotherapy of lymphoma: potent cytotoxicity of anti-CD20/CD74 bispecific antibodies in mantle cell and other lymphomas. *Blood*. 2012;119(16):3767-3778.
208. Stanglmaier M, Faltin M, Ruf P, Bodenhausen A, Schroder P, Lindhofer H. Bi20 (fBTA05), a novel trifunctional bispecific antibody (anti-CD20 × anti-CD3), mediates efficient killing of B-cell lymphoma cells even with very low CD20 expression levels. *Int J Cancer*. 2008;123(5):1181-1189.
209. Boehrer S, Schroeder P, Mueller T, Atz J, Chow KU. Cytotoxic effects of the trifunctional bispecific antibody FBTA05 in ex-vivo cells of chronic lymphocytic leukaemia depend on immune-mediated mechanism. *Anti Cancer Drugs*. 2011;22(6):519-530.
210. Schuster FR, Stanglmaier M, Woessmann W, et al. Immunotherapy with the trifunctional anti-CD20 × anti-CD3 antibody FBTA05 (Lymphomun) in paediatric high-risk patients with recurrent CD20-positive B cell malignancies. *Br J Haematol*. 2015;169(1):90-102.
211. Gresser I, Berman L, De The G, Brouty-Boye D, Coppey J, Falcoff E. Interferon and murine leukemia. V. Effect of interferon preparations on the evolution of Rauscher disease in mice. *J Natl Cancer Inst*. 1968;41(2):505-522.
212. Gresser I, Bourali C. Exogenous interferon and inducers of interferon in the treatment Balb-c mice inoculated with RC19 tumour cells. *Nature*. 1969;223(5208):844-845.
213. Darnell JE Jr, Kerr IM, Stark GR. Jak-STAT pathways and transcriptional activation in response to IFNs and other extracellular signaling proteins. *Science*. 1994;264(5164):1415-1421.
214. Sen GC, Lengyel P. The interferon system. A bird's eye view of its biochemistry. *J Biol Chem*. 1992;267(8):5017-5020.
215. Talpaz M, Kantarjian HM, McCredie K, Trujillo JM, Keating MJ, Gutterman JU. Hematologic remission and cytogenetic improvement induced by recombinant human interferon alpha A in chronic myelogenous leukemia. *N Engl J Med*. 1986;314(17):1065-1069.
216. Talpaz M, Kantarjian HM, McCredie KB, Keating MJ, Trujillo J, Gutterman J. Clinical investigation of human alpha interferon in chronic myelogenous leukemia. *Blood*. 1987;69(5):1280-1288.
217. Italian Cooperative Study Group on Chronic Myeloid Leukemia; Tura S, Baccarani M, Zuffa E, et al. Interferon alfa-2a as compared with conventional chemotherapy for the treatment of chronic myeloid leukemia. *N Engl J Med*. 1994;330(12):820-825.
218. Appelbaum FR. Perspectives on the future of chronic myeloid leukemia treatment. *Semin Hematol*. 2001;38(3 suppl 8):35-42.
219. Freund M, von Wussow P, Diedrich H, et al. Recombinant human interferon (IFN) alpha-2b in chronic myelogenous leukaemia: dose dependency of response and frequency of neutralizing anti-interferon antibodies. *Br J Haematol*. 1989;72(3):350-356.
220. Kalidas M, Kantarjian H, Talpaz M. Chronic myelogenous leukemia. *J Am Med Assoc*. 2001;286(8):895-898.
221. Li MQ, Zhang M, Liao AJ, Liu ZG. Meta-analysis of imatinib mesylate with or without interferon for chronic-phase chronic myeloid leukemia. *Zhonghua Xue Ye Xue Za Zhi*. 2013;34(8):685-690.
222. Malagola M, Breccia M, Skert C, et al. Long term outcome of Ph+ CML patients achieving complete cytogenetic remission with interferon based therapy moving from interferon to imatinib era. *Am J Hematol*. 2014;89(2):119-124.
223. O'Brien SG, Guilhot F, Larson RA, et al. Imatinib compared with interferon and low-dose cytarabine for newly diagnosed chronic-phase chronic myeloid leukemia. *N Engl J Med*. 2003;348(11):994-1004.
224. Quesada JR, Reuben J, Manning JT, Hersh EM, Gutterman JU. Alpha interferon for induction of remission in hairy-cell leukemia. *N Engl J Med*. 1984;310(1):15-18.
225. Golomb HM, Jacobs A, Fefer A, et al. Alpha-2 interferon therapy of hairy-cell leukemia: a multicenter study of 64 patients. *J Clin Oncol*. 1986;4(6):900-905.
226. VanderMolen LA, Steis RG, Duffey PL, et al. Low- versus high-dose interferon alfa-2a in relapsed indolent non-Hodgkin's lymphoma. *J Natl Cancer Inst*. 1990;82(3):235-238.
227. Greipp PR, Witzig T. Biology and treatment of myeloma. *Curr Opin Oncol*. 1996;8(1):20-27.
228. Kirkwood J. Cancer immunotherapy: the interferon-alpha experience. *Semin Oncol*. 2002;29(3 suppl 7):18-26.
229. Salmon SE, Crowley JJ, Grogan TM, Finley P, Pugh RP, Barlogie B. Combination chemotherapy, glucocorticoids, and interferon alfa in the treatment of multiple myeloma: a Southwest Oncology Group study. *J Clin Oncol*. 1994;12(11):2405-2414.
230. Ludwig H, Cohen AM, Polliack A, et al. Interferon-alpha for induction and maintenance in multiple myeloma: results of two multicenter randomized trials and summary of other studies. *Ann Oncol*. 1995;6(5):467-476.
231. Cooper MR, Dear K, McIntyre OR, et al. A randomized clinical trial comparing melphalan/prednisone with or without interferon alfa-2b in newly diagnosed patients with multiple myeloma: a Cancer and Leukemia Group B study. *J Clin Oncol*. 1993;11(1):155-160.
232. Alexanian R, Dimopoulos MA. Management of multiple myeloma. *Semin Hematol*. 1995;32(1):20-30.
233. Tomiyama J, Kudo H, Nakamura N, et al. Clinical-study of multiple-myeloma in the elderly. *Oncol Rep*. 1995;2(4):669-673.
234. Watanabe N, Narita M, Yokoyama A, et al. Type I IFN-mediated enhancement of anti-leukemic cytotoxicity of gammadelta T cells expanded from peripheral blood cells by stimulation with zoledronate. *Cytotherapy*. 2006;8(2):118-129.
235. Safdar A, Rodriguez GH, Lichtiger B, et al. Recombinant interferon gamma1b immune enhancement in 20 patients with hematologic malignancies and systemic opportunistic infections treated with donor granulocyte transfusions. *Cancer*. 2006;106(12):2664-2671.
236. Kiladjian JJ, Cassinat B, Chevret S, et al. Pegylated interferon-alfa-2a induces complete hematologic and molecular responses with low toxicity in polycythemia vera. *Blood*. 2008;112(8):3065-3072.
237. Morgan DA, Ruscetti FW, Gallo R. Selective in vitro growth of T lymphocytes from normal human bone marrows. *Science*. 1976;193(4257):1007-1008.
238. Ruscetti FW, Morgan DA, Gallo RC. Functional and morphologic characterization of human T cells continuously grown in vitro. *J Immunol*. 1977;119:131-138.
239. Gillis S, Smith KA. Long term culture of tumour-specific cytotoxic T cells. *Nature*. 1977;268(5616):154-156.

240. Baker PE, Gillis S, Smith KA. Monoclonal cytolytic T-cell lines. *J Exp Med*. 1979;149(1):273-278.
241. Gillis S, Union NA, Baker PE, Smith KA. The in vitro generation and sustained culture of nude mouse cytolytic T-lymphocytes. *J Exp Med*. 1979;149(6):1460-1476.
242. Lotze MT, Grimm EA, Mazumder A, Strausser JL, Rosenberg SA. Lysis of fresh and cultured autologous tumor by human lymphocytes cultured in T-cell growth factor. *Cancer Res*. 1981;41(11 pt 1):4420-4425.
243. Taniguchi T, Matsui H, Fujita T, et al. Structure and expression of a cloned cDNA for human interleukin-2. *Biotechnology*. 1983;24:304-309.
244. Smith KA. The interleukin 2 receptor. *Ann Rev Cell Biol*. 1989;5:397-425.
245. Siegel JP, Puri RK. Interleukin-2 toxicity. *J Clin Oncol*. 1991;9(4):694-704.
246. Koreth J, Matsuoka K, Kim HT, et al. Interleukin-2 and regulatory T cells in graft-versus-host disease. *N Engl J Med*. 2011;365(22):2055-2066.
247. Matsuoka K, Koreth J, Kim HT, et al. Low-dose interleukin-2 therapy restores regulatory T cell homeostasis in patients with chronic graft-versus-host disease. *Sci Transl Med*. 2013;5(179):179ra143.
248. Fang J, Hu C, Hong M, et al. Prophylactic effects of interleukin-2 receptor antagonists against graft-versus-host disease following unrelated donor peripheral blood stem cell transplantation. *Biol Blood Marrow Transplant*. 2012;18(5):754-762.
249. Petrosiute A, Auletta JJ, Lazarus HM. Achieving graft-versus-tumor effect in brain tumor patients: from autologous progenitor cell transplant to active immunotherapy. *Immunotherapy*. 2012;4(11):1139-1151.
250. Gale RP, Champlin RE. How does bone-marrow transplantation cure leukaemia? *Lancet*. 1984;2(8393):28-30.
251. Odom LF, August CS, Githens JH, et al. Remission of relapsed leukaemia during a graft-versus-host reaction. A "graft-versus-leukaemia reaction" in man? *Lancet*. 1978;2(8089):537-540.
252. Barrett J, Malkovska V. The graft-versus-leukemia effect. *Curr Opin Oncol*. 1996;8(2):89-95.
253. Del Papa B, Ruggeri L, Urbani E, et al. Clinical-grade-expanded regulatory T cells prevent graft-versus-host disease while allowing a powerful T cell-dependent graft-versus-leukemia effect in murine models. *Biol Blood Marrow Transplant*. 2017;23(11):1847-1851.
254. Dickinson AM, Norden J, Li S, et al. Graft-versus-Leukemia effect following hematopoietic stem cell transplantation for leukemia. *Front Immunol*. 2017;8:496.
255. Kessels HW, Wolkers MC, Schumacher TN. Adoptive transfer of T-cell immunity. *Trends Immunol*. 2002;23(5):264-269.
256. Petrungaro A, Gentile M, Mazzone C, et al. Ponatinib-induced graft-versus-host disease/graft-versus-leukemia effect in a patient with Philadelphia-positive acute lymphoblastic leukemia without the T315I mutation relapsing after allogeneic transplant. *Chemotherapy*. 2017;62(6):353-356.
257. Boyiadzis M, Arora M, Klein JP, et al. Impact of chronic graft-versus-host disease on late relapse and survival on 7,489 patients after myeloablative allogeneic hematopoietic cell transplantation for leukemia. *Clin Cancer Res*. 2015;21(9):2020-2028.
258. Goodell V, Salazar LG, Urban N, et al. Antibody immunity to the p53 oncogenic protein is a prognostic indicator in ovarian cancer. *J Clin Oncol*. 2006;24(5):762-768.
259. Furugaki K, Pokorna K, Le Pogam C, et al. DNA vaccination with all-trans retinoic acid treatment induces long-term survival and elicits specific immune responses requiring CD4+ and CD8+ T-cell activation in an acute promyelocytic leukemia mouse model. *Blood*. 2010;115(3):653-656.
260. Qin Y, Tian H, Wang G, Lin C, Li Y. A BCR/ABL-hIL-2 DNA vaccine enhances the immune responses in BALB/c mice. *BioMed Res Int*. 2013;2013:136492.
261. Maraninchi D, Gluckman E, Blaise D, et al. Impact of T-cell depletion on outcome of allogeneic bone-marrow transplantation for standard-risk leukaemias. *Lancet*. 1987;2(8552):175-178.
262. Hallett WH, Murphy WJ. Natural killer cells: biology and clinical use in cancer therapy. *Cell Mol Immunol*. 2004;1(1):12-21.
263. Giralt S, Hester J, Huh Y, et al. CD8-depleted donor lymphocyte infusion as treatment for relapsed chronic myelogenous leukemia after allogeneic bone marrow transplantation. *Blood*. 1995;86(11):4337-4343.
264. Johnson BD, Truitt RL. Delayed infusion of immunocompetent donor cells after bone marrow transplantation breaks graft-host tolerance allows for persistent antileukemic reactivity without severe graft-versus-host disease. *Blood*. 1995;85(11):3302-3312.
265. Nimer SD, Giorgi J, Gajewski JL, et al. Selective depletion of CD8+ cells for prevention of graft-versus-host disease after bone marrow transplantation. A randomized controlled trial. *Transplantation*. 1994;57(1):82-87.
266. Altman JD, Moss PA, Goulder PJ, et al. Phenotypic analysis of antigen-specific T lymphocytes. *Science*. 1996;274(5284):94-96.
267. Mutis T, Gillespie G, Schrama E, Falkenburg JH, Moss P, Goulmy E. Tetrameric HLA class I-minor histocompatibility antigen peptide complexes demonstrate minor histocompatibility antigen-specific cytotoxic T lymphocytes in patients with graft-versus-host disease. *Nat Med*. 1999;5(7):839-842.
268. Morecki S, Slavin S. Toward amplification of a graft-versus-leukemia effect while minimizing graft-versus-host disease. *J Hematother Stem Cell Res*. 2000;9(3):355-366.
269. Tiberghien P, Reynolds CW, Keller J, et al. Ganciclovir treatment of herpes simplex thymidine kinase-transduced primary T lymphocytes: an approach for specific in vivo donor T-cell depletion after bone marrow transplantation? *Blood*. 1994;84(4):1333-1341.
270. Litvinova E, Maury S, Boyer O, et al. Graft-versus-leukemia effect after suicide-gene-mediated control of graft-versus-host disease. *Blood*. 2002;100(6):2020-2025.
271. Di Stasi AD, Tey S, Dotti G, et al. Inducible apoptosis as a safety switch for adoptive cell therapy. *N Engl J Med*. 2011;365(18):1673-1683.
272. Sykes M, Harty MW, Szot GL, Pearson DA. Interleukin-2 inhibits graft-versus-host disease-promoting activity of CD4+ cells while preserving CD4- and CD8-mediated graft-versus-leukemia effects. *Blood*. 1994;83(9):2560-2569.
273. Falkenburg JH, Faber LM, van den Elshout M, et al. Generation of donor-derived antileukemic cytotoxic T-lymphocyte responses for treatment of relapsed leukemia after allogeneic HLA-identical bone marrow transplantation. *J Immunother Emphasis Tumor Immunol*. 1993;14(4):305-309.
274. Kochenderfer JN, Dudley ME, Carpenter RO, et al. Donor-derived CD19-targeted T cells cause regression of malignancy persisting after allogeneic hematopoietic stem cell transplantation. *Blood*. 2013;122(25):4129-4139.
275. Shimoni A, Giralt S, Khouri I, Champlin R. Allogeneic hematopoietic transplantation for acute and chronic myeloid leukemia: non-myeloablative preparative regimens and induction of the graft-versus-leukemia effect. *Curr Oncol Rep*. 2000;2(2):132-139.
276. Burroughs L, Storb R. Low-intensity allogeneic hematopoietic stem cell transplantation for myeloid malignancies: separating graft-versus-leukemia effects from graft-versus-host disease. *Curr Opin Hematol*. 2005;12(1):45-54.
277. Weisdorf D, Zhang MJ, Arora M, Horowitz MM, Rizzo JD, Eapen M. Graft-versus-host disease induced graft-versus-leukemia effect: greater impact on relapse and disease-free survival after reduced intensity conditioning. *Biol Blood Marrow Transplant*. 2012;18(11):1727-1733.
278. Bar M, Sandmaier BM, Inamoto Y, et al. Donor lymphocyte infusion for relapsed hematological malignancies after allogeneic hematopoietic cell transplantation: prognostic relevance of the initial CD3+ T cell dose. *Biol Blood Marrow Transplant*. 2013;19(6):949-957.
279. Innes AJ, Beattie R, Sergeant R, et al. Escalating-dose HLA-mismatched DLI is safe for the treatment of leukaemia relapse following alemtuzumab-based myeloablative allo-SCT. *Bone Marrow Transplant*. 2013;48(10):1324-1328.
280. Peggs KS, Thomson K, Hart DP, et al. Dose-escalated donor lymphocyte infusions following reduced intensity transplantation: toxicity, chimerism, and disease responses. *Blood*. 2004;103(4):1548-1556.
281. Schmid C, Labopin M, Nagler A, et al. Donor lymphocyte infusion in the treatment of first hematological relapse after allogeneic stem-cell transplantation in adults with acute myeloid leukemia: a retrospective risk factors analysis and comparison with other strategies by the EBMT Acute Leukemia Working Party. *J Clin Oncol*. 2007;25(31):4938-4945.
282. Giralt SA, Kolb HJ. Donor lymphocyte infusions. *Curr Opin Oncol*. 1996;8(2):96-102.
283. Collins RH Jr, Shpilberg O, Drobyski WR, et al. Donor leukocyte infusions in 140 patients with relapsed malignancy after allogeneic bone marrow transplantation. *J Clin Oncol*. 1997;15(2):433-444.
284. Kolb HJ, Mittermuller J, Clemm C, et al. Donor leukocyte transfusions for treatment of recurrent chronic myelogenous leukemia in marrow transplant patients. *Blood*. 1990;76(12):2462-2465.
285. Lubbert M, Bertz H, Wasch R, et al. Efficacy of a 3-day, low-dose treatment with 5-azacytidine followed by donor lymphocyte infusions in older patients with acute myeloid leukemia or chronic myelomonocytic leukemia relapsed after allografting. *Bone Marrow Transplant*. 2010;45(4):627-632.
286. Schroeder T, Czibere A, Platzbecker U, et al. Azacitidine and donor lymphocyte infusions as first salvage therapy for relapse of AML or MDS after allogeneic stem cell transplantation. *Leukemia*. 2013;27(6):1229-1235.
287. Schroeder T, Rachlis E, Bug G, et al. Treatment of acute myeloid leukemia or myelodysplastic syndrome relapse after allogeneic stem cell transplantation with azacitidine and donor lymphocyte infusions—a retrospective multicenter analysis from the German Cooperative Transplant Study Group. *Biol Blood Marrow Transplant*. 2015;21(4):653-660.
288. Steinmann J, Bertz H, Wasch R, et al. 5-Azacytidine and DLI can induce long-term remissions in AML patients relapsed after allograft. *Bone Marrow Transplant*. 2015;50(5):690-695.
289. Bejanyan N, Weisdorf DJ, Logan BR, et al. Survival of patients with acute myeloid leukemia relapsing after allogeneic hematopoietic cell transplantation: a center for international blood and marrow transplant research study. *Biol Blood Marrow Transplant*. 2015;21(3):454-459.
290. Motabi IH, Ghobadi A, Liu J, et al. Chemotherapy versus hypomethylating agents for the treatment of relapsed acute myeloid leukemia and myelodysplastic syndrome after allogeneic stem cell transplant. *Biol Blood Marrow Transplant*. 2016;22(7):1324-1329.
291. Huisman C, de Weger RA, de Vries L, Tilanus MG, Verdonck LF. Chimerism analysis within 6 months of allogeneic stem cell transplantation predicts relapse in acute myeloid leukemia. *Bone Marrow Transplant*. 2007;39(5):285-291.
292. Lee HC, Saliba RM, Rondon G, et al. Mixed T lymphocyte chimerism after allogeneic hematopoietic transplantation is predictive for relapse of acute myeloid leukemia and myelodysplastic syndromes. *Biol Blood Marrow Transplant*. 2015;21(11):1948-1954.
293. Peggs KS, Kayani I, Edwards N, et al. Donor lymphocyte infusions modulate relapse risk in mixed chimeras and induce durable salvage in relapsed patients after T-cell-depleted allogeneic transplantation for Hodgkin's lymphoma. *J Clin Oncol*. 2011;29(8):971-978.
294. de Lima M, Bonamino M, Vasconcelos Z, et al. Prophylactic donor lymphocyte infusions after moderately ablative chemotherapy and stem cell transplantation for hematological malignancies: high remission rate among poor prognosis patients at the expense of graft-versus-host disease. *Bone Marrow Transplant*. 2001;27(1):73-78.
295. Jedlickova Z, Schmid C, Koenecke C, et al. Long-term results of adjuvant donor lymphocyte transfusion in AML after allogeneic stem cell transplantation. *Bone Marrow Transplant*. 2016;51(5):663-667.
296. Bar BM, Schattenberg A, Mensink EJ, et al. Donor leukocyte infusions for chronic myeloid leukemia relapsed after allogeneic bone marrow transplantation. *J Clin Oncol*. 1993;11(3):513-519.
297. Drobyski WR, Keever CA, Roth MS, et al. Salvage immunotherapy using donor leukocyte infusions as treatment for relapsed chronic myelogenous leukemia after allogeneic bone marrow transplantation: efficacy and toxicity of a defined T-cell dose. *Blood*. 1993;82(8):2310-2318.

298. Molldrem JJ, Lee PP, Wang C, et al. Evidence that specific T lymphocytes may participate in the elimination of chronic myelogenous leukemia. *Nat Med.* 2000;6(9):1018-1023.
299. Ruggeri L, Capanni M, Urbani E, et al. Effectiveness of donor natural killer cell alloreactivity in mismatched hematopoietic transplants. *Science.* 2002;295(5562):2097-2100.
300. Soiffer RJ, Alyea EP, Hochberg E, et al. Randomized trial of CD8+ T-cell depletion in the prevention of graft-versus-host disease associated with donor lymphocyte infusion. *Biol Blood Marrow Transplant.* 2002;8(11):625-632.
301. Schmidt-Wolf IG, Negrin RS, Kiem HP, Blume KG, Weissman IL. Use of a SCID mouse/human lymphoma model to evaluate cytokine-induced killer cells with potent antitumor cell activity. *J Exp Med.* 1991;174(1):139-149.
302. Groh V, Rhinehart R, Randolph-Habecker J, Topp MS, Riddell SR, Spies T. Costimulation of CD8alphabeta T cells by NKG2D via engagement by MIC induced on virus-infected cells. *Nat Immunol.* 2001;2(3):255-260.
303. Karimi M, Cao TM, Baker JA, Verneris MR, Soares L, Negrin RS. Silencing human NKG2D, DAP10, and DAP12 reduces cytotoxicity of activated CD8+ T cells and NK cells. *J Immunol.* 2005;175(12):7819-7828.
304. Baker J, Verneris MR, Ito M, Shizuru JA, Negrin RS. Expansion of cytolytic CD8(+) natural killer T cells with limited capacity for graft-versus-host disease induction due to interferon gamma production. *Blood.* 2001;97(10):2923-2931.
305. Laport GG, Sheehan K, Baker J, et al. Adoptive immunotherapy with cytokine-induced killer cells for patients with relapsed hematologic malignancies after allogeneic hematopoietic cell transplantation. *Biol Blood Marrow Transplant.* 2011;17(11):1679-1687.
306. McClune BL, Ahn KW, Wang HL, et al. Allotransplantation for patients age >/=40 years with non-Hodgkin lymphoma: encouraging progression-free survival. *Biol Blood Marrow Transplant.* 2014;20(7):960-968.
307. Shook DR, Triplett BM, Srinivasan A, et al. Successful allogeneic hematopoietic cell engraftment after a minimal conditioning regimen in children with relapsed or refractory solid tumors. *Biol Blood Marrow Transplant.* 2013;19(2):291-297.
308. Kharbanda S, Smith AR, Hutchinson SK, et al. Unrelated donor allogeneic hematopoietic stem cell transplantation for patients with hemoglobinopathies using a reduced-intensity conditioning regimen and third-party mesenchymal stromal cells. *Biol Blood Marrow Transplant.* 2014;20(4):581-586.
309. Kurosawa S, Yakushijin K, Yamaguchi T, et al. Recent decrease in non-relapse mortality due to GVHD and infection after allogeneic hematopoietic cell transplantation in non-remission acute leukemia. *Bone Marrow Transplant.* 2013;48(9):1198-1204.
310. Rosenberg SA, Lotze MT, Muul LM, et al. Observations on the systemic administration of autologous lymphokine-activated killer cells and recombinant interleukin-2 to patients with metastatic cancer. *N Engl J Med.* 1985;313(23):1485-1492.
311. Rosenberg SA, Packard BS, Aebersold PM, et al. Use of tumor-infiltrating lymphocytes and interleukin-2 in the immunotherapy of patients with metastatic melanoma. A preliminary report. *N Engl J Med.* 1988;319(25):1676-1680.
312. Rosenstein M, Yron I, Kaufmann Y, Rosenberg SA. Lymphokine-activated killer cells: lysis of fresh syngeneic natural killer-resistant murine tumor cells by lymphocytes cultured in interleukin 2. *Cancer Res.* 1984;44(5):1946-1953.
313. Grimm EA, Ramsey KM, Mazumder A, Wilson DJ, Djeu JY, Rosenberg SA. Lymphokine-activated killer cell phenomenon. II. Precursor phenotype is serologically distinct from peripheral T lymphocytes, memory cytotoxic thymus-derived lymphocytes, and natural killer cells. *J Exp Med.* 1983;157(3):884-897.
314. Phillips JH, Lanier LL. Dissection of the lymphokine-activated killer phenomenon. Relative contribution of peripheral blood natural killer cells and T lymphocytes to cytolysis. *J Exp Med.* 1986;164(3):814-825.
315. Rosenberg SA, Lotze MT, Muul LM, et al. A progress report on the treatment of 157 patients with advanced cancer using lymphokine-activated killer cells and interleukin-2 or high-dose interleukin-2 alone. *N Engl J Med.* 1987;316(15):889-897.
316. Rosenberg SA, Lotze MT, Yang JC, et al. Experience with the use of high-dose interleukin-2 in the treatment of 652 cancer patients. *Ann Surg.* 1989;210(4):474-484, discussion 484-475.
317. Kimura H, Yamaguchi Y. A phase III randomized study of interleukin-2 lymphokine-activated killer cell immunotherapy combined with chemotherapy or radiotherapy after curative or noncurative resection of primary lung carcinoma. *Cancer.* 1997;80(1):42-49.
318. Rosenberg SA, Spiess P, Lafreniere R. A new approach to the adoptive immunotherapy of cancer with tumor-infiltrating lymphocytes. *Science.* 1986;233(4770):1318-1321.
319. Chacon JA, Sarnaik AA, Chen JQ, et al. Manipulating the tumor microenvironment ex vivo for enhanced expansion of tumor-infiltrating lymphocytes for adoptive cell therapy. *Clin Cancer Res.* 2015;21(3):611-621.
320. Chacon JA, Wu RC, Sukhumalchandra P, et al. Co-stimulation through 4-1BB/CD137 improves the expansion and function of CD8(+) melanoma tumor-infiltrating lymphocytes for adoptive T-cell therapy. *PLoS One.* 2013;8(4):e60031.
321. Hall M, Liu H, Malafa M, et al. Expansion of tumor-infiltrating lymphocytes (TIL) from human pancreatic tumors. *J Immunother Cancer.* 2016;4:61.
322. Fisher B, Packard BS, Read EJ, et al. Tumor localization of adoptively transferred indium-111 labeled tumor infiltrating lymphocytes in patients with metastatic melanoma. *J Clin Oncol.* 1989;7(2):250-261.
323. Griffith KD, Read EJ, Carrasquillo JA, et al. In vivo distribution of adoptively transferred indium-111-labeled tumor infiltrating lymphocytes and peripheral blood lymphocytes in patients with metastatic melanoma. *J Natl Cancer Inst.* 1989;81(22):1709-1717.
324. Rosenberg SA, Yannelli JR, Yang JC, et al. Treatment of patients with metastatic melanoma with autologous tumor-infiltrating lymphocytes and interleukin 2. *J Natl Cancer Inst.* 1994;86(15):1159-1166.
325. Andersen R, Donia M, Ellebaek E, et al. Long-lasting complete responses in patients with metastatic melanoma after adoptive cell therapy with tumor-infiltrating lymphocytes and an attenuated IL2 regimen. *Clin Cancer Res.* 2016;22(15):3734-3745.
326. Rosenberg SA, Yang JC, Sherry RM, et al. Durable complete responses in heavily pretreated patients with metastatic melanoma using T-cell transfer immunotherapy. *Clin Cancer Res.* 2011;17(13):4550-4557.
327. Baldan V, Griffiths R, Hawkins RE, Gilham DE. Efficient and reproducible generation of tumour-infiltrating lymphocytes for renal cell carcinoma. *Br J Cancer.* 2015;112(9):1510-1518.
328. Balermpas P, Michel Y, Wagenblast J, et al. Tumour-infiltrating lymphocytes predict response to definitive chemoradiotherapy in head and neck cancer. *Br J Cancer.* 2014;110(2):501-509.
329. Lee N, Zakka LR, Mihm MC Jr, Schatton T. Tumour-infiltrating lymphocytes in melanoma prognosis and cancer immunotherapy. *Pathology.* 2016;48(2):177-187.
330. Noble F, Mellows T, McCormick Matthews LH, et al. Tumour infiltrating lymphocytes correlate with improved survival in patients with oesophageal adenocarcinoma. *Cancer Immunol Immunother.* 2016;65(6):651-662.
331. Ward MJ, Thirdborough SM, Mellows T, et al. Tumour-infiltrating lymphocytes predict for outcome in HPV-positive oropharyngeal cancer. *Br J Cancer.* 2014;110(2):489-500.
332. Wansom D, Light E, Thomas D, et al. Infiltrating lymphocytes and human papillomavirus-16—associated oropharyngeal cancer. *Laryngoscope.* 2012;122(1):121-127.
333. Sarnaik AA, Hamid O, Khushalani NI, et al. Lifileucel, a tumor-infiltrating lymphocyte therapy, in metastatic melanoma. *J Clin Oncol.* 2021;39(24):2656-2666.
334. Creelan BC, Wang C, Teer JK, et al. Tumor-infiltrating lymphocyte treatment for anti-PD-1-resistant metastatic lung cancer: a phase 1 trial. *Nat Med.* 2021;27(8):1410-1418.
335. Riddell SR, Greenberg PD. Principles for adoptive T cell therapy of human viral diseases. *Annu Rev Immunol.* 1995;13:545-586.
336. Riddell SR, Watanabe KS, Goodrich JM, Li CR, Agha ME, Greenberg PD. Restoration of viral immunity in immunodeficient humans by the adoptive transfer of T cell clones. *Science.* 1992;257(5067):238-241.
337. Walter EA, Greenberg PD, Gilbert MJ, et al. Reconstitution of cellular immunity against cytomegalovirus in recipients of allogeneic bone marrow by transfer of T-cell clones from the donor. *N Engl J Med.* 1995;333(16):1038-1044.
338. Rosenberg SA. Progress in the development of immunotherapy for the treatment of patients with cancer. *J Intern Med.* 2001;250(6):462-475.
339. Rosenberg SA. Progress in human tumour immunology and immunotherapy. *Nature.* 2001;411(6835):380-384.
340. Yee C, Riddell SR, Greenberg PD. Prospects for adoptive T cell therapy. *Curr Opin Immunol.* 1997;9(5):702-708.
341. Heslop HE, Slobod KS, Pule MA, et al. Long-term outcome of EBV-specific T-cell infusions to prevent or treat EBV-related lymphoproliferative disease in transplant recipients. *Blood.* 2010;115(5):925-935.
342. Haque T, Wilkie GM, Jones MM, et al. Allogeneic cytotoxic T-cell therapy for EBV-positive posttransplantation lymphoproliferative disease: results of a phase 2 multicenter clinical trial. *Blood.* 2007;110(4):1123-1131.
343. Bollard CM, Gottschalk S, Torrano V, et al. Sustained complete responses in patients with lymphoma receiving autologous cytotoxic T lymphocytes targeting Epstein-Barr virus latent membrane proteins. *J Clin Oncol.* 2014;32(8):798-808.
344. Bollard CM, Tripic T, Cruz CR, et al. Tumor-specific T-cells engineered to overcome tumor immune evasion induce clinical responses in patients with relapsed Hodgkin lymphoma. *J Clin Oncol.* 2018;36(11):1128-1139.
345. Roche PA, Furuta K. The ins and outs of MHC class II-mediated antigen processing and presentation. *Nat Rev Immunol.* 2015;15(4):203-216.
346. Roeser JC, Leach SD, McAllister F. Emerging strategies for cancer immunoprevention. *Oncogene.* 2015;34(50):6029-6039.
347. Kochenderfer JN, Feldman SA, Zhao Y, et al. Construction and preclinical evaluation of an anti-CD19 chimeric antigen receptor. *J Immunother.* 2009;32(7):689-702.
348. Kochenderfer JN, Yu Z, Frasheri D, Restifo NP, Rosenberg SA. Adoptive transfer of syngeneic T cells transduced with a chimeric antigen receptor that recognizes murine CD19 can eradicate lymphoma and normal B cells. *Blood.* 2010;116(19):3875-3886.
349. Imai C, Mihara K, Andreansky M, et al. Chimeric receptors with 4-1BB signaling capacity provoke potent cytotoxicity against acute lymphoblastic leukemia. *Leukemia.* 2004;18(4):676-684.
350. Magnani CF, Tettamanti S, Alberti G, et al. Transposon-based CAR T cells in acute leukemias: where are we going? *Cells.* 2020;9(6):1337.
351. Bouhassira DC, Thompson JJ, Davila ML. Using gene therapy to manipulate the immune system in the fight against B-cell leukemias. *Expert Opin Biol Ther.* 2015;15(3):403-416.
352. Eshhar Z. Tumor-specific T-bodies: towards clinical application. *Cancer Immunol Immunother.* 1997;45(3-4):131-136.
353. Rafiq S, Hackett CS, Brentjens RJ. Engineering strategies to overcome the current roadblocks in CAR T cell therapy. *Nat Rev Clin Oncol.* 2020;17(3):147-167.
354. Boissel L, Betancur M, Lu W, et al. Comparison of mRNA and lentiviral based transfection of natural killer cells with chimeric antigen receptors recognizing lymphoid antigens. *Leuk Lymphoma.* 2012;53(5):958-965.
355. Davila ML, Riviere I, Wang X, et al. Efficacy and toxicity management of 19-28z CAR T cell therapy in B cell acute lymphoblastic leukemia. *Sci Transl Med.* 2014;6(224):224ra225.
356. Maude SL, Frey N, Shaw PA, et al. Chimeric antigen receptor T cells for sustained remissions in leukemia. *N Engl J Med.* 2014;371(16):1507-1517.
357. Lee DW, Kochenderfer JN, Stetler-Stevenson M, et al. T cells expressing CD19 chimeric antigen receptors for acute lymphoblastic leukaemia in children and young adults: a phase 1 dose-escalation trial. *Lancet.* 2015;385(9967):517-528.
358. Brentjens RJ, Davila ML, Riviere I, et al. CD19-targeted T cells rapidly induce molecular remissions in adults with chemotherapy-refractory acute lymphoblastic leukemia. *Sci Transl Med.* 2013;5(177):177ra138.

359. Kochenderfer JN, Dudley ME, Kassim SH, et al. Chemotherapy-refractory diffuse large B-cell lymphoma and indolent B-cell malignancies can be effectively treated with autologous T cells expressing an anti-CD19 chimeric antigen receptor. *J Clin Oncol*. 2015;33(6):540-549.
360. Porter DL, Levine BL, Kalos M, Bagg A, June CH. Chimeric antigen receptor-modified T cells in chronic lymphoid leukemia. *N Engl J Med*. 2011;365(8):725-733.
361. Neelapu SS, Locke FL, Bartlett NL, et al. Axicabtagene ciloleucel CAR T-cell therapy in refractory large B-cell lymphoma. *N Engl J Med*. 2017;377(26):2531-2544.
362. Maude SL, Laetsch TW, Buechner J, et al. Tisagenlecleucel in children and young adults with B-cell lymphoblastic leukemia. *N Engl J Med*. 2018;378(5):439-448.
363. Abramson JS, Palomba ML, Gordon LI, et al. Lisocabtagene maraleucel for patients with relapsed or refractory large B-cell lymphomas (TRANSCEND NHL 001): a multicentre seamless design study. *Lancet*. 2020;396(10254):839-852.
364. Porter DL, Hwang WT, Frey NV, et al. Chimeric antigen receptor T cells persist and induce sustained remissions in relapsed refractory chronic lymphocytic leukemia. *Sci Transl Med*. 2015;7(303):303ra139.
365. Brentjens RJ, Riviere I, Park JH, et al. Safety and persistence of adoptively transferred autologous CD19-targeted T cells in patients with relapsed or chemotherapy refractory B-cell leukemias. *Blood*. 2011;118(18):4817-4828.
366. Melenhorst JJ, Chen GM, Wang M, et al. Decade-long leukaemia remissions with persistence of CD4 + CAR T cells. *Nature*. 2022;602(7897):503-509.
367. Frey N, Shaw PA, Hexner E, et al. Optimizing chimeric antigen receptor T-cell therapy for adults with acute lymphoblastic leukemia. *J Clin Oncol*. 2020;38(5):415-422.
368. Kalos M, Levine BL, Porter DL, et al. T cells with chimeric antigen receptors have potent antitumor effects and can establish memory in patients with advanced leukemia. *Sci Transl Med*. 2011;3(95):95ra73.
369. Grupp SA, Kalos M, Barrett D, et al. Chimeric antigen receptor-modified T cells for acute lymphoid leukemia. *N Engl J Med*. 2013;368(16):1509-1518.
370. Fry TJ, Shah NN, Orentas RJ, et al. CD22-targeted CAR T cells induce remission in B-ALL that is naive or resistant to CD19-targeted CAR immunotherapy. *Nat Med*. 2018;24(1):20-28.
371. Schuster SJ, Svoboda J, Chong EA, et al. Chimeric antigen receptor T cells in refractory B-cell lymphomas. *N Engl J Med*. 2017;377(26):2545-2554.
372. Locke FL, Neelapu SS, Bartlett NL, et al. Phase 1 results of ZUMA-1: a multicenter study of KTE-C19 anti-CD19 CAR T cell therapy in refractory aggressive lymphoma. *Mol Ther*. 2017;25(1):285-295.
373. Jacobson C, Chavez JC, Sehgal AR, et al. Primary analysis of Zuma-5: a phase 2 study of axicabtagene ciloleucel (Axi-Cel) in patients with relapsed/refractory (R/R) indolent non-hodgkin lymphoma (iNHL). *Blood*. 2020;136(suppl 1):40-41.
374. Wang M, Munoz J, Goy A, et al. KTE-X19 CAR T-cell therapy in relapsed or refractory mantle-cell lymphoma. *N Engl J Med*. 2020;382(14):1331-1342.
375. Shah BD, Ghobadi A, Oluwole OO, et al. KTE-X19 for relapsed or refractory adult B-cell acute lymphoblastic leukaemia: phase 2 results of the single-arm, open-label, multicentre ZUMA-3 study. *Lancet*. 2021;398(10299):491-502.
376. Siddiqi T, Soumerai JD, Dorritie KA, et al. Phase 1 TRANSCEND CLL 004 study of lisocabtagene maraleucel in patients with relapsed/refractory CLL or SLL. *Blood*. 2022;139(12):1794-1806. doi:10.1182/blood.2021011895
377. Locke FL, Miklos DB, Jacobson CA, et al. Axicabtagene Ciloleucel as second-line therapy for large B-cell lymphoma. *N Engl J Med*. 2022;386(7):640-654. doi:10.1056/NEJMoa2116133
378. Kamdar M, Solomon SR, Arnason JE, et al. Lisocabtagene maraleucel (liso-cel), a CD19-directed chimeric antigen receptor (CAR) T cell therapy, versus standard of care (SOC) with salvage chemotherapy (CT) followed by autologous stem cell transplantation (ASCT) as second-line (2L) treatment in patients (Pts) with relapsed or refractory (R/R) large B-cell lymphoma (LBCL): results from the randomized phase 3 Transform study. *Blood*. 2021;138(suppl 1):91.
379. Bishop MR, Dickinson M, Purtill D, et al. Second-line tisagenlecleucel or standard care in aggressive B-cell lymphoma. *N Engl J Med*. 2021;386(7):629-639. doi:10.1056/NEJMoa2116596
380. Garfall AL, Maus MV, Hwang WT, et al. Chimeric antigen receptor T cells against CD19 for multiple myeloma. *N Engl J Med*. 2015;373(11):1040-1047.
381. Mikkilineni L, Kochenderfer JN. Chimeric antigen receptor T-cell therapies for multiple myeloma. *Blood*. 2017;130(24):2594-2602.
382. Munshi NC, Anderson LD, Shah N, et al. Idecabtagene Vicleucel in relapsed and refractory multiple myeloma. *N Engl J Med*. 2021;384(8):705-716.
383. Berdeja JG, Madduri D, Usmani SZ, et al. Ciltacabtagene autoleucel, a B-cell maturation antigen-directed chimeric antigen receptor T-cell therapy in patients with relapsed or refractory multiple myeloma (CARTITUDE-1): a phase 1b/2 open-label study. *Lancet*. 2021;398(10297):314-324.
384. Mikkilineni L, Kochenderfer JN. CAR T cell therapies for patients with multiple myeloma. *Nat Rev Clin Oncol*. 2021;18:71-84.
385. Brudno JN, Somerville RP, Shi V, et al. Allogeneic T cells that express an anti-CD19 chimeric antigen receptor induce remissions of B-cell malignancies that progress after allogeneic hmatopoietic stem-cell transplantation without causing graft-versus-host disease. *J Clin Oncol*. 2016;34(10):1112-1121.
386. Cruz CR, Micklethwaite KP, Savoldo B, et al. Infusion of donor-derived CD19-redirected virus-specific T cells for B-cell malignancies relapsed after allogeneic stem cell transplant: a phase 1 study. *Blood*. 2013;122(17):2965-2973.
387. Depil S, Duchateau P, Grupp S, Mufti G, Poirot L. 'Of-the-shelf' allogeneic CAR T cells: development and challenges. *Nat Rev Drug Discov*. 2020;19(3):185-199.
388. Benjamin R, Graham C, Yallop D, et al. Genome-edited, donor-derived allogeneic anti-CD19 chimeric antigen receptor T cells in paediatric and adult B-cell acute lymphoblastic leukaemia: results of two phase 1 studies. *Lancet*. 2020;396(10266):1885-1894.
389. Daher M, Rezvani K. Outlook for new CAR-based therapies with a focus on CAR NK cells: what lies beyond CAR-engineered T cells in the race against cancer. *Cancer Discov*. 2021;11(1):45-58.
390. Liu E, Marin D, Banerjee P, et al. Use of CAR-transduced natural killer cells in CD19-positive lymphoid tumors. *N Engl J Med*. 2020;382(6):545-553.
391. Biederstädt A, Rezvani K. Engineering the next generation of CAR-NK immunotherapies. *Int J Hematol*. 2021;114(5):554-571.
392. Barrett DM, Singh N, Porter DL, Grupp SA, June CH. Chimeric antigen receptor therapy for cancer. *Annu Rev Med*. 2014;65:333-347.
393. Lee DW, Santomasso BD, Locke FL, et al. ASTCT consensus grading for cytokine release syndrome and neurologic toxicity associated with immune effector cells. *Biol Blood Marrow Transplant*. 2019;25(4):625-638.
394. Hu Y, Sun J, Wu Z, et al. Predominant cerebral cytokine release syndrome in CD19-directed chimeric antigen receptor-modified T cell therapy. *J Hematol Oncol*. 2016;9(1):70.
395. Maus MV, Alexander S, Bishop MR, et al. Society for Immunotherapy of Cancer (SITC) clinical practice guideline on immune effector cell-related adverse events. *J Immuother Cancer*. 2020;8(2):e001511.
396. Kochenderfer JN, Dudley ME, Feldman SA, et al. B-cell depletion and remissions of malignancy along with cytokine-associated toxicity in a clinical trial of anti-CD19 chimeric-antigen-receptor-transduced T cells. *Blood*. 2012;119(12):2709-2720.
397. Berger TR, Maus MV. Mechanisms of response and resistance to CAR T cell therapies. *Curr Opin Immunol*. 2021;69:56-64.
398. Bachanova V, Cooley S, Defor TE, et al. Clearance of acute myeloid leukemia by haploidentical natural killer cells is improved using IL-2 diphtheria toxin fusion protein. *Blood*. 2014;123(25):3855-3863.
399. Miller JS, Soignier Y, Panoskaltsis-Mortari A, et al. Successful adoptive transfer and in vivo expansion of human haploidentical NK cells in patients with cancer. *Blood*. 2005;105(8):3051-3057.
400. Armand P. Immune checkpoint blockade in hematologic malignancies. *Blood*. 2015;125(22):3393-3400.
401. Ansell SM, Lesokhin AM, Borrello I, et al. PD-1 blockade with nivolumab in relapsed or refractory Hodgkin's lymphoma. *N Engl J Med*. 2015;372(4):311-319.
402. Armand P, Shipp MA, Ribrag V, et al. Programmed death-1 blockade with pembrolizumab in patients with classical hodgkin lymphoma after brentuximab vedotin failure. *J Clin Oncol*. 2016;34(31):3733-3739.
403. Lesokhin AM, Ansell SM, Armand P, et al. Preliminary results of a phase I study of Nivolumab (BMS-936558) in patients with relapsed or refractory lymphoid malignancies. *Blood*. 2014;124(21):291.
404. Juarez-Salcedo LM, Sandoval-Sus J, Sokol L, Chavez JC, Dalia S. The role of anti-PD-1 and anti-PD-L1 agents in the treatment of diffuse large B-cell lymphoma: the future is now. *Crit Rev Oncol Hematol*. 2017;113:52-62.
405. Kwong YL, Chan TSY, Tan D, et al. PD1 blockade with pembrolizumab is highly effective in relapsed or refractory NK/T-cell lymphoma failing l-asparaginase. *Blood*. 2017;129(17):2437-2442.
406. Khodadoust M, Rook AH, Porcu P. Pembrolizumab for treatment of relapsed/refractory mycosis fungoides and Sezary Syndrome: clinical efficacy in CITN multicenter phase 2 study. *Blood*. 2016;128:181.
407. Ansell SM, Hurvitz SA, Koenig PA, et al. Phase I study of ipilimumab, an anti-CTLA-4 monoclonal antibody, in patients with relapsed and refractory B-cell non-Hodgkin lymphoma. *Clin Cancer Res*. 2009;15(20):6446-6453.
408. Davids MS, Kim HT, Bachireddy P, et al. Ipilimumab for patients with relapse after allogeneic transplantation. *N Engl J Med*. 2016;375(2):143-153.
409. June CH, Sadelain M. Chimeric antigen receptor therapy. *N Engl J Med*. 2018;379:64-73.

Chapter 72 ■ Gene Therapy for Hematopoietic Stem Cell Disorders

ANDRE LAROCHELLE

INTRODUCTION

The blood-forming system is organized in an irreversible hierarchy including rare hematopoietic stem cells (HSCs), a larger population of more restricted progenitor cells and a vast pool of mature cells with defined functions. Unlike more mature cells, HSCs have an extensive proliferative capacity, an ability to differentiate to produce mature progeny of all myeloid and lymphoid blood cell lineages, and a self-renewal capacity to replace the cells that became progressively committed to differentiation. Because of these unique properties, HSCs have the remarkable ability to reconstitute and maintain a functional hematopoietic system for the lifetime of an individual. Hematopoietic stem and progenitor cells can be readily enriched for clinical and laboratory applications via selection of cells expressing the surface marker CD34.

Allogeneic transplantation of HSCs is employed in the clinic for the therapeutic correction of numerous inherited and acquired hematologic disorders whereby an individual carrying a normal genotype serves as the stem cell donor. However, this approach suffers from significant drawbacks, including the need for toxic myeloablative conditioning regimens, the limited availability of human leukocyte antigen (HLA)-matched donors, and the risks of complications such as graft-versus-host-disease or graft rejection. The molecular characterization of inherited human diseases over the past several decades has stimulated scientists and clinicians to envision genetic therapy as a new and exciting possibility.[1] Gene therapy, which utilizes a patient's own (autologous) HSCs, also offers the prospect of a curative, one-time therapy for a variety of congenital disorders while overcoming the shortcomings of allogeneic transplantation.[2-7]

Granulocyte colony–stimulating factor (G-CSF)–mobilized peripheral blood (MPB) is the preferred source of HSCs and has outcompeted bone marrow (BM) for HSC-based therapies.[8] Umbilical cord blood (UCB) represents an alternative source of HSCs commonly used in preclinical investigations, but limited cell dose has precluded its wide clinical utility.[9] Enrichment of HSCs from these various sources is essential to better understand their unique biology and identify novel therapeutic strategies targeting these cells. In humans, hematopoietic stem and progenitors are enriched within a cellular population expressing the CD34 cell surface marker, and the CD34$^+$CD38$^-$CD45RA$^-$CD90$^+$CD49f$^+$ phenotype is customarily accepted to define a cell population further enriched in HSCs.[10-12]

This chapter will review the fundamental features of gene transfer technologies and their applications in preclinical and clinical HSC gene therapy trials. The pace of the field is rapid, and many details may become obsolete, but the central concepts should remain relevant to any future gene therapy applications.

DEFINITIONS

What Is Gene Therapy?

Gene therapy can be generally defined as the transfer of a gene or genetic material (DNA or RNA) into a cell with therapeutic intent. The genotype of the cell is thus altered, with subsequent gene expression altering the phenotype of the cell. The therapeutic agent is the gene product, generally a protein, or less frequently RNA, for example, ribozymes or antisense molecules. This is in contrast to conventional therapies that act by directly altering the phenotype, even if the defect is genetic. For instance, the conventional approach to treat hemophilia is by directly replacing the defective or missing gene product by infusion of an exogenously manufactured or isolated factor. Gene therapy strategies instead aim at altering the underlying genetic abnormality to circumvent the need for these therapies. Various types of gene therapy have been described based on the target cells (somatic vs germ cells), modes of correction (in vivo vs ex vivo gene therapy), or approaches of correction (gene addition vs gene editing).

Somatic Versus Germ Cell Gene Therapy

To date, efforts have focused on somatic therapy, with genotypic alteration of only the diseased target tissue. Manipulation of germ cells, with transmission of altered genetic material to subsequent generations, is not yet feasible in humans, but the profound ethical and societal implications need to be addressed through the political process before the technology progresses further.[13] The recent development of induced pluripotent stem cells (iPSCs), whose behavior is analogous to embryonic stem cells (ESCs) but can be derived from somatic cells, has introduced the possibility of genetic manipulation of autologous pluripotent stem cells, circumventing the ethical issues surrounding ESCs.[14]

Ex Vivo Versus In Vivo Gene Therapy

In ex vivo gene therapy, cells are removed from the body, genetically engineered, and returned to the patient. This type of ex vivo manipulation avoids genetic alteration of nontarget cells and is less likely to generate an inflammatory or immune response or be hindered by inactivation of the gene transfer vehicle by complements. It has been used in all HSC gene therapy clinical trials to date. Other cellular targets for ex vivo transduction have included lymphocytes, hepatocytes, keratinocytes, tumor cells, and muscle progenitor cells. However, it is inconvenient and expensive, and only a small proportion of the intended target cell population can be explanted at one time. For less accessible cells or tissues, such as liver, differentiated muscle cells, airway epithelium, vascular endothelium, retinal pigment epithelium, and neurons, in vivo (or in situ) mode of gene delivery can be used in which the gene transfer vehicle is introduced directly in the affected tissue. This approach is often limited by the difficulty of tissue access and by the inability to transduce the majority of cells. An alternative and ideal in vivo strategy would allow intravenous injection of a vector followed by rapid and safe specific transduction of target cells around the body. At this time, there are no clinical examples of this in vivo approach for HSC gene therapy.

Gene Addition Versus Gene Editing Therapy

Current gene transfer methods predominantly rely on viral vector–mediated gene addition to enable either permanent genomic insertion or extrachromosomal (episomal) maintenance of a new therapeutic coding within the target cells.[15-17] The recent emergence of programmable engineered nuclease technologies provides a promising alternative to integrating viral vectors by facilitating precise gene correction or the site-specific integration of a therapeutic transgene cassette into a defined sequence within the target cell genome.[18,19] The term gene or genome editing has been coined for this approach. The ability to precisely edit cellular genomes would obviate the concerns of insertional mutagenesis inevitably associated with integrating vectors (see sections below), would drive expression of the corrected gene from endogenous promoters, and extend gene therapies to disorders requiring replacement of abnormal gene products rather than simple gene addition. Current approaches of genome editing are described below.

Gene Transfer Vectors and Transduction

The vehicle for transferring new genetic material into a target cell is called a *gene transfer vector*. At a minimum, a vector contains the gene or genes of interest along with regulatory elements such as promoters or enhancers that govern expression of the gene product. A vector may be a simple particle consisting of a fragment of DNA encapsulated within a liposome or conjugated to proteins that facilitate uptake into cells, or may be a more complex viral vector, capitalizing on the ability of viruses to enter cells easily and express genes robustly. Characteristics of the major vector systems are summarized in *Table 72.1*, and will be detailed in subsequent sections. The successful

Table 72.1. Gene Transfer Vector Systems

Vector System	Integration	Cell Cycle Dependence	Insert Size Limit	Clinical Experience	Advantages	Disadvantages	Major Applications
Murine retrovirus	Yes	Yes	8–10 kb	Extensive	Stable producer lines; No viral genes in vector; Low immunogenicity; Well-understood biology; Efficient entry and integration in many cell types; Proven clinical safety	Low titer, fragile vector; Requirement for cycling; Erratic expression; Insertional mutagenesis	Ex vivo: HSCs, lymphocytes, tumor cells, hepatocytes, myoblasts; In vivo: producer cell or vector injection into tumors
HIV-based lentivirus	Yes	No	8–10 kb	Moderate	Faithful delivery of complex genes; Well understood; Efficient entry and integration; Pseudotyping allows broad tissue range	Production labor intensive; Erratic expression; Insertional mutagenesis; Recombination with wild-type HIV	Ex vivo: HSCs, lymphocytes, tumor cells, nondividing cells
Foamy virus	Yes	Yes	Up to 12 kb	None	Nonpathogenic in humans; Backbone contains insulators allowing use of strong internal promoters; Efficient transduction of HSCs with minimal ex vivo culture time; Broad host and cell type tropism without pseudotyping	Production labor intensive; Insertional mutagenesis but safer integration profile than murine retrovirus and lentivirus	Ex vivo: HSCs; In vivo: HPCs
Adenovirus	No	No	8–10 kb	Moderate	High titer, stable vector; High-level transgene expression; Efficient entry into many cell types	No stable producer lines; Potential for recombination and replication-competent virus; Multiple viral genes expressed from vector; High immunogenicity (may be an advantage as a vaccine vector); Pre-existing immunity; Inflammatory response	In vivo: Pulmonary epithelium, tumor cells, muscle, liver
AAV	Yes—inefficient	Yes—controversial	4.5 kb	Minimal	Stable vector, extra- and intracellularly; High titer; High-level transgene expression; No expressed viral genes in vector	No stable producer cell lines; High percentage of defective particles; Requirement for helper adenovirus during production; Very limited insert size; Pre-existing immunity	Undefined
Naked DNA	No	No	No limit	Moderate	Ease of production; High level of safety; No extraneous expressed vector genes; No immunogenicity of vector	Inefficient cell entry, uptake into nucleus; Poor stability within cell; Low-level expression	In vivo: tissues accessible to injection, for transient expression or vaccination
Facilitated DNA (liposomes, polylysine conjugates, inactivated adenovirus, etc)	No	No	No limit	Moderate	Same as naked DNA plus: Can be targeted to specific cell types; More efficient uptake and intracellular stability	No mechanism for persistence	Same as naked DNA, plus in vivo tumor cells, vascular endothelium

Abbreviations: AAV, adeno-associated virus; HIV, human immunodeficiency virus; HSCs, hematopoietic stem cells; kb, kilobases.

interaction of a viral vector with a target cell, leading to an alteration in that cell's genotype, is termed transduction. Introduction of DNA or RNA into cells using nonviral approaches is termed transfection.

Replication-Defective Vectors

Vector production procedures are unique to each system, but a number of considerations are common to all, namely those developed for clinical use. A clinical vector must be feasible and practical to produce safely at pharmaceutical grade.[20,21] To prevent indiscriminate spread of viral genomes, most viral vectors designed for clinical applications must be rendered replication-defective meaning that once a viral vector enters a target cell, the cell will produce no new viral particles.

Multiplicity of Infection

High-titer vector preparations, containing a high concentration of functional vector particles, are also very important, allowing exposure of target cells to the highest possible multiplicity of infection (MOI), defined as the ratio of vector particles to target cells; this increases the probability of successful vector-cell interaction.

Transductional Targeting by Pseudotyping

A number of important steps must occur between exposure of a target cell to a vector and successful transduction of that cell, with persistence of the transferred genetic material in the correct cellular compartment and expression of the gene of interest or transgene. The vector must cross the plasma membrane efficiently and without damaging the cell. Nonviral vectors may cross the plasma membrane without the need for cell surface receptors. However, most viral vectors enter cells via specific receptors, and an important consideration for efficient transduction is the number of functional receptors on the proposed target cell for the vector being used.[22] Approaches to redirect retroviral particles entry to different cell surface receptors for gene therapy purposes are described as transductional targeting. One strategy for altering the tropism of viral vectors involves the genetic modification of viral envelope glycoproteins. Another process commonly used in HSC gene therapy, called pseudotyping, redirects gene transfer vectors by substituting alternative native (nonengineered) viral envelope proteins during the vector production process.[23-26]

Integrating and Episomal Vectors

After crossing the plasma membrane, the vector must then travel through the cytoplasm and cross the nuclear membrane in order to enter the nucleus and utilize the cell's transcriptional machinery for expression of the transgene. Nuclear entry of some vectors may be dependent on mitosis, with temporary breakdown of the nuclear membrane; others carry nuclear localization determinants that result in specific conveyance across the intact membrane. The transferred genetic material may integrate permanently into the target cell's own chromosomal DNA, ensuring passage of the new gene to all daughter cells with every cell division. The need for integration depends on the target cell and therapeutic application; it is absolutely required for gene transfer into HSCs where the transgene must be transmitted to all progeny cells, but is superfluous for cellular targets such as neurons or muscle cells that are not mitotic.

Alternatively, the gene may remain episomal, or nonintegrated. Some vectors are very stable as nuclear episomes, with prolonged persistence of transgene expression as long as the cell does not undergo mitosis. Unless the episome can reproduce itself, cell division will eventually dilute out episomal DNA, limiting the application of nonintegrating vectors to nonmitotic tissues or to situations requiring only transient expression.

Constitutive or Tissue-Specific Transgene Expression (Transcriptional Targeting)

The level of transgene expression necessary for the desired therapeutic effect and the ability to restrict expression to specific target cell types are important factors to consider. The level of expression is very important to determine during in vitro and animal experiments and varies greatly depending on the target cell type and the proposed clinical application. Unless a transgene is integrated at its endogenous genomic locus, transcriptional promoters must be included within the vector to allow sufficient expression. Often, lineage or tissue-specific promoter and enhancer elements are used to limit expression to a particular cell lineage derived from a target cell population.[27-29] For instance, hemoglobin gene regulatory sequences are required to drive transgene expression specifically in erythroid cells for genetic correction of globin disorders. This process of transcriptional targeting does not obviate the need for transductionally targeted vectors. Instead, its use will likely be most beneficial in combination with transductional targeting by providing an additional safety feature to protect normal tissues from collateral damage that can occur when toxic transgenes are inaccurately delivered.

In other situations, constitutive control elements that can drive transcription continuously in most cell types can be used. Genetic control elements that are inducible, or turned on by some exogenous manipulation such as the administration of an antibiotic, can be included in gene transfer vectors.[30,31] Endogenous cellular factors may shut off expression of transferred genes in some situations.[32,33] These factors have not been fully elucidated and vary from vector to vector. Silencing of transferred genes via methylation of vector sequences is one possible mechanism.[34]

Genotoxicity and Insertional Mutagenesis

As discussed in sections below, several HSC gene therapy trials have reported serious adverse events resulting from the genetic intervention. In affected patients, leukemia was triggered by insertional mutagenesis, that is, integration of retroviral vectors into chromosomal DNA of HSCs within or near genes that favor clonal competition, such as proto-oncogenes or tumor suppressor genes. In other patients, there was clear evidence of genotoxicity, indicated by numerous common integrations sites that were detected near such growth-promoting genes. However, these individuals did not develop leukemia or other cancers. The disease background appears to be a crucial factor in the leukemogenic potential of gene therapy. Thus, all insertional mutagenesis events are associated with genotoxicity, but not all genotoxic events lead to insertional mutagenesis.

GENE DELIVERY SYSTEMS IN HSCs

Nonviral Vectors

Use of purified transgene DNA with the necessary control sequences is the simplest approach to gene transfer.[21,35] These nonviral methods of gene delivery have been classified conceptually into physical delivery methods, chemical approaches, transposon, and episomal self-replicating systems (Figure 72.1).

Physical Delivery Methods

Direct DNA microinjection into individual cells is the least complex physical delivery method. However, it is restricted by the inability to inject sufficient HSCs for clinical applications. Electroporation, a technique in which an electrical field is applied to cells to increase the permeability of their membrane, is the most utilized physical approach, but its high toxicity in primary HSCs has limited its use. More recently, an electroporation platform that delivers more tailored electrical pulses has shown high-performance delivery of proteins, RNA, and small size DNA in HSCs with less toxicity. Namely, it has demonstrated benefits in genome-editing studies by delivering macromolecules (proteins, RNA, DNA oligonucleotides) with high efficiency and reduced toxicity.

Other physical approaches can introduce naked DNA into cells or tissues. Biolistic gene guns involve bombardment of the cell membrane with gold microparticles complexed to DNA.[36-40] Jet injection technology is based on jets of high velocity to introduce DNA in vivo by penetration of the skin and underlying tissues, such as tumors. Ultrasound exposure has also been shown to increase plasmid transfection efficiency in vitro via sonoporation, an acoustic-based process whereby short-lived pores are formed in the plasma membrane to facilitate DNA entry.

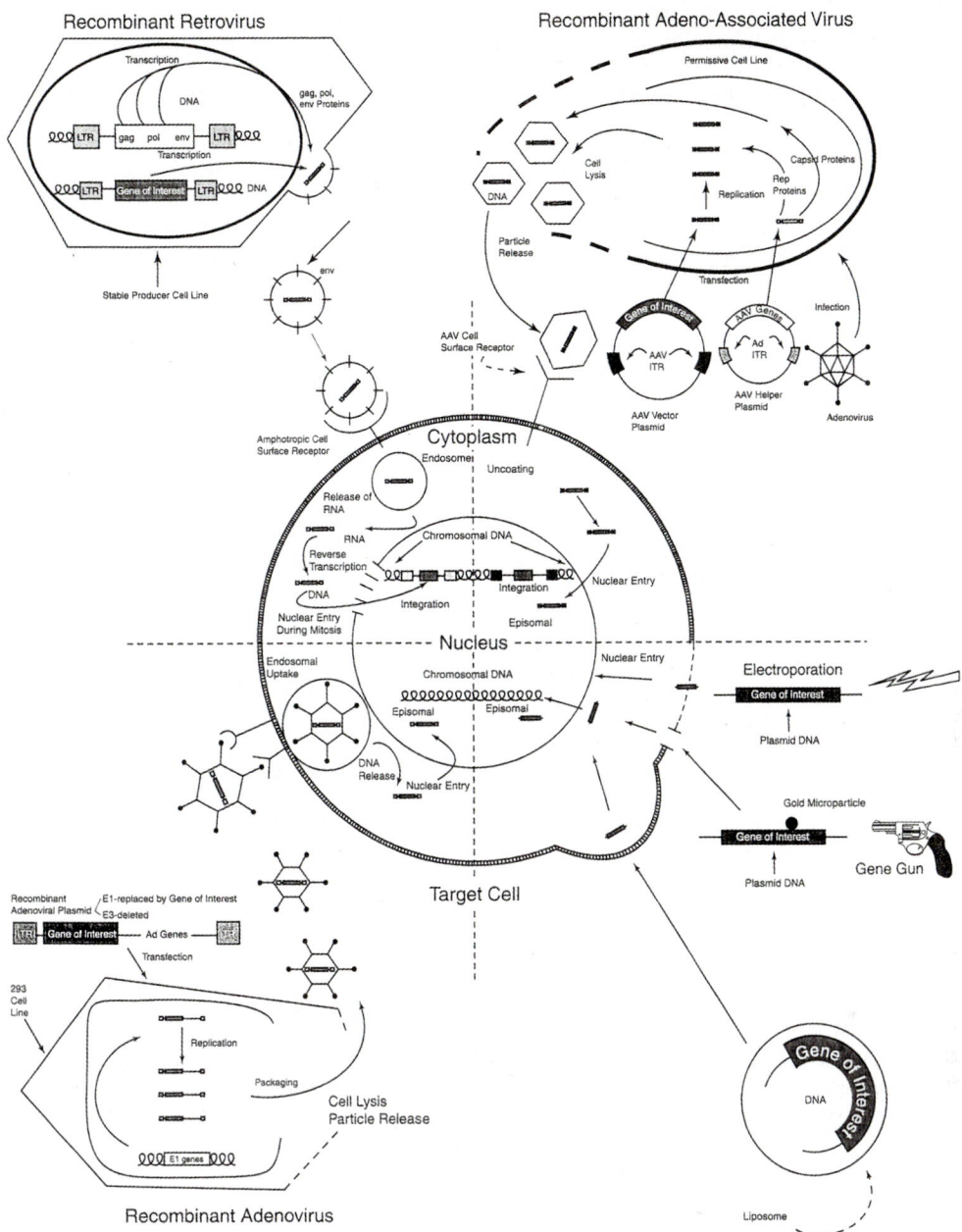

FIGURE 72.1 Schematic representation of transduction of a generic target cell by the four major gene transfer vector systems. The same "gene of interest" is shown being transferred with each vector. AAV, adeno-associated virus; Ad, adenovirus; ITR, inverted terminal repeat; LTR, long terminal repeat.

Chemical Delivery Methods

Chemical methods have also been explored for delivering large fragments of DNA into cells. Liposomes, composed of phospholipid bilayers enclosing an aqueous space loaded with DNA, can directly fuse with the plasma membrane, releasing DNA into the cytoplasm.[41-44] The development of cationic liposomes has improved cellular uptake of plasmid DNA and has circumvented cytoplasmic degradation.[45,46] In aqueous solution, these positively charged liposomes bind with up to 100% of negatively charged DNA without size restrictions and can deliver DNA to the cell nucleus, albeit inefficiently, where it remains primarily episomal.[47] If administered in vivo, liposomes demonstrate no target cell tropism and are rapidly cleared by the reticuloendothelial system. However, after intravenous injection of cationic liposomes, long-term low-level persistence of vector sequences in many murine organs has been demonstrated.[48,49]

Physical and chemical gene delivery methods offer, over their viral counterparts, the advantage of ease of preparation, decreased production costs, and they cannot generate potentially dangerous replication-competent infectious particles.[21,50] Transduction is also not dependent on target cell cycling, and no viral proteins are present to induce an antivector immune response. There are no size constraints. However, they have been hampered by a lower transduction efficiency than with viral systems. Also, most importantly, transgene integration is poor and persistent expression rare, limiting utility to situations requiring only transient transgene expression. Thus, the need for integration has precluded extensive investigation of these systems for hematopoietic applications requiring long-term expression. Recent advances in non–viral gene engineering may supersede these methods for gene-modified cell therapies, including transposons and episomal self-replicating systems.

Transposon Systems

The transposon system has attracted attention for its ability to efficiently transfer genes into a variety of cell types. DNA transposons are naturally occurring nonviral vehicles found in the genomes of lower organisms, capable of moving genetic material from place to place within the genome. Tc1-type transposons, initially found in nematodes and drosophila, can enter the genomes of vertebrates and humans. In the mid-1990s, a Tc1-like transposon was reconstructed from fish and coined the term *Sleeping Beauty* (SB) transposon. The SB system uses a transposon with an expression cassette replacing the transposase gene; the transposon can be mobilized when SB transposase is supplied *in trans* from a second plasmid.[51,52] With recent improvements to the SB system, including the development of optimized transposons and hyperactive SB variants, the vectorization of transposase, and transposon as mRNA and DNA minicircles to enhance performance and facilitate vector production, this approach may offer a practical nonviral vector for delivering genes into genomes of human cells, including HSCs.[53]

Episomal Self-Replicating Systems

Self-replicating *Epstein-Barr virus* (EBV)–based vector plasmids incorporate both the viral latent origin of replication (oriP) and the EBV nuclear antigen 1, which permit replication and retention in dividing cells. These vectors can also accommodate very large transgenes and regulatory sequences, which are also desirable characteristics for many applications. However, because EBV is a causative agent of infectious mononucleosis as well as various malignancies in human, it raises some concerns about safety.

Small circular vectors containing scaffold/matrix attachment regions (S/MARs) have also been exploited for episomal replication. Incorporation of these S/MARs sequences in the vector plasmid allows attachment of episomal DNA into the nuclear matrix. This facilitates both stability and replication, and consequently the transgene persists with the cells.

Artificial chromosome vectors are also considered as potential gene transfer vectors. This approach is based on the assembly of DNA components to approximate normal chromosomes that can be transferred to daughter cells. Artificial chromosomes can be constructed by the assembly of structural chromosomal elements, such as centromere, oriP, and telomeres, in a functional molecule (the "bottom-up" approach) or by size reduction of natural chromosomes (the "top-down" approach). These molecules offer the advantages of autonomous replication at 1 to 2 copies per cells and allow insertion of entire gene (exons and introns) with the proper regulatory elements. Because they are independent of other chromosomes, they are not expected to result in insertional mutagenesis. However, simple and efficient techniques to transfer these molecules into cells still have to be developed before their clinical potential can be explored.[54]

Viral Vectors

At present, all approved clinical gene therapy trials use viral vectors for delivery of therapeutic genes to HSCs. Modification of retroviruses represents the mainstay for the production replication-incompetent gene transfer vectors. The *Retroviridae* family of viruses has been divided into three subfamilies, primarily based on pathogenicity: Oncovirinae (e.g., Moloney murine leukemia virus [MMLV]), Lentivirinae (e.g., human immunodeficiency virus types 1 and 2 [HIV-1]), and Spumavirinae (e.g., human foamy virus). These retroviruses can infect mammalian cells via sophisticated and specific mechanisms for cell attachment, penetration, integration, survival, and replication. As detailed below, gene transfer vectors based on the natural life cycle of these highly infectious retroviruses offer several important advantages for delivering genes into various cell types, including HSCs, but also pose potential risks. Other viruses, including adenoviruses, adeno-associated viruses (AAVs), and herpesviruses, also have recognized advantages as gene transfer vectors but, unlike retroviruses, their inability to integrate into the host genome restrict potential applications in HSC gene therapy.

Gamma-Retroviral Vectors

Murine retroviruses of the *Oncovirinae* subfamily were the basis of the first practical viral vector system and are referred to as retroviral or γ-retroviral (γ-RV) vectors.[55-57] These retroviruses consist of two single strands of linear viral RNA bound to protein core and coated by a lipid envelope that is acquired from the plasma membrane of the infected cell upon viral release. The linear RNA genome can contain 2 to 9 kilobases (kb) of coding and regulatory sequences, flanked on each end by sequences termed long terminal repeats (LTRs) that permit integration into chromosomes and contain strong promoter/enhancer elements that normally drive expression of full-length viral RNA genomes, or via alternative splicing, the individual retroviral genes. These simple murine retroviruses contain only three genes necessary for viral replication and packaging: gag (group-specific antigens), encoding the viral core proteins; pol, encoding the viral DNA polymerase and endonuclease; and env, encoding the viral envelope glycoproteins.

Virus particles interact with a specific cell surface receptor via the *env* gene product. These receptors are large, widely expressed proteins involved in phosphate transport and other cellular homeostatic functions.[22] The *amphotropic receptor* is found on both rodent and primate cells and is the entry site for most murine retroviral vectors directed at human cells.[58-60] This leads to internalization of the virus particles and removal of the viral envelope protein (uncoating).

The virus core is then released within the cellular cytoplasm where its RNA is reverse transcribed to double-stranded (ds) DNA via the pol gene product. The dsDNA enters the nucleus of the infected cell and integrates into the host cell DNA, using the virally encoded endonuclease (pol gene). The LTR sequences allow random integration of the viral dsDNA into the host chromosomes. The integrated retroviral genome, or provirus, relies on the host cell's transcriptional machinery for expression of proviral genes and production of full-length viral RNA. The gag, pol, and env gene products are packaged along with the new viral RNA into viral particles, dependent on the presence of a packaging (ψ) sequence in the viral RNA, and viral particles are released from the cell via budding through the plasma membrane, without damaging the infected cell.

Recombinant retroviral vectors are constructed by removing the gag, pol, and env gene sequences from the viral nucleic acid backbone and replacing them with up to 7 to 8 kb of a gene or genes of interest, retaining only the LTRs and the packaging signal (ψ).[61] The resulting recombinant viral vector can integrate and express the gene or genes of interest, but cannot replicate and produce new retrovirus within the target cell, because of the lack of gag, pol, and env genes within its genome. Thus, it is termed replication defective. *Figure 72.1* diagrams the steps involved in making a retroviral vector. A packaging cell line is created by introducing two plasmids containing *gag-pol* and *env* sequences, respectively, but no ψ sequence into an immortalized cell line such as NIH3T3 or HEK293. The lack of the ψ sequence prevents these helper genes from being packaged into viral particles. A third plasmid containing the recombinant vector sequences (LTRs flanking the transgene or genes) is then introduced into these cells to create a producer cell line. Full-length vector RNA is transcribed from the vector plasmid sequences and packaged into viral particles using the gag, pol, and env proteins encoded by helper plasmid sequences. In this way, producer cell lines release helper-free replication-defective vector particles containing the recombinant genome into the culture supernatant. These particles contain the full-length vector RNA, consisting of the viral LTRs flanking the transgene or genes, and the env, gag, and pol proteins, but since they do not contain any actual gag, pol, or env viral gene sequences, no further infectious virus can be made after infection of the target cell.

The utility of retroviral vectors has been demonstrated in clinical trials. However, important drawbacks have limited their utility or required significant modifications to increase safety and efficacy. The potential for generation of replication-competent wild-type viruses within packaging cell lines is a significant safety concern.[20,62] This can theoretically occur through recombination between the vector and helper sequences in the packaging cell line, resulting in the transfer of an intact ψ packaging sequence into the helper plasmids containing the gag-pol and env genes. The presence of replication-competent virus could allow spread of vector and helper particles indiscriminately to nontarget cells in vivo, thus greatly increasing the risk of insertional mutagenesis by repeated infection of susceptible cell populations.[62,63] The absolute need for avoidance of replication competent viral particles in clinical vector preparations was inadvertently demonstrated when high-grade lymphomas occurred in rhesus monkeys transplanted with hematopoietic stem cells transduced with a vector preparation contaminated with high levels of replication-competent virus.[64] Several strategies have been used to prevent propagation of wild-type viruses able to replicate and spread in target cells. The chance of recombination between vector and helper genomes is reduced by decreasing homology between vector and helper genomes, and separating each helper function onto independent plasmids within the packaging cells. These safety-modified packaging lines, such as PA317, PG13, or GPe86, have been used in multiple clinical trials without evidence of helper-virus contamination or in vivo productive infection. In addition, sensitive systems for detecting replication-competent virus have been developed and are part of regulatory requirements for all gene therapy clinical trials.[20,65-67] A number of investigators have used packaging cell lines derived from human instead of murine cells to make producer cell lines, in hopes that lower levels of endogenous retroviral sequences in human cells would also decrease recombination events and thus replication-competent viral contamination.[68,69]

Even in the absence of wild-type virus, an important shortcoming of retroviral-based vectors, well illustrated in the French trial of gene therapy for X-linked severe combined immunodeficiency (SCID-X1), relates to the risk of insertion of replication-defective viral vectors into genomic sites capable of contributing to transformation. This event and the resulting reassessment of the risks of gene therapy using integrating vectors are reviewed in detail below. Additional shortcomings of retroviral vectors include limited space available in a viral particle for new genetic material and density of amphotropic receptors on certain target cell types too low to allow efficient transduction.[70] Thus, redirection of receptor specificity via pseudotyping with alternative envelope proteins is often required.

Requirement for active and rapid cell division is another important drawback of MMLV-based gene transfer vectors for use in quiescent HSC targets.[71] Active growth stimulation ex vivo by three or more cytokines for 3 to 4 days is required to coax HSCs in the S phase of the cell cycle and allow vectors to enter the nucleus and stably integrate into the host genome. Vector particles are unstable and degrade quickly in solution or within cells if cell division allowing nuclear entry and integration does not occur. While stimulation of early hematopoietic cells improves gene transfer efficiency, it may have detrimental effects by precipitating terminal differentiation or inhibiting homing and engraftment. Hematopoietic stem cells in G2/S/M phase of the cell cycle engraft poorly compared to cells in G0 and G1. This difficulty has focused interest on the development of lentiviral (LV) vectors, which can transduce nondividing cells without prolonged ex vivo stimulation.

Lentiviral Vectors

Unlike vectors based on standard retroviruses, LV vectors harbor a preintegration complex that appears more stable and able to cross an intact nuclear membrane, thus allowing transduction of nondividing cells such as hematopoietic stem cells. However, it is also generally agreed that cells must exit G0 and enter G1 for efficient transduction by HIV-1 based vectors. Other features of HIV-based vectors have also stimulated interest. Specifically, the superior faithful delivery of non-rearranged genes with complex regulatory elements has facilitated the long-awaited delivery of the human β-globin gene along with large portions of the complex locus control region (LCR).[72]

Similar to retroviral vectors, relatively high-titer vectors can be produced with a packaging cell line created by transient transfection of multiple helper plasmids (gag-pol, env, and the regulatory proteins rev-tat) and a vector containing the gene of interest into an immortalized cell line. For clinical applications, vectors must be produced, concentrated, and purified, usually by tangential flow filtration and ultracentrifugation, under current good manufacturing practices in certified laboratories. Because of safety concerns regarding recombination with endogenous HIV, a safety or "self-inactivating (SIN)" feature was incorporated in these vectors by eliminating a portion of the 3′-LTR, which on proviral integration replaces and thus inactivates the 5′-LTR.[73] For these SIN vectors, the efficiency of transgene expression is highly dependent on the addition of a ubiquitous internal promoters, such as the murine stem cell virus, the human elongation factor-1α, human phosphoglycerate kinase (PGK), spleen focus-forming virus (SFFV), gibbon-ape leukemia virus (GALV), or the hybrid chicken actin promoter containing the CMV enhancer region (CAG).[74-76]

Wild-type HIV-1 virions infect cells that express the CD4 receptor and an appropriate coreceptor. Expansion of the cellular tropism of HIV-1–based vectors has been accomplished by pseudotyping.[77] The MMLV amphotropic envelope used in most clinical gene therapy trials employing standard retroviral vectors was also chosen in early experiments with HIV-derived vectors.[75] However, its receptor, Pit-2, is only present at very low levels on HSCs, correlating with the low efficiency of LV transduction in this cell type.[70] Screening of an extensive panel of pseudotyped MMLV-based vectors using animal models established the superiority of the *GALV*, the cat endogenous retroviral glycoprotein (*RD114*), and the vesicular stomatitis virus-G protein (*VSV-G*) for the transduction of HSCs.[78-81] However, pseudotyping of LV vectors with alternate envelope proteins, namely GALV and RD114, has proven more difficult due to refractory residues within the cytoplasmic tail of both envelopes that limits their cleavage by LV proteases. To improve the LV packaging efficiency of GALV and RD114, chimeras of each envelope have been constructed by replacing the tail region of GALV and RD114 with the corresponding region from MMLV. The resulting chimeras, GALV-TR and RD114-TR, have been shown to pseudotype LV vectors with increased efficiency.[82-84]

In contrast to native GALV and RD114, VSV-G is efficiently incorporated in HIV-1 virions. VSV-G pseudotyping confers high vector particle stability, allowing for repeated freeze-thaw cycles and concentration by ultracentrifugation to titers exceeding 10^9 particles/mL.[24,75,85] Pseudotypes based on VSV-G have broad tropism long thought to be conferred by interaction with phosphatidylserine (PS), a ubiquitous cellular lipid, but the role of PS as a cell "receptor" for VSV-G particles has been refuted.[86] When directly compared to amphotropic or RD114-pseudotyped LV vectors using preclinical assays, vectors bearing the VSV-G envelope protein showed higher efficiency of transduction in human repopulating cells.[87] Toxicity of the VSV-G protein to cells in which it is expressed is perhaps the most significant shortcoming of this envelope protein. However, success has been obtained in deriving a stable packaging cell line by expressing VSV-G from a tetracycline-inducible promoter and this methodology has been used clinically.[88-90]

Envelope proteins made chimeric by the addition of a ligand, such as the early-acting cytokines stem cell factor (SCF) and thrombopoietin (TPO), have been explored as a mechanism for specifically targeting LV vectors to primitive hematopoietic cells expressing the SCF receptor *c-kit*. These vectors could be used for in vivo targeted gene delivery to HSCs, eliminating the risk of inducing cell differentiation and loss of the homing/engraftment potential of these cells as observed in ex vivo–targeted HSC gene delivery approaches. The selective transduction of HSCs by VSV-G/TPO/SCF–displaying vectors was demonstrated by their capacity to promote selective transduction of human long-term repopulating HSCs in an immuno-deficient murine model.[91] However, the fusion glycoprotein VSV-G in VSV-G/TPO/SCF–codisplaying LV vectors is sensitive to human immune/complement system, rendering these vectors unsuited for in vivo gene deliver.[84] Recently, complement-resistant vectors capable of specifically targeting the very rare immature progenitor cells in an immuno-deficient murine model were produced by substituting VSV-G for the complement-resistant glycoprotein mutant RD114-TR.[92] Completely obviating ex vivo manipulation of HSCs may be of particular interest for gene therapy of BM failure (BMF) syndromes for which the number of stem cells is limited. This approach has not yet been utilized in clinical settings.

Foamy Viral Vectors

Vectors based on FV represent an alternative approach for the genetic manipulation of HSCs. Unlike retroviral and LV vectors, FV backbone includes insulator sequences that remarkably reduce genotoxic potential, as shown in immortalization assays even when strong viral promoter-enhancers (e.g., SFFV) were used.[93] Hence, FV are considered ideal for situations where high transgene expression, necessitating strong promoters, is required for a therapeutic effect, with minimal risk of activating growth-promoting genes nearby the sites of integration. In comparative studies of integration site patterns in CD34+ cells, FV also had a safer integration profile than retroviral and LV vectors, with no preferences to integrate into genes.[94-97] In addition, unlike other retroviruses, wild-type FV are nonpathogenic in humans,[98,99] they include a large packaging capacity (up to 12 kb), and have a broad host and cell-type tropism.[100] Foamy viruses are cell cycle dependent for stable integration into the host genome. However, an interesting feature of foamy virus biology that clearly distinguishes foamy viruses from other Retroviridae is the occurrence of reverse transcription within the maturing foamy virus capsid, most likely prior to egress.[101-103] This replicative feature means that a certain percentage of packaged foamy virus vector genomes are competent for DNA integration upon transduction, thus dramatically shortening the necessary exposure time of target cells to vector, as well as the overall duration of ex vivo culture. This is significant as it allows the transduction of freshly thawed HSCs in the absence of pre stimulation and prolonged culture in the presence of vector, cellular manipulations that can decrease the total number of repopulating HSCs.[104]

A method for the production of helper free vectors stocks has been described[105] and third-generation vectors have been developed for preclinical applications using processes similar to those described above for other retroviruses. For instance, FV vectors were employed to phenotypically correct CD18 integrin deficiency in a canine model of leukocyte adhesion deficiency (LAD),[94] gp91phox deficiency in a mouse model of X-chronic granulomatous disease (CGD),[106] and hemolytic anemia in a canine model of pyruvate kinase deficiency.[107] However, major obstacles for scale-up of FV vector production and purification, including the limited stability of FV vectors in the absence of serum complicating subsequent purification steps, their sensitivity of shear forces, and the necessity to freeze in dimethyl sulfoxide have precluded large-scale manufacturing deeded for clinical application.

Adenoviral Vectors

Adenoviruses are nonenveloped double-stranded large DNA viruses.[108] The linear adenovirus genome contains 36 kb with an inverted terminal repeat (ITR) of 100 to 165 base pairs at each terminus. A set of early genes encode for regulatory proteins that serve to initiate cell proliferation, DNA replication, and downmodulation of host immune defenses, while the late genes encode for structural proteins. Adenovirus readily crosses the plasma membrane of many cell types, whether replicating or not, via receptor-mediated endocytosis[109] through the receptor, common to two distinct viral pathogens, coxsackie B and adenovirus 2 and 5, termed the coxsackie and adenovirus receptor.[110] Adenovirus escapes the endosome by altering the pH and then enters the nucleus where it remains as a linear episome (*Figure 72.1*). In permissive cells, adenovirus replicates and then enters a lytic cycle, destroying the host cell and releasing daughter viral particles. At least 57 human adenovirus serotypes have been identified which are further divided into subgroups A-G, based on similarities in tropism. Most serotypes are known to cause mild respiratory, gastrointestinal, and conjunctival infections in immunocompetent humans; no associated malignancies in humans have been reported, although some serotypes can transform cells in culture. The human embryonic kidney cell line HEK293 was, in fact, immortalized by transfection of kidney cells with sheared adenovirus serotype 5 DNA; the E1 gene that is integrated into the cellular genomic DNA is apparently responsible for the immortalization of the cell line.

Recombinant adenovirus vectors have been engineered from adenovirus (usually serotype 5) by the removal of the E1 and E3 genes (regulating replication and immune recognition) and replacement by the gene or genes of interest. They can accept relatively large foreign nuclei acid inserts, with a theoretical limit established at 7 to 8 kb.[111-115] High-titer adenovirus vectors, up to 10^{13} plaque-forming units per mL, can be reliably packaged through the use of a HEK293 cell line, which provide the helper or replication E1 genes. Adenoviruses show considerable stability and are thus amenable to subsequent purification and concentration procedures. The final product is a replication defective adenovirus vector which is free of helper or wild type virus that can efficiently transduce both dividing and nondividing cells.[113] These vectors do not integrate into the target cell genome, avoiding insertional mutagenesis and resulting in only transient transgene expression in proliferative tissues. Because of the tropism of adenovirus for epithelial cells, these vectors were initially investigated for the treatment of pulmonary diseases and diseases in which liver gene transfer is desirable.[116,117]

Transient transgene expression may also result from host cellular and humoral immune responses directed at either transgene-encoded antigens or adenovirus proteins expressed from the large portions of the adenovirus genome retained in these vectors.[118,119] Another concern is inflammation resulting from in vivo transduction of certain cell types, especially airway epithelium.[120] In vivo use may also be compromised by pre-existing or new antiviral neutralizing antibodies, limiting the efficacy of repeated dosing, which may be required for applications directed at mitotic tissues.[121] Gutless adenoviral vectors, in which essentially all viral genes are removed, were developed to circumvent antiadenoviral immunity. Unfortunately, although these vectors have little except the capsid proteins to mark themselves as foreign, there is evidence that they can trigger innate immunity by recognition through the toll-like receptor 9 pathway in target cells.[122] Further technical issues that are important include the decreased efficiency of vector production as more viral genes are deleted, since these functions need to be provided by accessory plasmids through transfection of vector producing cells. Hence, these highly deleted vectors are often called "helper-dependent." Specific dosage schedules (e.g., neonatal or embryonic exposure) or coadministration of immune modulators such as cyclosporine or IL12 may also prevent sensitization.[123-127]

Another strategy being explored is use of different vectors based on adenovirus serotypes other than adenovirus 5. One survey of unusual group B and group D adenovirus serotypes that might be considered for use as HIV vaccines indicates that in a target population in sub-Saharan Africa the existing immunity to adenovirus serotypes 11, 35, and 50 from group B and adenovirus serotypes 26, 48, and 49 from group D are substantially less than that of the commonly studied adenovirus 5 serotype from group C.[128] By employing alternatives to adenovirus 5, it might be possible to get around the barrier of pre-existing antivector antibodies for vaccination efforts. Further, it might be possible to alternate the vector type with subsequent vaccinations to thwart neutralizing antiadenovirus immunity to the vaccine vector. Recently, investigators developing HIV vaccination strategies have reported an adenovirus 41 serotype vector that can express HIV envelope protein.[129] The adenovirus 41 serotype virus is an enterotropic pathogen that causes diarrhea in its wild-type form; the use of a gene transfer vector with tropism for a mucosal surface may present advantages for vaccination against HIV, a pathogen that is normally encountered by the host in the mucosa.

The fact that most adenoviral gene transfer results in transient transgene expression (in contrast to retroviral-mediated gene transfer) has hampered their clinical use for HSC disorders. They have been investigated for disorders not requiring permanent expression of a missing protein, such as hemophilia, ornithine transcarbamoylase (OTC)-deficiency, or alpha-1-antitrypsin inhibitor deficiency, and cystic fibrosis.[130-132] In the latter application, despite the demonstration that airway cells could be transduced with these vectors in vivo with correction of the chloride transport defect, clinical utility has been precluded by the harmful immune and inflammatory responses noted above.

The most dramatic demonstration of immune response to these vectors came with the tragic death of an 18-year-old subject with relatively mild manifestations of OTC deficiency who volunteered for a Phase I dose escalation gene therapy trial and received a catheter-directed infusion of a high dose of an adenoviral vector encoding the corrective gene into the hepatic artery. This fatal adverse event was mediated in a large part by the "cytokine storm" and resultant systemic immune response that led to widespread capillary leak multiorgan failure.[133] Subsequently, many clinical gene therapy trials were temporarily put on hold and the maximum doses of adenovirus (or other) vectors to be given to humans were scaled back as a precautionary measure. Furthermore, a number of issues with respect to the pace of clinical gene therapy trials, the informed consent process, subject eligibility, reporting of adverse events, and oversight of clinical gene therapy trials were raised, and measures to increase the protection of research subjects were uniformly instituted across all gene therapy trials.[134,135] The active immune response induced by adenoviral vectors is also being explored as a possible advantage for adenovirus vectors when they are used to transduce tumor cells with cytokines or other immune modulators for tumor vaccine protocols.[136-138]

Adeno-Associated Virus Vectors

AAVs are small non–enveloped single-stranded DNA (ssDNA) viruses in the parvovirus family, dependovirus subfamily, that require a helper virus (typically a double-stranded DNA virus such as adenovirus or herpes simplex virus) for production of new viral particles.[139-141] The linear AAV genome is approximately 4.7 kb long and consists of two homologous ITRs of 145 bp flanking two groups of genes: the rep or nonstructural genes and the cap or structural genes. There are at least eight naturally occurring serotypes of AAV that differ mainly on the basis of their external capsid proteins. AAV-2 is the best characterized serotype. AAV-2 enters host cells primarily through interaction with the heparin sulfate proteoglycan protein on the cell surface, and by interaction with the $\alpha_V\beta5$ integrin and fibroblast growth factor receptor proteins.[142,143] AAV has oncoprotective and HIV-suppressive properties, and is not known to cause disease in humans or other animals.[144-146] Prior infection with AAV-2 in humans is common: seroepidemiological studies demonstrate that 80% of the adult population has antibodies.[140,147]

After cell entry mediated by the capsid protein, wild-type AAV integrates within the host chromosome.[148] Integration of multiple copies in tandem occurs in a site-specific manner within a relatively small area on chromosome 19; this site specificity appears to require rep protein.[149,150] Specifics of replication and integration are less well understood than for retroviruses.

Recombinant AAV (rAAV) vector DNA contains the AAV ITRs flanking a gene of interest replacing the rep and cap genes (*Figure 72.1*). This plasmid is introduced into a cell line permissive for adenovirus, along with a helper plasmid containing the AAV rep and cap genes but no ITRs. Upon exposure to adenovirus or transfection with adenovirus genes such as E4 (particularly open reading frame 6), the cell line packages the recombinant vector sequences using the rep and cap gene products produced by the helper plasmid, and recombinant vector particles are released as the producer cells lyse.[151-155] rAAV vectors have size constraints: vector sequences longer than 115% of the wild-type length are not packaged or encapsidated efficiently. Very high titers of rAAV particles can be produced, but often a significant percentage of capsids are empty or otherwise defective.

The need for replication-competent adenovirus during AAV vector production has complicated the manufacturing process, since the adenovirus must be inactivated or (preferably) removed before use. However, independent reports have described that introducing only the specific adenovirus genes necessary for AAV replication into producer cell lines reconstitutes the adenovirus helper functions and rendered the cell permissive for AAV production, avoiding live adenovirus.[156-158] The inability to harvest AAV vector without actual lysis and death of the producer cells also complicates production of pure and defined vector preparations. Generation of stable packaging cell lines is also hindered because the AAV rep gene product harms most cell types; but recently producer cell lines expressing rep from an inducible promoter have been isolated.[159,160] Another approach to avoid the issue of helper virus contamination is to transfect cells with multiple plasmids that separately encode the desired transgene nucleic acid as well as the structural and replication proteins.[161,162] An approach for large-scale production of AAV in insect cells (sf9) has been described.[163] Similar to rAAV production in mammalian cells, insect cells require both cis and trans factors from AAV for replication, packaging, and particle formation. These factors are provided by three baculovirus (BV) constructs including Bac-VP, Bac-Rep, and Bac-GOI encoding for capsid proteins, replication proteins, and the gene of interest, respectively. rAAV produced via the BV system has been administered in a Phase II human clinical trial for the treatment of lipoprotein lipase deficiency.[164]

Despite a great deal of initial enthusiasm for the use of AAV as a clinical gene transfer vector, more recent data suggest that integration of the recombinant vectors into target cell chromosomes is very inefficient, arguing against the use of AAV for most applications requiring stable integration in hematopoietic cells and their progeny.[155,165,166] Several laboratories have reported high transduction efficiency of both human and murine hematopoietic progenitors, as assayed by PCR or transgene expression analysis on individual colony-forming cell (CFC).[166-168] These are difficult to interpret, however, given the stability of the AAV vector DNA and the very high efficiency of transient expression of transgenes for days to weeks without integration.[165,167,168] Site-specific integration in chromosome 19, very desirable to avoid random insertional mutagenesis, does not occur with the rAAV vectors, presumably due to lack of rep protein in the vector particle.[166] Many cell types can be efficiently transduced, including nondividing cells such as neurons, but integration and increased efficiency of transduction still appear to depend on cell division or other DNA-disrupting events, although this conclusion is very controversial.[169-173]

Recently, there has been a great deal of interest in use of vectors based on serotypes other than AAV-2, especially AAV-6, considered the most efficient serotype for HSC transduction, as well as AAV-8 and AAV-9. Use of AAV-6 has gained popularity recently by facilitating robust delivery of essential CRISPR genome-editing components in HSCs. It is possible that a number of other parvoviruses can be developed as vectors, including AAV-3, nonpathogenic strains of B19, or novel autonomous parvoviruses isolated from nonhuman primates or other animal species.[174-176] These viruses are similar to AAV, but some, such as B19, never integrate. Self-complimentary AAV vectors based upon serotypes with high efficiency delivery to liver cells have been utilized recently to deliver factor IX as a potential treatment for hemophilia B in the canine model with correction of the bleeding abnormalities.[177,178] These results supported the first successful clinical trials in humans.[179]

Other Vectors

Herpes viruses are large DNA viruses with marked neurotropism, generating intense interest in their potential as vectors targeted at the nervous system.[180-183] They can accommodate very large DNA sequences (up to 30 kb). More recently, these vectors have been reported to transduce some types of hematopoietic cells, including monocytes, leukemic blasts, and progenitor cells.[184,185] However, these vectors result in only transient expression in dividing cells, and cause cytotoxicity, limiting clinical utility, at least for hematologic applications.

Vaccinia virus, a large DNA virus that replicates cytoplasmically, has also been considered for gene therapy applications.[186,187] It can accommodate very large transgenes (up to 30 kb) and expresses these genes at very high levels, but expression is transient, and production of replication-incompetent vectors has not yet been possible. Very high immunogenicity limits most clinical applications, but may be advantageous for in vivo vaccination with vaccinia-transduced tumor cells.[187-190]

BV, specifically *Autographa californica* multiple nucleopolyhedrovirus, is a large dsDNA virus recently proposed as a potential therapeutic vector.[191] Vectors based on BV offer advantages including a large packaging capacity of inserts at least 38 kb in size, a nonreplicating, nonintegrating life cycle in mammalian cells and, importantly, wild-type BV has not been associated with disease in humans. BV can transduce many immortalized cell lines,[192] and its potential for the delivery of large donor DNA and gene editing tools is under evaluation for HSC gene therapy applications.

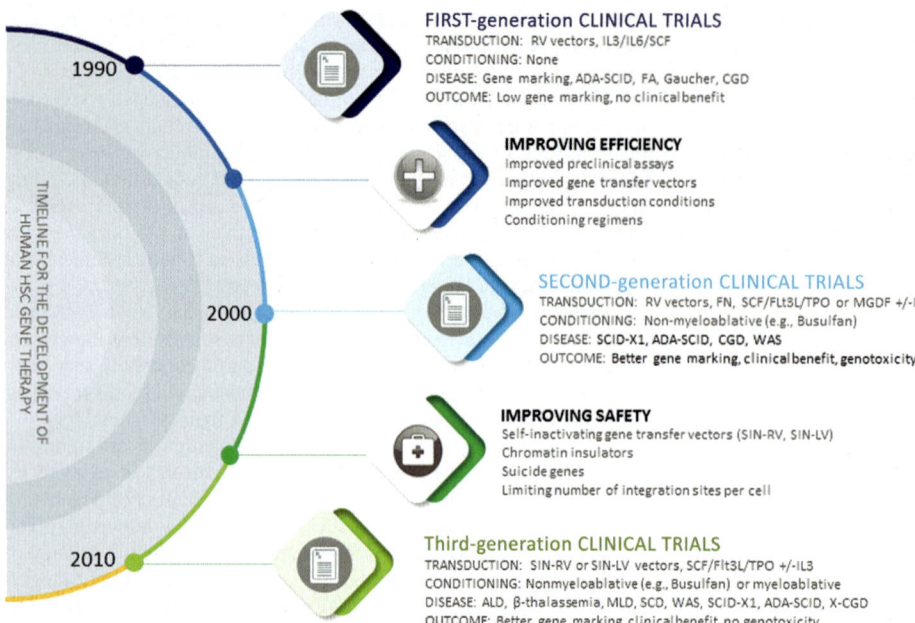

FIGURE 72.2 Timeline for the development of human gene therapy protocols targeting hematopoietic stem cells (HSCs). The main phases in the evolution of HSC gene therapy clinical trials are ordered chronologically. The principal features defining each phase are outlined. ADA, adenosine deaminase; ALD, adrenoleukodystrophy; BM, bone marrow; CB, cord blood; CGD, chronic granulomatous disease; FA, Fanconi anemia; Flt3L, *fms*-related tyrosine kinase 3 ligand; FN, fibronectin; HIV, human immunodeficiency virus; IL3, interleukin 3; IL6, interleukin 6; LSK, Lin⁻, Sca1⁺, Kit⁺; LV, lentivirus; MGDF, megakaryocyte growth and development factor; MLD, metachromatic leukodystrophy; MPB, mobilized peripheral blood; RV, retrovirus; SCF, stem cell factor; SCD, sickle cell disease; SCID, severe combined immunodeficiency disease; SIN, self-inactivating; TPO, thrombopoietin; WAS, Wiskott-Aldrich syndrome.

FIRST-GENERATION HSC GENE THERAPY TRIALS

The first-generation gene therapy clinical trials targeting HSCs began 3 decades ago (*Figure 72.2* and *Table 72.2*). Gene transfer protocols employed in these early trials were adapted from techniques developed in the mouse in the 1980s. Because long-term in vivo reconstitution after transplantation is the only relevant assay for HSCs, and experimental transplantation studies are impractical in humans, murine models were used to test gene transfer efficiency of marker genes (e.g., neomycin resistance gene, neo^R) in HSCs using retroviral vectors. Such in vivo reconstitution studies in the mouse have established that retroviral vectors can efficiently transfer and express new genes in primitive HSCs capable of reconstituting all lymphoid and myeloid tissues.[211-213]

Relevance of these data to human HSCs was tested using human in vitro CFC assays that detect committed progenitor cells and long-term bone marrow culture (LTBMC) assays that detect a cell capable of maintaining production of CFC for at least 5 weeks on a layer of stromal cells. Notwithstanding the fact that progenitors do not have the same biological properties as stem cells, investigators were initially encouraged when high gene transfer efficiency (up to 100%) was observed in these in vitro progenitor assays using gene transfer vectors and transduction conditions comparable to those employed in the mouse.[214-216]

The ability of retroviral vectors to permanently introduce marker genes into murine cells with lifelong repopulating ability led investigators to test whether this approach was feasible when clinically relevant genes were used. Genetic disorders with high morbidity and mortality and with no effective conventional treatments were considered prime candidates for preclinical evaluation. Demonstration of correction of glucocerebrosidase (GC) and adenosine deaminase (ADA) deficiency after retroviral vector-mediated gene transfer into progenitors from patients with Gaucher disease[217] and ADA-SCID,[218] respectively, provided even further impetus to regulators and investigators to initiate a first generation of human HSC gene transfer clinical trials, including gene marking studies and gene therapy trials with therapeutic intent.

Gene Marking Trials

The first human clinical gene transfer trials used retroviral vectors carrying nontherapeutic marker genes and were critical for establishing proof of principle and allaying safety concerns.[219,220] In these trials, retroviral vectors were used as tools for marking HSCs. Because of the largely random nature of integration of retroviruses, each cell in an infected population carries the integrated retrovirus at a different location. These unique, readily identifiable integrations sites provide a genetic tag to follow the progeny of HSCs after in vivo reconstitution of an ablated recipient.

Patients already undergoing autologous transplantation as therapy for an underlying malignancy received genetically marked hematopoietic stem and progenitor cells to determine whether reinfused tumor cells contribute to relapse after autologous transplantation and to establish if transduced HSCs could contribute to long-term hematopoietic reconstitution.[193-195,221,222] Genetically marked tumor cells were unequivocally demonstrated in several patients at the time of relapse, suggesting that the reinfused marrow had contributed to progression, and that investigation of therapeutic purging strategies was worthwhile. The presence of the marker gene was also followed in non–malignant hematopoietic cells. Gene-marked cells contributed for only 0.1% to 1% of the total BM but detection of the marker gene in T cells and B cells for as long as 18 months after transplantation was consistent with low-level transduction of primitive hematopoietic cells with multilineage capacity.

In a similar marking study, investigators determined that autologous BM used for transplantation in patients with chronic myelogenous leukemia (CML) following intensive therapy also contained cells that contributed to relapse.[196] Other gene marking trials involving patients with multiple myeloma,[197,199,201] breast cancer,[197,199] follicular lymphoma,[200] and acute myeloid leukemia (AML)[198] failed to show stable levels of marked cells of more than 0.1% after transplantation with autologous gene marked grafts, contrasting with the high levels marking observed in preclinical mouse models. Though valuable in the early stages, the perceived level of risk related to retroviral-marking clinical trials was altered dramatically after the reports of leukemias in patients receiving retrovirus-mediated gene therapy (see subsequent sections below), and given the lack of any possible benefit to the patient related to use of marking vectors, this type of trial has been completely abandoned.

Gene Therapy Trials With Therapeutic Intent

Despite the low efficiencies of gene transfer into long-term repopulating HSCs achieved in early human marking trials, several phase I/II clinical trials investigating the transfer of potentially therapeutic genes were initiated (*Table 72.2*). Important information was obtained on both the safety and feasibility of stem cell engraftment without ablation, and although these initial trials were largely disappointing, there were glimmers of hope regarding clinical benefit.

Table 72.2. First-, Second-, and Third-Generation HSC Gene Therapy Clinical Trials

Reference	Indication	Gene	CD34+ Cells	Transduction			Outcome	
				Cytokines and FN	Duration (MOI)	Vector	Conditioning	Gene Marking (# Patients)	Insertional Mutagenesis (# Patients)

First-Generation HSC Gene Therapy Clinical Trials

Reference	Indication	Gene	CD34+ Cells	Cytokines and FN	Duration (MOI)	Vector	Conditioning	Gene Marking (# Patients)	Insertional Mutagenesis (# Patients)
193	Gene marking (AML)	neo^R	BM	No cytokines No FN	P: 0 h T: 6 h (MOI = 10)	γ-RV Ampho env MLV-LTR promoter	Busulfan Cyclophosphamide	Low long-term gene marking	No
194	Gene marking (AML, neuroblastoma)	neo^R	BM	No cytokines No FN	P: 0 h T: 6 h (MOI = 10)	γ-RV Ampho env MLV-LTR promoter	Bu/Cy (AML) Carboplatin/Etoposide (neuroblastoma)	Low long-term gene marking	No
195	Gene marking (Neuroblastoma)	neo^R	BM MNC	No cytokines No FN	P: 0 h T: 6 h (MOI = 10)	γ-RV Ampho env MLV-LTR promoter	Carboplatin Etoposide	Low long-term gene marking	No
196	Gene marking (CML)	neo^R	BM	No cytokines No FN	P: 0 h T: 6 h (MOI = 10)	γ-RV Ampho env MLV-LTR promoter	TBI Cyclophosphamide Etoposide	Low long-term gene marking	No
197	Gene marking (MM and BC)	neo^R	BM MPB	IL3, SCF +/− IL6 No FN	P: 0 h T: 72 h	γ-RV Ampho env MLV-LTR promoter	Melphalan/TBI (MM) or ICE chemotherapy (BC)	Low long-term gene marking	No
198	Gene marking (AML and ALL)	neo^R	BM	No cytokines No FN	P: 0 h T: 4 h	γ-RV Ampho env MLV-LTR promoter	Busulfan Cyclophosphamide	Low long-term gene marking	No
199	Gene marking (MM and BC)	neo^R	BM MPB	No cytokines +/− Stroma No FN	P: 0 h T: 6-72 h	γ-RV Ampho env MLV-LTR promoter	Melphalan/TBI (MM) or ICE chemotherapy (BC)	Low long-term gene marking	No
200	Gene marking (NHL)	neo^R	BM MPB	No cytokines No FN	P: 0 h T: 6 h (MOI = 10)	γ-RV Ampho env MLV-LTR promoter	TBI Cyclophosphamide Etoposide	Low long-term gene marking	No
201	Gene marking (MM)	neo^R	BM MPB	IL3, IL6, SCF, bFGF No FN	P: 0 h T: 12 h (MOI = 5)	γ-RV Ampho env MLV-LTR promoter	Melphalan	Low long-term gene marking	No
202	ADA-SCID	ADA	BM	Co-culture No cytokines No FN	P: 0 h T: 72 h	γ-RV Ampho env MLV-LTR promoter	No conditioning	Low long-term gene marking	No
203,204	ADA-SCID	ADA	CB	IL3, IL6, SCF FN	P: 0 h T: 72 h	γ-RV Ampho env MLV-LTR promoter	No conditioning	Low long-term gene marking	No
205	CGD	NCF1 (P47phox)	MPB	PIXY321, G-CSF No FN	P: 18 h T: 72 h	γ-RV Ampho env MLV-LTR promoter	No conditioning	Low long-term gene marking	No
206	Breast CA Ovarian CA Glioblastoma	MDR1	BM MPB	IL3, IL6, SCF FN	P: 48 h T: 24 h	γ-RV Ampho env MLV-LTR promoter	High dose chemotherapy	Low long-term gene marking	No

Ref	Disease	Source	Cytokines	Timing	Vector	Conditioning	Outcome	Adverse Events
207	Gaucher	BM, MPB	IL3, IL6, SCF, No FN	P: 0 h, T: 72 h	γ-RV, Ampho env, MLV-LTR promoter	No conditioning	Low long-term gene marking	No
208	HIV	BM	IL3, IL6, SCF, +/− FN	P: 0 h, T: 72 h	γ-RV, Ampho env, MLV-LTR promoter	No conditioning	Low long-term gene marking	No
209	Breast CA	BM, MPB	IL3, IL6, SCF, No FN	P: 0 h, T: 72 h	γ-RV, Ampho env, MLV-LTR promoter	ICE chemotherapy	Low long-term gene marking	No
210	FA	BM, MPB	IL3, IL6, SCF, No FN	P: 0 h, T: 72 h	γ-RV, Ampho env, MLV-LTR promoter	No conditioning	Low long-term gene marking	No

Second-Generation HSC Gene Therapy Clinical Trials

Ref	Disease	Source	Cytokines	Timing	Vector	Conditioning	Outcome	Adverse Events
395–397	SCID-X1	BM	SCF, Flt3L, MGDF, IL3, FN	P: 24 h, T: 72 h	γ-RV, Ampho env, MLV-LTR promoter	No conditioning	Correction of SCID-X1 (9/10)	T-ALL (4/9) LMO2, CCND2, BMI1 gene insertions[412,413,617]
374	Germ cell tumors	MPB	SCF, IL6 or SCF, MGDF, G-CSF, FN	P: 48 h, T: 48 h	γ-RV, Ampho env, HaMSV-LTR promoter	Etoposide 2250 mg/m², Carboplatin 2100 mg/m²	Low long-term gene marking (6/11)	No
404	ADA-SCID	BM	SCF, Flt3L, TPO, IL3, FN	P: 24 h, T: 72 h	γ-RV, Ampho env, MLV-LTR promoter	Busulfan 4 mg/Kg	Correction of ADA-SCID (2/2)	No
618,619	HIV (Phase I)	MPB	MGDF, SCF, +/− FN	P: 18 h, T: 72 h (MOI = 5)	γ-RV, Ampho env, MLV-LTR promoter	No conditioning	Low long-term gene marking (10/10)	No
398–400	SCID-X1	BM	SCF, Flt3L, TPO, IL3, FN	P: 40 h, T: 56 h	γ-RV, GALV env, MLV-LTR promoter	No conditioning	Correction of SCID-X1 (10/10)	T-ALL (1/10) LMO2 gene insertion[415]
402	SCID-X1	BM	SCF, Flt3L, MGDF, IL3, FN	P: 24 h, T: 72 h	γ-RV, Ampho env, MLV-LTR promoter	No conditioning	Failure to correct SCID-X1 in older patients (2/2)	No
424	X-CGD	MPB	SCF, Flt3L, TPO, IL3, FN	P: 36 h, T: 72 h	γ-RV, Ampho env, SFFV-LTR promoter	Busulfan 8 mg/Kg	Correction of X-CGD (2/2)	MDS (2/2) MDS1-EVI1, PRDM16, SETBP1 gene insertions[427,428]
406	ADA-SCID	BM	SCF, Flt3L, TPO, IL3, FN	P: 40 h, T: 56 h	γ-RV, GALV env, SFFV-LTR promoter	Melphalan 140 mg/m²	Correction of ADA-SCID (1/1)	No
401	SCID-X1	MPB	SCF, Flt3L, TPO, IL3, FN	P: 16 h, T: 96 h (MOI = 1–2)	γ-RV, GALV env, MLV-LTR promoter	No conditioning	Clinical improvement (3/3)	No

(Continued)

Table 72.2. First-, Second-, and Third-Generation HSC Gene Therapy Clinical Trials (Continued)

Reference	Indication	Gene	CD34+ Cells	Transduction Cytokines and FN	Transduction Duration (MOI)	Transduction Vector	Conditioning	Outcome Gene Marking (# Patients)	Outcome Insertional Mutagenesis (# Patients FN)
619,620	HIV (Phase II)	Anti-HIV1 ribozyme	MPB	MGDF, SCF FN	P: 36 h T: 48 h (MOI = 5)	γ-RV Ampho env MLV-LTR promoter	No conditioning	Lower HIV-1 viral load (10/10)	No
403	ADA-SCID	ADA	BM	SCF, Flt3L, TPO, IL3 FN	P: 24 h T: 72 h	γ-RV Ampho env MLV-LTR promoter	Busulfan 4 mg/Kg	Correction of ADA-SCID (9/10)	No
434,435	WAS	WAS	MPB	SCF, Flt3L, TPO, IL3 No FN	P: 48 h T: 48 h (MOI = 5)	γ-RV GALV env MPSV promoter	Busulfan 8 mg/Kg	Correction of WAS (9/10)	T-ALL (6/9) AML (1/9) LMO2 (T-ALL) and MN1 or MDS1 for AML + other gene insertions[435]
425	X-CGD	CYBB (gp91phox)	MPB	SCF, Flt3L, TPO, IL3 FN	P: 18 h T: 96 h (MOI = 2)	γ-RV Ampho env MLV-LTR promoter	Busulfan 10 mg/Kg	Long-term clinical benefits (2/3)	No
426	X-CGD	CYBB (gp91phox)	MPB	SCF, Flt3L, TPO, IL3 FN	P: 40 h T: 40 h (MOI = 1–2)	γ-RV Ampho env MLV-LTR promoter	Fludarabine 120 mg/m² Busulfan 1.6 mg/Kg	Short-term clinical benefit (2/2)	No
409	ADA-SCID	ADA	BM	SCF, Flt3L, TPO, IL3 FN	P: 40 h T: 56 h	γ-RV GALV env SFFV-LTR promoter	Melphalan 140 mg/Kg or Busulfan 4 mg/Kg	Correction ADA-SCID (4/6)	No

Third-Generation HSC Gene Therapy Clinical Trials

Reference	Indication	Gene	CD34+ Cells	Transduction Cytokines and FN	Transduction Duration (MOI)	Transduction Vector	Conditioning	Outcome Gene Marking (# Patients)	Outcome Insertional Mutagenesis (# Patients FN)
309	X-ALD	ABCD1	MPB	SCF, Flt3L, MGDF, IL3, FN	P: 19 h T: 17 h (MOI = 25)	SIN-HIV-1 VSV-G env MND promoter	Busulfan 16 mg/Kg Cyclophos 200 mg/Kg	Halt progression of X-ALD (2/2)	No
464	X-ALD	ABCD1	MPB	Not disclosed	Not disclosed	SIN-HIV-1 (Lenti-D) VSV-G env MND promoter	Busulfan ~16 mg/Kg Cyclophos 200 mg/Kg	Halt progression of X-ALD (15/17)	No
465	β-thalassemia	β-globin	BM	SCF, Flt3L, TPO, IL3 FN	P: 34 h T: 18 h	SIN-HIV-1 (HPV569) VSV-G env β-globin promoter β-LCR	Busulfan ~12.8 mg/Kg	Correction of β-thalassemia phenotype (1/1)	Clonal dominance HMGA2 insertion (1/1)
471	β-thalassemia	β-globin	MPB	Not disclosed	Not disclosed	SIN-HIV-1 (BB305) VSV-G env β-globin promoter β-LCR	Busulfan ~12.8 mg/Kg (PK-adjusted dose)	Correction/improved β-thalassemia phenotype (22/22)	No

Ref	Disease	Gene	Source	Cytokines	Transduction	Vector	Conditioning	Outcome	Adverse events
472	β-thalassemia	β-globin	MPB	Not disclosed	Not disclosed	SIN-HIV-1 (BB305) VSV-G env β-globin promoter β-LCR	Busulfan ~12.8 mg/Kg (PK-adjusted dose)	Correction/improved β-thalassemia phenotype (22/22)	No
474	β-thalassemia	β-globin	MPB	SCF, Flt3L, TPO, IL3	Not disclosed	SIN-HIV-1 (GLOBE) VSV-G env β-globin promoter β-LCR	Treosulfan-Thiotepa (PK-adjusted dose)	Correction/improved β-thalassemia phenotype (7/7)	No
475	β-thalassemia	β-globin	MPB	SCF, Flt3L, TPO, IL3	P: 18-24 h T: 36-48 h	SIN-HIV-1 (TNS9.3.55) VSV-G env β-globin promoter β-LCR	Busulfan Nonmyeloablative (PK-adjusted dose)	Improved β-thalassemia phenotype (4/4)	No
476	SCD	β-globin	BM	SCF, Flt3, TPO, FN	P: 24 h T: 24 h (MOI~80)	SIN-HIV-1 (BB305) VSV-G β-globin promoter β-LCR	Busulfan 12.8 mg/Kg	Correction/improved SCD phenotype (1/1)	No
477	SCD	β-globin	MPB	Not disclosed	Not disclosed	SIN-HIV-1 VSV-G β-globin promoter β-LCR	Busulfan Myeloablative (PK-adjusted dose)	Correction/improved SCD phenotype (group C) (25/25)	No Clonal dominance VAMP4 insertion (1/7 in group A)
484,485	MLD	ARSA	BM	SCF, Flt3, TPO, IL3 FN	P: 24 h T: 2 × 14 h (MOI = 100)	SIN-HIV-1 VSV-G hPGK promoter	Busulfan q6 h × 4 d (PK-adjusted dose)	Prevention or halt progression of MLD (8/9)	No
486	MLD	ARSA	BM MPB	Not disclosed	Not disclosed	SIN-HIV-1 VSV-G hPGK promoter	Busulfan Myeloablative (PK-adjusted dose)	Prevention or halt progression of MLD (26/29)	No
491	Hurler syndrome	IDUA	MPB	SCF, Flt3, TPO, IL3 FN	P: 22 h T: 14 h (MOI = 100)	SIN-HIV-1 VSV-G hPGK promoter	Busulfan, Fludarabine Rituximab Myeloablative (PK-adjusted dose)	Prevention or halt progression of Hurler (8/8)	No
496	Fabry disease	GLA	MPB	SCF, Flt3, TPO, IL3 FN	P: 24 h T: 2 × 14 h (MOI = 100)	SIN-HIV-1 VSV-G EF-1α promoter	Melphalan Nonmyeloablative	Correction/improved Fabry disease phenotype (0/5)	No
497	Moderate WAS (children)	WAS	BM MPB	SCF, Flt3, TPO, IL3 FN	P: 24 h T: 2 × 12 h (MOI = 100)	SIN-HIV-1 VSV-G WAS promoter	Fludarabine 60 mg/m² Busulfan 9.6 mg/Kg	Correction/improved WAS phenotype (3/3)	No
498,499	Severe WAS (children)	WAS	BM MPB	SCF, Flt3, TPO, IL3 FN	P: 24 h T: 2 × 18 h	SIN-HIV-1 VSV-G WAS promoter	Fludarabine 120 mg/m² Busulfan 12 mg/Kg ± Alemtuzumab	Correction/improved WAS phenotype (8/9)	No
500	Severe WAS (adult)	WAS	MPB	SCF, Flt3, TPO, IL3 FN	P: 17 h T: 2 × 17 h	SIN-HIV-1 VSV-G WAS promoter	Fludarabine 120 mg/m² Busulfan 9.6 mg/Kg	Correction/improved WAS phenotype (1/1)	No

(Continued)

Table 72.2. First-, Second-, and Third-Generation HSC Gene Therapy Clinical Trials (Continued)

Reference	Indication	Gene	CD34+ Cells	Transduction Cytokines and FN	Transduction Duration (MOI)	Transduction Vector	Conditioning	Outcome Gene Marking (# Patients)	Outcome Insertional Mutagenesis (# Patients)
503	SCID-X1	IL2Rγ	BM	SCF, Flt3L, MGDF, IL3 FN	P: 24 h T: 72 h	SIN-γ-RV Ampho EFS promoter	Busulfan (variable doses)	Correction/improved SCID-X1 phenotype (7/9)	No
88	SCID-X1	IL2Rγ	MPB	SCF, Flt3, TPO, IL3 FN	P: 16 h T: 2 × 7 h	SIN-HIV-1 VSV-G EF1α promoter	Busulfan 6 mg/Kg	Correction/improved SCID-X1 phenotype (5/5)	No
504	ADA-SCID	ADA	BM MPB	Not disclosed	Not disclosed	SIN-HIV-1 VSV-G EFS promoter	Busulfan 4 mg/Kg	Correction/improved ADA-SCID phenotype (49/50)	No
505	X-CGD	CYBB (gp91phox)	MPB	SCF, Flt3, TPO, IL3	P: 16 h T: 2 × 24 h	SIN-HIV-1 VSV-G CatG/Cfes promoter	Busulfan Myeloablative (PK-adjusted dose)	Correction/improved X-CGD phenotype (6/9)	No
506	FA	FANCA	MPB	SCF, Flt3, TPO, IL3, anti-TNFα, NAC, hypoxia FN	P: 8–10 h T: 12–14 h	SIN-HIV-1 VSV-G hPGK promoter	No conditioning	Correction/improved FA phenotype (4/4)	No

Abbreviations: ABCD1, ATP-binding cassette subfamily D, member 1; ADA, adenosine deaminase; ALD, adrenoleukodystrophy; ALL, acute lymphoblastic leukemia; AML, acute myelogenous leukemia; Ampho, amphotropic; ARSA, arylsulfatase; AUC, area under the curve; BC, breast cancer; bFGF, basic fibroblast growth factor; BM, bone marrow; BMI1, B lymphoma MLV insertion region 1 homolog; Bu, busulfan; CatG/Cfes, CTSG gene encoding cathepsin G and the FES gene encoding Cfes; CB, cord blood; CCND2, cyclin D2; CGD, chronic granulomatous disease; CA, cancer; CML, chronic myelogenous leukemia; Cy, cyclophosphamide; CYBB, cytochrome B β-chain; EF-1α, elongation factor-1α promoter; EFS, short form elongation factor-1α promoter; Env, envelope; EVI1, ecotropic virus integration site 1 protein homolog; FA, Fanconi anemia; FANCA, Fanconi anemia complementation group A; FANCC, Fanconi anemia complementation group C; Flt3L, fms-related tyrosine kinase 3 ligand; FN, fibronectin; GALV, gibbon-ape-leukemia-virus; GC, glucocerebrosidase; G-CSF, granulocyte-colony stimulating factor; GLA, α-galactosidase A; HaMSV, Harvey murine sarcoma virus; HIV, human immunodeficiency virus; HMGA2, high mobility group AT-hook 2; ICE, ifosfamide, carboplatin, etoposide; hPGK, human phosphoglycerate kinase; IDUA, α-L-iduronidase; IL2Rγ, interleukin 2 receptor γ chain; IL3, interleukin 3; IL6, interleukin 6; LCR, locus control region; LMO2, LIM domain only 2; LTR, long-terminal repeat; MDR1, multidrug resistance gene 1; MDS, myelodysplastic syndrome; MGDF, megakaryocyte growth and development factor; MLD, metachromatic leukodystrophy; MLV, murine leukemia virus; MM, multiple myeloma; MNC, mononuclear cells; MND, myeloproliferative sarcoma virus enhancer, negative control region deleted, dl587rev primer binding site substituted; MOI, multiplicity of infection; MPB, mobilized peripheral blood; MPSV, myeloproliferative sarcoma virus; NAC, N-acetylcysteine; neo^R, neomycin resistance; NCF1, neutrophil cytosolic factor 1; NHL, non-Hodgkin lymphoma; P, prestimulation; Phox, phagocyte oxidase; PK, pharmacokinetics; PRDM16, PR domain containing 16; RRED, rev-responsive element decoy; RV, retroviruses; SCD, sickle cell disease; SCF, stem cell factor; SCID, severe combined immunodeficiency disease; SETBP1, SET-binding protein 1; SFFV, spleen focus-forming virus; SIN, self-inactivating; T, transduction; T-ALL, T-lineage acute lymphoblastic leukemia; TBI, total body irradiation; TNFα, tumor necrosis factor-α; TPO, thrombopoietin; VSV-G, vesicular stomatitis virus-G protein; WAS, Wiskott-Aldrich syndrome.

Severe Combined Immunodeficiency Disease

SCID due to ADA deficiency has been a prototype target disease for gene therapy since the initial development of retroviral vectors.[223] When first tested in preclinical murine models, stable expression of functional human ADA was demonstrated in all hematopoietic lineages at levels near endogenous murine levels in reconstituted mouse transplants.[224-229] The efficiencies of gene transfer and ADA levels achieved in these preclinical models, together with the anticipated in vivo selective survival advantage of transduced T cells, were thought to be predictive of successful correction of lymphoid dysfunction in patients with ADA deficiency.[6]

Children with ADA-deficient SCID were the subjects of the first clinical trial utilizing a vector carrying a therapeutic gene directed at T-lymphocyte targets. HSCs would be theoretically preferable to T cells as gene correction targets in this and other immunodeficiency disorders, because of the potential for permanent and complete reconstitution of the T-cell repertoire. To address this hypothesis directly, two ADA-deficient children received autologous BM and mature lymphocytes transduced with two different retroviral vectors carrying the therapeutic ADA gene and the neo^R gene and then repeatedly reinfused without conditioning.[203] In the first year after initiation of these infusions, vector-containing T cells originating from the transduced T cells were observed, but with time, there was a shift to vector-containing T cells originating from transduced BM cells. The proportion of gene-corrected clonable T cells was 2% to 4%, and analysis of T-cell–receptor gene rearrangements indicated a wide repertoire of corrected clones. A surprisingly high number of marrow myeloid colonies resistant to neomycin were also reported, despite lack of conditioning, suggesting an in vivo selective advantage for gene-corrected cells of all lineages.

For genetic disorders diagnosed in utero, the use of UCB cells as targets for gene transduction represents an exciting alternative approach.[230,231] Cord blood contains greater numbers of primitive reconstituting cells with higher proliferative potential and increased susceptibility to retroviral transduction. Moreover, early treatment is crucial in diseases that progress to irreversible damage before a child is old enough to allow collection of MPB or BM cells.[232] Three infants diagnosed in utero with ADA deficiency allowed the testing of this concept, and CB was collected at the time of delivery. The cells were CD34 enriched and transduced with an ADA/neo^R retroviral vector and infused in the absence of conditioning.[204] Vector sequences were initially detected in circulating myeloid and lymphoid cells at low levels of <0.1% in all three children for >18 months. As expected, if corrected lymphocytes have an in vivo advantage, 4 years after the newborns were given infusions of transduced autologous CB CD34+ cells, the frequency of gene-containing T lymphocytes rose to 1% to 10%, whereas the frequencies of other hematopoietic and lymphoid cells containing the gene remained <0.1%. Cessation of polyethylene glycol–conjugated ADA enzyme replacement in one subject led to a decline in immune function, despite the persistence of gene-containing T lymphocytes. Thus, despite the long-term engraftment of transduced HSCs and selective accumulation of gene-containing T lymphocytes, this study indicated that improved gene transfer and expression were needed to attain a therapeutic effect.[203]

Fanconi Anemia

Fanconi anemia (FA) is another genetic disorder of the hematopoietic system evaluated as possible candidate for gene therapy. This congenital syndrome is characterized by BMF, physical anomalies, and an increased susceptibility to leukemias. Etiologically, loss-of-function mutations in any one of at least 23 genes critical for protection against genomic instability have been associated with FA. Cells from these patients are abnormally sensitive to chemically induced DNA cross-linking. Allogeneic HSC transplantation remains the only long-term treatment option for the hematologic manifestations of FA. The general hypersensitivity and poor tolerance to chemotherapy and radiation therapy remains the greatest challenge for the design and utilization of transplantation regimens for patients with FA. Reduced intensity conditioning regimens with the avoidance of alkylating agents and marked reduction of total body irradiation doses improved the rate of immediate toxicities and reduced graft failures. However, donor availability and long-term risk for secondary malignancies still remain significant problems for HSC transplantation as a curative treatment of FA-associated BMF.[233,234] Oxymetholone, danazol, or other androgens have been successfully used to stabilize or even improve FA-associated cytopenias. About half to two third of patients with FA will at least respond transiently to androgens, but side effects, particularly in young patients, often prevent prolonged therapy.[235-239]

With the cloning and sequencing of FA complementation groups, a genetic approach was investigated for this disorder.[240] Phenotypic correction of this abnormality in cells from one patient group was successful after transduction with viral vectors carrying the Fanconi complementation group C gene (*FANCC*).[241,242] An in vivo survival advantage for gene-corrected primitive cells and their progeny has made FA an attractive candidate disease for HSC gene therapy. Even a very low efficiency of transduction results in gradual in vivo expansion of corrected stem and progenitor cell populations. A clinical trial testing this hypothesis using G-CSF-MPB CD34+ cells as targets yielded disappointing results, in part because of the very poor mobilization in these subjects,[243] yet engraftment with corrected progenitor cells was demonstrated.[210] However, classic ex vivo HSC gene therapy approaches are often viewed as impractical for patients with FA and other inherited BMF disorders because sufficient autologous HSCs for genetic modification are unavailable in these disorders. Instead, the appealing concept of generating iPSCs from an individual patient, correcting the genetic defect and differentiating the disease-free iPSCs into a theoretically infinite supply of transplantable autologous HSCs, may offer an ideal new therapeutic option for these disorders, but multiple obstacles still thwart clinical translation of this approach.

Gaucher Disease

Gaucher disease is an inherited deficiency of the lysosomal enzyme GC and the associated accumulation of glucocerebroside in the lysosomes of macrophages results in multisystem damage, including hepatosplenomegaly, gradual replacement of BM, skeletal deterioration, and neuropathology in some cases of Gaucher disease. Correction of enzyme deficiency in macrophages by HSC gene therapy has been considered an attractive therapeutic option for these patients. Mouse BM transplant models have been invaluable for initial evaluation of retrovirus-based gene transfer vectors developed for Gaucher disease.[244-249] These studies established the feasibility of efficient transfer of the GC gene to normal mouse HSCs and long-term expression in their progeny after reconstitution, strengthening the rationale for gene therapy as a treatment option for Gaucher disease.

Modeling preclinical murine transplantation models, gene therapy was attempted for Gaucher disease.[207] Similar to previous gene therapy trials, no conditioning was used in these patients prior to infusion of G-CSF mobilized or BM CD34+ cells transduced with standard retroviral vectors carrying a normal GC cDNA. Unlike results obtained in the mouse, low numbers of gene corrected cells were again detected, with little or no expression and no disease correction following transplantation.

Chronic Granulomatous Disease

CGD results from mutations in any one of four genes encoding the essential subunits of the phagocytic antimicrobial system NADPH phagocyte oxidase (phox),[250] including gp91^{phox}, p22^{phox}, p47^{phox}, and p67^{phox}, rendering individuals born with CGD particularly susceptible to bacterial and fungal microorganisms. Retrovirus-based gene transfer vectors were first tested in two CGD knockout mouse models.[251-253] These studies indicated that gene transfer into murine HSCs is feasible and that partial reconstitution of NADPH oxidase activity achieved after retroviral gene transfer can improve host defense if an adequate number of phagocytes exhibit enzyme activity.

In a subsequent clinical trial for an autosomal recessive form of CGD,[205] five patients received transduced G-CSF MPB CD34+ cells without preconditioning. Corrected granulocytes were detected in the peripheral blood of all individuals for up to 6 months after infusion, but the levels (0.004%-0.05%) were below the desired 5% to 10% required for therapeutic effects.

Lessons From First-Generation HSC Gene Therapy Trials—Improving Efficacy

While the first-generation human gene therapy trials established proof of principle of transduction of long-term repopulating HSCs, they uniformly failed to reach and maintain therapeutically relevant levels of genetically modified cells. These observations refocused efforts on developing more relevant assays for the target HSCs, better gene transfer vectors, improved ex vivo transduction conditions, and acceptable conditioning regimens to increase gene transfer efficiencies in human HSCs.

Preclinical Assays to Investigate Gene Transfer Into Human HSCs

The recognition of differences in HSC behavior between mice and humans and the disappointing results in the early human HSC gene therapy clinical trials underscored the need for alternative assays similar to those available in mice that permit direct identification and characterization of human long-term HSCs and their susceptibility to gene transfer.

Since prolonged follow-up of in vivo hematopoiesis is the most reliable parameter to identify human HSCs, large animals are more adapted than mice for evaluation of gene transfer to long-term repopulating cells, given their lifespan and their size, allowing repetitive blood and marrow sampling. The group of Esmail Zanjani, capitalizing on the immunologically tolerant environment of the fetal sheep between 50 and 60 days of gestation, successfully showed engraftment and persistence of human cells several years after intraperitoneal administration in utero of primitive human hematopoietic cells from CB or BM.[254-256] Among fetuses reaching maturity, at least 50% showed long-term persistence of human cells and demonstration that retrovirally transduced human cells could be detected,[257] suggesting transduction of primitive human HSCs. However, the procedure was hampered by low-level engraftment, a high rate of fetal loss, and impracticality for most research groups.

Given their phylogenetic proximity to humans, nonhuman primates, including baboons and old-world rhesus macaques, have been employed extensively for the preclinical testing of promising gene therapy strategies.[258,259] The cross-reactivity of reagents employed for human application adds to the practicality of these models. In contrast to murine studies, much lower levels of gene-modified circulating cells were reported using similar vector systems and transduction conditions, generally <0.01% to 1%.[260-263] These results were very similar to data obtained in first generation clinical trials, validating the importance of large animal models for the optimization of gene therapy strategies in humans.

The canine autologous transplantation model has also been used to test retroviral gene transfer strategies. Successful transduction of G-CSF–mobilized peripheral-blood engrafting cells was first demonstrated in the dog, as was the importance of partially or fully ablative conditioning radiation or chemotherapy for detectable engraftment with transduced primitive hematopoietic cells.[264-266] Cross-reactivity of human reagents has proven more problematic in the dog model, yet continued progress in this model has led to clinically relevant gene transfer technique.[267,268] Recently, further progress in this model has allowed the attainment of very high levels of genetically modified cells, approaching 100%.[267,269-273] The value of the dog model as a large-animal model is further strengthened by the presence of several disease states that mimic those in humans, which could allow stringent preclinical testing, as recently shown in a canine model of LAD[94] and pyruvate kinase deficiency.[107]

Large-animal models thus became a focus, but outbred animals introduce significant experimental variability and the high costs limit the breadth of experiments that can be performed. For this reason, a competitive repopulation model in which each animal serves as its own control has been utilized for the majority of subsequent comparative studies. In this model, hematopoietic progenitors are isolated and divided equally for transduction under two (or more) distinct experimental conditions using marking vectors that can be distinguished in vivo following reconstitution.

Although results from the large animal models have correlated better with results from early human clinical trials, the rhesus and canine experiments are expensive, slow, and technically difficult, not allowing large-scale testing of new approaches. Over the past 30 years, xenograft mouse models have gained in popularity, in part due to access, and investigators have begun to employ engraftment of transduced human hematopoietic cell populations in immunodeficient mice as an alternative experimental model.[274-278] Initially, large numbers of human BM cells were intravenously injected into sublethally irradiated mice lacking a functional immune system to prevent rejection of the injected human cells, including severe-combined immunodeficient (Scid) and beige/nude/xid (bnx) mice.[279,280] With regular treatment of engrafted Scid mice with a combination of human hematopoietic cytokines, human BM cells that migrated to the mouse marrow and spleen gave rise to a small but sustained pool of myeloid progenitors and B cells for several months, indicating that the engraftment was long-term and multipotent, fulfilling two key criteria used to define HSCs.

The Scid mouse used in these initial studies can spontaneously generate murine T and B cells with age and has high levels of natural killer (NK) cell activity, both impeding efficient and prolonged xenograft. To improve upon the available immunodeficient mouse strains, the Scid mutation was backcrossed onto the non–obese diabetic (NOD) background.[281] The resultant NOD-Scid mouse had reduced innate immunity and superior engraftment of human hematopoietic cells. However, further improvements were sought due to the high incidence of spontaneous thymic lymphomas that shortened their lifespan, a striking preferential development of human B cells after transplantation, and a persistence of murine NK cells resulting in a lack of human T- and NK-cell differentiation in this strain. By reducing or abolishing NK activity in NOD-Scid mice, a new strain, NSG (or NOG) mice, was developed and is a widely used humanized mouse model for gene therapy preclinical testing.[282-285] However, NSG mice require preconditioning and adoptive transfer of large numbers of HSCs to enable high levels of human cell chimerism.[285,286] To address these limitations, the NOD, B6.SCID IL-2rg$^{-/-}$KitW41/W41 (NBSGW) immunodeficient mouse strain was developed by adding KitW41/W41 alleles onto the NSG background.[287] This allele affords a competitive advantage to transplanted HSCs through a loss-of-function mutation of the tyrosine kinase motif of the SCF receptor, c-Kit, in recipient HSCs. A recent study demonstrated successful engraftment of NBSGW mice without pretransplant conditioning using HSCs sourced from human CB, BM, and MPB.[287]

The immunodeficient mouse model assays a human cell population, operationally defined as Scid-repopulating cells (SRCs), that is distinct from hematopoietic progenitors identified using in vitro methodology, including LTBMC-initiating cells and CFC.[216] Using a gene marking approach similar to that used in mouse transplant studies and early clinical trials, Guenechea et al[288] showed that individual engrafted and marked human SRCs could produce a large clone of differentiated progeny with engraftment potential in secondary NOD-Scid recipients, demonstrating the proliferative and self-renewal capacity of SRCs, respectively. Although this study did not contain a direct analysis of individual lineages, a subsequent investigation by the same group[12] successfully tracked self-renewal and multilineage output of single human cells purified using a complex set of markers (CD34$^+$CD38$^-$CD45RA$^-$CD90$^+$CD49f$^+$ Rho^{lo}) for at least 8 months after transplantation in NSG mice. Together, these studies fulfilled the proliferative, self-renewal, and multipotential criteria previously used to define murine HSCs, providing a compelling characterization of human HSCs. Although, in practical terms, the above studies served to validate the murine xenotransplant model as a sound surrogate assay system for human HSCs, the predictive value of these xenograft models remains questionable, as a direct comparison of engraftment of genetically modified autologous baboon cells in both the baboon, and the NOD/SCID mouse suggests distinct populations contributing to hematopoiesis, with short-term progenitors only read out in the immunodeficient mouse.[289]

Improved Gene Transfer Vectors

The dependence of standard retroviral vector systems on cell cycling for efficient transduction is thought to have contributed to the poor transduction efficiency in quiescent HSCs in first-generation clinical trials. Thus, as detailed in sections above, alternative viral vector systems have been explored. The need for integration has precluded extensive investigation of non–viral delivery systems for hematopoietic applications requiring long-term expression.

In recent years, LV-based vectors have attracted attention for their potential to transduce nondividing cells. Given the established lack of predictability of standard murine transplantation models for evaluation of HSC transduction efficiency in humans, investigators initially chose the murine xenotransplant assay to validate the ability of HIV-1–based vectors to efficiently transduce human hematopoietic cells, including CD34+ cells and the more primitive CD34+CD38− subset. Several groups reported efficient gene transfer of SRC derived from human CB,[290-294] BM,[290] and MPB[295,296] under conditions where standard retroviral vectors were ineffective. High-level GFP transgene expression in SRC capable of secondary[294] and tertiary[293] multilineage repopulation in NOD-Scid mice suggested transduction of primitive human HSCs with pluripotential, proliferative, and self-renewing capabilities.

Demonstration of the utility of HIV-1–based LV vectors to transduce hematopoietic cells with long-term repopulating potential was initially met with limited success in rhesus macaques[297,298] and baboons.[299] These old world monkeys were found to possess cellular antiviral factors responsible for the observed resistance to HIV-1 infection. In contrast, HIV-1–based LV vectors could mediate efficient gene transfer to long-term repopulating cells in the canine[269] and pigtailed macaque models.[300] The restriction to HIV-1 infection in rhesus macaques was alleviated by modification of HIV-1–based vectors[301-303] or by the use of an alternative LV vector based on the simian immunodeficiency virus.[304-308]

Despite the lack of predictability of standard murine transplantation studies for evaluation of gene transfer into human HSCs, mouse disease models developed by gene targeting or arising from spontaneous gene mutations may represent the only available option for preclinical testing of the impact of gene transfer vectors on disease phenotype; large animal disease models do not exist for most disorders treated by gene therapy, and for a number of orphan diseases that are common targets of gene transfer protocols, it is impractical to obtain biospecimens from a large cohort of patients to perform preclinical murine xenotransplant efficacy studies. All disorders with active HSC gene therapy clinical trials have employed murine models of human diseases to evaluate efficacy of LV vectors for correction of disease phenotype, including adrenoleukodystrophy (ALD),[309] Wiskott-Aldrich syndrome (WAS),[310-315] β-thalassemia,[316-319] SCID,[320-324] and CGD.[325]

One strategy to increase the efficiency of gene transfer entails the inclusion of selectable genes in vectors to confer an in vivo advantage to transduced cells. Successful in vivo selection has previously been documented in murine HSC transplantation models using several drug resistance genes, including multidrug resistance protein-1 (MDR-1),[326,327] dihydrofolate reductase (DHFR),[328] and O^6-methylguanine-DNA methyltransferase (MGMT).[329-331] However, in more clinically relevant large-animal models, in vivo selection using DHFR[332] and MDR-1[333,334] was variable and transient, with levels of gene-modified cells returning to baseline within a few weeks. MGMT is one of the most promising drug resistance genes that encodes for the DNA repair protein O^6-alkylguanine-DNA-alkyl-transferase. This protein confers resistance to the cytotoxic effects of alkylating agents, including nitrosoureas [e.g., BCNU] and temozolomide. Incorporation of a mutant form of MGMT in the gene transfer retroviral vectors can facilitate a greater selective advantage for primitive hematopoietic cells containing the vector after in vivo administration of an alkylating agent. In vivo selection of HSCs using MGMT was successfully achieved in murine,[330,331] nonhuman primate[272,335] and canine models,[271,272,336,337] and in human NOD/SCID-repopulating cells.[338,339] However, results in large animals were not uniformly positive.[306] While no evidence of leukemic transformation was seen using this approach, the risks of cumulative genotoxicity resulting from the combined use of alkylating agents and retroviral vectors must be considered.

Positive selection of transduced cells in vitro before reinfusion is another strategy to increase repopulation with gene-modified cells. Vectors containing genes for various cell surface proteins have allowed flow cytometric sorting of successfully transduced cells. A number of studies have utilized the human cell surface protein CD24, or the murine homolog heat-stable antigen (HSA). There is limited sequence homology between the murine and human forms, and non–cross-reactive antibodies are available for selection. Their small size takes up little space in the vector construct. Murine marrow cells transduced with a vector containing human CD24 and sorted before reinfusion resulted in greatly increased long-term reconstitution with vector-containing cells.[340] A vector expressing murine HSA allowed enrichment for transduced human progenitor cells.[341] However, CD24 and HSA are GPI-linked surface proteins, a class of proteins that has been shown to be transferred from cell to cell both in vitro and in vivo, clouding the specificity of this marker and raising concerns about ectopic expression of these genes in vivo.[165,340,341]

Retroviral vectors carrying a truncated, nonfunctional form of the human nerve growth factor receptor have also been developed as a selectable marker for use on hematopoietic targets, because hematopoietic cells do not express this receptor. The introduction of new cell-surface proteins has the theoretical disadvantage of altering trafficking or cell-cell interactions upon infusion of transduced cells. Alternative cytoplasmic markers such as green fluorescent protein (GFP) and mutated murine protein are naturally fluorescent, avoiding the need for preselection antibody staining.[342] However, prolonged stable expression of these proteins has proved difficult, and these proteins may exhibit toxicity in primary mammalian cells.[343,344] The use of selection for GFP after retroviral-mediated transduction in the non–human primate model to increase engraftment by genetically modified cells resulted in increased short-term engraftment only, raising another concern that expression of transferred genes may be more efficient in differentiated rather than stem cells, effectively enriching for progenitors with only short-term potential.[345]

In most diseases considered to be suitable targets for gene therapy, corrected cells do not themselves have an inherent growth advantage, providing an impetus to arm retroviral vectors with genes capable of conferring a selective growth advantage to transduced HSCs and their progeny. For example, mouse HSCs transduced with the homeobox gene *HOXB4* possess more than 10-fold greater repopulating ability than that of nontransduced BM.[346] Further, transgenic overexpression of the antiapoptotic protein Bcl-2 results in increased HSC numbers,[347] and expression of a truncated form of the human erythropoietin (EPO) receptor can augment HSC engraftment through the use of exogenous EPO.[348] Blau et al have utilized inactive monomeric signaling domains derived from receptors such as EPO or TPO to permit controlled growth of genetically modified cells through the use of chemical inducers of dimerization.[349,350] Another approach involves selective enrichment of genetically modified cells using vectors encoding a fusion protein between the growth-signaling portion of the G-CSF receptor and the hormone-binding domain of the estrogen receptor. This strategy allows controlled growth of genetically modified cells using exogenous estrogen, and preclinical testing in the nonhuman primate demonstrated the feasibility of this approach.[351,352]

However, the risks of combining integrating vectors and growth-promoting genes for clinical applications have been highlighted in large animal model preclinical studies. Investigators transduced monkey CD34+ cells with either a HOXB4-expressing vector or a control vector expressing only a marker gene and analyzed the competitive repopulating ability of these cells in vivo. As hoped, there was a very significant advantage for the *HOXB4*-transduced cells early following engraftment of the monkeys, but in contrast to mouse studies, a much less significant advantage for the *HOXB4*-transduced cells was observed long-term after transplantation.[353] However, approximately 2 years after transplant, they reported the first instances of leukemia linked to HOXB4 expression, both in the original group of monkeys and in dogs that received cells transduced with HOXB4-expressing vectors.[354] Myelodysplasia in two additional nonhuman primates was subsequently reported in association with retroviral vector–mediated insertional mutagenesis and overexpression of HOXB4.[355] Overall, these studies strongly indicated that overexpression of HOXB4 using integrating retroviral vectors is too risky for clinical applications.

Improved Ex Vivo Transduction Conditions

Various procedures have been refined by different laboratories to optimize retrovirus-mediated transduction in HSCs. A delicate balance must be reached to reconcile the needs for cell cycling for productive transduction without impairing the repopulating ability of HSCs. The current consensus based on large animal and murine xenograft models favors a transduction step in the presence of an early-acting cytokine cocktail composed of SCF, Flt-3L, and TPO, with the optional addition of interleukin (IL)-3. The mechanism of action of these early acting cytokines is generally related to their effect on cell cycle status but they have also been proposed to enhance transduction by downregulating proteasome activity in HSCs.[356,357] Transduction with standard retroviral vectors is typically performed over 72 hours with an obligatory 24-hour cytokine–mediated prestimulation step to favor cell cycling. For LV vectors, a 24-hour prestimulation followed by a single 24-hour transduction in serum-free medium with cytokines has been proposed as an optimal protocol for transduction of human CD34+ cells using the humanized NSG mouse xenograft model.[358,359]

The function of HSCs depends upon the signals from surrounding stromal cells (e.g., fibroblasts, osteoblasts) and extracellular matrix molecules (e.g., fibronectin) found within the highly specialized BM microenvironment. In murine studies, coculture of the hematopoietic target cells with the fibroblast-derived retroviral producer cells has been shown to be the most efficient gene transfer method. However, this approach is inappropriate for use in human clinical trials because of the risk of coinfusing the producer cells into patients along with the transduced hematopoietic cells.

To expand clinical applicability of murine gene transfer protocols, several investigators showed increased gene transfer to human hematopoietic cells adherent to autologous or allogeneic BM stromal cells using in vitro assays.[360-362] Similarly, addition of autologous stromal cells during the transduction period promoted gene transfer into HSCs in the rhesus macaque model.[363] However, the technical difficulties associated with extensive scale-up have limited widespread clinical application of this approach. Moritz et al. took a different tactic by transducing human hematopoietic cells cultured in vessels coated with the chemotrypic 35-kd carboxy-terminal fragment of human fibronectin (FN35) and noted enhanced transduction by retroviral vectors.[364] A recombinant version of this fragment (CH-296), commercially available as RetroNectin (Takara Biomedical, Otsu, Japan), was shown to enhance gene transfer in human CD34+ cells by colocalization of the cells with the vector,[365-367] unless an excess of retroviral particles was used during transduction.[368] The colocalization of vectors and target cells can be enhanced using spinoculation, a neologism coined to describe low speed centrifugation used at the start of transduction to augment gene transfer.[369] The enhancement effect achieved with fibronectin was also attributed to biological effects on HSCs, such as preservation of repopulating potential[366,370-372] and decreased apoptosis.[373] Extensive preclinical studies showed successful gene transfer into murine long-term repopulating stem cells as well as into human and nonhuman primate CD34+ cells derived from BM, CB, or MPB when transduction was performed in vitro[373-376] or in vivo[376] with retroviral vectors and RetroNectin. Correspondingly, in all recent clinical gene therapy trials showing therapeutic benefits, retroviral transduction of human CD34+ cells was conducted in the presence of human recombinant fibronectin.

Conditioning Regimens to Enhance Engraftment of Genetically Corrected HSCs

Engraftment of HSCs is a competitive process between endogenous and infused stem cells. For disorders such as SCID, a growth advantage conferred on genetically corrected cells enables engraftment without conditioning. However, for the majority of disorders in which HSC gene transfer may be applicable, no such advantage to the modified cells is conferred. Instead, most investigators have relied on toxic myeloablative conditioning to damage or destroy endogenous stem cells and thus provide a competitive advantage to the infused genetically modified stem cells. In preclinical models[363] and in patients with malignancies,[194,197,199] myeloablative regimens have been used routinely to enable engraftment of gene-modified primitive hematopoietic cells. However, many of the diseases that could be targeted by gene therapy are chronic, indolent disorders in which the risks of myeloablative regimens may outweigh the potential benefits.

Reduced intensity (nonmyeloablative) conditioning regimens were tested in preclinical models to assess engraftment of marked HSCs while reducing transplant-related toxicities. Engraftment of corrected cells can be achieved in mice in the absence of conditioning by using extremely large BM grafts, but this approach is not clinically feasible.[357-361] Moderate-dose irradiation or antimetabolite-based nonmyeloablative conditioning allowed correction of CGD[253,377-380] and SCID-X1[381] in mouse models of these disorders. Alternative conditioning strategies to promote engraftment of infused HSCs with increased safety have been investigated in mice and are of potential relevance for gene therapy applications. For instance, HSC mobilization with AMD3100, a CXCR4 antagonist with a favorable safety profile in clinical studies, was shown to vacate niches in the mouse BM microenvironment, suggesting possible application as preparative regimen for stem cell transplantation.[382] However, in a prospective pilot trial, AMD3100 given in combination with G-CSF to infants with SCID prior to infusion of CD34+ cells failed to overcome physical barriers to donor HSC engraftment.[383] In a series of experiments, administration of a monoclonal antibody (mAb) that blocks c-kit, the receptor for SCF, transiently reduced endogenous murine stem cells, facilitating engraftment with donor HSCs in immunodeficient Rag2$^{-/-}$/γc$^{-/-}$ mice, but not in immunocompetent mice.[384] Combination of this antibody with low-dose irradiation profoundly decreased endogenous repopulating activity, enabling efficient and durable engraftment of fresh or LV-transduced BM cells in wild-type and CGD mice.[385] Combining blockade of c-kit and CD47, a myeloid-specific immune checkpoint, extended anti-c-kit conditioning to fully immunocompetent mice. The combined treatment led to elimination of >99% of host HSCs and robust multilineage blood reconstitution after HCT.[386] Similarly, c-kit mAb in combination with 5-azacytidine significantly enhanced HSC depletion and donor engraftment in immunocompetent mice.[387] Recently, administration a single dose of c-kit-antibody-drug conjugate (c-kit-ADC) to saporin also enabled safe and effective HSC engraftment with preservation of immunity in preclinical murine model.[388]

In large animal models, no engraftment with genetically modified cells has been observed without conditioning. In one study using a nonmyeloablative regimen, 12% gene marked leukocytes persisted in the peripheral blood of a rhesus macaque for up to 33 weeks after transplant.[389] In other studies, autologous transplantation of transduced HSCs in nonhuman primates conditioned with low-dose irradiation or busulfan have generally resulted in low but measurable (~1%) long-term marking,[307,390-393] providing proof of principle that partial marrow cytoreduction allows engraftment of gene-modified cells without significant toxicity. A possible concern, however, is the unexpected finding that in partially ablated recipient mice, where the BM is a more competitive environment for repopulation compared to the fully ablated marrow, HSCs carrying survival- or proliferation-activating LV insertions had an advantage for engraftment, perhaps increasing the risk of leukemic progression.[394]

Optimized Gene Therapy Protocols

Preclinical studies and the clinical experience gained from first-generation HSC gene therapy trials have led to an optimized protocol

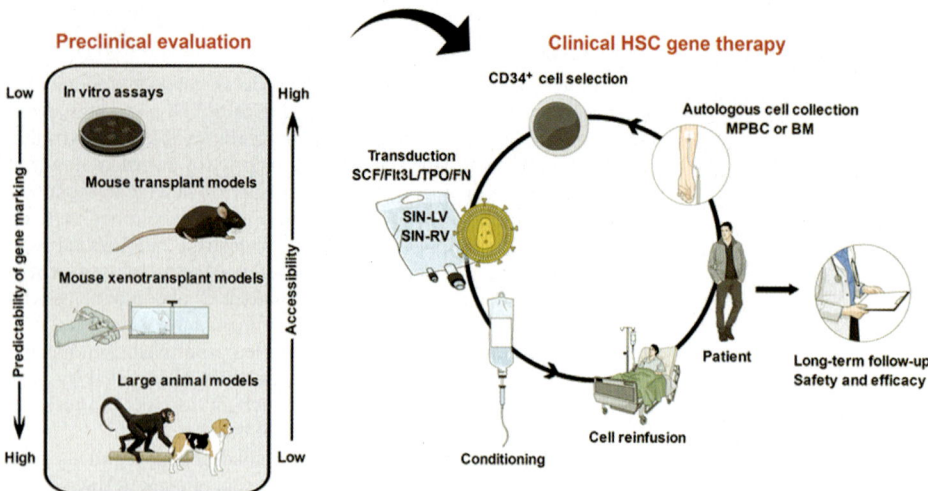

FIGURE 72.3 **Approach for the genetic manipulation of hematopoietic stem cells (HSCs).** The left panel compares the predictive value and accessibility of various preclinical models in the evaluation of gene transfer efficiency of vectors used in HSC gene therapy trials. The right panel depicts the optimized protocol for transduction of hematopoietic stem and progenitor cells, as used in recent clinical trials. BM, bone marrow; Flt3L, *fms*-related tyrosine kinase 3 ligand; FN, fibronectin; IL3, interleukin 3; LV, lentivirus; MLV, murine leukemia virus; MPB, mobilized peripheral blood; RV, retrovirus; SCF, stem cell factor; SIN, self-inactivating; TPO, thrombopoietin.

for ex vivo manipulation of HSCs that has been employed with success in recent clinical trials (*Figure 72.3*). Cells expressing the CD34 cell surface marker are purified from BM harvests or G-CSF-MPB cell collections. Following a brief (24 hours) ex vivo culture in conditions that favor cell cycle transition from G_0 to G_1 (e.g., culture medium supplemented with SCF, Flt3L, and TPO), the CD34+ cells are incubated on a surface coated with the C-terminal fragment of fibronectin in the presence of the same cytokines for an additional 72 hours with standard retroviral vectors or, preferably, for an additional 24 hours with VSV-G-pseudotyped SIN HIV-1–based vectors expressing the desired therapeutic gene from an internal promoter. For disorders in which corrected cells do not have a competitive repopulating advantage over uncorrected endogenous HSCs and their progeny, the patient is conditioned with a reduced intensity or myeloablative regimen prior to intravenous reinfusion of the treated cells. After autologous transplantation, transduced cells home to the BM where they initiate hematopoiesis. Transduction efficiency and safety of the procedure are evaluated by periodic collection of peripheral blood samples over extended periods of time.

SECOND-GENERATION HSC GENE THERAPY TRIALS

Optimized gene transfer protocols were rapidly applied with retroviral vectors in a second generation of HSC gene therapy clinical trials, with actual therapeutic intent, for immunodeficiency disorders, including SCID-X1, ADA-SCID, CGD, and WAS (*Figure 72.2* and *Table 72.2*).

Severe Combined Immunodeficiency Disease
The First Clinical Successes

The first HSC gene therapy trial demonstrating unequivocal clinical benefit was led by Fischer and Cavazzana-Calvo at the Necker Hospital in France.[395-397] Eleven boys with SCID-X1 were treated, and each patient received autologous CD34+ BM cells, transduced with a standard retroviral vector expressing the corrective *IL2Rγ* gene, and reinfused without conditioning because of the growth advantage conferred on genetically corrected cells previously observed with this disease. Rapid functional B and T cell immune reconstitution and clinical improvement were observed in all but one child. The same vector insertion site could be detected in both myeloid and lymphoid cells, suggesting that at least some true HSCs had been corrected. A similar gene therapy trial was also conducted in London on ten children with SCID-X1. All patients experienced substantial immunological recovery and in most patients this was accompanied by recovery of humoral immunity and withdrawal of immunoglobin supplementation.[398-400] In separate clinical trials targeting older patients with SCID-X1, minimal clinical improvement was detected in 2 of 3 preadolescents despite effective transduction and engraftment of G-CSF mobilized CD34+ cells,[401] and complete failure of gene therapy in two adult patients was reported after transplantation of transduced BM CD34+ cells.[402]

Sustained engraftment of engineered HSCs, associated with improvement in immune function, restoration of functional thymopoiesis, and effective metabolic detoxification, was also reported in patients with SCID resulting from ADA enzyme deficiency following transplantation of BM-derived transduced CD34+ cells using optimized protocols.[403-411] Most could stop immunoglobulin replacement therapy, showing ability to mount specific antibody response after vaccination and/or infections (e.g., chickenpox). The treatment provided significant and sustained reduction in severe infection rate after gene therapy, continued physical growth, and improved quality of life. On the other hand, there was no indication that gene therapy had an impact on incidence of neurological issues typically present in ADA-SCID patients.[405]

Insertional Mutagenesis in SCID-X1 Patients Treated by HSC Gene Therapy

Unfortunately, the elation after this success was short-lived; two SCID-X1 patients in the French trial developed a precipitous rise in T-cell counts which progressed to overt leukemia, 3 years following infusion of gene-corrected autologous CD34+ cells.[412] Retroviral integration site analysis in the leukemia cells from both patients demonstrated vector insertions within or just upstream of the *LMO2* gene, activating expression.[413] LMO2 is a transcription factor required for fetal hematopoietic development and was already known to be activated by chromosomal translocations in some cases of spontaneous childhood T cell leukemia.[414] Since that time, an additional two of the eleven SCID-X1 patients enrolled in the French trial and one of ten patients enrolled in the SCID-X1 trial in England have developed clonal vector-associated T cell leukemias.[396,415] Strikingly, four of the five patients had vector insertions activating *LMO2*, and the fifth had a vector insertion activating the *CCND2* gene, encoding cyclin D, a protein known to control cell cycle entry and to be associated with cancer when dysregulated. One of the patients has died of complications related to the leukemic process and its treatment, while the others have been successfully treated with chemotherapy.

The first report of these adverse events in 2003 resulted in a rapid response from investigators and regulatory agencies worldwide, with most gene therapy trials utilizing integrating MLV-derived retroviral vectors to transduce HSCs put on hold. The occurrence of these events was not predicted. Prior to the sequencing of the murine and human genomes, retroviral insertion was thought to be random, based on the lack of any specific motif at the few insertion sites that had been mapped. It was predicted that just one or a few insertions into a cell's genome was unlikely to activate a proto-oncogene, based on the size of the genome and assumed random insertion.[416] Vector-containing leukemias and lymphomas had previously been reported in animal models utilizing HSC gene transfer, but were attributed to contamination by replication-competent viruses in a non–human primate study, resulting in multiple proviral insertions and eventual activation of a proto-oncogene, or overexpression of a signaling receptor in a murine model.[64,417]

There was initially an intense focus on whether specific aspects of SCID-X1 patients themselves or constitutive expression of the *IL2rγ* transgene predisposed to vector-associated leukemia. One murine study suggested a greatly increased risk of leukemia when an *Il2rγ* transgene was overexpressed, and another reported a nonrandom relationship between activation of the *Lmo2* and *Il2rγ* genes and leukemias and lymphomas in susceptible neonatal mice.[418,419] Other unique aspects of the SCID-X1 clinical situation were proposed to have contributed to increasing risk, including the rapid expansion of lymphoid progenitors and mature T cells into an "empty" lymphoid compartment, very high doses of transduced CD34+ cells, and impaired antitumor immunity. A large survey of rhesus macaques, dogs, and baboons transplanted with CD34+ cells transduced with standard retroviral vectors containing marker genes or drug resistance genes failed to document any hematologic abnormalities, or progression to clonal or oligoclonal hematopoiesis, with a median follow-up of over 3 years.[420] And it is of interest that there have been no vector-related clonal expansions or malignant transformations detected in patients receiving transduced T cells, or undergoing in vivo gene therapy targeting hepatocytes, muscle cells, or other nonhematopoietic targets. It appears that HSCs are much more susceptible than differentiated cells to vector-related tumorigenesis.[421]

Insertional Mutagenesis in a Patient With ADA-SCID Treated by HSC Gene Therapy

The safety profile has been generally favorable for patients enrolled in ADA gene therapy trials.[407,411,422,423] In a cohort of 15 ADA-SCID children treated with γ-retroviral vectors, all but one patient had viral insertion sites within and/or near potentially oncogenic loci (e.g., *MECOM*, *LMO2*), but clones with these inserts were stable for several years. Only a benign clonal dominance was reported in a patient, likely due to a gene corrected NK cell–mediated response to chronic EBV viremia.[423]

With more than 2 decades of positive safety and efficacy data collected from ADA-SCID children,[405] ex vivo HSC gene therapy based on the single infusion of autologous CD34+ cells transduced with retroviral vectors encoding for the human ADA cDNA sequence was approved for licensure by the European Medicines Agency (EMA) in May 2016, under the commercial name of *Strimvelis*. This advanced therapy medicinal product was the first ex vivo HSC gene therapy to receive regulatory approval anywhere in the world. This milestone in the development of personalized medicine was made possible by a joint effort between GlaxoSmithKline, Orchard Therapeutics Ltd and the Italian Telethon Foundation and San Raffaele Scientific Institute where the medicinal product was originally developed. However, one recipient of this gene therapy recently developed a T-cell leukemia several years after treatment, representing the first case of insertional oncogenesis leading to a lymphoproliferative disorder in ADA-SCID patients.

Chronic Granulomatous Disease

In an attempt to genetically correct the defect in CGD patients, investigators obtained G-CSF-MPB CD34+ cells from two CGD patients and, using a vector similar to that used in the SCID-X1 trials, inserted a corrective copy of one gp91^{phox} gene needed to make a functional NADPH oxidase.[424] Unlike other CGD trials,[205,425,426] 3 weeks after the cells were reinfused into the patients, a surprisingly large fraction of circulating myeloid cells, more than 20%, carried the corrective gene. Initially the patients did very well, clearing chronic infections after engrafting with corrected cells.

Several months after transplantation, this sustained engraftment of functionally corrected cells with therapeutically relevant levels of NADPH oxidase was unexpectedly followed by further in vivo expansion of cell clones in the myeloid lineage, eventually reaching levels of 60% to 70%. This expansion was found to be almost entirely accounted for by contributions from clones with insertions in the *MDS1/EVI1* (also known as *MECOM*) locus.[424] A progressive decline in blood counts was eventually observed in both CGD patients at 15 and 28 months, respectively, after gene therapy,[427,428] consistent with progression to clonal myelodysplasia/myeloid leukemia, derived from one of their *MDS1/EVI1* clones, and associated with a secondary loss of chromosome 7 in the malignant cells.[428] Despite the persistent high frequency of vector-corrected neutrophils, expression of NADPH oxidase dropped precipitously in both subjects over time. The silencing of NADPH oxidase occurred through progressive CpG methylation of the promoter contained in the LTR of the vector. These events led to a series of infections and eventual death of one patient. The second subject was referred for unrelated donor stem cell transplantation while still infection free.

Wiskott-Aldrich Syndrome

WAS is an X-linked complex primary immunodeficiency disorder caused by mutations in the gene that encodes the WAS protein (WASP).[429] It is characterized by an increased susceptibility to recurrent infections associated with adaptive and innate immune deficiency, thrombocytopenia, eczema, and autoimmunity.[430,431] The generation of two WASP-deficient mice has facilitated preclinical safety and efficacy studies of retroviral vectors for the treatment of WAS. In one study,[432] vector-mediated WASP expression was shown to correct the T-cell defect in WASP− mice. In another study, investigators demonstrated rescue of T-cell signaling and amelioration of colitis upon transplantation of transduced WAS HSCs in mice.[433]

These preclinical models supported the development of gene therapy approaches for WAS. In 2010, a German group reported long-term (up to 5 years) correction of WAS in 9 of 10 patients through standard retroviral infection of G-CSF (and in some cases plerixafor) mobilized CD34+ cells transfused after busulfan-induced transient myelosuppression. Success of the procedure was evidenced by a decreased frequency and severity of infections and resolution of signs and symptoms of autoimmunity, including autoimmune hemolytic anemia, thrombocytopenia, neutropenia, and eczema. Analysis of retroviral insertion sites revealed >140,000 unambiguous integration sites and a polyclonal pattern of hematopoiesis in all patients early after gene therapy.[434,435]

Of 9 patients who showed sustained engraftment and multilineage correction of WASP expression, 7 patients developed leukemia as a complication of the treatment between 16 and 60 months after treatment, including 6 subjects with T-cell acute lymphoblastic leukemia (T-ALL) and one with AML.[435] In all patients with T-ALL, an increase of a cell clone harboring an integration site upstream of *LMO2* could be observed at the onset of leukemia, the same gene locus activated by vector insertion in most of the SCID-X1 patients who developed T-ALL. One to eight additional integrations sites were retrieved within the leukemic clone. Notably, an integration upstream of *TAL1* and an integration upstream of *LYL1* were detected. Both genes are known proto-oncogenes that were already described in T-ALL formation.[436] Cytogenetic analysis revealed additional genetic alterations, such as chromosomal translocations. All 6 patients with T-ALL were treated with conventional chemotherapy followed by HSC transplantation. Three remain in complete remission but two individuals developed secondary AML and one succumbed to progressive leukemia. The seventh patient was diagnosed with AML 39 months after gene therapy, associated with a dominant clone with vector integration of the *MDS1* oncogene. The patient was treated with chemotherapy and remains in remission after HSC transplantation.[435]

Lessons From Second-Generation Clinical Trials—Improving Safety

Second-generation HSC gene therapy clinical trials using optimized protocols led to the first clinical triumphs. However, serious adverse events, some fatal, in these trials emphasized the dangers of gene therapy which were no longer merely theoretical, and have had significant repercussions from regulatory, clinical, and scientific standpoints. Even though the number of individuals who have safely received genetic material in the form of vectors or vector modified cells now numbers in the many thousands, suggesting that current gene transfer approaches generally carry a low risk to subjects, only a small minority of these patients likely had clinical benefit with persistence of genetically modified cells. Risks must therefore be considered in this context. Well-designed pilot clinical trials in patients with sufficient disease severity to justify participation in a potentially risky protocol and a level of understanding allowing authentic informed consent became the most relevant path forward for gene therapy, no matter how many careful preclinical studies have been performed.

Replication-Defective Gene Transfer Vectors Can Contribute to Malignant Transformation

Gene therapy researchers have recognized that insertion of a vector proviral form into the genome can lead to dysregulated gene expression and thus potentially promote malignant transformation via several different mechanisms, as detailed in *Figure 72.4* and discussed in detail in a number of reviews[437,438]: (1) *Enhancer gene activation*: MMLV proviral LTR contains a strong promoter and enhancer, able to activate expression of upstream or downstream genes (proto-oncogenes) at distances as large as 90 kb. Internal promoters or enhancers, included within vectors to enhance transgene expression, can also activate nearby genes; (2) *Promoter fusion*: Retroviral insertions that replace or fuse endogenous regulatory (promoter) regions with those from the retrovirus can result in dysregulated expression of the target gene; (3) *Insertional inactivation of a tumor-repressor gene*: An exon interrupted by retroviral insertion could generate inactive transcripts by nonsense or frameshift mutations. Alleles on both chromosomes can be inactivated by a single retroviral insertion; and (4) *Hybrid transcript with altered splicing*: Proviral insertions downstream from genes might generate transcripts with novel 30 untranslated regions, owing to altered polyadenylation signaling. In this case, unstable hybrid mRNAs would be improperly spliced and/or translated.

The risk of insertion by replication-defective vectors into genomic sites capable of contributing to transformation was initially estimated to be extremely low,[439] based on the assumption that proviral integration into the genome was random and that most cells had only one insertion per cell.[57,440] Concurrent with these adverse events, the entire human and murine genome sequences were published and new technologies, such as linear amplification–mediated PCR, were developed that permitted large-scale mapping of vector insertion sites. Detailed large-scale mapping studies in cell lines and in primary hematopoietic cells revealed clear biases in integration site preferences for both standard retroviral and LV vectors. MMLV retroviral vectors were more likely to integrate near transcription start sites of genes, and LV vectors were likely to integrate in gene-rich regions and within actual genes.[441-443] Modeling based on the size of our genome, the 10 kb gene activation window for retroviral integration, and the estimate that there are 1000 proto-oncogenes give a probability of an insertional event within 10 kb of a potential proto-oncogene as 0.001 to 0.01.[444] However, it is likely that only a few genes might be open to the retroviral integration machinery at each stage in a cell's development, potentially owing to the chromatin environment around differentially expressed genes.[444]

Integration patterns were also assessed over time in mice, large animals and patients receiving transduced cells. Murine studies using high-titer retroviral vectors and performing much longer follow-up than previous studies documented a high rate of progression to clonal or oligoclonal hematopoiesis, specifically from clones with insertions into proto-oncogenes or other growth-altering loci, and frequent leukemias in secondary and tertiary recipients of transduced cells, associated with insertions into proto-oncogenes.[445,446] A rhesus macaque transplanted 5 years previously with retroviral vector–transduced CD34+ cells developed a clonal myeloid leukemia containing a vector insertion in the antiapoptotic gene *BCL2A1*.[447] A large-scale survey of retroviral vector insertion sites in long-term repopulating cells of rhesus macaques uncovered one locus that was markedly overrepresented, with nine independent insertions into the *MDS1/EVI1* proto-oncogene, accounting for 2% of all insertions mapped.[443] Proviral insertions at this locus were also identified in immortalized myeloid cell lines generated in vitro from retroviral vector transduced primary murine BM cells.[448]

Approaches to Decrease the Risk of Insertional Mutagenesis

Use of standard retroviral vectors with strong enhancers in their LTRs is no longer considered prudent for HSC-targeted gene therapy. The clinical adverse events and laboratory findings strongly support the need for long-term toxicity assessment in predictive preclinical models, development of vector systems less likely to activate or otherwise alter the behavior of adjacent genes, and careful risk-benefit analysis of gene therapy target diseases and patient populations.

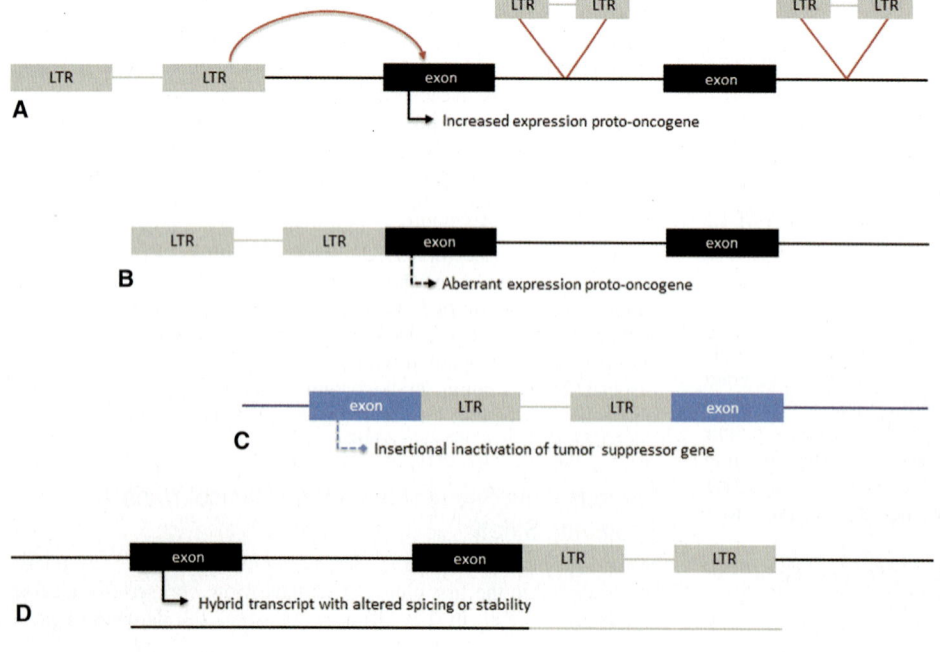

FIGURE 72.4 Mechanisms of gene dysregulation and oncogenesis via vector integration into genomic DNA. The reverse-transcribed retroviral or lentiviral DNA permanently integrates into the genome and can disrupt endogenous gene expression via a number of mechanisms. The integrated vector consists of two identical long terminal repeats (LTR) that contain a strong enhancer and a promoter. A, If the vector lands upstream, downstream, or within an intron of a proto-oncogene, the LTR enhancer can upregulate expression of the proto-oncogene. B, If the vector integrates within the first exon of a proto-oncogene, a constitutively expressed fusion transcript can result, with loss of endogenous control of expression. C, Vector integration within an exon can completely inactivate expression of a tumor suppressor gene via production of a truncated or fusion transcript. D, Vector integration can disrupt normal exon/intron or isoform splicing, resulting in an aberrantly regulated transcript, and upregulation of a proto-oncogene or downregulation of a tumor suppressor gene.

The serious adverse events related to insertional mutagenesis have reinforced interest in SIN gene transfer vectors lacking enhancer-promoter sequences in the LTRs as a means to reduce the probability of activating an adjacent proto-oncogene. Both retroviral and LV vectors with the SIN feature have been produced and shown to combine the desired properties of high efficiency and increased biosafety.[449]

The insertion pattern of LV vectors was considered potentially safer, given that transcription start sites are not targeted and thus less likely to activate surrounding genes. A lower rate of leukemic transformation or cellular immortalization with HIV as compared to standard MLV-based retroviral vectors has been reported using several preclinical models, and long-term follow-up of nonhuman primates receiving LV vector–transduced cells has not revealed any clonal dominance.[305,450,451] As detailed below (see third-generation of HSC gene therapy clinical trials), highly polyclonal patterns have thus far persisted long term in several patients who received HIV vector–transduced CD34+ cells.

Novel vectors based on foamy viruses have not been tested yet in clinical settings. However, the foamy virus backbone includes insulator DNA sequences that, as shown in preclinical immortalization assays, remarkably reduce genotoxic potential, even when strong viral promoter-enhancers (e.g., SFFV) were used (414-fold and 30-fold reduction compared to γ-RV and LV vectors, respectively).[93] In comparative studies of integration site patterns in CD34+ cells, FV vectors also had a safer integration profile than γ-RV or LV vectors, with no preferences to integrate into genes.[94-97]

There are several other approaches to increase the safety of integrating vectors. Chromatin insulators, similar to those naturally occurring in foamy viruses, were initially identified in the DNase I hypersensitive site 4 of the LCR of the chicken β-globin locus (cHS4) and can isolate the activity of a region of chromatin from the surrounding genome. These insulators can be incorporated in gene transfer vectors to mitigate or eliminate the risks of insertional mutagenesis.[452-454] However, the cHS4 insulator consumes precious space in viral vectors, and its incorporation often results in diminished vector titers. More recently, human insulators with high functional potency have been identified.[455] The elements are small and can be efficiently accommodated by viral vectors with no detrimental effects on viral vectors. They substantially decreased the risk of tumor formation in a cancer-prone animal model and may increase safety in gene therapy using viral vector.

It has also been suggested that all integrating vectors carry suicide genes, such as the gene-encoding herpes simplex thymidine kinase (tk), which would allow for an exogenous mission abort signal, via administration of ganciclovir, if evidence for unchecked clonal growth appears following gene therapy. However, killing efficiency is rarely greater than 90%. Furthermore, the tk gene is prone to mutate into an unresponsive state in vivo. The efficacy and safety of an alternative inducible caspase-9 (iCasp9) suicide gene[456] incorporated in a retroviral vector was also tested in a non–human primate transplantation model.[457] Following stable engraftment of iCasp9 expressing hematopoietic cells in rhesus macaques, administration of AP1903, a chemical inducer of dimerization able to activate iCasp9, specifically eliminated vector-containing cells in all hematopoietic lineages long term, suggesting activity at the HSC level. However, incomplete ablation (between 75% and 94%) of vector-containing cells was observed, perhaps linked to lower iCasp9 expression in residual cells. Thus, because many clones and subclones could persist with both tk and iCasp9 systems, these approaches are unlikely to be effective as a treatment for unchecked clonal proliferation.

In addition to improving safety of integrating retroviral and LV vectors, multiple alternative approaches are investigated. As described elsewhere in this chapter, the SB transposon is a potential nonviral method for genetic addition.[53] However, because of the random nature of SB transposon integration, it is still unclear whether its use will decrease the risk of insertional mutagenesis. As described in more detail below, gene-editing approaches could provide the ideal option to eliminate the risk of insertional mutagenesis, either by replacing an endogenous gene by a correct copy, by site-restricted integration of a gene of interest in an innocuous location, or targeted correction of mutations. Nonintegrating vectors would eliminate the risks of insertional mutagenesis, but their use in HSC gene therapy has been hampered by low level of transfection efficiency and lack of sustained expression. As detailed above, gene transfer systems that replicate as episomes, including EBV-based plasmids, S/MARs, and chromosomal vectors, are an attractive approach to allow passage of the vector into daughter cells without the risks associated with chromosomal integration.[458] These nonviral approaches depend on the development of more efficient and less toxic methods of transfection of large DNA molecules within primary cells before they can be of clinical utility.

One other aspect to consider is the number of integration events transplanted into patients. It is probable that multiple insertions into single cells will result in a disproportionate increase in the risk of insertional mutagenesis. Most models of tumorigenesis indicate that multiple hits are required for full cellular transformation; therefore, it is reasonable to aim for one integrant per cell. However, with the development of gene transfer vectors with a higher efficiency of integration and higher titers (allowing superior MOI), cells with more than one integrant are unavoidable. This could fuel dangerous transformations by contributing additional hits, potentially activating unchecked growth according to the multistep model of tumor initiation and progression.[459]

A separate, but related, aspect of gene therapy that can be controlled is target-cell dose. Because increasing the number of cells administered to patients also results in more retroviral insertions the patient is exposed to, researchers have proposed to limit cell doses to the lowest amount expected to result in adequate engraftment. However, this approach has several drawbacks. First, cell dose restriction is unlikely to reduce the net number of insertions administered by a factor of more than 2 to 5. Each patient would still receive millions of transduced cells, each with the potential to transform after accumulating further genetic damage. Second, even though the lower limits for an effective cell dose for gene-modified autologous CD34+ cells have not been formally studied, there is a clear dose effect, with CD34+ cell dosages under 1 to 2 million per kilogram body weight leading to poorer engraftment and disease correction. This is of particular relevance for patients undergoing gene therapy for whom non–myeloablative conditioning regimens are used. In this setting, competition from endogenous HSCs will prevent adequate engraftment of smaller doses of genetically modified cells, unless the transduced cells have a marked selective advantage, such as in SCID-X1 and FA. Third, the use of a limiting cell dose might also confer replicative stress to the smaller number of transduced HSC or progenitor clones, increasing the likelihood of additional genetic events, which could lead to full transformation in co-operation with vector insertion events. Modifications to gene transfer vectors discussed above, including the addition of in vivo selectable genes such as MGMT or the addition of genes that enhance engraftment and HSC function such as HOXB4, are now considered too risky.

THIRD-GENERATION GENE THERAPY CLINICAL TRIALS

Third-generation HSC gene therapy trials have emerged, supported by preclinical data suggesting that SIN and HIV-based gene transfer vectors may be safer and more efficient for transduction of HSCs than standard vectors based on γ-retroviruses.[292,300,305,438,460-463] This new generation of clinical trials has demonstrated efficacy while maintaining, thus far, a high safety profile in peroxisomal disorders, hemoglobinopathies, lysosomal storage diseases (LSDs), immunodeficiencies, inherited BM failure disorders, and HIV-associated lymphoma (*Figure 72.2* and *Table 72.2*).

Peroxisomal Disorders

The first use of an LV vector for HSC gene therapy was reported for the treatment of two children with X-linked ALD, a disorder caused by mutations in *ABCD1* (ATP-binding cassette, subfamily D, member 1), which encodes the peroxisomal half-transporter ALD protein.[309]

Deficiency of this transporter leads to abnormal breakdown of very-long-chain fatty acids, a process that predominantly affects adrenal and nervous system tissues. This is also the first study using a conventional myeloablative conditioning regimen before reinfusion of the genetically manipulated G-CSF MPB CD34+ cells. Functional myelomonocytic cells derived from corrected CD34+ cells migrated into the patient's central nervous system (CNS) to replace diseased microglia cells. At 24 and 30 months posttransplantation, both patients had highly polyclonal reconstitution of hematopoiesis and normal levels of ALD protein, which appeared to retard the progressive cerebral demyelination process. No evidence of genotoxicity has yet been reported in this trial.

Following this initial proof-of-principle study, a subsequent multicenter phase II/III LV-based HSC gene therapy trial enrolled 17 subjects with early-stage cerebral ALD to further investigate safety and efficacy.[464] As in the previous study, autologous CD34+ cells were collected from the patients by apheresis, transduced with LV vectors (designated Lenti-D) and reinfused after myeloablative conditioning. With an average of 29.4 months of follow-up, 15 of 17 patients were alive and free of major functional disabilities with expression of ALD protein in peripheral blood leukocytes. Two patients had neurologic disease progression and later died. Importantly, there was no evidence of insertional mutagenesis, and no preferential integration was detected in or near genes that have previously been involved in serious adverse events associated with gene therapy (e.g., *LMO2*).

Hemoglobinopathies
β-thalassemia

Cavazzana-Calvo and colleagues[465] have provided another example of the clinical potential of gene therapy using LV vectors by treating an 18-year-old male patient suffering from transfusion-dependent β^E/β^0-thalassemia. CD34+ cells were isolated from the individual's BM and transduced with a SIN LV vector (HPV569) containing a functional β-globin gene with an engineered T87Q amino acid substitution ($\beta^{A(T87Q)}$) that is distinguishable from normal adult β-globin (β^A) by high-performance liquid chromatography (HPLC) analysis. This substitution allows precise quantification of vector-derived therapeutic globin expression in vivo. Compared to previous trials, a conditioning regimen with higher doses of busulfan was used in this study. The levels of genetically modified cells gradually rose up to 11% at 33 months posttransplant with concomitant increases in levels of the normal β-globin protein and improved production and quality of normal RBCs. Remarkably, a year after treatment, the patient no longer needed RBC transfusions. This therapeutic benefit, however, was observed in the setting of clonal expansion resulting from integration of LV vectors in the high mobility group AT-hook 2 (*HMGA2*) gene.[466] The known association between HMGA2 overexpression and benign/malignant neoplasias initially raised concerns.[466-468] Fortunately, the clonal expansion eventually regressed after several years without transformation.[469] Marked expansion of a single corrected clone, persisting without malignant transformation for many years, has also been documented in an early[470] and more recent[423] ADA-SCID gene therapy trials, suggesting that clonal expansion does not irrevocably progress to malignancy.

To expand on this proof-of-concept study, investigators enrolled 22 additional adolescent or adult subjects with transfusion-dependent β-thalassemia in two companion phase 1/2 clinical trials (HGB-204 and HGB-205).[471] The LV vector used in these studies (LentiGlobin BB305, Bluebird Bio, Inc) was an HPV569-derivative without the cHS4 insulator sequences. Protocol-related features, including improved manufacturing of the gene therapy vector, enhanced RBC transfusion series before CD34+ cell harvest and optimized busulfan dosing, resulted in increased integrated vector copy numbers (VCNs) per cell and overall clinical efficacy. In several treated patients, hemoglobin levels reached or approached normal ranges. Fifteen subjects stopped receiving RBC transfusions several months after gene therapy, including three patients with a β^0/β^0 or equivalent disease genotype, and reduction in volume or number of transfusions was noted in the other patients. Genome-wide mapping of vector integration sites showed a highly polyclonal pattern. Unlike findings in the single patient previously treated with a much lower dose of vector-transduced hematopoietic cells,[465] no clonal dominance was observed and safety issues attributable to the gene transfer vector were not reported in this study. To further enhance VCN and average hemoglobin levels after infusion of the gene-modified cell product (labeled "betibeglogene autotemcel" or "beti-cel"), a refined CD34+ cell transduction process was developed and evaluated in a multicenter phase 3 study (HGB-207).[472] An interim analysis was reported on a total of 22 evaluable patients with transfusion-dependent β-thalassemia and a non-β^0/β^0 genotype, including 7 subjects younger than 12 years of age. Most (20 of 22) patients achieved the primary endpoint of transfusion independence with an average hemoglobin of 11.7 g/dL primarily derived from the therapeutic HbA^{T87Q} (median 8.7 g/dL). Although all patients experienced at least one adverse event during or after beti-cel infusion, including grade 3 thrombocytopenia in 2 patients, clonal predominance or insertional oncogenesis was not observed. In 2019, the EMA conditionally approved LentiGlobin BB305 for transfusion-dependent non-β^0/β^0 thalassemia in patients 12 years and older, representing the first approved gene therapy for this disease.[473] In 2020, the gene modified cellular product (i.e., autologous CD34+ cells encoding $\beta^{A(T87Q)}$) became commercially available as ZYNTEGLO in several member states of the European Union as well as the United Kingdom, Iceland, Liechtenstein, and Norway, but the roll-out suffered from issues with manufacturing, COVID-19 pandemic restrictions, safety concerns (see "Sickle Cell Disease" below), and significant pricing pushback in Europe. The US FDA previously granted beti-cel orphan drug status and breakthrough therapy designation, but the therapy has not yet received approval in the United States.

Other clinical studies of LV vector–mediated gene therapy in patients with β-thalassemia also showed evidence of clinical safety and efficacy. In the phase 1/2 TIGET-BTHAL study,[474] nine patients with β^0 or severe β^+ mutations received a myeloablative conditioning regimen followed by intrabone administration of autologous MPB HSCs genetically modified with the GLOBE lentiviral vector (Orchard Therapeutics). Efficacy outcome was reported for seven patients with >12 months of follow-up. Transfusion reduction was observed in the three adults treated in this study, whereas complete transfusion independence was achieved in three of four children. Sustained clonal complexity was demonstrated in hematopoietic lineages, with no evidence of oligoclonality or exhaustion. In the phase 1 study conducted at the Memorial Sloan Kettering Clinical Center (MSKCC), four adult subjects with transfusion-dependent β-thalassemia (β^0/β^0 or β^0/β^+ genotype) received autologous MPB CD34+ cells genetically corrected using the TNS9.3.55 LV vectors.[475] To minimize short- and long-term toxicity, reduced intensity conditioning with busulfan was used in this study. Transfusion requirements were diminished after gene therapy but not abrogated in any of the four treated patients. The low transduction efficiency in the cell product (median VCN 0.15) rather than the conditioning intensity precluded achieving transfusion independence in this cohort of patients. The lower level of transduction achieved in CD34+ cells with TNS9.3.55 was explained by significant impurities in the vector lot that precluded increasing the MOI, emphasizing the importance of an HPLC purification step during vector manufacturing. The combined data from the HGB, GLOBE, and MSKCC studies suggest that VCN less than 0.3 in vivo will only result in reduction of transfusion needs in patients with severe genotypes. Monitoring of vector integration sites in patients revealed a polyclonal profile without excessive dominance, but mapping of integration sites 4 to 7 years posttransplant indicated marked skewing toward cancer-related genes, such as UBR2 and STAT3. Although all clones are, to date, clinically benign, careful long-term monitoring of clonal expansions is critical in these patients.

Sickle Cell Disease

Sickle cell disease (SCD) results from a single amino acid substitution in adult β-globin. Sickle hemoglobin polymerizes on deoxygenation, reducing the deformability of red blood cells. It affects ~90,000 people in the United States who suffer significant neurological, lung, and kidney damage, as well as severe chronic pain episodes that adversely impact on quality of life. While current medical therapies (namely hydroxyurea) for SCD can reduce short-term morbidity, the inevitable progressive deterioration in organ function results in a significant decrease in quality of health with early mortality.

Sustained correction of SCD was recently reported in a single patient who received HSC gene therapy at the Necker Children's Hospital in Paris.[476] Bone marrow CD34+ cells were transduced with the same LentiGlobin BB305 vector used in gene therapy studies for β-thalassemia. The modified β-globin gene encoded by this vector ($β^{A(T87Q)}$) produces an antisickling hemoglobin. The subject underwent nonmyeloablative conditioning with busulfan before cell reinfusion. After 15 months of follow-up, the level of therapeutic antisickling β-globin remained high (approximately 50% of β-like–globin chains) without recurrence of sickle crises and with correction of the biologic hallmarks of the disease. Serial monitoring of integration sites in peripheral blood samples showed a consistently polyclonal profile without detection of a dominant clone.

A subsequent multicenter phase 1/2 clinical trial (HGB-206) utilizing the same LV vector evolved across three consecutive cohorts (groups A, B, C). In group C, a total of 35 patients with SCD ($β^s/β^s$, $β^s/β^0$, or $β^s/β^+$ genotype) were treated using a gene therapy process optimized based on findings in cohorts A and B, including enhanced transfusion regimen before HSC collection, refined manufacturing of LentiGlobin BB305 to improve transduction efficiency, myeloablative busulfan conditioning, and substitution of BM harvests with HSCs collected after plerixafor mobilization and apheresis to increase quality and dose of autologous CD34+ cells while mitigating risks of vaso-occlusive crises during collection.[477,478] With a follow-up of 3.7 to 37.5 months, sustained the production of HbA^{T87Q} in approximately 85% of RBCs was observed in all 25 subjects followed for at least 6 months. The treatment normalized hemoglobin levels, reduced markers of hemolysis, and led to resolution of severe vaso-occlusive events. Three patients had transient nonserious events related or possibly related to the treatment, including leukopenia, hypotension, and febrile neutropenia. Trisomy 8 was identified by FISH analysis in one subject 6 months after cell infusion, but no evidence of malignancies was reported in this or other patients treated in this cohort. In contrast, two participants enrolled in the initial cohort (group A) of the HGB-206 study were diagnosed with AML.[479-482] In one patient, the tumor cells lacked LV vector sequences.[479] Integration site analysis in leukemic cells of the second subject identified a dominant clone with vector insertion within the vesicle-associated membrane protein 4 (VAMP4) gene. However, the leukemia was thought to be unlikely related to vector integration given the nononcogenic nature of VAMP4, the location of the insertion within a noncoding region of the gene, the limited expression of VAMP4 in blast cells, and the detection of VAMP4 insertions in other SCD patients who had no sequelae.[481] Evolution to leukemia in these patients was likely multifactorial, including the poor cell doses achieved in the initial group A, the risks of leukemogenic mutations after genotoxic conditioning, and the inherent predisposition of SCD patients to malignant transformation.[480,482]

Lysosomal Storage Diseases
Metachromatic Leukodystrophy
Metachromatic leukodystrophy (MLD) is an autosomal recessive LSD caused by a deficiency of arylsulfatase A (ARSA) enzyme, affecting sphingolipid metabolism. Insufficient ARSA causes accumulation of the enzyme substrate sulfatide in oligodendrocytes, microglia, and certain neurons of the CNS, and in Schwann cells and macrophages of the peripheral nervous system. This build-up of sulfatides leads to widespread demyelination and neurodegeneration, as evidenced by progressive motor and cognitive impairment.[483]

In recent years, LV HSC gene therapy has provided clinical benefit to patients with MLD. Preliminary results of a phase I/II clinical trial were initially reported for three presymptomatic (late infantile, LI) patients, indicating stable engraftment of transduced HSCs with reconstitution of ARSA activity in all hematopoietic lineages as well as the cerebrospinal fluid (CSF).[484] These observations provided indirect evidence that HSC-derived cells had migrated to the CNS and produce the enzyme locally. Longer follow-up of these and additional MLD patients (total nine patients), some with early clinical manifestations (early juvenile, EJ), was subsequently reported.[485] For most treated patients, gross motor performance and neurocognitive development were similar to that of normally developing children. With regards to CNS involvement, the massive demyelination and severe atrophy observed in untreated patients were undetectable in most patients who underwent HSC gene therapy. Overall, these data indicated safe and effective LV-based gene therapy for MLD in the LI population and early promising observations in the broader EJ group of MLD patients.

In a follow-up study, a gene therapy ("atidarsagene autotemcel," arsa-cel) containing BM or MPB autologous CD34+ cells transduced ex vivo with an LV vector encoding human ARSA was administered to 29 subjects with presymptomatic or early symptomatic disease ($n = 16$ LI, $n = 13$ EJ) after myeloablative busulfan conditioning.[486,487] Efficacy was measured based on improvement in total gross motor function compared with an untreated natural history cohort of 31 patients of similar age and disease subtype, as well as ARSA activity in peripheral blood cells compared to baseline. Three patients died, two from progressive disease and one had a stroke, but the other children either maintained the ability to walk or progressively acquired motor skills within the predicted range of healthy subjects, including four patients who transiently developed anti-ARSA antibodies. Other treatment benefits, including cognitive development, delay of central or peripheral demyelination, and brain atrophy, were primarily observed in subjects treated before symptom onset. Consistent with these clinical observations, ARSA concentration was normal or elevated in the peripheral blood and CSF in both LI and EJ patients at 24 months posttreatment. Side effects were primarily related to busulfan toxicity or the underlying disease; no evidence of clonal dominance or proliferation was documented. Arsa-cel was approved for medical use in the European Union and in the United Kingdom under the brand name "Libmeldy" and is under investigation in the United States.

Hurler Syndrome
Glycosaminoglycans (GAGs) or mucopolysaccharides are long polysaccharides that undergo step-wise catabolism by lysosomal hydrolases within cells. In mucopolysaccharidosis type IH (MPSIH, Hurler syndrome), a rare autosomal recessive disorder characterized by deficiency in α-L-iduronidase (IDUA), lysosomal accumulation of GAGs leads to gradual cellular and multiorgan dysfunction. The clinical phenotype of children with Hurler syndrome includes progressive neurocognitive deterioration, musculoskeletal abnormalities, visual and hearing impairment, pulmonary and cardiac disease, and hepatomegaly. Without treatment, death is generally observed within the first decade of life.[488] Enzyme replacement therapy with recombinant human laronidase modifies the natural history of the disease in less affected patients, but does not reverse skeletal manifestations and, because the enzyme does not cross the blood-brain barrier, CNS conditions do not improve. Allogeneic HSC transplantation is the treatment of choice. Tissue-resident myeloid cells replaced after transplantation provide a stable endogenous source of IDUA to improve phenotype. However, the inherent complications associated with allogeneic transplant and the persistence or progression of cognitive and skeletal abnormalities over time impact patients' quality of life.[489,490]

In a recent phase 1/2 study, eight MPSIH patients with mild cognitive impairment underwent autologous transplant of gene-corrected MPB CD34+ cells using LV vectors encoding the PGK promoter–driven human IDUA cDNA.[491] A myeloablative conditioning regimen comprised of rituximab, busulfan, and fludarabine was used to promote engraftment of infused cells. Compared to IDUA concentrations achieved after allogenic transplantation, the potent PGK regulatory sequence used in this study allowed production of suraphysiologic levels of IDUA, resulting in more rapid and efficient reduction of GAG storage systemically. Although follow-up was short (1.5-2.9 years), all patients were alive at the time of analysis and displayed stable cognitive performance, continued motor development, reduced joint stiffness, and normal growth. Consistent with LV vector integration site profile in other studies, a stable polyclonal repertoire was observed in all patients and no evidence of insertional mutagenesis was documented. Overall, this study provided the first demonstration of safety and efficacy of HSC gene therapy in patients with Hurler syndrome, but the true impact of this treatment will require much longer monitoring of this patient cohort.

Fabry Disease

Fabry disease is an X-linked inborn error of the glycosphingolipid pathway.[492] Loss-of-function mutations within the coding or intervening sequences of the GLA gene result in deficiency of the lysosomal hydrolase α-galactosidase A (α-Gal A). Insufficient α-Gal A activity causes lysosomal accumulation of globotriaosylceramide (Gb_3) and of the hydrophilic deacylated derivative globotriaosylsphingosine (lyso-Gb_3) in various cells and tissues. Patients with Fabry disease may display a spectrum of clinical manifestations. In the classic (type 1) form of the disease, affected males present with severe neuropathic pain, dermatologic manifestations, gastrointestinal symptoms, corneal opacities, kidney function impairment, and progressive cardiac and cerebrovascular involvement.[493] Recombinant α-Gal A and migalastat hydrochloride, an oral pharmacologic chaperone that facilitates trafficking of residual α-Gal A to lysosomes, are therapeutic options for eligible individuals.[494,495] However, the required biweekly infusion of α-Gal A is intrusive, not curative and associated with considerable costs.

In a pilot study of five adult subjects with type 1 phenotype Fabry disease, MPB HSCs were transduced ex vivo using an LV vector containing a codon optimized cDNA of human GLA under the regulatory control of the EF-1α promoter.[496] Due to the chronic nature of Fabry disease and significant comorbidities in these patients, a reduced-intensity melphalan-based conditioning regimen was chosen to minimize toxicities. The overall safety profile was favorable, but characterization of LV vector insertion sites was not performed in this interim analysis. In peripheral blood cells, VNC was initially between 0.5 and 1.1 per diploid genome but gradually declined over time. Similarly, α-Gal A enzymatic activity in both plasma and leukocytes slowly waned after reaching normal or supraphysiologic levels in the first 100 days of treatment. Plasma and urine lyso-Gb_3 levels decreased in most patients but rose in subjects who chose to discontinue α-Gal A enzyme replacement after gene therapy. A more intense preparative regimen, as used in most other HSC gene therapy studies, could enable superior engraftment of transduced long-term repopulating HSCs and phenotypic correction, but likely at the expense of increased toxicities in this patient population.

Immunodeficiencies
Wiskott-Aldrich Syndrome

Although several occurrences of viral enhancer–mediated insertional mutagenesis were observed in WAS second generation HSC gene therapy clinical trials using γ-RV vectors, more recent studies using a SIN-LV vector (LV-w1.6 WASp) have demonstrated significant clinical benefit in children with WAS without evidence of oncogenic transformation or sustained clonal dominance.[497,498] Long-term follow-up (4-9 years after gene therapy) for patients treated in one study[498] and two additional subjects enrolled after the first report indicated persistence of gene-corrected cells in the absence of serious treatment-associated adverse events.[499] The same vector was also successfully used in a severely affected adult WAS patient without safe HSC transplant options.[500] Following reduced intensity conditioning, there was rapid engraftment and expansion of a polyclonal pool of transgene-positive functional T cells, and sustained gene marking in myeloid and B cell lineages, with associated clinical benefit up to 20 months of observation, indicating that LV vector gene therapy is a viable option when an allogeneic transplant procedure could present an unacceptable risk.

X-linked SCID

To improve the safety profile of gene therapy for SCID-X1 while maintaining the clinical efficacy observed in previous trials, the original retroviral vector was modified to create a SIN γ-RV vector carrying the same IL2Rγ cDNA under the control of the weak EF1α promoter.[501,502] This vector was used in an international study with participating centers in Paris, London, Boston, Cincinnati, and Los Angeles.[503] In contrast to the first SCID-X1 trials, this trial was restricted to children for whom the prognosis after allogeneic HCT would have been poor, due to severe, ongoing, treatment-refractory infections. All patients received transduced BM-derived CD34+ cells without preparative regimen. After up to 48 months of follow-up, eight of the nine patients were alive and well; one death at 4 months after gene therapy was attributed to an overwhelming adenoviral infection, well before full reconstitution by genetically modified T cells. Of the remaining eight patients, seven displayed full T cell reconstitution and normalized T cell proliferation, but no B cell correction. A retroviral integration site analysis of the patients' peripheral blood mononuclear cells revealed significantly less clustering within proto-oncogenes and genes involved in the serious adverse events in previous gene therapy trials. These data indicate that modified SIN retroviral vectors are efficacious in the treatment of SCID-X1 and may have a better safety profile.

In other trials for SCID-X1 conducted at the NIH and St. Jude Children's Hospital, investigators used an LV vector gene therapy approach to treat five older children with persistent immune dysfunction despite haploidentical HSC transplantation in infancy.[88] This study included the first use of SIN-LV vectors in SCID-X1, the first use of busulfan conditioning in that disease, and the first use of an LV vector manufactured from a stable producer cell line.[90] All patients achieved clinically relevant selective expansion of gene-marked T cells. Importantly, in contrast to other SCID-X1 trials conducted without conditioning, gene-corrected NK and B cells reconstitution was also observed, and associated with sustained restoration of humoral responses to immunization and overall clinical improvement with up to 3 years of follow-up. Because vector-related mutagenesis did not appear until 3 to 4 years after gene therapy in other SCID-X1 trials, insertional mutagenesis cannot be definitely excluded in this trial, although the absence of clonal dominance thus far, as in other HSC gene therapy trials using LV vectors, is reassuring.

Adenosine Deaminase-Severe Combined Immunodeficiency Disease

A total of 50 children or teenagers with ADA-SCID were treated with an investigational LV vectorbased gene therapy (OTL-101) in the United States and United Kingdom.[504] The prospective phase 1/2 studies utilized marrow or MPB autologous CD34+ HSCs transduced ex vivo with a SIN LV vector engineered with a codon-optimized human ADA cDNA under the control of the short-form elongation factor-1α promoter (EFS-ADA LV). Patients were treated with low dose busulfan conditioning before gene therapy and continued PEG-ADA enzyme replacement therapy until 30 days after treatment for continued protection against infections during immune reconstitution. In contrast, enzyme replacement must be discontinued before allogeneic HSC transplantation to limit expansion of host T cells and the potential for graft-versus-host disease. At a follow-up of 24 to 36 months, all patients were alive but one child failed to engraft and received rescue allogeneic HSC transplantation and another subject reinitiated enzyme replacement therapy due insufficient engraftment of transduced HSCs resulting in low ADA activity levels. The other patients showed sustained levels of gene marking in all leukocyte populations, including short-lived granulocytes, indicating stable engraftment of genetically modified long-term repopulating HSCs. Consistent with a selective advantage conferred on mature lymphocytes carrying the functional ADA transgene, VCNs gradually increased in these cells after treatment. Accordingly, significant immunological and metabolic recovery was observed, with improved T cell counts, increased serum immunoglobulin levels reflective of enhanced B cell function, and marked reduction in rates of severe infections. No evidence of clonal expansion, leukoproliferative complications, fatal, or life-threatening events were reported in these studies, adding to the growing evidence for the safety of LV vectors.

X-Chronic Granulomatous Disease

To minimize mutagenic risks observed in previous gene therapy trials for X-CGD,[424,428] a SIN LV vector (G1XCGD) was developed and optimized by incorporation of a novel chimeric cathepsin G/Cfes promoter to drive expression of the CYBB cDNA-encoded gp91phox at high levels in phagocytes.[505] Two phase 1/2 clinical trials conducted in the United States and United Kingdom enrolled a combined cohort of nine children or young adults with X-CGD. Both investigations were open-label study of autologous marrow or MPB CD34+ cells transduced with the G1XCGD and infused in these patients after myeloablative busulfan conditioning. Two patients died within 3 months of gene therapy due to pre-existing disease-related conditions. Sustained persistence of 16% to 46% oxidase-positive neutrophils, measured by dihydrorhodamine (DHR) assay, was observed in six of seven surviving patients at 24 months; CGD-related prophylactic antibiotic or antifungal treatment was discontinued in these subjects. The gradual decline in DHR+ neutrophils in one pediatric patient was attributed to poor engraftment of long-term repopulating HSCs, possibly due to CGD-associated inflammatory processes and concomitant myelosuppressive drug therapy. There was no evidence of transcriptional silencing of the integrated LV vector genome, as observed in an earlier X-CGD studies utilizing γ-retroviral vectors.[424,428] Nevertheless, all seven surviving individuals have remained free of new infectious complications up to 36 months after cell infusion. Consistent with the DHR assay in neutrophils, VCN remained stable in six patients over the course of follow-up. In the absence of survival or proliferative advantage of mature gene-corrected neutrophils, similar VCNs were measured in other cell lineages, with the exception of T cells, likely reflecting a lack of lymphodepletion following busulfan-based conditioning in these patients. Longitudinal analysis of integration site distributions documented a highly polyclonal population of gene-modified cells and no clone at genes of concern in the previous clinical trial (e.g., MDS/EVI1) expanded to comprise more than 0.3% of the total cellular population in any hematopoietic lineage.

Inherited Bone Marrow Failure Syndromes
Fanconi Anemia

In a phase 1/2 clinical study in Spain (FANCOLEN-1), mobilized CD34+ cells were obtained from four pediatric subjects (aged 3-6 years) with FANCA before the development of severe BM failure. Cells were transduced with the PGK-FANCA.WPRE* LV vector and reinfused to the patients without any cytotoxic preparative regimen.[506] Despite very low cell doses (<500,000 CD34+ cells/Kg) and the absence of pretransplant conditioning, a slow but sustained engraftment of autologous gene-corrected HSCs was observed in all patients over a period of 18 to 30 months. Corrected hematopoietic cells displayed reversion of their characteristic FA phenotype, as demonstrated by the progressive increase in mitomycin C resistance of marrow progenitor cells and decrease sensitivity of peripheral blood T cells to the DNA cross-linking agent diepoxybutane. Longitudinal analysis of vector integration sites showed polyclonal reconstitution pattern with successive contribution of marked clones over time. Integrations were not identified within genes (e.g., LMO2, CCND2, and MECOM) previously associated with insertional oncogenesis, and leukemic transformation was not observed in this study. However, at the time of analysis, no evident increase in peripheral blood counts had been observed in any patient. While this study presents the first evidence of long-term engraftment of gene modified HSCs in FA patients, infusion of higher numbers of transduced HSCs in combination with non–genotoxic conditioning regimen will likely be required to enable robust hematopoietic reconstitution in the these patients.

HIV-Associated Lymphoma

Recently, the transplantation of allogeneic HSCs with an HIV-resistant genotype based on a naturally occurring 32-bp deletion in the gene for the HIV coreceptor *chemokine receptor 5* (Δ32CCR5), used in conjunction with myeloablative therapy for leukemia, resulted in apparent elimination of HIV in the recipient.[507,508] This so-called "Berlin patient case" provided proof of concept that replacing a susceptible immune system with a genetically modified, virus-resistant one can result in reduced viral load and perhaps offer an approach to prevent progression to AIDS. While the frequency and logistics of finding matched allogeneic homozygous Δ32CCR5 donors precludes widespread use of this strategy, this case renewed excitement for the therapeutic potential of transplanting autologous HSCs genetically modified to render their progeny HIV resistant.

Multiple HSC gene therapy strategies have been proposed to inhibit HIV in vivo.[509] Because of its proven efficacy in the Berlin case, CCR5 has been a primary target of HSC gene therapy. Several approaches have been used to inhibit functional expression of CCR5, including the introduction of siRNA,[510,511] ribozymes,[512,513] trans-dominant forms of CCR5,[514] and single-chain intracellular antibodies.[515,516] As discussed below, CCR5 inactivation using novel genome-editing technologies is also an area of research that has generated intense interest. An alternative strategy for HSC modification involves insertion of a gp41-derived peptide (C46) to inhibit HIV entry. In an in vivo macaque model, T cells derived from C46-expressing HSCs were protected from subsequent HIV challenge, but only 4% to 7% of T cells were genetically modified.[517] Concern has also been raised that C46-based HSC gene therapy might be associated with the development of viral resistance. As reviewed elsewhere,[509] additional antiviral factors that prevent *viral replication* have been suggested as candidates for expression via HSC gene therapy–based approaches: (1) Genome disruption (e.g., evolved recombinases); (2) Gene expression inhibition (TAR decoys, anti-Tat ribozymes); (3) RNA export inhibition (trans-dominant, Rev); and (4) Viral release or infectivity factors (TRIM5α, APOBECs, tetherin).

Because of the extensive experience with standard small-molecule antiretroviral drugs indicating that combination therapy is necessary to prevent the emergence of viral resistance to these agents, HSC-based gene therapies also combine two or more antiviral genes to provide sufficient genetic barrier to prevent viral resistance. For instance, a recent study used a combination of a tat/rev shRNA, a TAR decoy, and a CCR5-targeting ribozyme to modify CD34+ HSCs in patients undergoing transplantation for HIV-associated lymphoma.[513] Given the low frequency of modified cells (<0.2% of circulating PBMC), no clinical benefit was observed. Improved approaches will allow the determination of the minimal marking efficiency required for clinical benefit and the relative benefits of various therapeutic gene combinations. Two clinical trials combining various genetic approaches are ongoing in the United States (NCT00569985, NCT02797470).

NEW PERSPECTIVES AND ONGOING CHALLENGES
Genome Editing

In recent years, transformative advances have emerged to more precisely edit cellular genomes, possibly obviating some of the safety and efficacy concerns associated with integrating vectors described above. Such strategies can be exploited in HSC gene therapy to correct disease-causing mutations, to allow safe targeted knock in of a therapeutic gene, or to provide a cell with a new feature, such as the resistance to a pathogen, through a targeted gene knockout.

Approaches for Genome Editing

Tools for the targeted modification of cellular genomes include zinc finger nucleases (ZFNs), homing endonucleases, transcription activator–like effector nucleases (TALENs), megaTALs, and RNA-guided nucleases based on type II bacterial clustered, regularly interspaced, short palindromic repeats (CRISPR), and the CRISPR-associated protein 9 (Cas9), known as CRISPR/Cas9.[518,519] The unifying activity for all of these tools is their nuclease activity, which is the ability to bind a specific sequence anywhere in the genome and introduce DNA double-strand breaks (DSBs) that are repaired by endogenous cellular mechanisms.

The CRISPR/Cas9 system offers the greatest flexibility for targeted gene therapy because of its specificity and ease of design. It consists of the Cas9 endonuclease, most commonly derived from *Streptococcus pyogenes* (SpCas9), and a 100-nucleotide chimeric single guide RNA (sgRNA) that targets the nuclease to a specific region of the genome. This sgRNA is generated by fusing two small RNAs required for target recognition and cleavage, CRISPR RNA (crRNA) and trans activating crRNA, via a linker loop (*Figure 72.5*). Target identification relies first on identification of a 3-base pair protospacer adjacent motif (PAM) and then base-pairing between a 20-nucleotide stretch of the sgRNA and the DNA target site, which triggers Cas9 to cleave both DNA strands. Possible outcomes of the approach include (1) Targeted gene knock-out by creating insertions or deletions (indels) at the site of the break through mutagenic nonhomologous end-joining (NHEJ) and (2) Targeted gene knock-in or knock-out, or precise change of a genomic sequence through homologous recombination (HR) using an exogenously introduced donor DNA template (*Figure 72.5*).

Challenges and New Advances to Genome Editing in HSCs

In primary human HSCs, the low mitotic index presents an impediment to gene editing via HR, which predominates in the S and G2 phases of the cell cycle, as compared to more efficient NHEJ in noncycling cells. With current approaches, low levels of targeted integration via HR have been reported in human HSCs.[520] Moreover, delivery of the Cas9/gRNA components and of bulky exogenous homologous DNA donor template for targeted gene addition and correction can result in pronounced cytotoxicity to HSCs.

New strategies to advance the current state of CRISPR-Cas9–mediated targeted gene delivery in HSCs have been proposed. For instance, sgRNAs modified at both termini with 2′ O-methyl 3′ phosphorothioate[521] enhanced genome-editing efficiencies in primary HSCs, perhaps by stabilizing the sgRNAs. Improved methods of delivery of Cas9 and sgRNA have also been reported, initially based on plasmids,[522] to RNA-based approaches,[521] to more recently described protocols based on precomplexed Cas9/sgRNA ribonucleoproteins (RNPs).[523] The RNP delivery system reduces stimulation of innate immunity that recognizes naked DNA and RNA, which can be associated with increased toxicity and reduced editing efficiencies in HSCs. Delivery of donor templates for homology-directed repair after DSBs has relied on electroporation, integrase defective lentiviral vectors (IDLVs),[520,524] or recombinant adeno-associated virus type 6 (AAV-6).[525-528] Delivery is efficient (up to 10%) and nontoxic using small single-stranded oligonucleotides (ssODNs), usually by electroporation. However, ssODNs can only be used to mediate precise nucleotide changes; they do not allow targeted addition of larger gene cassettes.[88,524,529-531] To insert large gene cassettes, electroporation is too toxic in HSCs and current literature suggests that rAAV6 is superior to IDLV.[532] However, a more comprehensive comparison is still needed to directly compare the latter two platforms.

The nuclease activity of Cas9 can be triggered when there is imperfect complementarity between the sgRNA sequence and an off-target site, particularly if mismatches are distal to the PAM sequence. For clinical translation of CRISPR-Cas9, defining the frequencies and locations of unintended nuclease-induced off-target mutations is important. Various approaches for detection of off-target effects have been described, including BLESS (direct in situ breaks labeling, enrichment on streptavidin, and next generation sequencing),[533,534] HTGTS (high-throughput, genome-wide, translocation sequencing),[535] GUIDE-Seq,[536,537] Digenome-Seq, and CIRCLE-Seq.[538,539] Even though reports have suggested possible extensive off-target effect for Cas9,[540] the magnitude of this effect remains controversial. Several strategies have been proposed to enhance Cas9 specificity, such as

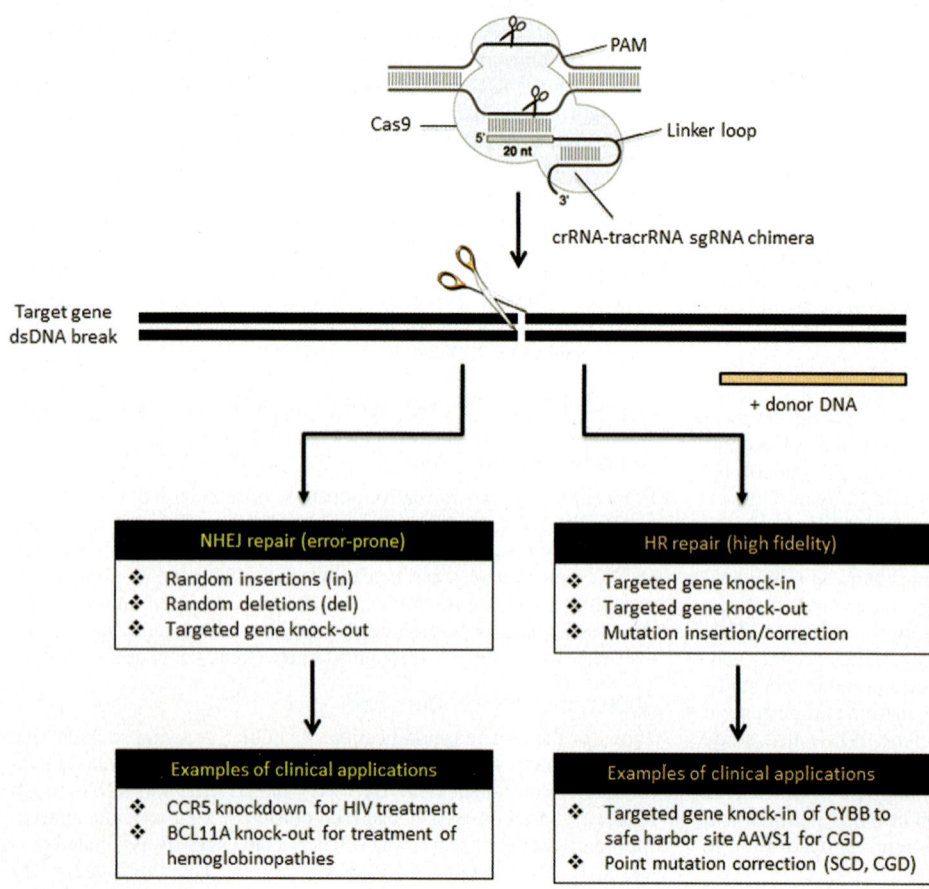

FIGURE 72.5 Genome editing with CRISPR/Cas9. A 100-nucleotide sgRNA targets the Cas9 endonuclease to a specific region of the genome. Target identification relies first on identification of a 3-base pair PAM sequence and then base-pairing between a 20-nucleotide stretch of the sgRNA and the DNA target site, which triggers Cas9 to cleave both DNA strands. dsDNA breaks are repaired by endogenous cellular mechanisms, including the error-prone NHEJ and the high fidelity HR pathways. Possible outcomes of this approach are indicated together with examples of clinical applications. AAVS1, adeno-associated virus integration site 1; CCR5, C-C chemokine receptor type 5; CGD, chronic granulomatous disease; CRISPR, clustered regularly interspaced short palindromic repeats; crRNA, CRISPR RNA; CYBB, cytochrome B β-chain; dsDNA, double-stranded DNA; HR, homologous recombination; NHEJ, nonhomologous end-joining; PAM, protospacer adjacent motif; SCD, sickle cell disease; sgRNA, single guide RNA; tracrRNA, trans-activating crRNA.

reducing the amount of active Cas9 in the cell,[541-543] using Cas9 nickase mutants to create a pair of juxtaposed ssDNA nicks,[544,545] truncating the guide sequence at the 5' end,[546] using a pair of catalytically inactive Cas9 nucleases, each fused to a FokI nuclease domain,[547,548] or using structure-guided protein engineering to improve the specificity of Cas9.[549]

Alternative strategies to manipulate cellular genomes that do not rely on double-stranded DNA cleavage and repair, including base editors,[550-553] prime editors,[554] and transposases/recombinases,[555-558] were also developed in recent years.[559] These approaches might be more effective than methods based on HR repair for HSC disorders. Base editing directly converts targeted base pairs and offers a promising therapeutic strategy for genetic disorders caused by point mutations. Adenine base editors (ABEs) and cytosine base editors (CBEs) can mediate targeted A/T to G/C or C/G to T/A base pair changes, respectively. They contain two primary components generally tethered to each other via a short linker: (1) An sgRNA-guided catalytically dead Cas9 nuclease (dCas9) or nickase Cas9 (nCas9) that can bind DNA but cannot make DSBs and (2) An ADA for ABE or cytidine deaminase for CBE for direct chemical conversion of the target bases. Cas binding exposes a small segment of ssDNA in an R-loop that then serves as substrate for the DNA modifying enzymes for base editing. The scope of base editing tools has been extensively broadened to allow higher efficiency, specificity, and accessibility to previously inaccessible genetic loci. However, they do not allow correction of DNA insertions or deletions, and efficient cellular delivery of the large components of base editors remains a significant challenge in hematopoietic stem cells.

Prime editing (PE) was developed as a more versatile system to enable correction of any point mutations, as well as short insertions (up to 44 bp) and deletions (up to 80 bp) and combinations of substitutions, insertions, and deletions.[554,559-561] PE is comprised of two primary modules: (1) An engineered reverse transcriptase (RT) fused to a Cas9 nickase that cuts only one strand of a DNA molecule, avoiding the formation of a DSB and (2) A PE gRNA (pegRNA) that contains a sequence complementary to the target DNA and a 3' extension encoding the desired edit. The PE complex binds one strand of the target DNA locus and nicks the opposite strand. This exposes a 3' DNA flap which binds to the primer binding site within the pegRNA. This RNA/DNA hybrid primes reverse transcription of the RNA template within the pegRNA extension. The edited 3' flap displaces the variant unedited DNA strand and is ultimately incorporated into the genome. This refined molecular tool is likely to advance therapeutic genome engineering. However, application of the PE system to primary HSCs presents inherent difficulties. For instance, even in its simplest form, it is large and highly modular, posing challenges for efficient cellular delivery. Moreover, targeted deletion, replacement, or integration of large genomic sequences cannot be mediated by the PE system. A variant of this approach, termed twin prime editing (twin PE), was recently developed to facilitate targeted integration of gene-sized DNA segments in transformed cell lines,[562] but the feasibility of this method in HSCs remains to be established.

Clinical Applications of Genome Editing in HSCs

Therapeutic genome-editing strategies based on activation of the NHEJ DSB repair pathways are more efficient than homology-directed repair mechanisms in HSCs. However, only rare HSC genetic disorders, such as SCD and β-thalassemia, can be cured by NHEJ-mediated incorporation of frameshift indels for disruption of open reading frames. Subjects with β-hemoglobinopathies who coinherit mutations causing hereditary persistence of fetal hemoglobin (HPFH), a benign condition where individuals display an unusually high expression of HbF, often present milder clinical symptoms.[563-565] Because HbF is normally silenced in adulthood by BCL11A,[566,567] disruption of coding or regulatory regions of the BCL11A gene are a promising tactic to induce HbF in patients' autologous HSCs and ameliorate clinical phenotype. To investigate this strategy, genome-editing approaches (ZFNs, TALENs, and CRISPR/Cas9) were initially used in preclinical studies to target exon 2 of BCL11A.[568] Unexpectedly, BCL11A was found to play a critical role in HSCs and BCL11A-deficient HSCs had markedly reduced engraftment potential after transplantation, limiting the potential clinical applicability of this approach.[569,570] This problem could be circumvented by targeting GATAA enhancer motif of BCL11A instead, likely because of residual BCL11A with this approach.[570] Cas9/sgRNA genome-editing strategies were also used to genetically recreate HPFH in human HSCs[571,572] with a robust rescue of the sickling phenotype found under hypoxic conditions.[571] Although encouraging, both studies failed to show long-term engraftment edited HSCs in the BM following long-term transplantation.

Based on these preclinical observations, the first evidence of clinical efficacy of NHEJ-based CRISPR genome editing in HSCs was reported in two patients, one with SCD and one with β-thalassemia, by disrupting a portion of the erythroid-control element of BCL11A in MPB CD34+ cells.[573] The cellular product (CTX001) was prepared by electroporation of an RNP complex targeting the BCL11A enhancer, and administered to each patient after busulfan-based myeloablative conditioning. After more than 1 year of follow-up, both patients had high BCL11A allelic editing frequencies in peripheral blood (~60%) and BM cells (~80%). No off-target editing was observed at any of the sites nominated by GUIDE-seq and by sequence homology. Both subjects experienced adverse events after receiving CTX001, including pneumonia, veno-occlusive liver disease with sinusoidal obstruction syndrome, sepsis, and cholelithiasis. All events resolved with treatment and both patients were clinically well at the time of last follow-up with marked increases in fetal hemoglobin distributed pancellularly, transfusion independence, and (in the patient with SCD) elimination of vaso-occlusive episodes.

Preclinical studies employing HR-based genome editing strategies have also been reported in β-hemoglobinopathies and X-linked CGD. The first reports used ZFNs[524] or CRISPR/Cas9[529,530] to revert the SCD-causing E6V point mutation to a wild-type sequence. While HR frequencies of 10% to 20% were observed in more mature progenitor cells in vitro, HR was much less efficient (0.2%-2%) in long-term repopulating cells measured after transplantation in NSG mice. In a subsequent report, improved HR frequencies (up to 7.5%) were observed after transplantation, by combining the delivery of Cas9/sgRNA RNP complexes by electroporation, and homologous donor template using rAAV6.[526] Enrichment scheme of targeted HSCs using reporters[526] or a marker-free methodology[531] can result in significant increase in gene-edited cells after transplantation, but the number of cells required is impractical for clinical applications.

Genome-editing technologies have also been employed in preclinical studies for correction of the defective CYBB gene in X-linked CGD. Using CD34+ cells from subjects with CGD, investigators used ZFN-based targeted gene addition to overexpress CYBB within the AAVS1 safe harbor site. They showed 6% to 16% human cell marking following engraftment into NSG mice, and functional correction in 15% of ex vivo–derived neutrophils of cells. Notably, use of a synthetic MND promoter, rather than an endogenous promoter at the AAVS1 site, was required to obtain robust functional correction. The same researchers showed high efficiency correction of the X-CGD C676T disease-causing mutation using electroporation (MaxCyte Systems) for the delivery of Cas9/sgRNA (as RNA) and ssODN donor template. Sequence-confirmed repair in >20% of hematopoietic stem and progenitor cells from these patients restored function in myeloid cells differentiated from these progenitors in vitro. Importantly, long-term (20 weeks) persistence of gene-edited cells (10%) was observed after transplantation, providing the highest demonstrated levels of HR in HSCs. Although promising, the ssODN strategy is limited in that it can only be applied to specific single point mutations.

Expansion of Genetically Modified HSCs

Low transduction efficiency of gene transfer vectors or low efficacy of HR-guided genome editing of primitive human HSCs may preclude sorting for a marker gene after genetic manipulation if, after sorting, too few stem cells remain to allow safe and rapid hematopoietic reconstitution; this is especially problematic after ablative chemotherapy. In addition, application of ex vivo gene therapy approaches requires sufficient number of cells to transduce. In some conditions, such as FA, the reduced numbers of HSCs limit the potential to treat through gene therapy. A potential solution to these issues would be HSC ex vivo expansion prior to reinfusion. However, when ex vivo–cultured cells compete against endogenous stem cells in a nonablative model, a significant engraftment defect is evident,[574,575] indicating that true long-term repopulating cells cannot be expanded efficiently or even maintained ex vivo using current culture conditions.[363,576-579] A number of small molecules have been identified that may support modest degrees of HSC expansion,[580,581] but the ideal drug or combination has not yet been reported that is capable of expanding human HSCs to a clinically meaningful extent (>10-fold) to improve the outcomes from gene therapy.

Derivation of Genetically Corrected HSCs From iPSCs

With Yamanaka's landmark reprogramming of adult somatic cells into iPSCs in 2006,[14] the appealing concept of generating iPSCs from an individual patient, correcting the genetic defect, and differentiating the disease-free iPSCs into a theoretically infinite supply of transplantable autologous HSCs arose. The proof of principle of using iPSC technologies to cure hematopoietic disorders attributed to a genetic defect has been performed in animal models[582-586] but obstacles still thwart clinical translation of this approach.

Several "directed differentiation" protocols have been proposed to facilitate the emergence of human HSCs from iPSCs.[587-591] These approaches aim at recapitulating hematopoietic development in vitro based on timed addition of cytokines and morphogens. Cells derived via directed differentiation display characteristics of primitive hematopoietic cells obtained from in vivo sources, including expression of HSC markers (e.g., CD34) and multilineage hematopoietic potential in clonogenic assays.[592] However, despite recent promising reports,[593,594] efficient derivation of functional HSCs with a robust capability for definitive in vivo engraftment and multilineage potential remains challenging.[595-599] Current protocols are thought to recapitulate the "primitive" wave of hematopoiesis during development. In this wave, the yolk sac transiently gives rise to nucleated glycophorin A+ ($CD235a^+$) red blood cells expressing embryonic hemoglobin, as well as primitive macrophages and megakaryocytes in the embryo. Only a later "definitive" wave of hematopoiesis, occurring intraembryonically in the aorta-gonad-mesonephros region in mammals and in particular the ventral wall of the dorsal aorta, provides HSCs with long-term repopulating potential.[600] This wave is not dependably reproduced by current in vitro iPSC differentiation approaches. In addition, the scale-up of these protocols to generate sufficient cells for clinical transplantation has not been addressed. At present, most differentiation protocols are based on embryoid body formation or coculture on OP9 cell lines. Translation of these iPSC-based approaches to a larger physiologic transplantation system would require liters of culture media and several grams of cytokines, rendering current approaches impractical and cost-ineffective for clinical applications. Therefore, new strategies to advance the current state of de novo HSC generation are needed for eventual clinical application.

Use of Purified HSCs

All HSC gene therapy clinical trials have used selected $CD34^+$ cells to enrich HSCs from collected BM or apheresis products. This approach reduces by at least 50-fold the number of cells and therefore the amount of vector needed for ex vivo transduction. Further purification based on surface markers that identify a more HSC-enriched population than bulk $CD34^+$ cells, such as $CD34^+CD38^-$ or $CD34^+CD90^+$, would further reduce by several folds the volumes of vector needed.[601] Because additional purification steps will likely come at the cost of additional cell losses of HSC,[602] an optimal compromise between enrichment and recovery will need to be struck.

Novel Pretransplant Conditioning Regimens

Conditioning has been demonstrated to be fundamental for appropriate engraftment of gene corrected cells.[603] Reduced intensity conditioning with busulfan has been well tolerated by patients in the short term. However, to reduce the risk of long-term sequelae of chemotherapy,[479] novel conditioning approaches are currently under investigation. The use of monoclonal antibodies, either alone or conjugated to an internalizing toxin, to target specific antigens on hematopoietic cells has been proposed as a tractable alternative, especially in contexts such as ex vivo autologous gene therapy. Efficient clearance of marrow has been demonstrated in preclinical models using CD45- or CD117-targeting antibodies conjugated to nonselective toxins.[384-386,388,604-606] By more selectively targeting and depleting HSCs in the BM, these strategies could allow robust, multilineage engraftment of autologous gene-corrected HSCs with minimal toxicity to nonhematopoietic tissues. This will be of particular relevance for more compromised patients, with pre-existing organ damage or for those with a milder phenotype when risks of conventional conditioning regimen would not be acceptable.

In Vivo Gene Therapy

All HSC gene therapy studies to date have relied on HSC harvest and ex vivo transduction before reinfusion. Ideally, suitable approaches will be developed that allow direct in vivo transduction of HSCs. By avoiding ex vivo HSC manipulation, the risk of cell loss through differentiation leading to homing/engraftment defects would be eliminated. Conceivably, in vivo gene therapy could also target most HSCs. Importantly, the need for toxic pretransplant conditioning regimens would be bypassed. Finally, the technical complexity and high cost of current ex vivo HSC gene therapy, barriers to a widespread application of this technology, would be circumvented with a simpler injection or infusion of gene transfer vectors.

As described in the section below, the most important problem posed by in vivo HSC gene therapy is the innate and adaptive immune responses potentially triggered by the gene transfer vectors. It is thought that AAVs trigger a weaker immune response than other vectors based on adenoviruses or LVs, but a direct comparison of the vector systems is unavailable. Another drawback of in vivo gene therapy is the requirement for higher doses of gene transfer vectors. This is due to vector sequestration by the reticuloendothelial system and the transduction of other cells in the body. Development of suitable targeted vectors could resolve this issue. Other technologies are being tested for the in vivo delivery of gene-editing agents, including lipid/polymer nanoparticles[607] and, more recently, viral like particles.[608,609] While promising, these strategies still require rigorous safety and efficacy testing before its widespread clinical application becomes a reality.

Immune Responses to Vectors and Transgenes

Immune responses against vector proteins or the transgene-encoded protein itself in a genetically null recipient have been the focus of intensive investigation. For in vivo vector administration, pre-existing immunity to a vector such as adenovirus is at least a theoretical concern. Repeated in vivo administration of complex vectors clearly stimulates an active immune response to vector proteins and greatly hinders success. The expression of viral genes remaining in the vector sequences could also stimulate an immune response against transduced target cells. This is not a problem for retroviral vectors; as well, newer modifications of adenoviral vectors have been developed that no longer contain or express residual adenoviral genes.[610,611] Non–human marker genes such as the neomycin resistance gene or viral suicide genes such as HSV-tk included in vectors for positive or negative selection may also induce an immune response.[612] Finally, the therapeutic gene product itself may induce an immune response if the patient completely lacks the endogenous gene product or the transgenic protein is processed or posttranslationally modified.[118]

Foreign genes expressed by HSCs and their progeny may be capable of inducing tolerance even across MHC barriers. Evidence was provided in a murine model of allogeneic skin graft survival.[613] Documentation in mice of very long-term persistence of expression of completely xenogeneic genes such as human GC also suggests that immune responses against genes introduced via repopulating stem cells will not induce immune responses.[244,614] On the other hand, immune responses to a retroviral vector–introduced transgene in the canine MPS-1 autologous transplantation model have been shown to limit efficiency.[615] Long-term persistence of genetically modified cells at clinically relevant levels can be achieved after very low dose irradiation with 100 cGy, even when highly immunogenic genes are transferred. Large animal testing in the nonhuman primate confirmed these observations, with equivalent levels of long-term engraftment of cells transduced with either a vector encoding the neo^R gene or a vector carrying but not expressing this gene product, but the overall levels of engraftment were much lower.[616]

Various methods of immunosuppression have been at least partially successful in avoiding immune rejection of transduced cells. Neonatal exposure to vector has allowed repeated treatments with adenoviral vectors.[126] Treatment with cyclosporine, cyclophosphamide, or IL-12 have all been reported to prolong survival of transduced cells.[123-127] But these general pharmacologic approaches are not desirable or practical for most gene therapy applications, which are attractive only if they prevent life-long reliance on toxic pharmacologic agents. Instead, improved vector design and possible inclusion of antirejection mechanisms in the vectors themselves are more attractive approaches.

CONCLUSIONS

Following a roller coaster ride, it is fair to impart that the field of HSC gene therapy has delivered on its promise 30 years ago to produce a new therapeutic option for patients with inherited blood disorders. The field owes a debt of gratitude to the brave families who enrolled their children on clinical trials, together with the clinicians who led this work and provided vital learning for the adjacent fields for the future. With the hope of bringing far-reaching curative treatments to patients with inherited HSC disorders, the next chapter of gene editing will be compelling to follow.

References

1. Blau HM, Springer ML. Gene therapy – a novel form of drug delivery. *N Engl J Med*. 1995;333(18):1204-1207.
2. Brenner MK. Gene transfer to hematopoietic cells. *N Engl J Med*. 1996;335(5):337-339.
3. Dunbar CE. Gene transfer to hematopoietic stem cells: implications for gene therapy of human disease. *Annu Rev Med*. 1996;47:11-20.
4. Dunbar CE, Emmons RV. Gene transfer into hematopoietic progenitor and stem cells: progress and problems. *Stem Cells*. 1994;12(6):563-576.
5. Hanania EG, Kavanagh J, Hortobagyi G, Giles RE, Champlin R, Deisseroth AB. Recent advances in the application of gene therapy to human disease. *Am J Med*. 1995;99(5):537-552.
6. Karlsson S. Treatment of genetic defects in hematopoietic cell function by gene transfer. *Blood*. 1991;78(10):2481-2492.
7. Yu M, Poeschla E, Wong-Staal F. Progress towards gene therapy for HIV infection. *Gene Ther*. 1994;1(1):13-26.
8. Hopman RK, DiPersio JF. Advances in stem cell mobilization. *Blood Rev*. 2014;28(1):31-40.
9. Ballen KK, Gluckman E, Broxmeyer HE. Umbilical cord blood transplantation: the first 25 years and beyond. *Blood*. 2013;122(4):491-498.
10. Huntsman HD, Bat T, Cheng H, et al. Human hematopoietic stem cells from mobilized peripheral blood can be purified based on CD49f integrin expression. *Blood*. 2015;126(13):1631-1633.
11. Majeti R, Park CY, Weissman IL. Identification of a hierarchy of multipotent hematopoietic progenitors in human cord blood. *Cell Stem Cell*. 2007;1(6):635-645.
12. Notta F, Doulatov S, Laurenti E, Poeppl A, Jurisica I, Dick JE. Isolation of single human hematopoietic stem cells capable of long-term multilineage engraftment. *Science*. 2011;333(6039):218-221.
13. Peters T. "Playing God" and germline intervention. *J Med Philos*. 1995;20(4):365-386.
14. Takahashi K, Yamanaka S. Induction of pluripotent stem cells from mouse embryonic and adult fibroblast cultures by defined factors. *Cell*. 2006;126(4):663-676.
15. Capecchi MR. Altering the genome by homologous recombination. *Science*. 1989;244(4910):1288-1292.
16. Camerini-Otero RD, Hsieh P. Homologous recombination proteins in prokaryotes and eukaryotes. *Annu Rev Genet*. 1995;29:509-552.
17. Stasiak A. Getting down to the core of homologous recombination. *Science*. 1996;272(5263):828-829.
18. Li H, Yang Y, Hong W, Huang M, Wu M, Zhao X. Applications of genome editing technology in the targeted therapy of human diseases: mechanisms, advances and prospects. *Signal Transduct Target Ther*. 2020;5:1.
19. Gaj T, Gersbach CA, Barbas CF III. ZFN, TALEN, and CRISPR/Cas-based methods for genome engineering. *Trends Biotechnol*. 2013;31(7):397-405.
20. Cornetta K, Morgan RA, Anderson WF. Safety issues related to retroviral-mediated gene transfer in humans. *Hum Gene Ther*. 1991;2(1):5-14.
21. Cooper MJ. Noninfectious gene transfer and expression systems for cancer gene therapy. *Semin Oncol*. 1996;23(1):172-187.
22. Miller AD. Cell-surface receptors for retroviruses and implications for gene transfer. *Proc Natl Acad Sci U S A*. 1996;93(21):11407-11413.
23. Yang Y, Vanin EF, Whitt MA, et al. Inducible, high-level production of infectious murine leukemia retroviral vector particles pseudotyped with vesicular stomatitis virus G envelope protein. *Hum Gene Ther*. 1995;6(9):1203-1213.
24. Burns JC, Friedmann T, Driever W, Burrascano M, Yee JK. Vesicular stomatitis virus G glycoprotein pseudotyped retroviral vectors: concentration to very high titer and efficient gene transfer into mammalian and nonmammalian cells. *Proc Natl Acad Sci U S A*. 1993;90(17):8033-8037.
25. Hopkins N. High titers of retrovirus (vesicular stomatitis virus) pseudotypes, at last. *Proc Natl Acad Sci U S A*. 1993;90(19):8759-8760.
26. Kasahara N, Dozy AM, Kan YW. Tissue-specific targeting of retroviral vectors through ligand-receptor interactions. *Science*. 1994;266(5189):1373-1376.
27. Holland CA, Anklesaria P, Sakakeeny MA, Greenberger JS. Enhancer sequences of a retroviral vector determine expression of a gene in multipotent hematopoietic progenitors and committed erythroid cells. *Proc Natl Acad Sci U S A*. 1987;84(23):8662-8666.
28. Miller JL, Walsh CE, Ney PA, Samulski RJ, Nienhuis AW. Single-copy transduction and expression of human gamma-globin in K562 erythroleukemia cells using recombinant adeno-associated virus vectors: the effect of mutations in NF-E2 and GATA-1 binding motifs within the hypersensitivity site 2 enhancer. *Blood*. 1993;82(6):1900-1906.
29. Wu X, Holschen J, Kennedy SC, Ponder KP. Retroviral vector sequences may interact with some internal promoters and influence expression. *Hum Gene Ther*. 1996;7(2):159-171.
30. Hofmann A, Nolan GP, Blau HM. Rapid retroviral delivery of tetracycline-inducible genes in a single autoregulatory cassette. *Proc Natl Acad Sci U S A*. 1996;93(11):5185-5190.
31. Gossen M, Freundlieb S, Bender G, Muller G, Hillen W, Bujard H. Transcriptional activation by tetracyclines in mammalian cells. *Science*. 1995;268(5218):1766-1769.
32. Williams DA, Lim B, Spooncer E, Longtine J, Dexter TM. Restriction of expression of an integrated recombinant retrovirus in primary but not immortalized murine hematopoietic stem cells. *Blood*. 1988;71(6):1738-1743.
33. Lu M, Maruyama M, Zhang N, Levine F, Friedmann T, Ho AD. High efficiency retroviral-mediated gene transduction into CD34+ cells purified from peripheral blood of breast cancer patients primed with chemotherapy and granulocyte-macrophage colony-stimulating factor. *Hum Gene Ther*. 1994;5(2):203-208.
34. Challita PM, Kohn DB. Lack of expression from a retroviral vector after transduction of murine hematopoietic stem cells is associated with methylation in vivo. *Proc Natl Acad Sci U S A*. 1994;91(7):2567-2571.
35. Zhang WW, Fujiwara T, Grimm EA, Roth JA. Advances in cancer gene therapy. *Adv Pharmacol*. 1995;32:289-341.
36. Yang NS, Sun WH. Gene gun and other non-viral approaches for cancer gene therapy. *Nat Med*. 1995;1(5):481-483.
37. Johnston SA, Tang DC. Gene gun transfection of animal cells and genetic immunization. *Methods Cell Biol*. 1994;43:353-365.
38. Woffendin C, Yang ZY, Udaykumar, et al. Nonviral and viral delivery of a human immunodeficiency virus protective gene into primary human T cells. *Proc Natl Acad Sci U S A*. 1994;91(24):11581-11585.
39. Klein RM, Wolf ED, Wu R, Sanford JC. High-velocity microprojectiles for delivering nucleic acids into living cells. 1987. *Biotechnology*. 1992;24:384-386.
40. Yang NS, Burkholder J, Roberts B, Martinell B, McCabe D. In vivo and in vitro gene transfer to mammalian somatic cells by particle bombardment. *Proc Natl Acad Sci U S A*. 1990;87(24):9568-9572.
41. Mannino RJ, Gould-Fogerite S. Liposome mediated gene transfer. *Biotechniques*. 1988;6(7):682-690.
42. Shigekawa K, Dower WJ. Electroporation of eukaryotes and prokaryotes: a general approach to the introduction of macromolecules into cells. *Biotechniques*. 1988;6(8):742-751.
43. Chen CA, Okayama H. Calcium phosphate-mediated gene transfer: a highly efficient transfection system for stably transforming cells with plasmid DNA. *Biotechniques*. 1988;6(7):632-638.
44. Andreason GL, Evans GA. Introduction and expression of DNA molecules in eukaryotic cells by electroporation. *Biotechniques*. 1988;6(7):650-660.
45. Farhood H, Gao X, Son K, et al. Cationic liposomes for direct gene transfer in therapy of cancer and other diseases. *Ann N Y Acad Sci*. 1994;716:23-34, discussion -5.
46. Felgner PL, Tsai YJ, Sukhu L, et al. Improved cationic lipid formulations for in vivo gene therapy. *Ann N Y Acad Sci*. 1995;772:126-139.
47. Labat-Moleur F, Steffan AM, Brisson C, et al. An electron microscopy study into the mechanism of gene transfer with lipopolyamines. *Gene Ther*. 1996;3(11):1010-1017.
48. Zhu N, Liggitt D, Liu Y, Debs R. Systemic gene expression after intravenous DNA delivery into adult mice. *Science*. 1993;261(5118):209-211.
49. Baudard M, Flotte TR, Aran JM, et al. Expression of the human multidrug resistance and glucocerebrosidase cDNAs from adeno-associated vectors: efficient promoter activity of AAV sequences and in vivo delivery via liposomes. *Hum Gene Ther*. 1996;7(11):1309-1322.
50. Ledley FD. Nonviral gene therapy: the promise of genes as pharmaceutical products. *Hum Gene Ther*. 1995;6(9):1129-1144.
51. Izsvak Z, Chuah MK, Vandendriessche T, Ivics Z. Efficient stable gene transfer into human cells by the Sleeping Beauty transposon vectors. *Methods*. 2009;49(3):287-297.
52. Mates L, Chuah MK, Belay E, et al. Molecular evolution of a novel hyperactive Sleeping Beauty transposase enables robust stable gene transfer in vertebrates. *Nat Genet*. 2009;41(6):753-761.

53. Kebriaei P, Izsvak Z, Narayanavari SA, Singh H, Ivics Z. Gene therapy with the sleeping beauty transposon system. *Trends Genet.* 2017;33(11):852-870.
54. Grimes BR, Warburton PE, Farr CJ. Chromosome engineering: prospects for gene therapy. *Gene Ther.* 2002;9(11):713-718.
55. Gunzburg WH, Salmons B. Development of retroviral vectors as safe, targeted gene delivery systems. *J Mol Med.* 1996;74(4):171-182.
56. Miller AD. Retroviral vectors. *Curr Top Microbiol Immunol.* 1992;158:1-24.
57. Coffin JM, ed. *Retroviridae: The Viruses and Their Replication.* Lippincott-Raven; 1996.
58. Kozak SL, Siess DC, Kavanaugh MP, Miller AD, Kabat D. The envelope glycoprotein of an amphotropic murine retrovirus binds specifically to the cellular receptor/phosphate transporter of susceptible species. *J Virol.* 1995;69(6):3433-3440.
59. Miller DG, Edwards RH, Miller AD. Cloning of the cellular receptor for amphotropic murine retroviruses reveals homology to that for gibbon ape leukemia virus. *Proc Natl Acad Sci U S A.* 1994;91(1):78-82.
60. Kavanaugh MP, Miller DG, Zhang W, et al. Cell-surface receptors for gibbon ape leukemia virus and amphotropic murine retrovirus are inducible sodium-dependent phosphate symporters. *Proc Natl Acad Sci U S A.* 1994;91(15):7071-7075.
61. Mann R, Mulligan RC, Baltimore D. Construction of a retrovirus packaging mutant and its use to produce helper-free defective retrovirus. *Cell.* 1983;33(1):153-159.
62. Boris-Lawrie K, Temin HM. The retroviral vector. Replication cycle and safety considerations for retrovirus-mediated gene therapy. *Ann N Y Acad Sci.* 1994;716:59-70, discussion 1.
63. Kurth R. Risk potential of the chromosomal insertion of foreign DNA. *Ann N Y Acad Sci.* 1995;772:140-151.
64. Donahue RE, Kessler SW, Bodine D, et al. Helper virus induced T cell lymphoma in nonhuman primates after retroviral mediated gene transfer. *J Exp Med.* 1992;176(4):1125-1135.
65. Miller AD, Buttimore C. Redesign of retrovirus packaging cell lines to avoid recombination leading to helper virus production. *Mol Cell Biol.* 1986;6(8):2895-2902.
66. Miller AD. Retrovirus packaging cells. *Hum Gene Ther.* 1990;1(1):5-14.
67. Markowitz D, Goff S, Bank A. A safe packaging line for gene transfer: separating viral genes on two different plasmids. *J Virol.* 1988;62(4):1120-1124.
68. Ory DS, Neugeboren BA, Mulligan RC. A stable human-derived packaging cell line for production of high titer retrovirus/vesicular stomatitis virus G pseudotypes. *Proc Natl Acad Sci U S A.* 1996;93(21):11400-11406.
69. Rigg RJ, Chen J, Dando JS, Forestell SP, Plavec I, Bohnlein E. A novel human amphotropic packaging cell line: high titer, complement resistance, and improved safety. *Virology.* 1996;218(1):290-295.
70. Orlic D, Girard LJ, Jordan CT, Anderson SM, Cline AP, Bodine DM. The level of mRNA encoding the amphotropic retrovirus receptor in mouse and human hematopoietic stem cells is low and correlates with the efficiency of retrovirus transduction. *Proc Natl Acad Sci U S A.* 1996;93(20):11097-11102.
71. Miller DG, Adam MA, Miller AD. Gene transfer by retrovirus vectors occurs only in cells that are actively replicating at the time of infection. *Mol Cell Biol.* 1990;10(8):4239-4242.
72. May C, Rivella S, Callegari J, et al. Therapeutic haemoglobin synthesis in beta-thalassaemic mice expressing lentivirus-encoded human beta-globin. *Nature.* 2000;406(6791):82-86.
73. Yu SF, von Ruden T, Kantoff PW, et al. Self-inactivating retroviral vectors designed for transfer of whole genes into mammalian cells. *Proc Natl Acad Sci U S A.* 1986;83(10):3194-3198.
74. Shimada T, Fujii H, Mitsuya H, Nienhuis AW. Targeted and highly efficient gene transfer into CD4+ cells by a recombinant human immunodeficiency virus retroviral vector. *J Clin Invest.* 1991;88(3):1043-1047.
75. Naldini L, Blomer U, Gallay P, et al. In vivo gene delivery and stable transduction of nondividing cells by a lentiviral vector. *Science.* 1996;272(5259):263-267.
76. Reiser J, Harmison G, Kluepfel-Stahl S, Brady RO, Karlsson S, Schubert M. Transduction of nondividing cells using pseudotyped defective high-titer HIV type 1 particles. *Proc Natl Acad Sci U S A.* 1996;93(26):15266-15271.
77. Cronin J, Zhang XY, Reiser J. Altering the tropism of lentiviral vectors through pseudotyping. *Curr Gene Ther.* 2005;5(4):387-398.
78. Kelly PF, Vandergriff J, Nathwani A, Nienhuis AW, Vanin EF. Highly efficient gene transfer into cord blood nonobese diabetic/severe combined immunodeficiency repopulating cells by oncoretroviral vector particles pseudotyped with the feline endogenous retrovirus (RD114) envelope protein. *Blood.* 2000;96(4):1206-1214.
79. Porter CD, Collins MK, Tailor CS, et al. Comparison of efficiency of infection of human gene therapy target cells via four different retroviral receptors. *Hum Gene Ther.* 1996;7(8):913-919.
80. Movassagh M, Desmyter C, Baillou C, et al. High-level gene transfer to cord blood progenitors using gibbon ape leukemia virus pseudotype retroviral vectors and an improved clinically applicable protocol. *Hum Gene Ther.* 1998;9(2):225-234.
81. Marandin A, Dubart A, Pflumio F, et al. Retrovirus-mediated gene transfer into human CD34+38low primitive cells capable of reconstituting long-term cultures in vitro and nonobese diabetic-severe combined immunodeficiency mice in vivo. *Hum Gene Ther.* 1998;9(10):1497-1511.
82. Bouard D, Sandrin V, Boson B, et al. An acidic cluster of the cytoplasmic tail of the RD114 virus glycoprotein controls assembly of retroviral envelopes. *Traffic.* 2007;8(7):835-847.
83. Christodoulopoulos I, Cannon PM. Sequences in the cytoplasmic tail of the gibbon ape leukemia virus envelope protein that prevent its incorporation into lentivirus vectors. *J Virol.* 2001;75(9):4129-4138.
84. Sandrin V, Boson B, Salmon P, et al. Lentiviral vectors pseudotyped with a modified RD114 envelope glycoprotein show increased stability in sera and augmented transduction of primary lymphocytes and CD34+ cells derived from human and nonhuman primates. *Blood.* 2002;100(3):823-832.
85. Bartz SR, Rogel ME, Emerman M. Human immunodeficiency virus type 1 cell cycle control: vpr is cytostatic and mediates G2 accumulation by a mechanism which differs from DNA damage checkpoint control. *J Virol.* 1996;70(4):2324-2331.
86. Coil DA, Miller AD. Phosphatidylserine is not the cell surface receptor for vesicular stomatitis virus. *J Virol.* 2004;78(20):10920-10926.
87. Kim YS, Wielgosz MM, Hargrove P, et al. Transduction of human primitive repopulating hematopoietic cells with lentiviral vectors pseudotyped with various envelope proteins. *Mol Ther.* 2010;18(7):1310-1317.
88. De Ravin SS, Wu X, Moir S, et al. Lentiviral hematopoietic stem cell gene therapy for X-linked severe combined immunodeficiency. *Sci Transl Med.* 2016;8(335):335ra57.
89. Greene MR, Lockey T, Mehta PK, et al. Transduction of human CD34+ repopulating cells with a self-inactivating lentiviral vector for SCID-X1 produced at clinical scale by a stable cell line. *Hum Gene Ther Methods.* 2012;23(5):297-308.
90. Throm RE, Ouma AA, Zhou S, et al. Efficient construction of producer cell lines for a SIN lentiviral vector for SCID-X1 gene therapy by concatemeric array transfection. *Blood.* 2009;113(21):5104-5110.
91. Verhoeyen E, Wiznerowicz M, Olivier D, et al. Novel lentiviral vectors displaying "early-acting cytokines" selectively promote survival and transduction of NOD/SCID repopulating human hematopoietic stem cells. *Blood.* 2005;106(10):3386-3395.
92. Frecha C, Costa C, Negre D, et al. A novel lentiviral vector targets gene transfer into human hematopoietic stem cells in marrow from patients with bone marrow failure syndrome and in vivo in humanized mice. *Blood.* 2012;119(5):1139-1150.
93. Goodman M, Arumugam PI, Pillis D, et al. Foamy virus backbone has insulator properties which remarkably reduce its genotoxicity potential. *Blood.* 2016;128(22):1002.
94. Bauer TR Jr, Allen JM, Hai M, et al. Successful treatment of canine leukocyte adhesion deficiency by foamy virus vectors. *Nat Med.* 2008;14(1):93-97.
95. Beard BC, Keyser KA, Trobridge GD, et al. Unique integration profiles in a canine model of long-term repopulating cells transduced with gammaretrovirus, lentivirus, or foamy virus. *Hum Gene Ther.* 2007;18(5):423-434.
96. Everson EM, Olzsko ME, Leap DJ, Hocum JD, Trobridge GD. A comparison of foamy and lentiviral vector genotoxicity in SCID-repopulating cells shows foamy vectors are less prone to clonal dominance. *Mol Ther Methods Clin Dev.* 2016;3:16048.
97. Trobridge GD, Miller DG, Jacobs MA, et al. Foamy virus vector integration sites in normal human cells. *Proc Natl Acad Sci U S A.* 2006;103(5):1498-1503.
98. Mergia A, Heinkelein M. Foamy virus vectors. *Curr Top Microbiol Immunol.* 2003;277:131-159.
99. Russell DW, Miller AD. Foamy virus vectors. *J Virol.* 1996;70(1):217-222.
100. Yu SF, Baldwin DN, Gwynn SR, Yendapalli S, Linial ML. Human foamy virus replication: a pathway distinct from that of retroviruses and hepadnaviruses. *Science.* 1996;271(5255):1579-1582.
101. Yu SF, Sullivan MD, Linial ML. Evidence that the human foamy virus genome is DNA. *J Virol.* 1999;73(2):1565-1572.
102. Moebes A, Enssle J, Bieniasz PD, et al. Human foamy virus reverse transcription that occurs late in the viral replication cycle. *J Virol.* 1997;71(10):7305-7311.
103. Roy J, Rudolph W, Juretzek T, et al. Feline foamy virus genome and replication strategy. *J Virol.* 2003;77(21):11324-11331.
104. Gothot A, van der Loo JC, Clapp DW, Srour EF. Cell cycle-related changes in repopulating capacity of human mobilized peripheral blood CD34(+) cells in non-obese diabetic/severe combined immune-deficient mice. *Blood.* 1998;92(8):2641-2649.
105. Trobridge GD, Russell DW. Helper-free foamy virus vectors. *Hum Gene Ther.* 1998;9(17):2517-2525.
106. Chatziandreou I, Siapati EK, Vassilopoulos G. Genetic correction of X-linked chronic granulomatous disease with novel foamy virus vectors. *Exp Hematol.* 2011;39(6):643-652.
107. Trobridge GD, Beard BC, Wu RA, Ironside C, Malik P, Kiem HP. Stem cell selection in vivo using foamy vectors cures canine pyruvate kinase deficiency. *PLoS One.* 2012;7(9):e45173.
108. Shenk T. Adenoviridae: The viruses and their replication. In: Fields BN, Knipe DM, Howley PM, eds. *Fields Virology.* Lippincott-Raven; 1996:2111-2148.
109. Huang S, Kamata T, Takada Y, Ruggeri ZM, Nemerow GR. Adenovirus interaction with distinct integrins mediates separate events in cell entry and gene delivery to hematopoietic cells. *J Virol.* 1996;70(7):4502-4508.
110. Bergelson JM, Cunningham JA, Droguett G, et al. Isolation of a common receptor for Coxsackie B viruses and adenoviruses 2 and 5. *Science.* 1997;275(5304):1320-1323.
111. Berns KI, Giraud C. Adenovirus and adeno-associated virus as vectors for gene therapy. *Ann N Y Acad Sci.* 1995;772:95-104.
112. Berkner KL. Expression of heterologous sequences in adenoviral vectors. *Curr Top Microbiol Immunol.* 1992;158:39-66.
113. Wilson JM. Adenoviruses as gene-delivery vehicles. *N Engl J Med.* 1996;334(18):1185-1187.
114. Brody SL, Crystal RG. Adenovirus-mediated in vivo gene transfer. *Ann N Y Acad Sci.* 1994;716:90-101, discussion 101-103.
115. Siegfried W. Perspectives in gene therapy with recombinant adenoviruses. *Exp Clin Endocrinol.* 1993;101(1):7-11.
116. Rosenfeld MA, Collins FS. Gene therapy for cystic fibrosis. *Chest.* 1996;109(1):241-252.
117. Rosenfeld MA, Yoshimura K, Trapnell BC, et al. In vivo transfer of the human cystic fibrosis transmembrane conductance regulator gene to the airway epithelium. *Cell.* 1992;68(1):143-155.
118. Tripathy SK, Black HB, Goldwasser E, Leiden JM. Immune responses to transgene-encoded proteins limit the stability of gene expression after injection of replication-defective adenovirus vectors. *Nat Med.* 1996;2(5):545-550.

119. Yang Y, Su Q, Wilson JM. Role of viral antigens in destructive cellular immune responses to adenovirus vector-transduced cells in mouse lungs. *J Virol.* 1996;70(10):7209-7212.
120. Crystal RG, McElvaney NG, Rosenfeld MA, et al. Administration of an adenovirus containing the human CFTR cDNA to the respiratory tract of individuals with cystic fibrosis. *Nat Genet.* 1994;8(1):42-51.
121. Yang Y, Li Q, Ertl HC, Wilson JM. Cellular and humoral immune responses to viral antigens create barriers to lung-directed gene therapy with recombinant adenoviruses. *J Virol.* 1995;69(4):2004-2015.
122. Cerullo V, Seiler MP, Mane V, et al. Toll-like receptor 9 triggers an innate immune response to helper-dependent adenoviral vectors. *Mol Ther.* 2007;15(2):378-385.
123. Yang Y, Trinchieri G, Wilson JM. Recombinant IL-12 prevents formation of blocking IgA antibodies to recombinant adenovirus and allows repeated gene therapy to mouse lung. *Nat Med.* 1995;1(9):890-893.
124. Dai Y, Schwarz EM, Gu D, Zhang WW, Sarvetnick N, Verma IM. Cellular and humoral immune responses to adenoviral vectors containing factor IX gene: tolerization of factor IX and vector antigens allows for long-term expression. *Proc Natl Acad Sci U S A.* 1995;92(5):1401-1405.
125. Fang B, Eisensmith RC, Wang H, et al. Gene therapy for hemophilia B: host immunosuppression prolongs the therapeutic effect of adenovirus-mediated factor IX expression. *Hum Gene Ther.* 1995;6(8):1039-1044.
126. Walter J, You Q, Hagstrom JN, Sands M, High KA. Successful expression of human factor IX following repeat administration of adenoviral vector in mice. *Proc Natl Acad Sci U S A.* 1996;93(7):3056-3061.
127. Smith TA, White BD, Gardner JM, Kaleko M, McClelland A. Transient immunosuppression permits successful repetitive intravenous administration of an adenovirus vector. *Gene Ther.* 1996;3(6):496-502.
128. Abbink P, Lemckert AA, Ewald BA, et al. Comparative seroprevalence and immunogenicity of six rare serotype recombinant adenovirus vaccine vectors from subgroups B and D. *J Virol.* 2007;81(9):4654-4663.
129. Lemiale F, Haddada H, Nabel GJ, Brough DE, King CR, Gall JG. Novel adenovirus vaccine vectors based on the enteric-tropic serotype 41. *Vaccine.* 2007;25(11):2074-2084.
130. Zabner J, Couture LA, Gregory RJ, Graham SM, Smith AE, Welsh MJ. Adenovirus-mediated gene transfer transiently corrects the chloride transport defect in nasal epithelia of patients with cystic fibrosis. *Cell.* 1993;75(2):207-216.
131. Crystal RG, Jaffe A, Brody S, et al. A phase 1 study, in cystic fibrosis patients, of the safety, toxicity, and biological efficacy of a single administration of a replication deficient, recombinant adenovirus carrying the cDNA of the normal cystic fibrosis transmembrane conductance regulator gene in the lung. *Hum Gene Ther.* 1995;6(5):643-666.
132. Crystal RG, Mastrangeli A, Sanders A, et al. Evaluation of repeat administration of a replication deficient, recombinant adenovirus containing the normal cystic fibrosis transmembrane conductance regulator cDNA to the airways of individuals with cystic fibrosis. *Hum Gene Ther.* 1995;6(5):667-703.
133. Raper SE, Chirmule N, Lee FS, et al. Fatal systemic inflammatory response syndrome in a ornithine transcarbamylase deficient patient following adenoviral gene transfer. *Mol Genet Metab.* 2003;80(1-2):148-158.
134. Wilson JM. Lessons learned from the gene therapy trial for ornithine transcarbamylase deficiency. *Mol Genet Metab.* 2009;96(4):151-157.
135. Yarborough M, Sharp RR. Public trust and research a decade later: what have we learned since Jesse Gelsinger's death? *Mol Genet Metab.* 2009;97(1):4-5.
136. Descamps V, Duffour MT, Mathieu MC, et al. Strategies for cancer gene therapy using adenoviral vectors. *J Mol Med.* 1996;74(4):183-189.
137. Clayman GL, el-Naggar AK, Roth JA, et al. In vivo molecular therapy with p53 adenovirus for microscopic residual head and neck squamous carcinoma. *Cancer Res.* 1995;55(1):1-6.
138. Caruso M, Pham-Nguyen K, Kwong YL, et al. Adenovirus-mediated interleukin-12 gene therapy for metastatic colon carcinoma. *Proc Natl Acad Sci U S A.* 1996;93(21):11302-11306.
139. Flotte TR, Carter BJ. Adeno-associated virus vectors for gene therapy. *Gene Ther.* 1995;2(6):357-362.
140. Berns KI. Parvoviridae: the viruses and their replication. In: Fields BN, ed. *Fields Virology.* Lippincott-Raven; 1996:2173-2198.
141. Bartlett JS, Samulski RJ. Genetics and biology of adeno-associated virus. In: Kaplitt MG, Loewy AD, eds. *Viral Vectors: Gene Therapy and Neuroscience Applications.* Academic Press; 1995:55-73.
142. Summerford C, Samulski RJ. Membrane-associated heparan sulfate proteoglycan is a receptor for adeno-associated virus type 2 virions. *J Virol.* 1998;72(2):1438-1445.
143. Summerford C, Bartlett JS, Samulski RJ. AlphaVbeta5 integrin: a co-receptor for adeno-associated virus type 2 infection. *Nat Med.* 1999;5(1):78-82.
144. Mayor HD. Defective parvoviruses may be good for your health! *Prog Med Virol.* 1993;40:193-205.
145. Hermonat PL. Inhibition of H-ras expression by the adeno-associated virus Rep78 transformation suppressor gene product. *Cancer Res.* 1991;51(13):3373-3377.
146. Antoni BA, Rabson AB, Miller IL, Trempe JP, Chejanovsky N, Carter BJ. Adeno-associated virus Rep protein inhibits human immunodeficiency virus type 1 production in human cells. *J Virol.* 1991;65(1):396-404.
147. Georg-Fries B, Biederlack S, Wolf J, zur Hausen H. Analysis of proteins, helper dependence, and seroepidemiology of a new human parvovirus. *Virology.* 1984;134(1):64-71.
148. Cheung AK, Hoggan MD, Hauswirth WW, Berns KI. Integration of the adeno-associated virus genome into cellular DNA in latently infected human Detroit 6 cells. *J Virol.* 1980;33(2):739-748.
149. Samulski RJ, Zhu X, Xiao X, et al. Targeted integration of adeno-associated virus (AAV) into human chromosome 19. *EMBO J.* 1991;10(12):3941-3950.
150. Linden RM, Ward P, Giraud C, Winocour E, Berns KI. Site-specific integration by adeno-associated virus. *Proc Natl Acad Sci U S A.* 1996;93(21):11288-11294.
151. Kotin RM. Prospects for the use of adeno-associated virus as a vector for human gene therapy. *Hum Gene Ther.* 1994;5(7):793-801.
152. Muzyczka N. Use of adeno-associated virus as a general transduction vector for mammalian cells. *Curr Top Microbiol Immunol.* 1992;158:97-129.
153. Samulski RJ, Chang LS, Shenk T. Helper-free stocks of recombinant adeno-associated viruses: normal integration does not require viral gene expression. *J Virol.* 1989;63(9):3822-3828.
154. Tratschin JD, Miller IL, Smith MG, Carter BJ. Adeno-associated virus vector for high-frequency integration, expression, and rescue of genes in mammalian cells. *Mol Cell Biol.* 1985;5(11):3251-3260.
155. Shaughnessy E, Lu D, Chatterjee S, Wong KK. Parvoviral vectors for the gene therapy of cancer. *Semin Oncol.* 1996;23(1):159-171.
156. Collaco RF, Cao X, Trempe JP. A helper virus-free packaging system for recombinant adeno-associated virus vectors. *Gene.* 1999;238(2):397-405.
157. Grimm D, Kern A, Rittner K, Kleinschmidt JA. Novel tools for production and purification of recombinant adenoassociated virus vectors. *Hum Gene Ther.* 1998;9(18):2745-2760.
158. Xiao X, Li J, Samulski RJ. Production of high-titer recombinant adeno-associated virus vectors in the absence of helper adenovirus. *J Virol.* 1998;72(3):2224-2232.
159. Tamayose K, Hirai Y, Shimada T. A new strategy for large-scale preparation of high-titer recombinant adeno-associated virus vectors by using packaging cell lines and sulfonated cellulose column chromatography. *Hum Gene Ther.* 1996;7(4):507-513.
160. Qiao C, Li J, Skold A, Zhang X, Xiao X. Feasibility of generating adeno-associated virus packaging cell lines containing inducible adenovirus helper genes. *J Virol.* 2002;76(4):1904-1913.
161. Cao L, Liu Y, During MJ, Xiao W. High-titer, wild-type free recombinant adeno-associated virus vector production using intron-containing helper plasmids. *J Virol.* 2000;74(24):11456-11463.
162. Grimm D, Kay MA, Kleinschmidt JA. Helper virus-free, optically controllable, and two-plasmid-based production of adeno-associated virus vectors of serotypes 1 to 6. *Mol Ther.* 2003;7(6):839-850.
163. Cecchini S, Negrete A, Kotin RM. Toward exascale production of recombinant adeno-associated virus for gene transfer applications. *Gene Ther.* 2008;15(11):823-830.
164. Gaudet D, Methot J, Dery S, et al. Efficacy and long-term safety of alipogene tiparvovec (AAV1-LPLS447X) gene therapy for lipoprotein lipase deficiency: an open-label trial. *Gene Ther.* 2013;20(4):361-369.
165. Anderson SM, Yu G, Giattina M, Miller JL. Intercellular transfer of a glycosylphosphatidylinositol (GPI)-linked protein: release and uptake of CD4-GPI from recombinant adeno-associated virus-transduced HeLa cells. *Proc Natl Acad Sci U S A.* 1996;93(12):5894-5898.
166. Goodman S, Xiao X, Donahue RE, et al. Recombinant adeno-associated virus-mediated gene transfer into hematopoietic progenitor cells. *Blood.* 1994;84(5):1492-1500.
167. Miller JL, Donahue RE, Sellers SE, Samulski RJ, Young NS, Nienhuis AW. Recombinant adeno-associated virus (rAAV)-mediated expression of a human gamma-globin gene in human progenitor-derived erythroid cells. *Proc Natl Acad Sci U S A.* 1994;91(21):10183-10187.
168. Zhou SZ, Broxmeyer HE, Cooper S, Harrington MA, Srivastava A. Adeno-associated virus 2-mediated gene transfer in murine hematopoietic progenitor cells. *Exp Hematol.* 1993;21(7):928-933.
169. Podsakoff G, Wong KK Jr, Chatterjee S. Efficient gene transfer into nondividing cells by adeno-associated virus-based vectors. *J Virol.* 1994;68(9):5656-5666.
170. Russell DW, Miller AD, Alexander IE. Adeno-associated virus vectors preferentially transduce cells in S phase. *Proc Natl Acad Sci U S A.* 1994;91(19):8915-8919.
171. Alexander IE, Russell DW, Miller AD. DNA-damaging agents greatly increase the transduction of nondividing cells by adeno-associated virus vectors. *J Virol.* 1994;68(12):8282-8287.
172. Russell DW, Alexander IE, Miller AD. DNA synthesis and topoisomerase inhibitors increase transduction by adeno-associated virus vectors. *Proc Natl Acad Sci U S A.* 1995;92(12):5719-5723.
173. Fisher-Adams G, Wong KK Jr, Podsakoff G, Forman SJ, Chatterjee S. Integration of adeno-associated virus vectors in CD34+ human hematopoietic progenitor cells after transduction. *Blood.* 1996;88(2):492-504.
174. Brown KE, Green SW, Young NS. Goose parvovirus – an autonomous member of the dependovirus genus? *Virology.* 1995;210(2):283-291.
175. Muramatsu S, Mizukami H, Young NS, Brown KE. Nucleotide sequencing and generation of an infectious clone of adeno-associated virus 3. *Virology.* 1996;221(1):208-217.
176. Brown KE, Green SW, O'Sullivan MG, Young NS. Cloning and sequencing of the simian parvovirus genome. *Virology.* 1995;210(2):314-322.
177. Niemeyer GP, Herzog RW, Mount J, et al. Long-term correction of inhibitor-prone hemophilia B dogs treated with liver-directed AAV2-mediated factor IX gene therapy. *Blood.* 2009;113(4):797-806.
178. Sabatino DE, Lange AM, Altynova ES, et al. Efficacy and safety of long-term prophylaxis in severe hemophilia A dogs following liver gene therapy using AAV vectors. *Mol Ther.* 2011;19(3):442-449.
179. Nathwani AC, Tuddenham EG, Rangarajan S, et al. Adenovirus-associated virus vector-mediated gene transfer in hemophilia B. *N Engl J Med.* 2011;365(25):2357-2365.
180. Breakefield XO, DeLuca NA. Herpes simplex virus for gene delivery to neurons. *N Biol.* 1991;3(3):203-218.
181. Ali M, Lemoine NR, Ring CJ. The use of DNA viruses as vectors for gene therapy. *Gene Ther.* 1994;1(6):367-384.

182. Glorioso JC, DeLuca NA, Fink DJ. Development and application of herpes simplex virus vectors for human gene therapy. *Annu Rev Microbiol.* 1995;49:675-710.
183. Glorioso J, Bender MA, Fink D, DeLuca N. Herpes simplex virus vectors. *Mol Cell Biol Hum Dis Ser.* 1995;5:33-63.
184. Weir JP, Dacquel EJ, Aronovitz J. Herpesvirus vector-mediated gene delivery to human monocytes. *Hum Gene Ther.* 1996;7(11):1331-1338.
185. Dilloo D, Rill D, Entwistle C, et al. A novel herpes vector for the high-efficiency transduction of normal and malignant human hematopoietic cells. *Blood.* 1997;89(1):119-127.
186. Moss B. Poxvirus expression vectors. *Curr Top Microbiol Immunol.* 1992;158:25-38.
187. Whitman ED, Tsung K, Paxson J, Norton JA. In vitro and in vivo kinetics of recombinant vaccinia virus cancer-gene therapy. *Surgery.* 1994;116(2):183-188.
188. Qin HX, Chatterjee SK. Construction of recombinant vaccinia virus expressing GM-CSF and its use as tumor vaccine. *Gene Ther.* 1996;3(1):59-66.
189. Hodge JW, Abrams S, Schlom J, Kantor JA. Induction of antitumor immunity by recombinant vaccinia viruses expressing B7-1 or B7-2 costimulatory molecules. *Cancer Res.* 1994;54(21):5552-5555.
190. Lattime EC, Lee SS, Eisenlohr LC, Mastrangelo MJ. In situ cytokine gene transfection using vaccinia virus vectors. *Semin Oncol.* 1996;23(1):88-100.
191. Ono C, Okamoto T, Abe T, Matsuura Y. Baculovirus as a tool for gene delivery and gene therapy. *Viruses.* 2018;10(9).
192. Chen CY, Lin CY, Chen GY, Hu YC. Baculovirus as a gene delivery vector: recent understandings of molecular alterations in transduced cells and latest applications. *Biotechnol Adv.* 2011;29(6):618-631.
193. Brenner MK, Rill DR, Moen RC, et al. Gene-marking to trace origin of relapse after autologous bone-marrow transplantation. *Lancet.* 1993;341(8837):85-86.
194. Brenner MK, Rill DR, Holladay MS, et al. Gene marking to determine whether autologous marrow infusion restores long-term haemopoiesis in cancer patients. *Lancet.* 1993;342(8880):1134-1137.
195. Rill DR, Santana VM, Roberts WM, et al. Direct demonstration that autologous bone marrow transplantation for solid tumors can return a multiplicity of tumorigenic cells. *Blood.* 1994;84(2):380-383.
196. Deisseroth AB, Zu Z, Claxton D, et al. Genetic marking shows that Ph+ cells present in autologous transplants of chronic myelogenous leukemia (CML) contribute to relapse after autologous bone marrow in CML. *Blood.* 1994;83(10):3068-3076.
197. Dunbar CE, Cottler-Fox M, O'Shaughnessy JA, et al. Retrovirally marked CD34-enriched peripheral blood and bone marrow cells contribute to long-term engraftment after autologous transplantation. *Blood.* 1995;85(11):3048-3057.
198. Cornetta K, Srour EF, Moore A, et al. Retroviral gene transfer in autologous bone marrow transplantation for adult acute leukemia. *Hum Gene Ther.* 1996;7(11):1323-1329.
199. Emmons RV, Doren S, Zujewski J, et al. Retroviral gene transduction of adult peripheral blood or marrow- derived CD34+ cells for six hours without growth factors or on autologous stroma does not improve marking efficiency assessed in vivo. *Blood.* 1997;89(11):4040-4046.
200. Bachier CR, Giles RE, Ellerson D, et al. Hematopoietic retroviral gene marking in patients with follicular non-Hodgkin's lymphoma. *Leuk Lymphoma.* 1999;32(3–4):279-288.
201. Alici E, Bjorkstrand B, Treschow A, et al. Long-term follow-up of gene-marked CD34+ cells after autologous stem cell transplantation for multiple myeloma. *Cancer Gene Ther.* 2007;14(3):227-232.
202. Bordignon C, Notarangelo LD, Nobili N, et al. Gene therapy in peripheral blood lymphocytes and bone marrow for ADA- immunodeficient patients. *Science.* 1995;270(5235):470-475.
203. Kohn DB, Hershfield MS, Carbonaro D, et al. T lymphocytes with a normal ADA gene accumulate after transplantation of transduced autologous umbilical cord blood CD34+ cells in ADA-deficient SCID neonates. *Nat Med.* 1998;4(7):775-780.
204. Kohn DB, Weinberg KI, Nolta JA, et al. Engraftment of gene-modified umbilical cord blood cells in neonates with adenosine deaminase deficiency. *Nat Med.* 1995;1(10):1017-1023.
205. Malech HL, Maples PB, Whiting-Theobald N, et al. Prolonged production of NADPH oxidase-corrected granulocytes after gene therapy of chronic granulomatous disease. *Proc Natl Acad Sci U S A.* 1997;94(22):12133-12138.
206. Hesdorffer C, Ayello J, Ward M, et al. Phase I trial of retroviral-mediated transfer of the human MDR1 gene as marrow chemoprotection in patients undergoing high-dose chemotherapy and autologous stem-cell transplantation. *J Clin Oncol.* 1998;16(1):165-172.
207. Dunbar CE, Kohn DB, Schiffmann R, et al. Retroviral transfer of the glucocerebrosidase gene into CD34+ cells from patients with Gaucher disease: in vivo detection of transduced cells without myeloablation. *Hum Gene Ther.* 1998;9(17):2629-2640.
208. Kohn DB, Bauer G, Rice CM, et al. A clinical trial of retroviral-mediated transfer of a rev-responsive element decoy gene into CD34(+) cells from the bone marrow of human immunodeficiency virus-1-infected children. *Blood.* 1999;94(1):368-371.
209. Cowan KH, Moscow JA, Huang H, et al. Paclitaxel chemotherapy after autologous stem-cell transplantation and engraftment of hematopoietic cells transduced with a retrovirus containing the multidrug resistance complementary DNA (MDR1) in metastatic breast cancer patients. *Clin Cancer Res.* 1999;5(7):1619-1628.
210. Liu JM, Kim S, Read EJ, et al. Engraftment of hematopoietic progenitor cells transduced with the Fanconi anemia group C gene (FANCC). *Hum Gene Ther.* 1999;10(14):2337-2346.
211. Dick JE, Magli MC, Huszar D, Phillips RA, Bernstein A. Introduction of a selectable gene into primitive stem cells capable of long-term reconstitution of the hemopoietic system of W/Wv mice. *Cell.* 1985;42(1):71-79.
212. Keller G, Paige C, Gilboa E, Wagner EF. Expression of a foreign gene in myeloid and lymphoid cells derived from multipotent haematopoietic precursors. *Nature.* 1985;318(6042):149-154.
213. Lemischka IR, Raulet DH, Mulligan RC. Developmental potential and dynamic behavior of hematopoietic stem cells. *Cell.* 1986;45(6):917-927.
214. Cassel A, Cottler-Fox M, Doren S, Dunbar CE. Retroviral-mediated gene transfer into CD34-enriched human peripheral blood stem cells. *Exp Hematol.* 1993;21(4):585-591.
215. Hughes PF, Eaves CJ, Hogge DE, Humphries RK. High-efficiency gene transfer to human hematopoietic cells maintained in long-term marrow culture. *Blood.* 1989;74(6):1915-1922.
216. Larochelle A, Vormoor J, Hanenberg H, et al. Identification of primitive human hematopoietic cells capable of repopulating NOD/SCID mouse bone marrow: implications for gene therapy. *Nat Med.* 1996;2(12):1329-1337.
217. Fink JK, Correll PH, Perry LK, Brady RO, Karlsson S. Correction of glucocerebrosidase deficiency after retroviral-mediated gene transfer into hematopoietic progenitor cells from patients with Gaucher disease. *Proc Natl Acad Sci U S A.* 1990;87(6):2334-2338.
218. Bordignon C, Mavilio F, Ferrari G, et al. Transfer of the ADA gene into bone marrow cells and peripheral blood lymphocytes for the treatment of patients affected by ADA-deficient SCID. *Hum Gene Ther.* 1993;4(4):513-520.
219. Cai Q, Rubin JT, Lotze MT. Genetically marking human cells--results of the first clinical gene transfer studies. *Cancer Gene Ther.* 1995;2(2):125-136.
220. Rosenberg SA, Aebersold P, Cornetta K, et al. Gene transfer into humans--immunotherapy of patients with advanced melanoma, using tumor-infiltrating lymphocytes modified by retroviral gene transduction. *N Engl J Med.* 1990;323(9):570-578.
221. Rill DR, Buschle M, Foreman NK, et al. Retrovirus-mediated gene transfer as an approach to analyze neuroblastoma relapse after autologous bone marrow transplantation. *Hum Gene Ther.* 1992;3(2):129-136.
222. Rill DR, Moen RC, Buschle M, et al. An approach for the analysis of relapse and marrow reconstitution after autologous marrow transplantation using retrovirus-mediated gene transfer. *Blood.* 1992;79(10):2694-2700.
223. Blaese RM. What is the status of gene therapy for primary immunodeficiency?. *Immunol Res.* 2007;38(1-3):274-284.
224. Kaleko M, Garcia JV, Osborne WR, Miller AD. Expression of human adenosine deaminase in mice after transplantation of genetically-modified bone marrow. *Blood.* 1990;75(8):1733-1741.
225. Lim B, Apperley JF, Orkin SH, Williams DA. Long-term expression of human adenosine deaminase in mice transplanted with retrovirus-infected hematopoietic stem cells. *Proc Natl Acad Sci U S A.* 1989;86(22):8892-8896.
226. Moore KA, Fletcher FA, Villalon DK, Utter AE, Belmont JW. Human adenosine deaminase expression in mice. *Blood.* 1990;75(10):2085-2092.
227. Osborne WR, Hock RA, Kaleko M, Miller AD. Long-term expression of human adenosine deaminase in mice after transplantation of bone marrow infected with amphotropic retroviral vectors. *Hum Gene Ther.* 1990;1(1):31-41.
228. van Beusechem VW, Kukler A, Einerhand MP, et al. Expression of human adenosine deaminase in mice transplanted with hemopoietic stem cells infected with amphotropic retroviruses. *J Exp Med.* 1990;172(3):729-736.
229. Wilson JM, Danos O, Grossman M, Raulet DH, Mulligan RC. Expression of human adenosine deaminase in mice reconstituted with retrovirus-transduced hematopoietic stem cells. *Proc Natl Acad Sci U S A.* 1990;87(1):439-443.
230. Lu L, Shen RN, Broxmeyer HE. Stem cells from bone marrow, umbilical cord blood and peripheral blood for clinical application: current status and future application. *Crit Rev Oncol Hematol.* 1996;22(2):61-78.
231. Gluckman E. Umbilical cord blood biology and transplantation. *Curr Opin Hematol.* 1995;2(6):413-416.
232. Lu L, Xiao M, Shen RN, Grigsby S, Broxmeyer HE. Enrichment, characterization, and responsiveness of single primitive CD34 human umbilical cord blood hematopoietic progenitors with high proliferative and replating potential. *Blood.* 1993;81(1):41-48.
233. Smith AR, Wagner JE. Current clinical management of Fanconi anemia. *Expet Rev Hematol.* 2012;5(5):513-522.
234. Dalle JH, Peffault de Latour R. Allogeneic hematopoietic stem cell transplantation for inherited bone marrow failure syndromes. *Int J Hematol.* 2016;103(4):373-379.
235. Diamond LK, Shahidi NT. Treatment of aplastic anemia in children. *Semin Hematol.* 1967;4(3):278-288.
236. Dufour C, Svahn J. Fanconi anaemia: new strategies. *Bone Marrow Transplant.* 2008;41(Suppl 2):S90-S95.
237. Paustian L, Chao MM, Hanenberg H, et al. Androgen therapy in Fanconi anemia: a retrospective analysis of 30 years in Germany. *Pediatr Hematol Oncol.* 2016;33(1):5-12.
238. Scheckenbach K, Morgan M, Filger-Brillinger J, et al. Treatment of the bone marrow failure in Fanconi anemia patients with danazol. *Blood Cells Mol Dis.* 2012;48(2):128-131.
239. Shahidi NT, Diamond LK. Testosterone-induced remission in aplastic anemia of both acquired and congenital types. Further observations in 24 cases. *N Engl J Med.* 1961;264:953-967.
240. Strathdee CA, Gavish H, Shannon WR, Buchwald M. Cloning of cDNAs for Fanconi's anaemia by functional complementation. *Nature.* 1992;356(6372):763-767.
241. Walsh CE, Grompe M, Vanin E, et al. A functionally active retrovirus vector for gene therapy in Fanconi anemia group C. *Blood.* 1994;84(2):453-459.
242. Walsh CE, Nienhuis AW, Samulski RJ, et al. Phenotypic correction of Fanconi anemia in human hematopoietic cells with a recombinant adeno-associated virus vector. *J Clin Invest.* 1994;94(4):1440-1448.
243. Croop JM, Cooper R, Fernandez C, et al. Mobilization and collection of peripheral blood CD34+ cells from patients with Fanconi anemia. *Blood.* 2001;98(10):2917-2921.

244. Correll PH, Colilla S, Dave HP, Karlsson S. High levels of human glucocerebrosidase activity in macrophages of long-term reconstituted mice after retroviral infection of hematopoietic stem cells. *Blood.* 1992;80(2):331-336.
245. Correll PH, Fink JK, Brady RO, Perry LK, Karlsson S. Production of human glucocerebrosidase in mice after retroviral gene transfer into multipotential hematopoietic progenitor cells. *Proc Natl Acad Sci U S A.* 1989;86(22):8912-8916.
246. Correll PH, Kew Y, Perry LK, Brady RO, Fink JK, Karlsson S. Expression of human glucocerebrosidase in long-term reconstituted mice following retroviral-mediated gene transfer into hematopoietic stem cells. *Hum Gene Ther.* 1990;1(3):277-287.
247. Nolta JA, Sender LS, Barranger JA, Kohn DB. Expression of human glucocerebrosidase in murine long-term bone marrow cultures after retroviral vector-mediated transfer. *Blood.* 1990;75(3):787-797.
248. Ohashi T, Boggs S, Robbins P, et al. Efficient transfer and sustained high expression of the human glucocerebrosidase gene in mice and their functional macrophages following transplantation of bone marrow transduced by a retroviral vector. *Proc Natl Acad Sci U S A.* 1992;89(23):11332-11336.
249. Weinthal J, Nolta JA, Yu XJ, Lilley J, Uribe L, Kohn DB. Expression of human glucocerebrosidase following retroviral vector-mediated transduction of murine hematopoietic stem cells. *Bone Marrow Transplant.* 1991;8(5):403-412.
250. Jirapongsananuruk O, Niemela JE, Malech HL, Fleisher TA. CYBB mutation analysis in X-linked chronic granulomatous disease. *Clin Immunol.* 2002;104(1):73-76.
251. Bjorgvinsdottir H, Ding C, Pech N, Gifford MA, Li LL, Dinauer MC. Retroviral-mediated gene transfer of gp91phox into bone marrow cells rescues defect in host defense against Aspergillus fumigatus in murine X-linked chronic granulomatous disease. *Blood.* 1997;89(1):41-48.
252. Dinauer MC, Li LL, Bjorgvinsdottir H, Ding C, Pech N. Long-term correction of phagocyte NADPH oxidase activity by retroviral-mediated gene transfer in murine X-linked chronic granulomatous disease. *Blood.* 1999;94(3):914-922.
253. Mardiney M III, Jackson SH, Spratt SK, Li F, Holland SM, Malech HL. Enhanced host defense after gene transfer in the murine p47phox- deficient model of chronic granulomatous disease. *Blood.* 1997;89(7):2268-2275.
254. Zanjani ED, Almeida-Porada G, Flake AW. The human/sheep xenograft model: a large animal model of human hematopoiesis. *Int J Hematol.* 1996;63(3):179-192.
255. Zanjani ED, Flake AW, Rice H, Hedrick M, Tavassoli M. Long-term repopulating ability of xenogeneic transplanted human fetal liver hematopoietic stem cells in sheep. *J Clin Invest.* 1994;93(3):1051-1055.
256. Zanjani ED, Pallavicini MG, Ascensao JL, et al. Engraftment and long-term expression of human fetal hemopoietic stem cells in sheep following transplantation in utero. *J Clin Invest.* 1992;89(4):1178-1188.
257. Porada CD, Tran ND, Almeida-Porada G, et al. Transduction of long-term-engrafting human hematopoietic stem cells by retroviral vectors. *Hum Gene Ther.* 2002;13(7):867-879.
258. Donahue RE, Dunbar CE. Update on the use of nonhuman primate models for preclinical testing of gene therapy approaches targeting hematopoietic cells. *Hum Gene Ther.* 2001;12(6):607-617.
259. Van Beusechem VW, Valerio D. Gene transfer into hematopoietic stem cells of nonhuman primates. *Hum Gene Ther.* 1996;7(14):1649-1668.
260. van Beusechem VW, Kukler A, Heidt PJ, Valerio D. Long-term expression of human adenosine deaminase in rhesus monkeys transplanted with retrovirus-infected bone-marrow cells. *Proc Natl Acad Sci U S A.* 1992;89(16):7640-7644.
261. van Beusechem VW, Bart-Baumeister JA, Hoogerbrugge PM, Valerio D. Influence of interleukin-3, interleukin-6, and stem cell factor on retroviral transduction of rhesus monkey CD34+ hematopoietic progenitor cells measured in vitro and in vivo. *Gene Ther.* 1995;2(4):245-255.
262. Bodine DM, Moritz T, Donahue RE, et al. Long-term in vivo expression of a murine adenosine deaminase gene in rhesus monkey hematopoietic cells of multiple lineages after retroviral mediated gene transfer into CD34+ bone marrow cells. *Blood.* 1993;82(7):1975-1980.
263. Xu LC, Karlsson S, Byrne ER, et al. Long-term in vivo expression of the human glucocerebrosidase gene in nonhuman primates after CD34+ hematopoietic cell transduction with cell-free retroviral vector preparations. *Proc Natl Acad Sci U S A.* 1995;92(10):4372-4376.
264. Schuening FG, Kawahara K, Miller AD, et al. Retrovirus-mediated gene transduction into long-term repopulating marrow cells of dogs. *Blood.* 1991;78(10):2568-2576.
265. Kiem HP, Darovsky B, von Kalle C, et al. Retrovirus-mediated gene transduction into canine peripheral blood repopulating cells. *Blood.* 1994;83(6):1467-1473.
266. Barquinero J, Kiem HP, von Kalle C, et al. Myelosuppressive conditioning improves autologous engraftment of genetically marked repopulating cells in dogs. *Blood.* 1995;85(5):1195-1201.
267. Goerner M, Bruno B, McSweeney PA, Buron G, Storb R, Kiem HP. The use of granulocyte colony-stimulating factor during retroviral transduction on fibronectin fragment CH-296 enhances gene transfer into hematopoietic repopulating cells in dogs. *Blood.* 1999;94(7):2287-2292.
268. Kiem HP, McSweeney PA, Bruno B, et al. Improved gene transfer into canine hematopoietic repopulating cells using CD34-enriched marrow cells in combination with a gibbon ape leukemia virus-pseudotype retroviral vector. *Gene Ther.* 1999;6(6):966-972.
269. Horn PA, Keyser KA, Peterson LJ, et al. Efficient lentiviral gene transfer to canine repopulating cells using an overnight transduction protocol. *Blood.* 2004;103(10):3710-3716.
270. Kiem HP, Allen J, Trobridge G, et al. Foamy-virus-mediated gene transfer to canine repopulating cells. *Blood.* 2007;109(1):65-70.
271. Neff T, Beard BC, Peterson LJ, Anandakumar P, Thompson J, Kiem HP. Polyclonal chemoprotection against temozolomide in a large-animal model of drug resistance gene therapy. *Blood.* 2005;105(3):997-1002.
272. Neff T, Horn PA, Peterson LJ, et al. Methylguanine methyltransferase-mediated in vivo selection and chemoprotection of allogeneic stem cells in a large-animal model. *J Clin Invest.* 2003;112(10):1581-1588.
273. Neff T, Horn PA, Valli VE, et al. Pharmacologically regulated in vivo selection in a large animal. *Blood.* 2002;100(6):2026-2031.
274. Bock TA, Orlic D, Dunbar CE, Broxmeyer HE, Bodine DM. Improved engraftment of human hematopoietic cells in severe combined immunodeficient (SCID) mice carrying human cytokine transgenes. *J Exp Med.* 1995;182(6):2037-2043.
275. Dick JE. Immune-deficient mice as models of normal and leukemic human hematopoiesis. *Cancer Cells.* 1991;3(2):39-48.
276. Dick JE, Kamel-Reid S, Murdoch B, Doedens M. Gene transfer into normal human hematopoietic cells using in vitro and in vivo assays. *Blood.* 1991;78(3):624-634.
277. Larochelle A, Vormoor J, Lapidot T, et al. Engraftment of immune-deficient mice with primitive hematopoietic cells from beta-thalassemia and sickle cell anemia patients: implications for evaluating human gene therapy protocols. *Hum Mol Genet.* 1995;4(2):163-172.
278. Nolta JA, Hanley MB, Kohn DB. Sustained human hematopoiesis in immunodeficient mice by cotransplantation of marrow stroma expressing human interleukin-3: analysis of gene transduction of long-lived progenitors. *Blood.* 1994;83(10):3041-3051.
279. Kamel-Reid S, Dick JE. Engraftment of immune-deficient mice with human hematopoietic stem cells. *Science.* 1988;242(4886):1706-1709.
280. Lapidot T, Pflumio F, Doedens M, Murdoch B, Williams DE, Dick JE. Cytokine stimulation of multilineage hematopoiesis from immature human cells engrafted in SCID mice. *Science.* 1992;255(5048):1137-1141.
281. Shultz LD, Schweitzer PA, Christianson SW, et al. Multiple defects in innate and adaptive immunologic function in NOD/LtSz-scid mice. *J Immunol.* 1995;154(1):180-191.
282. Hiramatsu H, Nishikomori R, Heike T, et al. Complete reconstitution of human lymphocytes from cord blood CD34+ cells using the NOD/SCID/gammacnull mice model. *Blood.* 2003;102(3):873-880.
283. Ito M, Hiramatsu H, Kobayashi K, et al. NOD/SCID/gamma(c)(null) mouse: an excellent recipient mouse model for engraftment of human cells. *Blood.* 2002;100(9):3175-3182.
284. Ito R, Katano I, Ida-Tanaka M, et al. Efficient xenoengraftment in severe immunodeficient NOD/Shi-scid IL2Rgammanull mice is attributed to a lack of CD11c+B220+CD122+ cells. *J Immunol.* 2012;89(9):4313-4320.
285. Shultz LD, Lyons BL, Burzenski LM, et al. Human lymphoid and myeloid cell development in NOD/LtSz-scid IL2R gamma null mice engrafted with mobilized human hemopoietic stem cells. *J Immunol.* 2005;174(10):6477-6489.
286. McDermott SP, Eppert K, Lechman ER, Doedens M, Dick JE. Comparison of human cord blood engraftment between immunocompromised mouse strains. *Blood.* 2010;116(2):193-200.
287. McIntosh BE, Brown ME, Duffin BM, et al. B6.SCID Il2rgamma−/− Kit(W41/W41) (NBSGW) mice support multilineage engraftment of human hematopoietic cells. *Stem Cell Rep.* 2015;4(2):171-180.
288. Guenechea G, Gan OI, Dorrell C, Dick JE. Distinct classes of human stem cells that differ in proliferative and self-renewal potential. *Nat Immunol.* 2001;2(1):75-82.
289. Horn PA, Thomasson BM, Wood BL, Andrews RG, Morris JC, Kiem HP. Distinct hematopoietic stem/progenitor cell populations are responsible for repopulating NOD/SCID mice compared with nonhuman primates. *Blood.* 2003;102(13):4329-4335.
290. Guenechea G, Gan OI, Inamitsu T, et al. Transduction of human CD34+ CD38-bone marrow and cord blood-derived SCID-repopulating cells with third-generation lentiviral vectors. *Mol Ther.* 2000;1(6):566-573.
291. Liu Y, Hangoc G, Campbell TB, et al. Identification of parameters required for efficient lentiviral vector transduction and engraftment of human cord blood CD34(+) NOD/SCID-repopulating cells. *Exp Hematol.* 2008;36(8):947-956.
292. Miyoshi H, Smith KA, Mosier DE, Verma IM, Torbett BE. Transduction of human CD34+ cells that mediate long-term engraftment of NOD/SCID mice by HIV vectors. *Science.* 1999;283(5402):682-686.
293. Piacibello W, Bruno S, Sanavio F, et al. Lentiviral gene transfer and ex vivo expansion of human primitive stem cells capable of primary, secondary, and tertiary multilineage repopulation in NOD/SCID mice. Nonobese diabetic/severe combined immunodeficient. *Blood.* 2002;100(13):4391-4400.
294. Woods NB, Fahlman C, Mikkola H, et al. Lentiviral gene transfer into primary and secondary NOD/SCID repopulating cells. *Blood.* 2000;96(12):3725-3733.
295. Benhamida S, Pflumio F, Dubart-Kupperschmitt A, et al. Transduced CD34+ cells from adrenoleukodystrophy patients with HIV-derived vector mediate long-term engraftment of NOD/SCID mice. *Mol Ther.* 2003;7(3):317-324.
296. Tesio M, Gammaitoni L, Gunetti M, et al. Sustained long-term engraftment and transgene expression of peripheral blood CD34+ cells transduced with third-generation lentiviral vectors. *Stem Cells.* 2008;26(6):1620-1627.
297. An DS, Kung SK, Bonifacino A, et al. Lentivirus vector-mediated hematopoietic stem cell gene transfer of common gamma-chain cytokine receptor in rhesus macaques. *J Virol.* 2001;75(8):3547-3555.
298. An DS, Wersto RP, Agricola BA, et al. Marking and gene expression by a lentivirus vector in transplanted human and nonhuman primate CD34(+) cells. *J Virol.* 2000;74(3):1286-1295.
299. Horn PA, Morris JC, Bukovsky AA, et al. Lentivirus-mediated gene transfer into hematopoietic repopulating cells in baboons. *Gene Ther.* 2002;9(21):1464-1471.
300. Trobridge GD, Beard BC, Gooch C, et al. Efficient transduction of pigtailed macaque hematopoietic repopulating cells with HIV-based lentiviral vectors. *Blood.* 2008;111(12):5537-5543.

301. Uchida N, Washington KN, Hayakawa J, et al. Development of a human immunodeficiency virus type 1-based lentiviral vector that allows efficient transduction of both human and rhesus blood cells. *J Virol.* 2009;83(19):9854-9862.
302. Rits MA, van Dort KA, Munk C, Meijer AB, Kootstra NA. Efficient transduction of simian cells by HIV-1-based lentiviral vectors that contain mutations in the capsid protein. *Mol Ther.* 2007;15(5):930-937.
303. Kootstra NA, Munk C, Tonnu N, Landau NR, Verma IM. Abrogation of postentry restriction of HIV-1-based lentiviral vector transduction in simian cells. *Proc Natl Acad Sci U S A.* 2003;100(3):1298-1303.
304. Hanawa H, Hematti P, Keyvanfar K, et al. Efficient gene transfer into rhesus repopulating hematopoietic stem cells using a simian immunodeficiency virus-based lentiviral vector system. *Blood.* 2004;103(11):4062-4069.
305. Kim YJ, Kim YS, Larochelle A, et al. Sustained high-level polyclonal hematopoietic marking and transgene expression 4 years after autologous transplantation of rhesus macaques with SIV lentiviral vector-transduced CD34+ cells. *Blood.* 2009;113(22):5434-5443.
306. Larochelle A, Choi U, Shou Y, et al. In vivo selection of hematopoietic progenitor cells and temozolomide dose intensification in rhesus macaques through lentiviral transduction with a drug resistance gene. *J Clin Invest.* 2009;119(7):1952-1963.
307. Tarantal AF, Giannoni F, Lee CC, et al. Nonmyeloablative conditioning regimen to increase engraftment of gene-modified hematopoietic stem cells in young rhesus monkeys. *Mol Ther.* 2012;20(5):1033-1045.
308. Verhoeyen E, Relouzat F, Cambot M, et al. Stem cell factor-displaying simian immunodeficiency viral vectors together with a low conditioning regimen allow for long-term engraftment of gene-marked autologous hematopoietic stem cells in macaques. *Hum Gene Ther.* 2012;23(7):754-768.
309. Cartier N, Hacein-Bey-Abina S, Bartholomae CC, et al. Hematopoietic stem cell gene therapy with a lentiviral vector in X-linked adrenoleukodystrophy. *Science.* 2009;326(5954):818-823.
310. Astrakhan A, Sather BD, Ryu BY, et al. Ubiquitous high-level gene expression in hematopoietic lineages provides effective lentiviral gene therapy of murine Wiskott-Aldrich syndrome. *Blood.* 2012;119(19):4395-4407.
311. Blundell MP, Bouma G, Calle Y, Jones GE, Kinnon C, Thrasher AJ. Improvement of migratory defects in a murine model of Wiskott-Aldrich syndrome gene therapy. *Mol Ther.* 2008;16(5):836-844.
312. Bosticardo M, Draghici E, Schena F, et al. Lentiviral-mediated gene therapy leads to improvement of B-cell functionality in a murine model of Wiskott-Aldrich syndrome. *J Allergy Clin Immunol.* 2011;127(6):1376-1384 e5.
313. Charrier S, Stockholm D, Seye K, et al. A lentiviral vector encoding the human Wiskott-Aldrich syndrome protein corrects immune and cytoskeletal defects in WASP knockout mice. *Gene Ther.* 2005;12(7):597-606.
314. Dupre L, Marangoni F, Scaramuzza S, et al. Efficacy of gene therapy for Wiskott-Aldrich syndrome using a WAS promoter/cDNA-containing lentiviral vector and nonlethal irradiation. *Hum Gene Ther.* 2006;17(3):303-313.
315. Marangoni F, Bosticardo M, Charrier S, et al. Evidence for long-term efficacy and safety of gene therapy for Wiskott-Aldrich syndrome in preclinical models. *Mol Ther.* 2009;17(6):1073-1082.
316. Imren S, Payen E, Westerman KA, et al. Permanent and panerythroid correction of murine beta thalassemia by multiple lentiviral integration in hematopoietic stem cells. *Proc Natl Acad Sci U S A.* 2002;99(22):14380-14385.
317. Negre O, Fusil F, Colomb C, et al. Correction of murine beta-thalassemia after minimal lentiviral gene transfer and homeostatic in vivo erythroid expansion. *Blood.* 2011;117(20):5321-5331.
318. Persons DA, Allay ER, Sawai N, et al. Successful treatment of murine beta-thalassemia using in vivo selection of genetically modified, drug-resistant hematopoietic stem cells. *Blood.* 2003;102(2):506-513.
319. Zhao H, Pestina TI, Nasimuzzaman M, Mehta P, Hargrove PW, Persons DA. Amelioration of murine beta-thalassemia through drug selection of hematopoietic stem cells transduced with a lentiviral vector encoding both gamma-globin and the MGMT drug-resistance gene. *Blood.* 2009;113(23):5747-5756.
320. Almarza E, Rio P, Meza NW, et al. Characteristics of lentiviral vectors harboring the proximal promoter of the vav proto-oncogene: a weak and efficient promoter for gene therapy. *Mol Ther.* 2007;15(8):1487-1494.
321. Benjelloun F, Garrigue A, Demerens-de Chappedelaine C, et al. Stable and functional lymphoid reconstitution in artemis-deficient mice following lentiviral artemis gene transfer into hematopoietic stem cells. *Mol Ther.* 2008;16(8):1490-1499.
322. Mostoslavsky G, Fabian AJ, Rooney S, Alt FW, Mulligan RC. Complete correction of murine Artemis immunodeficiency by lentiviral vector-mediated gene transfer. *Proc Natl Acad Sci U S A.* 2006;103(44):16406-16411.
323. Zhang F, Thornhill SI, Howe SJ, et al. Lentiviral vectors containing an enhancer-less ubiquitously acting chromatin opening element (UCOE) provide highly reproducible and stable transgene expression in hematopoietic cells. *Blood.* 2007;110(5):1448-1457.
324. Zhou S, Mody D, DeRavin SS, et al. A self-inactivating lentiviral vector for SCID-X1 gene therapy that does not activate LMO2 expression in human T cells. *Blood.* 2010;116(6):900-908.
325. Barde I, Laurenti E, Verp S, et al. Lineage- and stage-restricted lentiviral vectors for the gene therapy of chronic granulomatous disease. *Gene Ther.* 2011;18(11):1087-1097.
326. Podda S, Ward M, Himelstein A, et al. Transfer and expression of the human multiple drug resistance gene into live mice. *Proc Natl Acad Sci U S A.* 1992;89(20):9676-9680.
327. Sorrentino BP, Brandt SJ, Bodine D, et al. Selection of drug-resistant bone marrow cells in vivo after retroviral transfer of human MDR1. *Science.* 1992;257(5066):99-103.
328. Allay JA, Persons DA, Galipeau J, et al. In vivo selection of retrovirally transduced hematopoietic stem cells. *Nat Med.* 1998;4(10):1136-1143.
329. Davis BM, Koc ON, Gerson SL. Limiting numbers of G156A O(6)-methylguanine-DNA methyltransferase-transduced marrow progenitors repopulate nonmyeloablated mice after drug selection. *Blood.* 2000;95(10):3078-3084.
330. Ragg S, Xu-Welliver M, Bailey J, et al. Direct reversal of DNA damage by mutant methyltransferase protein protects mice against dose-intensified chemotherapy and leads to in vivo selection of hematopoietic stem cells. *Cancer Res.* 2000;60(18):5187-5195.
331. Sawai N, Zhou S, Vanin EF, Houghton P, Brent TP, Sorrentino BP. Protection and in vivo selection of hematopoietic stem cells using temozolomide, O6-benzylguanine, and an alkyltransferase-expressing retroviral vector. *Mol Ther.* 2001;3(1):78-87.
332. Persons DA, Allay JA, Bonifacino A, et al. Transient in vivo selection of transduced peripheral blood cells using antifolate drug selection in rhesus macaques that received transplants with hematopoietic stem cells expressing dihydrofolate reductase vectors. *Blood.* 2004;103(3):796-803.
333. Hibino H, Tani K, Ikebuchi K, et al. The common marmoset as a target preclinical primate model for cytokine and gene therapy studies. *Blood.* 1999;93(9):2839-2848.
334. Licht T, Haskins M, Henthorn P, et al. Drug selection with paclitaxel restores expression of linked IL-2 receptor gamma -chain and multidrug resistance (MDR1) transgenes in canine bone marrow. *Proc Natl Acad Sci U S A.* 2002;99(5):3123-3128.
335. Beard BC, Trobridge GD, Ironside C, McCune JS, Adair JE, Kiem HP. Efficient and stable MGMT-mediated selection of long-term repopulating stem cells in nonhuman primates. *J Clin Invest.* 2010;120(7):2345-2354.
336. Gerull S, Beard BC, Peterson LJ, Neff T, Kiem HP. In vivo selection and chemoprotection after drug resistance gene therapy in a nonmyeloablative allogeneic transplantation setting in dogs. *Hum Gene Ther.* 2007;18(5):451-456.
337. Gori JL, Beard BC, Ironside C, Karponi G, Kiem HP. In vivo selection of autologous MGMT gene-modified cells following reduced-intensity conditioning with BCNU and temozolomide in the dog model. *Cancer Gene Ther.* 2012;19(8):523-529.
338. Pollok KE, Hartwell JR, Braber A, et al. In vivo selection of human hematopoietic cells in a xenograft model using combined pharmacologic and genetic manipulations. *Hum Gene Ther.* 2003;14(18):1703-1714.
339. Zielske SP, Reese JS, Lingas KT, Donze JR, Gerson SL. In vivo selection of MGMT(P140K) lentivirus-transduced human NOD/SCID repopulating cells without pretransplant irradiation conditioning. *J Clin Invest.* 2003;112(10):1561-1570.
340. Pawliuk R, Kay R, Lansdorp P, Humphries RK. Selection of retrovirally transduced hematopoietic cells using CD24 as a marker of gene transfer. *Blood.* 1994;84(9):2868-2877.
341. Medin JA, Migita M, Pawliuk R, et al. A bicistronic therapeutic retroviral vector enables sorting of transduced CD34+ cells and corrects the enzyme deficiency in cells from Gaucher patients. *Blood.* 1996;87(5):1754-1762.
342. Cheng L, Fu J, Tsukamoto A, Hawley RG. Use of green fluorescent protein variants to monitor gene transfer and expression in mammalian cells. *Nat Biotechnol.* 1996;14(5):606-609.
343. Hanazono Y, Yu JM, Dunbar CE, Emmons RV. Green fluorescent protein retroviral vectors: low titer and high recombination frequency suggest a selective disadvantage. *Hum Gene Ther.* 1997;8(11):1313-1319.
344. Persons DA, Allay JA, Allay ER, et al. Retroviral-mediated transfer of the green fluorescent protein gene into murine hematopoietic cells facilitates scoring and selection of transduced progenitors in vitro and identification of genetically modified cells in vivo. *Blood.* 1997;90(5):1777-1786.
345. Kiem HP, Rasko JE, Morris J, Peterson L, Kurre P, Andrews RG. Ex vivo selection for oncoretrovirally transduced green fluorescent protein-expressing CD34-enriched cells increases short-term engraftment of transduced cells in baboons. *Hum Gene Ther.* 2002;13(8):891-899.
346. Thorsteinsdottir U, Sauvageau G, Humphries RK. Enhanced in vivo regenerative potential of HOXB4-transduced hematopoietic stem cells with regulation of their pool size. *Blood.* 1999;94(8):2605-2612.
347. Domen J, Weissman IL. Hematopoietic stem cells need two signals to prevent apoptosis; BCL-2 can provide one of these, Kitl/c-Kit signaling the other. *J Exp Med.* 2000;192(12):1707-1718.
348. Kirby S, Walton W, Smithies O. Hematopoietic stem cells with controllable tEpoR transgenes have a competitive advantage in bone marrow transplantation. *Blood.* 2000;95(12):3710-3715.
349. Blau CA, Neff T, Papayannopoulou T. Cytokine prestimulation as a gene therapy strategy: implications for using the MDR1 gene as a dominant selectable marker. *Blood.* 1997;89(1):146-154.
350. Jin L, Asano H, Blau CA. Stimulating cell proliferation through the pharmacologic activation of c-kit. *Blood.* 1998;91(3):890-897.
351. Hanazono Y, Nagashima T, Shibata H, et al. InVivo expansion of gene-modified hematopoietic cells by the selective amplifier gene in a nonhuman primate model. *Blood.* 2000;96(11):524a.
352. Ito K, Ueda Y, Kokubun M, et al. Development of a novel selective amplifier gene for controllable expansion of transduced hematopoietic cells. *Blood.* 1997;90(10):3884-3892.
353. Zhang XB, Beard BC, Beebe K, Storer B, Humphries RK, Kiem HP. Differential effects of HOXB4 on nonhuman primate short- and long-term repopulating cells. *PLoS Med.* 2006;3(5):e173.
354. Zhang XB, Beard BC, Trobridge GD, et al. High incidence of leukemia in large animals after stem cell gene therapy with a HOXB4-expressing retroviral vector. *J Clin Invest.* 2008;118(4):1502-1510.
355. Murnane R, Zhang XB, Hukkanen RR, Vogel K, Kelley S, Kiem HP. Myelodysplasia in 2 pig-tailed macaques (*Macaca nemestrina*) associated with retroviral vector-mediated insertional mutagenesis and overexpression of HOXB4. *Vet Pathol.* 2011;48(5):999-1001.

356. Leuci V, Mesiano G, Gammaitoni L, et al. Transient proteasome inhibition as a strategy to enhance lentiviral transduction of hematopoietic CD34(+) cells and T lymphocytes: implications for the use of low viral doses and large-size vectors. *J Biotechnol*. 2011;156(3):218-226.
357. Santoni de Sio FR, Cascio P, Zingale A, Gasparini M, Naldini L. Proteasome activity restricts lentiviral gene transfer into hematopoietic stem cells and is down-regulated by cytokines that enhance transduction. *Blood*. 2006;107(11):4257-4265.
358. Millington M, Arndt A, Boyd M, Applegate T, Shen S. Towards a clinically relevant lentiviral transduction protocol for primary human CD34 hematopoietic stem/progenitor cells. *PLoS One*. 2009;4(7):e6461.
359. Uchida N, Hsieh MM, Hayakawa J, Madison C, Washington KN, Tisdale JF. Optimal conditions for lentiviral transduction of engrafting human CD34+ cells. *Gene Ther*. 2011;18(11):1078-1086.
360. Moore KA, Deisseroth AB, Reading CL, Williams DE, Belmont JW. Stromal support enhances cell-free retroviral vector transduction of human bone marrow long-term culture-initiating cells. *Blood*. 1992;79(6):1393-1399.
361. Wells S, Malik P, Pensiero M, Kohn DB, Nolta JA. The presence of an autologous marrow stromal cell layer increases glucocerebrosidase gene transduction of long-term culture initiating cells (LTCICs) from the bone marrow of a patient with Gaucher disease. *Gene Ther*. 1995;2(8):512-520.
362. Xu LC, Kluepfel-Stahl S, Blanco M, Schiffmann R, Dunbar C, Karlsson S. Growth factors and stromal support generate very efficient retroviral transduction of peripheral blood CD34+ cells from Gaucher patients. *Blood*. 1995;86(1):141-146.
363. Tisdale JF, Hanazono Y, Sellers SE, et al. Ex vivo expansion of genetically marked rhesus peripheral blood progenitor cells results in diminished long-term repopulating ability. *Blood*. 1998;92(4):1131-1141.
364. Moritz T, Patel VP, Williams DA. Bone marrow extracellular matrix molecules improve gene transfer into human hematopoietic cells via retroviral vectors. *J Clin Invest*. 1994;93(4):1451-1457.
365. Carstanjen D, Dutt P, Moritz T. Heparin inhibits retrovirus binding to fibronectin as well as retrovirus gene transfer on fibronectin fragments. *J Virol*. 2001;75(13):6218-6222.
366. Hanenberg H, Xiao XL, Dilloo D, Hashino K, Kato I, Williams DA. Colocalization of retrovirus and target cells on specific fibronectin fragments increases genetic transduction of mammalian cells. *Nat Med*. 1996;2(8):876-882.
367. Lei P, Bajaj B, Andreadis ST. Retrovirus-associated heparan sulfate mediates immobilization and gene transfer on recombinant fibronectin. *J Virol*. 2002;76(17):8722-8728.
368. Relander T, Brun A, Hawley RG, Karlsson S, Richter J. Retroviral transduction of human CD34+ cells on fibronectin fragment CH-296 is inhibited by high concentrations of vector containing medium. *J Gene Med*. 2001;3(3):207-218.
369. Kotani H, Newton PB III, Zhang S, et al. Improved methods of retroviral vector transduction and production for gene therapy. *Hum Gene Ther*. 1994;5(1):19-28.
370. Dao MA, Hashino K, Kato I, Nolta JA. Adhesion to fibronectin maintains regenerative capacity during ex vivo culture and transduction of human hematopoietic stem and progenitor cells. *Blood*. 1998;92(12):4612-4621.
371. Sagar BM, Rentala S, Gopal PN, Sharma S, Mukhopadhyay A. Fibronectin and laminin enhance engraftibility of cultured hematopoietic stem cells. *Biochem Biophys Res Commun*. 2006;350(4):1000-1005.
372. Yokota T, Oritani K, Mitsui H, et al. Growth-supporting activities of fibronectin on hematopoietic stem/progenitor cells in vitro and in vivo: structural requirement for fibronectin activities of CS1 and cell-binding domains. *Blood*. 1998;91(9):3263-3272.
373. Donahue RE, Sorrentino BP, Hawley RG, An DS, Chen IS, Wersto RP. Fibronectin fragment CH-296 inhibits apoptosis and enhances ex vivo gene transfer by murine retrovirus and human lentivirus vectors independent of viral tropism in nonhuman primate CD34+ cells. *Mol Ther*. 2001;3(3):359-367.
374. Abonour R, Williams DA, Einhorn L, et al. Efficient retrovirus-mediated transfer of the multidrug resistance 1 gene into autologous human long-term repopulating hematopoietic stem cells. *Nat Med*. 2000;6(6):652-658.
375. Hanenberg H, Hashino K, Konishi H, Hock RA, Kato I, Williams DA. Optimization of fibronectin-assisted retroviral gene transfer into human CD34+ hematopoietic cells. *Hum Gene Ther*. 1997;8(18):2193-2206.
376. Lee HJ, Lee YS, Kim HS, et al. Retronectin enhances lentivirus-mediated gene delivery into hematopoietic progenitor cells. *Biologicals*. 2009;37(4):203-209.
377. Barese C, Pech N, Dirscherl S, et al. Granulocyte colony-stimulating factor prior to nonmyeloablative irradiation decreases murine host hematopoietic stem cell function and increases engraftment of donor marrow cells. *Stem Cells*. 2007;25(6):1578-1585.
378. Goebel WS, Pech NK, Dinauer MC. Stable long-term gene correction with low-dose radiation conditioning in murine X-linked chronic granulomatous disease. *Blood Cells Mol Dis*. 2004;33(3):365-371.
379. Goebel WS, Pech NK, Meyers JL, Srour EF, Yoder MC, Dinauer MC. A murine model of antimetabolite-based, submyeloablative conditioning for bone marrow transplantation: biologic insights and potential applications. *Exp Hematol*. 2004;32(12):1255-1264.
380. Goebel WS, Yoder MC, Pech NK, Dinauer MC. Donor chimerism and stem cell function in a murine congenic transplantation model after low-dose radiation conditioning: effects of a retroviral-mediated gene transfer protocol and implications for gene therapy. *Exp Hematol*. 2002;30(11):1324-1332.
381. Huston MW, van Til NP, Visser TP, et al. Correction of murine SCID-X1 by lentiviral gene therapy using a codon-optimized IL2RG gene and minimal pretransplant conditioning. *Mol Ther*. 2011;19(10):1867-1877.
382. Chen J, Larochelle A, Fricker S, Bridger G, Dunbar CE, Abkowitz JL. Mobilization as a preparative regimen for hematopoietic stem cell transplantation. *Blood*. 2006;107(9):3764-3771.
383. Dvorak CC, Horn BN, Puck JM, et al. A trial of plerixafor adjunctive therapy in allogeneic hematopoietic cell transplantation with minimal conditioning for severe combined immunodeficiency. *Pediatr Transplant*. 2014;18(6):602-608.
384. Czechowicz A, Kraft D, Weissman IL, Bhattacharya D. Efficient transplantation via antibody-based clearance of hematopoietic stem cell niches. *Science*. 2007;318(5854):1296-1299.
385. Xue X, Pech NK, Shelley WC, Srour EF, Yoder MC, Dinauer MC. Antibody targeting KIT as pretransplantation conditioning in immunocompetent mice. *Blood*. 2010;116(24):5419-5422.
386. Chhabra A, Ring AM, Weiskopf K, et al. Hematopoietic stem cell transplantation in immunocompetent hosts without radiation or chemotherapy. *Sci Transl Med*. 2016;8(351):351ra105.
387. Bankova AK, Pang WW, Velasco BJ, Long-Boyle JR, Shizuru JA. 5-Azacytidine depletes HSCs and synergizes with an anti-CD117 antibody to augment donor engraftment in immunocompetent mice. *Blood Adv*. 2021;5(19):3900-3912.
388. Czechowicz A, Palchaudhuri R, Scheck A, et al. Selective hematopoietic stem cell ablation using CD117-antibody-drug-conjugates enables safe and effective transplantation with immunity preservation. *Nat Commun*. 2019;10(1):617.
389. Huhn RD, Tisdale JF, Agricola B, Metzger ME, Donahue RE, Dunbar CE. Retroviral marking and transplantation of rhesus hematopoietic cells by nonmyeloablative conditioning. *Hum Gene Ther*. 1999;10(11):1783-1790.
390. Brenner S, Whiting-Theobald NL, Linton GF, et al. Concentrated RD114-pseudotyped MFGS-gp91phox vector achieves high levels of functional correction of the chronic granulomatous disease oxidase defect in NOD/SCID/beta-microglobulin−/− repopulating mobilized human peripheral blood CD34+ cells. *Blood*. 2003;102(8):2789-2797.
391. Kahl CA, Tarantal AF, Lee CI, et al. Effects of busulfan dose escalation on engraftment of infant rhesus monkey hematopoietic stem cells after gene marking by a lentiviral vector. *Exp Hematol*. 2006;34(3):369-381.
392. Kang EM, Hsieh MM, Metzger M, et al. Busulfan pharmacokinetics, toxicity, and low-dose conditioning for autologous transplantation of genetically modified hematopoietic stem cells in the rhesus macaque model. *Exp Hematol*. 2006;34(2):132-139.
393. Rosenzweig M, MacVittie TJ, Harper D, et al. Efficient and durable gene marking of hematopoietic progenitor cells in nonhuman primates after nonablative conditioning. *Blood*. 1999;94(7):2271-2286.
394. Sadat MA, Dirscherl S, Sastry L, et al. Retroviral vector integration in post-transplant hematopoiesis in mice conditioned with either submyeloablative or ablative irradiation. *Gene Ther*. 2009;16(12):1452-1464.
395. Cavazzana-Calvo M, Hacein-Bey S, de Saint Basile G, et al. Gene therapy of human severe combined immunodeficiency (SCID)-X1 disease. *Science*. 2000;288(5466):669-672.
396. Hacein-Bey-Abina S, Hauer J, Lim A, et al. Efficacy of gene therapy for X-linked severe combined immunodeficiency. *N Engl J Med*. 2010;363(4):355-364.
397. Hacein-Bey-Abina S, Le Deist F, Carlier F, et al. Sustained correction of X-linked severe combined immunodeficiency by ex vivo gene therapy. *N Engl J Med*. 2002;346(16):1185-1193.
398. Gaspar HB, Cooray S, Gilmour KC, et al. Long-term persistence of a polyclonal T cell repertoire after gene therapy for X-linked severe combined immunodeficiency. *Sci Transl Med*. 2011;3(97):97ra79.
399. Gaspar HB, Parsley KL, Howe S, et al. Gene therapy of X-linked severe combined immunodeficiency by use of a pseudotyped gammaretroviral vector. *Lancet*. 2004;364(9452):2181-2187.
400. Schwarzwaelder K, Howe SJ, Schmidt M, et al. Gammaretrovirus-mediated correction of SCID-X1 is associated with skewed vector integration site distribution in vivo. *J Clin Invest*. 2007;117(8):2241-2249.
401. Chinen J, Davis J, De Ravin SS, et al. Gene therapy improves immune function in preadolescents with X-linked severe combined immunodeficiency. *Blood*. 2007;110(1):67-73.
402. Thrasher AJ, Hacein-Bey-Abina S, Gaspar HB, et al. Failure of SCID-X1 gene therapy in older patients. *Blood*. 2005;105(11):4255-4257.
403. Aiuti A, Cattaneo F, Galimberti S, et al. Gene therapy for immunodeficiency due to adenosine deaminase deficiency. *N Engl J Med*. 2009;360(5):447-458.
404. Aiuti A, Slavin S, Aker M, et al. Correction of ADA-SCID by stem cell gene therapy combined with nonmyeloablative conditioning. *Science*. 2002;296(5577):2410-2413.
405. Cicalese MP, Ferrua F, Castagnaro L, et al. Update on the safety and efficacy of retroviral gene therapy for immunodeficiency due to adenosine deaminase deficiency. *Blood*. 2016;128(1):45-54.
406. Gaspar HB, Bjorkegren E, Parsley K, et al. Successful reconstitution of immunity in ADA-SCID by stem cell gene therapy following cessation of PEG-ADA and use of mild preconditioning. *Mol Ther*. 2006;14(4):505-513.
407. Cicalese MP, Ferrua F, Castagnaro L, et al. Gene therapy for adenosine deaminase deficiency: a comprehensive evaluation of short- and medium-term safety. *Mol Ther*. 2018;26(3):917-931.
408. Candotti F, Shaw KL, Muul L, et al. Gene therapy for adenosine deaminase-deficient severe combined immune deficiency: clinical comparison of retroviral vectors and treatment plans. *Blood*. 2012;120(18):3635-3646.
409. Gaspar HB, Cooray S, Gilmour KC, et al. Hematopoietic stem cell gene therapy for adenosine deaminase-deficient severe combined immunodeficiency leads to long-term immunological recovery and metabolic correction. *Sci Transl Med*. 2011;3(97):97ra80.
410. Shaw KL, Garabedian E, Mishra S, et al. Clinical efficacy of gene-modified stem cells in adenosine deaminase-deficient immunodeficiency. *J Clin Invest*. 2017;127(5):1689-1699.
411. Reinhardt B, Habib O, Shaw KL, et al. Long-term outcomes after gene therapy for adenosine deaminase severe combined immune deficiency. *Blood*. 2021;138(15):1304-1316.

412. Hacein-Bey-Abina S, von Kalle C, Schmidt M, et al. A serious adverse event after successful gene therapy for X-linked severe combined immunodeficiency. *N Engl J Med*. 2003;348(3):255-256.
413. Hacein-Bey-Abina S, Von Kalle C, Schmidt M, et al. LMO2-associated clonal T cell proliferation in two patients after gene therapy for SCID-X1. *Science*. 2003;302(5644):415-419.
414. Boehm T, Foroni L, Kaneko Y, Perutz MF, Rabbitts TH. The rhombotin family of cysteine-rich LIM-domain oncogenes: distinct members are involved in T-cell translocations to human chromosomes 11p15 and 11p13. *Proc Natl Acad Sci U S A*. 1991;88(10):4367-4371.
415. Howe SJ, Mansour MR, Schwarzwaelder K, et al. Insertional mutagenesis combined with acquired somatic mutations causes leukemogenesis following gene therapy of SCID-X1 patients. *J Clin Invest*. 2008;118(9):3143-3150.
416. Cornetta K. Safety aspects of gene therapy. *Br J Haematol*. 1992;80(4):421-426.
417. Li Z, Dullmann J, Schiedlmeier B, et al. Murine leukemia induced by retroviral gene marking. *Science*. 2002;296(5567):497.
418. Woods NB, Bottero V, Schmidt M, von Kalle C, Verma IM. Gene therapy: therapeutic gene causing lymphoma. *Nature*. 2006;440(7088):1123.
419. Dave UP, Jenkins NA, Copeland NG. Gene therapy insertional mutagenesis insights. *Science*. 2004;303(5656):333.
420. Kiem HP, Sellers S, Thomasson B, et al. Long-term clinical and molecular follow-up of large animals receiving retrovirally transduced stem and progenitor cells: No progression to clonal hematopoiesis or leukemia. *Mol Ther*. 2004;9(3):389-395.
421. Newrzela S, Cornils K, Li Z, et al. Resistance of mature T cells to oncogene transformation. *Blood*. 2008;112(6):2278-2286.
422. Biasco L, Ambrosi A, Pellin D, et al. Integration profile of retroviral vector in gene therapy treated patients is cell-specific according to gene expression and chromatin conformation of target cell. *EMBO Mol Med*. 2011;3(2):89-101.
423. Cooper AR, Lill GR, Shaw K, et al. Cytoreductive conditioning intensity predicts clonal diversity in ADA-SCID retroviral gene therapy patients. *Blood*. 2017;129(19):2624-2635.
424. Ott MG, Schmidt M, Schwarzwaelder K, et al. Correction of X-linked chronic granulomatous disease by gene therapy, augmented by insertional activation of MDS1-EVI1, PRDM16 or SETBP1. *Nat Med*. 2006;12(4):401-409.
425. Kang EM, Choi U, Theobald N, et al. Retrovirus gene therapy for X-linked chronic granulomatous disease can achieve stable long-term correction of oxidase activity in peripheral blood neutrophils. *Blood*. 2010;115(4):783-791.
426. Kang HJ, Bartholomae CC, Paruzynski A, et al. Retroviral gene therapy for X-linked chronic granulomatous disease: results from phase I/II trial. *Mol Ther*. 2011;19(11):2092-2101.
427. Dunbar CE, Larochelle A. Gene therapy activates EVI1, destabilizes chromosomes. *Nat Med*. 2010;16(2):163-165.
428. Stein S, Ott MG, Schultze-Strasser S, et al. Genomic instability and myelodysplasia with monosomy 7 consequent to EVI1 activation after gene therapy for chronic granulomatous disease. *Nat Med*. 2010;16(2):198-204.
429. Derry JM, Ochs HD, Francke U. Isolation of a novel gene mutated in Wiskott-Aldrich syndrome. *Cell*. 1994;78(4):635-644.
430. Notarangelo LD, Miao CH, Ochs HD. Wiskott-Aldrich syndrome. *Curr Opin Hematol*. 2008;15(1):30-36.
431. Puck JM, Candotti F. Lessons from the Wiskott-Aldrich syndrome. *N Engl J Med*. 2006;355(17):1759-1761.
432. Strom TS, Turner SJ, Andreansky S, et al. Defects in T-cell-mediated immunity to influenza virus in murine Wiskott-Aldrich syndrome are corrected by oncoretroviral vector-mediated gene transfer into repopulating hematopoietic cells. *Blood*. 2003;102(9):3108-3116.
433. Klein C, Nguyen D, Liu CH, et al. Gene therapy for Wiskott-Aldrich syndrome: rescue of T-cell signaling and amelioration of colitis upon transplantation of retrovirally transduced hematopoietic stem cells in mice. *Blood*. 2003;101(6):2159-2166.
434. Boztug K, Schmidt M, Schwarzer A, et al. Stem-cell gene therapy for the Wiskott-Aldrich syndrome. *N Engl J Med*. 2010;363(20):1918-1927.
435. Braun CJ, Boztug K, Paruzynski A, et al. Gene therapy for Wiskott-Aldrich syndrome--long-term efficacy and genotoxicity. *Sci Transl Med*. 2014;6(227):227ra33.
436. Nagel S, Venturini L, Meyer C, et al. Multiple mechanisms induce ectopic expression of LYL1 in subsets of T-ALL cell lines. *Leuk Res*. 2010;34(4):521-528.
437. Baum C. Parachuting in the epigenome: the biology of gene vector insertion profiles in the context of clinical trials. *EMBO Mol Med*. 2011;3(2):75-77.
438. Nienhuis AW, Dunbar CE, Sorrentino BP. Genotoxicity of retroviral integration in hematopoietic cells. *Mol Ther*. 2006;13(6):1031-1049.
439. Moolten FL, Cupples LA. A model for predicting the risk of cancer consequent to retroviral gene therapy. *Hum Gene Ther*. 1992;3(5):479-486.
440. Coffin JM. Retrovirus restriction revealed. *Nature*. 1996;382(6594):762-763.
441. Schroder AR, Shinn P, Chen H, Berry C, Ecker JR, Bushman F. HIV-1 integration in the human genome favors active genes and local hotspots. *Cell*. 2002;110(4):521-529.
442. Wu X, Li Y, Crise B, Burgess SM. Transcription start regions in the human genome are favored targets for MLV integration. *Science*. 2003;300(5626):1749-1751.
443. Hematti P, Hong BK, Ferguson C, et al. Distinct genomic integration of MLV and SIV vectors in primate hematopoietic stem and progenitor cells. *PLoS Biol*. 2004;2(12):e423.
444. Baum C, Dullmann J, Li Z, et al. Side effects of retroviral gene transfer into hematopoietic stem cells. *Blood*. 2003;101(6):2099-2113.
445. Kustikova O, Fehse B, Modlich U, et al. Clonal dominance of hematopoietic stem cells triggered by retroviral gene marking. *Science*. 2005;308(5725):1171-1174.
446. Kustikova OS, Geiger H, Li Z, et al. Retroviral vector insertion sites associated with dominant hematopoietic clones mark "stemness" pathways. *Blood*. 2007;109(5):1897-1907.
447. Seggewiss R, Pittaluga S, Adler RL, et al. Acute myeloid leukemia is associated with retroviral gene transfer to hematopoietic progenitor cells in a rhesus macaque. *Blood*. 2006;107(10):3865-3867.
448. Du Y, Jenkins NA, Copeland NG. Insertional mutagenesis identifies genes that promote the immortalization of primary bone marrow progenitor cells. *Blood*. 2005;106(12):3932-3939.
449. Schambach A, Bohne J, Chandra S, et al. Equal potency of gammaretroviral and lentiviral SIN vectors for expression of O6-methylguanine-DNA methyltransferase in hematopoietic cells. *Mol Ther*. 2006;13(2):391-400.
450. Modlich U, Navarro S, Zychlinski D, et al. Insertional transformation of hematopoietic cells by self-inactivating lentiviral and gammaretroviral vectors. *Mol Ther*. 2009;17(11):1919-1928.
451. Montini E, Cesana D, Schmidt M, et al. The genotoxic potential of retroviral vectors is strongly modulated by vector design and integration site selection in a mouse model of HSC gene therapy. *J Clin Invest*. 2009;119(4):964-975.
452. Evans-Galea MV, Wielgosz MM, Hanawa H, Srivastava DK, Nienhuis AW. Suppression of clonal dominance in cultured human lymphoid cells by addition of the cHS4 insulator to a lentiviral vector. *Mol Ther*. 2007;15(4):801-809.
453. Li CL, Xiong D, Stamatoyannopoulos G, Emery DW. Genomic and functional assays demonstrate reduced gammaretroviral vector genotoxicity associated with use of the cHS4 chromatin insulator. *Mol Ther*. 2009;17(4):716-724.
454. Ryu BY, Evans-Galea MV, Gray JT, Bodine DM, Persons DA, Nienhuis AW. An experimental system for the evaluation of retroviral vector design to diminish the risk for proto-oncogene activation. *Blood*. 2008;111(4):1866-1875.
455. Liu M, Maurano MT, Wang H, et al. Genomic discovery of potent chromatin insulators for human gene therapy. *Nat Biotechnol*. 2015;33(2):198-203.
456. Di Stasi A, Tey SK, Dotti G, et al. Inducible apoptosis as a safety switch for adoptive cell therapy. *N Engl J Med*. 2011;365(18):1673-1683.
457. Barese CN, Felizardo TC, Sellers SE, et al. Regulated apoptosis of genetically modified hematopoietic stem and progenitor cells via an inducible caspase-9 suicide gene in rhesus macaques. *Stem Cells*. 2015;33(1):91-100.
458. Conese M, Auriche C, Ascenzioni F. Gene therapy progress and prospects: episomally maintained self-replicating systems. *Gene Ther*. 2004;11(24):1735-1741.
459. Woods NB, Muessig A, Schmidt M, et al. Lentiviral vector transduction of NOD/SCID repopulating cells results in multiple vector integrations per transduced cell: risk of insertional mutagenesis. *Blood*. 2003;101(4):1284-1289.
460. Baum C. Insertional mutagenesis in gene therapy and stem cell biology. *Curr Opin Hematol*. 2007;14(4):337-342.
461. Case SS, Price MA, Jordan CT, et al. Stable transduction of quiescent CD34(+)CD38(−) human hematopoietic cells by HIV-1-based lentiviral vectors. *Proc Natl Acad Sci U S A*. 1999;96(6):2988-2993.
462. Mazurier F, Gan OI, McKenzie JL, Doedens M, Dick JE. Lentivector-mediated clonal tracking reveals intrinsic heterogeneity in the human hematopoietic stem cell compartment and culture-induced stem cell impairment. *Blood*. 2004;103(2):545-552.
463. Uchida N, Sutton RE, Friera AM, et al. HIV, but not murine leukemia virus, vectors mediate high efficiency gene transfer into freshly isolated G0/G1 human hematopoietic stem cells. *Proc Natl Acad Sci U S A*. 1998;95(20):11939-11944.
464. Eichler F, Duncan C, Musolino PL, et al. Hematopoietic stem-cell gene therapy for cerebral adrenoleukodystrophy. *N Engl J Med*. 2017;377(17):1630-1638.
465. Cavazzana-Calvo M, Payen E, Negre O, et al. Transfusion independence and HMGA2 activation after gene therapy of human beta-thalassaemia. *Nature*. 2010;467(7313):318-322.
466. Ikeda K, Mason PJ, Bessler M. 3'UTR-truncated Hmga2 cDNA causes MPN-like hematopoiesis by conferring a clonal growth advantage at the level of HSC in mice. *Blood*. 2011;117(22):5860-5869.
467. Inoue N, Izui-Sarumaru T, Murakami Y, et al. Molecular basis of clonal expansion of hematopoiesis in 2 patients with paroxysmal nocturnal hemoglobinuria (PNH). *Blood*. 2006;108(13):4232-4236.
468. Murakami Y, Inoue N, Shichishima T, et al. Deregulated expression of HMGA2 is implicated in clonal expansion of PIGA deficient cells in paroxysmal nocturnal haemoglobinuria. *Br J Haematol*. 2012;156(3):383-387.
469. Mansilla-Soto J, Riviere I, Boulad F, Sadelain M. Cell and gene therapy for the beta-thalassemias: advances and prospects. *Hum Gene Ther*. 2016;27(4):295-304.
470. Schmidt M, Carbonaro DA, Speckmann C, et al. Clonality analysis after retroviral-mediated gene transfer to CD34+ cells from the cord blood of ADA-deficient SCID neonates. *Nat Med*. 2003;9(4):463-468.
471. Thompson AA, Walters MC, Kwiatkowski J, et al. Gene therapy in patients with transfusion-dependent beta-thalassemia. *N Engl J Med*. 2018;378(16):1479-1493.
472. Locatelli F, Thompson AA, Kwiatkowski JL, et al. Betibeglogene autotemcel gene therapy for non-beta(0)/beta(0) genotype beta-thalassemia. *N Engl J Med*. 2022;386(5):415-427.
473. Harrison C. First gene therapy for beta-thalassemia approved. *Nat Biotechnol*. 2019;37(10):1102-1103.
474. Marktel S, Scaramuzza S, Cicalese MP, et al. Intrabone hematopoietic stem cell gene therapy for adult and pediatric patients affected by transfusion-dependent ss-thalassemia. *Nat Med*. 2019;25(2):234-241.
475. Boulad F, Maggio A, Wang X, et al. Lentiviral globin gene therapy with reduced-intensity conditioning in adults with beta-thalassemia: a phase 1 trial. *Nat Med*. 2022;28(1):63-70.
476. Ribeil JA, Hacein-Bey-Abina S, Payen E, et al. Gene therapy in a patient with sickle cell disease. *N Engl J Med*. 2017;376(9):848-855.
477. Kanter J, Walters MC, Krishnamurti L, et al. Biologic and clinical efficacy of LentiGlobin for sickle cell disease. *N Engl J Med*. 2022;386(7):617-628.
478. Tisdale JF, Pierciey FJ Jr, Bonner M, et al. Safety and feasibility of hematopoietic progenitor stem cell collection by mobilization with plerixafor followed by apheresis vs bone marrow harvest in patients with sickle cell disease in the multi-center HGB-206 trial. *Am J Hematol*. 2020;95(9):E239-E42.

479. Hsieh MM, Bonner M, Pierciey FJ, et al. Myelodysplastic syndrome unrelated to lentiviral vector in a patient treated with gene therapy for sickle cell disease. *Blood Adv.* 2020;4(9):2058-2063.
480. Leonard A, Tisdale JF. A pause in gene therapy: reflecting on the unique challenges of sickle cell disease. *Mol Ther.* 2021;29(4):1355-1356.
481. Goyal S, Tisdale J, Schmidt M, et al. Acute myeloid leukemia case after gene therapy for sickle cell disease. *N Engl J Med.* 2022;386(2):138-147.
482. Jones RJ, DeBaun MR. Leukemia after gene therapy for sickle cell disease: insertional mutagenesis, busulfan, both, or neither. *Blood.* 2021;138(11):942-947.
483. Penati R, Fumagalli F, Calbi V, Bernardo ME, Aiuti A. Gene therapy for lysosomal storage disorders: recent advances for metachromatic leukodystrophy and mucopolysaccaridosis I. *J Inherit Metab Dis.* 2017;40(4):543-554.
484. Biffi A, Montini E, Lorioli L, et al. Lentiviral hematopoietic stem cell gene therapy benefits metachromatic leukodystrophy. *Science.* 2013;341(6148):1233158.
485. Sessa M, Lorioli L, Fumagalli F, et al. Lentiviral haemopoietic stem-cell gene therapy in early-onset metachromatic leukodystrophy: an ad-hoc analysis of a non-randomised, open-label, phase 1/2 trial. *Lancet.* 2016;388(10043):476-487.
486. Fumagalli F, Calbi V, Natali Sora MG, et al. Lentiviral haematopoietic stem-cell gene therapy for early-onset metachromatic leukodystrophy: long-term results from a non-randomised, open-label, phase 1/2 trial and expanded access. *Lancet.* 2022;399(10322):372-383.
487. Kurtzberg J. Gene therapy offers new hope for children with metachromatic leukodystrophy. *Lancet.* 2022;399(10322):338-339.
488. McKusick VA, Howell RR, Hussels IE, Neufeld EF, Stevenson RE. Allelism, non-allelism, and genetic compounds among the mucopolysaccharidoses. *Lancet.* 1972;1(7758):993-996.
489. Muenzer J, Wraith JE, Clarke LA. International consensus panel on M, and treatment of mucopolysaccharidosis I. Mucopolysaccharidosis I: management and treatment guidelines. *Pediatrics.* 2009;123(1):19-29.
490. Bay L, Amartino H, Antacle A, et al. New recommendations for the care of patients with mucopolysaccharidosis type I. *Arch Argent Pediatr.* 2021;119(2):e121-e8.
491. Gentner B, Tucci F, Galimberti S, et al. Hematopoietic stem- and progenitor-cell gene therapy for Hurler syndrome. *N Engl J Med.* 2021;385(21):1929-1940.
492. Brady RO, Gal AE, Bradley RM, Martensson E, Warshaw AL, Laster L. Enzymatic defect in Fabry's disease. Ceramidetrihexosidase deficiency. *N Engl J Med.* 1967;276(21):1163-1167.
493. Germain DP. Fabry disease. *Orphanet J Rare Dis.* 2010;5:30.
494. Eng CM, Guffon N, Wilcox WR, et al. Safety and efficacy of recombinant human alpha-galactosidase A replacement therapy in Fabry's disease. *N Engl J Med.* 2001;345(1):9-16.
495. Germain DP, Hughes DA, Nicholls K, et al. Treatment of Fabry's disease with the pharmacologic chaperone migalastat. *N Engl J Med.* 2016;375(6):545-555.
496. Khan A, Barber DL, Huang J, et al. Lentivirus-mediated gene therapy for Fabry disease. *Nat Commun.* 2021;12(1):1178.
497. Aiuti A, Biasco L, Scaramuzza S, et al. Lentiviral hematopoietic stem cell gene therapy in patients with Wiskott-Aldrich syndrome. *Science.* 2013;341(6148):1233151.
498. Hacein-Bey Abina S, Gaspar HB, Blondeau J, et al. Outcomes following gene therapy in patients with severe Wiskott-Aldrich syndrome. *J Am Med Assoc.* 2015;313(15):1550-1563.
499. Magnani A, Semeraro M, Adam F, et al. Long-term safety and efficacy of lentiviral hematopoietic stem/progenitor cell gene therapy for Wiskott-Aldrich syndrome. *Nat Med.* 2022;28(1):71-80.
500. Morris EC, Fox T, Chakraverty R, et al. Gene therapy for Wiskott-Aldrich syndrome in a severely affected adult. *Blood.* 2017;130(11):1327-1335.
501. Thornhill SI, Schambach A, Howe SJ, et al. Self-inactivating gammaretroviral vectors for gene therapy of X-linked severe combined immunodeficiency. *Mol Ther.* 2008;16(3):590-598.
502. Zychlinski D, Schambach A, Modlich U, et al. Physiological promoters reduce the genotoxic risk of integrating gene vectors. *Mol Ther.* 2008;16(4):718-725.
503. Hacein-Bey-Abina S, Pai SY, Gaspar HB, et al. A modified gamma-retrovirus vector for X-linked severe combined immunodeficiency. *N Engl J Med.* 2014;371(15):1407-1417.
504. Kohn DB, Booth C, Shaw KL, et al. Autologous ex vivo lentiviral gene therapy for adenosine deaminase deficiency. *N Engl J Med.* 2021;384(21):2002-2013.
505. Kohn DB, Booth C, Kang EM, et al. Lentiviral gene therapy for X-linked chronic granulomatous disease. *Nat Med.* 2020;26(2):200-206.
506. Rio P, Navarro S, Wang W, et al. Successful engraftment of gene-corrected hematopoietic stem cells in non-conditioned patients with Fanconi anemia. *Nat Med.* 2019;25(9):1396-1401.
507. Hutter G, Nowak D, Mossner M, et al. Long-term control of HIV by CCR5 Delta32/Delta32 stem-cell transplantation. *N Engl J Med.* 2009;360(7):692-698.
508. Allers K, Hutter G, Hofmann J, et al. Evidence for the cure of HIV infection by CCR5Delta32/Delta32 stem cell transplantation. *Blood.* 2011;117(10):2791-2799.
509. Kiem HP, Jerome KR, Deeks SG, McCune JM. Hematopoietic-stem-cell-based gene therapy for HIV disease. *Cell Stem Cell.* 2012;10(2):137-147.
510. Kim SS, Peer D, Kumar P, et al. RNAi-mediated CCR5 silencing by LFA-1-targeted nanoparticles prevents HIV infection in BLT mice. *Mol Ther.* 2010;18(2):370-376.
511. Shimizu S, Hong P, Arumugam B, et al. A highly efficient short hairpin RNA potently down-regulates CCR5 expression in systemic lymphoid organs in the humanized BLT mouse model. *Blood.* 2010;115(8):1534-1544.
512. Feng Y, Leavitt M, Tritz R, et al. Inhibition of CCR5-dependent HIV-1 infection by hairpin ribozyme gene therapy against CC-chemokine receptor 5. *Virology.* 2000;276(2):271-278.
513. DiGiusto DL, Krishnan A, Li L, et al. RNA-based gene therapy for HIV with lentiviral vector-modified CD34(+) cells in patients undergoing transplantation for AIDS-related lymphoma. *Sci Transl Med.* 2010;2(36):36ra43.
514. Luis Abad J, Gonzalez MA, del Real G, et al. Novel interfering bifunctional molecules against the CCR5 coreceptor are efficient inhibitors of HIV-1 infection. *Mol Ther.* 2003;8(3):475-484.
515. Swan CH, Buhler B, Steinberger P, Tschan MP, Barbas CF III, Torbett BE. T-cell protection and enrichment through lentiviral CCR5 intrabody gene delivery. *Gene Ther.* 2006;13(20):1480-1492.
516. Steinberger P, Andris-Widhopf J, Buhler B, Torbett BE, Barbas CF III. Functional deletion of the CCR5 receptor by intracellular immunization produces cells that are refractory to CCR5-dependent HIV-1 infection and cell fusion. *Proc Natl Acad Sci U S A.* 2000;97(2):805-810.
517. Trobridge GD, Wu RA, Beard BC, et al. Protection of stem cell-derived lymphocytes in a primate AIDS gene therapy model after in vivo selection. *PLoS One.* 2009;4(11):e7693.
518. Dever DP, Porteus MH. The changing landscape of gene editing in hematopoietic stem cells: a step towards Cas9 clinical translation. *Curr Opin Hematol.* 2017;24(6):481-488.
519. Lux CT, Scharenberg AM. Therapeutic gene editing safety and specificity. *Hematol Oncol Clin North Am.* 2017;31(5):787-795.
520. Genovese P, Schiroli G, Escobar G, et al. Targeted genome editing in human repopulating haematopoietic stem cells. *Nature.* 2014;510(7504):235-240.
521. Hendel A, Bak RO, Clark JT, et al. Chemically modified guide RNAs enhance CRISPR-Cas genome editing in human primary cells. *Nat Biotechnol.* 2015;33(9):985-989.
522. Mandal PK, Ferreira LM, Collins R, et al. Efficient ablation of genes in human hematopoietic stem and effector cells using CRISPR/Cas9. *Cell Stem Cell.* 2014;15(5):643-652.
523. Gundry MC, Brunetti L, Lin A, et al. Highly efficient genome editing of murine and human hematopoietic progenitor cells by CRISPR/Cas9. *Cell Rep.* 2016;17(5):1453-1461.
524. Hoban MD, Cost GJ, Mendel MC, et al. Correction of the sickle cell disease mutation in human hematopoietic stem/progenitor cells. *Blood.* 2015;125(17):2597-2604.
525. De Ravin SS, Reik A, Liu PQ, et al. Targeted gene addition in human CD34+ hematopoietic cells for correction of X-linked chronic granulomatous disease. *Nat Biotech.* 2016;34(4):424-429.
526. Dever DP, Bak RO, Reinisch A, et al. CRISPR/Cas9 beta-globin gene targeting in human haematopoietic stem cells. *Nature.* 2016;539(7629):384-389.
527. Sather BD, Romano Ibarra GS, Sommer K, et al. Efficient modification of CCR5 in primary human hematopoietic cells using a megaTAL nuclease and AAV donor template. *Sci Transl Med.* 2015;7(307):307ra156.
528. Wang J, Exline CM, DeClercq JJ, et al. Homology-driven genome editing in hematopoietic stem and progenitor cells using ZFN mRNA and AAV6 donors. *Nat Biotechnol.* 2015;33(12):1256-1263.
529. DeWitt MA, Magis W, Bray NL, et al. Selection-free genome editing of the sickle mutation in human adult hematopoietic stem/progenitor cells. *Sci Transl Med.* 2016;8(360):360ra134.
530. Hoban MD, Lumaquin D, Kuo CY, et al. CRISPR/Cas9-Mediated correction of the sickle mutation in human CD34+ cells. *Mol Ther.* 2016;24(9):1561-1569.
531. Agudelo D, Duringer A, Bozoyan L, et al. Marker-free coselection for CRISPR-driven genome editing in human cells. *Nat Methods.* 2017;14(6):615-620.
532. Wang J, DeClercq JJ, Hayward SB, et al. Highly efficient homology-driven genome editing in human T cells by combining zinc-finger nuclease mRNA and AAV6 donor delivery. *Nucleic Acids Res.* 2016;44(3):e30.
533. Ran FA, Cong L, Yan WX, et al. In vivo genome editing using *Staphylococcus aureus* Cas9. *Nature.* 2015;520(7546):186-191.
534. Crosetto N, Mitra A, Silva MJ, et al. Nucleotide-resolution DNA double-strand break mapping by next-generation sequencing. *Nat Methods.* 2013;10(4):361-365.
535. Frock RL, Hu J, Meyers RM, Ho YJ, Kii E, Alt FW. Genome-wide detection of DNA double-stranded breaks induced by engineered nucleases. *Nat Biotechnol.* 2015;33(2):179-186.
536. Tsai SQ, Topkar VV, Joung JK, Aryee MJ. Open-source guideseq software for analysis of GUIDE-seq data. *Nat Biotechnol.* 2016;34(5):483.
537. Tsai SQ, Zheng Z, Nguyen NT, et al. GUIDE-seq enables genome-wide profiling of off-target cleavage by CRISPR-Cas nucleases. *Nat Biotechnol.* 2015;33(2):187-197.
538. Tsai SQ, Nguyen NT, Malagon-Lopez J, Topkar VV, Aryee MJ, Joung JK. CIRCLE-seq: a highly sensitive in vitro screen for genome-wide CRISPR-Cas9 nuclease off-targets. *Nat Methods.* 2017;14(6):607-614.
539. Kim D, Bae S, Park J, et al. Digenome-seq: genome-wide profiling of CRISPR-Cas9 off-target effects in human cells. *Nat Methods.* 2015;12(3):237-243, 1 p following 243.
540. Schaefer KA, Wu WH, Colgan DF, Tsang SH, Bassuk AG, Mahajan VB. Unexpected mutations after CRISPR-Cas9 editing in vivo. *Nat Methods.* 2017;14(6):547-548.
541. Zetsche B, Gootenberg JS, Abudayyeh OO, et al. Cpf1 is a single RNA-guided endonuclease of a class 2 CRISPR-Cas system. *Cell.* 2015;163(3):759-771.
542. Hsu PD, Scott DA, Weinstein JA, et al. DNA targeting specificity of RNA-guided Cas9 nucleases. *Nat Biotechnol.* 2013;31(9):827-832.
543. Davis KM, Pattanayak V, Thompson DB, Zuris JA, Liu DR. Small molecule-triggered Cas9 protein with improved genome-editing specificity. *Nat Chem Biol.* 2015;11(5):316-318.
544. Mali P, Aach J, Stranges PB, et al. CAS9 transcriptional activators for target specificity screening and paired nickases for cooperative genome engineering. *Nat Biotechnol.* 2013;31(9):833-838.
545. Ran FA, Hsu PD, Lin CY, et al. Double nicking by RNA-guided CRISPR Cas9 for enhanced genome editing specificity. *Cell.* 2013;154(6):1380-1389.
546. Fu Y, Foden JA, Khayter C, et al. High-frequency off-target mutagenesis induced by CRISPR-Cas nucleases in human cells. *Nat Biotechnol.* 2013;31(9):822-826.

547. Guilinger JP, Thompson DB, Liu DR. Fusion of catalytically inactive Cas9 to FokI nuclease improves the specificity of genome modification. *Nat Biotechnol.* 2014;32(6):577-582.
548. Tsai SQ, Wyvekens N, Khayter C, et al. Dimeric CRISPR RNA-guided FokI nucleases for highly specific genome editing. *Nat Biotechnol.* 2014;32(6):569-576.
549. Slaymaker IM, Gao L, Zetsche B, Scott DA, Yan WX, Zhang F. Rationally engineered Cas9 nucleases with improved specificity. *Science.* 2016;351(6268):84-88.
550. Gaudelli NM, Komor AC, Rees HA, et al. Programmable base editing of A*T to G*C in genomic DNA without DNA cleavage. *Nature.* 2017;551(7681):464-471.
551. Komor AC, Kim YB, Packer MS, Zuris JA, Liu DR. Programmable editing of a target base in genomic DNA without double-stranded DNA cleavage. *Nature.* 2016;533(7603):420-424.
552. Rees HA, Liu DR. Base editing: precision chemistry on the genome and transcriptome of living cells. *Nat Rev Genet.* 2018;19(12):770-788.
553. Yang B, Yang L, Chen J. Development and application of base editors. *CRISPR J.* 2019;2(2):91-104.
554. Anzalone AV, Randolph PB, Davis JR, et al. Search-and-replace genome editing without double-strand breaks or donor DNA. *Nature.* 2019;576(7785):149-157.
555. Chaikind B, Bessen JL, Thompson DB, Hu JH, Liu DR. A programmable Cas9-serine recombinase fusion protein that operates on DNA sequences in mammalian cells. *Nucleic Acids Res.* 2016;44(20):9758-9770.
556. Chen SP, Wang HH. An engineered Cas-transposon system for programmable and site-directed DNA Transpositions. *CRISPR J.* 2019;2(6):376-394.
557. Klompe SE, Vo PLH, Halpin-Healy TS, Sternberg SH. Transposon-encoded CRISPR-Cas systems direct RNA-guided DNA integration. *Nature.* 2019;571(7764):219-225.
558. Strecker J, Ladha A, Gardner Z, et al. RNA-guided DNA insertion with CRISPR-associated transposases. *Science.* 2019;365(6448):48-53.
559. Anzalone AV, Koblan LW, Liu DR. Genome editing with CRISPR-Cas nucleases, base editors, transposases and prime editors. *Nat Biotechnol.* 2020;38(7):824-844.
560. Chen PJ, Hussmann JA, Yan J, et al. Enhanced prime editing systems by manipulating cellular determinants of editing outcomes. *Cell.* 2021;184(22):5635.e29-5652.e29.
561. Nelson JW, Randolph PB, Shen SP, et al. Engineered pegRNAs improve prime editing efficiency. *Nat Biotechnol.* 2022;40(3):402-410.
562. Anzalone AV, Gao XD, Podracky CJ, et al. Programmable deletion, replacement, integration and inversion of large DNA sequences with twin prime editing. *Nat Biotechnol.* 2021;40(5):731-740.
563. Sankaran VG, Xu J, Byron R, et al. A functional element necessary for fetal hemoglobin silencing. *N Engl J Med.* 2011;365(9):807-814.
564. Forget BG. Molecular basis of hereditary persistence of fetal hemoglobin. *Ann N Y Acad Sci.* 1998;850:38-44.
565. Dover GJ, Brusilow S, Samid D. Increased fetal hemoglobin in patients receiving sodium 4-phenylbutyrate. *N Engl J Med.* 1992;327(8):569-570.
566. Bauer DE, Kamran SC, Lessard S, et al. An erythroid enhancer of BCL11A subject to genetic variation determines fetal hemoglobin level. *Science.* 2013;342(6155):253-257.
567. Canver MC, Smith EC, Sher F, et al. BCL11A enhancer dissection by Cas9-mediated in situ saturating mutagenesis. *Nature.* 2015;527(7577):192-197.
568. Bjurstrom CF, Mojadidi M, Phillips J, et al. Reactivating fetal hemoglobin expression in human adult erythroblasts through BCL11A knockdown using targeted endonucleases. *Mol Ther Nucleic Acids.* 2016;5:e351.
569. Liu P, Keller JR, Ortiz M, et al. Bcl11a is essential for normal lymphoid development. *Nat Immunol.* 2003;4(6):525-532.
570. Chang KH, Smith SE, Sullivan T, et al. Long-term engraftment and fetal globin Induction upon BCL11A gene editing in bone-marrow-derived CD34+ hematopoietic stem and progenitor cells. *Mol Ther Methods Clin Dev.* 2017;4:137-148.
571. Traxler EA, Yao Y, Wang YD, et al. A genome-editing strategy to treat beta-hemoglobinopathies that recapitulates a mutation associated with a benign genetic condition. *Nat Med.* 2016;22(9):987-990.
572. Ye L, Wang J, Tan Y, et al. Genome editing using CRISPR-Cas9 to create the HPFH genotype in HSPCs: an approach for treating sickle cell disease and beta-thalassemia. *Proc Natl Acad Sci U S A.* 2016;113(38):10661-10665.
573. Frangoul H, Altshuler D, Cappellini MD, et al. CRISPR-Cas9 gene editing for sickle cell disease and beta-thalassemia. *N Engl J Med.* 2021;384(3):252-260.
574. Peters SO, Kittler EL, Ramshaw HS, Quesenberry PJ. Murine marrow cells expanded in culture with IL-3, IL-6, IL-11, and SCF acquire an engraftment defect in normal hosts. *Exp Hematol.* 1995;23(5):461-469.
575. van der Loo JC, Ploemacher RE. Marrow- and spleen-seeding efficiencies of all murine hematopoietic stem cell subsets are decreased by preincubation with hematopoietic growth factors. *Blood.* 1995;85(9):2598-2606.
576. Spangrude GJ, Brooks DM, Tumas DB. Long-term repopulation of irradiated mice with limiting numbers of purified hematopoietic stem cells: in vivo expansion of stem cell phenotype but not function. *Blood.* 1995;85(4):1006-1016.
577. Sellers S, Tisdale J, Agricola B, Kato I, Donahue R, Dunbar C. Genetically-marked rhesus peripheral blood progenitor cells (PBPC) ex vivo expanded in the presence of fibronectin 296 contribute to both short and long term engraftment. *Blood.* 2000;96(11):589a.
578. Li CL, Johnson GR. Stem cell factor enhances the survival but not the self-renewal of murine hematopoietic long-term repopulating cells. *Blood.* 1994;84(2):408-414.
579. Bodine DM, Seidel NE, Zsebo KM, Orlic D. In vivo administration of stem cell factor to mice increases the absolute number of pluripotent hematopoietic stem cells. *Blood.* 1993;82(2):445-455.
580. Boitano AE, Wang J, Romeo R, et al. Aryl hydrocarbon receptor antagonists promote the expansion of human hematopoietic stem cells. *Science.* 2010;329(5997):1345-1348.
581. Fares I, Chagraoui J, Gareau Y, et al. Cord blood expansion. Pyrimidoindole derivatives are agonists of human hematopoietic stem cell self-renewal. *Science.* 2014;345(6203):1509-1512.
582. Garcon L, Ge J, Manjunath SH, et al. Ribosomal and hematopoietic defects in induced pluripotent stem cells derived from Diamond Blackfan anemia patients. *Blood.* 2013;122(6):912-921.
583. Gross B, Pittermann E, Reinhardt D, Cantz T, Klusmann JH. Prospects and challenges of reprogrammed cells in hematology and oncology. *Pediatr Hematol Oncol.* 2012;29(6):507-528.
584. Hanna J, Wernig M, Markoulaki S, et al. Treatment of sickle cell anemia mouse model with iPS cells generated from autologous skin. *Science.* 2007;318(5858):1920-1923.
585. Liu GH, Suzuki K, Li M, et al. Modelling Fanconi anemia pathogenesis and therapeutics using integration-free patient-derived iPSCs. *Nat Commun.* 2014;5:4330.
586. Raya A, Rodriguez-Piza I, Guenechea G, et al. Disease-corrected haematopoietic progenitors from Fanconi anaemia induced pluripotent stem cells. *Nature.* 2009;460(7251):53-59.
587. Daniel MG, Pereira CF, Lemischka IR, Moore KA. Making a hematopoietic stem cell. *Trends Cell Biol.* 2016;26(3):202-214.
588. Easterbrook J, Fidanza A, Forrester LM. Concise review: programming human pluripotent stem cells into blood. *Br J Haematol.* 2016;173(5):671-679.
589. Ebina W, Rossi DJ. Transcription factor-mediated reprogramming toward hematopoietic stem cells. *EMBO J.* 2015;34(7):694-709.
590. Rowe RG, Mandelbaum J, Zon LI, Daley GQ. Engineering hematopoietic stem cells: Lessons from development. *Cell Stem Cell.* 2016;18(6):707-720.
591. Vo LT, Daley GQ. De novo generation of HSCs from somatic and pluripotent stem cell sources. *Blood.* 2015;125(17):2641-2648.
592. Bhatia M. Hematopoiesis from human embryonic stem cells. *Ann N Y Acad Sci.* 2007;1106:219-222.
593. Gori JL, Butler JM, Chan YY, et al. Vascular niche promotes hematopoietic multipotent progenitor formation from pluripotent stem cells. *J Clin Invest.* 2015;125(3):1243-1254.
594. Sugimura R, Jha DK, Han A, et al. Haematopoietic stem and progenitor cells from human pluripotent stem cells. *Nature.* 2017;545(7655):432-438.
595. Amabile G, Welner RS, Nombela-Arrieta C, et al. In vivo generation of transplantable human hematopoietic cells from induced pluripotent stem cells. *Blood.* 2013;121(8):1255-1264.
596. Doulatov S, Vo LT, Chou SS, et al. Induction of multipotential hematopoietic progenitors from human pluripotent stem cells via respecification of lineage-restricted precursors. *Cell Stem Cell.* 2013;13(4):459-470.
597. Ledran MH, Krassowska A, Armstrong L, et al. Efficient hematopoietic differentiation of human embryonic stem cells on stromal cells derived from hematopoietic niches. *Cell Stem Cell.* 2008;3(1):85-98.
598. Risueno RM, Sachlos E, Lee JH, et al. Inability of human induced pluripotent stem cell-hematopoietic derivatives to downregulate microRNAs in vivo reveals a block in xenograft hematopoietic regeneration. *Stem Cells.* 2012;30(2):131-139.
599. Tian X, Woll PS, Morris JK, Linehan JL, Kaufman DS. Hematopoietic engraftment of human embryonic stem cell-derived cells is regulated by recipient innate immunity. *Stem Cells.* 2006;24(5):1370-1380.
600. Ditadi A, Sturgeon CM, Keller G. A view of human haematopoietic development from the Petri dish. *Nat Rev Mol Cell Biol.* 2017;18(1):56-67.
601. Zonari E, Desantis G, Petrillo C, et al. Efficient ex vivo engineering and expansion of highly purified human hematopoietic stem and progenitor cell populations for gene therapy. *Stem Cell Rep.* 2017;8(4):977-990.
602. Baldwin K, Urbinati F, Romero Z, et al. Enrichment of human hematopoietic stem/progenitor cells facilitates transduction for stem cell gene therapy. *Stem Cells.* 2015;33(5):1532-1542.
603. Bernardo ME, Aiuti A. The role of conditioning in hematopoietic stem cell gene therapy. *Hum Gene Ther.* 2016;27(10):741-748.
604. Chandrakasan S, Jayavaradhan R, Ernst J, et al. KIT blockade is sufficient for donor hematopoietic stem cell engraftment in Fanconi anemia mice. *Blood.* 2017;129(8):1048-1052.
605. Palchaudhuri R, Saez B, Hoggatt J, et al. Non-genotoxic conditioning for hematopoietic stem cell transplantation using a hematopoietic-cell-specific internalizing immunotoxin. *Nat Biotechnol.* 2016;34(7):738-745.
606. Srikanthan MA, Humbert O, Haworth KG. Effective multi-lineage engraftment in a mouse model of fanconi anemia using non-genotoxic antibody-based conditioning. *Mol Ther Methods Clin Dev.* 2020;17:455-464.
607. Musunuru K, Chadwick AC, Mizoguchi T, et al. In vivo CRISPR base editing of PCSK9 durably lowers cholesterol in primates. *Nature.* 2021;593(7859):429-434.
608. Banskota S, Raguram A, Suh S, et al. Engineered virus-like particles for efficient in vivo delivery of therapeutic proteins. *Cell.* 2022;185(2):250-265 e16.
609. Mangeot PE, Risson V, Fusil F, et al. Genome editing in primary cells and in vivo using viral-derived Nanoblades loaded with Cas9-sgRNA ribonucleoproteins. *Nat Commun.* 2019;10(1):45.
610. Amalfitano A, Begy CR, Chamberlain JS. Improved adenovirus packaging cell lines to support the growth of replication-defective gene-delivery vectors. *Proc Natl Acad Sci U S A.* 1996;93(8):3352-3356.
611. Clemens PR, Kochanek S, Sunada Y, et al. In vivo muscle gene transfer of full-length dystrophin with an adenoviral vector that lacks all viral genes. *Gene Ther.* 1996;3(11):965-972.
612. Riddell SR, Elliott M, Lewinsohn DA, et al. T-cell mediated rejection of gene-modified HIV-specific cytotoxic T lymphocytes in HIV-infected patients. *Nat Med.* 1996;2(2):216-223.
613. Sykes M, Sachs DH, Nienhuis AW, Pearson DA, Moulton AD, Bodine DM. Specific prolongation of skin graft survival following retroviral transduction of bone marrow with an allogeneic major histocompatibility complex gene. *Transplantation.* 1993;55(1):197-202.

614. Ally BA, Hawley TS, McKall-Faienza KJ, et al. Prevention of autoimmune disease by retroviral-mediated gene therapy. *J Immunol*. 1995;155(11):5404-5408.
615. Shull R, Lu X, Dube I, et al. Humoral immune response limits gene therapy in canine MPS I. *Blood*. 1996;88(1):377-379.
616. Kang EM, Hanazano Y, Frare P, et al. Persistent low-level engraftment of rhesus peripheral blood progenitor cells transduced with the fanconi anemia c gene after conditioning with low-dose irradiation. *Mol Ther*. 2001;3(6):911-919.
617. Hacein-Bey-Abina S, Garrigue A, Wang GP, et al. Insertional oncogenesis in 4 patients after retrovirus-mediated gene therapy of SCID-X1. *J Clin Invest*. 2008;118(9):3132-3142.
618. Amado RG, Mitsuyasu RT, Rosenblatt JD, et al. Anti-human immunodeficiency virus hematopoietic progenitor cell-delivered ribozyme in a phase I study: myeloid and lymphoid reconstitution in human immunodeficiency virus type-1-infected patients. *Hum Gene Ther*. 2004;15(3):251-262.
619. Mitsuyasu RT, Zack JA, Macpherson JL, Symonds GP. Phase I/II clinical trials using gene-modified adult hematopoietic stem cells for HIV: Lessons Learnt. *Stem Cells Int*. 2011;2011:393698.
620. Mitsuyasu RT, Merigan TC, Carr A, et al. Phase 2 gene therapy trial of an anti-HIV ribozyme in autologous CD34+ cells. *Nat Med*. 2009;15(3):285-292.

Section 2 ■ THE ACUTE LEUKEMIAS

Chapter 73 ■ Molecular Genetics of Acute Leukemia

RIDAS JUSKEVICIUS • UTPAL P. DAVÉ • MARY ANN THOMPSON

INTRODUCTION

Acute leukemia results when a normal hematopoietic stem or progenitor cell sequentially acquires mutations that confer clonal growth advantage. This clonal evolution model of cancer development involves gain of function of oncogenes and loss of function of tumor suppressor genes that cooperate to induce fulminant disease. The earliest view of the genome of acute leukemia was provided by cytogeneticists who karyotyped leukemic blasts, revealing recurrent chromosomal translocations. Cloning these translocation breakpoints led to the identification of genes whose altered activity could be directly linked to leukemogenesis. More recently, the genomes of acute leukemias have been probed at an unprecedented depth by next-generation sequencing (NGS), revealing various lesions at the base pair level, such as amplifications, insertions/deletions, and point mutations, that can deregulate oncogene or tumor suppressor gene function. Acute leukemias of either myeloid, B-cell, or T-cell origin (i.e. acute myeloid leukemia [AML], B-cell acute lymphoblastic leukemia [B-ALL], T-cell acute lymphoblastic leukemia [T-ALL]) have been classified by the World Health Organization (WHO) according to the presence of recurrent chromosomal rearrangements that affect the choice of therapy and have significant prognostic value. Acute leukemias without recurrent chromosomal rearrangement have been traditionally classified by their cell of origin, but recently these leukemias have been subjected to whole genome analyses revealing the presence of novel recurrent molecular lesions. As clinical data mature, the list of genes deregulated by mechanisms other than chromosomal rearrangement are being incorporated into new classification schemes. In this chapter, we focus on the more common recurrent genetic abnormalities found in acute leukemias, with special emphasis on how the genetic defects inform our concept of leukemia pathogenesis. We provide specific examples where the genetic lesions have led to the development of targeted therapies with fewer side effects than traditional cytotoxic chemotherapy. This is truly an exciting time for hematologic oncology, where laboratory findings have direct relevance to current treatment modalities.

Reasons for Studying Molecular Genetics of Acute Leukemia

A major reason for understanding the molecular genetics of acute leukemia is to develop novel molecular-directed treatments for acute leukemia. The paradigm for the translation of basic research knowledge to clinical treatment has been chronic myeloid leukemia (CML). The first leukemia to be associated with a recurrent translocation, t(9;22) (q34;q11) (the Philadelphia chromosome),[1] CML was also the first leukemia where the product of the translocation, BCR::ABL1, was characterized.[2] In addition, CML was the first leukemia for which a specific molecular inhibitor, imatinib (Gleevec), was designed.[3] As many specific recurring molecular lesions underlying acute leukemias have been recently discovered, chemical compounds targeting these lesions have also been developed. Many of these molecular drugs are already being used in the clinic, and research and clinical trials are currently underway to further increase the armamentarium of targeted molecular therapies.[4]

An additional benefit of being able to identify the molecular lesions in a given acute leukemia is the ability to carry out more accurate risk stratification of newly diagnosed patients. Numerous clinical studies have correlated clinical prognosis and response to therapy with the set of genes that are altered in a patient's leukemic blasts. Results from the initial cytogenetic and molecular studies on a patient's leukemic blasts are used to stratify the leukemia as favorable, intermediate, or unfavorable, as listed in *Tables 73.1* and *73.2* for adult AML and pediatric B-cell ALL, respectively. Finally, the particular array of mutated genes in the leukemic blasts provides a very sensitive method for determining efficacy of treatment by using these aberrant molecular markers to quantify minimal residual disease after treatment.

Another reason to study the molecular genetics of acute leukemia is to better understand the process of leukemogenesis itself. Over the years, study of readily available leukemic cells and study of the genes obviously dysregulated by recurrent translocations has driven many advances in understanding of gene regulation and oncogenesis. A large number of the genes altered by translocation encode transcriptional regulatory proteins that often preserve the original DNA binding specificity of one of the fusion partners but have altered properties of transcriptional activation or repression. The search to understand these altered properties has led to understanding of how transcriptional regulatory proteins modify chromatin structure to open up or inhibit the transcription of target genes. However, the genes that are recurrently mutated in acute leukemias also belong to other functional classes of proteins. Kinases that are rendered constitutively active by mutation can deregulate the cell's signal transduction pathways and lead to uncontrolled proliferation. Mutations in genes encoding proteins involved in modification of histones or methylation of DNA can lead to altered expression of groups of genes that can have effects as dramatic as those caused by mutations in transcription factors. Additional functional categories of products of genes that are recurrently mutated in leukemia are nuclear pore proteins, spliceosome proteins, and cohesins. This chapter will focus on the mechanisms by which mutations in genes in each of these major functional classes may contribute to the pathogenesis of leukemia. If we understand the mechanism by which "driver" mutations work, we may be able to reverse or inhibit their actions and develop novel treatment modalities for leukemia.

Multiple Hit Model of Leukemia

Another theme that emerges from the study of the molecular genetics of leukemia is that usually more than one genetic hit is necessary for the development of leukemia.[9] This principle has been repeatedly demonstrated in mouse models where introduction of the fusion gene found in acute leukemia into the mouse genome by transgenic technology or retroviral transduction results in predisposition to acute leukemia with long latency, unless the accumulation of additional genetic hits is facilitated by treatment with a mutagenic agent. The multistep model of carcinogenesis is not limited to leukemias, and is reviewed in Hanahan and Weinberg's recent update[10] of the original paper[11] first outlining the six hallmarks of cancer. These hallmarks, now updated to eight, are properties that cancer cells must acquire through multiple mutations in order to become malignant: sustained proliferative signaling, evading growth suppression, enabling replicative immortality, resisting cell death, inducing angiogenesis, activating invasion and metastasis, avoiding immune destruction, and deregulating cellular energetics.[10] In the field of leukemia research, attention has been focused on deregulation of proliferation (class I mutations) and a block in differentiation (class II mutations).[9] The block in differentiation is visually striking under the microscope, as blasts have morphologic

Table 73.1. Risk Groups in Adult AML Based on Cytogenetic and Molecular Analysis

Risk Profile	Genetic Abnormality	Other Mutations
Favorable	t(8;21)(q22;q22.1); *RUNX1::RUNX1T1* inv (16)(p13.1;q22) *or* t(16;16)(p13.1;q22); *CBFB::MYH11* Mutated *NPM1* without *FLT3*-ITD or with *FLT3*-ITD[low,a] Biallelic or single bZIP mutated CEBPA	Any mutation or combination thereof not classified as intermediate or adverse
Intermediate	Mutated *NPM1* and *FLT3*-ITD[high,a] Wild-type *NPM1* without *FLT3*-ITD or with *FLT3*-ITD[low,a] (without adverse-risk genetic lesions) t(9;11);(p21.3;q23.3); *MLLT3::KMT2A* Cytogenetic abnormality not classified as favorable or adverse	Any mutation or combination thereof not classified as favorable or adverse
Adverse	t(6;9);(p23;q34.1); *DEK::NUP214* t(v;11q23.3); *KMT2A* rearranged t(9;22)(q34.1;q11.2); *BCR::ABL1* inv (3)(q21.3q26.2) or t(3;3)(q21.3;q26.2); *GATA2,MECOM(EVI1)* -5 or del(5q); -7; -17/abn(17p) Complex karyotype, monosomal karyotype[b] Wild-type *NPM1* and *FLT3*-ITD[high,a] Mutated *RUNX1* Mutated *ASXL1* Mutated *TP53*	Any mutation or combination thereof not classified as favorable or intermediate

Adapted from Döhner H, Estey E, Grimwade D, et al. Diagnosis and management of AML in adults: 2017 ELN recommendations from an international expert panel. *Blood*. 2017;129(4): 424-447. Copyright © 2017 American Society of Hematology. With permission.

[a]Low, low allelic ratio (<0.5); high, high allelic ratio (>0.5); semiquantitative assessment of *FLT3*-ITD allelic ratio (using DNA fragment analysis) is determined as the ratio of the area under the curve "*FLT3*-ITD" divided by area under the curve "*FLT3*-wild type"; recent studies indicate that AML with *NPM1* mutation and *FLT3*-ITD low allelic ratio may also have a more favorable prognosis.[5-7]

[b]Complex karyotype defined as three or more unrelated chromosome abnormalities in the absence of one of the WHO-designated recurring translocations or inversions. Monosomal karyotype defined by the presence of one single monosomy (excluding loss of X or Y) in association with at least one additional monosomy or structural chromosome abnormality (excluding core-binding factor AML).[8]

characteristics of hematopoietic stem cells (HSCs) (*Figure 73.1*). However, what is relevant to leukemogenesis is that HSCs have self-renewal properties. Many of the well-characterized recurrent translocations in acute leukemia produce fusion genes that encode mutant transcription factors that can no longer activate the genes required for differentiation. However, some translocations (notably *BCR:ABL1*), and some of the genes most commonly affected by point mutations (*FLT3*) encode kinases that cause deregulated proliferation.[9] Through

Table 73.2. Risk Groups in Pediatric B-ALL Based on Cytogenetic and Molecular Analysis

Risk Group	Cytogenetic or Molecular Abnormality	Target Genes
Favorable	t(12;21)(p13;q22)	*ETV6::RUNX1*
	High hyperdiploidy (51-67 chromosomes)	Usually chromosomes 4, 10, 17, 18
	DUX4 rearrangements	*IGH::DUX4, ERG::DUX4*; may have associated *IKZF1* deletions
Intermediate	Trisomy 21–associated B-ALL	
	t(1;19)(q23;p13)	*TCF3::PBX1*
	Low hyperdiploidy (47-50 chromosomes)	
	ZNF384 rearrangements	*EP300::ZNF384*
	iAMP21	*RUNX1* (at least 5 copies by FISH)
	*PAX5*alt and *PAX5*P80R	*PAX5*
	NUTM1-rearranged	*NUTM1* and multiple partners
Unfavorable	Ph-like B-ALL	Multiple kinase genes Rearrangements involving *CRLF2, ABL1/2, CSF1R, PDGFRB, EPOR, JAK2*
	t(9;22)(q34;q11) (may be intermediate with TKI therapy)	*BCR::ABL1*
	KMT2A (MLL) translocations t(4;11)(q21;q23) is particularly unfavorable	*KMT2A* and multiple partners *KMT2A::AFF1*
	ETV6-RUNX1-like	
	MEF2D rearrangements	*MEF2D* and multiple fusion partners
	t(17;19) (q22;p13)	*TCF::HLF*
	Hypodiploidy (<44 chromosomes)	

From Iacobucci I, Kimura S, Mullighan CG. Biologic and therapeutic implications of genomic alterations in acute lymphoblastic leukemia. *J Clin Med*. 2021;10:3972-3996; Moorman AV. New and emerging prognostic and predictive genetic biomarkers in B-cell precursor acute lymphoblastic leukemia. *Haematologica*. 2016;101:407-416; Tasian SK, Hunger SP. Genomic characterization of paediatric acute lymphoblastic leukaemia: an opportunity for precision medicine therapeutics *Br J Haematol*. 2017;176:867-882.

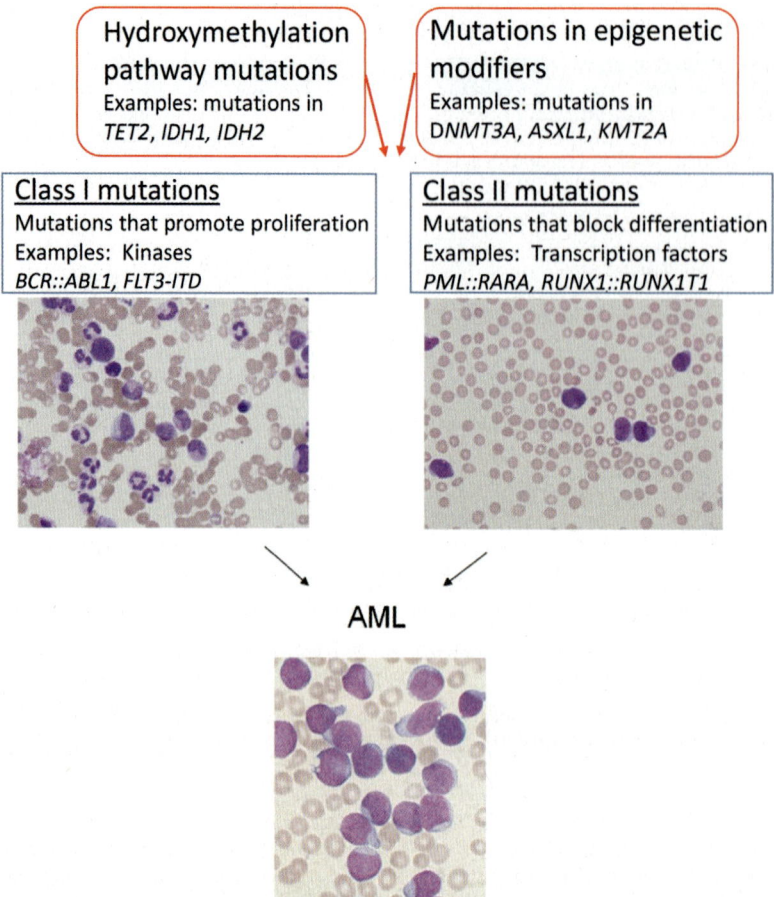

FIGURE 73.1 **Multiple mutations are necessary for the development of acute myeloid leukemia (AML).** The original two-step model of leukemogenesis proposed that most AMLs have a mutation or translocation in a gene that promotes proliferation (class I mutation), as well as a mutation or translocation that alters a gene whose product promotes differentiation (class II mutation) (blue boxes). Whole genome sequencing has identified mutations in a variety of genes in other functional classes, such as genes involved in hydroxymethylation pathways and epigenetic modification of DNA and histones (red boxes). The combination of all of these mutations results in AML, shown in the bottom photograph of myeloid blasts. The photograph under "class I mutations" is a peripheral blood smear from a patient with chronic myeloid leukemia; the photograph under "class II mutations" is a peripheral blood smear from a patient with acute promyelocytic leukemia. (This figure is based upon Kelly LM, Gilliland DG. Genetics of myeloid leukemias. *Annu Rev Genomics Hum Genet*. 2002;3:179-198; Shih AH, Abdel-Wahab O, Patel JP, Levine RL, et al. The role of mutations in epigenetic regulators in myeloid malignancies. *Nat Rev Cancer*. 2012;12:599-612.)

the new advances in technology outlined in the next section scientists have discovered a host of additional gene mutations that occur in leukemia, suggesting more than two hits in the path toward leukemia. In addition, further layers of regulation at the epigenetic level have been demonstrated by the number of genes mutated in leukemia that are active in modification of histones, in regulation of DNA methylation, or hydroxymethylation of nucleotides (*Figure 73.1*).

Advances in Technology: A Genomic Perspective of Acute Leukemia

The tremendous advances in technology in the last few years have revolutionized our ability to analyze individual genomes (*Table 73.3*). As mentioned above, G-banding of chromosomes was our first view of the leukemia genome and is still highly informative in identifying translocations, aneuploidy, and other gross chromosomal rearrangements (>4 Mb).[26,28] More focused analyses such as interphase fluorescent in situ hybridization (FISH) have improved the resolution of standard cytogenetics so that amplifications or deletions of 100 kb may be visualized.[21] In the last 15 years, oligonucleotides covering the entire human genome have been printed onto arrays allowing hybridization of fluorescently labeled leukemic and control genomic DNA.[22,23] This array comparative genomic hybridization (CGH) can identify copy number variation (CNV) and has been powerfully employed in identifying recurrent deletions and amplifications in acute leukemias. Similar microarrays were designed to cover common single-nucleotide polymorphisms (SNPs) for genotyping purposes, but they too have been used to identify CNVs, particularly copy number neutral loss of heterozygosity (also known as uniparental disomy) in leukemia.[24,29,30] Array CGH and SNP arrays display the human genome as small probes and will not detect balanced translocations. Most excitingly, major advances in whole genome sequencing now provide single base pair resolution so that point mutations across the genome may readily be identified.[12] These powerful technologies are readily deployed in the diagnosis of acute leukemia and provide a complete genomic perspective of the disease; however, there are important caveats. Human genomes are full of rare and common structural variants and SNPs.[31-35] Therefore, mutations can only be interpreted as being acquired in leukemogenesis if they are shown to be absent in normal somatic tissue. Thus, matched normal somatic tissue is frequently subjected to the same genomic analyses as leukemic blasts.

The sequence of the human genome was completed in 2001 at 90% coverage after 10 years of collaborative and arduous work from multiple laboratories for a cost of 1 billion dollars. As of 2017, a highly accurate reference sequence, currently at build 38 (https://www.ncbi.nlm.nih.gov/grc/human) is available.[36-38] At this writing, a sample human genome can be sequenced in less than a week for less than a thousand dollars.[39] This remarkably short processing time and reduction in cost were made possible by massively

Table 73.3. Resolution of Technologies Available to Identify Genetic Alterations in Acute Leukemia

Technique	Resolution	Molecular Lesion	References
Whole genome sequencing	1 bp	Point mutations, amplifications, insertions, deletions, translocations	12,13
Whole exome sequencing	1 bp	Point mutations, amplifications, deletions	14,15
Transcriptome sequencing	1 bp	Gene expression, fusion transcript detection, point mutations	16,17
Gene expression microarray	-	Gene expression	18-20
Interphase FISH	100 kb	Focal amplifications or deletions	21
Array comparative genomic hybridization	100 kb amplification 3-5 Mb deletion	Amplifications, deletions	22,23
SNP array	100 kb	Amplifications, deletions	23-25
Cytogenetics/karyotyping	3-4 Mb	Amplifications, deletions, translocations	26,27

parallel sequencing technologies, collectively known as next-generation sequencing (NGS).[40] The original draft human genome sequence was generated by Sanger sequencing or dideoxynucleotide chain termination and capillary electrophoresis, first-generation technologies. In next-generation technologies, the addition of nucleotides occurs in parallel on multiple DNA strands and is multiplexed frequently on microchips or beads.[41] This has resulted in an incredible information glut, and the burden has shifted toward efficient bioinformatics analysis. A number of publicly available genomic sequencing and other data repositories and web-based bioinformatics tools with robust online data-driven analysis platforms have become available, which allow cancer researchers and bioinformaticians to search, download, and share cancer data for analysis. One example of such platform is an effort toward shared cancer genomic data by the National Cancer Institute (NCI), the University of Chicago, the Ontario Institute for Cancer Research, and Leidos Biomedical Research. This information system contains genomic data that are harmonized using uniform analytic pipelines, as well as diagnostic, histologic, and clinical outcome data from NCI-funded projects such as The Cancer Genome Atlas (TCGA) and the Therapeutically Applicable Research to Generate Effective Treatments (TARGET) program (https://gdc.cancer.gov/).[42-44] Some of the complexity of genome assembly can be avoided by targeted sequencing or whole exome sequencing. Here, capture technologies utilize DNA hybridization to purify all the exons of a given genome. These are then fully sequenced; of course, in this case the mutations discovered are limited to the coding regions of the genome, missing mutations within regulatory regions that may also be present. Besides mutation analysis, NGS technology has expedited our ability to define whole genome chromatin marks,[45] CpG methylation,[45,46] microRNAs,[47] and noncoding RNAs.[48] For chromatin analysis, immunopurification can enrich for genomic DNA that is associated with specific histone marks that denote active or inactive gene expression. These tools are important in analyzing the effects of mutant leukemia proteins that modify histone residues. More recently, the tremendous proliferation of high-throughput experimental and computational technologies has enabled the advancement in understanding of the three-dimensional (3D) genome organization and function,[49,50] including genome folding. Genome folding forms loops that bring enhancers and target genes into close proximity, and we now know that enhancers function within these hierarchical chromatin structures, including topologically associated domains (TADs) and chromatin loops. Investigating disease-associated mutations and rearrangements in the context of the 3D genome may lead to a better understanding of why certain translocations occur repeatedly.[51]

In 2008 the entire genome sequence of a cytogenetically normal patient with AML was completed for the first time.[52] In 2009 and 2010 further refined techniques were used to sequence a second AML genome to a higher level of coverage (98%)[53] and depth.[54] In each patient, multiple acquired somatic mutations were identified by comparison with normal skin from the same patient. Screening of a large panel of AML samples for novel coding region mutations identified in the two sequenced genomes demonstrated two recurrently mutated genes not previously thought to be involved in leukemogenesis: *IDH1* (mutated in 16% of cytogenetically normal AML samples)[53] and *DNMT3A* (mutated in 22% of AML samples).[54] This early result showed the power of whole genome sequencing. A recent landmark study by the TCGA Research Network comprehensively analyzed genomes of 200 patients with de novo AML and found an average of five mutations per patient in genes that are recurrently mutated in AML.[55] The TCGA study also found that a total of 23 genes were significantly mutated, as defined by using the significantly mutated gene test in the Mutational Significance in Cancer (MuSiC) suite of tools, and 237 genes were mutated in two or more samples. The significantly mutated genes were organized into several functional categories that are relevant for pathogenesis, including transcription factor fusions (18% of cases), the gene encoding nucleophosmin (*NPM1*) (27%), tumor-suppressor genes (16%), DNA-methylation-related genes (44%), signaling genes (59%), chromatin-modifying genes (30%), myeloid transcription factor genes (22%), cohesin-complex genes (13%), and spliceosome-complex genes (14%). Almost all samples had at least one nonsynonymous mutation in one of these categories of genes.[55,56] Cooperation and mutual exclusivity patterns of these mutations were demonstrated, suggesting a strong biologic relationship between several of the categories of genes (*Figure 73.2*). In general, mutually exclusive mutations tend to reflect genes that are involved in the same pathway; therefore, an additional mutation in the same pathway would not give a selective advantage. However, gene mutations that commonly co-occur suggest that those gene products, often from different pathways, may collaborate in leukemogenesis. This and other studies indicate that most AML cases are characterized by clonal heterogeneity at diagnosis with the presence of both founding clone and at least one subclone.[55] The complexity of mutations in genes and the functional gene categories that contribute to the leukemic phenotype can be visually appreciated in *Figure 73.2*, a summary of co-occurrence and mutual exclusivity of mutations in patients with AML.[56-58]

As high-throughput NGS-based technology became widely available and less expensive; analysis of the genomic data generated from thousands of people without hematologic malignancy revealed acquired somatic mutations in leukemia-associated genes (most commonly in *DNMT3A*, *TET2*, and *ASXL1*). The frequency of these mutations increases with age (age-related clonal hematopoiesis). The term clonal hematopoiesis (CH) of indeterminate potential (CHIP) was also proposed to describe individuals with hematologic malignancy-associated somatic mutation but without other diagnostic criteria for hematologic malignancy.[59] Interestingly, CHIP is associated not only with an increased risk of developing hematologic malignancies but also with other cancers and a higher all-cause mortality.[60-63] In more recent studies including healthy volunteers and individuals aged >80 years using sensitive targeted error-corrected sequencing, CH, defined as mutations with >1% of variant allele frequency occurring in driver

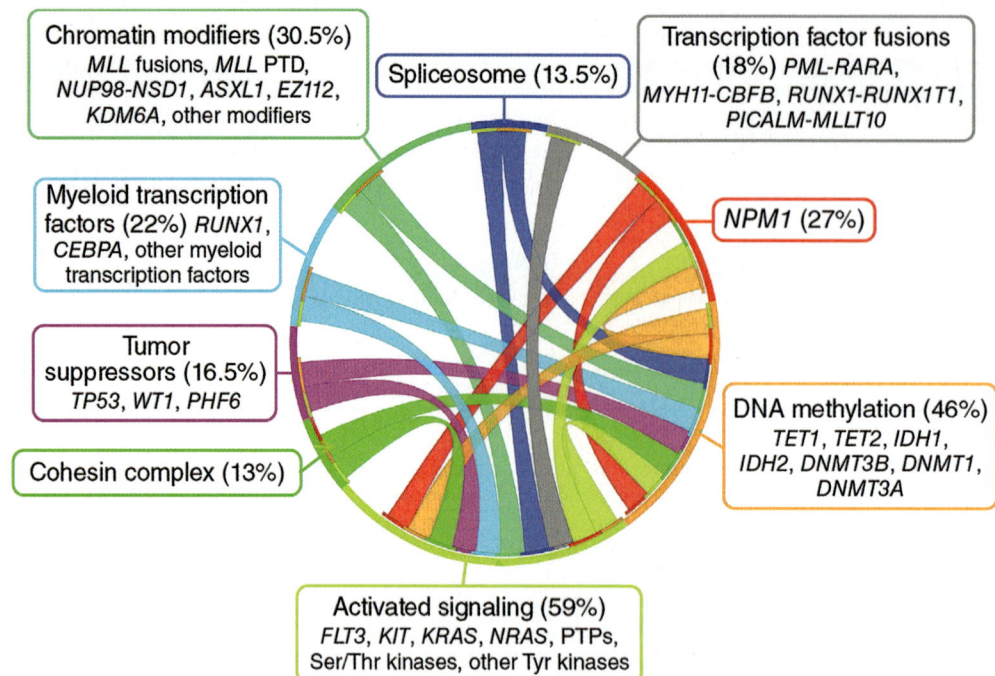

FIGURE 73.2 Circos plot showing a panoramic view of genetic events contributing to the pathogenesis of AML. Nine functional categories have been identified for mutated genes that show complex patterns of cooperation and mutual exclusivity. Ribbons connecting distinct categories of gene abnormalities within this plot reflect the associations between mutations in different pathways, whereas mutually exclusive alterations may exist between genes in the same pathway. Each AML case may have several gene mutations in different functional categories. PTPs, protein tyrosine phosphatases; *MLL* PTD, *MLL* partial tandem duplication. (Reprinted by permission from Nature: Chen SJ, Shen Y, Chen Z. A panoramic view of acute myeloid leukemia. *Nat Genet.* 2013;45(6):586-587. Copyright © 2013 Springer Nature.)

genes or genes known to be mutated in myeloid neoplasms, was present in the majority of individuals (62%) aged > 80 years and close to 40% of healthy volunteers >50 years old.[64,65] The risk of progression from CHIP to hematologic malignancy is thought to be approximately 0.5% to 1% per year. In this sense CHIP is similar to other premalignant hematologic clonal disorders, such as monoclonal gammopathy of undetermined significance (MGUS) and monoclonal B lymphocytosis (MBL). Unlike MGUS and MBL the spectrum of hematologic malignancies that may develop after CHIP include myeloid, lymphoid, and plasma cell neoplasms, which indicates that premalignant clones arise in multipotent stem cells.[60] The risk of evolution of CH to hematologic neoplasm appears to be dependent on the mutational profile of CH, with mutations in driver genes other than TET2 and DNMT3A associated with higher risk of evolution to a neoplastic process and higher risk of death.[60,61,65,66]

ACUTE MYELOID LEUKEMIA

Classification

AML is classified according to WHO Classification of Tumours of Haematopoietic and Lymphoid Tissues, the 4th edition of which underwent revision in 2016,[67,68] but new classifications are in the works at the time of preparing this chapter. In general, most patients with AML can be grouped into two broad and currently imprecisely defined biologically and clinically meaningful groups, de novo AML and secondary AML (s-AML). A subset of AML in the WHO classification is entitled "acute myeloid leukemia with recurrent genetic abnormalities"[67,68] (see *Table 73.4*). These recurrent translocations occur most often in de novo AML but are not restricted to this category. Another major category of AML in the WHO classification framework is "AML with myelodysplasia-related changes,"[67] where genetic mutations and chromosomal deletions occur secondary to the mutator phenotype of the underlying myelodysplastic syndrome (MDS). AML arising in the setting of prior cytotoxic therapy comprises a proportion of s-AML cases and is classified under the WHO category "Therapy-related myeloid neoplasms."[67,68] The precise biologic definition of the s-AML category is lacking and has been a subject of recent investigations.

Table 73.4. WHO Classification of Acute Myeloid Leukemia[6,67]

AML with recurrent genetic abnormalities (translocations and mutations)
AML with t(8;21)(q22;q22.1); *RUNX1::RUNX1T1*
AML with inv(16)(p13.1q22) or t(16;16)(p13.1;q22); *CBFB::MYH11*
Acute promyelocytic leukemia (APL) with t(15;17)(q22;q12); *PML::RARA*
AML with t(9;11)(p21.3;q23.3); *MLLT3::KMT2A*
AML with t(6;9)(p23;q34.1); *DEK::NUP214*
AML with inv(3)(q21.3q26.2) or t(3;3)(q21.3;q26.2); *GATA2,MECOM*
AML (megakaryoblastic) with t(1;22)(p13.3;q13.3); *RBM15::MKL1*
AML with *BCR::ABL1*
AML with mutated *NPM1*
AML with biallelic mutations of *CEBPA*
AML with mutated *RUNX1*
AML with myelodysplasia-related changes
Therapy-related myeloid neoplasms
AML, NOS
AML with minimal differentiation
AML without maturation
AML with maturation
Acute myelomonocytic leukemia
Acute monoblastic/monocytic leukemia
Pure erythroid leukemia
Acute megakaryoblastic leukemia
Acute basophilic leukemia
Acute panmyelosis with myelofibrosis
Myeloid sarcoma
Myeloid proliferations related to Down syndrome
Transient abnormal myelopoiesis (TAM)
Myeloid leukemia associated with Down syndrome

Adapted with permission from Swerdlow SH. *International Agency for Research on Cancer, World Health Organization. WHO Classification of Tumours of Haematopoietic and Lymphoid Tissues.* Revised 4th ed. International Agency for Research on Cancer; 2017:10; Adapted from Arber DA, Orazi A, Hasserjian R, et al. The 2016 revision to the World Health Organization classification of myeloid neoplasms and acute leukemia. *Blood.* 2016;127(20):2391-405. Copyright © 2016 American Society of Hematology. With permission.

Earlier whole genome sequencing studies based on bulk tumor cell analysis as well as more recent single-cell and sorted stem cell–based studies have clarified our understanding of the clonal evolution from MDS to AML. Walter et al. compared seven sets of samples from patients for whom there were paired samples of normal skin, preleukemic bone marrow diagnosed as MDS, and bone marrow involved by s-AML.[69] In each genome there were 304 to 872 somatic point mutants in coding regions or consensus splice site regions, and those point mutations with translational consequences comprised an average of 24 mutations per genome. These functional mutations occurred in a total of 168 genes over the 7 genomes. The strength of the study was that the number of mutations allowed study of clonal evolution from MDS to s-AML. A majority of the cells in the MDS sample contained the same cluster of mutations, meaning that, before blasts were even detected morphologically, the marrow was involved by a clonal process. At the s-AML stage, all the samples contained several clones, all of which had the original set of mutations but which were defined by acquisition of new sets of mutations as well. Presumably most of these somatic mutations are "passenger" mutations, but the multiplicity of mutations tracked adds credence to the description of clonal evolution.[69] In a more recent study Chen et al. examined the dynamics of clonal evolution in progression of MDS to s-AML by targeted single cell deep sequencing of fractionated phenotypically defined malignant stem cells (MDS-SC, AML-SC), premalignant stem cells (pre-MDS-SC, pre-AML-SC) as well as blast populations (MDS blasts, AML blasts) using longitudinal, paired samples from patients with MDS who had later progressed to s-AML.[70] The study found that stem cells at the MDS stage, including pre-MDS-SC, had a significantly higher subclonal complexity compared with blast cells and contained a large number of aging-related variants. The results of this study revealed a pattern of nonlinear, parallel clonal evolution, with distinct subclones within pre-MDS-SC and MDS-SC contributing to generation of MDS blasts or progression to AML, respectively (see Figure 73.3). In most cases studied, the dominant clone at the s-AML

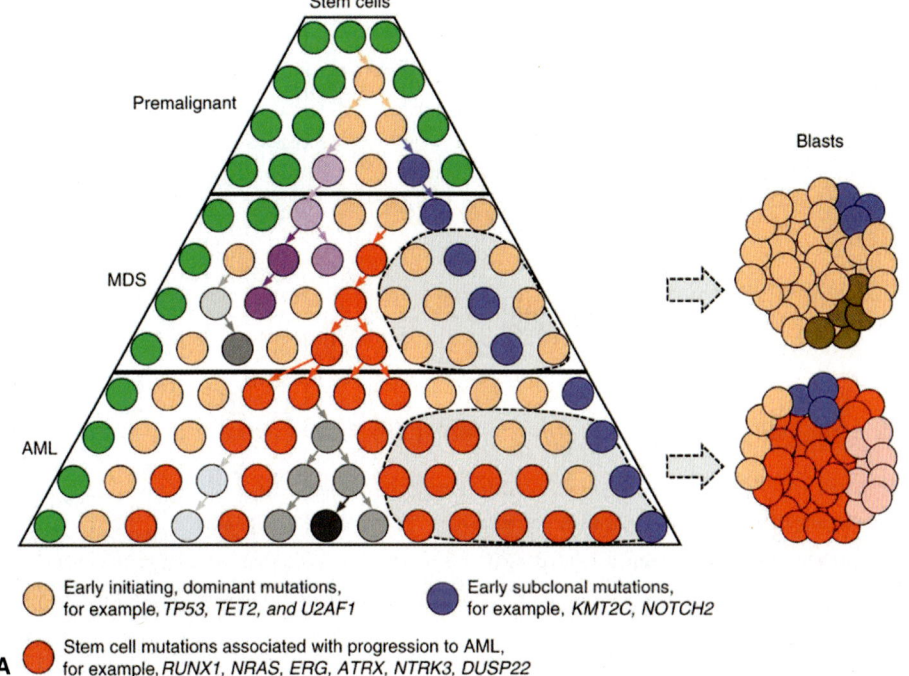

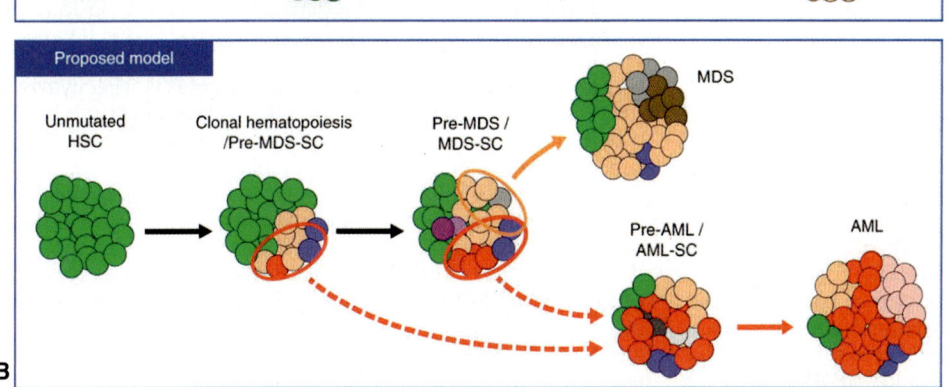

FIGURE 73.3 Proposed model of subclonal evolution of stem cells during the progression of MDS to s-AML. A, Accumulation of mutations in stem cell compartments gives rise to a highly diverse subclonal architecture (indicated by different colors) in MDS stem cells (MDS-SC). Certain subclones (orange, for example, with *TP53*, *TET2*, or *U2AF1* mutations, "clonal hematopoiesis") provide a shared basis for both MDS development (MDS blasts) as well as the formation of pre-AML-SC and AML-SC. However, pre-MDS- and MDS-SC acquire different additional mutations that then drive MDS blast formation or progression to s-AML, respectively, in a nonlinear and rather parallel manner in all patients studied. In majority of cases studied, the dominant clone at the s-AML stage originated from a clone (red, for example, with *RUNX1*, *NRAS*, or *ERG* and *ATRX* mutations) that was detectable in pre-MDS and/or MDS-SC but was undetectable in MDS blast cells. These results indicate that MDS-SC leading to the generation of MDS blasts can be different from those contributing to the progression to s-AML. B, Schematics of different models of MDS and s-AML development and progression. In comparison with the linear model (top), which suggests serial mutation accumulation during disease progression, the data support a model of parallel clonal evolution at the stem cell level during development of MDS and progression to s-AML (bottom). All cases in this study showed a highly diverse pool of (pre-)MDS-SC as the basis of MDS and s-AML development; in the majority of cases there was very early branching at the (pre-) MDS-SC level toward progression to AML-SC, leading to distinct clonal composition between MDS and AML bulk cells; and three of seven patients showed a pattern of slightly later branching (dashed red arrows) leading to more similar clonal composition between MDS and AML bulk cells compared with the early-branching cases. (Reprinted by permission from Nature: Chen J, Kao YR, Sun D, et al. Myelodysplastic syndrome progression to acute myeloid leukemia at the stem cell level. Nat Med. 2019;25(1):103-110. Copyright © 2018 Springer Nature.)

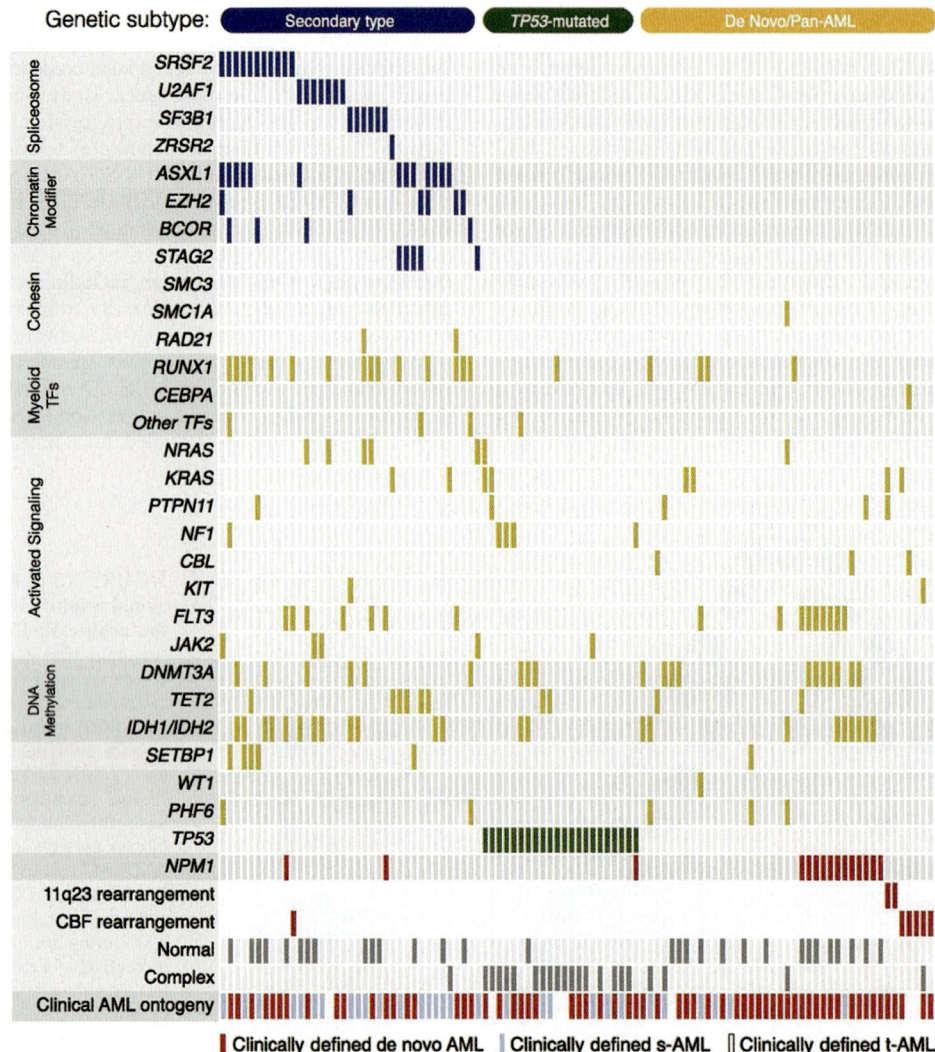

FIGURE 73.4 Comparison of mutations in MDS, secondary AML, and treatment-related AML. Mutations in an unselected cohort of patients with AML with a comutation plot showing nonsynonymous mutations in individual genes, grouped into categories, as labeled on the left. Mutations are depicted by colored bars, and each column represents 1 of the 105 sequenced samples. Blue gene mutations have >95% specificity for s-AML, red gene mutations have >95% specificity for de novo AML, *TP53* mutations are green, and yellow genes are pan-AML. Genetic ontogeny groups are labeled on the top. (Reprinted from Lindsley RC, Mar BG, Mazzola E, et al. Acute myeloid leukemia ontogeny is defined by distinct somatic mutations. *Blood*. 2015;125(9):1367-1376. Copyright © 2015 American Society of Hematology. With permission.)

stage originated from a clone that was detectable in pre-MDS and/or MDS-SC but was undetectable in MDS blast cells. In other words, the results of this study indicate that MDS-SC leading to the generation of MDS blasts can be different from those contributing to AML blasts upon the progression to s-AML.[70]

A study by Lindsley et al investigated the genetic basis of AML ontogeny by targeted mutational analysis of 194 patients with well-defined s-AML or therapy-related AML (t-AML) and 105 unselected AML patients.[71] They compared the spectrum of genetic lesions in their s-AML cohort with 180 cases of de novo non-M3 AML reported in TCGA, analyzing all genetic data through the same computational pipeline, and they identified three distinct mutually exclusive patterns of mutations (*Figure 73.4*). First, mutations in eight genes including *SRSF2*, *SF3B1*, *U2AF1*, *ZRSR2*, *ASXL1*, *EZH2*, *BCOR*, and *STAG2*, most belonging to spliceosome and chromatin modifier functional classes, had >95% specificity for s-AML as compared with de novo AML (called "secondary type" mutations). The mutations in these genes are commonly seen in MDS, appear early in leukemogenesis, and persist in clonal remissions, as was indicated by serial sample analysis from individual patients. Second, they identified three abnormalities that were significantly underrepresented in s-AML compared with de novo AML, which included *NPM1* mutations, *KMT2A*(*MLL*)/11q23 rearrangements, and core binding factor (CBF) rearrangements ("de novo–type" alterations). Third, cases with mutations in *TP53* have been associated with a distinct clinical phenotype including complex karyotype, therapy resistance, and very poor survival.[71] The more recent study by Gao et al. showed similar distinct patterns of mutational distribution in de novo AML vs s-AML.[72] *TP53* mutations are present in approximately 10% to 12% of patients with AML and MDS. *TP53* is located on chromosome 17p13 and is essential for cell cycle control and DNA damage response. It has been shown that some *TP53* mutations have a dominant negative effect and typically occur in founding clones that expand following cytotoxic stress, but the exact mechanism driving leukemogenesis in *TP53*-mutated cases is unknown. Mutant *TP53* is strongly associated with large structural and complex chromosomal aberrations as illustrated by the occurrence of complex karyotypes, which is associated with reduced overall survival in myeloid malignancies. The prior and recent studies indicate that the group of AML and MDS with excess blasts (MDS-EB) patients with *TP53* mutations represent a clinically distinct category of MDS/AML usually associated with complex karyotype and uniformly poor outcomes. Thus, separation of this group of cases into MDS and AML based on arbitrary blast percentage is no longer practical, as it has been shown repeatedly that mutant *TP53* AML and

MDS-EB do not differ with respect to molecular characteristics and survival. This group also includes therapy-related cases of AML/MDS as *TP53* mutations occur with higher frequency in therapy-related disease. Therefore, the argument can be made that TP53-mutated AML/MDS represents a clinically and biologically distinct disease category, which should be reflected in the next updated classification of AML and MDS.[73,74] The results of these studies provide more precise genomic characterization of secondary AML (most cases falling into the WHO category of "AML with myelodysplasia-related changes," which may or may not have clinical evidence of prior MDS) as compared with de novo disease.

In the subsequent sections, we will focus on the function of the genes that are repeatedly altered in AML, either by involvement in recurring translocations or by mutation. An understanding of the function of these gene products is essential for understanding the rationale of current classes of targeted therapies, which are opening up new possibilities for less toxic and more effective treatment of AML.

Transcription Factors
PML::RARA

One of the most elegant examples of the interaction between clinical and molecular advances in the treatment of acute leukemia is acute promyelocytic leukemia (APL). The association between the t(15;17)(q22;q21) and the characteristic morphology of APL (hypergranular blasts with frequent Auer rods or microgranular variant with dumbbell-shaped nuclei) has been known for a long time. The initial report from China[75] that all-trans retinoic acid (ATRA) could induce complete remission in patients with APL actually preceded the discovery that the t(15;17) involved the retinoic acid receptor-α gene (*RARα*) on chromosome 17.[76-78]

Of five translocations associated with APL, the most common is t(15;17)(q22;q21), in which the 5' portion of the fusion protein is encoded by the *PML* (ProMyelocytic Leukemia) gene from 15q22 and the 3' portion is encoded by the *RARA* gene from 17q21. The *RARA* gene is a ligand-dependent steroid receptor that mediates the effects of the ligand, retinoic acid (RA), on the cell. The breakpoint is invariant in intron 2 of *RARA*, yielding the C-terminal portion of the fusion protein, which includes the DNA-binding, ligand-binding, dimerization, and repression domains of RARα. There are three major breakpoints in the *PML* gene. The most common generates *PML(L)::RARA*, which includes the first six exons of *PML* encoding 554 amino acids of PML.[79]

The wild-type RARα is a nuclear receptor that acts as a transcription factor and binds to retinoic acid response elements (RAREs) in the promoters of many genes, including genes important in myeloid differentiation. RARα binds as a heterodimer with retinoid X receptor protein (RXR) and acts as a transcriptional repressor until ligand (RA) binding occurs, changing the conformation of the protein and resulting in transcriptional activation.[80] Target genes important for myeloid differentiation include colony-stimulating factors (granulocyte colony-stimulating factor [G-CSF]), colony-stimulating factor receptors (G-CSFRs), neutrophil granule proteins, cell-surface adhesion molecules, regulators of the cell cycle, regulators of apoptosis, and transcription factors (reviewed in reference 81). In the absence of retinoic acid, the wild-type RARα, present as a heterodimer with RXR on the RARE, binds to the corepressor proteins SMRT, N-CoR, mSin3, and histone deacetylases. Deacetylation of the histones at the target gene promoter results in transcriptional repression. Ligand binding at physiologic concentrations of ATRA causes a conformational change that results in release of corepressors and recruitment of a coactivator complex (SRC-1), which associates with histone acetyltransferases (*Figure 73.5A*).[82] Acetylation of the histones at the target gene promoter is associated with transcriptional activation (reviewed in reference 81).

In APL, the PML::RARα protein binds to RAREs with similar affinity to the RARα protein and is able to heterodimerize with RXR. It acts in a dominant negative manner, competing with wild-type RARα for binding to the RAREs. It binds corepressor proteins in the absence of ligand (via the RARα portion of the protein). However, physiologic levels of ATRA (10^{-9} M) are not able to convert PML::RARα into a transcriptional activator; pharmacologic concentrations are required (10^{-6} M; *Figure 73.5B*).[82,83] This provides the mechanistic basis for the efficacy of treatment of patients with APL with ATRA to induce differentiation of the promyelocytes.

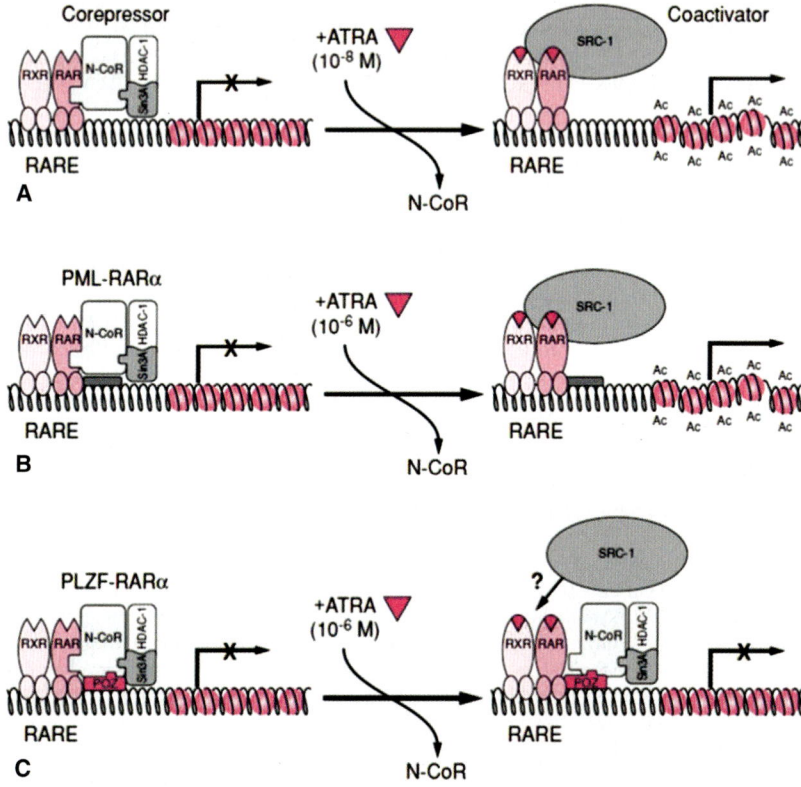

FIGURE 73.5 Model for the role of nuclear corepressors and retinoid acid receptor α (RARα) fusion proteins in the pathogenesis and treatment of acute promyelocytic leukemia. A, In the absence of all-trans retinoic acid (ATRA), RARα, promyelocytic leukemia (PML)::RARα, and promyelocytic leukemia zinc finger (PLZF)::RARα associate with the N-CoR/sin3A/HDAC1 corepressor complex, which deacetylates histone tails, resulting in a compressed chromatin and transcriptional repression. Binding of ATRA at a physiologic concentration induces a conformational change in RARα, causing release of the corepressor complex and binding of coactivator (SRC-1) with histone acetyltransferase activity. Acetylation (Ac) of histone tails opens up the chromatin, facilitating transcriptional activation. B, In the case of PML::RARα protein, pharmacologic doses of ATRA are required to achieve dissociation of the N-CoR repressor complex. C, Because of additional interactions of the PLZF moiety of PLZF::RARα fusion protein with corepressors, they do not dissociate even in the presence of pharmacologic doses of ATRA. Therefore, the chromatin still remains in the repressed state. (Reprinted from Guidez F, Ivins S, Zhu J, et al. Reduced retinoic acid-sensitivities of nuclear receptor corepressor binding to PML- and PLZF-RARα underlie molecular pathogenesis and treatment of acute promyelocytic leukemia. *Blood*. 1998;91(8):2634-2642. Copyright © 1998 American Society of Hematology. With permission.)

Understanding of the mechanism of the response of APL to ATRA was furthered by studies of an alternative translocation, t(11;17)(q23;q21), which is rarely seen in patients with APL.[84] Patients with this translocation are resistant to treatment with pharmacologic doses of ATRA. The fusion partner gene *ZBTB16* on chromosome 11q23 encodes promyelocytic zinc finger (PLZF), a transcriptional repressor. PLZF interacts with NCoR, SMRT, mSin3A, and HDAC1 via the POZ/BTB domain[85,86] and therefore contributes a second binding site for corepressor proteins. Therefore, although pharmacologic doses of ATRA induce release of corepressors from the RARα portion of the fusion protein, the corepressors binding to PLZF are unaffected (*Figure 73.5C*).[81,87] Significantly, concomitant treatment of cells with HDAC inhibitors such as Trichostatin A (TSA) restores ATRA sensitivity, since TSA inhibits the deacetylase activity of the corepressors on the PLZF moiety.[83,86]

Wild-type PML protein is normally localized in subnuclear PML oncogenic domains, also called nuclear bodies (NBs), in which other nuclear factors colocalize.[88] PML may act as a tumor suppressor protein and is involved in growth suppression as well as in induction of apoptosis (reviewed in reference 81). Although it does not bind DNA directly, it influences transcription by interacting with both CBP,[89] a transcriptional activator, and HDACs, transcriptional repressors, possibly within the NBs. The protein encoded by the *PML::RARA* fusion transcript resulting from the t(15;17) is delocalized from the NBs to a microspeckled nuclear pattern.[90]

Whole genome sequencing of de novo and relapsed APL patients demonstrated approximately eight nonsilent somatic mutations per exome.[91] In de novo APL cases, mutations in *FLT3*, *WT1*, *NRAS*, and *KRAS* were predominant. In relapsed APL there were frequent mutations in *RARA* and *PML*, with *RARA* mutations predominating in cases with a history of ATRA treatment and *PML* mutations associated with arsenic trioxide treatment. In addition, in relapsed APL, there were mutations in *ARID1A* and *ARID1B*, members of the SWI/SNF chromatin remodeling complex.[91]

Core Binding Factor Translocations

CBF AMLs refer to AMLs characterized by the recurring structural abnormalities of t(8;21)(q22;q22), involving *RUNX1* and *RUNX1T1*, and inv(16)(p13.1q22), involving *CBFB* and *MYH11*. Together, these comprise 30% of pediatric AML cases and 15% of adult AML cases.[92] The *RUNX1* (Runt-related transcription factor 1, formerly called *AML1*) gene, cloned from the t(8;21)(q22;q22) breakpoint,[93,94] is mutated in another 3% of AML. The activity of the murine counterpart of RUNX1 was first described as part of the CBF complex, which binds to a core enhancer sequence of the Molony leukemia virus long terminal repeat.[95] Another component of CBF, the non-DNA-binding CBFβ, was found to be associated with inversion 16 in M4 AML.[96] Finally, the fusion partner of *RUNX1* in t(8;21), named *RUNX1T1*, or *ETO* (eight-twenty-one), also encodes a transcriptional regulator.[97] A gene related to *RUNX1T1*, *MTG16*, is involved in yet another translocation involving *RUNX1*, t(16;21).[98]

The CBF complex recruits additional transcription factors and regulates hematopoietic differentiation. The CBFs are essential for hematopoietic development. Gene deletion of either *Runx1*[99] or *Cbfβ*[100] in mice results in fetal death at E11.5 to 12.5. These embryos lack all fetal hematopoiesis. Further transgenic experiments have demonstrated that RUNX1 is essential for development of HSCs in the aorta/gonadal/mesodermal (AGM) region, the source of definitive hematopoiesis.[101] The essential role of RUNX1 in hematopoietic development appears to be through its function as a transcriptional activator. It regulates lymphoid genes such as B-cell tyrosine kinase, T-cell receptor α and β,[102] cytokines (interleukin-3 [IL-3],[103] GM-CSF[104]), and granulocyte proteins (MPO, neutrophil elastase[105]).

RUNX1 is located at chromosome 21q22.3 and is encoded by 12 exons over 260 kb of DNA. The N-terminal portion of the protein contains the runt homology domain (RHD), which is homologous to the *Drosophila runt* protein[106] and is responsible for the official HUGO name, *RUNX1*. This is the DNA-binding domain, and it is mutated in familial platelet disorder (FPD) and in AML associated with *RUNX1* mutations.[107,108] CBFβ interacts via this domain and changes the conformation of RUNX1 to increase DNA binding affinity.[109]

The *ETO* gene, now called *RUNX1T1*, was cloned from the t(8;21) fusion[93] and is the mammalian homolog of the *Drosophila nervy* gene.[110] RUNX1T1 does not appear to bind DNA specifically on its own. However, it may act as a corepressor protein.[111] It associates with N-CoR and mSin3A and directly binds to class I HDACs.[112]

In the t(8;21), the *RUNX1* gene is fused to the *RUNX1T1* gene on chromosome 8. The breakpoint in the *RUNX1* locus is between exons 5 and 6,[113] yielding a fusion protein with the N-terminal 177aa of RUNX1,[93] which contains the DNA-binding domain.[114] The breakpoint in the *RUNX1T1* gene occurs in the introns between the first two alternative exons of *RUNX1T1*, resulting in the inclusion of almost all of the coding region for RUNX1T1 in the fusion transcript.[93]

The RUNX1::RUNX1T1 protein specifically binds to the same DNA-binding site as RUNX1 and can heterodimerize with CBFβ.[115] Therefore, the RUNX1::RUNX1T1 protein can act as a dominant negative inhibitor of wild-type RUNX1. However, cotransfection experiments demonstrated that RUNX1::RUNX1T1 can also function as an active transcriptional repressor.[116] The ability of RUNX1::RUNX1T1 to act as a transcriptional repressor depends on its association with HDACs (via RUNX1T1), since the HDAC inhibitor TSA can abrogate effects of RUNX1::RUNX1T1 on the cell cycle.[112] Targets of RUNX1::RUNX1T1 repression are presumed to include genes important for granulocyte differentiation. In addition, RUNX1::RUNX1T1 represses the tumor suppressor genes *P14ARF* and *NF1*.[117,118] P14ARF stabilizes TP53 by antagonizing MDM2, an inhibitor of TP53.[119] Therefore, repression of *P14ARF* reduces the checkpoint control path of TP53 and may be a key event in t(8;21) leukemogenesis. Surprisingly, expression of RUNX1::RUNX1T1 in myeloid progenitor cells inhibits cell cycle progression. However, this may contribute to leukemogenesis by allowing time for accumulation of mutations in a cell immune from TP53-induced apoptosis due to inactivation of P14ARF.[117]

Finally, inversion 16, present in about 8% of AML cases, involves the CBF complex member *CBFB* and is associated with a morphologically distinct subset of AML, M4Eo. M4Eo is a myelomonocytic leukemia with abnormal eosinophils that have dark purple as well as orange granules.[67] This cytogenetic abnormality in which the *CBFB* gene is fused to the smooth muscle myosin heavy-chain gene, *MYH11*, results in fusion of the first 165aa of CBFβ to the C-terminal coiled-coil region of smooth muscle myosin heavy-chain protein (SMMHC).[96] A C-terminal region of SMMHC is necessary for the activity of CBFβ::SMMHC as a transcriptional corepressor, and this region also associates with mSin3a and HDAC8. Presumably CBFβ::SMMHC, which cannot bind DNA on its own, interacts with RUNX1 to form a transcriptional repressor complex.[120]

A number of experiments demonstrate that the CBF translocations are necessary but not sufficient for induction of leukemia. Support for the hypothesis that genetic mutations besides a mutant *RUNX1* locus are necessary for development of acute leukemia comes from the study of patients with familial platelet disorder with propensity to develop AML (FPD/AML). These patients have mutations in one allele of *RUNX1*.[121] They have defective platelets and progressive pancytopenia and develop myelodysplasia and a high incidence of AML with age. However, secondary mutations appear to be necessary before progression to AML occurs.

The presence of additional mutations in CBF leukemia has been addressed directly by NGS experiments. In one experiment comparing patients with *RUNX1::RUNX1T1* and *CBFB::MYH11*, an average of 11.86 somatic mutations with functional consequences were present in *RUNX1::RUNX1T1* cases and 7.74 somatic mutations were present in *CBFB::MYH11* cases (see *Figure 73.6*).[92] Sixty-six percent of mutations were in kinase pathway genes such as *NRAS*, *KIT*, *FLT3*, *KRAS*, *PTPN11*, *NF1*, and *CCND2*.[92] *KIT* mutations were found in 45% of t(8;21) and 33% of inv(16) cases and required a mutant allelic ratio of 35% or greater to confer a worse prognosis.[92]

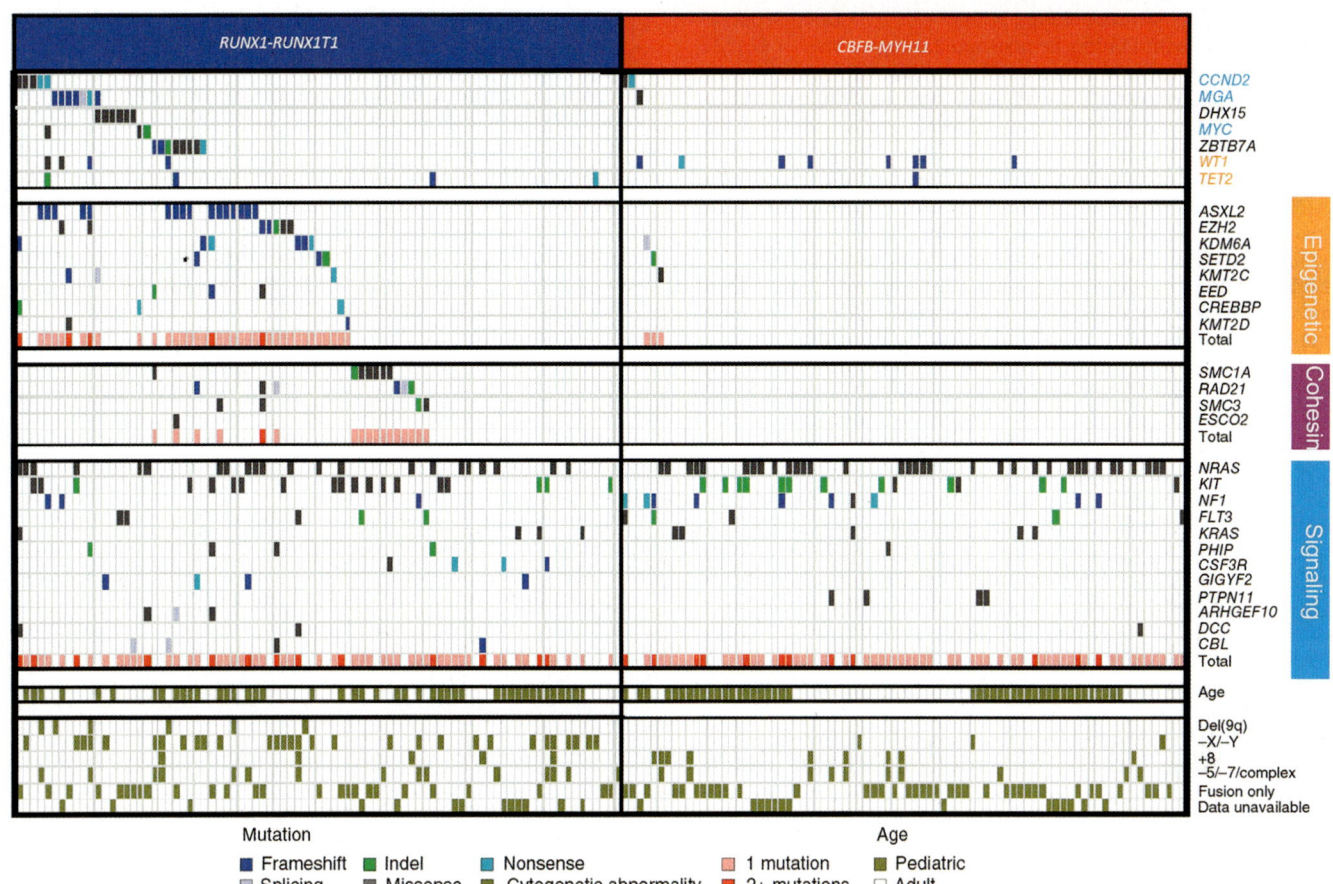

FIGURE 73.6 Comparison of mutational landscape of *RUNX1::RUNX1T1* AML and *CBFB::MYH11* AML. Mutational data are from 165 CBF::AML cases sequenced by whole genome (17) or whole exome (148) sequencing. Signaling, epigenetic, and cohesin genes are separated into functional groups indicated on the right. Cytogenetic abnormalities and patient age group (adult or pediatric) are shown along the bottom. Mutations in both epigenetic and cohesin genes are significantly enriched in *RUNX1::RUNX1T1* AML. (Reprinted by permission from Nature: Faber ZJ, Chen X, Gedman AL, et al. The genomic landscape of core-binding factor acute myeloid leukemias. *Nat Genet*. 2016;48(12):1551-1556. Copyright © 2016 Springer Nature.)

CCAAT/Enhancer Binding Protein-α

CCAAT/Enhancer Binding Protein-α (CEBPA) is a transcription factor that is essential for granulocytic differentiation.[122,123] Mice with a genetic knockout of *Cebpa* have a complete block in the transition from common myeloid progenitor to the granulocyte/monocyte progenitor, as well as increased repopulating activity of HSCs.[124] Cytogenetically silent mutations of *CEBPA* have been identified in about 10% of AML cases.[125] In addition, mutations in other leukemic oncogenes often lead to *CEBPA* downregulation. For example, the RUNX1::RUNX1T1 fusion transcription factor represses the *CEBPA* promoter.[126] *FLT3*-ITD activation of ERK leads to modification of CEBPA, which reduces its activity.[127] In addition, the *CEBPA* promoter is methylated in half of AML cases.[128]

The importance of *CEBPA* in granulocyte differentiation is demonstrated by the lack of mature granulocytes in *CEBPA* knockout mice,[129] while its conditional expression triggers granulocyte differentiation in bipotential precursors.[130] CEBPA transactivates the genes for G-CSF and GM-CSF receptors and several granulocyte-specific proteins. The *CEBPA* gene produces two proteins, p42 and p30, using alternative start sites. The p42 isoform promotes proliferation arrest, whereas the p30 isoform promotes myeloid specification.[131] Mutations in *CEBPA* are of two types: C-terminal bZIP domain mutations and N-terminal truncating mutations that lead to enhanced production of the 30-kD protein.[132-134] The former type inhibits dimerization and DNA binding. The latter type dimerizes with the long form but inhibits transactivation by the dimer, functioning in a dominant negative manner. In two-thirds of AML with *CEBPA* gene mutations, one allele has an N-terminal mutation and the other allele has a C-terminal variant. Several families with familial AML have been documented to have germline *CEBPA* N-terminal mutations, and progression to AML has been shown to correlate with a somatic mutation in the C terminus.[135] *CEBPA* mutations most often occur in intermediate-risk AML with normal cytogenetics, and these patients have a significantly improved outcome.[125] Interestingly, mutation of *CEBPA* at both alleles is associated with a better overall survival than mutation of *CEBPA* at a single allele.[136] Furthermore, more recent studies suggest that the site of the *CEBPA* mutation matters, with bZIP in-frame mutations but not TAD or other types of mutations being associated with a favorable outcome even when found as a single allele mutation.[137,138] The majority of patients (86.7%) with *CEBPA*-mutated AML have additional mutations, most commonly in *TET2* (29.2%), *GATA2* (28.3%), *DNMT3A* (18.8%), *FLT3*-ITD (16.3%), *NPM1* and *NRAS* (12.9% each), and *WT1* (12.5%).[137,138] Overall, the spectrum of comutations seen with *CEBPA* single mutant bZIP was more comparable with that of patients with *CEBPA* biallelic mutations and differed markedly from the comutations seen with the *CEBPA* single mutant TAD group, the latter being more similar to patients with *CEBPA* wild type.[137]

GATA1/GATA2

GATA1 is a zinc finger transcription factor that regulates erythroid and megakaryocytic differentiation. Mouse models have demonstrated that GATA1 is essential for erythropoiesis.[139] In *Gata1*-null mice, megakaryocytes do not undergo terminal differentiation but instead expand dramatically. Familial missense mutations in *GATA1* result in a syndrome of dyserythropoietic anemia and thrombocytopenia. Approximately 10% of patients with Down syndrome (DS) develop transient abnormal myelopoiesis (TAM) in the neonatal period (usually in the first week, almost always within the first 2 months of life), and these patients have mutations in *GATA1*.[140,141] Deep sequencing of neonates with DS has demonstrated a higher rate of *GATA1* mutation (20%) than is reflected in the incidence of TAM.[142] About one-third of patients with DS with TAM later develop acute megakaryoblastic leukemia (AMkL) within 5 years, and identical *GATA1* mutations have been identified in the AMkL blasts as were present in the TAM. A large study demonstrated that there is no difference in the *GATA1* mutations present in patients who just developed TAM compared with patients who went on to AMkL.[143]

Genomic sequencing studies comparing patients with TAM, DS-AMkL, and non-DS-AMkL has yielded interesting information about additional mutations involved in the development of AMkL. The mean number of nonsilent mutations in TAM was 1.7, with uniform detection of *GATA1* mutations, suggesting that the mutation of *GATA1* as well as the effects of trisomy 21 were sufficient to drive TAM. However, in DS-AMkL, besides the identical *GATA1* mutation there were an average of 4.8 additional nonsilent mutations.[144] The recurrent mutations detected in DS-AMkL fall in three major classes: mutations in cohesins or *CTCF* (65%), mutations in epigenetic regulators such as *EZH2* (45%), and mutations in *RAS* and other signal-transducing molecules (47%).[144] CTCF is a zinc finger protein, which is involved in long-range gene expression regulation, such as DNA loop formation.[144] EZH2 is a subunit of the Polycomb repressive complex 2 (PRC2) that is involved in methylation of histone H3lysine 27 (H3K27me); this gene was mutated in 33% of DS-AMkL cases.[144] The variant allele frequency of these mutations is high in DS-AMkL, suggesting that they are involved early on in the expansion of subclones that already have the *GATA1* mutation.[144]

AMkL in DS is sensitive to cytosine arabinoside/anthracycline-based chemotherapy, with event-free survival rates of 80% to 100%.[145] Interestingly, a putative target of GATA1 regulation is cytidine deaminase (*CDA*), which inactivates ara-C by deamination to the inactive uridine-arabinoside. Presumably failure of mutant GATA1 to transactivate *CDA* increases the efficacy of ara-C treatment.[146]

Epigenetic Factors Modifying Chromatin and DNA
Overview of Epigenetic Factors

The overall structure of the human epigenome in normal human cells and the relevant mutations that alter the cancer epigenome are depicted in *Figure 73.7*. Epigenetics refers to inherited information that is not directly dependent on DNA sequence. Here we will also include in the topic of epigenetic modification those changes that can influence gene expression during development and differentiation, as well as in oncogenesis. It is important to understand the basis of these modifications, as many of the genes that are mutated in acute leukemia encode proteins that carry out epigenetic modifications. Epigenetic modifications include DNA methylation, histone modifications, and RNA-based mechanisms (reviewed in Ref. 147). DNA methylation occurs at CpG sequences, and many genes have CpG islands, groups of up to 100 bp with high CpG content near promoters. Hypermethylation of the CpG islands usually causes silencing of genes, and in general cancer cells have been found to have an overall state of hypomethylation but increased hypermethylation at CpG islands.[148] This may be the mechanism by which tumor suppressor genes are silenced.[148] The nucleosome, the basic unit of chromatin, consists of 146 to 147 base pairs of DNA wound around a histone octamer composed of one H2A-H2B tetramer and two H3-H4 dimers.[149] The histones can be modified by methylation, acetylation, and other less common chemical modifications. These modifications affect the interaction of the histone N- and C-termini with the DNA strand and thereby affect the openness of the chromatin and, ultimately, gene expression. The histone modifications also affect which additional protein complexes can bind to the histones to effect further modifications or to promote DNA methylation. In general, histone acetylation is associated with gene activation. Acetylation of lysine residues in histones (most commonly H3K4, H3K9, H3K27, H3K36, H3K79, H4K5, H4K12, and H4K20) reduces the positive charge of the lysines that interact with

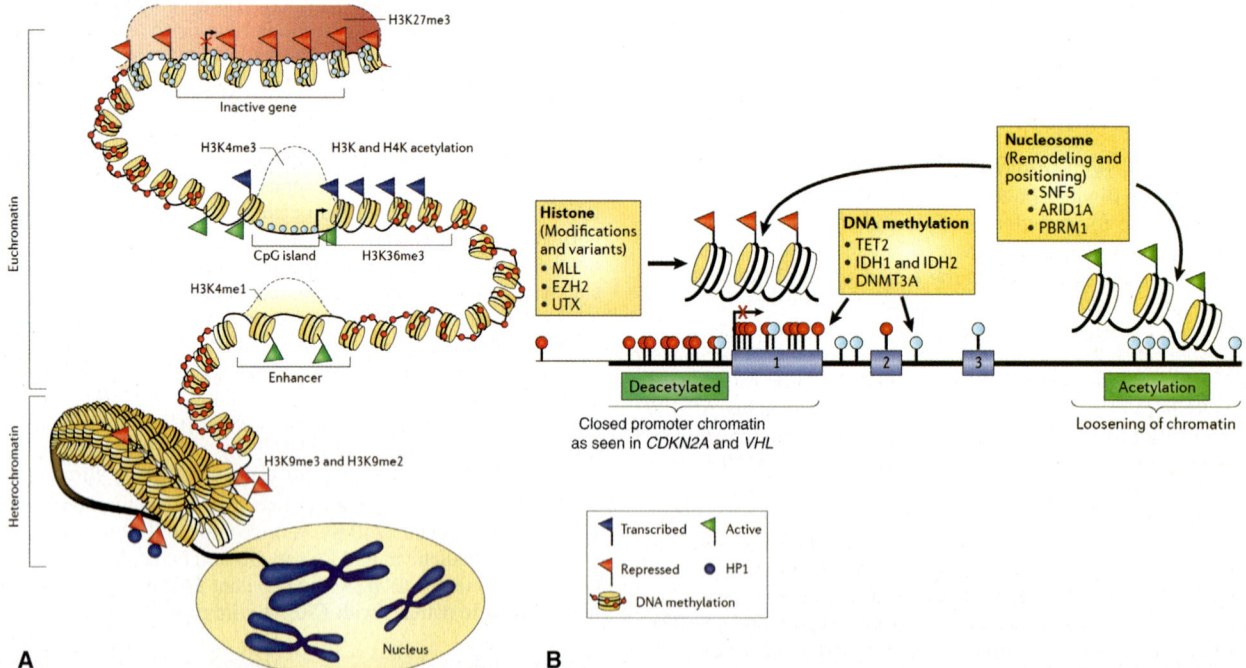

FIGURE 73.7 Model of the epigenome in normal and cancer cells. A, Normal human cells with inactive and active genes in euchromatin and packed heterochromatin. A silenced gene at the top (red X over arrow indicating transcription start site [TSS]) has repressive histone modifications (me = methylation) indicated by the red flags, mediated by the Polycomb group (red cloud). As a result, nucleosomes are positioned over the TSS. In the middle of the picture an actively transcribed gene has active histone methylation and acetylation marks at the promoter (green flags), and the promoter CpG island is unmethylated (pale blue circles). The TSS (arrow) is not occupied by nucleosomes. Elsewhere DNA is methylated (red circles). At the bottom is densely folded heterochromatin. B, Epigenetic changes in cancer cells. At left a hypothetical gene is silenced by repressive histone modifications (deacetylation), represented by red flags, and increased DNA methylation (red circles). An abnormally activated gene to the right shows abnormally acetylated histones (green flags) and demethylated CpG islands (blue circles). Genes commonly mutated in cancer whose products are involved in histone modification, DNA methylation, and nucleosome positioning are listed in the yellow boxes. (Reprinted by permission from Nature: Baylin SB, Jones PA. A decade of exploring the cancer epigenome - biological and translational implications. *Nat Rev Cancer*. 2011;11(10):726-734. Copyright © 2011 Springer Nature.)

the negatively charged phosphate groups of the DNA backbone. This change in charge reduces the tightness with which the histones bind the DNA, allowing more access by transcription factors to promoters and thereby resulting in increased gene transcription. The level of histone acetylation is regulated by the relative activity of histone acetyltransferases and histone deacetylases (HDACs).[150] Histone methylation, catalyzed by histone methyltransferase also occurs at lysine residues of histones H3 and H4, and the residues can be mono-, di-, or trimethylated. The effect of the methylation depends on the histone residue modified and the context. For example, methylation of H3K4 is enriched at enhancer, promoter, and transcription start sites and is considered a marker of gene activation, whereas methylation of H3K9 is associated with gene repression.[151] The pattern of histone acetylation and methylation and its effect on gene transcription is referred to as the histone code, with histone writers, erasers, and readers referring to the proteins that modify and interact with the histone modifications (reviewed in Ref. 152).

IDH1/IDH2 and TET2 Mutations

In the first whole genome sequencing of blasts from a patient with cytogenetically normal AML, mutations in isocitrate dehydrogenase 1 (*IDH1*) were detected and were found to be present in 16% of a panel of 80 cytogenetically normal AML samples.[53] In a further screen of AML DNA, it was found that *IDH1/IDH2* mutations are mutually exclusive with mutations in *TET2* (ten-eleven translocation 2) in de novo AML (*Figure 73.8*). AMLs with mutations in *IDH1* have similar patterns of DNA hypermethylation as AMLs with mutations in *TET2*, further suggesting a functional link between the products of these two genes.[153] The link became clear upon further investigation of the enzymatic activity of IDH1/IDH2 and TET1/TET2. Wild-type IDH1/IDH2 catalyzes production of α-ketoglutarate (α-KG), whereas the neomorphic enzymatic activity of mutant IDH1/IDH2 produces 2-hydroxyglutarate (2-HG). α-KG-dependent enzymes such as histone demethylases and TET1/TET2 are inhibited by 2-HG, which is structurally similar enough to α-KG that it can bind in place of α-KG and inhibit these enzymes.[154] The TET proteins catalyze the conversion of 5-methyl cytosine (5mC) to 5-hydroxymethyl cytosine (5hmC), a first step in demethylation of 5mC.[155] Experiments in which *TET2* genes containing mutations detected in AML cases are expressed in HEK293T tissue culture cells demonstrated decreased 5hmC and increased 5mC staining.[156] Therefore, mutations in *IDH1* and *TET2* both produce increased DNA methylation, mutant IDH1 by inhibiting TET2, and mutant TET2 by loss of its ability to convert 5mC to 5hmC.[153-155,157] The significance of these changes for pathogenesis of AML is demonstrated by experiments in which either stable expression of mutant IDH1 or shRNA-mediated knockdown of TET2 in primary mouse bone marrow cells resulted in increased C-KIT expression and decreased expression of the mature myeloid markers Mac-1 and Gr-1 by flow cytometric analysis.[153] Therefore, the hypermethylation and resultant silencing of genes as a result of *IDH1* and *TET2* mutations presumably inhibits myeloid differentiation and thereby promotes development of AML. Small-molecule inhibitors of IDH1 (Ivosidenib) and IDH2 (Enasidenib) are now in use[158]; these drugs prevent 2-HG production by the mutant IDH1/IDH2, thereby restoring proper enzymatic function to histone demethylases and TET2 and promoting normal histone and DNA methylation patterns.[154] Recent data indicate that the prognostic impact of mutations in *IDH1* and *TET2* in AML is context dependent with effects of a given mutation dependent on other comutated genes, patient's age, and the type of therapy.[57,159] Overall, a large meta-analysis demonstrated that presence of *TET2* mutations in AML is an unfavorable prognostic factor for overall survival and event-free survival.[160]

DNMT3A

One of the most frequently mutated genes in patients with cytogenetically normal AML is *DNMT3A*, encoding DNA methyltransferase 3 alpha (see *Figure 73.7B*), with an overall mutation rate of 23% in AML.[54] DNMT3A is a de novo methylase involved in methylation of CpG islands that occur near gene promoters.[161] The most commonly mutated site in DNMT3A is the R882 residue in the catalytic domain. The mutations detected in patients with AML map predominantly at the tetramer interface where they disrupt tetramerization of the DNMT3A molecules. Dimeric DNMT3A molecules still have methylase activity, but they dissociate from DNA more quickly than the wild type, so that fewer cytosines in a CpG island are methylated.[162] The effect on tetramerization explains why the *DNMT3A* mutations act in a dominant negative manner. Global methylation does not seem to be affected in DNA from AML with mutated *DNMT3A*, but analysis of DNA methylation by MeDIP-Chip (methylated DNA immunoprecipitation-Chip) in a matched set of DNAs from five patients with AML with mutated *DNMT3A* and five patients with AML with wild-type *DNMT3A* demonstrated 182 genomic sites where the DNA from patients with mutated *DNMT3A* was hypomethylated.[54] Studies of

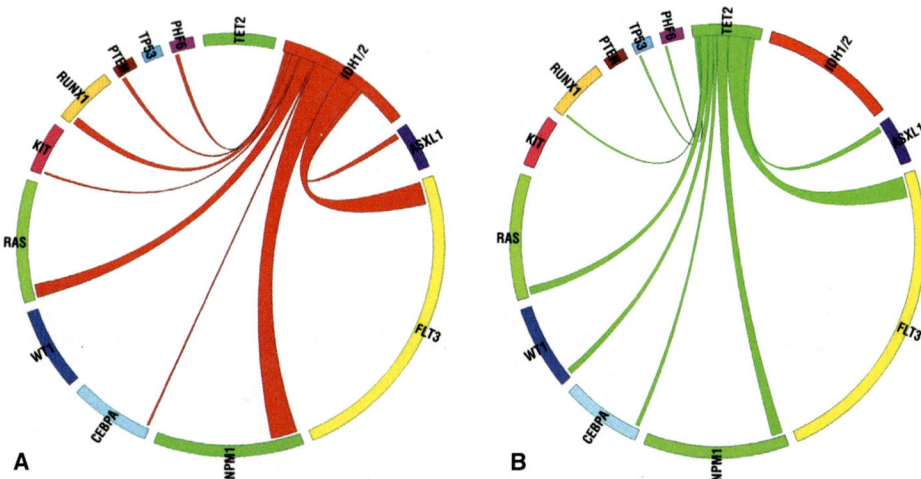

FIGURE 73.8 *IDH1/IDH2* **mutations are mutually exclusive with mutations in** *TET2* **in de novo AML.** A, Circos diagram revealing relative frequency and pairwise co-occurrences of mutations in *IDH1* and *IDH2* in a cohort of 385 patients with de novo AML. B, Circos diagram revealing relative frequency and pairwise co-occurrences of mutations in *TET2* in a cohort of 385 patients with de novo AML. (Reprinted from Figueroa ME, Abdel-Wahab O, Lu C, et al. Leukemic IDH1 and IDH2 mutations result in a hypermethylation phenotype, disrupt TET2 function, and impair hematopoietic differentiation. *Cancer Cell*. 2010;18:553-567. Copyright © 2010 Elsevier. With permission.)

DNA methylation in *Dnmt3a*-null murine HSCs demonstrated a complex story with poor correlation between changes in methylation sites and changes in gene expression comparing wild type with *Dnmt3a*-null HSCs. However, changes in gene expression patterns may be due to changes in methylation of regulatory regions of directly affected genes, whose expression then alters regulation of many other genes by mechanisms other than methylation. Transcriptional profiling of *Dnmt3a*-null HSCs did reveal that genes involved in the multipotency of normal HSCs were upregulated, whereas genes necessary for differentiation of the HSCs were downregulated. This suggests that the *DNMT3A* mutations may contribute to the block in differentiation that occurs in leukemic blasts.[163]

KMT2A (MLL)

A transcriptional activator that is characteristically rearranged in infant leukemia, therapy-related leukemia, and mixed-phenotype leukemia is the mixed lineage leukemia gene *KMT2A*, previously named *MLL*, which maps to chromosome 11q23 (reviewed in Ref. 164). The *KMT2A* gene consists of 34 exons over 100 kb encoding a 3969-aa protein.[164] *KMT2A* is the mammalian homolog of *trithorax*, a *Drosophila* transcriptional regulator that positively regulates homeobox genes.[165] Homeobox genes are a large family of genes that are developmental regulators essential for growth and differentiation. They were first identified in *Drosophila* during the study of genes whose mutations led to developmental abnormalities involving misassignment of body segment identity.[166] The mammalian homologs consist of 39 *HOX* genes, which are important in mammalian development and cell fate determination.[167] Wild-type KMT2A appears to be responsible for the downregulation of homeobox gene expression during development,[168-171] whereas the KMT2A fusion protein inappropriately activates *HOX* genes.[164] Wild-type KMT2A regulates *HOX* gene expression by methylation of histone H3 lysine (H3K4), requiring the SET domain, a protein domain shared by a number of transcriptional regulators with histone methyltransferase activity.[149] H3K4 methylation is associated with transcriptional activation.

KMT2A rearrangements involve approximately 10% of chromosomal rearrangements overall in patients with ALL, AML, and MDS and are associated with poor prognosis.[172] More than 60 different partner loci have been identified.[173] In pediatric and adult ALL, the most common translocation partners are the *AFF1(AF4)* gene at 4q21 in t(4;11), the *MLLT3(AF9)* gene at 9p21-22 in t(9;11), and the *MLLT1(ENL)* or *ELL* genes at 19p13.3 and 19p13.1, respectively, in t(11;19). Interestingly, the t(9;11) and t(11;19) are also associated with AML,[174] thus the older name mixed lineage leukemia (MLL), since the gene is involved with leukemias of both myeloid and lymphoid origins.

The breakpoints of 11q23 usually occur between exons 8 and 11 of *KMT2A*,[164] leaving approximately the N-terminal 1400 amino acids of the KMT2A/MLL protein.[175] The retained protein contains three AT-hook sequences thought to bind DNA at the minor groove,[176] the CxxC domain that specifically binds unmethylated DNA, and a lysine-rich RD2 region. The conserved C-terminal SET domain is routinely lost, although it is the domain that has the H3K4 histone methyltransferase activity that is the mechanism by which the wild-type protein activates *HOX* gene transcription.[164]

There has been much investigation as to the role of the multiplicity of fusion partners of *KMT2A*. Three of the most common fusion partners, *MLLT3(AF9)*, *AF10*, and *MLLT1(ENL)*, associate with DOT1L, which is a histone methyltransferase with a different activity than wild-type MLL, as it methylates histone H3 lysine 79 (H3K79me).[177,178] This histone modification is also associated with transcriptional activation. DOT1L is one of many proteins in a Dot.com complex, which consists of DOT1L, AF10, MLLT6(AF17), and MLLT1(ENL) (Figure 73.9).[164,177] Thus, the plethora of *KMT2A* fusion partners begin to make sense, as many of them normally associate together in complexes that regulate transcription. Therefore, the fusion protein associates with its usual partners, but the H3K79me marking occurs at different sites than usual, as the N-terminal KMT2A protein has the DNA-binding sites that bring the activating histone methyltransferase activity to KMT2A target genes. Demonstration of an abnormal increase in the H3K79 methylation pattern at target *HOXA* genes confirms this hypothesis.[172]

KMT2A rearrangements are associated with several unique types of leukemia. First, in infant acute leukemia (birth to 1 year), there is a 60% to 80% incidence of 11q23 rearrangement.[179] Second, in secondary acute leukemias developing after treatment with DNA topoisomerase II inhibitors, there is a 70% to 90% incidence of *KMT2A* rearrangements, particularly t(4;11)(q21;q23) and t(9;11)(p21-22;q23).[180,181] Topoisomerase II is an enzyme involved in unwinding of DNA during replication and transcription. It does so by producing double-stranded nicks in the DNA, after which the ends are rejoined by a ligase activity of topoisomerase II. Topoisomerase II inhibitors such as epipodophyllotoxins inhibit this ligase function so that DNA free ends accumulate, triggering apoptotic events. In *KMT2A* there are 11 sites similar to topoisomerase II consensus binding sites in the breakpoint cluster areas.[182] Therefore, if DNA free ends created by the topoisomerase II are incorrectly religated, translocations in *KMT2A* are likely to occur. Interestingly, infant leukemia with *KMT2A* translocations has a similar distribution of breakpoints, whereas sporadic cases of acute leukemia have more random breakpoints.[183] This observation has triggered speculation that in utero exposure to environmental topoisomerase II

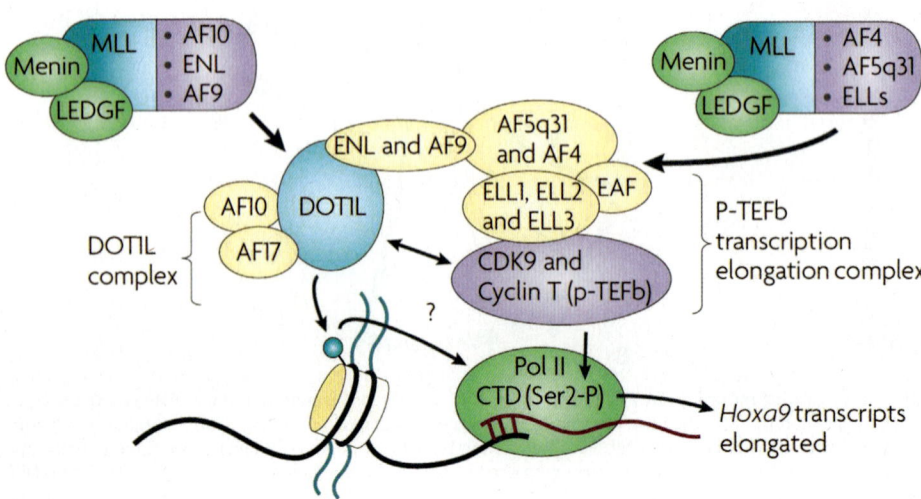

FIGURE 73.9 Proposed mechanism by which MLL (KMT2A) fusion proteins increase transcription of Hoxa9. MLL fusion proteins lose a large carboxy-terminal portion that includes the H3K4me3 writing methyltransferase SET domain, retain the chromatin-targeting property, and also acquire aberrant transactivation mechanisms through MLL fusion partners. On the left, A subset of MLL fusions MLL::AF10, MLL::ENL, and MLL::AF9 directly interact with DOT1L through the MLL fusion partner and induce the methylation of H3K79 at *Hoxa9*. Some other MLL fusions, MLL::AF4, MLL::AF5q31, and MLL::ELL, interact with and recruit the P-TEFb transcription elongation complexes to *HOXA9*. On the right, DOT1L complexes (DOT1L–AF10-AF17-ENL [or AF9]) associate with p-TEFb complexes through the shared component ENL. (Adapted by permission from Nature: Chi P, Allis CD, Wang GG. Covalent histone modifications—miswritten, misinterpreted and mis-erased in human cancers. *Nat Rev Cancer*. 2010;10(7):457-469. Copyright © 2010 Springer Nature.)

inhibitors such as flavonoids may have a role in the etiology of infant leukemia.[184]

Recently, a different type of *KMT2A* gene alteration involving an in-frame partial tandem duplication of exons 5 to 11 has been described in approximately 4% to 7% of patients with AML.[185] This occurs in the absence of visible chromosome abnormalities and is often associated with *FLT3* mutations.[185] This mutation retains the C-terminal SET domain, unlike all known *KMT2A* fusions resulting from balanced translocations. A mouse knock-in model replacing one copy of *KMT2A* with the *MLL*-PTD ($Mll^{PTD/WT}$ mice) results in overexpression of HOXA7, HOXA9, and HOXA10 in bone marrow, blood, and spleen.[186] Inspection of the promoter of *HOXA7* and *HOXA9* by chromatin immunoprecipitation assay demonstrates an increase in H3K4 methylation, as would be predicted due to the retention of the SET domain.

The latency of development of leukemia appears to be shorter for *KMT2A* rearrangements than for other leukemogenic rearrangements. In studies of twins who develop infant leukemia, those bearing a shared *KMT2A* rearrangement have a concordance of nearly 100% in the first year of life, whereas in twins sharing another rearrangement, the concordance is 25% and the time to development may be years instead of months.[187,188] Similarly, therapy-related leukemias based on *KMT2A* rearrangement occur sooner after therapy than those occurring after alkylating agents or radiation.[181,189] This suggests that the oncogenic fusion protein produced by the *KMT2A* rearrangement can deregulate the cell without the accumulation of many secondary mutations. Sequencing of infant B-ALL with a *KMT2A* rearrangement has one of the lowest somatic mutation rates (1.3 mutations per genome) of any sequenced cancer.[178] An additional reflection of the potency of *KMT2A* rearrangements is that they are a poor prognostic indicator in infant leukemia, ALL, and most AML cases.[179]

ASXL1

ASXL1 is another gene involved in epigenetic regulation that is one of the most frequently mutated genes in myeloid neoplasms as a whole and is generally associated with a poor prognosis.[190] It is mutated in 5% to 11% of patients with AML, particularly in older patients and secondary AML.[190] *ASXL1* (addition of sex combs-like 1), encoded on chromosome 20q11.21, interacts with mammalian BAP (BRCA1-associated protein) to form a Polycomb repressive deubiquitinase that removes ubiquitination of histone H2AK119. Wild-type ASXL1 also interacts with the PRC2 complex to induce methylation at H3K27 (H3K27me3), which has a repressive effect on gene expression, including repression of a subset of *HOXA* genes (reviewed in Ref. 190). In vitro studies of CD34+ bone marrow cells from *Asxl1*-knockout mice demonstrate global reduction of histone methylation (H3K27me3 and H3K4me3) and derepression of *HOX* genes.[191] However, many of the *ASXL1* mutations found in AML are gain-of-function mutations in which frameshift or nonsense mutations near the 5' end of the last exon produce a truncated C-terminal end of the ASXL1 protein.[192] These mutated ASXL1 proteins still appear to interfere with the PRC2 and result in decreased H3K27me3 methylation, leading to derepression of *HOXA* genes. Mouse experiments indicate that *ASXL1* mutations are not sufficient to induce myeloid transformation but that their effect on histone methylation increases susceptibility to myeloid leukemia.[190] *ASXL1* mutations most often occur in conjunction with *RUNX1* mutations[193] and are mutually exclusive with *DNMT3A*, *FLT3*-ITD, *NPM1*, and *SF3B1* mutations.[190]

EZH2

Mutations in *EZH2* (enhancer of zeste homologue 2), a H3K27 methyltransferase that is part of the enzymatic core of the PRC2 complex,[194] have been found in AML that is secondary to MDS or myeloproliferative diseases. These mutations result in loss of H3K27me3 and upregulation of *HOX* oncogenes, as well as several genes that confer chemoresistance (*FHL1* and *UBE2E1*).[161] Inhibitors of EZH2 activity in specific, and the PRC2 complex as a whole, are being investigated as a novel therapeutic approach for treatment of AML (reviewed in Ref. 194).

This enlarging group of genes involved in epigenetic regulation has led Shih et al to propose two additional categories of genes involved in the pathogenesis of AML besides the class I genes promoting proliferation and the class II genes promoting block in differentiation. These two additional categories are (1) mutations in genes involved in the hydroxymethylation pathway (*IDH1/IDH2*, *TET2*) and (2) mutations in genes involved in epigenetic modification (*DNMT3A*, *ASXL1*, *EZH2*, *KMT2A*)[58] (*Figure 73.1*).

Kinases

FLT3 Mutations

FLT3 may be the single most commonly mutated gene in AML (reviewed in Ref. 195), which is supported by the results from the TCGA study.[55] Originally cloned from CD34+ HSCs, it encodes a type III receptor tyrosine kinase. FLT3 ligand (FL) is a type I transmembrane protein that is expressed on the surface of support and hematopoietic cells in the bone marrow. It normally stimulates growth of immature myeloid cells and stem cells.[196] When FL ligand binds to the FLT3 receptor, FLT3 dimerizes and autophosphorylates intracytoplasmic tyrosine residues. The phosphorylated, activated FLT3 then activates downstream signal transduction pathways, including PI3K/AKT, MAPK/ERK, and STAT5[197,198] (*Figure 73.10* left). Several types of mutations in *FLT3* have been cloned from leukemic cells. The most common are internal tandem repeat (ITD) mutations, in which head-to-tail duplications of various lengths and positions occur in the juxtamembrane (JM) portion of the molecule.[199] These elongation mutations may occur due to DNA replication errors as a result of a

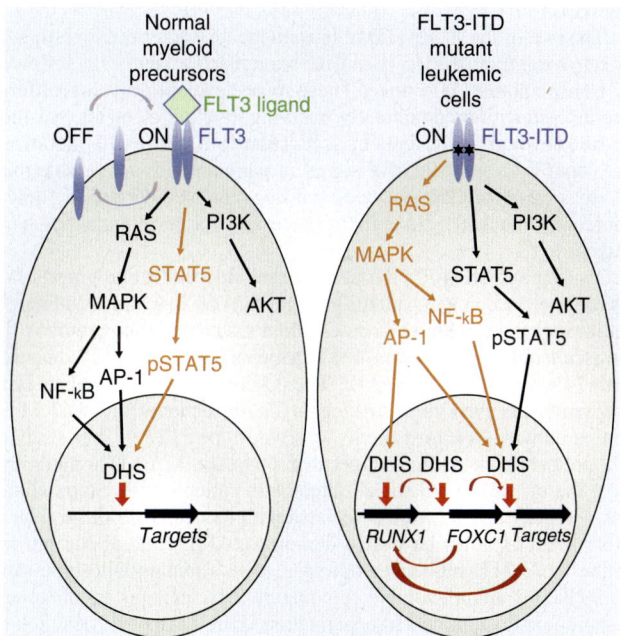

FIGURE 73.10 Interaction of normal and mutant FLT3 with downstream signaling pathways and transcription factors. Upon binding to the FLT3 ligand the FLT3 receptor dimerizes and undergoes activation by autophosphorylation of intracytoplasmic tyrosine residues, resulting in activation of downstream signal transduction pathways including MAPK/ERK/RAS, STAT5, and PI3K/AKT, affecting transcription factors such as NF-κB, AP-1, and pSTAT5, which bind at DNaseI hypersensitive sites (DHS) to regulate transcription (left). Mutations in *FLT3*, particularly internal tandem duplications (ITDs) in the juxtamembrane portion of the molecule result in mutant constitutively active protein that is able to dimerize and autophosphorylate in the absence of ligand. The *FLT3*-ITD mutations in AML are associated with aberrant signaling resulting in chronic activation of the MAPK inducible transcription factor AP-1, which induces and cooperates with RUNX1 to transactivate specific target genes mapped at FLT3-ITD-specific DHSs (right). (Reprinted from Cauchy P, James SR, Zacarias-Cabeza J, et al. Chronic Flt3-ITD signaling in acute myeloid leukemia is connected to a specific chromatin signature. *Cell Rep*. 2015;12(5):821-836. https://creativecommons.org/licenses/by/4.0/)

potential palindromic intermediate that may form at that site.[200] The JM domain is an autoinhibitory domain whose inhibitory function is usually relieved by autophosphorylation after ligand binding.[195] The in-frame insertions in the JM domain produce mutant proteins that are constitutively activated; they are able to dimerize and autophosphorylate in the absence of ligand.[200] In addition, insertion sites may be in the first tyrosine kinase domain (TKD1).[5] Other types of mutations include activation loop mutations, usually an Asp825Tyr substitution resulting from a point mutation in the second tyrosine kinase domain (TKD), producing constitutive activation of FLT3 (*FLT3*-TKD).[195]

Constitutive activation of FLT3 in AML with *FLT3*-ITD is associated with chronic activation of the MAPK signaling pathway. A recent study elegantly mapping DNase I hypersensitive sites and transcription factor–binding sites in samples of AML with *FLT3*-ITD demonstrates that the constitutively activated FLT3-ITD influences gene expression via the MAPK inducible transcription factor AP-1, which in turn upregulates the transcription factor RUNX1 and others to transcriptionally activate genes that promote growth and survival (*Figure 73.10* right).[201] This study shows how mutations in kinases can affect transcription factors and epigenetics, blurring the distinction between classes of mutations.

The overall frequency of *FLT3*-ITD in adult AML is 19% to 28% of patients, while in pediatric AML the frequency is somewhat lower at 10% to 15% (reviewed in Ref. 195). The frequency is highest in normal karyotype AML (up to 35%) but is very low in MDS and ALL. In contrast, the *FLT3*-TKD is reported in 7% of AML, 3% of MDS, and 3% of ALL patients.[202] *FLT3*-ITD is detected most frequently in APL, but it has been detected in all subtypes.[195] In addition, FLT3 is overexpressed at the mRNA and protein levels in many cases of AML and ALL.[203]

The role of the *FLT3*-ITD in leukemogenesis has been investigated by retroviral transduction of murine bone marrow stem cells followed by transplantation into mice. These mice develop a myeloproliferative disease with predominantly maturing myeloid elements, but they do not develop acute leukemia.[204] Therefore, the *FLT3* mutations may confer the proliferative signal in patients with acute leukemia, whereas a concomitant balanced translocation or other genetic defect confers the block in differentiation necessary for development of acute leukemia.[195]

The expression of *FLT3* is a significant independent prognostic factor for poor outcome in patients younger than 60 years. In a study of 91 pediatric patients with AML on Children's Cancer Group protocol, the remission induction rate was 40% in patients with *FLT3*-ITD compared with 74% with wild-type *FLT3*. The difference in event-free survival at 8 years was even more striking, at 7% for patients with *FLT3*-ITD compared with 44% for patients with wild-type *FLT3*.[205] In a study of 398 patients with AML younger than 60 years, *FLT3*-ITD mutations were the primary predictor of outcome in patients with intermediate-risk cytogenetics and were associated with reduced overall survival.[57] More recent studies have also demonstrated that the allelic burden of the *FLT3*-ITD influences outcome, with a mutant:wild type ratio >0.50 having an unfavorable outcome. In these patients an allogeneic hematopoietic stem cell transplantation (HSCT) may be beneficial.[5] The high allelic ratio may indicate loss of heterozygosity at the *FLT3* locus.[5] As with *BCR::ABL1* for CML, the implication of a mutant constitutively active tyrosine kinase receptor in the pathogenesis of AML opens up the possibility of identifying a selective kinase inhibitor as a specific treatment of patients with AML with a mutant *FLT3*. Several kinase inhibitors have been identified by inhibition of IL3-independent growth of cell lines expressing FLT3-ITD in culture.[206,207] In an early study a majority of patients achieved >50% reduction in peripheral blast count, but these reductions were transient, lasting several weeks to months. A study performed by Piloto et al[208] on resistant human cell lines developed through prolonged coculture with FLT3 tyrosine kinase inhibitors demonstrated that, although FLT3 phosphorylation was still inhibited, downstream signaling pathways were activated. In two cell lines, activating *NRAS* mutations were detected. No mutations in *FLT3* were detected. However, in other studies, single molecule real-time (SMRT) sequencing was used to demonstrate secondary *FLT3* kinase domain mutations in four of eight patients who relapsed after treatment with FLT3-TKI. From the crystal structure of FLT3 several of the mutations would force the molecule into an active kinase confirmation that is not recognized by the AC220 type II kinase inhibitor used in the study.[209] Second- and third-generation FLT3 inhibitors have been developed, including agents such as Gilteritinib, which has been shown to be more effective than salvage therapy in patients with relapsed or refractory *FLT3*-mutated AML.[210]

C-KIT Mutations

C-KIT is a gene encoding a tyrosine kinase receptor that was first identified as a cellular counterpart to the *v-kit* oncogene of the Hardy-Zukerman 4 feline sarcoma virus.[211] It is deregulated in AML, gastrointestinal stromal tumors, and germ cell tumors, among others. Physiologically, it is the receptor for stem cell factor (SCF), also known as Kit ligand, which is expressed by fibroblasts and endothelial cells. It is involved in the proliferation and differentiation of hematopoietic progenitors, melanocytes, and germ cells. SCF forms homodimers that cause dimerization and activation of C-KIT when it binds.

The gene encoding C-KIT is on chromosome 4q11 and consists of 21 exons. C-KIT is a type III receptor tyrosine kinase, similar in structure to PDGFRA/B and FLT3. The extracellular portion consists of five immunoglobulin-like domains, which are connected by a transmembrane domain to the intracellular portion, consisting of a JM domain, and two TKDs, separated by a kinase insert sequence and followed by a carboxy terminal tail. When ligand binding promotes dimerization, a conformational change occurs fostering interactions between the Ig-like domains 4 and 5 of the two adjacent C-KIT molecules. Further conformation changes promote autophosphorylation of the intracellular kinase domains. Crystallization of the active and inactive forms demonstrate that, in the inactive form the JM domain forms a loop inserting into the active site and therefore suppressing kinase activity. The initial transphosphorylation after dimerization alters the inhibitory conformation of this JM domain, allowing autophosphorylation to proceed on the kinase domains.[212]

C-KIT relies on several of the main signaling pathways for downstream signaling. These include class 1A of the phosphatidylinositol 3'-kinases (PI3'-kinases) and the serine/threonine kinase AKT downstream, which interferes with initiation of apoptosis. Activation of the SRC family of tyrosine kinases (SFK) is involved in the proliferative response to C-KIT activation, as well as prevention of apoptosis. MAP kinases, including ERK1/2, p38, and JNK are also activated downstream of C-KIT.[212]

Oncogenic mutations in *C-KIT* cause ligand-independent receptor phosphorylation and therefore constitutive activation. The oncogenic mutations are mainly in the JM domain, encoded by exon 11, and the second kinase domain, encoded by exon 17. Exon 17 is most commonly mutated in leukemia. In silico modeling of the most common mutation, D816V, may structurally alter the activation loop and also may alter the JM domain so that it can no longer act to inhibit the kinase domain.[213] The oncogenic mutations may also alter substrate specificity, leading to altered patterns of downstream signaling.[214]

C-KIT is expressed in most AMLs, as a reflection of the immature characteristics of the myeloblasts. Mutations in the *C-KIT* gene are seen particularly in CBF leukemias: 2-25% of t(8;21) cases and 30% of inv(16) cases. Usually these *KIT* mutations are in exon 17, either D816X or N822K. Both of these mutants are resistant to imatinib but sensitive to dasatinib.[212] The deleterious effect of a concomitant *C-KIT* mutation in CBF leukemias has been controversial. In a recent large study, *C-KIT* exon 17 mutation significantly influenced the relapse-free survival of patients with *RUNX1::RUNX1T1* but not patients with *CBFB::MYH11*.[215]

Nuclear Pore Proteins
Nucleophosmin

Nucleophosmin (NPM1) is a molecular chaperone that shuttles between cytoplasm and nucleus, which primarily resides in the nucleolus.[216] NPM1 has several major functions in cells; these include ribosome biogenesis, regulation of centrosome duplication during the cell cycle, potentiating the p53 stress response, interaction with the ARF tumor suppressor protein, and DNA repair functions (reviewed in Refs. 217-219). Mutations of *NPM1* have now been identified in 35% of adult AML with normal karyotype. The frequency is less (9%-27%) in pediatric AML with normal karyotype.[217,220,221] The *NPM1* mutation is stably expressed, being consistently present in leukemic blasts at relapse.[222] By inspection of variant allele frequencies, *NPM1* mutations precede the *FLT3* mutations that often co-occur in AML.

The wild-type NPM1 has two nuclear localization signals and two nuclear export signals (NESs) that mediate the nuclear-cytoplasmic shuttling of wild-type NPM1. Over 50 different mutations in *NPM1* have been found in patients with AML; all of these mutations cause changes in the C terminus of the NPM1 protein, including generation of a new NES motif, and loss of tryptophan residues 288 and 290 or 290 alone, causing unfolding of the C-terminal domain and disruption of binding to the nucleolus.[222,223] Presence of a mutation correlates absolutely with abnormal subcellular localization of NPM1, with relocation from its normal predominantly nucleolar location to the cytoplasm; this can be detected in tissue sections by immunohistochemistry. The mutation is always heterozygous, which may be related to the fact that homozygous mutant is embryonic lethal.[224] The mutant NPM1 appears to function in a dominant negative manner through heterodimerization with normal NPM1, to cause relocation of some of the normal NPM1, as well as the mutant NPM1, to the cytoplasm.[225]

The various mechanisms by which the cytoplasmically located NPM1 (NPM1c) promote leukemia are portrayed in *Figure 73.11*. One mechanism by which mutant NPM1 may promote leukemogenesis is by destabilizing the tumor suppressor protein P14ARF, which normally regulates the TP53 response by binding to MDM2, preventing degradation of TP53. P14ARF colocalizes with NPM1 to the nucleolus, and their interaction stabilizes P14ARF. Without this interaction and nuclear location, P19ARF (the mouse homologue) is more rapidly degraded by proteasomes. By this mechanism, mutant NPM1c may indirectly cause reduced TP53[218,222] (*Figure 73.11A*). In addition, the cytoplasmic NPM1c retains its ability to bind to cytoplasmic caspases 6 and 8, which may inhibit apoptosis, also enhancing leukemogenesis. Finally, NPM1 usually interacts with FBW7γ, an F-box protein that is part of the E3 ubiquitin ligase that degrades the MYC protein. When mutated NPM1c no longer holds FBW7γ in the nucleus, it is more rapidly degraded, thus indirectly increasing the levels of MYC protein (*Figure 73.11B*).[218]

NPM1 mutations occur most frequently in conjunction with *FLT3* and *DNMT3A* mutations, but they also have an increased incidence with *IDH1* and *IDH2* mutations (see *Figure 73.2*).[57,218,22.1] Several studies have shown that patients with *NPM1* mutations in the absence of *FLT3* mutations have a favorable response to chemotherapy.[221,223] This may be due to the role of wild-type NPM1 in DNA repair; if *NPM1* is mutated there is less efficient repair of DNA damage induced by chemotherapy.[219]

NUP214 (CAN)

Nucleoporin 214 (NUP214, previously known as CAN), is a nucleoporin, a member of the group of proteins making up the nuclear pore complex (NPC). The *NUP214* gene is encoded on chromosome 9 at band 9q34.1 and comprises 36 exons. It is detected in leukemias with several different fusion partners, most of which occur in T-ALL.[226] However, the *DEK::NUP214* fusion is a recurring translocation that has its own subdivision under AML in the WHO book. Although a rare type of AML (0.7%-1.8% of cases), it is distinctive in that more than half of the cases have basophilia; in addition, granulocytic and erythroid dysplasia is common. The prognosis is poor, and allogeneic stem cell transplant is the favored therapy.[227]

NUP214 participates in the cytoplasmic portion of the NPC and is considered an FG nucleoporin in reference to a domain consisting of repetitive stretches of phenylalanine-glycine motifs interspersed with charged residues that promote a disordered, unfolded conformation. These regions help the FG nucleoporin carry out its dual duties of restricting diffusion to small molecules (<40 kDa) and selective nucleocytoplasmic transport. NUP21 interacts with CRM1 (a major exportin for proteins) and NXF1 (nuclear RNA export factor 1, the major factor exporting mRNA). Genomic knockout of *Nup214* causes embryonic lethality in mice (reviewed in Ref. 228).

In the fusion protein DEK::NUP214, the majority of the FG domain is retained. As this is the portion of the NUP214 protein that interacts with CRM1, it is not surprising that experiments demonstrate that NUP214 fusion proteins sequester CRM1 into nuclear bodies. It is unclear whether selective or global dysregulation of CRM1-mediated export results (reviewed in Ref. 228).

The *DEK* gene is located at chromosome 6p22.3 and encodes an epigenetic regulator that has acidic domains that interact with lysine residues in histones H3 and H4 and thereby inhibits the activity of histone acetyltransferases such as p300/CBP and PCAF. Therefore, it acts as a negative regulator of transcription by hindering chromatin

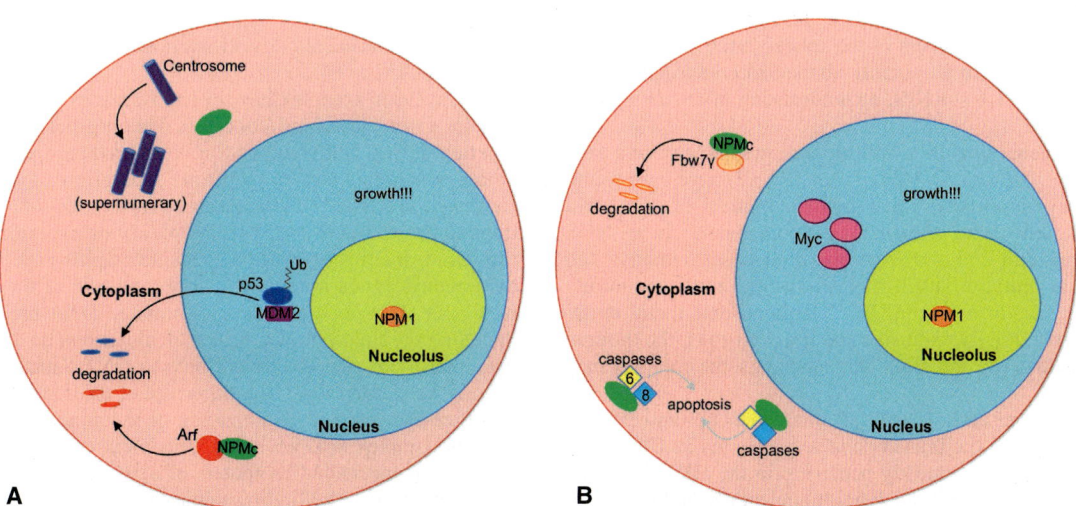

FIGURE 73.11 NPM1c and leukemogenesis. Wild-type NPM1 is shown as an orange oval in the nucleolus. Mutated NPM1 (NPM1c) is shown as a green oval in the cytoplasm. A, NPM1c sequesters ARF in the cytoplasm, causing its degradation. This facilitates p53 ubiquitination by MDM2, causing p53 degradation. In addition, reduced NPM1 leads to supernumerary centrosomes. B, NPM1c binds FBW7γ in the cytoplasm, causing its degradation. This allows MYC oncogene levels to increase in the nucleus. In addition, NPM1c inhibits caspase-6/-8, reducing apoptosis. (Reprinted by permission from Nature: Heath EM, Chan SM, Minden MD, et al. Biological and clinical consequences of NPM1 mutations in AML. *Leukemia*. 2017;31(4):798-807. Copyright © 2017 Springer Nature.)

relaxation.[229] The *DEK::NUP214* fusion gene retains much of the coding region of *DEK*, including the histone-binding region. If the DEK::NUP214 fusion protein causes aberrant hypoacetylation, a mechanism of leukemogenesis may be to silence genes important for hematopoietic differentiation.[228] In addition, it has been shown that DEK::NUP214 can upregulate *HOXA9/10* and *HOXB2/3* genes, which also leads to blocking of differentiation of early hematopoietic precursors.[230]

NUP98

NUP98 is another member of the NPC, normally present on both nuclear and cytoplasmic sides of the NPC, which has a role in protein and RNA export across the nuclear membrane.[231] *NUP98*, located on chromosome 11p15.4, is involved in over 25 fusions, primarily in pediatric AML. Although rare, this class of pediatric AML has an especially poor prognosis.[232] The most common fusion partners are *NUP98::NSD1* and *NUP98::JARID1A*. Both NDS1, a lysine methyltransferase, and JARID1A, a lysine demethylase, have plant homeodomain (PHD) finger domains that are retained in the C terminus of the fusion protein. A PHD finger is a protein domain that binds specifically to H3K2me3/2 motifs of Histone 3 (reviewed in Ref. 233). The N-terminal NUP98 portion of these fusion proteins has a role in transcriptional regulation, interacting with the histone acetylating proteins CBP/p300 and HDAC1.[234] A recent study defining the shared transcriptome of the most common NUP98 fusion proteins showed that the upregulated genes in common included regulators of self-renewal, including *HOX* genes as well as *MEIS1*.[234] Binding of H3K4me3/2 residues by the PHD domain of the NUP98 fusion protein was shown to be essential to persistent expression of these transcription factors that maintain a stem cell program of expression, thereby inhibiting differentiation and promoting leukemogenesis.[233,235] In addition, the cyclin dependent kinase CDK6 was highly upregulated by NUP98 fusion proteins; inhibition of this cell cycle regulator by kinase inhibitors may offer a targeted method of treating this category of AML with poor prognosis.[234]

Spliceosome Proteins

Another level of gene regulation that can be affected by mutations in AML is RNA splicing, the process where segments of precursor mRNA (pre-mRNA) are removed and the remaining pieces of RNA are religated to generate a mature mRNA. Usually this involves removal of introns, but many genes have alternatively spliced forms, with the different mature mRNA transcripts encoding proteins with different functions. Much is known about the canonical 5′ and 3′ splice site base pairs, as well as the branch-point sequence (BPS) and the polypyrimidine tract between the BPS and the 3′ splice site. These sites are recognized by members of the spliceosome, a metalloribozyme consisting of five small nuclear ribonucleoproteins (snRNPs): U1, U2, U4, U5, and U6 snRNPs, each consisting of an snRNA and multiple proteins.[236]

Mutations in genes encoding spliceosome components and auxiliary factors (*SF3B1*, *SRSF2*, *U2AF1*, and *ZRSR2*) have been found to have a positive predictive value for development of a myeloid neoplasm in patients with unexplained cytopenias.[237] In an NGS study of patients with AML, DNA from 20.7% cases demonstrated a splicing factor mutation at diagnosis, with the most commonly mutated splicing factor being *SRSF2*.[238] Spliceosome factor mutations are usually mutually exclusive and heterozygous, the thought being that more than one mutation in the spliceosome complex may be lethal.[237,238]

SF3B1 is a member of the U2snRNP complex that promotes binding of the U2snRNA to the branch point sequence via its C-terminal HEAT domain. Mutations, mostly occurring in the HEAT domain, cause utilization of aberrant branch-point nucleotides and cryptic 3′ splice sites (3′SS) (reviewed in Ref. 236). The U2AF heterodimer consists of U2AF1 and U2AF2; U2AF1 recognizes the 3′ SS and U2AF2 recognizes the polypyrimidine tract that is positioned between the branch point and the 3′SS. It is *U2AF1* that is more commonly mutated in myeloid neoplasms. The mutations occur in the first and second zinc finger domains of U2AF1, and each of the common mutations preferentially recognize different 3′ SS sequences, influencing splice site and therefore exon choices (reviewed in Ref. 236). SRSF2 is a member of the serine/arginine-rich (SR) family of proteins that bind to exonic splicing enhancer (ESE) sequences. Mutations in *SRSF2* cause the SRSF2 protein to bind ESE sequences that are C-rich preferentially to ESE sequences that are G-rich (reviewed in Ref. 236). Finally, *ZRSR2* encodes a protein involved in the minor spliceosome and binds to the 3′SS of U21-type introns (reviewed in Ref. 236).

RNA sequencing (RNA-seq) studies performed to delineate the extent of alternative splicing that occurs in AML with mutations in one of the splicing factor genes demonstrate that each splicing factor mutation results in a distinct differential isoform expression pattern. However, there is a limited overlap of alternatively spliced cancer-associated genes between the distinct isoform expression patterns. Overall, there is a decrease in splice junction usage, and there is a relative increase in alternative splicing of splicing factor genes themselves.[238] Several alternatively spliced target genes are particularly interesting. *SF3B1* mutations are commonly seen in MDS with ring sideroblasts, and one of the alternatively spliced genes encodes the iron transport protein ABCB7. The alternative splicing produces a premature termination codon, reducing the amount of intact transcript and resultant ABCB7 protein. Presumably this leads to the aberrant localization of iron in the erythroid precursors, producing the characteristic ring sideroblasts in the bone marrow of patients with an *SF3B1* mutation.[236,239] A functionally significant differential splicing event occurring in AML with an *SRSF2* mutation produces a defective isoform of EZH2 containing a "poison" exon that leads to nonsense-mediated decay of the EZH2 transcript and impaired hematopoietic differentiation.[240] Interestingly, *EZH2* mutations are mutually exclusive with *SRSF2* mutations in patients with AML.[241]

Cohesins

The cohesin complex is a multiprotein complex that forms a ring structure that interacts with the DNA helix. The ring is composed of a heterodimer of SMC1 and SMC3 (Structural Maintenance of the Chromosome genes), which form a V shape that is linked by RAD21 and bound to two helical repeat proteins STAG1 and STAG2 (*Figure 73.12A*; reviewed in Ref. 242). Mutations in four of the genes encoding these cohesin proteins (*SMC1A*, *SMC3*, *RAD21*, and *STAG2*) have been found in myeloid malignancies, and in particular are found in 12% of de novo AML and 20% of high-risk MDS and secondary AML.[55,243] Mutations in cohesin genes are commonly seen in DS-AMKL (*Figure 73.12B*)[244] and they are also associated with progression of the germline predisposition syndromes involving *GATA2*[245,246] or *RUNX1* mutations.[246,247] In these situations the cohesin gene mutations are not considered driver mutations but are associated with progression to AML.[242]

The cohesin complex has several functions. First, it plays a key role in sister chromatid cohesion, keeping the sister chromatids together during DNA replication, until anaphase when the cohesin complex is removed to facilitate separation of the chromatids (reviewed in Ref. 242). Interestingly, AML with cohesin gene mutations is not characterized by aneuploidy or hyperdiploidy, so disruption of this function of the cohesin complex may not be affected by a heterozygous mutation. The second role of the cohesin complex is in DNA repair of double-stranded DNA breaks by homologous recombination. The effect of mutations on this function of the cohesin complex may contribute to DNA damage in AML with cohesin gene mutations. The third role of the cohesin complex is in the three-dimensional organization of the genome. The role of the cohesin complex in DNA loop extrusion affects gene expression by looping enhancers and promoters of actively transcribed genes into nearby positions, facilitating enhancer-promoter interaction.[248,249] Therefore, mutation of cohesin complex genes may affect gene expression by interfering in this role. Experimental data suggest that cohesin complex dysregulation due to mutation may impair differentiation and maintain stem cell programs of expression in hematopoietic stem and progenitor cells (reviewed in Ref. 242).

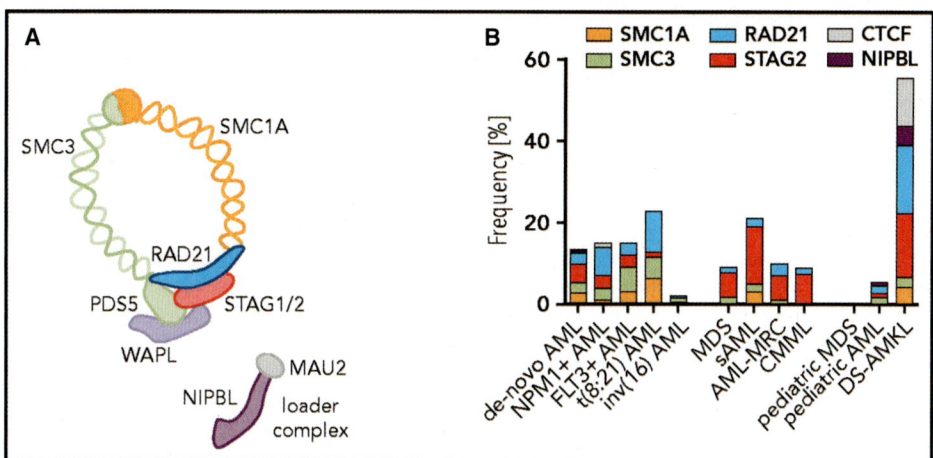

FIGURE 73.12 Cohesin complex mutations in myeloid malignancies. The core members of the cohesin complex ring and its loader complex are shown in (A). The frequency of mutations in the cohesin complex proteins according to AML diagnostic subgroup is shown in (B). AML-MRC, AML with myelodysplasia-related changes; CMML, chronic myelomonocytic leukemia; DS-AMKL, Down syndrome–associated acute megakaryoblastic leukemia. (Reprinted from Jann JC, Tothova Z. Cohesin mutations in myeloid malignancies. *Blood.* 2021;138:649-661. Copyright © 2021 American Society of Hematology. With permission.)

Risk Stratification of AML

A major purpose of molecular genetic testing performed on patients with AML is to have enough information for the assignment of the individual patient into a risk category, which informs prognostic outlook and dictates individualized therapeutic strategy. Optimal risk stratification allows deferring early aggressive therapies associated with significant treatment-related mortality, such as HSCT, when chemotherapy alone is likely to result in cure. On the other hand, patients with high-risk AML may benefit from early HSCT or be candidates for novel induction or targeted therapy approaches and posttransplant therapies. In addition, accurate identification of patients with uniformly poor outcomes regardless of initial therapeutic strategies and/or HSCT would allow consideration of those patients for novel clinical trials and/or palliative treatments focused on prolonging quality of life. Traditionally, risk stratification has been based on karyotype studies of leukemic blast cells (*Table 73.1*). Favorable cytogenetic abnormalities included rearrangements involving CBFs such as t(8;21) and inv(16), as well t(15;17). Deletions of chromosomes 5 and 7 or the presence of a complex karyotype were associated with poorer prognosis. Patients with a normal karyotype were classified as intermediate risk. The prognostic value of this cytogenetic classification has been confirmed in multiple studies over the last decades, some of which also led to identification of rarer abnormalities with adverse prognostic impact. However, many patients with AML (estimated at 50%) have a normal karyotype; therefore, therapeutic decision making for this group of patients is challenging. A decade ago directed sequencing of five genes implicated in leukemic transformation (*NPM1, FLT3, CEBPA, KMT2A, NRAS*) revealed at least one mutation in 84% of patients presenting with AML with normal karyotype (NK-AML). Further analyses suggested that patients with NK-AML can be assigned to meaningful prognostic groups based on patterns of mutations in these five genes.[250] This demonstrated the independent prognostic value of molecular analysis in NK-AML and for the first time led to incorporation of gene mutations into revised risk stratification guidelines.[251] Several notable subsequent studies have tested for mutations in a large number of patients with AML at diagnosis.[55,57] Most of the patients with AML (98%) had at least one somatic mutation. The frequency of recurrent gene mutations within functional groups is demonstrated in *Figure 73.2*, with Circos diagrams depicting the interrelationships between the mutations.[55,56] The diagrams visually convey the multiplicity of mutations that occur in most patients and demonstrate the patterns of co-occurring and mutually exclusive mutations. Some of the more important co-occurrences are *KIT* mutations and CBF alterations, co-occurrence of *IDH1/IDH2* mutations and *NPM1* mutations, and *DNMT3A* mutations with *NPM1*, *FLT3*, and *IDH1* mutations. As mentioned previously, *IDH1/IDH2* mutations do not occur in patients with *TET2* mutations (*Figure 73.8*). In addition, *IDH1/IDH2* and *WT1* mutations are mutually exclusive, as well as *DNMT3A* mutations and *KMT2A* translocations.[55,57] The most statistically significant predictors of overall survival are as follows: *FLT3*-ITD and *KMT2A* mutations are associated with reduced overall survival.[252-254] Biallelic as well as single bZIP in-frame *CEBPA* mutations[137,255,256] and CBF translocations are associated with improved overall survival. *PHF6* and *ASXL1* mutations are associated with reduced survival.[193,257] *IDH2* mutations (R140Q) have been associated with longer survival in younger patients (<60 years) compared with patients with wild-type *IDH2* genes.[57] In intermediate-risk AML, *FLT3*-ITD mutations are the primary factor influencing outcome. More recent studies have also demonstrated that the allelic burden of the *FLT3*-ITD influences outcome, with a mutant:wild type ratio > 0.50 having an unfavorable outcome.[5] In the cohort of patients analyzed by Patel et al, the group with favorable risk had a 3-year overall survival of 64%, whereas the group with intermediate risk had a 3-year overall survival of 42% and the group with adverse risk had a 12% overall survival. Multivariate analysis demonstrated that outcomes predicted from the risk stratification are independent of age, white blood cell (WBC), induction dose, transplantation status, and post-remission therapy.[57]

Grossman et al[258] developed a similar prognostic model based entirely on molecular mutational analysis rather than karyotype, in which they constructed an algorithm with 5 prognostic subgroups based upon analysis of 1000 patients for mutations in: *PML::RARA*, *RUNX1::RUNX1T1*, *CBFB::MYH11*, *FLT3*-ITD, *KMT2A*-PTD, *NPM1*, *CEBPA*, *RUNX1*, *ASXL1*, and *TP53*. The very favorable prognostic group (overall survival at 3 years of 82.9%) consisted of patients with *PML::RARA* rearrangement or *CEPBA* double mutations, and the very unfavorable group with an overall survival of 0% at 3 years consisted of patients with *TP53* mutations. *TP53*, a well-characterized tumor suppressor gene, is mutated in many cancers, and mutations in *TP53* are the basis of the cancer-prone Li-Fraumeni syndrome.[259] However, this study is the first to characterize the frequency of *TP53* mutations in AML (11.5%) and its prognostic significance.[258] Similar results were obtained by other recent studies including the TCGA AML study.[55] There have been some early attempts to use the ever-increasing amount of available molecular genetic data to construct purely genomic classification and prognostication of patients with AML.[159] *Table 73.1* shows the effects of gene mutations and the interplay with underlying cytogenetic changes on the revised risk stratification of the patients with AML.[260]

Despite the unprecedented technological advances over the recent years, which led to the generation of massive amount of genomic data, numerous questions remain. The translation of these data to actual understanding of the disease etiology and pathogenesis, new therapeutic strategies, and improved outcomes of patients diagnosed with AML has been slow. The particular combinations of genomic and clinical data with risk-adapted treatment strategies continue to change and evolve as the actual molecular mechanisms underlying the disease are elucidated by additional discoveries, new treatment trials, and additional patient cohorts, but the principle is important that risk stratification must take into account a multiplicity of genomic and possibly epigenomic events. The role of the molecular genetics diagnostic laboratory will certainly increase as new prognostically significant and cost-effective molecular genetic testing panels are developed and validated to perform on patients with AML at diagnosis. In addition, given the heterogeneity of the clinically important genomic lesions in AML requiring different testing modalities for their detection, new integrated analytical platforms with an ability to detect most or all genomic lesions underlying the specific disease may be developed.[261]

B-LYMPHOBLASTIC LEUKEMIA/LYMPHOMA

WHO Classification

Table 73.5 outlines the revised 4th edition WHO classification for B-cell acute lymphoblastic leukemia (B-ALL), which lists the major translocations and cytogenetic abnormalities that repeatedly occur in B-ALL and can be detected by routine cytogenetics or FISH.[227] The recent advent of NGS techniques has expanded the number of categories of B-ALL based on whole genome sequencing and RNA-seq studies that can detect cryptic rearrangements as well as point mutations (*Figure 73.13*).[262] These studies have subclassified the previous "B-other" category, and the specific mutations forming the basis of these new subcategories have also suggested new targeted therapies in certain cases.[262] In addition, transcriptome analysis and gene expression studies have identified additional categories with similar gene expression profiles but different genetic abnormalities (e.g., *BCR::ABL1*-like and *ETV6::RUNX1*-like categories[263-266]). Much progress in specific has been made in understanding the diverse genetic abnormalities found in *BCR::ABL1*-like B-ALL. This section will describe the genetic basis of the well-established categories of B-ALL based on recurrent translocations, as well as the new subcategories defined by NGS data.

Transcription Factors

PAX5

In a survey of 242 pediatric B-ALL cases by SNP array analysis, alterations in genes regulating B-lymphocyte differentiation were noted in 40% of B-ALL cases.[267] Mutations in genes necessary for B-cell differentiation are a perfect example of class II mutations that cause a block in cell differentiation in the classic model of acute leukemia pathogenesis (*Figure 73.1*). *Figure 73.14* demonstrates the position in B-cell development at which the major B-cell differentiation genes mutated in B-ALL have their normal effect. The B-cell differentiation genes found to be most commonly translocated or mutated include *EBF1*, *PAX5*, and *IKZF1*.[267]

PAX5 is essential for B-cell development, and it controls B-lineage-specific transcription of genes such as *CD19, CD79a, BLNK*, and *CD72*,[267] as well as repression of B-lineage inappropriate genes. In $Pax5^{-/-}$ mice B-cell development is arrested at the $B220^+$ pro-B-cell stage at the stage of V_H to DJ_H rearrangement, although these $Pax5^{-/-}$ pro-B cells maintain pluripotency.[268] PAX5 is a paired box domain (PRD) transcription factor, encoded by the *PAX5* gene at chromosome 9p13, and consists of 10 exons that encode a 391-amino-acid protein. In a recent integrated genomic analysis of 1988 cases of B-ALL spanning all ages, two subtypes involving PAX5 alterations were defined by distinct gene expression profiles. The PAX5-altered (PAX5alt) group comprised 7.4% of B-ALL cases and involved both rearrangements, mutations, and intragenic amplifications of PAX5.[269] Previously, 17 different fusion partners have been documented.[269] In all of the fusion proteins, the Paired box domain DNA-binding region and nuclear localization region are retained but the C-terminal transactivation domain is deleted.[270] Two of the most common *PAX5* fusion genes are *PAX5::ETV6* and *PAX5::FOXP1*.[270] The PAX5 fusion proteins may act as dominant negative molecules in conjunction with the wild-type PAX5 allele and in this way may repress genes whose products are necessary for B-cell differentiation. However, RNA-seq experiments comparing transcriptional targets of PAX5, PAX5::ETV6, and PAX5::FOXP1 demonstrate that only a small number of PAX5 target genes are actually repressed by the PAX5 fusion proteins. Rather, in the case of the fusion protein PAX5::ETV6, the Ets domain of ETV6 and the paired domain of PAX5 may cooperate to provide a distinct set of transcriptional targets. These targets include genes encoding proteins involved in cell migration and adhesion, intracellular signal transducers, and pre-BCR signaling.[270]

A second subtype of B-ALL involving PAX5 alteration but having a distinct gene expression profile is PAX5 p.Pro80Arg, found in 0.2% of B-ALL cases.[269] This mutation at aa80 is in the DNA-binding domain of the PAX5 transcription factor. Signaling pathway alterations are more common in this subset, including mutations in RAS pathway molecules or molecules involved in the JAK/STAT pathway, particularly IL7R.[269] In addition, the PAX5 p.Pro80Arg subtype almost always has biallelic *PAX5* alterations, either deletion of the wild-type *PAX5* allele, loss of heterozygosity, or mutation of the second *PAX5* allele.[269] Both B-ALL subtypes involving PAX5 have similar outcome data and are considered intermediate risk. However, due to the frequent signaling pathway alterations in the PAX5 p.Pro80Arg subtype, use of kinase inhibitors such as ruxolitinib is being considered as a treatment option.[269]

IKZF1

IKZF1 encodes IKAROS, a zinc-finger-containing transcription factor that is required for lymphoid lineage commitment. It is expressed in multipotent, self-renewing HSCs and is necessary for induction of genes important for the lymphoid lineage, as well as repression of genes responsible for self-renewal and multipotency in the differentiating progeny of HSCs[271] (see *Figure 73.14*). The importance of IKAROS in hematopoietic development is underscored by experiments in which $Ikzf1^{DN}$ mice lack all fetal and adult lymphoid cells.[272] *IKZF1* alterations occur in 15% of childhood B-ALL cases overall but are most common in Philadelphia chromosome–positive (Ph^+) B-ALL (70% of cases)[273] as well as Ph-like B-ALL (68% of cases).[274] Even in the poor-risk group of patients with Ph-like ALL, patients with an *IKZF1* mutation had a statistically significant decrease in 5-year event-free survival.[274] Deletions of *IKZF1* are usually of one allele, and the deletion most commonly involves exons 4 to 7.[267] Significantly, exons 4 to 6 encode the four N-terminal C2H2 zinc fingers responsible for DNA binding. Therefore, these deletions result in loss of the DNA-binding domain but preservation of the carboxy-terminal C2H2 zinc fingers responsible for dimerization and multimerization,[275] creating a

Table 73.5. WHO Classification of Precursor Lymphoid Neoplams[22,67]

B-lymphoblastic leukemia/lymphoma
B-lymphoblastic leukemia/lymphoma, not otherwise specified
B-lymphoblastic leukemia/lymphoma with recurrent genetic abnormalities
B-ALL with t(9;22)(q34;q11.2); *BCR::ABL1*
B-ALL with t(v;11q23); *KMT2A (MLL)* rearranged
B-ALL with t(12;21)(p13;q22); *ETV6::RUNX*
B-ALL with t(5;14)(q31;q32); *IL3::IGH*
B-ALL with t(1;19)(q23;p13.3); *TCF3::PBX1*
B-ALL with hyperdiploidy (>50 chromosomes)
B-ALL with hypodiploidy (<46 chromosomes)
B-ALL with iAMP21
B-ALL, *BCR::ABL1*-like
T-lymphoblastic leukemia/lymphoma
T-ALL, not otherwise specified
Early T-precursor ALL

Adapted with permission from Swerdlow SH. *International Agency for Research on Cancer, World Health Organization. WHO Classification of Tumours of Haematopoietic and Lymphoid Tissues*. Revised 4th ed. International Agency for Research on Cancer; 2017:11.

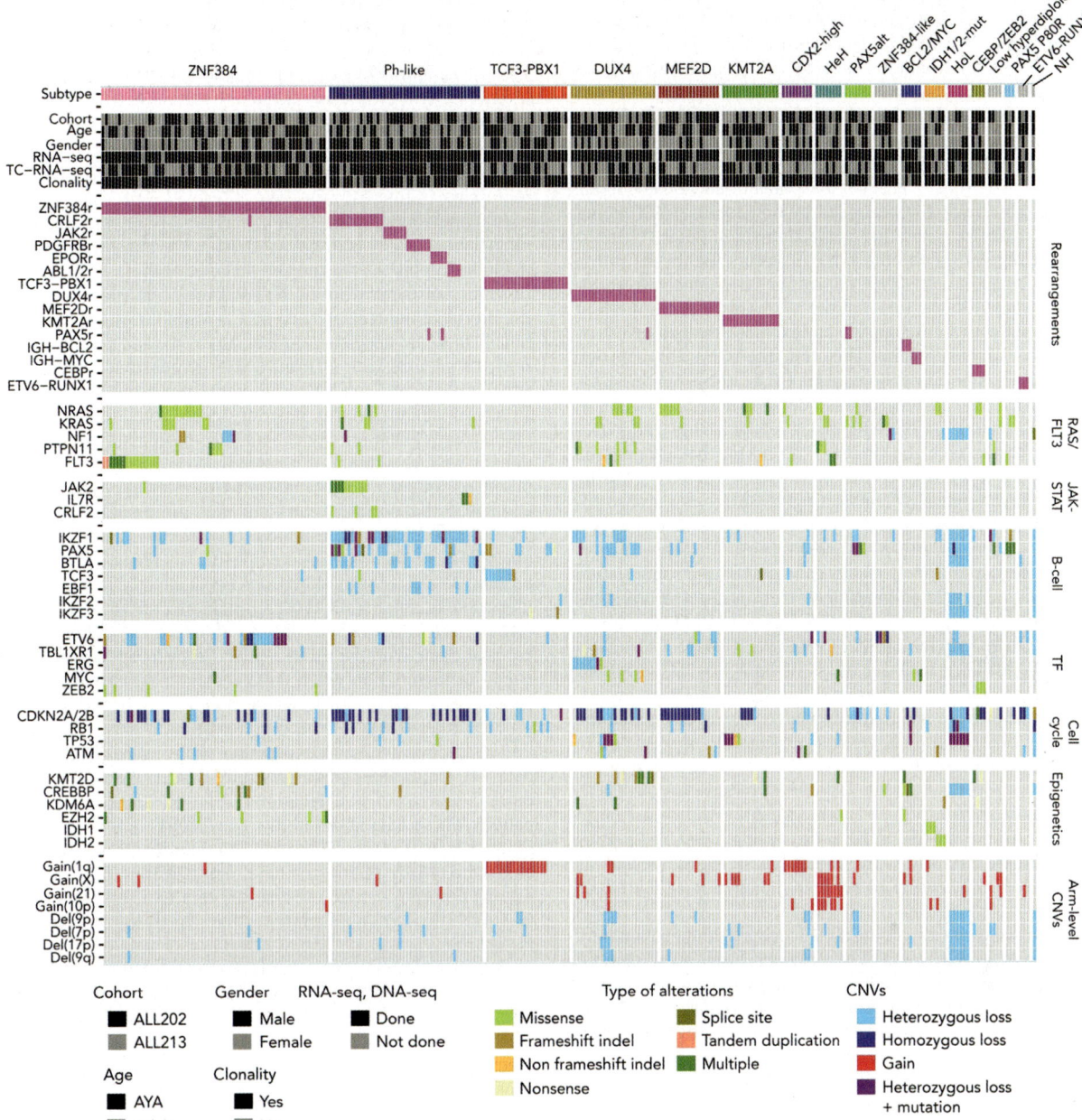

FIGURE 73.13 **B-ALL subtypes defined by RNA-seq and DNA-seq.** B-ALL subtypes were identified in adolescent, young adult, and adult populations (n = 262) by evaluation for genetic alterations (rearrangements, single nucleotide variants [SNVs], indels [insertions/deletions], and CNVs [copy number variants]). Each column represents variants detected in a single patient. Subtypes were defined by characteristic rearrangements (indicated by pink); gross chromosomal alterations (high-hyperdiploid [HeH], low-hypodiploid [HoL], low hyperdiploid, and near-haploid [NH]); mutations (*IDH1/IDH2*, *PAX5P80R*); and gene expression patterns (Cdx2-high, Ph-like, PAX5alt, and ZNF384-like). This particular study identified two new subgroups of B-ALL (CDX2-high and *IDH1/IDH2* mutated). (Adapted from Yasuda T, Sanada M, Kawazu M, et al. Two novel high-risk adult B-cell acute lymphoblastic leukemia subtypes with high expression of CDX2 and IDH1/2 mutations. *Blood*. 2022;139(12):1850-1862. Copyright © 2022 American Society of Hematology. With permission.)

dominant-negative molecule.[276] Gene expression analysis of cultured cells bearing mutations in the fourth zinc finger of *IKZF1* demonstrated upregulation of KIT, which is usually expressed in HSCs but not in mature B cells.[275] In addition, in B-ALL with *IKZF1* mutations, there is downregulation of *RAG* and *EBF1*, two genes whose products are involved in IgH VDJ recombination.[276] Therefore, downregulation of genes involved in normal B-cell differentiation, upregulation of genes expressed in self-renewing HSCs, and alterations in the interaction of the leukemic cells with the bone marrow stroma may all contribute to leukemogenesis in B-ALL with *IKZF1* deletion or mutation.[277]

TCF3(E2A) Translocations

A common translocation in childhood B-ALL, present in 5% of pre-B-ALL cases,[278] is the t(1;19)(q23;p13.3), which fuses the *TCF3* gene on chromosome 19p13.3 with the *PBX1* gene on chromosome 1q23.[266,279] The *TCF3* locus, previously known as *E2A*, encodes three transcripts, E12, E47, and E2-5, which are generated by alternative splicing.[280] They belong to class I of the basic helix-loop-helix (bHLH) family of transcription factors that bind to specific E-box (CANNTG) sequences in promoters and enhancers, the first of which was identified in the enhancer regions of the immunoglobulin heavy-chain and κ-chain genes.[280] Although TCF3 proteins are ubiquitous, they are preferentially expressed in B lymphocytes,[281] and E47 forms homodimers exclusively in B cells.[265] The requirement for TCF3 proteins in B-cell development is demonstrated by $E2a^{-/-}$ null mice, which exhibit a complete block in B-cell differentiation at the pre-pro-B-cell stage prior to immunoglobulin gene rearrangement[282,283] (see Figure 73.14).

PBX1 (Pre-B-cell leukemic homeoboX 1), identified as the fusion partner of TCF3 in t(1;19),[284] encodes a member of the homeodomain family of transcription factors, encoded by homeobox (HOX) genes and forms heterodimers with other homeodomain proteins.[285] In the t(1;19), the breakpoint on chromosome 19 occurs within the intron between exons 13 and 14 of TCF3, so that the N-terminal two-thirds of TCF3 are included in the fusion protein.[279] This includes both of the transcriptional activation domains but excludes the bHLH DNA-binding and dimerization domains. Therefore, the TCF3::PBX1 fusion protein depends on the homeodomain of PBX1 for DNA binding, with the presence of the TCF3 activation domains resulting in abnormally strong transactivation of target genes recognized by the PBX1 homeodomain.[286] One such gene is BMI-1,[287] a gene that is expressed in normal HSCs but whose expression normally decreases during hematopoietic development.[288] Interestingly, BMI-1 is a transcriptional repressor of the INK4A-ARF locus,[287] which encodes the two tumor suppressor genes P16INK4A and P14ARF.[289] Repression of P16INK4A by increased BMI-1 results in increased phosphorylation of Rb, promoting cell cycle progression to the S phase and proliferation.[290,291] The tumor suppressor P14ARF inhibits MDM2, a repressor of TP53[119]; therefore, inhibition of P14ARF by BMI-1 results in repression of TP53. Therefore, activation of BMI-1 by TCF3::PBX1 results in downregulation of two powerful tumor suppressor pathways.

Recent gene expression microarray analysis demonstrates that the kinases ZAP70, LCK, and SYK are transcriptionally upregulated in cells from conditional E2a::Pbx1 transgenic mice as well as primary B-ALL cells from patients with the TCF3::PBX1 translocation. These kinases are upstream from PLCγ2, which demonstrates increased phosphorylation in these TCF3::PBX1-expressing cells. The perturbation of this kinase pathway suggests that kinase inhibitors such as dasatinib are worth considering as possible therapy for TCF3::PBX1 B-ALL.[178]

Another translocation involving TCF3 occurs in approximately 1% of pediatric ALL, t(17;19)(q22;p13), which fuses TCF3 to HLF (hepatic leukemia factor).[292,293] Clinically, these patients are adolescents, they may present with disseminated intravascular coagulation and hypercalcemia, and they usually have a poor prognosis. HLF encodes a transcription factor of the basic leucine zipper (bZIP) family and is not usually expressed in hematopoietic cells.[294]

Core Binding Factors

RUNX1, a transcription factor required for the differentiation of HSCs (see Figure 73.14), is involved in a translocation that is present in 25% of pediatric B-ALL, t(12;21)(p13;q 22).[295] This translocation is associated with a good prognosis, although it is often missed by standard karyotype analysis. In this translocation, the N terminus of ETV6, formerly called TEL (translocation-ETS-leukemia), is fused to most of the coding region of RUNX1.[296] ETV6 acts as a transcriptional repressor.[297] Interestingly, the ETV6::RUNX1 translocation often occurs prenatally during fetal hematopoiesis. In one study of pediatric patients with ETV6::RUNX1 B-ALL, the translocation was present in Guthrie spots (DNA samples taken at birth) in 75% of patients.[298] In studies of twins with the ETV6::RUNX1 translocation, the latency time to development of leukemia is variable, suggesting that additional "hits" are necessary. In fact, an exome and genomic sequencing study of patients with ETV6::RUNX1 demonstrated an average of 11 structural variants and 14 coding point mutations per patient.[299] The structural variants, mostly deletions, were noted to have canonical or partial recombination signal sequence motifs surrounding the deletion, as well as addition of nontemplated sequence.[299] These are hallmarks of somatic recombination by the RAG endonucleases RAG1 and RAG2 that normally carry out VDJ joining in B cells. The majority of the deletions occur in the active promoter and enhancer regions where histone methylation at H3K4me3 is recognized by the RAG2 protein. The structural alterations occur mainly in genes previously identified as mutated in B-ALL, including ETV6, BTG1, TBL1XR1, PAX5, CDKN2A, NR3C2, RAG1, and BTLA.[299] Thus, the original prenatal clone with the ETV6::RUNX1 translocation is stalled in early B-cell differentiation when RAG recombinases are active, resulting in somatic alterations that include B-cell transcription factors such as PAX5, further stalling B-cell differentiation.[299,300]

Comprehensive gene expression profiling based upon RNA-seq data has identified a small group of B-ALL cases that do not have the ETV6::RUNX1 translocation but have a similar gene expression pattern. These data have led to a provisional subtype of B-ALL designated B-ALL with ETV6::RUNX1-like features. These cases are characterized by fusions or deletions in both ETV6 and IKZF1.[301] The ETV6::RUNX1-like subtype appears to also share the CD27^{pos}/CD44$^{low-neg}$ immunophenotype that characterizes ETV6::RUNX1 B-ALL.[302]

Another chromosomal alteration involving the RUNX1 locus that occurs in approximately 2% of pediatric patients with B-ALL is the intrachromosomal amplification of chromosome 21 (iAMP21). This is thought to be initiated by a breakage-fusion-bridge mechanism, creating a dicentric chromosome 21. This unstable structure is then susceptible to chromothripsis, a process of chromosome shattering and

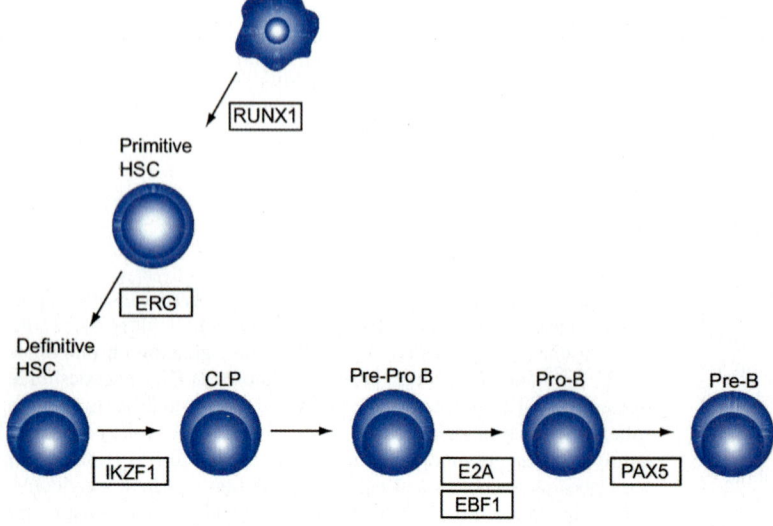

FIGURE 73.14 Normal function of the B-lineage transcription factors affected in B-ALL. The earliest critical function in hematopoiesis of each B-lineage transcription factor is indicated. RUNX1 is required for the emergence of primitive hematopoietic stem cells (HSCs) during development, and ERG is essential for definitive HSC maintenance. IKZF1 expression is necessary for formation of common lymphoid progenitors (CLPs), and E2A and EBF1 are necessary for pro-B cell generation. PAX 5 expression is required for generation of functional pre-B cells and maintaining B-cell identity. (Reprinted by permission from Nature: Tijchon E, Havinga J, van Leeuwen FN, et al. B-lineage transcription factors and cooperating gene lesions required for leukemia development. Leukemia. 2013;27(3):541-552. Copyright © 2012 Springer Nature.)

rearrangement.[303] There is a 6.6-mb common region of amplification (CRA) on chromosome 21 and in the majority of cases an associated 3.3-mb common region of deletion at the telomere. The amplification is usually detected by FISH using the RUNX1 probe and is defined as three or more extra RUNX1 signals on one chromosome, resulting in five or more RUNX1 signals per cell. Although RUNX1 is in the CRA, gene expression studies do not reveal increased transcription of RUNX1. This cytogenetic abnormality is associated with a complex karyotype and multiple mutations; however, clonal analysis indicates that the precipitating genetic event is the iAMP21 amplification.[304] The significance of recognizing this cytogenetic abnormality is that it is associated with a dismal prognosis if treated with standard chemotherapy. However, in recent studies treating these patients with high-risk chemotherapy regimens, there was no significant difference in overall survival.[303]

DUX4

DUX4, encoding a double-homeobox transcription factor, is located in a microsatellite repeat in the subtelomeric repeat unit on the long arm of chromosome 4.[305] Gene expression profiling has identified a subtype of B-ALL characterized by a DUX4::IGH translocation, in which the IGH enhancer drives elevated expression of DUX4. DUX4 is not expressed in normal B cells but is expressed in early embryonic development.[306] In an unusual example of transcriptional deregulation leading to B-ALL, DUX4::IGH translocation is associated with ERG dysregulation. ERG is an ETS-family transcription factor that is involved in normal hematopoietic regulation and has already been associated with T-ALL and AML. The overexpressed DUX4 binds to a DUX4-responsive element in ERG that promotes abnormal transcription of an ERG alt variant that starts from intron 6 of ERG.[305,307] The ERG alt retains the DNA-binding ETS and transactivation domains and acts as a dominant negative inhibitor of wild-type ERG. Further deregulation occurs by frequent deletion of the normal allele, possibly due to RAG-mediated activity.[305] Other mutations are associated with DUX4-rearranged B-ALL, including mutations in IKZF1, but nevertheless this subset of B-ALL has a favorable prognosis.[306]

MEF2D

RNA-seq analysis of 560 patients with B-ALL identified several not previously identified recurring rearrangements, including those involving MEF2D. MEF2D rearrangements, which are usually cryptic, are present in 4.1% of childhood cases (up to age 15 years), 6.5% of adolescent cases (age 16-20 years), and 2.7% of young adult cases.[308] MEF2D::BCL9 and MEF2D::HNRNPUL1 are the most common translocations, with five other fusion partners identified.[308,309] Most of these translocations involving MEF2D at chromosome 1q21-22 are cryptic. MEF2D (myocyte enhancer factor 2D), encoded at chromosome 1q21-22, is a MADS-box-type transcription factor, named for its conserved DNA-binding domain. B-ALL samples harboring any of the translocations involving MEF2D have a similar gene expression profile, thought to be due to the preservation of the amino terminus of the MEF2D protein, which contains the MADS-box in all of the translocations[308]; the role of the 3′ partner gene is unclear at this time. The gene expression profile is notable for downregulation of MEF2C and upregulation of GATA3, as well as HDAC9, a type II histone deacetylase.[308] This group of patients demonstrated additional genetic alterations, including an increased frequency of CDKN2A/CDKN2B deletions. Interestingly, these patients also have a distinct immunophenotype of the blasts, with low CD10 expression, high CD38 expression, cytoplasmic μ chain positivity, and variable expression of CD5.[309]

In mouse studies, Mef2c and Mef2d are highly expressed in B-cell development, as well as in other tissue types.[310] Knock-out experiments demonstrated that $Mef2c^{\Delta\Delta}$ or $Mef2d^{\Delta\Delta}$ mice displayed normal B-cell development, whereas double knock-out mice with deletion of both Mef2c and Mef2d demonstrated block of B-cell development at the pre-B-cell stage. Interestingly, since B-ALL cells with an MEF2D translocation demonstrate marked downregulation of MEF2C, these cells essentially lack normal MEF2D and MEF2C expression, which explains at least in part the block in differentiation in this B-ALL.[310]

It is important to identify patients with the usually cryptic MEF2D translocation, as they have a generally poor prognosis. They tend to be older patients with elevated WBC counts at presentation, a high incidence of relapse, and lack of response to stem cell transplant. As gene expression studies demonstrate elevated expression of HDAC9, an ex vivo study of the effect of HDAC inhibitors on leukemic cells in culture was undertaken and had promising results.[309]

ZNF384

Another class of translocations in B-ALL that are often cryptic involve the ZNF384 gene (zinc-finger protein 384) at chromosome 12p13.31 comprising 5% to 10% of other B leukemias (see Figure 73.13).[311] ZNF384 is also known as nuclear matrix protein 4 (NMP4), which is a regulator of ribosome biogenesis via its transcriptional repressor effect on genes including c-MYC and GADD34.[312] More than 10 fusion partners have been identified with ZNF384 in B-ALL and in B/myeloid mixed phenotype acute leukemia (MPAL).[313] The most commonly reported fusions are TCF3::ZNF384 and EP300::ZNF384; in each case ZNF384 forms the 3′ portion of the fusion and its entire coding region is fused in-frame with the partner gene.[314] This group of B-ALL cases has a characteristic immunophenotype with low expression of CD10 and aberrant expression of CD33 and/or CD13; in fact, this class of cytogenetic abnormality is one of the most commonly seen in B/myeloid MPAL.[314] The clinical characteristics seem to be influenced by the fusion partner, with TCF3::ZNF384-positive patients having a higher frequency of relapse.[314] In addition, cases without a ZNF384 fusion but with a similar transcriptome were found to have mutations affecting the last exon of ZNF384.[311]

CDX2

A recent study of 354 patients ages 15 to 64 years used RNA-seq and whole exome sequencing to further evaluate genetic events that may contribute to the poor outcome of adolescents, young adults, and adults with Ph-negative B-ALL. The study identified two novel high-risk B-ALL subtypes, one of which is characterized by overexpression of CDX2 (see Figure 73.13).[315] CDX2 is a homeobox gene that is normally expressed in early developmental hematopoiesis but not in normal HSCs. It has previously been shown to be expressed in patients with B-ALL with poor prognosis,[316] and it is also overexpressed in the majority of patients with AML. When Cdx2 is overexpressed in murine HSPCs, the Cdx2-transgenic mice develop MDS and progress to AML after acquisition of additional mutations.[317] CDX2 overexpression may not dysregulate other HOX family genes but instead appears to upregulate IGF1R and downregulate IGFBP7, which negatively regulates the IGF1 pathway.[315] There is a high incidence of chromosome 1q gain in the CDX2-high B-ALL subtype.[315]

Kinases

BCR::ABL1

The Philadelphia chromosome is the result of the t(9;22)(q34;q11) in which the 5′ domain of the BCR (breakpoint cluster region) gene from chromosome 22 is fused with the 3′ TKD of the ABL gene from chromosome 9. The Philadelphia chromosome is the resultant shortened chromosome 22. It is the most frequent recurring translocation in adult ALL, occurring in 15% to 30% of patients,[318] and also it is present in 5% of pediatric B-ALL.[319] It has been considered as an adverse prognostic factor in children and adults, although new risk-adapted therapeutic regimens that include tyrosine kinase inhibitors may improve the prognosis.

The BCR::ABL1 fusion gene is associated most commonly with CML. The pathogenesis of CML will be discussed in Chapter 83. A lymphoid blast crisis arising from CML may be difficult to distinguish from a Ph⁺ ALL. The size of the BCR::ABL1 fusion protein and whether it is restricted in expression to lymphoid cells may be helpful in making this distinction. The most common breakpoint region, the major breakpoint cluster region (M-bcr) spans almost 6 kb between exons 12 and 16 of BCR and results in a fusion protein of 210 kD, referred to as p210$^{BCR::ABL1}$.[320] A minor breakpoint, the m-bcr, is farther 5′, after exon 2 of *BCR*, resulting in a truncated fusion protein of 190 kD that contains only the first two exons of *BCR* (p190[BCR::ABL1]).[2] Interestingly, p210[BCR::ABL1] is much more common in CML and CML with lymphoid blast crisis, whereas p190[BCR::ABL1] is much more commonly expressed in Ph+ B-ALL. p190[BCR::ABL1] is present in 80% to 90% of pediatric Ph+ B-ALL and 50% of adult Ph+ B-ALL.[318] However, some cases of Ph+ B-ALL as well as CML contain both p190[BCR::ABL1] and p210[BCR::ABL1], which may be related to alternative splicing. Transgenic mice expressing p190[bcr::abl1] develop an aggressive leukemia restricted to pre–B cells, whereas transgenic mice expressing p210[bcr::abl1] develop a more chronic disease involving B and T cells and myeloid lineages.[321] In some cases of Ph+ B-ALL the aberrant fusion protein is present in lymphoid and myeloid marrow cells, whereas in other cases the aberrant fusion protein, usually p190[BCR::ABL1], is restricted to lymphoid cells. Those cases in which p210[BCR::ABL1] is present in both lymphoid and myeloid cells most likely represent a CML lymphoid blast crisis.[322]

Studies of BCR::ABL1 expression in CML have demonstrated the leukemogenic properties of BCR::ABL1 as a constitutive tyrosine kinase.[323] This constitutive kinase activates by phosphorylation of multiple downstream signal transduction intermediates, including RAS, PLCγ, and PI3 kinase.[324] Activation of these pathways results in proliferation and resistance to apoptosis.[325] Presumably similar mechanisms are at work in Ph+ B-ALL. Restriction of expression of BCR::ABL1 to the lymphoid lineage would explain the development of ALL. However, in those cases of Ph+ B-ALL in which BCR::ABL1 is expressed in the stem cell compartment, it is unclear why B-ALL has resulted instead of CML. A high percentage of Ph+ B-ALL, as well as B lymphoid blast crisis of CML, have concomitant mutations in *IKZF1*, as described above.[276,326,327]

Ph-Like B-ALL

In 2009 a gene expression profiling study of 190 children with newly diagnosed B-ALL demonstrated that 18% of the genetically unclassified cases had a gene expression pattern that clustered with *BCR::ABL1*-positive cases but did not have the *BCR::ABL1* translocation.[263] These patients also had an unfavorable outcome (59.5% 5-year disease-free survival) similar to the *BCR::ABL1*-positive cases. The presence of Ph-like B-ALL was an independent prognostic factor in each age group identified. The frequency of genomic alterations in kinase and cytokine receptor genes, both translocations and point mutations, identified in these patients by NGS was 91%. Subsequent studies have shown that Ph-like B-ALL comprises 10% of children with standard-risk B-ALL and 15% of children with high-risk B-ALL. The frequency increases with age, peaking in the young adult age group at 27% and declining in older patients with B-ALL.[274] Over 60 genetic alterations have been characterized in Ph-like B-ALL, with the common theme of activating cytokine receptor genes and kinase-signaling pathways, providing a therapeutic opportunity of using targeted therapies. The genetic alterations fall into five subgroups: (1) rearrangements of *CRLF* (47% of cases); (2) *ABL*-class gene rearrangements (*ABL1*, *ABL2*, *PDGFRB*, and *CSF1R*); (3) *JAK2* and *EPOR* rearrangements; (4) mutations or deletions activating JAK-STAT or MAPK signaling pathways; and (5) other rarer kinase alterations.[328] Rearrangement of *CRLF2* (discussed below) is the most common genetic alteration in Ph-like B-ALL. It is commonly associated with mutations in *JAK* genes, including the *JAK2* R683G mutation, a mutation different from the canonical *JAK2* V617F mutation and almost always seen in the context of a *CRLF2* aberration.[329] Fusions involving *ABL* genes always preserve the kinase domain, and clinical trials using imatinib and other tyrosine kinase inhibitors are underway.[330] *JAK2* is involved with over 20 different translocation partners, and these translocations preserve the JAK2 kinase domain; therefore, ruxolitinib and other JAK2 inhibitors are treatment possibilities; this class of drug is also being investigated for Ph-like B-ALL with *CRLF2* rearrangements.[331]

The poor prognosis of Ph-like B-ALL and the encouraging possibility of therapeutic agents such as TKIs and ruxolitinib make diagnosis of this subtype of B-ALL of utmost importance. Several different diagnostic approaches are currently in use. The COG uses a low-density microarray approach (LDA) based on the original characterization of this B-ALL subgroup by gene expression profiling. The most common LDA tests for expression of the following 15 genes: *IGJ*, *SPATS2L*, *MUC4*, *CRLF2*, *CA6*, *NRXN3*, *BMPR1B*, *GPR110*, *CHN2*, *SEMA6A*, *PON2*, *SLC2A5*, *S100Z*, *TP53INP1*, and *IFITM1*.[332] This is a screening tool for high-risk B-ALL cases likely to be Ph-like, and further molecular characterization requires additional NGS or RNA-seq evaluation to characterize the translocations involved.

Like Ph-positive B-ALL, concomitant *IKZF1* deletions are common in Ph-like B-ALL and are associated with a poor prognosis. The higher frequency of *IKZF1* deletions and IGH::*CRLF2* translocations in children of Hispanic/Latino background is associated with a higher death rate from B-ALL in this population.[330]

CRLF2

CRLF2 alterations occur in 8% of childhood B-ALL, 15% of high-risk B-ALL, and 15% of adult B-ALL and are generally associated with a worse prognosis, with higher rates of minimal residual disease at the end of induction therapy.[333] The *CRLF2* gene encodes a thymic stromal lymphopoietin receptor (TSLPR) subunit, which dimerizes with IL-7Rα to form the functional TSLPR, which binds the ligand thymic stromal lymphopoietin. *CRLF2* is encoded on Xp22.23 or Yp11.32. The most common structural alterations include translocation with the IGH gene (IGH::*CRLF2*) or an interstitial deletion resulting in a *CRLF2*::*P2RY8* fusion.[334] Both of these translocations result in constitutively active TSLPR. However, a structural translocation involving *CRLF2* accounts for only about half of the patients with high CRLF2 expression.[335] *IKZF1* deletions are associated with B-ALL with high CRLF2 expression; one study found *IKZF1* deletions in 43% of pediatric B-ALL with CRLF2 overexpression, and approximately 80% of Ph-like B-ALL with *CRLF2* rearrangement. As IKAROS binds to the promoter of *CRLF2* and acts as a transcriptional repressor, some mutations of *IKZF1* may abrogate its repressor function and result in overexpression of CRLF2.[18] The constitutive TSLPR activity brought about by the overexpression of CRLF2 activates several downstream signal transduction pathways, including JAK2, STAT4, and the PI3K/mTOR pathway. Therefore, signal transduction inhibitors of these pathways may be useful in treating this subset of high-risk B-ALL.[333]

Epigenetic Regulators

NUTM1

Fusions involving *NUTM1* (nuclear protein in testis midline carcinoma family 1) were identified in a study of 1223 B-ALL cases by RNA-seq, forming a unique gene expression pattern.[264] *NUTM1* fusions are found in 1% to 2% of childhood B-ALL and involve six different 5′ partners. The 3′ *NUTM1* fusion maintains most of its coding region, and increased expression of NUTM1 results. NUTM1 is usually expressed in the testis, and the gene has been implicated in fusions in nonhematopoietic tumors such as NUT midline carcinoma.[336] In this carcinoma, the BRD4-NUT fusion protein has been shown to recruit EP300, a histone acetyltransferase, to regions of chromatin, thereby activating them. Targets of activation have been shown to include proproliferative genes such as *MYC*.[336] In the B-ALL gene expression study,[264] the *NUTM1* fusion was associated with increased expression of *ZYG11A*, *HOXA9*, and genes in the NOTCH pathway. The possibility of treatment with HDAC inhibitors is being considered due to what is known about the function of NUTM1.[337]

IDH1/IDH2 Mutations

In the previously discussed study of high risk subtypes that may contribute to the poor outcome of adolescents, young adults, and adults with Ph-negative B-ALL, a small number of patients with poor outcomes were found to have *IDH1* and *IDH2* mutations (see *Figure 73.13*). As previously discussed, mutations in *IDH1* and *IDH2* result in production of 2-HG, which inhibits TET2 activity and results in increased methylation. In the *IDH1/IDH2*-mut subtype of B-ALL, aberrant DNA methylation of several genes was noted, including *ZEB2* and *MEF2C*, which may inhibit B-cell differentiation.[315]

T-LYMPHOBLASTIC LEUKEMIA/LYMPHOMA

Introduction

T-ALL is an uncommon acute leukemia but its genetics has been studied in considerable depth. The driver mutations in T-ALL were first identified by cloning the breakpoints at chromosomal translocations commonly found in T-ALL, often revealing oncogenes whose expression was deregulated by rearrangement with the promoters and enhancers of T-cell receptor genes.[338-341] Subsequently, it was shown that these same oncogenes may be overexpressed by mechanisms other than translocation.[19,342-345] Indeed, gene expression clustering based on these oncogene signatures has been highly informative in classifying T-ALL into distinct subtypes that relate to the cell of origin.[19,20,346] Whole exome sequencing and targeted sequencing have revealed numerous additional important mutations in T-ALL. As shown in Table 73.6, these oncogenes and tumor suppressor genes are divided into major gene classes. The *CDKN2A* locus encodes cell cycle regulatory genes, *P14ARF* and *P16INK4A*, and is the most commonly inactivated gene in human T-ALL.[338] *CDKN2A* is located on 9p21, which in one study of pediatric T-ALL showed homozygous deletion in 70% of patients.[267,341,347] *CDKN2A* is also inactivated by other mechanisms.[348,349] Deletions of 13q14.2, which include the *RB1* gene, occur in up to 12% of patients with T-ALL [267]; these deletions are found in patients with intact *CDKN2A*, an expected finding since both of these tumor suppressors act in the same pathway.[19,350] In addition, whole genome sequencing has characterized mutations that predominate in a particularly aggressive form of T-ALL, early T-cell precursor ALL (ETP-ALL).[351]

Transcription Factors

NOTCH1

The NOTCH pathway is mutated in the majority of patients with T-ALL. NOTCH1 is a regulatory protein that is important in many cell fate decisions, including commitment to T-cell lineage and choice of αβ lineage.[352-354] Uncommitted lymphoid precursors that enter the thymus from the bone marrow express the NOTCH1 receptor and are stimulated by the NOTCH ligand Delta-like 4 that is on the thymic epithelial cells in the thymic cortex. This activation of NOTCH1 promotes T-cell differentiation.[355] *NOTCH1* was first cloned from a t(7;9)(q34;q34) occurring in a patient with T-ALL that involved *NOTCH1* on chromosome 9q34 and the T-cell receptor β-chain gene on chromosome 7q34.[356] The t(7;9) turned out to be rare in T-ALL, but targeted sequencing revealed that over 60% of patients with T-ALL had activating mutations in *NOTCH1*.[357] NOTCH1 is synthesized as a single polypeptide protein that is cleaved in the Golgi at site S1 into two subunits, the ligand-binding N^{EC} (extracellular) and N^{TM} (transmembrane), which bind noncovalently at the heterodimerization domain. Upon ligand binding to N^{EC}, N^{TM} is cleaved at site S2 by a metalloprotease and cleaved at S3 by regulated intramembrane proteolysis catalyzed by a multiprotein enzyme, the gamma (γ) secretase (see Figure 73.15A).[358] The remaining intracellular portion, ICN1, translocates to the nucleus where it acts as a transcriptional regulator with the DNA-binding protein CSL and with coactivators of the Mastermind-like family (MAML).[359] The majority of the activating mutations in *NOTCH1* found in T-ALL occur in the heterodimerization domain or in the PEST domain (Figure 73.15B-G).[357] The PEST domain regulates the turnover of NOTCH1. Therefore, the heterodimerization domain mutants uncouple NOTCH1 activation from ligand binding and the PEST domain mutants increase NOTCH1 protein stability.[357] The NOTCH1/CSL complex has numerous transcriptional targets that affect diverse pathways required for cell transformation; among these *MYC* and *HES1* appear to be important for T-cell leukemogenesis.[360-363] The *FBXW7* gene is mutated in T-ALL and fits into the NOTCH pathway since it encodes a component of a multiprotein E3 ubiquitin ligase (SCF complex) that targets NOTCH1, MYC, and CCNE1 proteins for degradation.[364-366] Inactivating mutations in *FBXW7* are present in 9% to 16% of patients with T-ALL and are frequently mutually exclusive with *NOTCH1* mutations.[367,368] The unique proteolytic pathway leading to activated NOTCH1 can be targeted by small molecule inhibitors of the gamma secretase enzyme that is required for S3 cleavage.[369-371] Gamma secretase inhibitors have been in clinical testing for T-ALL but have induced significant gut toxicity due to the inhibition of NOTCH1 and NOTCH2 in intestinal epithelial cells causing them to assume a secretory phenotype.[372,373] Anti-NOTCH1 antibodies and inhibitors of downstream signaling intermediates are also under investigation as potential directed therapies.[355]

TAL1/SCL and LMO Factors

Class B bHLH transcription factors, *TAL1/SCL* (T-cell acute lymphoblastic leukemia 1/stem cell leukemia), *TAL2*, *LYL1*, and *OLIG2* are frequently deregulated in T-ALL.[341] The *TAL1/SCL* gene is deregulated in 30% of pediatric and 34% of adult T-ALL.[374] *TAL1* was originally cloned from a translocation, t(1;14)(p34;q11), present in 3% of patients with T-ALL.[375] In the translocation, the breakpoint is 5′ to the coding region of *TAL1/SCL* on chromosome 1, and the translocation places *TAL1/SCL* under the regulation of the T-cell receptor α/β gene on chromosome 14.[376,377] A second series of rearrangements that occur in 26% of patients with T-ALL result in deletion of 90 to 100 kb of DNA from the 5′ upstream region of *TAL1/SCL*, placing the gene under the control of the upstream constitutively active *SIL* promoter.[378] In both cases, the coding region of *TAL1/SCL* is intact, unlike the fusion proteins that are products of many translocations that occur in acute leukemias. Also, in some cases of T-ALL overexpression of TAL1/SCL occurs without gene rearrangement but by mutation in regulatory sequences.[379]

During development, TAL1/SCL is expressed in early hematopoietic elements, in both the yolk sac blood islands and the definitive blood cells of the AGM region and fetal liver.[380] Postnatally, it is expressed in erythroid, megakaryocyte, and mast cell lineages but not in T cells. In nonerythroid cells, TAL1/SCL is expressed in stem cells but is not expressed as the cells differentiate; however, in erythroid cells, TAL1 expression increases with early erythroid differentiation but decreases with terminal differentiation.[381] The essential role of *TAL1/SCL* in hematopoietic development is demonstrated in knockout mice where embryonic lethality occurs due to a total deficiency in hematopoietic progenitors.[382,383] Conditional gene targeting experiments using the Cre-lox system to delete *Tal1/Scl* in adult mice demonstrate that continued expression of TAL1/SCL is necessary for

Table 73.6. Functional Classes of Genes Mutated in T-Lymphoblastic Leukemia/Lymphoma

Gene Class	Gene Names
Cell cycle genes	*CDKN1B*, **CDKN2A**, **CDKN2B**, *RB1*, *TP53*
Notch and its targets	**NOTCH1**, *FBXW7*, *MYC*
Transcription factors	
BHLH and partners	*TAL1*, *TAL2*, *LYL1*, *OLIG2*, *LMO1-3*
Homeobox genes	*TLX1*, *TLX3*, *HOXA* cluster, *KMT2A (MLL)*, *CALM*
Others	*BCL11B*, *ETV6*, *GATA3*, *LEF1*, *MYB*, *RUNX1*, *WT1*, **PHF6**
Cytokine and signal transduction	*ABL1*, *FLT3*, *IL7R*, *JAK1*, *JAK3*, *LCK*, *NRAS*, *KRAS*, *IGF1R*, *DNM2*, *PI3KCA*, *PETN*, *PTPN2*, *STAT5B*
Chromatin modifiers	*DNMT3A*, *EZH2*, *EED*, *SUZ12*, *KDM6*, *UTX*
Translation and RNA stability	*CNOT3*, *mTOR*, *RPL10*, *RPS5*, *RPL11*

Genes expressed at a frequency of greater than or equal to 5% in pediatric and/or adult T-ALL were included. Genes in bold type are expressed at a frequency of greater than 25%.

Based upon Girardi T, Vicente C, Cools J, De Keersmaecker. The genetics and molecular biology of T-ALL. *Blood*. 2017;129:1113-1123; Gianni F, Belver L, Ferrando A. The genetics and mechanisms of T-cell acute lymphoblastic leukemia. *Cold Spring Harb Perspect Med*. 2020;10(3):a035246.

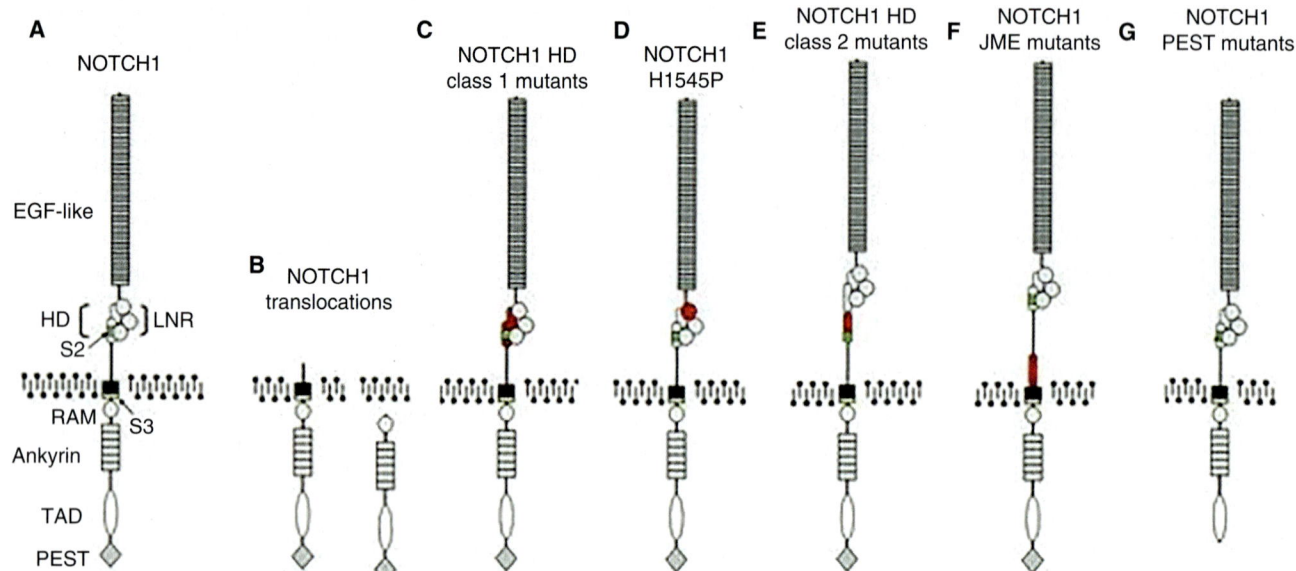

FIGURE 73.15 NOTCH1 mutations in T-ALL. A, Structure of the wild-type NOTCH1 receptor, with the functional domains identified as follows: EGF-like, EGF-like repeats; HD, heterodimerization domain; LNR, LNR repeats; RAM, RAM domain; Ankyrin, ankyrin repeats; TAD, transactivation domain; PEST, PEST domain. S2, metalloprotease cleavage site, and S3, g-secretase cleavage site, which is just interior to the transmembrane domain, depicted as a small black rectangle. B-G, *NOTCH1* mutations highlighted in red and their relationship to the functional domains. (Used with permission of American Society of Hematology from Ferrando AA. The role of NOTCH1 signaling in T-ALL. *Hematology Am Soc Hematol Educ Program.* 2009:353-361; permission conveyed through Copyright Clearance Center, Inc.)

erythrocyte and megakaryocyte differentiation but is not necessary for maintenance of HSCs.[384] Interestingly, the combined *Tal1/Lyl1* knockout revealed loss of hematopoiesis due to apoptosis, which could be rescued by *Lyl1* but not *Tal1*.[385]

TAL1/SCL, like LYL1, OLIG2, and TAL2, binds E box sequences in DNA by heterodimerizing with the class A bHLH transcription factor TCF3 (E2A), TCF4 (E2.2), or TCF12 (HEB). Tandem E boxes or E box GATA sequences can be bound by two TAL1/E2A heterodimers that are bridged by LIM domain Only 1 or 2 (LMO1/LMO2) proteins bound to LIM domain–binding protein 1 (LDB1).[386] Interestingly, *LMO1-3* genes are also important drivers of T-ALL, which can be deregulated by chromosomal rearrangements with T-cell receptor genes and other mechanisms.[387-389] Other TAL1 protein partners include GATA1 (erythroid progenitors), LDB1, coactivators p300 and pCAF, and corepressors mSin3A and HDAC1.[390,391] Interestingly, LMO2 can be coimmunoprecipitated with TAL1 from T-ALL cell lines,[392] and mice overexpressing both Tal1 and Lmo2 develop T-ALL with shorter latency than transgenic mice overexpressing either gene alone, providing evidence for cooperativity.[393-395] Studies suggest that TAL1 and LMO oncoproteins act in multisubunit complexes that are stabilized by LDB1.[396,397] Some transcriptional targets of activation or repression by TAL1/SCL have been identified in T-ALL.[398-401] Alternatively, TAL1 may act as a dominant negative inhibitor of the E2A transcription factors.[402,403] Human and murine T-ALLs induced by bHLH or *LMO* gene overexpression show repression of *TCF3* target genes.[404] LYL1, OLIG2, and TAL2 may all behave similar to TAL1 in that they cooperate with LMO proteins to regulate gene expression, although LYL1-overexpressing T-ALLs are more immature in the T-cell differentiation hierarchy than TAL1-overexpressing T-ALLs.[351,405-407] The expression of these bHLH genes was quantified in a large panel of T-ALLs showing mutually exclusive expression patterns, which also argues for functional redundancy in leukemia pathogenesis. Interestingly, LYL1 and TAL1 are also functionally redundant in the maintenance of adult hematopoietic stem and progenitor cells.[19,385]

Homeodomain Proteins

The homeobox genes are a major group of genes deregulated in T-ALL, mutually exclusive to the bHLH genes and LMO genes discussed above.[19] *TLX1* (*HOX11*) is overexpressed by chromosomal rearrangement or other mechanisms in 8% of pediatric and 20% of adult T-ALL.[374,408,409] *TLX3* (*HOX11L2*) is deregulated most commonly by a t(5;14)(q35;q32) in 19% of pediatric and 9% of adult T-ALL cases.[374,410,411] Finally, the *HOXA* gene cluster is deregulated in 5% of T-ALL cases by inv(7)(p15q34) and other transcriptional mechanisms.[412-414] TLX1-overexpressing T-ALLs have a distinctive block at the cortical stage of T-cell differentiation. Data from experiments using transgenic mice overexpressing TLX1 show that the protein may repress mitotic checkpoint genes, leading to aneuploidy, and may disrupt the normal factors needed for T-cell receptor α rearrangement.[415,416] *KMT2A* and its fusion partners *PICALM* and *AF10* are rearranged and overexpressed in 5% to 10% of T-ALL cases and may function by deregulating the expression of the *HOXA* gene cluster.[414,417-419]

Other transcription factors mutated in T-ALL include the *MYB* oncogene, which is duplicated in 8.4% of T-ALL cases as analyzed by array CGH and fiber FISH studies.[420,421] Array CGH, SNP arrays, and sequencing revealed deletion or missense mutation in the *BCL11B* gene in 9% of patients with T-ALL.[422] *Bcl11b* knockout mice show major defects in T-cell differentiation consistent with a role in T-cell progenitor transformation.[423]

Kinases

IL7R

T-ALL, like most acute leukemias, harbors mutations predominantly in transcription factors. These proteins are difficult therapeutic targets in comparison with cytokine receptors and signal transducing tyrosine kinases. Mutations in the latter group of genes are also involved in T-ALL pathogenesis as revealed by NGS studies. For example, gain-of-function mutations in the *IL7R* gene have been described in 5% to 10% of patients with T-ALL.[351,424,425] IL-7 signaling is necessary for normal T-cell development.[374] Some of the missense substitutions in *IL7R* introduce a cysteine residue in place of the wild-type amino acid in the JM domain. This creates a disulfide bond linking two receptors, resulting in constitutive phosphorylation of STAT5 and other downstream substrates.[425] The IL7R protein utilizes the nonreceptor tyrosine kinases JAK1 and JAK3 for signal transduction, and these too are mutated in 5% to 10% of T-ALL cases.[329,351,426,427] Activating mutations in *IL7R*, *JAK1*, *JAK3*, and/or *STAT5* are found in 20% to 30% of patients with T-ALL.[374] The presence of mutations in the JAK/STAT pathway has spurred preclinical studies evaluating the efficacy of using inhibitors such as ruxolitinib to treat T-ALL and overcome IL-7-induced glucocorticoid resistance.[428]

ETP-ALL

Mutations in signaling pathways are more common in ETP-ALL.[351,406] In contrast, *NOTCH1* mutations are less frequent in ETP-ALL cases.[351] ETP-ALL is derived from early T-cell precursors (DN1) that retain a degree of pluripotency.[429] They are defined by the following immunophenotype determined by flow cytometry: CD1a-, CD8-, CD5(negative to dim), positive for cytoplasmic CD3, negative for MPO, and positive for one or more stem cell or myeloid antigens (e.g., CD13, CD33, CD34, CD117, CD11b).[406,430] ETP-ALL comprises 11% to 12% of childhood T-ALL and 7.4% of adult T-ALL.[429] Whole genome sequencing has demonstrated a relative increase in mutations in cytokine receptor and Ras signaling genes (67%), inactivating mutations in genes disrupting T-cell development (58%), and mutations in histone-modifying genes (48%).[351] In addition, in a mutational analysis of adult ETP-ALL a higher rate of *DNMT3A* mutations (16%) was noted compared with normal T-ALL. The transcriptional profile is similar to myeloid HSCs. The ETP-ALL subtype has a worse prognosis than non-ETP-ALL when treated with conventional chemotherapy, although these numbers vary widely between series.[429] However, the prevalence of mutations in genes involved in signal transduction and in epigenetics implies that targeted therapies such as kinase inhibitors, demethylating agents, and histone deacetylase inhibitors may have a role in treatment of ETP-ALL.[431]

Epigenetic Factors Modifying Chromatin and DNA

DNMT3A and PRC2 Complex

A recent survey of mutations in epigenetic regulatory genes in pediatric cancer demonstrated that 56% of T-ALL cases have mutations in chromatin-modifying genes.[432] Mutations in *DNMT3A* have been identified in up to 18% of T-ALL.[433] Mutations in three core members of the polycomb repressive complex 2 (PRC2), *EZH2*, *SUZ12*, and *EED*, are detected in pediatric and adult T-ALL. The PRC2 complex causes H3K27me3 histone modification, which represses transcription. The *EZH2* and *SUZ12* mutations that occur in T-ALL are loss-of-function mutations, suggesting that the PRC2 has a tumor suppressor role in T-ALL. Interestingly, analysis of the transcriptional targets of NOTCH1 demonstrates that NOTCH1 binding to target genes such as *HES1* and *DTX1* is associated with reduced H3K27me3 in the promoters of those target genes.[434] Therefore, mutation of genes involved in the PRC2 complex would potentiate the leukemogenic effects of NOTCH1.

PHF6

An additional gene that is mutated in up to 30% of adult T-ALL cases[374] (see *Table 73.6*) is the plant homeodomain finger protein 6 (*PHF6*) gene, which is a chromatin adaptor protein. It contains two zinc finger domains (PZP/ZaP), two nuclear localization sequences, and a nucleolar localization sequence; as the latter suggest, it is localized in the nucleus and nucleolus. The PZP/ZaP domains are usually found in proteins that are involved in transcriptional regulation and chromatin modification. PHF6 has been shown to copurify with proteins that comprise the Nucleosome Remodeling and Deacetylation (NuRD) complex. In addition, it interacts with members of the PAF1 complex, which controls transcriptional elongation. One study has demonstrated that PHF6 binds to the *NOTCH1* and *RUNX1* promoters, which may be relevant to the role of mutant PHF6 in leukemogenesis. In addition, PHF6 is thought to participate in ribosome biogenesis, a function that correlates with its localization in the nucleolus.[435]

SUMMARY

This chapter has reviewed the major molecular genetic aberrations found in acute leukemias with a focus on well-known translocations as well as recently uncovered genomic landscapes made possible by rapid advances in NGS-based testing technologies and data analysis platforms. The function of the fusion proteins encoded by the translocated genes and the function of genes that are common sites of point mutations or deletions in acute leukemia are reviewed in the context of current understanding of the pathogenesis of leukemia, implications for novel targeted therapy, and prognosis. A fundamental theme has been alteration of transcriptional regulation. Study of the aberrant transcription factors resulting from translocations and mutations and epigenetic studies based on novel recently available technologies has increased our understanding of the importance of histone modification and DNA methylation in transcriptional regulation and chromatin organization. This knowledge has led to the development of demethylases and histone deacetylases as novel therapies. Study of mutated tyrosine kinases present in leukemia led to the first specifically engineered kinase inhibitor for the therapy of CML and Ph+ ALL. Kinase inhibitors have also been developed for the relatively common mutant FLT3 protein present in AML as well as for other less common kinase alterations, although appearance of subclones with mutations in the targeted kinases and in alternative signal transduction genes have made this avenue of treatment more difficult than originally thought. This is a truly exciting time for hematologic oncology, where discovery of genomic complexity and novel genomic lesions made possible by rapidly developing high-throughput genome interrogation technologies is helping with elucidation of the pathogenesis of acute leukemia, better risk stratification, and development of novel targeted therapeutic agents. Given the amount and the rate of the new genomic data generation in acute leukemias, a major challenge will be continued development of robust, user-friendly bioinformatics-based data analysis platforms with which to evaluate the new data. In addition, ongoing hypothesis-driven research undoubtedly will lead to increased understanding of leukemia pathogenesis and expansion of available effective targeted treatment strategies.

References

1. Nowell PC, Hungerford DA. A minute chromosome in human chronic granulocytic leukemia. *Science*. 1960;132:1497.
2. Kurzrock R, Shtalrid M, Romero P, et al. A novel c-abl protein product in Philadelphia-positive acute lymphoblastic leukaemia. *Nature*. 1987;325(6105):631-635.
3. Druker BJ, Talpaz M, Resta DJ, etal. Efficacy and safety of a specific inhibitor of the BCR-ABL tyrosine kinase in chronic myeloid leukemia. *N Engl J Med*. 2001;344(14):1031-1037.
4. Coombs CC, Tallman MS, Levine RL. Molecular therapy for acute myeloid leukaemia. *Nat Rev Clin Oncol*. 2016;13(5):305-318. doi:10.1038/nrclinonc.2015.210
5. Schlenk RF, Kayser S, Bullinger L, et al. Differential impact of allelic ratio and insertion site in FLT3-ITD-positive AML with respect to allogeneic transplantation. *Blood*. 2014;124(23):3441-3449.
6. Pratcorona M, Brunet S, Nomdedeu J, et al. Favorable outcome of patients with acute myeloid leukemia harboring a low-allelic burden FLT3-ITD mutation and concomitant NPM1 mutation: relevance to post-remission therapy. *Blood*. 2013;121(14):2734-2738. doi:10.1182/blood-2012-06-431122
7. Gale RE, Green C, Allen C, et al. The impact of FLT3 internal tandem duplication mutant level, number, size, and interaction with NPM1 mutations in a large cohort of young adult patients with acute myeloid leukemia. *Blood*. 2008;111(5):2776-2784. doi:10.1182/blood-2007-08-109090
8. Breems DA, Van Putten WLJ, De Greef GE, et al. Monosomal karyotype in acute myeloid leukemia: a better indicator of poor prognosis than a complex karyotype. *J Clin Oncol*. 2008;26(29):4791-4797. doi:10.1200/jco.2008.16.0259
9. Kelly LM, Gilliland DG. Genetics of myeloid leukemias. *Annu Rev Genom Hum Genet*. 2002;3:179-198.
10. Hanahan D, Weinberg RA. Hallmarks of cancer: the next generation. *Cell*. 2011;144(5)(5):646-674.
11. Hanahan D, Weinberg RA. The hallmarks of cancer. *Cell*. 2000;100(1):57-70.
12. Campbell PJ, Stephens PJ, Pleasance ED, et al. Identification of somatically acquired rearrangements in cancer using genome-wide massively parallel paired-end sequencing. *Nat Genet*. 2008;40(6):722-729.
13. Meyerson M, Gabriel S, Getz G. Advances in understanding cancer genomes through second-generation sequencing. *Nat Rev Genet*. 2010;11(10):685-696. doi:10.1038/nrg2841
14. Bamshad MJ, Ng SB, Bigham AW, et al. Exome sequencing as a tool for Mendelian disease gene discovery. *Nat Rev Genet*. 2011;12(11):745-755. doi:10.1038/nrg3031
15. Ng SB, Bigham AW, Buckingham KJ, et al. Exome sequencing identifies MLL2 mutations as a cause of Kabuki syndrome. *Nat Genet*. 2010;42(9):790-793. doi:10.1038/ng.646
16. Wang Z, Gerstein M, Snyder M. RNA-Seq: a revolutionary tool for transcriptomics. *Nat Rev Genet*. 2009;10(1):57-63. doi:10.1038/nrg2484
17. Mortazavi A, Williams BA, McCue K, Schaeffer L, Wold B. Mapping and quantifying mammalian transcriptomes by RNA-Seq. *Nat Methods*. 2008;5(7):621-628.

18. Alizadeh AA, Eisen MB, Davis RE, et al. Distinct types of diffuse large B-cell lymphoma identified by gene expression profiling. *Nature*. 2000;403(6769):503-511.
19. Ferrando AA, Neuberg DS, Staunton J, et al. Gene expression signatures define novel oncogenic pathways in T cell acute lymphoblastic leukemia. *Cancer Cell*. 2002;1(1):75-87.
20. Yeoh EJ, Ross ME, Shurtleff SA, et al. Classification, subtype discovery, and prediction of outcome in pediatric acute lymphoblastic leukemia by gene expression profiling. *Cancer Cell*. 2002;1(2):133-143.
21. Rautenstrauss BW, Liehr T. *FISH Technology. Springer Lab Manual*. x. Springer; 2002:494.
22. Bullinger L, Frohling S. Array-based cytogenetic approaches in acute myeloid leukemia: clinical impact and biological insights. *Semin Oncol*. 2012;39(1):37-46. doi:10.1053/j.seminoncol.2011.11.005
23. Gresham D, Dunham MJ, Botstein D. Comparing whole genomes using DNA microarrays. *Nat Rev Genet*. 2008;9(4):291-302. doi:10.1038/nrg2335
24. Gondek LP, Tiu R, O'Keefe CL, Sekeres MA, Theil KS, Maciejewski JP. Chromosomal lesions and uniparental disomy detected by SNP arrays in MDS, MDS/MPD, and MDS-derived AML. *Blood*. 2008;111(3):1534-1542. doi:10.1182/blood-2007-05-092304
25. Tiu RV, Gondek LP, O'Keefe CL, et al. Prognostic impact of SNP array karyotyping in myelodysplastic syndromes and related myeloid malignancies. *Blood*. 2011;117(17):4552-4560.
26. Godley LA, Cunningham J, Dolan ME, et al. An integrated genomic approach to the assessment and treatment of acute myeloid leukemia. *Semin Oncol*. 2011;38(2):215-224.
27. Grimwade D, Mrozek K. Diagnostic and prognostic value of cytogenetics in acute myeloid leukemia. *Hematol Oncol Clin North Am*. 2011;25(6):1135-1161, vii. doi:10.1016/j.hoc.2011.09.018
28. Rowley JD. Chromosomes in leukemia and beyond: from irrelevant to central players. *Annu Rev Genom Hum Genet*. 2009;10:1-18. doi:10.1146/annurev-genom-082908-150144
29. O'Keefe C, McDevitt MA, Maciejewski JP. Copy neutral loss of heterozygosity: a novel chromosomal lesion in myeloid malignancies. *Blood*. 2010;115(14):2731-2739. doi:10.1182/blood-2009-10-201848
30. Stirewalt DL, Pogosova-Agadjanyan EL, Tsuchiya K, Joaquin J, Meshinchi S. Copy-neutral loss of heterozygosity is prevalent and a late event in the pathogenesis of FLT3/ITD AML. *Blood Cancer J*. 2014;4:e208. doi:10.1038/bcj.2014.27
31. Marth GT, Yu F, Indap AR, et al. The functional spectrum of low-frequency coding variation. *Genome Biol*. 2011;12(9):R84. doi:10.1186/gb-2011-12-9-r84
32. Lander ES. Initial impact of the sequencing of the human genome. *Nature*. 2011;470(7333):187-197. doi:10.1038/nature09792
33. McCarroll SA. Copy number variation and human genome maps. *Nat Genet*. 2010;42(5):365-366. doi:10.1038/ng0510-365
34. Sebat J, Lakshmi B, Troge J, et al. Large-scale copy number polymorphism in the human genome. *Science*. 2004;305(5683):525-528. doi:10.1126/science.1098918
35. Sachidanandam R, Weissman D, Schmidt SC, et al. A map of human genome sequence variation containing 1.42 million single nucleotide polymorphisms. *Nature*. 2001;409(6822):928-933
36. International Human Genome Sequencing Consortium. Finishing the euchromatic sequence of the human genome. *Nature*. 2004;431(7011):931-945. doi:10.1038/nature03001
37. Lander ES, Linton LM, Birren B, et al. Initial sequencing and analysis of the human genome. *Nature*. 2001;409(6822):860-921. doi:10.1038/35057062
38. Venter JC, Adams MD, Myers EW, et al. The sequence of the human genome. *Science*. 2001;291(5507):1304-1351. doi:10.1126/science.1058040
39. Wetterstrand KA. *DNA Sequencing Costs: Data from the NHGRI Genome Sequencing Program (GSP)*; 2021.
40. Shendure J, Porreca GJ, Reppas NB, et al. Accurate multiplex polony sequencing of an evolved bacterial genome. *Science*. 2005;309(5741):1728-1732. doi:10.1126/science.1117389
41. Metzker ML. Sequencing technologies: the next generation. *Nat Rev Genet*. 2010;11(1):31-46.
42. Grossman RL, Heath AP, Ferretti V, et al. Toward a shared vision for cancer genomic data. *N Engl J Med*. 2016;375(12):1109-1112. doi:10.1056/NEJMp1607591
43. Zhang Z, Hernandez K, Savage J, et al. Uniform genomic data analysis in the NCI genomic data commons. *Nat Commun*. 2021;12(1):1226. doi:10.1038/s41467-021-21254-9
44. Heath AP, Ferretti V, Agrawal S, et al. The NCI genomic data commons. *Nat Genet*. 2021;53(3):257-262. doi:10.1038/s41588-021-00791-5
45. Baylin SB, Jones PA. A decade of exploring the cancer epigenome - biological and translational implications. *Nat Rev Cancer*. 2011;11(10):726-734. doi:10.1038/nrc3130
46. Esteller M. Cancer epigenomics: DNA methylomes and histone-modification maps. *Nat Rev Genet*. 2007;8(4):286-298. doi:10.1038/nrg2005
47. Kent OA, Mendell JT. A small piece in the cancer puzzle: microRNAs as tumor suppressors and oncogenes. *Oncogene*. 2006;25(46):6188-6196. doi:10.1038/sj.onc.1209913
48. Harries LW. Long non-coding RNAs and human disease. *Biochem Soc Trans*. 2012;40(4):902-906. doi:10.1042/BST20120020.
49. Roadmap Epigenomics Consortium, Kundaje A, Meuleman W, et al. Integrative analysis of 111 reference human epigenomes. *Nature*. 2015;518(7539):317-330. doi:10.1038/nature14248.
50. Schmitt AD, Hu M, Ren B. Genome-wide mapping and analysis of chromosome architecture. *Nat Rev Mol Cell Biol*. 2016;17(12):743-755. doi:10.1038/nrm.2016.104
51. Krijger PHL, de Laat W. Regulation of disease-associated gene expression in the 3D genome. *Nat Rev Mol Cell Biol*. 2016;17(12):771-782. doi:10.1038/nrm.2016.138
52. Ley TJ, Mardis ER, Ding L, et al. DNA sequencing of a cytogenetically normal acute myeloid leukaemia genome. *Nature*. 2008;456(7218):66-72.
53. Mardis ER, Ding L, Dooling DJ, et al. Recurring mutations found by sequencing an acute myeloid leukemia genome. *N Engl J Med*. 2009;361(11):1058-1066.
54. Ley TJ, Ding L, Walter MJ, et al. DNMT3A mutations in acute myeloid leukemia. *N Engl J Med*. 2010;363(25):2424-2433.
55. Cancer Genome Atlas Research Network; Ley TJ, Miller C, et al. Genomic and epigenomic landscapes of adult de novo acute myeloid leukemia. *N Engl J Med*. 2013;368(22):2059-2074. doi:10.1056/NEJMoa1301689.
56. Chen SJ, Shen Y, Chen Z. A panoramic view of acute myeloid leukemia. *Nat Genet*. 2013;45(6):586-587.
57. Patel JP, Gonen M, Figueroa ME, et al. Prognostic relevance of integrated genetic profiling in acute myeloid leukemia. *N Engl J Med*. 2012;366(12):1079-1089.
58. Shih AH, Abdel-Wahab O, Patel JP, Levine RL. The role of mutations in epigenetic regulators in myeloid malignancies. *Nat Rev Cancer*. 2012;12(9):599-612. doi:10.1038/nrc3343
59. Steensma DP, Bejar R, Jaiswal S, et al. Clonal hematopoiesis of indeterminate potential and its distinction from myelodysplastic syndromes. *Blood*. 2015;126(1):9-16. doi:10.1182/blood-2015-03-631747
60. Jaiswal S, Fontanillas P, Flannick J, et al. Age-related clonal hematopoiesis associated with adverse outcomes. *N Engl J Med*. 2014;371(26):2488-2498. doi:10.1056/NEJMoa1408617
61. Genovese G, Kähler AK, Handsaker RE, et al. Clonal hematopoiesis and blood-cancer risk inferred from blood DNA sequence. *N Engl J Med*. 2014;371(26):2477-2487.
62. Xie M, Lu C, Wang J, et al. Age-related mutations associated with clonal hematopoietic expansion and malignancies. *Nat Med*. 2014;20(12):1472-1478.
63. McKerrell T, Park N, Moreno T, et al. Leukemia-associated somatic mutations drive distinct patterns of age-related clonal hemopoiesis. *Cell Rep*. 2015;10(8):1239-1245. doi:10.1016/j.celrep.2015.02.005
64. Guermouche H, Ravalet N, Gallay N, et al. High prevalence of clonal hematopoiesis in the blood and bone marrow of healthy volunteers. *Blood Adv*. 2020;4(15):3550-3557. doi:10.1182/bloodadvances.2020001582
65. van Zeventer IA, Salzbrunn JB, de Graaf AO, et al. Prevalence, predictors, and outcomes of clonal hematopoiesis in individuals aged ≥80 years. *Blood Adv*. 2021;5(8):2115-2122.
66. Buscarlet M, Provost S, Zada YF, et al. DNMT3A and TET2 dominate clonal hematopoiesis and demonstrate benign phenotypes and different genetic predispositions. *Blood*. 2017;130(6):753-762.
67. *WHO Classification of Tumours of Haematopoietic and Lymphoid Tissues. World Health Organization Classification of Tumours*. IARC Press; 2008:325.
68. Arber DA, Orazi A, Hasserjian R, et al. The 2016 revision to the World Health Organization classification of myeloid neoplasms and acute leukemia. *Blood*. 2016;127(20):2391-2405.
69. Walter MJ, Shen D, Ding L, et al. Clonal architecture of secondary acute myeloid leukemia. *N Engl J Med*. 2012;366(12):1090-1098.
70. Chen J, Kao YR, Sun D, et al. Myelodysplastic syndrome progression to acute myeloid leukemia at the stem cell level. *Nat Med*. 2019;25(1):103-110. doi:10.1038/s41591-018-0267-4
71. Lindsley RC, Mar BG, Mazzola E, et al. Acute myeloid leukemia ontogeny is defined by distinct somatic mutations. *Blood*. 2015;125(9):1367-1376. doi:10.1182/blood-2014-11-610543
72. Gao Y, Jia M, Mao Y, et al. Distinct mutation landscapes between acute myeloid leukemia with myelodysplasia-related changes and de novo acute myeloid leukemia. *Am J Clin Pathol*. 2022;157(5):691-700. doi:10.1093/AJCP/AQAB172
73. Grob T, Al Hinai ASA, Sanders MA, et al. Molecular characterization of mutant TP53 acute myeloid leukemia and high-risk myelodysplastic syndrome. *Blood*. 2022;139(15):2347-2354. doi:10.1182/BLOOD.2021014472
74. Weinberg OK, Siddon AJ, Madanat YF, et al. TP53 mutation defines a unique subgroup within complex karyotype de novo and therapy-related MDS/AML. *Blood Adv*. 2022;6(9):2847-2853. doi:10.1182/bloodadvances.2021006239
75. Huang ME, Ye YC, Chen SR, et al. Use of all trans retinoic acid in the treatment of acute promyelocytic leukemia. *Blood*. 1988;72(2):567-572.
76. Borrow J, Goddard AD, Sheer D, Solomon E. Molecular analysis of acute promyelocytic leukemia breakpoint cluster region on chromosome 17. *Science*. 1990;249(4976):1577-1580.
77. de The H, Chomienne C, Lanotte M, Degos L, Dejean A. The t(15;17) translocation of acute promyelocytic leukaemia fuses the retinoic acid receptor alpha gene to a novel transcribed locus. *Nature*. 1990;347(6293):558-561.
78. Longo L, Pandolfi PP, Biondi A, et al. Rearrangements and aberrant expression of the retinoic acid receptor alpha gene in acute promyelocytic leukemias. *J Exp Med*. 1990;172(6):1571-1575.
79. Geng JP, Tong JH, Dong S, et al. Localization of the chromosome 15 breakpoints and expression of multiple PML-RAR alpha transcripts in acute promyelocytic leukemia: a study of 28 Chinese patients. *Leukemia*. 1993;7(1):20-26.
80. Schulman IG, Juguilon H, Evans RM. Activation and repression by nuclear hormone receptors--Hormone modulates an equilibrium between active and repressive states. *Mol Cell Biol*. 1996;16(7):3807-3813.
81. Melnick A, Licht JD. Deconstructing a disease: RARalpha, its fusion partners, and their roles in the pathogenesis of acute promyelocytic leukemia. *Blood*. 1999;93(10):3167-3215.
82. Guidez F, Ivins S, Zhu J, Soderstrom M, Waxman S, Zelent A. Reduced retinoic acid-sensitivities of nuclear receptor corepressor binding to PML- and PLZF-RARalpha underlie molecular pathogenesis and treatment of acute promyelocytic leukemia. *Blood*. 1998;91(8):2634-2642.
83. Lin RJ, Nagy L, Inoue S, Shao W, Miller WHJ, Evans RM. Role of the histone deacetylase complex in acute promyelocytic leukaemia. *Nature*. 1998;391(6669):811-814.

84. Licht J, Chomienne C, Goy A, et al. Clinical and molecular characterization of a rare syndrome of acute promyelocytic leukemia associated with translocation (11;17). *Blood*. 1995;85:1083.
85. David G, Alland L, Hong SH, Wong CW, DePinho RA, Dejean A. Histone deacetylase associated with mSin3A mediates repression by the acute promyelocytic leukemia-associated PLZF protein. *Oncogene*. 1998;16(19):2549-2556.
86. Grignani F, De Matteis S, Nervi C, et al. Fusion proteins of the retinoic acid receptor-alpha recruit histone deacetylase in promyelocytic leukaemia. *Nature*. 1998;391(6669):815-818.
87. He LZ, Guidez F, Tribioli C, et al. Distinct interactions of PML-RARalpha and PLZF-RARalpha with co-repressors determine differential responses to RA in APL. *Nat Genet*. 1998;18(2):126-135.
88. Zhong S, Muller S, Ronchetti S, Freemont PS, Dejean A, Pandolfi PP. Role of SUMO-1-modified PML in nuclear body formation. *Blood*. 2000;95(9):2748-2752.
89. Doucas V, Tini M, Egan DA, Evans RM. Modulation of CREB binding protein function by the promyelocytic (PML) oncoprotein suggests a role for nuclear bodies in hormone signaling. *Proc Natl Acad Sci U S A*. 1999;96(6):2627-2632.
90. Weis K, Rambaud S, Lavau C, et al. Retinoic acid regulates aberrant nuclear localization of PML-RAR alpha in acute promyelocytic leukemia cells. *Cell*. 1994;76(2):345-356.
91. Madan V, Shyamsunder P, Han L, et al. Comprehensive mutational analysis of primary and relapse acute promyelocytic leukemia. *Leukemia*. 2016;30(12):2430. doi:10.1038/leu.2016.237
92. Faber ZJ, Chen X, Gedman AL, et al. The genomic landscape of core-binding factor acute myeloid leukemias. *Nat Genet*. 2016;48(12):1551-1556. doi:10.1038/ng.3709
93. Erickson P, Gao J, Chang KS, et al. Identification of breakpoints in t(8;21) acute myelogenous leukemia and isolation of a fusion transcript, AML1/ETO, with similarity to Drosophila segmentation gene, runt. *Blood*. 1992;80(7):1825-1831.
94. Miyoshi H, Kozu T, Shimizu K, et al. The t(8;21) translocation in acute myeloid leukemia results in production of an AML1-MTG8 fusion transcript. *EMBO J*. 1993;12(7):2715-2721.
95. Golemis EA, Speck NA, Hopkins N. Alignment of U3 region sequences of mammalian type C viruses: identification of highly conserved motifs and implications for enhancer design. *J Virol*. 1990;64(2):534-542.
96. Liu P, Tarle SA, Hajra A, et al. Fusion between transcription factor CBF beta/PEBP2 beta and a myosin heavy chain in acute myeloid leukemia. *Science*. 1993;261(5124):1041-1044.
97. Erickson PF, Robinson M, Owens G, Drabkin HA. The ETO portion of acute myeloid leukemia t(8;21) fusion transcript encodes a highly evolutionarily conserved, putative transcription factor. *Cancer Res*. 1994;54(7):1782-1786.
98. Gamou T, Kitamura E, Hosoda F, et al. The partner gene of AML1 in t(16;21) myeloid malignancies is a novel member of the MTG8(ETO) family. *Blood*. 1998;91(11):4028-4037.
99. Okuda T, van Deursen J, Hiebert SW, Grosveld G, Downing JR. AML1, the target of multiple chromosomal translocations in human leukemia, is essential for normal fetal liver hematopoiesis. *Cell*. 1996;84(2):321-330.
100. Wang Q, Stacy T, Miller JD, et al. The CBFbeta subunit is essential for CBFalpha2 (AML1) function in vivo. *Cell*. 1996;87(4):697-708.
101. North T, Gu TL, Stacy T, et al. Cbfa2 is required for the formation of intra-aortic hematopoietic clusters. *Development*. 1999;126(11):2563-2575.
102. Libermann TA, Pan Z, Akbarali Y, et al. AML1 (CBFalpha2) cooperates with B cell-specific activating protein (BSAP/PAX5) in activation of the B cell-specific BLK gene promoter. *J Biol Chem*. 1999;274(35):24671-24676.
103. Uchida H, Zhang J, Nimer SD. AML1A and AML1B can transactivate the human IL-3 promoter. *J Immunol*. 1997;158(5):2251-2258.
104. Takahashi A, Satake M, Yamaguchi-Iwai Y, et al. Positive and negative regulation of granulocyte-macrophage colony-stimulating factor promoter activity by AML1-related transcription factor, PEBP2. *Blood*. 1995;86(2):607-616.
105. Nuchprayoon I, Meyers S, Scott LM, Suzow J, Hiebert S, Friedman AD. PEBP2/CBF, the murine homolog of the human myeloid AML1 and PEBP2 beta/CBF beta proto-oncoproteins, regulates the murine myeloperoxidase and neutrophil elastase genes in immature myeloid cells. *Mol Cell Biol*. 1994;14(8):5558-5568.
106. Levanon D, Negreanu V, Bernstein Y, Bar-Am I, Avivi L, Groner Y. AML1, AML2, and AML3, the human members of the runt domain gene-family: cDNA structure, expression, and chromosomal localization. *Genomics*. 1994;23(2):425-432.
107. Michaud J, Wu F, Osato M, et al. In vitro analyses of known and novel RUNX1/AML1 mutations in dominant familial platelet disorder with predisposition to acute myelogenous leukemia: implications for mechanisms of pathogenesis. *Blood*. 2002;99(4):1364-1372.
108. Osato M, Asou N, Abdalla E, et al. Biallelic and heterozygous point mutations in the runt domain of the AML1/PEBP2alphaB gene associated with myeloblastic leukemias. *Blood*. 1999;93(6):1817-1824.
109. Tahirov TH, Inoue-Bungo T, Morii H, et al. Structural analyses of DNA recognition by the AML1/Runx-1 Runt domain and its allosteric control by CBFbeta. *Cell*. 2001;104(5):755-767.
110. Feinstein PG, Kornfeld K, Hogness DS, Mann RS. Identification of homeotic target genes in Drosophila melanogaster including nervy, a proto-oncogene homologue. *Genetics*. 1995;140(2):573-586.
111. Melnick AM, Westendorf JJ, Polinger A, et al. The ETO protein disrupted in t(8;21)-associated acute myeloid leukemia is a corepressor for the promyelocytic leukemia zinc finger protein. *Mol Cell Biol*. 2000;20(6):2075-2086.
112. Amann JM, Nip J, Strom DK, et al. ETO, a target of t(8;21) in acute leukemia, makes distinct contacts with multiple histone deacetylases and binds mSin3A through its oligomerization domain. *Mol Cell Biol*. 2001;21(19):6470-6483.
113. de Greef GE, Hagemeijer A, Morgan R, et al. Identical fusion transcript associated with different breakpoints in the AML1 gene in simple and variant t(8;21) acute myeloid leukemia. *Leukemia*. 1995;9(2):282-287.
114. Licht JD. AML1 and the AML1-ETO fusion protein in the pathogenesis of t(8;21) AML. *Oncogene*. 2001;20(40):5660-5679.
115. Meyers S, Downing JR, Hiebert SW. Identification of AML-1 and the (8;21) translocation protein (AML-1/ETO) as sequence-specific DNA-binding proteins: the runt homology domain is required for DNA binding and protein-protein interactions. *Mol Cell Biol*. 1993;13(10):6336-6345.
116. Frank R, Zhang J, Uchida H, Meyers S, Hiebert SW, Nimer SD. The AML1/ETO fusion protein blocks transactivation of the GM-CSF promoter by AML1B. *Oncogene*. 1995;11(12):2667-2674.
117. Linggi B, Muller-Tidow C, van de Locht L, et al. The t(8;21) fusion protein, AML1-ETO, specifically represses the transcription of the p14^{ARF} tumor suppressor in acute myeloid leukemia. *Nat Med*. 2002;8(7):743-750.
118. Linggi BE, Brandt SJ, Sun ZW, Hiebert SW. Translating the histone code into leukemia. *J Cell Biochem*. 2005;96(5):938-950.
119. Zhang Y, Xiong Y, Yarbrough WG. ARF promotes MDM2 degradation and stabilizes p53: ARF-INK4a locus deletion impairs both the Rb and p53 tumor suppression pathways. *Cell*. 1998;92(6):725-734.
120. Durst KL, Lutterbach B, Kummalue T, Friedman AD, Hiebert SW. The inv(16) fusion protein associates with corepressors via a smooth muscle myosin heavy-chain domain. *Mol Cell Biol*. 2003;23(2):607-619.
121. Song W-J, Sullivan MG, Legare RD, et al. Haploinsufficiency of CBFA2 causes familial thrombocytopenia with propensity to develop acute myelogenous leukemia. *Nat Genet*. 1999;23(2):166-175.
122. Tenen DG, Hromas R, Licht JD, Zhang DE. Transcription factors, normal myeloid development, and leukemia. *Blood*. 1997;90(2):489-519.
123. Avellino R, Delwel R. Expression and regulation of C/EBPα in normal myelopoiesis and in malignant transformation. *Blood*. 2017;129(15):2083-2091. doi:10.1182/blood-2016-09-687822
124. Zhang P, Iwasaki-Arai J, Iwasaki H, et al. Enhancement of hematopoietic stem cell repopulating capacity and self-renewal in the absence of the transcription factor C/EBP alpha. *Immunity*. 2004;21(6):853-863.
125. Paz-Priel I, Friedman AD. C/EBPα dysregulation in AML and ALL. *Crit Rev Oncogene*. 2011;16:93-102.
126. Pabst T, Mueller BU, Harakawa N, et al. AML1-ETO downregulates the granulocytic differentiation factor C/EBPalpha in t(8;21) myeloid leukemia. *Nat Med*. 2001;7(4):444-451.
127. Radomska HS, Basseres DS, Zheng R, et al. Block of C/EBP alpha function by phosphorylation in acute myeloid leukemia with FLT3 activating mutations. *J Exp Med*. 2006;203(2):371-381.
128. Hackanson B, Bennett KL, Brena RM, et al. Epigenetic modification of CCAAT enhancer binding protein alpha expression in acute myeloid leukemia. *Cancer Res*. 2008;68(9):3142-3151.
129. Zhang DE, Zhang P, Wang ND, Hetherington CJ, Darlington GJ, Tenen DG. Absence of granulocyte colony-stimulating factor signaling and neutrophil development in CCAAT enhancer binding protein alpha-deficient mice. *Proc Natl Acad Sci U S A*. 1997;94(2):569-574.
130. Radomska HS, Huettner CS, Zhang P, Cheng T, Scadden DT, Tenen DG. CCAAT/enhancer binding protein alpha is a regulatory switch sufficient for induction of granulocytic development from bipotential myeloid progenitors. *Mol Cell Biol*. 1998;18(7):4301-4314.
131. Roe JS, Vakoc CR. C/EBPα: critical at the origin of leukemic transformation. *J Exp Med*. 2014;211(1):1-4. doi:10.1084/jem.20132530
132. Gombart AF, Hofmann WK, Kawano S, et al. Mutations in the gene encoding the transcription factor CCAAT/enhancer binding protein alpha in myelodysplastic syndromes and acute myeloid leukemias. *Blood*. 2002;99(4):1332-1340.
133. Pabst T, Mueller BU, Zhang P, et al. Dominant-negative mutations of CEBPA, encoding CCAAT/enhancer binding protein-alpha (C/EBPalpha), in acute myeloid leukemia. *Nat Genet*. 2001;27(3):263-270.
134. Preudhomme C, Sagot C, Boissel N, et al. Favorable prognostic significance of CEBPA mutations in patients with de novo acute myeloid leukemia: a study from the Acute Leukemia French Association (ALFA). *Blood*. 2002;100(8):2717-2723.
135. Pabst T, Eyholzer M, Haefliger S, Schardt J, Mueller BU. Somatic CEBPA mutations are a frequent second event in families with germline CEBPA mutations and familial acute myeloid leukemia. *J Clin Oncol*. 2008;26(31):5088-5093.
136. Grossmann V, Schnittger S, Kohlmann A, et al. A novel hierarchical prognostic model of AML solely based on molecular mutations. *Blood*. 2012;120(15):2963-2972. doi:10.1182/blood-2012-03-419622
137. Taube F, Georgi JA, Kramer M, et al. CEBPA mutations in 4708 patients with acute myeloid leukemia: differential impact of bZIP and TAD mutations on outcome. *Blood*. 2022;139(1):87-103.
138. Wakita S, Sakaguchi M, Oh I, et al. Prognostic impact of CEBPA bZIP domain mutation in acute myeloid leukemia. *Blood Adv*. 2022;6(1):238-247. doi:10.1182/bloodadvances.2021004292
139. Crispino JD, Horwitz MS. GATA factor mutations in hematologic disease. *Blood*. 2017;129(15):2103-2110. doi:10.1182/blood-2016-09-687889
140. Greene ME, Mundschau G, Wechsler J, et al. Mutations in GATA1 in both transient myeloproliferative disorder and acute megakaryoblastic leukemia of Down syndrome. *Blood Cells Mol Dis*. 2003;31(3):351-356.
141. Roy A, Roberts I, Norton A, Vyas P. Acute megakaryoblastic leukaemia (AMKL) and transient myeloproliferative disorder (TMD) in Down syndrome: a multi-step model of myeloid leukaemogenesis. *Br J Haematol*. 2009;147(1):3-12.
142. Roberts I, Alford K, Hall G, et al. GATA1-mutant clones are frequent and often unsuspected in babies with Down syndrome: identification of a population at risk of leukemia. *Blood*. 2013;122(24):3908-3917.
143. Alford KA, Reinhardt K, Garnett C, et al. Analysis of GATA1 mutations in down syndrome transient myeloproliferative disorder and myeloid leukemia. *Blood*. 2011;118(8):2222-2238.

144. Yoshida K, Toki T, Okuno Y, et al. The landscape of somatic mutations in Down syndrome-related myeloid disorders. *Nat Genet.* Nov 2013;45(11):1293-1299. doi:10.1038/ng.2759
145. Creutzig U, Reinhardt D, Diekamp S, Dworzak M, Stary J, Zimmermann M. AML patients with Down syndrome have a high cure rate with AML-BFM therapy with reduced dose intensity. *Leukemia.* 2005;19(8):1355-1360.
146. Muntean AG, Crispino JD. Differential requirements for the activation domain and FOG-interaction surface of GATA-1 in megakaryocyte gene expression and development. *Blood.* 2005;106(4):1223-1231.
147. Zhang Y, Sun Z, Jia J, et al. Overview of histone modification. *Adv Exp Med Biol.* 2021;1283:1-16.
148. Robertson KD. DNA methylation and human disease. *Nat Rev Genet.* 2005;6(8):597-610.
149. Jenuwein T, Allis CD. Translating the histone code. *Science.* 2001;293(5532):1074-1080.
150. Bannister AJ, Kouzarides T. Regulation of chromatin by histone modifications. *Cell Res.* 2011;21(3):381-395. doi:10.1038/cr.2011.22
151. Black JC, Van Rechem C, Whetstine JR. Histone lysine methylation dynamics: establishment, regulation, and biological impact. *Mol Cell.* 2012;48(4):491-507. doi:10.1016/j.molcel.2012.11.006
152. Zhao S, Allis CD, Wang GG. The language of chromatin modification in human cancers. *Nat Rev Cancer.* 2021;21(7):413-430. doi:10.1038/s41568-021-00357-x
153. Figueroa ME, Abdel-Wahab O, Lu C, et al. Leukemic IDH1 and IDH2 mutations result in a hypermethylation phenotype, disrupt TET2 function, and impair hematopoietic differentiation. *Cancer Cell.* 2010;18(6):553-567.
154. Xu W, Yang H, Liu Y, et al. Oncometabolite 2-hydroxyglutarate is a competitive inhibitor of α-ketoglutarate-dependent dioxygenases. *Cancer Cell.* 2011;19(1):17-30.
155. Williams K, Christensen J, Helin K. DNA methylation: TET proteins—guardians of CpG islands? *EMBO Rep.* 2011;13(1):28-35.
156. Ko M, Huang Y, Jankowska AM, et al. Impaired hydroxylation of 5-methylcytosine in myeloid cancers with mutant TET2. *Nature.* 2010;468(7325):839-843. doi:10.1038/nature09586
157. Lu C, Ward PS, Kapoor GS, et al. IDH mutation impairs histone demethylation and results in a block to cell differentiation. *Nature.* 2012;483(7390):474-478.
158. DiNardo CD, Stein EM, de Botton S, et al. Durable remissions with ivosidenib in IDH1-mutated relapsed or refractory AML. *N Engl J Med.* 2018;378(25):2386-2398.
159. Papaemmanuil E, Gerstung M, Bullinger L, et al. Genomic classification and prognosis in acute myeloid leukemia. *N Engl J Med.* 2016;374(23):2209-2221. doi:10.1056/NEJMoa1516192
160. Wang R, Gao X, Yu L. The prognostic impact of tet oncogene family member 2 mutations in patients with acute myeloid leukemia: a systematic-review and meta-analysis. *BMC Cancer.* 2019;19(1):389-389.
161. Huang HT, Figueroa ME. Epigenetic deregulation in myeloid malignancies. *Blood.* 2021;138(8):613-624. doi:10.1182/blood.2019004262
162. Holz-Schietinger C, Matje DM, Reich NO. Mutations in DNA methyltransferase (DNMT3A) observed in acute myeloid leukemia patients disrupt processive methylation. *J Biol Chem.* 2012;287(37):30941-30951.
163. Challen GA, Sun D, Jeong M, et al. DNMT3A is essential for hematopoietic stem cell differentiation. *Nat Genet.* 2011;44(1):23-31.
164. Muntean AG, Hess JL. The pathogenesis of mixed-lineage leukemia. *Annu Rev Pathol.* 2012;7:283-301.
165. Ingham PW. Trithorax and the regulation of homeotic gene expression in Drosophila: a historical perspective. *Int J Dev Biol.* 1998;42(3):423-429.
166. Gehring WJ, Affolter M, Burglin T. Homeodomain proteins. *Annu Rev Biochem.* 1994;63:487-526.
167. Maconochie M, Nonchev S, Morrison A, Krumlauf R. Paralogous Hox genes: function and regulation. *Annu Rev Genet.* 1996;30:529-556.
168. Ernst P, Fisher JK, Avery W, Wade S, Foy D, Korsmeyer SJ. Definitive hematopoiesis requires the mixed-lineage leukemia gene. *Dev Cell.* 2004;6(3):437-443.
169. Hess JL. MLL: a histone methyltransferase disrupted in leukemia. *Trends Mol Med.* 2004;10(10):500-507.
170. Yu BD, Hanson RD, Hess JL, Horning SE, Korsmeyer SJ. MLL, a mammalian trithorax-group gene, functions as a transcriptional maintenance factor in morphogenesis. *Proc Natl Acad Sci U S A.* 1998;95(18):10632-10636.
171. Yu BD, Hess JL, Horning SE, Brown GA, Korsmeyer SJ. Altered Hox expression and segmental identity in Mll-mutant mice. *Nature.* 1995;378(6556):505-508.
172. Krivtsov AV, Armstrong SA. MLL translocations, histone modifications and leukaemia stem-cell development. *Nat Rev Cancer.* 2007;7(11):823-833.
173. Meyer C, Kowarz E, Hofmann J, et al. New insights to the MLL recombinome of acute leukemias. *Leukemia.* 2009;23(8):1490-1499.
174. Bernt KM, Armstrong SA. Targeting epigenetic programs in MLL-rearranged leukemias. *Hematology Am Soc Hematol Educ Program.* 2011;2011:354-360.
175. Ernst P, Wang J, Korsmeyer SJ. The role of MLL in hematopoiesis and leukemia. *Curr Opin Hematol.* 2002;9(4):282-287.
176. Tkachuk DC, Kohler S, Cleary ML. Involvement of a homolog of Drosophila trithorax by 11q23 chromosomal translocations in acute leukemias. *Cell.* 1992;71(4):691-700.
177. Chi P, Allis CD, Wang GG. Covalent histone modifications--miswritten, misinterpreted and mis-erased in human cancers. *Nat Rev Cancer.* 2010;10(7):457-469.
178. Andersson AK, Ma J, Wang J, et al. The landscape of somatic mutations in infant MLL-rearranged acute lymphoblastic leukemias. *Nat Genet.* 2015;47(4):330-337. doi:10.1038/ng.3230
179. Rubnitz JE, Link MP, Shuster JJ, et al. Frequency and prognostic significance of HRX rearrangements in infant acute lymphoblastic leukemia; a Pediatric Oncology Group study. *Blood.* 1994;84(2):570-573.
180. Secker-Walker LM. General report on the European union concerted action workshop on 11q23, London, UK, may 1997. *Leukemia.* 1998;12(5):776-778.
181. Hunger SP, Tkachuk DC, Amylon MD, et al. HRX involvement in de novo and secondary leukemias with diverse chromosome 11q23 abnormalities. *Blood.* 1993;81(12):3197-3203.
182. Strissel PLRS, Rowley JD, Zeleznik-Le NJ. An in vivo topoisomerase II cleavage site and a NDase I hypersensitive site colocalize near exon 9 in the MLL breakpoint cluster region. *Blood.* 1998;92:3793-3803.
183. Cimino G, Rapanotti MC, Biondi A, et al. Infant acute leukemias show the same biased distribution of ALL1 gene breaks as topoisomerase II related secondary acute leukemias. *Cancer Res.* 1997;57(14):2879-2883.
184. Ross JA, Potter JD, Reaman GH, Pendergrass TW, Robison LL. Maternal exposure to potential inhibitors of DNA topoisomerase II and infant leukemia (United States): a report from the Children's Cancer Group. *Cancer Causes Control.* 1996;7(6):581-590.
185. Basecke J, Whelan JT, Griesinger F, Bertrand FE. The MLL partial tandem duplication in acute myeloid leukaemia. *Br J Haematol.* 2006;135(4):438-449.
186. Dorrance AM, Liu S, Yuan W, et al. Mll partial tandem duplication induces aberrant Hox expression in vivo via specific epigenetic alterations. *J Clin Invest.* 2006;116(10):2707-2716.
187. Ford AM, Bennett CA, Price CM, Bruin MC, Van Wering ER, Greaves MF. Fetal origins of the TEL-AML1 fusion gene in identical twins with leukemia. *Proc Natl Acad Sci U S A.* 1998;95(8):4584-4588.
188. Ford AM, Ridge SA, Cabrera ME, et al. In utero rearrangements in the trithorax-related oncogene in infant leukaemias. *Nature.* 1993;363(6427):358-360.
189. Super HJ, McCabe NR, Thirman MJ, et al. Rearrangements of the MLL gene in therapy-related acute myeloid leukemia in patients previously treated with agents targeting DNA-topoisomerase II. *Blood.* 1993;82(12):3705-3711.
190. Asada S, Fujino T, Goyama S, Kitamura T. The role of ASXL1 in hematopoiesis and myeloid malignancies. *Cell Mol Life Sci.* 2019;76(13):2511-2523.
191. Wang J, Li Z, He Y, et al. Loss of Asxl1 leads to myelodysplastic syndrome-like disease in mice. *Blood.* 2014;123(4):541-553. doi:10.1182/blood-2013-05-500272
192. Yang H, Kurtenbach S, Guo Y, et al. Gain of function of ASXL1 truncating protein in the pathogenesis of myeloid malignancies. *Blood.* 2018;131(3):328-341. doi:10.1182/blood-2017-06-789669
193. Paschka P, Schlenk RF, Gaidzik VI, et al. ASXL1 mutations in younger adult patients with acute myeloid leukemia: a study by the German-Austrian Acute Myeloid Leukemia Study Group. *Haematologica.* 2015;100(3):324-330. doi:10.3324/haematol.2014.114157.
194. Zeisig BB, So CWE. Therapeutic opportunities of targeting canonical and noncanonical PcG/TrxG functions in acute myeloid leukemia. *Annu Rev Genom Hum Genet.* 2021;22(1):103-125. doi:10.1146/annurev-genom-111120-102443
195. Gilliland DG, Griffin JD. The roles of FLT3 in hematopoiesis and leukemia. *Blood.* 2002;100(5):1532-1542.
196. Brasel K, Escobar S, Anderberg R, de Vries P, Gruss HJ, Lyman SD. Expression of the Flt3 receptor and its ligand on hematopoietic cells. *Leukemia.* 1995;9(7):1212-1218.
197. Brandts CH, Sargin B, Rode M, et al. Constitutive activation of Akt by Flt3 internal tandem duplications is necessary for increased survival, proliferation, and myeloid transformation. *Cancer Res.* 2005;65(21):9643-9650.
198. Mizuki M, Fenski R, Halfter H, et al. FLT3 mutations from patients with acute myeloid leukemia induce transformation of 32D cells mediated by the Ras and STAT5 pathways. *Blood.* 2000;96(12):3907-3914.
199. Nakao M, Yokota S, Iwai T, et al. Internal tandem duplication of the flt3 gene found in acute myeloid leukemia. *Leukemia.* 1996;10(12):1911-1918.
200. Kiyoi H, Towatari M, Yokota S, et al. Internal tandem duplication of the FLT3 gene is a novel modality of elongation mutation which causes constitutive activation of the product. *Leukemia.* 1998;12(9):1333-1337.
201. Cauchy P, James SR, Zacarias-Cabeza J, et al. Chronic FLT3-ITD signaling in acute myeloid leukemia is connected to a specific chromatin signature. *Cell Rep.* 2015;12(5):821-836.
202. Yamamoto Y, Kiyoi H, Nakano Y, et al. Activating mutation of D835 within the activation loop of FLT3 in human hematologic malignancies. *Blood.* 2001;97(8):2434-2439.
203. Sternberg DW, Licht JD. Therapeutic intervention in leukemias that express the activated fms-like tyrosine kinase 3 (FLT3): opportunities and challenges. *Curr Opin Hematol.* 2005;12(1):7-13.
204. Kelly LM, Liu Q, Kutok JL, Williams IR, Boulton CL, Gilliland DG. FLT3 internal tandem duplication mutations associated with human acute myeloid leukemias induce myeloproliferative disease in a murine bone marrow transplant model. *Blood.* 2002;99(1):310-318.
205. Meshinchi S, Woods WG, Stirewalt DL, et al. Prevalence and prognostic significance of Flt3 internal tandem duplication in pediatric acute myeloid leukemia. *Blood.* 2001;97(1):89-94.
206. Kelly LM, Yu JC, Boulton CL, et al. CT53518, a novel selective FLT3 antagonist for the treatment of acute myelogenous leukemia (AML). *Cancer Cell.* 2002;1(5):421-432.
207. Weisberg E, Boulton C, Kelly LM, et al. Inhibition of mutant FLT3 receptors in leukemia cells by the small molecule tyrosine kinase inhibitor PKC412. *Cancer Cell.* 2002;1(5):433-443.
208. Piloto O, Wright M, Brown P, Kim KT, Levis M, Small D. Prolonged exposure to FLT3 inhibitors leads to resistance via activation of parallel signaling pathways. *Blood.* 2007;109(4):1643-1652.
209. Smith CC, Wang Q, Chin CS, et al. Validation of ITD mutations in FLT3 as a therapeutic target in human acute myeloid leukaemia. *Nature.* 2012;485(7397):260-263.
210. Zhao JC, Agarwal S, Ahmad H, Amin K, Bewersdorf JP, Zeidan AM. A review of FLT3 inhibitors in acute myeloid leukemia. *Blood Rev.* 2022;52:100905. doi:10.1016/J.BLRE.2021.100905

211. Besmer P, Murphy JE, George PC, et al. A new acute transforming feline retrovirus and relationship of its oncogene v-kit with the protein kinase gene family. *Nature*. 1986;320(6061):415-421. doi:10.1038/320415a0
212. Lennartsson J, Rönnstrand L. Stem cell factor receptor/c-Kit: from basic science to clinical implications. *Physiol Rev*. 2012;92(4):1619-1649. doi:10.1152/PHYSREV.00046.2011
213. Laine E, Chauvot de Beauchêne I, Perahia D, Auclair C, Tchertanov L. Mutation D816V alters the internal structure and dynamics of c-KIT receptor cytoplasmic region: implications for dimerization and activation mechanisms. *PLoS Comput Biol*. 2011;7(6):e1002068.
214. Piao X, Paulson R, van der Geer P, Pawson T, Bernstein A. Oncogenic mutation in the Kit receptor tyrosine kinase alters substrate specificity and induces degradation of the protein tyrosine phosphatase SHP-1. *Proc Natl Acad Sci U S A*. 1996;93(25):14665-14669. doi:10.1073/pnas.93.25.14665
215. Ishikawa Y, Kawashima N, Atsuta Y, et al. Prospective evaluation of prognostic impact of KIT mutations on acute myeloid leukemia with RUNX1-RUNX1T1 and CBFB-MYH11. *Blood Adv*. 2020;4(1):66-75.
216. Ruggero D, Pandolfi PP. Does the ribosome translate cancer? *Nat Rev Cancer*. 2003;3(3):179-192.
217. Grisendi S, Pandolfi PP. NPM mutations in acute myelogenous leukemia. *N Engl J Med*. 2005;352(3):291-292.
218. Heath EM, Chan SM, Minden MD, Murphy T, Shlush LI, Schimmer AD. Biological and clinical consequences of NPM1 mutations in AML. *Leukemia*. 2017;31(4):798-807. doi:10.1038/leu.2017.30
219. Box JK, Paquet N, Adams MN, et al. Nucleophosmin: from structure and function to disease development. *BMC Mol Biol*. 2016;17(1):19. doi:10.1186/s12867-016-0073-9
220. Boissel N, Renneville A, Biggio V, et al. Prevalence, clinical profile, and prognosis of NPM mutations in AML with normal karyotype. *Blood*. 2005;106(10):3618-3620.
221. Falini B, Mecucci C, Tiacci E, et al. Cytoplasmic nucleophosmin in acute myelogenous leukemia with a normal karyotype. *N Engl J Med*. 2005;352(3):254-266.
222. Falini B, Bolli N, Liso A, et al. Altered nucleophosmin transport in acute myeloid leukaemia with mutated NPM1: molecular basis and clinical implications. *Leukemia*. 2009;23(10):1731-1743.
223. Falini B, Nicoletti I, Martelli MF, Mecucci C. Acute myeloid leukemia carrying cytoplasmic/mutated nucleophosmin (NPMc+ AML): biologic and clinical features. *Blood*. 2007;109(3):874-885.
224. Bolli N, De Marco MF, Martelli MP, et al. A dose-dependent tug of war involving the NPM1 leukaemic mutant, nucleophosmin, and ARF. *Leukemia*. 2009;23(3):501-509.
225. Falini B, Martelli MP, Bolli N, et al. Immunohistochemistry predicts nucleophosmin (NPM) mutations in acute myeloid leukemia. *Blood*. 2006;108(6):1999-2005.
226. Zhou MH, Yang QM. NUP214 fusion genes in acute leukemia (Review). *Oncol Lett*. 2014;8(3):959-962.
227. Swerdlow S, Campo E, Harris NL, et al. eds. *WHO Classification of Tumours of Haematopoietic and Lymphoid Tissues*. Revised 4th ed. IARC Press; 2017.
228. Mendes A, Fahrenkrog B. NUP214 in leukemia: it's more than transport. *Cells*. 2019;8(1):76-76.
229. Ko SI, Lee IS, Kim JY, et al. Regulation of histone acetyltransferase activity of p300 and PCAF by proto-oncogene protein DEK. *FEBS Lett*. 2006;580(13):3217-3222. doi:10.1016/j.febslet.2006.04.081
230. Qin H, Malek S, Cowell JK, Ren M. Transformation of human CD34+ hematopoietic progenitor cells with DEK-NUP214 induces AML in an immunocompromised mouse model. *Oncogene*. 2016;35(43):5686-5691.
231. Saito S, Yokokawa T, Iizuka G, Cigdem S, Okuwaki M, Nagata K. Function of Nup98 subtypes and their fusion proteins, Nup98-TopIIβ and Nup98-SETBP1 in nuclear-cytoplasmic transport. *Biochem Biophys Res Commun*. 2017;487(1):96-102. doi:10.1016/j.bbrc.2017.04.024
232. Struski S, Lagarde S, Bories P, et al. NUP98 is rearranged in 3.8% of pediatric AML forming a clinical and molecular homogenous group with a poor prognosis. *Leukemia*. 2017;31(3):565-572.
233. Wang GG, Song J, Wang Z, et al. Haematopoietic malignancies caused by dysregulation of a chromatin-binding PHD finger. *Nature*. 2009;459(7248):847-851. doi:10.1038/nature08036
234. Schmoellerl J, Barbosa IAM, Eder T, et al. CDK6 is an essential direct target of NUP98 fusion proteins in acute myeloid leukemia. *Blood*. 2020;136(4):387-400. doi:10.1182/blood.2019003267
235. Zhang Y, Guo Y, Gough SM, et al. Mechanistic insights into chromatin targeting by leukemic NUP98-PHF23 fusion. *Nat Commun*. 2020;11(1):3339. doi:10.1038/s41467-020-17098-4
236. Chen S, Benbarche S, Abdel-Wahab O. Splicing factor mutations in hematologic malignancies. *Blood*. 2021;138(8):599-612. doi:10.1182/blood.2019004260
237. Malcovati L, Gallì A, Travaglino E, et al. Clinical significance of somatic mutation in unexplained blood cytopenia. *Blood*. 2017;129(25):3371-3378. doi:10.1182/blood-2017-01-763425
238. Bamopoulos SA, Batcha AMN, Jurinovic V, et al. Clinical presentation and differential splicing of SRSF2, U2AF1 and SF3B1 mutations in patients with acute myeloid leukemia. *Leukemia*. 2020;34(10):2621-2634.
239. Nikpour M, Scharenberg C, Liu A, et al. The transporter ABCB7 is a mediator of the phenotype of acquired refractory anemia with ring sideroblasts. *Leukemia*. 2013;27(4):889-896. doi:10.1038/leu.2012.298
240. Kim E, Ilagan JO, Liang Y, et al. SRSF2 mutations contribute to myelodysplasia by mutant-specific effects on exon recognition. *Cancer Cell*. 2015;27(5):617-630. doi:10.1016/j.ccell.2015.04.006
241. Papaemmanuil E, Gerstung M, Malcovati L, et al. Clinical and biological implications of driver mutations in myelodysplastic syndromes. *Blood*. 2013;122(22):3616-3627; quiz 3699. doi:10.1182/blood-2013-08-518886
242. Jann JC, Tothova Z. Cohesin mutations in myeloid malignancies. *Blood*. 2021;138(8):649-661.
243. Kon A, Shih LY, Minamino M, et al. Recurrent mutations in multiple components of the cohesin complex in myeloid neoplasms. *Nat Genet*. 2013;45(10):1232-1237. doi:10.1038/ng.2731
244. Labuhn M, Perkins K, Matzk S, et al. Mechanisms of progression of myeloid preleukemia to transformed myeloid leukemia in children with down syndrome. *Cancer Cell*. 2019;36(3):340.
245. McReynolds LJ, Yang Y, Yuen Wong H, et al. MDS-associated mutations in germline GATA2 mutated patients with hematologic manifestations. *Leuk Res*. 01 2019;76:70-75. doi:10.1016/j.leukres.2018.11.013
246. Churpek JE, Pyrtel K, Kanchi KL, et al. Genomic analysis of germ line and somatic variants in familial myelodysplasia/acute myeloid leukemia. *Blood*. 2015;126(22):2484-2490.
247. Antony-Debré I, Duployez N, Bucci M, et al. Somatic mutations associated with leukemic progression of familial platelet disorder with predisposition to acute myeloid leukemia. *Leukemia*. 2016;30(4):999-1002.
248. Kagey MH, Newman JJ, Bilodeau S, et al. Mediator and cohesin connect gene expression and chromatin architecture. *Nature*. 2010;467(7314):430-435. doi:10.1038/nature09380
249. Rao SSP, Huang SC, Glenn St Hilaire B, et al. Cohesin loss eliminates all loop domains. *Cell*. 2017;171(2):305-320.e24. doi:10.1016/j.cell.2017.09.026
250. Schlenk RF, Dohner K, Krauter J, et al. Mutations and treatment outcome in cytogenetically normal acute myeloid leukemia. *N Engl J Med*. 2008;358(18):1909-1918.
251. Dohner H, Estey EH, Amadori S, et al. Diagnosis and management of acute myeloid leukemia in adults: recommendations from an international expert panel, on behalf of the European LeukemiaNet. *Blood*. 2010;115(3):453-474.
252. Frohling S, Schlenk RF, Breitruck J, et al. Prognostic significance of activating FLT3 mutations in younger adults (16 to 60 years) with acute myeloid leukemia and normal cytogenetics: a study of the AML Study Group Ulm. *Blood*. 2002;100(13):4372-4380. doi:10.1182/blood-2002-05-1440
253. Whitman SP, Maharry K, Radmacher MD, et al. FLT3 internal tandem duplication associates with adverse outcome and gene- and microRNA-expression signatures in patients 60 years of age or older with primary cytogenetically normal acute myeloid leukemia: a Cancer and Leukemia Group B study. *Blood*. 2010;116(18):3622-3626. doi:10.1182/blood-2010-05-283648
254. Balgobind BV, Raimondi SC, Harbott J, et al. Novel prognostic subgroups in childhood 11q23/MLL-rearranged acute myeloid leukemia: results of an international retrospective study. *Blood*. 2009;114(12):2489-2496. doi:10.1182/blood-2009-04-215152
255. Tarlock K, Lamble AJ, Wang YC, et al. CEBPA-bZip mutations are associated with favorable prognosis in de novo AML: a report from the Children's Oncology Group. *Blood*. 2021;138(13):1137-1147.
256. Taskesen E, Bullinger L, Corbacioglu A, et al. Prognostic impact, concurrent genetic mutations, and gene expression features of AML with CEBPA mutations in a cohort of 1182 cytogenetically normal AML patients: further evidence for CEBPA double mutant AML as a distinctive disease entity. *Blood*. 2011;117(8):2469-2475.
257. Schnittger S, Eder C, Jeromin S, et al. ASXL1 exon 12 mutations are frequent in AML with intermediate risk karyotype and are independently associated with an adverse outcome. *Leukemia*. 2013;27(1):82-91.
258. Grossmann V, Schnittger S, Kohlmann A, et al. A novel hierarchical prognostic model of AML solely based on molecular mutations. *Blood*. 2012;120(15):2963-2972.
259. Malkin D, Li FP, Strong LC, et al. Germ line p53 mutations in a familial syndrome of breast cancer, sarcomas, and other neoplasms. *Science*. 1990;250(4985):1233-1238.
260. Dohner H, Estey E, Grimwade D, et al. Diagnosis and management of AML in adults: 2017 ELN recommendations from an international expert panel. *Blood*. 2017;129(4):424-447.
261. McKerrell T, Moreno T, Ponstingl H, et al. Development and validation of a comprehensive genomic diagnostic tool for myeloid malignancies. *Blood*. 2016;128(1):e1-e9. doi:10.1182/blood-2015-11-683334
262. Iacobucci I, Kimura S, Mullighan CG. Biologic and therapeutic implications of genomic alterations in acute lymphoblastic leukemia. *J Clin Med*. 2021;10(17):3792. doi:10.3390/JCM10173792
263. Den Boer ML, van Slegtenhorst M, De Menezes RX, et al. A subtype of childhood acute lymphoblastic leukaemia with poor treatment outcome: a genome-wide classification study. *Lancet Oncol*. 2009;10(2):125-134.
264. Li JF, Dai YT, Lilljebjörn H, et al. Transcriptional landscape of B cell precursor acute lymphoblastic leukemia based on an international study of 1, 223 cases. *Proc Natl Acad Sci U S A*. 2018;115(50):E11711-E11720. doi:10.1073/PNAS.1814397115
265. Shen CP, Kadesch T. B-cell specific DNA binding by an E47 homodimer. *Mol Cell Biol*. 1995;15(8):4518-4524.
266. Hunger SP, Galili N, Carroll AJ, Crist WM, Link MP, Cleary ML. The t(1;19)(q23;p13) results in consistent fusion of E2A and PBX1 coding sequences in acute lymphoblastic leukemia. *Blood*. 1991;77(4):687-693.
267. Mullighan CG, Goorha S, Radtke I, et al. Genome-wide analysis of genetic alterations in acute lymphoblastic leukaemia. *Nature*. 2007;446(7137):758-764.
268. Nutt SL, Urbanek P, Rolink A, Busslinger M. Essential functions of Pax5 (BSAP) in pro-B cell development: difference between fetal and adult B lymphopoiesis and reduced V-to-DJ recombination at the IgH locus. *Genes Dev*. 1997;11(4):476-491.
269. Gu Z, Churchman ML, Roberts KG, et al. PAX5-driven subtypes of B-progenitor acute lymphoblastic leukemia. *Nat Genet*. 2019;51(2):296-307. doi:10.1038/s41588-018-0315-5
270. Smeenk L, Fischer M, Jurado S, et al. Molecular role of the PAX5-ETV6 oncoprotein in promoting B-cell acute lymphoblastic leukemia. *EMBO J*. 2017;36(6):718-735. doi:10.15252/embj.201695495

271. Ng SYM, Yoshida T, Zhang J, Georgopoulos K. Genome-wide lineage-specific transcriptional networks underscore IKAROS-dependent lymphoid priming in hematopoietic stem cells. *Immunity.* 2009;30(4):493-507.
272. Gounari F, Kee BL. Fingerprinting ikaros. *Nat Immunol.* 2013;14(10):1034-1035. doi:10.1038/ni.2709
273. Churchman ML, Mullighan CG. Ikaros: exploiting and targeting the hematopoietic stem cell niche in B-progenitor acute lymphoblastic leukemia. *Exp Hematol.* 2017;46:1-8.
274. Roberts KG, Li Y, Payne-Turner D, et al. Targetable kinase-activating lesions in Ph-like acute lymphoblastic leukemia. *N Engl J Med.* 2014;371(11):1005-1015.
275. Schjerven H, McLaughlin J, Arenzana TL, et al. Selective regulation of lymphopoiesis and leukemogenesis by individual zinc fingers of Ikaros. *Nat Immunol.* 2013;14(10):1073-1083.
276. Iacobucci I, Iraci N, Messina M, et al. IKAROS deletions dictate a unique gene expression signature in patients with adult B-cell acute lymphoblastic leukemia. *PLoS One.* 2012;7:409344.
277. Vitanza NA, Zaky W, Blum R, et al. Ikaros deletions in BCR-ABL-negative childhood acute lymphoblastic leukemia are associated with a distinct gene expression signature but do not result in intrinsic chemoresistance. *Pediatr Blood Cancer.* 2014;61(10):1779-1785. doi:10.1002/pbc.25119
278. Pui CH, Evans WE. Acute lymphoblastic leukemia. *N Engl J Med.* 1998;339(9):605-615.
279. Kamps MP, Look AT, Baltimore D. The human t(1;19) translocation in pre-B ALL produces multiple nuclear E2A-Pbx1 fusion proteins with differing transforming potentials. *Genes Dev.* 1991;5(3):358-368.
280. Murre C, McCaw PS, Baltimore D. A new DNA binding and dimerization motif in immunoglobulin enhancer binding, daughterless, MyoD, and myc proteins. *Cell.* 1989;56(5):777-783.
281. Rutherford MN, LeBrun DP. Restricted expression of E2A protein in primary human tissues correlates with proliferation and differentiation. *Am J Pathol.* 1998;153(1):165-173.
282. Bain F, Engel I, Robanus EC, et al. E2A deficiency leads to abnormaltieis in ab T-cell development and to rapid development of T-cell lymphomas. *Mol Cell Biol.* 1997;17:4782-4791.
283. Zhuang Y, Soriano P, Weintraub H. The helix-loop-helix gene E2A is required for B cell formation. *Cell.* 1994;79(5):875-884.
284. Nourse J, Mellentin JD, Galili N, et al. Chromosomal translocation t(1;19) results in synthesis of a homeobox fusion mRNA that codes for a potential chimeric transcription factor. *Cell.* 1990;60(4):535-545.
285. Chang CP, de Vivo I, Cleary ML. The Hox cooperativity motif of the chimeric oncoprotein E2a-Pbx1 is necessary and sufficient for oncogenesis. *Mol Cell Biol.* 1997;17(1):81-88.
286. LeBrun DP. E2A basic helix-loop-helix transcription factors in human leukemia. *Front Biosci.* 2003;8:s206-s222.
287. Smith KS, Chanda SK, Lingbeek M, et al. Bmi-1 regulation of INK4A-ARF is a downstream requirement for transformation of hematopoietic progenitors by E2a-Pbx1. *Mol Cell.* 2003;12(2):393-400.
288. Park I-K, Qian D, Kiel M, et al. Bmi-1 is required for maintenance of adult self-renewing haematopoietic stem cells. *Nature.* 2003;423(6937):302-305.
289. Chin L, Pomerantz J, DePinho RA. The INK4a/ARF tumor suppressor: one gene-two products-two pathways. *Trends Biochem Sci.* 1998;23:291-296.
290. Dyson N. The regulation of E2F by pRB-family proteins. *Genes Dev.* 1998;12(15):2245-2262.
291. Talluri S, Dick FA. Regulation of transcription and chromatin structure by pRB: here, there and everywhere. *Cell Cycle.* 2012;11(17):3189-3198.
292. Raimondi SC, Privitera E, Williams DL, et al. New recurring chromosomal translocations in childhood acute lymphoblastic leukemia. *Blood.* 1991;77(9):2016-2022.
293. Inaba T, Roberts WM, Shapiro LH, et al. Fusion of the leucine zipper gene HLF to the E2A gene in human acute B-lineage leukemia. *Science.* 1992;257(5069):531-534.
294. Hunger SP, Ohyashiki K, Toyama K, Cleary ML. Hlf, a novel hepatic bZIP protein, shows altered DNA-binding properties following fusion to E2A in t(17;19) acute lymphoblastic leukemia. *Genes Dev.* 1992;6(9):1608-1620.
295. Romana SP, Mauchauffe M, Le Coniat M, et al. The t(12;21) of acute lymphoblastic leukemia results in a tel-AML1 gene fusion. *Blood.* 1995;85(12):3662-3670.
296. Golub TR, Barker GF, Bohlander SK, et al. Fusion of the TEL gene on 12p13 to the AML1 gene on 21q22 in acute lymphoblastic leukemia. *Proc Natl Acad Sci U S A.* 1995;92(11):4917-4921.
297. Wang L, Hiebert SW. TEL contacts multiple co-repressors and specifically associates with histone deacetylase 3. *Oncogene.* 2001;20(28):3716-3725.
298. Greaves MF, Wiemels J. Origins of chromosome translocations in childhood leukaemia. *Nat Rev Cancer.* 2003;3(9):639-649. doi:10.1038/nrc1164
299. Papaemmanuil E, Rapado I, Li Y, et al. RAG-mediated recombination is the predominant driver of oncogenic rearrangement in ETV6-RUNX1 acute lymphoblastic leukemia. *Nat Genet.* 2014;46(2):116-125.
300. Kuiper RP, Waanders E. A RAG driver on the road to pediatric ALL. *Nat Genet.* 2014;46(2):96-98.
301. Lilljebjörn H, Henningsson R, Hyrenius-Wittsten A, et al. Identification of ETV6-RUNX1-like and DUX4-rearranged subtypes in paediatric B-cell precursor acute lymphoblastic leukaemia. *Nat Commun.* 2016;7:11790. doi:10.1038/NCOMMS11790
302. Zaliova M, Kotrova M, Bresolin S, et al. ETV6/RUNX1 -like acute lymphoblastic leukemia: a novel B-cell precursor leukemia subtype associated with the CD27/CD44 immunophenotype. *Genes Chromosomes Cancer.* 2017;56(8):608-616. doi:10.1002/gcc.22464
303. Harrison CJ. Blood Spotlight on iAMP21 acute lymphoblastic leukemia (ALL), a high-risk pediatric disease. *Blood.* 2015;125(9):1383-1386. doi:10.1182/blood-2014-08-569228
304. Rand V, Parker H, Russell LJ, et al. Genomic characterization implicates iAMP21 as a likely primary genetic event in childhood B-cell precursor acute lymphoblastic leukemia. *Blood.* 2011;117(25):6848-6855.
305. Zhang J, McCastlain K, Yoshihara H, et al. Deregulation of DUX4 and ERG in acute lymphoblastic leukemia. *Nat Genet.* 2016;48(12):1481-1489. doi:10.1038/NG.3691
306. Li J, Dai Y, Wu L, et al. Emerging molecular subtypes and therapeutic targets in B-cell precursor acute lymphoblastic leukemia. *Front Med.* 2021;15(3):347-371. doi:10.1007/S11684-020-0821-6
307. Dong X, Zhang W, Wu H, et al. Structural basis of DUX4/IGH-driven transactivation. *Leukemia.* 2018;32(6):1466-1476. doi:10.1038/S41375-018-0093-1
308. Gu Z, Churchman M, Roberts K, et al. Genomic analyses identify recurrent MEF2D fusions in acute lymphoblastic leukaemia. *Nat Commun.* 2016;7:13331. doi:10.1038/NCOMMS13331
309. Ohki K, Kiyokawa N, Saito Y, et al. Clinical and molecular characteristics of MEF2D fusion-positive B-cell precursor acute lymphoblastic leukemia in childhood, including a novel translocation resulting in MEF2D-HNRNPH1 gene fusion. *Haematologica.* 2019;104(1):128-137.
310. Herglotz J, Unrau L, Hauschildt F, et al. Essential control of early B-cell development by Mef2 transcription factors. *Blood.* 2016;127(5):572-581. doi:10.1182/BLOOD-2015-04-643270
311. Zaliova M, Winkowska L, Stuchly J, et al. A novel class of ZNF384 aberrations in acute leukemia. *Blood Adv.* 2021;5(21):4393-4397. doi:10.1182/bloodadvances.2021005318
312. Young SK, Shao Y, Bidwell JP, Wek RC. Nuclear matrix protein 4 is a novel regulator of ribosome biogenesis and controls the unfolded protein response via repression of Gadd34 expression. *J Biol Chem.* 2016;291(26):13780-13788. doi:10.1074/JBC.M116.729830
313. Hirabayashi S, Butler ER, Ohki K, et al. Clinical characteristics and outcomes of B-ALL with ZNF384 rearrangements: a retrospective analysis by the Ponte di Legno Childhood ALL Working Group. *Leukemia.* 2021;35(11):3272-3277. doi:10.1038/s41375-021-01199-0
314. Hirabayashi S, Ohki K, Nakabayashi K, et al. ZNF384 -related fusion genes define a subgroup of childhood B-cell precursor acute lymphoblastic leukemia with a characteristic immunotype. *Haematologica.* 2017;102(1):118-129. doi:10.3324/haematol.2016.151035
315. Yasuda T, Sanada M, Kawazu M, et al. Two novel high-risk adult B-cell acute lymphoblastic leukemia subtypes with high expression of CDX2 and IDH1/2 mutations. *Blood.* 2022;139(12):1850-1862.
316. Thoene S, Rawat VPS, Heilmeier B, et al. The homeobox gene CDX2 is aberrantly expressed and associated with an inferior prognosis in patients with acute lymphoblastic leukemia. *Leukemia.* 2009;23(4):649-655.
317. Vu T, Straube J, Porter AH, et al. Hematopoietic stem and progenitor cell-restricted Cdx2 expression induces transformation to myelodysplasia and acute leukemia. *Nat Commun.* 2020;11(1):3021.
318. Secker-Walker LM, Craig JM, Hawkins JM, Hoffbrand AV. Philadelphia positive acute lymphoblastic leukemia in adults: age distribution, BCR breakpoint and prognostic significance. *Leukemia.* 1991;5(3):196-199.
319. Uckun FM, Nachman JB, Sather HN, et al. Clinical significance of Philadelphia chromosome positive pediatric acute lymphoblastic leukemia in the context of contemporary intensive therapies: a report from the Children's Cancer Group. *Cancer.* 1998;83(9):2030-2039.
320. Kurzrock R, Gutterman JU, Talpaz M. The molecular genetics of Philadelphia chromosome-positive leukemias. *N Engl J Med.* 1988;319(15):990-998.
321. Voncken JW, Kaartinen V, Pattengale PK, Germeraad WT, Groffen J, Heisterkamp N. BCR/ABL p210 and p190 cause distinct leukemia in transgenic mice. *Blood.* 1995;86(12):4603-4611.
322. Radich JP. Philadelphia chromosome-positive acute lymphocytic leukemia. *Hematol Oncol Clin North Am.* 2001;15(1):21-36.
323. Laneuville P. Abl tyrosine protein kinase. *Semin Immunol.* 1995;7(4):255-266.
324. Pendergast AM, Quilliam LA, Cripe LD, et al. BCR-ABL-induced oncogenesis is mediated by direct interaction with the SH2 domain of the GRB-2 adaptor protein. *Cell.* 1993;75(1):175-185.
325. Faderl S, Talpaz M, Estrov Z, O'Brien S, Kurzrock R, Kantarjian HM. The biology of chronic myeloid leukemia. *N Engl J Med.* 1999;341(3):164-172.
326. Ribera JM. Advances in acute lymphoblastic leukemia in adults. *Curr Opin Oncol.* 2011;23(6):692-699.
327. Mullighan CG, Miller CB, Radtke I, et al. BCR-ABL1 lymphoblastic leukaemia is characterized by the deletion of Ikaros. *Nature.* 2008;453(7191):110-114.
328. Tran TH, Loh ML. Ph-like acute lymphoblastic leukemia. *Hematology Am Soc Hematol Educ Program.* 2016;2016(1):561-566. doi:10.1182/ASHEDUCATION-2016.1.561
329. Mullighan CG, Zhang J, Harvey RC, et al. JAK mutations in high-risk childhood acute lymphoblastic leukemia. *Proc Natl Acad Sci U S A.* 2009;106(23):9414-9418.
330. Iacobucci I, Roberts KG. Genetic alterations and therapeutic targeting of philadelphia-like acute lymphoblastic leukemia. *Genes.* 2021;12(5):687. doi:10.3390/GENES12050687
331. Harvey RC, Tasian SK. Clinical diagnostics and treatment strategies for Philadelphia chromosome-like acute lymphoblastic leukemia. *Blood Adv.* 2020;4(1):218-228.
332. Harvey RC, Kang H, Roberts KG, et al. Development and validation of a highly sensitive and specific gene expression classifier to prospectively screen and identify B-precursor acute lymphoblastic leukemia (ALL) patients with a Philadelphia chromosome-like ("Ph-like" or "BCR-ABL1-like") signat. *Blood.* 2013;122(21):826. doi:10.1182/blood.V122.21.826.826

333. Tasian SK, Doral MY, Borowitz MJ, et al. Aberrant STAT5 and PI3K/mTOR pathway signaling occurs in human CRLF2-rearranged B-precursor acute lymphoblastic leukemia. *Blood*. 2012;120(4):833-842.
334. Tasian SK, Loh ML. Understanding the biology of CRLF2-overexpressing acute lymphoblastic leukemia. *Crit Rev Oncog*. 2011;16(1-2):13-24.
335. Ge Z, Gu Y, Zhao G, et al. High CRLF2 expression associates with IKZF1 dysfunction in adult acute lymphoblastic leukemia without CRLF2 rearrangement. *Oncotarget*. 2016;7(31):49722-49732.
336. Alekseyenko AA, Walsh EM, Wang X, et al. The oncogenic BRD4-NUT chromatin regulator drives aberrant transcription within large topological domains. *Genes Dev*. 2015;29(14):1507-1523.
337. Mullighan CG. How advanced are we in targeting novel subtypes of ALL? *Best Pract Res Clin Haematol*. 2019;32(4):101095. doi:10.1016/j.beha.2019.101095
338. Rabbitts TH, Axelson H, Forster A, et al. Chromosomal translocations and leukaemia: a role for LMO2 in T cell acute leukaemia, in transcription and in erythropoiesis. *Leukemia*. 1997;11(suppl 3):271-272.
339. Raimondi SC. T-lineage acute lymphoblastic leukemia (T-ALL). *Atlas Genet Cytogenet Oncol Haematol*. 2007;11:69-81.
340. Armstrong SA, Look AT. Molecular genetics of acute lymphoblastic leukemia. *J Clin Oncol*. 2005;23(26):6306-6315.
341. De Keersmaecker K, Marynen P, Cools J. Genetic insights in the pathogenesis of T-cell acute lymphoblastic leukemia. *Haematologica*. 2005;90(8):1116-1127.
342. Ferrando AA, Look AT. Gene expression profiling in T-cell acute lymphoblastic leukemia. *Semin Hematol*. 2003;40(4):274-280.
343. Nagel S, Venturini L, Meyer C, et al. Multiple mechanisms induce ectopic expression of LYL1 in subsets of T-ALL cell lines. *Leuk Res*. 2010;34(4):521-528. doi:10.1016/j.leukres.2009.06.020
344. Mansour MR, Abraham BJ, Anders L, et al. Oncogene regulation. An oncogenic super-enhancer formed through somatic mutation of a noncoding intergenic element. *Science*. 2014;346(6215):1373-1377.
345. Rahman S, Magnussen M, León TE, et al. Activation of the *LMO2* oncogene through a somatically acquired neomorphic promoter in T-cell acute lymphoblastic leukemia. *Blood*. 2017;129(24):3221-3226.
346. Chiaretti S, Li X, Gentleman R, et al. Gene expression profile of adult T-cell acute lymphocytic leukemia identifies distinct subsets of patients with different response to therapy and survival. *Blood*. 2004;103(7):2771-2778. doi:10.1182/blood-2003-09-3243
347. Karrman K, Castor A, Behrendtz M, et al. Deep sequencing and SNP array analyses of pediatric T-cell acute lymphoblastic leukemia reveal NOTCH1 mutations in minor subclones and a high incidence of uniparental isodisomies affecting CDKN2A. *J Hematol Oncol*. 2015;8:42. doi:10.1186/s13045-015-0138-0
348. Okamoto A, Demetrick DJ, Spillare EA, et al. Mutations and altered expression of p16INK4 in human cancer. *Proc Natl Acad Sci U S A*. 1994;91(23):11045-11049.
349. Merlo A, Herman JG, Mao L, et al. 5' CpG island methylation is associated with transcriptional silencing of the tumour suppressor p16/CDKN2/MTS1 in human cancers. *Nat Med*. 1995;1(7):686-692.
350. Lowe SW, Sherr CJ. Tumor suppression by Ink4a-Arf: progress and puzzles. *Curr Opin Genet Dev*. 2003;13(1):77-83.
351. Zhang J, Ding L, Holmfeldt L, et al. The genetic basis of early T-cell precursor acute lymphoblastic leukaemia. *Nature*. 2012;481(7380):157-163.doi:10.1038/nature10725
352. Washburn T, Schweighoffer E, Gridley T, et al. Notch activity influences the alpha-beta versus gammadelta T cell lineage decision. *Cell*. 1997;88(6):833-843.
353. Sambandam A, Maillard I, Zediak VP, et al. Notch signaling controls the generation and differentiation of early T lineage progenitors. *Nat Immunol*. 2005;6(7):663-670.
354. Pui JC, Allman D, Xu L, et al. Notch1 expression in early lymphopoiesis influences B versus T lineage determination. *Immunity*. 1999;11(3):299-308.
355. Sanchez-Martin M, Ferrando A. The NOTCH1-MYC highway toward T-cell acute lymphoblastic leukemia. *Blood*. 2017;129(9):1124-1133. doi:10.1182/blood-2016-09-692582
356. Ellisen LW, Bird J, West DC, et al. TAN-1, the human homolog of the Drosophila notch gene, is broken by chromosomal translocations in T lymphoblastic neoplasms. *Cell*. 1991;66(4):649-661.
357. Weng AP, Ferrando AA, Lee W, et al. Activating mutations of NOTCH1 in human T cell acute lymphoblastic leukemia. *Science*. 2004;306(5694):269-271.
358. Aster JC, Pear WS, Blacklow SC. Notch signaling in leukemia. *Annu Rev Pathol*. 2008;3:587-613.
359. Roy M, Pear WS, Aster JC. The multifaceted role of Notch in cancer. *Curr Opin Genet Dev*. 2007;17(1):52-59.
360. Palomero T, Lim WK, Odom DT, et al. NOTCH1 directly regulates c-MYC and activates a feed-forward-loop transcriptional network promoting leukemic cell growth. *Proc Natl Acad Sci U S A*. 2006;103(48):18261-18266. doi:10.1073/pnas.0606108103
361. Sharma VM, Calvo JA, Draheim KM, et al. Notch1 contributes to mouse T-cell leukemia by directly inducing the expression of c-myc. *Mol Cell Biol*. 2006;26(21):8022-8031. doi:10.1128/mcb.01091-06
362. Weng AP, Millholland JM, Yashiro-Ohtani Y, et al. c-Myc is an important direct target of Notch1 in T-cell acute lymphoblastic leukemia/lymphoma. *Genes Dev*. 2006;20(15):2096-2109.
363. Wendorff AA, Koch U, Wunderlich FT, et al. Hes1 is a critical but context-dependent mediator of canonical Notch signaling in lymphocyte development and transformation. *Immunity*. 2010;33(5):671-684.
364. Reavie L, Della Gatta G, Crusio K, et al. Regulation of hematopoietic stem cell differentiation by a single ubiquitin ligase-substrate complex. *Nat Immunol*. 2010;11(3):207-215.
365. Welcker M, Clurman BE. FBW7 ubiquitin ligase: a tumour suppressor at the crossroads of cell division, growth and differentiation. *Nat Rev Cancer*. 2008;8(2):83-93. doi:10.1038/nrc2290
366. O'Neil J, Grim J, Strack P, et al. FBW7 mutations in leukemic cells mediate NOTCH pathway activation and resistance to gamma-secretase inhibitors. *J Exp Med*. 2007;204(8):1813-1824.
367. Thompson BJ, Buonamici S, Sulis ML, et al. The SCFFBW7 ubiquitin ligase complex as a tumor suppressor in T cell leukemia. *J Exp Med*. 2007;204(8):1825-1835.
368. Kox C, Zimmermann M, Stanulla M, et al. The favorable effect of activating NOTCH1 receptor mutations on long-term outcome in T-ALL patients treated on the ALL-BFM 2000 protocol can be separated from FBXW7 loss of function. *Leukemia*. 2010;24(12):2005-2013. doi:10.1038/leu.2010.203
369. Real PJ, Tosello V, Palomero T, et al. Gamma-secretase inhibitors reverse glucocorticoid resistance in T cell acute lymphoblastic leukemia. *Nat Med*. 2009;15(1):50-58. doi:10.1038/nm.1900
370. Weng AP, Nam Y, Wolfe MS, et al. Growth suppression of pre-T acute lymphoblastic leukemia cells by inhibition of notch signaling. *Mol Cell Biol*. 2003;23(2):655-664.
371. De Keersmaecker K, Lahortiga I, Mentens N, et al. In vitro validation of gamma-secretase inhibitors alone or in combination with other anti-cancer drugs for the treatment of T-cell acute lymphoblastic leukemia. *Haematologica*. 2008;93(4):533-542. doi:10.3324/haematol.11894
372. Tolcher AW, Messersmith WA, Mikulski SM, et al. Phase I study of RO4929097, a gamma secretase inhibitor of Notch signaling, in patients with refractory metastatic or locally advanced solid tumors. *J Clin Oncol*. 2012;30(19):2348-2353.
373. Krop I, Demuth T, Guthrie T, et al. Phase I pharmacologic and pharmacodynamic study of the gamma secretase (Notch) inhibitor MK-0752 in adult patients with advanced solid tumors. *J Clin Oncol*. 2012;30(19):2307-2313.
374. Girardi T, Vicente C, Cools J, De Keersmaecker K. The genetics and molecular biology of T-ALL. *Blood*. 2017;129(9):1113-1123. doi:10.1182/blood-2016-10-706465
375. Carroll AJ, Crist WM, Link MP, et al. The t(1;14)(p34;q11) is nonrandom and restricted to T-cell acute lymphoblastic leukemia: a Pediatric Oncology Group study. *Blood*. 1990;76(6):1220-1224.
376. Bernard OA, Guglielmi P, Jonveaux P, Cherif D. Two distinct mechanisms for the SCL gene activation in the t(1;14) translocation of T-cell leukemias. *Genes Chrom Cancer*. 1990;1:194-208.
377. Chen Q, Cheng J-T, Tasi LH, et al. The tal gene undergoes chromosome translocation in T cell leukemia and potentially encodes a helix-loop-helix protein. *EMBO J*. 1990;9(2):415-424.
378. Brown L, Cheng J-T, Chen Q, et al. Site-specific recombination of the tal-1 gene is a common occurrence in human T cell leukemia. *EMBO J*. 1990;9(10):3343-3351.
379. Xia Y, Brown L, Tsan JT, et al. The translocation (1;14)(p34;q11) in human T-cell leukemia: chromosome breakage 25 kilobase pairs downstream of the TAL1 protooncogene. *Genes Chromosomes Cancer*. 1992;4(3):211-216.
380. Labastie MC, Cortes F, Romeo PH, Dulac C, Peault B. Molecular identity of hematopoietic precursor cells emerging in the human embryo. *Blood*. 1998;92(8):3624-3635.
381. Cheng T, Shen H, Giokas D, Gere J, Tenen DG, Scadden DT. Temporal mapping of gene expression levels during the differentiation of individual primary hematopoietic cells. *Proc Natl Acad Sci U S A*. 1996;93(23):13158-13163.
382. Robb L, Lyons I, Li R, et al. Absence of yolk sac hematopoiesis from mice with a targeted disruption of the scl gene. *Proc Natl Acad Sci U S A*. 1995;92(15):7075-7079.
383. Shivdasani RA, Mayer EL, Orkin SH. Absence of blood formation in mice lacking the T-cell leukaemia oncoprotein tal-1/SCL. *Nature*. 1995;373(6513):432-434.
384. Mikkola HKA, Klintman J, Yang H, et al. Haematopoietic stem cells retain long-term repopulating activity and multipotency in the absence of stem-cell leukaemia SCL/tal-1 gene. *Nature*. 2003;421(6922):547-551.
385. Souroullas GP, Salmon JM, Sablitzky F, Curtis DJ, Goodell MA. Adult hematopoietic stem and progenitor cells require either Lyl1 or Scl for survival. *Cell Stem Cell*. 2009;4(2):180-186.
386. Layer JH, Alford CE, McDonald WH, Davé UP. LMO2 oncoprotein stability in T-cell leukemia requires direct LDB1 binding. *Mol Cell Biol*. 2016;36(3):488-506. doi:10.1128/MCB.00901-15
387. McCormack MP, Forster A, Drynan L, Pannell R, Rabbitts TH. The LMO2 T-cell oncogene is activated via chromosomal translocations or retroviral insertion during gene therapy but has no mandatory role in normal T-cell development. *Mol Cell Biol*. 2003;23(24):9003-9013.
388. Nam CH, Rabbitts TH. The role of LMO2 in development and in T cell leukemia after chromosomal translocation or retroviral insertion. *Mol Ther*. 2006;13(1):15-25. doi:10.1016/j.ymthe.2005.09.010
389. Van Vlierberghe P, Beverloo H, Buijs-Gladdines J, et al. Monoallelic or biallelic LMO2 expression in relation to the LMO2 rearrangement status in pediatric T-cell acute lymphoblastic leukemia. *Leukemia*. 2007;22(7):1434-1437.
390. Grutz GG, Bucher K, Lavenir I, Larson T, Larson RA, Rabbitts TH. The oncogenic T cell LIM-protein Lmo2 forms part of a DNA-binding complex specifically in immature T cells. *EMBO J*. 1998;17(16):4594-4605.
391. Osada H, Grutz GG, Axelson H, Forster A, Rabbitts TH. Association of erythroid transcription factors: complexes involving the LIM protein RBTN2 and the zinc-finger protein GATA1. *Proc Natl Acad Sci U S A*. 1995;92(21):9585-9589.
392. Valge-Archer VE, Forster A, Rabbitts TH. The LMO1 and LDB1 proteins interact in human T cell acute leukaemia with the chromosomal translocation t(1;14)(p15;q11). *Oncogene*. 1998;17:3199-3202.
393. Larson RC, Lavenir I, Larson TA, et al. Protein dimerization between Lmo2 (Rbtn2) and Tal1 alters thymocyte development and potentiates T cell tumorigenesis in transgenic mice. *EMBO J*. 1996;15(5):1021-1027.
394. Huang S, Qiu Y, Stein RW, Brandt SJ. p300 functions as a transcriptional coactivator for the TAL1/SCL oncoprotein. *Oncogene*. 1999;18(35):4958-4967.

395. Huang S, Brandt SJ. mSin3A regulates murine erythroleukemia cell differentiation through association with the TAL1 (or SCL) transcription factor. *Mol Cell Biol.* 2000;20(6):2248-2259.
396. Layer JH, Christy M, Placek L, Unutmaz D, Guo Y, Davé UP. LDB1 enforces stability on direct and indirect oncoprotein partners in leukemia. *Mol Cell Biol.* 2020;40(12):e00652-19. doi:10.1128/MCB.00652-19
397. Sun XJ, Wang Z, Wang L, et al. A stable transcription factor complex nucleated by oligomeric AML1-ETO controls leukaemogenesis. *Nature.* 2013;500(7460):93-97. doi:10.1038/nature12287
398. Ono Y, Fukuhara N, Yoshie O. Transcriptional activity of TAL1 in T cell acute lymphoblastic leukemia (T-ALL) requires RBTN1 or -2 and induces TALLA1, a highly specific tumor marker of T-ALL. *J Biol Chem.* 1997;272(7):4576-4581.
399. Ono Y, Fukuhara N, Yoshie O. TAL1 and LIM-only proteins synergistically induce retinaldehyde dehydrogenase 2 expression in T-cell acute lymphoblastic leukemia by acting as cofactors for GATA3. *Mol Cell Biol.* 1998;18(12):6939-6950.
400. Palomero T, Odom DT, O'Neil J, et al. Transcriptional regulatory networks downstream of TAL1/SCL in T-cell acute lymphoblastic leukemia. *Blood.* 2006;108(3):986-992. doi:10.1182/blood-2005-08-3482
401. Palii CG, Perez-Iratxeta C, Yao Z, et al. Differential genomic targeting of the transcription factor TAL1 in alternate haematopoietic lineages. *EMBO J.* 2011;30(3):494-509. doi:10.1038/emboj.2010.342
402. Park ST, Sun XH. The Tal1 oncoprotein inhibits E47-mediated transcription. Mechanism of inhibition. *J Biol Chem.* 1998;273(12):7030-7037.
403. O'Neil J, Shank J, Cusson N, Murre C, Kelliher M. TAL1/SCL induces leukemia by inhibiting the transcriptional activity of E47/HEB. *Cancer Cell.* 2004;5(6):587-596. doi:10.1016/j.ccr.2004.05.023
404. Dave UP, Akagi K, Tripathi R, et al. Murine leukemias with retroviral insertions at Lmo2 are predictive of the leukemias induced in SCID-X1 patients following retroviral gene therapy. *PLoS Genet.* 2009;5(5):e1000491. doi:10.1371/journal.pgen.1000491
405. Lin YW, Deveney R, Barbara M, et al. OLIG2 (BHLHB1), a bHLH transcription factor, contributes to leukemogenesis in concert with LMO1. *Cancer Res.* 2005;65(16):7151-7158.
406. Coustan-Smith E, Mullighan CG, Onciu M, et al. Early T-cell precursor leukaemia: a subtype of very high-risk acute lymphoblastic leukaemia. *Lancet Oncol.* 2009;10(2):147-156.
407. Asnafi V, Beldjord K, Libura M, et al. Age-related phenotypic and oncogenic differences in T-cell acute lymphoblastic leukemias may reflect thymic atrophy. *Blood.* 2004;104:4173-4180.
408. Ferrando AA, Herblot S, Palomero T, et al. Biallelic transcriptional activation of oncogenic transcription factors in T-cell acute lymphoblastic leukemia. *Blood.* 2004;103(5):1909-1911.
409. Ferrando AA, Neuberg DS, Dodge RK, et al. Prognostic importance of TLX1 (HOX11) oncogene expression in adults with T-cell acute lymphoblastic leukaemia. *Lancet.* 2004;363(9408):535-536.
410. Bernard OA, Busson-LeConiat M, Ballerini P, et al. A new recurrent and specific cryptic translocation, t(5;14)(q35;q32), is associated with expression of the Hox11L2 gene in T acute lymphoblastic leukemia. *Leukemia.* 2001;15(10):1495-1504.
411. Su XY, Della-Valle V, Andre-Schmutz I, et al. HOX11L2/TLX3 is transcriptionally activated through T-cell regulatory elements downstream of BCL11B as a result of the t(5;14)(q35;q32). *Blood.* 2006;108(13):4198-4201. doi:10.1182/blood-2006-07-032953
412. Cauwelier B, Cave H, Gervais C, et al. Clinical, cytogenetic and molecular characteristics of 14 T-ALL patients carrying the TCRbeta-HOXA rearrangement: a study of the Groupe Francophone de Cytogenetique Hematologique. *Leukemia.* 2007;21(1):121-128. doi:10.1038/sj.leu.2404410
413. Speleman F, Cauwelier B, Dastugue N, et al. A new recurrent inversion, inv(7)(p15q34), leads to transcriptional activation of HOXA10 and HOXA11 in a subset of T-cell acute lymphoblastic leukemias. *Leukemia.* 2005;19(3):358-366. doi:10.1038/sj.leu.2403657
414. Bergeron J, Clappier E, Cauwelier B, et al. HOXA cluster deregulation in T-ALL associated with both a TCRD-HOXA and a CALM-AF10 chromosomal translocation. *Leukemia.* 2006;20(6):1184-1187.
415. Dadi S, Le Noir S, Payet-Bornet D, et al. TLX homeodomain oncogenes mediate T cell maturation arrest in T-ALL via interaction with ETS1 and suppression of TCRα gene expression. *Cancer Cell.* 2012;21(4):563-576. doi:10.1016/j.ccr.2012.02.013
416. De Keersmaecker K, Ferrando AA. TLX1-induced T-cell acute lymphoblastic leukemia. *Clin Cancer Res.* 2011;17(20):6381-6386. doi:10.1158/1078-0432.CCR-10-3037
417. Dik WA, Brahim W, Braun C, et al. CALM-AF10+ T-ALL expression profiles are characterized by overexpression of HOXA and BMI1 oncogenes. *Leukemia.* 2005;19(11):1948-1957
418. Ferrando AA, Armstrong SA, Neuberg DS, et al. Gene expression signatures in MLL-rearranged T-lineage and B-precursor acute leukemias: dominance of HOX dysregulation. *Blood.* 2003;102(1):262-268. online:1-31.
419. Soulier J, Clappier E, Cayuela JM, et al. HOXA genes are included in genetic and biologic networks defining human acute T-cell leukemia (T-ALL). *Blood.* 2005;106(1):274-286.
420. O'Neil J, Tchinda J, Gutierrez A, et al. Alu elements mediate MYB gene tandem duplication in human T-ALL. *J Exp Med.* 2007;204(13):3059-3066. doi:10.1084/jem.20071637
421. Lahortiga I, De Keersmaecker K, Van Vlierberghe P, et al. Duplication of the MYB oncogene in T cell acute lymphoblastic leukemia. *Nat Genet.* 2007;39(5):593-595. doi:10.1038/ng2025
422. Gutierrez A, Kentsis A, Sanda T, et al. The BCL11B tumor suppressor is mutated across the major molecular subtypes of T-cell acute lymphoblastic leukemia. *Blood.* 2011;118(15):4169-4173.
423. Li L, Leid M, Rothenberg EV. An early T cell lineage commitment checkpoint dependent on the transcription factor Bcl11b. *Science.* 2010;329(5987):89-93. doi:10.1126/science.1188989
424. Shochat C, Tal N, Bandapalli OR, et al. Gain-of-function mutations in interleukin-7 receptor-alpha (IL7R) in childhood acute lymphoblastic leukemias. *J Exp Med.* 2011;208(5):901-908.
425. Zenatti PP, Ribeiro D, Li W, et al. Oncogenic IL7R gain-of-function mutations in childhood T-cell acute lymphoblastic leukemia. *Nat Genet.* 2011;43(10):932-939. doi:10.1038/ng.924
426. Flex E, Petrangeli V, Stella L, et al. Somatically acquired JAK1 mutations in adult acute lymphoblastic leukemia. *J Exp Med.* 2008;205(4):751-758. doi:10.1084/jem.20072182
427. Asnafi V, Le Noir S, Lhermitte L, et al. JAK1 mutations are not frequent events in adult T-ALL: a GRAALL study. *Br J Haematol.* 2010;148(1):178-179.
428. Delgado-Martin C, Meyer LK, Huang BJ, et al. JAK/STAT pathway inhibition overcomes IL7-induced glucocorticoid resistance in a subset of human T-cell acute lymphoblastic leukemias. *Leukemia.* 2017;31(12):2568-2576. doi:10.1038/leu.2017.136
429. Jain N, Lamb AV, O'Brien S, et al. Early T-cell precursor acute lymphoblastic leukemia/lymphoma (ETP-ALL/LBL) in adolescents and adults: a high-risk subtype. *Blood.* 2016;127(15):1863-1869.
430. Sin CF, Man PHM. Early T-cell precursor acute lymphoblastic leukemia: diagnosis, updates in molecular pathogenesis, management, and novel therapies. *Front Oncol.* 2021;11:750789.
431. Neumann M, Heesch S, Schlee C, et al. Whole-exome sequencing in adult ETP-ALL reveals a high rate of DNMT3A mutations. *Blood.* 2013;121(23):4749-4752. doi:10.1182/blood-2012-11-465138
432. Huether R, Dong L, Chen X, et al. The landscape of somatic mutations in epigenetic regulators across 1, 000 paediatric cancer genomes. *Nat Commun.* 2014;5:3630. doi:10.1038/ncomms4630
433. Peirs S, Van der Meulen J, Van de Walle I, et al. Epigenetics in T-cell acute lymphoblastic leukemia. *Immunol Rev.* 2015;263(1):50-67. doi:10.1111/imr.12237
434. Ntziachristos P, Tsirigos A, Van Vlierberghe P, et al. Genetic inactivation of the polycomb repressive complex 2 in T cell acute lymphoblastic leukemia. *Nat Med.* 2012;18(2):298-301. doi:10.1038/nm.2651
435. Todd MAM, Ivanochko D, Picketts DJ. PHF6 degrees of separation: the multifaceted roles of a chromatin adaptor protein. *Genes.* 2015;6(2):325-352. doi:10.3390/genes6020325
436. Tijchon E, Havinga J, van Leeuwen FN, Scheijen B. B-lineage transcription factors and cooperating gene lesions required for leukemia development. *Leukemia.* 2013;27(3):541-552. doi:10.1038/leu.2012.293

Chapter 74 ■ Diagnosis and Classification of the Acute Leukemias and Myelodysplastic Syndromes

DANIEL A. ARBER • ATTILIO ORAZI

INTRODUCTION

The diagnosis and classification of acute leukemias and myelodysplastic syndromes (MDSs) has grown increasingly complex,[1-3] and this complexity will increase with new classifications that are scheduled to be published in late 2022. Cases can no longer be fully classified by the use of only morphologic evaluation and cytochemical studies. Historic information such as the presence of Down syndrome, prior therapy, or prior MDS all impact the final diagnosis. Additionally, immunophenotypic studies are needed for many cases, and cytogenetic and molecular genetic studies are required for essentially all cases.

This increase in complexity in the evaluation of these neoplasms has resulted in more precise diagnostic categories and recognition that the broad categories of acute myeloid leukemia (AML), acute lymphoblastic leukemia (ALL), and MDS actually represent heterogeneous groups of diseases. The newer disease categories are more predictive of outcome than older classification systems, in part because of their ability to separate disease groups within each category.[4-7] Unfortunately, many physicians continue to use older terminology for these diseases on the basis of the French-American-British Cooperative Group (FAB) classification[8-11] of these neoplasms. Although the FAB classification provided firm diagnostic criteria and useful terminology for communication of findings using the methods available at the time, its use is no longer appropriate. The third (2001), fourth (2008), and revised fourth (2016) editions of the World Health Organization (WHO) classification of hematopoietic tumors have dramatically changed the approach to diagnosis of many of these neoplasms. As the time of this chapter, the 2016 WHO system is considered as the standard of care, but a 5th edition WHO classification and an alternative International Consensus Classification[12] of these neoplasms are in press or published. Modifications from the European LeukemiaNet group and others will certainly continue to aid in the refinement of our classification systems.[13-15] This evolution from the FAB to the WHO is reminiscent of changes in lymphoma classification with evolution from the Rappaport[16] and Kiel[17] classifications to the Working Formulation[18] to the Revised European American Lymphoma[19] classification and finally to the WHO classification.[2,3,20] Perhaps because the changes in lymphoma classification were more step wise with shorter time intervals between the changes than the leukemia classification changes, they have been more widely adopted. We no longer refer to diffuse large B-cell lymphoma as histiocytic lymphoma and should no longer refer to AML with t(8; 21)(q22;q22.1) as AML-M2, or to B-lymphoblastic leukemia with *BCR::ABL1* as ALL-L2.

Several discoveries have impacted the classification of these neoplasms and many of them are covered in great detail in other chapters, but genetic discoveries associated with the acute leukemias and MDSs are probably the most significant. The finding of recurrent cytogenetic abnormalities with prognostic significance impacts all of these diseases.[21-26] Although balanced translocations are more common in the acute leukemias, the presence of single and complex abnormalities in MDS has helped define disease prognosis as well as defining a specific disease category of MDS with isolated del(5q).[6,7] The more recent discoveries of specific gene mutations have further impacted both acute leukemia and MDS diagnosis.[15,27-33] Whereas many of these mutations have their greatest frequency in AMLs with a normal karyotype, others offer prognostic significance that complements other morphologic and karyotypic features and future classification systems will rely more heavily on mutation results.

The classification of AML and MDS has also been impacted greatly by the understanding of similarities between the two. The so-called myelodysplasia-related AML and de novo AML described by Head[34] helped lead to a new way of thinking about this disease, especially AML occurring in older patients.

This chapter highlights key classification issues in the acute leukemias and MDSs, which are discussed in detail in the chapters that follow.

DIAGNOSTIC EVALUATION

The diagnostic approach to acute leukemia and MDSs still begins with a morphologic evaluation, but requires careful integration of the morphologic findings with clinical information and relevant laboratory data, including cytogenetic and molecular results.[35] Laboratory data, particularly results of a recent complete blood count (CBC), must be reviewed with the samples. Morphologic evaluation requires a well-stained (usually Wright stained) peripheral blood (PB) smear prepared from a recent sample (less than 2 hours from procurement). A 200-cell manual differential count is required for PB smears. The bone marrow (BM) aspirate smears are best prepared at the bedside immediately after procurement and promptly stained usually with Wright's stain. The review of smears aspirate smears includes a 500-cell differential count. In patients with inaspirable marrow, touch preparation of the BM biopsy can be used in lieu of an aspirate smear. The BM biopsy is usually stained with hematoxylin and eosin (H&E) or Giemsa and is useful in many settings.[36] The morphologic assessment allows for the appropriate use of ancillary tests in these disorders. Details of the ancillary tests used for the workup of the various diseases are provided in Chapters 2 through 4 and will not be repeated here.

Cytochemical studies are still performed at many institutions and can often provide quick general information about the cell type of an acute leukemia (myeloid vs myeloperoxidase negative), but because more detailed and specific information can now be obtained by flow cytometry in the same time frame, the use of cytochemical studies has decreased. Immunophenotyping, usually by multicolor flow cytometry, is now standard for acute leukemias and is absolutely required to accurately diagnose the lymphoblastic leukemias.[8,13,14,37,38] In cases of acute leukemia with marrow fibrosis, as may occur with some acute megakaryoblastic leukemias and with acute panmyelosis with myelofibrosis (APMF) (see *Figure 74.1*), paraffin section immunohistochemistry performed on a BM trephine biopsy is essential.[39] The use of flow cytometry immunophenotyping in the MDSs is the subject of much study, and many centers have incorporated this technique into the evaluation of patients with potential MDS not only to help quantitate blood and marrow blast cell percentages but also to detect abnormal maturing cell populations.[13,40,41] These methods, however, do not replace morphologic evaluation, including morphologic blast cell counts on smears.

Cytogenetic studies should also be performed on all cases of suspected acute leukemia or MDS.[23,42,43] Although specific gene mutations and some structural abnormalities will be missed by this method, karyotype analysis currently provides the best overall assessment of chromosomal abnormalities and should not be supplanted by other studies. Fluorescence in situ hybridization (FISH) or polymerase chain reaction (PCR) studies are often helpful to detect cryptic abnormalities that may be missed by karyotype analysis and are often added in panels for suspected acute leukemia or MDS.[44] Finally, molecular studies for specific gene mutations are now routinely performed on samples from patients with these disorders, but when each mutation is studied individually, the specific tests performed should be ordered based on the findings of other studies. However, with the rapid growth of next-generation sequencing technology,[45] more cost-effective gene mutation panels have become available to reduce the need for selective testing.

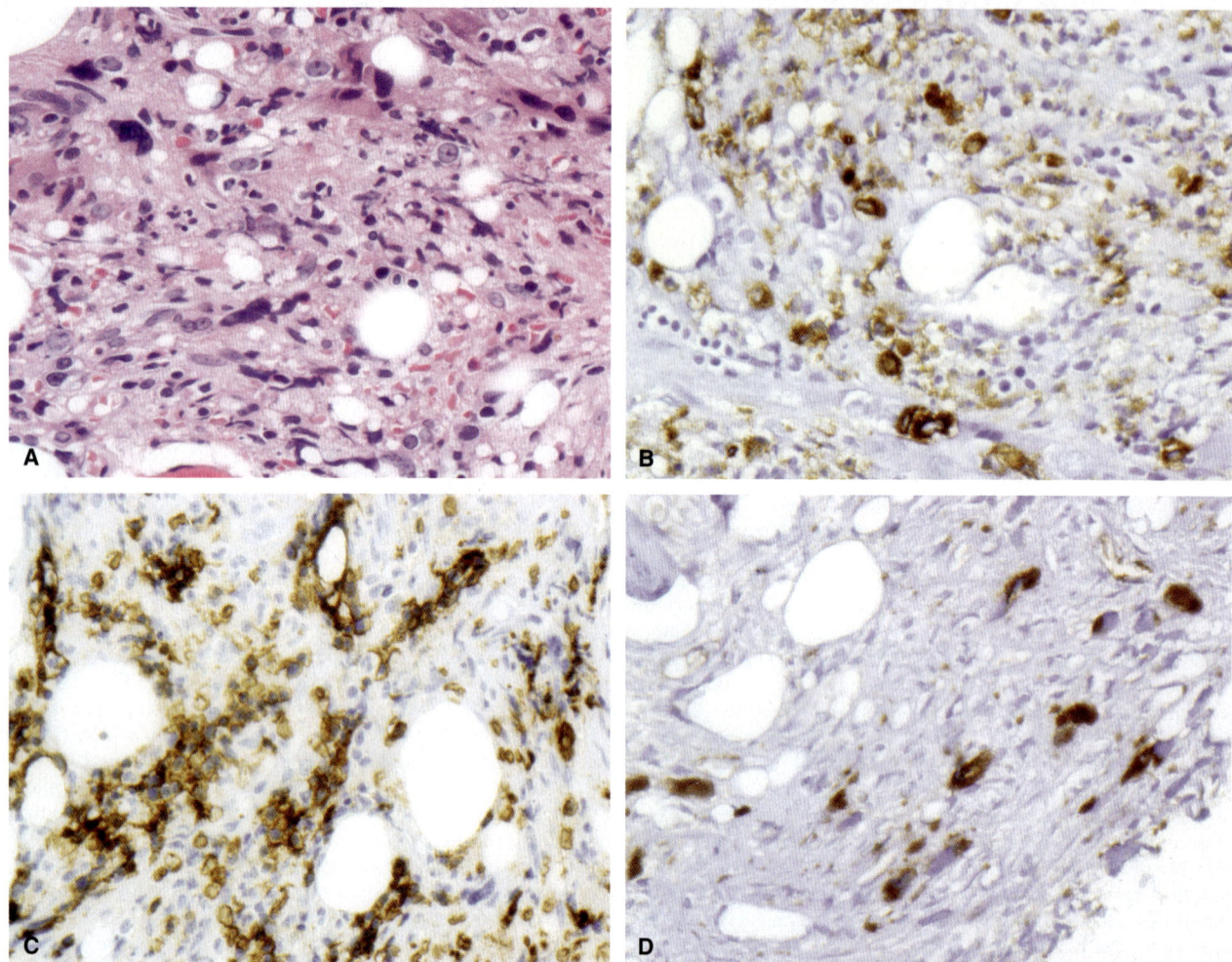

FIGURE 74.1 Acute panmyelosis with myelofibrosis illustrating the use of immunohistochemistry in diagnosis. The marrow is inaspirable due to marked marrow fibrosis (A) with a mixed cellular population that includes immature mononuclear cells. The cells show a mix of granulocyte precursors marking with myeloperoxidase (B), erythroid precursors marking with glycophorin B (C), and immature megakaryocytes marking with von Willebrand factor (D).

Once this broad array of studies is complete, the results should be incorporated into a single report with a final diagnosis. Because they cannot always be completed in the time interval needed to begin therapy, this approach requires the use of preliminary and amended reports. Because the modern classification relies on the use of cytogenetic studies and increasing numbers of disease groups are defined by mutation analysis, the diagnosis often needs to be refined, and thus amended, when these studies are complete.

MYELODYSPLASTIC SYNDROMES

Patients with MDS typically show persistent (>6 months) unexplained cytopenia(s). The vast majority of MDS patients present with anemia. Neutropenia and thrombocytopenia are less common presenting symptoms. Cytopenia levels are defined by common reference ranges.[46] However, they are considered pronounced with a hemoglobin level of less than 10 g/dL, an absolute neutrophil count of less than 1.8×10^9/L, and a platelet count of less than 100×10^9/L.[35,47] Because the presence of cytopenia(s) is required for the diagnosis, the most current and preferably previous CBCs have to be reviewed at the time of BM examination. Other pertinent data include medications, chemical exposure history, and previous and current illnesses because all of these can cause morphologic dysplasia indistinguishable from MDS. Comorbidities associated with morphologic dysplasia may include liver and kidney failure, autoimmune disorders, neoplasms, and systemic infections. In particular, morphologic evaluation is best performed when the patient is off medication.

Dysplastic features can be present in a single hematopoietic lineage (unilineage dysplasia) or involve all marrow populations (multilineage dysplasia) (*Figure 74.2*). At least 10% of all cells in a given lineage (erythroid, myeloid, megakaryocytic) have to be dysplastic for establishing the presence of MDS-associated dysplasia. The majority of MDS cases show dyserythropoiesis. PB shows normocytic, normochromic, or macrocytic anemia with macroovalocytes. Microcytosis can be present in rare cases of MDS (e.g., cases associated with congenital or acquired alpha thalassemia). The most common dysplastic features seen in erythroid precursors include nuclear abnormalities such as nuclear budding, nuclear fragmentation, irregular nuclear outlines, karyorrhexis, internuclear bridging, multinucleation, and megaloblastoid, coarsely condensed chromatin. Cytoplasmic vacuoles with coalescing vacuoles, defective hemoglobinization and increased numbers of ring sideroblasts can also be encountered. Similarly, dysgranulopoiesis is often manifested by abnormal nuclear features including hyposegmentation (pseudo–Pelger-Huët or monolobated neutrophils), hypersegmented and/or enlarged nuclei, nuclear sticks or fragments, macropolycytes, and abnormally condensed chromatin, which often coexists with nuclear hyposegmentation. Cytoplasmic features include hypogranulation, pseudo–Chediak-Higashi granules, and very rarely Auer rods. Hypogranulation occurs frequently and is related to the defective formation of secondary granules. Megakaryocyte morphology can be evaluated using both aspirate smear and the histologic sections (biopsy or clot section) with careful examination of at least 30 megakaryocytes.[35,47] Dysplastic features include nonlobated or hypolobated nuclei and multiple, widely separated nuclei including

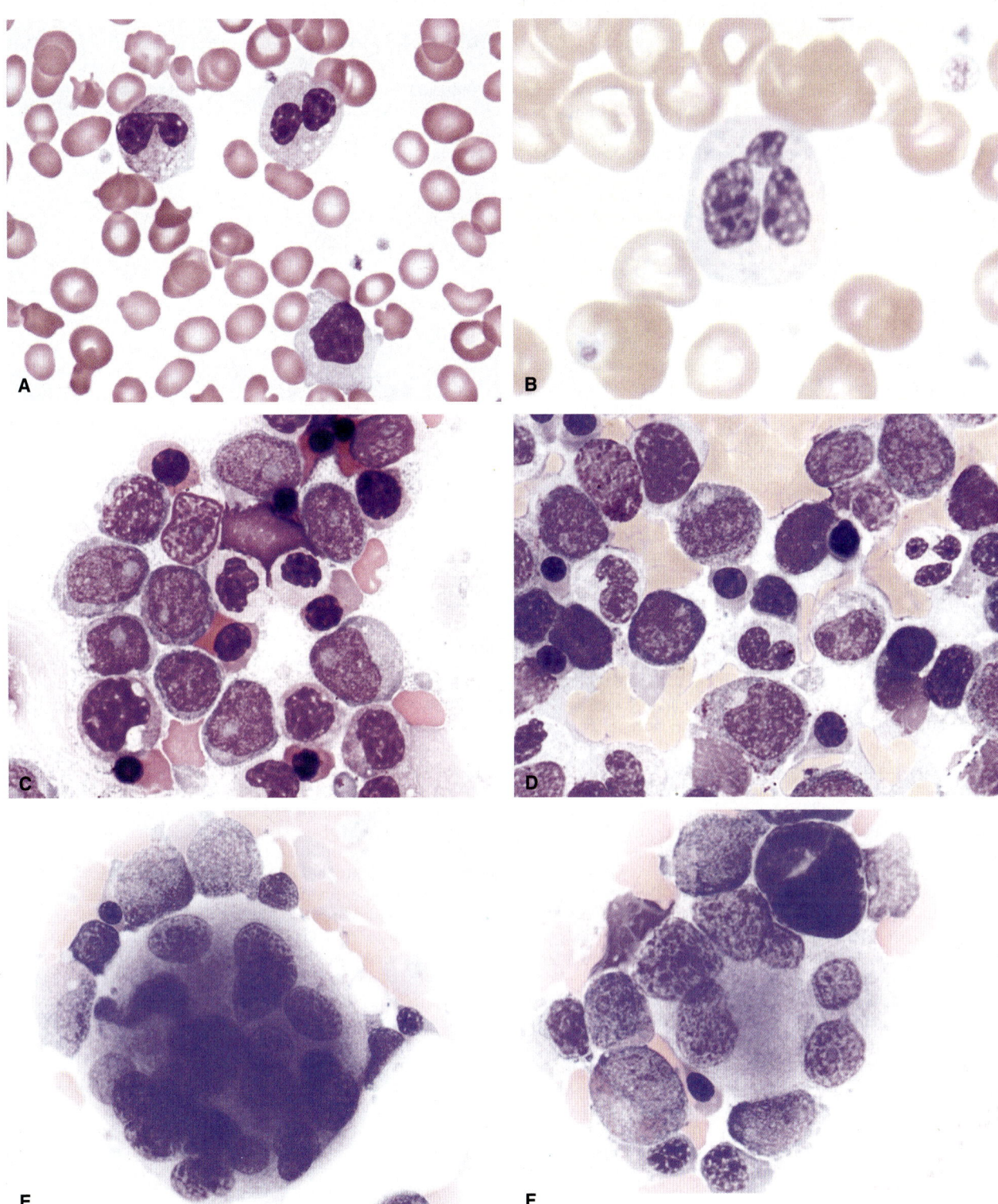

FIGURE 74.2 Dyspoietic changes in myelodysplastic syndrome and acute myeloid leukemia. Peripheral blood (A and B) and bone marrow (C and D) neutrophils may show cytoplasmic hypogranulation, clumped nuclear chromatin, and hyposegmentation, including pseudo–Pelger-Huët anomaly as shown in image (A). Dyserythropoiesis may include nuclear-cytoplasmic asynchrony and irregular nuclear shapes in the marrow erythroid precursors (C and D). Megakaryocyte changes include hypersegmented cells (E) and smaller, hypolobated cells (F).

"pawn ball" forms. Normal size or small megakaryocytes with a single (nonlobated) eccentrically placed nucleus are common in 5q-syndrome and in cases with abnormalities of chromosome 3. The latter also shows typically numerous bilobated forms. Megakaryocytic dysplasia is often associated with thrombocytopenia and platelets of variable size, including large forms occasionally showing hypogranulation.

The biopsy allows for the evaluation of cellularity, architectural features, fibrosis, and the presence of an associated, previously undiagnosed focal lesion such as mastocytosis, myeloma, metastatic neoplasm, or infection. In MDS marrows, the typical architectural organization is lost. Clusters of immature myeloid cells are frequently found in the center of the marrow space. This finding was originally termed abnormal localization of immature precursors (ALIPs) and is more frequently seen in cases of high-grade MDS. Based on pure morphology, ALIP included both blasts and promyelocytes clustering away from trabeculae. The proper identification of blasts both in clusters and scattered in the marrow is facilitated by CD34 immunohistochemistry, which is also useful to determine the overall number of blasts in cases with inaspirable marrows. The presence of CD34-positive cell clusters is a prognostically significant finding that is predominantly seen in high-risk MDS.[48] The BM biopsy is necessary for the assessment of BM fibrosis by a silver impregnation method (e.g., Gomori). Significant fibrosis occurs predominantly in high-risk and therapy-related MDS; however, it may also occur in low-risk disease. Finally, BM biopsy is critical for the exclusion of other hematologic and also nonhematologic diseases associated with unexplained cytopenia(s) which can clinically mimic MDS.

In addition to dysplasia, the evaluation of blasts constitutes a cornerstone of morphologic diagnosis of MDS. The optimal quality of BM aspirate and PB smears cannot be overemphasized.[35] The blast percentage is derived from a 500-cell differential count of marrow aspirate smear and a 200-cell differential count of PB smear, with both counts being essential for the subclassification of individual cases. In MDS, both agranular and granular (type I and type II) myeloblasts, and, if present, monoblasts, promonocytes, and megakaryoblasts are included in the blast category.[49] In the absence of an adequate BM aspirate smears (e.g., due to an inaspirable "dry tap" marrow), careful evaluation of the BM biopsy aided by a CD34 immunohistochemical stain can be used. The latter is particularly helpful in cases with significant marrow fibrosis or in hypoplastic marrows, which often yield hemodilute marrow aspirates.[50] Of note, blasts in MDS can rarely be negative for CD34; therefore, careful correlation with the visual blast identification is required in all cases. It is also important to emphasize that morphologic dysplasia is not equivalent to a diagnosis of MDS. Megakaryocytic and erythroid dysplasia are commonly seen in individuals in a variety of conditions. Nutritional deficiencies, heavy metal exposure, medications, and systemic diseases can produce morphologic changes resembling those seen in MDS. Therefore, as discussed previously, the correlation with clinical history is critical.

Cytogenetics is crucial and is also required for proper classification. The MDS-associated abnormalities are listed in *Table 74.1*. In addition, mutational analysis is an important additional tool in the prognostic assessment of MDS.[32,51] More than 90% of MDS have at least one myeloid neoplasms–associated mutation.[51,52] *SF3B1* mutation is currently considered as subtype defining for a subset of MDSs which were formerly recognized because of the presence of ring sideroblasts.[53] *TP53* biallelic mutations seem to identify a particularly aggressive subset of MDS patients.[54,55]

The 2016 WHO classification adopted new nomenclature for specific MDS disease groups and further refined the criteria for diagnosis and classification of MDS (*Table 74.2*). In general, the terms *refractory anemia* and *refractory cytopenia* have been replaced with *MDS*. Cases currently recognized as MDS with single lineage dysplasia (MDS-SLD) encompass patients with (mono) cytopenia or bicytopenia associated with unilineage dysplasia. Regardless of the lineage involved in MDS-SLD, blasts are absent or represent less than 1% of the PB differential count. Patients which would otherwise been considered as MDS-SLD or MDS with multilineage dysplasia (MDS-MLD) but with 1% blasts in PB or patients with unilineage dysplasia associated with pancytopenia are now classified as having unclassifiable MDS (MDS-U), owing to the uncertain but presumably more severe clinical significance of these findings.[3] Additionally, the category of MDS-U includes cytopenic patients lacking significant dysplasia, but presenting with cytogenetic abnormalities considered presumptive evidence of MDS.

The 2016 WHO classification acknowledged a subset of pediatric patients who present with cytopenia associated with dysplasia in at least two cell lines and marrow hypocellularity which has been included as a separate provisional category within the MDS group termed refractory cytopenia of childhood (RCC). This category encompasses children that have persistent cytopenia with less than 2%

Table 74.1. Recurrent Chromosomal Abnormalities and Their Frequency in Myelodysplastic Syndrome

Abnormality	Frequency (%)
Unbalanced	
+8	10
−7 or del(7q)	10
−5 or del(5q)	10
del(20q)	5-8
−Y	5
i(17q) or t(17q)	3-5
−13 or del(13q)	3
del(11q)	3
del(12q) or t(12q)	3
del(9q)	1-2
idic(X) (q13)	1-2
Balanced	
t(1; 3) (p36.3; q21.2)	1
t(2; 11) (p21; q23)	1
inv(3) (q21; q26.2)	1
t(6; 9) (p23; q34)	1

blasts in the PB and less than 5% blasts in the BM.[56,57] However, most of the RCC patients do not show mutations commonly seen in MDS in adults, while some shows constitutional genetic abnormalities; thus, their precise diagnostic categorization remains unclear.

Some subtypes or presentations of MDS are more challenging and will be discussed in more detail. MDS-U includes cases which do not fulfill criteria of other MDS subtypes. MDS-U can be diagnosed in patients fulfilling the following criteria: (1) patients who fit the criteria for a diagnosis of MDS-SLD or MDS-MLD, but in whom 1% blasts in the blood are found on at least two consecutive occasions; (2) patients with MDS with morphologic dysplasia limited to one hematopoietic lineage who present with pancytopenia; (3) patients with persistent cytopenia, no increase in blasts, and lacking diagnostic morphologic features of MDS (less than 10% dysplastic cells in any lineage), but with at least one clonal cytogenetic abnormality considered as a presumptive evidence of MDS. According to the 2016 WHO classification, if characteristic features of a specific subtype of MDS develop later in the course of the disease, the case initially classified as MDS-U should be reclassified accordingly. The prognosis of MDS-U varies and close follow-up is warranted.

Approximately 10% to 15% of MDS patients show a significant increase in reticulin fibers and/or collagen fibrosis at presentation.[58] MDS with fibrosis (MDS-F) is defined by the presence of significant fibrosis (at least 3+ reticulin fibrosis according to the Baumeister/Manoharan scoring system, or at least 2+ reticulin fibrosis according to the European consensus grading system).[47,58,59] In the past, select cases with 2+ reticulin fibrosis according to Baumeister/Manoharan scoring may have been classified as MDS-F. MDS-F should be subtyped according to the 2016 WHO classification, with the annotation to indicate the presence of fibrosis. The majority of MDS-F cases fall into the category of MDS with excess blasts (MDS-EBs). Therapy-related MDS cases frequently show significant marrow fibrosis, but are excluded from the MDS-F category in favor of placing them in a special entity of therapy-related myeloid neoplasms. The majority of MDS-F patients present with severe pancytopenia. Organomegaly is minimal or absent. The patients with MDS-F are reported to have shorter overall survival and disease-free survival times than those without fibrosis, even in the absence of excess blasts.[58,60,61] BM fibrosis is also associated with a poor outcome after BM transplantation.[62] BM

Table 74.2. The 2016 WHO Classification of MDS

Subtype	Blood Findings	Bone Marrow Findings
MDS with single lineage dysplasia	Unicytopenia or bicytopenia[a] <1% blasts	Unilineage dysplasia; ≥10% of the cells of the affected lineage are dysplastic <5% blasts <15% ring sideroblasts
MDS-RS with single lineage dysplasia	Anemia <1% blasts	Erythroid dysplasia only <5% blasts ≥15% ring sideroblasts (or ≥5% ring sideroblasts if *SF3B1* mutation is present)
MDS-RS with multilineage dysplasia	Cytopenia(s) <1% blasts No Auer rods	Dysplasia in ≥10% of cells in two or more myeloid Lineages <5% blasts No Auer rods ≥15% ring sideroblasts (or ≥5% ring sideroblasts if *SF3B1* mutation is present)
MDS with multilineage dysplasia	Cytopenia(s) No or rare blasts (<1%) No Auer rods	Dysplasia in ≥10% of cells in two or more myeloid Lineages <5% blasts No Auer rods <15% ring sideroblasts
MDS with excess blasts-1 (MDS-EB-1)	Cytopenias 2%-4% blasts No Auer rods	Unilineage or multilineage dysplasia 5%-9% blasts No Auer rods
MDS with excess blasts-2 (MDS-EB-2)	Cytopenias 5%-19% blasts ± Auer rods	Unilineage or multilineage dysplasia 10%-19% Blasts ± Auer rods[b]
Myelodysplastic syndrome, unclassified (MDS-U)	Cytopenias <1% or 1% blasts No Auer rods	Unequivocal dysplasia in <10% of cells in one or more myeloid cell lines associated with pancytopenia or MDS-associated cytogenetics or 1% circulating blasts <5% bone marrow blasts
MDS associated with isolated del(5q)	Anemia <1% blasts Platelet count usually normal or increased	Normal to increased megakaryocytes with hypolobated nuclei <5% blasts No Auer rods del(5q) alone or with one additional abnormality except −7 or del(7q)

Abbreviations: MDS, myelodysplastic syndrome; RS, ring sideroblasts.
[a]Bicytopenia may occasionally be observed. Cases with pancytopenia should be classified as MDS-U.
[b]If the diagnostic criteria for MDS are fulfilled and Auer rods are present, the patient should always be categorized as MDS-EB-2.

and PB often show trilineage dysplasia with excess blasts. There is prominent dysmegakaryopoiesis, often associated with increased numbers of megakaryocytes. Cellular streaming is frequently seen on H&E biopsy section and is indicative of significant fibrosis. CD34 immunostaining may be helpful in assessing the number of blasts because the aspirate smears are often inadequate in patients with fibrotic marrows. Differential diagnoses of MDS-F include other myelofibrotic myeloid neoplasms such as APMF, myeloproliferative, and myelodysplastic/myeloproliferative neoplasms. Similar to MDS-F, APMF, a subtype of AML-not otherwise specified (NOS), shows marked fibrosis, trilineage dysplasia, and dwarf megakaryocytes. The higher number of blasts (often in the range of 20%-25%), abrupt onset with fever and bone pain, and rapidly progressive course seen in APMF are helpful in establishing the definitive diagnosis.[39] Classic myeloproliferative neoplasms, such as primary myelofibrosis, can usually be easily distinguished from MDS-F by their morphologic characteristics (e.g., large-to-giant megakaryocytes with hypolobulated bulbous-shaped nuclei often tightly clustered together, lack of other myelodysplastic features) and by the presence of significant splenomegaly.[35,63,64]

Myelodysplastic/myeloproliferative neoplasms such as chronic myelomonocytic leukemia may show morphologic features similar to MDS, yet demonstrate laboratory and clinical features of a proliferative process such as elevated white blood cell (WBC) and monocytosis.

Hypoplastic MDS (h-MDS), which is defined by its low marrow cellularity (cellularity of less than 20% for patients older than 70 years of age and less than 30% for individuals younger than 70 years), accounts for 5% to 10% of MDS patients.[3,65] Similar to typical cases of MDS, h-MDS is a disease of the elderly. It is more common in women. h-MDS has a prognosis and rate of transformation to AML similar to the corresponding WHO-classified MDS subtypes. The major differential diagnosis of h-MDS is aplastic anemia.[65,66] The typically hemodilute marrow aspirates obtained from hypoplastic marrow limit the evaluation of cytologic features, and in this context, the information derived from BM biopsy/clot section is of paramount importance. The majority of patients with h-MDS present with dyserythropoiesis and no increase in blasts and are classified as MDS-SLD.[65,66] Dysgranulopoiesis, dysmegakaryopoiesis, and increase in blasts occur less frequently. Patients with h-MDS can show mast cell hyperplasia, interstitial lymphocytosis, and lymphoid follicles. In the absence of significant MLD and/or increased blast population, the distinction from aplastic anemia can be challenging. The presence of relatively more frequent megakaryocytes, mildly increased reticulin fibers, and focally increased CD34-positive cells all suggest h-MDS. The immunohistochemical stains for CD34 and megakaryocytic antigens (CD42b and CD61) and reticulin stain are recommended to highlight the presence of these features.[65,66] Additional findings such as immunophenotypic abnormalities by flow cytometry or the presence of select cytogenetic markers such as losses of chromosomes 5 and/or 7, which are uncommon in aplastic anemia, are also helpful. The applications of novel technologies may help to better differentiate aplastic anemia from h-MDS and aid in early detection of transformation in the former entity.[52,67] The diagnostic challenges might be related to the overlap in pathogenesis as demonstrated by the T-cell-mediated suppression of hematopoiesis or the coexistence of clones of paroxysmal nocturnal hemoglobinuria cells documented to occur in both diseases.[68]

Erythroid-predominant MDS (MDS-E) can also cause diagnostic difficulties. By the historic definition, these patients have less than 20% myeloblasts both as enumerated from the total marrow cellularity and from the nonerythroid BM population. The latter criteria were necessary to exclude a diagnosis of the erythroid/myeloid type of erythroleukemia, but because that category of AML has been excluded in the 2016 WHO classification, such cases are now diagnosed as MDS. In MDS-E, similar to other cases of MDS, myeloblasts are enumerated as a percentage of all BM cells and their number is used to classify cases into one of the MDS subtypes.[3,35] However, recent studies suggested that the alternative approach of calculating the percentage of myeloblasts as a proportion of nonerythroid cells might provide a more accurate assessment of overall prognosis in MDS-E.[69] If myeloblasts are calculated as a percentage of nonerythroid cells, the upgrade to a higher risk subtype of MDS occurs mainly between the categories of MDS-MLD and MDS-EB-1 and between MDS-EB-1 and MDS-EB-2. Until more evidence is published, it is currently recommended to use the standard WHO criteria, using myeloblast percentages based on all cells, to classify cases of MDS-E.

As briefly mentioned before, gene mutation analysis provides additional prognostic information in MDS,[32,33,51] but identical mutations may occur outside of the setting of MDS. Mutations occur more frequently in the elderly. Some may be present in otherwise healthy individuals and are termed clonal hematopoiesis of indeterminate potential (CHIP) and those associated with cytopenia are referred to as clonal cytopenia of undetermined significance (CCUS).[70,71]

CLONAL CYTOPENIA OF UNDETERMINED SIGNIFICANCE, A POTENTIAL PRE-MDS CONDITION

Clonal hematopoiesis is identified by the detection of somatic mutations or cytogenetic aberrations or copy number abnormalities on genetic testing. CHIP is defined by the presence of a somatic mutation in a myeloid neoplasm associated gene at a variant allele fraction (VAF) of at least 2% or by the presence of a clonal cytogenetic abnormality in a patient lacking a myeloid neoplasm or unexplained cytopenia. The presence of CHIP increases with age and is relatively common in individuals above the age of 60.

In CCUS, there is cytopenia but no other evidence of a myeloid neoplasm. The cytopenia is persistent and not due to another condition, that is, a concomitant comorbidity.[1] CCUS is considered a risk factor for the development of overt MDS.[71,72] Somatic mutation(s) can also occur in paroxysmal nocturnal hemoglobinuria and a subset of aplastic anemia, both of which may progress to MDS.

CCUS and other pre–malignant clonal cytopenias are distinguished from MDS by lack of dysplasia or increased blasts on PB and BM examination. A threshold VAF of ≥2% is recommended for CCUS and other clonal cytopenias, recognizing that certain mutations and high VAF are associated with higher risk of progression to MDS.[73] Further study is warranted to better define "high-risk" CCUS and its relationship to bona fide MDS.[74-76]

ACUTE MYELOID LEUKEMIA

The classification of AML has changed dramatically from the FAB classification[8,9,11] to the current classifications.[3] Whereas the FAB classification was based primarily on morphologic and cytochemical features of the blast cells, the WHO uses a combined approach to define prognostically significant and biologically relevant disease groups. Although many of the WHO categories rely heavily on cytogenetic findings, most still retain distinctive morphologic and immunophenotypic findings. The specific AML disease categories are listed in *Table 74.3*, and some of the distinctive morphologic and immunophenotypic features of specific types are illustrated in *Figures 74.1, 74.3, and 74.4* and described in *Table 74.4*.

For most cases, a blast cell count of 20% or more in either the PB or BM aspirate is necessary for a diagnosis of AML. For cases with one of three recurring genetic abnormalities *PML::RARA*; t(8; 21) (q22; q22.1) *RUNX1::RUNX1T1*; and inv(16) (p13.1q22) or t(16; 16) (p13.1; q22) *CBFB::MYH11*, however, a diagnosis of AML can be made with a lower blast count. These low blast count cases are uncommon and still have abnormal blood and marrow findings. The detection of the genetic abnormality would indicate AML over a diagnosis of MDS in these cases.

The WHO classification[1,3] defines AML types by recurring genetic abnormalities, by recognizing cases related to MDS, and by separating

Table 74.3. 2016 WHO Classification of Acute Myeloid Leukemia and Related Precursor Neoplasms

AML with Recurrent Genetic Abnormalities
AML with t(8; 21) (q22; q22.1) (*RUNX1::RUNX1T1*)
AML with inv(16) (p13.1q22) or t(16,16) (p13.1; q22) (*CBFB::MYH11*)
Acute promyelocytic leukemia with *PML::RARA*
AML with t(9; 11) (p22.3; q23.3) (*KMT2A::MLLT3*)
AML with t(6; 9) (p23; q34.1) (*DEK::NUP214*)
AML with inv(3) (q21.3q26.2) or t(3; 3) (q21.3; q26.2) (*GATA2, MECOM*)
AML (megakaryoblastic) with t(1; 22) (p13.3; q13.3) (*RBM1::MKL1*)
Provisional entity: AML with *BCR::ABL1*
AML with mutated *NPM1*
AML with biallelic mutations of *CEBPA*
Provisional entity: AML with mutated *RUNX1*
AML with myelodysplasia-related changes
Therapy-related myeloid neoplasms
AML, not otherwise specified
AML with minimal differentiation
AML without maturation
AML with maturation
Acute myelomonocytic leukemia
Acute monoblastic/monocytic leukemia
Pure erythroid leukemia
Acute megakaryocytic leukemia
Acute basophilic leukemia
Acute panmyelosis with myelofibrosis

Abbreviation: AML, acute myeloid leukemia.

diseases related to prior therapy or associated with Down syndrome. Cases that do not fall into any of those groups are placed in the AML-NOS group and can be subdivided by morphologic features. Many of these cases, however, have normal karyotypes, and the search for predictive markers to better categorize them is ongoing.[77,78] Many gene mutations that are not definitional of AML subtypes are still important for predicting prognosis and potential therapeutic targets.

The category of AML with recurring genetic abnormalities was expanded in the 2008 and 2016 WHO classifications to include more disease groups by incorporating disease-defining mutations. AML with biallelic mutations of *CEBPA* and AML with mutated *NPM1* are specific disease categories, and AML with mutated *RUNX1* is a provisional category on the basis of the hypothesis that these mutations are disease-defining events,[79-88] similar to the other recurring cytogenetic abnormalities in this category, and not merely secondary events that impact prognosis. Recently, it has become apparent that in-frame bZIP mutations of *CEBPA*, including those that are monoallelic, define the relevant biologic category in AML rather than any biallelic mutation of the gene.[89] AML with *BCR::ABL1*[90,91] was also added as a provisional entity in the 2016 WHO classification because of the potential for tyrosine kinase inhibitor therapy in this rare de novo disorder.

AML with myelodysplasia-related changes (AML-MRC) of the 2008 WHO classification (*Table 74.5*) was an expansion and revision of the category of AML with MLD in the 2001 classification. Certainly, cases of AML arising from MDS can lack sufficient background cells to diagnose multilineage dysplasia and the expansion of this category allows cases to be diagnosed as AML-MRC by demonstrating the presence of multilineage dysplasia, the presence of an MDS-associated cytogenetic abnormality (*Table 74.6*), a history of prior MDS or a

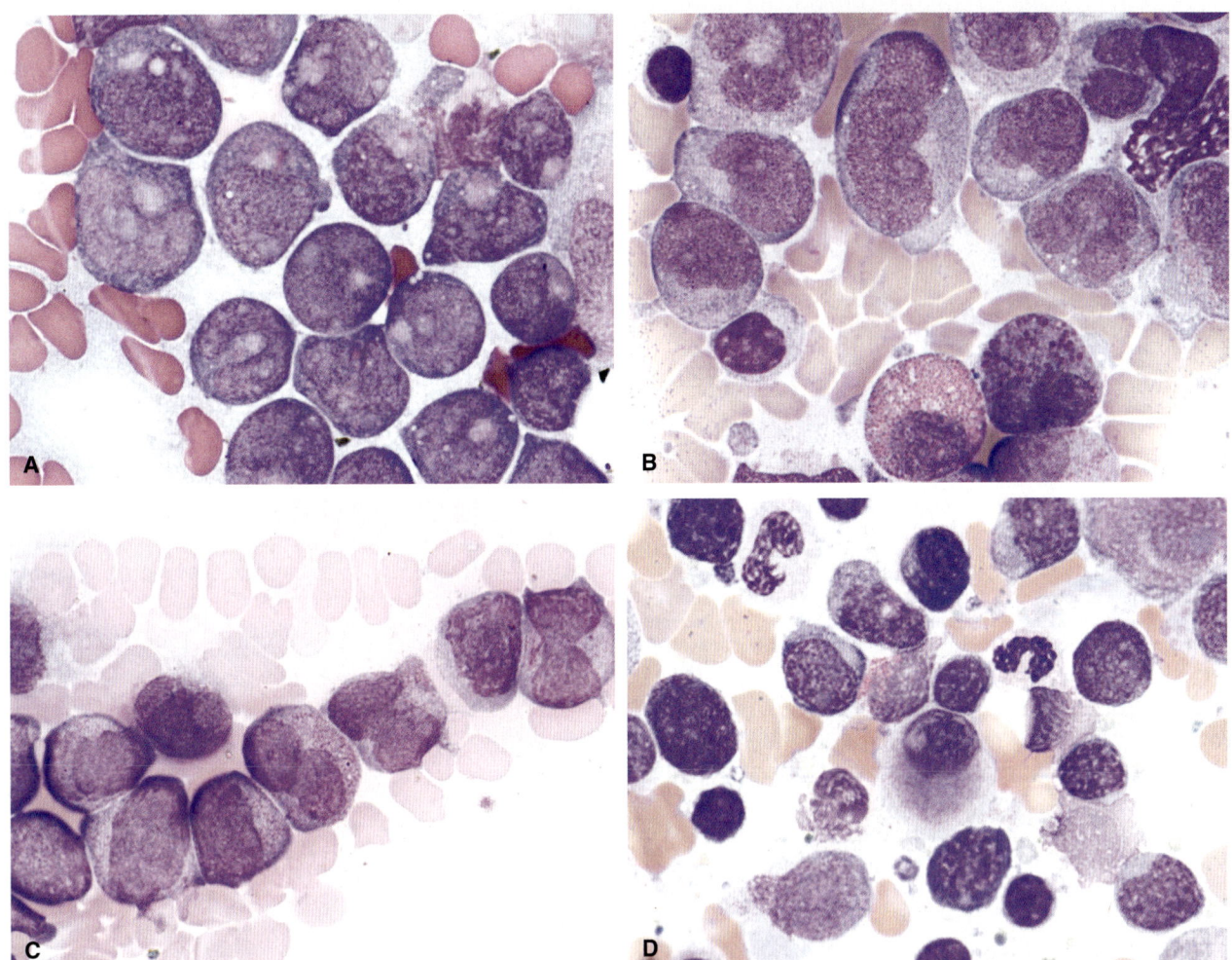

FIGURE 74.3 Morphologic features of more common acute myeloid leukemia types with recurrent cytogenetic abnormalities. A, Acute myeloid leukemia with t(8; 21) (q22; q22.1) (*RUNX1::RUNX1T1*) with blasts containing abundant cytoplasm with large granules and perinuclear clearing (hofs). B, Acute myeloid leukemia with inv(16) (p13.1q22) or t(16; 16) (p13.1; q22) (*CBFB::MYH11*) with an abnormal eosinophil containing large basophilic granules (lower right). C, Acute promyelocytic leukemia with *PML::RARA* typically shows blasts with bilobed nuclei, cytoplasmic granules and Auer rods (far right). D, Acute myeloid leukemia with inv(3) (q21.3; q26.2) (*GATA2, MECOM*) with background dyspoiesis and a small, nonlobated megakaryocyte (center).

Table 74.4. Distinctive Clinical, Morphologic, and Immunophenotypic Features of Acute Myeloid Leukemia Cytogenetic Subtypes

AML Subtype	Distinctive Features
AML with t(8; 21) (q22; q22.1) (*RUNX1::RUNX1T1*)	Granular blasts with perinuclear hofs, large salmon-colored granules, aberrant CD19 expression on CD34+ myeloblasts
AML with inv(16) (p13.1q22) or t(16; 16) (p13.1; q22) (*CBFB::MYH11*)	Presence of abnormal eosinophils with basophilic granules
Acute promyelocytic leukemia with *PML::RARA*	Bilobed nuclei with blasts lacking HLA-DR and usually CD34−
AML with t(6; 9) (p23; q34.1) (*DEK::NUP214*)	Multilineage dysplasia and associated basophilia
AML with inv(3) (q21.3q26.2) or t(3; 3) (q21.3; q26.2) (*GATA2, MECOM*)	Multilineage dysplasia and increased numbers of small mono- or bilobed megakaryocytes
AML (megakaryoblastic) with t(1; 22) (p13.3; q13.3) (*RBM15::MKL1*)	Infant without Down syndrome with CD41+ and CD61+ blasts. CD42b+ less frequent

Abbreviation: AML, acute myeloid leukemia.

myelodysplastic/myeloproliferative neoplasm, or a combination of such findings. This combined approach captures more cases of AML and defines a group with a particularly poor prognosis in adults. Cases with a normal karyotype and no history, but the presence of MLD, defined as two or more cell lines with 50% or more dysplastic cells, were the major area of controversy. Some large series failed to find prognostic significance for this group,[91,92] but other studies found multilineage dysplasia to independently predict a worse outcome compared with AML-NOS.[4,93] It is now more clear that multilineage dysplasia in de novo AML without MDS-related cytogenetic abnormalities, but with *NPM1* or biallelic *CEBPA* mutations, behaves more like the mutation-specific disease categories,[94-96] and such cases are no longer included in the AML-MRC category. The discovery of gene mutations associated with "secondary" AML[97,98] and the correlation of *TP53* mutations with therapy-related or MDS-related disease[99,100] are now allowing for gene mutation to further define this poor prognostic group and will alter the future diagnostic criteria for this group of AML patients.

Therapy-related myeloid neoplasms and the myeloid neoplasms associated with Down syndrome are also distinct from other AML types, and these also tend to show a continuum between cases with features of AML and MDS. For this reason, they are considered separate disease entities in the 2016 WHO classification, respectively, from the nontherapy- or Down-related leukemias. Cytogenetic and mutational findings in therapy-related myeloid neoplasms, however, remain prognostically significant.

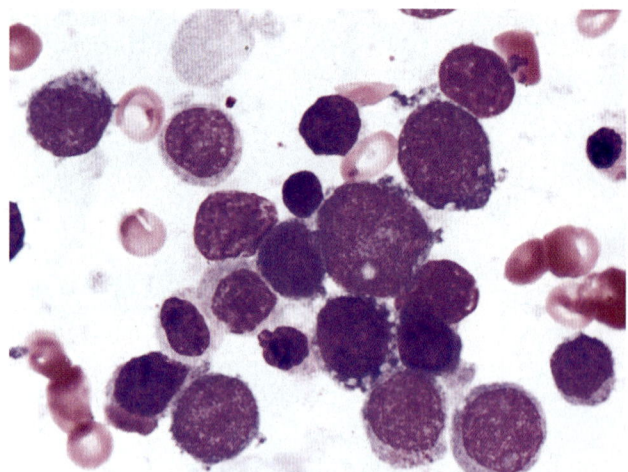

FIGURE 74.4 **Erythroid-rich myelodysplastic syndrome.** Over 50% erythroid precursors are present in the bone marrow with dyspoietic changes that include cytoplasmic vacuolization (lower center). In addition, scattered blasts, which mark as myeloblasts, are present in the background (upper left and lower right) representing over 20% of the nonerythroid cells in the marrow. Such cases were previously diagnosed as erythroid/myeloid type of acute erythroid leukemia, but are now considered as myelodysplastic syndrome.

Table 74.5. Criteria for Diagnosis of Acute Myeloid Leukemia With Myelodysplasia-Related Changes

1. At least 20% blasts in the blood or bone marrow
2. No history of prior cytotoxic therapy for other disease
3. Absence of a recurring chromosomal rearrangement as delineated in Table 74.3

AND, one or more of the following features:

1. Previous history of myelodysplastic syndrome or myelodysplastic/myeloproliferative disorder
2. Multilineage dysplasia (dyspoiesis in at least 50% of the elements from two or more lineages)[a]
3. Presence of an MDS-associated cytogenetic abnormality (see Table 74.6)

Abbreviation: MDS, myelodysplastic syndrome.
[a]This criterion cannot be used alone if a mutation of *NPM1* or a biallelic mutation of *CEBPA* is present.

Table 74.6. Cytogenetic Abnormalities Sufficient to Diagnose AML With Myelodysplasia-Related Changes when ≥20% Blasts Are Present in Blood or Bone Marrow in the Absence of Prior Cytotoxic Therapy

Complex Karyotype	≥3 Unrelated Chromosomal Abnormalities, Not Including Any Rearrangements That Would Define a Subtype of AML With Recurrent Cytogenetic Abnormalities	
Unbalanced abnormalities	−7/del(7q) del(5q)/t(5q) i(17q)/t(17p) −13/del(13q)	del(11q) del(12p)/t(12p) idic(X) (q13)
Balanced abnormalities	t(11; 16) (q23.3; p13.3) t(3; 21) (q26.2; q22.1) t(1; 3) (p36.3; q21.2) t(2; 11) (p21; q23.3)	t(5; 12) (q32; p13.2) t(5; 7) (q32; q11.2) t(5; 17) (q32; p13.2) t(5; 10) (q32; q21.2) t(3; 5) (q25.3; q35.1)

Abbreviation: AML, acute myeloid leukemia.

Table 74.7. European Leukemia Net Acute Myeloid Leukemia Risk Stratification by Genetics

Genetic Group	Subsets
Favorable	• t(8; 21) (q22; q22.1); *RUNX1::RUNX1T1* • inv(16) (p13.1q22) or t(16; 16) (p13.1; q22); *CBFB::MYH11* • Mutated *NPM1* without *FLT3*-ITD or with *FLT3*-ITD[low] • Biallelic mutated *CEBPA*
Intermediate-I	• Mutated *NPM1* and *FLT3*-ITD[high] • Wild-type *NPM1* without *FLT3*-ITD or with *FLT3*-ITD[low] • t(9; 11) (p22; q23.3); *KMT2A::MLLT3* • Cytogenetic abnormalities not classified as favorable or adverse
Adverse	• t(6; 9) (p23; q34.1); *DEK::NUP214* • t(v; 11) (v; q23.3); *KMT2A* rearranged • t(9; 22) (q34.1; q11.2); *BCR::ABL1* • inv(3) (q21.3q26.2) or t(3; 3) (q21.3; q26.2); *GATA2, MECOM* • −5 or del(5q); −7; −17/abn(17p) • Complex karyotype, monosomal karyotype • Wild-type *NPM1* and *FLT3*-ITD[high] • Mutated *RUNX1* • Mutated *ASXL1* • Mutated *TP53*

Abbreviation: ITD, internal tandem repeat.

The remaining cases are placed into the category of AML-NOS and this category includes many normal karyotype cases and cases that are diagnosed as AML with unique features. The subcategories of AML-NOS are of little clinical significance,[101] and mutation analysis is probably most important in this group. Selected mutations (*FLT3* and *KIT*) are included as prognostic markers for different AML types in the WHO classification. While the utility of *KIT* mutations is primarily in the core binding factor leukemias (those with t[8; 21][q22; q22.1] *RUNX1::RUNX1T1*; and inv[16][p13.1q22] or t[16; 16][p13.1; q22] *CBFB::MYH11*),[102] *FLT3* and *NPM1* mutations are prognostically predictive in most cases of AML-NOS.[30,79,80,103-106] In addition to the mutations included in the 2008 WHO classification, other mutations have been described and validated as potential prognostic markers.[29,107-110] Other frequently occurring or prognostically significant mutations in AML include *DNMT3A*, *IDH1*, *IDH2*, *TET2*, *RUNX1*, *TP53*, *ASXL1*, *NRAS*, and *WT1* and testing for many of these are now recommended for prognostic reasons or as potential therapeutic targets by different groups,[15,111] and this list will certainly grow. Table 74.7 demonstrates one approach to combining cytogenetic studies and mutation analysis to develop prognostic categories in AML, but this approach will have to be frequently updated to include new discoveries.[15]

Categories of AML-NOS that offer the greatest diagnostic challenge are probably pure erythroid leukemia and APMF. Acute erythroleukemia was historically divided into pure erythroid leukemia with over 80% erythroid cells and no myeloblasts or a mixed myeloid/erythroid type.[112] The latter type (*Figure 74.4*) had 50% or more BM erythroid precursors; and of the nonerythroid marrow cells, 20% or more myeloblasts. These cases, by definition, have less than 20% total myeloblasts and are now classified as MDS in the 2016 WHO classification.[113,114]

Only pure erythroid leukemia remains in the classification and is defined by the presence of over 80% erythroid cells with at least 30% normoblasts. APMF usually involves an inaspirable marrow with marked fibrosis and a mix of immature myeloid, erythroid, and megakaryocytic cells (*Figure 74.1*).[39,115] This rare disorder is also difficult to distinguish from MDS-F and may be related to such proliferations.

ACUTE LYMPHOBLASTIC LEUKEMIA

The diagnostic approach to ALL has also changed dramatically over time. Although the immunophenotype of ALL was not part of the FAB classification,[11] it is now essential for diagnosing these disorders. Also, the relationship between lymphoblastic lymphoma and ALL is

Table 74.8. 2016 WHO Classification of Precursor Lymphoid Neoplasms

B-lymphoblastic Leukemia/lymphoma, not otherwise specified
B-lymphoblastic leukemia/lymphoma with recurrent genetic abnormalities
B-lymphoblastic leukemia/lymphoma with t(9; 22) (q34.1; q11.2); *BCR::ABL1*
B-lymphoblastic leukemia/lymphoma with t(v; 11q23.3); *KMT2A* rearrangement
B-lymphoblastic leukemia/lymphoma with t(12; 21) (p13.2; q22.1); *ETV6::RUNX1*
B-lymphoblastic leukemia/lymphoma with hyperdiploidy
B-lymphoblastic leukemia/lymphoma with hypodiploidy
B-lymphoblastic leukemia/lymphoma with t(5; 14) (q31.1; q32.3); *IL3::IGH*
B-lymphoblastic leukemia/lymphoma with t(1; 19) (q23; p13.3); *TCF3::PBX1*
Provisional entity: B-lymphoblastic leukemia/lymphoma, *BCR::ABL1*-like
Provisional entity: B-lymphoblastic leukemia/lymphoma with iAMP21
T-lymphoblastic leukemia/lymphoma
Provisional entity: Early T-cell precursor lymphoblastic leukemia
Provisional entity: Natural killer cell lymphoblastic leukemia/lymphoma

now recognized, and these disorders are grouped together in the WHO classification. Cases diagnosed in the past as ALL with a mature B-cell phenotype (FAB L3) are no longer considered as ALL and are best classified as leukemic variants of the mature B-cell lymphomas.

Although morphologic evaluation is important in ALL to identify the presence of a blast cell proliferation, immunophenotyping must be performed because lymphoblasts cannot be distinguished reliably from undifferentiated myeloblasts by morphology alone. In fact some lymphoblasts will contain cytoplasmic granules that may incorrectly suggest myeloid lineage.[116] Cytochemical studies are also not sufficient for such a diagnosis, because the absence of myeloperoxidase or Sudan black B by these methods does not exclude undifferentiated myeloblasts and the detection of PAS-positive granules in blasts is not specific for lymphoblasts.

The 2016 WHO classification (see Table 74.8) includes cytogenetic subtypes of B-lymphoblastic leukemia and these studies are also essential for a complete diagnosis of ALL. There are no specific morphologic features for these ALL types (*Figure 74.5*), with the exception that the very rare ALL with t(5; 14) (q31.1; q32.3) (*IL3::IGH*) is associated with a marked proliferation of normal-appearing eosinophils.[73] Although there are no specific morphologic features in most of these disorders, there are some characteristic immunophenotypic features that provide clues to the diagnosis, some of which are listed in *Table 74.9*. Although many of these categories are defined by the detection of recurring cytogenetic abnormalities, the translocation of B-lymphoblastic leukemia/lymphoma with t(12; 21) (p13.2; q22.1) (*ETV6::RUNX1*) is cryptic,[117] and FISH or PCR testing must be performed to detect this category. Because this cytogenetic abnormality primarily occurs in children, routine molecular or FISH testing for this fusion is indicated in all pediatric B-ALL cases. Similarly, there are no morphologic clues to reliably distinguish T-lymphoblastic leukemia/lymphoma from B-lymphoblastic leukemia/lymphoma. Although nuclear convolutions are described as more common with a T-cell immunophenotype, this finding is not sufficiently reliable to replace immunophenotyping studies.

Although mutation studies are not part of the 2016 classification of ALL, numerous genetic alterations have been described in recent years for this disease and will further impact classification.[118] Interestingly, and in contrast to AML, many individual mutations in ALL have been shown not to have prognostic impact as a sole marker, but may define prognostic groups when they occur in combination.[119] *PAX5* mutations at 9p13 occur in approximately 30% of B-ALL cases and often occur in combination with other abnormalities, but this mutation alone does not appear to be clinically significant. In contrast, deletions of *IKZF1* at 7p12 often occur in combination with *PAX5* mutations and are seen in over 80% of patients with B-ALL with t(9; 22) (q34.1; q11.2) (*BCR::ABL1*). Even in the absence of the Philadelphia chromosome, children with this deletion (representing almost 30% of all Philadelphia chromosome-negative ALLs in one study) have a poor outcome that is similar to B-ALL with t(9; 22) (q34.1; q11.2). The poor prognosis of *IKZF1*-deleted ALL appears to be independent of age, WBC count, or cytogenetic subgroup.[120,121] Mutations of *JAK2*, found in approximately 8% of B-ALL cases, in combination with *IKZF1* deletions are associated with an even worse prognosis.[122,123]

A recurring cytogenetic abnormality involves *CRLF2* located at Xp22.3/Yp11.3 and most often translocated with IGH.[28,124] These translocations occur in 7% to 14% of B-ALL cases, but are associated with either ALL of Down syndrome or ALL in Hispanic patients. They are commonly associated with *JAK1* or *JAK2* mutations and *IKZF1* deletions and have a very poor prognosis.

Many of the above described findings, particularly *IKZF1* deletion, identify B-ALL cases that have a gene expression profile and clinical behavior similar to B-ALL with t(9; 22) (q34.1; q11.2) (*BCR::ABL1*), but lack this genetic event.[28,125,126] These cases of *BCR::ABL1*–like B-ALL

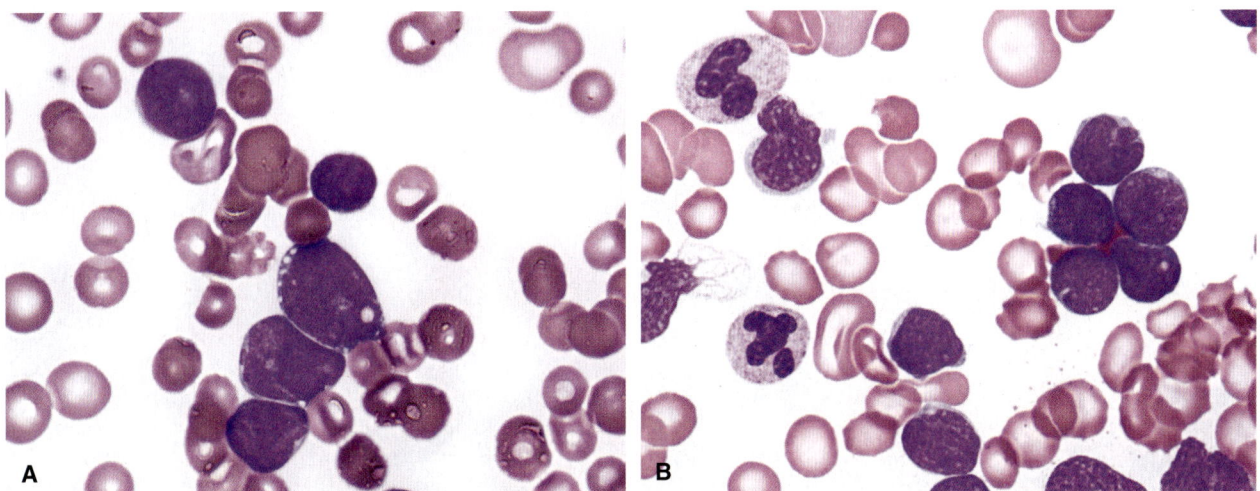

FIGURE 74.5 Acute lymphoblastic leukemia with blasts containing scant, agranular cytoplasm. The morphologic features are not specific and may also be present in minimally differentiated acute myeloid leukemia. Part (A) is from a case of B-lymphoblastic leukemia, not otherwise specified, whereas part (B) is from T-lymphoblastic leukemia, both showing similar morphologic changes.

Table 74.9. Distinctive Clinical, Morphologic, and Immunophenotypic Features of B-Lymphoblastic Leukemia Cytogenetic Subtypes

B-ALL Subtype	Distinctive Features
B-lymphoblastic leukemia/lymphoma with t(9; 22) (q34.1; q11.2); *BCR::ABL1*	Precursor B-cell lineage with aberrant expression of CD13, CD33, CD38, and CD25
B-lymphoblastic leukemia/lymphoma with t(v; 11q23.3); *KMT2A* rearrangement	CD10⁻ precursor B-cell lineage with aberrant CD15 expression
B-lymphoblastic leukemia/lymphoma with t(12; 21) (p13.2; q22.1); *ETV6::RUNX1*	Childhood leukemia with precursor B-cell lineage with CD34, bright CD10, and aberrant expression of CD13
B-lymphoblastic leukemia/lymphoma with t(5; 14) (q31.1; q32.3); *IL3::IGH*	Precursor B-cell lineage associated with marked eosinophilia
B-lymphoblastic leukemia/lymphoma with t(1; 19) (q23; p13.3); *TCF3::PBX1*	Precursor B-cell lineage lacking CD34 with cytoplasmic mu expression

are included as a provisional entity in the 2016 WHO classification, although the diagnostic criteria for this entity still need to be clarified.

Another provisional B-ALL entity in the 2016 WHO classification is B-ALL with intrachromosomal amplification of chromosome 21,[127] a childhood B-ALL type associated with a worse prognosis if not treated as high-risk ALL.

In contrast to AML, there is no category of ALL for therapy-related disease. Despite this, it is now recognized that ALL may occur after cytotoxic therapy although the relationship to the prior therapy and the leukemia may be underappreciated.[128,129] Most cases of therapy-related ALL are of precursor B lineage and some studies suggest that they are most often associated with *KMT2A* translocations involving 11q23.3.

Recurring cytogenetic abnormalities also occur in T-ALL, but are not included as diagnostic subcategories in the WHO classification. These translocations most often involve T-cell receptor genes at 7q32 (TRB) and 14q11 (TRA, TRD) and *TLX1*, *TLX3*, and *TAL1*, but many other genes may be involved in a smaller percentage of cases.[130,131] Prognostic significance has not been determined for many of these genetic changes, although *TLX1* translocations appear to confer a good prognosis. Mutations are also common in T-ALL, with mutations of *NOTCH1* found in 50% to 60% of adult and pediatric disease.[130-134] Mutations of *FBXW7*, a gene involved in NOTCH signaling, occur in 10% to 20% of cases.[132-134] Mutations of either gene appear to have some prognostic significance in children, at least predicting a favorable treatment response with protocols that include cranial irradiation, but appear to be of less significance in adult patients. *FLT3* mutations are rare in T-ALL, found in about 4% of cases.[135,136] However, these mutations are much more frequent in cases described as early T-cell precursor (ETP)-ALL, a provisional entity in the 2016 WHO Classification. These cases were considered to represent a particularly high-risk type of T-ALL,[135-137] but the prognostic significance of this finding in pediatric ALL is less clear with current therapy for T-ALL.[138] ETP-ALL expresses CD7, but lacks CD1a and CD8; shows only weak expression of CD5; expresses CD34, HLA-DR, and CD117; and often expresses myeloid-associated antigens such as CD13, CD33, and CD65s, but is myeloperoxidase negative. Some cases in the past were probably diagnosed as undifferentiated, mixed phenotype, or biphenotypic acute leukemia. Although often *FLT3* mutated, ETP-ALL typically lacks mutations of *NOTCH1* or *FBXW7*.[135]

ACUTE LEUKEMIAS OF AMBIGUOUS LINEAGE

Despite extensive immunophenotyping studies, a small subset of acute leukemias cannot be definitely classified as being derived from myeloid or lymphoid lineage.[139,140] These acute leukemias are either acute undifferentiated leukemias or mixed phenotype acute leukemias (MPALs) (Table 74.10). Acute undifferentiated leukemias have become extremely rare with modern immunophenotyping panels and are defined as lacking expression of markers specific for myeloid or lymphoid lineage. They often express nonspecific markers such as HLA-DR, CD34, CD38, CD7, or terminal deoxynucleotidyl transferase, but lack expression of cytoplasmic CD3, myeloperoxidase, cytoplasmic CD22, cytoplasmic CD79a, or strong expression of CD19, as well as markers of plasmacytoid dendritic cell tumors. No specific cytogenetic abnormalities are associated with these tumors.

The MPALs are slightly more common and are known by a variety of names that include mixed lineage acute leukemia, biphenotypic acute leukemia, and bilineal acute leukemia (Figure 74.6). The

Table 74.10. 2016 World Health Organization Classification of Acute Leukemias of Ambiguous Lineage

Acute Undifferentiated Leukemia
Mixed phenotype acute leukemia with t(9; 22) (q34.1; q11.2); *BCR::ABL1*
Mixed phenotype acute leukemia with t(v; 11q23.3); *KMT2A* rearranged
Mixed phenotype acute leukemia, B/myeloid, NOS
Mixed phenotype acute leukemia, T/myeloid, NOS

Abbreviation: NOS, not otherwise specified.

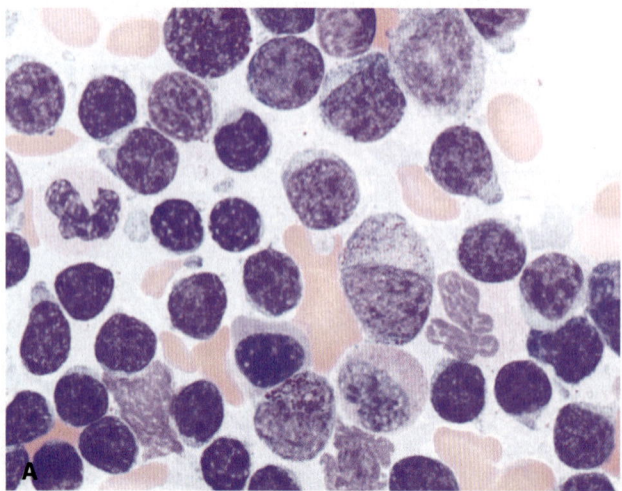
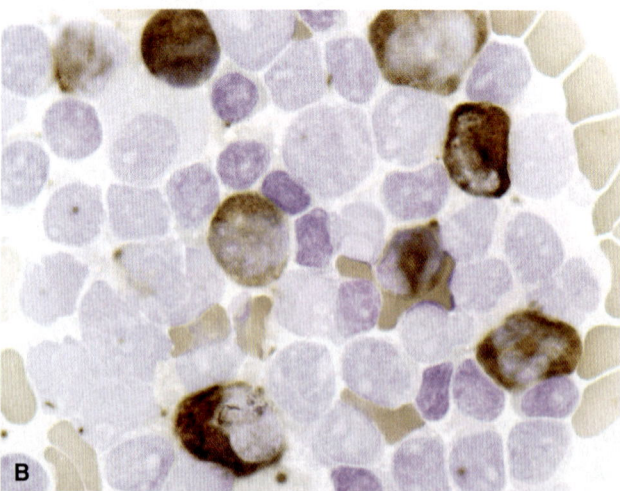

FIGURE 74.6 Mixed phenotype acute leukemia with a bilineal appearance. A mixture of small lymphocytes, small undifferentiated blast cells, and larger blasts with granular cytoplasm are present (A). The small blasts mark as B lymphoblasts, whereas the larger cells are myeloperoxidase positive by flow cytometry and cytochemistry (B).

Table 74.11. European Group for the Immunologic Classification of Leukemia Scoring System for Biphenotypic Acute Leukemia

Points/Lineage	B	T	Myeloid
2	CD79a Cytoplasmic IgM Cytoplasmic CD22	CD3 (membrane or cytoplasmic) TCR α/β TCR γ/δ	Myeloperoxidase
1	CD19 CD10 CD20	CD2 CD5 CD8 CD10	CD117 CD13 CD33 CD65s
0.5	TdT CD24	TdT CD7 CD1a	CD14 CD15 CD64

More than two points for an individual lineage is required.
Abbreviations: Ig, immunoglobulin; TCR, T-cell receptor; TdT, terminal deoxynucleotidyl transferase.

Table 74.12. 2016 WHO Criteria for Assigning Lineage for Mixed Phenotype Acute Leukemia

Lineage	Criteria
Myeloid	Myeloperoxidase or Monocytic differentiation (two or more: NSE, CD11c, CD14, CD64, lysozyme)
T lineage	Cytoplasmic or surface CD3
B lineage	Strong CD19 plus strong expression of at least one of CD79a, cCD22, CD10, or Weak CD19 plus strong expression of at least two of CD79a, cCD22, CD10

diagnostic criteria for these disorders have been vague in the past, and the frequency of diagnosis has increased with the use of multicolor flow cytometry using large panels of antibodies. Lineage infidelity is common in acute leukemias, and determining how many aberrant markers are sufficient to make a diagnosis of MPAL creates a challenge in many cases. A variety of diagnostic criteria have been proposed for these disorders, but the criteria proposed by the European Group for the Immunologic Classification of Leukemia (EGIL)[141,142] and the 2016 WHO[1] criteria are most often used, with the WHO criteria currently preferred. The EGIL criteria (Table 74.11) provided the ability to weigh the significance of different markers and reduced the number of cases diagnosed as MPAL. However, as new markers became available, the scoring system became less useful and it was not clear that the criteria resulted in a biologically distinct disease entity.

The WHO criteria (Table 74.12) are actually simpler to use, based on fewer markers, and specify two cytogenetic abnormalities (t[9;22][q34.1; q11.2] *BCR::ABL1*; t[v; 11q23.3] *KMT2A* rearranged) that are often reported in cases of MPAL. The WHO definition of MPAL does not separate cases with a single blast cell population showing a mixed phenotype (biphenotypic) from cases with two distinct blast cell populations (bilineal) because there is great overlap between these case types with some presenting with one pattern and relapsing with another. Although the two cytogenetic categories are similar to other acute leukemia categories in the WHO classification, it is not clear that these MPAL variants are distinct from other acute leukemias with the same cytogenetic abnormality (ie, MPAL with t[9; 22][q34.1; q11.2] *BCR::ABL1* vs ALL with t[9; 22][q34.1; q11.2] *BCR::ABL1*). The great variability of these disorders based on immunophenotype and recurring genetic changes suggest that immunophenotypic methods may not be the ideal means of classifying these tumors and future diagnostic methods may supplant this category in the future.

SUMMARY

The diagnostic evaluation for acute leukemia and MDSs has become increasingly complex, and the 2016 WHO classification has introduced new nomenclature and entities. A correct diagnosis requires careful coordination between the treating hematologist and hematopathologist to ensure that all sample types needed for diagnosis and prognosis are collected and appropriately tested. Because the various tests needed will be resulted at different times, consolidated reporting of all results using amended reports is suggested to ensure that all findings are interpreted in the context of the entire specimen.

References

1. Arber DA, Orazi A, Hasserjian R, et al. The 2016 revision to the World Health Organization classification of myeloid neoplasms and acute leukemia. *Blood*. 2016;127(20):2391-2405.
2. *WHO Classification of Tumours of Haematopoietic and Lymphoid Tissues*. In: Swerdlow SH, Campo E, Harris NL, et al., eds. IARC; 2008.
3. Swerdlow SH, Campo E, Harris NL, Jaffe ES, Pileri SA, Stein H, et al., eds. *WHO Classification Fo Tumours of Haematopoietic and Lymphoid Tissues*. IARC; 2017.
4. Weinberg OK, Seetharam M, Ren L, et al. Clinical characterization of acute myeloid leukemia with myelodysplasia-related changes as defined by the 2008 WHO classification system. *Blood*. 2009;113(9):1906-1908.
5. Arber DA, Stein AS, Carter NH, Ikle D, Forman SJ, Slovak ML. Prognostic impact of acute myeloid leukemia classification. Importance of detection of recurring cytogenetic abnormalities and multilineage dysplasia on survival. *Am J Clin Pathol*. 2003;119(5):672-680.
6. Muller-Berndorff H, Haas PS, Kunzmann R, Schulte-Monting J, Lubbert M. Comparison of five prognostic scoring systems, the French-American-British (FAB) and World Health Organization (WHO) classifications in patients with myelodysplastic syndromes: results of a single-center analysis. *Ann Hematol*. 2006;85(8):502-513.
7. Germing U, Strupp C, Kuendgen A, et al. Prospective validation of the WHO proposals for the classification of myelodysplastic syndromes. *Haematologica*. 2006;91(12):1596-1604.
8. Bennett JM, Catovsky D, Daniel MT, et al. Proposal for the recognition of minimally differentiated acute myeloid leukaemia (AML-M0). *Br J Haematol*. 1991;78:325-329.
9. Bennett JM, Catovsky D, Daniel MT, et al. Proposed revised criteria for the classification of acute myeloid leukemia. A report of the French-American-British Cooperative Group. *Ann Intern Med*. 1985;103(4):626-629.
10. Bennett JM, Catovsky D, Daniel MT, et al. Proposals for the classification of the myelodysplastic syndromes. *Br J Haematol*. 1982;51:189-199.
11. Bennett JM, Catovsky D, Daniel MT, et al. Proposals for the classification of the acute leukaemias. *Br J Haematol*. 1976;33:451-458.
12. Arber DA, Hasserjian RP, Orazi A, et al. Classification of myeloid neoplasms/acute leukemia: global perspectives and the international consensus classification approach. *Am J Hematol*. 2022;97(5):514-518.
13. van de Loosdrecht AA, Ireland R, Kern W, et al. Rationale for the clinical application of flow cytometry in patients with myelodysplastic syndromes: position paper of an International Consortium and the European LeukemiaNet Working Group. *Leuk Lymphoma*. 2013;54(3):472-475.
14. Bene MC, Nebe T, Bettelheim P, et al. Immunophenotyping of acute leukemia and lymphoproliferative disorders: a consensus proposal of the European LeukemiaNet Work Package 10. *Leukemia*. 2011;25(4):567-574.
15. Dohner H, Estey E, Grimwade D, et al. Diagnosis and management of AML in adults: 2017 ELN recommendations from an international expert panel. *Blood*. 2017;129(4):424-447.
16. Rappaport H. *Tumors of the Hematopoietic System*. Armed Forces Institute of Pathology; 1966:1-442.
17. Stansfeld AG, Diebold J, Kapanci Y, et al. Updated Kiel classification for lymphomas (letter). *Lancet*. 1988;1:292-293.
18. National Cancer Institute sponsored study of classifications of non-Hodgkin's lymphomas: summary and description of a working formulation for clinical usage. The Non-Hodgkin's Lymphoma Pathologic Classification Project. *Cancer*. 1982;49(10):2112-2135.
19. Harris NL, Jaffe ES, Stein H, et al. A revised European-American classification of lymphoid neoplasms: a proposal from the International Lymphoma Study Group. *Blood*. 1994;84(5):1361-1392.
20. Jaffe ES, Harris NL, Stein H, Vardiman JW. In: Jaffe ES, Harris NL, Stein H, Vardiman JW, eds. *Tumors of Haematopoietic and Lymphoid Tissues*. IARC press; 2001.
21. Raimondi SC, Chang MN, Ravindranath Y, et al. Chromosomal abnormalities in 478 children with acute myeloid leukemia: clinical characteristics and treatment outcome in a cooperative Pediatric Oncology Group study - POG 8821. *Blood*. 1999;94(11):3707-3716.
22. Rubnitz JE, Behm FG, Pui CH, et al. Genetic studies of childhood acute lymphoblastic leukemia with emphasis on p16, MLL, and ETV6 gene abnormalities: results of St Jude Total Therapy Study XII. *Leukemia*. 1997;11:1201-1206.
23. Moorman AV, Harrison CJ, Buck GA, et al. Karyotype is an independent prognostic factor in adult acute lymphoblastic leukemia (ALL): analysis of cytogenetic data from patients treated on the Medical Research Council (MRC) UKALLXII/Eastern Cooperative Oncology Group (ECOG) 2993 trial. *Blood*. 2007;109(8):3189-3197.

24. Grimwade D, Walker H, Harrison G, et al. The predictive value of hierarchical cytogenetic classification in older adults with acute myeloid leukemia (AML): analysis of 1065 patients entered into the United Kingdom Medical Research Council AML11 trial. *Blood*. 2001;98(5):1312-1320.
25. Grimwade D, Walker H, Oliver F, et al. The importance of diagnostic cytogenetics on outcome in AML: analysis of 1,612 patients entered into the MRC AML 10 trial. *Blood*. 1998;92(7):2322-2333.
26. Chessells JM, Swansbury GJ, Reeves B, Bailey CC, Richards SM. Cytogenetics and prognosis in childhood lymphoblastic leukaemia: results of MRC UKALL X. *Br J Haematol*. 1997;99:93-100.
27. Harvey RC, Mullighan CG, Wang X, et al. Identification of novel cluster groups in pediatric high-risk B-precursor acute lymphoblastic leukemia with gene expression profiling: correlation with genome-wide DNA copy number alterations, clinical characteristics, and outcome. *Blood*. 2010;116(23):4874-4884.
28. Harvey RC, Mullighan CG, Chen IM, et al. Rearrangement of CRLF2 is associated with mutation of JAK kinases, alteration of IKZF1, Hispanic/Latino ethnicity, and a poor outcome in pediatric B-progenitor acute lymphoblastic leukemia. *Blood*. 2010;115(26):5312-5321.
29. Marcucci G, Maharry K, Wu YZ, et al. IDH1 and IDH2 gene mutations identify novel molecular subsets within de novo cytogenetically normal acute myeloid leukemia: a Cancer and Leukemia Group B study. *J Clin Oncol*. 2010;28(14):2348-2355.
30. Baldus CD, Mrozek K, Marcucci G, Bloomfield CD. Clinical outcome of de novo acute myeloid leukaemia patients with normal cytogenetics is affected by molecular genetic alterations: a concise review. *Br J Haematol*. 2007;137(5):387-400.
31. Welch JS, Ley TJ, Link DC, et al. The origin and evolution of mutations in acute myeloid leukemia. *Cell*. 2012;150(2):264-278.
32. Bejar R, Stevenson K, Abdel-Wahab O, et al. Clinical effect of point mutations in myelodysplastic syndromes. *N Engl J Med*. 2011;364(26):2496-2506.
33. Papaemmanuil E, Cazzola M, Boultwood J, et al. Somatic SF3B1 mutation in myelodysplasia with ring sideroblasts. *N Engl J Med*. 2011;365(15):1384-1395.
34. Head DR. Revised classification of acute myeloid leukemia. *Leukemia*. 1996;10:1826-1831.
35. Komrokji RS, Bennett JM. Evolving classifications of the myelodysplastic syndromes. *Curr Opin Hematol*. 2007;14(2):98-105.
36. Orazi A. Histopathology in the diagnosis and classification of acute myeloid leukemia, myelodysplastic syndromes, and myelodysplastic/myeloproliferative diseases. *Pathobiology*. 2007;74(2):97-114.
37. Khalidi HS, Chang KL, Medeiros LJ, et al. Acute lymphoblastic leukemia. Survey of immunphenotype, French-American-British classification, frequency of myeloid antigen expression, and karyotypic abnormalities in 210 pediatric and adult cases. *Am J Clin Pathol*. 1999;111:467-476.
38. Kotylo PK, Seo IS, Smith FO, et al. Flow cytometric immunophenotypic characterization of pediatric and adult minimally differentiated acute myeloid leukemia (AML-M0). *Am J Clin Pathol*. 2000;113(2):193-200.
39. Orazi A, O'Malley DP, Jiang J, et al. Acute panmyelosis with myelofibrosis: an entity distinct from acute megakaryoblastic leukemia. *Mod Pathol*. 2005;18(5):603-614.
40. Stetler-Stevenson M, Arthur DC, Jabbour N, et al. Diagnostic utility of flow cytometric immunophenotyping in myelodysplastic syndrome. *Blood*. 2001;98(4):979-987.
41. Della Porta MG, Picone C, Pascutto C, et al. Multicenter validation of a reproducible flow cytometric score for the diagnosis of low-grade myelodysplastic syndromes: results of a European LeukemiaNET study. *Haematologica*. 2012;97(8):1209-1217.
42. Deeg HJ, Scott BL, Fang M, et al. Five-group cytogenetic risk classification, monosomal karyotype and outcome after hematopoietic cell transplantation for MDS or acute leukemia evolving from MDS. *Blood*. 2012;120(7):1398-1408.
43. Slovak ML, Kopecky KJ, Cassileth PA, et al. Karyotypic analysis predicts outcome of preremission and postremission therapy in adult acute myeloid leukemia: a Southwest Oncology Group/Eastern Cooperative Oncology Group Study. *Blood*. 2000;96(13):4075-4083.
44. Coleman JF, Theil KS, Tubbs RR, Cook JR. Diagnostic yield of bone marrow and peripheral blood FISH panel testing in clinically suspected myelodysplastic syndromes and/or acute myeloid leukemia: a prospective analysis of 433 cases. *Am J Clin Pathol*. 2011;135(6):915-920.
45. Patel JP, Gonen M, Figueroa ME, et al. Prognostic relevance of integrated genetic profiling in acute myeloid leukemia. *N Engl J Med*. 2012;366(12):1079-1089.
46. Greenberg PL, Tuechler H, Schanz J, et al. Cytopenia levels for aiding establishment of the diagnosis of myelodysplastic syndromes. *Blood*. 2016;128(16):2096-2097.
47. Valent P, Horny HP, Bennett JM, et al. Definitions and standards in the diagnosis and treatment of the myelodysplastic syndromes: consensus statements and report from a working conference. *Leuk Res*. 2007;31(6):727-736.
48. Verburgh E, Achten R, Maes B, et al. Additional prognostic value of bone marrow histology in patients subclassified according to the International Prognostic Scoring System for myelodysplastic syndromes. *J Clin Oncol*. 2003;21(2):273-282.
49. Goasguen JE, Bennett JM, Cox C, Hambley H, Mufti G, Flandrin G. Prognostic implication and characterization of the blast cell population in the myelodysplastic syndrome. *Leuk Res*. 1991;15(12):1159-1165.
50. Verhoef G, De Wolf-Peeters C, Kerim S, et al. Update on the prognostic implication of morphology, histology, and karyotype in primary myelodysplastic syndromes. *Hematol Pathol*. 1991;5(4):163-175.
51. Bejar R, Stevenson KE, Caughey BA, et al. Validation of a prognostic model and the impact of mutations in patients with lower-risk myelodysplastic syndromes. *J Clin Oncol*. 2012;30(27):3376-3382.
52. Caponetti GC, Bagg A. Mutations in myelodysplastic syndromes: core abnormalities and CHIPping away at the edges. *International journal of laboratory hematology*. 2020;42(6):671-684.
53. Malcovati L, Stevenson K, Papaemmanuil E, et al. SF3B1-mutant MDS as a distinct disease subtype: a proposal from the International Working Group for the Prognosis of MDS. *Blood*. 2020;136(2):157-170.
54. Bernard E, Nannya Y, Hasserjian RP, et al. Implications of TP53 allelic state for genome stability, clinical presentation and outcomes in myelodysplastic syndromes. *Nat Med*. 2020;26(10):1549-1556.
55. Weinberg OK, Siddon AJ, Madanat Y, et al. TP53 mutation defines a unique subgroup within complex karyotype de novo and therapy-related MDS/AML. *Blood Adv*. 2022;6(9):2847-2853.
56. Niemeyer CM, Baumann I. Classification of childhood aplastic anemia and myelodysplastic syndrome. *Hematology Am Soc Hematol Educ Program*. 2011;2011:84-89.
57. Baumann I, Fuhrer M, Behrendt S, et al. Morphological differentiation of severe aplastic anaemia from hypocellular refractory cytopenia of childhood: reproducibility of histopathological diagnostic criteria. *Histopathology*. 2012;61(1):10-17.
58. Lambertenghi-Deliliers G, Orazi A, Luksch R, Annaloro C. Myelodysplastic syndrome with increased marrow fibrosis: a distinct clinico-pathological entity. *Br J Haematol*. 1991;78:161-166.
59. Steensma DP, Hanson CA, Letendre L, Tefferi A. Myelodysplasia with fibrosis: a distinct entity? *Leuk Res*. 2001;25(10):829-838.
60. Buesche G, Teoman H, Wilczak W, et al. Marrow fibrosis predicts early fatal marrow failure in patients with myelodysplastic syndromes. *Leukemia*. 2008;22(2):313-322.
61. Della Porta MG, Malcovati L, Boveri E, et al. Clinical relevance of bone marrow fibrosis and CD34-positive cell clusters in primary myelodysplastic syndromes. *J Clin Oncol*. 2009;27(5):754-762.
62. Kroger N, Zabelina T, van Biezen A, et al. Allogeneic stem cell transplantation for myelodysplastic syndromes with bone marrow fibrosis. *Haematologica*. 2011;96(2):291-297.
63. Thiele J, Kvasnicka HM, Orazi A. Bone marrow histopathology in myeloproliferative disorders--current diagnostic approach. *Semin Hematol*. 2005;42(4):184-195.
64. Federmann B, Abele M, Rosero Cuesta DS, et al. The detection of SRSF2 mutations in routinely processed bone marrow biopsies is useful in the diagnosis of chronic myelomonocytic leukemia. *Hum Pathol*. 2014;45(12):2471-2479.
65. Orazi A, Albitar M, Heerema NA, Haskins S, Neiman RS. Hypoplastic myelodysplastic syndromes can be distinguished from acquired aplastic anemia by CD34 and PCNA immunostaining of bone marrow biopsy specimens. *Am J Clin Pathol*. 1997;107:268-274.
66. Bennett JM, Orazi A. Diagnostic criteria to distinguish hypocellular acute myeloid leukemia from hypocellular myelodysplastic syndromes and aplastic anemia: recommendations for a standardized approach. *Haematologica*. 2009;94(2):264-268.
67. Afable MG, IInd, Wlodarski M, Makishima H, et al. SNP array-based karyotyping: differences and similarities between aplastic anemia and hypocellular myelodysplastic syndromes. *Blood*. 2011;117(25):6876-6884.
68. Luzzatto L, Gianfaldoni G. Recent advances in biological and clinical aspects of paroxysmal nocturnal hemoglobinuria. *Int J Hematol*. 2006;84(2):104-112.
69. Wang SA, Tang G, Fadare O, et al. Erythroid-predominant myelodysplastic syndromes: enumeration of blasts from nonerythroid rather than total marrow cells provides superior risk stratification. *Mod Pathol*. 2008;21(11):1394-1402.
70. Steensma DP, Bejar R, Jaiswal S, et al. Clonal hematopoiesis of indeterminate potential and its distinction from myelodysplastic syndromes. *Blood*. 2015;126(1):9-16.
71. Malcovati L, Galli A, Travaglino E, et al. Clinical significance of somatic mutation in unexplained blood cytopenia. *Blood*. 2017;129(25):3371-3378.
72. Cargo CA, Rowbotham N, Evans PA, et al. Targeted sequencing identifies patients with preclinical MDS at high risk of disease progression. *Blood*. 2015;126(21):2362-2365.
73. Hogan TF, Koss W, Murgo AJ, Amato RS, Fontana JA, VanScoy FL. Acute lymphoblastic leukemia with chromosomal 5;14 translocation and hypereosinophilia: case report and literature review. *J Clin Oncol*. 1987;5(3):382-390.
74. Valent P, Orazi A, Steensma DP, et al. Proposed minimal diagnostic criteria for myelodysplastic syndromes (MDS) and potential pre-MDS conditions. *Oncotarget*. 2017;8(43):73483-73500.
75. Galli A, Todisco G, Catamo E, et al. Relationship between clone metrics and clinical outcome in clonal cytopenia. *Blood*. 2021;138(11):965-976.
76. van Zeventer IA, de Graaf AO, Wouters H, et al. Mutational spectrum and dynamics of clonal hematopoiesis in anemia of older individuals. *Blood*. 2020;135(14):1161-1170.
77. Mawad R, Estey EH. Acute myeloid leukemia with normal cytogenetics. *Curr Oncol Rep*. 2012;14(5):359-368.
78. Cancer Genome Atlas Research Network. Genomic and epigenomic landscapes of adult de novo acute myeloid leukemia. *N Engl J Med*. 2013;368(22):2059-2074.
79. Falini B, Nicoletti I, Martelli MF, Mecucci C. Acute myeloid leukemia carrying cytoplasmic/mutated nucleophosmin (NPMc+ AML): biologic and clinical features. *Blood*. 2007;109(3):874-885.
80. Thiede C, Koch S, Creutzig E, et al. Prevalence and prognostic impact of NPM1 mutations in 1485 adult patients with acute myeloid leukemia (AML). *Blood*. 2006;107(10):4011-4020.
81. Renneville A, Boissel N, Gachard N, et al. The favorable impact of CEBPA mutations in patients with acute myeloid leukemia is only observed in the absence of associated cytogenetic abnormalities and FLT3 internal duplication. *Blood*. 2009;113(21):5090-5093.
82. Preudhomme C, Sagot C, Boissel N, et al. Favorable prognostic significance of CEBPA mutations in patients with de novo acute myeloid leukemia: a study from the Acute Leukemia French Association (ALFA). *Blood*. 2002;100(8):2717-2723.
83. Pabst T, Mueller BU, Zhang P, et al. Dominant-negative mutations of CEBPA, encoding CCAAT/enhancer binding protein-alpha (C/EBPalpha), in acute myeloid leukemia. *Nat Genet*. 2001;27(3):263-270.
84. Wouters BJ, Lowenberg B, Erpelinck-Verschueren CA, van Putten WL, Valk PJ, Delwel R. Double CEBPA mutations, but not single CEBPA mutations, define a subgroup of acute myeloid leukemia with a distinctive gene expression profile that is uniquely associated with a favorable outcome. *Blood*. 2009;113(13):3088-3091.

85. Green CL, Koo KK, Hills RK, Burnett AK, Linch DC, Gale RE. Prognostic significance of CEBPA mutations in a large cohort of younger adult patients with acute myeloid leukemia: impact of double CEBPA mutations and the interaction with FLT3 and NPM1 mutations. *J Clin Oncol.* 2010;28(16):2739-2747.
86. Schnittger S, Dicker F, Kern W, et al. RUNX1 mutations are frequent in de novo AML with noncomplex karyotype and confer an unfavorable prognosis. *Blood.* 2011;117(8):2348-2357.
87. Tang JL, Hou HA, Chen CY, et al. AML1/RUNX1 mutations in 470 adult patients with de novo acute myeloid leukemia: prognostic implication and interaction with other gene alterations. *Blood.* 2009;114(26):5352-5361.
88. Mendler JH, Maharry K, Radmacher MD, et al. RUNX1 mutations are associated with poor outcome in younger and older patients with cytogenetically normal acute myeloid leukemia and with distinct gene and MicroRNA expression signatures. *J Clin Oncol.* 2012;30(25):3109-3118.
89. Tarlock K, Lamble AJ, Wang YC, et al. CEBPA-bZip mutations are associated with favorable prognosis in de novo AML: a report from the Children's Oncology Group. *Blood.* 2021;138(13):1137-1147.
90. Soupir CP, Vergilio JA, Dal Cin P, et al. Philadelphia chromosome-positive acute myeloid leukemia: a rare aggressive leukemia with clinicopathologic features distinct from chronic myeloid leukemia in myeloid blast crisis. *Am J Clin Pathol.* 2007;127(4):642-650.
91. Konoplev S, Yin CC, Kornblau SM, et al. Molecular characterization of de novo Philadelphia chromosome-positive acute myeloid leukemia. *Leuk Lymphoma.* 2013;54(1):138-144.
92. Miesner M, Haferlach C, Bacher U, et al. Multilineage dysplasia (MLD) in acute myeloid leukemia (AML) correlates with MDS-related cytogenetic abnormalities and a prior history of MDS or MDS/MPN but has no independent prognostic relevance: a comparison of 408 cases classified as "AML not otherwise specified" (AML-NOS) or "AML with myelodysplasia-related changes" (AML-MRC). *Blood.* 2010;116(15):2742-2751.
93. Park SH, Chi HS, Park SJ, Jang S, Park CJ. Clinical importance of morphological multilineage dysplasia in acute myeloid leukemia with myelodysplasia related changes. [Article in Korean]. *Korean J Lab Med.* 2010;30(3):231-238.
94. Falini B, Macijewski K, Weiss T, et al. Multilineage dysplasia has no impact on biologic, clinicopathologic, and prognostic features of AML with mutated nucleophosmin (NPM1). *Blood.* 2010;115(18):3776-3786.
95. Diaz-Beya M, Rozman M, Pratcorona M, et al. The prognostic value of multilineage dysplasia in de novo acute myeloid leukemia patients with intermediate-risk cytogenetics is dependent on NPM1 mutational status. *Blood.* 2010;116(26):6147-6148.
96. Bacher U, Schnittger S, Macijewski K, et al. Multilineage dysplasia does not influence prognosis in CEBPA-mutated AML, supporting the WHO proposal to classify these patients as a unique entity. *Blood.* 2012;119(20):4719-4722.
97. Lindsley RC, Mar BG, Mazzola E, et al. Acute myeloid leukemia ontogeny is defined by distinct somatic mutations. *Blood.* 2015;125(9):1367-1376.
98. Gao Y, Jia M, Mao Y, et al. Distinct mutation landscapes between acute myeloid leukemia with myelodysplasia-related changes and de novo acute myeloid leukemia. *Am J Clin Pathol.* 2021;157(5):691-700.
99. Ohgami RS, Ma L, Merker JD, et al. Next-generation sequencing of acute myeloid leukemia identifies the significance of TP53, U2AF1, ASXL1, and TET2 mutations. *Mod Pathol.* 2015;28(5):706-714.
100. Grob T, Al Hinai AS, Sanders MA, et al. Molecular characterization of mutant Tp53 acute myeloid leukemia and high-risk myelodysplastic syndrome. *Blood.* 2022;139(15):2347-2354.
101. Walter RB, Othus M, Burnett AK, et al. Significance of FAB subclassification of "acute myeloid leukemia, NOS" in the 2008 WHO classification: analysis of 5848 newly diagnosed patients. *Blood.* 2013;121(13):2424-2431.
102. Paschka P, Marcucci G, Ruppert AS, et al. Adverse prognostic significance of KIT mutations in adult acute myeloid leukemia with inv(16) and t(8;21): a Cancer and Leukemia Group B Study. *J Clin Oncol.* 2006;24(24):3904-3911.
103. Gale RE, Hills R, Pizzey AR, et al. Relationship between FLT3 mutation status, biologic characteristics, and response to targeted therapy in acute promyelocytic leukemia. *Blood.* 2005;106(12):3768-3776.
104. Schnittger S, Schoch C, Dugas M, et al. Analysis of FLT3 length mutations in 1003 patients with acute myeloid leukemia: correlation to cytogenetics, FAB subtype, and prognosis in the AMLCG study and usefulness as a marker for the detection of minimal residual disease. *Blood.* 2002;100(1):59-66.
105. Thiede C, Steudel C, Mohr B, et al. Analysis of FLT3-activating mutations in 979 patients with acute myelogenous leukemia: association with FAB subtypes and identification of subgroups with poor prognosis. *Blood.* 2002;99(12):4326-4335.
106. Suzuki T, Kiyoi H, Ozeki K, et al. Clinical characteristics and prognostic implications of NPM1 mutations in acute myeloid leukemia. *Blood.* 2005;106(8):2854-2861.
107. Metzeler KH, Maharry K, Radmacher MD, et al. TET2 mutations improve the new European LeukemiaNet risk classification of acute myeloid leukemia: a Cancer and Leukemia Group B study. *J Clin Oncol.* 2011;29(10):1373-1381.
108. Paschka P, Schlenk RF, Gaidzik VI, et al. IDH1 and IDH2 mutations are frequent genetic alterations in acute myeloid leukemia and confer adverse prognosis in cytogenetically normal acute myeloid leukemia with NPM1 mutation without FLT3 internal tandem duplication. *J Clin Oncol.* 2010;28(22):3636-3643.
109. Abbas S, Lugthart S, Kavelaars FG, et al. Acquired mutations in the genes encoding IDH1 and IDH2 both are recurrent aberrations in acute myeloid leukemia: prevalence and prognostic value. *Blood.* 2010;116(12):2122-2126.
110. Ley TJ, Ding L, Walter MJ, et al. DNMT3A mutations in acute myeloid leukemia. *N Engl J Med.* 2010;363:2424-2433.
111. Arber DA, Borowitz MJ, Cessna M, et al. Initial diagnostic workup of acute leukemia: guideline from the College of American Pathologists and the American Society of Hematology. *Arch Pathol Lab Med.* 2017;141(10):1342-1393.
112. Hasserjian RP, Zuo Z, Garcia C, et al. Acute erythroid leukemia: a reassessment using criteria refined in the 2008 WHO classification. *Blood.* 2010;115(10):1985-1992.
113. Arber DA, Hasserjian RP. Reclassifying myelodysplastic syndromes: what's where in the new WHO and why. *Hematology Am Soc Hematol Educ Program.* 2015;2015(1):294-298.
114. Arber DA. Revisiting erythroleukemia. *Curr Opin Hematol.* 2017;24(2):146-151.
115. Thiele J, Kvasnicka HM, Zerhusen G, et al. Acute panmyelosis with myelofibrosis: a clinicopathological study on 46 patients including histochemistry of bone marrow biopsies and follow-up. *Ann Hematol.* 2004;83(8):513-521.
116. Cerezo L, Shuster JJ, Pullen DJ, et al. Laboratory correlates and prognostic significance of granular acute lymphoblastic leukemia in children. A Pediatric Oncology Group study. *Am J Clin Pathol.* 1991;95(4):526-531.
117. Shurtleff SA, Buijs A, Behm FG, et al. TEL/AML1 fusion resulting from a cryptic t(12;21) is the most common genetic lesion in pediatric ALL and defines a subgroup of patients with an excellent prognosis. *Leukemia.* 1995;9(12):1985-1989.
118. Roberts KG, Mullighan CG. The biology of B-progenitor acute lymphoblastic leukemia. *Cold Spring Harb Perspect Med.* 2020;10(7):a034835.
119. Mullighan CG, Goorha S, Radtke I, et al. Genome-wide analysis of genetic alterations in acute lymphoblastic leukaemia. *Nature.* 2007;446(7137):758-764.
120. Mullighan CG, Su X, Zhang J, et al. Deletion of IKZF1 and prognosis in acute lymphoblastic leukemia. *N Engl J Med.* 2009;360(5):470-480.
121. Mullighan CG, Miller CB, Radtke I, et al. BCR-ABL1 lymphoblastic leukaemia is characterized by the deletion of Ikaros. *Nature.* 2008;453(7191):110-114.
122. Mullighan CG, Zhang J, Harvey RC, et al. JAK mutations in high-risk childhood acute lymphoblastic leukemia. *Proc Natl Acad Sci USA.* 2009;106(23):9414-9418.
123. Heerema NA, Carroll AJ, Devidas M, et al. Intrachromosomal amplification of chromosome 21 is associated with inferior outcomes in children with acute lymphoblastic leukemia treated in contemporary standard-risk children's oncology group studies: a report from the children's oncology group. *J Clin Oncol.* 2013;31(27):3397-3402.
124. Mullighan CG, Collins-Underwood JR, Phillips LA, et al. Rearrangement of CRLF2 in B-progenitor- and Down syndrome-associated acute lymphoblastic leukemia. *Nat Genet.* 2009;41(11):1243-1246.
125. Den Boer ML, van Slegtenhorst M, De Menezes RX, et al. A subtype of childhood acute lymphoblastic leukaemia with poor treatment outcome: a genome-wide classification study. *Lancet Oncol.* 2009;10(2):125-134.
126. Roberts KG, Li Y, Payne-Turner D, et al. Targetable kinase-activating lesions in Ph-like acute lymphoblastic leukemia. *N Engl J Med.* 2014;371(11):1005-1015.
127. Harrison CJ, Moorman AV, Schwab C, et al. An international study of intrachromosomal amplification of chromosome 21 (iAMP21): cytogenetic characterization and outcome. *Leukemia.* 2014;28(5):1015-1021.
128. Ishizawa S, Slovak ML, Popplewell L, et al. High frequency of pro-B acute lymphoblastic leukemia in adults with secondary leukemia with 11q23 abnormalities. *Leukemia.* 2003;17(6):1091-1095.
129. Chen W, Wang E, Lu Y, Gaal KK, Huang Q. Therapy-related acute lymphoblastic leukemia without 11q23 abnormality: report of six cases and a literature review. *Am J Clin Pathol.* 2010;133(1):75-82.
130. Graux C, Cools J, Michaux L, Vandenberghe P, Hagemeijer A. Cytogenetics and molecular genetics of T-cell acute lymphoblastic leukemia: from thymocyte to lymphoblast. *Leukemia.* 2006;20(9):1496-1510.
131. Kraszewska MD, Dawidowska M, Szczepanski T, Witt M. T-cell acute lymphoblastic leukaemia: recent molecular biology findings. *Br J Haematol.* 2012;156(3):303-315.
132. Clappier E, Collette S, Grardel N, et al. NOTCH1 and FBXW7 mutations have a favorable impact on early response to treatment, but not on outcome, in children with T-cell acute lymphoblastic leukemia (T-ALL) treated on EORTC trials 58881 and 58951. *Leukemia.* 2010;24(12):2023-2031.
133. Baldus CD, Thibaut J, Goekbuget N, et al. Prognostic implications of NOTCH1 and FBXW7 mutations in adult acute T-lymphoblastic leukemia. *Haematologica.* 2009;94(10):1383-1390.
134. Mansour MR, Sulis ML, Duke V, et al. Prognostic implications of NOTCH1 and FBXW7 mutations in adults with T-cell acute lymphoblastic leukemia treated on the MRC UKALLXII/ECOG E2993 protocol. *J Clin Oncol.* 2009;27(26):4352-4356.
135. Neumann M, Heesch S, Gokbuget N, et al. Clinical and molecular characterization of early T-cell precursor leukemia: a high-risk subgroup in adult T-ALL with a high frequency of FLT3 mutations. *Blood Cancer J.* 2012;2(1):e55.
136. Zaremba CM, Oliver D, Cavalier M, Fuda F, Karandikar NJ, Chen W. Distinct immunophenotype of early T-cell progenitors in T lymphoblastic leukemia/lymphoma may predict FMS-like tyrosine kinase 3 mutations. *Ann Diagn Pathol.* 2012;16(1):16-20.
137. Inukai T, Kiyokawa N, Campana D, et al. Clinical significance of early T-cell precursor acute lymphoblastic leukaemia: results of the Tokyo Children's Cancer Study Group Study L99-15. *Br J Haematol.* 2012;156(3):358-365.
138. Wood BL, Winter S, Dunsmore KP, et al. T-lymphoblastic leukemia (T-ALL) shows excellent outcome, lack of significance of the early Thymic precursor (ETP) immunophenotype, and validation of the prognostic value of End-Induction minimal residual disease (MRD) in children's oncology group (COG) study AALL0434. *Blood.* 2014;124:1.
139. Weinberg OK, Arber DA. Mixed-phenotype acute leukemia: historical overview and a new definition. *Leukemia.* 2010;24:1844-1851.
140. Bene MC, Porwit A. Acute leukemias of ambiguous lineage. *Semin Diagn Pathol.* 2012;29(1):12-18.
141. Bene MC, Castoldi G, Knapp W, et al. Proposal for the immunologic classification of acute leukemias. *Leukemia.* 1995;9:1783-1786.
142. European Group for the Immunological Classification of L. The value of c-kit in the diagnosis of biphenotypic acute leukemia. *Leukemia.* 1998;12(12):2038.

Chapter 75 ■ Acute Lymphoblastic Leukemia in Adults

EHAB ATALLAH • KRISTEN O'DWYER

INTRODUCTION

Acute lymphoblastic leukemia (ALL) is a neoplastic disease that results from the malignant transformation of B- or T-lineage progenitor cells at distinct stages of differentiation. In children, ALL is the most common malignancy, and considerable advances have led to the cure of most children with the disease.[1] Historically, treatment outcomes in adults have not been as favorable. Insight into the biologic heterogeneity of the disease has led to improved prognostic stratification, and the development of novel targeted therapies has finally provided additional therapeutic options. Dramatic advances in whole genome sequencing as well as sensitive methodologies to detect residual disease promise to further improve outcomes.

Patients with ALL present with signs and symptoms reflecting bone marrow as well as extramedullary involvement by leukemia, including but not limited to infection, malaise, ecchymosis, or bleeding, and in some cases bulky lymphadenopathy, a mediastinal mass, or pleural effusions, all of which can lead to life-threatening emergencies. Examination of the blood smear is often sufficient to suspect the diagnosis of ALL, but additional laboratory tests are essential for establishing a diagnosis, stratifying risk, and formulating an appropriate treatment plan. Current therapy for adults involves multiagent chemotherapy that starts with remission induction chemotherapy, followed by one or more cycles of chemotherapy consolidation and intensification, prophylaxis of the central nervous system (CNS), and prolonged maintenance lasting 2 to 3 years. With this multiagent, multicycle approach, between 30% and 60% of adults with ALL are cured of their disease.[2-4] Modifications to the frontline chemotherapy regimen, based on an appreciation of the high risk for disease relapse, have improved outcome for adult patients with ALL who have a mature B-cell phenotype (Burkitt leukemia),[5] those with the Philadelphia (Ph) chromosome,[6] as well as patients whose leukemia expresses CD20.[7] Improvement in outcomes for adolescents and young adult patients with Ph chromosome–negative B- and T-ALL has also been achieved, albeit without the addition of new therapies, but with the intensification of chemotherapy regimens that resemble pediatric ALL protocols.[8] Comorbidities remain a significant limitation to treatment intensity for the one-third of adults with ALL who are over the age of 60 years. A higher incidence of high-risk molecular abnormalities occur in adult patients, which predisposes them to inherent chemotherapy resistance and also accounts for the higher rates of relapse.

The need to reduce the risk of relapse after initial treatment is a major focus of current research efforts. Novel antibodies are being incorporated into the frontline regimens as a strategy to eradicate measurable residual disease (MRD). Chimeric antigen receptor (CAR) T-cell therapy for B-cell acute lymphoblastic leukemia (B-ALL)[9] and nelarabine for T-cell acute lymphoblastic leukemia (T-ALL)[10] have been effective in the relapsed setting and are under evaluation as part of the initial treatment to decrease relapse.

HISTORICAL BACKGROUND

During the past 70 years, the survival for children and young adults with ALL has changed dramatically; before the 1950 ALL was a universally incurable disease with an average survival of 3 months following the diagnosis. Today, almost 90% of children are cured with contemporary multiagent chemotherapy protocols.[11] The era of chemotherapy for the treatment of childhood ALL began with Sidney Farber and colleagues at Boston Children's Hospital, along with the crucial collaboration with chemist Yellapragada Subba Rao from the Lederle Laboratory.[12] Together, their 1947 report of temporary remissions with the use of folic acid antagonist, aminopterin, in children with acute leukemia paved the way. By 1950, O. H. Pearson and E. P. Eliel from Memorial Sloan Kettering published their first report of the efficacy of glucocorticoid hormone, cortisone, as a single agent in lymphoid malignancies and acute leukemia, even in patients who had developed resistance to aminopterin.[13] In the early 1950s, George Hitchings and Gertrude Elion developed compounds that blocked nucleic acid synthesis in cancer cells, among these compounds was the purine analogue, 6-mercaptopurine (6-MP), which proved active as monotherapy, but similar to the experience with aminopterin, the remission duration was short-lived, and all patients succumbed to the disease.[14] Also in the 1950s, James Holland, at the National Cancer Institute (NCI), developed a clinical protocol that combined daily methotrexate and 6-MP, based on the work by Lloyd Law (also at the NCI who had demonstrated in mice (mouse leukemia cell line, L2110) that combination chemotherapy was more effective than either drug used separately.[15,16] Dr. Holland, then at Roswell Park Memorial Institute, together with Emil "Tom" Frei and Emil Freireich at the NCI continued the studies of 6-MP and methotrexate and conducted the first randomized multicenter clinical trial for acute leukemia. That trial launched the Acute Leukemia Group B (ALBG), which later was named the Cancer and Leukemia Group B (CALGB) and served as the model for the cancer cooperative group structure in the United States.[17]

In the early 1960s, the St. Jude "total therapy" program for childhood ALL began under the leadership of Dr. Donald Pinkel. The first trials at St. Jude used combinations of the available chemotherapies (vincristine, asparaginase, cyclophosphamide, daunomycin, and cytarabine) instead of sequential administration of single agents as a strategy to overcome drug resistance and prolong hematologic remissions.[18-20] The outcomes with multiagent chemotherapy were superior to single-agent therapy, but still, few children experienced long-term survival. In the late 1960s and early1970s, the pivotal intervention of the use of cranial irradiation and intrathecal chemotherapy as effective prevention of leukemia relapse in the CNS prolonged survival.[21,22] Also, two important trials conducted in the 1970s demonstrated that intensification therapy soon after remission induction was responsible for improving survival.[23,24] The importance of combination chemotherapy administered in multiple components—remission induction, consolidation, intensification, maintenance, and CNS-directed therapy—was making a significant impact on survival.

Since the 1970s successive randomized clinical trials designed and performed by international cooperative cancer groups have clearly illustrated that incremental treatment modifications in successive cohorts of children have resulted in a steady improvement in survival outcome (see Chapter 77).[25-29] With further refinements of the chemotherapy protocols through successive clinical trials that have been tailored to patient's risk group, along with general improvement in supportive care, the chemotherapy approach has reached an optimal regimen, and approximately 90% of children with ALL are now cured of the disease in the developed world.[11,30]

The success demonstrated in the pediatric ALL trials led to similar approaches in the treatment of adults. Outcomes in consecutive cohorts of adults with ALL treated by the United Kingdom Acute Lymphoblastic Leukemia (UKALL) collaborative study group gradually improved as treatment was intensified and extended (Figure 75.1).[31] Compared with outcome improvements in childhood ALL, however, the degree of improvement in adults was only modest. The British Medical Research Council (MRC) initiated the pediatric UKALL trials in 1970 and included adults in UKALL I through V. The first trial, UKALL I, evaluated CNS prophylaxis but only enrolled 16

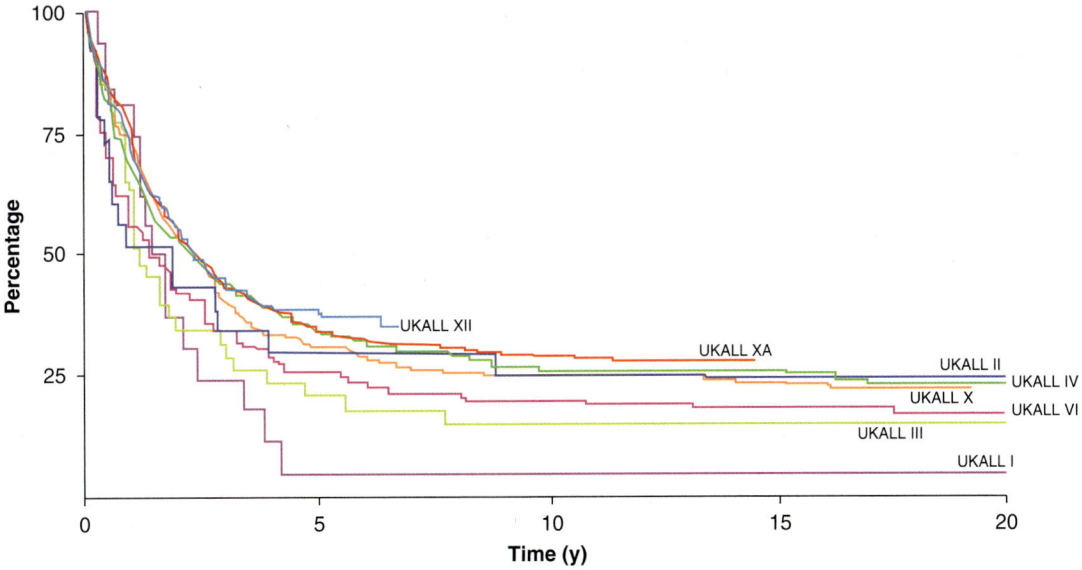

FIGURE 75.1 Overall survival in successive acute lymphoblastic leukemia patient cohorts. Adult patients with acute lymphoblastic leukemia treated by the UKALL collaborative study group. UKALL, UK Acute Lymphocytic Leukemia. (Reprinted from Durrant IJ, Richards SM, Prentice HG, et al. The Medical Research Council trials in adult acute lymphocytic leukemia. *Hematol Oncol Clin North Am.* 2000;14:1327-1352. Copyright © 2000 Elsevier. With permission.)

adults. Subsequent trials examined both the addition of active agents and more sustained intensive postremission therapy, and participation of adult patients progressively expanded. Survival for adults with ALL was still only 20% at the time the UKALL IX trial opened for patient accrual in 1980. It was the first trial in the series to enroll adults separately from children. UKALL IX and the subsequent trial, UKALL XA (1985), saw further, although minor, incremental improvement in the survival rate but provided important systematic analyses of prognostic indicators based on clinical, immunophenotypic, and cytogenetic characteristics.[31,32] The subsequent study, UKALL XII/Eastern Cooperative Oncology Group (ECOG) 2993, was the largest treatment study of newly diagnosed ALL in adults with a total enrollment of 1500 patients. It compared postremission chemotherapy with autologous or related donor allogeneic transplant. The complete remission (CR) rate was 90% in the 1646 Ph chromosome–negative patients, and overall survival (OS) at 5 years was 43%.[33] Patients up to age 50 years were eligible for allogeneic hematopoietic stem cell transplant (HSCT). Survival at 5 years was 54% for all Ph chromosome–negative patients with a donor, vs 44% for those without ($P = .007$) and 63% vs 52% for standard-risk patients ($P = .02$). There was no benefit to allogeneic transplant for high-risk or Ph chromosome–negative patients. Patients without a donor who underwent autologous transplant did no better than those who received chemotherapy alone. These series of studies, along with other national cooperative group studies of the CALGB and the German Multicenter Study Group for Adult ALL (GMALL) have led to remarkably similar long-term survival rates among adults who receive chemotherapy without transplant.[4,34,35] These outcomes are distinctly inferior to those achieved in the pediatric age group.

However, subsequent treatment approaches, detailed below in "Primary Therapy" section, have finally improved outcomes in adult ALL, with significantly higher survival rates in some patient categories.

PATHOPHYSIOLOGY

The cause of ALL is essentially unknown, and few clues can be derived from epidemiologic studies. The molecular pathogenesis of ALL is reviewed in Chapter 73. Points relevant to adult ALL concerning these issues are briefly highlighted in this chapter.

Epidemiology

The age-adjusted rate of new cases of ALL in the United States from 2015 to 2019 based on Surveillance, Epidemiology, and End Results (SEER) data is 1.8 per 100,000 individuals per year, and the number of deaths is 0.4 per 100,000.[36] There is a slight male predominance with a male to female ratio of 1.9:1.6. ALL is more common in Hispanics and whites and is less common in Asian/Pacific Islanders and blacks. Almost half of the 6600 new cases each year in the United States are diagnosed in persons younger than 20 years; the median age at diagnosis is 17 years (*Figure 75.2*). For 2012 to 2018, the estimated 5-year survival is 70.8%, primarily owing to the success in childhood ALL (*Figure 75.3*). The median age at death is 58 years, and the highest percent of deaths (16.4%) is among people aged 65 to 74 years.

Etiology

The cause of ALL in adults is largely unknown. Inherited factors and genetic predisposition syndromes, including Down syndrome, Fanconi anemia, and dyskeratosis congenita are more relevant to childhood ALL and account for less than 5% of cases.[37] These germline variants are not only important for susceptibility to ALL but also influence drug response and toxicities of ALL treatment. More common variants have been identified, albeit with weaker associations with ALL susceptibility. Rare cases of familial ALL have been identified to be caused by *TP53* mutations associated with the Li-Fraumeni syndrome. Approximately 50% of children with low-diploid ALL have this

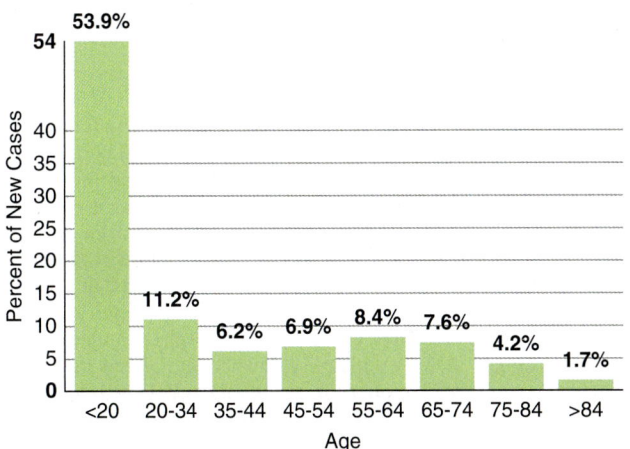

FIGURE 75.2 Percent of new cases by age group. Data from Acute lymphoblastic leukemia 2015 to 2019 (Surveillance, Epidemiology, and End Results [SEER] Program).

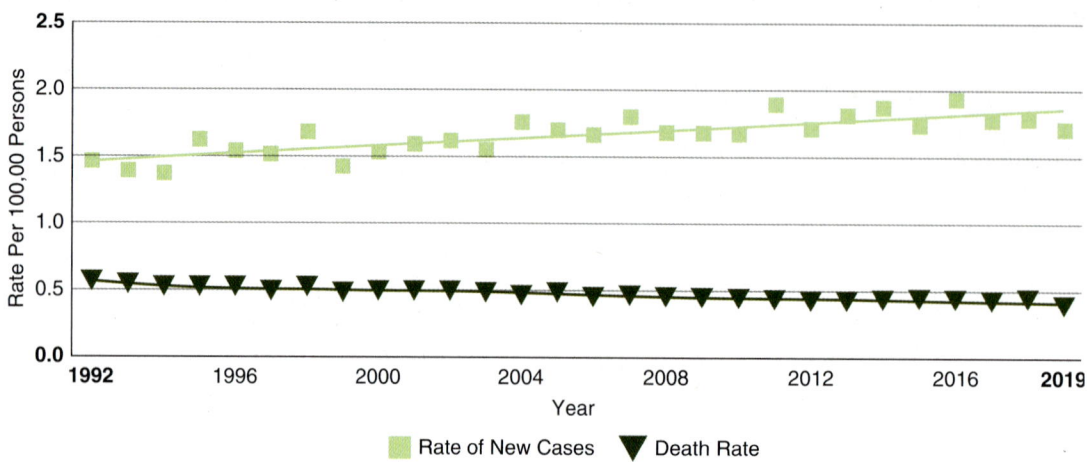

FIGURE 75.3 **New cases, deaths, and 5-year relative survival.** From SEER 9 incidence and US mortality, 1992 to 2019.

mutation.[38] Somewhat more relevant to adult ALL is the association between occupational exposure to low-dose ionizing radiation and a slightly increased risk for leukemia, although findings were inconsistent across populations.[39-41]

Among chemical environmental exposure, high-level benzene exposure that occurred before contemporary occupational safety standards is generally accepted as a cause of bone marrow aplasia, chromosome damage, and leukemia,[42] although its association with ALL remains inconclusive. Secondary acute leukemias occurring after exposure to chemotherapeutic agents are usually myeloid, although ALL has been observed in patients with antecedent malignancies as well as patients exposed to prior chemotherapy.[43]

Other theories for the etiology of ALL includes the Kinlen population mixing hypothesis and the Greaves delayed infection theory. Both theories suggest that leukemia originates as an uncommon response to an infection. The Kinlen population mixing hypothesis suggests that population mixing leads to a mix of susceptible (populations not previously exposed to the infective agent) and infected populations.[44] This leads to a rapid spread of the infective agent with leukemia occurring as an unusual reaction. The Greaves delayed infection hypothesis suggests a double hit theory for the development of childhood leukemia.[45] The first is an in utero acquisition of a genetic abnormality (most commonly *ETV6-RUNX1*) or chromosomal hyperdiploidy. Only 1% of children with these mutations develop ALL. The second hit is postulated to be an infection occurring later in childhood between the age of 2 and 6 years. Greaves theorizes that infections in the perinatal period are protective, while those occurring later in life lead to the development of leukemia in susceptible individuals who have a genetic abnormality.

Molecular Pathogenesis

Molecular abnormalities can be grouped according to the functional consequence of oncogenic mutation (see Chapter 73). Acquired constitutive activation of the ABL protein kinase by rearrangement with the *BCR* gene is an example of a mutation that confers a proliferative advantage. The fusion gene is the consequence of the t(9;22)(q34;q11) balanced chromosomal translocation, which is the most common cytogenetic abnormality in adult ALL, present in 10% to 35% of patients, depending on age.[46] ABL is a nonreceptor tyrosine protein kinase that enzymatically transfers phosphate molecules to substrate proteins, thereby activating downstream signal transduction pathways that are important in regulating cell growth and proliferation. Other gene rearrangements result in loss-of-function or gain-of-function mutations involving transcription factors that are important for normal hematopoietic development. An example is the t(12;21)(p12;q22) chromosomal translocation, leading to expression of the *ETV6-RUNX1* fusion (*TEL-AML1*).[47] Excluding numerical aberrations, *ETV6-RUNX1* is the most frequent cytogenetic abnormality in childhood ALL, although it is very uncommon in adults. Another general mechanism of cancer formation involves loss or inactivation of tumor-suppressor genes, many of which have key regulatory functions in controlling cell cycle progression. Stock et al investigated the incidence of cell cycle regulatory gene abnormalities in adult patients with de novo ALL.[48] Deletions, microdeletions, and gene rearrangements involving *RB1* (51%), *p16(INK4A)* (41%), and *TP53* (26%) were common. Concurrent abnormalities involving two or more of these genes were found in one-third of adult patients with ALL and were associated with significantly shorter median survival (8 vs 25 months).

Genome-wide gene expression arrays identified patients without the *BCR-ABL* transcript who had a prognostic profile similar to that of BCR-ABL ALL.[49] This Ph-negative (Ph−)-like group was present in 25% to 30% of young adults with ALL and had a similarly poor prognosis.[50] Molecular sequencing determined that 86% of cases had deletions in transcription factors regulating B-cell development, including IKAROS family zinc-finger 1 (IKZF1), paired box 5 (PAX5), early B-cell factor 1 (EBF1), ETV6, and RUNX1. Approximately 54% had alterations in cell cycle genes *CDKN2A/B*, *TP53*, and *RB1*. Almost all have kinase-activating alterations, and 46.8% had *CRLF2* overexpression including a subset with *JAK1/JAK2* mutations, resulting in overexpression of *CRLF2* protein, and enhanced signaling through JAK kinases.[51]

Aberrant expression of NOTCH1 has also been linked to ALL leukemogenesis in T-cell disease.[52] These patients are frequently MRD positive post induction, resulting in poor survival without transplant.[53] *NOTCH1* encodes a transmembrane receptor that regulates normal T-cell development. Upon proteolytic cleavage, NOTCH1 translocates to the nucleus and binds to a nuclear transcription factor, ultimately stimulating the transcription of target genes.

Activation of oncogenic transcription factors is a central feature of T-ALL, often by rearrangement with T-cell receptor loci. Moreover, more than 70% of cases are characterized by deletion of *CDKN2A/CDKN2B* tumor-suppressor loci.[54]

Early T-cell precursor (ETP)-ALL is recognized as a distinct subtype of T-ALL with a poor prognosis and is present in about 20% of adult T-cell disease.[55] It represents a progenitor cell leukemia, often with coexpression of myeloid markers. It is a genetically heterogeneous disease without distinct chromosomal aberrations, but several signaling pathways are typically mutated in ETP-ALL. Recognition of ETP-ALL in childhood ALL has led to intensification of therapy based on response and improved survival.[56] Retrospective analysis of outcomes in adults suggests that response-based risk stratification and therapy intensification including allogeneic HSCT can also overcome the poor prognosis.[57]

CLINICAL FEATURES

Although the clinical presentation is variable and may develop insidiously, adults diagnosed with ALL typically present with symptoms of only a few weeks duration. The symptoms generally reflect bone marrow failure or involvement of extramedullary sites by leukemia. Up to half of patients with ALL have fever or documented infections. One-third of patients have bleeding symptoms at diagnosis, which is less frequent than in patients presenting with acute myeloid leukemia (AML). Severe hemorrhage is uncommon. Fatigue, lethargy, dizziness, or even dyspnea and cardiac angina may reflect anemia in adults with ALL. Marrow expansion by leukemic blasts may produce bone pain and arthralgias, but marrow necrosis is much less frequently found in adults as compared with children who have ALL. Approximately 20% of adult patients have hepatomegaly, splenomegaly, or lymphadenopathy at diagnosis that can be appreciated on physical examination. Mediastinal masses are detected by chest radiographs or computed tomography scans primarily in patients with T-lineage ALL, who also frequently have pleural involvement and may complain of chest pain. Approximately 10% of patients with ALL will have CNS involvement at the time of initial diagnosis and may present with referable symptoms, such as headache, vomiting, neck stiffness, alteration in mental status, and focal neurologic abnormalities. Other sites of extramedullary involvement include testis, retina, and skin, although virtually any organ can be infiltrated by leukemic blast cells.[4,58,59]

LABORATORY FEATURES

In addition to a complete medical history and physical examination, patients with ALL should have laboratory tests to confirm the diagnosis, subcategorize the patient's disease for prognostic classification, and plan for appropriate therapy.[60] These studies include a bone marrow examination for morphologic assessment, immunophenotyping by flow cytometry, as well as cytogenetic and molecular profiling. The World Health Organization (WHO) classification was updated in 2022.[61] Morphologic, cytogenetic, and immunophenotypic characteristics of ALL are detailed in Chapter 74. This section emphasizes features pertinent to adults diagnosed with the disease.

Laboratory Evaluation

All patients should have a complete blood count with examination of the blood smear. A substantial number of adult patients with ALL have normal or only modestly elevated white blood cell (WBC) counts at the time of diagnosis. Hyperleukocytosis (>100 × 10^9/L) occurs in approximately 15% of patients and may exceed 200 × 10^9/L. Some degree of anemia is present in the majority of adults. Approximately one-third of patients have a platelet count less than 25 × 10^9/L, which is approximately the same proportion that present with bleeding symptoms. Circulating leukemic blasts may not be evident on examination of the blood smear in a significant number of patients. All patients should have electrolyte measurements, serum creatinine, hepatic enzymes, uric acid, calcium, and albumin. Metabolic abnormalities, including hyperuricemia, can occur, especially in patients with rapidly dividing leukemia cells and high tumor burden. Coagulation parameters are typically normal, but mild coagulopathy is seen more commonly in patients with T-lineage ALL. Disseminated intravascular coagulation is rarely observed, but therapy-related declines in anticoagulation factors, including fibrinogen, occur with L-asparaginase, a drug commonly used in the treatment of ALL, and baseline levels should, therefore, be obtained. Human leukocyte antigen (HLA) typing should be performed at the time of diagnosis in case of the need for allogeneic HSCT.

Radiographic Evaluation

A mediastinal mass may be detected with a chest radiograph. Computed tomography scans are necessary to detect extramedullary disease sites. A positron emission tomography scan is not routine for diagnostic purposes in ALL but may be useful in some cases to assess response to therapy.

Lumbar Puncture

A lumbar puncture should be performed at the time of diagnosis to examine the cerebral spinal fluid (CSF) for leukemia involvement. Intrathecal chemotherapy should be administered at the time of the first lumbar puncture. CNS involvement is traditionally defined as greater than 5 WBC/μL of CSF with morphologically unequivocal leukemic blasts on the cytocentrifuged specimen. Whether to perform a lumbar puncture in patients with a high circulating blast count is controversial, due to concerns of iatrogenic "seeding" of the CNS with leukemic cells. Studies in pediatric ALL have shown that, when the procedure is complicated by a traumatic tap, the finding of blast cells in the CSF occurs more frequently in children with higher presenting WBC count. Among the patients who had traumatic lumbar punctures, those with leukemic blasts in the CSF were more likely to have subsequent CNS relapse.[62] A traumatic lumbar puncture in a patient with circulating blasts can also make interpretation of the CSF difficult. There are limited data on the prognostic significance of traumatic lumbar puncture in adults with ALL.[63] For patients with thrombocytopenia at the time of the diagnostic lumbar puncture, the risk of a traumatic lumbar puncture can be decreased by administering a platelet transfusion.

Bone Marrow Evaluation

All patients with ALL should undergo a bone marrow aspiration and core biopsy procedure. The specimens must be submitted for histologic, cytogenetic, immunophenotypic, and molecular analysis. Morphologically, the marrow space is usually densely packed with leukemic blasts, accounting for greater than 90% of nucleated cells in many adult patients with ALL. As a result, the marrow biopsy sections are generally hypercellular, and in approximately 10% of adult patients with ALL, the normal marrow is completely replaced by leukemic blasts. A marrow that is replaced by blasts or with fibrosis may prevent a successful aspiration (a "dry tap"), and a touch imprint of the biopsy tissue then becomes useful in evaluating histologic features.

Cytogenetics

Historically, poor chromosomal morphology in ALL made banding studies challenging, and karyotypic abnormalities were not reliably detected in early studies. The implementation of modern metaphase spreading, banding, and molecular cytogenetic techniques now reveals prognostically significant abnormal karyotypes in most adult patients with ALL.[46] These molecular techniques include fluorescence in situ hybridization (FISH) using chromosome- and gene-specific probes for gene rearrangements that are difficult to identify. Age-related differences in the frequency of specific chromosomal abnormalities, including fewer occurrences of numerical chromosome abnormalities and a higher incidence of the Ph chromosome in adults, account for some of the observed difference in outcomes.

Because of the profound prognostic implication of the Ph chromosome and the treatment implication for use of a tyrosine kinase inhibitor (TKI), FISH testing for the Ph chromosome should be performed in all patients with newly diagnosed ALL. Molecular testing for the *BCR-ABL* gene rearrangement should be performed to identify the breakpoint. The Ph chromosome occurs when the *BCR* and *ABL* genes are juxtaposed within the so-called major breakpoint region. This transcribes a 7-kb messenger RNA that is expressed as a 210-kDa fusion protein, or p210$^{BCR-ABL}$. In ALL, a variant breakpoint location, which results in the smaller p190$^{BCR-ABL}$ oncoprotein, is commonly found. A polymerase chain reaction (PCR)-based laboratory test capable of detecting both the p210$^{BCR-ABL}$ and p190$^{BCR-ABL}$ gene transcripts should be performed in all newly diagnosed patients. Ph− like ALL is now recognized as a distinct entity with prognostic significance.[51] For patients with *BCR-ABL*-negative B-ALL, comprehensive analysis by karyotypic and FISH procedures should be performed. In addition, testing for the Ph-like signature should be performed. There is no universal agreement on the best method to detect the Ph-like signature. Methods to detect it include FISH, molecular testing and flow cytometry for CRLF2 overexpression, and DNA sequencing.[64]

Immunophenotype

Immunophenotyping is the characterization of antigens—either cell surface antigens or intracellular antigens—of a malignant cell. Muliparameter flow cytometry is the laboratory technique used to achieve the immunophenotyping using labeled antibodies that recognize the cellular antigens. The immunophenotype is central to establishing the diagnosis by definitively distinguishing acute leukemia as ALL or AML, to further classify ALL as either B or T lineage or mature B cell (Burkitt type), and to reveal the pattern of antigen expression to be used for minimal residual disease response assessments. In addition, with the use of targeted antibody therapy for B-ALL, it has become important to identify the presence or absence of specific antigens, CD19, CD20, and CD22, which may direct the treatment strategy. Hence, all patients should have their leukemic blasts characterized by immunophenotypic analysis. By current WHO classification, the majority of adult ALL cases involve the precursor lymphoid neoplasms (Table 75.1).[61] Approximately 75% of cases are B-ALL, and 25% are T-ALL. The common antigens for identification of B-lineage blasts are CD19, cytoplasmic CD79a, and cytoplasmic CD22. For T-lineage blasts, cytoplasmic CD3 and CD7 are the most common antigens. In clinical practice, panels of antibodies are used to examine the expression of up to 10 antigens to describe individual cases of leukemia.

In general, the immunophenotype for B- and T-ALL is believed to reflect the developmental stage at which lymphoid maturation arrest has occurred (pro-B, pre-B, immature B, and mature B, pro-T, pre-T, cortical T, mature T).[61] Among B-cell ALL and most T-cell cases, the immunophenotype per se does not have clinical significance. One exception is early thymic precursor (ETP) ALL. ETP ALL is a unique subtype of T-ALL that accounts for approximately 20% of adult T-ALL cases. It has a specific immunophenotype and distinctive clinical characteristics as compared with non-ETP ALL.[55,61] It is derived from immature thymocytes that are committed to the T lineage but that have undergone limited differentiation. The blasts are characterized by the lack of expression of CD1a, and CD8 and expression of at least one myeloid (CD13, CD33, HLA-DR) or stem cell marker (CD34/CD117), and dim CD5 expression (1 log lower expression than mature T cells or <75% positive).

Mixed-phenotype acute leukemia (MPAL) is a rare subset of acute leukemias of ambiguous lineage and account for <4% of acute leukemia cases. MPAL is defined by a blast population that expresses a specific combination of lineage-defining myeloid antigens and lineage-defining T- or B-lymphoid antigens'. Currently the genetic basis of most cases of MPAL is unknown, so most cases are classified by the WHO as one of the following lineage mixes: B/myeloid MPAL, T/myeloid MPAL, and MPAL not otherwise specified (NOS).[65] The WHO classification further categorizes MPAL by specific chromosome rearrangements involving the *BCR-ABL1* fusion and *KMNT2A* rearrangement (also known as *MLL*). An accurate diagnosis and classification is important clinically because MPAL is associated with a greater propensity for intrinsic resistance to chemotherapy and, thus, has a poor prognosis. The optimal treatment for MPAL remains uncertain, although retrospective analyses indicate that the outcomes for patients with MPAL are better when ALL-based chemotherapy regimens are used.[66] Allogeneic HSCT in first remission improves outcomes and is recommended for patients with MPAL.[67]

Next-Generation Sequencing

Identifying clonality by next-generation sequencing using high-throughput technology (HTS) is recommended for patients with newly diagnosed ALL when available. Patients achieving MRD negativity by HTS have a better prognosis compared with those with persistent disease.[68] This will be discussed later in greater detail.

DIFFERENTIAL DIAGNOSIS

The differential diagnosis of ALL in adult patients includes both malignant and nonmalignant diseases. Nonmalignant conditions that can mirror the clinical presentation of ALL include viral infections, particularly infectious mononucleosis, which can be associated with lymphocytosis, lymphadenopathy, and immune-mediated thrombocytopenia and anemia. Autoimmune disease, particularly juvenile rheumatoid arthritis, and osteomyelitis causing bone pain and arthralgias can mimic the acute symptomatic presentation of ALL. ALL can be distinguished from the lymphocytosis, lymphadenopathy, and hepatosplenomegaly associated with viral infections and autoimmune conditions by the presence of leukemic blasts in blood, bone marrow, or lymph node specimens.

The malignant diseases that should be considered in the evaluation of suspected ALL, particularly in the cases of bulky adenopathy or a mediastinal mass, include Hodgkin and non-Hodgkin lymphoma (i.e., primary mediastinal lymphoma, diffuse large B-cell lymphoma, and gray zone lymphoma), thymoma, B- or T-lineage lymphoblastic lymphoma, or germ cell tumor. ALL can be distinguished from lymphoma, thymoma, and germ cell tumor with the use of microscopy, but it often requires other methods including flow cytometry, immunohistochemistry, and FISH, karyotype analysis, and next-generation sequencing. Thus, biopsies of lymph nodes or a mediastinal mass should be excisional or large incisional to provide adequate tissue for diagnosis. Limited tissue sampling, that is, core needle biopsy or fine needle aspiration, can be insufficient for an accurate diagnosis. Precise classification of the potential lymphoid malignancies is critical because each of these malignancies requires a distinct cancer therapy administered with curative intent.

Lymphoblastic lymphoma is characterized by nodal involvement with lymphoblasts and <20% lymphoblasts in the bone marrow. ALL and lymphoblastic lymphoma (LBL) are considered the same disease and are often referred to as ALL/LBL.

Difficulty in making an accurate diagnosis of ALL may arise when patients present with an antecedent or overlapping period of pancytopenia before developing ALL, as has been sporadically reported.[69] It may be impossible to distinguish "aleukemic" pancytopenic ALL from aplastic anemia based on examination of the peripheral blood smear.

Table 75.1. 2022 WHO Classification for Precursor Leukemia/Lymphoma

Precursor B-cell Neoplasms
B-lymphoblastic leukemia/lymphoma, NOS
B-lymphoblastic leukemia/lymphoma with high hyperdiploidy
B-lymphoblastic leukemia/lymphoma with hypodiploidy
B-lymphoblastic leukemia/lymphoma with iAMP21
B-lymphoblastic leukemia/lymphoma with *BCR::ABL1* fusion
B-lymphoblastic leukemia/lymphoma with *BCR::ABL1*-like features
B-lymphoblastic leukemia/lymphoma with *KMT2A* rearrangement
B-lymphoblastic leukemia/lymphoma with *ETV6::RUNX1* fusion
B-lymphoblastic leukemia/lymphoma with *ETV6::RUNX1*-like features
B-lymphoblastic leukemia/lymphoma with *TCF3::PBX1* fusion
B-lymphoblastic leukemia/lymphoma with *IGH::IL3* fusion
B-lymphoblastic leukemia/lymphoma with *TCF3::HLF* fusion
B-lymphoblastic leukemia/lymphoma with other defined genetic abnormalities
Precursor T-cell Neoplasms
T-lymphoblastic leukemia/lymphoma
T-lymphoblastic leukemia/lymphoma, NOS
Early T-precursor lymphoblastic leukemia/lymphoma

Abbreviation: WHO, World Health Organization.
Adapted from Alaggio R, Hamador C, Anagnostopoulos I, et al. The 5th edition of the World Health Organization Classification of Haematolymphoid Tumours: Lymphoid Neoplasms. *Leukemia*. 2022;36(7):1720-1748. https://creativecommons.org/licenses/by/4.0/

Bone marrow evaluation and vigilant observation of the patient's clinical course are mandatory in these instances.

Patients in lymphoid blast crisis of CML are usually initially diagnosed in the chronic phase and later progress to acute leukemia. Characterization of the breakpoint region for patients with Philadelphia-positive (Ph+) ALL does not distinguish de novo ALL from CML lymphoid blast crisis because both p190$^{BCR-ABL}$ and p210$^{BCR-ABL}$ are found in even distribution in patients with Ph+ ALL. In the tyrosine kinase era, prognosis is similar for both fusion transcripts. Bone marrow examination may demonstrate evidence of CML in the background, which may help to differentiate ALL arising from CML or de novo ALL.[70]

PROGNOSTIC FACTORS

Many clinical and biologic characteristics previously identified as prognostic factors for adult patients with ALL have lost predictive value as therapy has evolved and become more intensive. Traditionally, age, WBC count at presentation, immunophenotype, and time to CR were strong predictors of disease-free survival (DFS) and OS. Chromosomal and genetic features remain important predictors of relapse[71]; however, risk models based on these features are imperfect and cannot provide definitive information for individual patient decisions. The presence of detectable (measurable) residual disease (MRD) after induction therapy is now recognized as the most important risk factor for relapse.[68,72,73] The German Multicenter Study Group for Adult ALL (GMALL) prospectively assessed MRD evaluation in two consecutive trials involving 1648 patients with standard- and high-risk disease. The complete response rate was 89% after induction, but the molecular CR rate prior to consolidation was only 70% in 580 evaluable patients in CR at day 71. Molecular failure after consolidation (week 16) had the greatest influence on continuous CR (CCR) after 5 years. The CCR rate was 74% for patients in molecular CR vs 35% for those with molecular persistence ($P < .0001$), and OS was 80% vs 42% ($P = .0001$), respectively. Many subsequent studies, not only in children but also in adults, have established the crucial role of MRD assessment. A meta-analysis of 16 studies including 2076 adults with ALL demonstrated a 10-year event-free survival (EFS) of 64% in those with undetectable MRD vs 21% in those with MRD positivity.[74] Treatment strategies based on MRD assessment have shown benefit in several small studies and is now routinely employed as a stratification factor or endpoint in trial designs.[75-77]

Clinical Features

Advanced age and high WBC count at the time of diagnosis are recognized as significant adverse prognostic factors in most adult ALL multicenter collaborative trials.[4,59] Both advanced age and high WBC count were inversely correlated with more frequent occurrences of CR, longer duration of CR, or better OS in either the majority or all of the collaborative studies. Advanced age was variably defined as greater than 30 or 35 years. When included in multivariate analysis as a continuous variable, increasing age predicted worse outcome across the entire age range, making it difficult to choose a cutoff separating standard-risk from high-risk patients. The cutoff for high WBC count was either 30×10^9/L or 50×10^9/L. In the trial conducted by the Cancer and Leukemia Group B (CALGB) study group, patients with advanced age (30-59 years) or high WBC count had an OS of 39% and 34%, respectively, compared with 69% and 59% for patients without these adverse prognostic factors.[4]

Laboratory Features
Immunophenotype

A specific immunophenotypic subgroup with prognostic value and therapeutic importance is the mature B-cell neoplasm, Burkitt leukemia. Burkitt leukemia is characterized by strong expression of surface immunoglobulin in addition to other markers common to B-lineage ALL, including CD10, CD19, CD20, and CD22. These patients respond poorly to standard ALL therapy, and outcome was dismal until brief, dose-intensified treatment programs were established as standard therapy (see Chapters 89 and 90). The substantial improvement in survival that resulted has negated the adverse prognostic value of this feature if patients are optimally managed.

T-ALL comprises approximately 20% to 30% of adult ALL cases.[78] It was previously considered an unfavorable prognostic subgroup, but changes to the frontline treatment regimens, along with intensification of treatment based on the persistence of MRD have improved outcomes.[78] Among cases of T-ALL, ETP ALL has been considered a high-risk subtype.[61] By a strategy first employed in pediatric patients, the Group for Research on Adult Acute Lymphoblastic Leukemia (GRAALL) used a pediatric-inspired regimen, including the use of allogeneic HSCT in patients who demonstrated early chemotherapy resistance.[57] Of the 47 patients with ETP, 22 demonstrated early resistance and underwent transplant with subsequent improved survival compared with those who did not undergo transplant. The benefit of allogeneic HSCT in the ETP patients eliminated the negative impact of intrinsic chemotherapy resistance such that OS rates were similar when compared with non-ETP patients.

Cytogenetics

Unfavorable cytogenetic abnormalities in adult ALL include *MLL* rearrangements including t(4;11) and t(9;11), present in 5% to 10% of cases, and hypodiploid karyotype, also present in 5% to 10% of cases. However, a much deeper understanding of the prognostic significance of specific chromosomal abnormalities is now possible because of the techniques allowing genetic and transcriptional profiling of these abnormalities.

In the UKALL XII/ECOG 2993 trial, 41 patients (5%) without an established translocation had a complex karyotype with five or more chromosomal abnormalities. Four patients were primary induction failures, and 19 of 37 CR patients relapsed. All but 3 of these 19 patients relapsed within 2 years of diagnosis, and 17 of 19 died. EFS and OS were significantly inferior in this group. These results established complex karyotype as a poor prognostic indicator.[46]

Ph+ ALL used to be considered a poor prognostic factor. However, the addition of TKIs such as imatinib, dasatinib, nilotinib, and ponatinib has dramatically improved the outcomes of those patients. The most frequent translocation in adults involving the *MLL* gene, located at chromosome band 11q23, is t(4;11)(q21;q23)/*KMT2A-AFF1* and is also associated with poor survival.[79] Individuals with the t(1;19)(q23;p13)/*TCF3-PBX1* translocation were found to have a 5-year EFS rate of only 53.6% and patients with hypodiploidy ranging from 30 to 39 chromosomes an EFS rate of 35.8%.

A significant advance in risk stratification is the identification of Ph chromosome–like ALL.[80,81] This subgroup represents 25% to 30% of adult ALL and is associated with a worse prognosis. It is recognized now as an entity (previously provisional entity) in the 5th edition of WHO classification of hematolymphoid tumors.[61] The gene expression profile of this subgroup significantly overlaps with Ph+ ALL and is characterized by activated kinase signaling, including the JAK/STAT and Ras pathways. Evidence is emerging that targeting these kinase pathways may be helpful to improve outcomes in this high-risk subtype.[82-84]

Genomic Profiling

Microarray profiling of gene expression and analysis of DNA copy number alterations, followed more recently by next-generation sequencing technologies, has allowed more comprehensive genomic classification of ALL. The ability to identify all inherited and somatic genetic alterations has provided crucial insights into specific genetic subtypes, leading to improved risk stratification and, in some cases, targeted approaches to therapy. These are discussed in detail in Chapter 73.

Response to Therapy

Response to therapy can be assessed by determination of time to attainment of CR, quantitation of early leukemic blast clearance, or detection of MRD. These measurements provide a direct assessment of biologic susceptibility to antileukemic agents, and as such, prognostic factors based on them have inherently high heuristic power. In addition, prospective evaluation of their utility as predictors of outcome in clinical trials has established that they also have high explanatory power.

Early Complete Remission

Failure to achieve CR within 4 weeks of starting treatment or after one course of induction chemotherapy has been considered an independent unfavorable prognostic factor, confirmed in most adult ALL studies. An exception is the international, multicenter UKALL XII/ECOG E2993 trial, which could not confirm its importance in its 1500 patient cohort.[85] Given that most patients achieve morphologic CR after induction, more sensitive measures of residual disease were developed and subsequently validated, as discussed in the subsequent section.

Early Leukemic Blast Clearance

Evaluation for persistence of leukemic blasts at even earlier time points, between days 7 and 21 of induction, was established as an important prognostic indicator for outcome in pediatric and adult ALL,[86-88] although risk-adapted therapy that results in later CR after consolidation often overcomes the negative predictive value of delayed blast clearance. Early persistence of leukemic blasts at 7 days after starting induction is thought to represent corticosteroid resistance. In contrast, persistence at time points after 21 days is considered a reflection of cytotoxic chemotherapy resistance. Numerous prospective studies in pediatric ALL have shown that a substantial unfavorable influence on outcome is associated with the morphologic detection of blood or marrow leukemic blasts persisting during induction therapy at day 7, day 21, or at other time points in between. Persistence of leukemia was usually defined as the finding of greater than 1×10^9/L blast cells in a peripheral blood sample or leukemic blasts greater than 5% of normal cells in a marrow specimen.

Pediatric protocols previously incorporated early treatment response assessment by a day 7 or day 14 bone marrow examination into risk classification, but now base therapy on MRD at later time points including post induction or post consolidation. The survival is optimal if negative MRD is achieved early after induction (day 29), but the prognosis can still be excellent if MRD becomes negative following dose adjustments with consolidation.

Measurable Residual Disease

Measurable residual disease (MRD) refers to the postremission persistence of leukemia that cannot be detected by morphologic assessment. Currently there are four main methods to identify MRD in patients with ALL, namely, multiparameter flow cytometry; real-time quantitative (RQ)-PCR for specific genes, for example, BCR-ABL1; allele-specific oligonucleotide RQ-PCR (ASO-PCR); and high-throughput sequencing for Ig/TCR rearrangements.[89] Flow cytometry, used in four or more color combinations, detects aberrant antigen expression on leukemic cells and can unambiguously distinguish one leukemic blast among more than 10^4 normal cells in 90% of all patients. This level of sensitivity is sufficient for prognostically significant MRD detection. In addition, flow cytometry is rapid and reliable and allows accurate quantitation, and the technical requirements for the assay are already in place at most centers, making it an attractive diagnostic tool. However, standardization across laboratories remains lacking.

RQ-PCR techniques, which can detect one leukemic blast in up to 10^6 normal cells are more sensitive than multi-parameter flow cytometry (MFC). The initial experience using PCR targets based on immunoglobulin and T-cell receptor gene rearrangements was limited by loss of sensitivity if consensus rather than patient-specific primers were used. However, RQ-PCR technology utilizing newer automated methods has proven to be technically simple, yielding precise and consistent quantitation of residual leukemic clones. Although ASO-PCR has been highly standardized in Europe, it still requires significant technical expertise and knowledge. Currently, high-throughput sequencing is considered the most sensitive assay. The clonoSEQ HTS technology is currently US Food and Drug Administration (FDA) approved in the United States; however, comparison with ASO-PCR and standardization is still needed before its widespread use.[90]

The prognostic utility of MRD detection was first described in studies conducted on children with ALL.[91-93] Studies assessing the predictive value of MRD have validated its importance in adults as well.[72,94,95] The kinetics of MRD clearance has also gained much attention with respect to predicting relapse risk. Among the 196 standard-risk patients with ALL monitored by quantitative PCR during their first year of treatment in the GMALL study, the 3-year relapse rate was 0% if MRD declined rapidly to lower than 10^{-4} at day 11, or below detection threshold at day 24, compared with a relapse rate of 94% if the MRD was at a level of 10^{-4} or higher until week 16.[95] Based on these results, they defined three risk groups based on MRD assessment in this otherwise homogeneous standard-risk group.

MRD assessment by RQ-PCR for BCR::ABL1 in patients with Ph-positive ALL has been shown to be prognostic during therapy, after completion of therapy and after HSCT. In studies combining intensive chemotherapy with a TKI (either ponatinib or dasatinib) the relapse-free survival (RFS) was 71% for patients who achieved a complete molecular response at 3 months.[96]

PRIMARY THERAPY

Current management strategies for adult patients with ALL require a careful assessment of relapse risk at the time treatment is initiated. Most adult patients with ALL with precursor B- or T-cell subtype and can be managed with established treatment programs that start with remission induction, followed by intensification/consolidation, CNS prophylaxis, and prolonged maintenance therapy. With modern multiagent regimens, up to 90% of patients achieve CR, and 30% to 60% can be cured. The need to improve DFS suggests that therapy should be tailored, particularly for patients who have an adverse prognostic profile. Risk-adapted therapy has proven remarkably effective for certain poor-risk groups, such as those with persistent MRD. Other patient groups known to have high risk for disease relapse should undergo allogeneic HSCT in first remission, given an appropriate donor. Considerable clinical data suggest that this strategy has been effective with Ph+ patients. The UKALL XII/ECOG E2993 trial also demonstrated the benefit of transplant in standard-risk patients under age 50 years.[33]

Differential approaches to subgroups of patients, including adolescent and young adult patients, defined as 15 to 39 years; older patients, defined as >60 years; patients with the Ph chromosome; and patients whose lymphoblasts express CD20 should also be taken into consideration. General issues relating to supportive care are also discussed in Chapter 70.

General Principles

On presentation, certain pretreatment considerations should be addressed before initiating therapy. These include not only genetic features but also comorbidities and goals of therapy. Leukemia therapy is guided by an estimate of relapse risk, although there is no formal risk assessment tool for adult ALL. Management decisions are complicated by conflicting outcome results for allogeneic HSCT in first remission.

Pretreatment Considerations

Attention should be paid to metabolic, infectious, and hematologic issues before starting leukemia-specific therapy. Hyperuricemia, hyperphosphatemia, and secondary hypocalcemia may be pronounced with high leukemic cell burden and require intravenous hydration and administration of allopurinol or rasburicase. Infections occur frequently in patients with newly diagnosed ALL, and patients presenting with fever, especially in the setting of neutropenia should be treated with broad-spectrum intravenous antibiotics while an infectious evaluation is completed. In addition to myelosuppression during intensive treatment blocks, ALL therapy suppresses cell-mediated immunity, and antimicrobial prophylaxis is recommended for prevention of herpes simplex virus, fungi or molds, and *Pneumocystis jiroveci* infections. For patients presenting with hyperleukocytosis (≥100 × 10^9/L), the clinical consequences can include dyspnea or hypoxia due to pulmonary leukostasis, headache or vision changes due to leukostasis effecting the CNS, and spontaneous tumor lysis. In symptomatic patients, leukapheresis can be performed to reduce the tumor burden. Alternatively, immediate administration of prednisone or vincristine can rapidly reduce the circulating blast count. In an adult series, the WBC count dropped from greater than 100 × 10^9/L to less than 1 × 10^9/L in 39% of patients given a 7-day course of prednisone immediately preceding remission induction chemotherapy.[58] Fertility preservation should be discussed with all patients of reproductive age, and patients should be referred to reproductive specialists for treatment recommendations and counseling.

Risk Assessment Model

There are no useful clinical staging or prognostic scoring systems for adult patients with ALL as there are for other hematologic malignancies, and there are no agreed-upon uniform risk criteria as there are for pediatric ALL. A prognostic model based on CALGB data suggested an additive effect of multiple adverse prognostic features on outcome, and conversely, those without any poor prognostic factors did exceptionally well with few relapses.[4] However, with conventional chemotherapy, a considerable number of standard-risk patients will relapse, and 20% to 25% of high-risk patients will remain disease free, thus highlighting the poor predictive power of risk stratification based only on clinical features at presentation.

Conversely, response to therapy, based on MRD detection, as a risk criterion for modulating therapy has been validated in several adult studies and in a recent meta-analysis.[76,77] In two consecutive GMALL trials (GMALL 06/99 and GMALL 07/03) involving 1648 patients, prospective MRD evaluation was used at several time points. The absence of MRD after consolidation therapy was highly predictive of CCR after 5 years (74% vs 35%) as well as OS (80% vs 42%). A multivariate analysis of prognostic factors, including age, immunophenotype, risk group, and MRD status after consolidation, found that only the MRD status was predictive of CCR after 5 years with a hazard ratio of 4.5 ($P < .0001$). Both age, with a hazard ratio of 1.3 ($P = .0007$), and MRD status, with a hazard ratio of 4.0 ($P < .0001$), influenced OS. In addition, patients with persistent MRD undergoing HSCT in first CR experienced higher rates of CCR than those without HSCT (66% vs 12%), which led to better survival (54% vs 33%).[76] A recent meta-analysis of 39 pediatric and adult studies that included more than 13,000 patients further supports the prognostic significance of MRD clearance, as survival benefit was demonstrated for all treatment protocols, MRD methods, timing of MRD assessment during protocol therapy, and MRD cut-points.[74] In general, persistent MRD after 16 weeks is an indication to consider HSCT in first remission.[97]

Remission Induction

The goal of remission induction therapy is hematologic CR, as defined by the eradication of morphologically detectable leukemia cells in blood and bone marrow and the return of normal hematopoiesis. The importance of achieving CR after induction was highlighted in a very large study of adult patients with ALL that demonstrated a 5-year OS rate of 45% in CR patients compared with 5% in patients who did not achieve CR.[85] Remission induction chemotherapy for adults with ALL is most commonly built around a backbone of vincristine and prednisone. Remission induction with these two drugs in combination produces CR in approximately half of patients with de novo ALL. The CR rate improves to 70% to 85% when an anthracycline is added, which was proven in a landmark CALGB trial to be superior to vincristine and prednisone alone.[98] Induction failures are evenly divided between refractory disease and toxicity-related mortality.

Many alterations to the basic induction regimen have been evaluated. A critical evaluation of the individual merits of these modifications is challenging. Improvement to hematologic CR rates that exceed 80% would be difficult to detect at a satisfactory level of significance. It is clear, however, that an MRD-undetectable CR is a more important goal because it correlates with improved survival. Modern treatment protocols are complex, and it is difficult to attribute outcome results to any one component or to make comparisons of significant findings between any two trials. For example, some modern induction protocols also incorporate L-asparaginase or cyclophosphamide or both, although neither has been proven by controlled trials to be beneficial in adult ALL when added to standard three-drug induction regimens. The one randomized trial with L-asparaginase found no improvement in frequency or duration of CR with the addition of L-asparaginase to doxorubicin, vincristine, and prednisone during induction.[99] Nonetheless, L-asparaginase has a mechanism of action that is close to being ALL specific, causes minimal myelosuppression, and has been shown to be efficacious in pediatric ALL. Consequently, contemporary clinical trials for young adult patients incorporate L-asparaginase in the induction regimen.[8] An Italian Gruppo Italiano Malattie Ematologiche dell' Adulto (GIMEMA) trial randomized adult patients with ALL to induction with daunorubicin, vincristine, prednisone, and L-asparaginase with or without cyclophosphamide.[58] The rate and durability of remission, as well as OS, did not differ between the two randomized treatment groups or for any subtype analyzed. In contrast, other studies have suggested a benefit with the inclusion of cyclophosphamide during induction, especially for patients with T-ALL.[4]

Dose-intensified anthracycline and high-dose cytarabine induction regimens have been evaluated as alternatives to traditional induction protocols. These treatment programs were intended to improve outcome by inducing rapid reduction of leukemic cell mass to achieve early CR but have not resulted in significant benefit. Todeschini et al. generated considerable interest with reports from two sequential trials showing that dose escalation of daunorubicin to 225 mg/m² and, subsequently, to 270 mg/m² significantly improved DFS.[100] Multicenter implementation of this protocol by the GIMEMA group, however, failed to reproduce the earlier experience based on an interim analysis of 460 of 501 total patients enrolled.[101]

Dexamethasone has been substituted for prednisone in standard-risk pediatric patients in a large, randomized trial.[102] The use of dexamethasone achieved a 34% reduction in relapse risk as well as a significant decrease in isolated CNS relapse. There was no benefit in high-risk patients. However, dexamethasone is associated with an increased risk of avascular necrosis in children and adolescents. Current pediatric protocols use prednisone for all children >10 years during induction and dexamethasone for those ≤10 years. In the adult population no difference in OS was found between dexamethasone and prednisolone.[103]

Granulocyte colony-stimulating factor started after completion of the first few days of ALL induction chemotherapy did not improve survival or ultimate outcome in randomized trials. It did, however, shorten the duration of neutropenia by 5 to 6 days and appeared to reduce the incidence of associated complications, particularly infections, and is frequently utilized as a supportive measure.[34]

Intensification/Consolidation Therapy

Postremission intensification or consolidation therapy after the attainment of CR is standard treatment for adult patients with ALL. This therapy refers to the administration of non-cross-resistant drugs aimed at eliminating residual leukemia to prevent relapse as well as the emergence of drug-resistant cells. Various myelosuppressive drugs have been used for intensification/consolidation including high-dose methotrexate, high-dose cytarabine, cyclophosphamide, and etoposide, as well as nonmyelosuppressive drugs such as vincristine and L-asparaginase. The doses of the different drugs are given according to various schedules depending on the specific protocol. Owing to the heterogeneity of approaches, it is difficult to assess the effect of any individual drug used during intensification, and only a general assessment of the overall value of intensification can be made.[104] A randomized trial in childhood ALL clearly demonstrated that administration of both early (given immediately after CR) and late (week 20) intensification therapies was better than either early or late intensification alone and better than no intensification at all.[105] Results from comparative trials in adults have been less clear, however, and again highlight the difficulty of comparing findings from discordantly designed studies. The pediatric study was conducted by the British UKALL study group, which also enrolled adult patients in a concurrent trial using essentially identical treatment regimens.[106] There was a significant decrease in relapse incidence for adult patients who received the early intensification block, but this was not reflected by a statistically significant improvement in DFS, possibly because of an increased number of deaths during remission. Likewise, two GIMEMA studies randomizing adult patients with ALL to intensive vs standard consolidation and maintenance saw no advantage in DFS for intensified postremission treatment.[58,107] No benefit was observed with extending consolidation started early in the postremission period from 1 to 4 consecutive months.[108] Adding two myelosuppressive consolidation courses patterned after AML, "3 + 7" daunorubicin and cytarabine, to maintenance alone made no difference in the duration of remission.[109] Lastly, very late intensification given at 6 or 11 months after CR, in two separate trials, led to no reduction in relapse compared with standard postremission therapy alone.[110,111]

In contrast, clinical data from nonrandomized trials provide evidence that adult patients with ALL benefit from intensification.[4,35] In the CALGB study, patients who achieved CR received two blocks of early intensification in addition to an 8-week late intensification therapy. The reported medians of remission duration and survival, 29 and 36 months, respectively, were substantially better than those observed in prior CALGB trials that did not use intensification blocks.[4] Outcomes better than historical comparison groups were reported by the GMALL studies that consolidated remission patients with a late "reinduction" of drugs identical to initial therapy given 21 weeks after starting treatment.[35,112]

One notable example of the benefit of an individual drug used as consolidation therapy is the use of the bispecific T-cell engager antibody blinatumomab. Single-agent blinatumomab has been shown to be very effective in eliminating MRD in B-cell ALL and improving outcomes.[104] Blinatumomab was used to treat 116 adult patients with ALL in hematologic CR, but who still had MRD ($\geq 10^{-3}$), resulting in a 78% complete MRD response. These patients had longer RFS (23.6 vs 5.7 months, $P = .002$) and OS (38.9 vs 12.5 months, $P = .002$) compared with MRD nonresponders.[104]

Maintenance Therapy

Like postremission intensification, the value of long-term, continuous maintenance therapy for adult ALL has not been established by randomized trials as it has for pediatric ALL.[113] Patterned after the childhood ALL experience, maintenance therapy usually consists of daily 6-mercaptopurine and weekly methotrexate for a total treatment period of 2 to 3 years. There is no information from adult ALL trials regarding the proper duration of maintenance therapy, but children who receive less than 18 months of therapy have worse outcome. The addition of monthly pulses of vincristine and prednisone reduced relapses in controlled childhood ALL studies and has been adopted in some adult maintenance therapy regimens. From a mechanism-of-action perspective, it may be that long-term drug exposure is required to eradicate residual, slowly dividing, or drug-resistant ALL clones.

Relatively strong evidence that adult patients with ALL benefit from maintenance therapy comes from a number of studies showing inferior outcome when prolonged maintenance was completely omitted.[114,115] A US cooperative study group investigated high-dose cytarabine intensification followed by eight cycles of multiagent consolidation.[116] Without maintenance, the median duration of remission was 10 months, and the DFS at 4 years was only 13%.

Central Nervous System Therapy

CNS prophylaxis is essential in the treatment of ALL. Approximately one-third of adult patients will develop CNS involvement at relapse without prophylactic therapy.[117] The advantage of CNS prophylaxis in adult ALL was established by the Southeastern Cancer Group in a randomized trial comparing cranial irradiation plus intrathecal methotrexate vs no prophylaxis.[118] CNS prophylaxis may involve combinations of intrathecal chemotherapy, cranial irradiation, and systemic administration of drugs with high CNS bioavailability, such as high-dose methotrexate, high-dose cytarabine, intensive asparaginase, and dexamethasone. Although the best combination of modalities and the preferred timing has not been established in controlled trials, a number of different approaches have all proved equally effective. Cranial irradiation between 1800 and 2400 cGy plus intrathecal methotrexate started after achievement of CR has been used as CNS prophylaxis, with CNS relapse rates between 0% and 11%.[4,119] Similar results were achieved in other studies that were able to omit cranial irradiation by starting intrathecal chemotherapy concurrent with induction and incorporating high-dose methotrexate or high-dose cytarabine or both.[2]

Adult patients with ALL with CNS involvement at diagnosis require additional CNS-directed therapy because it can adversely impact survival. In the UKALL XII/ECOG E2993 trial evaluating postremission therapies, OS at 10 years was inferior in patients with CNS disease at diagnosis compared with those without (34% vs 29%, $P = .03$).[120] Up to 10% of adults present with CNS leukemia at the time of diagnosis.[4,121,122] The treatment of CNS leukemia has generally involved early and repeated dosing of intrathecal chemotherapy started during induction therapy.[2,122] The investigators at MD Anderson Cancer Center (MDACC) recommend twice weekly administrations, alternating intrathecal methotrexate and cytarabine, until the CSF showed no leukemic blasts, followed by the standard intrathecal prophylaxis regimen.[2]

Hematopoietic Stem Cell Transplantation

Allogeneic HSCT in first remission can improve outcome for certain adult patients with ALL with high-risk features. Historical outcome data from most uncontrolled individual trials indicate DFS between 40% and 60% with matched sibling allogeneic HSCT,[123] and the DFS with chemotherapy alone is estimated at 35% to 50%.[33,124] However, the definition of high-risk disease varies considerably between studies. In an early transplant study, high-risk inclusion criteria were defined as age greater than 30 years, a WBC count greater than 25×10^9/L, failure to achieve morphologic CR within 6 weeks of starting induction, or the presence of unfavorable cytogenetic abnormalities. This study reported a DFS rate of 61%, albeit in a selected patient population.[125]

Registry data from the International Bone Marrow Transplant Registry (IBMTR) provide additional information. Registry data are useful in limiting the influence of selection bias and heterogeneity between patient groups at different institutions, especially when based on large patient numbers. Reporting on 243 adult patients with high-risk ALL undergoing sibling donor allogeneic HSCT, the 5-year estimate of DFS was 39%.[126] Treatment-related mortality (37%) exceeded disease relapse (30%) as the cause of treatment failure. Several comparisons of IBMTR data with outcome after standard therapy have been reported.[127] In these indirect comparisons with historical control groups, allogeneic HSCT in first CR proved superior for survival as a result of protection from relapse.

The first study providing controlled outcome data for allogeneic HSCT vs standard therapy was the French Leucémie Aiguë Lymphoblastique de l'Adulte (LALA)-87.[128] The study genetically randomized adult patients with ALL to sibling donor allogeneic HSCT in first CR vs consolidation and maintenance chemotherapy, regardless of risk category. Risk categorization was based on criteria set by the German study group.[122] Allogeneic HSCT was found to be significantly superior to standard therapy but only for high-risk patients. DFS at 10 years for these patients was 44% with allogeneic HSCT vs 11% for conventional therapy. For standard-risk patients, DFS with allogeneic HSCT was similar (49%) but no better than conventional therapy (43%). The subsequent LALA-94 study also favored allogeneic HSCT over standard chemotherapy for high-risk patients, with respective 5-year OS rates of 51% and 21%.[3] Conversely, the benefit of allogeneic HSCT from a related donor in first CR in standard-risk patients was demonstrated in the UKALL XII/ECOG E2993 trial but was not seen in high-risk patients.[33,129]

Allogeneic HSCT (see Chapter 106) has become more available owing to the ability to use reduced-intensity preparative regimens for patients who were previously ineligible, including in older patients

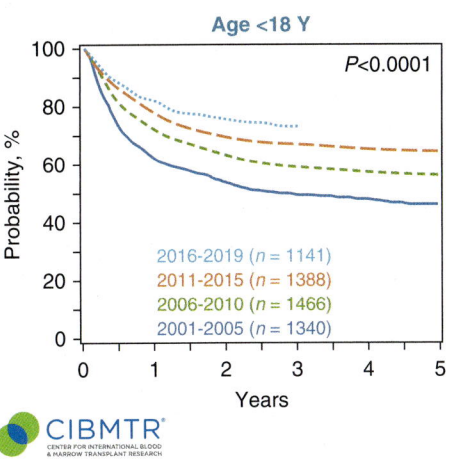
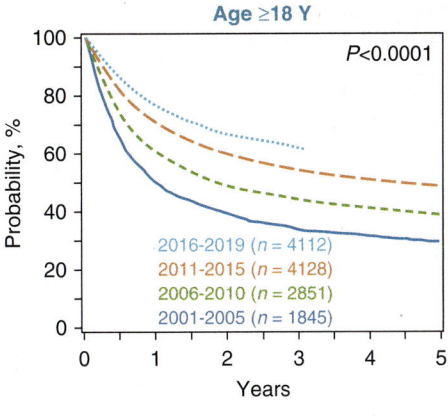

FIGURE 75.4 Trends in survival after allogeneic HSCTs for acute lymphoblastic leukemia, in the United States 2001 to 2019. From CIBMTR: Center for International Blood & Marrow Transplant Research.

and those with comorbidities, and from expanding types of alternative donors, including unrelated donors, umbilical cord, and mismatched family members. Weisdorf et al reported the outcome of 517 patients, ranging in age from 0 to 51 years, with high-risk ALL, including relapsed status and the t(4;11) and t(1;19) translocations, who received matched unrelated donor allogeneic HSCT in first or second CR. Transplant-related mortality was 42%, but relapse at 5 years was only 14% for those transplanted in first CR and 25% for those in second CR. The 5-year probability of DFS rates for those transplanted in first and second CR was 44% and 36%, respectively.[129] Similarly, in a large European study, 5-year DFS did not differ between patients receiving a graft from a matched related or unrelated donor as long as the HSCT occurred in first CR (42% vs 45%, respectively).[130] Treatment-related mortality also did not differ between the two donor types of HSCT.

There is little role for autologous HSCT as an option for postremission therapy in ALL. The French LALA-87 group performed a trial, parallel to the allogeneic HSCT study, that randomly assigned patients younger than 50 years who did not have a matched sibling donor to autologous HSCT vs standard therapy, regardless of disease risk.[128] Conventional therapy was found to be equivalent to autologous HSCT for standard-risk patients. The LALA-94 study compared the outcomes of high-risk patients with ALL who were assigned to allogeneic HSCT if they had a HLA-identical sibling or randomized to autologous HSCT vs standard therapy if they did not. Autologous HSCT conferred no advantage over chemotherapy in this high-risk population, and the respective 5-year OS rates of 32% and 21% were not significantly different in statistical analysis.[129] In the UKALL XII/ECOG E2993 trial, conventional chemotherapy was superior to autologous transplant, with a 46% vs 37% 5-year survival.[33]

A trial genetically randomizing adult patients in first CR to sibling donor allogeneic vs autologous HSCT found the former superior by a substantial margin.[131] The French Groupe Ouest-Est des Leucémies Aiguës et Maladies du Sang (GOELAL02) trial prospectively compared matched sibling allogeneic HSCT in first CR with autologous HSCT following sequential reinduction in patients who had no HLA-matched sibling donor or who were older than 50 years. Matched sibling HSCT significantly improved the 6-year OS (75% vs 40% after autologous HSCT).[132]

Outcomes reported from individual trials show highly variable long-term DFS of 15% to 45% after sibling donor allogeneic HSCT in second or greater CR.[133,134] Registry data from the Center for International Blood & Marrow Transplant Research (CIBMTR) show a 3-year survival estimate of 45%.[135] Unlike allogeneic HSCT for adult ALL in first remission, however, relapse outranked treatment-related mortality as the cause of treatment failure.

Allogeneic HSCT for active disease appears to yield inferior results. Results for individual trials reporting sibling donor allogeneic HSCT for untreated refractory or relapsed disease indicate DFS of 12% to 43%, although the higher figure is from a single center reporting on only 21 patients. The CIBMTR reported a 3-year OS of 37% in 249 patients. Not surprisingly, worse outcomes characterized transplantation performed for advanced disease (in or after second CR) or with high tumor burden (in relapse).

Overall, the outcome of allo-HSCT in adult patients with ALL has markedly improved over the last 2 decades (*Figure 75.4*). The 3-year survival probability is 34% vs 62% for the time period 2001 to 2005 vs 2016 to 2019.[135]

For the interested reader, an extensive review of HSCT trials is provided by the American Society of Blood and Marrow Transplantation's evidence-based review.[136] The advancements of targeted antibody therapy and chimeric antigen receptor T-cell therapy for relapsed ALL, TKI therapy for Ph-positive B-ALL, pediatric inspired regimens for young adult patients with B- and T-ALL, and the monitoring of MRD throughout the course of treatment have required the field to consider afresh the role, timing, and sequence of HSCT in the treatment of ALL.

B-cell Acute Lymphoblastic Leukemia

Almost all modern multiagent, multiphasic adult ALL treatment protocols are variations on the same basic treatment theme. The remission induction regimens are built around the three-drug combination of vincristine, prednisone or dexamethasone, and an anthracycline, most commonly daunorubicin. The Italian GIMEMA ALL 0288 protocol added cyclophosphamide, and the US CALGB 8811 protocol added both cyclophosphamide and L-asparaginase to the induction regimen.[4,58] The hyperfractionated cyclophosphamide, vincristine, doxorubicin, and dexamethasone (hyper-CVAD) regimen developed at MDACC alternates cycles of CVAD with high doses of methotrexate and cytosine arabinoside.[2] For young adult patients, pediatric-inspired protocols use a four-drug induction regimen (daunorubicin, vincristine, prednisone, and L-asparaginase).[8]

For those who achieve remission, induction is followed by various intensification or consolidation treatment blocks, generally completed within 6 months of starting treatment. Prolonged maintenance with 6-mercaptopurine and methotrexate is continued for a total of 2 or 3 years of scheduled therapy. Intermittent pulses of vincristine and prednisone are also given during maintenance in many protocols. Intrathecal treatment with ara-C, methotrexate, and/or dexamethasone is used as CNS relapse prophylaxis, and cranial radiation is included in some protocols.

Two prospective randomized trials have evaluated the addition of rituximab to standard-of-care chemotherapy for Ph-negative B-ALL. The GRAALL-2005-R trial demonstrated a superior EFS with the randomized addition of rituximab to induction, consolidation, intensification, and maintenance (16-18 doses throughout all phases of protocol treatment) for adults <60 years of age whose blasts expressed CD20 in at least 20% of the leukemic cell population.[7] The addition of rituximab improved EFS from 43% to 55% after 4 years of follow-up, largely because of a reduction in the cumulative incidence of relapse. However, the UKALL14 trial, which randomly assigned all patients (regardless of CD20 cell surface expression) to standard-of-care chemotherapy or standard-of-care chemotherapy plus four doses of rituximab during induction therapy only, did not demonstrate an improvement in EFS.[137]

The US CALGB 8811 trial demonstrated an 85% CR rate, median remission duration of 29 months, and DFS rate of 46% but with relatively short median follow-up of 43 months.[4] Six percent failed therapy due to death during induction, and an additional 7% due to refractory disease. Intensification of standard induction with cyclophosphamide was felt to contribute to favorable outcome with T-ALL but contributed to myelosuppression, requiring dose reduction in patients older than 60 years and hospital stays averaging 26 days during the induction phase. Prospective karyotype and immunophenotypic data were collected from patients on this and subsequent CALGB protocols for analysis of prognostic markers and were reported separately.[138,139] The German GMALL 02/84 trial evaluated sequential blocks of intensive induction and consolidation therapy that extended for nearly a year before beginning maintenance. CNS therapy was aggressive and incorporated intrathecal chemotherapy and cranial irradiation, as well as systemic high-dose cytarabine and methotrexate. International application of this treatment protocol confirmed the high CR rate and DFS of 39%, as reported by Hoelzer et al.[140,141]

The MRC UKALL XA trial was designed to evaluate the benefit of postremission therapy with early and late intensification blocks.[32] CR was achieved in 88% of adult patients, and DFS at 5 years was 28%. As previously mentioned, there was a reduction in relapse for patients randomized to receive the early intensification block, but this did not lead to a superior DFS rate. Additional analyses of this patient cohort describing clinical, immunophenotypic, and cytogenetic prognostic factors were detailed in separate reports.[59]

The GIMEMA ALL 0288 trial tested the prognostic value of response to preinduction prednisone and the efficacies of cyclophosphamide inclusion during induction followed by intensification of postremission therapy. An 82% CR rate was observed in 794 adult patients with ALL, which was not better among patients randomized to receive cyclophosphamide during induction.[58] The response to prednisone was shown to have prognostic significance. Prednisone responders had an OS rate of 33% at 8 years compared with 17% among nonresponders. The DFS rate was 29%, which was no better for patients who were randomized to an additional eight-drug consolidation after intensification, as opposed to proceeding directly to maintenance therapy.

In a single-institution study of 288 patients, dose-intensive hyper-CVAD courses alternating with high-dose methotrexate and cytarabine, with concomitant intrathecal CNS prophylaxis, achieved a CR rate of 92%. With a median follow-up of 63 months, the 5-year DFS and OS rates were both 38%,[2] demonstrating activity comparable with other established protocols.

Several retrospective analyses and prospective single-arm trials of adolescent and young adult (AYA) patients with ALL have demonstrated improved survival outcomes for AYA patients when treated with a pediatric ALL protocol that included intensification of the nonmyelosuppressive elements of treatment—glucocorticoids, vincristine, and L-asparaginase—and prolonged CNS prophylaxis and maintenance therapy.[8,142-147] The CALGB 10403 trial was the largest prospective trial designed in the United States to test the use of an intensive pediatric regimen. The 3-year OS was 73% with the pediatric regimen used in CALGB 10403 and represented a significant improvement in outcome in comparison with the historical controls, among whom the long-term OS was estimated at 46%.[8]

T-cell Acute Lymphoblastic Leukemia

T-ALL is less common than B-ALL. Treatment regimens for T-ALL are similar to those used for B-ALL. Unlike in patients with B-ALL where anti-CD20 and CD19 antibodies are effective therapies, currently there are no antibodies effective in the treatment of patients with T-ALL.[148,149] Early precursor T-ALL represents approximately 35% of cases of adult T-ALL and is associated with higher relapse rates. It is associated with germline mutations in cytokine receptor and Ras signaling pathways. Specific targeted therapies are being explored in trials. Intensification of therapy, including the use of allogeneic HSCT, improves survival, and patients with ETP-ALL should be evaluated for allogeneic HSCT after first CR.[56,57] Otherwise, the decision for HSCT in CR1 is dependent on the achievement of MRD after 12 to 14 weeks.

Patients with T-ALL are more likely to have CNS involvement. In the UKALL XII/ECOG E2993 trial, these patients had an inferior 5-year OS (42% vs 29%).[120] Both higher-dose methotrexate and PEG-asparaginase are typically used in T-ALL regimens.

Nelarabine has been evaluated in the frontline therapy of pediatric patients with T-ALL. The Children's Oncology Group AALL0434 trial, the largest trial (n = 1895) ever conducted for newly diagnosed T-ALL and T-LBL, involved a randomization at several time points of nelarabine vs no nelarabine in addition to standard chemotherapy. Not only were the overall results outstanding (4-year DFS and OS 84.3% and 90.2%, respectively), but those who received nelarabine had superior 4-year DFS (88.9% vs 83.3%, P = .0332, respectively).[150] Nelarabine in combination with hyper-CVAD did not lead to an improvement in CR duration or survival in all patients with T-ALL.[151] On further analysis, nelarabine improved the outcome of patients with non-ETP ALL. The 5-year OS was 83% for patients who received hyper-CVAD + nelarabine vs 38% with hyper-CVAD alone. The UKALL14 randomized adult patients with T-ALL to standard of care (SOC) vs SOC + three doses of nelarabine. There was no difference in OS, RFS, or toxicity between both arms.[152] In the UKALL14, patients received only 3 doses compared with 30 doses with the pediatric AALL0434, which could account for the different outcomes seen between UKALL14 and the AALL0433.

Philadelphia Chromosome–Positive Acute Lymphoblastic Leukemia

Ph+ ALL accounts for approximately 25% of adult cases[153] and has historically been associated with a poor prognosis.[46] However, the addition of TKIs and allogeneic HSCT has led to >70% 5-year OS rates.[96] Retrospective analyses suggest that the use of TKIs posttransplant decreases risk of relapse.[154] Finally, these targeted therapies have been used successfully in older patients, in some cases with minimal chemotherapy, with responses comparable with traditional chemotherapy regimens.[155]

Patients with Ph+ ALL tend to be older, with an incidence of nearly 50% in those 50 years or older. In the pre-TKI era, fewer than 25% achieved long-term remission with conventional chemotherapy. Earlier experiences with standard ALL induction chemotherapy demonstrated that most patients achieved CR, but few were long-term survivors owing to relapse. The median duration of survival ranged from 8 to 16 months, and DFS did not exceed 10%.[153,156]

A paradigm shift in the treatment of patients with Ph+ ALL occurred with the introduction in 2001 of the oral BCR::ABL1 TKI imatinib mesylate, with a response rate of 70% as a single agent.[157] Although imatinib monotherapy in relapsed or refractory disease resulted in disappointingly poor durability,[158] its integration into combination chemotherapy induction regimens followed by immediate postremission allogeneic HSCT has improved survival.[159] This is highlighted by an analysis of 2694 patients in the SEER database with pre-B-ALL diagnosed between 2010 and 2014 that demonstrated no significant difference in OS between the 206 patients with Ph+ pre B-ALL and the 2488 patients with Ph− disease.[160] The value of incorporating imatinib into chemotherapy regimens in the treatment of newly diagnosed Ph+ or BCR::ABL1-positive adult patients with ALL was demonstrated in a large study that enrolled patients between 1993 and 2008. In all, 266 patients with Ph+ ALL were enrolled in the pre-imatinib era, and 175 after imatinib became available and was incorporated into the treatment plan.[161] The CR rates were 82% and 92% (P = .004) and OS at 4 years was 22% and 38% (P = .003), respectively. Importantly, in the pre-imatinib era, only 31% of patients received an allogeneic HSCT vs 46% in the imatinib cohort. Finally, when including imatinib, concurrent administration with chemotherapy appears to be superior to an alternating schedule,[162] and attention to CNS prophylaxis remains paramount given its poor CNS penetrance.[163]

Table 75.2. Select High- and Lower-Intensity Regimens With Newly Diagnosed Philadelphia Chromosome–Positive ALL

	Age	N	CR (%)	MRD <0.1%	MRD uMRD	Allo (%)	DFS (y)	OS (y)	Median F/U
Dasatinib									
+Prednisone[155]	≥ 18	53	100	52	15	34	51(2)	69(2)	24.8 m
+Hyper-CVAD[166]	≥18 and ≤60 y	94	88	NR	NR	44	6 (3)	69(3)	36
+Hyper-CVAD[167]	>18	72	96	28	65	17	43 (5)	46 (5)	67
+Blinatumomab[168]	≥ 18	63	98	17*	55	38	88	95	18m
Ponatinib									
+Chemotherapy[169]	18-60	30	100			90	70 (3)	96 (3)	24m
+Hyper-CVAD[170]	≥18	76	100	97	83	20	70 (3)	76 (3)	36
+Blinatumomab[171]	>18	19	100	NR	87	0	100 (1)	100 (1)	14m

Abbreviations: Allo, allogeneic stem cell transplantation; CR, complete remission; DFS, disease-free survival; F/U, follow-up; MRD, measurable residual disease; N, number of patients; NR, not reported; OS, overall survival; uMRD, undetectable MRD.

The second-generation (dasatinib, nilotinib) and third-generation (ponatinib) TKIs have also shown efficacy when used either as single agents or in combination with chemotherapy in this patient population.[155,164,165]

Several studies have evaluated administering dasatinib with TKIs given in combination with steroids alone, in combination with chemotherapy, and most recently in combination with blinatumomab (Table 75.2). Dasatinib with steroids was administered to 53 newly diagnosed patients, and all patients achieved complete hematologic response.[155] Although the results of this trial show that significantly fewer toxic regimens that include TKIs and largely omit chemotherapy can achieve very high CR rates, relapses are almost inevitable unless a patient undergoes subsequent allogeneic HSCT. In a phase II study of dasatinib with hyper-CVAD in previously untreated Ph+ patients, 96% of 72 patients achieved CR.[167] With a median follow-up of 48 months in the surviving patients, 50% were alive and 43% remained in CR. This was followed by a large intergroup trial that demonstrated an 88% CR rate among 94 patients, with 41 undergoing subsequent allogeneic HSCT.[166] The 12-month RFS and OS after transplant were 71% and 87%, respectively. Dasatinib in combination with blinatumomab was administered to 63 patients. Patients initially received steroids + dasatinib for a total of 85 days. Following that patients had to receive two cycles of blinatumomab and may receive up to 5 cycles. With a median follow-up of 18 months, the OS was 95% and DFS was 88%. Of note, only 24 patients proceeded to receive an allograft.[168] An ongoing US intergroup trial is comparing chemotherapy + TKI vs blinatumomab + TKI in patients with newly diagnosed Ph+ ALL.

Nilotinib was combined with standard cytotoxic chemotherapy to treat 90 patients with Ph+ ALL.[172] The CR rate was 91%, and 57 patients received an allogeneic HSCT. The 2-year RFS was 72% for the 82 patients who achieved CR. The significant molecular remission rates achieved with either dasatinib- or nilotinib-based chemotherapy regimens raise the question of whether allogeneic HSCT adds additional benefit, as it does when imatinib-based regimens are used.[173]

Ponatinib is another ABL inhibitor and has activity against all known ABL mutations, including the resistant T315I mutation. In a phase II trial, 76 patients with newly diagnosed Ph+ ALL were treated with hyper-CVAD plus ponatinib.[170] All patients responded, and only 20% proceeded to allo-HSCT.[6] The 5-year EFS was 68%. The 5-year OS of patients treated with combination chemotherapy + ponatinib (73%) was better than that of patients treated with combination chemotherapy + dasatinib (42%).[96] In another study, 30 patients received standard chemotherapy + ponatinib followed by allo-HSCT. Of the 30 patients enrolled, 26 proceeded to allo-HSCT. The overall 3-year EFS and OS was 70% and 96%, respectively.[169]

Ponatinib given in combination with blinatumomab was administered to 19 patients with newly diagnosed ALL. With 14 months of follow-up, the OS and DFS was 100%.[171]

Allogeneic HSCT in first CR has long been the recommended treatment for patients with Ph+ ALL, but the success of the TKIs has brought the role of transplant into question in some patients, particularly if the patient achieves a molecular remission. The benefits of transplantation previously derived from the myeloablative therapy combined with the graft-vs-leukemia effect. In the prospective, multicenter LALA-94 trial of 154 patients with Ph+ ALL, both the absence of MRD and the presence of allogeneic HSCT were independent predictors of DFS and OS.[174] In the study of 267 patients with Ph+ ALL in the prospective, multicenter trial UKALL XII/ECOG E2993, the actuarial 5-year relapse risk was lowest for those undergoing allogeneic HSCT (32%) compared with those treated only with chemotherapy or with autologous HSCT (81%).[161] Recipients of allogeneic transplants experienced higher EFS and OS rates at 5 years (36% and 42%, respectively) compared with their counterparts (17% and 19%, respectively).

These data are in contrast to the data combining hyper-CVAD + ponatinib. Of the 76 patients enrolled, 15 patients underwent HSCT in first CR. The 3-year overall survival was 70% vs 87% for those who did compared with those who did not undergo HSCT.[170] Although the numbers are small, it does bring into question the utility of HSCT in this patient population.[6]

The use of TKIs for posttransplant maintenance is motivated by the observation that MRD following HSCT for Ph+ ALL portends imminent relapse.[175] Imatinib given in this setting was found to be effective in suppressing frank relapse in one study, inducing molecular negativity in 52% of 27 patients for the duration of treatment.[175] Relapse was observed if imatinib was unable to achieve molecular remission or in those who discontinued imatinib. DFS rates in those achieving molecular remission were 91% at 12 months and 54% at 24 months, compared with 8% at 12 months for those with remaining MRD. The only randomized study examined the use of imatinib postallogeneic HSCT using two approaches. One arm included 26 patients who received imatinib post allogeneic HSCT; in the second arm of 29 patients, imatinib was started only if MRD was detected at some point post transplant. Although the median treatment duration in both arms was short (201 and 127 days, respectively), the OS at 5 years was 80% and 75%, respectively. These results suggest a benefit of even short-term posttransplant treatment. The current recommendation is for treatment for 1 year of MRD negativity. The reported use of dasatinib or nilotinib has been limited to very small numbers of patients.

Acute Lymphoblastic Leukemia in Older Patients

One-third of adults diagnosed with ALL are older than 60 years according to US prevalence data.[36] Advanced age is itself an adverse prognostic factor for ALL, and survival decreases continuously with increasing age. Although older age is independently predictive of inferior outcome, a number of factors can be identified that may account for the poor prognosis. Elderly patients with ALL tend to have worse performance status, in part, reflecting comorbid medical conditions. The GMALL reported high rates of diabetes, cardiovascular disease, and chronic pulmonary disease in older adults, such that two-thirds had at least one significant comorbid medical condition.[176] These patients have limited tolerance for intensive therapy, contributing to a high rate of treatment-related morbidity and mortality.[177] Disease features reflecting the underlying biology of the leukemia likely have an influence as well. Elderly patients are more likely to be Ph+ or have other unfavorable cytogenetic abnormalities, be underrepresented in the more favorable T-cell subgroup, and have disease refractory to standard chemotherapy drugs used to treat ALL.[178,179]

In addition, toxicities of standard chemotherapy drugs, including cytarabine neurotoxicity, anthracycline cardiac failure, steroid hyperglycemia, and vincristine neuropathy and constipation, are more prevalent in the elderly. Several groups have described treatment outcome for these patients, and the results are summarized in *Table 75.3*.[180] In the CALGB 8811 trial involving 759 patients, the CR rate and 3-year OS rates were 57% and 12%, respectively, for those aged 60 years and above. Treatment intensity was less than for younger patients owing to significant toxicities. In contrast, younger patients achieved CR rates and 3-year OS rates of 81% and 38%, respectively.[4]

Older patients with ALL given no therapy may not survive more than a few weeks. Palliative therapy, usually moderate-dose prednisone and intermittent vincristine, has been used. Modest responses were observed, with survival extending to a few months. A retrospective review of one cooperative group member institution's 13-year experience revealed that only half of their patients with ALL older than 60 years were enrolled in their active study protocol.[181] Several groups uniformly treated fairly large cohorts (40-60) of elderly patients with "age-adjusted" chemotherapy programs. Impressive CR rates were sometimes observed, and median survival extended to 12 to 14 months. Data from major collaborative groups treating selected, elderly patients with ALL suggest that 40% to 70% may achieve CR with intensive therapy.[180] Resistant disease and toxic deaths were frequent, with OS at 3 years less than 20%.

New therapeutic options for older patients are now available that may be more efficacious with less toxicity.[182] Targeted therapies against CD19, CD20, CD22, and BCR::ABL1 offer the possibilities of more favorable outcomes. The largest experience to date has been with the oral TKIs in Ph+ ALL. Several studies evaluated the role of TKIs in newly diagnosed patients aged 55 years or greater with regimens including imatinib, nilotinib, dasatinib or ponatinib.[158,183-187] CR rates were at least 96%, with short-term OS (at 1-1.5 years) of 57% to 74% and 5-year OS of 36% in the largest study.

Results of blinatumomab given with maintenance chemotherapy in older patients with ALL were encouraging. Overall 66% of patients achieved CR and the 3-year OS and DFS was 37%.[188]

Combining the novel antibody-drug conjugate inotuzumab (discussed in subsequent section) with low-intensity chemotherapy followed by blinatumomab has led to significant improvement of outcome in older patients with AML in one study. Patients older than 60 years received mini-hyper-CVAD + inotuzumab followed by blinatumomab. Of the 69 patients evaluable for response, 98% responded. With a median follow-up of 56 months, the 5-year OS was 47%. The decrease in OS was still highly influenced by treatment-related mortality (32%) especially in patients >70 years old (20/29 patients).[189]

Much remains to be learned about treating older patients with ALL. With the use of oral TKIs and recently approved monoclonal antibodies, outcomes are improving for this population for which there remains an unmet need. As such, older patients should be referred for investigational protocols at study centers whenever feasible.

SALVAGE THERAPY

The prospect of salvage therapy for refractory or relapsing disease will eventually have to be considered for many adult patients with ALL. Primary resistance to induction chemotherapy reported by collaborative trials ranges from 8% to 15%.[4,58,85] Although most patients achieve a first CR, only 30% to 50% become long-term survivors, and the principal cause of treatment failure is disease relapse. Although a second or salvaged CR can be obtained for some with chemotherapy, the durability of remission is likely short unless an allogeneic HSCT is subsequently performed, and, even then, remission duration is limited for most patients.[190]

There have been many efforts to characterize the biologic and clinical features of disease relapse in adult patients with ALL. Thomas et al reviewed the presenting characteristics at relapse in patients referred for therapy at a single institution over a 17-year period.[191] The duration of CR was less than 1 year in 61%. Essentially, all patients had marrow relapses, although one-third had concurrent extramedullary involvement, including CNS leukemia in 16%. In other studies, the cytogenetic, immunophenotypic, and molecular changes at relapse compared with initial presentation were examined.[192] Clonal cytogenetic changes were the most common finding. Half of the cytogenetic findings were believed to represent clonal evolution, and the remainder were karyotypic changes. Immunophenotypic changes were twice as likely in patients with T-ALL vs B-ALL and were marked by gain or loss of one or two antigens but no complete shift from B- to T-lineage ALL, or vice versa. Neither the presence of a karyotypic shift nor an immunophenotypic shift adversely influenced survival from the time of relapse. Patterns of persistence and clearance of *BCR::ABL1* transcripts also characterize the assessment of MRD and appear to predict relapse in Ph+ ALL (see section "Measurable Residual Disease").

Table 75.3. Treatment Outcome in Elderly Patients With Acute Lymphoblastic Leukemia

Study	Year	Age (y)	N	Complete Remission (%)	Induction Mortality (%)	Survival (%)
SWOG 8419	1985	>50	85	41	37	9 at 3 y
CALGB 8811	1988	≥60	129	57	NR	12 at 3 y
GIMEMA ALL-028	1988	50-60	121	68	NR	15 at 8 y
MD Anderson	1992	≥60	44	80	16	17 at 5 y
MRC UKALL XII/ECOG 2993	1993	55-65	100	73	18	21 at 5 y
SWOG 9400	1995	50-65	43	63	NR	23 at 5 y
PETHEMA ALL-96	1996	≥55	33	58	36	39 at 2 y
SWOG1318	2022	≥65	29	66	3	37 at 3 y
Mini-Hyper-CVAD + inotuzumab ± blinatumomab	2022	≥60	69	99	52	47 at 5 y

Abbreviations: ALL, acute lymphoblastic leukemia; CALGB, Cancer and Leukemia Group B; ECOG, Eastern Cooperative Oncology Group; GIMEMA, Gruppo Italiano Malattie Ematologiche dell' Adulto; MRC, Medical Research Council; NR, not reported; PETHEMA, Programa para el Estudio de la Terapéutica en Hemopatía Maligna; SWOG, Southwest Oncology Group; UKALL, United Kingdom Acute Lymphoblastic Leukemia.

Chemotherapy

Reinduction of remission, or attainment of a *first* CR for refractory patients, can be expected in slightly more than half of patients with salvage chemotherapy. However, in the majority, remissions do not extend beyond 3 to 6 months and long-term survival is well below 10%, whether or not postremission therapy is given. In general, single-agent chemotherapy is inferior to multiagent protocols.

Salvage regimens based on high-dose cytarabine, which have been extensively studied, produce CR rates that vary widely but have occasionally exceeded 70%. Additional drugs have included an anthracycline, mitoxantrone, fludarabine, and bortezomib. Commonly used regimens include FLAG-ida (fludarabine, cytarabine, G-CSF, and idarubicin),[193] augmented hyper-CVAD,[194] and high-dose cytarabine.[195]

In a large single-institution review, Thomas et al described treatment outcome for 314 adult patients with relapsed or refractory ALL who received various salvage therapy regimens. Overall CR was achieved in 31%.[191] Patients with long first remissions received the customary frontline study salvage regimen, which varied depending on the study period, whereas patients resistant to or relapsing on therapy were treated with new drug combinations. Patients with primary refractory disease and those with relapsed disease were found to achieve CR equally well. Death occurred without achieving remission in 21%. Patients with long first CR duration (>2 years) were more likely to achieve CR and have longer durations of second remission. For the entire group, the median durations of remission and survival from the start of salvage therapy were 6 and 5 months, respectively. Although salvage regimens in resistant or relapsed disease offer only modest effects with short duration, they allow a bridge to allogeneic HSCT or CAR T-cell therapy, which have curative potential for select patients who achieve remission.

The treatment of patients with relapsed Ph+ ALL depends on the TKI used as part of the initial treatment regimens and the development of point mutations within the ABL kinase domain. In patients who had imatinib as the first-line therapy with no evidence of the T315I mutation, dasatinib would be an option. In patients who received dasatinib as initial therapy or who harbor the T315I mutation, ponatinib is the TKI of choice.[196] In a phase II study, ponatinib showed considerable activity in patients resistant to second-generation TKIs. A major hematologic response was observed in 36% of the 122 patients with Ph+ ALL and the T315I mutation.[197]

The novel antibody conjugate, inotuzumab, and the bispecific antibody, blinatumomab, discussed in the subsequent section, are now approved and clearly are superior to standard chemotherapy approaches for relapsed or refractory disease.[198,199] With more patients achieving remission after salvage therapy with these agents, more are able to receive potentially curative therapies, including allogeneic HSCT or CAR T-cell therapy.

Nelarabine was approved for the treatment of refractory or relapsed T-ALL or T-LBL in patients who have undergone at least two prior chemotherapy treatments. As a prodrug, it is converted to the deoxyguanosine analog, 9-β-D-arabinofuranosylguanine (ara-G), which selectively induces apoptosis in T cells by incorporating its phosphorylated form into DNA and inhibiting synthesis. Two phase II studies of single-agent nelarabine demonstrated CR rates of up to 23% in patients with refractory or relapsed T-ALL or T-LBL. Neurotoxicity is the dose-limiting toxicity,[10] for which close patient monitoring is strongly encouraged.

Antibodies

Two antibody therapeutics have improved the outcomes in ALL. Inotuzumab ozogamicin is an anti-CD22 calicheamicin conjugate with significant activity, even in heavily pretreated individuals. In a phase II experience, 49 previously treated patients received a 1-hour infusion of study drug every 3 to 4 weeks for one to five courses. Nine patients achieved a CR with an additional 19 with a bone marrow complete response. Nineteen had resistant disease. Duration of response was short, with median OS of 5.1 months in all patients and 7.9 months in the 28 responding patients.[200] A second study reported a 68% CR/CRi rate with 33% of patients able to proceed to allogeneic HSCT.[201] A phase III study of inotuzumab vs standard intensive therapy for relapsed ALL enrolled 326 patients.[198] Analysis of outcomes of the first 218 patients showed higher CR rates, MRD negativity, and duration of remission for those who received inotuzumab (80.7%, 78.4%, and 4.6 months vs 29.4%, 28.1%, and 3.1 months, respectively). Analysis of survival for all 326 patients showed longer progression-free survival and OS for those who received inotuzumab (5 and 7.7 months vs 1.8 and 6.7 months, respectively). In addition, a multicenter retrospective study confirmed the efficacy of inotuzumab in the nonclinical trial setting.[202] Owing to the significant efficacy observed, randomized trials are underway incorporating inotuzumab in frontline regimens.

Blinatumomab is a bispecific single-chain antibody that binds both cytotoxic $CD3^+$ T lymphocytes and CD19 on the surface of the B-cell leukemic blast. In a phase II trial of patients with B-ALL with persistent or relapsed MRD, 80% of patients responded. With a median follow-up of 33 months, the hematologic RFS of the 20 evaluable patients was 61%. These long-lasting remissions would be unusual for patients with MRD-detectable disease. A second, larger study enrolled 116 patients in first remission but with MRD-detectable disease.[104] The MRD clearance rate was 78% with RFS of 54% with median follow-up of 30 months. Complete MRD responders achieved longer RFS (23.6 vs 5.7 months; $P = .003$) and OS (38.9 vs 12.5 months; $P = .002$) compared with MRD nonresponders. Similar encouraging results were seen in another study that enrolled patients who were MRD+ up to 3 months after starting induction therapy in newly diagnosed patients or 1 month after salvage therapy.[203] These results demonstrate that persistent MRD is a modifiable risk factor. Subsequent studies enrolled patients with overt hematologic relapse. Two phase II trials demonstrated efficacy and safety of blinatumomab in patients with relapsed/refractory ALL.[204,205] Long-term pooled analysis demonstrated plateau of survival at 3 years with approximately 30% of patients alive in CR. Of the patients who received an HSCT in CR, 37% were alive at 3 years.[206]

A randomized phase III trial in patients with relapsed or refractory B-ALL compared blinatumomab with standard-of-care chemotherapy.[199] OS was significantly longer in the 271 patients who received blinatumomab than in the 134 patients who received chemotherapy (median 7.7 vs 4.0 months). Remission rates (44% vs 25%; $P < .001$), EFS (6-month estimates 31% vs 12%), and duration of remission (7.3 vs 4.6 months) were also superior with blinatumomab. In addition, a multicenter retrospective study confirmed the efficacy of blinatumomab in the nonclinical trial setting.[207]

On the basis of this promising activity, blinatumomab is currently being evaluated in the frontline setting in a study that has completed accrual and results are still pending.

Blinatumomab is also an option for relapsed Ph+ ALL. After its initial approval for patients with relapsed Ph− ALL, a phase II trial was conducted in relapsed patients with Ph+ ALL who had progressed after at least one second-generation TKI or were intolerant of these agents and had received imatinib as well. Thirty-six percent of the 45 patients achieved CR including 4 of 10 patients with the T315I mutation. A complete MRD response was seen in 88% of those with CR.[208]

A randomized trial of rituximab in 209 newly diagnosed patients with CD20-positive B-ALL demonstrated a superior 30-month EFS in those who received rituximab.[7] The estimated 2-year EFS rates were 65% and 52%, respectively, establishing the addition of rituximab to standard chemotherapy regimens as standard of care for patients with CD20-positive ALL.

Additional Agents/Novel Therapies

Clofarabine is a deoxyadenosine analog that was approved by the FDA for the treatment of pediatric patients (ages 1-21 years) with relapsed or refractory ALL. It demonstrated activity as a single agent, with a 30% overall response rate, in a phase II study of 61 heavily pretreated children.[147] It is not approved for adult patients with ALL. Multiple hematological malignancies, including ALL,[209,210] are dependent on BCL-2 activity for survival. Venetoclax is currently the only approved BCL-2 inhibitor. This agent has demonstrated activity in patients with ALL. Venetoclax, in combination with various chemotherapy regimens, was administered to patients with relapsed or refractory T-ALL. Of the 10 evaluable patients, 6 achieved a CR. There is some thought that ALL cells may be able to bypass BCL-2 inhibition by dependency on MCL-1 or BCL-XL. Based on that, ongoing studies combining venetoclax with the BCL-XL inhibitor, navitoclax, have shown promising results.[211] In one study, 60% of patients with relapsed refractory ALL achieved a CR. More importantly, 13 patients (28%) proceeded to allo-HSCT or CAR-T cell therapy.[212] Daratumumab, a CD38 antibody demonstrated preclinical activity in xenograft models of T-ALL.[213] Since then several studies reported efficacy of daratumumab for patients with T-ALL.[214-219] In a multicenter retrospective study, 20% of patients with relapsed refractory T-ALL responded to daratumumab.[218] Targeting CD38 with a bispecific antibody is currently being evaluated in patients with T-ALL.[220]

CD19-Directed Chimeric Antigen Receptor T-cell Therapy

CAR T-cell therapy (see Chapter 71) is now a proven treatment approach for children and adults with relapsed B-ALL. Phase I/II trials of CAR T-cell therapy in children and young adults (<25 years) have demonstrated overall response rates of 81% and an undetectable MRD rate of 100%. Long-term sustained remissions have been reported in a subgroup of these patients with a 12-month RFS of approximately 60% and OS of 76%.[221,222] Based on these data, in August 2017, the FDA approved tisagenlecleucel, the anti-CD19 CAR T-cell product, for pediatric and young adult patients with refractory B-ALL or in second or greater relapse.[223]

For adult patients with relapsed B-ALL, the phase I data from single-institution trials of anti-CD19 CAR T-cell therapy demonstrate similar efficacy with CR rates of 62% to 83% and median EFS of 6.1 months and median OS of 12.9 months.[224-226] The first multicenter phase II trial (ZUMA-3) for adult patients demonstrated an overall response rate of 71%. The rate of undetectable MRD for responding patients was 97%.[226] The median OS for all treated patients was 18.2 months and was not reached in responding patients.[227] This trial led to the FDA approval in October 2021 of brexucabtagene autoleucel for adult patients (>18 years) with relapsed/refractory B-ALL.

The unique toxicities associated with anti-CD-19-directed CAR T-cell therapy include the cytokine release syndrome (CRS) and immune effector cell–associated neurotoxicity syndrome (ICANS), which result from binding of the CAR T-cell product to the target ALL blast and subsequent immune activation and CAR T-cell expansion. Clinically, CRS manifests as fever, rigors, tachycardia, hypotension, hypoxia, and tachypnea, and these symptoms can progress to life-threatening hemodynamic instability, capillary leak syndrome, and coagulopathy. The neurologic symptoms of ICANS include headache, tremor, delirium, impaired consciousness, and speech impairment. ICANS can be severe with seizures, and fatal events of cerebral edema have occurred.[228]

Historically, allogeneic HSCT has been the only curative treatment for relapsed ALL. Whether additional consolidation therapy in the form of allogeneic HSCT is required for all patients following CAR T-cell therapy has not been determined and remains an important unanswered clinical question. Randomized clinical trials will be required to determine the optimal consolidation approach for ALL in CR2.[229]

SUMMARY AND FUTURE DIRECTIONS

The management of ALL has dramatically changed over the last decade. Chemotherapy followed by stem cell transplantation was considered the standard of care for most patients with ALL. With the marked improvement in prognostication and therapies, we can better tailor therapy for most patients thereby reducing morbidity and mortality. Better molecular characterization can identify patients for whom more intensive up-front therapy may be beneficial. Combining better up-front prognostication with MRD assessment further refines the prognostic classification. In addition, immunotherapy with antibodies (naked, conjugated, or bispecific) and CAR T cells have not only markedly improved the outcome but also decreased toxicity therapy allowing older more frail patients to receive therapy. As these new therapies move to the frontline setting, we hope that the cure for all patients with ALL is on the horizon.

ACKNOWLEDGMENT

This chapter is dedicated to Steven E. Coutre, MD, dedicated physician, insightful collaborator, cherished colleague, and friend.

References

1. Hunger SP, Mullighan CG. Acute lymphoblastic leukemia in children. *N Engl J Med.* 2015;373:1541-1552.
2. Kantarjian H, Thomas D, O'Brien S, et al. Long-term follow-up results of hyper-fractionated cyclophosphamide, vincristine, doxorubicin, and dexamethasone (Hyper-CVAD), a dose-intensive regimen, in adult acute lymphocytic leukemia. *Cancer.* 2004;101(12):2788-2801.
3. Thomas X, Boiron JM, Huguet F, et al. Outcome of treatment in adults with acute lymphoblastic leukemia: analysis of the LALA-94 trial. *J Clin Oncol.* 2004;22(20):4075-4086.
4. Larson RA, Dodge RK, Burns CP, et al. A five-drug remission induction regimen with intensive consolidation for adults with acute lymphoblastic leukemia: cancer and leukemia group B study 8811. *Blood.* 1995;85(8):2025-2037.
5. Hoelzer D, Walewski J, Dohner H, et al. Improved outcome of adult Burkitt lymphoma/leukemia with rituximab and chemotherapy: report of a large prospective multicenter trial. *Blood.* 2014;124(26):3870-3879.
6. Jabbour E, Haddad FG, Short NJ, Kantarjian H. Treatment of adults with Philadelphia chromosome-positive acute lymphoblastic leukemia-from intensive chemotherapy combinations to chemotherapy-free regimens: a review. *JAMA Oncol.* 2022;8(9):1340-1348.
7. Maury S, Chevret S, Thomas X, et al. Rituximab in B-lineage adult acute lymphoblastic leukemia. *N Engl J Med.* 2016;375(11):1044-1053.
8. Stock W, Luger SM, Advani AS, et al. A pediatric regimen for older adolescents and young adults with acute lymphoblastic leukemia: results of CALGB 10403. *Blood.* 2019;133(14):1548-1559.
9. Sheykhhasan M, Manoochehri H, Dama P. Use of CAR T-cell for acute lymphoblastic leukemia (ALL) treatment: a review study. *Cancer Gene Ther.* 2022;29(8-9):1080-1096.
10. DeAngelo DJ, Yu D, Johnson JL, et al. Nelarabine induces complete remissions in adults with relapsed or refractory T-lineage acute lymphoblastic leukemia or lymphoblastic lymphoma: Cancer and Leukemia Group B study 19801. *Blood.* 2007;109(12):5136-5142.
11. Pui CH, Yang JJ, Hunger SP, et al. Childhood acute lymphoblastic leukemia: progress through collaboration. *J Clin Oncol.* 2015;33(27):2938-2948.
12. Farber S, Diamond LK. Temporary remissions in acute leukemia in children produced by folic acid antagonist, 4-aminopteroyl-glutamic acid. *N Engl J Med.* 1948;238(23):787-793.
13. Pearson OH, Eliel LP. Use of pituitary adrenocorticotropic hormone (ACTH) and cortisone in lymphomas and leukemias. *J Am Med Assoc.* 1950;144(16):1349-1353.
14. Skipper HE, Thomson JR, Elion GB, Hitchings GH. Observations on the anticancer activity of 6-mercaptopurine. *Cancer Res.* 1954;14(4):294-298.
15. Law LW. Effects of combinations of antileukemic agents on an acute lymphocytic leukemia of mice. *Cancer Res.* 1952;12:871-878.
16. Green MR, George SL, Schilsky RL; Cancer and Leukemia Group B. Tomorrow's cancer treatments today: the first 50 years of the Cancer and Leukemia Group B. *Semin Oncol.* 2008;35(5):470-483.
17. Frei E III, Holland JF, Schneiderman MA, et al. A comparative study of two regimens of combination chemotherapy in acute leukemia. *Blood.* 1958;13(12):1126-1148.
18. Pinkel D. Five-year follow-up of "total therapy" of childhood lymphocytic leukemia. *J Am Med Assoc.* 1971;216(4):648-652.
19. Pinkel D, Hernandez K, Borella L, et al. Drug dosage and remission duration in childhood lymphocytic leukemia. *Cancer.* 1971;27(2):247-256.
20. Rivera GK, Pinkel D, Simone JV, Hancock ML, Crist WM. Treatment of acute lymphoblastic leukemia. 30 years' experience at St. Jude Children's Research Hospital. *N Engl J Med.* 1993;329(18):1289-1295.
21. Aur RJ, Simone J, Hustu HO, et al. Central nervous system therapy and combination chemotherapy of childhood lymphocytic leukemia. *Blood.* 1971;37(3):272-281.
22. Aur RJ, Simone JV, Hustu HO, Verzosa MS. A comparative study of central nervous system irradiation and intensive chemotherapy early in remission of childhood acute lymphocytic leukemia. *Cancer.* 1972;29(2):381-391.
23. Henze G, Langermann HJ, Bramswig J, et al. The BFM 76/79 acute lymphoblastic leukemia therapy study (author's transl). Article in German. *Klin Pädiatr.* 1981;193(3):145-154.
24. Sallan SE, Hitchcock-Bryan S, Gelber R, Cassady JR, Frei E III, Nathan DG. Influence of intensive asparaginase in the treatment of childhood non-T-cell acute lymphoblastic leukemia. *Cancer Res.* 1983;43(11):5601-5607.
25. Clavell LA, Gelber RD, Cohen HJ, et al. Four-agent induction and intensive asparaginase therapy for treatment of childhood acute lymphoblastic leukemia. *N Engl J Med.* 1986;315(11):657-663.
26. Gaynon PS, Steinherz PG, Bleyer WA, et al. Intensive therapy for children with acute lymphoblastic leukaemia and unfavourable presenting features. Early conclusions of study CCG-106 by the Childrens Cancer Study Group. *Lancet.* 1988;2(8617):921-924.

27. Riehm H, Feickert HJ, Schrappe M, Henze G, Schellong G. Therapy results in five ALL-BFM studies since 1970: implications of risk factors for prognosis. *Haematol Blood Transfus*. 1987;30:139-146.
28. Riehm H, Gadner H, Henze G, et al. Results and significance of six randomized trials in four consecutive ALL-BFM studies. *Haematol Blood Transfus*. 1990;33:439-450.
29. Raimondi SC, Privitera E, Williams DL, et al. New recurring chromosomal translocations in childhood acute lymphoblastic leukemia. *Blood*. 1991;77(9):2016-2022.
30. Hunger SP, Lu X, Devidas M, et al. Improved survival for children and adolescents with acute lymphoblastic leukemia between 1990 and 2005: a report from the Children's Oncology Group. *J Clin Oncol*. 2012;30(14):1663-1669.
31. Durrant IJ, Richards SM, Prentice HG, Goldstone AH. The Medical Research Council trials in adult acute lymphocytic leukemia. *Hematol Oncol Clin North Am*. 2000;14(6):1327-1352.
32. Secker-Walker LM, Prentice HG, Durrant J, Richards S, Hall E, Harrison G. Cytogenetics adds independent prognostic information in adults with acute lymphoblastic leukaemia on MRC trial UKALL XA. MRC Adult Leukaemia Working Party. *Br J Haematol*. 1997;96(3):601-610.
33. Goldstone AH, Richards SM, Lazarus HM, et al. In adults with standard-risk acute lymphoblastic leukemia, the greatest benefit is achieved from a matched sibling allogeneic transplantation in first complete remission, and an autologous transplantation is less effective than conventional consolidation/maintenance chemotherapy in all patients: final results of the International ALL Trial (MRC UKALL XII/ECOG E2993). *Blood*. 2008;111:1827-1833.
34. Larson RA, Dodge RK, Linker CA, et al. A randomized controlled trial of filgrastim during remission induction and consolidation chemotherapy for adults with acute lymphoblastic leukemia: CALGB study 9111. *Blood*. 1998;92(5):1556-1564.
35. Gokbuget N, Hoelzer D, Arnold R, et al. Treatment of Adult ALL according to protocols of the German Multicenter Study Group for Adult ALL (GMALL). *Hematol Oncol Clin North Am*. 2000;14:1307-1325, ix.
36. Cancer Stat Facts: Leukemia—Acute Lymphocytic Leukemia (ALL). https://seer.cancer.gov/statfacts/html/alyl.html
37. Moriyama T, Relling MV, Yang JJ. Inherited genetic variation in childhood acute lymphoblastic leukemia. *Blood*. 2015;125(26):3988-3995.
38. Qian M, Cao X, Devidas M, et al. TP53 germline variations influence the predisposition and prognosis of B-cell acute lymphoblastic leukemia in children. *J Clin Oncol*. 2018;36(6):591-599.
39. Cardis E, Vrijheid M, Blettner M, et al. Risk of cancer after low doses of ionising radiation: retrospective cohort study in 15 countries. *Br Med J*. 2005;331(7508):77.
40. Liu JJ, Freedman DM, Little MP, et al. Work history and mortality risks in 90, 268 US radiological technologists. *Occup Environ Med*. 2014;71(12):819-835.
41. Kim BH, Kwon YJ, Ju YS, et al. The work-relatedness at a case of acute lymphoblastic leukemia in a radiation oncologist. *Ann Occup Environ Med*. 2017;29:28.
42. Khalade A, Jaakkola MS, Pukkala E, Jaakkola JJK. Exposure to benzene at work and the risk of leukemia: a systematic review and meta-analysis. *Environ Health*. 2010;9:31.
43. Saygin C, Kishtagari A, Cassaday RD, et al. Therapy-related acute lymphoblastic leukemia is a distinct entity with adverse genetic features and clinical outcomes. *Blood Adv*. 2019;3(24):4228-4237.
44. Kinlen LJ. Epidemiological evidence for an infective basis in childhood leukaemia. *Br J Cancer*. 1995;71:1-5.
45. Greaves M, Cazzaniga V, Ford A. Can we prevent childhood Leukaemia? *Leukemia*. 2021;35(5):1258-1264.
46. Moorman AV, Harrison CJ, Buck GAN, et al. Karyotype is an independent prognostic factor in adult acute lymphoblastic leukemia (ALL): analysis of cytogenetic data from patients treated on the Medical Research Council (MRC) UKALLXII/Eastern Cooperative Oncology Group (ECOG) 2993 trial. *Blood*. 2007;109(8):3189-3197.
47. Moriyama T, Metzger ML, Wu G, et al. Germline genetic variation in ETV6 and risk of childhood acute lymphoblastic leukaemia: a systematic genetic study. *Lancet Oncol*. 2015;16:1659-1666.
48. Stock W, Tsai T, Golden C, et al. Cell cycle regulatory gene abnormalities are important determinants of leukemogenesis and disease biology in adult acute lymphoblastic leukemia. *Blood*. 2000;95(7):2364-2371.
49. Harvey RC, Mullighan CG, Wang X, et al. Identification of novel cluster groups in pediatric high-risk B-precursor acute lymphoblastic leukemia with gene expression profiling: correlation with genome-wide DNA copy number alterations, clinical characteristics, and outcome. *Blood*. 2010;116(23):4874-4884.
50. Roberts KG, Li Y, Payne-Turner D, et al. Targetable kinase-activating lesions in Ph-like acute lymphoblastic leukemia. *N Engl J Med*. 2014;371(11):1005-1015.
51. Roberts KG, Gu Z, Payne-Turner D, et al. High frequency and poor outcome of Philadelphia chromosome-like acute lymphoblastic leukemia in adults. *J Clin Oncol*. 2017;35(4):394-401.
52. Weng AP, Ferrando AA, Lee W, et al. Activating mutations of NOTCH1 in human T cell acute lymphoblastic leukemia. *Science*. 2004;306(5694):269-271.
53. Roberts KG, Mullighan CG. Genomics in acute lymphoblastic leukaemia: insights and treatment implications. *Nat Rev Clin Oncol*. 2015;12(6):344-357.
54. Hebert J, Cayuela JM, Berkeley J, Sigaux F. Candidate tumor-suppressor genes MTS1 (p16INK4A) and MTS2 (p15INK4B) display frequent homozygous deletions in primary cells from T- but not from B-cell lineage acute lymphoblastic leukemias. *Blood*. 1994;84(12):4038-4044.
55. Coustan-Smith E, Mullighan CG, Onciu M, et al. Early T-cell precursor leukaemia: a subtype of very high-risk acute lymphoblastic leukaemia. *Lancet Oncol*. 2009;10(2):147-156.
56. Conter V, Arico M, Valsecchi MG, et al. Long-term results of the Italian Association of Pediatric Hematology and Oncology (AIEOP) acute lymphoblastic leukaemia studies, 1982-1995. *Leukemia*. 2000;14(12):2196-2204.
57. Bond J, Graux C, Lhermitte L, et al. Early response-based therapy stratification improves survival in adult early thymic precursor acute lymphoblastic leukemia: a group for research on adult acute lymphoblastic leukemia study. *J Clin Oncol*. 2017;35(23):2683-2691.
58. Annino L, Vegna ML, Camera A, et al. Treatment of adult acute lymphoblastic leukemia (ALL): long-term follow-up of the GIMEMA ALL 0288 randomized study. *Blood*. 2002;99(3):863-871.
59. Chessells JM, Hall E, Prentice HG, Durrant J, Bailey CC, Richards SM. The impact of age on outcome in lymphoblastic leukaemia; MRC UKALL X and XA compared: a report from the MRC Paediatric and Adult Working Parties. *Leukemia*. 1998;12(4):463-473.
60. Arber DA, Borowitz MJ, Cessna M, et al. Initial diagnostic workup of acute leukemia: guideline from the College of American Pathologists and the American Society of Hematology. *Arch Pathol Lab Med*. 2017;141(10):1342-1393.
61. Alaggio R, Amador C, Anagnostopoulos I, et al. The 5th edition of the World Health Organization classification of haematolymphoid tumours: lymphoid neoplasms. *Leukemia*. 2022;36(7):1720-1748.
62. Gajjar A, Harrison PL, Sandlund JT, et al. Traumatic lumbar puncture at diagnosis adversely affects outcome in childhood acute lymphoblastic leukemia. *Blood*. 2000;96(10):3381-3384.
63. Atallah E, O'Brien S, Kaled S, et al. Traumatic lumbar puncture (TLP) is not associated with worse outcome in adults with acute lymphocytic leukemia (ALL) or burkitt-type leukemia/lymphoma (BLL) receiving hyper-CVAD regimens. *Blood*. 2007;110:4346.
64. Conant JL, Czuchlewski DR. BCR-ABL1-like B-lymphoblastic leukemia/lymphoma: review of the entity and detection methodologies. *Int J Lab Hematol*. 2019;41(suppl 1):126-130.
65. Alexander TB, Gu Z, Iacobucci I, et al. The genetic basis and cell of origin of mixed phenotype acute leukaemia. *Nature*. 2018;562(7727):373-379.
66. Wolach O, Stone RM. How I treat mixed-phenotype acute leukemia. *Blood*. 2015;125(16):2477-2485.
67. Munker R, Brazauskas R, Wang HL, et al. Allogeneic hematopoietic cell transplantation for patients with mixed phenotype acute leukemia. *Biol Blood Marrow Transplant*. 2016;22(6):1024-1029.
68. Short NJ, Kantarjian HM, Ravandi F, et al. High-sensitivity next-generation sequencing MRD assessment in ALL identifies patients at very low risk of relapse. *Blood Adv*. 2022;6(13):4006-4014.
69. Nakamori Y, Takahashi M, Moriyama Y, et al. The aplastic presentation of adult acute lymphoblastic leukemia. *Br J Haematol*. 1986;62(4):782-783.
70. Jaso J, Thomas DA, Cunningham K, et al. Prognostic significance of immunophenotypic and karyotypic features of Philadelphia positive B-lymphoblastic leukemia in the era of tyrosine kinase inhibitors. *Cancer*. 2011;117:4009-4017.
71. Paietta E, Roberts KG, Wang V, et al. Molecular classification improves risk assessment in adult BCR-ABL1-negative B-ALL. *Blood*. 2021;138(11):948-958.
72. Beldjord K, Chevret S, Asnafi V, et al. Oncogenetics and minimal residual disease are independent outcome predictors in adult patients with acute lymphoblastic leukemia. *Blood*. 2014;123(24):3739-3749.
73. Gokbuget N, Dombret H, Giebel S, et al. Minimal residual disease level predicts outcome in adults with Ph-negative B-precursor acute lymphoblastic leukemia. *Hematology*. 2019;24(1):337-348.
74. Berry DA, Zhou S, Higley H, et al. Association of minimal residual disease with clinical outcome in pediatric and adult acute lymphoblastic leukemia: a meta-analysis. *JAMA Oncol*. 2017;3(7):e170580.
75. Topp MS, Kufer P, Gokbuget N, et al. Targeted therapy with the T-cell-engaging antibody blinatumomab of chemotherapy-refractory minimal residual disease in B-lineage acute lymphoblastic leukemia patients results in high response rate and prolonged leukemia-free survival. *J Clin Oncol*. 2011;29:2493-2498.
76. Gokbuget N, Kneba M, Raff T, et al. Adult patients with acute lymphoblastic leukemia and molecular failure display a poor prognosis and are candidates for stem cell transplantation and targeted therapies. *Blood*. 2012;120(9):1868-1876.
77. Bassan R, Spinelli O, Oldani E, et al. Improved risk classification for risk-specific therapy based on the molecular study of minimal residual disease (MRD) in adult acute lymphoblastic leukemia (ALL). *Blood*. 2009;113(18):4153-4162.
78. Marks DI, Paietta EM, Moorman AV, et al. T-cell acute lymphoblastic leukemia in adults: clinical features, immunophenotype, cytogenetics, and outcome from the large randomized prospective trial (UKALL XII/ECOG 2993). *Blood*. 2009;114(25):5136-5145.
79. Lafage-Pochitaloff M, Baranger L, Hunault M, et al. Impact of cytogenetic abnormalities in adults with Ph-negative B-cell precursor acute lymphoblastic leukemia. *Blood*. 2017;130(16):1832-1844.
80. Mullighan CG, Su X, Zhang J, et al. Deletion of IKZF1 and prognosis in acute lymphoblastic leukemia. *N Engl J Med*. 2009;360(5):470-480.
81. Den Boer ML, van Slegtenhorst M, De Menezes RX, et al. A subtype of childhood acute lymphoblastic leukaemia with poor treatment outcome: a genome-wide classification study. *Lancet Oncol*. 2009;10(2):125-134.
82. Wells J, Jain N, Konopleva M. Philadelphia chromosome-like acute lymphoblastic leukemia: progress in a new cancer subtype. *Clin Adv Hematol Oncol*. 2017;15(7):554-561.
83. Cario G, Leoni V, Conter V, Baruchel A, Schrappe M, Biondi A. BCR-ABL1-like acute lymphoblastic leukemia in childhood and targeted therapy. *Haematologica*. 2020;105(9):2200-2204.
84. Tanasi I, Ba I, Sirvent N, et al. Efficacy of tyrosine kinase inhibitors in Ph-like acute lymphoblastic leukemia harboring ABL-class rearrangements. *Blood*. 2019;134(16):1351-1355.

85. Rowe JM, Buck G, Burnett AK, et al. Induction therapy for adults with acute lymphoblastic leukemia: results of more than 1500 patients from the international ALL trial. MRC UKALL XII/ECOG E2993. *Blood*. 2005;106(12):3760-3767.
86. Lauten M, Möricke A, Beier R, et al. Prediction of outcome by early bone marrow response in childhood acute lymphoblastic leukemia treated in the ALL-BFM 95 trial: differential effects in precursor B-cell and T-cell leukemia. *Haematologica*. 2012;97(7):1048-1056.
87. Cortes J, Fayad L, O'Brien S, Keating M, Kantarjian H. Persistence of peripheral blood and bone marrow blasts during remission induction in adult acute lymphoblastic leukemia confers a poor prognosis depending on treatment intensity. *Clin Cancer Res*. 1999;5(9):2491-2497.
88. Steinherz PG, Gaynon PS, Breneman JC, et al. Cytoreduction and prognosis in acute lymphoblastic leukemia – the importance of early marrow response: report from the Childrens Cancer Group. *J Clin Oncol*. 1996;14(2):389-398.
89. Bruggemann M, Kotrova M. Minimal residual disease in adult ALL: technical aspects and implications for correct clinical interpretation. *Hematology Am Soc Hematol Educ Program*. 2017;2017(1):13-21.
90. Bartram J, Patel B, Fielding AK. Monitoring MRD in ALL: methodologies, technical aspects and optimal time points for measurement. *Semin Hematol*. 2020;57(3):142-148.
91. Cave H, van der Werff ten Bosch J, Suciu S, et al. Clinical significance of minimal residual disease in childhood acute lymphoblastic leukemia. European Organization for Research and Treatment of Cancer – Childhood Leukemia Cooperative Group. *N Engl J Med*. 1998;339(9):591-598.
92. Coustan-Smith E, Sancho J, Behm FG, et al. Prognostic importance of measuring early clearance of leukemic cells by flow cytometry in childhood acute lymphoblastic leukemia. *Blood*. 2002;100(1):52-58.
93. van Dongen JJ, Seriu T, Panzer-Grumayer ER, et al. Prognostic value of minimal residual disease in acute lymphoblastic leukaemia in childhood. *Lancet*. 1998;352(9142):1731-1738.
94. Patel B, Rai L, Buck G, et al. Minimal residual disease is a significant predictor of treatment failure in non T-lineage adult acute lymphoblastic leukaemia: final results of the international trial UKALL XII/ECOG2993. *Br J Haematol*. 2010;148(1):80-89.
95. Bruggemann M, Raff T, Flohr T, et al. Clinical significance of minimal residual disease quantification in adult patients with standard-risk acute lymphoblastic leukemia. *Blood*. 2006;107(3):1116-1123.
96. Sasaki Y, Kantarjian HM, Short NJ, et al. Genetic correlates in patients with Philadelphia chromosome-positive acute lymphoblastic leukemia treated with Hyper-CVAD plus dasatinib or ponatinib. *Leukemia*. 2022;36(5):1253-1260.
97. Hoelzer D. Monitoring and managing minimal residual disease in acute lymphoblastic leukemia. *Am Soc Clin Oncol Educ Book*. 2013;2013:290-293.
98. Gottlieb AJ, Weinberg V, Ellison RR, et al. Efficacy of daunorubicin in the therapy of adult acute lymphocytic leukemia: a prospective randomized trial by cancer and leukemia group B. *Blood*. 1984;64(1):267-274.
99. Nagura E, Kimura K, Yamada K, et al. Nation-wide randomized comparative study of doxorubicin, vincristine and prednisolone combination therapy with and without L-asparaginase for adult acute lymphoblastic leukemia. *Cancer Chemother Pharmacol*. 1994;33(5):359-365.
100. Todeschini G, Tecchio C, Meneghini V, et al. Estimated 6-year event-free survival of 55% in 60 consecutive adult acute lymphoblastic leukemia patients treated with an intensive phase II protocol based on high induction dose of daunorubicin. *Leukemia*. 1998;12(2):144-149.
101. Mancini M, Scappaticci D, Cimino G, et al. A comprehensive genetic classification of adult acute lymphoblastic leukemia (ALL): analysis of the GIMEMA 0496 protocol. *Blood*. 2005;105(9):3434-3441.
102. Bostrom BC, Sensel MR, Sather HN, et al. Dexamethasone versus prednisone and daily oral versus weekly intravenous mercaptopurine for patients with standard-risk acute lymphoblastic leukemia: a report from the Children's Cancer Group. *Blood*. 2003;101(10):3809-3817.
103. Labar B, Suciu S, Willemze R, et al. Dexamethasone compared to prednisolone for adults with acute lymphoblastic leukemia or lymphoblastic lymphoma: final results of the ALL-4 randomized, phase III trial of the EORTC Leukemia Group. *Haematologica*. 2010;95(9):1489-1495.
104. Gokbuget N, Dombret H, Bonifacio M, et al. Blinatumomab for minimal residual disease in adults with B-cell precursor acute lymphoblastic leukemia. *Blood*. 2018;131(14):1522-1531.
105. Chessells JM, Bailey C, Richards SM. Intensification of treatment and survival in all children with lymphoblastic leukaemia: results of UK Medical Research Council trial UKALL X. Medical Research Council Working Party on Childhood Leukaemia. *Lancet*. 1995;345(8943):143-148.
106. Durrant IJ, Prentice HG, Richards SM. Intensification of treatment for adults with acute lymphoblastic leukaemia: results of U.K. Medical research Council randomized trial UKALL XA. Medical Research Council Working Party on Leukaemia in Adults. *Br J Haematol*. 1997;99(1):84-92.
107. Mandelli F, Annino L, Rotoli B. The GIMEMA ALL 0183 trial: analysis of 10-year follow-up. GIMEMA Cooperative Group, Italy. *Br J Haematol*. 1996;92(3):665-672.
108. Stryckmans P, De Witte T, Marie JP, et al. Therapy of adult ALL: overview of 2 successive EORTC studies. (ALL-2 & ALL-3). The EORTC Leukemia Cooperative Study Group. *Leukemia*. 1992;6(suppl 2):199-203.
109. Ellison RR, Mick R, Cuttner J, et al. The effects of postinduction intensification treatment with cytarabine and daunorubicin in adult acute lymphocytic leukemia: a prospective randomized clinical trial by Cancer and Leukemia Group B. *J Clin Oncol*. 1991;9(11):2002-2015.
110. Ribera JM, Ortega JJ, Oriol A, et al. Late intensification chemotherapy has not improved the results of intensive chemotherapy in adult acute lymphoblastic leukemia. Results of a prospective multicenter randomized trial (PETHEMA ALL-89). Spanish Society of Hematology. *Haematologica*. 1998;83(3):222-230.
111. Omura GA, Vogler WR, Martelo O, Gordon DS, Bartolucci AA. Late intensification therapy in adult acute lymphoid leukemia: long-term follow-up of the Southeastern Cancer Study Group Experience. *Leuk Lymphoma*. 1994;15(1-2):71-78.
112. Hoelzer D, Thiel E, Loffler H, et al. Intensified therapy in acute lymphoblastic and acute undifferentiated leukemia in adults. *Blood*. 1984;64(1):38-47.
113. Childhood ALL Collaborative Group. Duration and intensity of maintenance chemotherapy in acute lymphoblastic leukaemia: overview of 42 trials involving 12 000 randomised children. *Lancet*. 1996;347(9018):1783-1788.
114. Dekker AW, van't Veer MB, Sizoo W, et al. Intensive postremission chemotherapy without maintenance therapy in adults with acute lymphoblastic leukemia. Dutch Hemato-Oncology Research Group. *J Clin Oncol*. 1997;15(2):476-482.
115. Wernli M, Tichelli A, von Fliedner V, et al. Intensive induction/consolidation therapy without maintenance in adult acute lymphoblastic leukaemia: a pilot assessment. Working Party on Leukaemia of the Swiss Group for Epidemiologic and Clinical Cancer Research (SAKK). *Br J Haematol*. 1994;87(1):39-43.
116. Cassileth PA, Andersen JW, Bennett JM, et al. Adult acute lymphocytic leukemia: the eastern cooperative oncology group experience. *Leukemia*. 1992;6(suppl 2):178-181.
117. Cortes J. Central nervous system involvement in adult acute lymphocytic leukemia. *Hematol Oncol Clin North Am*. 2001;15(1):145-162.
118. Omura GA, Moffitt S, Vogler WR, Salter MM. Combination chemotherapy of adult acute lymphoblastic leukemia with randomized central nervous system prophylaxis. *Blood*. 1980;55(2):199-204.
119. Durrant IJ, Richards SM. Results of medical research Council trial UKALL IX in acute lymphoblastic leukaemia in adults: report from the Medical Research Council Working Party on Adult Leukaemia. *Br J Haematol*. 1993;85(1):84-92.
120. Lazarus HM, Richards SM, Chopra R, et al. Central nervous system involvement in adult acute lymphoblastic leukemia at diagnosis: results from the International ALL Trial MRC UKALL XII/ECOG E2993. *Blood*. 2006;108(2):465-472.
121. Cortes J, O'Brien SM, Pierce S, Keating MJ, Freireich EJ, Kantarjian HM. The value of high-dose systemic chemotherapy and intrathecal therapy for central nervous system prophylaxis in different risk groups of adult acute lymphoblastic leukemia. *Blood*. 1995;86(6):2091-2097.
122. Hoelzer D, Thiel E, Loffler H, et al. Prognostic factors in a multicenter study for treatment of acute lymphoblastic leukemia in adults. *Blood*. 1988;71(1):123-131.
123. El Fakih R, Ahmed S, Alfraih F, Hanbali A. Hematopoietic cell transplantation for acute lymphoblastic leukemia in adult patients. *Hematol Oncol Stem Cell Ther*. 2017;10(4):252-258.
124. Gupta V, Richards S, Rowe J; Acute Leukemia Stem Cell Transplantation Trialists' Collaborative Group. Allogeneic, but not autologous, hematopoietic cell transplantation improves survival only among younger adults with acute lymphoblastic leukemia in first remission: an individual patient data meta-analysis. *Blood*. 2013;121(2):339-350.
125. Chao NJ, Forman SJ, Schmidt GM, et al. Allogeneic bone marrow transplantation for high-risk acute lymphoblastic leukemia during first complete remission. *Blood*. 1991;78(8):1923-1927.
126. Barrett AJ, Horowitz MM, McCarthy DM, Kanfer E, Bortin MM. Bone marrow transplantation for acute lymphoblastic leukaemia in first and second remission. *Bone Marrow Transplant*. 1989;4(suppl 1):247-249.
127. Zhang MJ, Hoelzer D, Horowitz MM, et al. Long-term follow-up of adults with acute lymphoblastic leukemia in first remission treated with chemotherapy or bone marrow transplantation. The Acute Lymphoblastic Leukemia Working Committee. *Ann Intern Med*. 1995;123(6):428-431.
128. Sebban C, Lepage E, Vernant JP, et al. Allogeneic bone marrow transplantation in adult acute lymphoblastic leukemia in first complete remission: a comparative study. French Group of Therapy of Adult Acute Lymphoblastic Leukemia. *J Clin Oncol*. 1994;12:2580-2587.
129. Weisdorf D, Bishop M, Dharan B, et al. Autologous versus allogeneic unrelated donor transplantation for acute lymphoblastic leukemia: comparative toxicity and outcomes. *Biol Blood Marrow Transplant*. 2002;8(4):213-220.
130. Kiehl MG, Kraut L, Schwerdtfeger R, et al. Outcome of allogeneic hematopoietic stem-cell transplantation in adult patients with acute lymphoblastic leukemia: no difference in related compared with unrelated transplant in first complete remission. *J Clin Oncol*. 2004;22(14):2816-2825.
131. Attal M, Blaise D, Marit G, et al. Consolidation treatment of adult acute lymphoblastic leukemia: a prospective, randomized trial comparing allogeneic versus autologous bone marrow transplantation and testing the impact of recombinant interleukin-2 after autologous bone marrow transplantation. BGMT Group. *Blood*. 1995;86(4):1619-1628.
132. Hunault M, Harousseau JL, Delain M, et al. Better outcome of adult acute lymphoblastic leukemia after early genoidentical allogeneic bone marrow transplantation (BMT) than after late high-dose therapy and autologous BMT: a GOELAMS trial. *Blood*. 2004;104(10):3028-3037.
133. Doney K, Fisher LD, Appelbaum FR, et al. Treatment of adult acute lymphoblastic leukemia with allogeneic bone marrow transplantation. Multivariate analysis of factors affecting acute graft-versus-host disease, relapse, and relapse-free survival. *Bone Marrow Transplant*. 1991;7(6):453-459.
134. Wingard JR, Piantadosi S, Santos GW, et al. Allogeneic bone marrow transplantation for patients with high-risk acute lymphoblastic leukemia. *J Clin Oncol*. 1990;8(5):820-830.

135. Auletta J, Kou J, Chen M, Shaw B. Current use and outcome of hematopoietic stem cell transplantation: CIBMTR summary slides. 2021. http://www.cibmtr.org
136. Oliansky DM, Larson RA, Weisdorf D, et al. The role of cytotoxic therapy with hematopoietic stem cell transplantation in the treatment of adult acute lymphoblastic leukemia: update of the 2006 evidence-based review. *Biol Blood Marrow Transplant.* 2012;18(1):16-17.
137. Marks DI, Kirkwood AA, Rowntree CJ, et al. Addition of four doses of rituximab to standard induction chemotherapy in adult patients with precursor B-cell acute lymphoblastic leukaemia (UKALL14): a phase 3, multicentre, randomised controlled trial. *Lancet Haematol.* 2022;9(4):e262-e275.
138. Wetzler M, Dodge RK, Mrozek K, et al. Prospective karyotype analysis in adult acute lymphoblastic leukemia: the cancer and leukemia Group B experience. *Blood.* 1999;93(11):3983-3993.
139. Czuczman MS, Dodge RK, Stewart CC, et al. Value of immunophenotype in intensively treated adult acute lymphoblastic leukemia: cancer and leukemia Group B study 8364. *Blood.* 1999;93(11):3931-3939.
140. Bosco I, Teh A. Outcome of treatment in adult acute lymphoblastic leukaemia in an Asian population: comparison with previous multicentre German study. *Leukemia.* 1995;9(6):951-954.
141. Hoelzer D, Thiel E, Ludwig WD, et al. Follow-up of the first two successive German multicentre trials for adult ALL (01/81 and 02/84). German Adult ALL Study Group. *Leukemia.* 1993;7(Suppl 2):S130-S134.
142. Stock W, La M, Sanford B, et al. What determines the outcomes for adolescents and young adults with acute lymphoblastic leukemia treated on cooperative group protocols? A comparison of Children's Cancer Group and Cancer and Leukemia Group B studies. *Blood.* 2008;112(5):1646-1654.
143. Boissel N, Auclerc MF, Lhéritier V, et al. Should adolescents with acute lymphoblastic leukemia be treated as old children or young adults? Comparison of the French FRALLE-93 and LALA-94 trials. *J Clin Oncol.* 2003;21(5):774-780.
144. de Bont JM, Holt Bv d, Dekker AW, van der Does-van den Berg A, Sonneveld P, Pieters R. Significant difference in outcome for adolescents with acute lymphoblastic leukemia treated on pediatric vs adult protocols in the Netherlands. *Leukemia.* 2004;18(12):2032-2035.
145. Ram R, Wolach O, Vidal L, Gafter-Gvili A, Shpilberg O, Raanani P. Adolescents and young adults with acute lymphoblastic leukemia have a better outcome when treated with pediatric-inspired regimens: systematic review and meta-analysis. *Am J Hematol.* 2012;87(5):472-478.
146. Huguet F, Leguay T, Raffoux E, et al. Pediatric-inspired therapy in adults with Philadelphia chromosome-negative acute lymphoblastic leukemia: the GRAALL-2003 study. *J Clin Oncol.* 2009;27(6):911-918.
147. DeAngelo DJ, Stevenson KE, Dahlberg SE, et al. Long-term outcome of a pediatric-inspired regimen used for adults aged 18-50 years with newly diagnosed acute lymphoblastic leukemia. *Leukemia.* 2015;29(3):526-534.
148. Marks DI, Rowntree C. Management of adults with T-cell lymphoblastic leukemia. *Blood.* 2017;129(9):1134-1142.
149. Vadillo E, Dorantes-Acosta E, Pelayo R, Schnoor M. T cell acute lymphoblastic leukemia (T-ALL): new insights into the cellular origins and infiltration mechanisms common and unique among hematologic malignancies. *Blood Rev.* 2018;32(1):36-51.
150. Dunsmore KP, Winter SS, Devidas M, et al. Children's oncology group AALL0434: a phase III randomized clinical trial testing nelarabine in newly diagnosed T-cell acute lymphoblastic leukemia. *J Clin Oncol.* 2020;38(28):3282-3293.
151. Abaza Y, M Kantarjian H, Faderl S, et al. Hyper-CVAD plus nelarabine in newly diagnosed adult T-cell acute lymphoblastic leukemia and T-lymphoblastic lymphoma. *Am J Hematol.* 2018;93(1):91-99.
152. Rowntree CJ, Kirkwood AA, Clifton-Hadley L, et al. First analysis of the UKALL14 randomized trial to determine whether the addition of nelarabine to standard chemotherapy improves event free survival in adults with T-cell acute lymphoblastic leukaemia (CRUK/09/006). *Blood.* 2021;138:366.
153. Secker-Walker LM, Craig JM, Hawkins JM, Hoffbrand AV. Philadelphia positive acute lymphoblastic leukemia in adults: age distribution, BCR breakpoint and prognostic significance. *Leukemia.* 1991;5(3):196-199.
154. Giebel S, Czyz A, Ottmann O, et al. Use of tyrosine kinase inhibitors to prevent relapse after allogeneic hematopoietic stem cell transplantation for patients with Philadelphia chromosome-positive acute lymphoblastic leukemia: a position statement of the Acute Leukemia Working Party of the European Society for Blood and Marrow Transplantation. *Cancer.* 2016;122(19):2941-2951.
155. Foa R, Vitale A, Vignetti M, et al. Dasatinib as first-line treatment for adult patients with Philadelphia chromosome-positive acute lymphoblastic leukemia. *Blood.* 2011;118(25):6521-6528.
156. Faderl S, Kantarjian HM, Thomas DA, et al. Outcome of Philadelphia chromosome-positive adult acute lymphoblastic leukemia. *Leuk Lymphoma.* 2000;36(3-4):263-273.
157. Druker BJ, Sawyers CL, Kantarjian H, et al. Activity of a specific inhibitor of the BCR-ABL tyrosine kinase in the blast crisis of chronic myeloid leukemia and acute lymphoblastic leukemia with the Philadelphia chromosome. *N Engl J Med.* 2001;344(14):1038-1042.
158. Ottmann OG, Wassmann B, Pfeifer H, et al. Imatinib compared with chemotherapy as front-line treatment of elderly patients with Philadelphia chromosome-positive acute lymphoblastic leukemia (Ph+ALL). *Cancer.* 2007;109(10):2068-2076.
159. Lee S, Kim YJ, Min CK, et al. The effect of first-line imatinib interim therapy on the outcome of allogeneic stem cell transplantation in adults with newly diagnosed Philadelphia chromosome-positive acute lymphoblastic leukemia. *Blood.* 2005;105(9):3449-3457.
160. Igwe IJ, Yang D, Merchant A, et al. The presence of Philadelphia chromosome does not confer poor prognosis in adult pre-B acute lymphoblastic leukaemia in the tyrosine kinase inhibitor era - a surveillance, epidemiology, and end results database analysis. *Br J Haematol.* 2017;179(4):618-626.
161. Fielding AK, Rowe JM, Buck G, et al. UKALLXII/ECOG2993: addition of imatinib to a standard treatment regimen enhances long-term outcomes in Philadelphia positive acute lymphoblastic leukemia. *Blood.* 2014;123(6):843-850.
162. Wassmann B, Pfeifer H, Goekbuget N, et al. Alternating versus concurrent schedules of imatinib and chemotherapy as front-line therapy for Philadelphia-positive acute lymphoblastic leukemia (Ph+ ALL). *Blood.* 2006;108(5):1469-1477.
163. Pfeifer H, Wassmann B, Hofmann WK, et al. Risk and prognosis of central nervous system leukemia in patients with Philadelphia chromosome-positive acute leukemias treated with imatinib mesylate. *Clin Cancer Res.* 2003;9(13):4674-4681.
164. Ottmann OG, Larson RA, Kantarjian HM, et al. Phase II study of nilotinib in patients with relapsed or refractory Philadelphia chromosome – positive acute lymphoblastic leukemia. *Leukemia.* 2013;27(6):1411-1413.
165. Sanford DS, Kantarjian H, O'Brien S, Jabbour E, Cortes J, Ravandi F. The role of ponatinib in Philadelphia chromosome-positive acute lymphoblastic leukemia. *Expert Rev Anticancer Ther.* 2015;15(4):365-373.
166. Ravandi F, Othus M, O'Brien SM, et al. US intergroup study of chemotherapy plus dasatinib and allogeneic stem cell transplant in Philadelphia chromosome positive ALL. *Blood Adv.* 2016;1(3):250-259.
167. Ravandi F, O'Brien SM, Cortes JE, et al. Long-term follow-up of a phase 2 study of chemotherapy plus dasatinib for the initial treatment of patients with Philadelphia chromosome-positive acute lymphoblastic leukemia. *Cancer.* 2015;121(23):4158-4164.
168. Foa R, Bassan R, Vitale A, et al. Dasatinib-blinatumomab for ph-positive acute lymphoblastic leukemia in adults. *N Engl J Med.* 2020;383(17):1613-1623.
169. Ribera JM, García-Calduch O, Ribera J, et al. Ponatinib, chemotherapy, and transplant in adults with Philadelphia chromosome-positive acute lymphoblastic leukemia. *Blood Adv.* 2022;6(18):5395-5402.
170. Jabbour E, Short NJ, Ravandi F, et al. Combination of hyper-CVAD with ponatinib as first-line therapy for patients with Philadelphia chromosome-positive acute lymphoblastic leukaemia: long-term follow-up of a single-centre, phase 2 study. *Lancet Haematol.* 2018;5(12):e618-e627.
171. Short NJ, Kantarjian HM, Konopleva M et al. Combination of ponatinib and blinatumomab in Philadelphia chromosome-positive acute lymphoblastic leukemia: early results from a phase II study. *J Clin Oncol* 2021; 39: 7001.
172. Kim DY, Joo YD, Lim SN, et al. Nilotinib combined with multiagent chemotherapy for newly diagnosed Philadelphia-positive acute lymphoblastic leukemia. *Blood.* 2015;126(6):746-756.
173. Mizuta S, Matsuo K, Yagasaki F, et al. Pre-transplant imatinib-based therapy improves the outcome of allogeneic hematopoietic stem cell transplantation for BCR-ABL-positive acute lymphoblastic leukemia. *Leukemia.* 2011;25(1):41-47.
174. Dombret H, Gabert J, Boiron JM, et al. Outcome of treatment in adults with Philadelphia chromosome-positive acute lymphoblastic leukemia – results of the prospective multicenter LALA-94 trial. *Blood.* 2002;100(7):2357-2366.
175. Wassmann B, Pfeifer H, Stadler M, et al. Early molecular response to posttransplantation imatinib determines outcome in MRD+ Philadelphia-positive acute lymphoblastic leukemia (Ph+ ALL). *Blood.* 2005;106(2):458-463.
176. Gökbuget N. Treatment of older patients with acute lymphoblastic leukemia. *Hematology Am Soc Hematol Educ Program.* 2016;2016(1):573-579.
177. Hurria A, Lichtman SM. Clinical pharmacology of cancer therapies in older adults. *Br J Cancer.* 2008;98(3):517-522.
178. Thomas X, Olteanu N, Charrin C, Lheritier V, Magaud JP, Fiere D. Acute lymphoblastic leukemia in the elderly: the Edouard Herriot Hospital experience. *Am J Hematol.* 2001;67(2):73-83.
179. Moorman AV, Chilton L, Wilkinson J, Ensor HM, Bown N, Proctor SJ. A population-based cytogenetic study of adults with acute lymphoblastic leukemia. *Blood.* 2010;115(2):206-214.
180. Yilmaz M, Kantarjian H, Jabbour E. Treatment of acute lymphoblastic leukemia in older adults: now and the future. *Clin Adv Hematol Oncol.* 2017;15(4):266-274.
181. Legrand O, Marie JP, Marjanovic Z, et al. Prognostic factors in elderly acute lymphoblastic leukaemia. *Br J Haematol.* 1997;97(3):596-602.
182. Luskin MR. Acute lymphoblastic leukemia in older adults: curtain call for conventional chemotherapy? *Hematology Am Soc Hematol Educ Program.* 2021;2021(1):7-14.
183. Martinelli G, Papayannidis C, Piciocchi A, et al. INCB84344-201: ponatinib and steroids in frontline therapy for unfit patients with Ph+ acute lymphoblastic leukemia. *Blood Adv.* 2022;6(6):1742-1753.
184. Rousselot P, Coudé MM, Gokbuget N, et al. Dasatinib and low-intensity chemotherapy in elderly patients with Philadelphia chromosome-positive ALL. *Blood.* 2016;128(6):774-782.
185. Ottmann OG, Pfeifer H, Cayuela J-M, et al. Nilotinib (Tasigna®) and low intensity chemotherapy for first-line treatment of elderly patients with BCR-ABL1-positive acute lymphoblastic leukemia: final results of a prospective multicenter trial (EWALL-PH02). *Blood.* 2018;132:31-31.
186. Vignetti M, Fazi P, Cimino G, et al. Imatinib plus steroids induces complete remissions and prolonged survival in elderly Philadelphia chromosome–positive patients with acute lymphoblastic leukemia without additional chemotherapy: results of the Gruppo Italiano Malattie Ematologiche dell'Adulto (GIMEMA) LAL0201-B protocol. *Blood.* 2007;109(9):3676-3678.
187. Delannoy A, Delabesse E, Lhéritier V, et al. Imatinib and methylprednisolone alternated with chemotherapy improve the outcome of elderly patients with Philadelphia-positive acute lymphoblastic leukemia: results of the GRAALL AFR09 study. *Leukemia.* 2006;20(9):1526-1532.

188. Advani AS, Moseley A, O'Dwyer KM, et al. SWOG 1318: a phase II trial of blinatumomab followed by pomp maintenance in older patients with newly diagnosed Philadelphia chromosome-negative B-cell acute lymphoblastic leukemia. *J Clin Oncol.* 2022;40(14):1574-1582.
189. Short NJ, Kantarjian H, Ravandi F, et al. Updated results from a phase II study of mini-hyper-CVD plus inotuzumab ozogamicin, with or without blinatumomab, in older adults with newly diagnosed Philadelphia chromosome-negative B-cell acute lymphoblastic leukemia. *Blood.* 2021;138:3400-3400.
190. Fielding AK, Richards SM, Chopra R, et al. Outcome of 609 adults after relapse of acute lymphoblastic leukemia (ALL); an MRC UKALL12/ECOG 2993 study. *Blood.* 2007;109(3):944-950.
191. Thomas DA, Kantarjian H, Smith TL, et al. Primary refractory and relapsed adult acute lymphoblastic leukemia: characteristics, treatment results, and prognosis with salvage therapy. *Cancer.* 1999;86(7):1216-1230.
192. Chucrallah AE, Stass SA, Huh YO, Albitar M, Kantarjian HM. Adult acute lymphoblastic leukemia at relapse. Cytogenetic, immunophenotypic, and molecular changes. *Cancer.* 1995;76(6):985-991.
193. Specchia G, Pastore D, Carluccio P, et al. FLAG-IDA in the treatment of refractory/relapsed adult acute lymphoblastic leukemia. *Ann Hematol.* 2005;84(12):792-795.
194. Faderl S, Thomas DA, O'Brien S, et al. Augmented hyper-CVAD based on dose-intensified vincristine, dexamethasone, and asparaginase in adult acute lymphoblastic leukemia salvage therapy. *Clin Lymphoma Myeloma Leuk.* 2011;11(1):54-59.
195. Rosen PJ, Rankin C, Head DR, et al. A phase II study of high dose ARA-C and mitoxantrone for treatment of relapsed or refractory adult acute lymphoblastic leukemia. *Leuk Res.* 2000;24(3):183-187.
196. Branford S, Rudzki Z, Walsh S, et al. High frequency of point mutations clustered within the adenosine triphosphate-binding region of BCR/ABL in patients with chronic myeloid leukemia or Ph-positive acute lymphoblastic leukemia who develop imatinib (STI571) resistance. *Blood.* 2002;99(9):3472-3475.
197. Cortes JE, Kim DW, Pinilla-Ibarz J, et al. A phase 2 trial of ponatinib in Philadelphia chromosome-positive leukemias. *N Engl J Med.* 2013;369(19):1783-1796.
198. Kantarjian HM, DeAngelo DJ, Stelljes M, et al. Inotuzumab ozogamicin versus standard therapy for acute lymphoblastic leukemia. *N Engl J Med.* 2016;375(8):740-753.
199. Kantarjian H, Stein A, Gokbuget N, et al. Blinatumomab versus chemotherapy for advanced acute lymphoblastic leukemia. *N Engl J Med.* 2017;376(9):836-847.
200. Kantarjian H, Thomas D, Jorgensen J, et al. Results of inotuzumab ozogamicin, a CD22 monoclonal antibody, in refractory and relapsed acute lymphocytic leukemia. *Cancer.* 2013;119(15):2728-2736.
201. DeAngelo DJ, Stock W, Stein AS, et al. Inotuzumab ozogamicin in adults with relapsed or refractory CD22-positive acute lymphoblastic leukemia: a phase 1/2 study. *Blood Adv.* 2017;1(15):1167-1180.
202. Badar T, Szabo A, Wadleigh M, et al. Real-world outcomes of adult B-cell acute lymphocytic leukemia patients treated with inotuzumab ozogamicin. *Clin Lymphoma Myeloma Leuk.* 2020;20(8):556.e2-560.e2.
203. Jabbour EJ, Short NJ, Jain N, et al. Blinatumomab is associated with favorable outcomes in patients with B-cell lineage acute lymphoblastic leukemia and positive measurable residual disease at a threshold of 10^{-4} and higher. *Am J Hematol.* 2022;97(9):1135-1141.
204. Topp MS, Gokbuget N, Zugmaier G, et al. Phase II trial of the anti-CD19 bispecific T cell-engager blinatumomab shows hematologic and molecular remissions in patients with relapsed or refractory B-precursor acute lymphoblastic leukemia. *J Clin Oncol.* 2014;32(36):4134-4140.
205. Topp MS, Gokbuget N, Stein AS, et al. Safety and activity of blinatumomab for adult patients with relapsed or refractory B-precursor acute lymphoblastic leukaemia: a multicentre, single-arm, phase 2 study. *Lancet Oncol.* 2015;16(1):57-66.
206. Topp MS, Gokbuget N, Zugmaier G, et al. Long-term survival of patients with relapsed/refractory acute lymphoblastic leukemia treated with blinatumomab. *Cancer.* 2021;127(4):554-559.
207. Badar T, Szabo A, Advani A, et al. Real-world outcomes of adult B-cell acute lymphocytic leukemia patients treated with blinatumomab. *Blood Adv.* 2020;4(10):2308-2316.
208. Martinelli G, Boissel N, Chevallier P, et al. Complete hematologic and molecular response in adult patients with relapsed/refractory Philadelphia chromosome-positive B-precursor acute lymphoblastic leukemia following treatment with blinatumomab: results from a phase II, single-arm, multicenter study. *J Clin Oncol.* 2017;35(16):1795-1802.
209. Alford SE, Kothari A, Loeff FC, et al. BH3 inhibitor sensitivity and bcl-2 dependence in primary acute lymphoblastic leukemia cells. *Cancer Res.* 2015;75(7):1366-1375.
210. Seyfried F, Demir S, Hörl RL, et al. Prediction of venetoclax activity in precursor B-ALL by functional assessment of apoptosis signaling. *Cell Death Dis.* 2019;10(8):571.
211. Seyfried F, Stirnweiß FU, Niedermayer A, et al. Synergistic activity of combined inhibition of anti-apoptotic molecules in B-cell precursor ALL. *Leukemia.* 2022;36(4):901-912.
212. Pullarkat VA, Lacayo NJ, Jabbour E, et al. Venetoclax and navitoclax in combination with chemotherapy in patients with relapsed or refractory acute lymphoblastic leukemia and lymphoblastic lymphoma. *Cancer Discov.* 2021;11(6):1440-1453.
213. Bride KL, Vincent TL, Im SY, et al. Preclinical efficacy of daratumumab in T-cell acute lymphoblastic leukemia. *Blood.* 2018;131(9):995-999.
214. Voruz S, Blum S, de Leval L, Schoumans J, Solly F, Spertini O. Daratumumab and venetoclax in combination with chemotherapy provide sustained molecular remission in relapsed/refractory CD19, CD20, and CD22 negative acute B lymphoblastic leukemia with KMT2A-AFF1 transcript. *Biomark Res.* 2021;9(1):92.
215. Ofran Y, Ringelstein-Harlev S, Slouzkey I, et al. Daratumumab for eradication of minimal residual disease in high-risk advanced relapse of T-cell/CD19/CD22-negative acute lymphoblastic leukemia. *Leukemia.* 2020;34(1):293-295.
216. Zhang Y, Xue S, Liu F, Wang J. Daratumumab for quick and sustained remission in post-transplant relapsed/refractory acute lymphoblastic leukemia. *Leuk Res.* 2020;91:106332.
217. Ganzel C, Kharit M, Duksin C, Rowe JM. Daratumumab for relapsed/refractory Philadelphia-positive acute lymphoblastic leukemia. *Haematologica.* 2018;103(10):e489-e490.
218. Cerrano M, Bonifacio M, Olivi M, et al. Daratumumab with or without chemotherapy in relapsed and refractory acute lymphoblastic leukemia. A retrospective observational Campus ALL study. *Haematologica.* 2022;107(4):996-999.
219. Punatar S, Gokarn A, Nayak L, et al. Long term outcome of a patient with relapsed refractory early thymic precursor acute lymphoblastic leukemia treated with daratumumab. *Am J Blood Res.* 2021;11(5):528-533.
220. Murthy GSG, Kearl T, Cui W, et al. A phase 1 study of CD38-bispecific antibody (XmAb18968) for patients with CD38 expressing relapsed/refractory acute myeloid leukemia and T-cell acute lymphoblastic leukemia. *J Clin Oncol.* 2022;40:TPS7070.
221. Maude SL, Frey N, Shaw PA, et al. Chimeric antigen receptor T cells for sustained remissions in leukemia. *N Engl J Med.* 2014;371(16):1507-1517.
222. Maude SL, Laetsch TW, Buechner J, et al. Tisagenlecleucel in children and young adults with B-cell lymphoblastic leukemia. *N Engl J Med.* 2018;378(5):439-448.
223. O'Leary MC, Lu X, Huang Y, et al. FDA approval summary: tisagenlecleucel for treatment of patients with relapsed or refractory B-cell precursor acute lymphoblastic leukemia. *Clin Cancer Res.* 2019;25(4):1142-1146.
224. Brentjens RJ, Davila ML, Riviere I, et al. CD19-targeted T cells rapidly induce molecular remissions in adults with chemotherapy-refractory acute lymphoblastic leukemia. *Sci Transl Med.* 2013;5(177):177ra38.
225. Lee DW, Kochenderfer JN, Stetler-Stevenson M, et al. T cells expressing CD19 chimeric antigen receptors for acute lymphoblastic leukaemia in children and young adults: a phase 1 dose-escalation trial. *Lancet.* 2015;385(9967):517-528.
226. Shah BD, Bishop MR, Oluwole OO, et al. KTE-X19 anti-CD19 CAR T-cell therapy in adult relapsed/refractory acute lymphoblastic leukemia: ZUMA-3 phase 1 results. *Blood.* 2021;138:11-22.
227. Shah BD, Ghobadi A, Oluwole OO, et al. KTE-X19 for relapsed or refractory adult B-cell acute lymphoblastic leukaemia: phase 2 results of the single-arm, open-label, multicentre ZUMA-3 study. *Lancet.* 2021;398(10299):491-502.
228. Lee DW, Santomasso BD, Locke FL, et al. ASTCT consensus grading for cytokine release syndrome and neurologic toxicity associated with immune effector cells. *Biol Blood Marrow Transplant.* 2019;25(4):625-638.
229. Frey NV. Relapsed ALL: CAR T vs transplant vs novel therapies. *Hematology Am Soc Hematol Educ Program.* 2021;2021:1-6.

Chapter 76 ■ Acute Myeloid Leukemia in Adults

ASHKAN EMADI • MARIA R. BAER

Acute myeloid leukemia, previously also called *acute myelogenous leukemia* and *acute nonlymphocytic leukemia*, is a hematopoietic neoplasm characterized by the presence of a malignant clone of myeloid cells with maturation arrest at the level of blast.

AML may follow a myelodysplastic syndrome (MDS) (Chapter 80) or a myeloproliferative neoplasm (MPN) (Chapters 81-84). AML should be distinguished from acute lymphoblastic leukemia (ALL) (Chapter 75), in which blasts are of lymphoid rather than myeloid lineage. AML should also be distinguished from chronic myelogenous leukemia (CML) (Chapter 82), in which, in the initial phase of the disease, myeloid cells are expanded but do not exhibit maturation arrest. Chapter 78 addresses the presentation of and therapy for AML in children. Chapter 79 addresses the biology, presentation, and management of the acute promyelocytic leukemia (APL) subtype of AML in adults and children.

In this chapter, epidemiologic, clinical, biologic, cytogenetic, and molecular features of adult AML are addressed in the context of prognosis and therapeutic principles.

HISTORICAL PERSPECTIVE

The terms "*weisses blut*" and "leukhemia" were first used by Virchow in 1845 and 1847, "acute leukemia" was first described in 1857, and leukemias were divided into "myeloid" and "lymphocytic" by Naegeli in 1900.[1] Acute monoblastic leukemia was described in 1913,[2] acute erythroleukemia in 1917,[3] acute megakaryocytic leukemia in 1931,[4] and APL in 1947.[5]

Numerous cytogenetic abnormalities, both structural and numerical, have been identified in AML, beginning with the t(8;21)[6] and t(15;17)[7] translocations in 1973 and 1977, respectively. inv(16) was described in 1983.[8] Diverse molecular abnormalities have also been described in AML. Internal tandem duplication (ITD) of the fms-like tyrosine kinase 3 (*FLT3*) receptor tyrosine kinase gene was initially described in 1996[9] and mutation in the nucleophosmin 1 (*NPM1*) gene in 2005.[10]

The French-American-British (FAB) cooperative group developed the initial classification of AML in 1976[11] based on morphology and subsequently expanded it to incorporate immunophenotype, notably to include minimally differentiated disease with myeloid antigen expression.[12] The World Health Organization (WHO) classification, initially published in 1997 and updated in 2016[13] and 2022,[14] incorporates clinical, cytogenetic, and molecular data. It defines new AML subtypes based on several recurring structural cytogenetic and molecular abnormalities and also distinguishes therapy-related myeloid neoplasms (t-MN) and AML with myelodysplasia-related changes (AML-MRC). The International Consensus Classification of Myeloid Neoplasms and Acute Leukemias was published in 2022.[15] The European LeukemiaNet (ELN) developed and has serially updated a prognostic classification of AML incorporating cytogenetic and molecular data.[16,17]

The "7 + 3" cytosine arabinoside and anthracycline remission induction chemotherapy regimen was initially published in 1973,[18] and high-dose cytosine arabinoside (HiDAC) consolidation therapy in 1989.[19] These have remained the mainstay of AML therapy, while improvements in outcome have largely reflected improved supportive care, treatment stratification based on cytogenetic and molecular data, and advent of and improvements in allogeneic hematopoietic stem cell transplantation (allo-HSCT). However, after decades without new drug approvals for AML, there has been a spate of novel agents introduced for this disease in the recent past and, between 2017 and 2022, ten new drugs were approved by the US Food and Drug Administration (FDA), including eight molecularly targeted therapies.

EPIDEMIOLOGY

AML is the acute leukemia with the highest incidence rate in adults and accounts for 80% to 90% of adult acute leukemia cases.[20] It is estimated that 20,240 individuals (11,230 men and 9010 women) were diagnosed with AML and 11,400 died of AML in the United States in 2021.[21] AML accounts for 1.1% of all new cancer cases and 1.9% of all cancer deaths in the United States.[20] The lifetime risk of AML based on rates from 2016 through 2018 is approximately 0.5% in both men and women.[20] *Figure 76.1* illustrates the estimated numbers of new patients with AML and their survival and mortality in the United States from 1997 to 2021.

The rate of new cases of AML is 4.3 per 100,000 men and women per year in the United States.[20] The incidence of AML increases with age, with mean patient age of 68 years at diagnosis. An increased incidence of AML in the elderly over time is likely related to a combination of improved diagnosis, recognition of AML after MDS, longer survival of patients who receive chemotherapy or radiation for solid or other hematologic neoplasms, and longer life expectancy.[22]

The overall 5-year relative survival for AML from 2011 through 2017 in 18 Surveillance Epidemiology and End Results (SEER) geographic areas was 29.5%.[20] In 2018, there were an estimated 66,988 individuals living with AML in the United States.[20]

RISK FACTORS

AML arising following cytotoxic therapy for prior malignancies or benign conditions, termed therapy-related AML (t-AML), therapy-related myeloid neoplasm (t-MN)[13] or myeloid neoplasms post cytotoxic therapy (MN-pCT),[14] is an increasing problem in the face of successful therapy for solid and other hematological malignancies, and decreasing the risk of this devastating complication is an important goal in the evolution of oncology treatment regimens and strategies. Epidemiologic studies have also identified occupational, environmental, lifestyle, and genetic factors that increase the risk of AML.[23-25]

Therapy-Related AML

Antineoplastic therapy is associated with an increased risk of subsequent development of AML, and AML diagnosed following cytotoxic therapy for a prior malignant or benign condition is considered to be t-AML. Of note, the WHO classification groups t-AML and t-MDS as t-MN[13] or, more recently, MN-pCT.[14]

MN-pCT presentation and treatment response differ based on the setting in which it arises and the likely causative agent. MN-pCT most commonly develops following treatment with alkylating agents or topoisomerase II inhibitors, but nucleoside analogues, anti-tubulins and radiation are also associated with MN-pCT.[26-28] Most MN-pCT occur 3 to 10 years after initial therapy, with a longer latency for alkylating agents (5-9 years) than for topoisomerase II inhibitors (6 months to 5 years).[26,28] Alkylating agents cause chromosome deletions and unbalanced translocations, most commonly involving chromosomes 5 and/or 7, frequently in complex karyotypes (three or more unrelated cytogenetic abnormalities).[27] Topoisomerase II inhibitors inhibit a critical enzyme involved in DNA replication, leading to balanced chromosomal translocations usually involving 11q23, and less frequently 21q22, with the formation of fusion genes.[29] The role of clonal hematopoiesis of indeterminate potential (CHIP) in the development of MN-pCT is discussed in Chapter 81.

The prognosis for MN-pCT is poor, with a median survival of 7 to 10 months and usually less than 10% 5-year survival.[27] Alkylating agent-associated MN-pCT, generally characterized by deletions or

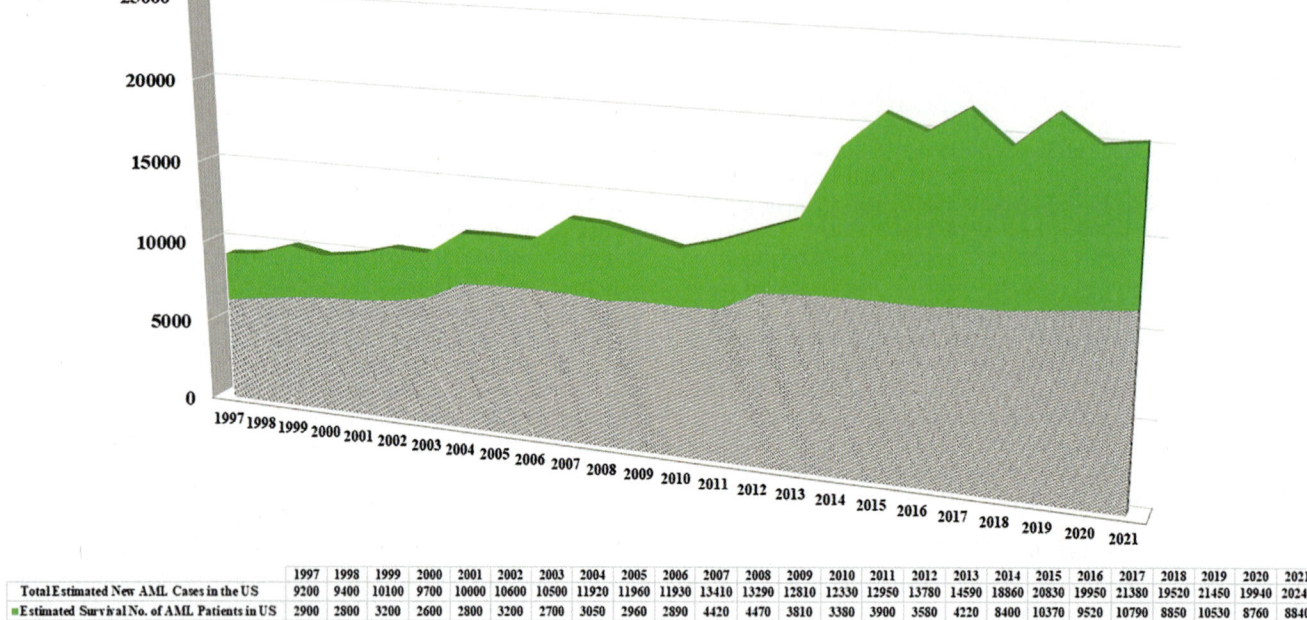

FIGURE 76.1 AML incidence and mortality in the United States 1997 to 2021.

monosomies of chromosomes 5 and/or 7 or complex karyotypes, as noted above, frequently evolves from MDS to AML and has a low complete remission (CR) rate and short disease-free (DFS) and overall survival (OS). In contrast, topoisomerase II–associated MN-pCT, most commonly with 11q23 translocations, typically presents as AML without prior MDS and has a high CR rate, but short DFS and OS. More rarely, patients treated with antineoplastic agents may develop t-AML with t(8;21), inv(16) or t(15;17).[28,30] An initial report suggested similar prognosis for t-AML and de novo AML with t(8;21) or inv(16),[31] while a subsequent report suggested a worse outcome for t-AML than for de novo AML with t(8;21).[32]

TP53 mutations are also common in MN-pCT and are associated with poor outcomes.[33,34] Data from an elegant genetic analysis of patients with *TP53*-mutated MN-pCT at serial time points suggested that cytotoxic therapy does not directly induce *TP53* mutations but rather that rare hematopoietic stem/progenitor cells carrying age-related *TP53* mutations are resistant to chemotherapy and therefore expand preferentially after treatment.[35]

Alkylating agent–associated t-AML has been extensively described. Cumulative drug dose is a primary determinant in causing leukemia, but alkylators differ in their leukemogenicity. Mechlorethamine and melphalan are more leukemogenic than cyclophosphamide. Alkylating agent–associated t-AML was initially best characterized following treatment of Hodgkin lymphoma, one of the first malignancies for which curative therapy was developed,[36-38] but has now been described after therapy for multiple neoplasms including, but not limited to, breast cancer, multiple myeloma, ovarian cancer, and non-Hodgkin lymphoma,[28,39-41] as well as in nonneoplastic disorders such as rheumatologic diseases.[28] Leukemia onset after alkylating agent exposure has ranged from 1 to 28 years and is most commonly in the 5- to 9-year range.[42] Up to two-thirds of patients who develop leukemia have a preceding myelodysplastic phase that lasts approximately 6 months, and increase in the mean corpuscular volume, or macrocytosis, may be an early myelodysplastic change.[42,43] Clonal cytogenetic abnormalities are often complex; the most common single abnormality is monosomy 7 (−7), followed by del(5q) and −5.[42] In addition, with the increased use of autologous transplantation (auto-HSCT) as salvage therapy for lymphomas, MN-pCT is being recognized in 5% to 15% of patients and is most commonly associated with complex karyotypes and/or chromosome 5 and/or 7 abnormalities and with poor outcomes.[28,44]

Topoisomerase II inhibitors, particularly etoposide and teniposide, were recognized as leukemogenic agents in survivors of lung cancer,[45,46] germ cell cancer,[47] ALL,[48] neuroblastoma,[49] and osteosarcoma[50] in the 1980s. Large cumulative doses and prolonged courses have been implicated in increasing the risk of leukemia. The latency period is short, with most cases occurring between 6 months and 5 years after initial therapy. There is no myelodysplastic phase, and the majority of cases are myelomonocytic or monoblastic. The most common cytogenetic abnormalities are translocations of chromosome band 11q23 rearranging the histone-lysine N-methyltransferase 2A (*KMT2A*) gene, previously designated mixed-lineage leukemia (*MLL*) and acute lymphoblastic leukemia 1 (*ALL-1*).[42] Over 40 partner genes that encode different proteins are involved in *KMT2A* translocations. AML with 11q23 translocations after topoisomerase II inhibitor therapy tends to be chemosensitive, but patients are rarely long-term survivors because of a high relapse rate.[42]

Breast cancer may be treated with both alkylating agents and topoisomerase II inhibitors, as well as anti-tubulins. Cytogenetic abnormalities in MN-pCT after breast cancer therapy are heterogenous and include those associated with alkylating agent and with topoisomerase II inhibitor therapy.[51] Use of granulocyte colony-stimulating factor (G-CSF) was implicated in increasing the risk of MN-pCT following breast cancer adjuvant therapy,[51-53] and radiation therapy may also contribute.[51,54-56]

Nucleoside analogues have also been implicated in MN-pCT. Fludarabine in chronic lymphocytic leukemia is associated with AML, particularly when combined with chlorambucil[57] or mitoxantrone.[58] Nucleoside analogues are also associated with an increased risk of t-AML in Waldenström macroglobulinemia.[59] Azathioprine has been associated with MN-pCT, frequently with chromosome 7 abnormalities, in patients with rheumatologic disorders and in solid organ transplant recipients.[60,61] 6-Mercaptopurine is also associated with t-AML.[62] In addition, MDS/AML with dysplasia and chromosome 7 abnormalities after treatment of de novo AML may represent MN-pCT associated with cytarabine.[63]

MN-pCT is well documented following therapy for APL with diverse chemotherapy drugs. Many of these cases have chromosome 5 and/or 7 abnormalities, but others have 11q23 translocations, and miscellaneous other abnormalities are also seen.[64] The incidence should decrease with decreasing use of chemotherapy drugs to treat APL (Chapter 79).

Although less so than chemotherapy, radiation therapy is leukemogenic, as evidenced by an increased leukemia risk in patients receiving radiation in the past for ankylosing spondylitis,[65] menorrhagia,[66] tinea capitis,[67] and peptic ulcer disease.[68] The risk of leukemia (latency period of 2-11 years) is approximately two times higher in patients who have received either radium implants or external beam radiation for cervical, ovarian, or endometrial cancer.[69-71] Similarly, a 2-fold increase in risk has been reported in patients with breast cancer receiving adjuvant radiotherapy, compared with a 10-fold increase in risk after chemotherapy, while combined radiation and chemotherapy resulted in a 17-fold risk.[51,56] Radiation therapy has been associated with only a small increase in risk of leukemia in patients with Hodgkin and non-Hodgkin lymphomas, unless it is extensive and encompasses a large volume of bone marrow.[38,72]

Patients with MN-pCT following radiation alone have a lower incidence of high-risk karyotypes and longer survival than those with MN-pCT following chemotherapy or chemotherapy and radiation, suggesting that postradiation AML may warrant a therapeutic approach similar to de novo AML.[73]

Medical exposure to radioactivity is leukemogenic. In a meta-analysis, the relative risk of leukemia in thyroid cancer survivors treated with radioactive iodine (RAI) was 2.5.[74] A standardized incidence ratio of 5.68 was reported in patients with low-risk (T1N0) well-differentiated thyroid cancer treated with RAI, with excess risk significantly greater in patients less than 45 years.[75]

Occupational Exposures

Occupational exposures are risk factors for the development of AML. An increased risk of AML has been reported in workers manufacturing, or exposed to, rubber, paint, embalming fluids, pesticides, ethylene oxide, petroleum, poultry, munitions, automobiles, nuclear power, plastics, and electrical wiring, as well as gasoline station attendants, beauticians, barbers, and cosmetologists.[76] Most of these reports are based on retrospective and cross-sectional studies, which makes establishing causal relationships difficult. The older literature also implicated employment in shoe-making, painting, furniture manufacturing or repair, paper mills, clothing or textile industry, chemical manufacturing, printing, nursing, and biological laboratories,[76] but enforcement of regulations limiting occupational exposures has likely altered the occupational risk profile. In a matched case-control analysis using California Cancer Registry data from 1988 to 2007, industries with a statistically significant increased AML risk were construction, agriculture and forestry, and animal slaughtering and processing, and occupations with a statistically significant increased AML risk included agricultural workers, fishers and fishing workers, nurses, psychiatric and home health aides, and janitors and building cleaners.[77] Of note, an association with hobbies has not been reported.[76]

The most fully characterized chemical exposure associated with AML is to the aromatic hydrocarbon benzene.[78-80] Toxicity is related to cumulative dose, and the risk of leukemia was high before regulations limiting occupational exposures were put in place. Increased risk of AML with occupational benzene exposure was confirmed in a systematic review and meta-analysis,[81] and occupational benzene exposure was found to be associated with specific aneuploidies.[82]

Environmental Factors

Ionizing radiation is carcinogenic primarily via induction of DNA double-strand breaks. The risk of leukemia correlates with radiation dosage and age at exposure, with a more rapid peak early in life (<15 years), as well as a more rapid decline than in those exposed at older ages (*Figure 76.2*).[83]

Fallout from atomic tests and exposure to nuclear reactors have been a concern since the middle of the 20th century. Atomic bombs

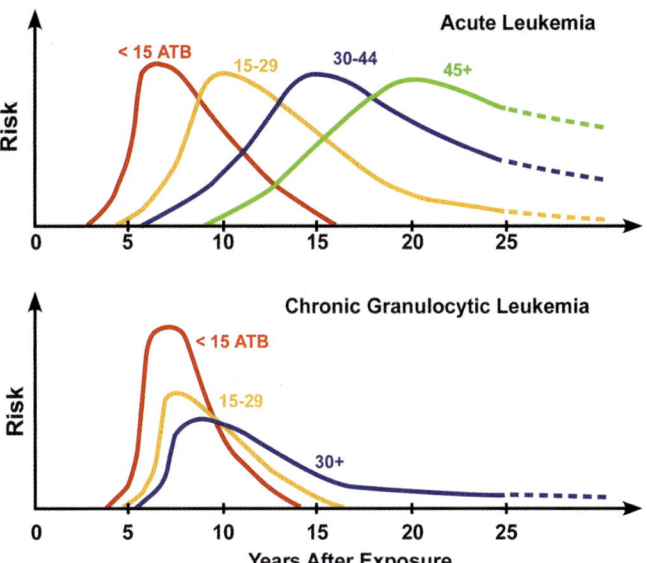

FIGURE 76.2 Effect of age at exposure and temporal pattern of developing leukemia according to cell type (acute vs chronic myeloid leukemia); ATB, at time of bomb.[83] (Reprinted from Folley JH, Borges W, Yamawaki T. Incidence of leukemia in survivors of the atomic bomb in Hiroshima and Nagasaki, Japan. *Am J Med*. 1952;13(3):311-321.)

were released over Hiroshima and Nagasaki in 1945, and an excess risk of leukemia was reported in 1952.[84] The excess relative rate of AML among Japanese atomic bomb survivors, per gray, was best described by a quadratic dose-response function that peaked approximately 10 years after exposure, but with the effect persisting for more than 5 decades.[85] Little radioactivity was released into the environment in the Three Mile Island nuclear meltdown, whereas there was extensive exposure to radioactivity after the Chernobyl nuclear accident,[86,87] and increased AML incidence was reported in Chernobyl clean-up workers.[88]

Lifestyle-Related Factors

Smoking has been repeatedly identified as a risk factor for AML.[89-95] Cigarette smoke contains more than 4000 chemical compounds, 60 of which have been found to be carcinogenic and leukemogenic, including benzene. Meta-analyses have estimated a relative risk for AML of 1.3 to 1.5 in smokers.[90,96] The risk of developing AML is two to three times higher in male smokers exceeding 20 pack-years.[89,97] Smokers of more than 40 cigarettes per day who develop AML have an increased incidence of unfavorable cytogenetic abnormalities, including −7/del(7q).[91,95]

Obesity has been reported as a risk factor for AML.[98-101] It was associated with a higher incidence of AML in both white and black male US veterans.[99] Similarly, the risk of AML was increased among women who reported being overweight or obese compared with women reporting normal weight (relative risks, 1.9 and 2.4) among over 40,000 women ages 55 to 69 years in the Iowa Women's Health Study.[100] Findings were similar in a Canadian population.[98] A proposed mechanistic explanation for the increased risk of AML associated with obesity is fatty acid–binding protein 4 (FABP4) increasing DNA methyltransferase 1 (DNMT1)-dependent DNA methylation.[102]

Finally, use of permanent, but not nonpermanent, dark hair dye has been associated with AML.[103]

Heritable Genetic Factors

Germline mutations associated with myeloid neoplasms, categorized in the 2016 WHO classification,[13] are listed in *Table 76.1*.

Another approach to categorizing germline mutations associated with leukemias is to distinguish those associated with leukemias and other cancers and those associated only with leukemias.[104] Diseases resulting from germline mutations associated with increased risk of leukemias and other cancers include Bloom syndrome (*BLM* gene),

Table 76.1. Classification of Myeloid Neoplasms With Germ Line Predisposition

Myeloid neoplasms with germ line predisposition without a preexisting disorder or organ dysfunction
AML with germ line CEBPA mutation
Myeloid neoplasms with germ line DDX41 mutation*
Myeloid neoplasms with germ line predisposition and preexisting platelet disorders
Myeloid neoplasms with germ line RUNX1 mutation*
Myeloid neoplasms with germ line ANKRD26 mutation*
Myeloid neoplasms with germ line ETV6 mutation*
Myeloid neoplasms with germ line predisposition and other organ dysfunction
Myeloid neoplasms with germ line GATA2 mutation
Myeloid neoplasms associated with BM failure syndromes
Myeloid neoplasms associated with telomere biology disorders
JMML associated with neurofibromatosis, Noonan syndrome or Noonan syndrome-like disorders
Myeloid neoplasms associated with Down syndrome*

*Lymphoid neoplasms also reported.

Fanconi anemia (*FANCA-P* gene), constitutional mismatch repair deficiency, dyskeratosis congenita, Diamond-Blackfan anemia, neurofibromatosis (*NF1* gene), and Noonan (*PTPN11* gene), Rothmund-Thomson (*RECQL4* gene), Li-Fraumeni (*TP53* gene) and Werner (*WRN* gene) syndromes. Of note, most of the genes mutated in these syndromes encode proteins involved in DNA damage response or DNA repair. Germline mutations associated only with leukemias include mutations in *ANKRD26* (*ANKRD26*-related thrombocytopenia); *CEBPA, DDX41, ELANE, HAX1, G6PC3* (the latter three associated with congenital neutropenia); *ETV6, GATA2, MPL* (congenital amegakaryocytic thrombocytopenia); *RBM8A* (thrombocytopenia absent radius syndrome); *RUNX1; SBDS* (Shwachman-Diamond syndrome); *SRP72*; Down syndrome; and familial monosomy 7 syndrome. Heritable syndromes associated with increased risk of AML are usually recognized in childhood and are discussed in Chapter 78.

Polymorphisms in genes encoding detoxifying enzymes and DNA repair proteins have also been associated with incidence of AML, as well as with treatment outcomes. Glutathione S-transferases (GSTs), including GSTM, GSTP, and GSTT, are detoxification enzymes involved in metabolism of carcinogens. A meta-analysis of the association of *GST* polymorphisms with risk of AML supported a significant risk of AML in the presence of null genotypes of *GSTM1* and *GSTT*.[105] Associations with treatment outcomes were also suggested.[106,107] Polymorphisms in the *RAD51* and *XRCC3* genes, encoding proteins involved in repair of DNA double-strand breaks by homologous recombination, have been associated with increased risk of development of AML.[108] Other work implicates polymorphisms of the XRCC1 gene, encoding a protein involved in base excision repair,[109] and of RAD51[110] in risk of t-AML, and polymorphisms in the xeroderma pigmentosum group D (XPD) DNA repair gene, encoding a protein involved in nucleotide excision repair, in AML with del(5q) and del(7q) chromosome deletions.[111]

Clonal Hematopoiesis

Clonal hematopoiesis describes the presence of a genetically distinct population of hematopoietic cells that share one or more acquired mutation(s) differentiating them from other hematopoietic cells. Clonal hematopoiesis may be identified in healthy persons with no or minimal hematologic abnormalities[112] and is associated with increased risk of hematologic malignancies, as well as of cardiovascular disease.[113] For a complete discussion of clonal hematopoiesis, please see Chapter 81.

The incidence of clonal hematopoiesis increases with age. Whole-exome sequencing of DNA in peripheral blood cells from approximately 12,400 individuals, unselected for cancer or hematologic abnormalities, matched with a national health outcome registry, identified clonal hematopoiesis in 10% of people older than 65 years but in only 1% of persons younger than 50 years.[114] Somatic mutations in three genes (*DNMT3A, ASXL1, TET2*) were frequently identified in the expanded clones.[114] Clonal hematopoiesis was identified as a strong risk factor for subsequent hematologic neoplasms (hazard ratio [HR], 13; 95% confidence interval [CI], 6-29).[114] Approximately 40% of hematologic neoplasms in this cohort occurred in persons who had clonality in DNA sampled more than 6 months before the first diagnosis of cancer.[114] In addition, blood cells of >2% of approximately 2700 individuals in The Cancer Genome Atlas and ~5% of those older than 70 years contained mutations potentially representing premalignant events that cause clonal hematopoietic expansion and a premalignant state. Nine genes (*DNMT3A, TET2, JAK2, ASXL1, TP53, GNAS, PPM1D, BCORL1, SF3B1*) were recurrently mutated.[115]

Single-cell analyses in AML demonstrated the presence of preleukemic hematopoietic stem cell clones with multiple mutations in some patients.[116]

Lymphomyeloid clonal hematopoiesis, defined by the presence of *DNMT3A* mutations in both the myeloid and T-lymphoid compartments, was found in diagnostic, CR, and relapse samples of 40 of 170 patients with AML and was associated with CHIP many years before AML, older age, secondary AML, and mutations in the *TET2, RUNX1*, and *EZH2* genes.[117] In ~80% of patients with AML with lymphomyeloid clonal hematopoiesis, the preleukemic clone persisted after chemotherapy and was the launching clone for relapse.[117] Long-term survival of patients with lymphomyeloid clonal hematopoiesis was only observed after allo-HSCT.[117]

Presence of clonal hematopoiesis may interfere with determination of minimal/measurable residual disease (MRD) by molecular genetic techniques post treatment in patients with AML. Hematopoietic clones that are detected in patients with AML in CR may represent true residual AML, early recurrent AML, a separate MDS clone, clonal hematopoiesis that is ancestral to the AML, or independent or newly emerging clones of uncertain leukemogenic potential.[118] In one report, postremission clonal hematopoiesis was identified in ~50% of patients with AML and persisted long-term in ~90% of trackable patients in spite of consolidation and maintenance therapies, but was eradicated in 95% of patients who underwent allo-HSCT.[119] Interestingly, postremission clonal hematopoiesis had little effect on relapse risk, nonrelapse mortality, or incidence of atherosclerotic cardiovascular disease, suggesting that, while residual clonal hematopoietic stem cells are commonly unaffected by consolidation and maintenance therapies, they may not impact clinical outcomes.[119]

Post-allo-HSCT clones can be donor-derived, with potential to initiate a new myeloid disorder clonally unrelated to the original AML of the recipient.[118]

CLINICAL PRESENTATION

Bone Marrow Failure

AML presenting symptoms and signs in most patients are related to failure of normal hematopoiesis, resulting in anemia, neutropenia, and thrombocytopenia. The most common symptoms are nonspecific fatigue, malaise, weakness, and dyspnea caused by anemia. Other constitutional symptoms are uncommon. Bone pain, most frequently back pain, occurs in less than 20% of patients. Fever is the presenting feature in 20% and may result from infection due to neutropenia or from leukemia itself, although infection must be presumed and treated. Hemorrhagic signs and symptoms are found in up to 50% of patients at diagnosis. Petechiae and mucosal bleeding, including epistaxis and gum bleeding, correlate with the severity of thrombocytopenia, while ecchymoses generally correlate with the presence of disseminated intravascular coagulation (DIC), which is common in APL and may also occur in other AML subtypes. Gastrointestinal and urinary bleeding and menorrhagia do not usually result from thrombocytopenia alone, and anatomic causes should be suspected and investigated at an appropriate time.

Hyperleukocytosis

Hyperleukocytosis, arbitrarily defined as a blood blast count greater than 100,000/mm³, occurs most commonly in monocytic AML subtypes (FAB M4/5) and in AML with FLT3-ITD.[120] Hyperleukocytosis is a medical emergency because it is associated with leukostasis in the lungs and the central nervous system (CNS),[120-122] which is usually rapidly fatal. Pulmonary leukostasis manifests as dyspnea, tachypnea, rales, interstitial infiltrates, and respiratory failure. CNS leukostasis manifests as headaches, blurred vision, somnolence, obtundation, ischemic stroke, and intracerebral hemorrhage. Coronary artery blockage resulting in massive myocardial infarction due to leukostasis has been reported in *FLT3*-ITD AML.[123] In patients with AML with blood blast count approaching, or above, 100,000/mm³, the white blood cell (WBC) count must be rapidly lowered using hydroxycarbamide (hydroxyurea) with or without leukapheresis, and definitive therapy must be initiated as rapidly as possible.

Extramedullary AML

Extramedullary leukemia is found in up to half of patients with AML, mostly in monocytic subtypes. In one series of newly diagnosed patients with AML, sites of involvement included lymph nodes (12%), spleen (7%), liver (5%), skin (5%), gingivae (4%), and CNS (1%).[124]

In multivariable analysis adjusted for known prognostic factors such as cytogenetic risk and WBC count, the presence of extramedullary leukemia did not have independent prognostic significance.[124]

Myeloid Sarcoma

Myeloid sarcoma, previously termed *granulocytic sarcoma*, *myeloblastoma*, or *chloroma*, is an extramedullary tumor that occurs in 2% to 14% of patients with AML.[125,126] The term *chloroma* derives from a green appearance caused by expression of myeloperoxidase. Myeloid sarcoma may precede or occur at the time of diagnosis of AML, or at relapse, including after allo-HSCT. It also occurs with MDS or MPN, usually predicting transformation to AML. Sites include orbit and paranasal sinuses, gastrointestinal or genitourinary tract, breast, cervix, salivary glands, mediastinum, pleura, peritoneum, and bile duct.[125]

Biopsy is required for diagnosis, and the diagnosis is suggested by presence of eosinophilic myelocytes in hematoxylin and eosin–stained biopsy sections. Imprint preparations can be helpful. The diagnosis can be made if Auer rods are detected or if myeloid origin is confirmed by cytochemical or immunohistochemical methods. Although myeloid sarcomas are radiosensitive, they are managed with systemic chemotherapy in most cases, even in the absence of bone marrow involvement.[127,128]

Central Nervous System Leukemia

The incidence of CNS disease at diagnosis of AML is difficult to determine because lumbar puncture is not generally performed in asymptomatic patients, in contrast to the practice in ALL.[129] In a large retrospective series, CNS involvement was reported in ~1% of patients with AML at diagnosis.[124] CNS disease was reported to develop in up to 16% of adults with AML during follow-up in an early series,[129] but routine use of HiDAC, which crosses the blood-brain barrier, in consolidation therapy has decreased the incidence of CNS leukemia in AML, as evidenced by a ~2% incidence in a subsequent review of 410 patients.[130]

CNS disease is associated with hyperleukocytosis and monocytic AML subtypes.[131] It presents with headache, nausea, and/or cranial nerve palsies, particularly involving cranial nerves V, VI, and VII. Ocular involvement may result in blindness and suggests meningeal involvement. Intracerebral masses were reported in AML with inv(16),[132] but they are also now uncommon with use of HiDAC consolidation chemotherapy. Prophylactic CNS therapy is not given routinely to adult patients with AML, but some clinicians advocate prophylaxis in patients with monocytic subtype or presenting white cell counts greater than 100,000 cells/mm³. Diagnostic lumbar puncture with prophylactic intrathecal chemotherapy may also be advocated prior to allo-HSCT. AML CNS involvement may be treated with HiDAC, cranial irradiation, and/or intrathecal methotrexate/cytarabine.[127] Cranial irradiation should be used to treat CNS AML with cranial nerve involvement, and should be initiated emergently.

Leukemia Cutis

Leukemic skin infiltration, or leukemia cutis, occurs in ~10% of patients with AML, most commonly in those with monocytic subtypes. Skin lesions can be nodular (*Figure 76.3*), violaceous, raised, and palpable and are generally painless. Lesions may be widespread or localized. Skin lesions may precede the diagnosis of AML or may occur concurrently with AML at diagnosis or relapse or as an isolated extramedullary relapse. Biopsy distinguishes leukemia cutis from benign skin lesions associated with AML, including Sweet syndrome[130] and pyoderma gangrenosum,[131] which are typically painful and respond to corticosteroids. Leukemia cutis is radiosensitive, but patients should usually be treated with systemic chemotherapy.[135]

Gingival Infiltration

Gum infiltration is characteristic of acute monocytic leukemia[136] and regresses with systemic therapy.[137] Patients may initially present for dental evaluation because of gingival hypertrophy (*Figure 76.4*).[138]

Other Extramedullary Manifestations of AML

Gastrointestinal symptoms include perirectal abscess and typhlitis, a necrotizing colitis related to leukemic infiltration of the bowel wall. Management of typhlitis is supportive, including antibiotics and nasogastric suction, but surgical intervention is sometimes unavoidable.[139] Cardiac abnormalities are usually related to electrolyte imbalances, particularly hypokalemia, but may result from direct involvement of the conduction system or infiltration of vessel walls.[123]

LABORATORY FINDINGS

Presenting blood counts vary widely in AML.[140] The WBC count is elevated in more than half of patients but is greater than 100,000 cells/mm³ in less than 20%. Blasts are usually present in the peripheral blood smear or in a buffy coat smear. Auer rods and Phi bodies, which are

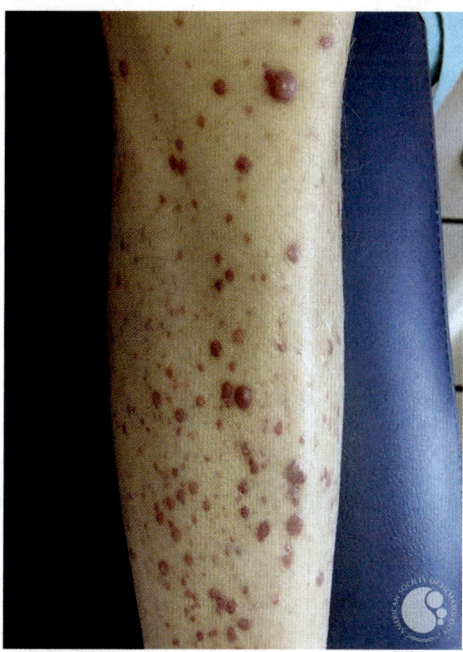

FIGURE 76.3 Leukemia cutis manifesting as subcutaneous nodules. Used with permission of American Society of Hematology from American Society of Hematology Image Bank [Author: Nidia P. Zapata, MD; Ramiro Espinoza-Zamora. Published July 3, 2018]; permission conveyed through Copyright Clearance Center, Inc.

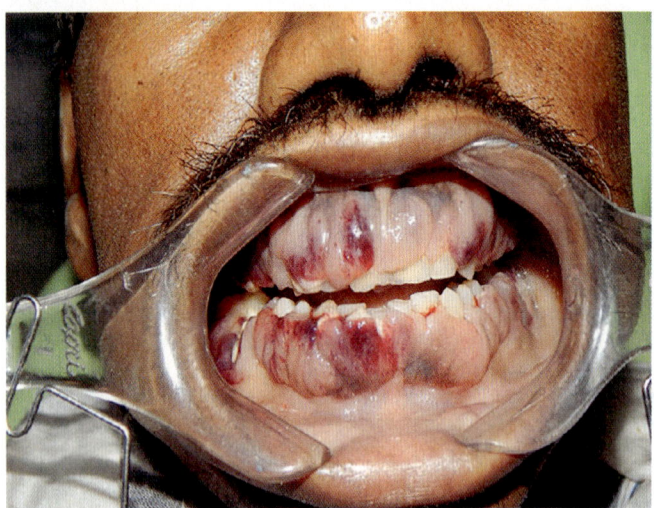

FIGURE 76.4 Gingival hypertrophy in a patient with AML.[138] (Reprinted with permission from Bhambal AM, Shrivastava H, Naik SP, et al. Oral manifestations of systemic leukemia-first sign of presentation. *J Indian Soc Periodontol*. 2021;25(4):347-349. Copyright © 2021 Journal of Indian Society of Periodontology.)

fusiform or spindle-shaped rods similar to Auer rods that require special stains for hydroperoxidase,[141] are considered pathognomonic of AML.

Cytopenias result from hematopoietic failure and contribute to symptoms and signs. Anemia is predominantly normochromic and normocytic. Reticulocytopenia is generally present, but nucleated red blood cells may be seen. Neutropenia is present in most patients with AML. Thrombocytopenia is usually present and may be severe at diagnosis. Thrombocytosis is rarely identified and is characteristic of AML with abnormalities of the long arm of chromosome 3(3q) involving the MDS1 and EVI1 complex locus protein EVI1 (*MECOM*) gene (formerly called *EVI1*).

Hyperleukocytosis, arbitrarily defined as a blood blast count greater than 100,000/mm³, occurs most commonly in monocytic AML subtypes and in AML with FLT3-ITD[120,121] and is a medical emergency because it is associated with leukostasis in the lungs and the CNS and potentially other organs, as discussed in section "Clinical Presentation."

DIC is more common in AML than in ALL and is most common in APL (Chapter 79). The incidence of DIC in AML other than APL is 10% to 30%.[142] DIC is thought to be caused by release of tissue factor–like procoagulants from the azurophilic granules in AML cells. DIC is manifested clinically by bruising and, when severe, by bleeding from multiple sites. Laboratory findings include thrombocytopenia, prolonged prothrombin time and partial thromboplastin time, hypofibrinogenemia, elevated fibrin split products and D-dimers, and deficiency of coagulation factors, including factor V and factor VIII.[143]

Hyperuricemia is noted in up to 50% of patients with AML and can also be associated with tumor lysis.[144] Hydration and administration of recombinant urate oxidase (rasburicase) for markedly elevated uric acid levels, or elevated uric acid levels with renal insufficiency, can prevent complications of tumor lysis that may occur with initiation of chemotherapy, most often in the setting of hyperleukocytosis. Allopurinol (or febuxostat, if allopurinol-allergic) also needs to be initiated and should be initiated in all patients when chemotherapy is initiated to prevent hyperuricemia associated with cytoreduction.

Serum lactate dehydrogenase levels may be elevated, particularly in monocytic disease, but to a lesser degree than in ALL.

Hypokalemia may result from potassium uptake by rapidly proliferating AML cells or from proximal renal tubular damage caused by elevated levels of lysozyme, particularly in monocytic disease. Hyperkalemia can occur in association with tumor lysis. With improved agents to treat hyperuricemia, hyperphosphatemia with or without hypocalcemia is the most common abnormality associated with renal failure during induction chemotherapy. Patients with AML may have hypocalcemia,[145] but hypercalcemia is very rare.[146]

BIOLOGIC FEATURES

Much of what is known about AML biology relates to cytogenetic and molecular findings, which are discussed in the next section. Here we discuss general biologic considerations.

The clonal nature of AML is confirmed by the presence of clonal cytogenetic abnormalities[147] and/or molecular abnormalities[148] in the majority of cases. As noted above, in one report, postremission clonal hematopoiesis was identified in ~50% of patients with AML and persisted long-term in ~90% of trackable patients in spite of consolidation and maintenance therapies, but was eradicated in 95% of patients who underwent allo-HSCT.[119] However, postremission clonal hematopoiesis had little effect on relapse risk.

AML cells usually have immunophenotypes that distinguish them from normal myeloid progenitor cells. Abnormalities include asynchronous myeloid antigen expression, antigen overexpression, loss of antigen expression, and coexpression of nonmyeloid antigens.[149] These findings are consistent with aberrant differentiation rather than arrest of normal differentiation. The ability to distinguish AML cells from normal marrow cells based on aberrant immunophenotypes enables detection of residual disease by flow cytometry in many cases.[150-152] Detection of residual or recurrent blasts by multiparameter flow cytometry at diverse time points following therapy predicts adverse outcome.[150,151-155] Immunophenotypes at relapse of AML commonly demonstrate gain or loss of one or more antigens and/or changes in antigen density.[156,157]

The proliferative characteristics of AML cells, including percentage of S-phase cells, S-phase duration and total cell cycle time, are highly variable,[158-160] and proliferation may be either slower or faster than that of normal myeloid cells. A high proliferative rate may be associated with rapid regrowth of leukemia following marrow aplasia after chemotherapy,[159] whereas slowly proliferating AML cells may be chemoresistant.[161]

Resistance to apoptosis induction contributes to both leukemogenesis and drug resistance in AML.[162] Chemotherapy kills malignant cells through activation of mitochondria-mediated apoptosis, and altered apoptotic pathways are a mechanism of resistance to chemotherapy. AML cells overexpress Bcl-2 and other antiapoptotic proteins, including Bcl-x(L), Mcl-1, XIAP, and survivin,[163,164] which may be upregulated by the effects of stromal cells[163] and cytokines.[165] Overexpression of antiapoptotic proteins blocks permeabilization of the mitochondrial outer membrane.[166] Mitochondrial readiness for apoptosis, or "mitochondrial priming," measured by an assay called BH3 profiling, has been shown to be a determinant of both initial response to induction chemotherapy and relapse.[167,168] Moreover, differential priming between malignant myeloblasts and normal hematopoietic stem cells supports a mitochondrial basis for the therapeutic index for chemotherapy.[167] Recent incorporation of the Bcl-2 inhibitor venetoclax into AML treatment regimens has improved treatment efficacy (see section "Targeted Therapies").

It is generally accepted that AML relapse is caused by survival and persistence of rare chemotherapy-resistant leukemia stem cells (LSCs) or leukemia-initiating cells.[169] Transplantation of AML cells into immune-deficient mice demonstrated that LSCs are present at a frequency of 1 in 250,000 cells in the peripheral blood of patients with AML, are usually enriched in the CD34+CD38- cell fraction,[170] and lack expression of CD71 and HLA-DR[171] but express CD123.[172] These cells are primarily nonproliferative.[173]

LSCs cannot be distinguished from normal hematopoietic stem cells based on the CD34+CD38- phenotype,[174] but intermediate levels of aldehyde dehydrogenase (ALDH) enzyme activity can distinguish CD34+CD38− LSCs, capable of engrafting immunodeficient mice, from normal HSCs, which have higher ALDH activity. Presence of CD34+CD38−ALDH^{intermediate} leukemia cells in CR after induction chemotherapy correlates with cytogenetic and molecular risk groups and is associated with subsequent relapse.[175,176]

Deep sequencing of AML cell genomes from patients at diagnosis and at relapse suggested two major clonal evolution patterns at AML relapse: (1) gain of new mutations by the founding clone in the primary tumor or (2) expansion of a subclone of the founding clone surviving initial chemotherapy, with gain of additional mutations.[177] Single-cell RNA sequencing from matched patient diagnosis and relapse samples showed changes in cellular networks involving metabolism, apoptosis, and chemokine signaling during AML progression.[178] Analysis of whole genome sequencing and deep-coverage single-cell RNA sequencing of more than 142,500 high-quality cells from diagnosis and relapse samples from six patients with normal karyotype AML demonstrated that transcriptional changes were significantly correlated with genetic changes, although independent transcriptional adaptation was also observed, suggesting that clonal evolution does not necessarily account for all relevant biological alterations.[179]

CYTOGENETIC ABNORMALITIES

Cytogenetic abnormalities were first described in AML in the 1960s, and with technical improvements, abnormal karyotypes were reported in 55% to 78% of AML cases in adults.[180,181] Approximately 55% of patients with AML with chromosome changes have a single cytogenetic abnormality, including 15% to 20% with gain or loss of a single chromosome as the only change, and the remaining 45% with two or more changes. The most common recurring cytogenetic abnormalities in non-APL AML in adults include t(8;21)(q22;q22.1), resulting in *RUNX1-RUNX1T1* rearrangement; inv(16)(p13.1q22) or t(16;16)(p13.1;q22), resulting in *CBFB-MYH11* rearrangement; t(9;11)(p22;q23), resulting in the *KMT2A-MLLT3* rearrangement; t(6;9)(p23;q34), resulting in *DEK-NUP214* rearrangement; inv(3) (q21q26.2) or t(3;3)(q21;q26.2), resulting in *RPN1-MECOM* rearrangement; and +8, +21, del(5q), −5, and −7.[180] Karyotyping of metaphase spreads is still the primary approach to identification of cytogenetic abnormalities, but refinement by incorporation of next-generation sequencing–based techniques or replacement by these techniques is being explored.[181,182] Whole-genome sequencing of 235 AML patient samples detected all 40 recurrent translocations and 91 copy number alterations that had been identified by cytogenetic analysis[183] and also identified new clinically relevant genomic events in 40 of 235 patients (17%).[183] Prospective sequencing of samples obtained from another 117 consecutive patients with AML provided new genetic information in 29 patients (25%) and altered the risk category for 19 patients (16%).[183]

Correlation of cytogenetic abnormalities and clinicopathologic data led to the recognition of distinct subtypes of AML and helped to identify prognostic groups.[180,184] The best described subtypes of AML are defined by recurring structural chromosome abnormalities, which primarily consist of balanced translocations, tend to correlate with morphology, and are predictive of treatment outcomes.

Approximately 10% of patients with AML present with t(8;21); most are children and young adults. Myeloid sarcoma is common. AML with t(8;21) has blasts with maturation, often with azurophilic granules and occasionally with very large granules (pseudo–Chédiak-Higashi granules),[185] typically with prominent Auer rods, marrow eosinophilia, and cytoplasmic globules and vacuoles (*Figure 76.5*). In addition to myeloid antigens, the natural killer cell–associated antigen CD56 and the B-cell antigen CD19 are frequently expressed.[185] The two genes involved in t(8;21) are *RUNX1* (previously called *AML1*, *CBFα*, and *PEBP2αB*) at 21q22, encoding the α subunit of the heterodimeric transcription factor core binding factor (CBF), and *RUNX1T1* (previously called *ETO* and *MTG8*) at 8q22.[186,187] They form a fusion gene on the derivative chromosome 8, which may be detected even in patients in long-term CR, indicating its low value as a marker for minimal residual disease.[188] t(8;21) usually occurs in de novo AML and generally predicts a favorable outcome, with a >80% CR rate and a long CR duration (5-year DFS 55%-70%), particularly after HiDAC consolidation therapy.[189] Some mutations of the growth factor receptor KIT in t(8;21) AML identify a subgroup of patients with leukocytosis (median 30,000/mm³), a higher incidence of extramedullary disease (33%), and a worse prognosis.[190] Expression of the CD56 antigen on AML cells with t(8;21) is also associated with

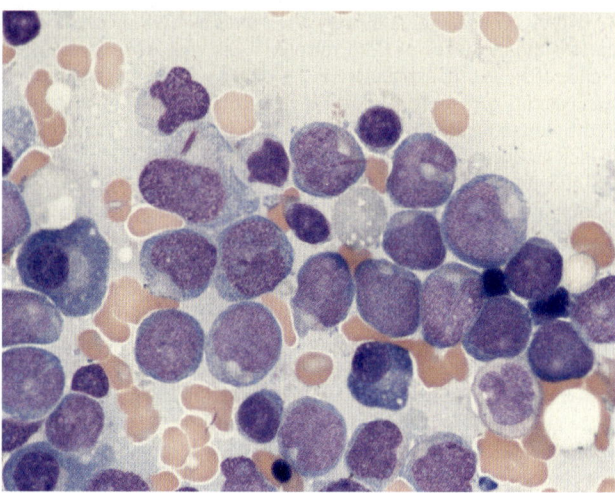

FIGURE 76.5 AML with t(8;21), Wright-stained bone marrow smear. Blasts with maturing myeloid maturation. (Courtesy of Dr. Qing Chen, University of Maryland.)

shorter DFS.[191] Because of high survival rates after multiple cycles of HiDAC consolidation, allo-HSCT is usually reserved for second CR (CR2), although a prospective multicenter study suggested that allo-HSCT can significantly improve clinical outcomes of subsets of patients with t(8;21).[190,192,193]

inv(16) (p13;q22) or t(16;16)(p13.1;q22) is present in approximately 5% to 10% of AML and is associated with peripheral monocytosis and monoblastic infiltration of the bone marrow (*Figure 76.6*). Organomegaly is common, with splenomegaly in 30% of patients. Hyperleukocytosis (>100,000/mm³) is present in 20% to 25% of patients.[194] Extramedullary disease occurs in 20% to 30% of patients.[194] The immature eosinophils have a monocytoid nucleus and a mixture of eosinophilic and large atypical basophilic granules. AML with inv(16) expresses the panmyeloid marker CD13 and the stem cell antigen CD34 and frequently expresses the T-lymphoid marker CD2, along with HLA-DR, with variable expression of other myeloid/monocytic markers, including CD11b, CD11c, CD14, and CD33. The two genes involved are *MYH11*, which encodes the smooth muscle myosin heavy chain, and *CBFβ* (also known as *PEBP2β*), which encodes the β subunit of the heterodimeric transcription factor CBF.[195,196] The 81% to 93% CR rate and 48% to 63% DFS of AML with inv(16) or t(16;16) after induction and HiDAC consolidation represent a better outcome than for most other AML subtypes,[197] so, as with t(8;21), allo-HSCT is usually reserved for

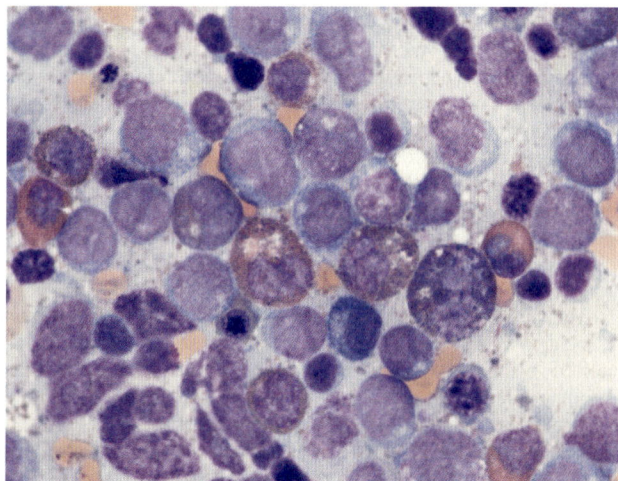

FIGURE 76.6 AML with inv(16), Wright-stained bone marrow smear. In addition to myeloblasts and monoblasts, abnormal eosinophils with large basophilic granules are characteristic of this type of AML. (Courtesy of Dr. Qing Chen, University of Maryland.)

CR2. HiDAC consolidation therapy also serves as CNS prophylaxis and decreases the incidence of CNS relapse.[132] As with AML with t(8;21), presence of some c-*KIT* mutations is associated with an increased relapse rate in patients with AML with inv(16) or t(16;16).[198] MRD can be monitored by quantitative reverse transcription polymerase chain reaction (RT-PCR) to identify patients at increased risk of relapse.[199-201]

11q23 translocations are common in MN-pCT arising following treatment with topoisomerase II inhibitors,[26,42] but they can also occur in de novo AML and are associated with monocytic differentiation. 11q23 translocations are characterized molecularly by rearrangement of the lysine methyltransferase 2A (*KMT2A*) gene (previously called *MLL* and *ALL-1*) at 11q23. *KMT2A* gene rearrangements may arise from aberrant nonhomologous end joining of DNA double-strand breaks. The normal KMT2A protein is proteolytically cleaved and functions as a transcriptional repressor or activator. Chimeric proteins that are generated from *KMT2A* rearrangements include the N-terminal region of KMT2A, which is involved in protein-protein interactions and transcriptional repression.[202] More than 40 different translocation partner genes for *KMT2A* have been identified. In t(9;11), t(10;11), and t(11;19), the amino terminus of the *KMT2A* gene is fused to one of three homologous genes, *AF9*, *AF10*, or *ENL*, from chromosomes 9q22, 10p12, and 19p13, respectively.[203] t(6;11)(q27;q23), resulting in rearrangement of *KMT2A* and the afadin gene (*AFDN*), has a particularly dismal prognosis.[204] In contrast to the short DFS associated with other *KMT2A* translocations, DFS of patients with de novo t(9;11) has varied among studies, placing it in the intermediate prognostic group.[205-207] Allo-HSCT in first CR has resulted in significant improvement in OS and relapse-free survival (RFS) of patients with AML with 11q23 translocations.[208]

t(6;9)(p21;q34) is a rare (<1%) cytogenetic abnormality in AML that is associated with young age, basophilia, FAB M2 or M4 subtype, and poor response to therapy.[209] The genes involved are the *DEK* gene on chromosome 6p23 and the 214-kDa nucleoporin gene, NUP214 (previously *CAN*), on chromosome 9p34.[210] *FLT3*-ITD is frequently present in AML with t(6;9)(p21;q34).[211] Outcomes are poor but are improved by allo-HSCT.[211]

AML with inv(3)(q21q26) or t(3;3)(q21;q26) typically presents with a normal platelet count or thrombocytosis, represents 1% to 3% of de novo AML, may follow MDS, and has a very poor prognosis.[212] In AML with inv(3)/t(3;3), repositioning of a GATA2 enhancer element leads to both overexpression of the MDS1 and EVI1 complex locus protein EVI1 (*MECOM*) gene, formerly called *EVI1* (ecotropic viral integration site 1), and haploinsufficiency of GATA2.[213] Other rare balanced rearrangements involving 3q26 include t(3;21)(q26;q22), t(3;12)(q26;p13), and t(2;3)(p15;22;q26). *MECOM* overexpression is also found in 10% of AML without 3q26 abnormalities and predicts poor treatment outcome.[214]

Structural abnormalities involving chromosomes 5q and/or 7q, monosomy 5 and/or 7, and complex karyotypes, defined by presence of three or more unrelated numerical and/or structural chromosome abnormalities, are frequently seen in AML arising from MDS and in t-AML after alkylating agent therapy.[27,42] These abnormalities, whether in de novo AML or t-AML, are associated with low CR rates and short DFS and OS. Other numerical chromosomal abnormalities associated with poor treatment outcome include +11, +13, and +21.

The monosomal karyotype (MK), defined by the presence of at least two autosomal monosomies or a single monosomy associated with at least one additional structural chromosomal abnormality, is present in approximately 10% of adult AML, increases in incidence with age, and is associated with a particularly dismal prognosis, with less than 5% 4-year OS, compared with approximately 25% in patients with complex, but nonmonosomal, karyotypes.[215] Allo-HSCT has resulted in limited improvement in outcome, to 25% 4-year OS.[216] MK+ AML is associated with deletions or mutations in the *TP53* gene in approximately 70% of patients, leading to a chromosome instability pattern known as chromothripsis, which is particularly associated with dismal prognosis.[217]

Presence of marker chromosomes, which can arise from chromothripsis, or chromosome fragmentation in a single catastrophic event, is particularly associated with dismal prognosis in AML.[217]

MOLECULAR ABNORMALITIES

AML is characterized by recurrent molecular abnormalities that confer constitutive and/or aberrant signaling through one or more pathways in the complex signaling network that regulates hematopoiesis. Genes with recurrent mutations in AML have been categorized into eight functional categories (*Table 76.2*), with an average of five recurrent gene mutations in AML cases.[218,219]

Prognosis in AML, particularly with a normal karyotype, is now routinely assessed with molecular markers.[220,221] Importantly, the therapeutic implications of targeting different signaling pathways are being exploited, with several small molecules and biological agents approved or in development (see "Therapy" section). It is of paramount importance to pay attention to whether specific mutations within each gene are pathogenic, benign, or variants of unknown significance.

FLT3 Mutations

FLT3 (*fms*-like tyrosine kinase 3) is a receptor tyrosine kinase that is expressed on hematopoietic progenitor cells and is activated by binding of FLT3 ligand (FL), inducing dimerization, tyrosine kinase activation, receptor autophosphorylation, and phosphorylation of downstream signaling proteins in the RAS/MAPK and PI3K/Akt pathways, thereby stimulating proliferation and inhibiting apoptosis.[222] FLT3 is expressed on AML cells in most cases, and mutations can be detected by genomic PCR amplification and gel electrophoresis in approximately 30% of cases. The most common *FLT3* mutation, present in approximately 25% of patients with AML,[223-227] is a small in-frame ITD in the *FLT3* gene that results in duplication of an amino acid sequence within the juxtamembrane domain of the receptor, which disrupts its autoinhibitory activity, resulting in constitutive tyrosine kinase activation (*Figure 76.7*).

FLT3-ITD signaling is also aberrant. In addition to activating the RAS/MAPK and PI3K/Akt pathways, *FLT3*-ITD activates signal transducer and activator of transcription (STAT) 5 and downstream effectors, including Pim-1 kinase.[223,228-230] Other effects include myeloid maturation arrest by virtue of suppression of the C/EBPα and PU.1 transcription factors[231] and antiapoptotic effects by virtue of phosphorylation and inactivation of the proapoptotic protein BAD by Pim-1.[232]

FLT3-ITD is associated with high peripheral blast count and normal karyotype. The presence of *FLT3*-ITD does not affect CR rate but predicts high relapse rate and short DFS and thus identifies a poor-risk subset of patients with cytogenetically normal AML.[223-225,233-235]

Table 76.2. Categories of Genes With Recurrent Mutations in AML[218]

Functional Class	Genes	Frequency
Signaling and kinase pathways	*FLT3, KRAS, NRAS, KIT, PTPN11, NF1*	59%
Nucleophosmin	*NPM1*	27%
Tumor suppressors	*TP53, WT1, PHF6*	16%
DNA methylation-related	*DNMT3A, IDH1, IDH2, TET2*	44%
Chromatin modification	*KMT2A, ASXL1, EZH2, KDM6A*	30%
Transcription factors	*CEBPA, RUNX1, GATA2*	18%
Spliceosome complex	*SRSF2, SF3B1, U2AF1, ZRSR2*	14%
Cohesin complex	*RAD21, STAG1, STAG2, SMC1A, SMC3*	13%

Used with permission of American Society of Hematology from DiNardo CD, Cortes JE. Mutations in AML: prognostic and therapeutic implications. *Hematology Am Soc Hematol Educ Program*. 2016;2016(1):348-355; permission conveyed through Copyright Clearance Center, Inc.

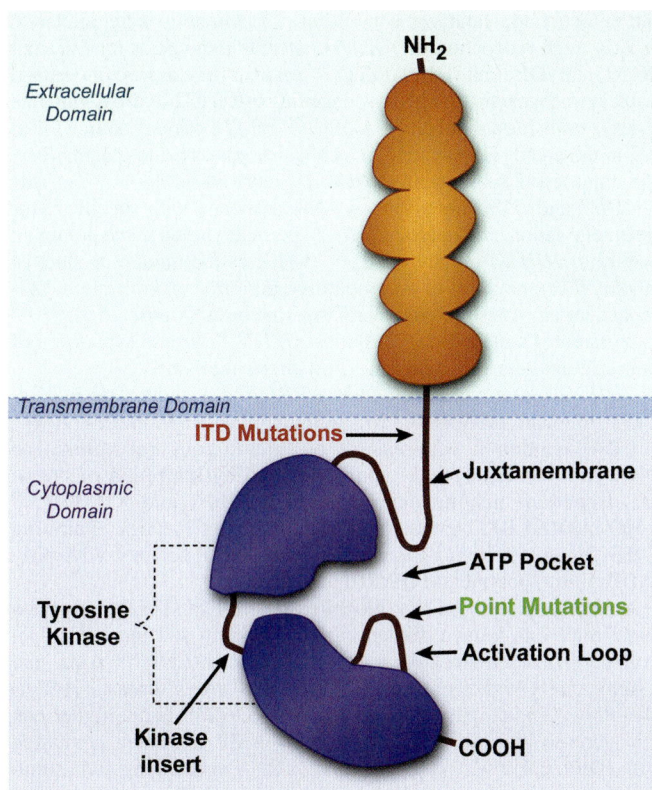

FIGURE 76.7 Simplified diagram of the FLT3 receptor: It contains 993 amino acids and consists of an extracellular ligand-binding domain with five immunoglobulin-like domains, a single transmembrane domain, and a cytoplasmic domain, which comprises a juxtamembrane domain followed by the tyrosine kinase domain. Internal tandem duplications (ITD) in the juxtamembrane domain and point mutations within the activation loop constitutively activate FLT3 signaling. (Drawing by Tim Gilfilen, Medical Art Group, Vanderbilt University.)

Prognosis of patients with *FLT3*-ITD is further worsened by higher ITD to wild-type allelic ratio, or larger base insertion length resulting in larger size of the ITD.[235] Of note, however, when the effect of *FLT3*-ITD/*FLT3* wild type (*FLT3*[wt]) ratio was analyzed in relation to *NPM1* mutation (*NPM1*[mut]) in patients with intermediate-risk karyotype AML treated with intensive chemotherapy, among *NPM1*[mut] patients, *FLT3*[wt] and low ratio (<0.5) subgroups showed similar OS, relapse risk, and leukemia-free survival, whereas high ratio (≥0.5) patients had a worse outcome, while in *NPM1*[wt] AML, *FLT3*-ITD subgroups had a higher risk of relapse and shorter OS than *FLT3*[wt] patients.[236]

FLT3-ITD AML has a high frequency of new structural chromosome abnormalities at relapse, suggesting a role of genomic instability in the genesis of relapse, associated with increased reactive oxygen species–mediated DNA double-strand breaks and error-prone DNA repair.[237] In addition, FL expression increases significantly during induction and consolidation chemotherapy, and AML blasts with *FLT3*-ITD remain highly responsive to FL at relapse, suggesting a potential role of FL in promoting relapse.[238]

Relapse continues to be the main reason for treatment failure in *FLT3*-ITD AML, with a 3-year incidence of approximately 65% with chemotherapy vs approximately 40% with allo-HSCT (see "Hematopoietic Stem Cell Transplantation" section).[239] In multiple studies allo-HSCT in CR1 is significantly associated with superior RFS and OS compared with consolidation chemotherapy in patients with *FLT3*-ITD AML, independent of *FLT3*-ITD allelic ratio and *NPM1* mutation status.[240]

Point mutations in the *FLT3* DNA sequence occur in 5% of AML[227] predominantly in the aspartic acid (D) residue at amino acid position 835, p.Asp835, and in the isoleucine (I) residue at amino acid position 836, p.Ile836,[224] in the tyrosine kinase domain (FLT3-TKD), causing constitutive activation. *FLT3* point mutations are not associated with aberrant signaling[241] and are less prognostically unfavorable than *FLT3*-ITDs.

The FLT3/multikinase inhibitor midostaurin was approved by the FDA for use with chemotherapy in newly diagnosed patients with FLT3 mutations in 2017[242] and the more potent and specific FLT3 inhibitor gilteritinib for relapsed and refractory (R/R) AML with *FLT3* mutations in 2018.[243] These and several other FLT3 inhibitors are currently being evaluated in preclinical studies and in clinical trials in AML in frontline, R/R, and maintenance settings (see "Therapy" section).

NPM1 Mutation

Mutations in exon 12 of the *NPM* or *NPM1* (nucleophosmin) gene are among the most common gene mutations in AML, present in up to half of AML cases with normal karyotypes.[244-247] *NPM1* mutations are associated with prolonged event-free survival (EFS) and OS.[244] Co-occurrence of *NPM1* with *FLT3*-ITD, but not with other mutations, negates their favorable prognosis.[235,245,246,248-250] Nucleophosmin is a nucleocytoplasmic shuttling protein that regulates the p53 tumor suppressor pathway, and *NPM1* mutations in AML cells result in cytoplasmic localization of the protein, which can be demonstrated by immunohistochemistry.[10] The mechanistic roles of *NPM1* in the pathogenesis of AML and in treatment response have not been fully elucidated, and targeted therapies have not been developed.

An RT-PCR assay was used to detect MRD in over 2500 samples obtained from approximately 350 patients with *NPM1*[mut] AML who had undergone intensive treatment in a British clinical trial.[251] Approximately 15% of patients had persistence of NPM1[mut] transcripts in blood after the second chemotherapy cycle, and this was associated with an approximately 5-fold greater risk of relapse and death after 3 years of follow-up, compared with patients without these transcripts. Importantly, relapse could be reliably predicted by a rising level of NPM1[mut] transcripts on serial monitoring of MRD.[251] In another study, 4-year cumulative incidence of relapse after double induction therapy was 53% in RT-PCR-positive patients, compared with 6.5% in patients who achieved NPM1[mut] transcript RT-PCR negativity ($P < .001$), and OS was much longer (90% vs 51%; $P = .001$) in RT-PCR-negative patients.[252]

In a single-center retrospective study of ~9000 patients with de novo AML, of ~6500 samples tested for *NPM1*, ~1980 were *NPM1*-mutated (30%).[253] The *NPM1* mutation was more common in younger (<60 years) compared with older patients (36% vs 27%, $P < .0001$) and was associated with normal karyotype in 87% of patients.[253] Within *NPM1*-mutated patients, the most commonly co-mutated genes were *DNMT3A* (45%), *FLT3*-ITD (41%), *TET2* (23%), *NRAS* (20%), *IDH2* (R140, 19%), and *IDH1* (14%).[253]

TP53 Mutations

The *TP53* gene on chromosome 17p encodes the p53 tumor suppressor protein, which binds to DNA and activates transcription to induce cell cycle arrest, apoptosis, or DNA repair in response to diverse cellular stresses. In unstressed cells, p53 undergoes targeted degradation via MDM2, a substrate recognition factor for ubiquitin-dependent proteolysis. Alterations in *TP53* are oncogenic as they result in loss of function of the protein and gain of transforming potential.[254] Germline mutations in *TP53* cause Li-Fraumeni syndrome, a hereditary cancer predisposition disorder associated with early-onset cancers.[255,256] *TP53* is the most frequently mutated gene in the cancer genome, with mutations in approximately half of all cancers.[257] Approximately two-thirds of *TP53* mutations are missense mutations and several recurrent missense mutations are common, including substitutions at codons R158, R175, R248, R273, and R282.[257,258] Recurrent missense mutations in *TP53* inactivate its ability to bind DNA and activate transcription of target genes.[259-261]

Mutations in the *TP53* gene have a frequency of 10% in de novo AML but a much higher frequency (40%-50%) in t-AML.[35] *TP53* mutations, or *TP53* mutations and 17p loss of heterozygosity combined, have independent negative prognostic effects on survival in AML.[262,263] They are associated with abnormalities of chromosomes

5 and/or 7, and complex karyotypes.[263,264] The chemotherapy response rate in *TP53*-mutated AML is low, and OS is short.[263] Initial efficacy of hypomethylating agents in AML with *TP53* mutation was reported, but OS remains short.[265] In addition, comparison between *TP53*-mutated and *TP53* wild-type bone marrow samples revealed higher expression of IFNG, FOXP3, immune checkpoints, markers of immune senescence, and phosphatidylinositol PI3K-Akt and NF-κB signaling intermediates in the *TP53*-mutated samples, and thus, *TP53* mutation might be a predictive biomarker for response to immunotherapeutics.[264]

MDM2 inhibitors/antagonists are under active investigations as a novel treatment option for AML with wild-type *TP53*.[266,267]

DNA Methylation–Related Genes: *DNMT3A*, *IDH1*, *IDH2*, *TET2*

Chromatin conformation can be impacted by addition of a methyl group to the C-5 position of cytosine. Cytosine methylation occurs when cytosine (C) is followed by guanosine (G) in CpG pairs (p indicates phosphodiester bond). When CpG dinucleotides in the genome cluster together, they form CpG islands, which are located proximal to gene promoter regions or in other intergenic areas. DNA methylation is catalyzed by the DNA methyltransferase (DNMT) family of enzymes, which transfer a methyl group from S-adenosyl methionine to DNA. Hypermethylation of CpG islands in the promoters of tumor suppressor genes is common in many cancers.

In 2010, Ley et al. found mutations in *DNMT3A* in 22% of 281 patients with de novo AML, predominantly with intermediate-risk cytogenetic profiles.[268] The precise effects of these mutations have not yet been elucidated. *FLT3*, *NPM1*, and *IDH1* mutations were significantly enriched in samples with *DNMT3A* mutations. *DNMT3A* mutations were independently associated with shorter median OS (12.3 vs 41.1 months, $P < .001$). In several subsequent studies, *DNMT3A* mutations were present in approximately 20% of older patients with normal-karyotype AML and were associated with higher WBC and platelet counts, and concurrent mutations in the *NPM1*, *FLT3*, and *IDH1* or *IDH2* genes, and were not associated with a lower CR rate, but independently predicted a higher relapse rate and shorter OS.[269-272]

DNMT3A mutations were significantly more frequent in younger patients (51% vs 40%, $P = .0012$); DNMT3A-R882 mutations were more frequent than non-R882 in younger patients (58% vs 42% in patients <60 years), and non-R882 was more common in older patients, compared with R882 (61% vs 39%, $P < .0001$).[253]

TET hydroxylase enzymes are involved in DNA hypomethylation and demethylation by α-ketoglutarate-dependent conversion of 5-methylcytosine to 5-hydroxymethylcytosine (alcohol moiety), followed by further oxidation to 5-formylcytosine (aldehyde moiety) and to 5-carboxylcytosine (acid moiety) (*Figure 76.8*).[273-275] Mutations in the *TET2* gene were identified in 24% of AML with preceding MDS or MPN, or MN-pCT.[276] Heterozygous *TET2* mutations were found in 7.6% of younger adult patients with AML in a subsequent series and were not associated with response to chemotherapy or OS.[277]

Mutations in the isocitrate dehydrogenase genes *IDH1* or *IDH2* (*IDH*mut) are present in approximately 20% of de novo AML,[219] most commonly with a normal karyotype, and are an unfavorable prognostic factor according to most studies.[278-282] While wild-type *IDH* in cytosol and mitochondria catalyzes conversion of isocitrate to α-ketoglutarate (α-KG), with production of NADPH, altered amino acids in *IDH1*mut (R132) and *IDH2*mut (R140 or R172) reside in the catalytic pocket and result in a neoenzymatic activity, converting α-KG to 2-hydroxyglutarate (2-HG), with consumption of NADPH.[283-285] The primary source for α-KG in these cells is glutamine, which is first converted to glutamate by glutaminase and subsequently to α-KG (*Figure 76.8*).[286]

IDH1 and *IDH2* mutations in AML associate with specific cytosine methylation, and aberrant DNA hypermethylation is the dominant feature of *IDH1/2*-mutant AML.[287] 2-HG, as the unique product of mutant *IDH* enzymes, is a competitive inhibitor of multiple α-KG-dependent enzymes including TET hydroxylases (*Figure 76.9*).[288,289] Expression of mutant *IDH1/2* and loss of *TET2* increase expression of stem cell markers and impair myeloid differentiation.[287]

IDH1/2 mutations can induce a BRCAness phenotype in clinically relevant models of different neoplasms, including AML, via 2-HG-induced suppression of homologous recombination DNA double-strand break repair mediated by inhibition of the α-KG-dependent histone demethylases KDM4A and KDM4B.[290] 2-HG-induced BRCAness suggests a treatment strategy exploiting 2-HG-dependent homologous recombination deficiency with poly (ADP-ribose) polymerase (PARP) inhibitors.[290]

It has been reported that global expression of *IDH2*mut in transgenic mice can induce dilated cardiomyopathy and muscular dystrophy.[291] In a retrospective study, patients with *IDH1*mut AML had a significantly higher prevalence of coronary artery disease (26% vs 6%, $P = .002$) and patients with *IDH1*mut/*IDH2*mut had a higher risk for decrease in cardiac function during AML treatment compared with IDH1/IDH2 wild-type patients.[292] RNA sequencing and immunostaining of cardiomyocytes showed that the 2-HG oncometabolite exacerbated anthracycline cardiotoxicity.[292]

The IDH2 inhibitor enasidenib was approved by the FDA in 2017, and the IDH1 inhibitor *ivosidenib in 2018, and a second IDH1 inhibitor, olutasidenib, in 2022*.[293] Several other IDH inhibitors are being evaluated in clinical trials in AML in frontline and R/R settings (see "Therapy" section).

The additional sex comb-like 1 (*ASXL1*) gene encodes an enhancer of trithorax and polycomb proteins that functions as a transcriptional activator or repressor in different cells. *ASXL1* mutations are 5 times more common in older (≥60 years) than in younger patients (16.2% vs 3.2%; $P < .001$) and are associated with wild-type *NPM1*, absence of *FLT3*-ITD and mutated *CEBPA*, and with inferior CR rate, DFS, EFS, and OS in older patients.[294]

Other Mutations

Mutations in the *CEBPA* (CCAAT/enhancer binding protein-alpha) gene,[295] encoding a transcription factor essential for myeloid differentiation, are present in approximately 10% of patients with AML overall and 15% of those with a normal karyotype.[296–297] Mutations at the *CEBPA* C terminus generate dysfunctional proteins, while frameshift mutations in the *CEBPA* N terminus create a dominant negative shorter protein. Biallelic *CEBPA* mutations in AML are associated with better prognosis than unmutated or monoallelic mutated *CEBPA*.[298-300] Presence of biallelic mutated *CEBPA* without other mutations defines a favorable risk category according to 2017 ELN risk stratification.

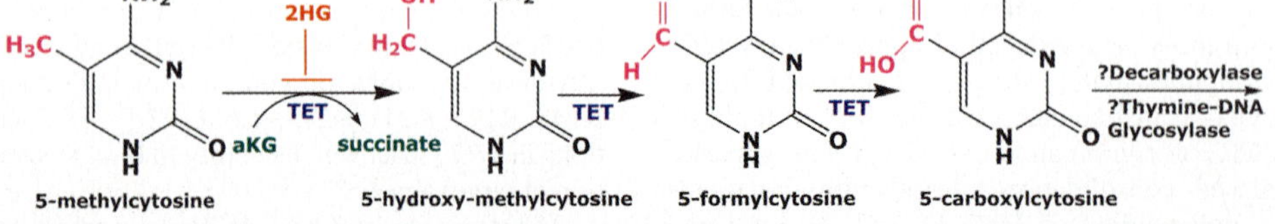

FIGURE 76.8 DNA demethylation reactions mediated by the effect of TET enzymes and 2-HG. 5-Methylcytosine in DNA is partially converted to 5-hydroxymethylcytosine by the TET (ten eleven translocation) dioxygenases. In DNA 5-hydroxymethylcytosines are oxidized to aldehyde (5-formylcytosine) and acid (5-carboxylcytosine) by TET enzymes. TET enzymes use α-KG as coenzyme. 2-HG produced by IDH mutant enzyme inhibits these reactions mediated by TET enzymes. The ultimate outcome is aberrant hypermethylation of DNA. (Drawing by Ashkan Emadi, MD, PhD, University of Maryland Greenebaum Comprehensive Cancer Center.)

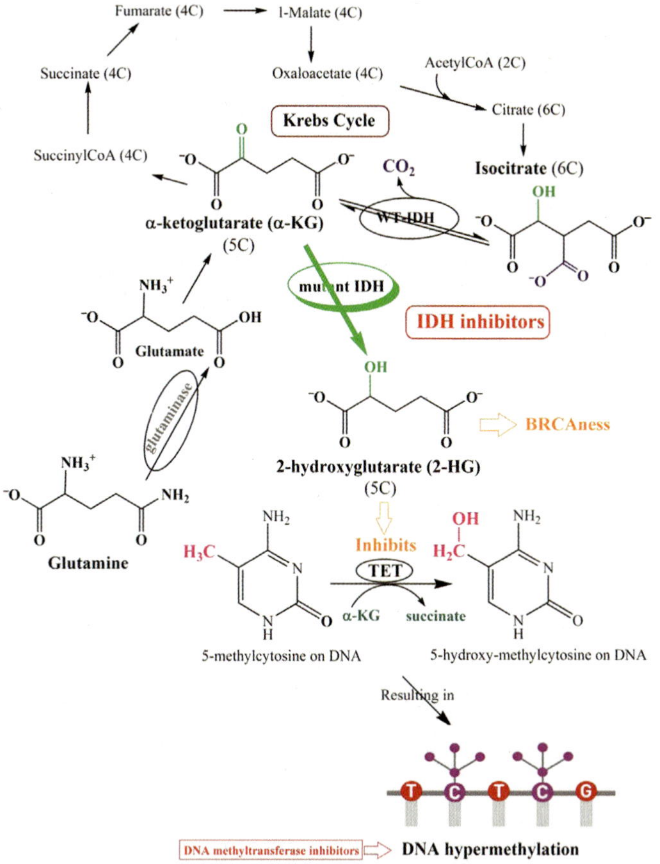

FIGURE 76.9 Biochemical reactions related to wild-type and mutant IDH enzymes. In normal cells, IDH catalyzes loss of one carboxyl (CO_2, purple) group from isocitrate and oxidizes its hydroxyl group (OH, green) to ketone (oxidative decarboxylation). The product is α-KG. The same enzymes can catalyze the conversion of α-KG to isocitrate via a reduction carboxylation reaction. In cells with mutant *IDH*, α-KG cannot be converted to isocitrate, and instead it is reduced to a new molecule, 2-HG. 2-HG is a competitive inhibitor of multiple α-KG-dependent enzymes including histone demethylases, prolyl hydroxylases, and TET hydroxylases. 2-HG also induces a state of BRCAness as manifested by a homologous recombination (HR) defect that makes leukemia cells sensitive to poly(adenosine 5′-diphosphate–ribose) polymerase (PARP) inhibitors. Glutamine is the primary source for α-KG, which is replenished via conversion of glutamine to glutamate by glutaminase. Glutamate can be converted to α-KG either by transamination or by oxidation processes. (Drawing by Ashkan Emadi, MD, PhD, University of Maryland Greenebaum Comprehensive Cancer Center.)

The *KRAS* proto-oncogene encodes a GTPase that functions in signal transduction and is a member of the RAS superfamily, which also includes *NRAS* and *HRAS*. RAS proteins mediate transmission of growth signals from the cell surface to the nucleus via the PI3K/Akt/mTOR and RAS/RAF/MEK/ERK pathways, which regulate cell division, differentiation, and survival.[301-303] *RAS* mutations occur in 10% to 44% of AML, but rarely with *FLT3* mutations, and have not consistently predicted prognosis.[227,233] Activation of the RAS/Raf/MEK/ERK pathway has also been demonstrated in AML, promoting AML cell survival and inhibiting apoptosis.[304,305] Acquired *RAS* mutations are a mechanism of resistance to FLT3 inhibitors.[306] The majority of *KRAS* mutations consist of point mutations occurring at G12, G13, and Q61. Mutations at A59, K117, and A146 have also been observed but are less frequent.[257,307] Currently, no therapies are approved for AML with *KRAS* aberrations. However, the *KRAS* G12C inhibitor sotorasib was granted FDA approval for previously treated patients with non–small cell lung cancer with *KRAS* G12C mutations.

Mutations in the *WT1* (Wilms tumor 1) gene occur in AML in 5% to 10% of patients, with equal distribution in cytogenetically normal and abnormal AML.[308] Both positive[309] and negative[310] prognostic impact of *WT1* gene mutation has been reported in AML. The *WT1* mutation in AML was found to be associated with overexpression of CD96, an LSC-specific marker, and of genes involved in gene regulation (e.g., *KMT2A*, *PML*, and *SNRPN*) and proliferative and metabolic processes (e.g., *INSR*, *IRS2*, and *PRKAA1*).[311]

The *RUNX1* gene, located on chromosome 21 at band q22.12, encodes a transcription factor that is involved in benign and malignant hematopoiesis. The t(8;21) translocation, present in 10% of AML cases, results in a RUNX1 and RUNX1T1 fusion protein. *RUNX1* mutations are identified in 6% to 13% of patients with AML and are more common in older patients and in men. *RUNX1* mutation is a poor prognostic factor, with resistance to chemotherapy and inferior EFS, RFS, and OS.[312-314] Germline RUNX1 mutation is a risk factor for development of AML (discussed in "Risk Factors" section).

KIT, like FLT3, is a receptor tyrosine kinase. Some *KIT* mutations are found in approximately a third of cases of AML with t(8;21) or inv(16) in adults, and their presence is associated with shorter DFS in this otherwise prognostically favorable cytogenetic subset.[315,316] The individual *KIT* mutations have distinct prognoses in adult t(8;21) AML; exon 17 D816 and D820 mutations carry an adverse prognosis, whereas exon 17 N822 and exon 8 mutations have a similar prognosis to wild type.[317] *KIT* mutations have been incorporated into the ELN prognostic classification.[16,318] KIT inhibitors are beginning to be tested in conjunction with chemotherapy in t(8;21) and inv(16) AML.[319]

Table 76.3. 2016 WHO Classification of AML and Related Neoplasms[13]

AML with recurrent genetic abnormalities
AML with t(8;21)(q22;q22.1); RUNX1-RUNX1T1
AML with inv(16)(p13.1q22) or t(16;16)(p13.1;q22); CBFB-MYH11
APL with PML-RARA
AML with t(9;11)(p21.3;q23.3); MLLT3-KMT2A
AML with t(6;9)(p23;q34.1); DEK-NUP214
AML with inv(3)(q21.3q26.2) or t(3;3)(q21.3;q26.2); GATA2, MECOM
AML (megakaryoblastic) with t(1;22)(p13.3;q13.3); RBM15-MKL1
Provisional entity: AML with BCR-ABL1
AML with mutated NPM1
AML with biallelic mutations of CEBPA
Provisional entity: AML with mutated RUNX1
AML with myelodysplasia-related changes
Therapy-related myeloid neoplasms
AML, NOS
AML with minimal differentiation
AML without maturation
AML with maturation
Acute myelomonocytic leukemia
Acute monoblastic/monocytic leukemia
Pure erythroid leukemia
Acute megakaryoblastic leukemia
Acute basophilic leukemia
Acute panmyelosis with myelofibrosis
Myeloid sarcoma
Myeloid proliferations related to Down syndrome
Transient abnormal myelopoiesis
Myeloid leukemia associated with Down syndrome

Reprinted from Arber DA, Orazi A, Hasserjian R, et al. The 2016 revision to the World Health Organization classification of myeloid neoplasms and acute leukemia. *Blood*. 2016;127(20):2391-2405. Copyright © 2016 American Society of Hematology. With permission.

CLASSIFICATION OF ACUTE MYELOID LEUKEMIA

FAB Classification

The FAB classification identified eight subtypes of AML based on morphology and cytochemical staining, with immunophenotypic data in some instances (Chapter 74).[12] Four types (M0, M1, M2, M3) were predominantly granulocytic and differed according to the extent of maturation. M4 was both granulocytic and monocytic, with at least 20% monocytic cells, whereas M5 was predominantly monocytic (at least 80% monocytic cells). M6 showed primarily erythroid differentiation and M7 was acute megakaryocytic leukemia (AMgL), identified by megakaryocyte antigens demonstrated by flow cytometry or immunohistochemistry.

World Health Organization Classification

The WHO classification evolved from the FAB classification to also include clinical, immunophenotypic, cytogenetic, and, most recently, molecular features.[13,14,320,321] Importantly, AML is defined by presence of 20% or more blasts, thus including cases with 20% to 30% blasts, which were categorized as MDS in the FAB classification.[322] In addition, in the WHO classification presence of recurrent cytogenetic abnormalities that are characteristic of AML, including (8;21)(q22;q22), inv(16)(p13;q22) or t(16;16)(p13q22), t(15;17)(q22;q12), or translocations involving 11q23, established the diagnosis of AML, even if the bone marrow contains less than 20% blasts (*Table 76.3*). In 2022, characteristic rearrangements involving *KMT2A*, *MECOM* and *NUP98* were added. The 2022 WHO classification recognizes the following categories: AML with recurrent genetic abnormalities, AML with myelodysplasia-related changes, MN-pCT, and AML not otherwise categorized (NOS), with morphologic subtypes, and myeloid sarcoma and myeloid proliferations related to Down syndrome. AML, myelodysplasia-related (AML-MR), previously called AML with myelodysplasia-related changes (AML-MRC), is defined as a neoplasm with ≥20% blasts expressing a myeloid immunophenotype and harboring specific cytogenetic and molecular abnormalities associated with MDS, arising de novo or following a known history of MDS or MDS/MPN. Myelodysplasia-related cytogenetic abnormalities include complex karyotype, −5/del(5q), −7/del(7q), del(11q), del(12p) and −13/del(13q) del(17p)/i(17q) and idic(X)(q13). Myelodysplasia-related molecular abnormalities include mutations in a set of 8 genes—*SRSF2*, *SF3B1*, *U2AF1*, *ZRSR2*, *ASXL1*, *EZH2*, *BCOR* or *STAG2*.

International Consensus Classification of Myeloid Neoplasms and Acute Leukemias

The International Consensus Classification of Myeloid Neoplasms and Acute Leukemias (ICC) was also published in 2022,[15] also to integrate morphologic, clinical, and genomic data.

European LeukemiaNet Classification

The ELN classification of AML was initially published in 2010 and was updated in 2017 and 2022 publication.[16,17,318] This classification, which has been widely adopted, integrates cytogenetic and molecular data to define favorable, intermediate, and unfavorable genetic groups. It has evolved and will undoubtedly continue to as knowledge accumulates about the significance of cytogenetic and molecular changes and the relative benefits of novel therapies. The 2017 classification is shown in *Table 76.4*.

PROGNOSIS

Prognostic factors affecting the OS of patients with AML include patient-specific and disease-specific features.

Patient-specific Prognostic Factors

Age is a powerful patient-specific prognostic factor, with older adults (65 years or older) having worse outcomes than younger adults.[323]

Table 76.4. 2017 ELN Risk Stratification by Genetics[16,a]

Favorable	t(8;21)(q22;q22.1); *RUNX1-RUNX1T1*
	inv(16)(p13.1q22) or t(16;16)(p13.1;q22); *CBFB-MYH11*
	Mutated *NPM1* without *FLT3*-ITD or with *FLT3*-ITD^{lowb}
	Biallelic mutated *CEBPA*
Intermediate	Mutated *NPM1* and *FLT3*-ITD^{highb}
	Wild-type *NPM1* without *FLT3*-ITD or with *FLT3*-ITD^{lowb} (without adverse-risk genetic lesions)
	t(9;11)(p21.3;q23.3); *MLLT3-KMT2A*^{c}
	Cytogenetic abnormalities not classified as favorable or adverse
Adverse	t(6;9)(p23;q34.1); *DEK-NUP214*
	t(v;11q23.3); *KMT2A* rearranged
	t(9;22)(q34.1;q11.2); *BCR-ABL1*
	inv(3)(q21.3q26.2) or t(3;3)(q21.3; q26.2); *GATA2,MECOM(EVI1)*
	−5 or del(5q); −7; −17/abn(17p)
	Complex karyotype,^{d} monosomal karyotype^e
	Wild-type *NPM1* and *FLT3*-ITD^{highb}
	Mutated *RUNX1*^{f}
	Mutated *ASXL1*^{f}
	Mutated *TP53*^{g}

^{a}Prognostic impact of a marker is treatment-dependent and may change with new therapies.
^{b}Low, low allelic ratio (<0.5); high, high allelic ratio (≥0.5); semiquantitative assessment of FLT3-ITD allelic ratio (using DNA fragment analysis) is determined as ratio of the area under the curve "FLT3-ITD" divided by area under the curve "FLT3-wild type"; recent studies indicate that AML with NPM1 mutation and FLT3-ITD low allelic ratio may also have a more favorable prognosis and patients should not routinely be assigned to allogeneic HCT.
^{c}The presence of t(9;11)(p21.3;q23.3) takes precedence over rare, concurrent adverse-risk gene mutations.
^{d}Three or more unrelated chromosome abnormalities in the absence of one of the WHO-designated recurring translocations or inversions, that is, t(8;21), inv(16) or t(16;16), t(9;11), t(v;11)(v;q23.3), t(6;9), inv(3) or t(3;3); AML with BCR-ABL1.
^{e}Defined by the presence of one single monosomy (excluding loss of X or Y) in association with at least one additional monosomy or structural chromosome abnormality (excluding core-binding factor AML).
^{f}These markers should not be used as an adverse prognostic marker if they co-occur with favorable-risk AML subtypes.
^{g}TP53 mutations are significantly associated with AML with complex and monosomal karyotype.

Figure 76.10 summarizes percent of deaths by age group for AML in the United States.[20] The median age at death for AML is 73 years.[20]

The clinical state of the patient, as reflected in performance status and comorbid conditions, also affects outcome.[324] A diminished capability to perform activities of daily living (Barthel Index) was reported to be independently correlated with decreased OS in patients with AML or high-risk MDS treated with either DNA methyltransferase inhibitors or best supportive care.[325]

In a comparison of survival between ~25,500 non-Hispanic white and black adults with AML using SEER data and ~1300 black and white patients with AML treated on frontline Alliance for Clinical Trials in Oncology clinical trials, black patients had shorter OS than white patients in both databases. Black race was an independent prognostic factor for poor survival. The disparity between black and white patients was especially pronounced in black patients younger than 60 years, after adjusting for socioeconomic (SEER) and molecular (Alliance) factors.[326]

Cytogenetic and Molecular Prognostic Factors

Chromosomal aberrations are the strongest leukemia-related risk factors for outcome of patients with AML after conventional intensive

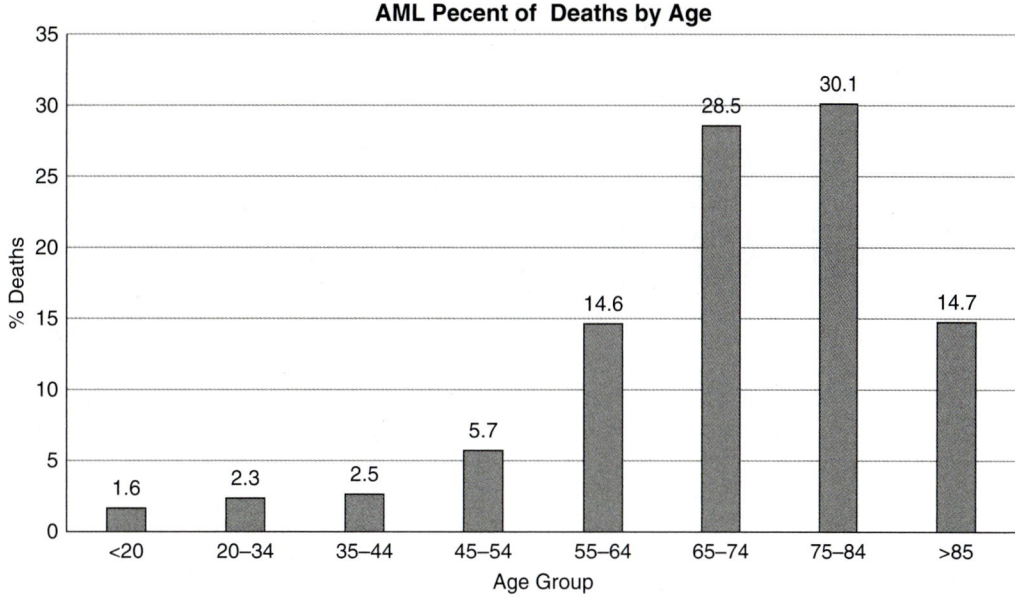

FIGURE 76.10 Percent of AML deaths by age in the United States.[20]

chemotherapy. Balanced translocations involving the CBF transcription factors, including t(8;21), inv(16), and t(16;16), confer favorable risk. In a study of approximately 6000 patients with AML,[327] the following chromosomal aberrations were correlated with poorer outcomes: abnormal(3q) (excluding t(3;5)(q25;q34)), inv(3)(q21q26)/t(3;3)(q21;q26), abnormal(5q)/del(5q), −5, −7, abnormal(7q)/del(7q), t(v;11q23) (excluding t(9;11)(p21-22;q23) and t(11;19)(q23;p13)), t(9;22)(q34;q11), −17, abnormal(17p) and complex cytogenetic abnormalities with at least three unrelated aberrations excluding t(8;21), inv(16), and t(16;16). MK, defined by presence of at least two autosomal monosomies or a single monosomy associated with at least one additional structural abnormality, is also a strong adverse prognostic factor, independent of the presence of a complex karyotype.[328]

Molecular abnormalities are also strong prognostic and predictive biomarkers in AML, especially with normal karyotype. Based on patterns of co-mutation in 1540 patients with AML, Papaemmanuil and coworkers established a Bayesian statistical model to categorize AML into 12 subtypes (Table 76.5) that are mutually exclusive, each with distinct diagnostic features and clinical outcomes (Figure 76.11).[148] They identified 5234 driver mutations in 76 genes or genomic regions, with ≥2 drivers identified in 86% of the patients. In addition to already defined AML subtypes, three heterogeneous genomic categories emerged: AML with mutations in genes encoding chromatin, RNA-splicing regulators, or both (18% of patients); AML with TP53 mutations, chromosomal aneuploidies, or both (13% of patients); and AML with IDH2-R172 mutations (1% of patients). Patients with chromatin-spliceosome and TP53-aneuploidy AML had poor outcomes, with the

Table 76.5. Main Genomic Subtypes of AML (Left Column) With Frequency (%) of Specific Co-occurring Gene Mutations or Genetic Abnormalities (Right Column)

Genomically Determined AMLs	Accompanied Gene Mutations or Genetic Abnormalities (% Co-occurrence)
Favorable	
AML with t(15;17)(q22; q12); PML-RARA	FLT3-ITD (35), WT1 (17)
AML with inv(16) (p13.1q22) or t(16;16) (p13.1;q22); CBFB-MYH11	NRAS (53), +8/8q (16), +22 (16), KIT (15), FLT3-TKD (15)
AML with t(8;21)(q22; q22); RUNX1-RUNX1T1	KIT (38), −Y (33), −9q (18)
AML with biallelic CEBPA mutations	NRAS (30), WT1 (21), GATA2 (20)
AML with NPM1 mutation	DNMT3A (54), FLT3-ITD (39), NRAS (19), TET2 (16), PTPN11 (15)
AML with IDH2-R172 mutations and no other class-defining lesions	DNMT3A (67), +8/8q (17)
Unfavorable	
AML with TP53 mutations, chromosomal aneuploidy, or both	Complex karyotype (68), −5/5q (47), −7/7q (44), TP53 (44), −17/17p (31), −12/12p (17), +8/8q (16)
AML with mutated chromatin, RNA-splicing genes, or both	RUNX1 (39), MLL-PTD (25), SRSF2 (22), DNMT3A (20), ASXL1 (17), STAG2 (16), NRAS (16), TET2 (15), FLT3-ITD (15)
AML with MLL fusion genes; t(x;11)(x;q23)	NRAS (23)
AML with inv(3) (q21q26.2) or t(3;3) (q21;q26.2); GATA2, MECOM(EVI1)	−7 (85), KRAS (30), NRAS (30), PTPN11 (30), ETV6 (15), PHF6 (15), SF3B1 (15)
AML with t(6;9)(p23; q34); DEK-NUP214	FLT3-ITD (80), KRAS (20)
AML with driver mutations but no detected class-defining lesions	FLT3-ITD (39), DNMT3A (16)

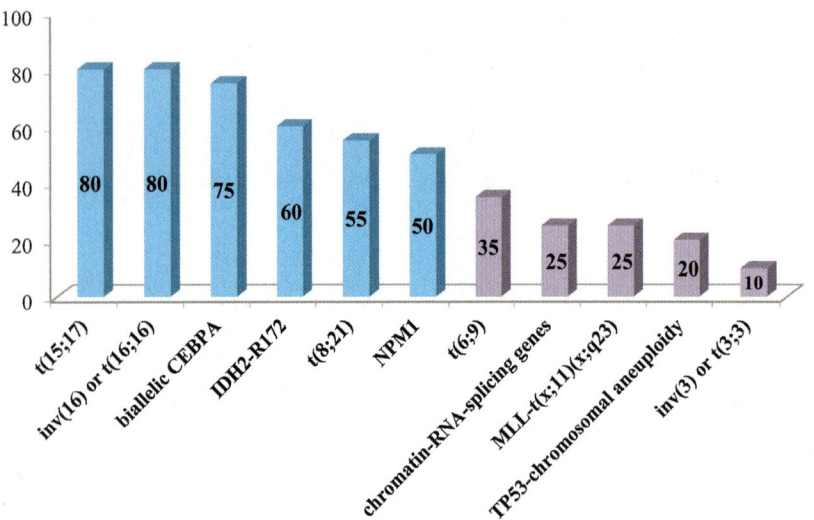

FIGURE 76.11 Probability of 6-year overall survival of patients with AML on the basis of genomically determined subgroup.[148] (Drawing by Ashkan Emadi, MD, PhD, University of Maryland Greenebaum Comprehensive Cancer Center.)

various class-defining mutations contributing independently and additively to outcome (*Figure 76.11*; *Table 76.5*).

Table 76.6 demonstrates an example of the interplay among four commonly mutated genes (*FLT3*-ITD, *NRAS*, *NPM1*, *DNMT3A*) in adult patients with AML and how they influence OS. For example, in *NPM1* wild-type AML, regardless of *DNMT3A* mutational status, presence or absence of *FLT3*-ITD or *NRAS* does not affect the 6-year OS. On the other hand, the 6-year OS in *NPM1* and *DNMT3A* mutant AML with *FLT3*-ITD is 20%, compared with 60% in the absence of *FLT3*-ITD.

Other Disease-Specific Prognostic Factors

Patients with secondary AML, defined by a preceding bone marrow disorder, including MDS or MPN, or with t-AML, have inferior response and survival compared with those with de novo AML.[329,330] Morphologic dysplasia is unfavorable, likely by virtue of association with unfavorable karyotypes.[331] Hyperleukocytosis correlates with shorter OS[332] due to both increased induction deaths[333] and association with *FLT3*-ITD.[227]

Measurable (Minimal) Residual Disease as a Prognostic Factor

MRD detection by multiparameter flow cytometry assessment of leukemia-associated immunophenotype (LAIP) is a sensitive assay and is approaching readiness for use in clinical practice. Buccisano and colleagues detected LAIPs in 86% of 143 adult patients with AML at diagnosis, and MRD status detected by flow cytometry after consolidation therapy was associated with survival in patients with favorable or intermediate cytogenetic risk.[334] These investigators then studied 135 consecutive adult patients with de novo AML. LAIPs were detected by multiparameter flow cytometry in 120 patients (89%) at presentation, with 100 (83%) achieving morphologic CR after induction and undergoing MRD monitoring. A cutoff value of 0.035% residual leukemia cells was used to discriminate MRD-negative from MRD-positive cases after both induction and consolidation. After induction 35% of patients (35/100) were MRD-negative and 65% (65/100) were MRD-positive, predicting relapse, RFS, and OS. In another study, adult patients with AML in CR but with an MRD level >0.1% after induction therapy were at high risk of relapse in a multivariate analysis.[335] MRD by flow cytometry in patients with AML in CR or CRi before allo-HSCT was independently associated with shorter OS following transplantation.[336]

MRD by RT-PCR has also been extensively investigated, with most of the known abnormalities currently lacking strong clinical correlations with the assays in use. In CBF leukemias, <3-log reduction in MRD level after induction and one cycle of consolidation compared with diagnosis was an independent prognostic factor for relapse in a prospective French intergroup trial.[337] PCR negativity for NPM1 post induction and upon completion of therapy was demonstrated to be a favorable prognostic factor, with superior OS.[252] Cutoff levels of >1 mutant NPM1 copy per 100 ABL1 copies after chemotherapy and >10 mutant NPM1 copies per 100 ABL1 copies after allo-HSCT were independently associated with poorer survival.[338]

THERAPY

Initial Management

Before initiation of therapy, diagnosis must be conclusively established. Diagnostic studies must include immunophenotyping, which will also enable future measurements of MRD by flow cytometry in most cases. In addition, AML samples must be sent for cytogenetic

Table 76.6. The Effect of Presence or Absence of *FLT3*-ITD or *NRAS* Codon 12/13 Mutations on Approximate 6-Year Overall Survival (%) of Patients With AML With Wild Type (WT) or Mutant *NPM1* or *DNMT3A*

			NPM1			
			Wild Type		Mutant	
			DNMT3A			
			Wild Type	Mutant	Wild Type	Mutant
FLT3-ITD	Present		No effect (*P* = .1) (40%)	No effect (*P* = .9) (25%)	40%	20%
	Absent				55% (*P* = .2)	60% (*P* = .009)
NRAS G12/13	present		No effect (*P* = .8) (40%)	No effect (*P* = 1.0) (30%)	60% (*P* = .5)	75% (*P* = .0007)
	absent				50%	40%

analysis and myeloid mutation studies. In many instances cytogenetic data will be used in the choice of initial therapy; notably, the safety of awaiting cytogenetic data to choose intensive vs nonintensive initial therapy in older patients with AML has been demonstrated.[339] A Leukemia and Lymphoma Society–sponsored clinical trial, Beat AML, confirmed the feasibility of using rapid (7-day) molecular, as well as cytogenetic, testing to enable stratified/molecularly targeted therapy in newly diagnosed older patients with AML.[340] For younger patients, rapidly testing for *FLT3* mutations enables use of a FLT3 inhibitor with induction and consolidation chemotherapy, with midostaurin having been FDA-approved in this setting.[341] Pretreatment cytogenetic and molecular data will also be used to assist in decisions about allo-HSCT following response to initial therapy and to determine eligibility for clinical trials of molecularly targeted therapies in patients who do not respond to initial therapy. Blood should also be sent for HLA typing for all patients who are potential candidates for allo-HSCT.

Patients' performance status and pretreatment comorbidities should be assessed and recorded in order to assist in decisions about therapeutic approach, especially in older patients, and potential eligibility for allo-HSCT. There is consensus about the importance of these assessments, but there is not a uniform approach to performing them.[342] Social support is also an important component of initial assessment.

In patients with hyperleukocytosis, the WBC count must be rapidly lowered to minimize the risk of leukostasis. Therapeutic measures include administration of large doses (e.g., 6 g daily) of hydroxycarbamide (hydroxyurea), leukapheresis, and rapid initiation of induction therapy.[220,343,344] No controlled clinical trials have defined the optimal management of hyperleukocytosis, but some retrospective data support the use of leukapheresis.[345] Some studies suggest that leukapheresis is associated with decreased early mortality and improved CR rates but not with improved survival.[344,346] A systematic review and meta-analysis of 13 two-arm, retrospective studies with 1743 patients (486 leukapheresis and 1257 nonleukapheresis patients) did not find evidence of a short-term mortality benefit for leukapheresis.[347] A large, multicenter, international study with the aim of investigating the short- and long-term clinical outcomes of leukapheresis in patients with AML retrospectively collected data from 779 patients with newly diagnosed AML with WBC >50,000/mm^3 who presented to 12 centers in the United States and Europe from 2006 to 2017 and received intensive chemotherapy.[348] Clinical leukostasis was reported in 27% of patients, and leukapheresis was used in 113 patients (15%). Use of leukapheresis did not significantly impact 30-day mortality, achievement of composite CR, or OS in multivariate analysis based on available data or in analysis based on multiple imputation.[348] Owing to temporary impact, lack of improvement of survival, and associated complications and logistic burden, the routine use of leukapheresis was not recommended; hydroxyurea should be administered, and induction therapy should be initiated as rapidly as possible.[120]

Red blood cell transfusions should be minimized initially in patients with hyperleukocytosis, as overcorrection of the hemoglobin level may increase blood viscosity and worsen leukostasis. A hemoglobin goal of 7 to 8 g/dL, but not higher, is generally appropriate. In contrast, platelet transfusions are needed to decrease the risk of hemorrhage, especially because the platelet count may be overestimated in the setting of hyperleukocytosis, as blast cell fragments may be counted as platelets. In addition, patients with hyperleukocytosis may also have DIC. An initial platelet count goal of 50,000/mm^3 is optimal in the setting of hyperleukocytosis and/or DIC. Patients who present with hyperleukocytosis frequently have *FLT3*-ITD and may have a higher risk of relapse following initial response to therapy even in the absence of *FLT3*-ITD.[349] These patients should be rapidly characterized with regard to presence of *FLT3*-ITD, and they should also be HLA-typed at diagnosis and should be evaluated for allo-HSCT.

Endpoints of AML Treatment

In patients receiving remission induction chemotherapy, early assessment of efficacy is performed by sampling the bone marrow approximately 14 days following initiation of chemotherapy, during pancytopenia. The morphologic leukemia-free state[350] desired at this time point is defined by presence of <5% blasts in an aspirate sample with marrow spicules and with a count of at least 200 nucleated cells and absence of blasts with Auer rods. A bone marrow biopsy performed at the same time allows bone marrow cellularity to be determined and allows evaluation for clusters of blasts. Patients with clear residual AML at the time of early assessment are unlikely to go on to achieve remission, and additional or alternative therapy should be considered. Persistent detection of AML cells with the pretreatment phenotype by flow cytometry in bone marrow that is morphologically leukemia-free is considered persistence of leukemia, although therapeutic decisions about reinduction therapy in clinical trials have generally not been based on flow cytometry findings. If presence of residual leukemia is questionable, a bone marrow aspirate and biopsy should be repeated approximately 7 days later.[350]

Peripheral blood blast clearance within 6 days after starting conventional cytotoxic induction therapy has also been suggested to be independently associated with improved survival.[351] A retrospective study of 164 patients with AML undergoing induction with cytarabine and anthracycline and with detectable peripheral blood blasts at diagnosis investigated the rate of clearance of peripheral blood blasts as an early measure of chemosensitivity.[352] Peripheral blood blast rate of clearance (PBB-RC) was defined as the percentage of the absolute peripheral blood blast count on the day of diagnosis that was cleared with each day of therapy, on average, until day 14 or the day of peripheral blood blast clearance.[352] Each 5% increase in PBB-RC approximately doubled the likelihood of day 14 bone marrow clearance (OR = 1.81; 95% CI: 1.24-2.64, $P < .005$). PBB-RC was also associated with improved CR rates (OR per 5% = 1.97; 95% CI: 1.27-3.01, $P < .005$) and OS (HR per 5% = 0.67; 95% CI: 0.52-0.87). The study concluded that PBB-RC during induction chemotherapy is predictive of day 14 bone marrow clearance, CR, and OS and can therefore serve as a prognostic marker for clinical outcomes in AML.[352]

The definition of CR has evolved.[350] The term CR generally refers to morphologic CR, defined by presence of <5% blasts by morphological examination of a bone marrow aspirate sample with marrow spicules and with a count of at least 200 nucleated cells, and absolute neutrophil count (ANC) ≥ 1000/mm^3, platelet count ≥100,000/mm^3, absence of leukemic blasts in the peripheral blood by morphological examination, and absence of extramedullary leukemia. For response assessment of extramedullary disease, imaging and invasive testing should be limited to sites involved by AML at baseline that cannot be evaluated by physical examination. The date of marrow sampling demonstrating CR is assigned as the CR date. In clinical trials, absence of data is generally considered failure to achieve CR.[353] Hematological relapse is defined as marrow blasts >5% by morphology, reappearance of blasts in the peripheral blood by morphology, or development of extramedullary disease. The duration of remission is defined as the time from CR to hematological relapse or death from any cause, whichever comes first.

CR with partial hematological recovery (CRh) was first introduced in 2014 with the accelerated approval of blinatumomab for treatment of relapsed or refractory CD19-positive B-cell ALL.[354] CRh defines the absence of leukemia and adequate neutrophil and platelet recovery as a functionally important endpoint. CRh is defined by <5% bone marrow blasts by morphological examination, absence of leukemic blasts in the peripheral blood by morphological examination, absence of extramedullary leukemia, and presence of *both* ANC ≥500/mm^3 and platelet count ≥50,000/mm^3. CRh as a clinical endpoint may be particularly applicable to molecularly targeted agents (e.g., *FLT3, IDH1, IDH2* inhibitors). CRh might be used as a palliative endpoint, and in this context the actual endpoint is CR + CRh, and adequate follow-up is required to establish meaningful duration of CR + CRh.[353]

Complete remission with incomplete recovery (CRi) is defined as <5% bone marrow blasts, no evidence of extramedullary disease, absence of blasts in the peripheral blood by morphologic examination, and ANC ≥1000/mm^3 or platelet count ≥100,000/mm^3. It is important to note that there is no lower limit of ANC or platelet counts for CRi. For example, a patient with <5% bone marrow blasts and no evidence of disease elsewhere and neutrophil count greater than 1000/mm^3

but platelet count less than 10,000/mm³ is in CRi, even though the patient is platelet transfusion-dependent and is at significant risk for a hemorrhagic event. Also, a patient with <5% bone marrow blasts and no evidence of disease elsewhere and platelet count ≥100,000/mm³ but neutrophil count less than 100/mm³ is in CRi, even though the patient is severely neutropenic and is at significant risk of infectious complications. Similarly, complete remission with incomplete platelet recovery (CRp) is defined as CR but with residual thrombocytopenia with platelet count <100,000/mm³, with no lower limit for the platelet count. Generally, regulatory agencies do not consider CRi or CRp as acceptable endpoints for drug approval.

Cytogenetic remission (CRc) has been proposed as a separate category of CR, indicating reversion to a normal marrow karyotype at CR in patients with an abnormal karyotype at diagnosis of AML.[350] Persistence of abnormal metaphases in morphologically normal marrows of patients with AML following recovery from induction chemotherapy is associated with relapse and with shorter survival.[355] It is important to specify how many metaphases were examined.

Molecular CR (CRm) is also relevant in some subtypes of AML. The prognostic significance of CRm achievement determined by PCR is clearly established for APL with *PML-RARα*,[356,357] and CRm is recognized as a therapeutic objective in APL. In contrast, the significance of CRm in the subsets of AML is still controversial, particularly in AML with t(8;21), in which *RUNX1-RUNX1T1* transcripts may continue to be detected in patients in long-term morphologic CR.[358] It is important to establish and specify the sensitivities of assays used in assessing CRm. Analysis of comprehensive genomic data from 71 patients with AML by whole-genome or exome sequencing and targeted deep sequencing showed that detection of persistent leukemia-associated mutations in at least 5% of marrow cells in day 30 CR samples was associated with a significantly increased risk of relapse and shorter OS.[359]

Partial remission (PR) is defined by attainment of the blood count criteria for CR, and a decrease of at least 50% in the percentage of blasts in the bone marrow aspirate, to 5% to 25%, or less than 5% blasts in the marrow with presence of Auer rods.[350] As with CRi and CRp, PR is not considered an acceptable endpoint for drug approval by the regulatory agencies.[353]

Transfusion independence, defined as the absence of red blood cell and platelet transfusions for a prespecified period of time during continued treatment, is a palliative endpoint that has been utilized for approval of drugs that are relatively nontoxic and nonmyelosuppressive.[353] Transfusion independence should be durable and be supported by evidence showing an impact of the treatment on the endpoint, reflecting antileukemic activity. Transfusion independence should be evaluated as a response achieved in the subgroup of patients who were transfusion-dependent at baseline (i.e., conversion from transfusion dependence to transfusion independence with treatment) separately from the subgroup of patients who were transfusion-independent at baseline (i.e., maintenance of transfusion independence with treatment). Transfusion dependence at baseline is based on the receipt of any packed red blood cell or platelet transfusions within at least 4 weeks prior to the start of anti-AML therapy.

Patients are assessed for response to induction chemotherapy at the time of blood count recovery. Induction treatment failure is defined as failure to achieve morphological CR.[353] Remission induction treatment failure can be divided into at least three categories (*Table 76.7*).[350] Patients who survive at least 7 days after completion of treatment and have persistent AML in marrow and/or blood are said to have treatment failure due to drug resistance. In addition, relative drug resistance is defined by marrow aplasia but subsequent regrowth of leukemia within 4 to 6 weeks. Patients who survive at least 7 days after completion of treatment and die while cytopenic and with a posttreatment marrow demonstrating aplasia or hypoplasia within 7 days of death are said to have treatment failure due to hypoplastic death. In addition, regeneration failure is defined by marrow hypocellularity persisting for >42 days. Finally, patients with treatment failure of indeterminate cause include those who die less than 7 days after completion of treatment, die 7 or more days after completion of treatment whose blood did not show persistent leukemia and whose marrow was not examined post treatment, or die without completing treatment.

Time-to-event efficacy endpoints used commonly for AML clinical trials include OS, EFS, and RFS. OS is defined as the time from start of treatment or time of pretreatment randomization to the date of death from any cause. EFS is defined as the time from start of treatment or pretreatment randomization to the date of induction treatment failure, relapse for those who have induction therapy success (e.g., CR), or death from any cause, whichever comes first. For patients who are alive and in remission at the data cutoff, EFS should be censored at the last assessment date. RFS is defined as the time from start of treatment or time of pretreatment randomization to the date of relapse or the date of death from any cause, whichever comes first. For patients alive and in remission at the data cutoff, RFS should be censored at the last assessment date. RFS may be an acceptable endpoint in studies of consolidation or maintenance treatments.

Table 76.7. Types of Failure in Therapy for Acute Myeloid Leukemia

Drug resistance
No response based on persistence of blasts and absence of hypocellularity (usually day 14)
Relative drug resistance: subsequent regrowth of leukemia within 4-6 wk
Complications from aplasia
Regeneration failure: marrow remains hypocellular for >6 wk
Hypoplastic death (within 4 wk)
Indeterminate cause of death if death occurs within 2-3 wk of initiating therapy
Hematologic remission but persistent disease
Myelodysplasia, extramedullary disease; cytogenetic, flow cytometric, or molecular disease

Overview of Treatment

For 5 decades, the standard treatment of patients with AML has been conventional intensive cytotoxic chemotherapy for induction and consolidation, with or without postremission allo-HSCT. The only intent of treatment was cure. Long-term remission and cure are feasible for a fraction of patients with AML and, indeed, in recent years the cure rate has increased with cytotoxic agents with or without targeted or immunotherapeutic agents, with or without allo-HSCT (see "Epidemiology" section). However, for many patients with AML with poor performance status or organ impairment at diagnosis, cytotoxic chemotherapy is considered to be associated with excessive risk of inducing life-threatening or fatal complications. In the past, older or medically unfit patients were offered only palliative treatments or no treatment at all. However, in the last 2 decades, the advent of less toxic and better tolerated new classes of anti-AML therapeutics targeting epigenetic alterations or particular genomic mutations has provided alternatives to cytotoxic drugs for the treatment of AML. These newer therapies may extend survival without expectation of cure. Improving survival can be a meaningful benefit for patients who would live for only days or weeks without treatment. This approach also extends to patients who might tolerate intensive chemotherapy but are unlikely to respond due to adverse cytogenetic and/or molecular changes.

Treatment of AML with cytotoxic therapy is divided into two phases, remission induction therapy and postremission therapy (*Figure 76.12*). The goal of induction therapy is attainment of a CR, which, except in APL, usually requires a period of marrow aplasia, or a "morphologic leukemia-free state," following chemotherapy. Serial changes in peripheral blood counts during induction therapy include clearance of blasts from the blood, followed by pancytopenia requiring red blood cell and platelet transfusion support and management of complications of neutropenia, followed by increases in neutrophil and platelet counts and eventual resolution of anemia.

Chapter 76: Acute Myeloid Leukemia in Adults

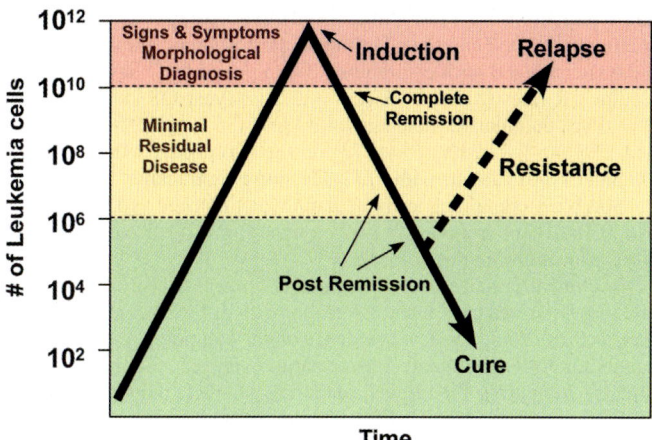

FIGURE 76.12 Phases of therapy. The diagnosis of AML can be made when the leukemia cell number is >10^{10} in the body. Induction therapy achieves a morphologic CR and is followed by postremission therapy with the goal of cure. If cells develop mechanisms of resistance, relapse occurs.

Postremission therapy is therapy administered after patients achieve CR. Its goal is to prolong CR and to maximize the probability of cure by preventing or delaying recurrence of AML. Postremission therapy may consist of intensification, consolidation, and/or maintenance therapies. Intensification may include allo-HSCT, or much less commonly auto-HSCT, while consolidation involves either a regimen similar to that used in induction or the use of drugs at higher dosages than in induction, and maintenance therapy is less intensive and less myelosuppressive than induction.[360] Particular considerations with regard to choice of treatment in older patients with AML are discussed below, as is treatment of AML diagnosed during pregnancy.

Remission Induction Chemotherapy

The most common induction chemotherapy regimens in AML involve the use of cytarabine and an anthracycline. Cytarabine, also known as cytosine arabinoside or ara-C, synthesized in 1959,[361] has been the most effective and universally used chemotherapeutic agent in the treatment of AML. Structurally, its arabinose sugar moiety is epimeric with ribose at the 2′-position. This difference prevents transformation of cytidylate to 2′-deoxycytidylate after conversion of ara-C to the ara-C triphosphate (ara-CTP) nucleotide. Other mechanisms of action of ara-C include induction of miscoding after incorporation into DNA and RNA, and inhibition of DNA-dependent DNA polymerase. Cytarabine is incorporated into DNA during DNA synthesis and is therefore only effective in cells in the S-phase of the cell cycle (*Figure 76.13*). In contrast, anthracyclines do not depend on the cell cycle. They possess potent antimitotic and cytotoxic activity, which is achieved by forming complexes with DNA, inhibiting topoisomerase II activity, inhibiting DNA polymerase activity, affecting regulation of gene expression, and producing DNA-damaging free radicals. Synergy exists between cytarabine and anthracyclines, with different mechanisms of action, and combination chemotherapy produces better results in AML.

Ara-C is usually administered as a continuous infusion of 100 to 200 mg/m²/d for 7 days, with an anthracycline given by intravenous push daily on the first 3 days, a combination called 7 + 3. Studies performed by the Cancer and Leukemia Group B (CALGB) cooperative group in the 1980s established the efficacy of this regimen for newly diagnosed patients with AML, and since then it has been the most commonly used induction regimen for treatment of adult patients with AML.[362-365]

Continuous infusion of ara-C at a dose of 100 mg/m² was shown to be superior to pulse doses of 100 mg/m² every 12 hours.[362] 7 + 3 was shown to be superior to the same drugs given over 5 and 2 days

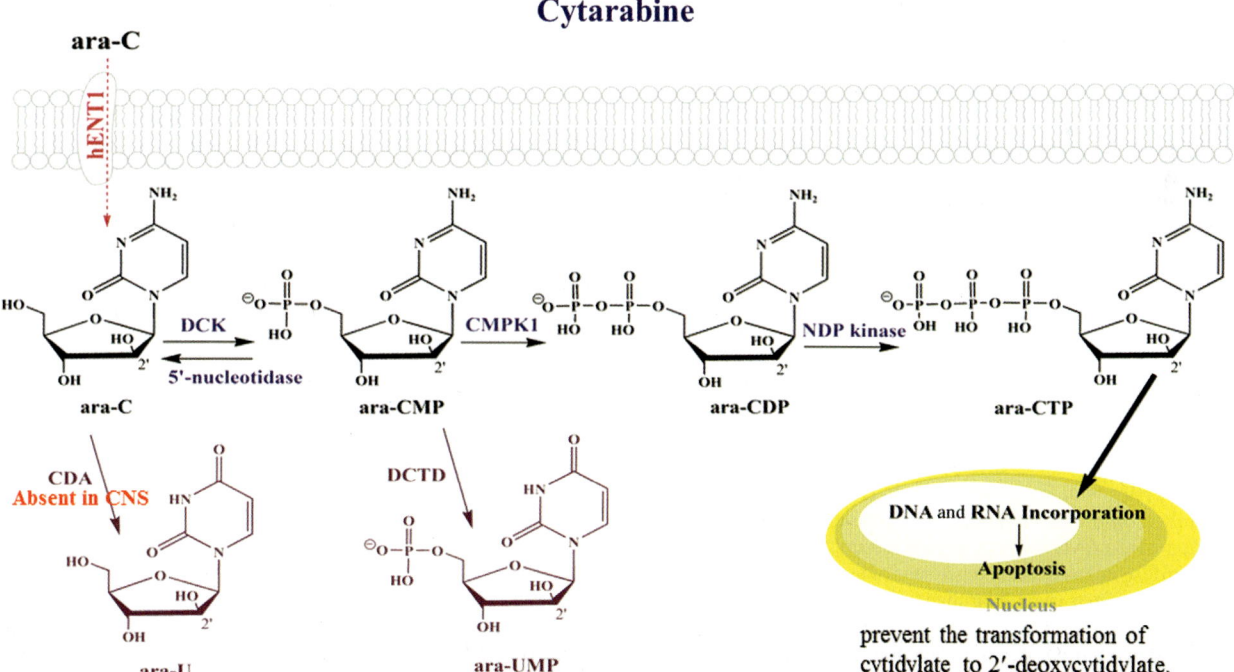

FIGURE 76.13 Cytarabine. After entering the cells via hENT1, ara-C is phosphorylated in a stepwise fashion at the 5′ position of arabinoside. Phosphorylation is mediated initially by deoxycytidine kinase (DCK) to convert ara-C to ara-C monophosphate (ara-CMP), then by deoxycytidylate kinase (CMPK1) to ara-C diphosphate and finally by nucleoside diphosphate (NDP) kinase to the active metabolite, ara-CTP. The intracellular concentration of ara-CTP is directly correlated with the therapeutic effect of ara-C. Inactivation of ara-C can occur through ara-CMP dephosphorylation by 5′-nucleotidase back to ara-C. Deaminase enzymes can convert and inactivate ara-C and ara-CMP to ara-uracil (ara-U) and ara-U monophosphate, respectively. Clinical efficacy of cytarabine depends heavily on dose and schedule because of its short half-life. At concentrations <1 micromolar, which are achieved with 100 to 200 mg/m² daily administration, the influx of cytarabine (ara-C) into the cells is strongly correlated with the number of nucleoside transporters (e.g., hENT1) per leukemic blast, but at plasma concentrations of >10 to 15 micromolar, which are achieved with high-dose ara-C (2000-3000 mg/m² over 2-3 hours repeated every 12 hours for 3-5 days), the drug diffuses freely into the cell, and cellular accumulation and retention of ara-CTP are adequate. Ara-C, cytarabine; Ara-CDP, Ara-C diphosphate; Ara-CMP, Ara-C monophosphate; Ara-CTP, Ara-C triphosphate; Ara-U, Ara-uracil; Ara-UMP, Ara-U monophosphate.

(5 + 2), respectively,[362] and appeared to be equivalent to "10 + 3."[364] The anthracycline most commonly used in 7 + 3 is daunorubicin, and its dose has ranged between 30 and 90 mg/m^2 in different studies. In early studies, daunorubicin 45 mg/m^2 daily was compared with 30 mg/m^2 daily in the 7 + 3 regimen, demonstrating higher CR rates with 45 mg/m^2 in patients younger than 60 years.[363] A single course of 7 + 3 ara-C and daunorubicin (45 mg/m^2) therapy produced a CR rate in the range of 40% to 50%. When a second course of ara-C and daunorubicin (either 5 + 2 or 7 + 3) was administered to patients with morphologic evidence of persistent leukemia in the bone marrow on day 14, the overall CR rate increased to 50% to 85%. The highest response rates (70%-85%) are seen in patients under 60 years of age with de novo AML.

Two phase 3 randomized clinical trials from the United States and South Korea confirmed the clinical benefit of daunorubicin dose intensification (90 mg/m^2 vs 45 mg/m^2) in the 7 + 3 regimen in patients younger than 60 years with previously untreated AML.[366,367] In the US study, 90 mg/m^2, compared with 45 mg/m^2, daunorubicin resulted in a significantly higher CR rate (71% vs 57%) and longer OS (median, 23.7 vs 15.7 months). Long-term follow-up of this study (median, ~80 months among survivors) showed that 90 mg/m^2 daunorubicin was associated with improved OS in all subgroups of patients, with a hazard ratio (HR) for death of 0.74 (P = .001) for the entire population, 0.66 (P = .002) for patients <50 years, 0.51 (P = .03) for patients with favorable cytogenetics, 0.68 (P = .01) for patients with intermediate cytogenetics, 0.66 (P = .04) for patients with unfavorable cytogenetics, 0.61 (P = .009) for patients with FLT3-ITD, 0.62 (P = .02) for patients with DNMT3A mutations, and 0.50 (P = .002) for patients with NPM1 mutations.[368] In addition, the presence of an NPM1 mutation was associated with a more favorable outcome only in patients receiving 90 mg/m^2 daunorubicin.[368] The rates of serious adverse events including cardiac toxicities were similar in the two groups.[366] In the study conducted in South Korea,[367] the CR rate was also significantly higher (83% vs 72%) with 90 mg/m^2, compared with 45 mg/m^2, daunorubicin. With approximately 4.5 years median follow-up, both OS (47% vs 35%) and EFS (41% vs 28%) were significantly better with 90 mg/m^2. The advantage of higher-dose daunorubicin was observed in patients with intermediate-risk cytogenetics but not in those with unfavorable karyotypes or high-risk molecular profiles. Toxicities were similar in the two groups.

Another clinical trial tested the potential benefit of high-dose daunorubicin in older patients receiving intensive chemotherapy.[369] Newly diagnosed patients with AML 60 years and older received the 7 + 3 regimen, consisting of cytarabine 200 mg/m^2 and daunorubicin either 45 mg/m^2 or 90 mg/m^2, followed by a second cycle of 1000 mg/m^2 cytarabine every 12 hours for 6 days. CR rates (64% vs 54%) and rates of CR after the first cycle of induction therapy (52% vs 35%) were significantly higher in the group that received 90 mg/m^2 daunorubicin. Thirty-day mortality rates, hematologic toxicities, and moderate, severe, or life-threatening adverse events did not differ significantly between the two groups. OS rates were similar in the two groups. Patients 60 to 65 years had higher CR (73% vs 51%), EFS (29% vs 14%), and OS (38% vs 23%) rates with 90 mg/m^2, compared with 45 mg/m^2, daunorubicin, while a difference was not seen in those over 65 years, with the exception of the favorable cytogenetic group, who benefited from daunorubicin dose intensification regardless of age.

In three randomized trials, idarubicin (12 mg/m^2) daily for 3 days with ara-C tended to produce a higher CR rate than daunorubicin and ara-C, more often required only one cycle to induce remission and was associated with better survival in some trials.[370-372] A meta-analysis suggested that idarubicin (10-12 mg/m^2) compared with daunorubicin (45-60 mg/m^2) in the 7 + 3 regimen was superior for achievement of CR.[373] In a randomized trial in patients with AML between 50 and 70 years, idarubicin produced a higher CR rate than high-dose daunorubicin (80 mg/m^2/day for 3 days).[374] Substitution of idarubicin with either fludarabine or topotecan in combination with ara-C for treatment of newly diagnosed AML or refractory anemia with excess blasts in transformation resulted in lower CR rates and shorter EFS and OS.[375] A phase 3 randomized clinical trial in approximately 300 younger adult patients with newly diagnosed AML comparing idarubicin (12 mg/m^2/d for 3 days) vs high-dose daunorubicin (90 mg/m^2/d for 3 days) combined with cytarabine (200 mg/m^2/d for 7 days) reported similar CR rates (81% vs 75%, P = .224), 4-year OS (51% vs 55%, P = .756), cumulative incidence of relapse (35% vs 25%, P = .194), and EFS (45% vs 51%, P = .772) on the two arms.[376] Interestingly, OS and EFS of patients with FLT3-ITD were significantly better in the daunorubicin-containing arm (median OS not reached vs 15.5 months, P = .030; EFS not reached vs 11.9 months, P = .028). Toxicity profiles were also similar in the two arms.[376]

In clinical practice and sometimes in clinical trials, daunorubicin and idarubicin are used interchangeably with different conversion factors, as there is no high-level evidence on the equipotency of these two agents for AML treatment. A systematic review of 15 clinical studies directly comparing the clinical outcomes of AML induction therapy utilizing daunorubicin and idarubicin estimated daunorubicin/idarubicin equipotency ratio at 5.90/1.0 (95% CI 1.7-20.7).[377] To validate the estimate from the meta-analysis biologically, in vitro tests comparing anti-AML activity of daunorubicin and idarubicin against six AML cell lines and two primary AML cells from patients with different cytogenetic and molecular characteristics were conducted and the equipotency dose ratio between daunorubicin and idarubicin was 4.06 to 1.0 (95% CI 3.64-4.49). Combining the estimates from the meta-analysis and the in vitro data using inverse-variance weighting suggested that the best estimate of the daunorubicin/idarubicin equipotent ratio is 4.1/1.0 (95% CI 3.9-4.3).[377]

Other studies have tested addition of a third agent to the 7 + 3 regimen. Addition of etoposide to 7 + 3 at 75 mg/m^2/d for 7 days ("7 + 3 + 7") did not improve CR rates and was associated with more mucositis, but it did improve median CR duration (18 vs 12 months), while OS was similar.[378] A three-drug induction regimen known as ADE, consisting of ara-C 100 mg/m^2/day for 7 days and both daunorubicin 90 mg/m^2 and etoposide 100 mg/m^2 daily for 3 days, was tested by CALGB in previously untreated patients with de novo AML less than 60 years, without excess cardiotoxicity, and with a CR rate of 75% and median DFS and OS of 1.34 and 1.86 years.[379]

Fludarabine has been extensively studied in AML because of preclinical[380] and clinical data demonstrating that its administration prior to ara-C sensitizes leukemic blasts to ara-C by enhancing ara-CTP formation.[381] The observation that administration of G-CSF with fludarabine further enhanced this effect[382] led to the design of a regimen consisting of fludarabine with high-dose cytarabine and G-CSF (FLAG) with or without idarubicin.[383,384] In one clinical trial patients with AML receiving two courses of FLAG-Ida and two courses of HiDAC had an 8-year survival of 63% for intermediate risk and 95% for favorable risk.[385] A 652-patient Polish Adult Leukemia Group randomized multicenter trial in patients with AML up to 60 years demonstrated that addition of cladribine, but not fludarabine, to 7 + 3 induction chemotherapy prolonged survival.[386] Patients received 7 + 3 alone (cytarabine 200 mg/m^2 on days 1-7 as a continuous infusion plus daunorubicin 60 mg/m^2 daily infusion on days 1-3) or 7 + 3 plus 3-hour infusions of cladribine 5 mg/m^2 daily on days 1 to 5 of 7 + 3 or 30-minute infusions of fludarabine 25 mg/m^2 daily on days 1 to 5. Consolidation chemotherapy included HiDAC and allo-HSCT or 2-year maintenance chemotherapy, based on relapse risk. Both the CR rates (68% vs 56% vs 59%) and 3-year OS rates (45% vs 33% vs 35%) were significantly improved by addition of cladribine to the 7 + 3 regimen, compared with 7 + 3 alone and 7 + 3 + fludarabine, respectively. Toxicity did not differ significantly in the three arms. Patients with unfavorable karyotypes also benefited from 7 + 3 + cladribine.

Several studies have incorporated HiDAC in induction therapy, but these trials did not show an efficacy advantage for HiDAC when compared with intermediate-/standard-dose cytarabine and patients in the HiDAC group generally experienced higher rates of serious toxicities.[387] On the basis of these data, use of HiDAC for induction chemotherapy for newly diagnosed AML is not generally recommended, unless in special circumstances.

A number of phase 3 trials using granulocyte-monocyte colony-stimulating factor and G-CSF in induction therapy consistently showed more rapid neutrophil recovery, which usually resulted in fewer infections and shorter hospitalizations, but no improvement in CR rates, relapse rates, or OS.[388-395] Two randomized trials evaluating the role of G-CSF after consolidation therapy showed decreases in the duration of severe neutropenia and a decreased rate of infection but no effect on CR duration or OS.[394,396] Based on these data, routine use of myeloid growth factors in AML is not recommended.

CPX-351 (Vyxeos) is a liposomal formulation of daunorubicin and cytarabine at a fixed 1:5 molar ratio, which was suggested to have synergistic cytotoxicity in AML cells in vitro and in vivo.[397] The liposomes migrate to and persist in the bone marrow in AML-bearing mice, are taken up by leukemia cells to a greater extent than by normal bone marrow cells, and undergo intracellular degradation, releasing cytarabine and daunorubicin intracellularly. In an initial clinical trial in older adults with untreated AML, a planned analysis of the secondary AML subgroup demonstrated an improved response rate (58% vs 32%, $P = .06$) and prolonged EFS (HR 0.59, $P = .08$) and OS (HR 0.46, $P = .01$).[398]

In 2017, the FDA and the European Medicine Agency (EMA) approved CPX-351 for the treatment of adults with newly diagnosed secondary AML, including t-AML and AML-MRC,[397] based on a randomized (1:1), multicenter, open-label, phase 3 clinical trial that was conducted across 39 academic and regional cancer centers in the United States and Canada, which compared CPX-351 with cytarabine (100 mg/m^2/d) and daunorubicin (60 mg/m^2/d) (7 + 3) in 309 patients 60 to 75 years of age with newly diagnosed t-AML (20%) or AML-MRC (79%).[399] Approximately one-third of patients had been previously treated with a hypomethylating agent for MDS, and more than 50% had unfavorable karyotypes. CPX-351 (daunorubicin 44 mg/m^2 and cytarabine 100 mg/m^2) liposome was given intravenously on days 1, 3, and 5 and on days 1 and 3 for a second induction in patients with <50% reduction in percent blasts. For consolidation, the CPX-351 dose was daunorubicin 29 mg/m^2 and cytarabine 65 mg/m^2 liposome on days 1 and 3. All patients on the CPX-351 arm and 97% of those on the 7 + 3 arm received at least one cycle of induction, and 32% on the CPX-351 arm and 21% on the 7 + 3 arm received at least one cycle of consolidation. Compared with 7 + 3 control, CPX-351 produced a higher CR rate (38% vs 26%, $P = .036$) and showed superiority in OS (median survival, (95% CI); 9.6 (6.6, 11.9) vs 5.9 (5.0, 7.8) months, with an HR (95% CI) of 0.69 (0.52, 0.90), $P = .005$).[397,399]

In the prospectively planned analysis of final 5-year follow-up results of the phase 3 study, at a median follow-up of approximately 60 months for both groups, median OS was 9.3 months with CPX-351 and 6 months with 7 + 3 (HR 0.70, 95% CI 0.6-0.9).[400] The 5-year OS was 18% (95% CI 12%-25%) with CPX-351 and 8% (4%-13%) with 7 + 3.[400] The most common cause of death in both groups was progressive leukemia. In a subsequent multicenter, observational study in adults with newly diagnosed t-AML or AML-MRC, the frequency of infusion-related reactions with CPX-351 was confirmed to be low.[401]

AML in Pregnancy

Although development of AML during pregnancy is rare, occurring in less than 1 in 10,000 pregnancies, it represents a major quandary in patient management.[402-404] Transmission of leukemia from mother to fetus is extremely unusual.[405,406] Diagnosis of AML is less common in the first trimester than in the second or third trimesters, occurring in 14% in a series of 59 patients.[407] Teratogenic effects of chemotherapy are more common in the first trimester and appear to be minimal in the second and third trimesters.[404,408,409] Options in the first trimester include therapeutic abortion or supportive therapy until the second trimester. Acute leukemia during the first trimester should generally be treated promptly, as in nonpregnant patients, but induction therapy should be initiated after pregnancy termination. Chemotherapy with intensive supportive care can result in a successful outcome for the fetus and the mother with leukemia in the second or third trimester,[403,404,409,410] usually without a need to terminate the pregnancy. Fetuses exposed to antileukemia therapy in utero may have slight growth retardation as well as transient myelosuppression if treatment is given near delivery, but they generally have normal growth and development in childhood.[411,412] The choice of induction chemotherapy is similar to that in nonpregnant patients. Delivery should optimally occur during a noncytopenic period.[413]

Postremission Therapy

In the absence of postremission therapy, the probability of cure is approximately zero,[414] with a median time to relapse of 6 months for all patients. Therefore, postremission therapy is essential, with the goals of decreasing and attempting to eliminate residual disease, delaying relapse, and increasing the likelihood of cure. While additional therapy clearly is required beyond induction therapy, utilizing drugs at similar doses to those used in induction therapy, with or without maintenance therapy, did not have a major impact on survival in AML, with only 15% to 25% of adults having prolonged survival after consolidation or maintenance therapy administered through 1980. Therefore higher-dose therapy was studied and adopted.

Consolidation Therapy

The antileukemic effect of cytarabine depends on dosage and schedule (*Figure 76.13*). HiDAC (1000-3000 mg/m^2 every 12-24 hours, for 4-12 doses) is one of the most commonly used consolidation regimens for patients with AML after achievement of CR. HiDAC crosses the blood-brain barrier and helps prevent CNS relapse, but cerebellar toxicity may develop, particularly in patients ≥60 years or with impaired renal function.[415] Lengthening the duration of administration from 1 hour to 3 hours or decreasing the dose from 3000 mg/m^2 to 1500 mg/m^2 or 1000 mg/m^2 lessens the risk of cerebellar toxicity by decreasing peak concentrations. HiDAC should not be administered to patients with creatinine clearance less than 40 to 45 mL/min. Patients receiving HiDAC must be tested for cerebellar toxicity before each dose, and subsequent doses of HiDAC must be withheld if cerebellar toxicity is documented or suspected; the ara-C dose must then be decreased, and HiDAC also cannot be administered as part of any subsequent therapy. Conjunctivitis and a painful, blistering erythematous rash involving the palms and soles are common side effects following HiDAC. Administration of corticosteroid eyedrops may prevent conjunctivitis, which is caused by secretion of ara-C administered at high doses into tears.

Wolff et al. reported the efficacy of HiDAC/daunorubicin intensification in AML, with a projected 49% survival that was age-dependent (83%, 50%, and 23% for age groups 25 or less, 26-45, and more than 45 years, respectively).[19]

In a landmark clinical trial, CALGB randomly assigned 596 patients in CR1 after 7 + 3 to four courses of postremission chemotherapy using one of three ara-C dose schedules: HiDAC at 3000 mg/m^2 over 3 hours every 12 hours on days 1, 3, and 5 (6 doses), intermediate-dose ara-C at 400 mg/m^2/d for 5 days by continuous infusion, or lower-dose ara-C at 100 mg/m^2 for 5 days by continuous infusion.[416] The estimated probabilities of remaining in CR at 4 years for patients up to 60 years were 44%, 29%, and 24% for the three treatments, respectively ($P = .002$), but there were no differences among the arms in patients over age 60 years, with a probability of 16% or less of remaining in CR. These results clearly show that consolidation with HiDAC improves DFS in younger patients in CR1. Multiple (four) cycles may be required to obtain the maximum benefit of HiDAC consolidation.[416,417]

The efficacy of HiDAC consolidation therapy also varies by cytogenetic group. In an analysis of cytogenetic correlates in the above CALGB three-arm consolidation study,[416] HiDAC consolidation had the greatest impact in the favorable cytogenetic group, with 78% of patients remaining in CR at 5 years, compared with 40% of those with a normal karyotype and 21% of those with other abnormalities.[418] The favorable impact of repetitive cycles of HiDAC in AML with the favorable karyotypes t(8;21) and inv(16) was confirmed in a series focusing on patients with those abnormalities.[419] In addition, patients up to 60 years with a normal karyotype had 5-year DFS rates of 41% and 45% following four cycles of HiDAC or ara-C 400 mg/m^2 consolidation or one cycle of HiDAC/etoposide followed by auto-HSCT.[420] Of note, these studies antedated the availability of molecular data.

In addition, a large ($n = 781$) Japanese prospective randomized trial compared four courses of conventional multiagent chemotherapy with three courses of HiDAC alone (2000 mg/m² twice daily for 5 days) as postremission therapy for AML in adult patients younger than 65 years in CR1.[421] Five-year DFS (43% vs 39%) and OS (58% vs 56%) were similar for HiDAC and multiagent chemotherapy, but in patients with favorable cytogenetic risk, 5-year DFS (57% vs 39%) and OS (75% vs 66%) were significantly better with HiDAC. Infections were more frequent in the HiDAC group.

In summary, for younger adults with favorable cytogenetic (and molecular) findings, HiDAC intensification alone (four cycles using CALGB doses and schedule) is often considered the best treatment. For younger adults with intermediate-prognosis cytogenetic and molecular findings, reasonable choices include HiDAC consolidation or allo-HSCT. For older patients who have a good performance status and an available donor and meet age and health criteria, allo-HSCT should be considered, and a modified HiDAC regimen can be used for those without transplant options or opting not to pursue transplant. Because no postremission chemotherapy regimen is established as superior to others in older patients, participation in clinical trials is recommended. For patients who have adverse prognostic features including unfavorable karyotypes or molecular findings (see "Prognosis" section) and who have an available donor and meet age and health criteria, allo-HSCT is considered the treatment of choice in CR1, although allo-HSCT outcomes for many of these patients are also poor (see "Hematopoietic Stem Cell Transplantation" section).

Maintenance Therapy

Maintenance therapy is low-dose therapy administered with the goal of prolonging the duration of remission and survival. In AML, in contrast to ALL, decades of investigations with cytotoxic chemotherapy, immunotherapy, and targeted small molecule therapy have provided only limited evidence in favor of maintenance therapy.[422] However, the landscape of maintenance therapy for AML changed with FDA approval of oral azacitidine (Onureg) in 2020.[423]

Oral azacitidine was approved for continued treatment of adult patients with AML who achieve first CR or CRi following intensive induction chemotherapy and are not able to complete intensive consolidation therapy with curative intent,[424] based on the multicenter, randomized, double-blind, placebo-controlled phase 3 QUZAR clinical trial.[424] Eligible patients were over 55 years and within 4 months of achieving first CR or CRi with intensive induction chemotherapy with or without consolidation therapy and were not candidates for allo-HSCT at the time of screening.[424] A total of 472 patients with AML were randomized 1:1 to receive oral azacitidine 300 mg ($n = 238$) or placebo ($n = 234$) orally on days 1 through 14 of 28-day cycles. Randomization was stratified by age at the time of induction therapy (55-64 vs ≥65 years), cytogenetic risk category (intermediate vs poor), prior history of MDS or chronic myelomonocytic leukemia, and whether patients had received consolidation therapy.

Baseline demographic and disease characteristics were balanced between the oral azacitidine and placebo arms, with median age 68 years (range, 55-86), >90% with Eastern Cooperative Oncology Group (ECOG) performance status 0 or 1, de novo AML in ~90%, and cytogenetic risk status at diagnosis intermediate for ~85% of patients and poor for ~15% in both groups. In the oral azacitidine arm 79% of patients had achieved CR and 21% CRi after induction, compared with 84% CR and 16% CRi in the placebo arm, and numbers of consolidation courses were similar on both arms.[424] Median OS from the time of randomization was significantly longer with oral azacitidine than with placebo (24.7 vs 14.8 months; $P < .0009$) (*Figure 76.14*).[424]

Median RFS was also significantly longer with oral azacitidine than with placebo (10.2 vs 4.8 months; $P < .001$). Benefits of oral azacitidine with respect to OS and RFS were demonstrated in most subgroups defined by baseline characteristics and in both CR and CRi patients. The most common adverse events in both groups were grade 1 or 2 gastrointestinal toxicities. Common grade 3 or 4 adverse events were neutropenia in 41% of patients on oral azacitidine and 24% on placebo and thrombocytopenia in 22% and 21%.[424]

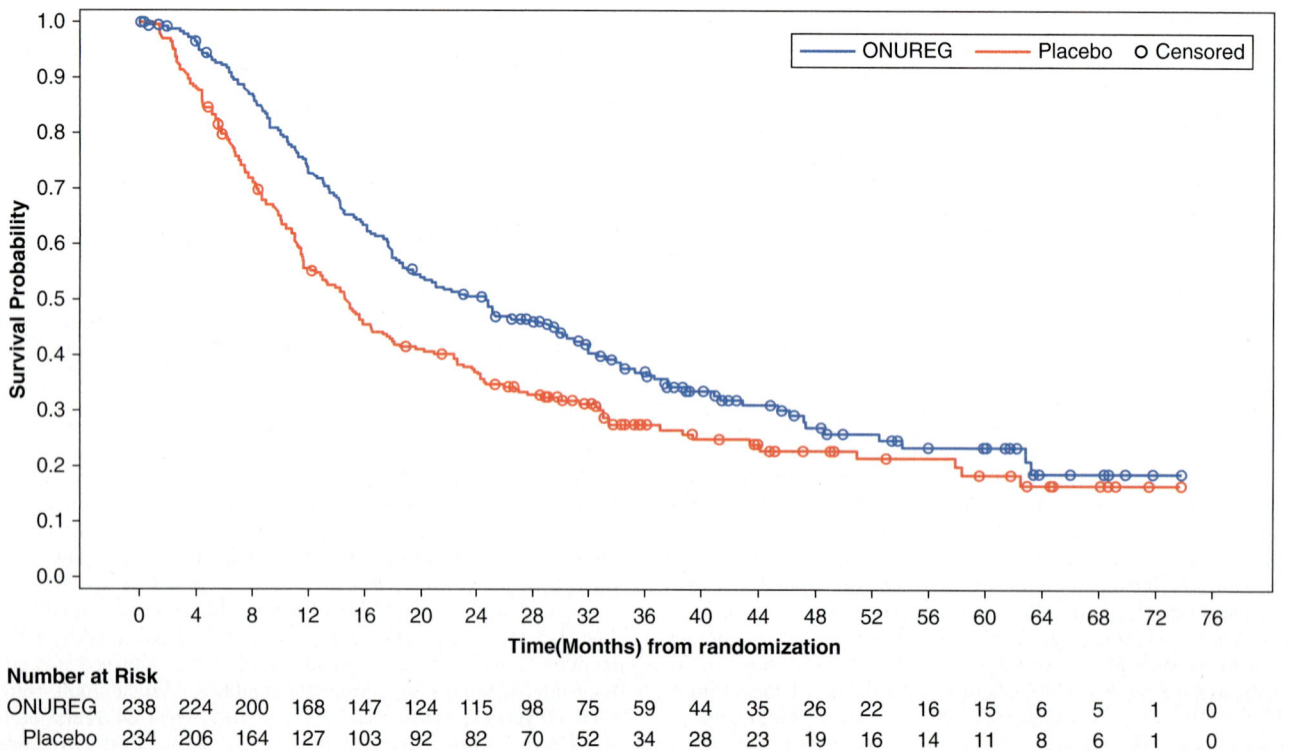

FIGURE 76.14 Kaplan-Meier curve for overall survival in the intention-to-treat population in the QUZAR study comparing oral azacitidine and placebo maintenance for patients with AML in first CR or CRi.[424]

Initial Treatment of AML in Patients Unfit for Cytotoxic Chemotherapy

There is consensus about the importance of assessing fitness for cytotoxic chemotherapy, particularly in older patients, but there is not a uniform approach to assessment.[342] The decision with regard to whether a patient with newly diagnosed AML is fit or unfit for cytotoxic chemotherapy should be based on performance status and comorbidities, rather than strictly on chronological age. There should be an attempt to assess premorbid performance status, rather than only current performance status, which may be acutely, and reversibly, worsened by complications of AML, such as anemia and fever/infection. Social support is also an important component of initial assessment, as is patient preference. Likelihood of response to cytotoxic chemotherapy based on disease characteristics, including karyotype and molecular abnormalities, also factors into the choice of initial therapy. In addition, given that remissions are typically short in older patients with AML, and particularly those without favorable karyotypes, likely feasibility of reduced-intensity allo-HSCT if remission is achieved may also be considered in the initial treatment decision.[425]

The FDA has accepted 75 years as an upper age limit for inclusion in trials of intensive chemotherapy and encourages use of no upper age limit for trials of nonintensive treatments for AML.[353] Newly diagnosed patients with AML deemed unfit for cytotoxic chemotherapy should optimally be treated on a clinical trial testing a treatment aimed at improving outcome. Outside of a clinical trial, the most common approach is treatment with a DNA methyltransferase inhibitor (DNMTi), also termed demethylating agent or hypomethylating agent. Clinical trials often combine a new agent with a DNMTi. New agents may target specific molecular abnormalities, or more universal biological features of AML, such as resistance to apoptosis.

A current clinical trial, Beat AML, sponsored by the Leukemia and Lymphoma Society, is testing the feasibility of using cytogenetic and molecular data available within 7 days from sample receipt to enable testing of targeted therapies in newly diagnosed older (≥60 years) patients with AML.[340] In an initial report, a total of 487 patients with suspected AML were enrolled in the Beat AML study; 395 were eligible. Median age was 72 years (range 60-92 years; 38% ≥75 years).[339] Cytogenetic and molecular analyses were completed within 7 days for 374 patients (95%); 224 (57%) enrolled on a Beat AML substudy and 103 elected standard of care, consisting of 7 + 3 or a DNMTi. Thirty-day mortality was lower and OS was significantly longer for patients enrolled on the Beat AML substudies.[340]

DNA Methyltransferase Inhibitor Therapy

The DNMTis decitabine and azacitidine have significant activity in newly diagnosed patients with AML unfit for chemotherapy.

Decitabine has efficacy in AML and is well tolerated and is therefore currently in widespread use to treat AML in previously untreated patients who are "unfit for chemotherapy."[426-431] Cashen et al[426] treated 55 previously untreated older patients with AML with decitabine 20 mg/m^2 intravenously daily for 5 days every 4 weeks. Importantly, decitabine was continued until disease progression or an unacceptable adverse event occurred; patients received a median of three (range, 1-25) cycles. The overall response rate was 25% (CR rate, 24%). Thirty-day mortality rate was 7% and median OS was 7.7 months. The most common toxicities were myelosuppression, neutropenic fever, and fatigue. In a phase 2, multicenter study of decitabine in the same schedule as first-line therapy in 227 older patients with AML,[427] 30 (13%) achieved CR, 29 (13%) achieved PR, and 60 (26%) had a lesser antileukemic effect. Median OS was 5.5 months and 1-year survival rate, 28%. Toxicities were predominantly hematologic. In a subsequently reported multicenter, randomized, open-label, phase 3 trial, 485 older patients with newly diagnosed AML were randomly assigned 1:1 to 5-day decitabine or either supportive care or low-dose cytarabine (LDAC).[428] The primary endpoint was OS, and the secondary endpoint was rate of CR plus CRp. The primary analysis after 396 deaths (82%) showed a nonsignificant increase in median OS with decitabine, 7.7 vs 5.0 months ($P = .108$). An unplanned analysis after 446 deaths (92%) showed a survival benefit for decitabine ($P = .037$). The most common drug-related adverse events with decitabine were thrombocytopenia (27%) and neutropenia (24%). Decitabine was approved for treatment of AML in Europe based on the results of this study. It is not approved as monotherapy for treatment of AML in the United States, but it is in widespread use off-label. As with decitabine in treatment of MDS, in order to sustain response, treatment of AML should continue on an ongoing basis, until disease progression.

Decitabine is also used in a 10-day regimen for AML.[429-431] The 10-day decitabine regimen produced response rates of 64% (47% CR and 17% CRi), 40% (CR), and 42% (31% CR and 11% CRi) in three series in untreated patients with AML unfit for chemotherapy.[429-431] Survival in responders was 481 days (approximately 16 months) and 19.4 months in the two series in which it was analyzed.[430,431] In contrast, the 10-day decitabine regimen produced a CR rate of only 16% in patients with R/R AML.[430] Welch et al reported marrow blast clearance in 53 of 116 (46%) AML and MDS patients treated with the 10-day decitabine regimen, with responses in 29 of 43 (67%) with unfavorable karyotypes and 21 of 21 patients with *TP53* mutations.[265]

Azacitidine also has efficacy in AML. Fenaux et al reported its activity in patients with AML with 20% to 30% marrow blasts who were treated on a randomized trial for MDS defined by FAB criteria, including 20% to 30% marrow blasts.[432] Older patients with AML ($n = 113$, median age 70 years) were randomly assigned to receive azacitidine ($n = 55$) or conventional care regimens (CCRs) ($n = 58$), including 47% best supportive care, 34% LDAC, and 19% intensive chemotherapy. At a median follow-up of 20.1 months, median OS for azacitidine-treated patients was 24.5 months compared with 16.0 months for CCR-treated patients ($P = .005$), and 2-year OS rates were 50% and 16%, respectively ($P = .001$). Azacitidine was associated with fewer total days in hospital than CCR ($P < .0001$). Another multicenter, 1:1 randomized, open-label, phase 3 trial evaluated azacitidine ($n = 241$) vs CCR ($n = 247$), including standard induction chemotherapy, LDAC, or supportive care, in 488 patients age ≥65 years with newly diagnosed AML with >30% bone marrow blasts.[433] Median OS was 10.4 months with azacitidine vs 6.5 months with CCR (stratified log-rank $P = .1009$). One-year survival rates with azacitidine and CCR were 47% and 34%, respectively. A prespecified analysis censoring patients who received AML treatment after discontinuing study drug showed median OS with azacitidine vs CCR of 12.1 vs 6.9 months (stratified log-rank $P = .0190$).

Outcomes of 671 patients 65 years and older with newly diagnosed AML treated with intensive chemotherapy ($n = 557$) or azacitidine- or decitabine-based therapy ($n = 114$) at MD Anderson Cancer Center between 2000 and 2010 were retrospectively reviewed.[434] Both groups were balanced according to cytogenetics and performance status. CR rates with chemotherapy and DNMTi therapy were 42% and 28%, respectively ($P = .001$), but 2-year RFS rates (28% vs 39%, $P = .843$) and median survival (6.7 vs 6.5 months, $P = .413$) were similar in the two groups. Decitabine was associated with improved median OS compared with azacitidine (8.8 vs 5.5 months, $P = .03$). Multivariate analysis identified older age, adverse cytogenetic risk, poor performance status, elevated creatinine, peripheral blood and bone marrow blasts, and hemoglobin, but not type of AML therapy, as independent prognostic factors for survival. The conclusion was that DNMTi therapy is associated with similar survival rates as intensive chemotherapy in older patients with newly diagnosed AML.

Given the efficacy of DNMTi therapy in AML, other novel agents, including targeted agents, are frequently tested in combination regimens with decitabine or azacitidine.

Targeted Therapies
BCL-2 Inhibitor

The BCL-2 inhibitor venetoclax is an orally bioavailable small molecule that specifically inhibits binding of BIM (BCL-2-like protein 11) and BAX proteins to BCL-2, resulting in activation of the proapoptotic protein BAK, which triggers apoptosis via mitochondrial outer membrane permeabilization and activation of caspases.[435] In 2018, venetoclax was approved by the FDA for use in combination with a DNMTi, azacitidine or decitabine, or LDAC for treatment of newly diagnosed adult patients with AML 75 years or older or with comorbidities precluding use of intensive induction chemotherapy.[436]

Modest single-agent anti-AML activity was initially demonstrated in a phase 2, single-arm study evaluating venetoclax 800 mg daily in patients with R/R AML or untreated AML unfit for intensive chemotherapy.[168] The overall response rate was 19%. Common adverse events included all grades nausea, diarrhea, and vomiting, as well as grade 3 and 4 febrile neutropenia and hypokalemia.[168] Some predictive biomarkers for response consistent with BCL-2 dependency were suggested, including *IDH1/2* mutations and results of BH3 profiling. The tolerability and preliminary efficacy of venetoclax combined with decitabine or azacitidine in elderly newly diagnosed patients with AML was investigated in a phase 1b study.[437] The recommended phase 2 dose was 400 mg daily. Of 57 patients, 4 (7%) died of sepsis, bacteremia, lung infection, or respiratory failure within 30 days of the first venetoclax dose, and 35 (61%; 95% CI 48-74) achieved CR or CRi.[437]

Subsequently, venetoclax was studied in adults with newly diagnosed AML who were older than 75 years or who were considered unfit for intensive induction chemotherapy based on ECOG performance status 2 to 3, severe cardiac or pulmonary comorbidity, moderate hepatic impairment, creatinine clearance <45 mL/min, and/or other comorbidity. VIALE-A was a randomized (2:1), double-blind, placebo-controlled, multicenter clinical trial evaluating the efficacy and safety of venetoclax vs placebo in combination with azacitidine.[438] Patients received venetoclax 400 mg orally once daily on days 1 to 28, following completion of a ramp-up dosing schedule, or placebo in combination with azacitidine 75 mg/m^2 daily either intravenously or subcutaneously on days 1 to 7 of each 28-day cycle. Once a bone marrow examination confirmed <5% myeloblasts following cycle 1 treatment, venetoclax or placebo was interrupted for up to 14 days or until ANC ≥500/mm^3 and platelet count ≥50,000/mm^3. Venetoclax or placebo was resumed on the same day as azacitidine following interruption. Patients continued treatment until disease progression or unacceptable toxicity. A total of 431 patients (median age 76 years in both groups; range, 49-91) were randomized: 286 to venetoclax + azacitidine and 145 to placebo + azacitidine. In both groups, approximately 55% of patients had ECOG performance status 0 or 1 and ~40% had ECOG performance status 2. AML was de novo in ~75% of patients in both arms, with 60% to 65% intermediate and 35% to 40% poor cytogenetic risk. The primary efficacy endpoint was OS.[438] At a median follow-up of 20.5 months, median OS was 14.7 months in the venetoclax + azacitidine arm and 9.6 months in the placebo + azacitidine arm ($P < .001$) (*Figure 76.15*).[438] The CR rate was also higher with venetoclax + azacitidine than with the control regimen (37% vs 18%; $P < .001$), with a longer median CR duration for venetoclax + azacitidine (18 vs 13.4 months, respectively), and the CR + CRh rate was also higher (65% vs 23%; $P < .001$).[438] Approximately 50% of patients with blood or platelet transfusion dependence at baseline became transfusion-independent in the venetoclax + azacitidine arm during any consecutive ≥56-day postbaseline period, compared with 27% in the placebo + azacitidine arm. Nausea of any grade occurred in 44% of patients in the venetoclax + azacitidine arm and 35% in the control arm. Key hematologic and infectious adverse events on azacitidine + venetoclax or placebo included grade 3 or higher thrombocytopenia (45% and 38%), neutropenia (42% and 28%), and febrile neutropenia (in 42% and 19%).[438]

The efficacy of venetoclax (400 mg orally once daily) in combination with azacitidine (75 mg/m^2 either intravenously or subcutaneously on days 1-7 of each 28-day cycle; $n = 29$) or decitabine (20 mg/m^2 intravenously on days 1-5 of each 28-day cycle; $n = 31$) in patients with newly diagnosed AML at least 65 years old and ineligible for intensive chemotherapy was evaluated in a nonrandomized, open-label clinical trial.[438] Median age was 74 years, with poor-risk cytogenetics in 49% of patients. Once a bone marrow examination confirmed <5% myeloblasts following cycle 1 treatment, venetoclax could be interrupted for up to 14 days to allow ANC recovery to ≥500/mm^3. The CR + CRi rate was 76% for venetoclax + azacitidine (median duration of remission not reached (NR), 95% CI: 5.6 –NR) and 71% for venetoclax + decitabine (median duration of remission 12.5 months, 95% CI: 5.1 –NR).[436]

VIALE-C was a randomized, double-blind, placebo-controlled, multicenter clinical trial evaluating the efficacy and safety of venetoclax (600 mg orally once daily on days 1-28 following completion of the ramp-up dosing schedule) vs placebo in combination with LDAC (20 mg/m^2 subcutaneously once daily on days 1-10 of each 28-day cycle) in adults ≥18 years with newly diagnosed AML ineligible for intensive chemotherapy.[440] Once a bone marrow examination confirmed <5% myeloblasts with cytopenias following cycle 1 treatment, venetoclax or placebo was interrupted up to 14 days or until ANC ≥500/mm^3 and platelet count ≥50,000/mm^3. Venetoclax or placebo was resumed on the same day as LDAC. Baseline demographic and disease characteristics were balanced between the two arms. Patients ($n = 211$) were randomized 2:1 to venetoclax ($n = 143$) or placebo ($n = 68$), plus LDAC. In both arms, median age was 76 years and ECOG performance status was 0 or 1 in 50% of patients. Primary end point was OS. Planned primary analysis showed a 25% reduction in risk of death with venetoclax + LDAC vs placebo + LDAC ($P = .114$), although not statistically significant; median OS was 7.2 vs 4.1 months. Unplanned analysis with 6 months additional follow-up demonstrated median OS of 8.4 months for the venetoclax arm ($P = .04$).[440] The CR rate in the venetoclax + LDAC arm was 27%), and the CR rate in the placebo + LDAC arm was 7.4%. The CR + CRh rate was 47% (95% CI: 39%–55%) in the venetoclax + LDAC arm and 15% (95% CI: 7.3%–25%) in the placebo + LDAC arm.[436] EFS was 4.7 months (95% CI: 3.7–6.4) vs 2.0 months (95% CI: 1.6–3.1).

While venetoclax in combination with DNMTis has produced encouraging results for newly diagnosed patients with AML, venetoclax efficacy is less in patients with R/R AML,[441] either as a monotherapy[168] or in combination with DNMTis,[442] underscoring the importance of developing novel rational combination therapies. Venetoclax combinations with cytotoxic chemotherapy[443,444] and with novel agents[445,446] are being investigated in AML.

FLT3 Inhibitors

As detailed above, mutations in *FLT3* resulting in constitutive signaling are common in AML, including ITD in the juxtamembrane domain in ~25% of patients and point mutations in the tyrosine kinase domain (TKD) in ~5%. Patients with AML with *FLT3*-ITD have a high relapse rate and short RFS and OS after chemotherapy. Constitutive FLT3 signaling resulting from *FLT3* mutations causes ligand-independent cell survival, proliferation, and resistance to apoptosis, and it was therefore hypothesized that inhibiting FLT3 signaling would produce cytotoxicity and clinical responses. *FLT3* mutations were the first "actionable" mutations in AML and the first molecular target for which an inhibitor was approved by the FDA.[242]

FLT3 inhibitors are classified into first and second generation based on their specificity for FLT3.[447] First-generation inhibitors, including midostaurin, sunitinib, and sorafenib, inhibit multiple other receptor tyrosine kinases in addition to FLT3. They may have enhanced antileukemia efficacy by virtue of inhibiting targets downstream of FLT3 or in parallel signaling pathways, or other targets in AML cells. However, off-target activities also cause toxicities. In contrast, second-generation FLT3 inhibitors, including quizartinib, crenolanib, and gilteritinib, were derived from rational drug development and are more specific and more potent against FLT3 and have fewer toxicities associated with off-target effects. However, second-generation FLT3 inhibitors generally do not have efficacy against targets downstream of FLT3 or in parallel signaling pathways. AML with *FLT3*-ITD is characterized by coexistence of multiple leukemic clones and sometimes low allelic burden of the FLT3 mutation at diagnosis, while FLT3-mutant allelic burden is higher at relapse,[448] potentially supporting efficacy of second-generation inhibitors in relapsed AML with FLT3 mutations, while first-generation inhibitors may have efficacy by inhibiting multiple targets in AML at diagnosis.

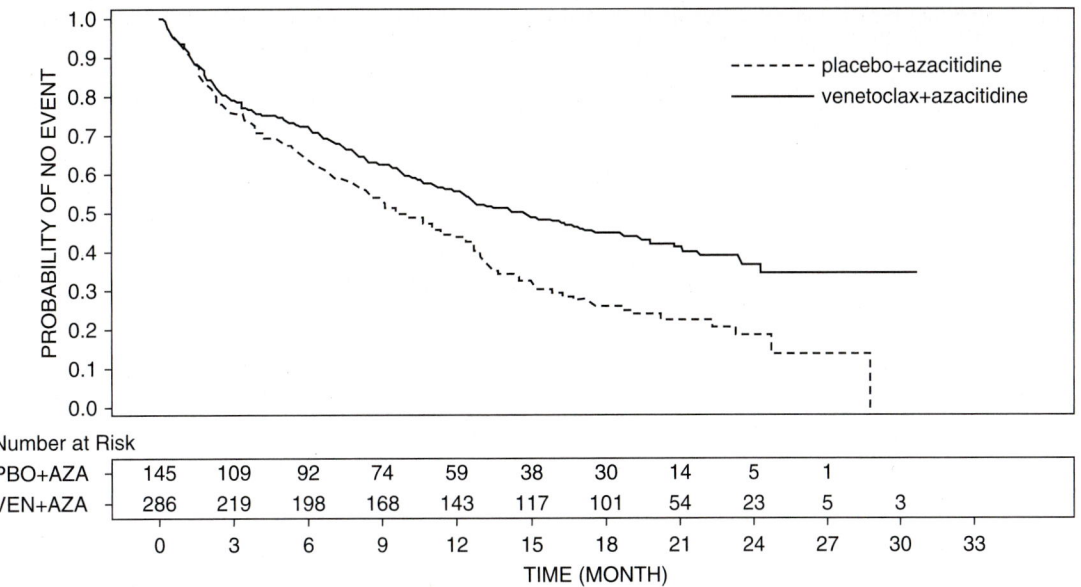

FIGURE 76.15 Kaplan-Meier curve for overall survival in the intention-to-treat population in VIALE-A study comparing venetoclax + azacitidine with placebo + azacitidine for newly diagnosed older or medically unfit patients with AML.

FLT3 inhibitors are also classified into types I and II based on their mechanism of interaction with FLT3.[447] Type I inhibitors bind to the ATP-binding site when the receptor is active, while type II inhibitors interact with a hydrophobic region immediately adjacent to the ATP-binding site that is only accessible when the receptor is in the inactive conformation, and they prevent receptor activation. D835 is the most common site for TKD mutations, and D835 mutations favor the active conformation. Consequently, type I inhibitors inhibit FLT3 signaling in AML cells with either ITD or TKD mutations, while type II inhibitors inhibit FLT3 with ITD, but not with TKD mutations, although some D835 mutations preserve sensitivity.[449] Importantly, development of D835 mutations in FLT3-ITD is a mechanism of acquired, or secondary, resistance to type II FLT3 inhibitors.[450] Type I inhibitors include sunitinib, midostaurin, crenolanib, and gilteritinib, while type II inhibitors include sorafenib, quizartinib, and ponatinib.

Midostaurin (Rydapt), a first-generation type I FLT3 inhibitor, was approved by the FDA in April 2017 for treatment of adults with newly diagnosed AML with FLT3-ITD or TKD mutations, in combination with cytarabine and daunorubicin induction and HiDAC consolidation chemotherapy and as subsequent maintenance therapy. Approval was based on a randomized, double-blind, placebo-controlled trial in 717 patients 18 to 59 years with previously untreated AML with FLT3 mutations.[341] Patients were randomly assigned to receive either midostaurin or placebo. Induction therapy consisted of cytarabine 200 mg/m^2 and daunorubicin 60 mg/m^2 as a 7 + 3 regimen, and consolidation therapy was four cycles of HiDAC, 3000 mg/m^2 over 3 hours every 12 hours on days 1, 3, and 5. The dose of midostaurin was 50 mg twice daily with food on days 8 to 21 of each induction and consolidation cycle, then 50 mg with food as single-agent maintenance therapy for up to 12 months. CR rates were similar on both arms (59% and 54%), but OS was significantly longer in the midostaurin arm than in the placebo arm (HR for death, 0.78; one-sided P = .009), as was EFS (HR for event or death, 0.78; one-sided P = .002). In both the primary analysis and an analysis in which data for patients who underwent transplantation were censored, the benefit of midostaurin was consistent for patients with FLT3-ITD with high (>0.7) or low (0.05-0.7) allelic ratios or with FLT3-TKD mutations.[341]

Sorafenib is a first-generation type II FLT3 inhibitor that also inhibits RAF, vascular endothelial growth factor receptors (VEGFR)-1,2,3, platelet-derived growth factor receptor (PDGFR)-β, KIT, and RET and is FDA-approved for treatment of renal, hepatocellular, and thyroid carcinomas. As a type II FLT3 inhibitor, sorafenib should be active against FLT3-ITD but not against most TKD mutations, including D835 mutations. Sorafenib monotherapy decreased marrow blasts in 12 of 13 patients with R/R AML with FLT3-ITD in a phase 2 clinical trial, with mean response duration of 72 days; notably, new D835 TKD mutations emerged in four of six patients studied at progression.[451] Importantly, sorafenib monotherapy has shown efficacy in treating relapsed FLT3-ITD AML, including after allo-HSCT.[452] Sorafenib can be safely administered as post-HSCT maintenance therapy, with a maximum tolerated dose of 400 mg twice daily,[453] and its efficacy in preventing post-HSCT relapse is being studied. Data on efficacy of sorafenib with chemotherapy have been inconsistent. In a randomized, double-blind, placebo-controlled phase 2 trial of sorafenib after induction and consolidation chemotherapy and as 12-month maintenance therapy in patients with AML 18 to 60 years with or without FLT3 mutations, median EFS was 21 vs 9 months with sorafenib vs placebo, and 3-year EFS 40% vs 22% (P = .013), although differences in patients with FLT3-ITD AML were not statistically significant.[454] In a randomized clinical trial in previously untreated patients with AML over 60 years, sorafenib after induction and consolidation chemotherapy was associated with increased toxicities and did not improve EFS or OS, including in patients with FLT3 mutations.[455] However, 1-year OS doubled vs historical controls (62% vs 30%; P < .0001) in newly diagnosed adults 60 years and older with ITD or TKD mutations receiving sorafenib on days 1 to 7 of induction and days 1 to 28 of consolidation chemotherapy and as 1-year maintenance therapy. Sorafenib maintenance therapy was associated with diarrhea, fatigue, transaminitis, and hand-foot syndrome.[456]

Quizartinib is a second-generation type II FLT3 inhibitor with potent activity and selectivity against AML with FLT3-ITD, but not TKD, mutations. In a phase 1 trial in patients with R/R AML,[457] the maximum tolerated dose was 200 mg daily, with prolonged QT interval as the dose-limiting toxicity. Quizartinib produced CR or CRi in 53% and 14% of patients with FLT3-ITD and wild-type FLT3, respectively, with median response duration and survival of 13.3 and 14 weeks. Quizartinib was then evaluated in a phase 2 trial in patients with R/R AML with FLT3-ITD.[458] Blast counts decreased sufficiently to allow allo-HSCT in 35% of patients, and allo-HSCT prolonged OS. Quizartinib was studied in QuANTUM-R, a randomized (2:1), controlled, multicenter phase 3 trial for adult patients with R/R FLT3-ITD AML after standard therapy with or without allo-HSCT. Patients received quizartinib (60 mg [30 mg lead-in] orally once daily) or investigator's choice of preselected chemotherapy: subcutaneous LDAC; mitoxantrone, etoposide, and cytarabine (MEC); or granulocyte colony-stimulating factor, fludarabine, cytarabine, and idarubicin (FLAG-Ida).[459] Overall 367 patients were enrolled; 245 received quizartinib and 122 salvage chemotherapy. Median OS was 6.2 months (5.3-7.2) for quizartinib and 4.7 months (4.0-5.5) for chemotherapy ($P = .02$).[459] The most common greater than grade 3 nonhematological treatment-emergent adverse events for quizartinib and chemotherapy were sepsis and septic shock (19% for both arms). There were 80 (33%) treatment-emergent deaths on quizartinib and 16 (17%) on chemotherapy.[459] While the Ministry of Health, Labor, and Welfare of Japan approved quizartinib for treatment of adult patients with R/R *FLT3*-ITD, the FDA has not granted approval to quizartinib. Quizartinib is being further studied in combination with chemotherapy in older and younger patients with newly diagnosed or R/R AML with *FLT3*-ITD, and as maintenance therapy after allo-HSCT.[460] Development of FLT3 point mutations, most commonly at D835, is a mechanism of acquired resistance to quizartinib.[450]

Gilteritinib is a second-generation type I FLT3 inhibitor, with activity in AML with *FLT3*-ITD or TKD mutations. In a phase 1/2 trial in adults with R/R AML,[461] gilteritinib was well tolerated. At least 90% FLT3 phosphorylation inhibition was seen by day 8 in most patients receiving a daily dose of 80 mg or higher. The overall response rate in patients with *FLT3* mutations receiving ≥80 mg daily was 52% (CR = 11%, CRp = 6%, CRi = 24%, PR = 11%). Median time to best response was 7.2 weeks, and median response duration was 20 weeks. The efficacy of gilteritinib (120 mg orally once daily) was then assessed in the ADMIRAL study, a randomized (2:1), controlled, multicenter phase 3 trial that included adult patients with R/R AML with *FLT3*-ITD, D835, or I836 mutations.[462] Of 371 eligible patients, 247 were randomly assigned to gilteritinib and 124 to salvage chemotherapy. In 2018, the FDA approved gilteritinib for the treatment of adult patients with R/R AML with a *FLT3* mutation as detected by an FDA-approved test,[243] based on the first interim analysis ($n = 138$) demonstrating the efficacy of gilteritinib on the basis of the rate of CR + CRh (21%, 95% CI: 15, 29), duration of CR + CRh (4.6 months, 95% CI: 2.8, 15.8), and rate of conversion from transfusion dependence to transfusion independence.[243] The two primary end points were OS and the percentage of patients who achieved CR or CRh. OS on the gilteritinib arm was significantly longer than that on the chemotherapy arm (9.3 vs 5.6 months; $P < .001$) (*Figure 76.16*).[462] Median EFS was 2.8 months for gilteritinib and 0.7 months for chemotherapy. The percentage of patients who achieved CR or CRh was 34% in the gilteritinib group and 15% in the chemotherapy group. Adverse events greater than grade 3 and serious adverse events occurred less frequently with gilteritinib than with chemotherapy; the most common greater than grade 3 adverse events in the gilteritinib arm were febrile neutropenia (46%), anemia (41%), and thrombocytopenia (23%).[462]

Analysis of baseline and progression samples from patients treated on clinical trials of gilteritinib showed that the most common mechanism of resistance to gilteritinib is treatment-emergent activating mutations in RAS/MAPK pathway signaling, most commonly in *NRAS* or *KRAS*. The second most common mechanism of resistance to gilteritinib is the development of secondary (i.e., additional to ITD) *FLT3*-F691L gatekeeper mutations.[306]

IDH Inhibitors

The biochemistry and metabolic, genetic, and epigenetic features of IDH1 and IDH2 wild-type and mutant enzymes are summarized in the "Molecular Abnormalities" section and in *Figures 76.8* and *76.9*.

In 2017, the FDA approved enasidenib for the treatment of adult patients with R/R AML with an *IDH2* mutation as detected by an FDA-approved test.[463] The recommended dose is 100 mg orally once daily until disease progression or unacceptable toxicity. Enasidenib is a small molecule inhibitor of the IDH2 enzyme, which targets the IDH2^{mut} variants R140Q, R172S, and R172K at approximately 40-fold lower concentrations (i.e., more potency) than the wild-type enzyme in vitro. In preclinical studies in mouse xenograft models of *IDH2*^{mut} AML, inhibition of the mutant IDH2 enzyme by enasidenib resulted in diminishing 2-HG levels and induction of myeloid differentiation. In patients with *IDH2*^{mut} AML, enasidenib reduced blast counts, increased percentages of mature myeloid cells, and decreased 2-HG levels. Enasidenib was approved based on an open-label, single-arm, multicenter, two-cohort clinical trial (Study AG221-C-001) of 199 adult patients with a median age of 68 years with relapsed (48%) or refractory (52%) AML with *IDH2*-R140 (78%) or *IDH2*-R172 (22%) mutations who received 100 mg daily dose until disease progression or unacceptable toxicity.[464] Efficacy of enasidenib was demonstrated based on the rates of CR (19%, 95% CI 13%-25%) plus CRh (4%, 95% CI 2%-8%), with median duration of CR + CRh 8.2 months (95% CI, 4.3-19.4) and a 34% rate of conversion from red blood cell and platelet transfusion dependence to independence. Median follow-up was 6.6 months (range, 0.4-27.7 months). Similar CR + CRh rates were observed in patients with either R140 or R172 mutation.[463] Enasidenib is also approved for the same indication in Australia and Canada.

The phase 3 international, multicenter, open-label, randomized clinical trial (IDHENTIFY study) comparing the efficacy and safety of enasidenib vs continuous 28-day cycles of best supportive care only, azacitidine subcutaneously plus best supportive care, LDAC subcutaneously plus best supportive care, or intermediate-dose cytarabine intravenously plus best supportive care, in patients aged 60 years or older with relapsed (after 2nd or 3rd line) or refractory AML with an IDH2 mutation did not meet the primary endpoint of OS.

In 2018, the FDA approved ivosidenib, a small molecule inhibitor of the IDH1 enzyme for treatment of *IDH1*-mutated R/R AML.[465] The efficacy of ivosidenib was assessed in an open-label, single-arm, multicenter clinical trial (Study AG120-C-001) of 174 adult patients with R/R AML with an *IDH1*-R132 mutation.[466] Ivosidenib was given orally at a starting dose of 500 mg daily until disease progression, development of unacceptable toxicity, or allo-HSCT; the latter occurred in 21 patients (12%). Median number of prior therapies was 2 (range 1-6) and approximately 25% of patients had had prior allo-HSCT.[466] Efficacy was established on the basis of the CR + CRh rate (33%, 95% CI: 26, 40), duration of CR + CRh (8.2 months, 95% CI: 5.6, 12), and rate of conversion from transfusion dependence to transfusion independence (37%).[465]

In 2019, based on data on 28 adult patients with newly diagnosed AML with an *IDH1* mutation,[467] the FDA extended the indication of ivosidenib to treatment of newly diagnosed *IDH1*-mutated AML in patients ≥75 years old or with comorbidities precluding use of intensive induction chemotherapy.[465] Importantly, 46% of these patients had received prior DNMTis for an antecedent hematologic disorder. The CR + CRh rate was 42% (95% CI: 26%, 61%); CR 30% (95% CI: 16%, 49%). Median durations of CR + CRh and CR were not reached; 62% and 78% of patients remained in remission at 1 year. With median follow-up of approximately 2 years (range, 0.6-40.9 months), median OS was 12.6 months (95% CI, 4.5-25.7). Of 21 transfusion-dependent patients at baseline, 9 (43%) became transfusion-independent.[467] A second IDH1 inhibitor, olutasidenib, in 2022.[293]

Isocitrate dehydrogenase differentiation syndrome is a potentially fatal (in ~5% of patients) clinical entity, occurring in approximately 20% of patients with *IDH1*^{mut}/*IDH2*^{mut} AML treated with *IDH1* or *IDH2* inhibitor.[468] Leukocytosis is present in 60% to 80% of cases.[469] Symptoms and signs of differentiation syndrome may include fever, dyspnea, hypoxia, pulmonary infiltrates, pleural or pericardial effusions, rapid weight gain or peripheral edema, hypotension, and hepatic, renal, or multiorgan dysfunction. Median time to onset of differentiation syndrome is approximately 3 weeks after the initiation of an IDH inhibitor, but it may occur up to 3 months after the start of treatment.[468] Baseline bone marrow blasts ≥48% and peripheral blood blasts ≥25% (for ivosidenib) and 15% (for enasidenib) are associated with increased risk of differentiation syndrome.[468] If differentiation syndrome is suspected, prompt initiation of corticosteroid therapy (dexamethasone 10 mg twice daily) is required and should continue until symptom resolution.[469] If symptoms do not respond within 48 hours, IDH inhibitor should be temporarily discontinued until resolution. Hydroxycarbamide may be used for cytoreduction.

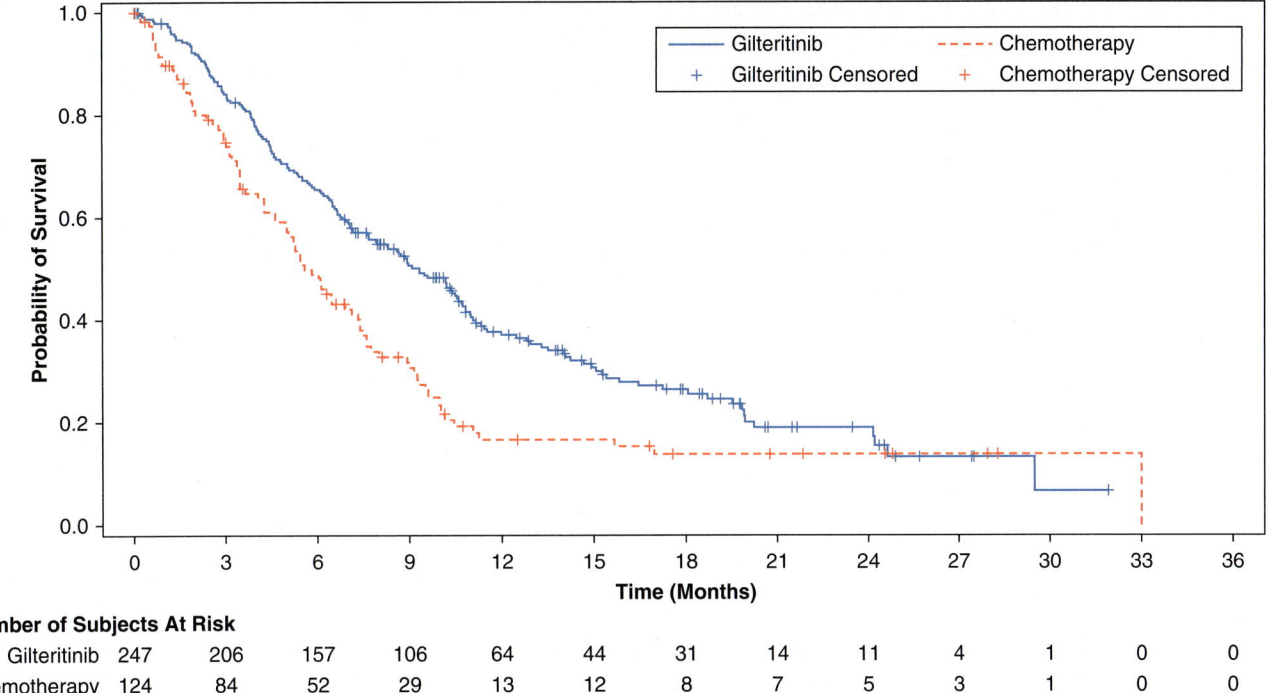

FIGURE 76.16 Kaplan-Meier curve for overall survival in the intention-to-treat population in the ADMIRAL study comparing gilteritinib with salvage chemotherapy for patients with relapsed or refractory AML with *FLT3* mutations (*FLT3* ITD, D835, or I836).

Hedgehog Pathway Inhibitor

In 2018, the FDA approved glasdegib in combination with LDAC for treatment of newly diagnosed AML in adult patients ≥75 years or with comorbidities precluding use of intensive induction chemotherapy.[470] Glasdegib is an inhibitor of the Hedgehog pathway and binds to and inhibits Smoothened, a transmembrane protein involved in hedgehog signal transduction.

The efficacy of glasdegib in combination with LDAC was evaluated in a multicenter, open-label, randomized clinical trial (Study BRIGHT AML 1003).[471] The study evaluated 115 patients ≥55 years with newly diagnosed AML who met at least one of the following criteria: age > 75 years, severe cardiac disease, baseline ECOG performance status 2, or baseline serum creatinine > 1.3 mg/dL. Patients were randomized 2:1 to receive glasdegib (100 mg daily) with LDAC (20 mg) subcutaneously twice daily on days 1-10 of a 28-day cycle ($n = 77$) or LDAC alone in 28-day cycles ($n = 38$) until disease progression or unacceptable toxicity. Patients were stratified by cytogenetic risk (good/intermediate or poor).[471] Baseline demographic and disease characteristics were balanced between the two arms.[471] Efficacy was established on the basis of OS. With a median follow-up of approximately 20 months, glasdegib with LDAC was superior to LDAC alone (median survival, 8.3 vs 4.3 months, $P = .0002$).[470] CR rates were 18% (14 of 77) with glasdegib + LDAC and 3% (1 out of 38) with LDAC alone. Glasdegib can cause embryo-fetal death or severe birth defects when administered to a pregnant woman; pregnancy test before its administration is mandatory. Glasdegib causes QTc interval prolongation >500 milliseconds in 5% of patients and severe muscle/leg spasms, also in 5%.

Gemtuzumab Ozogamicin

In early studies in AML, unconjugated monoclonal antibodies targeting CD14, CD15, and CD33 produced low response rates (<10%).[472,473] Consequently, investigators turned to conjugated antibody therapy, with CD33 one of the best studied targets, as it is expressed on AML cells in 90% of cases[156] but not on normal hematopoietic stem cells. The best studied anti-CD33 antibody conjugate is gemtuzumab ozogamicin (GO, Mylotarg), a recombinant humanized anti-CD33 monoclonal antibody attached to calicheamicin, an antibiotic that binds to the minor groove of DNA, causing double-strand breaks and apoptosis.[474]

When two 9 mg/m² GO doses were given over 4 hours 14 days apart to patients with CD33⁺ AML in untreated first relapse in phase 2 trials, the overall response rate was 26%, including 13% CR and 13% CRp.[475,476] Response rates did not differ based on age or duration of CR1. Median OS was 4.9 months for all patients and 12.6 months for responders. Severe myelosuppression occurred, reflecting expression of CD33 on mature myeloid cells, but sepsis (17%) and pneumonia (8%) were relatively uncommon.[476]

GO was subsequently also tested as frontline therapy. A 33% + 5% CR + CRp rate was seen in patients with AML 61 to 75 years of age who were not candidates for cytotoxic chemotherapy.[477] Addition of GO to different induction and consolidation chemotherapy regimens resulted in no overall difference in CR rate or survival, but survival benefit was demonstrated for patients with favorable-risk cytogenetic findings.[478]

GO was approved by the FDA for treatment of patients ≥60 years with CD33-positive AML in first relapse in May 2000 under the Accelerated Approval regulations. Postmarketing reports of fatal anaphylaxis, tumor lysis, adult respiratory distress syndrome, and hepatic veno-occlusive disease (VOD) required labeling revisions and initiation of a surveillance program.[474] Under accelerated approval, additional clinical trials are required after approval to confirm the drug's benefit. If those trials fail to confirm clinical benefit, the FDA can withdraw the drug from the market. A confirmatory clinical trial was designed and initiated in 2004 to determine whether adding GO to standard chemotherapy would improve survival of patients with AML. The trial was stopped early when no clinical benefit was observed and after a greater number of deaths occurred in patients who received GO compared with chemotherapy alone. GO was withdrawn from the market in June 2010.

Over the next 7 years, several clinical trials were reported with different doses and schedules of administration. In 2017, the FDA granted full approval to GO for treatment of newly diagnosed CD33⁺ AML in adults as well as R/R CD33⁺ AML in adults and in pediatric patients 2 years and older.[479] Approval of GO for newly diagnosed CD33+ AML in combination with chemotherapy was based on the results of a multicenter, randomized, open-label phase 3 study of 271 patients with newly diagnosed de novo AML age 50 to 70 years, who were randomized (1:1) to receive induction therapy consisting of cytarabine 200 mg/m^2 and daunorubicin 60 mg/m^2 as a 7 + 3 regimen with (n = 135) or without (n = 136) GO 3 mg/m^2 (up to maximum of one 5 mg vial) on days 1, 4, and 7 (ALFA-0701 study). Patients who did not achieve a response after first induction could receive a second induction with cytarabine and daunorubicin alone. Patients who achieved a response received two consolidation courses including 60 mg/m^2 of daunorubicin on day 1 of consolidation course 1 and days 1 and 2 of consolidation course 2 plus HiDAC 1000 mg/m^2 over 3 hours every 12 hours days 1 to 4, with or without GO 3 mg/m^2 on day 1, according to their initial randomization. For patients who achieved CR and planned to proceed to allo-HSCT, an interval of at least 2 months between the last dose of GO and transplantation was recommended because of concern for VOD. In this ALFA-0701 trial, median patient age was 62 years and baseline characteristics were balanced between treatment arms. Approximately 65% and 70% of patients had favorable/intermediate-risk and 27% and 21% had adverse-risk disease by the ELN and cytogenetic risk classifications, respectively. Median EFS was 17.3 months on the GO arm vs 9.5 months on the control arm (P < .001), Figure 76.17.[479,480]

A meta-analysis of five randomized trials showed that addition of GO to remission induction therapy improved survival in core-binding factor AML, with an absolute survival benefit of 20.7% (P = .0006), even though CR rates were not higher with GO-containing regimens. The largest benefits were observed in the studies that used lower (3 mg/m^2) or fractionated (3 mg/m^2 on days 1, 3, and 5: ALFA trial) doses of GO, rather than GO 6 mg/m^2.[481]

GO is also approved as monotherapy based on a multicenter, randomized (1:1), open-label phase 3 study comparing it with best supportive care (BSC), including standard supportive care measures and hydroxyurea or other antimetabolites for palliative purposes for patients with newly diagnosed AML either >75 years or 61 to 75 years with WHO performance status ≥2 or unwilling to receive intensive chemotherapy (Study AML-19). For induction, GO was given on day 1 (6 mg/m^2) and day 8 (3 mg/m^2). Patients continued therapy with up to eight courses of GO (2 mg/m^2 on day 1 every 4 weeks) in the absence of disease progression or significant toxicities. Median patient age was 77 years and baseline characteristics were balanced between treatment arms, except for more patients with favorable/intermediate-risk cytogenetics on the GO arm (n = 118; 50%) than the BSC arm (n = 119; 38%). Median OS was 4.9 months on the GO arm vs 3.6 months on the BSC arm (HR for OS 0.69, two-sided P = .005).[479]

GO was approved as monotherapy for treatment of adults with CD33+ AML in first relapse based on a single-arm (n = 57), open-label phase 2 study (MyloFrance-1). Forty-four patients (78%) had intermediate-risk and 12 (22%) poor-risk cytogenetics. Patients with secondary AML or previous auto- or allo-HSCT were excluded. For induction, GO was given on days 1, 4, and 7 (3 mg/m^2). Consolidation consisted of HiDAC (3000 mg/m^2 for patients <55 years and 1000 mg/m^2 for patients ≥55 years) every 12 hours on days 1 to 3. Fifteen patients (26%) achieved CR after a single course of GO, with a median CR1 duration of 10 months.[479]

Immunotherapy

Immunotherapeutic interventions are being explored in different treatment settings for patients with AML, including induction, post induction for clearance of minimal residual disease, post consolidation, and relapsed or refractory. Postconsolidation immunotherapy with interleukin-2 and histamine dihydrochloride, both administered subcutaneously, significantly improved 3-year leukemia-free survival.[482]

T-cell-based immunotherapy for AML includes bispecific and dual antigen receptor-targeting antibodies (targeted to CD33, CD123, CLL-1, and other antigens), chimeric antigen receptor (CAR) T-cell therapies, and T-cell immune checkpoint inhibitors targeting PD-1, PD-L1, CTLA-4, and TIM3,[483] allo-HSCT, donor lymphocyte infusion post allo-HSCT, and haploidentical NK cell infusion, CSL362 (unconjugated antibody targeting CD123), AMG330 (bispecific T-cell engaging antibody targeting CD33 and CD3), MGD006 (dual affinity retargeting antibody targeting CD123 and CD3), CD16x33 BiKE (bispecific killer cell engager antibody against CD16 and CD33), CART33 (chimeric

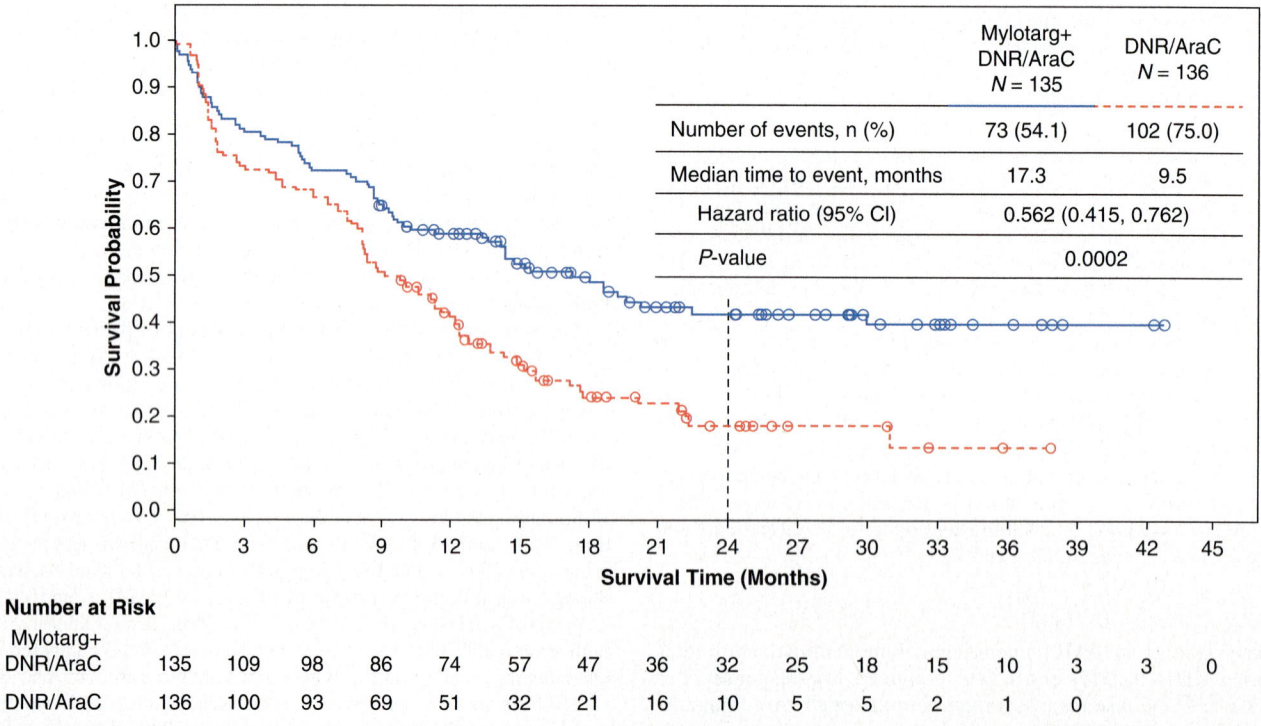

FIGURE 76.17 Kaplan-Meier curve of event-free survival from study ALFA-0701 comparing cytarabine and daunorubicin with or without gemtuzumab ozogamicin (GO; Mylotarg). Data are not censored for HSCT. Abbreviations: ALFA, Acute Leukemia French Association; DNR/AraC, daunorubicin + cytarabine; N, total number of patients in the treatment arm.

antigen receptor-transduced T cells targeting CD33), CART123 (chimeric antigen receptor-transduced T cells targeting CD123), WT1 peptide vaccine, and WT1-specific CD8+ T-cell infusion.

Flotetuzumab, a bispecific DART antibody-based molecule targeting CD3ε and CD123, was evaluated in a multicenter, open-label, phase 1/2 study in 88 adults with relapsed or refractory AML (42 in a dose-finding segment and 46 at the recommended phase 2 dose [RP2D] of 500 ng/kg/d).[484] The most frequent adverse events were grade 1 to 2 infusion-related reactions and cytokine release syndrome, which were successfully managed by stepwise dosing during week 1, pretreatment dexamethasone, prompt use of tocilizumab, a monoclonal antibody against the interleukin-6 receptor, and temporary dose reductions/interruptions. Clinical benefit was observed in patients with primary induction failure or early (<6 months) relapse, with a CR + CRh rate of 27% among 30 patients treated at the RP2D,[484] and median OS 10.2 months (range, 1.87-27.27), with 6- and 12-month survival rates of 75% (95% CI, 0.450-1.05) and 50% (95% CI, 0.154-0.846) in patients who achieved CR or CRh.[484] Interestingly, patients with relapsed or refractory AML with TP53 mutation or loss had a CR rate of 47% (7 of 15) and had a significantly higher tumor inflammation signature, including FOXP3, CD8, inflammatory chemokine, and PD1 gene expression scores, at baseline compared with nonresponders.[264]

Relapsed and Refractory AML

Approximately half of younger patients and a majority (>85%) of older patients with AML will either not achieve a CR (i.e., primary refractory) or will relapse. The percentage of patients who have refractory AML is at least 20% but varies depending on age, cytogenetics, and mutations.[485] Table 76.8 shows the European Prognostic Index (EPI) scoring system for patients with R/R AML.[486] Prognostic groups: favorable (EPI 1 to 6 points; OS of 70% at 1 year and 46% at 5 years); intermediate (EPI 7-9 points; OS of 49% at 1 year and 18% at 5 year); poor (EPI 10-14 points; OS of 16% at 1 year and 4% at 5 years).

To date, there is no standard regimen for induction of a CR2. Dose escalation and use of non-cross-resistant regimens have been helpful in inducing CR2. Cytarabine has been used in doses ranging from 1000 to 3000 mg/m² every 12 to 24 hours for 3 to 6 days, alone or in combination with other agents, including anthracyclines, etoposide, clofarabine, fludarabine, cladribine, GO, L-asparaginase, mitoxantrone, and topotecan (Table 76.9).[487-497] HiDAC alone resulted in a CR rate of 40%, compared with 56% in patients receiving HiDAC with an anthracycline.[487]

Capizzi and colleagues reported synergy between HiDAC and asparaginase in the treatment of adults with R/R AML.[489] In this CALGB study, the investigators randomly assigned 195 adult patients with refractory or first-relapse AML to receive HiDAC 3000 mg/m² as a 3-hour intravenous infusion every 12 hours for four doses, followed by 6000 U/m² intramuscular asparaginase administered at hour 42, or HiDAC alone, with treatment repeated on day 8.[489] Median patient age was 52 years. The CR rate on the HiDAC plus asparaginase arm was 40%, compared with 24% on the HiDAC arm (P = .02). Median OS was also longer with HiDAC + asparaginase compared with HiDAC (19.6 vs 15.9 weeks; P = .046). Toxicity was comparable on the two treatment arms.[485] In a retrospective single-center study of patients with R/R AML, HiDAC, mitoxantrone, and pegaspargase (HAM-pegA) appeared superior to cladribine, high-dose cytarabine, filgrastim, and mitoxantrone (CLAG-M).[498]

Single-agent clofarabine resulted in a 30% CR rate in a phase 2 single-arm clinical trial in patients with R/R AML.[499] A phase 3 prospective randomized trial (n = 320) in patients >55 years with R/R AML compared the combination of clofarabine plus ara-C with ara-C alone.[500] The CR rate (41% for the combination vs 16% for ara-C alone, P = .001) was higher with the combination regimen, but OS as the primary endpoint did not differ between the two arms (6.6 months for the combination vs 6.4 months in the ara-C arm).

In recent years, the DNMTis azacitidine and decitabine have been extensively used as monotherapy or in combination with conventional or novel/targeted therapeutic agents to treat R/R AML, albeit with lower response rates than in previously untreated disease.[501,502]

Table 76.8. Prognostic Scoring Systems for Patients With Refractory/Relapsed AML[486]

Factor	Points
CR1 duration (months)	
>18	0
7-18	3
<6	5
Cytogenetics at diagnosis	
t(16;16) or inv(16)	0
t(8;21)	3
Other	5
Age at first relapse (years)	
<35	0
36-45	1
>45	2
Stem cell transplantation before first relapse	
No	0
Yes	2

All patients with R/R AML are candidates for clinical trials with novel therapies (see "Therapy" section). Allo-HSCT is superior to chemotherapy for patients with R/R disease, but many patients are not candidates for transplant due to age, comorbidities, or lack of an appropriate donor (see "Hematopoietic Stem Cell Transplantation" section). Although patients with a matched related donor can be offered allo-HSCT in early relapse, there is an advantage and sometimes a necessity to administer additional chemotherapy to lessen the leukemia burden before transplantation, particularly if there is a delay in obtaining a donor (i.e., unrelated) or if a nonmyeloablative approach is utilized (see "Hematopoietic Stem Cell Transplantation" section). Auto-HSCT is also an alternative for patients in CR2, but it is probably inferior to allo-HSCT and is not usually recommended.

The probability of CR2 depends on duration of CR1 and cytogenetics, and CR2s are generally shorter than CR1s.[503-505] CR2 was achieved in 55% to 60% of patients with initial CR > 1 year, compared with 33% to 46% with CR < 1 year,[504,506] and in 80% to 88%, 18% to 49%, and 0% to 30% of patients with favorable-, intermediate- and poor-risk cytogenetics, respectively.[503,507]

HEMATOPOIETIC STEM CELL TRANSPLANTATION

HSCT is the focus of Chapter 105. Considerations specific to AML are briefly discussed here.

AML has replaced CML as the most common disease treated with allo-HSCT due to the success of tyrosine kinase inhibitors in treating CML. Allo-HSCT is thought to have excellent efficacy in treating AML due to both the effect of high-dose chemotherapy with or without whole body irradiation utilized in the conditioning regimen and the immunologic graft-vs-leukemia (GVL) effect.[508] Allo-HSCT is associated with the lowest relapse rates, but patient age, disease status, cytogenetics, mutations, prior therapy, comorbidities, performance status, and timing and type of transplant determine its outcome. Primary problems with allo-HSCT have been lack of suitable donors and high mortality caused by organ toxicity, infections, and graft-vs-host disease (GVHD). A recently published systematic review concluded that allo-HSCT provides a survival benefit in patients with intermediate- and high-risk AML and is currently part of standard clinical care.[509]

The donor pool is expanding, with increased availability of unrelated donors and umbilical cord transplants in adults and with innovative immunosuppression, including posttransplant cyclophosphamide, to allow HLA-mismatched donors.[510] Use of haplotype-matched

Table 76.9. List of a Few Conventional Salvage Chemotherapy Regimens and Their Reported CR Rates When Used in Patients With Relapsed/Refractory AML

Regimen	Agents	CR (%)	Treatment-Related or 30-Day Mortality (%)
HiDAC-based regimens			
HiDAC	Cytarabine 3 g/m^3 every 12 h days 1-6	32-47	12-15
HAM	Cytarabine 1-3 g/m^2 days 1-4 (8 doses) Mitoxantrone 10 mg/m^2 days 2-5	53	15-20
HAM-A	Cytarabine 1-3 g/m^2 days 1-3 (5 doses) Mitoxantrone 6 mg/m^2 days 1-3 Pegasparaginase 2000-2500/m^2 units day 4	41	14
FLA	Fludarabine 30 mg/m^2 days 1-5 Cytarabine 2 g/m^2 days 1-5	61	7
FLAD	Fludarabine 30 mg/m^2 days 1-3 Cytarabine 2 g/m^2 days 1-3 Liposomal daunorubicin 100 mg/m^2 days 1-3	53	7.5
FLAG/FLAG-IDA	Fludarabine 30 mg/m^2 days 1-5 Cytarabine 2 g/m^2 days 1-5 G-CSF 5 µg/kg day 0 until ANC recovery	48-55	10-11
	Fludarabine 30 mg/m^2 days 1-5 Cytarabine 2 g/m^2 days 1-5 G-CSF 300 µg day 0 until ANC recovery Idarubicin 8 mg/m^2 days 1-3	63	17
CLAG/CLAG-M	Cladribine 5 mg/m^2 days 2-6 Cytarabine 2 g/m^2 days 2-6 G-CSF 300 µg days 1-6	38-50	0-17
	Cladribine 5 mg/m^2 days 1-5 Cytarabine 2 g/m^2 days 1-5 G-CSF 300 µg days 0-5 Mitoxantrone 10 mg/m^2 days 1-3	50-58 (53% after first course)	0-7
MEC	Mitoxantrone 6 mg/m^2 days 1-6 Etoposide 80 mg/m^2 days 1-6 Cytarabine 1 g/m^2 days 1-6	59-66	3-6
	Mitoxantrone 8 mg/m^2 days 1-5 Etoposide 100 mg/m^2 days 1-5 Cytarabine 1 mg/m^2 days 1-5	18-24	7-11
MEC/Decitabine	Decitabine 20 mg/m^2 days 1-10 Mitoxantrone 8 mg/m^2 days 16-20 Etoposide 100 mg/m^2 days 16-20 Cytarabine 1 mg/m^2 days 16-20	30-50	20
EMA-86	Etoposide 200 mg/m^2 CI days 8-10 Mitoxantrone 12 mg/m^2 days 1-3 Cytarabine 500 mg/m^2 CI days 1-3 & 8-10	60	11
MAV	Mitoxantrone 10 mg/m^2 days 4-8 Cytarabine 100 mg/m^2 CI days 1-8 Etoposide 100-120 mg/m^2 days 4-8	58	11
FLAM	Flavopiridol 50 mg/m^2 days 1-3 Cytarabine 2 g/m^2/72 h starting day 6 Mitoxantrone 40 mg/m^2 day 9	28-43	5-28
Hybrid FLAM	Flavopiridol 30 mg/m^2 bolus, 60 mg/m^2 over 4 h days 1-3 Cytarabine 2 g/m^2/72 h starting day 6 Mitoxantrone 40 mg/m^2 day 9	40	9
Non-HiDAC-based regimens			
Clofarabine	Clofarabine 22.5-40 mg/m^2 days 2-6	28-51	6.2-13
HAA	Homoharringtonine 4 mg/m^2 days 1-3 Cytarabine 150 mg/m^2 days 1-7 Aclarubicin 12 mg/m^2 days 1-7	76-80	0
Vyxeos	CPX 351 101 U/m^2 days 1, 3, and 5	23-37 (CR + CRi = 49%)	7-13

CI, continuous infusion.

donors is particularly relevant to minority patients, for whom matched unrelated donors are less frequently available.

Age is no longer an absolute contraindication to allo-HSCT with the use of nonmyeloablative conditioning regimens (Figure 76.18),[511] which allow older patients and those with comorbid illnesses to undergo allo-HSCT with lower early mortality, albeit with a higher relapse rate. Because nonmyeloablative allo-HSCT has less antileukemic effect, it relies on the GVL effect. The 3-year DFS for AML utilizing reduced-intensity conditioning has been 30% to 66%.[512] A CALGB prospective multicenter phase 2 study assessed the efficacy of reduced-intensity conditioning allo-HSCT in 114 patients ages 60 to 74 years (median, 65 years) with AML in CR1.[513] Two-year DFS and OS were 42% and 48%, respectively, for the entire group, and 40% and 50% for the 52% of patients who had unrelated donors ($P > .05$). These outcomes were superior to those of historical older patients treated without allo-HSCT. Several studies have explored the feasibility of posttransplant treatment with DNMTis,[514,515] with the ultimate goal of preventing early relapse, before establishment of GVL.

Although there is general agreement that allo-HSCT offers the best option for preventing relapse in patients with AML with intermediate- or poor-risk cytogenetics, its overall impact on survival and the optimal timing and method of stem cell transplantation (related vs unrelated; myeloablative vs reduced intensity) remain unresolved issues. Myeloablative conditioning is preferred in eligible patients and a haploidentical related donor is preferred over a cord blood unit in the absence of an HLA-identical related or unrelated donor.[509]

In most trials utilizing allo-HSCT in CR1 for patients without favorable cytogenetics, 5-year DFS is 45% to 75% using a matched related donor (Figure 76.19).[516,517] There has been a significant decline in transplant-related mortality to less than 10% for patients in CR1 in some reports due to a decrease in deaths from GVHD, infections, and organ toxicity; this decline in transplant-related mortality has led to improved survival in CR1 patients but not in patients in relapse or CR2 (Figure 76.19).[518]

The role of HSCT in the treatment of AML has been investigated in several prospective clinical trials.[519-524] In four major prospective trials, involving approximately 2700 patients with AML in CR1, only 71% of eligible patients received allo-HSCT, and only 47% of the remainder were randomized. Intent-to-treat analyses comparing survival between donor and no-donor are recommended to assess the impact of allo-HSCT in prospective trials. In three large prospective trials, EORTC-GIMEMA favored the donor arm for poor-risk cytogenetics, MRC 10 favored the donor arm for intermediate-risk cytogenetics, and HOVON-SAKK favored the donor arm for both risk groups.[520,522,523] A systematic review and meta-analysis of clinical trials involving more than 3500 patients with AML in CR1 including prospective biologic assignment reported a significant survival advantage for allo-HSCT compared with non-allo-HSCT in the treatment of patients with AML with intermediate and unfavorable cytogenetics, but not with favorable cytogenetics.[525]

Transplant in CR1 is generally not recommended for patients with favorable-risk disease (Table 76.3). This includes patients with the t(8;21) and inv(16)/t(16;16) cytogenetic abnormalities, although some KIT mutations confer intermediate risk to these patients.[191,197,526] AML with NPM1 mutation without FLT3-ITD is also considered favorable-risk disease. However, in a recent series patients with NPM1 mutations underwent allo-HSCT if they had matched sibling donors,[527] and the 3-year RFS was 71% vs 47% for 77 and 227 patients with and without donors, although OS was similar, likely reflecting successful salvage treatment after relapse. In another study, 2-year leukemia-free survival following allo-HSCT in 156 patients with normal karyotype and mutated NPM1 without FLT3-ITD was 75% following transplant in CR1, 51% in CR2, and 30% for advanced disease ($P < .0001$).[528] Finally, in another study, among 44 patients 18 to 60 years old with AML with NPM1 mutations but nonfavorable AML according to the ELN classification and with MRD measurement available in CR1 who underwent allo-HSCT in CR1, allo-HSCT significantly improved outcome in patients with a <4-log reduction in NPM1 mutation blood MRD, but not in patients with greater reduction in MRD in CR1.[529] This study suggested that blood NPM1 mutation MRD can be used to determine the likelihood of benefitting from allo-HSCT in CR1.

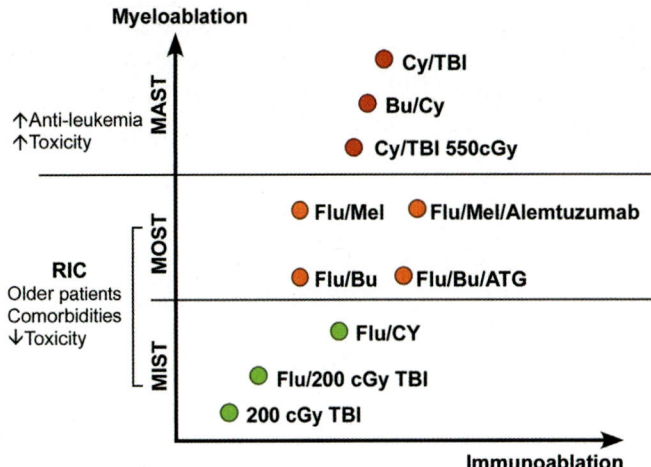

FIGURE 76.18 Diagram showing intensity of different regimens. The horizontal axis indicates the degree of immunoablation, and the vertical axis that of myeloablation. ATG, antithymocyte globulin; Bu, busulfan; CY, cyclophosphamide; Flu, fludarabine; MAST, myeloablative stem cell transplantation (SCT); Mel, melphalan; MIST, minimal-intensity SCT; MOST, moderate-intensity SCT; RIC, reduced-intensity SCT; TBI, total-body irradiation. (Adapted by permission from Nature: Kassim AA, Chinratanalab W, Ferrara JLM, Mineishi S. Reduced-intensity allogeneic hematopoietic stem cell transplantation for acute leukemias: 'what is the best recipe?' *Bone Marrow Transplant*. 2005;36(7):565-574. Copyright © 2005 Springer Nature.)

As detailed above, *FLT3*-ITD is the most important adverse prognostic factor in cytogenetically normal AML. A retrospective, single-institution study suggested that performing allo-HSCT in early CR1 could improve long-term outcomes for *FLT3*-ITD AML,[530] with comparable 4-year OS for 31 *FLT3*-ITD patients and 102 patients with wild-type *FLT3*. The role of allo-HSCT in CR1 was subsequently studied in 61 patients in relation to the allelic ratio of *FLT3*-ITD and presence or absence of *NPM1* mutations in the Study Alliance Leukemia AML2003 trial. *FLT3*-ITD AML was grouped into high- and low-ratio (HR-ITD and LR-ITD) using a predefined cutoff ratio of 0.8. OS ($P = .004$) and EFS ($P = .02$) were significantly improved in patients with HR-ITD AML who underwent allo-HSCT as consolidation treatment, compared with consolidation chemotherapy. Patients with LR-ITD AML and wild-type *NPM1* who underwent allo-HSCT in CR1 had longer OS ($P = .02$) and EFS ($P = .02$), whereas allo-HSCT in CR1 did not have a significant impact on OS and EFS in patients with LR-ITD AML and concomitant *NPM1* mutation.[240] Finally, in a retrospective analysis, 26 patients with AML with *FLT3*-ITD treated with the FLT3 multikinase inhibitor sorafenib as maintenance therapy after allo-HSCT in CR1 were compared with 55 patients who did not receive sorafenib.[531] Sorafenib was associated with improved 2-year progression-free survival (82% vs 53%, $P = .0081$) and lower 2-year cumulative incidence of relapse (8% vs 38%, $P = .0077$). In multivariate analysis, sorafenib significantly improved OS (HR, 0.26, $P = .021$) and progression-free survival (HR, 0.25, $P = .016$). Two-year nonrelapse mortality (10% vs 9%, $P = .82$) and 1-year chronic GVHD rate (56% vs 37%, $P = .28$) did not differ. Therefore, based on the current literature, allo-HSCT is the standard of care for patients with AML with *FLT3*-ITD with high allelic ratios and for patients with low allelic ratios without *NPM1* mutations, and posttransplant FLT3 inhibitor maintenance therapy appears to confer further benefit. Several FLT3 inhibitors are currently in clinical trials in the post-allo-HSCT setting.

The impact of combinations of *NPM1*, *FLT3*-ITD, and *CEBPα* mutations on outcome of allo-HSCT in CR1 was examined in 702 adults with cytogenetically normal AML.[532] Two-year OS from allo-HSCT was 81 ± 5% in $NPM1^{mut}/FLT3^{wt}$, 75 ± 3% in $NPM1^{wt}/FLT3^{wt}$, 66 ± 3% in $NPM1^{mut}/FLT3$-ITD, and 54 ± 7% in $NPM1^{wt}/FLT3$-ITD ($P = .003$). Analysis of *CEBPα* among patients with $NPM1^{wt}/FLT3^{wt}$ revealed excellent results in patients both with $CEBPα^{mut}$ and a triple-negative genotype, with 2-year OS of 100% and 77 ± 3%, respectively.

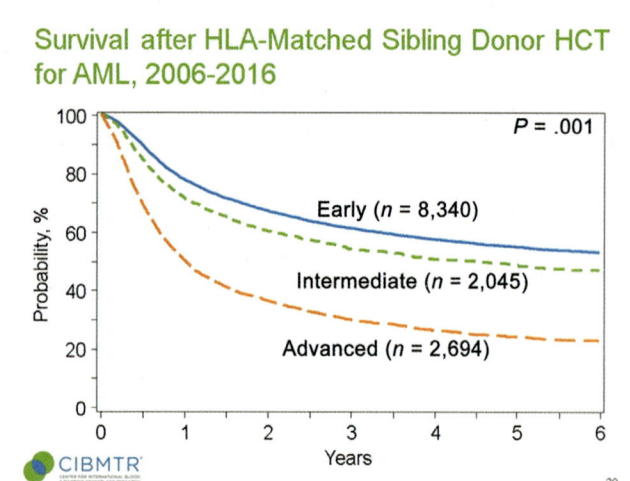
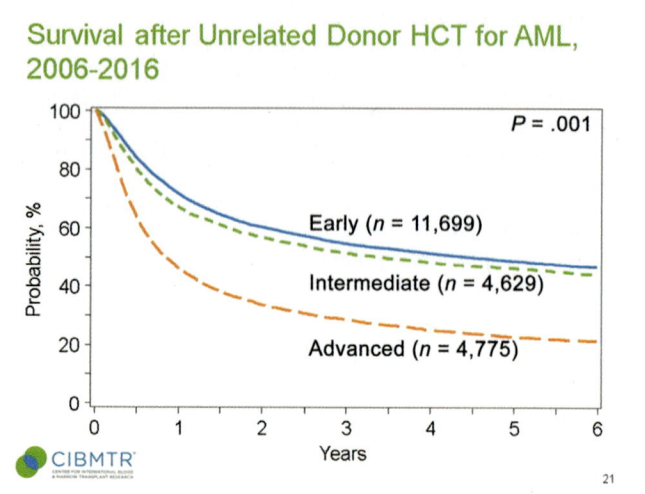

FIGURE 76.19 Center for International Blood and Marrow Transplant Research (CIBMTR) data for 34,221 patients receiving an HLA-matched sibling (n = 13,118) or unrelated donor (n = 21,103) transplant for AML between 2006 and 2016. Their disease status at the time of transplant and the donor type are the major predictors of posttransplant survival. The 3-year probabilities of survival after HLA-matched sibling transplant in this cohort were 59% ± 1%, 52% ± 1%, and 27% ± 1% for patients with early, intermediate, and advanced disease, respectively. The probabilities of survival after an unrelated donor transplant were 52% ± 1%, 49% ± 1%, and 26% ± 1% for patients with early, intermediate, and advanced disease, respectively.

As described in the above section on "Cytogenetic Abnormalities", *KMT2A* (previously *MLL*) translocations are generally prognostically unfavorable by virtue of association with short DFS, although survival of patients with de novo t(9;11) has varied among studies, placing it in an intermediate prognostic group. In 159 patients with 11q23/*KMT2A*-rearranged AML, mostly t(9;11), t(11;19), t(6;11), and t(10;11), allografted in CR1 (n = 138) or CR2, 2-year OS, leukemia-free survival, relapse incidence, and nonrelapse mortality were 56 ± 4%, 51 ± 4%, 31 ± 3%, and 17 ± 4%, respectively.[533] Outcomes were more favorable in patients with t(9;11) and t(11;19), compared with t(10;11) and t(6;11) (2-year OS: 64 ± 6% and 73 ± 10% vs 40 ± 13% and 24 ± 11%, respectively; $P < .0001$). Multivariate analysis for OS identified t(6;11), t(10;11), age>40 years and CR2 as unfavorable.

As detailed above, outcomes for AML with MK and/or *TP53* mutations are very poor. While MK and TP53 mutations therefore serve as indications for allo-HSCT, outcomes after allo-HSCT are also poor. Based on Center for International Blood and Marrow Transplant Research data, MK+ AML (n = 240) was associated with similar transplantation-related mortality (HR, 1.01; $P = .90$) but higher disease relapse (HR, 1.98; $P < .01$) and worse survival (HR, 1.67; $P < .01$) compared with other cytogenetically defined AML (n = 3360).[534] The strong negative impact of MK was observed in all age groups and with both myeloablative and reduced-intensity conditioning regimens. In another study, *TP53* mutations were found in 40 of 97 patients (41%) with AML and adverse-risk cytogenetics who underwent allo-HSCT in three randomized trials, and 3-year probabilities of OS and EFS were 10% and 8% ($P = .002$ and $P = .007$) for patients with *TP53* mutations, compared with 33% and 24% for patients with wild-type *TP53*, and *TP53* mutation had a negative impact on OS (HR, 1.7; $P = .066$) in multivariate analysis.[535] Thus the benefit of transplant in these two groups with very poor outcomes is unclear, and novel approaches must be sought and studied in clinical trials.

Despite improvements in HLA matching and supportive care, results of transplants from matched unrelated donors have been thought to be inferior to those from matched siblings in CR1.[536] However, recent reports have indicated equivalent survival for sibling and unrelated donor transplants for AML, particularly for patients in early relapse or CR2, for whom DFS is 20% to 40% (*Figure 76.20*). Approximately one-third of patients who do not achieve remission after initial induction therapy but achieve remission with subsequent therapy and proceed to allo-HSCT can have prolonged DFS.[537]

Finally, two recent studies from the Fred Hutchinson Cancer Research Center have demonstrated the impact of pre-alloSCT MRD on allo-HSCT outcome. In the first study, 359 consecutive adults with AML who underwent myeloablative allo-HSCT had pretransplant bone marrow aspirates analyzed by 10-color multiparametric flow cytometry, with any level of residual disease considered MRD-positive.[538] Three-year relapse estimates were 67% in 76 patients in MRD-positive morphologic remission and 65% in 48 patients with active AML, compared with 22% in 235 patients in MRD-negative remission, and 3-year OS estimates were 26%, 23%, and 73%. These results supported the use of MRD-based, rather than morphology-based, disease assessment pre-allo-HSCT. In a second study, this group examined peritransplant MRD dynamics in 279 adults receiving myeloablative allo-HSCT in CR1 or CR2 who underwent 10-color multiparametric flow cytometry (MFC) analyses of marrow aspirates before and 28 ± 7 days after transplantation.[539] MFC-detectable MRD before (n = 63) or after (n = 16) transplantation identified patients with high relapse risk and poor survival. Importantly, MRD-positive patients before transplantation had a high relapse risk regardless of whether they cleared MFC-detectable disease with conditioning.

Exome sequencing analysis on paired samples obtained at diagnosis of AML and at relapse from 15 patients who relapsed after allo-HSCT (from an HLA-matched sibling, HLA-matched unrelated donor, or HLA-mismatched unrelated donor) and from 20 patients who relapsed after chemotherapy showed that the variety of mutations gained and lost at relapse was similar.[540] AML relapse post transplant was not associated with acquisition of previously unknown mutations or structural variations in immune-related genes.[540] In contrast, RNA sequencing showed dysregulation of pathways involved in adaptive and innate immunity, including downregulation of HLA-DPA1, HLA-DPB1, HLA-DQB1, and HLA-DRB1 to levels that were 3 to 12 times lower than in paired samples at diagnosis.[540]

CONCLUSION

AML is the leukemia with the highest incidence rate in adults and accounts for 80% to 90% of adult acute leukemia cases. Numerous cytogenetic abnormalities, both structural and numerical, and diverse molecular abnormalities in defined functional classes have been described in AML and form the basis for assignment of prognosis, choice of treatment approach, and, increasingly, targeted therapies. 7 + 3 cytosine arabinoside and anthracycline remission induction chemotherapy and

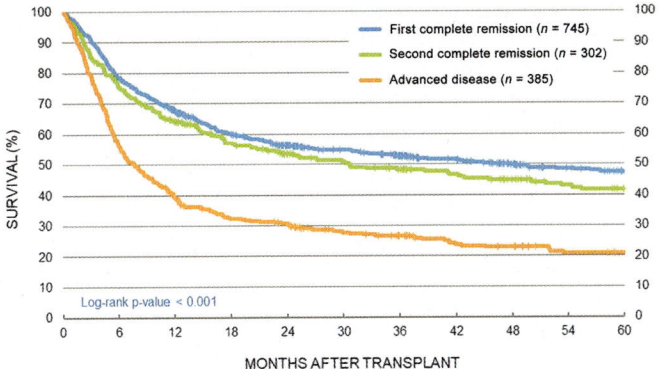

FIGURE 76.20 Survival of patients >18 years undergoing unrelated donor bone marrow transplants with myeloablative preparative regimens for AML by disease status, 2005 to 2014. Survival is significantly longer for transplants in CR1 or CR2 compared with more advanced disease. (Courtesy of National Marrow Donor Program®/Be The Match®.)

HiDAC consolidation therapy have remained the mainstay of AML therapy, while improvements in outcome have largely reflected improved supportive care, treatment stratification based on cytogenetic and molecular data, and allo-HSCT. However, after decades without new drug approvals for AML, ten new drugs have been approved since 2017, including eight molecularly targeted therapies. Additional novel targeted therapies and immunotherapies are in development.

References

1. Piller G. Leukaemia – a brief historical review from ancient times to 1950. *Br J Haematol*. 2001;112(2):282-292.
2. Reschad H, Schilling-Torgau V. Ueber eine neue leukamie durch echte uebergangsformen (splenozyten-leukamie) und ihre bedeutung fur die selbstandigkeit dieser zellen. *Munch Med Wochenschr*. 1913;60:1981.
3. DiGuglielmo G. Ricerche di hematologia: I. Una casa di eritroleucemia. *Folia Med*. 1917;13:386.
4. Von Boros J, Karenyi A. Uber einem fall von akuter megakaryoblastenleukamie, zugleich einige bemerkungen zum problem der akuten leukamie. *Z Klin Med*. 1931;118:697-718.
5. Hilstad LK. Acute promyelocytic leukemia. *Acta Med Scand*. 1947;159:189-194.
6. Rowley JD. Identification of a translocation with quinacrine fluorescence in a patient with acute leukemia. *Ann Genet*. 1973;16(2):109-112.
7. Rowley JD, Golomb HM, Dougherty C. 15/17 translocation, a consistent chromosomal change in acute promyelocytic leukaemia. *Lancet*. 1977;1(8010):549-550.
8. Le Beau MM, Larson RA, Bitter MA, Vardiman JW, Golomb HM, Rowley JD. Association of an inversion of chromosome 16 with abnormal marrow eosinophils in acute myelomonocytic leukemia. A unique cytogenetic-clinicopathological association. *N Engl J Med*. 1983;309(11):630-636.
9. Nakao M, Yokota S, Iwai T, et al. Internal tandem duplication of the flt3 gene found in acute myeloid leukemia. *Leukemia*. 1996;10(12):1911-1918.
10. Falini B, Mecucci C, Tiacci E, et al. Cytoplasmic nucleophosmin in acute myelogenous leukemia with a normal karyotype. *N Engl J Med*. 2005;352(3):254-266.
11. Bennett JM, Catovsky D, Daniel MT, et al. Proposals for the classification of the acute leukaemias. French-American-British (FAB) co-operative group. *Br J Haematol*. 1976;33(4):451-458.
12. Bennett JM, Catovsky D, Daniel MT, et al. Proposal for the recognition of minimally differentiated acute myeloid leukaemia (AML-M0). *Br J Haematol*. 1991;78(3):325-329.
13. Arber DA, Orazi A, Hasserjian R, et al. The 2016 revision to the World Health Organization classification of myeloid neoplasms and acute leukemia. *Blood*. 2016;127(20):2391-2405.
14. Khoury JD, Solary E, Abla O, et al. The 5th edition of the World Health Organization classification of haematolymphoid tumours: Myeloid and histiocytic/dendritic neoplasms. *Leukemia*. 2022;36(7):1703-1719.
15. Arber DA, Orazi A, Hasserjian RP, et al. International consensus classification of myeloid neoplasms and acute leukemias: Integrating morphologic, clinical, and genomic data. *Blood*. 2022;140(11):1200-1228.
16. Dohner H, Estey E, Grimwade D, et al. Diagnosis and management of AML in adults: 2017 ELN recommendations from an international expert panel. *Blood*. 2017;129(4):424-447.
17. Döhner H, Wei AH, Appelbaum FR, et al. Diagnosis and management of AML in adults: 2022 recommendations from an international expert panel on behalf of the ELN. *Blood*. 2022;140(12):1345-1377.
18. Yates JW, Wallace HJ Jr, Ellison RR, Holland JF. Cytosine arabinoside (NSC-63878) and daunorubicin (NSC-83142) therapy in acute nonlymphocytic leukemia. *Cancer Chemother Rep*. 1973;57(4):485-488.
19. Wolff SN, Herzig RH, Fay JW, et al. High-dose cytarabine and daunorubicin as consolidation therapy for acute myeloid leukemia in first remission: long-term follow-up and results. *J Clin Oncol*. 1989;7(9):1260-1267.
20. Howlader N, Noone AM, Krapcho M, et al. *SEER Cancer Statistics Review, 1975-2018*. National Cancer Institute. https://seercancergov/csr/1975_2018/. 2021; based on November 2020 SEER data submission, posted to the SEER web site, April 2021.
21. Siegel RL, Miller KD, Fuchs HE, Jemal A. Cancer statistics, 2021. *CA Cancer J Clin*. 2021;71(1):7-33.
22. Emadi A, Karp JE. The state of the union on treatment of acute myeloid leukemia. *Leuk Lymphoma*. 2014;55(11):2423-2425.
23. Sandler DP, Ross JA. Epidemiology of acute leukemia in children and adults. *Semin Oncol*. 1997;24(1):3-16.
24. Linet MS, Devesa SS. Epidemiology of leukemia: overview and patterns of occurrence. In: Henderson ES, Lister TA, Greaves MF, eds. *Leukemia*. W.B. Saunders; 2002:131-151.
25. Deschler B, Lubbert M. Acute myeloid leukemia: epidemiology and etiology. *Cancer*. 2006;107(9):2099-2107.
26. Karp JE, Smith MA. The molecular pathogenesis of treatment-induced (secondary) leukemias: foundations for treatment and prevention. *Semin Oncol*. 1997;24(1):103-113.
27. Larson RA, Le Beau MM. Therapy-related myeloid leukaemia: a model for leukemogenesis in humans. *Chem Biol Interact*. 2005;153-154:187-195.
28. Smith SM, Le Beau MM, Huo D, et al. Clinical-cytogenetic associations in 306 patients with therapy-related myelodysplasia and myeloid leukemia: the University of Chicago series. *Blood*. 2003;102(1):43-52.
29. Olney HJ, Mitelman F, Johansson B, Mrozek K, Berger R, Rowley JD. Unique balanced chromosome abnormalities in treatment-related myelodysplastic syndromes and acute myeloid leukemia: report from an international workshop. *Genes Chromosomes Cancer*. 2002;33(4):413-423.
30. Andersen MK, Pedersen-Bjergaard J. Therapy-related MDS and AML in acute promyelocytic leukemia. *Blood*. 2002;100(5):1928-1929; author reply 1929.
31. Quesnel B, Kantarjian H, Bjergaard JP, et al. Therapy-related acute myeloid leukemia with t(8;21), inv(16), and t(8;16): a report on 25 cases and review of the literature. *J Clin Oncol*. 1993;11(12):2370-2379.
32. Gustafson SA, Lin P, Chen SS, et al. Therapy-related acute myeloid leukemia with t(8;21) (q22;q22) shares many features with de novo acute myeloid leukemia with t(8;21)(q22;q22) but does not have a favorable outcome. *Am J Clin Pathol*. 2009;131(5):647-655.
33. Christiansen DH, Andersen MK, Pedersen-Bjergaard J. Mutations with loss of heterozygosity of p53 are common in therapy-related myelodysplasia and acute myeloid leukemia after exposure to alkylating agents and significantly associated with deletion or loss of 5q, a complex karyotype, and a poor prognosis. *J Clin Oncol*. 2001;19(5):1405-1413.
34. Shih AH, Chung SS, Dolezal EK, et al. Mutational analysis of therapy-related myelodysplastic syndromes and acute myelogenous leukemia. *Haematologica*. 2013;98(6):908-912.
35. Wong TN, Ramsingh G, Young AL, et al. Role of TP53 mutations in the origin and evolution of therapy-related acute myeloid leukaemia. *Nature*. 2015;518(7540):552-555.
36. Pedersen-Bjergaard J, Specht L, Larsen SO, et al. Risk of therapy-related leukaemia and preleukaemia after Hodgkin's disease. Relation to age, cumulative dose of alkylating agents, and time from chemotherapy. *Lancet*. 1987;2(8550):83-88.
37. Green DM, Hyland A, Barcos MP, et al. Second malignant neoplasms after treatment for Hodgkin's disease in childhood or adolescence. *J Clin Oncol*. 2000;18(7):1492-1499.
38. Swerdlow AJ, Barber JA, Hudson GV, et al. Risk of second malignancy after Hodgkin's disease in a collaborative British cohort: the relation to age at treatment. *J Clin Oncol*. 2000;18(3):498-509.
39. Chaplain G, Milan C, Sgro C, Carli PM, Bonithon-Kopp C. Increased risk of acute leukemia after adjuvant chemotherapy for breast cancer: a population-based study. *J Clin Oncol*. 2000;18(15):2836-2842.
40. Bergsagel DE, Bailey AJ, Langley GR, MacDonald RN, White DF, Miller AB. The chemotherapy on plasma-cell myeloma and the incidence of acute leukemia. *N Engl J Med*. 1979;301(14):743-748.
41. Greene MH, Boice JD Jr, Greer BE, Blessing JA, Dembo AJ. Acute nonlymphocytic leukemia after therapy with alkylating agents for ovarian cancer: a study of five randomized clinical trials. *N Engl J Med*. 1982;307(23):1416-1421.
42. Pedersen-Bjergaard J, Christiansen DH, Andersen MK, Skovby F. Causality of myelodysplasia and acute myeloid leukemia and their genetic abnormalities. *Leukemia*. 2002;16(11):2177-2184.
43. Pedersen-Bjergaard J, Philip P. Two different classes of therapy-related and de-novo acute myeloid leukemia? *Cancer Genet Cytogenet*. 1991;55(1):119-124.
44. Micallef IN, Lillington DM, Apostolidis J, et al. Therapy-related myelodysplasia and secondary acute myelogenous leukemia after high-dose therapy with autologous hematopoietic progenitor-cell support for lymphoid malignancies. *J Clin Oncol*. 2000;18(5):947-955.
45. Johnson DH, Porter LL, List AF, Hande KR, Hainsworth JD, Greco FA. Acute nonlymphocytic leukemia after treatment of small cell lung cancer. *Am J Med*. 1986;81(6):962-968.
46. Ratain MJ, Kaminer LS, Bitran JD, et al. Acute nonlymphocytic leukemia following etoposide and cisplatin combination chemotherapy for advanced non-small-cell carcinoma of the lung. *Blood*. 1987;70(5):1412-1417.
47. Whitlock JA, Greer JP, Lukens JN. Epipodophyllotoxin-related leukemia. Identification of a new subset of secondary leukemia. *Cancer*. 1991;68(3):600-604.
48. Pui CH, Behm FG, Raimondi SC, et al. Secondary acute myeloid leukemia in children treated for acute lymphoid leukemia. *N Engl J Med*. 1989;321(3):136-142.
49. Weh HJ, Hossfeld DK. 12p-chromosome in patients with acute myelocytic leukemia or myelodysplastic syndromes following exposure to mutagenic agents. *Cancer Genet Cytogenet*. 1986;19(3-4):355-356.

50. Fenaux P, Jouet JP, Bauters F, Lai JL, Lepelley P. Translocation t(9;11)(p21;q23) with acute myelomonocytic leukemia after chemotherapy for osteosarcoma: good response to antileukemic drugs. *J Clin Oncol.* 1987;5(8):1304-1305.
51. Smith RE, Bryant J, DeCillis A, Anderson S; National Surgical Adjuvant Breast and Bowel Project Experience. Acute myeloid leukemia and myelodysplastic syndrome after doxorubicin-cyclophosphamide adjuvant therapy for operable breast cancer: the National Surgical Adjuvant Breast and Bowel Project Experience. *J Clin Oncol.* 2003;21(7):1195-1204.
52. Le Deley MC, Suzan F, Cutuli B, et al. Anthracyclines, mitoxantrone, radiotherapy, and granulocyte colony-stimulating factor: risk factors for leukemia and myelodysplastic syndrome after breast cancer. *J Clin Oncol.* 2007;25(3):292-300.
53. Hershman D, Neugut AI, Jacobson JS, et al. Acute myeloid leukemia or myelodysplastic syndrome following use of granulocyte colony-stimulating factors during breast cancer adjuvant chemotherapy. *J Natl Cancer Inst.* 2007;99(3):196-205.
54. Boice JD Jr, Bigbee WL, Mumma MT, Blot WJ. Cancer mortality in counties near two former nuclear materials processing facilities in Pennsylvania, 1950-1995. *Health Phys.* 2003;85(6):691-700.
55. Boice JD Jr, Bigbee WL, Mumma MT, Blot WJ. Cancer incidence in municipalities near two former nuclear materials processing facilities in Pennsylvania. *Health Phys.* 2003;85(6):678-690.
56. Curtis RE, Boice JD Jr, Stovall M, et al. Risk of leukemia after chemotherapy and radiation treatment for breast cancer. *N Engl J Med.* 1992;326(26):1745-1751.
57. Morrison VA, Rai KR, Peterson BL, et al. Therapy-related myeloid leukemias are observed in patients with chronic lymphocytic leukemia after treatment with fludarabine and chlorambucil: results of an intergroup study, cancer and leukemia group B 9011. *J Clin Oncol.* 2002;20(18):3878-3884.
58. Carney DA, Westerman DA, Tam CS, et al. Therapy-related myelodysplastic syndrome and acute myeloid leukemia following fludarabine combination chemotherapy. *Leukemia.* 2010;24(12):2056-2062.
59. Leleu X, Soumerai J, Roccaro A, et al. Increased incidence of transformation and myelodysplasia/acute leukemia in patients with Waldenstrom macroglobulinemia treated with nucleoside analogs. *J Clin Oncol.* 2009;27(2):250-255.
60. Kwong YL. Azathioprine: association with therapy-related myelodysplastic syndrome and acute myeloid leukemia. *J Rheumatol.* 2010;37(3):485-490.
61. Ertz-Archambault N, Kosiorek H, Taylor GE, et al. Association of therapy for autoimmune disease with myelodysplastic syndromes and acute myeloid leukemia. *JAMA Oncol.* 2017;3(7):936-943.
62. Bo J, Schroder H, Kristinsson J, et al. Possible carcinogenic effect of 6-mercaptopurine on bone marrow stem cells: relation to thiopurine metabolism. *Cancer.* 1999;86(6):1080-1086.
63. Arana-Yi C, Block AW, Sait SN, Ford LA, Barcos M, Baer MR. Therapy-related myelodysplastic syndrome and acute myeloid leukemia following treatment of acute myeloid leukemia: possible role of cytarabine. *Leuk Res.* 2008;32(7):1043-1048.
64. Montesinos P, Gonzalez JD, Gonzalez J, et al. Therapy-related myeloid neoplasms in patients with acute promyelocytic leukemia treated with all-trans-retinoic Acid and anthracycline-based chemotherapy. *J Clin Oncol.* 2010;28(24):3872-3879.
65. Smith PG, Doll R. Mortality among patients with ankylosing spondylitis after a single treatment course with x rays. *Br Med J.* 1982;284(6314):449-460.
66. Inskip PD, Kleinerman RA, Stovall M, et al. Leukemia, lymphoma, and multiple myeloma after pelvic radiotherapy for benign disease. *Radiat Res.* 1993;135(1):108-124.
67. Ron E, Modan B, Boice JD Jr. Mortality after radiotherapy for ringworm of the scalp. *Am J Epidemiol.* 1988;127(4):713-725.
68. Griem ML, Kleinerman RA, Boice JD Jr, Stovall M, Shefner D, Lubin JH. Cancer following radiotherapy for peptic ulcer. *J Natl Cancer Inst.* 1994;86(11):842-849.
69. Boice JD Jr, Blettner M, Kleinerman RA, et al. Radiation dose and leukemia risk in patients treated for cancer of the cervix. *J Natl Cancer Inst.* 1987;79(6):1295-1311.
70. Curtis RE, Boice JD Jr, Stovall M, et al. Relationship of leukemia risk to radiation dose following cancer of the uterine corpus. *J Natl Cancer Inst.* 1994;86(17):1315-1324.
71. Kaldor JM, Day NE, Pettersson F, et al. Leukemia following chemotherapy for ovarian cancer. *N Engl J Med.* 1990;322(1):1-6.
72. Kaldor JM, Day NE, Clarke EA, et al. Leukemia following Hodgkin's disease. *N Engl J Med.* 1990;322(1):7-13.
73. Nardi V, Winkfield KM, Ok CY, et al. Acute myeloid leukemia and myelodysplastic syndromes after radiation therapy are similar to de novo disease and differ from other therapy-related myeloid neoplasms. *J Clin Oncol.* 2012;30(19):2340-2347.
74. Sawka AM, Thabane L, Parlea L, et al. Second primary malignancy risk after radioactive iodine treatment for thyroid cancer: a systematic review and meta-analysis. *Thyroid.* 2009;19(5):451-457.
75. Iyer NG, Morris LGT, Tuttle RM, Shaha AR, Ganly I. Rising incidence of second cancers in patients with low-risk (T1N0) thyroid cancer who receive radioactive iodine therapy. *Cancer.* 2011;117(19):4439-4446.
76. Terry PD, Shore DL, Rauscher GH, Sandler DP. Occupation, hobbies, and acute leukemia in adults. *Leuk Res.* 2005;29(10):1117-1130.
77. Tsai RJ, Luckhaupt SE, Schumacher P, Cress RD, Deapen DM, Calvert GM. Acute myeloid leukemia risk by industry and occupation. *Leuk Lymphoma.* 2014;55(11):2584-2591.
78. Vigliani EC. Leukemia associated with benzene exposure. *Ann N Y Acad Sci.* 1976;271:143-151.
79. Pyatt D. Benzene and hematopoietic malignancies. *Clin Occup Environ Med.* 2004;4(3):529-555, vii.
80. Glass DC, Gray CN, Jolley DJ, et al. Leukemia risk associated with low-level benzene exposure. *Epidemiology.* 2003;14(5):569-577.
81. Khalade A, Jaakkola MS, Pukkala E, Jaakkola JJK. Exposure to benzene at work and the risk of leukemia: a systematic review and meta-analysis. *Environ Health.* 2010;9:31.
82. Zhang L, Lan Q, Guo W, et al. Chromosome-wide aneuploidy study (CWAS) in workers exposed to an established leukemogen, benzene. *Carcinogenesis.* 2011;32(4):605-612.
83. Folley JH, Borges W, Yamawaki T. Incidence of leukemia in survivors of the atomic bomb in Hiroshima and Nagasaki, Japan. *Am J Med.* 1952;13(3):311-321.
84. Pierce DA, Shimizu Y, Preston DL, Vaeth M, Mabuchi K. Studies of the mortality of atomic bomb survivors. report 12, part I. Cancer: 1950-1990. 1996. *Radiat Res.* 2012;178(2):AV61-AV87.
85. Richardson D, Sugiyama H, Nishi N, et al. Ionizing radiation and leukemia mortality among Japanese Atomic Bomb Survivors, 1950-2000. *Radiat Res.* 2009;172(3):368-382.
86. Boice JD Jr, Holm LE. Radiation risk estimates for leukemia and thyroid cancer among Russian emergency workers at Chernobyl. *Radiat Environ Biophys.* 1997;36(3):213-214.
87. Littlefield LG, McFee AF, Salomaa SI, et al. Do recorded doses overestimate true doses received by Chernobyl cleanup workers? Results of cytogenetic analyses of Estonian workers by fluorescence in situ hybridization. *Radiat Res.* 1998;150(2):237-249.
88. Gluzman D, Imamura N, Sklyarenko L, Nadgornaya V, Zavelevich M, Machilo V. Malignant diseases of hematopoietic and lymphoid tissues in Chernobyl clean-up workers. *Hematol J.* 2005;5(7):565-571.
89. Garfinkel L, Boffetta P. Association between smoking and leukemia in two American Cancer Society prospective studies. *Cancer.* 1990;65(10):2356-2360.
90. Brownson RC, Novotny TE, Perry MC. Cigarette smoking and adult leukemia. A meta-analysis. *Arch Intern Med.* 1993;153(4):469-475.
91. Sandler DP, Shore DL, Anderson JR, et al. Cigarette smoking and risk of acute leukemia: associations with morphology and cytogenetic abnormalities in bone marrow. *J Natl Cancer Inst.* 1993;85(24):1994-2003.
92. Pasqualetti P, Festuccia V, Acitelli P, Collacciani A, Giusti A, Casale R. Tobacco smoking and risk of haematological malignancies in adults: a case-control study. *Br J Haematol.* 1997;97(3):659-662.
93. Bjork J, Albin M, Mauritzson N, Stromberg U, Johansson B, Hagmar L. Smoking and acute myeloid leukemia: associations with morphology and karyotypic patterns and evaluation of dose-response relations. *Leuk Res.* 2001;25(10):865-872.
94. Pogoda JM, Preston-Martin S, Nichols PW, Ross RK. Smoking and risk of acute myeloid leukemia: results from a Los Angeles County case-control study. *Am J Epidemiol.* 2002;155(6):546-553.
95. Bjork J, Johansson B, Broberg K, Albin M. Smoking as a risk factor for myelodysplastic syndromes and acute myeloid leukemia and its relation to cytogenetic findings: a case-control study. *Leuk Res.* 2009;33(6):788-791.
96. Doll R. Cancers weakly related to smoking. *Br Med Bull.* 1996;52(1):35-49.
97. Severson RK, Davis S, Heuser L, Daling JR, Thomas DB. Cigarette smoking and acute nonlymphocytic leukemia. *Am J Epidemiol.* 1990;132(3):418-422.
98. Kasim K, Levallois P, Abdous B, Auger P, Johnson KC. Lifestyle factors and the risk of adult leukemia in Canada. *Cancer Causes Control.* 2005;16(5):489-500.
99. Samanic C, Gridley G, Chow WH, Lubin J, Hoover RN, Fraumeni JF Jr. Obesity and cancer risk among white and black United States veterans. *Cancer Causes Control.* 2004;15(1):35-43.
100. Ross JA, Parker E, Blair CK, Cerhan JR, Folsom AR. Body mass index and risk of leukemia in older women. *Cancer Epidemiol Biomarkers Prev.* 2004;13(11 pt 1):1810-1813.
101. Strom SS, Oum R, Elhor Gbito KY, Garcia-Manero G, Yamamura Y. De novo acute myeloid leukemia risk factors: a Texas case-control study. *Cancer.* 2012;118(18):4589-4596.
102. Yan F, Shen N, Pang JX, et al. Fatty acid-binding protein FABP4 mechanistically links obesity with aggressive AML by enhancing aberrant DNA methylation in AML cells. *Leukemia.* 2017;31(6):1434-1442.
103. Rauscher GH, Shore D, Sandler DP. Hair dye use and risk of adult leukemia. *Am J Epidemiol.* 2004;160(1):19-25.
104. Porter CC. Germ line mutations associated with leukemias. *Hematology Am Soc Hematol Educ Program.* 2016;2016(1):302-308.
105. Das P, Shaik AP, Bammidi VK. Meta-analysis study of glutathione-S-transferases (GSTM1, GSTP1, and GSTT1) gene polymorphisms and risk of acute myeloid leukemia. *Leuk Lymphoma.* 2009;50(8):1345-1351.
106. Voso MT, D'Alo F, Putzulu R, et al. Negative prognostic value of glutathione S-transferase (GSTM1 and GSTT1) deletions in adult acute myeloid leukemia. *Blood.* 2002;100(8):2703-2707.
107. Voso MT, Hohaus S, Guidi F, et al. Prognostic role of glutathione S-transferase polymorphisms in acute myeloid leukemia. *Leukemia.* 2008;22(9):1685-1691.
108. Seedhouse C, Faulkner R, Ashraf N, Das-Gupta E, Russell N. Polymorphisms in genes involved in homologous recombination repair interact to increase the risk of developing acute myeloid leukemia. *Clin Cancer Res.* 2004;10(8):2675-2680.
109. Seedhouse C, Bainton R, Lewis M, Harding A, Russell N, Das-Gupta E. The genotype distribution of the XRCC1 gene indicates a role for base excision repair in the development of therapy-related acute myeloblastic leukemia. *Blood.* 2002;100(10):3761-3766.
110. Jawad M, Seedhouse CH, Russell N, Plumb M. Polymorphisms in human homeobox HLX1 and DNA repair RAD51 genes increase the risk of therapy-related acute myeloid leukemia. *Blood.* 2006;108(12):3916-3918.
111. Smith AG, Worrillow LJ, Allan JM. A common genetic variant in XPD associates with risk of 5q- and 7q-deleted acute myeloid leukemia. *Blood.* 2007;109(3):1233-1236.
112. Midic D, Rinke J, Perner F, et al. Prevalence and dynamics of clonal hematopoiesis caused by leukemia-associated mutations in elderly individuals without hematologic disorders. *Leukemia.* 2020;34(8):2198-2205.

113. Jaiswal S, Fontanillas P, Flannick J, et al. Age-related clonal hematopoiesis associated with adverse outcomes. *N Engl J Med*. 2014;371(26):2488-2498.
114. Genovese G, Kähler AK, Handsaker RE, et al. Clonal hematopoiesis and blood-cancer risk inferred from blood DNA sequence. *N Engl J Med*. 2014;371(26):2477-2487.
115. Xie M, Lu C, Wang J, et al. Age-related mutations associated with clonal hematopoietic expansion and malignancies. *Nat Med*. 2014;20(12):1472-1478.
116. Jan M, Snyder TM, Corces-Zimmerman MR, et al. Clonal evolution of preleukemic hematopoietic stem cells precedes human acute myeloid leukemia. *Sci Transl Med*. 2012;4(149):149ra118.
117. Thol F, Klesse S, Kohler L, et al. Acute myeloid leukemia derived from lympho-myeloid clonal hematopoiesis. *Leukemia*. 2017;31(6):1286-1295.
118. Hasserjian RP, Steensma DP, Graubert TA, Ebert BL. Clonal hematopoiesis and measurable residual disease assessment in acute myeloid leukemia. *Blood*. 2020;135(20):1729-1738.
119. Tanaka T, Morita K, Wang F, et al. Clonal dynamics and clinical implications of post-remission clonal hematopoiesis in acute myeloid leukemia (AML). *Blood*. 2021;138(18):1733-1739.
120. Baer MR. Management of unusual presentations of acute leukemia. *Hematol Oncol Clin North Am*. 1993;7(1):275-292.
121. Bunin NJ, Pui CH. Differing complications of hyperleukocytosis in children with acute lymphoblastic or acute nonlymphoblastic leukemia. *J Clin Oncol*. 1985;3(12):1590-1595.
122. McKee LC Jr, Collins RD. Intravascular leukocyte thrombi and aggregates as a cause of morbidity and mortality in leukemia. *Medicine*. 1974;53(6):463-478.
123. Thornton KA, Levis M. Images in clinical medicine. FLT3 Mutation and acute myelogenous leukemia with leukostasis. *N Engl J Med*. 2007;357(16):1639.
124. Ganzel C, Manola J, Douer D, et al. Extramedullary disease in adult acute myeloid leukemia is common but lacks independent significance: analysis of patients in ECOG-ACRIN cancer research group trials, 1980-2008. *J Clin Oncol*. 2016;34(29):3544-3553.
125. Wiernik PH. *Extramedullary Manifestations of Adult Leukemia*. BC Decker; 2001.
126. Pileri SA, Ascani S, Cox MC, et al. Myeloid sarcoma: clinico-pathologic, phenotypic and cytogenetic analysis of 92 adult patients. *Leukemia*. 2007;21(2):340-350.
127. Byrd JC, Edenfield WJ, Shields DJ, Dawson NA. Extramedullary myeloid cell tumors in acute nonlymphocytic leukemia: a clinical review. *J Clin Oncol*. 1995;13(7):1800-1816.
128. Almond LM, Charalampakis M, Ford SJ, Gourevitch D, Desai A. Myeloid sarcoma: presentation, diagnosis, and treatment. *Clin Lymphoma Myeloma Leuk*. 2017;17(5):263-267.
129. Peterson BA, Brunning RD, Bloomfield CD, et al. Central nervous system involvement in acute nonlymphocytic leukemia. A prospective study of adults in remission. *Am J Med*. 1987;83(3):464-470.
130. Castagnola C, Nozza A, Corso A, Bernasconi C. The value of combination therapy in adult acute myeloid leukemia with central nervous system involvement. *Haematologica*. 1997;82(5):577-580.
131. Cassileth PA, Sylvester LS, Bennett JM, Begg CB. High peripheral blast count in adult acute myelogenous leukemia is a primary risk factor for CNS leukemia. *J Clin Oncol*. 1988;6(3):495-498.
132. Holmes R, Keating MJ, Cork A, et al. A unique pattern of central nervous system leukemia in acute myelomonocytic leukemia associated with inv(16)(p13q22). *Blood*. 1985;65(5):1071-1078.
133. Cohen PR, Talpaz M, Kurzrock R. Malignancy-associated Sweet's syndrome: review of the world literature. *J Clin Oncol*. 1988;6(12):1887-1897.
134. Schwaegerle SM, Bergfeld WF, Senitzer D, Tidrick RT. Pyoderma gangrenosum: a review. *J Am Acad Dermatol*. 1988;18(3):559-568.
135. Baer MR, Barcos M, Farrell H, Raza A, Preisler HD. Acute myelogenous leukemia with leukemia cutis. Eighteen cases seen between 1969 and 1986. *Cancer*. 1989;63(11):2192-2200.
136. da Silva Santos PS, Fontes A, de Andrade F, de Sousa SC. Gingival leukemic infiltration as the first manifestation of acute myeloid leukemia. *Otolaryngol Head Neck Surg*. 2010;143(3):465-466.
137. Mani A, Lee DA. Images in clinical medicine. Leukemic gingival infiltration. *N Engl J Med*. 2008;358(3):274.
138. Bhambal AM, Shrivastava H, Naik SP, Nair P, Saawarn N. Oral manifestations of systemic leukemia-first sign of presentation. *J Indian Soc Periodontol*. 2021;25(4):347-349.
139. Keidan RD, Fanning J, Gatenby RA, Weese JL. Recurrent typhlitis. A disease resulting from aggressive chemotherapy. *Dis Colon Rectum*. 1989;32(3):206-209.
140. Boggs DR, Wintrobe MM, Cartwright GE. The acute leukemias. Analysis of 322 cases and review of the literature. *Medicine*. 1962;41:163-225.
141. Hanker JS, Laszlo J, Moore JO. The light microscopic demonstration of hydroperoxidase-positive Phi bodies and rods in leukocytes in acute myeloid leukemia. *Histochemistry*. 1978;58(4):241-252.
142. Yanada M, Matsushita T, Suzuki M, et al. Disseminated intravascular coagulation in acute leukemia: clinical and laboratory features at presentation. *Eur J Haematol*. 2006;77(4):282-287.
143. Ribeiro RC, Pui CH. The clinical and biological correlates of coagulopathy in children with acute leukemia. *J Clin Oncol*. 1986;4(8):1212-1218.
144. O'Regan S, Carson S, Chesney RW, Drummond KN. Electrolyte and acid-base disturbances in the management of leukemia. *Blood*. 1977;49(3):345-353.
145. Schenkein DP, O'Neill WC, Shapiro J, Miller KB. Accelerated bone formation causing profound hypocalcemia in acute leukemia. *Ann Intern Med*. 1986;105(3):375-378.
146. Gewirtz AM, Stewart AF, Vignery A, Hoffman R. Hypercalcaemia complicating acute myelogenous leukaemia: a syndrome of multiple aetiologies. *Br J Haematol*. 1983;54(1):133-141.
147. Yunis JJ, Bloomfield CD, Ensrud K. All patients with acute nonlymphocytic leukemia may have a chromosomal defect. *N Engl J Med*. 1981;305(3):135-139.
148. Papaemmanuil E, Gerstung M, Bullinger L, et al. Genomic classification and prognosis in acute myeloid leukemia. *N Engl J Med*. 2016;374(23):2209-2221.
149. Terstappen LW, Safford M, Konemann S, et al. Flow cytometric characterization of acute myeloid leukemia. Part II. Phenotypic heterogeneity at diagnosis. *Leukemia*. 1992;6(1):70-80.
150. Venditti A, Buccisano F, Del Poeta G, et al. Level of minimal residual disease after consolidation therapy predicts outcome in acute myeloid leukemia. *Blood*. 2000;96(12):3948-3952.
151. San Miguel JF, Vidriales MB, Lopez-Berges C, et al. Early immunophenotypical evaluation of minimal residual disease in acute myeloid leukemia identifies different patient risk groups and may contribute to postinduction treatment stratification. *Blood*. 2001;98(6):1746-1751.
152. Kern W, Voskova D, Schoch C, Hiddemann W, Schnittger S, Haferlach T. Determination of relapse risk based on assessment of minimal residual disease during complete remission by multiparameter flow cytometry in unselected patients with acute myeloid leukemia. *Blood*. 2004;104(10):3078-3085.
153. Feller N, van der Pol MA, van Stijn A, et al. MRD parameters using immunophenotypic detection methods are highly reliable in predicting survival in acute myeloid leukaemia. *Leukemia*. 2004;18(8):1380-1390.
154. Buccisano F, Maurillo L, Gattei V, et al. The kinetics of reduction of minimal residual disease impacts on duration of response and survival of patients with acute myeloid leukemia. *Leukemia*. 2006;20(10):1783-1789.
155. Gianfaldoni G, Mannelli F, Baccini M, Antonioli E, Leoni F, Bosi A. Clearance of leukaemic blasts from peripheral blood during standard induction treatment predicts the bone marrow response in acute myeloid leukaemia: a pilot study. *Br J Haematol*. 2006;134(1):54-57.
156. Baer MR, Stewart CC, Dodge RK, et al. High frequency of immunophenotype changes in acute myeloid leukemia at relapse: implications for residual disease detection (Cancer and Leukemia Group B Study 8361). *Blood*. 2001;97(11):3574-3580.
157. Buccisano F, Maurillo L, Del Principe MI, et al. Prognostic and therapeutic implications of minimal residual disease detection in acute myeloid leukemia. *Blood*. 2012;119(2):332-341.
158. Raza A, Maheshwari Y, Preisler HD. Differences in cell cycle characteristics among patients with acute nonlymphocytic leukemia. *Blood*. 1987;69(6):1647-1653.
159. Raza A, Preisler HD, Day R, et al. Direct relationship between remission duration in acute myeloid leukemia and cell cycle kinetics: a leukemia intergroup study. *Blood*. 1990;76(11):2191-2197.
160. Brons PP, Haanen C, Boezeman JB, et al. Proliferation patterns in acute myeloid leukemia: leukemic clonogenic growth and in vivo cell cycle kinetics. *Ann Hematol*. 1993;66(5):225-233.
161. Smeets ME, Raymakers RA, Vierwinden G, et al. Idarubicin DNA intercalation is reduced by MRP1 and not Pgp. *Leukemia*. 1999;13(9):1390-1398.
162. Schimmer AD, Hedley DW, Penn LZ, Minden MD. Receptor- and mitochondrial-mediated apoptosis in acute leukemia: a translational view. *Blood*. 2001;98(13):3541-3553.
163. Konopleva M, Zhao S, Hu W, et al. The anti-apoptotic genes Bcl-X(L) and Bcl-2 are over-expressed and contribute to chemoresistance of non-proliferating leukaemic CD34+ cells. *Br J Haematol*. 2002;118(2):521-534.
164. Carter BZ, Milella M, Tsao T, et al. Regulation and targeting of antiapoptotic XIAP in acute myeloid leukemia. *Leukemia*. 2003;17(11):2081-2089.
165. Turzanski J, Grundy M, Russell NH, Pallis M. Interleukin-1beta maintains an apoptosis-resistant phenotype in the blast cells of acute myeloid leukaemia via multiple pathways. *Leukemia*. 2004;18(10):1662-1670.
166. Del Poeta G, Bruno A, Del Principe MI, et al. Deregulation of the mitochondrial apoptotic machinery and development of molecular targeted drugs in acute myeloid leukemia. *Curr Cancer Drug Targets*. 2008;8(3):207-222.
167. Vo TT, Ryan J, Carrasco R, et al. Relative mitochondrial priming of myeloblasts and normal HSCs determines chemotherapeutic success in AML. *Cell*. 2012;151(2):344-355.
168. Konopleva M, Pollyea DA, Potluri J, et al. Efficacy and biological correlates of response in a phase II study of venetoclax monotherapy in patients with acute myelogenous leukemia. *Cancer Discov*. 2016;6(10):1106-1117.
169. Felipe Rico J, Hassane DC, Guzman ML. Acute myelogenous leukemia stem cells: from bench to bedside. *Cancer Lett*. 2013;338(1):4-9.
170. Lapidot T, Sirard C, Vormoor J, et al. A cell initiating human acute myeloid leukaemia after transplantation into SCID mice. *Nature*. 1994;367(6464):645-648.
171. Blair A, Hogge DE, Sutherland HJ. Most acute myeloid leukemia progenitor cells with long-term proliferative ability in vitro and in vivo have the phenotype CD34(+)/CD71(-)/HLA-DR. *Blood*. 1998;92(11):4325-4335.
172. Jordan CT, Upchurch D, Szilvassy SJ, et al. The interleukin-3 receptor alpha chain is a unique marker for human acute myelogenous leukemia stem cells. *Leukemia*. 2000;14(10):1777-1784.
173. Guan Y, Gerhard B, Hogge DE. Detection, isolation, and stimulation of quiescent primitive leukemic progenitor cells from patients with acute myeloid leukemia (AML). *Blood*. 2003;101(8):3142-3149.
174. Eppert K, Takenaka K, Lechman ER, et al. Stem cell gene expression programs influence clinical outcome in human leukemia. *Nat Med*. 2011;17(9):1086-1093.
175. Gerber JM, Smith BD, Ngwang B, et al. A clinically relevant population of leukemic CD34(+)CD38(-) cells in acute myeloid leukemia. *Blood*. 2012;119(15):3571-3577.
176. Gerber JM, Zeidner JF, Morse S, et al. Association of acute myeloid leukemia's most immature phenotype with risk groups and outcomes. *Haematologica*. 2016;101(5):607-616.
177. Ding L, Ley TJ, Larson DE, et al. Clonal evolution in relapsed acute myeloid leukaemia revealed by whole-genome sequencing. *Nature*. 2012;481(7382):506-510.

178. Stetson LC, Balasubramanian D, Ribeiro SP, et al. Single cell RNA sequencing of AML initiating cells reveals RNA-based evolution during disease progression. *Leukemia.* 2021;35(10):2799-2812.
179. Petti AA, Khan SM, Xu Z, et al. Genetic and transcriptional contributions to relapse in normal karyotype acute myeloid leukemia. *Blood Cancer Discov.* 2022;3(1):32-49.
180. Grimwade D, Walker H, Harrison G, et al. The predictive value of hierarchical cytogenetic classification in older adults with acute myeloid leukemia (AML): analysis of 1065 patients entered into the United Kingdom Medical Research Council AML11 trial. *Blood.* 2001;98(5):1312-1320.
181. Mareschal S, Palau A, Lindberg J, et al. Challenging conventional karyotyping by next-generation karyotyping in 281 intensively treated patients with AML. *Blood Adv.* 2021;5(4):1003-1016.
182. Mack EKM, Marquardt A, Langer D, et al. Comprehensive genetic diagnosis of acute myeloid leukemia by next-generation sequencing. *Haematologica.* 2019;104(2):277-287.
183. Duncavage EJ, Schroeder MC, O'Laughlin M, et al. Genome sequencing as an alternative to cytogenetic analysis in myeloid cancers. *N Engl J Med.* 2021; 384(10):924-935.
184. Brunning RD, Vardiman J, Matutes E. Acute myeloid leukemia. In: Jaffe E, Harris N, Stein H, Vardiman J, eds. *World Health Organization Classification of Tumours. Pathology and Genetics. Tumours of Haematopoietic and Lymphoid Tissues.* IARC Press; 2001:75-107.
185. Hurwitz CA, Raimondi SC, Head D, et al. Distinctive immunophenotypic features of t(8;21)(q22;q22) acute myeloblastic leukemia in children. *Blood.* 1992;80(12):3182-3188.
186. Nisson PE, Watkins PC, Sacchi N. Transcriptionally active chimeric gene derived from the fusion of the AML1 gene and a novel gene on chromosome 8 in t(8;21) leukemic cells. *Cancer Genet Cytogenet.* 1992;63(2):81-88.
187. Peterson LF, Zhang DE. The 8;21 translocation in leukemogenesis. *Oncogene.* 2004;23(24):4255-4262.
188. Kusec R, Laczika K, Knöbl P, et al. AML1/ETO fusion mRNA can be detected in remission blood samples of all patients with t(8;21) acute myeloid leukemia after chemotherapy or autologous bone marrow transplantation. *Leukemia.* 1994;8(5):735-739.
189. Byrd JC, Dodge RK, Carroll A, et al. Patients with t(8;21)(q22;q22) and acute myeloid leukemia have superior failure-free and overall survival when repetitive cycles of high-dose cytarabine are administered. *J Clin Oncol.* 1999;17(12):3767-3775.
190. Schnittger S, Kohl TM, Haferlach T, et al. KIT-D816 mutations in AML1-ETO-positive AML are associated with impaired event-free and overall survival. *Blood.* 2006;107(5):1791-1799.
191. Baer MR, Stewart CC, Lawrence D, et al. Expression of the neural cell adhesion molecule CD56 is associated with short remission duration and survival in acute myeloid leukemia with t(8;21)(q22;q22). *Blood.* 1997;90(4):1643-1648.
192. Zhu HH, Zhang XH, Qin YZ, et al. MRD-directed risk stratification treatment may improve outcomes of t(8;21) AML in the first complete remission: results from the AML05 multicenter trial. *Blood.* 2013;121(20):4056-4062.
193. Kayser S, Kramer M, Martinez-Cuadron D, et al. Characteristics and outcome of patients with core binding factor acute myeloid leukemia and FLT3-ITD: results from an international collaborative study. *Haematologica.* 2022;107(4):836-843.
194. Billstrom R, Ahlgren T, Bekassy AN, et al. Acute myeloid leukemia with inv(16) (p13q22): involvement of cervical lymph nodes and tonsils is common and may be a negative prognostic sign. *Am J Hematol.* 2002;71(1):15-19.
195. Liu PP, Hajra A, Wijmenga C, Collins FS. Molecular pathogenesis of the chromosome 16 inversion in the M4Eo subtype of acute myeloid leukemia. *Blood.* 1995;85(9):2289-2302.
196. Poirel H, Radford-Weiss I, Rack K, et al. Detection of the chromosome 16 CBF beta-MYH11 fusion transcript in myelomonocytic leukemias. *Blood.* 1995;85(5):1313-1322.
197. Delaunay J, Vey N, Leblanc T, et al. Prognosis of inv(16)/t(16;16) acute myeloid leukemia (AML): a survey of 110 cases from the French AML Intergroup. *Blood.* 2003;102(2):462-469.
198. Paschka P, Marcucci G, Ruppert AS, et al. Adverse prognostic significance of KIT mutations in adult acute myeloid leukemia with inv(16) and t(8;21): a Cancer and Leukemia Group B Study. *J Clin Oncol.* 2006;24(24):3904-3911.
199. Buonamici S, Ottaviani E, Testoni N, et al. Real-time quantitation of minimal residual disease in inv(16)-positive acute myeloid leukemia may indicate risk for clinical relapse and may identify patients in a curable state. *Blood.* 2002;99(2):443-449.
200. Perea G, Lasa A, Aventin A, et al. Prognostic value of minimal residual disease (MRD) in acute myeloid leukemia (AML) with favorable cytogenetics [t(8;21) and inv(16)]. *Leukemia.* 2006;20(1):87-94.
201. Stentoft J, Hokland P, Ostergaard M, Hasle H, Nyvold CG. Minimal residual core binding factor AMLs by real time quantitative PCR—initial response to chemotherapy predicts event free survival and close monitoring of peripheral blood unravels the kinetics of relapse. *Leuk Res.* 2006;30(4):389-395.
202. Harper DP, Aplan PD. Chromosomal rearrangements leading to MLL gene fusions: clinical and biological aspects. *Cancer Res.* 2008;68(24):10024-10027.
203. Nakamura T, Alder H, Gu Y, et al. Genes on chromosomes 4, 9, and 19 involved in 11q23 abnormalities in acute leukemia share sequence homology and/or common motifs. *Proc Natl Acad Sci U S A.* 1993;90(10):4631-4635.
204. Blum W, Mrozek K, Ruppert AS, et al. Adult de novo acute myeloid leukemia with t(6;11)(q27;q23): results from Cancer and Leukemia Group B Study 8461 and review of the literature. *Cancer.* 2004;101(6):1420-1427.
205. Mrozek K, Heinonen K, Lawrence D, et al. Adult patients with de novo acute myeloid leukemia and t(9;11)(p22;q23) have a superior outcome to patients with other translocations involving band 11q23: a cancer and leukemia group B study. *Blood.* 1997;90(11):4532-4538.
206. Byrd JC, Mrozek K, Dodge RK, et al. Pretreatment cytogenetic abnormalities are predictive of induction success, cumulative incidence of relapse, and overall survival in adult patients with de novo acute myeloid leukemia: results from Cancer and Leukemia Group B (CALGB 8461). *Blood.* 2002;100(13):4325-4336.
207. Schoch C, Schnittger S, Klaus M, Kern W, Hiddemann W, Haferlach T. AML with 11q23/MLL abnormalities as defined by the WHO classification: incidence, partner chromosomes, FAB subtype, age distribution, and prognostic impact in an unselected series of 1897 cytogenetically analyzed AML cases. *Blood.* 2003;102(7):2395-2402.
208. Chen Y, Kantarjian H, Pierce S, et al. Prognostic significance of 11q23 aberrations in adult acute myeloid leukemia and the role of allogeneic stem cell transplantation. *Leukemia.* 2013;27(4):836-842.
209. Soekarman D, von Lindern M, Daenen S, et al. The translocation (6;9) (p23;q34) shows consistent rearrangement of two genes and defines a myeloproliferative disorder with specific clinical features. *Blood.* 1992;79(11):2990-2997.
210. Ageberg M, Drott K, Olofsson T, Gullberg U, Lindmark A. Identification of a novel and myeloid specific role of the leukemia-associated fusion protein DEK-NUP214 leading to increased protein synthesis. *Genes Chromosomes Cancer.* 2008;47(4):276-287.
211. Kayser S, Hills RK, Luskin MR, et al. Allogeneic hematopoietic cell transplantation improves outcome of adults with t(6;9) acute myeloid leukemia: results from an International Collaborative Study. *Haematologica.* 2020;105(1):161-169.
212. Lugthart S, Groschel S, Beverloo HB, et al. Clinical, molecular, and prognostic significance of WHO type inv(3)(q21q26.2)/t(3;3)(q21;q26.2) and various other 3q abnormalities in acute myeloid leukemia. *J Clin Oncol.* 2010;28(24):3890-3898.
213. Katayama S, Suzuki M, Yamaoka A, et al. GATA2 haploinsufficiency accelerates EVI1-driven leukemogenesis. *Blood.* 2017;130(7):908-919.
214. Groschel S, Lugthart S, Schlenk RF, et al. High EVI1 expression predicts outcome in younger adult patients with acute myeloid leukemia and is associated with distinct cytogenetic abnormalities. *J Clin Oncol.* 2010;28(12):2101-2107.
215. Medeiros BC, Othus M, Fang M, Roulston D, Appelbaum FR. Prognostic impact of monosomal karyotype in young adult and elderly acute myeloid leukemia: the Southwest Oncology Group (SWOG) experience. *Blood.* 2010;116(13):2224-2228.
216. Fang M, Storer B, Estey E, et al. Outcome of patients with acute myeloid leukemia with monosomal karyotype who undergo hematopoietic cell transplantation. *Blood.* 2011;118(6):1490-1494.
217. Bochtler T, Granzow M, Stolzel F, et al. Marker chromosomes can arise from chromothripsis and predict adverse prognosis in acute myeloid leukemia. *Blood.* 2017;129(10):1333-1342.
218. DiNardo CD, Cortes JE. Mutations in AML: prognostic and therapeutic implications. *Hematology Am Soc Hematol Educ Program.* 2016;2016(1):348-355.
219. Cancer Genome Atlas Research Network, Ley TJ, Miller C, et al. Genomic and epigenomic landscapes of adult de novo acute myeloid leukemia. *N Engl J Med.* 2013;368(22):2059-2074.
220. Bienz M, Ludwig M, Leibundgut EO, et al. Risk assessment in patients with acute myeloid leukemia and a normal karyotype. *Clin Cancer Res.* 2005;11(4):1416-1424.
221. Mrozek K, Marcucci G, Paschka P, Whitman SP, Bloomfield CD. Clinical relevance of mutations and gene-expression changes in adult acute myeloid leukemia with normal cytogenetics: are we ready for a prognostically prioritized molecular classification? *Blood.* 2007;109(2):431-448.
222. Gilliland DG, Griffin JD. The roles of FLT3 in hematopoiesis and leukemia. *Blood.* 2002;100(5):1532-1542.
223. Kiyoi H, Ohno R, Ueda R, Saito H, Naoe T. Mechanism of constitutive activation of FLT3 with internal tandem duplication in the juxtamembrane domain. *Oncogene.* 2002;21(16):2555-2563.
224. Thiede C, Steudel C, Mohr B, et al. Analysis of FLT3-activating mutations in 979 patients with acute myelogenous leukemia: association with FAB subtypes and identification of subgroups with poor prognosis. *Blood.* 2002;99(12):4326-4335.
225. Kottaridis PD, Gale RE, Frew ME, et al. The presence of a FLT3 internal tandem duplication in patients with acute myeloid leukemia (AML) adds important prognostic information to cytogenetic risk group and response to the first cycle of chemotherapy: analysis of 854 patients from the United Kingdom Medical Research Council AML 10 and 12 trials. *Blood.* 2001;98(6):1752-1759.
226. Stirewalt DL, Kopecky KJ, Meshinchi S, et al. Size of FLT3 internal tandem duplication has prognostic significance in patients with acute myeloid leukemia. *Blood.* 2006;107(9):3724-3726.
227. Frohling S, Schlenk RF, Breitruck J, et al. Prognostic significance of activating FLT3 mutations in younger adults (16 to 60 years) with acute myeloid leukemia and normal cytogenetics: a study of the AML Study Group Ulm. *Blood.* 2002;100(13):4372-4380.
228. Mizuki M, Fenski R, Halfter H, et al. Flt3 mutations from patients with acute myeloid leukemia induce transformation of 32D cells mediated by the Ras and STAT5 pathways. *Blood.* 2000;96(12):3907-3914.
229. Spiekermann K, Bagrintseva K, Schwab R, Schmieja K, Hiddemann W. Overexpression and constitutive activation of FLT3 induces STAT5 activation in primary acute myeloid leukemia blast cells. *Clin Cancer Res.* 2003;9(6):2140-2150.
230. Brandts CH, Sargin B, Rode M, et al. Constitutive activation of Akt by Flt3 internal tandem duplications is necessary for increased survival, proliferation, and myeloid transformation. *Cancer Res.* 2005;65(21):9643-9650.
231. Zheng R, Friedman AD, Levis M, Li L, Weir EG, Small D. Internal tandem duplication mutation of FLT3 blocks myeloid differentiation through suppression of C/EBPalpha expression. *Blood.* 2004;103(5):1883-1890.
232. Kim KT, Levis M, Small D. Constitutively activated FLT3 phosphorylates BAD partially through pim-1. *Br J Haematol.* 2006;134(5):500-509.
233. Stirewalt DL, Kopecky KJ, Meshinchi S, et al. FLT3, RAS, and TP53 mutations in elderly patients with acute myeloid leukemia. *Blood.* 2001;97(11):3589-3595.

234. Boissel N, Cayuela JM, Preudhomme C, et al. Prognostic significance of FLT3 internal tandem repeat in patients with de novo acute myeloid leukemia treated with reinforced courses of chemotherapy. *Leukemia.* 2002;16(9):1699-1704.
235. Gale RE, Green C, Allen C, et al. The impact of FLT3 internal tandem duplication mutant level, number, size, and interaction with NPM1 mutations in a large cohort of young adult patients with acute myeloid leukemia. *Blood.* 2008;111(5):2776-2784.
236. Pratcorona M, Brunet S, Nomdedeu J, et al. Favorable outcome of patients with acute myeloid leukemia harboring a low-allelic burden FLT3-ITD mutation and concomitant NPM1 mutation: relevance to post-remission therapy. *Blood.* 2013;121(14):2734-2738.
237. Gourdin TS, Zou Y, Ning Y, et al. High frequency of rare structural chromosome abnormalities at relapse of cytogenetically normal acute myeloid leukemia with FLT3 internal tandem duplication. *Cancer Genet.* 2014;207(10-12):467-473.
238. Sato T, Yang X, Knapper S, et al. FLT3 ligand impedes the efficacy of FLT3 inhibitors in vitro and in vivo. *Blood.* 2011;117(12):3286-3293.
239. Oran B, Cortes J, Beitinjaneh A, et al. Allogeneic transplantation in first remission improves outcomes irrespective of FLT3-ITD allelic ratio in FLT3-ITD-positive acute myelogenous leukemia. *Biol Blood Marrow Transplant.* 2016;22(7):1218-1226.
240. Ho AD, Schetelig J, Bochtler T, et al. Allogeneic stem cell transplantation improves survival in patients with acute myeloid leukemia characterized by a high allelic ratio of mutant FLT3-ITD. *Biol Blood Marrow Transplant.* 2016;22(3):462-469.
241. Choudhary C, Schwable J, Brandts C, et al. AML-associated Flt3 kinase domain mutations show signal transduction differences compared with Flt3 ITD mutations. *Blood.* 2005;106(1):265-273.
242. Food and Drug Administration. *Midostaurin Label*; 2017. Accessed December 20, 2022. https://www.accessdata.fda.gov/drugsatfda_docs/label/2021/207997s008lbledt.pdf
243. Food and Drug Administration. *Gilteritinib Label*; 2018. Accessed December 20, 2022. https://www.accessdata.fda.gov/drugsatfda_docs/label/2022/211349s003lbl.pdf
244. Boissel N, Renneville A, Biggio V, et al. Prevalence, clinical profile, and prognosis of NPM mutations in AML with normal karyotype. *Blood.* 2005;106(10):3618-3620.
245. Schnittger S, Schoch C, Kern W, et al. Nucleophosmin gene mutations are predictors of favorable prognosis in acute myelogenous leukemia with a normal karyotype. *Blood.* 2005;106(12):3733-3739.
246. Dohner K, Schlenk RF, Habdank M, et al. Mutant nucleophosmin (NPM1) predicts favorable prognosis in younger adults with acute myeloid leukemia and normal cytogenetics: interaction with other gene mutations. *Blood.* 2005;106(12):3740-3746.
247. Thiede C, Koch S, Creutzig E, et al. Prevalence and prognostic impact of NPM1 mutations in 1485 adult patients with acute myeloid leukemia (AML). *Blood.* 2006;107(10):4011-4020.
248. Verhaak RGW, Goudswaard CS, van Putten W, et al. Mutations in nucleophosmin (NPM1) in acute myeloid leukemia (AML): association with other gene abnormalities and previously established gene expression signatures and their favorable prognostic significance. *Blood.* 2005;106(12):3747-3754.
249. Schlenk RF, Dohner K, Krauter J, et al. Mutations and treatment outcome in cytogenetically normal acute myeloid leukemia. *N Engl J Med.* 2008;358(18):1909-1918.
250. Haferlach C, Mecucci C, Schnittger S, et al. AML with mutated NPM1 carrying a normal or aberrant karyotype show overlapping biologic, pathologic, immunophenotypic, and prognostic features. *Blood.* 2009;114(14):3024-3032.
251. Hills RK, Ivey A, Grimwade D; UK National Cancer Research Institute NCRI AML Working Group. Assessment of minimal residual disease in standard-risk AML. *N Engl J Med.* 2016;375(6):e9-e433.
252. Kronke J, Schlenk RF, Jensen KO, et al. Monitoring of minimal residual disease in NPM1-mutated acute myeloid leukemia: a study from the German-Austrian acute myeloid leukemia study group. *J Clin Oncol.* 2011;29(19):2709-2716.
253. Cappelli LV, Meggendorfer M, Dicker F, et al. DNMT3A mutations are over-represented in young adults with NPM1 mutated AML and prompt a distinct co-mutational pattern. *Leukemia.* 2019;33(11):2741-2746.
254. Muller PAJ, Vousden KH. Mutant p53 in cancer: new functions and therapeutic opportunities. *Cancer Cell.* 2014;25(3):304-317.
255. Olivier M, Hollstein M, Hainaut P. TP53 mutations in human cancers: origins, consequences, and clinical use. *Cold Spring Harb Perspect Biol.* 2010;2(1):a001008.
256. Guha T, Malkin D. Inherited TP53 mutations and the Li-fraumeni syndrome. *Cold Spring Harb Perspect Med.* 2017;7(4):a026187.
257. Cerami E, Gao J, Dogrusoz U, et al. The cBio cancer genomics portal: an open platform for exploring multidimensional cancer genomics data. *Cancer Discov.* 2012;2(5):401-404.
258. Cancer Genome Atlas Research Network, Weinstein JN, Collisson EA, et al. The cancer genome Atlas pan-cancer analysis project. *Nat Genet.* 2013;45(10):1113-1120.
259. Olivier M, Eeles R, Hollstein M, Khan MA, Harris CC, Hainaut P. The IARC TP53 database: new online mutation analysis and recommendations to users. *Hum Mutat.* 2002;19(6):607-614.
260. Petitjean A, Achatz MIW, Borresen-Dale AL, Hainaut P, Olivier M. TP53 mutations in human cancers: functional selection and impact on cancer prognosis and outcomes. *Oncogene.* 2007;26(15):2157-2165.
261. Rivlin N, Brosh R, Oren M, Rotter V. Mutations in the p53 tumor suppressor gene: important milestones at the various steps of tumorigenesis. *Genes Cancer.* 2011;2(4):466-474.
262. Parkin B, Erba H, Ouillette P, et al. Acquired genomic copy number aberrations and survival in adult acute myelogenous leukemia. *Blood.* 2010;116(23):4958-4967.
263. Rucker FG, Schlenk RF, Bullinger L, et al. TP53 alterations in acute myeloid leukemia with complex karyotype correlate with specific copy number alterations, monosomal karyotype, and dismal outcome. *Blood.* 2012;119(9):2114-2121.
264. Vadakekolathu J, Lai C, Reeder S, et al. TP53 abnormalities correlate with immune infiltration and associate with response to flotetuzumab immunotherapy in AML. *Blood Adv.* 2020;4(20):5011-5024.
265. Welch JS, Petti AA, Miller CA, et al. TP53 and decitabine in acute myeloid leukemia and myelodysplastic syndromes. *N Engl J Med.* 2016;375(21):2023-2036.
266. Khurana A, Shafer DA. MDM2 antagonists as a novel treatment option for acute myeloid leukemia: perspectives on the therapeutic potential of idasanutlin (RG7388). *Onco Targets Ther.* 2019;12:2903-2910.
267. Konopleva M, Martinelli G, Daver N, et al. MDM2 inhibition: an important step forward in cancer therapy. *Leukemia.* 2020;34(11):2858-2874.
268. Ley TJ, Ding L, Walter MJ, et al. DNMT3A mutations in acute myeloid leukemia. *N Engl J Med.* 2010;363(25):2424-2433.
269. Thol F, Damm F, Ludeking A, et al. Incidence and prognostic influence of DNMT3A mutations in acute myeloid leukemia. *J Clin Oncol.* 2011;29(21):2889-2896.
270. Hou HA, Kuo YY, Liu CY, et al. DNMT3A mutations in acute myeloid leukemia: stability during disease evolution and clinical implications. *Blood.* 2012;119(2):559-568.
271. Markova J, Michkova P, Burckova K, et al. Prognostic impact of DNMT3A mutations in patients with intermediate cytogenetic risk profile acute myeloid leukemia. *Eur J Haematol.* 2012;88(2):128-135.
272. Renneville A, Boissel N, Nibourel O, et al. Prognostic significance of DNA methyltransferase 3A mutations in cytogenetically normal acute myeloid leukemia: a study by the Acute Leukemia French Association. *Leukemia.* 2012;26(6):1247-1254.
273. Ito S, Shen L, Dai Q, et al. Tet proteins can convert 5-methylcytosine to 5-formylcytosine and 5-carboxylcytosine. *Science.* 2011;333(6047):1300-1303.
274. He YF, Li BZ, Li Z, et al. Tet-mediated formation of 5-carboxylcytosine and its excision by TDG in mammalian DNA. *Science.* 2011;333(6047):1303-1307.
275. Ko M, Huang Y, Jankowska AM, et al. Impaired hydroxylation of 5-methylcytosine in myeloid cancers with mutant TET2. *Nature.* 2010;468(7325):839-843.
276. Delhommeau F, Dupont S, Della Valle V, et al. Mutation in TET2 in myeloid cancers. *N Engl J Med.* 2009;360(22):2289-2301.
277. Gaidzik VI, Paschka P, Spath D, et al. TET2 mutations in acute myeloid leukemia (AML): results from a comprehensive genetic and clinical analysis of the AML study group. *J Clin Oncol.* 2012;30(12):1350-1357.
278. Marcucci G, Maharry K, Wu YZ, et al. IDH1 and IDH2 gene mutations identify novel molecular subsets within de novo cytogenetically normal acute myeloid leukemia: a Cancer and Leukemia Group B study. *J Clin Oncol.* 2010;28(14):2348-2355.
279. Paschka P, Schlenk RF, Gaidzik VI, et al. IDH1 and IDH2 mutations are frequent genetic alterations in acute myeloid leukemia and confer adverse prognosis in cytogenetically normal acute myeloid leukemia with NPM1 mutation without FLT3 internal tandem duplication. *J Clin Oncol.* 2010;28(22):3636-3643.
280. Abbas S, Lugthart S, Kavelaars FG, et al. Acquired mutations in the genes encoding IDH1 and IDH2 both are recurrent aberrations in acute myeloid leukemia: prevalence and prognostic value. *Blood.* 2010;116(12):2122-2126.
281. Zou Y, Zeng Y, Zhang DF, Zou SH, Cheng YF, Yao YG. IDH1 and IDH2 mutations are frequent in Chinese patients with acute myeloid leukemia but rare in other types of hematological disorders. *Biochem Biophys Res Commun.* 2010;402(2):378-383.
282. Patel JP, Gonen M, Figueroa ME, et al. Prognostic relevance of integrated genetic profiling in acute myeloid leukemia. *N Engl J Med.* 2012;366(12):1079-1089.
283. Dang L, White DW, Gross S, et al. Cancer-associated IDH1 mutations produce 2-hydroxyglutarate. *Nature.* 2009;462(7274):739-744.
284. Chou WC, Hou HA, Chen CY, et al. Distinct clinical and biologic characteristics in adult acute myeloid leukemia bearing the isocitrate dehydrogenase 1 mutation. *Blood.* 2010;115(14):2749-2754.
285. Ward PS, Patel J, Wise DR, et al. The common feature of leukemia-associated IDH1 and IDH2 mutations is a neomorphic enzyme activity converting alpha-ketoglutarate to 2-hydroxyglutarate. *Cancer Cell.* 2010;17(3):225-234.
286. Gross S, Cairns RA, Minden MD, et al. Cancer-associated metabolite 2-hydroxyglutarate accumulates in acute myelogenous leukemia with isocitrate dehydrogenase 1 and 2 mutations. *J Exp Med.* 2010;207(2):339-344.
287. Figueroa ME, Abdel-Wahab O, Lu C, et al. Leukemic IDH1 and IDH2 mutations result in a hypermethylation phenotype, disrupt TET2 function, and impair hematopoietic differentiation. *Cancer Cell.* 2010;18(6):553-567.
288. Chowdhury R, Yeoh KK, Tian YM, et al. The oncometabolite 2-hydroxyglutarate inhibits histone lysine demethylases. *EMBO Rep.* 2011;12(5):463-469.
289. Emadi A. At the crossroads: tumor metabolism and epigenetics. *Sci Transl Med.* 2011;3(82):ec68.
290. Sulkowski PL, Corso CD, Robinson ND, et al. 2-Hydroxyglutarate produced by neomorphic IDH mutations suppresses homologous recombination and induces PARP inhibitor sensitivity. *Sci Transl Med.* 2017;9(375):eaal2463.
291. Akbay EA, Moslehi J, Christensen CL, et al. D-2-hydroxyglutarate produced by mutant IDH2 causes cardiomyopathy and neurodegeneration in mice. *Genes Dev.* 2014;28(5):479-490.
292. Kattih B, Shirvani A, Klement P, et al. IDH1/2 mutations in acute myeloid leukemia patients and risk of coronary artery disease and cardiac dysfunction-a retrospective propensity score analysis. *Leukemia.* 2021;35(5):1301-1316.
293. Watts JM, Baer MR, Yang J, et al. Olutasidenib alone or with azacitidine in IDH1-mutated acute myeloid leukaemia and myelodysplastic syndrome: phase 1 results of a phase 1/2 trial. *Lancet Haematol.* 2022:S2352-3026(22)00292-7.
294. Metzeler KH, Becker H, Maharry K, et al. ASXL1 mutations identify a high-risk subgroup of older patients with primary cytogenetically normal AML within the ELN favorable genetic category. *Blood.* 2011;118(26):6920-6929.
295. Pabst T, Mueller BU, Zhang P, et al. Dominant-negative mutations of CEBPA, encoding CCAAT/enhancer binding protein-alpha (C/EBPalpha), in acute myeloid leukemia. *Nat Genet.* 2001;27(3):263-270.

296. Preudhomme C, Sagot C, Boissel N, et al. Favorable prognostic significance of CEBPA mutations in patients with de novo acute myeloid leukemia: a study from the Acute Leukemia French Association (ALFA). *Blood*. 2002;100(8):2717-2723.
297. Frohling S, Schlenk RF, Stolze I, et al. CEBPA mutations in younger adults with acute myeloid leukemia and normal cytogenetics: prognostic relevance and analysis of cooperating mutations. *J Clin Oncol*. 2004;22(4):624-633.
298. Green CL, Koo KK, Hills RK, Burnett AK, Linch DC, Gale RE. Prognostic significance of CEBPA mutations in a large cohort of younger adult patients with acute myeloid leukemia: impact of double CEBPA mutations and the interaction with FLT3 and NPM1 mutations. *J Clin Oncol*. 2010;28(16):2739-2747.
299. Dufour A, Schneider F, Metzeler KH, et al. Acute myeloid leukemia with biallelic CEBPA gene mutations and normal karyotype represents a distinct genetic entity associated with a favorable clinical outcome. *J Clin Oncol*. 2010;28(4):570-577.
300. Marcucci G, Maharry K, Radmacher MD, et al. Prognostic significance of, and gene and microRNA expression signatures associated with, CEBPA mutations in cytogenetically normal acute myeloid leukemia with high-risk molecular features: a Cancer and Leukemia Group B Study. *J Clin Oncol*. 2008;26(31):5078-5087.
301. Pylayeva-Gupta Y, Grabocka E, Bar-Sagi D. RAS oncogenes: weaving a tumorigenic web. *Nat Rev Cancer*. 2011;11(11):761-774.
302. Karnoub AE, Weinberg RA. Ras oncogenes: split personalities. *Nat Rev Mol Cell Biol*. 2008;9(7):517-531.
303. Scott AJ, Lieu CH, Messersmith WA. Therapeutic approaches to RAS mutation. *Cancer J*. 2016;22(3):165-174.
304. Milella M, Estrov Z, Kornblau SM, et al. Synergistic induction of apoptosis by simultaneous disruption of the Bcl-2 and MEK/MAPK pathways in acute myelogenous leukemia. *Blood*. 2002;99(9):3461-3464.
305. Lunghi P, Tabilio A, Dall'Aglio PP, et al. Downmodulation of ERK activity inhibits the proliferation and induces the apoptosis of primary acute myelogenous leukemia blasts. *Leukemia*. 2003;17(9):1783-1793.
306. McMahon CM, Ferng T, Canaani J, et al. Clonal selection with RAS pathway activation mediates secondary clinical resistance to selective FLT3 inhibition in acute myeloid leukemia. *Cancer Discov*. 2019;9(8):1050-1063.
307. Allegra CJ, Rumble RB, Hamilton SR, et al. Extended RAS gene mutation testing in metastatic colorectal carcinoma to predict response to anti-epidermal growth factor receptor monoclonal antibody therapy: American society of clinical oncology provisional clinical opinion update 2015. *J Clin Oncol*. 2016;34(2):179-185.
308. Shen Y, Zhu YM, Fan X, et al. Gene mutation patterns and their prognostic impact in a cohort of 1185 patients with acute myeloid leukemia. *Blood*. 2011;118(20):5593-5603.
309. Miglino M, Colombo N, Pica G, et al. WT1 overexpression at diagnosis may predict favorable outcome in patients with de novo non-M3 acute myeloid leukemia. *Leuk Lymphoma*. 2011;52(10):1961-1969.
310. Virappane P, Gale R, Hills R, et al. Mutation of the Wilms' tumor 1 gene is a poor prognostic factor associated with chemotherapy resistance in normal karyotype acute myeloid leukemia: the United Kingdom Medical Research Council Adult Leukaemia Working Party. *J Clin Oncol*. 2008;26(33):5429-5435.
311. Becker H, Marcucci G, Maharry K, et al. Mutations of the Wilms tumor 1 gene (WT1) in older patients with primary cytogenetically normal acute myeloid leukemia: a Cancer and Leukemia Group B study. *Blood*. 2010;116(5):788-792.
312. Tang JL, Hou HA, Chen CY, et al. AML1/RUNX1 mutations in 470 adult patients with de novo acute myeloid leukemia: prognostic implication and interaction with other gene alterations. *Blood*. 2009;114(26):5352-5361.
313. Gaidzik VI, Bullinger L, Schlenk RF, et al. RUNX1 mutations in acute myeloid leukemia: results from a comprehensive genetic and clinical analysis from the AML study group. *J Clin Oncol*. 2011;29(10):1364-1372.
314. Mendler JH, Maharry K, Radmacher MD, et al. RUNX1 mutations are associated with poor outcome in younger and older patients with cytogenetically normal acute myeloid leukemia and with distinct gene and MicroRNA expression signatures. *J Clin Oncol*. 2012;30(25):3109-3118.
315. Wang YY, Zhou GB, Yin T, et al. AML1-ETO and C-KIT mutation/overexpression in t(8;21) leukemia: implication in stepwise leukemogenesis and response to Gleevec. *Proc Natl Acad Sci U S A*. 2005;102(4):1104-1109.
316. Kohl TM, Schnittger S, Ellwart JW, Hiddemann W, Spiekermann K. KIT exon 8 mutations associated with core-binding factor (CBF)-acute myeloid leukemia (AML) cause hyperactivation of the receptor in response to stem cell factor. *Blood*. 2005;105(8):3319-3321.
317. Qin YZ, Zhu HH, Jiang Q, et al. Heterogeneous prognosis among KIT mutation types in adult acute myeloid leukemia patients with t(8;21). *Blood Cancer J*. 2018;8(8):76.
318. Dohner H, Estey EH, Amadori S, et al. Diagnosis and management of acute myeloid leukemia in adults: recommendations from an international expert panel, on behalf of the European LeukemiaNet. *Blood*. 2010;115(3):453-474.
319. Marcucci G, Geyer S, Laumann K, et al. Combination of dasatinib with chemotherapy in previously untreated core binding factor acute myeloid leukemia: CALGB 10801. *Blood Adv*. 2020;4(4):696-705.
320. Vardiman JW, Harris NL, Brunning RD. The World Health Organization (WHO) classification of the myeloid neoplasms. *Blood*. 2002;100(7):2292-2302.
321. Vardiman JW. The World Health Organization (WHO) classification of tumors of the hematopoietic and lymphoid tissues: an overview with emphasis on the myeloid neoplasms. *Chem Biol Interact*. 2010;184(1-2):16-20.
322. Estey E, Thall P, Beran M, Kantarjian H, Pierce S, Keating M. Effect of diagnosis (refractory anemia with excess blasts, refractory anemia with excess blasts in transformation, or acute myeloid leukemia [AML]) on outcome of AML-type chemotherapy. *Blood*. 1997;90(8):2969-2977.
323. Appelbaum FR, Gundacker H, Head DR, et al. Age and acute myeloid leukemia. *Blood*. 2006;107(9):3481-3485.
324. Kantarjian H, O'Brien S, Cortes J, et al. Results of intensive chemotherapy in 998 patients age 65 years or older with acute myeloid leukemia or high-risk myelodysplastic syndrome: predictive prognostic models for outcome. *Cancer*. 2006;106(5):1090-1098.
325. Deschler B, Ihorst G, Platzbecker U, et al. Parameters detected by geriatric and quality of life assessment in 195 older patients with myelodysplastic syndromes and acute myeloid leukemia are highly predictive for outcome. *Haematologica*. 2013;98(2):208-216.
326. Bhatnagar B, Kohlschmidt J, Mrozek K, et al. Poor survival and differential impact of genetic features of black patients with acute myeloid leukemia. *Cancer Discov*. 2021;11(3):626-637.
327. Grimwade D, Hills RK, Moorman AV, et al. Refinement of cytogenetic classification in acute myeloid leukemia: determination of prognostic significance of rare recurring chromosomal abnormalities among 5876 younger adult patients treated in the United Kingdom Medical Research Council trials. *Blood*. 2010;116(3):354-365.
328. Breems DA, Van Putten WLJ, De Greef GE, et al. Monosomal karyotype in acute myeloid leukemia: a better indicator of poor prognosis than a complex karyotype. *J Clin Oncol*. 2008;26(29):4791-4797.
329. Hoyle CF, de Bastos M, Wheatley K, et al. AML associated with previous cytotoxic therapy, MDS or myeloproliferative disorders: results from the MRC's 9th AML trial. *Br J Haematol*. 1989;72(1):45-53.
330. Kayser S, Dohner K, Krauter J, et al. The impact of therapy-related acute myeloid leukemia (AML) on outcome in 2853 adult patients with newly diagnosed AML. *Blood*. 2011;117(7):2137-2145.
331. Haferlach T, Schoch C, Loffler H, et al. Morphologic dysplasia in de novo acute myeloid leukemia (AML) is related to unfavorable cytogenetics but has no independent prognostic relevance under the conditions of intensive induction therapy: results of a multiparameter analysis from the German AML Cooperative Group studies. *J Clin Oncol*. 2003;21(2):256-265.
332. Chang H, Brandwein J, Yi QL, Chun K, Patterson B, Brien B. Extramedullary infiltrates of AML are associated with CD56 expression, 11q23 abnormalities and inferior clinical outcome. *Leuk Res*. 2004;28(10):1007-1011.
333. Greenwood MJ, Seftel MD, Richardson C, et al. Leukocyte count as a predictor of death during remission induction in acute myeloid leukemia. *Leuk Lymphoma*. 2006;47(7):1245-1252.
334. Buccisano F, Maurillo L, Spagnoli A, et al. Cytogenetic and molecular diagnostic characterization combined to postconsolidation minimal residual disease assessment by flow cytometry improves risk stratification in adult acute myeloid leukemia. *Blood*. 2010;116(13):2295-2303.
335. Terwijn M, van Putten WLJ, Kelder A, et al. High prognostic impact of flow cytometric minimal residual disease detection in acute myeloid leukemia: data from the HOVON/SAKK AML 42A study. *J Clin Oncol*. 2013;31(31):3889-3897.
336. Walter RB, Gooley TA, Wood BL, et al. Impact of pretransplantation minimal residual disease, as detected by multiparametric flow cytometry, on outcome of myeloablative hematopoietic cell transplantation for acute myeloid leukemia. *J Clin Oncol*. 2011;29(9):1190-1197.
337. Jourdan E, Boissel N, Chevret S, et al. Prospective evaluation of gene mutations and minimal residual disease in patients with core binding factor acute myeloid leukemia. *Blood*. 2013;121(12):2213-2223.
338. Shayegi N, Kramer M, Bornhauser M, et al. The level of residual disease based on mutant NPM1 is an independent prognostic factor for relapse and survival in AML. *Blood*. 2013;122(1):83-92.
339. Sekeres MA, Elson P, Kalaycio ME, et al. Time from diagnosis to treatment initiation predicts survival in younger, but not older, acute myeloid leukemia patients. *Blood*. 2009;113(1):28-36.
340. Burd A, Levine RL, Ruppert AS, et al. Precision medicine treatment in acute myeloid leukemia using prospective genomic profiling: feasibility and preliminary efficacy of the Beat AML Master Trial. *Nat Med*. 2020;26(12):1852-1858.
341. Stone RM, Mandrekar SJ, Sanford BL, et al. Midostaurin plus chemotherapy for acute myeloid leukemia with a FLT3 mutation. *N Engl J Med*. 2017;377(5):454-464.
342. Rao AV. Fitness in the elderly: how to make decisions regarding acute myeloid leukemia induction. *Hematology Am Soc Hematol Educ Program*. 2016;2016(1):339-347.
343. Lichtman MA, Rowe JM. Hyperleukocytic leukemias: rheological, clinical, and therapeutic considerations. *Blood*. 1982;60(2):279-283.
344. Thiebaut A, Thomas X, Belhabri A, Anglaret B, Archimbaud E. Impact of preinduction therapy leukapheresis on treatment outcome in adult acute myelogenous leukemia presenting with hyperleukocytosis. *Ann Hematol*. 2000;79(9):501-506.
345. Bug G, Anargyrou K, Tonn T, et al. Impact of leukapheresis on early death rate in adult acute myeloid leukemia presenting with hyperleukocytosis. *Transfusion*. 2007;47(10):1843-1850.
346. Giles FJ, Shen Y, Kantarjian HM, et al. Leukapheresis reduces early mortality in patients with acute myeloid leukemia with high white cell counts but does not improve long-term survival. *Leuk Lymphoma*. 2001;42(1-2):67-73.
347. Bewersdorf JP, Giri S, Tallman MS, Zeidan AM, Stahl M. Leukapheresis for the management of hyperleukocytosis in acute myeloid leukemia-A systematic review and meta-analysis. *Transfusion*. 2020;60(10):2360-2369.
348. Stahl M, Shallis RM, Wei W, et al. Management of hyperleukocytosis and impact of leukapheresis among patients with acute myeloid leukemia (AML) on short- and long-term clinical outcomes: a large, retrospective, multicenter, international study. *Leukemia*. 2020;34(12):3149-3160.
349. Rollig C, Ehninger G. How I treat hyperleukocytosis in acute myeloid leukemia. *Blood*. 2015;125(21):3246-3252.
350. Cheson BD, Bennett JM, Kopecky KJ, et al. Revised recommendations of the international working group for diagnosis, standardization of response criteria, treatment

outcomes, and reporting standards for therapeutic trials in acute myeloid leukemia. *J Clin Oncol*. 2003;21(24):4642-4649.
351. Arellano M, Pakkala S, Langston A, et al. Early clearance of peripheral blood blasts predicts response to induction chemotherapy in acute myeloid leukemia. *Cancer*. 2012;118(21):5278-5282.
352. Holtzman NG, El Chaer F, Baer MR, et al. Peripheral blood blast rate of clearance is an independent predictor of clinical response and outcomes in acute myeloid leukaemia. *Br J Haematol*. 2020;188(6):881-887.
353. Food and Drug Administration. *Guidance for Industry (Draft Guidance); Acute Myeloid Leukemia: Developing Drugs and Biological Products for Treatment*; 2020. https://www.fda.gov/media/140821/download
354. Food and Drug Administration. *Blinatumomab Label*; 2014. Accessed December 20, 2022. https://www.accessdata.fda.gov/drugsatfda_docs/label/2022/125557s021lbl.pdf
355. Marcucci G, Mrozek K, Ruppert AS, et al. Abnormal cytogenetics at date of morphologic complete remission predicts short overall and disease-free survival, and higher relapse rate in adult acute myeloid leukemia: results from cancer and leukemia group B study 8461. *J Clin Oncol*. 2004;22(12):2410-2418.
356. Diverio D, Rossi V, Avvisati G, et al. Early detection of relapse by prospective reverse transcriptase-polymerase chain reaction analysis of the PML/RARalpha fusion gene in patients with acute promyelocytic leukemia enrolled in the GIMEMA-AIEOP multicenter "AIDA" trial. GIMEMA-AIEOP Multicenter "AIDA" Trial. *Blood*. 1998;92(3):784-789.
357. Jurcic JG, Nimer SD, Scheinberg DA, DeBlasio T, Warrell RP Jr, Miller WH Jr. Prognostic significance of minimal residual disease detection and PML/RARalpha isoform type: long-term follow-up in acute promyelocytic leukemia. *Blood*. 2001;98(9):2651-2656.
358. Jurlander J, Caligiuri MA, Ruutu T, et al. Persistence of the AML1/ETO fusion transcript in patients treated with allogeneic bone marrow transplantation for t(8;21) leukemia. *Blood*. 1996;88(6):2183-2191.
359. Klco JM, Miller CA, Griffith M, et al. Association between mutation clearance after induction therapy and outcomes in acute myeloid leukemia. *J Am Med Assoc*. 2015;314(8):811-822.
360. Bloomfield CD. Post-remission therapy in acute myeloid leukemia. *J Clin Oncol*. 1985;3(12):1570-1572.
361. Cohen SS. Introduction to the biochemistry of D-arabinosyl nucleosides. *Prog Nucleic Acid Res Mol Biol*. 1966;5:1-88.
362. Rai KR, Holland JF, Glidewell OJ, et al. Treatment of acute myelocytic leukemia: a study by cancer and leukemia group B. *Blood*. 1981;58(6):1203-1212.
363. Yates J, Glidewell O, Wiernik P, et al. Cytosine arabinoside with daunorubicin or adriamycin for therapy of acute myelocytic leukemia: a CALGB study. *Blood*. 1982;60(2):454-462.
364. Preisler H, Davis RB, Kirshner J, et al. Comparison of three remission induction regimens and two postinduction strategies for the treatment of acute nonlymphocytic leukemia: a cancer and leukemia group B study. *Blood*. 1987;69(5):1441-1449.
365. Dillman RO, Davis RB, Green MR, et al. A comparative study of two different doses of cytarabine for acute myeloid leukemia: a phase III trial of Cancer and Leukemia Group B. *Blood*. 1991;78(10):2520-2526.
366. Fernandez HF, Sun Z, Yao X, et al. Anthracycline dose intensification in acute myeloid leukemia. *N Engl J Med*. 2009;361(13):1249-1259.
367. Lee JH, Joo YD, Kim H, et al. A randomized trial comparing standard versus high-dose daunorubicin induction in patients with acute myeloid leukemia. *Blood*. 2011;118(14):3832-3841.
368. Luskin MR, Lee JW, Fernandez HF, et al. Benefit of high-dose daunorubicin in AML induction extends across cytogenetic and molecular groups. *Blood*. 2016;127(12):1551-1558.
369. Lowenberg B, Ossenkoppele GJ, van Putten W, et al. High-dose daunorubicin in older patients with acute myeloid leukemia. *N Engl J Med*. 2009;361(13):1235-1248.
370. Wiernik PH, Banks PL, Case DC Jr, et al. Cytarabine plus idarubicin or daunorubicin as induction and consolidation therapy for previously untreated adult patients with acute myeloid leukemia. *Blood*. 1992;79(2):313-319.
371. Vogler WR, Velez-Garcia E, Weiner RS, et al. A phase III trial comparing idarubicin and daunorubicin in combination with cytarabine in acute myelogenous leukemia: a Southeastern Cancer Study Group Study. *J Clin Oncol*. 1992;10(7):1103-1111.
372. Berman E, Heller G, Santorsa J, et al. Results of a randomized trial comparing idarubicin and cytosine arabinoside with daunorubicin and cytosine arabinoside in adult patients with newly diagnosed acute myelogenous leukemia. *Blood*. 1991;77(8):1666-1674.
373. A systematic collaborative overview of randomized trials comparing idarubicin with daunorubicin (or other anthracyclines) as induction therapy for acute myeloid leukaemia. AML Collaborative Group. *Br J Haematol*. 1998;103(1):100-109.
374. Gardin C, Turlure P, Fagot T, et al. Postremission treatment of elderly patients with acute myeloid leukemia in first complete remission after intensive induction chemotherapy: results of the Multicenter Randomized Acute Leukemia French Association (ALFA) 9803 trial. *Blood*. 2007;109(12):5129-5135.
375. Estey EH, Thall PF, Cortes JE, et al. Comparison of idarubicin + ara-C-fludarabine + ara-C-and topotecan + ara-C-based regimens in treatment of newly diagnosed acute myeloid leukemia, refractory anemia with excess blasts in transformation, or refractory anemia with excess blasts. *Blood*. 2001;98(13):3575-3583.
376. Lee JH, Kim H, Joo YD, et al. Prospective randomized comparison of idarubicin and high-dose daunorubicin in induction chemotherapy for newly diagnosed acute myeloid leukemia. *J Clin Oncol*. 2017;35(24):2754-2763.
377. Adige S, Lapidus RG, Carter-Cooper BA, et al. Equipotent doses of daunorubicin and idarubicin for AML: a meta-analysis of clinical trials versus in vitro estimation. *Cancer Chemother Pharmacol*. 2019;83(6):1105-1112.
378. Bishop JF, Lowenthal RM, Joshua D, et al. Etoposide in acute nonlymphocytic leukemia. Australian leukemia study group. *Blood*. 1990;75(1):27-32.
379. Kolitz JE, George SL, Marcucci G, et al. P-glycoprotein inhibition using valspodar (PSC-833) does not improve outcomes for patients younger than age 60 years with newly diagnosed acute myeloid leukemia: cancer and Leukemia Group B study 19808. *Blood*. 2010;116(9):1413-1421.
380. Gandhi V, Estey E, Keating MJ, Plunkett W. Biochemical modulation of arabinosylcytosine for therapy of leukemias. *Leuk Lymphoma*. 1993;(10 suppl):109-114.
381. Gandhi V, Estey E, Keating MJ, Plunkett W. Fludarabine potentiates metabolism of cytarabine in patients with acute myelogenous leukemia during therapy. *J Clin Oncol*. 1993;11(1):116-124.
382. Gandhi V, Estey E, Du M, Nowak B, Keating MJ, Plunkett W. Modulation of the cellular metabolism of cytarabine and fludarabine by granulocyte-colony-stimulating factor during therapy of acute myelogenous leukemia. *Clin Cancer Res*. 1995;1(2):169-178.
383. de la Rubia J, Regadera A, Martin G, et al. FLAG-IDA regimen (fludarabine, cytarabine, idarubicin and G-CSF) in the treatment of patients with high-risk myeloid malignancies. *Leuk Res*. 2002;26(8):725-730.
384. Virchis A, Koh M, Rankin P, et al. Fludarabine, cytosine arabinoside, granulocyte-colony stimulating factor with or without idarubicin in the treatment of high risk acute leukaemia or myelodysplastic syndromes. *Br J Haematol*. 2004;124(1):26-32.
385. Burnett AK, Russell NH, Hills RK, et al. Optimization of chemotherapy for younger patients with acute myeloid leukemia: results of the medical research council AML15 trial. *J Clin Oncol*. 2013;31(27):3360-3368.
386. Holowiecki J, Grosicki S, Giebel S, et al. Cladribine, but not fludarabine, added to daunorubicin and cytarabine during induction prolongs survival of patients with acute myeloid leukemia: a multicenter, randomized phase III study. *J Clin Oncol*. 2012;30(20):2441-2448.
387. Lowenberg B, Pabst T, Vellenga E, et al. Cytarabine dose for acute myeloid leukemia. *N Engl J Med*. 2011;364(11):1027-1036.
388. Stone RM, Berg DT, George SL, et al. Granulocyte-macrophage colony-stimulating factor after initial chemotherapy for elderly patients with primary acute myelogenous leukemia. Cancer and Leukemia Group B. *N Engl J Med*. 1995;332(25):1671-1677.
389. Zittoun R, Suciu S, Mandelli F, et al. Granulocyte-macrophage colony-stimulating factor associated with induction treatment of acute myelogenous leukemia: a randomized trial by the European Organization for Research and Treatment of Cancer Leukemia Cooperative Group. *J Clin Oncol*. 1996;14(7):2150-2159.
390. Lowenberg B, Boogaerts MA, Daenen SM, et al. Value of different modalities of granulocyte-macrophage colony-stimulating factor applied during or after induction therapy of acute myeloid leukemia. *J Clin Oncol*. 1997;15(12):3496-3506.
391. Lowenberg B, Suciu S, Archimbaud E, et al. Use of recombinant GM-CSF during and after remission induction chemotherapy in patients aged 61 years and older with acute myeloid leukemia: final report of AML-11, a phase III randomized study of the Leukemia Cooperative Group of European Organisation for the Research and Treatment of Cancer and the Dutch Belgian Hemato-Oncology Cooperative Group. *Blood*. 1997;90(8):2952-2961.
392. Rowe JM, Andersen JW, Mazza JJ, et al. A randomized placebo-controlled phase III study of granulocyte-macrophage colony-stimulating factor in adult patients (> 55 to 70 years of age) with acute myelogenous leukemia: a study of the Eastern Cooperative Oncology Group (E1490). *Blood*. 1995;86(2):457-462.
393. Dombret H, Chastang C, Fenaux P, et al. A controlled study of recombinant human granulocyte colony-stimulating factor in elderly patients after treatment for acute myelogenous leukemia. AML Cooperative Study Group. *N Engl J Med*. 1995;332(25):1678-1683.
394. Heil G, Hoelzer D, Sanz MA, et al. A randomized, double-blind, placebo-controlled, phase III study of filgrastim in remission induction and consolidation therapy for adults with de novo acute myeloid leukemia. The International Acute Myeloid Leukemia Study Group. *Blood*. 1997;90(12):4710-4718.
395. Godwin JE, Kopecky KJ, Head DR, et al. A double-blind placebo-controlled trial of granulocyte colony-stimulating factor in elderly patients with previously untreated acute myeloid leukemia: a Southwest oncology group study (9031). *Blood*. 1998;91(10):3607-3615.
396. Harousseau JL, Witz B, Lioure B, et al. Granulocyte colony-stimulating factor after intensive consolidation chemotherapy in acute myeloid leukemia: results of a randomized trial of the Groupe Ouest-Est Leucemies Aigues Myeloblastiques. *J Clin Oncol*. 2000;18(4):780-787.
397. Food and Drug Administration. *Vyxeos Label*; 2017. Accessed December 20, 2022. https://www.accessdata.fda.gov/drugsatfda_docs/label/2022/209401s011lbl.pdf
398. Lancet JE, Cortes JE, Hogge DE, et al. Phase 2 trial of CPX-351, a fixed 5:1 molar ratio of cytarabine/daunorubicin, vs cytarabine/daunorubicin in older adults with untreated AML. *Blood*. 2014;123(21):3239-3246.
399. Lancet JE, Uy GL, Cortes JE, et al. CPX-351 (cytarabine and daunorubicin) liposome for injection versus conventional cytarabine plus daunorubicin in older patients with newly diagnosed secondary acute myeloid leukemia. *J Clin Oncol*. 2018;36(26):2684-2692.
400. Lancet JE, Uy GL, Newell LF, et al. CPX-351 versus 7+3 cytarabine and daunorubicin chemotherapy in older adults with newly diagnosed high-risk or secondary acute myeloid leukaemia: 5-year results of a randomised, open-label, multicentre, phase 3 trial. *Lancet Haematol*. 2021;8(7):e481-e491.
401. Jacoby MA, Finn L, Emadi A, et al. Frequency of infusion-related reactions with CPX-351 treatment in an observational study in adults with newly diagnosed therapy-related AML or AML with myelodysplasia-related changes (AML-MRC). *Leuk Lymphoma*. 2021;62(10):2539-2542.
402. Juarez S, Cuadrado Pastor JM, Feliu J, Gonzalez Baron M, Ordonez A, Montero JM. Association of leukemia and pregnancy: clinical and obstetric aspects. *Am J Clin Oncol*. 1988;11(2):159-165.
403. Reynoso EE, Shepherd FA, Messner HA, Farquharson HA, Garvey MB, Baker MA. Acute leukemia during pregnancy: the Toronto Leukemia Study Group experience with long-term follow-up of children exposed in utero to chemotherapeutic agents. *J Clin Oncol*. 1987;5(7):1098-1106.

404. Brell J, Kalaycio M. Leukemia in pregnancy. *Semin Oncol*. 2000;27(6):667-677.
405. Dildy GA III, Moise KJ Jr, Carpenter RJ Jr, Klima T. Maternal malignancy metastatic to the products of conception: a review. *Obstet Gynecol Surv*. 1989;44(7):535-540.
406. Honore LH, Brown LB. Intervillous placental metastasis with maternal myeloid leukemia. *Arch Pathol Lab Med*. 1990;114(5):450.
407. Feliu J, Juarez S, Ordonez A, Garcia-Paredes ML, Gonzalez-Baron M, Montero JM. Acute leukemia and pregnancy. *Cancer*. 1988;61(3):580-584.
408. Doll DC, Ringenberg QS, Yarbro JW. Antineoplastic agents and pregnancy. *Semin Oncol*. 1989;16(5):337-346.
409. Greenlund LJ, Letendre L, Tefferi A. Acute leukemia during pregnancy: a single institutional experience with 17 cases. *Leuk Lymphoma*. 2001;41(5-6):571-577.
410. Chelghoum Y, Vey N, Raffoux E, et al. Acute leukemia during pregnancy: a report on 37 patients and a review of the literature. *Cancer*. 2005;104(1):110-117.
411. Aviles A, Diaz-Maqueo JC, Talavera A, Guzman R, Garcia EL. Growth and development of children of mothers treated with chemotherapy during pregnancy: current status of 43 children. *Am J Hematol*. 1991;36(4):243-248.
412. Resnik R. Cancer during pregnancy. *N Engl J Med*. 1999;341(2):120-121.
413. Shapira T, Pereg D, Lishner M. How I treat acute and chronic leukemia in pregnancy. *Blood Rev*. 2008;22(5):247-259.
414. Cassileth PA, Begg CB, Bennett JM, et al. A randomized study of the efficacy of consolidation therapy in adult acute nonlymphocytic leukemia. *Blood*. 1984;63(4):843-847.
415. Herzig RH, Herzig GP, Wolff SN, Hines JD, Fay JW, Phillips GL. Central nervous system effects of high-dose cytosine arabinoside. *Semin Oncol*. 1987;14(2 suppl 1):21-24.
416. Mayer RJ, Davis RB, Schiffer CA, et al. Intensive postremission chemotherapy in adults with acute myeloid leukemia. Cancer and Leukemia Group B. *N Engl J Med*. 1994;331(14):896-903.
417. Weick JK, Kopecky KJ, Appelbaum FR, et al. A randomized investigation of high-dose versus standard-dose cytosine arabinoside with daunorubicin in patients with previously untreated acute myeloid leukemia: a Southwest Oncology Group study. *Blood*. 1996;88(8):2841-2851.
418. Bloomfield CD, Lawrence D, Byrd JC, et al. Frequency of prolonged remission duration after high-dose cytarabine intensification in acute myeloid leukemia varies by cytogenetic subtype. *Cancer Res*. 1998;58(18):4173-4179.
419. Byrd JC, Ruppert AS, Mrozek K, et al. Repetitive cycles of high-dose cytarabine benefit patients with acute myeloid leukemia and inv(16)(p13q22) or t(16;16)(p13;q22): results from CALGB 8461. *J Clin Oncol*. 2004;22(6):1087-1094.
420. Farag SS, Ruppert AS, Mrozek K, et al. Outcome of induction and postremission therapy in younger adults with acute myeloid leukemia with normal karyotype: a cancer and leukemia group B study. *J Clin Oncol*. 2005;23(3):482-493.
421. Miyawaki S, Ohtake S, Fujisawa S, et al. A randomized comparison of 4 courses of standard-dose multiagent chemotherapy versus 3 courses of high-dose cytarabine alone in postremission therapy for acute myeloid leukemia in adults: the JALSG AML201 Study. *Blood*. 2011;117(8):2366-2372.
422. Reville PK, Kadia TM. Maintenance therapy in AML. *Front Oncol*. 2020;10:619085.
423. Food and Drug Administration. *Oral Azacitidine Label*; 2020. Accessed December 20, 2022. https://www.accessdata.fda.gov/drugsatfda_docs/label/2020/214120s000lbl.pdf
424. Wei AH, Dohner H, Pocock C, et al. Oral azacitidine maintenance therapy for acute myeloid leukemia in first remission. *N Engl J Med*. 2020;383(26):2526-2537.
425. Ossenkoppele G, Lowenberg B. How I treat the older patient with acute myeloid leukemia. *Blood*. 2015;125(5):767-774.
426. Cashen AF, Schiller GJ, O'Donnell MR, DiPersio JF. Multicenter, phase II study of decitabine for the first-line treatment of older patients with acute myeloid leukemia. *J Clin Oncol*. 2010;28(4):556-561.
427. Lubbert M, Ruter BH, Claus R, et al. A multicenter phase II trial of decitabine as first-line treatment for older patients with acute myeloid leukemia judged unfit for induction chemotherapy. *Haematologica*. 2012;97(3):393-401.
428. Kantarjian HM, Thomas XG, Dmoszynska A, et al. Multicenter, randomized, open-label, phase III trial of decitabine versus patient choice, with physician advice, of either supportive care or low-dose cytarabine for the treatment of older patients with newly diagnosed acute myeloid leukemia. *J Clin Oncol*. 2012;30(21):2670-2677.
429. Blum W, Garzon R, Klisovic RB, et al. Clinical response and miR-29b predictive significance in older AML patients treated with a 10-day schedule of decitabine. *Proc Natl Acad Sci U S A*. 2010;107(16):7473-7478.
430. Ritchie EK, Feldman EJ, Christos PJ, et al. Decitabine in patients with newly diagnosed and relapsed acute myeloid leukemia. *Leuk Lymphoma*. 2013;54(9):2003-2007.
431. Bhatnagar B, Duong VH, Gourdin TS, et al. Ten-day decitabine as initial therapy for newly diagnosed patients with acute myeloid leukemia unfit for intensive chemotherapy. *Leuk Lymphoma*. 2014;55(7):1533-1537.
432. Fenaux P, Mufti GJ, Hellstrom-Lindberg E, et al. Azacitidine prolongs overall survival compared with conventional care regimens in elderly patients with low bone marrow blast count acute myeloid leukemia. *J Clin Oncol*. 2010;28(4):562-569.
433. Dombret H, Seymour JF, Butrym A, et al. International phase 3 study of azacitidine vs conventional care regimens in older patients with newly diagnosed AML with >30% blasts. *Blood*. 2015;126(3):291-299.
434. Quintas-Cardama A, Ravandi F, Liu-Dumlao T, et al. Epigenetic therapy is associated with similar survival compared with intensive chemotherapy in older patients with newly diagnosed acute myeloid leukemia. *Blood*. 2012;120(24):4840-4845.
435. Souers AJ, Leverson JD, Boghaert ER, et al. ABT-199, a potent and selective BCL-2 inhibitor, achieves antitumor activity while sparing platelets. *Nat Med*. 2013;19(2):202-208.
436. Food and Drug Administration. *Venetoclax Label*; 2018. Accessed December 20, 2022. https://www.accessdata.fda.gov/drugsatfda_docs/label/2022/208573s027lbl.pdf
437. DiNardo CD, Pratz KW, Letai A, et al. Safety and preliminary efficacy of venetoclax with decitabine or azacitidine in elderly patients with previously untreated acute myeloid leukaemia: a non-randomised, open-label, phase 1b study. *Lancet Oncol*. 2018;19(2):216-228.
438. DiNardo CD, Jonas BA, Pullarkat V, et al. Azacitidine and venetoclax in previously untreated acute myeloid leukemia. *N Engl J Med*. 2020;383(7):617-629.
439. DiNardo CD, Pratz K, Pullarkat V, et al. Venetoclax combined with decitabine or azacitidine in treatment-naive, elderly patients with acute myeloid leukemia. *Blood*. 2019;133(1):7-17.
440. Wei AH, Montesinos P, Ivanov V, et al. Venetoclax plus LDAC for newly diagnosed AML ineligible for intensive chemotherapy: a phase 3 randomized placebo-controlled trial. *Blood*. 2020;135(24):2137-2145.
441. Winters AC, Gutman JA, Purev E, et al. Real-world experience of venetoclax with azacitidine for untreated patients with acute myeloid leukemia. *Blood Adv*. 2019;3(20):2911-2919.
442. DiNardo CD, Rausch CR, Benton C, et al. Clinical experience with the BCL2-inhibitor venetoclax in combination therapy for relapsed and refractory acute myeloid leukemia and related myeloid malignancies. *Am J Hematol*. 2018;93(3):401-407.
443. DiNardo CD, Lachowiez CA, Takahashi K, et al. Venetoclax combined with FLAG-IDA induction and consolidation in newly diagnosed and relapsed or refractory acute myeloid leukemia. *J Clin Oncol*. 2021;39(25):2768-2778.
444. Garcia JS, Kim HT, Murdock HM, et al. Adding venetoclax to fludarabine/busulfan RIC transplant for high risk MDS and AML is feasible, safe, and active. *Blood Adv*. 2021;5(24):5536-5545.
445. Emadi A, Kapadia B, Bollino D, et al. Venetoclax and pegcrisantaspase for complex karyotype acute myeloid leukemia. *Leukemia*. 2021;35(7):1907-1924.
446. Zhou FJ, Zeng CX, Kuang W, et al. Metformin exerts a synergistic effect with venetoclax by downregulating Mcl-1 protein in acute myeloid leukemia. *J Cancer*. 2021;12(22):6727-6739.
447. Larrosa-Garcia M, Baer MR. FLT3 inhibitors in acute myeloid leukemia: current status and future directions. *Mol Cancer Ther*. 2017;16(6):991-1001.
448. Pratz KW, Sato T, Murphy KM, Stine A, Rajkhowa T, Levis M. FLT3-mutant allelic burden and clinical status are predictive of response to FLT3 inhibitors in AML. *Blood*. 2010;115(7):1425-1432.
449. Smith CC, Lin K, Stecula A, Sali A, Shah NP. FLT3 D835 mutations confer differential resistance to type II FLT3 inhibitors. *Leukemia*. 2015;29(12):2390-2392.
450. Smith CC, Wang Q, Chin CS, et al. Validation of ITD mutations in FLT3 as a therapeutic target in human acute myeloid leukaemia. *Nature*. 2012;485(7397):260-263.
451. Man CH, Fung TK, Ho C, et al. Sorafenib treatment of FLT3-ITD(+) acute myeloid leukemia: favorable initial outcome and mechanisms of subsequent nonresponsiveness associated with the emergence of a D835 mutation. *Blood*. 2012;119(22):5133-5143.
452. Metzelder SK, Schroeder T, Finck A, et al. High activity of sorafenib in FLT3-ITD-positive acute myeloid leukemia synergizes with allo-immune effects to induce sustained responses. *Leukemia*. 2012;26(11):2353-2359.
453. Chen YB, Li S, Lane AA, et al. Phase I trial of maintenance sorafenib after allogeneic hematopoietic stem cell transplantation for fms-like tyrosine kinase 3 internal tandem duplication acute myeloid leukemia. *Biol Blood Marrow Transplant*. 2014;20(12):2042-2048.
454. Rollig C, Serve H, Huttmann A, et al. Addition of sorafenib versus placebo to standard therapy in patients aged 60 years or younger with newly diagnosed acute myeloid leukaemia (SORAML): a multicentre, phase 2, randomised controlled trial. *Lancet Oncol*. 2015;16(16):1691-1699.
455. Serve H, Krug U, Wagner R, et al. Sorafenib in combination with intensive chemotherapy in elderly patients with acute myeloid leukemia: results from a randomized, placebo-controlled trial. *J Clin Oncol*. 2013;31(25):3110-3118.
456. Uy GL, Mandrekar SJ, Laumann K, et al. A phase 2 study incorporating sorafenib into the chemotherapy for older adults with FLT3-mutated acute myeloid leukemia: CALGB 11001. *Blood Adv*. 2017;1(5):331-340.
457. Cortes JE, Kantarjian H, Foran JM, et al. Phase I study of quizartinib administered daily to patients with relapsed or refractory acute myeloid leukemia irrespective of FMS-like tyrosine kinase 3-internal tandem duplication status. *J Clin Oncol*. 2013;31(29):3681-3687.
458. Levis MJ, Martinelli G, Perl AE, et al. The benefit of treatment with quizartinib and subsequent bridging to HSCT for FLT3-ITD(+) patients with AML. *J Clin Oncol*. 2014;32(15).
459. Cortes JE, Khaled S, Martinelli G, et al. Quizartinib versus salvage chemotherapy in relapsed or refractory FLT3-ITD acute myeloid leukaemia (QuANTUM-R): a multicentre, randomised, controlled, open-label, phase 3 trial. *Lancet Oncol*. 2019;20(7):984-997.
460. Takahashi T, Usuki K, Matsue K, et al. Efficacy and safety of quizartinib in Japanese patients with FLT3-ITD positive relapsed or refractory acute myeloid leukemia in an open-label, phase 2 study. *Int J Hematol*. 2019;110(6):665-674.
461. Perl AE, Altman JK, Cortes J, et al. Selective inhibition of FLT3 by gilteritinib in relapsed or refractory acute myeloid leukaemia: a multicentre, first-in-human, open-label, phase 1-2 study. *Lancet Oncol*. 2017;18(8):1061-1075.
462. Perl AE, Martinelli G, Cortes JE, et al. Gilteritinib or chemotherapy for relapsed or refractory FLT3-mutated AML. *N Engl J Med*. 2019;381(18):1728-1740.
463. Food and Drug Administration. *Enasidenib Label*; 2017. https://wwwaccessdatafdagov/drugsatfda_docs/label/2020/209606s004lblpdf
464. Stein EM, DiNardo CD, Pollyea DA, et al. Enasidenib in mutant IDH2 relapsed or refractory acute myeloid leukemia. *Blood*. 2017;130(6):722-731.

465. Food and Drug Administration. *Ivosidenib Label*; 2018. Accessed December 20, 2022. https://www.accessdata.fda.gov/drugsatfda_docs/label/2022/211192s009lbl.pdf
466. DiNardo CD, Stein EM, de Botton S, et al. Durable remissions with ivosidenib in IDH1-mutated relapsed or refractory AML. *N Engl J Med*. 2018;378(25):2386-2398.
467. Roboz GJ, DiNardo CD, Stein EM, et al. Ivosidenib induces deep durable remissions in patients with newly diagnosed IDH1-mutant acute myeloid leukemia. *Blood*. 2020;135(7):463-471.
468. Norsworthy KJ, Mulkey F, Scott EC, et al. Differentiation syndrome with ivosidenib and enasidenib treatment in patients with relapsed or refractory IDH-mutated AML: a U.S. Food and drug administration systematic analysis. *Clin Cancer Res*. 2020;26(16):4280-4288.
469. Fathi AT, DiNardo CD, Kline I, et al. Differentiation syndrome associated with enasidenib, a selective inhibitor of mutant isocitrate dehydrogenase 2: analysis of a phase 1/2 study. *JAMA Oncol*. 2018;4(8):1106-1110.
470. Food and Drug Administration. *Glasdegib Label*; 2018. Accessed December 20, 2022. https://www.accessdata.fda.gov/drugsatfda_docs/label/2020/210656s002s004lbl.pdf
471. Cortes JE, Heidel FH, Fiedler W, et al. Survival outcomes and clinical benefit in patients with acute myeloid leukemia treated with glasdegib and low-dose cytarabine according to response to therapy. *J Hematol Oncol*. 2020;13(1):92.
472. Caron PC, Jurcic JG, Scott AM, et al. A phase 1B trial of humanized monoclonal antibody M195 (anti-CD33) in myeloid leukemia: specific targeting without immunogenicity. *Blood*. 1994;83(7):1760-1768.
473. Scheinberg DA, Lovett D, Divgi CR, et al. A phase I trial of monoclonal antibody M195 in acute myelogenous leukemia: specific bone marrow targeting and internalization of radionuclide. *J Clin Oncol*. 1991;9(3):478-490.
474. van Der Velden VH, te Marvelde JG, Hoogeveen PG, et al. Targeting of the CD33-calicheamicin immunoconjugate Mylotarg (CMA-676) in acute myeloid leukemia: in vivo and in vitro saturation and internalization by leukemic and normal myeloid cells. *Blood*. 2001;97(10):3197-3204.
475. Bross PF, Beitz J, Chen G, et al. Approval summary: gemtuzumab ozogamicin in relapsed acute myeloid leukemia. *Clin Cancer Res*. 2001;7(6):1490-1496.
476. Larson RA, Sievers EL, Stadtmauer EA, et al. Final report of the efficacy and safety of gemtuzumab ozogamicin (Mylotarg) in patients with CD33-positive acute myeloid leukemia in first recurrence. *Cancer*. 2005;104(7):1442-1452.
477. Amadori S, Suciu S, Stasi R, et al. Gemtuzumab ozogamicin (Mylotarg) as single-agent treatment for frail patients 61 years of age and older with acute myeloid leukemia: final results of AML-15B, a phase 2 study of the European Organisation for Research and Treatment of Cancer and Gruppo Italiano Malattie Ematologiche dell'Adulto Leukemia Groups. *Leukemia*. 2005;19(10):1768-1773.
478. Burnett AK, Hills RK, Milligan D, et al. Identification of patients with acute myeloblastic leukemia who benefit from the addition of gemtuzumab ozogamicin: results of the MRC AML15 trial. *J Clin Oncol*. 2011;29(4):369-377.
479. Food and Drug Administration. *Gemtuzumab Ozogamicin*; 2017. Accessed December 20, 2022. https://www.accessdata.fda.gov/drugsatfda_docs/label/2020/761060s004lbl.pdf
480. Lambert J, Pautas C, Terre C, et al. Gemtuzumab ozogamicin for de novo acute myeloid leukemia: final efficacy and safety updates from the open-label, phase III ALFA-0701 trial. *Haematologica*. 2019;104(1):113-119.
481. Hills RK, Castaigne S, Appelbaum FR, et al. Addition of gemtuzumab ozogamicin to induction chemotherapy in adult patients with acute myeloid leukaemia: a meta-analysis of individual patient data from randomised controlled trials. *Lancet Oncol*. 2014;15(9):986-996.
482. Brune M, Castaigne S, Catalano J, et al. Improved leukemia-free survival after postconsolidation immunotherapy with histamine dihydrochloride and interleukin-2 in acute myeloid leukemia: results of a randomized phase 3 trial. *Blood*. 2006;108(1):88-96.
483. Daver N, Alotaibi AS, Bucklein V, Subklewe M. T-cell-based immunotherapy of acute myeloid leukemia: current concepts and future developments. *Leukemia*. 2021;35(7):1843-1863.
484. Uy GL, Aldoss I, Foster MC, et al. Flotetuzumab as salvage immunotherapy for refractory acute myeloid leukemia. *Blood*. 2021;137(6):751-762.
485. Ravandi F, Cortes J, Faderl S, et al. Characteristics and outcome of patients with acute myeloid leukemia refractory to 1 cycle of high-dose cytarabine-based induction chemotherapy. *Blood*. 2010;116(26):5818-5823; quiz 6153.
486. Breems DA, Van Putten WLJ, Huijgens PC, et al. Prognostic index for adult patients with acute myeloid leukemia in first relapse. *J Clin Oncol*. 2005;23(9):1969-1978.
487. Herzig RH, Lazarus HM, Wolff SN, Phillips GL, Herzig GP. High-dose cytosine arabinoside therapy with and without anthracycline antibiotics for remission reinduction of acute nonlymphoblastic leukemia. *J Clin Oncol*. 1985;3(7):992-997.
488. Evans C, Winkelstein A, Rosenfeld CS, Zeigler ZR, Shadduck RK. High-dose cytosine arabinoside and L-asparaginase therapy for poor-risk adult acute nonlymphocytic leukemia. A retrospective study. *Cancer*. 1990;65(12):2624-2630.
489. Capizzi RL, Davis R, Powell B, et al. Synergy between high-dose cytarabine and asparaginase in the treatment of adults with refractory and relapsed acute myelogenous leukemia – a Cancer and Leukemia Group B Study. *J Clin Oncol*. 1988;6(3):499-508.
490. Carella AM, Cascavilla N, Greco MM, et al. Treatment of "poor risk" acute myeloid leukemia with fludarabine, cytarabine and G-CSF (flag regimen): a single center study. *Leuk Lymphoma*. 2001;40(3-4):295-303.
491. Tedeschi A, Montillo M, Strocchi E, et al. High-dose idarubicin in combination with Ara-C in patients with relapsed or refractory acute lymphoblastic leukemia: a pharmacokinetic and clinical study. *Cancer Chemother Pharmacol*. 2007;59(6):771-779.
492. Schimmer AD, Estey EH, Borthakur G, et al. Phase I/II trial of AEG35156 X-linked inhibitor of apoptosis protein antisense oligonucleotide combined with idarubicin and cytarabine in patients with relapsed or primary refractory acute myeloid leukemia. *J Clin Oncol*. 2009;27(28):4741-4746.
493. Stone RM, Moser B, Sanford B, et al. High dose cytarabine plus gemtuzumab ozogamicin for patients with relapsed or refractory acute myeloid leukemia: Cancer and Leukemia Group B study 19902. *Leuk Res*. 2011;35(3):329-333.
494. Prebet T, Etienne A, Devillier R, et al. Improved outcome of patients with low- and intermediate-risk cytogenetics acute myeloid leukemia (AML) in first relapse with gemtuzumab and cytarabine versus cytarabine: results of a retrospective comparative study. *Cancer*. 2011;117(5):974-981.
495. Tse E, Leung AYH, Sim J, et al. Clofarabine and high-dose cytosine arabinoside in the treatment of refractory or relapsed acute myeloid leukaemia. *Ann Hematol*. 2011;90(11):1277-1281.
496. Larson SM, Campbell NP, Huo D, et al. High dose cytarabine and mitoxantrone: an effective induction regimen for high-risk acute myeloid leukemia (AML). *Leuk Lymphoma*. 2012;53(3):445-450.
497. Becker PS, Kantarjian HM, Appelbaum FR, et al. Retrospective comparison of clofarabine versus fludarabine in combination with high dose cytarabine with or without granulocyte colony-stimulating factor as salvage therapies for acute myeloid leukemia. *Haematologica*. 2013;98(1):114-118.
498. Patzke CL, Duffy AP, Duong VH, et al. Comparison of high-dose cytarabine, mitoxantrone, and pegaspargase (HAM-pegA) to high-dose cytarabine, mitoxantrone, cladribine, and filgrastim (CLAG-M) as first-line salvage cytotoxic chemotherapy for relapsed/refractory acute myeloid leukemia. *J Clin Med*. 2020;9(2):E536.
499. Kantarjian H, Gandhi V, Cortes J, et al. Phase 2 clinical and pharmacologic study of clofarabine in patients with refractory or relapsed acute leukemia. *Blood*. 2003;102(7):2379-2386.
500. Faderl S, Wetzler M, Rizzieri D, et al. Clofarabine plus cytarabine compared with cytarabine alone in older patients with relapsed or refractory acute myelogenous leukemia: results from the CLASSIC I Trial. *J Clin Oncol*. 2012;30(20):2492-2499.
501. Motabi IH, Ghobadi A, Liu J, et al. Chemotherapy versus hypomethylating agents for the treatment of relapsed acute myeloid leukemia and myelodysplastic syndrome after allogeneic stem cell transplant. *Biol Blood Marrow Transplant*. 2016;22(7):1324-1329.
502. Bose P, Vachhani P, Cortes JE. Treatment of relapsed/refractory acute myeloid leukemia. *Curr Treat Options Oncol*. 2017;18(3):17.
503. Weltermann A, Fonatsch C, Haas OA, et al. Impact of cytogenetics on the prognosis of adults with de novo AML in first relapse. *Leukemia*. 2004;18(2):293-302.
504. Thalhammer F, Geissler K, Jager U, et al. Duration of second complete remission in patients with acute myeloid leukemia treated with chemotherapy: a retrospective single-center study. *Ann Hematol*. 1996;72(4):216-222.
505. Kern W, Haferlach T, Schnittger S, Ludwig WD, Hiddemann W, Schoch C. Karyotype instability between diagnosis and relapse in 117 patients with acute myeloid leukemia: implications for resistance against therapy. *Leukemia*. 2002;16(10):2084-2091.
506. Hiddemann W, Schleyer E, Uhrmeister C, et al. High-dose versus intermediate-dose cytosine arabinoside in combination with mitoxantrone for the treatment of relapsed and refractory acute myeloid leukemia—preliminary clinical and pharmacological data of a randomized comparison. *Cancer Treat Rev*. 1990;17(2-3):279-285.
507. Kern W, Haferlach T, Schoch C, et al. Early blast clearance by remission induction therapy is a major independent prognostic factor for both achievement of complete remission and long-term outcome in acute myeloid leukemia: data from the German AML Cooperative Group (AMLCG) 1992 Trial. *Blood*. 2003;101(1):64-70.
508. Horowitz MM, Gale RP, Sondel PM, et al. Graft-versus-leukemia reactions after bone marrow transplantation. *Blood*. 1990;75(3):555-562.
509. Dholaria B, Savani BN, Hamilton BK, et al. Hematopoietic cell transplantation in the treatment of newly diagnosed adult acute myeloid leukemia: an evidence-based review from the American society of transplantation and cellular therapy. *Transplant Cell Ther*. 2021;27(1):6-20.
510. Ciurea SO, Zhang MJ, Bacigalupo AA, et al. Haploidentical transplant with post-transplant cyclophosphamide vs matched unrelated donor transplant for acute myeloid leukemia. *Blood*. 2015;126(8):1033-1040.
511. Kassim AA, Chinratanalab W, Ferrara JLM, Mineishi S. Reduced-intensity allogeneic hematopoietic stem cell transplantation for acute leukemias: 'what is the best recipe?'. *Bone Marrow Transplant*. 2005;36(7):565-574.
512. Cornelissen JJ, Lowenberg B. Role of allogeneic stem cell transplantation in current treatment of acute myeloid leukemia. *Hematology Am Soc Hematol Educ Program*. 2005;2005:151-155.
513. Devine SM, Owzar K, Blum W, et al. Phase II study of allogeneic transplantation for older patients with acute myeloid leukemia in first complete remission using a reduced-intensity conditioning regimen: results from cancer and leukemia group B 100103 (alliance for clinical trials in oncology)/blood and marrow transplant clinical trial network 0502. *J Clin Oncol*. 2015;33(35):4167-4175.
514. Pusic I, Choi J, Fiala MA, et al. Maintenance therapy with decitabine after allogeneic stem cell transplantation for acute myelogenous leukemia and myelodysplastic syndrome. *Biol Blood Marrow Transplant*. 2015;21(10):1761-1769.
515. Craddock C, Jilani N, Siddique S, et al. Tolerability and clinical activity of post-transplantation azacitidine in patients allografted for acute myeloid leukemia treated on the RICAZA trial. *Biol Blood Marrow Transplant*. 2016;22(2):385-390.
516. McGlave PB, Haake RJ, Bostrom BC, et al. Allogeneic bone marrow transplantation for acute nonlymphocytic leukemia in first remission. *Blood*. 1988;72(5):1512-1517.
517. Blume KG, Forman SJ, O'Donnell MR, et al. Total body irradiation and high-dose etoposide: a new preparatory regimen for bone marrow transplantation in patients with advanced hematologic malignancies. *Blood*. 1987;69(4):1015-1020.

518. Bacigalupo A, Sormani MP, Lamparelli T, et al. Reducing transplant-related mortality after allogeneic hematopoietic stem cell transplantation. *Haematologica.* 2004;89(10):1238-1247.
519. Zittoun RA, Mandelli F, Willemze R, et al. Autologous or allogeneic bone marrow transplantation compared with intensive chemotherapy in acute myelogenous leukemia. European Organization for Research and Treatment of Cancer (EORTC) and the gruppo italiano malattie ematologiche maligne dell'Adulto (GIMEMA) leukemia cooperative groups. *N Engl J Med.* 1995;332(4):217-223.
520. Burnett AK, Wheatley K, Goldstone AH, et al. The value of allogeneic bone marrow transplant in patients with acute myeloid leukaemia at differing risk of relapse: results of the UK MRC AML 10 trial. *Br J Haematol.* 2002;118(2):385-400.
521. Harousseau JL, Cahn JY, Pignon B, et al. Comparison of autologous bone marrow transplantation and intensive chemotherapy as postremission therapy in adult acute myeloid leukemia. The Groupe Ouest Est Leucemies Aigues Myeloblastiques (GOELAM). *Blood.* 1997;90(8):2978-2986.
522. Cornelissen JJ, van Putten WLJ, Verdonck LF, et al. Results of a HOVON/SAKK donor versus no-donor analysis of myeloablative HLA-identical sibling stem cell transplantation in first remission acute myeloid leukemia in young and middle-aged adults: benefits for whom? *Blood.* 2007;109(9):3658-3666.
523. Suciu S, Mandelli F, de Witte T, et al. Allogeneic compared with autologous stem cell transplantation in the treatment of patients younger than 46 years with acute myeloid leukemia (AML) in first complete remission (CR1): an intention-to-treat analysis of the EORTC/GIMEMAAML-10 trial. *Blood.* 2003;102(4):1232-1240.
524. Cassileth PA, Harrington DP, Appelbaum FR, et al. Chemotherapy compared with autologous or allogeneic bone marrow transplantation in the management of acute myeloid leukemia in first remission. *N Engl J Med.* 1998;339(23):1649-1656.
525. Koreth J, Schlenk R, Kopecky KJ, et al. Allogeneic stem cell transplantation for acute myeloid leukemia in first complete remission: systematic review and meta-analysis of prospective clinical trials. *J Am Med Assoc.* 2009;301(22):2349-2361.
526. Cairoli R, Beghini A, Grillo G, et al. Prognostic impact of c-KIT mutations in core binding factor leukemias: an Italian retrospective study. *Blood.* 2006;107(9):3463-3468.
527. Rollig C, Bornhauser M, Kramer M, et al. Allogeneic stem-cell transplantation in patients with NPM1-mutated acute myeloid leukemia: results from a prospective donor versus no-donor analysis of patients after upfront HLA typing within the SAL-AML 2003 trial. *J Clin Oncol.* 2015;33(5):403-410.
528. Bazarbachi A, Labopin M, Kharfan-Dabaja MA, et al. Allogeneic hematopoietic cell transplantation in acute myeloid leukemia with normal karyotype and isolated Nucleophosmin-1 (NPM1) mutation: outcome strongly correlates with disease status. *Haematologica.* 2016;101(1):e34-e37.
529. Balsat M, Renneville A, Thomas X, et al. Postinduction minimal residual disease predicts outcome and benefit from allogeneic stem cell transplantation in acute myeloid leukemia with NPM1 mutation: a study by the acute leukemia French association group. *J Clin Oncol.* 2017;35(2):185-193.
530. DeZern AE, Sung A, Kim S, et al. Role of allogeneic transplantation for FLT3/ITD acute myeloid leukemia: outcomes from 133 consecutive newly diagnosed patients from a single institution. *Biol Blood Marrow Transplant.* 2011;17(9):1404-1409.
531. Brunner AM, Li S, Fathi AT, et al. Haematopoietic cell transplantation with and without sorafenib maintenance for patients with FLT3-ITD acute myeloid leukaemia in first complete remission. *Br J Haematol.* 2016;175(3):496-504.
532. Schmid C, Labopin M, Socie G, et al. Outcome of patients with distinct molecular genotypes and cytogenetically normal AML after allogeneic transplantation. *Blood.* 2015;126(17):2062-2069.
533. Pigneux A, Labopin M, Maertens J, et al. Outcome of allogeneic hematopoietic stem-cell transplantation for adult patients with AML and 11q23/MLL rearrangement (MLL-r AML). *Leukemia.* 2015;29(12):2375-2381.
534. Pasquini MC, Zhang MJ, Medeiros BC, et al. Hematopoietic cell transplantation outcomes in monosomal karyotype myeloid malignancies. *Biol Blood Marrow Transplant.* 2016;22(2):248-257.
535. Middeke JM, Herold S, Rucker-Braun E, et al. TP53 mutation in patients with high-risk acute myeloid leukemia treated with allogeneic haematopoietic stem cell transplantation. *Br J Haematol.* 2016;172(6):914-922.
536. Sierra J, Storer B, Hansen JA, et al. Unrelated donor marrow transplantation for acute myeloid leukemia: an update of the Seattle experience. *Bone Marrow Transplant.* 2000;26(4):397-404.
537. Cook G, Clark RE, Crawley C, et al. The outcome of sibling and unrelated donor allogeneic stem cell transplantation in adult patients with acute myeloid leukemia in first remission who were initially refractory to first induction chemotherapy. *Biol Blood Marrow Transplant.* 2006;12(3):293-300.
538. Araki D, Wood BL, Othus M, et al. Allogeneic hematopoietic cell transplantation for acute myeloid leukemia: time to move toward a minimal residual disease-based definition of complete remission? *J Clin Oncol.* 2016;34(4):329-336.
539. Zhou Y, Othus M, Araki D, et al. Pre- and post-transplant quantification of measurable ('minimal') residual disease via multiparameter flow cytometry in adult acute myeloid leukemia. *Leukemia.* 2016;30(7):1456-1464.
540. Christopher MJ, Petti AA, Rettig MP, et al. Immune escape of relapsed AML cells after allogeneic transplantation. *N Engl J Med.* 2018;379(24):2330-2341.

Chapter 77 ■ Acute Lymphoblastic Leukemia in Children

MAUREEN M. O'BRIEN • ALIX E. SEIF • STEPHEN P. HUNGER

INTRODUCTION

Acute lymphoblastic leukemia (ALL) is the most common childhood cancer, comprising approximately 20% of all malignancies and the majority of pediatric leukemias (77% for children under 15 years).[1] Approximately 32 children per 1,000,000 are newly diagnosed with ALL each year in the United States. The incidence of childhood ALL has increased by approximately 1% per year for reasons that are poorly understood.[1,2] Survival rates have improved dramatically, from less than 10% in the 1960s to 67% following the discovery of the need to treat presymptomatic central nervous system (CNS) disease in the early 1970s to over 90% for children diagnosed in the United States between 2006 and 2009 (Figure 77.1).[3,4] These improvements are the direct result of decades of study of children enrolled on cooperative group clinical trials, such as those run by the Children's Oncology Group (COG) in North America and the Berlin-Frankfurt-Münster (BFM) group in Western Europe. These studies have led to an increased understanding of how disease presentation, biology, and response to therapy may be used to tailor treatment to risk of relapse and have established standardized treatment regimens, thus allowing children diagnosed anywhere in the developed world to receive very similar and highly effective therapy. However, because ALL is the most common childhood cancer, the incidence of relapsed ALL is nearly as high as newly diagnosed acute myeloid leukemia (AML) and higher than most childhood non-CNS solid tumors. Although tremendous successes have been achieved in treating childhood ALL, relapsed ALL remains a significant challenge with a high fatality rate despite intensive therapy.[5]

RISK FACTORS FOR DEVELOPMENT OF CHILDHOOD ACUTE LYMPHOBLASTIC LEUKEMIA

ALL is more common in boys and in children of Hispanic ethnicity or White race compared to Black or Asian children (Figure 77.2). A pronounced peak in incidence occurs between ages 1 and 5 years. Children with certain genetic syndromes have an increased risk of developing childhood ALL. Down syndrome (DS) is the most common chromosomal anomaly and carries an increased risk of ALL (see Children with Down Syndrome and Acute Lymphoblastic Leukemia section). Genetic syndromes with defects in DNA repair also confer an increased risk of developing ALL (Table 77.1).[6] Germline alterations in B-cell development genes that are commonly somatically mutated in ALL have been identified in individual patients via genome-wide association studies (GWASs) as well as in several rare kindreds with familial ALL.[7-9] Mutations in a number of other genes and intragenic regions modestly increase the risk of developing ALL.[10] Similarly, children bearing a rare Robertsonian translocation of chromosomes 15 and 21 have a dramatically increased risk of developing ALL with intrachromosomal amplification of chromosome 21 (iAMP21).[11] However, in one study of over 1100 patients with a variety of childhood cancers, children with leukemia were least likely to have a germline mutation identified, with a prevalence of only 4.4%.[8]

There are few environmental risk factors with strong associations with the development of ALL. Prenatal exposure to ionizing radiation is associated with an increased risk of ALL development[12,13]; however, outside of isolated environmental disasters and with the introduction

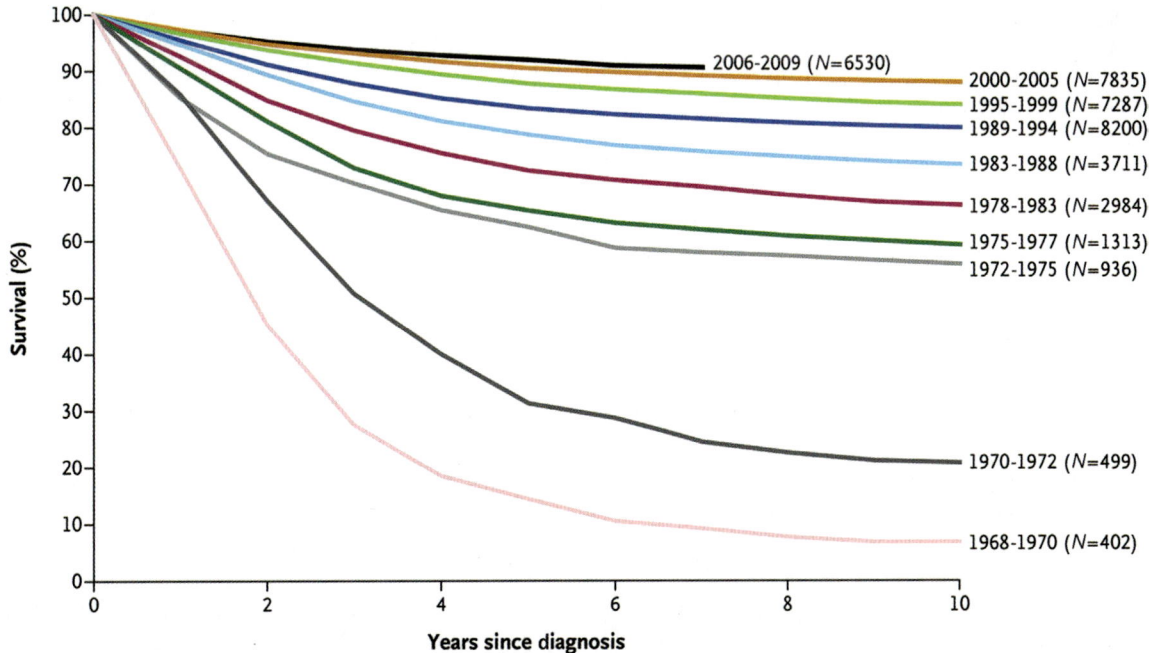

FIGURE 77.1 Improvements in acute lymphoblastic leukemia (ALL) survival over time. Overall survival rates have improved dramatically as a result of breakthroughs in therapy following cooperative group trials. Survival was less than 10% in the 1960s and rose to 67% following the discovery of the need to treat presymptomatic central nervous system disease in the early 1970s. Children diagnosed in the United States between 2000 and 2005 experienced overall survival of 90.4%. (From Hunger SP, Mullighan CG. Acute lymphoblastic leukemia in children. N Engl J Med. 2015;373(16):1541-1552. Copyright © 2015 Massachusetts Medical Society. Reprinted with permission from Massachusetts Medical Society.)

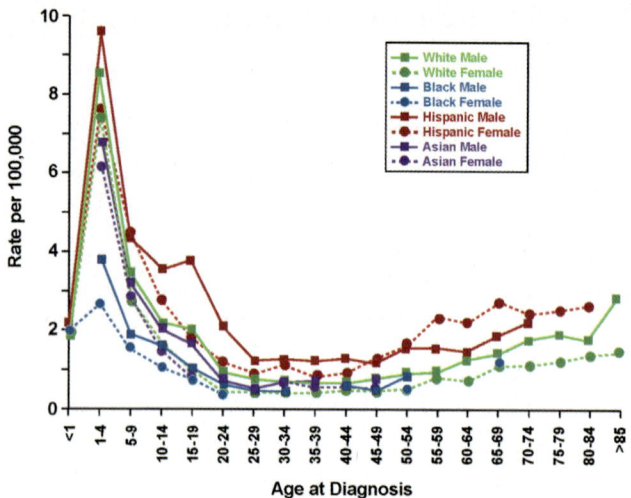

FIGURE 77.2 Acute lymphoblastic leukemia (ALL) incidence by age, sex, and race/ethnicity (SEER Cancer Statistics, 2000-2009). ALL is more common in boys than girls. Ethnicity and race also predict ALL risk, with Hispanic children having the highest incidence rates, followed by White and Asian children. Black children have a comparatively decreased risk of developing ALL. A pronounced peak in incidence occurs between ages 1 and 5 years that may reflect evolution of prenatal preleukemic clones into ALL, at least among children with the most common "first hit" genetic mutations. Absent lines are because of insufficient data.

Table 77.1. Germline Risk Factors for Development of ALL

ALL-Predisposition Syndromes		
Affected Gene	Associated Syndrome	Physical Signs
TP53	Li-Fraumeni syndrome	• None
ATM	Ataxia-telangiectasia	• Progressive ataxia • Oculocutaneous telangiectasias • Failure to thrive • Mask-like facies • Recurrent infections • Developmental delay
NBN	Nijmegen breakage syndrome	• Microcephaly • Prominent midface • Receding mandible • Café au lait spots • Recurrent infections • Marrow failure
BLM	Bloom syndrome	• Short stature • Immunodeficiency • Malar rash • Microcephaly • High-pitched voice • Hypogonadism
PAX5	Familial ALL syndrome	• None
ETV6	Familial ALL syndrome	• Thrombocytopenia
IKZF1	Early-onset immunodeficiency	• Abnormalities in multiple hematopoietic lineages, including T, B, myeloid, and dendritic cells
Germline single-nucleotide variants increasing ALL risk		
ARID5B	N/A	N/A
BAK1	N/A	N/A
CDKN2A	N/A	N/A
CEBPE	N/A	N/A
ELK3	N/A	N/A
ERG	N/A	N/A
GATA3	N/A	N/A
IGF2BP1	N/A	N/A
IKZF3	N/A	N/A
LHPP	N/A	N/A
PIP4K2A	N/A	N/A
RUNX1	N/A	N/A

Abbreviations: ALL, acute lymphoblastic leukemia; N/A, none.

of current practices requiring screening for pregnancy prior to radiography, these exposures do not account for the increasing incidence of pediatric ALL.[3] The observation that children with ALL have cells with ALL-associated mutations identifiable in samples obtained at birth many years before developing ALL speaks to the prenatal origin of many cases of ALL.[14-16] Furthermore, in a sample of healthy children, these mutated cells are detected at a prevalence several orders of magnitude higher than pediatric ALL incidence rates, demonstrating that only a small subset of children with ALL-associated mutations detectable at birth go on to develop ALL.[17] Immune activation in early life can lead to the depletion of preleukemic cells experimentally,[18] and delayed infections can lead to increased penetrance of fulminant leukemia in ALL-predisposition models.[19] Children with ALL were nearly four times as likely as healthy controls to have evidence of in utero cytomegalovirus (CMV) exposure, and congenital CMV polymerase chain reaction positivity was especially prevalent in Hispanic children.[20] These findings lend support to the hypothesis that delayed exposure to strong immune stimuli, exposure to immunosuppressive infections, or an abnormal immune response to infections among children in developed countries may play a role in the increasing incidence of ALL.[21]

PRESENTING CLINICAL FEATURES

The presenting signs and symptoms of ALL are related to marrow or extramedullary infiltration by leukemia cells. Some children may develop a slow, subacute process over weeks or months, whereas others experience rapid clinical changes. Symptoms as a result of cytopenias, such as pallor, lethargy, malaise, fevers, and recurrent infections, as well as petechiae, purpura, and spontaneous bruising or bleeding, are common.[22] Lymphoblast proliferation may also cause diffuse or localized lymphadenopathy and hepatosplenomegaly. Fevers often occur because of inflammation caused by the leukemic blasts and resolve shortly after initiation of chemotherapy, but fever in a child with newly diagnosed or suspected leukemia may also be a sign of a serious infection.[22] Abdominal symptoms, such as anorexia/weight loss, abdominal pain, and distension, are present in up to 30% of children at initial presentation.[22] Bone or joint pain is reported by 11% to 59% of children at diagnosis.[22,23] Musculoskeletal pain may be caused by marrow expansion, lytic lesions, compression fractures, or arthritis.[24]

Rarely, children are diagnosed with ALL incidentally, with 6% presenting with no clinical signs or symptoms.[22] Because ALL has significant clinical overlap with other syndromes, such as juvenile idiopathic arthritis (JIA), ALL may be difficult to distinguish from JIA in a child presenting with joint or back pain, limp, fevers, elevated inflammatory markers, and subtle cytopenias without circulating blasts.[23] Leukopenia, low-normal platelet count, and nighttime pain are relatively sensitive and specific for ALL, particularly when all are present.[23] Because empiric steroid treatment for JIA may partially treat or mask ALL, a bone marrow (BM) evaluation may be required prior to initiating JIA therapy that includes corticosteroids.

Children with T-cell ALL (T-ALL) are predisposed to bulky adenopathy, with one-third presenting with mediastinal thymic masses.[25] Less than 5% of children have CNS involvement at diagnosis, and only a small minority are symptomatic.[26] T-ALL is more likely than

B-cell ALL (B-ALL) to have CNS involvement and to present with neurologic deficits, such as signs of increased intracranial pressure or cranial nerve palsies.[26] Overt testicular involvement presents as painless, hard, nodular testicular enlargement in 1% to 2% of boys at diagnosis.[27] Leukemia cutis is present in 1.8% of pediatric patients with newly diagnosed ALL and is more common in B-ALL or ALL arising in infants.[28] Rarely, involvement of other extramedullary organs may cause clinical complications leading to an ALL diagnosis, such as pancreatitis, pericardial effusion, or epiglottitis.

PRESENTING LABORATORY AND RADIOGRAPHIC FEATURES

Laboratory evaluation for suspected ALL begins with a complete blood count. White blood cell (WBC) counts are elevated in 58% of patients at diagnosis, low in 27%, and within the normal range in 15%.[29] In most patients, blasts are apparent on the peripheral blood smear, but some present with cytopenias without circulating blasts. Approximately 13% of patients with ALL present with hyperleukocytosis (WBC count $\geq 100 \times 10^9$/L).[30] Children with T-ALL are more likely to present with elevated WBC counts: 59% have WBC $\geq 50 \times 10^9$/L and 46% with $\geq 100 \times 10^9$/L.[25] In contrast to children with AML, most children with markedly elevated lymphoblast counts do not experience side effects of leukostasis, such as respiratory compromise or spontaneous CNS hemorrhages, although they are at risk for metabolic derangements because of tumor lysis syndrome (TLS).[30] Most patients will present with a reticulocytopenic anemia (mean hematocrit 23%) and thrombocytopenia, with 59% presenting with platelet counts $<50 \times 10^9$/L; however, cytopenias may be mild.[29]

Careful attention to metabolic derangements at presentation and with treatment initiation is crucial because of the risk of development of TLS. Rapid cell turnover leads to the release of cytoplasmic contents, thus producing hyperuricemia, hyperkalemia, hyperphosphatemia, and secondary hypocalcemia.[31] These can cause acute renal failure from formation of urate or calcite crystals in the renal tubules and may be exacerbated by leukemic kidney involvement or ureteral compression by lymph nodes. Uncontrolled electrolyte abnormalities can lead to arrhythmias, seizures, and sudden death. Laboratory-defined TLS occurs in approximately 21% of patients presenting with ALL, and clinical TLS (TLS with evidence of renal injury, arrhythmia, or other clinical signs) occurs in 5%. A proposed risk classification system defines high-risk features as presenting WBC count $\geq 100 \times 10^9$/L, lactate dehydrogenase over twice the upper limit of normal, evidence of renal dysfunction at presentation, or elevated uric acid, phosphorus, or potassium.[31] All other patients with ALL are considered at intermediate risk (IR) of TLS, with an expected incidence of 1% to 5%. All patients with ALL should be started on preventive hydration without alkalinization, receive allopurinol, and have frequent laboratory monitoring. Some patients may require hyperhydration (2-3 L/m²/d) with diuretics to prevent fluid overload and to help with potassium excretion. Treatment with recombinant urate oxidase (rasburicase) may be indicated in children at high risk for TLS or with hyperuricemia.[31,32]

Although many children have circulating blasts that enable phenotypic diagnosis of leukemia, a BM aspiration and/or biopsy should be performed if medically safe. In ALL, the marrow is typically hypercellular with effacement of normal hematopoietic precursors and fat deposits by a homogeneous population of lymphoid blasts. These cells are then evaluated for morphology, immunophenotype by flow cytometry, and cytogenetic and molecular features. Initial staging for ALL requires sampling of the cerebrospinal fluid (CSF). Diagnostic evaluation includes a cell count and cytocentrifugation of a controlled CSF volume to enable more sensitive detection of leukemic blasts in the CSF. The degree of CNS involvement is defined as CNS1: WBC < 5/μL and no blasts on cytocentrifugation; CNS2: WBC < 5/μL with blasts present on cytocentrifugation; and CNS3: WBC ≥ 5/μL and blasts on morphology or cytocentrifugation, or clinical or radiographic signs of neurologic involvement. CSF flow cytometry is under investigation to improve detection of occult CNS involvement and risk stratification.[33] Owing to risks of CNS hemorrhage and introducing peripheral blasts into a chemotherapy sanctuary site, transfusions to achieve platelet counts ≥50 to 100×10^9/L and to correct coagulopathies, and performance of the lumbar puncture by an experienced provider are advised.

Some ALL patients present with anterior mediastinal adenopathy, which can cause cough, dyspnea (particularly when supine), or signs of superior vena cava syndrome. A chest radiograph should be performed in all children with newly diagnosed or suspected ALL, especially before administering sedation for diagnostic procedures. Additional radiographic findings are predominantly orthopedic, occurring in 40% to 75%.[24] Lytic lesions are most common (13.5%), followed by radiolucent metaphyseal bands, or "leukemic lines," in 9.8%. Diffuse osteopenia, periosteal reactions, and pathologic fractures also occur at presentation.

RISK FACTORS AND RISK STRATIFICATION FOR TREATMENT ALLOCATION

The goal of contemporary ALL risk stratification is to maximize the chance for cure while minimizing acute and long-term toxicity related to treatment. Identification of specific risk factors that predict outcome is critical to the allocation of patients to treatment regimens of appropriate intensity. For some patients, minimization of therapy may be possible, whereas for others, cure requires intensive treatments that may include hematopoietic stem cell transplantation (HCT) in first complete remission (CR1). Over decades, various prognostic factors have been identified including clinical characteristics, laboratory values, genomic alterations in leukemic blasts, and early response to treatment. Because therapy is the most important factor that influences outcome, the relative prognostic significance of different characteristics varies based on treatment strategy. Prognostic features must be rigorously evaluated in prospective clinical trials before they are adopted for formal risk stratification and treatment assignment and then reevaluated in the context of new therapies. Although this strategy has been extremely successful in pediatric ALL, relapses continue to occur in patients who are classified as low risk by current algorithms, demonstrating that further improvements are needed in risk stratification and therapy.

Clinical Features and Immunophenotype

Several clinical features are associated with the risk of relapse, most prominently older age and higher WBC count at the time of initial diagnosis. Consensus conferences held in 1985 and 1993 developed the National Cancer Institute (NCI) criteria that categorized most children with B-ALL into a standard risk (NCI-SR; ages 1-9 years with WBC count $< 50 \times 10^9$/L) subgroup with expected event-free survival (EFS) at that time of about 80% and a high-risk (NCI-HR; ≥10 years and/or with WBC count $\geq 50 \times 10^9$/L) subgroup with expected EFS about 65%.[34,35] Even with the addition of other prognostic features and improvements in outcome over subsequent decades, these clinical features remain prognostic in B-ALL today. Infants less than 1 year have poor outcomes driven by the high incidence of translocations involving the 11q23 mixed lineage leukemia (*MLL* or *KMT2A*) gene,[36,37] whereas older infants who lack *KMT2A* rearrangement have outcomes similar to children with HR B-ALL.[38] Among NCI-HR patients, older age is associated with inferior outcomes, with older adolescents and young adults with B-ALL having an inferior outcome to children and teenagers younger than 13 to 16 years.[39]

About 85% of childhood ALL cases are B-ALL that express surface markers of precursor B cells (CD19, CD22, CD79a, and others) without expression of surface immunoglobulin (IG), whereas about 15% of cases are T-ALL defined by cytoplasmic expression of CD3. As noted earlier, the clinical features of T-ALL differ from those of B-ALL. Historically, T-ALL immunophenotype was associated with a significantly inferior treatment outcome to B-ALL, but in recent eras, survival is similar for T-ALL and high-risk B-ALL.[4,40] Unlike B-ALL, NCI risk does not reliably predict outcome for patients with T-ALL.[41]

Regarding extramedullary disease, the 3% to 5% of patients with overt CNS leukemia (CNS3) are considered high risk, requiring intensification of CNS-directed therapy. Traumatic lumbar punctures (red blood cells > 10×10^9/L) with blasts as well as CNS2 status have been associated with inferior outcomes in some studies; as a result, some cooperative groups intensify intrathecal (IT) chemotherapy for these patients.[42,43] Overt testicular leukemia was an adverse prognostic factor in older trials, but is not with more effective contemporary therapy that enables most patients to be treated successfully with intensified systemic chemotherapy without testicular irradiation.[27,44]

Sentinel Cytogenetic and Molecular Genetic Alterations

Several leukemia-specific genetic alterations are associated with outcome in B-ALL and are frequently integrated into risk stratification algorithms.[45] Two common alterations are strong predictors of favorable outcomes: *ETV6-RUNX1* fusion produced by a cryptic t(12;21)(p13;q22) and high hyperdiploidy (>50-53 chromosomes), particularly when trisomies of chromosomes 4 and 10 are present (Table 77.2).[46-48] Other alterations are associated with poor outcome in B-ALL, and some trials allocate patients with these lesions to treatment with intensified cytotoxic chemotherapy, novel agents, or allogeneic HCT. The rare t(17;19) (q22;p13)/*TCF3-HLF* fusion and extreme hypodiploidy, defined as less than 44 chromosomes, have dismal outcomes and are often considered indications for allogeneic HCT in CR1.[49,50] Molecular profiling of hypodiploid ALL identified two subgroups: near-haploid ALL (24-31 chromosomes) harboring alterations targeting receptor tyrosine kinase and Ras pathway signaling, whereas 90% of low-hypodiploid ALL (32-39 chromosomes) had *TP53* mutations with half of these present in the germline, suggesting children with this rare ALL subtype should be evaluated for Li-Fraumeni syndrome.[51]

iAMP21 is a complex structural alteration of one copy of chromosome 21 comprising multiple regions of gain, amplification, inversion, and deletion with a common region of highest level amplification spanning 5.1 Mb that includes the *RUNX1* locus.[52] iAMP21 is identified by fluorescence in situ hybridization demonstrating ≥5 *RUNX1* signals (four or more on a derivative chromosome). Patients with iAMP21 have an inferior outcome when treated less intensively,[53,54] but when treated more intensively have outcomes similar to other HR B-ALL patients.[52,55] Thus, NCI-SR B-ALL patients with iAMP21 are often assigned to high-risk treatment protocols.

KMT2A rearrangements (*KMT2A*-R) occur in most infants with ALL (see Infants with Acute Lymphoblastic Leukemia section) and about 3% of older children. Most noninfant patients with *KMT2A*-R have NCI-HR features, and multiple fusion partners are reported, including the t(4;11) in about half of cases. In the past, *KMT2A*-R was associated with a poor outcome, and noninfants with *KMT2A*-R or the t(4;11) were often assigned to high-risk therapies, sometimes including HCT in CR1. With contemporary treatment protocols, the independent prognostic import of *KMT2A*-R is less clear, and treatment intensity in this subset is based on early treatment response.[45]

One of the most well-established very high-risk features is the presence of the t(9;22) (q34;q11) translocation, resulting in *BCR-ABL1* fusion, or "Philadelphia chromosome" (Ph+ ALL; 3% of B-ALL).[56] Outcomes for Ph+ ALL patients have dramatically improved with the addition of tyrosine kinase inhibitors (TKIs) targeting ABL1 to intensive chemotherapy backbones (discussed in detail in the subsequent

Table 77.2. Recurrent Sentinel Genetic Lesions in B-ALL

Genetic Alteration	Incidence in B-ALL	Prognostic Implication	Treatment
t(12;21) (p13;q22), *ETV6-RUNX1*	20%-25%	Favorable	NCI-risk group/response-based chemotherapy
High hyperdiploidy (>50-53 chromosomes) and/or trisomy of chromosomes 4 and 10	20%-25%	Favorable	NCI-risk group/response-based chemotherapy
t(1;19) (q23;p13), *TCF3-PBX1*	6%	Neutral	NCI-risk group/response-based chemotherapy
Hypodiploidy (<44 chromosomes)	1%-2%	Unfavorable	Consider allogeneic HCT in CR1
t(9;22) (q34;q11), *BCR-ABL1*	3%-5%	Unfavorable	Chemotherapy + ABL TKI; HCT in CR1 for poor responders
Ph-like ALL with fusions involving ABL class (*ABL1*, *ABL2*, *CSF1R*, *PDGFRB*) genes	<5%	Unfavorable	Consider clinical trial with chemotherapy + ABL TKI
Ph-like ALL with *JAK2* fusions	~1%	Unfavorable	Consider clinical trial with chemotherapy + JAK2 TKI
Ph-like ALL with *IGH-CRLF2* or *P2RY8-CRLF2*	2%-5%	Unfavorable in HR ALL	Consider clinical trial with chemotherapy + JAK2 TKI
t(17;19) (q22;p13), *TCF3-HLF*	<1%	Unfavorable	Consider allogeneic HCT in CR1
iAMP21	2%	Unfavorable	NCI-HR chemotherapy
KMT2A rearrangement	Varies by age	Unfavorable	NCI-HR chemotherapy
DUX4 rearranged	3%-4%	Favorable	NCI-risk group/response-based chemotherapy
ZNF384 rearranged	1%-2%	Intermediate	NCI-risk group/response-based chemotherapy
MEF2D rearranged	<3%	Intermediate	NCI-risk group/response-based chemotherapy
PAX5alt	5%	Intermediate	NCI-risk group/response-based chemotherapy
PAX5-P80 R	1%-2%	Intermediate	NCI-risk group/response-based chemotherapy
ETV6-RUNX1 like	1%-2%	Unfavorable	NCI-risk group/response-based chemotherapy
NUTM1 rearranged	<1%	Unknown	NCI-risk group/response-based chemotherapy
IKZF1 N159Y	<1%	Unknown	NCI-risk group/response-based chemotherapy
BCL2-, *MYC*-, or *BCL6*-rearranged	<1%	Unknown	NCI-risk group/response-based chemotherapy

Abbreviations: B-ALL, B-cell acute lymphoblastic leukemia; CR1, first complete remission; HCT, hematopoietic stem cell transplantation; HR, high risk; NCI, National Cancer Institute; TKI, tyrosine kinase inhibitor.

section).[57] More recently, a subgroup of patients with leukemic blast gene expression signature similar to Ph+ ALL but without BCR-ABL1 fusion has been defined.[58,59] This Philadelphia chromosome–like (Ph-like) subset accounts for 15% of NCI-HR B-ALL patients and is independently associated with poor outcome.[58,60] Deletions and sequence mutations in IKZF1 are associated with Ph-like ALL and with inferior outcomes in numerous retrospective studies; however, most groups do not currently use IKZF1 alterations for risk stratification and treatment allocation.[58,60,61] A significant percentage of patients with Ph-like ALL and/or IKZF1 alterations have genomic rearrangements that cause overexpression of the CRLF2 gene (CRLF2-R) that encodes a cytokine receptor.[62] The prognostic import of CRLF2-R or CRLF2 protein overexpression is controversial and likely context dependent and has not been incorporated into risk stratification algorithms at this time.[63,64] In recent years, many new genetic subtypes of B-ALL have been defined by next-generation sequencing studies, with the prognostic significant of most not known currently.[65]

Early Treatment Response

Clinical trials performed in the 1980s identified peripheral blood blast clearance following a 7-day prophase of prednisone (PRED) and a single dose of IT methotrexate (MTX) and the percentage of blasts remaining in the BM after 7 to 14 days of multiagent chemotherapy to be highly predictive of EFS and overall survival (OS).[66,67]

Numerous studies have demonstrated that detection of minimal residual disease (MRD), by either multiparametric flow cytometric (MFC) analysis of leukemia-associated antigens or polymerase chain reaction detection of leukemia-specific IG and T-cell receptor (TCR) rearrangements, is highly prognostic.[68,69] MRD detection early in the treatment of ALL is highly prognostic of outcome and currently is a key variable to determine the intensity of postinduction therapy for most cooperative groups. In the COG P9900 series of clinical trials, end-of-induction (EOI) BM MRD (*Figure 77.3A*) and day 8 peripheral blood MRD were the most powerful predictors of outcome in a multivariable analysis.[70] However, MRD is not the sole predictor of outcome in this model; NCI-risk group and genetic factors also remain prognostic, justifying a risk stratification approach that integrates clinical and genetic features with early MRD response. Other major cooperative groups have also adopted response-based treatment algorithms using MRD measurements at early specific time points with EOI MRD ≥ 0.01% associated with inferior outcomes.[71,72] Earlier MRD assessments can also be highly prognostic. The Associazione Italiana Ematologica Oncologia Pediatrica (AIEOP)-BFM 2000 trial showed that detection of ≥1 blast/μL in peripheral blood at day 8 predicted a cumulative incidence of relapse (CIR) of 12% compared to 2% in children who had <1 blast/μL.[73]

Importantly, use of MRD to allocate patients to intensified postinduction therapy can improve outcomes. The COG AALL0331 SR B-ALL trial allocated children with EOI MRD ≥0.1% to HR therapy with the augmented BFM regimen and these patients had a 6-year continuous complete remission rate of 86%.[74] Similarly, early MRD negativity can identify very low-risk patients, who can receive deintensified therapy without a loss of efficacy.[75] High-throughput sequencing (HTS) of IG/TCR rearrangements is roughly a log more sensitive than MFC MRD. Patients with negative MFC MRD but positive HTS MRD at EOI had worse EFS than those with negative MRD by both methods.[76] Recent studies have also shown the importance of MRD evaluation at time points beyond induction. In the AIEOP-BFM 2000 trial, patients with B-ALL and EOI MRD ≥0.1% (time point 1 [TP1]) were deemed MRD-HR if they remained MRD positive at day 84 (TP2) and MRD-IR if they became MRD negative at TP2. The MRD-HR patients had a two-fold higher CIR compared with MRD-IR patients (42.4% vs 23%, $P < .001$) at 7 years.[71] In the COG AALL0232 HR B-ALL trial, patients with positive EOI MRD who became MRD negative (<0.01%) by the end-of-consolidation (EOC) phase about 3 months postdiagnosis had 5-year disease-free survival (DFS) rate of 79% compared to 39% for those with persistent EOC MRD ≥0.01% ($P < .0001$; *Figure 77.3B*).[72] Thus, negative EOI MRD is prognostic for favorable outcomes, whereas the presence of detectable MRD at EOC is highly prognostic for poor outcomes, although late MRD-positivity may not portend as poor an outcome for SR B-ALL as it does for HR B-ALL.[77] Early MRD response is also the most important prognostic factor in T-ALL because clinical features (other than overt CNS leukemia) and cytogenetics have limited value in risk stratification. For T-ALL patients, MRD at about 3 months postdiagnosis (TP2) appears most prognostic.[78]

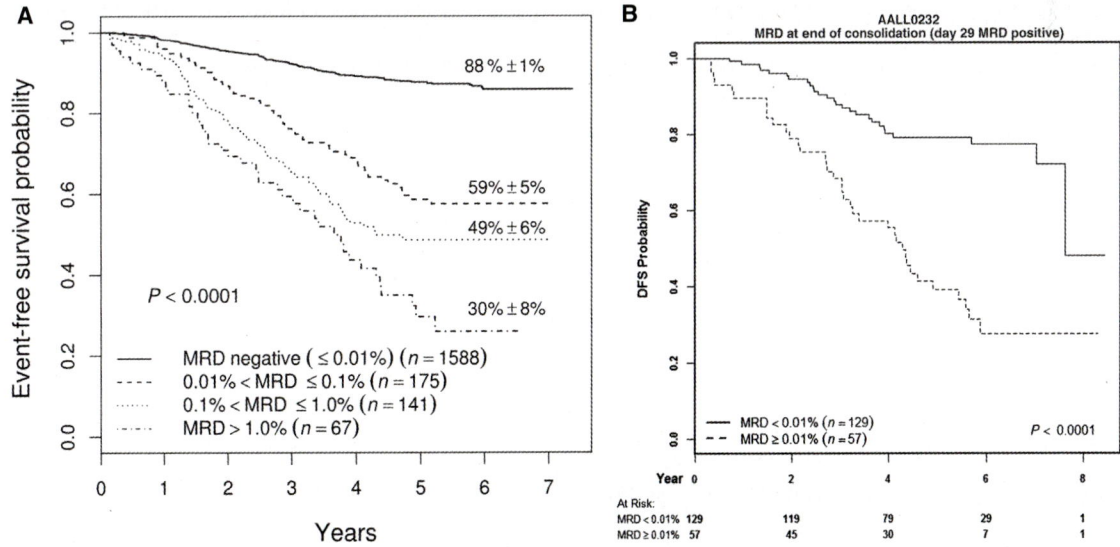

FIGURE 77.3 Event-free survival (EFS) by end-of-induction (EOI) and end-of-consolidation minimal residual disease (MRD). A, EOI MRD shows a strong dose effect in predicting long-term EFS when treatment is not modified based on MRD. In the Children's Oncology Group (COG) P9900 series studies, high-level MRD (>1%) was associated with only 30% 5-year EFS and even low-positive MRD (0.01% < MRD ≤ 0.1%) predicted a significant decrement in EFS down to 59% from 88% in MRD-negative patients. B, In the COG high-risk ALL study AALL0232, patients whose EOI MRD was ≥0.1% but had negative (<0.01%) MRD at the end of consolidation had very good 5-year disease-free survival (DFS) of 79%, whereas those who remained positive fared much worse with DFS 39%. (A, Reprinted from Borowitz MJ, Devidas M, Hunger SP, et al. Clinical significance of minimal residual disease in childhood acute lymphoblastic leukemia and its relationship to other prognostic factors: a Children's Oncology Group study. *Blood*. 2008;111(12):5477-5485. Copyright © 2008 American Society of Hematology. With permission. B, Reprinted from Borowitz MJ, Wood BL, Devidas M, et al. Prognostic significance of minimal residual disease in high risk B-ALL: a report from Children's Oncology Group study AALL0232. *Blood*. 2015;126(8):964-971. Copyright © 2015 American Society of Hematology. With permission.)

Induction failure has traditionally been defined by the persistence of leukemic blasts in blood, BM (5% or more marrow blasts), or any extramedullary site after 4 to 6 weeks of remission induction therapy and is observed in 2.4% of patients. Outcomes for this group of patients are historically poor with 10-year EFS 32%, and their therapy is often intensified with allogeneic HCT in CR1, which is particularly beneficial for patients with T-ALL.[79,80] In the era of MRD, the definitions of induction failure are also evolving. On the United Kingdom Acute Lymphoblastic Leukemia (UKALL) 2003 study, 1.9% of patients had induction failure by morphology, with a 5-year EFS of 50.7%.[81] An additional 2.3% of patients with morphologic remissions had EOI MRD ≥5%, and these patients had comparable EFS to the morphologic induction failure group at 47%. Conversely, a small group of patients had M2 marrows by morphology with negative MRD and had EFS 100%. A similar finding using COG data showed a significant EFS reduction among B-ALL patients with morphologic remission and MRD ≥ 5% but no significant difference for patients with T-ALL.[82] These and other findings have prompted new proposed definitions of remission and relapse.[83]

TREATMENT

Improved survival for ALL has resulted from a combination of refinement in CNS-directed therapy, optimization of intensity of standard chemotherapy agents, improved risk allocation with the incorporation of MRD testing, introduction of targeted therapies such as TKIs for the treatment of Ph+ ALL, and better supportive care. Ongoing studies seek to further refine elements of ALL therapy including MRD detection, optimal duration of maintenance therapy, further reductions in the use of cranial irradiation, and incorporation of highly active immunotherapies and other targeted therapies into frontline treatment regimens. Challenges still remain for certain high-risk ALL subgroups, including infants with KMT2A-R, adolescent and young adults (AYAs), and children with unfavorable blast cytogenetics, induction failure or persistence of MRD, DS, T-ALL, and relapsed ALL.

Primary Treatment

The mainstay of ALL treatment is 2 to 3 years of multiagent chemotherapy generally divided into induction, consolidation/intensification, and maintenance/continuation phases of treatment (*Figure 77.4*). Postinduction treatment intensity is risk stratified based on clinical features, genetic lesions, and response to induction therapy, including MRD. Following the achievement of remission, consolidation therapy blocks are administered to provide presymptomatic CNS treatment and improve the depth of remission. Additional postinduction intensification blocks are administered to eradicate residual leukemic clones. The goal of maintenance therapy is the preservation of remission by administration of lower intensity continuous therapy over a prolonged time frame.

Remission Induction

Current induction therapy includes 3 to 5 systemic agents over 4 to 6 weeks. Although most children will achieve remission with vincristine and a corticosteroid alone, the addition of an asparaginase product with or without an anthracycline raises the remission induction rate to 98% to 99%.[84] The COG treats children with NCI-SR B-ALL with a three-drug (vincristine, dexamethasone [DEX], and pegaspargase) induction regimen over 4 weeks and reserves the addition of an anthracycline for patients with NCI-HR B-ALL and all T-ALL; however, other groups use four- to five-drug induction regimens for all patients.[4,85-87] A three-drug induction for NCI-SR B-ALL has proven very effective provided children receive later intensification of therapy.[88] With contemporary supportive care measures, induction death rates are typically 1% to 2%.

Corticosteroids are the cornerstone of induction therapy.[89] Advantages of DEX compared to PRED include better CNS penetration and greater in vitro activity, and multiple trials in NCI-SR patients suggest an advantage for DEX in both improving EFS and decreasing risk of CNS relapse.[90,91] Studies using DEX to PRED ratio of 1:5 to 1:7 have shown a benefit for DEX, whereas those with DEX to PRED ratio exceeding 1:7 have shown similar outcomes.[89,92,93] In NCI-HR B-ALL, the COG AALL0232 trial compared four-drug induction with PRED 60 mg/m²/d on days 1 to 28 vs DEX 10 mg/m²/d on days 1 to 14. For patients younger than 10 years, DEX during induction had superior EFS when combined with high-dose MTX (HD-MTX) during interim maintenance (IM).[94] No benefit of DEX was observed for patients aged 10 years and older, and DEX was associated with a much higher risk of osteonecrosis (ON) in the older age group. Based on these results, within the COG, DEX is used as the induction steroid for children with NCI-HR B-ALL and age less than 10 years, whereas PRED is used for those 10 years and older within the context of a four-drug induction.

Following a PRED prophase, the AIEOP-BFM 2000 trial randomized patients to either DEX (10 mg/m²/d) or PRED (60 mg/m²/d) for 3 weeks plus tapering in induction.[95] DEX decreased 5-year CIR, particularly extramedullary, but the benefit was partially counterbalanced by a higher induction-related death rate, resulting in a significant benefit in 5-year EFS (83.9% for DEX and 80.8% for PRED) but

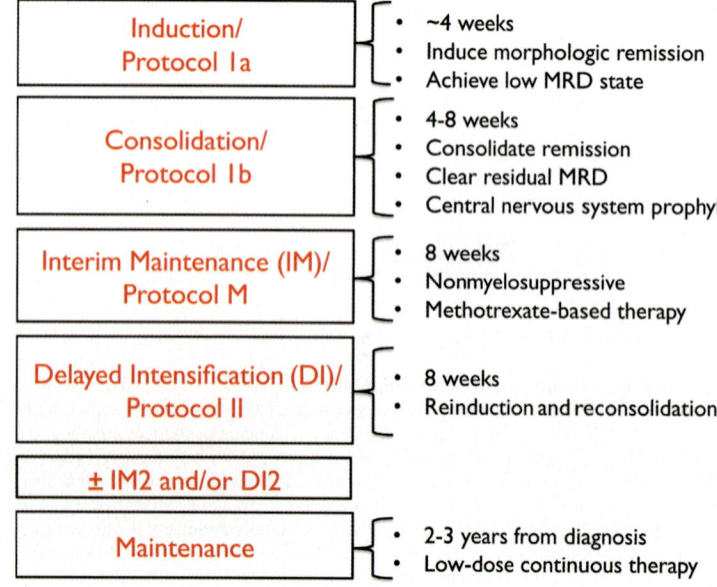

FIGURE 77.4 Phases of BFM- and COG-based pediatric ALL chemotherapy. Although individual blocks of chemotherapy vary across cooperative groups, the standard phases of therapy include an induction of remission, a consolidation block intended to treat presymptomatic central nervous system leukemia and "deepen" remission, postconsolidation blocks to eliminate residual leukemic clones, and prolonged, lower intensity maintenance blocks to preserve remission. ALL, acute lymphoblastic leukemia; BFM, Berlin-Frankfurt-Münster; COG, Children's Oncology Group; MRD, minimal residual disease.

no difference in 5-year OS (90.3% with DEX and 90.5% with PRED) in the total cohort.[95] However, a significant OS benefit of DEX was observed for patients with T-ALL. Despite concerns about increased toxicity with DEX including ON and higher induction death rates when combined with an anthracycline, DEX 6 mg/m^2/d × 28 days was well tolerated in the UKALL 2003 study within the context of a four-drug induction.[96]

Asparaginase has been a critical element of most induction regimens for ALL since the 1970s. Asparaginase deaminates asparagine to form aspartate, resulting in asparagine depletion with preferential toxicity for lymphoblasts, which are dependent on exogenous asparagine in vivo.[97] Three different formulations of asparaginase have mainly been used to date: native *Escherichia coli* L-asparaginase, polyethylene glycol conjugated *E. coli* L-asparaginase (pegaspargase), and *Erwinia chrysanthemi* L-asparaginase.[98] Pegaspargase is now used almost universally in children with ALL in North America and Europe; advantages of this formulation include its long half-life, which allows less frequent dosing, reduced immunogenicity, and more rapid blast clearance.[99] Asparaginase appears to be a critical component of therapy for T-ALL because studies suggest additional asparaginase may improve outcomes, including UKALL 2003, Dana Farber Cancer Institute (DFCI) consortium trials, and St. Jude Children's Research Hospital (SJCRH) Total Therapy XV.[87,96,100]

Presymptomatic Central Nervous System Therapy

Presymptomatic treatment of the CNS is an essential component of effective ALL therapy. In the 1960s, most children with ALL could attain remission with chemotherapy, but almost all relapsed within 6 to 12 months with about half of these relapses isolated to the CNS. The groundbreaking series of early Total Therapy trials at SJCRH demonstrated that administration of 24 Gy craniospinal and then 24 Gy cranial radiation therapy (CRT) with IT MTX resulted in 50% of patients achieving long-term DFS.[101,102] As concerns about the long-term sequelae from CRT have increased, there has been a growing trend to reduce both the CRT dose and the number of children who receive this treatment modality.[103,104] In a meta-analysis of patients treated on 47 trials, effective systemic therapy, including intravenous (IV) MTX and protracted IT chemotherapy, had comparable outcomes to CRT.[105] Analysis of 16,623 patients aged 1 to 18 years with newly diagnosed ALL treated between 1996 and 2007 by 10 cooperative groups demonstrated that CRT was associated with a reduced risk of relapse only in the small subgroup of CNS3 patients.[106] Some groups have eliminated CRT for all children with ALL without decline in outcomes using regimens with triple IT chemotherapy, DEX, and intermediate- or HD-MTX,[107,108] while most other groups deliver CRT to the subset of patients with CNS3 disease. In T-ALL, due to the higher incidence of CNS relapse, prophylactic CRT has continued to be given to significant proportion of patients in some cooperative groups. Recently, the incorporation of nelarabine was associated with a marked reduction in CNS relapse suggesting that this agent may allow omission of prophylactic CRT in more patients.[109]

Postinduction Intensification

Postinduction intensification is essential for all patients with ALL; however, there is not a consensus on an optimal regimen or duration of therapy.[84] Most contemporary ALL protocols include a delayed intensification (DI) phase. In 1970, investigators from the BFM group introduced a 3-month intensive induction/early intensification phase called Protocol I, in which four-drug induction was followed with a treatment block, including cyclophosphamide, cytarabine, and 6-mercaptopurine (6-MP).[110] In 1976, a second intensification phase with reinduction and reconsolidation (Protocol II) was added. Outcomes improved compared to historical controls, including significant benefit for higher risk patients. EFS rates were similar whether Protocol II followed immediately after Protocol I or after 2 months' delay, but morbidity was decreased when Protocol II was delayed.[111] In North America, Protocol II was termed "delayed intensification" (DI), and a series of studies established the benefit of DI therapy for both NCI-SR and NCI-HR patients.[88]

The CCG "augmented BFM" regimen used stronger and more prolonged postinduction intensification that included two DI phases and added three 2-week courses of nonmyelosuppressive vincristine and L-asparaginase during the periods of myelosuppression that invariably follow the cyclophosphamide, cytarabine, and thiopurine pulses in consolidation (Protocol Ib) and reconsolidation (Protocol IIb). Two courses of five Capizzi I pulses with vincristine, IV MTX, and L-asparaginase replaced the two IM courses of oral 6-MP and MTX between consolidation and DI #1 and between DI #1 and DI #2.[112] High-risk patients treated on the CCG 1882 trial with >25% marrow blasts on day 7 had a 5-year DFS rate 75% for the augmented regimen compared to 55% for standard BFM therapy ($P < .001$).[67]

Subsequently, the CCG-1961 trial demonstrated for NCI-HR patients with rapid initial responses to induction therapy (<25% blasts on day 7), the stronger intensification components of the augmented BFM regimen significantly improved 5-year EFS (81% vs 72%) and OS (89% vs 83%).[113] However, longer intensification with two IM and DI phases added no benefit. A second DI phase also provided no benefit to NCI-SR B-ALL patients who were rapid responders on the CCG-1991 trial.[114] The impact of intensified consolidation for NCI-SR B-ALL patients was evaluated in the COG AALL0331 trial that demonstrated no benefit for augmented BFM-based consolidation compared to standard consolidation with oral 6-MP and IT MTX for SR-average patients.[74] Based on these trials, current standard COG therapy backbones include a single DI phase for all patients and augmented consolidation for high-risk B-ALL and all T-ALL patients.

The optimal dose, route of administration, and schedule of MTX as a critical component of postinduction intensification have been studied by several groups. For NCI-SR B-ALL patients, the CCG-1991 trial showed a benefit for escalating IV MTX without leucovorin rescue compared to oral MTX during IM.[114] For NCI-HR B-ALL patients, the COG AALL0232 trial demonstrated the benefit of 24-hour HD-MTX infusions followed by leucovorin rescue (5-year EFS rate 79.6%) compared to escalating IV MTX and pegaspargase without leucovorin rescue (C-MTX; 5-year EFS rate 75.2%, $P = .008$).[94] HD-MTX decreased both marrow and CNS relapses. In contrast, C-MTX was superior to HD-MTX for patients with T-ALL treated on COG AALL0434, with estimated 5-year DFS 91.5% for C-MTX and 85.3% for HD-MTX ($P = .005$).[40]

Asparaginase is an essential element of most ALL intensification regimens. A series of DFCI ALL consortium trials demonstrated superior outcomes for patients receiving at least 26 weeks of continuous weekly asparaginase therapy postinduction and similar efficacy and toxicity for IV pegaspargase every 2 weeks compared to weekly intramuscular native *E. coli* L-asparaginase for 30 weeks.[115,116] Management of asparaginase-related complications is critical because patients who do not receive the full planned doses have inferior outcomes.[117,118] Clinical hypersensitivity occurs in 20% to 30% of patients receiving native *E. coli* L-asparaginase and is less common with pegaspargase.[97] Clinical hypersensitivity is associated with the formation of neutralizing antiasparaginase antibodies that reduce drug activity, although neutralizing antibodies may also develop in the absence of a clinically evident allergic reaction (silent inactivation). Some patients with clinical hypersensitivity may be successfully managed with desensitization including premedication and very slow ramp up of infusion concentration and rate[119]; however, for those patients with neutralizing antibodies, continued asparaginase therapy with the same formulation is ineffective.[120] Serum asparaginase activity (SAA) level is a surrogate for asparagine depletion and allows the identification of patients with neutralizing antibodies. Although the optimal SAA to define activity remains under investigation, currently, a trough level ≥0.1 IU/mL is considered adequate for sufficient asparagine depletion.[120] For patients with hypersensitivity to pegaspargase, *E. chrysanthemi* asparaginase is recommended as an alternative because it is antigenically distinct from *E. coli*–derived formulations, although its half-life is much shorter than that of pegaspargase (0.65 vs 5.73 days) requiring more frequent administration.[97,121] Administration of six doses of *E. chrysanthemi* asparaginase on a three times per week schedule (Mon-Wed-Fri) in place of one dose of pegaspargase achieves adequate nadir SAA.[122] Due to recurring drug shortages of *E. chrysanthemi* asparaginase, an alternate preparation, recombinant crisantaspase produced in *Pseudomonas fluorescens*, has been developed[123] and was recently approved by the US Food and Drug Administration (FDA).

Therapeutic drug monitoring of asparaginase is useful in the management of clinical allergy with published guidelines based on SAA as specific time points as well as prospectively for identification of silent inactivation.[120] In the DFCI 00-01 trial, patients who received individualized asparaginase dosing (ID) adjusted every 3 weeks based on nadir SAA had superior 5-year EFS (90% vs 82%; $P = .04$) compared with patients who received standard fixed dosing (FD) with similar frequency of asparaginase-related toxicity.[118] This improvement is attributed to the prospective identification of patients with silent inactivation on the ID arm who then switched asparaginase preparations, whereas on the FD arm, the asparaginase preparation was changed only for clinical allergy.

Maintenance Therapy

Early trials in ALL demonstrated that the chance of long-term remission was increased with administration of prolonged maintenance therapy with daily 6-MP and weekly MTX.[124] In modern ALL therapy, maintenance generally consists of daily oral 6-MP and weekly oral or parenteral MTX, with or without intermittent pulses of 5 to 7 days of a corticosteroid and 1 to 2 doses of vincristine, and with or without extended periodic IT therapy. Most regimens continue maintenance therapy for a minimum of 2 years from the time remission is achieved although optimal duration remains uncertain.[125] Some patient subgroups may be effectively treated with even shorter durations of maintenance therapy. The Tokyo L92-13 trial used intensified early treatment followed by 6 months of maintenance therapy with all treatment stopped 1 year after diagnosis; some patient subsets (*ETV6-RUNX1+* and *TCF3-PBX1+*) fared extremely well with this strategy, whereas others (high hyperdiploidy) did not.[126] Thus, the optimal duration of maintenance therapy may differ for different patient subgroups, or based on the composition of premaintenance chemotherapy. Most cooperative groups no longer use sex-specific duration of therapy.[125]

Both 6-MP and MTX have significant interindividual variation in bioavailability and cellular pharmacokinetics, so body surface area–derived doses are poorly related to drug exposure and not predictive of relapse.[127] WBC and/or ANC during maintenance therapy are used to guide dosing, as myelosuppression is associated with reduced relapse rate.[128,129] Accumulation of the 6-MP metabolite thioguanine nucleotides (TGN) in erythrocytes can be used a marker of nonadherence but is not superior to degree of myelosuppression for dose titration during maintenance.[128] In contrast, higher levels of TGN incorporated into DNA (DNA-TG) in circulating normal leukocytes have been associated with reduced relapse rate.[130] Attempts to increase TGN exposure by increasing 6-MP dosing, using parenteral administration, or substituting 6 thioguanine (6-TG) did not demonstrate clinical advantage, and prolonged administration of 6-TG during maintenance was associated with significant hepatic toxicity.[90,131,132] One strategy under investigation to increase DNA-TG is the addition of low-dose 6-TG to 6-MP/MTX maintenance therapy.[133] 6-MP–related toxicities in maintenance include hypoglycemia in young children, hepatic toxicity, nausea, and pancreatitis, all of which have been linked to skewed 6-MP metabolism with overproduction of the hepatotoxic metabolite 6-methyl mercaptopurine.[134-136] Coadministration of allopurinol has been demonstrated to be effective in mitigating these side effects, with the caveat that marked dose reduction of 6-MP is necessary to avoid severe myelosuppression.[137]

Thiopurine methyltransferase (*TPMT*) genotype influences 6-MP and 6-TG metabolism. Reduction in thiopurine dose is required for the rare patients (~1/300) with homozygous *TPMT* deficiency because of the risk of life-threatening myelosuppression with standard doses.[138] Patients with heterozygous *TPMT* deficiency (~10% of Caucasians) are at higher risk of myelosuppression with standard thiopurine doses but can also often tolerate full-dose 6-MP or 6-TG. A germline coding variant in *NUDT15* is highly associated with intolerance of 6-MP; the variant is most common in East Asians and Hispanics. Of children homozygous for either *TPMT* or *NUDT15* variants or heterozygous for both, 100% required ≥50% 6-MP dose reduction.[139] Additional *NUDT15* variants have subsequently been identified and may be incorporated in future trials similarly to *TPMT* genotyping.[140]

Until recently, 6-MP and MTX have generally been administered in the evening, based on early reports that the risk of relapse was several-fold higher for patients who reported taking 6-MP and MTX in the morning compared with patients on evening schedule.[141] In addition, most groups recommended that both 6-MP and MTX be taken on an empty stomach because of reduced bioavailability when administered with food, in particular milk because of xanthine oxidase content.[142] However, recent studies did not find any impact on relapse rate of administering 6-MP/MTX with food or on a morning vs evening schedule, suggesting that dose titration based on myelosuppression eliminates the impact of these factors.[143,144] As a result, some groups now advocate administration of 6-MP at the same time each day, with or without food.

Complex administration rules designed to improve drug exposure, such as fasting, may paradoxically lead to poor outcomes by contributing to nonadherence. Patients with 6-MP nonadherence (mean adherence rate < 95%) were at a 2.7-fold increased risk of relapse compared with patients with a mean adherence rate of 95% or greater.[145] Among adherers, high intraindividual variability in Ery-6-TGN levels contributed to increased relapse risk (hazard ratio, 4.4). Furthermore, adherers with varying Ery-6-TGN levels had varying 6-MP dose intensity and more 6-MP drug interruptions. Thus, while adherence to prescribed 6-MP during maintenance is critical, adherent patients who had frequent prescribed dose interruptions or adjustments also had inferior outcomes, suggesting that overly aggressive dose escalation attempts resulting in neutropenia with drug interruption may be detrimental. Adherence intervention studies are underway; a randomized trial comparing a multicomponent intervention to education alone did not improve the proportion of patients with >95% 6-MP adherence, but did identify adolescents with low baseline adherence as the target group for future studies.[146]

The benefit of vincristine and corticosteroid pulses during maintenance is controversial within the context of contemporary intensive therapy. Furthermore, there has been growing concern about the potential toxicities of pulse therapy, including ON, mood disturbances, obesity, and peripheral neuropathy. Although studies from earlier treatment eras showed a benefit for vincristine/corticosteroid pulses in maintenance, a review involving more than 5000 children with ALL has called the benefit of pulse therapy into question with current regimens where early therapy has been intensified.[147,148] In a multicenter randomized trial in children treated with a BFM-based regimen for IR ALL, no benefit for the addition of six pulses of vincristine and DEX during maintenance therapy was observed.[149] The COG AALL0932 trial demonstrated outstanding outcomes for children with NCI SR B-ALL who received pulses every 12 weeks rather than every 4 weeks during maintenance.[150] For younger children, when pulses are used in maintenance therapy, DEX is preferred because of the outcome benefits that have been reported, whereas PRED is used for older patients in some groups because of the concerns for a heightened risk of ON with DEX.[151]

UNIQUE PATIENT SUBGROUPS

Philadelphia Chromosome-Positive Acute Lymphoblastic Leukemia

The Philadelphia chromosome is present in 3% to 5% of pediatric ALL cases and about 25% of adult ALL. Unlike in chronic myeloid leukemia (CML), the breakpoint in Ph+ ALL usually occurs in intron 1, or minor breakpoint region of *BCR*, resulting in a 190-kDa protein (p190) in 90% of ALL cases, whereas a small subset of patients bear the CML-associated translocation involving the major breakpoint cluster region between exons 16 and 17 and generating a larger fusion protein (p210).[152] Prior to the development of targeted TKIs, outcomes for pediatric Ph+ ALL were very poor, with a 7-year EFS 32% and OS 44.9%, despite intensive chemotherapeutic regimens and a majority of children undergoing HCT in CR1.[56] The addition of imatinib (340 mg/m^2/d) to an intensive chemotherapy backbone on the COG trial AALL0031 resulted in markedly improved survival with 5-year EFS and OS approaching 70%, and a biologic assignment to HCT showed no benefit over imatinib plus chemotherapy.[57]

Postinduction imatinib on the high-risk BFM backbone had similar outcomes in a European intergroup study (EsPhALL).[153] The second-generation TKI dasatinib was studied on COG AALL0622 and demonstrated comparable outcomes to AALL0031 and the EsPhALL. The Chinese CCCG-ALL-2015 trial randomized children with Ph+ ALL to chemotherapy plus either imatinib (300 mg/m^2/d) or dasatinib (80 mg/m^2/d) and found significantly better EFS with dasatinib.[154] However, the outcome of the imatinib arm on this trial was poorer than expected and it is unclear whether dasatinib should replace imatinib in pediatric Ph+ ALL.[155]

Based on these and other trials, the outlook for Ph+ ALL is now much better than it was in the pre-TKI era; most patients will have a good response to intensive chemotherapy plus imatinib or dasatinib, defined as becoming MRD negative by 3 months postdiagnosis and can attain good outcomes without HCT in CR1.[155] The patients who remain MRD positive at 3 months have a significantly inferior outcome, and most groups consider them to be candidates for HCT in CR1.

Philadelphia Chromosome–Like Acute Lymphoblastic Leukemia

The leukemic blasts in Ph-like ALL have a gene expression signature that is highly similar to that of patients with Ph+ ALL, but lack the pathognomonic t(9;22) and *BCR-ABL1* fusion.[59,156] Similar to Ph+ ALL, these leukemic blasts commonly have deletions or point mutations in *IKZF1*, which encodes the critical lymphoid transcription factor IKAROS and is associated with poor outcomes.[59,157] A number of studies have shown that patients with Ph-like ALL have a significantly inferior outcome to other ALL patients.[58,60] The prevalence of Ph-like ALL increases with age, from 10% among children with NCI-SR B-ALL and 13% among those with NCI-HR B-ALL to 21% among adolescents and 27% among young adults. Outcomes are poor for all age groups and worsen with increasing age, with 5-year EFS rates of 58.2% for children with NCI-HR ALL, 41.0% for adolescents, and 24.1% for young adults.[58]

Detailed genomic studies of Ph-like ALL have shown that these leukemias have a variety of sentinel genomic alterations, almost all of which activate cytokine receptor and growth factor signaling.[58] Approximately half of the Ph-like patients had rearrangements involving the *CRLF2* gene at Xp22.3/Yp11.3. CRLF2 heterodimerizes with the interleukin-7 (IL7) receptor-α chain to form the receptor for thymic stromal lymphopoietin.[158] *CRLF2* is deregulated by rearrangement to the immunoglobulin heavy chain locus (*IGH-CRLF2*) or by a deletion of the PAR1 pseudoautosomal region upstream of the *CRLF2* locus that results in *P2RY8-CRLF2* fusion transcript that encodes full-length CRLF2.[62,159,160] CRLF2 overexpression is accompanied by activating *JAK1* or *JAK2* mutations in approximately 50% of cases, most commonly JAK2-R683G, resulting in constitutive activation of CRLF2/JAK-STAT signaling.[161,162] Activating JAK mutations are rarely seen in the absence of *CRLF2* abnormalities and appear to be a critical cooperating event in leukemogenesis.[163] In addition to JAK2 mutations, various other genomic alterations that activate JAK-STAT signaling have been described, including *JAK2* fusions with a variety of partner genes, truncating rearrangements of the erythropoietin receptor gene (*EPOR*) with genes including the *IGH* or *IGK* loci that result in overexpression and activation of receptor signaling, mutations that constitutively activate cytokine receptors including *IL7R*, *FLT3*, and *IL2RB* (encoding IL2 receptor subunit β), and mutations that impair function of negative regulators of JAK-STAT signaling (SH2B adaptor protein 3, *SH2B3* that encodes the JAK2-negative regulator LNK).[158,164-166] Preclinical data suggest that many Ph-like ALL cases containing genomic alterations involving *CRLF2*, *JAK1*, *JAK2*, *EPOR*, and *IL7R* are sensitive to JAK2 inhibitors, such as ruxolitinib.[167-169]

The other major classes of genomic alterations present in Ph-like ALL are translocations and interstitial deletions identified in approximately 15% of Ph-like ALL patients that create "ABL class" fusion genes involving *ABL1*, *ABL2*, *CSF1R*, or *PDGFRB*.[58,158] These rearrangements encode chimeric proteins that include the intact carboxy-terminal TK domain of the ABL class kinase joined in-frame to the amino terminus of the protein encoded by the fusion partner. These ABL class fusions phenocopy BCR-ABL1 in experimental models because their overexpression allows growth factor–dependent murine B-cell lines to survive and grow in the absence of exogenous growth factor, and cells containing these fusions die rapidly upon exposure to ABL class TKIs, such as imatinib and dasatinib.[58]

Clinically, the ABL class fusions are often associated with very poor early response, with *PDGFRB* fusions enriched in patients who fail to enter remission after induction chemotherapy.[58,170] There have been a number of case reports of patients with Ph-like ALL and ABL class fusions who had poor responses to chemotherapy but responded rapidly to addition of imatinib/dasatinib.[58,170-173] Taken together, these observations suggest that there are significant opportunities to develop clinical trials testing-targeted therapy in genetically defined subsets of Ph-like ALL, modeled after the successful combination of TKI plus chemotherapy for Ph+ ALL.[158] Several small studies have shown early evidence that adding imatinib or dasatinib to chemotherapy in patients with ABL-class fusions improves outcome.[174]

T-Lymphoblastic Leukemia/Lymphoma

T-ALL is immunophenotypically and genetically distinct from B-ALL, and often has a different clinical presentation and time to response to therapy. T-ALL is more prevalent in boys, Black children, and with increasing age,[4] and is more likely to present with a high WBC count and CNS or mediastinal involvement. Historically, T-ALL was observed to have a worse prognosis than B-ALL when treated with standard-risk approaches, but with therapeutic intensification, outcomes are similar to or better than those of children with high-risk B-ALL.[4,85,87] Unfortunately, outcomes for relapsed T-ALL are dismal, with less than 10% long-term survival,[5] and identification of high-risk patients and risk-adapted intensification to maximize cure rates for T-ALL with initial therapy is essential.

NCI risk is less prognostic in T-ALL than for B-ALL; however, there are some features at presentation that may be of prognostic value. Favorable features include CNS1 status, and the presence of *NOTCH1* or *FBXW7* mutations.[41] The presence of CNS2 or 3 status, testicular disease, or early T-cell precursor (ETP) phenotype confers IR status, while *RAS* or *PTEN* mutations, the lack of biallelic T-cell receptor gamma rearrangements, and potentially a very high WBC count (>200 × 10^3/μL) at diagnosis may all be unfavorable characteristics. However, the rarity of T-ALL compared to B-ALL leads to variable strengths of association across studies, resulting in conflicting findings.

Response to therapy is a robust prognostic indicator for T-ALL. While most B-ALL patients achieve an MRD-negative remission by EOI, a substantive proportion of patients with T-ALL have persistent disease at EOI but can still have favorable outcomes if they become MRD negative by EOC. In the ALL-AIEOP-BFM 2000 trial,[78] patients who were MRD negative (<0.01%) at both TP1 (day 33) and TP2 (day 78) were classified as standard risk; those who were positive at one or both time points but at a level <0.1% at TP2 were IR; and patients who had positive MRD ≥0.1% at TP2, were PRED poor responders, or had induction failure were assigned to high risk. With this stratification approach, IR T-ALL patients had a 7-year EFS of 80.6%, which was closer to the standard-risk EFS of 91.1% than to the high-risk EFS of 49.8%. Patients who remained MRD positive at TP2 had cumulative incidence of relapse ranging from 26% to 45% depending on level of detectable MRD, compared to <15% risk of relapse in patients who were MRD negative at TP2, irrespective of MRD at TP1. These data strongly suggest that the EOC is the most critical time point for identifying T-ALL patients at high risk of treatment failure. The excellent outcomes of patients who do achieve negative MRD by EOI were used to deintensify postinduction therapy on the UKALL2003 trial, with a resulting 5-year EFS of 93% (95% CI 87.2%-99%).[175] Other cooperative groups have confirmed the excellent prognosis of a good early response, with negative MRD at day 19 predicting favorable outcomes at SJCRH[68] and at day 29 in the COG phase 3 T-ALL trial AALL0434.[109]

ETP ALL was initially described in 2009 as a T-ALL subtype with immunophenotypic absence of CD1a and CD8 expression, with weak CD5 and at least one nonmyeloperoxidase myeloid lineage or stem cell marker.[176] Thirty ETP ALL patients had a dismal 10-year survival estimate of 19% and were observed to have delayed clearance of blasts compared to the non-ETP cohort, with high EOI MRD. More recent studies have demonstrated a more favorable outcome for this group of patients. On the UKALL 2003 study, children with ETP ALL had a statistically insignificant 10% lower survival than non-ETP patients but were noted to have EFS 76.7% and OS 82.4%, both far better than the survival rates observed in the initial St. Jude study.[177] Similarly, both the COG AALL0434 T-ALL trial and the AIEOP confirmed the slower initial response to therapy, but showed comparable survival outcomes among patients with ETP ALL and those with T-ALL receiving contemporary therapy.[109,178]

The use of DEX rather than PRED and intensification of asparaginase therapy are associated with improved outcomes in T-ALL. In the AIEOP-BFM 2000 trial, for patients with good initial PRED responses, DEX during induction was associated with three-fold reduction in the incidence of relapse compared to PRED and demonstrated an improvement in 5-year OS (91.4% vs 82.6%; $P = .036$).[95] Subsequently, the UKALL 2003 trial demonstrated a 5-year EFS 84.6% and OS 90.9% for newly diagnosed T-ALL patients.[96] This trial incorporated DEX 6 mg/m²/d for 28 days during induction and during the monthly maintenance steroid pulses for all patients, a risk-adapted intensification approach for consolidation, and Capizzi-style escalating MTX with pegaspargase during IM for high-risk patients, rather than oral MTX.[179]

The optimal dose and route of MTX in T-ALL remain under investigation. HD-MTX has been commonly used.[180] The COG AALL0434 trail used a four-drug PRED-based induction, with randomizations to Capizzi vs HD-MTX in IM. Overall outcomes were outstanding, and contrary to the findings in B-ALL, Capizzi MTX was superior to HD-MTX for patients with T-ALL.[40] The majority of patients in this trial received prophylactic CRT, so it remains to be determined whether HD-MTX is beneficial in T-ALL regimens that omit CRT.

Owing to the increased propensity for CNS involvement and relapse in T-ALL, reduction of the use of CRT in T-ALL has been more challenging than for B-ALL. Some cooperative groups have successfully replaced CRT in the majority of or all T-ALL patients with early aggressive IT chemotherapy and intensification of systemic agents that cross the blood-brain barrier, including DEX during induction, multiple courses of HD-MTX, and intensified asparaginase therapy.[107,108,181] Serial UKALL trials eliminated CRT in all T-ALL patients. In UKALL 2003, using DEX as the induction and maintenance steroid for all patients and extra doses of pegaspargase, but without HD-MTX, and with IT MTX rather than intrathecal triple chemotherapy, the incidences of isolated CNS and overall CNS relapse were 3% and 4%, respectively.[175] A recent single-arm meta-analysis of data from 10 cooperative groups did not find a benefit to CRT in T-ALL except for children with CNS3 status,[106] providing additional impetus to efforts to decrease or eliminate the use of CRT in children with T-ALL.

Given the very poor salvage rate of T-ALL following relapse, there is a great interest in testing whether new agents can improve cure rates for newly diagnosed T-ALL patients. Nelarabine, a prodrug of AraG, showed a very high response rate as a single agent in children with relapsed and refractory T-ALL but was associated with significant, often severe, and sometimes fatal CNS toxicity in this setting.[182] The COG added this agent cautiously to children with newly diagnosed T-ALL and showed in AALL0434 that it was safe to add nelarabine to augmented BFM therapy and improved EFS significantly with a major impact being reduction in CNS relapses.[109] The COG has recently completed AALL1231, which tested the proteasome inhibitor bortezomib in T-ALL patients, over 90% of whom did not receive CRT (NCT02112916).

Adolescents and Young Adults With Acute Lymphoblastic Leukemia

AYA patients (age 15 years and older) with ALL have inferior outcomes compared to younger children. In COG trials from 2000 to 2005, the 5-year OS rates were 74.5% for adolescents (15-19 years) and 91.7% for younger children.[4] In a review of outcomes for older adolescents (15-18 years) treated on four consecutive SJCRH trials studies), the AYA patients had significantly inferior EFS/OS on the first 3 trials but comparable outcomes to younger patients on the Total XV trial (5-year EFS 86.4% vs 87.4%).[183]

The etiology of the inferior outcomes for AYA patients with ALL is multifactorial, including lower incidence of favorable genetic abnormalities and higher incidence of unfavorable features, including T-cell immunophenotype, Ph+ ALL, and Ph-like ALL.[58,184] In parallel, AYA patients experience increased treatment-related toxicity compared to younger children, including ON, vincristine-induced neuropathy, and asparaginase-related toxicities, which may result in chemotherapy delays and dose reductions that impact outcome.[185] Finally, AYA patients have significant challenges with adherence to oral treatment regimens.[186]

AYA patients may be treated at pediatric or adult centers depending on local patterns of referral and hospital policies. Treatment strategies have historically differed significantly with adult centers typically using intensive myelosuppressive regimens with allogeneic HCT in first remission, whereas pediatric regimens are based on the BFM therapy backbone, including high cumulative doses of vincristine, corticosteroids, and asparaginase, and early CNS prophylaxis.[187] Retrospective studies have demonstrated superior outcomes for AYA patients treated with "pediatric-type" regimens with EFS rates approaching 70% compared to 30% to 45% for "adult-type" regimens.[39,188] Prospective studies from the United States and European cooperative groups as well as a large meta-analysis confirmed these results with EFS rates greater than 60% for AYAs treated with pediatric regimens.[189-191] The US Intergroup Study C10403 prospectively treated AYA patients younger than 40 years with the standard arm of COG AALL0232 with PRED induction and escalating IV MTX during IM and found manageable toxicities with 3-year EFS 59% and OS 73%.[192] Survival outcomes for patients receiving postremission chemotherapy on C10403 were superior compared to myeloablative HCT in CR1.[193] For AYA patients treated with pediatric regimens, the indications for allogeneic HCT in CR1 should be the same as those for younger children (see Hematopoietic Stem Cell Transplantation section).[187,194]

Infants With Acute Lymphoblastic Leukemia

ALL presenting in the first year of life is a rare but devastating diagnosis. In the United States, approximately 100 to 125 new cases of ALL are diagnosed in children <1 year annually, representing approximately 3% of all childhood ALL.[1] Infants are more likely than older children to present with adverse clinical features, including organomegaly, high WBC counts, and CNS disease.[195] A significant percentage of infant ALL is CD10 negative, which is indicative of leukemic transformation occurring in an immature lymphoid progenitor cell, and KMT2A-R are present in 70% to 75% of patients.[37,195-197] Outcomes for this group of patients are historically very poor, with the highest risk patients presenting at a young age (<6 months in Interfant and Japanese Infant Leukemia/Lymphoma Study Group [JILSG] studies and <3 months in COG trials), with a high WBC count (>300 × 10⁹/L per Interfant and >50 × 10⁹/L per COG), with CNS disease (JILSG), and with KMT2A-R (all groups).[37,195-198] Most infants are able to achieve CRs[196]; however, high relapse rates and treatment-related mortality (TRM) lead to poor survival. Multiple collaborative groups demonstrate EFS <50% for all KMT2A-R infants, with high-risk infants achieving only 15% to 20% EFS.[196,197,199,200] Infants with ALL are also at increased risk of infectious complications, because of, in part, prolonged, severe lymphopenia, and may require special monitoring for immune dysfunction and supportive care to prevent life-threatening infections.[201] *KMT2A*-R ALL cells nearly universally overexpress the FLT3 tyrosine kinase and demonstrate preclinical sensitivity to inhibition by lestaurtinib both alone and in combination with traditional cytotoxic chemotherapy.[202] These observations led to COG AALL0631 that tested addition of lestaurtinib to intensive chemotherapy in infants with *KMT2A*-R ALL, but lestaurtinib did not improve outcomes.[200] Interfant-06 randomized infants with *KMT2A*-R ALL to receive postinduction intensification with ALL or AML type therapy and found no overall benefit for AML therapy.[199] The COG AALL15P1 pilot study (NCT02828358) tested use of five-day azacitidine blocks prior to all postinduction cycles on the Interfant-06 backbone; results of that trial are not yet available.

Children With Down Syndrome and Acute Lymphoblastic Leukemia

Constitutional trisomy 21, or DS, is the most common chromosomal disorder, occurring in 1 to 2 per 1000 live births. Approximately 2% to 3% of children with ALL have DS, indicating a 20- to 40-fold relative risk of developing ALL compared to the general population.[203] Almost all cases of DS-ALL are B lineage with T-ALL rarely observed in children with DS. Trisomy 21 is a common somatic mutation observed in non–DS-associated ALL (non–DS-ALL), suggesting that the polysomic 21 facilitates leukemia development. Children with DS have a variety of immunodeficiencies, including B-cell lymphopenia.[204] Experimental mouse models of DS demonstrate a relative expansion of precursors at the pre- and pro-B cell stage compared to the later pro- and pre-B cell populations, and these precursors are more sensitive to IL7-driven expansion than wild-type B-cell precursors.[205] Up to 60% of children with DS-ALL have associated somatic *CRLF2*, *IKZF1*, and *JAK2* mutations or overexpression; all are deleterious mutations in non-DS populations, but the prognostic impacts of all but *IKZF1* are unclear in DS-ALL.[206-208] Children with DS-ALL are less likely than children with non–DS-ALL to carry favorable prognostic genetic markers such as *ETV6-RUNX1* fusion or high hyperdiploidy; although when they do, they are associated with a favorable outcome.[209]

Outcomes for children with DS-ALL are generally worse than those for the general population with ALL. The Ponte di Legno group published a retrospective analysis of 16 international trials comparing children with DS-ALL to those with non–DS-ALL.[209] Children with DS-ALL had decreased OS (74% vs 89%, $P < .0001$) and EFS (64% vs 81%, $P < .0001$) compared to the non–DS-ALL cohort, related both to higher relapse rates (26% vs 15%, $P < .0001$) and to a higher incidence (7% vs 2% in the non–DS-ALL cohort, $P < .0001$) of TRM. Infections are the major cause of TRM in this group,[209] and in many studies, the biggest independent risk factor for the development of infectious TRM is DS.[210] Importantly, while TRM in non–DS-ALL tends to occur during intensive phases of treatment, children with DS-ALL experience serious infectious complications even during maintenance therapy.[210] Children with DS-ALL are also more susceptible to noninfectious toxicity, with particular sensitivity to MTX unexplained by pharmacokinetic differences.[211] Despite this excess toxicity, children with DS-ALL have lower utilization of antiemetics and analgesics, suggesting a need for extra attention to symptom relief in this vulnerable population.[212]

TREATMENT AFTER RELAPSE

Biology of Relapse

With modern therapies, the CIR is approximately 10% to 15%,[4,71,78] although this risk differs substantially based on clinical risk factors, genetic subtype, and MRD response. Recent genome-wide analyses have yielded important insights into the biology of relapse. The driver sentinel translocations (*BCR-ABL1*, *ETV6-RUNX1*, *TCF3-PBX1*, etc.) are likely very early, perhaps even initiating, events in leukemogenesis and are almost always retained at relapse.[213] Whole exome sequencing studies have shown a mean of 10 to 20 non–silent somatic-coding region mutations per case at diagnosis, and about three times this many present at relapse.[214,215] These mutations cluster in genes encoding proteins involved in specific pathways, most commonly those related to B-cell development/differentiation, the TP53/RB tumor suppressor pathway, Ras signaling, and transcription factors.[214-216] The majority, but not all, point mutations are retained, but a minority is lost at relapse including some mutations in potentially targetable signaling pathways, such as the Ras and JAK/STAT pathways. Some genes are mutated more frequently at relapse, including *CREBBP*, *SETD2*, *WHSC1*, *TP53*, *USH2A*, *NRAS*, *IKZF1*, and *NT5C2* and the majority of relapse-specific alterations occur in genes involved in drug response.[214,215,217-220] *NT5C2* is particularly interesting because it encodes for a 5′-nucleotidase, and the mutant forms confer resistance to nucleoside analog therapies with drugs, such as 6-MP and 6-TG, which are the backbone of maintenance therapy. *NT5C2* mutations are rarely seen at initial diagnosis and even deep sequencing with high read depth generally does not identify mutant clones in diagnostic samples. Mutations in this gene are enriched in cases that relapse early, often during maintenance therapy while receiving daily 6-MP.

Detailed studies have shown that almost all cases of ALL harbor multiple subclones at initial diagnosis.[213,214] In most cases, the dominant subclone present at diagnosis is eradicated by therapy, and relapse occurs as a result of evolution in one of the minor subclones present at diagnosis.[214] This suggests that targeted therapies may be most effective if directed against early/initiating events that are present in all leukemia cells at diagnosis.

Relapse Risk Stratification

Risk factors present at diagnosis and at the time of ALL relapse are associated with survival following relapse. A multivariate analysis of data from COG studies conducted between 1988 and 2002 showed children who at initial diagnosis were <1 or ≥10 years, were NCI high risk, had CNS disease, or who had T-ALL fared significantly worse, as did boys.[5] A retrospective analysis of Nordic Society for Pediatric Hematology and Oncology (NOPHO) data additionally identified unfavorable cytogenetics and DS as poor prognostic factors for children being treated for relapse.[221] However, time to relapse/duration of first remission is the strongest prognostic indicator across multiple cooperative group studies, even among the highest risk groups, such as infants with ALL.[5,221-223] Location of relapse is also associated with survival, and children who experience relapses isolated to the so-called "sanctuary sites" that are relatively protected from chemotherapy and immune surveillance, mainly the CNS and the testes, have better outcomes than children who experience marrow relapses.[5] As such, treatment intensity is tailored to timing, immunophenotype, and location of relapse.

Response to reinduction therapy is also a strong predictor of outcome following ALL relapse. Children experiencing early marrow relapses (<36 months from diagnosis) are more likely to have detectable MRD ≥0.01% at the end of reinduction than those with late relapses (75% vs 51%, respectively, $P = .0375$), and MRD was strongly associated with outcome, with 1-year EFS 80% in MRD-negative patients vs 58% in those who were MRD positive ($P < .0005$).[224] Early relapses with positive end-of-reinduction MRD have a particularly dismal prognosis, with a 3-year OS 19%; in the COG AALL07P1 study, there were no survivors among the 30 patients with very early relapses (<18 months) and positive MRD.[225] The COG AALL0433 trial evaluated late marrow/combined relapses and found no prognostic difference between MRD 0.01% to 0.1% and MRD ≥0.1%.[226] End-of-reinduction MRD was a strong predictor of outcomes, with patients with MRD <0.1% having a 3-year EFS of 84.9% vs 53.7% for those with MRD ≥0.1%. Similar survival outcomes and lack of prognostic value of MRD beyond a sensitivity of 0.1% were identified in the ALL REZ-BFM 2002 study.[227] Novel therapies designed to circumvent chemoresistance in these persistent clones, such as the immunotherapy blinatumomab, are more effective than standard cytotoxic chemotherapy at eliminating MRD in high- and intermediate relapses.[228] Cooperative groups currently incorporate timing, location, and response to reinduction therapy to stratify relapses into risk groups (Table 77.3). In the future, a better understanding of genetic risk factors at relapse may help refine prognosis and lead to mutation-tailored therapy.[229]

Table 77.3. Relapse Risk Stratification by Study Group

Children's Oncology group	
Low	• Late marrow/combined (≥36 mo) + MRD < 0.1% • Late IEM (≥18 mo) + MRD < 0.1%
Intermediate	• Late marrow/combined (≥36 mo) + MRD ≥ 0.1% • Late IEM (≥18 mo) + MRD ≥ 0.1%
High	• Early marrow/combined (<36 mo) • Early IEM (<18 mo) • Any T-ALL relapse
Berlin-Frankfurt-Münster	
S1	• Late IEM (>6 mo from end of therapy)
S2	• Early IEM (≥18 mo from diagnosis and <6 mo from end of therapy) • Very early IEM (<18 mo from diagnosis) • Late marrow/combined non–T-ALL (>6 mo from end of therapy) • Early combined non–T-ALL (≥18 mo from diagnosis and <6 mo from end of therapy)
S3	• Early marrow non–T-ALL (≥18 mo from diagnosis and <6 mo from end of therapy)
S4	• Very early marrow/combined (<18 mo from diagnosis) • Any T-ALL marrow relapse
St Jude Children's Research Hospital	
Standard	• Any IEM + MRD < 0.01% • Late marrow/combined (≥6 mo from end of therapy) + MRD < 0.01%
High	• Early marrow/combined (<6 mo from end of therapy) • Any MRD ≥ 0.01% • Any T-ALL relapse

Abbreviations: HCT, hematopoietic stem cell transplantation; IEM, isolated extramedullary relapse; MRD, minimal residual disease; T-ALL, T-cell acute lymphoblastic leukemia.

Treatment of Bone Marrow Relapse

Currently most reinduction regimens for first relapse rely upon drugs used in frontline therapy. Postinduction therapy is typically consolidated either with intensification cycles, with or without CRT, followed by maintenance/continuation therapy for low-risk patients, or with HCT for higher risk patients. Attempts at dose intensification have not demonstrated significant benefits. Pediatric Oncology Group (POG) 9411 evaluated intensified asparaginase dosing during reinduction and added ifosfamide/etoposide and idarubicin/high-dose cytarabine to consolidation and continuation without improvement in outcomes compared to legacy data.[230] The COG AALL01P2 trial used a four-drug reinduction regimen similar to high-risk induction regimens with weekly vincristine, pegaspargase, a 4-week course of PRED, and doxorubicin, and established a three-block intensive chemotherapy including a four-drug reinduction block with vincristine, pegaspargase, PRED, and doxorubicin.[224] Among children with early marrow relapses (<36 months from diagnosis), CR2 was achieved in 68% with 12-month EFS 35%, while for those with late relapses (≥36 months) 96% achieved CR2 with 12-month EFS 80%. The UKALL R3 study substituted two five-day pulses of high-dose DEX for the PRED in the COG protocol and randomized patients to idarubicin vs the anthracenedione mitoxantrone.[231] The study demonstrated a clear advantage of mitoxantrone in both 3-year progression free survival (PFS) (64.6% vs 35.9%, P = .0004) and OS (69.0% vs 45.2%, P = .004) with all subgroups (B cell, T cell, timing and location of relapse, age at relapse, and cytogenetic risk factors) demonstrating a benefit from inclusion of mitoxantrone in reinduction, although rates of EOI MRD were not different by treatment arm. Of note, significant toxicity has been observed with the mitoxantrone-based reinduction block, limiting its use in combination with novel agents.[232] The COG AALL1331 phase 3 trial for first relapse of B-ALL incorporated a slightly modified UKALL R3 chemotherapy backbone and randomized higher risk patients (early relapse or MRD > 0.1% after reinduction) to chemotherapy or two cycles of blinatumomab followed by HCT and showed a significant improvement in both EFS and OS with blinatumomab, in part due to reduced toxicity allowing more patients to proceed to HCT.[228] In parallel, a phase 3 randomized trial comparing one cycle of blinatumomab vs the third block of consolidation chemotherapy in children found improved MRD clearance and EFS as well as fewer adverse events for the blinatumomab arm.[233] For patients with late marrow relapse with favorable MRD response to reinduction, the results of AALL1331 are pending. See HCT and Immunotherapy sections for additional discussions of management of relapsed B-ALL.

Treatment of Isolated Extramedullary Relapse

The CNS is the most common extramedullary site of relapse, occurring in 3% to 8% of patients, typically between 1 and 3 years after diagnosis; risk factors include T-cell immunophenotype, hyperleukocytosis, high-risk genetic abnormalities, and the presence of leukemic cells in the CSF at the time of diagnosis.[43] CNS relapse may present clinically with signs of increased intracranial pressure, such as headache or vomiting, as well as cranial nerve palsies. In North America, where almost all patients receive maintenance IT therapy, most CNS relapses occurring during treatment are discovered incidentally.[43] The second most common site of extramedullary relapse is the testes, accounting for approximately 5% of B-ALL relapses, although this rate is decreasing.[5] At least half of testicular relapses occur more than 3 years from diagnosis, and later relapses have better prognosis.[234]

Many patients with "isolated" extramedullary (IEM) relapse have submicroscopic BM involvement at the time of relapse, and the most common site of subsequent relapse is in the marrow, making systemic therapy a critical component of curative therapy for extramedullary relapse.[235] Local control of CNS or testicular sites can usually be obtained and maintained with chemotherapy and radiation therapy. CNS blasts may be cleared with weekly or twice-weekly IT therapy administered concurrently with systemic reinduction therapy followed by intensive systemic therapy and CRT with dosing 18 to 24 Gy.[236] Overall, at least 50% of patients achieve long-term survival after CNS relapse; however, time to relapse is prognostic. For isolated CNS relapse, 5-year survival rates are superior for those with late (≥36 months) relapse (78.2%) compared to early (<18 months) relapse (43.5%) or intermediate (18 to <36 months) relapse (68%; P < .0001).[5]

For patients with late isolated CNS relapse, HCT in CR2 is not indicated as a result of good long-term outcomes with intensive chemotherapy and CRT alone. POG 9412 evaluated a regimen of intensive systemic chemotherapy and delayed CRT (18 Gy cranial for patients with CR1 duration >18 months and 24 Gy cranial/15 Gy spinal for those with CR1 duration <18 months), which resulted in CR2 rate of 97.4% and overall 1-year EFS 70% with superior outcomes for late (77.7%) vs early relapses (51.6%, P = .027).[237] Subsequently, COG AALL02P2 evaluated the strategy of increasing chemotherapy intensity and decreasing the dose of CRT to 12 Gy for patients with late isolated CNS relapse, but the study was terminated early when outcomes were inferior to POG 9412.[238] Therefore, 18 Gy remains the recommended CRT dose. In contrast, for those with early isolated CNS relapse, EFS rates are only ~45%, leading many to recommend consolidation with HCT, while others have found that outcomes for this subgroup of patients are similar with radiation plus either HCT or chemotherapy.[239-241] Chimeric antigen receptor (CAR)-T cell therapy has demonstrated efficacy in clearance of CNS disease in small case series and is under investigation in first CNS relapse for B-ALL (NCT04276870).[242]

Late isolated testicular relapse is generally treated with intensive chemotherapy and local control with either radiation therapy or orchiectomy.[240] Although testicular irradiation is effective for disease control, the long-term consequences are significant. In adults, testicular irradiation doses greater than 4 to 6 Gy may result in persistent azoospermia, and doses greater than 20 Gy may compromise Leydig cell function in children, resulting in elevated luteinizing hormone, decreased testosterone, and delayed puberty.[243] In an attempt to decrease the use of testicular irradiation, COG AALL02P2 evaluated a strategy of intensified chemotherapy with 24 Gy testicular radiation only for those with persistent testicular disease confirmed on biopsy at the EOI. Outcomes were excellent with 5-year EFS 65% and OS 73%.[244] About three-quarters of patients were treated without testicular irradiation and outcomes were similar for those patients and the subgroup that received irradiation due to persistent testicular leukemia at end induction. The subgroup of 16 patients with late isolated testicular relapse treated on the ALL-REZ BFM-90 trial with chemotherapy plus 24 Gy radiation to the involved testis and 15 Gy to the contralateral testis achieved a 10-year EFS of 93%.[223] The optimal therapy for patients with late isolated testicular relapse to balance survival with preservation of gonadal function and fertility remains under investigation.

HEMATOPOIETIC STEM CELL TRANSPLANTATION

The risks of short- and long-term morbidity, mortality, and relapse post-HCT remain high despite improvements in supportive care, so a clear understanding of which children are most likely to benefit from this procedure is crucial. However, interpretation of HCT data is challenging because of a paucity of large collaborative randomized pediatric studies, as well as heterogeneity of analyses and pre-HCT treatment allocations. Many decisions regarding who should undergo HCT remain based on expert recommendations rather than randomized clinical trial data, but cooperative groups are working to incorporate HCT into clinical trials for newly diagnosed and relapsed pediatric ALL patients to standardize pre-HCT therapy and collect more unbiased data on HCT outcomes.

Only 25% of children will have a human leukocyte antigen (HLA)–matched sibling donor (MSD) available. Improvements in HLA typing resolution, graft-vs-host disease (GVHD) prophylaxis and treatment, and supportive care have essentially equalized survival following MSD and unrelated donor (URD) transplants.[245] Furthermore, the availability of umbilical cord blood (UCB) donor transplants and techniques to modify allografts from haploidentical donors has expanded the donor pool for children with ALL who might benefit from HCT.[246,247] For children lacking a suitable URD, modern era survival outcomes following UCB or haploidentical transplants are comparable both to each other and to MSD or URD outcomes.[246,248,249] A better understanding of the cell populations responsible for graft-vs-leukemia (GVL) may influence donor selection in the future. The role of natural killer cells in mediating ALL-directed GVL is underscored by the superior outcomes seen after transplantation with allografts from donors with activating killer immunoglobulin-like receptor mismatches.[250-252]

In addition to donor selection, the level of disease prior to HCT and selection of preparative regimen can affect HCT outcomes. Detectable MRD prior to HCT markedly increases the risk of relapse. Recent studies have delineated risk by MRD level and evaluated whether pre-HCT intensification can improve outcomes. Augmentation of therapeutic intensity and incorporation of novel agents, such as blinatumomab, have eliminated detectable MRD in over 60% of patients with positive MRD at the end of reinduction on NOPHO and COG studies.[228,253] ASCT0431 identified 0.1% as a predictive threshold for pre-HCT baseline MRD.[254] An Italian study found that patients with negative MRD had a 10-year EFS of 73%, while patients with detectable MRD <0.1% had EFS of 39%, and those with MRD ≥0.1% had EFS of 18%.[255] Patients transplanted in CR1 with low-level MRD had EFS comparable to the MRD-negative group, while patients in ≥CR2 with low-level MRD had comparable survival to the high-MRD group. Importantly, among patients with MRD detectable by next-generation sequencing of IG rearrangements prior to HCT, development of acute GVHD lowers the risk of relapse, suggesting ALL is susceptible to GVL.[256] Similarly, preemptive rapid reduction of prophylactic immunosuppressive therapy or infusion of donor lymphocytes has improved outcomes in small studies of patients with rising mixed donor chimerism or detectable MRD post-HCT, in one study equalizing the EFS of children with and without posttransplant MRD.[257,258] Because of the significant risk of late toxicity after total body irradiation (TBI), particularly in young children, the European BMT consortium FORUM study randomized children with ALL over age 4 to TBI and etoposide vs busulfan/treosulfan, thiotepa, and fludarabine to evaluate noninferiority of the radiation-free regimen.[259] This study closed early due to inferiority of the chemotherapy-only regimens, with 2-year OS 91% and EFS 86% for TBI and OS 75% and EFS 58% for chemotherapy conditioning. This advantage remained significant in multivariate analyses for both MRD-positive and MRD-negative patients at the time of HCT. However, small studies allocating HTS/NGS MRD-negative patients to non-TBI-based HCT have had promising outcomes, suggesting there may be cohorts who may be able to avoid TBI.[260]

Consensus indications for transplant of ALL in CR1 are evolving. Historical indications for HCT in CR1 recommended by an expert panel from the American Society of Blood and Marrow Transplantation, such as hypodiploidy and induction failure, are now being reconsidered based on more recent data.[261] Children with hypodiploid ALL showed no benefit to transplant in CR1, even among children with persistent EOI MRD.[262] In addition, evidence for both B and T-ALL that the EOC timepoint may be more predictive of outcomes than EOI has led to recent HR ALL and T-ALL trials permitting children with induction failure to remain on study and proceed with intensified chemotherapy and randomized interventions, as long as they achieve MRD-negative remissions by EOC.

Outcomes for other historically very high-risk subgroups, such as Ph+ ALL, have been markedly improved by targeted therapies and are no longer indications for HCT in CR1, except in case of slow response to frontline therapy. The international collaborative study AALL1631 (NCT01460160) only allocates children with Ph+ ALL who have persistent MRD ≥0.05% at the EOI IB to HCT and has introduced post-HCT imatinib maintenance. Infants with KMT2A-R ALL in the Interfant-99 trial who were <6 months at diagnosis and had presenting WBC ≥300 × 10⁹/L had superior 5-year DFS 60.1% and OS 65.6% compared to those who received intensified chemotherapy alone (DFS 46.8%, $P = .03$, and OS 48.6%, $P = .02$).[37] On the successor trial, Interfant 06, only 46% of HR infants were able to undergo HCT due to relapse and nonrelapse mortality events; among patients who had HCT, 6-year EFS was 44%, supporting a potential role for HCT in this group.[199]

Data regarding when HCT is indicated for ALL in CR2 are more robust than for CR1. Eapen and colleagues reported outcomes of children who experienced early marrow relapses (<36 months from diagnosis) between 1991 and 1997 and attained CR2, showing MSD transplant was associated with a decreased risk of relapse and improved 8-year leukemia-free survival (LFS) (41%) compared to treatment with chemotherapy alone (23%).[263] In contrast, those relapsing ≥36 months from diagnosis had no significant benefit when allocated to transplant. The BFM also demonstrated a benefit to allogeneic HCT for children experiencing early marrow or T-ALL relapses over chemoradiotherapy alone (10-year EFS 40% vs 20%, $P < .005$).[223] COG AALL0433 assigned children with intermediate-risk relapses (early IEM or late marrow/combined) to HCT if they had an MSD available.[226] For the IEM patients, DFS was 71.4% for HCT vs 28.6% for chemotherapy and cranial radiation alone. Patients with marrow/combined relapses showed an EFS advantage for HCT among children with negative MRD at end of reinduction. However, 3-year OS was >90% for both arms; thus, children who become MRD negative are not recommended to undergo HCT unless they experience a second relapse. There was no benefit to HCT among children with persistent MRD at end of reinduction; however, subsequent studies continue to allocate these children to HCT, with a focus on reducing the pre-HCT MRD using novel agents.[228] Since late IEM relapse outcomes are very good with chemotherapy alone, most cooperative groups only recommend transplant for patients with detectable MRD at the end of reinduction. Outcomes for children with relapsed T-ALL are dismal; however, for those who are able to undergo HCT in CR2, survival approaches those of children with early marrow relapse of B-ALL, with 3-year OS 48% and EFS 46%.[264] Children who undergo HCT in third or higher remission also have dismal outcomes, with LFS only as high as 30%; however, salvage with HCT is possible.[265] Future directions will include evaluation of posttransplant maintenance or targeted therapies, as well as how best to monitor, interpret, and manage MRD in the posttransplant setting.

PRECISION MEDICINE FOR ACUTE LYMPHOBLASTIC LEUKEMIA

Kinase Inhibitors

The dramatic improvement in outcome for patients with Ph+ ALL with the addition of the ABL class TKIs imatinib and dasatinib to cytotoxic chemotherapy has become a model for incorporation of targeted agents into the treatment for other ALL subgroups. International cooperative trials in pediatric Ph+ ALL seek to define the optimal TKI and chemotherapy backbones to maximize outcomes and minimize toxicity. In Ph-like ALL, approximately 12% of patients have fusions involving *ABL1*, *ABL2*, *CSF1R*, or *PDGFRB* and responses to ABL1 TKIs have been reported.[58,171-173] Several small studies have shown early evidence that adding imatinib or dasatinib to chemotherapy in patients with ABL-class fusions improves outcome.[174,266,267] For the Ph-like ALL patients with mutations affecting the CRLF2/JAK/STAT pathway, JAK inhibition may be effective,[164,168,169] and COG AALL1521 (NCT02723994) is evaluating the addition of the oral JAK1/2 inhibitor ruxolitinib to standard augmented modified BFM chemotherapy. Aberrant activation of JAK/STAT pathway is also observed in the ETP subtype of T-ALL, and ruxolitinib demonstrated activity in patient-derived murine xenograft models of ETP ALL, independent of JAK/STAT pathway mutations.[167]

Activation of the Ras signaling pathway because of mutations in *NRAS*, *KRAS*, *PTPN11*, *FLT3*, and *NF1* occurs in about 35% of newly diagnosed ALL cases with high frequency in Ph-like ALL, *KMT2A*-R, DS-ALL, and iAMP21.[58,268-271] Ras pathway mutations are present in 40% of patients at relapse, and are associated with early relapse, CNS involvement, and chemoresistance.[272,273] MEK kinase inhibitors, including trametinib and selumetinib, have demonstrated activity in primary samples, but their optimal use remains under investigation.[269,272,273]

Proteasome Inhibitors

Bortezomib is a selective inhibitor of the ubiquitin proteasome pathway with activity in ALL and demonstrates synergy with DEX and anthracyclines.[274-276] In T-ALL, activated Notch1 leads to activation of the NF-κB pathway, and bortezomib decreases expression of both, leading to interest in proteasome inhibitors for this subgroup of patients.[277] In clinical trials, bortezomib combined with a four-drug reinduction platform had an overall response rate of 80% in patients with multiply relapsed B-ALL.[278] Infectious toxicities were significant, and antifungal and antibacterial prophylaxis was mandated midway through the study. This regimen was evaluated in patients with first relapse on COG AALL07P1, and 11 of 17 patients with first relapse of T-ALL achieved CR2 at the end of Block 1 compared to 1 of 7 (17%) T-ALL patients treated with chemotherapy alone.[224,225] Bortezomib was studied in the COG AALL1231 trial for newly diagnosed T-ALL patients, but the trial was closed early when the results of AALL0434 became available, so the role of proteasome inhibition in this setting has not been defined.[279] Carfilzomib, a second-generation irreversible proteasome inhibitor, is currently under investigation in relapsed pediatric ALL in combination with reinduction chemotherapy (NCT02303821).[280]

Epigenetic Regulators

The histone deacetylase inhibitor vorinostat and the DNA methyltransferase inhibitor decitabine reverse aberrant gene expression and methylation profiles in relapsed blasts and induce chemosensitivity in primary patient samples and ALL cell lines.[281,282] While the combination of decitabine plus vorinostat administered prior to intensive reinduction chemotherapy with the ALLR3 backbone was not feasible due to infectious toxicity,[283] pharmacodynamic studies showed potent in vivo modulation of epigenetic marks, suggesting that this strategy might be effective with a different chemotherapy backbone. In infant ALL, epigenetic priming with azacitidine was safe in combination with the Interfant-06 chemotherapy backbone (COG AALL15P1; NCT02828358).[284] Genome-wide histone methylation studies revealed that the abnormal expression of *KMT2A* fusion target genes is associated with high levels of H3K79 methylation which is catalyzed by disruptor of telomeric-silencing 1-like (DOT1L).[285,286] Unfortunately, while small molecule inhibitors of DOT1L have preclinical activity in *KMT2A*-R leukemias, clinical trials have demonstrated modest single-agent responses and challenging pharmacologic properties.[287,288] More recently, inhibition of the interaction between Menin (*MEN1*) and *KMT2A* was highly effective in patient-derived xenograft models of *KMT2A*-R ALL, and clinical trials are underway (NCT04811580).[289]

BCL-2 Family Inhibitors

Members of the B-cell lymphoma 2 (BCL2) protein family function as key regulators of the intrinsic apoptosis pathway; inhibitors of this pathway promote apoptosis by directly releasing proapoptotic proteins and triggering mitochondrial outer membrane permeabilization and caspase activation.[290] Venetoclax (Bcl-2 inhibitor) and navitoclax (Bcl-X_L inhibitor) have significant activity in preclinical models of ALL as well as synergy in combination, although dosing of navitoclax is limited by on-target thrombocytopenia.[291-293] In a phase 1 trial for children with multiple relapsed or refractory ALL, venetoclax combined with steroid/vincristine/asparaginase had an objective response rate of 56%, consistent with the ability of venetoclax to overcome glucocorticoid resistance.[294,295] In a phase 1 trial for adults and children, safe dosing for the combination of venetoclax and navitoclax was identified and the CR rate was 60%.[296] Clinical trials incorporating venetoclax are in development for newly diagnosed infant ALL and relapsed T-ALL given demonstrated activity in these challenging populations,[297,298] and patients with ALL with the *TCF3-HLF* fusion are eligible for a clinical trial combining induction chemotherapy with venetoclax (NCT03236857).

Immunotherapies

Identification and targeting of tumor-specific antigens using unconjugated antibodies, antibodies conjugated to drugs or toxins, antibodies that link leukemia cells to effector cells, or engineered antigen receptors are currently in development for chemorefractory leukemias (*Figure 77.5*), and many have shown very promising clinical responses in pediatric ALL. Candidate antigen targets are expressed on normal tissues as well as on malignant cells, limiting the number of safely targeted epitopes because of on-target/off-tissue toxicities. In the case of B-ALL, the B cell aplasia resulting from targeting normal B cells expressing antigens, such as CD19 or CD22, results in a mild immunodeficiency, clinically similar to X-linked agammaglobulinemia and manageable with prophylactic IG replacement.

Unconjugated antibodies bind to surface markers on target cells, marking the target cell for clearance by cytolytic effector cells via antibody-dependent cell-mediated cytotoxicity (ADCC). Rituximab, ofatumumab, and obinutuzumab are all unconjugated antibodies targeting CD20, which is expressed in a subset of B-ALL. Epratuzumab is a CD22-targeted antibody that modulates B-cell activation rather than inducing a direct cytolytic effect by ADCC.[299] This agent was tested in children with relapsed ALL in combination with reinduction chemotherapy in the COG ADVL04P2 trial.[300] Although the study failed to meet predefined endpoint of improving CR rates, there was a suggestion of benefit in children with late marrow relapse compared to historical controls treated on the non-epratuzumab arm of COG AALL01P2.[300] This agent is now being tested in a randomized trial for relapsed ALL in Europe (NCT01802814).

Inotuzumab is an antibody conjugate consisting of a humanized anti-CD22 monoclonal antibody conjugated to the calicheamicin analog ozogamicin. The adult phase 3 INOVATE study demonstrated a remarkable improvement in response rates (CR/CRi with incomplete hematologic recovery—73.8% vs 30.9% inotuzumab vs standard

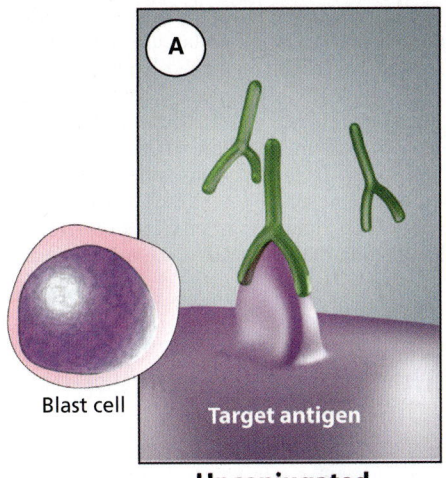
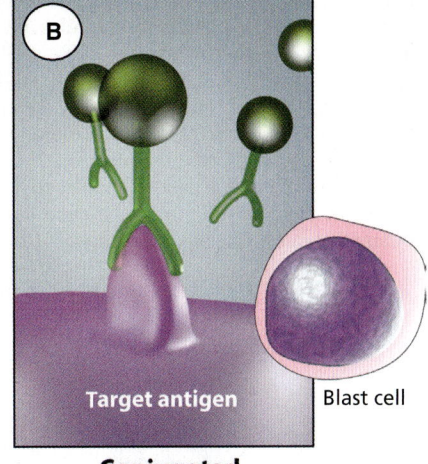
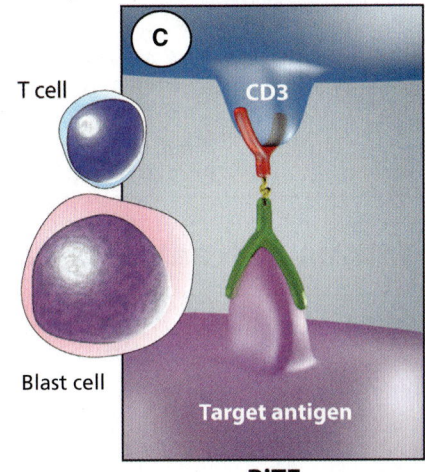

FIGURE 77.5 **Current immunotherapeutic approaches.** A, Unconjugated antibodies targeting tumor-specific antigens mark a target cell for destruction by cytotoxic effector cells or directly inhibit immune cell function. Clinically available agents relevant to pediatric ALL include rituximab, ofatumumab, and obinutuzumab, all targeting CD20 and epratuzumab (CD22). B, Conjugated antibodies bind tumor antigens, delivering a cytotoxin directly to the target cell. Inotuzumab ozogamicin is a CD22-targeted antibody conjugated to a calicheamicin analog. C, Bispecific T-cell engager (BiTE) molecules are engineered antibodies designed to bind a T cell receptor and a target antigen, bringing T cells in proximity to antigen-expressing malignant cells, such as the CD19-targeted BiTE antibody blinatumomab. D, Chimeric antigen receptor (CAR)–modified T cells are engineered to express a chimeric protein combining an antibody receptor with a T-cell receptor and costimulatory molecule. CAR T cells targeting CD19 and CD22 are currently in clinical trials. ALL, acute lymphoblastic leukemia. (Copyright © Sue Seif, MA, CMI, used with permission.)

chemotherapy, $P < .001$) and significantly prolonged PFS and OS, with liver toxicity, including hepatic veno-occlusive disease, as the major toxicity.[301] Similar impressive activity has been observed in pediatrics.[302] The COG is currently testing inotuzumab in a phase II trial for relapsed ALL (AALL1621; NCT02981628) and in a phase III trial for newly diagnosed high-risk ALL patients that are MRD negative at the EOC therapy (AALL1732; NCT03959085).

Several approaches to induce direct antileukemic T-cell responses are currently in clinical use in children with B-ALL. Blinatumomab is a bispecific T-cell engager (BiTE) that binds both CD3 and CD19, bringing T cells in proximity to CD19-expressing malignant and normal B cells, resulting in perforin-mediated cytotoxic killing of CD19+ cells.[303] A multi-institutional pediatric phase I/II study demonstrated an overall CR rate of 32%, with a 56% CR rate in children with <50% marrow blasts and 33% among those with higher levels of marrow blasts.[304] Over half of the responders achieved MRD-negative remissions. Two recent randomized trials have shown that blinatumomab is highly effective in children with relapsed B-ALL. As discussed above (see Treatment of Bone Marrow Relapse), COG AALL1331 demonstrated that two 4-week cycles of blinatumomab was more effective than two blocks of intensive chemotherapy with improved DFS and OS, markedly lower rates of serious toxicity, and improved rates of MRD-negative remissions.[228] A parallel European multiconsortium study for high-risk relapsed B-ALL included patients who received induction and two consolidation cycles per investigators' discretion, with randomization to chemotherapy or blinatumomab for the third consolidation cycle.[233] In this trial, blinatumomab was associated with higher EFS and OS, superior rates of MRD negativity, and a reduction in serious adverse events. Among patients who proceeded to allogeneic HCT, those who received blinatumomab had a lower proportion of relapse-associated deaths (6.3%) compared to the chemotherapy-only group (21.1%), suggesting the use of a treatment approach that may circumvent chemoresistance results in a lower disease burden at the time of HCT, thereby improving outcomes. Blinatumomab was approved for relapsed/refractory B-ALL by the European Medicines Agency in 2015 and by the US FDA in 2018. Blinatumomab is now being tested in the COG AALL1731 (NCT03914625) trial for newly diagnosed standard risk B-ALL.

CAR T cells targeting CD19 have produced remarkable responses with MRD-negative remissions obtained in up to 90% of patients with heavily pretreated, highly chemorefractory leukemia, most of whom have relapsed post-HCT.[305,306] Long-term follow-up of the FDA-approved tisagenlecleucel product resulted in a 12-month EFS of 50% and OS 76%, with very few patients receiving HCT.[305] Tisagenlecleucel is notable for its prolonged persistence in vivo, with 83% of responders having persistent B-cell aplasia at 6 months after infusion. Consolidation of CAR T cell therapy with HCT results in excellent long-term outcomes in other studies, with 5-year EFS after HCT of 61.9%.[306] Owing to concern for eventual CAR T cell loss, many centers use this therapy as a bridge to HCT for children; however, for a patient who has already experienced HCT and may not be willing or able to undergo a second transplant, CAR T cells may offer prolonged freedom from disease with a lower risk of permanent toxic injury than HCT. Tisagenlecleucel is now being tested in a COG-Novartis phase 2 trial for children with HR B-ALL who have MRD persisting through EOC (AALL1721; NCT03876769).

There are several mechanisms for treatment failure or relapse following BiTE and/or CAR T cell therapy (*Figure 77.6*). Immune checkpoints such as programmed death ligand-1 attenuate T-cell responses by inducing anergy and T-cell exhaustion and represent another mechanism of immune escape for these targeted cellular immunotherapies. Checkpoint markers have been identified on blasts in patients with resistance to blinatumomab, which may potentially be circumvented by the addition of checkpoint inhibitors, such as pembrolizumab or nivolumab.[307,308] The ongoing COG AALL1821 phase 2 trial (NCT04546399) randomizes patients with first relapse of B-ALL to blinatumomab ± nivolumab. The strong immune pressure of CAR T cells can select target cells with mutations in the CD19 locus recognized by the scFv of the engineered T cell, resulting in a "CD19-negative" relapse. These account for up to 74% of relapses after CD19-directed CAR T cell treatment.[309] Loss of B-cell aplasia is strongly associated with CD19-positive relapses but not with

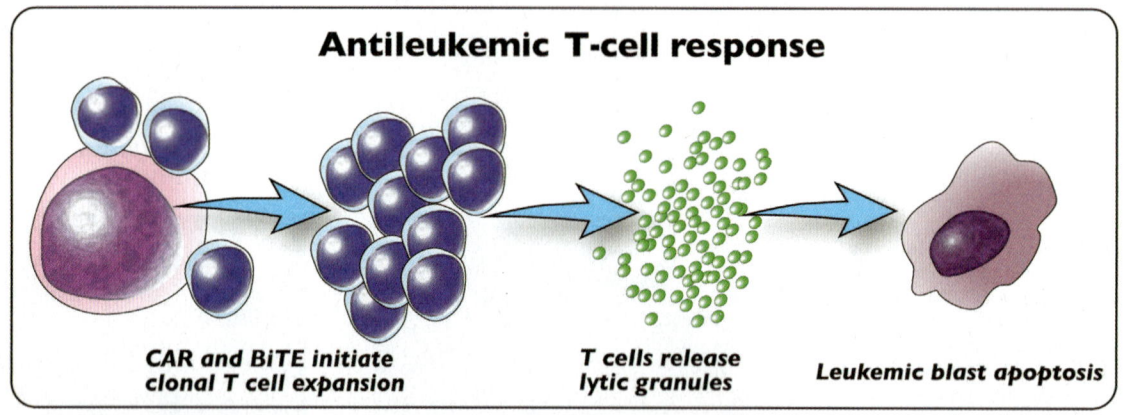

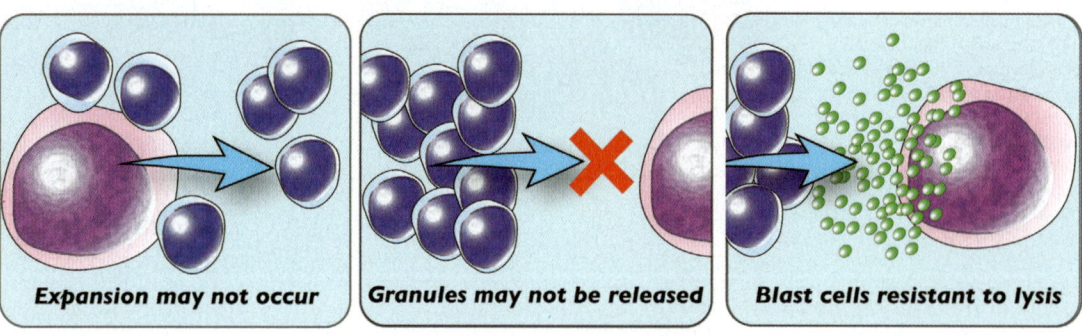

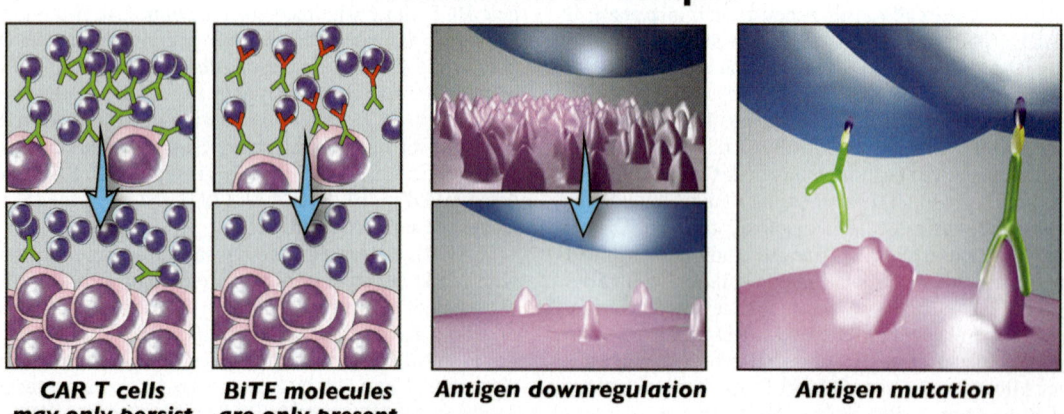

FIGURE 77.6 Mechanisms of failure and relapse after T-cell–based immunotherapies. T-cell–based immunotherapies rely on target recognition, leading to T-cell clonal expansion. The expanded T cells then release toxic granules to kill the target cells, which then undergo apoptosis. Failure to achieve remission may be seen with poor T-cell expansion in vivo, impaired T-cell lytic function, or target cell resistance to cytotoxic killing. CAR T cells may only persist for weeks to months in some cases, leading to relapse after loss of immune surveillance. Similarly, blinatumomab has a very short half-life, and relapses may occur once the molecule is no longer present to bring the T cells and their targets in close physical approximation. Immune escape occurs when a clone with downregulated or mutated target antigens develops. BiTE, bispecific T-cell engager; CAR, chimeric antigen receptor. (Copyright © Sue Seif, MA, CMI, used with permission.)

CD19-negative relapse. Prior blinatumomab exposure may be a risk factor for antigen-negative immune escape. For patients who experience CD19-negative relapses, targeting CD22 with inotuzumab or with a CD22-directed CAR T cell may be effective at reinducing remission, and bispecific CD19/CD22 CAR T cells are currently in clinical development.[310,311] Children whose leukemia has underlying myeloid/lymphoid plasticity, as with KMT2A rearrangements, can experience lineage switch following CAR T cell immune pressure.[312] Optimal strategies for addressing this relapse mechanism are not yet defined. Finally, while most children are able to undergo successful collections for CAR T cell manufacture, nearly 20% have inadequate T cell numbers or quality after multiple rounds of intensive lympholytic chemotherapy.[305] In these cases, URD T cells may be genetically modified both with a lentiviral CAR and using approaches such as transcription activator-like effector nucleases to prevent expression of alloreactive TCRs.[313] This approach results in an "off-the-shelf" or universal CAR T cell product that has promising efficacy in early phase studies. Finally, approaches to prolong persistence of CAR T cells include a fully humanized CAR molecule to reduce the risk of rejection due to immune responses against xenogeneic antigens.[314]

B-ALL was the ideal starting point for development of targeted immunotherapies. Targeting T-ALL has more inherent challenges, as elimination of all T cells would result in a fatal immunodeficiency. There are a variety of CAR T cell trials targeting T cell markers expressed only on activated or subset T cells, such as CD5 (NCT03081910) and CD7 (NCT03690011). Impressive early results have recently been published with allogeneic CD7-directed CAR T cells for relapsed/refractory T-ALL.[315] CD38 is often expressed on T-ALL blasts and may be a promising target for antibody or cellular therapy. Daratumumab, an unconjugated anti-CD38 antibody, has been evaluated extensively in multiple myeloma and has shown preclinical efficacy in T-ALL patient–derived xenografts.[316] This agent is currently being evaluated in combination with standard chemotherapy in children and young adults with relapsed or refractory ALL (NCT03384654).

TOXICITIES AND LATE EFFECTS OF THERAPY FOR ACUTE LYMPHOBLASTIC LEUKEMIA

Quality of Life

Survivors of childhood ALL are more likely to have chronic medical conditions than their unaffected siblings, with a 3.7-fold risk of a severe or life-threatening condition and a 2.8-fold risk of reporting multiple health conditions.[317] Even for those reporting coping well with late effects, a sense of frailty can persist in patient-reported outcomes.[318] As a group, they are also less likely to be employed, get married, graduate from high school, or carry health insurance than their healthy siblings, particularly if they were diagnosed at a younger age, underwent CRT, or experienced a relapse.[317,319,320] Cranial radiation is consistently associated with more overall late effects, including effects on health-related quality of life (HRQOL); however, the introduction of hyperfractionated CRT, in which a standard dose is delivered in multiple small fractions, is associated with improved rates of living independently and engagement in a long-term relationship.[321] Nonetheless, long-term survivors of ALL generally report very good HRQOL compared to healthy adults.[322]

Neuropsychologic Sequelae

Children undergoing therapy for ALL are at risk for neurocognitive deficits later in life. Deficits in memory, attention, and processing speed are well described, and survivors are also at increased risk of sensory deficits, coordination problems, motor problems, seizures, and headaches compared to healthy sibling controls.[103] Poor cognitive function is associated with lower HRQOL scores, and attention deficits can lead to poor social functioning.[323,324] Childhood cancer survivors are significantly more likely to be placed into special education programs and to have lower household incomes than healthy siblings.[325]

Exposure to CRT, particularly at a young age, is associated with significantly slower and less accurate processing compared to population norms, even at lower doses used for treatment (18 Gy) or prophylaxis (12 Gy) of CNS leukemia.[326] A study of very long-term survivors (average 20 years after diagnosis) demonstrated decreased verbal and performance intelligence quotient for patients who had received prior irradiation compared to healthy population controls, as well as memory and motor deficits.[327] Survivors with CRT exposure are also more likely to experience clinically significant anxiety-depression, inattention-hyperactivity, and social withdrawal than their healthy siblings.[325]

Contemporary ALL treatment regimens seek to avoid CRT exposure to minimize risks of late effects. However, this is accomplished by intensified CNS-directed systemic therapy and IT chemotherapy, and these chemotherapy-only regimens are also associated with long-term cognitive effects. High-dose IV MTX has been implicated in high rates of leukoencephalopathy (68%) detectable up to 7.7 years after the end of therapy,[328] and longitudinal studies of survivors of high-intensity CNS-directed chemotherapy demonstrated persistent mild-to-moderate attention and processing deficits that predicted poor academic performance 2 years off therapy.[329] DEX is more likely to cause impaired memory, attention, and executive function than PRED in nonirradiated long-term and very long-term survivors.[104] Risk factors for neurocognitive late effects after chemotherapy include younger age at diagnosis, higher dexamethasone and MTX exposures, as well as genetic variants in COMT, APOE, monoamine oxidase, and folic acid metabolic pathways.[330] Underlying cognitive dysfunction, as with DS, and adverse socioeconomic factors are also associated with worse neurocognitive outcomes.[330,331] Exposure to repeated general anesthesia for procedures such as lumbar punctures has also been associated with a decline in neurocognitive function.[332] In addition to direct toxicity to neurons and glial cells, investigators have identified additional mechanisms underlying neurocognitive toxicity such as vascular injury, inflammation, reduced telomerase activity, and epigenetic changes.[333] These discoveries may lead to biomarkers that can identify vulnerable individuals or subclinical changes that would lead to interventions to prevent further injury, and late effects of novel therapies with known acute neurotoxicities, such as blinatumomab and CD19-directed CAR T cells, need to be determined. A variety of hospital-, school-, and home-based interventions have been shown to improve cognitive testing, school performance, and graduation rates.[334]

Secondary Malignant Neoplasms

Children exposed to cytotoxic chemotherapy and radiation are at increased risk of developing secondary malignant neoplasms (SMN) compared to the general population. The Childhood Cancer Survivor Study (CCSS) reported a cumulative incidence of SMNs of 3.8% in a cohort of 6148 survivors of childhood ALL diagnosed between 1970 and 1999.[335] Incidence is highest among children who received HR-ALL therapy and has declined since the 1980s; children receiving SR-ALL therapy in the 1990s had no increase in SMN incidence over the general population. In a cohort of 5006 children with ALL treated on BFM trials between 1979 and 1995, the median time from initiation of primary ALL therapy to SMN was 6 years (range 11 months-15 years) and varied by SMN: median time to AML was 3.8 years (range 1-11.5) and CNS tumors 7.9 years (range 4-13).[336] A long-term follow-up study of children treated on CCG protocols revealed a 52-fold increased risk of AML in children treated for ALL compared to the general population; however, this risk declined after the first 5 years from therapy, and no cases were detected more than 10 years after the end of therapy.[337] Cumulative incidences of CNS tumors, soft-tissue sarcomas, and carcinomas continue to increase over time.[336-338] In a 25-year follow-up study of CCSS patients diagnosed between 1970 and 1986, 81% of all SMN occurred in people who had received radiation therapy as children.[317] Over half of these SMNs were CNS tumors, and radiation exposure was associated with twice the cumulative incidence as in unexposed patients. In addition to radiation exposure, increasing radiation dose, female sex, and younger age at diagnosis are associated with higher rates of SMN.[337,338] Genetic predispositions may increase the risk of development of SMN. *TPMT* polymorphisms were associated with a trend toward an increased risk of CNS tumors in radiation-exposed children in the SJCRH study.[338]

Osteonecrosis

ON (avascular necrosis of bone) occurs in 5% to 10% of patients.[339,340] The incidence of symptomatic ON increases dramatically with age, affecting 20% to 30% of those age 10 to 20 years at the time of treatment, with females affected more frequently and at younger ages than males.[339,341] Affected patients have three sites of involvement on average, and 80% have at least two sites of involvement.[339] The most common sites of involvement are the hips and knees each in about one-third of patients, shoulders in about 10%, and ankles, elbows, and wrists in <10% (Figure 77.7).[339] Severity of ON ranges from asymptomatic to debilitating, including pain, reduction in joint mobility, joint degeneration, and collapse.[342]

The pathogenesis of ON is multifactorial and thought to be caused by ischemia due to microvascular thrombi and extravascular lipid deposition that compromises intramedullary blood flow. During revascularization, bone resorption by osteoclasts results in demineralization and trabecular thinning with subsequent mechanical collapse.[343] The primary modality for diagnosis of ON is magnetic resonance imaging, and long-term joint outcome is associated with the extent of articular surface involved; in the hip, the worst prognosis was associated with lesions occupying more than 30% of the femoral head volume with 80% of hips with these lesions collapsed within 2 years of diagnosis and 50% requiring arthroplasty.[344]

Therapeutic options are limited. Small case series report improvements in pain with bisphosphonate therapy or surgical core decompression, but the impact on progression of joint degeneration is unknown, and a recent follow-up of patients enrolled in UKALL 2003 showed that core decompression of the femoral head did not improve the rates of femoral head survival.[345-347] Joint collapse frequently requires surgical intervention with total joint replacement. With 10 to 15 years of follow-up, 38% of patients diagnosed with symptomatic ON underwent joint replacement surgery, most commonly of the hips or knees.[339]

Corticosteroids are the component of ALL therapy that contribute most greatly to risk of ON, with increased risk with greater exposure to more potent formulations. Incidence of ON increases with the use of DEX, particularly in older patients, which is partially mitigated by treatment regimens with discontinuous dosing. The CCG-1961 study found that alternate-week DEX (days 1-7 and 15-21 rather than 1-21) during the DI phase significantly reduced the incidence of ON compared to continuous dosing schedules with incidence rates of 8.7% vs 17%, respectively ($P = .0005$).[339] In COG AALL0232 trial for NCI-HR B-ALL patients aged 10 years and older, the 5-year cumulative incidence of ON was 24.3% for DEX and 15.9% for PRED ($P = .001$) during induction.[94] Low albumin, elevated lipids, and poor DEX clearance are associated with ON, and may be caused by inherited genetic factors as well as interactions between DEX and asparaginase.[348] Hypertension may also be a modifiable risk factor for ON development.[349] Genetic polymorphisms associated with ON risk are under active investigation, with recent studies implicating a role for glutamate signaling in the pathogenesis of ON.[350] Self-reported and genetically

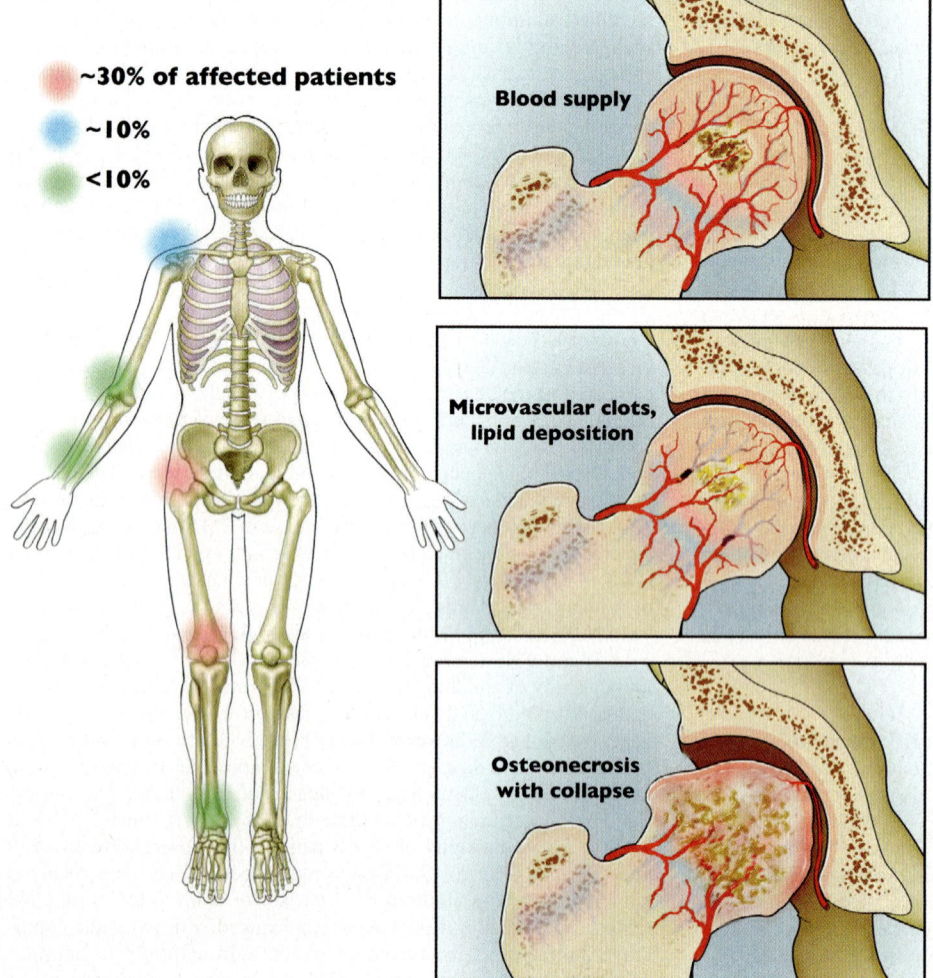

FIGURE 77.7 Primary sites and pathophysiology of osteonecrosis. The pathogenesis of osteonecrosis is thought to be due to ischemia caused by microvascular thrombi and extravascular lipid deposition, which compromises intramedullary blood flow. During revascularization, bone resorption by osteoclasts results in demineralization and trabecular thinning with subsequent mechanical collapse. The most common sites of involvement are the hips and knees each in about one-third of patients, shoulders in about 10%, and ankles, elbows, and wrists in <10%. (Copyright © Sue Seif, MA, CMI, used with permission.)

defined Black and Hispanic patients had significantly lower rates of ON development than whites in the DFCI 05-001 trial.[351]

Cardiac Toxicity

Childhood exposure to anthracyclines and anthracenediones is associated with an increased risk of late cardiotoxicity, with detectable abnormalities in contractility and afterload occurring in over half of patients who receive cumulative doses exceeding 250 mg/m^2.[352,353] In addition to higher doses, younger age at exposure and female sex are associated with an increased risk of cardiotoxicity.[353,354] However, even in patients who receive the lowest doses of anthracyclines, up to 30% of patients experience subclinical decrements in cardiac function.[353]

The free radical scavenger dexrazoxane has been used to decrease oxidative stress on cardiomyocytes in children with ALL, resulting in fewer elevations in cardiac troponin T and brain natriuretic peptide, biomarkers predictors of late cardiomyopathy.[355,356] The POG study P9407 randomized children with T-ALL to receive dexrazoxane following doxorubicin doses (cumulative dose 360 mg/m^2).[357] Those on the dexrazoxane arm experienced fewer elevations in troponin and were less likely to have abnormal left ventricular fractional shortening, wall thickness, and thickness to dimension ratio than children in the doxorubicin-only arm at 3 years after treatment. There were no differences in EFS or OS between the two groups.[357,358]

CAR T cells can induce severe cytokine release syndrome that leads to left ventricular dysfunction and heart failure.[359] Risk factors for cardiotoxicity in children include blasts >25% on marrow biopsy and lower pre-CAR T cell infusion cardiac function. While cardiac function generally returns to baseline in most of these children, the long-term consequences of severe immune activation are unknown.

Work is ongoing to define the genetic risk factors for anthracycline-induced cardiotoxicity. Gene variants involved in anthracycline transportation, metabolism and excretion, sarcomere structure and function, cardiac remodeling, reactive oxygen species generation, and DNA double strand break repairs have all been implicated.[360] In addition to chemoprevention with dexrazoxane, lifestyle interventions, such as programs to encourage physical activity, may be beneficial to children treated for ALL.[361]

Endocrinologic Late Effects

Late effects of ALL therapy include an array of endocrine abnormalities. Survivors of childhood ALL are at increased risks of both obesity and being underweight, particularly if they were overweight or underweight at the time of diagnosis.[362] Female sex, younger age at diagnosis, and radiation exposure were consistently associated with increased risk across studies.[362] Children with ALL who live in neighborhoods with high area deprivation indices are also at an increased risk for obesity.[363] Among ALL survivors, 43% had evidence of sarcopenic obesity, characterized by an increased adipose tissue: lean muscle mass ratio, which can result in premature frailty and decreased HRQOL scores.[364] GWAS has identified gene variants that were enriched among patients with increased body mass index measurements who were (LINC00856) or were not (EMR1 intron) exposed to CRT, suggesting an interaction effect.[365] Self-reported thyroid dysfunction is also observed in survivors of childhood ALL at an increased rate compared to healthy siblings, and a Scandinavian study showed survivors of childhood ALL had a 2.3-fold increased relative risk of hyperthyroidism compared to the general population.[366,367] Linear growth is impaired in survivors of childhood ALL with a median reduction in expected adult height of 6.2 ± 3.2 cm in adults who had received 18 Gy of cranial radiation; children who were not exposed to cranial radiation also experienced modest decreases in final adult height.[368,369] Growth hormone replacement has been shown to be safe and effective at allowing pediatric ALL survivors to achieve comparable adult heights to those predicted at diagnosis, with no evidence of increased risk of disease recurrence.[370] Among survivors who received chemotherapy alone, self-reported age at menarche was similar to unaffected siblings; however, cranial radiation was associated with early menarche (<10 years; odds ratio 6.2), particularly when the exposure occurred at a young age.[371] Female survivors who received CRT around the time of menarche have decreased relative fertility compared to healthy siblings, as well as a prolonged time to first pregnancy.[372] Boys who undergo treatment for ALL as children may have decreased sperm counts, with CRT and cyclophosphamide exposure as risk factors. The St. Jude Lifetime Cohort Study found that boys who had CRT ≤26 Gy had no increased risk of azoospermia or oligospermia compared to boys who had no CRT.[373] However, diagnosis at age 5 to 9 years or cumulative cyclophosphamide equivalent doses ≥8 g/m^2 increased this risk significantly. Monitoring of endocrine late effects is of crucial importance because many of these sequelae may have significant negative impacts on HRQOL and can be treated with pharmacologic and behavioral interventions.

HEALTH DISPARITIES AND INEQUITIES IN ALL

For decades, patients from historically marginalized racial and ethnic backgrounds have consistently experienced worse survival. Since 1975, the stark differences in 5- and 10-year OS for Black vs white children under age 15 years have narrowed, with Black children experiencing almost double the improvements in annual percentage change in OS compared to white children.[374] However, while white AYA patients with ALL have experienced markedly improved OS, survival for Black AYAs has lagged significantly. Hispanic/Latino patients with ALL have more modest disparities in OS compared to white children but again have greater differences in outcomes among AYA patients.[374] In the current era, EFS and OS for Black and white patients with SR-ALL are similar.[375] In contrast, Black patients with HR-ALL had a nearly four-fold increased hazard of death and three-fold increased hazard of relapse or death compared to white patients in a model adjusted for race, sex, and public insurance.[375]

Genetic ancestry may explain a portion of the observed differences, as patients with Native American genetic ancestry are the most likely group to have ALL with CRLF2-R and lower rates of ETV6-RUNX1.[376] Patients with African genetic ancestry are more likely to have TCF3-PBX1 fusions and less likely to have favorable DUX4 alterations or hyperdiploidy than patients of Asian or European ancestry. However, even after controlling for biological risk factors, patients with Native American or African genetic ancestry have worse EFS, OS, and CIR than patients of Asian or European ancestry.[376] Among 24,979 children with ALL treated on COG trials, Hispanic and non-Hispanic Black patients had worse survival than non-Hispanic white or non-Hispanic Asian patients.[377] Adjustment for race-ethnicity, socioeconomic status proxied by insurance status, and disease prognosticators attenuated most of the increased hazard for Hispanic patients, but non-Hispanic Black patients persisted in having worse EFS even after adjusting for these factors (hazard ratio 1.32, $P < .0001$).[377]

Analyses focusing on adverse social determinants of health (SDOH) beyond demographic data commonly captured by clinical trials have uncovered additional factors mediating poor outcomes among patients from historically marginalized backgrounds. Residence in high-poverty areas conferred worse OS and was associated with 92% of relapses occurring early compared to only 48% in patients from the lowest poverty areas.[378] Notably, this did not differ by race or ethnicity. Texas cancer registry data indicate that among Hispanic patients, living in a Hispanic enclave or in an area with a high deprivation score was independently associated with a 30% to 67% increase in hazard of mortality.[379,380] Mediation analyses can determine relative contributions of direct and indirect factors associated with race and ethnicity on the outcomes. For example, using SEER data, Black patients with ALL had a 1.43-fold increased mortality risk ($P < .01$). The indirect effect of race on survival operating through the SDOH pathway had a hazard ratio of 1.17 ($P < .01$), thus accounting for 44% of the observed effect of race on outcome. Among Hispanic patients, SDOH accounted for 31% of the increased hazard of mortality.[381] Efforts to expand access to novel relapse therapies, such as targeted immunotherapies and alternative donor transplantation, are paramount, as Black and Hispanic patients are both more likely to experience relapse and barriers to accessing optimal care.[382]

CONCLUSION

The diagnosis, risk stratification, and treatment of children and adolescents with ALL have continued to evolve, such that a significant majority is cured with frontline chemotherapy regimens. For patients with favorable outcomes, ongoing research is investigating strategies to decrease acute and chronic toxicity while maintaining high cure rates. Advances in the understanding of the biology of ALL subtypes, such as Ph-like ALL, have improved risk stratification and allowed investigation of novel targeted agents for patients in these subgroups. The advent of novel immunotherapies, in particular CD19-targeted therapies, has offered effective options for patients with relapsed B-ALL, and their role in newly diagnosed very high-risk patients is now under investigation. Research efforts will continue to focus on those patient subgroups for whom outcomes with current therapies remain poor, including infants with *KMT2A*-R, T-ALL patients with relapse, B-ALL patients with early marrow relapse, and AYA patients.

References

1. Linabery AM, Ross JA. Trends in childhood cancer incidence in the U.S. (1992-2004). *Cancer.* 2008;112(2):416-432.
2. Smith MA, Seibel NL, Altekruse SF, et al. Outcomes for children and adolescents with cancer: challenges for the twenty-first century. *J Clin Oncol.* 2010;28(15):2625-2634.
3. Smith M, Ries L, Gurney J, Ross J. Leukemia. In: Ries L, Smith M, Gurney J, et al, eds. *Cancer Incidence and Survival Among Children and Adolescents: United States SEER Program 1975-1995.* National Cancer Institute, SEER Program; 1999:17-34. NIH Pub. No. 99-4649.
4. Hunger SP, Lu X, Devidas M, et al. Improved survival for children and adolescents with acute lymphoblastic leukemia between 1990 and 2005: a report from the children's oncology group. *J Clin Oncol.* 2012;30(14):1663-1669.
5. Nguyen K, Devidas M, Cheng SC, et al. Factors influencing survival after relapse from acute lymphoblastic leukemia: a Children's Oncology Group study. *Leukemia.* 2008;22(12):2142-2150.
6. Kratz CP, Stanulla M, Cave H. Genetic predisposition to acute lymphoblastic leukemia: overview on behalf of the I-BFM ALL host genetic variation working group. *Eur J Med Genet.* 2016;59(3):111-115.
7. Shah S, Schrader KA, Waanders E, et al. A recurrent germline PAX5 mutation confers susceptibility to pre-B cell acute lymphoblastic leukemia. *Nat Genet.* 2013;45(10):1226-1231.
8. Zhang J, Walsh MF, Wu G, et al. Germline mutations in predisposition genes in pediatric cancer. *N Engl J Med.* 2015;373(24):2336-2346.
9. Churchman ML, Qian M, Te Kronnie G, et al. Germline genetic IKZF1 variation and predisposition to childhood acute lymphoblastic leukemia. *Cancer Cell.* 2018;33(5):937-948 e938.
10. Pui CH, Nichols KE, Yang JJ. Somatic and germline genomics in paediatric acute lymphoblastic leukaemia. *Nat Rev Clin Oncol.* 2019;16(4):227-240.
11. Li Y, Schwab C, Ryan S, et al. Constitutional and somatic rearrangement of chromosome 21 in acute lymphoblastic leukaemia. *Nature.* 2014;508(7494):98-102.
12. Doll R, Wakeford R. Risk of childhood cancer from fetal irradiation. *Br J Radiol.* 1997;70:130-139.
13. Preston DL, Kusumi S, Tomonaga M, et al. Cancer incidence in atomic bomb survivors. Part III. Leukemia, lymphoma and multiple myeloma, 1950-1987. *Radiat Res.* 1994;137(2 suppl):S68-S97.
14. Gale KB, Ford AM, Repp R, et al. Backtracking leukemia to birth: identification of clonotypic gene fusion sequences in neonatal blood spots. *Proc Natl Acad Sci U S A.* 1997;94(25):13950-13954.
15. Taub JW, Konrad MA, Ge Y, et al. High frequency of leukemic clones in newborn screening blood samples of children with B-precursor acute lymphoblastic leukemia. *Blood.* 2002;99(8):2992-2996.
16. Wiemels JL, Ford AM, Van Wering ER, Postma A, Greaves M. Protracted and variable latency of acute lymphoblastic leukemia after TEL-AML1 gene fusion in utero. *Blood.* 1999;94(3):1057-1062.
17. Mori H, Colman SM, Xiao Z, et al. Chromosome translocations and covert leukemic clones are generated during normal fetal development. *Proc Natl Acad Sci U S A.* 2002;99(12):8242-8247.
18. Fidanza M, Seif AE, DeMicco A, et al. Inhibition of precursor B-cell malignancy progression by toll-like receptor ligand-induced immune responses. *Leukemia.* 2016;30(10):2116-2119.
19. Martin-Lorenzo A, Hauer J, Vicente-Duenas C, et al. Infection exposure is a causal factor in B-cell precursor acute lymphoblastic leukemia as a result of Pax5-inherited susceptibility. *Cancer Discov.* 2015;5(12):1328-1343.
20. Francis SS, Wallace AD, Wendt GA, et al. In utero cytomegalovirus infection and development of childhood acute lymphoblastic leukemia. *Blood.* 2017;129(12):1680-1684.
21. Greaves M. Infection, immune responses and the aetiology of childhood leukaemia. *Nat Rev Cancer.* 2006;6(3):193-203.
22. Clarke RT, Van den Bruel A, Bankhead C, Mitchell CD, Phillips B, Thompson MJ. Clinical presentation of childhood leukaemia: a systematic review and meta-analysis. *Arch Dis Child.* 2016;101(10):894-901.
23. Jones OY, Spencer CH, Bowyer SL, Dent PB, Gottlieb BS, Rabinovich CE. A multicenter case-control study on predictive factors distinguishing childhood leukemia from juvenile rheumatoid arthritis. *Pediatrics.* 2006;117(5):e840-e844.
24. Sinigaglia R, Gigante C, Bisinella G, Varotto S, Zanesco L, Turra S. Musculoskeletal manifestations in pediatric acute leukemia. *Journal of pediatric orthopedics.* 2008;28(1):20-28.
25. Arico M, Basso G, Mandelli F, et al. Good steroid response in vivo predicts a favorable outcome in children with T-cell acute lymphoblastic leukemia. The Associazione Italiana Ematologia Oncologia Pediatrica (AIEOP). *Cancer.* 1995;75(7):1684-1693.
26. Ingram LC, Fairclough DL, Furman WL, et al. Cranial nerve palsy in childhood acute lymphoblastic leukemia and non-Hodgkin's lymphoma. *Cancer.* 1991;67(9):2262-2268.
27. Sirvent N, Suciu S, Bertrand Y, Uyttebroeck A, Lescoeur B, Otten J. Overt testicular disease (OTD) at diagnosis is not associated with a poor prognosis in childhood acute lymphoblastic leukemia: results of the EORTC CLG Study 58881. *Pediatr Blood Cancer.* 2007;49(3):344-348.
28. Millot F, Robert A, Bertrand Y, et al. Cutaneous involvement in children with acute lymphoblastic leukemia or lymphoblastic lymphoma. The children's leukemia cooperative group of the European Organization of Research and Treatment of Cancer (EORTC). *Pediatrics.* 1997;100(1):60-64.
29. Boggs DR, Wintrobe MM, Cartwright GE. The acute leukemias. Analysis of 322 cases and review of the literature. *Medicine.* 1962;41:163-225.
30. Bunin NJ, Pui CH. Differing complications of hyperleukocytosis in children with acute lymphoblastic or acute nonlymphoblastic leukemia. *J Clin Oncol.* 1985;3(12):1590-1595.
31. Coiffier B, Altman A, Pui CH, Younes A, Cairo MS. Guidelines for the management of pediatric and adult tumor lysis syndrome: an evidence-based review. *J Clin Oncol.* 2008;26(16):2767-2778.
32. Pui CH, Mahmoud HH, Wiley JM, et al. Recombinant urate oxidase for the prophylaxis or treatment of hyperuricemia in patients with leukemia or lymphoma. *J Clin Oncol.* 2001;19(3):697-704.
33. Thastrup M, Marquart HV, Levinsen M, et al. Flow cytometric detection of leukemic blasts in cerebrospinal fluid predicts risk of relapse in childhood acute lymphoblastic leukemia: a Nordic Society of Pediatric Hematology and Oncology study. *Leukemia.* 2020;34(2):336-346.
34. Mastrangelo R, Poplack D, Bleyer A, Riccardi R, Sather H, D'Angio G. Report and recommendations of the Rome workshop concerning poor-prognosis acute lymphoblastic leukemia in children: biologic bases for staging, stratification, and treatment. *Med Pediatr Oncol.* 1986;14(3):191-194.
35. Smith M, Bleyer A, Crist W, Murphy S, Sallan SE. Uniform criteria for childhood acute lymphoblastic leukemia risk classification. *J Clin Oncol.* 1996;14(2):680-681.
36. Pui CH, Behm FG, Downing JR, et al. 11q23/MLL rearrangement confers a poor prognosis in infants with acute lymphoblastic leukemia. *J Clin Oncol.* 1994;12(5):909-915.
37. Mann G, Attarbaschi A, Schrappe M, et al. Improved outcome with hematopoietic stem cell transplantation in a poor prognostic subgroup of infants with mixed-lineage-leukemia (MLL)-rearranged acute lymphoblastic leukemia: results from the Interfant-99 Study. *Blood.* 2010;116(15):2644-2650.
38. De Lorenzo P, Moorman AV, Pieters R, et al. Cytogenetics and outcome of infants with acute lymphoblastic leukemia and absence of MLL rearrangements. *Leukemia.* 2014;28(2):428-430.
39. Stock W, La M, Sanford B, et al. What determines the outcomes for adolescents and young adults with acute lymphoblastic leukemia treated on cooperative group protocols? A comparison of Children's Cancer Group and Cancer and Leukemia Group B studies. *Blood.* 2008;112(5):1646-1654.
40. Winter SS, Dunsmore KP, Devidas M, et al. Improved survival for children and young adults with T-lineage acute lymphoblastic leukemia: results from the children's oncology group AALL0434 methotrexate randomization. *J Clin Oncol.* 2018;36(29):2926-2934.
41. Teachey DT, Pui CH. Comparative features and outcomes between paediatric T-cell and B-cell acute lymphoblastic leukaemia. *Lancet Oncol.* 2019;20(3):e142-e154.
42. Burger B, Zimmermann M, Mann G, et al. Diagnostic cerebrospinal fluid examination in children with acute lymphoblastic leukemia: significance of low leukocyte counts with blasts or traumatic lumbar puncture. *J Clin Oncol.* 2003;21(2):184-188.
43. Pui CH, Howard SC. Current management and challenges of malignant disease in the CNS in paediatric leukaemia. *Lancet Oncol.* 2008;9(3):257-268.
44. Hijiya N, Liu W, Sandlund JT, et al. Overt testicular disease at diagnosis of childhood acute lymphoblastic leukemia: lack of therapeutic role of local irradiation. *Leukemia.* 2005;19(8):1399-1403.
45. Tasian SK, Hunger SP. Genomic characterization of paediatric acute lymphoblastic leukaemia: an opportunity for precision medicine therapeutics. *Br J Haematol.* 2017;176(6):867-882.
46. Moorman AV, Ensor HM, Richards SM, et al. Prognostic effect of chromosomal abnormalities in childhood B-cell precursor acute lymphoblastic leukaemia: results from the UK Medical Research Council ALL97/99 randomised trial. *Lancet Oncol.* 2010;11(5):429-438.
47. Paulsson K, Forestier E, Andersen MK, et al. High modal number and triple trisomies are highly correlated favorable factors in childhood B-cell precursor high hyperdiploid acute lymphoblastic leukemia treated according to the NOPHO ALL 1992/2000 protocols. *Haematologica.* 2013;98(9):1424-1432.
48. Maloney K, McGavran L, Murphy J, et al. TEL-AML1 fusion identifies a subset of children with standard risk acute lymphoblastic leukemia who have an excellent prognosis when treated with therapy that includes a single delayed intensification. *Leukemia.* 1999;13(11):1708-1712.
49. Hunger SP. Chromosomal translocations involving the E2A gene in acute lymphoblastic leukemia: clinical features and molecular pathogenesis. *Blood.* 1996;87(4):1211-1224.

50. Nachman JB, Heerema NA, Sather H, et al. Outcome of treatment in children with hypodiploid acute lymphoblastic leukemia. *Blood*. 2007;110(4):1112-1115.
51. Holmfeldt L, Wei L, Diaz-Flores E, et al. The genomic landscape of hypodiploid acute lymphoblastic leukemia. *Nat Genet*. 2013;45(3):242-252.
52. Harrison CJ, Moorman AV, Schwab C, et al. An international study of intrachromosomal amplification of chromosome 21 (iAMP21): cytogenetic characterization and outcome. *Leukemia*. 2014;28(5):1015-1021.
53. Attarbaschi A, Mann G, Panzer-Grumayer R, et al. Minimal residual disease values discriminate between low and high relapse risk in children with B-cell precursor acute lymphoblastic leukemia and an intrachromosomal amplification of chromosome 21: the Austrian and German acute lymphoblastic leukemia Berlin-Frankfurt-Munster (ALL-BFM) trials. *J Clin Oncol*. 2008;26(18):3046-3050.
54. Heerema NA, Carroll AJ, Devidas M, et al. Intrachromosomal amplification of chromosome 21 is associated with inferior outcomes in children with acute lymphoblastic leukemia treated in contemporary standard-risk children's oncology group studies: a report from the children's oncology group. *J Clin Oncol*. 2013;31(27):3397-3402.
55. Moorman AV, Robinson H, Schwab C, et al. Risk-directed treatment intensification significantly reduces the risk of relapse among children and adolescents with acute lymphoblastic leukemia and intrachromosomal amplification of chromosome 21: a comparison of the MRC ALL97/99 and UKALL2003 trials. *J Clin Oncol*. 2013;31(27):3389-3396.
56. Arico M, Schrappe M, Hunger SP, et al. Clinical outcome of children with newly diagnosed Philadelphia chromosome-positive acute lymphoblastic leukemia treated between 1995 and 2005. *J Clin Oncol*. 2010;28(31):4755-4761.
57. Schultz KR, Bowman WP, Aledo A, et al. Improved early event-free survival with imatinib in Philadelphia chromosome-positive acute lymphoblastic leukemia: a children's oncology group study. *J Clin Oncol*. 2009;27(31):5175-5181.
58. Roberts KG, Li Y, Payne-Turner D, et al. Targetable kinase-activating lesions in Ph-like acute lymphoblastic leukemia. *N Engl J Med*. 2014;371(11):1005-1015.
59. Mullighan CG, Su X, Zhang J, et al. Deletion of IKZF1 and prognosis in acute lymphoblastic leukemia. *N Engl J Med*. 2009;360(5):470-480.
60. van der Veer A, Waanders E, Pieters R, et al. Independent prognostic value of BCR-ABL1-like signature and IKZF1 deletion, but not high CRLF2 expression, in children with B-cell precursor ALL. *Blood*. 2013;122(15):2622-2629.
61. Boer JM, van der Veer A, Rizopoulos D, et al. Prognostic value of rare IKZF1 deletion in childhood B-cell precursor acute lymphoblastic leukemia: an international collaborative study. *Leukemia*. 2016;30(1):32-38.
62. Harvey RC, Mullighan CG, Chen IM, et al. Rearrangement of CRLF2 is associated with mutation of JAK kinases, alteration of IKZF1, Hispanic/Latino ethnicity, and a poor outcome in pediatric B-progenitor acute lymphoblastic leukemia. *Blood*. 2010;115(26):5312-5321.
63. Ensor HM, Schwab C, Russell LJ, et al. Demographic, clinical, and outcome features of children with acute lymphoblastic leukemia and CRLF2 deregulation: results from the MRC ALL97 clinical trial. *Blood*. 2011;117(7):2129-2136.
64. Chen IM, Harvey RC, Mullighan CG, et al. Outcome modeling with CRLF2, IKZF1, JAK, and minimal residual disease in pediatric acute lymphoblastic leukemia: a Children's Oncology Group study. *Blood*. 2012;119(15):3512-3522.
65. Gu Z, Churchman ML, Roberts KG, et al. PAX5-driven subtypes of B-progenitor acute lymphoblastic leukemia. *Nat Genet*. 2019;51(2):296-307.
66. Schrappe M, Reiter A, Zimmermann M, et al. Long-term results of four consecutive trials in childhood ALL performed by the ALL-BFM study group from 1981 to 1995. Berlin-Frankfurt-Munster. *Leukemia*. 2000;14(12):2205-2222.
67. Nachman JB, Sather HN, Sensel MG, et al. Augmented post-induction therapy for children with high-risk acute lymphoblastic leukemia and a slow response to initial therapy. *N Engl J Med*. 1998;338(23):1663-1671.
68. Pui CH, Pei D, Raimondi SC, et al. Clinical impact of minimal residual disease in children with different subtypes of acute lymphoblastic leukemia treated with Response-Adapted therapy. *Leukemia*. 2017;31(2):333-339.
69. Flohr T, Schrauder A, Cazzaniga G, et al. Minimal residual disease-directed risk stratification using real-time quantitative PCR analysis of immunoglobulin and T-cell receptor gene rearrangements in the international multicenter trial AIEOP-BFM ALL 2000 for childhood acute lymphoblastic leukemia. *Leukemia*. 2008;22(4):771-782.
70. Borowitz MJ, Devidas M, Hunger SP, et al. Clinical significance of minimal residual disease in childhood acute lymphoblastic leukemia and its relationship to other prognostic factors: a Children's Oncology Group study. *Blood*. 2008;111(12):5477-5485.
71. Conter V, Bartram CR, Valsecchi MG, et al. Molecular response to treatment redefines all prognostic factors in children and adolescents with B-cell precursor acute lymphoblastic leukemia: results in 3184 patients of the AIEOP-BFM ALL 2000 study. *Blood*. 2010;115(16):3206-3214.
72. Borowitz MJ, Wood BL, Devidas M, et al. Prognostic significance of minimal residual disease in high risk B-ALL: a report from Children's Oncology Group study AALL0232. *Blood*. 2015;126(8):964-971.
73. Schumich A, Maurer-Granofszky M, Attarbaschi A, et al. Flow-cytometric minimal residual disease monitoring in blood predicts relapse risk in pediatric B-cell precursor acute lymphoblastic leukemia in trial AIEOP-BFM ALL 2000. *Pediatr Blood Cancer*. 2019;66(5):e27590.
74. Maloney KW, Devidas M, Wang C, et al. Outcome in children with standard-risk B-cell acute lymphoblastic leukemia: results of children's oncology group trial AALL0331. *J Clin Oncol*. 2020;38(6):602-612.
75. Sidhom I, Shaaban K, Youssef SH, et al. Reduced-intensity therapy for pediatric lymphoblastic leukemia: impact of residual disease early in remission induction. *Blood*. 2021;137(1):20-28.
76. Wood B, Wu D, Crossley B, et al. Measurable residual disease detection by high-throughput sequencing improves risk stratification for pediatric B-ALL. *Blood*. 2018;131(12):1350-1359.
77. Rau RE, Dai Y, Devidas M, et al. Prognostic impact of minimal residual disease at the end of consolidation in NCI standard-risk B-lymphoblastic leukemia: a report from the Children's Oncology Group. *Pediatr Blood Cancer*. 2021;68(4):e28929.
78. Schrappe M, Valsecchi MG, Bartram CR, et al. Late MRD response determines relapse risk overall and in subsets of childhood T-cell ALL: results of the AIEOP-BFM-ALL 2000 study. *Blood*. 2011;118(8):2077-2084.
79. Balduzzi A, Valsecchi MG, Uderzo C, et al. Chemotherapy versus allogeneic transplantation for very-high-risk childhood acute lymphoblastic leukaemia in first complete remission: comparison by genetic randomisation in an international prospective study. *Lancet*. 2005;366(9486):635-642.
80. Schrappe M, Hunger SP, Pui CH, et al. Outcomes after induction failure in childhood acute lymphoblastic leukemia. *N Engl J Med*. 2012;366(15):1371-1381.
81. O'Connor D, Moorman AV, Wade R, et al. Use of minimal residual disease assessment to redefine induction failure in pediatric acute lymphoblastic leukemia. *J Clin Oncol*. 2017;35(6):660-667.
82. Gupta S, Devidas M, Loh ML, et al. Flow-cytometric vs. -morphologic assessment of remission in childhood acute lymphoblastic leukemia: a report from the Children's Oncology Group (COG). *Leukemia*. 2018;32(6):1370-1379.
83. Buchmann S, Schrappe M, Baruchel A, et al. Remission, treatment failure, and relapse in pediatric ALL: an international consensus of the Ponte-di-Legno Consortium. *Blood*. 2021;139(12):1785-1793. doi:10.1182/blood.2021012328
84. Pui CH, Mullighan CG, Evans WE, Relling MV. Pediatric acute lymphoblastic leukemia: where are we going and how do we get there? *Blood*. 2012;120(6):1165-1174.
85. Moricke A, Zimmermann M, Reiter A, et al. Long-term results of five consecutive trials in childhood acute lymphoblastic leukemia performed by the ALL-BFM study group from 1981 to 2000. *Leukemia*. 2010;24(2):265-284.
86. Mitchell C, Richards S, Harrison CJ, Eden T. Long-term follow-up of the United Kingdom medical research council protocols for childhood acute lymphoblastic leukaemia, 1980-2001. *Leukemia*. 2010;24(2):406-418.
87. Silverman LB, Stevenson KE, O'Brien JE, et al. Long-term results of Dana-Farber Cancer Institute ALL Consortium protocols for children with newly diagnosed acute lymphoblastic leukemia (1985-2000). *Leukemia*. 2010;24(2):320-334.
88. Gaynon PS, Angiolillo AL, Carroll WL, et al. Long-term results of the children's cancer group studies for childhood acute lymphoblastic leukemia 1983-2002: a Children's Oncology Group Report. *Leukemia*. 2010;24(2):285-297.
89. Inaba H, Pui CH. Glucocorticoid use in acute lymphoblastic leukaemia. *Lancet Oncol*. 2010;11(11):1096-1106.
90. Bostrom BC, Sensel MR, Sather HN, et al. Dexamethasone versus prednisone and daily oral versus weekly intravenous mercaptopurine for patients with standard-risk acute lymphoblastic leukemia: a report from the Children's Cancer Group. *Blood*. 2003;101(10):3809-3817.
91. Mitchell CD, Richards SM, Kinsey SE, et al. Benefit of dexamethasone compared with prednisolone for childhood acute lymphoblastic leukaemia: results of the UK Medical Research Council ALL97 randomized trial. *Br J Haematol*. 2005;129(6):734-745.
92. Igarashi S, Manabe A, Ohara A, et al. No advantage of dexamethasone over prednisolone for the outcome of standard- and intermediate-risk childhood acute lymphoblastic leukemia in the Tokyo Children's Cancer Study Group L95-14 protocol. *J Clin Oncol*. 2005;23(27):6489-6498.
93. Domenech C, Suciu S, De Moerloose B, et al. Dexamethasone (6 mg/m2/day) and prednisolone (60 mg/m2/day) were equally effective as induction therapy for childhood acute lymphoblastic leukemia in the EORTC CLG 58951 randomized trial. *Haematologica*. 2014;99(7):1220-1227.
94. Larsen EC, Devidas M, Chen S, et al. Dexamethasone and high-dose methotrexate improve outcome for children and young adults with high-risk B-acute lymphoblastic leukemia: a report from children's oncology group study AALL0232. *J Clin Oncol*. 2016;34(20):2380-2388.
95. Moricke A, Zimmermann M, Valsecchi MG, et al. Dexamethasone vs prednisone in induction treatment of pediatric ALL: results of the randomized trial AIEOP-BFM ALL 2000. *Blood*. 2016;127(17):2101-2112.
96. Vora A, Goulden N, Mitchell C, et al. Augmented post-remission therapy for a minimal residual disease-defined high-risk subgroup of children and young people with clinical standard-risk and intermediate-risk acute lymphoblastic leukaemia (UKALL 2003): a randomised controlled trial. *Lancet Oncol*. 2014;15(8):809-818.
97. Asselin B, Rizzari C. Asparaginase pharmacokinetics and implications of therapeutic drug monitoring. *Leuk Lymphoma*. 2015;56(8):2273-2280.
98. Asselin BL, Whitin JC, Coppola DJ, Rupp IP, Sallan SE, Cohen HJ. Comparative pharmacokinetic studies of three asparaginase preparations. *J Clin Oncol*. 1993;11(9):1780-1786.
99. Panetta JC, Gajjar A, Hijiya N, et al. Comparison of native E. coli and PEG asparaginase pharmacokinetics and pharmacodynamics in pediatric acute lymphoblastic leukemia. *Clin Pharmacol Ther*. 2009;86(6):651-658.
100. Pui CH, Pei D, Campana D, et al. A revised definition for cure of childhood acute lymphoblastic leukemia. *Leukemia*. 2014;28(12):2336-2343.
101. Simone JV, Aur RJ, Hustu HO, Verzosa M, Pinkel D. Combined modality therapy of acute lymphocytic leukemia. *Cancer*. 1975;35(1):25-35.
102. Simone J, Aur RJ, Hustu HO, Pinkel D. "Total therapy" studies of acute lymphocytic leukemia in children. Current results and prospects for cure. *Cancer*. 1972;30(6):1488-1494.
103. Goldsby RE, Liu Q, Nathan PC, et al. Late-occurring neurologic sequelae in adult survivors of childhood acute lymphoblastic leukemia: a report from the Childhood Cancer Survivor Study. *J Clin Oncol*. 2010;28(2):324-331.
104. Krull KR, Brinkman TM, Li C, et al. Neurocognitive outcomes decades after treatment for childhood acute lymphoblastic leukemia: a report from the St Jude lifetime cohort study. *J Clin Oncol*. 2013;31(35):4407-4415.

105. Richards S, Pui CH, Gayon P. Childhood Acute Lymphoblastic Leukemia Collaborative Group. Systematic review and meta-analysis of randomized trials of central nervous system directed therapy for childhood acute lymphoblastic leukemia. *Pediatr Blood Cancer*. 2013;60(2):185-195.
106. Vora A, Andreano A, Pui CH, et al. Influence of cranial radiotherapy on outcome in children with acute lymphoblastic leukemia treated with contemporary therapy. *J Clin Oncol*. 2016;34(9):919-926.
107. Pui CH, Campana D, Pei D, et al. Treating childhood acute lymphoblastic leukemia without cranial irradiation. *N Engl J Med*. 2009;360(26):2730-2741.
108. Veerman AJ, Kamps WA, van den Berg H, et al. Dexamethasone-based therapy for childhood acute lymphoblastic leukaemia: results of the prospective Dutch Childhood Oncology Group (DCOG) protocol ALL-9 (1997-2004). *Lancet Oncol*. 2009;10(10):957-966.
109. Dunsmore KP, Winter SS, Devidas M, et al. Children's oncology group AALL0434: a phase III randomized clinical trial testing nelarabine in newly diagnosed T-cell acute lymphoblastic leukemia. *J Clin Oncol*. 2020;38(28):3282-3293.
110. Riehm H, Gadner H, Henze G, et al. Results and significance of six randomized trials in four consecutive ALL-BFM studies. *Haematol Blood Transfus*. 1990;33:439-450.
111. Henze G, Langermann HJ, Ritter J, Schellong G, Riehm H. Treatment strategy for different risk groups in childhood acute lymphoblastic leukemia: a Report from the BFM Study Group. *Haematol Blood Transfus*. 1981;26:87-93.
112. Capizzi RL. Asparaginase-methotrexate in combination chemotherapy: schedule-dependent differential effects on normal versus neoplastic cells. *Cancer Treat Rep*. 1981;65(suppl 4):115-121.
113. Seibel NL, Steinherz PG, Sather HN, et al. Early postinduction intensification therapy improves survival for children and adolescents with high-risk acute lymphoblastic leukemia: a report from the Children's Oncology Group. *Blood*. 2008;111(5):2548-2555.
114. Matloub Y, Bostrom BC, Hunger SP, et al. Escalating intravenous methotrexate improves event-free survival in children with standard-risk acute lymphoblastic leukemia: a report from the Children's Oncology Group. *Blood*. 2011;118(2):243-251.
115. Silverman LB, Gelber RD, Dalton VK, et al. Improved outcome for children with acute lymphoblastic leukemia: results of Dana-Farber Consortium Protocol 91-01. *Blood*. 2001;97(5):1211-1218.
116. Place AE, Stevenson KE, Vrooman LM, et al. Intravenous pegylated asparaginase versus intramuscular native *Escherichia coli* L-asparaginase in newly diagnosed childhood acute lymphoblastic leukaemia (DFCI 05-001): a randomised, open-label phase 3 trial. *Lancet Oncol*. 2015;16(16):1677-1690.
117. Gupta S, Wang C, Raetz EA, et al. Impact of asparaginase discontinuation on outcome in childhood acute lymphoblastic leukemia: a report from the children's oncology group. *J Clin Oncol*. 2020;38(17):1897-1905.
118. Vrooman LM, Stevenson KE, Supko JG, et al. Postinduction dexamethasone and individualized dosing of *Escherichia Coli* L-asparaginase each improve outcome of children and adolescents with newly diagnosed acute lymphoblastic leukemia: results from a randomized study—Dana-Farber Cancer Institute ALL Consortium Protocol 00-01. *J Clin Oncol*. 2013;31(9):1202-1210.
119. Swanson HD, Panetta JC, Barker PJ, et al. Predicting success of desensitization after pegaspargase allergy. *Blood*. 2020;135(1):71-75.
120. van der Sluis IM, Vrooman LM, Pieters R, et al. Consensus expert recommendations for identification and management of asparaginase hypersensitivity and silent inactivation. *Haematologica*. 2016;101(3):279-285.
121. Pieters R, Hunger SP, Boos J, et al. L-asparaginase treatment in acute lymphoblastic leukemia: a focus on Erwinia asparaginase. *Cancer*. 2011;117(2):238-249.
122. Salzer WL, Asselin B, Supko JG, et al. Erwinia asparaginase achieves therapeutic activity after pegaspargase allergy: a report from the Children's Oncology Group. *Blood*. 2013;122(4):507-514.
123. Maese L, Rau RE, Raetz EA, et al. Open-label, multicenter, phase 2/3 study of Recombinant Crisantaspase produced in Pseudomonas Fluorescens (RC-P) in patients with Acute Lymphoblastic Leukemia (ALL) or Lymphoblastic Lymphoma (LBL) following hypersensitivity to *Escherichia coli*-derived asparaginases. *Blood*. 2019;134(suppl_1):2586.
124. Rivera GK, Pinkel D, Simone JV, Hancock ML, Crist WM. Treatment of acute lymphoblastic leukemia. 30 years' experience at St. Jude Children's Research Hospital. *N Engl J Med*. 1993;329(18):1289-1295.
125. Teachey DT, Hunger SP, Loh ML. Optimizing therapy in the modern age: differences in length of maintenance therapy in acute lymphoblastic leukemia. *Blood*. 2021;137(2):168-177.
126. Kato M, Ishimaru S, Seki M, et al. Long-term outcome of 6-month maintenance chemotherapy for acute lymphoblastic leukemia in children. *Leukemia*. 2017;31(3):580-584.
127. Balis FM, Holcenberg JS, Poplack DG, et al. Pharmacokinetics and pharmacodynamics of oral methotrexate and mercaptopurine in children with lower risk acute lymphoblastic leukemia: a joint children's cancer group and pediatric oncology branch study. *Blood*. 1998;92(10):3569-3577.
128. Schmiegelow K, Nielsen SN, Frandsen TL, Nersting J. Mercaptopurine/Methotrexate maintenance therapy of childhood acute lymphoblastic leukemia: clinical facts and fiction. *J Pediatr Hematol Oncol*. 2014;36(7):503-517.
129. Schmiegelow K, Nersting J, Nielsen SN, et al. Maintenance therapy of childhood acute lymphoblastic leukemia revisited-should drug doses be adjusted by white blood cell, neutrophil, or lymphocyte counts? *Pediatr Blood Cancer*. 2016;63(12):2104-2111.
130. Nielsen SN, Grell K, Nersting J, et al. DNA-thioguanine nucleotide concentration and relapse-free survival during maintenance therapy of childhood acute lymphoblastic leukaemia (NOPHO ALL2008): a prospective substudy of a phase 3 trial. *Lancet Oncol*. 2017;18(4):515-524.
131. Stork LC, Matloub Y, Broxson E, et al. Oral 6-mercaptopurine versus oral 6-thioguanine and veno-occlusive disease in children with standard-risk acute lymphoblastic leukemia: report of the Children's Oncology Group CCG-1952 clinical trial. *Blood*. 2010;115(14):2740-2748.
132. Vora A, Mitchell CD, Lennard L, et al. Toxicity and efficacy of 6-thioguanine versus 6-mercaptopurine in childhood lymphoblastic leukaemia: a randomised trial. *Lancet*. 2006;368(9544):1339-1348.
133. Larsen RH, Utke Rank C, Grell K, et al. Increments in DNA-thioguanine level during thiopurine enhanced maintenance therapy of acute lymphoblastic leukemia. *Haematologica*. 2021;106(11):2824-2833. doi:10.3324/haematol.2020.278166
134. Cohen G, Cooper S, Sison EA, Annesley C, Bhuiyan M, Brown P. Allopurinol use during pediatric acute lymphoblastic leukemia maintenance therapy safely corrects skewed 6-mercaptopurine metabolism, improving inadequate myelosuppression and reducing gastrointestinal toxicity. *Pediatr Blood Cancer*. 2020;67(11):e28360.
135. Miller MB, Brackett J, Schafer ES, Rau RE. Prevention of mercaptopurine-induced hypoglycemia using allopurinol to reduce methylated thiopurine metabolites. *Pediatr Blood Cancer*. 2019;66(4):e27577.
136. Zerra P, Bergsagel J, Keller FG, Lew G, Pauly M. Maintenance treatment with low-dose mercaptopurine in combination with allopurinol in children with acute lymphoblastic leukemia and mercaptopurine-induced pancreatitis. *Pediatr Blood Cancer*. 2016;63(4):712-715.
137. Conneely SE, Cooper SL, Rau RE. Use of allopurinol to mitigate 6-mercaptopurine associated gastrointestinal toxicity in acute lymphoblastic leukemia. *Front Oncol*. 2020;10:1129.
138. Relling MV, Gardner EE, Sandborn WJ, et al. Clinical pharmacogenetics implementation consortium guidelines for thiopurine methyltransferase genotype and thiopurine dosing: 2013 update. *Clin Pharmacol Ther*. 2013;93(4):324-325.
139. Yang JJ, Landier W, Yang W, et al. Inherited NUDT15 variant is a genetic determinant of mercaptopurine intolerance in children with acute lymphoblastic leukemia. *J Clin Oncol*. 2015;33(11):1235-1242.
140. Moriyama T, Nishii R, Perez-Andreu V, et al. NUDT15 polymorphisms alter thiopurine metabolism and hematopoietic toxicity. *Nat Genet*. 2016;48(4):367-373.
141. Rivard GE, Infante-Rivard C, Hoyoux C, Champagne J. Maintenance chemotherapy for childhood acute lymphoblastic leukaemia: better in the evening. *Lancet*. 1985;2(8467):1264-1266.
142. de Lemos ML, Hamata L, Jennings S, Leduc T. Interaction between mercaptopurine and milk. *J Oncol Pharm Pract*. 2007;13(4):237-240.
143. Schmiegelow K, Glomstein A, Kristinsson J, Salmi T, Schroder H, Bjork O. Impact of morning versus evening schedule for oral methotrexate and 6-mercaptopurine on relapse risk for children with acute lymphoblastic leukemia. Nordic Society for Pediatric Hematology and Oncology (NOPHO). *J Pediatr Hematol Oncol*. 1997;19(2):102-109.
144. Clemmensen KK, Christensen RH, Shabaneh DN, et al. The circadian schedule for childhood acute lymphoblastic leukemia maintenance therapy does not influence event-free survival in the NOPHO ALL92 protocol. *Pediatr Blood Cancer*. 2014;61(4):653-658.
145. Bhatia S, Landier W, Hageman L, et al. Systemic exposure to thiopurines and risk of relapse in children with acute lymphoblastic leukemia: a children's oncology group study. *JAMA Oncol*. 2015;1(3):287-295.
146. Bhatia S, Hageman L, Chen Y, et al. Effect of a daily text messaging and directly supervised therapy intervention on oral mercaptopurine adherence in children with acute lymphoblastic leukemia: a randomized clinical trial. *JAMA Netw Open*. 2020;3(8):e2014205.
147. Eden T, Pieters R, Richards S. Childhood Acute Lymphoblastic Leukaemia Collaborative Group. Systematic review of the addition of vincristine plus steroid pulses in maintenance treatment for childhood acute lymphoblastic leukaemia: an individual patient data meta-analysis involving 5,659 children. *Br J Haematol*. 2010;149(5):722-733.
148. Bleyer WA, Sather HN, Nickerson HJ, et al. Monthly pulses of vincristine and prednisone prevent bone marrow and testicular relapse in low-risk childhood acute lymphoblastic leukemia: a report of the CCG-161 study by the Childrens Cancer Study Group. *J Clin Oncol*. 1991;9(6):1012-1021.
149. Conter V, Valsecchi MG, Silvestri D, et al. Pulses of vincristine and dexamethasone in addition to intensive chemotherapy for children with intermediate-risk acute lymphoblastic leukaemia: a multicentre randomised trial. *Lancet*. 2007;369(9556):123-131.
150. Angiolillo AL, Schore RJ, Kairalla JA, et al. Excellent outcomes with reduced frequency of vincristine and dexamethasone pulses in standard-risk B-lymphoblastic leukemia: results from children's oncology group AALL0932. *J Clin Oncol*. 2021;39(13):1437-1447.
151. Mattano LA, Jr, Sather HN, Trigg ME, Nachman JB. Osteonecrosis as a complication of treating acute lymphoblastic leukemia in children: a report from the Children's Cancer Group. *J Clin Oncol*. 2000;18(18):3262-3272.
152. Suryanarayan K, Hunger SP, Kohler S, et al. Consistent involvement of the bcr gene by 9;22 breakpoints in pediatric acute leukemias. *Blood*. 1991;77(2):324-330.
153. Biondi A, Schrappe M, De Lorenzo P, et al. Imatinib after induction for treatment of children and adolescents with Philadelphia-chromosome-positive acute lymphoblastic leukaemia (EsPhALL): a randomised, open-label, intergroup study. *Lancet Oncol*. 2012;13(9):936-945.
154. Shen S, Chen X, Cai J, et al. Effect of dasatinib vs imatinib in the treatment of pediatric Philadelphia chromosome-positive acute lymphoblastic leukemia: a randomized clinical trial. *JAMA Oncol*. 2020;6(3):358-366.
155. Slayton WB, Schultz KR, Silverman LB, Hunger SP. How we approach Philadelphia chromosome-positive acute lymphoblastic leukemia in children and young adults. *Pediatr Blood Cancer*. 2020;67(10):e28543.
156. Den Boer ML, van Slegtenhorst M, De Menezes RX, et al. A subtype of childhood acute lymphoblastic leukaemia with poor treatment outcome: a genome-wide classification study. *Lancet Oncol*. 2009;10(2):125-134.
157. Kuiper RP, Waanders E, van der Velden VH, et al. IKZF1 deletions predict relapse in uniformly treated pediatric precursor B-ALL. *Leukemia*. 2010;24(7):1258-1264.
158. Tasian SK, Loh ML, Hunger SP. Philadelphia chromosome-like acute lymphoblastic leukemia. *Blood*. 2017;130(19):2064-2072.

159. Mullighan CG, Collins-Underwood JR, Phillips LA, et al. Rearrangement of CRLF2 in B-progenitor- and Down syndrome-associated acute lymphoblastic leukemia. *Nat Genet.* 2009;41(11):1243-1246.
160. Russell LJ, Capasso M, Vater I, et al. Deregulated expression of cytokine receptor gene, CRLF2, is involved in lymphoid transformation in B-cell precursor acute lymphoblastic leukemia. *Blood.* 2009;114(13):2688-2698.
161. Hertzberg L, Vendramini E, Ganmore I, et al. Down syndrome acute lymphoblastic leukemia, a highly heterogeneous disease in which aberrant expression of CRLF2 is associated with mutated JAK2: a report from the International BFM Study Group. *Blood.* 2010;115(5):1006-1017.
162. Yoda A, Yoda Y, Chiaretti S, et al. Functional screening identifies CRLF2 in precursor B-cell acute lymphoblastic leukemia. *Proc Natl Acad Sci U S A.* 2010;107(1):252-257.
163. Mullighan CG, Zhang J, Harvey RC, et al. JAK mutations in high-risk childhood acute lymphoblastic leukemia. *Proc Natl Acad Sci U S A.* 2009;106(23):9414-9418.
164. Iacobucci I, Li Y, Roberts KG, et al. Truncating erythropoietin receptor rearrangements in acute lymphoblastic leukemia. *Cancer Cell.* 2016;29(2):186-200.
165. Perez-Garcia A, Ambesi-Impiombato A, Hadler M, et al. Genetic loss of SH2B3 in acute lymphoblastic leukemia. *Blood.* 2013;122(14):2425-2432.
166. Shochat C, Tal N, Bandapalli OR, et al. Gain-of-function mutations in interleukin-7 receptor-alpha (IL7R) in childhood acute lymphoblastic leukemias. *J Exp Med.* 2011;208(5):901-908.
167. Maude SL, Dolai S, Delgado-Martin C, et al. Efficacy of JAK/STAT pathway inhibition in murine xenograft models of early T-cell precursor (ETP) acute lymphoblastic leukemia. *Blood.* 2015;125(11):1759-1767.
168. Maude SL, Tasian SK, Vincent T, et al. Targeting JAK1/2 and mTOR in murine xenograft models of Ph-like acute lymphoblastic leukemia. *Blood.* 2012;120(17):3510-3518.
169. Tasian SK, Doral MY, Borowitz MJ, et al. Aberrant STAT5 and PI3K/mTOR pathway signaling occurs in human CRLF2-rearranged B-precursor acute lymphoblastic leukemia. *Blood.* 2012;120(4):833-842.
170. Schwab C, Ryan SL, Chilton L, et al. EBF1-PDGFRB fusion in pediatric B-cell precursor acute lymphoblastic leukemia (BCP-ALL): genetic profile and clinical implications. *Blood.* 2016;127(18):2214-2218.
171. Kobayashi K, Miyagawa N, Mitsui K, et al. TKI dasatinib monotherapy for a patient with Ph-like ALL bearing ATF7IP/PDGFRB translocation. *Pediatr Blood Cancer.* 2015;62(6):1058-1060.
172. Perwein T, Strehl S, Konig M, et al. Imatinib-induced long-term remission in a relapsed RCSD1-ABL1-positive acute lymphoblastic leukemia. *Haematologica.* 2016;101(8):e332-e335.
173. Weston BW, Hayden MA, Roberts KG, et al. Tyrosine kinase inhibitor therapy induces remission in a patient with refractory EBF1-PDGFRB-positive acute lymphoblastic leukemia. *J Clin Oncol.* 2013;31(25):e413-e416.
174. Tanasi I, Ba I, Sirvent N, et al. Efficacy of tyrosine kinase inhibitors in Ph-like acute lymphoblastic leukemia harboring ABL-class rearrangements. *Blood.* 2019;134(16):1351-1355.
175. Vora A, Wade R, Mitchell CD, Goulden N, Richards S. Improved outcome for children and young adults with T-cell acute lymphoblastic leukaemia (ALL): results of the United Kingdom medical research council (MRC) trial UKALL 2003. *Blood.* 2008;112(11):908.
176. Coustan-Smith E, Mullighan CG, Onciu M, et al. Early T-cell precursor leukaemia: a subtype of very high-risk acute lymphoblastic leukaemia. *Lancet Oncol.* 2009;10(2):147-156.
177. Patrick K, Wade R, Goulden N, et al. Outcome for children and young people with Early T-cell precursor acute lymphoblastic leukaemia treated on a contemporary protocol, UKALL 2003. *Br J Haematol.* 2014;166(3):421-424.
178. Conter V, Valsecchi MG, Buldini B, et al. Early T-cell precursor acute lymphoblastic leukaemia in children treated in AIEOP centres with AIEOP-BFM protocols: a retrospective analysis. *Lancet Haematol.* 2016;3(2):e80-e86.
179. Vora A, Goulden N, Wade R, et al. Treatment reduction for children and young adults with low-risk acute lymphoblastic leukaemia defined by minimal residual disease (UKALL 2003): a randomised controlled trial. *Lancet Oncol.* 2013;14(3):199-209.
180. Asselin BL, Devidas M, Wang C, et al. Effectiveness of high-dose methotrexate in T-cell lymphoblastic leukemia and advanced-stage lymphoblastic lymphoma: a randomized study by the Children's Oncology Group (POG 9404). *Blood.* 2011;118(4):874-883.
181. Hofmans M, Suciu S, Ferster A, et al. Results of successive EORTC-CLG 58 881 and 58 951 trials in paediatric T-cell acute lymphoblastic leukaemia (ALL). *Br J Haematol.* 2019;186(5):741-753.
182. Berg SL, Blaney SM, Devidas M, et al. Phase II study of nelarabine (compound 506U78) in children and young adults with refractory T-cell malignancies: a report from the Children's Oncology Group. *J Clin Oncol.* 2005;23(15):3376-3382.
183. Pui CH, Pei D, Campana D, et al. Improved prognosis for older adolescents with acute lymphoblastic leukemia. *J Clin Oncol.* 2011;29(4):386-391.
184. Nachman J. Clinical characteristics, biologic features and outcome for young adult patients with acute lymphoblastic leukemia. *Br J Haematol.* 2005;130(2):166-173.
185. Bukowinski AJ, Burns KC, Parsons K, Perentesis JP, O'Brien MM. Toxicity of cancer therapy in adolescents and young adults (AYAs). *Semin Oncol Nurs.* 2015;31(3):216-226.
186. Butow P, Palmer S, Pai A, Goodenough B, Luckett T, King M. Review of adherence-related issues in adolescents and young adults with cancer. *J Clin Oncol.* 2010;28(32):4800-4809.
187. Curran E, Stock W. How I treat acute lymphoblastic leukemia in older adolescents and young adults. *Blood.* 2015;125(24):3702-3710.
188. Boissel N, Auclerc MF, Lheriter V, et al. Should adolescents with acute lymphoblastic leukemia be treated as old children or young adults? Comparison of the French FRALLE-93 and LALA-94 trials. *J Clin Oncol.* 2003;21(5):774-780.
189. Hocking J, Schwarer AP, Gasiorowski R, et al. Excellent outcomes for adolescents and adults with acute lymphoblastic leukemia and lymphoma without allogeneic stem cell transplant: the FRALLE-93 pediatric protocol. *Leuk Lymphoma.* 2014;55(12):2801-2807.
190. DeAngelo DJ, Stevenson KE, Dahlberg SE, et al. Long-term outcome of a pediatric-inspired regimen used for adults aged 18-50 years with newly diagnosed acute lymphoblastic leukemia. *Leukemia.* 2015;29(3):526-534.
191. Ram R, Wolach O, Vidal L, Gafter-Gvili A, Shpilberg O, Raanani P. Adolescents and young adults with acute lymphoblastic leukemia have a better outcome when treated with pediatric-inspired regimens: systematic review and meta-analysis. *Am J Hematol.* 2012;87(5):472-478.
192. Stock W, Luger SM, Advani AS, et al. A pediatric regimen for older adolescents and young adults with acute lymphoblastic leukemia: results of CALGB 10403. *Blood.* 2019;133(14):1548-1559.
193. Wieduwilt MJ, Stock W, Advani A, et al. Superior survival with pediatric-style chemotherapy compared to myeloablative allogeneic hematopoietic cell transplantation in older adolescents and young adults with Ph-negative acute lymphoblastic leukemia in first complete remission: analysis from CALGB 10403 and the CIBMTR. *Leukemia.* 2021;35(7):2076-2085.
194. Seftel MD, Neuberg D, Zhang MJ, et al. Pediatric-inspired therapy compared to allografting for Philadelphia chromosome-negative adult ALL in first complete remission. *Am J Hematol.* 2016;91(3):322-329.
195. Hilden JM, Dinndorf PA, Meerbaum SO, et al. Analysis of prognostic factors of acute lymphoblastic leukemia in infants: report on CCG 1953 from the Children's Oncology Group. *Blood.* 2006;108(2):441-451.
196. Dreyer ZE, Hilden JM, Jones TL, et al. Intensified chemotherapy without SCT in infant ALL: results from COG P9407 (Cohort 3). *Pediatr Blood Cancer.* 2015;62(3):419-426.
197. Pieters R, Schrappe M, De Lorenzo P, et al. A treatment protocol for infants younger than 1 year with acute lymphoblastic leukaemia (Interfant-99): an observational study and a multicentre randomised trial. *Lancet.* 2007;370(9583):240-250.
198. Tomizawa D, Koh K, Hirayama M, et al. Outcome of recurrent or refractory acute lymphoblastic leukemia in infants with MLL gene rearrangements: a report from the Japan Infant Leukemia Study Group. *Pediatr Blood Cancer.* 2009;52(7):808-813.
199. Pieters R, De Lorenzo P, Ancliffe P, et al. Outcome of infants younger than 1 year with acute lymphoblastic leukemia treated with the interfant-06 protocol: results from an international phase III randomized study. *J Clin Oncol.* 2019;37(25):2246-2256.
200. Brown PA, Kairalla JA, Hilden JM, et al. FLT3 inhibitor lestaurtinib plus chemotherapy for newly diagnosed KMT2A-rearranged infant acute lymphoblastic leukemia: Children's Oncology Group trial AALL0631. *Leukemia.* 2021;35(5):1279-1290.
201. Geerlinks AV, Issekutz T, Wahlstrom JT, et al. Severe, persistent, and fatal T-cell immunodeficiency following therapy for infantile leukemia. *Pediatr Blood Cancer.* 2016;63(11):2046-2049.
202. Brown P, Levis M, McIntyre E, Griesemer M, Small D. Combinations of the FLT3 inhibitor CEP-701 and chemotherapy synergistically kill infant and childhood MLL-rearranged ALL cells in a sequence-dependent manner. *Leukemia.* 2006;20(8):1368-1376.
203. Mezei G, Sudan M, Izraeli S, Kheifets L. Epidemiology of childhood leukemia in the presence and absence of Down syndrome. *Cancer Epidemiol.* 2014;38(5):479-489.
204. Verstegen RH, Kusters MA, Gemen EF, Vries DE. Down syndrome B-lymphocyte subpopulations, intrinsic defect or decreased T-lymphocyte help. *Pediatr Res.* 2010;67(5):563-569.
205. Lane AA, Chapuy B, Lin CY, et al. Triplication of a 21q22 region contributes to B cell transformation through HMGN1 overexpression and loss of histone H3 Lys27 trimethylation. *Nat Genet.* 2014;46(6):618-623.
206. Attarbaschi A, Morak M, Cario G, et al. Treatment outcome of CRLF2-rearranged childhood acute lymphoblastic leukaemia: a comparative analysis of the AIEOP-BFM and UK NCRI-CCLG study groups. *Br J Haematol.* 2012;158(6):772-777.
207. Blink M, Buitenkamp TD, van den Heuvel-Eibrink MM, et al. Frequency and prognostic implications of JAK 1-3 aberrations in Down syndrome acute lymphoblastic and myeloid leukemia. *Leukemia.* 2011;25(8):1365-1368.
208. Buitenkamp TD, Pieters R, Gallimore NE, et al. Outcome in children with Down's syndrome and acute lymphoblastic leukemia: role of IKZF1 deletions and CRLF2 aberrations. *Leukemia.* 2012;26(10):2204-2211.
209. Buitenkamp TD, Izraeli S, Zimmermann M, et al. Acute lymphoblastic leukemia in children with Down syndrome: a retrospective analysis from the Ponte di Legno study group. *Blood.* 2014;123(1):70-77.
210. O'Connor D, Bate J, Wade R, et al. Infection-related mortality in children with acute lymphoblastic leukemia: an analysis of infectious deaths on UKALL2003. *Blood.* 2014;124(7):1056-1061.
211. Buitenkamp TD, Mathot RA, de Haas V, Pieters R, Zwaan CM. Methotrexate-induced side effects are not due to differences in pharmacokinetics in children with Down syndrome and acute lymphoblastic leukemia. *Haematologica.* 2010;95(7):1106-1113.
212. Salazar EG, Li Y, Fisher BT, et al. Supportive care utilization and treatment toxicity in children with Down syndrome and acute lymphoid leukaemia at free-standing paediatric hospitals in the United States. *Br J Haematol.* 2016;174(4):591-599.
213. Mullighan CG, Phillips LA, Su X, et al. Genomic analysis of the clonal origins of relapsed acute lymphoblastic leukemia. *Science (New York, NY).* 2008;322(5906):1377-1380.
214. Ma X, Edmonson M, Yergeau D, et al. Rise and fall of subclones from diagnosis to relapse in pediatric B-acute lymphoblastic leukaemia. *Nat Commun.* 2015;6:6604.
215. Mar BG, Bullinger LB, McLean KM, et al. Mutations in epigenetic regulators including SETD2 are gained during relapse in paediatric acute lymphoblastic leukaemia. *Nat Commun.* 2014;5:3469.

216. Zhang J, Mullighan CG, Harvey RC, et al. Key pathways are frequently mutated in high-risk childhood acute lymphoblastic leukemia: a report from the Children's Oncology Group. *Blood*. 2011;118(11):3080-3087.
217. Meyer JA, Wang J, Hogan LE, et al. Relapse-specific mutations in NT5C2 in childhood acute lymphoblastic leukemia. *Nat Genet*. 2013;45(3):290-294.
218. Tzoneva G, Perez-Garcia A, Carpenter Z, et al. Activating mutations in the NT5C2 nucleotidase gene drive chemotherapy resistance in relapsed ALL. *Nat Med*. 2013;19(3):368-371.
219. Li B, Brady SW, Ma X, et al. Therapy-induced mutations drive the genomic landscape of relapsed acute lymphoblastic leukemia. *Blood*. 2020;135(1):41-55.
220. Waanders E, Gu Z, Dobson SM, et al. Mutational landscape and patterns of clonal evolution in relapsed pediatric acute lymphoblastic leukemia. *Blood Cancer Discov*. 2020;1(1):96-111.
221. Oskarsson T, Soderhall S, Arvidson J, et al. Relapsed childhood acute lymphoblastic leukemia in the Nordic countries: prognostic factors, treatment and outcome. *Haematologica*. 2016;101(1):68-76.
222. Driessen EM, de Lorenzo P, Campbell M, et al. Outcome of relapsed infant acute lymphoblastic leukemia treated on the interfant-99 protocol. *Leukemia*. 2016;30(5):1184-1187.
223. Tallen G, Ratei R, Mann G, et al. Long-term outcome in children with relapsed acute lymphoblastic leukemia after time-point and site-of-relapse stratification and intensified short-course multidrug chemotherapy: results of trial ALL-REZ BFM 90. *J Clin Oncol*. 2010;28(14):2339-2347.
224. Raetz EA, Borowitz MJ, Devidas M, et al. Reinduction platform for children with first marrow relapse of acute lymphoblastic Leukemia: a Children's Oncology Group Study[corrected]. *J Clin Oncol*. 2008;26(24):3971-3978.
225. Horton TM, Whitlock JA, Lu X, et al. Bortezomib reinduction chemotherapy in high-risk ALL in first relapse: a report from the Children's Oncology Group. *Br J Haematol*. 2019;186(2):274-285.
226. Lew G, Chen Y, Lu X, et al. Outcomes after late bone marrow and very early central nervous system relapse of childhood B-acute lymphoblastic leukemia: a report from the Children's Oncology Group phase III study AALL0433. *Haematologica*. 2021;106(1):46-55.
227. Eckert C, Groeneveld-Krentz S, Kirschner-Schwabe R, et al. Improving stratification for children with late bone marrow B-cell acute lymphoblastic leukemia relapses with refined response classification and integration of genetics. *J Clin Oncol*. 2019;37(36):3493-3506.
228. Brown PA, Ji L, Xu X, et al. Effect of postreinduction therapy consolidation with blinatumomab vs chemotherapy on disease-free survival in children, adolescents, and young adults with first relapse of B-cell acute lymphoblastic leukemia: a randomized clinical trial. *JAMA*. 2021;325(9):833-842.
229. Irving JA, Enshaei A, Parker CA, et al. Integration of genetic and clinical risk factors improves prognostication in relapsed childhood B-cell precursor acute lymphoblastic leukemia. *Blood*. 2016;128(7):911-922.
230. Kelly ME, Lu X, Devidas M, et al. Treatment of relapsed precursor-B acute lymphoblastic leukemia with intensive chemotherapy: POG (Pediatric Oncology Group) study 9411 (SIMAL 9). *J Pediatr Hematol Oncol*. 2013;35(7):509-513.
231. Parker C, Waters R, Leighton C, et al. Effect of mitoxantrone on outcome of children with first relapse of acute lymphoblastic leukaemia (ALL R3): an open-label randomised trial. *Lancet*. 2010;376(9757):2009-2017.
232. Sun W, Orgel E, Malvar J, et al. Treatment-related adverse events associated with a modified UK ALLR3 induction chemotherapy backbone for childhood relapsed/refractory acute lymphoblastic leukemia. *Pediatr Blood Cancer*. 2016;63(11):1943-1948.
233. Locatelli F, Zugmaier G, Rizzari C, et al. Effect of blinatumomab vs chemotherapy on event-free survival among children with high-risk first-relapse B-cell acute lymphoblastic leukemia: a randomized clinical trial. *JAMA*. 2021;325(9):843-854.
234. Wofford MM, Smith SD, Shuster JJ, et al. Treatment of occult or late overt testicular relapse in children with acute lymphoblastic leukemia: a Pediatric Oncology Group study. *J Clin Oncol*. 1992;10(4):624-630.
235. Hagedorn N, Acquaviva C, Fronkova E, et al. Submicroscopic bone marrow involvement in isolated extramedullary relapses in childhood acute lymphoblastic leukemia: a more precise definition of "isolated" and its possible clinical implications, a collaborative study of the Resistant Disease Committee of the International BFM study group. *Blood*. 2007;110(12):4022-4029.
236. Ritchey AK, Pollock BH, Lauer SJ, Andejeski Y, Barredo J, Buchanan GR. Improved survival of children with isolated CNS relapse of acute lymphoblastic leukemia: a pediatric oncology group study. *J Clin Oncol*. 1999;17(12):3745-3752.
237. Barredo JC, Devidas M, Lauer SJ, et al. Isolated CNS relapse of acute lymphoblastic leukemia treated with intensive systemic chemotherapy and delayed CNS radiation: a pediatric oncology group study. *J Clin Oncol*. 2006;24(19):3142-3149.
238. Hastings C, Chen Y, Devidas M, et al. Late isolated central nervous system relapse in childhood B-cell acute lymphoblastic leukemia treated with intensified systemic therapy and delayed reduced dose cranial radiation: a report from the Children's Oncology Group study AALL02P2. *Pediatr Blood Cancer*. 2021;68(12):e29256.
239. Eapen M, Zhang MJ, Devidas M, et al. Outcomes after HLA-matched sibling transplantation or chemotherapy in children with acute lymphoblastic leukemia in a second remission after an isolated central nervous system relapse: a collaborative study of the Children's Oncology Group and the Center for International Blood and Marrow Transplant Research. *Leukemia*. 2008;22(2):281-286.
240. Locatelli F, Schrappe M, Bernardo ME, Rutella S. How I treat relapsed childhood acute lymphoblastic leukemia. *Blood*. 2012;120(14):2807-2816.
241. Masurekar AN, Parker CA, Shanyinde M, et al. Outcome of central nervous system relapses in childhood acute lymphoblastic leukaemia–prospective open cohort analyses of the ALLR3 trial. *PLoS One*. 2014;9(10):e108107.
242. Rubinstein JD, Krupski C, Nelson AS, O'Brien MM, Davies SM, Phillips CL. Chimeric antigen receptor T cell therapy in patients with multiply relapsed or refractory extramedullary leukemia. *Biol Blood Marrow Transplant*. 2020;26(11):e280-e285.
243. Sklar CA, Robison LL, Nesbit ME, et al. Effects of radiation on testicular function in long-term survivors of childhood acute lymphoblastic leukemia: a report from the Children Cancer Study Group. *J Clin Oncol*. 1990;8(12):1981-1987.
244. Barredo JC, Hastings C, Lu X, et al. Isolated late testicular relapse of B-cell acute lymphoblastic leukemia treated with intensive systemic chemotherapy and response-based testicular radiation: a Children's Oncology Group study. *Pediatr Blood Cancer*. 2018;65(5):e26928.
245. Balduzzi A, Dalle JH, Wachowiak J, et al. Transplantation in children and adolescents with acute lymphoblastic leukemia from a matched donor versus an HLA-identical sibling: is the outcome comparable? Results from the international BFM ALL SCT 2007 study. *Biol Blood Marrow Transplant*. 2019;25(11):2197-2210.
246. Locatelli F, Merli P, Pagliara D, et al. Outcome of children with acute leukemia given HLA-haploidentical HSCT after alphabeta T-cell and B-cell depletion. *Blood*. 2017;130(5):677-685.
247. Mehta RS, Holtan SG, Wang T, et al. GRFS and CRFS in alternative donor hematopoietic cell transplantation for pediatric patients with acute leukemia. *Blood Adv*. 2019;3(9):1441-1449.
248. Klein OR, Buddenbaum J, Tucker N, et al. Nonmyeloablative haploidentical bone marrow transplantation with post-transplantation cyclophosphamide for pediatric and young adult patients with high-risk hematologic malignancies. *Biol Blood Marrow Transplant*. 2017;23(2):325-332.
249. Zhang MJ, Davies SM, Camitta BM, et al. Comparison of outcomes after HLA-matched sibling and unrelated donor transplantation for children with high-risk acute lymphoblastic leukemia. *Biol Blood Marrow Transplant*. 2012;18(8):1204-1210.
250. Bari R, Rujkijyanont P, Sullivan E, et al. Effect of donor KIR2DL1 allelic polymorphism on the outcome of pediatric allogeneic hematopoietic stem-cell transplantation. *J Clin Oncol*. 2013;31(30):3782-3790.
251. Oevermann L, Michaelis SU, Mezger M, et al. KIR B haplotype donors confer a reduced risk for relapse after haploidentical transplantation in children with ALL. *Blood*. 2014;124(17):2744-2747.
252. Babor F, Peters C, Manser AR, et al. Presence of centromeric but absence of telomeric group B KIR haplotypes in stem cell donors improve leukaemia control after HSCT for childhood ALL. *Bone Marrow Transplant*. 2019;54(11):1847-1858.
253. Ifversen M, Turkiewicz D, Marquart HV, et al. Low burden of minimal residual disease prior to transplantation in children with very high risk acute lymphoblastic leukaemia: the NOPHO ALL2008 experience. *Br J Haematol*. 2019;184(6):982-993.
254. Pulsipher MA, Langholz B, Wall DA, et al. The addition of sirolimus to tacrolimus/methotrexate GVHD prophylaxis in children with ALL: a phase 3 Children's Oncology Group/Pediatric Blood and Marrow Transplant Consortium trial. *Blood*. 2014;123(13):2017-2025.
255. Lovisa F, Zecca M, Rossi B, et al. Pre- and post-transplant minimal residual disease predicts relapse occurrence in children with acute lymphoblastic leukaemia. *Br J Haematol*. 2018;180(5):680-693.
256. Pulsipher MA, Carlson C, Langholz B, et al. IgH-V(D)J NGS-MRD measurement pre- and early post-allotransplant defines very low- and very high-risk ALL patients. *Blood*. 2015;125(22):3501-3508.
257. Horn B, Wahlstrom JT, Melton A, et al. Early mixed chimerism-based preemptive immunotherapy in children undergoing allogeneic hematopoietic stem cell transplantation for acute leukemia. *Pediatr Blood Cancer*. 2017;64(8):10.1002/pbc.26464. doi:10.1002/pbc.26464
258. Rettinger E, Merker M, Salzmann-Manrique E, et al. Pre-emptive immunotherapy for clearance of molecular disease in childhood acute lymphoblastic leukemia after transplantation. *Biol Blood Marrow Transplant*. 2017;23(1):87-95.
259. Peters C, Dalle JH, Locatelli F, et al. Total body irradiation or chemotherapy conditioning in childhood ALL: a multinational, randomized, noninferiority phase III study. *J Clin Oncol*. 2021;39(4):295-307.
260. Friend BD, Bailey-Olson M, Melton A, et al. The impact of total body irradiation-based regimens on outcomes in children and young adults with acute lymphoblastic leukemia undergoing allogeneic hematopoietic stem cell transplantation. *Pediatr Blood Cancer*. 2020;67(2):e28079.
261. Oliansky DM, Camitta B, Gaynon P, et al. Role of cytotoxic therapy with hematopoietic stem cell transplantation in the treatment of pediatric acute lymphoblastic leukemia: update of the 2005 evidence-based review. *Biol Blood Marrow Transplant*. 2012;18(4):505-522.
262. McNeer JL, Devidas M, Dai Y, et al. Hematopoietic stem-cell transplantation does not improve the poor outcome of children with hypodiploid acute lymphoblastic leukemia: a report from children's oncology group. *J Clin Oncol*. 2019;37(10):780-789.
263. Eapen M, Raetz E, Zhang MJ, et al. Outcomes after HLA-matched sibling transplantation or chemotherapy in children with B-precursor acute lymphoblastic leukemia in a second remission: a collaborative study of the Children's Oncology Group and the Center for International Blood and Marrow Transplant Research. *Blood*. 2006;107(12):4961-4967.
264. Burke MJ, Verneris MR, Le Rademacher J, et al. Transplant outcomes for children with T cell acute lymphoblastic leukemia in second remission: a report from the center for international blood and marrow transplant research. *Biol Blood Marrow Transplant*. 2015;21(12):2154-2159.
265. Nemecek ER, Ellis K, He W, et al. Outcome of myeloablative conditioning and unrelated donor hematopoietic cell transplantation for childhood acute lymphoblastic leukemia in third remission. *Biol Blood Marrow Transplant*. 2011;17(12):1833-1840.

266. Moorman AV, Schwab C, Winterman E, et al. Adjuvant tyrosine kinase inhibitor therapy improves outcome for children and adolescents with acute lymphoblastic leukaemia who have an ABL-class fusion. *Br J Haematol.* 2020;191(5):844-851.
267. Cario G, Leoni V, Conter V, et al. Relapses and treatment-related events contributed equally to poor prognosis in children with ABL-class fusion positive B-cell acute lymphoblastic leukemia treated according to AIEOP-BFM protocols. *Haematologica.* 2020;105(7):1887-1894.
268. Case M, Matheson E, Minto L, et al. Mutation of genes affecting the RAS pathway is common in childhood acute lymphoblastic leukemia. *Cancer Res.* 2008;68(16):6803-6809.
269. Kerstjens M, Driessen EM, Willekes M, et al. MEK inhibition is a promising therapeutic strategy for MLL-rearranged infant acute lymphoblastic leukemia patients carrying RAS mutations. *Oncotarget.* 2017;8(9):14835-14846.
270. Nikolaev SI, Garieri M, Santoni F, et al. Frequent cases of RAS-mutated Down syndrome acute lymphoblastic leukaemia lack JAK2 mutations. *Nat Commun.* 2014;5:4654.
271. Ryan SL, Matheson E, Grossmann V, et al. The role of the RAS pathway in iAMP21-ALL. *Leukemia.* 2016;30(9):1824-1831.
272. Irving J, Matheson E, Minto L, et al. Ras pathway mutations are prevalent in relapsed childhood acute lymphoblastic leukemia and confer sensitivity to MEK inhibition. *Blood.* 2014;124(23):3420-3430.
273. Oshima K, Khiabanian H, da Silva-Almeida AC, et al. Mutational landscape, clonal evolution patterns, and role of RAS mutations in relapsed acute lymphoblastic leukemia. *Proc Natl Acad Sci U S A.* 2016;113(40):11306-11311.
274. Houghton PJ, Morton CL, Kolb EA, et al. Initial testing (stage 1) of the proteasome inhibitor bortezomib by the pediatric preclinical testing program. *Pediatr Blood Cancer.* 2008;50(1):37-45.
275. Horton TM, Gannavarapu A, Blaney SM, D'Argenio DZ, Plon SE, Berg SL. Bortezomib interactions with chemotherapy agents in acute leukemia in vitro. *Cancer Chemother Pharmacol.* 2006;58(1):13-23.
276. Junk S, Cario G, Wittner N, et al. Bortezomib treatment can overcome glucocorticoid resistance in childhood B-cell precursor acute lymphoblastic leukemia cell lines. *Klin Pädiatr.* 2015;227(3):123-130.
277. Koyama D, Kikuchi J, Hiraoka N, et al. Proteasome inhibitors exert cytotoxicity and increase chemosensitivity via transcriptional repression of Notch1 in T-cell acute lymphoblastic leukemia. *Leukemia.* 2014;28(6):1216-1226.
278. Messinger YH, Gaynon PS, Sposto R, et al. Bortezomib with chemotherapy is highly active in advanced B-precursor acute lymphoblastic leukemia: therapeutic Advances in Childhood Leukemia & Lymphoma (TACL) Study. *Blood.* 2012;120(2):285-290.
279. Teachey DT, O'Connor D. How I treat newly diagnosed T-cell acute lymphoblastic leukemia and T-cell lymphoblastic lymphoma in children. *Blood.* 2020;135(3):159-166.
280. Wartman LD, Fiala MA, Fletcher T, et al. A phase I study of carfilzomib for relapsed or refractory acute myeloid and acute lymphoblastic leukemia. *Leuk Lymphoma.* 2016;57(3):728-730.
281. Bhatla T, Wang J, Morrison DJ, et al. Epigenetic reprogramming reverses the relapse-specific gene expression signature and restores chemosensitivity in childhood B-lymphoblastic leukemia. *Blood.* 2012;119(22):5201-5210.
282. Stumpel DJ, Schneider P, Seslija L, et al. Connectivity mapping identifies HDAC inhibitors for the treatment of t(4;11)-positive infant acute lymphoblastic leukemia. *Leukemia.* 2012;26(4):682-692.
283. Burke MJ, Lamba JK, Pounds S, et al. A therapeutic trial of decitabine and vorinostat in combination with chemotherapy for relapsed/refractory acute lymphoblastic leukemia. *Am J Hematol.* 2014;89(9):889-895.
284. Guest E, Kairalla J, Devidas M, et al. American Society of Pediatric Hematology/Oncology (ASPHO) 2021 Paper and poster abstracts. *Pediatr Blood Cancer.* 2021;68(suppl 3):e29060.
285. Chen CW, Armstrong SA. Targeting DOT1L and HOX gene expression in MLL-rearranged leukemia and beyond. *Exp Hematol.* 2015;43(8):673-684.
286. Bernt KM, Zhu N, Sinha AU, et al. MLL-rearranged leukemia is dependent on aberrant H3K79 methylation by DOT1L. *Cancer Cell.* 2011;20(1):66-78.
287. Daigle SR, Olhava EJ, Therkelsen CA, et al. Potent inhibition of DOT1L as treatment of MLL-fusion leukemia. *Blood.* 2013;122(6):1017-1025.
288. Klaus CR, Iwanowicz D, Johnston D, et al. DOT1L inhibitor EPZ-5676 displays synergistic antiproliferative activity in combination with standard of care drugs and hypomethylating agents in MLL-rearranged leukemia cells. *J Pharmacol Exp Ther.* 2014;350(3):646-656.
289. Krivtsov AV, Evans K, Gadrey JY, et al. A menin-MLL inhibitor induces specific chromatin changes and eradicates disease in models of MLL-rearranged leukemia. *Cancer Cell.* 2019;36(6):660-673 e611.
290. Kale J, Osterlund EJ, Andrews DW. BCL-2 family proteins: changing partners in the dance towards death. *Cell Death Differ.* 2018;25(1):65-80.
291. Kang MH, Kang YH, Szymanska B, et al. Activity of vincristine, L-ASP, and dexamethasone against acute lymphoblastic leukemia is enhanced by the BH3-mimetic ABT-737 in vitro and in vivo. *Blood.* 2007;110(6):2057-2066.
292. Lock R, Carol H, Houghton PJ, et al. Initial testing (stage 1) of the BH3 mimetic ABT-263 by the pediatric preclinical testing program. *Pediatr Blood Cancer.* 2008;50(6):1181-1189.
293. Wilson WH, O'Connor OA, Czuczman MS, et al. Navitoclax, a targeted high-affinity inhibitor of BCL-2, in lymphoid malignancies: a phase 1 dose-escalation study of safety, pharmacokinetics, pharmacodynamics, and antitumour activity. *Lancet Oncol.* 2010;11(12):1149-1159.
294. Place AE, Karol SE, Forlenza CJ, et al. Pediatric patients with relapsed/refractory acute lymphoblastic leukemia harboring heterogeneous genomic profiles respond to venetoclax in combination with chemotherapy. *Blood.* 2020;136(suppl 1):37-38.
295. Autry RJ, Paugh SW, Carter R, et al. Integrative genomic analyses reveal mechanisms of glucocorticoid resistance in acute lymphoblastic leukemia. *Nat Cancer.* 2020;1(3):329-344.
296. Pullarkat VA, Lacayo NJ, Jabbour E, et al. Venetoclax and navitoclax in combination with chemotherapy in patients with relapsed or refractory acute lymphoblastic leukemia and lymphoblastic lymphoma. *Cancer Discov.* 2021;11(6):1440-1453.
297. Khaw SL, Suryani S, Evans K, et al. Venetoclax responses of pediatric ALL xenografts reveal sensitivity of MLL-rearranged leukemia. *Blood.* 2016;128(10):1382-1395.
298. Richard-Carpentier G, Jabbour E, Short NJ, et al. Clinical experience with venetoclax combined with chemotherapy for relapsed or refractory T-cell acute lymphoblastic leukemia. *Clin Lymphoma Myeloma Leuk.* 2020;20(4):212-218.
299. Rossi EA, Goldenberg DM, Michel R, Rossi DL, Wallace DJ, Chang CH. Trogocytosis of multiple B-cell surface markers by CD22 targeting with epratuzumab. *Blood.* 2013;122(17):3020-3029.
300. Raetz EA, Cairo MS, Borowitz MJ, et al. Re-induction chemoimmunotherapy with epratuzumab in relapsed acute lymphoblastic leukemia (ALL): phase II results from Children's Oncology Group (COG) study ADVL04P2. *Pediatr Blood Cancer.* 2015;62(7):1171-1175.
301. Kantarjian HM, DeAngelo DJ, Stelljes M, et al. Inotuzumab ozogamicin versus standard of care in relapsed or refractory acute lymphoblastic leukemia: final report and long-term survival follow-up from the randomized, phase 3 INO-VATE study. *Cancer.* 2019;125(14):2474-2487.
302. Brivio E, Locatelli F, Lopez-Yurda M, et al. A phase 1 study of inotuzumab ozogamicin in pediatric relapsed/refractory acute lymphoblastic leukemia (ITCC-059 study). *Blood.* 2021;137(12):1582-1590.
303. Loffler A, Kufer P, Lutterbuse R, et al. A recombinant bispecific single-chain antibody, CD19 x CD3, induces rapid and high lymphoma-directed cytotoxicity by unstimulated T lymphocytes. *Blood.* 2000;95(6):2098-2103.
304. von Stackelberg A, Locatelli F, Zugmaier G, et al. Phase I/phase II study of blinatumomab in pediatric patients with relapsed/refractory acute lymphoblastic leukemia. *J Clin Oncol.* 2016;34(36):4381-4389.
305. Maude SL, Laetsch TW, Buechner J, et al. Tisagenlecleucel in children and young adults with B-cell lymphoblastic leukemia. *N Engl J Med.* 2018;378(5):439-448.
306. Shah NN, Lee DW, Yates B, et al. Long-term follow-up of CD19-CAR T-cell therapy in children and young adults with B-ALL. *J Clin Oncol.* 2021;39(15):1650-1659.
307. Feucht J, Kayser S, Gorodezki D, et al. T-cell responses against CD19+ pediatric acute lymphoblastic leukemia mediated by bispecific T-cell engager (BiTE) are regulated contrarily by PD-L1 and CD80/CD86 on leukemic blasts. *Oncotarget.* 2016;7(47):76902-76919.
308. Kohnke T, Krupka C, Tischer J, Knosel T, Subklewe M. Increase of PD-L1 expressing B-precursor ALL cells in a patient resistant to the CD19/CD3-bispecific T cell engager antibody blinatumomab. *J Hematol Oncol.* 2015;8:111.
309. Dourthe ME, Rabian F, Yakouben K, et al. Determinants of CD19-positive vs CD19-negative relapse after tisagenlecleucel for B-cell acute lymphoblastic leukemia. *Leukemia.* 2021;35(12):3383-3393. doi:10.1038/s41375-021-01281-7
310. Fry TJ, Shah NN, Orentas RJ, et al. CD22-targeted CAR T cells induce remission in B-ALL that is naive or resistant to CD19-targeted CAR immunotherapy. *Nat Med.* 2018;24(1):20-28.
311. Dai H, Wu Z, Jia H, et al. Bispecific CAR-T cells targeting both CD19 and CD22 for therapy of adults with relapsed or refractory B cell acute lymphoblastic leukemia. *J Hematol Oncol.* 2020;13(1):30.
312. Jacoby E, Nguyen SM, Fountaine TJ, et al. CD19 CAR immune pressure induces B-precursor acute lymphoblastic leukaemia lineage switch exposing inherent leukaemic plasticity. *Nat Commun.* 2016;7:12320.
313. Benjamin R, Graham C, Yallop D, et al. Genome-edited, donor-derived allogeneic anti-CD19 chimeric antigen receptor T cells in paediatric and adult B-cell acute lymphoblastic leukaemia: results of two phase 1 studies. *Lancet.* 2020;396(10266):1885-1894.
314. Myers RM, Li Y, Barz Leahy A, et al. Humanized CD19-targeted chimeric antigen receptor (CAR) T cells in CAR-naive and CAR-exposed children and young adults with relapsed or refractory acute lymphoblastic leukemia. *J Clin Oncol.* 2021;39(27):3044-3055.
315. Pan J, Tan Y, Wang G, et al. Donor-derived CD7 chimeric antigen receptor T cells for T-cell acute lymphoblastic leukemia: first-in-human, phase I trial. *J Clin Oncol.* 2021;39(30):3340-3351. JCO2100389.
316. Bride KL, Vincent TL, Im SY, et al. Preclinical efficacy of daratumumab in T-cell acute lymphoblastic leukemia. *Blood.* 2018;131(9):995-999.
317. Mody R, Li S, Dover DC, et al. Twenty-five-year follow-up among survivors of childhood acute lymphoblastic leukemia: a report from the Childhood Cancer Survivor Study. *Blood.* 2008;111(12):5515-5523.
318. Andres-Jensen L, Larsen HB, Johansen C, Frandsen TL, Schmiegelow K, Wahlberg A. Everyday life challenges among adolescent and young adult survivors of childhood acute lymphoblastic leukemia: an in-depth qualitative study. *Psycho Oncol.* 2020;29(10):1630-1637.
319. Holmqvist AS, Wiebe T, Hjorth L, Lindgren A, Ora I, Moell C. Young age at diagnosis is a risk factor for negative late socio-economic effects after acute lymphoblastic leukemia in childhood. *Pediatr Blood Cancer.* 2010;55(4):698-707.
320. Essig S, Li Q, Chen Y, et al. Risk of late effects of treatment in children newly diagnosed with standard-risk acute lymphoblastic leukaemia: a report from the Childhood Cancer Survivor Study cohort. *Lancet Oncol.* 2014;15(8):841-851.
321. Tang A, Alyman C, Anderson L, Hodson DI, Marjerrison S. Long-term social outcomes of hyperfractionated radiation on childhood ALL survivors. *Pediatr Blood Cancer.* 2016;63(8):1445-1450.

322. Harila MJ, Salo J, Lanning M, Vilkkumaa I, Harila-Saari AH. High health-related quality of life among long-term survivors of childhood acute lymphoblastic leukemia. *Pediatr Blood Cancer.* 2010;55(2):331-336.
323. Kunin-Batson A, Kadan-Lottick N, Neglia JP. The contribution of neurocognitive functioning to quality of life after childhood acute lymphoblastic leukemia. *Psycho Oncol.* 2014;23(6):692-699.
324. Moyer KH, Willard VW, Gross AM, et al. The impact of attention on social functioning in survivors of pediatric acute lymphoblastic leukemia and brain tumors. *Pediatr Blood Cancer.* 2012;59(7):1290-1295.
325. Jacola LM, Edelstein K, Liu W, et al. Cognitive, behaviour, and academic functioning in adolescent and young adult survivors of childhood acute lymphoblastic leukaemia: a report from the Childhood Cancer Survivor Study. *Lancet Psychiatr.* 2016;3(10):965-972.
326. Edelstein K, D'Agostino N, Bernstein LJ, et al. Long-term neurocognitive outcomes in young adult survivors of childhood acute lymphoblastic leukemia. *J Pediatr Hematol Oncol.* 2011;33(6):450-458.
327. Harila MJ, Winqvist S, Lanning M, Bloigu R, Harila-Saari AH. Progressive neurocognitive impairment in young adult survivors of childhood acute lymphoblastic leukemia. *Pediatr Blood Cancer.* 2009;53(2):156-161.
328. Duffner PK, Armstrong FD, Chen L, et al. Neurocognitive and neuroradiologic central nervous system late effects in children treated on Pediatric Oncology Group (POG) P9605 (standard risk) and P9201 (lesser risk) acute lymphoblastic leukemia protocols (ACCL0131): a methotrexate consequence? A report from the Children's Oncology Group. *J Pediatr Hematol Oncol.* 2014;36(1):8-15.
329. Jacola LM, Krull KR, Pui CH, et al. Longitudinal assessment of neurocognitive outcomes in survivors of childhood acute lymphoblastic leukemia treated on a contemporary chemotherapy protocol. *J Clin Oncol.* 2016;34(11):1239-1247.
330. Kesler SR, Sleurs C, McDonald BC, Deprez S, van der Plas E, Nieman BJ. Brain imaging in pediatric cancer survivors: correlates of cognitive impairment. *J Clin Oncol.* 2021;39(16):1775-1785.
331. Roncadin C, Hitzler J, Downie A, et al. Neuropsychological late effects of treatment for acute leukemia in children with Down syndrome. *Pediatr Blood Cancer.* 2015;62(5):854-858.
332. Banerjee P, Rossi MG, Anghelescu DL, et al. Association between anesthesia exposure and neurocognitive and neuroimaging outcomes in long-term survivors of childhood acute lymphoblastic leukemia. *JAMA Oncol.* 2019;5(10):1456-1463.
333. Williams AM, Cole PD. Biomarkers of cognitive impairment in pediatric cancer survivors. *J Clin Oncol.* 2021;39(16):1766-1774.
334. Gilleland Marchak J, Devine KA, Hudson MM, et al. Systematic review of educational supports of pediatric cancer survivors: current approaches and future directions. *J Clin Oncol.* 2021;39(16):1813-1823.
335. Dixon SB, Chen Y, Yasui Y, et al. Reduced morbidity and mortality in survivors of childhood acute lymphoblastic leukemia: a report from the childhood cancer survivor study. *J Clin Oncol.* 2020;38(29):3418-3429.
336. Loning L, Zimmermann M, Reiter A, et al. Secondary neoplasms subsequent to Berlin-Frankfurt-Munster therapy of acute lymphoblastic leukemia in childhood: significantly lower risk without cranial radiotherapy. *Blood.* 2000;95(9):2770-2775.
337. Bhatia S, Sather HN, Pabustan OB, Trigg ME, Gaynon PS, Robison LL. Low incidence of second neoplasms among children diagnosed with acute lymphoblastic leukemia after 1983. *Blood.* 2002;99(12):4257-4264.
338. Hijiya N, Hudson MM, Lensing S, et al. Cumulative incidence of secondary neoplasms as a first event after childhood acute lymphoblastic leukemia. *JAMA.* 2007;297(11):1207-1215.
339. Mattano LA, Jr, Devidas M, Nachman JB, et al. Effect of alternate-week versus continuous dexamethasone scheduling on the risk of osteonecrosis in paediatric patients with acute lymphoblastic leukaemia: results from the CCG-1961 randomised cohort trial. *Lancet Oncol.* 2012;13(9):906-915.
340. te Winkel ML, Pieters R, Hop WC, et al. Prospective study on incidence, risk factors, and long-term outcome of osteonecrosis in pediatric acute lymphoblastic leukemia. *J Clin Oncol.* 2011;29(31):4143-4150.
341. Patel B, Richards SM, Rowe JM, Goldstone AH, Fielding AK. High incidence of avascular necrosis in adolescents with acute lymphoblastic leukaemia: a UKALL XII analysis. *Leukemia.* 2008;22(2):308-312.
342. Ojala AE, Paakko E, Lanning FP, Lanning M. Osteonecrosis during the treatment of childhood acute lymphoblastic leukemia: a prospective MRI study. *Med Pediatr Oncol.* 1999;32(1):11-17.
343. Weinstein RS. Glucocorticoid-induced osteonecrosis. *Endocrine.* 2012;41(2):183-190.
344. Karimova EJ, Rai SN, Howard SC, et al. Femoral head osteonecrosis in pediatric and young adult patients with leukemia or lymphoma. *J Clin Oncol.* 2007;25(12):1525-1531.
345. Leblicq C, Laverdiere C, Decarie JC, et al. Effectiveness of pamidronate as treatment of symptomatic osteonecrosis occurring in children treated for acute lymphoblastic leukemia. *Pediatr Blood Cancer.* 2013;60(5):741-747.
346. Te Winkel ML, Pieters R, Wind EJ, Bessems JH, van den Heuvel-Eibrink MM. Management and treatment of osteonecrosis in children and adolescents with acute lymphoblastic leukemia. *Haematologica.* 2014;99(3):430-436.
347. Amin N, Kraft J, Fishlock A, et al. Surgical management of symptomatic osteonecrosis and utility of core decompression of the femoral head in young people with acute lymphoblastic leukaemia recruited into UKALL 2003. *Bone Joint Lett J.* 2021;103-B(3):589-596.
348. Kawedia JD, Kaste SC, Pei D, et al. Pharmacokinetic, pharmacodynamic, and pharmacogenetic determinants of osteonecrosis in children with acute lymphoblastic leukemia. *Blood.* 2011;117(8):2340-2347. quiz 2556.
349. Janke LJ, Van Driest SL, Portera MV, et al. Hypertension is a modifiable risk factor for osteonecrosis in acute lymphoblastic leukemia. *Blood.* 2019;134(12):983-986.
350. Karol SE, Yang W, Van Driest SL, et al. Genetics of glucocorticoid-associated osteonecrosis in children with acute lymphoblastic leukemia. *Blood.* 2015;126(15):1770-1776.
351. Yao S, Zhu Q, Cole PD, et al. Genetic ancestry and skeletal toxicities among childhood acute lymphoblastic leukemia patients in the DFCI 05-001 cohort. *Blood Adv.* 2021;5(2):451-458.
352. Chow EJ, Chen Y, Kremer LC, et al. Individual prediction of heart failure among childhood cancer survivors. *J Clin Oncol.* 2015;33(5):394-402.
353. Lipshultz SE, Colan SD, Gelber RD, Perez-Atayde AR, Sallan SE, Sanders SP. Late cardiac effects of doxorubicin therapy for acute lymphoblastic leukemia in childhood. *N Engl J Med.* 1991;324(12):808-815.
354. Lipshultz SE, Lipsitz SR, Mone SM, et al. Female sex and higher drug dose as risk factors for late cardiotoxic effects of doxorubicin therapy for childhood cancer. *N Engl J Med.* 1995;332(26):1738-1743.
355. Lipshultz SE, Miller TL, Scully RE, et al. Changes in cardiac biomarkers during doxorubicin treatment of pediatric patients with high-risk acute lymphoblastic leukemia: associations with long-term echocardiographic outcomes. *J Clin Oncol.* 2012;30(10):1042-1049.
356. Lipshultz SE, Rifai N, Dalton VM, et al. The effect of dexrazoxane on myocardial injury in doxorubicin-treated children with acute lymphoblastic leukemia. *N Engl J Med.* 2004;351(2):145-153.
357. Asselin BL, Devidas M, Chen L, et al. Cardioprotection and safety of dexrazoxane in patients treated for newly diagnosed T-cell acute lymphoblastic leukemia or advanced-stage lymphoblastic non-Hodgkin lymphoma: a report of the children's oncology group randomized trial pediatric oncology group 9404. *J Clin Oncol.* 2016;34(8):854-862.
358. Chow EJ, Asselin BL, Schwartz CL, et al. Late mortality after dexrazoxane treatment: a report from the children's oncology group. *J Clin Oncol.* 2015;33(24):2639-2645.
359. Burns EA, Gentille C, Trachtenberg B, Pingali SR, Anand K. Cardiotoxicity associated with anti-CD19 chimeric antigen receptor T-cell (CAR-T) therapy: recognition, risk factors, and management. *Diseases.* 2021;9(1):20.
360. Berkman AM, Hildebrandt MAT, Landstrom AP. The genetic underpinnings of anthracycline-induced cardiomyopathy predisposition. *Clin Genet.* 2021;100(2):132-143.
361. Lemay V, Caru M, Samoilenko M, et al. Prevention of long-term adverse health outcomes with cardiorespiratory fitness and physical activity in childhood acute lymphoblastic leukemia survivors. *J Pediatr Hematol Oncol.* 2019;41(7):e450-e458.
362. van Santen HM, Geskus RB, Raemaekers S, et al. Changes in body mass index in long-term childhood cancer survivors. *Cancer.* 2015;121(23):4197-4204.
363. Oluyomi A, Aldrich KD, Foster KL, et al. Neighborhood deprivation index is associated with weight status among long-term survivors of childhood acute lymphoblastic leukemia. *J Cancer Surviv.* 2021;15(5):767-775.
364. Marriott CJC, Beaumont LF, Farncombe TH, et al. Body composition in long-term survivors of acute lymphoblastic leukemia diagnosed in childhood and adolescence: a focus on sarcopenic obesity. *Cancer.* 2018;124(6):1225-1231.
365. Richard MA, Brown AL, Belmont JW, et al. Genetic variation in the body mass index of adult survivors of childhood acute lymphoblastic leukemia: a report from the Childhood Cancer Survivor Study and the St. Jude Lifetime Cohort. *Cancer.* 2021;127(2):310-318.
366. Chow EJ, Friedman DL, Stovall M, et al. Risk of thyroid dysfunction and subsequent thyroid cancer among survivors of acute lymphoblastic leukemia: a report from the Childhood Cancer Survivor Study. *Pediatr Blood Cancer.* 2009;53(3):432-437.
367. Clausen CT, Hasle H, Holmqvist AS, et al. Hyperthyroidism as a late effect in childhood cancer survivors - an Adult Life after Childhood Cancer in Scandinavia (ALiCCS) study. *Acta Oncol.* 2019;58(2):227-231.
368. Bongers ME, Francken AB, Rouwe C, Kamps WA, Postma A. Reduction of adult height in childhood acute lymphoblastic leukemia survivors after prophylactic cranial irradiation. *Pediatr Blood Cancer.* 2005;45(2):139-143.
369. Vandecruys E, Dhooge C, Craen M, Benoit Y, De Schepper J. Longitudinal linear growth and final height is impaired in childhood acute lymphoblastic leukemia survivors after treatment without cranial irradiation. *J Pediatr.* 2013;163(1):268-273.
370. Leung W, Rose SR, Zhou Y, et al. Outcomes of growth hormone replacement therapy in survivors of childhood acute lymphoblastic leukemia. *J Clin Oncol.* 2002;20(13):2959-2964.
371. Chow EJ, Friedman DL, Yasui Y, et al. Timing of menarche among survivors of childhood acute lymphoblastic leukemia: a report from the Childhood Cancer Survivor Study. *Pediatr Blood Cancer.* 2008;50(4):854-858.
372. Byrne J, Fears TR, Mills JL, et al. Fertility in women treated with cranial radiotherapy for childhood acute lymphoblastic leukemia. *Pediatr Blood Cancer.* 2004;42(7):589-597.
373. Green DM, Zhu L, Wang M, et al. Effect of cranial irradiation on sperm concentration of adult survivors of childhood acute lymphoblastic leukemia: a report from the St. Jude Lifetime Cohort Studydagger. *Hum Reprod.* 2017;32(6):1192-1201.
374. Kahn JM, Keegan TH, Tao L, Abrahão R, Bleyer A, Viny AD. Racial disparities in the survival of American children, adolescents, and young adults with acute lymphoblastic leukemia, acute myelogenous leukemia, and Hodgkin lymphoma. *Cancer.* 2016;122(17):2723-2730.
375. Walsh A, Chewning J, Li X, et al. Inferior outcomes for black children with high risk acute lymphoblastic leukemia and the impact of socioeconomic variables. *Pediatr Blood Cancer.* 2017;64(2):267-274.
376. Lee SHR, Antillon-Klussmann F, Pei D, et al. Association of genetic ancestry with the molecular subtypes and prognosis of childhood acute lymphoblastic leukemia. *JAMA Oncol.* 2022;8(3):354-363.
377. Gupta S, Teachey DT, Devidas M, et al. Racial, ethnic, and socioeconomic factors result in disparities in outcome among children with acute lymphoblastic leukemia

378. Bona K, Blonquist TM, Neuberg DS, Silverman LB, Wolfe J. Impact of socioeconomic status on timing of relapse and overall survival for children treated on dana-farber cancer Institute ALL consortium protocols (2000-2010). *Pediatr Blood Cancer*. 2016;63(6):1012-1018.
379. Schraw JM, Peckham-Gregory EC, Rabin KR, Scheurer ME, Lupo PJ, Oluyomi A. Area deprivation is associated with poorer overall survival in children with acute lymphoblastic leukemia. *Pediatr Blood Cancer*. 2020;67(9):e28525.
380. Schraw JM, Peckham-Gregory EC, Hughes AE, Scheurer ME, Pruitt SL, Lupo PJ. Residence in a Hispanic enclave is associated with inferior overall survival among children with acute lymphoblastic leukemia. *Int J Environ Res Publ Health*. 2021;18(17):9273.
381. Kehm RD, Spector LG, Poynter JN, Vock DM, Altekruse SF, Osypuk TL. Does socioeconomic status account for racial and ethnic disparities in childhood cancer survival? *Cancer*. 2018;124(20):4090-4097.
382. Winestone LE, Aplenc R. Disparities in survival and health outcomes in childhood leukemia. *Curr Hematol Malig Rep*. 2019;14(3):179-186.

(continued from previous) not fully attenuated by disease prognosticators: a children's oncology group (COG) study. *Blood*. 2021;138(suppl 1):211.

Chapter 78 ■ Acute Myeloid Leukemia in Children

JENNIFER L. KAMENS • DANIELLE SHIN • NORMAN LACAYO

HISTORICAL BACKGROUND

Acute myeloid leukemia (AML) represents a heterogeneous group of hematologic malignancies arising from the transformation and expansion of an early myeloid stem or progenitor cell into a dominant and subclonal architecture. The term *leukemia* originated with Virchow, who, in 1845, recognized a clinical entity characterized by too many white blood cells (WBCs), leading him to name the condition *white blood,* or *leukemia*. Of some historical interest is that Dr. John Hughes Bennett's report of a case of leukemia preceded Virchow's description by approximately 6 weeks.[1] However, Bennett had concluded that the condition was secondary to an infection and referred to it as *pyemia*. The term *myelogenous,* or *myeloid,* derives from the terms *myelos,* meaning marrow and *genesis,* meaning birth.

The original cases of Virchow and Bennett probably represented what we now know to be either chronic lymphocytic or myelogenous leukemia. The first likely case of acute leukemia was reported by Friedreich and was believed to be lymphocytic.[2] It would take the identification of the myeloblast as a precursor cell for granulocytes by Naegeli in 1900 to set the stage for the description of the first case of AML or what was originally termed *acute nonlymphocytic leukemia*.[3] Even during the first half of the 20th century, reports describing different types of myeloid leukemia made it clear that this was not one but a variety of distinct disorders, all deriving from a bone marrow precursor myeloblast. Initially, cases of monocytic leukemia were described, followed by myelomonocytic leukemia.[3,4] Cases of erythroleukemia, megakaryoblastic leukemia, and acute promyelocytic leukemia (APL) were subsequently described in 1917, 1931, and 1957, respectively.[5–7] During the mid-1970s, the French/American/British (FAB) classification system was developed and defined the major categories of AML as M1 through M7.[8] More recently, the World Health Organization (WHO) provided a new classification system that utilizes genetic, immunophenotypic, biologic, and clinical features in addition to morphology.

The description and classification of AML moved more rapidly than the development of effective treatments. During the mid-1800s, Virchow used diet therapies, ferric iodide, and application of abdominal and foot baths.[1] In 1865, Lissauer used arsenic (Fowler solution) to treat patients with leukemia, but with little success.[1] Radiation therapy was used in the late 1800s, mostly as a form of palliation for chronic leukemias.[1] In 1938, Forkner stated, "Although leukemia is a fatal disease much can be done to add to the comfort, and promote the general health of sufferers from the chronic forms of the disease. Unfortunately acute leukemia does not respond satisfactorily to any form of treatment."[1] In 1948, Farber demonstrated that the use of the antimetabolite aminopterin could produce transient remissions in children with acute lymphoblastic leukemia (ALL).[9] The pioneering work resulted in the National Cancer Institute developing screening programs for other possible antitumor therapies during the 1950s. During the 1960s, several chemotherapeutic agents, particularly cytarabine and anthracyclines, were developed and used in the treatment of AML. During the 1970s, clinical trials demonstrated that combining these two agents would result in long-term remissions for 10% to 15% of patients with AML. The subsequent introduction of more intensive remission induction regimens and postremission therapy increased the need for more rigorous supportive care measures, and the development of bone marrow transplantation led to current cure rates of approximately 55% to 65%.[10,11]

Over the last few decades, increased understanding of leukemia cell biology, namely cytogenetic and molecular abnormalities by the use of whole exome sequencing (WES), whole genome sequencing (WGS), and RNA sequencing to detect fusion products, have led to refined prognostication and treatment stratification.[12,13] The ability to detect measurable residual disease (MRD; also referred to as minimal residual disease) and evaluate response to therapy far below the microscopic level has had significant impact on improving risk classification; however, it also illustrates the limit of risk stratification due to the diversity of clonal architecture on how it can be remodeled under therapeutic pressure into a responsive and drug resistant disease.[14,15] The current plateau (*Figure 78.1*) in survival represents a challenge in the design of clinical trials. Further advances may need to include prospective surveillance of clonal structure/substructure and opportunities to layer single or combination of targeted/untargeted therapies to maximize disease eradication and probability of cure.

EPIDEMIOLOGY

Approximately 6500 children <20 years of age develop acute leukemia annually in the United States, and AML represents approximately 15%, resulting in approximately 1000 new cases/year.[16] The remaining cases of acute leukemia in children and adolescents are ALL and rare subtypes. Essentially the opposite ratios exist for adults, with AML accounting for about 80% and ALL the remaining 20%. With the exception of a peak in incidence of AML in infants, the incidence of AML is relatively constant until early adolescence following which it continues to rise slowly through young adulthood, and beyond 50 years of age the incidence rises dramatically.[17,18]

The incidence of pediatric AML in the United States has been estimated to be 7.7 cases per million for children 0 to 14 years of age.[19] Overall, there is not much variation among different racial and ethnic groups. However, Hispanic children and young adults have been found to have the highest rates of APL.[20–22] As the incidence of childhood leukemia increases, especially in the Amerindian/Hispanic population, studies of inherited genomic predisposition features modulated by environmental factors are warranted.[23] There are differences among the annual incidence in children from different countries with some of highest rates reported in New Zealand.[24] The increasing incidence of secondary leukemia, resulting from chemotherapy and treatment for other malignancies, is a problem of increasing significance in pediatrics.[25–27]

CELLULAR AND MOLECULAR ORIGINS OF ACUTE MYELOID LEUKEMIA: HEMATOPOIETIC HIERARCHIES

The determination of the AML stem cell is not solely of biologic interest but has profound significance for understanding the causes of leukemia and potentially the development of curative therapies. Normal hematopoiesis occurs through a series of complex changes that facilitate multipotential hematopoietic stem cells to both expand and differentiate into various mature blood cell types. Because AML is derived from an abnormal immature hematopoietic precursor cell, these leukemias also have the capacity to expand and to show characteristics of limited differentiation. Thus, myeloid leukemias retain many of the molecular and cellular phenotypic characteristics of their normal hematopoietic origins, providing the means to distinguish subtypes of the disease and define potential leukemic stem cell compartments. For example, although most myeloid leukemia cells often express growth, survival, and differentiation receptors for specific cytokines such as KIT, FLT3, and granulocyte-macrophage colony-stimulating factor receptor, some subtypes also express more lineage-specific surface

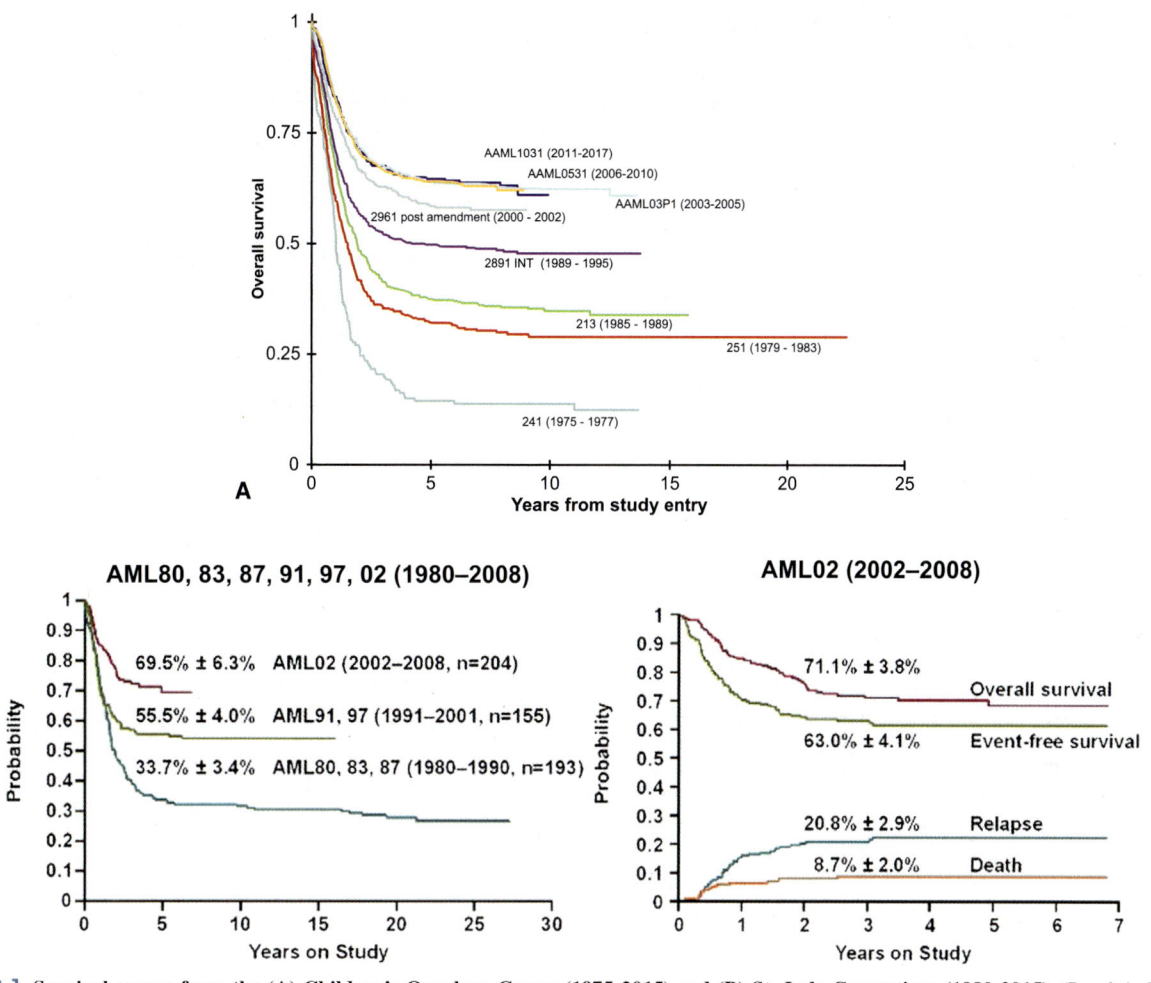

FIGURE 78.1 Survival curves from the (A) Children's Oncology Group (1975-2015) and (B) St. Jude Consortium (1980-2015). (Panel A. Used with permission. © Children's Oncology Group.)

receptors, such as those for granulocyte colony-stimulating factor (G-CSF) and erythropoietin. The same is true for the expression of differentiation markers that characterize various myeloid lineages such as megakaryoblastic, erythroid, or monocytic.

These diverse phenotypic characteristics of different subtypes suggest significant heterogeneity of both the genetic changes and the cell of origin in AML. Furthermore, identification of genetic hierarchy and temporal variegation in the clonal history of AML adds an additional dimension of complexity, with recapitulation of leukemogenesis at relapse via evolution and adaptation under genotoxic treatment pressure.[28,29]

Some of the earliest biologic tools used to define the cellular compartment in which leukemic stem cells arise included the use of X-linked glucose-6-phosphate dehydrogenase isoenzyme analysis in female patients with chronic myeloid leukemia (CML) and then AML.[30] Subsequently, karyotypic abnormalities were examined in the maturing colony-forming units to evaluate which lineage (colony-forming unit stem, colony-forming unit granulocyte-macrophage, colony-forming unit megakaryocyte, colony-forming unit granulocyte, colony-forming unit eosinophil, etc) contained the aberrant chromosomal marker.[31] These studies revealed that although CML arises in a very early pluripotential hematopoietic cell, there are cases of AML that arise in more mature cells.[32,33]

By depleting samples of AML with antibodies directed against lineage-specific surface antigens, a very small percentage of lineage-negative (Lin−) cells were isolated that had the capacity to generate AML at a higher percentage than more mature leukemic cells when transferred to immunodeficient mice. These leukemogenic CD34+, CD38−, Lin− cells (termed *self-renewing leukemia-initiating cells*) were in most cases rare, having a frequency of as few as 0.2 to 200/10^6 mononuclear cells.[34,35] Of further significance was that the frequency of the self-renewing leukemia-initiating cell (LIC) did not correlate with age, sex, or FAB classification, with the exception of some APL cases.[32] In APL, a significant percentage of cases appeared to be derived from a more committed progenitor cell.[36] Subsequent investigations identified both CD34+ and CD34− lineage-negative self-renewing LIC populations that were present at extremely low frequency, demonstrating that the AML stem cell is in many cases derived from a very immature hematopoietic precursor cell.[35]

When these results are placed into the context of the hematopoietic differentiation and developmental trajectory schema, one can conclude that there must be a primary genetic change that occurs in a very primitive self-renewing stem cell and that the nature of those genetic changes in part determines the subtype of AML. For example, a t(8;21) abnormality may lead to M1 AML with minimal differentiation, whereas an inv(16) abnormality may result in an M4Eo subtype. The initiating events may primarily affect the ability of the leukemic stem cell to differentiate along a specified trajectory, and retain the ability to self-replicate.[37,38] Subsequent genetic changes, such as mutation pathways regulating apoptosis, cell survival, cellular metabolism, and proliferation, may further change the phenotype as well as provide proliferative potential for the leukemia. There is also a growing body of literature suggesting that "leukemic stem cells" possess not only unique genetic and immunophenotypic features, but are also characterized by a distinct metabolic state with regard to oxidation status and preferential utilization of nutrient substrates which may also be amenable to therapeutic intervention.[39,40] These might be considered "driver" and "modifier" mutations, respectively. Mutations that do not affect the phenotype may be considered "passenger" mutations. This latter type of genetic change involves mostly secondary mutations that affect the function of growth and survival factor receptors, such as NRAS, KRAS, or KIT. By themselves, most single mutations are insufficient to cause leukemia. However, when present together in the same cell, they can cooperate and lead to the development of AML.

A slightly different alternative way of understanding the etiology of AML in the context of gene mutations is to consider genetic changes under the "two-hit" model. In this model, type I mutations confer a proliferative or survival advantage to cells, and type II mutations result in impaired differentiation and apoptosis of cells.[38] In this model, a driver mutation occurs in a hematopoietic stem cell, thus transforming it into a LIC. The mutation confers a survival advantage and the clone expands. When an additional driver mutation occurs within the cell of the expanding clone, this becomes the "founding" leukemia clone that is detected at presentation. In addition to the few driver mutations, leukemic cells will also have passenger mutations that were gained over time as the clone expanded. Additionally, each mutational event can also result in subclone outgrowth.[41]

Genome-wide sequencing has confirmed the above models but also revealed many additional subkaryotypic abnormalities that include gene mutations in proteins that regulate epigenetic patterning.[42–45] Furthermore, such studies have also helped to define the heterogeneity of AML and its clonal evolution during treatment, which can be influenced by exposure to chemotherapy, especially genotoxic agents. Additional mutations are gained from relapse to diagnosis. This can either occur in a dominant clone that preserves the many mutations present at diagnosis, or a subclone can expand and acquire a different mutational profile. Of interest, although many of the same mutations observed in adults with AML have been found in children with AML, there is a growing body of evidence that shows significant differences also exist. Döhner et al described eight functional categories of genes that are commonly mutated in adult AML (tyrosine kinase receptors, myeloid transcriptions factors, nucleocytoplasmic shuttling proteins, spliceosome gene complex, cohesion-complex gene mutations, epigenetic homeostasis, chromatin homeostasis, and tumor suppressor genes).[46–48] These results have important implications not only for understanding the etiology and pathogenesis of AML but also for the development of more effective treatments.

PREDISPOSING FACTORS AND PATHOPHYSIOLOGY

Inherited Predisposition Syndromes

Abnormal Chromosomal Number

Trisomy 21, or Down syndrome (DS), represents the most common inherited condition that predisposes to the development of myeloid proliferations of Down syndrome (MPDS). In this population the overall risk of developing leukemia has been estimated to be about 14-fold above that of the general population.[49,50] Although older children with DS have a similar frequency of ALL and AML, within the first 3 years of life, AML, and particularly acute megakaryoblastic leukemia (AMKL), predominates.

Infants with DS also have an increased predisposition to develop a condition known as *preleukemia* or *transient abnormal myelopoiesis* (TAM). Approximately 10% of newborns with DS develop TAM. Although clinically indistinguishable from congenital leukemia (Figure 78.2), TAM, as the name suggests, is usually self-resolving. It is important to note that even children who are mosaic for trisomy 21 but phenotypically normal share the increased risk of developing TAM and subsequent leukemia. Approximately 15% to 20% of children whose TAM resolves still develop AMKL.[51–57]

The close association of trisomy 21 with TAM and AMKL suggests that predisposing genetic events exist. *RUNX1*, which is located on chromosome 21 and known to be involved in some subtypes of AML, has been implicated etiologically, but no definitive evidence has yet demonstrated a specific mutation or gene dosage effect leading to AML. However, other investigations have demonstrated the interesting finding that TAM and AMKL are both characterized by mutations

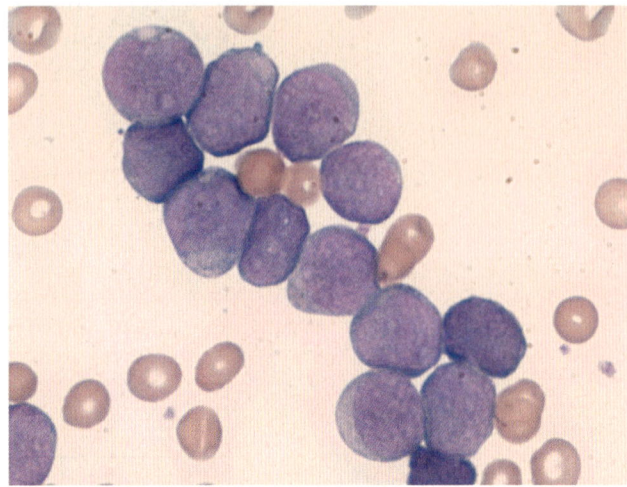

FIGURE 78.2 Photomicrograph of a peripheral blood smear from a patient with Down syndrome and transient abnormal myelopoiesis.

of the *GATA1* gene that result in the introduction of a premature stop codon, truncating *GATA1* before the amino-terminal activation domain and reducing its transcriptional activation ability.[51,52,58] The same *GATA1* mutation has been observed in the blasts from TAM as well as in AMKL. These results argue strongly that mutations in the GATA1 hematopoietic transcription factor are an early event in the development of TAM and AMKL in children with DS. However, it remains unclear why a majority of children with DS and TAM show regression of their disease.

An increased risk of developing AML in patients with Klinefelter syndrome (XXY) and Turner syndrome (XO) has also been reported, but the numbers of such cases are quite low.[59,60]

Inherited Marrow Failure and Chromosome Instability Syndromes

There are several inherited syndromes characterized by progressive marrow failure and cytopenias with a high frequency of myelodysplastic syndrome (MDS) and progression to AML. Fanconi anemia (FA) is an autosomal recessive inherited disorder with common congenital abnormalities that include skeletal abnormalities, short stature, microcephaly, cardiac abnormalities, genitourinary tract abnormalities, café-au-lait spots, and mental retardation. Patients with FA have an estimated 15,000 times greater risk than the general population for developing AML and an actuarial risk of MDS or AML of approximately 52% by 40 years of age. There are multiple gene defects that give rise to FA and affect distinct but functionally related proteins that regulate DNA repair; the mutations result in hypersensitivity to the genotoxic agents mitomycin C or diepoxybutane, and chromosomal instability.[61] Somatic mutations in several of the FA genes have also been observed in AML outside the setting of FA, thus further strengthening the link of these genes with predisposition for AML.[62,63]

Diamond-Blackfan anemia (DBA) is another inherited syndrome characterized by congenital anemia, skeletal and urogenital abnormalities,[53] and an increased risk of developing MDS and AML. An association of mutations and/or deletions in both small and large ribosomal subunit protein encoding genes has established DBA as a ribosomopathy. In addition to showing an increased frequency of AML, patients with DBA appear to have a predisposition to other cancers, making DBA a true cancer predisposition syndrome.

Severe congenital neutropenia (Kostmann syndrome) represents an important inherited cytopenia of the granulocytic lineage with an increased risk of MDS/AML that increases with age.[64] Introduction of G-CSF for the treatment of patients with Kostmann syndrome has been linked to the development of AML. However, it is possible that patients on G-CSF may survive for longer periods, raising the possibility that the development of AML is secondary to an intrinsically increased risk of leukemia in patients with Kostmann syndrome or a combination of this predisposition and G-CSF stimulation. Mutations in the elastase gene have been associated with both cyclic neutropenias and Kostmann syndrome.[65] The detection of somatic activating mutations of the G-CSF receptor has been observed before the development of overt AML in patients with Kostmann syndrome.[66,67]

Shwachman-Diamond syndrome, another inherited syndrome characterized by neutropenia is also associated with pancreatic insufficiency, skeletal abnormalities, and an increased incidence of MDS and AML.[63,68] Patients with dyskeratosis congenita, an inherited disorder due to mutations in genes involved in telomere maintenance, can present with and have an increased risk of MDS and AML.[69]

An increased risk of AML has also been demonstrated for individuals with inherited syndromes involving the platelet lineage including congenital amegakaryocytic thrombocytopenia (defects in the CFFA2 gene and thrombopoietin receptor gene, C-MPL), autosomal dominant macrothrombocytopenia (Fechtner syndrome, MYH9 gene), and familial platelet disorder with propensity to myeloid malignancy (germline mutations in the RUNX1/CEPB-alpha gene).[70]

Germline mutations in the RAS/mitogen-activated protein kinase pathway result in multiple syndromes with overlapping phenotypes that are all associated with a higher risk of leukemia, specifically juvenile myelomonocytic leukemia (JMML). These syndromes, known as "RASopathies" include neurofibromatosis type I (NF1), Noonan syndrome (NS), Costello, Noonan-like CBL, Legius, and cardio-facial cutaneous syndromes.[71] NF1 is caused by mutations in the neurofibromin gene, encoding a RAS-inactivating GTPase, and closely associated with an increased incidence of JMML and AML.[71,] NS, caused by mutations in the PTPN11 gene, which encodes a SHP-2 tyrosine phosphatase, also has an increased predisposition to JMML.[72,73] Importantly, many children with NS can have a transient JMML-like syndrome that can resolve spontaneously.[74] Mutations in CBL, encoding an E3 ubiquitin ligase, have been reported to be associated with a dominant inheritance and result in a clinical phenotype as well as a predisposition to JMML.[71–75]

Germline syndromes characterized by defects in DNA repair have also been shown to have an increased risk of developing leukemia, although more commonly of the lymphoid lineage. Patients with Li-Fraumeni syndrome and Bloom syndrome, with defects in TP53 and the BLM helicase gene, respectively, have also been reported to have a propensity to develop leukemia, including AML.[76–81]

Twins and Familial Cases

Key insights regarding the developmental origins of AML have also come from studies of twin pairs. The increased frequency of both AML and ALL in siblings of patients with leukemia has been recognized since the early 1920s. The risk for identical twins is high when leukemia first develops during infancy; in most cases, transmission has been shown to be the result of transplacental transfer. Transmission rates have been reported to be 20% to 30%, although other investigators have concluded transmission rates may approach 100%.[82–85] There is also a high concordance of timing of the onset of leukemia. Molecular studies have demonstrated that identical molecular defects characterized the leukemia in twins.[86]

Clinical follow-up is therefore essential in identical twins when one of them is diagnosed with acute leukemia. The clinically unaffected twin should be followed approximately every 1 to 2 months until approximately 2 years of age with physical examinations and peripheral blood cell counts, with bone marrow evaluation performed only when clinically indicated. The risk of developing acute leukemia for nonidentical twins has been estimated to be a two- to fourfold increase until about 6 years of age, after which the risk becomes similar to that of the general population. Nontwin familial cases of AML are rare and often associated with constitutional translocations, such as t(7;20) and t(3;6) or monosomy 7. Familial MDS/AML secondary to GATA2 mutations has also been described.[79,84,85,87]

In contrast, AML in older adults is likely results from the slow, gradual acquisition of mutations over many decades, as demonstrated by growing understanding of the phenomenon of clonal hematopoiesis (CH), also referred to as age-related clonal hematopoiesis (ARCH) or clonal hematopoiesis of indeterminate potential (CHIP, see Chapter 80: The Myelodysplastic Syndromes), which describes the presence of expanded clones of cells harboring AML-associated mutations in adults without overt hematologic disease. Specific CH mutations have been shown to lead to an increased risk of both AML as well as cardiovascular disease, and the early detection and management of this clinical entity is an area of active study.[88–91] The implications of CH for the development of pediatric disease remain unclear, although it has long been known that AML-associated translocations can be detected in the neonatal blood spot, also known as the Guthrie card, obtained from a heelstick at birth even in cases where the patient did not develop AML until later in childhood.[83]

Acquired Predisposition

In addition to the inherited bone marrow failure syndromes, acquired aplastic anemia can also be idiopathic or immune-mediated and, as such, patients may acquire predisposition to AML. Patients with severe aplastic anemia (SAA) treated with immunosuppressive agents, such as cyclosporin A and antithymocyte globulin or cyclophosphamide, as well as with recombinant human G-CSF have been reported to have up to a 20% risk of developing MDS or AML. Acquired aplastic anemia also has a close association with paroxysmal nocturnal hemoglobinuria, which is itself associated with an increased risk of developing MDS and AML although less frequently than SAA.[92,93] Although AML arising in patients with MDS is a relatively common event in adults, MDS is rare in children and may differ in biologic and clinical characteristics from that observed in adults. Acquired chromosomal abnormalities such as monosomy 7 may predispose individuals to developing MDS and AML and may be[94,95] linked to exogenous exposures.[96]

Environmental Factors

Just as inherited defects in DNA damage repair lead to increased risk of developing AML, exposure to DNA damaging agents can have similar consequences. For example, in the period after the atomic bombs were dropped on Nagasaki and Hiroshima, an approximately 20-fold increase in myeloid leukemia was documented, with a peak incidence between 6 and 8 years.[97–99] The absence of a documented increase in leukemia in children exposed prenatally to the radiation of the atomic bombs has been reported[100] and may be consistent with the absence of definitive evidence that prenatal exposure to x-rays increases leukemia risk.[101] There is no convincing evidence that ultrasound or the effects of living near high-voltage power lines predispose individuals to leukemia, although reports differ in their conclusions.[102,103]

While chemotherapy represents an obvious and intentional exposure to genotoxic stress for the purpose of treating cancer, there has also been a concerted research effort to better understand the role of maternal and environmental exposures in the development of childhood AML. For instance, there is an association between women treated with topoisomerase II inhibitors and the development of AML, specifically mixed lineage leukemia (KMT2A/MLL) rearrangements in offspring in case control studies in populations across the world.[104,105]

A significant association of dose response of prenatal alcohol consumption and the development of AML in offspring[91] has also been documented. However, not all reports have agreed on the strength of such associations. Parental smoking of tobacco or marijuana has also been associated with an increased incidence of AML in offspring, although there are reports[94,95] with dissenting conclusions. Some reports have also linked cigarette smoking in adults to an increased incidence of AML, making antismoking preventive counseling important, particularly during teenage years.[96,97] Other potential environmental exposures that have been studied are petroleum products, benzene, pesticides, and[98,99] herbicides. Although these studies have not focused on children, in some instances, such as with organophosphate pesticides, children may[100] be at greater risk for accumulating higher levels of these chemicals, so further epidemiological studies are needed as these environmental risk factors may yield insight into geographic and socioeconomic disparities.

An increasingly worrisome group of patients are those who develop AML as a result of chemotherapeutic exposures for treatment of their primary cancer or even nonmalignant conditions. There are three genetic types related to prior chemotherapy: alkylator related with abnormalities of 5, 7 and complex often with a preceding MDS phase, the topo inhibitors with 11q23 abnormalities and acute monocytic presentation at 2 to 5 years, and favorable cytogenetics.

For example, exposure to alkylating agents, commonly used to treat patients with brain tumors, lymphomas, and other solid tumors, results in an increased incidence of secondary AML, with a peak incidence at 4 to 5 years but with an at-risk period extending 12 years.[106–108] Exposure to topoisomerase I inhibitors, including anthracyclines, and topoisomerase II inhibitors, including epipodophyllotoxins such as etoposide, is also etiologically linked to the development of AML.[109,110] Whereas cumulative dose and schedule of drug delivery may play important roles in the development of AML[111] nearly any exposures to such genotoxic agents can result in secondary AML, as demonstrated in a child initially treated for neuroblastoma.[112,113] The development of secondary AML in patients treated first for primary cancers may be one of the most compelling reasons to develop alternative and less genotoxic approaches to therapy.

PRESENTATION

The clinical presentation of AML varies greatly with systemic symptoms and severity of illness usually being a result of leukemia cells' replacement of normal hematopoietic progenitors in the bone marrow as well as their infiltration into various organs. Approximately 10^{12} leukemia cells have been estimated to be present at the time of diagnosis. The leukemic blasts can invade extramedullary sites, such as soft tissues, skin (leukemia cutis), gingiva, orbit, and neuraxis. Patients typically present with signs and symptoms of neutropenia, anemia, and thrombocytopenia. On occasion, other systems may be involved at presentation and demand immediate attention, as in the case of coagulopathy seen most commonly in APL, spinal cord compression from chloromas, or end-organ damage of brain and lungs due to hyperleukocytosis. In such critical cases, it is important to provide directed and supportive treatment even before a diagnosis is known. For example, in cases of suspected APL with significant coagulopathy emergent intervention with aggressive blood product support and administration of all-trans retinoic acid (ATRA) is warranted, emergently, even before the diagnosis is confirmed (see Chapter 79 on Acute Promyelocytic Leukemia).

The total WBC count may be low, normal, or high depending upon the number of circulating leukemic cells. The absolute neutrophil count is often less than 0.5×10^9/L and is associated with an increased risk of infections, often life threatening. Blood cultures and broad-spectrum intravenous antibiotic coverage are indicated in any newly diagnosed patient with leukemia and fever. Anemia results in fatigue, lethargy, decreased exercise tolerance, headache, and pallor. The median hemoglobin is approximately 70 g/L, with a range of 25 to 140 g/L. Although uncommon at the time of presentation, severe anemia, usually normocytic and normochromic, can result in hemodynamic instability or congestive heart failure (CHF). Evidence of red cell fragmentation may be seen in cases presenting with disseminated intravascular coagulation (DIC). Unless there is bleeding or evidence of hemodynamic instability, the transfusion of packed red blood cells should usually be done slowly to prevent precipitating or worsening CHF; and in the case of hyperleukocytosis avoid increased viscosity of blood.

Thrombocytopenia often leads to bruising and petechiae, and occasionally overt hemorrhage into the gastrointestinal track, lungs, or central nervous system (CNS). Nearly 75% of patients present with a platelet count $<100 \times 10^9$/L.[114] Thrombocytopenia may cause petechiae, purpura, mucosal bleeding, and, rarely, CNS and pulmonary hemorrhage. Thrombocytopenia is exacerbated by coagulopathy, especially in the M3 (APL) and M5 AML subtypes. APL blasts express high levels tissue factor (TF; FVII), which results in a consumptive coagulopathy and resultant fibrinolysis leading to DIC. Tissue factor (TF) promoter is activated by the retinoic acid receptor alpha (RARA) oncoprotein expressed in APL blasts, as well as APL cell apoptosis. Although the mechanism for DIC is not known in M5 AML, there is convincing evidence that expression of annexin II, a receptor for fibrinolytic proteins, facilitates plasminogen activation by associating plasminogen and its activator, tissue plasminogen activator, at the APL (M3) leukemic blast cell surface.[115,116]

Patients with peripheral blast counts $>100 \times 10^9$/L should be monitored closely as patients with a blast count $>200 \times 10^9$/L are at risk for CNS stroke due to hyperviscosity, and may benefit from low-dose chemotherapy or leukapheresis to drop the blast count rapidly.[117] Similarly, pulmonary insufficiency may occur in patients with very high leukemia blast counts. Approximately 5% of patients with AML have CNS disease at diagnosis (CNS3), 10% of patients have blasts in the cerebrospinal fluid (CSF) secondary to a traumatic lumbar puncture (LP) if RBCs are present; and a smaller percentage present with CNS chloromas.[118] These patients may have headaches, cranial nerve palsies, focal neurologic deficits, and rarely seizures. Approximately 50% of patients have hepatosplenomegaly and lymphadenopathy. Gingival hyperplasia and leukemia cutis are less frequent but particularly characteristic of myeloid leukemia with monocytic differentiation.

DIAGNOSTIC WORKUP

Differential Diagnosis

The differential diagnosis of AML is broad, including both malignant and nonmalignant conditions. Juvenile rheumatoid arthritis, infectious mononucleosis, aplastic anemia, congenital and acquired cytopenias, and the transient abnormal myelopoiesis of DS infants may all mimic AML. AML may be mistaken for MDS or chronic leukemias, including CML, chronic myelomonocytic leukemia, and JMML. Undifferentiated leukemia or L2 ALL may be morphologically difficult to distinguish from megakaryoblastic AML. Metastatic rhabdomyosarcoma or neuroblastoma in the bone marrow may appear as megakaryoblastic or monoblastic AML, especially in the neonate.

Diagnostic Workup

The diagnosis of AML is typically made on bone marrow aspirate examination, with special stains, flow cytometry, karyotyping, FISH, and molecular testing of DNA and RNA by WES, WGS, and RNAseq providing important additional data for risk stratification. Cytogenetic and molecular analyses are critical not only in assisting in definitive diagnosis, but also provide important prognostic information and are used in treatment stratification. On occasion, definitive diagnosis is difficult either because of technical difficulties in obtaining an adequate specimen or because of conflicting data. Repeat marrow aspirate and biopsy may provide a specimen adequate for diagnosis. Touch preparations of the bone marrow biopsy may be used in cases in which bone marrow aspiration is difficult. Increasingly, a diagnosis can be made from peripheral blood using multiparameter flow cytometry, although in some instances significant differences in antigen expression may exist on leukemic blasts in the bone marrow compared to the peripheral blood.

Investigation of the CSF is considered necessary in children at baseline, as children with CNS involvement require additional CNS-directed therapy. However, in patients with severe bleeding or coagulopathy, the diagnostic LP should be postponed until significant risk of bleeding has resolved. In some current protocols the diagnostic LP is delayed to day 8 of induction, to reduce the incidence of blast contamination into the CSF space. CNS positivity is generally defined as $>5 \times 10^6$/L WBCs in the CSF on a nonbloody tap. To avoid a traumatic tap it should be performed by the most experienced clinician, and with a pencil-point spinal needle. In addition to complete blood counts and differential, electrolytes with complete renal and hepatic function, coagulation testing should be performed.

Next-generation sequencing (NGS) and RNAseq at diagnosis, as a reference for risk stratification and a more sensitive and specific mode of MRD assessment during therapy, may become a standard way of tracking mutations and cryptic translocations during therapy. NGS studies are under study in Children's Oncology Group (COG) and St. Jude frontline AML studies to evaluate their use for MRD monitoring and prognosis.[119]

ACUTE MYELOID LEUKEMIA SUBTYPES

Both FAB[8] and WHO[120] classification systems have been used by clinicians treating pediatric AML patients. The FAB classification system may be especially relevant in regions where genetic sequencing platforms are difficult to access. Generally, both classification systems apply equally well to pediatric and adult patients (Table 78.1). The FAB AML subtypes M0, M1, and M2 correspond to AML that is minimally differentiated, without maturation, and with maturation, respectively; these are more common in older rather than younger children, with frequencies in children 10 to 15 years of age very similar to reported adult frequencies.[121,122] On the other hand, FAB subtypes M5 (acute monocytic leukemia) and M7 (AMKL) are significantly more common in younger children.[121] Likewise, the increased frequency of M7 AML in young patients is mostly due to the high rate of the M7 subtype in patients with DS.[123,124] M0 AML is defined as AML without morphologic signs of differentiation and by expression of CD13, CD33, and CD117 (c-KIT) and myeloperoxidase by flow cytometry or electron microscopy.

Younger children (<2 years of age) are less likely to have t(8;21) and t(15;17) but more frequently have chromosome abnormalities involving 11q23 (KMT2A). KMT2A is a promiscuous fusion partner and to date nearly 100 translocation partners have been identified. The cytogenetic features t(8;21) and inv(16)/t(16;16) are known as core binding factor (CBF) lesions and identify patients with a more favorable prognosis when treated with standard chemotherapy.

More recently the classification of AML in children is based on the WHO[120] system defined by cytogenetics; however, this will continue to evolve based on newly defined molecular subtypes derived from the NIH (National Institutes of Health)-sponsored AML TARGET (therapeutically applicable research to generate effective treatments) project (Figure 78.3).[1,3] State-of-the-art therapy and clinical trials require comprehensive cytogenetic and molecular testing for risk stratification, and measurement of minimal residual disease by multiparameter flow cytometry or more sensitive polymerase chain reaction (PCR), or clinical applications of NGS techniques currently in development as a research test as specified in a clinical trial.[119,125]

THERAPY FOR PATIENTS WITH NEWLY DIAGNOSED ACUTE MYELOID LEUKEMIA

Background

Pediatric AML protocols begin with a remission-induction regimen, followed by a course of consolidation or intensification courses that may include hematopoietic cell transplantation (HCT). This relatively brief but intensive approach has yielded an approximately 60% to 70% chance of overall survival (OS) across different cooperative group

Table 78.1. Comparison of Key Characteristics of Acute Myeloid Leukemia (AML) in Pediatric vs Adult Patients

Characteristic	Pediatric ≤21 y	Adults >21 and <55-60 y
Cytogenetics	Higher frequency favorable risk cytogenetics	Greater percent of unfavorable cytogenetics and drug-resistant markers
Antecedent AML predisposing disorders	Rare (some inherited predisposition)	Common (MDS, MPN, and therapy-related)
Subtype	More M4/M5, DS, TMD	Less M4/M5, no DS or TMD
Extramedullary disease	More CNS disease/leukemia cutis	Uncommon except in monocytic lineage
Induction	ADE	"7 and 3" standard
Remission rates (after 2 courses)	85%-90%	60%-80%
CNS prophylaxis	Yes	Not routine
HCT	Only for high-risk patients	For some intermediate- and most high-risk patients
APL treatment	ATRA at 25 mg/m^2	ATRA at 45 mg/m^2
Gene mutations		
FLT3-ITD	10%-20%	20%-50%
FLT3-TKD or ALM	5%-7%	5%-7%
KIT	25% in t(8;21)	17% in CBF
N-RAS	20%	10%
PTPN11	5%-21% (infants)	Rare
WT1	13% (CN-AML)	10% (normal karyotype)
NPM1	5%-10% (14%-22% in CN-AML)	35% (53% in CN-AML)
CEBPA	5% (14% in CN-AML)	10% in CN-AML
IDH1 or 2	1%-2%	12%-15%
TET2	Rare	16%
DNMT3A	Rare	20%
Overall survival	Approximately 60%-65%	Approximately 30%-40%
Late complications	Growth, endocrine, cardiac, neurocognitive, secondary malignancies	Secondary malignancies

Abbreviations: ADE, Ara-C, daunomycin and etoposide; APL, acute promyelocytic leukemia; ATRA, all-trans retinoic acid; CBF, core binding factor; CN-AML, cytogenetically normal AML; CNS, central nervous system; DS, down syndrome; HCT, hematopoietic cell transplantation; MDS, myelodysplastic syndrome; MPN, myeloproliferative neoplasm; TMD, transient myeloproliferative disorder.
Adapted from Arceci RJ, Meshinchi S, Rosenblat TL, Jurcic JG, Tallman MS. Childhood, adolescent and young adult acute myeloid leukemias. In: Cairo MS, Perkins SL, eds. Hematological Malignancies in Children, Adolescents and Young Adults. World Scientific Publishing; 2012 and Creutzig U, van den Heuvel-Eibrink MM, Gibson B, et al. Diagnosis and management of acute myeloid leukemia in children and adolescents: recommendations from an international expert panel. Blood. 2012;120(16):3187-3205. doi:10.1182/blood-2012-03-362608

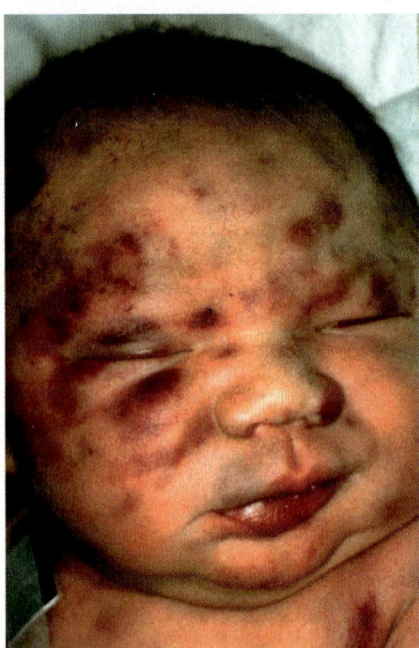

FIGURE 78.3 Leukemia cutis in an infant with congenital leukemia. (Reprinted with permission from Arceci RJ, Weinstein HJ. Neoplasia. In: MacDonald MG, Mullett MD, Seshia MM, eds. *Avery's Neonatology: Pathophysiology and Management of the Newborn.* Lippincott Williams & Wilkins; 2005:1444-1468.)

protocols.[15,126–129] Although there is general agreement that pediatric AML therapy should be based on the use of anthracyclines and cytarabine, pediatric cooperative groups differ in their induction regimens and the use of HCT in the postremission period. Risk stratification based on cytogenetic and molecular lesions, as well as response to therapy, is being used to refine prognostic and therapeutic approaches, including the introduction of targeted agents. The heterogeneity of AML as noted in the introduction is the likely explanation for the plateau in survival after last 2 decades (see survival curves *Figure 78.1*).

Induction Therapy

The primary goal of induction therapy is to achieve a remission of disease. Historically, this is defined in the United States as peripheral blood count recovery with a normal or slightly hypocellular marrow with fewer than 5% leukemic blasts and no evidence of extramedullary disease. An increasingly important additional marker of response is the eradication of detectable MRD, which is evaluated by either multidimensional flow cytometry or molecular testing using PCR. Cooperative groups in the United States currently use eradication of MRD for defining remission status following induction therapy.[14,15,129]

The first significant successful remission-induction regimen for patients with AML included 7 days of continuous infusion Ara-C at 100 mg/m^2/d and 3 initial days of an anthracycline, such as daunorubicin, at 45 mg/m^2 to 60 mg/m^2/d. This regimen resulted in remission rates of between 60% and 70% in children and young adults.[130] However, several approaches have been utilized to improve on these remission rates, including altering the schedule and doses of Ara-C and anthracyclines, as well as the introduction of additional agents. Furthermore, supportive care measures, such as the preemptive use of broad-spectrum antibiotics and/or blood product transfusions, have proven to reduce significantly remission induction mortality and thus have improved remission rates.

Despite the different approaches taken by the cooperative groups, several important conclusions can be made. First, remission quality, now defined as undetectable MRD at the end of induction, modifies relapse risk, and more intensive induction regimens may provide deeper remissions with lower relapse rates and improved OS.[14,15,129] The issue of induction intensification was nicely demonstrated in the Children's Cancer Group (CCG)-2891 study, in which the intensively timed DCTER (dexamethasone, cytarabine, thioguanine, etoposide, and daunorubicin) arm had a similar morphologic induction success rate compared to the standard timing regimen, but the relapse rate for the intensively timed arm was lower regardless of postinduction therapy.[127] However, more intensive induction regimens also carry greater treatment-related morbidity and mortality that can diminish the net benefit of such intensive therapy. In general, trials using a very intensive induction regimen noted an initial toxic death rate of approximately 15%, which decreases to usually less than 5% with acquired treatment experience.[131–133]

This high induction mortality rate has been reduced in several studies by mandated supportive care guidelines (see the section "Supportive Care"). Although escalating the economic cost of AML therapy, these supportive care guidelines are critical for improved outcomes. In the CCG, these guidelines mandated early initiation of broad-spectrum antibiotics, including vancomycin at the first febrile episode, early initiation of treatment doses of antifungal agents after 3 to 5 days of persistent fevers, hospitalization until granulocyte recovery, strict hand washing, and use of high-efficiency particulate-air-filtered rooms whenever possible. Institution of these guidelines lowered toxic mortality to approximately 5% across cooperative group trials.[134]

Various trials have also tried to answer additional remission induction questions, including (1) determining the optimal dose and schedule of cytarabine,[135,136] (2) determining the optimal anthracycline and dose, and (3) determining what agents can be added to the cytarabine and anthracycline backbone to improve outcomes. Although dose intensification of cytarabine has not been demonstrated to improve remission induction rates, higher doses appear to confer lower rates of leukemia relapse in adults with CBF AML.[130,137] Becton et al reported the Pediatric Oncology Group (POG)-9421 trial that randomized patients to standard vs high-dose cytarabine in induction therapy.[138]

Debate continues over the optimal anthracycline choice in induction. The Berlin-Frankfurt-Munster (BFM) group showed evidence that idarubicin was superior to daunorubicin in induction as shown in the AML-BFM 93, which compared 60 mg/m^2/d daunorubicin with 12 mg/m^2/d idarubicin for 3 days each, combined with cytarabine and etoposide during induction.[139–141]

And a meta-analysis by the Medical Research Council (MRC)/Institute for Cancer Research of randomized idarubicin/daunorubicin comparisons suggested that idarubicin is superior.[142] The CCG-2941 and COG-2961 trials showed that idarubicin was too toxic to be used in sequential courses of intensively timed IdaDCTER therapy.[132–134]

The MRC AML-12 trial randomized daunorubicin, Ara-C, and etoposide (ADE) vs mitoxantrone, Ara-C, etoposide (MAE) as induction regimens. Although the MAE regimen showed a decrease in the relapse rate compared to the ADE-treated group, the increased risk of treatment-related mortality led to no overall benefit in disease-free survival (DFS) or OS.[114,143] Anthracyclines remain a standard of AML therapy due to their efficacy; however, concerns about cardiotoxicity and late effects have led to the use of liposomal daunorubicin in Europe. More recently, in adults the use of liposomal combination of cytarabine and daunorubicin at a 5:1 molar ratio appears to be as or more active and less toxic than the combined use of nonliposomal cytarabine and daunorubicin.[144] This liposomal combination is currently under study randomized against ADE in the COG study AAML1831.

Whereas the addition of other agents to the "7 and 3" backbone has helped increase induction rates from 70% to 85%, no randomized trial has demonstrated the superiority of a particular agent, or combination of agents, over any other combination. Specifically, the MRC-10 trial tested 6-thioguanine vs etoposide with daunomycin and cytarabine and found no statistically significant difference between the two induction regimens. In an attempt to introduce a novel, non-cross-resistant agent into induction therapy, the COG AAML03P1 trial demonstrated that gemtuzumab ozogamicin (GO) can be safely added to a backbone of induction cytarabine, daunorubicin, and etoposide, resulting in a remission rate of 83.5% after 1 cycle of therapy.[128,145,146] Following the establishment of the safety of GO, the COG AAML0531 trial randomized patients to receive GO and demonstrated that its addition resulted in improved event-free survival (EFS) and decreased relapse risk; however, an OS advantage was not observed. This may have been partly due to higher toxic mortality among patients receiving GO.[147] The French cooperative group randomized trial demonstrated an improvement in OS as well as relapse-free survival with the addition of GO.[148] A randomized study from the MRC demonstrated no change in remission rates or OS with the addition of GO, but an OS advantage for patients with CBF AML was observed.[149] No advantage was observed in a Nordic Society of Pediatric Hematology and Oncology (NOPHO) trial randomizing GO in the postremission setting.[150]

In summary, current pediatric AML induction regimens successfully induce remission in approximately 85% of patients using a variety of induction strategies. The improvements in induction remission rates have come primarily from intensification of therapy, either by adding additional agents to the "7 and 3" backbone or from dose intensification.[151–153] Although successful, it appears unlikely that further dose escalation or intensification will significantly improve remission rates. Thus, a central remission induction question now centers on the selection and safe integration of other novel agents, which includes immunotherapeutic strategies such as GO, or other anti-CD33 monoclonal antibody conjugates, or bispecific T-cell engager antibodies, in order to increase antileukemic activity with less toxicity than conventional chemotherapy.[145,146,154] In addition, agents that inhibit the BCL2 family of proteins to lower the apoptotic threshold without genotoxic effects are in early-phase testing,[155] and may be candidates to test with a "7 and 3" backbone as a pilot pediatric study AML23 by the St. Jude AML consortium (personal communication). Readers are referred to the following sources for updated recommendations on the standard of care for induction in pediatric AML for the COG and St. Jude AML consortiums.[156,157]

Postremission Therapy

Once a complete remission (CR) has been achieved, including undetectable flow-MRD status, additional therapy is required to avoid disease relapse. Various combinations and numbers of courses of therapy have been tested. Risk stratification using cytogenetic,[158] molecular, and disease response allows for more appropriate postremission therapeutic strategies in biologically distinct subsets of patients and identifies patients who can benefit the most from more intensive consolidation strategies, namely allogeneic hematopoietic stem cell transplantation (allo-HCT, or haplo-HCT).[159]

Dose and Duration

Although agreement exists on the role of cytarabine-based intensification therapy, especially for CBF myeloid leukemias in which additional courses of cytarabine appear to decrease relapse risk significantly, the optimal number of cycles of intensification chemotherapy is not known.[160–164] The published pediatric AML trials have used either 2 or 3 courses of consolidation therapy, for a total of 4 or 5 courses of therapy.[143,] The MRC AML-10 trial randomized patients to either auto-HCT transplant or no further therapy and demonstrated a decreased relapse risk in patients receiving auto-HCT. However, the addition of auto-HCT was associated with significant morbidity and mortality, thus abrogating any OS advantage.[165] The CCG-2961 trial gave patients a total of 3 courses of chemotherapy with a resulting OS of 57% following changes in supportive care recommendations.[132] The MRC AML-12 trial randomized patients to a total of 4 vs 5 courses of chemotherapy with an OS of 81% vs 78%, respectively, at 5 years (P = .5).[143] The question of duration and intensity of consolidation therapy from recent North American trials (AAML1031 and St. Jude AML08) are under analysis but preliminary results suggest that low-risk patients (CBF AML) may benefit from 5 courses of chemotherapy.

The use of maintenance therapy with relatively low-dose chemotherapy has been currently abandoned with the exception of BFM studies, which in part base this choice on the results of BFM-87, in which a maintenance phase was beneficial to a low-risk group of patients who did not receive HCT. However, when only randomized patients were analyzed, no significant difference in outcome was observed.[166,167] Other cooperative groups, however, have shown that maintenance therapy is associated with a decrease in both EFS and OS when compared to shorter, more intensive regimens, with relapsed disease being more resistant to subsequent therapies.[168,169]

Hematopoietic Cell Transplantation

Sustained improvements in chemotherapeutic regimens and supportive care have continued to reduce the need for patients to receive allogeneic HCT. Furthermore, several studies have shown equivalent OS when compared to chemotherapy; most cooperative groups have thus omitted autologous HCT from consideration in order potentially to avoid greater short- and long-term toxicities.[166,170] However, with equivalency of overall outcome between autologous HCT and chemotherapy, one might also conclude that either approach would be a reasonable, evidenced-based recommendation.[171] In addition, alternative approaches to transplantation, such as the use of nonablative or intensity-reduced allogeneic or haplo-identical HCT with and without manipulation of T-cell subsets, perform well in comparison to more conventional approaches.

Key questions are whether allogeneic HCT provides an overall improvement in survival and quality of life compared to chemotherapy-only treatment approaches. In order to answer these questions, it has been necessary to define risk groups more carefully in terms of outcome and potential for benefit from HCT. In addition, there are some subtypes of high-risk AML that may not benefit from HCT; thus early-phase studies are needed for these patients. More recently, several studies have demonstrated that risk classification allows for identification of certain subgroups of patients that benefit from consolidation HCT. In addition, whereas most trials have analyzed outcomes on whether patients did or did not have an HLA-matched donor, the improved success with matched unrelated donor (MUD) HCT has led to outcome analysis based on availability of the best HLA-matched donor.

Many trials have shown that allogeneic HCT results in an improved DFS compared to chemotherapy or autologous HCT.[172,173] However, HCT has not usually resulted in an improved EFS or OS, reflecting the associated increased treatment-related mortality. Such results suggest that HCT may benefit some groups more than others. Several studies have attempted to define such subgroups more precisely.

Based on the MRC AML-10 cytogenetic and response-based risk stratification, OS at 5 years from the time of relapse was 57%, 14%, and 8% for good, standard, and poor risk groups, respectively; this led to the conclusion that allogeneic HCT should not be done in good risk AML in CR1. Although outcomes from MRC AML-10 also suggested that allo-HCT in first remission was improved for patients with intermediate- and high-risk AML, combined data from the MRC AML-10 and 12 trials showed no statistically significant benefit for these groups of patients compared to chemotherapy alone. BFM trials and POG-8821 and 9421 studies showed comparable results although in the POG trials a detailed subgroup stratification was not done.[114,123,143,149]

Analysis of postremission treatment of 1464 children less than age 21 years on five consecutive CCG trials from 1979 to 1996 has shown an advantage to those patients assigned a HCT in terms of OS (P = .026), DFS (P = .005), and relapse rate (P < .001).[167] Subgroup analysis demonstrated that HCT was associated with improved survival for patients with WBC greater than 50,000/μL and for those with normal karyotype, but was not beneficial for patients with AML characterized by good-risk cytogenetics, such as inv(16) or t(8;21).

A more detailed analysis of the MRC AML-12 outcomes has reported no advantage of HCT for patients in the good and intermediate groups, but a statistically significant advantage for relapse-free survival and OS for a subset of patients with high-risk AML; for example, in the 12% of patients defined as having poor-risk AML, HCT was associated with an OS of 41% compared to 10% for those who received only chemotherapy (P = .001).[114]

A high *FLT3-ITD* (internal tandem duplication) mutant to normal allele frequency has been uniformly associated with a poor prognosis when patients are treated with standard chemotherapeutic regimens alone with DFS of approximately 20% to 30%.[174–177] In POG-9421 gene expression analysis in a small cohort of patients (n = 42) segregated *FLT3*-ITD and *TKD* (tyrosine kinase domain mutation) patients with intermediate and poor outcome, reflecting the heterogeneity of AML in the setting of a powerful prognostic factor such as *FLT3* mutation.[178] Several studies have demonstrated an advantage of HCT for patients with a high mutant allele frequency of *FLT3*-ITD mutations.[179,180] Data from the CCG-2941 and 2961 trials showed a borderline significant difference in relapse for patients with *FLT3-ITD* positive AML who received a allogeneic matched sibling donor HCT (27% ± 27%) compared to those treated with only chemotherapy (65% ± 15%, P = .05). However, OS at 4 years from the end of the second course of treatment was not significantly different (64% ± 29% for those with *FLT3-ITD* AML who received an allogeneic HCT and 48% ± 17% for those treated with chemotherapy [P = .4]).[175,179–181] Importantly, no difference was seen in low allelic ratio patients according to consolidation treatment strategy. Patients with *FLT3-ITD* have high levels of CD33 expression and the use of induction GO followed by consolidation HCT in this group is associated with improved DFS of 65% and reduced relapse.[182] Currently, most ongoing clinical trials for children and young adults assign allogeneic HCT for patients with high mutant *FLT3-ITD* to normal allelic ratio, often in the context of additional targeted therapy directed toward inhibition of the mutant *FLT3* receptor.[182–188]

Patients with AML characterized by alterations in CBF t(8;21), inv(16), t(16;16) have an approximately 80% OS with chemotherapy alone and, thus, HCT is recommended only in CR2.[189,190] Similarly, children and young adults with APL have an OS of 75% to 95%, depending on risk group, with combinations of chemotherapy plus ATRA and arsenic.[191,192] Thus, HCT is not usually recommended in CR1 for these patients, but instead in some cases following CR2 or refractory disease, in which case allogeneic, and in some instances autologous, HCT results in an approximately 70% OS.[189,193,194]

KMT2A-rearranged AML represents an extremely heterogeneous group of leukemias associated with variable outcomes according to the 11q23 translocation partner. For example, an international trial has reported that survival is 100%, 63%, 27%, and 22% for patients with the t(1;11), the t(9;11), the t(4;11), and the t(6;11), respectively.[195] Because of the wide variability of outcomes along with small numbers of patients with *KMT2A/MLL* subtypes as well as no prospective definitive data that demonstrate HCT improves outcome in this group of patients, most cooperative group clinical trials have not used allogeneic HCT in CR1.[143] An intention-to-treat analysis of the AML-BFM 98 study has suggested an improved OS with allogeneic MSD HCT for patients with 11q23 rearrangements.[142] Consolidation HCT in CR1 could be considered for patients with *KMT2A* subtypes associated with poor prognosis in multiple studies, including t(6;11) and t(10;11).[195] Patients with poor-risk *KMT2A* rearrangements have been shown to have improved survival when treated with HCT.[196]

AML characterized by a normal karyotype represents a large percentage of cases and is a molecularly heterogeneous group. For example, nucleophosmin member 1 (*NPM1*) mutations are associated with an improved outcome, although not necessarily in the presence of high mutant *FLT3-ITD* to normal allelic ratio.[197] AML with *CEBPA* mutations is usually associated with normal karyotype AML and improved OS, thus making HCT undesirable in CR1.[46] Point mutations involving *KIT*, *RAS*, or *WT1* (Wilms tumor 1) have not yet been definitively shown to improve outcome although some data exist linking them to a poorer prognosis.[198] Furthermore, patients with AML and high-risk cytogenetics, such as monosomy 7 or del(5q)- and -5, are recommended to have HCT in CR1 (Table 78.2).

The COG AML clinical trial AAML0531 stratified patients to receive allogeneic HCT in first remission only for those predicted high risk of treatment failure based on unfavorable cytogenetic, molecular characteristics and elevated end-of-induction MRD levels.[147] In contrast, the AML-BFM 2004 clinical trial restricted allogeneic HCT to patients in second CR or refractory AML, based on results from their AML-BFM 98 study showing no improvement in DFS or OS for high-risk patients receiving allogeneic HCT.[199,200] Although the optimal timing for allogeneic HCT has not been determined, most cooperative groups recommend a HCT following the second or third course of chemotherapy, based in part due to the time involved in obtaining HLA typing. The use of MUDs, single- or double-cord blood donor, or nonablative approaches for HCT in CR1 are not as clearly established as MSD or haploidentical HCT donors, but are increasingly used to provide potential curative treatment for patients with recurrent AML.[170,192,201,202]

Table 78.2. Risk Groups Defined by Cytogenetic, Molecular Alterations, and Minimal Residual Disease (MRD)

Low Risk/Low Risk 1: (HCT not recommended)
- t(8;21), inv16, CEBPA biallelic mutation, NPM1 AND flow-MRD <0.05% after induction 1
- t(15;17) [treated on APL-specific protocol with own specified low- and high-risk categories]
- *GATA1* (Down syndrome)

Low Risk 2/Intermediate Risk:
- absence of low- and high-risk features
- t(9;11)
- t(8;21), inv16, CEBPA biallelic mutation, NPM1 AND flow-MRD ≥0.05% and negative for unfavorable risk markers
- t(8;21), inv16/t(16;16) and coexisting KIT exon 17 mutation and negative for unfavorable risk factors
- *FLT3*-ITD/wild-type allelic ratio >0.1 without bZIP CEBPa or NPM1 AND flow-MRD <0.05% at end of induction 1
- flow-MRD <0.05% at end of induction 1 and no favorable or unfavorable prognostic markers
- Presence of non-FLT3-ITD activating mutations with flow-MRD <0.05%

High Risk: (candidate for HCT)
- MRD≥0.1% after induction 1
- *FLT3*-ITD/wild-type allelic ratio >0.1 without bZIP CEBPa or NPM1 AND flow-MRD ≥0.05% at end of induction 1
- Presence of non-FLT3-ITD activating mutations with flow-MRD ≥0.05%
- RAM phenotype
- *WT1/FLT3*-ITD
- inv(3)(q21q26.2)/t(3;3)(q21.3q26.2); [RPN1-MECOM]
- t(3;21)(26/2;q22); [RUNX1-MECOM]
- t(3;5)(q25;q34); [NPM1-MLF1]
- t(6;9)(p22.3;q34/1); [DEK-NUP214 = MLL-MLLT2]
- t(8;16)(p11/2;p13.3); [KAT6A-CREBBP] if 90 d or older.
- t(16;21)(p11.2;q22.2); [FUS-ERG]
- t(4;11)(q21;q23.3); [KMT2A-AFF1 = MLL-MLLT2]
- t(6;11); [KMT2A-AFDN = MLL-MLLT4]]
- t(10;11)(p12.3;q23.3); [KMT2A-MLLT10]
- t(10;11)(p12.1;q23.3); [KMT2A-ABI1]
- t(11;19)(q23/3;p13.3); [KMT2A-MLLT1 = MLL-ENL]
- t(5;11)(q35;p15.5); [NUP98-NSD1]
- t(7;11)(p15.4;p15); [NUP98-HOXA9]
- t(11;12)(p15; p13); [NUP98-KDM5A] or any NUP98 partner
- t(7;12)(q36;p13); [ETV6-HLXB] or any ETV6 partner
- t(X;11)(q24;q23); [SEPT6-KMT2A]
- inv(16)(p13.3q24.3); [CBFA2T3-GLIS2]
- Deletion 12p, 12p13.2 rearrangement; [ETV6-any partner gene]
- 10p12.3 rearrangement; [MLLT10-any partner gene]
- AML with minimal differentiation
- Acute erythroid leukemia
- Acute megakaryoblastic leukemia (AMKL) with *KMT2A* rearrangements
- t(1;22) in non-DS
- t(9;22)
- Complex karyotype
- Refractory anemia with excessive blasts and >10% bone marrow blasts (RAEB-2)
- AML arising from MDS
- Monosomy 7, monosomy 5, 5q- [loss of EGR1]
- Treatment-related (secondary) AML

Summary of Therapy for Patients With Newly Diagnosed Acute Myeloid Leukemia

Despite some differences in their approaches, most pediatric cooperative groups share a common treatment strategy based on anthracyclines and cytarabine and risk stratified use of HCT. OS at 5 years for children with AML is in the 65% to 70% range, with some patients doing significantly better and others worse based on cytogenetic, molecular, and response characteristics. Patients with molecular lesions amenable to therapeutic targeting, namely *FLT3*-ITD mutations with FLT3 inhibitors, can receive tyrosine kinase inhibitors in conjunction with chemotherapy. Further, immunotherapeutic strategies and their role in upfront therapy, including CD33 targeting, liposomal option for "7 + 3," are the focus of much investigation. As more children and adolescents are long-term survivors, increased attention is also now being paid to survivorship issues.

THERAPY FOR PATIENTS WITH RELAPSED/REFRACTORY DISEASE

Despite AML treatment intensification, recurrent and/or refractory disease remain the major causes of treatment failure. Re-induction regimens typically use high-dose cytarabine, even if prior therapy has included substantial cytarabine exposure. With the addition of agents such as mitoxantrone, etoposide, fludarabine, cladribine, or clofarabine to cytarabine, azacytidine, or decitabine window followed by fludarabine and cytarabine, and more recently venetoclax to a backbone of cytarabine and idarubicin, approximately 50% to 70% of patients with relapsed or refractory disease achieve CR, depending on the time of their relapse relative to their therapy.[203–208] There is evidence that the combination of fludarabine, idarubicin, and cytarabine (FLAG-Ida) has a high remission-induction rate. However, the toxicity associated with this regimen is also substantial.[206,208] Subsequent studies evaluating fludarabine + cytarabine compared to fludarabine, cytarabine, and the liposomal version of daunorubicin found no benefit with the addition of an anthracycline to remission rates or survival.[209] However, for patients with CBF AML the addition of an anthracycline to salvage therapy resulted in improved survival. The combination of mitoxantrone and high-dose cytarabine used in the CCG-2951 study achieved a 76% overall remission rate.[210] Several adult trials have demonstrated that GO may be safely combined with several chemotherapy regimens for AML re-induction therapy. The COG AAML00P2 trial demonstrated that GO could be safely combined with either cytarabine/mitoxantrone or with cytarabine/L-asparaginase. However, exposure to GO, particularly at single-agent doses, <3 months prior to HCT increases the risk of severe veno-occlusive disease (VOD) during HCT; however, use of defibrotide greatly improves the management of post-HCT of VOD.[211–213]

Patients with refractory or relapsed AML will require an allogeneic HCT from either a related or an unrelated donor to achieve a long-term cure.[200,214] Conditioning regimens are quite variable, and randomized and prospective trials are rare. Because many investigators are reluctant to give conditioning regimens that include total-body irradiation to young children, the balance between risks and benefits of total-body irradiation-containing regimens for relapsed AML is largely based on retrospective comparative reports. Donor sources have included MUD, HLA-matched and HLA-mismatched cord blood (single or double) donors, haploidentical donors as well as KIR-mismatched unrelated or haploidentical donors.

Although the use of cord blood units and haploidentical grafts makes alternative donors available for almost every patient, fully matched sibling donor is usually the preferred source. Patients with detectable MRD at the time of transplant experienced lower rates of relapse following cord blood transplant as compared to unrelated donors, including matched and mismatched.[215] Haploidentical grafts may be associated with higher rates of graft-vs-host disease, as well as higher rates of viral infections and posttransplant lymphoproliferative disease as a result of the intensive immunosuppressive transplant regimens used.[216]

Despite the increased risks of toxicity, infectious complications, and graft-vs-host disease associated with the allogeneic transplant typically used for relapsed or refractory AML, between 20% and 50% of patients may achieve long-term survival.[215,217] Cure is significantly affected by the duration of first CR, with shorter CR1 (e.g., <6 months off therapy or while on therapy) being associated with lower OS.[218] Leukemia karyotype may also modify the probability of achieving CR with relapsed and/or refractory AML.[219] Overall, patients with AML characterized by such high-risk features have a 3-year survival of <20%, whereas patients with initial CR lasting >1 year may have a 30% to 40% 3-year survival. However, the rate of cure for patients with relapsed CBF AML shows an excellent survival rate following CR2 and allogeneic HCT. Clinicians can seek information on precision oncology studies for relapse and refractory AML at https://www.lls.org/dare-to-dream/pedal.

SUPPORTIVE CARE

Current AML treatments are among the most intensive used in children with cancer, and cause a wide variety of severe complications. AML treatment-related morbidity and mortality significantly affect OS of patients, both through treatment delays and deaths due to toxicity. Thus, patients with AML should be cared for by physicians and nurses experienced in AML therapy in institutions with appropriate laboratory, radiology, blood banking, and surgical services.

Standardization of supportive care, as shown by Riley et al, may reduce treatment-related mortality by 50%.[131] AML supportive care guidelines typically focus on infection prophylaxis and treatment, although hematologic support is also critical. Fever and neutropenia in patients with AML constitute a medical emergency. After obtaining blood cultures, broad-spectrum antibiotic therapy should be instituted rapidly. Coverage for penicillin-resistant *Streptococcus viridans* and gram-negative organisms should be given, and anaerobic coverage should be added if clinically indicated. Local microbial resistance patterns should dictate selection of initial antibiotics, although broad-spectrum antibiotics are typically included in the initial antibiotic selection. Patients should remain on broad-spectrum coverage until their neutropenia shows signs of resolution with recovery of hematopoiesis. Vancomycin use may be limited to 24 to 48 hours until a resistant *S. viridans* infection has been excluded.[219,220] Although patients with AML are at risk for a wide range of bacterial infections, gram-negative organisms occur frequently at diagnosis, and α-hemolytic streptococcus (*S. viridans*) is often seen after intensive high-dose cytarabine containing consolidation regimens.[220–222] In many centers and protocols the use of levofloxacin prophylaxis is used during periods of profound and extended neutropenia.[223]

Empiric antifungal therapy should begin if fever persists for >3 to 5 days after initiation of antibiotic therapy or with recurrent fever. Voriconazole has recently emerged as the first-line choice for antifungal coverage due its broad activity and efficacy, particularly against aspergillosis. Caspofungin can also be used as can amphotericin B, which is often utilized as second-line to its significant side effect profile.[224] Given the availability of new antifungal agents, the selection of the appropriate antifungal agent is guided by culture results, which may require confirmatory diagnostic testing, including biopsy or bronchial alveolar lavage. Radiographic findings of lesions can be difficult to biopsy and in those cases treatment with empiric therapy until resolution of findings should be the standard. Note that strict hand-washing guidelines, mandated hospitalization until neutrophil recovery, and use of high-efficiency particulate-air-filtered rooms whenever possible all significantly decrease the incidence, morbidity, and mortality of infections in pediatric AML patients.

Multiple studies, including the recently reported BFM 98 trial, have demonstrated that G-CSF may decrease the length of neutropenia and the length of hospital stay, but it does not appear to alter severe toxicity or infection rates.[225–227] Unlike studies in adults, G-CSF treatment in patients with hypercellular day 7 bone marrows on CCG-2891 had a statistically significantly improved remission rate and OS, although the introduction of G-CSF in this study was not randomized.[228]

There has been no randomized study showing the advantage of using growth factors. However, in clinical practice when facing a patient requiring pressor support in the setting of suspected or identified infection, some clinicians may initiate growth factor support.

Prophylaxis against opportunistic infections is also an important supportive care issue. Although *Pneumocystis jirovecii* is rare in pediatric patients with AML, prophylaxis with trimethoprim-sulfamethoxazole is often given. *S. viridans* sepsis may be prevented by penicillin prophylaxis in centers where *S. viridans* remains penicillin-sensitive. Penicillin resistance, however, is becoming more frequently detected. High-efficiency particulate-air-filtration has been shown to diminish *Aspergillus* infection in marrow transplant patients and likely benefits AML patients who experience prolonged periods of neutropenia and immunosuppression.[229] In addition to management of infectious complications, the preemptive use of blood products has also been shown to play a critical role in the successful treatment of patients with AML.[230–232] Recently developed NGS and bioinformatics techniques provide rapid serum detection of over a thousand bacteria, DNA viruses, yeasts, molds and protozoa. Ongoing early clinical trials will define its application to reduce or prevent infectious disease morbidity and mortality in the treatment of AML patients.[233]

LATE EFFECTS OF THERAPY

Although intensive AML protocols cure a substantial fraction of children with AML, the late effects of these therapies can be significant. Several investigators have reported on AML late effects, but population-based follow-up studies of recent intensive therapies are lacking and remain a critically needed area of research.[234–236] Leung et al, reporting on 77 patients surviving more than 10 years from diagnosis, observed that increasing radiation dose as well as younger age at diagnosis and timing of radiation therapy were risk factors for growth delay, infertility, academic difficulties, cataracts, and hypothyroidism. Patients receiving total-body irradiation had lower cumulative anthracycline doses (204 mg/m^2 vs 335 mg/m^2) but did not have a lower rate of cardiomyopathy, suggesting an interaction of radiation and anthracyclines.[236] An analysis of a cohort of infants with leukemia treated by chemotherapy and then HCT indicated that 59% had growth hormone deficiency, 35% had hypothyroidism, 24% had osteochondromas, 24% had decreased bone mineral density, and 59% had dyslipidemias.[237] Temming et al reported on results from the United Kingdom that there was a 13.7% and 17.4% prevalence of early and late cardiotoxicity in childhood AML survivors treated with chemotherapy.[238] Patients who survive AML therapy also have a significantly increased rate of secondary malignancies.[239] However, primary disease relapse and therapy-related morbidity decrease EFS significantly more than secondary AML.

A population-based study involving children treated on NOPHO clinical trials demonstrated overall equivalent usage of health care services compared to their siblings, although there was a significant increase in use of prescription medications, especially for asthma in the leukemia survivors.[240] A Childhood Cancer Survivor Study analysis of 272 5-year survivors of AML showed excellent resiliency and health in this group with significant concerns relating to secondary malignant neoplasms (the majority of which were in the setting of radiation exposure) as well as lower socioeconomic achievement compared to siblings. In addition, half of the survivors reported at least one chronic medical problem and were considered at increased risk for a severe or life-threatening condition compared to their siblings.[241] Since nearly all infants, children, and adolescents with AML are treated in the inpatient setting, with typically intravenous administration of chemotherapy less attention has been paid to disparities in outcome. As more focus in placed in this important area of investigation, there is evidence of disparity of in-hospital mortality, disparity in access and enrollment into clinical trials. These disparities are likely a combination of biologic features of the disease, and socioeconomic factors. We expect that prospective research in this important area will inform on how to address disparities in outcome, and more importantly in access of care at pediatric oncology centers.[242,243]

MANAGEMENT OF PATIENTS WITH DOWN SYNDROME

The majority of leukemias in children with DS are lymphoid, although DS children comprise 10% of pediatric AML patients and thus represent the most frequently genetic disorder associated with the development of AML[244] (*Figure 78.2*). Furthermore, there is an up to 20-fold risk of developing leukemia in children with DS or mosaicism for trisomy 21. Approximately 5% of newborns with DS experience TAM, previously referred to as transient myeloproliferative disorder.[244] Although TAM will usually spontaneously resolve over the course of several weeks to months, about 10% to 20% of these infants will go on to develop AML, mostly of the megakaryoblastic subtype (AMKL). The leukemic blasts in TAM and DS AMKL express exon 2 mutations of *GATA1* and originate from fetal liver hematopoietic precursors.[245] Infants with TAM may have symptoms due to the abnormal myeloproliferation including hydrops fetalis, organomegaly, and hepatic fibrosis.

Because of the spontaneous remissions observed in DS patients with TAM, close observation is usually the first approach to management. However, when life-threatening signs and symptoms occur, often a result of hyperleukocytosis and organomegaly, treatment approaches can include exchange transfusion and/or low-dose cytarabine arabinoside for 3 to 7 days until improvement of symptoms.[244,246]

In cases where young children with DS develop AML, they often experience favorable outcomes compared to non-DS patients and are treated with less intensive chemotherapy regimens.[247–249] However, age at the time of diagnosis is an important prognostic factor in children with DS and AML, with children older than 4 years having a significantly worse 4-year EFS of 28% compared to the greater than 85% for younger patients.[250] Older patients with DS and AML are often now treated on conventional AML protocols, albeit with mixed results. Significant improvements in therapy are needed for this group of patients.[251,252] However, because of the excellent prognosis of younger patients with DS and AML, the goal of trials continues to be directed toward reducing the intensity of therapy, and, particularly, anthracycline exposure as well as risk of severe infections. The COG study AAML0434 showed that (1) flow cytometry MRD is a new prognostic factor for clinical outcome; and that (2) a 25% reduction in cumulative daunorubicin did not impact outcome; prospective studies are in progress.[253]

MANAGEMENT OF PATIENTS WITH NON–DOWN SYNDROME INHERITED SYNDROMES

Patients with inherited syndromes, such as those characterized by DNA repair defects, usually are not able to tolerate the effects of chemotherapy or radiation treatment as well as other children with AML. For example, patients with FA require substantial dose reductions in chemotherapeutic drugs as well as bone marrow transplantation regimens, but such patients can sometimes be cured of their AML. However, chemotherapy to cytoreduce leukemia burden followed by reduced-intensity regimens is therefore recommended for such patients. Treatments used in elderly AML patients that use epigenetic agents such as azacytidine and venetoclax, due to their low intensity and low toxicity, warrant further study in these patients.[254–257] Patients with other familial cancer predisposition syndromes, such as those with germline *CEBPA* mutations, or Kostmann syndrome, who develop AML, can also be effectively treated with allogeneic HCT.[258,259]

MANAGEMENT OF INFANTS WITH ACUTE MYELOID LEUKEMIA

Congenital leukemia is defined as that which occurs in the first month of life. Approximately two-thirds of patients present with leukemia cutis, giving a "blueberry muffin" baby appearance that may also be seen in metastatic neuroblastoma or rhabdomyosarcoma and histiocytosis (Figure 78.4). Hepatosplenomegaly is also typically present, but lymphadenopathy less so; CNS involvement is present in 50% of cases that included performance of an LP. The WBC count is typically elevated, and the majority of reported congenital myeloid leukemias have been of the M5 subtype. A majority of congenital AML cases have abnormal cytogenetic findings, with approximately one-fourth of cases having 11q23 (KMT2A) abnormalities.[260,261] Similarly, AML in infants (usually considered as being less than 12 months of age) is also characterized by a high predominance of KMT2A rearrangements.[262] There are many fusion products identified by RNAseq that are found in infant AML.[13,263]

Although spontaneous remissions have been reported in neonates with AML,[264] OS tends to be poor, with an OS of 24% at 2 years in the most comprehensive review.[260,261] For these neonates and infants, conventional approaches to therapy using AML regimens used in older children are typically used, but with dose adjustments.[262] This is in part due to the immaturity of organs as well as the immune system, resulting in significant treatment-related toxicities, including death, requiring significant supportive care compared to noninfants with acute leukemia.[262,265] For instance, the AML-BFM studies have suggested the dose reduction of cytarabine arabinoside because of the reduced clearance in children younger than 2 years.[266] With such intensive, although in part modified, AML-directed regimens, the survival for infants can be similar to that reported in older children, that is, in the 65% to 75% range for 5-year OS.[114,132,262] The role of transplantation in infants remains unclear.

MANAGEMENT OF ACUTE PROMYELOCYTIC LEUKEMIA

Before the introduction of differentiation targeted therapy, APL had a significantly poor outcome (see Chapter 79). The use of ATRA, directed against the fusion proteins characteristically involving the RARA formed as a result of the usual t(15;17) chromosomal translocation, reversed this scenario.[267,268] OS at 5 years is now in the 75% to 95% range depending upon the presence of different risk factors when patients are treated with combination regimens that include ATRA, arsenic trioxide (ATO), and chemotherapy.[192,269–272] Other RARA fusion proteins occur less frequently and display varying sensitivity to ATRA. An important consideration in treating patients with APL is to evaluate their initial risk status. Patients who present with APL and a WBC >10,000/μL are considered in most studies to have high-risk disease, especially with regard to severe coagulopathy up front and are usually treated with more intense regimens.[273,274] The presence of FLT3-ITD mutation might predict early death in pediatric patients with APL[275] and a low FLT3-ITD to normal FLT3 allele ratio has been reported to be associated with an improved prognosis in APL.[276]

The therapy for APL is essentially identical for pediatric and adult patients. This has resulted in pediatric patients being exposed to significant amounts of anthracyclines as well as higher doses of ATRA. For instance, a conventional dose of ATRA at 45 mg/m^2 is usually employed in adult trials, and results in a 90% or greater CR rate when used alone or in combination with chemotherapy.[277,278] This type of treatment in children has been associated with increased toxicities, such as pseudotumor cerebri and "APL differentiation syndrome," which can occur in up to 25% of patients and is characterized by fever, respiratory distress, pulmonary infiltrates, pleural/pericardial effusions, fluid overload, hypotension, and acute renal failure.[279] A dose of 25 mg/m^2 of ATRA appears to be equally effective and is thus recommended in most pediatric trials.[192,280] The recognition of this syndrome and early treatment with corticosteroids and temporary cessation of ATRA is critical. The effective use of prophylactic corticosteroids has been reported for patients with presenting WBC counts of >5000/μL.[279]

Since high doses of anthracyclines can have particularly significant adverse consequences to cardiac function in children, an ongoing goal for APL trials in pediatrics, and adults, has been to reduce overall anthracycline exposure. The introduction of ATO as a single agent in APL lead to CR rates of up to 85% in patients with relapsed disease, and provided a significant alternative to anthracyclines.[281–283] In addition, several studies have shown excellent results when testing ATO in combination with chemotherapy along with ATRA. The use of ATRA for induction therapy followed by 6 months of maintenance with arsenic has been reported to achieve a 3-year OS of 86%.[284] The combined use of ATRA, arsenic, and immunotargeted therapy with anti-CD33-calicheamicin monoclonal antibody (gemtuzumab ozogamicin) GO has also been reported.[285,286]

Recent trials have demonstrated that the combination of upfront ATRA + ATO alone for patients with low-risk APL (WBC <10,000/μL) is at least equivalent to chemotherapy combinations.[287] This trial completely eliminated anthracyclines from low-risk patients, but also eliminated the 2-year maintenance antimetabolite therapy. Importantly, higher rates of QTc prolongation and hepatic toxicity were seen in the ATRA + ATO cohort, although in most cases this did not affect therapy.[287]

The COG AAML0631 trial reduced anthracycline exposure to 355 mg/m^2 of daunorubicin equivalents for standard-risk patients with negative MRD at the end of induction and to 455 mg/m^2 for high-risk patients and standard-risk patients who have MRD after the third treatment course. The current COG AAML1331 trial is evaluating the ATRA + ATO induction and consolidation strategy in low-risk pediatric patients, currently considered the standard of care in adults. For patients with high-risk disease in the latter trial, anthracyclines are still being used in induction therapy only, as well as for patients who do not achieve an appropriate response.[288]

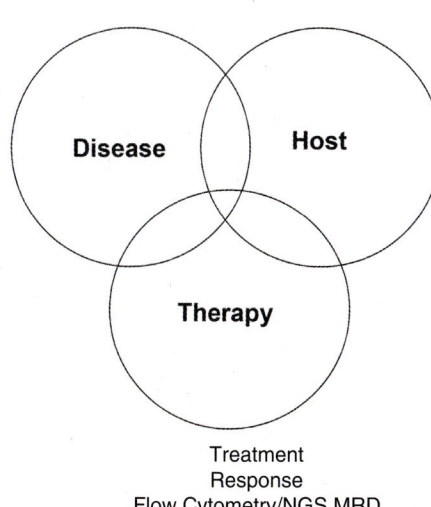

FIGURE 78.4 Relationship of prognostic factors in pediatric acute myeloid leukemia. See text for details. FAB, French/American/British classification; MRD, measurable residual disease; PCR, polymerase chain reaction; WBC, white blood cell.

The use of intrathecal (IT) chemotherapy as prophylaxis in patients with APL remains unclear. Some studies have suggested that the incidence of CNS relapse is higher in patients treated with ATRA or with high-risk APL; however, definitive data demonstrating that IT prophylaxis reduces extramedullary relapse have not been reported.[289] Overall, the incidence of extramedullary relapse in patients with APL is about 3% to 5%.[290] Most pediatric trials continue to include some IT prophylaxis, although IT chemotherapy is not standard in adult trials. Most recommendations support awaiting resolution of all coagulopathy before proceeding with a diagnostic LP.

Patients with high-risk APL make up a large percentage of the approximately 15% to 20% of patients with APL who experience relapse of their leukemia. The detection of molecular relapse, which can be detected much earlier than hematologic, in adults has also proven to be advantageous.[291,292] Patients who received an additional course of therapy with ATO were alive at 2 years compared to 78% who underwent either allogeneic or autologous HCT.[293] Thus, some type of HCT as consolidation therapy for patients with relapsed APL is usually recommended. A study from the European APL Group reported that the 7-year OS for adults was significantly better for those who received autologous HCT compared to those receiving an allogeneic HCT (60% vs 52%, respectively; $P = .04$); this difference was in large part due to the increased treatment-related toxicity with allogeneic HCT.[294] Another important consideration, however, is whether there is any bone marrow molecular evidence of residual APL, at the time of stem cell harvest for autologous HCT. Meloni et al reported that all patients whose autologous graft was positive by RT-PCR for RARA fusion transcript relapsed within 9 months of autologous HCT.[295] Thus, autologous HCT may be beneficial for patients who achieve a molecular remission before graft harvest, whereas for those with residual disease, an allogeneic HCT is the best treatment strategy.[296,297]

A significant and unresolved challenge in both children and adults with APL is the prevention of early death due to hemorrhagic complications, which can occur in about 3% of patients.[298] The pathogenesis of the underlying coagulopathy in APL is complex, involving the release of activators of both coagulation and fibrinolysis by the leukemic cells. Early detection and initiation of antileukemic treatment along with aggressive supportive care measures to control the coagulopathy are essential.[299] When a diagnosis of APL is suspected, ATRA should be started immediately, even before confirmation of the diagnosis with detection of PML-RARA transcript, and can always be discontinued if alternative therapy is required.

GRANULOCYTIC SARCOMA

Granulocytic sarcoma, myeloid sarcoma, extramedullary AML, and chloroma all refer to AML presenting as a solid tumor from the localized proliferation of malignant myeloblasts. These may occur anywhere in the body, but are most commonly seen in skin, bones, or paraspinal/epidural sites. Chloromas may be present in up to about 5% of cases and are most frequently associated with AML characterized by the t(8;21) chromosomal translocation, but also can be seen in other subtypes, especially in infants with myelomonocytic or monocytic AML.[300] Patients may also present, albeit it rarely, with a chloroma and no detectable bone marrow or other systemic involvement.[300,301] Biopsy of a chloroma with special immunohistochemical staining for myeloid markers, FISH, and cytogenetics for AML-related alterations as well as flow immunophenotyping should be done as such lesions can be confused with lymphomas or bone and soft-tissue sarcomas.

The management of patients presenting with chloromas should be similar to that of patients with AML as defined by conventional risk groups. A CCG study reported that EFS and local recurrence rates were similar for patients treated with chemotherapy alone compared to chemotherapy plus radiation to the chloroma(s).[302] Radiation therapy may thus be reserved in cases where a chloroma does not respond to intensive AML-directed chemotherapy.[300,302] In the upfront setting the presence of extramedullary disease has no impact on prognosis.[303] However, in some studies it has been found to be a favorable feature, although this may be due to the strong association between the favorable CBF AML features and presence of chloromas.[118]

MIXED PHENOTYPE ACUTE LEUKEMIA

Biphenotypic, bilineage, bilineal, or mixed phenotype acute leukemia (MPAL) refer to leukemias which co-express proteins that are characteristically restricted during differentiation to either the lymphoid or myeloid lineage. The WHO classification has referred to these leukemias as having ambiguous lineage, with biphenotypic referring to one population of leukemic blasts that co-express myeloid and lymphoid antigens and bilineage referring to two distinct populations of leukemic blasts of different lineages. Usually more than one lineage marker from the opposite lineage is considered to be necessary to call the leukemia biphenotypic. Aberrant expression of lymphoid-associated or myeloid-associated proteins have not been shown to have prognostic significance in a subset of ALL and AML.[304] A report by Alexander et al shows that MPAL T/Myeloid and MPAL B/Myeloid are genetically distinct.[305]

There remains some debate on the optimal treatment of children with mixed lineage leukemia. Treatment strategies directed at the dominant phenotype have resulted in reasonable outcomes, although CR rates and survival with these strategies remain lower than ALL.[306-308] A study by Rubnitz et al found that a majority of patients with myeloid phenotype did not have a favorable response to AML induction therapy but did respond to salvage ALL therapy. Therefore starting with ALL therapy, even if a predominantly myeloid phenotype is considered a reasonable strategy and salvage AML therapy can be utilized in the setting of inadequate response.[309] This approach was recently validated in an MPAL cohort analysis from the COG.[310] Although these leukemias are often considered to arise from earlier progenitors and thus difficult to cure with chemotherapy alone, HCT may not be required in a significant number of cases, especially for those with response to upfront therapy.[305,311]

SECONDARY OR THERAPY-RELATED ACUTE MYELOID LEUKEMIA

Therapy-related AML (t-AML) is most commonly related to exposure to specific chemotherapeutic agents, such as alkylating agents or topoisomerase inhibitors, as well as radiation.[25,312,313] The goal of treatment should be to achieve a CR and then proceed to allogeneic HCT with the best available donor, including haploidentical donors. In addition to genotoxic exposures, there may also be predisposing genetic susceptibilities, such as polymorphisms in drug detoxification and DNA repair enzymes.[314-316] Depending on the level of exposures and predisposing factors, the risk for developing t-AML for patients undergoing treatment for solid tumors is between 0.4% and 2%.[317]

CR rates and OS are usually lower for patients with t-AML compared to those with de novo AML.[318,319] A high nonrelapse mortality has also been reported for this group of patients undergoing HCT. Adverse or high-risk cytogenetic abnormalities and molecular alterations are more frequently observed in t-AML.[313] Although this is not always possible, re-induction regimens should ideally include chemotherapeutic agents not previously used to reduce the risk of leukemia cross-resistance. However, novel agents and regimens available through clinical trials should be strongly considered if available. The relatively poor outcome for such patients increases the importance of determining more effective and less toxic treatments for patients with first malignancies.

PROGNOSTIC FACTORS

One of the greatest challenges in the treatment of patients with AML has been the identification of risk factors that could be used to more precisely direct treatment. Such risk or prognostic factors include those of the host and the disease as well as the treatment that is used (*Figure 78.5*). The limited ability to identify and act on such factors has

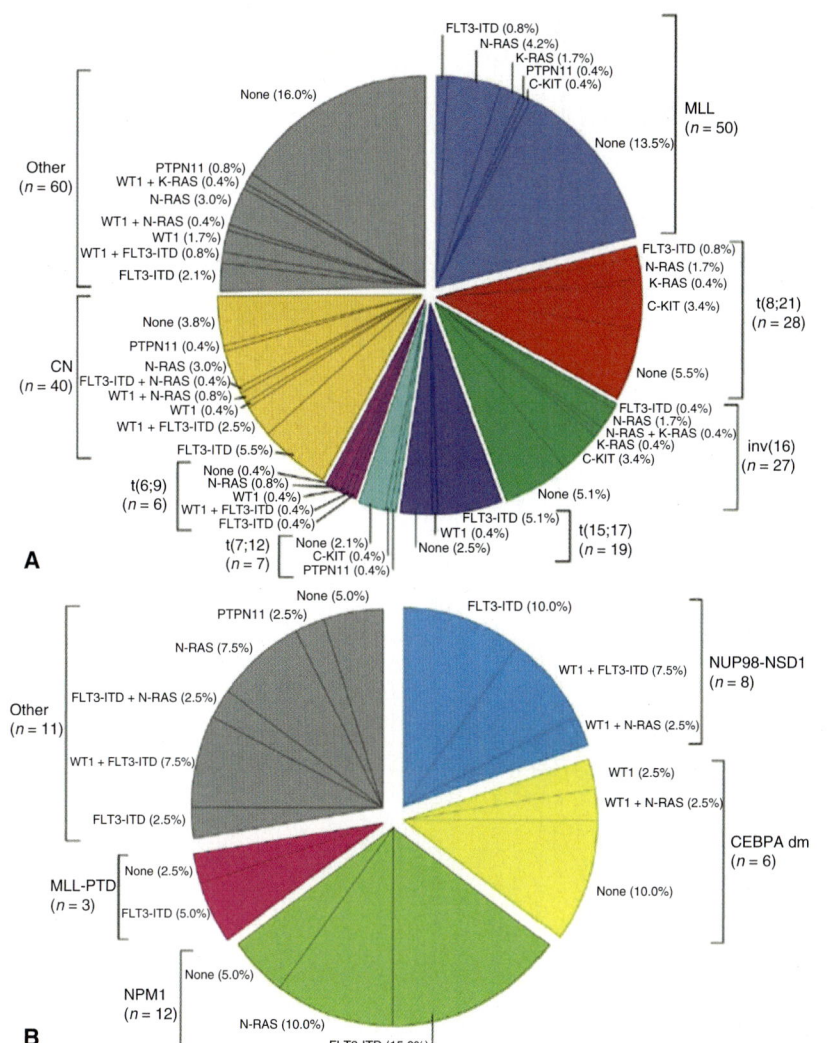

FIGURE 78.5 Pie chart representations of cytogenetic abnormalities and gene mutations alone and in combination in pediatric acute myeloid leukemia. A, Data shown for all subtypes. B, Detailed data apply to only cytogenetically normal (CN) AML. The data are based on 237 pediatric patients with de novo AML. The different pie slices indicate the percentage of patients whose AML had one or more mutations as noted. (Reprinted from Creutzig U, van den Heuvel-Elbrink MM, Gibson B, et al. Diagnosis and management of acute meyloid leukemia in children and adolescents: recommendations from an international expert panel. *Blood*. 2012;120(16):3187-3205. Copyright © 2012 American Society of Hematology. With permission.)

relegated AML treatment to a population-based approach; however, there has been a continuous effort to improve prognostication. Recent advances in genomic sequencing aimed at identifying biomarkers as well as enhanced diagnostic methodologies to determine response to therapy have led to more refined therapeutic approaches. As NGS methodologies for minimal residual disease are studies retrospectively, additional studies on leukemia stem cell signatures[320,321] under investigation as well as pharmacologic sensitivities based on polygenomic response scores for cytarabine and gemtuzumab ozogomycin appear promising.[322–324] This remains a significant area of research with the goal that future therapeutic approaches will be more individualized.

Host Factors

Among the host factors, patient age, race, ethnicity, and specific constitutional abnormalities are most strongly correlated with outcome. The impact of age remains an area of debate as in general, patient age is inversely related to treatment outcome. This relationship was clearly demonstrated in the MRC AML-10 trial and was confirmed in MRC AML-12, in which infants, despite worse toxicity, had higher survival rates than older children.[214,325,326] The CCG-2891 trial as well as St. Jude AML91, AML97, and AML02 trials also demonstrated a benefit of young age.[15,127,327] However, some of the higher risk biologic features are more prevalent in older children and adolescents and age was not found to be an independent risk factor in AML-BFM trials.[262,326] These differences may in part be due to treatment effects (*Table 78.3*). Several studies have suggested that older children have higher rates of toxicity with chemotherapy; this may be especially true in overweight and obese children.[334–336]

In CCG studies, race has consistently been a predictor of outcome, specifically with African-Americans having a poorer outcome than whites,[337] although this has not been observed in other studies.[338,339] The importance of body weight has also been underscored by a report from the CCG-2961 study, in which there was a twofold greater risk of treatment-related toxic deaths associated with patients who were ≤10th percentile or >95% percentile.[335]

Whereas the pharmacogenetic basis of treatment response is poorly understood, homozygous deletions of the *GST* theta gene, a detoxifying phase II enzyme, have been reported to be associated with decreased survival (52% vs 40%; $P = .05$).[340] This difference in survival is due to an excess of toxicity in patients who are *GST* theta null (24% vs 12%; $P = .05$).

Patients with constitutional abnormalities also have altered risk of treatment response. Most notably, patients with trisomy 21 who are less than 4 years of age may experience more therapy-related toxicity with conventional, dose-intensive AML regimens, but have higher survival rates than patients with a normal constitutional karyotype when less intensive regimens are used.[244,341] Patients with other constitutional abnormalities, particularly FA, have increased toxicity with standard AML therapy and for this reason any suspicion of underlying marrow failure or FA should be investigated and excluded prior to initiation of intensive AML therapy. The underlying ineffective hematopoiesis leading to cytopenias limits their ability to recover normal hematopoiesis after AML therapy. As a result, these patients are generally excluded from standard AML protocols.

Table 78.3. Treatment Outcomes From Selected Pediatric Group Trials

Study	Years	# of Patients[a]	Early Death (%)	CR Rate (%)	CR Evaluation after Course #	Anthracyclines (mg/m²)[c]	Cytarabine (g/m²)	Etoposide (g/m²)	5-y EFS %	SE	5-y OS %	SE	Reference
POG-8821	1988-1993	511	3.9	77	2	360	55.7	2.25	31	2	40	2	152
CCG-2891	1989-1995	750	4.0	77	2	350	28.3	1.9	34	3	45	3	
MRC-AML 10	1988-1995	303	4	93	4	550	10.6	0.5-1.5	49		58		
PINDA-92	1992-1998	151	21	74	NS	350	7.64	0.45	36		37		328
LAME-91	1991-1998	247	6	91	2	460	9.8-13.4	0.4	48	4	62	4	
TCCSG M91-13/M96-14	1991-1998	192	4	88	NS	495	69.4-99.4	3.75-5.75	56		62		
BFM-93	1993-1998	427	7	82	4	300-400	23-41	0.95	50	2	57	2	151
CCG 2961	1996-1999	901	6	83	2	360	15.2-19.6	1.6	42	3	52	4	132
EORTC-CLG 58921	1993-2000	166	1	84	2	380	23-29	1.35	49	4	62	4	170
GATLA-AML90	1993-2000	179	20	70	NS	300	41.1	1.45	31	4	41	4	329
AIEOP LAM-92	1992-2001	160	6	89	2	Not provided	Not provided	Not provided	54	4	60	4	162
NOPHO-AML 93	1993-2001	223	2	92	3	300-375	49.6-61.3	1.6	50	3	66	3	164
MRC-AML 12	1995-2002	504	4	92	4	300-610	4.6-34.6	1.5	54		63		142,143,330
AML99	2000-2002	260	2	94	2	300-375	59.4-78.4	3.15-3.2	61	3	75	3	331
BFM-98	1998-2004	430	3	88	4	420	41-47	0.95	51	3	61	2	332
SJCRH AML02[b]	2002-2008	230	1	94	2	300-550	34-48	1-1.5	63	4	71	4	15
COG AAML03P1[b]	2003-2005	350	3	83	2	300-480	21.6-45.6	1-1.75	53	6	66	5	146

Results are reported for only those trials that had 150 patients and information provided for each of the column headings. All numbers and percentages were rounded to the lowest value if less than 0.5 and to the next upper integer if ≥0.5.

Abbreviations: AIEOP LAM, Associazione Italiana di Ematologia e Oncologia Pediatrica Leucemia Acuta Mieloide; BFM, Berlin-Frankfurt-Munster; CCG, Children's Cancer Group; COG, Children's Oncology Group; CR, complete remission; EFS, event-free survival; EORTC-CLG, European Organization for Research and Treatment of Cancer Children's Leukemia Group; GATLA-AML, Argentine Group for the Treatment of Acute Leukemia; LAME, Leucemie Aigue Myeloblastique Enfant; MRC-AML, United Kingdom's Medical Research Council Acute Myelogenous Leukemia Study; NOPHO-AML, Nordic Society of Pediatric Hematology and Oncology-Acute Myeloid Leukemia; NS, not specified; OS, overall survival; PINDA, National Program for Antineoplastic Drugs for Children; POG, Pediatric Oncology Group; SJCRH, St. Jude Children's Research Hospital; TCCSG, Tokyo Children's Cancer Study Group.

[a]Ages include patients from 0 up to and including age 15 years; BFM-98 included patients from 0 to less than 17 years of age; number of patients excludes patients with Down syndrome; CCG-2961 included patients from 0 to 21 years of age.

[b]SJCRH AML02 and the COG AAML03P1 have EFS and OS at 3-year follow-up; COG AAML03P1 enrolled patients ≥1 month and ≤21 years of age.

[c]Anthracycline conversions were according to daunorubicin equivalents, including idarubicin 5X, mitoxantrone 5X, doxorubicin 1X. Another conversion factor for idarubicin and mitoxantrone that has been used is 3X.

Reprinted with permission from Pui CH, Carroll WL, Meshinchi S, et al. Biology, risk stratification, and therapy of pediatric acute leukemias: an update. J Clin Oncol. 2011;29(5):551-565. Copyright © 2011 by American Society of Clinical Oncology.

Disease-Associated Factors—Clinical

Several characteristics of leukemia including initial WBC count and FAB morphology have been associated with outcome; however, recent studies demonstrate that it is the underlying cytogenic and molecular features of the disease that explain the prognostic impact of these features. Like age, initial WBC blast count is inversely related to outcome. An initial WBC count <20 × 10^9/L is associated with a favorable prognosis, whereas an initial WBC count >100 × 10^9/L has been associated with an unfavorable prognosis in both the MRC and BFM trials. In the CCG-2891 study, patients with a WBC count >330 × 10^9/L had an unfavorable prognosis, with an EFS of 7%, due to early death, induction failure, and relapse.[127] However, in the BFM trials, very high leukemia blast counts at diagnosis were not associated with a worse DFS, but with increased risk of early death and decreased induction remission.[342] High leukemia blast counts are now known to be associated with biologic factors, such as *FLT3-ITD* mutations.

CNS involvement, which occurs in about 5% to 10% of children with AML, has not been shown to result in decreased remission rates or survival, although there may be an increase of isolated CNS relapse.[343,344] Of note, of patients with chloromatous disease, those with orbital involvement have been reported to have an improved outcome.[118]

Morphologic classification schemes once used to assign risk to subtypes of AML were replaced by the most recent WHO[120] classification based on molecular and biologic features, and a new WHO classification in progress will add more biologic features that are associated with poor outcome as RNAseq technology accurately informs risk stratification. However, in income poor countries, the FAB classification remains important. In the past this classification group has been associated with treatment outcome, but different studies have found different associations. The BFM group reported that patients with FAB M1-M4 had improved survival over patients with either M0 or M5-7.[345] However, in both MRC-10 and CCG-2891, the M5 FAB subtype was associated with favorable prognosis. FAB M7 in non-trisomy 21 patients has been associated with poor survival in CCG studies. Lastly, FAB subtypes M1/M2 have been historically associated with a favorable prognosis but have a higher representation of favorable-risk cytogenetics changes. One historical exception may be with APL, where today the early morphologic recognition with rapid FISH confirmation of t(15;17) and initiation of treatment can have important clinical consequences.

The cytogenetics karyotype of the leukemia blasts is a robust predictor of outcome. Patients with t(15;17), t(8;21), and inv(16) fare better than patients with other cytogenetic findings.[346] Patients with monosomy 7 or 5 do poorly, as do patients with complex karyotypes, although the concomitant presence of monosomy 7 or 5 with complex karyotypes has made it difficult to discriminate between the contributions of other chromosomal changes.[347]

Disease-Associated Characteristics—Cytogenetics/Molecular

The detection of recurrent chromosomal rearrangements in AML has been used to decide on probable risk of treatment failure since the 1990s. Importantly, the cytogenetic alterations observed in pediatric AML are very different from adult AML. Chromosomal translocations involving CBF are associated with a favorable prognosis, such as the t(8;21)(q22;q22) and inv(16)(p13.1q22) or t(16;16)(p13;q22), and account for approximately 20% to 25% of pediatric AML. Contemporary studies demonstrate that patients with CBF AML have an approximate OS of 80% to 85% with contemporary chemotherapy regimens and do not require HCT in CR1.[15,143,147] Although these CBF leukemias are often considered together as a single group, there are important differences. For instance, the AML-BFM group has reported that reduction of intensity of treatment by omitting a high-dose Ara-C and mitoxantrone course during induction led to a decreased EFS and OS for patients with AML with t(8;21) but not inv(16).[346] AML characterized by t(8;21) is slightly more common than inv(16) and is also associated in about 20% of cases with the occurrence of chloromas and expression of CD19 and CD56 antigens.[348,349] The inv(16) translocation is associated with the FAB M4 morphologic subtype.

The t(15;17)(q22;q21) translocation resulting in the *PML-RARA* gene fusion occurs in about 5% to 10% of pediatric AML and, as discussed above, is associated with excellent OS using APL-directed therapies. APL with t(11;17), which involves the *PLZF* instead of the *PML* gene, has been associated with decreased sensitivity to ATRA.[350]

Rearrangements of the *MLL* or *KMT2A* gene at chromosome band 11q23 occur in 15% to 20% of pediatric AML, making them the most commonly observed cytogenetic abnormality.[190,347]

Many fusion partners have been reported, importantly the specific fusion gene generated from *KMT2A* rearrangements have different impacts on outcomes. For example, patients with AML having a t(1;11)(q21;q23) have a favorable prognosis, whereas those with t(4;11), t(10;11), and t(6;11) have poor outcomes, while the t(9;11) has an intermediate prognosis.[351,352] When combined with the core-binding factor leukemias, including APL, *KMT2A*-rearranged AML represents approximately 50% of pediatric AML.

Several large studies have defined other chromosomal abnormalities as being associated with unfavorable outcomes. Monosomy 7 or abnormalities of 7q, when recurrent genetic changes are excluded,[353] are rare and represent about 3% of pediatric AML. Of note, AML with del(7q) has been reported to have a better prognosis (5-year OS of 51%) compared to monosomy 7 (5-year OS of 30%).[190,347,353] Chromosomal 5q- portends a poor prognosis in adults but is exceedingly rare in childhood AML. Complex karyotypes, usually defined as the presence of three or more chromosome abnormalities in the absence of one of the WHO-noted recurring chromosomal translocations or inversions, are generally associated with unfavorable outcomes regardless of whether good prognosis changes are observed.[190,347]

Studies from the MRC and BFM AML groups have reported that abnormalities of chromosome 12p, often associated with 12p13 rearrangements that involve the *ETV6* gene, are associated with an unfavorable prognosis.[190,347] Other poor prognostic cytogenetic changes include t(7;12), t(6;9), and -17/abn(17p).[354,355] Rearrangements involving the 3q26 locus that includes the *EVI1* gene, including t(3;3)(q21;26), have been reported to be a very poor prognostic factor in adults but are extremely rare in children.[354,356] However, increased expression of EVI1 in children with *MLL*-rearranged leukemia, monosomy 7 or megakaryoblastic morphology, has been reported to predict an intermediate or unfavorable prognosis.[357–359] Although these cytogenetic features indicate a poor prognosis, the therapeutic implications are less clear. HCT in CR1 is generally recommended for all high-risk AML; however, the benefit of HCT over chemotherapy has not been definitively shown.[360]

Cytogenetic abnormalities are very common in infant AML, with *KMT2A* rearrangements being the most common. Pediatric AMKL is a rare subtype of AML and when it occurs in non-DS patients has a high prevalence of cytogenetic abnormalities, including cryptic fusions not detected with conventional karyotype with distinct prognostic features. Patients with *KMT2A* rearrangements, *CBFA2T3-GLIS2* (inv(16)(p13.3a24.3)), and *NUP98-KDM5A* translocations, and monosomy 7 have been found to have a poor OS of approximately 30% to 40%.[361,362] This was in contrast to patients with the *RBM15-MKL1* (t(1;22)(p13;q13)) translocation, which has an intermediate outcome of approximately 60%.[361,363,364]

Alterations in the *NUP* genes, *NUP98* and *NUP214*, are a recurring alteration in pediatric AML and often predict poor outcomes. The *DEK-NUP214* (t(6;9)) fusion is associated with poor prognosis and is highly associated with *FLT3-ITD*. NUP98 rearrangements have been described with the increased use of genomic sequencing and occur in approximately 10% to 15% of what has been labeled as cytogenetically normal pediatric AML.[187,365] *NUP98* fusions result in aberrant HOXA and B expression and likely results in epigenetic dysregulation with aberrant histone modification.[365,366] *NUP98-NSD1* fusions are associated with a poor prognosis with an OS of approximately 30% to 35%.[188,365] This is especially true in patients with dual *NUP98-NSD1-FLT3-ITD* mutations who have very high rates of induction failure of approximately 70% and an OS of approximately 25% to 30%.[365,367]

Although *NUP98-NSD1* fusions are the most common recurring *NUP98* translocation, multiple translocation partners have been identified, including *HOXD13*, *JARID1A*, *PHF23*, and *DDX10*.[187]

Approximately 20% of children with AML have essentially normal cytogenetics and thus cannot be stratified into risk groups based on such criteria. Molecular studies have helped to further determine patients with more or less favorable AML in this group. Receptor tyrosine kinase pathways that play key roles in regulating cellular proliferation, growth, and survival are the most common type of somatic mutation in AML. Internal tandem duplications in the juxtamembrane region of the FLT3 tyrosine kinase receptor, called *FLT3*-ITD mutations, increase in prevalence with age and occur in approximately 15% of children, with a prevalence of 20% in adolescents and young adults, and about 25% of adults. High mutant to normal allelic ratios have been shown to predict a poor prognosis across several large studies in children and adults.[368] Mutations may also occur in the tyrosine kinase domain of FLT3 (*FLT3-TKD*), and occur in 5% to 7% of pediatric AML and have not been shown to portend an adverse prognosis.[369] Although FLT3-ITD mutations with allelic ratio at and greater than 0.4 were associated with poor outcome, current clinical trials institute on-study use of FLT3 inhibitors regardless of allelic ratio, in order to treat presumed subclonal populations that may result in recurrent disease. The results of current studies will inform in the future if this approach results in improved outcome. *FLT3* mutations have also been reported to be present in up to 40% of children and adults with APL, and appear to be associated with the microgranular variant, hyperleukocytosis, and early death in children.[276,370] Mutations in the KIT tyrosine kinase receptor occur in up to 25% of patients with CBF AML. Studies in adults have reported these mutations to define a higher risk subgroups of CBF AML; however, an inferior survival among this group of patients has not been universally reported.[371,372] Alterations in RAS signaling, both through NRAS and KRAS, are common events but these are often found to be subclonal events acquired late in leukemogenesis and of no prognostic impact.[373,374] *NRAS* and *KRAS* mutations have been reported in approximately 15% to 20% of pediatric AML, and up to 20% in adult AML.[375,376]

Mutations in the *NPM1*, a component of nuclear to cytoplasmic transport complexes, tend to increase chemosensitivity and are associated with improved outcomes with 5-year EFS of about 70%.[196] Notably, when *NPM1* mutations occur in the presence of HAR *FLT3*-ITD mutations, they do not appear to ameliorate an unfavorable prognosis. The absence of high-risk molecular lesions with normal karyotype and mutations of NPM1 are now considered low-risk in current risk stratification schemas as there is nearly a universal overlap of mutant NPM1 and no other mutations when FLT3-ITD mutations are absent.[377,378]

CEBPA mutations occur in approximately 6% of pediatric AML and are usually associated with normal karyotype AML and favorable prognosis.[47,379,380] Biallelic mutations of *CEBPA* define a distinct subtype of AML with a favorable prognosis.[381,382]

Mutations in the *WT1* gene occur in about 10% of pediatric AML and are usually associated with normal karyotypes, but can be associated with *FLT3*-ITD in approximately 40% of cases.[383] *WT1* mutations in some studies are associated with poor 5-year OS; however, it is possible that the large overlap with *FLT3*-ITD may account for the poor outcome as not all studies have identified *WT1* mutations as an independent prognostic factor in multivariate analysis.[174,198] Patients with dual *WT1/FLT3-ITD* mutations have lower rates of CR and a very poor 5-year OS of approximately 20%. Interestingly, *WT1* single-nucleotide polymorphism (SNP) of rs16754 in exon 7 has been reported to be present on a major allele in 28% of patients and to be associated with an improved 5-year OS of 62% compared to 44% for AML not containing the SNP.[384] However, this has not been seen in all studies.[385]

Mutations in regulators of epigenetic patterning are common in adult AML, but in contrast are rare in pediatric AML. For instance, whereas mutations of *TET2* on chromosome 4q24 have been reported in about 12% of adult AML (about 23% in normal cytogenetic AML) and portend a poor prognosis,[386–388] these mutations occur in only about 6% of pediatric AML and may be, however, similarly associated with poorer prognosis.[44,389] Mutations of the *IDH1* (isocitrate dehydrogenase) gene interestingly produce a gain-of-function activity that in turn results in increased levels of 2-hydroxyglutarate and aberrantly hypermethylated promoter CpG sites.[390,391] Although *IDH1/2* mutations occur in approximately 25% to 30% of adult AML, they have been identified in only approximately 3% to 5% of pediatric AML.[392–394] Poor outcome has been associated with *IDH1/2* mutations in adults, but this has not been demonstrated in multivariate analyses from pediatric trials.[45,393] A minor SNP at rs11554137 associated with *IDH1*, found in about 10% of pediatric patients with AML, was not correlated with outcome.[394] Although mutations of the DNA methyltransferase encoding gene, *DNMT3A*, may occur in up to 20% of adult AML and have been associated with poor prognosis,[42,395] such mutations are exceedingly rare in pediatric AML.[44,396,397] *Figure 78.6* summarizes cytogenetic abnormalities and gene mutations in pediatric AML.

Despite the acknowledgment of the increasing heterogeneity of AML based on genetic, RNA expression, and epigenetic patterns, a complete understanding of what predicts response or resistance to therapy is lacking. For now early response to therapy is the best biomarker yet not specific for prediction of outcome. Initially conventional morphologic assessment of early response to therapy was utilized; however, the application of flow-cytometric immunophenotyping or molecular methods has demonstrated substantially better sensitivity and predictability.[398,399] MRC AML studies have demonstrated that 94% of children with AML have informative immunophenotypes that could identify AML blasts from normal hematopoietic progenitors. The 3-year RFS for those patients with MRD less than 0.1% at the end of induction was 64% compared to 14% for those with MRD values of greater than 0.5%. Note that MRD assessment retained its significance in a multivariate analysis that included such factors as age, WBC, cytogenetics, and *FLT3*-ITD status.[400] A study from SJCRH demonstrated by flow cytometry that MRD values at the end of induction of 1% or higher was the most significant adverse prognostic factor for EFS and OS.[15] Using four-color multiparameter flow cytometry, COG reported from the AAML0531 study that an MRD value at the end of induction greater than 0.1% predicted a DFS at 3 years of 34% compared to 60% for patients without detectable MRD.[14] The prognostic utility of MRD currently at 0.02% with state-of-the-art flow-cytometry hardware and software appears to have the most utility in intermediate risk patients and can assist in risk stratification to inform therapeutic allocation, especially in redefining two major stratification categories as low and high risk.

Genomic alterations, although somewhat limited by the heterogeneous nature of AML, monitored by PCR-based approaches to detect MRD have also been employed. Several reports have shown that increasing levels of t(8;21) or inv(16) transcripts portend relapse.[401,402] Detection of the t(15;17) fusion gene on consecutive testing during remission is associated with a high risk of relapse, although this assay is not very informative at the end of APL induction therapy as the majority of patients will still have detectable fusion transcripts at that time.[400]

Comprehensive Genomic Profiling

Over the past decade, advances in NGS technologies have revolutionized the ability to interrogate cancer genomes. The biologic insights that have emerged from studies utilizing NGS technology have already begun to have clinical impact in pediatric AML. For example, the identification of cryptic translocations *CBFA2T3-GLIS2* and *NUP98-NSD1* that have gone undetected with conventional karyotyping is now recognized as a poor prognostic feature and affects risk stratification and treatment strategies. This technology (1) identifies markers for disease monitoring, (2) furthers understanding of leukemogenesis and (3) may inform patient-specific therapeutic intervention(s). Such examples highlight the importance of clinical comprehensive genomic sequencing platforms in pediatric AML. Already comprehensive NGS platforms for clinical use that focus on hematologic malignancies, with a turnaround of a few days to weeks, are used in both de novo and relapsed settings. The information that often identifies multiple

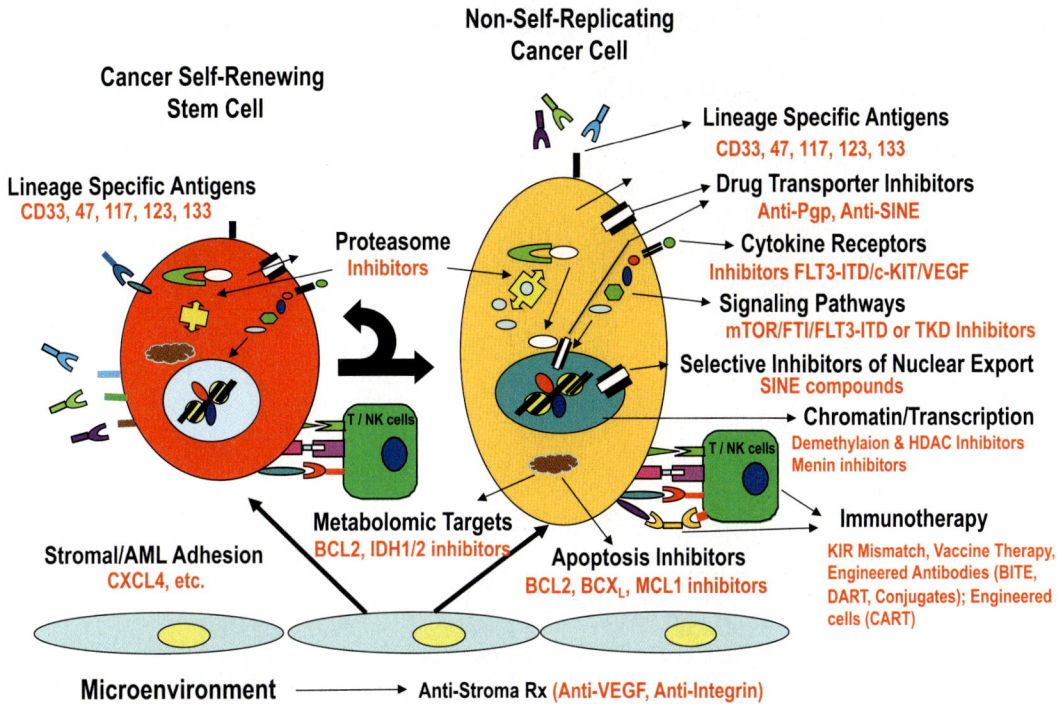

FIGURE 78.6 Therapeutic targets being tested in acute myelogenous leukemia (AML). The schema shows different pathways and/or approaches that have been or are being tested in clinical trials, including those that may affect the leukemia-initiating cell.

somatic mutations per patient is accelerating at a rapid pace and presents its own unique set of challenges. As comprehensive genomic information regarding individual patients' leukemia becomes more readily available, it is unclear how treating physicians can identify driver vs passenger mutations, hierarchy of target mutations, and how to accurately choose targets for therapeutic intervention outside the context of an early-phase clinical trial.[403] The availability of these technologies commercially complicate the power of clinical trials as physicians, upon the finding of adverse genetic factors, may remove likely high-risk patients from clinical trials, thus reducing the power of these trials to identify the efficacy of new drug combinations.

Future Therapeutic Challenges

Although chemotherapy dose intensification with or without HCT has significantly improved the outcome of patients with AML, the limits of the associated morbidity and mortality have been reached and preclude further intensification. Furthermore, it is likely that beyond CBF AMLs, the use of dose-intense genotoxic therapy may accelerate clonal evolution and adaptation to the detriment of the patient. Therefore, future therapeutic advances need to deliver greater leukemic cell killing (1) without additional collateral toxicity to normal tissues, and (2) without genotoxic stress that drives evolution and adaptation of LIC into more aggressive, drug-resistant subclones that raise the risk of relapse.

Novel therapeutic strategies have been focused on development of targeted agents that (1) inhibit leukemia survival, growth dependent pathways, and immune-evasive drug resistance mechanisms; and (2) immunotherapeutic strategies aimed at leukemia-specific targets without genotoxic effects that evade classical drug resistance mechanisms (*Figure 78.7*).

Targeted therapies are directed toward specific molecular pathways that lead to increased leukemic cell survival, proliferation, and drug resistance. Some of these targets may be prognostic factors, but this is certainly not a requirement, as some key pathways that drive leukemia may not necessarily be predictive of outcome in the context of conventional and novel chemotherapeutic approaches.

In part because of advances in understanding the genetic defects and their molecular consequences in AML, there are many potential therapeutic targets that are under study. However, the continuous expansion of big "molecular" data makes it particularly challenging to distinguish mutations and overlapping pathways that drive leukemic development and behavior, especially behavior that allows acquisition of new mutations that drive adaptation and proliferation of leukemia with increasing drug resistance.

Ideally, molecularly targeted therapies should be leukemia-specific. Examples of this approach include strategies targeting the unique fusion proteins that result from distinctive chromosomal translocations or the use of agents that would specifically exploit a mutation in aberrantly activated kinase pathways. The use of FLT3 inhibitors, specifically gilteritinib under study in the COG study AAML1831, and the approval of midostaurin in adult AML is the canonical example of this strategy in AML—when this feature is indeed a "driver" mutation. Other therapies directed at chromatin remodeling and reprogramming gene expression involve inhibitors of DNA methyltransferases as well as histone-modifying enzymes. The latter abnormalities are more common in adult than pediatric AML. Some preclinical studies suggest the LIC compartment is not sensitive to demethylating agents,[404] but its targeting has not been studied in a randomized fashion, and it is unknown if target/off-target effects are of therapeutic benefit when added to conventional chemotherapy. Additional approaches are aimed at targeting pathways or molecular targets that are shared by tumor cells and normal cells, but on which leukemic cells are more dependent in terms of their survival and proliferation. Such strategies might include inhibition of antiapoptotic pathways dependent on BCL2 and BCL_{XL} expression has shown activity in relapsed pediatric AML, the inhibition of activated RAS and its downstream pathways, and regulation of protein localization and degradation. Although inhibitors of the P-glycoprotein cell membrane transporter have not demonstrated clinical activity in adults and children,[138] a new type of selective inhibitors of nuclear export (SINE compounds) at the cell nuclear membrane have shown activity in early-phase trials. It remains to be seen if there will be any role for these new agents in frontline studies of de novo

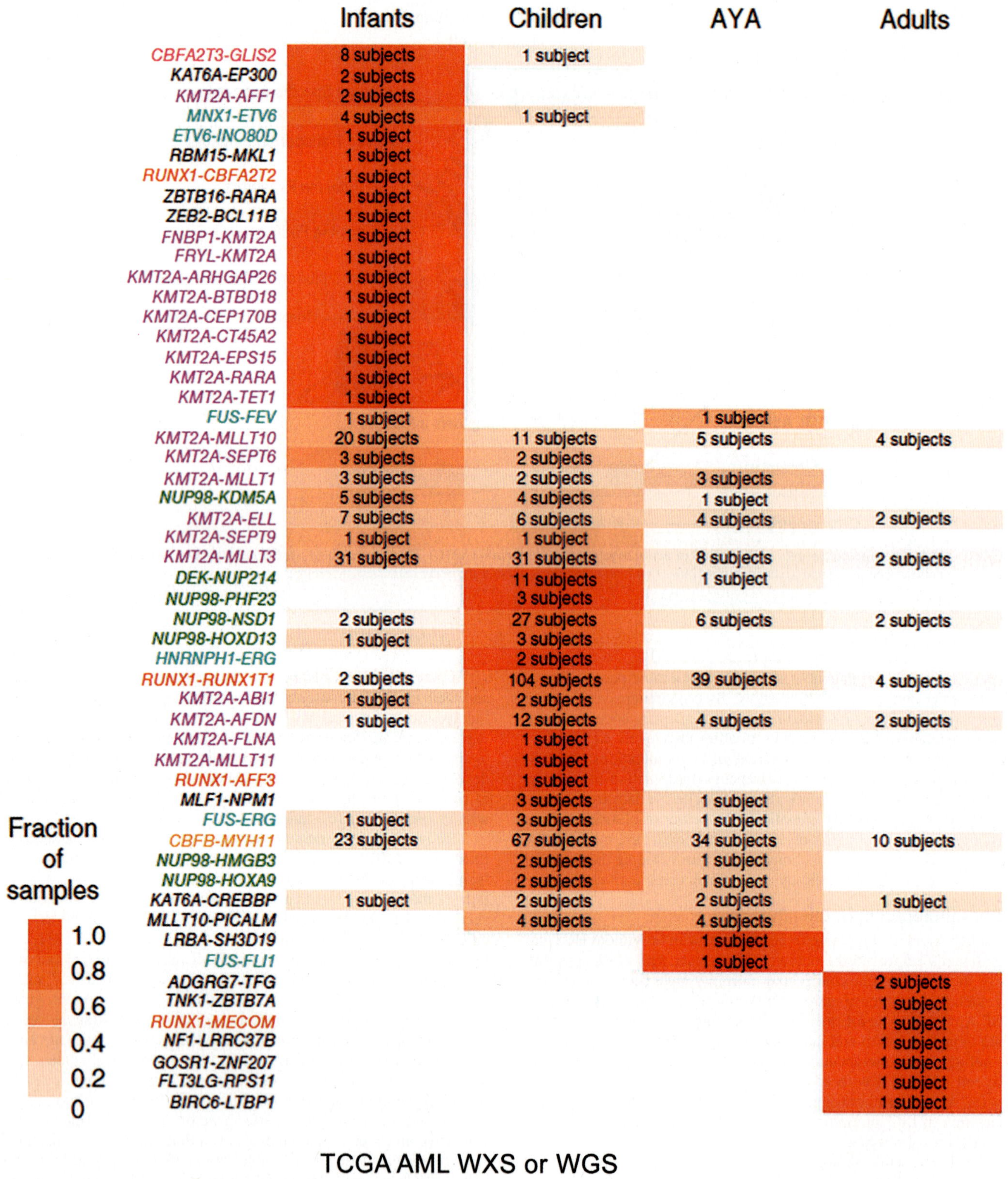

	Infants	Children	AYA	Adults
CBFA2T3-GLIS2	8 subjects	1 subject		
KAT6A-EP300	2 subjects			
KMT2A-AFF1	2 subjects			
MNX1-ETV6	4 subjects	1 subject		
ETV6-INO80D	1 subject			
RBM15-MKL1	1 subject			
RUNX1-CBFA2T2	1 subject			
ZBTB16-RARA	1 subject			
ZEB2-BCL11B	1 subject			
FNBP1-KMT2A	1 subject			
FRYL-KMT2A	1 subject			
KMT2A-ARHGAP26	1 subject			
KMT2A-BTBD18	1 subject			
KMT2A-CEP170B	1 subject			
KMT2A-CT45A2	1 subject			
KMT2A-EPS15	1 subject			
KMT2A-RARA	1 subject			
KMT2A-TET1	1 subject			
FUS-FEV	1 subject		1 subject	
KMT2A-MLLT10	20 subjects	11 subjects	5 subjects	4 subjects
KMT2A-SEPT6	3 subjects	2 subjects		
KMT2A-MLLT1	3 subjects	2 subjects	3 subjects	
NUP98-KDM5A	5 subjects	4 subjects	1 subject	
KMT2A-ELL	7 subjects	6 subjects	4 subjects	2 subjects
KMT2A-SEPT9	1 subject	1 subject		
KMT2A-MLLT3	31 subjects	31 subjects	8 subjects	2 subjects
DEK-NUP214		11 subjects	1 subject	
NUP98-PHF23		3 subjects		
NUP98-NSD1	2 subjects	27 subjects	6 subjects	2 subjects
NUP98-HOXD13	1 subject	3 subjects		
HNRNPH1-ERG		2 subjects		
RUNX1-RUNX1T1	2 subjects	104 subjects	39 subjects	4 subjects
KMT2A-ABI1	1 subject	2 subjects		
KMT2A-AFDN	1 subject	12 subjects	4 subjects	2 subjects
KMT2A-FLNA		1 subject		
KMT2A-MLLT11		1 subject		
RUNX1-AFF3		1 subject		
MLF1-NPM1		3 subjects	1 subject	
FUS-ERG	1 subject	3 subjects	1 subject	
CBFB-MYH11	23 subjects	67 subjects	34 subjects	10 subjects
NUP98-HMGB3		2 subjects	1 subject	
NUP98-HOXA9		2 subjects	1 subject	
KAT6A-CREBBP	1 subject	2 subjects	2 subjects	1 subject
MLLT10-PICALM		4 subjects	4 subjects	
LRBA-SH3D19			1 subject	
FUS-FLI1			1 subject	
ADGRG7-TFG				2 subjects
TNK1-ZBTB7A				1 subject
RUNX1-MECOM				1 subject
NF1-LRRC37B				1 subject
GOSR1-ZNF207				1 subject
FLT3LG-RPS11				1 subject
BIRC6-LTBP1				1 subject

Fraction of samples: 1.0, 0.8, 0.6, 0.4, 0.2, 0

TCGA AML WXS or WGS

FIGURE 78.7 Novel cryptic age-specific distributions of validated gene fusions identified by the AML TARGET project.

pediatric AML.[405] Another group of drugs that target the metabolic pathways of AML cells may have a role in a small subset of pediatric AML.[392]

Specific and selective targeted therapies are currently being tested in both adult and pediatric patients with AML. However, recent data demonstrate that even molecularly targeted therapies are not often as specific as initial results would suggest and that leukemia resistance commonly develops or is already present at the initiation of treatment, which leads in turn to the selection of resistant leukemic clones, including LICs. Although targeted therapies hold significant hope for improved antileukemic activity and for potentially sparing normal tissues from damage, there are clearly significant hurdles to overcome: first, how to define the key leukemogenic molecular pathways, and second, how to optimize the use of specific and selected targeted agents in combinations that will address cellular responses and feedback mechanisms of resistance.

Immunotherapy is emerging as a major pillar of therapy and include a variety of agents such as antibodies, antibody drug conjugates (ADCs), antibodies that are bispecific T-cell or NK-cell engagers or dual-affinity re-targetting, selected T cell subsets,[406] and chimeric antigen receptor T cells (CARTs). Anti-CD33 therapy has demonstrated that cell surface antigen targeting is a useful and potentially very significant therapeutic modality in AML and second-generation ADCs or CARTs against CD33 as well as CD123, and immune checkpoint inhibitors are currently being investigated in adults, and soon in children.[407-410] It is important to consider that many of the antigens expressed on AML blasts are also expressed on normal HSCs; therefore significant and dose limiting myelosuppression is a concern for many agents, especially for immune checkpoint inhibitors and T-cell engagers that depend on functioning T cells. Although this may limit the utility of some agents in chemotherapeutic regimens, these agents may still offer significant antileukemic benefit when used upfront after diagnosis in the case of immunoconjugates, in the setting of MRD or maintenance phase after immunosuppressive chemotherapy, or pre-HCT as part of a nongenotoxic conditioning regimen. It is also important to consider any off-target effects on nonhematopoietic tissues that also express the target antigens. Immunotherapies, namely CART cells, show significant clinical activity in relapsed ALL; however, AML presents a distinct challenge due to its heterogeneity as well as coexpression of many AML surface antigens on hematopoietic stem cells. Upcoming preclinical and clinical studies will define the optimal use and supportive care for immunotherapies in AML.

For the next decade physicians who treat relapsed and refractory pediatric AML should consult and support the Leukemia Lymphoma Society and the COG LLS PEDAL program that will feature precision medicine early-phase therapies for childhood acute leukemia (https://www.lls.org/dare-to-dream/pedal), as well as efforts by other pediatric cancer consortia and institutions testing new combination therapies.

ACKNOWLEDGMENT

Robert J. Arceci, MD, PhD, was a national and international mentor in the field of Pediatric Hematology-Oncology. He was an inspiration to many leaders in pediatric AML and Langerhans cell histiocytosis. We dedicate this chapter to him and all he inspired to continue his work.

References

1. Gunz FW. The dread leukemias and the lymphomas: their nature and their prospects. In: Wintrobe MM, ed. *Blood, Pure and Eloquent*. McGraw-Hill Book Company; 1980:511-548.
2. Friedreich N. Ein neue fall von leukamie. *Virchows Arch Path Anat*. 1857;12:37.
3. Naegli O. Ueber rotes knochenmark und myeloblasten. *Dtsch Med Wochenschr*. 1900;26:287.
4. Reschad H, Schilling-Torgau V. Ueber eine neue leukamie durch echte uebergangsformen (splenozyten-leukamie) und ihre bedeutung Fur die selbstandigkeit dieser zellen. *Munch Med Wochenschr*. 1913;60:1981.
5. DiGuglielmo G. Ricerche di hematologia: I. Una casa di eritroleucemia. *Folia Med*. 1917;13:386.
6. Hilstad LK. Acute promyelocytic leukemia. *Acta Med Scand*. 1957;159:189.
7. Von Boros J, Karenyi A. Uber einem fall von akuter megakaryoblastenleukamie: zugleich einige bemerkungen zum problem der akuten leukamie. *Z Klin Med*. 1931;118:697.
8. Bennett JM, Catovsky D, Daniel MT, et al. Proposals for the classification of the acute leukaemias. French-American-British (FAB) co-operative group. *Br J Haematol*. 1976;33(4):451-458.
9. Farber S, Diamond LK, Mercer RD, Sylvester RF, Wolff JA. Temporary remissions in acute leukemia in children produced by folic acid antagonist, 4-aminopteroyl-glutamic acid (Aminopterin). *N Engl J Med*. 1948;238:787-793.
10. Arceci RJ. Progress and controversies in the treatment of pediatric acute myelogenous leukemia. *Curr Opin Hematol*. 2002;9(4):353-360.
11. Clark JJ, Smith FO, Arceci RJ. Update in childhood acute myeloid leukemia: recent developments in the molecular basis of disease and novel therapies. *Curr Opin Hematol*. 2003;10(1):31-39.
12. Gamis AS, Alonzo TA, Perentesis JP, Meshinchi S; COG Acute Myeloid Leukemia Committee. Children's Oncology Group's 2013 blueprint for research: acute myeloid leukemia. *Pediatr Blood Cancer*. 2013;60(6):964-971. doi:10.1002/pbc.24432
13. Bolouri H, Farrar JE, Triche T Jr, et al. The molecular landscape of pediatric acute myeloid leukemia reveals recurrent structural alterations and age-specific mutational interactions. *Nat Med*. 2018;24(4):526.
14. Loken MR, Alonzo TA, Pardo L, et al. Residual disease detected by multidimensional flow cytometry signifies high relapse risk in patients with de novo acute myeloid leukemia: a report from Children's Oncology Group. *Blood*. 2012;120(8):1581-1588. doi:10.1182/blood-2012-02-408336
15. Rubnitz JE, Inaba H, Dahl G, et al. Minimal residual disease-directed therapy for childhood acute myeloid leukaemia: results of the AML02 Multicentre Trial. *Lancet Oncol*. June 2010;11(6):543-552. doi:10.1016/S1470-2045(10)70090-5
16. Ward E, Robbins A, Kohler B, Jemal A. Childhood and adolescent cancer statistics, 2014. *CA Cancer J Clin*. 2014;64:83-103. doi:10.3322/caac.21219
17. Juliusson G, Antunovic P, Derolf A, et al. Age and acute myeloid leukemia: real world data on decision to treat and outcomes from the Swedish Acute Leukemia Registry. *Blood*. 2009;113(18):4179-4187. doi:10.1182/blood-2008-07-172007
18. Bhatia S, Neglia JP. Epidemiology of childhood acute myelogenous leukemia. *J Pediatr Hematol Oncol*. 1995;17(2):94-100.
19. Puumala SE, Ross JA, Aplenc R, Spector LG. Epidemiology of childhood acute myeloid leukemia. *Pediatr Blood Cancer*. 2013;60(5):728-733. doi:10.1002/pbc.24464
20. Gurney JG, Severson RK, Davis S, Robison LL. Incidence of cancer in children in the United States. Sex, race, and 1 year age-specific rates by histologic type. *Cancer*. 1995;75:2186-2195.
21. Glazer ER, Perkins CI, Young JL Jr, Schlag RD, Campleman SL, Wright WE. Cancer among Hispanic children in California, 1988-1994: comparison with non-Hispanic white children. *Cancer*. 1999;86(6):1070-1079.
22. Matasar MJ, Ritchie EK, Consedine N, Magai C, Neugut AI. Incidence rates of acute promyelocytic leukemia among Hispanics, blacks, Asians, and non-Hispanic whites in the United States. *Eur J Cancer Prev*. 2006;15(4):367-370.
23. Metayer C, Zhang L, Wiemels JL, et al. Tobacco smoke exposure and the risk of childhood acute lymphoblastic and myeloid leukemias by cytogenetic subtype. *Cancer Epidemiol Biomarkers Prev*. 2013;22(9):1600-1611. doi:10.1158/1055-9965.epi-13-0350
24. Stiller CA. Epidemiology and genetics of childhood cancer. *Oncogene*. 2004;23(38):6429-6444.
25. Verma D, O'Brien S, Thomas D, et al. Therapy-related acute myelogenous leukemia and myelodysplastic syndrome in patients with acute lymphoblastic leukemia treated with the hyperfractionated cyclophosphamide, vincristine, doxorubicin, and dexamethasone regimens. *Cancer*. 2009;115(1):101-106. doi:10.1002/cncr.24005
26. Le Deley MC, Leblanc T, Shamsaldin A, et al. Risk of secondary leukemia after a solid tumor in childhood according to the dose of epipodophyllotoxins and anthracyclines: a case-control study by the Societe Francaise d'Oncologie Pediatrique. *J Clin Oncol*. 2003;21(6):1074-1081.
27. Sandoval C, Pui CH, Bowman LC, et al. Secondary acute myeloid leukemia in children previously treated with alkylating agents, intercalating topoisomerase II inhibitors, and irradiation. *J Clin Oncol*. 1993;11(6):1039-1045.
28. Fialkow PJ. Stem cell origin of human myeloid blood cell neoplasms. *Verh Dtsch Ges Pathol*. 1990;74:43-47.
29. Hirsch P, Zhang Y, Tang R, et al. Genetic hierarchy and temporal variegation in the clonal history of acute myeloid leukaemia. *Nat Commun*. 2016;7:12475. doi:10.1038/ncomms12475
30. Fialkow PJ, Gartler SM, Yoshida A. Clonal origin of chronic myelocytic leukemia in man. *Proc Natl Acad Sci U S A*. 1967;58:1468.
31. Bonnet D. Normal and leukaemic stem cells. *Br J Haematol*. 2005;130(4):469-479. doi:10.1111/j.1365-2141.2005.05596.x
32. Bonnet D, Dick JE. Human acute myeloid leukemia is organized as a hierarchy that originates from a primitive hematopoietic cell. *Nat Med*. 1997;3(7):730-737.
33. Masetti R, Castelli I, Astolfi A, et al. Genomic complexity and dynamics of clonal evolution in childhood acute myeloid leukemia studied with whole-exome sequencing. *Oncotarget*. 2016;7(35):56746-56757. doi:10.18632/oncotarget.10778
34. Sirard C, Lapidot T, Vormoor J, et al. Normal and leukemic SCID-repopulating cells (SRC) coexist in the bone marrow and peripheral blood from CML patients in chronic phase, whereas leukemic SRC are detected in blast crisis. *Blood*. 1996;87(4):1539-1548.
35. Terpstra W, Prins A, Ploemacher RE, et al. Long-term leukemia-initiating capacity of a CD34-subpopulation of acute myeloid leukemia. *Blood*. 1996;87(6):2187-2194.
36. Turhan AG, Lemoine FM, Debert C, et al. Highly purified primitive hematopoietic stem cells are PML-RARA negative and generate nonclonal progenitors in acute promyelocytic leukemia. *Blood*. 1995;85(8):2154-2161.
37. Ley TJ, Mardis ER, Ding L, et al. DNA sequencing of a cytogenetically normal acute myeloid leukaemia genome. *Nature*. 2008;456(7218):66-72. doi:10.1038/nature07485
38. Gilliland DG, Griffin JD. The roles of FLT3 in hematopoiesis and leukemia. *Blood*. 2002;100(5):1532-1542. doi:10.1182/blood-2002-02-0492
39. Lagadinou ED, Sach A, Callahan K, et al. BCL-2 inhibition targets oxidative phosphorylation and selectively eradicates quiescent human leukemia stem cells. *Cell Stem Cell*. 2013;12(3):329-341. doi:10.1016/j.stem.2012.12.013
40. Jones CL, Stevens BM, D'Alessandro A, et al. Inhibition of amino acid metabolism selectively targets human leukemia stem cells. *Cancer Cell*. 2018;34(5):724.e4-740.e4. doi:10.1016/j.ccell.2018.10.005
41. Welch JS, Ley TJ, Link DC, et al. The origin and evolution of mutations in acute myeloid leukemia. *Cell*. 2012;150(2):264-278. doi:10.1016/j.cell.2012.06.023
42. Ley TJ, Ding L, Walter MJ, et al. DNMT3A mutations in acute myeloid leukemia. *N Engl J Med*. 2010;363(25):2424-2433. doi:10.1056/NEJMoa1005143
43. Ding L, Ley TJ, Larson DE, et al. Clonal evolution in relapsed acute myeloid leukaemia revealed by whole-genome sequencing. *Nature*. 2012;481(7382):506-510. doi:10.1038/nature10738
44. Ho PA, Kutny MA, Alonzo TA, et al. Leukemic mutations in the methylation-associated genes DNMT3A and IDH2 are rare events in pediatric AML: a report

from the Children's Oncology Group. *Pediatr Blood Cancer*. 2011;57(2):204-209. doi:10.1002/pbc.23179
45. Ho PA, Alonzo TA, Kopecky KJ, et al. Molecular alterations of the IDH1 gene in AML: a children's oncology group and southwest oncology group study. *Leukemia*. 2010;24(5):909-913. doi:10.1038/leu.2010.56
46. Ho PA, Alonzo TA, Gerbing RB, et al. Prevalence and prognostic implications of CEBPA mutations in pediatric acute myeloid leukemia (AML): a report from the Children's Oncology Group. *Blood*. 2009;113(26):6558-6566. doi:10.1182/blood-2008-10-184747
47. Balgobind BV, Hollink IH, Arentsen-Peters ST, et al. Integrative analysis of type-I and type-II aberrations underscores the genetic heterogeneity of pediatric acute myeloid leukemia. *Haematologica*. 2011;96(10):1478-1487. doi:10.3324/haematol.2010.038976
48. Dohner H, Weisdorf DJ, Bloomfield CD. Acute myeloid leukemia. *N Engl J Med*. 2015;373(12):1136-1152. doi:10.1056/NEJMra1406184
49. Ross JA, Spector LG, Robison LL, Olshan AF. Epidemiology of leukemia in children with Down syndrome. *Pediatr Blood Cancer*. 2005;44(1):8-12.
50. Groet J, McElwaine S, Spinelli M, et al. Acquired mutations in GATA1 in neonates with Down's syndrome with transient myeloid disorder. *Lancet*. 2003;361(9369):1617-1620.
51. Massey GV, Zipursky A, Chang MN, et al. A prospective study of the natural history of transient leukemia (TL) in neonates with Down syndrome (DS): Children's Oncology Group (COG) study POG-9481. *Blood*. 2006;107(12):4606-4613. doi:10.1182/blood-2005-06-2448
52. Bhatnagar N, Nizery L, Tunstall O, Vyas P, Roberts I. Transient abnormal myelopoiesis and AML in down syndrome: an update. *Curr Hematol Malig Rep*. 2016;11(5):333-341. doi:10.1007/s11899-016-0338-x
53. Izraeli S, Vora A, Zwaan CM, Whitlock J. How I treat ALL in Down's syndrome: pathobiology and management. *Blood*. 2014;123(1):35-40. doi:10.1182/blood-2013-07-453480
54. Rainis L, Bercovich D, Strehl S, et al. Mutations in exon 2 of GATA1 are early events in megakaryocytic malignancies associated with trisomy 21. *Blood*. 2003;102(3):981-986.
55. Evans EJ, DeGregori J. Dissecting stepwise mutational impairment of megakaryopoiesis in a model of Down syndrome-associated leukemia. *J Clin Invest*. 2022;132(14). doi:10.1172/JCI161659
56. Hasle H, Kline RM, Kjeldsen E, et al. Germline GATA1s-generating mutations predispose to leukemia with acquired trisomy 21 and Down syndrome-like phenotype. *Blood*. 2022;139(21):3159-3165. doi:10.1182/blood.2021011463
57. de Castro CPM, Cadefau M, Cuartero S. The mutational landscape of myeloid leukaemia in down syndrome. *Cancers (Basel)*. 2021;13(16). doi:10.3390/cancers13164144
58. Hitzler J, Zipursky A. GATA 1 mutations as clonal markers of minimal residual disease in acute megakaryoblastic leukemia of Down syndrome—a new tool with significant potential applications. *Leuk Res*. November 2005;29(11):1239-1240.
59. Geraedts JP, Ford CE, Briet E, Hartgrink-Groeneveld CA, den Ottolander GJ. Klinefelter syndrome: predisposition to acute non-lymphocytic leukaemia? *Lancet*. 1980;1(8177):1092.
60. Wertelecki W, Shapiro JR. 45,XO Turner's syndrome and leukaemia. *Lancet*. 1970;1(7650):789-790.
61. Alter BP, Giri N, Savage SA, et al. Malignancies and survival patterns in the National Cancer Institute inherited bone marrow failure syndromes cohort study. *Br J Haematol*. 2010;150(2):179-188. doi:10.1111/j.1365-2141.2010.08212.x
62. Auerbach AD. Fanconi anemia and its diagnosis. *Mutat Res*. 2009;668(1-2):4-10. doi:10.1016/j.mrfmmm.2009.01.013
63. Alter BP. Diagnosis, genetics, and management of inherited bone marrow failure syndromes. *Hematology Am Soc Hematol Educ Program*. 2007;2007:29-39. doi:10.1182/asheducation-2007.1.29
64. Jeha S, Chan KW, Aprikyan AG, et al. Spontaneous remission of granulocyte colony-stimulating factor- associated leukemia in a child with severe congenital neutropenia. *Blood*. 2000;96(10):3647-3649.
65. Zeidler C, Schwinzer B, Welte K. Congenital neutropenias. *Rev Clin Exp Hematol*. 2003;7(1):72-83.
66. Steele JM, Sung L, Klaassen R, et al. Disease progression in recently diagnosed patients with inherited marrow failure syndromes: a Canadian Inherited Marrow Failure Registry (CIMFR) report. *Pediatr Blood Cancer*. 2006;47(7):918-925.
67. Hunter MG, Avalos BR. Granulocyte colony-stimulating factor receptor mutations in severe congenital neutropenia transforming to acute myelogenous leukemia confer resistance to apoptosis and enhance cell survival. *Blood*. 2000;95(6):2132-2137.
68. Tamary H, Alter BP. Current diagnosis of inherited bone marrow failure syndromes. *Pediatr Hematol Oncol*. 2007;24(2):87-99. doi:10.1080/08880010601123240
69. Alter BP, Giri N, Savage SA, Rosenberg PS. Cancer in dyskeratosis congenita. *Blood*. 2009;113(26):6549-6557. doi:10.1182/blood-2008-12-192880
70. Hayashi Y, Harada Y, Harada H. Myeloid neoplasms and clonal hematopoiesis from the RUNX1 perspective. *Leukemia*. 05 2022;36(5):1203-1214. doi:10.1038/s41375-022-01548-7
71. Niemeyer CM. RAS diseases in children. *Haematologica*. 2014;99(11):1653-1662. doi:10.3324/haematol.2014.114595
72. de Vries AC, Zwaan CM, van den Heuvel-Eibrink MM. Molecular basis of juvenile myelomonocytic leukaemia. *Haematologica*. 2010;95(2):179-182. doi:10.3324/haematol.2009.016865
73. Tartaglia M, Niemeyer CM, Fragale A, et al. Somatic mutations in PTPN11 in juvenile myelomonocytic leukemia, myelodysplastic syndromes and acute myeloid leukemia. *Nat Genet*. 2003;34(2):148-150.
74. Shiba N, Kato M, Park MJ, et al. CBL mutations in juvenile myelomonocytic leukemia and pediatric myelodysplastic syndrome. *Leukemia*. 2010;24(5):1090-1092. doi:10.1038/leu.2010.49
75. Locatelli F, Niemeyer CM. How I treat juvenile myelomonocytic leukemia. *Blood*. 2015;125(7):1083-1090. doi:10.1182/blood-2014-08-550483
76. Poppe B, Van Limbergen H, Van Roy N, et al. Chromosomal aberrations in Bloom syndrome patients with myeloid malignancies. *Cancer Genet Cytogenet*. 2001;128(1):39-42.
77. Owen CJ, Toze CL, Koochin A, et al. Five new pedigrees with inherited RUNX1 mutations causing familial platelet disorder with propensity to myeloid malignancy. *Blood*. 2008;112(12):4639-4645. doi:10.1182/blood-2008-05-156745
78. Matheny CJ, Speck ME, Cushing PR, et al. Disease mutations in RUNX1 and RUNX2 create nonfunctional, dominant-negative, or hypomorphic alleles. *EMBO J*. 2007;26(4):1163-1175. doi:10.1038/sj.emboj.7601568
79. Wlodarski MW, Collin M, Horwitz MS. GATA2 deficiency and related myeloid neoplasms. *Semin Hematol*. 2017;54(2):81-86. doi:10.1053/j.seminhematol.2017.05.002
80. Lynch HT, Weisenburger DD, Quinn-Laquer B, et al. Family with acute myelocytic leukemia, breast, ovarian, and gastrointestinal cancer. *Cancer Genet Cytogenet*. 2002;137(1):8-14. doi:S016546080200537X
81. Alter BP. Bone marrow failure syndromes in children. *Pediatr Clin North Am*. 2002;49(5):973-988.
82. Greaves MF, Maia AT, Wiemels JL, Ford AM. Leukemia in twins: lessons in natural history. *Blood*. 2003;102(7):2321-2333.
83. Wiemels J. Chromosomal translocations in childhood leukemia: natural history, mechanisms, and epidemiology. *J Natl Cancer Inst Monogr*. 2008;(39):87-90. doi:10.1093/jncimonographs/lgn006
84. Kurita S, Kamei Y, Ota K. Genetic studies on familial leukemia. *Cancer*. 1974;34:1098.
85. Markkanen A, Ruutu T, Rasi V, Franssila K, Knuutila S, de la Chapelle A. Constitutional translocation t(3;6)(p14;p11) in a family with hematologic malignancies. *Cancer Genet Cytogenet*. 1987;25(1):87-95.
86. Greaves M. Pre-natal origins of childhood leukemia. *Rev Clin Exp Hematol*. 2003;7(3):233-245.
87. Minelli A, Maserati E, Giudici G, et al. Familial partial monosomy 7 and myelodysplasia: different parental origin of the monosomy 7 suggests action of a mutator gene. *Cancer Genet Cytogenet*. 2001;124(2):147-151.
88. Smeets MF, Tan SY, Xu JJ, et al. Initiates myeloid bias and myelodysplastic/myeloproliferative syndrome from hemopoietic stem cells. *Blood*. 2018;132(6):608-621. doi:10.1182/blood-2018-04-845602
89. Buscarlet M, Provost S, Zada YF, et al. Lineage restriction analyses in CHIP indicate myeloid bias for. *Blood*. 2018;132(3):277-280. doi:10.1182/blood-2018-01-829937
90. Severson EA, Riedlinger GM, Connelly CF, et al. Detection of clonal hematopoiesis of indeterminate potential in clinical sequencing of solid tumor specimens. *Blood*. 2018;131(22):2501-2505. doi:10.1182/blood-2018-03-840629
91. Shlush LI. Age-related clonal hematopoiesis. *Blood*. 2018;131(5):496-504. doi:10.1182/blood-2017-07-746453
92. Nouri AM, Dorey E, Davis CL, Rohatiner A, Lister TA, Oliver RT. Generation of cytotoxic T lymphocytes from peripheral blood of leukaemic patients. *Cancer Immunol Immunother*. 1993;37(1):47-53.
93. Ohara A, Kojima S, Hamajima N, et al. Myelodysplastic syndrome and acute myelogenous leukemia as a late clonal complication in children with acquired aplastic anemia. *Blood*. 1997;90(3):1009-1013.
94. Bagby GC, Meyers G. Myelodysplasia and acute leukemia as late complications of marrow failure: future prospects for leukemia prevention. *Hematol Oncol Clin North Am*. 2009;23(2):361-376. doi:10.1016/j.hoc.2009.01.006
95. Luna-Fineman S, Shannon KM, Atwater SK, et al. Myelodysplastic and myeloproliferative disorders of childhood: a study of 167 patients. *Blood*. 1999;93(2):459-466.
96. Maris JM, Wiersma SR, Mahgoub N, et al. Monosomy 7 myelodysplastic syndrome and other second malignant neoplasms in children with neurofibromatosis type 1. *Cancer*. 1997;79(7):1438-1446.
97. Ichimaru M, Ishimaru T, Belsky JL. Incidence of leukemia in atomic bomb survivors belonging to a fixed cohort in Hiroshima and Nagasaki. 1950-1971: radiation dose, years after exposure, age at exposure, and type of leukemia. *J Radiat Res*. 1978;19:262.
98. Ichimaru M, Tomonaga M, Amenomori T, Matsuo T. Atomic bomb and leukemia. *J Radiat Res*. 1991;32(suppl 2):14-19.
99. Kato H, Schull WJ. Studies of the mortality of A-bomb survivors: mortality, 1950-1978. Part I. Cancer mortality. *Radiat Res*. 1982;90:395.
100. Shimizu Y, Schull WI, Kato H. Cancer risk among atomic bomb survivors: the RERF Life Span Study. *J Am Med Assoc*. 1990;264:601-604.
101. Jablon S, Kato H. Childhood cancer in relation to prenatal exposure to atomic-bomb radiation. *Lancet*. 1970;2(7681):1000-1003.
102. Wakeford R, Little MP. Childhood cancer after low-level intrauterine exposure to radiation. *J Radiol Prot*. 2003;22(3A):A123-A127.
103. Linet MS, Hatch EE, Kleinerman RA, et al. Residential exposure to magnetic fields and acute lymphoblastic leukemia in children. *N Engl J Med*. 1997;337(1):1-7.
104. Alexander FE, Patheal SL, Biondi A, et al. Transplacental chemical exposure and risk of infant leukemia with MLL gene fusion. *Cancer Res*. 2001;61(6):2542-2546.
105. Strick R, Strissel PL, Borgers S, Smith SL, Rowley JD. Dietary bioflavonoids induce cleavage in the MLL gene and may contribute to infant leukemia. *Proc Natl Acad Sci U S A*. 2000;97(9):4790-4795.
106. Baehring JM, Marks PW. Treatment-related myelodysplasia in patients with primary brain tumors. *Neuro Oncol*. 2012;14(5):529-540. doi:10.1093/neuonc/nos068
107. Haupt R, Fears TR, Rosso P, et al. Increased risk of secondary leukemia after single-agent treatment with etoposide for Langerhans' cell histiocytosis. *Pediatr Hematol Oncol*. 1994;11(5):499-507.
108. Schneider DT, Hilgenfeld E, Schwabe D, et al. Acute myelogenous leukemia after treatment for malignant germ cell tumors in children. *J Clin Oncol*. 1999;17(10):3226-3233.

109. Stine KC, Saylors RL, Sawyer JR, Becton DL. Secondary acute myelogenous leukemia following safe exposure to etoposide. *J Clin Oncol.* 1997;15(4):1583-1586.
110. Ogami A, Morimoto A, Hibi S, et al. Secondary acute promyelocytic leukemia following chemotherapy for non-Hodgkin's lymphoma in a child. *J Pediatr Hematol Oncol.* 2004;26(7):427-430. doi:00043426-200407000-00005
111. Pui CH, Ribeiro RC, Hancock ML, et al. Acute myeloid leukemia in children treated with epipodophyllotoxins for acute lymphoblastic leukemia. *N Engl J Med.* 1991;325(24):1682-1687.
112. Megonigal MD, Cheung NK, Rappaport EF, et al. Detection of leukemia-associated MLL-GAS7 translocation early during chemotherapy with DNA topoisomerase II inhibitors. *Proc Natl Acad Sci U S A.* 2000;97(6):2814-2819.
113. Pegram LD, Megonigal MD, Lange BJ, et al. t(3;11) translocation in treatment-related acute myeloid leukemia fuses MLL with the GMPS (GUANOSINE 5' MONOPHOSPHATE SYNTHETASE) gene. *Blood.* 2000;96(13):4360-4362.
114. Burnett AK, Hills RK, Milligan DW, et al. Attempts to optimize induction and consolidation treatment in acute myeloid leukemia: results of the MRC AML12 trial. *J Clin Oncol.* 2010;28(4):586-595. doi:10.1200/JCO.2009.22.9088
115. Wang J, Weiss I, Svoboda K, Kwaan HC. Thrombogenic role of cells undergoing apoptosis. *Br J Haematol.* 2001;115(2):382-391.
116. Yan J, Wang K, Dong L, et al. PML/RARalpha fusion protein transactivates the tissue factor promoter through a GAGC-containing element without direct DNA association. *Proc Natl Acad Sci U S A.* 2010;107(8):3716-3721. doi:10.1073/pnas.0915006107
117. Rollig C, Ehninger G. How I treat hyperleukocytosis in acute myeloid leukemia. *Blood.* 2015;125(21):3246-3252. doi:10.1182/blood-2014-10-551507
118. Johnston DL, Alonzo TA, Gerbing RB, Lange BJ, Woods WG. Superior outcome of pediatric acute myeloid leukemia patients with orbital and CNS myeloid sarcoma: a report from the Children's Oncology Group. *Pediatr Blood Cancer.* 2012;58(4):519-524. doi:10.1002/pbc.23201
119. Young AL, Challen GA, Birmann BM, Druley TE. Clonal haematopoiesis harbouring AML-associated mutations is ubiquitous in healthy adults. *Nat Commun.* 2016;7:12484. doi:10.1038/ncomms12484
120. Arber DA, Orazi A, Hasserjian R, et al. The 2016 revision to the World Health Organization classification of myeloid neoplasms and acute leukemia. *Blood.* 2016;127(20):2391-2405. doi:10.1182/blood-2016-03-643544
121. Webb DK, Harrison G, Stevens RF, Gibson BG, Hann IM, Wheatley K. Relationships between age at diagnosis, clinical features, and outcome of therapy in children treated in the Medical Research Council AML 10 and 12 trials for acute myeloid leukemia. *Blood.* 2001;98(6):1714-1720.
122. Haferlach T, Schoch C, Loffler H, et al. Morphologic dysplasia in de novo acute myeloid leukemia (AML) is related to unfavorable cytogenetics but has no independent prognostic relevance under the conditions of intensive induction therapy: results of a multiparameter analysis from the German AML Cooperative Group studies. *J Clin Oncol.* 2003;21(2):256-265.
123. Raimondi SC, Chang MN, Ravindranath Y, et al. Chromosomal abnormalities in 478 children with acute myeloid leukemia: clinical characteristics and treatment outcome in a cooperative pediatric oncology group study-POG 8821. *Blood.* 1999;94(11):3707-3716.
124. Kaspers GJ. Pediatric acute myeloid leukemia. *Expet Rev Anticancer Ther.* 2012;12(3):405-413. doi:10.1586/era.12.1
125. Klco JM, Miller CA, Griffith M, et al. Association between mutation clearance after induction therapy and outcomes in acute myeloid leukemia. *J Am Med Assoc.* 2015;314(8):811-822, doi:10.1001/jama.2015.9643
126. Creutzig U, Ritter J, Zimmermann M, et al. Improved treatment results in high-risk pediatric acute myeloid leukemia patients after intensification with high-dose cytarabine and mitoxantrone: results of Study Acute Myeloid Leukemia-Berlin-Frankfurt-Munster 93. *J Clin Oncol.* 2001;19(10):2705-2713.
127. Woods WG, Kobrinsky N, Buckley JD, et al. Timed-sequential induction therapy improves postremission outcome in acute myeloid leukemia: a report from the Children's Cancer Group. *Blood.* 1996;87(12):4979-4989.
128. Cooper TM, Franklin J, Gerbing RB, et al. AAML03P1, a pilot study of the safety of gemtuzumab ozogamicin in combination with chemotherapy for newly diagnosed childhood acute myeloid leukemia: a report from the Children's Oncology Group. *Cancer.* 2012;118(3):761-769. doi:10.1002/cncr.26190
129. Creutzig U, van den Heuvel-Eibrink MM, Gibson B, et al. Diagnosis and management of acute myeloid leukemia in children and adolescents: recommendations from an international expert panel. *Blood.* 2012;120(16):3187-3205. doi:10.1182/blood-2012-03-362608
130. Weick JK, Kopecky KJ, Appelbaum FR, et al. A randomized investigation of high-dose versus standard-dose cytosine arabinoside with daunorubicin in patients with previously untreated acute myeloid leukemia: a Southwest Oncology Group study. *Blood.* 1996;88(8):2841-2851.
131. Riley LC, Hann IM, Wheatley K, Stevens RF. Treatment-related deaths during induction and first remission of acute myeloid leukaemia in children treated on the Tenth Medical Research Council acute myeloid leukaemia trial (MRC AML10). The MCR Childhood Leukaemia Working Party. *Br J Haematol.* 1999;106(2):436-444.
132. Lange BJ, Smith FO, Feusner J, et al. Outcomes in CCG-2961, a children's oncology group phase 3 trial for untreated pediatric acute myeloid leukemia: a report from the children's oncology group. *Blood.* 2008;111(3):1044-1053. doi:10.1182/blood-2007-04-084293
133. Lange BJ, Dinndorf P, Smith FO, et al. Pilot study of idarubicin-based intensive-timing induction therapy for children with previously untreated acute myeloid leukemia: Children's Cancer Group Study 2941. *J Clin Oncol.* 2004;22(1):150-156.
134. Lange BJ, Smith FO, Feusner J, et al. Outcomes in CCG-2961, a Children's Oncology Group phase 3 trial for untreated pediatric acute myeloid leukemia (AML): a report from the Children's Oncology Group. *Blood.* 2008;111(3):1044-1053.
135. Bloomfield CD, Lawrence D, Byrd JC, et al. Frequency of prolonged remission duration after high-dose cytarabine intensification in acute myeloid leukemia varies by cytogenetic subtype. *Cancer Res.* 1998;58(18):4173-4179.
136. Byrd JC, Dodge RK, Carroll A, et al. Patients with t(8;21)(q22;q22) and acute myeloid leukemia have superior failure-free and overall survival when repetitive cycles of high-dose cytarabine are administered. *J Clin Oncol.* 1999;17(12):3767-3775.
137. Bishop JF, Matthews JP, Young GA, et al. A randomized study of high-dose cytarabine in induction in acute myeloid leukemia. *Blood.* 1996;87(5):1710-1717.
138. Becton D, Dahl GV, Ravindranath Y, et al. Randomized use of cyclosporin A (CsA) to modulate P-glycoprotein in children with AML in remission: pediatric oncology group study 9421. *Blood.* 2006;107(4):1315-1324.
139. Lowenthal RM, Bradstock KF, Matthews JP, et al. A phase I/II study of intensive dose escalation of cytarabine in combination with idarubicin and etoposide in induction and consolidation treatment of adult acute myeloid leukemia. Australian Leukaemia Study Group (ALSG). *Leuk Lymphoma.* 1999;34(5-6):501-510.
140. Creutzig U, Ritter J, Zimmermann M, et al. Idarubicin improves blast cell clearance during induction therapy in children with AML: results of study AML-BFM 93. AML-BFM Study Group. *Leukemia.* 2001;15(3):348-354.
141. Wheatley K. Meta-analysis of randomized trials of idarubicin (IDAR) or metozantrone (Mito) versus daunorubicin (DNR) as induction therapy for acute myeloid leukaemia (AML). *Blood.* 1995;86:43A.
142. Gibson BE, Wheatley K, Hann IM, et al. Treatment strategy and long-term results in paediatric patients treated in consecutive UK AML trials. *Leukemia.* 2005;19(12):2130-2138.
143. Gibson BE, Webb DK, Howman AJ, De Graaf SS, Harrison CJ, Wheatley K. Results of a randomized trial in children with Acute Myeloid Leukaemia: medical research council AML12 trial. *Br J Haematol.* 2011;155(3):366-376. doi:10.1111/j.1365-2141.2011.08851.x
144. Cortes JE, Goldberg SL, Feldman EJ, et al. Phase II, multicenter, randomized trial of CPX-351 (cytarabine:daunorubicin) liposome injection versus intensive salvage therapy in adults with first relapse AML. *Cancer.* 2015;121(2):234-242. doi:10.1002/cncr.28974
145. Sievers EL. Targeted therapy of acute myeloid leukemia with monoclonal antibodies and immunoconjugates. *Cancer Chemother Pharmacol.* 2000;(46 suppl):S18-S22.
146. Cooper TM, Franklin J, Gerbing RB, et al. A pilot study of the safety and efficacy of gemtuzumab ozogamicin in combination with chemotherapy for newly diagnosed childhood acute myeloid leukemia: a report from the Children's Oncology Group. *Cancer.* 2012;118(3):761-769.
147. Gamis AS, Alonzo TA, Meshinchi S, et al. Gemtuzumab ozogamicin in children and adolescents with de novo acute myeloid leukemia improves event-free survival by reducing relapse risk: results from the randomized phase III Children's Oncology Group trial AAML0531. *J Clin Oncol.* 2014;32(27):3021-3032. doi:10.1200/jco.2014.55.3628
148. Castaigne S, Pautas C, Terre C, et al. Effect of gemtuzumab ozogamicin on survival of adult patients with de-novo acute myeloid leukaemia (ALFA-0701): a randomised, open-label, phase 3 study. *Lancet.* 2012;379(9825):1508-1516. doi:10.1016/s0140-6736(12)60485-1
149. Burnett AK, Hills RK, Milligan D, et al. Identification of patients with acute myeloblastic leukemia who benefit from the addition of gemtuzumab ozogamicin: results of the MRC AML15 trial. *J Clin Oncol.* 2011;29(4):369-377. doi:10.1200/JCO.2010.31.4310
150. Hasle H, Abrahamsson J, Forestier E, et al. Gemtuzumab ozogamicin as postconsolidation therapy does not prevent relapse in children with AML: results from NOPHO-AML 2004. *Blood.* 2012;120(5):978-984. doi:10.1182/blood-2012-03-416701
151. Creutzig U, Zimmermann M, Ritter J, et al. Treatment strategies and long-term results in paediatric patients treated in four consecutive AML-BFM trials. *Leukemia.* 2005;19(12):2030-2042.
152. Ravindranath Y, Chang M, Steuber CP, et al. Pediatric Oncology Group (POG) studies of Acute Myeloid Leukemia (AML): a review of four consecutive childhood AML trials conducted between 1981 and 2000. *Leukemia.* 2005;19(12):2101-2116. doi:10.1038/sj.leu.2403927
153. Alonzo TA, Wells RJ, Woods WG, et al. Postremission therapy for children with acute myeloid leukemia: the children's cancer group experience in the transplant era. *Leukemia.* 2005;19(6):965-970.
154. Masarova L, Kantarjian H, Garcia-Mannero G, Ravandi F, Sharma P, Daver N. Harnessing the immune system Against leukemia: monoclonal antibodies and checkpoint strategies for AML. *Adv Exp Med Biol.* 2017;995:73-95. doi:10.1007/978-3-319-53156-4_4
155. Airiau K, Prouzet-Mauleon V, Rousseau B, et al. Synergistic cooperation between ABT-263 and MEK1/2 inhibitor: effect on apoptosis and proliferation of acute myeloid leukemia cells. *Oncotarget.* 2016;7(1):845-859. doi:10.18632/oncotarget.6417
156. Aplenc R, Meshinchi S, Sung L, et al. Bortezomib with standard chemotherapy for children with acute myeloid leukemia does not improve treatment outcomes: a report from the Children's Oncology Group. *Haematologica.* 07 2020;105(7):1879-1886. doi:10.3324/haematol.2019.220962
157. Rubnitz JE, Lacayo NJ, Inaba H, et al. Clofarabine can replace anthracyclines and etoposide in remission induction therapy for childhood acute myeloid leukemia: the AML08 multicenter, randomized phase III trial. *J Clin Oncol.* 2019;37(23):2072-2081. doi:10.1200/JCO.19.00327
158. Grimwade D, Walker H, Oliver F, et al. The importance of diagnostic cytogenetics on outcome in AML: analysis of 1,612 patients entered into the MRC AML 10 trial. The Medical Research Council Adult and Children's Leukaemia Working Parties. *Blood.* 1998;92(7):2322-2333.

159. Locatelli F, Merli P, Pagliara D, et al. Outcome of children with acute leukemia given HLA-haploidentical HSCT after αβ T-cell and B-cell depletion. *Blood.* 2017;130(5):677-685. doi:10.1182/blood-2017-04-779769
160. Ribeiro RC, Razzouk BI, Pounds S, Hijiya N, Pui CH, Rubnitz JE. Successive clinical trials for childhood acute myeloid leukemia at St Jude Children's Research Hospital, from 1980 to 2000. *Leukemia.* 2005;19(12):2125-2129. doi:10.1038/sj.leu.2403872
161. Kardos G, Zwaan CM, Kaspers GJ, et al. Treatment strategy and results in children treated on three Dutch Childhood Oncology Group acute myeloid leukemia trials. *Leukemia.* 2005;19(12):2063-2071. doi:10.1038/sj.leu.2403873
162. Pession A, Rondelli R, Basso G, et al. Treatment and long-term results in children with acute myeloid leukaemia treated according to the AIEOP AML protocols. *Leukemia.* 2005;19(12):2043-2053.
163. Dluzniewska A, Balwierz W, Armata J, et al. Twenty years of Polish experience with three consecutive protocols for treatment of childhood acute myelogenous leukemia. *Leukemia.* 2005;19(12):2117-2124. doi:10.1038/sj.leu.2403892
164. Lie SO, Abrahamsson J, Clausen N, et al. Long-term results in children with AML: NOPHO-AML Study Group—report of three consecutive trials. *Leukemia.* 2005;19(12):2090-2100.
165. Burnett AK, Goldstone AH, Stevens RM, et al. Randomised comparison of addition of autologous bone-marrow transplantation to intensive chemotherapy for acute myeloid leukaemia in first remission: results of MRC AML 10 trial. UK Medical Research Council Adult and Children's Leukaemia Working Parties. *Lancet.* 1998;351(9104):700-708.
166. Creutzig U, Bender-Gotze C, Klingebiel T, et al. Comparison of chemotherapy alone with allogeneic bone marrow transplantation in first full remission in children with acute myeloid leukemia in the AML-BFM-83 and AML-BFM-87 studies – matched pair analysis. *Klin Pädiatr.* 1992;204(4):246-252.
167. Smith FO, Alonzo TA, Gerbing RB, Woods WG, Arceci RJ. Long-term results of children with acute myeloid leukemia: a report of three consecutive phase III trials by the Children's Cancer Group. CCG 251, CCG 213 and CCG 2891. *Leukemia.* 2005;19(12):2054-2062.
168. Perel Y, Auvrignon A, Leblanc T, et al. Treatment of childhood acute myeloblastic leukemia: dose intensification improves outcome and maintenance therapy is of no benefit – multicenter studies of the French LAME (Leucemie Aigue Myeloblastique Enfant) Cooperative Group. *Leukemia.* 2005;19(12):2082-2089.
169. Perel Y, Auvrignon A, Leblanc T, et al. Impact of addition of maintenance therapy to intensive induction and consolidation chemotherapy for childhood acute myeloblastic leukemia: results of a prospective randomized trial, LAME 89/91. Leucamie Aique Myeloide Enfant. *J Clin Oncol.* 2002;20(12):2774-2782.
170. Entz-Werle N, Suciu S, van der Werff ten Bosch J, et al. Results of 58872 and 58921 trials in acute myeloblastic leukemia and relative value of chemotherapy vs allogeneic bone marrow transplantation in first complete remission: the EORTC Children Leukemia Group report. *Leukemia.* 2005;19(12):2072-2081. doi:10.1038/sj.leu.2403932
171. Oliansky DM, Rizzo JD, Aplan PD, et al. The role of cytotoxic therapy with hematopoietic stem cell transplantation in the therapy of acute myeloid leukemia in children: an evidence-based review. *Biol Blood Marrow Transplant.* 2007;13(1):1-25.
172. Woods WG, Kobrinsky N, Buckley J, et al. Intensively timed induction therapy followed by autologous or allogeneic bone marrow transplantation for children with acute myeloid leukemia or myelodysplastic syndrome: a Childrens Cancer Group Pilot Study. *J Clin Oncol.* 1993;11(8):1448-1457.
173. Ravindranath Y, Yeager AM, Chang MN, et al. Autologous bone marrow transplantation versus intensive consolidation chemotherapy for acute myeloid leukemia in childhood. Pediatric Oncology Group. *N Engl J Med.* 1996;334(22):1428-1434.
174. Meshinchi S, Arceci RJ. Prognostic factors and risk-based therapy in pediatric acute myeloid leukemia. *Oncol.* 2007;12(3):341-355.
175. Zwaan CM, Meshinchi S, Radich JP, et al. FLT3 internal tandem duplication in 234 children with acute myeloid leukemia: prognostic significance and relation to cellular drug resistance. *Blood.* 2003;102(7):2387-2394.
176. Meshinchi S, Alonzo TA, Gerbing R, Lange B, Radich JP. FLT3 internal tandem duplication is a prognostic factor for poor outcome in pediatric AML; a CCG-1961 study [abstract]. *Blood.* 2003;102(11):335a.
177. Gale RE, Hills R, Kottaridis PD, et al. No evidence that FLT3 status should be considered as an indicator for transplantation in acute myeloid leukemia (AML): an analysis of 1135 patients, excluding acute promyelocytic leukemia, from the UK MRC AML10 and 12 trials. *Blood.* 2005;106(10):3658-3665.
178. Lacayo NJ, Meshinchi S, Kinnunen P, et al. Gene expression profiles at diagnosis in de novo childhood AML patients identify FLT3 mutations with good clinical outcomes. *Blood.* 2004;104(9):2646-2654. doi:10.1182/blood-2003-12-4449
179. Bornhauser M, Illmer T, Schaich M, Soucek S, Ehninger G, Thiede C. Improved outcome after stem-cell transplantation in FLT3/ITD-positive AML. *Blood.* 2007;109(5):2264-2265.
180. Meshinchi S, Arceci RJ, Sanders JE, et al. Role of allogeneic stem cell transplantation in FLT3/ITD-positive AML. *Blood.* 2006;108(1):400-401.
181. Doubek M, Muzik J, Szotkowski T, et al. Is FLT3 internal tandem duplication significant indicator for allogeneic transplantation in acute myeloid leukemia? An analysis of patients from the Czech Acute Leukemia Clinical Register (ALERT). *Neoplasma.* 2007;54(1):89-94.
182. Tarlock K, Alonzo TA, Gerbing RB, et al. Gemtuzumab ozogamicin reduces relapse risk in FLT3/ITD acute myeloid leukemia: a report from the children's oncology group. *Clin Cancer Res.* 2016;22(8):1951-1957. doi:10.1158/1078-0432.ccr-15-1349
183. Schlenk RF, Kayser S, Bullinger L, et al. Differential impact of allelic ratio and insertion site in FLT3-ITD-positive AML with respect to allogeneic transplantation. *Blood.* 2014;124(23):3441-3449. doi:10.1182/blood-2014-05-578070
184. Chisholm KM, Heerema-McKenney AE, Choi JK, et al. Acute erythroid leukemia is enriched in NUP98 fusions: a report from the Children's Oncology Group. *Blood Adv.* 2020;4(23):6000-6008. doi:10.1182/bloodadvances.2020002712
185. Mohanty S, Jyotsana N, Sharma A, et al. Targeted inhibition of the NUP98-NSD1 fusion oncogene in acute myeloid leukemia. *Cancers (Basel).* 2020;12(10):2766. doi:10.3390/cancers12102766
186. Kivioja JL, Thanasopoulou A, Kumar A, et al. Dasatinib and navitoclax act synergistically to target NUP98-NSD1. *Leukemia.* 2019;33(6):1360-1372. doi:10.1038/s41375-018-0327-2
187. Bisio V, Zampini M, Tregnago C, et al. NUP98-fusion transcripts characterize different biological entities within acute myeloid leukemia: a report from the AIEOP-AML group. *Leukemia.* 2017;31(4):974-977. doi:10.1038/leu.2016.361
188. Struski S, Lagarde S, Bories P, et al. NUP98 is rearranged in 3.8% of pediatric AML forming a clinical and molecular homogenous group with a poor prognosis. *Leukemia.* 2017;31(3):565-572. doi:10.1038/leu.2016.267
189. Oliansky DM, Appelbaum F, Cassileth PA, et al. The role of cytotoxic therapy with hematopoietic stem cell transplantation in the therapy of acute myelogenous leukemia in adults: an evidence-based review. *Biol Blood Marrow Transplant.* 2008;14(2):137-180. doi:10.1016/j.bbmt.2007.11.002
190. Harrison CJ, Hills RK, Moorman AV, et al. Cytogenetics of childhood acute myeloid leukemia: United Kingdom Medical Research Council Treatment trials AML 10 and 12. *J Clin Oncol.* 2010;28(16):2674-2681. doi:10.1200/JCO.2009.24.8997
191. Ortega JJ, Madero L, Martin G, et al. Treatment with all-trans retinoic acid and anthracycline monochemotherapy for children with acute promyelocytic leukemia: a multicenter study by the PETHEMA Group. *J Clin Oncol.* 2005;23(30):7632-7640. doi:10.1200/JCO.2005.01.3359
192. Bally C, Fadlallah J, Leverger G, et al. Outcome of acute promyelocytic leukemia (APL) in children and adolescents: an analysis in two consecutive trials of the European APL Group. *J Clin Oncol.* 2012;30(14):1641-1646. doi:10.1200/JCO.2011.38.4560
193. Chen AR, Alonzo TA, Woods WG, Arceci RJ. Current controversies: which patients with acute myeloid leukaemia should receive a bone marrow transplantation? – an American view. *Br J Haematol.* 2002;118(2):378-384.
194. Burnett AK, Wheatley K, Goldstone AH, et al. The value of allogeneic bone marrow transplant in patients with acute myeloid leukaemia at differing risk of relapse: results of the UK MRC AML 10 trial. *Br J Haematol.* 2002;118(2):385-400.
195. Balgobind BV, Raimondi SC, Harbott J, et al. Novel prognostic subgroups in childhood 11q23/MLL-rearranged acute myeloid leukemia: results of an international retrospective study. *Blood.* 2009;114(12):2489-2496. doi:10.1182/blood-2009-04-215152
196. Groschel S, Schlenk RF, Engelmann J, et al. Deregulated expression of EVI1 defines a poor prognostic subset of MLL-rearranged acute myeloid leukemias: a study of the German-Austrian Acute Myeloid Leukemia Study Group and the Dutch-Belgian-Swiss HOVON/SAKK Cooperative Group. *J Clin Oncol.* 2013;31(1):95-103. doi:10.1200/jco.2011.41.5505
197. Brown P, McIntyre E, Rau R, et al. The incidence and clinical significance of nucleophosmin mutations in childhood AML. *Blood.* 2007;110(3):979-985.
198. Ho PA, Zeng R, Alonzo TA, et al. Prevalence and prognostic implications of WT1 mutations in pediatric acute myeloid leukemia (AML): a report from the Children's Oncology Group. *Blood.* 2010;116(5):702-710. doi:10.1182/blood-2010-02-268953
199. Klusmann JH, Reinhardt D, Zimmermann M, et al. The role of matched sibling donor allogeneic stem cell transplantation in pediatric high-risk acute myeloid leukemia: results from the AML-BFM 98 study. *Haematologica.* 2012;97(1):21-29. doi:10.3324/haematol.2011.051714
200. Niewerth D, Creutzig U, Bierings MB, Kaspers GJ. A review on allogeneic stem cell transplantation for newly diagnosed pediatric acute myeloid leukemia. *Blood.* 2010;116(13):2205-2214. doi:10.1182/blood-2010-01-261800
201. Beier R, Albert MH, Bader P, et al. Allo-SCT using BU, CY and melphalan for children with AML in second CR. *Bone Marrow Transplant.* 2012;48(5):651-656. doi:10.1038/bmt.2012.204
202. Milano F, Gooley T, Wood B, et al. Cord-blood transplantation in patients with minimal residual disease. *N Engl J Med.* 2016;375(10):944-953. doi:10.1056/NEJMoa1602074
203. Leahey A, Kelly K, Rorke LB, Lange B. A phase I/II study of idarubicin (Ida) with continuous infusion fludarabine (F-ara-A) and cytarabine (ara-C) for refractory or recurrent pediatric acute myeloid leukemia (AML). *J Pediatr Hematol Oncol.* 1997;19(4):304-308.
204. Martinelli G, Testoni N, Zuffa E, et al. FLANG (fludarabine + cytosine arabinoside + novantrone + G-CSF) induces partial remission in lymphoid blast transformation of Ph+ chronic myelogenous leukaemia. *Leuk Lymphoma.* 1996;22(1-2):173-176.
205. Thomas MB, Koller C, Yang Y, et al. Comparison of fludarabine-containing salvage chemotherapy regimens for relapsed/refractory acute myelogenous leukemia. *Leukemia.* 2003;17(5):990-993, doi:10.1038/sj.leu.2402862
206. Fleischhack G, Graf N, Hasan C, et al. IDA-FLAG (idarubicin, fludarabine, high dosage cytarabine and G-CSF)– an effective therapy regimen in treatment of recurrent acute myelocytic leukemia in children and adolescents. Initial results of a pilot study. *Klin Pädiatr.* 1996;208(4):229-235.
207. Miano M, Pistorio A, Putti MC, et al. Clofarabine, cyclophosphamide and etoposide for the treatment of relapsed or resistant acute leukemia in pediatric patients. *Leuk Lymphoma.* 2012;53(9):1693-1698. doi:10.3109/10428194.2012.663915
208. Quarello P, Berger M, Rivetti E, et al. FLAG-liposomal doxorubicin (Myocet) regimen for refractory or relapsed acute leukemia pediatric patients. *J Pediatr Hematol Oncol.* 2012;34(3):208-216. doi:10.1097/MPH.0b013e3182427593
209. Kaspers GJ, Zimmermann M, Reinhardt D, et al. Improved outcome in pediatric relapsed acute myeloid leukemia: results of a randomized trial on liposomal daunorubicin by the International BFM Study Group. *J Clin Oncol.* 2013;31(5):599-607. doi:10.1200/jco.2012.43.7384

210. Wells RJ, Adams MT, Alonzo TA, et al. Mitoxantrone and cytarabine induction, high-dose cytarabine, and etoposide intensification for pediatric patients with relapsed or refractory acute myeloid leukemia: Children's Cancer Group Study 2951. *J Clin Oncol.* 2003;21(15):2940-2947.
211. Arceci RJ, Sande J, Lange B, et al. Safety and efficacy of gemtuzumab ozogamicin in pediatric patients with advanced CD33+ acute myeloid leukemia. *Blood.* 2005;106(4):1183-1188.
212. Karagun BS, Akbas T, Erbey F, Sasmaz İ, Antmen B. The prophylaxis of hepatic veno-occlusive disease/sinusoidal obstruction syndrome with defibrotide after hematopoietic stem cell transplantation in children: single center experience. *J Pediatr Hematol Oncol.* 2022;44(1):e35-e39. doi:10.1097/MPH.0000000000002379
213. Corbacioglu S, Kernan NA, Pagliuca A, Ryan RJ, Tappe W, Richardson PG. Incidence of anicteric veno-occlusive disease/sinusoidal obstruction syndrome and outcomes with defibrotide following hematopoietic cell transplantation in adult and pediatric patients. *Biol Blood Marrow Transplant.* 2020;26(7):1342-1349. doi:10.1016/j.bbmt.2020.03.011
214. Webb DK, Wheatley K, Harrison G, Stevens RF, Hann IM. Outcome for children with relapsed acute myeloid leukaemia following initial therapy in the Medical Research Council (MRC) AML 10 trial. MRC Childhood Leukaemia Working Party. *Leukemia.* 1999;13(1):25-31.
215. Davies SM, Ruggieri L, DeFor T, et al. Evaluation of KIR ligand incompatibility in mismatched unrelated donor hematopoietic transplants. Killer immunoglobulin-like receptor. *Blood.* 2002;100(10):3825-3827.
216. Peters C, Matthes-Martin S, Fritsch G, et al. Transplantation of highly purified peripheral blood CD34+ cells from HLA-mismatched parental donors in 14 children: evaluation of early monitoring of engraftment. *Leukemia.* 1999;13(12):2070-2078.
217. Davies SM, Wagner JE, Defor T, et al. Unrelated donor bone marrow transplantation for children and adolescents with aplastic anaemia or myelodysplasia. *Br J Haematol.* 1997;96(4):749-756.
218. Estey EH. Treatment of relapsed and refractory acute myelogenous leukemia. *Leukemia.* 2000;14(3):476-479.
219. Tavernier E, Le QH, Elhamri M, Thomas X. Salvage therapy in refractory acute myeloid leukemia: prediction of outcome based on analysis of prognostic factors. *Leuk Res.* 2003;27(3):205-214.
220. Johannsen KH, Handrup MM, Lausen B, Schroder H, Hasle H. High frequency of streptococcal bacteraemia during childhood AML therapy irrespective of dose of cytarabine. *Pediatr Blood Cancer.* 2013;60(7):1154-1160. doi:10.1002/pbc.24448
221. Lewis V, Yanofsky R, Mitchell D, et al. Predictors and outcomes of viridans group streptococcal infections in pediatric acute myeloid leukemia: from the Canadian infections in AML research group. *Pediatr Infect Dis J.* 2014;33(2):126-129. doi:10.1097/inf.0000000000000058
222. Gamis AS, Howells WB, DeSwarte-Wallace J, Feusner JH, Buckley JD, Woods WG. Alpha hemolytic streptococcal infection during intensive treatment for acute myeloid leukemia: a report from the Children's Cancer Group Study CCG-2891. *J Clin Oncol.* 2000;18(9):1845-1855.
223. Maser B, Pelland-Marcotte MC, Alexander S, Sung L, Gupta S. Levofloxacin prophylaxis in hospitalized children with leukemia: a cost-utility analysis. *Pediatr Blood Cancer.* 10 2020;67(10):e28643. doi:10.1002/pbc.28643
224. Lehrnbecher T, Phillips R, Alexander S, et al. Guideline for the management of fever and neutropenia in children with cancer and/or undergoing hematopoietic stem-cell transplantation. *J Clin Oncol.* 2012;30(35):4427-4438. doi:10.1200/JCO.2012.42.7161
225. Dombret H, Sutton L, Duarte M, et al. Combined therapy with all-trans-retinoic acid and high-dose chemotherapy in patients with hyperleukocytic acute promyelocytic leukemia and severe visceral hemorrhage. *Leukemia.* 1992;6(12):1237-1242.
226. Estey E, Thall P, Andreeff M, et al. Use of granulocyte colony-stimulating factor before, during, and after fludarabine plus cytarabine induction therapy of newly diagnosed acute myelogenous leukemia or myelodysplastic syndromes: comparison with fludarabine plus cytarabine without granulocyte colony-stimulating factor. *J Clin Oncol.* 1994;12(4):671-678.
227. Heil G, Hoelzer D, Sanz MA, et al. A randomized, double-blind, placebo-controlled, phase III study of filgrastim in remission induction and consolidation therapy for adults with de novo acute myeloid leukemia. The International Acute Myeloid Leukemia Study Group. *Blood.* 1997;90(12):4710-4718.
228. Alonzo TA, Kobrinsky NL, Aledo A, Lange BJ, Buxton AB, Woods WG. Impact of granulocyte colony-stimulating factor use during induction for acute myelogenous leukemia in children: a report from the Children's Cancer Group. *J Pediatr Hematol Oncol.* 2002;24(8):627-635.
229. Sherertz RJ, Belani A, Kramer BS, et al. Impact of air filtration on nosocomial Aspergillus infections. Unique risk of bone marrow transplant recipients. *Am J Med.* 1987;83(4):709-718.
230. Rebulla P, Finazzi G, Marangoni F, et al. The threshold for prophylactic platelet transfusions in adults with acute myeloid leukemia. Gruppo Italiano Malattie Ematologiche Maligne dell'Adulto. *N Engl J Med.* 1997;337(26):1870-1875. doi:10.1056/NEJM199712253372602
231. Hebert PC. Anemia and red cell transfusion in critical care. Transfusion requirements in critical care investigators and the Canadian critical care trials group. *Minerva Anestesiol.* 1999;65(5):293-304.
232. Inaba H, Gaur AH, Cao X, et al. Feasibility, efficacy, and adverse effects of outpatient antibacterial prophylaxis in children with acute myeloid leukemia. *Cancer.* 2014;120(13):1985-1992. doi:10.1002/cncr.28688
233. Abril MK, Barnett AS, Wegermann K, et al. Diagnosis of *Capnocytophaga canimorsus* sepsis by whole-genome next-generation sequencing. *Open Forum Infect Dis.* 2016;3(3):ofw144. doi:10.1093/ofid/ofw144
234. Liesner RJ, Leiper AD, Hann IM, Chessells JM. Late effects of intensive treatment for acute myeloid leukemia and myelodysplasia in childhood. *J Clin Oncol.* 1994;12(5):916-924.
235. Leahey AM, Teunissen H, Friedman DL, Moshang T, Lange BJ, Meadows AT. Late effects of chemotherapy compared to bone marrow transplantation in the treatment of pediatric acute myeloid leukemia and myelodysplasia. *Med Pediatr Oncol.* 1999;32(3):163-169.
236. Leung W, Hudson MM, Strickland DK, et al. Late effects of treatment in survivors of childhood acute myeloid leukemia. *J Clin Oncol.* 2000;18(18):3273-3279.
237. Perkins JL, Kunin-Batson AS, Youngren NM, et al. Long-term follow-up of children who underwent hematopoietic cell transplant (HCT) for AML or ALL at less than 3 years of age. *Pediatr Blood Cancer.* 2007;49(7):958-963. doi:10.1002/pbc.21207
238. Temming P, Qureshi A, Hardt J, et al. Prevalence and predictors of anthracycline cardiotoxicity in children treated for acute myeloid leukaemia: retrospective cohort study in a single centre in the United Kingdom. *Pediatr Blood Cancer.* 2011;56(4):625-630. doi:10.1002/pbc.22908
239. Leone G, Fianchi L, Voso MT. Therapy-related myeloid neoplasms. *Curr Opin Oncol.* 2011;23(6):672-680. doi:10.1097/CCO.0b013e32834bcc2a
240. Molgaard-Hansen L, Glosli H, Jahnukainen K, et al. Quality of health in survivors of childhood acute myeloid leukemia treated with chemotherapy only: a NOPHO-AML study. Research Support, Non-U.S. Gov't. *Pediatr Blood Cancer.* 2011;57(7):1222-1229. doi:10.1002/pbc.22931
241. Mulrooney DA, Dover DC, Li S, et al. Twenty years of follow-up among survivors of childhood and young adult acute myeloid leukemia: a report from the Childhood Cancer Survivor Study. *Cancer.* 2008;112(9):2071-2079. doi:10.1002/cncr.23405
242. Castellanos MI, Dongarwar D, Wanser R, et al. In-hospital mortality and racial disparity in children and adolescents with acute myeloid leukemia: a population-based study. *J Pediatr Hematol Oncol.* 2022;44(1):e114-e122. doi:10.1097/MPH.0000000000002204
243. Winestone LE, Getz KD, Rao P, et al. Disparities in pediatric acute myeloid leukemia (AML) clinical trial enrollment. *Leuk Lymphoma.* 2019;60(9):2190-2198. doi:10.1080/10428194.2019.1574002
244. Gamis AS. Acute myeloid leukemia and Down syndrome evolution of modern therapy—state of the art review. *Pediatr Blood Cancer.* 2005;44(1):13-20.
245. Li Z, Godinho FJ, Klusmann JH, Garriga-Canut M, Yu C, Orkin SH. Developmental stage-selective effect of somatically mutated leukemogenic transcription factor GATA1. *Nat Genet.* 2005;37(6):613-619. doi:10.1038/ng1566
246. Klusmann JH, Creutzig U, Zimmermann M, et al. Treatment and prognostic impact of transient leukemia in neonates with Down syndrome. *Blood.* 2008;111(6):2991-2998. doi:10.1182/blood-2007-10-118810
247. Ravindranath Y, Abella E, Krischer JP, et al. Acute myeloid leukemia (AML) in Down's syndrome is highly responsive to chemotherapy: experience on Pediatric Oncology Group AML Study 8498. *Blood.* 1992;80(9):2210-2214.
248. Creutzig U, Ritter J, Vormoor J, et al. Myelodysplasia and acute myelogenous leukemia in Down's syndrome. A report of 40 children of the AML-BFM Study Group. *Leukemia.* 1996;10(11):1677-1686.
249. Gamis AS, Woods WG, Alonzo TA, et al. Increased age at diagnosis has a significantly negative effect on outcome in children with Down syndrome and acute myeloid leukemia: a report from the Children's Cancer Group Study 2891. *J Clin Oncol.* 2003;21(18):3415-3422.
250. Gamis AS, Alonzo TA, Gerbing RB, et al. Natural history of transient myeloproliferative disorder clinically diagnosed in Down syndrome neonates: a report from the Children's Oncology Group Study A2971. *Blood.* 2011;118(26):6752-6759, quiz 6996. doi:10.1182/blood-2011-04-350017
251. O'Brien MM, Taub JW, Chang MN, et al. Cardiomyopathy in children with Down syndrome treated for acute myeloid leukemia: a report from the Children's Oncology Group Study POG 9421. *J Clin Oncol.* 2008;26(3):414-420. doi:10.1200/JCO.2007.13.2209
252. Hassler A, Bochennek K, Gilfert J, et al. Infectious complications in children with acute myeloid leukemia and down syndrome: analysis of the prospective multicenter trial AML-BFM 2004. *Pediatr Blood Cancer.* 2016;63(6):1070-1074. doi:10.1002/pbc.25917
253. Taub JW, Berman JN, Hitzler JK, et al. Improved outcomes for myeloid leukemia of Down syndrome: a report from the Children's Oncology Group AAML0431 trial. *Blood.* 2017;129(25):3304-3313. doi:10.1182/blood-2017-01-764324
254. Davies SM, Khan S, Wagner JE, et al. Unrelated donor bone marrow transplantation for Fanconi anemia. *Bone Marrow Transplant.* 1996;17(1):43-47.
255. Gluckman E, Wagner JE. Hematopoietic stem cell transplantation in childhood inherited bone marrow failure syndrome. *Bone Marrow Transplant.* 2008;41(2):127-132. doi:10.1038/sj.bmt.1705960
256. Ruggeri A, de Latour RP, Rocha V, et al. Double cord blood transplantation in patients with high risk bone marrow failure syndromes. *Br J Haematol.* 2008;143(3):404-408. doi:10.1111/j.1365-2141.2008.07364.x
257. Zanis-Neto J, Ribeiro RC, Medeiros C, et al. Bone marrow transplantation for patients with Fanconi anemia: a study of 24 cases from a single institution. *Bone Marrow Transplant.* 1995;15(2):293-298.
258. Stelljes M, Corbacioglu A, Schlenk RF, et al. Allogeneic stem cell transplant to eliminate germline mutations in the gene for CCAAT-enhancer-binding protein alpha from hematopoietic cells in a family with AML. *Leukemia.* 2011;25(7):1209-1210. doi:10.1038/leu.2011.64
259. Fukano R, Nagatoshi Y, Shinkoda Y, et al. Unrelated bone marrow transplantation using a reduced-intensity conditioning regimen for the treatment of Kostmann syndrome. *Bone Marrow Transplant.* 2006;38(9):635-636. doi:10.1038/sj.bmt.1705492
260. Ishii E, Oda M, Kinugawa N, et al. Features and outcome of neonatal leukemia in Japan: experience of the Japan infant leukemia study group. *Pediatr Blood Cancer.* 2006;47(3):268-272.

261. Bresters D, Reus AC, Veerman AJ, van Wering ER, van der Does-van den Berg A, Kaspers GJ. Congenital leukaemia: the Dutch experience and review of the literature. *Br J Haematol.* 2002;117(3):513-524.
262. Creutzig U, Zimmermann M, Bourquin JP, et al. Favorable outcome in infants with AML after intensive first- and second-line treatment: an AML-BFM study group report. *Leukemia.* 2012;26(4):654-661. doi:10.1038/leu.2011.267
263. Bolouri H, Ries R, Pardo L, et al. A B-cell developmental gene regulatory network is activated in infant AML. *PLoS One.* 2021;16(11):e0259197. doi:10.1371/journal.pone.0259197
264. Grundy RG, Martinez A, Kempski H, Malone M, Atherton D. Spontaneous remission of congenital leukemia: a case for conservative treatment. *J Pediatr Hematol Oncol.* 2000;22(3):252-255.
265. Hutson JR, Weitzman S, Schechter T, Arceci RJ, Kim RB, Finkelstein Y. Pharmacokinetic and pharmacogenetic determinants and considerations in chemotherapy selection and dosing in infants. *Expet Opin Drug Metab Toxicol.* 2012;8(6):709-722. doi:10.1517/17425255.2012.680884
266. Periclou AP, Avramis VI. NONMEM population pharmacokinetic studies of cytosine arabinoside after high-dose and after loading bolus followed by continuous infusion of the drug in pediatric patients with leukemias. *Cancer Chemother Pharmacol.* 1996;39(1-2):42-50.
267. Huang ME, Ye YC, Chen SR, et al. All-trans retinoic acid with or without low dose cytosine arabinoside in acute promyelocytic leukemia. Report of 6 cases. *Chin Med J.* 1987;100(12):949-953.
268. Huang ME, Ye YC, Chen SR, et al. Use of all-trans retinoic acid in the treatment of acute promyelocytic leukemia. *Blood.* 1988;72(2):567-572.
269. Avvisati G, Lo-Coco F, Paoloni FP, et al. AIDA 0493 protocol for newly diagnosed acute promyelocytic leukemia: very long-term results and role of maintenance. *Blood.* 2011;117(18):4716-4725. doi:10.1182/blood-2010-08-302950
270. Sanz MA, Montesinos P, Rayon C, et al. Risk-adapted treatment of acute promyelocytic leukemia based on all-trans retinoic acid and anthracycline with addition of cytarabine in consolidation therapy for high-risk patients: further improvements in treatment outcome. *Blood.* 2010;115(25):5137-5146. doi:10.1182/blood-2010-01-266007
271. Tallman M, Douer D, Gore S, et al. Treatment of patients with acute promyelocytic leukemia: a consensus statement on risk-adapted approaches to therapy. Consensus Development Conference. *Clin Lymphoma Myeloma Leuk.* 2010;10(suppl 3):S122-S126. doi:10.3816/CLML.2010.s.023
272. Li EQ, Xu L, Zhang ZQ, et al. Retrospective analysis of 119 cases of pediatric acute promyelocytic leukemia: comparisons of four treatment regimes. *Exp Ther Med.* July 2012;4(1):93-98. doi:10.3892/etm.2012.546
273. Yanada M, Matsushita T, Asou N, et al. Severe hemorrhagic complications during remission induction therapy for acute promyelocytic leukemia: incidence, risk factors, and influence on outcome. *Eur J Haematol.* 2007;78(3):213-219. doi:10.1111/j.1600-0609.2006.00803.x
274. Tallman MS, Abutalib SA, Altman JK. The double hazard of thrombophilia and bleeding in acute promyelocytic leukemia. *Semin Thromb Hemost.* 2007;33(4):330-338. doi:10.1055/s-2007-976168
275. Kutny MA, Moser BK, Laumann K, et al. FLT3 mutation status is a predictor of early death in pediatric acute promyelocytic leukemia: a report from the Children's Oncology Group. *Pediatr Blood Cancer.* 2012;59(4):662-667. doi:10.1002/pbc.24122
276. Schnittger S, Bacher U, Haferlach C, Kern W, Alpermann T, Haferlach T. Clinical impact of FLT3 mutation load in acute promyelocytic leukemia with t(15;17)/PML-RARA. *Haematologica.* 2011;96(12):1799-1807. doi:10.3324/haematol.2011.049007
277. Mann G, Reinhardt D, Ritter J, et al. Treatment with all-trans retinoic acid in acute promyelocytic leukemia reduces early deaths in children. *Ann Hematol.* 2001;80(7):417-422.
278. Testi AM, Biondi A, Lo Coco F, et al. GIMEMA-AIEOPAIDA protocol for the treatment of newly diagnosed acute promyelocytic leukemia (APL) in children. *Blood.* 2005;106(2):447-453. doi:10.1182/blood-2004-05-1971
279. Wiley JS, Firkin FC. Reduction of pulmonary toxicity by prednisolone prophylaxis during all-trans retinoic acid treatment of acute promyelocytic leukemia. Australian Leukaemia Study Group. *Leukemia.* 1995;9(5):774-778.
280. Castaigne S, Lefebvre P, Chomienne C, et al. Effectiveness and pharmacokinetics of low-dose all-trans retinoic acid (25 mg/m^2) in acute promyelocytic leukemia. *Blood.* 1993;82(12):3560-3563.
281. Soignet SL, Maslak P, Wang ZG, et al. Complete remission after treatment of acute promyelocytic leukemia with arsenic trioxide. *N Engl J Med.* 1998;339(19):1341-1348.
282. Zhou J, Zhang Y, Li J, et al. Single-agent arsenic trioxide in the treatment of children with newly diagnosed acute promyelocytic leukemia. *Blood.* 2010;115(9):1697-1702. doi:10.1182/blood-2009-07-230805
283. Gore SD, Gojo I, Sekeres MA, et al. Single cycle of arsenic trioxide-based consolidation chemotherapy spares anthracycline exposure in the primary management of acute promyelocytic leukemia. *J Clin Oncol.* 2010;28(6):1047-1053. doi:10.1200/JCO.2009.25.5158
284. Asou N, Kishimoto Y, Kiyoi H, et al. A randomized study with or without intensified maintenance chemotherapy in patients with acute promyelocytic leukemia who have become negative for PML-RARalpha transcript after consolidation therapy: the Japan Adult Leukemia Study Group (JALSG) APL97 study. *Blood.* 2007;110(1):59-66. doi:10.1182/blood-2006-08-043992
285. Ravandi F, Estey E, Jones D, et al. Effective treatment of acute promyelocytic leukemia with all-trans-retinoic acid, arsenic trioxide, and gemtuzumab ozogamicin. *J Clin Oncol.* 2009;27(4):504-510. doi:10.1200/JCO.2008.18.6130
286. Estey EH, Giles FJ, Beran M, et al. Experience with gemtuzumab ozogamycin ("mylotarg") and all-trans retinoic acid in untreated acute promyelocytic leukemia. *Blood.* 2002;99(11):4222-4224.
287. Lo-Coco F, Avvisati G, Vignetti M, et al. Retinoic acid and arsenic trioxide for acute promyelocytic leukemia. *N Engl J Med.* 2013;369(2):111-121. doi:10.1056/NEJMoa1300874
288. Burnett AK, Russell NH, Hills RK, et al. Arsenic trioxide and all-trans retinoic acid treatment for acute promyelocytic leukaemia in all risk groups (AML17): results of a randomised, controlled, phase 3 trial. *Lancet Oncol.* 2015;16(13):1295-1305. doi:10.1016/s1470-2045(15)00193-x
289. Ravandi F Prophylactic intrathecal chemotherapy in acute promyelocytic leukemia (APL). *Leukemia.* 2004;18(4):879-880. doi:10.1038/sj.leu.2403306.
290. de Botton S, Sanz MA, Chevret S, et al. Extramedullary relapse in acute promyelocytic leukemia treated with all-trans retinoic acid and chemotherapy. *Leukemia.* 2006;20(1):35-41.
291. Lo-Coco F, Ammatuna E. Front line clinical trials and minimal residual disease monitoring in acute promyelocytic leukemia. *Curr Top Microbiol Immunol.* 2007;313:145-156.
292. Grimwade D, Jovanovic JV, Hills RK, et al. Prospective minimal residual disease monitoring to predict relapse of acute promyelocytic leukemia and to direct pre-emptive arsenic trioxide therapy. *J Clin Oncol.* 2009;27(22):3650-3658. doi:10.1200/JCO.2008.20.1533
293. Douer D, Hu W, Giralt S, Lill M, DiPersio J. Arsenic trioxide (trisenox) therapy for acute promyelocytic leukemia in the setting of hematopoietic stem cell transplantation. *Oncol.* 2003;8(2):132-140.
294. de Botton S, Fawaz A, Chevret S, et al. Autologous and allogeneic stem-cell transplantation as salvage treatment of acute promyelocytic leukemia initially treated with all-trans-retinoic acid: a retrospective analysis of the European acute promyelocytic leukemia group. *J Clin Oncol.* 2005;23(1):120-126.
295. Meloni G, Diverio D, Vignetti M, et al. Autologous bone marrow transplantation for acute promyelocytic leukemia in second remission: prognostic relevance of pretransplant minimal residual disease assessment by reverse-transcription polymerase chain reaction of the PML/RAR alpha fusion gene. *Blood.* 1997;90(3):1321-1325.
296. Ramadan SM, Di Veroli A, Camboni A, et al. Allogeneic stem cell transplantation for advanced acute promyelocytic leukemia in the ATRA and ATO era. *Haematologica.* 2012;97(11):1731-1735. doi:10.3324/haematol.2012.065714
297. Thirugnanam R, George B, Chendamarai E, et al. Comparison of clinical outcomes of patients with relapsed acute promyelocytic leukemia induced with arsenic trioxide and consolidated with either an autologous stem cell transplant or an arsenic trioxide-based regimen. *Biol Blood Marrow Transplant.* 2009;15(11):1479-1484. doi:10.1016/j.bbmt.2009.07.010
298. Choudhry A, DeLoughery TG. Bleeding and thrombosis in acute promyelocytic leukemia. *Am J Hematol.* 2012;87(6):596-603. doi:10.1002/ajh.23158
299. Breen KA, Grimwade D, Hunt BJ. The pathogenesis and management of the coagulopathy of acute promyelocytic leukaemia. *Br J Haematol.* 2012;156(1):24-36. doi:10.1111/j.1365-2141.2011.08922.x
300. Reinhardt D, Creutzig U. Isolated myelosarcoma in children – update and review. *Leuk Lymphoma.* 2002;43(3):565-574.
301. Landis DM, Aboulafia DM. Granulocytic sarcoma: an unusual complication of aleukemic myeloid leukemia causing spinal cord compression. A case report and literature review. *Leuk Lymphoma.* 2003;44(10):1753-1760.
302. Dusenbery KE, Howells WB, Arthur DC, et al. Extramedullary leukemia in children with newly diagnosed acute myeloid leukemia: a report from the Children's Cancer Group. *J Pediatr Hematol Oncol.* 2003;25(10):760-768.
303. Kobayashi R, Tawa A, Hanada R, Horibe K, Tsuchida M, Tsukimoto I. Extramedullary infiltration at diagnosis and prognosis in children with acute myelogenous leukemia. *Pediatr Blood Cancer.* 2007;48(4):393-398. doi:10.1002/pbc.20824
304. Smith FO, Lampkin BC, Versteeg C, et al. Expression of lymphoid-associated cell surface antigens by childhood acute myeloid leukemia cells lacks prognostic significance. *Blood.* 1992;79(9):2415-2422.
305. Alexander TB, Gu Z, Iacobucci I, et al. The genetic basis and cell of origin of mixed phenotype acute leukaemia. *Nature.* 10 2018;562(7727):373-379. doi:10.1038/s41586-018-0436-0
306. Al-Seraihy AS, Owaidah TM, Ayas M, et al. Clinical characteristics and outcome of children with biphenotypic acute leukemia. *Haematologica.* 2009;94(12):1682-1690. doi:10.3324/haematol.2009.009282
307. Mejstrikova E, Volejnikova J, Fronkova E, et al. Prognosis of children with mixed phenotype acute leukemia treated on the basis of consistent immunophenotypic criteria. *Haematologica.* 2010;95(6):928-935. doi:10.3324/haematol.2009.014506
308. Gerr H, Zimmermann M, Schrappe M, et al. Acute leukaemias of ambiguous lineage in children: characterization, prognosis and therapy recommendations. *Br J Haematol.* 2010;149(1):84-92. doi:10.1111/j.1365-2141.2009.08058.x
309. Rubnitz JE, Onciu M, Pounds S, et al. Acute mixed lineage leukemia in children: the experience of St Jude Children's Research Hospital. *Blood.* 2009;113(21):5083-5089. doi:10.1182/blood-2008-10-187351
310. Orgel E, Alexander TB, Wood BL, et al. Mixed-phenotype acute leukemia: a cohort and consensus research strategy from the Children's Oncology Group Acute Leukemia of Ambiguous Lineage Task Force. *Cancer.* 2020;126(3):593-601. doi:10.1002/cncr.32552
311. Alexander TB, Orgel E. Mixed phenotype Acute leukemia: current approaches to diagnosis and treatment. *Curr Oncol Rep.* 2021;23(2):22. doi:10.1007/s11912-020-01010-w
312. Barnard DR, Woods WG. Treatment-related myelodysplastic syndrome/acute myeloid leukemia in survivors of childhood cancer—an update. *Leuk Lymphoma.* 2005;46(5):651-663.
313. Larson RA. Etiology and management of therapy-related myeloid leukemia. *Hematology Am Soc Hematol Educ Program.* 2007;2007:453-459. doi:10.1182/asheducation-2007.1.453

314. Bolufer P, Collado M, Barragan E, et al. Profile of polymorphisms of drug-metabolising enzymes and the risk of therapy-related leukaemia. Br J Haematol. 2007;136(4):590-596. doi:10.1111/j.1365-2141.2006.06469.x
315. Ezoe S. Secondary leukemia associated with the anti-cancer agent, etoposide, a topoisomerase II inhibitor. Int J Environ Res Publ Health. 2012;9(7):2444-2453. doi:10.3390/ijerph9072444
316. Ding Y, Sun CL, Li L, et al. Genetic susceptibility to therapy-related leukemia after Hodgkin lymphoma or non-Hodgkin lymphoma: role of drug metabolism, apoptosis and DNA repair. Blood Cancer J. 2012;2(3):e58. doi:10.1038/bcj.2012.4
317. Schmiegelow K. Epidemiology of therapy-related myeloid neoplasms after treatment for pediatric acute lymphoblastic leukemia in the nordic countries. Mediterr J Hematol Infect Dis. 2011;3(1):e2011020. doi:10.4084/MJHID.2011.020
318. Aguilera DG, Vaklavas C, Tsimberidou AM, Wen S, Medeiros LJ, Corey SJ. Pediatric therapy-related myelodysplastic syndrome/acute myeloid leukemia: the MD Anderson Cancer Center experience. J Pediatr Hematol Oncol. 2009;31(11):803-811. doi:10.1097/MPH.0b013e3181ba43dc
319. Yokoyama H, Mori S, Kobayashi Y, et al. Hematopoietic stem cell transplantation for therapy-related myelodysplastic syndrome and acute leukemia: a single-center analysis of 47 patients. Int J Hematol. 2010;92(2):334-341. doi:10.1007/s12185-010-0640-7.
320. Elsayed AH, Rafiee R, Cao X, et al. A six-gene leukemic stem cell score identifies high risk pediatric acute myeloid leukemia. Leukemia. 03 2020;34(3):735-745. doi:10.1038/s41375-019-0604-8
321. Gbadamosi MO, Shastri VM, Elsayed AH, et al. A ten-gene DNA-damage response pathway gene expression signature predicts gemtuzumab ozogamicin response in pediatric AML patients treated on COGAAML0531 and AAML03P1 trials. Leukemia. 2022;36(8):2022-2031. doi:10.1038/s41375-022-01622-0
322. Elsayed AH, Cao X, Mitra AK, et al. Polygenic ara-C response score identifies pediatric patients with acute myeloid leukemia in need of chemotherapy augmentation. J Clin Oncol. 2022;40(7):772-783. doi:10.1200/JCO.21.01422
323. Fornerod M, Ma J, Noort S, et al. Integrative genomic analysis of pediatric myeloid-related acute leukemias identifies novel subtypes and prognostic indicators. Blood Cancer Discov. 2021;2(6):586-599. doi:10.1158/2643-3230.BCD-21-0049
324. Nguyen NHK, Wu H, Tan H, et al. Global proteomic profiling of pediatric AML: a pilot study. Cancers (Basel). 2021;13(13):3161. doi:10.3390/cancers13133161
325. Wheatley K, Burnett AK, Goldstone AH, et al. A simple, robust, validated and highly predictive index for the determination of risk-directed therapy in acute myeloid leukaemia derived from the MRC AML 10 trial. United Kingdom Medical Research Council's Adult and Childhood Leukaemia Working Parties. Br J Haematol. 1999;107(1):69-79.
326. Creutzig U, Buchner T, Sauerland MC, et al. Significance of age in acute myeloid leukemia patients younger than 30 years: a common analysis of the pediatric trials AML-BFM 93/98 and the adult trials AMLCG 92/99 and AMLSG HD93/98A. Cancer. 2008;112(3):562-571.
327. Rubnitz JE, Pounds S, Cao X, et al. Treatment outcome in older patients with childhood acute myeloid leukemia. Cancer. 2012;118(24):6253-6259. doi:10.1002/cncr.27659
328. Quintana J, Advis P, Becker A, et al. Acute myelogenous leukemia in Chile PINDA protocols 87 and 92 results. Leukemia. 2005;19(12):2143-2146. doi:10.1038/sj.leu.2403959
329. Armendariz H, Barbieri MA, Freigeiro D, Lastiri F, Felice MS, Dibar E. Treatment strategy and long-term results in pediatric patients treated in two consecutive AML-GATLA trials. Leukemia. 2005;19(12):2139-2142. doi:10.1038/sj.leu.2403854
330. Burnett AK, Hills RK, Green C, et al. The impact on outcome of the addition of all-trans retinoic acid to intensive chemotherapy in younger patients with nonacute promyelocytic acute myeloid leukemia: overall results and results in genotypic subgroups defined by mutations in NPM1, FLT3, and CEBPA. Blood. 2010;115(5):948-956. doi:10.1182/blood-2009-08-236588
331. Tsukimoto I, Tawa A, Horibe K, et al. Risk-stratified therapy and the intensive use of cytarabine improves the outcome in childhood acute myeloid leukemia: the AML99 trial from the Japanese Childhood AML Cooperative Study Group. J Clin Oncol. 2009;27(24):4007-4013. doi:10.1200/JCO.2008.18.7948
332. Creutzig U, Reinhardt D, Zimmermann M. Prognostic relevance of risk groups in the pediatric AML-BFM trials 93 and 98. Ann Hematol. 2004;83(suppl 1):S112-S116. doi:10.1007/s00277-004-0850-2
333. Creutzig U, Zimmermann M, Dworzak M, et al. Study AML-BFM 2004: improved survival in childhood acute myeloid leukemia without increased toxicity. ASH Annual Meeting Abstracts. 2010;116:181.
334. Lohmann DJ, Abrahamsson J, Ha SY, et al. Effect of age and body weight on toxicity and survival in pediatric acute myeloid leukemia: results from NOPHO-AML 2004. Haematologica. 2016;101(11):1359-1367. doi:10.3324/haematol.2016.146175
335. Lange BJ, Gerbing RB, Feusner J, et al. Mortality in overweight and underweight children with acute myeloid leukemia. J Am Med Assoc. January 12, 2005;293(2):203-211.
336. Canner J, Alonzo TA, Franklin J, et al. Differences in outcomes of newly diagnosed acute myeloid leukemia for adolescent/young adult and younger patients: a report from the Children's Oncology Group. Cancer. 2013;119(23):4162-4169. doi:10.1002/cncr.28250
337. Aplenc R, Alonzo TA, Gerbing RB, et al. Ethnicity and survival in childhood acute myeloid leukemia: a report from the Children's Oncology Group. Blood. 2006;108(1):74-80.
338. Rubnitz JE, Lensing S, Razzouk BI, Pounds S, Pui CH, Ribeiro RC. Effect of race on outcome of white and black children with acute myeloid leukemia: the St. Jude experience. Pediatr Blood Cancer. 2007;48(1):10-15. doi:10.1002/pbc.20878
339. Brady AK, Fu AZ, Earl M, et al. Race and intensity of post-remission therapy in acute myeloid leukemia. Leuk Res. 2011;35(3):346-350. doi:10.1016/j.leukres.2010.07.020
340. Davies SM, Robison LL, Buckley JD, Radloff GA, Ross JA, Perentesis JP. Glutathione S-transferase polymorphisms in children with myeloid leukemia: a Children's Cancer Group study. Cancer Epidemiol Biomarkers Prev. 2000;9(6):563-566.
341. Creutzig U, Reinhardt D, Diekamp S, Dworzak M, Stary J, Zimmermann M. AML patients with Down syndrome have a high cure rate with AML-BFM therapy with reduced dose intensity. Leukemia. 2005;19(8):1355-1360. doi:10.1038/sj.leu.2403814
342. Creutzig U, Zimmermann M, Ritter J, et al. Definition of a standard-risk group in children with AML. Br J Haematol. 1999;104(3):630-639.
343. Abbott BL, Rubnitz JE, Tong X, et al. Clinical significance of central nervous system involvement at diagnosis of pediatric acute myeloid leukemia: a single institution's experience. Leukemia. 2003;17(11):2090-2096. doi:10.1038/sj.leu.2403131
344. Johnston DL, Alonzo TA, Gerbing RB, Lange BJ, Woods WG. The presence of central nervous system disease at diagnosis in pediatric acute myeloid leukemia does not affect survival: a Children's Oncology Group study. Research Support, N.I.H., Extramural. Pediatr Blood Cancer. 2010;55(3):414-420.
345. Swerdlow SH, Campo E, Harris NL, et al. WHO Classification of Tumors of Haematopoetic and Lymphoid Tissues. International Agency for Research on Cancer; 2008.
346. Creutzig U, Zimmermann M, Bourquin JP, et al. Second induction with high-dose cytarabine and mitoxantrone: different impact on pediatric AML patients with t(8;21) and with inv(16). Blood. 2011;118(20):5409-5415. doi:10.1182/blood-2011-07-364661
347. von Neuhoff C, Reinhardt D, Sander A, et al. Prognostic impact of specific chromosomal aberrations in a large group of pediatric patients with acute myeloid leukemia treated uniformly according to trial AML-BFM 98. J Clin Oncol. 2010;28(16):2682-2689. doi:10.1200/JCO.2009.25.6321
348. Brown LM, Daeschner CD, Timms J, Crow W. Granulocytic sarcoma in childhood acute myelogenous leukemia. Pediatr Neurol. 1989;5(3):173-178.
349. Hurwitz CA, Raimondi SC, Head D, et al. Distinctive immunophenotypic features of t(8;21)(q22;q22) acute myeloblastic leukemia in children. Blood. 1992;80(12):3182-3188.
350. Licht JD, Chomienne C, Goy A, et al. Clinical and molecular characterization of a rare syndrome of acute promyelocytic leukemia associated with translocation (11;17). Blood. 1995;85(4):1083-1094.
351. Balgobind BV, Zwaan CM, Pieters R, Van den Heuvel-Eibrink MM. The heterogeneity of pediatric MLL-rearranged acute myeloid leukemia. Leukemia. 2011;25(8):1239-1248. doi:10.1038/leu.2011.90
352. Rubnitz JE, Raimondi SC, Tong X, et al. Favorable impact of the t(9;11) in childhood acute myeloid leukemia. J Clin Oncol. 2002;20(9):2302-2309.
353. Hasle H, Alonzo TA, Auvrignon A, et al. Monosomy 7 and deletion 7q in children and adolescents with acute myeloid leukemia: an international retrospective study. Blood. 2007;109(11):4641-4647.
354. Grimwade D, Hills RK, Moorman AV, et al. Refinement of cytogenetic classification in acute myeloid leukemia: determination of prognostic significance of rare recurring chromosomal abnormalities among 5876 younger adult patients treated in the United Kingdom Medical Research Council trials. Blood. 2010;116(5):354-365. doi:10.1182/blood-2009-11-254441
355. Tarlock K, Alonzo TA, Moraleda PP, et al. Acute myeloid leukaemia (AML) with t(6;9)(p23;q34) is associated with poor outcome in childhood AML regardless of FLT3-ITD status: a report from the Children's Oncology Group. Br J Haematol. 2014;166(2):254-259. doi:10.1111/bjh.12852
356. Levy ER, Parganas E, Morishita K, et al. DNA rearrangements proximal to the EVI1 locus associated with the 3q21q26 syndrome. Blood. 1994;83(5):1348-1354.
357. Lugthart S, Groschel S, Beverloo HB, et al. Clinical, molecular, and prognostic significance of WHO type inv(3)(q21q26.2)/t(3;3)(q21;q26.2) and various other 3q abnormalities in acute myeloid leukemia. J Clin Oncol. 2010;28(24):3890-3898. doi:10.1200/JCO.2010.29.2771
358. Balgobind BV, Lugthart S, Hollink IH, et al. EVI1 overexpression in distinct subtypes of pediatric acute myeloid leukemia. Leukemia. 2010;24(5):942-949. doi:10.1038/leu.2010.47
359. Shackelford D, Kenific C, Blusztajn A, Waxman S, Ren R. Targeted degradation of the AML1/MDS1/EVI1 oncoprotein by arsenic trioxide. Cancer Res. 2006;66(23):11360-11369. doi:10.1158/0008-5472.CAN-06-1774
360. Kelly MJ, Horan JT, Alonzo TA, et al. Comparable survival for pediatric acute myeloid leukemia with poor-risk cytogenetics following chemotherapy, matched related donor, or unrelated donor transplantation. Pediatr Blood Cancer. 2014;61(2):269-275. doi:10.1002/pbc.24739
361. de Rooij JD, Masetti R, van den Heuvel-Eibrink MM, et al. Recurrent abnormalities can be used for risk group stratification in pediatric AMKL: a retrospective intergroup study. Blood. 2016;127(26):3424-3430. doi:10.1182/blood-2016-01-695551
362. Gruber TA, Larson Gedman A, Zhang J, et al. An Inv(16)(p13.3q24.3)-encoded CBFA2T3-GLIS2 fusion protein defines an aggressive subtype of pediatric acute megakaryoblastic leukemia. Cancer Cell. 2012;22(5):683-697. doi:10.1016/j.ccr.2012.10.007
363. Carroll A, Civin C, Schneider N, et al. The t(1;22) (p13;q13) is nonrandom and restricted to infants with acute megakaryoblastic leukemia: a Pediatric Oncology Group Study. Blood. 1991;78(3):748-752.
364. Mercher T, Busson-Le Coniat M, Nguyen Khac F, et al. Recurrence of OTT-MAL fusion in t(1;22) of infant AML-M7. Genes Chromosomes Cancer. 2002;33(1):22-28.

365. Hollink IH, van den Heuvel-Eibrink MM, Arentsen-Peters ST, et al. NUP98/NSD1 characterizes a novel poor prognostic group in acute myeloid leukemia with a distinct HOX gene expression pattern. *Blood*. 2011;118(13):3645-3656. doi:10.1182/blood-2011-04-346643
366. Wang GG, Cai L, Pasillas MP, Kamps MP. NUP98-NSD1 links H3K36 methylation to Hox-A gene activation and leukaemogenesis. *Nat Cell Biol*. 2007;9(7):804-812. doi:10.1038/ncb1608
367. Ostronoff F, Othus M, Gerbing RB, et al. NUP98/NSD1 and FLT3/ITD coexpression is more prevalent in younger AML patients and leads to induction failure: a COG and SWOG report. *Blood*. 2014;124(15):2400-2407. doi:10.1182/blood-2014-04-570929
368. Meshinchi S, Stirewalt DL, Alonzo TA, et al. Structural and numerical variation of FLT3/ITD in pediatric AML. *Blood*. 2008;111(10):4930-4933. doi:10.1182/blood-2008-01-117770
369. Schnittger S, Schoch C, Dugas M, et al. Analysis of FLT3 length mutations in 1003 patients with acute myeloid leukemia: correlation to cytogenetics, FAB subtype, and prognosis in the AMLCG study and usefulness as a marker for the detection of minimal residual disease. *Blood*. 2002;100(1):59-66.
370. Arrigoni P, Beretta C, Silvestri D, et al. FLT3 internal tandem duplication in childhood acute myeloid leukaemia: association with hyperleucocytosis in acute promyelocytic leukaemia. *Br J Haematol*. 2003;120(1):89-92.
371. Shimada A, Taki T, Tabuchi K, et al. KIT mutations, and not FLT3 internal tandem duplication, are strongly associated with a poor prognosis in pediatric acute myeloid leukemia with t(8;21): a study of the Japanese Childhood AML Cooperative Study Group. *Blood*. 2006;107(5):1806-1809.
372. Pollard JA, Alonzo TA, Gerbing RB, et al. Prevalence and prognostic significance of KIT mutations in pediatric patients with core binding factor AML enrolled on serial pediatric cooperative trials for de novo AML. *Blood*. 2010;115(12):2372-2379. doi:10.1182/blood-2009-09-241075
373. Faber ZJ, Chen X, Gedman AL, et al. The genomic landscape of core-binding factor acute myeloid leukemias. *Nat Genet*. 2016;48(12):1551-1556. doi:10.1038/ng.3709
374. Bachas C, Schuurhuis GJ, Hollink IH, et al. High-frequency type I/II mutational shifts between diagnosis and relapse are associated with outcome in pediatric AML: implications for personalized medicine. *Blood*. 2010;116(15):2752-2758. doi:10.1182/blood-2010-03-276519
375. Meshinchi S, Stirewalt DL, Alonzo TA, et al. Activating mutations of RTK/ras signal transduction pathway in pediatric acute myeloid leukemia. *Blood*. 2003;102(4):1474-1479.
376. Berman JN, Gerbing RB, Alonzo TA, et al. Prevalence and clinical implications of NRAS mutations in childhood AML: a report from the Children's Oncology Group. *Leukemia*. 2011;25(6):1039-1042. doi:10.1038/leu.2011.31
377. Karlsson L, Nyvold CG, Soboli A, et al. Fusion transcript analysis reveals slower response kinetics than multiparameter flow cytometry in childhood acute myeloid leukaemia. *Int J Lab Hematol*. 2022;44(6):1094-1101. doi:10.1111/ijlh.13935
378. Noort S, Oosterwijk JV, Ma J, et al. Analysis of rare driving events in pediatric acute myeloid leukemia. *Haematologica*. 2023;108(1):48-60.
379. Liang DC, Shih LY, Huang CF, et al. CEBPalpha mutations in childhood acute myeloid leukemia. *Leukemia*. 2005;19(3):410-414.
380. Hollink IH, van den Heuvel-Eibrink MM, Arentsen-Peters ST, et al. Characterization of CEBPA mutations and promoter hypermethylation in pediatric acute myeloid leukemia. *Haematologica*. 2011;96(3):384-392. doi:10.3324/haematol.2010.031336
381. Wouters BJ, Lowenberg B, Erpelinck-Verschueren CA, van Putten WL, Valk PJ, Delwel R. Double CEBPA mutations, but not single CEBPA mutations, define a subgroup of acute myeloid leukemia with a distinctive gene expression profile that is uniquely associated with a favorable outcome. *Blood*. 2009;113(13):3088-3091. doi:10.1182/blood-2008-09-179895.
382. Tarlock K, Lamble AJ, Wang YC, et al. CEBPA-bZip mutations are associated with favorable prognosis in de novo AML: a report from the Children's Oncology Group. *Blood*. 2021;138(13):1137-1147. doi:10.1182/blood.2020009652
383. Ho PA, Kuhn J, Gerbing RB, et al. WT1 synonymous single nucleotide polymorphism rs16754 correlates with higher mRNA expression and predicts significantly improved outcome in favorable-risk pediatric acute myeloid leukemia: a report from the children's oncology group. *J Clin Oncol*. 2011;29(6):704-711. doi:10.1200/JCO.2010.31.9327
384. Damm F, Heuser M, Morgan M, et al. Single nucleotide polymorphism in the mutational hotspot of WT1 predicts a favorable outcome in patients with cytogenetically normal acute myeloid leukemia. *J Clin Oncol*. 2010;28(4):578-585. doi:10.1200/jco.2009.23.0342
385. Hollink IH, van den Heuvel-Eibrink MM, Zimmermann M, et al. No prognostic impact of the WT1 gene single nucleotide polymorphism rs16754 in pediatric acute myeloid leukemia. *J Clin Oncol*. 2010;28(28):e523-e526. doi:10.1200/JCO.2010.29.3860
386. Ko M, Huang Y, Jankowska AM, et al. Impaired hydroxylation of 5-methylcytosine in myeloid cancers with mutant TET2. *Nature*. 2010;468(7325):839-843. doi:10.1038/nature09586
387. Chou WC, Chou SC, Liu CY, et al. TET2 mutation is an unfavorable prognostic factor in acute myeloid leukemia patients with intermediate-risk cytogenetics. *Blood*. 2011;118(14):3803-3810. doi:10.1182/blood-2011-02-339747
388. Metzeler KH, Maharry K, Radmacher MD, et al. TET2 mutations improve the new European LeukemiaNet risk classification of acute myeloid leukemia: a Cancer and Leukemia Group B study. *J Clin Oncol*. 2011;29(10):1373-1381. doi:10.1200/JCO.2010.32.7742
389. Langemeijer SM, Jansen JH, Hooijer J, et al. TET2 mutations in childhood leukemia. *Leukemia*. 2011;25(1):189-192. doi:10.1038/leu.2010.243
390. Gross S, Cairns RA, Minden MD, et al. Cancer-associated metabolite 2-hydroxyglutarate accumulates in acute myelogenous leukemia with isocitrate dehydrogenase 1 and 2 mutations. *J Exp Med*. 2010;207(2):339-344. doi:10.1084/jem.20092506
391. Figueroa ME, Lugthart S, Li Y, et al. DNA methylation signatures identify biologically distinct subtypes in acute myeloid leukemia. *Cancer Cell*. 2010;17(1):13-27. doi:10.1016/j.ccr.2009.11.020.
392. Andersson AK, Miller DW, Lynch JA, et al. IDH1 and IDH2 mutations in pediatric acute leukemia. *Leukemia*. 2011;25(10):1570-1577. doi:10.1038/leu.2011.133
393. Green CL, Evans CM, Hills RK, Burnett AK, Linch DC, Gale RE. The prognostic significance of IDH1 mutations in younger adult patients with acute myeloid leukemia is dependent on FLT3/ITD status. *Blood*. 2010;116(15):2779-2782. doi:10.1182/blood-2010-02-270926
394. Ho PA, Kopecky KJ, Alonzo TA, et al. Prognostic implications of the IDH1 synonymous SNP rs11554137 in pediatric and adult AML: a report from the Children's Oncology Group and SWOG. *Blood*. 2011;118(17):4561-4566. doi:10.1182/blood-2011-04-348888.
395. Shah MY, Licht JD. DNMT3A mutations in acute myeloid leukemia. *Nat Genet*. 2011;43(4):289-290. doi:10.1038/ng0411-289
396. Hama A, Muramatsu H, Makishima H, et al. Molecular lesions in childhood and adult acute megakaryoblastic leukaemia. *Br J Haematol*. 2012;156(3):316-325. doi:10.1111/j.1365-2141.2011.08948.x
397. Hollink IH, Feng Q, Danen-van Oorschot AA, et al. Low frequency of DNMT3A mutations in pediatric AML, and the identification of the OCI-AML3 cell line as an in vitro model. *Leukemia*. 2012;26(2):371-373. doi:10.1038/leu.2011.210
398. Sievers EL, Lange BJ, Alonzo TA, et al. Immunophenotypic evidence of leukemia after induction therapy predicts relapse: results from a prospective Children's Cancer Group study of 252 patients with acute myeloid leukemia. *Blood*. 2003;101(9):3398-3406.
399. Coustan-Smith E, Ribeiro RC, Rubnitz JE, et al. Clinical significance of residual disease during treatment in childhood acute myeloid leukaemia. *Br J Haematol*. 2003;123(2):243-252.
400. Grimwade D, Lo Coco F. Acute promyelocytic leukemia: a model for the role of molecular diagnosis and residual disease monitoring in directing treatment approach in acute myeloid leukemia. *Leukemia*. 2002;16(10):1959-1973. doi:10.1038/sj.leu.2402721
401. Yin JA, Frost L. Monitoring AML1-ETO and CBFbeta-MYH11 transcripts in acute myeloid leukemia. *Curr Oncol Rep*. 2003;5(5):399-404.
402. Buonamici S, Ottaviani E, Testoni N, et al. Real-time quantitation of minimal residual disease in inv(16)-positive acute myeloid leukemia may indicate risk for clinical relapse and may identify patients in a curable state. *Blood*. 2002;99(2):443-449.
403. Farrar JE, Schuback HL, Ries RE, et al. Genomic profiling of pediatric acute myeloid leukemia reveals a changing mutational landscape from disease diagnosis to relapse. *Cancer Res*. 2016;76(8):2197-2205. doi:10.1158/0008-5472.can-15-1015
404. Craddock C, Quek L, Goardon N, et al. Azacitidine fails to eradicate leukemic stem/progenitor cell populations in patients with acute myeloid leukemia and myelodysplasia. *Leukemia*. 2013;27(5):1028-1036. doi:10.1038/leu.2012.312
405. Alexander TB, Lacayo NJ, Choi JK, Ribeiro RC, Pui CH, Rubnitz JE. Phase I study of selinexor, a selective inhibitor of nuclear export, in combination with fludarabine and cytarabine, in pediatric relapsed or refractory acute leukemia. *J Clin Oncol*. 2016;34(34):4094-4101. doi:10.1200/jco.2016.67.5066
406. Roncarolo MG, Gregori S, Bacchetta R, Battaglia M. Tr1 cells and the counterregulation of immunity: natural mechanisms and therapeutic applications. *Curr Top Microbiol Immunol*. 2014;380:39-68. doi:10.1007/978-3-662-43492-5_3
407. Laszlo GS, Estey EH, Walter RB. The past and future of CD33 as therapeutic target in acute myeloid leukemia. *Blood Rev*. 2014;28(4):143-153. doi:10.1016/j.blre.2014.04.001
408. Kung Sutherland MS, Walter RB, Jeffrey SC, et al. SGN-CD33A: a novel CD33-targeting antibody-drug conjugate using a pyrrolobenzodiazepine dimer is active in models of drug-resistant AML. *Blood*. 2013;122(8):1455-1463. doi:10.1182/blood-2013-03-491506
409. Han L, Jorgensen JL, Brooks C, et al. Antileukemia efficacy and mechanisms of action of SL-101, a novel anti-CD123 antibody conjugate, in acute myeloid leukemia. *Clin Cancer Res*. 2017;23(13):3385-3395. doi:10.1158/1078-0432.ccr-16-1904
410. Chhabra A, Ring AM, Weiskopf K, et al. Hematopoietic stem cell transplantation in immunocompetent hosts without radiation or chemotherapy. *Sci Transl Med*. 2016;8(351):351ra105. doi:10.1126/scitranslmed.aae0501

Chapter 79 ■ Acute Promyelocytic Leukemia

YASMIN M. ABAZA • MARTIN S. TALLMAN • JESSICA K. ALTMAN

INTRODUCTION

Acute promyelocytic leukemia (APL) is a rare and distinct subtype of acute myeloid leukemia (AML) accounting for 10% to 15% of all AML cases.[1] APL is characterized by a balanced reciprocal translocation between chromosomes 15 and 17 [t (15;17) (q24; q21)], which fuses the promyelocytic leukemia (PML) and the retinoic acid receptor α (RARα) genes together resulting in the formation of the chimeric oncoprotein, PML-RARα.[2] The PML-RARα fusion protein blocks myeloid differentiation at the promyelocytic stage while preventing apoptosis and promoting proliferation of leukemic progenitor cells.[3,4]

Once considered a highly fatal disease, all-trans retinoic acid (ATRA) has revolutionized the treatment of APL, decreasing the 4-week mortality rate from 38% to 16% and improving the 5-year overall survival (OS) rate from 20% to 75%, converting it to one of the most curable forms of AML.[5] ATRA induces terminal differentiation of promyelocytes along the granulocytic lineage through selective targeting and degradation of the PML-RARα protein via the proteasome pathway.[6-8] Emergence of ATRA resistance led to the introduction of arsenic trioxide (ATO), a second differentiating agent, in the treatment of APL.[9,10] ATO binds to the PML protein moiety of PML-RARα leading to its degradation thereby inducing partial differentiation and apoptosis of leukemic promyelocytes.[3] As a single agent, ATO demonstrated potent clinical activity achieving complete remission (CR) in more than 85% of patients with newly diagnosed and relapsed APL, previously treated with ATRA-containing regimens, inducing durable molecular remission.[11-16] Preclinical studies demonstrated synergy between ATRAs, which binds to the RARα moiety of PML-RARα, and ATO which was later on confirmed by numerous prospective clinical trials.[17-22]

Despite being a curable disease, early mortality remains the main cause of death in APL accounting for about 30% of all APL-related deaths.[23] Coagulopathy and bleeding complications are major causes of early mortality, underscoring the importance of immediate initiation of ATRA upon suspicion of APL prior to cytogenetic or molecular confirmation. Therefore, key elements for the proper management of APL include early diagnosis and treatment initiation, aggressive supportive care, and recognition and appropriate management of therapy-related complications.

EPIDEMIOLOGY

APL is a rare form of AML, comprising approximately 7% to 8% of adult AML cases with a median age of 47 years.[24] An increased incidence has been reported in Hispanic populations,[25,26] although some reports have debated this finding.[27] One group has reported an association with obesity.[28] Although relatively uncommon in children, clustering of cases in pediatric populations has been described, raising the issue of possible environmental exposure.[29] APL generally is not preceded by a myelodysplastic syndrome. The disease may, however, result because of prior cytotoxic therapy (see section below on treatment-related disease).

APPROACH TO PATIENTS WITH SUSPECTED APL

As in other acute leukemias, patients with APL typically display signs and symptoms associated with cytopenias. The hemorrhagic complications are, however, often out of proportion to the degree of thrombocytopenia reflecting the underlying biologic properties of the transformed promyelocytes. Signs and symptoms of hemorrhage may include petechiae, ecchymosis, subconjunctival hemorrhage, and visual changes due to retinal hemorrhages.

To prevent early mortality that is associated with APL, all patients with suspected APL should be immediately hospitalized and managed as a medical emergency even if the patient appears to be clinically stable.[30,31] Review of a peripheral blood smear often shows heavily granulated promyelocytes which is pathognomonic to this subtype of AML (Figure 79.1). ATRA and supportive care measures to counteract the life-threatening coagulopathy inherent with this disease must be initiated immediately upon clinical suspicion, even before genetic confirmation of the disease.

MORPHOLOGY AND DIAGNOSTIC APPROACH

To confirm the diagnosis of APL, a peripheral blood smear should be reviewed immediately and peripheral blood or bone marrow (BM) samples should be sent to the laboratory for morphologic, immunophenotypic, cytogenetic, and molecular analysis. Currently, we favor performing a BM biopsy in newly diagnosed patients. In the majority of cases, the BM aspirate is generally hypercellular consisting predominantly of abnormal promyelocytes. Blasts may be increased, but their number alone may not meet the minimal criteria by which classification systems such as the French-American-British or the World Health Organization define AML.[32,33] The malignant promyelocytes need to be considered as part of the total blast count to establish a diagnosis of AML. Malignant promyelocytes are heavily granulated with granules often obscuring the nucleus making the nucleocytoplasmic border somewhat indistinct.[32,33] In addition, the nucleus may be folded or bilobed.[32,33] The cytoplasm often contains vacuoles, and distinctive Auer rods are frequently visible and abundant.[32,33] Most APL cases will stain intensely with myeloperoxidase and Sudan black B stains which can aid in the confirmation of the diagnosis.[34,35]

Immunophenotypically, leukemic promyelocytes typically express the early myeloid marker, CD33, but lack human leukocyte antigen (HLA)-DR, a marker often associated with some earlier progenitor cells. The stem cell marker CD34 is generally not expressed, whereas the myeloid lineage marker CD13 is occasionally observed and is possibly associated with the development of differentiation syndrome (DS).[36] The T-cell marker CD7 is negative, as are the myelomonocytic markers CD11b and CD14. CD11b is also an indicator of myeloid maturation, and along with CD16, a surface marker found on granulocytes can be induced with differentiation therapy. It is important to emphasize that this immunophenotypic profile is characteristic but not diagnostic of APL.[37,38]

Since APL is defined by its distinct cytogenetics, rapid genetic confirmation of the diagnosis is mandatory and should be performed on BM samples, if possible, using conventional karyotyping, fluorescence in situ hybridization (FISH), and reverse-transcriptase polymerase chain reaction (RT-PCR). The balanced translocation between chromosomes 15 and 17 characterizes over 95% of cases of APL.[39,40] The breakpoints for the translocation usually occur at q22 loci on chromosome 15 and q21 on chromosome 17. The t(15;17) (q22;q21) is generally detected by conventional cytogenetic techniques and provides definitive evidence of the diagnosis of APL. The molecular consequence of this translocation results in the fusion of the RARα gene on chromosome 17 to the PML gene on chromosome 15 leading to the formation of the PML-RARα oncoprotein.[2,39,41,42] Although the break within the RARα gene is invariable within the second intron of the gene, the point of rearrangement within the PML gene can occur at two major breakpoints, resulting in three isoforms of the transcript. Breakpoints within PML intron 3 (BCR3) generally yield the short form of the messenger RNA transcript, whereas breakpoints within intron 6 (BCR1) result in the long form of the transcript.[43] Breakpoints

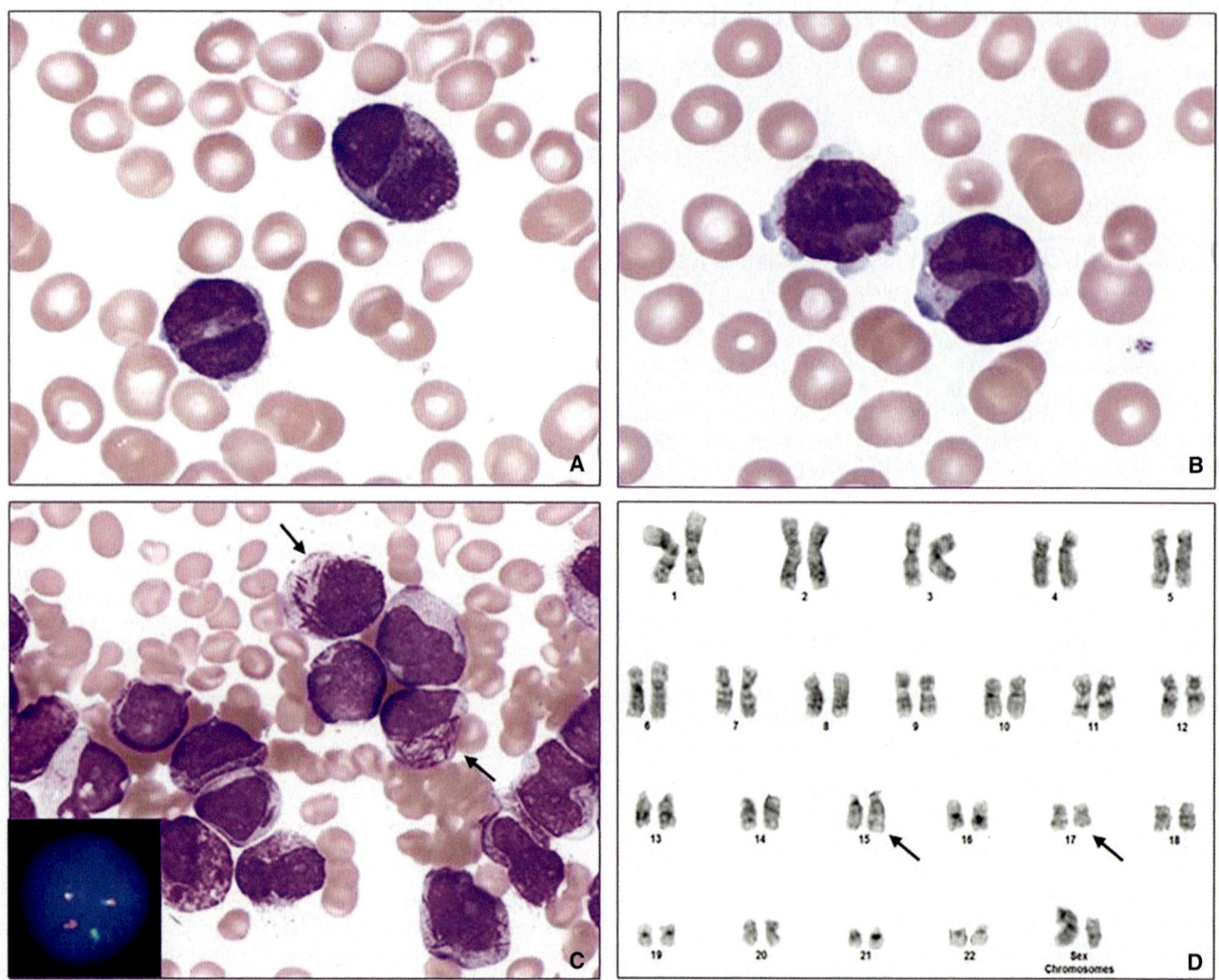

FIGURE 79.1 **Morphology of acute promyelocytic leukemia.** A, Hypergranular type. Peripheral blood smear shows abnormal promyelocytes/blasts with bilobed nuclei and cytoplasmic azurophilic granulation. B, Hypogranular type. Peripheral blood smear shows abnormal promyelocytes/blasts with paucity or absence of cytoplasmic granules. C, Bone marrow aspirate smear shows abundant abnormal promyelocytes/blasts, some with multiple Auer rods (arrows). Inset. Fluorescence in situ hybridization (FISH) analysis demonstrates fusion signals (yellow) of *PML* (orange) and *RARA* (green). D, Cytogenetic studies reveals t(15;17) (arrows) (q24;q21).

within intron 6 of *PML* can also occur at a second site (BCR2) and result in a transcript of variable length. These different isoforms of PML-RARα do not have any independent prognostic significance.[44] Detection of the PML-RARα fusion transcript, in peripheral blood or BM samples, using RT-PCR analysis is considered the gold standard for confirming the diagnosis of APL.[30,31,45] In addition to its high sensitivity and specificity, RT-PCR analysis plays a key role in defining the PML breakpoint location thus identifying the target needed for reliable monitoring of minimal residual disease (MRD).[30,31,45]

Although the t(15;17) is the defining cytogenetic abnormality in APL, additional chromosomal abnormalities can be found in 30% to 40% of patients and have no negative impact on prognosis.[21,46-49] Trisomy 8, isochromosome 17q, and deletion 9q are among the most frequently detected secondary chromosomal abnormalities reported in APL.[47,49] Up to 2% of APL patients will present with variant chromosomal translocations, such as t(11;17) and t(5;17), which are typically more resistant to ATRA and/or ATO-based regimens.[45,50]

The *FLT3* internal tandem duplication (ITD) mutation is the most frequently detected mutation in APL occurring in about 30% of patients.[21,51-53] The constitutive activation of the FLT3 receptor via this mutation is known to confer a proliferative and survival advantage to AML blasts.[54,55] In non-APL AML, this mutation occurs at a similar frequency and is generally associated with worse disease-free survival (DFS) and OS than that occurring in *FLT3-ITD* wild-type AML.[56,57] Unlike other subtypes of AML, the prognostic significance of *FLT3-ITD* in APL patients treated with ATRA plus chemotherapy remains controversial.[51] In a large meta-analysis assessing 11 studies including a total of 1063 patients with APL, *FLT3-ITD* was found to be associated with high white blood cell (WBC) count at diagnosis and inferior 3-year DFS and OS rates. Most of the patients included in this meta-analysis (10 of the 11 studies) were treated with ATRA plus chemotherapy.[58] However, recent studies have shown that the potential adverse impact of *FLT3-ITD* seen in patients treated with ATRA plus chemotherapy is abrogated by the incorporation of ATO in induction and consolidation.[59-61]

PATHOPHYSIOLOGY

Based on experimental data generated in cell lines, transgenic mice, and correlations with clinical treatment data, a model for leukemogenesis in APL has been developed.[62-66] On the most basic level, this hypothesis states that APL results from transcriptional dysregulation of differentiation produced by the PML-RARα gene product. In the normal cell, RARα plays an important role in modulating myeloid differentiation by virtue of its ability to recruit various nuclear corepressors like SMRT/N-CoR and mSin3. These transcription corepressors, in turn, bind various histone deacetylases, affecting chromatin conformation and resulting in the repression of transcription of target genes fundamental to the differentiation process. Under physiologic conditions, binding of retinoic acid causes dissociation of the corepressor complex, recruits transcriptional activators, and "opens" the chromatin, facilitating the transcription of the various target genes and allowing normal maturation. The PML-RARα fusion protein has an increased affinity for the N-CoR corepressor complex such that physiologic doses of RA ($<10^{-8}$ M) fail to produce a dissociation of the complex, resulting in continued transcriptional repression and a maturational block. Instead, suprapharmacologic doses achieved by the administration of ATRA are required to recapitulate the behavior of the wild-type receptor. In the promyelocytic leukemia zinc finger (PLZF)-RARα variant, there is a second binding site for the corepressor proteins within the PLZF portion of the fusion protein that is not sensitive to retinoic acid. Hence, even suprapharmacologic doses are unable to free the corepressor complex and permit the conformational changes in the histones necessary for permitting differentiation to occur. This may be an explanation for the clinical resistance of t(11;17) to ATRA and has led investigators to explore compounds like histone deacetylase inhibitors that bypass corepressor binding as defined by the activity of RARs and directly affect transcriptional activation.

Although the model of transcriptional repression through chromatin remodeling may rest on the interaction of the aberrant RARα fusion protein with key regulatory genetic elements, the primary partners in the molecular fusion proteins, namely, PML and PLZF, are important in leukemogenesis and may also serve to amplify the dysregulation of transcription.[62,67] PML does not directly bind DNA but has been found to regulate transcription through interaction with a number of transcription factors and repressors.[68-70] In the normal cell, PML is localized in discreet subnuclear structures called PML oncogenic domains or PML nuclear bodies (PNBs). These PNBs may functionally regulate transcription by either binding various transcription activators/repressors or sequestering them from circulating in the nucleoplasm, thereby preventing any interaction with other regulatory elements or by providing an environment where the various regulatory factors can interact or be modified. This function, in turn, may affect fundamental cellular processes such as growth, senescence, and apoptosis. PML-RAR disrupts the organization and function of the PNBs and displaces PML, forming a microspeckled pattern in the nucleus. Treatment with RA causes the PNBs to reorganize and presumably restores not only the structure, but also the functional activity.

Less is known regarding the function of PLZF in leukemogenesis. It also modulates transcriptional repression through multiple interactions with SMRT/N-CoR/mSin3/HDAC complexes and may localize in structures similar to the PNBs. Some of the mediators with which PLZF interacts are insensitive to modulation by RA, and these properties are retained in the PLZF-RAR fusion product, resulting in clinical ATRA resistance. More recent data provide evidence that PLZF-driven leukemogenesis is mediated by upregulation of eyes absent homolog 2 gene, which conferred aberrant self-renewal capacity on hematopoietic progenitor cells, providing a potential future therapeutic target in PLZF-RARA APL.[71]

In addition to providing an understanding of the underlying biology of leukemia with possible application to cancer as a whole, the molecular genetics of APL also provides a useful tool for the clinician in confirming the diagnosis and planning therapy. As discussed earlier, the vast majority of APL is characterized by t(15;17), resulting in a PML-RAR fusion product. These genetic changes are specific for APL and are easily detectable.

COAGULOPATHY AND BLEEDING

High early mortality and bleeding complications remain one of the major hurdles in the treatment of APL.[72,73] The pathophysiology of the coagulopathy associated with APL is very complex and broadly consists of disseminated intravascular coagulation (DIC) and hyperfibrinolysis.[74] DIC occurs through the increased release of the procoagulant, tissue factor (TF), which is highly expressed in APL cells.[75,76] TF forms a potent procoagulant complex with cell membrane phospholipids and factor VII triggering the coagulation cascade through the activation of factor X. Release of TF occurs during spontaneous and chemotherapy-induced death of APL cells. In addition, recent studies have demonstrated overexpression of the platelet-aggregating protein podoplanin on the surface of APL promyelocytes inducing platelet aggregation and consumption leading to thrombocytopenia and bleeding diathesis.[74,77] Primary and secondary hyperfibrinolysis, as well as nonspecific proteolysis, have also been found to play a major role in the pathogenesis of APL-induced coagulopathy particularly responsible for the increased risk of hemorrhagic complications. Annexin II, a cell-surface receptor for plasminogen and tissue plasminogen activator, is highly expressed on APL cells leading to the overproduction of plasmin and dysregulated fibrinolysis.[78,79] The potential for hemorrhage is further amplified by the depletion of the main inhibitor of plasmin, α_2-plasmin inhibitor, which is consumed in an effort to counter the increased production of plasmin. Collectively, these processes lead to the laboratory abnormalities seen in APL patients including prolongation of prothrombin time (PT), activated partial thromboplastin time (aPTT), and internationalized normal ratio (INR) for prothrombin time, low fibrinogen levels, and elevation in the fibrin degradation products (FDPs) and D-dimer levels, reflecting widespread disruption of the normal coagulation cascade.[80] These disturbances in coagulation and fibrinolysis lead to the bleeding diathesis, characteristic of this type of leukemia, and less commonly venous and arterial thrombotic complications.[81,82]

Management of APL-Associated Coagulopathy

Recognition and management of coagulopathy is of utmost importance when treating patients with APL due to the high rate of early mortality associated with this subtype of AML. Patients at high risk for fatal hemorrhagic complications include those with active bleeding, hypofibrinogenemia (<100 mg/dL), increase in D-dimers or FDP, along with prolonged PT, aPTT, or INR.[31,74] High peripheral blast count at presentation has been the only main predictor of early hemorrhagic deaths in APL.[67,83,84] ATRA is well known to rapidly improve APL-induced coagulopathy and therefore should be administered immediately, at first suspicion of APL, even before genetic confirmation of the diagnosis.[73]

Aggressive support with blood products is strongly recommended for all APL patients, regardless of risk, throughout the duration of induction therapy. Platelet transfusions should be given to maintain the platelet count above 30×10^9/L to 50×10^9/L, while cryoprecipitate and/or fresh frozen plasma should be administered to maintain serum fibrinogen of 100 to 150 mg/dL and INR less than 1.5.[18,21,30,31] Platelet counts and routine coagulation parameters, including PT, aPTT, INR, and fibrinogen levels, should be checked three to four times a day for the first several days until they become stable.[30,31] Invasive procedures such as central venous catheterization, lumbar puncture, and bronchoscopy, should be avoided before and during remission induction therapy, and certainly until coagulopathy has resolved, due to the high risk for hemorrhagic complications.[30,31] There is insufficient evidence to support the use of prothrombin complex concentrates and recombinant factor VIIa for the treatment of life-threatening hemorrhages in APL, especially given the increased thrombotic risk with these agents.[30,31,74]

Despite the wide availability of ATRA and dramatic improvement in outcomes, early mortality primarily due to intracerebral and pulmonary hemorrhages before and during induction therapy remains the main cause of treatment failure in APL.[73,85-89] In a large PETHEMA study, the majority of hemorrhagic deaths occurred early during AIDA (ATRA and idarubicin) induction with a median time to intracranial and pulmonary hemorrhage of 6 and 9 days, respectively.[83] Since a large proportion of patients with APL are managed in the community at institutions with limited experience in this disease entity, educating healthcare providers, including community oncologists, regarding the importance of early recognition of APL, prompt initiation of ATRA, and aggressive supportive care to counteract coagulopathy, is of utmost importance to improve patient outcomes.[31,73,90] In an attempt to reduce early mortality, Jillella and colleagues conducted a prospective study to assess the impact of education (through provision of simplified guidelines) and comanaging patients with APL at their local hospitals between the community oncologist and an APL expert in an academic institution.[90] Community oncologists contacted an APL expert at the first suspicion of APL and had regular communication throughout the induction period, with more frequent exchanges in the first 2 weeks.[90] This study showed a dramatic reduction in the induction mortality rate from about 30% to 8.5%.[90] These encouraging results suggest that this patient care strategy, which includes education and academic-community partnership, may be an effective model in the treatment of APL and is the basis of an ongoing national cooperative group study (ClinicalTrials.gov Identifier: NCT03253848).[23,90]

Thrombosis, both arterial and venous, is a more common complication in APL than previously appreciated with an incidence ranging from 5% to 20%.[74] Although ATRA rapidly reverses APL-induced coagulopathy, it was found to paradoxically increase the risk for thrombosis through exacerbation of the procoagulant state associated with the development of DS.[91] In a large prospective study conducted by the PETHEMA group (LPA2005 and LPA2012 trials), the incidence for thrombosis among 921 patient with APL was 13.4% (4.1% at presentation and 9.3% during induction) with catheter-related thrombosis (46%) being the most common site of thrombosis followed by deep vein thrombosis (17%), cerebral stroke (12%), pulmonary embolism (12%), and acute myocardial infarction (9%).[92] Elevated WBC count, BCR3 isoform, *FLT3-ITD*, and expression of CD2 and CD15 surface antigens have been identified as potential risk factors for the development of thrombosis in APL.[93] Use of antifibrinolytic agents, such as tranexamic acid, as prophylaxis against hemorrhagic complications has been associated with increased risk for thrombotic events without improvement in hemorrhagic mortality.[74] As a result, the prophylactic use of heparin, tranexamic acid, and other anticoagulant or antifibrinolytic agents to decrease the risk of bleeding or thrombosis associated with APL is prohibited outside the context of a clinical trial.[30,31] Treatment of severe thrombotic events using unfractionated or low-molecular-weight heparin should be done with extreme caution due to the high risk of hemorrhagic complications, especially in patients with cerebral strokes.[30,31,75] In cases of catheter-related thrombosis, the central venous line should be removed as soon as possible.[30,31,75]

TREATMENT OF ACUTE PROMYELOCYTIC LEUKEMIA

Over the past 3 decades, the combination of ATRA and ATO has drastically changed the landscape of APL therapy. Although APL was recognized as a distinct subtype of AML in 1957,[94] until the early 1990s APL was managed with standard cytotoxic chemotherapy, similar to other subtypes of AML. Anthracyclines are one of the most important cytotoxic agents used in the treatment of AML and several studies have demonstrated its significant clinical activity in APL with CR rates as high as 55% to 88%.[95-102] Although cytarabine is considered the backbone of AML treatment, it does not seem to play a clear role in the treatment of APL. A retrospective analysis of 62 patients with APL treated with either single-agent daunorubicin or in combination with cytarabine for induction therapy showed no difference in CR rates.[98] Similarly, a randomized study conducted by the GIMEMA cooperative group comparing induction with idarubicin alone and in combination with cytarabine in patients with newly diagnosed APL showed no difference in the CR rate or event-free survival (EFS) between both groups.[103] Despite the exquisite sensitivity of APL to anthracyclines, the long-term DFS in these patients did not exceed 40%.[95,96]

The introduction of ATRA fundamentally changed the treatment and outcome of APL. As a single agent, ATRA achieved CR rates of 70% to 85% comparable to that achieved using chemotherapy.[88,104] However, the high relapse rates again noted with the use of ATRA monotherapy prompted the development of multiple prospective clinical trials to assess the efficacy ATRA when given in combination with chemotherapy. The European APL group demonstrated superiority of concurrent ATRA plus chemotherapy (daunorubicin and cytarabine) compared to sequential ATRA followed by chemotherapy in patients with newly diagnosed APL with significant reduction in the relapse rate at 2 years from 16% in the sequential arm to 6% in patients who received concurrent therapy.[87,105] These results were confirmed by multiple large prospective studies that led to the establishment of concurrent ATRA plus chemotherapy as the new standard of care for the treatment of patients with newly diagnosed APL resulting in CR rates up to 95% with cure rates exceeding 80%.[31,61,85,105-116]

The potent single-agent activity of ATO and its preclinical synergy with ATRA led investigators at the Shanghai Institute of Hematology to conduct a randomized trial in which patients with newly diagnosed APL received ATRA monotherapy, ATO monotherapy, or ATRA plus ATO induction therapy followed by eight cycles of chemotherapy-based consolidation and maintenance therapy.[11-17,117] Although there was no difference in the CR rate among the three groups (≥90%), the combination of ATRA plus ATO was associated with a shorter remission induction time, significant reduction in disease burden, and a lower relapse rate when compared to ATRA or ATO monotherapy.[117] After a median follow-up of 70 months, the 5-year EFS and OS rates for patients treated with the combination regimen were 89% and 92%, respectively, confirming the abovementioned synergy and establishing the efficacy on this regimen in eradication of APL.[118]

To assess the role of ATO during consolidation, the North America Leukemia Intergroup Study (C9710) randomized 481 patients with untreated APL who received ATRA, daunorubicin, and cytarabine induction to receive ATRA plus daunorubicin consolidation with or without ATO. Regardless of risk category, the 3-year EFS and DFS rates were significantly higher for patients who received ATO consolidation compared to those who received ATRA plus daunorubicin alone (80% vs 63%; 90% vs 70%; respectively); there was also a nonstatistically significant improvement in the 3-year OS rate (86% vs 81%, $P = .07$).[119] Furthermore, the addition of ATO during consolidation overcame the negative impact of high-risk disease with comparable DFS rates to those with low-risk disease confirming the beneficial role of ATO during consolidation therapy.[119] A subsequent cooperative group study (S0521) assessed the need for maintenance therapy in patients with low-risk APL who achieved molecular CR after receiving ATRA, daunorubicin, and cytarabine induction followed by ATRA, daunorubicin, and ATO consolidation.[120] Sixty-eight patients in molecular CR were randomized to either observation or 1-year maintenance therapy with ATRA, 6-mercaptopurine, and methotrexate.[120] There were no relapses observed in either group of patients after a median follow-up of 3 years suggesting that incorporation of ATO in consolidation therapy may negate the need for maintenance therapy.[120]

Collectively, these encouraging results led to numerous large randomized and nonrandomized trials conducted to investigate the efficacy of ATRA plus ATO induction/consolidation in patients with newly diagnosed APL, in an attempt to further de-escalate treatment and eliminate the need of chemotherapy. Results of these trials are summarized in *Table 79.1* and discussed below in more detail. Although the CR rates achieved using ATRA plus ATO were comparable to that achieved using ATRA plus chemotherapy, induction mortality, deaths in CR, relapse rates, and development of therapy–related myeloid neoplasms (T-MN) were significantly higher with the use of ATRA plus chemotherapy.[20,122] Therefore, ATRA plus ATO approaches have been established as the new standard of care for the front-line treatment of APL.

To help risk stratify APL patients and develop a predictive model for relapse, Sanz at al conducted a combined analysis of newly diagnosed APL patients treated on both the GIMEMA and PETHEMA trials using ATRA plus chemotherapy. In this study, they identified three distinctive prognostic groups of APL patients: (1) low-risk group: presenting WBC count ≤10 × 10^9/L and platelet count >40 × 10^9/L; (2) intermediate-risk group: presenting WBC and platelet counts ≤10 × 10^9/L and ≤40 × 10^9/L, respectively; and (3) high-risk group: presenting WBC count >10 × 10^9/L, with statistically significant difference in relapse-free survival (RFS).[123] However, given the

Table 79.1. Summary of the Major Clinical Trials in the Treatment of Acute Promyelocytic Leukemia

Trial (Reference)	Risk Group (N)	Induction	Consolidation	Maintenance	GO Dose	Prophylactic Steroid Regimen	EFS (%) L/I	EFS (%) H	DFS (%) L/I	DFS (%) H	OS (%) L/I	OS (%) H
APL0406; Lo-Coco et al[20,120]	Low (112) Int (147)	ATRA + ATO vs ATRA + IDA	ATRA + ATO vs ATRA + IDA + MTZ	None for ATRA-ATO arm vs ATRA + MTX + 6-MP for AIDA arm	NA	Prednisone 0.5 mg/kg/day from day 1 until end of induction therapy	97.3 vs 80	NA	97.3 vs 82.6 4-year	NA	99.2 vs 92.6	NA
AML17; Burnett et al[22]	Low (177) High (56)	ATRA + ATO (+GO for high-risk) vs ATRA + IDA	ATRA + ATO vs ATRA + IDA + MTZ	None	6 mg/m2 x1 dose	None	92 vs 71	87 vs 64	97 vs 78 (not stratified by risk category) 4-year		95 vs 90	87 vs 84
MD Anderson; Abaza et al[21]	Low (133) High (54)	ATRA+ATO+(GO or IDA for high-risk or low-risk who develop leukocytosis)	ATRA + ATO	None	9 mg/m2 x1 dose	Methylprednisolone 50 mg IV daily x5 days, followed by rapid taper on day 6 in absence of DS	87	81	99 5-year	89	89	86
APML4; Iland et al[60,61]	L/I (101) High (23)	ATRA + ATO + IDA	ATRA + ATO	ATRA + MTX + 6-MP	NA	Prednisone 1 mg/kg/day from days 1-10 of induction or until WBC count < 1 × 10⁹/L or until resolution of DS (whichever occurs last)	92	83	96 5-year	95	96	87
C9710; Powell et al[119]	Low (136) Int (232) High (113)	ATRA + Ara-C + DNR	ATRA + DNR + ATO vs ATRA + DNR	ATRA vs ATRA+6-MP + MTX	NA	None	80 vs 63		90 vs 70		86 vs 81 3-year Not stratified by risk group	
SWOG S0535; Lancet et al[121]	High (70)	ATRA + ATO + GO	ATRA + ATO + GO + DNR	ATRA+6-MP + MTX	9 mg/m2 x1 dose	None	NA	78	NA	91 3-year	NA	86

Abbreviations: 6-MP: 6-mercaptopurine; AIDA: ATRA plus idarubicin; AML: acute myeloid leukemia; APL: acute promyelocytic leukemia; Ara-C: cytarabine; ATO: arsenic trioxide; ATRA: all-trans retinoic acid; DFS: disease-free survival; DNR: daunorubicin; EFS: event-free survival; GO: gemtuzumab ozogamicin; H: High; IDA: idarubicin; Int: intermediate; L/I: low/intermediate; MTX: methotrexate; MTZ: mitoxantrone; OS: overall survival.

similarities in treatment outcomes, low- and intermediate-risk APL are grouped together in the same risk category. Therefore, APL is categorized based on the presenting WBC count into two groups: low-risk APL (defined by a WBC count ≤ 10×10^9/L) and high-risk APL (WBC count > 10×10^9/L).[123] This method of risk stratification is the basis for the development of risk-adapted protocols for the treatment of patients with APL.

Treatment of Low-Risk APL

Two landmark phase 3, multicenter, randomized trials comparing ATRA plus ATO to ATRA plus chemotherapy in the frontline treatment of patients with low-risk APL showed noninferiority and potential superiority of ATRA plus ATO in this patient population.[20,22]

The first reported multicenter, randomized trial, conducted by Lo-Coco et al (the APL0406 study), compared ATRA plus chemotherapy (AIDA regimen) to ATRA plus ATO in 156 patients with newly diagnosed low-risk APL.[20] In the ATRA-ATO arm, patients received ATRA plus ATO for induction until CR or for a maximum of 60 days followed by consolidation therapy consisting of ATRA (45 mg/m²/d) 2 weeks on and 2 weeks off for a total of seven courses plus ATO (0.15 mg/kg/d) 5 d/ wk, 4 weeks on and 4 weeks off for a total of 4 cycles of therapy (total of 28 weeks after the CR date; Figure 79.2). This noninferiority study met its primary endpoint with a 2-year EFS rate of 98% vs 85% in the ATRA-ATO and ATRA-chemotherapy arms, respectively, with a statistically significant improvement in OS.[20] Although there were no significant differences in the 2-year DFS and cumulative incidence of relapse (CIR) rates in this initial report,[20] an extended series of this trial including 263 patients with a median follow-up of 40.6 months showed a statistically significant improvement in all analyzed outcomes including EFS (97.3% vs 80%), DFS (97.3% vs 82.6%), OS (99.2% vs 92.6%), and CIR (1.9% vs 13.9%) with ATRA-ATO compared to ATRA-chemotherapy.[122] Moreover, they reported higher rates of death in CR and development of T-MN in the ATRA-chemotherapy arm.[122] Long-term follow-up of the APL-0406 trial (median follow-up 66.4 months) confirmed durability of the responses achieved with ATRA-ATO and achievement of long-term benefits namely lower relapse rates and absence of T-MN, accounting for the improvement in survival observed with this regimen.[124]

Superiority of the ATRA-ATO regimen was subsequently demonstrated by a phase 3, multicenter, randomized trial (AML17) conducted in the United Kingdom comparing ATRA-ATO to ATRA-idarubicin in 235 patients with newly diagnosed APL regardless of risk stratification.[22] Patients with high-risk APL who were assigned to the ATRA-ATO arm were allowed to receive one dose of gemtuzumab ozogamicin (GO; 6 mg/m² intravenously).[22] The 4-year EFS (91% vs 70%), morphologic RFS (97% vs 78%), and CIR (1% vs 18%) rates were significantly improved in the ATRA-ATO group compared to ATRA-idarubicin arm.[22] Furthermore, the 4-year molecular RFS (98% vs 70%) and cumulative incidence of molecular relapse (0% vs 27%) were superior with ATRA-ATO compared to ATRA-chemotherapy supporting the use of this chemotherapy-free regimen in APL including high-risk patients.[22] In line with other studies, the 4-year cumulative incidence of T-MN was 0% in the ATRA-ATO group compared to 3% with the ATRA plus chemotherapy.[22]

Of note, in this study ATO was given at a dose of 0.3 mg/kg on days 1 to 5 of each course and at 0.25 mg/kg twice weekly in weeks 2 to 8 of cycle 1 of induction and weeks 2 to 4 of cycles 2 to 5 of consolidation.[22] This alternative ATO schedule may be the reason behind the lower incidence of grade 3 or 4 hepatotoxicity reported in this trial.[20,22] Moreover, the lower frequency of ATO administration provides a more convenient outpatient schedule which may improve compliance without jeopardizing patient outcomes.[20-22] This treatment schedule is an attractive alternative for patients who are unable to commit to the 5-day per week schedule which is more commonly used in clinical practice.[18-22,61]

Collectively, these results confirm the advantage of ATRA-ATO over ATRA-chemotherapy and establish this chemotherapy-free regimen as the new standard of care for front-line treatment of patients with low-risk APL.[20,22] In these studies, ATRA-ATO was associated with significantly less hematologic toxicity and fewer infections

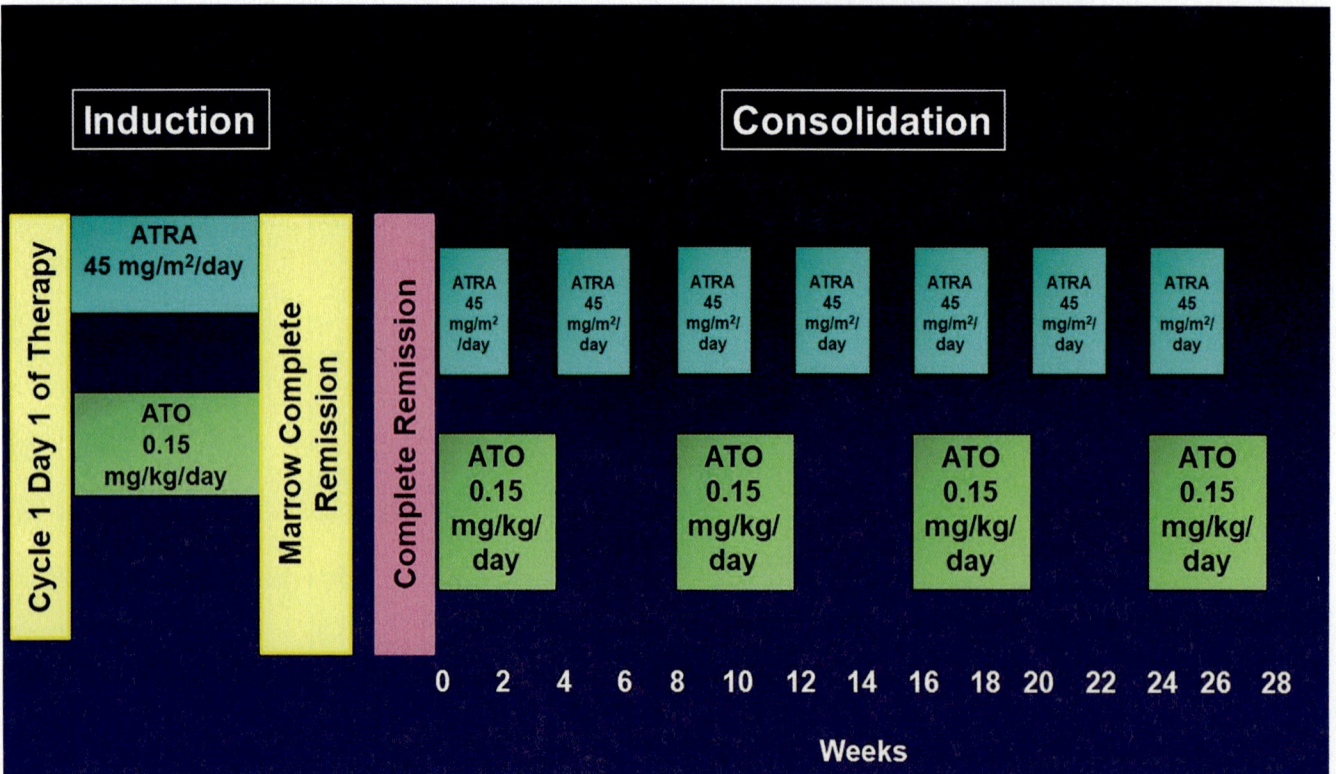

FIGURE 79.2 Treatment Schema for Low-Risk Acute Promyelocytic Leukemia using the APL0406 Regimen. ATO: arsenic trioxide; ATRA: all-trans retinoic acid.

compared to ATRA-chemotherapy, but there were higher rates of transient hepatotoxicity [aspartate transaminase/alanine transaminase elevation] and corrected QT (QTc) interval prolongation that were managed with temporary discontinuation of ATRA and/or ATO and subsequent dose adjustments.[20-22]

Treatment of High-Risk APL

Although ATRA plus ATO is now the standard of care for the treatment of low-risk APL, the optimal therapy of high-risk patients is not yet standardized (*Figure 79.3*). Elevated WBC count upon initial presentation further rises rapidly with the administration of ATRA leading to numerous complications including DS, hypoxemia, coagulopathy, and intracranial hemorrhage, emphasizing the importance of concomitant cytoreduction early during induction for these patients.

In the nonrandomized, phase 2, Australian APML4 study, 124 newly diagnosed APL patients, including 23 high-risk patients, were treated with ATRA-ATO plus idarubicin (age-adjusted 6-12 mg/m^2 on days 2, 4, 6, 8) induction followed by 2 consolidation cycles of ATRA-ATO, and then maintenance therapy with ATRA plus chemotherapy for 2 years.[61] For the entire cohort, the 2-year DFS rate was 97.5%, unaffected by the Sanz risk stratification, and the 2-year OS rate was 93%, comparable to other studies, suggesting the importance of using some anthracycline chemotherapy during induction to maximize long-term outcomes.[19,61] Long-term follow-up on the APML4 trial confirmed efficacy of this regimen in both low- and high-risk patients with no significant differences between the 5-year EFS (92% vs 83%), DFS (96% vs 95%), OS (96% vs 87%), and CIR (5% vs 5%) rates in both risk groups, respectively.[60]

To better assess the impact of adding ATO to induction and consolidation and eliminating chemotherapy from consolidation, Iland et al compared the results of the APML4 study to their preceding APML3 protocol which used ATRA/idarubicin based therapy only in both induction and consolidation.[61,125] Compared to historic control, there was statistically significant improvement in the 2-year relapse-free rate (98% vs 87%, $P = .006$) and 2-year DFS rate (98% vs 86%, $P = .003$) with the APML4 protocol. In multivariate analysis combining data from both the APML3 and APML4 studies, the superiority of incorporating ATO in induction/consolidation was maintained for DFS ($P = .0015$), EFS ($P = .0013$), and OS ($P = .022$) after adjusting for age and Sanz risk category.[60] Consistent with previous reports, these results further support the use of ATRA-ATO combination in the front-line treatment of APL and the omission of cytotoxic agents during consolidation.[61,125] Despite the small number of high-risk patients included in this trial, these promising results were the basis for approval of ATO in Australia for the treatment of patients with high-risk APL and this is one of the preferred regimens in the National Comprehensive Cancer Network (NCCN) guidelines for the treatment of patients with high-risk disease.[126]

GO is an anti-CD33 monoclonal antibody conjugated to the anthracycline antibiotic calicheamicin. GO is significantly active in APL due to the high expression CD33 on the surface of leukemic promyelocytes and was found to be safe and clinical active when combined to ATRA in patients with untreated APL.[127,128] Investigators from the MD Anderson Cancer Center (TX, USA) conducted three consecutive nonrandomized trials combining ATRA plus ATO (similar to Lo-Coco et al regimen)[20] with the addition of one dose of GO 9 mg/m^2 in patients with either high-risk disease (day 1 of therapy) or low-risk disease who develop leukocytosis (WBC > 10 × 10^9/L) within the first 4 weeks of ATRA/ATO induction therapy.[18,19,21] Due to intermittent lack of access to GO, patients were allowed to receive one dose of idarubicin 12 mg/m^2 instead. Collectively, 187 patients with newly diagnosed APL were treated with this regimen, including 54 patients with high-risk disease.[21] The CR rate for the entire cohort was 96% with an equal CR rate among low-risk and high-risk patients. Confirmed molecular remission was achieved in 98% of patients, of which 96% remained in molecular remission.[21] Among the high-risk patients, 83% received GO, 13% idarubicin, and 2% received both cytoreductive agents with induction therapy. The 5-year EFS, DFS, and OS rates for the entire cohort were 85%, 96%, and 88%, respectively.[21] When stratified by risk group, the 5-year EFS, DFS, and OS rates in patients with low-risk and high-risk disease were 87% versus 81%, 99% versus 89%, and 89% versus 86%, respectively.[21] Despite the small number of patients, there was no difference in the 5-year OS rate among high-risk patients who received cytoreduction with either GO or idarubicin.[21]

To confirm that ATRA-ATO-GO was not inferior to ATRA-chemotherapy, Burnett at al randomized 57 patients to receive either ATRA-ATO plus GO ($N = 30$) or ATRA plus idarubicin ($N = 27$).[22] Among the 30 patients randomized to the ATRA-ATO-GO arm, 28 patients (93%) received GO; the remaining two patients received anthracyclines due to lack of GO, with a 4-year OS rate of 89% in this group of high-risk patients.[22] There was no significant difference in

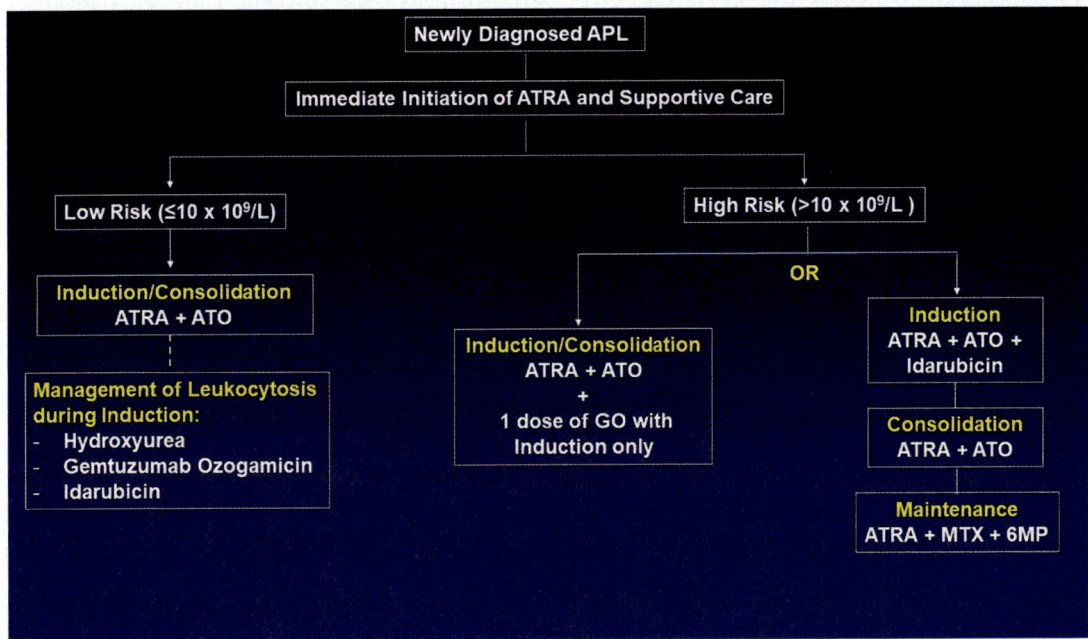

FIGURE 79.3 Treatment algorithm for newly diagnosed acute promyelocytic leukemia. 6-MP: 6-mercaptopurine; APL: acute promyelocytic leukemia; ATO: arsenic trioxide; ATRA: all-trans retinoic acid; GO: gemtuzumab ozogamicin.

the 4-year EFS (87% vs 64%; HR 0.34) or OS (87% vs 84%) among high-risk patients treated with either ATRA-ATO-GO or ATRA-chemotherapy, respectively.[22] Taken together, results published by MD Anderson and Burnett et al provide sufficient evidence that the ATRA-ATO-GO combination regimen is at least as effective as ATRA-chemotherapy in patients with high-risk disease.[21,22] Therefore, both ATRA-ATO-GO schedules, using GO at doses of either 6 mg/m^2 or 9 mg/m^2, are among the preferred regimens in the NCCN guidelines for the front-line treatment of high-risk patients.[126]

In the SWOG 0535 study, 73 patients with high-risk APL were induced with ATRA-ATO plus GO 9 mg/m^2 (given on day 1) followed by sequential consolidation consisting of 2 cycles of ATO, ATRA plus daunorubicin, and GO for a total of six consolidation cycles followed by 1-year maintenance with ATRA plus chemotherapy.[121] The 3-year EFS and OS rates reported on this study were 78% and 86%, respectively, confirming the effectiveness of chemotherapy-free ATRA-ATO-GO induction regimen.[121]

GO was unavailable for commercial use in the United States from 2010 to 2017. Since GO is not always readily accessible in all hospitals, routine use of ATRA-ATO-GO may be limited in routine clinical practice. When available, many experts recommend using ATRA-ATO-GO in the treatment of high-risk APL using either 6 mg/m^2 of 9 mg/m^2 of GO per the published data, due to the efficacy and safety of this regimen.[129] Extrapolating from the phase 3 ALFA-0701 trial conducted in older, de novo, non-APL AML patients, some experts suggest fractionating GO and giving it at doses of 3 mg/m^2 on days 1, 4, and 7 of induction therapy in patients with high-risk APL for a total cumulative dose of 9 mg/m^2.[129,130] Although this is an attractive alternative schedule of GO which has shown to be safe in non-APL AML, this schedule has not yet been tested in APL. In the absence of GO, idarubicin can be used in combination with ATRA-ATO induction following either the APML4 schedule (age-adjusted 6-12 mg/m^2 on days 2, 4, 6, 8) or the MD Anderson protocol (idarubicin 12 mg/m^2 on day 1); both regimens have been shown to be highly effective in the treatment of patients with high-risk APL.[21,61] Importantly, anthracycline-based regimens are associated with higher risk of T-MN, which although infrequent, is a severe complication associated with poor prognosis.[131] Major adverse events associated with the main agents used in the treatment of APL are summarized in Table 79.2.

Optimal Dose and Schedule for ATRA

Most of the prospective studies conducted in adult patients with APL used ATRA at a standard dose of 45 mg/m^2 given in two divided doses daily. In two pediatric studies using the AIDA regimen, ATRA given at a reduced dose of 25 mg/m^2/d was found to be associated with lower rates of pseudotumor cerebri and headaches with similar efficacy when compared to studies using the standard dose of ATRA.[132,133] Pharmacokinetic studies conducted in adult patients with APL showed no difference in the peak plasma concentrations or mean area under the concentration-time curves when patients were treated with ATRA at a dose 25 mg/m^2 or 45 mg/m^2 daily.[134,135] Among 12 adult patients with newly diagnosed APL who received single-agent ATRA at the reduced dose of 25 mg/m^2/d, 10 patients achieved CR and 2 died during induction supporting the clinical efficacy of the lower dose of ATRA.[134] These results were subsequently confirmed by a randomized study conducted by Shen et al, in which 95% of patients (19/20) with newly diagnosed APL induced with lower dose (25 mg/m^2/d) single-agent ATRA achieved CR.[117] Since almost all of the randomized controlled studies conducted in adult patients used the standard dose of ATRA (45 mg/m^2/d), experts in the field recommend using this dose when possible. However, the dose of ATRA may be reduced to 25 mg/m^2/d in patients who develop significant side effects related to ATRA.

Multiple studies including the APL0406, UK AML 17, and the MD Anderson studies used ATRA for 2 weeks every 4 weeks for a total of seven cycles during postremission consolidation.[18-22] Pharmacokinetic studies have shown a significant decline in both the peak plasma level and area under the concentration-time curve with continued ATRA administration which occurred early within the first 7 days of treatment. This decline was associated with an increase in the urinary excretion of ATRA metabolites suggesting that the accelerated plasma clearance of ATRA was due to increased drug catabolism.[136] A subsequent study showed that ATRA metabolites induce CYP26A1 expression, the main enzyme responsible of ATRA clearance, increasing the metabolism of ATRA thereby limiting its own therapeutic efficacy.[137] Enzyme activity returns to baseline within 7 days of ATRA discontinuation.[137] These pharmacokinetic findings were the basis behind the alternate week schedule of ATRA (7 days on followed by 7 days off) used in the second cycle of consolidation in the APML4 trial and during maintenance therapy in the North American Intergroup Study C9710.[60,61,119] Based on these observations, either schedule may be used for ATRA administration during consolidation.[129]

Maintenance Therapy

In the pre-ATO era, the role of maintenance therapy in the treatment of APL was controversial due to conflicting data from numerous randomized clinical trials. In the study conducted by Fenaux et al (European APL93 study), after ATRA/chemotherapy-based induction/consolidation, 289 patients were randomized for maintenance therapy between either no therapy, intermittent ATRA for 2 years, continuous low-dose chemotherapy for 2 years, or both ATRA/chemotherapy.[87] There was a statistically significant improvement in the 2-year relapse rate among patients randomized to chemotherapy versus no chemotherapy (11% vs 27%, P = .0002) and to those randomized to ATRA versus no ATRA (13% vs 25%).[87] OS was improved

Table 79.2. Overview of the Common Adverse Events Associated With Agents Used in the Treatment of Acute Promyelocytic Leukemia

Treatment Agent	Adverse Events
All-*trans*-retinoic acid	Differentiation syndrome Cytokine release syndrome Teratogenicity Elevation of liver function tests Arrhythmias Gastrointestinal abnormalities (e.g. nausea, vomiting, and diarrhea) Pseudotumor cerebri Hypertriglyceridemia Xeroderma and cheilitis
Arsenic Trioxide	Differentiation syndrome Corrected QT (QTc) prolongation Arrhythmias Hepatotoxicity Electrolyte disturbances Gastrointestinal abnormalities (e.g. nausea, vomiting, and diarrhea) Peripheral neuropathy
Gemtuzumab ozogamicin	Hepatotoxicity Veno-occlusive disease Infusion reaction Myelosuppression QTc prolongation Hypokalemia
Idarubicin	Cardiotoxicity (cardiomyopathy) Myelosuppression Arrhythmia Gastrointestinal abnormalities (e.g., nausea, vomiting, and diarrhea) Mucositis Alopecia Skin rash Elevation of liver function tests
Hydroxyurea	Myelosuppression Vasculitic ulcer Mucositis Gastrointestinal abnormalities (e.g., nausea, vomiting, and diarrhea)

in patients who received maintenance chemotherapy ($P = .01$) with a trend toward improvement in OS among those who received maintenance ATRA ($P = .22$).[87] These results we subsequently confirmed by the North American Intergroup APL trial in which 350 patients with newly diagnosed APL were randomized to either chemotherapy (daunorubicin and cytarabine) or ATRA for induction and then to either observation or ATRA maintenance after consolidation chemotherapy.[116] There was significant improvement in the 5-year DFS rate among patients randomized to ATRA compared to observation (61% vs 36%, $P < .0001$).[116]

In the study conducted by Avvisati et al (AIDA 0493 protocol), 586 patients in molecular CR after ATRA-idarubicin–based therapy were randomly assigned to 4 maintenance arms: chemotherapy (arm 1); ATRA alone (arm 2); chemotherapy plus ATRA (arm 3); and observation (arm 4).[111] In contrary to the APL93 and North American Intergroup APL studies, there was no difference in the 12-year DFS among the 4 maintenance arms (arm 1: 70.4%; arm 2: 69%; arm 3: 67.6%; arm 4: 69.1%) arguing against the need for maintenance therapy.[87,111,116]

All of these abovementioned studies were based on an ATRA/chemotherapy backbone without the incorporation of ATO. In the era of ATO-based regimens, there does not seem to be a need for maintenance therapy in the treatment of APL. In SWOG/ECOG/CALGB S0521 randomized noninferiority study, 68 patients with newly diagnosed low-risk APL who achieved molecular CR after ATRA-chemotherapy induction followed by ATO-chemotherapy consolidation, per the C9710 regimen, were randomized to either 1-year maintenance with ATRA-chemotherapy or observation.[119,120] Although the study was terminated prematurely due to slow accrual, there were no relapses in either arm with a median follow-up of 36 months arguing against the need of maintenance therapy with the incorporation of ATO during consolidation.[120] Furthermore, the APL0406, UK AML 17, and MD Anderson Cancer Center studies did not include maintenance therapy in their protocols and showed excellent long-term outcomes in both low- and high-risk patients.[20-22] Based on these data, there is no need for maintenance therapy in the treatment of patients with APL unless if the regimen that is chosen for treatment has maintenance therapy included in the treatment protocol, such as in the APML4 trial.[61,126] It is strongly recommended that patients be treated on an established regimen without mixing treatment strategies from different protocols unless there is a compelling reason (i.e. change in clinical status of patient preventing their ability to continue to be treated on their assigned regimen).

Supportive Care

Supportive care measures to mitigate and treat inherent coagulopathy, therapy-induced leukocytosis, and DS are discussed elsewhere in the chapter. Since ATO can prolong the QTc interval, electrocardiographic surveillance is recommended twice weekly coupled with aggressive electrolyte replacement to maintain potassium above 4 mEq/L and magnesium above 1.8 mg/dL.[30] Concomitant use of medications that prolong QTc, such as fluoroquinolones, azoles, and 5-HT3 receptor antagonists, should be avoided.[138] The QT interval should be corrected using formulas other than the classical Bazett correction, such as Fridericia, Hodges, and Framingham rate correction formulas, to avoid unnecessary interruptions in ATO therapy.[139] Patients who develop QT/QTc prolongation beyond 500 ms or experience syncope or arrhythmia should have all medications that may prolong the QTc interval discontinued and ATO temporarily held with aggressive electrolyte replacement.[30] Once the QT/QTc interval improves to about 460 ms, ATO may be restarted with a 50% dose reduction which can be gradually increased to full dose provided that the electrolytes are adequately replaced.[30]

Despite being minimally myelosuppressive, there is significant association between ATO therapy and herpes zoster (HZ) reactivation with the majority of cases occurring during the first 6 months of therapy.[140-142] This association is thought to be secondary to impaired cellular immunity induced by ATO.[140] In a recent study assessing the benefit of antiviral prophylaxis in 112 ATO treated patients with APL, HZ reactivation occurred in 11.6% of patients within 6 months of completing ATO therapy.[143] Compared to patients who did not receive antiviral prophylaxis, there was a significant reduction in the incidence of HZ reactivation with the use of antiviral prophylaxis (17.5% vs 4.1%, $P = .025$) with a number needed to treat of 7.7.[143] Therefore, routine use of antiviral prophylaxis should be considered in patients with APL receiving ATO.[140,143] Prophylaxis should preferably start prior to initiation of ATO therapy and continue for at least 6 months after completion of therapy.[140,143]

CENTRAL NERVOUS SYSTEM PROPHYLAXIS

As treatment outcomes improved with the introduction of ATRA to chemotherapy, central nervous system (CNS) relapse emerged as an area of concern especially among patients with high-risk disease and those who develop intracranial hemorrhage during induction.[144] Although some protocols included intrathecal chemotherapy for patients with high-risk disease, the role of CNS prophylaxis in the treatment of APL remains controversial due to the lack of prospective randomized data.[31] Furthermore, all the protocols that included CNS prophylaxis were from the pre-ATO era when only ATRA and chemotherapy were used in the treatment of APL.[129]

In a study conducted by Au et al, elemental ATO levels were measured in 67 paired cerebrospinal fluid (CSF) and plasma samples from 9 patients with APL on oral ATO. There was linear correlation between the levels of ATO in CSF and plasma ($P < .001$), with ATO detectable in CSF at therapeutically meaningful levels.[145] Since ATO crosses the blood-brain barrier, CNS prophylaxis was not included in any of the trials that used an ATRA-ATO combination regimen, such as APML4 study, UK AML17 trial, MD Anderson protocol, and the Intergroup SWOG 0535 trial.[18,19,21,22,61,121] High-risk patients treated on these four studies had low incidence of CNS relapse supporting protective effect of ATO.[21,22,61,121]

Therefore, there is no formal evidence to support the use of prophylactic intrathecal chemotherapy in the ATO era. However, if CNS prophylaxis is implemented, its use should be restricted to patients with high-risk APL and those who develop intracranial hemorrhage with induction. It should be emphasized that CNS prophylaxis should be postponed until after achievement of CR due to the high risk for hemorrhagic complications as previously mentioned.[30,31]

MANAGEMENT OF LEUKOCYTOSIS DURING INDUCTION IN LOW-RISK APL

Leukocytosis, defined as WBC count $>10 \times 10^9$/L, is a common side effect among patients with low-risk APL treated with ATRA-ATO which is considered a sign of differentiation and should not lead to the reclassification of patients to high-risk disease.[30] It typically develops 7 to 21 days from start of therapy (median, 8 days) and can be managed by either hydroxyurea or other potent anti-APL cytotoxic agents such as idarubicin or GO.[20,22,117]

In the APL0406 study, leukocytosis which developed during induction therapy was managed using hydroxyurea as follows: (1) WBC 10 to 50×10^9/L: 500 mg four times a day and (2) WBC $> 50 \times 10^9$/L: 1 g four times a day. Hydroxyurea was discontinued once WBC count was below 10×10^9/L. In this study, 47% of patients in the ATRA-ATO group and 24% in the ATRA-chemotherapy group ($P = .007$) developed leukocytosis which was successfully managed in all the cases with the use of hydroxyurea.[20] However, among the 133 patients with low-risk APL treated by the MD Anderson group using the ATRA-ATO combination regimen, 96 patients (72%) developed leukocytosis with induction with a median time of 10 days (range, 2-26 days) from start of therapy.[21] Out of these patients, only 60 (63%) received cytoreductive therapy (GO, $N = 51$; idarubicin, $N = 9$) at a median time of 8 days (range, 2-14 days) from start of treatment with rapid normalization of WBC count in all treated patients.[21] Due to the lack of difference in survival data between the two studies, the use of either hydroxyurea or cytotoxic agents, such as GO or idarubicin, is an acceptable method of count control during induction therapy.[20,21] In general, leukapheresis should be completely avoided in APL due to the high risk of precipitating fatal hemorrhages.[30]

Response Criteria and Monitoring

To assess response to therapy, all patients should have a BM aspirate and/or biopsy weekly starting 21 to 28 days after the start of induction therapy.[18,21] Once the BM shows less than 5% blasts and no abnormal promyelocytes (marrow CR), treatment with ATRA-ATO may be discontinued until patients achieve CR which is defined by absolute neutrophil and platelet counts greater than 1×10^9/L and 100×10^9/L, respectively.[18,19,21]

Importantly, due to the delayed differentiation of blasts noted with the use of ATRA-ATO, detection of cells positive for the t(15;17) using conventional cytogenetics or FISH or detectable PML-RARA transcripts using RT-PCR analysis is expected after induction therapy and should not be considered treatment failure.[30]

Burnett et al studied the kinetics of molecular remission by assessing the difference in the RT-PCR profiles between 26 patients who eventually relapsed and 79 patients who remained in CR.[146] Detection of a positive PCR after 3 cycles of therapy had a statistically significant increase in the risk of relapse compared to other time points and was the most predictive of worse OS.[146] Therefore, there is no clinical significance of RT-PCR positivity detected at the time of CR after induction therapy since with consolidation therapy these patients will achieve MRD negativity.[18]

Achievement of MRD negativity using RT-PCR for PML-RARA (which has sensitivity to detect PML-RARA transcripts at concentrations of about 10^{-4}) on BM samples at the end of consolidation is the most important MRD end point.[147] Patients with high-risk APL who achieve MRD negativity at the end of consolidation should continue to be monitored using RT-PCR analysis on BM specimens every 3 months for 2 to 3 years after completion of consolidation therapy.[18,147,148] This stringent schedule for MRD monitoring after consolidation is crucial for the early detection of molecular relapses and treatment initiation which is beneficial for patients with high-risk disease.[30,31,147,149,150] However, given the dramatic improvement in outcomes with the use of ATRA-ATO, post–consolidation MRD monitoring can be avoided in patients with low-risk APL who achieve MRD-negative CR after completion of consolidation, due to the extreme rarity of relapse.[30,147] Although longitudinal comparative analysis of paired peripheral blood and BM samples for MRD monitoring showed greater sensitivity of MRD assessment on BM, peripheral blood monitoring is acceptable and may be utilized for post–consolidation MRD monitoring.[147,151]

Patients who have positive RT-PCR tests, on either BM or peripheral blood, on two separate occasions 2 to 4 weeks apart are considered to have MRD-positive disease.[18,19,21,30,147] Patients who fail to achieve MRD negativity by the end of consolidation therapy are considered to have molecular persistent disease.[21,30,147] However, change in the status of the PML-RARA by RT-PCR from undetectable to detectable, confirmed by repeat testing 2 to 4 weeks apart, is consistent with molecular relapse.[21,30,147] Both molecular persistence and molecular relapse are treated in a similar manner and will be discussed in subsequent sections.

Treatment-Related Complications

Differentiation Syndrome

DS, formerly known as retinoic acid syndrome, is a common complication in patients with APL undergoing induction therapy with ATRA and/or ATO.[91,152] The full-blown syndrome consists of unexplained fever, weight gain, volume overload, hypotension, dyspnea with interstitial pulmonary infiltrates, acute renal failure, and pleuropericardial effusion.[153] The reported incidence of DS is very broad ranging from 2% to 27%.[36,91,152,154-156] Reasons behind this variation in the incidence of DS may be attributed to the different diagnostic criteria used for DS as well as differences in the induction therapy and supportive care measures used in the treatment of APL.[91,152] Although the pathogenesis of DS is complex and remains largely unclear, release of proinflammatory cytokines, increased vascular permeability, and endothelial damage by the differentiating promyelocytes appear to be the major drivers behind this syndrome.[152,157,158] Cytokine release syndrome leads to the development of systemic inflammatory response syndrome, which manifests with unexplained fever, myalgia, hypotension, tachypnea, tachycardia, and even shock.[91,153,158] Furthermore, the increased vascular permeability and endothelial damage with capillary leak syndrome can also lead to weight gain (>5 kg), fluid overload, dyspnea, hypoxia, hypotension, peripheral and pulmonary edema, effusion, acute renal failure, organ hypoperfusion, distributive shock, and eventually multiorgan failure.[152,153] Therefore, early recognition and treatment of DS is essential to prevent the increased morbidity and potential life-threatening complications of this phenomenon.

The PETHEMA group analyzed 183 patients with newly diagnosed APL treated with AIDA regimen who developed DS; 93 patients with severe; and 90 with moderate DS.[91] There was a significant increase in age, serum creatinine level, WBC count, and coagulopathy among patients who developed DS.[91] Patients developed DS at a median of 12 days from start of therapy (range, 0-46 day) with a bimodal pattern of distribution observed in which peaks occurred during the first and third weeks of therapy. Severe DS occurred early in therapy (median of 6 days) compared to moderate DS (median of 15 days).[91] Dyspnea, interstitial pulmonary infiltrates, unexplained fever, weight gain (>5 kg), pleuropericardial effusions, and renal failure were more frequently seen in patients with severe DS compared to those with moderate DS.[91] In addition, the frequency of hypotension was significantly higher in late (>7 days from start of therapy) compared to early severe DS.[91]

Despite the lack of universally standardized diagnostic criteria for DS, experts in the field prefer the diagnostic criteria and grading system published by Montesinos et al that uses the following signs and symptoms originally described by Frankel et al. dyspnea, unexplained fever (≥38°C), weight gain (>5 kg), unexplained hypotension, acute renal failure, and radiographic evidence of either pulmonary infiltrates or pleuropericardial effusion.[91,152,153] Of importance, authors of this study did not consider any isolated sign or symptom sufficient to diagnose DS and alternative medical conditions that could explain the clinical presentation should be excluded prior to diagnosis. Patients were classified into 2 grades of severity: moderate: 2 or 3 of these features and severe: patients with 4 or more of these signs or symptoms.[91]

Upon first suspicion of DS, all patients should be started immediately on intravenous dexamethasone at a dose of 10 mg twice daily, an approach associated with significant reduction in DS-related mortality.[20,36,91,107,153,154,156] For patients who are on prednisone prophylaxis (0.5 mg/kg), steroids need to be converted to treatment dose of dexamethasone per the APL0406 trial.[20] It is crucial to rule out conditions that may mimic or occur concomitantly with DS, such as infection/sepsis, volume overload, pulmonary embolism, exacerbation of congestive heart failure, drug-induced anaphylaxis, and diffuse alveolar hemorrhage.[152] Since in many cases it may be clinically difficult to confidently distinguish between these conditions and DS, empiric therapy for both DS and these medical conditions may be warranted using steroids, diuretics, antimicrobials, etc., as clinically indicated. Patients who fail to improve after 24 hours of intravenous dexamethasone should have the dose increased to 10 mg every 6 hours. ATRA-ATO therapy should be continued unless patients develop severe DS, significant organ dysfunction such as respiratory or renal failure, or do not respond to at least 24 hours of dexamethasone therapy. Once symptoms have completely resolved for at least 3 days,[20] dexamethasone may be discontinued (either tapered off slowly or abruptly stopped) and ATRA/ATO may be restarted if held.

Supportive care, as previously discussed, is a key element in the treatment of patients with APL, especially those who develop DS. Strict daily weights are essential for all patients during induction therapy since an increase of more than 5 kg from baseline is considered a surrogate marker for impending DS warranting aggressive diuresis.[91,159] It should be noted that DS is never seen beyond remission induction therapy once patients achieve CR.

Role of Corticosteroid Prophylaxis

The role of corticosteroids as prophylaxis for DS remains largely unclear with no definitive randomized data supporting its routine use during remission induction treatment of APL. There has also been extreme heterogeneity among trials regarding the regimen used for prophylaxis: (1) in the APL0406 study, prednisone 0.5 mg/kg/d from start of therapy until the end of induction[20]; (2) MD Anderson Cancer Center protocols used methylprednisolone 50 mg/d for 5 days followed by a rapid taper in the absence of DS[18,19,21]; and (3) in the APML4 study, prednisone 1 mg/kg/d was administered prophylactically for all patients for at least 10 days regardless of risk status.[61] On the other hand, the Intergroup C9710, UK AML 17, and the SWOG 0535 did not use prophylactic steroids.[22,119,121]

Montesinos et al compared the incidence of severe DS among patients with newly diagnosed APL treated on two consecutive studies by the PETHEMA Group (LPA96 and LPA 99) using AIDA-based regimens but different corticosteroid prophylaxis. In the LPA96 trial, only patients with a WBC count >5 × 10^9/L (before or during therapy) received intravenous dexamethasone prophylaxis at a dose of 10 mg every 12 hours for 7 days, while in the LPA99 study all patients regardless of risk received prophylaxis using prednisone 0.5 mg/kg/d for 15 days during remission induction therapy.[91] The incidence of severe DS was significantly lower in patients enrolled on the LPA99 trial compared to those treated on the LPA96 trial (11.3% vs 16.6%, respectively; $P = .07$) suggesting potential benefit from routine use of corticosteroid prophylaxis regardless of WBC count.[91] Furthermore, there was no difference in the infectious mortality between the LPA96 and LPA99 trials confirming the safety of systemic use of prednisone prophylaxis in these patients.[83] Therefore, despite the lack of prospective randomized trials supporting the universal use of corticosteroid prophylaxis, most experts recommend using corticosteroid prophylaxis for all APL patients receiving ATRA + ATO-based therapy due to the dual differentiation effect regardless of WBC count. If corticosteroid prophylaxis was not implemented at start of therapy, it should be initiated in patients who develop either WBC counts higher than 5 × 10^9/L or serum creatinine above 1.4 mg/dL at any time during remission induction therapy due to their high risk of developing DS.[157]

TREATMENT OF RELAPSE AND ROLE OF STEM CELL TRANSPLANTATION

There are two major types of relapses in APL: (1) hematologic relapse is defined by the presence of more than 5% blasts plus abnormal promyelocytes in the BM or evidence of extramedullary disease; (2) confirmed molecular relapse is defined as PML-RARA detected by RT-PCR analysis in two consecutive BM samples performed 2 to 4 weeks apart.[19,21]

With the introduction of the ATRA-ATO combination regimen, relapse rates have dramatically declined and do not exceed 4%, with the majority of relapses occurring among high-risk patients.[20-22]

Two retrospective studies have shown a survival benefit of early treatment initiation in patients who develop molecular relapse compared to those who are treated at the time of hematologic relapse.[149,150] Therefore, patients with molecular persistence or molecular relapse should be immediately offered salvage therapy. As a single agent, ATO has shown to be highly effective in the treatment of patients with relapsed APL with CR rates ranging from 85% to 100%, molecular remission rates from 70% to 86%, and an OS rate of 50% to 80% at 1 to 2 years.[12,16,160-163] However, in these studies, ATO was not included in the front-line treatment of these patients. Therefore, with the current routine use of ATO in the frontline treatment of APL, it remains unclear whether ATO will retain its activity in the relapsed setting.

Choice of salvage therapy depends on the initial front-line regimen used and the duration of first CR (CR1). Patients who remain in CR for more than 2 years prior to the first relapse may be treated using the same initial regimen used to achieve CR1.[30] Per NCCN guidelines, patients who develop late relapses (≥6 months) after an ATO-based regimen may be retreated using ATO ± ATRO ± GO.[126] Otherwise, patients with molecular persistence or relapse after ATRA-ATO may be offered ATRA plus chemotherapy as salvage therapy and vice versa.[30] GO is another very attractive agent to be considered in situations of molecular persistence or relapse given its high activity in APL. Lo-Coco et al treated 16 APL patients in molecular relapse using GO (6 mg/m² for 2 or 3 doses) with 14 patients (88%) achieving complete molecular remission.[164] Of these 14 responders, 7 remained in sustained complete molecular remission and 7 experienced molecular relapse; 2 of the latter group achieved another molecular remission with repeat GO therapy. In line with other studies, these results indicate that GO is highly effective in the treatment of molecularly relapsed patients including those with advanced, heavily pretreated disease.[164,165] According to the MD Anderson protocol, patients who develop a hematologic or molecular relapse or have molecular persistent disease were treated with GO (9 mg/m²) once every 4 to 5 weeks for 3 months while continuing ATRA-ATO therapy, or resuming in patients who discontinued therapy.[18,19,21] In patients who converted to MRD negativity, treatment with ATRA-ATO plus GO was continued for an additional 3 months.[18,19,21] Although GO is an attractive agent for salvage therapy, it is associated with high risk of veno-occlusive disease/sinusoidal obstructive syndrome in patients who proceed to hematopoietic stem cell transplantation (HSCT).

Regardless of the type of salvage regimen, the ultimate goal is to achieve molecular remission as a bridge to HSCT, which offers the best chance for cure.[30,166] The choice between autologous and allogenic HSCT depends on multiple factors such as age, donor availability, and MRD status, with no strict guidelines to aid in the decision-making. Autologous HSCT should be considered in patients with prolonged CR1 (>1 year) who achieve MRD negativity prior to stem cell collection since this approach is associated with favorable survival outcomes, better tolerability due to absence of graft-versus-host disease, and significantly lower treatment-related mortality, when compared to allogeneic HSCT.[31,167-171] Allogeneic HSCT should be recommended for patients who have multiply relapsed or refractory APL, have a short CR1 duration (<1 year), or are MRD positive at the time of transplant, due to the greater antileukemic activity provided by the graft-versus-leukemia effect.[31,167,172]

About 5% of all relapses in APL have a CNS component and therefore CNS involvement should be ruled out in patients who develop hematologic or molecular relapse.[31,173,174] Treatment of extramedullary relapses, particularly CNS relapses, is challenging due to paucity of data. Similar to other forms of leukemia, patients with CNS relapse are offered intrathecal chemotherapy, using methotrexate, cytarabine, and hydrocortisone, along with systemic therapy since CNS relapses are almost invariably accompanied with hematologic or molecular relapse.[31] Either ATRA-ATO or chemotherapy-based regimens with high CNS penetration, such as high-dose cytarabine, are acceptable salvage regimens in these patients. Preferably, patients should be offered autologous or allogeneic HSCT as consolidation therapy.[31]

SPECIAL CONSIDERATIONS

Therapy-Related APL

Therapy-related APL (t-APL) accounts for about 3% to 22% of cases of therapy-related AML (t-AML) and comprises up to 12% of all APL cases.[31,175] Median age at the time of diagnosis is 47 years with a slight female predominance.[175] Topoisomerase II inhibitors and radiation therapy are the most common inciting risk factors for the development of t-APL.[31,175] Unlike other forms of t-AML, t-APL occurs at a median of 2 years following the treatment of the primary antecedent condition (most commonly breast cancer, lymphoma, and genitourinary malignancies) without a preleukemic or myelodysplastic phase.[31,175] Interestingly, the risk of developing t-APL rapidly diminishes after the peak incidence at 2 years.[175] Similar to de novo APL, isolated t(15;17) is the sole cytogenetic abnormality in the majority of patients.[31,175] Furthermore, patients with t-APL should be treated identically as de novo APL with similar favorable outcomes.[31,175,176] Front-line treatment using ATRA-ATO has been shown to be effective in the treatment of t-APL.[176] In addition to its efficacy in t-APL, ATRA-ATO may be a preferred regimen in these patients where the use of anthracyclines may be limited by prior anthracycline exposure and cardiac toxicity.[30,31,176]

Treatment of the Elderly and Those Patients With Comorbidities

The superiority of ATRA-ATO over ATRA-chemotherapy in patients with low-risk APL allows treatment de-escalation with complete omission of chemotherapy in these patients sparing them the toxicities associated with the use of cytotoxic chemotherapy, such as myelosuppression, anthracycline-induced cardiotoxicity, and T-MN. This is particularly beneficial in patients who are unfit for chemotherapy due to older age or comorbidities which account for up to 20% of APL cases.[21,22,119] Of 104 older patients (≥60 years) with newly diagnosed APL treated on 2 successive PETHEMA studies (LPA96 and LPA99) using ATRA plus chemotherapy, there was a significant increase in the mortality rate in CR from 3% in patients younger than 70 years to 24% in those older than 70 year of age.[177] In the APML4 trial, exploratory subgroup analysis again showed an increased risk of early death in patients over the age of 70 compared to patients aged 70 years or younger [odds ratio 21.2, 95% CI 1.3-350); $P = .016$).[60] These results suggest the importance of using a chemotherapy-free regimen in older APL patients particularly since the incidence of low-risk disease is significantly higher in the elderly population compared to younger patients.[177]

The GIMEMA group recently published results of the amended AIDA 0493 protocol designed for patients with APL above 60 years of age, utilizing induction with ATRA plus idarubicin, followed by a single course of consolidation with idarubicin plus cytarabine and maintenance with intermittent ATRA.[178] Using this attenuated regimen, the 5-year OS and DFS rates were 76.1% and 64.6%, respectively.[178] These results are similar to those published by Abaza et al, which reported a 5-year OS and DFS rates of 74% and 97%, respectively, in elderly APL patients (≥60) treated with ATRA-ATO plus GO.[21]

Therefore, despite limited experience, ATRA-ATO plus GO (for high-risk patients) seems to be a very reasonable chemotherapy-free strategy for the front-line treatment of older and younger patients with severe comorbidities unfit for chemotherapy.[30] As with younger patients, the aim of therapy should be to achieve molecular remission at the end of consolidation due to the favorable nature of this disease.[31]

FUTURE DIRECTIONS

Administration of ATO intravenously 5 days a week for 4 consecutive weeks in an 8-week cycle for a total of 4 cycles of consolidation is associated with increased risk for noncompliance, burden on outpatient infusion centers, risk and expense of maintaining suitable vascular access, and increased medical costs with risk for financial toxicity. Therefore, there are huge efforts toward substitution with oral formulations of ATO that are bioequivalent to intravenous ATO.[179-181] There are data to suggest that oral ATO is associated with reduced cardiac toxicity, including QTc prolongation and ventricular arrhythmias, compared to intravenous ATO which may be attributed to the potentially favorable pharmacokinetic profile of the oral formulation.[182]

A randomized, multicenter, phase III noninferiority trial conducted in China compared oral arsenic (Realgar-*Indigo naturalis* formula, RIF) to intravenous ATO as both induction and maintenance therapies in patients with newly diagnosed APL.[180] Two hundred and forty-two patients with APL were randomly assigned to either oral RIF or intravenous ATO combined with low-dose ATRA (25 mg/m^2) during induction followed by three cycles of consolidation chemotherapy and maintenance therapy with sequential ATRA followed by either RIF or intravenous ATO for a total of 2 years.[180] With a median follow-up of 39 months, there was no significant difference in the 2-year DFS, CR rate, 3-year OS, or rates of adverse events between both groups confirming noninferiority of oral RIF plus ATRA as the front-line treatment in APL.[180] Authors of this study also showed a significant reduction in the medical costs and length of hospitalization during induction in APL patients treated with oral arsenic compared to intravenous ATO.[183]

To assess the activity of oral arsenic (RIF) plus ATRA without chemotherapy, Zhu et al conducted another single-center pilot study in which 20 patients with low-risk APL received oral arsenic plus ATRA induction/consolidation, using a schedule similar to Lo-Coco et al, with complete molecular response as the primary end point.[184] With a median follow-up of 14 months, all patients achieved hematologic CR at a median of 29.5 days and complete molecular remission at 6 months. Out of these 20 patients, 10 completed the induction therapy on an outpatient basis, without hospitalization. Patients resumed their normal lifestyle during consolidation therapy with near-normal quality of life.[184] Other novel oral formulations of ATO, including the encapsulated oral ATO (Phebra, Australia) and ORH-2014, have also shown comparable oral bioavailability to intravenous ATO and are potential oral options for the treatment of APL.[185,186]

Results of these studies suggest that oral formulations of ATO combined with ATRA have the strong potential to provide a more convenient, safe, and cost-effective measure for outpatient management of APL. Multicenter, prospective, randomized trials assessing the efficacy and safety of oral ATO combined with ATRA in patients with newly diagnosed APL are currently under way in the United States.

CONCLUSION

APL is a highly curable form of AML. Advances made in the treatment of APL have been one of the greatest success stories of AML history and a true testament to the power of translational research and development of targeted therapy. Despite these advances, early mortality due to coagulopathy and catastrophic bleeding remains the major cause of death in patients with APL, underscoring the importance of early diagnosis and treatment. National efforts are directed toward the development of a widely implemented patient care model through academic-community partnership with the aim of reducing induction mortality and improving patient outcomes. Future oral formulations of ATO provide the hope for a more convenient all-oral combination regimen for APL.

References

1. Tallman MS, Altman JK. Curative strategies in acute promyelocytic leukemia. *Hematology Am Soc Hematol Educ Program*. 2008;2008:391-399.
2. Kakizuka A, Miller WH, Jr, Umesono K, et al. Chromosomal translocation t(15;17) in human acute promyelocytic leukemia fuses RAR alpha with a novel putative transcription factor. *PML Cell*. 1991;66:663-674.
3. Shao W, Fanelli M, Ferrara FF, et al. Arsenic trioxide as an inducer of apoptosis and loss of PML/RAR alpha protein in acute promyelocytic leukemia cells. *J Natl Cancer Inst*. 1998;90:124-133.
4. Grignani F, Ferrucci PF, Testa U, et al. The acute promyelocytic leukemia-specific PML-RAR alpha fusion protein inhibits differentiation and promotes survival of myeloid precursor cells. *Cell*. 1993;74:423-431.
5. Sasaki K, Ravandi F, Kadia TM, et al. De novo acute myeloid leukemia: a population-based study of outcome in the United States based on the Surveillance, Epidemiology, and End Results (SEER) database, 1980 to 2017. *Cancer*. 2021;127:2049-2061.
6. Warrell RP, Jr, Frankel SR, Miller WH, Jr, et al. Differentiation therapy of acute promyelocytic leukemia with tretinoin (all-trans-retinoic acid). *N Engl J Med*. 1991;324:1385-1393.
7. Raelson JV, Nervi C, Rosenauer A, et al. The PML/RAR alpha oncoprotein is a direct molecular target of retinoic acid in acute promyelocytic leukemia cells. *Blood*. 1996;88:2826-2832.
8. Yoshida H, Kitamura K, Tanaka K, et al. Accelerated degradation of PML-retinoic acid receptor alpha (PML-RARA) oncoprotein by all-trans-retinoic acid in acute promyelocytic leukemia: possible role of the proteasome pathway. *Cancer Res*. 1996;56:2945-2948.
9. Castaigne S, Chomienne C, Daniel MT, et al. All-trans retinoic acid as a differentiation therapy for acute promyelocytic leukemia. I. Clinical results. *Blood*. 1990;76:1704-1709.
10. Chen ZX, Xue YQ, Zhang R, et al. A clinical and experimental study on all-trans retinoic acid-treated acute promyelocytic leukemia patients. *Blood*. 1991;78:1413-1419.
11. Shen ZX, Chen GQ, Ni JH, et al. Use of arsenic trioxide (As$_2$O$_3$) in the treatment of acute promyelocytic leukemia (APL): II. Clinical efficacy and pharmacokinetics in relapsed patients. *Blood*. 1997;89:3354-3360.
12. Soignet SL, Frankel SR, Douer D, et al. United States multicenter study of arsenic trioxide in relapsed acute promyelocytic leukemia. *J Clin Oncol*. 2001;19:3852-3860.

13. Ghavamzadeh A, Alimoghaddam K, Rostami S, et al. Phase II study of single-agent arsenic trioxide for the front-line therapy of acute promyelocytic leukemia. *J Clin Oncol*. 2011;29:2753-2757.
14. Mathews V, George B, Lakshmi KM, et al. Single-agent arsenic trioxide in the treatment of newly diagnosed acute promyelocytic leukemia: durable remissions with minimal toxicity. *Blood*. 2006;107:2627-2632.
15. Mathews V, George B, Chendamarai E, et al. Single-agent arsenic trioxide in the treatment of newly diagnosed acute promyelocytic leukemia: long-term follow-up data. *J Clin Oncol*. 2010;28:3866-3871.
16. Lazo G, Kantarjian H, Estey E, et al. Use of arsenic trioxide (As_2O_3) in the treatment of patients with acute promyelocytic leukemia: the M. D. Anderson experience. *Cancer*. 2003;97:2218-2224.
17. Lallemand-Breitenbach V, Guillemin MC, Janin A, et al. Retinoic acid and arsenic synergize to eradicate leukemic cells in a mouse model of acute promyelocytic leukemia. *J Exp Med*. 1999;189:1043-1052.
18. Estey E, Garcia-Manero G, Ferrajoli A, et al. Use of all-trans retinoic acid plus arsenic trioxide as an alternative to chemotherapy in untreated acute promyelocytic leukemia. *Blood*. 2006;107:3469-3473.
19. Ravandi F, Estey E, Jones D, et al. Effective treatment of acute promyelocytic leukemia with all-trans-retinoic acid, arsenic trioxide, and gemtuzumab ozogamicin. *J Clin Oncol*. 2009;27:504-510.
20. Lo-Coco F, Avvisati G, Vignetti M, et al. Retinoic acid and arsenic trioxide for acute promyelocytic leukemia. *N Engl J Med*. 2013;369:111-121.
21. Abaza Y, Kantarjian H, Garcia-Manero G, et al. Long-term outcome of acute promyelocytic leukemia treated with all-trans-retinoic acid, arsenic trioxide, and gemtuzumab. *Blood*. 2017;129:1275-1283.
22. Burnett AK, Russell NH, Hills RK, et al. Arsenic trioxide and all-trans retinoic acid treatment for acute promyelocytic leukaemia in all risk groups (AML17): results of a randomised, controlled, phase 3 trial. *Lancet Oncol*. 2015;16:1295-1305.
23. Lehmann S, Ravn A, Carlsson L, et al. Continuing high early death rate in acute promyelocytic leukemia: a population-based report from the Swedish Adult Acute Leukemia Registry. *Leukemia*. 2011;25:1128-1134.
24. Dores GM, Devesa SS, Curtis RE, Linet MS, Morton LM. Acute leukemia incidence and patient survival among children and adults in the United States, 2001-2007. *Blood*. 2012;119(1):34-43. doi:10.1182/blood-2011-04-347872
25. Guru Murthy GS, Szabo A, Michaelis L, et al. Improving outcomes of acute promyelocytic leukemia in the current era: analysis of the SEER database. *J Natl Compr Cancer Netw*. 2020;18(2):169-175. doi:10.6004/jnccn.2019.7351
26. Kamath GR, Tremblay D, Coltoff A, et al. Comparing the epidemiology, clinical characteristics and prognostic factors of acute myeloid leukemia with and without acute promyelocytic leukemia. *Carcinogenesis*. 2019;40(5):651-660. doi:10.1093/carcin/bgz014
27. Matasar MJ, Ritchie EK, Consedine N, Magai C, Neugut AI. Incidence rates of acute promyelocytic leukemia among Hispanics, blacks, Asians, and non-Hispanic whites in the United States. *Eur J Cancer Prev*. 2006;15(4):367-370. doi:10.1097/00008469-200608000-00011
28. Estey E, Thall P, Kantarjian H, Pierce S, Kornblau S, Keating M. Association between increased body mass index and a diagnosis of acute promyelocytic leukemia in patients with acute myeloid leukemia. *Leukemia*. 1997;11(10):1661-1664. doi:10.1038/sj.leu.2400783
29. Gilbert RD, Karabus CD, Mills AE. Acute promyelocytic leukemia. A childhood cluster. *Cancer*. 1987;59(5):933-935. doi:10.1002/1097-0142(19870301)59:5<933::aid-cncr2820590513>3.0.co;2-r
30. Sanz MA, Fenaux P, Tallman MS, et al. Management of acute promyelocytic leukemia: updated recommendations from an expert panel of the European LeukemiaNet. *Blood*. 2019;133:1630-1643.
31. Sanz MA, Grimwade D, Tallman MS, et al. Management of acute promyelocytic leukemia: recommendations from an expert panel on behalf of the European LeukemiaNet. *Blood*. 2009;113:1875-1891.
32. Bennett JM, Catovsky D, Daniel MT, et al. Proposals for the classification of the acute leukaemias. French-American-British (FAB) co-operative group. *Br J Haematol*. 1976;33:451-458.
33. Bennett JM, Catovsky D, Daniel MT, et al. Proposed revised criteria for the classification of acute myeloid leukemia. A report of the French-American-British Cooperative Group. *Ann Intern Med*. 1985;103:620-625.
34. Drewinko B, Bollinger P, Brailas C, et al. Flow cytochemical patterns of white blood cells in human haematopoietic malignancies. I. Acute leukaemias. *Br J Haematol*. 1987;66:27-36.
35. Krause JR, Stolc V, Kaplan SS, et al. Microgranular promyelocytic leukemia: a multiparameter examination. *Am J Hematol*. 1989;30:158-163.
36. Vahdat L, Maslak P, Miller WH, Jr, et al. Early mortality and the retinoic acid syndrome in acute promyelocytic leukemia: impact of leukocytosis, low-dose chemotherapy, PMN/RAR-alpha isoform, and CD13 expression in patients treated with all-trans retinoic acid. *Blood*. 1994;84:3843-3849.
37. Das Gupta A, Sapre RS, Shah AS, et al. Cytochemical and immunophenotypic heterogeneity in acute promyelocytic leukemia. *Acta Haematol*. 1989;81:5-9.
38. Paietta E, Andersen J, Gallagher R, et al. The immunophenotype of acute promyelocytic leukemia (APL): an ECOG study. *Leukemia*. 1994;8:1108-1112.
39. Larson RA, Kondo K, Vardiman JW, et al. Evidence for a 15;17 translocation in every patient with acute promyelocytic leukemia. *Am J Med*. 1984;76:827-841.
40. Rowley JD, Golomb HM, Dougherty C. 15/17 translocation, a consistent chromosomal change in acute promyelocytic leukaemia. *Lancet*. 1977;1:549-550.
41. de The H, Chomienne C, Lanotte M, et al. The t(15;17) translocation of acute promyelocytic leukaemia fuses the retinoic acid receptor alpha gene to a novel transcribed locus. *Nature*. 1990;347:558-561.
42. de The H, Lavau C, Marchio A, et al. The PML-RAR alpha fusion mRNA generated by the t(15;17) translocation in acute promyelocytic leukemia encodes a functionally altered RAR. *Cell*. 1991;66:675-684.
43. Guglielmi C, Martelli MP, Diverio D, et al. Immunophenotype of adult and childhood acute promyelocytic leukaemia: correlation with morphology, type of PML gene breakpoint and clinical outcome. A cooperative Italian study on 196 cases. *Br J Haematol*. 1998;102:1035-1041.
44. Gallagher RE, Willman CL, Slack JL, et al. Association of PML-RAR alpha fusion mRNA type with pretreatment hematologic characteristics but not treatment outcome in acute promyelocytic leukemia: an intergroup molecular study. *Blood*. 1997;90:1656-1663.
45. Sobas M, Talarn-Forcadell MC, Martinez-Cuadron D, et al. PLZF-RARalpha, NPM1-RARalpha, and other acute promyelocytic leukemia variants: the PETHEMA registry experience and systematic literature review. *Cancers (Basel)*. 2020;12:1313.
46. Hernandez JM, Martin G, Gutierrez NC, et al. Additional cytogenetic changes do not influence the outcome of patients with newly diagnosed acute promyelocytic leukemia treated with an ATRA plus anthracyclin based protocol. A report of the Spanish group PETHEMA. *Haematologica*. 2001;86:807-813.
47. Johansson B, Mertens F, Mitelman F. Secondary chromosomal abnormalities in acute leukemias. *Leukemia*. 1994;8:953-962.
48. Slack JL, Arthur DC, Lawrence D, et al. Secondary cytogenetic changes in acute promyelocytic leukemia–prognostic importance in patients treated with chemotherapy alone and association with the intron 3 breakpoint of the PML gene: a Cancer and Leukemia Group B study. *J Clin Oncol*. 1997;15:1786-1795.
49. Schoch C, Haase D, Haferlach T, et al. Incidence and implication of additional chromosome aberrations in acute promyelocytic leukaemia with translocation t(15;17)(q22;q21): a report on 50 patients. *Br J Haematol*. 1996;94:493-500.
50. Wang ZY, Chen Z. Acute promyelocytic leukemia: from highly fatal to highly curable. *Blood*. 2008;111:2505-2515.
51. Barragan E, Montesinos P, Camos M, et al. Prognostic value of FLT3 mutations in patients with acute promyelocytic leukemia treated with all-trans retinoic acid and anthracycline monochemotherapy. *Haematologica*. 2011;96:1470-1477.
52. Gale RE, Hills R, Pizzey AR, et al. Relationship between FLT3 mutation status, biologic characteristics, and response to targeted therapy in acute promyelocytic leukemia. *Blood*. 2005;106:3768-3776.
53. Schnittger S, Bacher U, Haferlach C, et al. Clinical impact of FLT3 mutation load in acute promyelocytic leukemia with t(15;17)/PML-RARA. *Haematologica*. 2011;96:1799-1807.
54. Choudhary C, Schwable J, Brandts C, et al. AML-associated Flt3 kinase domain mutations show signal transduction differences compared with Flt3 ITD mutations. *Blood*. 2005;106:265-273.
55. Grundler R, Miething C, Thiede C, et al. FLT3-ITD and tyrosine kinase domain mutants induce 2 distinct phenotypes in a murine bone marrow transplantation model. *Blood*. 2005;105:4792-4799.
56. Marcucci G, Maharry K, Whitman SP, et al. High expression levels of the ETS-related gene, ERG, predict adverse outcome and improve molecular risk-based classification of cytogenetically normal acute myeloid leukemia: a Cancer and Leukemia Group B Study. *J Clin Oncol*. 2007;25:3337-3343.
57. Schlenk RF, Dohner K, Krauter J, et al. Mutations and treatment outcome in cytogenetically normal acute myeloid leukemia. *N Engl J Med*. 2008;358:1909-1918.
58. Beitinjaneh A, Jang S, Roukoz H, et al. Prognostic significance of FLT3 internal tandem duplication and tyrosine kinase domain mutations in acute promyelocytic leukemia: a systematic review. *Leuk Res*. 2010;34:831-836.
59. Cicconi L, Divona M, Ciardi C, et al. PML-RARalpha kinetics and impact of FLT3-ITD mutations in newly diagnosed acute promyelocytic leukaemia treated with ATRA and ATO or ATRA and chemotherapy. *Leukemia*. 2016;30:1987-1992.
60. Iland HJ, Collins M, Bradstock K, et al. Use of arsenic trioxide in remission induction and consolidation therapy for acute promyelocytic leukaemia in the Australasian Leukaemia and Lymphoma Group (ALLG) APML4 study: a non-randomised phase 2 trial. *Lancet Haematol*. 2015;2:e357-e366.
61. Iland HJ, Bradstock K, Supple SG, et al. All-trans-retinoic acid, idarubicin, and IV arsenic trioxide as initial therapy in acute promyelocytic leukemia (APML4). *Blood*. 2012;120:1570-1580. quiz 1752.
62. Guidez F, Ivins S, Zhu J, Söderström M, Waxman S, Zelent A. Reduced retinoic acid-sensitivities of nuclear receptor corepressor binding to PML-and PLZF-RARα underlie molecular pathogenesis and treatment of acute promyelocytic leukemia. *Blood*. 1998;91:2634-2642.
63. Heinzel T, Lavinsky RM, Mullen TM, et al. A complex containing N-CoR, mSin3 and histone deacetylase mediates transcriptional repression. *Nature*. 1997;387:43-48.
64. Hong SH, David G, Wong CW, Dejean A, Privalsky ML. SMRT corepressor interacts with PLZF and with the PML-retinoic acid receptor alpha (RARalpha) and PLZF-RARalpha oncoproteins associated with acute promyelocytic leukemia. *Proc Natl Acad Sci U S A*. 1997;94:9028-9033.
65. Lin RJ, Nagy L, Inoue S, Shao W, Miller WH, Jr, Evans RM. Role of the histone deacetylase complex in acute promyelocytic leukaemia. *Nature*. 1998;391:811-814.
66. Utley RT, Ikeda K, Grant PA, et al. Transcriptional activators direct histone acetyltransferase complexes to nucleosomes. *Nature*. 1998;394:498-502.
67. He LZ, Guidez F, Tribioli C, et al. Distinct interactions of PML-RARalpha and PLZF-RARalpha with co-repressors determine differential responses to RA in APL. *Nat Genet*. 1998;18:126-135.
68. Rego EM, Wang ZG, Peruzzi D, He LZ, Cordon-Cardo C, Pandolfi PP. Role of promyelocytic leukemia (PML) protein in tumor suppression. *J Exp Med*. 2001;193:521-529.

69. Wang ZG, Delva L, Gaboli M, et al. Role of PML in cell growth and the retinoic acid pathway. *Science*. 1998;279:1547-1551.
70. Wang ZG, Ruggero D, Ronchetti S, et al. PML is essential for multiple apoptotic pathways. *Nat Genet*. 1998;20:266-272.
71. Ono R, Masuya M, Ishii S, Katayama N, Nosaka T. Eya2, a target activated by Plzf, is critical for PLZF-RARA-Induced Leukemogenesis. *Mol Cell Biol*. 2017;37:e00585-16.
72. Mantha S, Tallman MS, Devlin SM, et al. Predictive factors of fatal bleeding in acute promyelocytic leukemia. *Thromb Res*. 2018;164(suppl 1):S98-S102.
73. Park JH, Qiao B, Panageas KS, et al. Early death rate in acute promyelocytic leukemia remains high despite all-trans retinoic acid. *Blood*. 2011;118:1248-1254.
74. Sanz MA, Montesinos P. Advances in the management of coagulopathy in acute promyelocytic leukemia. *Thromb Res*. 2020;191(suppl 1):S63-S67.
75. Gouault Heilmann M, Chardon E, Sultan C, et al. The procoagulant factor of leukaemic promyelocytes: demonstration of immunologic cross reactivity with human brain tissue factor. *Br J Haematol*. 1975;30:151-158.
76. Zhu J, Guo WM, Yao YY, et al. Tissue factors on acute promyelocytic leukemia and endothelial cells are differently regulated by retinoic acid, arsenic trioxide and chemotherapeutic agents. *Leukemia*. 1999;13:1062-1070.
77. Lavallee VP, Chagraoui J, MacRae T, et al. Transcriptomic landscape of acute promyelocytic leukemia reveals aberrant surface expression of the platelet aggregation agonist Podoplanin. *Leukemia*. 2018;32:1349-1357.
78. Liu Y, Wang Z, Jiang M, et al. The expression of annexin II and its role in the fibrinolytic activity in acute promyelocytic leukemia. *Leuk Res*. 2011;35:879-884.
79. Menell JS, Cesarman GM, Jacovina AT, et al. Annexin II and bleeding in acute promyelocytic leukemia. *N Engl J Med*. 1999;340:994-1004.
80. Dombret H, Scrobohaci ML, Daniel MT, et al. In vivo thrombin and plasmin activities in patients with acute promyelocytic leukemia (APL): effect of all-trans retinoic acid (ATRA) therapy. *Leukemia*. 1995;9:19-24.
81. De Stefano V, Sora F, Rossi E, et al. The risk of thrombosis in patients with acute leukemia: occurrence of thrombosis at diagnosis and during treatment. *J Thromb Haemostasis*. 2005;3:1985-1992.
82. Mitrovic M, Suvajdzic N, Elezovic I, et al. Thrombotic events in acute promyelocytic leukemia. *Thromb Res*. 2015;135:588-593.
83. de la Serna J, Montesinos P, Vellenga E, et al. Causes and prognostic factors of remission induction failure in patients with acute promyelocytic leukemia treated with all-trans retinoic acid and idarubicin. *Blood*. 2008;111:3395-3402.
84. Mantha S, Goldman DA, Devlin SM, et al. Determinants of fatal bleeding during induction therapy for acute promyelocytic leukemia in the ATRA era. *Blood*. 2017;129:1763-1767.
85. Asou N, Adachi K, Tamura J, et al. Analysis of prognostic factors in newly diagnosed acute promyelocytic leukemia treated with all-trans retinoic acid and chemotherapy. Japan Adult Leukemia Study Group. *J Clin Oncol*. 1998;16:78-85.
86. Avvisati G, Lo Coco F, Diverio D, et al. AIDA (all-trans retinoic acid + idarubicin) in newly diagnosed acute promyelocytic leukemia: a Gruppo Italiano Malattie Ematologiche Maligne dell'Adulto (GIMEMA) pilot study. *Blood*. 1996;88:1390-1398.
87. Fenaux P, Chastang C, Chevret S, et al. A randomized comparison of all transretinoic acid (ATRA) followed by chemotherapy and ATRA plus chemotherapy and the role of maintenance therapy in newly diagnosed acute promyelocytic leukemia. The European APL Group. *Blood*. 1999;94:1192-1200.
88. Tallman MS, Andersen JW, Schiffer CA, et al. All-trans-retinoic acid in acute promyelocytic leukemia. *N Engl J Med*. 1997;337:1021-1028.
89. Breccia M, Latagliata R, Cannella L, et al. Early hemorrhagic death before starting therapy in acute promyelocytic leukemia: association with high WBC count, late diagnosis and delayed treatment initiation. *Haematologica*. 2010;95:853-854.
90. Jillella AP, Arellano ML, Gaddh M, et al. Comanagement strategy between academic institutions and community practices to reduce induction mortality in acute promyelocytic leukemia. *JCO Oncol Pract*. 2021;17:e497-e505.
91. Montesinos P, Bergua JM, Vellenga E, et al. Differentiation syndrome in patients with acute promyelocytic leukemia treated with all-trans retinoic acid and anthracycline chemotherapy: characteristics, outcome, and prognostic factors. *Blood*. 2009;113:775-783.
92. Falanga ARL, Montesinos P. Acute promyelocytic leukemia coagulopathy in oussama abla FLC. In: Sanz M, ed. *Acute Promyelocytic Leukemia*. Springer; 2018:55-70.
93. Breccia M, Avvisati G, Latagliata R, et al. Occurrence of thrombotic events in acute promyelocytic leukemia correlates with consistent immunophenotypic and molecular features. *Leukemia*. 2007;21:79-83.
94. Hillestad LK. Acute promyelocytic leukemia. *Acta Med Scand*. 1957;159:189-194.
95. Kantarjian HM, Keating MJ, Walters RS, et al. Acute promyelocytic leukemia. M.D. Anderson Hospital experience. *Am J Med*. 1986;80:789-797.
96. Marty M, Ganem G, Fischer J, et al. Acute promyelocytic leukemia: retrospective study of 119 patients treated with daunorubicin. [Article in French] *Nouv Rev Fr Hematol*. 1984;26:371-378.
97. Avvisati G, Mandelli F, Petti MC, et al. Idarubicin (4-demethoxydaunorubicin) as single agent for remission induction of previously untreated acute promyelocytic leukemia: a pilot study of the Italian cooperative group GIMEMA. *Eur J Haematol*. 1990;44:257-260.
98. Petti MC, Avvisati G, Amadori S, et al. Acute promyelocytic leukemia: clinical aspects and results of treatment in 62 patients. *Haematologica*. 1987;72:151-155.
99. Cunningham I, Gee TS, Reich LM, et al. Acute promyelocytic leukemia: treatment results during a decade at Memorial Hospital. *Blood*. 1989;73:1116-1122.
100. Fenaux P, Pollet JP, Vandenbossche-Simon L, et al. Treatment of acute promyelocytic leukemia: a report of 70 cases. *Leuk Lymphoma*. 1991;4:239-248.
101. Rodeghiero F, Avvisati G, Castaman G, et al. Early deaths and anti-hemorrhagic treatments in acute promyelocytic leukemia. A GIMEMA retrospective study in 268 consecutive patients. *Blood*. 1990;75:2112-2117.
102. Warrell RP, Jr, de The H, Wang ZY, et al. Acute promyelocytic leukemia. *N Engl J Med*. 1993;329:177-189.
103. Avvisati G, Petti MC, Lo-Coco F, et al. Induction therapy with idarubicin alone significantly influences event-free survival duration in patients with newly diagnosed hypergranular acute promyelocytic leukemia: final results of the GIMEMA randomized study LAP 0389 with 7 years of minimal follow-up. *Blood*. 2002;100:3141-3146.
104. Huang ME, Ye YC, Chen SR, et al. Use of all-trans retinoic acid in the treatment of acute promyelocytic leukemia. *Blood*. 1988;72:567-572.
105. Ades L, Guerci A, Raffoux E, et al. Very long-term outcome of acute promyelocytic leukemia after treatment with all-trans retinoic acid and chemotherapy: the European APL Group experience. *Blood*. 2010;115:1690-1696.
106. Lengfelder E, Reichert A, Schoch C, et al. Double induction strategy including high dose cytarabine in combination with all-trans retinoic acid: effects in patients with newly diagnosed acute promyelocytic leukemia. German AML Cooperative Group. *Leukemia*. 2000;14:1362-1370.
107. Mandelli F, Diverio D, Avvisati G, et al. Molecular remission in PML/RAR alpha-positive acute promyelocytic leukemia by combined all-trans retinoic acid and idarubicin (AIDA) therapy. Gruppo Italiano-Malattie Ematologiche Maligne dell'Adulto and Associazione Italiana di Ematologia ed Oncologia Pediatrica Cooperative Groups. *Blood*. 1997;90:1014-1021.
108. Fenaux P, Le Deley MC, Castaigne S, et al. Effect of all transretinoic acid in newly diagnosed acute promyelocytic leukemia. Results of a multicenter randomized trial. European APL 91 Group. *Blood*. 1993;82:3241-3249.
109. Sanz MA, Martin G, Rayon C, et al. A modified AIDA protocol with anthracycline-based consolidation results in high antileukemic efficacy and reduced toxicity in newly diagnosed PML/RARalpha-positive acute promyelocytic leukemia. PETHEMA group. *Blood*. 1999;94:3015-3021.
110. Asou N, Kishimoto Y, Kiyoi H, et al. A randomized study with or without intensified maintenance chemotherapy in patients with acute promyelocytic leukemia who have become negative for PML-RARalpha transcript after consolidation therapy: the Japan Adult Leukemia Study Group (JALSG) APL97 study. *Blood*. 2007;110:59-66.
111. Avvisati G, Lo-Coco F, Paoloni FP, et al. AIDA 0493 protocol for newly diagnosed acute promyelocytic leukemia: very long-term results and role of maintenance. *Blood*. 2011;117:4716-4725.
112. Burnett AK, Hills RK, Grimwade D, et al. Inclusion of chemotherapy in addition to anthracycline in the treatment of acute promyelocytic leukaemia does not improve outcomes: results of the MRC AML15 trial. *Leukemia*. 2013;27:843-851.
113. Lengfelder E, Haferlach C, Saussele S, et al. High dose ara-C in the treatment of newly diagnosed acute promyelocytic leukemia: long-term results of the German AMLCG. *Leukemia*. 2009;23:2248-2258.
114. Lo-Coco F, Avvisati G, Vignetti M, et al. Front-line treatment of acute promyelocytic leukemia with AIDA induction followed by risk-adapted consolidation for adults younger than 61 years: results of the AIDA-2000 trial of the GIMEMA Group. *Blood*. 2010;116:3171-3179.
115. Sanz MA, Montesinos P, Rayon C, et al. Risk-adapted treatment of acute promyelocytic leukemia based on all-trans retinoic acid and anthracycline with addition of cytarabine in consolidation therapy for high-risk patients: further improvements in treatment outcome. *Blood*. 2010;115:5137-5146.
116. Tallman MS, Andersen JW, Schiffer CA, et al. All-trans retinoic acid in acute promyelocytic leukemia: long-term outcome and prognostic factor analysis from the North American Intergroup protocol. *Blood*. 2002;100:4298-4302.
117. Shen ZX, Shi ZZ, Fang J, et al. All-trans retinoic acid/As2O3 combination yields a high quality remission and survival in newly diagnosed acute promyelocytic leukemia. *Proc Natl Acad Sci U S A*. 2004;101:5328-5335.
118. Hu J, Liu YF, Wu CF, et al. Long-term efficacy and safety of all-trans retinoic acid/arsenic trioxide-based therapy in newly diagnosed acute promyelocytic leukemia. *Proc Natl Acad Sci U S A*. 2009;106:3342-3347.
119. Powell BL, Moser B, Stock W, et al. Arsenic trioxide improves event-free and overall survival for adults with acute promyelocytic leukemia: North American Leukemia Intergroup Study C9710. *Blood*. 2010;116:3751-3757.
120. Coutre SE, Othus M, Powell B, et al. Arsenic trioxide during consolidation for patients with previously untreated low/intermediate risk acute promyelocytic leukaemia may eliminate the need for maintenance therapy. *Br J Haematol*. 2014;165:497-503.
121. Lancet JE, Moseley AB, Coutre SE, et al. A phase 2 study of ATRA, arsenic trioxide, and gemtuzumab ozogamicin in patients with high-risk APL (SWOG 0535). *Blood Adv*. 2020;4:1683-1689.
122. Platzbecker U, Avvisati G, Cicconi L, et al. Improved outcomes with retinoic acid and arsenic trioxide compared with retinoic acid and chemotherapy in non-high-risk acute promyelocytic leukemia: final results of the randomized Italian-German APL0406 trial. *J Clin Oncol*. 2017;35:605-612.
123. Sanz MA, Lo Coco F, Martin G, et al. Definition of relapse risk and role of nonanthracycline drugs for consolidation in patients with acute promyelocytic leukemia: a joint study of the PETHEMA and GIMEMA cooperative groups. *Blood*. 2000;96:1247-1253.
124. Cicconi L, Platzbecker U, Avvisati G, et al. Long-term results of all-trans retinoic acid and arsenic trioxide in non-high-risk acute promyelocytic leukemia: update of the APL0406 Italian-German randomized trial. *Leukemia*. 2020;34:914-918.
125. Iland H, Bradstock K, Seymour J, et al. Results of the APML3 trial incorporating all-trans-retinoic acid and idarubicin in both induction and consolidation as initial therapy for patients with acute promyelocytic leukemia. *Haematologica*. 2012;97:227-234.

126. National Comprehensive Cancer Network. *Acute Myeloid Leukemia (Version 3.2021).* 2021.
127. Takeshita A, Shinjo K, Naito K, et al. Efficacy of gemtuzumab ozogamicin on ATRA- and arsenic-resistant acute promyelocytic leukaemia (APL) cells. *Leukemia.* 2005;19:1306-1311.
128. Estey EH, Giles FJ, Beran M, et al. Experience with gemtuzumab ozogamycin ("mylotarg") and all-trans retinoic acid in untreated acute promyelocytic leukemia. *Blood.* 2002;99:4222-4224.
129. Osman AEG, Anderson J, Churpek JE, et al. Treatment of acute promyelocytic leukemia in adults. *J Oncol Pract.* 2018;14:649-657.
130. Castaigne S, Pautas C, Terre C, et al. Effect of gemtuzumab ozogamicin on survival of adult patients with de-novo acute myeloid leukaemia (ALFA-0701): a randomised, open-label, phase 3 study. *Lancet.* 2012;379:1508-1516.
131. Montesinos P, Gonzalez JD, Gonzalez J, et al. Therapy-related myeloid neoplasms in patients with acute promyelocytic leukemia treated with all-trans-retinoic acid and anthracycline-based chemotherapy. *J Clin Oncol.* 2010;28:3872-3879.
132. Ortega JJ, Madero L, Martin G, et al. Treatment with all-trans retinoic acid and anthracycline monochemotherapy for children with acute promyelocytic leukemia: a multicenter study by the PETHEMA Group. *J Clin Oncol.* 2005;23:7632-7640.
133. Testi AM, Biondi A, Lo Coco F, et al. GIMEMA-AIEOPAIDA protocol for the treatment of newly diagnosed acute promyelocytic leukemia (APL) in children. *Blood.* 2005;106:447-453.
134. Castaigne S, Lefebvre P, Chomienne C, et al. Effectiveness and pharmacokinetics of low-dose all-trans retinoic acid (25 mg/m2) in acute promyelocytic leukemia. *Blood.* 1993;82:3560-3563.
135. Chen GQ, Shen ZX, Wu F, et al. Pharmacokinetics and efficacy of low-dose all-trans retinoic acid in the treatment of acute promyelocytic leukemia. *Leukemia.* 1996;10:825-828.
136. Muindi JR, Frankel SR, Huselton C, et al. Clinical pharmacology of oral all-trans retinoic acid in patients with acute promyelocytic leukemia. *Cancer Res.* 1992;52:2138-2142.
137. Topletz AR, Tripathy S, Foti RS, et al. Induction of CYP26A1 by metabolites of retinoic acid: evidence that CYP26A1 is an important enzyme in the elimination of active retinoids. *Mol Pharmacol.* 2015;87:430-441.
138. Turner JR, Rodriguez I, Mantovani E, et al. Drug-induced proarrhythmia and torsade de pointes: a primer for students and practitioners of medicine and pharmacy. *J Clin Pharmacol.* 2018;58:997-1012.
139. Roboz GJ, Ritchie EK, Carlin RF, et al. Prevalence, management, and clinical consequences of QT interval prolongation during treatment with arsenic trioxide. *J Clin Oncol.* 2014;32:3723-3728.
140. Glass JL, Derkach A, Hilden P, et al. Arsenic trioxide therapy predisposes to herpes zoster reactivation despite minimally myelosuppressive therapy. *Leuk Res.* 2021;106:106569.
141. Au WY, Kwong YL. Frequent varicella zoster reactivation associated with therapeutic use of arsenic trioxide: portents of an old scourge. *J Am Acad Dermatol.* 2005;53:890-892.
142. Yamakura M, Tsuda K, Ugai T, et al. High frequency of varicella zoster virus reactivation associated with the use of arsenic trioxide in patients with acute promyelocytic leukemia. *Acta Haematol.* 2014;131:76-77.
143. Freyer CW, Peterson CE, Man Y, et al. Herpes zoster during arsenic trioxide therapy for acute promyelocytic leukemia. *Leuk Lymphoma.* 2021;62: 696-702.
144. Montesinos P, Diaz-Mediavilla J, Deben G, et al. Central nervous system involvement at first relapse in patients with acute promyelocytic leukemia treated with all-trans retinoic acid and anthracycline monochemotherapy without intrathecal prophylaxis. *Haematologica.* 2009;94:1242-1249.
145. Au WY, Tam S, Fong BM, et al. Determinants of cerebrospinal fluid arsenic concentration in patients with acute promyelocytic leukemia on oral arsenic trioxide therapy. *Blood.* 2008;112:3587-3590.
146. Burnett AK, Grimwade D, Solomon E, et al. Presenting white blood cell count and kinetics of molecular remission predict prognosis in acute promyelocytic leukemia treated with all-trans retinoic acid: result of the Randomized MRC Trial. *Blood.* 1999;93:4131-4143.
147. Schuurhuis GJ, Heuser M, Freeman S, et al. Minimal/measurable residual disease in AML: a consensus document from the European LeukemiaNet MRD Working Party. *Blood.* 2018;131:1275-1291.
148. Gallagher RE, Yeap BY, Bi W, et al. Quantitative real-time RT-PCR analysis of PML-RAR alpha mRNA in acute promyelocytic leukemia: assessment of prognostic significance in adult patients from intergroup protocol 0129. *Blood.* 2003;101:2521-2528.
149. Esteve J, Escoda L, Martin G, et al. Outcome of patients with acute promyelocytic leukemia failing to front-line treatment with all-trans retinoic acid and anthracycline-based chemotherapy (PETHEMA protocols LPA96 and LPA99): benefit of an early intervention. *Leukemia.* 2007;21:446-452.
150. Lo Coco F, Diverio D, Avvisati G, et al. Therapy of molecular relapse in acute promyelocytic leukemia. *Blood.* 1999;94:2225-2229.
151. Grimwade D, Jovanovic JV, Hills RK, et al. Prospective minimal residual disease monitoring to predict relapse of acute promyelocytic leukemia and to direct pre-emptive arsenic trioxide therapy. *J Clin Oncol.* 2009;27:3650-3658.
152. Stahl M, Tallman MS. Differentiation syndrome in acute promyelocytic leukaemia. *Br J Haematol.* 2019;187:157-162.
153. Frankel SR, Eardley A, Lauwers G, et al. The "retinoic acid syndrome" in acute promyelocytic leukemia. *Ann Intern Med.* 1992;117:292-296.
154. De Botton S, Dombret H, Sanz M, et al. Incidence, clinical features, and outcome of all trans-retinoic acid syndrome in 413 cases of newly diagnosed acute promyelocytic leukemia. The European APL Group. *Blood.* 1998;92:2712-2718.
155. Wiley JS, Firkin FC. Reduction of pulmonary toxicity by prednisolone prophylaxis during all-trans retinoic acid treatment of acute promyelocytic leukemia. Australian Leukaemia Study Group. *Leukemia.* 1995;9:774-778.
156. Tallman MS, Andersen JW, Schiffer CA, et al. Clinical description of 44 patients with acute promyelocytic leukemia who developed the retinoic acid syndrome. *Blood.* 2000;95:90-95.
157. Sanz MA, Montesinos P. How we prevent and treat differentiation syndrome in patients with acute promyelocytic leukemia. *Blood.* 2014;123:2777-2782.
158. Dubois C, Schlageter MH, de Gentile A, et al. Hematopoietic growth factor expression and ATRA sensitivity in acute promyelocytic blast cells. *Blood.* 1994;83:3264-3270.
159. Kota V, Kharkhanis P, Caprara CR, et al. Weight gain during induction therapy of acute promyelocytic leukemia patients: a preventable problem. *Blood.* 2017;130:5017.
160. Au WY, Lie AK, Chim CS, et al. Arsenic trioxide in comparison with chemotherapy and bone marrow transplantation for the treatment of relapsed acute promyelocytic leukaemia. *Ann Oncol.* 2003;14:752-757.
161. Shigeno K, Naito K, Sahara N, et al. Arsenic trioxide therapy in relapsed or refractory Japanese patients with acute promyelocytic leukemia: updated outcomes of the phase II study and postremission therapies. *Int J Hematol.* 2005;82:224-229.
162. Niu C, Yan H, Yu T, et al. Studies on treatment of acute promyelocytic leukemia with arsenic trioxide: remission induction, follow-up, and molecular monitoring in 11 newly diagnosed and 47 relapsed acute promyelocytic leukemia patients. *Blood.* 1999;94:3315-3324.
163. Raffoux E, Rousselot P, Poupon J, et al. Combined treatment with arsenic trioxide and all-trans-retinoic acid in patients with relapsed acute promyelocytic leukemia. *J Clin Oncol.* 2003;21:2326-2334.
164. Lo-Coco F, Cimino G, Breccia M, et al. Gemtuzumab ozogamicin (Mylotarg) as a single agent for molecularly relapsed acute promyelocytic leukemia. *Blood.* 2004;104:1995-1999.
165. Breccia M, Cimino G, Diverio D, et al. Sustained molecular remission after low dose gemtuzumab-ozogamicin in elderly patients with advanced acute promyelocytic leukemia. *Haematologica.* 2007;92:1273-1274.
166. Thirugnanam R, George B, Chendamarai E, et al. Comparison of clinical outcomes of patients with relapsed acute promyelocytic leukemia induced with arsenic trioxide and consolidated with either an autologous stem cell transplant or an arsenic trioxide-based regimen. *Biol Blood Marrow Transplant.* 2009;15:1479-1484.
167. Meloni G, Diverio D, Vignetti M, et al. Autologous bone marrow transplantation for acute promyelocytic leukemia in second remission: prognostic relevance of pretransplant minimal residual disease assessment by reverse-transcription polymerase chain reaction of the PML/RAR alpha fusion gene. *Blood.* 1997;90:1321-1325.
168. Yanada M, Tsuzuki M, Fujita H, et al. Phase 2 study of arsenic trioxide followed by autologous hematopoietic cell transplantation for relapsed acute promyelocytic leukemia. *Blood.* 2013;121:3095-3102.
169. Ferrara F, Finizio O, Izzo T, et al. Autologous stem cell transplantation for patients with acute promyelocytic leukemia in second molecular remission. *Anticancer Res.* 2010;30:3845-3849.
170. de Botton S, Fawaz A, Chevret S, et al. Autologous and allogeneic stem-cell transplantation as salvage treatment of acute promyelocytic leukemia initially treated with all-trans-retinoic acid: a retrospective analysis of the European acute promyelocytic leukemia group. *J Clin Oncol.* 2005;23:120-126.
171. Sanz J, Labopin M, Sanz MA, et al. Hematopoietic stem cell transplantation for adults with relapsed acute promyelocytic leukemia in second complete remission. *Bone Marrow Transplant.* 2020;56(6):1272-1280.
172. Tallman MS. Treatment of relapsed or refractory acute promyelocytic leukemia. *Best Pract Res Clin Haematol.* 2007;20:57-65.
173. de Botton S, Sanz MA, Chevret S, et al. Extramedullary relapse in acute promyelocytic leukemia treated with all-trans retinoic acid and chemotherapy. *Leukemia.* 2006;20:35-41.
174. Specchia G, Lo Coco F, Vignetti M, et al. Extramedullary involvement at relapse in acute promyelocytic leukemia patients treated or not with all-trans retinoic acid: a report by the Gruppo Italiano Malattie Ematologiche dell'Adulto. *J Clin Oncol.* 2001;19:4023-4028.
175. Rashidi A, Fisher SI. Therapy-related acute promyelocytic leukemia: a systematic review. *Med Oncol.* 2013;30:625.
176. Dayyani F, Kantarjian H, O'Brien S, et al. Outcome of therapy-related acute promyelocytic leukemia with or without arsenic trioxide as a component of frontline therapy. *Cancer.* 2011;117:110-115.
177. Sanz MA, Vellenga E, Rayon C, et al. All-trans retinoic acid and anthracycline monochemotherapy for the treatment of elderly patients with acute promyelocytic leukemia. *Blood.* 2004;104:3490-3493.
178. Latagliata R, Breccia M, Fazi P, et al. GIMEMA AIDA 0493 amended protocol for elderly patients with acute promyelocytic leukaemia. Long-term results and prognostic factors. *Br J Haematol.* 2011;154:564-568.
179. Au WY, Kumana CR, Kou M, et al. Oral arsenic trioxide in the treatment of relapsed acute promyelocytic leukemia. *Blood.* 2003;102:407-408.
180. Zhu HH, Wu DP, Jin J, et al. Oral tetra-arsenic tetra-sulfide formula versus intravenous arsenic trioxide as first-line treatment of acute promyelocytic leukemia: a multicenter randomized controlled trial. *J Clin Oncol.* 2013;31: 4215-4221.

181. Kumana CR, Au WY, Lee NS, et al. Systemic availability of arsenic from oral arsenic-trioxide used to treat patients with hematological malignancies. *Eur J Clin Pharmacol.* 2002;58:521-526.
182. Siu CW, Au WY, Yung C, et al. Effects of oral arsenic trioxide therapy on QT intervals in patients with acute promyelocytic leukemia: implications for long-term cardiac safety. *Blood.* 2006;108:103-106.
183. Jiang H, Liang GW, Huang XJ, et al. Reduced medical costs and hospital days when using oral arsenic plus ATRA as the first-line treatment of acute promyelocytic leukemia. *Leuk Res.* 2015;39:1319-1324.
184. Zhu HH, Huang XJ. Oral arsenic and retinoic acid for non-high-risk acute promyelocytic leukemia. *N Engl J Med.* 2014;371:2239-2241.
185. Iland H, Reynolds J, Boddy A., et al. *Comparative Bioavailability of a Novel Oral Formulation of Arsenic Trioxide in Patients Undergoing Consolidation Therapy for Acute Promyelocytic Leukemia: Final Analysis of the ALLG APML5 Trial.* EHA Learning Center; 2021. (abstr EP433), 2021.
186. Ravandi F, Koumenis I, Johri A, et al. Oral arsenic trioxide ORH-2014 pharmacokinetic and safety profile in patients with advanced hematologic disorders. *Haematologica.* 2020;105:1567-1574.

Chapter 80 ■ Myelodysplastic Syndromes

NAMRATA S. CHANDHOK • MIKKAEL A. SEKERES

INTRODUCTION

Myelodysplastic syndromes (MDS) are a heterogenous spectrum of clonal stem cell disorders characterized by varying degrees of peripheral blood cytopenias, bone marrow dysplasia in one or more myeloid lineages, and a predilection for transforming to acute myeloid leukemia (AML). Genetic defects such as point mutations, chromosomal aberrations, abnormal gene expression, and copy number alterations are common in MDS. Given its clonal origin, corruption of normal hematopoietic elements, and severe truncation of life expectancy, MDS is considered a cancer. It is strongly associated with aging, antecedent bone marrow disorders, and prior chemotherapy, radiation, or other toxic assaults on the bone marrow and evolves over years or decades.

The clinical presentation of MDS can be nonspecific; while many patients present with symptoms or complications of their cytopenias, such as fatigue from anemia or frequent infections due to neutropenia, others are diagnosed when cytopenias are noted incidentally on labs obtained during routine medical care. As a diverse pathologic grouping that is closely related to other myeloid neoplasms, MDS has a natural history that is also variable and ranges from relatively indolent clonal cytopenias that progress over years to rapid acquisition of deleterious mutations and ultimate conversion to AML. Since the initial classification of MDS as a pathologic entity in the 1980s by the French-American-British cooperative group (FAB), there have been significant advancements in our understanding of MDS pathobiology, classification, and management, which has accelerated in the past decade. Still, effective disease-modifying therapeutic options remain limited and almost all patients with MDS will succumb either to complications of the disease itself, such as infections or bleeding, or to transformation to AML.

In this chapter, we will summarize the epidemiology, pathogenesis, diagnostic assessment, risk-stratification, and risk adapted therapeutic strategies for the management of adult MDS.

MDS EPIDEMIOLOGY AND RISK FACTORS

While diagnostic criteria for MDS have changed over decades, at its core, the disease has remained centered on the premise of ineffective hematopoiesis and the clinical sequelae of this defect. The first descriptively identifiable case of MDS was published in 1900, involving a patient who died of a febrile illness and who had marrow failure with megaloblastic cellular maturation.[1] Links to leukemia and radiation were recognized long before the disorder was classified, first as "dysmyelopoetic syndromes" by the FAB cooperative group in 1976, and formally as MDS by the World Health Organization (WHO) in 2001.[2,3]

Due to the relatively recent establishment of the diagnosis, the evolving diagnostic criteria, and underreporting to population-based cancer registries due to misclassification of the disease, and underdiagnosis in older adults with cytopenias, MDS is likely underreported. The most recent Surveillance, Epidemiology, and End-results (SEER) 5-year incidence rate (2014-2018) estimates 3.1 cases per 100,000 women, and 5.8 cases per 100,000 men (4.5 per 100,000 overall, translating to approximately 20,000 cases yearly in the United States), while claims-based data suggest that at least 30,000 cases of MDS are diagnosed annually.[4,5] There is a strong link between aging and MDS, and the diagnosis of MDS in the absence of a toxic exposure or an underlying genetic predisposition is rare in people under the age of 50; the average age of diagnosis is approximately 71 years.[6,7]

Racial and ethnic variations in the diagnosis and natural history of MDS are becoming more recognized. Rates of myeloid malignancies are comparable in the United States and Western Europe, but the incidence of MDS seems to be lower in Asian counties, where age of diagnosis is younger and patients tend have more aggressive subtypes and higher risk (HR) disease.[8-10] Within the United States, minority patients are underrepresented in clinical trials, cancer databases and many have less access to care, which may contribute to lower incidence rates for MDS among Blacks in SEER. Blacks in the United States with MDS also may have poorer risk cytogenetics and mutations than whites.[11] Hispanic patients tend to be younger than whites at diagnosis, with a higher incidence in females, worse thrombocytopenia, and with poorer response to erythropoiesis-stimulating agents (ESAs), but with possibly better overall survival (OS).[12,13]

As previously noted, aging is the most important risk factor for developing MDS, and in 90% of cases, it is the only identifiable risk factor. Expected age-related accumulation of somatic mutations in DNA leads to clonal expansion in hematopoietic stem cells (HSCs), which can cooperate with subsequent acquired mutations and lead to development of clinically evident myeloid malignancies.[14] The remaining 10% to 15% of MDS diagnoses are considered secondary, or therapy-related, and may be linked to exposure to ionizing radiation, DNA damaging agents (such as DNA alkylating agents and topoisomerase inhibitors that are frequently used in chemotherapy), or toxic workplace or environmental exposures to carcinogens such as benzene or its derivatives (present in some lubricants, dyes, industrial detergents, pesticides, and cigarettes).

While it can be difficult to establish causality between a prior therapeutic or environmental exposure and the development of MDS in epidemiologic studies, assessment of patients with exposure to excessive environmental radiation related to the tragic atomic bombings of Hiroshima and Nagasaki and leading to high rates of MDS decades later have helped delineate differences between secondary and de novo MDS.[15,16] MDS is a multistep process in which molecular mutations lead to progressive compromise of blood counts as the clinical disease becomes evident. Previous treatment with DNA damaging agents, or environmental exposure to a compound like benzene, may represent one step in that process. Therapy-related MDS is considered a distinct clinical entity characterized by, but not limited to, high-risk cytogenetic and molecular abnormalities and acquired defects in the DNA damage response pathways.[17] Modifiable risk factors that have been associated with MDS include cigarette smoking, alcohol consumption, and agricultural exposures to chemicals.[18-20]

Finally, several hereditary, predisposing syndromes can lead to the development of MDS and, like therapy-related MDS, these patients represent a distinct clinical entity in the 2016 WHO classification system.[21] Patients presenting at a younger age without a clear toxic exposure should be evaluated for a hereditary predisposition, although some hereditary syndromes will present later in life. Genetic syndromes leading to MDS predisposition broadly fall into the categories of faulty DNA repair, transcription factor defects, ribosomal abnormalities, defective telomere maintenance, and abnormal RAS pathway signaling. Down syndrome, Fanconi anemia, Diamond-Blackfan anemia, Shwachman-Diamond syndrome, dyskeratosis congenita, Noonan syndrome, Bloom syndrome, and Treacher Collins syndrome, among others, are all associated with an increased risk of MDS, which may present as childhood MDS.[22] Pediatric MDS is rare, with an incidence rate of 1 to 4 patients per million yearly. The genetic drivers that characterize pediatric MDS are distinct from those seen in adults; somatic driver mutations in SETBP1, ASXL1, RUNX1, and RAS oncogenes are much more common in pediatric MDS, whereas mutations in TET2, DNMT3A, and TP53 and the spliceosome complex are more characteristic in adult MDS.[23]

Genetic disorders frequently do not have a syndromic presentation; manifestations can be subtle, with variable presentations within a family, and patients with germline mutations may initially present with manifestations of MDS as adults. For example, familial mutations in the zinc-finger transcription factor GATA2 that are associated with MDS development and immunodeficiency disorders were studied in a third-generation GATA2-mutated family. Family members presented with hematologic disorders from age 14 to 74 and presentations included mild pancytopenia, opportunistic infections, MDS with monosomy 7, non-Hodgkin lymphoma, Emberger syndrome (characterized by lymphedema and MDS), and acute leukemias.[24] Germline mutations in RUNX1, another hematopoietic transcription factor that is often associated with familial thrombocytopenia, led to MDS or AML in 35% of carriers.[25] CCAAT/Enhancer/Binding Protein/A is another important germline predisposition to myeloid malignancies, but this more commonly presents as AML. Finally, germline mutations in DDX41, a gene encoding a ribonucleic acid (RNA) helicase involved in cytoplasmic RNA recognition that is thought to act as a tumor suppressor, are among the most recently studied germline predispositions. The predisposition can remain quiescent for decades, and patients with these mutations tend to present with MDS as adults.[26,27] This particular mutation may also be associated with responsiveness to the drug lenalidomide.[26]

PATHOGENESIS OF MDS

MDS is driven by initiating genetic alterations that lead to clonal expansion and the subsequent acquisition of cooperating mutations, sometimes occurring over years or decades. These mutations ultimately result in dysregulated hematopoietic differentiation leading to dysplasia, impaired differentiation, and eventually cytopenias. Genetic defects such as chromosomal abnormalities, germline or somatic molecular mutations, abnormal gene expression, and copy number alterations are common in MDS. Earlier studies of MDS were focused on a few known mutations and recurrent cytogenetic abnormalities reflecting genetic instability in later stages of disease. In the past decade, advances in sequencing technology have led to a much deeper understanding of the MDS genome and the identification of approximately 50 genes that are recurrently mutated in 90% to 95% of MDS diagnoses.[28-32] The most common mutations are highlighted in *Table 80.1*. With the widespread adoption of targeted sequencing panels, it is now recognized that >80% of MDS patients harbor ≥1 known recurrently mutated genes that span varied functional categories including histone modification, chromatin remodeling, epigenetic regulation, RNA splicing, transcription, and kinase signaling networks.[30,31] On a population level, patients with molecular mutations leading to clonal hematopoiesis (but without clinical manifestations of dysregulated hematopoiesis—a process called clonal hematopoiesis of indeterminate potential or CHIP) have an increased risk of developing both lymphoid and myeloid malignancies, which supports the stem cell basis of MDS[33] (For a more detailed discussion of CHIP, please see Chapter 73). Following the initial clonal expansion, disease propagation and development of MDS involves a complex interplay among several factors including genetic and epigenetic alterations, the immune system and inflammation, and changes in the bone marrow microenvironment, a process that may occur over the span of years (*Figure 80.1*).

Molecular Pathogenesis of MDS

The acquisition of somatic mutations is expected with aging. However, not all molecular mutations have pathogenic potential; clonal hematopoiesis due to randomly acquired somatic mutations is generally "passenger mutations," often without clinical consequence. "Driver mutations" are mutations with pathogenic potential. These mutations lead to disease initiation, when mutated early in pathogenesis, or disease progression when they are late events. The most commonly mutated genes, within the context of the associated pathway, are briefly discussed below.

Epigenetic Regulators

Epigenetics refers to a heritable phenotype that is not encoded in the DNA sequence, but is transmitted through cell division. Epigenetics involves the transcriptional machinery, transcription factors, histone modifications, multi-protein chromatin-modifying complexes, and microRNAs and long noncoding RNAs.[34] Epigenetic changes may be a result of somatic mutations in genes encoding for epigenetic proteins or may be a consequence of epigenetic drift (a gradual divergence of the epigenome due to aging). Mutations affecting epigenetic modifier genes (*TET2, DNMT3A, IDH1/2, ASXL1, EZH2, and others*) are common early events in MDS initiation.

TET2 is a frequently mutated epigenetic regulator that can lead to DNA demethylation; mutations leading to the premature truncation of the enzyme's catalytic region leading to disrupted cellular activity can have a profound impact on cellular differentiation and proliferation.[35] *TET2* mutations are more common in low-risk MDS. The overall prognostic impact of this mutation is still unclear.

DNMT3A enzymes catalyze the transfer of methyl groups to specific CpG structures in DNA and are responsible for maintenance of the DNA methylation pattern, from the parental DNA strand to the daughter strand, during replication.[36] *DNMT3A* mutations, frequently seen in CHIP, are considered important for leukemia predisposition, as these mutations provide a growth advantage, but do not lead to the MDS phenotype in isolation when studied in animal models.[37,38] The inhibition of DNA methyltransferases is one of the potential mechanisms of action of the hypomethylating agents (HMAs) azacitidine (AZA) and decitabine, described in the treatment section.

IDH1/2 mutations are conserved hotspot mutations that lead to downstream alteration of isocitrate dehydrogenase (IDH) enzymatic activity, which normally catalyze the conversion of isocitrate to α-ketoglutarate and lead to the production of (R)-2-hydroxyglutarate.[39] These changes affect metabolism, hypoxic response, and shape the epigenetic landscape by inhibition of αKG-dependent lysine demethylases and inhibition of the TET family of 5-methylcytosine hydroxylases, inducing histone and DNA hypermethylation in different models.[40,41] Targeted inhibitors of *IDH1/2* are approved by the US Food and Drug Administration (FDA) for the treatment of relapsed/refractory AML with these mutations.

Pathogenic ASXL1 mutations are primarily truncating mutations that are thought to disrupt chromatin leading to transcriptional changes.[42] These mutations co-occur more frequently than expected by chance alone with certain mutations in splicing, transcriptional, and other epigenetic regulators, suggesting a cooperative role in pathogenesis.[30] They are uniformly associated with poor prognosis in myeloid malignancies.[43]

EZH2 encodes a histone methyltransferase that is crucial for epigenetic silencing of genes involved in stem cell renewal. Mutations in *EZH2* are usually seen without characteristics that are considered high risk by the Revised International Prognostic Scoring System (IPSS-R) (as discussed later) but are independently associated with a poorer prognosis.[44]

RNA-Splicing Machinery

Splicing dysfunction is a key contributor to MDS biology, and mutations in the slicing machinery occur in more than 50% of patients with MDS. The most common spliceosome mutations in MDS are *SF3B1, U2AF1, SRSF2, ZRSR2,* and *PRPF8*,[30,31] but *ZRSR2* and *PRPF8* are comparatively less common. Splicing factor mutations are thought to be loss-of-function mutations and do not frequently co-occur with other splicing factor mutations.

SF3B1 is important for the recognition and selection of the branch site in RNA splicing. Mutations in *SF3B1* lead to decreased fidelity to branch site selection, leading to alternative splicing events. SF3B1 mutations are associated morphologically with ring sideroblasts, as the mutation induces mis-splicing that has a downstream effect on the mitochondrial iron exporter responsible for maintaining iron homeostasis.[29,45] Recently, there has been a movement to create a distinct pathologic subtype for SF3B1-mutant MDS due to the characteristic genotype-phenotype association with MDS with ring sideroblasts, and the independent good prognostic value of these mutations.[46]

Table 80.1. Most Common Mutations in MDS

Mutational Class	Mutation	Frequency (%)	Prognostic Implication	Additional Information
RNA Splicing	Common early mutations that result in altered patterns of splicing			
	SF3B1	20-30	Favorable	Favorable risk, mutated in ~80% of patients with ringed sideroblasts
	SRSF2	10-15	Adverse	Enriched in CMML (commonly with TET2)
	U2AF1	8-12	Adverse	
	ZRSR2	5-8	Unclear	Enriched in HR-MDS (compared to LR-MDS)
Epigenetic Regulators	Common early mutations that result in altered DNA methylation/histone modification			
	TET2	20-30	Neutral	Enriched in HR-MDS (compared to LR-MDS), common in CMML (with SRSF2)
	DNMT3A	10-18	Neutral	
	IDH1/2	5-10	Likely Adverse	High risk of progression to AML
	ASXL1	15-25	Adverse	Enriched in HR-MDS (compared to LR-MDS)
	EZH2	5-10	Adverse	Enriched in CMML
	BCOR	<5	Unclear	
Cohesins	Cohesin complex mutations may drive MDS by aberrant transcription			
	STAG2	5-10	Unclear	Enriched in HR-MDS (compared to LR-MDS)
	RAD21	<5	Unclear	
	SMC3/SMC1A	<5	Unclear	
Transcription	Play a role in lineage-specific gene expression programs—MDS germline mutations are enriched in this group.			
	RUNX1	10-15	Adverse	Enriched in HR-MDS (compared to LR-MDS)
	ETV6	<5	Adverse	
	CUX1	<5	Unclear	
	GATA2	<5	Unclear	Enriched in HR-MDS (compared to LR-MDS)
Signaling	More commonly second mutations in MDS, enriched in other associated myeloid disorders			
	NRAS	5-10	Adverse	High risk of progression to AML
	KRAS		Unclear	Enriched in HR-MDS (compared to LR-MDS)
	CBL	<5	Likely Adverse	Enriched in chronic myelomonocytic leukemia
	JAK2	<5	Neutral	Enriched in myeloproliferative neoplasms
	FLT3	<5	Adverse	High risk of progression to AML
	KIT	<5	Unclear	Enriched in mast cell disorders
	FLT3	<5	Adverse	High risk of progression to AML
P53 pathway	These genes are central to cellular stress response and inactivation of tumor suppressors leads to genetic instability			
	TP53	5-12	Adverse	Enriched in HR-MDS (compared to LR-MDS), Frequently, therapy-related MDS, associated with complex karyotype
	PPM1D	<5	Adverse	Enriched in therapy related MDS

Abbreviations: AML, Acute myeloid leukemia; CMML, Chronic myelomonocytic leukemia; HR MDS, High-risk MDS; LR MDS, Low-risk MDS.

SRSF2 guides splice site selection for constitutive and alternatively spliced exons and introns. SRSF2 is the second most frequently mutated splicing factor. Differentially spliced genes due to mutations in SRSF2 are enriched for genes implicated in cancer progression, development, and apoptosis pathways, and these mutations are generally associated with worse prognosis.[47,48]

U2AF1 forms a complex with U2AF2 and together these proteins are responsible for 3′ splice site selection.[49] Mutations in U2AF1 mutations lead to mis-splicing events, and splicing patterns with this mutation are under investigation. U2AF1 mutations are associated with shorter OS and increased risk of transformation to AML.[50]

Transcriptional Factors

Hematopoietic transcription factors are recurrently mutated in MDS. While most of these mutations are somatic, loss-of-function mutations in RUNX1, GATA2, and ETV6 are frequently associated with inherited bone marrow failure disorders that carry a risk of MDS and AML.[51]

RUNX1 is part of a transcriptional complex that regulates important target genes in hematopoiesis, and *RUNX1* mutations (typically loss-of-function or dominant negative mutations) affect both the major functional domains of the protein.[52] These mutations are associated with a shorter survival, HR, and shorter latency for progression to AML.[53]

Tumor Suppressors

TP53 is a tumor suppressor gene that encodes a transcription factor involved in key cellular functions, including DNA damage response.[54] Mutations in the tumor suppressor TP53 are the most clinically significant mutations in MDS. Li-Fraumeni syndrome, caused by a germline

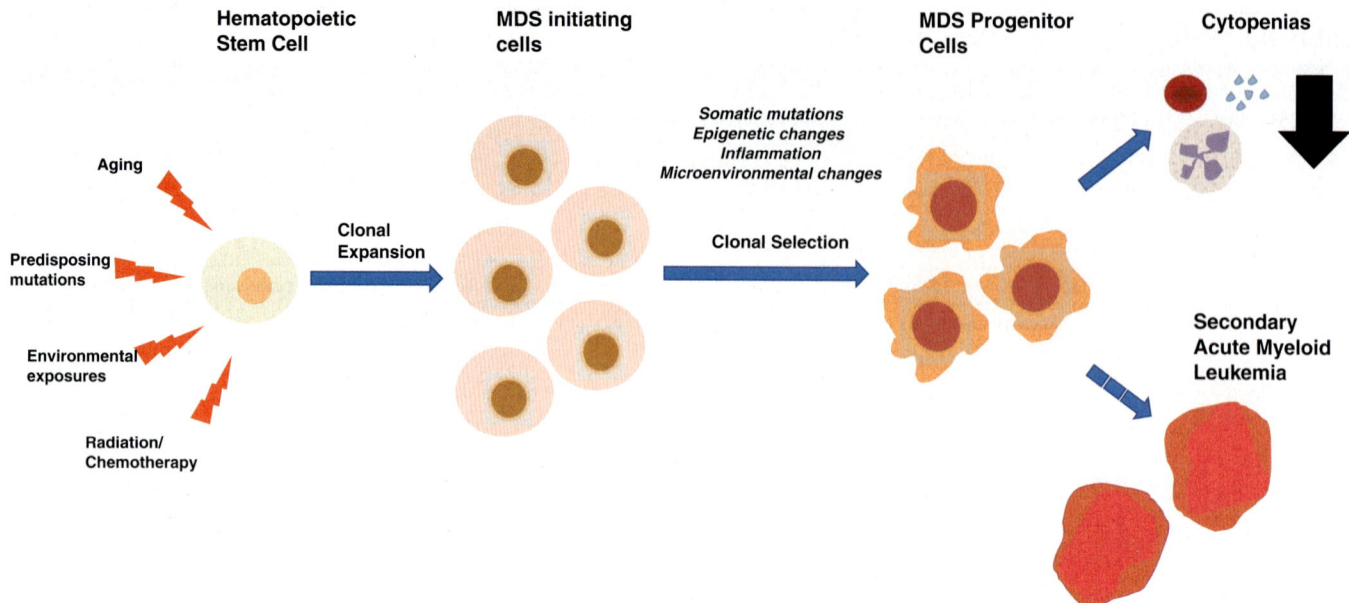

FIGURE 80.1 MDS pathogenesis. MDS, myelodysplastic syndrome.

pathogenic variant of TP53, is associated with many malignancies, including early development of MDS.[55] Somatic TP53 mutations are associated with genome instability, low platelet levels, a high blast count, and complex karyotype.[56,57] These mutations are common in patients with therapy-related MDS and, especially when associated with a complex karyotype, portend a poor prognosis.[57]

Cohesin Complex

The Cohesin complex STAG2, SMC3, SMC1A, and RAD21 proteins help maintain sister chromatid cohesion, thus preventing collapse of the replication fork. These proteins also help with homologous recombination-mediated DNA repair. Although the role of cohesins in MDS remains incompletely understood, cohesin mutations primarily thought to drive MDS pathogenesis by affecting long-range chromatin interactions that lead to altered gene expression.[58-60]

Signaling Pathway

Signaling pathways interact with each other to allow for coordinated myeloid differentiation in a stage- and lineage-specific manner. Defects in these pathways lead to uncontrolled proliferation and survival of hematopoietic progenitor cells.[61] Signaling pathway mutations in myeloid malignancies include janus kinase 2 (JAK2), CBL, FLT3, NRAS, KRAS, NF1, PTPN11, and others. These mutations are more commonly associated with other myeloid malignancies and may help in classification of patients who are morphologically equivocal. The MAPK family of protein kinases plays an important role in cellular programs like proliferation, differentiation, development, transformation, and apoptosis; mutations in pathway mutations involving NRAS, KRAS, NF1, and PTPN11 are more common in MDS, occurring in up to 10% of patients.[30,31] Acquisition of signaling pathway mutations, like FLT3 mutations, frequently leads to transformation from MDS to AML.

Other Key Factors in MDS Pathogenesis

Hematopoiesis is a tightly regulated process to ensure the balance between differentiation into all mature blood cell lineages (by repression of self-renewal pathways) and HSC renewal (by repression of differentiation pathways) that is necessary to sustain blood production over a person's lifespan. Aging is associated with reduced HSC regeneration capacity and skewing to the myeloid lineage, although with poorer output that predisposes to anemia and decreased immunity. Intrinsic HSC aging resulting in increased DNA damage, smaller clonal populations leading to decreased blood production, epigenetic drift, changes in metabolism resulting in increased oxidative stress, altered protein homeostasis, and changes in intrinsic signaling pathways collectively contribute to MDS pathogenesis. Microenvironmental changes such as inflammation and immune dysregulation also lead to altered hematopoiesis that can ultimately lead to MDS tumorigenesis. While there is ample evidence of chronic inflammation in the bone marrow and blood of patients with MDS, the mechanisms leading to pathogenesis are not well characterized.

CLINICAL PRESENTATION OF MDS

Peripheral blood cytopenias are commonly seen in general medical practice and often have an insidious onset in older adults, leading to a deficit in workup for etiology. Anemia is also the most common cytopenia noted in patients with MDS, and usually occurs over time, which improves tolerability by the patient. Therefore, patients with MDS frequently present with only vague symptoms such as fatigue, or no symptoms at all, unless they present after their compensatory mechanisms start to fail. Less common presentations include critically symptomatic anemia, bleeding from thrombocytopenia, neutropenic fever, constitutional symptoms, or other unexplained infectious processes and frequent infections. Organomegaly and related symptoms are unusual with MDS and should prompt an evaluation for a myeloproliferative neoplasm (MPN) or other malignancy.

While cytopenias are common in older patients, *they should not be considered a natural consequence of aging*. Therefore, patients with persistent cytopenias should have a comprehensive clinical evaluation to ascertain a cause for the cytopenia, such as evaluation for blood loss, nutritional deficiency, autoimmune or rheumatologic disorders, infectious processes, drugs (see differential diagnosis) to exclude alternate etiologies, and assess for clues that may point to a malignant disorder. For example, there is a high index of suspicion for myeloid malignancies in patients who have had prior exposure to chemotherapy, radiation, and environmental toxins in the presence of unexplained cytopenias. Patients with pancytopenia, bicytopenia, or any otherwise unexplained isolated cytopenia should be referred to a malignant hematologist for a bone marrow biopsy and additional workup. Diagnosing MDS can be challenging given "MDS mimics" and overlap between the diagnostic criteria of the various myeloid neoplasms and subtypes of MDS. Therefore, early involvement of a subspecialist and specialized hematopathologist is important to establish the diagnosis.

DIAGNOSIS AND CLASSIFICATION OF MDS

Minimum Diagnostic Criteria

As previously noted, MDS is a group of myeloid neoplasms that emerge from the clonal expansion of an abnormal hematopoietic progenitor cell leading to ineffective hematopoiesis and dysplasia. The minimum diagnostic criteria for MDS include at least one persistent and otherwise unexplained peripheral blood cytopenia, as well as a definitive finding on a bone marrow biopsy such as the presence of dysplasia in at least 10% of one or more myeloid lineage, the presence of increased myeloblasts (≥5%) or ring sideroblasts in the blood or bone marrow, or an MDS-defining cytogenetic abnormality (*Table 80.2*).

MDS were initially defined using the FAB criteria, but in the 21st century, the WHO classification, most recently updated in 2016, is the prevailing classification system. The 2016 WHO criteria made some modifications to the cytopenia and morphological changes and started to integrate genetic information in MDS diagnosis and classification, compared to previous iterations (*Table 80.3*).

ELEMENTS OF DIAGNOSTIC EVALUATION

Evaluation of Cytopenias

A complete blood count with differential can reveal cytopenias. Anemia is the most common cytopenia associated with MDS (occurring in approximately 80% of MDS patients) and is most frequently macrocytic or normocytic. Bicytopenia is common, and approximately half of all patients present with a concomitant neutropenia or thrombocytopenia. Less commonly, patients will present with isolated neutropenia or thrombocytopenia (approximately 6% of the time).[62] Certain ethnic patient populations may have a lower neutrophil count at baseline (Duffy-negative phenotype), highlighting the importance of comparing recent laboratory values with prior data to assess trends.

Morphologic Evaluation (Peripheral Smear and Bone Marrow Biopsy)

Historically, the diagnosis of MDS was largely reliant on morphologic findings in the blood and bone marrow, and morphologic classification was based on the degree of dysplasia, the presence or ring sideroblasts, or the presence of myeloblasts. Dysplasia refers to the abnormal morphology that may be detected on maturing bone marrow precursor cells (erythroid, granulocytic, and megakaryocytic). While a normal peripheral smear does not rule out MDS, an abnormal peripheral blood smear with evidence of dysplasia or excess blasts warrants strong consideration of MDS or other myeloid malignancies.

A bone marrow biopsy and aspirate are always necessary to confirm a diagnosis of MDS. The core biopsy is important to determine the marrow cellularity, marrow architecture, and detect possible marrow fibrosis, which has prognostic value (and may point to an overlap MDS/MPN diagnosis). The bone marrow aspirate allows for greater cellular evaluation of the myeloid compartment, but also informs the pathologist of inflammatory changes in the bone marrow, such as increased populations of lymphocytes, plasma cells, and mast cells, and is necessary to accurately determine blast percentage. The *WHO classification of Tumours of Haematopoietic and Lymphoid Tissues* guidelines recommend that 500 nucleated bone marrow cells and 200 from peripheral blood are evaluated to help characterize the dysplasia and distinguish among the various types of MDS. Biopsy and aspirate smear quality are crucial for accurate diagnosis, and poor-quality smears can lead to misinterpretation of the degree of dysplasia, particularly in the case of neutrophil granulation, which is critical to establish the diagnosis of MDS. It is also critical to consider reactive etiologies of dysplasia (see differential diagnosis) when assessing for MDS, as nonmalignant causes can lead to subtle dysplasia in more than 10% of the marrow cellularity and these changes are morphologically indistinguishable from a malignant process. Dysplasia may present as nuclear or cytoplasmic atypia or the presence of specific abnormal cellular morphology and inclusions. More specific measures of dysplasia include dysmegakaryopoiesis in the form of micromegakaryocytes, hypolobation, or multinucleation, the presence of mature neutrophils with hyposegmented nuclei, neutrophils with cytoplasmic hypogranulation, the presence of ring sideroblasts, or the presence of myeloblasts. Based on morphologic criteria, MDS is subclassified into 10 categories (*Table 80.3*).

Although morphology is fundamental for diagnosis of MDS and morphologic subsets have different natural histories, morphology can be subjective and by itself is insufficient to make prognostic predictions or to select therapy. In one report from the US National MDS Natural History Study, clinically meaningful disagreements between local and central pathologists about an MDS diagnosis occurred almost 20% of the time.[63] For example, in a patient who presents with a hypocellular marrow, it is challenging to distinguish between aplastic anemia and hypoplastic MDS based on morphology alone. Similarly, marrow hyperplasia and fibrosis can be associated with both MDS and MPNs.

Cytogenetics

Cytogenetics is a critical independent diagnostic and prognostic factor in MDS. Chromosomal abnormalities are seen in about 50% to 60% of patients with conventional karyotyping and are commonly partial or complete loss of a chromosome.[64] There is no specific cytogenetic pattern diagnostic of MDS, but karyotypic information may help differentiating between the closely related myeloid malignancies. Conventional karyotyping is considered the gold standard in the cytogenetic profiling and typically requires analysis of 20 metaphase cells, which may be difficult in MDS samples depending on growth characteristics.

Cytogenetic abnormalities are grouped based on their impact on prognosis (*Figure 80.2*), and this was the basis for the IPSS-R described in the next section. Cytogenetics can also impact therapy, most notably in patients with deletion of the long arm of chromosome 5. This is discussed further in the treatment section.

Flow Cytometry

Flow cytometry enables the evaluation of hematopoietic cells on a single cell level, and immunophenotypic abnormalities may be more sensitive than morphology in detecting myeloid dysplasia.[65] These abnormalities include abnormal intensity or lack of expression immunophenotypic abnormalities, asynchronous markers, or expression of lineage infidelity markers; no single immunophenotypic

---

Table 80.2. Minimal Diagnostic Criteria for MDS

Peripheral blood cytopenia (at Least one of the following for ≥6 months):
  i. Hemoglobin < 10 g/dL
  ii. Platelets < 100 × 10^9/L
  iii. Absolute Neutrophil Count; <1.8 × 10^9/L

Bone Marrow Findings (at least one of the following):
  i. The presence of dysplasia in at least 10% of cells in one or more major BM lineage(s) (erythroid, neutrophilic, megakaryocytic)
  ii. Increased ring sideroblasts (RS) of ≥15% (or ≥5% in the presence of a SF3B1 mutation)
  iii. Increased myeloid blasts of 5%-19% in dysplastic BM smears (in the absence of AML-specific gene rearrangements)
  iv. 2%-19% meyloblasts in peripheral blood smears
  v. An MDS-related karyotype

Exclude alternate explanations for blood and marrow findings
- AML defining lesions
- Alternate hematologic disorders or congenital disorders (e.g., myeloproliferative neoplasms, aplastic anemia/Fanconi anemia)
- Infections (e.g., HIV)
- Nutritional deficiencies (e.g., B_{12}, folate, copper)
- Autoimmune conditions (e.g., rheumatoid arthritis, systemic lupus erythematosus)
- Medication affects (e.g., chemotherapy)
- Alcohol abuse/illicit drug use

Abbreviations: AML, acute myeloid leukemia; BM, bone marrow; MDS, myelodysplastic syndrome.

Table 80.3. Classification of MDS per the 2016 Revision to the World Health Organization Classification of Myeloid Neoplasms and Acute Leukemia

Disease Classification	Defining Characteristics
MDS with single lineage dysplasia	One dysplastic lineage with on dysplasia in at least 10% of bone marrow cellularity with 1-2 cytopenias Less than 15% ringed sideroblasts OR less than 5% in the presence of an SF3B1 mutation Less than 5% bone marrow blasts/less than 1% peripheral blasts/No Auer rods/Does not meet criteria for MDS with isolated del(5q)
MDS with multilineage dysplasia	More than 1 dysplastic lineage with 2-3 cytopenias Less than 15% ringed sideroblasts OR less than 5% in the presence of an SF3B1 mutation Less than 5% bone marrow blasts/less than 1% peripheral blasts/No Auer rods/Does not meet criteria for MDS with isolated del(5q)
MDS with ring sideroblasts (MDS-RS)	
MDS-RS and single lineage dysplasia	One dysplastic lineage with dysplasia in at least 10% of bone marrow cellularity with 1-2 cytopenias. 15% (or greater) ringed sideroblasts OR 5% (or greater) ringed sideroblasts in the presence of an SF3B1 mutation Less than 5% bone marrow blasts/less than 1% peripheral blasts/No Auer rods/Does not meet criteria for MDS with isolated del(5q)
MDS-RS and multilineage dysplasia	More than 1 dysplastic lineage with 2-3 cytopenias 15% (or greater) ringed sideroblasts OR 5% (or greater) ringed sideroblasts in the presence of an SF3B1 mutation Less than 5% bone marrow blasts/less than 1% peripheral blasts/No Auer rods/Does not meet criteria for MDS with isolated del(5q)
MDS with isolated del(5q)	del(5q) alone or with 1 additional abnormality except—7 or del(7q) One or more dysplastic lineages with 1-2 cytopenias Less than 5% bone marrow blasts/less than 1% peripheral blasts/No Auer rods
MDS with excess blasts (MDS-EBs)	
MDS-EB-1	1-3 cytopenias 5%-9% bone marrow blasts or 2%-4% peripheral blasts/No Auer rods
MDS-EB-2	1-3 cytopenias 10%-19% bone marrow blasts or 5%-19% peripheral **blasts**/No Auer rods
MDS, unclassifiable	
With 1% blood blasts	1 or more dysplastic lineages in at least 10% of bone marrow cellularity with 1-3 cytopenias Less than 5% bone marrow blasts/more than 1% peripheral blasts/No Auer rods
With single lineage dysplasia and pancytopenia	1 dysplastic lineage in at least 10% of bone marrow cellularity with 3 cytopenias Less than 5% bone marrow blasts/less than 1% peripheral blasts/No Auer rods
Based on defining cytogenetic abnormality	No significant dysplastic features with 1-3 cytopenias in the presence of an MDS defining cytogenetic abnormality Less than 5% bone marrow blasts/less than 2% peripheral blasts/No Auer rods

Abbreviation: MDS, myelodysplastic syndrome.
Adapted from Arber DA, Orazi A, Hasserjian R, et al. The 2016 revision to the World Health Organization classification of myeloid neoplasms and acute leukemia. *Blood.* 2016;127(20):2391-2405. Copyright © 2016 American Society of Hematology. With permission.

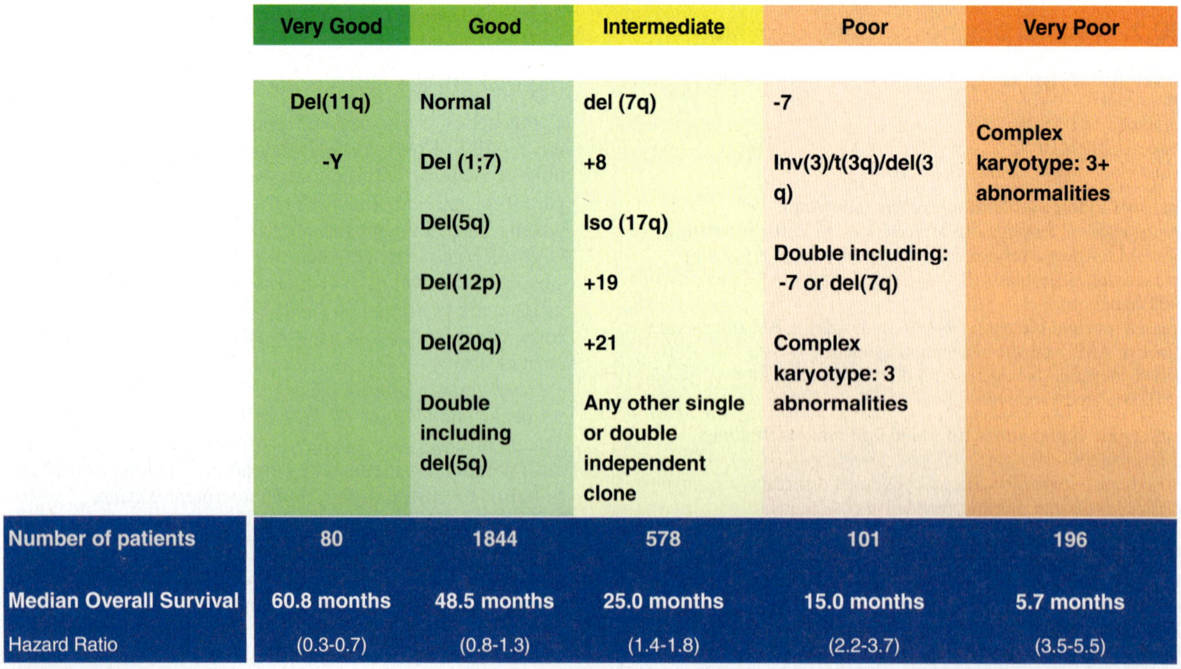

	Very Good	Good	Intermediate	Poor	Very Poor
	Del(11q) -Y	Normal Del (1;7) Del(5q) Del(12p) Del(20q) Double including del(5q)	del (7q) +8 Iso (17q) +19 +21 Any other single or double independent clone	-7 Inv(3)/t(3q)/del(3q) Double including: -7 or del(7q) Complex karyotype: 3 abnormalities	Complex karyotype: 3+ abnormalities
Number of patients	80	1844	578	101	196
Median Overall Survival	60.8 months	48.5 months	25.0 months	15.0 months	5.7 months
Hazard Ratio	(0.3-0.7)	(0.8-1.3)	(1.4-1.8)	(2.2-3.7)	(3.5-5.5)

FIGURE 80.2 Cytogenetics. (Adapted from Greenberg PL, Tuechler H, Schanz J, et al. Revised international prognostic scoring system for myelodysplastic syndromes. *Blood.* 2012;120:2454-2465.)

parameter is diagnostic of MDS, but combinations of such parameters can help discriminate MDS from other causes of cytopenias with high sensitivity and specificity.[66] Different scoring systems for flow cytometry have also revealed that higher numbers of cytometric aberrancies correlate with HR disease by IPSS, and that more cytometric defects in lower-risk MDS suggest an increased risk of progression. Based on these data, the International/European LeukemiaNet Working Group have proposed guidelines to integrate flow cytometry into the WHO classification, with adaptable parameters for areas with limited resources.[65] At present, flow cytometry is still considered experimental given lack of standardization among flow cytometry labs worldwide and is complementary to morphology and genetic results.

Molecular Analysis

More than 90% of patients with MDS are noted to have a clonal abnormality when cytogenetics are combined with gene sequencing.[31] Molecular analysis has only superficially been integrated into a formal diagnosis of MDS, with the integration of *SF3B1* mutations that define MDS with ring sideroblasts in patients with ≥5% ring sideroblasts. The presence of recurrent somatic mutations refines the diagnosis and prognosis and are increasingly guiding therapeutic decision-making (discussed in the treatment section).[30,32,67-71]

PROGNOSTIC ASSESSMENT

Prognosis in MDS is dependent on a constellation of features including degree of cytopenias, percentage of bone marrow blasts, karyotypic abnormalities, and molecular mutations. In addition, age, frailty, marrow fibrosis, lactic acid dehydrogenase, ferritin, and β2-microglobulin, among other factors, can further modify risk. Since 2012, the IPSS-R has been the standard risk-based clinical outcomes assessment tool based on key prognostic features that help guide therapy.[72] It is used essentially as a default staging system for MDS.

The original IPSS was developed in 1997 based upon assessment of a cohort of 880 patients that did not receive therapy, establishing four prognostic categories (low-, intermediate 1–, intermediate 2–, and high-risk disease) with significant differences in OS and risk of transformation to AML.[73] This static prognostic model, to be used only at MDS diagnosis, was based on the FAB morphologic criteria that classified bone marrow blasts up to 29% as MDS (as opposed to blasts up to 19% in the current WHO definition). Classically, patients with low and int-1 MDS were considered to have "lower risk" disease, while those with int-2 and high IPSS categorization were consider to have "higher risk" disease. The revised IPSS, or IPSS-R, adjusts for some of the limitations of the original IPSS, which underestimates the importance of severity of cytopenias and provides too much weight to the percentage of blasts at the expense of karyotypic alterations. The revised IPSS, or IPSS-R, summarized in *Table 80.4*, changes the cut-offs of cytopenias, percentage of marrow blasts, and includes the updated five-subgroup cytogenetic risk classification schema (see cytogenetics) to create five prognostic categories (very good, good, intermediate, poor, and very poor).[72] IPSS-R remains a static assessment developed in de novo MDS patients; it has been evaluated in treated patients who received ESAs, lenalidomide, and prior to hematopoietic cell transplantation (HCT), but is not predictive of outcomes in patients with secondary or therapy-related MDS.[74] Its accuracy deteriorates in patients who are about to receive or have already been treated with HMAs.[75] Using the IPSS-R, patients with a score ≤ 3.5 have "lower risk" disease, while those with a score > 3.5 have HR MDS.[76]

INTEGRATION OF GENETICS INTO PROGNOSTIC SYSTEMS

Increasingly, molecular data are being incorporated into prognostic scoring systems, as the importance of genetic mutations and their impact on risk has been recognized. That being said, the biologic impact of the site and type of mutation (location on the gene), hierarchy, variant allele frequency, and cooperative impact of multiple mutations add to the complexity of modifying clinical prognostic schemas. Finally, application of clinical context is important; for example, commonly mutated MDS genes like TET2, DNMT3a, and ASXL1 may be seen in older individuals with normal blood counts (CHIP).

Large series have demonstrated that a greater number of mutations are associated with poorer prognosis, and that on average, patients with three or more acquired mutations are predicted to have leukemia transformation within 2 years.[28,30] Mutations in TP53, EZH2, RUNX1, NRAS, and ASXL1 have been independently associated with adverse prognosis, whereas mutations in the splicing factor *SF3B1* are associated with favorable outcomes.[32,71,77-79] The TP53 mutation is poor risk, even with the favorable isolated del5q karyotypic abnormality,[80] and higher variant allele frequencies of TP53 are also associated with even worse outcomes.[81] Incorporating discrete molecular mutations into the IPSS and IPSS-R improves the accuracy of these schemas in predicting transformation to leukemia and death, and newer, machine learning approaches refine prognosis even further, and allow for dynamic application at any time during a patient's disease course.[71,82,83]

Comorbidities and Frailty

The IPSS-R provides a prognostic framework that helps stratify disease-associated prognosis, with age-adjusted calculation of risk integrated into the IPSS-RA. However, age is not a reliable metric for frailty, which refers to a state of vulnerability state created by a multidimensional loss of physiological reserve that includes energy, physical ability, cognition, and general health.[84] Patients with a severe comorbidity have up to a 50% decrease in survival, independent of age and IPSS risk group. Consequently, integrating frailty and the impact of comorbidities can improve prognostication, leading to improved clinical decision-making.[85] In particular, congestive heart failure, pulmonary and liver failure, infections, hemorrhage, and solid tumors are the main causes of nonleukemic death in MDS.[85-87]

Table 80.4. The Revised International Prognostic Scoring System (IPSS-R)

Prognostic variable	0	0.5	1	1.5	2	3	4
Cytogenetics	Very Good	-	Good	-	Intermediate	Poor	Very Poor
Bone Marrow Blast %	≤2	-	>2 - <5	-	5-10	>10	-
Hemoglobin	≥10	-	8 - <10	<8	-	-	-
Platelets	≥100	50 - <100	<50	-	-	-	-
Absolute Neutrophil Count	≥0.8	<0.8	-	-	-	-	-

Risk Category	Very Low	Low	Intermediate	High	Very High
Risk Score	≤1.5	>1.5-3	>3-4.5	>4.5-6	>6

Reprinted from Greenberg PL, Tuechler H, Schanz J, et al. Revised international prognostic scoring system for myelodysplastic syndromes. *Blood*. 2012;120(12):2454-2465. Copyright © 2012 American Society of Hematology. With permission.

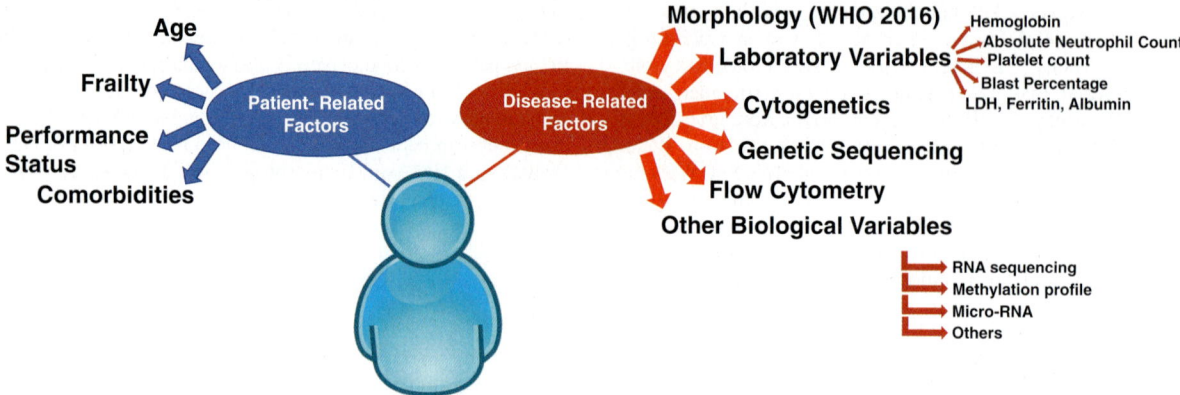

FIGURE 80.3 Prognostic factors in MDS. LDH, lactic acid dehydrogenase; MDS, myelodysplastic syndrome. (Adapted from Nazha A. The MDS genomics – prognosis symbiosis. *Hematology*. 2018;1:270-276.)

Historically, integration of these factors was left to the judgment of the provider or using universal tools such as the Charlson Comorbidity Index.[88] Efforts are being made to create MDS-specific comorbidity and frailty tools that can help standardize assessments.[85,89-91]

The prognostic factors in MDS are outlined in *Figure 80.3*.

TREATMENT OF MYELODYSPLASTIC SYNDROMES

Given the substantial genetic, pathologic, and clinical heterogeneity of MDS, along with competing comorbidities in an older population, therapy requires an individually tailored approach that is also sensitive to cytopenia trends and degree at presentation, patient symptoms, and expected disease trajectory. One limitation in this personalized approach is the degree to which the understanding of the biologic underpinnings of the disease has outstripped the limited number of available therapies. In general, treatment approaches are geared separately to those with lower risk and higher risk disease. In addition to risk, the patient's comorbid conditions and overall frailty should be considered (*Figure 80.4*).[89,92,93]

Lower Risk MDS

About two-thirds of all MDS patients will present with lower risk (LR-MDS): very low, low, or low-intermediate disease according to an IPSS-R score ≤3.5 points. These patients, by definition, often have a low bone marrow blast percentage, low number and depth of cytopenias, and relatively good karyotypic or molecular abnormalities. Certain mutations (TP53, EZH2, ASXL1, CBL, and U2AF1) also predict poorer outcomes than what is predicted by IPSS-R independent of lower risk IPSS-R assignment.[78,79]

Treatment goals for patients with lower-risk MDS include managing symptoms related to cytopenias (such as symptoms of anemia or thrombocytopenia), minimizing transfusions, improving or maintaining quality of life, and preventing disease progression. For patients with mild cytopenias who are minimally symptomatic without HR molecular or cytogenetic features, no therapy may be the best therapy, along with routine clinical/lab follow-up.

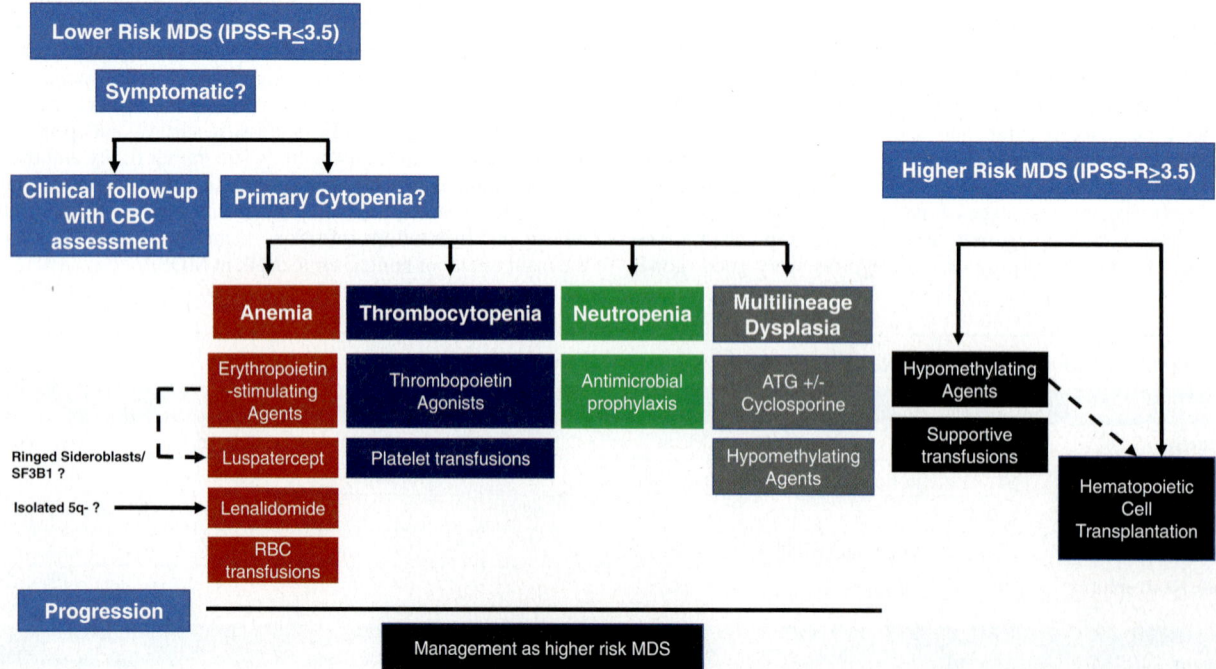

FIGURE 80.4 Outline for the MDS treatment algorithm. ATG, antithymocyte globulin; CBC, complete blood count; MDS, myelodysplastic syndrome; RBC, red blood cell. (Adapted from Sekeres M, Patel B. Lowering the boom on lower-risk myelodysplastic syndromes. *Hematology Am Soc Hematol Educ Program*. 2019;1:367-372.)

For patients requiring therapeutic intervention, the provider must consider the predominating cytopenia, endogenous erythropoietin (EPO) levels, the presence of del(5q), and, most importantly, the burden of disease as reflected by general health status and symptoms of hematopoietic insufficiency. Clinical trial enrollment, whenever available, should be strongly considered, and pretransplant workup and evaluation should be obtained in patients with a good performance status, poor risk features, and progression following the non–transplant therapeutic options discussed below. Initial management commonly includes the use of hematopoietic growth factors such as ESAs, myeloid growth factors, and thrombopoiesis-stimulating agents based on the primary cytopenia. Other therapeutic agents for lower risk disease include lenalidomide, which is most effective in patients with del5q, erythroid maturation agents such as luspatercept for MDS with ring sideroblasts, immunosuppressive approaches, and the HMAs AZA and decitabine (including oral decitabine/cedazuridine).

Features worrisome for progression, which should always prompt a repeat bone marrow and genetics assessment, include progressive cytopenias despite adequate therapy, clinical symptoms that are out of proportion to the cytopenias and are not explained by an alternate comorbid condition, clonal progression or acquisition of additional cytogenetic or molecular abnormalities, or new mutations associated with AML such as FLT3 or NPM1.

Anemia Management

Anemia is the most common cytopenia in MDS, caused primarily by abnormal maturation and differentiation of erythroid progenitors and increased destruction of abnormal erythroblasts, which leads to ineffective erythropoiesis. A cross-sectional survey of US hematologist/oncologists from 2005 to 2007 showed that the median hemoglobin at the time of MDS diagnosis was 9.1 g/dL.[94] In addition to fatigue, chronic anemia has been linked to cognitive and cardiopulmonary decline, exacerbation of the effects of frailty, and longer term complications. The degree of anemia in MDS is independently associated with reduced OS, poorer quality of life, and HR of nonleukemic death and cardiac death.[95-97]

Due to gradual progression in anemia, many MDS patients will tolerate lower hemoglobin levels, and not all patients with MDS will require therapy. There are no prospective data that have shown that early therapeutic intervention prevents clonal evolution or provides a survival advantage. Therefore, in patients without symptoms, continued active clinical surveillance is appropriate.

For patients who require therapy in the setting of lower risk disease, the most important biomarkers with respect to anemia management include serum EPO levels and the presence of isolated del(5q) in lower risk patients, as these are strong predictors of response to ESAs and lenalidomide, respectively. Anemia in patients with ring sideroblasts and SF3B1 mutations can be managed with the novel agent luspatercept.

Erythropoiesis-Stimulating Agents

ESAs are recombinant analogues of EPO, the endogenous glycoprotein that regulates erythropoiesis. ESAs are generally considered first-line agents to manage symptomatic anemia for patients with LR-MDS, and both recombinant EPO (short-acting agent) and darbepoetin (DAR) (long-acting agent) have been evaluated in numerous clinical studies, including phase III clinical trials.[98,99] Mechanistically, they are thought to target early stages of erythropoiesis by inhibiting apoptosis and stimulating EPO-responsive erythroid precursor proliferation, and by promoting erythroid maturation.[100]

Clinical trials of ESAs in lower risk MDS patients have demonstrated hematologic improvement and greater transfusion independence in up to 40% of patients, with most responses occurring within 3 months, and a duration of response that is typically a median of 12 to 15 months.[98,99,101-103] While there are specific recommendations on an optimal dosing schedule, higher doses of ESAs (EPO 60,000-80,000 U/wk and DAR 500 µg every two to 3 weeks) are considered standard for MDS.[99,104,105]

Patients most likely to benefit from ESA therapy include those with low transfusion requirements and low serum EPO levels (<500).[101,106] Lower transfusion requirement is defined as transfusion of 3 to 7 units of packed red blood cells (pRBCs) in a 16-week period.[107] Other factors that are predictive of improved response to ESAs include normal cytogenetics, normal flow cytometry, a less inflammatory microenvironment, normal myeloblast counts, and minimal prior transfusion dependence.[101,106,108-111] Patients with MDS with ring sideroblasts have a shorter median duration of response to ESAs compared to other subtypes.[112] The addition of granulocyte colony-stimulating factor to ESAs may rescue responses in 10% to 20% of cases, particularly in the presence of MDS with ring sideroblasts (MDS-RS).[113]

Luspatercept/Erythropoiesis-Maturating Agents

Luspatercept is a recombinant fusion protein (activin receptor type IIB fusion ligand trap) that binds transforming growth factor-beta ligands to reduce SMAD2 and SMAD3 signaling, a pathway that regulates cellular development and growth. This pathway suppression leads to late-stage erythroblast differentiation.[114] This first-in-class erythroid maturation agent received FDA and erythropoiesis-maturating agent (EMA) approval in 2020 for transfusion-dependent lower risk MDS patients with ring sideroblasts (MDS-RS), spliceosome mutations with a lower percentage of ring sideroblasts, or with myelodysplastic/MPN with ring sideroblasts and thrombocytosis.[115]

Therapy response, as measured by transfusion independence, was first seen in the single-arm phase 2 PACE MDS study. In this study, the transfusion independence rate in patients treated with the higher doses of luspatercept was 38%. Lower EPO levels corresponded with improved response; however, up to 43% of patients with EPO >500 U/L demonstrated measurable erythroid response. Mutations in SF3B1 were particularly predictive of improved response, with hematologic improvement in 77% of patients with *SF3B1* mutations.[116] In the phase 3 MEDALIST trial, luspatercept was compared to placebo in transfusion-dependent, LR-MDS patients with either ≥15% RS or ≥5% RS with SF3B1 mutation refractory to or unlikely to respond to ESA (based on high serum EPO levels). Approximately half of the patients (53%) in the luspatercept arm had hematologic improvement in erythrocytes, compared to 12% in the placebo arm; transfusion independence was achieved by 38% and 13%, respectively, for a median of 30.6 weeks was achieved in the luspatercept arm compared with 13.6 weeks in the placebo group.[117] Some improvement in thrombocytopenia and neutropenia was also noted in patients treated with luspatercept. This agent is now being tested vs ESA in the first-line setting irrespective of mutational status in low-risk MDS, in combination with ESAs and in HR MDS.

Lenalidomide

Lenalidomide, an analog of thalidomide, is considered an immunomodulatory agent that was approved by the US FDA in 2005 specifically for the treatment of lower-risk, transfusion-dependent MDS patients with the del(5q) cytogenetic abnormality.

Del5q is the most common cytogenetic abnormality in MDS and is considered a distinct clinical and pathological disease.[118] Lenalidomide modulates the function of an E3 ubiquitin ligase leading to the ubiquitination and degradation of several specific proteins, including the protein casein kinase 1a1 (CK1a). While cells tolerate decreased levels of CK1a in the setting of del5q (Ck1a is encoded by the CSNK1A1 gene on the long arm of chromosome 5, and protein levels are decreased in the setting of allelic haploinsufficiency), they are unable to tolerate the further decrease of CK1α that is degraded by lenalidomide, leading to synthetic lethality of del(5q) MDS population.[119,120]

Lenalidomide was initially studied in an unselected lower risk MDS population (MDS-001 study) and demonstrated a particular benefit in patients with an isolated deletion of the long arm of chromosome 5 that included band q31 (del5q).[121] Subsequent studies focused on MDS with del5q: MDS-003 (phase 2) and MDS-004 (phase 3).[122,123] In the randomized study, 61% of patients treated with lenalidomide (10 mg dose) on the phase 3 study achieved transfusion independent for 8 weeks or longer, and 56% achieved transfusion independence >26 weeks, vs 6% in the placebo arm. Median time to an erythroid response was 4.6 weeks and the median duration of response was 2.2 years.[124] Worsening neutropenia and thrombocytopenia are side effects that may occur within the first few months of therapy and correlate with eventual erythroid response.[125] Higher initial lenalidomide starting dose, and subsequent dose reduction due to cytopenias, was also associated with improved OS.[126]

Of the patients with del5q, patients with pretreatment thrombocytopenia, mutations in TP53, a complex karyotype that includes del5q, and those with excess marrow blasts tend to have a lower response rate to lenalidomide treatment than those lacking these characteristics.[122,127]

Lenalidomide has also been evaluated in an international phase 3 trial for patients without del5q (MDS-005) who were unresponsive or likely to be refractory to ESAs. Patients randomized to lenalidomide had a 27% transfusion independence response rate and a 33-week median duration of response.[128] Based on these data, lenalidomide may be considered for off-label use in selected patients without del5q.

Neutropenia Management

Neutropenia predisposes patients to life-threatening infections. In addition to quantitative defects in neutrophils, patients with MDS have functionally defective neutrophils, as well as impaired B-, T-, and NK-cell defects.[129-134] Isolated neutropenia is a less common presentation of MDS, but neutropenia with other cytopenias is seen in patients with multilineage dysplasia and as a consequence of therapy. Severe neutropenia (absolute neutrophil count $<0.5 \times 10^9$/L) at diagnosis has a negative prognostic impact in patients with lower risk MDS.[72,135]

Use of myeloid growth factors has not been shown convincingly to prevent infections, prolong survival, or improve the quality of life.[136] Prophylactic myeloid growth factor use is not recommended in MDS patients. While these drugs can be considered in patients who develop frequent infections, there are no concrete data to suggest that this approach leads to infection prevention.[137] Myeloid growth factors have been studied in the context of neutropenia stemming from primary MDS therapy (lenalidomide, HMAs). When used in this context, growth factors are commonly used for a short period of time until neutropenia resolves.[138] Myeloid growth factors support the proliferation and differentiation of a broad range of myeloid precursor cells, including leukemic blasts.[139]

Thrombocytopenia Management

Thrombocytopenia, which occurs more commonly in older adults and in those with higher risk disease, is seen in up to 65% of patients with MDS.[140] Severe thrombocytopenia (platelet $< 30 \times 10^9$/L) is much less common, but bleeding due to low platelet count and platelet dysfunction accounts for 10% to 20% of MDS deaths, making it the second most common cause of death for MDS patients.[140-142] Severity of thrombocytopenia has been associated with decreased OS, and the IPSS-R incorporates this information into prognostication.[143]

While the mechanisms contributing to thrombocytopenia in MDS are incompletely understood, inhibitory cytokine-mediated suppression of megakaryocytic differentiation, increased megakaryocytic apoptosis, and aberrant thrombopoietin (TPO) signaling affecting megakaryocytic development and increased immune mediated platelet destruction all contribute.[144] Precise platelet levels that lead to an increased risk of bleeding have not been well defined.[145] In a retrospective analysis of 2900 patients from the Duesseldorf MDS Registry, patients with HR MDS had more frequent hemorrhagic complications, and those with platelet levels lower than 100,000/μL had shortened survival due to an increased risk of bleeding (16% vs 8% for those with higher platelet levels) and HR of progression to AML. Platelet counts <20,000/μL were associated with spontaneous clinical signs of bleeding.[146]

In patients with lower-risk MDS, supportive care includes TPO growth factors and platelet transfusions. Higher risk patients are limited to transfusion support.

Thrombopoietin Growth Factors

The TPO receptor agonists romiplostim and eltrombopag are approved by the US FDA for the management of aplastic anemia, chronic immune thrombocytopenia, and liver disease. While considered off-label therapies, these agents have been independently evaluated in patients with MDS.

Romiplostim is a TPO mimetic; it a single chain peptide that binds to the TPO receptor leading to stimulation of JAK2, downstream signal transduction, and transcriptional activation, which leads to megakaryocyte proliferation and differentiation. This weekly subcutaneous agent was evaluated in a phase II study of 250 patients with low- or intermediate-1 risk MDS randomized to receive romiplostim or placebo. Patients randomized 2:1 to receive romiplostim had significantly higher platelet response rates of 36.5% (vs 3.6% in placebo) and lower clinically significant bleeding events than those receiving placebo. However, an interim analysis of this study was concerning for a potentially higher frequency of progression to AML and marrow fibrosis in patients receiving romiplostim,[147] particularly among those who started the study with excess blasts. Most patients had resolution blast percentage spikes upon cessation of romiplostim, and longer term follow-up of up to 5 years of patients treated on this study showed similar rates of leukemic transformation rate and mortality in both arms.[148]

Eltrombopag is an oral TPO receptor agonist that binds to TPO-R in a noncompetitive fashion leading to megakaryocytic proliferation and differentiation.[149] In a small, randomized study conducted in patients with lower-risk MDS, improved platelet counts were noted in 47% of patients treated with eltrombopag, with no difference in disease progression or progression to AML compared to patients receiving placebo.[150] Eltrombopag has also been evaluated in HR MDS patients treated with AZA, but in this setting, the combination resulted in increased progression to AML and worse platelet recovery than patients treated with AZA monotherapy.[151-153] A meta-analysis of six TPO trials in MDS reinforces the conclusion that, while there is no evidence of premature progression to AML in lower risk MDS patients, this assertion will need to be further explored prospectively.[154]

Based on these results, in clinical practice, eltrombopag or romiplostim can be considered for patients with lower risk MDS, but due to insufficient and controversial safety data, they should be avoided in patients with MDS with excess blasts.

Immunosuppressive Therapies

The use of immunosuppressive treatment (IST) for the management of patients with lower-risk MDS originates from studies in patients with severe aplastic anemia, in which treatment with antithymocyte globulin (ATG) led to hematopoietic recovery.[155] Similar to aplastic anemia, pancytopenia in MDS may result from immune dysregulation via lymphocyte-mediated stem cell destruction.[156,157] Patients with lower-risk MDS may have expansion of autoreactive cytotoxic T lymphocytes, and associated increase in proapoptotic inflammatory cytokines such as tumor necrosis factor alpha, perforin, and granzyme. This can lead to hematopoietic precursor death and suppression of normal hematopoiesis.[158-162]

The subset of lower risk MDS patients who will respond to IST is not well defined. Previously reported predictors of response include younger age, hypocellular marrow, blasts <5%, normal karyotype, HLA-DR positivity, and shorter duration of transfusion dependence, but these predictors have not been reproducible between studies, and do not hold up in multivariate analyses of predictors of response in a large cohort.[163-166] The role of somatic gene mutations on response to IST is also an area of ongoing investigation, with one recent study reporting that the presence of SF3B1 mutations adversely effected response.[167]

ATG is the best-studied IST agent both as monotherapy and in combination with other agents such as cyclosporine and prednisone.[156,168-171] Others include cyclosporine, alemtuzumab, and etanercept, though use is less common.[172-176]

Horse ATG is known to be superior to rabbit ATG in aplastic anemia and retrospective results suggest the same in MDS.[166,177] In the most selective study of horse ATG and cyclosporine in younger patients that incorporated HLA-DR15-positive status, BM cellularity <30%, and/or BM T-lymphocyte hyperfunction into its inclusion criteria, a total response rate of 77.5% with durable responses in a majority of the patients was reported.[178] These results are markedly higher than most studies that represent more typical MDS patients who are older and use more standard inclusion criteria for enrollment. The only phase 3 study randomized patients with MDS to horse ATG and oral cyclosporine or best supportive care and demonstrated a response rate of 29% for those receiving ATG compared to 9% in the control arm with a median 16.4-month duration of response.[170] A phase 2 study conducted in the United States showed a similar response rate and duration.[168] An international cohort study showed an overall response rate of 49% to IST regimens (43% of which included ATG) and median OS of 47 months, while a systematic review and meta-analysis of IST studies including treatment with ATG +/− cyclosporine showed an overall response rate of 42.5%, complete remission rate of 12.5%, and red blood cell (RBC) transfusion independence rate of 33.4%.[166,179] Taken together, IST should be considered in patients with anemia or multiple cytopenias, often following trial of other agents.

Hypomethylating Agents (Lower Risk)

The HMAs AZA and decitabine (and the oral decitabine/cedazuridine) are often used in patients with lower-risk MDS either when other agents have failed or for patients with multiple cytopenias. A randomized phase II trial comparing three-day schedules of AZA or decitabine for lower risk MDS conducted through the US MDS Clinical Research Consortium, most of whom were treatment naïve, reported high response rates to truncated dosing schedules (49% and 70%, respectively) with 32% and 16% of patients achieving transfusion independence, respectively, and with a median event-free survival of 18 months and a median OS that had not been reached after a median follow-up of 20 months.[180]

MDS Supportive Interventions

PRBC Transfusion Support

Transfusions of packed RBCs and platelets are an integral part of MDS management, and the goals of therapy are to improve acute and chronic symptoms of anemia and thrombocytopenia while minimizing the risk of complications caused by deficiencies. Unfortunately, a vast majority of MDS patients need RBC transfusions over the course of their therapy with many becoming RBC transfusion dependent, and up to 65% of patients will need ≥1 platelet transfusion.[181-183] Transfusion dependence is considered a negative prognostic factor in patients with MDS; transfusion-dependent patients have a shorter OS compared to transfusion-independent patients.[184,185] Transfusion-dependent MDS patients are at an HR of iron overload, transfusion reactions, transfusion-associated circulatory overload, alloimmunization, and report a decreased quality of life.[186]

At present there is no standardized approach to transfusions, and several individualized factors such as symptoms, cost, access, potential transfusion complications, symptomatic improvement with transfusion, and cardiovascular risks of both liberal and conservative transfusion parameters need to be considered in patient-provider joint decision-making. Transfusion parameters have historically been extrapolated from studies looking at patients with acute anemia, such as patients with cardiovascular disease; however, more recent studies are delineating optimal RBC transfusion support thresholds in patients with MDS,[187] with one identifying a hemoglobin level of 7.5 g/dL.[188]

Iron Chelation

Ineffective erythropoiesis and intravascular influx of iron via transfusions lead to iron overload in MDS. The detrimental effects of iron overload are well studied in several other hematologic disorders (hemochromatosis, sickle cell anemia, etc.), but the consequences in MDS are less clear. Iron chelation has not demonstrated OS benefit in a prospective randomized trial. The TELESTO study (a multicenter, randomized, double-blind, placebo-controlled trial) reported an improved event-free survival, but failed to show improvement in OS.[189] The reported survival benefit of iron chelation is derived primarily from single institution studies or observational data, therefore, while iron chelation can be considered in selected patients with lower risk MDS.[190,191]

Antimicrobial Prophylaxis

Infectious complications are significant, and among the main causes of death, in patients with MDS.[143,192-194] In addition to a defective immune response due to quantitative and functional disease–related neutropenia and due to treatment, iron overload may lead to an increased risk of both bacterial and fungal infections, although the data in this setting have been generated primarily in MDS patients with iron overload following allogeneic stem cell transplantation.[195-197] Antimicrobial prophylaxis may reduce the risk of infection in immunosuppressed patients. The American Society of Clinical Oncology/ Infectious Diseases Society of America guidelines for patients with cancer-related immunosuppression support the use of antibacterial prophylaxis with fluoroquinolones (levofloxacin is most studied in MDS), as well as antifungal prophylaxis with an oral triazole or parenteral echinocandin for patients at risk of profound, protracted neutropenia.[198] Acyclovir is also frequently used for antiviral prophylaxis, extrapolating from data in leukemia patients undergoing induction and post allogeneic transplant patients.[198,199]

Platelet Transfusion Support

For patients who are not candidates for TPO growth factors, platelet transfusions are often necessary. Platelet transfusions are not durable, and therefore logistically cumbersome. Platelets are also immunogenic, and in addition to routine transfusion-related risks, frequent platelet transfusions can lead to alloimmunization, and ultimately platelet transfusion refractoriness.

Higher Risk MDS

In general, patients with HR MDS have an extremely poor prognosis, with a median OS measured in less than 2 years. Thus, goals of therapy focus on prolonging life, delaying AML transformation, and improving patient-reported outcomes. Allogeneic HCT is the only curative intent therapy and should be considered for patients in patients with an otherwise good performance status, well-managed comorbidities, and a desire to undergo the procedure.

Hypomethylating Agents

HMAs are the cornerstone of therapy for patients with HR MDS. US FDA-approved HMAs include AZA, decitabine, and the oral formulation of decitabine plus cedazuridine.[200-202]

AZA is a pyrimidine nucleoside cytidine analog that has modulating effects on cellular differentiation, gene expression, and DNA synthesis and metabolism. It is known to inhibit DNA methyltransferase during DNA replication, which leads to reduced methylation of certain genes.[203] AZA is primarily incorporated into RNA and thus also inhibits the translation of proteins.

AZA was introduced into clinical care based on the (CALGB)-9221 study.[201] Prior to this study, there were no pharmacologic agents that could alter the natural history of MDS. Treatment with azacytidine 75 mg/m^2 for 7 consecutive days every 28 days was associated with an overall response rate of 60%, complete remission rate of 7%, and improvement in quality of life. In the follow-up AZA-001 study,[204] patients were randomly assigned to receive either azacytidine or conventional care regimens (60% of which was best supportive care, with the remaining 40% of patients on the conventional care arm receiving low-dose cytarabine or AML-type induction chemotherapy). Thirty-five percent of patients receiving azacytidine had a response according to the International Working Group criteria, and patients treated with AZA had a median OS that was significantly prolonged, at a median of 24.5 months, compared to 15 months in the conventional care group.

More recent registry studies and large cooperative group clinical trials show that OS with AZA is generally lower than reported on the AZA-MDS-001, with a median 12- to 20-month survival more typical.[205-208] Additional analysis of AZA-001 has also provided significant clues for the clinical management of patients with MDS. First, the median number of cycles with AZA in this group of patients was nine. It is believed that the duration of therapy is crucial for the survival advantage documented with this drug. Second, in a posthoc analysis, investigators studied the impact of age and AML blasts by

WHO category (20%-30% blasts) in patients treated with AZA-001. The results indicated that older individuals benefited significantly from therapy and that excess blasts were not a negative predictor of response.[209] When assessing cytogenetic predictors, multivariate analyses from the AZA-001 and other studies have demonstrated that autosomal monosomies such as deletion of chromosome 7 were associated with response to AZA therapy.[210,211] Higher responses for AZA and decitabine are also seen in patients with TP53 abnormalities, though they are not sustained.[208,212]

Decitabine, the other approved cytidine analog, differs from AZA in that it only integrates into DNA, whereas AZA integrates into both DNA and RNA.[213] Following various dose and schedule finding studies, a five-day schedule of decitabine 20 mg/m^2 every 28 days was established and found to have an overall response rate similar to that of AZA.[214,215] Unlike AZA, however, in a randomized phase III trial of patients with HR MDS comparing decitabine to best supportive care conducted in Europe, a beneficial effect of decitabine on OS or time to AML transformation was not demonstrated.[204,216] This is likely due to the dosing and schedule of decitabine used on study, as well as disease characteristics of patients treated on the decitabine study. There are no prospective studies comparing AZA and decitabine, but retrospective comparisons of decitabine vs AZA in 2025 HR- MDS patients using the SEER-Medicare linked database in the United States, as well as a Korean MDS registry study and several smaller analyses, have failed to show differences in survival based on the HMA received.[217,218]

The most recent development in HMA therapy for MDS is the FDA approval of oral decitabine and cedazuridine In the ASCERTAIN study, oral decitabine and cedazuridine taken once daily for five consecutive days of each 28-day cycle was shown to be bioequivalent to the decitabine 20 mg/m^2 5-day schedule.[202]

Who Will Respond?

Fewer than 50% of patients respond to HMAs, responses are rarely sustained, and outcomes after treatment failure are poor.[219,220] Improving patient selection that may distinguish responders from nonresponders would minimize unnecessary treatment-related toxicity, cost, and time lost on HMA therapy. There is no reliable biomarker of response to identify patients most likely to benefit from therapy. While the name "hypomethylating agent" suggests that responses may be tied to epigenetic aberrations in methylation, pretreatment global DNA methylation profiles or changes in methylation profiles with therapy do not neatly correlate with response.[221-228] The predictive capacity of mutations in genes involved in DNA methylation and epigenetic regulation (DNMT3A, TET2, IDH1, and IDH2, ASXL1, EZH2, and TET2) has also been assessed and appear to correlate with response, though not sustained response or improvement in OS.[229-232] As a heterogeneous disease with a complicated genomic landscape novel, machine learning integrative approaches, such as assessment of mutational combinations, as opposed to the role of single mutations, and their impact on response to therapy may be more representative of pathology, and improve response prediction accuracy.[233]

When HMAs Fail

For patients with progression on HMA therapy, outcomes are exceptionally poor and treatment options are limited.[234] Median survival is measured in months, though attempts have been made to distinguish better and worse risk groups post-HMAs.[235] In general, patients should be offered therapy within a clinical trial whenever possible. Efforts are being made to improve responses with combination therapies that include a backbone of HMAs and drugs targeting defective pathways in MDS.

Intensive Induction Chemotherapy

For younger, fitter patients who can be treated with curative intent with allogeneic transplantation, cytotoxic chemotherapy used in AML induction may be considered. The remission rates to induction in this setting are lower than in the case of de novo AML (~50%) with a short duration of response, requiring quick bridge to allogeneic HCT.[236,237] Several induction regimens, such as "7 + 3" (cytarabine and an anthracycline), FLAG-Ida (fludarabine, cytarabine, idarubicin, and G-CSF), and others, have been used. While response rates in HR MDS may be higher to intensive chemotherapy, this has not translated into a clear survival benefit compared to HMA-based therapy in any age group.[204,237-240] A subgroup analysis of patients with oligoblastic AML enrolled to the AZA-001 study comparing AZA to conventional care regimens showed that AZA was superior, with improvement in OS and several morbidity measures.[209] Other studies have shown that in older patients with HR MDS, aggressive induction therapy can lead to remission in 20% to 50% of patients, but induction mortality is high (30%-50%) and 1-year survival is poor.[237-240]

The role of less intensive induction regimens being used in AML, such as the combination of venetoclax, a BCL2 inhibitor, or pevonedistat, and Nedd8-activating enzyme inhibitor and AZA are now being evaluated in MDS.[241,242] One subgroup analysis of the IDH2 inhibitor enasidenib showed a response rate of 40% that was sustained for a median of 9 months in HR MDS patients with IDH2 mutations, and this may be an option for post-HMA failure.[243]

Hematopoietic Cell Transplantation

HCT is the only curative therapy for MDS. That being said, it is associated with significant morbidity and mortality, and appropriate patient selection is essential. Transplant has been underused in the management of MDS, particularly because older patients were historically considered transplant ineligible based purely on age or lack of insurance coverage and often did not undergo transplant evaluation.[94] However, recent (CIBMTR) data comparing the outcomes of MDS patients who underwent HCT aged 65 years or older with patients aged 55 to 64 years demonstrate similar OS, relapse free survival, nonrelapse mortality, and graft-vs-host disease risk, suggesting that chronologic age should not empirically deter from transplant.[244] Therefore, after careful consideration of performance status, frailty, comorbidities, HCT specific comorbidity index, and disease characteristics, "fit" older patients with HR disease, lower risk disease with adverse genetics, and patients with profound cytopenias for whom other available therapies have failed should be considered for HCT.[245]

Two decision analyses (one focusing on intensive, myeloablative HCT conditioning and the other on reduced intensity) have shown that patients with HR MDS live longer when treated with up-front HCT compared to conventional therapy. For lower-risk MDS patients, survival is maximized when HCT is delayed until other available treatment options are exhausted, or evolution to HR disease is impending.[246,247] Data are less clear with intermediate risk disease.[245,247,248] Reduced intensity conditioning (RIC) has a comparable OS to myeloablative conditioning (76% vs 63% respectively) at 2 years of follow-up that makes HCT even more accessible to older patients with some comorbidities by lowering the risk of transplant-related mortality.[249]

Disease characteristics that that portend poorer prognoses with transplant include patients with a higher blast burden (greater than 5%), HR karyotypes, HR mutations including ASXL1, RUNX1, JAK2, RAS pathway mutations, and most notably mutations in TP53.[56,69,250-256] In patients with these characteristics, clinical trials may be a better management strategy, emphasizing the role of thoughtful patient selection.

In HR disease, upfront HCT without any preceding therapy can be considered, particularly if blasts are not increased.[257] In patients with increased blasts, a cytoreductive strategy with HMAs or intensive chemotherapy as a bridge to transplant to reduce disease burden is common. With regard to choice of cytoreductive therapy, retrospective analyses adjusted for age, IPSS, donor, and conditioning intensity failed to show any benefit in outcomes for patients receiving intensive chemotherapy compared to HMA even when there was a higher proportion of patients with primary refractory disease in the HMA group.[258-261] This has not been prospectively studied, and therefore, due to the higher toxicity and mortality risk of intensive regimens, HMA therapy is preferred.

The VidazaAllo study comparing AZA induction followed by allogeneic stem cell transplantation vs continuous AZA treatment according to donor availability in older patients with newly diagnosed HR

MDS showed that about one-third of patients could not proceed with transplant due to progression while receiving debulking hypomethylating therapy.[262] In the CTN 1102 trial, 384 patients ages 50 to 75 years with HR MDS underwent biological randomization to HCT or no HCT. In the no transplant arm, over 25% of patients did not receive HMA therapy. A significant OS advantage was seen in older patients with int-2 and high IPSS risk de novo MDS who were RIC HCT candidates and had an HLA-matched donor, when compared with those without a donor. There are also data that show transplant outcomes are better in patients who respond to HMAs, and therefore, a better understanding of HMA response predictors, overall disease biology, and its influence on pretransplant therapy is needed.[263,264]

CONCLUSION

The field of MDS is rapidly evolving, with a plethora of scientific data that are leading to new and innovative clinical developments in the field. Unfortunately, our understanding of disease biology has outstripped the available therapies to meaningful alter the disease course. For most MDS patients, currently available therapies are only effective for a few years, highlighting the enormous potential for improvement. With improved disease classification and prognostication, as well novel therapeutic advances in clinical development, we hope to move beyond simply pushing the needle forward to completely revolutionizing care for patients with MDS.

References

1. Steensma DP. Historical perspectives on myelodysplastic syndromes. *Leuk Res*. 2012;36(12):1441-1452.
2. Bennett JM, Catovsky D, Daniel MT, et al. Proposals for the classification of the acute leukaemias French-American-British (FAB) Co-operative group. *Br J Haematol*. 1976;33(4):451-458.
3. Vardiman JW, Harris NL, Brunning RD. The World Health Organization (WHO) classification of the myeloid neoplasms. *Blood*. 2002;100(7):2292-2302.
4. SEER. *SEER MDS Incidence 2014-2018*. 2020.
5. Cogle CR, Craig BM, Rollison DE, List AF. Incidence of the myelodysplastic syndromes using a novel claims-based algorithm: high number of uncaptured cases by cancer registries. *Blood*. 2011;117(26):7121-7125.
6. Ma X, Does M, Raza A, Mayne ST. Myelodysplastic syndromes: incidence and survival in the United States. *Cancer*. 2007;109(8):1536-1542.
7. Sekeres MA. Epidemiology, natural history, and practice patterns of patients with myelodysplastic syndromes in 2010. *J Natl Compr Canc Netw*. 2011;9(1):57-63.
8. Visser O, Trama A, Maynadié M, et al. Incidence, survival and prevalence of myeloid malignancies in Europe. *Eur J Cancer*. 2012;48(17):3257-3266.
9. Jiang Y, Eveillard JR, Couturier MA, et al. Asian population is more Prone to develop high-risk myelodysplastic syndrome, concordantly with their propensity to exhibit high-risk cytogenetic aberrations. *Cancers*. 2021;13(3):481.
10. Miyazaki Y, Tuechler H, Sanz G, et al. Differing clinical features between Japanese and Caucasian patients with myelodysplastic syndromes: analysis from the international working group for prognosis of MDS. *Leuk Res*. 2018;73:51-57.
11. Nazha A, Al-Issa K, Przychodzen B, et al. Differences in genomic patterns and clinical outcomes between African-American and White patients with myelodysplastic syndromes. *Blood Cancer J*. 2017;7(9):e602.
12. Goksu SY, Ozer M, Goksu BB, et al. The impact of race and ethnicity on outcomes of patients with myelodysplastic syndromes: a population-based analysis. *Leuk Lymphoma*. 2022;63(7):1651-1659.
13. Ramadan H; Melody M; Steele A, et al. Racial disparities in patients with myelodysplastic syndrome (MDS): clinical and molecular depiction. *Blood*. 2016;128(22):1997.
14. Xie M, Lu C, Wang J, et al. Age-related mutations associated with clonal hematopoietic expansion and malignancies. *Nat Med*. 2014;20(12):1472-1478.
15. Iwanaga M, Hsu WL, Soda M, et al. Risk of myelodysplastic syndromes in people exposed to ionizing radiation: a retrospective cohort study of Nagasaki atomic bomb survivors. *J Clin Oncol*. 2010;29(4):428-434.
16. Taguchi M, Mishima H, Shiozawa Y, et al. Genome analysis of myelodysplastic syndromes among atomic bomb survivors in Nagasaki. *Haematologica*. 2020;105(2):358-365.
17. Kuendgen A, Nomdedeu M, Tuechler H, et al. Therapy-related myelodysplastic syndromes deserve specific diagnostic sub-classification and risk-stratification—an approach to classification of patients with t-MDS. *Leukemia*. 2021;35(3):835-849.
18. Du Y, Fryzek J, Sekeres MA, Taioli E. Smoking and alcohol intake as risk factors for myelodysplastic syndromes (MDS). *Leuk Res*. 2010;34(1):1-5.
19. Tong H, Hu C, Yin X, Yu M, Yang J, Jin J. A meta-analysis of the relationship between cigarette smoking and incidence of myelodysplastic syndromes. *PLoS One*. 2013;8(6):e67537.
20. Jin J; Yu M; Hu C, et al. Pesticide exposure as a risk factor for myelodysplastic syndromes: a meta-analysis based on 1,942 cases and 5,359 controls. *PLoS One*. 2014;9(10):e110750.
21. Furutani E, Shimamura A. Genetic predisposition to MDS: diagnosis and management. *Hematology*. 2019;2019(1):110-119.
22. Kennedy AL, Shimamura A. Genetic predisposition to MDS: clinical features and clonal evolution. *Blood*. 2019;133(10):1071-1085.
23. Locatelli F, Strahm B. How I treat myelodysplastic syndromes of childhood. *Blood*. 2018;131(13):1406-1414.
24. Hsu AP, McReynolds LJ, Holland SM. GATA2 deficiency. *Curr Opin Allergy Clin Immunol*. 2015;15(1):104-109.
25. Owen CJ, Toze CL, Koochin A, et al. Five new pedigrees with inherited RUNX1 mutations causing familial platelet disorder with propensity to myeloid malignancy. *Blood*. 2008;112(12):4639-4645.
26. Polprasert C, Schulze I, Sekeres MA, et al. Inherited and somatic defects in DDX41 in myeloid neoplasms. *Cancer Cell*. 2015;27(5):658-670.
27. Klco JM, Mulligan CG. Advances in germline predisposition to acute leukaemias and myeloid neoplasms. *Nat Rev Cancer*. 2021;21(2):122-137.
28. Bejar R, Stevenson K, Abdel-Wahab O, et al. Clinical effect of point mutations in myelodysplastic syndromes. *N Engl J Med*. 2011;364(26):2496-2506.
29. Yoshida K, Sanada M, Shiraishi Y, et al. Frequent pathway mutations of splicing machinery in myelodysplasia. *Nature*. 2011;478(7367):64-69.
30. Papaemmanuil E, Gerstung M, Malcovati L, et al. Clinical and biological implications of driver mutations in myelodysplastic syndromes. *Blood*. 2013;122(22):3616-3627. quiz 3699.
31. Haferlach T, Nagata Y, Grossmann V, et al. Landscape of genetic lesions in 944 patients with myelodysplastic syndromes. *Leukemia*. 2014;28(2):241-247.
32. Makishima H, Yoshizato T, Yoshida K, et al. Dynamics of clonal evolution in myelodysplastic syndromes. *Nat Genet*. 2017;49(2):204-212.
33. Jaiswal S, Fontanillas P, Flannick J, et al. Age-related clonal hematopoiesis associated with adverse outcomes. *N Engl J Med*. 2014;371(26):2488-2498.
34. Itzykson R, Fenaux P. Epigenetics of myelodysplastic syndromes. *Leukemia*. 2014;28(3):497-506.
35. Cimmino L, Abdel-Wahab O, Levine RL, Aifantis I. TET family proteins and their role in stem cell differentiation and transformation. *Cell Stem Cell*. 2011;9(3):193-204.
36. Bestor TH. Activation of mammalian DNA methyltransferase by cleavage of a Zn binding regulatory domain. *EMBO J*. 1992;11(7):2611-2617.
37. Bröske AM, Vockentanz L, Kharazi S, et al. DNA methylation protects hematopoietic stem cell multipotency from myeloerythroid restriction. *Nat Genet*. 2009;41(11):1207-1215.
38. Mayle A, Yang L, Rodriguez B, et al. Dnmt3a loss predisposes murine hematopoietic stem cells to malignant transformation. *Blood*. 2015;125(5):629-638.
39. Dang L, Su S-SM. Isocitrate dehydrogenase mutation and (R)-2-Hydroxyglutarate: from basic discovery to therapeutics development. *Annu Rev Biochem*. 2017;86(1):305-331.
40. Abla H, Sollazzo M, Gasparre G, Iommarini L, Porcelli AM. The multifaceted contribution of α-ketoglutarate to tumor progression: an opportunity to exploit? *Semin Cell Dev Biol*. 2020;98:26-33.
41. Waitkus MS, Diplas BH, Yan H. Biological role and therapeutic potential of IDH mutations in cancer. *Cancer Cell*. 2018;34(2):186-195.
42. Yang H, Kurtenbach S, Guo Y, et al. Gain of function of ASXL1 truncating protein in the pathogenesis of myeloid malignancies. *Blood*. 2018;131(3):328-341.
43. Gelsi-Boyer V, Brecqueville M, Devillier R, Murati A, Mozziconacci M-J, Birnbaum D. Mutations in ASXL1 are associated with poor prognosis across the spectrum of malignant myeloid diseases. *J Hematol Oncol*. 2012;5(1):12.
44. Nikoloski G, Langemeijer SM, Kuiper RP, et al. Somatic mutations of the histone methyltransferase gene EZH2 in myelodysplastic syndromes. *Nat Genet*. 2010;42(8):665-667.
45. Bondu S, Alary AS, Lefèvre C, et al. A variant erythroferrone disrupts iron homeostasis in SF3B1-mutated myelodysplastic syndrome. *Sci Transl Med*. 2019;11(500):eaav5467.
46. Malcovati L, Stevenson K, Papaemmanuil E, et al. SF3B1-mutant MDS as a distinct disease subtype: a proposal from the International Working Group for the Prognosis of MDS. *Blood*. 2020;136(2):157-170.
47. Wu SJ, Kuo YY, Hou HA, et al. The clinical implication of SRSF2 mutation in patients with myelodysplastic syndrome and its stability during disease evolution. *Blood*. 2012;120(15):3106-3111.
48. Hershberger CE, Daniels NJ, Padgett RA. Spliceosomal factor mutations and mis-splicing in MDS. *Best Pract Res Clin Haematol*. 2020;33(3):101199.
49. Merendino L, Guth S, Bilbao D, Martínez C, Valcárcel J. Inhibition of msl-2 splicing by Sex-lethal reveals interaction between U2AF35 and the 3′ splice site AG. *Nature*. 1999;402(6763):838-841.
50. Li B, Zou D, Yang S, Ouyang G, Mu Q. Prognostic significance of U2AF1 mutations in myelodysplastic syndromes: a meta-analysis. *J Int Med Res*. 2020;48(3):300060519891013.
51. Churpek JE, Bresnick EH. Transcription factor mutations as a cause of familial myeloid neoplasms. *J Clin Invest*. 2019;129(2):476-488.
52. Sood R, Kamikubo Y, Liu P. Role of RUNX1 in hematological malignancies. *Blood*. 2017;129(15):2070-2082.
53. Tsai SC, Shih LY, Liang ST, et al. Biological activities of RUNX1 mutants predict secondary acute leukemia transformation from chronic myelomonocytic leukemia and myelodysplastic syndromes. *Clin Cancer Res*. 2015;21(15):3541-3551.
54. Sill H, Zebisch A, Haase D. Acute myeloid leukemia and myelodysplastic syndromes with *TP53* aberrations—a distinct stem cell disorder. *Clin Cancer Res*. 2020;26(20):5304-5309.
55. Swaminathan M, Bannon SA, Routbort M, et al. Hematologic malignancies and Li-Fraumeni syndrome. *Cold Spring Harb Mol Case Stud*. 2019;5(1):003210.
56. Bernard E, Nannya Y, Hasserjian RP, et al. Implications of TP53 allelic state for genome stability, clinical presentation and outcomes in myelodysplastic syndromes. *Nat Med*. 2020;26(10):1549-1556.

57. Haase D, Stevenson KE, Neuberg D, et al. TP53 mutation status divides myelodysplastic syndromes with complex karyotypes into distinct prognostic subgroups. *Leukemia.* 2019;33(7):1747-1758.
58. Viny AD, Levine RL. Cohesin mutations in myeloid malignancies made simple. *Curr Opin Hematol.* 2018;25(2):61-66.
59. Sperling AS, Gibson CJ, Ebert BL. The genetics of myelodysplastic syndrome: from clonal haematopoiesis to secondary leukaemia. *Nat Rev Cancer.* 2017;17(1):5-19.
60. Thota S, Viny AD, Makishima H, et al. Genetic alterations of the cohesin complex genes in myeloid malignancies. *Blood.* 2014;124(11):1790-1798.
61. Zhang W, Liu HT. MAPK signal pathways in the regulation of cell proliferation in mammalian cells. *Cell Res.* 2002;12(1):9-18.
62. Kantarjian H, Giles F, List A, et al. The incidence and impact of thrombocytopenia in myelodysplastic syndromes. *Cancer.* 2007;109(9):1705-1714.
63. Zhang L, Stablein DM, Epling-Burnette P, et al. Diagnosis of myelodysplastic syndromes and related conditions: rates of discordance between local and central review in the NHLBI MDS natural history study. *Blood.* 2018;132 (suppl 1):4370.
64. Zahid MF, Malik UA, Sohail M, Hassan IN, Ali S, Shaukat MHS. Cytogenetic abnormalities in myelodysplastic syndromes: an overview. *Int J Hematol Oncol Stem Cell Res.* 2017;11(3):231-239.
65. Porwit A, van de Loosdrecht AA, Bettelheim P, et al. Revisiting guidelines for integration of flow cytometry results in the WHO classification of myelodysplastic syndromes-proposal from the International/European LeukemiaNet Working Group for Flow Cytometry in MDS. *Leukemia.* 2014;28(9):1793-1798.
66. Kussick SJ, Fromm JR, Rossini A, et al. Four-color flow cytometry shows strong concordance with bone marrow morphology and cytogenetics in the evaluation for myelodysplasia. *Am J Clin Pathol.* 2005;124(2):170-181.
67. Kwok B, Hall JM, Witte JS, et al. MDS-associated somatic mutations and clonal hematopoiesis are common in idiopathic cytopenias of undetermined significance. *Blood.* 2015;126(21):2355-2361.
68. Hansen JW, Westman MK, Sjö LD, et al. Mutations in idiopathic cytopenia of undetermined significance assist diagnostics and correlate to dysplastic changes. *Am J Hematol.* 2016;91(12):1234-1238.
69. Lindsley RC, Saber W, Mar BG, et al. Prognostic mutations in myelodysplastic syndrome after stem-cell transplantation. *N Engl J Med.* 2017;376(6):536-547.
70. Malcovati L, Papaemmanuil E, Ambaglio I, et al. Driver somatic mutations identify distinct disease entities within myeloid neoplasms with myelodysplasia. *Blood.* 2014;124(9):1513-1521.
71. Nazha A, Al-Issa K, Hamilton BK, et al. Adding molecular data to prognostic models can improve predictive power in treated patients with myelodysplastic syndromes. *Leukemia.* 2017;31(12):2848-2850.
72. Greenberg PL, Tuechler H, Schanz J, et al. Revised international prognostic scoring system for myelodysplastic syndromes. *Blood.* 2012;120(12):2454-2465.
73. Greenberg P, Cox C, LeBeau MM, et al. International scoring system for evaluating prognosis in myelodysplastic syndromes. *Blood.* 1997;89(6):2079-2088.
74. Nazha A, Seastone DP, Keng M, et al. The Revised International Prognostic Scoring System (IPSS-R) is not predictive of survival in patients with secondary myelodysplastic syndromes. *Leuk Lymphoma.* 2015;56(12):3437-3439.
75. Zeidan AM, Sekeres MA, Garcia-Manero G, et al. Comparison of risk stratification tools in predicting outcomes of patients with higher-risk myelodysplastic syndromes treated with azanucleosides. *Leukemia.* 2016;30(3):649-657.
76. Pfeilstöcker M, Tuechler H, Sanz G, et al. Time-dependent changes in mortality and transformation risk in MDS. *Blood.* 2016;128(7):902-910.
77. Malcovati L, Karimi M, Papaemmanuil E, et al. SF3B1 mutation identifies a distinct subset of myelodysplastic syndrome with ring sideroblasts. *Blood.* 2015;126(2):233-241.
78. Bejar R, Stevenson KE, Caughey BA, et al. Validation of a prognostic model and the impact of mutations in patients with lower-risk myelodysplastic syndromes. *J Clin Oncol.* 2012;30(27):3376-3382.
79. Bejar R, Papaemmanuil E, Haferlach T, et al. Somatic mutations in MDS patients are associated with clinical features and predict prognosis independent of the IPSS-R: analysis of combined datasets from the international working group for prognosis in MDS-molecular committee. *Blood.* 2015;126(23):907.
80. Lodé L, Ménard A, Flet L, et al. Emergence and evolution of TP53 mutations are key features of disease progression in myelodysplastic patients with lower-risk del(5q) treated with lenalidomide. *Haematologica.* 2018;103(4):e143-e146.
81. Sallman DA, Komrokji R, Vaupel C, et al. Impact of TP53 mutation variant allele frequency on phenotype and outcomes in myelodysplastic syndromes. *Leukemia.* 2016;30(3):666-673.
82. Nagata Y, Zhao R, Awada H, et al. Machine learning demonstrates that somatic mutations imprint invariant morphologic features in myelodysplastic syndromes. *Blood.* 2020;136(20):2249-2262.
83. Nazha A, Komrokji RS, Meggendorfer M, et al. A personalized prediction model to risk stratify patients with myelodysplastic syndromes. *Blood.* 2018;132(suppl 1):793.
84. Buckstein R, Wells RA, Zhu N, et al. Patient-related factors independently impact overall survival in patients with myelodysplastic syndromes: an MDS-CAN prospective study. *Br J Haematol.* 2016;174(1):88-101.
85. Naqvi K, Garcia-Manero G, Sardesai S, et al. Association of comorbidities with overall survival in myelodysplastic syndrome: development of a prognostic model. *J Clin Oncol.* 2011;29(16):2240-2246.
86. Della Porta MG, Malcovati L. Clinical relevance of extra-hematologic comorbidity in the management of patients with myelodysplastic syndrome. *Haematologica.* 2009;94(5):602-606.
87. Zipperer E, Pelz D, Nachtkamp K, et al. The hematopoietic stem cell transplantation comorbidity index is of prognostic relevance for patients with myelodysplastic syndrome. *Haematologica.* 2009;94(5):729-732.
88. Austin SR, Wong Y-N, Uzzo RG, Beck JR, Egleston BL. Why summary comorbidity measures such as the Charlson comorbidity index and elixhauser score work. *Med Care.* 2015;53(9):e65-e72.
89. Starkman R, Alibhai S, Wells RA, et al. An MDS-specific frailty index based on cumulative deficits adds independent prognostic information to clinical prognostic scoring. *Leukemia.* 2020;34(5):1394-1406.
90. Wan BA, Nazha A, Starkman R, et al. Revised 15-item MDS-specific frailty scale maintains prognostic potential. *Leukemia.* 2020;34(12):3434-3438.
91. Breccia M, Federico V, Loglisci G, et al. MDS-specific comorbidity index (MDS-CI) identifies overall survival differences in myelodysplastic syndrome patients. *Blood.* 2011;118(21):3793.
92. Abel GA, Buckstein R. Integrating frailty, comorbidity, and quality of life in the management of myelodysplastic syndromes. *Am Soc Clin Oncol Educ Book.* 2016;35:e337-e344.
93. Sorror ML, Sandmaier BM, Storer BE, et al. Comorbidity and disease status based risk stratification of outcomes among patients with acute myeloid leukemia or myelodysplasia receiving allogeneic hematopoietic cell transplantation. *J Clin Oncol.* 2007;25(27):4246-4254.
94. Sekeres MA, Schoonen WM, Kantarjian H, et al. Characteristics of US patients with myelodysplastic syndromes: results of six cross-sectional physician surveys. *J Natl Cancer Inst.* 2008;100(21):1542-1551.
95. Malcovati L, Della Porta MG, Strupp C, et al. Impact of the degree of anemia on the outcome of patients with myelodysplastic syndrome and its integration into the WHO classification-based Prognostic Scoring System (WPSS). *Haematologica.* 2011;96(10):1433-1440.
96. Buckstein R, Alibhai S, Lam A, et al. Transfusion dependence and low hemoglobin have the greatest impact on quality of life (QOL) in MDS patients: a tertiary care cross sectional and longitudinal study. *Blood.* 2009;114(22):2500.
97. Szende A, Schaefer C, Goss TF, et al. Valuation of transfusion-free living in MDS: results of health utility interviews with patients. *Health Qual Life Outcomes.* 2009;7:81.
98. Fenaux P, Santini V, Spiriti MAA, et al. A phase 3 randomized, placebo-controlled study assessing the efficacy and safety of epoetin-α in anemic patients with low-risk MDS. *Leukemia.* 2018;32(12):2648-2658.
99. Platzbecker U, Symeonidis A, Oliva EN, et al. A phase 3 randomized placebo-controlled trial of darbepoetin alfa in patients with anemia and lower-risk myelodysplastic syndromes. *Leukemia.* 2017;31(9):1944-1950.
100. Malik J, Kim AR, Tyre KA, Cherukuri AR, Palis J. Erythropoietin critically regulates the terminal maturation of murine and human primitive erythroblasts. *Haematologica.* 2013;98(11):1778-1787.
101. Hellström-Lindberg E, Gulbrandsen N, Lindberg G, et al. A validated decision model for treating the anaemia of myelodysplastic syndromes with erythropoietin + granulocyte colony-stimulating factor: significant effects on quality of life. *Br J Haematol.* 2003;120(6):1037-1046.
102. Golshayan AR, Jin T, Maciejewski J, et al. Efficacy of growth factors compared to other therapies for low-risk myelodysplastic syndromes. *Br J Haematol.* 2007;137(2):125-132.
103. Park S, Greenberg P, Yucel A, et al. Clinical effectiveness and safety of erythropoietin-stimulating agents for the treatment of low- and intermediate-1–risk myelodysplastic syndrome: a systematic literature review. *Br J Haematol.* 2019;184(2):134-160.
104. Balleari E, Filiberti RA, Salvetti C, et al. Effects of different doses of erythropoietin in patients with myelodysplastic syndromes: a propensity score-matched analysis. *Cancer Med.* 2019;8(18):7567-7576.
105. Gabrilove J, Paquette R, Lyons RM, et al. Phase 2, single-arm trial to evaluate the effectiveness of darbepoetin alfa for correcting anaemia in patients with myelodysplastic syndromes. *Br J Haematol.* 2008;142(3):379-393.
106. Wallvik J, Stenke L, Bernell P, Nordahl G, Hippe E, Hast R. Serum erythropoietin (EPO) levels correlate with survival and independently predict response to EPO treatment in patients with myelodysplastic syndromes. *Eur J Haematol.* 2002;68(3):180-185.
107. Platzbecker U, Fenaux P, Adès L, et al. Proposals for revised IWG 2018 hematological response criteria in patients with MDS included in clinical trials. *Blood.* 2019;133(10):1020-1030.
108. Rigolin GM, Porta MD, Ciccone M, et al. In patients with myelodysplastic syndromes response to rHuEPO and G-CSF treatment is related to an increase of cytogenetically normal CD34 cells. *Br J Haematol.* 2004;126(4):501-507.
109. Westers TM, Alhan C, Chamuleau ME, et al. Aberrant immunophenotype of blasts in myelodysplastic syndromes is a clinically relevant biomarker in predicting response to growth factor treatment. *Blood.* 2010;115(9):1779-1784.
110. Musto P, Matera R, Minervini MM, et al. Low serum levels of tumor necrosis factor and interleukin-1 beta in myelodysplastic syndromes responsive to recombinant erythropoietin. *Haematologica.* 1994;79(3):265-268.
111. Sekeres MA, Fu AZ, Maciejewski JP, Golshayan AR, Kalaycio ME, Kattan MW. A Decision analysis to determine the appropriate treatment for low-risk myelodysplastic syndromes. *Cancer.* 2007;109(6):1125-1132.
112. Hellström-Lindberg E, Negrin R, Stein R, et al. Erythroid response to treatment with G-CSF plus erythropoietin for the anaemia of patients with myelodysplastic syndromes: proposal for a predictive model. *Br J Haematol.* 1997;99(2):344-351.
113. Greenberg PL, Sun Z, Miller KB, et al. Treatment of myelodysplastic syndrome patients with erythropoietin with or without granulocyte colony-stimulating factor: results of a prospective randomized phase 3 trial by the Eastern Cooperative Oncology Group (E1996). *Blood.* 2009;114(12):2393-2400.
114. Kubasch AS, Fenaux P, Platzbecker U. Development of luspatercept to treat ineffective erythropoiesis. *Blood Adv.* 2021;5(5):1565-1575.
115. U. S. Food and Drug Administration. FDA approves luspatercept-aamt for anemia in adults with MDS. Published April 3, 2020. Accessed June 5, 2021. https://www.fda.gov/drugs/resources-information-approved-drugs/fda-approves-luspatercept-aamt-anemia-adults-mds

116. Platzbecker U, Germing U, Götze KS, et al. Luspatercept for the treatment of anaemia in patients with lower-risk myelodysplastic syndromes (PACE-MDS): a multicentre, open-label phase 2 dose-finding study with long-term extension study. *Lancet Oncol.* 2017;18(10):1338-1347.
117. Fenaux P, Platzbecker U, Mufti GJ, et al. Luspatercept in patients with lower-risk myelodysplastic syndromes. *N Engl J Med.* 2020;382(2):140-151.
118. Haase D, Germing U, Schanz J, et al. New insights into the prognostic impact of the karyotype in MDS and correlation with subtypes: evidence from a core dataset of 2124 patients. *Blood.* 2007;110(13):4385-4395.
119. List A, Ebert BL, Fenaux P. A decade of progress in myelodysplastic syndrome with chromosome 5q deletion. *Leukemia.* 2018;32(7):1493-1499.
120. Krönke J, Fink EC, Hollenbach PW, et al. Lenalidomide induces ubiquitination and degradation of CK1α in del(5q) MDS. *Nature.* 2015;523(7559):183-188.
121. List A, Kurtin S, Roe DJ, et al. Efficacy of lenalidomide in myelodysplastic syndromes. *N Engl J Med.* 2005;352(6):549-557.
122. Fenaux P, Giagounidis A, Selleslag D, et al. A randomized phase 3 study of lenalidomide versus placebo in RBC transfusion-dependent patients with Low-/Intermediate-1-risk myelodysplastic syndromes with del5q. *Blood.* 2011;118(14):3765-3776.
123. List A, Dewald G, Bennett J, et al. Lenalidomide in the myelodysplastic syndrome with chromosome 5q deletion. *N Engl J Med.* 2006;355(14):1456-1465.
124. List AF, Bennett JM, Sekeres MA, et al. Extended survival and reduced risk of AML progression in erythroid-responsive lenalidomide-treated patients with lower-risk del(5q) MDS. *Leukemia.* 2014;28(5):1033-1040.
125. Sekeres MA, Maciejewski JP, Giagounidis AA, et al. Relationship of treatment-related cytopenias and response to lenalidomide in patients with lower-risk myelodysplastic syndromes. *J Clin Oncol.* 2008;26(36):5943-5949.
126. Sekeres MA, Swern AS, Giagounidis A, et al. The impact of lenalidomide exposure on response and outcomes in patients with lower-risk myelodysplastic syndromes and del(5q). *Blood Cancer J.* 2018;8(10):90.
127. Mossner M, Jann JC, Nowak D, et al. Prevalence, clonal dynamics and clinical impact of TP53 mutations in patients with myelodysplastic syndrome with isolated deletion (5q) treated with lenalidomide: results from a prospective multicenter study of the German MDS study group (GMDS). *Leukemia.* 2016;30(9):1956-1959.
128. Santini V, Almeida A, Giagounidis A, et al. Randomized phase III study of lenalidomide versus placebo in RBC transfusion-dependent patients with lower-risk non-del(5q) myelodysplastic syndromes and ineligible for or refractory to erythropoiesis-stimulating agents. *J Clin Oncol.* 2016;34(25):2988-2996.
129. Boogaerts MA, Nelissen V, Roelant C, Goossens W. Blood neutrophil function in primary myelodysplastic syndromes. *Br J Haematol.* 1983;55(2):217-227.
130. Elghetany MT. Surface marker abnormalities in myelodysplastic syndromes. *Haematologica.* 1998;83(12):1104-1115.
131. Ito Y, Kawanishi Y, Shoji N, Ohyashiki K. Decline in antibiotic enzyme activity of neutrophils is a prognostic factor for infections in patients with myelodysplastic syndrome. *Clin Infect Dis.* 2000;31(5):1292-1295.
132. Marisavljević D, Kraguljac N, Rolović Z. Immunologic abnormalities in myelodysplastic syndromes: clinical features and characteristics of the lymphoid population. *Med Oncol.* 2006;23(3):385-391.
133. Okamoto T, Okada M, Mori A, et al. Correlation between immunological abnormalities and prognosis in myelodysplastic syndrome patients. *Int J Hematol.* 1997;66(3):345-351.
134. Shioi Y, Tamura H, Yokose N, Satoh C, Dan K, Ogata K. Increased apoptosis of circulating T cells in myelodysplastic syndromes. *Leuk Res.* 2007;31(12):1641-1648.
135. Cordoba I, Gonzalez-Porras JR, Such E, et al. The degree of neutropenia has a prognostic impact in low risk myelodysplastic syndrome. *Leuk Res.* 2012;36(3):287-292.
136. Hutzschenreuter F, Monsef I, Kreuzer KA, Engert A, Skoetz N. Granulocyte and granulocyte-macrophage colony stimulating factors for newly diagnosed patients with myelodysplastic syndromes. *Cochrane Database Syst Rev.* 2016;2:CD009310.
137. Steensma DP. Hematopoietic growth factors in myelodysplastic syndromes. *Semin Oncol.* 2011;38(5):635-647.
138. Greenberg PL, Stone RM, Al-Kali A, et al. Myelodysplastic syndromes, version 2.2017, NCCN clinical practice guidelines in oncology. *J Natl Compr Canc Netw.* 2017;15(1):60-87.
139. Metcalf D. The granulocyte-macrophage colony-stimulating factors. *Science.* 1985;229(4708):16.
140. Kantarjian HM; Giles F; List AF, et al. The incidence and impact of thrombocytopenia in myelodysplastic syndrome (MDS). *Blood.* 2006;108(11):2617.
141. Zeidman A, Sokolover N, Fradin Z, Cohen A, Redlich O, Mittelman M. Platelet function and its clinical significance in the myelodysplastic syndromes. *Hematol J.* 2004;5(3):234-238.
142. Nachtkamp K, Stark R, Strupp C, et al. Causes of death in 2877 patients with myelodysplastic syndromes. *Ann Hematol.* 2016;95(6):937-944.
143. Kao JM, McMillan A, Greenberg PL. International MDS risk analysis workshop (IMRAW)/IPSS reanalyzed: impact of cytopenias on clinical outcomes in myelodysplastic syndromes. *Am J Hematol.* 2008;83(10):765-770.
144. Li W, Morrone K, Kambhampati S, Will B, Steidl U, Verma A. Thrombocytopenia in MDS: epidemiology, mechanisms, clinical consequences and novel therapeutic strategies. *Leukemia.* 2016;30(3):536-544.
145. Alessandrino EP, Amadori S, Barosi G, et al. Evidence- and consensus-based practice guidelines for the therapy of primary myelodysplastic syndromes. A statement from the Italian Society of Hematology. *Haematologica.* 2002;87(12):1286-1306.
146. Neukirchen J, Blum S, Kuendgen A, et al. Platelet counts and haemorrhagic diathesis in patients with myelodysplastic syndromes. *Eur J Haematol.* 2009;83(5):477-482.
147. Giagounidis A, Mufti GJ, Fenaux P, et al. Results of a randomized, double-blind study of romiplostim versus placebo in patients with low/intermediate-1-risk myelodysplastic syndrome and thrombocytopenia. *Cancer.* 2014;120(12):1838-1846.
148. Kantarjian HM, Fenaux P, Sekeres MA, et al. Long-term follow-up for up to 5 years on the risk of leukaemic progression in thrombocytopenic patients with lower-risk myelodysplastic syndromes treated with romiplostim or placebo in a randomised double-blind trial. *Lancet Haematol.* 2018;5(3):e117-e126.
149. Erickson-Miller C; Delorme E; Giampa L, et al, Biological activity and selectivity for Tpo receptor of the orally bioavailable, small molecule Tpo receptor agonist, SB-497115. *Blood.* 2004;104(11):2912.
150. Oliva EN, Alati C, Santini V, et al. Eltrombopag versus placebo for low-risk myelodysplastic syndromes with thrombocytopenia (EQoL-MDS): phase 1 results of a single-blind, randomised, controlled, phase 2 superiority trial. *Lancet Haematol.* 2017;4(3):e127-e136.
151. Dickinson M, Cherif H, Fenaux P, et al. Azacitidine with or without eltrombopag for first-line treatment of intermediate- or high-risk MDS with thrombocytopenia. *Blood.* 2018;132(25):2629-2638.
152. Platzbecker U, Wong RS, Verma A, et al. Safety and tolerability of eltrombopag versus placebo for treatment of thrombocytopenia in patients with advanced myelodysplastic syndromes or acute myeloid leukaemia: a multicentre, randomised, placebo-controlled, double-blind, phase 1/2 trial. *Lancet Haematol.* 2015;2(10):e417-e426.
153. Mittelman M, Platzbecker U, Afanasyev B, et al. Eltrombopag for advanced myelodysplastic syndromes or acute myeloid leukaemia and severe thrombocytopenia (ASPIRE): a randomised, placebo-controlled, phase 2 trial. *Lancet Haematol.* 2018;5(1):e34-e43.
154. Dodillet H, Kreuzer KA, Monsef I, Skoetz N. Thrombopoietin mimetics for patients with myelodysplastic syndromes. *Cochrane Database Syst Rev.* 2017;9(9):Cd009883.
155. Gluckman E, Devergie A, Poros A, Degoulet P. Results of immunosuppression in 170 cases of severe aplastic anaemia. Report of the European Group of Bone Marrow Transplant (EGBMT). *Br J Haematol.* 1982;51(4):541-550.
156. Molldrem JJ, Caples M, Mavroudis D, Plante M, Young NS, Barrett AJ. Antithymocyte globulin for patients with myelodysplastic syndrome. *Br J Haematol.* 1997;99(3):699-705.
157. Molldrem JJ, Jiang YZ, Stetler-Stevenson M, Mavroudis D, Hensel N, Barrett AJ. Haematological response of patients with myelodysplastic syndrome to antithymocyte globulin is associated with a loss of lymphocyte-mediated inhibition of CFU-GM and alterations in T-cell receptor Vbeta profiles. *Br J Haematol.* 1998;102(5):1314-1322.
158. Sloand EM, Mainwaring L, Fuhrer M, et al. Preferential suppression of trisomy 8 compared with normal hematopoietic cell growth by autologous lymphocytes in patients with trisomy 8 myelodysplastic syndrome. *Blood.* 2005;106(3):841-851.
159. Benesch M, Platzbecker U, Ward J, Deeg HJ, Leisenring W. Expression of FLIP(Long) and FLIP(Short) in bone marrow mononuclear and CD34+ cells in patients with myelodysplastic syndrome: correlation with apoptosis. *Leukemia.* 2003;17(12):2460-2466.
160. Kochenderfer JN, Kobayashi S, Wieder ED, Su C, Molldrem JJ. Loss of T-lymphocyte clonal dominance in patients with myelodysplastic syndrome responsive to immunosuppression. *Blood.* 2002;100(10):3639-3645.
161. Chamuleau ME, Westers TM, van Dreunen L, et al. Immune mediated autologous cytotoxicity against hematopoietic precursor cells in patients with myelodysplastic syndrome. *Haematologica.* 2009;94(4):496-506.
162. Sugimori C, List AF, Epling-Burnette PK. Immune dysregulation in myelodysplastic syndrome. *Hematol Rep.* 2010;2(1):e1.
163. Haider M, Al Ali N, Padron E, et al. Immunosuppressive therapy: exploring an underutilized treatment option for myelodysplastic syndrome. *Clin Lymphoma Myeloma Leuk.* 2016;16:S44-S48.
164. Sloand EM, Wu CO, Greenberg P, Young N, Barrett J. Factors affecting response and survival in patients with myelodysplasia treated with immunosuppressive therapy. *J Clin Oncol.* 2008;26(15):2505-2511.
165. Saunthararajah Y, Nakamura R, Wesley R, Wang QJ, Barrett AJ. A simple method to predict response to immunosuppressive therapy in patients with myelodysplastic syndrome. *Blood.* 2003;102(8):3025-3027.
166. Stahl M, DeVeaux M, de Witte T, et al. The use of immunosuppressive therapy in MDS: clinical outcomes and their predictors in a large international patient cohort. *Blood Adv.* 2018;2(14):1765-1772.
167. Zhang Q, Haider M, Al Ali NH, et al. SF3B1 mutations negatively predict for response to immunosuppressive therapy in myelodysplastic syndromes. *Clin Lymphoma Myeloma Leuk.* 2020;20(6):400-406.e2.
168. Komrokji RS, Mailloux AW, Chen DT, et al. A phase II multicenter rabbit antithymocyte globulin trial in patients with myelodysplastic syndromes identifying a novel model for response prediction. *Haematologica.* 2014;99(7):1176-1183.
169. Killick SB, Mufti G, Cavenagh JD, et al. A pilot study of antithymocyte globulin (ATG) in the treatment of patients with 'low-risk' myelodysplasia. *Br J Haematol.* 2003;120(4):679-684.
170. Passweg JR, Giagounidis AA, Simcock M, et al. Immunosuppressive therapy for patients with myelodysplastic syndrome: a prospective randomized multicenter phase III trial comparing antithymocyte globulin plus cyclosporine with best supportive care--SAKK 33/99. *J Clin Oncol.* 2011;29(3):303-309.
171. Yazji S, Giles FJ, Tsimberidou AM, et al. Antithymocyte globulin (ATG)-based therapy in patients with myelodysplastic syndromes. *Leukemia.* 2003;17(11):2101-2106.
172. Chen S, Jiang B, Da W, Gong M, Guan M. Treatment of myelodysplastic syndrome with cyclosporin A. *Int J Hematol.* 2007;85(1):11-17.
173. Okamoto T, Okada M, Yamada S, et al. Good response to cyclosporine therapy in patients with myelodysplastic syndromes having the HLA-DRB1*1501 allele. *Leukemia.* 2000;14(2):344-346.
174. Sloand EM, Olnes MJ, Shenoy A, et al. Alemtuzumab treatment of intermediate-1 myelodysplasia patients is associated with sustained improvement in blood counts and cytogenetic remissions. *J Clin Oncol.* 2010;28(35):5166-5173.

175. Jonásova A, Neuwirtová R, Cermák J, et al. Cyclosporin A therapy in hypoplastic MDS patients and certain refractory anaemias without hypoplastic bone marrow. *Br J Haematol*. 1998;100(2):304-309.
176. Scott BL, Ramakrishnan A, Fosdal M, et al. Anti-thymocyte globulin plus etanercept as therapy for myelodysplastic syndromes (MDS): a phase II study. *Br J Haematol*. 2010;149(5):706-710.
177. Scheinberg P, Nunez O, Weinstein B, et al. Horse versus rabbit antithymocyte globulin in acquired aplastic anemia. *N Engl J Med*. 2011;365(5):430-438.
178. Xiao L, Qi Z, Qiusheng C, Li X, Luxi S, Lingyun W. The use of selective immunosuppressive therapy on myelodysplastic syndromes in targeted populations results in good response rates and avoids treatment-related disease progression. *Am J Hematol*. 2012;87(1):26-31.
179. Maximilian S, Jan Philipp B, Smith G, Rong W, Amer MZ. Use of immunosuppressive therapy for management of myelodysplastic syndromes: a systematic review and meta-analysis. *Haematologica*. 2020;105(1):102-111.
180. Jabbour E, Short NJ, Montalban-Bravo G, et al. Randomized phase 2 study of low-dose decitabine vs low-dose azacitidine in lower-risk MDS and MDS/MPN. *Blood*. 2017;130(13):1514-1522.
181. McQuilten ZK, Polizzotto MN, Wood EM, Sundararajan V. Myelodysplastic syndrome incidence, transfusion dependence, health care use, and complications: an Australian population-based study 1998 to 2008. *Transfusion*. 2013;53(8):1714-1721.
182. DeZern AE, Binder G, Rizvi S, et al. Patterns of treatment and costs associated with transfusion burden in patients with myelodysplastic syndromes. *Leuk Lymphoma*. 2017;58(11):2649-2656.
183. Cheok KPL, Chhetri R, Wee LYA, et al. The burden of immune-mediated refractoriness to platelet transfusions in myelodysplastic syndromes. *Transfusion*. 2020;60(10):2192-2198.
184. Hiwase DK, Singhal D, Strupp C, et al. Dynamic assessment of RBC-transfusion dependency improves the prognostic value of the revised-IPSS in MDS patients. *Am J Hematol*. 2017;92(6):508-514.
185. Malcovati L, Porta MG, Pascutto C, et al. Prognostic factors and life expectancy in myelodysplastic syndromes classified according to WHO criteria: a basis for clinical decision making. *J Clin Oncol*. 2005;23(30):7594-7603.
186. Ryblom H, Hast R, Hellström-Lindberg E, Winterling J, Johansson E. Self-perception of symptoms of anemia and fatigue before and after blood transfusions in patients with myelodysplastic syndromes. *Eur J Oncol Nurs*. 2015;19(2):99-106.
187. Stanworth SJ, Killick S, McQuilten ZK, et al. Red cell transfusion in outpatients with myelodysplastic syndromes: a feasibility and exploratory randomised trial. *Br J Haematol*. 2020;189(2):279-290.
188. Tanasijevic AM, Revette A, Klepin HD, et al. Consensus minimum hemoglobin level above which patients with myelodysplastic syndromes can safely forgo transfusions. *Leuk Lymphoma*. 2020;61(12):2900-2904.
189. Angelucci E, Li J, Greenberg P, et al. Iron chelation in transfusion-dependent patients with low- to intermediate-1-risk myelodysplastic syndromes: a randomized trial. *Ann Intern Med*. 2020;172(8):513-522.
190. Marlijn H, Ge Y, Saskia L, et al. On behalf of the, E. R. P., Impact of treatment with iron chelation therapy in patients with lower-risk myelodysplastic syndromes participating in the European MDS registry. *Haematologica*. 2020;105(3):640-651.
191. Leitch HA, Parmar A, Wells RA, et al. Overall survival in lower IPSS risk MDS by receipt of iron chelation therapy, adjusting for patient-related factors and measuring from time of first red blood cell transfusion dependence: an MDS-CAN analysis. *Br J Haematol*. 2017;179(1):83-97.
192. Toma A, Fenaux P, Dreyfus F, Cordonnier C. Infections in myelodysplastic syndromes. *Haematologica*. 2012;97(10):1459-1470.
193. Neukirchen J, Nachtkamp K, Schemenau J, et al. Change of prognosis of patients with myelodysplastic syndromes during the last 30 years. *Leuk Res*. 2015;39(7):679-683.
194. Goldberg SL, Chen E, Corral M, et al. Incidence and clinical complications of myelodysplastic syndromes among United States Medicare beneficiaries. *J Clin Oncol*. 2010;28(17):2847-2852.
195. Bullen JJ, Rogers HJ, Spalding PB, Ward CG. Natural resistance, iron and infection: a challenge for clinical medicine. *J Med Microbiol*. 2006;55(pt 3):251-258.
196. Pullarkat V, Blanchard S, Tegtmeier B, et al. Iron overload adversely affects outcome of allogeneic hematopoietic cell transplantation. *Bone Marrow Transplant*. 2008;42(12):799-805.
197. Pullarkat V. Objectives of iron chelation therapy in myelodysplastic syndromes: more than meets the eye? *Blood*. 2009;114(26):5251-5255.
198. Taplitz RA, Kennedy EB, Flowers CR. Antimicrobial prophylaxis for adult patients with cancer-related immunosuppression: ASCO and IDSA clinical practice guideline update summary. *J Oncol Pract*. 2018;14(11):692-695.
199. Bergmann OJ, Mogensen SC, Ellermann-Eriksen S, Ellegaard J. Acyclovir prophylaxis and fever during remission-induction therapy of patients with acute myeloid leukemia: a randomized, double-blind, placebo-controlled trial. *J Clin Oncol*. 1997;15(6):2269-2274.
200. Kantarjian H, Issa JP, Rosenfeld CS, et al. Decitabine improves patient outcomes in myelodysplastic syndromes: results of a phase III randomized study. *Cancer*. 2006;106(8):1794-1803.
201. Silverman LR, Demakos EP, Peterson BL, et al. Randomized controlled trial of azacitidine in patients with the myelodysplastic syndrome: a study of the cancer and leukemia group B. *J Clin Oncol*. 2002;20(10):2429-2440.
202. Garcia-Manero G, McCloskey J, Griffiths EA, et al. Pharmacokinetic exposure equivalence and preliminary efficacy and safety from a randomized cross over phase 3 study (ASCERTAIN study) of an oral hypomethylating agent ASTX727 (cedazuridine/decitabine) compared to IV decitabine. *Blood*. 2019;134(suppl_1):846.
203. Kaminskas E, Farrell A, Abraham S, et al. Approval summary: azacitidine for treatment of myelodysplastic syndrome subtypes. *Clin Cancer Res*. 2005;11(10):3604-3608.
204. Fenaux P, Mufti GJ, Hellstrom-Lindberg E, et al. Efficacy of azacitidine compared with that of conventional care regimens in the treatment of higher-risk myelodysplastic syndromes: a randomised, open-label, phase III study. *Lancet Oncol*. 2009;10(3):223-232.
205. Mozessohn L, Cheung MC, Fallahpour S, et al. Azacitidine in the 'real-world': an evaluation of 1101 higher-risk myelodysplastic syndrome/low blast count acute myeloid leukaemia patients in Ontario, Canada. *Br J Haematol*. 2018;181(6):803-815.
206. Zeidan AM, Stahl M, DeVeaux M, et al. Counseling patients with higher-risk MDS regarding survival with azacitidine therapy: are we using realistic estimates? *Blood Cancer J*. 2018;8(6):55.
207. Prebet T, Sun Z, Figueroa ME, et al. Prolonged administration of azacitidine with or without entinostat for myelodysplastic syndrome and acute myeloid leukemia with myelodysplasia-related changes: results of the US Leukemia Intergroup trial E1905. *J Clin Oncol*. 2014;32(12):1242-1248.
208. Sekeres MA, Othus M, List AF, et al. Randomized phase II study of azacitidine alone or in combination with lenalidomide or with vorinostat in higher-risk myelodysplastic syndromes and chronic myelomonocytic leukemia: North American Intergroup study SWOG S1117. *J Clin Oncol*. 2017;35(24):2745-2753.
209. Fenaux P, Mufti GJ, Hellström-Lindberg E, et al. Azacitidine prolongs overall survival compared with conventional care regimens in elderly patients with low bone marrow blast count acute myeloid leukemia. *J Clin Oncol*. 2010;28(4):562-569.
210. Raj K, John A, Ho A, et al. CDKN2B methylation status and isolated chromosome 7 abnormalities predict responses to treatment with 5-azacytidine. *Leukemia*. 2007;21(9):1937-1944.
211. Lübbert M, Wijermans P, Kunzmann R, et al. Cytogenetic responses in high-risk myelodysplastic syndrome following low-dose treatment with the DNA methylation inhibitor 5-aza-2'-deoxycytidine. *Br J Haematol*. 2001;114(2):349-357.
212. Welch JS, Petti AA, Miller CA, et al. TP53 and decitabine in acute myeloid leukemia and myelodysplastic syndromes. *N Engl J Med*. 2016;375(21):2023-2036.
213. Derissen EJ, Beijnen JH, Schellens JH. Concise drug review: azacitidine and decitabine. *Oncol*. 2013;18(5):619-624.
214. Steensma DP, Baer MR, Slack JL, et al. Multicenter study of decitabine administered daily for 5 days every 4 weeks to adults with myelodysplastic syndromes: the alternative dosing for outpatient treatment (ADOPT) trial. *J Clin Oncol*. 2009;27(23):3842-3848.
215. Kantarjian H, Oki Y, Garcia-Manero G, et al. Results of a randomized study of 3 schedules of low-dose decitabine in higher-risk myelodysplastic syndrome and chronic myelomonocytic leukemia. *Blood*. 2007;109(1):52-57.
216. Lübbert M, Suciu S, Baila L, et al. Low-dose decitabine versus best supportive care in elderly patients with intermediate- or high-risk myelodysplastic syndrome (MDS) ineligible for intensive chemotherapy: final results of the randomized phase III study of the European Organisation for Research and treatment of cancer leukemia group and the German MDS study group. *J Clin Oncol*. 2011;29(15):1987-1996.
217. Zeidan AM, Davidoff AJ, Long JB, et al. Comparative clinical effectiveness of azacitidine versus decitabine in older patients with myelodysplastic syndromes. *Br J Haematol*. 2016;175(5):829-840.
218. Lee YG, Kim I, Yoon SS, et al. Comparative analysis between azacitidine and decitabine for the treatment of myelodysplastic syndromes. *Br J Haematol*. 2013;161(3):339-347.
219. Fenaux P, Ades L. Review of azacitidine trials in Intermediate-2-and High-risk myelodysplastic syndromes. *Leuk Res*. 2009;33:S7-S11.
220. Prébet T, Gore SD, Esterni B, et al. Outcome of high-risk myelodysplastic syndrome after azacitidine treatment failure. *J Clin Oncol*. 2011;29(24):3322-3327.
221. Shen L, Kantarjian H, Guo Y, et al. DNA methylation predicts survival and response to therapy in patients with myelodysplastic syndromes. *J Clin Oncol*. 2010;28(4):605-613.
222. Yan P, Frankhouser D, Murphy M, et al. Genome-wide methylation profiling in decitabine-treated patients with acute myeloid leukemia. *Blood*. 2012;120(12):2466-2474.
223. Tobiasson M, Abdulkadir H, Lennartsson A, et al. Comprehensive mapping of the effects of azacitidine on DNA methylation, repressive/permissive histone marks and gene expression in primary cells from patients with MDS and MDS-related disease. *Oncotarget*. 2017;8(17):28812-28825.
224. Meldi K, Qin T, Buchi F, et al. Specific molecular signatures predict decitabine response in chronic myelomonocytic leukemia. *J Clin Invest*. 2015;125(5):1857-1872.
225. Voso MT, Fabiani E, Piciocchi A, et al. Role of BCL2L10 methylation and TET2 mutations in higher risk myelodysplastic syndromes treated with 5-azacytidine. *Leukemia*. 2011;25(12):1910-1913.
226. Fandy TE, Herman JG, Kerns P, et al. Early epigenetic changes and DNA damage do not predict clinical response in an overlapping schedule of 5-azacytidine and entinostat in patients with myeloid malignancies. *Blood*. 2009;114(13):2764-2773.
227. Follo MY, Finelli C, Mongiorgi S, et al. Reduction of phosphoinositide-phospholipase C beta1 methylation predicts the responsiveness to azacitidine in high-risk MDS. *Proc Natl Acad Sci U S A*. 2009;106(39):16811-16816.
228. Gawlitza AL, Speith J, Rinke J, et al. 5-Azacytidine modulates CpG methylation levels of EZH2 and NOTCH1 in myelodysplastic syndromes. *J Cancer Res Clin Oncol*. 2019;145(11):2835-2843.
229. Itzykson R, Kosmider O, Cluzeau T, et al. Impact of TET2 mutations on response rate to azacitidine in myelodysplastic syndromes and low blast count acute myeloid leukemias. *Leukemia*. 2011;25(7):1147-1152.

230. Traina F, Visconte V, Elson P, et al. Impact of molecular mutations on treatment response to DNMT inhibitors in myelodysplasia and related neoplasms. *Leukemia.* 2014;28(1):78-87.
231. Jung SH, Kim YJ, Yim SH, et al. Somatic mutations predict outcomes of hypomethylating therapy in patients with myelodysplastic syndrome. *Oncotarget.* 2016;7(34):55264-55275.
232. Bejar R, Lord A, Stevenson K, et al. TET2 mutations predict response to hypomethylating agents in myelodysplastic syndrome patients. *Blood.* 2014;124(17):2705-2712.
233. Nazha A, Sekeres MA, Bejar R, et al. Genomic biomarkers to predict resistance to hypomethylating agents in patients with myelodysplastic syndromes using artificial intelligence. *JCO Precis Oncol.* 2019;2019(3):1-11.
234. Santini V. How I treat MDS after hypomethylating agent failure. *Blood.* 2019;133(6):521-529.
235. Aziz N, Rami SK, Guillermo G-M, et al. The efficacy of current prognostic models in predicting outcome of patients with myelodysplastic syndromes at the time of hypomethylating agent failure. *Haematologica.* 2016;101(6):e224-e227.
236. Beran M, Shen Y, Kantarjian H, et al. High-dose chemotherapy in high-risk myelodysplastic syndrome: covariate-adjusted comparison of five regimens. *Cancer.* 2001;92(8):1999-2015.
237. de Witte T, Suciu S, Peetermans M, et al. Intensive chemotherapy for poor prognosis myelodysplasia (MDS) and secondary acute myeloid leukemia (sAML) following MDS of more than 6 months duration. A pilot study by the Leukemia Cooperative Group of the European Organisation for Research and Treatment in Cancer (EORTC-LCG). *Leukemia.* 1995;9(11):1805-1811.
238. Kantarjian H, O'Brien S, Cortes J, et al. Results of intensive chemotherapy in 998 patients age 65 years or older with acute myeloid leukemia or high-risk myelodysplastic syndrome: predictive prognostic models for outcome. *Cancer.* 2006;106(5):1090-1098.
239. Knipp S, Hildebrand B, Kündgen A, et al. Intensive chemotherapy is not recommended for patients aged >60 years who have myelodysplastic syndromes or acute myeloid leukemia with high-risk karyotypes. *Cancer.* 2007;110(2):345-352.
240. Cortes J, Kantarjian H, Albitar M, et al. A randomized trial of liposomal daunorubicin and cytarabine versus liposomal daunorubicin and topotecan with or without thalidomide as initial therapy for patients with poor prognosis acute myelogenous leukemia or myelodysplastic syndrome. *Cancer.* 2003;97(5):1234-1241.
241. DiNardo CD, Jonas BA, Pullarkat V, et al. Azacitidine and venetoclax in previously untreated acute myeloid leukemia. *N Engl J Med.* 2020;383(7):617-629.
242. Sekeres MA, Watts J, Radinoff A, et al. Randomized phase 2 trial of pevonedistat plus azacitidine versus azacitidine for higher-risk MDS/CMML or low-blast AML. *Leukemia.* 2021;35(7):2119-2124.
243. Stein EM, Fathi AT, DiNardo CD, et al. Enasidenib in patients with mutant IDH2 myelodysplastic syndromes: a phase 1 subgroup analysis of the multicentre, AG221-C-001 trial. *Lancet Haematol.* 2020;7(4):e309-e319.
244. Atallah E, Logan B, Chen M, et al. Comparison of patient Age groups in transplantation for myelodysplastic syndrome: the medicare coverage with evidence development study. *JAMA Oncol.* 2020;6(4):486-493.
245. de Witte T, Bowen D, Robin M, et al. Allogeneic hematopoietic stem cell transplantation for MDS and CMML: recommendations from an international expert panel. *Blood.* 2017;129(13):1753-1762.
246. Koreth J, Pidala J, Perez WS, et al. Role of reduced-intensity conditioning allogeneic hematopoietic stem-cell transplantation in older patients with de novo myelodysplastic syndromes: an international collaborative decision analysis. *J Clin Oncol.* 2013;31(21):2662-2670.
247. Cutler CS, Lee SJ, Greenberg P, et al. A decision analysis of allogeneic bone marrow transplantation for the myelodysplastic syndromes: delayed transplantation for low-risk myelodysplasia is associated with improved outcome. *Blood.* 2004;104(2):579-585.
248. Alessandrino EP, Porta MG, Malcovati L, et al. Optimal timing of allogeneic hematopoietic stem cell transplantation in patients with myelodysplastic syndrome. *Am J Hematol.* 2013;88(7):581-588.
249. Kröger N, Iacobelli S, Franke G-N, et al. Dose-reduced versus standard conditioning followed by allogeneic stem-cell transplantation for patients with myelodysplastic syndrome: a prospective randomized phase III study of the EBMT (RICMAC trial). *J Clin Oncol.* 2017;35(19):2157-2164.
250. Runde V, de Witte T, Arnold R, et al. Bone marrow transplantation from HLA-identical siblings as first-line treatment in patients with myelodysplastic syndromes: early transplantation is associated with improved outcome. Chronic Leukemia Working Party of the European Group for Blood and Marrow Transplantation. *Bone Marrow Transplant.* 1998;21(3):255-261.
251. Deeg HJ, Storer B, Slattery JT, et al. Conditioning with targeted busulfan and cyclophosphamide for hemopoietic stem cell transplantation from related and unrelated donors in patients with myelodysplastic syndrome. *Blood.* 2002;100(4):1201-1207.
252. van Gelder M, de Wreede LC, Schetelig J, et al. Monosomal karyotype predicts poor survival after allogeneic stem cell transplantation in chromosome 7 abnormal myelodysplastic syndrome and secondary acute myeloid leukemia. *Leukemia.* 2013;27(4):879-888.
253. Koenecke C, Göhring G, de Wreede LC, et al. Impact of the revised International Prognostic Scoring System, cytogenetics and monosomal karyotype on outcome after allogeneic stem cell transplantation for myelodysplastic syndromes and secondary acute myeloid leukemia evolving from myelodysplastic syndromes: a retrospective multicenter study of the European Society of Blood and Marrow Transplantation. *Haematologica.* 2015;100(3):400-408.
254. Bejar R, Stevenson KE, Caughey B, et al. Somatic mutations predict poor outcome in patients with myelodysplastic syndrome after hematopoietic stem-cell transplantation. *J Clin Oncol.* 2014;32(25):2691-2698.
255. Della Porta MG, Gallì A, Bacigalupo A, et al. Clinical effects of driver somatic mutations on the outcomes of patients with myelodysplastic syndromes treated with allogeneic hematopoietic stem-cell transplantation. *J Clin Oncol.* 2016;34(30):3627-3637.
256. Yoshizato T, Nannya Y, Atsuta Y, et al. Genetic abnormalities in myelodysplasia and secondary acute myeloid leukemia: impact on outcome of stem cell transplantation. *Blood.* 2017;129(17):2347-2358.
257. Schroeder T, Wegener N, Lauseker M, et al. Comparison between upfront transplantation and different pretransplant cytoreductive treatment approaches in patients with high-risk myelodysplastic syndrome and secondary acute myelogenous leukemia. *Biol Blood Marrow Transplant.* 2019;25(8):1550-1559.
258. Alessandrino EP, Della Porta MG, Pascutto C, Bacigalupo A, Rambaldi A. Should cytoreductive treatment Be performed before transplantation in patients with high-risk myelodysplastic syndrome? *J Clin Oncol.* 2013;31(21):2761-2762.
259. Damaj G, Duhamel A, Robin M, et al. Impact of Azacitidine Before Allogeneic Stem-Cell Transplantation for Myelodysplastic Syndromes: a Study by the Société Française de Greffe de Moelle et de Thérapie-Cellulaire and the Groupe-Francophone des Myélodysplasies. *J Clin Oncol.* 2012;30(36):4533-4540.
260. Gerds AT, Gooley TA, Estey EH, Appelbaum FR, Deeg HJ, Scott BL. Pretransplantation therapy with azacitidine vs induction chemotherapy and post-transplantation outcome in patients with MDS. *Biol Blood Marrow Transplant.* 2012;18(8):1211-1218.
261. Potter VT, Iacobelli S, van Biezen A, et al. Comparison of intensive chemotherapy and hypomethylating agents before allogeneic stem cell transplantation for advanced myelodysplastic syndromes: a study of the myelodysplastic syndrome subcommittee of the chronic malignancies working party of the European Society for Blood and Marrow Transplant Research. *Biol Blood Marrow Transplant.* 2016;22(9):1615-1620.
262. Kroeger N; Sockel K; Wolschke C, et al. Prospective multicenter phase 3 study comparing 5-azacytidine (5-aza) induction followed by allogeneic stem cell transplantation versus continuous 5-aza according to donor availability in elderly MDS patients (55-70 years) (VidazaAllo study). *Blood.* 2018;132:208.
263. Yahng SA, Kim M, Kim TM, et al. Better transplant outcome with pre-transplant marrow response after hypomethylating treatment in higher-risk MDS with excess blasts. *Oncotarget.* 2016;8(7):12342-12354.
264. Nakamura R, Saber W, Martens MJ, et al. Biologic assignment trial of reduced-intensity hematopoietic cell transplantation based on donor availability in patients 50-75 years of age with advanced myelodysplastic syndrome. *J Clin Oncol.* 2021;39(30):3328-3339.
265. Arber DA, Orazi A, Hasserjian R, et al. The 2016 revision to the World Health Organization classification of myeloid neoplasms and acute leukemia. *Blood.* 2016;127(20):2391-2405.

Suggested Reading

266. Arber DA, Orazi A, Hasserjian R, et al. The 2016 revision to the World Health Organization classification of myeloid neoplasms and acute leukemia. *Blood.* 2016;127(20):2391-2405.
267. Greenberg PL, Tuechler H, Schanz J, et al. Revised international prognostic scoring system for myelodysplastic syndromes. *Blood.* 2012;120(12):2454-2465.

Chapter 81 ■ Clonal Hematopoiesis of Indeterminate Potential and Myeloid Diseases

MRINAL M. PATNAIK • PINKAL DESAI

INTRODUCTION

Clonal hematopoiesis (CH) is defined by the acquisition of somatic mutations in hematopoietic stem and progenitor cells (HSPCs), with the potential to expand based on clonal selection pressures and clonal evolutionary dynamics. There are an estimated 150,000 to 200,000 hematopoietic stem cells (HSCs) in the human body. With each HSC cycling once every few months, at least one pathogenic variant on an average can be expected to accumulate every decade of human life.[1-4] While most mutations result in passenger events, extinguishing over time, a subset of mutations can result in enhanced HSPC fitness, with potential to expand and evolve into hematopoietic neoplasms (*Figure 81.1*).

CH was first documented almost 2 decades ago. Researchers noted an age-dependent increase in nonrandom inactivation of the X chromosomes in females, with several of these women later being detected to have somatic *TET2* mutations.[5,6] With the advent of next-generation sequencing techniques (whole genome/exome sequencing, targeted exome, and amplicon-based sequencing assays) and with increased depth and accuracy of sequencing (error correction using unique molecular bar codes), a plethora of research defining the landscape, prevalence, clinical impact, and evolutionary patterns associated with CH has followed. While CH was not surprisingly associated with an increase in risk of hematological neoplasms, its association with increased all-cause mortality, largely related to an increased risk of cardiovascular disease, was striking.[7] In this chapter we discuss the prevalence, clinical associations, biology, and pathophysiology of CH.

DEFINITIONS

a. Clonal hematopoiesis: is defined by the acquisition of somatic mutations in HSPC in apparently healthy individuals, without underlying hematological neoplasms, with the potential to expand over time, under the influence of clonal selection pressures.[8]
b. Clonal hematopoiesis of indeterminate potential (CHIP): is operationally defined as CH involving leukemia-associated somatic driver mutations in HSPC, with the mutation(s) having a variant allele fraction (VAF) ≥ 2%, without an underlying hematological neoplasm, and without persistent cytopenias.[8]
c. Clonal cytopenias of undetermined significance (CCUS): is defined by unexplained and persistent cytopenia(s) in one or more peripheral blood cell lineages, with evidence for somatic leukemia-associated driver mutations, or mosaic chromosomal alterations (mCAs) in HSPC, without overt features of an underlying hematological neoplasm.
d. Clonal expansion: is defined by the propagation of a mutant clone with enhanced fitness secondary to the nature of the somatic mutation/copy number alteration in the HSPC and related dynamic clonal selection pressures.

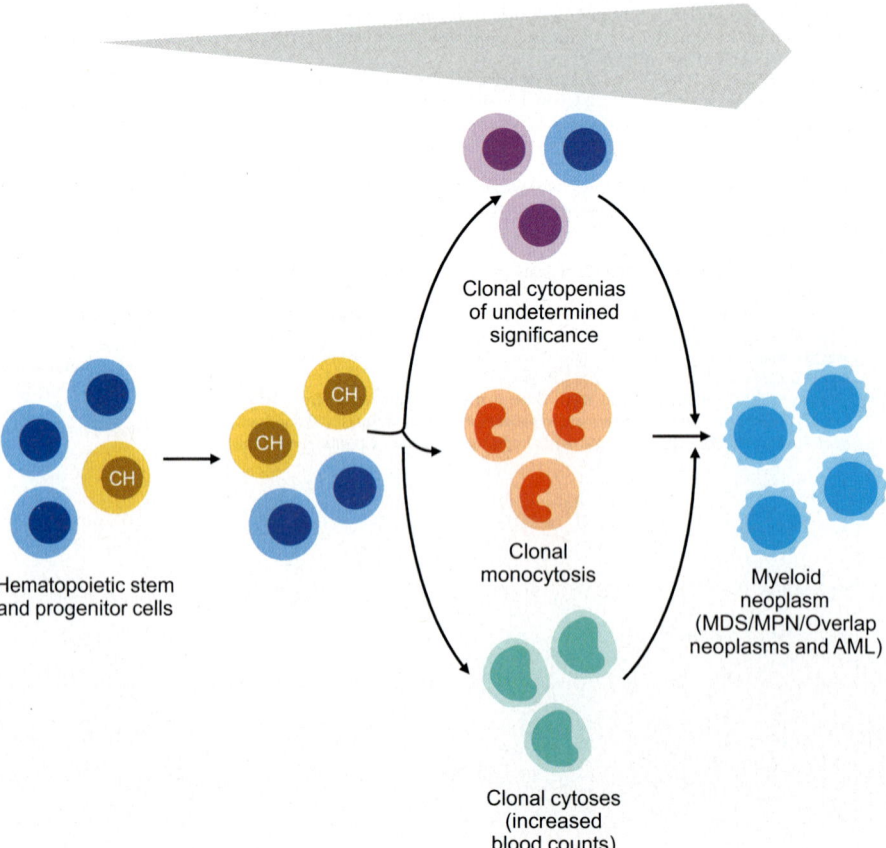

FIGURE 81.1 The role of inflammation and aging in clonal hematopoiesis (CH). Within the context of an aged microenvironment, inflammation leads to the selection of hematopoietic stem and progenitor cells with somatic mutations that confer relative fitness. These mutant clones in turn can then propagate the pervasive inflammation, leading to clonal progression to hematological neoplasms such as myelodysplastic syndromes (MDS), myeloproliferative neoplasms (MPN), and acute myeloid leukemia (AML).

e. Mosaic chromosomal alterations: These are age-related DNA changes (gene deletions, duplications, copy neutral loss of heterozygosity) in HSPC that are associated with clonal expansions and aberrations of blood cell counts and are associated with an increased risk for hematological neoplasms.
f. Variant allele fraction (VAF): This is defined as the percentage of sequence reads observed matching a specific sequence variant observed, expressed as a proportion of the overall coverage at that specific locus.
g. Copy Neutral Loss of Heterozygosity: also referred to as uniparental disomy. This is defined as the loss of heterozygosity generated by the duplication of a maternal (unimaternal) or paternal (unipaternal) chromosome or chromosomal region and concurrent loss of the other allele.

BIOLOGY OF CH/CHIP

With aging, somatic mutations accumulate in several cells and organ systems including HSPC, skin, and esophagus. While most mutations are relatively indolent with minimal clonal potential, mutations involving oncogenic driver genes, including epigenetic regulator genes, tend to have a high propensity for clonal selection and propagation. Based on epidemiological data, greater than 75% of CH/CHIP mutations in the normal aging population involve two enzymes regulating DNA methylation with opposing biochemical functions: DNA methyltransferase 3 alpha (*DNMT3A*, a cytosine methylator involved in iterative DNA methylation) and TET methylcytosine dioxygenase 2 (*TET2*, a demethylator, involved in iterative DNA hydroxymethylation).[7,9] Despite having opposite effects on DNA methylation, *DNMT3A* and *TET2* mutations in the context of CH/CHIP lead to similar clinical outcomes and are associated with increased all-cause mortality (hazard ratio [HR]: 1.4; 95% confidence interval [CI]: 1.1-1.8).[9] In addition to having opposite biochemical impacts on DNA methylation, mouse models have shown a differential impact on hematopoiesis. In *Tet2* knock-out mice, a clear myelomonocytic bias was observed in progenitors, while in *Dnmt3a* knock-out mice, a clear erythroid bias has been noted and linked to differential methylation (hyper- or hypomethylated) of CpG sites within transcription factor binding motifs.[10]

One of the strongest risk factors for CH/CHIP is aging, with cross-sectional studies showing the prevalence of CHIP to be nearly ubiquitous in octogenarians.[11-13] Additional risk factors that have been described contributing to CHIP development and propagation include inflammation, male sex, cigarette smoking, germline predisposition states, and exposures to chemotherapy or ionizing radiation.[14-17] While the association between CHIP and the risk of developing hematological neoplasms is clear (HR: 11-13), the rate of progression and factors that lead to clonal evolution remain to be defined (currently broadly approximated at between 0.5%-1%, per year).[9,18] In addition to nucleotide variants used to define CHIP, there are emerging data showing that mCAs/somatic copy number alterations and their co-occurrence with CHIP mutations are associated with a higher risk of clonal evolution and all-cause mortality.[19] It is important to keep in mind that CHIP is not a binary variable and that clonal evolution is dependent on the type of mutation, mutation VAF, co-occurring mutations, cell intrinsic and extrinsic clonal selection pressures, and the host microenvironment.[15,16,20-22] This is exemplified by the fact that mutations in *TP53* (DNA damage response) or *U2AF1* (spliceosome assembly) lead to an increased risk of acute myeloid leukemia (AML) (HR range 7.9-47.2), while mutations in *DNMT3A* and *TET2* are associated with HRs of 1.4 and 1.6, respectively, with the HR for *DNMT3A* mutations with VAF >10% being 4.8, respectively.[23,24] In addition, while the *DNMT3A* R882 hot spot mutation is common in myeloid neoplasms such as myelodysplastic syndromes and AML, it is infrequent in CHIP, suggesting that certain mutational hot spots have a higher likelihood of clonal evolution in comparison with others, based on how they impact the function of the gene. Interestingly, in patients with myeloproliferative neoplasms (MPNs), oncogenic *JAK2* mutations have been identified many years prior to diagnosis, with computational work suggesting that these mutations might in fact be acquired in utero, during embryonic development, gradually progressing over several years before clinical manifestation.[25,26] Recently, somatic mutations and mCAs, specifically predisposing to the development of lymphoid neoplasms, have been described and annotated as lymphoid-CHIP.[27] The striking association between CHIP and cardiovascular disease is thought to be secondary to a CHIP-derived inflammatory environment and associated endothelial cell dysfunction. Studies have shown an elevated risk for coronary artery disease (HR: 2.0, 95% CI: 1.1-1.8) and stroke (HR: 2.6; 95% CI: 1.4-4.8) in patients with CH/CHIP.[9] Patients with CHIP also have a worse prognosis in the context of congestive heart failure and transfemoral aortic valve implantation (*Figure 81.2*).[28-33]

CHIP AND INFLAMMATION

Patients with CHIP have been shown to have higher levels of cytokines such as TNF-alpha, IL-1b, and IL-6 (*Figure 81.2*), changes characterized as promoting an inflammatory milieu. This is thought to be secondary to the impact of CH mutations on inflammatory cell types and in macrophage-mediated inflammasome activation (mediated through NLRP3). This process is clearly interdependent, with CHIP giving rise to inflammation and inflammation selectively propagating HSPC clones that have been conferred selective fitness due to CHIP mutations. This is supported by the fact that, in response to inflammatory stimuli (chronic mycobacterial infections or administration of proinflammatory IFN-gamma), $DNMT3A^{-/-}$ HSCs undergo a substantial clonal expansion.[34] Similarly, increased inflammation via bacterial stimuli results in the proliferation of *TET2*-deficient HSPC.[35] Patients with HIV (human immunodeficiency virus) infection, a known chronic inflammatory condition, have higher a prevalence of CHIP,[36] in addition to patients with ulcerative colitis,[37] rheumatoid arthritis,[38] and other inflammatory diseases.[39,40] Conversely, patients with structural somatic variants indicative of CH are predisposed to the development of infections.[41] Furthermore, patients with CHIP who developed COVID-19 were more likely to have more severe outcomes.[42] Evidence has shown that CHIP effects are likely secondary to a deregulated inflammatory environment, termed "the inflammasome" and altered endothelial cell function.[43,44] For instance, *TET2*-deficient macrophages were shown to be proinflammatory leading to increased atherosclerosis, $Tet2^{-/-}$ mice have higher levels of plasma TNF-alpha, and *TET2*-deficient stem and progenitor cells have TNF-alpha resistance.[44,45] Loss of *TET2* results in the upregulation of IL-6 when stimulated.[46] In *TET2*-deficient cells, studies have shown increased inflammatory cytokines including IL-6, TNF-α, and IL-1β[31,44,45,47] and *DNMT3A* inactivation promoted increase of CXCL1, CXCL2, IL-6, and CCL5.[48] CHIP has also been associated with an increased incidence of gout, and *DNMT3A* CHIP has been associated with osteoporosis.

CHIP AND AML RISK IN POPULATION STUDIES

While large-scale whole genome and exome studies showed that CHIP increased the risk of hematologic cancers and that this risk was 50× higher in patients with high VAF (>10%) mutations,[9,18] specific data on AML risk were demonstrated by several case control studies of pre-AML samples and controls using targeted deep sequencing methodologies (*Table 81.1*).[13,23,24] These studies demonstrated that, in healthy participants, not exposed to chemotherapy/radiation, CH mutations were found several years prior to diagnosis of AML (median 9-10 years) and were enriched in participants who eventually developed AML compared with controls (odds ratio [OR]: 4.86; 95% CI: 3.07-7.77; P:3.8×10^{-13}) (*Table 81.1*). The most common mutations in the pre-AML participants included *DNMT3A, TP53, TET2, SRSF2, IDH2, SF3B1, JAK2,* and *ASXL1*. Since individuals who never developed AML also harbored CH mutations in the common DAT genes, distinguishing patterns that predict AML in terms of specific gene, clone size, clonal behavior over time, and clonal complexity are important if early detection strategies are to be implemented.

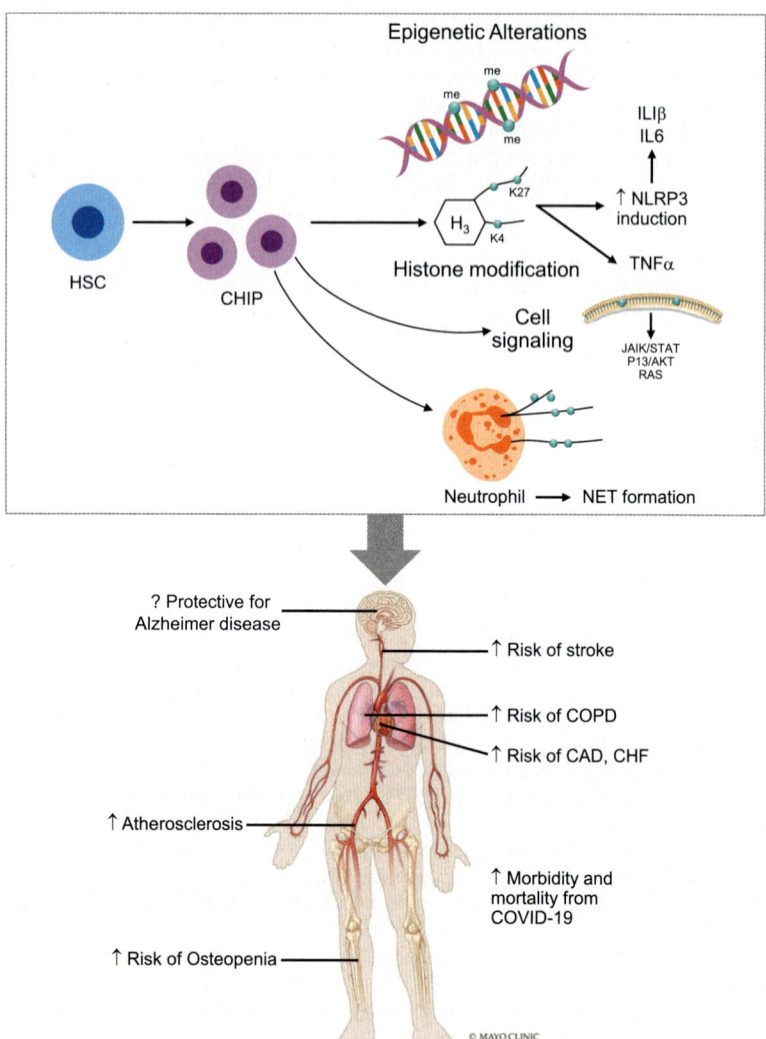

FIGURE 81.2 Biological and clinical impact of clonal hematopoiesis in patients. A, Biological impact of CH with different somatic mutations resulting in alterations in DNA methylation (*DNMT3A*, *TET2*), chromatin and histone modifications (*ASXL1*), cell signaling (*JAK2*), and neutrophil function (NET, neutrophil extracellular traps). These alterations often lead to an inflammatory state mediated by increased cytokine production and inflammasome activation. B, Clinical impact of CH with largely deleterious effects including an increased risk of stroke, cardiovascular disease, and osteoporosis among others. Potential benefits, including a reduced risk for Alzheimer disease, have also been described. CAD, coronary artery disease; CHF, congestive heart failure; COPD, chronic obstructive pulmonary disease.

Mutation-Specific Risk

Mutations in *TP53* and *IDH1* or *IDH2* demonstrate the highest risk for AML (*Table 81.1*), even at smaller VAF sizes of >0.5%-1% and regardless of the specific changes in the DNA-binding domain of *TP53* gene as a result of the mutation. Some studies suggest the AML risk in these mutations to be absolute, other studies suggest a very high, but not absolute, risk in the follow-up time that the participants were observed in the cohorts. Importantly, *IDH* mutations are associated with a long latency of up to 20 years prior to the development of AML, with rising VAFs associated with faster times to overt disease.[24] Conversely, *TP53* mutations are associated with shorter latency to AML development (OR: 5.24, 95% CI: 1.9-14.49, $P = .001$). *DNMT3A* and *TET2* are the most prevalent mutations in individuals with CH, accounting for 45% to 55% and 10% to 30% of all CH mutations, respectively.[51,52] Although the presence of *DNMT3A* and *TET2* CH mutations is associated with an increased risk of AML (*Table 81.1*), the vast majority of *DNMT3A* and *TET2* CH do not progress to AML. Clonal size (>10% VAF) and complexity confer a higher risk for AML, particularly the presence of two or more variants in *DNMT3A* and *TET2* (*DNMT3A* 2 + vs 1 variants OR 12.6 vs 2.1, *TET2* 2 + vs 1 variants OR 69.3 vs 3.29),[24] while participants who did not develop AML mostly had isolated mutations in *DNMT3A* and *TET2*. Interestingly, while *DNMT3A* R882 mutations are a common subtype (65%) in AML,[53] their prevalence is lower in CH (18%).[13,24] The data on progression to AML with R882 mutations are mixed with some studies demonstrating no difference in AML risk with R882 vs other *DNMT3A* variants[23,24] and some showing an increased risk with R882 mutations (*Table 81.1*).[13] *ASXL1* mutations are the 3rd most common in age related CH, with opposing data with regards to their risk for AML development.

Spliceosome mutations (*SRSF2*, *U2AF1*, *SF3B1*, *ZRSR2*) are the other high-risk CH group for AML risk (OR: 7.43, 95% CI: 1.71-32.22, $P = .002$)[24] (*Table 81.1*), with *U2AF1* mutations being associated with a higher risk compared with other spliceosome mutations, and are seen relatively more commonly in younger patients (60.3 vs 77.3 years, $P = 1.7 \times 10^{-4}$).[23] The AML risk with spliceosome mutations seems independent of clone size.[23,24] Lastly, *JAK2-V617F* is also associated with increased risk for AML transformation (OR: 6.1, 95% CI: 1.2-61.1, $P = .03$) (*Table 81.1*).[23,24]

Clonal Complexity

Apart from specific risk conferred by the high-risk mutations, clonal complexity, defined as the presence of more than one CH mutation, is another important factor in AML risk. Clonal complexity increases with aging and is linked to not only an increased risk of AML but also a shorter latency to AML diagnosis (OR 9.01, 95% CI: 4.1-21.4, $P = 9.7 \times 10^{-10}$) (*Table 81.1*). It remains unknown whether the risk of AML is different if multiple mutations arise from different clones, or from serial acquisition of new mutations in a single clone.

Table 81.1. Studies of CH and Myeloid Cancer Risk

Type of Study	Effect Size	De Novo or Therapy Related
Desai et al[24] Observational case control study (188 cases and 181 controls) (Women's Health Initiative)	Risk of AML with presence of CH: OR: 4.86, 95% CI: 3.07-7.77, $P = 3.8 \times 10^{-13}$ Risk of AML with clonally complex CH: OR: 9.01, 95% CI: 4.1-21.4, $P = 9.7 \times 10^{-10}$ Mutation-specific risk: TP53: OR: 47.2; 95% CI: 2.5-879.1 $P < .001$ IDH (including IDH1 and IDH2): OR: 28.5; 95% CI: 1.45-562.81 $P < .001$ Spliceosome genes (including SF3B1, SRSF2, and U2AF1): OR: 7.4; 95% CI: 1.71-32.2 $P = .002$ TET2: OR: 5.8; 95% CI: 2.6-12.9 $P < .001$ DNMT3A: OR: 2.6; 95% CI: 1.5-4.5 $P < .001$	De novo
Young et al[13] Population-based case control study 35 cases and 70 controls (Nurses Health Study)	Individuals with mutations with VAF>=0.01 increased risk of AML OR: 5.4, 95% CI: 1.8-16.6, $P = .003$ Mutation-specific risk: DNMT3A R822H: OR: 14.0, 95% CI: 1.7-113.8; $P = .01$ DNMT3A R882H or R882C: OR: 7.3, 95% CI: 1.5-34.7; $P = .01$ JAK2 V617F: OR: 8.0; 95% CI: 0.9-71.6; $P = .06$	De novo
Abelson et al[23] Population-based case control study 95 cases and 414 controls (EPIC study)	Splicing factor mutations in pre-AML cases vs controls: OR: 17.5; 95% CI: 8.1-40.4; $P = 5.2 \times 10^{-16}$ Mutation-specific risk: TP53 (HR: 12.5; 95% CI: 5.0-160.5) $P = 1.35 \times 10^{-37}$ U2AF1 (HR: 7.9; 95% CI: 4.1-192.2) $P = 2.6 \times 10^{-35}$	De novo
Genovese et al[18] (n = 12,380) (Swedish cohort) Observational study	Hematologic malignancy risk with CH: HR: 12.9, 95% CI: 5.8-28.7, $P < .001$	De novo
Jaiswal et al[9] (n = 17,182) (Multiple cohorts)	Hematologic malignancy risk with CH: HR: 11.1; 95% CI: 3.9-32.6, $P < .001$)	De novo
Saiki et al[19] Observational cohort (Japan Biobank cohort, n = 11,234)	Risk for hematologic malignancy mortality for SNVs: HR: 2.84, 95% CI: 2.14-3.78 $P = 2.9 \times 10^{-7}$ HR for CNAs: 2.64, 95% CI: 1.94-3.60 $P = 8.2 \times 10^{-7}$	De novo
Niroula et al[27] Observational cohort (UK biobank, n = 55,383)	Risk of myeloid malignancy with CH: HR: 7.0, 95% CI: 5.0-9.8; $P < .001$ Risk of myeloid malignancy with mCA: HR: 28.9, 95% CI: 24.2-34.4, $P < .001$	De novo
Gao et al[22] Cancer-treated cohort, single-institution study, n = 32,442	Risk of t-MN with mCA: HR: 14; 95% CI: 6-33; $P < .001$	Therapy-related AML
Gillis et al[49] (13 cases vs 56 controls) Nested case control study	Risk of t-MN with CH: OR: 5.75, 95% CI: 1.52-25.09, $P = .013$	Therapy related
Takahashi et al[50] 14 patients and 54 controls Retrospective case control study	CH increased risk of t-MN (HR: 13.7; $P = .013$) Risk of t-MN with CH at 5 y (CH: 30% [95% CI: 16%-51%] vs no CH: 7% [95% CI: 2%-21%], $P = .016$) t-MN incidence in patients with vs not at 10 y (Validation cohort, external): (CH: 29% [95% CI: 8%-53%] vs no CH: 0% [95% CI: 0%-0%], $P = .0009$)	Therapy related

Clone Size

Except for IDH and TP53 mutations, the risk of AML is higher for VAF ≥ 10% vs < 10% (DNMT3A [OR: 4.8 vs 2.5, $P = .002$], TET2 [OR: 20.4 vs 3.6, $P = .004$], and spliceosome genes [OR: 14.1 vs 3.4, $P = .019$]) (Table 81.1).[24] Regardless, most clones increased in VAF up to the time of AML diagnosis. The risk of AML proportionately increases with increasing VAF.[23] One study did not show any difference in VAF in any genes among those who progressed to AML vs not, but that may be due to smaller size of the study and differences in blood collection time points prior to AML diagnosis.[13]

CH AS RISK FACTOR FOR THERAPY-RELATED MYELOID NEOPLASM

Therapy-related myeloid neoplasms (t-MNs) arise due to DNA damage from chemotherapy and/or radiation and are associated with treatment resistance and poor overall survival. CH increases the risk for t-MN and is thought to occur due to chemotherapy or radiation-related stress, leading to the expansion of previously present CH mutations or, rarely, creation of new ones, although the latter is not thought to be common and may be related to the inability to detect subclonal mutations at low frequencies that expand post chemotherapy/radiation.[54] However, additional steps in mutagenesis are likely needed for transformation and influenced by germline risk,[54] immune deregulation, and inflammation in addition to stochastic drifts. Like CH in normal healthy populations, CH in patients with cancer is also associated with older age and smoking.[16,17] Exposure to prior chemotherapy and radiation is linked to higher likelihood of having CH and a higher clonal complexity of CH compared with patients with cancer who did not undergo such therapy (OR: 1.3, $P = 1 \times 10^{-6}$), particularly the presence of classic mutations that are found at the time of diagnosis of t-MN, that is, TP53 and PPM1D. The most common CH mutations in patients with cancer include DNMT3A, TET2, PPM1D, ASXL1, ATM, and TP53.

Initial evidence of CH as a risk factor for t-MN came from case controls studies of patients undergoing chemotherapy for other malignancies that demonstrated that CH prevalence was increased at baseline before administration of chemotherapy in patients who eventually developed t-MN compared with those who did not (Table 81.1),[49,50] with the cumulative incidence of t-MN at 10 years follow-up being 29% in patients with CH vs 0% in patients without CH ($P = .009$). While the incidence of t-MN in cancer survivors is 2% to 5%, in survivors with CH, it can be as high as 30%.[50,55] Subsequently, the presence of CH at the time of autologous transplantation has also been associated with increased risk of t-MN[55] (Table 81.2).[59] Autologous transplantation is unique in the sense that it combines the hematopoietic stress of chemotherapy in addition to a prolonged postchemotherapy competitive state where resistant clones can populate a relatively empty stem cell compartment.

The effect of VAF on risk of t-MN is not straightforward, with contradicting results from different studies. Limited data in patients with serial samples after chemotherapy show that some clones remained stable, some increased, and some decreased over time.[21] While TP53 and PPM1D CH are the most implicated in t-MN risk, other mutations are also prevalent[60] and not all expansion of CH clones lead to t-MN and not all TP53 or PPM1D clones go on to develop t-MN. Also, certain clones present may demonstrate differential growth or attrition over time, suggesting that CH may be oligoclonal.[21] Interestingly, the presence of CH has been linked to worse outcomes overall in advanced solid tumors resulting from progression of the primary tumor as well. The mechanism of this relationship is unknown, but it may be linked to alterations in the tumor microenvironment.[61] These data may evolve with different tumor types, and indeed a recent study in metastatic colon cancer found better survival in patients with CH compared with those who did not have CH.[62]

TP53 CH and t-MN Risk

Mutations in TP53 are known to be present in normal healthy populations with no exposure to chemotherapy.[9,18,63] Given that in patients who eventually develop TP53-mutated t-MN TP53 clones are typically detected prior to exposure to chemotherapy,[49] it is hypothesized that since these clones are generally chemotherapy resistant, they may have selective advantage in the postchemotherapy state.[60,64]

Table 81.2. Studies of Association of CH, Cytopenia, and Myeloid Cancer Risk

Type of Study	Effect Size
Galli et al[56] Cohort study	CCUS and risk of myeloid cancer overall, HR: 4.9, $P < .001$ 1 somatic mutation: HR: 2.8, $P = .045$ 2 or more somatic mutations: HR: 7.9, $P < .001$ Mutation-specific risk of myeloid cancer in patients with CCUS: Spliceosome mutations: HR: 7.4, $P < .005$ ASXL1 HR: 4.2, $P < .005$ TET2 HR: 3.7, $P < .005$
Malcovati et al[57] Prospective cohort Learning cohort: 683 patients Validation cohort: 190 patients	HR for 1 or more somatic mutations and risk of myeloid neoplasms: 13.9, 95% CI: 5.40-35.91, $P < .001$ Negative predictive value for no mutations and risk of myeloid neoplasm: 0.76 (95% CI: 0.70-0.81) Positive predictive value for 1 or more somatic mutations and risk of myeloid neoplasms: 0.81 (95% CI: 0.76-0.84) Positive predictive value for 2 or more somatic mutations and risk of myeloid neoplasms: 0.88 (95% CI: 0.84-0.92)
Van Zeventer et al[58] $N = 167{,}729$ from Lifelines cohort 676 cases and 1:1 matched controls Case control Population based	Anemia increased with increasing age, each year older: (OR: 1.07; 95% CI: 1.05-1.09; $P < 0.001$) With anemia who had CH: 46.6% and those without anemia who had CH: 39.1%, $P = .007$) TP53 more likely in patients with anemia than controls (OR: 2.67; 95% CI: 1.23-6.29; $P = .009$) SF3B1 more likely in patients with anemia than controls (OR: 2.47; 95% CI: 0.88-7.88; $P = .071$)

As somatic TP53 mutations are present in 50% of patients with a complex karyotype,[65-71] it is likely that the path to progression from TP53 CH to t-MN likely involves somatic copy number alterations.[72] Indeed, patients with TP53 CH have demonstrated subclonal chromosome 5 and 7 copy number variations years before the diagnosis of t-MN, suggesting the possibility that TP53 clones precede the development of cytogenetic abnormalities in t-MN.

PPM1D and t-MN Risk

Similar to TP53, PPM1D mutations are enriched in t-MN (20%)[14] and in patients exposed to chemotherapy, while the population frequency of PPM1D CH remains low.[73] PPM1D mutations are associated with exposure to platinum, etoposide, cytarabine, and doxorubicin chemotherapeutic agents[14,17] and usually not seen in the context of radiation therapy. PPM1D mutations are thought to inhibit p53-mediated apoptosis via a regulatory feedback loop with p53.[73,74] Unlike TP53, where the mutation forms the bulk of the tumor, PPM1D mutations are generally present in relatively small VAFs, suggesting different pathways to leukemogenesis. With regards to modern therapies, PARP inhibitors have been linked to increased risk of t-MN (1%-3%), which becomes particularly important when given in the front-line setting with a prolonged maintenance for curative intent. TP53 mutations have been known to be enriched at baseline in patients who developed t-MN after PARPi therapy compared with those who did not (OR: 5.2; 95% CI: 1.6-16; $P = .009$).[75] While platinum chemotherapy has been linked to increased TP53 and PPM1D CH and can bias the association of PARPi with t-MN,[76] the reported incidence of t-MN in patients treated with PARPi is higher than in patients treated with other modalities.

MCA AND MYELOID CANCER RISK

Like single nucleotide variants (SNVs) in several genes that are generally recognized as classic CH mutations, mCAs are also relatively common and, like classic CH, increase with age, associate with male sex, and have been linked to several CH-like disease outcomes.[19,27] Population-based studies have found co-occurrence of SNVs in the classic CH genes with mCA in approximately 16% of participants with CH SNVs and 7% overall (Table 81.1).[19] This co-occurrence with SNVs is more than that would be expected by chance, and SNVs in TP53, TET2, JAK2, SF3B1, and U2AF1 seem to correlate more closely with mCA. In addition, mCA prevalence is also more common in clonally complex CH SNVs as well as high VAF SNVs, suggesting that it is the genomic instability that exists with high-risk CH that abets the mCA co-occurrence. However, it is still not proven which event occurs first. The presence of mCAs in population studies has been linked to increased risk of mortality from hematologic malignancies both independently and in the presence of CH (Table 81.1).[19,27] This risk was seen for both myeloid and lymphoid neoplasms and more so when the CH SNVs and mCA led to biallelic alterations at the same gene locus, giving further evidence that these biallelic alterations are important in the pathogenesis of myeloid malignancies and occur early in the course of the disease biology.

The significance of copy number alterations in patients undergoing chemotherapy for solid malignancies has also been studied. As in population studies, CNAs/mCA are linked to older age (OR: 1.8, $P < .001$), male sex (OR: 1.3, $P = .012$), radiation exposure (OR: 1.7, $P = .022$), and Caucasian heritage (OR: 1.5, $P = .033$) but, unlike SNVs, not linked to smoking or chemotherapy (OR: 0.9, $P = .56$) (Table 81.1).[22] Co-occurrence of SNVs and CNVs followed a cis-alteration, where both occurred in overlapping locus in the allele and commonly occurred in conjunction with mutations in DNMT3A, TET2, JAK2, MPL, EZH2, TP53, and ATM, leading to a biallelic alteration (more common). In addition, 9% of co-occurrence followed a trans-alteration leading to cooperating functional relationships with SNVs (e.g., TP53 CH with complex aneuploidies). When paired samples were available before and at the time of leukemia diagnosis, these composite genotypes were found to be present at the time of transformation as well suggesting an interplay between SNVs and CNVs in the evolution of myeloid malignancies.

CH AND MYELOPROLIFERATIVE NEOPLASMS

MPNs are a group of myeloid disorders characterized by high blood counts, elevation in inflammatory cytokines, and increased risk of thrombosis. These disorders are largely characterized by mutations in *JAK2* V617F, *CALR,* and *MPL,* which activate the JAK/STAT pathway. Many European population-based studies have shown that the presence of *JAK2* CH is common in the general population (3%) and 20 times more common than *CALR* CH. Interestingly, in MPN,[77] this difference in prevalence is less obvious (4×),[78-80] suggesting that there may be more variability in penetrance of *JAK2* CH toward conversion to MPN than *CALR*. Both *JAK2* and *CALR* CH are associated with higher platelet counts in population databases, but *JAK2* V617F CH is specifically linked to a higher thrombosis risk even prior to disease progression. This effect can be seen even at low VAFs (2%).[77] Like CH in the classic DTA genes, *JAK2* V617F CH may be affected by having a proinflammatory state and a positive feedback loop might be responsible for progression to MPN.[81,82] A proinflammatory state as characterized by elevated neutrophil counts is associated with higher thrombosis risk in MPN. Evidence supporting this is the observation that having the loss of function IL-6 receptor variant is associated with reduced risk of MPN overall and in participants with *JAK2* V617F CH mutation.[81] With mounting evidence that *JAK2* CH maybe acquired in early childhood and of the prolonged phase of clonal growth before diagnosis of MPN, along with the prominent role of inflammation in the associated thrombosis risk with both *JAK2*+ CH and MPN, risk factors that govern the clonal growth trajectories and ultimately the risk of MPN are of immense clinical significance.

CLONAL HEMATOPOIESIS AND CLONAL CYTOPENIAS UNCERTAIN SIGNIFICANCE

The presence of CHIP at high VAFs (>10%) has been associated with increased red cell distribution width (RDW). In fact, the presence of increased RDW (>14) was associated with an increased the risk of AML in a large electronic health database ($P = .0016$).[23] Using machine learning with an algorithm that incorporated RDW and blood counts, AML could be predicted 6 to 12 months prior to diagnosis with a sensitivity of 25% and specificity of 98.2% according to one study. While this remains to be validated, there are several studies that have evaluated CH when it presents with cytopenias (CCUS).

CH is found at a higher prevalence in older patients with anemia regardless of whether the cause of anemia is unknown or related to chronic inflammation compared with age-matched controls without anemia.[58] Moreover, VAF >5% in patients with anemia were associated with a lower overall survival, in comparison to anemia patients with VAF <5% (Table 81.2).[58] If all unexplained cytopenias are considered, approximately 30% of patients have CH (a condition called CCUS) (Table 81.2).[56] CCUS is associated with increased risk of progression to myeloid neoplasms (HR for one somatic mutation: 2.8, hazard ratio for two or more somatic mutations: 7.9), and this progression risk is increased with the presence of *ASXL1*, spliceosome, and *TET2* mutations as well as a higher VAF.[56] In patients with cytopenias, having no mutations had a negative predictive value of 0.75 for myeloid neoplasms, while the positive predictive value of one or more mutations was 0.81 and two or more mutations was 0.88 (Table 81.2).[57]

Because patients with CCUS have the same overall survival as those with low-grade MDS[83] and the spectrum of mutations in CCUS is like low-grade MDS, comparisons between CCUS and MDS is of clinical interest if early treatment is to be contemplated. Indeed, patients with CCUS with dysplasia and patients with CCUS without dysplasia did not differ significantly with respect to degree of cytopenias, bone marrow cellularity, or abnormal phenotypic features. However, patients with CCUS with dysplasia have more mutations typical of myeloid neoplasms (e.g., more spliceosome genes) than CCUS without dysplasia (Table 81.2).[83] CCUS with dysplasia that does not meet WHO-defined dysplasia required for MDS diagnosis may in future be defined as MDS if certain classic mutations are present (e.g., *SF3B1*).

CH AND AML OUTCOMES

As CH is a risk factor for both de novo AML and t-MN, the implication of the presence of these mutations once the disease sets in is of clinical significance. After AML induction, most CH mutations persist even in complete remission, and current induction strategies do not eliminate CH clones. Reassuringly, persistence of the classic DTA (*DNMT3A, TET2, ASXL1*) in remission is not associated with worse AML outcomes overall (Table 81.3).[84,87] However, these data are evolving with a more recent study showing that, when measured in remission and just prior to allogeneic stem cell transplantation, persistence of canonical *DNMT3A* and *ASXL1* mutations had significantly higher cumulative incidence of relapse ($P = .01$) and worse overall survival ($P = .04$) than persistent noncanonical *DNMT3A* and *ASXL1* mutations.[88] For non-DTA mutations, there may be differential effects. In patients with *NPM1* mutations, persistence of non-DTA mutations at the time of complete molecular remission (for *NPM1* mutation) was

Table 81.3. CH and Its Impact on HSCT Outcomes

Type of Study	Effect Size	Type of Transplant
Heini et al[84] 110 patients with AML	Overall survival HR: 0.79, 95% CI: 0.41-1.51, $P = .440$ Progression-free survival HR: 0.75, 95% CI: 0.42-1.33, $P = .287$	Autologous SCT
Frick et al[85] $N = 500$ HSPC donors	Overall survival HR: 0.88, 95% CI: 0.65-1.321, $P = .434$ Risk of chronic GVHD with CHIP HR: 1.73, 95% CI: 1.21-2.49, $P = .003$ Patients with CHIP who underwent HSCT in noncomplete relapse lower risk of CIR/P: HR: 0.49; 95% CI: 0.27-0.88; $P = .019$ Patients with DNMT3A mutation who underwent HSCT in noncomplete relapse lower risk of CIR/P: HR: 0.34; 95% CI: 0.15-0.81; $P = .015$	Allogeneic SCT
Gibson et al[55] $N = 401$ patients with non-Hodgkin lymphoma who underwent ASCT Cohort study	Nucleoside analogue and risk of t-MN (HR: 2.9; 95% CI: 1.1-7.3; $P = .03$) Lifetime dose of cyclophosphamide greater than 10 g/m² (SHR: 4.6; range:1.7-12.5; $P = .003$) CHIP and risk of t-MN (SHR: 3.7; range:1.4-9.9; $P = .009$) CHIP and lower overall survival: 5 year 59.9% for those with CHIP vs 72.4% with no CHIP and 10 y survival with CHIP 30.4% and without CHIP 60.9% (HR: 1.8; 95% CI: 1.4-2.8; $P=.001$)	Autologous SCT
Newell et al[86] $N = 290$ 15 cases with CH from donor 45 controls Case control	Patients with CH from donor increased risk of GVHD that required immunosuppressive treatment ($P = .045$) Time to neutrophil or platelet engraftment was not significantly different between those with CH and those without ($P = .729$) No patients with CH from donor had relapse but 15.6% of control cohort had relapse $P = .176$	Allogeneic SCT

SHR, subdistribution hazard ratio.

associated with a worse relapse risk.[89] Contrasting to this, another study showed that persistence of non-DTA CH mutations in remission does not negatively impact relapse or death post remission (P = .174 and P = .827).[90]

CHIP AND HEMATOPOIETIC STEM CELL TRANSPLANT OUTCOMES

Donor-derived CH in the presence of allogeneic stem cell transplantation is of obvious interest as HSCs are subjected to rapid proliferation and bone marrow reconstitution along with an altered bone marrow microenvironment. As a result, donor-derived CH clones may not only have differential rates of reconstitution of the bone marrow but may also impact graft-vs-host disease (GVHD) and graft-vs-leukemia effect. The presence of donor CH has been associated with slower count recovery in allogeneic transplant recipients.[91] However, several studies have now shown no adverse outcomes in terms of survival and relapse when donor CH was identified retrospectively after allogeneic HSCT. In fact, the presence of donor CH was associated with reduced rates of relapse when the disease was not in remission at the time of transplant. This effect was thought to be due to an increased incidence of chronic GVHD among patients who had *DNMT3A* CH derived from the donors[85] (Table 81.3). Donor *TET2* and *ASXL1* CH has also similarly been linked to longer survival.[92] While most data exist for the more common DTA CH, data on *TP53* and *PPM1D* CH that has been implicated in t-MN are lacking and its effect on survival and leukemia relapse post allogeneic HSCT is unknown. Of particular interest is the incidence of donor cell leukemia, which is thought to occur due to rapid expansion of donor CH in the setting of hematopoietic recovery in an inflammatory and altered bone marrow microenvironment.[93,94] Despite the theoretical possibility, rates of donor cell leukemia in recipients of donor-derived CH seems very low.

In contrast to allogeneic HSCT, where a relatively healthy stem cell population reconstitutes the bone marrow, autologous transplant (ASCT) combines the effect of cytotoxic chemotherapy-induced stress on stem cells that then reconstitute the bone marrow and thus chemoresistant CH clones may have a proliferation advantage and consequently a higher risk of t-MN. In patients undergoing ASCT for non-Hodgkin lymphoma, the presence of CH was associated with a 10-year cumulative incidence of t-MN of 7.6%, with 7.4% and 14.1% incidence at 5- and 10-year follow-up, respectively, compared with 1.7% and 4.3% at 5 and 10 years in patients without baseline CH (P = .002) (Table 81.2).[55] *TP53* and *PPM1D* mutations were the most implicated in addition to clonal complexity (cumulative incidence of 25% at 10 years for CH with more than one mutation, compared with 9.9% for patients with only one CH mutation, P < .001). The inferior outcomes after ASCT in patients with CH is not limited just to increased t-MN risk as the nonrelapse mortality from cardiovascular diseases is also higher in CHIP carriers (10-year overall survival, 30.4% vs 60.9% in CHIP-negative and CHIP-positive participants, respectively; P < .001).[55] These data have implications in guiding physicians when alternative treatment options are available.

CH IN ACQUIRED AND INHERITED BONE MARROW FAILURE SYNDROMES

Acquired Aplastic Anemia

Since acquired aplastic anemia (AA) is associated with stem cell attrition, CH clones arising in this situation might have a survival advantage. This is reflected in the fact that patients with AA have a 10% to 15% 10-year risk of MDS/AML,[95] which is higher than that in normal populations. In fact, 47% of patients with AA undergoing immunosuppressive therapy (IST) are reported to harbor CH mutations.[96] Increased clonal complexity and acquisition of new clones usually precede the development of MDS/AML,[96,97] but not all expansions of CH mutations lead to MDS/AML, and complex interactions between stem cell attrition and immune factors likely play a role in malignant transformation. While the patterns of *DNMT3A* and *ASXL1* mutations closely resemble age-related CH in normal populations with increasing clonal size with time, *BCOR* and *PIGa* mutations are uniquely seen in AA and largely remain stable. Paradoxically, these mutations are linked to improved survival (HR: 0.27, 0.09-0.78; P = .016) and better response to IST.[96] In fact, CH clones are known to rapidly expand after IST use (P < .001)[96] and yet not progress to MDS/AML.

Inherited Bone Marrow Failure Syndromes

If CH clones in AA are associated with increased risk of MDs/AML, inherited bone marrow failure syndromes are more unique. These germline states give age-related CH a longer time to expand, and CH clones might function as an escape mechanism for transient hematopoiesis. This is exactly what has been seen in patients with Shwachman-Diamond syndrome (SDS) and Diamond-Blackfan anemia (DBA) where ribosomal stress and increased *TP53*-driven apoptosis lead to bone marrow failure.[98,99] Clones harboring CH mutations in *TP53* have an advantage in these conditions, leading to transient rescue of hematopoiesis but higher risk of MDS/AML.[98] This is reflected in the higher occurrence of *TP53* mutations in patients with SDS (48%) and also at the time of AML diagnosis[100,101] as well as a higher risk of AML in general (36% of patients with SDS develop AML by age 30 years).[102] *TP53* CH mutations are also known to occur in DBA, but with lower rates of progression to MDS/AML, with a cumulative incidence of 5% by 46 years of age.[103]

The mechanisms by which specific CH clones play a role in expansion and AML/MDS risk depends on the underlying mechanism of bone marrow failure. For example, patients with Fanconi anemia who progress to MDS/AML have a complex karyotype at diagnosis but without *TP53* mutations (in de novo AML *TP53* mutations and complex karyotype co-occur commonly) and CH mutations in *RUNX1* as well as chromosomal abnormalities in 3q+ and monosomy 7/del (7q) ultimately drive the risk of MDS/AML risk.[104-106] Similarly, in patients with severe congenital neutropenia, while somatic *CSF3R* mutations are common, it is the acquisition of *RUNX1* mutations that are strongly associated with AML evolution.[107]

CONCLUSIONS

CH has firmly been established as a precursor for myeloid malignancies with a long latency between establishment of CH and the occurrence of myeloid malignancies. This risk is not absolute, and many factors lead to malignant transformation including type and complexity of CH as well as extrinsic (environment, chemotherapy, and radiation) and intrinsic (inflammation, aging, germline genetics) clonal selection pressures. A deeper understanding of these risk factors is important for identifying patients with high risk for malignant transformation, which would then lead to potential methods of abrogation of disease progression. In addition, establishment of biologic pathways that are mutation or person specific and aid in malignant transformation are also important to identify from a therapeutic standpoint. Generalized population screening is not recommended at this time point for CH. However, incidentally, discovered CH either in the setting of low blood counts (CCUS), prior to transplant, or at the time of visceral malignancy diagnosis presents with unique management decisions for physicians. CH clinics are now established in several institutions, and monitoring of patients with known CH is already underway. Treatment of CH is not recommended at this point outside of clinical trials, and decisions regarding alteration of treatment for other cancers (chemotherapy/radiation) should be based on careful discussions with oncologists, patients, and the specific risk vs benefit ratio for any decision. Regardless, as more evidence mounts, prevention of myeloid cancers is likely to take center stage in the coming years.

References

1. Welch JS, Ley TJ, Link DC, et al. The origin and evolution of mutations in acute myeloid leukemia. *Cell.* 2012;150(2):264-278.
2. Lee-Six H, Obro NF, Shepherd MS, et al. Population dynamics of normal human blood inferred from somatic mutations. *Nature.* 2018;561(7724):473-478.
3. Scala S, Aiuti A. In vivo dynamics of human hematopoietic stem cells: novel concepts and future directions. *Blood Adv.* 2019;3(12):1916-1924.

4. Osorio FG, Rosendahl Huber A, Oka R, et al. Somatic mutations reveal lineage relationships and age-related mutagenesis in human hematopoiesis. *Cell Rep*. 2018;25(9):2308.e4-2316.e4.
5. Busque L, Mio R, Mattioli J, et al. Nonrandom X-inactivation patterns in normal females: lyonization ratios vary with age. *Blood*. 1996;88(1):59-65.
6. Busque L, Patel JP, Figueroa ME, et al. Recurrent somatic TET2 mutations in normal elderly individuals with clonal hematopoiesis. *Nat Genet*. 2012;44(11):1179-1181.
7. Jaiswal S, Natarajan P, Silver AJ, et al. Clonal hematopoiesis and risk of atherosclerotic cardiovascular disease. *N Engl J Med*. 2017;377(2):111-121.
8. Jaiswal S, Ebert BL. Clonal hematopoiesis in human aging and disease. *Science*. 2019;366(6465):eaan4673.
9. Jaiswal S, Fontanillas P, Flannick J, et al. Age-related clonal hematopoiesis associated with adverse outcomes. *N Engl J Med*. 2014;371(26):2488-2498.
10. Izzo F, Lee SC, Poran A, et al. DNA methylation disruption reshapes the hematopoietic differentiation landscape. *Nat Genet*. 2020;52(4):378-387.
11. van Zeventer IA, Salzbrunn JB, de Graaf AO, et al. Prevalence, predictors, and outcomes of clonal hematopoiesis in individuals aged ≥80 years. *Blood Adv*. 2021;5(8):2115-2122.
12. Young AL, Challen GA, Birmann BM, Druley TE. Clonal haematopoiesis harbouring AML-associated mutations is ubiquitous in healthy adults. *Nat Commun*. 2016;7:12484.
13. Young AL, Tong RS, Birmann BM, Druley TE. Clonal hematopoiesis and risk of acute myeloid leukemia. *Haematologica*. 2019;104(12):2410-2417.
14. Hsu JI, Dayaram T, Tovy A, et al. PPM1D mutations drive clonal hematopoiesis in response to cytotoxic chemotherapy. *Cell Stem Cell*. 2018;23(5):700-713.e6.
15. King KY, Huang Y, Nakada D, Goodell MA. Environmental influences on clonal hematopoiesis. *Exp Hematol*. 2020;83:66-73.
16. Bolton KL, Ptashkin RN, Gao T, et al. Cancer therapy shapes the fitness landscape of clonal hematopoiesis. *Nat Genet*. 2020;52(11):1219-1226.
17. Coombs CC, Zehir A, Devlin SM, et al. Therapy-related clonal hematopoiesis in patients with non-hematologic cancers is common and associated with adverse clinical outcomes. *Cell Stem Cell*. 2017;21(3):374-382.e4.
18. Genovese G, Kahler AK, Handsaker RE, et al. Clonal hematopoiesis and blood-cancer risk inferred from blood DNA sequence. *N Engl J Med*. 2014;371(26):2477-2487.
19. Saiki R, Momozawa Y, Nannya Y, et al. Combined landscape of single-nucleotide variants and copy number alterations in clonal hematopoiesis. *Nat Med*. 2021;27(7):1239-1249.
20. Watson CJ, Papula AL, Poon GYP, et al. The evolutionary dynamics and fitness landscape of clonal hematopoiesis. *Science*. 2020;367(6485):1449-1454.
21. Arends CM, Galan-Sousa J, Hoyer K, et al. Hematopoietic lineage distribution and evolutionary dynamics of clonal hematopoiesis. *Leukemia*. 2018;32(9):1908-1919.
22. Gao T, Ptashkin R, Bolton KL, et al. Interplay between chromosomal alterations and gene mutations shapes the evolutionary trajectory of clonal hematopoiesis. *Nat Commun*. 2021;12(1):338.
23. Abelson S, Collord G, Ng SWK, et al. Prediction of acute myeloid leukaemia risk in healthy individuals. *Nature*. 2018;559(7714):400-404.
24. Desai P, Mencia-Trinchant N, Savenkov O, et al. Somatic mutations precede acute myeloid leukemia years before diagnosis. *Nat Med*. 2018;24(7):1015-1023.
25. Van Egeren D, Escabi J, Nguyen M, et al. Reconstructing the lineage histories and differentiation trajectories of individual cancer cells in myeloproliferative neoplasms. *Cell Stem Cell*. 2021;28(3):514.e9-523.e9.
26. Williams N, Lee J, Moore L, et al. Driver mutation acquisition in utero and childhood followed by lifelong clonal evolution underlie myeloproliferative neoplasms. *Blood*. 2020;136:LBA-1.
27. Niroula A, Sekar A, Murakami MA, et al. Distinction of lymphoid and myeloid clonal hematopoiesis. *Nat Med*. 2021;27(11):1921-1927.
28. Dorsheimer L, Assmus B, Rasper T, et al. Association of mutations contributing to clonal hematopoiesis with prognosis in chronic ischemic heart failure. *JAMA Cardiol*. 2019;4(1):25-33.
29. Assmus B, Cremer S, Kirschbaum K, et al. Clonal haematopoiesis in chronic ischaemic heart failure: prognostic role of clone size for DNMT3A- and TET2-driver gene mutations. *Eur Heart J*. 2021;42(3):257-265.
30. Pascual-Figal DA, Bayes-Genis A, Diez-Diez M, et al. Clonal hematopoiesis and risk of progression of heart failure with reduced left ventricular ejection fraction. *J Am Coll Cardiol*. 2021;77(14):1747-1759.
31. Sano S, Oshima K, Wang Y, et al. Tet2-Mediated clonal hematopoiesis accelerates heart failure through a mechanism involving the IL-1β/NLRP3 Inflammasome. *J Am Coll Cardiol*. 2018;71(8):875-886.
32. Mas-Peiro S, Hoffmann J, Fichtlscherer S, et al. Clonal haematopoiesis in patients with degenerative aortic valve stenosis undergoing transcatheter aortic valve implantation. *Eur Heart J*. 2020;41(8):933-939.
33. Cremer S, Kirschbaum K, Berkowitsch A, et al. Multiple somatic mutations for clonal hematopoiesis are associated with increased mortality in patients with chronic heart failure. *Circ Genom Precis Med*. 2020;13(4):e003003.
34. Hormaechea-Agulla D, Matatall KA, Le DT, et al. Chronic infection drives Dnmt3a-loss-of-function clonal hematopoiesis via IFNgamma signaling. *Cell Stem Cell*. 2021;28(8):1428.e6-1442.e6.
35. Meisel R, Hinterleitner R, Pacis A, et al. Microbial signals drive pre-leukaemic myeloproliferation in a Tet2-deficient host. *Nature*. 2018;557(7706):580-584.
36. Dharan NJ, Yeh P, Bloch M, et al; ARCHIVE Study Group. HIV is associated with an increased risk of age-related clonal hematopoiesis among older adults. *Nat Med*. 2021;27(6):1006-1011.
37. Zhang CRC, Nix D, Gregory M, et al. Inflammatory cytokines promote clonal hematopoiesis with specific mutations in ulcerative colitis patients. *Exp Hematol*. 2019;80:36-41 e3.
38. Savola P, Kelkka T, Rajala HL, et al. Somatic mutations in clonally expanded cytotoxic T lymphocytes in patients with newly diagnosed rheumatoid arthritis. *Nat Commun*. 2017;8:15869.
39. Arends CM, Weiss M, Christen F, et al. Clonal hematopoiesis in patients with anti-neutrophil cytoplasmic antibody-associated vasculitis. *Haematologica*. 2020;105(6):e264-e267.
40. Bekele DI, Patnaik MM. Autoimmunity, clonal hematopoiesis, and myeloid neoplasms. *Rheum Dis Clin North Am*. 2020;46(3):429-444.
41. Zekavat SM, Lin SH, Bick AG, et al. Hematopoietic mosaic chromosomal alterations increase the risk for diverse types of infection. *Nat Med*. 2021;27(6):1012-24.
42. Bolton KL, Koh Y, Foote MB, et al. Clonal hematopoiesis is associated with risk of severe Covid-19. *Nat Commun*. 2021;12(1):5975.
43. Abplanalp WT, Mas-Peiro S, Cremer S, John D, Dimmeler S, Zeiher AM. Association of clonal hematopoiesis of indeterminate potential with inflammatory gene expression in patients with severe degenerative aortic valve stenosis or chronic postischemic heart failure. *JAMA Cardiol*. 2020;5(10):1170-1175.
44. Abegunde SO, Buckstein R, Wells RA, Rauh MJ. An inflammatory environment containing TNFα favors Tet2-mutant clonal hematopoiesis. *Exp Hematol*. 2018;59:60-65.
45. Cull AH, Snetsinger B, Buckstein R, Wells RA, Rauh MJ. Tet2 restrains inflammatory gene expression in macrophages. *Exp Hematol*. 2017;55:56-70 e13.
46. Zhang Q, Zhao K, Shen Q, et al. Tet2 is required to resolve inflammation by recruiting Hdac2 to specifically repress IL-6. *Nature*. 2015;525(7569):389-393.
47. Ichiyama K, Chen T, Wang X, et al. The methylcytosine dioxygenase Tet2 promotes DNA demethylation and activation of cytokine gene expression in T cells. *Immunity*. 2015;42(4):613-626.
48. Sano S, Oshima K, Wang Y, Katanasaka Y, Sano M, Walsh K. CRISPR-mediated gene editing to assess the roles of Tet2 and Dnmt3a in clonal hematopoiesis and cardiovascular disease. *Circ Res*. 2018;123(3):335-341.
49. Gillis NK, Ball M, Zhang Q, et al. Clonal haemopoiesis and therapy-related myeloid malignancies in elderly patients: a proof-of-concept, case-control study. *Lancet Oncol*. 2017;18(1):112-121.
50. Takahashi K, Wang F, Kantarjian H, et al. Preleukaemic clonal haemopoiesis and risk of therapy-related myeloid neoplasms: a case-control study. *Lancet Oncol*. 2017;18(1):100-111.
51. Buscarlet M, Provost S, Zada YF, et al. DNMT3A and TET2 dominate clonal hematopoiesis and demonstrate benign phenotypes and different genetic predispositions. *Blood*. 2017;130(6):753-762.
52. Heuser M, Thol F, Ganser A. Clonal hematopoiesis of indeterminate potential. *Dtsch Arztebl Int*. 2016;113(18):317-322.
53. Cancer Genome Atlas Research Network; Ley TJ, Miller C, Ding L, et al. Genomic and epigenomic landscapes of adult de novo acute myeloid leukemia. *N Engl J Med*. 2013;368(22):2059-2074.
54. Desai P, Roboz GJ. Clonal Hematopoiesis and therapy related MDS/AML. *Best Pract Res Clin Haematol*. 2019;32(1):13-23.
55. Gibson CJ, Lindsley RC, Tchekmedyian V, et al. Clonal hematopoiesis associated with adverse outcomes after autologous stem-cell transplantation for lymphoma. *J Clin Oncol*. 2017;35(14):1598-1605.
56. Galli A, Todisco G, Catamo E, et al. Relationship between clone metrics and clinical outcome in clonal cytopenia. *Blood*. 2021;138(11):965-976.
57. Malcovati L, Gallì A, Travaglino E, et al. Clinical significance of somatic mutation in unexplained blood cytopenia. *Blood*. 2017;129(25):3371-3378.
58. van Zeventer IA, de Graaf AO, Wouters HJCM, et al. Mutational spectrum and dynamics of clonal hematopoiesis in anemia of older individuals. *Blood*. 2020;135(14):1161-1170.
59. Soerensen JF, Aggerholm A, Kerndrup GB, et al. Clonal hematopoiesis predicts development of therapy-related myeloid neoplasms post-autologous stem cell transplantation. *Blood Adv*. 2020;4(5):885-892.
60. Wong TN, Miller CA, Jotte MRM, et al. Cellular stressors contribute to the expansion of hematopoietic clones of varying leukemic potential. *Nat Commun*. 2018;9(1):455.
61. Kleppe M, Comen E, Wen HY, et al. Somatic mutations in leukocytes infiltrating primary breast cancers. *NPJ Breast Cancer*. 2015;1:15005.
62. Arends C.M., Dimitriou S, Stahler A., et al. Clonal hematopoiesis is associated with improved survival in patients with metastatic colorectal cancer from the FIRE-3 trial. *Blood*. 2022;139(10):1593-1597.
63. Xie M, Lu C, Wang J, et al. Age-related mutations associated with clonal hematopoietic expansion and malignancies. *Nat Med*. 2014;20(12):1472-1478.
64. Wong TN, Ramsingh G, Young AL, et al. Role of TP53 mutations in the origin and evolution of therapy-related acute myeloid leukaemia. *Nature*. 2015;518(7540):552-555.
65. Rücker FG, Schlenk RF, Bullinger L, et al. TP53 alterations in acute myeloid leukemia with complex karyotype correlate with specific copy number alterations, monosomal karyotype, and dismal outcome. *Blood*. 2012;119(9):2114-2121.
66. Papaemmanuil E, Gerstung M, Bullinger L, et al. Genomic classification and prognosis in acute myeloid leukemia. *N Engl J Med*. 2016;374(23):2209-2221.
67. Metzeler KH, Herold T, Rothenberg-Thurley M, et al; AMLCG Study Group. Spectrum and prognostic relevance of driver gene mutations in acute myeloid leukemia. *Blood*. 2016;128(5):686-698.
68. Volkert S, Kohlmann A, Schnittger S, Kern W, Haferlach T, Haferlach C. Association of the type of 5q loss with complex karyotype, clonal evolution, TP53 mutation status, and prognosis in acute myeloid leukemia and myelodysplastic syndrome. *Genes Chromosomes Cancer*. 2014;53(5):402-410.
69. Sebaa A, Ades L, Baran-Marzack F, et al. Incidence of 17p deletions and TP53 mutation in myelodysplastic syndrome and acute myeloid leukemia with 5q deletion. *Genes Chromosomes Cancer*. 2012;51(12):1086-1092.
70. Kadia TM, Jain P, Ravandi F, et al. TP53 mutations in newly diagnosed acute myeloid leukemia: clinicomolecular characteristics, response to therapy, and outcomes. *Cancer*. 2016;122(22):3484-3491.

71. Lindsley RC, Mar BG, Mazzola E, et al. Acute myeloid leukemia ontogeny is defined by distinct somatic mutations. *Blood*. 2015;125(9):1367-1376.
72. Welch JS. Patterns of mutations in TP53 mutated AML. *Best Pract Res Clin Haematol*. 2018;31(4):379-383.
73. Kahn JD, Miller PG, Silver AJ, et al. PPM1D-truncating mutations confer resistance to chemotherapy and sensitivity to PPM1D inhibition in hematopoietic cells. *Blood*. 2018;132(11):1095-1105.
74. Dudgeon C, Shreeram S, Tanoue K, et al. Genetic variants and mutations of PPM1D control the response to DNA damage. *Cell Cycle*. 2013;12(16):2656-2664.
75. Kwan TT, Oza AM, Tinker AV, et al. Preexisting TP53-variant clonal hematopoiesis and risk of secondary myeloid neoplasms in patients with high-grade ovarian cancer treated with rucaparib. *JAMA Oncol*. 2021;7(12):1772-1781.
76. Swisher EM, Harrell MI, Norquist BM, et al. Somatic mosaic mutations in PPM1D and TP53 in the blood of women with ovarian carcinoma. *JAMA Oncol*. 2016;2(3):370-372.
77. Cordua S, Kjaer L, Skov V, Pallisgaard N, Hasselbalch HC, Ellervik C. Prevalence and phenotypes of *JAK2* V617F and *calreticulin* mutations in a Danish general population. *Blood*. 2019;134(5):469-479.
78. Karantanos T, Chaturvedi S, Braunstein EM, et al. Sex determines the presentation and outcomes in MPN and is related to sex-specific differences in the mutational burden. *Blood Adv*. 2020;4(12):2567-2576.
79. Lundberg P, Karow A, Nienhold R, et al. Clonal evolution and clinical correlates of somatic mutations in myeloproliferative neoplasms. *Blood*. 2014;123(14):2220-2228.
80. Nangalia J, Massie CE, Baxter EJ, et al. Somatic CALR mutations in myeloproliferative neoplasms with nonmutated JAK2. *N Engl J Med*. 2013;369(25):2391-2405.
81. Pedersen KM, Çolak Y, Ellervik C, Hasselbalch HC, Bojesen SE, Nordestgaard BG. Loss-of-function polymorphism in *IL6R* reduces risk of *JAK2*V617F somatic mutation and myeloproliferative neoplasm: a Mendelian randomization study. *EClinicalMedicine*. 2020;21:100280.
82. Hasselbalch HC. Perspectives on chronic inflammation in essential thrombocythemia, polycythemia vera, and myelofibrosis: is chronic inflammation a trigger and driver of clonal evolution and development of accelerated atherosclerosis and second cancer? *Blood*. 2012;119(14):3219-3225.
83. Jajosky AN, Sadri N, Meyerson HJ, et al. Clonal cytopenia of undetermined significance (CCUS) with dysplasia is enriched for MDS-type molecular findings compared to CCUS without dysplasia. *Eur J Haematol*. 2021;106(4):500-507.
84. Heini AD, Porret N, Zenhaeusern R, Winkler A, Bacher U, Pabst T. Clonal hematopoiesis after autologous stem cell transplantation does not confer adverse prognosis in patients with AML. *Cancers (Basel)*. 2021;13(13):3190.
85. Frick M, Chan W, Arends CM, et al. Role of donor clonal hematopoiesis in allogeneic hematopoietic stem-cell transplantation. *J Clin Oncol*. 2019;37(5):375-385.
86. Newell LF, Williams T, Liu J, et al. Engrafted donor-derived clonal hematopoiesis after allogenic hematopoietic cell transplantation is associated with chronic graft-versus-host disease requiring immunosuppressive therapy, but no adverse impact on overall survival or relapse. *Transplant Cell Ther*. 2021;27(8):662 e1-e9.
87. Jongen-Lavrencic M, Grob T, Hanekamp D, et al. Molecular minimal residual disease in acute myeloid leukemia. *N Engl J Med*. 2018;378(13):1189-1199.
88. Jentzsch M, Grimm J, Bill M, et al. Measurable residual disease of canonical versus non-canonical DNMT3A, TET2, or ASXL1 mutations in AML at stem cell transplantation. *Bone Marrow Transplant*. 2021;56(10):2610-2612.
89. Cappelli LV, Meggendorfer M, Baer C, et al. Indeterminate and oncogenic potential: CHIP vs CHOP mutations in AML with NPM1 alteration. *Leukemia*. 2022;36(2):394-402.
90. Tanaka T, Morita K, Loghavi S, et al. Clonal dynamics and clinical implications of postremission clonal hematopoiesis in acute myeloid leukemia. *Blood*. 2021;138(18):1733-1739.
91. Gibson CJ, Kennedy JA, Nikiforow S, et al. Donor-engrafted CHIP is common among stem cell transplant recipients with unexplained cytopenias. *Blood*. 2017;130(1):91-94.
92. Grimm J, Bill M, Jentzsch M, et al. Clinical impact of clonal hematopoiesis in acute myeloid leukemia patients receiving allogeneic transplantation. *Bone Marrow Transplant*. 2019;54(8):1189-1197.
93. Gondek LP, Zheng G, Ghiaur G, et al. Donor cell leukemia arising from clonal hematopoiesis after bone marrow transplantation. *Leukemia*. 2016;30(9):1916-1920.
94. Yasuda T, Ueno T, Fukumura K, et al. Leukemic evolution of donor-derived cells harboring IDH2 and DNMT3A mutations after allogeneic stem cell transplantation. *Leukemia*. 2014;28(2):426-428.
95. Li H. A statistical framework for SNP calling, mutation discovery, association mapping and population genetical parameter estimation from sequencing data. *Bioinformatics*. 2011;27(21):2987-2993.
96. Yoshizato T, Dumitriu B, Hosokawa K, et al. Somatic mutations and clonal hematopoiesis in aplastic anemia. *N Engl J Med*. 2015;373(1):35-47.
97. Kulasekararaj AG, Jiang J, Smith AE, et al. Somatic mutations identify a subgroup of aplastic anemia patients who progress to myelodysplastic syndrome. *Blood*. 2014;124(17):2698-2704.
98. Schaefer EJ, Lindsley RC. Significance of clonal mutations in bone marrow failure and inherited myelodysplastic syndrome/acute myeloid leukemia predisposition syndromes. *Hematol Oncol Clin North Am*. 2018;32(4):643-655.
99. Elghetany MT, Alter BP. p53 protein overexpression in bone marrow biopsies of patients with shwachman-diamond syndrome has a prevalence similar to that of patients with refractory anemia. *Arch Pathol Lab Med*. 2002;126(4):452-455.
100. Xia J, Miller CA, Baty J, et al. Somatic mutations and clonal hematopoiesis in congenital neutropenia. *Blood*. 2018;131(4):408-416.
101. Lindsley RC, Saber W, Mar BG, et al. Prognostic mutations in myelodysplastic syndrome after stem-cell transplantation. *N Engl J Med*. 2017;376(6):536-547.
102. Donadieu J, Delhommeau F. TP53 mutations: the dawn of Shwachman clones. *Blood*. 2018;131(4):376-377.
103. Vlachos A, Rosenberg PS, Atsidaftos E, Alter BP, Lipton JM. Incidence of neoplasia in Diamond Blackfan anemia: a report from the Diamond Blackfan Anemia Registry. *Blood*. 2012;119(16):3815-3819.
104. Quentin S, Cuccuini W, Ceccaldi R, et al. Myelodysplasia and leukemia of Fanconi anemia are associated with a specific pattern of genomic abnormalities that includes cryptic RUNX1/AML1 lesions. *Blood*. 2011;117(15):e161-e170.
105. Cioc AM, Wagner JE, MacMillan ML, DeFor T, Hirsch B. Diagnosis of myelodysplastic syndrome among a cohort of 119 patients with Fanconi anemia: morphologic and cytogenetic characteristics. *Am J Clin Pathol*. 2010;133(1):92-100.
106. Tönnies H, Huber S, Kuhl JS, Gerlach A, Ebell W, Neitzel H. Clonal chromosomal aberrations in bone marrow cells of Fanconi anemia patients: gains of the chromosomal segment 3q26q29 as an adverse risk factor. *Blood*. 2003;101(10):3872-3874.
107. Skokowa J, Steinemann D, Katsman-Kuipers JE, et al. Cooperativity of RUNX1 and CSF3R mutations in severe congenital neutropenia: a unique pathway in myeloid leukemogenesis. *Blood*. 2014;123(14):2229-2237.

Section 3 ■ MYELOPROLIFERATIVE DISORDERS

Chapter 82 ■ Pathology of the Myeloproliferative Neoplasms

TRACY I. GEORGE • DEVON S. CHABOT-RICHARDS

INTRODUCTION

The myeloproliferative neoplasms (MPNs) are characterized by a proliferation of myeloid cells in the bone marrow.[1] This chapter reviews the pathology of the myeloproliferative diseases, including pertinent clinical, laboratory, histologic, cytogenetic, and molecular genetic findings necessary for the classification of these disorders. Both MPNs and myelodysplastic/myeloproliferative neoplasms (MDS/MPNs) are clonal neoplasms with typical increased marrow cellularity, maturation of cell lineages, and organomegaly. The MPNs also share effective hematopoiesis and varying amounts of marrow fibrosis, but generally differ by which myeloid cell lineage dominates hematopoiesis. The MDS/MPNs overlap features of both myeloproliferative and myelodysplastic disorders, with varying degrees of effective hematopoiesis and myelodysplasia. Pathogenic gene mutations have been discovered in many of these disease processes, often affecting tyrosine kinase signaling pathways.[2-6] Not only has this helped further our understanding of these complex disorders, but also identification of aberrant kinase signaling cascades has led to targeted small molecule tyrosine kinase inhibitors (TKIs), such as imatinib, being used successfully in the treatment of certain diseases. Thus, the diagnosis and classification of the MPNs and overlap disorders requires correlation of morphology with clinical, hematologic, and molecular genetic findings.[7] An abbreviated overview of select myeloid neoplasms, including the myeloproliferative diseases (Table 82.1), correlates each disease with its corresponding identified aberrant tyrosine kinase or related gene involved in the pathogenesis of the disorder and corresponding molecular genetic findings. In categorizing these disorders, separation of the MPNs from the overlap MDS/MPNs is recognized by the presence of dysplasia in the latter syndromes. Of the MPNs, there are the four common disorders: chronic myeloid leukemia (CML), with its characteristic 9;22 translocation and BCR::ABL1 fusion protein, and three non-CML MPNs: polycythemia vera (PV), essential thrombocythemia (ET), and primary myelofibrosis (PMF). These common non-CML MPNs (PV, ET, PMF) share a high incidence of the acquired point mutation (V617F) in the JAK2 kinase,[8-11] a cytoplasmic tyrosine kinase important in hematopoietic proliferation. This mutation is associated with constitutive JAK-STAT activation in cell lines and MPN-like disorders in mouse models,[4,12] and occurs in stem cells in humans with PV predisposing toward erythroid hyperplasia.[13,14] Other JAK2 mutations in exon 12 have also been described in patients with PV.[15] ET and PMF are both associated with mutations in CALR and MPL. Identification of mutations in JAK2, CALR, and MPL can be helpful in confirming the diagnosis of MPN and can provide prognostic information.[16] More than 50% of patients with PV, ET or PMF harbor additional mutations including TET2, ASXL1, DNMT3A, and others, which may influence both phenotype and prognosis.[17] The order in which mutations are acquired also plays a significant role.[18]

The MPNs also include a number of uncommon or atypical disorders. These uncommon MPNs include chronic eosinophilic leukemia not otherwise specified (CEL) and chronic neutrophilic leukemia (CNL). CNL has been associated with mutation in CSF3R, the gene encoding granulocyte colony-stimulating factor. Several atypical MPNs and MDS-MPNs with eosinophilia are now also recognized as associated with specific molecular abnormalities, including rearrangements of PDGFRA, PDGFRB, FGFR1, or PCM1::JAK2. These disorders are now classified according to their molecular abnormality[19] rather than as subtypes of other MPNs. The presence of these genetic abnormalities is not merely academic, as these rearrangements can predict response to targeted therapies. For example, MPNs with eosinophilia and FIP1L1::PDGFRA can contain proliferations of CD25-positive mast cells that are sensitive to imatinib and other TKIs, whereas systemic mastocytosis (SM) with KIT D816V mutations (and dense proliferations of CD25-positive mast cells) is resistant to imatinib.[20,21] The latter patients may respond to second-generation TKIs initially developed for imatinib-resistant CML patients or FLT3 inhibitors developed for patients with acute myeloid leukemia (AML), as these drugs have activity against multiple tyrosine kinases.[22,23] FGFR1 rearranged cases often present with T-lymphoblastic leukemia/lymphoma or AML and are resistant to treatment with TKIs. PCM1::JAK2 rearranged neoplasia is a provisional entity added to this category in the 2016 update to the World Health Organization (WHO) and can present in a similar fashion to PMF or rarely as lymphoblastic leukemia. These cases show response to JAK2 inhibitors. The development of new tyrosine kinase pathway-targeted small molecule inhibitors is likely to accelerate further the molecular classification of MPNs.

The overlap MDS/MPNs, according to the WHO classification, include chronic myelomonocytic leukemia (CMML), juvenile myelomonocytic leukemia (JMML), and atypical CML (aCML). Myelodysplastic/myeloproliferative neoplasm with ring sideroblasts and thrombocytosis (MDS/MPN-RS-T) also fits within this overlap group, sharing features of dysplasia and MPN and showing frequent

Table 82.1. Myeloid Neoplasms With Associated Tyrosine Kinases and Genetic Abnormalities

Myeloproliferative Neoplasms		
CML	BCR::ABL1	t(9;22)(q34;q11); BCR::ABL1
Non-CML MPN		
PV	JAK2	JAK2 V617F, JAK2 exon 12
ET	JAK2, MPL, CALR	JAK2 V617F
PMF	JAK2, MPL, CALR	JAK2 V617F
CNL	CSF3R	
Uncommon non-CML MPNs and other myeloid neoplasms		
Myeloid neoplasms with eosinophilia	PDGFRA	del(4q12); FIP1L1::PDGFRA
	PDGFRB	t(5;12); ETV6::PDGFRB
	FGFR1	8p11 abnormalities
	PCM1::JAK2	t(8;9)(p22;p24.1)
SM	KIT	KIT D816V
Myelodysplastic/Myeloproliferative Syndromes		
JMML	KRAS, NRAS, NF1, PTPN11, CBL	
MDS/MPN-RS-T	JAK2, SF3B1	JAK2 V617F

Abbreviations: CML, chronic myeloid leukemia; CNL, chronic neutrophilic leukemia; ET, essential thrombocythemia; JMML, juvenile myelomonocytic leukemia; MDS/MPN-RS-T, myelodysplastic/myeloproliferative neoplasm with ring sideroblasts and thrombocytosis; PMF, primary myelofibrosis; PV, polycythemia vera; SM, systemic mastocytosis.

association with mutations in *SF3B1*. These diseases most commonly show normal karyotypes; however, there are recurrent molecular findings including mutations in *SRSF2, TET2, ASXL1, SETBP1, CBL,* and *EZH2. CSF3R* mutations are rare in these overlap disorders and can be used to support an alternate diagnosis of CNL. *ASXL1* mutation is associated with aggressive disease and poor prognosis in CMML.

MYELOPROLIFERATIVE NEOPLASMS

The traditional classification of the common MPNs is based on which cell line is most proliferative (i.e., granulocytic, erythroid, and megakaryocytic) and the amount of marrow fibrosis, combined with clinical, laboratory, and cytogenetic/molecular genetic features (*Table 82.2*). As a consequence of excess cell proliferation with effective maturation, there is resulting leukocytosis, erythrocytosis, and/or thrombocytosis. Subsequent hepatosplenomegaly follows because of sequestration of excess cells, extramedullary hematopoiesis, or infiltration by neoplastic cells. Although this initial dysregulated proliferation may manifest as an indolent disorder, these clonal stem cell disorders all have the potential for evolution. This manifests as either a stepwise increase in fibrosis to an end-stage myelofibrosis with bone marrow failure or as an increase in blasts, transforming through an accelerated phase (10%-19% blasts) to overt acute leukemia (20% or more blasts). The MPNs differ in the incidence of this evolution and transformation.

Chronic Myeloid Leukemia

Chronic myeloid leukemia, BCR::ABL1 positive (CML)[24,25] is the most common of the MPNs and can occur at any age, although it is uncommon in children. The average age at diagnosis is 50 to 60 years with a slightly increased male-to-female ratio. CML is defined by the presence of the Philadelphia chromosome or molecular genetic evidence of the *BCR::ABL1* fusion. In contrast to the t(9;22) of acute leukemias, which are usually associated with the p190 BCR::ABL1 fusion protein, CML almost always demonstrates the "major breakpoint" e13a2 translocation, which produces the p210 fusion protein. The rare p230 fusion protein is typical of the rare neutrophilic form of CML, which is discussed later. CML is primarily a proliferation of granulocytic cells, although the Philadelphia chromosome can be found in different cell types. This expansion of myeloid cells typically involves the blood, bone marrow, spleen, and liver. Extramedullary involvement may be seen during the blast phase of the disease. The typical clinical course of CML is an indolent chronic phase followed by either blast crisis or progression to an accelerated phase with subsequent blast crisis.

The peripheral blood findings are those of a leukocytosis with granulocytes at all stages of maturation (*Figure 82.1*). Segmented neutrophils may show abnormal nuclear segmentation but overt dysplasia is not present. Myelocytes and metamyelocytes are present in high numbers in the peripheral blood with concomitant basophilia in up to 20% of cells in the chronic phase and often eosinophilia. Abnormal basophils with "washed-out" granules may be identified. Platelets are usually elevated. Mild absolute monocytosis may also be present. A bone marrow biopsy should be performed in all new diagnoses of CML to confirm the phase of the disease. The bone marrow is markedly hypercellular with cellularity approaching 100% in most untreated cases (*Figure 82.2*). The myeloid-to-erythroid ratio of the bone marrow is increased, often >10:1. An atypical megakaryocytic hyperplasia is present, with clustering of small, hypolobated forms. Some degree of reticulin fibrosis is usually demonstrated in these cases, and marked increases in reticulin and collagen marrow fibrosis are associated with accelerated phase and decreased survival.[26] Pseudo-Gaucher histiocytes are common in CML, reportedly present in 37% to 70% of cases.[27] Leukemoid reactions, in patients with infectious or other reactive conditions, may demonstrate features similar to CML. These reactive proliferations, however, do not usually show the basophilia, degree of marrow cellularity, or megakaryocyte clustering characteristic of CML. However, cytogenetic or molecular genetic studies are indicated if the differential diagnosis includes CML.

CML usually presents in the *chronic phase*, which is essentially defined by the lack of features of accelerated phase or blast phase. Marrow blasts are usually <5%, but may range up to 9%. The natural course of the disease is progression from chronic phase to a more aggressive phase of the disease within 3 to 5 years. Any one of a variety of parameters defines the *accelerated phase* of CML, but the criteria are inconsistent in the literature.[28,29] WHO criteria (*Table 82.3*) require the presence of either 10% to 19% blasts in the peripheral blood or bone marrow, the presence of specific additional chromosomal abnormalities or development of any new clonal abnormality, elevations of basophils to 20% or more of blood cells, persistent thrombocytosis (>1000 × 10^9/L) or thrombocytopenia (<100 × 10^9/L), persistent or increasing white blood cell (WBC) (>10 × 10^9/L), persistent or increasing splenomegaly, or evidence of resistance to TKI therapy including mutations in *BCR::ABL1*.[30] Cytogenetic abnormalities sufficient for diagnosis of the accelerated phase include an extra Philadelphia chromosome, trisomy 8, i(17q), trisomy 19, complex karyotype, or abnormalities involving 3q26.2.[25,31,32] Any new clonal abnormality that develops while the patient is on therapy can also be used. In addition, megakaryocytic proliferation in sheets and clusters

Table 82.2. Select Molecular Genetic, Morphologic, Laboratory, and Clinical Findings in the Common Myeloproliferative Neoplasms

Disease	Molecular Findings	Blood Smear	Bone Marrow	Fibrosis	Splenomegaly	Other
CML	*BCR::ABL1*	Leukocytosis with immature granulocytes, basophilia	Marked myeloid hyperplasia with prominence of neutrophils and myelocytes	Variable	++	
PV	*JAK2* V617F *JAK2* exon 12	Normo- or hypochromic anemia, may have thrombocytosis and mild basophilia	Panmyelosis ± erythroid hyperplasia, atypical megakaryocytic hyperplasia	Increased in spent phase	++	Low EPO
PMF	*JAK2* V617F *MPL* *CALR*	Leukoerythroblastic with dacrocytes, giant and bizarre platelets	Panmyelosis with atypical megakaryocytic hyperplasia, dysplastic and bizarre megakaryocytes	Marked in fibrotic phase	+++	
ET	*JAK2* V617F *MPL* *CALR*	Thrombocytosis, often with abnormal platelets and megakaryocytic nuclei	Atypical megakaryocytic hyperplasia with large/giant forms	Minimal	–/+	

Abbreviations: –/+, borderline; ++, moderate; +++, severe; CML, chronic myeloid leukemia; EPO, erythropoietin; ET, essential thrombocythemia; PMF, primary myelofibrosis; PV, polycythemia vera.
Adapted from George TI, Arber DA. Pathology of the myeloproliferative diseases. *Hematol Oncol Clin North Am.* 2003;17(5):1101-1127, Copyright © 2003 Elsevier. With permission.

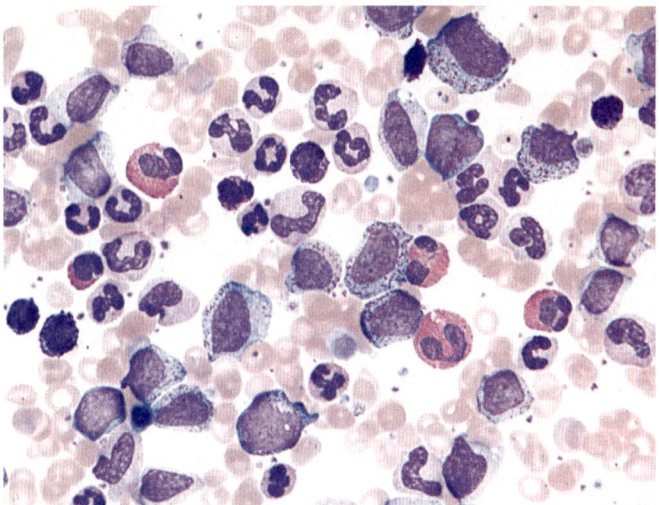

FIGURE 82.1 Chronic myeloid leukemia. The peripheral blood demonstrates neutrophilia with prominent left-shift, eosinophilia, and basophilia. Typically numerous myelocytes and segmented neutrophils predominate. Wright-Giemsa, ×500.

Table 82.3. WHO Criteria for Accelerated Phase of Chronic Myeloid Leukemia

Blasts 10%-19% in blood or marrow
Peripheral blood basophilia ≥ 20%
Additional clonal cytogenetic abnormalities in Ph+ cells at diagnosis including a second Ph, trisomy 8, iso17q, trisomy 19, complex karyotype, or abnormalities of 3q26.2
Any new clonal abnormality in Ph+ cells occurring on therapy
Persistent thrombocytopenia (<100 × 10^9/L) unrelated to treatment
Persistent thrombocytosis (>1000 × 10^9/L) unresponsive to therapy
Increasing splenomegaly and/or increasing WBC count unresponsive to therapy

Provisional response-to-TKI criteria
  Hematological resistance to the first TKI
  Any hematological, cytogenetic, or molecular indications of resistance to two sequential TKIs
  Occurrence of two or more mutations in *BCR::ABL1* during TKI therapy

The diagnosis requires one or more of the listed criteria.
Abbreviations: TKI, tyrosine kinase inhibitor; WBC, white blood cell; WHO, World Health Organization.

associated with marked fibrosis and/or marked granulocytic dysplasia has also been described as suggestive of an accelerated phase.[33]

Blast phase, or blast crisis, of CML is defined by the presence of 20% or more blasts in the peripheral blood or bone marrow (*Figure 82.3*).[30] Large clusters of blasts on the bone marrow biopsy or development of extramedullary myeloid tumors (myeloid or granulocytic sarcomas, chloromas) is also sufficient for blast phase using the WHO criteria.[33] In addition, any finding of lymphoblasts in a patient with CML may indicate progression to the blast phase.

Detection of t(9;22)(q34;q11) by karyotype analysis, fluorescence in situ hybridization (FISH), or molecular methods such as reverse transcriptase-polymerase chain reaction (RT-PCR) are essential for the diagnosis of CML. Detection of this abnormality confirms the clonal or neoplastic nature of the proliferation and excludes reactive conditions and other MPNs that may mimic CML. Baseline quantitation of *BCR::ABL1* transcripts by RT-PCR is essential for therapeutic monitoring, even if FISH or cytogenetic studies are positive. Molecular response is defined as the absence of detectable transcripts by standard RT-PCR techniques. The International Scale allows standardization of molecular monitoring across laboratories.

Immunophenotyping studies add little in the chronic phase of CML, but are helpful in defining the blast cell population of accelerated and blast phases of this disease.[34,35] In particular, the presence of any lymphoblast population is concerning for lymphoblastic transformation. The majority of blast crisis cases will express myeloid-associated antigens without lymphoid markers and are easily classified as *myeloid blast phase* by immunophenotyping studies; however, some myeloid blast phase cases may be myeloperoxidase negative by cytochemistry. Although most blast transformations of CML are proliferations of myeloblasts, approximately one-third of cases are *lymphoid blast crises* (*Figure 82.4*). The vast majority of lymphoid blast phase cases are of precursor B-cell lineage, but rare T-cell blast phase cases occur. Lymphoid blast crisis is reported to have a better prognosis than myeloid blast crisis, and lymphoid blast crisis has traditionally been defined as a blast cell proliferation that is terminal deoxynucleotidyl transferase positive. More detailed immunophenotyping of these cases usually demonstrates expression of other precursor B-cell markers, such as CD19 and CD10, but expression of myeloid-associated

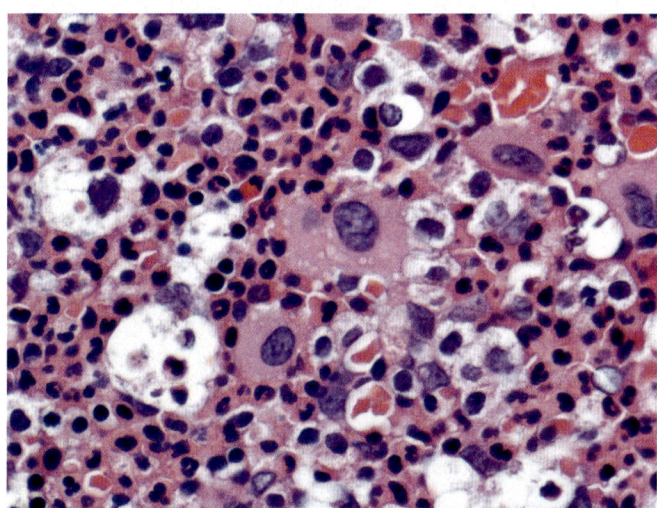

FIGURE 82.2 Chronic myeloid leukemia (CML). The bone marrow biopsy is hypercellular with myeloid and megakaryocytic hyperplasia. Note the clusters of small hypolobated megakaryocytes typical of CML. Hematoxylin and eosin, ×500.

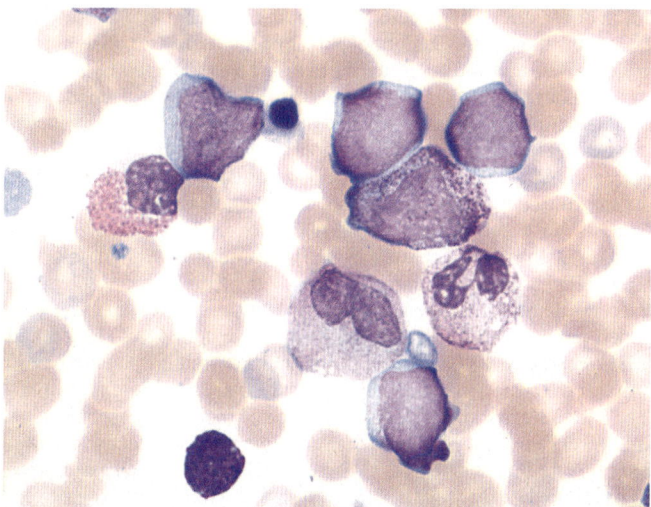

FIGURE 82.3 Myeloid blast phase of chronic myeloid leukemia (CML). Peripheral blood smear showing numerous agranular blasts on a background of neutrophils, immature granulocytes, eosinophils, and basophils. When blasts are the dominant cell present, the background changes of CML may be subtle or obscured. Wright-Giemsa, ×1000.

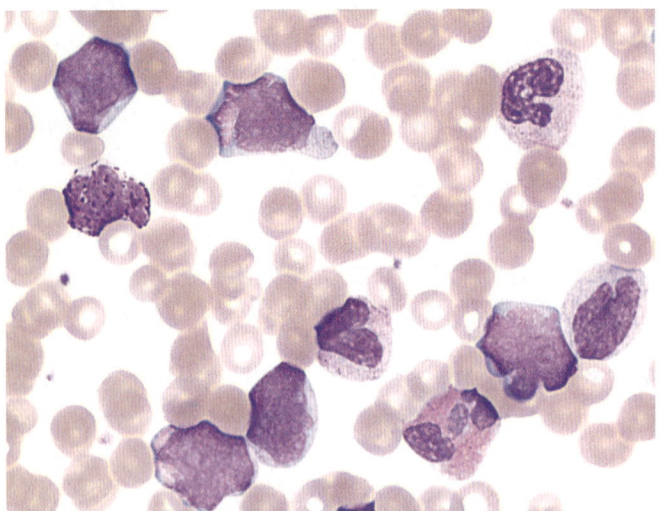

FIGURE 82.4 Lymphoid blast phase of chronic myeloid leukemia (CML). Peripheral blood smear shows intermediate-sized blasts with high nuclear-to-cytoplasmic ratios, a very small amount of basophilic cytoplasm, irregular and clefted nuclear contours, and immature chromatin. The background shows features of CML. Flow cytometry demonstrated a B-lymphoblastic immunophenotype. Wright-Giemsa, ×1000.

antigens, such as CD13 and CD33, is also common. Cases with a lymphoid immunophenotype lacking myeloperoxidase, irrespective of the expression of other myeloid antigens, have an improved survival[35] and are probably best classified as lymphoid blast crises. A small proportion of CML blast crises are mixed phenotype, which must be distinguished from de novo mixed phenotype acute leukemia, a subset of which also has the BCR::ABL1 gene rearrangement.

Typically, patients with all phases of CML are treated with a TKI, imatinib, which directly blocks the effects of the BCR::ABL1 fusion protein.[36] Imatinib results in a clinical, morphologic, and at least partial cytogenetic remission in most patients, with reduction in marrow cellularity, normalization of the myeloid-to-erythroid ratio, and normalization of megakaryocyte number and morphology.[37-41] The peripheral blood is the first to respond to imatinib therapy with a normalization of the WBC and platelet counts, a decrease in basophils, and normal-appearing platelets occurring after about 2 months of therapy. During therapy, the hemoglobin level tends to decrease slightly, and a subset of patients may develop neutropenia or thrombocytopenia. Bone marrow hypercellularity gradually decreases and by 8 to 11 months the marrow is normocellular or hypocellular with a normal or decreased myeloid-to-erythroid ratio in most patients. Even in the chronic phase, bone marrow blasts and megakaryocytes decrease, and the number of hypolobated megakaryocytes and the presence of megakaryocyte clustering become less common as the marrow cellularity decreases. This therapy has also been reported to gradually eliminate the marrow fibrosis that is prominent in some cases of CML.[37,38,42] Patients with accelerated or blast phases of CML show similar changes with rapid decreases in peripheral blood and bone marrow blast cell counts.[37] Two-thirds of patients treated in the chronic phase tolerate imatinib therapy well and experience an excellent and sustained remission.[40,41] More recently, the development of second and third generation TKIs (dasatinib, nilotinib, bosutinib, ponatinib) has proven effective in many patients who fail or are not tolerant of imatinib. These drugs show better cytogenetic and molecular response rates and lower rates of progression than imatinib and are effective alternatives for frontline therapy.[43-45] Whereas TKIs are now well established as frontline therapy, stem cell transplantation (SCT) remains an effective curative option, although the risks are not insignificant. SCT is therefore now employed as salvage therapy depending on patient age and comorbidities and presence of an acceptable donor.[46]

Neutrophilic-chronic myeloid leukemia appears to be a less aggressive variant of CML in which t(9;22) codes for a 230-kDa BCR::ABL1 fusion protein.[47] This disease is associated with a proliferation of more mature granulocytes, usually at the segmented neutrophil stage of development. These patients have less severe clinical symptoms and are slower to progress to a blastic stage. This CML variant has been shown in one study to have low levels of p230 BCR::ABL1 messenger RNA and undetectable protein product, which may explain the milder phenotype in these patients.[48]

Philadelphia chromosome-negative CML is not recognized in the 2016 WHO classification and such a diagnosis should be made with caution. Cryptic BCR::ABL1 translocations may occur that cannot be identified by routine karyotype analysis. When this is suspected, molecular genetic studies, such as FISH or RT-PCR analysis, are indicated. When these studies are negative, other diagnostic considerations must be entertained. A review of cytogenetic and molecular genetic Philadelphia chromosome-negative CML cases has resulted in most being reclassified as CMML or aCML.[49]

Polycythemia Vera

Polycythemia vera is a clonal proliferation, usually occurring in elderly patients with a male predominance, that presents as an expansion of the RBC mass.[50-52] This expansion is secondary to increased red cell production from dysregulated erythropoiesis. An acquired *JAK2* V617F mutation in exon 14 is detected in 95% to 97% of patients with PV,[53,54] with exon 12 mutations accounting for most *JAK2* V617F-negative cases.[14,55] The WHO 2016 criteria for PV include *JAK2* mutations as a major criterion for diagnosis (Table 82.4).[15,17] These mutations produce a PV-like disease in mice[14,55] and involve a stem cell in humans predisposing toward erythroid differentiation.[8] Typically, the spleen is enlarged and erythropoietin levels are decreased in this disease, and decreased erythropoietin may be used as a diagnostic criterion in the absence of *JAK2* mutation.[56] The presence of a *JAK2* mutation allows for the exclusion of a reactive erythrocytosis, but is not diagnostic of PV, as *JAK2* mutations occur in approximately one-half of patients with ET and PMF, as well as involving atypical MPNs and overlap MDS/MPNs at lower levels.[53,57,58]

Two morphologic phases of PV are well described.[59] The *polycythemic phase* typically shows elevations of red blood cells (RBCs), WBCs, and platelets. The hemoglobin should be greater than 16.5 g/dL in men and 16.0 g/dL in women or the hematocrit should be greater than 49% in men and 48% in women. Other evidence of red cell mass greater than 25% of the mean normal predicted value may also be accepted in regions with significantly different red cell parameters, such as at high altitude. Slight elevations in the peripheral blood basophil count may be present, but are not as elevated as is usually seen in CML. A neutrophilia with left-shifted granulocytes is commonly seen. Platelet counts can exceed 600×10^9/L, which may cause confusion with ET. It is not uncommon for patients to have associated iron deficiency with microcytic RBCs; absent stainable iron on marrow examination is typical.[59] Bone marrow morphologic features are also included in the diagnostic criteria and bone marrow biopsy

Table 82.4. WHO Criteria for the Diagnosis of Polycythemia Vera

Major criteria
• Hemoglobin >16.5 g/dL or hematocrit >49% in men, >16.0 g/dL or 48% in women or evidence of increased red cell mass[a]
• Hypercellular bone marrow with panmyelosis with pleomorphic mature megakaryocytes
• *JAK2* V617F or exon 12 mutation

Minor criterion
• Low serum erythropoietin level

Diagnosis requires the presence of all three major criteria or the first two major and the minor criterion.
Abbreviation: WHO, World Health Organization.
[a]Hemoglobin or hematocrit >25% of mean normal predicted value for age, sex, and altitude of residence.

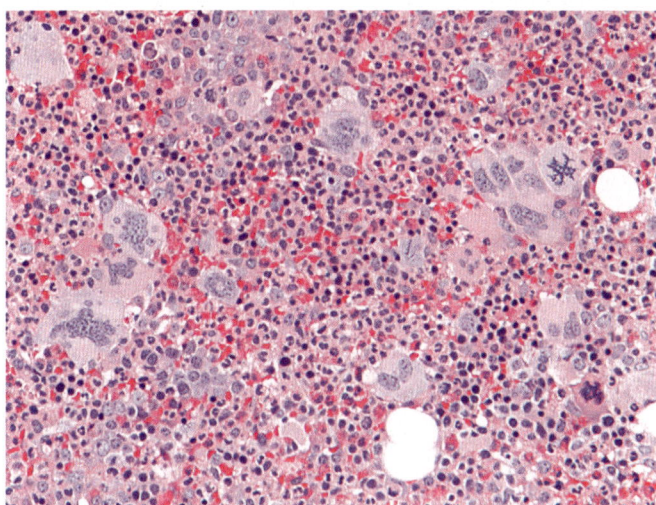

FIGURE 82.5 Polycythemia vera. The bone marrow biopsy from a patient with polycythemia vera is hypercellular, with panmyelosis, an increased number of erythroid precursors, and pleomorphic megakaryocytes in loose clusters. Hematoxylin and eosin, ×200.

should be performed in all patients at diagnosis to evaluate fibrosis. The bone marrow is usually moderately hypercellular with trilineage proliferation (*Figure 82.5*). In contrast to the other MPNs, however, the erythroid series may be relatively increased. Loose clusters of pleomorphic megakaryocytes are prominent, with very small and giant megakaryocytes adjacent to each other. Marrow fibrosis may be minimal in this stage of the disease.[60,61] Reactive lymphoid aggregates are also common.[62]

The *spent phase* or *post-polycythemic myelofibrosis phase* of PV can be diagnosed after a previously documented PV and is associated with marked (grade 2-3) marrow fibrosis and shows peripheral blood and bone marrow changes that are similar or identical to those seen in PMF; with leukoerythroblastic peripheral blood changes, anemia, splenomegaly, and marrow fibrosis (*Figure 82.6*). Patients may also

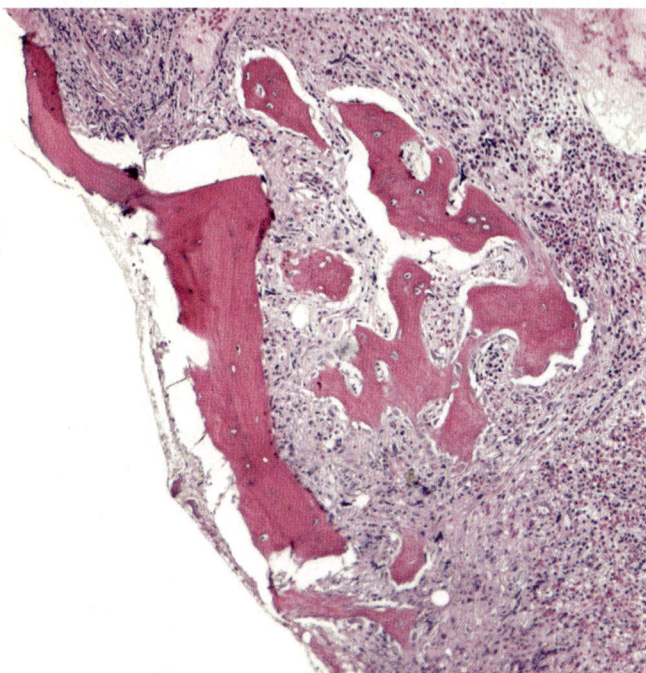

FIGURE 82.6 Post-polycythemic phase of polycythemia vera. Bone marrow biopsy showing increased fibrosis and osteosclerosis. Hematoxylin and eosin, ×400.

develop constitutional symptoms. Differentiation between these two diseases may not be possible without a history of the earlier phase of PV (*Figure 82.7*). Approximately 10% of PV patients will transform to AML within 15 years and up to half will develop acute leukemia over 20 years (*Figure 82.8*).[63] Rare cases of myelodysplastic transformation are also reported in the literature, which appear to be treatment related.[64]

An absolute erythrocytosis is the feature that separates PV from other MPNs,[65] and red cell mass may be decreased in PV patients with concurrent iron deficiency; thus, studies may have to be repeated after iron therapy. Reactive or secondary polycythemias must also be excluded and these may be related to smoking, lung and renal disease, erythropoietin-producing tumors, congenital conditions causing erythropoietin overproduction, and exogenous administration of erythropoietin or testosterone. Although these secondary polycythemias can be distinguished by their lack of *JAK2* mutations, not all idiopathic erythrocytoses that meet neither criterion for PV or secondary polycythemia are well understood.[66] Some of these idiopathic erythrocytoses represent PV with recently described exon 12 or 14 *JAK2* mutations, whereas others are still being investigated.[14,55] Studies have emphasized the value of bone marrow histology in distinguishing between early-stage PV and reactive polycythemias. The atypical megakaryocytic hyperplasia of PV is not seen in secondary polycythemias. These reactive conditions tend to show only a borderline increase in cellularity, with an altered interstitial compartment containing increased deposition of cellular debris within histiocytic cells, hemosiderin-laden macrophages, and perivascular plasmacytosis.[60,61]

Karyotypic abnormalities may be detected in up to half of cases of PV, with chromosome 20q deletions being the most common.[67,68] These abnormalities, however, are not specific to PV.[69] Various other point mutations occur in association with polycythemias, particularly in the congenital or familial forms.[70] Progenitor cells from patients with PV are hypersensitive to several growth factors, and in vitro detection of endogenous erythroid colonies occurs in PV. Although the predictive value of clonogenic stem cell assays in certain defined settings may be high (97%),[71] their availability is limited and these assays are difficult to standardize. Thus, these assays are now infrequently used in the routine diagnosis of PV.[72]

Primary Myelofibrosis

Primary myelofibrosis, also known as chronic idiopathic myelofibrosis, occurs in elderly patients and usually presents with leukocytosis, massive splenomegaly, and marrow fibrosis.[73-75] The peripheral blood changes include the presence of large teardrop-shaped RBCs (dacrocytes), leukocytosis with a granulocyte left-shift that often includes rare myeloblasts, and thrombocytosis with giant platelets that are larger than a RBC (*Figure 82.9*). Basophilia may be present and bare megakaryocyte nuclei are often seen in the blood and bone marrow. A leukoerythroblastic peripheral blood smear may be seen in the fibrotic, or overt, stage of PMF. Although spleen enlargement occurs with many MPNs, the splenomegaly of PMF is striking and may cause severe discomfort and wasting syndromes. The bone marrow may be hypercellular, particularly early in the disease when marrow fibrosis is less prominent, in the *early/prefibrotic phase* of PMF. Reticulin and collagen fibrosis is minimal to absent in early/prefibrotic PMF. The myeloid-to-erythroid ratio is slightly increased with both increased granulocytes and decreased erythropoiesis, and megakaryocytes are increased. Atypical megakaryocyte clustering is prominent, with clusters of medium-sized to giant megakaryocytes often adjacent to sinuses and bony trabeculae. The megakaryocytes are atypical with hyperchromatic megakaryocytic nuclei and coarse lobulations.[76-78] The differential diagnosis between the prefibrotic stage of PMF and ET can be quite difficult, but abnormal megakaryopoiesis is most helpful in establishing the diagnosis of PMF, although other features including bone marrow cellularity (increased markedly in the cellular phase of PMF) and left-shifted myeloid hyperplasia (usual in PMF) are also useful.[79-84] Most patients are diagnosed with overt PMF in the *fibrotic stage*, and show marked marrow fibrosis of at least MF = 2 (*Figure 82.10*), which may include collagen fibrosis. Interestingly,

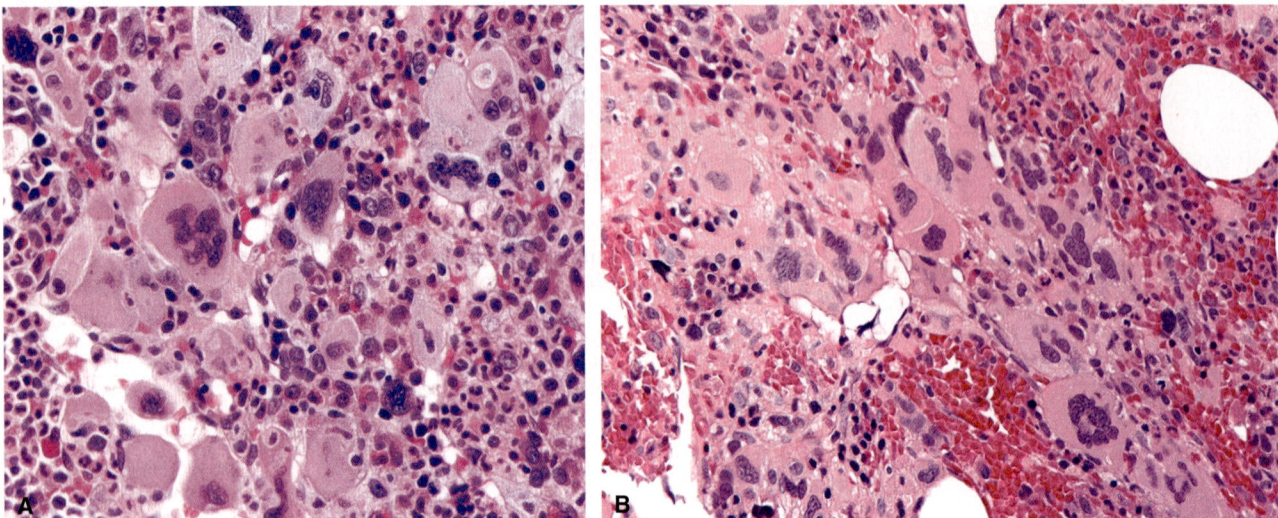

FIGURE 82.7 **The post-polycythemic phase of polycythemia vera shows bone marrow changes (A) indistinguishable from those of the fibrotic stage of primary myelofibrosis (B).** Both bone marrow biopsies are hypercellular with atypical megakaryocyte clustering, including hyperchromatic enlarged megakaryocytes amid a fibrotic background. Hematoxylin and eosin, ×400.

this accompanying fibrosis is reactive, whereas clonal studies have shown that the trilineage hematopoietic proliferation is monoclonal.[85] Clusters of atypical megakaryocytes remain prominent in association with the fibrosis, and megakaryocyte clusters in sinusoids may be evident. The sinuses are often dilated with intrasinusoidal hematopoiesis. Sclerosis of bone trabeculae also occurs in many patients with broad irregular trabeculae, which can occupy much of the marrow biopsy (*Figure 82.10D*). Lymphoid aggregates, of predominantly T cells, occur commonly in association with PMF.

Ancillary studies are required to exclude the Philadelphia chromosome of CML, and approximately 60% of PMF patients will have an acquired *JAK2* V617F mutation.[53] *CALR* mutations have been identified in 25% of PMF patients and are associated with an improved survival compared to *JAK2*-mutated cases. *MPL* mutations have also been seen in 6% to 7%; some of these patients lacked the *JAK2* mutation whereas others occurred concurrently.[86,87] The remainder of cases are designated "triple negative." These patients have inferior leukemia-free survival compared to *JAK2*- and *CALR*-mutated cases. In addition, mutations in other myeloid neoplasm associated genes may be present. Mutations in *ASXL1*, *SRSF2*, and *IDH1* and *IDH2* are associated with inferior prognosis compared to cases without mutation. Studies report that 35% to 61% of patients will demonstrate a cytogenetic abnormality, with deletions of chromosomal arms 20q and 13q most common, as well as der(6)t(1;6)(q21-23;p21.3).[74,88-91] Other ancillary studies are of limited utility with the exception of immunophenotyping of blasts in cases that undergo blastic transformation.

The Italian criteria for myelofibrosis focused on the fibrotic phase of the disease, requiring diffuse fibrosis of the marrow, among other features.[92] The 2016 update to the WHO diagnostic criteria for early/prefibrotic PMF requires three major and one of four minor criteria.[16] The first major criterion addresses bone marrow histology and requires proliferation of atypical megakaryocytes with hypercellularity for age, and granulocytic proliferation and frequent decreased erythropoiesis. Myelofibrosis must be grade 1 or less and minor reactive fibrosis should be excluded. The two additional required major criteria are the demonstration of *JAK2*, *CALR*, or *MPL* mutation or other clonal marker, and the exclusion of other MPNs, MDS, and *BCR::ABL1*-positive CML (*Table 82.5*). One of four minor criteria must also be met, including (a) anemia not caused by another condition,

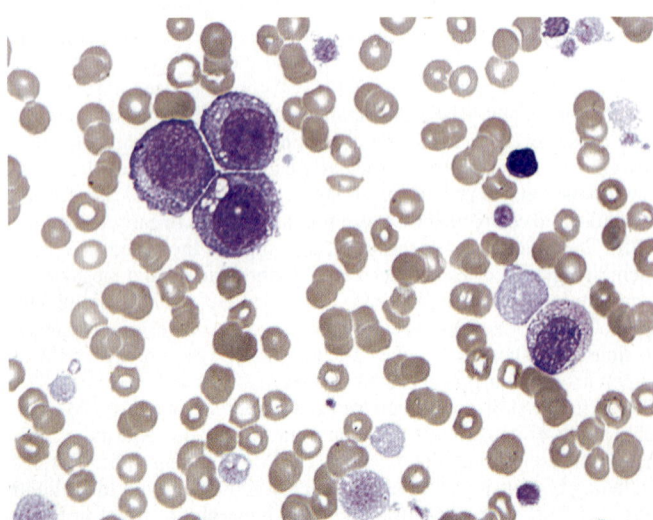

FIGURE 82.8 **Transformation of polycythemia vera.** Peripheral blood smear shows numerous giant platelets, including hypogranular forms, a myelocyte, a lymphocyte, and a cluster of three blasts. Wright-Giemsa, ×600.

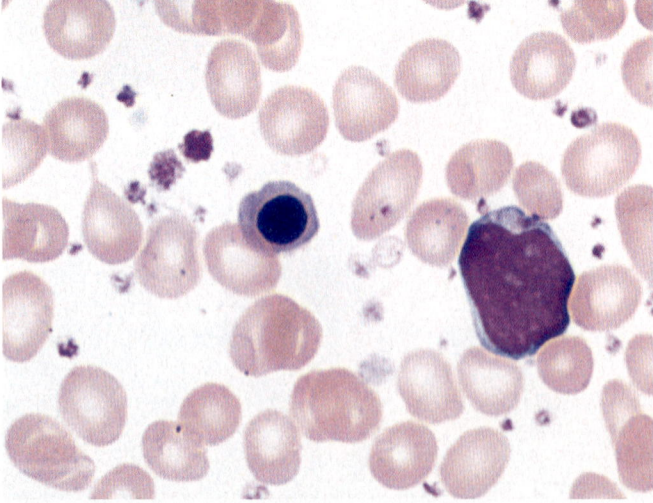

FIGURE 82.9 **Primary myelofibrosis.** The peripheral blood changes of myelofibrosis show the characteristic findings of leukoerythroblastosis with rare blasts, nucleated red blood cells, large platelets, and teardrop-shaped red cells (dacrocytes). Wright-Giemsa, ×1000.

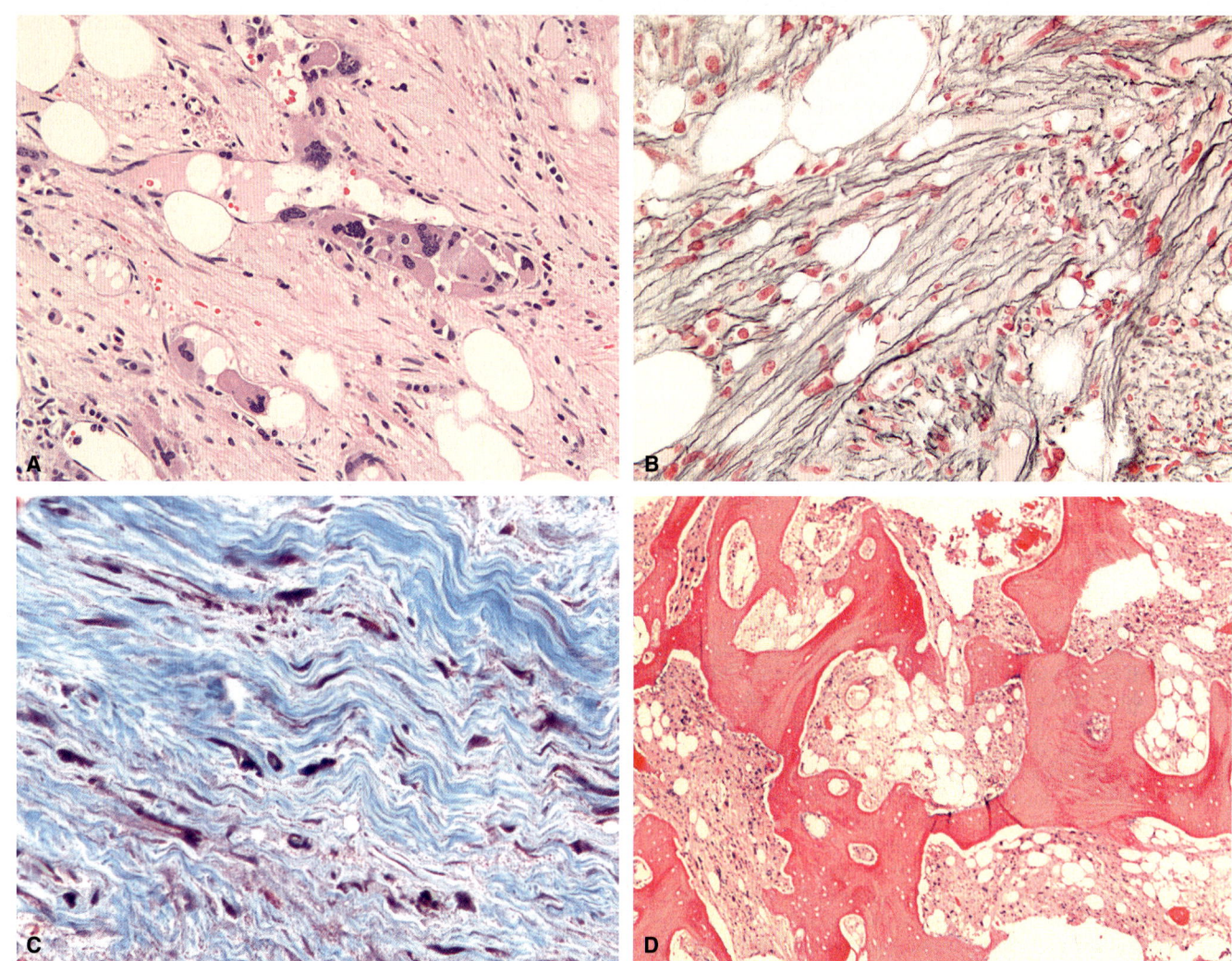

FIGURE 82.10 Bone marrow changes of fibrotic phase primary myelofibrosis. Fibrosis and intrasinusoidal clusters of atypical megakaryocytes are evident in (A). Hematoxylin and eosin, ×200. Diffusely increased coarse reticulin fibrosis is shown in (B). Reticulin stain, ×500. Coarse collagen fibrils are demonstrated in (C). Masson trichrome, ×500. Late-stage osteosclerotic changes are noted in (D). Hematoxylin and eosin, ×50.

Table 82.5. WHO Criteria for Prefibrotic Primary Myelofibrosis

Major criteria
- Atypical megakaryocytic hyperplasia, without fibrosis >grade 1, megakaryocytic atypia and marrow hypercellularity with granulocytic hyperplasia and erythroid hypoplasia
- Exclusion of WHO criteria for PV, CML, MDS, or other myeloid neoplasms
- *JAK2*, *CALR*, or *MPL* mutation or presence of another clonal marker or absence of reactive fibrosis

Minor criteria
- Anemia
- Leukocytosis
- Splenomegaly
- Increased LDH

Diagnosis requires all three major criteria and one minor criterion.
Abbreviations: CML, chronic myeloid leukemia; LDH, lactate dehydrogenase; MDS, myelodysplastic syndrome; MPN, myeloproliferative neoplasm; PV, polycythemia vera; WHO, World Health Organization.

(b) leukocytosis ≥11 × 10^9/L, (c) palpable splenomegaly, or (d) increased LDH. As described earlier, the megakaryocytic atypia is quite marked with loose to tight clusters of megakaryocytes, including a wide variation in size with hyperchromatic, irregularly folded or bulbous nuclei, as well as abnormal nuclear-to-cytoplasmic ratios.[78,93] A diagnosis of fibrotic, or overt, PMF has the additional major criterion of reticulin and/or collagen fibrosis grade 2 or 3 and the minor criterion of leukoerythroblastosis.[16]

Median survival for patients with PMF varies from 17.5 to 1.8 years for low- to high-risk subgroups,[94] using the Dynamic International Prognostic Scoring System plus with the following eight risk factors: age > 65 years, constitutional symptoms, RBC transfusion need, hemoglobin < 10 g/dL, leukocyte count > 25 × 10^9/L, circulating blasts ≥ 1%, platelet count > 100 × 10^9/L, and an unfavorable karyotype.[95] The most frequent causes of death are complications of marrow failure (22%), including anemia, infection, and hemorrhage; transformation to AML (15%); and complications related to massive splenomegaly (11%).[88] At present, there are few therapeutic options for PMF.[96] Ruxolitinib can be helpful in controlling symptoms. Allogeneic SCT provides a chance for cure, but the morbidity and mortality in PMF can be significant.[97]

Essential Thrombocythemia

Essential thrombocythemia is a bone marrow proliferation characterized primarily by an elevation in peripheral blood platelets, often over 1000×10^9/L. The 2016 update to the WHO classification requires cases to meet either four major criteria or three major and one minor criterion for diagnosis. The four major criteria are a platelet count $\geq 450 \times 10^9$/L; bone marrow biopsy showing mainly megakaryocyte proliferation with enlarged, mature megakaryocytes with hyperlobated nuclei and with no significant increase or left-shift of granulopoiesis or erythropoiesis and no or minor reticulin fibrosis; not meeting criteria for another MPN including *BCR::ABL1+* CML, MDS, or another myeloid neoplasm; and mutation of *JAK2*, *MPN*, or *CALR* (Table 82.6).[16] The minor criterion is presence of another marker of clonality or absence of reactive thrombocytosis, for example iron deficiency, splenectomy, surgery, infection, inflammation, connective tissue disease, metastatic cancer, and lymphoproliferative diseases. *JAK2* mutations are found in 60% of patients with ET, *CALR* in 20% to 25%, and *MPL* in 3%, with rare cases positive for more than one mutation.[58,98]

Even with strict adherence to diagnostic criteria, a subset of cases may not represent true neoplasia.[99] Patients with the nonclonal form of the disease may include those with congenital abnormalities of the thrombopoietin gene, and appear to be at a decreased risk of developing thrombosis.[99,100] These cases show similar peripheral blood and bone marrow features.

The thrombocytosis in ET is usually accompanied by abnormal large platelets. If leukocytosis is present, it is usually mild without the prominent left-shift or associated increase in basophils seen in CML. The marrow is normocellular to moderately hypercellular with increased numbers of megakaryocytes occurring in loose clusters or distributed throughout the marrow (*Figure 82.11*). The megakaryocytes tend to be large with abundant cytoplasm and multilobated nuclei,[101] larger than those seen in reactive conditions and CML.[80] The myeloid-to-erythroid ratio is near normal and granulopoiesis and erythropoiesis are not increased. Marrow fibrosis is absent or minimal. The absence of fibrosis can be useful to delineate cases of ET from prefibrotic PMF.

The most frequent significant complications of ET are thrombosis and hemorrhage.[102] In high-risk patients, these complications are significantly reduced with low-dose aspirin, hydroxyurea, and anagrelide therapy.[103,104] Transformation to acute leukemia or progression to overt myelofibrosis is uncommon,[105,106] provided the diagnosis is made with careful adherence to 2016 WHO criteria in order to differentiate ET from early PMF.[83] A diagnosis of post-ET myelofibrosis should only be considered if there is a clearly documented history of previous ET with later development of bone marrow fibrosis and symptoms associated with PMF. Therapy-related myeloid neoplasms may occur in ET patients treated with chemotherapy, particularly alkylating agents.[105] When compared with anagrelide, a medication with no known mutagenic potential, hydroxyurea showed no increased risk of leukemogenesis.[103] To date, there are no convincing data demonstrating that the rate of leukemic transformation in ET is attributable to hydroxyurea.

There is considerable overlap between ET and PMF.[73,80,107] In one retrospective study of 120 patients,[107] of a group of 43 "true" ET, only one developed an increase in reticulin fibrosis on subsequent serial bone marrow biopsies; this group also showed an 80% probability of lacking splenomegaly. Serial bone marrow biopsies on the other patients identified prefibrotic PMF, with 65 of 77 patients in this group evolving into overt myelofibrosis/osteosclerosis. Survival analysis confirmed better prognosis of the ET group compared to the PMF group. Thus, in the gray area of ET and the early or cellular phase of PMF, bone marrow morphology plays an important role in discriminating between these two entities, and sequential biopsies may allow for definitive classification in difficult cases. Reactive causes of megakaryocyte hyperplasia and thrombocytosis also must be excluded. Red cell mass studies may be necessary to exclude cases of PV with associated thrombocytosis that might mimic ET. Whereas the presence of *JAK2* V617F, *MPL*, or *CALR* mutation will not distinguish among the non-CML MPNs presenting with thrombocytosis, the presence of mutations will exclude reactive thrombocytosis.[108]

The value of other ancillary studies in ET is similar to CML. The detection of clonal cytogenetic abnormalities is useful in determining that the morphologic changes represent a neoplastic rather than a reactive process. Although the vast majority of cases do not demonstrate cytogenetic abnormalities, abnormalities such as del(20q), trisomy 8, and many others have been reported in ET.[109] Cases with morphologic features of ET but with *BCR::ABL1* should be considered unusual variants of CML.[110] However, both the development of a new *BCR::ABL1* clone in patients with a preexisting *JAK2*-positive MPN and the development of a *JAK2* V617F clone in patients with CML have also been reported.[111]

Cases that present with features of ET but show ring sideroblasts on iron stain should be diagnosed as MDS/MPNs with ring sideroblasts and thrombocytosis, described in the following text.[112-114]

Chronic Eosinophilic Leukemia

Chronic eosinophilic leukemia, not otherwise specified is an MPN in which the predominant finding is an eosinophilic proliferation in the blood and marrow (*Figure 82.12*). The peripheral blood shows a sustained proliferation of eosinophils $\geq 1.5 \times 10^9$/L and the bone marrow is hypercellular with proliferation of eosinophil precursors. Other myeloid neoplasms with eosinophilia (CML, AML with inv[16]/t[16;16], and neoplasms involving *PDGFRA*, *PDGFRB* or *FGFR1* or with *PCM1::JAK2*) are excluded. Causes of reactive

Table 82.6. WHO Criteria for Essential Thrombocythemia

Major criteria
- Sustained platelet count $\geq 450 \times 10^9$/L
- Bone marrow biopsy showing proliferation of enlarged mature megakaryocytes with hyperlobulated nuclei, without significant increase or left-shift of granulopoiesis or erythropoiesis, reticulin fibrosis $\leq$ grade 1
- Exclusion of WHO criteria for PV, CML, MDS, or other myeloid neoplasm
- *JAK2*, *CALR*, or *MPL* mutation

Minor criterion
- Presence of another clonal marker or absence of reactive causes of thrombocytosis

Diagnosis requires all four major criteria or the first three major criteria and the minor criterion.

Abbreviations: CML, chronic myeloid leukemia; MDS, myelodysplastic syndrome; PMF, primary myelofibrosis; PV, polycythemia vera; WHO, World Health Organization.

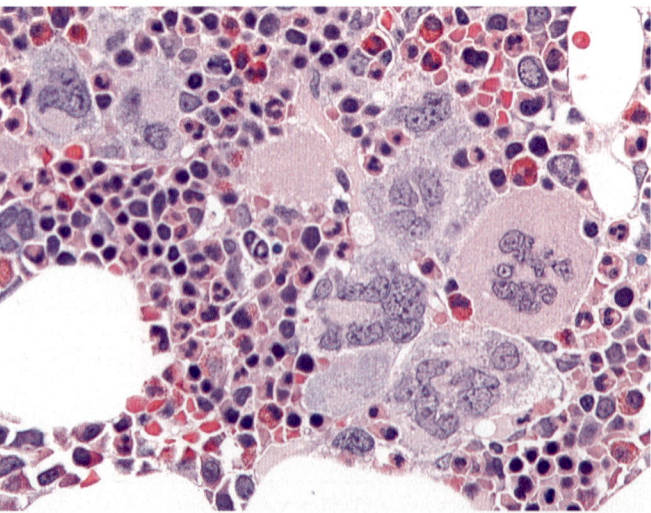

FIGURE 82.11 Essential thrombocythemia. Bone marrow biopsy is mildly hypercellular with atypical megakaryocyte clustering. The megakaryocytes are enlarged with abundant cytoplasm and distinct nuclear lobations. Hematoxylin and eosin, ×500.

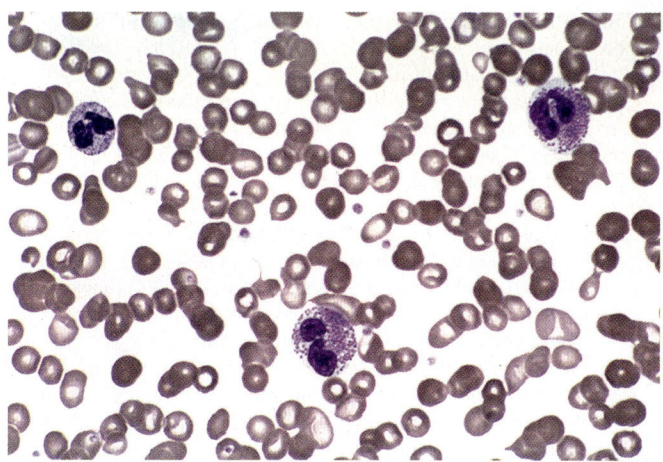

FIGURE 82.12 Chronic eosinophilic leukemia, not otherwise specified. Peripheral blood smear showing increased numbers of normal-appearing eosinophils. Wright-Giemsa, ×600.

physiologic eosinophilia, including allergic disease, collagen vascular disease, medication hypersensitivity, pulmonary eosinophilic disease, adrenal insufficiency, parasite infections, other nonmyeloid malignancies, or an aberrant or clonal T-cell population, should also be excluded. The latter refers to lymphocyte-variant hypereosinophilia, in which a clonal T-cell population produces cytokines resulting in a reactive eosinophilia.[115,116] The 2016 update to the WHO diagnostic criteria requires either a clonal cytogenetic or molecular abnormality, or an elevation in blasts ≥2% in the blood or ≥5% in the marrow (but less than 20%).[16] Some cases without clonal cytogenetic abnormalities have demonstrated molecular evidence of clonality or are clonal by analysis of X-chromosome inactivation patterns.[117]

The diagnosis of idiopathic hypereosinophilic syndrome (HES) is recommended for those cases without any evidence of either a primary myeloproliferative or secondary eosinophilia. Idiopathic HES is defined as eosinophilia ≥1.5 × 10^9/L on two separate occasions more than 1 month apart without an identifiable cause, with evidence of organ damage, or tissue evidence of >20% eosinophils, otherwise extensive eosinophil infiltration, or deposition of eosinophil granule proteins.[118] Patients with idiopathic HES may subsequently develop a myeloid malignancy or acquire a clonal abnormality. Eosinophilic tissue damage may affect any organ system, including skin, pulmonary, gastrointestinal, and cardiac,[118] presumably related to release of eosinophil granule contents. In the absence of organ damage, the term hypereosinophilia of undetermined significance is preferred.

The diagnostic algorithm for hypereosinophilia should include a bone marrow examination with cytogenetic studies for those patients whose workup is negative for secondary causes of eosinophilia.[116] Rather than CEL, a finding of *PDGFRA*, *PDGFRB*, *FGFR1*, or *PCM1::JAK2* rearrangements should indicate a diagnosis of these specific disorders.[19,119-122] As standard cytogenetics will not detect the *FIP1L1::PDGFRA* fusion gene, this must be accomplished by either FISH or RT-PCR.[123]

Chronic Neutrophilic Leukemia

Chronic neutrophilic leukemia is a rare myeloproliferative disorder that requires the demonstration of mutations in *CSF3R* and exclusion of reactive leukocytoses and other MPNs.[124-128] WHO diagnostic criteria are: peripheral blood leukocytosis ≥25 × 10^9/L with neutrophils and band forms comprising ≥80% without dysgranulopoiesis, immature granulocytes <10%, and myeloblasts only rarely observed, and monocytes <1 × 10^9/L; bone marrow myeloid hyperplasia with normal maturation, myeloblasts <5%; no Philadelphia chromosome or *BCR::ABL1*; no rearrangement of *PDGFRA*, *PDGFRB*, or *FGFR1*, and no *PCM1::JAK2*; no evidence of another MPN (PV, PMF, ET); and presence of *CSF3R* T618I or other activating mutation.[16] If *CSF3R* mutation is not present, other cytogenetic or molecular evidence of clonality is acceptable or splenomegaly and persistent neutrophilia must be present without identifiable cause of secondary neutrophilia. Common causes of reactive neutrophilia include chronic infection and inflammation, medication, and other neoplasms. In particular, plasma cell neoplasms can be associated with neutrophilia and must be excluded.

Mutations in *CSF3R*, the gene encoding the granulocyte colony-stimulating factor, are associated with aberrant activation. The most common mutation is T618I, affecting the proximal membrane region of the receptor. Other *CSF3R* mutations, including truncating mutations, have also been identified.[126] While *JAK2* mutations have been reported in CNL, mutations in *CALR* and *MPL* are very rare. Mutations in *SETBP1* are very rare in CNL and should prompt consideration of an alternate diagnosis. Cytogenetics are abnormal in less than 20% of patients and have included trisomy 9, deletion of 11q, deletion of 20q, and trisomy 21.[129] Prognosis is usually indolent. When progression occurs, it is typically characterized by slowly increasing neutrophil count, splenomegaly, and thrombocytopenia; however, reports of transformation to acute leukemia are documented.[130,131] Treatment with ruxolitinib has shown efficacy in CNL with those patients harboring the *CSF3R* T618I mutation most likely to respond.[132]

Systemic Mastocytosis

Mastocytosis includes a variety of disorders that are characterized by the presence of mast cell aggregates in tissue sections, ranging from isolated indolent proliferations to aggressive systemic disorders.[133,134] The WHO classification of mastocytosis (*Table 82.7*) separates cutaneous from systemic and localized forms of the disease.[135] Subclassification of SM subtypes requires correlation with clinical, laboratory, and molecular features (*Table 82.8*). In tissue or bone marrow biopsy sections, mast cells can range from aggregates of round cells with fine granular pink abundant cytoplasm to more spindled cells with associated fibrosis. Mast cells are often accompanied by eosinophils and small lymphocytes, even plasma cells, and may be overlooked because of these cellular components. On bone marrow aspirate smears, mast cells are most easily identified in the central portion of marrow particles as round or spindled cells with fine basophilic granules that obscure the nucleus. Nuclei may be round to oval in shape, with irregular nuclear contours yielding "dumbbell-shaped" forms. Immature mast cell features tend to correlate with the more aggressive clinical syndromes, but morphology alone is not adequate for classification.

A diagnosis of SM requires detection of multiple dense mast cell aggregates in bone marrow or other extracutaneous tissue sections (major criterion) and one minor criterion or, in the absence of tissue section aggregates, identification of three minor criteria (*Table 82.9*). Further subclassification of SM requires correlation with clinical, morphologic, and laboratory findings designated as "B" or "C" findings (*Table 82.8*).[135] The subdivisions include indolent systemic mastocytosis (ISM), smoldering mastocytosis (SSM), SM with an associated hematologic neoplasm (SM-AHN), aggressive systemic mastocytosis

Table 82.7. WHO Classification of Mastocytosis

Cutaneous mastocytosis
• Maculopapular cutaneous mastocytosis/urticaria pigmentosa
• Diffuse cutaneous mastocytosis
• Mastocytoma of skin
SM
• ISM
• Smoldering SM
• SM with an associated hematologic neoplasm
• ASM
• Mast cell leukemia
Mast cell sarcoma

Abbreviations: ASM, aggressive systemic mastocytosis; ISM, indolent systemic mastocytosis; SM, systemic mastocytosis; WHO, World Health Organization.

Table 82.8. WHO B and C Findings in Systemic Mastocytosis

B findings
- >30% of bone marrow mast cells in focal dense aggregates and serum total tryptase level >200 ng/mL
- Signs of dysplasia or myeloproliferation in nonmast cell lineage, but insufficient criteria for a definitive diagnosis of a myeloid neoplasm by WHO, with normal or only slightly abnormal blood counts
- Hepatomegaly without liver function impairment, and/or palpable splenomegaly without hypersplenism, and/or palpable or visceral lymphadenopathy

C findings
- Bone marrow dysfunction manifested by 1+ cytopenias (ANC < 1.0×10^9/L, Hgb < 10 g/dL, or PLT < 100×10^9/L)
- Palpable hepatomegaly with impairment of liver function, ascites, and/or portal hypertension
- Skeletal involvement with large-sized osteolysis and/or pathologic fractures
- Palpable splenomegaly with hypersplenism
- Malabsorption with weight loss resulting from gastrointestinal mast cell infiltrates

Abbreviations: ANC, absolute neutrophil count; Hgb, hemoglobin; PLT, platelet count; WHO, World Health Organization.

(ASM), and mast cell leukemia. ISM, the most common form of systemic mast cell disease, meets criteria for SM with one or fewer B findings without C findings and no evidence of another hematologic malignancy. Skin lesions are usually present. In the absence of skin lesions in ISM, a diagnosis of bone marrow mastocytosis can be rendered. SSM is diagnosed when two or more B findings are present. SM-AHN is defined just as the name states and occurs in approximately one-third of systemic mast cell disease patients. Typically, the associated clonal, hematologic disease is a myeloid malignancy. MDS, MPNs, MDS/MPN, AML, and CEL have all been described as associated myeloid malignancies. Associated lymphoid malignancies may occur less frequently, including plasma cell myeloma, chronic lymphocytic leukemia, acute lymphoblastic leukemia, and hairy cell leukemia. It is the associated hematologic malignancy that determines the prognosis of these patients. In rare cases, mast cell disease is not identified at initial diagnosis but becomes apparent later in the disease. ASM includes criteria for SM and includes one or more of the C findings (Table 82.8), which indicates organ dysfunction secondary to mast cell infiltration. These patients have a very short survival of weeks to months. A variant termed *lymphadenopathic mastocytosis with eosinophilia* will present with lymphadenopathy and eosinophilia, but those cases with a *PDGFRA* rearrangement are excluded. Finally, *mast cell leukemia* is a type of SM with diffuse marrow infiltration with 20% or more mast cells in the bone marrow aspirate smear.[136] This is an aggressive disease with similar prognosis as found in ASM. New multikinase inhibitors, such as midostaurin and avapritinib, inhibit the KIT tyrosine kinase pathway and have shown promising responses and improve overall survival and progression-free survival while improving quality of life.[137,138]

Special stains, including toluidine blue and chloroacetate esterase, will mark normal mast cells, but more specific immunophenotypic markers now exist. Mast cells express CD33, CD43, CD68, CD117, and tryptase, with tryptase being the most lineage-specific of these markers. Neoplastic mast cells express CD25, CD2, and/or CD30, detectable either by immunohistochemistry or by flow cytometry.[139,140] A typical immunohistochemical panel of CD25 (if negative, then CD30), CD117, and tryptase is recommended for most cases to confirm cell lineage and aberrant immunophenotype. In the bone marrow, immunohistochemistry can be performed on the core biopsy and will show paratrabecular aggregates of mast cells with associated fibrosis in SM (Figure 82.13). As bone marrow aspirates may yield hemodilute samples due to fibrosis with fewer mast cells for analysis, flow cytometry immunophenotyping may require a higher number of events for adequate immunophenotypic characterization of mast cells present.[141]

The most common genetic abnormality in mastocytosis is a point mutation of the tyrosine kinase receptor gene *KIT* resulting in a substitution of valine for aspartate at codon 816 of exon 17, Asp816Val, or D816V.[135,142-144] D816V is found in over 90% of patients with SM.[135] Other mutations include tyrosine or phenylalanine substitutions for aspartate at codon 816 and lysine for glutamic acid at codon 839.[145] *KIT* mutations, including D816V, are not specific for mastocytosis and have been reported in other diseases.[146,147]

A proliferation of mast cells with eosinophilia that is associated with the *FIP1L1::PDGFRA* fusion gene[148,149] is now classified with *myeloid and lymphoid neoplasms with eosinophilia and abnormalities of PDGFRA, PDGFRB, or FGFR1* or with *PCM1::JAK2*, discussed in the following section.

MYELOID AND LYMPHOID NEOPLASMS WITH EOSINOPHILIA AND REARRANGEMENT OF *PDGFRA*, *PDGFRB*, OR *FGFR1* OR WITH *PCM1::JAK2*

This category is composed of rare myeloid as well as lymphoid neoplasms that share eosinophilia and recently recognized acquired genetic mutations within a specific group of genes resulting in an aberrant tyrosine kinase within a pluripotent hematopoietic stem cell.[19,116] Eosinophilia may be absent in some cases. The genes involved are the platelet-derived growth factor receptor-α (*PDGFRA*) on chromosome 4q12, platelet-derived growth factor receptor-β (*PDGFRB*) at 5q32, fibroblast growth factor receptor 1 (*FGFR1*) at 8p11.2, and *PCM1::JAK2* rearrangement. The associated diseases may present with features of an MPN (CEL or SM), MDS/MPN (CMML), AML, T-lymphoblastic leukemia/lymphoma, or more rarely, B-lymphoblastic leukemia/lymphoma. The clinical significance in recognizing these rare but distinct entities is their response to TKIs and JAK inhibitors.

Myeloid and Lymphoid Neoplasms With *PDGFRA* Rearrangement

The most common *PDGFRA* rearrangement is *FIP1L1::PDGFRA*, formed by a cryptic deletion at 4q12; however, at least six other partners have been described. This fusion gene has been identified in a subset of patients with CEL and also in patients with features similar to SM with eosinophilia, but has also been described in AML and T-lymphoblastic lymphoma.

Patients are young men with eosinophilia and a subset may present with elevated serum tryptase levels.[148] A prevalence of 14% of the *FIP1L1::PDGFRA* fusion gene has been reported in patients with primary eosinophilia.[150] Morphologic findings are those of a hypercellular marrow with a myeloid hyperplasia and marked eosinophilia; fibrosis is typically present (Figure 82.14). Although in some cases

Table 82.9. Modified WHO Criteria for Systemic Mastocytosis

Major criterion
- Multifocal, dense mast cell infiltrates (≥15 cells) in bone marrow biopsy or extracutaneous tissue sections

Minor criteria
- >25% spindled, immature, or atypical mast cells in tissue sections or bone marrow aspirate smears
- Detection of *KIT* mutation at codon 816
- Expression of CD25 and/or CD30, with or without CD2
- Serum total tryptase persistently >20 ng/mL (unless associated with a myeloid neoplasm)

Diagnosis requires major and one minor or three minor criteria.
Abbreviation: WHO, World Health Organization.

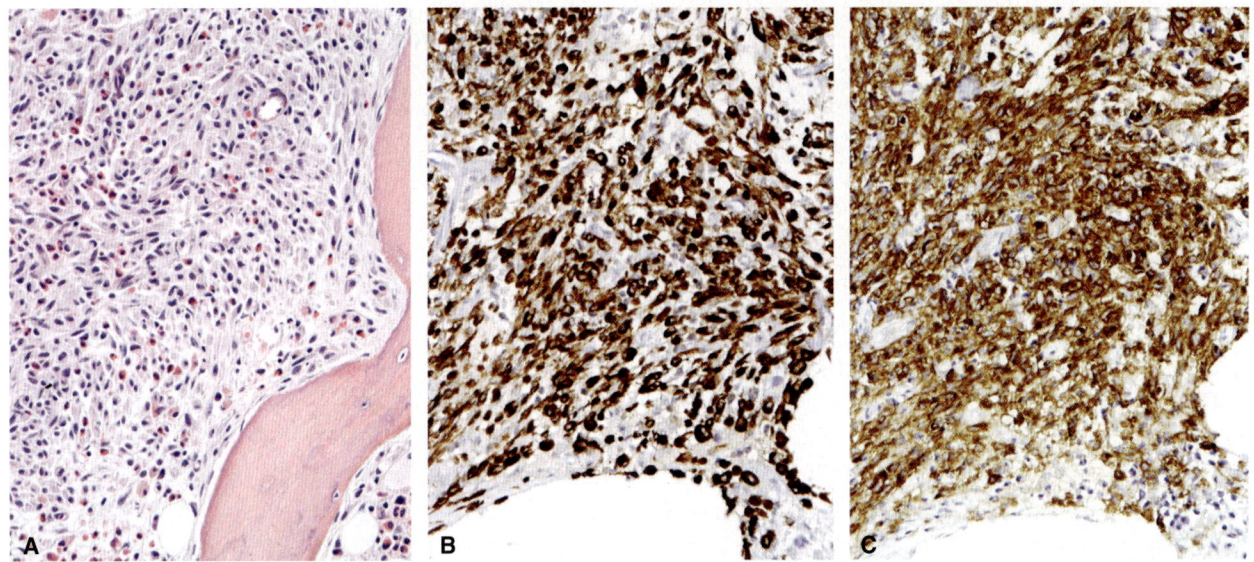

FIGURE 82.13 Aggressive systemic mastocytosis. Bone marrow biopsy shows a paratrabecular nodule of spindled mast cells admixed with scattered eosinophils (A). Mast cells are highlighted by tryptase (B) and CD25 (C). Hematoxylin and eosin, ×200.

there is no abnormal mast cell infiltrate[150]; in other cases, tryptase or CD117 immunostaining typically identifies loose, ill-defined mast cell aggregates that are difficult to appreciate on hematoxylin and eosin sections (Figure 82.14),[148] which does not technically meet WHO criteria for mastocytosis. Mast cells show a similar aberrant immunophenotype with CD25 coexpression and demonstrate *CHIC2* deletion, a marker for the *FIP1L1::PDGFRA* fusion gene,[149] but do not have the *KIT* D816V mutation. Recognition and awareness of this *FIP1L1::PDGFRA* myeloid neoplasm involving eosinophilia and mast cell proliferations but lacking *KIT* mutations should avoid misclassification as CEL or SM.[116,119] The importance of the *FIP1L1::PDGFRA* translocation is underscored by its responsiveness to imatinib with rapid and complete hematologic remissions.[20,151,152]

Myeloid Neoplasms With *PDGFRB* Rearrangement

The most common *PDFGRB* rearrangement is t(5;12)(q32;p13.2) with production of the fusion oncogene, *ETV6::PDGFRB*, resulting in constitutive activation of the kinase domain of *PDGFRB*.[120-122] Translocations involving at least 25 other fusion partners for *PDGFRB* have also been described.[153] The disease associated with *ETV6::PDGFRB* presents with features suggestive of CMML with eosinophilia (Figure 82.15). The variant translocations have been associated with features of CMML, CEL, and chronic basophilic leukemia, as well as a Ph-negative MPN resembling CML or aCML. Not all cases have an associated eosinophilia. Isolated cases with features of JMML or transformed AML have been reported. The chronic myeloid

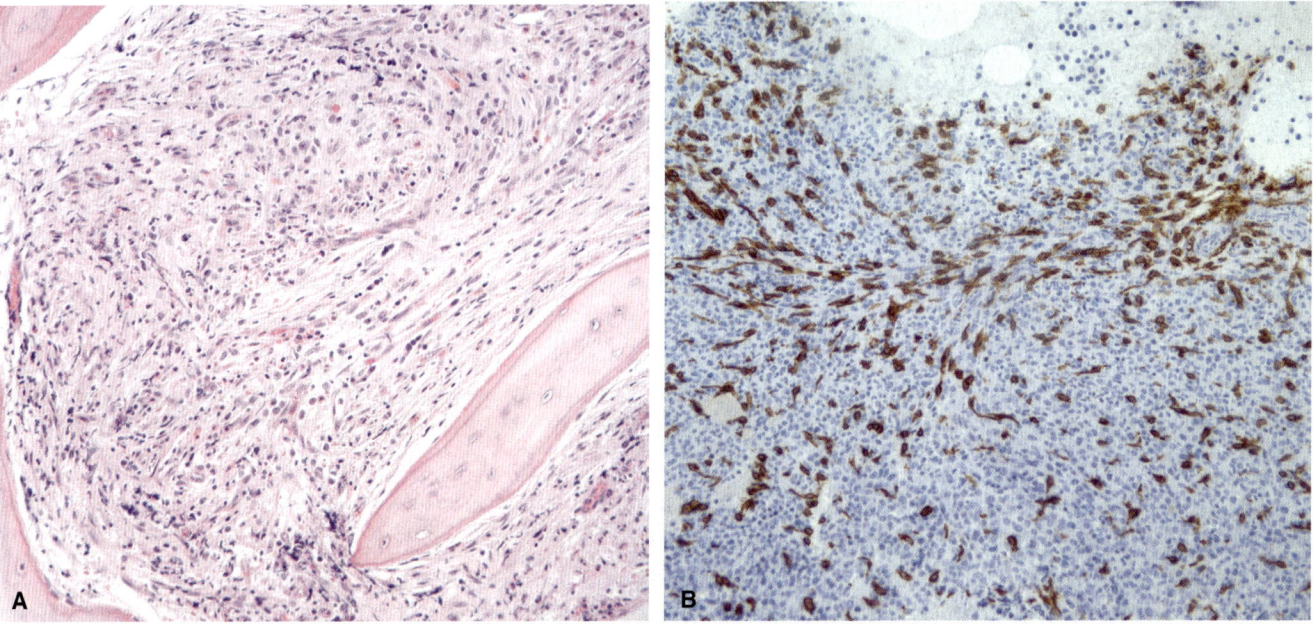

FIGURE 82.14 Chronic eosinophilic leukemia with *PDGFRA*. The bone marrow biopsy is striking for marked fibrosis that accompanies a hypercellular marrow with eosinophilia (A). Hematoxylin and eosin, ×200. A loose infiltrate of mast cells is seen using immunohistochemistry directed against CD117, which was not readily visible on hematoxylin and eosin–stained sections of the bone marrow biopsy (B). CD117, ×200.

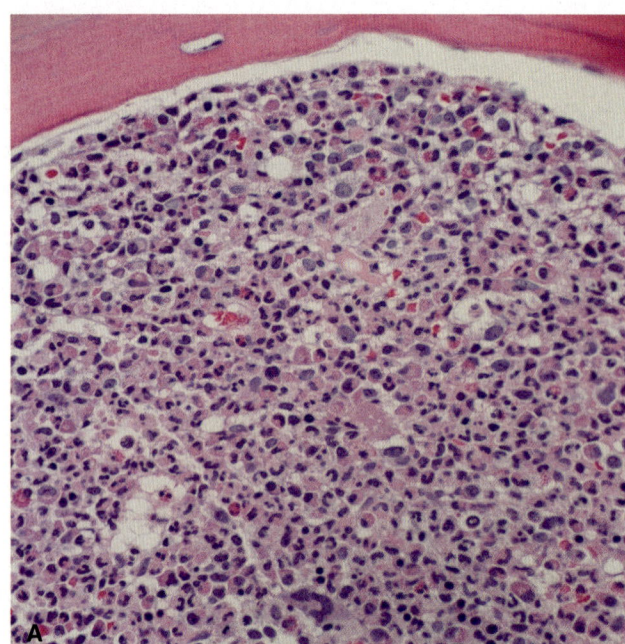
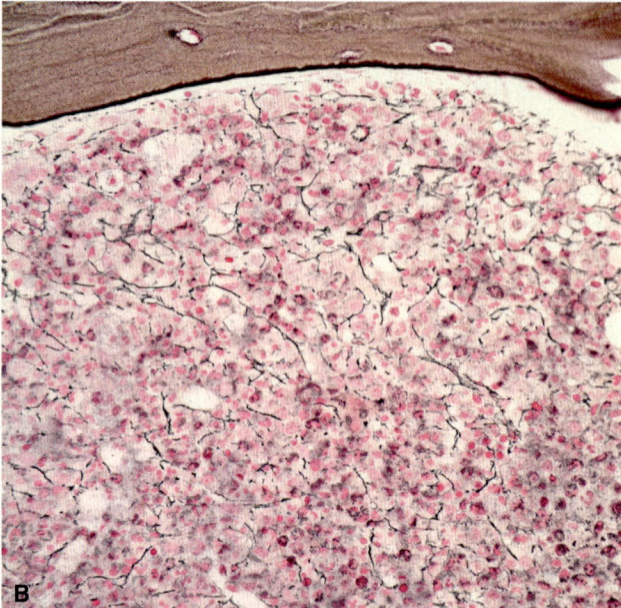

FIGURE 82.15 **Myeloid neoplasm with eosinophilia with** *PDGFRB*. The bone marrow biopsy is hypercellular with a granulocytic hyperplasia and marrow eosinophilia (A). Hematoxylin and eosin, ×400. Increased coarse reticulin fibrosis is present (B). Reticulin stain, ×400.

neoplasms with *PDGFRB* rearrangements appear to be aggressive, with a high risk of acute transformation. Similar to rearrangements of *PDGFRA*, diseases with rearrangements of *PDGFRB* are sensitive to TKI therapy.

Myeloid and Lymphoid Neoplasms With *FGFR1* Rearrangement

Hematologic neoplasms associated with rearrangements of the *FGFR1* gene of chromosome band 8p11 are heterogeneous. Although they most often present with T-lymphoblastic leukemia or AML with eosinophilia, they may manifest as T-lymphoblastic lymphoma, B-lymphoblastic or mixed lineage acute leukemia, or less commonly B-lymphoblastic lymphoma or CEL.[154-157] Those cases presenting with features of CEL have an increased risk of transformation to AML or myeloid sarcoma. Regardless of the presenting neoplasm, patients usually have eosinophilia in the blood, marrow, or both. The *FGFR1* gene most commonly fuses with the *ZMYM2* gene of 13q12 for a t(8;13)(p11;q12), but other translocations are frequent.[158,159] Unlike the neoplasms involving *PDGFRA* and *PDGFRB*, neoplasms with *FGFR1* rearrangements are associated with a poor prognosis; pemigatinib, a TKI with activity against FGFR1, has recently received orphan drug designation for treatment of patients with myeloid and lymphoid neoplasms with *FGFR1* rearrangements.[160]

Myeloid and Lymphoid Neoplasms With *PCM1::JAK2*

Hematologic neoplasms with t(8;9)(p22;p24.1); *PCM1::JAK2* rearrangements are rare diseases that present with eosinophilia and bone marrow findings, which resemble an MPN.[161,162] There is erythroid predominance with left-shift, lymphoid aggregates, and variable fibrosis.[161,162] This can infrequently present with features of MDS, MDS/MPN, or B-lymphoblastic leukemia. These diseases respond to *JAK2* inhibition.

MYELODYSPLASTIC/MYELOPROLIFERATIVE NEOPLASMS: MYELODYSPLASTIC NEOPLASMS WITH PROLIFERATIVE EVOLUTION

Some proliferations have features of both an MPN and MDS.[163] These disorders may present with cytopenias and dysplastic changes of any cell line, similar to the myelodysplastic syndromes, as well features more commonly associated with myeloproliferative disorders including leukocytosis, hypercellular marrow with fibrosis, and organomegaly. The presence of fibrosis alone in a case that is otherwise typical of myelodysplasia is not sufficient for diagnosis of these diseases. In addition, patients with a long history of MPN who subsequently develop dysplasia are not classified in this group. The MDS/MPNs are CMML, aCML (myelodysplastic syndrome with proliferative evolution and neutrophilia), JMML, MDS/MPN with ring sideroblasts and thrombocytosis (myelodysplastic syndrome with proliferative evolution, *SF3B1* mutation, and thrombocytosis), and MDS/MPN-unclassifiable (myelodysplastic neoplasm with proliferative evolution, not otherwise specified). Features that are helpful in differentiating the chronic phase of CML from aCML and CMML in adults are listed in *Table 82.10*.

Chronic Myelomonocytic Leukemia

Chronic myelomonocytic leukemia was originally defined as a myelodysplastic syndrome in the French-American-British classification, but is now best classified as a mixed MDS/MPN using the WHO classification.[16,164] Patients often have both dysplastic changes and leukocytosis with splenomegaly. The disease can be divided into *myelodysplastic* and *myeloproliferative subtypes* based on the WBC level, with $\geq 13 \times 10^9$/L considered proliferative and $<13 \times 10^9$/L considered dysplastic.[165] Constitutional symptoms including fever, weight loss, and night sweats are more frequent in the myeloproliferative group, while fatigue, infection, and bleeding are more common in the myelodysplastic subtype.[166-169]

The diagnosis of CMML requires the presence of both $\geq 1 \times 10^9$/L and $\geq 10\%$ of monocytes in the peripheral blood (*Table 82.11*). The monocytes may be abnormal in appearance.[170] Promonocytes, with more immature nuclear chromatin, delicate nuclear folding or creasing, and abundant gray or basophilic cytoplasm and fine granules, may be present in the blood, but monoblasts are usually rare to absent. Much controversy surrounds the definition of a promonocyte, and distinguishing a promonocyte from a monoblast or a mature monocyte can be difficult, even in the most experienced of laboratories. A consensus guideline has been developed, which defines morphologic criteria to help standardize the differentiation of monoblasts and promonocytes from immature and mature monocytes based on nuclear and cytoplasmic features.[171] Monoblasts have smooth nuclear

Table 82.10. The Differential Diagnosis of Chronic-Phase CML, Atypical CML, and CMML in Adults

Feature	CML	Atypical CML	CMML
BCR::ABL1	positive	negative	negative
WBC	+++	++	+
Basophils[a]	≥2%	<2%	<2%
Monocytes[a]	<3%	3%-10%	Usually >10%
Immature granulocytes[a]	>20%	10%-20%	<10%
Granulocyte dysplasia	–	++	+
Marrow erythroid hyperplasia	–	–	+

Only CML is distinguished by the presence of the Philadelphia chromosome or BCR::ABL1. CML typically has a higher WBC count than either CMML or atypical CML, with occasional WBC counts of >200 × 10^9/L. A prominent basophilia is also more characteristic of CML, although a mild basophilia may occur in either atypical CML or CMML. A marked monocytosis is more typical of CMML than either CML or atypical CML. CML also shows a marked left-shift in granulocytes on the peripheral blood smear compared to atypical CML or CMML; however, increased circulating blasts may occur in atypical CML compared with CML or CMML. Atypical CML also shows the most prominent granulocytic dysplasia. Finally, a bone marrow erythroid hyperplasia occurs more often in CMML than in de novo CML or atypical CML.

Abbreviations: +, mildly elevated; ++, moderately elevated; +++, markedly elevated; CML, chronic myeloid leukemia, chronic phase; CMML, chronic myelomonocytic leukemia; WBC, white blood cell count.

Adapted from George TI, Arber DA. Pathology of the myeloproliferative diseases. Hematol Oncol Clin North Am. 2003;17(5):1101-1127. Copyright © 2003 Elsevier. With permission.

[a]Refers to peripheral blood.

contours, fine nuclear chromatin, prominent nucleoli, and basophilic cytoplasm with only rare azurophilic granules. In promonocytes, the nuclei show folds or indentations, but retain fine chromatin and prominent nucleoli. They may have greater cytoplasmic granulation. Mature monocytes have lobulated nuclei with condensed nuclear chromatin and no nucleoli, and gray cytoplasm.

The peripheral blood in CMML (*Figure 82.16*) may demonstrate cytopenias and dysplastic changes similar to the myelodysplastic syndromes, or dysplastic changes may be minimal. Cases showing dysplastic changes tend to have a WBC count <13 × 10^9/L and are associated with *RUNX1* mutations and have a worse prognosis.[120] A subset of patients presents with eosinophilia of >1.5 × 10^9/L and rearrangements of *PDGFRA*, *PDGFRB*, or *FGFR1*, or with *PCM1::JAK2*.[122,172] This CMML with eosinophilia variant is now classified with the myeloid and lymphoid neoplasms with eosinophilia and abnormalities of *PDGFRA*, *PDGFRB*, or *FGFR1* or with *PCM1::JAK2*, although the designation of CMML should be included with the diagnosis.[173] Although an elevated peripheral blood monocyte count is necessary for the diagnosis of CMML, such a diagnosis should never be made without examination of the bone marrow. Some AMLs with monocytic differentiation may show peripheral blood changes similar to CMML because of maturation of the blast cell population in the peripheral blood. The bone marrow of CMML is

Table 82.11. WHO Criteria for Chronic Myelomonocytic Leukemia

Persistent peripheral blood monocytes >1.0 × 10^9/L and monocytes >10%
Blasts + promonocytes <20% in blood and marrow
Not meeting criteria for another MPN
No rearrangement of *PDGFRA*, *PDGFRB*, *FGFR1*, or *PCM1::JAK2*
Dysplasia in one or more myeloid lineages[a]

Abbreviations: MPN, myeloproliferative neoplasm; WHO, World Health Organization.
[a]If minimal to absent myelodysplasia, the diagnosis also requires either of the following criteria: acquired, clonal cytogenetic or molecular abnormality; or persistent monocytosis for at least 3 months and exclusion of all other causes of monocytosis.

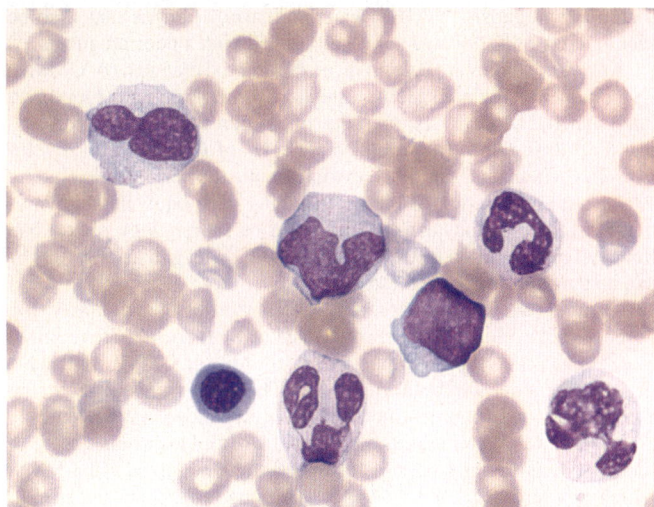

FIGURE 82.16 Chronic myelomonocytic leukemia. Peripheral blood smear with monocytes demonstrating abundant pale cytoplasm containing fine granulation, and folded nuclei with delicate chromatin and small nucleoli. Dysplastic hypogranular neutrophils, a single blast, and a nucleated red cell are also present. Wright-Giemsa, ×1000.

usually hypercellular and may demonstrate monocytic or granulocytic hyperplasia (*Figure 82.17*). When granulocytic hyperplasia is prominent, it may be difficult to distinguish the abnormal monocyte population from myelocytes. Erythroid precursors and megakaryocytes may demonstrate prominent dysplastic changes, but often these cell types are normal in appearance. Ring sideroblasts are present in increased numbers in some cases and may be associated with *SF3B1* mutation. Blasts and promonocytes may be elevated up to 19%. When bone marrow blasts and promonocytes are ≥20%, the case should be diagnosed as AML. CMML is graded by blast count in the peripheral blood and bone marrow. Cases where blasts are <2% in the blood and <5% in the marrow are designated CMML-0, a new category in the 2016 update to the WHO classification. Cases with 2% to 4% blasts in the blood and 5% to 9% in the marrow are designated CMML-1, whereas cases with 5% to 19% blasts in the blood or 10% to 19% in the marrow are diagnosed as CMML-2. The presence of Auer rods will also designate a case as CMML-2. Cases with significantly different blast counts in the blood and bone marrow should be graded in the highest applicable category. Multiple studies have shown that increased blasts correlate

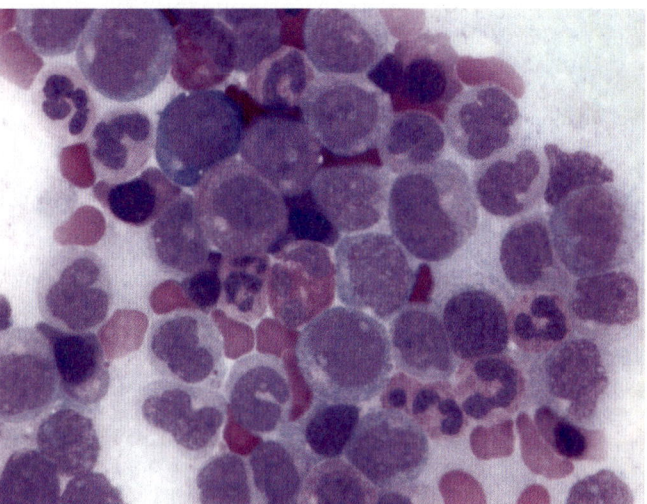

FIGURE 82.17 Chronic myelomonocytic leukemia. Bone marrow aspirate shows a monocytic and left-shifted myeloid hyperplasia. Wright-Giemsa, ×1000.

with poor prognosis.[168,174-177] Variable marrow fibrosis may also be seen in up to 50% of cases, and is associated with a poor prognosis.[178]

Ancillary studies are helpful in the differential diagnosis of CMML. Cytochemistry for nonspecific esterase on the peripheral blood and bone marrow confirms the presence of an increase in monocytes and can help differentiate abnormal monocytes of CMML from myelocytes in CML and aCML. Flow cytometry may be helpful in excluding AML, but enumeration of blasts (including blast-equivalents, monoblasts, and promonocytes) must be based on morphology rather than flow cytometry. Blasts in CMML may be CD34 negative, and CD117 can be a useful marker in these cases.

Cytogenetic and molecular genetic studies, particularly the absence of the Philadelphia chromosome or *BCR::ABL1*, are required to exclude CML. Approximately 20% to 40% of CMML will have detectable clonal abnormalities.[179-181] The most frequent recurring cytogenetic abnormalities include trisomy 8, monosomy 7/deletion (7q), structural abnormalities of 12p, and i(17q). Isochromosome 17q has been identified as a possible distinct subtype of mixed MDS/MPN, which is addressed later.[182] *JAK2* mutations have been detected in ~3% of patients.[183]

The most commonly mutated genes in CMML are *ASXL1* and *TET2*, which are also seen in clonal hematopoiesis, and *SRSF2*. Mutations of *RAS* are detected in approximately one-third of CMML cases. RAS pathway mutations as well as mutations in *ASXL1*, *RUNX1*, and *SETBP1* are associated with a poor prognosis. Mutations occur less frequently in *SETBP1*, *RUNX1*, *CBL*, *IDH1*, *IDH2*, and *EZH2*.[184]

The differential diagnosis between *BCR::ABL1*-negative aCML and CMML may be difficult, but is critical given the worse prognosis of patients with aCML when compared to CMML. CMML may be distinguished from aCML by peripheral blood features,[165] but some overlap with aCML may occur (*Table 82.10*). Monocytes are slightly elevated in aCML, but do not usually exceed 10%, whereas monocytes in CMML are usually >10%. Also, the degree of granulocyte dysplasia in CMML is not as pronounced as is usually seen in aCML. aCML demonstrates an increase in immature granulocytes, including blasts, promyelocytes, and myelocytes, of up to 20% in the peripheral blood; these cell types are almost always below 10% in the blood of patients with CMML.

Atypical Chronic Myeloid Leukemia, *BCR::ABL1* Negative (Myelodysplastic Neoplasm With Proliferative Evolution and Neutrophilia)

Atypical chronic myeloid leukemia is a misnomer with no relation to CML.[165,185] When this diagnosis is considered, CML should be excluded by standard cytogenetics karyotype and PCR or FISH for *BCR::ABL1*, as should rearrangements of *PDGFRA*, *PDGFRB*, *FGFR1*, or *PCM1::JAK2*. This rare MDS/MPN affects elderly patients with an apparent male predominance. Patients have an elevated WBC count with predominantly granulocytic cells, anemia, and normal or decreased platelets. Patients with aCML may have an initial presentation more typical of myelodysplasia with leukopenia, later developing leukocytosis.[186] The WBCs are left-shifted with immature granulocytes, including blasts, promyelocytes, and myelocytes, representing >10% of cells (*Figure 82.18*). Monocytes are usually not increased and must be <10% of peripheral blood cells. In contrast to usual CML, basophilia is not prominent, usually <2% of peripheral WBCs. The bone marrow is hypercellular, with an elevated myeloid-to-erythroid ratio, and marrow fibrosis may be prominent. There is dysplasia of the granulocyte lineage, with or without dysplasia in other lineages. Granulocytes may show pseudo–Pelger-Huët changes and cytoplasmic hypogranularity. Dyserythropoiesis and megakaryocyte dysplasia are common but not required for diagnosis and megakaryocytes may be reduced in number with associated thrombocytopenia. aCML is an aggressive disease, with progression occurring within 2 years.[187-190] There must be no evidence of cytogenetic abnormalities that define other diseases. Patients may develop acute leukemia or bone marrow failure secondary to marked fibrosis. Cytogenetic and molecular genetic studies are essential in the diagnosis of aCML, to exclude abnormalities diagnostic of other diseases such as CML.

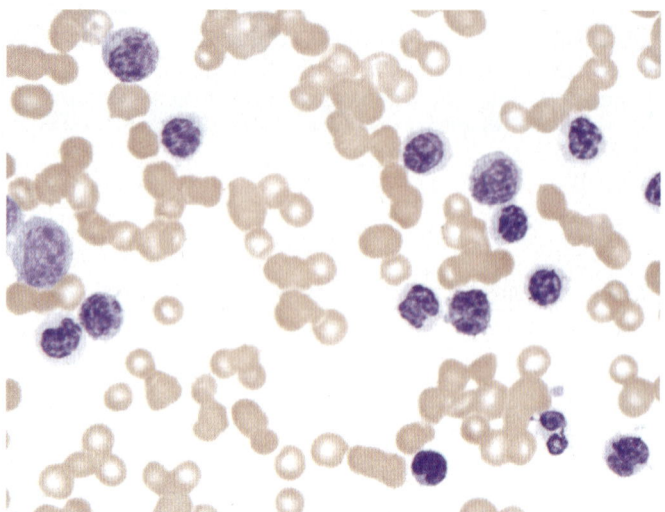

FIGURE 82.18 Atypical chronic myeloid leukemia. The peripheral blood smear shows leukocytosis and marked thrombocytopenia. Granulocytes are left-shifted and dysplastic with hypolobated nuclei and hypogranular cytoplasm. Wright-Giemsa, ×600.

There are no defining cytogenetic abnormalites known at this time for aCML, although +8, +13, del(12p), del(20)(q11), and i(17q) have been reported. The majority of cases, up to 80%, have normal karyotype.[187-189,191] Rare cases with features of aCML containing t(5;10)(q33;q22) have been described in which the fusion gene *PDGFRB::CCDC6* is expressed,[192,193] but these should now be considered cases of myeloid neoplasms with *PDGFRB* rearrangement. In addition, three cases have been shown to have t(4;22)(q12;q11).[194] *SETBP1* and *ETNK1* mutations are seen in up to a third of cases, but mutations in *CSF3R* are very rare and their presence should prompt an evaluation for CNL.[195] Other common mutations include *KRAS*, *NRAS*, *SRSF2*, *ASXL1*, *EZH2*, and *TET2*.[186] Other ancillary studies, particularly immunophenotyping studies, are usually not helpful unless an elevation in blasts is present.

Juvenile Myelomonocytic Leukemia

Juvenile myelomonocytic leukemia[196] is a childhood MDS/MPN that includes childhood leukemias previously classified as CMML, juvenile CML, and infantile monosomy 7 syndrome. JMML, although rare,[197-199] is the most common MDS/MPN of children.[200-204] Children with JMML are more often boys and develop the disease by age 4 years in most cases. There is a significant association with germline predisposition, including in neurofibromatosis, Noonan syndrome, and other genetic disorders. The children usually have marked elevations of fetal hemoglobin for their age. Skin lesions often precede the diagnosis, and these children present with an elevated WBC count, composed of granulocytes and monocytes, which may be identical to CMML of adults (*Figure 82.19*). Thrombocytopenia is also often present and organomegaly is common. Dysplastic changes and marrow hypercellularity are typical (*Figure 82.20*), similar to adult CMML. Overlap with features of adult aCML also occurs and the criteria for aCML and CMML are probably not appropriate in children.[205] JMML must also be differentiated from infection, which can present with similar clinical and morphologic findings.[206] Criteria (*Table 82.12*) for the diagnosis of JMML describe typical clinical findings of hepatosplenomegaly, lymphadenopathy, pallor, fever, and skin rash.[196,207] Laboratory criteria include the absence of t(9;22), monocytosis of >1 × 10⁹/L, and <20% bone marrow blast cells. Genetic studies are absolutely required for diagnosis and include evaluation for somatic mutations in *PTPN11*, *KRAS*, and *NRAS*; germline mutation of *NF1* (or clinical diagnosis of neurofibromatosis type 1), *PTPN11*, *NRAS*, *KRAS*, and *CBL*; and loss of heterozygosity of *CBL*.[208] *Infantile monosomy 7 syndrome* is clinically similar to JMML and may represent a subgroup of JMML patients, however, a subset of these patients will have germline *SAMD9* or *SAMD9L* mutations and may be better classified as MIRAGE syndrome or ataxia pancytopenia syndrome.[209] Cytogenetic

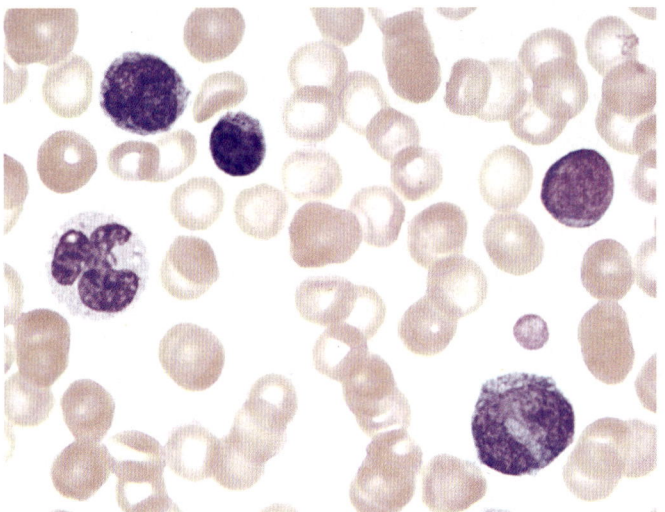

FIGURE 82.19 Juvenile myelomonocytic leukemia. Peripheral blood smear shows left-shifted leukocytosis and dysplastic monocytosis. A small blast is above a sparsely granulated lone platelet adjacent to a monocyte. Two dysplastic monocytes on the upper left contrast with a lymphocyte. Wright-Giemsa, ×1000. (Reprinted with permission from Tkachuk DC, Hirschmann JV, eds. *Wintrobe's Atlas of Clinical Hematology*. Wolters Kluwer Health/Lippincott Williams & Wilkins; 2007; *Figure 4.52*.)

Table 82.12. WHO Criteria for Juvenile Myelomonocytic Leukemia

I. Clinical and hematologic criteria (all required)
Peripheral blood monocytes > 1.0×10^9/L
Blasts + promonocytes <20% in blood and marrow
Splenomegaly
Absence of Philadelphia chromosome or *BCR::ABL1* fusion gene
II. Genetic criteria (1 sufficient or see III)
Somatic mutation of *PTPN11*, *KRAS*, or *NRAS*
NF1 mutation or clinical diagnosis of neurofibromatosis 1
Germline *CBL* mutation and loss of heterozygosity
III. Patients without genetic criteria
Monosomy 7 or other chromosomal abnormality or any two or more of • Hemoglobin F increased for age • Myeloid or erythroid precursors in the peripheral blood • GM-CSF hypersensitivity in colony assay • Hyperphosphorylation of STAT5

Abbreviations: GM-CSF, granulocyte-macrophage colony-stimulating factor; WHO, World Health Organization.

abnormalities other than monosomy 7, which may occur with any of the myelodysplastic syndromes, are not specific for JMML.[210] There is also an association between JMML and neurofibromatosis type 1, as well as with Noonan syndrome, leading to a markedly increased risk of developing JMML.[202,208,211] Abnormalities of the *NF1* gene lead to loss of neurofibromin, a guanosine triphosphatase (GTPase)-activating protein for *RAS*, resulting in deregulation of the normal RAS signaling pathways, with subsequent selective hypersensitivity of myeloid progenitor cells to granulocyte-macrophage colony-stimulating factor (GM-CSF).[212,213] The increased prevalence of JMML in Noonan syndrome is linked to germline mutations in the *PTPN11* gene, a gene that encodes SHP-2, required for RAS-dependent functions; these mutations also induce hypersensitivity of myeloid progenitors to GM-CSF.[214] Germline *KRAS*, *NRAS*, and *CBL* mutations can also lead to JMML. In addition to germline mutations, JMML can result from somatic mutations in *PTPN11*, *NRAS*, *KRAS*, and *CBL*. While germline mutations in these genes are associated with a favorable clinical course, somatic mutations are associated with aggressive disease and treatment with stem cell transplant is often recommended.[196] Given the aggressive clinical course of JMML with current treatment regimens,[200,201,204,215] work has focused on targeting the RAS pathway, which may result in new therapies.[216,217]

Myelodysplastic/Myeloproliferative Neoplasm With Ring Sideroblasts and Thrombocytosis (Myelodysplastic Neoplasm With Proliferative Evolution, *SF3B1* Mutation, and Thrombocytosis)

Previously included in the WHO as a provisional category is *myelodysplastic/myeloproliferative neoplasm with ring sideroblasts and thrombocytosis (MDS/MPN-RS-T)*.[16,112-114,163,218] These cases have no sex predilection or specific cytogenetic abnormality and must be differentiated from the 5q-syndrome. The bone marrow contains ≥15% ring sideroblasts with an accompanying atypical megakaryocytic proliferation; megakaryocytes often resemble those seen in PMF or ET (*Figure 82.21*). Anemia with erythroid dysplasia is present. The platelet counts are $≥450 \times 10^9$/L. *SF3B1* spliceosome gene is mutated in the

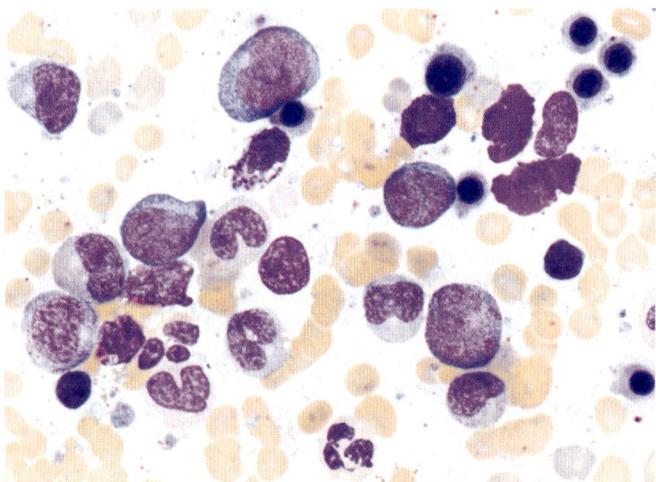

FIGURE 82.20 Juvenile myelomonocytic leukemia. Bone marrow aspirate shows numerous erythroid precursors and left-shifted immature myeloid cells with dysplasia. Wright-Giemsa, ×600.

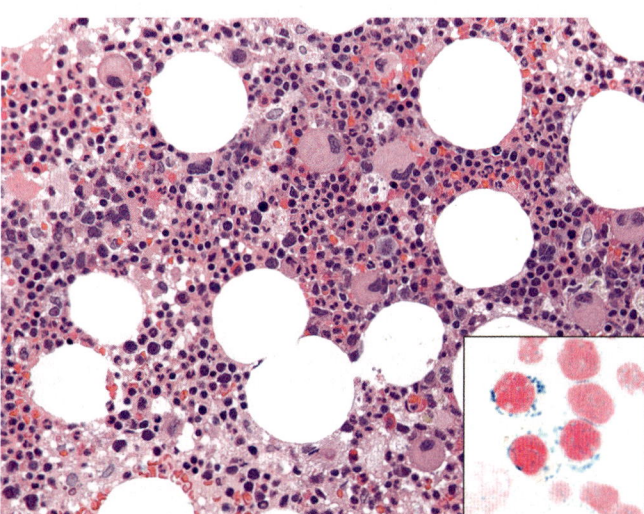

FIGURE 82.21 Myelodysplastic/myeloproliferative neoplasm with ring sideroblasts and thrombocytosis. The bone marrow biopsy shows dysplastic megakaryocytes, small hypolobated forms, and micromegakaryocytes, in a hypercellular marrow, with the inset demonstrating numerous ring sideroblasts. Hematoxylin and eosin, ×400. Prussian blue stain, ×1000.

majority of these cases and is associated with the morphologic finding of ring sideroblasts.[219,220] *JAK2* mutations are found in a majority of cases; *CALR* and *MPL* mutations are rarely seen.

Myelodysplastic/Myeloproliferative Neoplasm, Unclassifiable (Myelodysplastic Neoplasm With Proliferative Evolution, Not Otherwise Specified)

Some cases with features of both MDS and MPN do not fit well into any of the previously mentioned categories. Many of these cases have typical features of myelodysplasia, as well as an atypical finding more suggestive of a myeloproliferative disorder, such as marked marrow fibrosis and hypercellularity or organomegaly. Such cases may be termed *myelodysplastic/myeloproliferative disease, unclassifiable*, with a comment describing the atypical findings.[195] For example, an MDS/MPN associated with *isochromosome 17q* that occurs in adults with a male predominance associated with severe hyposegmentation of neutrophil nuclei, monocytosis, and a high rate of transformation to AML has been described.[182] Diseases with molecular markers diagnostic of other diseases should not be included in this category. For example, myeloid neoplasms with abnormalities of chromosome 3q21q26 often show granulocytic dysplasia accompanied by thrombocytosis with micromegakaryocytes on bone marrow histology.[221-226] These cases usually have a poor prognosis and should not be placed in the unclassifiable mixed MDS/MPN category. Rather, they should be classified in the appropriate MDS or AML category.

CONCLUSION

The classification of myeloid neoplasms now includes MPNs; neoplasms with eosinophilia and abnormalities of *PDGFRA*, *PDGFRB* or *FGFR1* or with *PCM:JAK2*, MDS/MPNs, MDS; and AMLs. MPNs and MDS/MPNs, both clonal stem cell diseases, share myeloproliferative features including typically hypercellular marrows, cell lineage maturation, and organomegaly. The MPNs generally differ by which myeloid cell lineage dominates hematopoiesis, and the main players include CML, PV, ET, and PMF. The new category of myeloid and lymphoid neoplasms with eosinophilia and abnormalities of *PDGFRA*, *PDGFRB* or *FGFR1* or with *PCM1::JAK2* represents another significant step forward in the molecular classification of neoplastic diseases. This category is also highly clinically relevant, because of the responsiveness of the *PDGFRA*- and *PDGFRB*-associated neoplasms to TKI therapy. The MDS/MPNs also show dysplastic features and variable amounts of effective hematopoiesis; these disorders include CMML, JMML, aCML, and MDS/MPN-RS-T. Given the mix of morphology among these diseases, correlation with clinical, hematologic, and cytogenetic/molecular genetic findings is imperative for precise classification.

References

1. Tremblay D, Yacoub A, Hoffman R. Overview of myeloproliferative neoplasms: history, pathogenesis, diagnostic criteria, and complications. *Hematol Oncol Clin North Am*. 2021;35:159-176.
2. Deininger MW, Goldman JM, Melo JV. The molecular biology of chronic myeloid leukemia. *Blood*. 2000;96:3343-3356.
3. Shannon K, Van Etten RA. JAKing up hematopoietic proliferation. *Cancer Cell*. 2005;7:291-293.
4. Levine RL, Gilliland DG. JAK-2 mutations and their relevance to myeloproliferative disease. *Curr Opin Hematol*. 2007;14:43-47.
5. Kota J, Caceres N, Constantinescu SN. Aberrant signal transduction pathways in myeloproliferative neoplasms. *Leukemia*. 2008;22:1828-1840.
6. Vainchenker W, Delhommeau F, Constantinescu SN, Bernard OA. New mutations and pathogenesis of myeloproliferative neoplasms. *Blood*. 2011;118:1723-1735.
7. George TI, Arber DA. Pathology of the myeloproliferative diseases. *Hematol Oncol Clin North Am*. 2003;17:1101-1127.
8. Levine RL, Wadleigh M, Cools J, et al. Activating mutation in the tyrosine kinase JAK2 in polycythemia vera, essential thrombocythemia, and myeloid metaplasia with myelofibrosis. *Cancer Cell*. 2005;7:387-397.
9. Baxter EJ, Scott LM, Campbell PJ, et al. Acquired mutation of the tyrosine kinase JAK2 in human myeloproliferative disorders. *Lancet*. 2005;365:1054-1061.
10. James C, Ugo V, Le Couedic JP, et al. A unique clonal JAK2 mutation leading to constitutive signalling causes polycythaemia vera. *Nature*. 2005;434:1144-1148.
11. Kralovics R, Passamonti F, Buser AS, et al. A gain-of-function mutation of JAK2 in myeloproliferative disorders. *N Engl J Med*. 2005;352:1779-1790.
12. Oh ST, Gotlib J. JAK2 V617F and beyond: role of genetics and aberrant signaling in the pathogenesis of myeloproliferative neoplasms. *Expert Rev Hematol*. 2010;3:323-337.
13. Jamieson CH, Gotlib J, Durocher JA, et al. The JAK2 V617F mutation occurs in hematopoietic stem cells in polycythemia vera and predisposes toward erythroid differentiation. *Proc Natl Acad Sci U S A*. 2006;103:6224-6229.
14. Chen E, Beer PA, Godfrey AL, et al. Distinct clinical phenotypes associated with JAK2V617F reflect differential STAT1 signaling. *Cancer Cell*. 2010;18:524-535.
15. Scott LM, Tong W, Levine RL, et al. JAK2 exon 12 mutations in polycythemia vera and idiopathic erythrocytosis. *N Engl J Med*. 2007;356:459-468.
16. Arber D, Orazi A, Hasserjian R, et al. The 2016 revision to the World Health Organization classification of myeloid neoplasms and acute leukemia. *Blood*. 2016;127:2391-2405.
17. Grinfeld J, Nangalia EJ, Baxter DC, et al. Classification and personalized prognosis in myeloproliferative neoplasms. *N Engl J Med*. 2018;379:1416-1430.
18. Ortman CA, Kent DG, Nangalia J, et al. Effect of mutation order on myeloproliferative neoplasms. *N Engl J Med*. 2015;372:601-612.
19. Bain BJ, Gilliland DG, Horny H-P, et al. Myeloid and lymphoid neoplasms with eosinophilia and abnormalities of PDGFRA, PDGFRB, or FGFR1. In: Swerdlow SH, Campo E, Harris NL, et al, eds. *WHO Classification of Tumours of Haematopoietic and Lymphoid Tissues*; IARC Press; 2008:68-73.
20. Cools J, DeAngelo DJ, Gotlib J, et al. A tyrosine kinase created by fusion of the PDGFRA and FIP1L1 genes as a therapeutic target of imatinib in idiopathic hypereosinophilic syndrome. *N Engl J Med*. 2003;348:1201-1214.
21. Ma Y, Zeng S, Metcalfe DD, et al. The c-KIT mutation causing human mastocytosis is resistant to STI571 and other KIT kinase inhibitors; kinases with enzymatic site mutations show different inhibitor sensitivity profiles than wild-type kinases and those with regulatory-type mutations. *Blood*. 2002;99:1741-1744.
22. Verstovsek S, Tefferi A, Cortes J, et al. Phase II study of dasatinib in Philadelphia chromosome-negative acute and chronic myeloid diseases, including systemic mastocytosis. *Clin Cancer Res*. 2008;14:3906-3915.
23. Gotlib J, Berube C, Growney JD, et al. Activity of the tyrosine kinase inhibitor PKC412 in a patient with mast cell leukemia with the D816V KIT mutation. *Blood*. 2005;106:2865-2870.
24. Jabbour E, Kantarjarjian H. Chronic myeloid leukemia: 2018 update on diagnosis, therapy and monitoring. *Am J Hematol*. 2018;93:442-459.
25. Sawyers CL. Chronic myeloid leukemia. *N Engl J Med*. 1999;340:1330-1340.
26. Thiele J, Kvasnicka HM, Titius BR, et al. Histological features of prognostic significance in CML–an immunohistochemical and morphometric study (multivariate regression analysis) on trephine biopsies of the bone marrow. *Ann Hematol*. 1993;66:291-302.
27. Busche G, Majewski H, Schlue J, et al. Frequency of pseudo-Gaucher cells in diagnostic bone marrow biopsies from patients with Ph-positive chronic myeloid leukaemia. *Virchows Arch*. 1997;430:139-148.
28. Arlin ZA, Silver RT, Bennett JM. Blastic phase of chronic myeloid leukemia (blCML): a proposal for standardization of diagnostic and response criteria. *Leukemia*. 1990;4:755-757.
29. Ross DW, Brunning RD, Kantarjian HM, et al. A proposed staging system for chronic myeloid leukemia. *Cancer*. 1993;71:3788-3791.
30. Vardiman JW, Melo JV, Baccarani M, Thiele J. Chronic myelogenous leukemia, BCR-ABL1 positive. In: Swerdlow SH, Campo E, Harris NL, et al, eds. *WHO Classification of Tumours of Haematopoietic and Lymphoid Tissues*. IARC Press; 2008:32-37.
31. Brunning RD, McKenna RW. *Tumors of the Bone Marrow*. Armed Forces Institute of Pathology; 1994.
32. Mitelman F, Levan G, Nilsson PG, et al. Non-random karyotypic evolution in chronic myeloid leukemia. *Int J Cancer*. 1976;18:24-30.
33. Mitelman F. The cytogenetic scenario of chronic myeloid leukemia. *Leuk Lymphoma*. 1993;11(suppl 1):11-15.
34. Khalidi HS, Brynes RK, Medeiros LJ, et al. The immunophenotype of blast transformation of chronic myelogenous leukemia: a high frequency of mixed lineage phenotype in "lymphoid" blasts and a comparison of morphologic, immunophenotypic, and molecular findings. *Mod Pathol*. 1998;11:1211-1221.
35. Cervantes F, Villamor N, Esteve J, et al. "Lymphoid" blast crisis of chronic myeloid leukaemia is associated with distinct clinicohaematological features. *Br J Haematol*. 1998;100:123-128.
36. Kantarjian H, Sawyers C, Hochhaus A, et al. Hematologic and cytogenetic responses to imatinib mesylate in chronic myelogenous leukemia. *N Engl J Med*. 2002;346:645-652.
37. Hasserjian RP, Boecklin F, Parker S, et al. ST1571 (imatinib mesylate) reduces bone marrow cellularity and normalizes morphologic features irrespective of cytogenetic response. *Am J Clin Pathol*. 2002;117:360-367.
38. Braziel RM, Launder TM, Druker BJ, et al. Hematopathologic and cytogenetic findings in imatinib mesylate-treated chronic myelogenous leukemia patients: 14 months' experience. *Blood*. 2002;100:435-441.
39. Druker BJ, Guilhot F, O'Brien SG, et al. Five-year follow-up of patients receiving imatinib for chronic myeloid leukemia. *N Engl J Med*. 2006;355:2408-2417.
40. Gambacorti-Passerini C, Antolini L, Mahon FX, et al. Multicenter independent assessment of outcomes in chronic myeloid leukemia patients treated with imatinib. *J Natl Cancer Inst*. 2011;103:553-561.
41. Palandri F, Castagnetti F, Alimena G, et al. The long-term durability of cytogenetic responses in patients with accelerated phase chronic myeloid leukemia treated with imatinib 600 mg: the GIMEMA CML Working Party experience after a 7-year follow-up. *Haematologica*. 2009;94:205-212.
42. Beham-Schmid C, Apfelbeck U, Sill H, et al. Treatment of chronic myelogenous leukemia with the tyrosine kinase inhibitor STI571 results in marked regression of bone marrow fibrosis. *Blood*. 2002;99:381-383.

43. Ibrahim AR, Clark RE, Holyoake TL, et al. Second-generation tyrosine kinase inhibitors improve the survival of patients with chronic myeloid leukemia in whom imatinib therapy has failed. *Haematologica*. 2011;96:1779-1782.
44. Saglio G, Kantarjian H, Holyoake T, et al. Proceedings of the third global workshop on chronic myeloid leukemia. *Clin Lymphoma Myeloma Leuk*. 2010;10:443-451.
45. Zhou T, Medeiros LJ, Hu S. Chronic myeloid leukemia: beyond BCR-ABL1. *Curr Hematol Malig Rep*. 2018;13:435-445.
46. Radich J. Stem cell transplant for chronic myeloid leukemia in the imatinib era. *Semin Hematol*. 2010;47:354-361.
47. Pane F, Frigeri F, Sindona M, et al. Neutrophilic-chronic myeloid leukemia: a distinct disease with a specific molecular marker (BCR/ABL with C3/A2 junction). *Blood*. 1996;88:2410-2414.
48. Verstovsek S, Lin H, Kantarjian H, et al. Neutrophilic-chronic myeloid leukemia: low levels of p230 BCR/ABL mRNA and undetectable BCR/ABL protein may predict an indolent course. *Cancer*. 2002;94:2416-2425.
49. Wiedemann LM, Karhi KK, Shivji MK, et al. The correlation of breakpoint cluster region rearrangement and p210 phl/abl expression with morphological analysis of Ph-negative chronic myeloid leukemia and other myeloproliferative diseases. *Blood*. 1988;71:349-355.
50. Michiels JJ, De Raeve H, Berneman Z, et al. The 2001 World Health Organization and updated European clinical and pathological criteria for the diagnosis, classification, and staging of the Philadelphia chromosome-negative chronic myeloproliferative disorders. *Semin Thromb Hemost*. 2006;32:307-340.
51. Polycythemia vera: the natural history of 1213 patients followed for 20 years. Gruppo Italiano Studio Policitemia. *Ann Intern Med*. 1995;123:656-664.
52. Putter JS, Seghatchian. Polycythaemia vera: molecular genetics, diagnostics and therapeutics. *Vox Sang*. 2021;116:617-627.
53. Tefferi A, Gilliland DG. The JAK2V617F tyrosine kinase mutation in myeloproliferative disorders: status report and immediate implications for disease classification and diagnosis. *Mayo Clin Proc*. 2005;80:947-958.
54. Pardanani A, Lasho TL, Finke C, et al. Prevalence and clinicopathologic correlates of JAK2 exon 12 mutations in JAK2V617F-negative polycythemia vera. *Leukemia*. 2007;21:1960-1963.
55. Scott LM. The JAK2 exon 12 mutations: a comprehensive review. *Am J Hematol*. 2011;86:668-676.
56. Johansson P, Safai-Kutti S, Lindstedt G, et al. Red cell mass, spleen size and plasma erythropoietin in polycythaemia vera and apparent polycythaemia. *Acta Haematol*. 2002;108:1-7.
57. Steensma DP, Dewald GW, Lasho TL, et al. The JAK2 V617F activating tyrosine kinase mutation is an infrequent event in both "atypical" myeloproliferative disorders and myelodysplastic syndromes. *Blood*. 2005;106:1207-1209.
58. Jones AV, Kreil S, Zoi K, et al. Widespread occurrence of the JAK2 V617F mutation in chronic myeloproliferative disorders. *Blood*. 2005;106:2162-2168.
59. Ellis JT, Peterson P, Geller SA, et al. Studies of the bone marrow in polycythemia vera and the evolution of myelofibrosis and second hematologic malignancies. *Semin Hematol*. 1986;23:144-155.
60. Thiele J, Kvasnicka HM, Zankovich R, et al. The value of bone marrow histology in differentiating between early stage polycythemia vera and secondary (reactive) polycythemias. *Haematologica*. 2001;86:368-374.
61. Thiele J, Kvasnicka HM, Muehlhausen K, et al. Polycythemia rubra vera versus secondary polycythemias. A clinicopathological evaluation of distinctive features in 199 patients. *Pathol Res Pract*. 2001;197:77-84.
62. Thiele J, Zirbes TK, Kvasnicka HM, et al. Focal lymphoid aggregates (nodules) in bone marrow biopsies: differentiation between benign hyperplasia and malignant lymphoma—a practical guideline. *J Clin Pathol*. 1999;52:294-300.
63. Murphy S. Diagnostic criteria and prognosis in polycythemia vera and essential thrombocythemia. *Semin Hematol*. 1999;36:9-13.
64. Najean Y, Deschamps A, Dresch C, et al. Acute leukemia and myelodysplasia in polycythemia vera. A clinical study with long-term follow-up. *Cancer*. 1988;61:89-95.
65. Tefferi A. The rise and fall of red cell mass measurement in polycythemia vera. *Curr Hematol Rep*. 2005;4:213-217.
66. Finazzi G, Gregg XT, Barbui T, et al. Idiopathic erythrocytosis and other non-clonal polycythemias. *Best Pract Res Clin Haematol*. 2006;19:471-482.
67. Diez-Martin JL, Graham DL, Petitt RM, et al. Chromosome studies in 104 patients with polycythemia vera. *Mayo Clin Proc*. 1991;66:287-299.
68. Asimakopoulos FA, Gilbert JG, Aldred MA, et al. Interstitial deletion constitutes the major mechanism for loss of heterozygosity on chromosome 20q in polycythemia vera. *Blood*. 1996;88:2690-2698.
69. Asimakopoulos FA, Green AR. Deletions of chromosome 20q and the pathogenesis of myeloproliferative disorders. *Br J Haematol*. 1996;95:219-226.
70. Prchal JF, Prchal JT. Molecular basis for polycythemia. *Curr Opin Hematol*. 1999;6:100-109.
71. Zwicky C, Theiler L, Zbaren K, et al. The predictive value of clonogenic stem cell assays for the diagnosis of polycythaemia vera. *Br J Haematol*. 2002;117:598-604.
72. Streiff MB, Smith B, Spivak JL. The diagnosis and management of polycythemia vera in the era since the Polycythemia Vera Study Group: a survey of American Society of Hematology members' practice patterns. *Blood*. 2002;99:1144-1149.
73. Thiele J, Kvasnicka HM, Werden C, et al. Idiopathic primary osteo-myelofibrosis: a clinico-pathological study on 208 patients with special emphasis on evolution of disease features, differentiation from essential thrombocythemia and variables of prognostic impact. *Leuk Lymphoma*. 1996;22:303-317.
74. Tefferi A. Myelofibrosis with myeloid metaplasia. *N Engl J Med*. 2000;342:1255-1265.
75. Tefferi A. Primary Myelofibrosis: 2021 update on diagnosis, risk–stratification and management. *Am J Hematol*. 2021;96:145-162.
76. Michiels JJ, Thiele J. Clinical and pathological criteria for the diagnosis of essential thrombocythemia, polycythemia vera, and idiopathic myelofibrosis (agnogenic myeloid metaplasia). *Int J Hematol*. 2002;76:133-145.
77. Thiele J, Kvasnicka HM, Zankovich R, et al. Early-stage idiopathic (primary) myelofibrosis—current issues of diagnostic features. *Leuk Lymphoma*. 2002;43:1035-1041.
78. Thiele J, Kvasnicka HM. Hematopathologic findings in chronic idiopathic myelofibrosis. *Semin Oncol*. 2005;32:380-394.
79. Thiele J, Kvasnicka HM, Boeltken B, et al. Initial (prefibrotic) stages of idiopathic (primary) myelofibrosis (IMF)—a clinicopathological study. *Leukemia*. 1999;13:1741-1748.
80. Thiele J, Kvasnicka HM, Diehl V, et al. Clinicopathological diagnosis and differential criteria of thrombocythemias in various myeloproliferative disorders by histopathology, histochemistry and immunostaining from bone marrow biopsies. *Leuk Lymphoma*. 1999;33:207-218.
81. Thiele J, Kvasnicka HM, Zankovich R, et al. Relevance of bone marrow features in the differential diagnosis between essential thrombocythemia and early stage idiopathic myelofibrosis. *Haematologica*. 2000;85:1126-1134.
82. Thiele J, Kvasnicka HM. Clinicopathological criteria for differential diagnosis of thrombocythemias in various myeloproliferative disorders. *Semin Thromb Hemost*. 2006;32:219-230.
83. Barbui T, Thiele J, Passamonti F, et al. Survival and disease progression in essential thrombocythemia are significantly influenced by accurate morphologic diagnosis: an international study. *J Clin Oncol*. 2011;29:3179-3184.
84. Thiele J, Kvasnicka HM, Müllauer L, et al. Essential thrombocythemia versus early primary myelofibrosis: a multicenter study to validate the WHO classification. *Blood*. 2011;117:5710-5718.
85. Jacobson RJ, Salo A, Fialkow PJ. Agnogenic myeloid metaplasia: a clonal proliferation of hematopoietic stem cells with secondary myelofibrosis. *Blood*. 1978;51:189-194.
86. Lasho TL, Pardanani A, McClure RF, et al. Concurrent MPL515 and JAK2V 617F mutations in myelofibrosis: chronology of clonal emergence and changes in mutant allele burden over time. *Br J Haematol*. 2006;135:683-687.
87. Pardanani AD, Levine RL, Lasho T, et al. MPL515 mutations in myeloproliferative and other myeloid disorders: a study of 1182 patients. *Blood*. 2006;108:3472-3476.
88. Dupriez B, Morel P, Demory JL, et al. Prognostic factors in agnogenic myeloid metaplasia: a report on 195 cases with a new scoring system. *Blood*. 1996;88:1013-1018.
89. Dingli D, Grand FH, Mahaffey V, et al. Der(6)t(1;6)(q21-23;p21.3): a specific cytogenetic abnormality in myelofibrosis with myeloid metaplasia. *Br J Haematol*. 2005;130:229-232.
90. Reilly JT, Snowden JA, Spearing RL, et al. Cytogenetic abnormalities and their prognostic significance in idiopathic myelofibrosis: a study of 106 cases. *Br J Haematol*. 1997;98:96-102.
91. Tefferi A, Meyer RG, Wyatt WA, et al. Comparison of peripheral blood interphase cytogenetics with bone marrow karyotype analysis in myelofibrosis with myeloid metaplasia. *Br J Haematol*. 2001;115:316-319.
92. Barosi G, Ambrosetti A, Finelli C, et al. The Italian consensus conference on diagnostic criteria for myelofibrosis with myeloid metaplasia. *Br J Haematol*. 1999;104:730-737.
93. Thiele J, Kvasnicka HM, Vardiman J. Bone marrow histopathology in the diagnosis of chronic myeloproliferative disorders: a forgotten pearl. *Best Pract Res Clin Haematol*. 2006;19:413-437.
94. Tefferi A, Lasho TL, Jimma T, et al. One thousand patients with primary myelofibrosis: the mayo clinic experience. *Mayo Clin Proc*. 2012;87:25-33.
95. Gangat N, Caramazza D, Vaidya R, et al. DIPSS plus: a refined Dynamic International Prognostic Scoring System for primary myelofibrosis that incorporates prognostic information from karyotype, platelet count, and transfusion status. *J Clin Oncol*. 2011;29:392-397.
96. Tefferi A. How I treat myelofibrosis. *Blood*. 2011;117:3494-3504.
97. Ballen KK, Shrestha S, Sobocinski KA, et al. Outcome of transplantation for myelofibrosis. *Biol Blood Marrow Transplant*. 2010;16:358-367.
98. Vannucchi AM, Antonioli E, Guglielmelli P, et al. Characteristics and clinical correlates of MPL 515W>L/K mutation in essential thrombocythemia. *Blood*. 2008;112:844-847.
99. Harrison CN, Gale RE, Machin SJ, et al. A large proportion of patients with a diagnosis of essential thrombocythemia do not have a clonal disorder and may be at lower risk of thrombotic complications. *Blood*. 1999;93:417-424.
100. Nimer SD. Essential thrombocythemia: another "heterogeneous disease" better understood? *Blood*. 1999;93:415-416.
101. Thiele J, Schneider G, Hoeppner B, et al. Histomorphometry of bone marrow biopsies in chronic myeloproliferative disorders with associated thrombocytosis—features of significance for the diagnosis of primary (essential) thrombocythaemia. *Virchows Arch A Pathol Anat Histopathol*. 1988;413:407-417.
102. Besses C, Cervantes F, Pereira A, et al. Major vascular complications in essential thrombocythemia: a study of the predictive factors in a series of 148 patients. *Leukemia*. 1999;13:150-154.
103. Harrison CN, Campbell PJ, Buck G, et al. Hydroxyurea compared with anagrelide in high-risk essential thrombocythemia. *N Engl J Med*. 2005;353:33-45.
104. Cortelazzo S, Finazzi G, Ruggeri M, et al. Hydroxyurea for patients with essential thrombocythemia and a high risk of thrombosis. *N Engl J Med*. 1995;332:1132-1136.
105. Sterkers Y, Preudhomme C, Lai JL, et al. Acute myeloid leukemia and myelodysplastic syndromes following essential thrombocythemia treated with hydroxyurea: high proportion of cases with 17p deletion. *Blood*. 1998;91:616-622.
106. Mesa RA, Silverstein MN, Jacobsen SJ, et al. Population-based incidence and survival figures in essential thrombocythemia and agnogenic myeloid metaplasia: an Olmsted County Study, 1976-1995. *Am J Hematol*. 1999;61:10-15.

107. Thiele J, Kvasnicka HM, Schmitt-Graeff A, et al. Follow-up examinations including sequential bone marrow biopsies in essential thrombocythemia (ET): a retrospective clinicopathological study of 120 patients. *Am J Hematol.* 2002;70:283-291.
108. Tefferi A, Pardanani A. Mutation screening for JAK2V617F: when to order the test and how to interpret the results. *Leuk Res.* 2006;30:739-744.
109. Steensma DP, Tefferi A. Cytogenetic and molecular genetic aspects of essential thrombocythemia. *Acta Haematol.* 2002;108:55-65.
110. Aviram A, Blickstein D, Stark P, et al. Significance of BCR-ABL transcripts in bone marrow aspirates of Philadelphia-negative essential thrombocythemia patients. *Leuk Lymphoma.* 1999;33:77-82.
111. Hussein K, Bock O, Theophile K, et al. Chronic myeloproliferative diseases with concurrent BCR-ABL junction and JAK2V617F mutation. *Leukemia.* 2008;22(5):1059-1062.
112. Case records of the Massachusetts General Hospital. Weekly clinicopathological exercises. Case 17-1992. Repeated bouts of hematochezia in an 80-year-old hypertensive man. *N Engl J Med.* 1992;326:1137-1146.
113. Gupta R, Abdalla SH, Bain BJ. Thrombocytosis with sideroblastic erythropoiesis: a mixed myeloproliferative myelodysplastic syndrome. *Leuk Lymphoma.* 1999;34:615-619.
114. Koike T, Uesugi Y, Toba K, et al. 5q-syndrome presenting as essential thrombocythemia: myelodysplastic syndrome or chronic myeloproliferative disorders? *Leukemia.* 1995;9:517-518.
115. Roufousse F, Cogan E, Goldman M. Recent advances in pathogenesis and management of hypereosinophilic syndromes. *Allergy.* 2004;59:673-689.
116. Shomali W, Gotlib J. World Health Organization-defined eosinophilic disorders: 2019 update on diagnosis, risk stratification, and management. *Am J Hematol.* 2019;94:1149-1167.
117. Chang HW, Leong KH, Koh DR, et al. Clonality of isolated eosinophils in the hypereosinophilic syndrome. *Blood.* 1999;93:1651-1657.
118. Reiter A, Gotlib J. Myeloid neoplasms with eosinophilia. *Blood.* 2017;129:704-714.
119. Gotlib J, Cools J, Malone JM, III, et al. The FIP1L1-PDGFRalpha fusion tyrosine kinase in hypereosinophilic syndrome and chronic eosinophilic leukemia: implications for diagnosis, classification, and management. *Blood.* 2004;103:2879-2891.
120. Cervera N, Itzykson R, Coppin E, et al. Gene mutations differently impact the prognosis of the myelodysplastic and myeloproliferative classes of chronic myelomonocytic leukemia. *Am J Hematol.* 2014;89:604-609.
121. Berkowicz M, Rosner E, Rechavi G, et al. Atypical chronic myelomonocytic leukemia with eosinophilia and translocation (5;12). A new association. *Cancer Genet Cytogenet.* 1991;51:277-278.
122. Golub TR, Barker GF, Lovett M, et al. Fusion of PDGF receptor beta to a novel ets-like gene, tel, in chronic myelomonocytic leukemia with t(5;12) chromosomal translocation. *Cell.* 1994;77:307-316.
123. Cools J, Stover EH, Gilliland DG. Detection of the FIP1L1-PDGFRA fusion in idiopathic hypereosinophilic syndrome and chronic eosinophilic leukemia. *Methods Mol Med.* 2006;125:177-187.
124. Elliott MA, Dewald GW, Tefferi A, et al. Chronic neutrophilic leukemia (CNL): a clinical, pathologic and cytogenetic study. *Leukemia.* 2001;15:35-40.
125. Elliott MA, Hanson CA, Dewald GW, et al. WHO-defined chronic neutrophilic leukemia: a long-term analysis of 12 cases and a critical review of the literature. *Leukemia.* 2005;19:313-317.
126. Maxson JE, Gotlib J, Pollyea DA, et al. Oncogenic CSF3R mutations in chronic neutrophilic leukemia and atypical CML. *N Engl J Med.* 2013;368:1781-1790.
127. Pardanani A, Lasho TL, Laborde RR, et al. CSF3R T618I is a highly prevalent and specific mutation in chronic neutrophilic leukemia. *Leukemia.* 2013;27:1870-1873.
128. Bain BJ, Brunning RD, Vardiman JW, et al. Chronic neutrophilic leukemia. In: Swerdlow SH, Campo E, Harris NL, eds. *WHO Classification of Tumours of Haematopoietic and Lymphoid Tissues.* IARC Press; 2008:38-39.
129. Bench AJ, Nacheva EP, Champion KM, et al. Molecular genetics and cytogenetics of myeloproliferative disorders. *Baillieres Clin Haematol.* 1998;11:819-848.
130. Hasle H, Olesen G, Kerndrup G, et al. Chronic neutrophil leukaemia in adolescence and young adulthood. *Br J Haematol.* 1996;94:628-630.
131. Katsuki K, Shinohara K, Takeda K, et al. Chronic neutrophilic leukemia with acute myeloblastic transformation. *Jpn J Clin Oncol.* 2000;30:362-365.
132. Dao KT, Gotlib J, Deininger MMN, et al. Efficacy of ruxolitinib in patients with chronic neutrophilic leukemia and atypical chronic myeloid leukemia. *J Clin Oncol.* 2020;38:1006-1018.
133. Tzankov A, Duncavage E, Craig FE, et al. Mastocytosis. *Am J Clin Pathol.* 2021;155:239-266.
134. Reiter A, George TI, Gotlib J. New developments in diagnosis, prognostication, and treatment of advanced mastocytosis. *Blood.* 2020;135:1365-1376.
135. Valent P, Akin C, Metcalfe DD. Mastocytosis 2016: updated WHO classification and novel emerging treatment concepts. *Blood.* 2017;129:1420-1427.
136. Georgin-Lavialle S, Lhermitte L, Dubreuil P, et al. Mast cell leukemia. *Blood.* 2013;121:1285-1295.
137. Gotlib J, Kluin-Nelemans H, George TI, et al. Efficacy and safety of Midostaurin in advanced systemic mastocytosis. *N Engl J Med.* 2016;374:2530-2541.
138. DeAngelo D, Radia DH, George TI, et al. Safety and efficacy of avapritinib in advanced systemic mastocytosis: the phase 1 EXPLORER trial. *Nat Med.* 2021;27:2183-2191.
139. Sotlar K, Horny HP, Simonitsch I, et al. CD25 indicates the neoplastic phenotype of mast cells: a novel immunohistochemical marker for the diagnosis of systemic mastocytosis (SM) in routinely processed bone marrow biopsy specimens. *Am J Surg Pathol.* 2004;28:1319-1325.
140. Morgado JM, Perbellini O, Johnson RC, et al. CD30 expression by bone marrow mast cells from different diagnostic variants of systemic mastocytosis. *Histopathology.* 2013;63:780-787.
141. Escribano L, Diaz-Agustin B, Lopez, et al. Immunophenotypic analysis of mast cells in mastocytosis: when and how to do it. Proposals of the Spanish network on mastocytosis (REMA). *Cytometry B Clin Cytom.* 2004;58:1-8.
142. Longley BJ, Tyrrell L, Lu S. Somatic c-KIT activating mutation in urticaria pigmentosa and aggressive mastocytosis: establishment of clonality in a human mast cell neoplasm. *Nat Genet.* 1996;12:312-314.
143. Nagata H, Worobec AS, Oh CK. Identification of a point mutation in the catalytic domain of the protooncogene c-kit in peripheral blood mononuclear cells of patients who have mastocytosis with an associated hematologic disorder. *Proc Natl Acad Sci U S A.* 1995;92:10560-10564.
144. Furitsu T, Tsujimura T, Tono T. Identification of mutations in the coding sequence of the proto-oncogene c-kit in a human mast cell leukemia cell line causing ligand-independent activation of c-kit product. *J Clin Invest.* 1993;92:1736-1744.
145. Tefferi A, Gilliland DG. Oncogenes in myeloproliferative disorders. *Cell Cycle.* 2007;6:550-566.
146. Lasota J, Miettinen M. Clinical significance of oncogenic KIT and PDGFRA mutations in gastrointestinal stromal tumours. *Histopathology.* 2008;53:245-266.
147. Beghini A, Ripamonti CB, Cairoli R, et al. KIT activating mutations: incidence in adult and pediatric acute myeloid leukemia, and identification of an internal tandem duplication. *Haematologica.* 2004;89:920-925.
148. Klion AD, Noel P, Akin C, et al. Elevated serum tryptase levels identify a subset of patients with a myeloproliferative variant of idiopathic hypereosinophilic syndrome associated with tissue fibrosis, poor prognosis, and imatinib responsiveness. *Blood.* 2003;101:4660-4666.
149. Pardanani A, Ketterling RP, Brockman SR, et al. CHIC2 deletion, a surrogate for FIP1L1-PDGFRA fusion, occurs in systemic mastocytosis associated with eosinophilia and predicts response to imatinib mesylate therapy. *Blood.* 2003;102:3093-3096.
150. Pardanani A, Brockman SR, Paternoster SF, et al. FIP1L1-PDGFRA fusion: prevalence and clinicopathologic correlates in 89 consecutive patients with moderate to severe eosinophilia. *Blood.* 2004;104:3038-3045.
151. Gleich GJ, Leiferman KM, Pardanani A, et al. Treatment of hypereosinophilic syndrome with imatinib mesilate. *Lancet.* 2002;359:1577-1578.
152. Ault P, Cortes J, Koller C, et al. Response of idiopathic hypereosinophilic syndrome to treatment with imatinib mesylate. *Leuk Res.* 2002;26:881-884.
153. Bain BJ, Fletcher SH. Chronic eosinophilic leukemias and the myeloproliferative variant of the hypereosinophilic syndrome. *Allergy Clin North Am.* 2007;27:377-388.
154. Macdonald D, Aguiar RC, Mason PJ, et al. A new myeloproliferative disorder associated with chromosomal translocations involving 8p11: a review. *Leukemia.* 1995;9:1628-1630.
155. Abruzzo LV, Jaffe ES, Cotelingam JD, et al. T-cell lymphoblastic lymphoma with eosinophilia associated with subsequent myeloid malignancy. *Am J Surg Pathol.* 1992;16:236-245.
156. Macdonald D, Reiter A, Cross NC. The 8p11 myeloproliferative syndrome: a distinct clinical entity caused by constitutive activation of FGFR1. *Acta Haematol.* 2002;107:101-107.
157. Walz C, Chase A, Schoch C, et al. The t(8;17)(p11;q23) in the 8p11 myeloproliferative syndrome fuses MYO18A to FGFR1. *Leukemia.* 2005;19:1005-1009.
158. Reiter A, Sohal J, Kulkarni S, et al. Consistent fusion of ZNF198 to the fibroblast growth factor receptor-1 in the t(8;13)(p11;q12) myeloproliferative syndrome. *Blood.* 1998;92:1735-1742.
159. Xiao S, Nalabolu SR, Aster JC, et al. FGFR1 is fused with a novel zinc-finger gene, ZNF198, in the t(8;13) leukaemia/lymphoma syndrome. *Nat Genet.* 1998;18:84-87.
160. Gerds AT, Gotlib J, Bose P, et al. Myeloid/lymphoid neoplasms with eosinophilia and TK fusion genes, version 3.2021, NCCN clinical practice guidelines in oncology. *J Natl Compr Cancer Netw.* 2020;18:1248-1269.
161. Tang G, Sydney Sir Philip JK, Weinberg O, et al. Hematopoietic neoplasms with 9p24/JAK2 rearrangement: a multicenter study. *Mod Pathol.* 2019;32:490-498.
162. Pozdnyakova O, Orazi A, Kelemen K, et al. Myeloid/lymphoid neoplasms associated with eosinophilia and rearrangements of PDGFRA, PDGFRB, or FGFR1 or with PCM1-JAK2. *Am J Clin Pathol.* 2021;155:160-178.
163. Neuwirtova R, Mocikova K, Musilova J, et al. Mixed myelodysplastic and myeloproliferative syndromes. *Leuk Res.* 1996;20:717-726.
164. Orazi A, Bennett JM, Germing U, et al. Chronic myelomonocytic leukemia. In: Swerdlow SH, Campo E, Harris NL, et al, eds. *WHO Classification of Tumours of Haematopoietic and Lymphoid Tissues.* IARC Press; 2017:82-86.
165. Bennett JM, Catovsky D, Daniel MT, et al. The chronic myeloid leukaemias: guidelines for distinguishing chronic granulocytic, atypical chronic myeloid, and chronic myelomonocytic leukaemia. Proposals by the French-American-British Cooperative Leukaemia Group. *Br J Haematol.* 1994;87:746-754.
166. Germing U, Gattermann N, Minning H, et al. Problems in the classification of CMML—dysplastic versus proliferative type. *Leuk Res.* 1998;22:871-878.
167. Voglova J, Chrobak L, Neuwirtova R, et al. Myelodysplastic and myeloproliferative type of chronic myelomonocytic leukemia—distinct subgroups or two stages of the same disease? *Leuk Res.* 2001;25:493-499.
168. Onida F, Kantarjian HM, Smith TL, et al. Prognostic factors and scoring systems in chronic myelomonocytic leukemia: a retrospective analysis of 213 patients. *Blood.* 2002;99:840-849.
169. Gonzalez-Medina I, Bueno J, Torrequebrada A, et al. Two groups of chronic myelomonocytic leukaemia: myelodysplastic and myeloproliferative. Prognostic implications in a series of a single center. *Leuk Res.* 2002;26:821-824.
170. Kouides PA, Bennett JM. Morphology and classification of the myelodysplastic syndromes and their pathologic variants. *Semin Hematol.* 1996;33:95-110.
171. Goasguen JE, Bennett JM, Bain BJ, et al. Morphological evaluation of monocytes and their precursors. *Haematologica.* 2009;94:994-997.

172. Sawyers CL, Denny CT. Chronic myelomonocytic leukemia: tel-a-kinase what Ets all about. *Cell.* 1994;77:171-173.
173. Valent P, Orazi A, Savona MR. Proposed diagnostic criteria for classical chronic myelomonocytic leukemia (CMML), CMML variants, and pre-CMML conditions. *Haematologica.* 2019;104:1935-1949.
174. Fenaux P, Beuscart R, Lai JL, et al. Prognostic factors in adult chronic myelomonocytic leukemia: an analysis of 107 cases. *J Clin Oncol.* 1988;6:1417-1424.
175. Chronic myelomonocytic leukemia: single entity or heterogeneous disorder? A prospective multicenter study of 100 patients. Groupe Francais de Cytogenetique Hematologique. *Cancer Genet Cytogenet.* 1991;55:57-65.
176. Storniolo AM, Moloney WC, Rosenthal DS, et al. Chronic myelomonocytic leukemia. *Leukemia.* 1990;4:766-770.
177. Tefferi A, Hoagland HC, Therneau TM, et al. Chronic myelomonocytic leukemia: natural history and prognostic determinants. *Mayo Clin Proc.* 1989;64:1246-1254.
178. Petrova-Drus K, Chiu A, Margolskee E. Bone marrow fibrosis in chronic myelomonocytic leukemia is associated with increased megakaryopoiesis, splenomegaly, and with a shorter median time to disease progression. *Oncotarget.* 2017;8:103274-103282.
179. Toyama K, Ohyashiki K, Yoshida Y, et al. Clinical implications of chromosomal abnormalities in 401 patients with myelodysplastic syndromes: a multicentric study in Japan. *Leukemia.* 1993;7:499-508.
180. Haase D, Fonatsch C, Freund M, et al. Cytogenetic findings in 179 patients with myelodysplastic syndromes. *Ann Hematol.* 1995;70:171-187.
181. Fenaux P, Morel P, Lai JL. Cytogenetics of myelodysplastic syndromes. *Semin Hematol.* 1996;33:127-138.
182. McClure RF, Dewald GW, Hoyer JD, et al. Isolated isochromosome 17q: a distinct type of mixed myeloproliferative disorder/myelodysplastic syndrome with an aggressive clinical course. *Br J Haematol.* 1999;106:445-454.
183. Gur HD, Loghavi S, Garcia-Manero G. Chronic myelomonocytic leukemia with fibrosis is a distinct disease subset with myeloproliferative features and frequent JAK2 p.V617F mutations. *Am J Surg Pathol.* 2018;45:799-806.
184. Mughal TI, Cross NC, Padron E, et al. An international MDS/MPN working group's perspective and recommendations on molecular pathogenesis, diagnosis and clinical characterization of myelodysplastic/myeloproliferative neoplasms. *Haematologica.* 2015;100:1117-1130.
185. Dobrovic A, Morley AA, Seshadri R, et al. Molecular diagnosis of Philadelphia negative CML using the polymerase chain reaction and DNA analysis: clinical features and course of M-bcr negative and M-bcr positive CML. *Leukemia.* 1991;5:187-190.
186. Sadigh S, Hasserjian RP, Hobbs G. Distinguishing atypical chronic myeloid leukemia from other Philadelphia-negative chronic myeloid neoplasms. *Hematology.* 2020;27:122-127.
187. Hernandez JM, del Canizo MC, Cuneo A, et al. Clinical, hematological and cytogenetic characteristics of atypical chronic myeloid leukemia. *Ann Oncol.* 2000;11:441-444.
188. Costello R, Sainty D, Lafage-Pochitaloff M, et al. Clinical and biological aspects of Philadelphia-negative/BCR-negative chronic myeloid leukemia. *Leuk Lymphoma.* 1997;25:225-232.
189. Martiat P, Michaux JL, Rodhain J. Philadelphia-negative (Ph-) chronic myeloid leukemia (CML): comparison with Ph+ CML and chronic myelomonocytic leukemia. The Groupe Francais de Cytogenetique Hematologique. *Blood.* 1991;78:205-211.
190. Shepherd PC, Ganesan TS, Galton DA. Haematological classification of the chronic myeloid leukaemias. *Baillieres Clin Haematol.* 1987;1:887-906.
191. Oscier D. Atypical chronic myeloid leukemias. *Pathol Biol (Paris).* 1997;45:587-593.
192. Schwaller J, Anastasiadou E, Cain D, et al. H4(D10S170), a gene frequently rearranged in papillary thyroid carcinoma, is fused to the platelet-derived growth factor receptor beta gene in atypical chronic myeloid leukemia with t(5;10)(q33;q22). *Blood.* 2001;97:3910-3918.
193. Siena S, Sammarelli G, Grimoldi MG, et al. New reciprocal translocation t(5;10) (q33;q22) associated with atypical chronic myeloid leukemia. *Haematologica.* 1999;84:369-372.
194. Baxter EJ, Hochhaus A, Bolufer P, et al. The t(4;22)(q12;q11) in atypical chronic myeloid leukaemia fuses BCR to PDGFRA. *Hum Mol Genet.* 2002;11:1391-1397.
195. Wang SA, Hasserjian RP, Fox PS. Atypical chronic myeloid leukemia is clinically distinct from unclassifiable myelodysplastic/myeloproliferative neoplasms. *Blood.* 2014;123:2645-2651.
196. Gupta AK, Meena JP, Chopra A. Juvenile myelomonocytic leukemia-a comprehensive review and recent advances in management. *Am J Blood Res.* 2021;11:1-21.
197. Jackson GH, Carey PJ, Cant AJ, et al. Myelodysplastic syndromes in children. *Br J Haematol.* 1993;84:185-186.
198. Hasle H, Kerndrup G, Jacobsen BB. Childhood myelodysplastic syndrome in Denmark: incidence and predisposing conditions. *Leukemia.* 1995;9:1569-1572.
199. Hasle H, Wadsworth LD, Massing BG, et al. A population-based study of childhood myelodysplastic syndrome in British Columbia, Canada. *Br J Haematol.* 1999;106:1027-1032.
200. Sasaki H, Manabe A, Kojima S, et al. Myelodysplastic syndrome in childhood: a retrospective study of 189 patients in Japan. *Leukemia.* 2001;15:1713-1720.
201. Hasle H, Arico M, Basso G, et al. Myelodysplastic syndrome, juvenile myelomonocytic leukemia, and acute myeloid leukemia associated with complete or partial monosomy 7. European Working Group on MDS in Childhood (EWOG-MDS). *Leukemia.* 1999;13:376-385.
202. Luna-Fineman S, Shannon KM, Atwater SK, et al. Myelodysplastic and myeloproliferative disorders of childhood: a study of 167 patients. *Blood.* 1999;93:459-466.
203. Arico M, Biondi A, Pui CH. Juvenile myelomonocytic leukemia. *Blood.* 1997;90:479-488.
204. Niemeyer CM, Arico M, Basso G, et al. Chronic myelomonocytic leukemia in childhood: a retrospective analysis of 110 cases. European Working Group on Myelodysplastic Syndromes in Childhood (EWOG-MDS). *Blood.* 1997;89:3534-3543.
205. Hasle H, Kerndrup G. Atypical chronic myeloid leukaemia and chronic myelomonocytic leukaemia in children. *Br J Haematol.* 1995;89:428-429.
206. Pinkel D. Differentiating juvenile myelomonocytic leukemia from infectious disease. *Blood.* 1998;91:365-367.
207. Emanuel PD. Myelodysplasia and myeloproliferative disorders in childhood: an update. *Br J Haematol.* 1999;105:852-863.
208. Locatelli F, Niemeyer CM. How I treat juvenile myelomonocytic leukemia. *Blood.* 2015;125:1083-1090.
209. Inaba T, Honda H, Matsui H. The enigma of monosomy 7. *Blood.* 2018;131:2891-2898.
210. Flotho C, Valcamonica S, Mach-Pascual S, et al. RAS mutations and clonality analysis in children with juvenile myelomonocytic leukemia (JMML). *Leukemia.* 1999;13:32-37.
211. Tartaglia M, Niemeyer CM, Fragale A, et al. Somatic mutations in PTPN11 in juvenile myelomonocytic leukemia, myelodysplastic syndromes and acute myeloid leukemia. *Nat Genet.* 2003;34:148-150.
212. Largaespada DA, Brannan CI, Jenkins NA, et al. Nf1 deficiency causes Ras-mediated granulocyte/macrophage colony stimulating factor hypersensitivity and chronic myeloid leukaemia. *Nat Genet.* 1996;12:137-143.
213. Bollag G, Clapp DW, Shih S, et al. Loss of NF1 results in activation of the Ras signaling pathway and leads to aberrant growth in haematopoietic cells. *Nat Genet.* 1996;12:144-148.
214. Loh ML, Vattikuti S, Schubbert S, et al. Mutations in PTPN11 implicate the SHP-2 phosphatase in leukemogenesis. *Blood.* 2004;103:2325-2331.
215. Woods WG, Barnard DR, Alonzo TA, et al. Prospective study of 90 children requiring treatment for juvenile myelomonocytic leukemia or myelodysplastic syndrome: a report from the Children's Cancer Group. *J Clin Oncol.* 2002;20:434-440.
216. Iversen PO, Emanuel PD, Sioud M. Targeting Raf-1 gene expression by a DNA enzyme inhibits juvenile myelomonocytic leukemia cell growth. *Blood.* 2002;99:4147-4153.
217. Emanuel PD, Snyder RC, Wiley T, et al. Inhibition of juvenile myelomonocytic leukemia cell growth in vitro by farnesyltransferase inhibitors. *Blood.* 2000;95:639-645.
218. Streeter RR, Presant CA, Reinhard E. Prognostic significance of thrombocytosis in idiopathic sideroblastic anemia. *Blood.* 1977;50:427-432.
219. Malcovati L, Papaemmanuil E, Bowen D, et al. Clinical significance of SF3B1 mutations in myelodysplastic syndromes and myelodysplastic/myeloproliferative neoplasms. *Blood.* 2011;118:6239-6246.
220. Cazzola M, Rossi M, Malcovati L. Biologic and clinical significance of somatic mutations of SF3B1 in myeloid and lymphoid neoplasms. *Blood.* 2013;121:260-269.
221. Norrby A, Ridell B, Swolin B, et al. Rearrangement of chromosome no. 3 in a case of preleukemia with thrombocytosis. *Cancer Genet Cytogenet.* 1982;5:257-263.
222. Carroll AJ, Poon MC, Robinson NC, et al. Sideroblastic anemia associated with thrombocytosis and a chromosome 3 abnormality. *Cancer Genet Cytogenet.* 1986;22:183-187.
223. Jotterand Bellomo M, Parlier V, Muhlematter D, et al. Three new cases of chromosome 3 rearrangement in bands q21 and q26 with abnormal thrombopoiesis bring further evidence to the existence of a 3q21q26 syndrome. *Cancer Genet Cytogenet.* 1992;59:138-160.
224. Grigg AP, Gascoyne RD, Phillips GL, et al. Clinical, haematological and cytogenetic features in 24 patients with structural rearrangements of the Q arm of chromosome 3. *Br J Haematol.* 1993;83:158-165.
225. Fonatsch C, Gudat H, Lengfelder E, et al. Correlation of cytogenetic findings with clinical features in 18 patients with inv(3)(q21q26) or t(3;3)(q21;q26). *Leukemia.* 1994;8:1318-1326.
226. Secker-Walker LM, Mehta A, Bain B. Abnormalities of 3q21 and 3q26 in myeloid malignancy: a United Kingdom Cancer Cytogenetic Group study. *Br J Haematol.* 1995;91:490-501.

Chapter 83 ■ Chronic Myeloid Leukemia

EHAB ATALLAH • MICHAEL W. DEININGER

HISTORICAL PERSPECTIVE

Chronic myeloid leukemia (CML), although a rare disease, has disproportionately impacted hematology/oncology and modern medicine. The story began in the 1830s with Alfred Francois Donné of Paris who pioneered the use of microscopy in medicine and was the first to describe the different types of blood cells. When asked to examine a blood sample of a 44-year-old woman suffering from a painless left-abdominal mass, he noticed the excess of white cells and speculated that the patient's blood may contain pus.[1,2] Donné also organized a *Cours de Microscopie*, which was attended by Edinburgh pathologist John Hughes Bennet who in 1845 published a "Case of Hypertrophy of the Spleen and Liver in which Death Took Place from Suppuration of the Blood".[3] Only a few weeks later Rudolf Virchow of Berlin reported on a very similar case in an article titled "Weisses Blut" (white blood).[4] It is likely that both patients suffered from CML and presented with its most typical clinical features: leukocytosis and splenomegaly. While Bennett believed that the new disease represented an infection, Virchow recognized the neoplastic nature of the process and coined the term "leukemia," from the Greek words "λευκον αιμα," which mean "white blood." The ensuing academic dispute was eventually settled cordially: Virchow acknowledged Bennett's priority of discovery and Bennett that leukemia is a neoplastic rather than an infectious process. The next leap forward came in 1872, when Ernst Neumann established the bone marrow as the origin of leukemia and of blood cells in general.[5] The following 100 years saw progress in understanding leukemia, with perhaps the most notable advance being the recognition of myeloid vs lymphoid disease. In 1951, William Dameshek posited that CML belongs to a larger group of related disorders characterized by increased numbers of differentiated blood cells as the result of enhanced proliferation of the bone marrow, which he accordingly named myeloproliferative disorders.[6]

Just as better microscopes had enabled the first description of leukemia, improvements in chromosome banding led to a breakthrough by Philadelphia cytogeneticists Peter Nowell and David Hungerford. In 1960, they described an abnormally small G-group chromosome in metaphase spreads from several patients with CML.[7] Ironically, in a now mostly forgotten manuscript, a team from Edinburgh led by Ishbel Tough reported similar findings just a few months later.[8] This first consistent karyotypic abnormality associated with cancer settled the debate as to whether DNA or proteins transmitted the neoplastic phenotype to the next generation of cells. The discovery team anticipated that this minute chromosome in CML might represent the first in a long list of cancer chromosomes, and thus referred to it as the Ph[1] chromosome, now more commonly known as Ph. The presence of Ph in all CML cells was indicative of their clonal origin from a single parental cell. Formal proof for this notion was lacking until Fred Fialkow demonstrated X-chromosome inactivation in CML neutrophils by uniform glucose-6-phosphate dehydrogenase isoenzyme expression.[9] This was consistent with inactivation of either a maternal or paternal X chromosome in all cells rather than the random inactivation characteristic of polyclonal tissues.[9]

In 1973, Janet Rowley, working at the University of Chicago, recognized that Ph was not just a shortened chromosome 22, but was in fact the product of a reciprocal translocation between chromosomes 9 and 22.[10] Over the following 25 years, the molecular anatomy and consequences of t(9;22) were revealed with increasing resolution. Work from several laboratories identified the genes juxtaposed by t(9;22) to form a fusion gene on Ph.[11,12] The chromosome 9 partner was found to be *ABL1* (formerly *ABL*), the human homolog of v-abl oncogene of the Abelson murine leukemia virus (A-MuLV).[13] On the derivative chromosome 22, *ABL1* sequences consistently translocated to the same genetic region, which became known as the "breakpoint cluster region" (*BCR*), a name that was subsequently used to describe the new gene fused upstream of *ABL1*.[14] The next discoveries were that BCR-ABL1, similar to mouse v-Abl, is a constitutively active tyrosine kinase and that kinase activity is required for cellular transformation.[15] Lastly, retroviral expression of BCR-ABL1 in mouse bone marrow cells was found to induce a CML-like disease, another milestone in the history of cancer research.[16]

Therapy developed slowly. Arsenicals, in use for cancer treatment since ancient times, were the only CML therapy available in the 19th century, usually in the form of Fowler solution, which contained potassium arsenite. The German physician Heinrich Lissauer is credited with the first publication on the remarkable efficacy of Fowler solution in a patient with leukemia.[17] In an 1882 *Lancet* paper, Conan Doyle, the author of the Sherlock Holmes detective stories, published on a patient with the clinical presentation of CML who achieved a partial response to arsenic.[18] It seems the reviewers of his paper gave him a pass on novelty, since the use of arsenic for cancer therapy had been described by the poet Valmiki in the Indian Ramayana in approximately 500 BC. In the 1920s, splenic irradiation was used for symptomatic relief and remained the mainstay of therapy for the first half of the 20th century. In 1959, busulfan was introduced as the first drug that reliably controlled white blood cell counts in CML and, 10 years later, hydroxyurea premiered as the first intervention that significantly prolonged survival.[19] Despite these advances, a cure remained elusive until the late 1970s, when the Seattle group reported the disappearance of Ph in CML patients who underwent HCT.[20] Soon after that, interferon (IFN)-α was found to induce durable complete cytogenetic responses (CCyRs) and long-term survival in 10% to 20% of patients.[21] In 1992, Alexander Levitzki proposed inhibiting ABL1 with small molecules called tyrphostins as a potentially useful approach to treat leukemias driven by *ABL1* oncogenes.[22] At about the same time, Alois Matter, Jürg Zimmermann, and Nick Lydon at Ciba-Geigy had synthesized a compound called GCP57148B, now known as imatinib, that inhibited ABL1 and a restricted set of other tyrosine kinases at submicromolar concentrations.[23] Of note, GCP57148B's anti-ABL activity was the serendipitous byproduct of a drug development effort to identify inhibitors of platelet-derived growth factor receptor (PDGFR) for cardiovascular indications. Clinical trials led by Brian Druker from Oregon Health & Science University, very much in the face of skepticism by the manufacturer, rapidly established imatinib's unprecedented activity in patients with CML and revolutionized CML therapy.[24-26] Solving the crystal structure of ABL1 in complex with imatinib provided the foundation for subsequent studies into the autoregulation of ABL1 kinase activity and its disruption in BCR-ABL1.[27-29] These studies were of fundamental importance for understanding kinases and their regulation in physiological and aberrant signal transduction. Despite imatinib's general efficacy, subsets of patients developed resistance, frequently due to point mutations in BCR-ABL1, stimulating the development of subsequent generations of tyrosine kinase inhibitors (TKIs).[30-32] Dasatinib, nilotinib, and bosutinib are second-generation (2G) TKIs with increased activity against BCR-ABL1 that were initially developed to overcome imatinib resistance but have since gained approval for frontline therapy.[33-35] Two additional TKIs have enriched the therapeutic armamentarium. Ponatinib is a third-generation TKI whose use is limited to specific sets of resistant patients.[36,37] The latest development is asciminib, an allosteric inhibitor that mimics the physiological autoinhibition of ABL1.[38,39] Despite the unprecedented efficacy of TKIs, once CML has progressed to the blast phase (BP), allogeneic stem cell transplant is still the recommendation for all eligible patients.

There is compelling evidence that CML stem cells are not dependent on BCR-ABL1 kinase activity.[40] Nonetheless, starting with the Stop Imatinib (STIM) trial, a plethora of studies has demonstrated that approximately 50% of patients with deep molecular responses (defined as reduction of *BCR-ABL1* transcripts by at least 4 logs) maintain remission even after discontinuation of TKIs, a state termed treatment-free remission (TFR).[41] While survival remains the universal goal for all CML patients, TFR has gained much traction as a treatment goal for selected patient populations, particularly young individuals.[42]

The unprecedented success of TKIs in CML treatment has established a paradigm for molecularly targeted therapy that informs approaches in other types of cancer. However, many scientific, clinical, and societal questions remain. Despite improved understanding of blast phase CML (BP-CML) at the molecular level, no fundamentally new treatments have emerged beyond chemotherapy followed by HCT, and the prognosis remains poor. At the opposite extreme, increasing the proportion of TFR eligible patients and improving the success rate will be crucial to minimize long-term TKI toxicity. However, as the biological underpinnings of TFR have remained elusive, rational approaches to improve current results are lacking. Last but not least, the exorbitant costs of TKIs, particularly in the United States, raise ethical and societal questions that cannot be answered on medical grounds alone.[43] Again, CML has prepared the ground for fundamental discussions far beyond what one might expect from an orphan disease.

PATHOPHYSIOLOGY

It is thought that CML originates from a single hematopoietic cell that has acquired Ph. In contrast to acute myeloid leukemia (AML)–associated fusion genes like *MOZ-TIF2*, *BCR-ABL1* does not confer self-renewal capacity, implying that the initial translocation event must occur in a multipotent hematopoietic stem cell (HSC) already endowed with this critical property.[44] *BCR-ABL1* is detected in cells of all hematopoietic lineages. For unknown reasons, the *BCR-ABL1*–induced cellular expansion predominantly targets the myeloid progenitor cell compartment, giving rise to the clinical phenotype, while many newly diagnosed patients have mostly Ph⁻ stem cells.[45] Consequently, the hierarchical organization of hematopoiesis is maintained during the chronic phase, and a substantial number of Ph⁻ stem cells are available to reconstitute the system if CML hematopoiesis is therapeutically suppressed. Both factors are important for the response to TKIs. The salient biologic features of CML cells are increased proliferation, resistance to apoptosis, perturbed interaction with bone marrow stromal cells, and genetic instability.[46]

BCR-ABL1 Translocation and Fusion Gene

Ph is the result of a reciprocal translocation between the long arms of chromosomes 9 and 22 (t[9;22][q34;q11]).[10] As a result of this translocation, genetic sequences from the *ABL1* gene on 9q34 are fused downstream of the *BCR* gene on 22q11 (*Figure 83.1A* and *B*). With rare exceptions, breaks in chromosome 22 localize to one of three *BCR*s and determine the portions of *BCR* retained in the *BCR-ABL1* fusion mRNA and protein. In contrast, the chromosome 9 breaks occur over a large genetic region, 5′ of *ABL1* exon Ib, 3′ of *ABL1* exon Ia, or most commonly between the two alternative first *ABL1* exons. Rare exceptions aside, splicing consistently leads to fusion mRNAs that encompass *ABL1* exons 2 to 11 (*Figure 83.1C*).[47] Breakpoints in the minor *BCR* (m-*BCR*) give rise to an e1a2 fusion mRNA and p190$^{BCR-ABL}$, which is found in two-thirds of Ph⁺ acute lymphoblastic leukemia (ALL) cases. The very rare p190$^{BCR-ABL}$ positive CML is associated with monocytosis and exhibits a more aggressive clinical course.[48] The origin and biology of p190$^{BCR-ABL}$-positive CML is mysterious. Either m-*BCR* rearrangements are much less likely to occur in HSCs than the major *BCR* (M-*BCR*) rearrangements typical of CML, or the cell of origin is different, or a yet unknown concomitant somatic mutation creates a state conducive to transformation by p190$^{BCR-ABL}$. In an overwhelming majority of CML patients, the break occurs in the M-*BCR*, generating e13a2 or e14a2 fusion mRNAs (formerly referred to as b2a2 and b3a2) and a p210$^{BCR-ABL}$ fusion protein. p230$^{BCR-ABL}$, the largest of the fusion proteins, corresponds to a break in the micro *BCR*, an e19a2 fusion mRNA, and is associated with neutrophilic predominance and possibly less aggressive disease.[49] Besides the major types of *BCR-ABL1* fusion mRNAs, there are rare variants whose main clinical significance is that they can give rise to misleading reverse transcription polymerase chain reaction (RT-PCR) results.[50-52] Approximately two-thirds of CML cases also express the reciprocal *ABL1-BCR* mRNA, but there is no definitive evidence that this influences disease biology or prognosis.[53,54] However, absence of *ABL1-BCR* mRNA is evidence for deletions flanking the breakpoints in *BCR*, *ABL1*, or both. For unknown reasons, the deletions are associated with significantly reduced survival in patients treated with IFN-α, but their adverse impact is reduced or abolished by TKI therapy.[55,56]

BCR and ABL1 Proteins and Their Contribution to Cellular Transformation

BCR is a ubiquitously expressed 160 kDa cytoplasmic protein with several functional domains (*Figure 83.2A*). The N-terminus contains a coiled-coil motif that allows for dimerization, which is critical for activation of ABL1 kinase in the BCR-ABL1 fusion protein.[57] Further down from 3′ there are: a serine/threonine kinase motif whose only recognized substrate is Bap-1, a member of the 14-3-3 family of proteins, and *dbl*-like and pleckstrin-homology domains.[58,59] It is thought that these domains stimulate the exchange of GTP for Guanosine diphosphate (GDP) on Rho guanidine exchange factors.[59] The C-terminus of BCR contains a putative site for calcium-dependent lipid binding and a GTPase activating function (RAC-GAP). The latter regulates activity of RAC, a small GTPase of the RAS superfamily that regulates actin polymerization and an NADPH oxidase in phagocytic cells.[60,61] Despite these diverse functions, *Bcr* null mice are viable and fertile and the only recognizable defect is an increased oxidative burst in neutrophils, suggesting redundancy of signaling pathways.[62] BCR can be phosphorylated on several tyrosine residues, most importantly tyrosine 177, which binds GRB2, an adapter molecule involved in activation of the RAS pathway in CML cells.[63,64] The Rho-GEF and RAC-GAP functions of BCR retained in p210$^{BCR-ABL}$ but missing from p190$^{BCR-ABL}$ are thought to attenuate the disease and cause a phenotypic shift from lymphoid to myeloid leukemia (*Figure 83.2C*).[59,65,66] Recent work has shown that the protein networks entertained by p190$^{BCR-ABL1}$ and p210$^{BCR-ABL1}$ are profoundly different, and the differences have been attributed to the retention of the PH domain in p210$^{BCR-ABL1}$.[67] It remains unclear how this impacts lineage commitment and why HSCs are susceptible to transformation by p210$^{BCR-ABL}$, while p190$^{BCR-ABL1}$ targets pre-B cells.[68] Although it has been suggested that BCR may negatively regulate BCR-ABL1–induced leukemogenesis,[69] incidence and biology of p190$^{BCR-ABL1}$-induced leukemia are identical in *Bcr*$^{-/-}$ mice compared to wild-type mice, indicating that BCR is not essential for Ph⁺ leukemia.[70]

ABL1, the human homolog of the v-*abl* oncogene of the A-MuLV,[13] encodes a non–receptor tyrosine kinase.[71] The 145-kDa ABL1 protein is ubiquitously expressed and exhibits two isoforms arising from alternative splicing of the first exon.[72] The N-terminal region contains three SRC-homology domains (SH1–SH3). SH1 carries the tyrosine kinase function, while the SH2 and SH3 domains engage in protein-protein interactions (*Figure 83.2B*).[73] Additionally, proline-rich sequences in the center of ABL1 interact with SH3 domains of other proteins such as Crk.[74] The C-terminus contains nuclear localization, DNA-binding,[75] and actin-binding motifs.[76] Diverse functions have been attributed to ABL1, which include negative regulation of cell cycle and proliferation,[76,77] response to genotoxic stress,[78-82] and integrin signaling.[80] Gain of function in the germline is also detrimental, as shown by a recent report of mutations in the myristate binding pocket that confer constitutive kinase activation and are associated with cardiac and skeletal defects.[83] The emerging picture is complex and perhaps ABL1 could best be characterized as a cellular module that integrates signals from various extra- and intracellular sources to influence decisions regarding cell cycle and apoptosis. *Abl1*$^{-/-}$ mice have a severe phenotype,

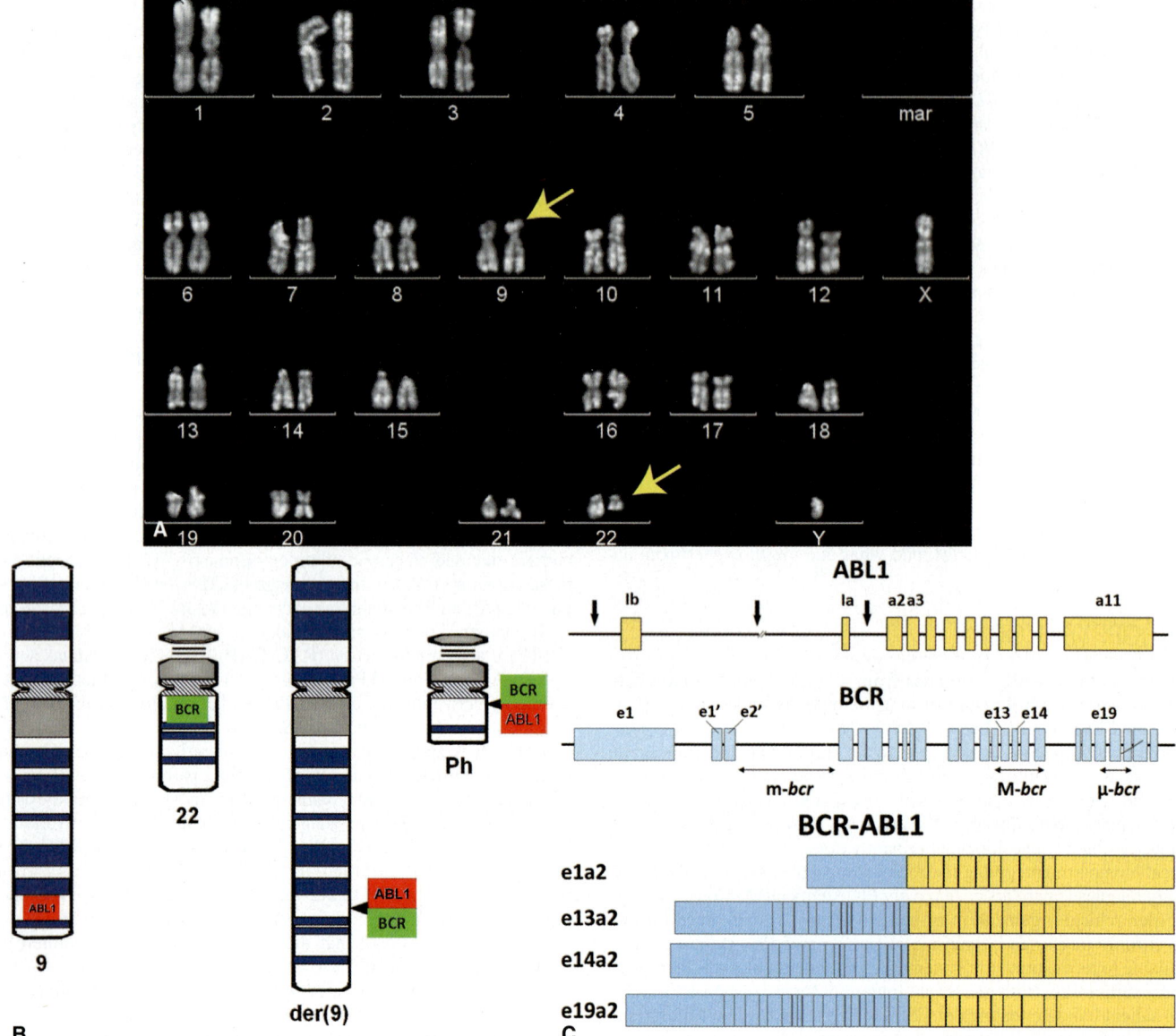

FIGURE 83.1 A, Metaphase karyogram of a newly diagnosed man with CML. The yellow arrows indicate the derivative chromosome 9 and the Philadelphia chromosome (Ph). B, Schematic of chromosomes 9, 22 and the derivatives resulting from t(9;22) (q34;q11). C, Molecular anatomy of the BCR-ABL1 translocation (upper panels). Genomic loci of ABL1 and BCR with exon numbering. The three breakpoint cluster regions in BCR are also indicated. (lower panel). Fusion mRNAs derived from the chimeric genes. Note that the e13a2 and e14a2 fusion mRNAs were previously referred to as b2a2 and b3a2, respectively.

including high perinatal mortality, runting, and skeletal and immune system defects.[84,85] Mice null for *Abl1* and the *Abl*-related gene (formerly *Arg*, now *Abl2*) are embryonically lethal owing to absence of neurulation.[86] The latter observation raised considerable concerns about the potential side effects of ABL inhibitors that were fortunately not confirmed clinically.

Constitutive Kinase Activation in the BCR-ABL1 Fusion Protein

In contrast to ABL1, a tightly regulated nuclear kinase, BCR-ABL1 is constitutively active and localized to the cytoplasm. The mechanism by which the replacement of the ABL1 N-terminus with BCR sequences leads to kinase activation has been probed by mutagenesis and X-ray crystallography.[87] A critical feature is the coiled-coil domain of BCR that promotes dimerization, which allows for an initial transphosphorylation event, followed by autophosphorylation of additional tyrosine residues to fully activate the kinase.[88] Other proteins with the ability to form dimers can substitute for BCR, such as ETV6 and NUP214 that form ABL1 fusion genes associated with an myeloproliferative neoplasm (MPN) or ALL.[89,90] The N-terminal "cap" region of ABL1, when myristoylated, binds a hydrophobic pocket at the base of the kinase domain. The resulting conformation resembles a latch that seems to hold the kinase in an inactive state.[28,29,91] However, small molecules binding to the myristate pocket can inhibit kinase activity, indicating that the concept of a "mechanical" latch is too simplistic. Rather than that, an allosteric mechanism controls kinase activity that does not require the ABL1 N-terminal sequences and hence is preserved and amenable to therapeutic targeting in BCR-ABL1.[38,92] How precisely information is communicated from the myristate pocket to the catalytic site is unknown. Recent data suggest that reverse signaling is also possible, as mutations in the adenosine triphosphate (ATP) site can influence binding of small molecules to the myristate pocket.[93] Additional levels of regulation exist: certain residues within the SH2 domain participate in the regulation of kinase activity,[94] and trans-acting binding partners such as the ABL1 interacting proteins have been implicated as physiological inhibitors.[95,96]

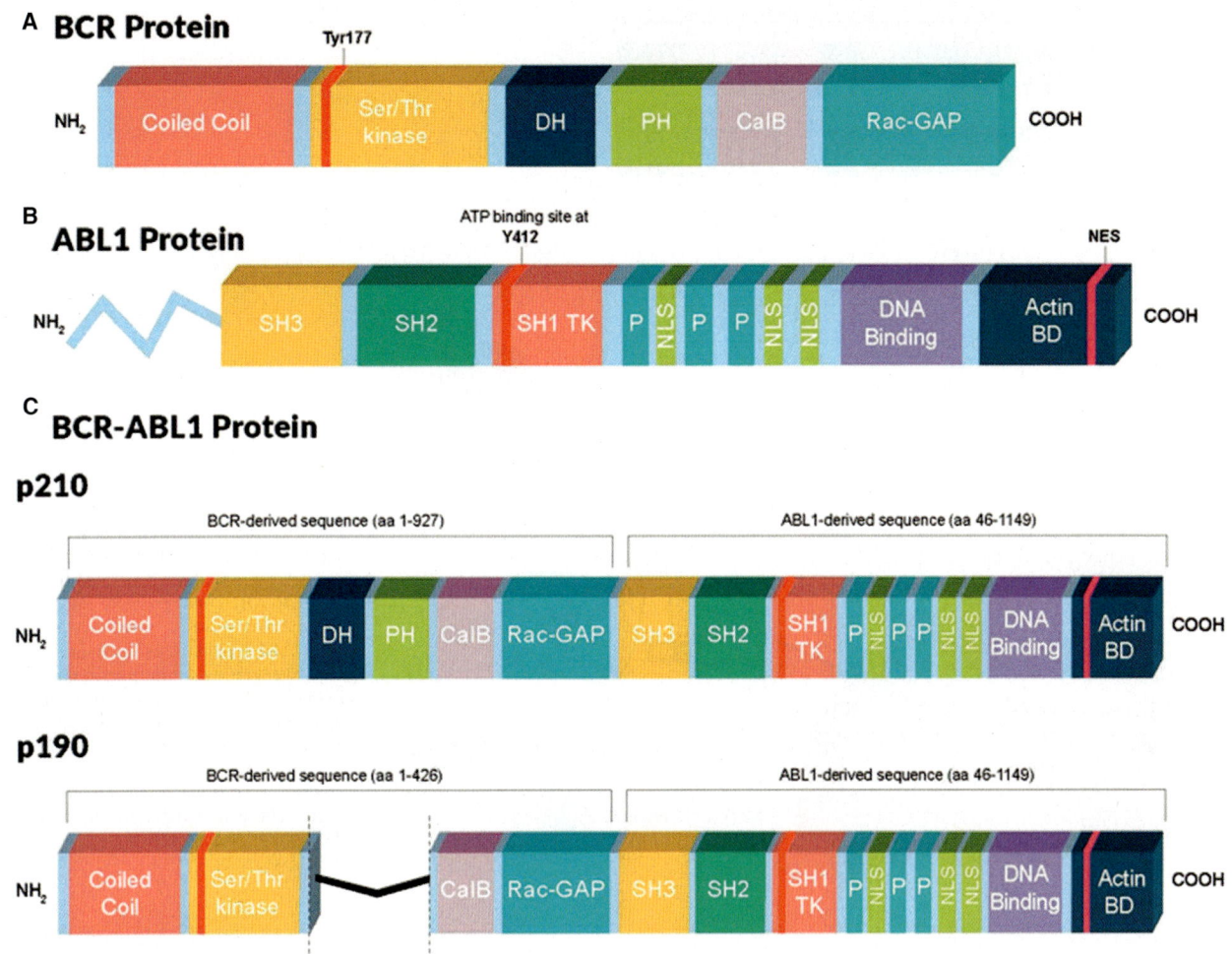

FIGURE 83.2 **Structural domains and signaling motifs in BCR, ABL1, and BCR-ABL1 proteins.** A, BCR protein. Shown are the N-terminal coiled coil (oligomerization), serine/threonine kinase, Dbl-like domain (DH), pleckstrin homology (PH) domain, calcium-binding domain (CalB), and Rac-GAP domain. B, ABL1 protein. Shown are SRC homology domains 1 to 3 (SH1-3), proline-rich motifs (P), nuclear localization signals (NLS), DNA-binding domain, and actin-binding domain. C, p210BCR-ABL1 and p190BCR-ABL1 proteins. Note that p210BCR-ABL1 retains the DH and PH domains, which are missing from p190BCR-ABL1.

Signaling Pathways in BCR-ABL1 Transformed Cells

Two decades of intense research have identified multiple BCR-ABL1 substrates, binding partners, and downstream signaling molecules involved in the process of cellular transformation (*Figure 83.3*). Much effort has been directed at linking these pathways to the specific pathologic features that characterize CML cells, such as increased proliferation or genetic instability leading to disease progression. A comprehensive review of the multiple pathways implicated in BCR-ABL1 transformation is beyond the scope of this chapter. Studies of mice with homozygous deletions of signaling proteins have identified very few pathway components with a truly essential role for BCR-ABL1–induced leukemia, speaking to the extensive redundancy of the transformation network.

Phosphatidylinositol-3 Kinase

In BCR-ABL1 expressing cells, phosphatidylinositol-3 kinase (PI3K) is activated by at least two different mechanisms. The first requires autophosphorylation of BCR-ABL1 tyrosine 177 (Y177), which generates a docking site for the GRB2 adapter protein, which in turn recruits GAB2, another adapter, into a complex that activates PI3K.[97,98] Consistent with a critical role for the Y177/GRB2/GAB2 axis, mutation of tyrosine 177 to phenylalanine or lack of GAB2 abrogates myeloid leukemia in murine models.[98] Alternatively, PI3K can be activated by complex formation between the p85 regulatory subunit of PI3K, CBL, and CRKL, which bind to the SH2 and proline-rich domains of BCR-ABL1.[99] The main downstream outlet of PI3K is the serine-threonine kinase AKT, a major conduit for oncogenic signals in different cancer types. In CML cells, AKT enhances survival by suppressing activity of the forkhead O transcription factors (FOXO), as well as phosphorylation and inactivation of proapoptotic proteins like BAD.[100,101] Additionally, PI3K promotes proteasomal degradation of p27, a cyclin-dependent kinase inhibitor, through upregulation of SKP2, the F-Box recognition protein of SCF^{SKP2} E3 ubiquitin ligase. Accordingly, the absence of SKP2 from leukemia cells prolongs survival in a murine CML model.[102] Furthermore, AKT activates mTOR, which phosphorylates ribosomal proteins p70S6 kinase (S6K) and 4E-BP1. S6K, a serine/threonine kinase, phosphorylates multiple substrates that collectively promote cell proliferation. Phosphorylated mTOR has been shown to inactivate 4EBP-1, releasing the translation initiation factor eIF4E from inhibition to enhance protein synthesis.[103,104]

RAS/Mitogen-Activated Protein Kinase Pathways

Phosphorylation of tyrosine 177 with recruitment of GRB2 and SOS promotes exchange of GTP for GDP on RAS.[97,105] In its GTP-bound form, RAS activates the serine-threonine kinase RAF-1,[106,107] which subsequently activates mitogen-activated protein kinase. Other small GTPases like RAC1/2 have also been implicated in BCR-ABL1 signaling.[108] Lack of RAC1/2 has been shown to delay *BCR-ABL1* leukemia in a mouse model.[109]

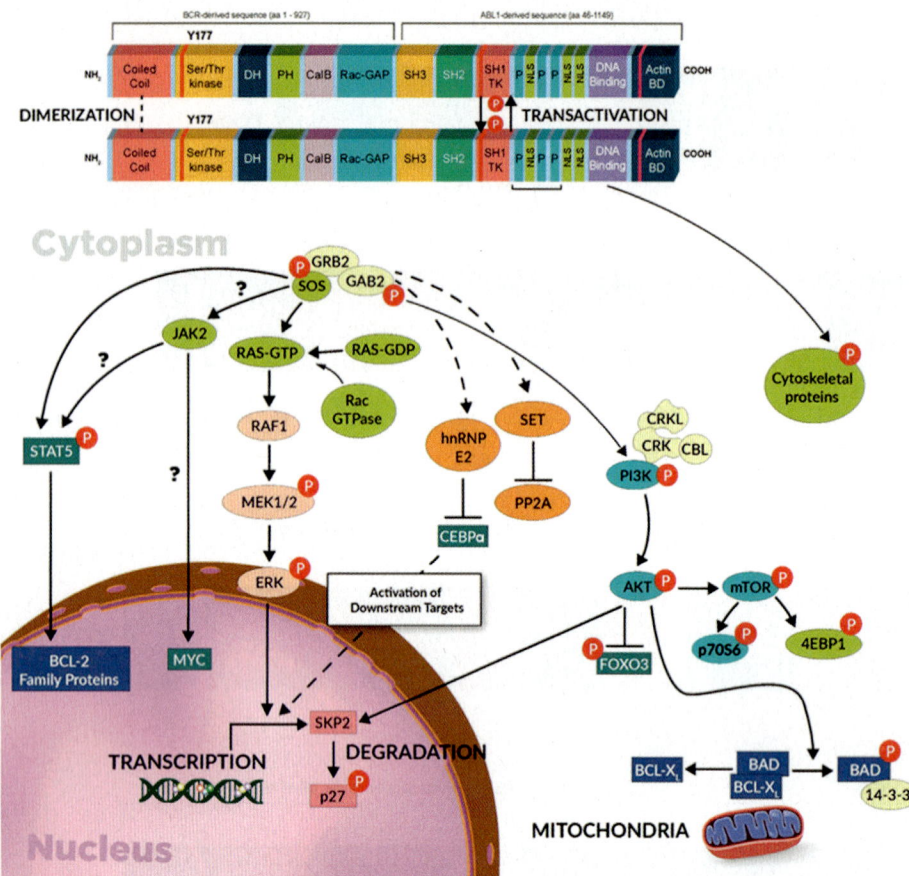

FIGURE 83.3 Simplified representation of signaling pathways activated in CML cells. Autophosphorylation generates binding sites on BCR-ABL1 that promote interaction with intermediary proteins, some of which are also BCR-ABL1 substrates such as CRKL and CBL, generating a multimeric complex. The BCR-ABL1 signaling complexes activate multiple downstream pathways that inhibit apoptosis, enhance proliferation, perturb adhesion and migration, and confer instability. Few of these downstream mediators are required for BCR-ABL's ability to transform cells, indicating that the signaling network is highly redundant. For details, see text.

Janus Kinase/Signal Transducer and Activator of Transcription Pathway

The transcription factor signal transducer and activator of transcription 5 (STAT5) is constitutively tyrosine-phosphorylated in CML cells. Initial experiments in mice failed to demonstrate a critical role for STAT5.[110] However, it was subsequently established that the mice used in this study were not null for *Stat5*, but expressed an N-terminally deleted protein with partially retained function. While STAT5 is not required for the initiation of CML, there is convincing evidence that it plays a rate-limiting role in leukemogenesis.[111,112] In fact, absence of only STAT5A or overexpression of a dominant-negative STAT5 mutant in the bone marrow attenuates CML.[113] The principal consequence of STAT5 activation is inhibition of apoptosis by enhancing transcription of antiapoptotic proteins like MCL-1 and BCL-XL.[114] Importantly, conditional deletion of STAT5 prevents the establishment of active CML in mice, but does not eliminate the BCR-ABL1 expressing cells.[111] BCR-ABL1 may activate STAT5 through direct phosphorylation or indirectly by promoting phosphorylation by HCK or Janus kinase 2 (JAK2).[115,116] There is controversy about the role of JAK2 in *BCR-ABL1*–induced leukemia. Previous studies had suggested that JAK2 plays an important if not essential role,[117] but a recent report using conditional knockout technology showed that murine CML does not require JAK2.[118]

Cytoskeletal Proteins

BCR-ABL1 phosphorylates several proteins involved in adhesion and migration, including focal adhesion kinase, CRKL, paxillin, p130CAS, and HEF1.[119-124] Although details remain to be elucidated, it is thought that this may explain why integrin-mediated adhesion of CML progenitors to bone marrow stroma and extracellular matrix is defective. Alternatively, integrin functions may be compromised through activation of RAS or BCR-ABL1 binding to F-actin.[97,125] Given that adhesion of integrins inhibits proliferation of hematopoietic progenitors, the defect in integrin function may contribute to the premature circulation as well as the abnormal proliferation of Ph+ progenitor cells.[126]

DNA Damage Surveillance and Repair Pathways

The fact that untreated chronic phase CML (CP-CML) invariably progresses to BP-CML is testimony to the profound dysregulation of DNA repair in CML. A central finding is the two- to sixfold increase in reactive oxygen species (ROS) in CML CD34+ cells compared to normal controls, which is particularly pronounced in BP-CML cells.[127-129] ROS generate oxidized bases and double-strand breaks (DSBs). It was estimated that CML cells may contain up to eight times more oxidized bases and DSBs than normal cells.[130] It was generally thought that ROS generation in CML cell is controlled by BCR-ABL1 through activation of PI3K. However, recent mouse work has shown that this may not be the case in CML stem cells, which continue to accumulate ROS-induced DNA damage despite TKI inhibition of BCR-ABL1.[131,132] An additional mutagenic mechanism operational in lymphoid BP cells is activation of activation-induced cytidine deaminase, which promotes point mutations.[133]

The consequences of increased DNA damage are greatly aggravated by impairment of DNA damage surveillance and repair. Multiple mechanisms have been implicated, and many but not all these mechanisms are BCR-ABL1 dependent. For example, BCR-ABL1 has been shown to impair the intra-S-phase cell cycle checkpoint through suppression of checkpoint kinase 1, either by inhibition of the nuclear protein kinase ATR[134] or downregulation of BRCA1, a substrate of ataxia telangiectasia mutated.[135] Nonhomologous end-joining (NHEJ) and homologous recombination (HR), critical DSB repair pathways, are also deregulated in CML. For instance, the catalytic subunit of DNA-dependent protein kinase is downregulated in CD34+ CML progenitors, leading to error-prone NHEJ.[136] Furthermore,

BCR-ABL1 upregulates RAD51.[137] As a result, DSB repair upon challenge with cytotoxic agents and induced ROS is shifted toward a rapid but low-fidelity pathway, thus promoting chronic oxidative DNA damage. Lastly, telomere length is correlated with time to disease progression.[138]

Cycling cells have access to a range of DNA repair mechanisms, including HR, single strand annealing, transcription-associated homologous recombination and NHEJ. In contrast, quiescent cells have limited options, using mostly NHEJ (*Figure 83.4A*). There are differences in the usage of the various DNA repair pathways between LSCs and HSCs that in the future may provide individualized therapeutic opportunities, based on the principle of synthetic lethality. For instance, BRCA1/2 is frequently downregulated in CML. Additionally, some cases have downregulated one of the components of D-NHEJ, rendering them vulnerable to a combination of PARP inhibitors such as olaparib and inhibitors of RAD51, while cycling HSCs can resort to BRCA1/2-based HR, and quiescent HSCs to D-NHEJ (*Figure 83.4B and C*).[139,140] There is little evidence that TKIs themselves cause DNA damage, although imatinib was reported to induce centrosome abnormalities in vitro.[141] Conflicting data have been reported regarding the risk of second (nonhematologic) malignancies in CML patients on TKIs, but there is consensus that any excess incidence is related to CML rather than TKI therapy.[142,143] Similarly, there is no evidence that the clonal cytogenetic abnormalities in Ph-negative cells (CCA/Ph−) detected in 5% to 10% of CML patients with a cytogenetic response to TKI therapy are induced by TKIs.[144]

CML Hematopoiesis

In contrast to acute leukemia, the hierarchical structure of hematopoiesis is initially maintained in CML. Maturation is delayed, but cellular function is mostly normal, evidenced by the fact that CP-CML patients are not at increased risk of infection or bleeding. Although *BCR-ABL1* is present in cells of all hematopoietic lineages, including B cells and T cells, the thrust of *BCR-ABL1*–induced cellular expansion targets the myeloid progenitor cell compartment, which is almost exclusively Ph+.[145] In contrast, in most newly diagnosed patients, the majority of the most primitive cells (defined as long-term culture initiating cells, long-term culture initiating cells or quiescent CD34+ cells) are partially or even predominantly Ph−.[45] These normal HSCs are the basis for cytogenetic and molecular responses to therapy. The cause of the myeloid bias is incompletely understood. One possible explanation is that BCR-ABL1 alone is insufficient to overcome the powerful metabolic growth restraint placed on lymphoid precursor cells, which is thought to minimize the risk of malignant transformation during V(D)J rearrangement or T cell receptor diversification.[146]

What distinguishes LSCs from HSCs has been the topic of intense research. The ultimate diagnostic test for stemness is functional—the ability of a cell to generate progeny of all lineages in vivo, while phenotypic markers are only surrogates. As such, the terms HSC and LSC frequently denote populations of cells that are enriched for functionally defined "true" stem cells, but not pure populations. For instance, in many studies stem cells are conveniently defined as lineage−CD34+CD38−, but <10% of these cells are functional stem cells. Thus far no universal immunophenotypic marker has been identified that separates LSCs from HSCs, but strategies using multiple markers have achieved considerable enrichment for BCR-ABL+ cells. The issue is complicated by the fact that some, but not all, markers are regulated by BCR-ABL1 kinase activity, and that TKIs predominantly eliminate proliferating LSCs with a late myeloid signature, while relatively sparing the most primitive LSCs.[147] Consequently, the immunophenotype of LSCs in untreated CML patients is different from that in patients with residual disease on TKIs. Some clinical features of CML can be linked to biological aberrancies of LSCs. For instance, LSCs exhibit reduced integrin-mediated adhesion to bone marrow stroma and abnormal migration to CXCL12 (SDF1), which may account for leukocytosis and extramedullary hematopoiesis in the spleen and liver.[148,149] Transcriptomic profiling of CD34+38− cells showed that quiescent LSCs are primed to proliferate compared to HSCs, explaining their hypersensitivity to cytokines such as interleukin-3 and granulocyte colony stimulating factor.[150,151]

A question of considerable clinical importance is whether CML stem cells are dependent on BCR-ABL1 or not. The fact that residual *BCR-ABL1+* cells remain detectable by PCR in most patients on TKIs has been interpreted as evidence for persistence of LSCs despite continued suppression of BCR-ABL1 kinase activity. Consistent with this, primitive CML cells survive TKI treatment ex vivo.[40,152] However, recent data have revealed that long-lived B cells and less frequently T cells account for most of the positive PCR results in patients in TFR, while granulocytes are consistently *BCR-ABL1−*. These data do not prove that multipotent CML stem cells are absent, but they explain the puzzling observation of positive PCR results in patients with stable TFR for years. Conceptually, the central question is whether an LSC with kinase-disabled BCR-ABL1 is equal to a normal HSC or is still "re-wired." The latter could happen through at least three mechanisms. First there is compelling data that some BCR-ABL1 functions are kinase independent.[102,126] Whether these functions alone are sufficient to support long-term survival of LSCs is unknown. Second, epigenetic reprogramming as a result of exposure to unopposed BCR-ABL1 kinase activity could persist even when BCR-ABL1 is no longer active.[153] Third, the presence of a large multidomain protein like BCR-ABL1 may interfere with physiological signaling, for instance, through sequestration of adaptor proteins. Indeed, considerable evidence has accumulated to suggest that LSCs exhibit specific vulnerabilities that may be exploitable therapeutically, either alone or in combination with TKIs (*Table 83.1*). Although several pathways, such as β-catenin, PP2A, and JAK2, are supported by multiple independent studies, translation of these data into clinical trials has been slow and conclusive data regarding clinical efficacy are mostly missing.

A wealth of data on BCR-ABL1 signaling has been amassed, yet a complete picture is still elusive. As conventional approaches have

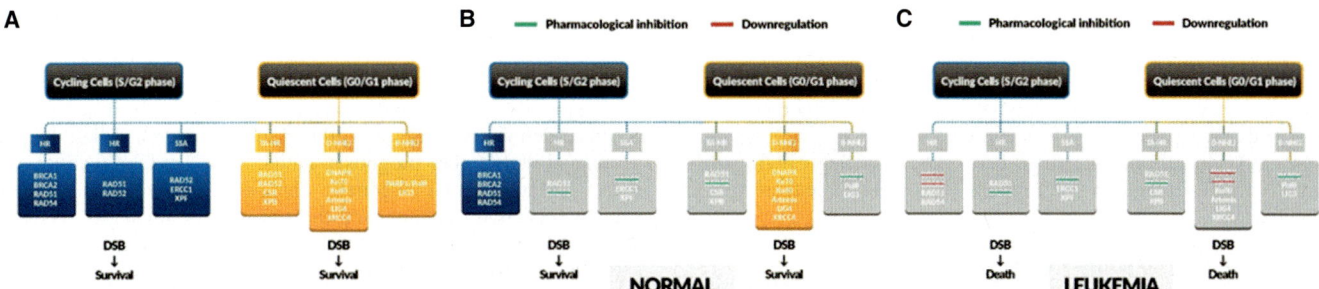

FIGURE 83.4 DNA repair pathways in cycling and quiescent HSCs and LSCs. A, Fully active DNA repair. B, Cycling HSCs maintain BRCA1/2-dependent homologous recombination (HR) upon inhibition of RAD52-dependent HR, single-strand annealing and transcription-dependent homologous recombination and DNA-PK–dependent nonhomologous end joining (D-NHEJ) upon PARP inhibition of B-NHEJ with drugs such as olaparib. C, Cycling and HSCs from some patients downregulate BRCA1/2 and/or components of the D-NHEJ (DNA-PK, Ku70, Ku80, LIG4), respectively, and become susceptible to synthetically lethal combinations of RAD52 and PARP inhibitors. DSB, double strand break.

Table 83.1. Pathways Implicated in the Survival of CML Stem Cells

Pathway	Publications	Clinical Trial	Status	Final Report
WNT/β-Catenin	Zhao et al *Cancer Cell* 2007[154]; McWeeney et al *Blood* 2010[155]; Heidel et al *Cell Stem Cell* 2012[155]; Schürch et al *JCI* 2012[157]; Lim et al *PNAS* 2013[158]; Zhang et al *Blood* 2013[159]; Eiring et al *Leukemia* 2015[160]; Agarwal et al *Blood* 2017[161]	No	NA	NA
HDAC	Zhang et al *Cancer Cell* 20109[162]	Panobinostat	Lack of efficacy	No
Hedgehog	Dierks et al *Cancer Cell* 2008[163]; Zhao et al *Nature* 2009[164]	LDE225+NIL BMS-833923+DAS	Terminated Terminated	No No
5-Lipoxygenase	Chen et al *Nat Genet.* 2009[165]	Zileuton+IM	Terminated	No
BCL6	Hurtz et al *JExMed.* 2011[166]	No	NA	NA
MYC	Ravie et al *Cancer Cell* 2013[167]; Abraham et al *Nature* 2016[168]	No	NA	NA
PP2A	Neviani et al *JCI* 2013[169]; Lai et al *Sci Trans Med*[170]	No	NA	NA
SIRT1	Li et al *Cancer Cell* 2012[171]	No	NA	NA
PRMT5	Jin et al *JCI* 2016[172]	No	NA	NA
Rad52	Cramer-Morales et al *Blood* 2013[139]	No	NA	NA
PIM2	Ma et al *PNAS* 2019[173]	No	NA	NA
BCL2	Goff et al *Cancer Stem Cell* 2013[174]	Venetoclax+DAS	Recruiting	NA
PPRγ	Prost et al *Nature* 2015[175]	Pioglitazone	Potentially active	Rousselot et al *Cancer* 2017[176]
Autophagy	Bellodi et al *JCI* 2009[177]; Baqero et al *Blood* 2019[178]	Chloroquine	Modest activity	Horne et al *Leukemia* 2020[179]
PML	Ito et al *Nature* 2008[180]	Arsenic trioxide	Terminated or not reported	NA
JAK2/STAT3/STAT5	Ye et al *Blood* 2006[113]; Traer et al *Leukemia* 2012[181]; Neviani et al *JCI* 2013[169]; Gallipoli et al *Blood* 2014[182]; Eiring et al *Leukemia* 2015[160]	Ruxolitinib+TKI	Potentially active	Sweet et al *Leuk Res* 2018[183]
Mitochondrial protein translation	Kuntz et al *Nat Med* 2017[184]	No	No	NA
TGFβ	Naka et al *Nature* 2010[185]	No	No	NA
Musashi2	Ito et al *Nature* 2010[186]	No	No	NA
ADAR1	Jiang et al *PNAS* 2013[187]	No	No	NA
EZH2	Scott et al *Cancer Discov* 2016[188]; Xie et al *Cancer Discov* 2016[189]			
ASXL1	Branford et al *Blood* 2018[190]			
TET2	Kreuzer KA et al. *Br J Haemotol* 2001[191]			
WT1	Roche-Lestienne et al *Leukemia* 2011[192]			

Abbreviations: DAS, dasatinib; IM, imatinib; NA, not applicable; NIL, nilotinib.
Modified from Eiring AM, Deininger MW. Individualizing kinase-targeted cancer therapy: the paradigm of chronic myeloid leukemia. *Genome Biol.* 2014;15(9):461. http://creativecommons.org/licenses/by/4.0/

typically focused on single pathways, efforts are now underway to characterize more comprehensively BCR-ABL1 signaling complexes by quantitative genomics.[67,193] These data suggest that cellular processes in CML rely on integrated networks rather than single pathways, which cooperate to fully realize BCR-ABL1's leukemogenic potential.

Transformation to Blast Phase

As the chronic phase of CML is compatible with life, one could argue that the main objective in CML therapy is to prevent transformation to BP-CML, an acute leukemia with myeloid (M-BP) or, less commonly, pre B cell phenotype (L-BP). A host of genetic alterations has been associated with transformation to BP (*Figure 83.5*). CCA/Ph+ is present in 70% to 80% of cases and includes various nonrandom abnormalities. Classically, +8, +Ph, i(17q), and +19 were considered as "major route" abnormalities, although this is not a universally accepted definition.[194] Several other recurrent abnormalities are also associated with a poor prognosis, including −7 and 3q26 abnormalities.[195] Many other cytogenetic changes have been described in smaller subsets of patients, and their prognostic impact is less well established. This notwithstanding, the acquisition of any CCA/Ph+ in a patient on TKI therapy is consistent with a diagnosis of accelerated phase CML (AP-CML) irrespective of other disease features.[42] Next-generation sequencing (NGS) has revealed point mutations, indels, and fusion genes in addition to BCR-ABL1 (*Figure 83.5*). For example, inactivating mutations of *RUNX1* occur in ~25% of M-BP cases, respectively, while ~55% of L-BP cases have inactivating mutations in *IKZF1*.[190,196,197]

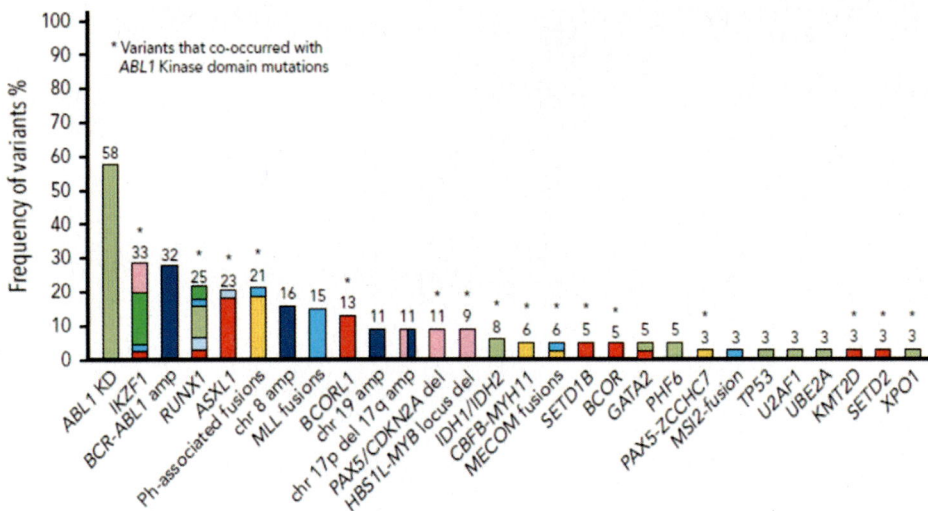

FIGURE 83.5 Somatic mutations associated with blast phase CML. (Reprinted from Branford S, Wang P, Yeung DT, et al. Integrative genomic analysis reveals cancer-associated mutations at diagnosis of CML in patients with high-risk disease. *Blood.* 2018;132(9):948-961. Copyright © 2018 American Society of Hematology. With permission.)

BCR-ABL1 expression tends to increase with progression to BP. In some patients, rising *BCR-ABL1* mRNA levels are associated with duplication of Ph, but in the majority, this seems to result from transcriptional upregulation due to as yet unknown mechanisms.[198] The increase in BCR-ABL1 expression promotes expression of SET, which inhibits the tumor suppressor phosphatase PP2A by forming a complex with the PP2A catalytic subunit. As PP2A activates SHP-1 to dephosphorylate BCR-ABL1 and other important substrates, reduced PP2A activity increases BCR-ABL1 activity, further enhancing the signal in a positive feedback loop.[169] Reduced SHP-1 activity has been associated with resistance to TKIs, emphasizing the importance of this pathway.[199] In addition to SET, cancerous inhibitor of PP2A (CIP2A) was implicated in PP2A inhibition in CML and high CIP2A activity is associated with a high risk of transformation to BP.[200]

The most salient feature of transformation from the chronic to the BP is the loss of terminal differentiation capacity. Rare patients acquire AML-type translocations such as *CBFβ-MYH11* at the time of transformation.[201] Mutant RUNX1 functions in a dominant-negative fashion to block neutrophil differentiation.[202] In most M-BC patients, myeloid differentiation is impaired due to suppression of CAAT enhancer binding protein α (C/EBPα), which is the result of enhanced expression of the RNA-binding protein heterogeneous nuclear ribonucleoprotein E2 (hnRNP-E2), which inhibits C/EBPα translation. Two mechanisms underlie the increased expression and activity of hnRNP-E2. First the increase in BCR-ABL1 activity promotes expression of hnRNP-E2.[203] Second, miR-328, which binds to hnRNP-E2 to block its activity, is downregulated.[204] Disruption of other myeloid transcription factors such as C/EBPβ and overexpression of MECOM (EVI-1) have also been implicated in blastic transformation.[205-207] With the loss of differentiation capacity, the organization of CML hematopoiesis is disrupted, as granulocyte-macrophage progenitor cells acquire self-renewal capacity, possibly by activation of nuclear β-catenin, undermining the hierarchical structure of chronic phase hematopoiesis.[208] Various mechanisms have been implicated in β-catenin activation, including stabilization by BCR-ABL1 tyrosine phosphorylation, inactivation of glycogen synthase kinase 3β by mis-splicing, and activation of MNK family kinases.[158,209,210] Transformation to L-BC, which has almost invariably a pre B cell phenotype, is caused by inactivation of transcription factors that are critical for orderly B cell development, such as IKZF1 or PAX-5. An important physiological function of these transcription factors is to impose a metabolic restraint on developing B cells that limits the risk of malignant transformation during antigen receptor diversification.[146] Interestingly, the types of structural rearrangements in L-BC suggest that they originate from aberrant RAG-mediated recombination.[211]

The variability of somatic mutations associated with BP-CML is consistent with conversion of multiple aberrancies into a relatively uniform phenotype. Recent multiomic work has implicated epigenetic dysregulation as the overarching mechanism. Specifically, downregulation of polycomb repressive complex 2 (PRC2) and upregulation of PRC1 activity may explain phenotypic conversion despite heterogeneous upstream mutations.[197] In this framework, histone and DNA methylation work hand in hand to achieve profound epigenetic reprogramming, consistent with the frequent mutation of epigenetic regulators observed in multiple studies.[190,212] PRC2 directs BP DNA hypermethylation, which in turn silences myeloid differentiation and tumor suppressor genes through epigenetic switching, while PRC1 represses an overlapping and distinct set of genes, including BP tumor suppressors. This may provide a rationale for therapeutic opportunities that are broadly applicable, for instance, the combination of EZH2 (PRC2) and BMI1 (PRC1) inhibitors.

CLINICAL FEATURES

Epidemiology

With an annual incidence of 1.3 to 1.6 per 10^5 population, CML accounts for 15% to 20% of cases of leukemia in adults. Males are more commonly affected, but there is no geographic, ethnic, or familial predisposition. The only well-established risk factor is exposure to ionizing radiation, evident by the increased CML incidence in survivors of the atomic bomb explosions in Japan and patients who were treated with radiotherapy or exposed to thorotrast, an α-emitting contrast medium used in the 1930s.[213-215] From 2004 to 2009, the median age at diagnosis in the United States was 64 years.[216] The prevalence of CML is increasing owing to reduced mortality, particularly in high-risk patients.[217] For the United States, estimates are 144,000 in 2030 and 181,000 in 2050, when prevalence is predicted to approach a plateau.[218] At that point, CML will become the most prevalent myeloid neoplasm, with considerable implications for health care economics.

Clinical Presentation
Signs and Symptoms

CML may present with fatigue, weight loss, fever, night sweats, bone pain, abdominal pain, and fullness.[219] Severe constitutional symptoms raise concerns about advanced disease. Splenomegaly may cause moderate discomfort, shoulder pain, or abdominal fullness; severe, sharp pain should raise suspicion of splenic infarction or rupture, rare but potentially life-threatening CML complications.[219] Excessively high white blood cell counts can lead to leukostasis, especially in case

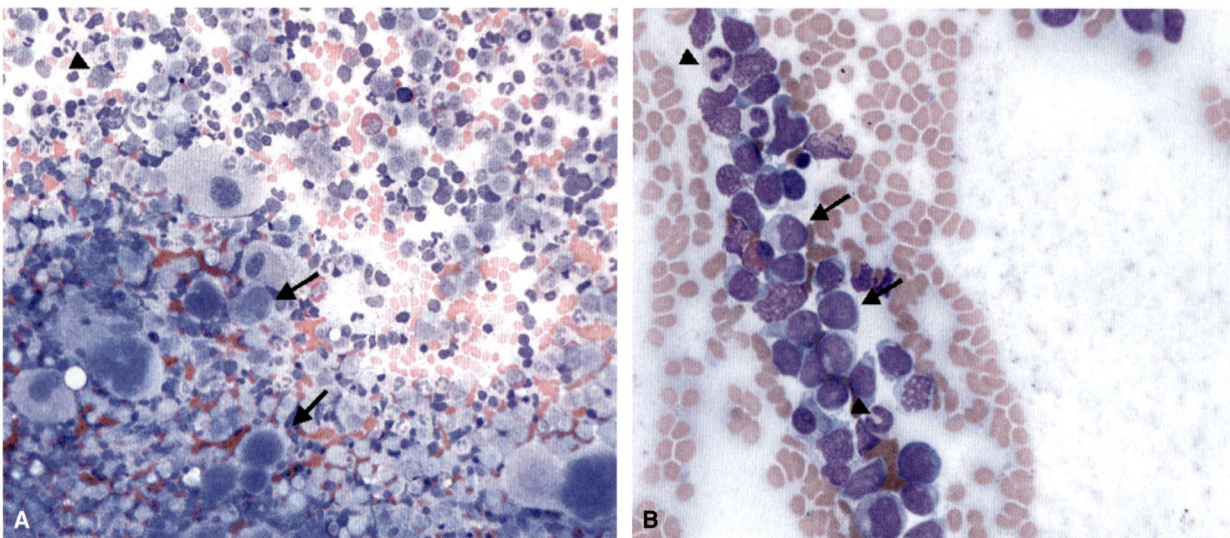

FIGURE 83.6 A, Bone marrow aspirate in chronic phase chronic myeloid leukemia (magnification ×20). Note the hypercellularity and the predominance of granulopoiesis. Maturation is preserved, with only occasional blasts (arrowhead). Numerous megakaryocytes, many of them small with hypolobulated nuclei (micromegakaryocytes), form sheets and clusters (arrows). B, Bone marrow aspirate in a patient with blast phase. Most of the cells are immature blasts (arrows), with only occasional cells still exhibiting differentiation (arrowheads). (Courtesy of Dr Marc Loriaux, Department of Pathology, Oregon Health & Science University, USA.)

of a high proportion of blasts in the differential. Clinically, leukostasis may manifest as priapism, chest pain, respiratory compromise, neurological deficits, or visual impairment. Physical exam may reveal splenomegaly and sometimes hepatomegaly, while involvement of other extramedullary sites is uncommon. Extramedullary disease other than hepatosplenomegaly is uncommon at presentation, and if suspected, must be verified histologically. Some reactive lymphadenopathy may occur, but significant lymph node enlargement requires a biopsy to rule out blastic transformation. An immature cellular infiltrate (chloroma) indicates BP, but if there is differentiation, it can be difficult to distinguish true extramedullary disease from an inflammatory process that recruits CML cells. There are no signs or symptoms that are pathognomonic for CML. In developed countries, many patients are diagnosed incidentally, when an abnormal complete count blood obtained for an unrelated reason leads to a diagnostic workup.

Disease Phases

CML evolves in stages termed CP-CML, AP-CML, and BP-CML. In the Western world, most patients present in CP-CML, while more advanced disease at diagnosis is common in developing countries. CP-CML is characterized by left-shifted granulocytosis with maintained terminal differentiation, frequently accompanied by basophilia and sometimes eosinophilia. Thrombocytosis and mild anemia are also common. Dysplasia is not a feature of CML and raises the question of alternative diagnoses, such as atypical CML.[220] Bone marrow aspirate and histology are hypercellular for age but demonstrate complete cellular maturation (*Figure 83.6A*). A typical finding is small, monolobated megakaryocytes (micromegakaryocytes). Mild reticulin fibrosis may be present, but severe reticulin fibrosis is uncommon and may be associated with poorer outcomes.[221] Without effective therapy, CP-CML inexorably progresses to BP-CML, which can exhibit a pre-B-lymphoid (25%), myeloid (70%), or indeterminate (5%) phenotype (*Figure 83.6B*).[222] BP-CML can develop rapidly or over a period of years through the intermediary stage of AP-CML. A variety of clinical and laboratory features have been used to define AP-CML, making comparison of results between different studies difficult. Today, the criteria used in the clinical trials leading to approval of imatinib are widely accepted (*Table 83.2*).[223] The exception is clonal cytogenetic evolution (CCA/Ph+). While there is agreement that CCA/Ph+ on treatment is diagnostic of AP-CML and therapy failure, this is not yet universally accepted for newly diagnosed patients.[224] Recent studies showed that these patients have inferior outcomes even in the absence

Table 83.2. Definition of Accelerated Phase

MDACC	European LeukemiaNet	WHO
PB blasts 15%-29%	Clonal chromosome abnormalities in Ph+ cells (CCA/Ph+), major route, on treatment	PB or BM blasts 10%-19%
PB blasts + promyelocytes ≥30%		
PB basophils ≥20%	PB basophils ≥20%	PB basophils ≥20%
Platelets ≤100 × 109/L (unrelated to therapy)	Platelets ≤100 × 109/L (unrelated to therapy)	Platelets ≤100 × 109/L (unrelated to therapy) or >1000 × 109/L (unresponsive to therapy)
Splenomegaly (unresponsive to therapy)		Increasing spleen size and increasing WBC unresponsive to therapy
Cytogenetic evolution on treatment	Clonal chromosome abnormalities in Ph+ cells (CCA/Ph+), major route, on treatment	Additional clonal chromosomal abnormalities in Ph+ cells at diagnosis that include "major route" abnormalities (second Ph, trisomy 8, isochromosome 17q, trisomy 19), complex karyotype, or abnormalities of 3q26.2
		Any new clonal chromosomal abnormality in Ph+ cells that occurs during therapy

Abbreviations: BM, Bone marrow; MDACC, MD Anderson Cancer Center; PB, peripheral blood of any other features of AP-CML, raising the question of whether the criteria should be revised.[192] A blast count of ≥30% in the blood or bone marrow or extramedullary blastic leukemic infiltrates (chloroma) in tissues other than liver or spleen define BP-CML. Gene expression profiling has revealed that AP-CML and BP-CML are closely related to each other, suggesting that CML is a two-phase rather than a three-phase disease.[225] Although data are sparse, newly diagnosed AP-CML responds very well to TKIs, suggesting that separating AP as a distinct disease state is no longer justified. Upcoming revisions of the World Health Organization and European Leukemia Net (ELN) definitions may no longer include AP-CML. The hope is that more consistent criteria will be developed in the future that encompass relevant clinical and molecular findings, such as somatic mutations detected by NGS.[226]

Risk Scores

Several prognostication systems have been developed to subclassify CP-CML. The oldest, developed by Joseph Sokal, uses a formula based on age, blast count in the blood, platelet count, and spleen size (in cm palpated below the left costal margin). Scores of <0.8, 0.8 to 1.2, and >1.2 define low, intermediate, and high risk.[227] Although the Sokal score was derived from a cohort of patients treated with busulfan-based chemotherapy, it has been applied successfully to risk-stratify patients treated with IFN or TKIs.[228,229] Subsequently, Hasford developed a score optimized for patients on IFN.[230] Owing to the efficacy of TKIs, the impact of a CML diagnosis on overall survival has been greatly reduced, diminishing the precision of scores using overall survival as an endpoint irrespective of causality. CML-specific survival scores such as the EUTOS long-term survival scores are designed to overcome this shortcoming.[231] As with the definitions of disease phases, molecular markers may eventually replace clinical risk scores.[226]

DIAGNOSIS AND INITIAL WORKUP

Clinical Evaluation

A complete history and physical exam are mandatory. Constitutional symptoms raise concerns about more aggressive disease. Spleen size must be documented. Despite its inaccuracy, this simple clinical test has remained a significant component of most CML risk scores.[227,230,231] Imaging studies such as abdominal ultrasound or computed tomography are not necessary unless there is suspicion of additional abdominal pathology. In the absence of an algorithm to convert imaging-based measurements of spleen size into clinical measurements, these data cannot be used to calculate risk scores. Extramedullary disease other than hepatosplenomegaly is uncommon at presentation, and if suspected, must be verified histologically.

Laboratory Tests

Complete Blood Count

A complete blood count (CBC) with manual white blood cell differential count is usually the first diagnostic step or the first abnormal finding in an otherwise asymptomatic patient. The diagnosis of CML is suspected based on the morphology of a Wright-Giemsa–stained blood smear. Typical features of CML include left-shifted granulopoiesis, and the examiner may identify the full spectrum of granulocytic precursors including blasts and promyelocytes, basophilia, and sometimes eosinophilia and thrombocytosis. Some automated cell counters do not provide the percentage of promyelocytes and/or basophils, which are required to determine the phase of disease. Since all risk scores to stratify CP-CML are based on pretherapeutic values, it is important to document the counts before initiating treatment. Flow cytometry is indicated only if AP/BP is suspected. Problems can arise in cases of discrepancies between morphologic and immunophenotypic blast counts, which are usually based on CD34 expression. In our practice, morphologic blast counts take precedence over flow cytometry, but there is currently no universally accepted rule.

Bone Marrow Aspirate and Biopsy

Bone marrow morphology studies at presentation are essential to establish disease phase. Unfortunately, many patients do not have a bone marrow aspirate at diagnosis, and in some of these, AP/BP may be overlooked, resulting in undertreatment. Whether all patients should have a biopsy is debatable, and practice varies considerably from country to country. We routinely perform a biopsy at diagnosis to identify the occasional patient with nests of blasts undetected by cytology. This is particularly important in patients with an aggressive presentation and those with inadequate aspirates or dry taps. As for peripheral blood, flow cytometry is not typically indicated.

Bone Marrow Karyotyping

Metaphase karyotyping of bone marrow cells using G- or R-banding must be performed at diagnosis. In 95% of CML patients, the *BCR-ABL1* fusion gene will be evident as Ph, sometimes as part of complex translocations involving additional chromosomes. These complex translocations do not seem to affect the outcome of patients on TKI therapy, and they must not be confused with clonal cytogenetic abnormalities in Ph⁺ cells (CCA/Ph⁺). As a rule, a minimum of 20 metaphase spreads are analyzed. Rare patients have a silent Ph that is not identified by karyotyping; in these patients, molecular testing is required to establish the diagnosis of CML. Another important piece of information from karyotyping is CCA/Ph⁺, since these patients have inferior progression-free and overall survival on TKI therapy, even in the absence of other features suggestive of AP.[195]

Fluorescence In Situ Hybridization

Fluorescence in situ hybridization (FISH) uses fluorescent DNA probes that hybridize to *BCR* and *ABL1* genetic regions adjacent to the translocation breakpoints—typically red fluorescence to label *ABL1* and green fluorescence to label *BCR*. Most FISH assays in current use identify both *BCR-ABL1* (on Ph) and *ABL1-BCR* fusion signals (on the derivative chromosome 9) and have low false-positive and -negative rates.[232] In contrast to karyotyping, FISH is usually performed on interphase nuclei, which increases sensitivity as 200 to 500 nuclei can be analyzed routinely. FISH is an excellent test to establish the diagnosis of CML in cases of silent Ph, but it should not routinely replace karyotyping, as CCA/Ph⁺ will be missed. Modern FISH probes also identify deletions in *ABL1* adjacent to the translocation breakpoint, which confer an adverse prognosis to patients treated with IFN and second-line imatinib, but not to patients on frontline TKI therapy.[55,56,233] Altogether, FISH at diagnosis does not add actionable information in addition to standard karyotyping and its routine use in addition to conventional karyotyping is not justified. However, as a negative result by FISH has a very high positive predictive value for a CCyR by karyotyping, FISH is an extremely useful test to monitor patients with atypical BCR-ABL1 transcripts that are not detected by standard quantitative PCR (qPCR) assays.[234]

Reverse Transcription Polymerase Chain Reaction

The main use of *qualitative* PCR is to identify a *BCR-ABL1* fusion mRNA in patients with suspected CML who are Ph⁻ by metaphase karyotyping. As such, this technique provides the same information as FISH. If qualitative RT-PCR is used to ascertain the presence of a *BCR-ABL1* translocation, it is important to make sure that the assay detects all types of *BCR-ABL1* transcripts, including atypical transcripts.[235] qPCR assays will detect most types of *BCR-ABL1* mRNA transcripts but depending on test design will miss e1a2 and atypical transcripts. Thus, qPCR is not indicated to establish the diagnosis of CML, while it is used routinely to monitor patients on therapy. A detailed discussion of qPCR for *BCR-ABL1* is provided in the section on monitoring response.

Differential Diagnosis

MPNs such as atypical CML, chronic myelomonocytic leukemia, chronic neutrophilic leukemia, MPN associated with rearrangements within the *PDGFRs*, or fibroblast growth factor receptor 3 genes can be indistinguishable from CML on morphologic and clinical grounds alone. Conversely, some CML patients present with a disease that resembles essential thrombocythemia or primary myelofibrosis.[220] Given the profound therapeutic implications, it is mandatory to ascertain the presence or absence of *BCR-ABL1* in every patient with MPN. Once Ph or *BCR-ABL1* has been demonstrated, the diagnosis is CML, irrespective of the particular MPN morphology.[220] Tests like the leukocyte alkaline phosphatase score (low in CML, high in leukemoid reactions) or vitamin B_{12} levels (high in CML) have been superseded by molecular tests and are of historical interest only. CML may present in lymphoid or myeloid BP and these cases can be difficult to distinguish from de novo Ph+ ALL or Ph+ AML, a rare and sometimes disputed entity.[220] Residual left-shifted but maturing granulocytic precursors, basophilia and splenomegaly, point to a prior CP-CML. A *BCR* breakpoint in the m-*BCR* with e1a2 *BCR-ABL1* transcript establishes a diagnosis of Ph+ ALL for all practical purposes.

MONITORING RESPONSE TO THERAPY

Once treatment is initiated, response is measured by clinical, hematologic, cytogenetic, and eventually molecular parameters. These different levels of response reflect the decrease of leukemia burden (*Figure 83.7*).

Complete Hematologic Response

Complete hematologic response (CHR) requires the normalization of white blood cell and platelet counts as well as the white blood cell differential. Normalization of hemoglobin is not part of the CHR definition. Additionally, all CML-related clinical symptoms must have resolved, and the spleen should not be palpable. While the latter requirement is stringent and precise, bulky splenomegaly is often slow to resolve and the significance of persistent minimal splenomegaly in patients who meet all other CHR criteria is unknown. The term "major hematologic response" is sometimes used to describe response in patients with AP/BP who clear blasts from the blood and have less than 5% of blasts in the bone marrow but lack reconstitution of peripheral blood counts.

Cytogenetic Response

At least 20 metaphases must be karyotyped to assess cytogenetic response. A partial cytogenetic response (PCyR) is present if 35% or less of these metaphases are Ph+, and a CCyR if all are Ph−. The 35% definition of PCyR reflects the lower bound of the 95% confidence interval around 50% Ph+ metaphases based on analysis of 20 metaphases. CCyR and PCyR combined are referred to as major cytogenetic response. Some studies also report minor (36%-65% Ph+) and minimal (66%-95% Ph+) cytogenetic response, but these response levels have limited clinical significance.

Molecular Response

qPCR is widely used for monitoring of patients on TKI therapy or after allogeneic stem cell transplantation. The previous use of numerous different technologies led to efforts aimed at harmonization of *BCR-ABL1* testing. An exhaustive discussion of qPCR monitoring is beyond the scope of this chapter and the reader is referred to comprehensive reviews of the subject and current best practice recommendations.[236-239]

Compared to metaphase karyotyping and FISH, qPCR has a much greater dynamic range, which may span up to 5 logs. However, this sensitivity is reached only if the sample is of optimal quality. Thus, reliable laboratories report the sensitivity achieved for a given sample to enable correct interpretation of results. Not all housekeeping genes are equally suitable as control genes for normalization of RNA input. Acceptable choices include *ABL1, BCR, GUS,* and *G6PD*.[236] β-Actin is not suitable owing to high-level expression that may conceal degradation of the sample.

In clinical practice, it is often necessary to decide whether a rise of *BCR-ABL1* mRNA is significant and should trigger a more extensive workup. The most important factor is the quality of the test, which determines the extent of intertest variation and, as such, the optimal compromise between sensitivity and specificity.[240] Current recommendation is that a fivefold rise in transcript level be regarded as significant.[42] In excellent laboratories, this may decrease to 2-fold,[241] while in poor laboratories even 10-fold rises may not be dependable. For the clinician, it is important to know the performance of the laboratory to ascertain correct interpretation of test results. qPCR is more reproducible at high levels of *BCR-ABL1* than at low levels. Thus, in case of rising *BCR-ABL1* mRNA levels, it is good clinical practice to repeat the test before rushing to conclusions, particularly if the changes occur at a low level.

A breakthrough was the introduction of the international scale (IS), which allows for the expression of values from different laboratories

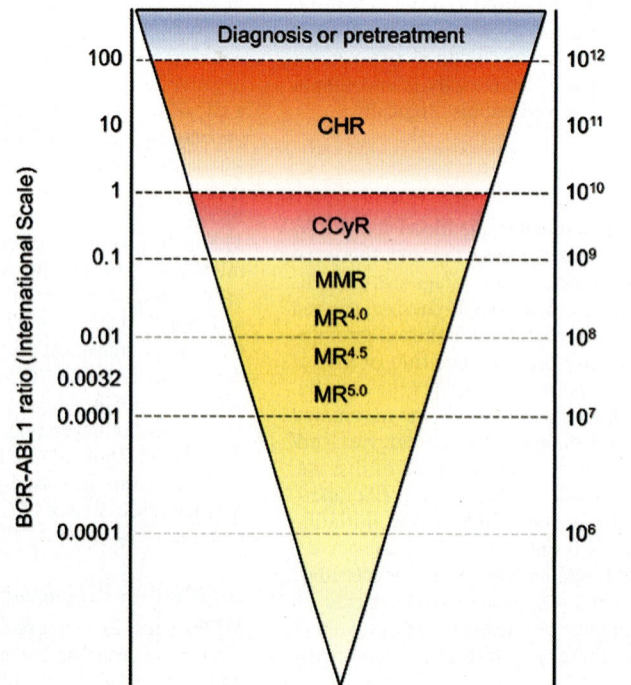
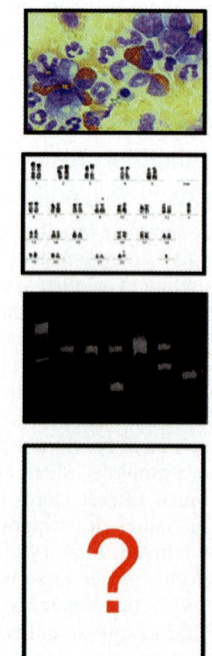

FIGURE 83.7 Reduction of leukemia burden with increasing depth of response. Estimates are that at least 1012 chronic myeloid leukemia cells may be present at diagnosis. Complete hematologic response (CHR) is the first therapeutic objective. A complete cytogenetic response (CCyR) is equivalent to approximately 2-log reduction of disease burden and a major molecular response (MMR) to 3-log reduction, compared to a standardized baseline (not to the individual patient's initial disease burden). Reductions of BCR-ABL1 transcripts by 4-log or more are referred to as deep molecular response (DMR). MR4.5 or—in the best laboratories—MR5.0 are currently the detection limits for clinical testing.

and different assays on a uniform scale. To express their individual values on the IS, laboratories obtain a series of standards to calculate a lab-specific conversion factor.[239,242,243] Key anchoring points of the IS are (1) 100%, which is equivalent to the average *BCR-ABL1* mRNA expression of a cohort of patients treated on the International Randomized Study of Interferon and STI571 (IRIS) study[244] and (2) a level of 0.1% IS, corresponding to a 3-log reduction compared to this baseline and referred to as a major molecular response (MMR). Achievement of MMR on TKI therapy is an important milestone that portends a good prognosis. Further reductions of *BCR-ABL1* mRNA by 4 or 4.5 logs are referred to as MR^4 or MR$^{4.5}$, respectively. An important feature of the IS is that values are directly comparable between different laboratories, enabling continuity. The percent BCR-ABL1 corresponds to MR only if expressed on the IS. This is of practical importance. Mistaking data expressed on some obscure percentage scale as IS results can give a patient false reassurance about their response to TKIs, and the use of non-IS tests is discouraged. Additionally, one must be aware that the fold reductions of *BCR-ABL1* expressed on IS refer to a standardized baseline, not to the patient's individual baseline, thus representing an absolute measurement of leukemia burden. Residual leukemia levels are underestimated if the patient-specific baseline is used in patients with high levels of *BCR-ABL1* mRNA at diagnosis. Since this correlates with more advanced disease, this is exactly the group of patients where overestimating response may have dire consequences.[198] On the other hand, recent reports showed that calculation of the individual reduction of *BCR-ABL1* mRNA may add valuable prognostic information.[245,246] Since the accurate measurement of high initial *BCR-ABL* mRNA expression is possible only with control genes other than *ABL1*, applying this finding in practice requires detailed knowledge of the specific PCR test used. A complete molecular response (CMR) had been defined as undetectable *BCR-ABL1* mRNA by qPCR or nested PCR. However, as a negative PCR test reflects not only the level of residual leukemia, but also the sensitivity of the PCR test and the quality of the sample, there is no universal definition of CMR, and the term should be avoided. Recently, the term "deep molecular response" was introduced to denote a more than 4-log reduction of *BCR-ABL1* transcripts, which is a prerequisite for a trial of TFR.

BCR-ABL1 Mutation Testing

BCR-ABL1 mutations are an important mechanism of TKI resistance and mutation testing is indicated in patients with evidence of clinical resistance. Mutation testing at diagnosis was previously recommended for patients presenting in AP/BP but has a low yield and is not indicated. Similarly, the benefit of mutation surveillance in high-risk patients remains to be determined prospectively, and both are not recommended in the updated recommendations of the ELN and National Comprehensive Cancer Network (NCCN).[42,247] Direct (Sanger) sequencing of *BCR-ABL1* amplicons to identify mutant alleles is still widely used. While the sensitivity of Sanger sequencing is limited to 20% to 30% of mutant allele, clones detected at this level are likely to be clinically relevant and inform TKI selection. Retrospective studies indicate that earlier mutation detection using assays with a sensitivity of 1% to 5% can inform the choice of salvage TKI to avoid selection of resistant clones.[248] In contrast, detection of *BCR-ABL1* kinase domain mutations by very sensitive assays such as allele-specific PCR does not predict failure and is not useful clinically.[249] The clinical importance of low-level mutations also depends on the TKI used for salvage and may be overcome with third-generation drugs like ponatinib.[250] Many laboratories have moved to NGS, which reliably calls 1% to 5% mutant alleles.[250]

THERAPY

Cytotoxic Agents and Interferon

Busulfan, an alkylating agent with considerable HSC toxicity, was the first drug that effectively controlled white blood cell and platelet counts, but is rarely used today except as part of conditioning regimens in allogeneic stem cell transplantation.[19] Chronic busulfan exposure is associated with pulmonary fibrosis, and proper dosing can be challenging owing to prolonged cytopenias. Hydroxyurea, a ribonucleotide reductase inhibitor, is indicated as an effective method for lowering white blood cell counts until the diagnosis of CML is confirmed. Since, at conventional doses, hydroxyurea acts predominantly on the more mature progenitor cells, cytopenias are usually short-lived and therapy is easily adjusted based on CBCs. IFN was the first drug therapy that induced durable cytogenetic responses, albeit only in a small minority of patients and for reasons that remain incompletely understood. Combinations with cytarabine, which has single agent activity in CML, were the standard of care in the 1990s.[251,252] Omacetaxine (formerly known as homoharringtonine) was approved in the United States for the treatment of adult patients with CP-CML or AP-CML with resistance and/or intolerance to two or more TKIs. Omacetaxine is a protein synthesis inhibitor that is administered subcutaneously. Key toxicity is myelosuppression.[253]

Tyrosine Kinase Inhibitors

TKIs are the standard of care for newly diagnosed CML patients in all disease phases. Imatinib, dasatinib, nilotinib, and bosutinib are approved for the first-line treatment of CML. Ponatinib is approved for patients with the T315I mutation or for whom no other TKI is indicated. These TKIs are distinguished by their potency, activity against *BCR-ABL1* mutants (discussed in detail below), spectrum of activity against kinases other than *BCR-ABL1*, and side effect profiles (Tables 83.3 and 83.4). Today's treatment algorithms are based on the results of a series of clinical trials, starting with a phase 1 imatinib study initiated in 1998 (Table 83.5) (Figure 83.8).

Imatinib

A phase 1 trial of imatinib in CML patients who had failed conventional therapy demonstrated activity in all disease phases. Importantly, cytogenetic responses were seen, particularly in CP-CML.[25,26] No maximum tolerated dose was identified. Based on cytogenetic responses, an initial dose of 400 mg daily was selected for phase 2 studies in CP, AP, and BP. These trials confirmed the phase 1 results and led to approval of imatinib for patients who had failed IFN owing to resistance or intolerance.[254-257] CP-CML responses were mostly durable, but there was a high failure rate in advanced CML, which led to an increase of the starting dose to 600 mg imatinib daily. Approval for frontline use in newly diagnosed patients followed in 2003 based on the results of the IRIS study, which compared imatinib 400 mg daily vs a combination of IFN and cytarabine. This trial showed imatinib to be vastly superior in all major endpoints, most importantly in progression-free survival.[244] Crossover was permitted for resistance or intolerance and occurred almost exclusively in patients failing IFN. The fact that many of these patients were effectively salvaged by imatinib may explain why no difference in overall survival between the two experimental arms was observed.[229,244] A 10-year update of the IRIS trial reported an estimated overall survival of 83.3% for patients treated with imatinib up-front vs 78.8% for the control arm.[258] Subsequent phase 3 studies of imatinib in newly diagnosed CP-CML patients mainly addressed the question of the optimal dose and the role of combinations with IFN and cytarabine. Single-arm studies in comparison with historical controls had suggested higher rates of CCyR and MMR for 800 mg imatinib daily, commonly referred to as high-dose imatinib.[259,260] However, this was not uniformly confirmed in prospective randomized studies. The Tyrosine Kinase Inhibitor Optimization and Selectivity Study trial compared 400 vs 800 mg imatinib daily in newly diagnosed patients irrespective of Sokal risk, and an Italian study compared the identical doses in high-Sokal-risk patients. Both studies failed in their primary endpoint, improved MMR, or CCyR at 12 months at the higher dose.[261,262] The German CML IV study reported superior rates of MMR at 12 months for 800 mg imatinib daily (59% vs 44%, $P < .001$).[263] In this study, imatinib dosing was more flexible and was maximized based on the individual patient's tolerability, resulting in a median dose of 627 mg daily. Similarly, the US Intergroup reported higher MMR rates at

Table 83.3. Tyrosine Kinase Inhibitors Approved for the First-Line Treatment of CML

Inhibitor	Imatinib	Nilotinib	Dasatinib	Bosutinib
Binding mode	Inactive conformation (type II)	Inactive conformation (type II)	Active conformation (type I)	Active conformation (type I)
IC_{50} native BCR-ABL expressing cells [nM]	260	13	0.8	41.6
IC_{50} ABL substrate phosphorylation [nM]	280	15	0.6	2.4
Additional targets	KIT, PDGFRA/B, CSF1R, LCK	KIT, PDGFRA/B	SRC family and multiple other kinases	SRC family, CAMK2G, TEC family, STE20 family; inactive against KIT and PDGFR
Dose	400 mg once daily (CP-CML) 600 mg once daily (AP-CML, BP-CML)	300 mg twice daily (CP-CML, newly diagnosed) 400 mg twice daily (CP-CML, AP-CML resistant to imatinib)	100 mg once daily (CP-CML) 140 mg once daily (AP-CML, BP-CML resistant to imatinib)	400 mg daily
Adverse events in newly diagnosed patients irrespective of relation to drug (only grades 3 and 4)	Fluid retention 62 (3) Superficial edema 60 (2) Other fluid retention reactions 7 (1) Nausea 50 (1) Muscle cramps 49 (2) Musculoskeletal pain 47 (5) Diarrhea 45 (3) Rash 40 (3) Fatigue 39 (2) Headache 37 (<1) Joint pain 31 (3) Abdominal pain 37 (4) Nasopharyngitis 31 (0) Hemorrhage 29 (2) GI hemorrhage 2 (<1) CNS hemorrhage 0.2 (0) Myalgia 24 (2) Vomiting 23 (2) Dyspepsia 19 (0) Cough 20 (<1) Pharyngolaryngeal pain 18 (<1) Upper respiratory tract infection 21 (<1) Dizziness 19 (<1) Pyrexia 18 (<1) Weight gain 16 (2) Insomnia 15 (0) Depression 15 (<1) Influenza 14 (<1) Bone pain 11 (2) Constipation 11 (<1)	Rash 33 (2) Pruritus 29 (1) Nausea 31 (1) Diarrhea 22 (3) Constipation 21 (<1) Vomiting 21 (<1) Abdominal pain 11 (1) Headache 31 (3) Fatigue 28 (1) Pyrexia 14 (1) Asthenia 14 (0) Edema, peripheral 11 (0) Arthralgia 18 (2) Myalgia 14 (2) Pain in extremity 13 (1) Bone pain 11 (<1) Muscle spasms 11 (<1) Back pain 10 (<1) Cough 17 (<1) Dyspnea 11 (1) Nasopharyngitis 16 (<1)	Fluid retention 23 (1) Pleural effusion 12 (<1) Superficial localized edema 10 (0) Generalized edema 3 (0) Congestive heart failure/cardiac dysfunctions 2 (<1) Pericardial effusion 2 (<1) Pulmonary hypertension 1 (0) Pulmonary edema <1 (0) Diarrhea 18 (<1) Headache 12 (0) Musculoskeletal pain 12 (0) Rash 11 (0) Nausea 9 (0) Fatigue 8 (<1) Myalgia 6 (0) Hemorrhage 6 (1) Gastrointestinal bleeding 2 (1) Other bleeding 5 (0) Vomiting 5 (0) Muscle inflammation 4 (0)	Diarrhea 84 (9) Nausea 44 (1) Rash 44 (9) Vomiting 35 (3) Abdominal pain 23 (1) Upper abdominal pain 19 (0) Fatigue 22 (1) Pyrexia 21 (<1) Cough 16 (0) Headache 16 (0) Edema 15 (<1) Arthralgia 14 (<1)

Abbreviations: AP, accelerated phase; BP, blast phase; CML, chronic myeloid leukemia; CNS, central nervous system; CP, chronic phase; GI, gastrointestinal; PDGFR, platelet-derived growth factor receptor.

12 months for patients treated with 800 vs 400 mg imatinib (53% vs 35%, P = .049) as well as superior progression-free and overall survival.[264] Again, dosing was flexible and aimed at keeping patients on study. Lastly, the French SPIRIT study reported higher MMR rates at 12 months (49% vs 38%) for patients treated with 600 vs 400 mg imatinib daily.[265] Thus, the optimal dose of imatinib may be approximately 600 mg daily, equal to the recommended dose for AP/BP. It is tempting to speculate that the results of 600 mg imatinib daily in first-line therapy may come close to those of 2G TKIs, but prospective data are unavailable. Given the large price differential between generic imatinib and 2G TKIs, this information would be of great practical importance.[266]

Dasatinib

An initial phase 1 study on CML patients in all disease phases who had failed imatinib owing to resistance or intolerance revealed considerable activity upon treatment with dasatinib.[31] This study was followed by a series of phase 2 trials that tested dasatinib in larger cohorts of patients in the different disease phases, and two-dose optimization studies that tested 100 vs 140 mg daily administered as a single dose or in two separate doses.[267-271] From these studies, 100 mg dasatinib once daily for CP-CML, and 140 mg once daily for AP and BP, emerged as the recommended doses. Dasatinib was subsequently compared with imatinib 400 mg in a phase 3 study (DASatinib vs Imatinib Study In treatment-Naive CML patients, DASISION) in newly diagnosed CP-CML patients and proved superior in the primary endpoint, CCyR at 12 months, as well as several secondary endpoints, including MMR at 12 months.[33] Progression events were reduced, but the difference did not reach statistical significance, and no difference in overall survival was observed. Based on the DASISION trial, dasatinib was approved for use in newly diagnosed CML patients. A 60-month follow-up was recently reported and confirmed the superior molecular responses with dasatinib, but also the lack of an overall survival benefit.[272]

Table 83.4. Tyrosine Kinase Inhibitors Approved for Salvage Treatment of CML

Inhibitor	Ponatinib	Asciminib
Binding mode	Inactive conformation (type II)	allosteric inhibitor that binds a myristoyl site
IC_{50} native BCR-ABL expressing cells [nM]	0.5	0.25
IC_{50} ABL substrate phosphorylation [nM]	0.37	NA
Additional targets	SRC family, FGFR family, RET, FLT3, KIT, PDGFR, and multiple other kinases	None
Dose	15-45 mg once daily	Non T315I: 40 mg bid or 80 mg daily T315I: 200 mg bid
Adverse events in patients treated for failure of previous therapy (only grades 3 and 4) Bosutinib: irrespective of relation to drug Ponatinib: treatment-related adverse events	Rash 40 (4) Dry skin 39 (2) Abdominal pain 27 (7) Headache 23 (2) Fatigue 19 (1) Constipation 20 (1) Myalgia 17 (1) Arthralgia 17 (2) Nausea 14 (<1) Pancreatitis 7 (6) Hypertension 9 (2) Dyspnea 5 (1) Cardiac failure 1 (<1)[a]	Headache 25 (1.9) Diarrhea 18 (11.5) Hypertension 18 (11.5) Nausea 18 (11.5) Fatigue 16 (10.3) Nasopharyngitis 15 (9.6) Arthralgia 14 (9) Rash 11 (7.1) Vomiting 11 (7.1) Back pain 10 (6.4) Cough 10 (6.4) Dizziness 10 (6.4) Increased amylase 9 (5.8) Increased ALT 6 (3.8) Increased AST 6 (3.8)

Abbreviation: CML, chronic myeloid leukemia.
[a]Irrespective of the relationship of the events to treatment, as ascribed by the investigators, 7.1% of patients had cardiovascular events, 3.6% had cerebrovascular vents, and 4.9% had peripheral vascular events. Two patients discontinued ponatinib after the occurrence of one event. Of the remaining patients, 36% had one or more additional events. Cardiovascular, cerebrovascular, and peripheral vascular serious adverse events that were related to treatment were observed in 2.0%, 0.4%, and 0.4% of patients, respectively. Regardless of the relationship to treatment, 5.1% of the patients had cardiovascular serious adverse events, 2.4% had cerebrovascular serious adverse events, and 2.0% had peripheral vascular serious adverse events.

Nilotinib

An initial phase 1 study tested nilotinib in a cohort of CML and Ph+ ALL patients who had failed imatinib owing to resistance or intolerance. Considerable activity was seen in CP and AP, while results in BP were less impressive.[32] Subsequent phase 2 studies led to approval of nilotinib 400 mg twice daily for patients with CP-CML and AP-CML who had failed prior imatinib therapy.[273,274] Although the results of nilotinib in BP-CML are comparable to those of dasatinib, the drug is not approved for this indication.[275] Nilotinib (300 or 400 mg twice daily) was then compared to imatinib in the Evaluating Nilotinib Efficacy and Safety in Clinical Trials–Newly Diagnosed (ENESTnd) study, with MMR at 12 months as the major endpoint.[34]

Table 83.5. Results of TKI Therapy in Major Front-Line Studies

Trial	N =	Treatment	CCyR	MMR	MR4.5	TFS	OS
IRIS (18 mo)	553	IM 400 mg/d	74% (est. at 18 mo)	57% (est. at 12 mo)[a]	NA/NR	96.7% (at 18 mo)	97.2% (est. at 18 mo)
IRIS (18 mo)	553	IM 400 mg/d	74% (est. at 18 mo)	57% (est. at 12 mo)[a]	NA/NR	96.7% (at 18 mo)	97.2% (est. at 18 mo)
IRIS (60 mo)	553	IM 400 mg/d	87% (est. at 60 mo)	NA/NR	NA/NR	93% (at 60 mo)	89% (est. at 60 mo)
IRIS (10.9 y)	553	IM 400 mg/d	83% (at 10.9 y)	NA/NR	NA/NR	92% (at 10.9 y)	83.3% (at 10.9 y)
TOPS (42 mo)	157	IM 400 mg/d	80.3% (by 42 mo)	51.6% (at 42 mo)	NA/NR	94.4% (est. at 48 mo)	94.0% (est. at 48 mo)
	319	IM 800 mg/d	81.5% (by 42 mo)	50.2% (at 42 mo)	NA/NR	95.8% (est. at 48 mo)	93.4% (est. at 48 mo)
ENESTnd (10 years)	282	NIL 600 mg/d	NA/NR	77.0% (by 60 mo)	53.5% (by 60 mo)	96.3% (est. by 60 mo)	93.7% (est. by 60 mo)
	281	NIL 800 mg/d	NA/NR	77.2% (by 60 mo)	52.3% (by 60 mo)	97.8% (est. by 60 mo)	96.2% (est. by 60 mo)
	283	IM 400 mg/d	NA/NR	60.4% (by 60 mo)	31.4% (by 60 mo)	92.6% (est. by 60 mo)	91.7% (est. by 60 mo)
DASISION (60 mo)	259	DAS 100 mg/d	NA/NR	76% (by 60 mo)	33% (by 60 mo)	95.4% (by 60 mo)	91% (est. by 60 mo)
	260	IM 400 mg/d	NA/NR	64% (by 60 mo)	42% (by 60 mo)	92.7% (by 60 mo)	90% (est. by 60 mo)
BFORE (~15 mo)	246[b]	BOS 400 mg/d	77.4% (by 12 mo)	73.9% (at 60 mo)	47.4% (at 60 mo)	93.3% (by 60 mo)[c]	94.5% (est. by 60 mo)
	241[b]	IM 400 mg/d	66.4% (by 12 mo)	64.6% (by 60 mo)	36.6% (at 60 mo)	90.7% (by 60 mo)[c]	94.6% (est. by 60 mo)

Abbreviations: CCyR, complete cytogenetic response; est., estimated; MMR, major molecular response; MR4.5, ≥4.5-log reduction of BCR-ABL1 transcripts; NA/NR, not available/or nor reported; OS, overall survival, TFS, transformation (to accelerated or blast phase)-free survival; TKI, tyrosine kinase inhibitor.
[a]Only patients with CCyR had qPCR monitoring.
[b]Five of these patients (bosutinib, n = 3; imatinib, n = 2) met AP criteria solely on the basis of basophil count within 2 weeks after random assignment. All five of these patients continued to receive the study drug; four achieved MMR.
[c]Four patients (1.6%) receiving bosutinib and six patients (2.5%) receiving imatinib experienced disease progression to AP or BP during treatment.

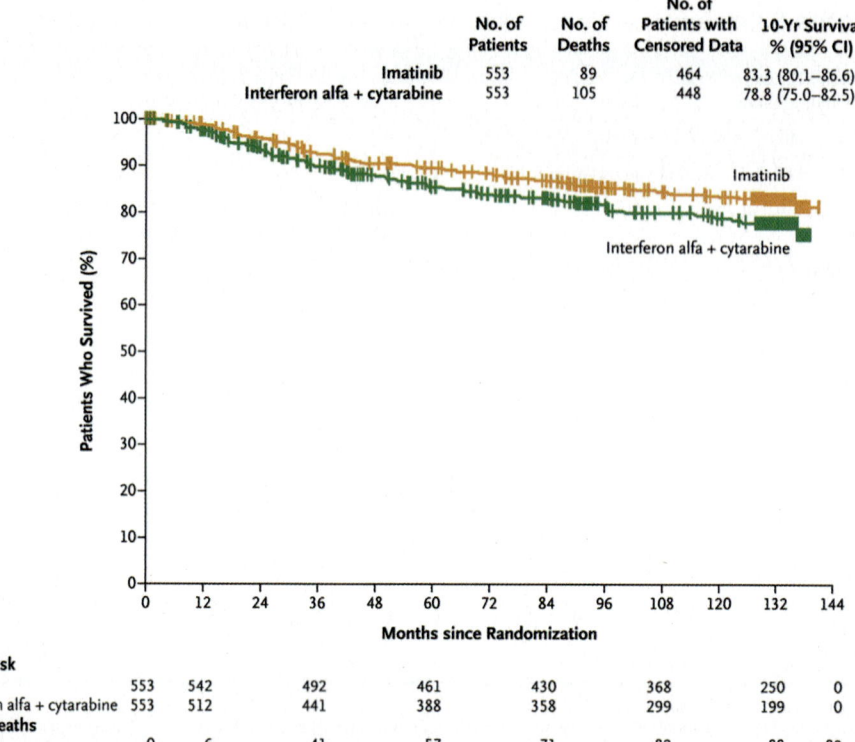

FIGURE 83.8 Overall survival of patients treated on the International Randomized Study of Interferon study at 10.9 years of follow-up.

This study showed both experimental arms superior to the standard arm. Importantly, progression-free survival was improved with nilotinib. The results of the ENESTnd study led to approval of nilotinib (300 mg twice daily) for frontline therapy in newly diagnosed patients with CP-CML. A 10-year follow-up month follow-up was recently reported and confirmed the superior molecular responses with nilotinib as well as a reduced rate of transformation to accelerated and BPs, but no significant difference in overall survival.[276]

Bosutinib

Based on the results of a phase 1 and subsequent phase 2 study in patients who had failed imatinib and in some cases also dasatinib or nilotinib, bosutinib was approved for salvage therapy in all phases of CML.[275] In contrast, a phase 3 study comparing bosutinib 500 mg daily vs imatinib 400 mg daily (Bosutinib Efficacy and Safety in Newly Diagnosed Chronic Myeloid Leukemia trial) failed in its primary endpoint, CCyR at 12 months, possibly due to overly aggressive treatment discontinuation for manageable adverse events.[276] MMR rates at 12 months were superior to those of imatinib. Results from a repeat phase 3 trial comparing 400 mg bosutinib vs 400 mg imatinib demonstrated superiority of bosutinib 400 mg daily over imatinib 400 mg daily in terms of MMR at 12 months and CCyR by 12 months and led to the approval of bosutinib for patients with newly diagnosed CML.[35]

Ponatinib

This TKI was developed to address the unmet need of patients with the T315I mutation. An initial phase 1 and a large phase 2 study (Ponatinib Ph+ ALL and CML Evaluation [PACE]) demonstrated efficacy in patients who had failed other TKIs, including patients with the T315I mutation, other BCR-ABL1 mutations, or no mutations.[36,37] Considering that most patients had been treated with several TKIs prior to ponatinib, results were excellent and appeared to be superior to those observed with dasatinib or nilotinib in the second-line setting. As a result, ponatinib was approved for patients who had failed other therapies. A phase 3 study (Evaluation of Ponatinib vs Imatinib in Chronic Myeloid Leukemia) was initiated comparing imatinib 400 mg vs ponatinib 45 mg. This trial was stopped when a significant incidence of cardiovascular, cerebrovascular, and peripheral vascular events was reported with longer follow-up of the phase 1 and PACE trials.[279] These observations led to a transient suspension of commercial ponatinib in the United States, but not in Europe. Ponatinib is now available for CP-CML with resistance or intolerance to at least two prior kinase inhibitors and A/BP-CML for whom no other kinase inhibitors are indicated. According to the package insert, the recommended starting dose is 45 mg, but dose reductions are common upon achievement of CCyR or MMR to reduce adverse events (AEs), particularly arterial occlusive events. This empirical practice was validated by the OPTIC trial, which randomized CP-CML patients with failure to at least two TKIs or with the T315I mutation between 45, 30, and 15 mg ponatinib daily at treatment initiation. The dose was reduced to 15 mg as soon as patients achieved BCR-ABL1 <1%. At 12 months, 60%, 25%, and 11% of patients with T315I who received ponatinib 45 mg, 30, and 15 mg, respectively, achieved BCR-ABL1 ≤1%. For patients without a T315I mutation, response rates were 48%, 38%, and 30%. The OPTIC trial clearly demonstrated that the optimal initial dose for patients with a T315I mutation is 45 mg. Patients without a T315I mutation may derive benefit also with an initial dose of 30 mg. Irrespective of this, the ponatinib dose should be reduced to 15 mg as soon as patients achieve BCR-ABL1 ≤1%.[280]

Asciminib

Unlike all other approved TKIs, asciminib is an allosteric inhibitor that binds to the myristoyl pocket of BCR-ABL1 kinase.[38] The initial phase I trial enrolled CML patients who had failed at least two TKIs.[39] No MTD dose of was reached. The rates of CHR, CCyR, and MMR were 92%, 54%, and 48%. In patients with T315I, asciminib 200 mg bid was administered to 52 patients. Of the 49 patients not in MMR at enrollment, 23 (46.9%) achieved MMR. These responses were durable with 46.9% of patients still in MMR at 96 weeks.[281] The phase 1 trial was followed by a randomized phase III trial of asciminib 40 mg bid vs bosutinib 400 mg daily in patients with failure to at least 2 TKIs, but without the T315I mutation.[282] At week 24, the MMR rate was higher for asciminib (25.5%) compared to bosutinib (13.2%), meeting the primary endpoint of the study.

Drug Combinations

Imatinib has been tested in combination with multiple cytotoxic agents and signal transduction inhibitors, mostly in the setting of resistance. In the frontline setting, data are limited to combinations with cytarabine and IFN. In the SPIRIT study, 400 mg imatinib daily was compared with 600 mg daily as well as 400 mg daily combined with pegylated IFN or cytarabine, with MMR at 12 months as the major endpoint.[265] Patients in the IFN/imatinib arm had significantly higher rates of MMR than all other arms of the study (57% vs 38% at 12 months for the comparison with imatinib 400 mg daily). Importantly, these data were confirmed by a smaller Scandinavian study.[283] Thus far, no differences in overall and progression-free survival have been reported, and IFN/imatinib combinations should be considered experimental. Imatinib and other TKIs were combined with AML-type multiagent chemotherapy in patients with myeloid BP, and with ALL-type chemotherapy in patients with lymphoid BP with acceptable toxicity. Imatinib also demonstrated activity when combined with hypomethylating agents in TKI-resistant CML.[284] Unfortunately, all these studies were single-armed, and the evidence supporting the addition of chemotherapy to TKIs is limited.

Tyrosine Kinase Inhibitor Toxicity

TKIs cause a number of acute and chronic adverse events (*Tables 83.3* and *83.4*). Some toxicities overlap, particularly myelosuppression, which is thought to reflect a lack of normal hematopoiesis available for reconstitution of hematopoiesis upon TKI suppression of the CML clone, but most are nonoverlapping and tend not to recur if an alternate TKI is selected.[285] This provides the clinician with multiple choices but has also lowered the threshold for switching TKIs for relatively minor side effects, and consequently rapid exhaustion of options. On the other hand, chronic side effects impair quality of life, compliance, and as a consequence, outcomes, and must be managed carefully, as even a relatively minor degree of nonadherence impairs outcomes.[286] While most TKI-induced adverse events are nonfatal and reversible, or very rare, cardiovascular toxicity is a relatively common and potentially life-threatening adverse event first recognized in patients treated with ponatinib.[36,37,279] However, cardiovascular risk is also increased with nilotinib, mandating a careful and individualized consideration of risk and benefit.[276,287,288] Although ponatinib and nilotinib are the TKIs most often associated with cardiovascular toxicity, it is likely that all approved TKIs increase cardiovascular risk, except for imatinib and possibly asciminib, although the number of patients treated with asciminib and their follow-up is too limited to be certain. Unique among the BCR-ABL1 TKIs, dasatinib is associated with pulmonary hypertension.[289,290] The pathophysiology underlying vascular events in patients on BCR-ABL1 TKIs is incompletely understood and likely different across various agents and vascular beds. Detailed reviews of this subject provide an overview and preliminary clinical guidance.[291,292] It will be important to delineate whether cardiovascular TKI toxicity is the result of off or on target effects. If the latter is the case, this will constitute a natural barrier for improving BCR-ABL1 inhibition to optimize efficacy.

APPROACH TO THE NEWLY DIAGNOSED CHRONIC PHASE PATIENT

Selection of Frontline Tyrosine Kinase Inhibitor

Once staging and risk assessment are complete, the question is how to choose among the four approved TKIs. Selection is influenced by several considerations, not all of which are strictly medical. As of 2022, there is no significant difference in overall survival between patients treated with imatinib vs dasatinib, nilotinib, or bosutinib. However, key molecular endpoints such as MMR and CMR are achieved faster and at a higher rate with the newer TKIs.[272,276] It remains possible that with more follow-up, a relatively small but significant advantage in overall survival will become apparent. One would need to balance this gain against the long and very impressive safety record of imatinib and the risk of long-term toxicity with 2G TKIs. The risk/benefit assessment would change in favor of a 2G TKI if there was a substantial increase in the numbers of patients entering TFR. An important factor to consider is the risk score. Although molecular responses with dasatinib, nilotinib, and bosutinib are superior across all risk categories, progression to AP/BP is very rare in low-risk patients treated with imatinib. Conversely, high-risk patients may benefit disproportionately from 2G TKIs.[276,293]

Lastly, the patient's past medical history is critical for TKI selection. Diabetes, pancreatitis, cardiovascular disease, and QT prolongation are contraindications for nilotinib,[32] while a history of pleural effusions, heart failure, or gastrointestinal bleeding argues against dasatinib.[31] Peripheral edema is frequently aggravated by imatinib.[244] Bosutinib is associated with a high incidence of hepatic toxicity.[277] In many cases, there are no firm contraindications against any one of the four TKIs, and it can be a matter of trial and error to identify the drug with the optimal tolerability in a given patient. In some patients, compatibility with lifestyle may favor once-daily dosing to optimize regimen adherence. Medication cost has become a major consideration with the approval of generic imatinib. There is no evidence that generic products marketed in the European Union or North America are less active than the brand name drug, but reduced activity has been reported for generic imatinib sold in developing countries.[294,295]

Optimizing drug therapy for newly diagnosed patients in a general way will require a CML management strategy rather than a single-drug approach. Important questions will need to be answered in well-designed prospective studies. For example, can 2G TKIs be used as an induction therapy, followed in good responders by low-cost/low-risk-maintenance imatinib? Or could patients be started on imatinib and switch to a 2G TKI if an early response assessment reveals an unsatisfactory response?

Monitoring Patients on Therapy

Regardless of the TKI selected for initial therapy, weekly CBCs are indicated until blood counts are stable, at which point intervals are extended. Cytopenias are common during the initial phase of treatment and may require dose interruption and/or reduction. In most cases, cytopenias are transient, reflecting therapeutic effects on leukemic hematopoiesis, when residual normal hematopoiesis is still suppressed. Algorithms have been proposed to optimize dose intensity, while avoiding prolonged myelosuppression.[296] Additionally, complete metabolic profiles (including lipase in the case of nilotinib) must be done periodically to monitor for liver and pancreatic toxicity as well as electrolyte imbalances. Monitoring by qPCR every 3 months is recommended if there is access to a reliable lab and results are expressed on the IS. Once stable MMR or even CMR has been achieved, these intervals can be extended to 6 months.[42] Although no exact data are available, it is likely that many rises of *BCR-ABL1* levels in patients with well-controlled CML reflect nonadherence or drug interactions. Repeat bone marrow biopsy is only recommended if there is no reliable qPCR or there is suspicion of progression to AP/BP-CML. FISH for *BCR-ABL1* on peripheral blood interphases should be used only if there is no access to reliable qPCR. An expert panel convened by the ELN has recommended milestones of response on TKI therapy, which have been widely accepted internationally, although minor differences remain compared to the NCCN guidelines.[42,297] The ELN milestones are defined time points in which responses are classified as optimal, warning, and failure (*Table 83.6*). Warning signs may trigger clinical actions such as an increased density of surveillance.

CCA/Ph⁻ are detected in 3% to 10% of patients with a cytogenetic response to TKIs.[144] Although these chromosomal abnormalities resemble those seen in MDS, the survival of patients with CCA/Ph⁻ is identical to that of other CML patients with a comparable cytogenetic response, and routine marrow karyotyping is not indicated if blood counts are stable.[298] The exception to this rule is chromosome 7 abnormalities that are associated with a considerable risk of

Table 83.6. BCR-ABL 1 Response Milestones in Chronic Phase CML Patients Treated With TKIs

Evaluation Time	Optimal	Warnings	Failure
Baseline	NA	High risk or CCA/Ph$^+$, major route	NA
3 mo	BCR-ABL1 ≤ 10%	>10%	>10% if confirmed within 1-3 mo
6 mo	≤1%	1%-10%	>10%
12 mo	≤0.1%	0.1%-1%	>1%
Then, and at any time	≤0.1%	>0.1%-1%	>1%, resistance mutations, high-risk ACA

Abbreviations: ACA, Additional cytogenetic abnormalities; CML, chronic myeloid leukemia; NA, not applicable; TKIs, tyrosine kinase inhibitors.
Adapted from Hochhaus A, Baccarani M, Silver RT, et al. European LeukemiaNet 2020 recommendations for treating chronic myeloid leukemia. *Leukemia.* 2020;34(4):966-984. http://creativecommons.org/licenses/by/4.0/

progression to MDS or AML.[224,299] A clinical challenge arises when TKI suppression of the proliferative yet functional BCR-ABL1–positive cell clone allows other, less functional and more aggressive clones to dominate.[300]

APPROACH TO THE PATIENT PRESENTING IN ACCELERATED PHASE/BLAST PHASE

As presentation of CML in AP or BP is uncommon in the developed world, there are limited data for this group of patients. Patients meeting currently used criteria for AP present a decision challenge. It is our practice to start these patients on a 2G TKI or ponatinib, perform HLA typing, and obtain a transplant consult, followed by close monitoring with qPCR and bone marrow biopsy/aspirate including karyotyping and flow cytometry. Patients who meet response criteria for CP-CML continue TKIs, while we recommend transplant to those who do not, provided they are good transplant candidates. Shared decision-making is key in ambiguous situations. In the case of BP, TKIs are usually combined with AML- or ALL-type multiagent chemotherapy. The use of chemotherapy in this setting is based on limited data, and potential benefits need to be weighed carefully against toxicity.[301,302] All patients presenting with BP should be strongly considered for an allogeneic stem cell transplant, with TKI therapy used to restore a second chronic phase and bridge the time to transplant. Whether or not to proceed to allograft in a BP patient who attained a very good response to TKIs can pose a challenging clinical decision and it is wise to discuss this eventuality prior to starting TKI therapy. Transplant risk, comorbidities, and the patient's personal preferences are critical decision factors.

RESISTANCE TO TYROSINE KINASE INHIBITORS

TKI resistance is grouped into primary and secondary (acquired) resistance. At a mechanistic level, resistance can be classified as BCR-ABL1 dependent or BCR-ABL1 independent. In BCR-ABL1–dependent resistance, there is reactivation of BCR-ABL1 kinase, which implies that responses may be recaptured if BCR-ABL1 inhibition is restored. In BCR-ABL1–independent resistance, alternative growth and survival pathways substitute for BCR-ABL1 kinase activity.[303]

BCR-ABL1 Kinase Domain Mutations

The most common mechanism of BCR-ABL1 reactivation is mutations in the kinase domain of BCR-ABL1 that impair drug binding through steric hindrance or by stabilizing a kinase conformation from which a given inhibitor is excluded.[30,303,304] The spectrum of mutations conferring clinical resistance is broadest for imatinib, reflecting its relatively low potency. Hot spots include the ATP-binding loop (p-loop; for example, Q252H, Y253(H/F), and E255(K/V)), activation loop (e.g., H396P), and T315, which controls access to a hydrophobic pocket in the catalytic site and is frequently referred to as the gatekeeper residue.[305] Compared to imatinib, 2G TKIs exhibit a much more contracted spectrum of resistance mutations, and in aggregate cover all clinical mutations except T315I. This is since all first-generation and 2G TKIs make a hydrogen bond with T315 and require access to the catalytic site hydrophobic pocket. In contrast, ponatinib skirts T315I through a rigid triple carbon bond,[306] and asciminib binds an allosteric pocket distant from the ATP-binding site.[38] Kinase domain mutations are more common in acquired resistance than in primary resistance and in AP/BP-CML than in CP-CML.[307] Biochemical and cell proliferation data are used to rank kinase domain mutations according to the degree of TKI resistance they confer (*Table 83.7*).[305,308] Although these data are based on in vitro studies, they tend to correlate with clinical responses.[309,310] For several other mutants, the difference in sensitivity is sufficient to support the use of one specific TKI over another (*Table 83.7*). Altogether, however, the value of genotyping is mostly to avoid selecting an inactive TKI, while the presence of a "sensitive" mutation does not guarantee a clinical response. An in-depth discussion of the many reported mutations and their sensitivity profiles is beyond the scope of this chapter and the reader is referred to detailed reviews of this subject.[303,305,308,311] Studies in cell lines have implicated overexpression of BCR-ABL1 by gene amplification or transcriptional upregulation, but the importance of these findings for clinical resistance is less clear.[312] All TKIs are substrates for various efflux pumps, including ABCB1 (MDR1), and several polymorphisms have been correlated with the depth of response.[313] One study showed that overexpression of MDR1 may be sufficient to protect CML stem and progenitor cells, until they acquire a BCR-ABL1 kinase domain mutation that is able to drive overt resistance.[314]

Activation of Alternative Signaling Pathways

In contrast to kinase domain mutations, BCR-ABL1 kinase–independent resistance is less well understood and involves multiple different mechanisms. For example, activation of SRC family kinases, MAP kinase, STAT5, SYK, and PI3K have all been associated with TKI resistance despite sustained inhibition of BCR-ABL1.[315-318] Extrinsic factors such as cytokines derived from the bone marrow stroma may also play a role.[181,319] Targeting these diverse pathways is challenging.

APPROACH TO THE PATIENT WITH TYROSINE KINASE INHIBITOR RESISTANCE

Failure to achieve therapeutic milestones or a loss of response from a given level suggests TKI resistance and should trigger a careful evaluation. The first call of order is to assess medication adherence through a thorough history. Drug level testing may be useful in select cases, but is not widely available, and patients have been found to make up for skipped doses during the last few days prior to the office visit.[286] Drug interactions should be considered, especially in patients on multiple comedications. It is particularly important to include herbal preparations and other over-the-counter remedies—for example, St John wort, which can drastically lower imatinib plasma concentrations.[320] A realistic view is that drug interactions are almost impossible to predict in patients on polypharmacy, and the situation is even more complicated in cases of impaired renal or hepatic function. If nonadherence or drug interactions appear unlikely, a complete resistance workup is indicated, including physical exam, CBC, bone marrow aspirate and biopsy, bone marrow metaphase karyotyping, and *BCR-ABL1* mutation analysis. TKI resistance defines a high-risk situation and should be approached as a diagnosis with significant clinical implications. Key pieces of information derived from this workup are disease phase, *BCR-ABL1* mutation status, and karyotype, including CCA/Ph+.

Patients with resistance to imatinib can be managed with a 2G TKI alone if they are in chronic phase. The selection of dasatinib, nilotinib, or bosutinib is based on past medical history to avoid specific side effects and the type of *BCR-ABL1* mutation (if present, Table 83.7). It is good practice to have the patient evaluated or reevaluated by a transplant center. Analogous to newly diagnosed patients, patients on second-line TKIs must be assessed at regular intervals to determine whether their response meets expectations. One study reported significantly superior overall and event-free survival for patients with <10% BCR-ABL1 at 3 months, which in multivariate analysis superseded all other prognostic factors.[321] Patients with CCyR at 12 months had excellent overall survival. In view of the limited data regarding the prognostic significance of milestones in second-line TKI therapy, the ELN recommends using the well-established framework for first-line TKI therapy.[42] Patients who fail frontline or second-line dasatinib, nilotinib, or bosutinib are at high risk, even if still in CP and should be considered for ponatinib or asciminib, balancing the risks of the disease vs the risks of cardiovascular toxicity.[37] Switching between 2G TKIs is effective only in patients who fail 2G inhibitors owing to nonhematologic toxicity and in cases with a specific *BCR-ABL1* mutation that is effectively covered with the alternative 2G TKI.[321] Patients with the T315I mutation are candidates for ponatinib or asciminib. Omacetaxine has some activity in these patients, but responses are not durable.[322] Patients who progress to AP/BP on imatinib are managed with the appropriate second- or third-line TKI, in the case of

Table 83.7. Sensitivity of BCR-ABL1 Kinase Domain Mutants to Approved Tyrosine Kinase Inhibitors

Location of Mutation	Mutation	IC_{50}-fold Increase (WT = 1)				
		Imatinib	Bosutinib	Dasatinib	Nilotinib	Ponatinib
	Parental	10.8	38.3	568.3	38.4	570.0
	WT	1	1	1	1	1
P-loop	M244V	0.9	0.9	2.0	1.2	3.2
	L248R	14.6	22.9	12.5	30.2	6.2
	L248V	3.5	3.5	5.1	2.8	3.4
	G250E	6.9	4.3	4.4	4.6	6.0
	Q252H	1.4	0.8	3.1	2.6	6.1
	Y253F	3.6	1.0	1.6	3.2	3.7
	Y253H	8.7	0.6	2.6	36.8	2.6
	E255K	6.0	9.5	5.6	6.7	8.4
	E255V	17.0	5.5	3.4	10.3	12.9
C-helix	D276G	2.2	0.6	1.4	2.0	2.1
	E279K	3.6	1.0	1.6	2.0	3.0
	E279L	0.7	1.1	1.3	1.8	2.0
ATP-binding region	V299L	1.5	26.1	8.7	1.3	0.6
	T315A	1.7	6.0	58.9	2.7	0.4
	T315I	17.5	45.4	75.0	39.4	3.0
	T315V	12.2	29.3	738.8	57.0	2.1
	F317L	2.6	2.4	4.5	2.2	0.7
	F317R	2.3	33.5	114.8	2.3	4.9
	F317V	0.4	11.5	21.3	0.5	2.3
SH2-contact	M343T	1.2	1.1	0.9	0.8	0.9
	M351T	1.8	0.7	0.9	0.4	1.2
Substrate binding region	F359I	6.0	2.9	3.0	16.3	2.9
	F359V	2.9	0.9	1.5	5.2	4.4
A-loop	L384M	1.3	0.5	2.2	2.3	2.2
	H396P	2.4	0.4	1.1	2.4	1.4
	H396R	3.9	0.8	1.6	3.1	5.9
C-terminal lobe	F486S	8.1	2.3	3.0	1.9	2.1
	L248R 1 F359I	11.7	39.3	13.7	96.2	17.7
Sensitive	≤2					
Moderately resistant	2.1 – 10					
Highly resistant	>10					

Abbreviation: ATP, adenosine triphosphate; WT, wild type.
From Eiring AM, Deininger MW. Individualizing kinase-targeted cancer therapy: the paradigm of chronic myeloid leukemia. *Genome Biol.* 2014;15(9):461. Copyright © 2014, Eiring and Deininger. Adapted with permission from Redaelli S, Mologni L, Rostagno R, et al. Three novel patient-derived BCR/ABL mutants show different sensitivity to second and third generation tyrosine kinase inhibitors. *Am J Hematol.* 2012;87(11):E125-8. Copyright © 2012 Wiley Periodicals, Inc.

BP typically combined with chemotherapy. All eligible patients in this category should be offered an allogeneic stem cell transplant, with the second-line TKI used as a bridge.

With the availability of multiple different TKIs, an individual patient's disease course reflects the sequencing of therapies based on tolerance, response, resistance, and availability/cost. In this complex landscape, the data to support decision-making become progressively weaker with each line of therapy, and referral to a specialized center should be considered in ambiguous cases.

TREATMENT-FREE REMISSION

After initial caution and skepticism, discontinuation of TKI therapy (commonly referred to as a TFR) has recently become part of routine CML management and practice guidelines.[42,247] The first large prospective study (*Stop Im*atinib—STIM trial) included patients in the first chronic phase who had been negative for *BCR-ABL1* by qPCR for at least 2 years. At 24 months' median follow-up, approximately 40% of patients maintained responses without TKI treatment, sometimes with intermittent low-level positivity by qPCR, while 60% had clear molecular recurrence of CML.[41] Interestingly, almost all failures occurred within 6 months, and patients with recurrence universally responded to retreatment, suggesting that TFR is a safe approach if patients are monitored closely. An update of the study at 5 years of follow-up revealed remarkably stable results, suggesting that patients destined to experience recurrence identify themselves early on.[323] The STIM results were confirmed in numerous subsequent studies, with even higher rates of successful TFR when less stringent criteria were used to define recurrence, such as MMR.[324-327] TFR is associated with improved quality of life and considerable savings to healthcare systems.[328] Other trials validated the TFR concept in patients treated with 2G TKIs.[329-331] TFR represents a major conceptual shift in CML treatment goals. Since many patients have intermittent or even permanent molecular evidence of CML, an operational definition of cure is required, conceding that complete eradication of the CML clone may not be possible or even necessary to achieve long-term survival without active disease. The safety of TFR is predicated on appropriate selection of patients and high-quality molecular monitoring. Unfortunately, there are no biomarkers or other parameters that reliably predict successful TFR candidates. Positive correlations with duration of TKI therapy and deep molecular response were reported with some consistency, and several studies have implicated immunologic parameters, but much of the clinical variation remains unexplained.[41,325,332,333] In countries with highly fragmented healthcare systems like the United States, the concern is that some patients will be lost to follow-up and eventually CML outcomes may be impaired. While TFR has clearly left the experimental realm, this should not discourage the enrollment of patients on prospective trials.

ALLOGENEIC STEM CELL TRANSPLANTATION

Allogeneic HSC transplantation was the first treatment modality that restored Ph⁻ hematopoiesis and induced durable responses.[20] CML is more susceptible to immunotherapy in an allogeneic setting than most other hematologic cancers. Donor leukocyte infusions were first used in CML patients and demonstrated not only the effectiveness of this approach, but also substantiated the existence of a graft-vs-leukemia effect.[334] Prior to the introduction of imatinib, allografting was recommended to all eligible patients, and even today it is still regarded as the only therapy capable of eradicating the CML clone. Risk scores for allografting in CML were developed by the European Group for Blood and Marrow Transplantation (EBMT) in the preimatinib era and identified disease duration of >12 months, more advanced disease, higher age, unrelated donor type, and the combination of a male recipient with a female donor as adverse prognostic factors (*Table 83.8*).[335] Disease phase had the greatest impact on outcome. Although somewhat historical, the EBMT score is still useful for prognostication, but major improvements such as molecular HLA typing likely reduce or eliminate the impact of some of these parameters.

Table 83.8. AlloHSCT Risk Factors and EBMT Risk Score

Risk Factor	Score and Description
Disease phase	0 if CP; 1 if AP; 2 if BP
Age	0 if <20 y; 1 if 20-40 y; 2 if >40 y
Interval from diagnosis	0 if ≤1 y; 1 if >1 y
Donor type	0 if HLA-identical sibling; 1 in any other instance
Donor-recipient sex match	1 if female donor and male recipient; 0 for any other match

The EBMT risk score was based on 3142 patients treated with AlloHSCT between 1989 and 1997, prior to the introduction of tyrosine kinase inhibitors. For low-risk patients (ie, risk score of 0-2), the transplantation-related mortality was 31% in the original cohort; however, in a more recent cohort of patients who underwent transplantation between 2000 and 2003, transplantation-related mortality was reduced to 17%. For the patients with a risk score of 3 to 4, transplantation-related mortality was approximately 50%, and it was approximately 70% for the patients with a risk score of 5 to 6.93. Abbreviations: AlloHSCT, allogeneic hematopoietic stem cell transplantation; AP, accelerated phase; BP, blast phase; CP, chronic phase; EBMT, European Group for Blood and Marrow Transplantation.
Adapted from Gratwohl A, Hermans J, Goldman JM, et al. Risk assessment for patients with chronic myeloid leukemia before allogeneic blood or marrow transplantation. Chronic Leukemia Working Party of the European Group for Blood and Marrow Transplantation. *Lancet*. 1998;352:1087-1092.

Only one study prospectively compared allotransplant vs drug therapy. Newly diagnosed patients with CP-CML were biologically randomized to a matched sibling transplant vs IFN-based drug therapy, the best nontransplant treatment available when the trial was initiated.[336] Patients managed with drug therapy had superior survival, with the biggest difference observed in low-risk patients. After approximately 8 years, the survival curves crossed, suggesting that transplant would be superior in the long run if IFN was the alternative. An update of this study with 10-year follow-up showed comparable overall survival, but transplanted patients with very low transplant risk score did better than patients managed with nontransplant therapy.[337] Given the efficacy of TKIs in the frontline setting, and that early transplant-related mortality is clearly higher than the risk of early disease progression, allotransplant is no longer justifiable in newly diagnosed patients with CP-CML.[42] There is consensus that allotransplant should be offered to patients with BP and those who progress to AP while on TKI therapy. Good transplant risk patients in chronic phase who fail a 2G TKI should also be considered, although ponatinib is also an option in patients with low cardiovascular risk. Fortunately, there is no evidence that imatinib or other TKIs prior to allografting negatively impact the outcome. On the contrary, for unknown reasons, imatinib prior to allotransplant may reduce chronic graft-vs-host disease and possibly relapse risk.[338-340] Results from the German CML study group reassert the importance of transplanting patients while they are still in chronic phase: three-year overall survival was 91% for patients transplanted in CP after failing imatinib vs 59% for patients transplanted after progressing to AP/BP.[341] There is an emerging consensus that bone marrow is preferred over peripheral blood stem cells (PBSCs) in patients with CP-CML, where graft-vs-host disease is a greater concern than disease control.[342] PBSCs are preferred for patients with transformation to AP/BP, even if they have achieved a second CP. High relapse risk patients should receive a TKI posttransplant, with selection based on *BCR-ABL1* mutation analysis at the time of resistance. Given the high median age at the time of diagnosis, many patients will be eligible only for reduced intensity conditioning regimens. An in-depth discussion of the various conditioning regimens, selection of bone marrow vs PBSCs, and posttransplant immunosuppression is presented elsewhere.

FUTURE PERSPECTIVES

Transformation to BP is rare in the era of TKIs, but the prognosis for patients crossing this threshold remains dismal, even with highly potent TKIs such as ponatinib.[36] Although ponatinib blocks all single

BCR-ABL1 mutants, responses in BP are rarely maintained regardless of *BCR-ABL1* mutational status.[36,37] *In vitro* studies have shown that compound mutations, that is, the presence of two point mutations in the same BCR-ABL1 molecule, confer high-level ponatinib resistance if they include T315I and the same may occur in vivo.[343] *In vitro* data indicate that combining ponatinib with asciminib restores efficacy, but this has not been tested in patients.[93] The fact that a substantial subset of patients with ponatinib resistance have no detectable *BCR-ABL1* kinase domain mutations and CCyR and MMR rates tend to be lower in patients without mutations implicates BCR-ABL1–independent mechanisms in resistance.[344] As with refractory AML, it seems that we are approaching a ceiling on what can be achieved by concentrating on the leukemia cells, and future research must take into consideration leukemia cell intrinsic mechanisms as well as extrinsic protective factors provided by the microenvironment.

At the other extreme of the disease spectrum, most patients responding to TKIs continue to harbor residual leukemia cells, evident either as low-level qPCR positivity or as recurrence in the case of TKI discontinuation, a state often referred to as disease persistence. *Ex vivo* studies on cells from patients in CMR have identified Ph+ cells both in progenitor and primitive long-term culture-initiating cells, and the frequency of leukemia stem cells in the CD34+CD38− fraction was estimated at 0.59% ± 0.1% based on xenograft studies in immunodeficient mice.[345,346] There is convincing evidence that persistent CML cells are not (or are not solely) dependent on BCR-ABL1 kinase activity for their survival.[40,152] Several pathways have been implicated in mediating survival despite inhibition of BCR-ABL1 activity, including Wnt/β-catenin, PML, Hedgehog, Alox5, BCL6, MYC, and PP2A, among others.[154,163-166,168,180,181,347-349] Extrinsic factors may play a key role in activating these pathways, providing a sanctuary to residual CML cells.

Significant efforts are being directed toward identifying therapeutic targets to eradicate residual CML. The biggest challenge is that many potential targets have important roles in normal hematopoiesis or development in general, limiting the therapeutic windows of targeted therapies. As a comprehensive review of this topic is beyond the scope of this chapter, the reader is referred to recent reviews of the subject.[350] From a clinical perspective, the observation that a fraction of patients in TFR continue to harbor detectable residual leukemia indicates that we need to reconsider the definition of cure in the context of CML. Perhaps, one should define cure as a risk of active CML that is not different from that of the general population, irrespective of whether the CML clone has been eliminated or not. Although elimination is impossible to prove, it is tempting to speculate that some patients in long-term TFR have reached this point. Potential mechanisms are that the CML clone, once reduced to very low levels by TKI treatment, is extinguished by the immune system or eliminated by stochastic processes.[350] Another explanation is that the BCR-ABL1 is expressed by long-lived B cells.[351] The current reality is, however, that a majority of patients will require long-term TKI therapy to maintain responses and avoid progression, testimony that CML is far from being a problem of the past.

ACKNOWLEDGMENTS

This work was supported by R01CA257602, R01CA254354, and R21CA256128. We are grateful to our partners Jutta and Amy for their unwavering support and encouragement.

References

1. Thorburn AL. Alfred Francois Donne, 1801-1878, discoverer of Trichomonas vaginalis and of leukaemia. *Br J Vener Dis.* 1974;50(5):377-380.
2. Donne A. *Cours de Microscopie.* Bailliere; 1844.
3. Bennett JH. Case of hypertrophy of the spleen and liver in which death took place from suppuration of the blood. *Edinb Med Surg J.* 1845;64:413-423.
4. Virchow R. Weisses Blut. *Froriep's Notizen.* 1845;36:151-156.
5. Neumann E. *Ein Fall von Leuk„mie mit Erkrankung des Knochenmarks.* Archive der Heilkunde; 1870.
6. Dameshek W. Some speculations on the myeloproliferative syndromes. *Blood.* 1951;6(4):372-375.
7. Nowell P, Hungerford D. A minute chromosome in human chronic granulocytic leukemia. *Science.* 1960;132:1497.
8. Baikie AG, Court-Brown WM, Buckton KE, Harnden DG, Jacobs PA, Tough IM. A possible specific chromosome abnormality in human chronic myeloid leukaemia. *Nature.* 1960;188:1165-1166.
9. Fialkow PJ, Gartler SM, Yoshida A. Clonal origin of chronic myelocytic leukemia in man. *Proc Natl Acad Sci U S A.* 1967;58(4):1468-1471.
10. Rowley JD. A new consistent chromosomal abnormality in chronic myelogenous leukaemia identified by quinacrine fluorescence and Giemsa staining. *Nature.* 1973;243(5405):290-293.
11. Groffen J, Stephenson JR, Heisterkamp N, de Klein A, Bartram CR, Grosveld G. Philadelphia chromosomal breakpoints are clustered within a limited region, bcr, on chromosome 22. *Cell.* 1984;36(1):93-99.
12. Bartram CR, de Klein A, Hagemeijer A, et al. Translocation of c-abl oncogene correlates with the presence of a Philadelphia chromosome in chronic myelocytic leukaemia. *Nature.* 1983;306(5940):277-280.
13. Abelson HT, Rabstein LS. Lymphosarcoma: virus-induced thymic-independent disease in mice. *Cancer Res.* 1970;30(8):2213-2222.
14. Heisterkamp N, Groffen J, Stephenson JR, et al. Chromosomal localization of human cellular homologues of two viral oncogenes. *Nature.* 1982;299(5885):747-749.
15. Lugo TG, Pendergast AM, Muller AJ, Witte ON. Tyrosine kinase activity and transformation potency of bcr-abl oncogene products. *Science.* 1990;247(4946):1079-1082.
16. Daley GQ, Van Etten RA, Baltimore D. Induction of chronic myelogenous leukemia in mice by the P210bcr/abl gene of the Philadelphia chromosome. *Science.* 1990;247(4944):824-830.
17. Lissauer H. Zwei Faelle von Leucaemie. *Berl Klin Wochenschr.* 1865;2:403-405.
18. Cowan Doyle A. Notes on a case of leukocythaemia. *Lancet.* 1882;119(3056):490.
19. Hehlmann R, Heimpel H, Hasford J, et al. Randomized comparison of interferon-alpha with busulfan and hydroxyurea in chronic myelogenous leukemia. The German CML Study Group. *Blood.* 1994;84(12):4064-4077.
20. Fefer A, Cheever MA, Thomas ED, et al. Disappearance of Ph1-positive cells in four patients with chronic granulocytic leukemia after chemotherapy, irradiation and marrow transplantation from an identical twin. *N Engl J Med.* 1979;300(7):333-337.
21. Talpaz M, Kantarjian H, Kurzrock R, Trujillo JM, Gutterman JU. Interferon-alpha produces sustained cytogenetic responses in chronic myelogenous leukemia. Philadelphia chromosome-positive patients. *Ann Intern Med.* 1991;114(7):532-538.
22. Anafi M, Gazit A, Gilon C, Ben-Neriah Y, Levitzki A. Selective interactions of transforming and normal abl proteins with ATP, tyrosine-copolymer substrates, and tyrphostins. *J Biol Chem.* 1992;267(7):4518-4523.
23. Buchdunger E, Zimmermann J, Mett H, et al. Selective inhibition of the platelet-derived growth factor signal transduction pathway by a protein-tyrosine kinase inhibitor of the 2-phenylaminopyrimidine class. *Proc Natl Acad Sci U S A.* 1995;92(7):2558-2562.
24. Druker BJ, Tamura S, Buchdunger E, et al. Effects of a selective inhibitor of the Abl tyrosine kinase on the growth of Bcr-Abl positive cells. *Nat Med.* 1996;2(5):561-566.
25. Druker BJ, Sawyers CL, Kantarjian H, et al. Activity of a specific inhibitor of the BCR-ABL tyrosine kinase in the blast crisis of chronic myeloid leukemia and acute lymphoblastic leukemia with the Philadelphia chromosome. *N Engl J Med.* 2001;344(14):1038-1042.
26. Druker BJ, Talpaz M, Resta DJ, et al. Efficacy and safety of a specific inhibitor of the BCR-ABL tyrosine kinase in chronic myeloid leukemia. *N Engl J Med.* 2001;344(14):1031-1037.
27. Schindler T, Bornmann W, Pellicena P, Miller WT, Clarkson B, Kuriyan J. Structural mechanism for STI-571 inhibition of abelson tyrosine kinase. *Science.* 2000;289(5486):1938-1942.
28. Nagar B, Hantschel O, Young MA, et al. Structural basis for the autoinhibition of c-Abl tyrosine kinase. *Cell.* 2003;112(6):859-871.
29. Hantschel O, Nagar B, Guettler S, et al. A myristoyl/phosphotyrosine switch regulates c-Abl. *Cell.* 2003;112(6):845-857.
30. Gorre ME, Mohammed M, Ellwood K, et al. Clinical resistance to STI-571 cancer therapy caused by BCR-ABL gene mutation or amplification. *Science.* 2001;293(5531):876-880.
31. Talpaz M, Shah NP, Kantarjian H, et al. Dasatinib in imatinib-resistant Philadelphia chromosome-positive leukemias. *N Engl J Med.* 2006;354(24):2531-2541.
32. Kantarjian H, Giles F, Wunderle L, et al. Nilotinib in imatinib-resistant CML and Philadelphia chromosome-positive ALL. *N Engl J Med.* 2006;354(24):2542-2551.
33. Kantarjian H, Shah NP, Hochhaus A, et al. Dasatinib versus imatinib in newly diagnosed chronic-phase chronic myeloid leukemia. *N Engl J Med.* 2010;362(24):2260-2270.
34. Saglio G, Kim DW, Issaragrisil S, et al. Nilotinib versus imatinib for newly diagnosed chronic myeloid leukemia. *N Engl J Med.* 2010;362(24):2251-2259.
35. Cortes JE, Gambacorti-Passerini C, Deininger MW, et al. Bosutinib versus imatinib for newly diagnosed chronic myeloid leukemia: results from the randomized BFORE trial. *J Clin Oncol.* 2018;36(3):231-237.
36. Cortes JE, Kantarjian H, Shah NP, et al. Ponatinib in refractory Philadelphia chromosome-positive leukemias. *N Engl J Med.* 2012;367(22):2075-2088.
37. Cortes JE, Kim DW, Pinilla-Ibarz J, et al. A phase 2 trial of ponatinib in Philadelphia chromosome-positive leukemias. *N Engl J Med.* 2013;369(19):1783-1796.
38. Wylie AA, Schoepfer J, Jahnke W, et al. The allosteric inhibitor ABL001 enables dual targeting of BCR-ABL1. *Nature.* 2017;543(7647):733-737.
39. Hughes TP, Mauro MJ, Cortes JE, et al. Asciminib in chronic myeloid leukemia after ABL kinase inhibitor failure. *N Engl J Med.* 2019;381(24):2315-2326.
40. Corbin AS, Agarwal A, Loriaux M, Cortes J, Deininger MW, Druker BJ. Human chronic myeloid leukemia stem cells are insensitive to imatinib despite inhibition of BCR-ABL activity. *J Clin Invest.* 2011;121(1):396-409.
41. Mahon FX, Rea D, Guilhot J, et al. Discontinuation of imatinib in patients with chronic myeloid leukaemia who have maintained complete molecular remission for at least 2 years: the prospective, multicentre Stop Imatinib (STIM) trial. *Lancet Oncol.* 2010;11(11):1029-1035.

42. Hochhaus A, Baccarani M, Silver RT, et al. European LeukemiaNet 2020 recommendations for treating chronic myeloid leukemia. *Leukemia.* 2020;34(4):966-984.
43. Experts in Chronic Myeloid Leukemia. The price of drugs for chronic myeloid leukemia (CML) is a reflection of the unsustainable prices of cancer drugs: from the perspective of a large group of CML experts. *Blood.* 2013;121(22):4439-4442.
44. Huntly BJ, Shigematsu H, Deguchi K, et al. MOZ-TIF2, but not BCR-ABL, confers properties of leukemic stem cells to committed murine hematopoietic progenitors. *Cancer Cell.* 2004;6(6):587-596.
45. Petzer AL, Eaves CJ, Lansdorp PM, Ponchio L, Barnett MJ, Eaves AC. Characterization of primitive subpopulation of normal and leukemic cells present in the blood of patients with newly diagnosed as well as established chronic myeloid leukemia. *Blood.* 1996;88(6):2162-2171.
46. Deininger MW, Goldman JM, Melo JV. The molecular biology of chronic myeloid leukemia. *Blood.* 2000;96(10):3343-3356.
47. Melo JV. The diversity of BCR-ABL fusion proteins and their relationship to leukemia phenotype. *Blood.* 1996;88(7):2375-2384.
48. Verma D, Kantarjian HM, Jones D, et al. Chronic myeloid leukemia (CML) with P190 BCR-ABL: analysis of characteristics, outcomes, and prognostic significance. *Blood.* 2009;114(11):2232-2235.
49. Pane F, Frigeri F, Sindona M, et al. Neutrophilic chronic myeloid leukemia: a distinct disease with a specific molecular marker (BCR/ABL with C3/A2 junction). *Blood.* 1996;88(7):2410-2414.
50. Hochhaus A, Reiter A, Skladny H, et al. A novel BCR-ABL fusion gene (e6a2) in a patient with Philadelphia chromosome-negative chronic myelogenous leukemia. *Blood.* 1996;88(6):2236-2240.
51. Al-Ali HK, Leiblein S, Kovacs I, Hennig E, Niederwieser D, Deininger M. CML with an e1a3 BCR-ABL fusion: rare, benign, and a potential diagnostic pitfall. *Blood.* 2002;100(3):1092-1093.
52. Demehri S, Paschka P, Schultheis B, et al. e8a2 BCR-ABL: more frequent than other atypical BCR-ABL variants? *Leukemia.* 2005;19(4):681-684.
53. Melo JV, Gordon DE, Cross NC, Goldman JM. The ABL-BCR fusion gene is expressed in chronic myeloid leukemia. *Blood.* 1993;81(1):158-165.
54. Huntly BJ, Bench AJ, Delabesse E, et al. Derivative chromosome 9 deletions in chronic myeloid leukemia: poor prognosis is not associated with loss of ABL-BCR expression, elevated BCR-ABL levels, or karyotypic instability. *Blood.* 2002;99(12):4547-4553.
55. Huntly BJ, Guilhot F, Reid AG, et al. Imatinib improves but may not fully reverse the poor prognosis of patients with CML with derivative chromosome 9 deletions. *Blood.* 2003;102(6):2205-2212.
56. Quintas-Cardama A, Kantarjian H, Talpaz M, et al. Imatinib mesylate therapy may overcome the poor prognostic significance of deletions of derivative chromosome 9 in patients with chronic myelogenous leukemia. *Blood.* 2005;105(6):2281-2286.
57. McWhirter JR, Galasso DL, Wang JY. A coiled-coil oligomerization domain of Bcr is essential for the transforming function of Bcr-Abl oncoproteins. *Mol Cell Biol.* 1993;13(12):7587-7595.
58. Maru Y, Witte ON. The BCR gene encodes a novel serine/threonine kinase activity within a single exon. *Cell.* 1991;67(3):459-468.
59. Harnois T, Constantin B, Rioux A, Grenioux E, Kitzis A, Bourmeyster N. Differential interaction and activation of Rho family GTPases by p210bcr-abl and p190bcr-abl. *Oncogene.* 2003;22(41):6445-6454.
60. Diekmann D, Brill S, Garrett MD, et al. Bcr encodes a GTPase-activating protein for p21rac. *Nature.* 1991;351(6325):400-402.
61. Diekmann D, Nobes CD, Burbelo PD, Abo A, Hall A. Rac GTPase interacts with GAPs and target proteins through multiple effector sites. *EMBO J.* 1995;14(21):5297-5305.
62. Voncken JW, van Schaick H, Kaartinen V, et al. Increased neutrophil respiratory burst in bcr-null mutants. *Cell.* 1995;80(5):719-728.
63. Liu J, Campbell M, Guo JQ, et al. BCR/ABL tyrosine kinase is autophosphorylated or transphosphorylates P160 BCR on tyrosine predominantly within the first BCR exon. *Oncogene.* 1993;8(1):101-109.
64. Ma G, Lu D, Wu Y, Liu J, Arlinghaus RB. Bcr phosphorylated on tyrosine 177 binds Grb2. *Oncogene.* 1997;14(19):2367-2372.
65. Kin Y, Li G, Shibuya M, Maru Y. The Dbl homology domain of BCR is not a simple spacer in P210BCR-ABL of the Philadelphia chromosome. *J Biol Chem.* 2001;276(42):39462-39468.
66. Demehri S, O'Hare T, Eide CA, et al. The function of the pleckstrin homology domain in BCR-ABL-mediated leukemogenesis. *Leukemia.* 2010;24(1):226-229.
67. Reckel S, Hamelin R, Georgeon S, et al. Differential signaling networks of Bcr-Abl p210 and p190 kinases in leukemia cells defined by functional proteomics. *Leukemia.* 2017;31(7):1502-1512.
68. Castor A, Nilsson L, Astrand-Grundstrom I, et al. Distinct patterns of hematopoietic stem cell involvement in acute lymphoblastic leukemia. *Nat Med.* 2005;11(6):630-637.
69. Wu Y, Ma G, Lu D, et al. Bcr: a negative regulator of the Bcr-Abl oncoprotein. *Oncogene.* 1999;18(31):4416-4424.
70. Voncken JW, Kaartinen V, Groffen J, Heisterkamp N. Bcr/Abl associated leukemogenesis in bcr null mutant mice. *Oncogene.* 1998;16(15):2029-2032.
71. Konopka JB, Watanabe SM, Witte ON. An alteration of the human c-abl protein in K562 leukemia cells unmasks associated tyrosine kinase activity. *Cell.* 1984;37(3):1035-1042.
72. Bernards A, Rubin CM, Westbrook CA, Paskind M, Baltimore D. The first intron in the human c-abl gene is at least 200 kilobases long and is a target for translocations in chronic myelogenous leukemia. *Mol Cell Biol.* 1987;7(9):3231-3236.
73. Laneuville P. Abl tyrosine protein kinase. *Semin Immunol.* 1995;7(4):255-266.
74. Feller SM, Ren R, Hanafusa H, Baltimore D. SH2 and SH3 domains as molecular adhesives: the interactions of Crk and Abl. *Trends Biochem Sci.* 1994;19(11):453-458.
75. Kipreos ET, Wang JY. Cell cycle-regulated binding of c-Abl tyrosine kinase to DNA. *Science.* 1992;256(5055):382-385.
76. Sawyers CL, McLaughlin J, Goga A, Havlik M, Witte O. The nuclear tyrosine kinase c-Abl negatively regulates cell growth. *Cell.* 1994;77(1):121-131.
77. Kipreos ET, Wang JY. Differential phosphorylation of c-Abl in cell cycle determined by cdc2 kinase and phosphatase activity. *Science.* 1990;248(4952):217-220.
78. Baskaran R, Wood LD, Whitaker LL, et al. Ataxia telangiectasia mutant protein activates c-Abl tyrosine kinase in response to ionizing radiation. *Nature.* 1997;387(6632):516-519.
79. Yuan ZM, Utsugisawa T, Ishiko T, et al. Activation of protein kinase C delta by the c-Abl tyrosine kinase in response to ionizing radiation. *Oncogene.* 1998;16(13):1643-1648.
80. Lewis JM, Baskaran R, Taagepera S, Schwartz MA, Wang JY. Integrin regulation of c-Abl tyrosine kinase activity and cytoplasmic-nuclear transport. *Proc Natl Acad Sci U S A.* 1996;93(26):15174-15179.
81. Kharbanda S, Pandey P, Jin S, et al. Functional interaction between DNA-PK and c-Abl in response to DNA damage. *Nature.* 1997;386(6626):732-735.
82. Yuan ZM, Huang Y, Ishiko T, et al. Regulation of Rad51 function by c-Abl in response to DNA damage. *J Biol Chem.* 1998;273(7):3799-3802.
83. Wang X, Charng WL, Chen CA, et al. Germline mutations in ABL1 cause an autosomal dominant syndrome characterized by congenital heart defects and skeletal malformations. *Nat Genet.* 2017;49(4):613-617.
84. Schwartzberg PL, Stall AM, Hardin JD, et al. Mice homozygous for the ablm1 mutation show poor viability and depletion of selected B and T cell populations. *Cell.* 1991;65(7):1165-1175.
85. Tybulewicz VL, Crawford CE, Jackson PK, Bronson RT, Mulligan RC. Neonatal lethality and lymphopenia in mice with a homozygous disruption of the c-abl proto-oncogene. *Cell.* 1991;65(7):1153-1163.
86. Koleske AJ, Gifford AM, Scott ML, et al. Essential roles for the Abl and Arg tyrosine kinases in neurulation. *Neuron.* 1998;21(6):1259-1272.
87. Zhao X, Ghaffari S, Lodish H, Malashkevich VN, Kim PS. Structure of the Bcr-Abl oncoprotein oligomerization domain. *Nat Struct Biol.* 2002;9(2):117-120.
88. Smith KM, Yacobi R, Van Etten RA. Autoinhibition of Bcr-abl through its SH3 domain. *Mol Cell.* 2003;12(1):27-37.
89. Golub TR, Goga A, Barker GF, et al. Oligomerization of the ABL tyrosine kinase by the Ets protein TEL in human leukemia. *Mol Cell Biol.* 1996;16(8):4107-4116.
90. Graux C, Cools J, Melotte C, et al. Fusion of NUP214 to ABL1 on amplified episomes in T-cell acute lymphoblastic leukemia. *Nat Genet.* 2004;36(10):1084-1089.
91. Pluk H, Dorey K, Superti-Furga G. Autoinhibition of c-Abl. *Cell.* 2002;108(2):247-259.
92. Adrian FJ, Ding Q, Sim T, et al. Allosteric inhibitors of Bcr-abl-dependent cell proliferation. *Nat Chem Biol.* 2006;2(2):95-102.
93. Eide CA, Zabriskie MS, Savage Stevens SL, et al. Combining the allosteric inhibitor asciminib with ponatinib suppresses emergence of and restores efficacy against highly resistant BCR-ABL1 mutants. *Cancer Cell.* 2019;36(4):431-443.e435.
94. Grebien F, Hantschel O, Wojcik J, et al. Targeting the SH2-kinase interface in Bcr-Abl inhibits leukemogenesis. *Cell.* 2011;147(2):306-319.
95. Dai Z, Pendergast AM. Abi-2, a novel SH3-containing protein interacts with the c-Abl tyrosine kinase and modulates c-Abl transforming activity. *Genes Dev.* 1995;9(21):2569-2582.
96. Dai Z, Quackenbush RC, Courtney KD, et al. Oncogenic Abl and Src tyrosine kinases elicit the ubiquitin- dependent degradation of target proteins through a Ras-independent pathway. *Genes Dev.* 1998;12(10):1415-1424.
97. Chu S, Li L, Singh H, Bhatia R. BCR-tyrosine 177 plays an essential role in Ras and Akt activation and in human hematopoietic progenitor transformation in chronic myelogenous leukemia. *Cancer Res.* 2007;67(14):7045-7053.
98. Sattler M, Mohi MG, Pride YB, et al. Critical role for Gab2 in transformation by BCR/ABL. *Cancer Cell.* 2002;1(5):479-492.
99. Gaston I, Johnson KJ, Oda T, et al. Coexistence of phosphotyrosine-dependent and -independent interactions between Cbl and Bcr-Abl. *Exp Hematol.* 2004;32(1):113-121.
100. Komatsu N, Watanabe T, Uchida M, et al. A member of Forkhead transcription factor FKHRL1 is a downstream effector of STI571-induced cell cycle arrest in BCR-ABL-expressing cells. *J Biol Chem.* 2003;278(8):6411-6419.
101. Neshat MS, Raitano AB, Wang HG, Reed JC, Sawyers CL. The survival function of the Bcr-Abl oncogene is mediated by Bad-dependent and -independent pathways: roles for phosphatidylinositol 3-kinase and Raf. *Mol Cell Biol.* 2000;20(4):1179-1186.
102. Agarwal A, Mackenzie RJ, Besson A, et al. BCR-ABL1 promotes leukemia by converting p27 into a cytoplasmic oncoprotein. *Blood.* 2014;124(22):3260-3273.
103. Markova B, Albers C, Breitenbuecher F, et al. Novel pathway in Bcr-Abl signal transduction involves Akt-independent, PLC-gamma1-driven activation of mTOR/p70S6-kinase pathway. *Oncogene.* 2010;29(5):739-751.
104. Ly C, Arechiga AF, Melo JV, Walsh CM, Ong ST. Bcr-Abl kinase modulates the translation regulators ribosomal protein S6 and 4E-BP1 in chronic myelogenous leukemia cells via the mammalian target of rapamycin. *Cancer Res.* 2003;63(18):5716-5722.
105. Kardinal C, Konkol B, Lin H, et al. Chronic myelogenous leukemia blast cell proliferation is inhibited by peptides that disrupt Grb2-SoS complexes. *Blood.* 2001;98(6):1773-1781.
106. Marais R, Light Y, Paterson HF, Marshall CJ. Ras recruits Raf-1 to the plasma membrane for activation by tyrosine phosphorylation. *Embo J.* 1995;14(13):3136-3145.
107. Salomoni P, Wasik MA, Riedel RF, et al. Expression of constitutively active Raf-1 in the mitochondria restores antiapoptotic and leukemogenic potential of a transformation-deficient BCR/ABL mutant. *J Exp Med.* 1998;187(12):1995-2007.
108. Thomas EK, Cancelas JA, Zheng Y, Williams DA. Rac GTPases as key regulators of p210-BCR-ABL-dependent leukemogenesis. *Leukemia.* 2008;22(5):898-904.

109. Thomas EK, Cancelas JA, Chae HD, et al. Rac guanosine triphosphatases represent integrating molecular therapeutic targets for BCR-ABL-induced myeloproliferative disease. *Cancer Cell.* 2007;12(5):467-478.
110. Sexl V, Piekorz R, Moriggl R, et al. Stat5a/b contribute to interleukin 7-induced B-cell precursor expansion, but abl- and bcr/abl-induced transformation are independent of stat5. *Blood.* 2000;96(6):2277-2283.
111. Walz C, Ahmed W, Lazarides K, et al. Essential role for Stat5a/b in myeloproliferative neoplasms induced by BCR-ABL1 and JAK2(V617F) in mice. *Blood.* 2012;119(15):3550-3560.
112. Hoelbl A, Schuster C, Kovacic B, et al. Stat5 is indispensable for the maintenance of bcr/abl-positive leukaemia. *EMBO Mol Med*;2010;2(3):98-110.
113. Ye D, Wolff N, Li L, Zhang S, Ilaria RL, Jr. STAT5 signaling is required for the efficient induction and maintenance of CML in mice. *Blood.* 2006;107(12):4917-4925.
114. Klejman A, Schreiner SJ, Nieborowska-Skorska M, et al. The Src family kinase Hck couples BCR/ABL to STAT5 activation in myeloid leukemia cells. *Embo J.* 2002;21(21):5766-5774.
115. Frank DA, Varticovski L. BCR/abl leads to the constitutive activation of Stat proteins, and shares an epitope with tyrosine phosphorylated Stats. *Leukemia.* 1996;10(11):1724-1730.
116. Ilaria RL, Jr, Van Etten RA. P210 and P190(BCR/ABL) induce the tyrosine phosphorylation and DNA binding activity of multiple specific STAT family members. *J Biol Chem.* 1996;271(49):31704-31710.
117. Samanta AK, Lin H, Sun T, Kantarjian H, Arlinghaus RB. Janus kinase 2: a critical target in chronic myelogenous leukemia. *Cancer Res.* 2006;66(13):6468-6472.
118. Hantschel O, Warsch W, Eckelhart E, et al. BCR-ABL uncouples canonical JAK2-STAT5 signaling in chronic myeloid leukemia. *Nat Chem Biol.* 2012;8(3):285-293.
119. Gotoh A, Miyazawa K, Ohyashiki K, et al. Tyrosine phosphorylation and activation of focal adhesion kinase (p125FAK) by BCR-ABL oncoprotein. *Exp Hematol.* 1995;23(11):1153-1159.
120. Salgia R, Li JL, Lo SH, et al. Molecular cloning of human paxillin, a focal adhesion protein phosphorylated by P210BCR/ABL. *J Biol Chem.* 1995;270(10):5039-5047.
121. Salgia R, Pisick E, Sattler M, et al. p130CAS forms a signaling complex with the adapter protein CRKL in hematopoietic cells transformed by the BCR/ABL oncogene. *J Biol Chem.* 1996;271(41):25198-25203.
122. Sattler M, Salgia R, Shrikhande G, et al. Differential signaling after beta1 integrin ligation is mediated through binding of CRKL to p120(CBL) and p110(HEF1). *J Biol Chem.* 1997;272(22):14320-14326.
123. Uemura N, Griffin JD. The adapter protein Crkl links Cbl to C3G after integrin ligation and enhances cell migration. *J Biol Chem.* 1999;274(53):37525-37532.
124. Oda T, Heaney C, Hagopian JR, Okuda K, Griffin JD, Druker BJ. Crkl is the major tyrosine-phosphorylated protein in neutrophils from patients with chronic myelogenous leukemia. *J Biol Chem.* 1994;269(37):22925-22928.
125. Verfaillie CM, Hurley R, Zhao RC, Prosper F, Delforge M, Bhatia R. Pathophysiology of CML: do defects in integrin function contribute to the premature circulation and massive expansion of the BCR/ABL positive clone? *J Lab Clin Med.* 1997;129(6):584-591.
126. Ramaraj P, Singh H, Niu N, et al. Effect of mutational inactivation of tyrosine kinase activity on BCR/ABL-induced abnormalities in cell growth and adhesion in human hematopoietic progenitors. *Cancer Res.* 2004;64(15):5322-5331.
127. Cramer K, Nieborowska-Skorska M, Koptyra M, et al. BCR/ABL and other kinases from chronic myeloproliferative disorders stimulate single-strand annealing, an unfaithful DNA double-strand break repair. *Cancer Res.* 2008;68(17):6884-6888.
128. Nowicki MO, Falinski R, Koptyra M, et al. BCR/ABL oncogenic kinase promotes unfaithful repair of the reactive oxygen species-dependent DNA double-strand breaks. *Blood.* 2004;104(12):3746-3753.
129. Koptyra M, Falinski R, Nowicki MO, et al. BCR/ABL kinase induces self-mutagenesis via reactive oxygen species to encode imatinib resistance. *Blood.* 2006;108(1):319-327.
130. Perrotti D, Jamieson C, Goldman J, Skorski T. Chronic myeloid leukemia: mechanisms of blastic transformation. *J Clin Invest.* 2010;120(7):2254-2264.
131. Sattler M, Verma S, Shrikhande G, et al. The BCR/ABL tyrosine kinase induces production of reactive oxygen species in hematopoietic cells. *J Biol Chem.* 2000;275(32):24273-24278.
132. Bolton-Gillespie E, Schemionek M, Klein HU, et al. Genomic instability may originate from imatinib-refractory chronic myeloid leukemia stem cells. *Blood.* 2013;121(20):4175-4183.
133. Feldhahn N, Henke N, Melchior K, et al. Activation-induced cytidine deaminase acts as a mutator in BCR-ABL1-transformed acute lymphoblastic leukemia cells. *J Exp Med.* 2007;204(5):1157-1166.
134. Melo JV, Barnes DJ. Chronic myeloid leukaemia as a model of disease evolution in human cancer. *Nat Rev Cancer.* 2007;7(6):441-453.
135. Risch HA, McLaughlin JR, Cole DE, et al. Population BRCA1 and BRCA2 mutation frequencies and cancer penetrances: a kin-cohort study in Ontario, Canada. *J Natl Cancer Inst.* 2006;98(23):1694-1706.
136. Deutsch E, Dugray A, AbdulKarim B, et al. BCR-ABL down-regulates the DNA repair protein DNA-PKcs. *Blood.* 2001;97(7):2084-2090.
137. Slupianek A, Hoser G, Majsterek I, et al. Fusion tyrosine kinases induce drug resistance by stimulation of homology-dependent recombination repair, prolongation of G(2)/M phase, and protection from apoptosis. *Mol Cell Biol.* 2002;22(12):4189-4201.
138. Brummendorf TH, Holyoake TL, Rufer N, et al. Prognostic implications of differences in telomere length between normal and malignant cells from patients with chronic myeloid leukemia measured by flow cytometry. *Blood.* 2000;95(6):1883-1890.
139. Cramer-Morales K, Nieborowska-Skorska M, Scheibner K, et al. Personalized synthetic lethality induced by targeting RAD52 in leukemias identified by gene mutation and expression profile. *Blood.* 2013;122(7):1293-1304.
140. Slupianek A, Dasgupta Y, Ren SY, et al. Targeting RAD51 phosphotyrosine-315 to prevent unfaithful recombination repair in BCR-ABL1 leukemia. *Blood.* 2011;118(4):1062-1068.
141. Fabarius A, Giehl M, Frank O, et al. Induction of centrosome and chromosome aberrations by imatinib in vitro. *Leukemia.* 2005;19(9):1573-1578.
142. Gambacorti-Passerini C, Antolini L, Mahon FX, et al. Multicenter independent assessment of outcomes in chronic myeloid leukemia patients treated with imatinib. *J Natl Cancer Inst.* 2011;103(7):553-561.
143. Gunnarsson N, Stenke L, Hoglund M, et al. Second malignancies following treatment of chronic myeloid leukaemia in the tyrosine kinase inhibitor era. *Br J Haematol.* 2015;169(5):683-688.
144. Bumm T, Muller C, Al Ali HK, et al. Emergence of clonal cytogenetic abnormalities in Ph- cells in some CML patients in cytogenetic remission to imatinib but restoration of polyclonal hematopoiesis in the majority. *Blood.* 2003;101(5):1941-1949.
145. Takahashi N, Miura I, Saitoh K, Miura AB. Lineage involvement of stem cells bearing the Philedelphia chromosome in chronic myeloid leukemia in the chronic phase as shown by a combination of fluorescence-activated cell sorting and fluorescence in situ hybridization. *Blood.* 1998;92(12):4758-4763.
146. Chan LN, Chen Z, Braas D, et al. Metabolic gatekeeper function of B-lymphoid transcription factors. *Nature.* 2017;542(7642):479-483.
147. Warfvinge R, Geironson L, Sommarin MNE, et al. Single-cell molecular analysis defines therapy response and immunophenotype of stem cell subpopulations in CML. *Blood.* 2017;129(17):2384-2394.
148. Jiang Y, Zhao RC, Verfaillie CM. Abnormal integrin-mediated regulation of chronic myelogenous leukemia CD34+ cell proliferation: BCR/ABL up-regulates the cyclin-dependent kinase inhibitor, p27Kip, which is relocated to the cell cytoplasm and incapable of regulating cdk2 activity. *Proc Natl Acad Sci U S A.* 2000;97(19):10538-10543.
149. Peled A, Hardan I, Trakhtenbrot L, et al. Immature leukemic CD34+CXCR4+ cells from CML patients have lower integrin-dependent migration and adhesion in response to the chemokine SDF-1. *Stem Cell.* 2002;20(3):259-266.
150. Schemionek M, Elling C, Steidl U, et al. BCR-ABL enhances differentiation of long-term repopulating hematopoietic stem cells. *Blood.* 2010;115(16):3185-3195.
151. Graham SM, Vass JK, Holyoake TL, Graham GJ. Transcriptional analysis of quiescent and proliferating CD34+ human hemopoietic cells from normal and chronic myeloid leukemia sources. *Stem Cell.* 2007;25(12):3111-3120.
152. Hamilton A, Helgason GV, Schemionek M, et al. Chronic myeloid leukemia stem cells are not dependent on Bcr-Abl kinase activity for their survival. *Blood.* 2012;119(6):1501-1510.
153. Pellicano F, Copland M, Jorgensen HG, Mountford J, Leber B, Holyoake TL. BMS-214662 induces mitochondrial apoptosis in chronic myeloid leukemia (CML) stem/progenitor cells, including CD34+38- cells, through activation of protein kinase Cbeta. *Blood.* 2009;114(19):4186-4196.
154. Zhao C, Blum J, Chen A, et al. Loss of beta-catenin impairs the renewal of normal and CML stem cells in vivo. *Cancer Cell.* 2007;12(6):528-541.
155. McWeeney SK, Pemberton LC, Loriaux MM, Vartanian K, Willis SG, Yochum G, Wilmot B, Turpaz Y, Pillai R, Druker BJ, Snead JL, MacPartlin M, O'Brien SG, Melo JV, Lange T, Harrington CA, Deininger MW. A gene expression signature of CD34+ cells to predict major cytogenetic response in chronic-phase chronic myeloid leukemia patients treated with imatinib. *Blood.* 2010;115(2):315-325. doi: 10.1182/blood-2009-03-210732
156. Heidel FH, Bullinger L, Feng Z, Wang Z, Neff TA, Stein L, Kalaitzidis D, Lane SW, Armstrong SA. Genetic and pharmacologic inhibition of β-catenin targets imatinib-resistant leukemia stem cells in CML. *Cell Stem Cell.* 2012;10(4):412-424. doi: 10.1016/j.stem.2012.02.017.
157. Schürch C, Riether C, Matter MS, Tzankov A, Ochsenbein AF. CD27 signaling on chronic myelogenous leukemia stem cells activates Wnt target genes and promotes disease progression. *J Clin Invest.* 2012;122(2):624-638. doi: 10.1172/JCI45977
158. Lim S, Saw TY, Zhang M, et al. Targeting of the MNK-eIF4E axis in blast crisis chronic myeloid leukemia inhibits leukemia stem cell function. *Proc Natl Acad Sci U S A.* 2013;110(25):E2298-E2307.
159. Zhang B, Li M, McDonald T, Holyoake TL, Moon RT, Campana D, Shultz L, Bhatia R. Microenvironmental protection of CML stem and progenitor cells from tyrosine kinase inhibitors through N-cadherin and Wnt-β-catenin signaling. *Blood.* 2013;121(10):1824-1838. doi: 10.1182/blood-2012-02-412890
160. Eiring AM, Khorashad JS, Anderson DJ, Yu F, Redwine HM, Mason CC, Reynolds KR, Clair PM, Gantz KC, Zhang TY, Pomicter AD, Kraft IL, Bowler AD, Johnson K, Partlin MM, O'Hare T, Deininger MW. β-Catenin is required for intrinsic but not extrinsic BCR-ABL1 kinase-independent resistance to tyrosine kinase inhibitors in chronic myeloid leukemia. *Leukemia.* 2015;29(12):2328-2337. doi: 10.1038/leu.2015.196
161. Agarwal P, Zhang B, Ho Y, Cook A, Li L, Mikhail FM, Wang Y, McLaughlin ME, Bhatia R. Enhanced targeting of CML stem and progenitor cells by inhibition of porcupine acyltransferase in combination with TKI. *Blood.* 2017;129(8):1008-1020. doi: 10.1182/blood-2016-05-714089
162. Zhang B, Strauss AC, Chu S, Li M, Ho Y, Shiang KD, Snyder DS, Huettner CS, Shultz L, Holyoake T, Bhatia R. Effective targeting of quiescent chronic myelogenous leukemia stem cells by histone deacetylase inhibitors in combination with imatinib mesylate. *Cancer Cell.* 2010;17(5):427-442. doi: 10.1016/j.ccr.2010.03.011
163. Dierks C, Beigi R, Guo GR, et al. Expansion of Bcr-Abl-positive leukemic stem cells is dependent on Hedgehog pathway activation. *Cancer Cell.* 2008;14(3):238-249.
164. Zhao C, Chen A, Jamieson CH, et al. Hedgehog signalling is essential for maintenance of cancer stem cells in myeloid leukaemia. *Nature.* 2009;458(7239):776-779.
165. Chen Y, Hu Y, Zhang H, Peng C, Li S. Loss of the Alox5 gene impairs leukemia stem cells and prevents chronic myeloid leukemia. *Nat Genet.* 2009;41(7):783-792.

166. Hurtz C, Hatzi K, Cerchietti L, et al. BCL6-mediated repression of p53 is critical for leukemia stem cell survival in chronic myeloid leukemia. *J Exp Med.* 2011;208(11):2163-2174.
167. Reavie L, Buckley SM, Loizou E, Takeishi S, Aranda-Orgilles B, Ndiaye-Lobry D, Abdel-Wahab O, Ibrahim S, Nakayama KI, Aifantis I. Regulation of c-Myc ubiquitination controls chronic myelogenous leukemia initiation and progression. *Cancer Cell.* 2013;23(3):362-375. doi: 10.1016/j.ccr.2013.01.025
168. Abraham SA, Hopcroft LE, Carrick E, et al. Dual targeting of p53 and c-MYC selectively eliminates leukaemic stem cells. *Nature.* 2016;534(7607):341-346.
169. Neviani P, Santhanam R, Trotta R, et al. The tumor suppressor PP2A is functionally inactivated in blast crisis CML through the inhibitory activity of the BCR/ABL-regulated SET protein. *Cancer Cell.* 2005;8(5):355-368.
170. Lai D, Chen M, Su J, Liu X, Rothe K, Hu K, Forrest DL, Eaves CJ, Morin GB, Jiang X. Response to Comment on "PP2A inhibition sensitizes cancer stem cells to ABL tyrosine kinase inhibitors in BCR-ABL+ human leukemia". *Sci Transl Med.* 2019;11(501):eaav0819. doi: 10.1126/scitranslmed.aav0819
171. Li L, Wang L, Li L, Wang Z, Ho Y, McDonald T, Holyoake TL, Chen W, Bhatia R. Activation of p53 by SIRT1 inhibition enhances elimination of CML leukemia stem cells in combination with imatinib. *Cancer Cell.* 2012;21(2):266-281. doi: 10.1016/j.ccr.2011.12.020
172. Jin Y, Zhou J, Xu F, Jin B, Cui L, Wang Y, Du X, Li J, Li P, Ren R, Pan J. Targeting methyltransferase PRMT5 eliminates leukemia stem cells in chronic myelogenous leukemia. *J Clin Invest.* 2016;126(10):3961-3980. doi: 10.1172/JCI85239
173. Ma L, Pak ML, Ou J, Yu J, St Louis P, Shan Y, Hutchinson L, Li S, Brehm MA, Zhu LJ, Green MR. Prosurvival kinase PIM2 is a therapeutic target for eradication of chronic myeloid leukemia stem cells. *Proc Natl Acad Sci U S A.* 2019;116(21):10482-10487. doi: 10.1073/pnas.1903550116
174. Goff DJ, Court Recart A, Sadarangani A, Chun HJ, Barrett CL, Krajewska M, Leu H, Low-Marchelli J, Ma W, Shih AY, Wei J, Zhai D, Geron I, Pu M, Bao L, Chuang R, Balaian L, Gotlib J, Minden M, Martinelli G, Rusert J, Dao KH, Shazand K, Wentworth P, Smith KM, Jamieson CA, Morris SR, Messer K, Goldstein LS, Hudson TJ, Marra M, Frazer KA, Pellecchia M, Reed JC, Jamieson CH. A Pan-BCL2 inhibitor renders bone-marrow-resident human leukemia stem cells sensitive to tyrosine kinase inhibition. *Cell Stem Cell.* 2013;12(3):316-328. doi: 10.1016/j.stem.2012.12.011
175. Prost S, Relouzat F, Spentchian M, Ouzegdouh Y, Saliba J, Massonnet G, Beressi JP, Verhoeyen E, Raggueneau V, Maneglier B, Castaigne S, Chomienne C, Chrétien S, Rousselot P, Leboulch P. Erosion of the chronic myeloid leukaemia stem cell pool by PPARγ agonists. *Nature.* 2015;525(7569):380-383. doi: 10.1038/nature15248
176. Rousselot P, Prost S, Guilhot J, Roy L, Etienne G, Legros L, Charbonnier A, Coiteux V, Cony-Makhoul P, Huguet F, Cayssials E, Cayuela JM, Relouzat F, Delord M, Bruzzoni-Giovanelli H, Morisset L, Mahon FX, Guilhot F, Leboulch P; French CML Group. Pioglitazone together with imatinib in chronic myeloid leukemia: A proof of concept study. *Cancer.* 2017;123(10):1791-1799. doi: 10.1002/cncr.30490
177. Bellodi C, Lidonnici MR, Hamilton A, Helgason GV, Soliera AR, Ronchetti M, Galavotti S, Young KW, Selmi T, Yacobi R, Van Etten RA, Donato N, Hunter A, Dinsdale D, Tirrò E, Vigneri P, Nicotera P, Dyer MJ, Holyoake T, Salomoni P, Calabretta B. Targeting autophagy potentiates tyrosine kinase inhibitor-induced cell death in Philadelphia chromosome-positive cells, including primary CML stem cells. *J Clin Invest.* 2009;119(5):1109-1123. doi: 10.1172/JCI35660. Erratum in: *J Clin Invest.* 2013;123(8):3634.
178. Baquero P, Dawson A, Mukhopadhyay A, Kuntz EM, Mitchell R, Olivares O, Ianniciello A, Scott MT, Dunn K, Nicastri MC, Winkler JD, Michie AM, Ryan KM, Halsey C, Gottlieb E, Keaney EP, Murphy LO, Amaravadi RK, Holyoake TL, Helgason GV. Targeting quiescent leukemic stem cells using second generation autophagy inhibitors. *Leukemia.* 2019;33(4):981-994. doi: 10.1038/s41375-018-0252-4
179. Horne GA, Stobo J, Kelly C, Mukhopadhyay A, Latif AL, Dixon-Hughes J, McMahon L, Cony-Makhoul P, Byrne J, Smith G, Koschmieder S, BrÜmmendorf TH, Schafhausen P, Gallipoli P, Thomson F, Cong W, Clark RE, Milojkovic D, Helgason GV, Foroni L, Nicolini FE, Holyoake TL, Copland M. A randomised phase II trial of hydroxychloroquine and imatinib versus imatinib alone for patients with chronic myeloid leukaemia in major cytogenetic response with residual disease. *Leukemia.* 2020 ;34(7):1775-1786. doi: 10.1038/s41375-019-0700-9
180. Ito K, Bernardi R, Morotti A, et al. PML targeting eradicates quiescent leukaemia-initiating cells. *Nature.* 2008;453(7198):1072-1078.
181. Traer E, MacKenzie R, Snead J, et al. Blockade of JAK2-mediated extrinsic survival signals restores sensitivity of CML cells to ABL inhibitors. *Leukemia.* 2012;26(5):1140-1143.
182. Gallipoli P, Cook A, Rhodes S, Hopcroft L, Wheadon H, Whetton AD, Jørgensen HG, Bhatia R, Holyoake TL. JAK2/STAT5 inhibition by nilotinib with ruxolitinib contributes to the elimination of CML CD34+ cells in vitro and in vivo. Blood. 2014;124(9):1492-1501. doi: 10.1182/blood-2013-12-545640
183. Sweet K, Hazlehurst L, Sahakian E, Powers J, Nodzon L, Kayali F, Hyland K, Nelson A, Pinilla-Ibarz J. A phase I clinical trial of ruxolitinib in combination with nilotinib in chronic myeloid leukemia patients with molecular evidence of disease. *Leuk Res.* 2018;74:89-96. doi: 10.1016/j.leukres.2018.10.002
184. Kuntz EM, Baquero P, Michie AM, Dunn K, Tardito S, Holyoake TL, Helgason GV, Gottlieb E. Targeting mitochondrial oxidative phosphorylation eradicates therapy-resistant chronic myeloid leukemia stem cells. *Nat Med.* 2017;23(10):1234-1240. doi: 10.1038/nm.4399
185. Naka K, Hoshii T, Muraguchi T, Tadokoro Y, Ooshio T, Kondo Y, Nakao S, Motoyama N, Hirao A. TGF-beta-FOXO signalling maintains leukaemia-initiating cells in chronic myeloid leukaemia. *Nature.* 2010 ;463(7281):676-680. doi: 10.1038/nature08734.
186. Ito T, Kwon HY, Zimdahl B, Congdon KL, Blum J, Lento WE, Zhao C, Lagoo A, Gerrard G, Foroni L, Goldman J, Goh H, Kim SH, Kim DW, Chuah C, Oehler VG, Radich JP, Jordan CT, Reya T. Regulation of myeloid leukaemia by the cell-fate determinant Musashi. *Nature.* 2010;466(7307):765-768. doi: 10.1038/nature09171
187. Jiang Q, Crews LA, Barrett CL, Chun HJ, Court AC, Isquith JM, Zipeto MA, Goff DJ, Minden M, Sadarangani A, Rusert JM, Dao KH, Morris SR, Goldstein LS, Marra MA, Frazer KA, Jamieson CH. ADAR1 promotes malignant progenitor reprogramming in chronic myeloid leukemia. *Proc Natl Acad Sci U S A.* 2013;110(3):1041-1046. doi: 10.1073/pnas.1213021110
188. Scott MT, Korfi K, Saffrey P, Hopcroft LE, Kinstrie R, Pellicano F, Guenther C, Gallipoli P, Cruz M, Dunn K, Jorgensen HG, Cassels JE, Hamilton A, Crossan A, Sinclair A, Holyoake TL, Vetrie D. Epigenetic Reprogramming Sensitizes CML Stem Cells to Combined EZH2 and Tyrosine Kinase Inhibition. *Cancer Discov.* 2016;6(11):1248-1257. doi: 10.1158/2159-8290.CD-16-0263
189. Xie H, Peng C, Huang J, Li BE, Kim W, Smith EC, Fujiwara Y, Qi J, Cheloni G, Das PP, Nguyen M, Li S, Bradner JE, Orkin SH. Chronic Myelogenous Leukemia- Initiating Cells Require Polycomb Group Protein EZH2. *Cancer Discov.* 2016;6(11):1237-1247. doi: 10.1158/2159-8290.CD-15-1439.
190. Branford S, Wang P, Yeung DT, et al. Integrative genomic analysis reveals cancer-associated mutations at diagnosis of CML in patients with high-risk disease. *Blood.* 2018;132(9):948-961.
191. Kreuzer KA, Saborowski A, Lupberger J, Appelt C, Na IK, le Coutre P, Schmidt CA. Fluorescent 5'-exonuclease assay for the absolute quantification of Wilms' tumour gene (WT1) mRNA: implications for monitoring human leukaemias. *Br J Haematol.* 2001;114(2):313-318. doi: 10.1046/j.1365-2141.2001.02912.x. PMID: 11529849.
192. Roche-Lestienne, C., Marceau, A., Labis, E. et al. Mutation analysis of TET2, IDH1, IDH2 and ASXL1 in chronic myeloid leukemia. *Leukemia.* 2011;25:1661-1664 doi:10.1038/leu.2011.139
193. Brehme M, Hantschel O, Colinge J, et al. Charting the molecular network of the drug target Bcr-Abl. *Proc Natl Acad Sci U S A.* 2009;106(18):7414-7419.
194. Johansson B, Fioretos T, Mitelman F. Cytogenetic and molecular genetic evolution of chronic myeloid leukemia. *Acta Haematol.* 2002;107(2):76-94.
195. Fabarius A, Leitner A, Hochhaus A, et al. Impact of additional cytogenetic aberrations at diagnosis on prognosis of CML: long-term observation of 1151 patients from the randomized CML Study IV. *Blood.* 2011;118(26):6760-6768.
196. Mullighan CG, Williams RT, Downing JR, Sherr CJ. Failure of CDKN2A/B (INK4A/B-ARF)-mediated tumor suppression and resistance to targeted therapy in acute lymphoblastic leukemia induced by BCR-ABL. *Genes Dev.* 2008;22(11):1411-1415.
197. Ko TK, Javed A, Lee KL, et al. An integrative model of pathway convergence in genetically heterogeneous blast crisis chronic myeloid leukemia. *Blood.* 2020;135(26):2337-2353.
198. Elmaagacli AH, Beelen DW, Opalka B, Seeber S, Schaefer UW. The amount of BCR-ABL fusion transcripts detected by the real-time quantitative polymerase chain reaction method in patients with Philadelphia chromosome positive chronic myeloid leukemia correlates with the disease stage. *Ann Hematol.* 2000;79(8):424-431.
199. Esposito N, Colavita I, Quintarelli C, et al. SHP-1 expression accounts for resistance to imatinib treatment in Philadelphia chromosome-positive cells derived from patients with chronic myeloid leukemia. *Blood.* 2011;118(13):3634-3644.
200. Lucas CM, Harris RJ, Giannoudis A, Copland M, Slupsky JR, Clark RE. Cancerous inhibitor of PP2A (CIP2A) at diagnosis of chronic myeloid leukemia is a critical determinant of disease progression. *Blood.* 2011;117(24):6660-6668.
201. Wu Y, Slovak ML, Snyder DS, Arber DA. Coexistence of inversion 16 and the Philadelphia chromosome in acute and chronic myeloid leukemias: report of six cases and review of literature. *Am J Clin Pathol.* 2006;125(2):260-266.
202. Gerritsen M, Yi G, Tijchon E, et al. RUNX1 mutations enhance self-renewal and block granulocytic differentiation in human in vitro models and primary AMLs. *Blood Adv.* 2019;3(3):320-332.
203. Perrotti D, Cesi V, Trotta R, et al. BCR-ABL suppresses C/EBPalpha expression through inhibitory action of hnRNP E2. *Nat Genet.* 2002;30(1):48-58.
204. Eiring AM, Harb JG, Neviani P, et al. miR-328 functions as an RNA decoy to modulate hnRNP E2 regulation of mRNA translation in leukemic blasts. *Cell.* 2010;140(5):652-665.
205. Guerzoni C, Bardini M, Mariani SA, et al. Inducible activation of CEBPB, a gene negatively regulated by BCR/ABL, inhibits proliferation and promotes differentiation of BCR/ABL-expressing cells. *Blood.* 2006;107(10):4080-4089.
206. Cuenco GM, Ren R. Both AML1 and EVI1 oncogenic components are required for the cooperation of AML1/MDS1/EVI1 with BCR/ABL in the induction of acute myelogenous leukemia in mice. *Oncogene.* 2004;23(2):569-579.
207. De Weer A, Poppe B, Cauwelier B, et al. EVI1 activation in blast crisis CML due to juxtaposition to the rare 17q22 partner region as part of a 4-way variant translocation t(9;22). *BMC Cancer.* 2008;8:193.
208. Jamieson CH, Ailles LE, Dylla SJ, et al. Granulocyte-macrophage progenitors as candidate leukemic stem cells in blast-crisis CML. *N Engl J Med.* 2004;351(7):657-667.
209. Coluccia AM, Vacca A, Dunach M, et al. Bcr-Abl stabilizes beta-catenin in chronic myeloid leukemia through its tyrosine phosphorylation. *EMBO J.* 2007;26(5):1456-1466.
210. Abrahamsson AE, Geron I, Gotlib J, et al. Glycogen synthase kinase 3beta missplicing contributes to leukemia stem cell generation. *Proc Natl Acad Sci USA.* 2009;106(10):3925-3929.
211. Thomson DW, Shahrin NH, Wang PPS, et al. Aberrant RAG-mediated recombination contributes to multiple structural rearrangements in lymphoid blast crisis of chronic myeloid leukemia. *Leukemia.* 2020;34(8):2051-2063.
212. Nteliopoulos G, Bazeos A, Claudiani S, et al. Somatic variants in epigenetic modifiers can predict failure of response to imatinib but not to second-generation tyrosine kinase inhibitors. *Haematologica.* 2019;104(12):2400-2409.
213. Tanaka K, Takechi M, Hong J, et al. 9;22 translocation and bcr rearrangements in chronic myelocytic leukemia patients among atomic bomb survivors. *J Radiat Res.* 1989;30(4):352-358.

214. Corso A, Lazzarino M, Morra E, et al. Chronic myelogenous leukemia and exposure to ionizing radiation - a retrospective study of 443 patients. *Ann Hematol.* 1995;70(2):79-82.
215. Van Kaick G, Wesch H, Luhrs H, Liebermann D, Kaul A. Neoplastic diseases induced by chronic alpha-irradiation: epidemiological, biophysical and clinical results of the German Thorotrast Study. *J Radiat Res Tokyo.* 1991;32(suppl 2):20-33.
216. SEER. Vol. 2012. https://seer.cancer.gov/statfacts/html/cmyl.html
217. Corm S, Roche L, Micol JB, et al. Changes in the dynamics of the excess mortality rate in chronic phase-chronic myeloid leukemia over 1990-2007: a population study. *Blood.* 2011;118(16):4331-4337.
218. Huang X, Cortes J, Kantarjian H. Estimations of the increasing prevalence and plateau prevalence of chronic myeloid leukemia in the era of tyrosine kinase inhibitor therapy. *Cancer.* 2012;118(12):3123-3127.
219. Sawyers CL. Chronic myeloid leukemia. *N Engl J Med.* 1999;340(17):1330-1340.
220. Arber DA, Orazi A, Hasserjian R, et al. The 2016 revision to the World Health Organization classification of myeloid neoplasms and acute leukemia. *Blood.* 2016;127(20):2391-2405.
221. Thiele J, Kvasnicka HM, Schmitt-Graeff A, et al. Bone marrow features and clinical findings in chronic myeloid leukemia: a comparative, multicenter, immunohistological and morphometric study on 614 patients. *Leuk Lymphoma.* 2000;36(3-4):295-308.
222. Hehlmann R. How I treat CML blast crisis. *Blood.* 2012;120(4):737-747.
223. Kantarjian HM, Talpaz M. Definition of the accelerated phase of chronic myelogenous leukemia. *J Clin Oncol.* 1988;6(1):180-182.
224. Baccarani M, Deininger MW, Rosti G, et al. European LeukemiaNet recommendations for the management of chronic myeloid leukemia: 2013 *Blood.* 2013;122(6):872-884.
225. Radich JP, Dai H, Mao M, et al. Gene expression changes associated with progression and response in chronic myeloid leukemia. *Proc Natl Acad Sci U S A.* 2006;103(8):2794-2799.
226. Mitchell B, Deininger M. Techniques for risk stratification of newly diagnosed patients with chronic myeloid leukemia. *Leuk Lymphoma.* 2011;52(suppl 1):4-11.
227. Sokal JE, Cox EB, Baccarani M, et al. Prognostic discrimination in "good-risk" chronic granulocytic leukemia. *Blood.* 1984;63(4):789-799.
228. Bonifazi F, de Vivo A, Rosti G, et al. Chronic myeloid leukemia and interferon-alpha: a study of complete cytogenetic responders. *Blood.* 2001;98(10):3074-3081.
229. Druker BJ, Guilhot F, O'Brien SG, et al. Five-year follow-up of patients receiving imatinib for chronic myeloid leukemia. *N Engl J Med.* 2006;355(23):2408-2417.
230. Hasford J, Pfirrmann M, Hehlmann R, et al. A new prognostic score for survival of patients with chronic myeloid leukemia treated with interferon alfa. Writing Committee for the Collaborative CML Prognostic Factors Project Group. *J Natl Cancer Inst.* 1998;90(11):850-858.
231. Hasford J, Baccarani M, Hoffmann V, et al. Predicting complete cytogenetic response and subsequent progression-free survival in 2060 patients with CML on imatinib treatment: the EUTOS score. *Blood.* 2011;118(3):686-692.
232. Sinclair PB, Green AR, Grace C, Nacheva EP. Improved sensitivity of BCR-ABL detection: a triple-probe three-color fluorescence in situ hybridization system. *Blood.* 1997;90(4):1395-1402.
233. Sinclair PB, Nacheva EP, Leversha M, et al. Large deletions at the t(9;22) breakpoint are common and may identify a poor-prognosis subgroup of patients with chronic myeloid leukemia. *Blood.* 2000;95(3):738-743.
234. Testoni N, Marzocchi G, Luatti S, et al. Chronic myeloid leukemia: a prospective comparison of interphase fluorescence in situ hybridization and chromosome banding analysis for the definition of complete cytogenetic response—a study of the GIMEMA CML WP. *Blood.* 2009;114(24):4939-4943.
235. Cross NC, Melo JV, Feng L, Goldman JM. An optimized multiplex polymerase chain reaction (PCR) for detection of BCR-ABL fusion mRNAs in haematological disorders. *Leukemia.* 1994;8(1):186-189.
236. Hughes T, Deininger M, Hochhaus A, et al. Monitoring CML patients responding to treatment with tyrosine kinase inhibitors: review and recommendations for harmonizing current methodology for detecting BCR-ABL transcripts and kinase domain mutations and for expressing results. *Blood.* 2006;108(1):28-37.
237. Cross NC, Hochhaus A, Müller MC. Molecular monitoring of chronic myeloid leukemia: principles and interlaboratory standardization. *Ann Hematol.* 2015;94(suppl 2):S219-S225.
238. Cross NC, White HE, Müller MC, Saglio G, Hochhaus A. Standardized definitions of molecular response in chronic myeloid leukemia. *Leukemia.* 2012;26(10):2172-2175.
239. Branford S, Fletcher L, Cross NC, et al. Desirable performance characteristics for BCR-ABL measurement on an international reporting scale to allow consistent interpretation of individual patient response and comparison of response rates between clinical trials. *Blood.* 2008;112(8):3330-3338.
240. Press RD, Willis SG, Laudadio J, Mauro MJ, Deininger MW. Determining the rise in BCR-ABL RNA that optimally predicts a kinase domain mutation in patients with chronic myeloid leukemia on imatinib. *Blood.* 2009;114(13):2598-2605.
241. Branford S, Rudzki Z, Parkinson I, et al. Real-time quantitative PCR analysis can be used as a primary screen to identify patients with CML treated with imatinib who have BCR-ABL kinase domain mutations. *Blood.* 2004;104(9):2926-2932.
242. White H, Deprez L, Corbisier P, et al. A certified plasmid reference material for the standardisation of BCR-ABL1 mRNA quantification by real-time quantitative PCR. *Leukemia.* 2015;29(2):369-376.
243. Muller MC, Saglio G, Lin F, et al. An international study to standardize the detection and quantitation of BCR-ABL transcripts from stabilized peripheral blood preparations by quantitative RT-PCR. *Haematologica.* 2007;92(7):970-973.
244. O'Brien SG, Guilhot F, Larson RA, et al. Imatinib compared with interferon and low-dose cytarabine for newly diagnosed chronic-phase chronic myeloid leukemia. *N Engl J Med.* 2003;348(11):994-1004.

245. Hanfstein B, Shlyakhto V, Lauseker M, et al. Velocity of early BCR-ABL transcript elimination as an optimized predictor of outcome in chronic myeloid leukemia (CML) patients in chronic phase on treatment with imatinib. *Leukemia.* 2014;28(10):1988-1992.
246. Branford S, Yeung DT, Parker WT, et al. Prognosis for patients with CML and >10% BCR-ABL1 after 3 months of imatinib depends on the rate of BCR-ABL1 decline. *Blood.* 2014;124(4):511-518.
247. National Comprehensive Cancer Network. *Chronic Myeloid Leukemia.* Version: 2. (2022).
248. Parker WT, Lawrence RM, Ho M, et al. Sensitive detection of BCR-ABL1 mutations in patients with chronic myeloid leukemia after imatinib resistance is predictive of outcome during subsequent therapy. *J Clin Oncol.* 2011;29(32):4250-4259.
249. Willis SG, Lange T, Demehri S, et al. High-sensitivity detection of BCR-ABL kinase domain mutations in imatinib-naive patients: correlation with clonal cytogenetic evolution but not response to therapy. *Blood.* 2005;106(6):2128-2137.
250. Deininger MW, Hodgson JG, Shah NP, et al. Compound mutations in BCR-ABL1 are not major drivers of primary or secondary resistance to ponatinib in CP-CML patients. *Blood.* 2016;127(6):703-712.
251. Guilhot F, Chastang C, Michallet M, et al. Interferon alfa-2b combined with cytarabine versus interferon alone in chronic myelogenous leukemia. French Chronic Myeloid Leukemia Study Group. *N Engl J Med.* 1997;337(4):223-229.
252. Baccarani M, Rosti G, de Vivo A, et al. A randomized study of interferon-alpha versus interferon-alpha and low-dose arabinosyl cytosine in chronic myeloid leukemia. *Blood.* 2002;99(5):1527-1535.
253. Cortes J, Lipton JH, Rea D, et al. Phase 2 study of subcutaneous omacetaxine mepesuccinate after TKI failure in patients with chronic-phase CML with T315I mutation. *Blood.* 2012;120(13):2573-2580.
254. Kantarjian H, Sawyers C, Hochhaus A, et al. Hematologic and cytogenetic responses to imatinib mesylate in chronic myelogenous leukemia. *N Engl J Med.* 2002;346(9):645-652.
255. Talpaz M, Silver RT, Druker BJ, et al. Imatinib induces durable hematologic and cytogenetic responses in patients with accelerated phase chronic myeloid leukemia: results of a phase 2 study. *Blood.* 2002;99(6):1928-1937.
256. Ottmann OG, Druker BJ, Sawyers CL, et al. A phase 2 study of imatinib in patients with relapsed or refractory Philadelphia chromosome-positive acute lymphoid leukemias. *Blood.* 2002;100(6):1965-1971.
257. Sawyers CL, Hochhaus A, Feldman E, et al. Imatinib induces hematologic and cytogenetic responses in patients with chronic myelogenous leukemia in myeloid blast crisis: results of a phase II study. *Blood.* 2002;99(10):3530-3539.
258. Hochhaus A, Larson RA, Guilhot F, et al. Long-term outcomes of imatinib treatment for chronic myeloid leukemia. *N Engl J Med.* 2017;376(10):917-927.
259. Cortes J, Giles F, O'Brien S, et al. Result of high-dose imatinib mesylate in patients with Philadelphia chromosome: positive chronic myeloid leukemia after failure of interferon-alpha. *Blood.* 2003;102(1):83-86.
260. Kantarjian H, Talpaz M, O'Brien S, et al. High-dose imatinib mesylate therapy in newly diagnosed Philadelphia chromosome-positive chronic phase chronic myeloid leukemia. *Blood.* 2004;103(8):2873-2878.
261. Castagnetti F, Palandri F, Amabile M, et al. Results of high-dose imatinib mesylate in intermediate Sokal risk chronic myeloid leukemia patients in early chronic phase: a phase 2 trial of the GIMEMA CML Working Party. *Blood.* 2009;113(15):3428-3434.
262. Cortes JE, Baccarani M, Guilhot F, et al. Phase III, randomized, open-label study of daily imatinib mesylate 400 mg versus 800 mg in patients with newly diagnosed, previously untreated chronic myeloid leukemia in chronic phase using molecular end points: tyrosine kinase inhibitor optimization and selectivity study. *J Clin Oncol.* 2010;28(3):424-430.
263. Hehlmann R, Lauseker M, Jung-Munkwitz S, et al. Tolerability-adapted imatinib 800 mg/d versus 400 mg/d versus 400 mg/d plus Interferon-{alpha} in newly diagnosed chronic myeloid leukemia. *J Clin Oncol.* 2011;29(12):1634-1642.
264. Deininger MW, Kopecky KJ, Radich JP, et al. Imatinib 800 mg daily induces deeper molecular responses than imatinib 400 mg daily: results of SWOG S0325, an intergroup randomized PHASE II trial in newly diagnosed chronic phase chronic myeloid leukaemia. *Br J Haematol.* 2014;164(2):223-232.
265. Preudhomme C, Guilhot J, Nicolini FE, et al. Imatinib plus peginterferon alfa-2a in chronic myeloid leukemia. *N Engl J Med.* 2010;363(26):2511-2521.
266. Hoffmann VS, Hasford J, Deininger M, Cortes J, Baccarani M, Hehlmann R. Systematic review and meta-analysis of standard-dose imatinib vs. high-dose imatinib and second generation tyrosine kinase inhibitors for chronic myeloid leukemia. *J Cancer Res Clin Oncol.* 2017;143(7):1311-1318.
267. Hochhaus A, Kantarjian HM, Baccarani M, et al. Dasatinib induces notable hematologic and cytogenetic responses in chronic-phase chronic myeloid leukemia after failure of imatinib therapy. *Blood.* 2007;109(6):2303-2309.
268. Cortes J, Rousselot P, Kim DW, et al. Dasatinib induces complete hematologic and cytogenetic responses in patients with imatinib-resistant or -intolerant chronic myeloid leukemia in blast crisis. *Blood.* 2007;109(8):3207-3213.
269. Guilhot F, Apperley J, Kim DW, et al. Dasatinib induces significant hematologic and cytogenetic responses in patients with imatinib-resistant or -intolerant chronic myeloid leukemia in accelerated phase. *Blood.* 2007;109(10):4143-4150.
270. Shah NP, Kantarjian HM, Kim DW, et al. Intermittent target inhibition with dasatinib 100 mg once daily preserves efficacy and improves tolerability in imatinib-resistant and -intolerant chronic-phase chronic myeloid leukemia. *J Clin Oncol.* 2008;26(19):3204-3212.
271. Kantarjian HM, Hochhaus A, Saglio G, et al. Nilotinib versus imatinib for the treatment of patients with newly diagnosed chronic phase, Philadelphia chromosome-positive, chronic myeloid leukaemia: 24-month minimum follow-up of the phase 3 randomised ENESTnd trial. *Lancet Oncol.* 2011;12(9):841-851.

272. Cortes JE, Saglio G, Kantarjian HM, et al. Final 5-year study results of DASISION: the dasatinib versus imatinib study in treatment-naive chronic myeloid leukemia patients trial. *J Clin Oncol*. 2016;34(20):2333-2340.
273. Le CP, Ottmann OG, Giles F, et al. Nilotinib (formerly AMN107), a highly selective BCR-ABL tyrosine kinase inhibitor, is active in patients with imatinib-resistant or -intolerant accelerated-phase chronic myelogenous leukemia. *Blood*. 2008;111(4):1834-1839.
274. Kantarjian HM, Giles F, Gattermann N, et al. Nilotinib (formerly AMN107), a highly selective BCR-ABL tyrosine kinase inhibitor, is effective in patients with Philadelphia chromosome-positive chronic myelogenous leukemia in chronic phase following imatinib resistance and intolerance. *Blood*. 2007;110(10):3540-3546.
275. Giles FJ, Kantarjian HM, le Coutre PD, et al. Nilotinib is effective in imatinib-resistant or -intolerant patients with chronic myeloid leukemia in blastic phase. *Leukemia*. 2012;26(5):959-962.
276. Kantarjian HM, Hughes TP, Larson RA, et al. Long-term outcomes with frontline nilotinib versus imatinib in newly diagnosed chronic myeloid leukemia in chronic phase: ENESTnd 10-year analysis. *Leukemia*. 2021;35(2):440-453.
277. Cortes JE, Kantarjian HM, Brummendorf TH, et al. Safety and efficacy of bosutinib (SKI-606) in chronic phase Philadelphia chromosome-positive chronic myeloid leukemia patients with resistance or intolerance to imatinib. *Blood*. 2011;118(17):4567-4576.
278. Cortes JE, Kim DW, Kantarjian HM, et al. Bosutinib versus imatinib in newly diagnosed chronic-phase chronic myeloid leukemia: results from the BELA trial. *J Clin Oncol*. 2012;30(28):3486-3492.
279. Lipton JH, Chuah C, Guerci-Bresler A, et al. Ponatinib versus imatinib for newly diagnosed chronic myeloid leukaemia: an international, randomised, open-label, phase 3 trial. *Lancet Oncol*. 2016;17(5):612-621.
280. Cortes JE, Apperley J, Lomaia E, et al. OPTIC primary analysis: a dose-optimization study of 3 starting doses of ponatinib (PON). *J Clin Oncol*. 2021;39(15_suppl):7000.
281. Cortes JE, Hughes TP, Mauro MJ, et al. Asciminib, a first-in-class STAMP inhibitor, provides durable molecular response in patients (pts) with chronic myeloid leukemia (CML) harboring the T315I mutation: primary efficacy and safety results from a phase 1 trial. *Blood*. 2020;136(suppl 1):47-50.
282. Réa D, Mauro MJ, Boquimpani C, et al. A phase 3, open-label, randomized study of asciminib, a STAMP inhibitor, vs bosutinib in CML after 2 or more prior TKIs. *Blood*. 2021;138(21):2031-2041.
283. Simonsson B, Gedde-Dahl T, Markevarn B, et al. Combination of pegylated IFN-alpha2b with imatinib increases molecular response rates in patients with low- or intermediate-risk chronic myeloid leukemia. *Blood*. 2011;118(12):3228-3235.
284. Ruggiu M, Oberkampf F, Ghez D, et al. Azacytidine in combination with tyrosine kinase inhibitors induced durable responses in patients with advanced phase chronic myelogenous leukemia. *Leuk Lymphoma*. 2018;59(7):1659-1665.
285. Khoury HJ, Goldberg SL, Mauro MJ, et al. Cross-intolerance with dasatinib among imatinib-intolerant patients with chronic phase chronic myeloid leukemia. *Clin Lymphoma Myeloma Leuk*. 2016;16(6):341-349 e341.
286. Marin D, Bazeos A, Mahon FX, et al. Adherence is the critical factor for achieving molecular responses in patients with chronic myeloid leukemia who achieve complete cytogenetic responses on imatinib. *J Clin Oncol*. 2010;28(14):2381-2388.
287. Kim TD, Rea D, Schwarz M, et al. Peripheral artery occlusive disease in chronic phase chronic myeloid leukemia patients treated with nilotinib or imatinib. *Leukemia*. 2013;27(6):1316-1321.
288. Giles FJ, Mauro MJ, Hong F, et al. Rates of peripheral arterial occlusive disease in patients with chronic myeloid leukemia in the chronic phase treated with imatinib, nilotinib, or non-tyrosine kinase therapy: a retrospective cohort analysis. *Leukemia*. 2013;27(6):1310-1315.
289. Montani D, Bergot E, Gunther S, et al. Pulmonary arterial hypertension in patients treated by dasatinib. *Circulation*. 2012;125(17):2128-2137.
290. Weatherald J, Chaumais MC, Savale L, et al. Long-term outcomes of dasatinib-induced pulmonary arterial hypertension: a population-based study. *Eur Respir J*. 2017;50(1):1700217.
291. Valent P, Hadzijusufovic E, Schernthaner GH, Wolf D, Rea D, le Coutre P. Vascular safety issues in CML patients treated with BCR/ABL1 kinase inhibitors. *Blood*. 2015;125(6):901-906.
292. Moslehi JJ, Deininger M. Tyrosine kinase inhibitor-associated cardiovascular toxicity in chronic myeloid leukemia. *J Clin Oncol*. 2015;33(35):4210-4218.
293. Hochhaus A, Saglio G, Hughes TP, et al. Long-term benefits and risks of frontline nilotinib vs imatinib for chronic myeloid leukemia in chronic phase: 5-year update of the randomized ENESTnd trial. *Leukemia*. 2016;30(5):1044-1054.
294. Abou Dalle I, Kantarjian H, Burger J, et al. Efficacy and safety of generic imatinib after switching from original imatinib in patients treated for chronic myeloid leukemia in the United States. *Cancer Med*. 2019;8(15):6559-6565.
295. de Lemos ML, Kyritsis V. Clinical efficacy of generic imatinib. *J Oncol Pharm Pract*. 2015;21(1):76-79.
296. Deininger MW, O'Brien SG, Ford JM, Druker BJ. Practical management of patients with chronic myeloid leukemia receiving imatinib. *J Clin Oncol*. 2003;21(8):1637-1647.
297. Deininger MW, Shah NP, Altman JK, et al. Chronic myeloid leukemia, version 2.2021, NCCN clinical practice guidelines in oncology. *J Natl Compr Canc Netw*. 2020;18(10):1385-1415.
298. Deininger MW, Cortes J, Paquette R, et al. The prognosis for patients with chronic myeloid leukemia who have clonal cytogenetic abnormalities in philadelphia chromosome-negative cells. *Cancer*. 2007;110(7):1509-1519.
299. Karimata K, Masuko M, Ushiki T, et al. Myelodysplastic syndrome with Ph negative monosomy 7 chromosome following transient bone marrow dysplasia during imatinib treatment for chronic myeloid leukemia. *Intern Med*. 2011;50(5):481-485.
300. Khorashad JS, Tantravahi SK, Yan D, et al. Rapid conversion of chronic myeloid leukemia to chronic myelomonocytic leukemia in a patient on imatinib therapy. *Leukemia*. 2016;30(11):2275-2279.
301. Fruehauf S, Topaly J, Buss EC, et al. Imatinib combined with mitoxantrone/etoposide and cytarabine is an effective induction therapy for patients with chronic myeloid leukemia in myeloid blast crisis. *Cancer*. 2007;109(8):1543-1549.
302. Copland M, Slade D, McIlroy G, et al. Ponatinib with fludarabine, cytarabine, idarubicin, and granulocyte colony-stimulating factor chemotherapy for patients with blast-phase chronic myeloid leukaemia (MATCHPOINT): a single-arm, multicentre, phase 1/2 trial. *Lancet Haematol*. 2022;9(2):e121-e132.
303. O'Hare T, Zabriskie MS, Eiring AM, Deininger MW. Pushing the limits of targeted therapy in chronic myeloid leukaemia. *Nat Rev Cancer*. 2012;12(8):513-526.
304. Shah NP, Nicoll JM, Nagar B, et al. Multiple BCR-ABL kinase domain mutations confer polyclonal resistance to the tyrosine kinase inhibitor imatinib (STI571) in chronic phase and blast crisis chronic myeloid leukemia. *Cancer Cell*. 2002;2(2):117-125.
305. Eiring AM, Deininger MW. Individualizing kinase-targeted cancer therapy: the paradigm of chronic myeloid leukemia. *Genome Biol*. 2014;15(9):461.
306. O'Hare T, Shakespeare WC, Zhu X, et al. AP24534, a pan-BCR-ABL inhibitor for chronic myeloid leukemia, potently inhibits the T315I mutant and overcomes mutation-based resistance. *Cancer Cell*. 2009;16(5):401-412.
307. Soverini S, Colarossi S, Gnani A, et al. Contribution of ABL kinase domain mutations to imatinib resistance in different subsets of Philadelphia-positive patients: by the GIMEMA Working Party on Chronic Myeloid Leukemia. *Clin Cancer Res*. 2006;12(24):7374-7379.
308. O'Hare T, Eide CA, Deininger MW. Bcr-Abl kinase domain mutations, drug resistance, and the road to a cure for chronic myeloid leukemia. *Blood*. 2007;110(7):2242-2249.
309. Muller MC, Cortes JE, Kim DW, et al. Dasatinib treatment of chronic-phase chronic myeloid leukemia: analysis of responses according to preexisting BCR-ABL mutations. *Blood*. 2009;114(24):4944-4953.
310. Hughes T, Saglio G, Branford S, et al. Impact of baseline BCR-ABL mutations on response to nilotinib in patients with chronic myeloid leukemia in chronic phase. *J Clin Oncol*. 2009;27(25):4204-4210.
311. Apperley JF. Part I: mechanisms of resistance to imatinib in chronic myeloid leukaemia. *Lancet Oncol*. 2007;8(11):1018-1029.
312. Mahon FX, Deininger MW, Schultheis B, et al. Selection and characterization of BCR-ABL positive cell lines with differential sensitivity to the tyrosine kinase inhibitor STI571: diverse mechanisms of resistance. *Blood*. 2000;96(3):1070-1079.
313. Dulucq S, Bouchet S, Turcq B, et al. Multidrug resistance gene (MDR1) polymorphisms are associated with major molecular responses to standard-dose imatinib in chronic myeloid leukemia. *Blood*. 2008;112(5):2024-2027.
314. Eadie LN, Hughes TP, White DL. ABCB1 overexpression is a key initiator of resistance to tyrosine kinase inhibitors in CML cell lines. *PLoS One*. 2016;11(8):e0161470.
315. Donato NJ, Wu JY, Stapley J, et al. BCR-ABL independence and LYN kinase overexpression in chronic myelogenous leukemia cells selected for resistance to STI571. *Blood*. 2003;101(2):690-698.
316. Burchert A, Wang Y, Cai D, et al. Compensatory PI3-kinase/Akt/mTor activation regulates imatinib resistance development. *Leukemia*. 2005;19(10):1774-1782.
317. Warsch W, Kollmann K, Eckelhart E, et al. High STAT5 levels mediate imatinib resistance and indicate disease progression in chronic myeloid leukemia. *Blood*. 2011;117(12):3409-3420.
318. Gioia R, Leroy C, Drullion C, et al. Quantitative phosphoproteomics revealed interplay between Syk and Lyn in the resistance to nilotinib in chronic myeloid leukemia cells. *Blood*. 2011;118(8):2211-2221.
319. Wang Y, Cai D, Brendel C, et al. Adaptive secretion of granulocyte-macrophage colony-stimulating factor (GM-CSF) mediates imatinib and nilotinib resistance in BCR/ABL+ progenitors via JAK-2/STAT-5 pathway activation. *Blood*. 2007;109(5):2147-2155.
320. Frye RF, Fitzgerald SM, Lagattuta TF, Hruska MW, Egorin MJ. Effect of St John's wort on imatinib mesylate pharmacokinetics. *Clin Pharmacol Ther*. 2004;76(4):323-329.
321. Milojkovic D, Apperley JF, Gerrard G, et al. Responses to second-line tyrosine kinase inhibitors are durable: an intention-to-treat analysis in chronic myeloid leukemia patients. *Blood*. 2012;119(8):1838-1843.
322. Cortes JE, Kantarjian HM, Rea D, et al. Final analysis of the efficacy and safety of omacetaxine mepesuccinate in patients with chronic- or accelerated-phase chronic myeloid leukemia: results with 24 months of follow-up. *Cancer*. 2015;121(10):1637-1644.
323. Etienne G, Guilhot J, Rea D, et al. Long-term follow-up of the French Stop imatinib (STIM1) study in patients with chronic myeloid leukemia. *J Clin Oncol*. 2017;35(3):298-305.
324. Rousselot P, Charbonnier A, Cony-Makhoul P, et al. Loss of major molecular response as a trigger for restarting tyrosine kinase inhibitor therapy in patients with chronic-phase chronic myelogenous leukemia who have stopped imatinib after durable undetectable disease. *J Clin Oncol*. 2014;32(5):424-430.
325. Ross DM, Branford S, Seymour JF, et al. Safety and efficacy of imatinib cessation for CML patients with stable undetectable minimal residual disease: results from the TWISTER study. *Blood*. 2013;122(4):515-522.
326. Saussele S, Richter J, Guilhot J, et al. Discontinuation of tyrosine kinase inhibitor therapy in chronic myeloid leukaemia (EURO-SKI): a prespecified interim analysis of a prospective, multicentre, non-randomised, trial. *Lancet Oncol*. 2018:19(6):747-757.
327. Atallah E, Schiffer CA. Discontinuation of tyrosine kinase inhibitors in chronic myeloid leukemia: when and for whom? *Haematologica*. 2020;105:2738-2745.
328. Atallah E, Schiffer CA, Radich JP, et al. Assessment of outcomes after stopping tyrosine kinase inhibitors among patients with chronic myeloid leukemia: a nonrandomized clinical trial. *JAMA Oncol*. 2021;7(1):42-50.
329. Imagawa J, Tanaka H, Okada M, et al. Discontinuation of dasatinib in patients with chronic myeloid leukaemia who have maintained deep molecular response

329. for longer than 1 year (DADI trial): a multicentre phase 2 trial. *Lancet Haematol.* 2015;2(12):e528-e535.
330. Shah NP, García-Gutiérrez V, Jiménez-Velasco A, et al. Dasatinib discontinuation in patients with chronic-phase chronic myeloid leukemia and stable deep molecular response: the DASFREE study. *Leuk Lymphoma.* 2020;61(3):650-659.
331. Ross DM, Masszi T, Gómez Casares MT, et al. Durable treatment-free remission in patients with chronic myeloid leukemia in chronic phase following frontline nilotinib: 96-week update of the ENESTfreedom study. *J Cancer Res Clin Oncol.* 2018;144(5):945-954.
332. Ilander M, Olsson-Strömberg U, Schlums H, et al. Increased proportion of mature NK cells is associated with successful imatinib discontinuation in chronic myeloid leukemia. *Leukemia.* 2017;31(5):1108-1116.
333. Schütz C, Inselmann S, Saussele S, et al. Expression of the CTLA-4 ligand CD86 on plasmacytoid dendritic cells (pDC) predicts risk of disease recurrence after treatment discontinuation in CML. *Leukemia.* 2017;31(4):829-836.
334. Kolb HJ, Mittermuller J, Clemm C, et al. Donor leukocyte transfusions for treatment of recurrent chronic myelogenous leukemia in marrow transplant patients. *Blood.* 1990;76(12):2462-2465.
335. Gratwohl A, Hermans J, Goldman JM, et al. Risk assessment for patients with chronic myeloid leukaemia before allogeneic blood or marrow transplantation. Chronic Leukemia Working Party of the European Group for Blood and Marrow Transplantation. *Lancet.* 1998;352(9134):1087-1092.
336. Hehlmann R, Berger U, Pfirrmann M, et al. Drug treatment is superior to allografting as first-line therapy in chronic myeloid leukemia. *Blood.* 2007;109(11):4686-4692.
337. Gratwohl A, Pfirrmann M, Zander A, et al. Long-term outcome of patients with newly diagnosed chronic myeloid leukemia: a randomized comparison of stem cell transplantation with drug treatment. *Leukemia.* 2016;30(3):562-569.
338. Deininger M, Schleuning M, Greinix H, et al. The effect of prior exposure to imatinib on transplant-related mortality. *Haematologica.* 2006;91(4):452-459.
339. Oehler VG, Gooley T, Snyder DS, et al. The effects of imatinib mesylate treatment before allogeneic transplantation for chronic myeloid leukemia. *Blood.* 2007;109(4):1782-1789.
340. Lee SJ, Kukreja M, Wang T, et al. Impact of prior imatinib mesylate on the outcome of hematopoietic cell transplantation for chronic myeloid leukemia. *Blood.* 2008;112(8):3500-3507.
341. Saussele S, Lauseker M, Gratwohl A, et al. Allogeneic hematopoietic stem cell transplantation (allo SCT) for chronic myeloid leukemia in the imatinib era: evaluation of its impact within a subgroup of the randomized German CML Study IV. *Blood.* 2010;115(10):1880-1885.
342. Zhang H, Chen J, Que W. Allogeneic peripheral blood stem cell and bone marrow transplantation for hematologic malignancies: meta-analysis of randomized controlled trials. *Leuk Res.* 2012;36(4):431-437.
343. Zabriskie MS, Eide CA, Tantravahi SK, et al. BCR-ABL1 compound mutations combining key kinase domain positions confer clinical resistance to ponatinib in Ph chromosome-positive leukemia. *Cancer Cell.* 2014;26(3):428-442.
344. Zhao H, Deininger MW. Declaration of Bcr-Abl1 independence. *Leukemia.* 2020;34(11):2827-2836.
345. Chu S, McDonald T, Lin A, et al. Persistence of leukemia stem cells in chronic myelogenous leukemia patients in prolonged remission with imatinib treatment. *Blood.* 2011;118(20):5565-5572.
346. Chomel JC, Bonnet ML, Sorel N, et al. Leukemic stem cell persistence in chronic myeloid leukemia patients with sustained undetectable molecular residual disease. *Blood.* 2011;118(13):3657-3660.
347. Perrotti D, Neviani P. Protein phosphatase 2A (PP2A), a drugable tumor suppressor in Ph1(+) leukemias. *Cancer Metastasis Rev.* 2008;27(2):159-168.
348. Holyoake TL, Vetrie D. The chronic myeloid leukemia stem cell: stemming the tide of persistence. *Blood.* 2017;129(12):1595-1606.
349. Deininger M. Hematology: curing CML with imatinib--a dream come true? *Nat Rev Clin Oncol.* 2011;8(3):127-128.
350. Zhao H, Deininger M. Eradicating residual chronic myeloid leukaemia: basic research lost in translation. *Lancet Haematol.* 2021;8(2):e101-e104.
351. Pagani IS, Dang P, Saunders VA, et al. Lineage of measurable residual disease in patients with chronic myeloid leukemia in treatment-free remission. *Leukemia.* 2020;34(4):1052-1061.

Chapter 84 ■ Polycythemia Vera

LAURA C. MICHAELIS • ROBERT T. MEANS JR

DEFINITION AND HISTORY

Polycythemia vera (PV), also called *polycythemia rubra vera*, is a chronic clonal myeloproliferative disorder characterized by a striking absolute increase in the number of red blood cells and in the total blood volume, and usually by leukocytosis, thrombocytosis, and splenomegaly. The bone marrow is typically hypercellular and exhibits hyperplasia of myeloid, erythroid, and megakaryocyte lineages. Key events in the history of this disorder, from the first recognition of noncardiac polycythemia by Vaquez in 1892 through Osler's recognition of isolated case reports indicating a previously undescribed disease to the demonstration of clonality and molecular mechanisms in recent years, are outlined in *Table 84.1*.[1] While the disease may be indolent for years, the condition does have significant health consequences that impact life expectancy—predominantly the risks of thrombotic, fibrotic, or leukemic events.

EPIDEMIOLOGY

The age-standardized incidence rate of PV in the United States between 2002 and 2016 was 1.55 per 100,000 person-years, with a male and female predominance ratio of 1.57.[2] Although male predominance is consistently observed in different populations, this difference appears to be less marked in younger patients and in patients older than 70 years.[3-5] The prevalence of disease is estimated at about 22 to 57 per 100,000 person-years with a 5-year relative survival of 84% to 89%.

PV tends to be a disease of older individuals, with median age at diagnosis 65 years in the United States, and similar peak incidence observed in other populations.[3-5] The incidence increases with age: incidence at age 20 is less than 1 per million person-years, increasing to approximately 10 per million for persons in their 60s and peaking around 50 per million person-years at age 80.

Racial and ethnic factors influence the incidence of PV. The incidence of PV in African Americans and in persons of Hispanic or Asian/Pacific ancestry is approximately 60% of that found in Americans of white European ancestry. Ashkenazi Jews in Northern Israel exhibit a higher incidence of PV than do their neighbors of Arab or Sephardic Jewish origins.[3,6]

Six percent of the patients enrolled in the protocols of the Polycythemia Vera Study Group (PVSG) reported relatives with PV, and similar findings have been reported in other large series.[7,8] There is growing investigation into the role that inherited genetic abnormalities may play in the lifetime risk for MPNs. Individuals with a first-degree relative affected by an MPN are up to 7 times more likely than unaffected controls to develop an MPN.[5] The exact proportion of MPNs arising out of a familial syndrome or germline predisposition is unknown, but estimated to be 5% to 10%.[9-11] Germline predisposition may be very complex, and variants may affect the risk of later development of MPN as well as disease phenotype, outcome, and response to therapy.[11,12] There is an association between PV and being a blood donor: this may simply reflect that persons with elevated hemoglobin (Hb) concentrations not yet diagnosed with PV may be better able to donate blood and encouraged to do so by physicians.[8]

CLINICAL FEATURES

Many of the symptoms and signs of PV can be attributed in large part to the expanded total blood volume and to the slowing of the blood flow because of increased blood viscosity, as discussed in Chapter 45. There may be a substantial lag in the time to diagnosis, as the symptoms may be mild or erratic. Patients may complain of headache, dizziness, tinnitus, visual disturbances, dyspnea, lassitude, or weakness. Although the color of the skin is often acknowledged to have been abnormal for a long time, this complaint alone rarely brings the patient to the physician. Skin and mucous membrane hemorrhages are common; these, or a sense of fullness or swelling in the abdomen owing to enlargement of the spleen, may be the initial symptoms. The lack of specificity of symptoms may in fact contribute to the delay in diagnosis. On the other hand, some patients have no complaints whatsoever, and polycythemia is discovered incidentally. *Table 84.2* lists the frequency of common symptoms and physical findings in patients with PV.

Table 84.1. Key Events in the History of PV

Year(s)	Event
1892	Description of polycythemia and splenomegaly in the absence of heart disease (Vaquez)
1902	Distinction between true polycythemia reflecting increased red cell mass and erythrocytosis from decreased plasma volume (Vaquez and Quiserne)
1903	Recognition of polycythemia, plethora, and splenomegaly as a distinct clinical syndrome and first summary of cases (Osler)
1904	Recognition of platelet and white cell abnormalities in PV (Türk)
1951	Recognition of concept of myeloproliferative disorders (Dameshek)
1967–1987	Polycythemia Vera Study Group: diagnostic criteria and multicenter clinical trials (Wasserman and colleagues)
1976	Demonstration of clonal/stem cell origin of PV (Adamson and Fialkow)
1980s	Description of erythropoietin-independent/erythropoietin hypersensitive erythroid colony formation (multiple investigators)
2005	Description of *JAK2* V617F mutation in majority of PV cases (multiple investigators)
2014	Ruxolitinib approved by the US Food and Drug Administration (FDA) for the treatment of patients with polycythemia vera who have had an inadequate response to or are intolerant of hydroxyurea.
2019	Ropeginterferon-alfa-2b-njft approved by European regulators for the treatment of adults with polycythemia vera

Abbreviation: PV, polycythemia vera.
Modified from Means RT. Perspective: Osler's 1903 paper on polycythemia vera. *Am J Med Sci*. 2008;335(6):418-419.

Table 84.2. Physical Findings and Symptoms in Polycythemia Vera

Physical Findings	Frequency (%)
Splenomegaly	70
Skin plethora	67
Conjunctival plethora	59
Engorged vessels in the optic fluid	46
Hepatomegaly	40
Systolic blood pressure > 140 mm Hg	72
Diastolic blood pressure > 90 mm Hg	32
Symptoms	
Headache	48
Weakness	47
Pruritus	43
Dizziness	43
Diaphoresis	33
Visual disturbances	31
Weight loss	29
Paresthesias	29
Dyspnea	26
Joint symptoms	26
Epigastric discomfort	24

Data from Berlin NI. Diagnosis and classification of the polycythemias. *Semin Hematol.* 1975;12(4):339-351.

Skin and Mucous Membranes

Early reports of what was eventually recognized as PV frequently described the patients as "cyanotic." The color of the face was not cyanotic but was more "ruddy," as might be produced by severe sunburn or a profound blush. The face might appear swollen. The abnormal coloring is most striking in the lips, cheeks, tip of the nose, ears, and neck (*Figure 84.1*); the skin of the trunk is usually not particularly affected. The skin capillaries are distended, and the capillary loops are enlarged. These findings are not unique to PV but are also observed in patients with an elevated hematocrit (Hct) from secondary erythrocytosis. However, this impressive presentation is rarely encountered at present because patients typically come to medical attention earlier than they did historically.

Ecchymoses and purpura of various sizes may occur as the disease progresses. Red or dark violet spots or brownish pigmentation of the skin may be found, and a great variety of skin lesions have been observed, including dry skin, eczema, acneiform or urticarial changes, acne rosacea, acne urticaria, urticaria pigmentosa, and neutrophilic dermatosis (Sweet syndrome).[13,14] The eyes may appear bloodshot. The mucous membranes may be a deep raspberry red, and epistaxis and/or gingival bleeding may occur.

A common complaint is aquagenic pruritus, intense itching after exposure to water (most typically in a bath or shower). This may be the initial presentation of PV and is reported in up to 60% of PV patients younger than 40 years.[15,16] The itching may be so troublesome that bathing with hot or even warm water is avoided. The reaction is less frequent after the use of cold water. This complaint tends to disappear as the polycythemia is managed.[17] Reddening, swelling, and pain in the digits (erythromelalgia) may occur and are typically associated with extreme platelet elevations.[18]

Cardiovascular System

Cardiac symptoms are not particularly prominent, and cardiac hypertrophy is typically absent. Electrocardiograms may show prolonged QT duration.[19] Echocardiography may show evidence of pulmonary hypertension and impaired myocardial performance index.[20,21] PV occurs in an older patient population, the population generally considered to be at higher risk for myocardial infarction, and the extent to which PV increases this risk is unclear.[22] Increased blood viscosity related to polycythemia, however, may contribute to symptoms in patients with atherosclerotic cardiovascular disease.[23,24] Thrombotic events, in both the arterial and venous circulations, are common in patients with PV. In all, 19% of the 1213 patients followed by the Gruppo Italiano Studio Policitemia (GISP) experienced a thrombotic event. Of these, 50.5% of nonfatal thrombotic events were documented as having occurred in the arterial circulation and 38.5% in the venous circulation. More than 80% of fatal thromboses were arterial.[4] Other abnormalities of the venous system include varicosities and phlebitis. Moderate or significant thickening of the peripheral arteries is found in patients with PV, and coronary thrombosis, claudication without occlusion, arterial occlusion with gangrene, acroparesthesia, Raynaud phenomenon, and thromboangiitis obliterans have been described.[25,26] Coronary risk factors, independent of PV, should be assessed as a key element of risk stratification in this condition.

One of the most interesting research developments in the last decade has been the delineation of non–malignant health consequences of clonal hematopoiesis of indeterminant potential (CHIP).[27] A full review of this condition is included in Chapter 82. Among the common mutations in CHIP are ones that also occur in PV, including *TET2, DNMT3a,* and *ASXL1*. Given this finding, research is beginning to accumulate about the contribution of molecular mutations to atherosclerotic events in PV.[28] Atherosclerotic plaque stability, impaired efferocytosis, and the increased formation of neutrophil extracellular traps are all described as important effector mechanisms for increased atherothrombosis with the JAK V617F mutation.[29] For additional information, the reader is directed to the following reviews of CHIP and atherosclerosis.[30-33]

As noted in *Table 84.2*, hypertension is relatively common in patients with PV. It is unclear whether this reflects the increased incidence of hypertension in the middle aged and elderly, a consequence of blood viscosity, or of molecular interactions that have yet to be described. Certainly, improvement of blood viscosity by reduction of the red cell volume aids in the control of blood pressure. In addition, management of hypertension may decrease overall risk for cardiovascular and cerebral events, as such intervention does in the wider population.

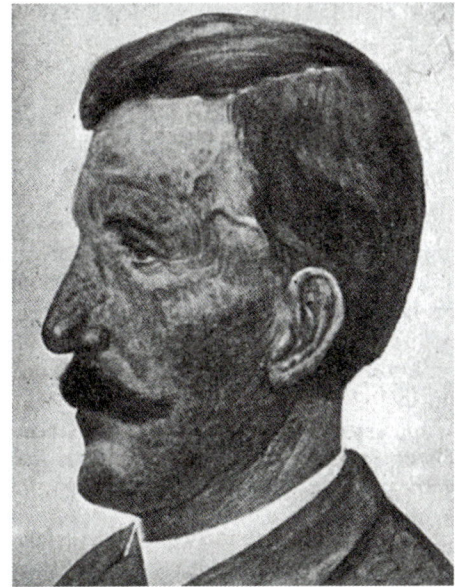

FIGURE 84.1 Photograph of a drawing (original in color) of one of Osler's original patients.

Gastrointestinal System

In addition to nonspecific gastrointestinal symptoms such as sensations of fullness, thirst, gas pains, and constipation, patients with PV have an increased frequency of peptic ulcer, gastrointestinal bleeding, or thrombosis of mesenteric vessels. When compared with dyspeptic controls, PV patients have a three- to fourfold greater frequency of upper gastrointestinal erosions or ulcers. The frequency of *Helicobacter pylori* infection is increased in PV patients.[34]

Massive hemorrhage from varices in the esophagus, stomach, or bowel may be observed.[35] Thrombosis in the mesenteric veins and arteries may be mistaken for peritonitis or the perforation of an ulcer. Hepatomegaly is common (*Table 84.2*), and cirrhosis has been reported.[36] *Mosse syndrome* is a term applied by some to the coexistence of cirrhosis and PV. Budd-Chiari syndrome also occurs,[37] with particularly increased risk in patients with a concurrent hypercoagulable state. The diagnosis of PV may be "masked" in cases of splanchnic venous thrombosis (SVT). In these cases, the World Health Organization (WHO) classification defines patients with an SVT associated with a JAK2 mutation, but not meeting the WHO-listed criteria for PV as MPN-U, which also includes cases with the so-called "masked" PV.[38]

Splenomegaly

Palpable splenomegaly occurs in more than two-thirds of PV patients (*Table 84.2*). The size of the spleen varies greatly between individual patients and occasionally may extend to the pelvic brim. Upon physical exam, it is typically noted to be firm. Patients may experience pain in the splenic region, and after infarction, a friction rub can be heard in this area. The general assumption is that polycythemia antedates the enlargement of the spleen and that engorgement of this organ with blood and extramedullary hematopoiesis are the major contributors to splenomegaly.[39]

Respiratory System

Dyspnea on severe exertion is common, and hoarseness is usual with markedly elevated Hb concentrations. Chest radiographs may reveal prominent vascular markings. It has long been established that the vast majority of patients with PV have normal arterial oxygen saturation, even when the Hb levels were high, indicating that the high viscosity of the blood does not prevent normal blood oxygenation; oxygen dissociation studies are also normal.[40]

In a 2020 analysis of a large data set, researchers found that after adjusting for age, gender, race, diabetes, tobacco use, previous history of tumor, previous history of pulmonary embolism, chronic lung disease, and chronic kidney disease, patients with PV have a threefold higher risk for pulmonary arterial hypertension compared to the general population.[41]

Genitourinary System

Renal disease is very uncommon in PV and etiology is difficult to tease out if associated with hypertension or concomitant thrombosis. In one series reviewing chronic renal disease in myeloproliferative disorders, only 6% of PV patients had estimated glomerular filtration rates <45 mL/min/1.73 m^2. Glomerulonephritis, particularly membranoproliferative glomerulonephritis, is occasionally reported.[42,43]

Neuromuscular System

Headache is the most common neurologic symptom, but lassitude, vertigo and giddiness, transitory syncope, insomnia, weakness, and a sensation of fullness in the head, tinnitus, and numbness and tingling in the fingers (less often in the feet) are also common. These symptoms frequently reflect increased viscosity and may improve with phlebotomy. The cerebrospinal fluid pressure may be increased.[44]

Visual disturbances are common and include transitory dimness of vision, or even temporary blindness, scotomas, specks and bright points in front of the field of vision, diplopia, and temporary paralysis of one of the eye muscles. On examination of the eye grounds, the vessels may be engorged, tortuous, and irregular in diameter; the veins may be dark purple; and the retina deeply colored. Papilledema and embolism of the central retinal artery have been reported.[45]

Central nervous system thrombosis is among the most serious complications of PV. Central nervous system vascular events represented 30% of the nonfatal thrombotic events and 10.3% of deaths observed in the GISP study.[4] In the European collaboration study on low-dose aspirin in polycythemia vera (ECLAP) study, there were 23 nonfatal, nonhemorrhagic strokes recorded among the 1638 patients with PV enrolled.[46]

Pain in the limbs may be troublesome and severe but is uncommon given the current early recognition of disease and initiation of treatment for highly symptomatic patients. It has been attributed to pressure on the bone by swollen, hyperplastic bone marrow. Unusual paresthesias may be encountered, but anatomic evidence of spinal cord changes has not typically been found at autopsy.

BLOOD AND LABORATORY FINDINGS

Hematologic Findings

Erythrocytes

Hb concentration is typically in the range of 18 to 24 g/dL at diagnosis. The current diagnostic criteria require men to have an Hb recorded at above 16.5 g/dL and women over 16 g/dL or Hcts of more than 49% in men and 48% in women.[47] The individual erythrocytes usually appear normal. Slight anisocytosis may be evident, but poikilocytosis is unusual. Polychromatophilia and, occasionally, basophilic stippling may be found. An occasional normoblast may be observed in the blood smear and, in the presence of a relatively normal or definitely increased red cell count, should arouse suspicion of PV. The reticulocyte percentage is not significantly increased, but absolute numbers may be elevated because of elevated red blood cell counts. After hemorrhage, however, the reticulocyte percentage may be increased, and other immature forms of the red cell series may be encountered. If blood loss (from phlebotomy or from a pathologic source) occurs repeatedly, iron-deficient erythropoiesis may develop. This raises an interesting semantic point: these patients are iron deficient in that iron stores are absent, but the total body iron content, including the iron present as Hb in red cells, may be normal.

Leukocytes

Leukocyte count is often elevated, with mean in one series at 13.5×10^9/L.[48] More than one-quarter of patients have leukocyte counts greater than 15.0×10^9/L.[49] The myeloid leukocytes are both relatively and absolutely increased, metamyelocytes are increased in number, and 1% or 2% myelocytes, sometimes more, are found. Myeloblasts are usually not observed in the peripheral circulation. If they are observed, particular care needs to be taken to ensure that the underlying diagnosis is not primary myelofibrosis (MF). Basophil, eosinophil, or monocyte concentrations may be increased and provide a marker of an underlying myeloproliferative disorder. A total leukocyte count greater than 12.5 to 15.0×10^9/L is a risk factor for thrombosis,[50] and a large study looking at more than 1500 patients with PV found that, in multivariable analysis, survival was adversely affected by older age, leukocytosis greater than 15.0×10^9/L, venous thrombosis, and abnormal karyotype.[51] One retrospective study looked at the WBC counts as measured in patients at 10 academic centers. They found that high WBC was not linked to thrombosis but was an indication of disease progression.[52]

Platelets

The platelet count frequently is increased, usually in the range of 500 to 1000×10^9/L, but counts as high as 3000 and even 6000×10^9/L have been reported.[53] Conventional coagulation parameters are usually normal, but the clot may retract poorly. An artifactual elevation of prothrombin time and activated partial thromboplastin time may be observed in patients with erythrocytosis. The standard citrated tube used for coagulation studies contains a fixed quantity of anticoagulant for a fixed volume of blood. In polycythemia, there is a relative reduction of plasma, meaning that there will be excess anticoagulant for the volume of plasma. Functional assays of coagulation factors will thus be prolonged without clinical consequence. Platelets may appear to be abnormally large or even bizarrely shaped, and megakaryocyte fragments sometimes are seen in the blood smear.

Total Blood Volume

The total blood volume characteristically is increased. The enormous increase in blood volume, which distends even the smaller vessels of the whole body, no doubt accounts for many of the symptoms of this disease. In a group of 30 patients in whom the Hct was 0.55 or greater, the total red cell volume, measured by the ^{32}P-labeled red cell method, was 38.8 to 91.9 mL/kg body weight as compared with the normal average of 29.9 mL/kg.[54] In two-thirds of this patient group, the plasma volumes were below the lower limits of normal, and in no patient was the plasma volume above normal. Because of the variations in plasma volume, the packed cell volume (or Hct) gives only an approximate indication of the size of the red cell mass. In the past, measurement of the red cell mass was commonly used in diagnosis. This method is rarely employed at present.[55]

Other Laboratory Findings

The viscosity of the blood may be five to eight times greater than normal.[56] The degree of abnormality varies with the relative quantity of red corpuscles. The erythrocyte sedimentation rate of polycythemic blood is low.[57] As mentioned earlier, estimated glomerular filtration rate is usually normal. Hyperuricemia is common and may be associated with secondary gout. Spurious hyperkalemia has been noted when platelets or leukocytes are greatly increased in number.[58] A vitamin B_{12}–binding protein, which may be an altered form of transcobalamin I, has been found in the plasma of patients with PV and in a variety of conditions involving leukocytosis.[59] Unsaturated B_{12}–binding capacity and serum B_{12} are typically increased.[60] Plasma homocysteine levels in polycythemic patients are higher than nonpolycythemic subjects but still in the normal range.[61]

Serum erythropoietin concentration is typically low in PV and may be elevated in secondary polycythemia. A low serum erythropoietin concentration is one of the WHO diagnostic criteria for PV.[47]

Bleeding-associated defects reported in PV include altered von Willebrand factor multimers and acquired von Willebrand syndrome (AVWS).[62,63] Studies by thromboelastography and whole-blood rotational thromboelastometry suggest a hypercoagulable platelet phenotype.[64,65] Patients with PV and thrombosis exhibit a greater frequency of procoagulant abnormalities in antithrombin III, protein C, and protein S, and resistance to activated protein C than do PV patients without thrombosis.[66] Studies of prothrombin and factor V gene polymorphisms with a thrombotic diathesis showed no increased incidence of these abnormalities in PV patients. However, polymorphisms of the Pl^{A2} allele of platelet glycoprotein IIIa were associated with increased arterial thrombosis in PV and essential thrombocythemia (ET) patients.[67]

Bone Marrow

Bone marrow examination was not one of the parameters included in the PVSG criteria for the diagnosis of PV. However, both currently accepted diagnostic requirements for PV, the WHO criteria and the European Clinical and Pathological (ECP) criteria, formally include bone marrow examination (*Table 84.3*).

The marrow is typically hypercellular (*Figure 84.2*), but normal cellularity is noted at the time of diagnosis in some cases. Hyperplasia involves the marrow elements and displaces marrow fat. In several series, the mean cellularity of the marrow was 80% to 90% compared to approximately 30% in normal subjects and 40% in patients with secondary erythrocytosis.[68-70]

An increase in megakaryocyte number and size is well documented in association with PV. The ratio of the different cell types in the marrow is not strikingly different from normal. Clumps of pronormoblasts and basophilic erythroblasts are seen, and the percentage of nucleated red cells may be moderately elevated. Myelocyte and myeloblast numbers may be greater than normal, and an increase in eosinophils and basophils may be found.[71]

Iron pigment is absent from the marrow in more than 90% of patients, even when phlebotomy has not been performed.[72] Increased marrow iron stores have been suggested as a morphologic hallmark favoring a secondary form of erythrocytosis over PV.[71] An increase in marrow reticulin levels and/or fibrosis has often been reported, but an increase was observed in only 11% to 15% of patients studied early in the course of their disease. The increase in reticulin correlates with the degree of marrow cellularity.[72] Marrow vascularity may be increased in PV and other myeloproliferative disorders. In patients with a high degree of fibrosis, the diagnosis of MF should be entertained. The diagnosis of diagnosis of post-PV MF requires the presence of ≥grade 2 fibrosis, concomitant with progressive splenomegaly, anemia, leukoerythroblastosis, or constitutional symptoms.[73]

Cytogenetics

Characteristic cytogenetic abnormalities in PV are presented in *Table 84.4*.[74,75] Cytogenetic abnormalities occur only in the minority of patients with PV at diagnosis, approximately 20 percent.[76] Patients evaluated during a clinical course not associated with progression had cytogenetic abnormalities in 25% to 35% of cases.[77] However, patients who progressed to myeloid metaplasia, MF, or acute

Table 84.3. World Health Organization for Diagnosis of Polycythemia Vera

WHO
Major Criteria
Hb > 16.5 g/dL male/16.0 g/dL female or Hct >49% male/48% women or RCM > 125% of mean predicted value
Bone marrow hypercellular for age with trilineage growth, including prominent erythroid, granulocytic, and megakaryocyte proliferation with pleomorphic mature megakaryocytes
JAK2 V617F or *JAK2* exon 12 mutation
Minor Criterion
Subnormal serum erythropoietin level
Diagnosis requires all three major criteria or the first two major criteria and the minor criterion, unless there is sustained erythrocytosis (Hb > 18.5 g/dL or Hct >55.5% male/Hb > 16.5 g/dL or Hct > 49.5% female) in which case only the minor criterion and major criterion 3 are required.

Abbreviations: Hb, hemoglobin; Hct, hematocrit; LAP, leukocyte alkaline phosphatase; PV, polycythemia vera; RCM, red cell mass.
Reprinted from Arber DA, Orazi A, Hasserjian R, et al. The 2016 revision to the World Health Organization classification of myeloid neoplasms and acute leukemia. *Blood.* 2016;127(20):2391-2405. Copyright © 2016 American Society of Hematology. With permission.

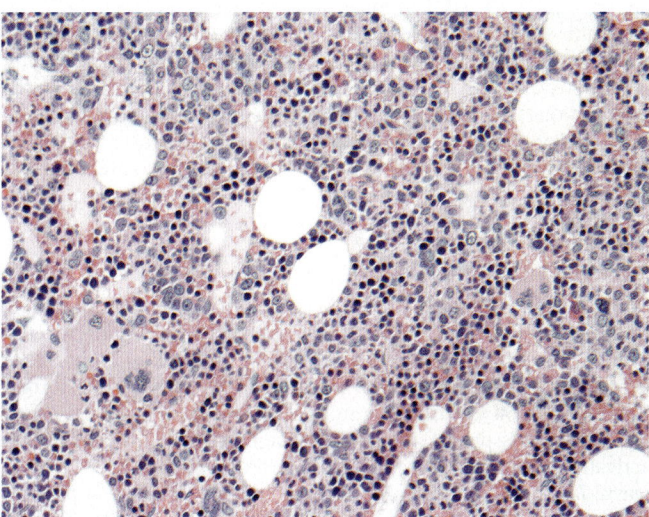

FIGURE 84.2 Bone marrow biopsy from a patient with polycythemia vera showing hypercellularity and hyperplasia of myeloid, erythroid, and megakaryocyte series (×1000).

Table 84.4. Frequency of Abnormal Cytogenetics by Polycythemia Vera Disease Stage in Two Series

		Frequency (Expressed as Percentage of Patients)				
Reference	Patient Number	At Diagnosis	Polycythemia Vera	Myelofibrosis	Myeloid Metaplasia	Acute Leukemia/ Myelodysplasia
(56)	64	17	32	85	75	75
(57)	37	14	25	40	78	100

leukemia/myelodysplastic syndrome had abnormal cytogenetics in 75% to 100% of evaluations. Abnormal cytogenetics is established as a risk factor for decreased survival in PV.[78]

PATHOGENESIS

Clonality

In view of the increased production and turnover of erythrocytes, neutrophils, and platelets as well as the hypercellular marrow, hematopoiesis in PV is abnormal at a multipotent progenitor or stem cell level. Evidence supporting this hypothesis was provided by one study of two female patients with PV who were heterozygous for X-linked glucose-6-phosphate dehydrogenase deficiency.[79] In these patients, tissues not affected by PV (skin fibroblasts and lymphocytes) possessed both A-type and B-type glucose-6-phosphate dehydrogenase isozymes, as expected. Red blood cells, granulocytes, and platelets contained only one isozyme (type A), however, thus demonstrating a probable clonal origin of this disorder at a pluripotent hematopoietic progenitor level. In one other patient, most B lymphocytes were also from the disease clone, indicating involvement of an earlier hematopoietic progenitor that had differentiation potential for the lymphoid as well as the myeloid, erythroid, and megakaryocytic series.[80]

Molecular Genetic Features

The observation that patients with myeloproliferative disorders frequently have a gain-of-function mutation on the short arm of chromosome 9, in which the valine at position 617 of the Janus kinase 2 gene is replaced by phenylalanine (*JAK2* V617F),[81-84] has had transformational impact on the approach to the diagnosis of PV and on investigation into its pathogenesis. This mutation results in constitutive activation of tyrosine kinase signaling through the *JAK/STAT* pathways. *JAK2* V617F is present in approximately 95% of PV patients at diagnosis. However, it is not pathognomonic for PV, inasmuch as a significant proportion of patients with essential thrombocytosis and MF also have the *JAK2* V617F mutation. The majority of PV patients who lack the *JAK2* V617F mutation have alternate mutations in exon 12 of the *JAK2* gene.[85] Exon 12 mutations may be associated with a marrow morphology showing isolated erythocytosis.[86,87]

As outlined by the discovering researchers, the V617F mutation results in constitutive JAK2 kinase activity by interfering with the inhibitory activity of the JAK2 pseudokinase domain. Subsequently, multiple downstream targets are aberrantly activated. This downstream activation is mediated by activator of transcription (STAT) protein signaling and, to a lesser extent, via mitogen-activated protein kinase and phosphoinositide 3-kinase signaling pathways. The consequence is overactive myeloid cell proliferation and differentiation.[88] The fact that this single mutation can be present in three phenotypically distinct diseases (ET, primary MF, and PV) is under intense study and may be a result of cell-extrinsic factors, that is, serum erythropoietin levels, iron stores, or cell-intrinsic consequences of differential STAT1 activation. Allelic burden has been linked to the final phenotype in PV.[89] The specific phenotype seen with *JAK2* V617F mutations is effected by concurrent expression of other genes (*TET2, PRV1,* and *IDH1* or *IDH2*) and by the *JAK2* haplotype.[90] *JAK2* V617F expression correlates with the expression of erythrocyte adhesion molecules, such as laminin α_5 and Lu/BCAM, which may also play a role in the atherosclerotic events associated with the mutation.[29,91,92] Following leukemic transformation of *JAK2* V617F expressing PV, blasts that do not express a *JAK2* mutation are common. *TP53* and *RUNX1* mutations are predictors of leukemic transformation in PV.[93]

Although mice expressing *JAK2* V617F have a clinical phenotype resembling a myeloproliferative disorder,[94] *JAK2* mutations may not always be the initiating event in the molecular cascade leading to PV.[95] It has been shown in some patients to be preceded by other mutational events.[89,96] In a fascinating development, published in 2022, researchers from the Wellcome Sanger Institute reported on whole genome sequencing of 1013 clonal hematopoietic colonies from 12 patients with myeloproliferative neoplasms.[97] The results demonstrated that driver mutations may occur extremely early in life, even in utero. Subsequent rates of expansion were highly heterogeneous. The authors also show that additional driver mutations accelerate expansion. The reader is referred to several reviews for additional detail.[98-101] It is not only the hematopoietic clones that have impact on disease development, but likely the bone marrow niche as well. A growing body of evidence is examining the role of the immune landscape in MPNs.[102]

The thrombopoietin receptor (Mpl) has been reported to be markedly decreased or absent on the platelets of PV patients and also of some individuals with MF.[103] It has been suggested that this abnormality in Mpl expression and function is both a marker for PV and, through suppression of apoptosis, a potential pathophysiologic contributor.[104] Updates on this research has demonstrated that Mpl surface expression is reduced secondary to abnormal posttranslational glycosylation and premature destruction of JAK2. Murine experiments support the role of MPL expression and polycythemia phenotype and point to potential therapeutic avenues that exploit this growth-factor axis.[105,106]

PRV-1 (CD177) is a gene of the urokinase plasminogen activator receptor superfamily, which is highly expressed in granulocytes from PV patients but not from patients with other chronic myeloproliferative disorders or from normal individuals.[107] *PRV-1* expression is highly correlated with expression of the *JAK2* V617F mutation.[108]

Hematopoietic Growth Factors and Hematopoiesis

A hallmark of PV (and other myeloproliferative disorders as well) is erythroid progenitor colony formation in vitro without the addition of exogenous erythropoietin, the phenomenon called *endogenous erythroid colonies* (EECs) or sometimes *erythropoietin-independent colony formation*.[109] This phenomenon has been observed with progenitors cultured from the marrow or the blood of PV patients.[109,110] This can be a consequence of true erythropoietin independence or of exquisite sensitivity to erythropoietin, which would permit a response to the extremely small quantities of erythropoietin present in the serum used in culture media. Studies using antibodies capable of blocking the erythropoietin receptor suggest that erythroid burst-forming units fall into two categories: those that exhibit a normal response to erythropoietin and those that are truly erythropoietin independent.[111] In addition to interleukin-3 and erythropoietin, erythroid progenitors from PV patients have been reported to exhibit hypersensitivity to interleukin-3, granulocyte-macrophage colony-stimulating factor, interleukin-1, stem cell factor, and insulin-like growth factor-1.[112] EEC formation is also associated with expression of JAK2 and the apoptosis regulators STAT5 and/or Bcl-xL.[113,114]

DIAGNOSIS

The two widely accepted criteria for PV are the WHO criteria and the ECP criteria.[47,115,116] The ECP criteria are strongly oriented toward morphologic and molecular diagnostic criteria, and separate PV into overt PV (having a high red cell mass) and early PV. Both WHO and ECP criteria may be less applicable to childhood PV.[117] The WHO criteria are outlined in *Table 84.3*.

The diagnostic approach to erythrocytosis outlined in Chapter 45 is based on the WHO criteria (*Table 84.3*), which includes patients who do not exhibit marked erythrocytosis (Hb 16.6-18.5 g/dL in men or 16.1-16.5 in women). However, a patient with polycythemia manifested by sustained erythrocytosis at a high level (Hb > 18.5 g/dL male/16.5 g/dL female) should undergo testing for *JAK2* V617F as the first step. If positive, the patient presumably has PV, although a low erythropoietin concentration is required for confirmation. In this case, the diagnosis can be made without bone marrow examination. In other circumstances, the WHO criteria require a bone marrow biopsy is required to demonstrate hypercellularity for age, panmyelosis and megakaryocytic proliferation. Given the higher risk associated with karyotypic abnormalities, cytogenetic assessment is also warranted at diagnosis.

In *JAK2* V617F-negative patients, testing for alternate *JAK2* mutations can be considered. As noted earlier, it has been suggested that *JAK2* exon 12 mutations identify a specific subset of PV characterized by "pure" erythrocytosis, with few or no abnormalities in the white blood cell or platelet lineages. Long-term follow-up of patients with exon 12 mutations demonstrates similar outcomes to those with the V617F mutation.[87,118]

If *JAK2* V617F is not present, then one must determine whether features are suggestive of PV by bone marrow examination and serum erythropoietin determination, or if one should proceed to identify an etiology of secondary polycythemia. Some clinical situations, such as distinguishing *JAK2* V617F-positive essential thrombocytosis with concurrent secondary polycythemia from PV, may be challenging to sort out. Next generation sequencing of myeloid genes may help to determine the presence of a clonal disorder. Several reviews have been published recently that include diagnostic algorithms that may be useful for consultation.[38,119,120]

NATURAL HISTORY

The clinical picture of PV is characterized by the complications of polycythemia-induced hyperviscosity, expanded blood volume, and thrombosis. The occurrence and severity of these complications is significantly affected by therapy and is discussed under specific therapeutic modalities.

Two other significant complications that may be observed late in the course of PV are[1] the development of myeloid metaplasia with MF and[2] transformation to acute leukemia. Old series suggested that up to 25% of patients with PV developed a progressive reduction in erythrocyte survival, decreased erythropoiesis, progressive splenomegaly, and MF, but these rates were confounded by treatment modalities at the time.[121] A recent review on this topic suggests clinically significant MF has an incidence of 4.9% to 6% 10 years after diagnosis and 6% to 14% at 15 years after diagnosis.[93] The range of values reflects both the retrospective nature of the studies reviewed and the different management strategies applied and the different demographics of the populations reported. Extramedullary hematopoiesis takes place in the spleen and liver associated with a rising leukocyte count with increased immature myeloid forms and the teardrop and nucleated red cells characteristic of MF and myeloid metaplasia appear in the blood. Splenomegaly may be massive and sufficient to cause symptoms. Some patients develop progressive anemia and thrombocytopenia and die of a variety of intercurrent complications in the "spent" or "burnt-out" phase of myeloid metaplasia.[122] In some patients, acute leukemia develops. This may evolve out of post–PV myeloid metaplasia or occurs without preceding evidence of myeloid metaplasia or MF. The incidence of this has been reported to range from 2.3% to 14.7% at 10 years and 5.5% to 18% at 15 years.[51,93] Risk factors for leukemia transformation include older age, anemia, leukocytosis, thrombocytopenia, and thrombocytosis >1000 × 10^9/L or abnormal karyotype.[123-126]

The ability to predict which patients with PV will transform to acute leukemia has significant clinical utility, although, at the current time, there is no therapy with data to prove reduction in this risk. Molecular mutations have been explored to determine predictive features and several groups have proposed classifications systems. In one of these studies, both *TP53* mutations and mutations in the chromatin/spliceosome (including *ASXL1*, *EZH2*, and *SRSF2*) were associated with a higher risk of leukemic evolution.[126] In another study, PV which included mutations of *SRSF2* constituted a high-risk group.[78]

In recent study, French researchers analyzed patients with either PV or ET who had progressed to acute leukemia and had DNA samples available. Of their cohort, 24 had PV, with a time to leukemic transformation ranging from 2 to 30 years. They were able to define (using the combined ET and PV cohort) three groups of patients, molecularly defined, which corresponded to a shorter time to transformation, an intermediate time to transformation, and a longer time to transformation. The median time to transformation was 3, 10, and 21 years for the short-term, intermediate, and long-term groups, respectively.[123]

A number of other diseases have been reported in association with PV. It is unclear whether these represent coincidence or an actual pathophysiologic relationship. The potential role of inflammatory activation in the natural history of the myeloproliferative disorders suggests common pathogenesis with disorders such as polymyalgia rheumatic, inflammatory bowel disease, and juvenile rheumatoid arthritis.[127]

Risk Stratification

When considering therapy for what may be an indolent disease, risk stratification methods become crucial. Overall survival of PV patients is decreased compared to age- and sex-matched controls. Some of the earliest reported series on patients estimated median survival of untreated PV patients to be less than 2 years. However, in the current era, median survival after diagnosis is reported to be 14 years in all PV patients and 24 years in patients diagnosed before age 60.[128] *Table 84.5* gives the causes of death from three large series of PV patients.[4,129,130] Acute leukemia and other malignancies, hemorrhage, and MF/myeloid metaplasia represent 2% to 4% of patient deaths. To date, no intervention has proved able to reproducibly decrease the risk for leukemic or myelofibrotic transformation.

As mentioned above, there have been efforts to incorporate molecular mutations into the prognostic models for PV.[78] Studies in PV patients have confirmed the negative prognostic consequences of karyotypic abnormalities, higher WBC counts, and certain non-JAK2 mutations including SRSF2 and IDH2. Notably, more than half of PV

Table 84.5. Causes of Death in Polycythemia Vera Patients

Cause of Death	PVSG[88] (%)	GISP[3] (%)	ECLAP[89] (%)
Thrombosis/thromboembolism	31	29.7	26
Acute myeloid leukemia	19	14.6	12.5
Other malignancy	15	15.5	20
Hemorrhage	6	2.6	4
Myelofibrosis/myeloid metaplasia	4	2.6	0.5
Other	25	35.0	37

Abbreviations: ECLAP, European Collaborative on Low-Dose Aspirin in Polycythemia Vera; GISP, Gruppo Italiano Studio Policitemia; PVSG, Polycythemia Vera Study Group.

patients may have DNA sequence variants/mutations discovered when sequencing is performed for myeloid panels. These often include TET2, ASXL1, and LNK. Other adverse mutations (SRSF2, IDH2, RUNX1, U2AF1) are used in models like the mutation-enhanced international prognostic model-PV.[78] In this model, age over 67, leukocytosis, abnormal karyotype, and presence of SRSF2 mutation were used to discriminate median survivals as long at 24 years and as short as 3.2 years. This model has not been extensively validated, so at the current time NGS is not routinely used in clinical practice. This may change as more is learned and additional therapies become available.

However, thrombotic and cardiovascular events are the leading cause of death, and therefore, the current risk stratification system relies on data that are aimed at preventing these outcomes. The most important predictors of cardiovascular events are age older than 65 years and a history of thrombosis.[130] Among 665 with PV seen at the Mayo Clinic between 1967 and 2017, 79 (12%) were ages ≤40 years, 226 (34%) ages 41 to 60, and 360 (54%) ages > 60, with corresponding median survivals of 37, 22, and 10 years.[131,132]

The JAK2 V617F allele burden appears to identify patients at higher risk for major vascular events and evolution to MF, inasmuch as it also identifies patients more likely to have marked leukocytosis,[133] that may be the basis for the increased thrombotic risk.[134-136]

The purpose of risk stratification is to estimate the likelihood of thrombotic complications, which is estimated to occur in approximately 26% of patients followed for a median of 20 years, and only intervene when appropriate. Accordingly, conventional risk stratification in PV includes two risk categories: high-risk (either age > 60 years or thrombosis history or both) and low-risk (neither risk factor). Current standard of care is for cytoreductive therapy to be utilized in the management of high-risk patients.[130,137] The ECLAP study[133] of 1638 patients with PV confirmed both age and thrombotic history as the most critical risk factors for arterial thrombotic events and found that antiplatelet therapy was more effective than cytoreduction in protection against cardiovascular events. Subsequent research has shown that prior arterial events, diabetes, hyperlipidemia, and hypertension are risk factors for arterial thrombosis in this population and that previous venous event, age ≥ 65 years, leukocytosis, and prior major hemorrhage are risk factors for venous events.[138-140]

At the current time, when determining the need for cytoreductive therapy, the clinician is best guided by the history of arterial and venous thromboses and advanced age. Cardiovascular risk factors should be mitigated with appropriate lipid control, antihypertensive medications, management of diabetes, and aspirin.[38,55,134,137] There are some clinical situations when cytoreduction may be instituted in patients who do not meet high-risk criteria, with an understanding that our current risk stratification is based on the risk for thrombosis. These examples include patients with disease-related symptoms.[141] There is also growing debate on whether we should institute interferon therapy in asymptomatic, low-risk patients based on evidence that this therapy can reduce the JAK2 V617F allelic burden.[142] This debate is explored later in this chapter.

TREATMENT

The objective of therapy in PV is to produce a reduction in the red cell mass by methods that (a) permit the longest survival; (b) are associated with fewest significant complications, allowing the patient maximum quality of life; and (c) are least expensive and inconvenient for the patient.

Phlebotomy and Antiplatelet Agents

Phlebotomy offers prompt and effective reduction of the red cell mass and blood volume to an Hct < 45%—which has been determined in the CYTO-PV study to better protect against death from cardiovascular causes or thrombotic events than a protocol that aims for an Hct of 45% to 50%.[143] The goal of phlebotomy is to induce a state of iron deficiency with a normal Hb concentration that will itself suppress erythrocytosis. Many, perhaps even most, patients can be maintained in an essentially normal state by phlebotomy together with aspirin (discussed later). The advantages of phlebotomy are that it is inexpensive, requires extremely limited technical support, and allows rapid control of symptoms. Criticisms of phlebotomy are the potential problem of venous access in elderly patients, and that it does not address leukocytosis or thrombocytosis (and may occasionally exacerbate the latter). Phlebotomy also, intentionally, creates an iron-deficient state with the potential for symptoms such as cognitive impairment, fatigue, and leg cramps.[141]

Studies by the PVSG demonstrated a survival advantage in PV patients treated with phlebotomy compared with patients treated with radioactive phosphorus, or chlorambucil.[144] The apparent advantage of phlebotomy was undercut by an increased risk of thrombosis. Thrombosis-free cumulative survival was significantly worse in the phlebotomy arm ($P = .015$), with the increased risk predominantly limited to the first 3 years of therapy. An initial study using a high-dose antiplatelet regimen (aspirin 300 mg and dipyridamole 75 mg three times daily) was stopped early because of excessive thrombosis, hemorrhage, and death in the phlebotomy/aspirin/dipyridamole arm.[144] Subsequent small studies supported the efficacy and safety of aspirin at doses of 40 to 325 mg/d, and the ECLAP study randomized 518 patients to aspirin 100 mg/d or placebo, and followed them for at least a year. Median time since the diagnosis of PV was <5 years. Patients in the aspirin group had no increased bleeding incidence and had a decrease in combined endpoints, including nonfatal stroke, nonfatal myocardial infarction, pulmonary embolism, and major venous thrombosis. However, there was no impact on cardiovascular mortality or overall mortality.[133] The efficacy may have been underestimated in this study because optimum control of the Hct appears not to have been obtained in most patients (median Hct 48%). In a large retrospective study, patients treated with antithrombotic agents such as aspirin and phlebotomy to keep the Hct < 48%, and who did not receive alkylating agents, had survival that did not differ from that of healthy age-matched controls.[145]

The goal of phlebotomy should be to maintain the Hct in the normal range (42%-44% for men and 39%-42% for women). The Cytoreductive Therapy in Polycythemia Vera Collaborative Group has recently reported that patients treated with an Hct goal of less than 45% had significantly lower cardiovascular mortality and fewer major thrombotic events than patients in the 45% to 50% Hct range. Patients with Hcts < 45% obtained their target with phlebotomy with or without cytoreductive drugs as needed.[143] In elderly patients, patients with known cardiovascular disease or hospitalized patients with severe symptoms, phlebotomy should be initiated cautiously, using either frequent small-volume phlebotomy (100-150 mL every day or on alternate days) or in larger (500 mL) volumes weekly or every other week if tolerated using fluid replacement so that the patient remains isovolemic. Excessively aggressive initial phlebotomy may compromise blood pressure and oxygen delivery to tissue in patients with established cardiovascular disease.[146] After the Hct falls to < 55%, or more than 750 to 1000 mL of blood have been removed, phlebotomy of 250 to 500 mL can generally be carried out safely at biweekly or monthly intervals, as clinically indicated.

Occasionally, one can consider the administration of iron during phlebotomy to prevent the "symptoms" of iron deficiency. However, this defeats the long-term purpose of phlebotomy, which is to establish a state of iron deficiency that will restrict red cell production. While there are historical data that iron-deficient PV patients have no greater symptoms compared to other PV patients in a comparable state of disease control,[147] a recent trial contradicted this finding and demonstrated a relationship between traditional aggressive therapy for PV and increased symptom burden with prolonged therapy.[148] It is an obligation of the physician to monitor for disease-related and treatment-related symptoms.

Some researchers have argued that rather than Hct, the therapeutic aim should be for a RBC mass of 5 g/dL in microcytic men and 4.5 g/dL in microcytic woman.[149] This argument rests on the discordance that results between Hct and RBC mass in patients who are microcytic. As patients may still be at risk for cardiovascular events with elevated

RBC mass and normal Hct, following RBC mass may be beneficial. This may be a challenging prospect in the more proliferative PV patient unless cytoreductive therapy is utilized.

Aspirin is generally given in daily doses of 80 to 100 mg. Some authors have suggested that twice-daily administration of low-dose aspirin may be considered in individuals with very high cardiovascular risk.[134] In individuals with a bleeding diathesis, aspirin may be contraindicated. Such patients and individuals with platelet counts >1000 × 10^9/L should be evaluated for AVWS (see Chapter 53). Aspirin should be withheld until cytoreductive therapy brings AVWS under control.

Cytoreductive Therapy

Cytoreductive therapy should be considered in patients at high risk for thrombotic events. The most significant risk factors are age >60 years and/or a personal history of thrombosis, but other potential risk factors include general cardiovascular risk factors (tobacco use, hypertension, diabetes, and significant dyslipidemia).[100] Static or stable leukocytosis and marked thrombocytosis can be considered risk factors but of themselves are probably not major indications for therapy. However, evidence of active myeloproliferation (progressive leukocytosis and/or thrombocytosis, and progressive splenomegaly) may prompt initiation of treatment.

There is a growing debate about whether not cytoreductive therapy with pegylated interferon should be initiated for individuals with traditionally low-risk disease by the parameters of age and a personal history of thrombosis.[141,150] The arguments in favor of such an approach are generally that there is no evidence that phlebotomy alone is sufficient to *predictably and steadily* maintain an Hct level under the target of 45%–the goal established by the CYTO-PV study.[143] Some practitioners also argue that in "low-risk" PV patients, the rate of major arterial and venous embolic events is 2%/year—which is too high to tolerate.[142] Those who advocate for employing interferon in a low-risk population also point to the need to control leukocytosis and the reduction in quality of life that may occur with repeated phlebotomy. Finally, there are data that pegylated interferon, over time, may substantially reduce the mutant allelic burden in PV.[38,150-152] This has not been systematically investigated in a low-risk population and we are yet to understand the benefits of such reduction to outcomes. However, the disease-modifying activity of a relatively low-risk intervention has compelled many to argue in favor of utilizing this even in low-risk, asymptomatic patients.

These reasons formed the rationale for the low-PV trial.[142] In this phase II study, patients were randomly assigned to standard therapy (phlebotomy plus low-dose aspirin) vs standard therapy plus ropeginterferon-Alfa-2b-njft (roPEG-IFN). In this trial, all patients were both under the age of 60 years and had not had a prior thrombotic event, that is, classically considered to have low-risk disease. A total of 127 patients were enrolled, 63 on standard therapy and 64 on the experimental arm. At 12 months, patients who received roPEG-IFN in addition to phlebotomy and aspirin achieved superior outcomes including Hct control, decreased phlebotomy need, increased ferritin, and normalization of non–erythrocyte cell lines. The experimental arm patients did have higher rates of fever and fatigue, although the other symptoms of PV were improved in the experimental arm.

To address the question of whether patients with low risk should be exposed to cytoreduction, an expert panel was recently convened by the European Leukemia Net (ELN).[137] They used stringent evidence review criteria and asked (1) what benefits should be expected from cytoreductive therapy drugs over phlebotomy in patients with low-risk PV, (2) which patients with low-risk PV might benefit from cytoreductive drugs, and (3) which cytoreductive drugs should be preferred in low-risk patients. A careful reading of this report is recommended to understand the nuances to the recommendations. The majority of the panel *recommended* cytoreductive therapy for low-risk patients with poor tolerance to phlebotomy (strictly defined as recurrent episodes of postphlebotomy syncope despite appropriate preventive interventions or blood phobia leading to avoidance behavior despite counseling, or severe difficulties in venous access), for those with symptomatic progressive splenomegaly (if transformation to MF has been ruled out) or for those with a leukocyte count >20 × 10^9 cells per L confirmed at 3 months. This panel also felt there was sufficient evidence to *consider* cytoreductive drugs in patients with progressive and persistent leukocytosis (not meeting the criteria above), extreme thrombocytosis, or unexplained bleeding or inadequate Hct control despite phlebotomies.[137] As of this writing, the National Comprehensive Cancer Network (NCCN) guidelines recommend cytoreductive therapy in low-risk PV for individuals requiring frequent phlebotomies, those with splenomegaly, progressive leukocytosis, or thrombocytosis or if there is significant fatigue, night sweats, weight loss or pruritus. At this point, there remains substantial debate over whether or not asymptomatic, low-risk PV patients should be exposed to interferon for the sole potential benefit of JAK2 allelic reduction.[150]

Hydroxyurea

The non–alkylating myelosuppressive agent hydroxyurea remains the most frequently prescribed cytoreductive agent PV.[38,55,134] At appropriate doses, it can control erythrocyte, leukocyte, and platelet counts for patients. While hydroxyurea can rapidly reduce leukocyte and platelet counts, supplemental phlebotomy may occasionally be necessary to reduce the red cell mass.[144] As a rule, neutropenia or thrombocytopenia corrects rapidly after cessation or reduction of hydroxyurea dose. For the same reason, however, missing a few days of therapy may be associated with recurrence of leukocytosis or thrombocytosis—a rebound that may be alarming to patients.

When looking at the preponderance of evidence, it has been argued that statistical associations have not implicated hydroxyurea monotherapy as leukemogenic. The incidence of leukemia in patients treated long term with hydroxyurea appears to be very low and similar to that observed in patients treated with phlebotomy alone.[144] However, as one researcher wrote "a lack of association is difficult to definitively disprove," especially in a relatively uncommon disease.[153] Response to hydroxyurea has been associated with a decline in *JAK2* V617F expression by some but not all investigators.[154,155] Alvarez-Larran and colleagues identified the frequency of manifestations of hydroxyurea intolerance or resistance in a large group of PV patients.[154] In 3.3% of patients, hydroxyurea failed to eliminate the need for phlebotomy, and 1.6% showed continuing active myeloproliferation with 0.8% having resistant splenomegaly. Nine percent had nonhematologic toxicity. Approximately 1.7% developed cytopenias requiring dose reduction before hydroxyurea had achieved maximum benefit. These patients were more likely to develop MF or leukemia.

The usual starting dose of hydroxyurea is 500 mg either once or twice daily and is adjusted according to clinical requirements. Several authors recommend titrating to keep the platelets in the normal range; however, there are no controlled data to support a restrictive control of platelets. The development of leg ulcers, particularly over the malleoli of the ankles, is an idiosyncratic adverse effect requiring drug cessation.

Interferon

Recombinant human interferon-α is an agent with clear efficacy in PV.[38,55,134] Even prior to the pegylated formulation being used, data demonstrated that interferon appeared to control leukocytosis and thrombocytosis and to reduce or eliminate the need for phlebotomy in a significant proportion of patients as well as improving pruritus.[156,157] Similar results have been reported for pegylated interferon in less highly selected patients outside the clinical trials setting.[158] Several studies have demonstrated that pegylated interferon-α can decrease the expression of *JAK2* V617F, and even, in some cases producing complete molecular response, rather than simply controlling abnormal blood counts.[151,159-161]

There have been several randomized studies recently published on the use of either pegylated interferon or the newer, longer-acting formulation ropeginterferon. The Myeloproliferative Disease Research Consortium (MPD-RC) 112 randomized treatment-naïve patients with either high-risk PV or ET to hydroxyurea or peginterferon-alpha-2a (PEG-INF; PEGASYS).[162] The primary endpoint was the comparison of CR rates after 12 months of treatment, with CR defined as a platelet count <400 × 10⁹/L, Hct < 45% without phlebotomy for patients with PV only, white blood cell count <10 × 10⁹/L, resolution of splenomegaly, and resolution of disease-related symptoms. The primary endpoint was achieved in 37% and 35% of patients treated with hydroxyurea and PEG-IFN, respectively ($P = .80$). While the study was originally designed to include 300 patients, it was stopped after 168 patients were enrolled, when supply of pegylated interferon was stopped. Median weekly dose of hydroxyurea was 6708 mg and 89.4 µg for PEG-INF and there was no significant difference in the percentage of patients treated for 12 months or longer. Reductions in *JAK2* V617F VAF were observed in most patients treated with hydroxyurea or PEG-INF. The median *JAK2* V617F level decreased through month 24 in the PEG-IFN arm but increased in the hydroxyurea arm after that time.

This study can be viewed as similar to the PROUD-PV and CONTINUOUS-PV[163] studies of roPEG-IFN-α-2b (roPEG-IFN; BESREMi) vs hydroxyurea, though the MPD-RC study was disadvantaged by the early halt to accrual. Concerns about tolerability of interferon led to development of a newer formulation of pegylated interferon with the addition of proline in the N-terminal end and with a longer half-life and a limited isoform profile.[152] The PROUD-PV study was a phase III randomized study that included two populations of patients with PV: hydroxyurea-naïve patients and patients currently treated or pretreated with hydroxyurea for less than 3 years, not responding to hydroxyurea treatment. At 60 months, the complete hematologic response rates were 56% and 44% in the roPEG-IFN and hydroxyurea arms, respectively. In the fifth year of treatment, 81.8% of patients in the roPEG-IFN arm vs. 63.2% in the hydroxyurea arm were free of phlebotomy. Molecular response was like what was seen in the MPD-RC study. Between the 12th and 60th month of treatment, a further, significant reduction in the *JAK2* V617F allelic burden was noted in patients on roPEG-IFN, with an opposite trend among those treated with hydroxyurea. Discontinuation due to adverse events was similar, 4% and 8% in the hydroxyurea and RoPEG-IFN arms, respectively. RoPEG-IFN was approved by the European Medicines Agency in 2019 for patients with PV and no splenomegaly and by the US Food and Drug Administration in 2021 for the same patient population, without mention of spleen size.

Some patients will have tolerability issues with interferon, even the novel pegylated versions.[13,38] In the MPD-RC study, the most common nonhematologic adverse events were fatigue, headache, flulike symptoms, and injection-site reactions. There is now, with the approval of RoPEG-IFN and the publication of the phase III MPD-RC study, documentation that allows for physician to follow dose-adjustment guidelines for these medications.

The question whether interferon is first- or second-line therapy in PV is not fully answered. Many hematologists are becoming more comfortable with using interferon as first-line therapy, especially in younger patients. It certainly makes sense to consider PEG-IFN or RoPEG-IFN in individuals of childbearing years.[164] As evidence develops about the clinical health consequences of a decrease in *JAK2* V617F allele burden, it may become more important to set this up as a treatment goal for patients with PV. One of the significant challenges in the field at this time is understanding which surrogate markers are most important to measure if our goals are improving the quality and length of life for PV patients.[150]

JAK2 Inhibitors

The *JAK2* inhibitor ruxolitinib has been demonstrated to improve symptoms and quality of life in PV patients,[165] particularly those whose disease phenotype is closer on the spectrum to MF. Several studies reported high efficacy of ruxolitinib in PV patients refractory to hydroxyurea compared to several other alternative agents. The RESPONSE trial[166] had a composite endpoint of Hct control and reduction in spleen volume. The RESPONSE-2 trial[167] included patients without splenomegaly and the primary outcome was Hct control only. In the 5-year follow-up to RESPONSE-2, investigators noted that most of the best-available therapy patients had crossed over to the investigational arm. With a dose of 10 mg twice daily, the median Hct level was under 45%, with fewer phlebotomies required for the RUX-treated group. The most common grade 3 to 4 adverse events among those treated with ruxolitinib were hypertension and thrombocytopenia. On the basis of such studies, ruxolitinib was approved by the US Food and Drug Administration for the treatment of PV patients intolerant of or unresponsive to hydroxyurea. In patients with a history of hepatitis B, ruxolitinib can lead to reactivation and an increase in viral load.

Alkylating Agents

Alkylating agents have been standard cytoreductive agents in PV for many years. Many of the agents employed fell into disuse through a poor toxicity to efficacy ratio. Busulfan may have potential benefit as a second-line agent in specific cases.[134,168] It can be argued that an increase in leukemic risk in PV patients from alkylating agents above that intrinsic to the disease is not clearly established, but other established effects, such as impairment of fertility, suggest that it may be prudent to limit its use to older patients.

Approach to Treatment

Guidelines for the treatment of PV have been published.[55,134,141,150] *Table 84.6* reflects these guidelines as well as the authors' experience.

All patients should have phlebotomy to control the circulating red cell mass and, unless contraindicated, aspirin 80 to 100 mg daily to reduce thrombotic risk. Cytoreductive therapy should be added in high-risk patients. The best-established markers of a high-risk state are age greater than 60 years and/or a personal history of thrombosis. Other factors that may inform a decision to initiate cytoreduction include progressive increases in leukocyte or platelets or worsening

Table 84.6. Treatment Algorithm for Polycythemia Vera Patients

Patient Group	Modality	Comments
All patients	Phlebotomy with aspirin 80-100 mg/d	Phlebotomy target: Hct 41%-44% men, 39%-42% women. Patients with a history of bleeding or platelets >1000 × 10⁹/L should be evaluated for AVWS. Aspirin may be contraindicated if bleeding diathesis present
High-risk patients	Cytoreduction	
First line	Hydroxyurea or interferon (standard or pegylated)	Interferon may be preferred in younger patients or women of childbearing potential
Second-line therapy in patients refractory to or intolerant of first line		
	Interferon (standard or pegylated)	If treated with hydroxyurea initially
	Ruxolitinib	May be particularly helpful in patients with splenomegaly, weight loss, or severe fatigue
	Busulfan	

Abbreviations: AVWS, acquired von Willebrand syndrome; Hct, hematocrit.
Modified from Besses C, Alvarez-Larran A. How to treat essential thrombocythemia and polycythemia vera. *Clin Lymphoma Myeloma Leuk*. 2016;16(suppl):S114-S123.

splenomegaly or severe symptoms, as outlined above and in the recent ELN guidelines.[137] Some very healthy patients in whom age is the only high-risk factor can be managed effectively with phlebotomy and aspirin only. The reader is also referred to the NCCN guidelines, which are regularly updated to reflect the consensus of physicians working in United States designated cancer centers.[169]

Hydroxyurea and pegylated interferon are generally the initial cytoreductive agents of choice. The latter is generally attractive in younger patients. The order of second-line agents in *Table 84.6* reflects the authors' preferences.

Special Topics
Pruritus

Pruritus, particularly after exposure to hot water, can be a significant symptom impairing quality of life in PV patients. The mechanism is unclear and has been attributed to mast cell activation with histamine release.[170] In patients who would not otherwise be treated with cytoreduction, symptoms can be controlled in many cases by strong antihistamines, by cimetidine, or by serotonin release inhibitors. For patients whose symptoms are not relieved, hydroxyurea, interferon, or ruxolitinib can decrease pruritus.[15,165] In refractory cases, responses have been demonstrated with phototherapy, either psoralen–ultraviolet A or ultraviolet B therapy, but given the efficacy of ruxolitinib in refractory cases, this is rarely needed currently. The most effective management of pruritus is establishing good hematologic control of PV.

Hyperuricemia

Because of the excessive urinary load of uric acid excreted by patients with myeloproliferative disorders, urate may be precipitated in the kidneys, leading to stone formation or nephropathy. An effective means of reducing uric acid production in patients with PV, other than by myelosuppression, is with the administration of allopurinol, 300 mg/d. This agent is most useful during the short periods at the initiation of cytoreductive therapy when cell turnover is likely to be high and the avoidance of uric acid deposition is a major concern.

Surgery

Patients with poorly controlled PV are at increased risk for complications of elective surgery. Complications primarily involve thrombotic events, but bleeding may also be noted.[171] Patient who are in a stable state of good hematologic control have a lower complication rate. Attention should also be paid to thrombosis prophylaxis.[172] In newly diagnosed patients who have not yet achieved a normal Hct, elective surgery may be deferred until hematologic control is obtained. Traditionally, it was recommended that patients have a 4-month interval of well-maintained count; however, this recommendation antedates modern cytoreductive therapy and may be an overestimate. In more urgent surgery, normal blood counts should be obtained as quickly as possible using phlebotomy with volume replacement, hydroxyurea, and/or cytapheresis to control the platelet count if necessary, and should be maintained as long as possible pre- and postoperatively.

References

1. Means RT, Jr. Perspective: Osler's 1903 paper on polycythemia vera. *Am J Med Sci.* 2008;335(6):418-419.
2. Verstovsek S, Yu J, Scherber RM, et al. Changes in the incidence and overall survival of patients with myeloproliferative neoplasms between 2002 and 2016 in the United States. *Leuk Lymphoma.* 2022;63(3):694-702.
3. Srour SA, Devesa SS, Morton LM, et al. Incidence and patient survival of myeloproliferative neoplasms and myelodysplastic/myeloproliferative neoplasms in the United States, 2001-12. *Br J Haematol.* 2016;174(3):382-396.
4. Polycythemia vera: the natural history of 1213 patients followed for 20 years. Gruppo Italiano Studio Policitemia. *Ann Intern Med.* 1995;123(9):656-664.
5. Shallis RM, Zeidan AM, Wang R, Podoltsev NA. Epidemiology of the Philadelphia chromosome-negative classical myeloproliferative neoplasms. *Hematol Oncol Clin North Am.* 2021;35(2):177-189.
6. Chaiter Y, Brenner B, Aghai E, Tatarsky I. High incidence of myeloproliferative disorders in Ashkenazi Jews in northern Israel. *Leuk Lymphoma.* 1992;7(3):251-255.
7. Brubaker LH, Wasserman LR, Goldberg JD, et al. Increased prevalence of polycythemia vera in parents of patients on polycythemia vera study group protocols. *Am J Hematol.* 1984;16(4):367-373.
8. Anderson LA, Duncombe AS, Hughes M, Mills ME, Wilson JC, McMullin MF. Environmental, lifestyle, and familial/ethnic factors associated with myeloproliferative neoplasms. *Am J Hematol.* 2012;87(2):175-182.
9. Rumi E, Passamonti F, Picone C, et al. Disease anticipation in familial myeloproliferative neoplasms. *Blood.* 2008;112(6):2587-2588. author reply 8-9.
10. Rumi E, Cazzola M. Advances in understanding the pathogenesis of familial myeloproliferative neoplasms. *Br J Haematol.* 2017;178(5):689-698.
11. Masselli E, Pozzi G, Carubbi C, Vitale M. The genetic makeup of myeloproliferative neoplasms: role of germline variants in defining disease risk, phenotypic diversity and outcome. *Cells.* 2021;10(10):2597.
12. McMullin MF, Anderson LA. Aetiology of myeloproliferative neoplasms. *Cancers (Basel).* 2020;12(7):1810.
13. Bluefarb SM. Cutaneous manifestations of polycythemia vera. *Q Bull Northwest Univ Med Sch.* 1955;29(1):8-17.
14. Gomez Vazquez M, Sanchez-Aguilar D, Peteiro C, Toribio J. Sweet's syndrome and polycythaemia vera. *J Eur Acad Dermatol Venereol.* 2005;19(3):382-383.
15. Saini KS, Patnaik MM, Tefferi A. Polycythemia vera-associated pruritus and its management. *Eur J Clin Invest.* 2010;40(9):828-834.
16. Najean Y, Mugnier P, Dresch C, Rain JD. Polycythaemia vera in young people: an analysis of 58 cases diagnosed before 40 years. *Br J Haematol.* 1987;67(3):285-291.
17. Lelonek E, Matusiak L, Wrobel T, Szepietowski JC. Aquagenic pruritus in polycythemia vera: a cross-sectional study. *J Am Acad Dermatol.* 2021;85(1):211-213.
18. Michiels JJ, Berneman Z, Schroyens W, et al. Platelet-mediated erythromelalgic, cerebral, ocular and coronary microvascular ischemic and thrombotic manifestations in patients with essential thrombocythemia and polycythemia vera: a distinct aspirin-responsive and coumadin-resistant arterial thrombophilia. *Platelets.* 2006;17(8):528-544.
19. Kayrak M, Acar K, Gul EE, et al. Electrocardiographic findings in patients with polycythemia vera. *Int J Med Sci.* 2012;9(1):93-102.
20. Kayrak M, Acar K, Gul EE, et al. Assessment of left ventricular myocardial performance by tissue Doppler echocardiography in patients with polycythemia vera. *Echocardiography.* 2011;28(9):948-954.
21. Reisner SA, Rinkevich D, Markiewicz W, Tatarsky I, Brenner B. Cardiac involvement in patients with myeloproliferative disorders. *Am J Med.* 1992;93(5):498-504.
22. Venegoni P, Cyprus G. Polycythemia and the heart. A review. *Tex Heart Inst J.* 1994;21(3):198-201.
23. Piccirillo G, Fimognari FL, Valdivia JL, Marigliano V. Effects of phlebotomy on a patient with secondary polycythemia and angina pectoris. *Int J Cardiol.* 1994;44(2):175-177.
24. Gordeuk VR, Key NS, Prchal JT. Re-evaluation of hematocrit as a determinant of thrombotic risk in erythrocytosis. *Haematologica.* 2019;104(4):653-658.
25. Cucuianu A, Stoia M, Farcas A, et al. Arterial stenosis and atherothrombotic events in polycythemia vera and essential thrombocythemia. *Rom J Intern Med.* 2006;44(4):397-406.
26. Varma S, Sharma A, Malhotra P, Kumari S, Jain S, Varma N. Thrombotic complications of polycythemia vera. *Hematology.* 2008;13(6):319-323.
27. Jaiswal S, Ebert BL. Clonal hematopoiesis in human aging and disease. *Science.* 2019;366(6465):eaan4673.
28. Wang W, Liu W, Fidler T, et al. Macrophage inflammation, erythrophagocytosis, and accelerated atherosclerosis in Jak2 (V617F) mice. *Circ Res.* 2018;123(11):e35-e47.
29. Libby P, Molinaro R, Sellar RS, Ebert BL. Jak-ing up the Plaque's lipid coreand even more. *Circ Res.* 2018;123(11):1180-1182.
30. Zuriaga MA, Fuster JJ. Clonal hematopoiesis and atherosclerotic cardiovascular disease: a primer. *Clin Investig Arterioscler.* Published online 2021.
31. Björkegren JLM, Lusis AJ. Atherosclerosis: recent developments. *Cell.* 2022;185(10):1630-1645.
32. Fidler TP, Xue C, Yalcinkaya M, et al. The AIM2 inflammasome exacerbates atherosclerosis in clonal haematopoiesis. *Nature.* 2021;592(7853):296-301.
33. Jaiswal S, Natarajan P, Silver AJ, et al. Clonal hematopoiesis and risk of atherosclerotic cardiovascular disease. *N Engl J Med.* 2017;377(2):111-121.
34. Torgano G, Mandelli C, Massaro P, et al. Gastroduodenal lesions in polycythaemia vera: frequency and role of *Helicobacter pylori*. *Br J Haematol.* 2002;117(1):198-202.
35. Yan M, Geyer H, Mesa R, et al. Clinical features of patients with Philadelphia-negative myeloproliferative neoplasms complicated by portal hypertension. *Clin Lymphoma Myeloma Leuk.* 2015;15(1):e1-e5.
36. Ameredes HT, Joyce JM, Fecher A, Landreneau R, Keenan R, Jackson T. Scintigraphic diagnosis of pleuroperitoneal communication in cirrhosis secondary to polycythemia vera. *Clin Nucl Med.* 2003;28(4):332-333.
37. Goldstein G, Maor J, Kleinbaum Y, Palumbo M, Sidi Y, Salomon O. Budd-Chiari syndrome in very young adult patients with polycythemia vera: report of case series with good outcome with direct thrombin inhibitor treatment. *Blood Coagul Fibrinolysis.* 2013;24(8):848-853.
38. Tefferi A, Vannucchi AM, Barbui T. Polycythemia vera: historical oversights, diagnostic details, and therapeutic views. *Leukemia.* 2021;35(12):3339-3351.
39. Calabresi P, Meyer OO. Polycythemia vera. I. Clinical and laboratory manifestations. *Ann Intern Med.* 1959;50(5):1182-1202.
40. Bader RA, Bader ME, Duberstein JL. Polycythemia vera and arterial oxygen saturation. *Am J Med.* 1963;34:435-439.
41. Stempel JM, Gopalakrishnan A, Krishnamoorthy P, et al. Pulmonary arterial hypertension in hospitalized patients with polycythemia vera (from the national inpatient database). *Am J Cardiol.* 2021;143:154-157.
42. Christensen AS, Moller JB, Hasselbalch HC. Chronic kidney disease in patients with the Philadelphia-negative chronic myeloproliferative neoplasms. *Leuk Res.* 2014;38(4):490-495.

43. Said SM, Leung N, Sethi S, et al. Myeloproliferative neoplasms cause glomerulopathy. *Kidney Int*. 2011;80(7):753-759.
44. Kremer M, Lambert CD, Lawton N. Progressive neurological deficits in primary polycythaemia. *Br Med J*. 1972;3(5820):216-218.
45. Ahn BY, Choi KD, Choi YJ, Jea SY, Lee JE. Isolated monocular visual loss as an initial manifestation of polycythemia vera. *J Neurol Sci*. 2007;258(1-2):151-153.
46. Finazzi G, low-dose aspirin in polycythemia (ECLAP). A prospective analysis of thrombotic events in the European collaboration study on low-dose aspirin in polycythemia (ECLAP). *Pathol Biol (Paris)*. 2004;52(5):285-288.
47. Arber DA, Orazi A, Hasserjian R, et al. The 2016 revision to the World Health Organization classification of myeloid neoplasms and acute leukemia. *Blood*. 2016;127(20):2391-2405.
48. Dan K, Yamada T, Kimura Y, et al. Clinical features of polycythemia vera and essential thrombocythemia in Japan: retrospective analysis of a nationwide survey by the Japanese Elderly Leukemia and Lymphoma Study Group. *Int J Hematol*. 2006;83(5):443-449.
49. Gangat N, Wolanskyj AP, Schwager SM, Hanson CA, Tefferi A. Leukocytosis at diagnosis and the risk of subsequent thrombosis in patients with low-risk essential thrombocythemia and polycythemia vera. *Cancer*. 2009;115(24):5740-5745.
50. De Stefano V, Za T, Rossi E, et al. Leukocytosis is a risk factor for recurrent arterial thrombosis in young patients with polycythemia vera and essential thrombocythemia. *Am J Hematol*. 2010;85(2):97-100.
51. Tefferi A, Rumi E, Finazzi G, et al. Survival and prognosis among 1545 patients with contemporary polycythemia vera: an international study. *Leukemia*. 2013;27(9):1874-1881.
52. Ronner L, Podoltsev N, Gotlib J, et al. Persistent leukocytosis in polycythemia vera is associated with disease evolution but not thrombosis. *Blood*. 2020;135(19):1696-1703.
53. Kessler CM, Klein HG, Havlik RJ. Uncontrolled thrombocytosis in chronic myeloproliferative disorders. *Br J Haematol*. 1982;50(1):157-167.
54. Berlin NI, Lawrence JH, Gartland J. Blood volume in polycythemia as determined by P32 labeled red blood cells. *Am J Med*. 1950;9(6):747-751.
55. Spivak JL. How I treat polycythemia vera. *Blood*. 2019;134(4):341-352.
56. Hershko C, Carmeli D. The effect of packed cell volume, hemoglobin content and red cell count on whole blood viscosity. *Acta Haematol*. 1970;44(3):142-154.
57. Streichman S, Avdi N, Joffe G, Matathias L, Tatarsky I. Some characteristics of circulating erythrocytes in polycythaemia vera: common features with normal young and foetal red blood cells. *Scand J Haematol*. 1986;36(1):33-38.
58. Fukasawa H, Furuya R, Kato A, et al. Pseudohyperkalemia occurring in a patient with chronic renal failure and polycythemia vera without severe leukocytosis or thrombocytosis. *Clin Nephrol*. 2002;58(6):451-454.
59. Carmel R. Vitamin B 12-binding protein abnormality in subjects without myeloproliferative disease. I. Elevated serum vitamin B 12-binding capacity levels in patients with leucocytosis. *Br J Haematol*. 1972;22(1):43-51.
60. Rachmilewitz B, Manny N, Rachmilewitz M. The transcobalamins in polycythaemia vera. *Scand J Haematol*. 1977;19(5):453-462.
61. Gisslinger H, Rodeghiero F, Ruggeri M, et al. Homocysteine levels in polycythaemia vera and essential thrombocythaemia. *Br J Haematol*. 1999;105(2):551-555.
62. Castaman G, Lattuada A, Ruggeri M, Tosetto A, Mannucci PM, Rodeghiero F. Platelet von Willebrand factor abnormalities in myeloproliferative syndromes. *Am J Hematol*. 1995;49(4):289-293.
63. Mital A, Prejzner W, Swiatkowska-Stodulska R, Hellmann A. Factors predisposing to acquired von Willebrand syndrome during the course of polycythemia vera - retrospective analysis of 142 consecutive cases. *Thromb Res*. 2015;136(4):754-757.
64. Giaccherini C, Verzeroli C, Marchetti M, et al. PO-26—whole blood rotational thromboelastometry (ROTEM) to detect hypercoagulability in patients with myeloproliferative neoplasm (MPN). *Thromb Res*. 2016;140(suppl 1):S185-S186.
65. Rusak T, Ciborowski M, Uchimiak-Owieczko A, Piszcz J, Radziwon P, Tomasiak M. Evaluation of hemostatic balance in blood from patients with polycythemia vera by means of thromboelastography: the effect of isovolemic erythrocytapheresis. *Platelets*. 2012;23(6):455-462.
66. Bucalossi A, Marotta G, Bigazzi C, Galieni P, Dispensa E. Reduction of antithrombin III, protein C, and protein S levels and activated protein C resistance in polycythemia vera and essential thrombocythemia patients with thrombosis. *Am J Hematol*. 1996;52(1):14-20.
67. Afshar-Kharghan V, Lopez JA, Gray LA, et al. Hemostatic gene polymorphisms and the prevalence of thrombotic complications in polycythemia vera and essential thrombocythemia. *Blood Coagul Fibrinolysis*. 2004;15(1):21-24.
68. Ellis JT, Peterson P, Geller SA, Rappaport H. Studies of the bone marrow in polycythemia vera and the evolution of myelofibrosis and second hematologic malignancies. *Semin Hematol*. 1986;23(2):144-155.
69. Thiele J, Kvasnicka HM, Zankovich R, Diehl V. The value of bone marrow histology in differentiating between early stage Polycythemia vera and secondary (reactive) Polycythemias. *Haematologica*. 2001;86(4):368-374.
70. Kvasnicka HM, Orazi A, Thiele J, et al. European LeukemiaNet study on the reproducibility of bone marrow features in masked polycythemia vera and differentiation from essential thrombocythemia. *Am J Hematol*. 2017;92(10):1062-1067.
71. Lundberg LG, Lerner R, Sundelin P, Rogers R, Folkman J, Palmblad J. Bone marrow in polycythemia vera, chronic myelocytic leukemia, and myelofibrosis has an increased vascularity. *Am J Pathol*. 2000;157(1):15-19.
72. Thiele J, Kvasnicka HM, Muehlhausen K, Walter S, Zankovich R, Diehl V. Polycythemia rubra vera versus secondary polycythemias. A clinicopathological evaluation of distinctive features in 199 patients. *Pathol Res Pract*. 2001;197(2):77-84.
73. Barosi G, Mesa RA, Thiele J, et al. Proposed criteria for the diagnosis of post-polycythemia vera and post-essential thrombocythemia myelofibrosis: a consensus statement from the international working group for myelofibrosis research and treatment. *Leukemia*. 2008;22(2):437-438.
74. Diez-Martin JL, Graham DL, Petitt RM, Dewald GW. Chromosome studies in 104 patients with polycythemia vera. *Mayo Clin Proc*. 1991;66(3):287-299.
75. Swolin B, Weinfeld A, Westin J. A prospective long-term cytogenetic study in polycythemia vera in relation to treatment and clinical course. *Blood*. 1988;72(2):386-395.
76. Gangat N, Strand J, Lasho TL, et al. Cytogenetic studies at diagnosis in polycythemia vera: clinical and JAK2V617F allele burden correlates. *Eur J Haematol*. 2008;80(3):197-200.
77. Sever M, Quintás-Cardama A, Pierce S, Zhou L, Kantarjian H, Verstovšek S. Significance of cytogenetic abnormalities in patients with polycythemia vera. *Leuk Lymphoma*. 2013;54(12):2667-2670.
78. Tefferi A, Guglielmelli P, Lasho TL, et al. Mutation-enhanced international prognostic systems for essential thrombocythaemia and polycythaemia vera. *Br J Haematol*. 2020;189(2):291-302.
79. Adamson JW, Fialkow PJ, Murphy S, Prchal JF, Steinmann L. Polycythemia vera: stem-cell and probable clonal origin of the disease. *N Engl J Med*. 1976;295(17):913-916.
80. Raskind WH, Jacobson R, Murphy S, Adamson JW, Fialkow PJ. Evidence for the involvement of B lymphoid cells in polycythemia vera and essential thrombocythemia. *J Clin Invest*. 1985;75(4):1388-1390.
81. Baxter EJ, Scott LM, Campbell PJ, et al. Acquired mutation of the tyrosine kinase JAK2 in human myeloproliferative disorders. *Lancet*. 2005;365(9464):1054-1061.
82. James C, Ugo V, Le Couédic J-P, et al. A unique clonal JAK2 mutation leading to constitutive signalling causes polycythaemia vera. *Nature*. 2005;434(7037):1144-1148.
83. Kralovics R, Passamonti F, Buser AS, et al. A gain-of-function mutation of JAK2 in myeloproliferative disorders. *N Engl J Med*. 2005;352(17):1779-1790.
84. Levine RL, Wadleigh M, Cools J, et al. Activating mutation in the tyrosine kinase JAK2 in polycythemia vera, essential thrombocythemia, and myeloid metaplasia with myelofibrosis. *Cancer Cell*. 2005;7(4):387-397.
85. Scott LM, Tong W, Levine RL, et al. JAK2 exon 12 mutations in polycythemia vera and idiopathic erythrocytosis. *N Engl J Med*. 2007;356(5):459-468.
86. Villafuerte FC, Corante N. Chronic mountain sickness: clinical aspects, etiology, management, and treatment. *High Alt Med Biol*. 2016;17(2):61-69.
87. Bernardi M, Ruggeri M, Albiero E, Madeo D, Rodeghiero F. Isolated erythrocytosis in V617F negative patients with JAK2 exon 12 mutations: report of a new mutation. *Am J Hematol*. 2009;84(4):258-260.
88. Nangalia J, Green AR. Myeloproliferative neoplasms: from origins to outcomes. *Hematology Am Soc Hematol Educ Program*. 2017;2017(1):470-479.
89. Li J, Kent DG, Chen E, Green AR. Mouse models of myeloproliferative neoplasms: JAK of all grades. *Dis Model Mech*. 2011;4(3):311-317.
90. Tefferi A. Novel mutations and their functional and clinical relevance in myeloproliferative neoplasms: JAK2, MPL, TET2, ASXL1, CBL, IDH and IKZF1. *Leukemia*. 2010;24(6):1128-1138.
91. Wautier MP, El Nemer W, Gane P, et al. Increased adhesion to endothelial cells of erythrocytes from patients with polycythemia vera is mediated by laminin alpha5 chain and Lu/BCAM. *Blood*. 2007;110(3):894-901.
92. Wautier JL, Wautier MP. Cellular and molecular aspects of blood cell-endothelium interactions in vascular disorders. *Int J Mol Sci*. 2020;21(15):5315.
93. Cerquozzi S, Tefferi A. Blast transformation and fibrotic progression in polycythemia vera and essential thrombocythemia: a literature review of incidence and risk factors. *Blood Cancer J*. 2015;5(11):e366.
94. Zaleskas VM, Krause DS, Lazarides K, et al. Molecular pathogenesis and therapy of polycythemia induced in mice by JAK2 V617F. *PLoS One*. 2006;1:e18.
95. Kralovics R, Teo SS, Li S, et al. Acquisition of the V617F mutation of JAK2 is a late genetic event in a subset of patients with myeloproliferative disorders. *Blood*. 2006;108(4):1377-1380.
96. Ortmann CA, Kent DG, Nangalia J, et al. Effect of mutation order on myeloproliferative neoplasms. *N Engl J Med*. 2015;372(7):601-612.
97. Williams N, Lee J, Mitchell E, et al. Life histories of myeloproliferative neoplasms inferred from phylogenies. *Nature*. 2022;602(7895):162-168.
98. Mitchell E, Spencer Chapman M, Williams N, et al. Clonal dynamics of haematopoiesis across the human lifespan. *Nature*. 2022;606(7913):343-350.
99. Fabre MA, de Almeida JG, Fiorillo E, et al. The longitudinal dynamics and natural history of clonal haematopoiesis. *Nature*. 2022;606(7913):335-342.
100. Lee J, Godfrey AL, Nangalia J. Genomic heterogeneity in myeloproliferative neoplasms and applications to clinical practice. *Blood Rev*. 2020;42:100708.
101. Constantinescu SN, Vainchenker W, Levy G, Papadopoulos N. Functional consequences of mutations in myeloproliferative neoplasms. *Hemasphere*. 2021;5(6):e578.
102. Strickland M, Quek L, Psaila B. The immune landscape in BCR-ABL negative myeloproliferative neoplasms: inflammation, infections and opportunities for immunotherapy. *Br J Haematol*. 2022;196(5):1149-1158.
103. Moliterno AR, Hankins WD, Spivak JL. Impaired expression of the thrombopoietin receptor by platelets from patients with polycythemia vera. *N Engl J Med*. 1998;338(9):572-580.
104. Moliterno AR, Spivak JL. Posttranslational processing of the thrombopoietin receptor is impaired in polycythemia vera. *Blood*. 1999;94(8):2555-2561.
105. Spivak JL, Merchant A, Williams DM, et al. Thrombopoietin is required for full phenotype expression in a JAK2V617F transgenic mouse model of polycythemia vera. *PLoS One*. 2020;15(6):e0232801.
106. Spivak JL, Moliterno AR. The thrombopoietin receptor, MPL, is a therapeutic target of Opportunity in the MPN. *Front Oncol*. 2021;11:641613.
107. Temerinac S, Klippel S, Strunck E, et al. Cloning of PRV-1, a novel member of the uPAR receptor superfamily, which is overexpressed in polycythemia rubra vera. *Blood*. 2000;95(8):2569-2576.

108. Cario H, Goerttler PS, Steimle C, Levine RL, Pahl HL. The JAK2V617F mutation is acquired secondary to the predisposing alteration in familial polycythaemia vera. *Br J Haematol.* 2005;130(5):800-801.
109. Reid CD, Fidler J, Kirk A. Endogenous erythroid clones (EEC) in polycythaemia and their relationship to diagnosis and the response to treatment. *Br J Haematol.* 1988;68(4):395-400.
110. Mladenovic J, Adamson JW. Characteristics of circulating erythroid colony-forming cells in normal and polycythaemic man. *Br J Haematol.* 1982;51(3):377-384.
111. Kralovics R, Prchal JT. Haematopoietic progenitors and signal transduction in polycythaemia vera and primary thrombocythaemia. *Baillieres Clin Haematol.* 1998;11(4):803-818.
112. Kralovics R, Sokol L, Prchal JT. Absence of polycythemia in a child with a unique erythropoietin receptor mutation in a family with autosomal dominant primary polycythemia. *J Clin Invest.* 1998;102(1):124-129.
113. Lee SA, Kim JY, Choi Y, Kim Y, Kim HO. Application of mutant JAK2V617F for in vitro generation of red blood cells. *Transfusion.* 2016;56(4):837-843.
114. Garçon L, Rivat C, James C, et al. Constitutive activation of STAT5 and Bcl-xL overexpression can induce endogenous erythroid colony formation in human primary cells. *Blood.* 2006;108(5):1551-1554.
115. Michiels JJ, Bernema Z, Van Bockstaele D, De Raeve H, Schroyens W. Current diagnostic criteria for the chronic myeloproliferative disorders (MPD) essential thrombocythemia (ET), polycythemia vera (PV) and chronic idiopathic myelofibrosis (CIMF). *Pathol Biol (Paris).* 2007;55(2):92-104.
116. Michiels JJ, De Raeve H, Berneman Z, et al. The 2001 World Health Organization and updated European clinical and pathological criteria for the diagnosis, classification, and staging of the Philadelphia chromosome-negative chronic myeloproliferative disorders. *Semin Thromb Hemost.* 2006;32(4 pt 2):307-340.
117. Teofili L, Giona F, Martini M, et al. The revised WHO diagnostic criteria for Ph-negative myeloproliferative diseases are not appropriate for the diagnostic screening of childhood polycythemia vera and essential thrombocythemia. *Blood.* 2007;110(9):3384-3386.
118. Tondeur S, Paul F, Riou J, et al. Long-term follow-up of JAK2 exon 12 polycythemia vera: a French Intergroup of Myeloproliferative Neoplasms (FIM) study. *Leukemia.* 2021;35(3):871-875.
119. Gangat N, Szuber N, Pardanani A, Tefferi A. JAK2 unmutated erythrocytosis: current diagnostic approach and therapeutic views. *Leukemia.* 2021;35(8):2166-2181.
120. Passamonti F, Maffioli M. Update from the latest WHO classification of MPNs: a user's manual. *Hematology Am Soc Hematol Educ Program.* 2016;2016(1):534-542.
121. Lawrence JH, Winchell HS, Donald WG. Leukemia in polycythemia vera. Relationship to splenic myeloid metaplasia and therapeutic radiation dose. *Ann Intern Med.* 1969;70(4):763-771.
122. Silverstein MN. The evolution into and the treatment of late stage polycythemia vera. *Semin Hematol.* 1976;13(1):79-84.
123. Luque Paz D, Jouanneau-Courville R, Riou J, et al. Leukemic evolution of polycythemia vera and essential thrombocythemia: genomic profiles predict time to transformation. *Blood Adv.* 2020;4(19):4887-4897.
124. Tefferi A, Mudireddy M, Mannelli F, et al. Blast phase myeloproliferative neoplasm: Mayo-AGIMM study of 410 patients from two separate cohorts. *Leukemia.* 2018;32(5):1200-1210.
125. Finazzi G, Caruso V, Marchioli R, et al. Acute leukemia in polycythemia vera: an analysis of 1638 patients enrolled in a prospective observational study. *Blood.* 2005;105(7):2664-2670.
126. Grinfeld J, Nangalia J, Baxter EJ, et al. Classification and personalized prognosis in myeloproliferative neoplasms. *N Engl J Med.* 2018;379(15):1416-1430.
127. Hasselbalch HC, Bjørn ME. MPNs as inflammatory diseases: the evidence, consequences, and Perspectives. *Mediators Inflamm.* 2015;2015:102476.
128. Tefferi A, Guglielmelli P, Larson DR, et al. Long-term survival and blast transformation in molecularly annotated essential thrombocythemia, polycythemia vera, and myelofibrosis. *Blood.* 2014;124(16):2507-2513.
129. Wasserman LR, Balcerzak SP, Berk PD, et al. Influence of therapy on causes of death in polycythemia vera. *Trans Assoc Am Phys.* 1981;94:30-38.
130. Marchioli R, Finazzi G, Landolfi R, et al. Vascular and neoplastic risk in a large cohort of patients with polycythemia vera. *J Clin Oncol.* 2005;23(10):2224-2232.
131. Szuber N, Mudireddy M, Nicolosi M, et al. 3023 Mayo clinic patients with myeloproliferative neoplasms: risk-stratified comparison of survival and outcomes data among disease subgroups. *Mayo Clin Proc.* 2019;94(4):599-610.
132. Szuber N, Vallapureddy RR, Penna D, et al. Myeloproliferative neoplasms in the young: Mayo Clinic experience with 361 patients age 40 years or younger. *Am J Hematol.* 2018;93(12):1474-1484.
133. Landolfi R, Marchioli R, Kutti J, et al. Efficacy and safety of low-dose aspirin in polycythemia vera. *N Engl J Med.* 2004;350(2):114-124.
134. Tefferi A, Barbui T. Polycythemia vera and essential thrombocythemia: 2021 update on diagnosis, risk-stratification and management. *Am J Hematol.* 2020;95(12):1599-1613.
135. Barbui T, Carobbio A, Ferrari A. Leukocytosis and thrombosis in polycythemia vera: can clinical trials settle the debate? *Blood Adv.* 2019;3(23):3951-3952.
136. Carobbio A, Ferrari A, Masciulli A, Ghirardi A, Barosi G, Barbui T. Leukocytosis and thrombosis in essential thrombocythemia and polycythemia vera: a systematic review and meta-analysis. *Blood Adv.* 2019;3(11):1729-1737.
137. Marchetti M, Vannucchi AM, Griesshammer M, et al. Appropriate management of polycythaemia vera with cytoreductive drug therapy: European LeukemiaNet 2021 recommendations. *Lancet Haematol.* 2022;9(4):e301-e311.
138. Barbui T, Carobbio A, Rumi E, et al. In contemporary patients with polycythemia vera, rates of thrombosis and risk factors delineate a new clinical epidemiology. *Blood.* 2014;124(19):3021-3023.
139. Barbui T, Vannucchi AM, Carobbio A, et al. The effect of arterial hypertension on thrombosis in low-risk polycythemia vera. *Am J Hematol.* 2017;92(1):E5-E6.
140. Cerquozzi S, Barraco D, Lasho T, et al. Risk factors for arterial versus venous thrombosis in polycythemia vera: a single center experience in 587 patients. *Blood Cancer J.* 2017;7(12):662.
141. How J, Hobbs G. Management issues and controversies in low-risk patients with essential thrombocythemia and polycythemia vera. *Curr Hematol Malig Rep.* 2021;16(5):473-482.
142. Barbui T, Vannucchi AM, De Stefano V, et al. Ropeginterferon alfa-2b versus phlebotomy in low-risk patients with polycythaemia vera (Low-PV study): a multicentre, randomised phase 2 trial. *Lancet Haematol.* 2021;8(3):e175-e184.
143. Marchioli R, Finazzi G, Specchia G, et al. Cardiovascular events and intensity of treatment in polycythemia vera. *N Engl J Med.* 2013;368(1):22-33.
144. Berk PD, Wasserman LR, Fruchtman SM, Goldberg JD. Treatment of polycythemia vera: a summary of trials conducted by the Polycythemia Vera Study Group. In: Wasserman LR, ed. *Polycythemia Vera and the Myeloproliferative Disorders.* WB Saunders; 1995:166-194.
145. Crisa E, Venturino E, Passera R, et al. A retrospective study on 226 polycythemia vera patients: impact of median hematocrit value on clinical outcomes and survival improvement with anti-thrombotic prophylaxis and non-alkylating drugs. *Ann Hematol.* 2010;89(7):691-699.
146. Kiraly JF III, Feldmann JE, Wheby MS. Hazards of phlebotomy in polycythemic patients with cardiovascular disease. *JAMA.* 1976;236(18):2080-2081.
147. Rector WG, Jr, Fortuin NJ, Conley CL. Non-hematologic effects of chronic iron deficiency. A study of patients with polycythemia vera treated solely with venesections. *Medicine (Baltimore).* 1982;61(6):382-389.
148. Scherber RM, Geyer HL, Dueck AC, et al. The potential role of hematocrit control on symptom burden among polycythemia vera patients: insights from the CYTO-PV and MPN-SAF patient cohorts. *Leuk Lymphoma.* 2017;58(6):1481-1487.
149. Silver RT, Gjoni S. The hematocrit value in polycythemia vera: caveat utilitor. *Leuk Lymphoma.* 2015;56(5):1540-1541.
150. Gotlib J. Treatment and clinical endpoints in polycythemia vera: seeking the best obtainable version of the truth. *Blood.* 2022;139(19):2871-2881.
151. Kiladjian JJ, Cassinat B, Chevret S, et al. Pegylated interferon-alfa-2a induces complete hematologic and molecular responses with low toxicity in polycythemia vera. *Blood.* 2008;112(8):3065-3072.
152. Gisslinger H, Kralovics R, Gisslinger B, et al. AOP2014, a novel Peg-proline-interferon alpha-2b with improved pharmacokinetic properties, is safe and well tolerated and shows promising efficacy in patients with polycythemia vera (PV). *Blood.* 2012;120(21):175.
153. Cuthbert D, Stein BL. Therapy-associated leukemic transformation in myeloproliferative neoplasms - what do we know? *Best Pract Res Clin Haematol.* 2019;32(1):65-73.
154. Besses C, Alvarez-Larran A, Martinez-Aviles L, et al. Modulation of JAK2 V617F allele burden dynamics by hydroxycarbamide in polycythaemia vera and essential thrombocythaemia patients. *Br J Haematol.* 2011;152(4):413-419.
155. Antonioli E, Carobbio A, Pieri L, et al. Hydroxyurea does not appreciably reduce JAK2 V617F allele burden in patients with polycythemia vera or essential thrombocythemia. *Haematologica.* 2010;95(8):1435-1438.
156. Lengfelder E, Berger U, Hehlmann R. Interferon alpha in the treatment of polycythemia vera. *Ann Hematol.* 2000;79(3):103-109.
157. Elliott MA, Tefferi A. Interferon-alpha therapy in polycythemia vera and essential thrombocythemia. *Semin Thromb Hemost.* 1997;23(5):463-472.
158. Gowin K, Jain T, Kosiorek H, et al. Pegylated interferon alpha-2a is clinically effective and tolerable in myeloproliferative neoplasm patients treated off clinical trial. *Leuk Res.* 2017;54:73-77.
159. Quintas-Cardama A, Kantarjian H, Manshouri T, et al. Pegylated interferon alfa-2a yields high rates of hematologic and molecular response in patients with advanced essential thrombocythemia and polycythemia vera. *J Clin Oncol.* 2009;27(32):5418-5424.
160. Quintas-Cardama A, Abdel-Wahab O, Manshouri T, et al. Molecular analysis of patients with polycythemia vera or essential thrombocythemia receiving pegylated interferon alpha-2a. *Blood.* 2013;122(6):893-901.
161. Gowin K, Thapaliya P, Samuelson J, et al. Experience with pegylated interferon alpha-2a in advanced myeloproliferative neoplasms in an international cohort of 118 patients. *Haematologica.* 2012;97(10):1570-1573.
162. Mascarenhas J, Kosiorek HE, Prchal JT, et al. A randomized phase 3 trial of interferon-alpha vs hydroxyurea in polycythemia vera and essential thrombocythemia. *Blood.* 2022;139(19):2931-2941.
163. Gisslinger H, Klade C, Georgiev P, et al. Ropeginterferon alfa-2b versus standard therapy for polycythaemia vera (PROUD-PV and CONTINUATION-PV): a randomised, non-inferiority, phase 3 trial and its extension study. *Lancet Haematol.* 2020;7(3):e196-e208.
164. DeBaun MR. Hydroxyurea therapy contributes to infertility in adult men with sickle cell disease: a review. *Expert Rev Hematol.* 2014;7(6):767-773.
165. Mesa R, Verstovsek S, Kiladjian JJ, et al. Changes in quality of life and disease-related symptoms in patients with polycythemia vera receiving ruxolitinib or standard therapy. *Eur J Haematol.* 2016;97(2):192-200.
166. Verstovsek S, Vannucchi AM, Griesshammer M, et al. Ruxolitinib versus best available therapy in patients with polycythemia vera: 80-week follow-up from the RESPONSE trial. *Haematologica.* 2016;101(7):821-829.
167. Passamonti F, Palandri F, Saydam G, et al. Ruxolitinib versus best available therapy in inadequately controlled polycythaemia vera without splenomegaly (RESPONSE-2): 5-year follow up of a randomised, phase 3b study. *Lancet Haematol.* 2022;9(7):e480-e492.
168. Brodsky I. Busulphan treatment of polycythaemia vera. *Br J Haematol.* 1982;52(1):1-6.

169. Gerds A, Gotlib J, Ali H, et al. *Myeloproliferative neoplasms version 2. 2022. — April 13, 2022 2022 [updated April 2022. NCCN Guidelines]*. https://www.nccn.org/professionals/physician_gls/pdf/mpn.pdf
170. Buchanan JG, Ameratunga RV, Hawkins RC. Polycythemia vera and water-induced pruritus: evidence against mast cell involvement. *Pathology*. 1994;26(1):43-45.
171. Ruggeri M, Rodeghiero F, Tosetto A, et al. Postsurgery outcomes in patients with polycythemia vera and essential thrombocythemia: a retrospective survey. *Blood*. 2008;111(2):666-671.
172. Stein BL, Martin K. From Budd-Chiari syndrome to acquired von Willebrand syndrome: thrombosis and bleeding complications in the myeloproliferative neoplasms. *Hematology Am Soc Hematol Educ Program*. 2019;2019(1):397-406.

Chapter 85 ■ Myelofibrosis

ANDREW T. KUYKENDALL • SRDAN VERSTOVSEK • ERIC PADRON • RAMI KOMROKJI

DEFINITION

Myelofibrosis (MF) is a rare, serious myeloid malignancy classified as one of the Philadelphia chromosome negative (Ph[−]) myeloproliferative neoplasms (MPNs).[1]

MF is subdivided into primary MF (PMF) and secondary MF.[2] Secondary MF may arise from polycythemia vera (PV) or essential thrombocythemia (ET).[3]

Terms frequently used synonymously with PMF include chronic idiopathic MF (World Health Organization [WHO]), agnogenic myeloid metaplasia, MF with myeloid metaplasia, and idiopathic MF.[4,5]

The International Working Group for Myelofibrosis Research and Treatment (IWG-MRT) has defined MF as either PMF (de novo presenting disease) or post-PV or ET MF (MF transformation from prior PV or ET). Furthermore, patients with transformation to acute leukemia are referred to as PMF in blast phase or post-PV/ET MF in blast phase.[5]

The hallmark of MF neoplasm is an increase in mature blood cells, which arise from clonal expansion driven by genetic mutations in pluripotent cells of the bone marrow compartment. The response to this malignant myeloproliferative process is the secretion of multiple profibrogenic, angiogenic, and inflammatory cytokines that eventually results in polyclonal bone marrow fibrosis. The biologic hallmark of the disease is deregulation of Janus kinase-signal transducer and activator of transcription (JAK-STAT) pathway. MF is typically associated with progressive splenomegaly and, in many cases, with hepatomegaly, which can lead to other complications, such as portal hypertension or splenic infarcts, cytopenias, and an increased likelihood of transforming to the blast phase.[6,7]

HISTORICAL PERSPECTIVE

- **1879** First report of PMF was by Heuck.[8]
- **1935** Secondary myelofibrosis (post-PV MF) was described by Hirsch.[9]
- **1951** Dameshek coined the classification of PMF as a myeloproliferative disorder (MPD).[10]
- **1960** The Philadelphia chromosome abnormality t(9;22) (q32;q13) was described in chronic myeloid leukemia (CML) by Nowell and Hungerford.[11]
- **1978** PMF was characterized as a stem cell–derived clonal MPD associated with reactive MF by Fialkow's group.[12]
- **1992** The JAK-STAT pathway was described.[13]
- **2005** A few groups described a novel gain-of-function mutation in the gene encoding JAK2. The mutation is a single-nucleotide change, which results in a valine-to-phenylalanine substitution at codon 617 (JAK2 V617F) in over 98% of patients with PV and ~50% of those with either PMF or ET.[14-17]
- **2006** A mutation in the myeloproliferative leukemia (MPL) virus gene for the thrombopoietin receptor was described in ~5% of patients with PMF.[18] The mutation was a substitution of tryptophan to leucine at position 515 in the MPL gene sequence, MPL W515L. The "W" and "L" are the shorthand way to indicate which change occurred and resulted in the gene becoming abnormally active.[19]
- **2008** The WHO classification changed the term from MPD to MPN.[3]
- **2009** Other novel mutations were described for PMF in other genes, including ten-eleven-translocation-2 (TET2), additional sex combs like-1 (ASXL1), Casitas B-lineage lymphoma (CBL), isocitrate dehydrogenase (IDH) 1 and 2, and IKAROS family zinc finger-1 (IKZF1). These mutations occur in 0% to 17% of MPNs and are more common in chronic (TET2, ASXL1, and CBL) or juvenile (CBL) myelomonocytic leukemia, myelodysplastic syndromes (MDSs) (TET2 and ASXL1), and secondary acute myeloid leukemia (AML), including the blast phase of MPN.[20]
- **2011** The US Food and Drug Administration (FDA) approved the first JAK2 inhibitor, ruxolitinib, for the treatment of intermediate-risk or high-risk PMF or secondary MF.
- **2013** Calreticulin (CALR) gene mutations described in MPN.[21]
- **2016** The WHO classification revisions were PMF diagnostic criteria update and introduction of prefibrotic PMF category.[22]
- **2019** The FDA-approved fedratinib, a JAK2 inhibitor, for the treatment of intermediate-2 or high-risk PMF or secondary MF.

EPIDEMIOLOGY

PMF is a rare disease. The annual incidence of MF has been estimated to be 0.41 to 1.46 cases per 100,000 individuals.[23,24] The prevalence of MF in the United States has been estimated as 16,000 to 18,500 patients. MF is slightly more common in males and more common in older patients.[23] The median age of patients at the time of diagnosis is 67 years.[23] Among the Philadelphia chromosome negative MPNs (e.g., MF, PV, and ET), MF is the most symptomatic and carries the worst prognosis.

A higher incidence of PMF and related MPN has been suggested for persons of Jewish Ashkenazi ancestry.[25] Benzene, industrial solvents, and radiation exposure have been reported to be associated with increased risk of PMF.[26-28]

PATHOGENESIS

Current understanding suggests that PMF occurs secondary to acquired mutations that target the hematopoietic stem cell.[1,12,29] These mutations can, in some cases, predate the MPN diagnosis by decades.[30] As a result, ineffective hematopoiesis and proliferation of dysfunctional megakaryocytes are commonly seen in MF. The hallmark of the disease pathologically is bone marrow reticulin and collagen fibrosis, ineffective extramedullary hematopoiesis (EMH), and deregulated cytokine production.

The disease-initiating mutations remain unknown. Cytogenetic abnormalities originating on the progenitor cell level are well described in MF. In general, approximately half of patients with PMF display cytogenetic abnormalities that include del(20) (q11;q13), del(13) (q12;q22), trisomy 8, trisomy 9, del(12) (p11;p13), monosomy or deletions of chromosome 7, and partial trisomy 1q. None of these abnormalities is specific to PMF, although the presence of either del(13) (q12;q22) or der(6)t(1;6) (q21-23;p21-23) is strongly suggestive of PMF diagnosis. In one study of 826 patients with PMF, an abnormal karyotype was found in 42.6% of patients with del(20q) and del(13q) being the most common abnormalities, occurring in 23.3% and 18.2% of patients, respectively.[31] Molecular cytogenetics using fluorescence in situ hybridization did not reveal additional karyotypically occult cytogenetic lesions, but comparative genomic hybridization studies have disclosed gain of chromosome 9p as the most frequent abnormality occurring in 50% of patients.[32-35]

Somatic gene mutations are observed in 90% of MF patients, which include mutations in JAK-STAT pathway, epigenetic regulation, histone modification, and splicing and transcription factor mutations. The somatic mutations can be thought of as phenotype driver mutations such as JAK2 V617, MPL, or CALR, disease-initiating mutations such as TET-2 or DNMT3A, and mutations associated with disease progression like *ASXL1* or *SRSF2* mutations. The hierarchy or order of those mutations impacts the clinical phenotype.[36,37]

Deregulation of the JAK-STAT pathway is the key contributor to the clinical phenotype of the disease regardless of the presence or absence of the *JAK2* V617F mutation. The mutation described is not a disease-initiating abnormality. The JAK-STAT pathway plays a pivotal role in the differentiation and development of hematopoietic cells and the functioning of the immune system.[38] The JAK family comprises JAK1, JAK2, JAK3, and TYK2.[39] Cytokines and growth factors activate the extracellular portion of their cognate receptors,[39,40] which promote the recruitment of JAK proteins to associate closely with the intracellular portion of these receptors and the activation of the JAK proteins via phosphorylation (*Figure 85.1*). Phosphorylation of JAK proteins, in turn, leads to the phosphorylation and activation of several intracellular downstream signaling proteins, such as STAT proteins.[41] Phosphorylated STATs translocate to the nucleus and act as inducible nuclear transcription factors, which lead to transcriptional modulation and eventual expression of cellular, molecular, and (patho)physiologic actions that were promoted by the initial signal (ligand).

The dysregulation of the JAK-STAT signaling pathway in hematopoietic progenitor cells has been implicated in the pathogenesis of MF. JAK-STAT signaling in the pathogenesis of MF also relates to its role in mediating signaling from proinflammatory cytokines. These cytokines are elevated in environments of myeloproliferative disease and contribute to the debilitating symptoms of MPNs.[42] Somatic mutations that contribute to this dysregulated JAK-STAT activity include gain-of-function mutations directly in *JAK2*, or upstream signaling mutations such as the mutation of the thrombopoietin receptor (*MPL* W515L or K),[18] and loss of JAK regulation by mutations in the gene for the lymphocyte-specific adaptor protein (*LNK* exon 2 mutations).[43] Frameshift mutations of *CALR* have been found in the majority of PMF patients with wild-type *JAK2* and *MPL*[21,44] and drive JAK-STAT signaling through interaction with the extracellular portion of the thrombopoietin receptor.[45]

Mutations in *JAK2* that lead to the constitutive activation of the JAK-STAT pathway, namely, the *JAK2* V617F[14-16] and *JAK2* exon 12 mutations, have been identified, although this latter mutation was primarily identified in patients with PV.[46] *JAK2* V617F is the most common mutation occurring in a large proportion (50%-60%) of patients with PMF.[14,15] With *JAK2* activating mutations, the pathway becomes cytokine and growth factor independent; therefore, even in the absence of these ligands, the intracellular signaling proteins are constitutively active. Clonal expansion leads to an increased *JAK2* V617F allele burden and homozygosity, thus influencing disease phenotype and differentiation of PV and ET. *CALR* mutations are observed in 30% of PMF patients (two-thirds of *JAK2* V617F mutation negative). Thus far, *CALR* mutations have been frameshift mutations within exon 9, resulting in a mutant protein with a novel C-terminus. The most common

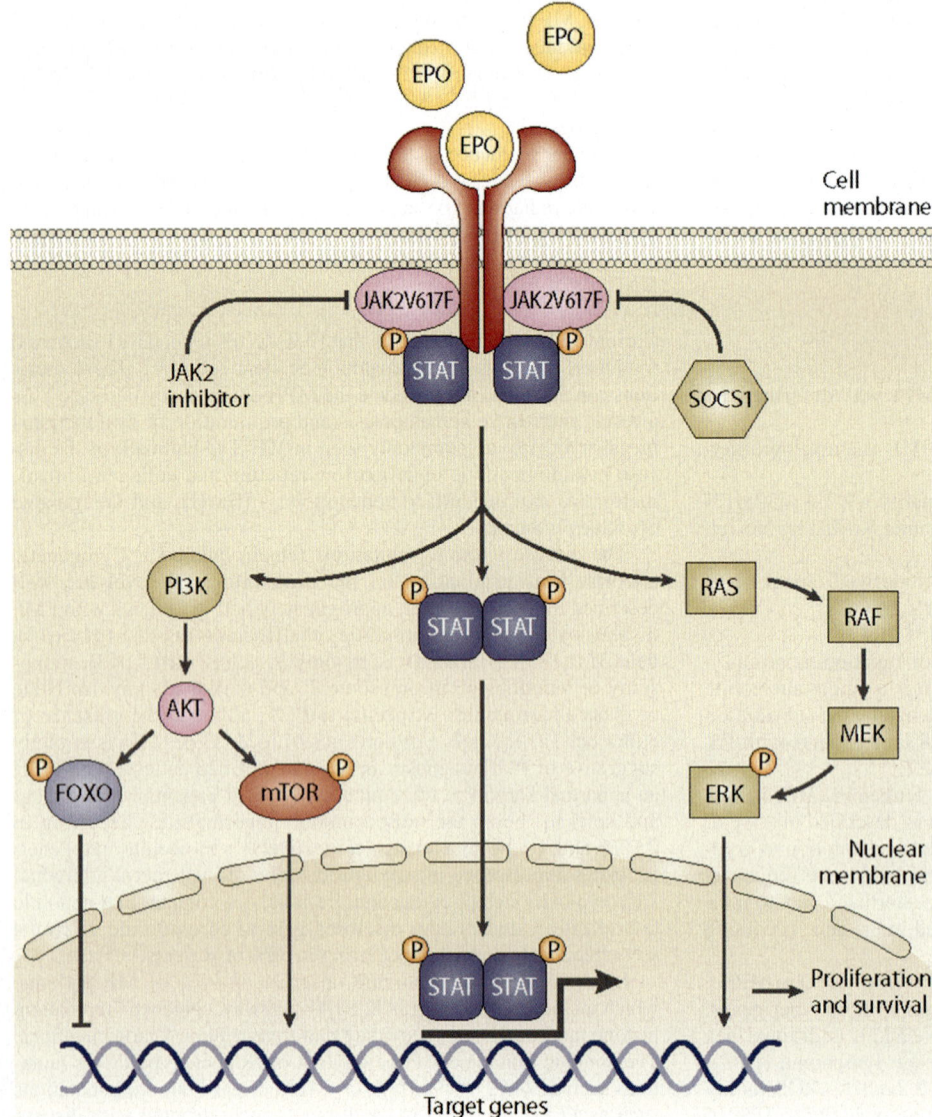

FIGURE 85.1 **The JAK-STAT signaling pathway.** Cytokines and growth factors bind to the extracellular receptor and induce a series of intracellular changes: (1) JAK proteins associate with the intracellular portion of the receptor and are phosphorylated; (2) phosphorylated JAK proteins in turn phosphorylate STAT proteins, which then phosphorylate other downstream proteins; and (3) phosphorylated STAT translocates into the nucleus and promotes the transcription of genes. Other proteins also regulate this signaling pathway, such as SOCS1, which prevents activation of this pathway. ERK, extracellular signal-regulated kinase; FOXO, forkhead O transcription factors; JAK, Janus kinase; MEK, MAPK/ERK kinase; mTOR, mammalian target of rapamycin; STAT, signal transducer and activator of transcription. (Reprinted by permission from Nature: Quintas-Cardama A, Kantarjian H, Cortes J, et al. Janus kinase inhibitors for the treatment of myeloproliferative neoplasias and beyond. *Nat Rev Drug Discov*. 2011;10(2):127-140. Copyright © 2011 Springer Nature.)

CALR mutation is a 52-base pair deletion (type 1) and is more often seen in PMF than type 2 (5-base pair insertion) mutations. While *CALR* mutations are associated with favorable outcomes, this may be limited to type 1 mutations.[21,44,47]

Megakaryocyte-derived transforming growth factor (TGF) β_1 has been identified as the primary cytokine that mediates many of the bone marrow stromal changes (i.e., collagen fibrosis, osteosclerosis, and angiogenesis) in PMF.[48,49] In mice, the PMF phenotype has been induced either by systemic overexpression of thrombopoietin (TPO^{high} mice) or by megakaryocyte lineage–restricted underexpression of the transcription factor GATA-1 (GATA-1^{low} mice). In both instances, the megakaryocytes display abnormal distribution of P-selectin that is believed to promote a pathologic interaction between megakaryocytes and neutrophils, resulting in the release of both fibrogenic and angiogenic cytokines, including TGF-β, platelet-derived growth factor, basic fibroblast growth factor, vascular endothelial growth factor, tissue inhibitors of matrix metalloproteinases, and neutrophil-derived elastase and other proteases.[50,51]

Another characteristic feature in PMF that accompanies the aberrant bone marrow stromal reaction involves peripheral blood expansion of both CD34-positive myeloid progenitors and endothelial cells.[52,53] Current consensus implicates both circulating progenitor cell trapping and abnormal cytokine stimulation of embryonic hematopoietic sites as mechanisms of hepatosplenic EMH in PMF.[54,55] Such a contention is supported by the high concordance between bone marrow and splenic tissue cytogenetic findings in PMF.[56]

Disease progression to blast phase (AML) is probably driven by additional clonal evolution and acquired mutations (see section "Disease Course").

CLINICAL FEATURES

Splenomegaly is a well-established clinical feature of MF with 85% or more of MF patients presenting with palpable splenomegaly at the time of diagnosis. One-third of patients will have marked splenomegaly (*Figure 85.2A*), and 50% of patients will also have hepatomegaly.[57,58] Spleen-related symptoms include abdominal discomfort, early satiety, and pain under the left ribs. Portal hypertension and variceal bleeding can be morbid complications of splenomegaly. Some patients may experience severe pain secondary to splenic infarcts.[59]

Constitutional symptoms are common and often debilitating. Disease burden as a result of such symptoms often interferes with daily quality of life (QoL). These symptoms include fatigue, pruritus, night sweats, fever and bone/muscle pain, and cachexia. The presence of constitutional symptoms is associated with worse outcome.

Cytopenias can dominate the course of the disease especially at the advanced stages. Two-thirds of patients may have anemia at diagnosis, and 20% are transfusion dependent.[60,61] Thrombocytopenia may be present in 21% to 37% and leukopenia in 7% to 22%.[62]

Some patients present with leukocytosis (41%-49% incidence) and/or thrombocytosis (13%-31%). Furthermore, >10% of patients may present with extreme thrombocytosis (platelet count > 1000×10^9/L), whereas >20% present with marked leukocytosis (leukocyte count > 20×10^9/L).[59] Patients with MF are also at risk for developing thrombohemorrhagic complications secondary to leukocytosis and/or thrombocytosis.[63]

Other potential symptoms and complications include ascites, portal hypertension, lymphadenopathy, pleural effusions, and nerve or cord compression secondary to EMH.[64]

The characteristic laboratory findings in MF may include peripheral blood leukoerythroblastosis, dacryocytosis, teardrop-shaped red blood cells (RBCs), circulating immature myeloid cells, increased serum lactate dehydrogenase (LDH), increased vitamin B_{12} levels, and hyperuricemia. The characteristic bone marrow aspirate and biopsy findings may be limited by the inability to collect an adequate bone marrow aspirate (the so-called dry tap). The clustering of atypical megakaryocytes, which may often be mistaken as dysplasia by an inexperienced pathologist, is a pathologic hallmark of myeloproliferative neoplasms (see *Figure 85.2B*).[65] Reticulin staining demonstrates

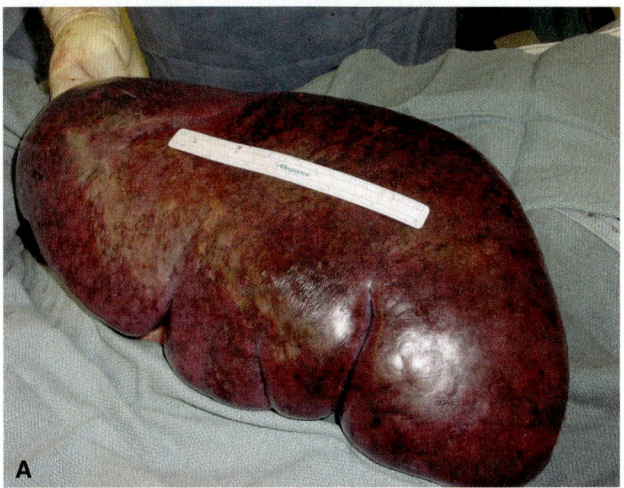

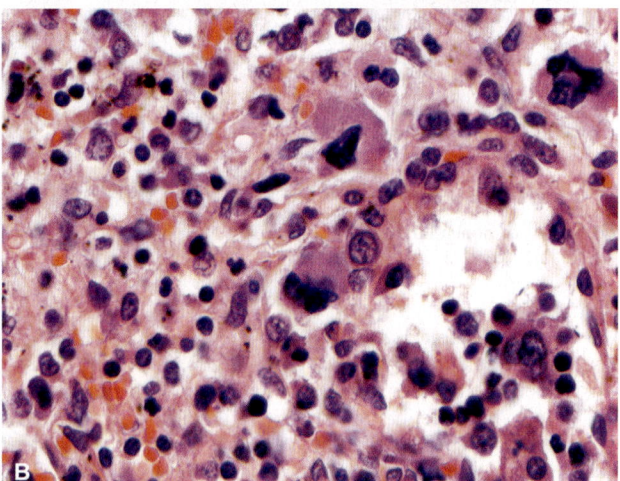

FIGURE 85.2 Splenomegaly due to extramedullary hematopoiesis in a patient with myelofibrosis. A, Massive splenomegaly. B, Chronic idiopathic myelofibrosis in the spleen. The red pulp shows extensive involvement by maturing myeloid and erythroid cells, as well as atypical megakaryocytes. Some of this abnormal extramedullary hematopoiesis is in a sinus at the lower right side of the figure.

an increased deposition of reticulin fibers. Collagen fibrosis can be appreciated and may be more disease specific compared to reticulin staining. In some early cases of MF, the bone marrow could only be hypercellular with no evidence of fibrosis.[7] *Figure 85.3* illustrates typical bone marrow findings in MF.

Circulating levels of CD34$^+$, hematopoietic stem cells, and progenitors are high in patients with MF compared with healthy patients as well as patients with other Philadelphia chromosome negative MPNs.[51]

DIAGNOSIS

The differential diagnosis of MF should include bone marrow fibrosis associated with nonneoplastic and neoplastic conditions (*Table 85.1*) including but not limited to CML, MDS, chronic myelomonocytic leukemia, lymphoma, or AML. The presence of *JAK2* or *MPL* mutation is a reliable screen to rule out reactive bone marrow fibrosis or a nonmyeloid malignancy. The diagnosis of PMF is facilitated using the WHO criteria, whereas post-PV or post-EF MF diagnosis is based on the IWG-MRT criteria (*Table 85.2*).[66,67]

PMF is typically characterized by the presence of morphologically bizarre megakaryocytes in clusters. However, it is important to note that the presence of apparent reticulin fibrosis is not essential for the diagnosis of PMF. Accordingly, there are two histologic variants of

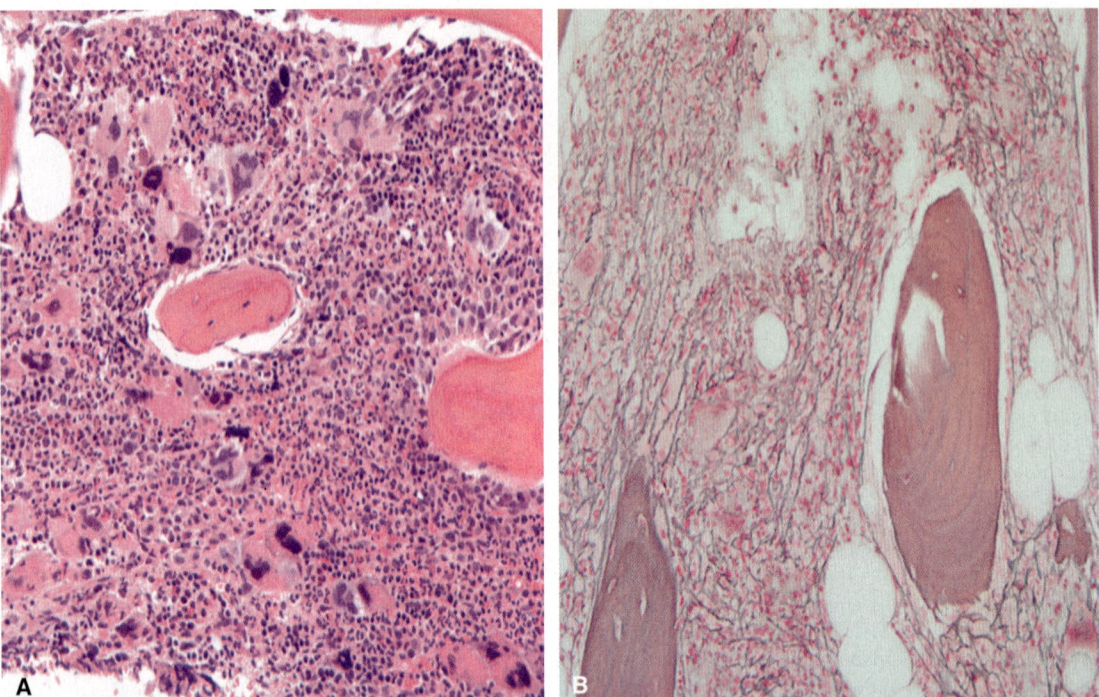

FIGURE 85.3 Bone marrow in myelofibrosis. A, Hypercellular bone marrow biopsy with megakaryocytic atypia. B, Reticulin stain demonstrating the presence of myelofibrosis.

PMF that have been included in the 2016 revision of the WHO classification of myeloid neoplasms: overt and prefibrotic.[66,68] Reticulin fibrosis is either absent or minimal in prefibrotic PMF, and it is thus possible to confuse prefibrotic PMF with ET. However, the bone marrow is markedly hypercellular, with both granulocytic and megakaryocytic proliferation in prefibrotic PMF, as opposed to a normocellular bone marrow with only megakaryocytic hyperplasia in ET. Further distinction is facilitated by the appreciation of subtle differences in megakaryocyte morphology; prefibrotic PMF megakaryocytes display defective maturation with prominent "cloudlike" hyperchromatic nuclei, whereas ET megakaryocytes appear mature although large in size, with well-lobulated (i.e., staghorn-like) nuclei.[69] Other distinguishing features between prefibrotic PMF and ET include the presence of myelophthisis and/or increased LDH in the former but not the latter. One distinct WHO category of AML (i.e., acute MF) can sometimes be confused with PMF. Patients with fibrotic AML, either AML M7 or other AML subtype, usually present with severe constitutional symptoms, pancytopenia, mild or no splenomegaly, and feature an increase in blood and bone marrow blasts that might not necessarily fulfill the required threshold for AML diagnosis.

DISEASE COURSE

MF is a progressive disease. Patients develop progressive splenomegaly and its related complications and suffer from debilitating disease burden symptoms such as cachexia, bone pain, and/or profound fatigue. Cytopenias can worsen during the course of the disease with more patients becoming RBC transfusion dependent and developing

Table 85.1. Differential Diagnosis for Bone Marrow Fibrosis

Hematologic Disorders		
Myeloid Disorders	**Lymphoid Disorders**	**Nonhematologic Disorders**
Primary myelofibrosis	Hairy cell leukemia	Metastatic cancer
Chronic myeloid leukemia	Hodgkin lymphoma	Autoimmune myelofibrosis
Myelodysplastic syndrome	Non-Hodgkin lymphoma	Systemic lupus erythematosus
Chronic myelomonocytic leukemia	Multiple myeloma	Kala-Azar (leishmaniasis)
Chronic eosinophilic leukemia		Tuberculosis
Systemic mastocytosis		Paget disease
Acute megakaryocytic leukemia		HIV infection
Other acute myeloid leukemias		Vitamin D–deficient rickets
Acute lymphocytic leukemia		Renal osteodystrophy
Acute myelofibrosis		Hyperparathyroidism
Malignant histiocytosis		Gray platelet syndrome
		Familial infantile myelofibrosis
		Idiopathic pulmonary hypertension

Table 85.2. WHO Criteria for Diagnosis of Primary and Post-ET/PV MF

WHO Criteria: Primary MF [Subdivided in 2016 Into Prefibrotic and Overt MF]	IWG Criteria: Post-ET MF and Post-PV MF
Major criteria (all required) • Megakaryocyte proliferation and atypia • Reticulin or collagen fibrosis [Present in overt MF; not present in prefibrotic MF] • Does not meet criteria for other myeloid disorders (e.g., PV, CML, MDS) • Driver mutation involving JAK2, MPL, CALR (or, in absence of these mutations, another clonal marker)	Major criteria (all required) • Previous diagnosis of ET or PV • Grade 2-3 bone marrow fibrosis (on 0-3 scale) or Grade 3-4 bone marrow fibrosis (on 0-4 scale)
Minor criteria (must have at least 1) • Increase in serum LDH • Palpable splenomegaly • Leukoerythroblastosis (not a minor criterion for prefibrotic MF) • Leukocytosis ≥ 11 × 10⁹/L • Anemia not attributed to a comorbid condition	Minor criteria (must meet 2) • ≥5 cm increase in palpable splenomegaly or new splenomegaly • Leukoerythroblastosis • One or more constitutional symptoms • Increase in serum LDH (post-ET MF only) • Anemia with Hgb ≥ 2 g/L decrease from baseline (post-ET MF only) • Anemia or sustained loss of requirement for either cytoreductive treatment or phlebotomy (post-PV MF only)

Abbreviations: CML, chronic myeloid leukemia; Hgb, hemoglobin; IWG, International Working Group; LDH, lactate dehydrogenase; MDS, myelodysplastic syndrome; Post-ET MF, post–essential thrombocythemia myelofibrosis; Post-PV MF, post–polycythemia vera myelofibrosis; WHO, World Health Organization.

thrombocytopenia and neutropenia. The rate of secondary AML transformation (or better termed blast phase MPN) is 10% to 15%. This is thought to occur due to the development of additional somatic mutations. Genes that have been linked to an increased risk of leukemic transformation include *IDH, RAS* (and *RAS*-pathway), *ASXL1, SRSF2, EZH2, TET2*, and *TP53*.[70-76] Blast phase MPN is very difficult to manage, and response to intensive chemotherapy is poor.[77] The major causes of death in PMF include infections (26%-29%), bleeding (11%-22%), heart failure (7%-15%), liver failure (3%-8%), and portal hypertension (6%).[78,79]

RISK STRATIFICATION AND PROGNOSIS

MF is a progressive hematologic disease, and its prognosis depends on several factors. The International Prognostic Scoring System (IPSS) estimates survival from the time of diagnosis using the following risk factors: (1) age 65 years or older; (2) anemia (hemoglobin < 100 g/L); (3) presence of constitutional symptoms; (4) leukocytosis (white blood cell count > 25 × 10⁹/L); and (5) circulating blasts of at least 1%.[80] Patients presenting with more than two of the aforementioned prognostic factors of MF have a median survival of less than 3 years, whereas patients without any of the factors have a median survival of more than 10 years. The presence of 0, 1, 2, and ≥3 factors using IPSS define low-, intermediate-1-, intermediate-2-, and high-risk disease, respectively.

Patient karyotype abnormality is also prognostic of survival. In a retrospective review of 200 MF patients, in comparison with trisomy 8 or a complex karyotype, patients with sole 13q deletion, 20q deletion, or trisomy 9 had an improved survival and no leukemia transformation.[81] In one study of 433 patients with PMF, a high-risk cytogenetic profile was when patients had a complex karyotype or sole or two abnormalities that included +8, −7/7q, i(17q), −5/5q−, 12p−, or 11q23 rearrangement, and a low-risk profile was when patients had normal karyotype, or sole abnormalities not present in the high-risk group, including +9, 13q−, 20q−, or chromosome 1 translocations/duplications.[82] The 5-year survival rates were 8% and 51%, respectively (Figure 85.4). In one study of 793 patients, 62 (8%) displayed an unfavorable karyotype by way of complex cytogenetics (n = 41) or sole trisomy 8 (n = 21).[83] The presence of monosomal karyotype in 41% of the patients with complex cytogenetics resulted in an extremely poor prognosis with a 2-year leukemic transformation rate of 29.4% and a median survival of only 6 months.

In an update to the IPSS, the Dynamic IPSS (DIPSS) was modified using the same prognostic factors from IPSS.[84] Unlike the IPSS, the DIPSS may be used at any time point in disease to estimate survival; contrary to IPSS, in DIPSS, the development of disease-related anemia carries two points. Most recently, the DIPSS was updated to the DIPSS-plus, which incorporates three more prognostic factors, including RBC transfusion dependence, platelet count < 100 × 10⁹/L, and unfavorable karyotype (Figure 85.5).[85] Table 85.3 summarizes risk stratification models in MF.

More recently, efforts have been made to incorporate somatic mutations into prognostic scoring systems. Studies have suggested that mutations involving *EZH2, SRSF2, ASXL1, IDH*, and *U2AF1* predict inferior outcomes.[71,86-88] Moreover, the number of these detrimental genes that are mutated was found to be prognostic as well.[72] Analysis of the recently discovered driving *CALR* mutation has suggested that its presence correlates with more favorable outcomes as compared to *JAK2*- and *MPL*-mutated cases of MF,[89,90] although this correlation may be limited to type 1 or type 1–like *CALR* mutations.[91] MF patients who lack a mutation in *JAK2, MPL*, and *CALR* (the so-called "triple-negative" patients) are thought to have an inferior prognosis. In a retrospective study of 617 patients, "triple-negative" patients were found to have a median overall survival (OS) of 3.2 years compared to median OS of 9.2, 9.1, and 17.7 years in *JAK2*-, *MPL*-, and *CALR*-mutated patients, respectively.[89] Based on this, two new scoring systems utilizing molecular data have been developed.[92,93] The first, mutation-enhanced IPSS developed for transplantation-age patients (MIPSS70), utilizes clinical and mutational data. Independent prognostic factors in this model include constitutional symptoms, hemoglobin < 100 g/L, leukocyte count > 25 × 10⁹/L, platelet count < 100 × 10⁹/L, circulating blasts ≥ 2%, fibrosis grade ≥ 2, absence of type 1 *CALR* mutation, presence of at least one high molecular risk (HMR) mutation among *ASXL1, EZH2, SRSF2, IDH1/2*, and ≥ 2 HMR mutated genes. This model created a three-tiered system. This model outperformed IPSS in predicting survival and was validated in an independent cohort of 211 patients.[92] Based upon this framework, subsequent models were developed to incorporate cytogenetic information (MIPSS70-plus), the prognostic significance of *U2AF1* Q157 mutations, and hemoglobin adjustments for sex and severity (MIPSS70-plus version 2.0).[94] An additional model eschewed clinical information in lieu of age and genomic data as its sole input in a genetically inspired prognostic scoring system (GIPSS). Cytogenetic risk groups were created with "very high" risk group defined as having single or multiple abnormalities of −7, i(17q), inv(3)/3q21, 12p−/12p11.2, 11q−/11q23, +21, or other autosomal trisomies not including +8/+9. Favorable-risk group was defined as normal karyotype or sole abnormalities of 13q−, +9, 20q−, chromosome 1 translocation/duplication, or sex chromosome abnormality including −Y. Unfavorable risk group was defined as all other abnormalities. In addition to cytogenetic risk groups, other parameters in the GIPSS model include absence of type 1 or type 1–like *CALR* mutation and presence of *ASXL1, SRSF2*, or *U2AF1* Q157 mutations. On the basis of the previous parameters, four risk groups were defined and validated by independent application to the two large cohorts that informed the model as well as to transplant-age patients.[93]

Notably, the vast majority of prognostic models have been developed in patients with PMF. They have been applied to patients with secondary MF occurring after a prior diagnosis of PV or ET, despite the fact that they are suboptimal to

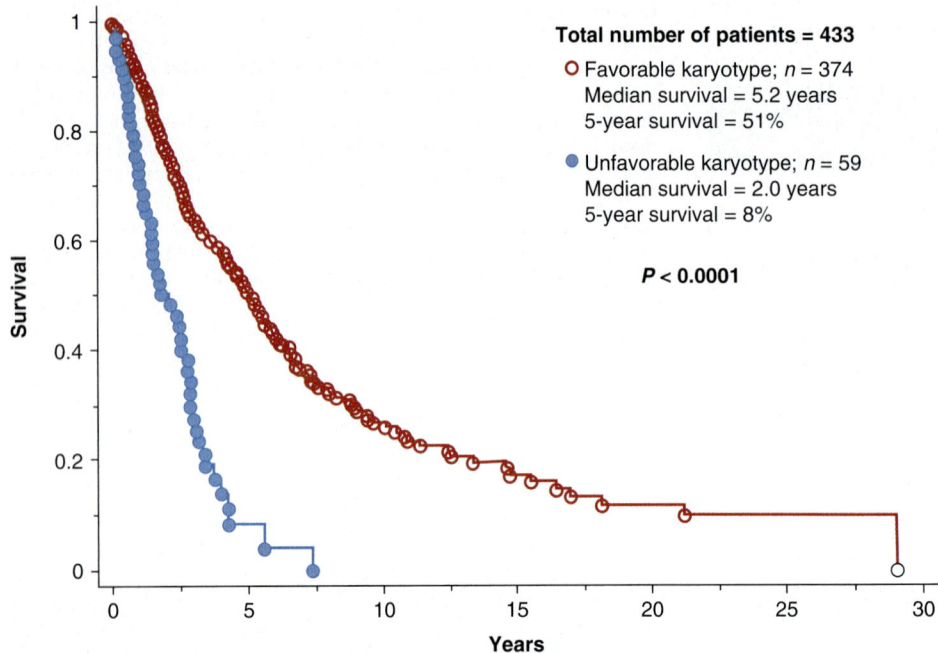

FIGURE 85.4 Survival data of patients with primary myelofibrosis stratified by two-tiered cytogenetic risk categorization: unfavorable (complex karyotype or sole or two abnormalities that include +8, −7/7q−, i[17q], inv[3], −5/5q−, 12p−, or 11q23 rearrangement) and favorable (all others including normal karyotype). (Reprinted by permission from Nature: Caramazza D, Begna KH, Gangat N, et al. Refined cytogenetic-risk categorization for overall and leukemia-free survival in primary myelofibrosis: a single center study of 433 patients. *Leukemia.* 2011;25(1):82-88. Copyright © 2010 Springer Nature.)

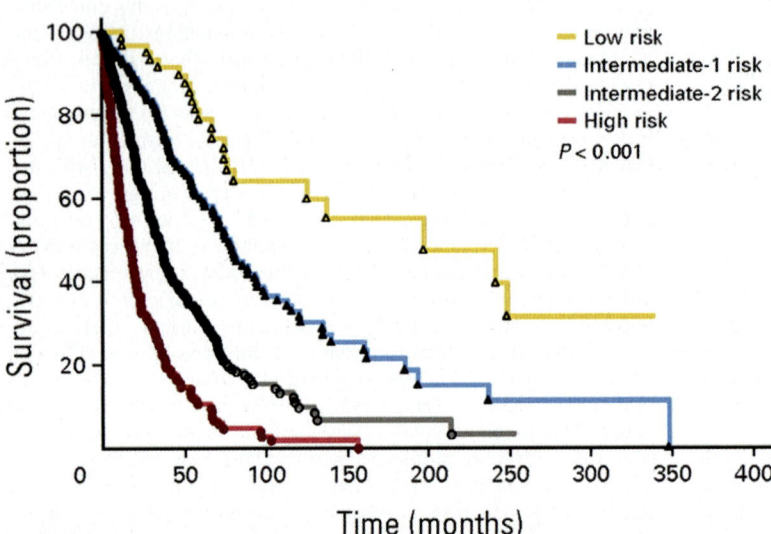

FIGURE 85.5 Survival data of 793 patients with primary myelofibrosis evaluated at time of their first Mayo Clinic referral and stratified by their Dynamic International Prognostic Scoring System (DIPSS) + karyotype + platelet count + transfusion status prognostic scores. Low risk, zero adverse points; $n = 66$; median survival, 185 months. Intermediate-1 risk, one adverse point; $n = 174$; median survival, 78 months. Intermediate-2 risk, two or three adverse points, $n = 360$; median survival, 35 months. High risk, four to six adverse points; $n = 193$; median survival, 16 months. (Reprinted with permission from Gangat N, Caramazza D, Vaidya R, et al. DIPSS plus: a refined dynamic international prognostic scoring system for primary myelofibrosis that incorporates prognostic information from karyotype, platelet count, and transfusion status. *J Clin Oncol.* 2011;29:392-397. Copyright © 2011 American Society of Clinical Oncology.)

predict survival in this group of patients.[95,96] To address this, a prognostic model was designed specifically for patients with MF occurring after a diagnosis of PV or ET. The Myelofibrosis Secondary to PV and ET-Prognostic Model (MYSEC-PM) incorporates age, hemoglobin < 110 g/L, platelet count < 150 × 10^9/L, circulating blasts ≥ 3%, *CALR*-unmutated genotype, and constitutional symptoms to stratify four risk groups with median survivals not reached in low-risk, 9.3 years in intermediate-1 risk, 4.5 years in intermediate-2 risk, and 2.0 years in high-risk patients. The MYSEC-PM outperformed the IPSS, even after incorporating *CALR* mutation status as a covariate.[97] This model has subsequently been validated in an independent patient cohort.[98] The ability to prognosticate and stratify severity of disease is critical in effectively counseling patients regarding expected outcome and define the most appropriate treatment strategies. Risk stratification allows the clinician to identify high-risk patients who may benefit from intensive therapy such as allogeneic stem cell transplant where benefit outweighs the risk. Lower risk MF patients or MF patients who are not transplant candidates are managed based on the presence of constitutional symptoms, symptomatic splenomegaly, or severe cytopenias.

Response Criteria and Assessment Tools

The IWG-MRT developed criteria for response to therapy in MF, modeled after other criteria, such as the IWG criteria for MDS.[99] Treatment responses are categorized as complete remission (CR), partial remission (PR), or clinical improvement. Revised response criteria by the IWG and European Leukemia Net have been proposed (*Table 85.4*).[99,100] The criteria for "clinical improvement" incorporate reduction in spleen size and improvements in anemia, platelet count, and neutrophil count. The CR and PR as surrogate markers of survival have not been validated, and it would be difficult to achieve CR or PR with currently available therapy apart from allogeneic hematopoietic cell transplantation (alloHCT).

Some clinical trials define spleen response as a ≥50% reduction in splenic size (length) as assessed by palpation (consistent with IWG-MRT criteria) or ≥35% reduction when assessed by imaging

Table 85.3. Risk Stratification Models in Myelofibrosis

Risk Factor	IPSS	DIPSS	DIPSS-Plus
Age > 65	X	X	X
Constitutional symptoms	X	X	X
Anemia (Hgb < 100 g/L)	X	X	X
WBC > 25 × 10^9/L	X	X	X
Circulating myeloblasts ≥ 1%	X	X	X
RBC transfusion dependence (TD)			X
Unfavorable karyotype, complex karyotype, or sole or 2 abnormalities that include +8, −7/7q−, i(17q), inv(3), −5/5q−, 12p−, or 11q23 rearrangement			X
Platelets < 100 × 10^9/L			X
Points	1 each	1 each except anemia = 2	1 for TD, unfavorable karyotype, and thrombocytopenia. 1, 2, 3 points assigned for DIPSS int-1, int-2, and high-risk status, respectively
Risk groups (sum points)	0 = Low 1 = Int-1 2 = Int-2 ≥3 = High risk	0 = Low 1-2 = Int-1 3-4 = Int-2 5-6 = High risk	0 = Low 1 = Int-1 2-3 = Int-2 ≥4 = High risk
Median overall survival	Low: 11.3 y Int-1: 7.9 y Int-2: 4 y High 2.3 y	Low: NR Int-1 14.2 y Int-2: 4 y High 1.5 y	Low: 15.4 Int-1 6.5 y Int-2: 2.9 y High 1.3 y

Abbreviations: X denotes variable included in prognostic model DIPSS, Dynamic IPSS; Int-1/2, intermediate-1/2; IPSS, International Prognostic Scoring System; NR, not reached.

(corresponding to an approximate ≥50% reduction in palpable spleen length, as shown in the phase I/II trial of ruxolitinib).[42] Evaluating changes in spleen size by palpation, however, may not be as objective as evaluating changes in spleen size by magnetic resonance imaging (MRI). In a phase II study evaluating the JAK inhibitor pacritinib (formerly known as SB1518), a 50% reduction in spleen size as assessed by palpation correlated with a 25% reduction in spleen size as assessed by MRI.[101] Thus, the use of objective measurements such as MRI or computed tomography (CT) to evaluate changes in spleen size may be more useful in evaluating response to therapy, especially in clinical trials. In practice, physical examination or ultrasound remain the most common tools utilized for spleen size assessment.

The Myelofibrosis Symptom Assessment Form (MFSAF) is a tool specifically developed to evaluate the presence and severity of MF-associated symptoms.[102] In a recent version of the MFSAF (v4.0), patients rate the presence and severity of splenomegaly-related symptoms (abdominal discomfort, pain under the ribs on left side, and early satiety), systemic symptoms (night sweats, pruritus, and bone pain), and fatigue using a scale of 0 (symptom not present) to 10 (symptom present and worst imaginable).[103]

Fatigue is a problematic symptom and is pervasive, persistently severe, and almost universally present in MF patients.[104] Moreover, it interferes with activities of daily living and QoL. Tools to evaluate fatigue include the Functional Assessment of Cancer Therapy Fatigue (FACT) Scale, the Brief Fatigue Inventory, the Cancer Linear Analog Scale, and the Patient Reported Outcomes Measurement Information System Fatigue Scale.[105,106] The FACT-Lym, which was developed for the assessment of symptoms in lymphoma patients, includes an evaluation of constitutional (or "B") symptoms, such as pruritus, bone/muscle pain, and fatigue.[107]

MANAGEMENT

The first step in disease management is risk stratification. For patients with intermediate-2-risk or high-risk disease, allogeneic stem cell transplant should be considered. If patients are nontransplant candidates or have lower risk disease, treatment is only for symptomatic patients (with constitutional and/or spleen-related symptoms) and those with severe cytopenias. The selection of treatment is based on the particular patient's characteristics. *Figure 85.6* summarizes a suggested algorithm for the management of PMF.

Treatment of Anemia

Treatment of anemia and resultant RBC transfusion dependency remain an unmet challenge for the management of PMF. Options for treatment include erythroid-stimulating agents (ESAs), steroids, androgens, or immunomodulatory drugs (IMiDs) that include thalidomide and lenalidomide. Novel single-agent and combination strategies to treat MF-related anemia are actively being investigated and include the erythroid maturation agent, luspatercept, which is approved for select patients with beta thalassemia and MDS with ring sideroblasts; momelotinib, a JAK1/JAK2/ACVR1 inhibitor; and pelabrasib (CPI-0610), a potent and selective bromodomain inhibitor.[108-110]

Subcutaneous erythropoietin (Epo) injections (40,000 U weekly) are safe and most suitable for patients with an endogenous serum Epo level <125 U/L. Response rate in such patients is estimated at 50% and might be even higher in transfusion-independent patients.[111] The median duration of response is only 1 year, and some patients experience further enlargement of their spleen during treatment with ESA.

Corticosteroid therapy (variable doses of prednisone, between 0.5 and 1.0 mg/kg/d) has been used in the past, with response rates that were higher in female patients (52%) compared to male patients (29%).[112] Similar response rates (i.e., 30%-40%) have also been observed with several androgen preparations, including testosterone enanthate (400-600 mg intramuscularly, weekly) and oral fluoxymesterone (10 mg per three times a day).[112] The addition of corticosteroids appears to increase the response rate observed with androgens, whereas the presence of a cytogenetic abnormality predicts a lower response rate.[113] Danazol produces a transient (average 5 months) response rate in PMF that is similar to that seen with other androgen preparations (i.e., ~30%-40% at a dose of 600 mg/d).[114]

Thalidomide and lenalidomide have each demonstrated a ~20% response rate.[115,116] Thalidomide is used at low doses (50 mg/d) and in combination with corticosteroids (prednisone, 15-30 mg/d for 3 months only),[117] and lenalidomide is clearly active in the presence of del(5)(q31).[116,118] A phase II clinical study using lenalidomide 10 mg

Table 85.4. Revised International Working Group for Myeloproliferative Neoplasms Research and Treatment and European Leukemia Net Response Criteria for Myelofibrosis

Response Categories	Required Criteria (for All Response Categories, Benefit Must Last for ≥12 wk in Order to Qualify as a Response)
Complete remission (CR)	*Bone marrow*[a]: Age-adjusted normocellularity; <5% blasts; ≤grade 1 myelofibrosis,[b] and *Peripheral blood:* Hemoglobin ≥ 100 g/L and <UNL; neutrophil count ≤ 1 × 10⁹/L and <UNL. Platelet count ≥ 100 × 10⁹/L and <UNL; <2% immature myeloid cells,[c] and *Clinical:* Resolution of disease symptoms; spleen and liver not palpable; no evidence of EMH.
Partial remission (PR)	*Peripheral blood:* Hemoglobin ≥ 100 g/L and <UNL; neutrophil count ≥ 1 × 10⁹/L and <UNL. Platelet count ≥ 100 × 10⁹/L and <UNL; <2% immature myeloid cells,[c] and *Clinical:* Resolution of disease symptoms; spleen and liver not palpable; No evidence of EMH, or *Bone marrow*[a]: Age-adjusted normocellularity; <5% blasts; = Grade 1 myelofibrosis,[b] and *Peripheral blood:* Hemoglobin ≥ 85 but < 100 g/L and <UNL; neutrophil count ≥1 × 10⁹/L and <UNL; Platelet count ≥ 50 but <100 × 10⁹/L and <UNL; <2% immature myeloid cells,[c] and *Clinical: Resolution of disease symptoms; the spleen and liver not palpable; no evidence of EMH.*
Clinical improvement (CI)	The achievement of anemia, spleen, or symptoms response without progressive disease or deterioration in anemia.[d]
Anemia response	*Transfusion-independent patients:* a ≥20 g/L increase in hemoglobin level.[e] *Transfusion-dependent patients:* becoming transfusion independent.[f]
Spleen response[g]	A baseline splenomegaly i.e. palpable at 5-10 cm, below the LCM, becomes not palpable,[h] or a baseline splenomegaly i.e. palpable at >10 cm, below the LCM, decreases by ≥50%[h] A baseline splenomegaly i.e. *palpable at <5 cm, below the LCM, is not eligible for spleen response.* A spleen response requires confirmation by MRI or CT showing ≥35% spleen volume reduction.
Symptoms response	A ≥50% reduction in the Myeloproliferative Neoplasm Symptom Assessment Form total symptom score (MPN-SAF TSS).[i]
Progressive disease[j]	Appearance of a new splenomegaly i.e. palpable at least 5 cm below the LCM, or A ≥100% increase in palpable distance, below LCM, for baseline splenomegaly of 5-10 cm, or a 50% increase in palpable distance, below LCM, for baseline splenomegaly of >10 cm, or leukemic transformation confirmed by a bone marrow blast count of ≥20%, or a peripheral blood blast count of ≥20% that lasts for at least 2 wk.
Stable disease	Belonging to none of the above-listed response categories.
Relapse	No longer meeting criteria for at least CI after achieving CR, PR, or CI, or loss of anemia response persisting for at least 1 mo, or loss of spleen response persisting for at least 1 mo
Guidelines for Assessing Treatment-induced Cytogenetic and Molecular Changes	
Cytogenetic remission	At least 10 metaphases must be analyzed for cytogenetic response evaluation, and requires confirmation by repeat testing within 6 mo window. *Complete response:* eradication of a preexisting abnormality. *Partial response:* ≥50% reduction in abnormal metaphases. (Partial response applies only to patients with at least 10 abnormal metaphases at baseline).
Molecular remission	Molecular response evaluation must be analyzed in peripheral blood granulocytes, and requires confirmation by repeat testing within 6 mo window. *Complete response:* eradication of a preexisting abnormality. *Partial response:* ≥50% decrease in allele burden. (Partial response applies only to patients with at least 20% mutant allele burden at baseline.)
Cytogenetic/molecular relapse	Reemergence of a preexisting cytogenetic or molecular abnormality i.e. confirmed by repeat testing.

Abbreviations: CT, computed tomography; EMH, extramedullary hematopoiesis (no evidence of EMH implies the absence of pathology, or imaging study-proven nonhepatosplenic EMH); LCM, left costal margin; MRI, magnetic resonance imaging; UNL, upper normal limit.
Modified from Tefferi A, Cervantes F, Mesa R, et al. Revised response criteria for myelofibrosis: International Working Group-Myeloproliferative Neoplasms Research and Treatment (IWG-MRT) & European LeukemiaNet (ELN) consensus report. *Blood.* 2013;122(8):1395-1398. Copyright © 2013 American Society of Hematology. With permission.
[a]Baseline and post–treatment bone marrow slides are to be stained at the same time and interpreted at one sitting by a central review process. Cytogenetic and molecular responses are not required for CR assignment.
[b]Grading of myelofibrosis is according to the European classification. (Thiele K, Kvasnicka HM, Facchetti F, Franco V, van der Walt J, Orazi A. European consensus on grading bone marrow fibrosis and assessment of cellularity. *Haematologica.* 2005;90:1128.)
[c]Immature myeloid cells constitute blasts + promyelocytes + myelocytes + metamyelocytes + nucleated red blood cells. In splenectomized patients, <5% immature myeloid cells is allowed.
[d]See *Table 85.4* for definitions of anemia response, spleen response, and progressive disease. Deterioration in anemia constitutes the occurrence of new transfusion dependency or a ≥20 g/L decrease in hemoglobin level from pretreatment baseline that lasts for at least 12 weeks.
[e]Applicable only to patients with baseline hemoglobin <100 g/L. In patients not meeting the strict criteria for transfusion dependency at the time of study enrollment (see below), but have received transfusions within the previous month, the pretransfusion hemoglobin level should be used as the baseline.
[f]Transfusion dependency before study enrollment is defined as transfusions of at least 6 U of packed red blood cells (PRBCs), in the 12 weeks prior to study enrollment, for a hemoglobin level of ≥85 g/L, in the absence of bleeding or treatment-induced anemia. In addition, the most recent transfusion episode must have occurred in the 28 days prior to study enrollment. Response in transfusion-dependent patients requires absence of any PRBC transfusions during any consecutive "rolling" 12-week interval during the treatment phase, capped by a hemoglobin level of ≥85 g/L.
[g]In splenectomized patients, palpable hepatomegaly is substituted with the same measurement strategy.
[h]Spleen or liver responses must be confirmed by imaging studies where a ≥35% reduction in spleen volume, as assessed by MRI or CT, is required. Furthermore, a ≥35% volume reduction in the spleen or liver, by MRI or CT, constitutes a response regardless of what is reported with physical examination.
[i]Symptoms are evaluated by the MPN-SAF TSS.[102] The MPN-SAF TSS is assessed by the patients themselves and includes fatigue, concentration, early satiety, inactivity, night sweats, itching, bone pain, abdominal discomfort, weight loss, and fevers. Scoring is from 0 (absent/as good as it can be) to 10 (worst imaginable/as bad as it can be) for each item. The MPN-SAF TSS is the sum of all the individual scores (0-100 scale). Symptoms response requires ≥50% reduction in the MPN-SAF TSS.
[j]Progressive disease assignment for splenomegaly requires confirmation by MRI or CT showing a ≥25% increase in spleen volume from baseline. Baseline values for both physical examination and imaging studies refer to pretreatment baseline and not to posttreatment measurements.

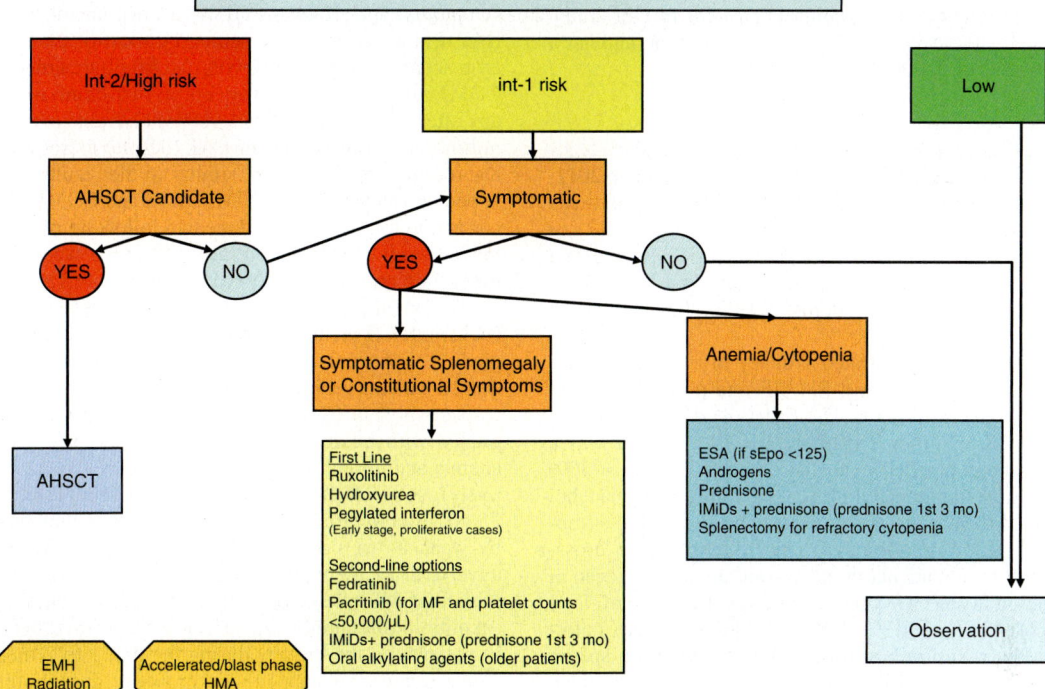

FIGURE 85.6 Suggested algorithm for management of myelofibrosis (MF). AHSCT, allogeneic hematopoietic stem cell transplantation; DIPSS, Dynamic IPSS; ESA, erythroid-stimulating agents; IMiDs, immunomodulatory drugs (lenalidomide or thalidomide); Int, intermediate; IPSS, International Prognostic Scoring System; sEpo, endogenous serum erythropoietin level.

(orally) PO daily for 21 days every 28 days (dose adjusted based on platelet count) combined with prednisone for 3 months (30 mg daily first month, 15 mg daily second month, and 15 mg every other day third month) reported a 30% hemoglobin response but not if patients had baseline thrombocytopenia or neutropenia.[119] Pomalidomide was also studied for anemia treatment in PMF.[120] In phase I/II studies, 0.5 mg was the recommended dose, and durable hemoglobin responses were reported in 25% of patients. A phase III placebo-controlled study failed to show benefit for pomalidomide in treating anemia in PMF. Outside the context of a clinical trial, we use lenalidomide in patients without baseline of thrombocytopenia/neutropenia and thalidomide if those are present.

Luspatercept is an activin receptor ligand trap that prevents the interaction between TGF-β superfamily ligands and the activin receptor. TGF-β signaling inhibits terminal erythroid differentiation through activation of Smad signaling and has also been implicated in the pathogenesis of bone marrow fibrosis.[108] This suggests that luspatercept, as well as other agents targeting TGF-β, may have particular efficacy in anemic patients with MF. The phase III, placebo-controlled INDEPENDENCE study (NCT04717414) is assessing the efficacy of luspatercept in patients with MF who are being treated with a JAK2 inhibitor and require RBC transfusions. Additionally, a substudy of the FREEDOM trial (NCT03755518) is assessing the safety and efficacy of luspatercept in combination with fedratinib in anemic MF patients who have been previously treated with ruxolitinib.

Treatment of Splenomegaly and/or Constitutional Symptoms

Splenomegaly-related symptoms and constitutional symptoms remain the most common indications for treatment. JAK2 inhibitors are particularly effective in managing these symptoms with ruxolitinib, fedratinib, and pacritinib being approved by the FDA as of March 2022.

Non-JAK2 inhibitor options for splenomegaly and/or constitutional symptoms include hydroxyurea, alkylating agents, purine analogs, interferon, IMiDs, azanucleosides, splenectomy, and splenic radiation. These options have been rendered largely obsolete after the emergence of JAK2 inhibitors and are currently utilized in the salvage setting. Azanucleosides have largely been relegated to use in accelerated and blast phases of MF; however, the combination of azacitidine and ruxolitinib has been associated with impressive spleen response rates in the chronic phase as well.[121]

Conventional Drug Therapy

Historically, hydroxyurea was considered the first-line therapy for decreasing splenomegaly, and the estimated patient response rate is less than 50%.[57] Limitations with hydroxyurea include lack of sustained improvements, rarity in inducing complete regression of the enlarged spleen, the requirement for high doses to induce a response, and the potential for cytopenias.[57] Other agents that may alleviate splenomegaly, but have their own risks, include oral alkylating agents such as melphalan (2.5 mg three times a week),[122] busulfan (2-6 mg/d with close monitoring of blood counts),[123] and intravenous cladribine (5 mg/m²/d in a 2-hour infusion for 5 consecutive days, repeated for 4-6 monthly cycles).[124]

Splenomegaly reduction was reported in 33% of patients with low-dose thalidomide combined with a prednisone taper.[117] Lenalidomide produced similar results in a separate study and was better tolerated in patients with adequate baseline neutrophils and platelets.[119]

Interferon

For the treatment of PMF, interferon-α has been evaluated; however, many clinical studies in PMF have been disappointing[125-127]; results of a prospective study of 17 low- and intermediate-1-risk patients treated with interferon-α reported that >80% of patients had either response or stable disease (2 patients with CR and 7 with PR).[128] Interferon-α may be considered in young, lower risk patients and is the treatment of choice in women of childbearing age contemplating pregnancy. Pegylated interferon may be an appealing choice for further study, inasmuch as it is given less frequently (usually once a week) and has a better toxicity profile than standard interferon.[129,130]

JAK 2 Inhibitors

There are several JAK2 inhibitors that were tested in clinical trials for the management of MF (Table 85.5).[101,131-136] In November 2011, ruxolitinib was approved by the FDA for the treatment of patients with intermediate-risk (both intermediate-1 and intermediate-2) or high-risk MF, including PMF, post-PV MF, and post-ET MF, marking the first MF disease-specific drug approval and the first in its class. Fedratinib received FDA approval in August 2019 for the treatment of intermediate-2 or high-risk MF.

Ruxolitinib treatment demonstrated efficacy in two large phase III studies in patients with PMF, post-PV MF, and post-ET MF and intermediate-2- or high-risk disease. The COntrolled MyeloFibrosis study with ORal JAK inhibitor Treatment I (COMFORT-I) was a double-blind, placebo-controlled phase III clinical study (n = 309) in which patients were randomized (1:1) to ruxolitinib or placebo. Patients randomized to placebo and experiencing worsening symptoms and splenomegaly were allowed to receive ruxolitinib ("crossover"). Significantly more patients in the ruxolitinib arm achieved at least a 35% reduction in spleen volume, as assessed by MRI or CT, vs placebo at week 24 (41.9% vs 0.7%, $P < .001$). Indeed, a great majority of patients in the ruxolitinib arm had some reduction in spleen volume.[131] Improvements in MF-associated symptoms were also achieved with ruxolitinib therapy. Symptom burden was assessed with the modified MFSAF v2.0 where 45.9% of patients in the ruxolitinib arm achieved a 50% or greater improvement in total symptom score by week 24 vs 5.3% in the placebo group ($P < .001$). Moreover, patients also experienced improvements in fatigue and QoL. At the 5-year data cutoff, 27.7% originally randomized to ruxolitinib remained on treatment.[137] Note that, despite a crossover study design (about three-quarters of placebo-treated patients received ruxolitinib upon disease worsening) in the intent-to-treat analysis, those patients randomized to ruxolitinib had improved survival over those initially randomized to placebo.[138]

In a separate open-label, randomized phase III study (COMFORT-II; $n < 219$), patients were randomized (2:1) to ruxolitinib or best available therapy (BAT). This study also allowed a crossover of patients from BAT to ruxolitinib for disease worsening.[132] Significantly more patients in the ruxolitinib arm (28%) achieved at least a 35% reduction in spleen volume versus BAT (0%) ($P < .001$) at week 48. Although most patients in the ruxolitinib arm had a reduction in spleen size, the majority of patients in the BAT arm had worsening splenomegaly. Patients in the ruxolitinib arm experienced improvements in global health status and functioning, as well as individual MF-related symptoms captured by the QLQ-C30 instrument, whereas those in the BAT arm experienced worsening by most of these measures. FACT-Lym scores also improved with ruxolitinib treatment. Similarly to the COMFORT-I study, most patients on ruxolitinib were still on the therapy after 2-year follow-up. A survival advantage of therapy with ruxolitinib versus therapy with BAT (despite a crossover to ruxolitinib) has recently been reported, similar to the results of COMFORT-I.[139] A pooled analysis of the COMFORT-I and COMFORT-II studies with correction for crossover and median follow-up of 3 years showed prolonged survival with ruxolitinib with OS at week 144 of 78% in the ruxolitinib arm compared to 61% in the control arm.[140]

The most common adverse drug effects in COMFORT-I and COMFORT-II included thrombocytopenia and anemia. The rates of grade 3 or 4 anemia and thrombocytopenia were greater in ruxolitinib-treated patients versus placebo (45.2% and 12.9% vs 19.2% and 1.3%, respectively) in COMFORT-I. Similarly, in COMFORT-II, patients treated with ruxolitinib versus BAT experienced more grade 3 or 4 anemia and thrombocytopenia (42% and 8% vs 31% and 7%, respectively). In COMFORT-I, the mean hemoglobin level reached a nadir of 95 g/L after approximately 8 to 12 weeks of therapy with an increase by week 24 to a new steady state of 101 g/dL. Non–hematologic adverse drug effects included ecchymosis, dizziness, and headache. Note that MF-related symptoms typically returned after 1 week of ruxolitinib discontinuation, strongly suggesting that close monitoring of patients on the therapy during the first 1 to 2 months (when most of the side effects happen) and proactive dose modification are very important, in order to deliver therapy in the best possible way and avoid unnecessary interruptions.

The starting dose of ruxolitinib depends on the baseline platelet count. For patients with a platelet count greater than 200×10^9/L, a dose of 20 mg twice daily is indicated, and 15 mg twice daily is indicated in patients with a platelet count between 100×10^9/L and 200×10^9/L. There are no contraindications to the use of ruxolitinib; however, experience with its use in patients with platelet count lower than 100×10^9/L is limited. It is prudent to use ruxolitinib in such patients at a reduced dose. A dose-finding study of ruxolitinib in thrombocytopenic MF patients demonstrated 10 mg twice daily dosing to be the maximum safe starting dose in patients with platelet count between 50×10^9/L and 100×10^9/L, though close monitoring is required as dose interruptions and modifications are frequently required in this group.[141] If thrombocytopenia develops during the course of treatment, the dosage should be reduced. The dosage may be increased to a maximum of 25 mg twice daily depending on patient response. If no reductions in splenomegaly or symptoms are observed

Table 85.5. Approved JAK Inhibitors and Those in Late-Stage development

JAK Inhibitor	Study/Status	Targets	Efficacy	Major Adverse Events
Ruxolitinib	Phase III Approved	JAK1/JAK2	Spleen response 42% >50% reduction in symptoms in 46%	Anemia Thrombocytopenia
Fedratinib	Phase III Approved	JAK2/FLT3	Spleen response 36% >50% reduction in symptoms in 36%	Anemia Thrombocytopenia Diarrhea Nausea Black box warning for encephalopathy
Pacritinib	Phase III Approved	JAK2/IRAK1/FLT3	Spleen response 19% >50% reduction in symptoms in 19%	Diarrhea Nausea
Momelotinib	Phase III Ongoing	JAK1/JAK2/ACVR1	Spleen response 27% >50% reduction in symptoms in 28% Lower rates of transfusion dependence	Diarrhea Nausea Neuropathy

Van Egeren D, Escabi J, Nguyen M, et al. Reconstructing the lineage histories and differentiation trajectories of individual cancer cells in myeloproliferative neoplasms. *Cell Stem Cell.* 2021;28(3):514-523 e9.

after 6 months, therapy should be discontinued. Ruxolitinib is nonspecific for *JAK2* V617F mutation; therefore, it may be useful in all patients with MF.

Fedratinib is an oral, JAK2/FLT3 inhibitor that demonstrated efficacy in JAK inhibitor–naïve MF patients in comparison to placebo and in MF patients previously treated with ruxolitinib. In a phase 3 trial (JAKARTA), patients were randomized to fedratinib 400 mg once daily, fedratinib 500 mg once daily, or placebo. Thirty-six percent of patients treated with fedratinib 400 mg daily achieved the primary end point of ≥35% reduction in spleen volume (with confirmatory imaging 4 weeks later) compared to 1% of patients in the placebo group. Similarly, a ≥50% reduction in total symptom score at week 24 was demonstrated in 36% of patients treated with fedratinib 400 mg daily compared to 7% in the placebo group.[142] Due to concerns with neurologic toxicity, specifically 7 suspected cases of Wernicke encephalopathy among 877 fedratinib-treated patients across 8 clinical trials, a clinical hold was placed on fedratinib in November 2013.

The clinical hold impaired long-term follow-up of the phase 3 JAKARTA study as well as primary analysis of the phase 2 JAKARTA2 study, a single-arm phase 2 study of fedratinib in patients previously treated with ruxolitinib. In this study, MF patients deemed to be resistant or intolerant to ruxolitinib were treated with fedratinib (400 mg daily) with a primary endpoint of ≥35% reduction in spleen volume at week 24. The trial enrolled 97 patients with the clinical hold occurring 2.5 months after completing accrual. Still, among 83 evaluable patients, 46 (55%) achieved a spleen response.[143] An updated analysis of JAKARTA2 using stringent criteria for ruxolitinib failure and intention-to-treat analysis principles demonstrated a revised spleen response rate of 31% in the intention-to-treat population and 30% in the stringent criteria cohort.[144]

Gastrointestinal adverse events commonly occur with fedratinib treatment with diarrhea, vomiting, and nausea of any grade occurring in 66%, 42%, and 64% of patients treated with fedratinib 400 mg daily in the phase 3 JAKARTA study compared to 16%, 5%, and 15% of patients treated with placebo. Grade ≥ 3 gastrointestinal events were rare; however, the frequency of events has led to recommendations for prophylactic antiemetics, coadministration with a high-fat meal, and as needed antidiarrheal medications. Grade ≥ 3 anemia and thrombocytopenia were also common, occurring in 43% and 17% of patients treated with fedratinib 400 mg daily in the JAKARTA study compared to 25% and 9%, respectively.[142]

Pacritinib, an oral JAK2/IRAK1/FLT3 inhibitor, has completed advanced phase trials in MF. In a phase II trial, treatment with pacritinib led to reduction in spleen volume of ≥35% in 31% of patients as determined by MRI and a ≥50% reduction in spleen size when measured by physical examination in 42% of patients. Critically, this response was seen without concomitant cytopenias that are commonly seen with ruxolitinib. The most common side effects were grade 1 or 2 diarrhea and nausea, which were seen in 69% and 49% of patients, respectively.[145] A phase III trial (PERSIST-I) comparing pacritinib to BAT demonstrated spleen volume reduction ≥35% at week 24 in 19% of pacritinib-treated patients as compared to 5% for BAT (*P* = .0003) in an intention-to-treat analysis. In patients with baseline platelet counts <100,000/μL and <50,000 μL, spleen responses were seen in 17% and 23% of patients treated with pacritinib, respectively, whereas no spleen responses were seen in cytopenic patients in the BAT arm. Moreover, 25% of RBC transfusion-dependent patients in the pacritinib arm achieved transfusion independency compared to 0% of BAT patients.[146] In February 2016, pacritinib was placed on a full clinical hold because of concerns around death and cardiac/hemorrhagic events seen in PERSIST-1. Another phase III trial (PERSIST-2) compared two different dosing schedules of pacritinib (200 mg PO twice a day and 400 mg daily) to BAT, including ruxolitinib, in MF patients with platelet counts <100,000/μL. At 24 weeks, ≥35% reduction in spleen volume was seen in 18% of pacritinib-treated patients (at either dose) versus 3% of BAT. Improvement in constitutional symptoms (≥50% reduction in total symptom score) was seen in 25% of pacritinib-treated patients as compared to 14% of BAT patients—a difference that did not reach statistical significance (*P* = .08). When the cohort of patients who received pacritinib on a twice-daily schedule was compared to BAT, significant improvement in spleen and symptom response was seen. Decreased RBC transfusion needs were seen in approximately 20% of patients in the pacritinib arms compared to 8% in the BAT arm. Grades 3 and 4 adverse events were comparable in this study across the three arms.[147] The FDA lifted the clinical hold on pacritinib in January 2017. In response to safety and dosing concerns, a dose-finding study (PAC203) of pacritinib was initiated that randomized MF patients who were intolerant of or resistant to ruxolitinib to pacritinib 100 mg daily, 100 mg twice per day, or 200 mg twice per day. Patients with a baseline platelet count <50 000/μL comprised 44% of the study population. Spleen responses were highest in the 200 mg twice per day group with symptom response rates being comparable across different dose levels. With the utilization of enhanced monitoring, eligibility criteria, and dose modifications, excess hemorrhagic or cardiac events did not occur at the 200 mg twice per day dose level.[148] On June 1, 2021, the FDA granted priority review to a new drug application for pacritinib, and on February 28, 2022, approved it as a treatment for patients with MF and platelet count <50,000/μL.

Splenectomy is associated with significant morbidity and mortality. The perioperative mortality of splenectomy in PMF is between 5% and 10%, and postsplenectomy complications occur in ~50% of patients: surgical-site bleeding, thrombosis, accelerated hepatomegaly, extreme thrombocytosis, and leukocytosis with excess blasts.[149] The indications for splenectomy include symptomatic portal hypertension (eg, variceal bleeding and ascites), drug-refractory marked splenomegaly that is either painful or associated with severe cachexia, and frequent RBC transfusions or refractory cytopenia.

Radiation provides transient (median response duration of 3-6 months) symptomatic relief of mechanical discomfort from hepatosplenomegaly. When it is employed, splenic irradiation is given in a total dose of 0.1 to 0.5 Gy in 5 to 10 fractions and is associated with a >10% mortality rate from consequences of cytopenias.[150] In our practice, we restrict the use of splenic radiation as a last resort for pure palliation for drug-refractory patients. Radiation therapy is most useful in patients with nonhepatosplenic EMH presenting with mass effect.[151] The thoracic vertebral column is the most frequent site of nonhepatosplenic EMH in PMF; other sites include the lymph nodes, the lung, pleura, small bowel, peritoneum, urogenital tract, and heart. When patients are symptomatic, such occurrences are effectively treated with low-dose radiation therapy (0.1-1 Gy in 5-10 fractions).[151]

Primary Myelofibrosis and Risk of Thrombosis

In a cohort of 707 patients, the cumulative rate of fatal and nonfatal cerebrovascular (CV) events was 7.2%, accounting for 1.75 events per 100 patient-years (2.23 events per 100 patient-years adjusted).[152] For nonfatal CV events, the cumulative rate was 6.6%; the incidences of myocardial infarction and peripheral arterial thrombosis were lower than those of stroke. There was a remarkably high rate of fatal (9 cases) and nonfatal (22 cases) venous thrombosis. In patients presenting with thrombosis at diagnosis or with a thrombotic history, the incidence of recurrences was 9%. In multivariable analysis, age and *JAK2* mutation were the only two risk factors to independently predict risk of thrombosis; and patients who were *JAK2* V617F mutated and presented with leukocytosis had the highest incidence of thrombosis (3.9% patient-years).

Management of Blast-Phase Primary Myelofibrosis

Treatment of the blast phase is typically met with limited success. In a retrospective analysis of 91 cases of blast-phase PMF seen at the Mayo Clinic, 98% of the patients died at a median of 2.6 months (range 0-24.2 months) from time of transformation into blast-phase PMF. Aggressive chemotherapy was no better than supportive care, and AML-like induction chemotherapy did not produce CR in any patient.[77] Allogeneic stem cell transplant may offer better long-term outcome in a small subset of patients.[153] Outside the context of a clinical trial, we use azanucleosides (azacitidine or decitabine) as an alternative to intensive chemotherapy for patients with accelerated phase or blast-phase PMF.[154] Two studies have assessed the combination of ruxolitinib and decitabine for the treatment of accelerated and blast-phase MPN with median OS of 7.9 and 6.9 months in each of these studies.[155,156]

The combination of azanucleosides and the B-cell lymphoma-2 (Bcl-2) inhibitor, venetoclax has emerged as a preferred option to treat AML in patients unfit for induction chemotherapy. However, the experience of using this combination in blast-phase MPN has not been as positive. Several retrospective analyses have demonstrated that clinical responses in blast phase MPN patients treated with azanucleoside-venetoclax combination are short lived, toxicity is significant, and OS has not been meaningfully improved.[157-160]

Allogeneic Hematopoietic Stem Cell Transplantation

AlloHCT remains the only curative option for patients with PMF. The decision and timing to proceed with HCT is a complex issue weighing potential benefits and substantial morbidity and mortality (for more details of HCT for MF, see Chapter 104).[161-166] The current recommendation is to consider if alloHCT is worth the risk in patients with PMF whose median survival is expected to be less than 5 years.[167] The consensus is to evaluate alloHCT for patients with a good performance status and no major comorbidities who are intermediate-2- or high-risk disease by risk stratification models. However, an argument can be made to allograft selected low- and intermediate-1 DIPSS risk patients who have had 5-year survivals following alloHCT over 80% and 60%, respectively, compared to median survivals of 7 and 2.5 years for intermediate-2- and high-risk patients, respectively.[168]

The use of reduced intensity conditioning (RIC) has expanded the availability of alloHCT in diseases such as PMF where most patients are of advanced age and harbor comorbidities. The nonrelapse mortality is lower, and the relapse rate is higher, but the disease-free survival of patients undergoing RIC tends to be similar to that of patients who receive myeloablative conditioning.[164] Alternative donors, particularly matched unrelated, are also allowing more patients to undergo alloHCT, and the results were initially inferior but are approaching those seen with matched sibling donors.[169]

The role of splenectomy for PMF prior to alloHCT is controversial. Splenectomized patients may engraft more quickly, but there is the problem of perioperative morbidity and mortality, and there are conflicting results about its effect on graft versus host disease (GVHD) and survival. Massive splenomegaly can resolve following alloHCT, including RIC-alloHCT.[170] Although splenectomy may be considered for an individual patient, pre-emptive splenectomy is not routinely recommended for patients with PMF undergoing HCT.

The role of JAK2 inhibitors prior to alloHCT in PMF is uncertain, but they could reduce spleen size and improve engraftment and could decrease the levels of inflammatory cytokines that might affect GVHD and prognosis post-alloHCT.[164] A retrospective assessment of patients receiving JAK2 inhibitors prior to transplant suggested they did not adversely impact posttransplant outcomes.[171] Clearing of *JAK2* V617F in the peripheral blood after alloHCT had a significantly reduced risk of relapse than patients who did not clear the mutation.[172] Clinical trials are warranted to determine the efficacy of JAK2 inhibition as a bridge to alloHCT, a strategy to delay HCT, or a therapy after HCT.

Emerging Therapies

Building upon an increased understanding of the biologic mechanisms that drive MF, multiple therapeutic agents have moved into late stages of development indicating that the treatment landscape for MF could be substantially transformed in the coming years. Agents currently in phase 3 trials include the bromodomain and extra-terminal domain inhibitor, pelabresib (formerly CPI-0610); the phosphatidylinositol-3-kinase-delta inhibitor, parsaclisib; the mouse double minute 2 inhibitor, navtemadlin (formerly KRT-232); the B-cell lymphoma-2 (Bcl-2) and Bcl-extra large inhibitor, navitoclax; the telomerase inhibitor, imetelstat; and the activin receptor ligand trap, luspatercept. Pelbabresib, parsaclisib, navitoclax, and luspatercept are being investigated in combination with JAK inhibitors, while navtemadlin and imetelstat are being investigated as single agents in the second-line setting.[173,174] These agents, in addition to the continued development of the JAK inhibitors pacritinib[175] and momelotinib,[176] have shown significant clinical activity in MF patients and aim to build upon the substantial, but limited, success of single-agent JAK inhibition.

SUMMARY

MF is a progressive MPN associated with significant disease burden, including splenomegaly, cytopenias, and constitutional symptoms that have an impact on patient survival and QoL. Over the past several years, important biologic aspects of the disease such as discovery of the JAK-STAT pathway dysregulation and multiple different mutations, leading to abnormal genetic and epigenetic regulation in MF, were found. After establishing the diagnosis, risk stratification is the most important next step. Allogeneic stem cell transplant remains the only curative option and should be offered for higher risk patients. The goals of medical therapy are mostly centered on improving splenomegaly, anemia, and very poor QoL. Treatment options remain limited, but the development of JAK inhibitors resulted in better control of the signs and symptoms of the disease and, therefore, improved patients' outlook. JAK inhibitors may serve as a building block for combination therapies that would significantly alter the biology of the disease.

ACKNOWLEDGMENTS

The authors recognize Ayalew Tefferi for his many contributions to the understanding and therapy of myelofibrosis.

References

1. Bose P, Masarova L, Amin HM, Verstovsek S. Philadelphia chromosome-negative myeloproliferative neoplasms. In: Kantarjian HM, Wolff RA, Rieber AG, eds. *The MD Anderson Manual of Medical Oncology*. 4th ed. McGraw Hill; 2022.
2. Tefferi A, Vainchenker W. Myeloproliferative neoplasms: molecular pathophysiology, essential clinical understanding, and treatment strategies. *J Clin Oncol*. 2011;29:573-582.
3. Tefferi A, Thiele J, Orazi A, et al. Proposals and rationale for revision of the World Health Organization diagnostic criteria for polycythemia vera, essential thrombocythemia, and primary myelofibrosis: recommendations from an ad hoc international expert panel. *Blood*. 2007;110:1092-1097.
4. Mesa RA. Navigating the evolving paradigms in the diagnosis and treatment of myeloproliferative disorders. *Hematology Am Soc Hematol Educ Program*. 2007;2007:355-362.
5. Mesa RA, Verstovsek S, Cervantes F, et al. Primary myelofibrosis (PMF), post polycythemia vera myelofibrosis (post-PV MF), post essential thrombocythemia myelofibrosis (post-ET MF), blast phase PMF (PMF-BP): consensus on terminology by the international working group for myelofibrosis research and treatment (IWG-MRT). *Leuk Res*. 2007;31:737-740.
6. Pardanani A, Vannucchi AM, Passamonti F, et al. JAK inhibitor therapy for myelofibrosis: critical assessment of value and limitations. *Leukemia*. 2011;25:218-225.
7. Tefferi A. Myelofibrosis with myeloid metaplasia. *N Engl J Med*. 2000;342:1255-1265.
8. Heuck G. Zwei Falle von Leukemie mit eigenthumlichen Blutresp. Knokenmarksbefund. *Arch Pathol Anat Physiol Virchows*.. 1879;78:475-496.
9. Hirsch R. Generalized osteosclerosis with chronic polycythemia vera. *Arch Pathol*. 1935;19:91-97.
10. Dameshek W. Some speculations on the myeloproliferative syndromes. *Blood*. 1951;6:372-375.
11. Nowell PC, Hungerford DA. Chromosome studies on normal and leukemic human leukocytes. *J Natl Cancer Inst*. 1960;25:85-109.
12. Jacobson RJ, Salo A, Fialkow PJ. Agnogenic myeloid metaplasia: a clonal proliferation of hematopoietic stem cells with secondary myelofibrosis. *Blood*. 1978;51:189-194.
13. Schindler C, Shuai K, Prezioso VR, et al. Interferon-dependent tyrosine phosphorylation of a latent cytoplasmic transcription factor. *Science*. 1992;257:809-813.
14. Levine RL, Wadleigh M, Cools J, et al. Activating mutation in the tyrosine kinase JAK2 in polycythemia vera, essential thrombocythemia, and myeloid metaplasia with myelofibrosis. *Cancer Cell*. 2005;7:387-397.
15. Baxter EJ, Scott LM, Campbell PJ, et al. Acquired mutation of the tyrosine kinase JAK2 in human myeloproliferative disorders. *Lancet*. 2005;365:1054-1061.
16. Kralovics R, Passamonti F, Buser AS, et al. A gain-of-function mutation of JAK2 in myeloproliferative disorders. *N Engl J Med*. 2005;352:1779-1790.
17. James C, Ugo V, Le Couedic JP, et al. A unique clonal JAK2 mutation leading to constitutive signalling causes polycythaemia vera. *Nature*. 2005;434:1144-1148.
18. Pikman Y, Lee BH, Mercher T, et al. MPLW515L is a novel somatic activating mutation in myelofibrosis with myeloid metaplasia. *PLoS Med*. 2006;3:e270.
19. Pardanani AD, Levine RL, Lasho T, et al. MPL515 mutations in myeloproliferative and other myeloid disorders: a study of 1182 patients. *Blood*. 2006;108:3472-3476.
20. Tefferi A. Novel mutations and their functional and clinical relevance in myeloproliferative neoplasms: JAK2, MPL, TET2, ASXL1, CBL, IDH and IKZF1. *Leukemia*. 2010;24:1128-1138.

21. Klampfl T, Gisslinger H, Harutyunyan AS, et al. Somatic mutations of calreticulin in myeloproliferative neoplasms. *N Engl J Med.* 2013;369:2379-2390.
22. Guglielmelli P, Pacilli A, Rotunno G, et al. Presentation and outcome of patients with 2016 WHO diagnosis of prefibrotic and overt primary myelofibrosis. *Blood.* 2017;129:3227-3236.
23. Rollison DE, Howlader N, Smith MT, et al. Epidemiology of myelodysplastic syndromes and chronic myeloproliferative disorders in the United States, 2001-2004, using data from the NAACCR and SEER programs. *Blood.* 2008;112:45-52.
24. Mesa RA, Silverstein MN, Jacobsen SJ, et al. Population-based incidence and survival figures in essential thrombocythemia and agnogenic myeloid metaplasia: an Olmsted County Study, 1976-1995. *Am J Hematol.* 1999;61:10-15.
25. Chaiter Y, Brenner B, Aghai E, et al. High incidence of myeloproliferative disorders in Ashkenazi Jews in northern Israel. *Leuk Lymphoma.* 1992;7:251-255.
26. Tondel M, Persson B, Carstensen J. Myelofibrosis and benzene exposure. *Occup Med (Lond).* 1995;45:51-52.
27. Honda Y, Delzell E, Cole P. An updated study of mortality among workers at a petroleum manufacturing plant. *J Occup Environ Med.* 1995;37:194-200.
28. Anderson RE, Hoshino T, Yamamoto T. Myelofibrosis with myeloid metaplasia in survivors of the atomic bomb in Hiroshima. *Ann Intern Med.* 1964;60:1-18.
29. Reeder TL, Bailey RJ, Dewald GW, et al. Both B and T lymphocytes may be clonally involved in myelofibrosis with myeloid metaplasia. *Blood.* 2003;101:1981-1983.
30. Van Egeren D, Escabi J, Nguyen M, et al. Reconstructing the lineage histories and differentiation trajectories of individual cancer cells in myeloproliferative neoplasms. *Cell Stem Cell.* 2021;28(3):514-523 e9.
31. Wassie E, Finke C, Gangat N, et al. A compendium of cytogenetic abnormalities in myelofibrosis: molecular and phenotypic correlates in 826 patients. *Br J Haematol.* 2015;169:71-76.
32. Tefferi A, Mesa RA, Schroeder G, et al. Cytogenetic findings and their clinical relevance in myelofibrosis with myeloid metaplasia. *Br J Haematol.* 2001;113:763-771.
33. Dingli D, Grand FH, Mahaffey V, et al. Der(6)t(1;6)(q21-23;p21.3): a specific cytogenetic abnormality in myelofibrosis with myeloid metaplasia. *Br J Haematol.* 2005;130:229-232.
34. Tefferi A, Meyer RG, Wyatt WA, Dewald GW. Comparison of peripheral blood interphase cytogenetics with bone marrow karyotype analysis in myelofibrosis with myeloid metaplasia. *Br J Haematol.* 2001;115:316-319.
35. Al-Assar O, Ul-Hassan A, Brown R, Wilson GA, Hammond DW, Reilly JT. Gains on 9p are common genomic aberrations in idiopathic myelofibrosis: a comparative genomic hybridization study. *Br J Haematol.* 2005;129:66-71.
36. Vainchenker W, Kralovics R. Genetic basis and molecular pathophysiology of classical myeloproliferative neoplasms. *Blood.* 2017;129:667-679.
37. Ortmann CA, Kent DG, Nangalia J, et al. Effect of mutation order on myeloproliferative neoplasms. *N Engl J Med.* 2015;372:601-612.
38. Pesu M, Laurence A, Kishore N, Zwillich SH, Chan G, O'Shea JJ. Therapeutic targeting of Janus kinases. *Immunol Rev.* 2008;223:132-142.
39. Quintas-Cardama A, Kantarjian H, Cortes J, Verstovsek S. Janus kinase inhibitors for the treatment of myeloproliferative neoplasias and beyond. *Nat Rev Drug Discov.* 2011;10:127-140.
40. Agrawal M, Garg RJ, Cortes J, Kantarjian H, Verstovsek S, Quintas-Cardama A. Experimental therapeutics for patients with myeloproliferative neoplasias. *Cancer.* 2011;117:662-676.
41. O'Sullivan LA, Liongue C, Lewis RS, Stephenson SE, Ward AC. Cytokine receptor signaling through the Jak-Stat-Socs pathway in disease. *Mol Immunol.* 2007;44:2497-2506.
42. Verstovsek S, Kantarjian H, Mesa RA, et al. Safety and efficacy of INCB018424, a JAK1 and JAK2 inhibitor, in myelofibrosis. *N Engl J Med.* 2010;363:1117-1127.
43. Vainchenker W, Delhommeau F, Constantinescu SN, Bernard OA. New mutations and pathogenesis of myeloproliferative neoplasms. *Blood.* 2011;118:1723-1735.
44. Nangalia J, Massie CE, Baxter EJ, et al. Somatic CALR mutations in myeloproliferative neoplasms with nonmutated JAK2. *N Engl J Med.* 2013;369:2391-2405.
45. Araki M, Yang Y, Masubuchi N, et al. Activation of the thrombopoietin receptor by mutant calreticulin in CALR-mutant myeloproliferative neoplasms. *Blood.* 2016;127(10):1307-1316.
46. Scott LM, Tong W, Levine RL, et al. JAK2 exon 12 mutations in polycythemia vera and idiopathic erythrocytosis. *N Engl J Med.* 2007;356:459-468.
47. Guglielmelli P, Rotunno G, Fanelli T, et al. Validation of the differential prognostic impact of type 1/type 1-like versus type 2/type 2-like CALR mutations in myelofibrosis. *Blood Cancer J.* 2015;5:e360.
48. Chagraoui H, Komura E, Tulliez M, Giraudier S, Vainchenker W, Wendling F. Prominent role of TGF-beta 1 in thrombopoietin-induced myelofibrosis in mice. *Blood.* 2002;100:3495-3503.
49. Vannucchi AM, Bianchi L, Cellai C, et al. Development of myelofibrosis in mice genetically impaired for GATA-1 expression (GATA-1(low) mice). *Blood.* 2002;100:1123-1132.
50. Schmitt A, Jouault H, Guichard J, Wendling F, Drouin A, Cramer EM. Pathologic interaction between megakaryocytes and polymorphonuclear leukocytes in myelofibrosis. *Blood.* 2000;96:1342-1347.
51. Xu M, Bruno E, Chao J, et al. Constitutive mobilization of CD34+ cells into the peripheral blood in idiopathic myelofibrosis may be due to the action of a number of proteases. *Blood.* 2005;105:4508-4515.
52. Massa M, Rosti V, Ramajoli I, et al. Circulating CD34+, CD133+, and vascular endothelial growth factor receptor 2-positive endothelial progenitor cells in myelofibrosis with myeloid metaplasia. *J Clin Oncol.* 2005;23:5688-5695.
53. Barosi G, Viarengo G, Pecci A, et al. Diagnostic and clinical relevance of the number of circulating CD34(+) cells in myelofibrosis with myeloid metaplasia. *Blood.* 2001;98:3249-3255.
54. Wolf BC, Neiman RS. Hypothesis: splenic filtration and the pathogenesis of extramedullary hematopoiesis in agnogenic myeloid metaplasia. *Hematol Pathol.* 1987;1:77-80.
55. O'Keane JC, Wolf BC, Neiman RS. The pathogenesis of splenic extramedullary hematopoiesis in metastatic carcinoma. *Cancer.* 1989;63:1539-1543.
56. Mesa RA, Li CY, Schroeder G, Tefferi A. Clinical correlates of splenic histopathology and splenic karyotype in myelofibrosis with myeloid metaplasia. *Blood.* 2001;97:3665-3667.
57. Mesa RA. How I treat symptomatic splenomegaly in patients with myelofibrosis. *Blood.* 2009;113:5394-5400.
58. Cervantes F, Pereira A, Esteve J, Cobo F, Rozman C, Montserrat E. The changing profile of idiopathic myelofibrosis: a comparison of the presenting features of patients diagnosed in two different decades. *Eur J Haematol.* 1998;60:101-105.
59. Jaroch MT, Broughan TA, Hermann RE. The natural history of splenic infarction. *Surgery.* 1986;100:743-750.
60. Strasser-Weippl K, Steurer M, Kees M, et al. Age and hemoglobin level emerge as most important clinical prognostic parameters in patients with osteomyelofibrosis: introduction of a simplified prognostic score. *Leuk Lymphoma.* 2006;47:441-450.
61. Dupriez B, Morel P, Demory JL, et al. Prognostic factors in agnogenic myeloid metaplasia: a report on 195 cases with a new scoring system. *Blood.* 1996;88:1013-1018.
62. Kreft A, Weiss M, Wiese B, et al. Chronic idiopathic myelofibrosis: prognostic impact of myelofibrosis and clinical parameters on event-free survival in 122 patients who presented in prefibrotic and fibrotic stages. A retrospective study identifying subgroups of different prognoses by using the RECPAM method. *Ann Hematol.* 2003;82:605-611.
63. Vannucchi AM. Management of myelofibrosis. *Hematology Am Soc Hematol Educ Program.* 2011;2011:222-230.
64. Abdel-Wahab OI, Levine RL. Primary myelofibrosis: update on definition, pathogenesis, and treatment. *Annu Rev Med.* 2009;60:233-245.
65. Tefferi A, Lasho TL, Jimma T, et al. One thousand patients with primary myelofibrosis: the mayo clinic experience. *Mayo Clin Proc.* 2012;87:25-33.
66. Arber DA, Orazi A, Hasserjian R, et al. The 2016 revision to the World Health Organization classification of myeloid neoplasms and acute leukemia. *Blood.* 2016;127(20):2391-2405.
67. Barosi G, Mesa RA, Thiele J, et al. Proposed criteria for the diagnosis of post-polycythemia vera and post-essential thrombocythemia myelofibrosis: a consensus statement from the International Working Group for Myelofibrosis Research and Treatment. *Leukemia.* 2008;22:437-438.
68. Thiele J, Kvasnicka HM, Tefferi A, et al. Primary myelofibrosis. In: Swerdlow SH, Campo E, Harris NL, et al., eds. *World Health Organization Classification of Tumors: Tumours of Haematopoietic and Lymphoid Tissues.* International Agency for Research on Cancer; 2008:44-47.
69. Thiele J, Kvasnicka HM. A critical reappraisal of the WHO classification of the chronic myeloproliferative disorders. *Leuk Lymphoma.* 2006;47:381-396.
70. Tefferi A, Jimma T, Sulai NH, et al. IDH mutations in primary myelofibrosis predict leukemic transformation and shortened survival: clinical evidence for leukemogenic collaboration with JAK2V617F. *Leukemia.* 2012;26:475-480.
71. Vannucchi AM, Lasho TL, Guglielmelli P, et al. Mutations and prognosis in primary myelofibrosis. *Leukemia.* 2013;27:1861-1869.
72. Guglielmelli P, Lasho TL, Rotunno G, et al. The number of prognostically detrimental mutations and prognosis in primary myelofibrosis: an international study of 797 patients. *Leukemia.* 2014;28:1804-1810.
73. Beer PA, Ortmann CA, Stegelmann F, et al. Molecular mechanisms associated with leukemic transformation of MPL-mutant myeloproliferative neoplasms. *Haematologica.* 2010;95:2153-2156.
74. Lundberg P, Karow A, Nienhold R, et al. Clonal evolution and clinical correlates of somatic mutations in myeloproliferative neoplasms. *Blood.* 2014;123:2220-2228.
75. Coltro G, Rotunno G, Mannelli L, Mannarelli C, Fiaccabrino S, Romagnoli S, et al. RAS/MAPK pathway mutations are associated with adverse survival outcomes and may predict resistance to JAK inhibitors in myelofibrosis. Presented at EHA Annual Meeting 2020(Abstract S211).
76. Santos FPS, Getta B, Masarova L, et al. Prognostic impact of RAS-pathway mutations in patients with myelofibrosis. *Leukemia.* 2020;34(3):799-810.
77. Mesa RA, Tefferi A. Survival and outcomes to therapy in leukemic transformation of myelofibrosis with myeloid metaplasia; a single institution experience with 91 patients. *Blood.* 2003;102:917a-918a.
78. Cervantes F, Pereira A, Esteve J, et al. Identification of "short-lived" and "long-lived" patients at presentation of idiopathic myelofibrosis. *Br J Haematol.* 1997;97:635-640.
79. Okamura T, Kinukawa N, Niho Y, Mizoguchi H. Primary chronic myelofibrosis: clinical and prognostic evaluation in 336 Japanese patients. *Int J Hematol.* 2001;73:194-198.
80. Cervantes F, Dupriez B, Pereira A, et al. New prognostic scoring system for primary myelofibrosis based on a study of the International Working Group for Myelofibrosis Research and Treatment. *Blood.* 2009;113:2895-2901.
81. Hussein K, Pardanani AD, Van Dyke DL, Hanson CA, Tefferi A. International prognostic scoring system-independent cytogenetic risk categorization in primary myelofibrosis. *Blood.* 2010;115:496-499.
82. Caramazza D, Begna KH, Gangat N, et al. Refined cytogenetic-risk categorization for overall and leukemia-free survival in primary myelofibrosis: a single center study of 433 patients. *Leukemia.* 2011;25:82-88.
83. Vaidya R, Caramazza D, Begna KH, et al. Monosomal karyotype in primary myelofibrosis is detrimental to both overall and leukemia-free survival. *Blood.* 2011;117:5612-5615.
84. Passamonti F, Cervantes F, Vannucchi AM, et al. A dynamic prognostic model to predict survival in primary myelofibrosis: a study by the IWG-MRT (International Working Group for Myeloproliferative Neoplasms Research and Treatment). *Blood.* 2010;115:1703-1708.

85. Gangat N, Caramazza D, Vaidya R, et al. DIPSS plus: a refined Dynamic International Prognostic Scoring System for primary myelofibrosis that incorporates prognostic information from karyotype, platelet count, and transfusion status. *J Clin Oncol.* 2010;29:392-397.
86. Guglielmelli P, Biamonte F, Score J, et al. EZH2 mutational status predicts poor survival in myelofibrosis. *Blood.* 2011;118:5227-5234.
87. Lasho TL, Jimma T, Finke CM, et al. SRSF2 mutations in primary myelofibrosis: significant clustering with IDH mutations and independent association with inferior overall and leukemia-free survival. *Blood.* 2012;120:4168-4171.
88. Tefferi A, Finke CM, Lasho TL, et al. U2AF1 mutation types in primary myelofibrosis: phenotypic and prognostic distinctions. *Leukemia.* 2018;32(10):2274-2278.
89. Rumi E, Pietra D, Pascutto C, et al. Clinical effect of driver mutations of JAK2, CALR, or MPL in primary myelofibrosis. *Blood.* 2014;124:1062-1069.
90. Tefferi A, Lasho TL, Finke CM, et al. CALR vs JAK2 vs MPL-mutated or triple-negative myelofibrosis: clinical, cytogenetic and molecular comparisons. *Leukemia.* 2014;28:1472-1477.
91. Tefferi A, Lasho TL, Tischer A, et al. The prognostic advantage of calreticulin mutations in myelofibrosis might be confined to type 1 or type 1-like CALR variants. *Blood.* 2014;124:2465-2466.
92. Guglielmelli P, Lasho TL, Rotunno G, et al. MIPSS70: mutation-enhanced international prognostic score system for transplantation-age patients with primary myelofibrosis. *J Clin Oncol.* 2017;36(4):310-318. doi:10.1200/JCO2017764886
93. Tefferi A, Guglielmelli P, Nicolosi M, et al. GIPSS: genetically inspired prognostic scoring system for primary myelofibrosis. *Leukemia.* 2018;32(7):1631-1642.
94. Tefferi A, Guglielmelli P, Lasho TL, et al. MIPSS70+ version 2.0: mutation and karyotype-enhanced international prognostic scoring system for primary myelofibrosis. *J Clin Oncol.* 2018;36(17):1769-1770.
95. Gowin K, Coakley M, Kosiorek H, Mesa R. Discrepancies of applying primary myelofibrosis prognostic scores for patients with post polycythemia vera/essential thrombocytosis myelofibrosis. *Haematologica.* 2016;101(10):e405-e406.
96. Harrison CN, Mead AJ, Panchal A, et al. Ruxolitinib vs best available therapy for ET intolerant or resistant to hydroxycarbamide. *Blood.* 2017;130(17):1889-1897.
97. Passamonti F, Giorgino T, Mora B, et al. A clinical-molecular prognostic model to predict survival in patients with post polycythemia vera and post essential thrombocythemia myelofibrosis. *Leukemia.* 2017;31(12):2726-2731.
98. Masarova L, Bose P, Pemmaraju N, et al. Validation of the myelofibrosis secondary to PV and ET-prognostic model in patients with post-polycythemia vera and post-essential thrombocythemia myelofibrosis: MD Anderson Cancer Center. *Blood.* 2017;130. (suppl 1):4205
99. Tefferi A, Barosi G, Mesa RA, et al. International Working Group (IWG) consensus criteria for treatment response in myelofibrosis with myeloid metaplasia, for the IWG for Myelofibrosis Research and Treatment (IWG-MRT). *Blood.* 2006;108:1497-1503.
100. Barosi G, Bordessoule D, Briere J, et al. Response criteria for myelofibrosis with myeloid metaplasia: results of an initiative of the European Myelofibrosis Network (EUMNET). *Blood.* 2005;106:2849-2853.
101. Komrokji RS, Wadleigh M, Seymour JF, et al. Results of a phase 2 study of pacritinib (SB1518), a novel oral JAK2 inhibitor, in patients with primary, post-polycythemia vera, and post-essential thrombocythemia myelofibrosis. *Blood.* 2011;118:282.
102. Mesa RA, Schwager S, Radia D, et al. The Myelofibrosis Symptom Assessment Form (MFSAF): an evidence-based brief inventory to measure quality of life and symptomatic response to treatment in myelofibrosis. *Leuk Res.* 2009;33:1199-1203.
103. Gwaltney C, Paty J, Kwitkowski VE, et al. Development of a harmonized patient-reported outcome questionnaire to assess myelofibrosis symptoms in clinical trials. *Leuk Res.* 2017;59:26-31.
104. Mesa RA, Niblack J, Wadleigh M, et al. The burden of fatigue and quality of life in myeloproliferative disorders (MPDs): an international Internet-based survey of 1179 MPD patients. *Cancer.* 2007;109:68-76.
105. Ahlberg K, Ekman T, Gaston-Johansson F, Mock V. Assessment and management of cancer-related fatigue in adults. *Lancet.* 2003;362:640-650.
106. Cella D, Yount S, Rothrock N, et al. The Patient-Reported Outcomes Measurement Information System (PROMIS): progress of an NIH Roadmap cooperative group during its first two years. *Med Care.* 2007;45:S3-S11.
107. Cella D, Webster K, Cashy J, et al. Development of a measure of health-related quality of life for non-Hodgkin's lymphoma clinical research: the functional assessment of cancer therapy - lymphoma (FACT-Lym). *Blood.* 2005;106:750.
108. Fenaux P, Kiladjian JJ, Platzbecker U. Luspatercept for the treatment of anemia in myelodysplastic syndromes and primary myelofibrosis. *Blood.* 2019;133(8):790-794.
109. Oh ST, Talpaz M, Gerds AT, et al. ACVR1/JAK1/JAK2 inhibitor momelotinib reverses transfusion dependency and suppresses hepcidin in myelofibrosis phase 2 trial. *Blood Adv.* 2020;4(18):4282-4291.
110. Mascarenhas J, Kremyanskaya M, Patriarca A, et al. BET inhibitor pelabresib (CPI-0610) combined with ruxolitinib in patients with myelofibrosis – JAK-inhibitor naïve or with suboptimal response to ruxolitinib – Preliminary data from the MANIFEST study. *HemaSphere.* 2022;6:S3:99-100, abstract S198.
111. Cervantes F, Alvarez-Larran A, Hernandez-Boluda JC, Sureda A, Torrebadell M, Montserrat E. Erythropoietin treatment of the anaemia of myelofibrosis with myeloid metaplasia: results in 20 patients and review of the literature. *Br J Haematol.* 2004;127:399-403.
112. Silverstein MN. *Agnogenic Myeloid Metaplasia.* Publishing Sciences Group; 1975:126.
113. Besa EC, Nowell PC, Geller NL, Gardner FH. Analysis of the androgen response of 23 patients with agnogenic myeloid metaplasia: the value of chromosomal studies in predicting response and survival. *Cancer.* 1982;49:308-313.
114. Cervantes F, Alvarez-Larran A, Domingo A, Arellano-Rodrigo E, Montserrat E. Efficacy and tolerability of danazol as a treatment for the anaemia of myelofibrosis with myeloid metaplasia: long-term results in 30 patients. *Br J Haematol.* 2005;129:771-775.
115. Elliott MA, Mesa RA, Li CY, et al. Thalidomide treatment in myelofibrosis with myeloid metaplasia. *Br J Haematol.* 2002;117:288-296.
116. Tefferi A, Cortes J, Verstovsek S, et al. Lenalidomide therapy in myelofibrosis with myeloid metaplasia. *Blood.* 2006;108:1158-1164.
117. Mesa RA, Steensma DP, Pardanani A, et al. A phase 2 trial of combination low-dose thalidomide and prednisone for the treatment of myelofibrosis with myeloid metaplasia. *Blood.* 2003;101:2534-2541.
118. Tefferi A, Lasho TL, Mesa RA, Pardanani A, Ketterling RP, Hanson CA. Lenalidomide therapy in del(5)(q31)-associated myelofibrosis: cytogenetic and JAK2V617F molecular remissions. *Leukemia.* 2007;21:1827-1828.
119. Quintas-Cardama A, Kantarjian HM, Manshouri T, et al. Lenalidomide plus prednisone results in durable clinical, histopathologic, and molecular responses in patients with myelofibrosis. *J Clin Oncol.* 2009;27:4760-4766.
120. Tefferi A, Verstovsek S, Barosi G, et al. Pomalidomide is active in the treatment of anemia associated with myelofibrosis. *J Clin Oncol.* 2009;27:4563-4569.
121. Masarova L, Verstovsek S, Hidalgo-Lopez JE, et al. A phase 2 study of ruxolitinib in combination with azacitidine in patients with myelofibrosis. *Blood.* 2018;132(16):1664-1674.
122. Petti MC, Latagliata R, Spadea T, et al. Melphalan treatment in patients with myelofibrosis with myeloid metaplasia. *Br J Haematol.* 2002;116:576-581.
123. Naqvi T, Baumann MA. Myelofibrosis: response to busulfan after hydroxyurea failure. *Int J Clin Pract.* 2002;56:312-313.
124. Tefferi A, Silverstein MN, Li CY. 2-Chlorodeoxyadenosine treatment after splenectomy in patients who have myelofibrosis with myeloid metaplasia. *Br J Haematol.* 1997;99:352-357.
125. Tefferi A, Elliot MA, Yoon SY, et al. Clinical and bone marrow effects of interferon alfa therapy in myelofibrosis with myeloid metaplasia. *Blood.* 2001;97:1896.
126. Barosi G, Liberato LN, Costa A, Ascari E. Cytoreductive effect of recombinant alpha interferon in patients with myelofibrosis with myeloid metaplasia. *Blut.* 1989;58:271-274.
127. Gilbert HS. Long-term treatment of myeloproliferative disease with interferon-alpha-2b: feasibility and efficacy. *Cancer.* 1998;83:1205-1213.
128. Silver RT, Vandris K, Goldman JJ. Recombinant interferon-alpha may retard progression of early primary myelofibrosis: a preliminary report. *Blood.* 2011;117:6669-6672.
129. Ianotto JC, Kiladjian JJ, Demory JL, et al. PEG-IFN-alpha-2a therapy in patients with myelofibrosis: a study of the French Groupe d'Etudes des Myelofibroses (GEM) and France Intergroupe des syndromes Myeloproliferatifs (FIM). *Br J Haematol.* 2009;146:223-225.
130. Hasselbalch HC, Kiladjian JJ, Silver RT. Interferon alfa in the treatment of Philadelphia-negative chronic myeloproliferative neoplasms. *J Clin Oncol.* 2011;29:e564-e565.
131. Verstovsek S, Mesa RA, Gotlib J, et al. A double-blind, placebo-controlled trial of ruxolitinib for myelofibrosis. *N Engl J Med.* 2012;366:799-807.
132. Harrison C, Kiladjian JJ, Al-Ali HK, et al. JAK inhibition with ruxolitinib versus best available therapy for myelofibrosis. *N Engl J Med.* 2012;366:787-798.
133. Pardanani A, Gotlib JR, Jamieson C, et al. Safety and efficacy of TG101348, a selective JAK2 inhibitor, in myelofibrosis. *J Clin Oncol.* 2011;29:789-796.
134. Pardanani A, George G, Lasho T, et al. A Phase I/II study of CYT387, an oral JAK-1/2 inhibitor, in myelofibrosis: significant response rates in anemia, splenomegaly, and constitutional symptoms. *Blood.* 2010;116:460.
135. Verstovsek S, Mesa R, Kloeker-Rhoades S, et al. Phase I study of the JAK2 V617F inhibitor, LY2784544, in patients with myelofibrosis (MF), polycythemia vera (PV), and essential thrombocythemia (ET). *Blood.* 2011;118:2814.
136. Barosi G. Myelofibrosis with myeloid metaplasia: diagnostic definition and prognostic classification for clinical studies and treatment guidelines. *J Clin Oncol.* 1999;17:2954-2970.
137. Verstovsek S, Mesa RA, Gotlib J, et al. Long-term treatment with ruxolitinib for patients with myelofibrosis: 5-year update from the randomized, double-blind, placebo-controlled, phase 3 COMFORT-I trial. *J Hematol Oncol.* 2017;10(1):55.
138. Verstovsek S, Kiladjian JJ, Mesa R, et al. Effect of ruxolitinib on the incidence of splenectomy in patients with myelofibrosis: a retrospective analysis of data from ruxolitinib clinical trials. *Blood.* 2012;120:2847.
139. Cervantes F, Kiladjian JJ, Niederwieser D, et al. Long-term safety, efficacy, and survival findings from COMFORT-II, a phase 3 study comparing ruxolitinib with best available therapy (BAT) for the treatment of myelofibrosis (MF). *Blood.* 2012;120:801.
140. Vannucchi AM, Kantarjian HM, Kiladjian JJ, et al. A pooled analysis of overall survival in COMFORT-I and COMFORT-II, 2 randomized phase III trials of ruxolitinib for the treatment of myelofibrosis. *Haematologica.* 2015;100:1139-1145.
141. Vannucchi AM, Te Boekhorst PAW, Harrison CN, et al. EXPAND, a dose-finding study of ruxolitinib in patients with myelofibrosis and low platelet counts: 48-week follow-up analysis. *Haematologica.* 2019;104(5):947-954.
142. Pardanani A, Harrison C, Cortes JE, et al. Safety and efficacy of fedratinib in patients with primary or secondary myelofibrosis: a randomized clinical trial. *JAMA Oncol.* 2015;1(5):643-651.
143. Harrison CN, Schaap N, Vannucchi AM, et al. Janus kinase-2 inhibitor fedratinib in patients with myelofibrosis previously treated with ruxolitinib (JAKARTA-2): a single-arm, open-label, non-randomised, phase 2, multicentre study. *Lancet Haematol.* 2017;4(7):e317-e324.
144. Harrison CN, Schaap N, Vannucchi AM, et al. Fedratinib in patients with myelofibrosis previously treated with ruxolitinib: an updated analysis of the JAKARTA2 study using stringent criteria for ruxolitinib failure. *Am J Hematol.* 2020;95(6):594-603.

145. Komrokji RS, Seymour JF, Roberts AW, et al. Results of a phase 2 study of pacritinib (SB1518), a JAK2/JAK2(V617F) inhibitor, in patients with myelofibrosis. *Blood.* 2015;125:2649-2655.
146. Mesa RA, Vannucchi AM, Mead A, et al. Pacritinib versus best available therapy for the treatment of myelofibrosis irrespective of baseline cytopenias (PERSIST-1): an international, randomised, phase 3 trial. *Lancet Haematol.* 2017;4(5):e225-e236.
147. Mascarenhas J, Hoffman R, Talpaz M, et al. Pacritinib vs best available therapy, including ruxolitinib, in patients with myelofibrosis: a randomized clinical trial. *JAMA Oncol.* 2018;4(5):652-659.
148. Gerds AT, Savona MR, Scott BL, et al. Determining the recommended dose of pacritinib: results from the PAC203 dose-finding trial in advanced myelofibrosis. *Blood Adv.* 2020;4(22):5825-5835.
149. Tefferi A, Mesa RA, Nagorney DM, Schroeder G, Silverstein MN. Splenectomy in myelofibrosis with myeloid metaplasia: a single-institution experience with 223 patients. *Blood.* 2000;95:2226-2233.
150. Elliott MA, Chen MG, Silverstein MN, Tefferi A. Splenic irradiation for symptomatic splenomegaly associated with myelofibrosis with myeloid metaplasia. *Br J Haematol.* 1998;103:505-511.
151. Koch CA, Li CY, Mesa RA, Tefferi A. Nonhepatosplenic extramedullary hematopoiesis: associated diseases, pathology, clinical course, and treatment. *Mayo Clin Proc.* 2003;78:1223-1233.
152. Barbui T, Carobbio A, Cervantes F, et al. Thrombosis in primary myelofibrosis: incidence and risk factors. *Blood.* 2010;115:778-782.
153. Kundranda MN, Tibes R, Mesa RA. Transformation of a chronic myeloproliferative neoplasm to acute myelogenous leukemia: does anything work? *Curr Hematol Malig Rep.* 2012;7:78-86.
154. Shahin OA, Chifotides HT, Bose P, Masarova L, Verstovsek S. Accelerated phase of myeloproliferative neoplasms. *Acta Haematologica.* 2021;144(5):484-499.
155. Rampal RK, Mascarenhas JO, Kosiorek HE, et al. Safety and efficacy of combined ruxolitinib and decitabine in accelerated and blast-phase myeloproliferative neoplasms. *Blood Adv.* 2018;2(24):3572-3580.
156. Bose P, Verstovsek S, Cortes JE, et al. A phase 1/2 study of ruxolitinib and decitabine in patients with post-myeloproliferative neoplasm acute myeloid leukemia. *Leukemia.* 2020;34(9):2489-2492.
157. King AC, Weis TM, Derkach A, et al. Multicenter evaluation of efficacy and toxicity of venetoclax-based combinations in patients with accelerated and blast phase myeloproliferative neoplasms. *Am J Hematol.* 2022;97(1):E7-E10.
158. Masarova L, DiNardo CD, Bose P, et al. Single-center experience with venetoclax combinations in patients with newly diagnosed and relapsed AML evolving from MPNs. *Blood Adv.* 2021;5(8):2156-2164.
159. Gangat N, Guglielmelli P, Szuber N, et al. Venetoclax and azacitidine or decitabine in blast-phase myeloproliferative neoplasms: a multicenter series of 32 consecutive cases. *Am J Hematol.* 2021;96(7):781-789.
160. Tremblay D, Feld J, Dougherty M, et al. Venetoclax and hypomethylating agent combination therapy in acute myeloid leukemia secondary to a myeloproliferative neoplasm. *Leuk Res.* 2020;98:106456.
161. Ballen KK, Shrestha S, Sobocinski KA, et al. Outcome of transplantation for myelofibrosis. *Biol Blood Marrow Transplant.* 2010;16:358-367.
162. Bacigalupo A, Soraru M, Dominietto A, et al. Allogeneic hemopoietic SCT for patients with primary myelofibrosis: a predictive transplant score based on transfusion requirement, spleen size and donor type. *Bone Marrow Transplant.* 2010;45:458-463.
163. Gupta V, Kroger N, Aschan J, et al. A retrospective comparison of conventional intensity conditioning and reduced-intensity conditioning for allogeneic hematopoietic cell transplantation in myelofibrosis. *Bone Marrow Transplant.* 2009;44:317-320.
164. Gupta V, Hari P, Hoffman R. Allogeneic hematopoietic cell transplantation for myelofibrosis in the era of JAK inhibitors. *Blood.* 2012;120:1367-1379.
165. McLornan DP, Mead AJ, Jackson G, Harrison CN. Allogeneic stem cell transplantation for myelofibrosis in 2012. *Br J Haematol.* 2012;157:413-425.
166. Ballen K. How to manage the transplant question in myelofibrosis. *Blood Cancer J.* 2012;2:e59.
167. Barbui T, Tefferi A, Vannucchi AM, et al. Philadelphia chromosome-negative classical myeloproliferative neoplasms: revised management recommendations from European LeukemiaNet. *Leukemia.* 2018;32(5):1057-1069.
168. Scott BL, Gooley TA, Sorror ML, et al. The dynamic international prognostic scoring system for myelofibrosis predicts outcomes after hematopoietic cell transplantation. *Blood.* 2012;119:2657-2664.
169. Kroger N, Zabelina T, Schieder H, et al. Pilot study of reduced-intensity conditioning followed by allogeneic stem cell transplantation from related and unrelated donors in patients with myelofibrosis. *Br J Haematol.* 2005;128:690-697.
170. Ciurea SO, Sadegi B, Wilbur A, et al. Effects of extensive splenomegaly in patients with myelofibrosis undergoing a reduced intensity allogeneic stem cell transplantation. *Br J Haematol.* 2008;141:80-83.
171. Shanavas M, Popat U, Michaelis LC, et al. Outcomes of allogeneic hematopoietic cell transplantation in patients with myelofibrosis with prior exposure to Janus kinase 1/2 inhibitors. *Biol Blood Marrow Transplant.* 2016;22(3):432-440.
172. Alchalby H, Badbaran A, Zabelina T, et al. Impact of JAK2V617F mutation status, allele burden, and clearance after allogeneic stem cell transplantation for myelofibrosis. *Blood.* 2010;116:3572-3581.
173. Kuykendall AT, Horvat NP, Pandey G, Komrokji R, Reuther GW. Finding a Jill for JAK: assessing past, present and future JAK inhibitor combination Approaches in myelofibrosis. *Cancers (Basel).* 2020;12(8):2278.
174. Chifotides HT, Bose P, Masarova L, Pemmaraju N, Verstovsek S. SOHO state of the art updates and next questions: Novel therapies in development for myelofibrosis. *Clin Lymphoma Myeloma Leuk.* 2022;22(4):210-223.
175. Mascarenhas J. Pacritinib for the treatment of patients with myelofibrosis and thrombocytopenia. *Expert Review Hematol.* 2022;15(8):671-684.
176. Chifotides HT, Bose P, Verstovsek S. Momelotinib: An emerging treatment for myelofibrosis patients with anemia. *J Hematol Oncol.*, 2022;15(1):7.

Chapter 86 ■ Eosinophilic Neoplasms and Hypereosinophilic Syndrome

JASON GOTLIB

HISTORICAL BACKGROUND

Paul Ehrlich's use of aniline dyes facilitated identification of the eosinophil as a unique leukocyte in 1879.[1] Reactive eosinophilias and eosinophilia-associated leukemias were recognized in the early- to mid-20th century. However, a nomenclature for unexplained eosinophilias was not formulated until 1968 when Hardy and Anderson originated the term *hypereosinophilic syndrome* (HES).[2] In 1975, Chusid and colleagues generated diagnostic criteria for (idiopathic) HES based on a small case series of patients: (1) persistent eosinophilia of 1.5×10^9/L for more than 6 months; (2) lack of evidence for parasitic, allergic, or other known causes of eosinophilia; and (3) signs and symptoms of organ involvement.[3] In the past 20 years, the evaluation of eosinophilic disorders has advanced from its descriptive roots to a more comprehensive approach that relies on a combination of histopathology, cytogenetics, molecular genetics, and immunophenotyping. Table 86.1 lists recent modern nosologic and clinicopathologic landmarks that reflect this evolution in the diagnosis and classification of eosinophilic disorders.

DEFINITION OF EOSINOPHILIA

Although minor differences may exist between laboratories, the upper limit of normal for the percent peripheral blood eosinophils is 5%, with a corresponding absolute eosinophil count (AEC) of approximately 0.5×10^9/L (500/mm^3).[3-5] The severity of hypereosinophilia (HE) has been stratified into mild, moderate, or severe (with AECs between the upper range of normal to 1.5×10^9/L (1500/mm^3), 1.5 to 5.0×10^9/L (1500-5000/mm^3), and $>5.0 \times 10^9$/L (>5000/mm^3), respectively. Alternatively, the singular term *hypereosinophilia* has been used to denote an AEC of $>1.5 \times 10^9$/L (>1500/mm^3).

EPIDEMIOLOGY

HES and chronic eosinophilic leukemia (CEL) are very uncommon disorders. Data obtained from the Surveillance, Epidemiology, and End Results (SEER) program during the years 2001 to 2005 revealed an age-adjusted incidence rate of 0.036 per 100,000.[6] A more recent analysis of CEL, not otherwise specified (NOS) in the SEER registry between 2004 and 2015 revealed a stable incidence of 0.4 cases/1,000,000 persons.[7] Eosinophilias with recurrent genetic abnormalities [platelet-derived growth factor receptor-α/β (*PDGFRA/B*) and fibroblast growth factor receptor-1 (*FGFR1*)] are yet even more rare, representing approximately 10% cases of initially unexplained eosinophilias in developed countries.[8] SEER identified a peak age range at diagnosis of 65 to 74 years, with cases uncommonly diagnosed in infants and children. The male to female ratio of HES/CEL is approximately 1.5:1, but *FIP1L1-PDGFRA*–positive disease is almost exclusively diagnosed in men, a phenomenon whose biologic basis remains unknown.[6,8]

EOSINOPHIL PHYSIOLOGY

Eosinophil-committed hematopoietic progenitors are identified within the CD34$^+$ progenitor population as interleukin-5 receptor (IL5R)$^+$/CCR3$^+$ cells.[9] Their production is tightly regulated by a network of eosinophilopoietic cytokines. IL-5, IL-3, and granulocyte-macrophage colony–stimulating factor are the most relevant to eosinophil physiology and are primarily responsible for the commitment, proliferation, and differentiation of hematopoietic progenitors into the eosinophil lineage.[4,10] These factors are elaborated by several cell types, including T lymphocytes, mast cells, and stromal cells, and bind to their respective receptors on eosinophils.[11] Migration of eosinophils from the circulation to tissues is mediated via interactions between endothelial cell adhesion molecules, such as intercellular adhesion molecule 1 and vascular cell adhesion molecule-1, and eosinophil surface integrins (e.g., the α1 and β2 integrins VLA-4 and CD18, respectively).[12] Eosinophil migration is influenced by several potent eosinophil chemoattractants, including leukotriene β4, complement fragment 5a, platelet-activating factor, RANTES, and eotaxins, which are ligands for the eosinophil receptor CCR3.[13-15] Although eosinophils serve as an essential component of the immune system's normal homeostatic function, including defense against infection and recruitment in response to allergy and inflammation, the potential for collateral

Table 86.1. Modern Classification and Clinicopathologic Landmarks in Eosinophilic Disorders

Year	Event
1968	Term *hypereosinophilic syndrome* coined by Hardy and Anderson
1975	Diagnostic criteria for HES established by Chusid and colleagues
1994	Characterization of the first *PDGFRB* rearrangement (*ETV6-PDGFRB*), t(5; 12) (q31-33; p13)
1994	First description of lymphocyte-variant hypereosinophilia
1998	Identification of rearrangement of the *FGFR1* gene as the basis for the 8p11 syndrome
2001	WHO diagnostic criteria for HES and CEL
2001-2002	Successful empiric treatment of HES patients with imatinib
2002	Characterization of the first *PDGFRA* rearrangement (*BCR-PDGFRA*), t(4; 22) (q12q11)
2003	Identification of the FIP1L1-PDGFRα fusion as the therapeutic target of imatinib
2003	Identification of *FIP1L1-PDGFRA* using the surrogate test "FISH for the *CHIC2* deletion"
2008	WHO criteria include the category of "Myeloid and lymphoid neoplasms with eosinophilia and abnormalities of *PDGFRA*, *PDGFRB*, or *FGFR1*"
2022	WHO and ICC Classifications for renamed category "Myeloid/lymphoid neoplasms with eosinophilia and tyrosine kinase gene fusions" which include rearranged *PDGFRA, PDGFRB, FGFR1, JAK2, FLT3,* and *ETV6::ABL1*

Abbreviations: CEL, chronic eosinophilic leukemia; *FGFR1*, fibroblast growth factor receptor-1; FISH, fluorescent in situ hybridization; HES, hypereosinophilic syndrome; ICC, International Consensus Classification; *PDGFRA*; platelet-derived growth factor receptor-α; *PDGFRB*, platelet-derived growth factor receptor-β; WHO, World Health Organization.

tissue injury exists because of mediators released from eosinophils undergoing marked or persistent activation. These biologically active molecules are released from intracellular granule compartments and include preformed substances, such as major basic protein, eosinophil peroxidase, eosinophil cationic protein, and eosinophil-derived neurotoxin.[4] Eosinophils also contain hydrolytic enzymes, such as acid phosphatase, catalase, arylsulfatase, and newly synthesized mediators, such as hydrogen peroxide, that can contribute to organ damage.[4]

MODERN CLASSIFICATION

In 2022, the fifth edition of the World Health Organization (WHO) classification and the new International Consensus Classification (ICC), primary eosinophilic neoplasms are included among the myeloproliferative neoplasms (MPNs), and also serve as a major category.[16,17] Both new classifications renamed the 2016 WHO major category of "Myeloid/lymphoid neoplasms with eosinophilia and rearrangement of *PDGFRA*, *PDGFRB*, or *FGFR1* or with *PCM1-JAK2*." to `Myeloid/lymphoid neoplasms with eosinophilia and tyrosine kinase gene fusions." This group now includes not only rearrangements involving *PDGFRA*, *PDGFRB*, and *FGFR1*, but all fusion genes involving *JAK2* (not just *PCM1*), as well as *FLT3*, and *ETV6::ABL1*. While eosinophilia is not an invariable feature of these neoplasms, it can serve as a pre-diagnostic checkpoint to consider these rare (and often overlooked) entities in the differential diagnosis.

Both the WHO and ICC classifications detailed similar diagnostic criteria for chronic eosinophilic leukemia.[16,17] The WHO classification removed the qualifier "NOS" and the time interval required to define sustained hypereosinophilia is reduced from 6 months to 4 weeks.[16] The ICC criteria for CEL are shown in *Table 86.3*.[17] Both classifications stress the importance of dysplastic bone marrow morphology as an important diagnostic criterion to distinguish CEL vs HES, with dysplastic megakaryocytes with or without dysplasia in other cell lineages and bone marrow fibrosis as common findings in CEL. In the absence of increased bone marrow or peripheral blood blasts, or a clonal cytogenetic abnormality and/or somatic mutation(s), bone marrow findings suggestive of the diagnosis can suffice in the presence of persistent eosinophilia provided other causes of eosinophilia have been ruled out. Although next-generation sequencing can be helpful in identifying somatic mutations, suggestive of CEL, these may alternatively represent clonal hematopoiesis of indeterminate potential and the presence of mutation(s) in isolation are not sufficient to diagnose CEL or most other myeloid neoplasms. The diagnostic criteria of HES, first formulated by Chusid and colleagues, are now formally outlined by the WHO[16] and ICC (*Table 86.3*),[17] but the original requirement that eosinophilia persists for more than 6 months is no longer consistently embraced. This relates to the faster-paced and more sophisticated evaluation of eosinophilia that is now feasible, and the recognition that early treatment can be critical to mitigating eosinophilia-mediated organ damage. The distinction between "idiopathic HE" and "idiopathic HES" reflects the requirement that organ damage be present in the latter. "Lymphocyte-variant HE" (*Table 86.4*) is a diagnostic entity that is referred to in the WHO and ICC classifications and should be considered before committing to the diagnosis of idiopathic HE or HES, which are diagnoses of exclusion.[16,17]

In 2011, members from the Working Conference on Eosinophil Disorders and Syndromes proposed a new terminology for eosinophilic syndromes.[19] In 2022, an updated consensus was published by the Working Conference.[20] The panel recommended the higher level term *hypereosinophilia* for persistent and marked eosinophilia (AEC > 1.5×10^9/L). In turn, HE subtypes were divided into a hereditary (familial) variant (HE_{FA}), HE of undetermined significance (HE_{US}), primary (clonal/neoplastic) HE produced by clonal/neoplastic eosinophils (HE_N), and secondary (reactive) HE (HE_R). HE_{US} was introduced as a novel term in lieu of "idiopathic HE." Any HE (not just idiopathic) associated with organ damage is referred to as "HES" with specific variants designated by subscripts (e.g., HES_{US}, HES_N, and HES_R). Additional recommendations advanced by the consensus panel are summarized in their report.[19]

DIAGNOSTIC EVALUATION FOR HYPEREOSINOPHILIA

In addition to a hematology consultation, a multidisciplinary evaluation, including allergy/immunology, dermatology, and infectious diseases/tropical medicine, may be required to identify the etiology of HE. The workup of HE (*Figure 86.1*) should commence with a thorough evaluation of reactive causes, with particular attention to comorbid health conditions, medications, and travel history/environmental exposures. Helminth infections are the most common cause of HE in developing countries, and hypersensitivity/atopy is the most frequent etiology in industrialized nations. In addition to infection and hypersensitivity conditions, other secondary causes of HE include connective tissue disorders (Churg-Strauss syndrome, granulomatosis with polyangiitis [Wegener], and systemic lupus erythematosus), solid or hematologic malignancies, metabolic disorders (e.g., adrenal insufficiency), eosinophilic pulmonary diseases, and rare entities such as familial eosinophilia,[21] hyperimmunoglobulin (Ig)E syndrome, Omenn syndrome, episodic angioedema and eosinophilia (Gleich syndrome), and eosinophilia-myalgia syndrome (possibly related to tryptophan ingestion and the historical epidemic of toxic-oil syndrome).[22,23]

In addition to a complete blood count with a white blood cell (WBC) count differential to measure the severity of eosinophilia, the initial laboratory workup for reactive causes of HE typically includes stool culture and serial ova and parasite testing, and sometimes serologic testing for specific parasites (e.g., strongyloides antibody). Testing for specific bacteria, fungi, or viruses may also be warranted in selected cases. The use of chest X-ray, electrocardiogram and/or echocardiography, and computed tomography scan of the chest or abdomen/pelvis is similarly guided by the patient's symptoms and physical examination findings. Imaging studies may help discern the basis for eosinophilia, establish the presence or severity of organ damage, and guide the need for tissue biopsy. For eosinophilic lung diseases, pulmonary function testing, bronchoscopy, and serologic tests (e.g., *Aspergillus* IgE to evaluate for allergic bronchopulmonary aspergillosis) may be obtained to further characterize lung involvement.

If secondary causes of eosinophilia are excluded, the workup should proceed to the evaluation of a primary bone marrow disorder. Bone marrow aspirate and trephine biopsy with cytogenetics and

Table 86.2. Primary Eosinophilic Neoplasms in the 2022 International Consensus Classification[a]

Myeloproliferative Neoplasms
Chronic myeloid leukemia
Polycythemia vera
Essential thrombocythemia

Primary myelofibrosis
    Early/prefibrotic primary myelofibrosis
    Overt primary myelofibrosis

Chronic neutrophilic leukemia
Chronic eosinophilic leukemia, not otherwise specified
MPN, unclassifiable
Myeloid/lymphoid neoplasms with eosinophilia and tyrosine kinase gene fusions
Myeloid/lymphoid neoplasm with *PDGFRA* rearrangement
Myeloid/lymphoid neoplasm with *PDGFRB* rearrangement
Myeloid/lymphoid neoplasm with *FGFR1* rearrangement
Myeloid/lymphoid neoplasm with *JAK2* rearrangement
Myeloid/lymphoid neoplasm with *FLT3* rearrangement
Myeloid/lymphoid neoplasm with *ETV6::ABL1*

[a]Primary eosinophilic neoplasms are noted in red font.
Adapted from Arber DA, Orazi A, Hasserjian RP, et al. International Consensus Classification of Myeloid Neoplasms and Acute Leukemias: integrating morphologic, clinical, and genomic data. *Blood*. 2022;140(11):1200-1228. Table 1. Copyright © American Society of Hematology. With permission.

Table 86.3. International Consensus Classification Diagnostic Criteria for Chronic Eosinophilic Leukemia, Not Otherwise Specified (CEL, NOS) and Idiopathic Hypereosinophilic Syndrome (HES)

Chronic Eosinophilic Leukemia, Not Otherwise Specified (CEL, NOS)
1. Peripheral blood hypereosinophilia (eosinophil count ≥ 1.5 x 10^9/L and eosinophils ≥ 10% of white blood cells)
2. Blasts constitute < 20% cells in peripheral blood and bone marrow, not meeting other diagnostic criteria for AML*
3. No tyrosine kinase gene fusion including *BCR::ABL1*, other *ABL1*, *PDGFRA*, *PDGFRB*, *FGFR1*, *JAK2*, or *FLT3* fusions
4. Not meeting criteria for other well-defined MPN; chronic myelomonocytic leukemia, or SM†
5. Bone marrow shows increased cellularity with dysplastic megakaryocytes with or without dysplastic features in other lineages and often significant fibrosis, associated with an eosinophilic infiltrate or increased blasts ≥ 5% in the bone marrow and/or ≥ 2% in the peripheral blood
6. Demonstration of a clonal cytogenetic abnormality and/or somatic mutation(s)‡
The diagnosis of CEL requires all 6 criteria.
Idiopathic Hypereosinophilic Syndrome (HES)
1. Persistent peripheral blood hypereosinophilia (eosinophil count ≥ 1.5 x 10^9/L and ≥ 10% eosinophils)**
2. Organ damage and/or dysfunction attributable to tissue eosinophilic infiltrate††
3. No evidence of a reactive, well-defined autoimmune disease or neoplastic condition/disorder underlying the hypereosinophilia
4. Exclusion of lymphocyte variant hypereosinophilic syndrome‡
5. Bone marrow morphologically within normal limits except for increased eosinophils
6. No molecular genetic clonal abnormality, with the caveat of clonal hematopoiesis of indeterminate potential (CHIP)
The diagnosis of iHES requires all 6 criteria.

*AML with recurrent genetic abnormalities with <20% blasts is excluded.
†Eosinophilia can be seen in association with SM. However, "true" CEL, NOS may occur as SM-AMN (SM with an associated myeloid malignancies). ‡In the absence of a clonal cytogenetic abnormality and/or somatic mutation(s) or increased blasts, bone marrow findings supportive of the diagnosis will suffice in the presence of persistent eosinophilia, provided other causes of eosinophilia having been excluded.
**Preferably a minimal duration of 6 months if documentation is available.
††Hypereosinophilia of uncertain significance has no tissue damage, but otherwise fulfills the same diagnostic criteria.
‡An abnormal T-cell population must be detected immunophenotypically with or without T-cell receptor clonality by molecular analysis.
Abbreviations: AML, acute myeloid leukemia; MPN, myeloproliferative neoplasm; SM, systemic mastocytosis.
Adapted from Arber DA, Orazi A, Hasserjian RP, et al. International Consensus Classification of Myeloid Neoplasms and Acute Leukemias: integrating morphologic, clinical, and genomic data. *Blood*. 2022;140(11):1200-1228. Tables 7 and 8. Copyright © American Society of Hematology. With permission.

immunophenotyping (with relevant iron and reticulin/trichrome stains) are useful to elucidate WHO-defined clonal myeloid neoplasms associated with eosinophilia, such as AML, specifically AML with inv(16)(p13.1; q22) or t(16; 16) (p13.1; q22), CML or other MPNs (e.g., SM), and overlap MDS/MPN disorders, such as chronic myelomonocytic leukemia (CMML).[18]

Multigene mutation panels are now more commonly employed to ascertain whether cases of idiopathic HE or HES may carry one or more pathogenic myeloid mutations, which could potentially define cases such as CEL-NOS. For example, among 426 patients in the German Registry with HE of unknown significance, *KIT* D816V and *JAK*2 V617F mutations were identified in 3% and 4% of patients, respectively.[24] Another study found myeloid mutations in 14 of 51 patients with a diagnosis of HES, including a single mutated gene in seven patients and two or more mutated genes in another seven patients. The most commonly mutated genes were *ASXL1* (43%), *TET2* (36%), *EZH2* (29%), *SETBP1* (22%), *CBL* (14%), and *NOTCH1* (14%).[25] Patients with HES ultimately found to have positive sequencing results exhibited a prognosis that was inferior to HES patients without mutation findings, but similar to patients with CEL-NOS.[25]

Myeloid malignancies primarily defined by eosinophilia include the aforementioned CEL-NOS and the category of myeloid/lymphoid neoplasms with eosinophilia and tyrosine kinase gene fusions. Diagnostic assessment of primary eosinophilia should begin with screening of the peripheral blood for the *FIP1L1-PDGFRA* gene fusion by interphase or metaphase fluorescence in situ hybridization (FISH).[26] Less commonly, reverse transcriptase-polymerase chain reaction (RT-PCR) is used to detect the fusion. FISH probes that hybridize between the *FIP1L1* and *PDGFRA* loci detect the 800-kb interstitial deletion on chromosome 4q12 that results in gene fusion. Because the *CHIC2* gene is located in this deleted genetic segment, the test has been referred to as "FISH for the *CHIC2* deletion."[27] If *FIP1L1-PDGFRA* screening is not available, serum tryptase has been used as a surrogate marker for *FIP1L1-PDGFRA*–positive disease because increased levels have been associated with the fusion or myeloproliferative forms of HE.[28] In contrast to *FIP1L1-PDGFRA*, which is not detectable by standard karyotyping, rearrangements involving *PDGFRB* and *FGFR1* can be inferred by cytogenetic analysis, represented by the breakpoints 5q31 to 33 (*PDGFRB*) and 8p11 to 12 (*FGFR1*), respectively.[16,17] Reciprocal chromosomal translocations involving the breakpoints 9p24 or 13q12 may relate to *JAK2* (e.g., *PCM1-JAK2*; *BCR-JAK2*) or *FLT3* (e.g., *ETV6-FLT3*) fusions, respectively, and have been associated with myeloid/lymphoid neoplasms with eosinophilia.[29,30] Knowledge of these breakpoints is critical because targeted therapy may have clinical efficacy against these constitutively activated tyrosine kinases. Bone marrow biopsy studies, as highlighted previously, should be performed to complement peripheral blood analyses.

If both secondary and primary causes of eosinophilias are excluded, lymphocyte-variant HE should be considered next in the diagnostic algorithm.[31] Patients with lymphocyte-variant HE often have cutaneous signs and symptoms as the primary disease manifestation. Although patients' skin disease can be symptomatic, the natural history of this condition is typically indolent, with rare patients progressing to T-cell lymphoma or Sézary syndrome. Progression has been associated with acquisition of cytogenetic abnormalities (e.g., partial 6q and 10p deletions, trisomy 7) in T cells and with proliferation of lymphocytes with the CD3−CD4+ phenotype.[32-35] This syndrome represents a mixture of clonal and reactive processes, resulting in the expansion of a clone of T lymphocytes that produce cytokines that drive eosinophilia.[31,36,37] Although these laboratory findings constitute basic elements of this syndrome, neither the WHO nor other consensus panels have established specific diagnostic criteria for this condition.[16-19] The finding of isolated T-cell clonality by PCR without

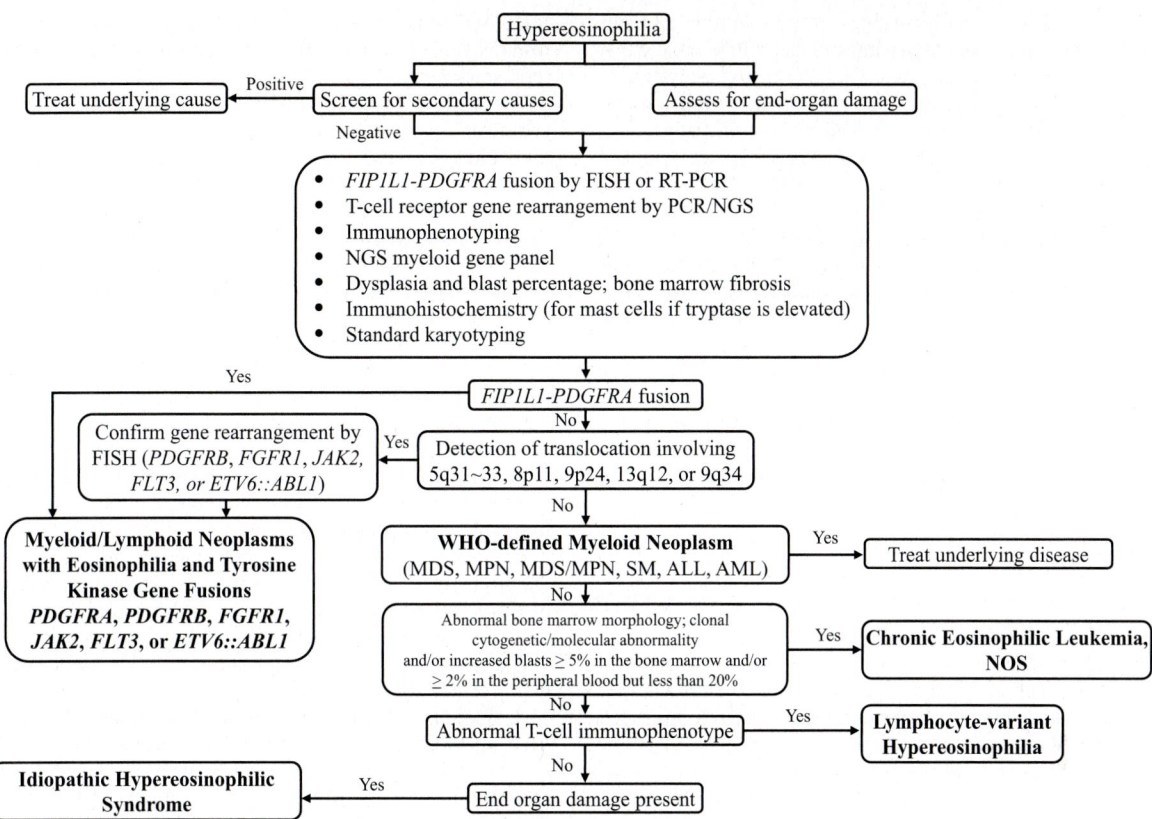

FIGURE 86.1 Diagnostic algorithm for hypereosinophilia. ALL, acute lymphoblastic leukemia; AML, acute myeloid leukemia; FGFR1, fibroblast growth factor receptor-1; FISH, fluorescence in situ hybridization; NOS, not otherwise specified; PDGFA/B, platelet-derived growth factor receptor-α/β; RT-PCR, reverse transcriptase-polymerase chain reaction. (Adapted from Shomali W, Gotlib J. World Health Organization-defined eosinophilic disorders: 2022 update on diagnosis, risk stratification, and management. *Am J Hematol.* 2022;97(1):129-148. Copyright © 2021 Wiley Periodicals LLC. Reprinted by permission of John Wiley & Sons, Inc.)

T-cell immunophenotypic abnormalities or demonstration of Th2 cytokine production is not sufficient to make a diagnosis of this variant.[36] In an analysis of patients diagnosed with HES, 18 (43%) of 42 subjects exhibited a clonal T-cell receptor gene rearrangement by PCR.[38] However, the biologic relevance of such clonal T-cell populations to eosinophilia was not established.[38] Therefore, whether such patients should still be referred to as HES, or as lymphocyte-variant HE, remains a matter of debate. Laboratory features that suggest this disorder are shown in *Table 86.4*.

BIOLOGY OF FIP1L1-PDGFRA

FIP1L1-PDGFRA can promote the proliferation and survival of eosinophils through the activation of several signaling pathways, such as phosphoinositide 3-kinase (PI3 kinase), ERK1/2, and STAT5.[26,39] The exact mechanism by which FIP1L1-PDGFRA preferentially affects eosinophils remains unclear. It was found that in vitro inhibition of JAK2 in the *FIP1L1-PDGFRA*–positive EOL-1 cell line, primary *FIP1L1-PDGFRA*–positive cells, and T674I *FIP1L1-PDGFRA*-imatinib–resistant cells, either by JAK2-specific short-interfering RNA or by the tyrphostin derivative AG490 (a JAK inhibitor), significantly reduced cellular proliferation and induced cellular apoptosis.[40] JAK2 inhibition also reduced PI3 kinase, AKT, and nuclear factor κB activity in a dose-dependent manner, and suppressed expression levels of c-myc and survivin.[40] The results suggest that JAK2 is activated by FIP1L1-PDGFRA and is required for cellular proliferation, possibly through induction of c-myc and survivin.

In one murine model, expression of the *FIP1L1-PDGFRA* fusion in bone marrow cells was not sufficient to cause eosinophilia, but only a general myeloproliferative disease.[41] However, in another murine model, the expression of *FIP1L1-PDGFRA* together with overexpression of IL-5, a potent eosinophilopoietic cytokine, mimicked more typical features of HES, such as tissue infiltration of eosinophils.[42]

Polymorphic variation at the IL-5 receptor-a (*IL5RA*) gene revealed an association between a single-nucleotide polymorphism in the 5′ untranslated region of *IL5RA* and the eosinophil count/presence of tissue infiltration in *FIP1L1-PDGFRA*–positive patients.[43] These data suggest that *FIP1L1-PDGFRA* alone is not sufficient to explain the development of HES/CEL and that additional factors, such as IL-5 signaling, may also be implicated in the disease phenotype.

The structure of the FIP1L1-PDGFRA fusion protein is similar to the structure of the ETV6-PDGFRA, ZMYM2-FGFR1 (formerly ZNF198-FGFR1), and BCR-ABL1 proteins, for which homotypic oligomerization mediated by domains within ETV6, ZMYM2, or BCR has been reported.[44-46] Oligomerization of the corresponding fusion proteins leads to the activation of the tyrosine kinase domains, which, in turn, activate

Table 86.4. Laboratory Findings in Lymphocyte-Variant Hypereosinophilia

1. Cytokine-producing abnormal T-lymphocyte population with aberrant immunophenotype
   a. Double-negative, immature T cells (e.g., CD3⁺CD4⁻CD8⁻), or
   b. Absence of CD3 (e.g., CD3⁻CD4⁺), a normal component of the T-cell receptor, or
   c. Elevated CD5 expression on CD3⁻CD4⁺ cells, or
   d. Loss of surface CD7 and/or expression of CD27
2. Reactive eosinophilia in response to T-lymphocyte secretion of eosinophilopoietic cytokines
3. Elevated serum IgE levels
4. Lymphocyte production of cytokines (e.g., IL-5, IL-4, IL-13) suggesting Th2 cytokine profile
5. Elevated production of TARC, a chemokine in Th2-mediated diseases

Abbreviations: IL, interleukin; TARC, thymus and activation-regulated chemokine; Th2, T cells with helper type 2.

downstream signaling pathways regulating cell proliferation and survival. In contrast, interruption of the juxtamembrane of PDGFRA, either as a result of mutations or duplications, causes constitutive activation of kinase activity.[47,48] This mechanism occurs with internal tandem duplications in *FLT3* and mutations of *KIT* in AML or gastrointestinal stromal tumors.[49,50] Fusion of FIP1L1 to the PDGFRA protein yields a constitutively active tyrosine kinase only if the juxtamembrane domain of PDGFRA is partially or completely removed.[51] The different breakpoints within the *PDGFRA* gene are tightly clustered, resulting in the removal of part of the juxtamembrane domain and activation of the kinase domain.[52] In contrast, with many PDGFRB fusions, the juxtamembrane is completely intact, and activation of PDGFRB kinase activity is obtained through oligomerization mediated by the fusion partner.

In addition to dysregulation of *PDGFRA* by fusion to *FIP1L1* or other partner genes, activating point mutations have been identified in *PDGFRA* in patients with HE.[50] Although there was variability in their transforming ability, injection of cells harboring these mutants into mice induced a leukemia-like disease. Imatinib treatment significantly decreased leukemic growth and prolonged survival.[53]

CLINICAL PRESENTATION AND PROGNOSIS

Clinicopathologic Features

Patients with *FIP1L1-PDGFRA*–associated eosinophilia present with features of an MPN: splenomegaly, hypercellular bone marrows, and clinicopathologic characteristics that overlap with systemic mast cell disease, including increased numbers of abnormal-appearing bone marrow mast cells, marrow fibrosis, and elevated serum tryptase levels (see *Figure 86.2*).[28,52] Soon after the discovery of the fusion, a debate arose regarding whether *FIP1L1-PDGFRA*–positive disease represents a subtype of SM rather than a primary eosinophilic neoplasm because atypical mast cells can be found in the marrows of these patients. Bone marrow biopsies of *FIP1L1-PDGFRA*–positive patients commonly demonstrate a loose, interstitial pattern of mast cells by tryptase immunostaining rather than the multifocal dense aggregates characteristic of *KIT* D816V-positive SM.[54] The mast cells often exhibit spindle-shaped morphology and aberrant surface expression of CD25, both WHO minor criteria for SM. However, in the 2008 WHO classification, this entity was not considered a subtype of SM, but instead was included in the new category "Myeloid and lymphoid neoplasms with eosinophilia and abnormalities of *PDGFRA*, *PDGFRB*, or *FGFR1*."[16] The distinction between *KIT* D816V-positive SM with eosinophilia (now more commonly referred to as SM-CEL) and *FIP1L1-PDGFRA*–positive eosinophilia was evaluated using several clinical and laboratory features.[55] In the *KIT* D816V-positive SM cohort, gastrointestinal symptoms, urticaria pigmentosa, thrombocytosis, median serum tryptase value, and the presence of dense marrow mast cell aggregates were significantly elevated or more frequently represented compared to patients with *FIP1L1-PDGFRA*–positive disease. Conversely, male sex, cardiac and pulmonary symptoms, median peak AEC, the eosinophil to tryptase ratio, and serum B12 levels were significantly elevated or more frequently represented in the *FIP1L1-PDGFRA*–positive group. A scoring system that incorporated these findings was devised that could reliably predict these two diagnostic entities.

Although *FIP1L1-PDGFRA* positivity is almost always associated with the phenotype of a chronic MPN, the fusion may be rarely found in AMLs or T-cell leukemias/lymphomas associated with eosinophilia.[56] In addition to the *FIP1L1-PDGFRA* fusion gene, 7 *PDGFRA* fusion genes, as well as >35 different *PDGFRB* genes, have been described in MPNs with eosinophilia (*Figure 86.3*).[57] Among 56,709 cytogenetically defined cases at the Mayo Clinic, only 25 (0.04%) exhibited the t(5;12) breakpoint.[58] The classic variant t(5;12) (q33; p13), likely representing the *ETV6-PDGFRB* gene fusion, was present in only four of these cases.[58] Despite the rare frequency (<<1%) of *PDGFRB* rearrangements in cytogenetically defined cases with features of CMML and other myeloid neoplasms (e.g., atypical CML, juvenile myelomonocytic leukemia, chronic basophilic leukemia, and MDS/MPN unclassifiable),[58] their recognition is critical given their responsiveness to imatinib. However, not all 5q31~q33 breakpoints represent the *PDGFRB* gene. For example, IL-3 (on chromosome 5q31) is fused to the Ig heavy chain gene (chromosome 14q32) in a subset of eosinophilia-associated B-cell acute lymphoblastic leukemias (ALLs).[59] In addition, in cases of MDS/AML with associated eosinophilia and a t(5; 12) (q31; p13), an *ETV6-ACS2* gene fusion was identified.[60] Finally, 16 fusion partners of *FGFR1* have been described, of which *ZMYM2* and *BCR* are the most common; these cases have been historically referred to as "8p11 myeloproliferative syndrome" or "stem cell leukemia/lymphoma" (*Figure 86.3*).[57]

Clinical Presentation

In two retrospective series of HES, eosinophilia was an incidental finding in 6% to 12% of patients with HE.[61,62] In a study of 188 patients, the mean peak eosinophil count was 6.6×10^9/L (range $1.5\text{-}400 \times 10^9$/L).[62] Primary marrow eosinophilias, also referred to as "myeloproliferative variants of eosinophilia," may be characterized by blood or bone marrow neutrophilia, basophilia, and myeloid immaturity. Eosinophil morphology can be normal or abnormal in marrow-derived eosinophilias and cannot be used as a distinguishing feature between reactive and primary eosinophilias. Marrow findings of Charcot-Leyden crystals, increased blasts, and fibrosis are found in a spectrum of eosinophilic myeloid neoplasms and are not unique to CEL-NOS or myeloid neoplasms with eosinophilia and rearrangements of *PDGRA/B* or *FGFR1*.[16,18]

Common nonhematologic signs and symptoms of HES include (in descending frequency) weakness and fatigue (26%), cough (24%), dyspnea (16%), myalgias or angioedema (14%), rash or fever (12%), and rhinitis (10%).[63] In follow-up of patients with sustained eosinophilia, skin involvement was the most frequent clinical manifestation (69% of patients), followed by pulmonary (44%) and gastrointestinal (38%) findings.[62] Cardiac sequelae (unrelated to hypertension, atherosclerosis, or rheumatic disease) were eventually identified in 20% of patients at follow-up (only 6% at the time of initial presentation).[62] *Table 86.5* presents the frequency and type of organ system involvement from three historical studies.[61,64,65]

Prognosis

Older case series identify cardiac disease as the primary etiology of premature death. A review of 57 HES cases published through 1973 reported a median survival of 9 months, and the 3-year survival rate was only 12%.[3] Patients usually presented with advanced disease, with congestive heart failure accounting for 65% of deaths at autopsy. In addition to cardiac involvement, peripheral blood blasts and a WBC count greater than 100×10^9/L were poor prognostic factors.[3] A later report of 40 HES patients cited a 5-year survival rate of 80%, decreasing to 42% at 15 years.[64] Factors predictive of a worse outcome included the presence of an MPN, corticosteroid-refractory HE, cardiac disease, male sex, and the height of eosinophilia.[64]

A Mayo Clinic retrospective review of 247 HES patients identified 23 subjects who died during the 19-year review period. The cause of death was identified in 15 (65%) patients and included cardiac dysfunction (33%), infection (20%), unrelated malignancy (20%), thromboembolic events (13%), and vascular disease (13%).[66] In a multivariate analysis of 98 patients with HES and idiopathic HE [62], age >60 years, hemoglobin <10 g/dL, cardiac involvement, and hepatosplenomegaly were associated with inferior overall survival (OS).[67] 11 patients (11%) harbored a pathogenetic mutation in one of the following genes: *TET2*, *ASXL1*, *KIT*, *IDH2*, *JAK2*, *SF3B1*, and *TP53*, but the presence of one of the mutations was only significant in a univariate analysis of survival.

WHO-defined CEL-NOS carries a poor prognosis. In a cohort of 10 patients, the median survival was 22.2 months, and 5 of 10 patients developed AML after median of 20 months following diagnosis.[68] Three of five patients who did not develop AML died with active disease; one patient underwent an allogeneic hematopoietic stem cell transplant and maintained a long-term remission; the remaining patient achieved a

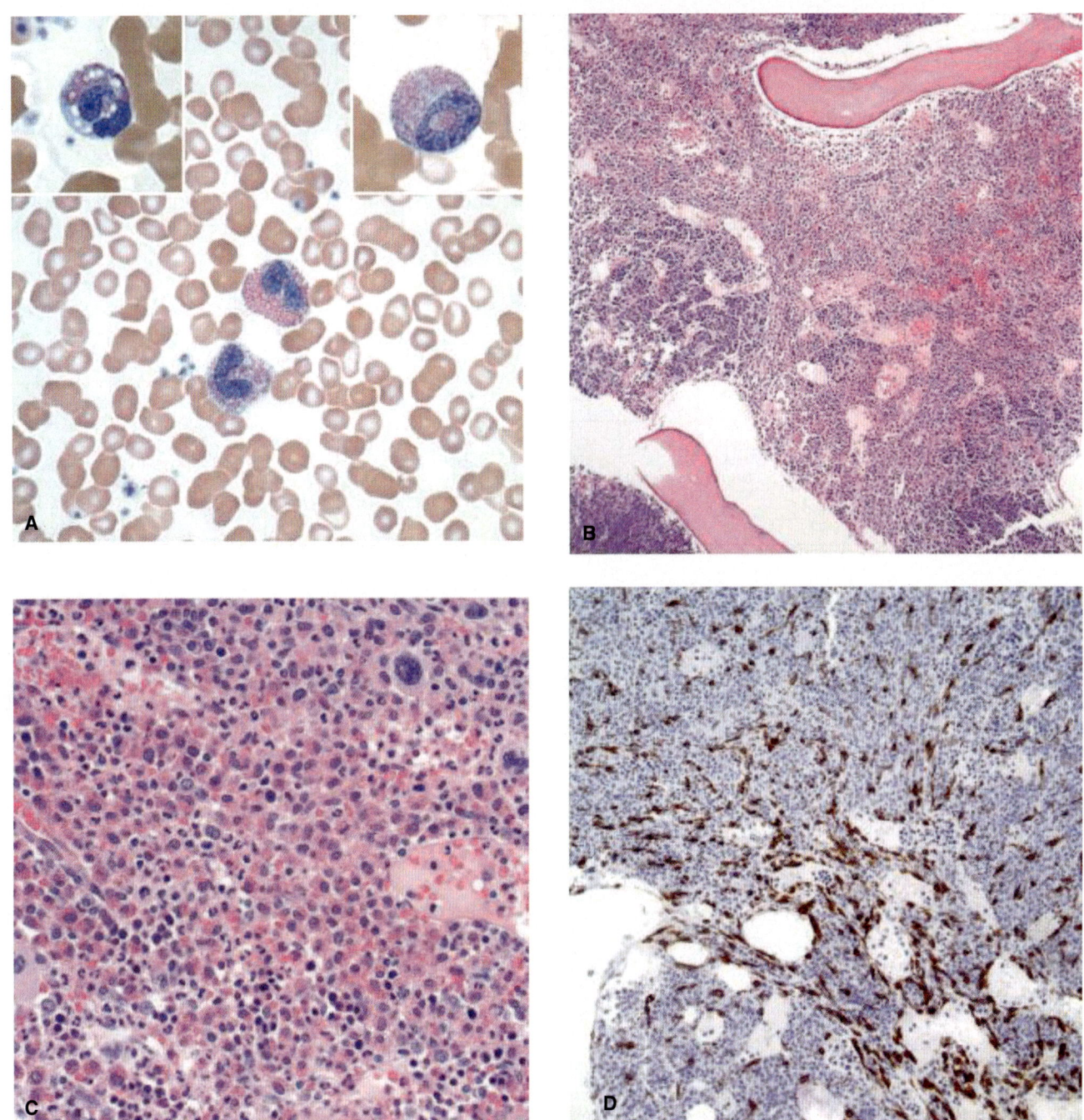

FIGURE 86.2 Histopathology of a *FIP1L1-PDGFRA*–positive myeloid neoplasm associated with eosinophilia. A peripheral eosinophilia is present with an absolute eosinophil count of 2.48 × 10⁹/L. Eosinophils include atypical forms with ring nuclei (inset, right), vacuolated cytoplasm (inset, left), as well as irregularly granulated eosinophils (A) Wright-Giemsa, ×1000. The bone marrow biopsy is hypercellular for age with dilated marrow sinuses, a feature associated with marrow fibrosis (B) hematoxylin and eosin, ×100. The bone marrow biopsy shows a myeloid hyperplasia with a marked eosinophilia (C) hematoxylin and eosin, ×400. Loose aggregates of mast cells are present in the bone marrow biopsy as shown by immunohistochemistry, but were not readily visible on hematoxylin- and eosin-stained sections (D) CD117, ×200. (Images provided courtesy of Dr. Tracy George.)

complete remission (CR) on imatinib and hydroxyurea.[68] In a second series of 17 CEL patients from Mayo Clinic, 18% of patients progressed to AML and the median overall survival was 16 months.[69]

The historical, shortened life expectancy related to heart damage provides a useful example of the consequences of eosinophil-mediated tissue injury. It is typically a stepwise process resulting from local infiltration and release of toxic mediators.[61,65] Damage to the endocardium can lead to local deposition of platelet thrombi, and subsequently to larger mural thrombi and increased risk of thromboembolic disease. With time, fibrous thickening of the endocardial lining and leaflets of the mitral and tricuspid valves can result in a restrictive cardiomyopathy and valvular insufficiency.[70,71] Advances in cardiac surgery have reduced morbidity and mortality related to eosinophil-mediated heart damage.

In WHO-defined myeloid malignancies, the prognostic importance of associated eosinophilia has only been studied in a few diseases. In a series of 123 patients with SM, eosinophilia was prevalent in 34% of cases, but was prognostically neutral and not affected by exclusion of *FIP1L1-PDGFRA*–positive cases.[72] In a study of 1008 patients with de novo MDS, eosinophilia (and basophilia) predicted a significantly reduced survival without having a significant impact on leukemia-free survival.[73] A retrospective analysis of 288 individuals

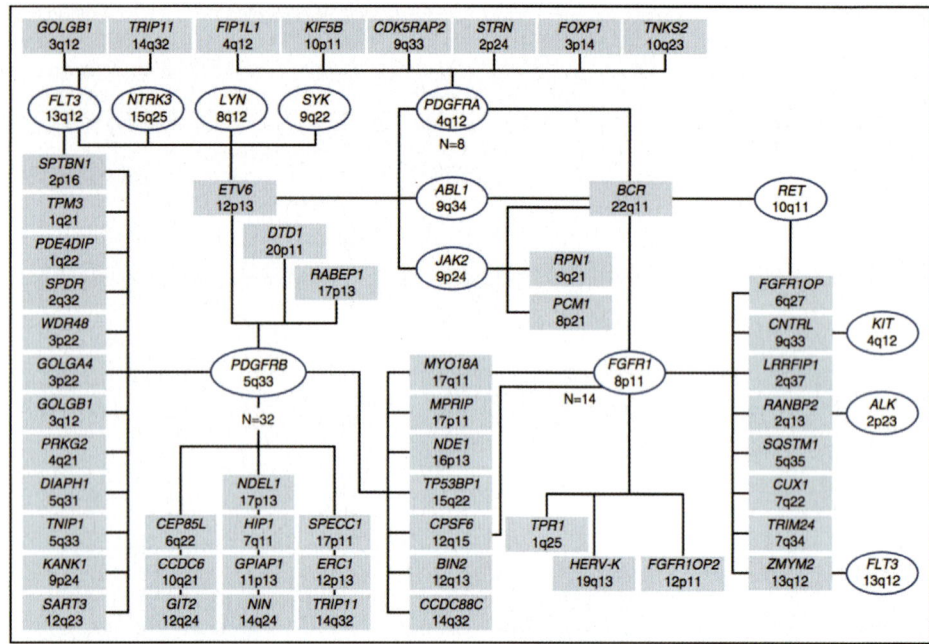

FIGURE 86.3 Fusion tyrosine kinase genes associated with myeloid/lymphoid neoplasms and eosinophilia. As of October 2016, 72 tyrosine kinase fusion genes had been described. (Figure courtesy of Professor Nicholas C. P. Cross. Reprinted from Reiter A, Gotlib J. Myeloid neoplasms with eosinophilia. *Blood.* 2017;129(6):704-714. Copyright © 2017 American Society of Hematology. With permission.)

Table 86.5. Organ Manifestations of Eosinophilic Neoplasms/Hypereosinophilic Syndromes

Organ System	Cumulative Frequency From Three Studies (%)[a]	Examples of Organ-Specific Manifestations
Hematologic	100	Leukocytosis with eosinophilia; neutrophilia, basophilia, myeloid immaturity, immature and/or dysplastic eosinophils; anemia, thrombocytopenia or thrombocytosis, increased marrow blasts, myelofibrosis
Cardiovascular	58	Cardiomyopathy, congestive heart failure, constrictive pericarditis, myocarditis, mural thrombi, valvular dysfunction, endomyocardial fibrosis, myocardial infarction, pericardial effusion, deep venous thrombosis, superficial thrombophlebitis
Dermatologic	56	Angioedema, urticaria, papules/nodules, dermatitis, plaques, (aquagenic) pruritus, erythroderma, mucosal ulcers, vesiculobullous lesions, microthrombi, vasculitis, Wells syndrome
Neurologic	54	Thromboembolic stroke, peripheral neuropathy, encephalopathy, dementia, epilepsy, cerebellar disease, eosinophilic meningitis, vertigo, paresthesia, change in mentation, aphasia, visual disturbances
Pulmonary	49	Pulmonary infiltrates, effusions, fibrosis, emboli, nodules/focal ground glass attenuation, acute respiratory distress syndrome, asthma, sinusitis, rhinitis, cough, dyspnea, recurrent upper respiratory tract infection
Spleen	43	Splenomegaly, hypersplenism, infarct
Liver/gallbladder	30	Hepatomegaly, focal or diffuse hepatic lesions on imaging, chronic active hepatitis, hepatic necrosis, Budd-Chiari syndrome, sclerosing cholangitis, cholecystitis, cholestasis
Ocular	23	Microthrombi, choroidal infarcts, retinal arteritis, episcleritis, keratoconjunctivitis sicca, Adie syndrome (pupillotonia)
Gastrointestinal	23	Ascites, diarrhea, gastritis, colitis, pancreatitis, abdominal pain, vomiting
Musculoskeletal/rheumatologic	–	Arthritis/arthralgias, effusions, bursitis, synovitis, Raynaud phenomena, digital necrosis, polymyositis/myopathy, myalgias
Renal	–	Acute renal failure with Charcot-Leyden crystalluria, nephrotic syndrome, immunotactoid glomerulopathy, crescentic glomerulonephritis

[a]Data from Fauci AS, Harley JB, Roberts WC, et al. The idiopathic hypereosinophilic syndrome. Clinical, pathophysiologic, and therapeutic considerations. *Ann Intern Med*. 1982;97:78-92; Lefebvre C, Bletry O, Degoulet P, et al. Prognostic factors of hypereosinophilic syndrome. Study of 40 cases. *Ann Med Interne (Paris)*. 1989;140:253-257; and Spry CJ, Davies J, Tai PC, et al. Clinical features of fifteen patients with the hypereosinophilic syndrome. *Q J Med*. 1983;52:1-22.
Adapted from Gotlib J, Cools J, Malone JM III, et al. The FIP1L1-PDGFRa fusion tyrosine kinase in hypereosinophilic syndrome and chronic eosinophilic leukemia: implications for diagnosis, classification, and management. *Blood*. 2004;103(8):2879-2891. Copyright © 2004 American Society of Hematology. With permission.

with newly diagnosed MDS revealed that significantly higher numbers of patients with eosinophilia or basophilia (compared to patients with neither) had chromosomal abnormalities carrying an intermediate or poor prognosis.[74] In addition, the OS rate was significantly lower, and a higher rate of evolution to AML was observed.[74] In a large cohort of 2350 patients with SM from the European Competence Network on Mastocytosis registry, 6.8% had mild eosinophilia and 3.1% had HE.[75] Eosinophilia/HE were mainly present in patients with advanced SM. Eosinophilia at diagnosis was associated with lower OS and progression-free survival (PFS), with 10-year OS of 19% for patients with HE, 70% for those with mild eosinophilia, and 88% for patients with a normal eosinophil count.[75]

Treatment of Patients With Genetically Defined Neoplasms

At the turn of the 21st century, no unique and recurrent clonal marker had been linked to eosinophilic neoplasms despite an ever-growing list of nonspecific chromosomal abnormalities (e.g., trisomy 8) having been cataloged.[76] In 2001, Schaller and Burkland described a male patient with HES who was resistant or intolerant to prior therapies, including corticosteroids, hydroxyurea, and interferon α (IFN-α).[77] The patient was treated with imatinib at least partly based on the rationale that the myeloproliferative features of HES could share a similar pathobiology to CML. After several days of imatinib therapy of 100 mg daily, the patient achieved a rapid and complete hematologic remission with resolution of peripheral blood eosinophilia just after 1 month of treatment. Shortly thereafter, a few case series established that imatinib at doses ranging from 100 to 400 mg daily could produce complete and rapid hematologic responses in patients with heavily pretreated refractory/relapsed HES or CEL.[78,79] In the landmark report published in 2003, the fusion tyrosine kinase FIP1L1-PDGFRα was ultimately identified as the therapeutic target of imatinib in responding patients.[26] At the same time, the *FIP1L1-PDGFRA* fusion was discovered in the imatinib-sensitive EOL-1 cell line by another group of investigators.[80]

Similar to the experience with CML, imatinib has transformed the prognosis of patients with the *FIP1L1-PDGFRA* fusion. In addition to rapid hematologic remissions, molecular remissions can be achieved in the majority of patients with doses in the range of 100 to 400 mg daily and 400 mg daily.[26,69,70] Although maintenance doses of 100 to 200 mg weekly may preserve ongoing molecular remissions in some patients, the optimal dose for maintaining response has not been defined.[81] Because of its good tolerability and safety profile, ongoing therapy with a starting dose of 100 to 400 mg is commonly employed.

The long-term prognosis of imatinib-treated patient with *FIP1L1-PDGFRA*–positive disease is outstanding. In an Italian prospective study of 27 patients followed for a median period of 25 months (range 15-60 months), patients were initially dosed at 100 mg daily and increased to 400 mg daily.[82] Complete hematologic remission was achieved in all patients within 1 month, and all patients became PCR negative for *FIP1L1-PDGFRA* after a median period of 3 months (range 1-10 months). Patients continuing imatinib remained PCR negative during a median follow-up period of 19 months (range 6-56+ months). Another European study prospectively assessed the natural history of molecular responses to imatinib doses of 100 to 400 mg daily.[83] Among 11 patients with high pretreatment transcript levels, all achieved a 3-log reduction in transcript levels by 1 year of therapy, and 9 of 11 patients achieved a molecular remission.

Despite in-depth and durable molecular remissions, discontinuation of imatinib usually leads to disease relapse. In a dose de-escalation trial of imatinib in five patients who had achieved a stable hematologic and molecular remission at 300 to 400 mg daily for at least 1 year, molecular relapse was observed in all patients after 2 to 5 months of either imatinib dose reduction or discontinuation.[84] Molecular remissions were reestablished with reinitiation of imatinib in all patients at a dose range of 100 to 400 mg daily. In a cohort of patients evaluated by the Mayo Clinic, hematologic relapse occurred only several weeks after discontinuation of imatinib in four patients.[85] Recent cohorts reported relapse rates (molecular or hematologic) of 33% to 57% in patients who discontinued imatinib, occurring within a median of 10 months.[86,87] Time to imatinib initiation and duration of imatinib treatment were independent factors of relapse after discontinuation of imatinib.[86] Molecular remissions could be re-established with reinduction of imatinib in most cases at a dose range of 100 to 400 mg daily. These data indicate that prolonged use of imatinib does not cure *FIP1L1-PDGFRA*–positive disease in most individuals, but that treatment-free remission may be feasible in selected patients.

As with CML, *FIP1L1-PDGFRA*–positive patients can develop resistance to imatinib, mostly involving the T674I mutation within the adenosine triphosphate–binding domain of PDGFRA.[26,88-90] T674I *PDGFRA* is analogous to the T315I *ABL1* mutation in CML, which confers pan-resistance to the tyrosine kinase inhibitors imatinib, dasatinib, and nilotinib. However, unlike CML, this secondary resistance is rare and is almost exclusively observed during advanced phases of the disease. In one study, it was found that the PDGFRA kinase domain contains a limited number of residues where exchanges critically interfere with the binding of and inhibition by available PDGFR kinase inhibitors.[91] This may be one explanation for the low frequency of imatinib resistance in these patients.

Options for second-line treatment for T674I imatinib resistance are limited. Reports have demonstrated either in vitro or in vivo activity of sorafenib, midostaurin, or nilotinib against the T674I mutant.[41,92-94] One patient with the *FIP1L1-PDGFRA* T674I mutation in blast crisis responded briefly to sorafenib, but this was followed by rapid emergence of a pan-resistant *FIP1L1-PDGFRA* D842V mutant, which is another default resistance mutation in this disease.[92] Avapritinib is approved by the Food and Drug Administration (FDA) for patients with gastrointestinal stromal tumors harboring *PDGFRA* D842V but has not been studied in patients with *FIP1L1-PDGFRA* fusion harboring this mutation, and T674I confers resistance to avapritinib.[95]

The ability of alternative tyrosine kinase inhibitors to elicit durable clinical remissions (despite in vitro data demonstrating inhibitory activity against mutated fusions) has been disappointing.[96] To date, the only report of primary resistance to imatinib in chronic phase *FIP1L1-PDGFRA*–positive disease has been attributed to the identification of two novel mutations, *PDGFRA* S601P and L629P.[97]

In patients with rearrangements of *PDGFRB* or *PDGFRA* variants other than *FIP1L1-PDGFRA*, case reports and series indicate that imatinib, usually at doses of 400 mg daily, can elicit durable hematologic and cytogenetic remissions.[98] FISH and conventional karyotyping can gauge cytogenetic responses to imatinib in *PDGFRB*-rearranged cases.

Although well tolerated, with a safety profile similar to imatinib used in CML, several cases have been reported in which *FIP1L1-PDGFRA*–positive patients treated with imatinib experienced cardiogenic shock.[99,100] It is, therefore, recommended that for patients with known cardiac disease or elevated troponin levels (possibly related to eosinophil-mediated damage of cardiac tissue), prophylactic steroids should be given for 7 to 10 days at the time of imatinib initiation.

Long-term follow-up (median 10.2 years) of *PDGFRB*-rearranged patients treated with imatinib for a median duration of 6.6 years showed a 96% response rate and a 10-year OS rate of 90%. None of the patients who achieved a complete cytogenetic ($n = 13$) or molecular ($n = 8$) remission lost their response or exhibited progression to blast crisis.[101] In the blast phase of *PDGFRA*- or *PDGFRB*-rearranged disease, imatinib can still be effective. In a case series of 17 patients with blast phase or myeloid sarcoma, 15 patients treated with imatinib monotherapy achieved durable complete hematologic and molecular remissions. Only 2 (12%) of 17 patients died after a median observation time of 65 months (range 7-106).[102]

The poor-prognosis *FGFR1*-rearranged neoplasms remain a therapeutic challenge. These diseases can present as chronic myeloid neoplasms (e.g. MDS, MPN, MDS/MPN overlap), blast phase disease (e.g., AML, T- or B-cell lymphoblastic lymphoma/leukemia, or mixed phenotype acute leukemia), and/or as extramedullary disease (EMD) of any lineage.[16,17,57,103] Patients with these stem cell neoplasms exhibit an aggressive course usually terminating in AML in 1 to 2 years.[16] The cumulative incidence of transformation to blast phase disease at 12 months has been reported to be almost 50%, and one-year survival rate from the development of blast crisis was 30%.[104] Chronic phase disease has typically been treated with hydroxyurea and multikinase inhibitors with anti-FGFR1 activity including midostaurin and ponatinib.[105-107] In one report, midostaurin inhibited the dysregulated *ZMYM2-FGFR1* fusion in vitro and elicited a hematologic response in a patient with this molecular abnormality.[105] Ponatinib has variable activity against the FGFR1 tyrosine kinase.[106,107] It was shown to be active in a patient with *BCR-FGFR1*–positive trilineage T/B/myeloid mixed phenotype acute leukemia where it produced marked reduction of bulky lymphadenopathy unresponsive to induction chemotherapy.[106] Reintroduction after allogeneic hematopoietic stem cell transplantation (HSCT) elicited a substantial reduction of minimal residual disease assayed by RT-PCR. In contrast, a German group found either no evidence for sustained hematologic or cytogenetic responses or progressive disease with either ponatinib or intensive chemotherapy in 7 *FGFR1*-rearranged patients.[107] Four of these patients underwent allogeneic HSCT and were reported in CMR and alive after a median time of 19 months (range, 8-36 months) after diagnosis and 13 months (range, 4-29 months) after allogeneic HSCT. Selective and potent inhibitors of FGFR1 are in development that may offer benefit for this patient group. The Chronic Malignancies Working Party of the European Society for Blood and Marrow Transplantation recently reported allogeneic transplantation results for 22 patients with *FGFR1*-rearranged myeloid/lymphoid neoplasms.[108] After a median follow-up of 4.1 years from transplant, the estimated five-year survival rate, PFS, nonrelapse mortality, and relapse incidence were 74%, 63%, 14%, and 23%, respectively. Death was due to relapse/progression ($n = 4$), graft-vs-host disease ($n = 2$), and organ toxicity ($n = 1$). Six patients experienced disease relapse at a median of 6.1 months (range: 2.3-119.6).[108] Two of these patients achieved a CR with ponatinib or pemigatinib (see below) and were alive at 34.5 and 37 months after relapse.

For blast phase disease, intensive chemotherapy with AML-type inductions or ALL-based regimens such as HyperCVAD (e.g., cyclophosphamide, vincristine, doxorubicin, and dexamethasone alternating with cycles of methotrexate and cytarabine) ± tyrosine kinase inhibition followed by early allogeneic HSCT is recommended for patients with *FGFR1*-rearranged disease.[109]

Notwithstanding allogeneic transplantation, the currently available treatments for MLN with *FGFR1* rearrangement often lead to only partial responses or short-lived complete clinical and cytogenetic responses. However, selective inhibitors of FGFR1 are in clinical development for these diseases and include futibatinib (selective inhibitor of FGFR1-4) and pemigatinib (selective inhibitor of FGFR1-3).[110,111] In a patient with a *PCM1-FGFR1* fusion, futibatinib 20 mg daily (dose reduced to 16 mg daily after 3 months for a grade 2 bullous rash) produced a durable, complete hematologic and cytogenetic remission which was ongoing after >18 months of therapy. Pemigatinib is approved for treating locally advanced or metastatic cholangiocarcinoma with an *FGFR2* fusion or other rearrangement.[112] Interim results of the ongoing phase 2 FIGHT-203 study were presented in 2021. The starting regimen of pemigatinib was 13.5 mg daily on an intermittent dosing schedule and was changed to 13.5 mg daily on a continuous schedule with a protocol amendment. Eighteen patients had chronic phase disease, 13 had some component of blast phase disease either in the bone marrow and/or an EMD, and 2 patients had treated MLN with persistent cytogenetic abnormality without marrow, blood, or EMD involvement. The average number of prior therapies was 1.6 (range, 0-6); 3 patients had prior HSCT. Responses were assessed by investigators and a Central Review Committee (CRC). Among 31 patients evaluable for clinical response, the CR rates were 64.5% per the investigators and 77.4% per the CRC. Among the 33 patients evaluable for cytogenetic response, the complete cytogenetic response rates were 72.7% per the investigators and 75.8% per the CRC. The most common hematologic treatment-emergent adverse event (TEAE) was anemia, reported in 35% of patients. Hyperphosphatemia, alopecia, and diarrhea were the most common nonhematologic TEAEs, reported in at least 50% of patients. Clinical and cytogenetic responses in patients with blast phase disease were less frequent and less durable than in the patients with chronic phase. However, 23% of the patients with blast phase disease were bridged to transplant. The longest duration of pemigatinib exposure was 192.4 weeks, with a median dosing duration of 29.3 weeks. At data cutoff, treatment was ongoing in 18 patients (53%). The most common reason for study drug discontinuation was transition to HSCT, followed by progressive disease. These data suggest that pemigatinib may offer a long-term treatment option for patients with *FGFR1*-rearranged disease ineligible for transplant or may facilitate bridging to transplant in eligible patients. Based on these data, the FDA approved pemigatinib for myeloid/lymphoid neoplasms with eosinophilia after 1 prior therapy in August 2022.

For patients with *JAK2* or *FLT3* rearrangements, there may be a role for small molecule inhibitors of FLT3 and JAK2. Two reports highlighted complete hematologic remissions and cytogenetic responses (one compete and one major) in two patients with CEL with the *PCM1-JAK2* fusion [t(8; 9) (p22; p24)] treated with the JAK1/JAK2 inhibitor ruxolitinib.[113,114]

Hematologic and cytogenetic remissions, however, can be variable in *JAK2*-rearranged patients, with some lasting only 1 to 2 years.[115,116] In a cohort of 9 patients, hematologic and cytogenetic remissions were achieved in 5/9 and 2/9 patients, respectively. Ruxolitinib was stopped in 6 patients because of primary resistance or progression, and therefore, allogeneic transplant should be considered early for suitable candidates.[117] Acquiring an *IKZF1* deletion and a switch from cytokine dependence to an activated B-cell receptor–like signaling phenotype were identified as putative mechanisms of resistance to ruxolitinib in a patient with a *BCR-JAK2* fusion and lymphoid blast transformation.[118] Similarly, in *FLT3*-rearranged cases, hematologic and cytogenetic responses have been observed with FLT3/multikinase inhibitors such as sorafenib, sunitinib, and gilteritinib, but durability can be brief, necessitating the consideration of HSCT.[119-121] For patients with myeloid/lymphoid neoplasms with rearranged *ABL1* (e.g., *ETV6-ABL1*), 2nd generation *ABL1* inhibitors (e.g., dasatinib, nilotinib) may elicit higher, more durable clinical responses.[115]

Treatment of Hypereosinophilic Syndrome and Chronic Eosinophilic Leukemia

For patients with hypereosinophilic syndrome and chronic eosinophilic leukemia, not otherwise specified, corticosteroids (e.g., prednisone 1 mg/kg) are recommended as the first-line treatment for HES. Steroids have potent antieosinophil activity and can produce rapid reductions in eosinophil count. In a retrospective analysis of 188 patients,[62] 141 HES patients on corticosteroids as first-line monotherapy achieved a CR or partial remission (PR) after 1 month, with duration of therapy ranging from 2 to 20 years and a median maintenance dose of 10 mg/d.[62] As symptoms improve and eosinophil counts normalize, a steroid taper can be instituted, particularly given the long-term treatment side effects of steroids. Hydroxyurea at 500 to 1000 mg daily is also an effective first-line option for HES, with the understanding that, like corticosteroids, hydroxyurea is palliative and does not change the natural course of the disease. Hydroxyurea can be used as monotherapy or in combination with corticosteroids. In the same retrospective study, 64 HES patients (34%) received hydroxyurea monotherapy, with 13 (72%) achieving CR or PR.[62] One should note that for CEL-NOS and steroid-refractory idiopathic HES, hydroxyurea has been used as either first- or second-line therapy.

IFN-α has been used effectively to induce hematologic and cytogenetic remissions in patients with HES and CEL-NOS who are either refractory to steroids or hydroxyurea, or administered in addition to corticosteroids as a steroid-sparing agent.[122-128] Of the 188 patients in a retrospective study, 46 were treated with IFN-α in combination with steroids, with response rates ranging from 50% to 75%, respectively.[62] IFN-α remissions have been associated with improvement in clinical symptoms as well as occasional improvement or reversion of end-organ injury, including hepatosplenomegaly and cardiac and thromboembolic complications.[108-124,127,128] The optimal starting or maintenance dose of IFN-α has not been well defined, but the initial dose required to control eosinophil counts often exceeds the doses required to sustain a remission. Initiation of therapy at 1 million units by subcutaneous injection three times weekly (tiw) and gradual escalation of the dose to 3 to 4 million units tiw or higher may be required to control the eosinophil count. Treatment of four HES patients with polyethylene glycol (PEG)-IFN-α-2b among a larger cohort of *BCR-ABL1*–negative MPN patients resulted in one CR and one PR, but side effects required that the initial study dose be reduced from 3 to 2 µg/kg/wk.[129] A lower starting dose of 90 µg/kg weekly (e.g., 1-1.5 µg/kg weekly) is better tolerated based on the experience of PEG-IFN-α-2a (Pegasys) in the MPNs polycythemia vera and essential thrombocythemia.[130,131] Side effects of short- and long-acting formulations of IFN-α are usually dose dependent and can include fatigue and flu-like symptoms, transaminitis, cytopenias, depression, hypothyroidism, and peripheral neuropathy. IFN-α is considered safe for use in pregnancy.

Second- and third-line agents for the treatment of HES have included vincristine, cyclophosphamide, etoposide, 2-chlorodeoxyadenosine alone or in combination with cytarabine, and cyclosporin-A.[132-141] Imatinib has been used empirically in *PDGFRA/PDGFRB* rearrangement-negative patients (e.g., with HES or CEL-NOS). At doses of 400 mg or higher,[142] partial hematologic responses are sometimes observed, but are more often transient and may reflect drug-related myelosuppression.

Similar to HES, patients with lymphocyte-variant HE are initially treated with corticosteroids. Refractory or relapsed disease may be considered for treatment with IFN-α or steroid-sparing immunosuppressive agents. Hydroxyurea and imatinib are less likely to demonstrate efficacy in this form of HE. Elevated serum IgE and thymus and activation-regulated chemokine levels have been associated with responsiveness to steroids.[62]

Antibody Approaches

Other treatment options for HES have included the anti-CD52 monoclonal antibody, alemtuzumab, based on the expression of the CD52 antigen on eosinophils. In patients with HES who were refractory to other therapies, infusion of alemtuzumab one to three times weekly produced a hematologic remission in 10 (91%) of 11 patients, but responses were not sustained when alemtuzumab was discontinued.[143] Patients with hematologic remission who received maintenance alemtuzumab therapy exhibited significantly longer time to progression than patients who were only observed. Eleven patients relapsed (only 1 while on maintenance), and 6 were rechallenged with alemtuzumab. 5 (83%) achieved a second hematologic remission after a median of 3.5 weeks, for a median duration of 123 weeks.[144]

Mepolizumab is an anti–IL-5, humanized monoclonal antibody that inhibits binding of IL-5 to the α chain of the IL5R found on eosinophils.[145] Mepolizumab was evaluated in a large, randomized, double-blinded, placebo-controlled trial of 85 HES patients (e.g., *FIP1L1-PDGFRA*–negative patients).[146] Patients were randomized to intravenous mepolizumab 750 mg or placebo every 4 weeks for 36 weeks. No adverse events were significantly more frequent with mepolizumab compared to placebo. A significantly higher proportion of mepolizumab-treated HES patients vs placebo was able to achieve the primary efficacy endpoint of a daily prednisone dose of <10 mg daily for at least 8 consecutive weeks. In a long-term follow-up of 78 patients treated for a mean exposure of 251 weeks (range 4-302 weeks), the median daily prednisone dose decreased from 20 to 0 mg in the first 24 weeks, and 62% of patients were prednisone free without other HES medications for ≥12 consecutive weeks.[147]

Results of the registrational, randomized, placebo-controlled trial of mepolizumab have been reported.[148] In this trial, a total of 108 patients (aged 12 years and older) with uncontrolled idiopathic HES (defined as at least 2 flares in the past 12 months and AEC of ≥1 × 10^9/L) were randomized (1:1) to receive mepolizumab (300 mg subcutaneous) or placebo every 4 weeks, in addition to their existing therapy, for 32 weeks. Mepolizumab significantly reduced the occurrence of flares (28% in mepolizumab group vs 53% in the placebo group had a flare or withdrew from the trial).[148] In addition, the time to first flare was 66% lower in the mepolizumab group. Both groups had similar rate of adverse events. This study led to the approval of mepolizumab (300 mg subcutaneous once every 4 weeks) in idiopathic HES in 2020.

Benralizumab is an anti–IL-5 receptor antibody that has been shown to reduce the annual asthma exacerbation rate in two phase III trials of patients with severe, uncontrolled eosinophilic asthma.[149,150] It was also effective as an oral glucocorticoid sparing therapy in adults with severe asthma in a randomized phase III trial,[151] and is currently FDA approved for adults with severe eosinophilic asthma. Benralizumab has been evaluated in 20 patients with *PDGFRA*-negative HES in a small randomized, double-blind, placebo-controlled, phase II trial.[152] Nine of 10 patients in the benralizumab arm met the primary endpoint of at least 50% reduction in the AEC at 12 weeks, in comparison to 3 of 10 patients who received placebo during the randomized phase ($P = .02$). Clinical and hematological responses were sustained for 48 weeks in 14 of 19 patients (74%) during the open phase of the trial, and the median duration of response was 84 weeks. The most common drug-related adverse events were headache and an elevated lactate dehydrogenase level, occurring in 32% of patients and resolved within 48 hours. One of the responders was previously treated unsuccessfully with mepolizumab. No response was seen in two patients with a *JAK2* V617F-positive CEL, and three out of four patients with lymphocyte variant HES relapsed after an initial response.[152] The lack of response of CEL to benralizumab is similar to the mepolizumab experience.[153] Benralizumab is currently undergoing a registrational phase III placebo-controlled study (clinicaltrials.gov identifier: NCT04191304).

Siglec-8 is an inhibitor receptor selectively expressed on eosinophils, mast cells, and basophils. Targeting siglec-8 with the antibody lirentelimab (AK002) is a novel approach that showed significant reduction in tissue eosinophils and symptoms in patients with eosinophilic gastritis and duodenitis and warrants evaluation in HES.[154,155] Dupilumab is an IL-4 receptor alpha antagonist indicated for the treatment of adult patients with moderate-to-severe atopic dermatitis, but is under study for various eosinophilic disorders including eosinophilic esophagitis and eosinophilic asthma.[156,157]

Allogeneic Stem Cell Transplantation

Allogeneic stem cell transplantation has been attempted for patients with aggressive disease with anecdotal benefit. Disease-free survival ranging from 8 months to 5 years has been reported,[158-162] with one patient relapsing at 40 months.[163] Allogeneic transplantation using nonmyeloablative-conditioning regimens has been reported in three patients, with remission duration of 3 to 12 months at the time of reported follow-up.[164,165] In one patient who underwent an allogeneic stem cell transplantation from a human leukocyte antigen–matched sibling, the patient was disease free at 3 years, and there was no evidence of the *FIP1L1-PDGFRA* fusion which was present at diagnosis.[166] Despite success in selected cases, the role of transplantation in HES is not well established.

Cardiac Surgery

Although less commonly used today, cardiac surgery has extended the life of patients with late-stage cardiac disease manifested by endomyocardial fibrosis, mural thrombosis, and valvular insufficiency.[61,63] Mitral and/or tricuspid valve repair or replacement[62,167-170] and endomyocardectomy for late-stage fibrotic heart disease[70,171] can improve cardiac function. Bioprosthetic devices are preferred over their mechanical counterparts because of the reduced frequency of valve thrombosis. Anticoagulants and antiplatelet agents have shown variable success in preventing recurrent thromboembolism.[172,173]

SUMMARY

Recognition of molecularly defined eosinophilias, whose pathobiology is linked to dysregulated tyrosine kinases, has transformed the classification and treatment of these diseases. The sensitivity of *PDGFRA/PDGFRB*-rearranged eosinophilic neoplasms to imatinib has reversed the course of these historically poor-prognosis diseases. Recent data with the selective inhibitor pemigatinib are encouraging for the poor-prognosis myeloid/lymphoid neoplasms with *FGFR1* fusion tyrosine kinases. In addition to small molecule inhibitors, antibody approaches (e.g. mepolizumab and benralizumab) offer effective therapeutic options beyond corticosteroids for lymphocyte-variant and idiopathic HES. Next-generation sequencing technologies should now be incorporated in the diagnostic evaluation of HES to facilitate the identification of molecular lesions that may offer opportunities for targeted therapy.

References

1. Perkins WH. Beitrage zur Kenntnis der granulirten Bindewebzellen und der eosinophilen Leukocythen. *Archiv Anat Physiol Physiol Abteil (Leipzig).* 1879:166-169.
2. Hardy WR, Anderson RE. The hypereosinophilic syndrome. *Ann Intern Med.* 1968;68:1220-1229.

3. Chusid MJ, Dale DC, West BC, et al. The hypereosinophilic syndrome. Analysis of fourteen cases with review of the literature. *Medicine (Baltim)*. 1975;54:1-27.
4. Rothenberg ME. Eosinophilia. *N Engl J Med*. 1998;338:1592-1600.
5. Brigden M, Graydon C. Eosinophilia detected by automated blood cell counting in ambulatory North American outpatients. Incidence and clinical significance. *Arch Pathol Lab Med*. 1997;121:963-967.
6. Crane MM, Chang CM, Kobayashi MG, et al. Incidence of myeloproliferative hypereosinophilic syndrome in the Unites States and an estimate of all hypereosinophilic syndrome incidence. *J Allergy Clin Immunol*. 2010;126:179-181.
7. Ruan GJ, Smith CJ, Day C, et al. A population-based study of chronic eosinophilic leukemia-not otherwise specified in the United States. *Am J Hematol*. Published online 2020. doi:10.1002/ajh.25906
8. Shomali W, Gotlib J. World Health Organization-defined eosinophilic disorders: 2022 update on diagnosis, risk stratification, and management. *Am J Hematol*. 2022;97:129-148.
9. Lamkhioued B, Abdelilah SG, Hamid Q, et al. The CCR3 receptor is involved in eosinophil differentiation and is up-regulated by Th2 cytokines in CD34+ progenitor cells. *J Immunol*. 2003;170:537-547.
10. Sanderson CJ. Interleukin-5, eosinophils, and disease. *Blood*. 1992;79:3101-3109.
11. Hogan SP, Rosenberg HF, Moqbel R, et al. Eosinophils: biological properties and role in health and disease. *Clin Exp Allergy*. 2008;38:709-750.
12. Schleimer RP, Sterbinsky SA, Kaiser J, et al. IL-4 induces adherence of human eosinophils and basophils but not neutrophils to endothelium: association with expression of VCAM-1. *J Immunol*. 1992;148:1086-1092.
13. Wardlaw AJ, Moqbel R, Cromwell O, et al. Platelet-activating factor: a potent chemotactic and chemokinetic factor for human eosinophils. *J Clin Invest*. 1986;78:1701-1706.
14. Forssman U, Uguccioni M, Loetscher P, et al. Eotaxin-2, a novel CC chemokine that is selective for the chemokine receptor CCR3, and acts like eotaxin on human eosinophil and basophil leukocytes. *J Exp Med*. 1997;185:2171-2176.
15. Kameyoshi Y, Dorschner A, Mallet AI, et al. Cytokine RANTES released by thrombin-stimulated platelets is a potent attractant for human eosinophils. *J Exp Med*. 1992;176:587-592.
16. Khoury JD, Solary E, Abia O, et al. The 5th edition of the World Health Organization classification of haematolymphoid tumours: Myeloid and histiocytic/dendritic neoplasms. *Leukemia*. 2022;36:1703-1719.
17. Arber DA, Orazi A, Hasserjian RP, et al. International consensus classification of myeloid neoplasms and acute leukemias: integrating morphologic, clinical, and genomic data. *Blood*. 2022;140;1200-1228.
18. Bain BJ, Gilliland DG, Horny HP, et al. Chronic eosinophilic leukaemia, not otherwise specified. In: Swerdlow S, Harris NL, Stein H, Jaffe ES, Theile J, Vardiman JW, eds. *World Health Organization Classification of Tumours. Pathology and Genetics of Tumours of Haematopoietic and Lymphoid Tissues*. IARC Press; 2008:51-53.
19. Valent P, Klion D, Horny HP, et al. Contemporary consensus proposal on criteria and classification of eosinophilic disorders and related syndromes. *J Allergy Clin Immunol*. 2012;130(3):607-612.
20. Valent P, Klion AD, Roufosse F, et al. Proposed refined diagnostic criteria and classification of eosinophil disorders and related syndromes. *Allergy*. 2022. doi:10.1111/all.15544.
21. Klion AD, Law MA, Riemenschneider W, et al. Familial eosinophilia: a benign disorder? *Blood*. 2004;103:4050-4055.
22. Amor B, Rajzbaum G, Poiraudeau S, et al. Eosinophilia-myalgia linked with L-tryptophan. *Lancet*. 1990;335:420-421.
23. Kilbourne EM, Rigau-Perez JG, Heath CW, Jr, et al. Clinical epidemiology of toxic-oil syndrome. Manifestations of a new illness. *N Engl J Med*. 1983;209:1408-1414.
24. Schwaab J, Umbach R, Metzgeroth G, et al. KIT D816V and JAK2 V617F mutations are seen recurrently in hypereosinophilia of unknown significance. *Am J Hematol*. 2015;90:774-777.
25. Wang SA, Tam W, Tsai AG, et al. Targeted next-generation sequencing identifies a subset of idiopathic hypereosinophilic syndrome with features similar to chronic eosinophilic leukemia, not otherwise specified. *Mod Pathol*. 2016;29:854-864.
26. Cools J, DeAngelo DJ, Gotlib J, et al. A tyrosine kinase created by fusion of the PDGFRA and FIP1L1 genes as a therapeutic target of imatinib in idiopathic hypereosinophilic syndrome. *N Engl J Med*. 2003;348:1201-1214.
27. Pardanani A, Ketterling RP, Brockman SR, et al. CHIC2 deletion, a surrogate for FIP1L1-PDGFRA fusion, occurs in systemic mastocytosis associated with eosinophilia and predicts response to imatinib mesylate therapy. *Blood*. 2003;102:3093-3096.
28. Klion AD, Noel P, Akin C, et al. Elevated serum tryptase levels identify a subset of patients with a myeloproliferative variant of idiopathic hypereosinophilic syndrome associated with tissue fibrosis, poor prognosis, and imatinib responsiveness. *Blood*. 2003;101:4660-4666.
29. Reiter A, Walz C, Watmore A, et al. The t(8;9)(p22;p24) is a recurrent abnormality in chronic and acute leukemia that fuses PCM1 to JAK2. *Cancer Res*. 2005;65:2662-2667.
30. Vu HA, Xinh PT, Masusa M, et al. FLT3 is fused to ETV6 in a myeloproliferative disorder with hypereosinophilia and a t(12;13) (p13;q12) translocation. *Leukemia*. 2006;20:1414-1421.
31. Roufosse F, Cogan E, Goldman M. Recent advances in pathogenesis and management of hypereosinophilic syndromes. *Allergy*. 2004;59:673-689.
32. Bank I, Amariglio N, Reshef A, et al. The hypereosinophilic syndrome associated with CD4+CD3–helper type 2 (Th2) lymphocytes. *Leuk Lymphoma*. 2001;42:123-133.
33. Simon HU, Plotz SG, Dummer R, Blaser K. Abnormal clones of T cells producing interleukin-5 in idiopathic hypereosinophilia. *N Engl J Med*. 1999;341:1112-1120.
34. Brugnoni D, Airo P, Tosoni C, et al. CD3–CD4+ cells with a Th2-like pattern of cytokine production in the peripheral blood of a patient with cutaneous T cell lymphoma. *Leukemia*. 1997;11:1983-1985.
35. Roumier AS, Grardel N, Lai JL, et al. Hypereosinophilia with abnormal T cells, trisomy 7, and elevated TARC serum level. *Haematologica*. 2003;88:ECR24.
36. Roufosse F. Hypereosinophilic syndrome variants: diagnostic and therapeutic considerations. *Haematologica*. 2009;94:1188-1193.
37. Cogan E, Schandene L, Crusiaux A, et al. Brief report: clonal proliferation of type 2 helper T cells in a man with the hypereosinophilic syndrome. *N Engl J Med*. 1994;330:535-538.
38. Helbig G, Wieczorkiewicz A, Dziaczkowska-Suszek J, et al. T-cell abnormalities are present at high frequencies in high frequencies in patients with hypereosinophilic syndrome. *Haematologica*. 2009;94:1236-1241.
39. Buitenhuis M, Verhagen LP, Cools J, et al. Molecular mechanisms underlying FIP1L1-PDGFRA-mediated myeloproliferation. *Cancer Res*. 2007;67:3759-3766.
40. Li B, Zhang G, Li C, et al. Identification of JAK2 as a mediator of FIP1L1-PDGFRA-induced eosinophil growth and function in CEL. *PLoS One*. 2012;7(4):e34912.
41. Cools J, Stover EH, Boulton CL, et al. PKC412 overcomes resistance to imatinib in a murine model of FIP1L1-PDGFRalpha-induced myeloproliferative disease. *Cancer Cell*. 2003;3:459-469.
42. Yamada Y, Rothenberg ME, Lee AW, et al. The FIP1L1-PDGFRA fusion gene cooperates with IL-5 to induce murine hypereosinophilic syndrome (HES)/chronic eosinophilic leukemia (CEL)-like disease. *Blood*. 2006;107:4071-4079.
43. Burgstaller S, Kreil S, Waghorn K, et al. The severity of FIP1L1-PDGFRA-positive chronic eosinophilic leukaemia is associated with polymorphic variation at the IL5RA locus. *Leukemia*. 2007;21:2428-2432.
44. Golub TR, Goga A, Barker GF, et al. Oligomerization of the ABL tyrosine kinase by the Ets protein TEL in human leukemia. *Mol Cell Biol*. 1996;16:4107-4116.
45. Xiao S, McCarthy JG, Aster JC, et al. ZNF198-FGFR1 transforming activity depends on a novel proline-rich ZNF198 oligomerization domain. *Blood*. 2000;96:699-704.
46. McWhirter JR, Galasso DL, Wang JY. A coiled-coil oligomerization domain of Bcr is essential for the transforming function of Bcr-Abl oncoproteins. *Mol Cell Biol*. 1993;13:7587-7595.
47. Chan PM, Ilangumaran S, La RJ, et al. Autoinhibition of the kit receptor tyrosine kinase by the cytosolic juxtamembrane region. *Mol Cell Biol*. 2003;23:3067-3078.
48. Griffith J, Black J, Faerman C, et al. The structural basis for autoinhibition of FLT3 by the juxtamembrane domain. *Mol Cell*. 2004;13:169-178.
49. Gilliland DG, Griffin JD. The roles of FLT3 in hematopoiesis and leukemia. *Blood*. 2002;100:1532-1542.
50. Heinrich MC, Corless CL, Demetri GD, et al. Kinase mutations and imatinib response in patients with metastatic gastrointestinal stromal tumor. *J Clin Oncol*. 2003;21:4342-4349.
51. Stover EH, Chen J, Folens C, et al. Activation of FIP1L1-PDGFRalpha requires disruption of the juxtamembrane domain of PDGFRalpha and is FIP1L1-independent. *Proc Natl Acad Sci USA*. 2006;103:8078-8083.
52. Gotlib J, Cools J, Malone JM, et al. The FIP1L1-PDGFRa fusion tyrosine kinase in hypereosinophilic syndrome and chronic eosinophilic leukemia: implications for diagnosis, classification, and management. *Blood*. 2004;103:2879-2891.
53. Elling C, Erben P, Walz C, et al. Novel imatinib-sensitive PDGFRA-activating point mutations in hypereosinophilic syndrome induce growth factor independence and leukemia-like disease. *Blood*. 2011;117:2935-2943.
54. Pardanani A, Brockman SR, Paternoster SF, et al. FIP1L1-PDGFRA fusion: prevalence and clinicopathologic correlates in 89 consecutive patients with moderate to severe eosinophilia. *Blood*. 2004;104:3038-3045.
55. Maric I, Robyn J, Metcalfe DD, et al. KIT D816V-associated systemic mastocytosis with eosinophilia and FIP1L1/PDGFRA-associated chronic eosinophilic leukemia are distinct entities. *J Allergy Clin Immunol*. 2007;120:680-687.
56. Metzgeroth G, Walz C, Score J, et al. Recurrent finding of the FIP1L1-PDGFRA fusion gene in eosinophilia-associated acute myeloid leukemia and lymphoblastic T-cell lymphoma. *Leukemia*. 2007;21:1183-1188.
57. Reiter A, Gotlib J. Myeloid neoplasms with eosinophilia. *Blood*. 2017;129:704-714.
58. Greipp PT, Dewald GW, Tefferi A. Prevalence, breakpoint distribution, and clinical correlates of t(5;12). *Cancer Genet Cytogenet*. 2004;153:170-172.
59. Meeker TC, Hardy D, Willman C, et al. Activation of the interleukin-3 gene by chromosome translocation in acute lymphoblastic leukemia with eosinophilia. *Blood*. 1990;76:285-289.
60. Yagasaki F, Jinnai I, Yoshida S, et al. Fusion of TEL/ETV6 to a novel ACS2 in myelodysplastic syndrome and acute myelogenous leukemia with t(5;12)(q31;p13). *Genes Chromosomes Cancer*. 1999;26:192-202.
61. Fauci AS, Harley JB, Roberts WC, et al. The idiopathic hypereosinophilic syndrome. Clinical, pathophysiologic, and therapeutic considerations. *Ann Intern Med*. 1982;97:78-92.
62. Ogbogu PU, Bochner BS, Butterfield JH, et al. Hypereosinophilic syndromes: a multicenter, retrospective analysis of clinical characteristics and response to therapy. *J Allergy Clin Immunol*. 2009;124:1319-1325.
63. Weller PF, Bubley GJ. The idiopathic hypereosinophilic syndrome. *Blood*. 1994;83:2759-2779.
64. Lefebvre C, Bletry O, Degoulet P, et al. Prognostic factors of hypereosinophilic syndrome. Study of 40 cases. *Ann Med Interne*. 1989;140:253-257.
65. Spry CJ, Davies J, Tai PC, et al. Clinical features of fifteen patients with the hypereosinophilic syndrome. *Q J Med*. 1983;52:1-22.
66. Podjasek HC, Butterfield JH. Mortality in hypereosinophilic syndrome: 19 years of experience at Mayo Clinic with a review of the literature. *Leuk Res*. 2013;37:392-395.

67. Pardanani A, Lasho T, Wassie E, et al. Predictors of survival in WHO-defined hypereosinophilic syndrome and idiopathic hypereosinophilia and the role of next-generation sequencing. *Leukemia*. 2016;30:1924-1926.
68. Helbig G, Soja A, Bartkowska-Chrobok A, et al. Chronic eosinophilic leukemia-not otherwise specified has a poor prognosis with unresponsiveness to conventional treatment and high risk of acute transformation. *Am J Hematol*. 2012;87:643-645.
69. Morsia E, Reichard K, Pardanani A, Tefferi A, Gangat N. WHO defined chronic eosinophilic leukemia, not otherwise specified (CEL, NOS): A contemporary series from the Mayo Clinic. *Am J Hematol*. 2020;95(7):E172-E174.
70. Tanino M, Kitamura K, Ohta G, et al. Hypereosinophilic syndrome with extensive myocardial involvement and mitral valve thrombus instead of mural thrombi. *Acta Pathol Jpn*. 1983;33:1233-1242.
71. Radford DJ, Garlick RB, Pohlner PG. Multiple valvular replacement for hypereosinophilic syndrome. *Cardiol Young*. 2002;12:67-70.
72. Pardanani A, Lim KH, Lasho TL, et al. Prognostically relevant breakdown of 123 patients with systemic mastocytosis associated with other myeloid malignancies. *Blood*. 2009;114:3769-3772.
73. Wimazal F, Germing U, Kundi M, et al. Evaluation of the prognostic significance of eosinophilia and basophilia in a larger cohort of patients with myelodysplastic syndromes. *Cancer*. 2010;116:2372-2381.
74. Matsushima T, Handa H, Yokohama A, et al. Prevalence and clinical characteristics of myelodysplastic syndrome with bone marrow eosinophilia or basophilia. *Blood*. 2003;101:3386-3390.
75. Kluin-Nelemans HC, Reiter A, Illerhaus A, et al. Prognostic impact of eosinophils in mastocytosis: analysis of 2350 patients collected in the ECNM Registry. *Leukemia*. 2020;34:1090-1101.
76. Gotlib J. Molecular classification and pathogenesis of eosinophilic disorders: 2005 update. *Acta Haematol*. 2005;114:7-25.
77. Schaller JL, Burkland GA. Case report: rapid and complete control of idiopathic hypereosinophilia with imatinib mesylate. *Med Gen Med*. 2001;3:9.
78. Gleich GJ, Leiferman KM, Pardanani A, et al. Treatment of hypereosinophilic syndrome with imatinib mesylate. *Lancet*. 2002;359:1577-1578.
79. Ault P, Cortes J, Koller C, et al. Response of idiopathic hypereosinophilic syndrome to treatment with imatinib mesylate. *Leuk Res*. 2002;26:881-884.
80. Griffin JH, Leung J, Bruner RJ, et al. Discovery of a fusion kinase in EOL-1 cells and idiopathic hypereosinophilic syndrome. *Proc Natl Acad Sci USA*. 2003;100:7830-7835.
81. Helbig G, Stella-Hołowiecka B, Majewski M, et al. A single weekly dose of imatinib is sufficient to induce and maintain remission of chronic eosinophilic leukaemia in FIP1L1-PDGFRA-expressing patients. *Br J Haematol*. 2008;141(2):200-204.
82. Baccarani M, Cilloni D, Rondoni M, et al. The efficacy of imatinib mesylate in patients with FIP1L1-PDGFRalpha-positive hypereosinophilic syndrome. Results of a multicenter prospective study. *Haematologica*. 2007;92:1173-1179.
83. Jovanovic JV, Score J, Waghorn K, et al. Low-dose imatinib mesylate leads to rapid induction of major molecular responses and achievement of complete molecular remission in FIP1L1-PDGFRA-positive chronic eosinophilic leukemia. *Blood*. 2007;109:4635-4640.
84. Klion AD, Robyn J, Maric I, et al. Relapse following discontinuation of imatinib mesylate therapy for FIP1L1/PDGFRA-positive chronic eosinophilic leukemia: implications for optimal dosing. *Blood*. 2007;110:3552-3556.
85. Pardanani A, Ketterling RP, Li CY, et al. FIP1L1-PDGFRA in eosinophilic disorders: prevalence in routine clinical practice, long-term experience with imatinib therapy, and a critical review of the literature. *Leuk Res*. 2006;30:965-970.
86. Rohmer J, Couteau-Chardon A, Trichereau J, et al. Epidemiology, clinical picture and long-term outcomes of FIP1L1-PDGFRA-positive myeloid neoplasm with eosinophilia: data from 151 patients. *Am J Hematol*. 2020;95(11):1314-1323.
87. Metzgeroth G, Schwaab J, Naumann N, et al. Treatment-free remission in FIP1L1-PDGFRA-positive myeloid/lymphoid neoplasms with eosinophilia after imatinib discontinuation. *Blood Adv*. 2020;4(3):440-443.
88. Von Bubnoff N, Sandherr M, Schlimok G, et al. Myeloid blast crisis evolving during imatinib treatment of an FIP1L1-PDGFRalpha-positive chronic myeloproliferative disease with prominent eosinophilia. *Leukemia*. 2004;19:286-287.
89. Ohnishi H, Kandabashi K, Maeda Y, et al. Chronic eosinophilic leukaemia with FIP1L1-PDGFRA fusion and T6741 mutation that evolved from Langerhans cell histiocytosis with eosinophilia after chemotherapy. *Br J Haematol*. 2006;134:547-549.
90. Lierman E, Michaux L, Beullens E, et al. FIP1L1-PDGFRalpha D842V, a novel panresistant mutant, emerging after treatment of FIP1L1-PDGFRalpha T674I eosinophilic leukemia with single agent sorafenib. *Leukemia*. 2009;23:845-851.
91. von Bubnoff N, Gorantla SP, Engh RA, et al. The low frequency of clinical resistance to PDGFR inhibitors in myeloid neoplasms with abnormalities of PDGFRA might be related to the limited repertoire of possible PDGFRA kinase domain mutations in vitro. *Oncogene*. 2011;30:933-943.
92. Lierman E, Folens C, Stover EH, et al. Sorafenib is a potent inhibitor of FIP1L1-PDGFRalpha and the imatinib-resistant FIP1L1-PDGFRalpha T674I mutant. *Blood*. 2006;108:1374-1376.
93. Stover EH, Chen J, Lee BH, et al. The small molecule tyrosine kinase inhibitor AMN107 inhibits TEL-PDGFRbeta and FIP1L1-PDGFRalpha in vitro and in vivo. *Blood*. 2005;106:3206-3213.
94. von Bubnoff N, Gorantla SP, Thone S, et al. The FIP1L1-PDGFRA T674I mutation can be inhibited by the tyrosine kinase inhibitor AMN107 (nilotinib). *Blood*. 2006;107:4970-4971.
95. Grunewald S, Klug LR, Mühlenberg T, et al. Resistance to avapritinib in PDGFRA-driven GIST is caused by secondary mutations in the PDGFRA kinase domain. *Cancer Discov*. 2021;11(1):108-125.
96. Metzgeroth G, Erben P, Martin H, et al. Limited clinical activity of nilotinib and sorafenib in FIP1L1-PDGFRA positive chronic eosinophilic leukemia with imatinib-resistant T674I mutation. *Leukemia*. 2012;26:162-164.
97. Simon D, Salemi S, Yousefi S, Simon HU. Primary resistance to imatinib in Fip1-like 1-platelet-derived growth factor receptor alpha-positive eosinophilic leukemia. *J Allergy Clin Immunol*. 2008;121:1054-1056.
98. Cross DM, Cross NC, Burgstaller S, et al. Durable responses to imatinib in patients with PDGFRB fusion gene-positive and BCR-ABL-negative chronic myeloproliferative disorders. *Blood*. 2007;109:61-64.
99. Pardanani A, Reeder T, Porrata L, et al. Imatinib therapy for hypereosinophilic syndrome and other eosinophilic disorders. *Blood*. 2003;101:3391-3397.
100. Pitini V, Arrigo C, Azzarello D, et al. Serum concentration of cardiac troponin T in patients with hypereosinophilic syndrome treated with imatinib is predictive of adverse outcomes. *Blood*. 2003;102:3456-3457.
101. Cheah CY, Burbury K, Apperley JF, et al. Patients with myeloid malignancies bearing PDGFRB fusion genes achieve durable long-term remissions with imatinib. *Blood*. 2014;123:3574-3577.
102. Metzgeroth G, Schwaab J, Gosenca D, et al. Long-term follow-up of treatment with imatinib in eosinophilia-associated myeloid/lymphoid neoplasms with PDGFR rearrangements in blast phase. *Leukemia*. 2013;27:2254-2256.
103. MacDonald D, Aguiar C, Mason PJ, Goldman JM, Cross NC. A new myeloproliferative disorder associated with chromosomal translocations involving 8p11: a review. *Leukemia*. 1995;9:1628-1630.
104. Umino K, Fujiwara S-I, Ikeda T, et al. Clinical outcomes of myeloid/lymphoid neoplasms with fibroblast growth factor receptor-1 (FGFR1) rearrangement. *Hematology*. 2018;23:470-477.
105. Chen J, DeAngelo DJ, Kutok JL, et al. PKC412 inhibits the zinc finger 198-fibroblast growth factor receptor 1 fusion tyrosine kinase and is active in treatment of stem cell myeloproliferative disorder. *Proc Natl Acad Sci USA*. 2004;101:14479-14484.
106. Khodadoust MS, Luo B, Medeiros BC, et al. Clinical activity of ponatinib in a patient with FGFR1-rearranged mixed phenotype acute leukemia. *Leukemia*. 2016;30:947-950.
107. Kreil S, Ades L, Bommer M, et al. Limited efficacy of ponatinib in myeloproliferative neoplasms associated with FGFR1 fusion genes. *Blood*. 2015;126:Abstract 2812.
108. Hernandez-Boluda J-C, Pereira A, Zinger N, et al. Allogeneic hematopoietic cell transplantation in patients with myeloid/lymphoid neoplasm with FGFR1-rearrangement: a study of the Chronic Malignancies Working Party of EBMT. *Bone Marrow Transplant*. 2022;57:416-422.
109. NCCN Clinical Practice Guidelines in Oncology. *Myeloid/lymphoid neoplasms with eosinophilia and tyrosine kinase fusion genes*. Version 4.2021https://www.nccn.org/guidelines/guidelines-detail?category=1&id=1505. Accessed April 2, 2022.
110. Kasbekar M, Nardi V, Dan Cin P, et al. Targeted FGFR inhibition results in a durable remission in an FGFR1-driven myeloid neoplasm with eosinophilia. *Blood Adv*. 2020;4:3136-3140.
111. Gotlib J, Kiladjian JJ, Vannucchi A, et al. A phase 2 study of pemigatinib (FIGHT-203; INCB054828) in patients with myeloid/lymphoid neoplasms (MLNs) with fibroblast growth factor receptor 1 (FGFR1) rearrangement (MLN^{FGFR1}). *Blood*. 2021;138(suppl 1):385. [Abstract].
112. Merz V, Zecchetto C, Melisi D. Pemigatinib, a potent inhibitor of FGFRs for the treatment of cholangiocarcinoma. *Future Oncol*. 2021;17:389-402.
113. Lierman E, Selleslag D, Smits S, et al. Ruxolitinib inhibits transforming JAK2 fusion proteins in vitro and induces complete cytogenetic remission in t(8;9)(p22;p24)/PCM1-JAK2-positive chronic eosinophilic leukemia. *Blood*. 2012;120:1529-1531.
114. Rumi E, Milosevic JD, Casetti I, et al. Efficacy of ruxolitinib in chronic eosinophilic leukemia associated with a PCM1-JAK2 fusion gene. *J Clin Oncol*. 2013;31:e269-e271.
115. Rumi E, Milosevic JD, Selleslag D, et al. Efficacy of ruxolitinib in myeloid neoplasms with PCM1-JAK2 fusion gene. *Ann Hematol*. 2015;94:1927-1928.
116. Schwaab J, Knut M, Haferlach C, et al. Limited duration of complete remission on ruxolitinib in myeloid neoplasms with PCM1-JAK2 and BCR-JAK2 fusion genes. *Ann Hematol*. 2015;94:233-238.
117. Schwaab J, Naumann N, Luebke J, et al. Response to tyrosine kinase inhibitors in myeloid neoplasms associated with PCM1-JAK2, BCR-JAK2 and ETV6-ABL1 fusion genes. *Am J Hematol*. 2020;95(7):824-833.
118. Chen JA, Hou Y, Roskin KM, et al. Lymphoid blast transformation in an MPN with BCR-JAK2 treated with ruxolitinib: putative mechanisms of resistance. *Blood Adv*. 2021;5:3492-3496.
119. Walz C, Erben P, Ritter M, et al. Response of ETV6-FLT3-positive myeloid/lymphoid neoplasm with eosinophilia to inhibitors of FMS-like tyrosine kinase 3. *Blood*. 2011;118:2239-2242.
120. Falchi L, Mehrotra M, Newberry KJ, et al. ETV6-FLT3 fusion gene-positive, eosinophilia-associated myeloproliferative neoplasm successfully treated with sorafenib and allogeneic stem cell transplant. *Leukemia*. 2014;28:2090-2092.
121. Spitzer B, Dela Cruz FS, Ibanez Sanchez GD, et al. ETV6-FLT3-positive myeloid/lymphoid neoplasm with eosinophilia presenting in an infant: an entity distinct from JMML. *Blood Adv*. 2021;5:1899-1902.
122. Quiquandon I, Claisse JF, Capiod JC, et al. Alpha-interferon and hypereosinophilic syndrome with trisomy 8: karyotypic remission. *Blood*. 1995;85:2284-2285.
123. Luciano L, Catalano L, Sarrantonio C, et al. aIFN–induced hematologic and cytogenetic remission in chronic eosinophilic leukemia with t(1;5). *Haematologica*. 1999;84:651-653.
124. Yamada O, Kitahara K, Imamura K, et al. Clinical and cytogenetic remission induced by interferon-a in a patient with chronic eosinophilic leukemia associated with a unique t(3;9;5) translocation. *Am J Hematol*. 1998;58:137-141.
125. Malbrain ML, Van den Bergh H, Zachee P. Further evidence for the clonal nature of the idiopathic hypereosinophilic syndrome: complete haematological and cytogenetic remission induced by interferon-alpha in a case with a unique chromosomal abnormality. *Br J Haematol*. 1996;92:176-183.
126. Butterfield JH, Gleich GJ. Response of six patients with idiopathic hypereosinophilic syndrome to interferon alpha. *J Allergy Clin Immunol*. 1994;94:1318-1326.

127. Ceretelli S, Capochiani E, Petrini M. Interferon-alpha in the idiopathic hypereosinophilic syndrome: consideration of five cases. *Ann Hematol.* 1998;77:161-164.
128. Yoon TY, Ahn GB, Chang SH. Complete remission of hypereosinophilic syndrome after interferon-alpha therapy: report of a case and literature review. *J Dermatol.* 2000;27:110-115.
129. Jabbour E, Kantarjian H, Cortes J, et al. PEG-IFN-a-2b therapy in BCR-ABL-negative myeloproliferative disorders. Final result of a phase 2 study. *Cancer.* 2007;110:2012-2018.
130. Kiladjian JJ, Cassinat B, Chevret S, et al. Pegylated interferon-alpha-2a induces complete hematologic and molecular responses with low toxicity in polycythemia vera. *Blood.* 2008;112:3065-3072.
131. Quintas-Cardama A, Kantarjian H, Manshouri T, et al. Pegylated interferon-alpha-2a yields high rates of hematologic and molecular response in patients with advanced essential thrombocythemia and polycythemia vera. *J Clin Oncol.* 2009;27:5418-5424.
132. Chusid MJ, Dale DC. Eosinophilic leukemia. Remission with vincristine and hydroxyurea. *Am J Med.* 1975;59:297-300.
133. Cofrancesco E, Cortellaro M, Pogliani E, et al. Response to vincristine treatment in a case of idiopathic hypereosinophilic syndrome with multiple clinical manifestations. *Acta Haematol.* 1984;72:21-25.
134. Sakamoto K, Erdreich-Epstein A, deClerck Y, et al. Prolonged clinical response to vincristine treatment in two patients with hypereosinophilic syndrome. *Am J Pediatr Hematol Oncol.* 1992;14:348-351.
135. Lee JH, Lee JW, Jang CS, et al. Successful cyclophosphamide therapy in recurrent eosinophilic colitis associated with hypereosinophilic syndrome. *Yonsei Med J.* 2002;43:267-270.
136. Smit AJ, van Essen LH, de Vries EG. Successful long-term control of idiopathic hypereosinophilic syndrome with etoposide. *Cancer.* 1991;67:2826-2827.
137. Bourrat E, Lebbe C, Calvo F. Etoposide for treating the hypereosinophilic syndrome. *Ann Intern Med.* 1994;121:899-900.
138. Ueno NT, Zhao S, Robertson LE, et al. 2-chlorodeoxyadenosine therapy for idiopathic hypereosinophilic syndrome. *Leukemia.* 1997;11:1386-1390.
139. Jabbour E, Verstovsek S, Giles F, et al. 2-chlorodeoxyadenosine and cytarabine combination therapy for idiopathic hypereosinophilic syndrome. *Cancer.* 2005;104:541-546.
140. Zabel P, Schlaak M. Cyclosporine for hypereosinophilic syndrome. *Ann Hematol.* 1991;62:230-231.
141. Nadarajah S, Krafchik B, Roifman C, et al. Treatment of hypereosinophilic syndrome in a child using cyclosporine: implication for a primary T-cell abnormality. *Pediatrics.* 1997;99:630-633.
142. Butterfield JH. Success of short-term, higher-dose imatinib mesylate to induce clinical response in FIP1L1-PDGFRalpha-negative hypereosinophilic syndrome. *Leuk Res.* 2009;33:1127-1129.
143. Verstovsek S, Tefferi A, Kantarjian H, et al. Alemtuzumab therapy for hypereosinophilic syndrome and chronic eosinophilic leukemia. *Clin Cancer Res.* 2009;15:368-373.
144. Strati P, Cortes J, Faderl S, et al. Long-term follow-up of patients with hypereosinophilic syndrome treated with Alemtuzumab, an anti-CD52 antibody. *Clin Lymphoma Myeloma Leuk.* 2013;13:287-291.
145. Hart TK, Cook RM, Zia-Amirhosseini P, et al. Preclinical efficacy and safety of mepolizumab (SB-240563), a humanized monoclonal antibody to IL-5, in cynomolgus monkeys. *J Allergy Clin Immunol.* 2001;108:250-257.
146. Rothenberg ME, Klion AD, Roufosse FE, et al. Treatment of patients with the hypereosinophilic syndrome with mepolizumab. *New Engl J Med.* 2008;358:1215-1228.
147. Roufosse FE, Kahn JE, Gleich GJ, et al. Long-term safety of mepolizumab for the treatment of hypereosinophilic syndromes. *J Allergy Clin Immunol.* 2013;131:461-467.
148. Roufosse F, Kahn JE, Rothenberg ME, et al. Efficacy and safety of mepolizumab in hypereosinophilic syndrome: a phase III, randomized, placebo-controlled trial. *J Allergy Clin Immunol.* 2020;146:1397-1405.
149. Bleecker ER, FitzGerald JM, Chanez P, et al. Efficacy and safety of benralizumab for patients with severe asthma uncontrolled with high-dosage corticosteroids and long-acting β2-agonists (SIROCCO): a randomised, multicenter, placebo-controlled phase 3 trial. *Lancet.* 2016;388:2115-2127.
150. FitzGerald JM, Bleecker ER, Nair P, et al. Benralizumab, an anti-interleukin-5 receptor α monoclonal antibody, as add-on treatment for patients with severe, uncontrolled, eosinophilic asthma (CALIMA): a randomised, double-blind, placebo-controlled phase 3 trial. *Lancet.* 2016;388:2128-2141.
151. Nair P, Wenzel S, Rabe KF, et al. Oral glucocorticoid-sparing effect of benralizumab in severe asthma. *N Engl J Med.* 2017;376:2448-2458.
152. Kuang FL, Legrand F, Makiya M, et al. Benralizumab for PDGFRA-negative hypereosinophilic syndrome. *N Engl J Med.* 2019;380:1336-1346.
153. Kuang FL, Fay MP, Ware J, et al. Long-term clinical outcomes of high-dose mepolizumab treatment for hypereosinophilic syndrome. *J Allergy Clin Immunol Pract.* 2018;6:1518-1527.e5.
154. Rasmussen HS, Chang AT, Tomasevic N, Bebbington C. A randomized, double-blind, placebo-controlled, ascending dose phase 1 study of AK002, a novel siglec-8 selective monoclonal antibody, in healthy subjects. *J Allergy Clin Immunol.* 2018;141:403.
155. Dellon ES, Peterson KA, Murray JA, et al. Anti-Siglec-8 antibody for eosinophilic gastritis and duodenitis. *N Engl J Med.* 2020;383:1624-1634.
156. Hirano I, Dellon ES, Hamilton JD, et al. Efficacy of dupilumab in a phase 2 randomized trial of adults with active eosinophilic esophagitis. *Gastroenterology.* 2020;158:111-122.
157. Castro M, Corren J, Pavord ID, et al. Dupilumab efficacy and safety in moderate-to-severe uncontrolled asthma. *N Engl J Med.* 2018;378:2486-2496.
158. Vazquez L, Caballero D, Cañizo CD, et al. Allogeneic peripheral blood cell transplantation for hypereosinophilic syndrome with myelofibrosis. *Bone Marrow Transplant.* 2000;25:217-218.
159. Chockalingam A, Jalil A, Shadduck RK, Lister J. Allogeneic peripheral blood stem cell transplantation for hypereosinophilic syndrome with severe cardiac dysfunction. *Bone Marrow Transplant.* 1999;23:1093-1094.
160. Basara N, Markova J, Schmetzer B, et al. Chronic eosinophilic leukemia: successful treatment with an unrelated bone marrow transplantation. *Leuk Lymphoma.* 1998;32:189-93.
161. Sigmund DA, Flessa HC. Hypereosinophilic syndrome: successful allogeneic bone marrow transplantation. *Bone Marrow Transplant.* 1995;15:647-648.
162. Esteva-Lorenzo FJ, Meehan KR, Spitzer TR, et al. Allogeneic bone marrow transplantation in a patient with hypereosinophilic syndrome. *Am J Hematol.* 1996;51:164-65.
163. Sadoun A, Lacotte L, Delwail V, et al. Allogeneic bone marrow transplantation for hypereosinophilic syndrome with advanced myelofibrosis. *Bone Marrow Transplant.* 1997;19:741-743.
164. Juvonen E, Volin L, Kopenen A, et al. Allogeneic blood stem cell transplantation following non-myeloablative conditioning for hypereosinophilic syndrome. *Bone Marrow Transplant.* 2002;29:457-458.
165. Ueno NT, Anagnostopoulos A, Rondon G, et al. Successful non-myeloablative allogeneic transplantation for treatment of idiopathic hypereosinophilic syndrome. *Br J Haematol.* 2002;119:131-34.
166. Halaburda K, Prejzner W, Szatkowski D, et al. Allogeneic bone marrow transplantation for hypereosinophilic syndrome: long-term follow-up with eradication of FIP1L1-PDGFRA fusion transcript. *Bone Marrow Transplant.* 2006;38(4)319-320.
167. Harley JB, McIntosh XL, Kirklin JJ, et al. Atrioventricular valve replacement in the idiopathic hypereosinophilic syndrome. *Am J Med.* 1982;73:77-81.
168. Hendren WG, Jones EL, Smith MD. Aortic and mitral valve replacement in idiopathic hypereosinophilic syndrome. *Ann Thorac Surg.* 1988;46:570-571.
169. Cameron J, Radford DJ, Howell J, et al. Hypereosinophilic heart disease. *Med J Aust.* 1985;143:408-410.
170. Weyman AE, Rankin R, King H. Loeffler's endocarditis presenting as mitral and tricuspid stenosis. *Am J Cardiol.* 1977;40:438-444.
171. Chandra M, Pettigrew RI, Eley JW, et al. Cine-MRI-aided endomyocardectomy in idiopathic hypereosinophilic syndrome. *Ann Thorac Surg.* 1996;62:1856-858.
172. Moore PM, Harley JB, Fauci AS. Neurologic dysfunction in the idiopathic hypereosinophilic syndrome. *Ann Intern Med.* 1985;102:109-14.
173. Johnston AM, Woodcock BE. Acute aortic thrombosis despite anticoagulant therapy in idiopathic hypereosinophilic syndrome. *J R Soc Med.* 1998;91:492-493.

Chapter 87 ■ Systemic Mastocytosis

DEAN D. METCALFE • JONATHAN J. LYONS • JASON GOTLIB

HISTORICAL BACKGROUND

Mastocytosis is a heterogeneous disease characterized by the abnormal growth and accumulation of mast cells in one or more organs. The first case of mastocytosis was reported in 1869 by Nettleship and Tay under the heading of "rare forms of urticarial." Cutaneous lesions were described as "brown cutaneous lesions that wheal after scratching"[1] and were termed *urticaria pigmentosa* (UP) (now referred to as maculopapular cutaneous mastocytosis [MPCM]) 1 year after this initial description.[2] The association between mast cells and mastocytosis was made in 1887, when Unna found that UP lesions were characterized by an increased number of mast cells in the dermis.[3]

Subsequent appreciation of the full clinical spectrum of these disorders has identified variants of mastocytosis that involve mast cell infiltration of visceral organs, and these forms of disease are collectively termed *systemic mastocytosis* (SM) as adopted by the World Health Organization.[4] It is now accepted that SM may present with or without skin lesions and may show an indolent or aggressive clinical course, in some cases complicated by a concomitant hematologic neoplasm, usually of myeloid origin, such as a myelodysplastic syndrome (MDS), myeloproliferative neoplasm (MPN), or overlap MDS/MPN. This has led to a further updated classification of mastocytosis based on hematologic findings, molecular markers, and serum levels of biomarkers like tryptase and the cluster designation (CD) markers such as CD25, thereby grouping patients into better-defined clinical categories.[4-6]

PATHOPHYSIOLOGY

The current understanding of the etiology of mastocytosis has evolved from concentrated research efforts in the 1990s that linked two key factors controlling mast cell growth and activity: stem cell factor (SCF) and the SCF receptor, KIT, and disruption of the normal function of KIT through activating mutations.[7]

Mastocytosis is thus recognized in the majority of cases to represent a clonal disorder of a pluripotent hematopoietic progenitor cell with the most common mutation consisting of an activating mutation at codon 816 in *KIT*.[7-10] This precursor is believed to be more primitive than precursors committed to either the neutrophil/macrophage or erythroid cell lineages, with the affected clone showing variable expansion in these lineages in the peripheral blood of patients with SM.[11] Thus, mastocytosis in such cases represents a somatic cell disorder that is confined to hematopoietic lineages. Although T cells and B cells of such mastocytosis patients carry a codon 816 mutation (such as p.D816V), unlike mast cells, these cells do not express surface KIT when mature, and thus may be less susceptible to the biologic effects of constitutively activated KIT.

Early research efforts in the area of mast cell biology concentrated on identifying the key biochemical pathways and mediators that accounted for the clinical sequelae seen in physiologic processes as a result of mast cell activation, including anaphylaxis and allergic diseases. Subsequent work by Kitamura et al[12,13] focused on murine models of mast cell deficiency via studies on mice that exhibited abnormal *Kit* (W/W^v mice)[12] and laid the foundation for suggesting the pathophysiologic basis of human mastocytosis was dysfunction involving the KIT-SCF axis.[13] Two predominant hypotheses thus emerged regarding the etiology of mastocytosis: (a) mastocytosis as a result of local overproduction of soluble SCF and (b) mastocytosis as a result of mutations in *KIT* and downstream signaling molecules that lead to cell proliferation. Over time, with the lack of evidence of significant overproduction of SCF in tissues[14] and with the identification of the p.D816V mutation in *KIT* in patients with mastocytosis,[7] the second hypothesis rose to prominence.

Human mast cells normally reside in tissues associated with epithelial surfaces, blood vessels, nerves, and glands, and are derived from CD34$^+$ pluripotential progenitor cells.[15,16] Except for a population of mast cells that reside in the bone marrow, mast cells complete maturation in peripheral tissues. During this maturation, mast cells downregulate CD34, but continue to express cell surface CD117.[15-17] Under normal physiologic conditions, mast cells and mast cell progenitors do not or only minimally express CD2, CD25, or CD30 on their cell surface. This expression pattern, however, is altered in most patients with mastocytosis.[18]

The *KIT* mutation p.D816V or another similar activating mutation in *KIT* is found in the majority of adults with SM. However, this single mutation cannot alone explain the multiple variants of mastocytosis. It is now generally accepted that *KIT* p.D816V plays an important and possibly causative role in indolent mastocytosis, where the pathologic hallmark is mast cell differentiation and clustering without signs of substantial proliferation. More advanced cases of mastocytosis exhibit additional genetic defects not specific to mastocytosis; for example, myeloid mutations such as *TET2*, *SRSF2*, *ASXL1*, *RUNX1*, *JAK2*, *EZH2*, *CBL*, or *NRAS*[19] that appear to contribute to the severity of disease and often reflect the presence of an associated myeloid neoplasm.

Human mast cells are heterogeneous in terms of morphologic, biochemical, and functional characteristics. These differences correlate with differences in their anatomic locations and, when perturbed in function, associate with specific clinical signs and symptoms. Clinical sequelae of mastocytosis are thus not only the result of organ infiltration but also the result of mast cell mediator release from spontaneous or induced mechanisms.

Mast cells are deemed to be long-lived cells, though it appears that at least some mast cells may proliferate locally in tissues in response to inflammatory or repair processes. In tissue sections, mast cells typically appear as either round or elongated cells, usually with a nonsegmented nucleus with moderate condensation of nuclear chromatin, and contain prominent cytoplasmic granules and lipid bodies. The cytoplasmic granules of mast cells contain heparin and chondroitin sulfate proteoglycans covalently linked to a protein core. Under appropriate conditions, the proteoglycan complexes stain metachromatically with basic dyes.

Human mast cells are characterized primarily as either mucosal (adaptive) or connective tissue (innate) mast cells, the former being more commonly located at mucosal locations, such as the mucosal surfaces of the respiratory system or lamina propria of the gastrointestinal (GI) tract, and containing a specific tryptase (thus a "T-type" mast cell). The latter are more commonly found within connective tissues of the skin, GI submucosa, and genitourinary tracts and contain both tryptase and a chymotryptase (TC mast cells).[20] Human mast cell granules also contain biologically active molecules, such as histamine, acid hydrolases, cathepsin G, and carboxypeptidase.[21] They are activated by a number of stimuli that are both FcεRI-dependent and FcεRI-independent. After activation, mast cells immediately release granule-associated mediators and generate lipid-derived substances that induce immediate allergic responses. Together, these mediators are deemed responsible for many of the clinical sequelae of the immediate hypersensitivity reaction, including pruritus, flushing, palpitations, and lightheadedness, also commonly reported in patients with mastocytosis.

Major lipid mediators produced on appropriate activation via immunoglobulin E (IgE) or non-IgE stimuli include prostaglandin D$_2$ and leukotriene C$_4$.[22] Mast cell activation is followed hours later by the synthesis and release of additional chemokines and cytokines, which then contribute to chronic inflammation. Growth factors, cytokines, and chemokines reported to be synthesized and released from mast cells include basic fibroblast growth factor, nerve growth factor, tumor necrosis factor, granulocyte-macrophage colony-stimulating factor, vascular endothelial growth factor, chemokines CCL2, CCL3 and CCL5, interleukin 2 (IL-2), IL-3, IL-4, IL-5, IL-6, IL-8 (CXCL8), IL-9, IL-10, IL-13, IL-16, and IL-31.[20,22]

Studies performed in rodents, nonhuman primates, and humans have shown that many aspects of mast cell development are critically regulated by SCF, produced by cells such as endothelial cells, fibroblasts, and mast cells.[20,22,23] SCF has been shown to work in concert with other growth factors, such as IL-3, IL-4, IL-5, IL-6, IL-9, and nerve growth factor, to induce optimal mast cell precursor proliferation and survival.[15,16,21] SCF has also been reported to be present in the lesional skin of patients with MPCM[24] but was not identified in blister fluids,[14] and has been reported within neoplastic mast cells.[25] SCF augments mast cell mediator release in response to stimulation by IgE and antigen.[23] Cells bearing mutated KIT on their surface have been shown to have an increased chemotactic response toward SCF.[26] SCF may influence the aggregation of mast cells, leading to mast cell lesions as found in SM within marrow.

The binding of SCF to KIT induces dimerization, with activation of intrinsic tyrosine kinase activity and autophosphorylation of the receptor. This, in turn, leads to exposure of specific recognition motifs for intracellular binding proteins containing SRC homology (SH2) domains, such as phospholipase Cγ-1, phosphatidylinositol-3' kinase, mitogen-activated kinase, and RAS protein.[21,27] Gain-of-function mutations in *KIT* are associated with constitutive tyrosine kinase activation and ligand-independent autophosphorylation of KIT, thereby giving affected mast cells an apparent survival advantage over wild-type cells.[21,28-30]

The *KIT* p.D816V mutation was first reported in peripheral blood mononuclear cells (PBMCs) of adult patients with mastocytosis with an associated hematologic neoplasm (AHN) and in patients with persistent mastocytosis and extensive disease. It is now known that this mutation is present in more than 80% of all patients with SM (>90% using highly sensitive assays such *KIT* p.D816V allele-specific polymerase chain reaction [PCR][31] or droplet digital PCR [ddPCR]) and in approximately 30% of children with cutaneous mastocytosis (CM).[7,8,30] Additional codon 816 mutations (p.D816Y, p.D816T, p.D816F, p.D816A, and p.D816H) as well as mutations elsewhere in *KIT*, such as p.D820G, p.V560G, p.F522C, p.V819I, p.K642E, and del419, have been reported in some patients with SM.[7,8,29,32-34] Finally, there are patients who do not have identifiable variants in *KIT* including about 70% of those who are diagnosed with well-differentiated SM, a rare morphologic variant that spans the WHO-defined subtypes of SM.

Additional mutations have been identified in patients with SM, are generally found in patients with more aggressive variants of disease, and are particularly enriched in SM patients with an associated myeloid neoplasm. These mutations affect genes including those that encode signaling molecules (*KRAS, NRAS, JAK2, CBL*), epigenetic regulators (*TET2, ASXL1, DNMT3A*), splicing factors (*SRSF2, SF3B1*), and genes encoding transcription factors (*RUNX1*).[35] In a proportion of patients with SM–acute myeloid leukemia (AML), the t(8;21)(q22;q22) *RUNX1-RUNX1T1* rearrangement is identified and can be found in both myeloblasts and neoplastic mast cells, implicating a pluripotent hematopoietic progenitor that gives rise to both disease components.[36,37] A subset of patients with eosinophilia and increased serum tryptase levels has been described; these patients carry the *Fip1-like-1–platelet-derived growth factor receptor-α* (*FIP1L1-PDGFRA*) fusion oncogene, which results from an approximately 800-kb interstitial deletion of chromosome 4q12.[38] The bone marrow of such patients may exhibit interstitial involvement by atypical mast cells that express CD25, but is not considered a subtype of SM by the WHO classification. Similarly, a rare case of SM and chronic basophilic leukemia was found secondary to a *PRKG2-PDGFRB* fusion.[39] A polymorphism in the gene for the IL-4 receptor α-chain has been shown to be associated with less extensive mast cell involvement, with disease usually localized to the skin.[40] In addition, the bone marrow cells of patients with mastocytosis have been found to constitutively express the antiapoptotic proteins BCL-XL and BCL-2,[41] which may explain the long survival of these cells and perhaps their resistance to chemotherapy-induced apoptosis.

Additional studies using gene expression analysis of bone marrow mast cells derived from patients with indolent SM (ISM) revealed that, compared with healthy controls, patients with mastocytosis displayed a highly consistent profile with 168 genes that were significantly upregulated or downregulated in patient samples.[42] No recurrent patterns of chromosomal changes have been consistently reported in patients with SM. The implications of these findings and the mutations noted above are that, at least in some patients with mastocytosis, the etiology of their disease may encompass a broader problem of chromosomal and/or genomic instability. For instance, tumor mast cell lines express persistently high telomerase activity throughout the cell cycle that does not appear to be dependent on intracellular signals or cell replication, in contrast to normal human progenitor mast cells that experience transient induction of telomerase activity that is dependent on growth factor-mediated signals, such as SCF-, IL-3-, and IL-6-mediated p38 mitogen-activated kinase and phosphatidylinositol-3' kinase.[43,44]

CLINICAL FEATURES

The clinical manifestations of mastocytosis are diverse and may be divided into those that are systemic or localized.[21,32,34] Systemic effects of this disorder are associated with the release of mast cell mediators into the circulation. Clinical signs and symptoms that comprise systemic mediator release are those reported with anaphylaxis and include flushing, pruritus, hypotension, syncope, palpitations, and tachycardia. GI symptoms are commonly associated with mastocytosis and include nausea, vomiting, abdominal cramping, bloating, and/or diarrhea. Peptic ulcer disease, which appears to reflect at least partially increased gastric acid secretion as a result of hyperhistaminemia, may occur in up to 50% of patients with systemic disease.[45] Malabsorption, although less common, tends to be mild, but when present, reflects more advanced disease. Local sequelae of mastocytosis are largely caused by the effects of mast cell collections at specific organ sites and may result in severe end-organ damage caused by infiltration of normal tissue with mast cells and subsequent fibrosis (e.g., end-stage liver disease caused by fibrosis and bone marrow failure).

For some patients, in particular those with advanced disease or with an AHN, the most bothersome complaints include severe and nonspecific constitutional symptoms of fatigue, weakness, anorexia, weight loss, low-grade fevers, night sweats, musculoskeletal pain, headaches, depression, altered attention span, irritability, and even subtle cognitive deficits such as mild memory loss. Some of these symptoms are attributable to ongoing chronic disease, whereas others may in part be a result of the central nervous system effects of mast cell mediators.

Attacks in some individuals are precipitated by stimuli, such as heat, cold, pressure, alcohol, medications (e.g., opiates, nonsteroidal anti-inflammatory agents, and estrogens), radiocontrast agents, and venoms. Reactions may be more severe in such patients (e.g., anaphylaxis after Hymenoptera stings) because of an expanded mast cell population.[22,46] Patients with aggressive disease also often present with lymphadenopathy, splenomegaly, or hepatomegaly that may or may not be symptomatic. One of the most difficult clinical scenarios of mastocytosis from a management perspective is the treatment of severe musculoskeletal pain and/or pathologic fractures. Besides local disruption of normal bone architecture, mast cell infiltration of bone may cause bone loss as a result of the secretion of heparin, IL-6, proteases, and other mediators, and from their paracrine effects on osteoclast function.

The most frequently involved organs in SM are the skin, bone marrow, lymph nodes, spleen, liver, and GI tract. Atopy (e.g., eczema and allergic rhinitis) and airway hyperreactivity (e.g., asthma) can occur concomitantly with mastocytosis and complicate management.

Updated criteria for the diagnosis of cutaneous and SM are provided in *Table 87.1*.[5] The diagnosis of SM requires that one major and one minor criterion or at least three minor criteria be present. Criteria for variants of SM are provided in *Table 87.2*.

The prognosis of patients with adult mastocytosis depends on the extent of disease and presence of an AHN. Patients with ISM have a life expectancy similar to age-matched controls and tend to remain within this category of disease; however, a small subset will progress to more aggressive forms of disease, such as SM-AHN or aggressive SM/mast cell leukemia (ASM/MCL). For children with isolated MPCM, at least 50% of cases are reported to resolve by adulthood.[47] Patients with SM-AHN have a median life expectancy of 2 years; however, within this group, there is substantial heterogeneity in prognosis that largely depends on the specific type and stage of the AHN and

Table 87.1. World Health Organization Diagnostic Criteria for Cutaneous and Systemic Mastocytosis

Cutaneous mastocytosis
Typical clinical findings of MPCM, DCM, or cutaneous mastocytoma, and typical infiltrates of mast cells in a multifocal or diffuse pattern on skin biopsy.

Systemic Mastocytosis
The diagnosis of SM is made if one major and one minor criteria are present, or if at least three minor criteria are met.

Major Criterion
Multifocal, dense infiltrates of mast cells (15 or more in aggregates) detected in sections of bone marrow and/or another extracutaneous organ.

Minor Criteria
a. In biopsy sections of bone marrow or other extracutaneous organs, more than 25% of the mast cells in the infiltrate are spindle shaped or have atypical morphology, or, of all mast cells in bone marrow aspirate smears, more than 25% are immature or atypical mast cells.
b. Detection of an activating mutation at codon 816 or elsewhere in *KIT* in bone marrow, blood, or another extracutaneous organ.
c. Mast cells in the bone marrow, blood, or another extracutaneous organ express CD25 or CD30, with or without CD2, in addition to normal mast cell markers.
d. Serum total tryptase persistently greater than 20 ng/mL in the absence of an unrelated clonal myeloid disorder or HaT.

Abbreviations: DCM, diffuse cutaneous mastocytosis; HaT, hereditary alpha-tryptasemia; MPCM, maculopapular cutaneous mastocytosis; SM, systemic mastocytosis; UP, urticaria pigmentosa.

Table 87.2. Consensus Criteria for Variants of Systemic Mastocytosis

Indolent systemic mastocytosis (ISM)
Meets criteria for SM (see *Table 87.1*). No more than one "B" finding, no "C" finding. Typical skin findings. For ISM without skin lesions, no or one "B" finding and/or basal serum tryptase equal to or greater than 125 ng/mL and/or dense SM infiltrates in an extramedullary organ. No C-finding, no criteria for MCL on an AHN

Bone marrow mastocytosis (BMM)
Meets criteria for SM, no skin lesions, no "B" or "C" findings, basal serum tryptase less than 125 ng/mL, no dense SM infiltrates in an extramedullary organ, no criteria for MCL, or AHN

Smoldering systemic mastocytosis (SSM)
As above for ISM, but with two or more "B" findings and no "C" findings, no criteria for MCL, or AHN

Systemic mastocytosis with associated hematologic neoplasm (SM-AHN)
Meets criteria for ISM or SM variant (BMM, SSM, ASM, MCL) and criteria for an associated, clonal hematologic non–mast cell lineage disorder, AHN (MDS, MPN, AML, lymphoma, or other hematologic neoplasm that meets the criteria for a distinct entity in the WHO classification).

Aggressive systemic mastocytosis (ASM)
Meets criteria for SM with one or more "C" findings. No evidence of mast cell leukemia or AHN. Usually without skin lesions. Mast cells on peripheral blood or bone marrow smears below 20% to exclude MCL.[a]

Mast cell leukemia (MCL)
Meets criteria for SM. Bone marrow typically shows a diffuse infiltration by atypical, immature mast cells. Bone marrow aspirate smears show 20% or more mast cells. Mast cells account for 10% or more of peripheral white blood cells. Variant: aleukemic mast cell leukemia as above, but less than 10% of white blood cells are mast cells. Usually without skin lesions.[a]

Mast cell sarcoma (MCS)
Localized mast cell tumor. No evidence of CM or SM. Immature atypical mast cells. Destructive growth pattern.[a]

"B" findings
1. Bone marrow biopsy showing greater than 30% infiltration by mast cells (focal, dense aggregates) and/or tryptase >200 ng/mL and/or *KIT* p.D816V VAF > 10% in marrow or peripheral blood leukocytes.
2. Signs of dysplasia or myeloproliferation in non–mast cell lineages, but insufficient criteria for definitive diagnosis of a hematopoietic neoplasm.
3. Hepatomegaly without impairment of liver function or ascites, and/or palpable splenomegaly without hypersplenism and without weight loss, and/or lymphadenopathy on palpation or imaging.

"C" findings
1. Bone marrow dysfunction manifested by one or more cytopenias (ANC < 1.0×10^9/L, Hb < 10 g/dL, or platelets < 100×10^9/L) caused by neoplastic mast cell infiltration.
2. Palpable hepatomegaly with elevated liver enzymes and ascites, and/or portal hypertension and/or cirrhotic liver.
3. Skeletal involvement with large-sized osteolysis (>2 cm lesions) and/or pathologic fractures.
4. Palpable splenomegaly with hypersplenism.
5. Malabsorption with hypoalbuminemia ± weight loss.

Abbreviations: AML, acute myeloid leukemia; GI, gastrointestinal; Hb, hemoglobin; MDS, myelodysplastic syndrome; MPN, myeloproliferative neoplasm; WHO, World Health Organization.
[a]See text for details.

response to cytoreductive therapy.[21,48] In one series, the median life expectancies of patients with ASM and MCL were 3.5 years and less than 6 months; however, their prognosis, similar to SM-AHN patients, is quite variable.[48] The term "chronic mast cell leukemia" has been used for those MCL patients without organ damage who may experience a more indolent course and relatively better survival.[49] Variables that have been associated with poor survival in adult patients include advanced age, weight loss, anemia, thrombocytopenia, hypoalbuminemia, and excess bone marrow blasts.[48] New risk stratification scoring systems provide a more refined assessment of prognosis, and are discussed below.

Cutaneous Mastocytosis

CM is more common in children and is diagnosed based on typical skin lesions, a positive Darier sign and absence of evidence of systemic involvement. In adults, CM is usually accompanied by systemic disease, but where staging is not yet complete including a marrow study, the provisional diagnosis is mastocytosis in the skin. CM is composed of three distinct clinical variants: MPCM, diffuse CM (DCM), and cutaneous mastocytoma (*Table 87.1*). MPCM is further subcategorized into two subvariants: polymorphic (MPCM-p) and monomorphic (MPCM-m).[5] The monomorphic variant consists of small maculopapular lesions, which are typically seen in adult patients. The polymorphic variant consists of larger lesions of variable size and shape and is seen mainly in children.

MPCM consists of reddish-brown macules, papules, or plaques that urticate (i.e., form a wheal and erythema with a distinct border when stroked [a positive Darier sign]). However, in a number of adult patients, cutaneous lesions are lacking, and other organs, particularly the bone marrow, when biopsied, support the diagnosis of SM. MPCM tends to occur in a generalized distribution, most commonly occurring over the trunk and generally sparing the face, scalp, palms, and soles. When abundant, they may form a cobblestone appearance. There appears to be no sex predilection or familial pattern of cutaneous disease, though mastocytosis of one form or another has been described in families, including several sets of twins.[47]

Histologically, MPCM lesions are composed of a collection of mast cells within the papillary dermis with variable extension throughout the reticular dermis and into the subcutaneous fat. An increase in dermal mast cells ≥10 times that of normal skin, in the absence of other pathology, is highly suggestive of MPCM.[47,50] Petechiae, ecchymoses, and telangiectasias may be present in or adjacent to the lesions. Blister formation and hemorrhage may occur, particularly in infants and young children. This complication is presumed to take place because of high local levels of mediators released from mast cells, but why this younger age group is more adversely affected is unknown. The onset of MPCM lesions tends to follow a biphasic curve, with one peak at 2.5 months of age and another at 26.5 years.[50] Of pediatric patients in whom MPCM occurs, approximately half lose these lesions by adolescence, especially the polymorphic form. The remaining patients generally have lighter macular lesions at previously involved sites. Pruritus is the most common symptom that accompanies MPCM. Between 15% and 30% of pediatric patients with skin lesions, especially of the monomorphic type, persist into adulthood.[51]

Although MPCM in adults may persist indefinitely, a subset of patients, estimated from 7% to 19% in published series, experience fading or resolution of cutaneous lesions over time.[52] Regression of MPCM in patients with ISM appears to parallel a decrease in disease severity in terms of constitutional symptoms, although bone marrow findings of ISM may remain. The absence or presence of the *KIT* p.D816V mutation in PBMCs does not necessarily predict the course of MPCM. Disease progression in patients with SM-AHN is, therefore, also monitored with serum tryptase levels and bone marrow biopsy findings rather than with changes in the number, distribution, or intensity of skin lesions.

DCM is a less frequent cutaneous manifestation and generally presents before the age of 3 years. It is characterized by a diffuse mast cell infiltration of the dermis, and the entire skin is generally involved. Darier sign is positive. DCM presents as a yellow-red-brown discoloration with a peau d'orange appearance, or as a generalized erythroderma in which severe edema gives the skin a doughy appearance. Additionally, yellow-cream-colored papules have been described that resemble xanthomas and pseudoxanthoma elasticum.[50] Only rarely does skin appear superficially normal in DCM. Dermatographism and formation of hemorrhagic blisters may occur. GI manifestations, such as diarrhea, flushing, and hypotension, may be associated, and such patients have an increased risk for more serious clinical sequelae, such as shock, significant GI bleeding, and death. DCM may resolve spontaneously by age 5 to 15 months, but when persistent, the skin may remain thickened and doughy and recalcitrant to treatment.

Isolated or multilocalized cutaneous mastocytomas are considered a variant of CM that may present at birth or more commonly within the first 3 months, often with spontaneous involution during childhood.[47,50] They are only rarely described in adults. They present as macules, plaques, or nodules and are formed by dermal collections of mast cells without cellular atypia. They are most commonly seen on the extremities and may involve the palms or soles. When systemic symptoms are present, they most commonly involve flushing. In young children with typical mastocytoma, testing for Darier sign is often avoided because of a risk to produce systemic reactions. Telangiectasia macularis eruptiva perstans is no longer considered a subtype of MPCM.[53]

Indolent Systemic Mastocytosis

ISM is characterized by mast cell involvement at various organ sites, although significant organ damage (C findings) is absent, and prognosis in these patients is generally favorable. The bone marrow is the most common site of extracutaneous mastocytosis, with the vast majority of adult patients with indolent disease demonstrating bone marrow mast cell infiltration.[54-56] The criteria for diagnosis of ISM are provided in *Table 87.2*.[5]

Characteristic bone marrow lesions of ISM are aggregates of mast cells, identified by anti-tryptase staining, although the diagnosis of ISM may be made in their absence if three minor diagnostic criteria are fulfilled.[5] Focal lesions are frequently observed in paratrabecular and perivascular areas and may be associated with adjacent T and B cells and/or eosinophil aggregates.[54,56] Mast cells in these patients show characteristic cytologic abnormalities, including cytoplasmic surface projections, eccentric oval nuclei, and a hypogranulated cytoplasm (atypical mast cell type I).[5] A representative bone marrow aspirate from a patient with ISM with characteristic morphologic features compared with a control bone marrow aspirate is shown in *Figure 87.1*. Clonal mast cells generally express CD2 or CD25, or both, on their cell surface, and a *KIT* p.D816V mutation.[5,18,55] The histopathology of associated lymphoid aggregates is similar to benign lymphoid aggregates associated with reactive bone marrow and not lymphoproliferative disease, the latter being uncommon in patients with ISM. In bone marrow extensively involved by mast cell infiltration, the bony trabeculae may be moderately to markedly thickened. On occasion, mast cell infiltrates may be masked by other cellular infiltrates associated with AHN. Thus, it is recommended to reapply the diagnostic criteria for SM after cytoreductive therapy to assess for the possible diagnosis of SM-AHN.

In contrast to adults with ISM, definitive marrow involvement in children is much less common. Here a bone marrow study is usually not recommended unless there are signs of SM or another hematologic neoplasm including abnormal peripheral blood indices, organomegaly, lymphadenopathy, elevated liver enzymes without a known disorder such as viral hepatitis, serum tryptase persistently above 20 ng/mL or an increased value (>11.4 ng/mL) in the absence of hereditary alpha-tryptasemia (HαT), or malabsorption with weight loss.[57] Identification of the *KIT* p.D816V mutation in peripheral blood by allele-specific qPCR or ddPCR has been reported to be negative in children with cutaneous disease only, but to be positive in approximately 85% of patients with both cutaneous and systemic/probable systemic disease.[58]

Isolated bone marrow mastocytosis (BMM) is a rare variant of SM that is distinctive in lacking cutaneous and multiorgan involvement.[4,5] The tryptase level in this group of patients is <125 ng/mL. There are

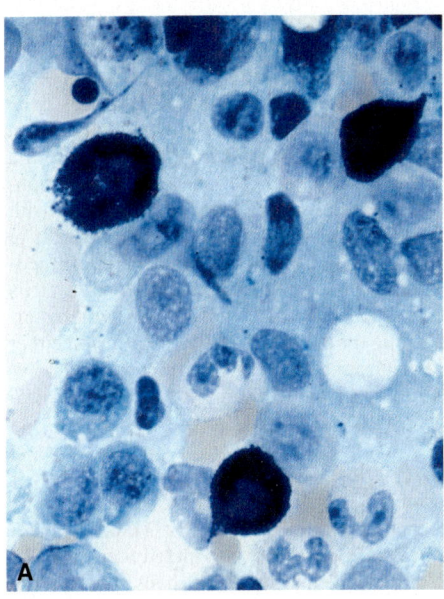 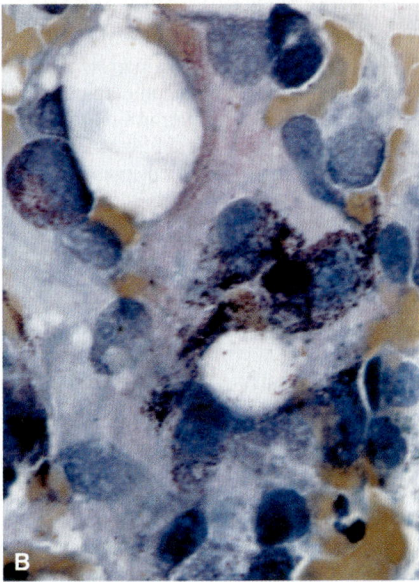

FIGURE 87.1 Morphologic features of mast cells from normal vs mastocytosis bone marrow aspirate. Panel A showing staining of a control bone marrow aspirate from an individual with aplastic anemia using toluidine blue stain (magnification, ×40). Panel B showing a hematoxylin and eosin stain of a bone marrow aspirate acquired from a patient with indolent systemic mastocytosis and illustrating representative spindle-shaped mast cells with an eccentric nucleus (magnification, ×40).

no dense mast cell infiltrates in an extramedullary organ, and no criteria for MCL or an AHN. These patients generally require no specific therapy, but this subvariant must be differentiated from ASM or MCL and prognosis is favorable. Those with BMM have a relatively high prevalence of IgE-mediated venom allergies and osteoporosis.

Smoldering Systemic Mastocytosis

Smoldering systemic mastocytosis (SSM) was previously categorized as a subtype of ISM,[5,59] but is now listed as a unique variant.[60] Unlike typical ISM, these patients manifest two or three B findings (but no C findings) (*Table 87.2*) and have a higher mast cell burden (e.g., bone marrow infiltration grade >30% [dense infiltrates] and serum tryptase >200 ng/mL). Although these patients have no overt myeloproliferative or myelodysplastic disease, they are at higher risk for progression to more aggressive forms of mastocytosis and carry a worse prognosis than those with ISM. Bone marrow lesions typically contain dense focal and diffuse mast cell infiltrates, and mast cells detected in such lesions may be immature. Markers of a poorer prognosis in this subvariant include a hypercellular bone marrow, hepatosplenomegaly or lymphadenopathy, and the presence of *KIT* p.D816V in multilineage cells of the peripheral blood.[61] Patients with SSM should thus be followed closely, with useful parameters to monitor including basal serum tryptase (BSL), alkaline phosphatase, and *KIT* p.D816V variant allele frequency in peripheral blood. In the new WHO classification, a KIT p.D816V variant allele frequency of ≥10% was added as a B-finding.[4]

Lymphadenopathy is present in a subset of patients with ISM, but is more commonly seen in those with more aggressive variants such as SSM. Peripheral lymphadenopathy has been reported in 26% of patients and central lymphadenopathy in 19% of patients at the time of the diagnosis of SM.[62] Hyperplasia of lymph nodes is the result of infiltration with mast cells, and approximately one-half of cases are associated with aggregates of eosinophils. Infiltrates are more commonly observed in the paracortex, follicles, medullary cords, and sinuses. Other histopathologic findings may include extramedullary hematopoiesis, small blood vessel proliferation in paracortical areas, and collagen fibrosis.[63] Patients who develop progressive lymphadenopathy, and especially if accompanied by peripheral blood abnormalities, should be closely monitored for evolution into a more aggressive systemic disorder.

Splenomegaly is categorized as a "B" finding and if hypersplenism is present, becomes a "C" finding.[5,60] A review of pathologic features of 16 spleens from patients with mastocytosis showed a paratrabecular distribution of mast cell infiltrates in 15 of 16 spleens. In addition, parafollicular, follicular, and diffuse infiltrates were noted in 10 (64%), 2 (4%), and 1 (7%) patients, respectively.[62] Varying degrees of trabecular and capsular fibrosis and eosinophilic hematopoiesis and plasmacytosis were seen, and 71% of all biopsies revealed extramedullary hematopoiesis. The prognostic significance of splenomegaly is seen with markedly increased splenic weights (>700 g) that have been reported to correlate with SM-AHN or ASM[64] and may be a contributing factor to the hematologic abnormalities observed in such patients.

Mast cell infiltration of the liver is a common finding in SM, although severe liver disease and hepatomegaly are relatively uncommon except, again, in patients with more aggressive forms of disease. Thus, hepatomegaly without impairment of liver function is a "B" finding and with impairment of liver function, which may be associated with ascites, becomes a "C" finding. In one study of 41 patients with mastocytosis, liver disease was reported in 61%.[65] Approximately one-half of the patients with liver disease in this series exhibited elevated liver function tests, either an elevated alkaline phosphatase, 5′ nucleotidase, or γ-glutamyl transpeptidase. Mast cell infiltration of the liver has been described in two distinct patterns: diffuse infiltration involving the cords and sinuses in the red pulp and focal infiltration in the white pulp of the liver. Hepatomegaly, infiltration of the liver by mast cells on liver biopsy, and hepatic fibrosis correlate with elevated levels of serum alkaline phosphatase. These findings are more commonly seen in patients with aggressive disease, ascites, and/or portal hypertension. As confirmed on liver biopsy, portal fibrosis and venopathy with subsequent veno-occlusive disease appear to be a result of vascular obstruction by mast cell infiltrates.[65] Fibrosis, including that which affects the liver, often accompanies mast cell proliferation and may be due to mast cell release of proinflammatory mediators, such as transforming growth factor-β.

GI symptoms reported in SM include abdominal pain, cramping, nausea, vomiting, diarrhea, and peptic ulcer disease. Malabsorption with hypoalbuminemia caused by mucosal mast cell infiltration is less commonly observed and may be associated with weight loss and is a "C" finding.[45,66] One prospective study revealed that 6 of 16 patients with SM had a significantly elevated basal acid secretion, with concomitantly low gastrin levels.[45] These data were found to be consistent with the hypothesis that histamine secreted by mast cells contributes to gastric hypersecretion. Subsequent studies have shown that biopsy of gastric tissues in mastocytosis patients with acid hypersecretion symptoms did not always demonstrate increased mast cell infiltrates, thereby suggesting that the hyperhistaminemia observed in such patients may be caused by oversecretion by all mast cells and not to an increased mast cell burden in the gastric tissues. GI disease is much less common in children, although GI bleeding is a potential complication with severe disease,[47] and abdominal cramping and diarrhea have also been reported.

Musculoskeletal pain in patients with SM has been well documented, although of uncertain etiology unless associated with osteopenia or osteoporosis, with more advanced cases of osteoporosis associated with pathologic fractures.[67-69] In some cases, osteoporosis or pathologic fractures or both may be the initial manifestation of mastocytosis.

In the evaluation of skeletal disease in mastocytosis, skeletal surveys may show focal or diffuse abnormalities, and the latter have been associated with more aggressive disease and a worse prognosis. The most commonly reported abnormalities are diffuse, poorly demarcated, sclerotic, and lucent areas involving the axial skeleton.[68] In addition to bone loss, patients with mastocytosis may exhibit concomitant abnormal bone formation, resulting in osteosclerosis. The presence of osteolytic lesions greater than or equal to 2 cm in diameter with clear clinical impact such as fractures and confirmed histology is a "C" finding.[5]

Occasionally, patients in whom bone involvement by mastocytosis is not seen on routine diagnostic evaluation and symptoms are not found to be attributable to any known cause may nonetheless report myalgias and arthralgias, often in concert with constitutional symptoms of fatigue, general weakness, and depression. Management of this patient subset may be particularly challenging and may require behavior modification practices as well as therapeutic intervention emphasizing nonnarcotic analgesics for adequate pain relief.

Systemic Mastocytosis With an AHN

A subset of patients with SM either presents with, or develops over time, a defined hematologic neoplasm including myeloid neoplasms and rarely lymphoid neoplasms (except those detected in a separate organ system). These patients are categorized as SM-AHN.[5,56,69,70] The term "SM-AHN" was introduced in the revised 2016 WHO classification, and is now used instead of the previous term "SM with an associated hematologic non-mast cell lineage disorder (SM-AHNMD)."[60] In the new International Consensus Classification, the term as been changed to 'SM-AMN', or SM with an associated myeloid neoplasm' reflecting the fact that almost all associated diseases are myeloid in nature.[6] Subdiagnostic clonal conditions such as monoclonal gammopathy of undetermined significance do not count as an AHN. Thus, among 138 consecutive reported cases with SM-AHN, 89% had an associated myeloid neoplasm: MPN (45%), chronic myelomonocytic leukemia (CMML; 29%), MDS (23%), and acute leukemia (3%).[71] Myeloma or lymphoma was rarely observed.[5,56,69,70] In all such patients, WHO criteria to diagnose an AHN as well as SM are applied with specific reference to the associated diagnostic entity.[5,71] The *KIT* p.D816V mutation has been identified in both neoplastic mast cells and in cells of the associated myeloid neoplasm (e.g., CMML) by laser microdissection.[72] Although the prognosis of SM-AHN frequently relates to the AHN component, the type and stage of the associated myeloid neoplasm need to be considered on an individual basis. For example, whereas the average overall median survival of SM-AHN was 24 months in one analysis, SM-MPN exhibited an average survival of 31 months compared to 15 months for SM-CMML and 13 months for SM-MDS.[73]

Management of these patients involves treating the disease component that is contributing to the immediate clinical sequelae, although it can be very challenging to dissect whether the SM or AHN component (or both) is the primary contributor to B and C findings. To this point, targeted organ biopsy may be useful for ascertaining the cause of organ damage and for decision-making regarding whether the patient's AHN can be observed, or requires more intensive treatment, such as chemotherapy, or consideration of bone marrow (stem cell) transplantation in suitable candidates (see section "Management").

Bone marrow findings that are more common with SM-AHN include a hypercellular bone marrow, dysplasia of myeloid or erythroid cell lineages, and an increased megakaryocyte number or megakaryocyte atypia. Fibrosis may be seen and is more frequent in patients with an associated hematologic disorder. Mast cells with bilobed nuclei, if seen on biopsy, portend a poor prognosis. Peripheral blood monocytosis and/or eosinophilia may reflect an associated CMML or chronic eosinophilic leukemia (CEL), respectively.

An imatinib-sensitive *FIP1L1-PDGFRA* fusion oncogene-positive group of myeloid neoplasms with eosinophilia may exhibit increased serum tryptase levels. Such patients display clinical and histologic features of a MPN (more rarely AML) with increased numbers of bone marrow mast cells in an interstitial pattern, but lack the pathognomonic aggregates of atypical mast cells characteristic of SM bone marrows on routine hematoxylin and eosin staining.[38,74] Similarly, an imatinib-sensitive *PRKG2-PDGFRB* fusion has been identified in a patient presenting with increased numbers of mast cells and peripheral basophilia.[39] The WHO classification[5,60] places these cases with *PDGFRA* or *PDGRFB* fusion genes with an increase in mast cells in the bone marrow in the major category of Myeloid/lymphoid neoplasms with eosinophilia and tyrosine kinase gene fusions.[4,6] It is thus recommended that all suspected mastocytosis cases with hypereosinophilia undergo screening for the *FIP1L1-PDGFRA* fusion either by fluorescence in situ hybridization or by reverse transcriptase polymerase chain reaction (RT-PCR) given the exquisite sensitivity of such cases to imatinib therapy.

Aggressive Systemic Mastocytosis

ASM is a variant of mastocytosis characterized by one or more "C" findings but with no evidence of an MCL or an AHN. MPCM is often absent. Abnormal myelopoiesis is observed with mixed focal and diffuse mast cell infiltration of the bone marrow. These cells may be atypical and may be associated with other peripheral blood abnormalities (initially often presenting with eosinophilia), hepatosplenomegaly, osteopenia and pathologic fractures, and life-threatening organ impairment.[5,75] A subset of cases appears to be associated with a prior history of malignant germ cell tumors.[76]

In some patients, bone marrow aspirates may reveal significant numbers of mast cells with bilobed or multilobed nuclei (high-grade morphology). Metachromatic blasts may also be detected. The peripheral blood smear may show cytopenias, leukocytosis, eosinophilia, or monocytosis.[77] Laboratory test abnormalities are frequently observed in such patients, with elevations in liver function, and serum alkaline phosphatase, and a prolonged prothrombin and partial thromboplastin time. Because of impaired hepatic function and a propensity for spontaneous mast cell degranulation, ASM patients with more advanced disease may be at high risk for spontaneous hemorrhage during periods of mast cell mediator release. Serum tryptase levels may be high and demonstrate wide fluctuations potentially due to spontaneous mast cell degranulation.

In most patients with ASM, the percentage of abnormal mast cells in the bone marrow smear is below 5%, which is a favorable prognostic sign. Mast cells must be below 20% to exclude MCL. Notably, in the less frequent ASM patients in whom mast cells comprise 5% to 19% of all nucleated bone marrow cells on a Giemsa-stained BM smear, termed "ASM in transformation," the prognosis is poor because many of these patients progress and transform to MCL or an ASM-AHN.[49]

Mast Cell Leukemia and MCL Variants

MCL is an unusual and rare variant of mastocytosis, with a generally poor prognosis.[5,48,49,78,79] MCL has been subdivided by some investigators into a few subtypes depending on the variable: (a) classical leukemic form with mast cells greater than or equal to 10% of all leukocytes in peripheral blood smears vs an aleukemic variant with mast cells less than 10% in peripheral blood smears; (b) primary (de novo MCL) vs secondary MCL (arising from a less advanced form of SM [e.g. ISM, SSM, or SM-AHN] or CM); (c) acute MCL with C-findings and chronic MCL where C-findings are not detected; and (d) MCL with or without AHN. In a multivariate analysis of 28 MCL patients, positivity for one or more of the high-risk mutations *SRSF2*, *ASXL1*, or *RUNX1* was the only independent poor risk factor for overall survival (OS).[79]

Challenges in diagnostic morphology related to the diagnosis of MCL partly relate to the fact that whereas a core biopsy may show a high burden of neoplastic mast cells (e.g., 70%-80% or higher) by immunohistochemical staining for CD117, tryptase, and CD25, the bone marrow aspirate may not always demonstrate a commensurate burden of neoplastic mast cells. This may relate to sampling, and/or difficulty in aspirating mast cells if the marrow is extensively involved by peri-aggregate fibrosis. The bone marrow typically shows a dense and diffuse infiltration of mast cells that display an immature, blastlike morphology with bilobed or multilobed nuclei; diffuse fibrosis is uncommon. Many of these mast cells express CD2 or CD25 or both.[5,80] *KIT* p.D816V may be detected in 80% of patients, but generally is found at a lower frequency than in ISM, ASM, and SM-AHN because alternative *KIT* p.D816 variants, non-exon 17 *KIT* mutations, or non-*KIT* molecular abnormalities may be contributing to disease progression. When MCL is accompanied by an AHN, peripheral blood abnormalities that may be observed include leukocytosis, monocytosis, eosinophilia, anemia, and/or thrombocytopenia, and one or both disease components may contribute to cytopenias. Like ASM, MCL patients are prone to bleeding diatheses, with or without signs of consumption or hyperfibrinolysis. The prognosis of MCL is generally very poor. A series of 342 consecutive patients included four patients with MCL whose prognosis was only 2 months.[48] Similarly, a literature review of 51 cases of MCL identified a median OS of 6 months with a range of 0.5 to 98 months, emphasizing the clinical heterogeneity of this subgroup.[8,9] In a recent ECNM registry series of 92 MCL patients, the largest published to date the median overall survival was 1.6 years.[81]

Myelomastocytic leukemia (MML) is in the differential diagnosis of MCL. In those with MML, criteria for SM are not met and neoplastic mast cells (greater than or equal to 10% in marrow or blood smears) are derived from neoplastic stem cells of an underlying myeloid neoplasm.[5] Some may be re-classified as MCL over time.

Mast Cell Sarcoma

Mast cell sarcoma (MCS) is a rare and ill-defined localized, malignant neoplasm composed of atypical mast cells with a high nucleus-to-cytoplasm ratio, nucleoli, and a hypogranulated cytoplasm. CM and SM criteria are not met. Mutations in *KIT* are usually absent. MCS may occur at any age in any organ system, and carries a highly unfavorable prognosis and is resistant to therapy. The cellular atypia described in MCS is comparable to the high-grade cytologic abnormalities found in MCL. It is characterized by local, destructive, sarcoma-like growth, with transformation to generalized involvement of multiple organ sites in its terminal phase. Cases described in the literature have included MCS of the larynx, the ascending colon, and an intracranial site.[82-84] This disorder may terminate as MCL. A MCS-like progression of SM including SM-AHN or MCL is occasionally observed in which instances *KIT* p.D816V is more likely to be detected.

Extracutaneous Mastocytoma

Extracutaneous mastocytoma is an extremely rare variant of mast cell disease, with most cases reported in the literature occurring in the lungs.[85] They are generally considered benign because of their low-grade histology consisting of mature mast cells, and lack of progression to aggressive disease or MCL. Because they may present similarly to MCS, they must be differentiated from the latter. Extracutaneous mastocytoma was removed as one of the mastocytosis subtypes in the revised 2016 WHO classification.[60]

Primary (Clonal) Mast Cell Activation Syndrome

Mast cell activation syndrome (MCAS) by consensus is defined as the occurrence of severe, episodic and recurrent symptoms induced by mast cell mediators such as tryptase, with concurrent involvement of at least two organ systems including the cutaneous, respiratory, GI and cardiovascular systems, and response to antimediator therapy. Primary (clonal) MCAS includes conditions characterized using MCAS criteria and with a population of clonal mast cells exhibiting an activating mutation in *KIT* and/or aberrant expression of CD25. This includes both mastocytosis (CM or SM) or the presence of clonal mast cells without CM/SM.[34] Patients with such findings have been identified within groups of patients diagnosed with idiopathic anaphylaxis and patients with anaphylaxis to stinging insects.[46,86,87] A suggestion has been made that some of the patients with clonal mast cells who do not currently meet the definition of SM may ultimately meet the diagnostic criteria for SM. Currently no natural history studies have been performed on such patients, thus those with clonal mast cells not meeting the diagnosis of SM could be considered to have a pre-SM condition (monoclonal mast cells of uncertain significance) akin to the relationship between monoclonal gammopathy of undetermined significance and multiple myeloma. For now, it is recommended that such patients have a yearly follow-up to include a physical examination to rule out evolving organomegaly or lymphadenopathy, a serum tryptase level to determine whether there is indirect evidence of an expanding mast cell compartment, and a complete blood count with differential and platelet count to help rule out an evolving hematologic disorder.

Secondary and Idiopathic MCAS

The term secondary MCAS is applied as a diagnosis for individuals who present with episodic allergic-like signs and symptoms, such as flushing, urticaria, or diarrhea, and where a medical evaluation reveals an allergy/hypersensitivity or other reactive condition as an etiology. The term idiopathic MCAS is applied to individuals having episodic symptoms due to release of mediators from mast cells without identified causes. Individuals with the diagnosis of both mastocytosis and an allergy with MCAS thus can be referred to as having mixed primary and secondary MCAS.

In the diagnosis of MCAS, mast cell mediators that may be documented to increase during an event include validated urinary markers (e.g., *N*-methylhistamine, prostaglandin D_2, and 11β-prostaglandin $F_2α$) or the validated serum marker tryptase.[88,89] Historically, a diagnostic threshold increase in tryptase consistent with mast cell degranulation is an increase over BST of 20% plus 2 ng/mL.[88,89] However, a recent study has demonstrated that this algorithm has low specificity among patients with elevated BST, including those with mastocytosis. In this study, an increase of 68.5% over BST was found to have improved specificity without affecting sensitivity.[90]

LABORATORY FINDINGS

The diagnosis of mastocytosis is based on the finding of confluent clusters of mast cells in affected organ sites or diffuse infiltration with replacement of normal tissue by mast cells, coupled with clinical signs and symptoms and laboratory tests that are consistent with mast cell disease.[5] Bone marrow biopsy in pediatric-onset cutaneous disease is generally not recommended unless there is evidence of significant systemic disease, such as unexplained peripheral blood abnormalities, hepatosplenomegaly, or lymphadenopathy.[57] In adult patients with CM and/or elevated serum total tryptase or when *KIT* p.D816V is identified in peripheral blood,[5] a bone marrow biopsy and aspiration should be considered. The decision to obtain a tissue biopsy specimen from the liver, spleen, GI tract, or lymph nodes should be based on a high suspicion of disease involvement and likelihood of yielding clinically useful information. Slight increases in mast cell numbers in target tissues (up to fourfold) are not diagnostic because they may reflect normal variation or inflammatory or reactive processes.

Examination of the bone marrow in patients with suspected mastocytosis includes an inspection of both the bone marrow biopsy and the aspirate. Immunohistochemical staining of the bone marrow biopsy with antibody directed to mast cell tryptase is the method of choice to visualize mast cells,[5,91,92] as shown in *Figure 87.2*. In most patients with SM, tryptase-positive infiltrates are composed of spindle-shaped mast cells. In these patients, SM can be diagnosed without additional tests, provided that major and minor SM criteria are met. In the case of patients with tryptase-positive round cell infiltrates where the infiltrates comprise >95% round cells and <5% spindle-shaped cells, application of additional immunohistochemistry markers to confirm the diagnosis of SM should be applied if possible (e.g., 2D7 or BB1) because basophils and sometimes myeloblasts also express tryptase.[34] The co-expression of CD25 with or without CD2 in CD117 (KIT)-positive mast cells by flow cytometry of bone marrow aspirates or by immunohistochemical analysis of bone marrow biopsies is generally accepted to be the most sensitive and specific method to support the diagnosis of SM.[22,34,52] CD30 is a cytoplasmic and membrane-bound antigen that was more recently identified on mast cells and has been added is a minor diagnostic criterion, joining CD25 and CD2.[5,93] Although it was originally reported as an immunohistochemical marker that was specific for more advanced forms of

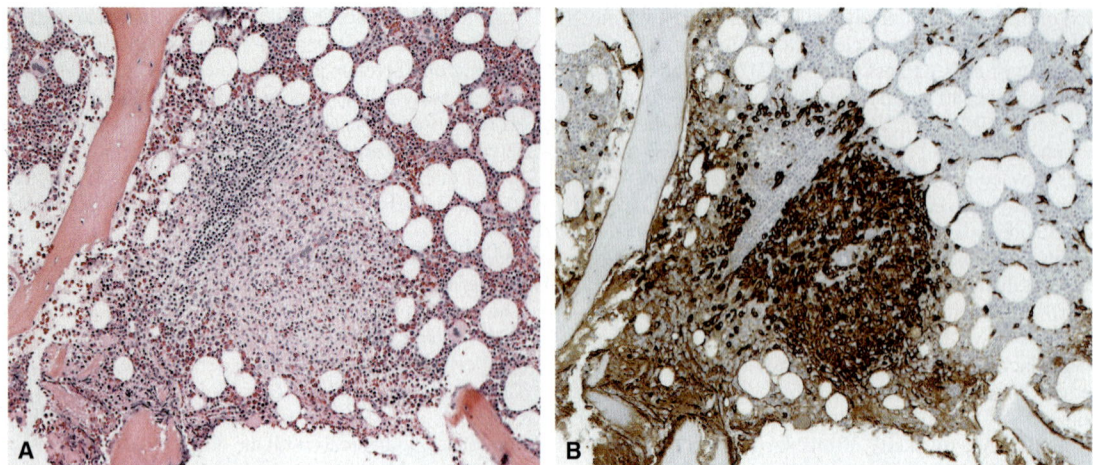

FIGURE 87.2 Bone marrow histopathology showing focal mast cell infiltrates in a bone marrow biopsy taken from a patient with indolent systemic mastocytosis. Panel A showing staining of a representative mast cell lesion with hematoxylin and eosin stain (magnification, ×10), and panel B showing staining of the same section with anti-tryptase antibody (magnification, ×10).

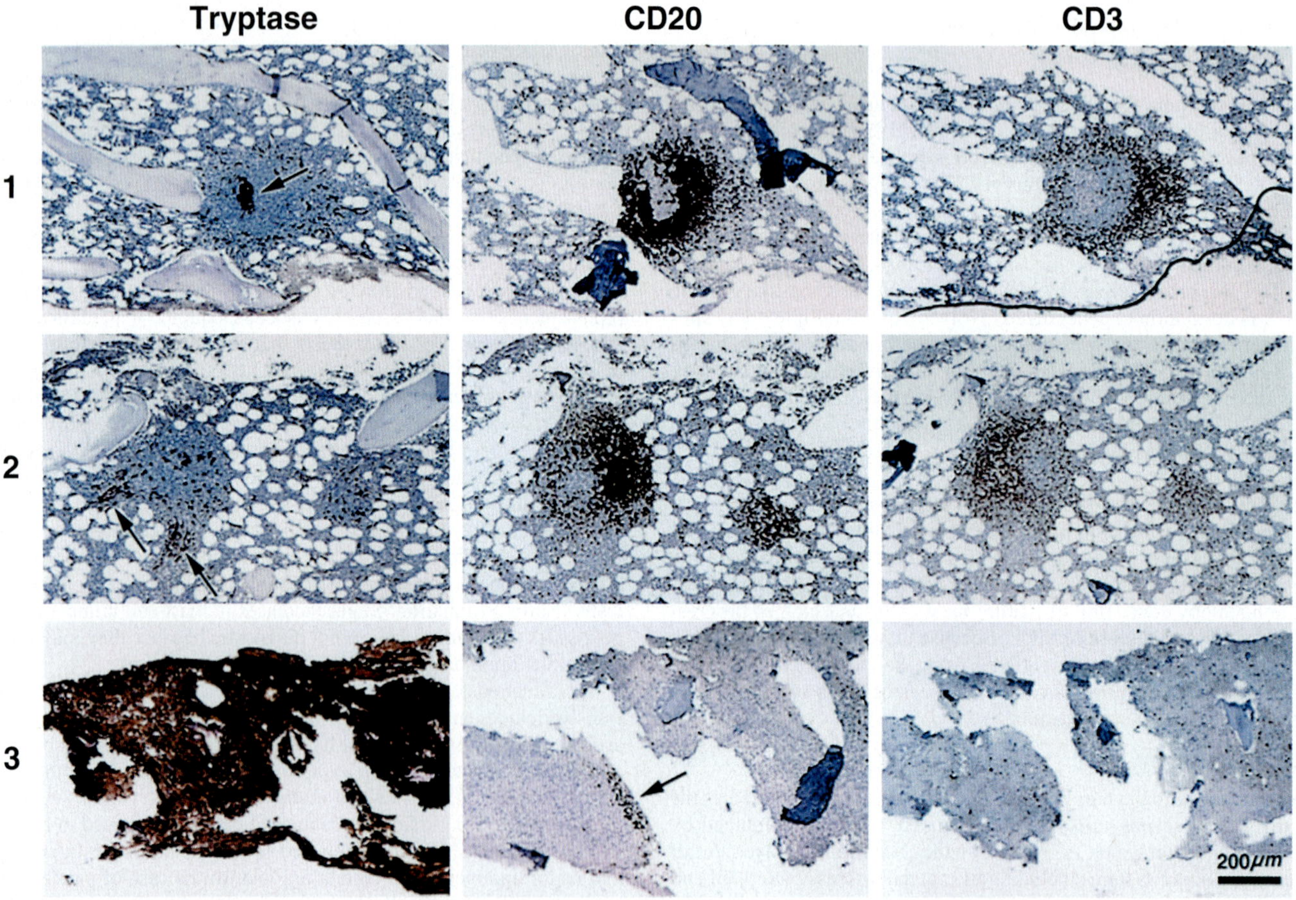

FIGURE 87.3 Immunohistochemical staining of lymphoid aggregates in two patients with a focal (1 and 2) and one patient with a diffuse (3) increase in mast cells. Antibodies are shown on top of each column. Nodular lesions shown in (1) and (2) contain a central core of mast cells (arrows) surrounded by B cells (CD20) and a peripheral rim of T cells (CD3). Diffuse mast cell infiltrates (3) are seen in association with a small B-cell collection (arrow) and scattered single T cells. The bar represents 200 μm. (From Akin C, Jaffe ES, Raffeld M, et al. An immunohistochemical study of the bone marrow lesions of systemic mastocytosis: expression of stem cell factor by lesional mast cells. *Am J Clin Pathol*. 2002;118(2):242-247. Reproduced by permission of American Society of Clinical Pathologists.)

SM,[92] other studies could detect CD30 by immunohistochemistry in less advanced forms of mast cell disease, including CM, as well as ISM and SSM.[94,95] CD123 is the α-subunit of the IL-3 receptor. It is reported to be expressed on neoplastic mast cells at 100%, 61%, 57%, and 0% in ASM, ISM, SM-AHN, and MCL, respectively.[96,97]

The cellular composition of lymphoid collections is evaluated by using lineage-specific antibodies against CD3 and CD20, respectively,[25] as shown in *Figure 87.3*. Other approaches commonly used include reticulin staining to detect fibrosis and Masson trichrome staining to evaluate the extent of collagen deposition.

The finding of clusters of confluent mast cells on bone marrow aspirate is consistent with SM; however, not all patients demonstrate this finding. Therefore, underestimation of the degree of mast cell infiltration through examination of an aspirate may be more common than appreciated, with aspirates compromised because of underlying marrow fibrosis and a resultant inability to obtain adequate marrow aspirate or spicules at fibrotic marrow sites. Surrogate disease markers in mastocytosis include serum or plasma tryptase levels, serum histamine and urinary histamine metabolites, or soluble CD117, CD25, and CD2.[98]

Total serum mast cell tryptase is the most commonly used surrogate marker for SM and is quantified using a commercial enzyme-linked immunosorbent assay. It has both high sensitivity and high specificity.[98-100] A total tryptase >20 ng/mL is suggestive of mastocytosis and is a minor criterion in the diagnosis of SM.[5,34] Median baseline levels in healthy individuals are approximately 4 ng/mL and generally less than 10 ng/mL. Tryptase levels ≤20 ng/mL have been detected in patients with CM and in those with limited systemic disease.[90,100] However, the use of this biomarker in the diagnosis of SM is complicated by the recent identification of the genetic trait HaT caused by increased copy number of the *TPSAB1* gene encoding alpha-tryptase resulting in elevated BST. HaT affects approximately 5% of the general populations of the United States and Europe and it is not yet determined how this could affect diagnostic criteria for systemic mastocytosis.[101] However, in general, higher tryptase values in patients with mastocytosis increase the likelihood of multiorgan involvement. Thus, the tryptase level is an important parameter in evaluating patients with suspected mastocytosis and is useful in assessing disease severity, activity, and progression.

Other mast cell mediators that are surrogate disease markers for mastocytosis include serum histamine and a 24-hour urine sampling for the urinary histamine metabolites, *N*-methylhistamine, and methylimidazole acetic acid. These tests are less commonly used with the availability of a commercial tryptase assay. Disadvantages of using blood and urinary histamine levels for the diagnosis and prognostication of patients with mastocytosis are the variability of histamine levels among healthy individuals and patients, difficulty in assay standardization, the problem of false-positive results as a result of presumed synthesis of histamine by bacteria in the urinary tract and the possibility of rare histamine-secreting carcinoids. Other variables that can alter results of histamine assays are prior ingestion of foods rich in histamine and improper storage of the urine sample. Because basophils also contain histamine, hematologic disorders presenting with basophilia or allergic events associated with basophil and/or mast cell activation also result in elevated histamine levels.

Various metabolites of arachidonic acid are also elevated in patients with mastocytosis. These include urinary PGD-M or 9α,11β-dihydroxy-15-oxo-2,2,18,19-tetranorprost-5-ene-1,20-dioxic acid, as well as plasma thromboxane B_2 and its metabolites. Because the source of prostaglandins and thromboxanes in mastocytosis is not exclusively limited to mast cells, reliance on assays that measure these metabolites is unlikely to be sufficiently specific for diagnostic purposes. However, if measured, elevations in one or more mast cell mediators raise the suspicion of mastocytosis and warrant further diagnostic evaluation.

The identification of genetic markers of mastocytosis, such as point mutations in *KIT*, helps support the diagnosis of mastocytosis. The identification of an activating mutation in *KIT* fulfills a minor diagnostic criterion in the diagnosis of mastocytosis.[5,102] Such mutations are more easily identified in patients with more severe disease because of the relative clonal expansion of cells derived from the neoplastic progenitor. Such mutations may be helpful in following disease progression by assessing their allele frequency over the patient's course and in response to therapy. Analysis for *KIT* mutations are best performed on bone marrow and, specifically, on sorted malignant mast cells to increase sensitivity. Inability to identify the presence of a point mutation at codon 816 in *KIT* or another activating mutation in *KIT*, particularly in peripheral blood, does not eliminate the possibility that cells bearing this mutation are present because the malignant clone may have not expanded to sufficient cell numbers to allow for detection of a mutation in *KIT*.[22] In patients with coexisting eosinophilia, peripheral blood should be examined for the presence of the *FIP1L1-PDGFRA* fusion gene by using fluorescence in situ hybridization (FISH) for the *CHIC2* gene deletion, or less commonly, RT-PCR for the fusion gene. Several techniques to detect *KIT* mutations have been reported, but current recommendations for the most sensitive assays include peptide nucleic acid-mediated PCR, or allele-specific PCR, or ddPCR.[31,34,102] When employing *KIT* mutations as a diagnostic criterion for SM, it is important to be aware that such mutations are also detectable in some patients with germ cell tumors or other non–mast cell tumors with or without coexisting SM.[34] Next-generation sequencing is becoming more routine in the evaluation of advanced forms of SM because genetic complexity often supervenes in these cases. Myeloid mutation panels can often detect one or more myeloid mutations in addition to an activating mutation in *KIT*, especially in patients with SM-AHN.[35] Because of the relatively lower sensitivity of myeloid mutation panels (~5%), screening for the *KIT* p.D816V mutation should be undertaken with one of the aforementioned higher sensitivity assays.[31,34,102]

Plasma IL-6 levels correlate with disease severity, in particular the extent of bone marrow pathology and presence of a non-mast cell hematologic disorder.[14,103] Additional surrogate markers that may also be useful in assessing more severe forms of mastocytosis, such as SM-AHN, and in following disease severity are the soluble receptors CD117 (KIT) and CD25 (the α-chain of the IL-2 receptor).[104] These receptors are expressed in both membrane-bound and soluble forms, with the latter being a result of proteolytic cleavage. Soluble forms of these receptors are more readily detectable in the circulation in patients with an increased mast cell burden and correlate with disease severity and bone marrow pathology. Soluble CD117 levels are also found to be elevated in some patients with AML and advanced MDS. Elevated serum levels of CD25 may be seen in patients with hairy cell leukemia, solid tumors, and a number of infectious and autoimmune diseases. A comparison of the plasma CD117 and tryptase levels for various categories of mastocytosis revealed that tryptase levels were more sensitive indicators of early disease, whereas elevated plasma CD117 levels demonstrated a stronger correlation with advanced disease.[104]

A dual-energy x-ray absorptiometry (DEXA) scan should be employed to monitor osteoporosis in those with mastocytosis. Sites commonly measured include the lumbar spine and hip. The diagnosis is established according to the WHO criteria defining osteopenia.[34] A physical examination, serum tryptase determination, and complete blood count should be recommended at yearly intervals in patients with stable ISM.[22,34]

PROGNOSTICATION USING GENETIC AND CLINICAL VARIABLES

Genetic characterization of cases of SM has provided more opportunities for improved prognostic characterization of patients with SM. Using next-generation sequencing of a panel of genes associated with myeloid malignancies (*ASXL1, CBL, ETV6, EZH2, IDH1/2, JAK2, KRAS, MLL-PTD, NPM1, NRAS, TP53, RUNX1, SRSF2, SF3B1, SETBP1, TET2,* and *U2AF1*), investigators identified additional molecular aberrations beyond *KIT* p.D816V in 24 of 27 patients (89%) with advanced SM (ASM, SM-AHN, and MCL) compared to 3 of 12 patients with ISM or SSM.[35] The most commonly mutated genes were *TET2, SRSF2, ASXL1, CBL,* and *RUNX1*. Patients with a mutation in one or more of these genes exhibited a worse prognosis compared to patients who only exhibited the *KIT* p.D816V mutation ($P = .019$).[35] A related analysis of 70 patients with advanced SM was undertaken to discern which mutations carried the most prognostic import. It was found that OS was adversely impacted by mutations in *SRSF2* ($P < .0001$), *ASXL1* ($P = .002$), and *RUNX1* ($P = .03$) on univariate analysis, but not by *TET2* or *JAK2* mutations.[105] In a multivariate analysis, *SRSF2* and *ASXL1* were the most predictive adverse indicators of OS, as well as number of mutated genes in the *SRSF2/ASXL1/RUNX1* (S/A/R) panel ($P < .0001$).[105]

Clinical and genetic information have been combined to develop prognostic scoring systems to gauge survival in SM. One group found that spleen volume ≥450 mL by magnetic resonance imaging and elevated level of serum alkaline phosphatase were each associated with inferior survival in a multivariate analysis among ISM and advanced SM patients combined.[106] Among advanced SM patients only, the variables of spleen volume >1200 mL, increased alkaline phosphatase, and mutation(s) in *SRSF2*, *ASXL1*, or *RUNX1* were significant adverse prognostic factors in a univariate analysis; however, in a multivariate analysis, only increased alkaline phosphatase and mutation in the *SRSF2/ASXL1/RUNX1* gene panel retained statistical significance. The 3-year OS was 76% for patients with 0 to 1 (intermediate risk, $n = 28$) features and 38% for patients with 2 (high risk, $n = 32$) parameters.[106] In an analysis of patients with advanced SM, it was found that age >60 years, hemoglobin <10 g/dL or transfusion dependence, platelet count <150 × 10^9/L, serum albumin <3.5 g/dL, and mutation of *ASXL1* were each associated with inferior survival in a multivariate analysis.[107] These investigators developed a "mutation-augmented prognostic scoring system" that stratified these patients with advanced SM into high-, intermediate-, and low-risk groups with respective median survivals of 5, 21 and 86 months.

Several prognostic scoring systems have now been formalized that include clinical variables with or without addition mutational data and are applicable to indolent disease, only advanced SM, or all forms of SM. These prognostic scoring systems are increasingly used to better risk stratify patents and are now incorporated into the National Comprehensive Care Network (NCCN) guidelines for systemic mastocytosis.[108]

International Prognostic Scoring System for Mastocytosis

The International Prognostic Scoring System for Mastocytosis (IPSM) was created based on a large cohort of patients with mastocytosis ($n = 1639$) derived from the European Competence Network on Mastocytosis (ECNM).[109] IPSM was validated in a cohort of 462 patients. Age > 60 years and alkaline phosphatase >100 U/L were identified as predictors of higher-grade mastocytosis and OS in patients with nonadvanced mastocytosis (CM, MIS, ISM, and SSM). Patients with nonadvanced SM were stratified into three risk groups (low, intermediate-risk 1 [INT-1], and intermediate-risk 2 [INT-2]) with significantly different OS (10-year OS rates were 87%, 52%, and 22%, respectively) and progression-free survival (PFS; 10-year PFS rates were 96%, 87%, and 76%, respectively). For patients with advanced SM, age > 60 years, tryptase > 125 ng/mL, leukocytes >16 × 10^9/L, hemoglobin < 11 g/dL, platelets < 100 × 10^9/L, and skin involvement were independent prognostic factors for OS. Patients with AdvSM were stratified into four risk groups (advanced SM 1 [AdvSM-1], advanced SM 2 [AdvSM-2], advanced SM 3 [AdvSM-3], and advanced SM 4 [AdvSM-4]). The OS for patients in risk groups AdvSM-1 and AdvSM-2 was similar to that of patients with nonadvanced mastocytosis in the INT-1 and INT-2 risk groups, respectively.

Mutation-Adjusted Risk Score

In the mutation-adjusted risk score (MARS) study of 383 patients with advanced SM,[110] the following variables retained significance as independent predictors of inferior OS: age greater than 60 years, hemoglobin less than 10 g/dL, platelets less than 100 × 10^9/L, the presence of one high-risk mutation (*SRSF2*, *ASXL1*, and/or *RUNX1* [S/A/R]), and the presence of >2 S/A/R mutations. A weighted score was developed by assigning 2 points for the presence of ≥2 S/A/R mutations and 1 point for each of the other adverse factors. Patients with advanced SM were stratified into three risk groups (low, intermediate, and high). The median OS was not reached for the low-risk group compared to 4 and 2 years, respectively, for the intermediate and high-risk groups.

The Mayo Alliance Prognostic Scoring System

In the Mayo Alliance Prognostic Scoring System (MAPS) analysis of 580 patients with SM,[111] clinical variables including age greater than 60 years, advanced SM (vs ISM/SSM), thrombocytopenia (platelets < 150 × 10^9/L), anemia (hemoglobin level below sex-adjusted normal), and increased alkaline phosphatase were identified as independent risk factors for survival. In addition, the presence of *ASXL1*, *RUNX1*, and *NRAS* mutations was independently associated with inferior survival. In the combined clinical and molecular risk factor analysis, the presence of high molecular risk mutations, advanced SM, thrombocytopenia, increased alkaline phosphatase, and age greater than 60 years retained prognostic significance. Patients with SM are stratified into four different risk groups (low, intermediate-1, intermediate-2, and high) with significantly different median survivals (not reached, 85, 36, and 12 months, respectively). The MAPS risk stratification is applicable only to advanced SM patients.

The Global Prognostic Score for Mastocytosis

In the global prognostic score for mastocytosis (GPSM) study,[112] prognostic parameters were examined in a discovery cohort of 422 patients with SM. The clinical variables that were prognostic for PFS were platelet count < 100 × 10^9/L, serum β2-microglobulin > 2.5 µg/mL, and serum baseline tryptase > 125 µg/L. The clinical variables that were prognostic for OS were hemoglobin <11 g/dL, serum alkaline phosphatase > 140 IU/L, and presence of *SRSF2*, *ASXL1*, *RUNX1*, or *DNMT3A* gene mutations. Using the GPSM-PFS ($n = 399$) and GPSM-OS ($n = 411$) models, patients were stratified into three risk groups (low-risk, intermediate-risk, and high-risk). The PFS at 5 years was 100%, 94%, and 47%, respectively, while the OS at 5 years was 100%, 94%, and 62%, respectively. These results were corroborated in a validation cohort of 853 patients. After patient stratification in the low-, intermediate- and high-risk groups using GPSM-PFS ($n = 670$) and GPSM-OS ($n = 768$) models, the 5-year PFS was 98%, 84%, and 43%, and the 5-year OS was 99%, 61%, and 30% respectively. A comparison of different scoring models showed that the GPSM-PFS model had a high prognostic capability, especially in patients with nonadvanced SM.[110] For patients with advanced SM, the GPSM-OS model and the IPSM model for advanced SM were the best predictive models, although other scoring systems such as MARS performed almost as well.

DIFFERENTIAL DIAGNOSIS

The differential diagnostic list of disorders for mastocytosis consists of those diseases that have a similar clinical presentation. These include hereditary or acquired angioedema, idiopathic flushing or anaphylaxis, carcinoid tumor, pheochromocytoma, and idiopathic capillary leak syndrome. Pheochromocytoma should be considered when episodic hypertension is a predominant clinical manifestation. Unexplained gastroduodenal disease should include evaluation for Zollinger-Ellison gastrinoma. *Helicobacter pylori* infection should be considered in all patients with gastric ulcers, including those diagnosed with mastocytosis.

DCM should be included in the differential diagnosis of neonatal blister disorders, such as pemphigoid. Extensive bullae with crusting may be the first presentation in an infant who later develops DCM.

A number of non–mast cell hematologic disorders, such as the MPNs (e.g., chronic myeloid leukemia) or lymphoma of the bone marrow, may present with an increased number of mast cells and, in some cases, immature mast cells on bone marrow biopsy, though circumscribed lesions are generally lacking in these disorders and the WHO criteria for diagnosis of primary mast cell disease are not met.[113,114] Diseases associated with bone marrow lesions on biopsy that appear similar to SM on gross analysis include primary myelofibrosis, angioimmunoblastic lymphadenopathy, eosinophilic fibrohistiocytoma, and "myelomastocytic leukemia."[113,115] A close evaluation of histopathologic specimens differentiates these disorders from mastocytosis, in part, on the basis of a general absence of mast cell infiltrates. Myelofibrosis can resemble mastocytosis when fibrosis is extensive and the marrow is diffusely infiltrated with an increased number of mast cells. The distinguishing feature between these two disorders is the greater absolute number of mast cells on bone marrow biopsy in mastocytosis. Although differentiation of mastocytosis from angioimmunoblastic lymphadenopathy may be made based on the presence of plasma cells and immunoblasts in the latter and absence of neovascularity in mastocytosis, differentiation of mastocytosis from fibrohistiocytoma is more difficult. Large histiocytic cells noted in eosinophilic fibrohistiocytic lesions have a similar appearance to the large mast cells seen in many mast cell lesions.[116]

Conditions with secondary changes in mast cell numbers have been observed at sites of pathology in autoimmune disorders, including systemic lupus erythematosus, rheumatoid arthritis, psoriatic arthritis, and scleroderma, with chronic liver or renal disease, and with infectious diseases, although in such cases, these increases are nominal.[21] On resolution of the infection, mast cell numbers generally return to normal. At sites of allergic inflammation, increases of mast cells fourfold or more over normal have been described.

MANAGEMENT

The treatment of all categories of mastocytosis involves control of symptoms by blocking the action of mast cell mediators, though several newer therapeutic strategies hold promise for more severe forms of the disease by targeting mast cell growth, development, and activation.[117-119] Because of the heterogeneous nature of disease manifestations in this group of disorders, therapy should be individualized to each patient's clinical presentation and prognosis. Cytoreductive therapy is typically not initiated in patients with ISM because this disease category has a favorable prognosis. A summary of treatment approaches for mastocytosis is provided in *Table 87.3*.

The treatment for most categories of mastocytosis includes H_1 and H_2 blockade with antihistamines for prophylaxis of hypotensive episodes, for control of cutaneous manifestations such as pruritus and flushing, and for gastric hypersecretion. Corticosteroids are used for more short-term control of malabsorption and ascites and for amelioration of anaphylaxis.[21,117,120,121] Nonsedating antihistamines have utility when patient sedation is a key concern and are now considered the agents of choice for pruritus and urticaria. Alternative approaches include administration of a nonsedating antihistamine during the day, with supplementation of one of the sedating antihistamines at bedtime for added symptom relief.

Addition of an H_2 antihistamine may be beneficial in cases in which insufficient symptom control is afforded by use of an H_1 antihistamine alone.[112,116] Aspirin has been used in some patients to treat flushing, tachycardia, and syncope. However, aspirin must be used with caution because it may cause vascular collapse in some patients with mastocytosis and may also exacerbate peptic ulcer disease. Alternative treatments that have been used for refractory mediator symptoms include the off-label antihistamine/mast cell stabilizer ketotifen, and the anti-IgE antibody omalizumab, which has also been used for anaphylaxis, as well as asthma. Generally, chemotherapy and splenectomy do not have a role in the treatment of cutaneous or indolent forms of mastocytosis. However, in selected SM patients with debilitating and refractory mediator symptoms, more aggressive treatment may be required.

For cutaneous manifestations of mastocytosis, other therapies may be beneficial in addition to antihistamines.[117] MPCM and DCM have been shown to be responsive to topical corticosteroids[122,123] and oral methoxypsoralen therapy with long-wave ultraviolet radiation; psoralen and ultraviolet A light have been used for both MPCM and DCM.[124-126] Indeed, some patients report a decrease in the number or intensity of cutaneous lesions after repeated exposure to natural sunlight.[127] Photochemotherapy or topical steroids, however, should only be used in instances of extensive cutaneous disease unresponsive to other therapy. Improvement with either therapy is transient in both MPCM and DCM.[127] In children with mastocytomas with associated severe systemic symptoms because of mast cell mediator release, surgical excision of the mastocytoma may be considered.[47] An alternative approach involves injection of the mastocytoma with corticosteroids to induce involution.[128] Occlusion dressings embedded with topical steroids with or without phototherapy, and both topical and oral forms of sodium cromoglycate have been used with reported benefit.[47] Other options for the treatment of CM not yet validated include the use of topical pimecrolimus, an immunomodulating agent used in the treatment of eczema.[129]

Management of GI symptoms should address the type and severity of symptoms. H_2 antihistamines are specifically used to treat gastric hypersecretion and peptic ulcer disease associated with mastocytosis. Proton pump inhibitors may be effective in decreasing diarrhea in addition to controlling gastric acid hypersecretion.[127] Antileukotrienes are effective in some patients in helping control symptoms of flushing, diarrhea, and abdominal cramping. Anticholinergics and orally administered cromolyn sodium may also be useful for control of diarrhea.[130] Intestinal absorption of cromolyn is limited (≤1%), and a number of weeks of therapy may be needed before clinical benefits are seen. The recommended adult dosage is 200 mg four times daily, and doses ranging from 60 mg daily to 100 mg four times daily have been used in children.[47,117] In addition to its efficacy in treating GI symptoms, cromolyn has been reported to decrease musculoskeletal pain and headaches and improve cognitive abilities.[117] Its purported mechanism of action is decrease in mast cell degranulation. As such, its use would not be expected to alter the natural course of the disease.

Malabsorption is generally managed with corticosteroids.[117] In adults, oral prednisone (40-60 mg/d) usually results in a decrease in malabsorption over 10 to 20 days, after which steroids can usually be tapered to as low as 15 to 20 mg every other day. A more difficult treatment dilemma, ascites, has also been shown to improve with systemic corticosteroids.[117] Again, in adults, treatment with prednisone, 40 to 60 mg/d, with tapering to an every-other-day dose, usually results in a decrease in ascites. A subgroup of patients with mastocytosis who develop ascites may also develop portal hypertension, which may be exceedingly difficult to manage and indicates a poor prognosis.[131] Management of portal hypertension includes consideration of a portacaval shunt.[132]

An important component of management of all categories of mastocytosis is patient avoidance of triggering factors such as alcohol and nonsteroidal anti-inflammatory agents in sensitive patients; pressure, friction, or extremes of temperature; and agents to which the patient is specifically allergic.[86,87,117] As with other syndromes in which patients may be at risk for severe type I hypersensitivity reactions, patients with mastocytosis should carry epinephrine-filled syringes and be skilled in self-administration. Epinephrine is used to treat acute episodes of hypotension.[117] Treatment of refractory hypotension and shock requires fluid resuscitative measures along with additional pharmacologic intervention. Because anaphylaxis can also be a feature of MCAS, these patients are candidates for similar therapy. The treatment of choice for life-threatening hymenoptera allergy/anaphylaxis is venom immunotherapy that should be undertaken with precautions using a multidisciplinary approach led by allergists. Similarly, perioperative management of anesthetics, which can precipitate immediate and delayed mast cell activation, requires consultation with the surgical, anesthesiology, and allergy teams to minimize the occurrence and severity of anaphylaxis. Pharmacologic agents that should be avoided if possible include β-adrenergic agents and α-adrenergic and cholinergic receptor antagonists. Serum tryptase levels should be obtained, and blood coagulation parameters monitored perioperatively and during anesthesia if a suspected mast cell degranulation event occurs.[133] General guidelines regarding anesthesia and analgesic management in patients with mastocytosis have been published.[134,135]

Osteoporosis in patients with mastocytosis may be underappreciated and, hence, undertreated. Recommended approaches to treatment include calcium supplementation, vitamin D, use of bisphosphonates and use the monoclonal RANK ligand inhibitor denosumab, and more aggressive therapies.[34,108,117] Narcotic analgesics should be used with care because these, particularly at high doses or in susceptible patients, have been suspected of potentiating mast cell degranulation, in addition to their addictive properties. Radiotherapy may have a palliative role in decreasing bone pain in isolated areas.[136] In severe cases or patients with drug intolerance, low-dose interferon-α2b may be appropriate because the literature indicates that interferon-α2b may have some efficacy in decreasing musculoskeletal pain and improving bone mineralization in patients with extensive bony involvement.[117] Patients with osteolysis and pathologic fractures are candidates for cytoreductive drugs (plus a bisphosphonate). The decision to initiate

Table 87.3. Suggested Therapy for Mastocytosis

FOR ALL VARIANTS: Hypotensive/anaphylaxis
Epinephrine (intramuscular [e.g., Epi-Pen])
More severe, frequent episodes: consider prophylaxis with H_1 and H_2 antihistamines ± corticosteroids

Cutaneous Disease
Antihistamines: $H_1 \pm H_2$
Corticosteroids
Psoralen and ultraviolet A light: consider for recalcitrant disease
Laser therapy: consider for MPCM

Gastrointestinal Disease
Peptic ulcer disease/gastroesophageal reflux: H_2 antihistamines, omeprazole
Abdominal cramping: cromolyn sodium
Diarrhea: anticholinergics, cromolyn sodium, omeprazole
Malabsorption: corticosteroids
Ascites: corticosteroids, consider a portacaval shunt

Bone Disease
Calcium supplementation ± vitamin D
Bisphosphonates
Consider denosumab; or estrogen therapy for postmenopausal women, testosterone replacement in men with low testosterone levels
Consider [PEG]-interferon-α in patients with severe bone disease and severe musculoskeletal pain
Radiotherapy: palliative therapy for severe, localized bone pain

Indolent Systemic Mastocytosis
No cytoreductive treatment (may rarely be indicated for refractory, debilitating mediator symptoms despite maximal therapy)

Smoldering systemic mastocytosis
In selected cases with disease progression, consider interferon-α, cladribine, and tyrosine kinase inhibitors

Systemic Mastocytosis With an Associated Hematologic Neoplasm
If indicated, treatment of the associated non-mast cell hematologic disorder
Avapritinib (for platelets ≥ 50 x 10⁹/L)
Midostaurin
[PEG]-Interferon-α ± corticosteroids
2-chlorodeoxyadenosine (2-CdA; Cladribine)
Therapy directed to the AHN (e.g., hydroxyurea, hypomethylating agents)
Hematopoietic stem cell transplantation
Clinical trial

Aggressive Systemic Mastocytosis
Avapritinib (for platelets ≥ 50 x 10⁹/L)
Midostaurin
Imatinib (if *KIT* p.D816V mutation-negative or *KIT* mutation status unknown)
[PEG]-Interferon-α ± corticosteroids
2-chlorodeoxyadenosine (2-CdA; Cladribine)
Hematopoietic stem cell transplantation
Clinical trial

Mast Cell Leukemia
Avapritinib (for platelets ≥ 50 x 10⁹/L)
Midostaurin
Cladribine
Multiagent induction-type chemotherapy
Hematopoietic stem cell transplantation
Clinical trial

Abbreviation: AHN, associated hematologic neoplasm.

treatment with interferon-α2b therapy should take into consideration side effects such as fever, malaise, nausea, and hypothyroidism, along with the small but well-described risk for anaphylaxis. Patients with mastocytosis who ultimately require joint replacement because of extensive bone loss generally tolerate these procedures well; however, such procedures do not obviate further decline in bone mass.[137]

Cytoreductive Therapy

For patients with ISM with debilitating and refractory mediator symptoms, SSM patients with rapid progression of B findings, and advanced SM patients with organ damage, cytoreductive therapy is used with the aim of reducing or reversing the neoplastic mast cell–related organ dysfunction. Interferon-α and cladribine have historically been used as first-line agents, with the latter favored in patients with kinetically active disease who require rapid debulking of mast cells. However, tyrosine kinase inhibitors have been increasingly used in patients with advanced SM, as well as more indolent forms of disease.[21,138]

Interferon-α

Interferon-α (IFN-α) with or without steroids has been employed as first-line cytoreductive therapy in more advanced forms of SM.[73,108,117,139] Because of its cytostatic mechanisms of action, IFN-α is generally not recommended for advanced SM cases where rapid debulking is required. The optimal dose and duration of therapy are unclear, and results are mixed. In general, interferon-α treatment appears to diminish skin findings and symptoms, decrease mast cell infiltration of the marrow, lessen osteoporosis, and ameliorate cytopenias.[140] The time to response may approach a year, and relapse after discontinuing interferon-α is common.[73] Furthermore, its use can be complicated by flu-like symptoms, fever, hypothyroidism, and cytopenias.[117] One group commonly starts with 1 to 3 million units subcutaneously three times per week, followed by gradual escalation to 3 to 5 million units thrice to five times weekly.[73] Prednisone 0.5 to 1 mg/kg is commonly used from the start and tapered as possible. Duration of therapy is determined by the response and absence of significant side effects. Pegylated forms of IFN-α have been used with increasing frequency because of their improved tolerability profile.

Cladribine

Cladribine (2-chlorodeoxyadenosine), a purine nucleoside analog, has been reported to reduce neoplastic mast cell burden and induce clinical remissions in patients with more aggressive forms of mastocytosis.[73,141,142] Cladribine is a reasonable therapeutic approach in treating those with aggressive forms of mastocytosis who need a rapid reduction in mast cell burden, or have interferon-α-resistant advanced disease or interferon intolerance. Potential toxicities include myelosuppression, lymphopenia, and opportunistic infections. Prophylactic antibiotics are recommended.

In 2015, one group published their long-term experience with cladribine in both ISM (n = 36) and advanced (n = 32) SM patients.[143] Cladribine was administered at a dose of 0.14 mg/kg as a 2-hour intravenous infusion or subcutaneously from 1 to 5 days, every 4 to 12 weeks. A median of 3.7 courses was administered (range 1-9). The overall response rate (ORR) was 72%; 92% of ISM patients responded compared to 50% of patients with advanced disease. Among patients with advanced SM, the complete response (CR), major response (MR), and partial response rates were 0%, 37.5%, and 12.5%, respectively. Significant decreases in serum tryptase levels were only observed in ISM patients, and changes in bone marrow mast cell burden were evaluated only in nine patients, making it difficult to draw conclusions regarding this histopathologic endpoint. Median durations of response were 3.71 (0.1-8) and 2.47 (0.5-8.6) years for ISM and advanced SM, respectively. Lymphopenia (82%), neutropenia (47%), and opportunistic (13%) infections were the most common grade 3/4 adverse events. Although cladribine demonstrates activity in early and advanced stages of SM, its use in ISM patients (even those with refractory mediator symptoms) needs to be approached very cautiously because of the potential for high-grade hematologic and nonhematologic toxicities in a population of patients with a life expectancy similar to that of an age-matched healthy population.

Tyrosine Kinase Inhibitors

Midostaurin

Midostaurin (*N*-benzoylstaurosporine; PKC412) is an inhibitor of multiple tyrosine kinases, including wild-type and p.D816V-mutated KIT, FLT3, PDGFR-α/β, and VEGFR2. In Ba/F3 cells transformed by *KIT* p.D816V, the IC_{50} of midostaurin was 30 to 40 nM, compared to greater than 1 μM with imatinib.[144] A 69% response rate in an investigator-initiated, phase 2 trial of 26 patients with advanced SM[145] led to a global, multicenter, open-label of midostaurin (100 mg twice daily on 28-day continuous cycles) in patients with ASM, MCL, and SM-AHN.[146]

The trial employed a steering committee and central pathology review to adjudicate eligibility, response, and histopathology.[146] Among 89 evaluable patients, the ORR was 60%, of which 75% were MRs. Responses were observed regardless of *KIT* p.D816V status, prior therapy, or the presence of an AHN. The median best reduction in serum tryptase level was −58%. In addition, the median change in bone marrow MC burden was -59%, and 57% of patients had a ≥50% reduction in the bone marrow mast cell burden. After a median follow-up of 26 months, the median duration of response (DOR) and median OS were 24.1 and 28.7 months, respectively. Median OS in responders was 44.4 months. Of the 16 patients with MCL, 8 responded, including 7 MR (44%); among MCL patients, the median DOR was not reached, with 3 MRs ongoing at 49, 33, and 19 months at the time of data cutoff. The median OS was 9.4 months among all patients with MCL, and was not reached among responding MCL patients. Symptoms and quality of life, measured by the Memorial Symptom Assessment Scale and Short-Form 12 survey, respectively, were significantly improved with midostaurin treatment. The drug was generally well tolerated with a manageable toxicity profile consisting mostly of GI side effects. These data support further exploration of midostaurin in combination with other agents with activity in advanced SM (e.g., cladribine), and evaluation of the drug in ISM patients with significant and refractory mast cell mediator-induced symptoms. Midostaurin was approved by the U.S. Midostaurin was approved by the Food and Drug Administration (FDA) and European Medicines Agency (EMA) in 2017, and represents the first drug approval for patients with advanced SM irrespective of *KIT* mutational status.

Avapritinib

Avapritinib is a selective and potent inhibitor of KIT p.D816V signaling in preclinical models. In the HMC1.2 cell line (both *KIT* p.V560G and p.D816V positive), avapritinib blocks phosphorylation of AKT and STAT3, and in mice xenografted with P815 mastocytoma cells, the drug induced dose-dependent tumor inhibition.[147] The phase I EXPLORER study and a prespecified interim analysis of the phase II PATHFINDER trial were recently published and supported the FDA approval of avapritinib for advanced SM in June 2021.[148,149] The EMA approved avapritinib as second line therapy for advanced SM in 2022.

The multicenter phase 1 EXPLORER trial accrued 69 patients into dose escalation ($n = 37$) and dose expansion ($n = 32$) cohorts.[148] Among the 53 patients evaluable using modified IWG-MRT-ECNM response criteria in the phase I trial, the ORR was 75%, consisting of a 36% complete remission rate with full or partial hematologic recovery. Response rates were 100%, 76%, and 69% in patients with ASM, SM-AHN, and MCL, respectively. Prior therapy, including midostaurin, and *S/A/R* mutation status did not impact response rate. A >50% reduction in bone marrow mast cells was observed in 92% of patients, and a >50% decrease in serum tryptase level was achieved in 99% of patients. Using a ddPCR with a sensitivity of 0.17%, avapritinib induced in-depth molecular remissions, with *KIT* p.D816V becoming undetectable in 30% of patients.

The most common adverse events (all grades/grade 3-4, %) were periorbital edema (69/2), anemia (55/30), diarrhea (45/1), nausea (44/3), thrombocytopenia (44/23), fatigue (41/9), and peripheral edema (40/0). Intracranial bleeding occurred in 13% overall, and in 1% of patients without severe thrombocytopenia. In the phase 2 PATHFINDER trial prespecified interim analysis of 32 evaluable AdvSM patients, avapritinib demonstrated an ORR of 75% and similar safety profile to the phase I study.[149] Only one case of intracranial bleeding occurred after mitigation procedures were implemented for thrombocytopenia.

Based on these trial data, the approved starting dose avapritinib for patients with advanced SM is 200 mg daily. This drug is not recommended for the treatment of patients with platelet counts less than 50×10^9/L due to the higher risk of intracranial bleeding in these patients. Avapritinib is also being evaluated in patients with indolent SM with high symptom burden in the double-blind, placebo-controlled, randomized PIONEER trial.

Additional tyrosine kinase inhibitors with activity against KIT p.D816V have entered clinical trial evaluation. The oral type 2 switch control kinase inhibitor ripretinib (DCC-2618; Deciphera Pharmaceuticals) exhibits activity against multiple *KIT* and *PDGFRA* mutants, with antineoplastic activity in preclinical models using *KIT* p.D816V-transfected mast cell lines.[150] Bezuclastinib (CGT9486) is an oral, highly selective tyrosine kinase inhibitor with potent activity against *KIT* p.D816V, which is also commencing trials in both indolent and advanced SM. BLU-263, also a highly selective KIT D816V inhibitor, is a derivative of avapritinib with less CNS penetration. It is currently being evaluated in indolent SM, with an advanced SM trial planned as monotherapy or in combination with azacitidine in SM with MDS or MDS/MPN.

Imatinib

Imatinib mesylate is currently FDA approved for adult patients with ASM without the *KIT* p.D816V mutation or with unknown *KIT* mutational status. Although imatinib lacks activity against KIT p.D816V in vitro and in vivo,[151-156] it has demonstrated clinical benefit in patients with alternative *KIT* mutations or wild-type *KIT*. For example, imatinib has elicited responses in cases of well-differentiated SM with either the p.F522C transmembrane *KIT* mutation[156] or wild-type *KIT*[157]; in a patient with familial SM carrying the germline *KIT* p.K509I mutation[158]; with deletion of codon 419 in exon 8 of *KIT* in pediatric CM[159]; and in a case of MCL with mutation in exon 9 of *KIT* (p.A502_Y503dup).[160]

Masitinib

Masitinib (AB1010) is an inhibitor of LYN, FYN, PDGFR-α/β, and wild-type KIT.[160] After an initial study II trial in patients with ISM or CM with symptoms unresponsive to prior therapy,[162] masitinib was studied in a phase 3, randomized, double-blind trial of 135 patients with ISM or SSM (108 subjects formally satisfied the WHO criteria for SM).[163] Subjects were randomized to oral masitinib or placebo. The primary endpoint of the study was based on a 75% or more improvement in one or more symptom categories: pruritus, flushing, depression, or fatigue.[163] Of the patients taking masitinib, 18.7% achieved this endpoint compared to 7.4% of patients taking placebo. At week 24, there was an 18% decrease in the serum tryptase level in the masitinib arm vs an increase in 2.2% in the placebo arm ($P < .0001$). Also, on masitinib treatment, UP lesions decreased by an average body surface area of 12.3% vs an increase in 15.9% in those taking placebo. Masitinib-associated clinical benefits were generally sustained during a 2-year extension period. Although treatment was generally well tolerated, there was an excess incidence of diarrhea, rash, and asthenia in 9%, 6%, and 4% of patients taking masitinib compared to placebo. In addition, 24% of masitinib-treated patients discontinued therapy because of an adverse event, compared with 10% in the placebo arm. In this population of lower risk SM patients who generally carry a normal life expectancy, these side effects need to be weighed against the potential palliative benefits of the drug. At the time of writing, masitinib remains investigational.

Dasatinib and Nilotinib

Although dasatinib exhibits in vitro activity against KIT p.D816V,[164,165] a case series and a phase 2 trial of the drug have shown limited activity in SM.[166,167] In a phase 2 trial of 33 ISM and advanced SM patients, 11 (33%) responded. Two CRs were recorded in patients without the *KIT* p.D816V mutation, including a patient with *JAK2* p.V617F-positive SM with associated primary myelofibrosis, and a patient with SM and concurrent chronic eosinophilic leukemia.[167] The other nine responses were of a symptomatic nature, without clinically significant reductions in either bone marrow mast cell burden or serum tryptase levels. Nilotinib was evaluated in an open-label phase 2 trial of 61 patients with SM; among the 37 patients with ASM, the ORR was 22%, and there were no CRs.[168]

Hematopoietic Stem Cell Transplantation

Historically, the experience with hematopoietic stem cell transplantation (HSCT) in advanced SM has been limited to a few case reports and small series.[169-172] In 2014, one group published a large, multicenter retrospective analysis on the outcomes of 57 patients with SM (SM-AHN, n = 38 [AML = 20]; ASM, n = 7; and MCL, n = 12) who underwent allogeneic HSCT.[173] These data are derived from the pre-KIT inhibitor era. Donor types consisted of human leukocyte antigen-matched identical (n = 34) and unrelated (n = 17) donors, umbilical cord blood (n = 2), haploidentical (n = 1), and 3 unknown. Responses were observed in 70% of patients, including 16% with a CR. The remaining 30% of responses were split between stable disease (21%) and primary refractory disease (9%). All 38 patients with SM-AHN achieved a CR regarding the AHN component, but 10 subsequently relapsed with AHN, and half of these patients died.

The median OS for all patients at 3 years was 57% for all patients, 74% for patients with SM-AHN, and 43% and 17% for ASM and MCL patients, respectively.[173] The strongest risk factor for worse OS was a diagnosis of MCL. In addition, lower survival was observed in patients undergoing reduced intensity vs myeloablative conditioning. However, patient age, donor age, donor type (sibling or unrelated donor), graft source (bone marrow or peripheral HSCT), *KIT* mutation status, karyotype, and total body irradiation used in myeloablative conditioning had no impact on OS or PFS. Treatment-related mortality at 6 months and 1 year was 11% and 20%, respectively, and was highest in MCL patients. Although a prospective trial is needed to better define the role of HSCT in advanced SM, these data suggest that transplantation can provide extended survival in selected patients, particularly for those with SM-AHN. The role of allogeneic HSCT in the era of KIT inhibitors has not been defined, including who are optimal candidates for transplant, and the role of KIT inhibition pre- and post-transplant.

Other Agents

Phase 1/2 trials of denileukin diftitox,[174] everolimus,[175] daclizumab,[176] thalidomide,[177] and lenalidomide[178] have shown limited or no activity in small case series of SM patients. Based on the expression of CD30 in SM, the anti-CD30 antibody drug immunoconjugate brentuximab vedotin was tested in advanced SM with CD30+ advanced SM. However, no responses were observed in a cohort of 10 patients.[179] Hydroxyurea has been used to control leukocytosis and splenomegaly in patients with an AHN, such as a MPN, MDS/MPN, CEL, or even AML. Splenectomy is less commonly employed in the modern therapy of SM, but has been considered historically in patients with progressive, symptomatic splenomegaly.[180] Multiagent, intensive chemotherapy is usually reserved for patients with MCL, especially for patients with kinetically active disease, but outcomes have generally been disappointing.[138] For patients with SM-associated AML, anthracycline plus cytarabine-based induction chemotherapy is the standard of care for patients who are suitable for high-intensity therapy.[138] In such cases, treatment of the AML almost always will take priority, and the finding of the *KIT* p.D816V mutation may provide an opportunity to consider the addition of KIT inhibitors such as midostaurin to the induction and consolidation phases of treatment. However, the safety and efficacy of this approach requires validation in clinical trials.

FUTURE THERAPEUTIC DIRECTIONS

Clinical trials are under development to investigate targets and pathways relevant to MC pathobiology. Potential approaches include use of JAK inhibitors (e.g., ruxolitinib), inhibitors of BCL-2 (e.g., venetoclax), and agonist antibodies against inhibitory receptors such as siglec-8 to induce MC apoptosis or decrease MC activation (e.g. AK002).[181] In addition, selective inhibitors of KIT p.D816V continue to enter trials. Given the genetic and clinical heterogeneity of advanced SM, combining therapeutics with nonoverlapping mechanisms of action, such as doublet and triplet chemoimmunotherapy approaches in chronic lymphocytic leukemia and multiple myeloma, is a rationale strategy to increase the response rate as well as the quality and DOR. This is a high priority for patients with SM-AHN where tandem therapies addressing the SM and AHN components are needed.[19]

DEVELOPMENT OF CLINICAL RESPONSE CRITERIA AND BIOLOGIC CORRELATES TO ASSESS THERAPEUTIC EFFICACY

Despite the emergence of novel pharmaceutical agents for the treatment of mastocytosis, assessment of response to therapy using uniform criteria that are objective, reproducible, and mastocytosis variant-specific remains the subject of discussion. Previous response criteria have been published,[34] and have now been supplanted by consensus international response criteria by the International Working Group in Myeloproliferative Neoplasms and Treatment (IWG-MRT) and ECNM that better characterize nonhematologic and hematologic organ damage findings, and lend more specificity to the severity of organ dysfunction that is required to be eligible for evaluation, as well as the thresholds which define clinical and histopathologic improvement.[182] The IWG-MRT-ECNM response criteria have been used to harmonize response evaluation between clinical trials, and are anchored to evaluating clinical improvement in SM-related organopathy. In addition to reversion of organ damage, changes in mast cell burden and serum tryptase levels are employed to categorize higher levels of response such as partial and complete remission. Modified IWG-MRT-ECNM response criteria were used in the trials of avapritinib in advanced SM[148,149] and are currently being adopted by most registrational studies aiming to receive approval of novel agents in this patient population. Because these criteria can be confounded by disparate responses between improvement in C-findings and reduction in objective measures of mast cell burden, efforts are ongoing to develop criteria that are anchored to changes in bone marrow mast cell percentage and serum tryptase level, for example "pure pathologic response" (PPR) criteria. In a post-hoc analysis of the EXPLORER trial, PPR criteria were more effective in discriminating OS compared to modified IWG-MRT-ECNM criteria.[183] PPR criteria are simple, can be utilized in clinical practice, increase the number of evaluable patients (even those without C-findings), and are applicable to all AdvSM patients with measurable disease burden (e.g. bone marrow mast cells and serum tryptase level).[184]

Efforts are currently being led by the ECNM to combine patient data from multiple collaborators into a central registry, which now enlists greater than 4000 patients and should provide the power to address questions that are otherwise not answerable given the orphan nature of SM.[185] The American Initiative in Mast Cell Diseases (AIM) is a nascent Pan-American organization whose objective is to bring together physician-scientists studying mast cell disorders and treating patients across the spectrum of subspecialties. AIM and ECNM plan to synergize efforts to address outstanding research and clinical questions to advance patient care.[186]

Current and future research efforts are underway to validate SM-specific patient-reported outcome tools to qualitatively and quantitatively measure patients' symptom burden and quality of life, an increasing focus of regulatory health agencies.[187] Biologic correlates of therapeutic response, such as changes in *KIT* mutant allele burden, changes in the mutational landscape of myeloid-associated genes by interrogation of circulating tumor DNA, and cytokine profiling, are now being incorporated into trials. Transcriptome and proteomic analysis of purified mast cells and cells derived from the associated AHN may also provide opportunities for individualized and molecularly tailored therapy.

Websites

The following websites provide updated information on mastocytosis: https://rarediseases.info.nih.gov/diseases/6987/mastocytosis and www.rarediseases.org.

References

1. Nettleship E, Tay W. Rare forms of urticaria. *Br Med J*. 1869;2:323-330.
2. Sanger A. An anomalous mottled rash, accompanied by pruritus, factious urticaria and pigmentation, "urticaria pigmentosa". *Trans Clin Soc Lond*. 1878;11:161-163.
3. Unna PG. Beitrage zur anatomic und pathogenese der urticaria simplex und pigmentosa. *Mschr Prakt Dermatol Suppl Dermatol Stud*. 1887;3:9.
4. Khoury JD, Solary E, Abia O, et al. The 5th edition of the World Health Organization classification of haematolymphoid tumours: Myeloid and histiocytic/dendritic neoplasms. *Leukemia*. 2022;36:1703-1719.
5. Valent P, Akin C, Hartmann K, et al. Updated diagnostic criteria and classification of mast cell disorders: A consensus proposal. *HemaSphere*. 2021;5(11):e646.
6. Arber DA, Orazi A, Hasserjian RP, et al. International Consensus Classification of myeloid neoplasms and acute leukemias: integrating morphologic, clinical, and genomic data. *Blood*. 2022;140:1200-1228.
7. Nagata H, Worobec AS, Oh CK, et al. Identification of a point mutation in the catalytic domain of the protooncogene c-kit in peripheral blood mononuclear cells of patients who have mastocytosis with an associated hematologic disorder. *Proc Natl Acad Sci U S A*. 1995;92:10560-10564.
8. Longley BJ, Tyrrell L, Lu SZ, et al. Somatic c-KIT activating mutation in urticaria pigmentosa and aggressive mastocytosis: establishment of clonality in a human mast cell neoplasm. *Nat Genet*. 1996;12:312-314.
9. Yavuz AS, Lipsky PE, Yavuz S, Metcalfe DD, Akin C. Evidence for the involvement of a hematopoietic progenitor cell in systemic mastocytosis from single-cell analysis of mutations in the c-kit gene. *Blood*. 2002;100:661-665.
10. Taylor ML, Sehgal D, Raffeld M, et al. Demonstration that mast cells, T cells, and B cells bearing the activating mutation D816V occur in clusters within the marrow of patients with mastocytosis. *J Mol Diagn*. 2004;6:335-342.
11. Akin C, Kirshenbaum AS, Semere T, Worobec AS, Scott LM, Metcalfe DD. Analysis of the surface expression of the c-kit Asp816Val activating mutation in T cells, B cells, and myelomonocytic cells in patients with mastocytosis. *Exp Hematol*. 2000;28:140-147.
12. Kitamura Y, Go S, Hatanaka K. Decrease in mast cells in W/W^v mice and their increase by bone marrow transplantation. *Blood*. 1978;52:447-452.
13. Sonoda T, Kitamura Y, Haku Y, Hara H, Mori KJ. Mast cell precursors in various haematopoietic colonies of mice produced in vivo and in vitro. *Br J Haematol*. 1983;53:611-620.
14. Brockow KC, Akin C, Huber M, Scott LM, Schwartz LB, Metcalfe DD. Levels of mast cell growth factors in plasma and in suction skin blister fluid in adults with mastocytosis: correlation with dermal mast cell numbers and mast cell tryptase. *J Allergy Clin Immunol*. 2002;109:82-88.
15. Kirshenbaum AS, Goff JP, Kessler SW, Mican JM, Zsebo KM, Metcalfe DD. Effects of IL-3 and stem cell factor on the appearance of human basophils and mast cells from CD34+ pluripotent progenitor cells. *J Immunol*. 1992;148:772-777.
16. Kirshenbaum AS, Goff JP, Semere T, Foster B, Scott LM, Metcalfe DD. Demonstration that human mast cells arise from a progenitor cell population that is CD34+, c-kit+, and expresses aminopeptidase N (CD13). *Blood*. 1999;94:2333-2342.
17. Kirshenbaum AS, Kessler SW, Goff JP, Metcalfe DD. Demonstration of the origin of human mast cells from CD34+ bone marrow progenitor cells. *J Immunol*. 1991;146:1410-1415.
18. Escribano L, Orfao A, Diaz-Agustin B, et al. Indolent systemic mast cell disease in adults: immunophenotypic characterization of bone marrow mast cells and its diagnostic implication. *Blood*. 1998;91:2731-2736.
19. Reiter A, George TI, Gotlib J. New developments in diagnosis, prognostication, and treatment of advanced systemic mastocytosis. *Blood*. 2020;135:1365-1376.
20. Bradding P, Saito S. Biology of mast cells and their mediators. In: Burkes AW, Holgate ST, O'Hehir RE, et al, eds. *Middleton's Allergy Principles and Practice*. 9th ed. Elsevier; 2020:215-242.
21. Metcalfe DD. Mast cells and mastocytosis. *Blood*. 2008;112:946-956.
22. Metz M, Brockow K, Metcalfe DD, Galli SJ. Mast cells, basophils and mastocytosis. In: Rich RR, Fleisher TA, Shearer WT, Schroeder HW, Frew AJ, Weyand CM, eds. *Clinical Immunology: Principles and Practice*. 4th ed. Elsevier; 2015:284-297.
23. Gilfillan AM, Peavy RD, Metcalfe DD. Amplification mechanisms for the enhancement of antigen mediated mast cell activation. *Immunol Res*. 2009;43:15-24.
24. Longley BJ, Jr, Morganroth GS, Tyrrell L, et al. Altered metabolism of mast-cell growth factor (c-kit ligand) in cutaneous mastocytosis. *N Engl J Med*. 1993;328:1302-1307.
25. Akin C, Jaffe ES, Raffeld M, et al. An immunohistochemical study of the bone marrow lesions of systemic mastocytosis. *Am J Clin Pathol*. 2002;118:242-247.
26. Taylor ML, Dastych J, Sehgal D, et al. The Kit-activating mutation D816V enhances stem cell factor-dependent chemotaxis. *Blood*. 2001;28:140-147.
27. Cruse G, Metcalfe DD, Olivera A. Functional deregulation of KIT: link to mast cell proliferative diseases and other neoplasms. *Immunol Allergy Clin North Am*. 2014;34:219-237.
28. Miettinen M, Lasota J. KIT (CD117): a review on expression in normal and neoplastic tissues, and mutations and their clinicopathologic correlation. *Appl Immunohistochem Mol Morphol*. 2005;13:205-220.
29. Furitsu T, Tsujimura T, Tono T, et al. Identification of mutations in the coding sequence of the proto-oncogene c-kit in a human mast cell leukemia cell line causing ligand-independent activation of c-kit product. *J Clin Invest*. 1993;92:1736-1744.
30. Nedoszytko B, Arock m, Lyons JJ, et al. Clinical impact of inherited and acquired genetic variants in mastocytosis. *Int J Mol Sci*. 2021;22(1):E511.
31. Kristensen T, Vestergaard H, Bindslev-Jensen C, et al. Sensitive KIT D816V mutation analysis of blood as a diagnostic test in mastocytosis. *Am J Hematol*. 2014;89:493-498.
32. Longley BJ, Jr, Metcalfe DD, Tharp M, et al. Activating and dominant inactivation c-KIT catalytic domain mutations in distinct clinical forms of human mastocytosis. *Proc Natl Acad Sci U S A*. 1999;96:1609-1614.
33. Carter MC, Metcalfe DD. Pediatric mastocytosis. *Arch Dis Child*. 2002;86:315-319.
34. Valent P, Akin C, Escribano L, et al. Standards and standardization in mastocytosis: consensus statement on diagnostics, treatment recommendations and response criteria. *Eur J Clin Invest*. 2007;37:435-453.
35. Schwaab J, Schnittger S, Sotlar K, et al. Comprehensive mutational profiling in advanced systemic mastocytosis. *Blood*. 2013;122(14):2460-2466.
36. Johnson RC, Savage NM, Chiang T, et al. Hidden mastocytosis in acute myeloid leukemia with t(8;21)(q22;q22). *Am J Clin Pathol*. 2013;140:525-535.
37. Pullarkat V, Bedell V, Kim Y, et al. Neoplastic mast cells in systemic mastocytosis associated with t(8;21) acute myeloid leukemia are derived from the leukemic clone. *Leuk Res*. 2007;31:261-265.
38. Cools J, DeAngelo DJ, Gotlib J, et al. A tyrosine kinase created by fusion of the PDGFRA and FIP1L1 genes as a therapeutic target of imatinib in idiopathic hypereosinophilic syndrome. *N Engl J Med*. 2003;348:1201-1214.
39. Lahortiga I, Akin C, Cools J, et al. Activity of imatinib in systemic mastocytosis with chronic basophilic leukemia and PRKG2-PDGFRB fusion. *Haematologica*. 2008;93:49-56.
40. Daley T, Metcalfe DD, Akin C. Association of the Q576R polymorphism in the interleukin-4 receptor alpha chain with indolent mastocytosis limited to the skin. *Blood*. 2001;98:880-882.
41. Mekori YA, Gilfillan AM, Akin C, Hartmann K, Metcalfe DD. Human mast cell apoptosis is regulated through Bcl-2 and Bcl-XL. *J Clin Immunol*. 2001;21:171-174.
42. D'Ambrosio C, Akin C, Wu Y, Magnusson MK, Metcalfe DD. Gene expression analysis in mastocytosis reveals a highly consistent profile with candidate molecular markers. *J Allergy Clin Immunol*. 2003;112:1162-1170.
43. Gupta R, Bain BJ, Knight CL. Cytogenetic and molecular genetic abnormalities in systemic mastocytosis. *Acta Haematol*. 2002;107:123-128.
44. Chaves-Dias C, Hundley TR, Gilfillan AM, et al. Induction of telomerase activity during development of human mast cells from peripheral blood CD34+ cells: comparisons with tumor mast cell lines. *J Immunol*. 2001;166:6647-6656.
45. Cherner JA, Jensen RT, Dubois A, O'Dorisio TM, Gardner JD, Metcalfe DD. Gastrointestinal dysfunction in systemic mastocytosis. *Gastroenterology*. 1988;95:657-667.
46. Rueff F, Placzek M, Przybilla B. Mastocytosis and hymenoptera venom allergy. *Curr Opin Allergy Clin Immunol*. 2006;6:284-288.
47. Castells M, Metcalfe DD, Escribano L. Diagnosis and treatment of cutaneous mastocytosis in children: practical recommendations. *Am J Clin Dermatol*. 2011;12:259-270.
48. Lim KH, Tefferi A, Lasho TL, et al. Systemic mastocytosis in 342 consecutive adults: survival studies and prognostic factors. *Blood*. 2009;113:5727-5736.
49. Valent P, Sotlar K, Sperr WR, et al. Refined diagnostic criteria and classification of mast cell leukemia (MCL) and myelomastocytic leukemia (MML): a consensus proposal. *Ann Oncol*. 2014;25:1691-1700.
50. Soter NA. Mastocytosis and the skin. *Hematol Oncol Clin North Am*. 2000;14:537-555.
51. Caplan R. The natural course of urticaria pigmentosa. Analysis and follow-up of 112 cases. *Arch Dermatol*. 1963;87:146-157.
52. Brockow K, Scott LM, Worobec AS, et al. Regression of urticaria pigmentosa in adult patients with systemic mastocytosis: correlation with clinical patterns of disease. *Arch Dermatol*. 2002;138:785-790.
53. Hartmann K, Escribano L, Grattan C, et al. Cutaneous manifestations in patients with mastocytosis: consensus report of the European competence network on mastocytosis; the American academy of allergy, asthma and immunology; and the European academy of allergology and clinical immunology. *J Allergy Clin Immunol*. 2016;137:35-45.
54. Horny HP, Valent P. Histopathological and immunohistochemical aspects of mastocytosis. *Int Arch Allergy Immunol*. 2002;127:115-117.
55. Akin C, Valent P, Escribano L. Urticaria pigmentosa and mastocytosis: the role of immunophenotyping in diagnosis and determining response to treatment. *Curr Allergy Asthma Rep*. 2006;6:282-288.
56. Lawrence JB, Friedman BS, Travis WD, Chinchilli VM, Metcalfe DD, Gralnick HR. Hematologic manifestations of systemic mast cell disease: a prospective study of laboratory and morphologic features and their relation to prognosis. *Am J Med*. 1991;91:612-624.
57. Carter MC, Metcalfe DD. Decoding the intricacies of the mast cell compartment. *Br J Haematol*. 2022;196(2):304-315.
58. Carter MC, Bai Y, Ruiz-Esteves N, et al. Detection of KIT D816V in peripheral blood of children with cutaneous mastocytosis suggests systemic disease. *Br J Haematol*. 2018;183:775-782.
59. Valent P, Akin C, Sperr WR, Horny HP, Metcalfe DD. Smouldering mastocytosis: a novel subtype of systemic mastocytosis with slow progression. *Int Arch Allergy Immunol*. 2002;127:137-139.
60. Arber DA, Orazi A, Hasserjian R, et al. The 2016 revision to the World Health Organization classification of myeloid neoplasms and acute leukemia. *Blood*. 2016;127:2391-2405.
61. Teodosio C, García-Montero AC, Jara-Acevedo M, et al. An immature immunophenotype of bone marrow mast cells predicts for multilineage D816V KIT mutation in systemic mastocytosis. *Leukemia*. 2012;26:951-958.
62. Travis WD, Li CY. Pathology of the lymph node and spleen in systemic mast cell disease. *Mod Pathol*. 1988;1:4-14.
63. Horny HP, Kaiserling E, Parwaresch MR, Lennert K. Lymph node findings in generalized mastocytosis. *Histopathology*. 1992;21:439-446.

64. Horny HP, Ruck MT, Kaiserling E. Spleen findings in generalized mastocytosis. A clinicopathologic study. *Cancer*. 1992;70:459-468.
65. Mican JM, Di Bisceglie AM, Fong TL, et al. Hepatic involvement in mastocytosis: clinicopathologic correlations in 41 cases. *Hepatology*. 1995;22:1163-1170.
66. Jensen RT. Gastrointestinal abnormalities and involvement in systemic mastocytosis. *Hematol Oncol Clin North Am*. 2000;14:579-623.
67. Chen CC, Andrich MP, Mican JM, Metcalfe DD. A retrospective analysis of bone scan abnormalities in mastocytosis: correlation with disease category and prognosis. *J Nucl Med*. 1994;35:1471-1475.
68. Horan RF, Austen KF. Systemic mastocytosis: retrospective review of a decade's clinical experience at the Brigham and Women's Hospital. *J Invest Dermatol*. 1991;96:5S-13S.
69. Travis WD, Li CY, Yam LT, Bergstralh EJ, Swee RG. Significance of systemic mast cell disease with associated hematologic disorders. *Cancer*. 1988;62:965-972.
70. Sperr WR, Horny HP, Lechner K, Valent P. Clinical and biological diversity of leukemias occurring in patients with mastocytosis. *Leuk Lymphoma*. 2000;37:473-486.
71. Pardanani A, Lim KH, Lasho TL, et al. Prognostically relevant breakdown of 123 patients with systemic mastocytosis associated with other myeloid malignancies. *Blood*. 2009;114:3769-3772.
72. Sotlar K, Fridrich C, Mall A, et al. Detection of c-kit point mutation Asp-816 → Val in microdissected pooled single mast cells and leukemic cells in a patient with systemic mastocytosis and concomitant chronic myelomonocytic leukemia. *Leuk Res*. 2002;26:979-984.
73. Pardanani A. Systemic mastocytosis in adults: 2019 update on diagnosis, risk stratification, and management. *Am J Hematol*. 2019;94:363-377.
74. Klion AD, Noel P, Akin C, et al. Elevated serum tryptase levels identify a subset of patients with a myeloproliferative variant of idiopathic hypereosinophilic syndrome associated with tissue fibrosis, poor prognosis, and imatinib responsiveness. *Blood*. 2003;101:4660-4666.
75. Valent P, Akin C, Sperr WR, et al. Aggressive systemic mastocytosis and related mast cell disorders: current treatment options and proposed response criteria. *Leuk Res*. 2003;27:635-641.
76. Travis WD, Li CY, Bergstralh EJ. Solid and hematologic malignancies in 60 patients with systemic mast cell disease. *Arch Pathol Lab Med*. 1989;113:365-368.
77. Valent P. Biology, classification and treatment of human mastocytosis. *Wien Klin Wochenschr*. 1986;39:385-397.
78. Georgin-Lavialle S, Lhermitte L, Dubreuil P, Chandesris MO, Hermine O, Damaj G. Mast cell leukemia. *Blood*. 2013;121:1285-1295.
79. Jawhar M, Schwaab J, Meggendorfer M, et al. The clinical and molecular diversity of mast cell leukemia with or without associated hematologic neoplasm. *Haematologica*. 2017;102:1035-1043.
80. Sperr WR, Escribano L, Jordan JH, et al. Morphologic properties of neoplastic mast cells: delineation of stages of maturation and implication for cytological grading of mastocytosis. *Leuk Res*. 2001;25:529-536.
81. Kennedy VE, Perkins C, Reiter A, et al. Mast cell leukemia: Clinical and molecular features and survival outcomes of patients in the ECNM registry. *Blood Adv*. 2022:bloodadvances.2022008292. doi:10.1182/bloodadvances.2022008292.
82. Horny HP, Parwaresch MR, Kaiserling E, et al. Mast cell sarcoma of the larynx. *J Clin Pathol*. 1986;39:596-602.
83. Kojima M, Nakamura S, Itoh H, et al. Mast cell sarcoma with tissue eosinophilia arising in the ascending colon. *Mod Pathol*. 1999;12:739-743.
84. Guenther PP, Huebner A, Sobottka SB, et al. Temporary response of localized intracranial mast cell sarcoma to combination chemotherapy. *J Pediatr Hematol Oncol*. 2001;23:134-138.
85. Kudo H, Morinaga S, Shimosato Y, et al. Solitary mast cell tumor of the lung. *Cancer*. 1988;61:2089-2094.
86. Bonadonna P, Perbellini O, Passalacqua G, et al. Clonal mast cell disorders in patients with systemic reactions to hymenoptera stings and increased serum tryptase levels. *J Allergy Clin Immunol*. 2009;123:680-686.
87. Akin C, Scott LM, Kocabas CN, et al. Demonstration of an aberrant mast cell population with clonal markers in a subset of patients with "idiopathic" anaphylaxis. *Blood*. 2007;110:2331-2333.
88. Akin C, Valent P, Metcalfe DD. Mast cell activation syndrome: proposed diagnostic criteria. *J Allergy Clin Immunol*. 2010;126:1099-1104.
89. Valent P, Akin C, Arock M, et al. Definitions, criteria, and global classification of mast cell disorders with special reference to mast cell activation syndromes: a consensus proposal. *Int Arch Allergy Immunol*. 2012;157:215-225.
90. Mateja A, Wang Q, Chovanec J, et al. Defining baseline variability of serum tryptase levels improves accuracy in identifying anaphylaxis. *J Allergy Clin Immunol*. Published online 2021. doi:10.1016/j.jaci.2021.08.007
91. Schwartz LB. Clinical utility of tryptase levels in systemic mastocytosis and associated hematologic disorders. *Leuk Res*. 2001;25:553-562.
92. Li CY. Diagnosis of mastocytosis: value of cytochemistry and immunohistochemistry. *Leuk Res*. 2001;25:537-541.
93. Sotlar K, Cerny-Reiterer S, Petat-Dutter K, et al. Aberrant expression of CD30 in neoplastic mast cells in high-grade mastocytosis. *Mod Pathol*. 2011;24:585-595.
94. Arredondo AR, Jennings CD, Shier L, et al. CD30 expression in mastocytosis. *Lab Invest*. 2011;91:285A-286A.
95. van Anrooij B, Kluin PM, Oude Elberink JN, Kluin-Nelemans JC. CD30 in systemic mastocytosis. *Immunol Allergy Clin North Am*. 2014;34(2):341-355.
96. Pardanani A, Lasho T, Chen D, et al. Aberrant expression of CD123 (interleukin-3 receptor-α) on neoplastic mast cells. *Leukemia*. 2015;29:1605-1608.
97. Pardanani A, Reichard KK, Zblewski D, et al. CD123 immunostaining patterns in systemic mastocytosis: differential expression in disease subgroups and potential prognostic value. *Leukemia*. 2016;30:914-918.
98. Akin C, Metcalfe DD. Surrogate markers of disease in mastocytosis. *Int Arch Allergy Immunol*. 2002;127:133-136.
99. Sperr WR, Jordan JH, Fiegl M, et al. Serum tryptase levels in patients with mastocytosis: correlation with mast cell burden and implication for defining the category of disease. *Int Arch Allergy Immunol*. 2002;128:136-141.
100. Valent P, Sperr WR, Sotlar K, et al. The serum tryptase test: an emerging robust biomarker in clinical hematology. *Expert Rev Hematol*. 2014;7:683-690.
101. Lyons JJ, Yu X, Hughes JD, et al. Elevated basal serum tryptase identifies a multisystem disorder associated with increased TPSAB1 copy number. *Nat Genet*. 2016;48:1564-1569.
102. Arock M, Sotlar K, Akin C, et al. KIT mutation analysis in mast cell neoplasms: recommendations of the European Competence Network on Mastocytosis. *Leukemia*. 2015;29:1223-1232.
103. Brockow K, Akin C, Huber M, Metcalfe DD. IL-6 levels predict disease variant and extent of organ involvement in patients with mastocytosis. *Clin Immunol*. 2005;115:216-223.
104. Akin C, Schwartz LB, Kitoh T, et al. Soluble stem cell factor receptor (CD117) and IL-2 receptor alpha chain (CD25) levels in the plasma of patients with mastocytosis: relationships to disease severity and bone marrow pathology. *Blood*. 2000;96:1267-1273.
105. Jawhar M, Schwaab J, Schnittger S, et al. Additional mutations in SRSF2, ASXL1, and/or RUNX1 identify a high-risk group of patients with KIT D816V(+) advanced systemic mastocytosis. *Leukemia*. 2016;30:136-143.
106. Jawhar M, Schwaab J, Hausmann D, et al. Splenomegaly, elevated alkaline phosphatase, and mutations in the SRSF2/ASXL1/RUNX1 gene panel are strong adverse prognostic markers in patients with systemic mastocytosis. *Leukemia*. 2016;30:2342-2350.
107. Pardanani A, Lasho T, Elala Y, et al. Next-generation sequencing in systemic mastocytosis: derivation of a mutation-augmented clinical prognostic model for survival. *Am J Hematol*. 2016;91:888-893.
108. Gotlib J, Gerds AT, Bose P, et al. Systemic mastocytosis, version 2.2019, NCCN clinical practice guidelines in oncology. *J Natl Compr Canc Netw*. 2018;16:1500-1537.
109. Sperr WR, Kundi M, Alvarez-Twose I, et al. International prognostic scoring system for mastocytosis (IPSM): a retrospective cohort study. *Lancet Haematol*. 2019;6:e638-e649.
110. Jawhar M, Schwaab J, Alvarez-Twose I, et al. MARS: mutation-adjusted risk score for advanced systemic mastocytosis. *J Clin Oncol*. 2019;37:2846-2856.
111. Pardanani A, Shah S, Mannelli F, et al. Mayo alliance prognostic system for mastocytosis: clinical and hybrid clinical-molecular models. *Blood Adv*. 2018;2:2964-2972.
112. Munoz-Gonzalez JI, Alvarez-Twose I, Jara-Acevedo M, et al. Proposed global prognostic score for systemic mastocytosis: a retrospective prognostic modelling study. *Lancet Haematol*. 2021;8:e194-e204.
113. Valent P, Sperr WR, Samorapoompichit P, et al. Myelomastocytic overlap syndromes: biology, criteria, and relationship to mastocytosis. *Leuk Res*. 2001;25:595-602.
114. Dunphy CH. Evaluation of mast cells in myeloproliferative disorders and myelodysplastic syndromes. *Arch Pathol Lab Med*. 2005;129:219-222.
115. Sperr WR, Drach J, Hauswirth AW, et al. Myelomastocytic leukemia: evidence for the origin of mast cells from the leukemic clone and eradication by allogeneic stem cell transplantation. *Clin Cancer Res*. 2005;11:6787-6792.
116. Te Velde J, Vismans FJ, Leenheers-Binnendijk L, Vos CJ, Smeenk D, Bijvoet OL. The eosinophilic fibrohistiocytic lesion of the bone marrow: a mastocellular lesion in bone disease. *Virchows Arch A Pathol Anat Histol*. 1978;377:277-285.
117. Worobec AS. Treatment of systemic mast cell disorders. *Hematol Oncol Clin North Am*. 2000;14:659-687.
118. Lim KH, Pardanani A, Butterfield JH, Li CY, Tefferi A. Cytoreductive therapy in 108 adults with systemic mastocytosis: outcome analysis and response prediction during treatment with interferon-alpha, hydroxyurea, imatinib mesylate or 2-chlorodeoxyadenosine. *Am J Hematol*. 2009;84:790-794.
119. Ustun C, DeRemer DL, Akin C. Tyrosine kinase inhibitors in the treatment of systemic mastocytosis. *Leuk Res*. 2011;35:1143-1152.
120. Frieri M, Alling DW, Metcalfe DD. Comparison of the therapeutic efficacy of cromolyn sodium with that of combined chlorpheniramine and cimetidine in systemic mastocytosis. Results of a double-blind clinical trial. *Am J Med*. 1985;78:9-14.
121. Escribano L, Akin C, Castells M, Schwartz LB. Current options in the treatment of mast cell mediator-related symptoms in mastocytosis. *Inflamm Allergy Drug Targets*. 2006;5:61-77.
122. Tebbe B, Stavropoulos PG, Krasagakis K, Orfanos CE. Cutaneous mastocytosis in adults. Evaluation of 14 patients with respect to systemic disease manifestations. *Dermatology*. 1998;197:101-108.
123. Higgins EM, Humphreys S, Duvivier AW. Urticaria pigmentosa 研 response to topical steroids. *Clin Exp Dermatol*. 1994;19:438-440.
124. Mackey S, Pride HB, Tyler WB. Diffuse cutaneous mastocytosis: treatment with oral psoralen plus UV-A. *Arch Dermatol*. 1996;132:1429-1430.
125. Stege H, Schopf E, Ruzicka T, Krutmann J. High-dose UVA1 for urticaria pigmentosa. *Lancet*. 1996;347:64.
126. Godt O, Proksch E, Streit V, Christophers E. Short- and long-term effectiveness of oral and bath PUVA therapy in urticaria pigmentosa and systemic mastocytosis. *Dermatology*. 1997;195:35-39.
127. Wilson TM, Metcalfe DD, Robyn J. Treatment of systemic mastocytosis. *Immunol Allergy Clin North Am*. 2006;26:549-573.
128. Allison MA, Schmidt CP. Urticaria pigmentosa. *Int J Dermatol*. 1997;36:321-325.
129. Correia O, Duarte AF, Quirino P, Azevedo R, Delgado L. Cutaneous mastocytosis: two pediatric cases treated with topical pimecrolimus. *Dermatol Online J*. 2010;16:8.

130. Achord JL, Langford H. The effect of cimetidine and propantheline on the symptoms of a patient with systemic mastocytosis. *Am J Med*. 1980;69:610-614.
131. Fonga-Djimi HS, Gottrand F, Bonnevalle M, Farriaux JP. A fatal case of portal hypertension complicating systemic mastocytosis in an adolescent. *Eur J Pediatr*. 1995;154:819-821.
132. Bonnet P, Smadja C, Szekely AM, et al. Intractable ascites in systemic mastocytosis treated by portal diversion. *Dig Dis Sci*. 1987;32:209-213.
133. Carter MC, Uzzaman A, Scott LM, Metcalfe DD, Quezado Z. Pediatric mastocytosis: routine anesthetic management for a complex disease. *Anesth Analg*. 2008;107:422-427.
134. Chaar CI, Bell RL, Duffy TP, Duffy AJ. Guidelines for safe surgery in patients with systemic mastocytosis. *Am Surg*. 2009;75:74-80.
135. Pardanani A. How I treat patients with indolent and smoldering mastocytosis (rare conditions but difficult to manage). *Blood*. 2013;121:3085-3094.
136. Johnstone PA, Mican JM, Metcalfe DD, DeLaney TF. Radiotherapy of refractory bone pain due to systemic mast cell disease. *Am J Clin Oncol*. 1994;17:328-330.
137. Moret H, Plihal E, Saudan Y. Case report of bone mastocytosis: total hip arthroplasty for osteoarthritis and open reduction for condylar fracture of the knee. *Clin Rheumatol*. 1994;13:619-623.
138. Valent P, Sperr WR, Akin C. How I treat patients with advanced systemic mastocytosis. *Blood*. 2010;116:5812-5817.
139. Casassus P, Caillat-Vigneron N, Martin A, et al. Treatment of adult systemic mastocytosis with interferon-alpha: results of a multicentre phase II trial on 20 patients. *Br J Haematol*. 2002;119:1090-1097.
140. Lehmann T, Beyeler C, Lammle B, et al. Case report: severe osteoporosis due to systemic mast cell disease – successful treatment with interferon alpha-2b. *Br J Rheumatol*. 1996;35:898-900.
141. Tefferi A, Li CY, Butterfield JH, Hoagland HC. Treatment of systemic mast cell disease with cladribine. *N Engl J Med*. 2001;344:307-309.
142. Kluin-Nelemans HC, Oldhoff JM, Van Doormaal JJ, et al. Cladribine therapy for systemic mastocytosis. *Blood*. 2003;102:4270-4276.
143. Barete S, Lortholary O, Damaj G, et al. Long-term efficacy and safety of cladribine (2-CdA) in adult patients with mastocytosis. *Blood*. 2015;126:1009-1016.
144. Gotlib J, Berube C, Growney JD, et al. Activity of the tyrosine kinase inhibitor PKC412 in a patient with mast cell leukemia with the D816V KIT mutation. *Blood*. 2005;106:2865-2870.
145. Gotlib J, DeAngelo DJ, George TI, et al. KIT inhibitor midostaurin exhibits a high rate of clinically meaningful and durable responses in advanced systemic mastocytosis: report of a fully accrued phase II trial. *Blood*. 2010;116:316.
146. Gotlib J, Kluin-Nelemans HC, George TI, et al. Efficacy and safety of midostaurin in advanced systemic mastocytosis. *N Engl J Med*. 2016;374:2530-2541.
147. Evans EK, Gardino AK, Kim JL, et al. A precision therapy against cancers driven by KIT/PDGFRA mutations. *Sci Transl Med*. 2017;9:eaao1690.
148. DeAngelo DJ, Radia DH, George TI, et al. Safety and efficacy of avapritinib in advanced systemic mastocytosis: the phase 1 EXPLORER trial. *Nature Med*. 2021;27(12):2183-2191.
149. Gotlib J, Reiter A, Radia D, et al. Efficacy and safety of avapritinib in patients with advanced systemic mastocytosis: an interim analysis of the phase 2 PATHFINDER trial. *Nature Med*. 2021;27(12):2192-2199.
150. Smith BD, Kaufman MD, Lu W-P, et al. Ripretinib (DCC-2618) is a switch control kinase inhibitor of a broad spectrum of oncogenic and drug-resistant KIT and PDGFRA variants. *Cancer Cell*. 2019;35:738.
151. Akin C, Brockow K, D'Ambrosio C, et al. Effects of tyrosine kinase inhibitor STI571 on human mast cells bearing wild-type or mutated c-kit. *Exp Hematol*. 2003;31:686-692.
152. Ma Y, Zeng S, Metcalfe DD, et al. The c-kit mutation causing human mastocytosis is resistant to STI571 and other kit kinase inhibitors; kinases with enzymatic site mutations show different inhibitor sensitivity profiles than wild-type kinases and those with regulatory-type mutations. *Blood*. 2002;99:1741-1744.
153. Ueda S, Ikeda H, Mizuki M, et al. Constitutive activation of c-kit by the juxtamembrane but not the catalytic domain mutations is inhibited selectively by tyrosine kinase inhibitors STI571 and AG1296. *Int J Hematol*. 2002;76:427-435.
154. Droogendijk HJ, Kluin-Nelemans HJ, van Doormaal JJ, Oranje AP, van de Loosdrecht AA, van Daele PL. Imatinib mesylate in the treatment of systemic mastocytosis: a phase II trial. *Cancer*. 2006;107:345-351.
155. Vega-Ruiz A, Cortes JE, Sever M, et al. Phase II study of imatinib mesylate as therapy for patients with systemic mastocytosis. *Leuk Res*. 2009;33:1481-1484.
156. Akin C, Fumo G, Yavuz AS, Lipsky PE, Neckers L, Metcalfe DD. A novel form of mastocytosis associated with a transmembrane c-kit mutation and response to imatinib. *Blood*. 2004;103:3222-3225.
157. Alvarez-Twose I, Gonzalez P, Morgado JM, et al. Complete response after imatinib mesylate therapy in a patient with well-differentiated systemic mastocytosis. *J Clin Oncol*. 2012;30:e126-e129.
158. Zhang LY, Smith ML, Schultheis B, et al. A novel K509I mutation of KIT identified in familial mastocytosis-in vitro and in vivo responsiveness to imatinib therapy. *Leuk Res*. 2006;30:373-378.
159. Hoffmann KM, Moser A, Lohse P, et al. Successful treatment of progressive cutaneous mastocytosis with imatinib in a 2-year-old boy carrying a somatic KIT mutation. *Blood*. 2008;112:1655-1657.
160. Mital A, Piskorz A, Lewandowski K, Wasąg B, Limon J, Hellmann A. A case of mast cell leukaemia with exon 9 KIT mutation and good response to imatinib. *Eur J Haematol*. 2011;86:531-535.
161. Dubreuil P, Letard S, Ciufolini M, et al. Masitinib (AB1010), a potent and selective tyrosine kinase inhibitor targeting KIT. *PLoS One*. 2009;4:e7258.
162. Paul C, Sans B, Suarez F, et al. Masitinib for the treatment of systemic and cutaneous mastocytosis with handicap: a phase 2a study. *Am J Hematol*. 2010;85:921-925.
163. Lortholary O, Chandesris MO, Bulai Livideanu C, et al. Masitinib for treatment of severely symptomatic indolent systemic mastocytosis: a randomised, placebo-controlled, phase 3 study. *Lancet*. 2017;389:612-620.
164. Schittenhelm MM, Shiraga S, Schroeder A, et al. Dasatinib (BMS-354825), a dual SRC/ABL kinase inhibitor, inhibits the kinase activity of wild-type, juxtambrane, and activation loop mutant KIT isoforms associated with human malignancies. *Cancer Res*. 2006;66(1):473-481.
165. Shah NP, Lee FY, Luo R, Jiang Y, Donker M, Akin C. Dasatinib (BMS-354825) inhibits KITD816V, an imatinib-resistant activating mutation that triggers neoplastic growth in most patients with systemic mastocytosis. *Blood*. 2006;108:286-291.
166. Purtill D, Cooney J, Sinniah R, et al. Dasatinib therapy for systemic mastocytosis: four cases. *Eur J Haematol*. 2008;80:456-458.
167. Verstovsek S, Tefferi A, Cortes J, et al. Phase II study of dasatinib in Philadelphia chromosome-negative acute and chronic myeloid diseases, including systemic mastocytosis. *Clin Cancer Res*. 2008;14:3906-3915.
168. Hochhaus A, Baccarani M, Giles FJ, et al. Nilotinib in patients with systemic mastocytosis: analysis of the phase 2, open-label, single-arm nilotinib registration study. *J Cancer Res Clin Oncol*. 2015;141:2047-2060.
169. Nakamura R, Chakrabarti S, Akin C, et al. A pilot study of nonmyeloablative allogeneic hematopoietic stem cell transplantation for advanced systemic mastocytosis. *Bone Marrow Transplant*. 2006;37:353-358.
170. Przepiorka D, Giralt S, Khouri I, Champlin R, Bueso-Ramos C. Allogeneic marrow transplantation for myeloproliferative disorders other than chronic myelogenous leukemia: review of forty cases. *Am J Hematol*. 1998;57:24-28.
171. Ronnov-Jessen D, Lovgreen Nielsen P, Horn T. Persistence of systemic mastocytosis after allogeneic bone marrow transplantation in spite of complete remission of the associated myelodysplastic syndrome. *Bone Marrow Transplant*. 1991;8:413-415.
172. Van Hoof A, Criel A, Louwagie A, Vanvuchelen J. Cutaneous mastocytosis after autologous bone marrow transplantation. *Bone Marrow Transplant*. 1991;8:151-153.
173. Ustun C, Reiter A, Scott BL, et al. Hematopoietic stem-cell transplantation for advanced systemic mastocytosis. *J Clin Oncol*. 2014;32:3264-3274.
174. Quintás-Cardama A, Kantarjian H, Verstovsek S. Treatment of systemic mastocytosis with denileukin diftitox. *Am J Hematol*. 2007;82:1124.
175. Parikh SA, Kantarjian HM, Richie MA, Cortes JE, Verstovsek S. Experience with everolimus (RAD001), an oral mammalian target of rapamycin inhibitor, in patients with systemic mastocytosis. *Leuk Lymphoma*. 2010;51:269-274.
176. Quintas-Cardama A, Amin HM, Kantarjian H, Verstovsek S. Treatment of aggressive systemic mastocytosis with daclizumab. *Leuk Lymphoma*. 2010;51:540-542.
177. Damaj G, Bernit E, Ghez D, et al. Thalidomide in advanced mastocytosis. *Br J Haematol*. 2008;141:249-253.
178. Kluin-Nelemans HC, Ferenc V, van Doormaal JJ, et al. Lenalidomide therapy in systemic mastocytosis. *Leuk Res*. 2009;33:e19-e22.
179. Gotlib J, Baird JH, George TI, et al. A phase 2 study of brentuximab vedotin in patients with CD30-positive advanced systemic mastocytosis. *Blood Adv*. 2019;3:2264-2271.
180. Friedman B, Darling G, Norton J, Hamby L, Metcalfe D. Splenectomy in the management of systemic mast cell disease. *Surgery*. 1990;107:94-100.
181. Youngblood BA, Brock EC, Leung J, et al. AK002, a humanized sialic acid-binding immunoglobulin-like lectin-8 antibody that induces antibody dependent cell-mediated cytotoxicity against human eosinophils and inhibits mast cell-mediated anaphylaxis in mice. *Int Arch Allergy Immunol*. 2019;180:91-102.
182. Gotlib J, Pardanani A, Akin C, et al. International working group-myeloproliferative neoplasms research and treatment (IWG-MRT) & European competence network on mastocytosis (ECNM) consensus response criteria in advanced systemic mastocytosis. *Blood*. 2013;121:2393-2401.
183. Gotlib J, Radia DH, George TI, et al. Pure pathologic response is associated with improved overall survival in patients with advanced systemic mastocytosis receiving avapritinib in the phase I EXPLORER study. *Blood*. 2020;136(suppl 1):37-38. [abstract].
184. Shomali W, Gotlib J. Response criteria in advanced systemic mastocytosis: evolution in the era of KIT inhibitors. *Int J Mol Sci*. 2021;22:2983.
185. Valent P, Oude Elberink JNG, Gorska A, et al. The data registry of the European Competence Network on Mastocytosis (ECNM): set up, projects, and perspectives. *J Allergy Clin Immunol Pract*. 2019;7:81.
186. Gotlib J, George TI, Carter MC, et al. Proceedings from the inaugural American initiative in mast cell diseases (AIM) investigator conference. *J Allergy Clin Immunol*. 2021;147:2043-2052.
187. Taylor F, Li X, Yip C, et al. Psychometric evaluation of the advanced systemic mastocytosis symptom assessment form (AdvSM-SAF). *Leuk Res*. 2021;108:106606.

Section 4 ■ LYMPHOPROLIFERATIVE DISORDERS

Chapter 88 ■ Diagnosis and Classification of Lymphomas

PEDRO HORNA • JI YUAN • REBECCA L. KING

SPECIMEN EVALUATION

Tissue Sampling and Processing

Precise assessment of hematopathologic specimens depends, in large part, on adequate sampling and proper handling of tissues, both of which may be influenced significantly by clinicians. Therefore, effective communication between the clinician and the pathologist is imperative for obtaining pertinent patient history and the proper specimen. The largest lymph node or mass lesion generally provides the most useful material for accurate diagnosis and should undergo surgical biopsy. Fresh tissue, moistened in a balanced solution, such as normal saline, should be sent intact to the surgical pathology laboratory without delay to maximize the immunophenotypic, genotypic, and karyotypic studies that are available and to minimize irreversible tissue artifacts. Frozen sections should be discouraged on small specimens, as lymphoid hyperplasia may appear indistinguishable from lymphomas, and freezing permanently distorts the tissue. Touch imprints are generally satisfactory for initial evaluation and for directing specimen workup.

Needle biopsy and aspiration cytology are playing an expanded role in the primary diagnosis and monitoring of patients with malignant lymphomas. The major advantages of these techniques include the following: (1) their relatively noninvasive nature and (2) the rapidity with which the cytology can be reviewed (minutes) and the aspirated cells immunophenotyped (2-3 hours by flow cytometry). With computed tomography guidance, lesions in the mediastinum and retroperitoneum or in any highly vascular organ or tissue can be sampled with minimal morbidity. Technical advances in flow cytometry and molecular biology continue to reduce the amount of tissue required to provide immunophenotypic and genetic data. Just as with lymph node and bone marrow biopsies, however, optimal information can be obtained only by close coordination between the clinician, the person performing the aspirate (radiologist or pathologist), and the hematopathologist providing ancillary diagnostic services. If the material is put into fixative, it cannot be used for flow cytometric phenotypic analysis or standard karyotypic studies.

The limitations of fine-needle aspiration (FNA) and needle biopsies include the following: (1) the possibility of missing focal lesions, (2) the difficulty in making a primary diagnosis of malignant lymphoma,[1] and (3) the difficulty in precisely classifying many lymphomatous and reactive processes in which the architectural features are of prominent diagnostic importance. For example, based only on an FNA and a small needle core biopsy, it may be impossible in certain circumstances to distinguish between small lymphocytic lymphoma (SLL) with prominent proliferation centers and diffuse large B-cell lymphoma (DLBCL); or between classic Hodgkin lymphoma (CHL) and a T-cell lymphoma with Hodgkin-like B immunoblasts. Furthermore, immunophenotypic, genetic, and molecular studies often do not completely resolve these difficult differential diagnoses. Despite these limitations, FNA and needle biopsies currently play a major role in the diagnosis and follow-up of many non-Hodgkin lymphomas (NHLs).

Morphologic Examination

Morphologic examination starts at low magnification to evaluate tissue architecture and patterns of infiltration. Lymphomas may cause partial or complete destruction of the normal architectural features of the lymph node. Growth patterns are generally described as nodular or diffuse. Lymphomas are often distributed within specific anatomic compartments of the lymph node, such as germinal centers, mantle or marginal zones, or the paracortical and medullary areas. The low magnification pattern of neoplastic cell distribution within the lymph node suggests the type of lymphoma present (*Figure 88.1*). High magnification is then used to examine cytologic features, such as the neoplastic cell types (e.g., centrocytes, centroblasts, immunoblasts, and plasmacytoid lymphocytes or plasma cells), because this information helps establish the classification and grade of the tumor. In some lymphomas, the composition of the reactive cell constituents also may be of diagnostic significance.

Immunophenotypic Analysis

Immunophenotypic analysis uses antibodies of variable specificity to detect cellular antigens (surface, cytoplasmic, or nuclear) in cell suspensions (flow cytometry) or in frozen or paraffin-embedded tissue sections (*Table 88.1*). These studies are often invaluable, because they help in distinguishing subtle lymphomatous infiltrates from reactive hyperplasia, can demonstrate the lineage of the neoplastic cell (e.g., B-cell, T cell, and natural killer [NK] cell), can provide data necessary for precise classification of some lymphomas (e.g., mantle cell lymphoma [MCL] vs SLL) (*Table 88.2*), can identify important nonlineage-related markers (e.g., CD15, CD30, and CD56), and can determine the proliferative rate of lymphomas. Immunoglobulin (Ig) light chain restriction is evidence of B-cell clonality, whereas aberrant B-cell or T-cell phenotypes infer clonality. Of note, small clonal B-cell or T-cell populations may be seen in reactive processes or clinically indolent clonal lymphoproliferations.[2-4] Thus, correlation of these studies with the morphologic features is essential to prevent misdiagnosis and clinical confusion.

Immunohistochemical studies on paraffin-embedded tissue permit direct visualization of antigens on the cells of interest. Leukocyte common antigen (CD45) is a reliable marker for identifying most hematopoietic or lymphoid neoplasms but can be negative in acute leukemias, plasma cell neoplasms, anaplastic large cell lymphoma

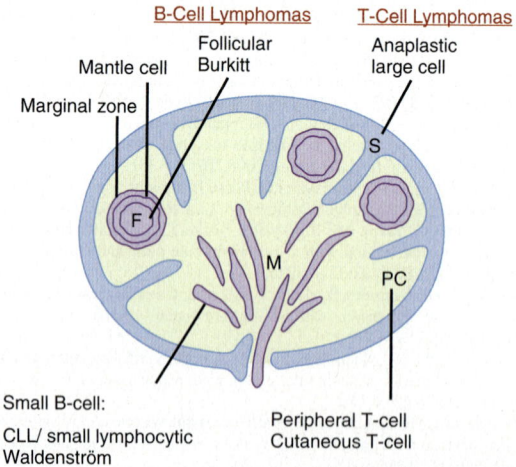

FIGURE 88.1 Sites of origin of malignant lymphomas in a lymph node according to anatomic and functional compartments of the immune system. CLL, chronic lymphocytic leukemia; F, follicles with germinal centers; M, medullary cords; PC, paracortex, or interfollicular areas; S, sinuses. (Adapted from Mann RB, Jaffe ES, Berard CW. Malignant lymphomas: a conceptual understanding of morphologic diversity: A review. *Am J Pathol*. 1979;94(1):105-191. Copyright © 1979 American Society for Investigative Pathology. With permission.)

Table 88.1. Immunophenotypic Markers Used in Diagnosis of Malignant Lymphomas

Antibody Designation	Reactivity	Examples of Lymphoid Neoplasms
CD1a	Thymocytes, dendritic cells, and epidermal Langerhans cells	T lymphoblastic leukemia/lymphoma and Langerhans cell histiocytosis
CD2	T cells and natural killer cells	T-cell and natural killer-cell lymphomas
CD3	T cells (surface and cytoplasmic) and natural killer (cytoplasmic only)	T-cell lymphomas and natural killer-cell lymphomas
CD4	Helper T cells, monocytes, and macrophages	T-cell lymphomas and diffuse large B-cell lymphoma with ALK expression (rare)
CD5	T cells and B-cell subset	T-cell lymphomas, chronic lymphocytic leukemia/small lymphocytic lymphoma, and mantle cell lymphoma
CD7	T cells and natural killer cells	T-cell and natural killer-cell lymphomas
CD8	Cytotoxic and suppressor cells T cells and natural killer cells	Cytotoxic T-cell lymphomas and natural killer cell lymphomas
CD10	Precursor B cells, B-cell subset (follicle center cells), and follicle center T-helper cells	B and some T lymphoblastic leukemias/lymphomas, follicular lymphoma, some diffuse large B-cell lymphomas, Burkitt lymphoma, and angioimmunoblastic T-cell lymphoma
CD11c	Monocytes, macrophages, neutrophils, dendritic cells	Hairy cell leukemia
CD15	Granulocytes, monocytes, Reed-Sternberg cells, activated lymphocytes, and some epithelial cells	Classic Hodgkin lymphomas
CD19	B cells	B-cell lymphomas
CD20	B cells	B-cell lymphomas and nodular lymphocyte predominant Hodgkin lymphoma
CD21	B-cell subset and follicular dendritic cells	Follicular dendritic cell meshworks in follicular lymphoma, nodular lymphocyte predominant Hodgkin lymphoma and angioimmunoblastic T-cell lymphoma
CD22	B-cell subset	Some B-cell lymphomas and hairy cell leukemia
CD23	Activated B-cells, mantle B-cells, and follicular dendritic cells	Chronic lymphocytic leukemia/small lymphocytic lymphoma. Primary mediastinal large B-cell lymphoma. Highlights follicular dendritic cell meshworks similar to CD21.
CD25	Activated T- and B-cells and activated macrophages	Adult T-cell leukemia/lymphoma, anaplastic large cell lymphoma, and hairy cell leukemia
CD30	Activated T- and B-cells and Reed-Sternberg cells	Classic Hodgkin lymphomas, anaplastic large cell lymphoma, some peripheral T-cell lymphomas, NOS, and some large B-cell lymphomas
CD38	Plasma cells, thymocytes, and activated T cells	Plasma cell neoplasms, B-cell lymphomas with plasmacytic differentiation, and some chronic lymphocytic leukemias/small lymphocytic lymphomas
CD43	T cells, granulocytes, and monocytes and macrophages	T-cell lymphomas, chronic lymphocytic leukemia/small lymphocytic lymphoma, mantle cell lymphoma, some marginal zone B-cell lymphomas, and Burkitt lymphoma
CD45	Leukocytes	Non-Hodgkin lymphomas and nodular lymphocyte predominant Hodgkin lymphoma
CD56	Natural killer cells and T-cell subset	Natural killer-cell lymphomas, some cytotoxic T-cell lymphomas, and plasma cell neoplasms
CD57	Natural killer cells and T-cell subset	Natural killer-cell lymphomas, some cytotoxic T-cell lymphomas, and diffuse large B-cell lymphoma with ALK expression (rare)
CD79a	B-cells	Most B-cell lymphomas and plasma cell neoplasms
CD103	Intestinal intraepithelial T cells	Enteropathy-associated T-cell lymphoma and hairy cell leukemia
CD138	Plasma cells	Plasma cell neoplasms and some B-cell lymphomas with plasmacytic differentiation
CD246 (ALK)	Neoplastic cells in anaplastic large cell lymphoma	ALK-positive anaplastic large cell lymphomas, and diffuse large B-cell lymphoma with ALK expression (rare)
BCL2	B-cell subset and T cells	Follicular lymphoma and most other B-cell and T-cell lymphomas
BCL6	Follicle center B cells	Follicular lymphoma and some diffuse large B-cell lymphomas
CXCL13	Follicle center T helper cells	Angioimmunoblastic T-cell lymphoma and nodular lymphocyte predominant Hodgkin lymphoma
Cyclin D1	Neoplastic mantle cells	Mantle cell lymphoma, hairy cell leukemia, and some plasma cell neoplasms
Epithelial membrane antigen	Epithelial cells and plasma cells	Anaplastic large cell lymphoma, nodular lymphocyte predominant Hodgkin lymphoma, plasmablastic lymphoma, and plasma cell neoplasms

Table 88.1. Immunophenotypic Markers Used in Diagnosis of Malignant Lymphomas (Continued)

Antibody Designation	Reactivity	Examples of Lymphoid Neoplasms
FoxP3	$CD4^+/CD25^+$ regulatory T cells	Adult T-cell leukemia/lymphoma
Granzyme A, B, and M	Natural killer cells and activated cytotoxic T cells	Natural killer cell and activated cytotoxic T-cell lymphomas
IgA, IgD, IgE, IgG, IgG4, and IgM	Immunoglobulin heavy chains	B-cell lymphomas and plasma cell neoplasms
IRTA1	Marginal zone B cells	Distinction of MZL from other small B cell lymphomas
Kappa and Lambda	Immunoglobulin light chains	B-cell lymphomas and plasma cell neoplasms
Ki-67/mib-1	Nuclear proliferation antigens	Indicator of cell proliferation rate in lymphomas; greater than 95% expression in Burkitt lymphoma
LEF1	B cells in CLL/SLL, normal T cells	CLL/SLL distinction from mantle cell lymphoma
MNDA	B cells in marginal zone lymphoma; normal myelomonocytic cells	Distinction from other small B cell lymphomas
MUM1	B-cells in terminal phase of differentiation, plasma cells, activated T cells, and Reed-Sternberg cells	Lymphoplasmacytic lymphoma, some diffuse large B-cell lymphomas, plasma cell neoplasms, some T-cell lymphomas, and Hodgkin lymphomas
PAX5	B cells and Reed-Sternberg cells	B-cell lymphomas, including Hodgkin lymphomas
SOX11	B cells in mantle cell lymphoma	Distinction from other small B cell lymphomas
T-cell receptor α/β	α/β T cells	Most T-cell lymphomas
T-cell receptor λ/δ	λ/σ T cells	Few T-cell lymphomas
TdT	Lymphoblasts	B and T lymphoblastic leukemias/lymphomas
TIA-1	Natural killer cells and cytotoxic T cells	Natural killer-cell and cytotoxic T-cell lymphomas

Abbreviations: ALK, anaplastic lymphoma kinase; CLL/SLL, chronic lymphocytic leukemia/small lymphocytic lymphoma; MZL, marginal zone lymphoma; NOS, not otherwise specified.

Table 88.2. Pathologic Features in the Differential Diagnosis of Small B-Cell Lymphomas

Lymphoma Type	Growth Pattern	Cytology	Immunophenotype			Surface Ig	Genetics
			CD5	CD10	CD23		
Follicular lymphoma	Nodular (follicular)	Lymphocytes with irregular cleaved nuclei (centrocytes) and admixed large cells (centroblasts)	−	+	−	Bright	t(14;18)(q32;q21) in >85%
Chronic lymphocytic leukemia/small lymphocytic lymphoma	Diffuse with proliferation centers	Small lymphocytes with round nuclei and scant cytoplasm	+	−	+	Weak IgM and IgD > IgG > IgA	None useful for diagnosis. See Chapter 92.
Lymphoplasmacytic lymphoma	Diffuse or interfollicular	Small lymphocytes, plasma cells, and plasmacytoid lymphocytes	−	−	−	Moderate IgM	*MYD88* L265P mutation *CXCR4*- WHIM mutation
Mantle cell lymphoma	Diffuse or vaguely nodular	Small lymphocytes with irregular nuclei, scant cytoplasm, and few admixed large cells	+	−	−	Moderate IgM and IgD; Lambda > kappa	t(11;14)(q13;q32)
Nodal marginal zone B-cell lymphoma	Interfollicular and perisinusoidal	Small lymphocytes with round, folded nuclei and abundant cytoplasm ± plasma cells	−	−	−	Moderate IgM	None specific.
Splenic marginal zone B-cell lymphoma	Nodular	Biphasic: inner core of small lymphocytes with irregular nuclei and scant cytoplasm; outer core of medium-size lymphocytes with round nuclei and abundant clear cytoplasm ± plasma cells	−	−	−	IgM ± IgD	Del 7q in subset
Extranodal marginal zone B-cell lymphoma of mucosa-associated lymphoid tissue	Diffuse	Small lymphocytes with round, folded nuclei and abundant cytoplasm ± plasma cells	−	−	−	IgM	*MALT1* translocations in subset

Abbreviations: Ig, immunoglobulin; +, positive; −, negative.

(ALCL), classic HLs, and large B-cell lymphomas with plasmablastic differentiation. Two markers that work well in paraffin, such as CD20 (pan-B-cell) and CD3 (pan-T cell), are adequate to categorize most NHLs as to their B-cell or T-cell lineage. Detection of light chain restriction is most easily achieved in B-cell lymphomas that have abundant cytoplasmic Ig (most lymphomas with plasmacytic differentiation and many large B-cell lymphomas). Nowadays, the widespread availability of fixation-sensitive antibodies and antigen retrieval protocols allows for a comprehensive immunohistochemical profiling of lymphomas in paraffin-embedded tissue.

Flow cytometry is a commonly used tool used for phenotyping most NHLs.[5,6] This technology permits the rapid analysis of large numbers of cells for the expression of multiple surface or cytoplasmic antigens, and is capable of detecting minimal residual disease.[6,7] In contrast to immunohistochemistry, Ig light chain expression is readily detected in most B-cell (surface) and plasma cell (cytoplasmic) populations; and studies for coexpression of more than one marker are easily accomplished (e.g., light chain restriction on $CD5^+/CD19^+$ B-cells). Data storage in "list mode" electronic files permits retrospective off-line multiparameter analysis of lymphocyte subpopulations. However, for most analyses, flow cytometry requires viable cell populations. The quality of the information produced by flow cytometry is directly related to the quality of the communication between the flow cytometrist and the pathologist. The basic question is: "Is the cell population of interest to the pathologist the same cell population analyzed by flow cytometry?"

Cytogenetic and Molecular Studies

Polymerase chain reaction (PCR)-based B-cell and T-cell receptor analysis of clonality provides a standardized, rapid and highly sensitive means of detecting clonal lymphoproliferations and their lineage.[8] This technology is particularly helpful for establishing B-cell or T-cell clonality in lymphoproliferations present in paraffin-embedded small biopsies, such as those obtained by endoscopy. PCR clonality testing is most useful when immunophenotypic studies are inconclusive and are the only practical way of proving B-cell or T-cell clonality. In this setting, positive results should be interpreted with caution and correlated with morphology and clinical features, as clonal B-cell and T-cell expansions may be seen in some reactive processes and indolent lymphoproliferations. PCR assays are also available to detect the presence of specific gene mutations (e.g., $MYD88^{L265P}$ and $BRAF^{V600E}$) of diagnostic utility in the work up of NHLs. In addition, PCR detection of somatic hypermutation on the variable region of the Ig heavy chain has shown to be important in the prognostic assessment of chronic lymphocytic leukemia (CLL).

Fluorescence in situ hybridization (FISH) applied to fresh or paraffin-embedded tissue allows for the detection of critical translocations in NHLs with a sensitivity that is much greater than conventional karyotyping.[9] FISH can be performed on very small specimens (e.g., smears and touch imprints) and may be completed in less than 24 hours.[10-12]

Recently, next-generation sequencing (NGS) technologies have provided an unparalleled insight into the genetic abnormalities of NHLs, with important findings relevant to the diagnosis, classification, risk stratification, and targeted therapy of selected diseases.[13] Already a number of NGS panels have become available to simultaneously detect mutations and/or translocations of a selected number of genes relevant to NHLs. The clinical applications of these findings are currently under investigation but have potential to provide important predictive and prognostic data in some lymphomas. Another application of NGS is the sequencing of variable regions of B- and T-cell receptor genes, which not only establishes the presence of a clonal lymphoproliferation but also provides a unique tumor-specific sequence that can be utilized for minimal residual disease assessment.[14,15]

Classification of Non-Hodgkin Lymphomas

For the clinician, pathologist, and basic scientist working in lymphoid neoplasia, the classification of NHLs is a persistent, confusing, and controversial problem. Several competing classification schemes have evolved, all with their supporters and detractors.

In the 1950s, Rappaport developed a classification system based on growth pattern (nodular or diffuse) and cytology of lymphocytes (well differentiated, poorly differentiated, undifferentiated, or histiocytic).[16] This scheme enjoyed enormous popularity because of its simplicity and reproducibility, but was superseded by classification schemes that reflected advances in cellular immunology. In the early 1970s, Lukes and Collins,[17] in the United States, and Lennert,[18] in Kiel, Germany, proposed NHL classifications that related morphology to lymphocyte lineage. Both recognized follicular structures as a histologic correlate of B-cell differentiation. Each subdivided follicular lymphomas (FLs) by the cytologic appearance of the predominant follicle center cell type: small and large cleaved cells in the Lukes-Collins classification (centrocytes in Kiel classification) and small and large noncleaved (transformed) cells in the Lukes-Collins classification (centroblasts in Kiel classification). For NHLs with diffuse growth patterns, immunophenotypic studies facilitated and, in many cases, were essential for precise classification.[19] In 1982, the Working Formulation (WF) was introduced in an attempt to provide a morphologic classification scheme with prognostic relevance.[20] Although the WF was an improvement over the earlier Rappaport classification, it had the same limitations as all purely morphologic classification schemes, separating biologically closely related lymphomas, and grouping together biologically unrelated entities. All consideration regarding immunophenotype was excluded, so that the WF did not foster recognition of new entities.

In 1994, the Revised European American Lymphoma (REAL) classification was proposed and listed well-defined, "real disease entities recognized and diagnosed in daily practice."[21] In 2001, the World Health Organization (WHO) classification[22] built on the REAL classification and corrected some of its deficiencies. The now widely accepted WHO classification was updated in 2008[23] and recently revised in 2017[24] to include recent cytogenetic and molecular findings as well as newly recognized rare disease entities. The WHO classification has many strong points, including its comprehensiveness and inclusion of virtually all lymphoid malignancies described to date (Table 88.3). It defines diseases by four features: morphology, immunophenotype, genetics, and clinical information. Accordingly, the major diagnostic criteria for each of the major groups of NHL and HL are presented in the following discussion. Because a separate chapter is dedicated to molecular genetics of lymphoma (Chapter 89), genetic information provided in this chapter is limited to what is routinely used in the setting of diagnosis and classification.

B-CELL LYMPHOMAS

Follicular Lymphoma
Background

The follicle center is the major site of B-cell differentiation and proliferation.[25,26] It may also serve as the site of lymphomagenesis of most B-cell lymphomas and HLs.[27] B-cells move into the follicle after they first encounter protein antigen in the paracortex, to begin a series of steps that ultimately produces plasma cells with high-affinity Ig and memory B cells. Morphologically, the follicular center reflects this biologic transformation by frequent mitoses and by its range of cell types, including centrocytes and larger centroblasts. Differentiation results in the Ig heavy chain class switching from IgM to IgG, IgA, or IgE, and in enhanced Ig synthesis. Proliferation produces the clonal expansion that is the basis of immunologic memory and an effective humoral immune response.

Somatic mutation in the Ig genes occurring during proliferation is followed by selection of B cells with surface Ig of optimal affinity for antigen. Successful interaction of B cells with antigen-bearing follicular dendritic cells triggers B-cell expression of BCL2 protein that saves the B-cell from apoptotic cell death.[28] Tingible body macrophages mark the death via apoptosis of B-cells not selected for survival. Somatic mutation may serve to identify those neoplasms that have arisen from B cells that have been exposed to antigen in the environment of the follicle. Most B-cell NHLs and HLs have extensive somatic mutations.[27,29,30]

Table 88.3. The Revised 4th Edition World Health Organization Classification of Lymphoid Neoplasms

Precursor B-cell Neoplasm	Precursor T-cell Neoplasm
B lymphoblastic leukemia/lymphoma	T lymphoblastic leukemia/lymphoma
Mature B-cell Neoplasms	**Mature T-cell and NK-cell Neoplasms**
Follicular lymphoma	Peripheral T-cell lymphoma, NOS
Chronic lymphocytic leukemia/small lymphocytic lymphoma	Angioimmunoblastic T-cell lymphoma
Mantle cell lymphoma	ALCL types: ALCL ALK+, ALCL ALK−, primary cutaneous ALCL, breast implant–associated ALCL
Lymphoplasmacytic lymphoma	T-cell prolymphocytic leukemia
Nodal marginal zone lymphoma	Extranodal NK/T-cell lymphoma, nasal type
Extranodal marginal zone lymphoma of mucosa-associated lymphoid tissue	Aggressive NK-cell leukemia
Splenic marginal zone lymphoma	Adult T-cell leukemia/lymphoma
Hairy cell leukemia	T-cell large granular lymphocytic leukemia
Rare small B-cell lymphoma types: Duodenal-type follicular lymphoma; pediatric-type follicular lymphoma; pediatric nodal marginal zone lymphoma; splenic diffuse red pulp small B-cell lymphoma; hairy cell leukemia variant; primary cutaneous follicle center lymphoma.	Chronic lymphoproliferative disorder of NK cells
B-cell prolymphocytic leukemia	Hepatosplenic T-cell lymphoma
DLBCL, NOS	Rare peripheral T-cell lymphomas: Follicular T-cell lymphoma; nodal peripheral T-cell lymphoma with T follicular helper phenotype; systemic EBV+ T-cell lymphoma of childhood.
T-cell/histiocyte-rich large B-cell lymphoma	Enteropathy-associated T-cell lymphoma
Primary mediastinal (thymic) large B-cell lymphoma	Monomorphic epitheliotropic intestinal T-cell lymphoma
Primary DLBCL of the CNS	Mycosis fungoides
EBV+ DLBCL, NOS	Sézary syndrome
High-grade B-cell lymphoma, with *MYC* and *BCL2* and/or *BCL6* rearrangements, and high-grade B-cell lymphoma, NOS.	Lymphomatoid papulosis
Rare large B-cell lymphoma types: DLBCL associated with chronic inflammation; lymphomatoid granulomatosis; intravascular large B-cell lymphoma; ALK-positive large B-cell lymphoma; plasmablastic lymphoma; HHV8+ DLBCL, NOS; primary effusion lymphoma; primary cutaneous DLBCL, leg type; large B-cell lymphoma with IRF4 rearrangement; Burkitt-like lymphoma with 11q aberration	Subcutaneous panniculitis-like T-cell lymphoma
Burkitt lymphoma	Primary cutaneous γδ T-cell lymphoma
Classic Hodgkin lymphoma	Rare cutaneous T-cell lymphoproliferations: primary cutaneous aggressive epidermotropic cytotoxic T-cell lymphoma, primary cutaneous acral CD8+ T-cell lymphoma; primary cutaneous CD4+ small/medium T-cell lymphoproliferative disorder; hydroa vacciniforme-like lymphoproliferative disorder.
Nodular lymphocyte predominant Hodgkin lymphoma	
B-cell lymphoma, unclassifiable, with features intermediate between DLBCL and classic Hodgkin lymphoma	

Not included are *in-situ* neoplasias, prelymphomatous proliferations, polymorphous EBV-positive lymphoproliferations and post-transplant lymphoproliferative disorders.
Abbreviations: ALCL, anaplastic large cell lymphoma; CNS, central nervous system; DLBCL, diffuse large B-cell lymphoma; EBV, Epstein-Barr virus; HHV-8, human herpes virus 8; NK, natural killer; NOS, not otherwise specified.

The recognition of the contribution of somatic mutation, receptor editing, and class switching in lymphomagenesis supports a major role for the follicle in neoplastic transformation.[27,31,32]

In addition to typical, adult-type FL, the WHO recognizes pediatric-type FL and primary cutaneous follicle center lymphoma (PCFCL) as distinct clinicopathologic entities. Additionally, duodenal-type FL[24] and testicular FL, which are subsets of adult-type FL, have unique features deserving of mention. These, along with in situ follicular neoplasia (ISFN), will be discussed here. ISFN itself has a low rate of progression, but may be associated with concurrent or prior overt FL.[33,34]

Morphology

FLs are recognized at low magnification by the effacement of nodal architecture by follicles that crowd one another and fill the cortex and the medulla (*Figure 88.2A*). Neoplastic follicles attempt to recapitulate their normal counterpart. However, morphologic differences are apparent, as mantle zones are usually attenuated, and tingible body macrophages seen in reactive follicles are often absent.

FLs, as with reactive follicles, are composed of varying proportions of small, angulated cells with irregular nuclei and condensed chromatin (centrocytes) and a variable number of larger centroblasts with oval nuclei (greater in size than a macrophage nucleus), dispersed chromatin, and multiple nucleoli that often abut the nuclear membrane. The number of centroblasts in an FL case forms the basis for grading the neoplasm (*Figure 88.2B* and *C*). Centroblasts are counted in 10 consecutive 400X microscopic fields and the mean number of centroblasts per 400X field is then determined. Grade is as follows: Grade 1 if less than/equal to 5 centroblasts per 400X field, Grade 2 between 6 and 15 centroblasts per 400X field, and Grade 3 more than 15 centroblasts per 400X field. Grade 3 is further subdivided into grade 3a and 3b,

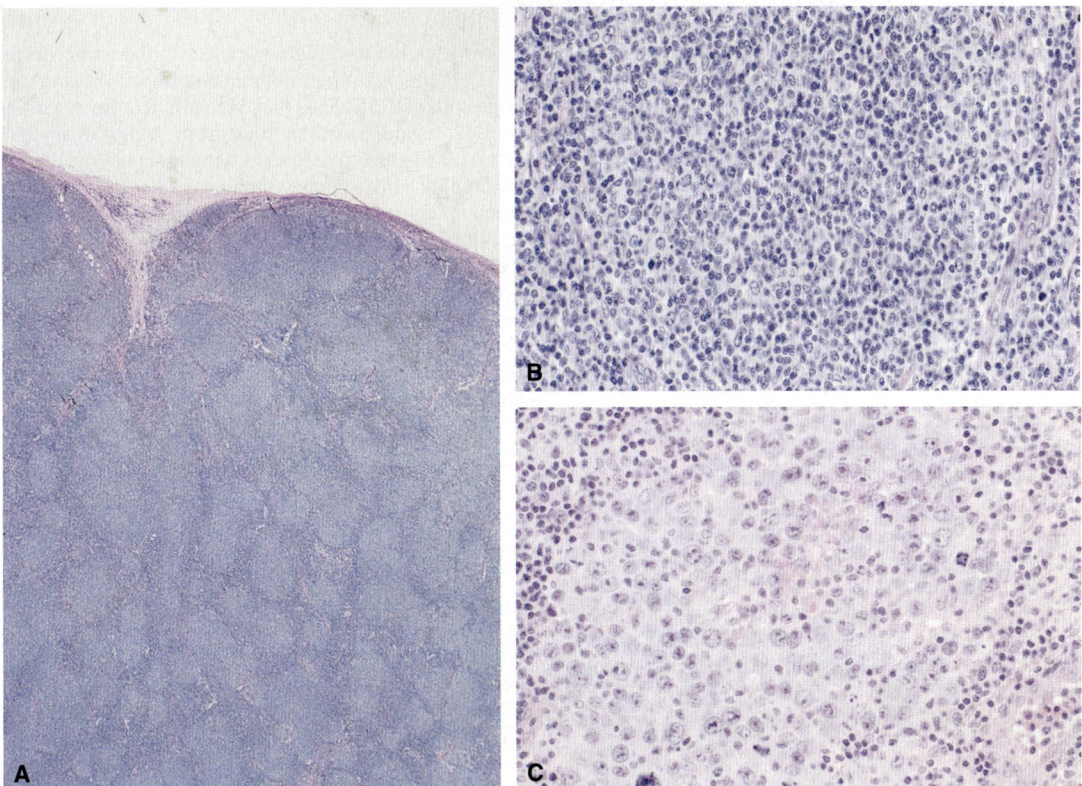

FIGURE 88.2 Lymph node: follicular lymphoma. A, Low magnification demonstrates effacement of architecture by a follicular proliferation producing a nodular pattern. B, In a higher magnification, the follicles are composed almost entirely of centrocytes (follicular lymphoma, grade 1), whereas in (C), from another patient, the follicles are dominated by centroblasts (follicular lymphoma, grade 3).

with grade 3b having essentially 100% centroblasts and grade 3a being composed of a mixture of both cell types. Because of lack of evidence to suggest clinical utility for splitting grades 1 and 2, the WHO classification now deems it preferable to use the designation "grade 1 to 2" for cases that meet grading criteria for either grade 1 or grade 2 FL.

In many cases, the neoplastic nodules are accompanied by a diffusely growing component, and in rare examples, FLs grow in a purely diffuse pattern. A subset of these predominantly diffuse cases arising commonly in inguinal lymph nodes show recurrent molecular and cytogenetic abnormalities and reproducible phenotypic and morphologic features.[35] A small number of FLs show differentiation to marginal zone–like cells with a "halo-like" distribution around neoplastic follicles. These marginal zone cells, although often CD10 and BCL2 protein negative, are genetically identical to the neoplastic cells of the follicles.[36]

A leukemic phase may be present in as many as 10% of patients with low-grade FLs. Circulating cells show nuclear irregularity and are immunophenotypically distinct from neoplastic cells of B-cell CLL/SLL or MCL.

Pediatric-type FL shows characteristic morphology with large, expansile follicles that may retain some morphologic features of reactive follicles including mantle zones and tingible body macrophages. PCFCL may show follicular growth, but often has a diffuse or vaguely serpiginous growth pattern. These latter two entities are not graded in the traditional method noted above, but are diagnosed as specific entities, when possible, based on clinicopathologic features.

Immunophenotype

FL expresses pan B-cell markers (CD20, CD19, PAX5, CD79a). FLs generally express bright surface Ig, but some grade 3 FLs are surface Ig negative. Most FLs express germinal center markers CD10 and BCL6, with some grade 3 FL showing CD10 loss. In cases where CD10 is negative, other germinal center markers such as GCET and LMO2 may be useful to support germinal center origin. FLs are almost always CD5−, but rare CD5+/CD10+ cases have been described that often exhibit atypical histopathology such as floral variants or patterns that may be confused with progressive transformation of germinal centers (PTGCs).[37,38] BCL2 is typically expressed within the neoplastic cells. This aberrant expression of BCL2 protein may be helpful in differentiating some follicular lymphoid hyperplasias from FL; however, overexpression of BCL2 protein does not help differentiate FLs from other NHLs. Additionally, BCL2 expression (and associated *BCL2* translocation discussed below) is not seen in all cases of FL, with negative cases more commonly exhibiting grade 3 histology. Both pediatric-type FL and PCFCL are, as a rule, BCL2-negative.

Ki-67 is typically low (<30%) in keeping with the indolent nature of the disease. However, some FLs with a low-grade histologic appearance may show a high proliferation index on Ki-67 staining.[39] These may behave more aggressively, although more data are needed.

Genetics

More than 85% of nodal FLs and 25% to 30% of DLBCLs have an IGH::BCL2 chromosomal abnormality. These numbers are lower in children and in patients with extranodal presentations (described below). In a small subset of FLs, especially those lacking the IGH::BCL2, there are translocations involving the *BCL6* gene at chromosome 3q27.

FLs with a predominantly diffuse growth pattern, often occurring in inguinal lymph nodes, may be negative for the t(14; 18)(q32; q21), and commonly show deletions at chromosome 1p36.[35] Pediatric-type FL must be negative for *BCL2::*IGH, by definition. In cutaneous lesions, the presence of an IGH::BCL2 should prompt strong consideration for cutaneous involvement by systemic FL, rather than PCFCL.

NGS studies have identified recurrently mutated genes in FL including *CREBBP, KMT2D, EZH2, BCL2,* and *TNFRSF14.*[40] However, the precise clinical utility of either targeted or whole exome NGS testing in FL remains to be established, and to date, these studies have limited utility in disease classification by the WHO.

Pediatric-type Follicular Lymphoma

The 2017 WHO recognizes pediatric-type FL as a distinct entity. Cases have been reported in adults as well as children.[41] Pediatric-type FL is rare, representing 1% to 2% of B-cell NHL in the pediatric age group. Patients with pediatric-type FL present with low-stage disease, typically involving lymph nodes in the head and neck region.[41,42]

The pediatric-type FL cases have characteristic histopathologic features that distinguish them from typical FL. These include large, expansile follicles with high proliferation rate, reminiscent of florid follicular hyperplasia.[35,41,43] The neoplastic follicles in pediatric-type FLs, are usually composed of medium-sized, blastoid cells that do not exactly resemble either centroblasts or centrocytes.[35,41,42] Caution must be taken in these cases first to recognize this as a lymphomatous process, and second to distinguish this cytologically from a high-grade process.

The follicles express CD10, BCL6, and are typically negative for BCL2 and MUM1. By definition, these cases must lack the t(14;18) IGH::BCL2 fusion.[24,35,41,42] High Ki-67 proliferation index (>30%) is also a diagnostic criterion of pediatric-type FL, but does not impart aggressive behavior.[42] Strict adherence to these diagnostic criteria is essential, because pediatric-type FL, whether in children or adults, may not require systemic therapy.[24,35,41,44]

Of note, there are rare FL cases that present in the testis, most often in children. These cases may be pathophysiologically distinct from pediatric-type FL because they have occasional *BCL6* rearrangements. However, they are phenotypically similar in that they often lack BCL2 expression and lack IGH::BCL2 rearrangements. These cases also have an indolent course.[41]

Duodenal-type Follicular Lymphoma

FL in the duodenum is often confined to that location. Because of its unique features, the WHO now recognizes duodenal-type FL as a distinct entity. These lesions typically involve the second portion of the duodenum, forming periampullary sessile polyps within the lamina propria. The lymphomas are low grade and are composed of CD10 and/or BCL6 positive, BCL2 positive tumor cells. As in gastric mucosa–associated lymphoid tissue (MALT) lymphomas, there is a high frequency of association with *Helicobacter pylori* and these tumors show restricted usage of IgVH4 genes.

Primary Cutaneous Follicle Center Lymphoma

PCFCL typically presents as localized plaques or nodules on the head and neck, and is usually not associated with systemic disease. As with other B-cell lymphomas in the skin, there is typically a Grenz zone without epidermotropism, and the lesional cells infiltrate the superficial dermis in a nodular, vaguely nodular, or diffuse fashion. Cytologically, these lesions are often composed of medium-sized centrocytes, which may have more open chromatin and a larger-cell appearance than typical nodal FL, but should not be confused for DLBCL. Like other FLs, these express the germinal center marker BCL6, although expression of CD10 is less common, and BCL2 is expected to be negative. Clinical correlation is required to distinguish these lesions from systemic FL involving the skin.

In Situ Follicular Neoplasia

Occasional patients with FL, usually with limited stage disease, have partial nodal involvement amidst residual reactive lymphoid follicles. This must be distinguished from what is termed ISFN (previously FL in situ).[33,45] In ISFN, there is no effacement of tissue architecture, but there is a cytologically and immunophenotypically aberrant B-cell population within the germinal centers. BCL2 expression is seen within CD10 and/or BCL6-positive germinal centers, clonality can be seen by flow cytometry or IHC, and IGH::BCL2 translocations can be present. It is critical to ensure that there is no infiltration of CD10 or BCL6-positive lymphocytes into the interfollicular areas of the lymph node, as this would be characteristic of an overt FL. These lesions have an uncertain malignant potential, with some patients harboring concurrent overt FL, and others never developing FL.

Transformation

Transformation to a higher grade lymphoma occurs in 20% to 60% of FL. Pathology reports should emphasize areas of diffuse growth of large cells (DLBCL), as they are sufficient for regarding the tumor as DLBCL regardless of the grade of the tumor in any residual follicles. Occasionally, the transformed lymphoma has cytologic characteristics resembling a high-grade lymphoma rather than a large cell lymphoma. Accompanying this change, the tumor cells can acquire the t(8;14)(q24;q32) involving *MYC* (8q24) and IGH (14q32), and along with the IGH::BCL2 or *BCL6* rearrangement would be classified as a high-grade B-cell lymphoma with *MYC* and *BCL2* and/or *BCL6* rearrangements ("double-hit/triple hit" lymphoma). Additionally, a controversial and rare form of transformation in which the tumor cells have a blast-like morphology and features more characteristic of B lymphoblastic leukemia/lymphoma has been recognized. These blastoid variants of transformed FL are aggressive clinically.[46]

Chronic Lymphocytic Leukemia/Small Lymphocytic Lymphoma

Background

CLL/SLL is a neoplasm of small round B-cells that usually have low-level surface Ig and a $CD5^+$/$CD23^+$ phenotype. SLL is the term used to describe the disease when lymph node involvement is the dominant feature. B-cell clones in the peripheral blood that measure below 5×10^9/L are termed "monoclonal B-cell lymphocytosis." Greater than 5×10^9/L clonal B cells must be present to diagnose CLL even if there is SLL, cytopenias, or disease-related symptoms.[24] Usually, CLL/SLL presents in elderly patients with a leukemic phase and generalized lymphadenopathy on routine physical examination. Bone marrow involvement is often extensive. Occasionally, patients present with bacterial infection related to hypogammaglobulinemia or with signs and symptoms secondary to anemia or thrombocytopenia that may have an autoimmune basis. CLL may occur in familial clusters with a decreasing age of onset from generation to generation.[47]

Morphology

In the peripheral blood and bone marrow, CLL typically shows lymphocytosis with small, round lymphocytes with condensed chromatin and scant cytoplasm. These cells often show multiple chromatin condensations in a "soccer ball" pattern. Bone marrow core biopsies can show involvement in an interstitial pattern, as well as nodular or diffuse sheets, with the latter having a worse prognosis.[48,49]

Lymph node architecture in SLL is totally effaced with loss of lymphoid follicles and obliteration of sinuses by an infiltrate of monomorphic small round lymphocytes with condensed chromatin and scant cytoplasm. Proliferation centers (collections of intermediate-size round lymphocytes with open chromatin and small nucleoli called paraimmunoblasts and prolymphocytes) are dispersed throughout the lymph node (*Figure 88.3*).[50] This feature is not seen in other small B-cell lymphomas. Morphologic features that correlate with a worse prognosis include prominent proliferation centers in lymph nodes or increased numbers (>10%) of prolymphocytes (intermediate-size lymphocytes with prominent central nucleoli) in the blood.[51,52]

Richter syndrome, which is the transformation of CLL/SLL to an aggressive lymphoma (usually DLBCL), occurs in less than 5% of patients.[53-55] Some SLL cases contain prominent, almost coalescing proliferation centers that at first may resemble a DLBCL. Recognition of the spectrum of small, medium, and larger lymphocytes present in these cases can help distinguish these cases from overt transformation. As mentioned above, some studies have found a correlation between prominent proliferation centers and more aggressive disease in CLL.[51]

Rarely, CLL/SLL can transform into CHL.[56] This must be distinguished from CLL/SLL with Reed-Sternberg (RS)–like cells, although the clinical significance of this distinction remains uncertain.[57] Both are often associated with Epstein-Barr virus (EBV) as detected by in situ hybridization.[58]

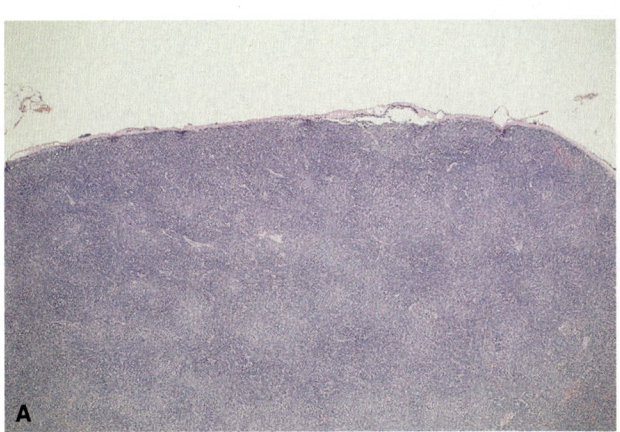
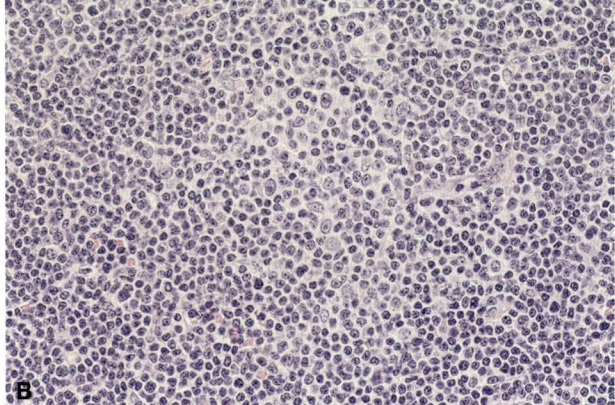

FIGURE 88.3 Lymph node: chronic lymphocytic leukemia/small lymphocytic lymphoma. A, Low magnification shows diffuse alteration of architecture, with pale areas corresponding to proliferation centers. B, A higher power of a proliferation center that is composed of intermediate-sized cells with small nucleoli that are surrounded by small round lymphocytes.

Immunophenotype

On immunophenotyping studies, CLL cells have weak surface Ig, which usually is IgM associated with IgD. Neoplastic lymphocytes coexpress the T-cell antigen CD5 with B-cell markers CD19, CD20 (weak), CD200, LEF1, and CD23. The tumor cells are negative for FMC7, CD10, SOX11, and cyclinD1. Phenotypically, SLL and CLL are identical. CD23 expression and FMC7, SOX11, and cyclinD1 negativity are helpful in the phenotypic separation of CLL/SLL from MCL, another CD5+ small B-cell neoplasm.

Genetics

FISH studies detect abnormalities of chromosomes 11, 12, 13, and 17 in almost two-thirds of patients with CLL/SLL. Molecular genetic studies divide CLL/SLL into two major groups based on the presence or absence of somatic mutation, which is now typically assessed by sequencing of the Ig heavy chain variable (IgVH) genes rather than by historical surrogates such as CD38 or ZAP20 expression. Mutation of IgVH genes correlates with the more favorable subgroup. *TP53* mutations are associated with poor prognosis and poor response to chemotherapy in CLL. The prognostic significance of the various molecular genetic abnormalities in CLL/SLL will be discussed at length in Chapter 89. Importantly, there are no genetic rearrangements that are diagnostic for CLL/SLL.

Lymphoplasmacytic Lymphoma
Background

Lymphoplasmacytic lymphomas (LPLs) are uncommon B-cell neoplasms composed of small lymphocytes, plasmacytoid lymphocytes, and plasma cells. These lymphomas often have marrow involvement and a leukemic phase. They are often associated with high levels of an IgM paraprotein (Waldenström macroglobulinemia). In at least 90% of cases, it is associated with mutations in the myeloid differentiation primary response gene 88 (*MYD88*).[59]

Morphology

In the lymph nodes and bone marrow, the cytologic features of LPL are similar. The infiltrate can be composed of varying proportions of small lymphocytes, plasmacytoid lymphocytes, and plasma cells. Dutcher bodies (cytoplasmic Ig inclusions that appear to be intranuclear) are common, as are reactive mast cells, and hemosiderin-laden macrophages. In lymph nodes, the infiltrate may spare the sinuses, and in bone marrow, aggregates may be paratrabecular.

Immunophenotype

Plasmacytoid lymphocytes and plasma cells contain abundant intracellular Ig, which usually is monotypic IgM without IgD. Rare cases express IgG or IgA.[60] Clonal plasma cells and lymphocytes can be identified in most cases. Lymphocytes express pan-B-cell markers CD19 and CD20 and are usually negative for CD5 and CD10, although exceptions occur. Plasma cells express CD138, CD38, and often retain expression of CD19 and CD45, unlike in myeloma.[61]

Genetics

MYD88 L265P mutations have been identified in at least 90% of cases of LPL. In addition to aiding in diagnosis, *MYD88* L265P may also have prognostic value and impact therapy selection.[62,63] Recurrent mutations in the C-X-C chemokine receptor type 4 gene, similar to those present in WHIM syndrome, have been identified in 30% to 40% of LPL cases.[62,63] Although the prognostic and diagnostic utility of this marker has yet to be fully elucidated, early studies suggest a role for predicting response to BTK inhibitors such as ibrutinib.[62,63]

Mantle Cell Lymphoma
Background

MCL is a B-cell lymphoma typically composed of small lymphocytes with irregular nuclear outlines that have a CD5+ and CD23− phenotype and overexpress cyclin D1. These lymphomas are usually widespread at diagnosis with generalized adenopathy and extensive bone marrow involvement. They may involve extranodal sites with one classic presentation being lymphomatous polyposis of the lower gastrointestinal tract. Presentation may be with a leukemic phase mimicking CLL.[64] Although historically considered to be a uniformly aggressive disease, a more indolent form characterized by non–nodal, leukemic disease, SOX11 negativity, and IGVH-mutated status is now recognized.[24,65-68]

Morphology

MCL is composed of small monomorphic lymphocytes with scant cytoplasm. MCLs usually have a diffuse growth pattern (*Figure 88.4A and B*) or surround reactive germinal centers in a mantle zone pattern. Extension of the lymphoma into the capsule and perinodal fat is common. The blastoid variant of MCL is characterized by nuclei with increased size, dispersed chromatin, small nucleoli, and frequent mitoses, and may mimic DLBCL or acute leukemia morphologically.

Immunophenotype

The neoplastic cell of MCL shares immunophenotypic features with normal mantle zone lymphocytes, including moderate amounts of surface IgM, usually with IgD. Neoplastic cells are generally CD5+ and CD10−, but a subset of MCLs has CD5− tumor cells, and rare cases may coexpress CD10 and CD5. MCLs usually mark with antibodies to pan-B-cell antigens (CD20, CD19, PAX5, CD79a). CD23 is negative or sometimes partially expressed, and FMC7 is positive in contrast to the tumor cells of CLL/SLL. Overexpression of cyclin

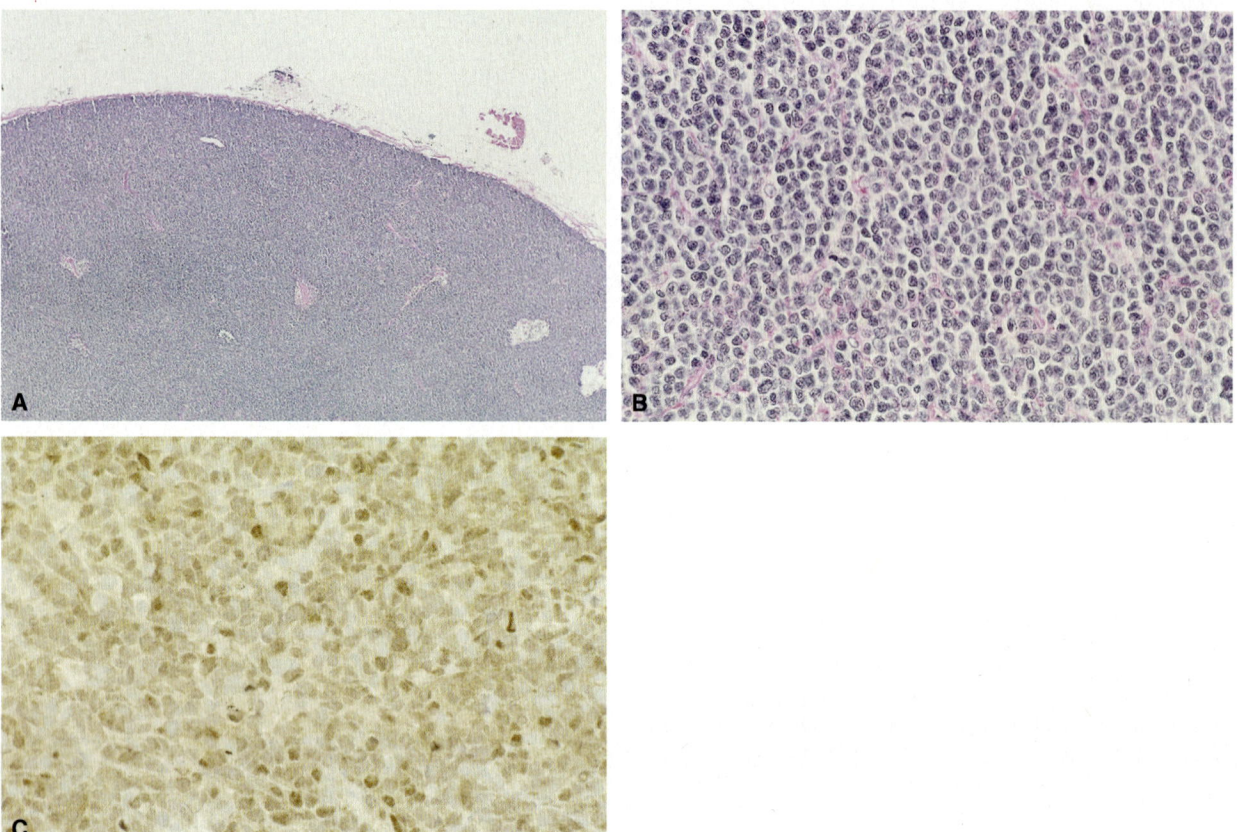

FIGURE 88.4 Lymph node: mantle cell lymphoma. A, Low magnification shows diffuse architectural effacement, which, on higher magnification in (B), is composed of sheets of small irregular lymphocytes with few large cells. C, Small lymphocytes exhibit nuclear staining for cyclin D1.

D1 is almost universal in MCL (*Figure 88.4C*). SOX11 is another specific marker for MCL, although a subset of cases may be negative.[69] MCL shows low intensity expression of CD200, and is most often LEF1-negative, both of which may aid in the distinction from CLL/SLL. High Ki-67 expression in MCL (>30%) is associated with a poor prognosis.[70,71]

Genetics

The prototypic abnormality in MCL is t(11;14)(q13;q32) involving the cyclinD1 gene (*CCND1*) and IGH. Rare cyclin D1-negative MCL exhibits a gene expression profile similar to cyclin D1-positive tumors including expression of SOX11.[72] These cases may show overexpression and translocations involving cyclin D2 or possibly in rare cases cyclin D3.[73] The specificity of these translocations, however, is uncertain. Almost one-third of patients with MCL have somatic mutation of their Ig heavy chain genes. The presence of somatic mutation is associated with nonnodal disease, lack of SOX11 expression, and a more indolent clinical course.[24,65-68]

TP53 mutations in MCL correlate with poor prognosis; assessing for *TP53* mutation status by molecular methods in MCL has become standard of care. As mentioned, there is a biologic subgroup of MCL with highly mutated IgVH genes which is associated with indolent, nonnodal disease. However, correlation with clinical findings and *TP53* status is warranted before assuming indolent behavior in MCL based on IgVH status.

In Situ Mantle Cell Neoplasia

As in FL, rare "in situ" MCLs, now termed in situ mantle cell neoplasia, have been recognized in which cyclin D1-positive cells fill unexpanded mantle zones without distortion of nodal architecture.[74] The clinical significance of this finding is uncertain, as not all of these patients will have overt MCL.

Nodal Marginal Zone Lymphoma
Background

Nodal marginal zone lymphomas (NMZLs) represent a rare, clinically and biologically heterogeneous entity. The diagnosis often rests on exclusion of other possible lymphomas, in particular, nodal involvement by splenic marginal zone lymphoma (SMZL) and extranodal marginal zone lymphoma.

NMZLs characteristically involve the interfollicular areas of lymph nodes and are composed predominantly of "monocytoid" small- and medium-sized lymphocytes of uniform size with distinct cell membranes that surround an abundant amount of pale cytoplasm. Nuclei are bland and oval to coffee bean in shape. In some cases, plasma cells are prominent. Admixed large lymphocytes are present, and mitotic activity is variable. Colonization of reactive follicles by the neoplastic cells may impart a nodular growth pattern and may make distinction from FL challenging.

A pediatric subtype of NMZL has been described, mainly in younger patients, in which the pattern of infiltration leads to a PTGC-like appearance.

Immunophenotype

Nodal marginal zone B-cell lymphomas express pan-B-cell antigens CD19, CD20, CD22, and CD79a and monotypic Ig (usually IgM without IgD). Most are BCL2 positive, and CD43 is variable. They are typically negative for CD5, CD10, BCL6, SOX11, LEF1, and cyclin D1. However, CD5 positive cases and BCL6 positive cases do occur, and may lead to misdiagnosis as another subtype of small BCL. More recently, immunohistochemical markers such as MNDA and IRTA1 have been shown to be expressed frequently in NMZL, and less often in FL.[75] These may aid in diagnosis, although neither are 100% sensitive or specific for MZL. Phenotypic features of the pediatric subtype are similar, although establishing light chain restriction and clonality becomes essential to exclude a reactive process in this setting.

Genetics

Although nonspecific, trisomy 3 is the most common cytogenetic abnormality associated with NMZL. Recently, sequencing to determine IGVH mutational status has revealed potential prognostic significance in this disease as well, with mutated cases having superior progression-free survival.[76] NGS studies have found mutations in *NOTCH2* commonly in NMZL, although the utility of this in diagnosis still remains uncertain.[77] As with the other small B-cell lymphomas, diagnosis continues to rely on morphologic and phenotypic features with data provided by genetics being supplemental but not independently diagnostic.

Splenic Marginal Zone B-cell Lymphoma

Background

SMZL is a rare disease accounting for approximately 1% of all lymphomas and approximately 20% of lymphoproliferative disorders in diagnostic splenectomy specimens. The main differential diagnosis within splenectomy specimens is with other, rare small B cell lymphomas of the spleen including hairy cell leukemia and others. As these entities are rare, the salient pathologic features useful in the differential diagnosis are summarized in *Table 88.4*. SMZL is a small B-cell lymphoma of the white pulp of the spleen that often involves the splenic hilar lymph nodes, bone marrow, and peripheral blood. The patients typically present with splenomegaly, B symptoms (fever, weight loss, and night sweats), abdominal pain, and cytopenias. A low level of monoclonal paraprotein can be detected in approximately one-half of the patients.

Morphology

The spleen is massively enlarged, weighing well over 1 kg in most cases. Microscopically, the most striking feature is a nodular infiltrate centered on the preexisting white pulp lymphoid follicles. The tumor has a biphasic pattern with an inner core of small lymphocytes and an outer margin of medium-sized lymphocytes. The inner central zone of small lymphocytes resembles normal mantle zone cells with scant cytoplasm and small irregular nuclei, clumped chromatin, and indistinct nucleoli. The lymphocytes occupying the marginal zone appear similar to normal splenic marginal zone lymphocytes. These have well-defined clear cytoplasm and round/oval nuclei with a more open chromatin pattern and indistinct nucleoli. Variable numbers of large lymphocytes with prominent nucleoli are also present in the marginal zone. Occasionally, plasmacytic differentiation within the marginal zone or in the center of the nodules can be observed. Bone marrow involvement is interstitial, rather than paratrabecular and frequently intrasinusoidal. Tumor cells in peripheral blood often have short villous projections.[80,81] This cytologic appearance is the reason why some cases of SMZL were previously called splenic lymphoma with villous lymphocytes. Transformation to large B-cell lymphoma occurs in as many as 15% of cases.

Immunophenotype

Neoplastic cells express pan-B-cell antigens CD19, CD20, CD22, and CD79a. They express surface Ig with monotypic IgM, with or without IgD. They are typically negative for CD5, CD10, BCL6, SOX11, LEF1, and cyclin D1. A variable number are positive for BCL2 protein. Unlike hairy cell leukemia, they are usually CD11c, CD103, and DBA.44 negative. The main challenge in the diagnosis of SMZL occurs when only a bone marrow specimen is available, as the morphologic and phenotypic features are nonspecific and overlap with other small BCLs.

Genetics

Allelic loss of 7q21 to 32 is seen in slightly less than one-half of patients.[82] Chromosomal translocations that are seen in other small B-cell lymphomas involving *CCND1*, *BCL2*, and *MALT1* are not present. NGS studies have identified mutations in *KLF2*, a member of the *KLF* family of zinc finger transcription factors, in 20% to 42% of SMZL, and in *NOTCH2* in 20% to 25% although again the diagnostic utility of these markers remains uncertain in the clinical setting.[83-86] *NOTCH2* mutations have been proposed as being prognostically relevant.[87] *KLF2* mutations may subdivide SMZL into two genetic groups: one with *KLF2* mutations, IGV1-2 rearrangements, and 7q deletion, and one without *KLF2* mutations, with higher rates of *MYD88* and *TP53* mutations.[86]

Extranodal Marginal Zone B-cell Lymphoma of Mucosa-Associated Lymphoid Tissue

Background

Extranodal marginal zone B-cell lymphoma or MALT lymphoma is the third most common type of NHL, accounting for 6% to 8% of all NHLs in the Western hemisphere. Although MALT lymphomas are clinically indolent, the disease is typically chronic, requiring long-term clinical surveillance and, often, repeated biopsies.

Most MALT lymphomas arise in mucosal sites devoid of organized lymphoid structures. Development of MALT lymphoma is often preceded by a chronic inflammatory process that leads to acquisition of lymphoid tissue.[88-98] This forms the background for the emergence of the lymphoma. The examples of chronic inflammatory processes that are associated with MALT lymphoma development are listed in *Table 88.5*.

The infectious process not only creates the microenvironment for development of the tumor but also the microenvironment necessary to sustain the tumor progression. Eradication of the infectious etiology has been shown to lead to remission in gastric, orbital, and cutaneous MALT lymphomas and is recognized as the first line of therapy, particularly for gastric MALT lymphoma.

Morphology

MALT lymphomas are cytologically low-grade lymphoid neoplasms and are thought to arise from the marginal zone B-cell compartment of the mucosal lymphoid follicles.[99] The cytologic features and the

Table 88.4. Differential Diagnosis of Splenic Small B Cell lymphomas

Lymphoma	Pattern in Spleen	Pattern in Bone Marrow	Useful Phenotypic Markers	Genetics
Splenic marginal zone lymphoma	White pulp nodules	Sinusoidal and interstitial	Negative for AnnexinA1, CD103, CD123	Del 7q *KLF2*, *NOTCH2*
Hairy cell leukemia	Diffuse red pulp Blood lakes	Interstitial	CD103+, CD11c+ CD25+, dim CyclinD1+, AnnexinA1+, CD123+	*BRAF* V600E
Splenic diffuse red pulp small B cell lymphoma[a]	Diffuse red pulp	Sinusoidal and interstitial	Usually negative for AnnexinA1, CD103, CD123	*BCOR*, *CCND3* mutations.[78,79]
Hairy cell leukemia variant[a]	Diffuse red pulp	Sinusoidal and interstitial	CD11c+, CD103+; Negative for CD25, CD123, CD200, AnnexinA1	*MAP2K1* mutations

[a]Considered provisional entities in the WHO (2017).

Table 88.5. Risk Factors for Extranodal Marginal Zone B-cell Lymphomas of Mucosa-Associated Lymphoid Tissue (MALT Lymphomas)

Site	Risk Factor
Stomach	*Helicobacter pylori*
Intestine	*Campylobacter jejuni*
Orbit	*Chlamydia psittaci*
Salivary gland	Hepatitis C virus, autoimmunity (Sjögren syndrome)
Thyroid	Autoimmunity (Hashimoto thyroiditis)
Skin	*Borrelia burgdorferi*

architecture of the tumor often mimic the features of normal mucosal organized lymphoid tissues such as intestinal Peyer patches. MALT lymphomas tend to remain localized at the site of origin for many years. When they disseminate, they tend to go to other mucosal sites, a phenomenon thought to be a result of homing programming. Transformation to large cell lymphoma occurs in a minority of cases.[100]

The lymphoma cells assume varied cytologic appearances. Characteristic are the centrocyte-like cells, small to medium-sized lymphocytes with irregular nuclei. Alternatively, the neoplastic cells may have a monocytoid appearance with abundant pale cytoplasm and distinct cell borders. The tumor cells also may resemble mature small lymphocytes. Scattered large cells are usually dispersed throughout the lymphoma. Variable numbers of plasma cells are frequently present, often adjacent to epithelium. In approximately one-third of cases, the plasma cells are part of the neoplastic clone and may show atypical features such as Dutcher bodies. Regardless of the neoplastic cells' appearance, they produce a diffuse infiltrate that invades epithelial structures, producing lymphoepithelial lesions (*Figure 88.5A* and *B*) and subsequent epithelial disruption.[101] Reactive lymphoid follicles are generally present, and the neoplastic lymphocytes may infiltrate and colonize them.[102]

Immunophenotype

MALT lymphomas express pan-B-cell antigens CD19, CD20, CD22, and CD79a. They are typically negative for CD5, CD10, BCL6, SOX11, LEF1, and cyclin D1. They may be CD43 positive. Newer markers such as MNDA and IRTA1 are frequently positive and may aid in distinguishing these from FL.[24]

MALT lymphomas express surface Ig, usually with monotypic IgM, although IgA and IgG positive cases also occur. Within cutaneous marginal zone lymphomas, two subsets have now been described: one with class-switched IgG expression (often IgG4) (~75%), and one with IgM expression (25%), with some morphologic differences noted between the two groups. While the IgM expressing cases show similar features to other MALT lymphomas, the class-switched cases may represent a distinct clinicopathologic subset characterized by frequent IgG4 expression, peripherally located plasma cells, more superficial dermal disease, and a Th2 cytokine profile.[103]

Genetics

The three major chromosomal translocations seen in MALT lymphomas are t(11;18)(q22;q21)/*BIRC3* (*API2*)::*MALT1*, t(14;18)(q32;q21)/*IGH*::*MALT1*, and t(1;14)(p22;q32)/*IGH*::*BCL10*.[100,104] Remarkably, these appear to promote lymphoma development by a common mechanism. This concordance results from the roles of both the adapter protein BCL10 and the caspase-like protein MALT1 in antigen receptor–mediated activation of nuclear factor kappa B (NF*k*B), a transcription factor that regulates the expression of genes involved in lymphocyte proliferation and survival.[105,106] t(11;18) identifies gastric MALT lymphomas that (1) present with advanced-stage disease, (2) do not respond to *Helicobacter pylori* eradication, and (3) are unlikely to transform to large cell lymphoma.[107,108] Importantly, MALT lymphomas do not carry t(11;14)(q13;q32)/*IGH*::*CCND1* or t(14;18)(q32;q21)/*IGH*::*BCL2* chromosomal abnormalities typical of MCL or FL, respectively.

Diffuse Large B-cell Lymphoma

DLBCLs are a morphologically, phenotypically, and genetically heterogeneous group of mature B-cell malignancies unified by the presence of large (nuclear size greater than the macrophage nuclei) neoplastic B-cells.[109] Comprising 30% to 40% of all lymphomas, they are the most common lymphoma type in the United States and Europe. A greater appreciation for their complexity has followed from recent clinical, pathologic, and biologic studies, so that the most recent WHO classification recognizes 17 subtypes of large B-cell lymphoma clinical entities.[24] The more common DLBCL entities are discussed below.

Diffuse Large B-cell Lymphoma, Not Otherwise Specified

DLBCL, not otherwise specified (NOS), occurs in all age groups, with an incidence that increases with age, and with a sight male predominance.[24,110] Though most DLBCL, NOS cases arise de novo, risk factors for DLBCL, NOS include immunosuppression and prior low-grade B-cell lymphoma. The most common presentation is as a bulky mass of lymph nodes, but up to 40% of cases arise in extranodal sites, including spleen or bone marrow. Staging bone marrows are involved in approximately 10% to 25% of cases. The pattern of bone marrow involvement may be concordant or discordant constituted by a lower grade lymphoma. The former is associated with an adverse outcome, while the prognostic significance of the latter remains controversial.[111,112]

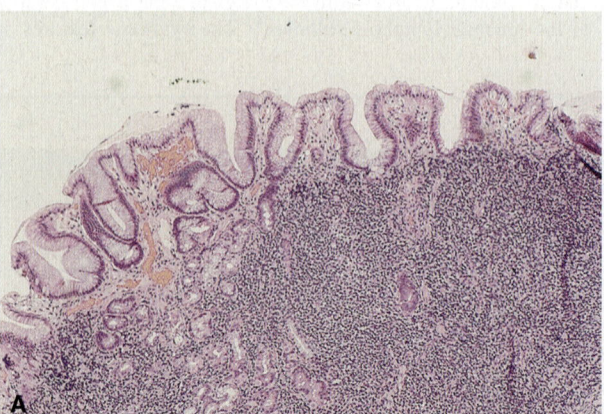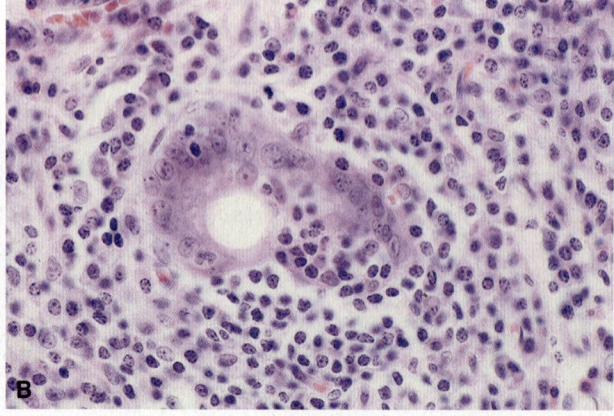

FIGURE 88.5 Stomach: extranodal marginal zone B-cell lymphoma of mucosa-associated lymphoid tissue. A, The submucosa contains a diffuse infiltrate of small lymphocytes. B, Centrocyte-like cells with moderate amounts of clear cytoplasm invade gastric glands, producing lymphoepithelial lesions.

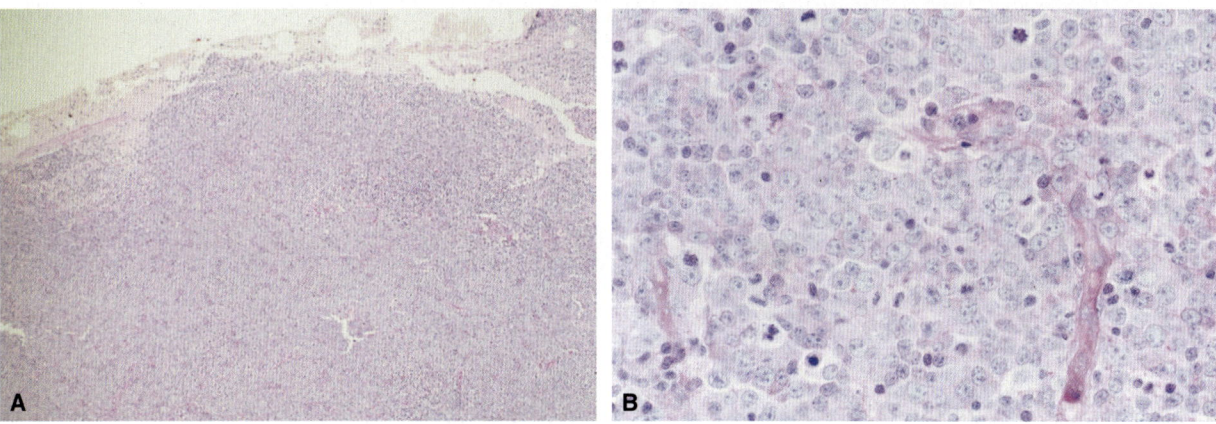

FIGURE 88.6 **Lymph node: diffuse large B-cell lymphoma.** A, On low magnification, a neoplastic large lymphocyte population diffusely effaces lymph node architecture. B, On high magnification, round nuclei, partially clumped chromatin, small nucleoli, and modest amounts of pale cytoplasm characterize the tumor cells. Note the apoptotic bodies and mitotic figures.

Morphology

Regardless of the anatomic site involved by DLBCL, NOS, the basic pathologic features are similar. The large neoplastic lymphoid cells grow in a purely diffuse pattern and efface the underlying tissue architecture (*Figure 88.6*). Tingible body macrophages, apoptotic bodies, mitotic figures, and zones of necrosis and/or fibrosis variably accompany the neoplastic cells. Traditionally, three cytologic variants have been recognized[24]: centroblastic, immunoblastic (*Figure 88.7*), and anaplastic. Rounded nuclei, dispersed chromatin, multiple small nucleoli, and modestly abundant basophilic cytoplasm characterize centroblastic DLBCL. These cells resemble the centroblasts of normal germinal centers. Round nuclei, with dispersed or marginated chromatin, prominent single centrally located nucleoli, and abundant cytoplasm usually eccentrically distributed relative to the nucleus are the cytologic features of immunoblastic DLBCL. A pleomorphic cell population that includes multinucleated tumor giant cells constitutes anaplastic DLBCL. Occasional DLBCLs have further cytologic diversity that includes signet ring cells, cells with multilobate nuclei, or spindle-shaped cells.

Immunophenotype

DLBCL cells express CD45 and a variety of pan-B-cell antigens, including CD19, CD20, CD22, CD79a, and PAX-5 in almost every case.[113] Ninety percent express light chain restricted surface Ig. Following rituximab (R) therapy, CD20 may be lost from the tumor cells,[114] in which case B-cell lineage is defined by expression of one or more of the other B-cell antigens. Variable subsets of DLBCL express CD10, BCL6, GCET1, LMO2, BCL2, IRF4 (MUM1), and FoxP1. The pattern of expression of these latter markers by immunohistochemistry variably correlates with germinal center (CD10, BCL6, GCET1, LMO2) or activated (IRF4 and FoxP1) B-cell derivation of the DLBCL as defined by gene expression profiling (GEP).[115] Germinal center B-cell (GCB)-type DLBCL is thought to have a better prognosis than activated B-cell (ABC)-type DLBCL, and so for practical purposes, several immunohistochemistry algorithms, Choi,[116] Hans,[117] Muris,[118] Nyman,[119] and Talley,[120] have been proposed by which GCB and ABC types are assigned (*Figure 88.8*).[121] Each has been shown to predict prognosis of R-CHOP-treated DLBCL patients in some, but not all studies. Subclassification of DLBCL as GCB or ABC type has also been shown useful for selecting optimal therapy, as certain agents such as bortezomib and ibrutinib preferentially benefit patients with DLBCL ABC-type. More recently, novel GEP technologies have been adapted to formalin-fixed paraffin-embedded tissue for ABC vs GCB typing in DLBCL, with demonstrated prognostic value.[122,123]

Coexpression of MYC and BCL2 by immunohistochemistry has been associated with an adverse prognosis, independent of the ABC or GCB type.[124-126] Although thresholds for positivity have been inconsistent in different studies, the recently revised WHO classification has suggested considering MYC/BCL2 coexpression when at least 40% of tumor cells are positive for MYC and 50% are positive for BCL2.[24]

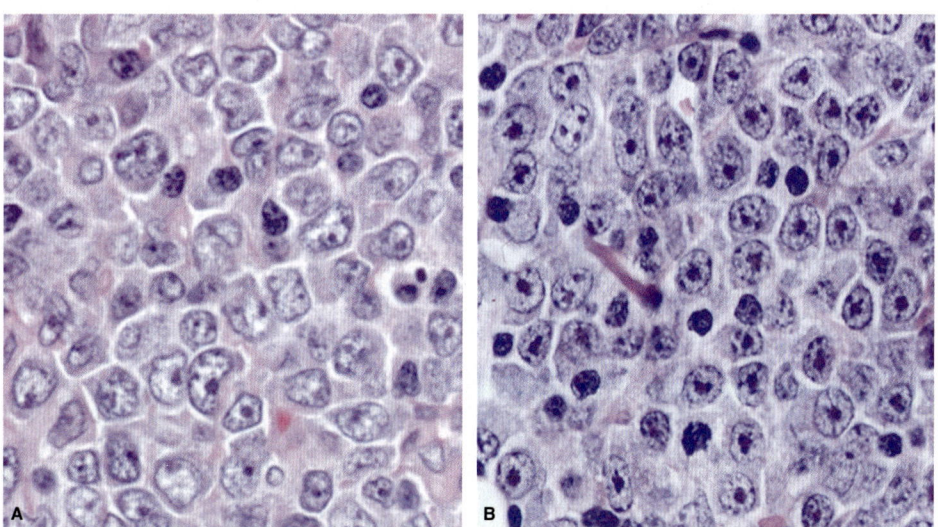

FIGURE 88.7 **Lymph node: cytologic variability in diffuse large B-cell lymphoma.** A, Centroblastic. B, Immunoblastic.

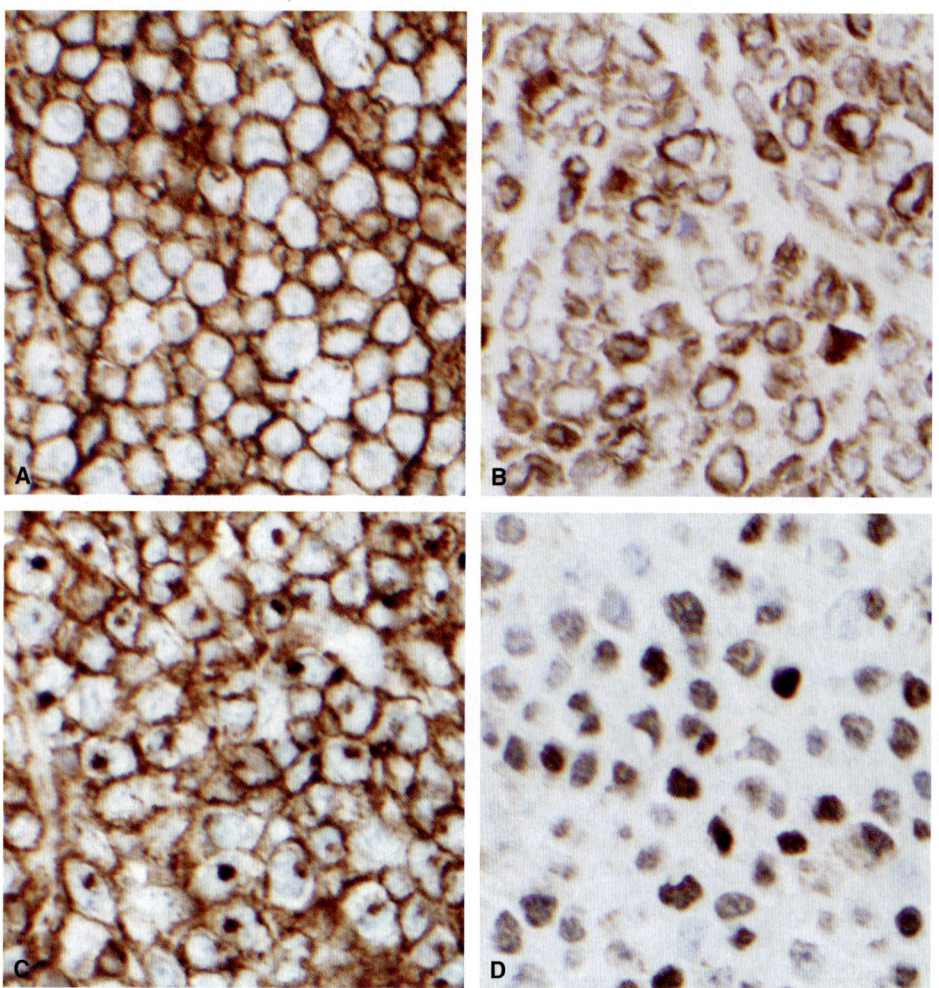

FIGURE 88.8 Lymph node: germinal center B-cell lymphoma phenotype. By the criteria of the Hans algorithm this DLBCL has a germinal center phenotype. Using immunohistochemistry on paraffin sections the neoplastic cells express: A, CD20. B, BCL2. C, CD10. D, BCL6. DLBCL, diffuse large B-cell lymphoma.

Of note, most DLBCLs with MYC and/or BCL2 overexpression do not have *MYC* or *BCL2* translocations (see Genetics section below).[127]

Approximately 5% of DLBCL cases express CD5.[128,129] These cases are distinguished from the blastoid variant of MCL because they are cyclin D1−. They tend to occur in older patients, are more frequent in women than in men, and tend to be disseminated at the time of diagnosis.[128,130] They are biologically distinct by genetic and GEP studies,[131,132] but are not recognized as a separate entity in the WHO classification.

Genetics

There is no single genetic abnormality that typifies DLBCL. Rather, a complex karyotype with genetic imbalances occurs in two-thirds of cases.[133] GCB type DLBCL commonly harbors a t(14;18); IGH::BCL2 (34%)[109]; and/or loss of *PTEN* (55%),[134] while ABC type DLBCL frequently bears *BCL6* translocations (62%),[135] *CDKN2A* deletion (30%),[136] and/or *BCL2* amplification (28%).[137] Recent advances in high-throughput methodologies have identified multiple gene mutations involving several signaling pathways. In particular, ABC-type DLBCLs are enriched for mutations in *PIM1*, *TNFAIP3*, *CD79A/B*, *CARD11*, *IRF4*, and *MYD88*, which are associated with activation of the B-cell receptor and toll-like receptor (TLR) signaling pathways resulting in NFkB activation. In contrast, GCB-type DLBCLs show frequent mutations of genes involved in epigenetic regulation, such as *MLL2*, *EZH2*, *CREBBP*, and *EP300*.[138,139] These and other recurrent genetic abnormalities and corresponding disrupted molecular pathways have been utilized to identify five or six distinct molecular subtypes of DLBCL of prognostic significance, best defined by multiplatform high-throughput genetic testing not yet readily applicable for routine diagnostics.[140-142]

High-Grade B-cell Lymphoma

A subset of large B-cell lymphomas (approximately 5%-10% of cases) show recurrent morphologic and/or cytogenetic characteristics that have been reproducibly associated with very poor response to standard rituximab, cyclophosphamide, doxorubicin, vincristine, prednisone (R-CHOP) therapy. These cases frequently have a blastoid appearance and intermediate cell size reminiscent of Burkitt lymphoma or lymphoblastic lymphoma. Cytogenetically, they often bear a *MYC* rearrangement in addition to a *BCL2* and/or *BCL6* rearrangement (high-grade B cell lymphoma with *MYC* and *BCL2* and/or *BCL6* rearrangements), for which they have been colloquially referred to as "double-hit" or "triple-hit" lymphomas. Most but not all cases show a germinal center phenotype with CD10 and/or BCL6 expression, and a high Ki-67 proliferation rate.[24,143-146] In the current WHO classification scheme, the category of high-grade B-cell lymphoma includes all "double-" and "triple-hit" large B-cell lymphomas (except for rare cases of FL and B lymphoblastic lymphoma), as well as cases termed "high-grade B cell lymphoma, not otherwise specified" (HGBCL-NOS), which have cytomorphology of medium sized, blastoid or Burkitt-like cells, but do not meet criteria for either Burkitt lymphoma or have double/triple-hit genetics.

Recognition of this heterogenous but consistently aggressive lymphoma subtype has led to widespread testing for double or triple-hit cytogenetics on all newly diagnosed large B-cell lymphomas by FISH, as the morphologic and immunophenotypic features of this genetically defined variant are often indistinguishable from DLBCL-NOS. In addition, careful evaluation of the morphologic and immunophenotypic features is required to adequately recognize high-grade B-cell lymphomas without double- or triple-hit cytogenetics (HGBCL-NOS), and to distinguish them for DLBCL-NOS, Burkitt lymphoma and B lymphoblastic leukemia/lymphoma. GEP by RNA sequencing might more accurately identify highly aggressive large B-cell lymphomas compared to routine morphology, immunohistochemistry, and FISH[147]; but the limited availability of this technology in diagnostic laboratories currently precludes its widespread implementation for disease classification.

T-cell/Histiocyte-Rich Large B-cell Lymphoma

The typical patient with THRLBCL presents with systemic symptoms and widespread disease involving lymph nodes and bone marrow with or without hepatosplenic involvement. THRLBCL occurs at a younger median age than DLBCL, NOS and has a decided male predominance.[24,148,149]

Morphology

In lymph nodes, a heterogeneous cell population diffusely effaces the architecture. Small lymphocytes and histiocytes in varying proportions dominate the histologic picture. In contrast, the neoplastic cells are in the minority and are singly distributed without clustering together or forming sheets. Centroblast-like, immunoblast-like, or pleomorphic cytologic features typify the neoplastic cells in most cases (*Figure 88.9*). Because the reactive elements dominate the histologic picture, the challenge in these cases is to recognize THRLBCL as lymphoma rather than a reactive process. In some cases, the neoplastic cells have characteristics similar to lymphocyte-predominant (LP) cells of nodular lymphocyte predominant Hodgkin lymphoma (NLPHL); in others, they resemble diagnostic RS cells of CHL. In these cases, the diagnostic challenge is to distinguish THRLBCL from HL. The phenotype of both the neoplastic cells and the reacting cell populations usually resolves the differential diagnostic problems.

Immunophenotype

The large neoplastic cells express CD45 and pan-B-cell antigens (CD19, CD20, CD22, and PAX5), are usually positive for BCL6, and variably express BCL2. They typically lack expression of classic Hodgkin cell–associated markers such as CD15 and CD30. The small background lymphocytes are CD3+ T cells and the histiocytes express CD68 and CD163. Virtually no small nonneoplastic CD20+ or IgD+ lymphocytes accompany the large cells and the lesions are usually devoid of both CD57/CD279 (PD-1) positive T cell rosettes surrounding the neoplastic B-cells and CD21+ follicular dendritic cell meshworks. These latter are immunoarchitectural features that may help to distinguish THRLBCL from NLPHL.[150]

Genetics

High-resolution karyotyping shows multiple non–specific genomic imbalances, including gains in 2p16.1, possibly associated with REL overexpression.[151] Copy gains or amplifications of PD-L1 and PD-L2 on 9p24.1 are encountered in approximately half of cases, resulting in overexpression of these ligands, which contribute to evasion of anti–tumor T-cell immunity.[152] As expected, these tumors have a gene expression profile enriched for a T cell/histiocytic host response.[153]

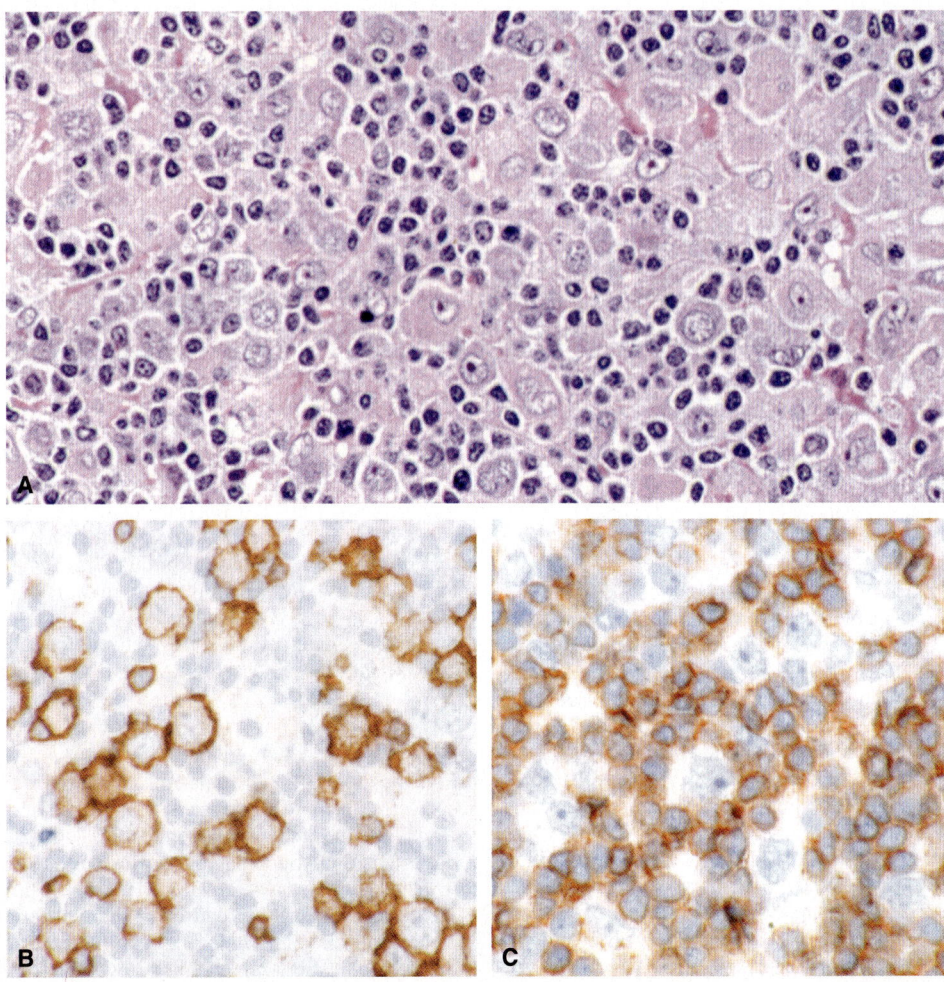

FIGURE 88.9 **Lymph node: T-cell/histiocyte-rich large B-cell lymphoma.** A, A mixture of small lymphocytes and histiocytes dominates the morphology. Occasional large neoplastic cells with rounded to lobulated nuclei, delicate chromatin, small nucleoli, and pale cytoplasm are present. Immunoperoxidase stains for (B) CD20 highlight the neoplastic cells and for (C) CD3 demonstrate staining in the nonneoplastic T-cells.

Primary Mediastinal (Thymic) Large B-cell Lymphoma

Primary mediastinal large B-cell lymphoma (PMBCL) is a biologically, clinically, and pathologically distinct lymphoma type thought to arise from a peculiar subset of intrathymic B-cells.[154] The tumor originates in the thymus and grows into a mediastinal mass that produces symptoms as it enlarges, infiltrates, and compresses local structures such as lung, pericardium, and superior vena cava. Women are affected more commonly than men and PMBCL typically occurs at a younger age (median, 35 years) than DLBCL, NOS.[154,155]

Morphology

A diffusely growing population of medium to large lymphoid cells effaces the architecture of the underlying thymus and infiltrates into adjacent anatomic sites. The tumor cells are variably accompanied by a richly vascular fibrous stroma that frequently circumscribes clusters of neoplastic cells. This can be a cause of diagnostic difficulty, because fibrosis itself and/or compression artifact introduced when biopsying a firm mass can obscure the tumor cells. PMBCL is cytologically characterized by case-to-case variability. Some examples are composed of cells resembling centroblasts; others contain a prominent population of immunoblast-like neoplastic cells. Cells with multilobated nuclei and varying amounts of clear cytoplasm or with features of RS or Hodgkin cells can constitute the neoplasm in some cases. This cytologic diversity is not of prognostic significance, but pathologists must appreciate it as part of the possible spectrum observed in PMBCL. A nonneoplastic population of T cells and histiocytes often accompanies and together with fibrosis can also potentially obscure the neoplastic cells. Finally, residual thymic Hassall corpuscles can be found in some cases.

Immunophenotype

The tumor cells express CD45, CD19, CD20, PAX5, and the transcription factors OCT2 and BOB1.[154] They are frequently positive for CD23,[156] BCL6, and IRF4 (MUM1), and either lack or show only variable immunoreactivity for CD30. They are typically negative for surface and cytoplasmic Ig and for CD15. Expression of CD23, MAL, PDL1, and PDL2 can be demonstrated in the majority of cases, unlike most cases of DLBCL-NOS. Stains for keratin highlight the residual thymic epithelial elements.

Genetics

PMBCL typically harbors translocations involving the major histocompatibility complex (MHC) class II transactivator *CIITA*, as well as gains in chromosomes 9p24[157] that include *JAK2*, *PDL1*, and *PDL2*.[158] These genetic lesions are only rarely seen in other types of DLBCL. Conversely, *BCL2* and *BCL6* translocations common in DLBCL are only rarely detected in PMBCL. Overexpression of PDL1 and PDL2 and downregulation of MHC class II molecules secondary to these chromosomal abnormalities are believed to inhibit T-cell activation in the tumor microenvironment, favoring immune escape of the malignant B-cells.

Other Considerations

In GEP studies, primary mediastinal large B cell lymphoma (PMLBCL) cases are more similar to cases of nodular sclerosis (NS) CHL than to DLBCL, NOS.[159-161] Both tumor types contain similar genetic abnormalities and have activation of the NF*k*B pathway, altered JAK/STAT signaling, and aberrant activation of the PI3K/AKT pathway. Thus, it is no surprise that morphologic and clinical overlap between PMBCL and nodular sclerosis classic Hodgkin lymphoma (NSHL) occurs. In most cases, sufficient sampling, careful microscopic observations, and application of immunohistochemical stains can readily distinguish these two from one another. However, in rare instances, PMBCL cannot be distinguished from NSHL. Recognition of this phenomenon has led the WHO to acknowledge a lymphoma category termed "*B-cell lymphoma, unclassifiable, with features intermediate between DLBCL and CHL*," or, colloquially, "gray zone lymphoma."[24,162] Cases in this provisional category appear to have a worse outcome than PMLBCL,[163] although the actual diagnostic criteria are incompletely defined. A diagnosis of "gray zone lymphoma" should be applied rarely and only for cases where an abundant tissue sample has been comprehensively evaluated by morphology and phenotype, and the distinction between PMBCL and CHL is still impossible.

Primary Diffuse Large B-cell Lymphoma of the Central Nervous System

This tumor is defined as a neoplasm of large B-cells exclusively involving the brain parenchyma, spinal cord, leptomeninges, or the eye (retina, vitreous, but not the soft tissues of the orbit).[24] Secondary brain involvement by systemic lymphoma, exclusive dural involvement, or a history of immunodeficiency/immunosuppression excludes the diagnosis of primary central nervous system lymphoma (PCNSL). The lymphomas may be unifocal (75%) or multifocal (25%) in the brain. Of patients who present with intraocular involvement, intraparenchymal brain involvement eventually develops in the majority, and about 20% of patients who present with intracerebral disease will develop intraocular involvement. Most patients with PCNSL are elderly. There is a slight male predominance.[164-166]

Morphology

PCNSLs preferentially involve perivascular spaces with varying degrees of infiltration into the brain parenchyma. The neoplastic cells usually have cytologic features of centroblasts or immunoblasts or a combination of both. Reactive astrocytes, activated microglial cells, and histiocytes complete the histologic picture. Preoperative corticosteroid therapy to reduce intracerebral edema prior to biopsy can cause intralesional necrosis or regression of the neoplasm. Sometimes tumor cell ghosts can be recognized within the necrotic areas suggesting the diagnosis, but in some cases, steroid therapy leaves behind only a mixture of small T-lymphocytes and histiocytes or sheets of foamy macrophages. Necrosis in a large B-cell lymphoma involving the central nervous system (CNS) is also relatively common in cases that are associated with EBV or with immunosuppression. Thus, necrotic areas in a large cell lymphoma involving the CNS should raise the question of prior corticosteroid therapy, underlying immunosuppression, or an association of the lesion with EBV, and the diagnosis/classification of the tumor adjusted accordingly.[24]

Immunophenotype

PCNSL cells are CD19+ and CD20+. They almost always express IRF4 and are positive for BCL6 in a substantial subset of the cases. Because they typically lack immunoreactivity for CD10 and are positive for IRF4, only a small subset of PCNSL have a GCB phenotype using the GCB vs non-GCB immunohistochemistry-based classifier algorithms.[167]

Genetics

Complex genomic imbalances are common in PCNSL cases, including frequent deletions of 9p21.3 (*CDKN2A/2B*) and 6q21 (human leukocyte antigen genes), in addition to loss of 6q21 (*PRDM1*) and 6q23(*TNFAIP3*).[168] *BCL6* translocations occur in 15% to 45% of cases with both IGH and non-Ig gene partners. Translocations involving *MYC* and *BCL2* are rare in this lymphoma type.[165,169] By NGS, PCNSL shows frequent mutations in *MYD88*, *CD79B*, *PIM1*, and *CARD11*.[168,170] Overall, the genetic alterations affect the B-cell receptor and TLR pathways, favoring activation of NF*k*B in a fashion similar to what has been described for ABC type DLBCL.

Epstein-Barr Virus–Positive Diffuse Large B-cell Lymphoma, Not Otherwise Specified

EBV-positive DLBCL was initially described in elderly patients exhibiting a more aggressive clinical behavior than EBV-negative cases.[171] More recently, EBV-positive DLBCL, NOS has also been documented in young patients with an overall survival similar to age-matched EBV negative DLBCL.[172,173] By definition, patients have no identifiable underlying cause for immunosuppression/immunodeficiency and the clinico-morphologic findings are not consistent with other specific EBV-positive large B-cell lymphoproliferations, such as lymphomatoid granulomatosis, mucocutaneous ulcer, primary effusion lymphoma, EBV-positive Burkitt lymphoma, EBV-positive CHL, or plasmablastic lymphoma. In elderly patients, it is presumed that age-related immune senescence allows latently infected EBV+ B-cells to escape from immune surveillance and proliferate to form these tumors. The physiopathology in younger patients is unknown. EBV-positive DLBCL, NOS increases in frequency with age, has a male predominance, and most frequently involves extranodal sites.[174,175]

Morphology
These tumors show a diffusely growing EBV-positive large B-cell population with varied cytomorphology that effaces the architecture of the underlying tissue.[176] Many cases are composed of a relatively monomorphic population of large lymphoid cells resembling centroblasts and immunoblasts with varying proportions of RS-like cells. The most abnormal-appearing neoplastic cells frequently surround areas of necrosis (*Figure 88.10A*). Other cases might resemble conventional DLBCL, NOS, THRLBCL and, less commonly, B-cell lymphoma unclassifiable with features intermediate between DLBCL and Hodgkin lymphoma (HL).

Immunophenotype
The neoplastic cells in EBV-positive DLBCL usually express CD45, CD19, CD20, PAX5, and IRF4 (*Figure 88.10B*). They typically exhibit an ABC phenotype and are often positive for CD30. The greater the number of neoplastic plasmacytoid and plasma cells contained in the tumor, the less frequently CD20 is expressed by the tumor and the more frequently IRF4+ and CD138+ cells constitute the tumor cell population. The ease with which light chain–restricted cytoplasmic Ig expression can be demonstrated also increases with increasing plasma cell differentiation in these tumors. By definition, the tumor cells are positive for EBV, most sensitively detected by in situ hybridization with probes that recognize EBV-encoded RNA (EBER) (*Figure 88.10C*). By immunohistochemistry, the neoplasms express EBV latent membrane protein (LMP)-1 in 94% of cases and Epstein-Barr nuclear antigen 2 in 28% of cases.[174]

Genetics
Insufficient numbers of cases have been studied to comment on recurring genetic abnormalities in these tumors.

Other Considerations
EBV-positive DLBCL has most recently been recognized as the most malignant end of a spectrum of EBV-related lymphoproliferative disorders occurring in adults. While it is outside the scope of this chapter to comment on the more benign entities, EBV reactivation with

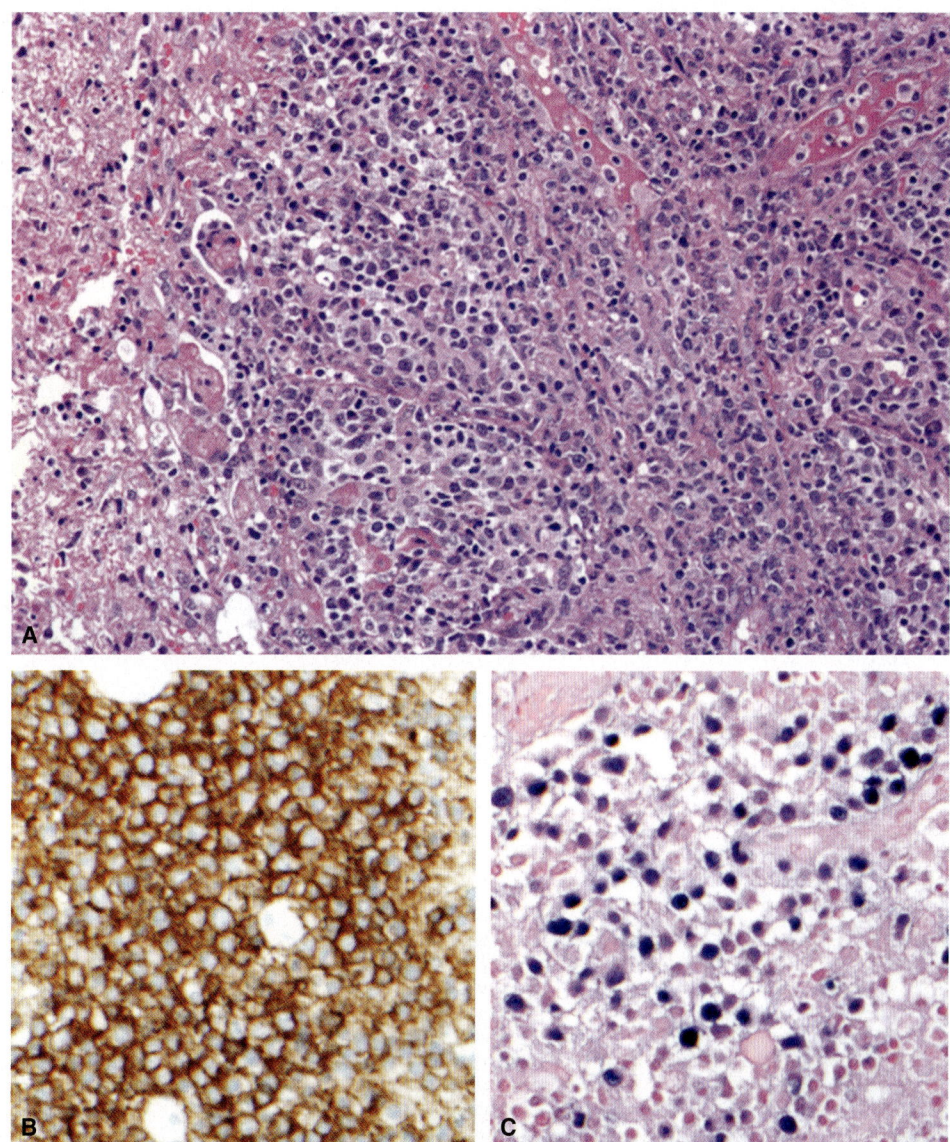

FIGURE 88.10 **Soft tissue: EBV-positive DLBCL.** A, The tumor diffusely effaces tissue architecture and is associated with necrosis (*left*). The neoplastic cells are medium size and large with hyperchromatic, irregular nuclei. They are positive for (B) CD20 by immunohistochemistry and for (C) EBER by in situ hybridization. DLBCL, diffuse large B-cell lymphoma; EBER, EBV-encoded RNA; EBV, Epstein-Barr virus.

reactive lymphoid hyperplasia, EBV-associated polymorphous extranodal lymphoproliferations (including mucocutaneous ulcer),[177] and polymorphous nodal EBV-associated lymphoproliferations all are within the differential diagnosis of EBV-positive DLBCL.[178] The differential diagnosis of EBV-related lesions in adults also includes posttransplant lymphoproliferative disorders and EBV-related lymphoproliferations that occur following immunomodulatory therapy for autoimmune diseases. They are morphologically and phenotypically similar to EBV-positive DLBCL. Except in the situation of pathologically and clinically overt DLBCL, consideration of the patient's history and following the clinical evolution of the lesion are important so that aggressive therapy is not prematurely instituted in EBV-associated lymphoproliferative disorders.

Rare Large B-cell Lymphoma Types

Some rare large B-cell lymphoma types have been described in the WHO classification[24] and are shown in *Table 88.6* and illustrated in *Figure 88.11*.

Burkitt Lymphoma

Burkitt lymphoma is a high-grade B-cell lymphoma composed of medium-sized, rapidly dividing lymphocytes. These lymphomas usually affect children and young adults and often present at extranodal sites. Less commonly, they have a leukemic phase. Three clinical forms are recognized: (1) endemic, which classically presents as jaw or facial masses in young boys in equatorial Africa; (2) sporadic, which may present at any age with frequent abdominal involvement; and (3) epidemic (immunodeficiency associated), such as in patients who are human immunodeficiency virus (HIV)–positive. All subtypes are characterized by chromosomal rearrangements involving the *MYC* oncogene that lead to its inappropriate expression in B-cells. The three forms have variable association with EBV infection, 100% in endemic Burkitt lymphomas, and 20% to 40% in sporadic and immunodeficiency-associated Burkitt lymphomas.[24,198-200]

Burkitt lymphomas typically have a diffuse growth pattern that is dominated on low magnification by the "starry sky" produced by tingible body macrophages (*Figure 88.12A*). Tumor cells may home into residual follicles and often have a cohesive appearance at the interface of tumor and soft tissue. Nuclear size is equivalent to that of endothelial cells or macrophages. The nuclei are round to oval with small nucleoli and a moderate amount of amphophilic cytoplasm. Mitoses are frequent (*Figure 88.12B*). On Wright-stained touch imprints, the neoplastic cells show remarkable nuclear homogeneity and the presence of characteristic vacuolated, basophilic cytoplasm.

Immunophenotypically, these lymphomas express pan-B-cell antigens, are CD10+ and BCL6+, and are negative for BCL2.[24] They have monotypic surface Ig (usually IgM) and are TdT−, indicating a mature B-cell phenotype. Ki-67/mib-1 staining shows greater than 95% of tumor cells are positive, which is consistent with a high growth fraction.

These tumors have reciprocal translocations involving the *MYC* oncogene mapped to chromosome 8q24, which is usually juxtaposed to the IGH gene on chromosome 14q32. The translocation less commonly involves the *K*-light chain (IGK; chromosome 2p12) or *λ*-light chain (IGL; chromosome 22q11) genes.[200] In endemic Burkitt lymphoma, the translocation breakpoints are located far upstream 5′ to *MYC* and in the joining region of IGH.[201] In the sporadic form, the breakpoints are immediately 5′ to *MYC* and in the switch region of IGH. In the immunodeficiency-associated cases, the breakpoints involve the first exon or intron of *MYC* and the switch region of IGH. Therefore, different mechanisms may generate the chromosomal breakpoints in the various forms of this lymphoma.[202]

Up to 20% of B-cell lymphomas with morphologic and immunophenotypic features of Burkitt lymphoma do not have a detectable *MYC* translocation. A minority of these cases have a specific chromosomal abnormality characterized by amplification or duplication of 11q23.2-23.3, and deletion of 11q23.1-ter.[203] These rare neoplasms are currently considered as a separate entity by the 2017 WHO classification as "Burkitt-like lymphoma with 11q aberration."[24] GEP may provide a more precise biologic definition of Burkitt lymphoma,[204,205] but this technique is not currently useful for daily clinical practice.

T-CELL AND NATURAL KILLER CELL LYMPHOMAS

T-cell and NK-cell lymphomas may be grouped together, because their normal counterparts apparently arise from a common progenitor cell that expresses CD3ε and is unable to develop into B cells.[206]

Table 88.6. Rare Large B-cell Lymphoma Types

Rare Large B-cell Lymphoma Type	Clinical Features	Morphology	Phenotype	Genetics
DLBCL associated with chronic inflammation[179-181]	• Elderly patients • M:F = 12:1 • Arises in sites associated with longstanding (>10 y) chronic inflammation (e.g., lung/pleura in tuberculosis patients or near prosthetic/chronically inflamed joints). • Most locally invasive and aggressive. A subset arise within fibrin deposits on pseudocysts or cardiovascular system and have an indolent behavior.	• Similar to DLBCL, NOS	• Most: CD19+, CD20+, PAX-5+ • Some: CD20−, IRF4+, CD138+ • Rare aberrant T-cell antigen expression • EBER+ almost all	• Complex clonal karyotype
Lymphomatoid granulomatosis[182,183]	• Predominantly adults • M:F = 2:1 • May be immunodeficiency related • Typically extranodal: lung (90%)-prototypic site, kidney, brain, liver, skin, others	• Angiocentric, angiodestructive lymphohistiocytic infiltrates associated with necrotic zones ("granulomatosis") • Varying proportion of large abnormal lymphocytes resembling centroblasts and immunoblasts and small lymphocytes	• Large lymphoid cells: CD19+, CD20±, EBER+ • Small lymphocytes: CD3+ T cells enriched in TIA-1 positive cytolytic lymphocytes	• Nondistinctive

(Continued)

Table 88.6. Rare Large B-cell Lymphoma Types (Continued)

Rare Large B-cell Lymphoma Type	Clinical Features	Morphology	Phenotype	Genetics
Intravascular large B-cell lymphoma[184,185]	• Predominantly adults • M:F = 1:1 • Protean clinical manifestations • Anatomic sites: disseminated, bone marrow, brain, lung, skin, kidney, others, but only rarely detectable in peripheral blood • Hemophagocytic syndrome (more common in Asian cases)	• Large neoplastic lymphoid cells resembling centroblasts or immunoblasts • Neoplastic cells confined to blood vessel lumens • Minimal or no extravascular infiltrates	• CD19+, CD20+ • CD5+ in 38%, CD10+ in 13%	• Insufficient studied cases
ALK-positive large B-cell lymphoma[186-188]	• Very rare • Predominantly adults, but described in children • M:F = 3:1 • Anatomic sites: lymph nodes most common, isolated cases reported in extranodal locations	• Preferentially involves lymph node sinuses • Cytologic features similar to immunoblasts/plasmablasts	• CD138+, IRF4+ • CD20− (most cases) • ALK+ (entity defining phenotype) • Cytoplasmic Ig light chain restriction and expression of IgH, usually IgA	• t(2; 17) (p23; q23); involves ALK and CLTC genes (most cases) • t(2; 5) (p23; q35) involves ALK and NPM genes • Other rare translocations/insertions involving ALK
Plasmablastic lymphoma[189,190]	• Predominantly adults • Male predominance • Underlying immunodeficiency in almost cases (HIV, immunomodulatory therapy for autoimmune diseases, organ transplant, immune senescence in elderly) • MUST exclude multiple myeloma in EBV negative cases • Anatomic sites: mostly extranodal (oral cavity, nasopharynx, orbit, skin, gastrointestinal, others)	• Diffuse sheets of cells with plasmablastic cytology (round nuclei, marginated chromatin, distinct central nucleoli, eccentrically distributed cytoplasm with a perinuclear hof) variably mixed with more "mature" plasma cells	• CD138+, CD38+, IRF4+ • CD20 and PAX-5- to minimally positive • Cytoplasmic Ig light chain restriction and expression of IgH, usually IgG • EBER+ (in most cases)	• Complex karyotype • MYC translocation usually with immunoglobulin genes in 50% of cases.
HHV8-positive DLBCL, NOS[191,192]	• HIV+ adults • Most commonly in the setting of HHV-8-associated multicentric Castleman disease • Severe immunodeficiency associated with asymmetric lymph node enlargement and/or splenomegaly • Also associated with concurrent Kaposi sarcoma	• Background of Castleman disease (regressively transformed germinal centers and interfollicular plasma cell sheets) • Progression from isolated immunoblast/plasmablast-like cells in follicular mantles (polyclonal) to aggregates of these cells (emergence of monoclonal proliferation) to sheets of overtly neoplastic large lymphoid cells that diffusely efface tissue architecture. Rare cases with disseminated disease at presentation.	• CD20±, CD138−, IRF4+ • Cytoplasmic Ig light chain restriction (almost always λ) and expression of IgH, almost always IgM • HHV-8+ (entity defining phenotype) • EBER−	• Insufficient studied cases
PEL[193-195]	• Epidemiology linked to cause for immunosuppression (found in almost all cases): young HIV+ males, solid organ transplant recipients, elderly patients with immune-related immunosenescence, often from Mediterranean countries with high HHV-8 prevalence • Pleural, pericardial, and abdominal cavities, minimal organ infiltration, rare lymph node or extranodal cases ("solid PEL")	• Immunoblastic/plasmablastic cytology, often with pleomorphic tumor giant cells and abundant apoptotic bodies in cytocentrifuge preparations or cell blocks made from involved fluids • Preferentially involve sinusoids in rare cases involving lymph nodes	• CD45+, CD19−, CD20−, CD79a− • Surface and cytoplasmic immunoglobulin negative • CD38+, CD138+, and IRF4+ • HHV-8+ (disease defining phenotype). • EBER+ (in most cases)	• Complex clonal karyotype
Primary cutaneous DLBCL, leg type.[196,197]	• Elderly patients • M:F = 1:3-4 • Most commonly in lower extremities. • Rapidly developing nodules or tumors.	• Diffuse monotonous sheets of large non–cleaved lymphoid cells with centroblastic or immunoblastic cytology.	• CD19+, CD20+. • Typically BCL6+, BCL2+, IRF4+, MYC+, and CD10−.	• Frequent translocations of BCL6 or MYC with IGH genes. MYD88 L265P mutation in 60% of cases.

Abbreviations: ALK, anaplastic lymphoma kinase; DLBCL, diffuse large B-cell lymphoma; EBER, Epstein-Barr virus-encoded RNA; HHV, human herpes virus; NK, natural killer; NOS, not otherwise specified; PEL, primary effusion lymphoma.

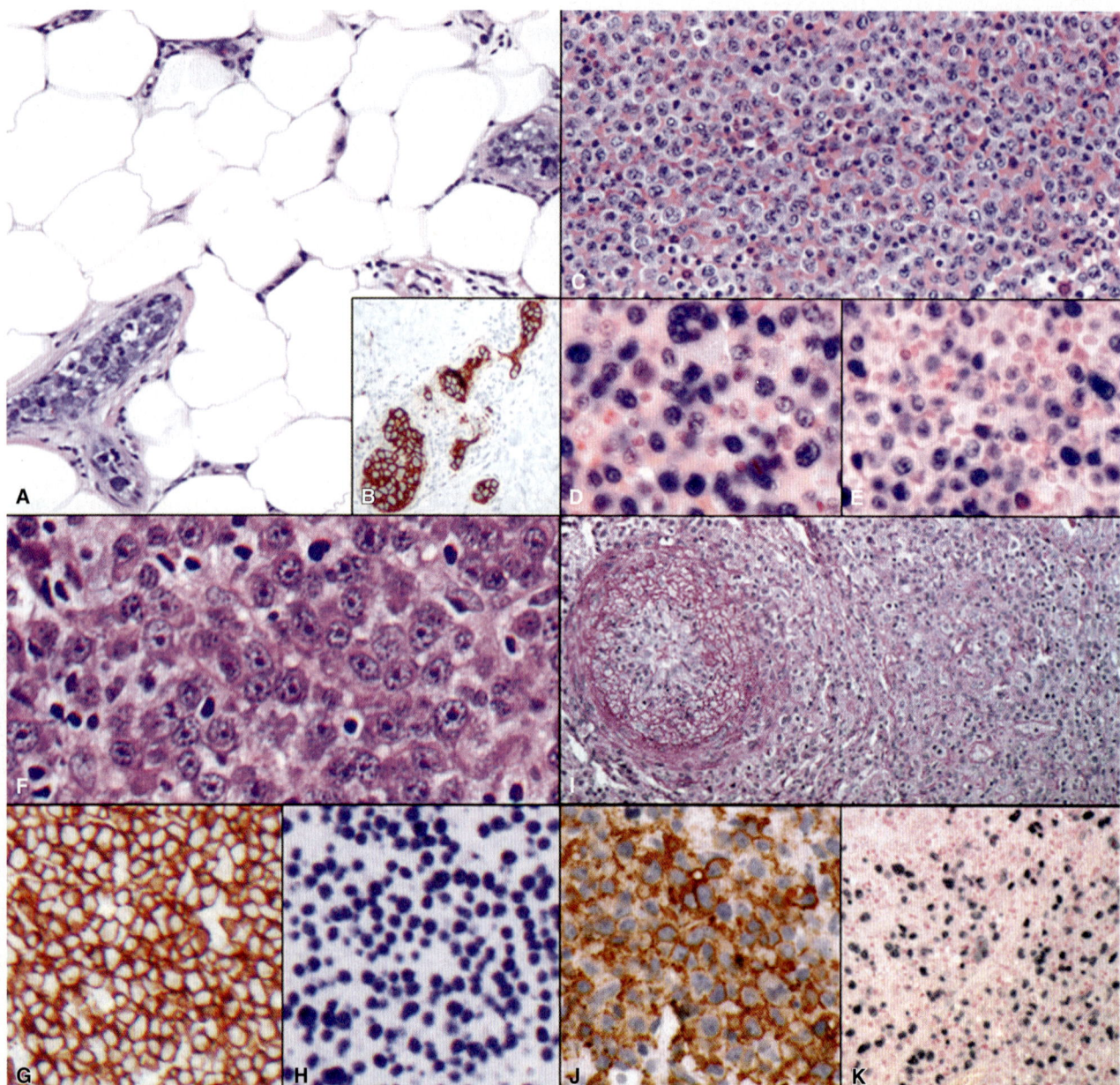

FIGURE 88.11 Various tissue sites: uncommon types of DLBCL. A and B, Intravascular large B-cell lymphoma. A, Large neoplastic cells fill vascular spaces in the subcutis and are positive for (B) CD20. C, D, and E, Primary effusion lymphoma. C, The cell block prepared from pleural fluid contains pleomorphic tumor cells characteristic for this entity. By in situ hybridization they are positive for (D) EBER and (E) HHV-8. F, G, and H, Plasmablastic lymphoma. F, Note the round nuclei, marginated chromatin, prominent nucleoli, and eccentric cytoplasm of the plasmablasts. They express (G) CD138 and are positive for (H) EBER. I, J and K, Lymphomatoid granulomatosis. I, In this periodic acid-Schiff-stained section, the angiocentric, angioinvasive growth pattern is highlighted. The tumor cells express (J) CD20 and are (K) EBER positive. DLBCL, diffuse large B-cell lymphoma; EBER, EBV-encoded RNA; HHV-8, human herpes virus-8.

Furthermore, some lymphomas from these two lymphoid lineages have considerable morphologic, immunologic, and clinical overlap. Overall, T and NK cell lymphomas are less common than B-cell malignancies, as they comprise approximately 10% of NHLs in the United States and Western Europe.[24]

The WHO classification divides T-cell and NK-cell neoplasms into precursor and mature categories.[24] The mature (peripheral) T-cell and NK-cell neoplasms are subdivided into those that are leukemic, cutaneous and extranodal, and nodal in origin. Most peripheral T-cell lymphomas (PTCLs) are postthymic malignancies that express T-cell receptor (TCR) α/β chains and are apparently derived from the adaptive (antigen-specific receptor-based) immune system (e.g., PTCL, NOS, angioimmunoblastic T-cell lymphoma [AITL], and systemic ALCL).[207] They generally arise in peripheral lymphoid organs from naïve, effector (regulatory [CD4+] and cytotoxic [CD8+]) or memory T cells.[208] NK-cell lymphomas and a small number of PTCLs that may be extrathymically derived are related to the innate (non–MHC-restricted) immune system.[207] The PTCLs in this group (e.g., hepatosplenic T-cell lymphoma [HSTCL], subcutaneous panniculitis-like T-cell lymphoma, and enteropathy-associated T-cell lymphoma [EATL]) tend to arise in mucosal or cutaneous sites, and often express TCR λ/δ chains, NK–cell-associated antigens, and cytotoxic granule–associated proteins, including granzyme M.[209-211]

Peripheral T- and NK-cell lymphomas are discussed in the following sections. T lymphoblastic leukemia (T-ALL) (Chapters 73, 74, and 76), T-cell prolymphocytic leukemia and T-cell large granular lymphocytic leukemia (Chapters 89 and 90), and mycosis fungoides (Chapter 94) are discussed elsewhere in this text.

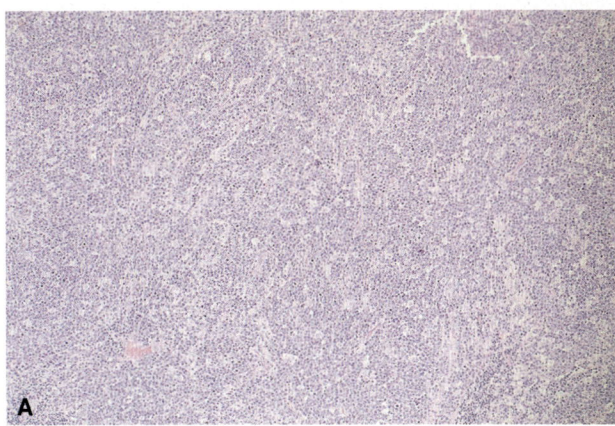
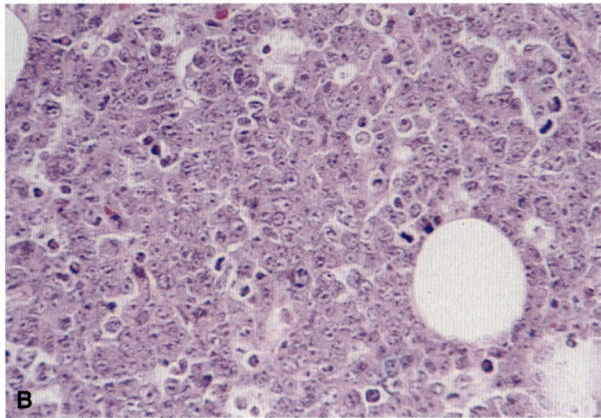

FIGURE 88.12 **Lymph node: Burkitt lymphoma.** A, The architecture is effaced by a diffuse infiltrate with a "starry sky" appearance. B, High magnification shows a monotonous population of small noncleaved lymphocytes with round to oval nuclei and variable cytoplasm. Mitotic figures are frequent. Numerous tingible body macrophages are present.

Peripheral T-cell Lymphoma, Not Otherwise Specified

Nearly one-third of PTCLs do not fit a distinctive type and are regarded as PTCL, NOS. These lymphomas are the most common nodal PTCL and are a heterogeneous category. They usually present in adults who have disseminated disease accompanied by B symptoms and poor performance status. There is generally a diffuse growth pattern, but rare cases may appear nodular.[209,212] A variety of the following morphologic features may also be seen: neoplastic lymphocytes of varying size that often have clear cytoplasm; large tumor cells that may have hyperlobated nuclei, may be multinucleate, or may resemble RS cells; frequent reactive epithelioid histiocytes; delicate connective tissue bands that segregate cells into clusters; and hypervascularity.[212] These lesions have diverse and often aberrant T-cell phenotypes.[213] Most express α/β TCRs and demonstrate TCR gene rearrangements.[214,215] Tumors with a cytotoxic lymphocyte phenotype or that are EBV+ appear to have a worse prognosis than other lymphomas in this category.[216,217] A recurrent t(5;9)(q31-q32;q22) chromosomal abnormality that fuses *ITK* to *SYK* has been identified in a very small number of PTCL, NOS that tend to have follicular involvement.[218] Rare cases of cytotoxic PTCL, NOS, with skin and bone marrow involvement, have a t(6;14)(p25;q11.2) that fuses *IRF4* to the TCR-alpha locus.[219] Otherwise, recurrent chromosomal translocations in PTCL, NOS have not been described. GEP has identified two major molecular subgroups PTCL-GATA3 and PTCL-TBX21, based on expression of *GATA3* or *TBX21(T-BET)*.[220,221] PTCL-GATA3 is associated with an inferior overall survival compared with PTCL-TBX21 subgroup. Loss of tumor suppressor gene *CDKN2A* has been shown a poor overall survival in the PTCL, NOS and PTCL-GATA3 subgroup.[222] An immunohistochemistry algorithm has been recently described to translate GEP classification to clinical practice using four commercially available antibodies specific for GATA3, CCR4, TBX21, and CXCR3.[223] The cutoff values for positivity are ≥20% for TBX21 or CXCR3 and ≥50% for GATA3 and CCR4. If the neoplastic T-cells express either TBX21 or CXCR3, it is classified as PTCL-TBX21 subtype. Cases with TBX21 and CXCR3 expression below the cutoffs, but with either GATA3 and CCR4 expression, are classified as PTCL-GATA3 subtype. This immunohistochemistry algorithm has been shown to reproduce the gene expression results in 85% of cases and has only variably been adopted into routine practice.

Lymphoepithelioid Lymphoma

Lymphoepithelioid (Lennert) lymphoma[224,225] is considered a specific morphologic variant among PTCL, NOS in the WHO classification.[226] The most striking histologic feature is the numerous clusters of epithelioid histiocytes that are relatively evenly dispersed throughout tissues obliterated by a lymphomatous infiltrate composed primarily of small neoplastic T cells. This moderately aggressive lymphoma must be distinguished from some cases of HL, B-cell lymphomas, and other PTCLs that are also accompanied by a high content of epithelioid histiocytes.[227-230] Misinterpretation as a reactive process may occur when attention is focused on the histiocytes rather than on the lymphoid infiltrate that destroys tissue architecture. When localized, Lennert lymphoma tends to involve the head and neck region, particularly cervical lymph nodes and sometimes the Waldeyer ring.

Angioimmunoblastic T-cell Lymphoma

AITL, the second most common nodal PTCL (approximately 20%), was first described in the 1970s as a clinical syndrome characterized by generalized lymphadenopathy, hepatosplenomegaly, anemia, and hypergammaglobulinemia.[231,232] The lymph node histology showed a number of distinctive features, including partial effacement of the architecture by a polymorphic inflammatory cell infiltrate, including large lymphocytes (immunoblasts), and marked vascular proliferation. Based on these histologic appearances, the disease was called a variety of terms, including immunoblastic lymphadenopathy, lymphogranulomatosis X, and angioimmunoblastic lymphadenopathy with dysproteinemia. Once the presence of clonal T-cell populations was established, the disease was renamed angioimmunoblastic T cell lymphoma.

Morphology

AITL is characterized by partial effacement of the lymph node architecture by a polymorphic inflammatory cell infiltrate predominantly within the paracortical areas (*Figure 88.13A*). In the original descriptions of AITL, absence of hyperplastic B-cell follicles was considered to be a characteristic feature. It is now recognized that the architectural changes in AITL fall into three overlapping patterns.[233,234] In pattern I (15% of the cases), there is partial preservation of the lymph node architecture. Hyperplastic B-cell follicles with poorly developed mantle zones and ill-defined borders are easily identifiable in the cortex of the lymph node. These merge into the expanded paracortex, containing a polymorphic infiltrate of small lymphocytes, immunoblasts, plasma cells, macrophages, and eosinophils within a prominent vascular network. Pattern II (25% of the cases) is characterized by loss of normal architecture except for the presence of occasional depleted follicles with concentrically arranged follicular dendritic cells. In some cases, follicular dendritic cell proliferation extending beyond the follicles can be identified. The rest of the lymph node shows a polymorphic inflammatory cell infiltrate with increased numbers of immunoblasts and vascular proliferation similar to that described for pattern I. In pattern III (60% of the cases), the normal architecture is completely effaced and no B-cell follicles can be identified. Prominent irregular proliferation of follicular dendritic cells can be seen in hematoxylin and eosin (H&E)–stained sections in some cases, and this is

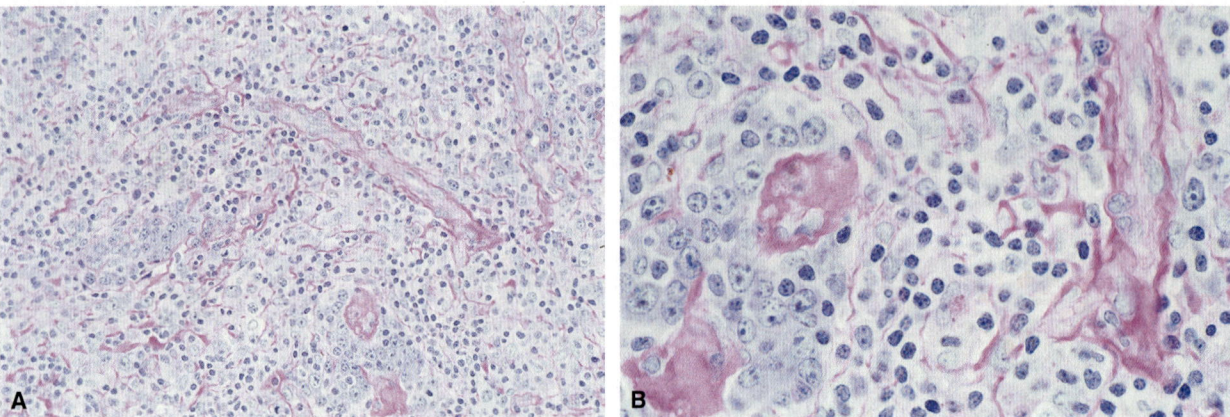

FIGURE 88.13 Lymph node: angioimmunoblastic T-cell lymphoma. A, There is a diffuse lymphoproliferation that is associated with prominent periodic acid-Schiff-staining blood vessels. B, Perivascular clusters of "clear cell" immunoblasts *(left)* are admixed with small lymphocytes and periodic acid-Schiff-staining blood vessels.

accompanied by extensive vascular proliferation and a polymorphic inflammatory cell infiltrate similar to that seen in patterns I and II. Approximately one-half of the cases contain perivascular collections of atypical medium-large lymphoid cells with clear or pale cytoplasm (*Figure 88.13B*), whereas cytologic features of malignancy may not be apparent in other cases. In a few instances where consecutive biopsies from the same patient have been reviewed, there appears to be a transition from pattern 1 to pattern 3 as the tumor progresses. This suggests that pattern 3 cases represent advanced disease.[233]

Although generalized lymphadenopathy is the main presenting sign, many of the patients have evidence of extranodal involvement at the time of diagnosis. The most frequently involved extranodal sites include the bone marrow, spleen, skin, and lungs. The histologic appearances in these sites are usually nonspecific but mimic some of the features described in the lymph node including increased vascularity and a polymorphic inflammatory cell infiltrate.[235-237] Cytologic features of malignancy can rarely be identified and tumor involvement can be shown only by immunohistochemistry and molecular clonality analysis. Therefore, the initial diagnosis of AITL rests on histologic examination of the lymph node.

Immunophenotype

Immunohistochemistry shows the expansion of the interfollicular areas by a diffuse infiltrate of CD3+ T cells. In most cases, CD4+ T cells dominate, but there is usually an intermixed population of CD8+ cells. B-cell markers CD20 and CD79a highlight the residual follicle center and mantle zone B-cells as well as many of the immunoblasts in the interfollicular areas. In some instances, these can be numerous, mimicking a large B-cell lymphoma or classic HL, though they are typically polytypic for Ig light chain expression. One of the most important immunophenotypic features in AITL is the expansion of the follicular dendritic cell meshwork that typically surrounds the paracortical small vessels. Although this is sometimes visible on H&E-stained sections, it is best demonstrated by staining for follicular dendritic cell markers such as CD21.[238,239]

The neoplastic cells of AITL express a number of T follicular helper (T_{FH}) cell markers, including BCL6, CD10, CD279 (PD-1), CXCL13, and ICOS, which can be utilized to differentiate AITL from other PTCLs, and is helpful for extranodal dissemination.[233,238,240-248] Though the number and degree of T_{FH} marker expression are variable among cases, the neoplastic T-cells are typically positive for at least two T_{FH} markers. Among them, CD279 and ICOS are the most sensitive markers, whereas CD10 and CXCL13 are the most specific markers. Initially, the tumor cells account for only a small fraction of the whole infiltrate (pattern 1). The cells are intimately related to the residual reactive B-cell follicles and the expanded follicular dendritic cell meshwork, some being located within the follicle centers and others surrounding the follicles. As the tumor progresses (patterns 2 and 3) the neoplastic cells spill into the interfollicular area but retain the intimate association with the follicular dendritic cell meshwork. This suggests that the follicular dendritic cell microenvironment may be important in tumor growth. Interestingly, follicular dendritic cells also express CXCL13, a chemokine critical for B-cell entry into follicle centers.

The majority of AITLs contain increased numbers of EBV-infected cells with immunoblastic or RS cell-like morphology. Double immunolabeling suggests that these are B-cells. Other lymphomas, particularly EBV-positive B-cell lymphomas, can occur with AITL metachronously or synchronously.[249,250]

Genetics

The overwhelming evidence indicates that there is a monoclonal T-cell population in the vast majority of AITLs. Interestingly, the presence of a B-cell clone can also be demonstrated in a subset of cases.[232] Such clones are thought to be expanded EBV-infected B-cell clones possibly secondary to underlying immunodeficiency/immune activation.

GEP has shown contributions by nonneoplastic elements as well as by the tumor cells. There is overexpression of B-cell–related and follicular dendritic cell–related genes and of genes related to the extracellular matrix and vasculature.[246] The tumor cell signature has overexpression of T_{FH} cell–associated genes.[246] *RHOA* G17V mutations occur in approximately 70% of AITLs and appear to be disease specific, whereas *TET2*, *DNMT3A*, and *IDH2* mutations, also common in AITL, are not disease specific.[221,251] However, recent study has showed chromosome 5 gain co-occurring with chromosome 21 gain and *IDH2*^{R172} mutation are specifically associated with AITL.[222] A missense mutation in *CD28* T195P occurs in approximately 10% of AITLs but appears highly specific.[252]

Other Nodal Lymphomas of T_{FH} Origin

The WHO 2017 introduced the concept of nodal T-cell lymphomas of T_{FH} phenotype to include not only AITL, but also other nodal T-cell lymphomas that express at least two T_{FH} markers and that were included previously among PTCL, NOS. These include follicular T-cell lymphoma and nodal PTCL with T-FH phenotype.[24]

Follicular T-cell lymphoma is rare and is characterized by intrafollicular or perifollicular aggregates of T cells with clear cytoplasm that have a follicular T_{FH} cell phenotype.[241] The resulting expansion of the lymphoid follicles may mimic FL or, sometimes, NLPHL. A t(5;9) (q31-q32;q22) is present in some cases.[218] Follicular T-cell lymphoma may progress morphologically to AITL in serial biopsies suggesting these lymphomas are a spectrum of a single biologic process.

Nodal PTCL of T_{FH} phenotype is essentially PTCL-NOS that expresses at least two, but ideally three T-FH markers. The characteristic histopathologic feature is an interfollicular growth of primarily small neoplastic T cells with clear cytoplasm. AITL-like features discussed above may be present, but are, by definition not well developed enough for a diagnosis of AITL.

Anaplastic Large Cell Lymphoma

ALCL, the third most common nodal PTCL (approximately 10%), is characterized by an infiltrate of pleomorphic large lymphocytes that express strong CD30, a T-cell activation–associated antigen.[253,254] As defined by the WHO classification, ALCL comprises three different clinicopathologic entities sharing similar morphology and immunophenotype but showing distinct clinical features. These are (1) systemic ALCL, ALK-positive[255]; (2) systemic ALCL, ALK-negative[256]; and (3) cutaneous ALCL, which is grouped among cases classified as "*primary cutaneous CD30-positive T-cell lymphoproliferative disorders.*"[257] Breast implant–associated ALCL is considered a provisional entity by the WHO classification.[258]

Anaplastic Lymphoma Kinase-Positive Anaplastic Large Cell Lymphoma

Systemic ALCL, ALK-positive is a moderately aggressive tumor that generally presents in young patients.[259,260] The lymphoma preferentially infiltrates nodal sinuses (*Figure 88.14A*) and extends into the paracortical region, often sparing secondary lymphoid follicles. The neoplastic large cells seem cohesive and usually have great variability in nuclear appearance, including some that are horseshoe- or doughnut shaped ("hallmark" cells) (*Figure 88.14B*) or are multinucleate with a resemblance to RS cells of HL.[261] Some have more monomorphous large cell cytology resembling centroblasts.[259] These features of the tumor cells are characteristic of the common variant of ALCL which accounts for 70% of cases. The common variant of ALCL may be misdiagnosed as metastatic carcinoma or histiocytic sarcoma because of the pleomorphic cytologic features of the tumor cells.[253,254] Small cell and lymphohistiocytic variants have been described, each comprising approximately 10% of ALCL.[262,263] The latter two variants may be misdiagnosed as an inflammatory process.

The tumor cells in ALCL are always CD30+, may express pan-T-cell antigens such as CD2 and CD3 and, frequently, cytotoxic granule–associated proteins.[210,264] Most cases express ALK oncoprotein, most frequently due to a t(2;5)(p23;q35.1) chromosomal abnormality.[265,266] This translocation fuses the *ALK* gene on chromosome 2 and the nucleophosmin (*NPM1*) gene on chromosome 5.[267] The fusion protein can be detected with a cytoplasmic and nuclear ALK staining pattern by immunohistochemistry.[268] Approximately 70% to 80% of ALK-positive ALCL have cytoplasmic and nuclear staining, whereas the remainder have cytoplasmic staining only, indicating variant translocations involving *ALK* and partner genes other than *NPM1*.[269-277]

Anaplastic Lymphoma Kinase–Negative Anaplastic Large Cell Lymphoma

Systemic ALCLs lacking ALK expression are morphologically and immunophenotypically very similar to ALK-positive ALCLs but they lack genetic abnormalities involving *ALK* and ALK protein expression. ALK-negative ALCLs also appear genetically distinct from ALK-positive ALCLs by comparative genomic hybridization and microarray GEP.[278-280] Furthermore, the patients are typically older and often have a worse prognosis compared to those with ALK-positive ALCLs.[281,282]

However, ALK-negative ALCLs are genetically heterogeneous, which affects patient outcome.[283] Approximately 30% of patients with ALK-negative ALCLs have a *DUSP22(IRF4)* rearrangement at 6p25.3, and they tend to have a prognosis similar to patients with ALK-positive ALCLs. *DUSP22*-rearranged ALCLs tend to have more doughnut cells and less pleomorphic cells than other ALK-negative ALCLs.[284] Approximately 8% of patients with ALK-negative ALCLs have a *TP63* rearrangement at 3q28, which has conferred a very poor prognosis. Patients with ALCLs that lack rearrangements of *ALK, DUSP22,* and *TP63* (triple-negative ALCLs) have a prognosis intermediate between those with ALK-negative ALCLs that have a *DUSP22* or a *TP63* rearrangement, a 5-year overall survival akin to that historically observed for ALK-negative ALCLs as a whole.

Primary Cutaneous Anaplastic Large Cell Lymphoma

Primary cutaneous ALCL is one end of the spectrum of primary cutaneous CD30-positive T-cell lymphoproliferative disorders. It typically occurs in adults who have localized disease at the time of diagnosis.[257] This form of ALCL is often indolent and may be an extension of lymphomatoid papulosis (LyP) type A or type C. The tumor cells generally resemble those of the common variant of primary systemic ALCL and express T-cell antigens. Primary cutaneous ALCL is usually epithelial membrane antigen negative and lacks t(2;5) and ALK expression, suggesting it has a different pathogenetic mechanism than that of primary systemic ALK-positive ALCL.[265] Approximately 20% of primary cutaneous ALCLs have *DUSP22 (IRF4)* translocations, an abnormality occasionally seen in LyP.[285]

Breast Implant–Associated Anaplastic Large Cell Lymphoma

ALCLs have been reported in seroma fluid or in capsules associated with silicone or saline breast implants.[286-288] The absolute risk of developing ALCL adjacent to breast implants is exceedingly low, and the tumors show little propensity for producing solid tumors or systemic disease despite being consistently ALK negative. This clonal

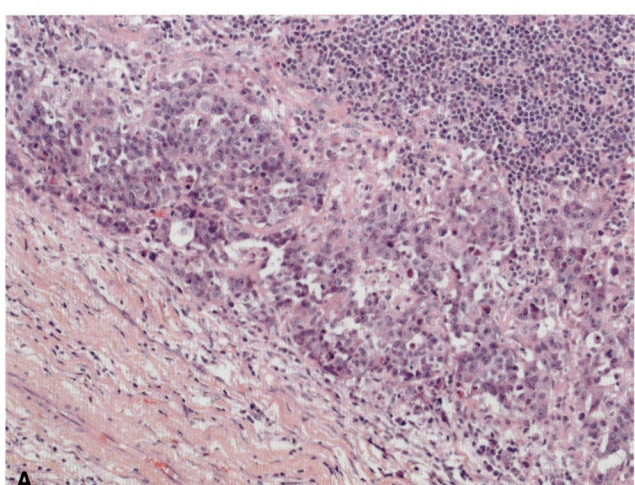
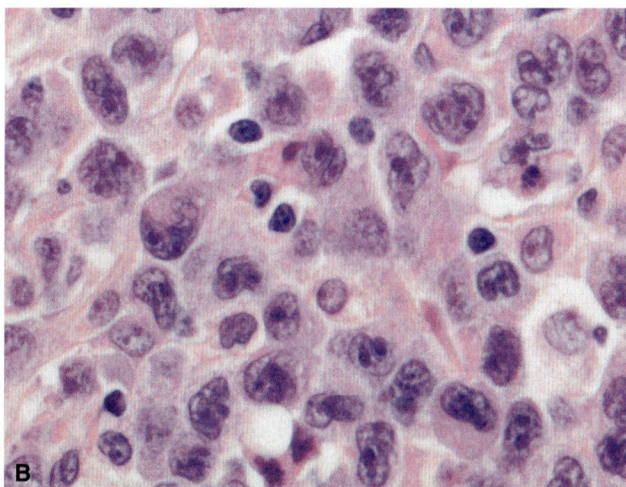

FIGURE 88.14 Lymph node: anaplastic large cell lymphoma. A, Tumor cell infiltrates with a cohesive appearance fill the sinuses, mimicking a metastatic carcinoma. B, The lymphoma is composed of pleomorphic large lymphocytes, some of which have the horseshoe- or bean-shaped nuclei that are characteristic of "hallmark" cells of anaplastic large cell lymphoma.

proliferation has an indolent clinical behavior when confined to the seroma and capsule; removal of the capsule may produce disease resolution. Patients who present with a breast mass or who have nodal involvement likely require systemic therapy. The morphologic and immunophenotypic features of breast implant–associated ALCL are similar to those of systemic ALK-negative ALCL. It shows activation of the JAK-STAT3 signaling pathway and is consistently negative for rearrangements of *ALK*, *DUSP22*, and *TP63*.[289]

Adult T-cell Leukemia/Lymphoma

Adult T-cell leukemia/lymphoma (ATLL) is a peripheral T-cell neoplasm caused by human T cell lymphotropic virus (HTLV)-1, and it is most prevalent where the retrovirus is endemic (southwestern Japan, central Africa, and the Caribbean basin). However, the incidence of the disease appears to be increasing in nonendemic areas due to spreading by carriers of the virus.[290] There is a long latency period for HTLV-1, and the lifetime risk of developing ATLL is <5% among those infected. ATLL occurs in adults and has four clinical subtypes: acute, chronic, lymphomatous, and smoldering.[291,292] Bone marrow infiltrates are interstitial or diffuse and may be less impressive than the degree of peripheral blood involvement. Circulating tumor cells have hyperlobate nuclei, sometimes with a cloverleaf shape. Lymph nodes are generally effaced by a diffuse infiltrate of pleomorphic lymphocytes of variable size, an appearance that may be difficult to distinguish from some PTCL, NOS by morphology alone. Cutaneous infiltrates may be difficult to distinguish from mycosis fungoides, because ATLL can have epidermotropism with formation of Pautrier microabscesses.[290] The neoplastic cells express T-cell antigens but often lack CD7. Most cases are CD4+, express the activation marker CD25 (interleukin-2 receptor), and are positive for FoxP3, a phenotype characteristic of regulatory T cells.[293] ATLL exhibits clonal TCR gene rearrangements and clonal integration of HTLV-1 genomes.[291] The virally encoded protein, Tax, activates numerous transcription factors and represses cell cycle–active proteins, resulting in persistent clonal proliferation of virally infected cells.

Hepatosplenic T-cell Lymphoma

HSTCL, a rare extranodal lymphoma comprising <1% of NHLs, probably arises from the cytotoxic γ/δ and α/β T cells of the splenic red pulp.[294] Despite the few descriptions of HSTCLs,[295-297] a fairly typical clinicopathologic picture has emerged for these neoplasms. Most cases involve young, adult men who present with B symptoms, massive hepatosplenomegaly, no lymphadenopathy, moderate anemia, and marked thrombocytopenia. Approximately 20% of HSTCLs arise in the setting of prolonged antigenic stimulation or chronic immunosuppression, such as following solid organ transplantation or treatment of inflammatory bowel disease.[297,298] The disease is aggressive, and most patients die within 2 years, even if a remission is achieved initially with therapy.

This lymphoma preferentially infiltrates the cords and sinuses of the splenic red pulp, hepatic sinusoids, and bone marrow sinuses. A leukemic phase may develop as the disease progresses. Tumor cells are generally small to intermediate in size, but some cases may have a predominance of large cells. There are condensed chromatin, indistinct nucleoli, and scant eosinophilic cytoplasm. Circulating tumor cells are generally agranular, but cytoplasmic granules have been detected by electron microscopy in some cases.[299] There may be an associated hemophagocytosis by benign histiocytes.[299] The characteristic phenotype is CD2+, CD3+, CD4−, CD5−, CD7+, and CD8−. Most reported cases express TCR γ/δ chains, but a subset has TCR α/β chains.[300] The TCR γ/δ cases are derived preferentially from the Vδ1 subset of γ/δ T cells. NK-cell–associated antigens, such as CD16 and CD56, are often detected.[296,299] The pattern of cytotoxic granule–associated protein expression, TIA-1+, granzyme M+, granzyme B−, and perforin−, is consistent with nonactivated cytotoxic T cells of the innate immune system.[211,296,297,299] HSTCLs also express killer cell Ig-like receptors (KIRs) consistent with a derivation from memory T cells, and their exhibiting multiple KIR isoforms (CD158a, CD158b, and CD158e) is unique among cytotoxic T-cell lymphomas.[301] TCR gene rearrangements are observed. Karyotypic studies often show isochromosome 7q that may be accompanied by trisomy 8 and loss of a sex chromosome.[296,297,300] HSTCL has a distinct molecular signature when compared with GEP of other T-cell lymphomas, and NGS of HSTCLs has begun to elucidate the mutational landscape of this lymphoma.[302,303]

Subcutaneous Panniculitis–Like T-cell Lymphoma

Subcutaneous panniculitis–like T-cell lymphoma usually presents as multiple erythematous subcutaneous nodules of variable size (0.5-12.0 cm) on the extremities or trunk, or both, of adults.[304-307] This moderately aggressive lymphoma tends to remain localized to the subcutis throughout the clinical course that may be complicated by a severe, and often fatal, hemophagocytic syndrome.

The lymphoma primarily involves the subcutaneous adipose tissue, where there is a lobular panniculitic infiltrate of pleomorphic lymphocytes of variable size. There may be tumor in the deep dermis, but the upper dermis and epidermis are spared. Karyorrhexis and fat necrosis are always present, as are benign histiocytes that often exhibit phagocytosis of nuclear debris or red blood cells. The lymphoma cells express a T-cell phenotype that may be aberrant. Only cases with α/β TCRs are accepted in this disease category.[304] Lymphomas that have a subcutaneous panniculitis–like growth pattern but express γ/δ TCRs are included in the cutaneous γ/δ T-cell lymphoma group among the primary cutaneous PTCL, rare subtypes category.[304] Subcutaneous panniculitis–like T-cell lymphomas often express CD8, contain cytotoxic granule-associated proteins, and may express NK-cell–associated antigens.[304,307] TCR gene rearrangements have been identified.[304,307]

Intestinal T-cell Lymphoma

Intestinal T-cell lymphoma (ITL) is a tumor of the intraepithelial lymphocytes most frequently arising as a complication of celiac disease, in which case it is termed *enteropathy-associated T-cell lymphoma (EATL)*.[308] ITLs that develop in patients who do not have features of celiac disease are termed *monomorphic epitheliotropic intestinal T-cell lymphoma (MEITL)*.[309] Most patients with ITLs are middle-aged to elderly; it is unusual for these lymphomas to present before 40 years of age. The most common presenting symptoms are abdominal pain and weight loss. Diarrhea is present less often but is not infrequent. There may be signs of acute obstruction or spontaneous perforation. The disease has an aggressive course, with most patients dying within a few years of diagnosis.

It is now realized that the pathology of the tumor shows a spectrum.[309-312] At one end of the spectrum, the lymphoma is limited to the intraepithelial lymphocyte population (intraepithelial EATL). No tumor mass or cytologic features of malignancy are seen, but there is often aberrant loss of CD8 expression and a monoclonal T-cell population by molecular analysis. These patients with EATLs frequently present with refractory celiac disease and demonstrate serologic findings of celiac disease. Some of these cases are complicated by multiple ulcers in the small intestinal mucosa (ulcerative jejunitis). Tumors cannot be identified by histology in the ulcer bases, which contain a mixed inflammatory cell infiltrate. TCR gene rearrangements can be demonstrated, however.[313] At the other end of the spectrum, the lymphoma presents as single or multiple tumor masses along the small intestine, most frequently in the jejunum. A clonally linked intraepithelial component is commonly present in the distant small intestinal mucosa, suggesting that the lymphoma has arisen from underlying aberrant intraepithelial lymphocytes. Histologically, the tumor cells are usually intermediate to large in size with oval to pleomorphic nuclei (formerly known as type I EATL). There is generally abundant clear to eosinophilic cytoplasm, and azurophilic cytoplasmic granules are occasionally observed on touch imprints of the tumor. Mitotic activity is usually brisk. The phenotype is variable but is often CD2+, CD3+, CD4−, CD5−, CD7+, CD8−/+, and TCRα/β positive. Some cases may be CD30+ and must be distinguished from ALCL. MEITLs, which lack an association with celiac disease, are composed of monomorphic small- to medium-sized lymphoid cells that express CD8 and CD56 with a TCRγ/δ phenotype (formerly known as type II EATL).

Comparative genomic hybridization has shown chromosomal imbalances in 87% of EATLs and MEITLs with gains at chromosome

9q being the most frequent by far.[314] EATLs demonstrate more frequent chromosomal gains of 1q and 5q than MEITLs.[314,315] Mutations in *STAT5B* and gains of the 8q24 locus involving *MYC* are frequent recurring abnormalities in MEITLs.[316,317] *SETD2* mutations, the most commonly mutated gene, provide survival/proliferation advantage to the lymphoma cells.[309]

Extranodal Natural Killer/T-cell Lymphoma, Nasal Type

Nasal NK/T-cell lymphomas occur in the nasopharyngeal or sinonasal areas and include cases with morphologic features described previously as *polymorphic reticulosis* and *lethal midline granuloma*. These lymphomas are often angiocentric, angioinvasive, and angiodestructive lesions composed of a polymorphic infiltrate of small lymphocytes and immunoblasts with variable cytologic atypia.[318,319] The lymphoid infiltrate often occludes vessels producing areas of ischemic necrosis. The clinical course is typically aggressive and prognosis is poor. These lymphomas are observed most frequently in East Asia and among the indigenous populations of Mexico, Central America, and South America. They are rare in ethnic Caucasians of the United States and Europe. Any age group can be affected.

Recent studies have shown these lymphomas can be true NK-cell lymphomas or cytotoxic PTCLs. Most cases express NK-cell–associated antigens, particularly CD56, and some contain azurophilic cytoplasmic granules on Romanowsky-type–stained smears or cytotoxic granule–associated proteins recognized by immunohistochemistry.[318-321] The true NK-cell lymphomas lack TCR gene rearrangements, whereas the few well-defined T-cell cases demonstrate clonal TCR gene rearrangements.[318-322] Determining T-cell vs NK-cell lineage is not essential for diagnosis. By definition, these are EBV-positive lymphomas.[319,321-323] Extranodal NK/T-cell lymphoma, nasal type, has a distinct molecular signature when compared with GEP of PTCL, NOS.[324]

Extranodal NK/T-cell lymphoma, nasal type, usually but not always exhibits involvement of the nasal cavity. Skin, soft tissue, gastrointestinal tract, and testis are the most frequent nonnasal extranodal sites involved.[325-327]

HODGKIN LYMPHOMA

Although HL has distinct clinical manifestations that help to define the disease, its simplest pathology definition is a neoplasm of RS cells and RS cell variants or Hodgkin cells (abbreviated as RS cells throughout this chapter) that are associated with an inflammatory response that often dominates the morphologic picture. This histopathologic definition, formulated by Jackson and Parker and further refined by Lukes, Butler, and Hicks, has formed the basis for reproducible diagnosis of this disease for many years. However, based on advances in the understanding of the biology of Hodgkin cells, the WHO modified the defining features of HL to include phenotypic criteria.[23,24] Although much work has been done on the genetics of HL, genetic testing, either by conventional cytogenetic or molecular modalities, is not part of the routine diagnosis of HL.

HL is subdivided into two major categories: NLPHL (5% of cases) and CHL (95% of cases). Both demonstrate a paucity of neoplastic B-cells within a background of reactive inflammatory cells, underscoring both the relatedness of these two entities to each other. In addition, clinically they are primarily nodal diseases that disseminate in a predictable manner to contiguous nodal regions distinct from other NHLs.

Classic Hodgkin Lymphoma
Morphology

The histopathologic features of CHL include architectural effacement of the involved tissue by a mixed cell infiltrate that includes RS cells as well as variants which are large neoplastic cells with some, but not all, of the features of RS cells (*Figure 88.15*). Each nucleus or nuclear lobe has a thick nuclear membrane with vesicular chromatin. Typically, large inclusion-like nucleoli surrounded by a perinucleolar halo are present. The cytoplasm is abundant, eosinophilic to

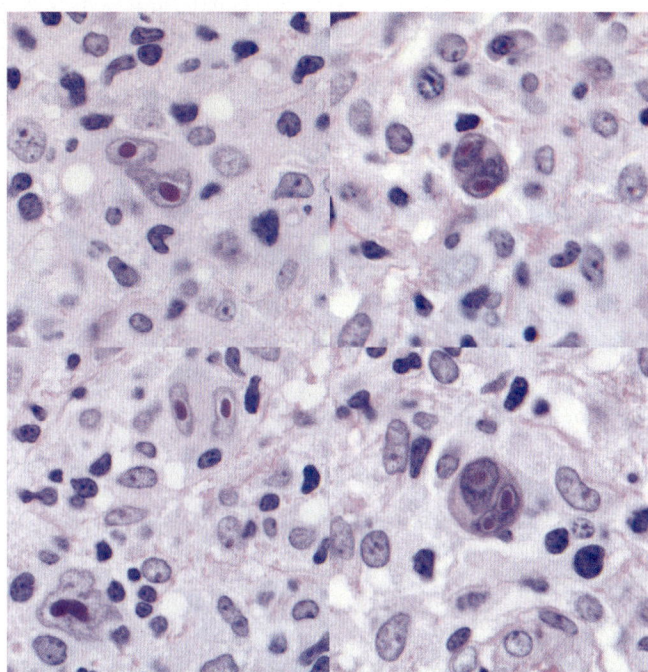

FIGURE 88.15 Lymph node: Classic Hodgkin lymphoma. This composite photograph highlights the features of diagnostic Reed-Sternberg cells: Multiple or bilobed nuclei, prominent inclusion-like nucleoli and abundant eosinophilic cytoplasm.

amphophilic and homogeneous throughout. "Lacunar" cells, named from the cytoplasmic retraction of the large tumor cells that occurs as an artifact of formalin fixation, may be seen. "Mummified" cells, tumor cells with dark, compact nuclear chromatin, may also be found throughout the infiltrate.

The admixed inflammatory cells are prominent including varying numbers of small lymphocytes, macrophages, plasma cells, eosinophils, neutrophils and fibroblasts.

The WHO classification recognizes four subtypes of CHL: mixed cellularity (MC), lymphocyte-rich (LR), nodular sclerosis (NS), and lymphocyte depleted (LD).[23,24] Once the essential diagnostic features are recognized, CHL is subclassified based upon the presence or absence of particular types of RS cell variants and upon the varying proportions of reacting host inflammatory cells and fibrosis.

Although the presence and phenotype of RS cells constitute defining features of CHL, cells that are cytologically (and phenotypically) identical to RS cells can be seen in reactive conditions, such as infectious mononucleosis and in other NHLs. Therefore, tissue architectural effacement and the inflammatory cells that accompany the Hodgkin cells are also critical criteria for the diagnosis of HL. Careful attention to the inflammatory cells, particularly the lymphocytes, helps the pathologist to distinguish HLs from NHLs containing RS-like cells. In the former, there is a dimorphism between the Hodgkin cells and the small bland appearing lymphocytes. NHLs with RS-like cells often contain a population of medium-size lymphocytes with cytological features, including nuclear irregularities and pleomorphism.

The presence of the prominent host response in HL also complicates separation of HL from benign, inflammatory processes. Granulomas containing multinucleated giant cells with or without central necrosis, abundant neutrophils, numerous eosinophils, granulation tissue, collagen deposition, and vascular proliferation are the hallmarks of the host immune response to a variety of infectious agents or can be seen in allergic reactions and autoimmune diseases. Extranodal tissues involved by CHL can contain these same features.

Nodular Sclerosis Subtype

NS CHL is the most common histologic type of CHL encountered in the United States accounting for 50% to 80% of cases.[23] In addition

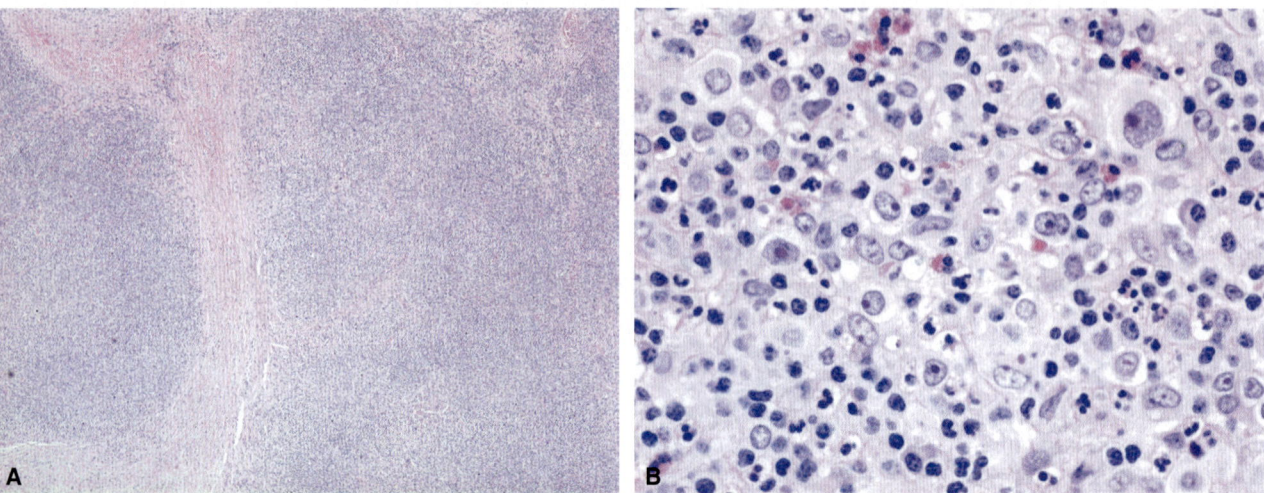

FIGURE 88.16 Lymph node: Classic Hodgkin lymphoma, nodular sclerosis subtype. A, Collagen band formation is illustrated, circumscribing the mixed cell infiltrates into nodules. B, Cytologic features of lacunar cells (upper right) are illustrated. Note the background population of small lymphocytes, neutrophils, eosinophils, and plasma cells.

to meeting the general criteria of HL (phenotypically characteristic RS cells and the appropriate inflammatory cellularity), two additional features define this subtype: collagen band formation that thickens the capsule and dissects through the lymph node parenchyma imparting a nodular appearance and presence of lacunar cells (*Figure 88.16*).[328] In some cases, the neoplastic cells cluster into large aggregates or sheets which are then surrounded by the typical inflammatory cells and fibrosis. These cases are termed "syncytial variant" and are significant mainly because of the potential for misdiagnosis of an NHL or non-hematologic malignancy.

Mixed Cellularity Subtype

MC CHL is the second most common subtype of CHL (20%-30% of cases).[23,294] In the most characteristic cases, RS cells and an admixture of lymphocytes, plasma cells, eosinophils, and macrophages diffusely efface lymph node architecture (*Figure 88.17*). RS cells are typically quite numerous. There may be a delicate collagen fibrosis between the cells, but collagen bands that thicken the lymph node capsule and define the borders of nodules are not present. In some cases, the diagnostic infiltrates of CHL occur between reactive germinal centers in an interfollicular pattern.[329] MC CHL often presents at higher stages than NS CHL[330] and is more likely to be associated with EBV and HIV infection.[331,332]

Lymphocyte-Rich Subtype

LR CHL is an uncommon subtype that accounts for approximately 5% of all CHL cases.[23] This subtype demonstrates neoplastic RS cells and variants in a background of predominantly small lymphocytes, with a distinct absence of eosinophils and neutrophils (*Figure 88.18*). This infiltrate grows in a nodular pattern created by an association with normal lymphoid follicles rather than bands of fibrosis. Often a residual germinal center can be found at the periphery of the nodule. Morphologically and clinically, this is the subtype of CHL that most closely resembles NLPHL.[333] LR CHL often presents at low stage and demonstrates a more indolent course, similar to NLPHL.[23,24,334] In cases with challenging histology, distinction between NLPHL and LR CHL is made based on the differing phenotypes of neoplastic cells.

Lymphocyte Depleted Subtype

LD CHL is the least common type of CHL (<1% of CHL) and most morphologically distinct subtype.[23,335] This subtype is

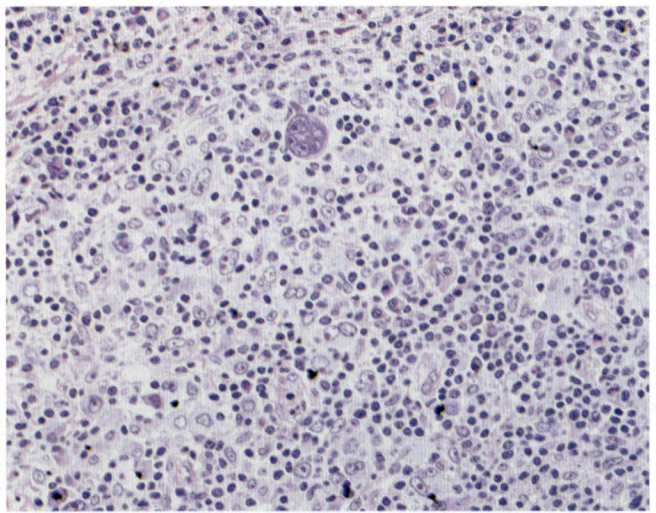

FIGURE 88.17 Lymph node: Classic Hodgkin lymphoma, mixed cellularity subtype. There are many large Hodgkin cells (variant RS cells), a diagnostic RS cell (upper center), and a background population of small lymphocytes, histiocytes, plasma cells, and eosinophils. RS, Reed-Sternberg.

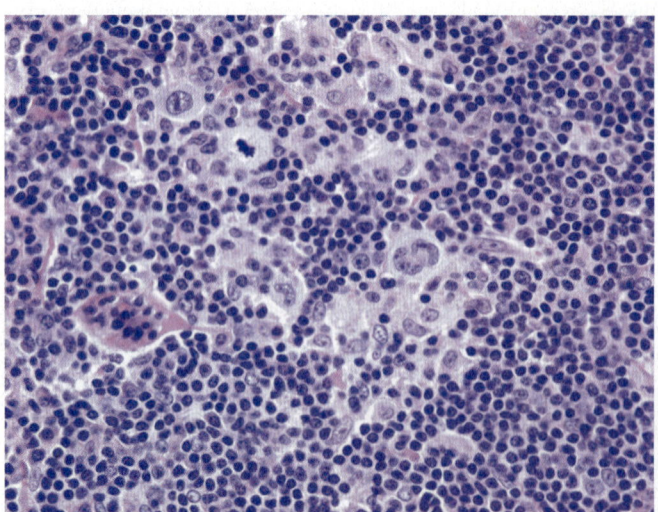

FIGURE 88.18 Lymph node: Classic Hodgkin lymphoma, lymphocyte-rich subtype. Few RS cells are present in a background of composed almost exclusively of small lymphocytes and histiocytes. RS, Reed-Sternberg.

Extranodal Involvement

Spleen, liver, and bone marrow are the most frequent sites of extranodal involvement by CHL. Bone marrow involvement by CHL is uncommon (5% cases at diagnosis). When involved, there are typically interstitial marrow nodules containing a mixed inflammatory infiltrate with widely scattered RS cells (*Figure 88.20*). Granulomas may be present. This paucity of neoplastic cells can make primary diagnosis of CHL in the BM challenging. The histologic subtype of CHL cannot be determined from the bone marrow findings, as all subtypes show similar patterns in the bone marrow.

Splenic involvement by CHL typically demonstrates multinodular, discrete tumor masses rather than diffuse red or white pulp involvement. Hepatic involvement shows periportal infiltrates.

Immunophenotype

Because of the relative paucity of neoplastic cells, and their large size, flow cytometry is not generally useful in the diagnosis of CHL. Regardless of subtype, the neoplastic cells in CHL share a consistent immunophenotype (*Figure 88.21*). RS cells and variants are known to derive from GCB cells based on the presence of clonal Ig gene rearrangements in microdissected tumor cells.[337] In keeping with their B-cell origin, RS cells express the B-cell transcription factor PAX5 albeit at lower levels than non–neoplastic B-cells. Other markers of B-cell lineage, however, are most often negative in RS cells. CD20 is usually negative, although it may be expressed dimly or in a subset of tumor cells in up to 40% of cases. CD19, CD79a, and the B-cell transcription factors OCT-2 and BOB.1 are likewise negative. As a result of the loss of these key B-cell transcription factors, and "crippling" point mutations in the Ig genes, RS cells typically lack expression of Ig.[337,338] Diagnostically useful antigens in CHL include CD30,

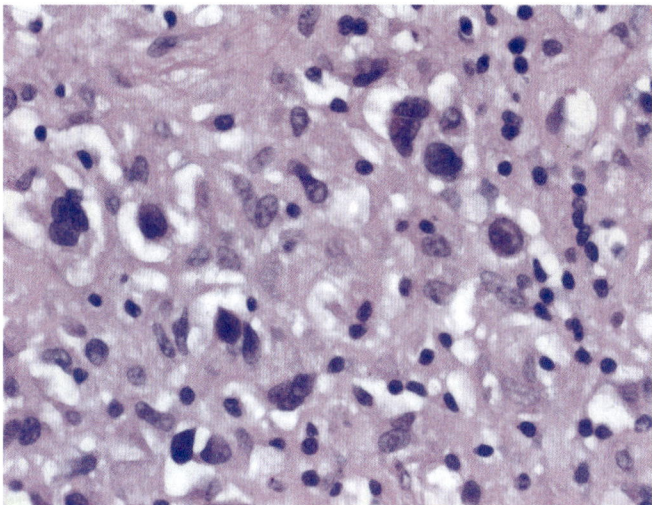

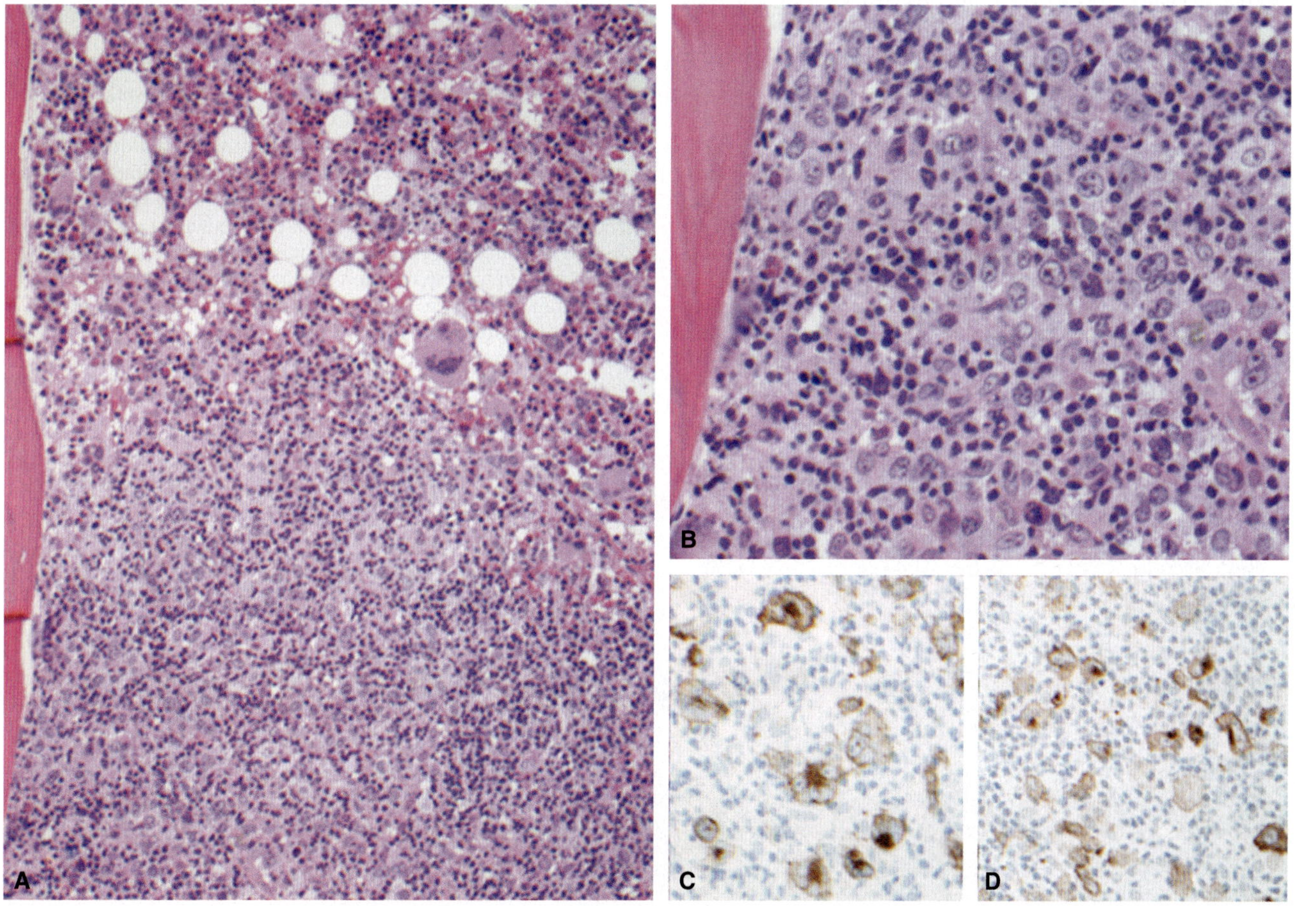

FIGURE 88.19 Lymph node: Classic Hodgkin lymphoma, lymphocyte depleted subtype with diffuse fibrosis. Hodgkin cells and a few small lymphocytes are present amid the disorganized collagen.

characterized by a predominance of RS cells and variants and relatively few background inflammatory cells. There may be a background of diffuse fibrosis as well. Often the RS cells are extremely pleomorphic, almost sarcomatoid appearing, which may lead to complications in diagnosis (*Figure 88.19*). This subtype is more common in patients with HIV,[336] and has a predilection for abdominal organs and lymph nodes.[23]

FIGURE 88.20 Bone marrow: Classic Hodgkin lymphoma. A, The bone marrow is focally replaced by Hodgkin lymphoma. B, Small lymphocytes, macrophages and Hodgkin cells (but no diagnostic Reed-Sternberg cells) are present in the infiltrates. Using paraffin-section immunohistochemistry, the Hodgkin cells express C. CD30 and D. CD15.

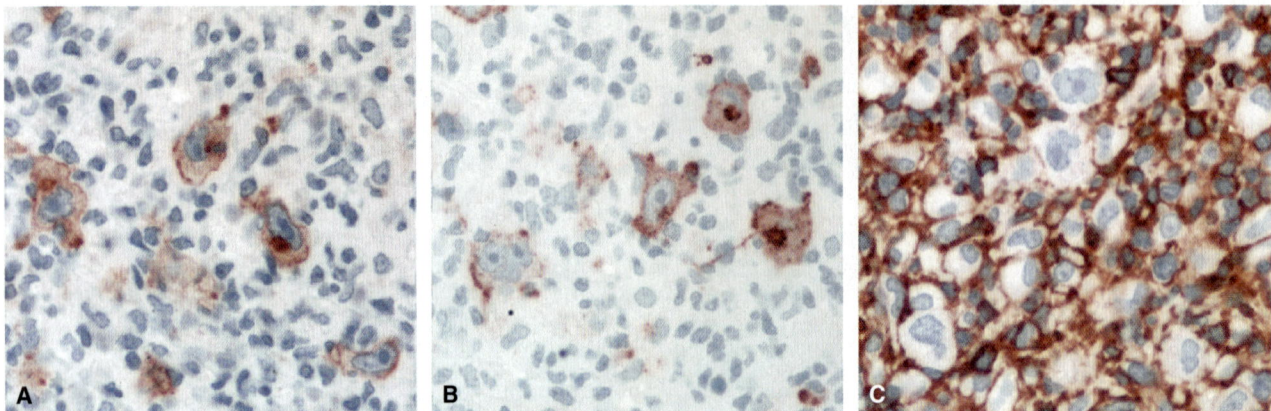

FIGURE 88.21 **Lymph node: Phenotypic features of Reed-Sternberg (RS) cells in classic Hodgkin lymphoma.** The large RS cells are positive for A, CD30, B, CD15 and are negative for C, CD45 in immunoperoxidase stains performed on paraffin sections.

which is strongly positive in RS cells with a distinct membrane and Golgi staining pattern in virtually all cases, and CD15, which is also expressed in the majority (75%-85% of cases).

In spite of their derivation from GCB cells, RS cells generally lack expression of germinal center antigens such as CD10 and BCL6. Newer germinal center markers, LMO2 and HGAL, however, are positive in 100% and 75% of CHL cases, respectively.[339,340] In keeping with the tendency of RS cells to lose lineage defining antigen expression, these cells are negative for the pan-hematopoietic marker CD45.

RS cells are EBV positive in up to 50% of cases with the highest frequency detected in the MC subtype.[331] The most sensitive method for detection of EBV in paraffin tissues is via in situ hybridization probes that recognize EBER. Typically, EBV in CHL exhibits a type II latency pattern with expression of LMP1 and in many instances LMP2A, but lacking EBNA2, glycoprotein 350/250, viral capsid antigen, and early membrane antigen.[341]

Genetics

Studies on the genetics of CHL were initially limited by the paucity of neoplastic cells within the tumors. However, in the late 1990s, it was confirmed by single-cell microdissection that RS cells in CHL represent a clonal process derived from GCB cells that harbor mutations in the Ig heavy chain genes that normally would be targeted for apoptosis.[337,342] Activation of the NF-kB pathway by various mutations likely plays a role in the inhibition of apoptosis as well as in cell proliferation in CHL.[343] More recently, aberrations in the MAP/ERK and JAK/STAT pathways, as well as mutations that contribute to an immunosuppressive tumor microenvironment (PD-L1 and PD-L2), have been found.[344]

The non–neoplastic inflammatory cells in CHL form a unique tumor microenvironment that is immunosuppressive and favorable to tumor growth. Conversion of tumor-supporting microenvironment to a tumor-inhospitable one by immune checkpoint PD1 inhibitors has shown encouraging efficacy in refractory or relapsed CHL.[345,346]

Nodular Lymphocyte Predominant Hodgkin Lymphoma
Morphology

The morphologic features of NLPHL include the presence of large neoplastic lymphocytes termed LP cells, and a host response rich in small lymphocytes and macrophages. LP cells have distinctly indented or lobulated nuclei (sometimes termed "popcorn cells" due to their appearance) delicate chromatin, small nucleoli, and pale staining cytoplasm. There is, however, a marked degree of overlap in cytology between the malignant cells of CHL and NLPHL.

The typical growth pattern of NLPHL is termed macronodular or macrofollicular (*Figure 88.22*). The nodules are formed by expanded follicular dendritic meshworks, are usually larger than reactive lymphoid follicles, and are composed of predominantly small mantle zone B-cells and small T cells. The neoplastic cells are dispersed in varying numbers within these nodules. Epithelioid macrophages can be present within the nodules, distributed singly or in small clusters, or they can satellite around the nodules in a wreath-like arrangement.

One additional histologic feature that may accompany NLPHL and also may be histologically confused for NLPHL is PTGCs. PTGC

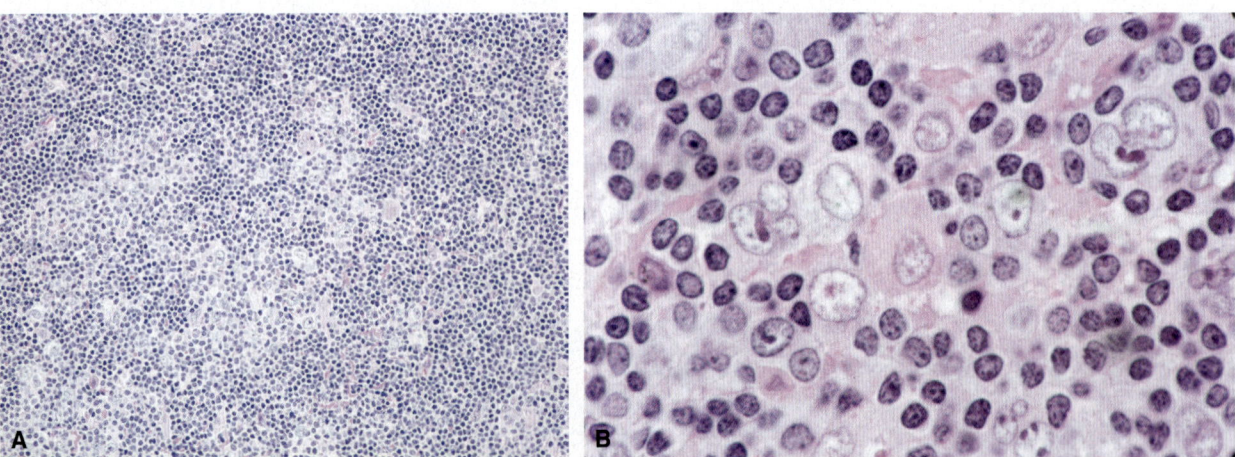

FIGURE 88.22 **Lymph node: Nodular lymphocyte–predominant Hodgkin lymphoma.** A, This nodule of NLPHL shows a few LP cells together with abundant small lymphocytes and a few histiocytes. B, Typical LP cells have lobulated nuclei, delicate chromatin, small nucleoli and delicate, pale cytoplasm. NLPHL, nodular lymphocyte predominant Hodgkin lymphoma.

is an unusual reactive pattern most frequently seen in florid follicular hyperplasia. The follicles in PTGC have a "darker" appearance because they are composed of a large proportion of small lymphocytes indistinguishable from mantle zone lymphocytes. Although small lymphocytes predominate, all PTGCs contain single and clustered germinal center cells, scattered tingible body macrophages, and expanded follicular dendritic cell mesh works. In contrast to the nodules of NLPHL, PTGCs do not tend toward confluence, do not efface lymph node architecture, and they do not contain LP cells. PTGC can be present in reactive lymph node specimens from patients prior to the development of NLPHL, concurrent with NLPHL, or following NLPHL, suggesting a relationship between these two conditions.[347] However, PTGC occurs much more frequently as a reactive process accompanying follicular lymphoid hyperplasia. Its presence does not de facto indicate the presence of NLPHL, nor does it necessarily predict for subsequent development of NLPHL.[348]

In early involvement by NLPHL, only a few nodules are present in the lymph node cortex accompanied by follicular lymphoid hyperplasia and progressively transformed germinal centers. In the most histologically advanced cases, the nodules coalesce, becoming confluent, such that almost all the tumor grows in a diffuse pattern with only focal nodularity. This variability in histology, as well as differences in cytologic composition, is reflected in the several different histologic patterns that have been described in NLPHL: classic B-cell–rich nodular, serpiginous nodular, nodular variant with prominent extranodular LP cells, T-cell rich nodular, and T-cell rich DLBCL like.[24] In fact, most cases present with several patterns in the same lymph node.[24] Recognition of areas within the tumor that show a diffuse growth pattern (T-cell rich DLBCL like) is important as these may reflect a more aggressive behavior.[349,350] Importantly, if any nodular areas remain within the tumor, even if the majority is diffuse, it is still considered NLPHL.[24,351] Of course, in cases with prominent diffuse growth, the differential diagnosis of T-cell/histiocyte rich large B-cell lymphoma (TCRLBL), or TCRLBL-like transformation of NLPHL may arise.[24,351] As such, adequate tissue sampling, typically excisional lymph node biopsy, is essential in this setting.

Bone marrow involvement by NLPHL is even less common than in CHL (<5% of cases).[24] Intertrabecular and paratrabecular aggregates of small lymphocytes admixed with macrophages and occasional LP cells typify bone marrow involvement by NLPHL.

NLPHL transforms to overt DLBCL in approximately 5% of cases.[352] These cases are characterized by sheets of large B-cells that help to distinguish them from TCRLBL, which has a diffuse growth pattern but with still a paucity of large B cells.[353]

Immunophenotype

LP cells have a distinctive and consistent phenotype, indicating GCB cell lineage (*Figure 88.23*). They are consistently positive for pan-B-cell antigens, such as CD19, CD20, CD22, CD79a, PAX-5, OCT2, BOB1, and J chain.[354] They are negative for CD30 and CD15, and positive for CD45 aiding in the distinction from CHL. BCL6 is positive, although CD10 is typically negative. While the heavy chain type expressed by LP cells is usually IgG, a subset of cases with unique histological and clinical attributes contains LP cells positive for IgD.[355] These cases typically occur in young males.

In most cases of NLPHL, the majority of the small lymphocytes accompanying the LP cells are polytypic IgD and IgM expressing B-cells. The small lymphocytes that are immediately adjacent to the

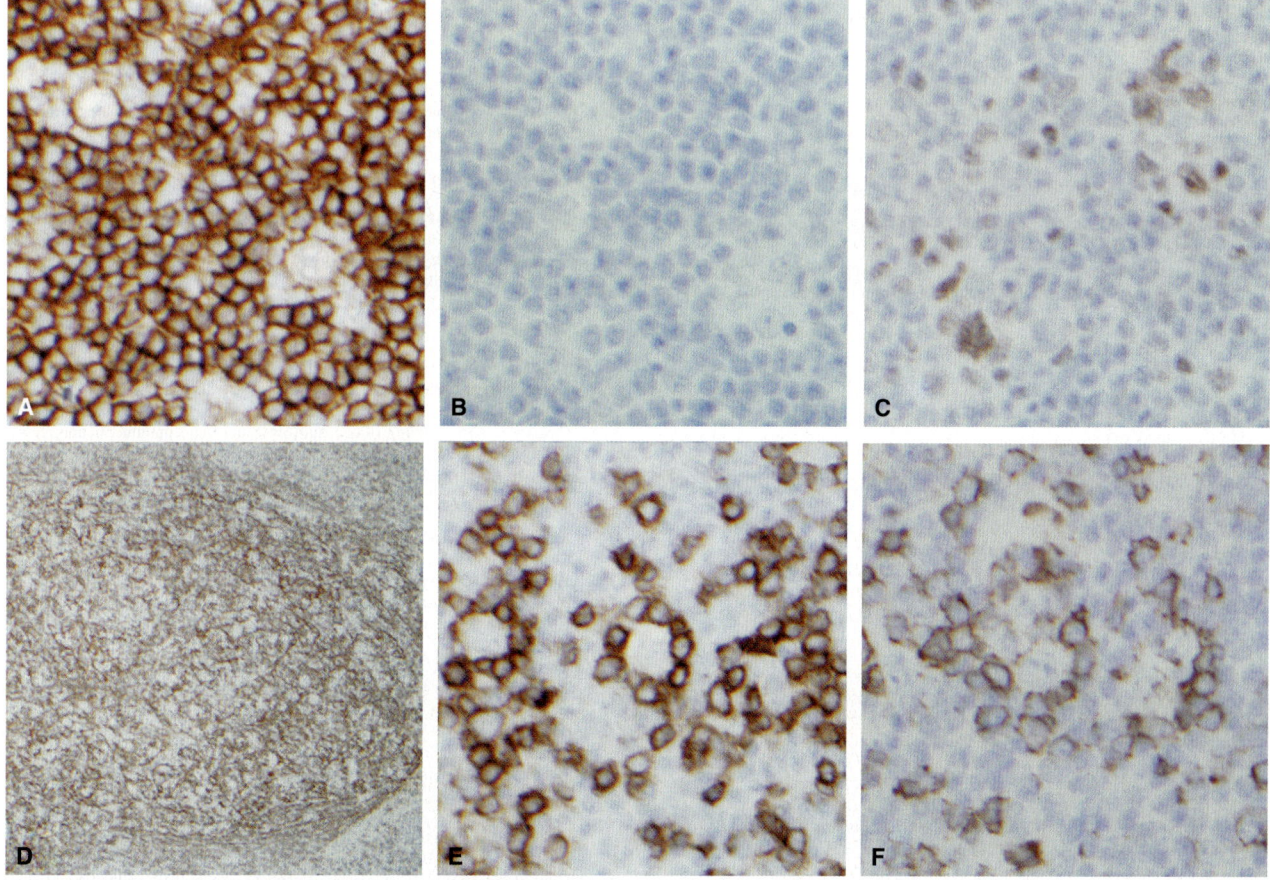

FIGURE 88.23 Lymph node: Immunoarchitecture of nodular lymphocyte predominant Hodgkin lymphoma. A, The LP cells and most of the background small lymphocytes are positive for CD20. B, The LP cells and small lymphocytes are CD30-negative. C, Nuclear positivity for BCL6 is present in the LP cells. D, CD21-positive follicular dendritic cells form a meshwork that defines the nodules. E, Small lymphocytes in the immediate vicinity of the LP cells, some forming rosettes around the tumor cells are CD3-positive and F, CD57-positive.

LP cells ("rosetting" around the LP cells) are T cells with a T-FH phenotype (CD279/PD-1, etc). Expanded meshworks of CD21 positive follicular dendritic cells form the immune-architectural background of the nodules of NLPHL.

Genetics

As with CHL, molecular and cytogenetic testing in NLPHL is mainly an investigative endeavor. Unlike in CHL where recurrent translocations are uncommon, BCL6 translocations can be found in approximately 50% of NLPHLs.[356] As with CHL, constitutive activation of the NF-kB pathway is critical to NLPHL pathogenesis, albeit by different mechanisms.[357]

References

1. Iqbal S, DePew ZS, Kurtin PJ, et al. Endobronchial ultrasound and lymphoproliferative disorders: a retrospective study. *Ann Thorac Surg*. 2012;94(6):1830-1834.
2. Chamberlain WD, Falta MT, Kotzin BL. Functional subsets within clonally expanded CD8(+) memory T cells in elderly humans. *Clin Immunol*. 2000;94(3):160-172.
3. Nam-Cha SH, San-Millan B, Mollejo M, et al. Light-chain-restricted germinal centres in reactive lymphadenitis: report of eight cases. *Histopathology*. 2008;52(4):436-444.
4. Kussick SJ, Kalnoski M, Braziel RM, Wood BL. Prominent clonal B-cell populations identified by flow cytometry in histologically reactive lymphoid proliferations. *Am J Clin Pathol*. 2004;121(4):464-472.
5. van Dongen JJ, Lhermitte L, Bottcher S, et al. EuroFlow antibody panels for standardized n-dimensional flow cytometric immunophenotyping of normal, reactive and malignant leukocytes. *Leukemia*. 2012;26(9):1908-1975.
6. Kaleem Z. Flow cytometric analysis of lymphomas: current status and usefulness. *Arch Pathol Lab Med*. 2006;130(12):1850-1858.
7. Rawstron AC, Villamor N, Ritgen M, et al. International standardized approach for flow cytometric residual disease monitoring in chronic lymphocytic leukaemia. *Leukemia*. 2007;21(5):956-964.
8. Langerak AW, Groenen PJ, Bruggemann M, et al. EuroClonality/BIOMED-2 guidelines for interpretation and reporting of Ig/TCR clonality testing in suspected lymphoproliferations. *Leukemia*. 2012;26(10):2159-2171.
9. Ventura RA, Martin-Subero JI, Jones M, et al. FISH analysis for the detection of lymphoma-associated chromosomal abnormalities in routine paraffin-embedded tissue. *J Mol Diagn*. 2006;8(2):141-151.
10. Safley AM, Buckley PJ, Creager AJ, et al. The value of fluorescence in situ hybridization and polymerase chain reaction in the diagnosis of B-cell non-Hodgkin lymphoma by fine-needle aspiration. *Arch Pathol Lab Med*. 2004;128(12):1395-1403.
11. Jorgensen JL. State of the Art Symposium: flow cytometry in the diagnosis of lymphoproliferative disorders by fine-needle aspiration. *Cancer*. 2005;105(6):443-451.
12. Dey P, Amir T, Al Jassar A, et al. Combined applications of fine needle aspiration cytology and flow cytometric immunphenotyping for diagnosis and classification of non Hodgkin lymphoma. *Cytojournal*. 2006;3:24.
13. Mullighan CG. Genome sequencing of lymphoid malignancies. *Blood*. 2013;122(24):3899-3907.
14. Kurtz DM, Green MR, Bratman SV, et al. Noninvasive monitoring of diffuse large B-cell lymphoma by immunoglobulin high-throughput sequencing. *Blood*. 2015;125(24):3679-3687.
15. Warren EH, Matsen FA, Chou J. High-throughput sequencing of B- and T-lymphocyte antigen receptors in hematology. *Blood*. 2013;122(1):19-22.
16. Rappaport H. Tumors of the hematopoietic system. In: Pathology UAFIo, ed. *Atlas of Tumor Pathology, Section 3, Fascicle 8*. US Armed Forces Institute of Pathology; 1966.
17. Lukes RJ, Collins RD. Immunologic characterization of human malignant lymphomas. *Cancer*. 1974;34(4 suppl):1488-1503.
18. Lennert K, Mohri N, Stein H, Kaiserling E. The histopathology of malignant lymphoma. *Br J Haematol*. 1975;31(s1):193-203.
19. Bloomfield CD, Gajl-Peczalska KJ, Frizzera G, Kersey JH, Goldman AI. Clinical utility of lymphocyte surface markers combined with the Lukes-Collins histologic classification in adult lymphoma. *N Engl J Med*. 1979;301(10):512-518.
20. Project TN-HsLPC. National Cancer Institute sponsored study of classifications of non-Hodgkin's lymphomas: summary and description of a working formulation for clinical usage. The Non-Hodgkin's Lymphoma Pathologic Classification Project. *Cancer*. 1982;49(10):2112-2135.
21. Harris NL, Jaffe ES, Stein H, et al. A revised European-American classification of lymphoid neoplasms: a proposal from the International Lymphoma Study Group. *Blood*. 1994;84(5):1361-1392.
22. Jaffe ES. *World Health Organization Classification of Tumours. Pathology and Genetics of Tumours of Haematopoietic and Lymphoid Tissues*. IARC Press; 2001.
23. Swerdlow S, Campo E, Harris N, et al, eds. *WHO Classification of Tumours of Haematopoietic and Lymphoid Tissues*. 4th ed. IARC Press; 2008.
24. Swerdlow S, Campo E, Harris N, et al, eds. *WHO Classification of Tumours of Haematopoietic and Lymphoid Tissues*. Revised 4th ed. IARC Press; 2017.
25. Liu YJ, Johnson GD, Gordon J, MacLennan IC. Germinal centres in T-cell-dependent antibody responses. *Immunol Today*. 1992;13(1):17-21.
26. Liu YJ, Banchereau J. The paths and molecular controls of peripheral B-cell development. *Immunologist*. 1996;4:55-66.
27. Kuppers R, Klein U, Hansmann ML, Rajewsky K. Cellular origin of human B-cell lymphomas. *N Engl J Med*. 1999;341(20):1520-1529.
28. Korsmeyer SJ. Bcl-2 initiates a new category of oncogenes: regulators of cell death. *Blood*. 1992;80(4):879-886.
29. Bahler DW, Levy R. Clonal evolution of a follicular lymphoma: evidence for antigen selection. *Proc Natl Acad Sci U S A*. 1992;89(15):6770-6774.
30. Zhu D, Hawkins RE, Hamblin TJ, Stevenson FK. Clonal history of a human follicular lymphoma as revealed in the immunoglobulin variable region genes. *Br J Haematol*. 1994;86(3):505-512.
31. Brauninger A, Hansmann ML, Strickler JG, et al. Identification of common germinal-center B-cell precursors in two patients with both Hodgkin's disease and non-Hodgkin's lymphoma. *N Engl J Med*. 1999;340(16):1239-1247.
32. Kuppers R, Dalla-Favera R. Mechanisms of chromosomal translocations in B cell lymphomas. *Oncogene*. 2001;20(40):5580-5594.
33. Jegalian AG, Eberle FC, Pack SD, et al. Follicular lymphoma in situ: clinical implications and comparisons with partial involvement by follicular lymphoma. *Blood*. 2011;118(11):2976-2984.
34. Pillai RK, Surti U, Swerdlow SH. Follicular lymphoma-like B cells of uncertain significance (in situ follicular lymphoma) may infrequently progress, but precedes follicular lymphoma, is associated with other overt lymphomas and mimics follicular lymphoma in flow cytometric studies. *Haematologica*. 2013;98(10):1571-1580.
35. Katzenberger T, Kalla J, Leich E, et al. A distinctive subtype of t(14;18)-negative nodal follicular non-Hodgkin lymphoma characterized by a predominantly diffuse growth pattern and deletions in the chromosomal region 1p36. *Blood*. 2009;113(5):1053-1061.
36. Yegappan S, Schnitzer B, Hsi ED. Follicular lymphoma with marginal zone differentiation: microdissection demonstrates the t(14;18) in both the follicular and marginal zone components. *Mod Pathol*. 2001;14(3):191-196.
37. Tiesinga JJ, Wu CD, Inghirami G. CD5+ follicle center lymphoma. Immunophenotyping detects a unique subset of "floral" follicular lymphoma. *Am J Clin Pathol*. 2000;114(6):912-921.
38. Barekman CL, Aguilera NS, Abbondanzo SL. Low-grade B-cell lymphoma with coexpression of both CD5 and CD10. A report of 3 cases. *Arch Pathol Lab Med*. 2001;125(7):951-953.
39. Wang SA, Wang L, Hochberg EP, Muzikansky A, Harris NL, Hasserjian RP. Low histologic grade follicular lymphoma with high proliferation index: morphologic and clinical features. *Am J Surg Pathol*. 2005;29(11):1490-1496.
40. Garcia-Alvarez M, Alonso-Alvarez S, Prieto-Conde I, et al. Genetic complexity impacts the clinical outcome of follicular lymphoma patients. *Blood Cancer J*. 2021;11(1):11.
41. Liu Q, Salaverria I, Pittaluga S, et al. Follicular lymphomas in children and young adults: a comparison of the pediatric variant with usual follicular lymphoma. *Am J Surg Pathol*. 2013;37(3):333-343.
42. Louissaint A, Jr, Ackerman AM, Dias-Santagata D, et al. Pediatric-type nodal follicular lymphoma: an indolent clonal proliferation in children and adults with high proliferation index and no BCL2 rearrangement. *Blood*. 2012;120(12):2395-2404.
43. Siddiqi IN, Friedman J, Barry-Holson KQ, et al. Characterization of a variant of t(14;18) negative nodal diffuse follicular lymphoma with CD23 expression, 1p36/TNFRSF14 abnormalities, and STAT6 mutations. *Mod Pathol*. 2016;29(6):570-581.
44. Louissaint A, Jr, Schafernak KT, Geyer JT, et al. Pediatric-type nodal follicular lymphoma: a biologically distinct lymphoma with frequent MAPK pathway mutations. *Blood*. 2016;128(8):1093-1100.
45. Cong P, Raffeld M, Teruya-Feldstein J, Sorbara L, Pittaluga S, Jaffe ES. In situ localization of follicular lymphoma: description and analysis by laser capture microdissection. *Blood*. 2002;99(9):3376-3382.
46. Natkunam Y, Warnke RA, Zehnder JL, Jones CD, Milatovich-Cherry A, Cornbleet PJ. Blastic/blastoid transformation of follicular lymphoma: immunohistologic and molecular analyses of five cases. *Am J Surg Pathol*. 2000;24(4):525-534.
47. Aoun P, Zhou G, Chan WC, et al. Familial B-cell chronic lymphocytic leukemia: analysis of cytogenetic abnormalities, immunophenotypic profiles, and immunoglobulin heavy chain gene usage. *Am J Clin Pathol*. 2007;127(1):31-38.
48. Jahic A, Iljazovic E, Arnautovic-Custovic A, Halilbasic A, Simendic V, Zabic A. Prognostic significance of bone-marrow pattern and immunophenotypic score in B-chronic lymphocytic leukemia at diagnosis. *Med Arh*. 2011;65(3):132-136.
49. Rozman C, Hernandez-Nieto L, Montserrat E, Brugues R. Prognostic significance of bone-marrow patterns in chronic lymphocytic leukaemia. *Br J Haematol*. 1981;47(4):529-537.
50. Müller-Hermelink HK, Montserrat E, Catovsky D, et al. Chronic lymphocytic leukemia/small lymphocytic lymphoma. In: Swerdlow SH, Campo E, Harris NL, et al, eds. *World Health Organization Classification of Tumours. WHO Classification of Tumours of Haematopoietic and Lymphoid Tissues*. 4th ed. IARC Press; 2008:180-182.
51. Ciccone M, Agostinelli C, Rigolin GM, et al. Proliferation centers in chronic lymphocytic leukemia: correlation with cytogenetic and clinicobiological features in consecutive patients analyzed on tissue microarrays. *Leukemia*. 2012;26(3):499-508.
52. Ben-Ezra J, Burke JS, Swartz WG, et al. Small lymphocytic lymphoma: a clinicopathologic analysis of 268 cases. *Blood*. 1989;73(2):579-587.
53. Nakamura N, Abe M. Richter syndrome in B-cell chronic lymphocytic leukemia. *Pathol Int*. 2003;53(4):195-203.
54. Robertson LE, Pugh W, O'Brien S, et al. Richter's syndrome: a report on 39 patients. *J Clin Oncol*. 1993;11(10):1985-1989.
55. Timar B, Fulop Z, Csernus B, et al. Relationship between the mutational status of VH genes and pathogenesis of diffuse large B-cell lymphoma in Richter's syndrome. *Leukemia*. 2004;18(2):326-330.
56. Choi H, Keller RH. Coexistence of chronic lymphocytic leukemia and Hodgkin's disease. *Cancer*. 1981;48(1):48-57.
57. Xiao W, Chen WW, Sorbara L, et al. Hodgkin lymphoma variant of Richter transformation: morphology, Epstein-Barr virus status, clonality, and survival analysis-with comparison to Hodgkin-like lesion. *Hum Pathol*. 2016;55:108-116.

58. Momose H, Jaffe ES, Shin SS, Chen YY, Weiss LM. Chronic lymphocytic leukemia/small lymphocytic lymphoma with Reed-Sternberg-like cells and possible transformation to Hodgkin's disease. Mediation by Epstein-Barr virus. *Am J Surg Pathol.* 1992;16(9):859-867.
59. Treon SP, Xu L, Yang G, et al. MYD88 L265P somatic mutation in Waldenstrom's macroglobulinemia. *N Engl J Med.* 2012;367(9):826-833.
60. King RL, Gonsalves WI, Ansell SM, et al. Lymphoplasmacytic lymphoma with a non-IgM paraprotein shows clinical and pathologic heterogeneity and may harbor MYD88 L265P mutations. *Am J Clin Pathol.* 2016;145(6):843-851.
61. Rosado FG, Morice WG, He R, Howard MT, Timm M, McPhail ED. Immunophenotypic features by multiparameter flow cytometry can help distinguish low grade B-cell lymphomas with plasmacytic differentiation from plasma cell proliferative disorders with an unrelated clonal B-cell process. *Br J Haematol.* 2015;169(3):368-376.
62. Treon SP, Tripsas CK, Meid K, et al. Ibrutinib in previously treated Waldenstrom's macroglobulinemia. *N Engl J Med.* 2015;372(15):1430-1440.
63. Treon SP, Cao Y, Xu L, Yang G, Liu X, Hunter ZR. Somatic mutations in MYD88 and CXCR4 are determinants of clinical presentation and overall survival in Waldenstrom macroglobulinemia. *Blood.* 2014;123(18):2791-2796.
64. Schlette E, Lai R, Onciu M, Doherty D, Bueso-Ramos C, Medeiros LJ. Leukemic mantle cell lymphoma: clinical and pathologic spectrum of twenty-three cases. *Mod Pathol.* 2001;14(11):1133-1140.
65. Sander B, Quintanilla-Martinez L, Ott G, et al. Mantle cell lymphoma – a spectrum from indolent to aggressive disease. *Virchows Arch.* 2016;468(3):245-257.
66. Ruan J, Martin P. Which patients with mantle cell lymphoma do not need aggressive therapy. *Curr Hematol Malig Rep.* 2016;11(3):234-240.
67. Jares P, Colomer D, Campo E. Molecular pathogenesis of mantle cell lymphoma. *J Clin Invest.* 2012;122(10):3416-3423.
68. Narurkar R, Alkayem N, Liu D. SOX11 is a biomarker for cyclin D1-negative mantle cell lymphoma. *Biomark Res.* 2016;4:6.
69. Mozos A, Royo C, Hartmann E, et al. SOX11 expression is highly specific for mantle cell lymphoma and identifies the cyclin D1-negative subtype. *Haematologica.* 2009;94(11):1555-1562.
70. Raty R, Franssila K, Joensuu H, Teerenhovi L, Elonen E. Ki-67 expression level, histological subtype, and the International Prognostic Index as outcome predictors in mantle cell lymphoma. *Eur J Haematol.* 2002;69(1):11-20.
71. Tiemann M, Schrader C, Klapper W, et al. Histopathology, cell proliferation indices and clinical outcome in 304 patients with mantle cell lymphoma (MCL): a clinicopathological study from the European MCL Network. *Br J Haematol.* 2005;131(1):29-38.
72. Fu K, Weisenburger DD, Greiner TC, et al. Cyclin D1-negative mantle cell lymphoma: a clinicopathologic study based on gene expression profiling. *Blood.* 2005;106(4):4315-4321.
73. Shiller SM, Zieske A, Holmes H III, Feldman AL, Law ME, Saad R. CD5-positive, cyclinD1-negative mantle cell lymphoma with a translocation involving the CCND2 gene and the IGL locus. *Cancer Genet.* 2011;204(3):162-164.
74. Richard P, Vassalo J, Valmary S, Missoury R, Delsol G, Brousset P. "In situ-like" mantle cell lymphoma: a report of two cases. *J Clin Pathol.* 2006;59(9):995-996.
75. van den Brand M, van Krieken JH. Recognizing nodal marginal zone lymphoma: recent advances and pitfalls. A systematic review. *Haematologica.* 2013;98(7):1003-1013.
76. Granai M, Amato T, Di Napoli A, et al. IGHV mutational status of nodal marginal zone lymphoma by NGS reveals distinct pathogenic pathways with different prognostic implications. *Virchows Arch.* 2020;477(1):143-150.
77. Spina V, Khiabanian H, Messina M, et al. The genetics of nodal marginal zone lymphoma. *Blood.* 2016;128(10):1362-1373.
78. Jallades L, Baseggio L, Sujobert P, et al. Exome sequencing identifies recurrent BCOR alterations and the absence of KLF2, TNFAIP3 and MYD88 mutations in splenic diffuse red pulp small B-cell lymphoma. *Haematologica.* 2017;102(10):1758-1766.
79. Curiel-Olmo S, Mondejar R, Almaraz C, et al. Splenic diffuse red pulp small B-cell lymphoma displays increased expression of cyclin D3 and recurrent CCND3 mutations. *Blood.* 2017;129(8):1042-1045.
80. Mollejo M, Camacho FI, Algara P, Ruiz-Ballesteros E, Garcia JF, Piris MA. Nodal and splenic marginal zone B cell lymphomas. *Hematol Oncol.* 2005;23(3-4):108-118.
81. Isaacson PG, Matutes E, Burke M, Catovsky D. The histopathology of splenic lymphoma with villous lymphocytes. *Blood.* 1994;84(11):3828-3834.
82. Mateo M, Mollejo M, Villuendas R, et al. 7q31-32 allelic loss is a frequent finding in splenic marginal zone lymphoma. *Am J Pathol.* 1999;154(5):1583-1589.
83. Arcaini L, Rossi D, Paulli M. Splenic marginal zone lymphoma: from genetics to management. *Blood.* 2016;127(17):2072-2081.
84. Martinez N, Almaraz C, Vaque JP, et al. Whole-exome sequencing in splenic marginal zone lymphoma reveals mutations in genes involved in marginal zone differentiation. *Leukemia.* 2014;28(6):1334-1340.
85. Piva R, Deaglio S, Fama R, et al. The Kruppel-like factor 2 transcription factor gene is recurrently mutated in splenic marginal zone lymphoma. *Leukemia.* 2015;29(2):503-507.
86. Clipson A, Wang M, de Leval L, et al. KLF2 mutation is the most frequent somatic change in splenic marginal zone lymphoma and identifies a subset with distinct genotype. *Leukemia.* 2015;29(5):1177-1185.
87. Campos-Martin Y, Martinez N, Martinez-Lopez A, et al. Clinical and diagnostic relevance of NOTCH2- and KLF2-mutations in splenic marginal zone lymphoma. *Haematologica.* 2017;102(8):e310-e312.
88. Wotherspoon AC, Ortiz-Hidalgo C, Falzon MR, Isaacson PG. Helicobacter pylori-associated gastritis and primary B-cell gastric lymphoma. *Lancet.* 1991;338(8776):1175-1176.
89. Parsonnet J, Hansen S, Rodriguez L, et al. *Helicobacter pylori* infection and gastric lymphoma. *N Engl J Med.* 1994;330(18):1267-1271.
90. Baginsky LA, Diss TC, Hongtao Y, Wren B, Qing Du M, Isaacson PG, Dogan A. Campylobacter jejuni infection in intestinal lymphoma: a strong association with immunoproliferative small intestinal disease. *Blood.* 2004;104(11):1369.
91. Lecuit M, Abachin E, Martin A, et al. Immunoproliferative small intestinal disease associated with Campylobacter jejuni. *N Engl J Med.* 2004;350(3):239-248.
92. Ferreri AJ, Guidoboni M, Ponzoni M, et al. Evidence for an association between Chlamydia psittaci and ocular adnexal lymphomas. *J Natl Cancer Inst.* 2004;96(8):586-594.
93. Ferreri AJ, Ponzoni M, Guidoboni M, et al. Regression of ocular adnexal lymphoma after Chlamydia psittaci-eradicating antibiotic therapy. *J Clin Oncol.* 2005;23(22):5067-5073.
94. Ambrosetti A, Zanotti R, Pattaro C, et al. Most cases of primary salivary mucosa-associated lymphoid tissue lymphoma are associated either with Sjogren syndrome or hepatitis C virus infection. *Br J Haematol.* 2004;126(1):43-49.
95. Hyjek E, Smith WJ, Isaacson PG. Primary B-cell lymphoma of salivary glands and its relationship to myoepithelial sialadenitis. *Hum Pathol.* 1988;19(7):766-776.
96. Goodlad JR, Davidson MM, Hollowood K, et al. Primary cutaneous B-cell lymphoma and Borrelia burgdorferi infection in patients from the Highlands of Scotland. *Am J Surg Pathol.* 2000;24(9):1279-1285.
97. Cerroni L, Zochling N, Putz B, Kerl H. Infection by Borrelia burgdorferi and cutaneous B-cell lymphoma. *J Cutan Pathol.* 1997;24(8):457-461.
98. Roggero E, Zucca E, Mainetti C, et al. Eradication of Borrelia burgdorferi infection in primary marginal zone B-cell lymphoma of the skin. *Hum Pathol.* 2000;31(2):263-268.
99. Isaacson PG, Spencer J. Malignant lymphoma of mucosa-associated lymphoid tissue. *Histopathology.* 1987;11(5):445-462.
100. Bacon CM, Du MQ, Dogan A. Mucosa-associated lymphoid tissue (MALT) lymphoma: a practical guide for pathologists. *J Clin Pathol.* 2007;60(4):361-372.
101. Papadaki L, Wotherspoon AC, Isaacson PG. The lymphoepithelial lesion of gastric low-grade B-cell lymphoma of mucosa-associated lymphoid tissue (MALT): an ultrastructural study. *Histopathology.* 1992;21(5):415-421.
102. Isaacson PG, Wotherspoon AC, Diss T, Pan LX. Follicular colonization in B-cell lymphoma of mucosa-associated lymphoid tissue. *Am J Surg Pathol.* 1991;15(9):819-828.
103. Carlsen ED, Swerdlow SH, Cook JR, Gibson SE. Class-switched primary cutaneous marginal zone lymphomas are frequently IgG4-positive and have features distinct from IgM-positive cases. *Am J Surg Pathol.* 2019;43(10):1403-1412.
104. Isaacson PG, Du MQ. MALT lymphoma: from morphology to molecules. *Nat Rev Cancer.* 2004;4(8):644-653.
105. Thome M. CARMA1, BCL-10 and MALT1 in lymphocyte development and activation. *Nat Rev Immunol.* 2004;4(5):348-359.
106. Lin X, Wang D. The roles of CARMA1, Bcl10, and MALT1 in antigen receptor signaling. *Semin Immunol.* 2004;16(6):429-435.
107. Liu H, Ye H, Ruskone-Fourmestraux A, et al. T(11;18) is a marker for all stage gastric MALT lymphomas that will not respond to H. pylori eradication. *Gastroenterology.* 2002;122(5):1286-1294.
108. Liu H, Ruskon-Fourmestraux A, Lavergne-Slove A, et al. Resistance of t(11;18) positive gastric mucosa-associated lymphoid tissue lymphoma to *Helicobacter pylori* eradication therapy. *Lancet.* 2001;357(9249):39-40.
109. Hsi ED. Update in large cell lymphoma: understanding the pathology report. *Hematology Am Soc Hematol Educ Program.* 2015;2015:605-617.
110. Diebold J, Anderson JR, Armitage JO, et al. Diffuse large B-cell lymphoma: a clinicopathologic analysis of 444 cases classified according to the updated Kiel classification. *Leuk Lymphoma.* 2002;43(1):97-104.
111. Brudno J, Tadmor T, Pittaluga S, Nicolae A, Polliack A, Dunleavy K. Discordant bone marrow involvement in non-Hodgkin lymphoma. *Blood.* 2016;127(8):965-970.
112. Shim H, Oh JJ, Park SH, et al. Prognostic impact of concordant and discordant cytomorphology of bone marrow involvement in patients with diffuse, large, B-cell lymphoma treated with R-CHOP. *J Clin Pathol.* 2013;66(5):420-425.
113. de Leval L, Harris NL. Variability in immunophenotype in diffuse large B-cell lymphoma and its clinical relevance. *Histopathology.* 2003;43(6):509-528.
114. Davis TA, Czerwinski DK, Levy R. Therapy of B-cell lymphoma with anti-CD20 antibodies can result in the loss of CD20 antigen expression. *Clin Cancer Res.* 1999;5(3):611-615.
115. Alizadeh AA, Eisen MB, Davis RE, et al. Distinct types of diffuse large B-cell lymphoma identified by gene expression profiling. *Nature.* 2000;403(6769):503-511.
116. Choi WW, Weisenburger DD, Greiner TC, et al. A new immunostain algorithm classifies diffuse large B-cell lymphoma into molecular subtypes with high accuracy. *Clin Cancer Res.* 2009;15(17):5494-5502.
117. Hans CP, Weisenburger DD, Vose JM, et al. A significant diffuse component predicts for inferior survival in grade 3 follicular lymphoma, but cytologic subtypes do not predict survival. *Blood.* 2003;101(6):2363-2367.
118. Muris JJ, Meijer CJ, Vos W, et al. Immunohistochemical profiling based on Bcl-2, CD10 and MUM1 expression improves risk stratification in patients with primary nodal diffuse large B cell lymphoma. *J Pathol.* 2006;208(5):714-723.
119. Nyman H, Adde M, Karjalainen-Lindsberg ML, et al. Prognostic impact of immunohistochemically defined germinal center phenotype in diffuse large B-cell lymphoma patients treated with immunochemotherapy. *Blood.* 2007;109(11):4930-4935.
120. Meyer PN, Fu K, Greiner TC, et al. Immunohistochemical methods for predicting cell of origin and survival in patients with diffuse large B-cell lymphoma treated with rituximab. *J Clin Oncol.* 2011;29(2):200-207.
121. Hwang HS, Park CS, Yoon DH, Suh C, Huh J. High concordance of gene expression profiling-correlated immunohistochemistry algorithms in diffuse large B-cell lymphoma, not otherwise specified. *Am J Surg Pathol.* 2014;38(8):1046-1057.

122. Scott DW, Mottok A, Ennishi D, et al. Prognostic significance of diffuse large B-cell lymphoma cell of origin determined by digital gene expression in formalin-fixed paraffin-embedded tissue biopsies. *J Clin Oncol*. 2015;33(26):2848-2856.
123. Scott DW, Wright GW, Williams PM, et al. Determining cell-of-origin subtypes of diffuse large B-cell lymphoma using gene expression in formalin-fixed paraffin-embedded tissue. *Blood*. 2014;123(8):1214-1217.
124. Hu S, Xu-Monette ZY, Tzankov A, et al. MYC/BCL2 protein coexpression contributes to the inferior survival of activated B-cell subtype of diffuse large B-cell lymphoma and demonstrates high-risk gene expression signatures: a report from the International DLBCL Rituximab-CHOP Consortium Program. *Blood*. 2013;121(20):4021-4031, quiz 4250.
125. Horn H, Ziepert M, Becher C, et al. MYC status in concert with BCL2 and BCL6 expression predicts outcome in diffuse large B-cell lymphoma. *Blood*. 2013;121(12):2253-2263.
126. Green TM, Young KH, Visco C, et al. Immunohistochemical double-hit score is a strong predictor of outcome in patients with diffuse large B-cell lymphoma treated with rituximab plus cyclophosphamide, doxorubicin, vincristine, and prednisone. *J Clin Oncol*. 2012;30(28):3460-3467.
127. Kluk MJ, Ho C, Yu H, et al. MYC immunohistochemistry to identify MYC-driven B-cell lymphomas in clinical practice. *Am J Clin Pathol*. 2016;145(2):166-179.
128. Yamaguchi M, Seto M, Okamoto M, et al. De novo CD5+ diffuse large B-cell lymphoma: a clinicopathologic study of 109 patients. *Blood*. 2002;99(3):815-821.
129. Alinari L, Gru A, Quinion C, et al. De novo CD5+ diffuse large B-cell lymphoma: adverse outcomes with and without stem cell transplantation in a large, multicenter, rituximab treated cohort. *Am J Hematol*. 2016;91(4):395-399.
130. Jain P, Fayad LE, Rosenwald A, Young KH, O'Brien S. Recent advances in de novo CD5+ diffuse large B cell lymphoma. *Am J Hematol*. 2013;88(9):798-802.
131. Kobayashi T, Yamaguchi M, Kim S, et al. Microarray reveals differences in both tumors and vascular specific gene expression in de novo CD5(+) and CD5(−) diffuse large B-Cell lymphomas. *Cancer Res*. 2003;63(1):60-66.
132. Tagawa H, Tsuzuki S, Suzuki R, et al. Genome-wide array-based comparative genomic hybridization of diffuse large B-cell lymphoma: comparison between CD5-positive and CD5-negative cases. *Cancer Res*. 2004;64(17):5948-5955.
133. Chaganti RS, Nanjangud G, Schmidt H, Teruya-Feldstein J. Recurring chromosomal abnormalities in non-Hodgkin's lymphoma: biologic and clinical significance. *Semin Hematol*. 2000;37(4):396-411.
134. Roschewski M, Staudt LM, Wilson WH. Diffuse large B-cell lymphoma-treatment approaches in the molecular era. *Nat Rev Clin Oncol*. 2014;11(1):12-23.
135. Shustik J, Han G, Farinha P, et al. Correlations between BCL6 rearrangement and outcome in patients with diffuse large B-cell lymphoma treated with CHOP or R-CHOP. *Haematologica*. 2010;95(1):96-101.
136. Jardin F, Jais JP, Molina TJ, et al. Diffuse large B-cell lymphomas with CDKN2A deletion have a distinct gene expression signature and a poor prognosis under R-CHOP treatment: a GELA study. *Blood*. 2010;116(7):1092-1104.
137. Kusumoto S, Kobayashi Y, Sekiguchi N, et al. Diffuse large B-cell lymphoma with extra Bcl-2 gene signals detected by FISH analysis is associated with a "non-Germinal center phenotype." *Am J Surg Pathol*. 2005;29(8):1067-1073.
138. Dubois S, Viailly PJ, Mareschal S, et al. Next-generation sequencing in diffuse large B-cell lymphoma highlights molecular divergence and therapeutic opportunities: a LYSA study. *Clin Cancer Res*. 2016;22(12):2919-2928.
139. Bohers E, Mareschal S, Bertrand P, et al. Activating somatic mutations in diffuse large B-cell lymphomas: lessons from next generation sequencing and key elements in the precision medicine era. *Leuk Lymphoma*. 2015;56(5):1213-1222.
140. Schmitz R, Wright GW, Huang DW, et al. Genetics and pathogenesis of diffuse large B-cell lymphoma. *N Engl J Med*. 2018;378(15):1396-1407.
141. Chapuy B, Stewart C, Dunford A, et al. Molecular subtypes of diffuse large B cell lymphoma are associated with distinct pathogenic mechanisms and outcomes. *Nature medicine*. 2018;24(5):679-690.
142. Sehn LH, Salles G. Diffuse large B-cell lymphoma. *N Engl J Med*. 2021;384(9):842-858.
143. McClure RF, Remstein ED, Macon WR, et al. Adult B-cell lymphomas with burkitt-like morphology are phenotypically and genotypically heterogeneous with aggressive clinical behavior. *Am J Surg Pathol*. 2005;29(12):1652-1660.
144. Wang W, Hu S, Lu X, Young KH, Medeiros LJ. Triple-hit B-cell lymphoma with MYC, BCL2, and BCL6 translocations/rearrangements: clinicopathologic features of 11 cases. *Am J Surg Pathol*. 2015;39(8):1132-1139.
145. Oki Y, Noorani M, Lin P, et al. Double hit lymphoma: the MD Anderson Cancer Center clinical experience. *Br J Haematol*. 2014;166(6):891-901.
146. Pillai RK, Sathanoori M, Van Oss SB, Swerdlow SH. Double-hit B-cell lymphomas with BCL6 and MYC translocations are aggressive, frequently extranodal lymphomas distinct from BCL2 double-hit B-cell lymphomas. *Am J Surg Pathol*. 2013;37(3):323-332.
147. Ennishi D, Jiang A, Boyle M, et al. Double-hit gene expression signature defines a distinct subgroup of germinal center B-cell-like diffuse large B-cell lymphoma. *J Clin Oncol*. 2019;37(3):190-201.
148. Achten R, Verhoef G, Vanuytsel L, De Wolf-Peeters C. Histiocyte-rich, T-cell-rich B-cell lymphoma: a distinct diffuse large B-cell lymphoma subtype showing characteristic morphologic and immunophenotypic features. *Histopathology*. 2002;40(1):31-45.
149. Lim MS, Beaty M, Sorbara L, et al. T-cell/histiocyte-rich large B-cell lymphoma: a heterogeneous entity with derivation from germinal center B cells. *Am J Surg Pathol*. 2002;26(11):1458-1466.
150. Nam-Cha SH, Roncador G, Sanchez-Verde L, et al. PD-1, a follicular T-cell marker useful for recognizing nodular lymphocyte-predominant Hodgkin lymphoma. *Am J Surg Pathol*. 2008;32(8):1252-1257.
151. Hartmann S, Doring C, Vucic E, et al. Array comparative genomic hybridization reveals similarities between nodular lymphocyte predominant Hodgkin lymphoma and T cell/histiocyte rich large B cell lymphoma. *Br J Haematol*. 2015;169(3):415-422.
152. Griffin GK, Weirather JL, Roemer MGM, et al. Spatial signatures identify immune escape via PD-1 as a defining feature of T-cell/histiocyte-rich large B-cell lymphoma. *Blood*. 2021;137(10):1353-1364.
153. Monti S, Savage KJ, Kutok JL, et al. Molecular profiling of diffuse large B-cell lymphoma identifies robust subtypes including one characterized by host inflammatory response. *Blood*. 2005;105(5):1851-1861.
154. Cazals-Hatem D, Lepage E, Brice P, et al. Primary mediastinal large B-cell lymphoma. A clinicopathologic study of 141 cases compared with 916 nonmediastinal large B-cell lymphomas, a GELA ("Groupe d'Etude des Lymphomes de l' Adulte") study. *Am J Surg Pathol*. 1996;20(7):877-888.
155. Jacobson JO, Aisenberg AC, Lamarre L, et al. Mediastinal large cell lymphoma. An uncommon subset of adult lymphoma curable with combined modality therapy. *Cancer*. 1988;62(9):1893-1898.
156. Calaminici M, Piper K, Lee AM, Norton AJ. CD23 expression in mediastinal large B-cell lymphomas. *Histopathology*. 2004;45(6):619-624.
157. Joos S, OtanoJoos MI, Ziegler S, et al. Primary mediastinal (thymic) B-cell lymphoma is characterized by gains of chromosomal material including 9p and amplification of the REL gene. *Blood*. 1996;87(4):1571-1578.
158. Wessendorf S, Barth TF, Viardot A, et al. Further delineation of chromosomal consensus regions in primary mediastinal B-cell lymphomas: an analysis of 37 tumor samples using high-resolution genomic profiling (array-CGH). *Leukemia*. 2007;21(12):2463-2469.
159. Renne C, Willenbrock K, Martin-Subero JI, et al. High expression of several tyrosine kinases and activation of the PI3K/AKT pathway in mediastinal large B cell lymphoma reveals further similarities to Hodgkin lymphoma. *Leukemia*. 2007;21(4):780-787.
160. Rosenwald A, Wright G, Leroy K, et al. Molecular diagnosis of primary mediastinal B cell lymphoma identifies a clinically favorable subgroup of diffuse large B cell lymphoma related to Hodgkin lymphoma. *J Exp Med*. 2003;198(6):851-862.
161. Savage KJ, Monti S, Kutok JL, et al. The molecular signature of mediastinal large B-cell lymphoma differs from that of other diffuse large B-cell lymphomas and shares features with classical Hodgkin lymphoma. *Blood*. 2003;102(12):3871-3879.
162. Traverse-Glehen A, Pittaluga S, Gaulard P, et al. Mediastinal gray zone lymphoma: the missing link between classic Hodgkin's lymphoma and mediastinal large B-cell lymphoma. *Am J Surg Pathol*. 2005;29(11):1411-1421.
163. Wilson WH, Pittaluga S, Nicolae A, et al. A prospective study of mediastinal gray-zone lymphoma. *Blood*. 2014;124(10):1563-1569.
164. Batchelor T, Loeffler JS. Primary CNS lymphoma. *J Clin Oncol*. 2006;24(8):1281-1288.
165. Montesinos-Rongen M, Siebert R, Deckert M. Primary lymphoma of the central nervous system: just DLBCL or not? *Blood*. 2009;113(1):7-10.
166. Tomlinson FH, Kurtin PJ, Suman VJ, et al. Primary intracerebral malignant lymphoma: a clinicopathological study of 89 patients. *J Neurosurg*. 1995;82(4):558-566.
167. Camilleri-Broet S, Criniere E, Broet P, et al. A uniform activated B-cell-like immunophenotype might explain the poor prognosis of primary central nervous system lymphomas: analysis of 83 cases. *Blood*. 2006;107(1):190-196.
168. Braggio E, Van Wier S, Ojha J, et al. Genome-Wide analysis uncovers novel recurrent alterations in primary central nervous system lymphomas. *Clin Cancer Res*. 2015;21(17):3986-3994.
169. Cady FM, O'Neill BP, Law ME, et al. Del(6)(q22) and BCL6 rearrangements in primary CNS lymphoma are indicators of an aggressive clinical course. *J Clin Oncol*. 2008;26(29):4814-4819.
170. Poulain S, Boyle EM, Tricot S, et al. Absence of CXCR4 mutations but high incidence of double mutant in CD79A/B and MYD88 in primary central nervous system lymphoma. *Br J Haematol*. 2015;170(2):285-287.
171. Ok CY, Papathomas TG, Medeiros LJ, Young KH. EBV-positive diffuse large B-cell lymphoma of the elderly. *Blood*. 2013;122(3):328-340.
172. Nicolae A, Pittaluga S, Abdullah S, et al. EBV-positive large B-cell lymphomas in young patients: a nodal lymphoma with evidence for a tolerogenic immune environment. *Blood*. 2015;126(7):863-872.
173. Uccini S, Al-Jadiry MF, Scarpino S, et al. Epstein-Barr virus-positive diffuse large B-cell lymphoma in children: a disease reminiscent of Epstein-Barr virus-positive diffuse large B-cell lymphoma of the elderly. *Hum Pathol*. 2015;46(5):716-724.
174. Asano N, Yamamoto K, Tamaru J, et al. Age-related Epstein-Barr virus (EBV)-associated B-cell lymphoproliferative disorders: comparison with EBV-positive classic Hodgkin lymphoma in elderly patients. *Blood*. 2009;113(12):2629-2636.
175. Shimoyama Y, Oyama T, Asano N, et al. Senile Epstein-Barr virus-associated B-cell lymphoproliferative disorders: a mini review. *J Clin Exp Hematop*. 2006;46(1):1-4.
176. Oyama T, Yamamoto K, Asano N, et al. Age-related EBV-associated B-cell lymphoproliferative disorders constitute a distinct clinicopathologic group: a study of 96 patients. *Clin Cancer Res*. 2007;13(17):5124-5132.
177. Dojcinov SD, Venkataraman G, Raffeld M, Pittaluga S, Jaffe ES. EBV positive mucocutaneous ulcer – a study of 26 cases associated with various sources of immunosuppression. *Am J Surg Pathol*. 2010;34(3):405-417.
178. Dojcinov SD, Venkataraman G, Pittaluga S, et al. Age-related EBV-associated lymphoproliferative disorders in the Western population: a spectrum of reactive lymphoid hyperplasia and lymphoma. *Blood*. 2011;117(18):4726-4735.
179. Cheuk W, Chan AC, Chan JK, Lau GT, Chan VN, Yiu HH. Metallic implant-associated lymphoma: a distinct subgroup of large B-cell lymphoma related to pyothorax-associated lymphoma? *Am J Surg Pathol*. 2005;29(6):832-836.
180. Nakatsuka S, Yao M, Hoshida Y, Yamamoto S, Iuchi K, Aozasa K. Pyothorax-associated lymphoma: a review of 106 cases. *J Clin Oncol*. 2002;20(20):4255-4260.
181. Petitjean B, Jardin F, Joly B, et al. Pyothorax-associated lymphoma: a peculiar clinicopathologic entity derived from B cells at late stage of differentiation and with occasional aberrant dual B- and T-cell phenotype. *Am J Surg Pathol*. 2002;26(6):724-732.

182. Colby TV. Current histological diagnosis of lymphomatoid granulomatosis. *Mod Pathol.* 2012;25(suppl 1):S39-S42.
183. Song JY, Pittaluga S, Dunleavy K, et al. Lymphomatoid granulomatosis—a single institute experience: pathologic findings and clinical correlations. *Am J Surg Pathol.* 2015;39(2):141-156.
184. Murase T, Nakamura S, Kawauchi K, et al. An Asian variant of intravascular large B-cell lymphoma: clinical, pathological and cytogenetic approaches to diffuse large B-cell lymphoma associated with haemophagocytic syndrome. *Br J Haematol.* 2000;111(3):826-834.
185. Ponzoni M, Ferreri AJ, Campo E, et al. Definition, diagnosis, and management of intravascular large B-cell lymphoma: proposals and perspectives from an international consensus meeting. *J Clin Oncol.* 2007;25(21):3168-3173.
186. Gascoyne RD, Lamant L, Martin-Subero JI, et al. ALK-positive diffuse large B-cell lymphoma is associated with Clathrin-ALK rearrangements: report of 6 cases. *Blood.* 2003;102(7):2568-2573.
187. Onciu M, Behm FG, Downing JR, et al. ALK-positive plasmablastic B-cell lymphoma with expression of the NPM-ALK fusion transcript: report of 2 cases. *Blood.* 2003;102(7):2642-2644.
188. Pan Z, Hu S, Li M, et al. ALK-positive large B-cell lymphoma: a clinicopathologic study of 26 cases with review of additional 108 cases in the literature. *Am J Surg Pathol.* 2017;41(1):25-38.
189. Colomo L, Loong F, Rives S, et al. Diffuse large B-cell lymphomas with plasmablastic differentiation represent a heterogeneous group of disease entities. *Am J Surg Pathol.* 2004;28(6):736-747.
190. Morscio J, Dierickx D, Nijs J, et al. Clinicopathologic comparison of plasmablastic lymphoma in HIV-positive, immunocompetent, and posttransplant patients: single-center series of 25 cases and meta-analysis of 277 reported cases. *Am J Surg Pathol.* 2014;38(7):875-886.
191. Isaacson PCE, Harris N. Large B-cell lymphoma arising in HHV8-associated multicentric Castleman disease. In: Swerdlow SH, Campo E, Harris NL, et al, eds. *World Health Organization Classification of Tumours. WHO Classification of Tumours of Haematopoietic and Lymphoid Tissues.* 4th ed. IARC Press; 2008.
192. Ferry JA, Sohani AR, Longtine JA, Schwartz RA, Harris NL. HHV8-positive, EBV-positive Hodgkin lymphoma-like large B-cell lymphoma and HHV8-positive intravascular large B-cell lymphoma. *Mod Pathol.* 2009;22(5):618-626.
193. Ansari MQ, Dawson DB, Nador R, et al. Primary body cavity-based AIDS-related lymphomas. *Am J Clin Pathol.* 1996;105(2):221-229.
194. Cesarman E, Chang Y, Moore PS, Said JW, Knowles DM. Kaposi's sarcoma-associated herpesvirus-like DNA sequences in AIDS-related body-cavity-based lymphomas. *N Engl J Med.* 1995;332(18):1186-1191.
195. Cesarman E, Nador RG, Aozasa K, Delsol G, Said JW, Knowles DM. Kaposi's sarcoma-associated herpesvirus in non-AIDS related lymphomas occurring in body cavities. *Am J Pathol.* 1996;149(1):53-57.
196. Hristov AC. Primary cutaneous diffuse large B-cell lymphoma, leg type: diagnostic considerations. *Arch Pathol Lab Med.* 2012;136(8):876-881.
197. Pham-Ledard A, Prochazkova-Carlotti M, Andrique L, et al. Multiple genetic alterations in primary cutaneous large B-cell lymphoma, leg type support a common lymphomagenesis with activated B-cell-like diffuse large B-cell lymphoma. *Mod Pathol.* 2014;27(3):402-411.
198. Raphael M, Gentilhomme O, Tulliez M, Byron PA, Diebold J. Histopathologic features of high-grade non-Hodgkin's lymphomas in acquired immunodeficiency syndrome. The French Study Group of Pathology for Human Immunodeficiency Virus-Associated Tumors. *Arch Pathol Lab Med.* 1991;115(1):15-20.
199. Magrath IT. African Burkitt's lymphoma. History, biology, clinical features, and treatment. *Am J Pediatr Hematol Oncol.* 1991;13(2):222-246.
200. Kornblau SM, Goodacre A, Cabanillas F. Chromosomal abnormalities in adult non-endemic Burkitt's lymphoma and leukemia: 22 new reports and a review of 148 cases from the literature. *Hematol Oncol.* 1991;9(2):63-78.
201. Shiramizu B, Barriga F, Neequaye J, et al. Patterns of chromosomal breakpoint locations in Burkitt's lymphoma: relevance to geography and Epstein-Barr virus association. *Blood.* 1991;77(7):1516-1526.
202. Hecht JL, Aster JC. Molecular biology of Burkitt's lymphoma. *J Clin Oncol.* 2000;18(21):3707-3721.
203. Salaverria I, Martin-Guerrero I, Wagener R, et al. A recurrent 11q aberration pattern characterizes a subset of MYC-negative high-grade B-cell lymphomas resembling Burkitt lymphoma. *Blood.* 2014;123(8):1187-1198.
204. Hummel M, Bentink S, Berger H, et al. A biologic definition of Burkitt's lymphoma from transcriptional and genomic profiling. *N Engl J Med.* 2006;354(23):2419-2430.
205. Dave SS, Fu K, Wright GW, et al. Molecular diagnosis of Burkitt's lymphoma. *N Engl J Med.* 2006;354(23):2431-2442.
206. Spits H, Lanier LL, Phillips JH. Development of human T and natural killer cells. *Blood.* 1995;85(10):2654-2670.
207. Jaffe ES. Pathobiology of peripheral T-cell lymphomas. *Hematology Am Soc Hematol Educ Program.* 2006:317-322.
208. Geissinger E, Bonzheim I, Krenacs L, et al. Nodal peripheral T-cell lymphomas correspond to distinct mature T-cell populations. *J Pathol.* 2006;210(2):172-180.
209. Macon WR, Williams ME, Greer JP, et al. Natural killer-like T-cell lymphomas: aggressive lymphomas of T-large granular lymphocytes. *Blood.* 1996;87(4):1474-1483.
210. Felgar RE, Macon WR, Kinney MC, Roberts S, Pasha T, Salhany KE. TIA-1 expression in lymphoid neoplasms. Identification of subsets with cytotoxic T lymphocyte or natural killer cell differentiation. *Am J Pathol.* 1997;150(6):1893-1900.
211. Krenacs L, Smyth MJ, Bagdi E, et al. The serine protease granzyme M is preferentially expressed in NK-cell, gamma delta T-cell, and intestinal T-cell lymphomas: evidence of origin from lymphocytes involved in innate immunity. *Blood.* 2003;101(9):3590-3593.
212. Waldron JA, Leech JH, Glick AD, Flexner JM, Collins RD. Malignant lymphoma of peripheral T-lymphocyte origin: immunologic, pathologic, and clinical features in six patients. *Cancer.* 1977;40(4):1604-1617.
213. Hastrup N, Ralfkiaer E, Pallesen G. Aberrant phenotypes in peripheral T cell lymphomas. *J Clin Pathol.* 1989;42(4):398-402.
214. Gaulard P, Bourquelot P, Kanavaros P, et al. Expression of the alpha/beta and gamma/delta T-cell receptors in 57 cases of peripheral T-cell lymphomas. Identification of a subset of gamma/delta T-cell lymphomas. *Am J Pathol.* 1990;137(3):617-628.
215. Bruggemann M, White H, Gaulard P, et al. Powerful strategy for polymerase chain reaction-based clonality assessment in T-cell malignancies report of the BIOMED-2 Concerted Action BHM4 CT98-3936. *Leukemia.* 2007;21(2):215-221.
216. Asano N, Suzuki R, Kagami Y, et al. Clinicopathologic and prognostic significance of cytotoxic molecule expression in nodal peripheral T-cell lymphoma, unspecified. *Am J Surg Pathol.* 2005;29(10):1284-1293.
217. Dupuis J, Emile JF, Mounier N, et al. Prognostic significance of Epstein-Barr virus in nodal peripheral T-cell lymphoma, unspecified: a Groupe d'Etude des Lymphomes de l'Adulte (GELA) study. *Blood.* 2006;108(13):4163-4169.
218. Streubel B, Vinatzer U, Willheim M, Raderer M, Chott A. Novel t(5;9)(q33;q22) fuses ITK to SYK in unspecified peripheral T-cell lymphoma. *Leukemia.* 2006;20(2):313-318.
219. Feldman AL, Law M, Remstein ED, et al. Recurrent translocations involving the IRF4 oncogene locus in peripheral T-cell lymphomas. *Leukemia.* 2009;23(3):574-580.
220. Iqbal J, Wright G, Wang C, et al. Gene expression signatures delineate biological and prognostic subgroups in peripheral T-cell lymphoma. *Blood.* 2014;123(19):2915-2923.
221. Wang T, Feldman AL, Wada DA, et al. GATA-3 expression identifies a high-risk subset of PTCL, NOS with distinct molecular and clinical features. *Blood.* 2014;123(19):3007-3015.
222. Heavican TB, Bouska A, Yu J, et al. Genetic drivers of oncogenic pathways in molecular subgroups of peripheral T-cell lymphoma. *Blood.* 2019;133(15):1664-1676.
223. Amador C, Greiner TC, Heavican TB, et al. Reproducing the molecular subclassification of peripheral T-cell lymphoma-NOS by immunohistochemistry. *Blood.* 2019;134(24):2159-2170.
224. Burke JS, Butler JJ. Malignant lymphoma with a high content of epitheloid histiocytes (Lennert's lymphoma). *Am J Clin Pathol.* 1976;66(1):1-9.
225. Patsouris E, Noel H, Lennert K. Histological and immunohistological findings in lymphoepithelioid cell lymphoma (Lennert's lymphoma). *Am J Surg Pathol.* 1988;12(5):341-350.
226. Campo E, Swerdlow SH, Harris NL, Pileri S, Stein H, Jaffe ES. The 2008 WHO classification of lymphoid neoplasms and beyond: evolving concepts and practical applications. *Blood.* 2011;117(19):5019-5032.
227. Patsouris E, Noel H, Lennert K. Lymphoplasmacytic/lymphoplasmacytoid immunocytoma with a high content of epithelioid cells. Histologic and immunohistochemical findings. *Am J Surg Pathol.* 1990;14(7):660-670.
228. Patsouris E, Noel H, Lennert K. Angioimmunoblastic lymphadenopathy – type of T-cell lymphoma with a high content of epithelioid cells. Histopathology and comparison with lymphoepithelioid cell lymphoma. *Am J Surg Pathol.* 1989;13(4):262-275.
229. Patsouris E, Noel H, Lennert K. Cytohistologic and immunohistochemical findings in Hodgkin's disease, mixed cellularity type, with a high content of epithelioid cells. *Am J Surg Pathol.* 1989;13(12):1014-1022.
230. Kojima M, Nakamura S, Motoori T, et al. Centroblastic and centroblastic-centrocytic lymphomas associated with prominent epithelioid granulomatous response without plasma cell differentiation: a clinicopathologic study of 12 cases. *Hum Pathol.* 1996;27(7):660-667.
231. Frizzera G, Moran EM, Rappaport H. Angio-immunoblastic lymphadenopathy with dysproteinaemia. *Lancet.* 1974;1(7866):1070-1073.
232. Dogan A, Attygalle AD, Kyriakou C. Angioimmunoblastic T-cell lymphoma. *Br J Haematol.* 2003;121(5):681-691.
233. Attygalle A, Al-Jehani R, Diss TC, et al. Neoplastic T cells in angioimmunoblastic T-cell lymphoma express CD10. *Blood.* 2002;99(2):627-633.
234. Ree HJ, Kadin ME, Kikuchi M, et al. Angioimmunoblastic lymphoma (AILD-type T-cell lymphoma) with hyperplastic germinal centers. *Am J Surg Pathol.* 1998;22(6):643-655.
235. Brown HA, Macon WR, Kurtin PJ, Gibson LE. Cutaneous involvement by angioimmunoblastic T-cell lymphoma with remarkable heterogeneous Epstein-Barr virus expression. *J Cutan Pathol.* 2001;28(8):432-438.
236. Seehafer JR, Goldberg NC, Dicken CH, Su WP. Cutaneous manifestations of angioimmunoblastic lymphadenopathy. *Arch Dermatol.* 1980;116(1):41-45.
237. Grogg KL, Morice WG, Macon WR. Spectrum of bone marrow findings in patients with angioimmunoblastic T-cell lymphoma. *Br J Haematol.* 2007;137(5):416-422.
238. Bagdi E, Krenacs L, Krenacs T, Miller K, Isaacson PG. Follicular dendritic cells in reactive and neoplastic lymphoid tissues: a reevaluation of staining patterns of CD21, CD23, and CD35 antibodies in paraffin sections after wet heat-induced epitope retrieval. *Appl Immunohistochem Mol Morphol.* 2001;9(2):117-124.
239. Jones D, Jorgensen JL, Shahsafaei A, Dorfman DM. Characteristic proliferations of reticular and dendritic cells in angioimmunoblastic lymphoma. *Am J Surg Pathol.* 1998;22(8):956-964.
240. Attygalle AD, Diss TC, Munson P, Isaacson PG, Du MQ, Dogan A. CD10 expression in extranodal dissemination of angioimmunoblastic T-cell lymphoma. *Am J Surg Pathol.* 2004;28(1):54-61.
241. de Leval L, Savilo E, Longtine J, Ferry JA, Harris NL. Peripheral T-cell lymphoma with follicular involvement and a CD4+/bcl-6+ phenotype. *Am J Surg Pathol.* 2001;25(3):395-400.
242. Ree HJ, Kadin ME, Kikuchi M, Ko YH, Suzumiya J, Go JH. Bcl-6 expression in reactive follicular hyperplasia, follicular lymphoma, and angioimmunoblastic T-cell lymphoma with hyperplastic germinal centers: heterogeneity of intrafollicular T-cells and their altered distribution in the pathogenesis of angioimmunoblastic T-cell lymphoma. *Hum Pathol.* 1999;30(4):403-411.

243. Grogg KL, Attygalle AD, Macon WR, Remstein ED, Kurtin PJ, Dogan A. Angioimmunoblastic T-cell lymphoma: a neoplasm of germinal-center T-helper cells? *Blood*. 2005;106(4):1501-1502.
244. Grogg KL, Attygalle AD, Macon WR, Remstein ED, Kurtin PJ, Dogan A. Expression of CXCL13, a chemokine highly upregulated in germinal center T-helper cells, distinguishes angioimmunoblastic T-cell lymphoma from peripheral T-cell lymphoma, unspecified. *Mod Pathol*. 2006;19(8):1101-1107.
245. Dupuis J, Boye K, Martin N, et al. Expression of CXCL13 by neoplastic cells in angio-immunoblastic T-cell lymphoma (AITL): a new diagnostic marker providing evidence that AITL derives from follicular helper T cells. *Am J Surg Pathol*. 2006;30(4):490-494.
246. de Leval L, Rickman DS, Thielen C, et al. The gene expression profile of nodal peripheral T-cell lymphoma demonstrates a molecular link between angioimmunoblastic T-cell lymphoma (AITL) and follicular helper T (TFH) cells. *Blood*. 2007;109(11):4952-4963.
247. Marafioti T, Paterson JC, Ballabio E, et al. The inducible T-cell co-stimulator molecule is expressed on subsets of T cells and is a new marker of lymphomas of T follicular helper cell-derivation. *Haematologica*. 2010;95(3):432-439.
248. Basha BM, Bryant SC, Rech KL, et al. Application of a 5 marker panel to the routine diagnosis of peripheral T-cell lymphoma with T-follicular helper phenotype. *Am J Surg Pathol*. 2019;43(9):1282-1290.
249. Attygalle AD, Kyriakou C, Dupuis J, et al. Histologic evolution of angioimmunoblastic T-cell lymphoma in consecutive biopsies: clinical correlation and insights into natural history and disease progression. *Am J Surg Pathol*. 2007;31(7):1077-1088.
250. Willenbrock K, Brauninger A, Hansmann ML. Frequent occurrence of B-cell lymphomas in angioimmunoblastic T-cell lymphoma and proliferation of Epstein-Barr virus-infected cells in early cases. *Br J Haematol*. 2007;138(6):733-739.
251. Ondrejka SL, Hsi ED. T-Cell lymphomas: updates in biology and diagnosis. *Surg Pathol Clin*. 2016;9(1):131-141.
252. Lee SH, Kim JS, Kim J, et al. A highly recurrent novel missense mutation in CD28 among angioimmunoblastic T-cell lymphoma patients. *Haematologica*. 2015;100(12):e505-e507.
253. Kinney MC, Higgins RA, Medina EA. Anaplastic large cell lymphoma: twenty-five years of discovery. *Arch Pathol Lab Med*. 2011;135(1):19-43.
254. Stein H, Foss HD, Durkop H, et al. CD30(+) anaplastic large cell lymphoma: a review of its histopathologic, genetic, and clinical features. *Blood*. 2000;96(12):3681-3695.
255. Falini B, Lamant-Rochaix L, Campo E, et al. Anaplastic large cell lymphoma, ALK-positive. In: Swerdlow SH, Campo E, Harris NL, et al, eds. *World Health Organization Classification of Tumours. WHO Classification of Tumours of Haematopoietic and Lymphoid Tissues*. Revised 4th ed. International Agency for Research on Cancer; 2017:413-418.
256. Feldman AL, Harris NL, Stein H, et al. Anaplasticlarge cell lymphoma, ALK-negative. In: Swerdlow SH, Campo E, Harris NL, et al, eds. *World Health Organization Classification of Tumours. WHO Classification of Tumours of Haematopoietic and Lymphoid Tissues*. 4th ed. International Agency for Research on Cancer; 2017:418-421. Revised.
257. Willemze R, Paulli M, Kadin ME. Primary cutaneous CD30-positive T-cell lymphoproliferative disorders. In: Swerdlow SH, Campo E, Harris NL, et al, eds. *World Health Organization Classification of Tumours. WHO Classification of Tumours of Haematopoietic and Lymphoid Tissues*. Revised 4th ed. International Agency for Research on Cancer; 2017:392-396.
258. Feldman AL, Harris NL, Stein H, et al. Breast implant-associated anaplastic large cell lymphoma. In: Swerdlow SH, Campo E, Harris NL, et al, eds. *World Health Organization Classification of Tumours. WHO Classification of Tumours of Haematopoietic and Lymphoid Tissues*. 4th ed. International Agency for Research on Cancer; 2017:421-422. Revised.
259. Kadin ME, Sako D, Berliner N, et al. Childhood Ki-1 lymphoma presenting with skin lesions and peripheral lymphadenopathy. *Blood*. 1986;68(5):1042-1049.
260. de Bruin PC, Beljaards RC, van Heerde P, et al. Differences in clinical behaviour and immunophenotype between primary cutaneous and primary nodal anaplastic large cell lymphoma of T-cell or null cell phenotype. *Histopathology*. 1993;23(2):127-135.
261. Chott A, Kaserer K, Augustin I, et al. Ki-1-positive large cell lymphoma. A clinicopathologic study of 41 cases. *Am J Surg Pathol*. 1990;14(5):439-448.
262. Pileri S, Falini B, Delsol G, et al. Lymphohistiocytic T-cell lymphoma (anaplastic large cell lymphoma CD30+/Ki-1+ with a high content of reactive histiocytes). *Histopathology*. 1990;16(4):383-391.
263. Kinney MC, Collins RD, Greer JP, Whitlock JA, Sioutos N, Kadin ME. A small-cell-predominant variant of primary Ki-1 (CD30)+ T-cell lymphoma. *Am J Surg Pathol*. 1993;17(9):859-868.
264. Krenacs L, Wellmann A, Sorbara L, et al. Cytotoxic cell antigen expression in anaplastic large cell lymphomas of T- and null-cell type and Hodgkin's disease: evidence for distinct cellular origin. *Blood*. 1997;89(3):980-989.
265. DeCoteau JF, Butmarc JR, Kinney MC, Kadin ME. The t(2;5) chromosomal translocation is not a common feature of primary cutaneous CD30+ lymphoproliferative disorders: comparison with anaplastic large-cell lymphoma of nodal origin. *Blood*. 1996;87(8):3437-3441.
266. Le Beau MM, Bitter MA, Larson RA, et al. The t(2;5)(p23;q35): a recurring chromosomal abnormality in Ki-1-positive anaplastic large cell lymphoma. *Leukemia*. 1989;3(12):866-870.
267. Morris SW, Kirstein MN, Valentine MB, et al. Fusion of a kinase gene, ALK, to a nucleolar protein gene, NPM, in non-Hodgkin's lymphoma. *Science*. 1994;263(5151):1281-1284.
268. Pulford K, Lamant L, Morris SW, et al. Detection of anaplastic lymphoma kinase (ALK) and nucleolar protein nucleophosmin (NPM)-ALK proteins in normal and neoplastic cells with the monoclonal antibody ALK1. *Blood*. 1997;89(4):1394-1404.
269. Touriol C, Greenland C, Lamant L, et al. Further demonstration of the diversity of chromosomal changes involving 2p23 in ALK-positive lymphoma: 2 cases expressing ALK kinase fused to CLTCL (clathrin chain polypeptide-like). *Blood*. 2000;95(10):3204-3207.
270. Lamant L, Dastugue N, Pulford K, Delsol G, Mariame B. A new fusion gene TPM3-ALK in anaplastic large cell lymphoma created by a (1;2)(q25;p23) translocation. *Blood*. 1999;93(9):3088-3095.
271. Hernandez L, Pinyol M, Hernandez S, et al. TRK-fused gene (TFG) is a new partner of ALK in anaplastic large cell lymphoma producing two structurally different TFG-ALK translocations. *Blood*. 1999;94(9):3265-3268.
272. Ma Z, Cools J, Marynen P, et al. Inv(2)(p23q35) in anaplastic large-cell lymphoma induces constitutive anaplastic lymphoma kinase (ALK) tyrosine kinase activation by fusion to ATIC, an enzyme involved in purine nucleotide biosynthesis. *Blood*. 2000;95(6):2144-2149.
273. Trinei M, Lanfrancone L, Campo E, et al. A new variant anaplastic lymphoma kinase (ALK)-fusion protein (ATIC-ALK) in a case of ALK-positive anaplastic large cell lymphoma. *Cancer Res*. 2000;60(4):793-798.
274. Tort F, Pinyol M, Pulford K, et al. Molecular characterization of a new ALK translocation involving moesin (MSN-ALK) in anaplastic large cell lymphoma. *Lab Invest*. 2001;81(3):419-426.
275. Meech SJ, McGavran L, Odom LF, et al. Unusual childhood extramedullary hematologic malignancy with natural killer cell properties that contains tropomyosin 4 – anaplastic lymphoma kinase gene fusion. *Blood*. 2001;98(4):1209-1216.
276. Lamant L, Gascoyne RD, Duplantier MM, et al. Non-muscle myosin heavy chain (MYH9): a new partner fused to ALK in anaplastic large cell lymphoma. *Genes Chromosomes Cancer*. 2003;37(4):427-432.
277. Feldman AL, Vasmatzis G, Asmann YW, et al. Novel TRAF1-ALK fusion identified by deep RNA sequencing of anaplastic large cell lymphoma. *Genes Chromosomes Cancer*. 2013;52(11):1097-1102.
278. Lamant L, de Reynies A, Duplantier MM, et al. Gene-expression profiling of systemic anaplastic large-cell lymphoma reveals differences based on ALK status and two distinct morphologic ALK+ subtypes. *Blood*. 2007;109(5):2156-2164.
279. Zettl A, Rudiger T, Konrad MA, et al. Genomic profiling of peripheral T-cell lymphoma, unspecified, and anaplastic large T-cell lymphoma delineates novel recurrent chromosomal alterations. *Am J Pathol*. 2004;164(5):1837-1848.
280. Thompson MA, Stumph J, Henrickson SE, et al. Differential gene expression in anaplastic lymphoma kinase-positive and anaplastic lymphoma kinase-negative anaplastic large cell lymphomas. *Hum Pathol*. 2005;36(5):494-504.
281. Falini B, Pileri S, Zinzani PL, et al. ALK+ lymphoma: clinico-pathological findings and outcome. *Blood*. 1999;93(8):2697-2706.
282. Gascoyne RD, Aoun P, Wu D, et al. Prognostic significance of anaplastic lymphoma kinase (ALK) protein expression in adults with anaplastic large cell lymphoma. *Blood*. 1999;93(11):3913-3921.
283. Parrilla Castellar ER, Jaffe ES, Said JW, et al. ALK-negative anaplastic large cell lymphoma is a genetically heterogeneous disease with widely disparate clinical outcomes. *Blood*. 2014;124(9):1473-1480.
284. King RL, Dao LN, McPhail ED, et al. Morphologic features of ALK-negative anaplastic large cell lymphomas with DUSP22 rearrangements. *Am J Surg Pathol*. 2016;40(1):36-43.
285. Wada DA, Law ME, Hsi ED, et al. Specificity of IRF4 translocations for primary cutaneous anaplastic large cell lymphoma: a multicenter study of 204 skin biopsies. *Mod Pathol*. 2011;24(4):596-605.
286. Miranda RN, Aladily TN, Prince HM, et al. Breast implant-associated anaplastic large-cell lymphoma: long-term follow-up of 60 patients. *J Clin Oncol*. 2014;32(2):114-120.
287. Roden AC, Macon WR, Keeney GL, Myers JL, Feldman AL, Dogan A. Seroma-associated primary anaplastic large-cell lymphoma adjacent to breast implants: an indolent T-cell lymphoproliferative disorder. *Mod Pathol*. 2008;21(4):455-463.
288. de Jong D, Vasmel WL, de Boer JP, et al. Anaplastic large-cell lymphoma in women with breast implants. *J Am Med Assoc*. 2008;300(17):2030-2035.
289. Oishi N, Brody GS, Ketterling RP, et al. Genetic subtyping of breast implant-associated anaplastic large cell lymphoma. *Blood*. 2018;132(5):544-547.
290. Jaffe ES, Blattner WA, Blayney DW, et al. The pathologic spectrum of adult T-cell leukemia/lymphoma in the United States. Human T-cell leukemia/lymphoma virus-associated lymphoid malignancies. *Am J Surg Pathol*. 1984;8(4):263-275.
291. Yoshida M, Seiki M, Yamaguchi K, Takatsuki K. Monoclonal integration of human T-cell leukemia provirus in all primary tumors of adult T-cell leukemia suggests causative role of human T-cell leukemia virus in the disease. *Proc Natl Acad Sci U S A*. 1984;81(8):2534-2537.
292. Shimoyama M. Diagnostic criteria and classification of clinical subtypes of adult T-cell leukaemia-lymphoma. A report from the Lymphoma Study Group (1984-1987). *Br J Haematol*. 1991;79(3):428-437.
293. Karube K, Ohshima K, Tsuchiya T, et al. Expression of FoxP3, a key molecule in CD4CD25 regulatory T cells, in adult T-cell leukaemia/lymphoma cells. *Br J Haematol*. 2004;126(1):81-84.
294. Falini B, Flenghi L, Pileri S, et al. Distribution of T cells bearing different forms of the T cell receptor gamma/delta in normal and pathological human tissues. *J Immunol*. 1989;143(8):2480-2488.
295. Farcet JP, Gaulard P, Marolleau JP, et al. Hepatosplenic T-cell lymphoma: sinusal/sinusoidal localization of malignant cells expressing the T-cell receptor gamma delta. *Blood*. 1990;75(11):2213-2219.
296. Cooke CB, Krenacs L, Stetler-Stevenson M, et al. Hepatosplenic T-cell lymphoma: a distinct clinicopathologic entity of cytotoxic gamma delta T-cell origin. *Blood*. 1996;88(11):4265-4274.
297. Belhadj K, Reyes F, Farcet JP, et al. Hepatosplenic gammadelta T-cell lymphoma is a rare clinicopathologic entity with poor outcome: report on a series of 21 patients. *Blood*. 2003;102(13):4261-4269.
298. Shale M, Kanfer E, Panaccione R, Ghosh S. Hepatosplenic T cell lymphoma in inflammatory bowel disease. *Gut*. 2008;57(12):1639-1641.
299. Salhany KE, Feldman M, Kahn MJ, et al. Hepatosplenic gammadelta T-cell lymphoma: ultrastructural, immunophenotypic, and functional evidence for cytotoxic T lymphocyte differentiation. *Hum Pathol*. 1997;28(6):674-685.

300. Macon WR, Levy NB, Kurtin PJ, et al. Hepatosplenic alphabeta T-cell lymphomas: a report of 14 cases and comparison with hepatosplenic gammadelta T-cell lymphomas. *Am J Surg Pathol.* 2001;25(3):285-296.
301. Morice WG, Macon WR, Dogan A, Hanson CA, Kurtin PJ. NK-cell-associated receptor expression in hepatosplenic T-cell lymphoma, insights into pathogenesis. *Leukemia.* 2006;20(5):883-886.
302. McKinney M, Moffitt AB, Gaulard P, et al. The genetic basis of hepatosplenic T-cell lymphoma. *Cancer Discov.* 2017;7(4):369-379.
303. Travert M, Huang Y, de Leval L, et al. Molecular features of hepatosplenic T-cell lymphoma unravels potential novel therapeutic targets. *Blood.* 2012;119(24):5795-5806.
304. Gaulard P, Berti E, Willemze R, et al. Primary cutaneous peripheral T-cell lymphomas, rare subtypes. In: Swerdlow SH, Campo E, Harris NL, et al, eds. *World Health Organization Classification of Tumours. WHO Classification of Tumours of Haematopoietic and Lymphoid Tissues.* International Agency for Research on Cancer; 2017:397-402.
305. Gonzalez CL, Medeiros LJ, Braziel RM, Jaffe ES. T-cell lymphoma involving subcutaneous tissue. A clinicopathologic entity commonly associated with hemophagocytic syndrome. *Am J Surg Pathol.* 1991;15(1):17-27.
306. Mehregan DA, Su WP, Kurtin PJ. Subcutaneous T-cell lymphoma: a clinical, histopathologic, and immunohistochemical study of six cases. *J Cutan Pathol.* 1994;21(2):110-117.
307. Salhany KE, Macon WR, Choi JK, et al. Subcutaneous panniculitis-like T-cell lymphoma: clinicopathologic, immunophenotypic, and genotypic analysis of alpha/beta and gamma/delta subtypes. *Am J Surg Pathol.* 1998;22(7):881-893.
308. Egan LJ, Walsh SV, Stevens FM, Connolly CE, Egan EL, McCarthy CF. Celiac-associated lymphoma. A single institution experience of 30 cases in the combination chemotherapy era. *J Clin Gastroenterol.* 1995;21(2):123-129.
309. Moffitt AB, Ondrejka SL, McKinney M, et al. Enteropathy-associated T cell lymphoma subtypes are characterized by loss of function of SETD2. *J Exp Med.* 2017;214(5):1371-1386.
310. Isaacson PG. Relation between cryptic intestinal lymphoma and refractory sprue. *Lancet.* 2000;356(9225):178-179.
311. Bagdi E, Diss TC, Munson P, Isaacson PG. Mucosal intra-epithelial lymphocytes in enteropathy-associated T-cell lymphoma, ulcerative jejunitis, and refractory celiac disease constitute a neoplastic population. *Blood.* 1999;94(1):260-264.
312. Cellier C, Delabesse E, Helmer C, et al. Refractory sprue, coeliac disease, and enteropathy-associated T-cell lymphoma. French Coeliac Disease Study Group. *Lancet.* 2000;356(9225):203-208.
313. Ashton-Key M, Diss TC, Pan L, Du MQ, Isaacson PG. Molecular analysis of T-cell clonality in ulcerative jejunitis and enteropathy-associated T-cell lymphoma. *Am J Pathol.* 1997;151(2):493-498.
314. Zettl A, Ott G, Makulik A, et al. Chromosomal gains at 9q characterize enteropathy-type T-cell lymphoma. *Am J Pathol.* 2002;161(5):1635-1645.
315. Deleeuw RJ, Zettl A, Klinker E, et al. Whole-genome analysis and HLA genotyping of enteropathy-type T-cell lymphoma reveals 2 distinct lymphoma subtypes. *Gastroenterology.* 2007;132(5):1902-1911.
316. Kucuk C, Jiang B, Hu X, et al. Activating mutations of STAT5B and STAT3 in lymphomas derived from gammadelta-T or NK cells. *Nat Commun.* 2015;6:6025.
317. Tomita S, Kikuti YY, Carreras J, et al. Genomic and immunohistochemical profiles of enteropathy-associated T-cell lymphoma in Japan. *Mod Pathol.* 2015;28(10):1286-1296.
318. Suzumiya J, Takeshita M, Kimura N, et al. Expression of adult and fetal natural killer cell markers in sinonasal lymphomas. *Blood.* 1994;83(8):2255-2260.
319. Van Gorp J, De Bruin PC, Sie-Go DM, et al. Nasal T-cell lymphoma: a clinicopathological and immunophenotypic analysis of 13 cases. *Histopathology.* 1995;27(2):139-148.
320. Chiang AK, Srivastava G, Lau PW, Ho FC. Differences in T-cell-receptor gene rearrangement and transcription in nasal lymphomas of natural killer and T-cell types: implications on cellular origin. *Hum Pathol.* 1996;27(7):701-707.
321. Pongpruttipan T, Sukpanichnant S, Assanasen T, et al. Extranodal NK/T-cell lymphoma, nasal type, includes cases of natural killer cell and αβ, γδ, and αβ/γδ T-cell origin: a comprehensive clinicopathologic and phenotypic study. *Am J Surg Pathol.* 2012;36(4):481-499.
322. Petrella T, Delfau-Larue MH, Caillot D, et al. Nasopharyngeal lymphomas: further evidence for a natural killer cell origin. *Hum Pathol.* 1996;27(8):827-833.
323. Chan JK, Yip TT, Tsang WY, et al. Detection of Epstein-Barr viral RNA in malignant lymphomas of the upper aerodigestive tract. *Am J Surg Pathol.* 1994;18(9):938-946.
324. Huang Y, de Reynies A, de Leval L, et al. Gene expression profiling identifies emerging oncogenic pathways operating in extranodal NK/T-cell lymphoma, nasal type. *Blood.* 2010;115(6):1226-1237.
325. Wong KF, Chan JK, Ng CS, Lee KC, Tsang WY, Cheung MM. CD56 (NKH1)-positive hematolymphoid malignancies: an aggressive neoplasm featuring frequent cutaneous/mucosal involvement, cytoplasmic azurophilic granules, and angiocentricity. *Hum Pathol.* 1992;23(7):798-804.
326. Nakamura S, Suchi T, Koshikawa T, et al. Clinicopathologic study of CD56 (NCAM)-positive angiocentric lymphoma occurring in sites other than the upper and lower respiratory tract. *Am J Surg Pathol.* 1995;19(3):284-296.
327. Totonchi KF, Engel G, Weisenberg E, Rhone DP, Macon WR. Testicular natural killer/t-cell lymphoma, nasal type, of true natural killer-cell origin. *Arch Pathol Lab Med.* 2002;126(12):1527-1529.
328. Stein H, von Wasielewski R, Poppema S, MacLennan KA, Guenova M. Nodular sclerosis classical Hodgkin lymphoma. In: Swerdlow SH, Campo E, Harris NL, et al, eds. *World Health Organization Classification of Tumours. WHO Classification of Tumours of Haematopoietic and Lymphoid Tissues.* International Agency for Research on Cancer; 2008:330.
329. Doggett RS, Colby TV, Dorfman RF. Interfollicular Hodgkin's disease. *Am J Surg Pathol.* 1983;7(2):145-149.
330. Diehl V, Klimm B, Re D. Hodgkin lymphoma. A curable disease: what comes next? *Eur J Haematol Suppl.* 2005;(66):6-13.
331. Kapatai G, Murray P. Contribution of the Epstein Barr virus to the molecular pathogenesis of Hodgkin lymphoma. *J Clin Pathol.* 2007;60(12):1342-1349.
332. Herndier BG, Sanchez HC, Chang KL, Chen YY, Weiss LM. High prevalence of Epstein-Barr virus in the Reed-Sternberg cells of HIV-associated Hodgkin's disease. *Am J Pathol.* 1993;142(4):1073-1079.
333. Shimabukuro-Vornhagen A, Haverkamp H, Engert A, et al. Lymphocyte-rich classical Hodgkin's lymphoma: clinical presentation and treatment outcome in 100 patients treated within German Hodgkin's Study Group trials. *J Clin Oncol.* 2005;23(24):5739-5745.
334. Diehl V, Sextro M, Franklin J, et al. Clinical presentation, course, and prognostic factors in lymphocyte-predominant Hodgkin's disease and lymphocyte-rich classical Hodgkin's disease: report from the European Task Force on Lymphoma Project on Lymphocyte-Predominant Hodgkin's Disease. *J Clin Oncol.* 1999;17(3):776-783.
335. Benkharroch D, Stein H, Peh SC. Lymphocyte-depleted classical Hodgkin lymphoma. In: Swerdlow S, Campo E, Harris N, et al, eds. *WHO Classification of Tumours of Haematopoietic and Lymphoid Tissues.* IARC; 2008:334.
336. Glaser SL, Clarke CA, Gulley ML, et al. Population-based patterns of human immunodeficiency virus-related Hodgkin lymphoma in the Greater San Francisco Bay Area, 1988-1998. *Cancer.* 2003;98(2):300-309.
337. Kanzler H, Kuppers R, Hansmann ML, Rajewsky K. Hodgkin and Reed-Sternberg cells in Hodgkin's disease represent the outgrowth of a dominant tumor clone derived from (crippled) germinal center B cells. *J Exp Med.* 1996;184(4):1495-1505.
338. Garcia-Cosio M, Santon A, Martin P, et al. Analysis of transcription factor OCT.1, OCT.2 and BOB.1 expression using tissue arrays in classical Hodgkin's lymphoma. *Mod Pathol.* 2004;17(12):1531-1538.
339. Natkunam Y, Hsi ED, Aoun P, et al. Expression of the human germinal center-associated lymphoma (HGAL) protein identifies a subset of classic Hodgkin lymphoma of germinal center derivation and improved survival. *Blood.* 2007;109(1):298-305.
340. Shams TM. High expression of LMO2 in Hodgkin, Burkitt and germinal center diffuse large B cell lymphomas. *J Egypt Natl Cancer Inst.* 2011;23(4):147-153.
341. Deacon EM, Pallesen G, Niedobitek G, et al. Epstein-Barr virus and Hodgkin's disease: transcriptional analysis of virus latency in the malignant cells. *J Exp Med.* 1993;177(2):339-349.
342. Kuppers R, Rajewsky K, Zhao M, et al. Hodgkin disease: Hodgkin and Reed-Sternberg cells picked from histological sections show clonal immunoglobulin gene rearrangements and appear to be derived from B cells at various stages of development. *Proc Natl Acad Sci U S A.* 1994;91(23):10962-10966.
343. Bargou RC, Emmerich F, Krappmann D, et al. Constitutive nuclear factor-kappaB-RelA activation is required for proliferation and survival of Hodgkin's disease tumor cells. *J Clin Invest.* 1997;100(12):2961-2969.
344. Steidl C, Connors JM, Gascoyne RD. Molecular pathogenesis of Hodgkin's lymphoma: increasing evidence of the importance of the microenvironment. *J Clin Oncol.* 2011;29(14):1812-1826.
345. Bair SM, Strelec LE, Feldman TA, et al. Outcomes and toxicities of programmed death-1 (PD-1) inhibitors in Hodgkin lymphoma patients in the United States: a real-World, multicenter retrospective analysis. *Oncol.* 2019;24(7):955-962.
346. Armand P, Engert A, Younes A, et al. Nivolumab for relapsed/refractory classic Hodgkin lymphoma after failure of Autologous hematopoietic cell transplantation: Extended follow-up of the multicohort single-arm phase II checkmate 205 trial. *J Clin Oncol.* 2018;36(14):1428-1439.
347. Hansmann ML, Fellbaum C, Hui PK, Moubayed P. Progressive transformation of germinal centers with and without association to Hodgkin's disease. *Am J Clin Pathol.* 1990;93:219-226.
348. Ferry JA, Zukerberg LR, Harris WL. Florid progressive transformation of germinal centers: a syndrome affecting young men without early progression to nodular lymphocyte predominance Hodgkin's disease. *Am J Surg Pathol.* 1992;16:252-258.
349. Hartmann S, Eichenauer DA, Plutschow A, et al. The prognostic impact of variant histology in nodular lymphocyte-predominant Hodgkin lymphoma: a report from the German Hodgkin Study Group (GHSG). *Blood.* 2013;122(26):4246-4252, quiz 4292.
350. Hartmann S, Doring C, Jakobus C, et al. Nodular lymphocyte predominant hodgkin lymphoma and T cell/histiocyte rich large B cell lymphoma – endpoints of a spectrum of one disease? *PLoS One.* 2013;8(11):e78812.
351. Harris NL. Shades of gray between large B-cell lymphomas and Hodgkin lymphomas: differential diagnosis and biological implications. *Mod Pathol.* 2013;26(suppl 1):S57-S70.
352. Hansmann ML, Stein H, Fellbaum C, Hui PK, Parwaresch MR, Lennert K. Nodular paragranuloma can transform into high-grade malignant lymphoma of B type. *Hum Pathol.* 1989;20:1169-1175.
353. Cotta CV, Coleman JF, Li S, Hsi ED. Nodular lymphocyte predominant Hodgkin lymphoma and diffuse large B-cell lymphoma: a study of six cases concurrently involving the same site. *Histopathology.* 2011;59(6):1194-1203.
354. McCune RC, Syrbu SI, Vasef MA. Expression profiling of transcription factors Pax-5, Oct-1, Oct-2, BOB.1, and PU.1 in Hodgkin's and non-Hodgkin's lymphomas: a comparative study using high throughput tissue microarrays. *Mod Pathol.* 2006;19(7):1010-1018.
355. Prakash S, Fountaine T, Raffeld M, Jaffe ES, Pittaluga S. IgD positive L&H cells identify a unique subset of nodular lymphocyte predominant Hodgkin lymphoma. *Am J Surg Pathol.* 2006;30(5):585-592.
356. Wlodarska I, Nooyen P, Maes B, et al. Frequent occurrence of BCL6 rearrangements in nodular lymphocyte predominance Hodgkin lymphoma but not in classical Hodgkin lymphoma. *Blood.* 2003;101(2):706-710.
357. Schumacher MA, Schmitz R, Brune V, et al. Mutations in the genes coding for the NF-κB regulating factors IκBα and A20 are uncommon in nodular lymphocyte-predominant Hodgkin's lymphoma. *Haematologica.* 2010;95(1):153-157.

Chapter 89 ■ Molecular Genetic Aspects of Non-Hodgkin Lymphomas

ANNETTE S. KIM • SCOTT B. LOVITCH • MARK A. MURAKAMI

INTRODUCTION

The lymphomas are a diverse group of mature lymphoid neoplasms with a wide range of cellular morphologies, histologic presentations, clinical presentations, cells of origin, etiologies, and responses to therapy. Owing to the protean manifestations, lymphomas remain a significant diagnostic challenge for hematopathologists. In fact, using morphology alone, the interpathologist consensus is 41% to 93%, depending on the diagnosis.[1] This lack of consensus is especially true of the T-cell lymphomas, which are even more varied in presentation than their B-cell counterparts. Incorporation of clinical history and immunophenotyping can improve the consensus, but pathognomonic diagnostic clues are often missing. Accordingly, molecular genetic findings are playing an ever-increasing role in the assessment of lymphomas.

The non-Hodgkin lymphomas (NHLs) represent 4.3% of all cancers with an overall annual incidence of 19.4/100,000 in the United States in 2018 (Figure 89.1), making it the sixth most common cancer in both males and females.[2-5] Despite their relatively high frequency in clinical practice, the NHLs have defied numerous attempts to classify them. Early classification schemes relied heavily upon morphology. However, as the classification of acute leukemias moved to emphasize the cell of origin, so too did lymphoma classifications attempt to identify a cell of origin and stage of maturation.

In fact, the researchers of the NHLs were pioneers in the discovery of molecular genetic underpinnings of hematolymphoid malignancies. The first reciprocal translocations that caused tumorigenesis were identified in 1958 in Burkitt lymphoma (BL), translocations involving the *MYC* oncogene.[6] These were followed in 1984 by the discovery of the t(14;18) in follicular lymphoma (FL).[7] However, overall the NHLs have lagged behind their leukemia counterparts in the identification of the molecular genetic causes of neoplasia. Although there is a wealth of new information on the molecular findings in NHLs, the World Health Organization classification scheme still largely relies upon cell of origin as the primary discriminator of the B-cell NHLs,[5,8,9] and T-cell lymphomas are even less well understood in general, with many of the classifications defined by the site of the tumor.[2,5] Cytogenetic and molecular genetic changes in NHLs, although often associated with a given type of lymphoma, cross diagnostic boundaries with few that are pathognomonic of a specific entity.[5,10,11]

However, new efforts in next-generation sequencing (NGS) and mutational analysis in general are elucidating new markers of disease. It is possible, however, that disease classification in the future of NHL will not be defined by single molecular aberrations but by pathways of dysregulation, which may be the focus of targeted therapeutics. Therefore, more global methods of assessing molecular genetic aberrations are becoming central in the diagnosis, prognosis, and treatment strategies for NHLs in the years to come.

OVERVIEW OF METHODOLOGIES

Commonly Used Techniques

One of the mainstays of molecular testing in lymphoid malignancies is the use of clonality testing. These methods are based upon the unique rearrangement of either the B-cell receptor (BCR), composed of an immunoglobulin (Ig) heavy chain and one of two light chains, or the T-cell receptor (TCR), heterodimers of either α/β subunits or γ/δ subunits. However, there are other recurrent reciprocal translocations that can also be assessed by polymerase chain reaction (PCR), quantitative real-time polymerase chain reaction (q-PCR), fluorescent in situ hybridization (FISH), or metaphase cytogenetics (MC). The latter two methodologies can also identify other structural or numeric aberrations as well. Lastly, the availability of NGS has led to the identification of many somatic alterations that may aid in the diagnosis, prognosis, disease monitoring, and therapy decision support. Gene naming conventions throughout the chapter follow the nomenclature recommendations set forth by the HUGO Gene Nomenclature Committee.[12] In addition, recurrent hotspot somatic variants will be referred to by their more well-known protein changes (p. nomenclature) rather than cDNA or gDNA changes (c. nomenclature) but are meant to encompass their DNA-level changes.

Clonality Testing

Immunoglobulin Gene Rearrangements

The expression of Ig is one of the defining characteristics of all mature B cells. At the earliest stages of B-cell ontogeny, recombination of the Ig heavy chain (IGH) can be detected, well before the expression of the complete heterotetrameric product composed of two heavy chains and two light chains on the surface of the B cell, where the light chain can be either kappa or lambda (Figure 89.2). The IGH locus on chromosome 14q32, the kappa locus (IGK) at 2p11, and the lambda locus (IGL) at 22q11 are all structured in a similar fashion to enable the unique somatic recombination of germline gene segments that create the antigen specificity of the final Ig protein heterotetramer. During this recombination process, individual variable regions (V regions), joining regions (J regions), and constant regions (C regions) are selected, which form the body of the final Ig chain and contribute to the antigen specificity. In addition, the IGH locus also contains diversity regions (D regions), for a final VDJC rearrangement (vs VJC for the light chains).[13]

Each gene segment is marked for potential recombination by a recombination signal sequence, which is acted upon by the recombination-activating genes 1 and 2 to create double-stranded DNA breaks that are recombined through nonhomologous end joining, with assistance from the DNA-bending proteins, HMG1 and HMG2. The D-J recombination is the first rearrangement of the IGH locus, followed by V-DJ and VDJ-C. At each recombination site, these double-stranded breaks can be further modified by being filled in with palindromic nucleotide insertions (P nucleotides), removal of one to two nucleotides through a random exonuclease activity, or further varied by the addition of N nucleotides that are not templated in the germline sequence through terminal deoxynucleotidyl transferase. These actions also contribute to the diversity of the Igs. The cut and modified ends of the coding sequence are then also repaired by nonhomologous end joining.[13]

The variable regions of all the Ig proteins form a canonical beta-sheet structure, which necessarily means that the majority of amino acids are paradoxically highly conserved.[14] These conserved regions are termed the framework regions, FR1-3 (Figure 89.3). Between these framework regions are the truly variable complementary determining regions (CDRs1-3), which encode sequences of approximately 10 amino acids that project from the tips of the beta-sheet as fingers reaching out to contact antigen. Therefore, although the IGH gene contains up to 200 different V regions (approximately 80 of which are widely used in human biology),[13] consensus primers can be constructed against the V regions that will permit the amplification of the gene across the VDJ recombination sites by PCR. Owing to the variability of the encompassed CDRs as well as the diversity created by the random exonuclease activity and N nucleotide addition, physiologic B cells should each have a distinctively sized PCR product and clonal populations should have identically sized PCR products. This forms the basis of the Ig gene rearrangement studies by PCR and

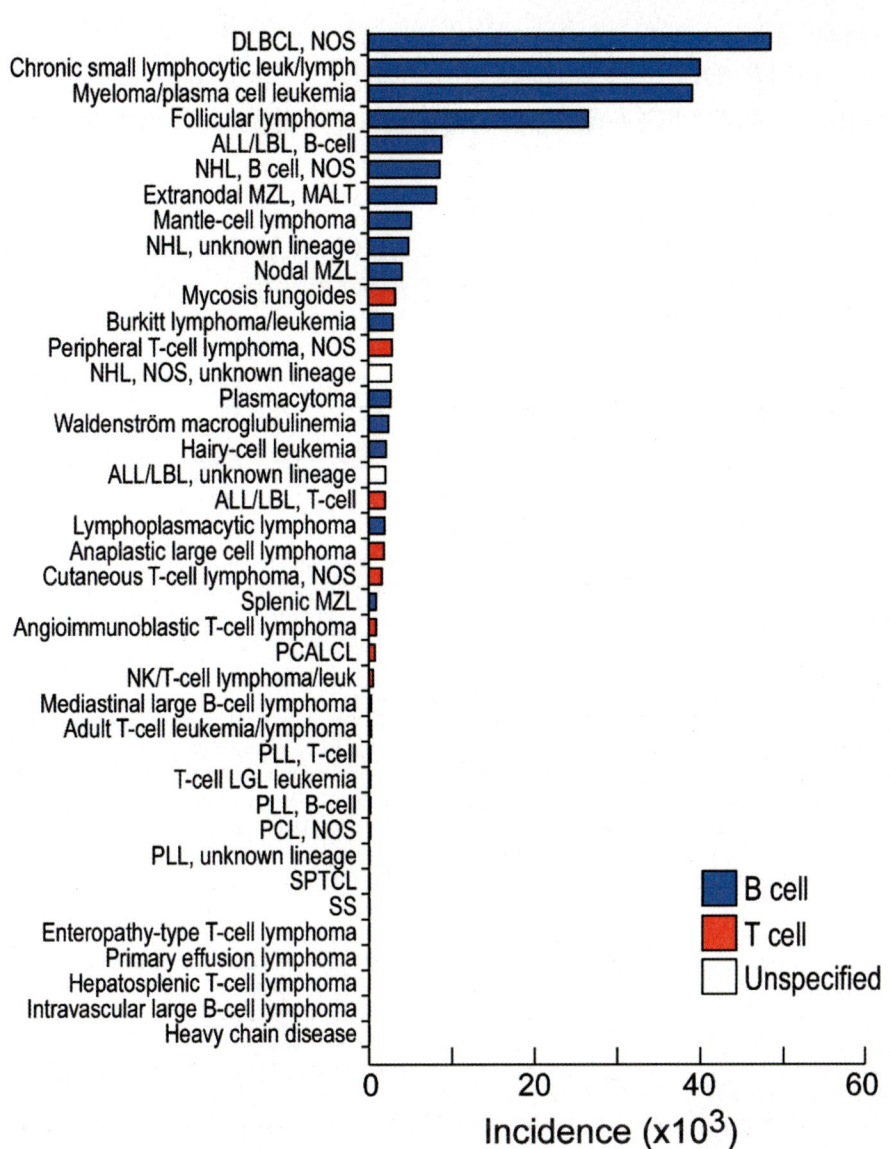

FIGURE 89.1 Surveillance epidemiology and end result (SEER) data for the incidence of non-Hodgkin lymphomas (blue, B-cell neoplasms; red, T-cell neoplasms; white, unspecified). (From Howlader N, Noone AM, Krapcho M, et al, eds. *SEER Cancer Statistics Review, 1975 to 2013.* 2016.)

NGS. Southern blot methods, which look for the unique rearrangements on unamplified DNA, have been considered the gold standard for gene rearrangement studies but have fallen into disuse with the ease of PCR-based methods and now NGS and will not be discussed further.

PCR primers may be constructed against any of the three framework regions. FR1 amplicons are longest of the three and may not be amplifiable when using formalin-fixed paraffin-embedded (FPPE) tissues that have undergone shearing during preservation (*Figure 89.3*). Indeed, it is critical for the assay to include sample amplification controls up to 400 bp in length if interrogating FR1 to ensure that the DNA is of adequate length/quality for PCR. Therefore, some laboratories choose to use only FR3 primers (coupled with J region primers) or a combination of FR3 and FR2 primers that have average sizes typically of 125 and 265 bp, respectively, using the frequently used BIOMED-2 primers.[15] However, somatic hypermutation (SHM), a normal physiologic process of the germinal center that can prevent the binding of individual primers should a mutation occur in the targeted "consensus" sequence, can limit the clinical sensitivity of limited sets of primers to detect clonal populations of B cells.[8,14] SHM may also result in unusually large amplicon sizes when SHM prevents reverse priming from the first available J region and switches to a later J. However, several commercial kits are now available that utilize multiplexed sets of primers against all the FRs, in the hopes that at least one primer will have an intact unmutated sequence to permit amplification of the unique PCR product.[15-18] In addition, primers against IGK and IGL can also be utilized, although the PCR products do not form a well-dispersed Gaussian distribution as in the case of the IGH assay, complicating their interpretation.[15]

Table 89.1 shows the range of clinical detection rates (clinical sensitivity) of multiplexed IGH PCR assays compiled from several published papers.[16-18] These data clearly demonstrate the high clinical detection rates for neoplasms of pre-germinal center B cells (pre-GCBs). However, the gene rearrangement assays have a lower clinical sensitivity for neoplasms of post-GCB cells and particularly of germinal center lesions, during which active SHM may be ongoing.[8,18] Therefore, combinations of primers of all three frameworks of IGH and for IGK are required to ensure reasonable clinical sensitivity across all B-cell neoplasms.[16-18] On the other hand, the detection of an apparently clonal population does not equate with neoplasia, as pseudoclonality can be seen in reactive conditions with a strong reaction to a particular antigen, or in cases of a limited B-cell repertoire.

Analytical sensitivity of the IGH PCR assay depends upon the number of polytypic background B cells. In cases of significant numbers of background polytypic B cells, the detection of a clonal peak rising above the Gaussian distribution of background B-cell rearrangements can achieve only 5% analytical sensitivity, although 1% can be reached in the absence of a polyclonal background (*Figure 89.4*). The

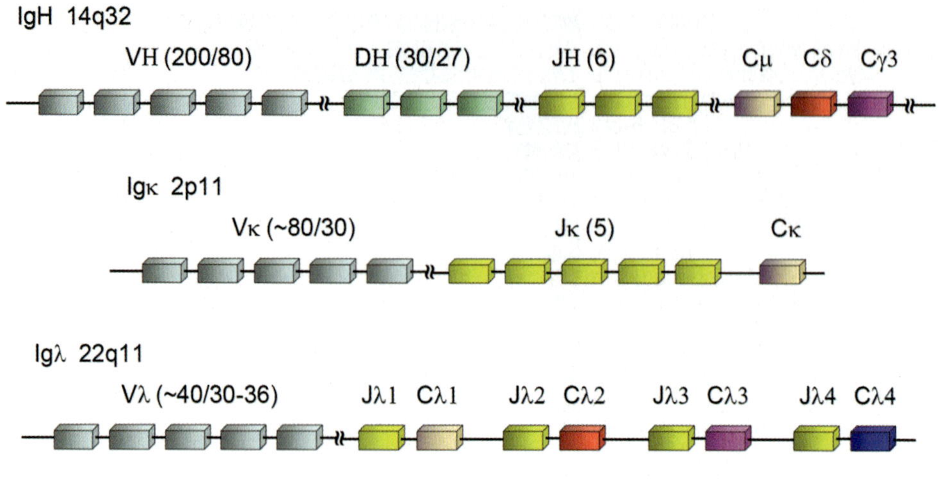

FIGURE 89.2 Immunoglobulin genes and their chromosomal organization. The number of subunits of each type (V, D, or J) is noted in parentheses as follows: total number of subunits/number of subunits in physiologic use.

analytical sensitivity can be increased by the design of allele-specific oligonucleotide (ASO) primers. However, this technique requires sequencing of the patient's specific clonal Ig rearrangement.

Deep sequencing through NGS methods has been clinically validated to detect rearrangements without allele-specific primers and has been developed as a method to determine clonality and to monitor measurable residual disease (MRD).[19,20] Commercial NGS methods for immunoglobulin gene rearrangements include DNA-based multiplex PCR method and, less commonly, RNA-based methods.[21] As with capillary electrophoresis, multiplexed primers can be generated against the leader region (upstream of FR1), FR1, 2, or 3, or combinations thereof as well as against the J region. Owing to the size of the leader amplicons, these primers require sequencing longer read lengths and are not amenable to use in FFPE tissue. NGS identifies clonal populations by sequence rather than by size and accordingly can readily identify clonal populations, even when they occur at a common size. Concordance is excellent with CE methods (96%-97% concordance when using FR1 or combined FR1/2/3 primers) with more clonal populations detected by NGS for the aforementioned reasons.[22] Owing to the ability to include heavily multiplexed primers and leader primers, SHM becomes less of an issue and clinical sensitivity can approach greater than 95% with just leader and FR1 primers, even with neoplasms such as FL and plasma cell neoplasms.[22] Analytically, NGS has the potential to detect extremely low levels of MRD, limited only by the prior knowledge of the clonal sequence and the expense of deep sequencing. Comparisons of NGS vs other MRD methods in B-cell precursor lymphoblastic leukemia (B-ALL) demonstrate 90% concordance with multiparametric flow cytometry and 96% concordance of ASO-PCR with NGS proving more analytically sensitive than flow cytometry in all discordant cases and in all but one case with ASO-PCR.[19,23] The utility of this method has also been demonstrated in mature B-cell neoplasms including plasma cell myeloma (MM) and chronic lymphocytic leukemia (CLL) with statistically significant stratification of disease-free survival in patients based upon MRD status by NGS IGH sequencing.[24,25] Circulating tumor DNA (ctDNA) monitoring of IGH gene rearrangements has also been to be clinically prognostic in diffuse large B-cell lymphoma (DLBCL) and FL but requires specific methods for error correction to detect such low levels of the rearrangements.[26,27] NGS can also be used to assign the V, D, and J subtypes and provide a SHM quantification.[28]

T-cell Gene Rearrangements

The TCR is a heterodimer of two proteins that form the functional receptor, either $\alpha\beta$ or $\gamma\delta$. During T-cell ontogeny, the γ (TRG) and δ (TRD) genes tend to rearrange first, so that the $\gamma\delta$ receptor is typically the first to be expressed. Subsequently the α (TRA) and β (TRB) genes rearrange, and ultimately 85% to 98% of mature peripheral T cells express the $\alpha\beta$ receptor.[19,29] Since the δ locus is embedded within the α gene on chromosome 14q11, the subsequent rearrangement of the α gene results in excision of the δ gene from the cell's DNA (*Figure 89.5*). However, the β and γ loci, although both on chromosome 7, are distinct (7q34 and 7p15, respectively), and the rearrangement of the γ loci is retained in $\alpha\beta$ T cells.

Like the immunoglobulin genes, the TCR genes are composed of V, D (β and δ genes only), J, and C regions (*Figure 89.5*). In contrast, there are no specific framework regions. Therefore, except for homology between a few of the V regions, separate V region primers are required to assess all physiologically relevant *TCR* gene rearrangements. Owing to the location of the *d* gene within the *a* gene, which limits its utility, the limited number of γ gene V regions (only Vγ1-11 are physiologically relevant of the 15 Vγ segments),[30] and the homology between the Vγ segments 1 to 8, which allows the use of a common primer for those segments, typically TRG is the common target of most clinical assays, with or without the addition of TRB assessment as well. While amplification controls, particularly for FFPE tissue, are important, they are not as critical as for the IGH assay since the target amplicons are typically smaller than 260 bp.[15]

The clinical sensitivity of the TRG assay is higher than for the corresponding Ig assay due to the absence of SHM of the TCR. However, the assay still does not detect 100% of all neoplastic rearrangements due to other acquired mutations, and the true clinical sensitivity is approximately 89% to 94%.[16,18,31,32] In cases of a known neoplastic

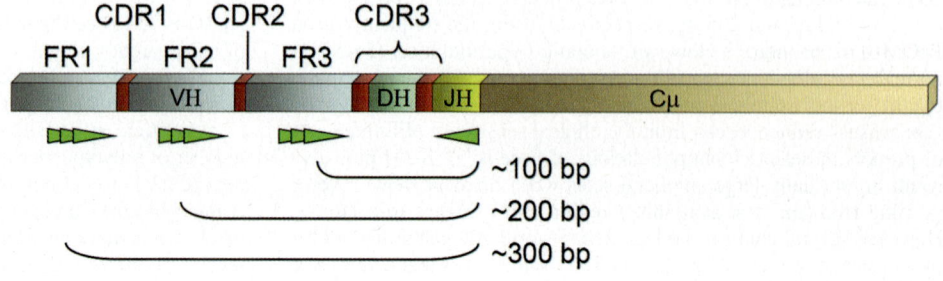

FIGURE 89.3 Schematic of an immunoglobulin gene rearrangement assay. Shown are the framework regions (FR1-3, light blue), complementary determining regions (CDRs, red; note CDR3 is composed of the DH region and the flanking variable junctions created by random exonuclease activity and N and P nucleotide insertions), and representations of potential locations of primers in the FRs noted (*bright green*). General sizes of polymerase chain reaction products are indicated.

Table 89.1. Clinical Sensitivities of the Immunoglobulin Gene Rearrangement Studies

Method	MCL	CLL	FL	DLBCL	MZL
IGH FR1	100	95-100	30-73	50-68	48-73
IGH FR2	98-100	91-100	30-76	58-61	66-85
IGH FR3	96-100	93-100	13-52	50	62-68
IGH FR1-3	100	100	37-84	79-88	86-88
IGK	75-94	96-100	60-63	58-61	62-68
IGK$_{de}$	50-75	61-67	57-59	46-58	48-54
all IGK	100	100	80-84	75-80	69-83
IGL	44-75	30-44	21-23	8-28	28-29
IGH FR1-3 and all IGK	100	100	100	96-98	95-100

Abbreviations: CLL, chronic lymphocytic leukemia; DLBCL, diffuse large B-cell lymphoma; FL, follicular lymphoma; IGH, immunoglobulin heavy chain; IGK, immunoglobulin kappa locus; IGL, immunoglobulin lambda locus; MCL, mantle cell lymphoma; MZL, marginal zone lymphoma.

From van Dongen JJ, Langerak AW, Bruggemann M, et al. Design and standardization of PCR primers and protocols for detection of clonal immunoglobulin and T-cell receptor gene recombinations in suspect lymphoproliferations: report of the BIOMED-2 Concerted Action BMH4-CT98-3936. *Leukemia*. 2003;17(12):2257-2317; Liu H, Bench AJ, Bacon CM, et al. A practical strategy for the routine use of BIOMED-2 PCR assays for detection of B- and T-cell clonality in diagnostic haematopathology. *Br J Haematol*. 2007;138(1):31-43; Evans PA, Pott C, Groenen PJ, et al. Significantly improved PCR-based clonality testing in B-cell malignancies by use of multiple immunoglobulin gene targets. Report of the BIOMED-2 Concerted Action BHM4-CT98-3936. *Leukemia*. 2007;21(2):207-214.

T-cell process, TRB assay can also be used to look for a clonal marker of disease. The analytical sensitivity of the TCR clonality assays is similar to that of the immunoglobulin assays, although for biologic reasons limited T-cell repertoires and use of the less common V9, V10, or V11 regions (compared with the V1-8 regions) can often lead to pseudoclonality or oligoclonality in certain tissues (such as skin), making it easy to overcall or undercall TCR clonality results.

NGS methods have also been developed for diagnostic and MRD purposes for the assessment of T-cell clonality.[19,20] NGS provides better clinical sensitivity and quantification of the clone frequency, which can be prognostically significant in diseases such as mycosis fungoides.[33,34] NGS has also been used in MRD assessment in T-cell precursor lymphoblastic leukemia (T-ALL) and has proven to be 10- to 100-fold more sensitive than multiparametric flow cytometry.[35] MRD can in theory be applied to other T-cell neoplasms as well, both in blood and in ctDNA, but is a less mature field than in the B-cell neoplasms.

Polymerase Chain Reaction

PCR is a commonly used method for template amplification due to its ease, versatility, and analytical sensitivity. The achievable levels of amplification are such that as few as 1 neoplastic cell can be detected out of 10^5 to 10^7 cells (0.001% to 0.00001% analytical sensitivity). Amplification also permits the use of this assay in small sample volumes. In addition, if the size of the targeted amplicon (product of the PCR reaction) is small, even partially sheared DNA, such as that obtained from FFPE tissue, is adequate for the assay. The high sensitivity of the assay also makes it ideal for the detection of MRD.

In this assay, forward and reverse primers (typically 15-25 bp in length) are generated against the target region. These primers may be specific for a mutated vs wild-type sequence (ASO) or may flank the area of interest (especially flanking areas of small insertions or deletions or flanking a translocation site) if there is a size difference in the mutant amplicon. If compatible conditions can be designed for multiple sets of primers, the PCR assay can be multiplexed. The template can consist of genomic DNA or mRNA that has been reverse transcribed into clonal DNA (cDNA).

PCR products, or amplicons, can be detected in several different ways. *Qualitative detection methods* include agarose gel electrophoresis and capillary electrophoresis, both of which allow the separation of amplicons by size. In the latter method, fluorescently tagged primers are used, which allows separation of the amplicons along the capillary tube and detection using a fluorescent camera as the separated products exit the tube. By using multiple different fluorophores on each primer set, even multiplexed assays can be analyzed by this method.

Quantitative detection methods can also be used, typically involving some version of q-PCR. In this technique, fluorescence is directly proportional to the amount of amplicon generated. This fluorescence can be generated by the intercalation of a fluorescent dye, such as SYBR green, or can be continuously generated during each cycle of amplification by the release of fluorescence during the extension step (e.g., TaqMan probes). Using premade dilutions of the desired amplicon to generate a standard curve, direct quantitation of the amount of the target in the sample can be made.

Fluorescent In Situ Hybridization

FISH is another molecular method of interrogating genomic aberrations. FISH utilizes longer probes than PCR (typically 200-400 bp in length), which bind in a complementary sequence-specific fashion to the intact chromatin of interphase cells.[36] FISH is commonly used to identify balanced translocations and can also identify copy number variations (CNVs) of large segments of chromatin. In the former case, both fusion probes (directed against both translocation partners) and break-apart probes (probes located adjacent to each other on either side of the putative breakpoint in the one known translocation partner) can be utilized (*Figure 89.6*), depending on the promiscuity of the known partner(s).

FISH, like PCR, is necessarily targeted and therefore biased by the subjective nature of which probes are selected for study (*Table 89.2*). Unlike PCR, FISH has low resolution of the sites of aberrancy, in the range of 2 to 5 kb (kilobase pairs).[36] The analytical sensitivity depends upon the nature of the probes utilized in the assay and the number of interphases assessed. However, typical analytical sensitivities range from 1% to 5% for 200 interphase cells evaluated. Translocations may be detected in FFPE samples (especially using fusion probes) as well as copy number gains, but FISH is not as sensitive for copy number losses in FFPE due to partial sectioning of the cell nuclei. Nevertheless, FISH remains a mainstay in the identification of genetic aberrances in lymphoid lesions due to the variety of breakpoints and translocation partners in these malignancies, which often limit the use of the highly targeted PCR methods.

Metaphase Cytogenetics

Conventional karyotyping, based upon MC, is a mainstay in hematopathology due to its unbiased and uniform genome-wide coverage (*Table 89.2*). Owing to the requirement to culture the cells to obtain metaphase spreads and the time-consuming microscopy to generate the karyotypes, the method takes several days. In addition, terminally differentiated cells, such as mature lymphocytes and plasma cells, do not readily undergo mitosis, and stimulation to induce mitoses may be required.[37,38]

The resolution of MC is low, 5 to 10 Mb (megabase pairs).[39] In addition, owing to the need to construct the individual karyotypes manually, even with the aid of computers, typically only 20 metaphases are examined, and the analytical sensitivity is therefore only approximately 10% (for balanced translocations, 2 of 20 metaphases must demonstrate the same abnormality for it to be considered a clonal change, and 3 metaphases must demonstrate the same CNV for it to be considered clonal).[40] Thus, this methodology is of limited utility in MRD testing and often is not helpful for lymphoid neoplasms with routine culture conditions.

Other Techniques
Somatic Hypermutation

SHM testing can be used both to identify clonal rearrangements of the IGH gene and to calculate the percent of nucleotides that have undergone SHM in the V regions of IGH. This assay has been used to understand the biology of many B-cell neoplasms but is standard of care for CLL/small lymphocytic lymphoma (SLL). Typically, a cutoff of 98% homology to germline is used to determine the mutational status, with

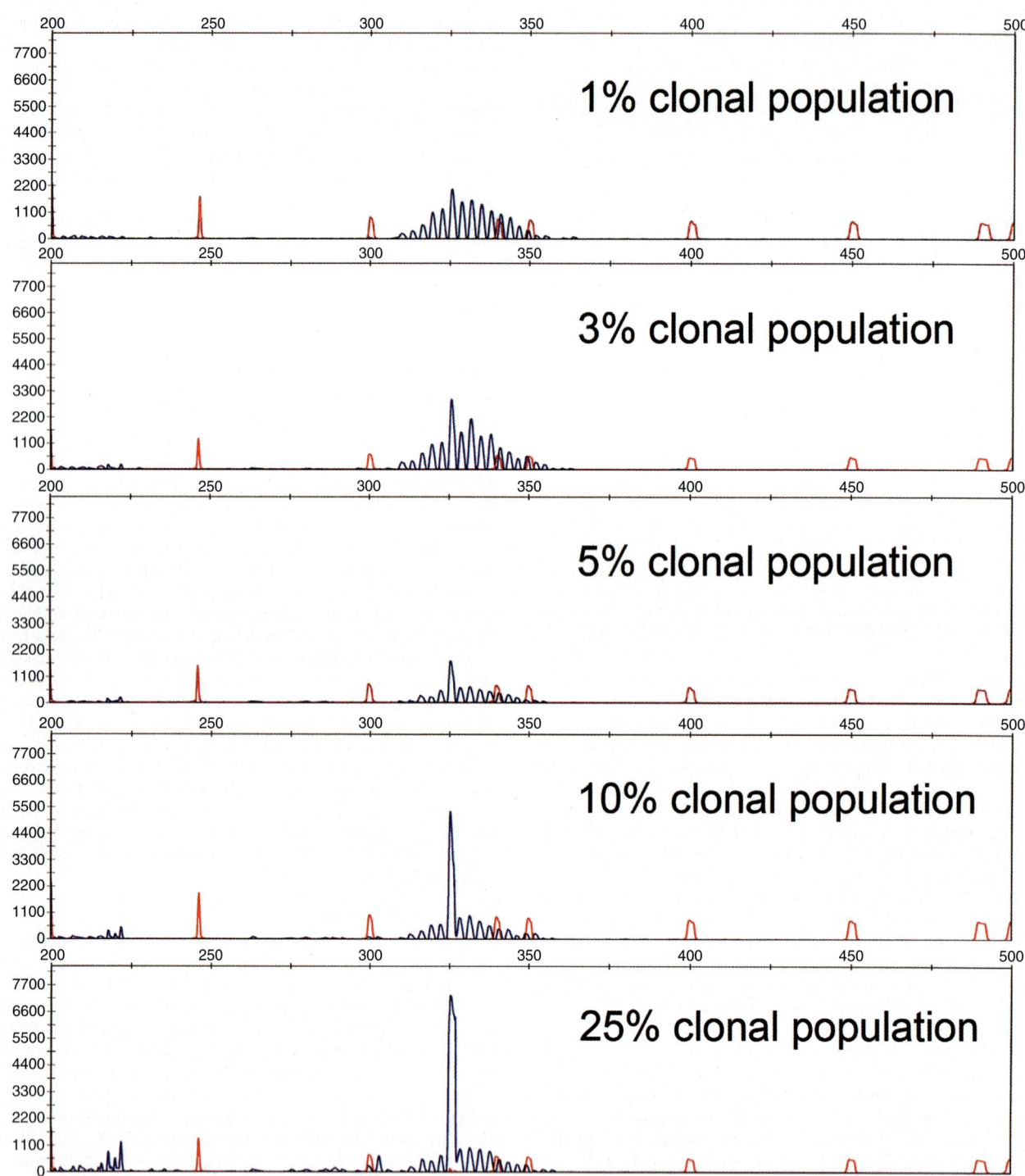

FIGURE 89.4 Analytical sensitivity of immunoglobulin gene rearrangement studies as illustrated by dilutions of a clonal population into a polyclonal background.

greater than 98% homology corresponding to the unmutated designation, which carries a poor prognosis in CLL.[41,42]

In SHM testing, typically FR1 primers or leader primers are used in conjunction with partner J_H primers.[43] PCR can be performed on either genomic DNA (gDNA) or cDNA and is best performed with more than one primer set to avoid false-negative results due to SHM. Utilization of gDNA is the easiest to perform since it involves the isolation of the more stable DNA from the samples and avoids a requisite reverse transcription step. However, cDNA is better for the identification of function rearrangements as well as double in-frame small insertions and deletions (indels) and Ig isotype assignment. After PCR, the amplicons can then be directly Sanger sequenced or can be cloned into a plasmid and then sequenced (to remove background polyclonal B cells). SHM testing can also be performed by NGS, which is rapidly becoming the method of choice. In either method, the bioinformatic alignment provides the percentage identity to germline as well as simultaneously provides the immunoglobulin family and subtype that are prognostically critical in several B-cell neoplasms. Care is required to align to the most up-to-date reference sequences and determine if the rearrangement is productive or not.

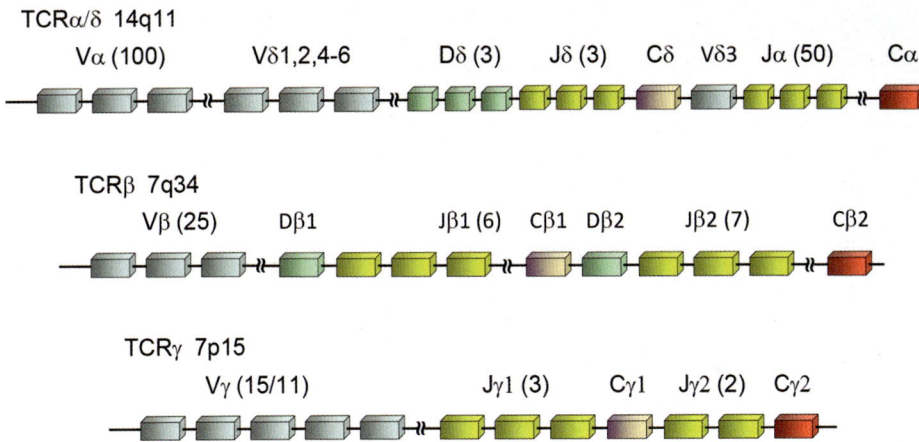

FIGURE 89.5 **T-cell receptor genes.** The number of subunits of each type (V, D, or J) is noted in parentheses as follows: total number of subunits/number of subunits in physiologic use.

Array Comparative Genomic Hybridization and Array Single Nucleotide Polymorphism

CGH was initially developed as a method to identify CNVs in patient tissues. The methodology is based upon the differential labeling of patient and control DNA, followed by competitively hybridizing those labeled samples to metaphase spreads. Areas of deletions would be seen as regions with a predominance of the control DNA fluorophore, whereas areas of duplications show a predominance of the patient DNA fluorophore. Owing to the limitations of metaphase spreads, the array format was developed to contain an array of probes that span the genome (*Figure 89.7*). The probes for array comparative genomic hybridization (aCGH) can be obtained from bacterial artificial chromosome–derived sequences, cDNA, or from oligonucleotides. Using this method, CNVs and unbalanced translocations can be interrogated uniformly throughout the genome at a resolution as low as 5 to 6 kb (kilobase pairs) in some cases (*Table 89.2*).[39,44,45] The analytical sensitivity varies from 2% to 30%.

By contrast, aSNP (array single nucleotide polymorphisms) is a single-color experiment that hybridizes labeled patient DNA or amplicons to an array composed of probes that are sequence specific to interrogate individual SNPs. Because these are designed to target specific SNPs at their nonrandom genomic locations, the genome coverage is not uniform and this method is not useful in identifying balanced translocations or in distinguishing germline from somatic changes.[39,44] However, aSNP is especially useful in the identification of copy neutral loss of heterozygosity (LOH) and uniparental disomy that are not assessed by aCGH. Analytical sensitivities are similar to those for aCGH. To leverage the advantages of both aSNP and aCGH, many commercial platforms are now available that combine the two array methods.

Owing to the challenges of obtaining metaphases in lymphoid neoplasms, aCGH was rapidly applied to the study of CLL, for which disease aCGH can identify clonal abnormalities in 100% of cases.[38] For comparison with FISH and MC, other studies have demonstrated the ability of aCGH to detect abnormalities in 12% of normal-karyotype CLL cases[38] and in 21% of cases where no aberration was detected by FISH.[46]

Metaphases are also difficult to obtain in plasma cell neoplasms, leading to the prominent role of FISH in the diagnosis and prognosis of myeloma. However, because FISH is targeted, it cannot provide an unbiased genome-wide assessment as can be achieved by aCGH. Gutierrez et al found CNVs by aCGH in 69% of patients with myeloma and that those patients had significantly decreased overall survival.[37] The prognostic significance of other specific loci, which include gains of 1q and 7q, have also been studied using aCGH.[47,48] The latter study also highlighted the utility of this method in paraffin-embedded tissue.

Next-Generation Sequencing

Whole genome sequencing (WGS) provides the theoretically optimal combination of uniform unbiased genome-wide coverage with nucleotide-level resolution for the discovery of acquired genetic aberrations in oncology (*Table 89.2*). The caveats, of course, center upon the cost and analysis of the potentially terabytes of data accumulated by a single WGS analysis. Prior to 2005, nearly all DNA sequencing

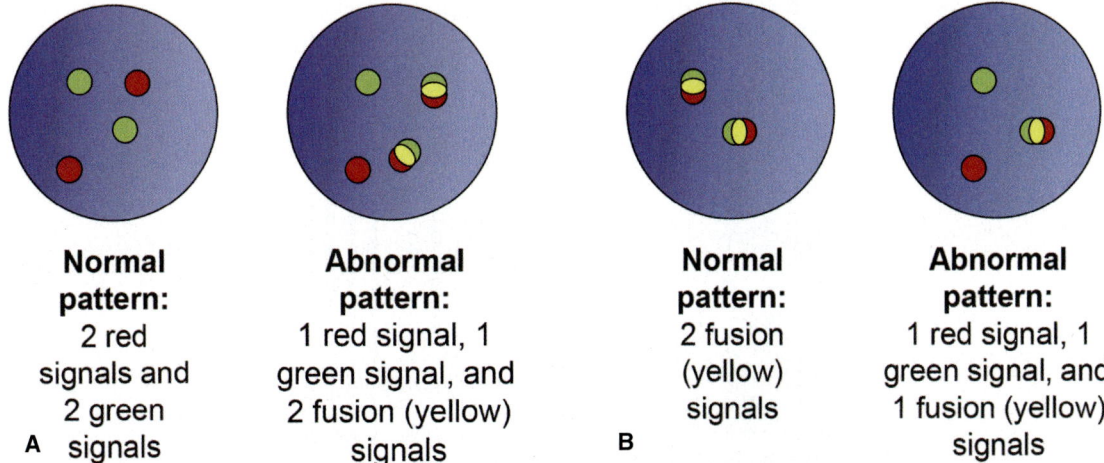

FIGURE 89.6 **Examples of FISH patterns.** A, Schematic of dual color dual fusion fluorescent in situ hybridization (FISH) probes. B, Schematic of break-apart FISH probes.

Table 89.2. Characteristics of Different Genome-wide Studies

Method	Resolution	Genome Coverage	Sensitivity	Detection of UPD and CN LOH	Detection of Balanced Translocations	Detection of Unbalanced Translocations	Utility in Screening New Lesions	Distinguish Different Individual Clones	Utilize Interphase DNA	Distinguish Somatic vs Germline Aberrations
aCGH	5-6 kb	Uniform	2%-30%	No	No	Yes	Yes	No	Yes	Yes
aSNP	25-50 kb	Not uniform	2%-30%	Yes	No	No	Yes	No	Yes	No
Conventional karyotyping	5-10 Mb	Uniform	10%[a]	No	Yes	Yes	Yes	Yes	No	No/Yes
FISH	2-5 kb	Targeted	1%-5%	No	Yes	No	No	Yes	Yes	No/Yes
PCR	Potentially single nucleotide aberrations	Targeted	Variable, potentially as low as 0.00001%	No	Possible	Possible	Yes	No	Yes	Possible
NGS	Potentially single nucleotide aberrations	Uniform or targeted	5%-10%	Possible	Possible	Possible	Yes	No	Yes	Possible

Abbreviations: aCGH, array comparative genomic hybridization; aSNP, array single nucleotide polymorphisms; CN LOH, copy neutral loss of heterozygosity; FISH, fluorescent in situ hybridization; NGS, next-generation sequencing; PCR, polymerase chain reaction; UPD, uniparental disomy.

[a]Clonality is typically defined as involving at least 2 of 20 metaphases.[28] For PCR and NGS methods, depending on the design of the assay/experiment, different questions may be answered. For instance, if normal and tumor tissues are examined for a particular mutation, somatic vs germline mutational status can be ascertained by PCR.

Portions adapted from Schwaenen C, Nessling M, Wessendorf S, et al. Automated array-based genomic profiling in chronic lymphocytic leukemia: development of a clinical tool and discovery of recurrent genomic alterations. *Proc Natl Acad Sci U S A.* 2004;101(4):1039-1044.

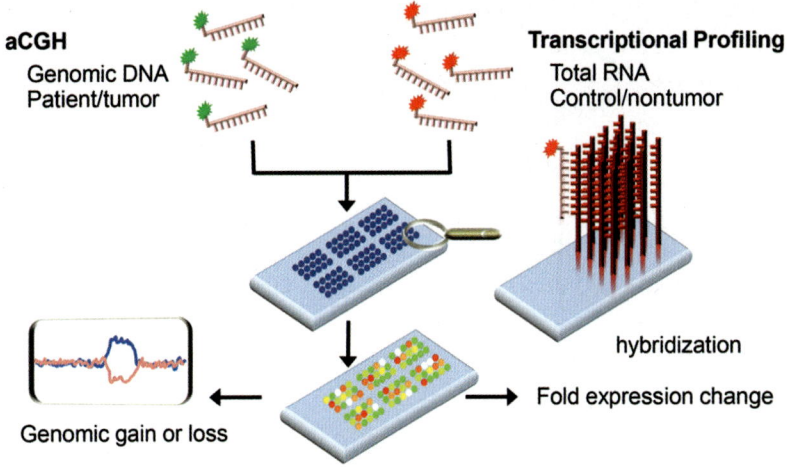

FIGURE 89.7 **Schematic of array comparative hybridization (aCGH) and transcriptional profiling using a dual-channel platform.** Patient and control genomic DNA (aCGH) or RNA (transcriptional profiling) are differentially labeled with fluorophores, then stoichiometrically mixed and allowed to hybridize to probes fixed to a solid surface. The relative amounts of fluorescence at each feature is measured to gain information about gains or losses in the patient sample compared with control (aCGH) or about over- or underexpression of genes (transcriptional profiling).

was performed using some variant of Sanger sequencing, a method by which sequencing was achieved by stochastic chain termination first described in 1977.[49] These Sanger-based methods typically required large quantities of input DNA since the DNA is needed to serve as the template for at least as many polymerase extension reactions as nucleotides to be sequenced. The polymerase products are separated by size to determine the sequence. This traditional sequencing is plagued by poor quality of the initial 15 to 40 bases of the sequence, and read lengths are limited to 500 to 1000 bases.[50]

All NGS methodologies are based on read-through sequence determination or sequence by synthesis (*Figure 89.8*).[50,51] Short DNA fragments are typically required for NGS (reads typically 150-250 bp in length). The shorter read length makes NGS amenable to the use of FFPE tissues, which are sheared to varying degrees during preservation.

For targeted sequencing, the most common modality in use for oncology somatic testing, the library preparation typically involves either a massively multiplexed amplification or DNA fragmentation followed by hybrid capture-based enrichment of the targeted regions. This library is modified to contain universal adapters ligated to the fragments that can be used for amplification steps, the addition of sample barcodes, as well as potentially unique molecular identifiers. These universal adapters also allow the targeted DNA regions to be immobilized in spatially fixed, typically on slides or beads, and then iteratively interrogated by the repeated addition of individual nucleotides.

Several methods of sequence detection are utilized by the various commercial platforms. The two most common clinical platforms involve cyclic reversible chain termination (such as used by Illumina platforms) or the detection of chemical by-products (such as used by the Ion Torrent platforms). Cyclic reversible termination uses dye-labeled nucleotides that contain protecting groups on the 3′ hydroxyl group preventing the addition of more than one nucleotide at a time; after detection of addition of a labeled nucleotide by the fluorophore dye, the protecting group and the dye are both chemically removed before the next nucleotide is added. By contrast, chemical by-product detection uses the detection of the release of pyrophosphate or H+ ion, which are chemically produced each time a nucleotide is added by the polymerase. The amount of by-product detected is directly proportional to the number of molecules of that nucleotide that is added. Targeted NGS panels are frequently used in the diagnosis and management of lymphoid neoplasms, although less commonly than in the myeloid neoplasms. Owing to the ubiquity of FFPE tissues acquired in the diagnosis of lymphoid neoplasms, the library preparation and sequencing methods must accommodate the sheared DNA and lower amounts of DNA obtained from FFPE. Accordingly, hybrid-capture methods are more accommodating of the lower-quality sheared DNA, despite the typically higher input requirements of these methods. Pathologist evaluation of the slides and circling of areas of highest tumor burden for microdissection is recommended. Diagnostic entities such as classic Hodgkin lymphoma or other lymphomas of rare neoplastic cells are not amenable to NGS without some sort of tumor cell enrichment. The analytical sensitivity for typical NGS can approach 5% tumor cells in a background of nonneoplastic cells.[52] However, newer deep sequencing methods involving error correction and/or unique molecular identifiers have been adapted for MRD and cell-free DNA (cfDNA) testing.[53] Using very high read depths, sensitivities of 0.0001% can be achieved.[19,20]

Gene content should be designed for the assessment of lymphoid neoplasms. While many pan-cancer panels have some relevant content for lymphomas, not all pan-cancer panels will have sufficient gene coverage for the appropriate workup of lymphoid neoplasms. Informatic pipelines are typically optimized for the detection of single nucleotide variants (SNVs) and small insertions or deletions (indels). Specialized informatics are required for the assessment of copy number variants (CNVs) and translocations. Translocations are, of course, highly recurrent in lymphoid neoplasms. In general, RNA-based NGS is the preferred method for translocation detection as it removes intronic regions, enabling targeting of more limited coding sequences. In addition, partner-agnostic baits allow the identification of unanticipated fusions of common, but promiscuous, targets. However, translocations of these IGH or TCR genes to other partners often involve noncoding enhancer or switch regions, precluding the use of RNA-based NGS. DNA-based NGS requires extensive tiling of amplicons or baited regions across the vast tracts of potential intronic breakpoints but is better, while still challenging, for these clonality purposes. Immunoglobulin and TCR gene VDJ rearrangements result in complex sequencing results and informatic requirements.

For most laboratories performing clinical testing, it appears that the current trend is to use one of the smaller desk-top sequencers with on-board bioinformatic pipelines to call the variants, although many larger commercial and academic laboratories have internally developed pipelines.[54,55] Most laboratories conduct tumor only sequencing, although a few sequence tumor-normal pairs. Recent studies analyzing the performance of NGS in proficiency testing demonstrate overall excellent performance of NGS in the detection of SNVs and small indels.[56-58]

Methods have been developed to conduct whole exome sequencing, targeted NGS, transcriptome sequencing (RNA-seq), sequencing of DNA methylation sites (bisulfite seq), miRNome sequencing (miRNA-seq), sequencing of immunoprecipitated DNA (ChIP-seq), and many others.[50] Many of these targeted RNA-seq-based platforms can also perform expression profiling by sequencing.

Transcriptional Profiling

Initially developed in the 1980s, transcriptional profiling was the first *omic* technology to see widespread utilization.[59] The majority of the

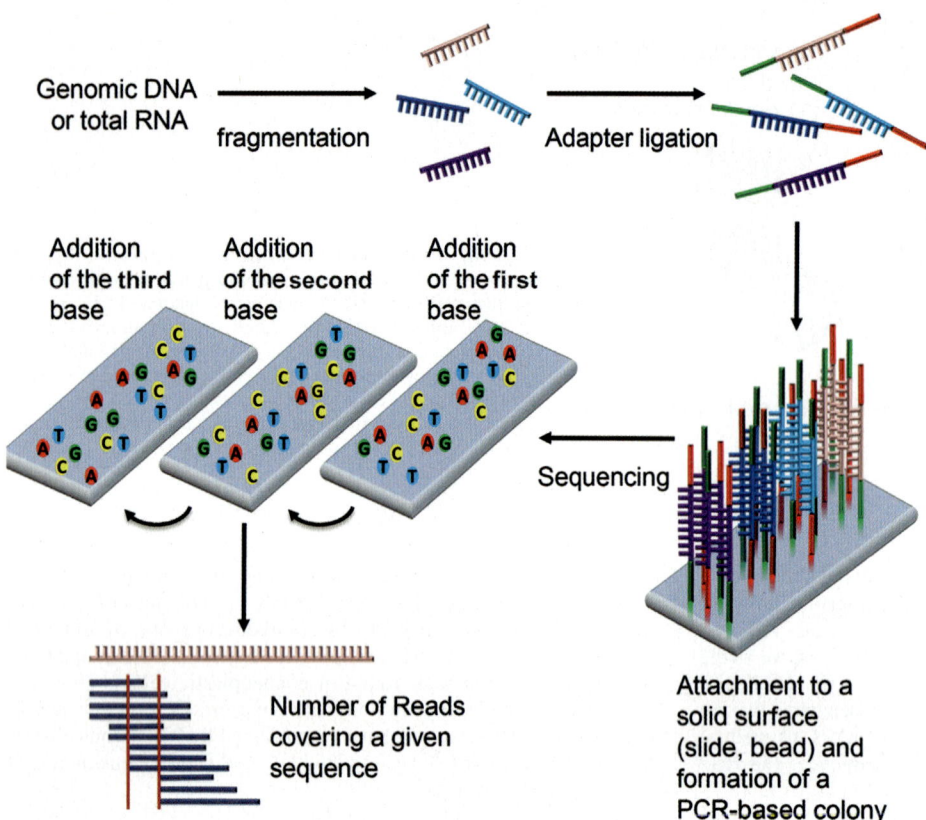

FIGURE 89.8 **Schematic of next-generation sequencing using dye-labeled nucleotides, which act as reversible chain terminators.** The DNA is first sheared and modified with adaptors. These adaptors can be used to immobilize the DNA fragments and serve as primers for polymerase chain reaction (PCR) amplification and for sequencing using the reversible chain terminators. The sequence of each fragment is determined, followed by the computational alignment of the fragments to construct the genomic sequence.

commercial platforms now use oligonucleotide probes rather than cDNA probes. Transcriptional profiling can be performed as either a single-channel or a dual-channel experiment (*Figure 89.7*).

This methodology does not capture the protein expression of various genes and any posttranslational modifications. In addition, when the mRNA levels are varied between two samples, it is impossible to determine in a single timepoint comparison whether the differences are due to primary changes at the DNA mutational level, primary changes at the transcriptional level, or secondary changes at the transcriptional level resulting from the true disease-causing aberration. In addition, the methodology has limited analytical sensitivity for small fold changes and limited clinical sensitivity if the reference samples are not chosen wisely.

Nonetheless, transcriptional profiling has led to significant discoveries in lymphoid malignancies. One main utility has been in the definition of prognostic subgroups. For example, its use in the study of SHM status in CLL led to the identification of ZAP70 expression as an independent poor prognostic marker.[60] Similarly, in DLBCL, transcriptional profiling has identified cell-of-origin prognostic subgroups: GCB-like with better prognosis, and activated B-cell (ABC) and type 3 DLBCL, which does not express either set of genes at a high level, the latter two subgroups with poorer prognosis.[61] Gene expression profiling studies have also been useful to demonstrate the similarities between primary mediastinal large B-cell lymphoma and classical Hodgkin lymphoma (cHL)-derived cell lines,[62] or between anaplastic large cell lymphoma (ALCL) and cHL.[63]

MicroRNAs, Epigenetic Changes

MicroRNAs

Both plants and animals have evolved microRNAs (miRNAs), single-stranded RNAs of approximately 19 to 22 nucleotides, as a mechanism for translational regulation. These miRNAs are encoded in the genome and are transcribed by DNA polymerase II. Following processing in both the nucleus and cytoplasm, the mature miRNA, mediated by the RNA-induced silencing complex, binds in a complementary fashion to the 3′ untranslated regions (3′-UTR) of target mRNAs to cause translational repression.

Physiologically, miRNAs play a key role in the tightly regulated development and identity of hematopoietic cells.[64-66] Thus, miRNAs, individually or in profiles, can be markers of tissue type through several methods: miRNA RT-PCR, microarrays, and NGS methods. Interestingly, the location of all miRNAs in the human genome is nonrandom. It has been demonstrated that miRNAs are concentrated by a factor of nine in genomic fragile sites and others that are commonly altered in cancer.[67] Thus, over half of 186 miRNAs evaluated in one study were located at cancer-associated genomic regions, such as regions of LOH, common breakpoints, and areas of amplification. These findings suggest that aberrant miRNA expression might be a common pathway in oncogenesis.

The commonly deleted region in CLL (13q14) contains two miRNAs, *miR-15a* and *miR-16-1*.[68-70] These are consequently downregulated in CLL, resulting in overexpression of their target mRNAs, *BCL2* and *MCL1*, and an overall antiapoptotic effect.[70] By contrast, *miR-155* has been identified as upregulated in a number of B-cell lymphomas. First identified in cases of childhood BL, expression of the pre-miRNA for *miR-155* was found to be upregulated in BL, DLBCL (associated with the ABC subtype), CLL, and marginal zone lymphoma.[71-73] The miRNA polycistron *miR-17-92*, located at 13q31, is also implicated in lymphomas such as DLBCL, FL, mantle cell lymphoma (MCL), and primary cutaneous B-cell lymphoma.[74]

Epigenetics

Epigenetics involves the heritable alterations in gene expression that are not caused by actual changes in the genomic sequence. Epigenetic changes occur through one of two main pathways. Methylation of the 5-position of cytosines, particularly in CpG-rich sites such as CpG islands, shores, and shelves, results in transcriptional repression. CpG islands are defined as regions >500 bp in length with a CG percentage >55% and an observed to expected CpG ratio of >65%.[75,76] Alternatively, posttranslational modification of the amino acids of histones via methylation or acetylation can result in heritable changes in histone structure and therefore the accessibility of the DNA to transcription. DNA methylation has been the better-examined epigenetic mechanism of the two, and methylome studies can be conducted via NGS, methylation arrays, and targeted methylation methods.

All methods to interrogate methylation status depend upon one of three main techniques.[77-79] Isoschizomer restriction enzyme–based methods rely upon the selective cleavage of either methylated or unmethylated sequences by specific restriction enzymes. A second method uses the chemistry of bisulfite to convert unmethylated cytosine to uracil, thereby causing a sequence change in unmethylated CpG sites but not in methylated sites. These differences can then be identified via sequencing or sequence-specific hybridization methods. Lastly, proteins that selectively bind to methylated CpG sites, whether the naturally occurring methylation binding protein or antibodies generated against CpG sites, can be used to pull down methylated fragments of DNA. All three techniques can be used to prepare samples for sequencing, arrays, or more targeted methods.

RECURRENT MOLECULAR ABERRANCIES IN B-CELL AND T-CELL NEOPLASMS

Tables 89.3 and 89.4 list many of the common reciprocal translocations found in B-cell and T-cell malignancies, respectively. Of note, many of the reciprocal translocations involve one of the immunoglobulin genes

Table 89.3. Common Chromosomal Translocations in B-Cell NHL

Translocation	Product	Disease Association
t(1;14)(p22;q32)	BCL10 overexpression (IGH)	MALT[a]
t(1;14)(q21;q32)	BCL9 overexpression (IGH)	B-LBL and others
t(1;14)(q21;q32)	FCRL4/5 overexpression (IGH)	Myeloma (<5%)
t(1;14)(q22;q32)	MUC1 overexpression (IGH)	DLBCL
t(1;22)(q23;q11)	FCGR2B overexpression (IGL)	Transformed FL
t(2;7)(p12;q21-q22)	CDK6	SMZL
t(2;14)(p16.1;q32)	BCL11A overexpression (IGH)	CLL, DLBCL
t(2;17)(p23;q23)	CLTC-ALK	ALK-positive LBCL
t(3;14)(q27;q32)/t(3;v)(q27;v)	BCL6 overexpression (IGH or IGK/IGL)	DLBCL (5%-10%) and others
t(3;14)(p14;q32)	FOXP1 overexpression (IGH)	MALT
t(4;14)(p16;q32)	WHSC1 (MMSET)::FGFR3 overexpression (IGH)	Myeloma (20%-25%)
t(5;14)(q23-q31;q32)	IL3 overexpression (IGH)	B-LBL
t(6;14)(p25-p23;q32)	IRF4 overexpression (IGH)	Myeloma (~20%)
t(6;14)(p21;q32)	CCND3 overexpression (IGH)	Myeloma (<5%), DLBCL, SMZL, MZL
t(6;14)(p22;q32)	ID4 overexpression (IGH)	B-LBL (<1%)
t(8;14)(q24;q32)/t(8;v)(q24;v)	MYC overexpression (IGH or IGK/IGL)	BL (>98%), DLBCL[a], FL[a], PLL, myeloma
t(8;14)(q11;q32)	CEBPD overexpression (IGH)	B-LBL (<1%)
t(9;14)(p13;q32)	PAX5 overexpression (IGH)	LPL (1%-2%), other neoplasms with plasmacytic differentiation, DLBCL
t(10;14)(q24;q32)	NFKB2 overexpression (IGH)	DLBCL
t(11;14)(q13;q32)	CCND1 overexpression (IGH)	MCL (>95%), PLL, SMZL, myeloma[b] (20%-25%)
t(11;14)(q23;q32)	PAFAH1B2 overexpression (IGH)	PMBCL
t(11;14)(q23;q32)	DDX6 overexpression (IGH)	DLBCL
t(11;18)(q22;q21)	BIRC3::MALT1 fusion	MALT[a]
t(12;14)(q23;q32)	CHST11 overexpression (IGH)	DLBCL, CLL (rare)
t(12;14)(q24;q32)	BCL7A	BL, myeloma
t(12;15)(q32;q11-13)	NBEAP1?	DLBCL
t(12;22)(p13;q11)	CCND2	CLL
t(14;16)(q32;q22-q23)	MAF overexpression (IGH)	Myeloma (20%-25%)
t(14;18)(q32;q21)	BCL2 overexpression (IGH)	FL (~80%), DLBCL (~20%)
t(14;18)(q32;q21)	MALT1 overexpression (IGH)	MALT
t(14;19)(q32;q13)	BCL3 overexpression (IGH)	CLL
t(14;19)(q32;q13)	CEBPA overexpression (IGH)	B-LBL (<1%)
t(14;20)(q32;q11-q13)	MAFB overexpression (IGH)	Myeloma

Abbreviations: B-LBL, B-lymphoblastic leukemia/lymphoma; BL, Burkitt lymphoma; CLL, chronic lymphocytic leukemia; DLBCL, diffuse large B-cell lymphoma; FL, follicular lymphoma; LBCL, large B-cell lymphoma; LPL, lymphoplasmacytic lymphoma; MALT, mucosa-associated lymphoid tissue; MCL, mantle cell lymphoma; PLL, prolymphocytic leukemia; PMBCL, primary mediastinal large B-cell lymphoma; SMZL, splenic marginal zone lymphoma.
[a]Indicates adverse prognostic significance in addition to diagnostic role.
[b]Indicates favorable prognostic significance in addition to diagnostic role.

Table 89.4. Common Chromosomal Translocations in T-Cell NHL

Translocation	Product	Disease Association
t(1;14)(p34;q11)/t(1;7)(p32;q34)	*TAL1* overexpression (TRD/*TRB*)	T-LBL (3%)
t(1;7)(p34;q34)	*LCK* overexpression (TRB)	T-LBL (1%)
t(2;5)(p23;q35)	*ALK1::NPM* fusion	ALCL (>80% of ALK-positive cases)
t(5;9)(q33;q22)	*ITK::SYK* fusion	AITL
t(5;14)(q35;q11)	*TLX3* overexpression (TRD)	T-LBL (1%)
t(6;7)(q23;q32-36)	*MYB* overexpression (TRB)	T-LBL (1%)
t(6;7)(p25.3;q32.2)	*DUSP22::FRA7H*	ALK-negative ALCL
t(7;7)(q34;p14/inv(7)(q35p14)	*HOXA* cluster overexpression (TRB)	T-LBL (5%)
t(7;9)(q34;q32)	*TAL2* overexpression (TRB)	T-LBL (1%)
t(7;9)(q34;q34)	*NOTCH1* overexpression (TRB)	T-LBL (1%)
t(7;12)(q34;p13)	*CCND2* overexpression (TRB)	T-LBL (1%)
t(7;19)(q34;p13)	*LYL1* overexpression (TRB)	T-LBL (1%)
iso(7q)	?	HTCL (>80%)
t(8;13)(p11;q12)	*FGFR1::ZNF198* fusion	Myeloproliferative neoplasm associated with T-LBL
t(8;14)(q24;q11)	*MYC* overexpression (TRD/A)	T-LBL (1%)
t(10;14)(q24;q11)/t(7;10)(q34;q11)	*TLX1* overexpression (TRD/B)	T-LBL (10%-30%)
t(11;14)(p13;q11)/t(7;11)(q34;p13)	*LMO2* overexpression (TRD/B)	T-LBL (3%)
t(11;14)(p15;q11)	*LMO1* overexpression (TRD)	T-LBL (2%)
t(14;14)(q11;q32)/inv14(q11q32)	*TCL1* overexpression (TRD/A)	T-PLL (70%-75%), T-LBL (<1%)
t(X;14)(q28;q11)	*MCTP1* overexpression (TRD/A)	T-PLL (~5%)

Abbreviations: AITL; angioimmunoblastic T-cell lymphoma; ALCL, anaplastic large cell lymphoma; HTCL, hepatosplenic T-cell lymphoma; T-LBL, T-lymphoblastic leukemia/lymphoma; T-PLL, T-cell prolymphocytic leukemia.

in the case of B-cell lymphomas (most commonly IGH on chromosome 14q32). A smaller proportion of T-cell lymphomas involve the TCRα/δ locus on chromosome 14q11. The ensuing text highlights the key known translocations and other genetic alterations identified in specific lymphoid neoplasms.

Mature Neoplasms of B Cells
Mantle Cell Lymphoma

MCL accounts for 5% to 6% of NHLs, occurring predominantly in males over the age of 55 years (male:female ratio of 4:1).[5] MCL is typically thought of as an aggressive disease that is often widespread at diagnosis, although more indolent cases, often with a more leukemic presentation, can have longer survival times (average 79 months rather than 36-60 months for typical cases).[80,81] Other morphologic variants, such as the pleomorphic or blastoid variants, tend to have poorer outcomes.[5]

Rearrangements. The hallmark cytogenetic aberration in MCL is the *CCND1::IGH* translocation that can be found in above 90% of cases of MCL.[82,83] In addition, this rearrangement can also be seen in 20% to 25% of plasma cell myelomas, and some cases of CLL or prolymphocytic leukemia (PLL), and splenic marginal zone lymphomas (SMZLs).[84-87] This translocation results in the overexpression of cyclin D1, which can be assessed via IHC, with greater than 90% sensitivity for the translocation.[87] However, overexpression of cyclin D1 is also associated with the above lymphoid neoplasms as well as in the proliferation centers of typical CLL and in some cases of hairy cell leukemia (HCL) that do not harbor the translocation.[88,89]

The t(11;14)(q13;q32) in MCL juxtaposes the *CCND1* gene on 11q13, which encodes for cyclin D1 with J$_H$ subunit of the IGH locus on 14q32. The translocation places the entire coding region of *CCND1* under regulation of the IGH enhancer, resulting in overexpression of the full cyclin D1 protein. Cyclin D1 associates with the cyclin-dependent kinases, CDK4 and CDK6, to form a complex that hyperphosphorylates the retinoblastoma protein (Rb).[90] When phosphorylated, Rb is unable to sequester and inhibit the function of E2F1 in promoting entry into S phase and promoting cell cycling (*Figure 89.9*). This increased proliferation is marked by Ki-67 IHC staining, with higher levels of Ki-67 portending a more aggressive disease (cutoffs vary from >40% to >60%).[91,92]

The majority of the *CCND1* breakpoints occur upstream or centromeric to the coding sequence (*Figure 89.10*). However, these breakpoint regions are spread out across approximately 120 kb.[93,94] Although there are three main regions of breakpoints, these are not tightly clustered. The major translocation cluster (MTC) spans an 80- to 100-bp region located the farthest upstream from the *CCND1* gene, accounting for 30% to 40% of translocations. This region was formerly known as the B-cell lymphoma/leukemia 1 region (*BCL1*), prior to the recognition that the gene responsible for the biology of MCL was the downstream *CCND1* gene. The minor translocation clusters (mTC1 and mTC2) lie closer to the *CCND1* coding sequence. In addition, occasional breakpoints 3′ to the coding sequence can be seen, especially in plasma cell myeloma. In addition to the translocations, deletions or point mutations in the 3′-UTR of *CCND1* mRNA have been identified in 5% to 10% of patients, which result in increased stability of the transcript, potentially due to inability of miR-16-1 to target the mRNA. The resultant increased half-life of the transcript is associated with increased proliferative rate and poor survival.[95,96] By contrast, 5′-UTR and first exon mutations in *CCND1* appear to be bystander mutations without prognostic significance.[97]

The wide distribution of these breakpoints explains the poor clinical sensitivity of PCR-based molecular assays for the t(11;14). The majority of PCR assays are designed to target just the MTC, resulting in a 30% to 40% clinical sensitivity with product sizes spanning 143 to 934 bp.[93] By contrast, FISH, with its large probes, has nearly 100% sensitivity for the rearrangement.[83,87] However, given the greater than

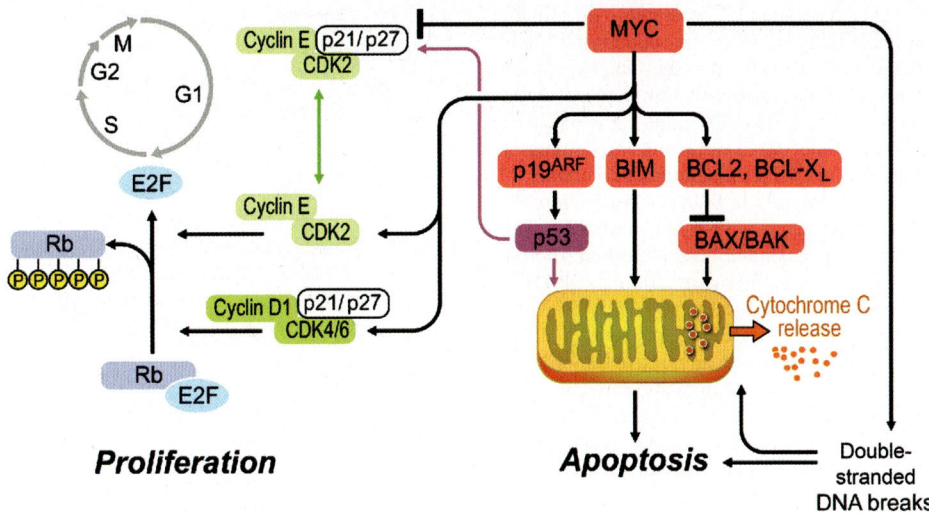

FIGURE 89.9 Apoptosis and proliferation pathways illustrating some of the roles of cyclin D1, MYC, and BCL2. Cyclin D1 associates with the cyclin-dependent kinases, CDK4 and CDK6, to form a complex that hyperphosphorylates the retinoblastoma protein (Rb). When phosphorylated, Rb is unable to sequester and inhibit the function of E2F1 in promoting entry into S phase and promoting cell cycling. MYC inhibits p21 and p27, inhibitors of the cyclin-dependent kinases, and promotes the expression of CDK2 and CDK4. MYC also inhibits several antiapoptotic proteins, such as BCL2. BCL2 forms a heterodimer with BAX, thereby preventing the formation of proapoptotic BAX/BAK homodimers. MYC also promotes the p19^{ARF} activation of p53-mediated apoptosis and cell cycle arrest through p21 and p27.

90% correlation of the presence of the translocation with IHC, in most cases IHC alone is required to make the diagnosis, with the caveat that other benign and neoplastic entities can have some cyclin D1 expression without harboring the t(11;14).

FISH and IHC, however, are not sufficiently sensitive for the detection of MRD. However, a clonal immunoglobulin gene rearrangement can be identified in the majority of cases of MCL (approaching 100% in some studies with a single set of FR3 primers).[16-18] The high clinical sensitivity of this test is due to the pre-germinal center naive B-cell origin of this neoplasm. More detailed analysis, however, reveals that 26% of cases of MCL do indeed exceed the 2% nonhomology with germline used to define SHM, with an average mutation rate of 1.51% for the 32 cases examined.[98] These cases tend to be negative for SOX11 (vide infra) with possible leukemic presentations. Using allele-specific primers, the utility of RT-PCR for IGH VDJ rearrangement assays (peripheral blood either MRD positive or negative) has been demonstrated in the prediction of progression-free survival.[99] These methods, however, have not yet achieved widespread clinical utilization.

Between 1% to 10% of cases of MCL are t(11;14)-negative, involving variant translocations. These are divided among cyclin D1 overexpression by rearrangement with the light chains as well as overexpression of cyclin D2 or D3 with the immunoglobulins: t(2;11)(p11;q13) (CCND1::IGK), t(11;22)(q13;q11) (CCND1::IGL), t(12;14)(p13;q32) (CCND2::IGH), t(2;12)(p11;p13) (CCND2::IGK), t(12;22)(p13;q21) (CCND2::IGL), and t(6;14)(p21;q32) (CCND3::IGH).[83] These cases may be difficult to diagnose using cyclin D1 FISH, although break apart of the CCND1 signal may be seen with the light chain variants and break apart of the IGH locus may be seen with either CCND2 or CCND3 recombinations with IGH. Strong expression of SOX11 by IHC has been identified in 90% of MCLs, including the t(11;14)-negative cases.[100,101] Expression of this transcription factor is negative in nearly all other mature B- and T-cell lymphomas, with the exception of some cases of BL, T-prolymphocytic leukemia (T-PLL), and lymphoblastic neoplasms, none of which are typically on a diagnostic differential with MCL.[102]

Copy number variations. Functional analyses have implicated cell-cycle progression, cell adhesion, and signal transduction as broad oncogenic processes in MCL. Approximately 20% to 30% of MCLs have deletions of the INK4a/ARF locus (CDKN2A) on 9p21.3, which encodes for both p14 and p16 in alternate reading frames.[103-106] These deletions are often homozygous. Other common aberrations identified by karyotyping, aSNP, or aCGH include (candidate genes and percentage of cases in parentheses): gains of 3q (32%-70%), 7p (5%-27%), 8q (MYC, 10%-32%), 12q (CDK4, 5%-30%), 15q (4%-26%), and 18q (BCL2, 7%-26%) and losses of 1p (CDKN2C/FAF1, 24%-52%), 6q (TNGAIP3/LATS1, 13%-37%), 8p (MCPH1, 7%-79%), 9p (CDKN2A/B, 7%-30%), 9q (5%-21%), 10p (3%-18%), 11q (ATM, 19%-37%), 13q (RB1, 17%-70%), and 17p (TP53%, 4%-30%).[83] Many of these changes are aberrations commonly associated with CLL, such as del(11q23), del(17p13), del(13q14), and may suggest some commonality in pathogenic pathways. Blastoid and pleomorphic MCL may harbor tetraploid cytogenetics as well as gains of 3q, 7p, and 12q, and losses of 9p21 (CDKN2A) and 17p (TP53).[83] By contrast, indolent cases of MCL often have t(11;14) as the sole abnormality.[83]

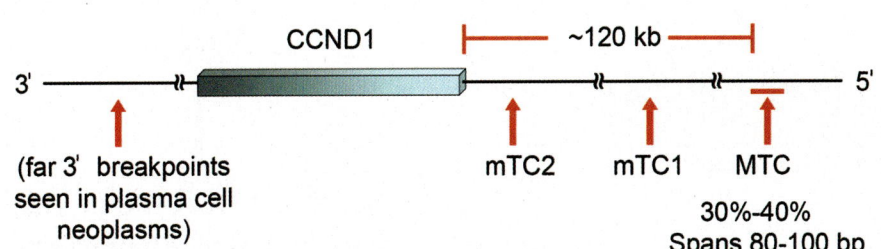

FIGURE 89.10 Location of breakpoint regions in the CCND1 gene and the frequency of the most common breakpoint in mantle cell lymphoma. MTC, major translocation cluster; mTC, minor translocation cluster.

Somatic variants. MCL is also commonly associated with somatic SNVs. A general theme is the striking heterogeneity underlying MCL, with relatively few genes mutated in >10% of cases. The exceptions are those drivers long known to play a role in this disease. *ATM, CCND1,* and *TP53* are mutated in ~50%, 30%, and 25% of cases, respectively, the former and the latter often occurring in conjunction with deletions of *ATM* and *TP53* resulting in biallelic dysfunction.[83,107-110] *ATM* mutations are seen exclusively in SOX11-positive tumors, while *CCND1* mutations are associated with *IGHV*-mutated cases. Additional significantly mutated genes have been identified, including mutations in *BIRC3, TLR2,* and the chromatin modifiers *WHSC1, MLL2,* and *MEF2B.* Furthermore, mutations in *NOTCH2* (5%, also seen in SMZL) as well as in *NOTCH1* (5%-12%, also characteristic of CLL) have been identified and associated with aggressive tumors with dismal prognosis.[102,111] These mutations are truncation mutations or small frameshift indels in the PEST domain, in particular the ΔCT variant, that result in decreased ubiquitination and increased NOTCH1 activity. Additional recurrently mutated genes found in MCL have included *RB1, POT1, MLL3,* and *SMARCA4.*[112]

Gene expression and methylation profiling. Gene expression profiling on a large series of patients with MCL has identified a characteristic signature of 20 genes which, not surprisingly, are associated with proliferation.[106] When this gene set was pared down to a minimal set of five genes (*RAN, MYC, TNFRSF10B, POLE2,* and *SLC29A2*), the profile by RT-PCR was able to predict survival.[113] Methylation profiling has been helpful in distinguishing MCL from CLL, identifying an MCL methylation profile demonstrating hypermethylation of developmental genes, in particular homeobox genes.[114,115]

Guidelines for Molecular Testing in Mantle Cell Lymphoma

Diagnosis	MRD
IHC for CyclinD1, Ki-67, p53	
Consider PCR or NGS for Ig gene rearrangement studies	Consider NGS for Ig gene rearrangement studies
Consider FISH for variant translocations or 17p13	
Consider IHC for SOX11	
Consider somatic variant testing for various prognostic markers such as *TP53, NOTCH1,* and *NOTCH2*	

Chronic Lymphocytic Leukemia/Small Lymphocytic Lymphoma

Accounting for only 6.7% of NHLs, CLL/SLL is nonetheless the most common adult chronic leukemia in Western countries.[5] The majority of these cases are leukemic (CLL), with the isolated lymphomatous presentation of SLL uncommon. Although considered to be overall an indolent disease, there is wide variability in clinical outcomes. A minority of cases can progress to large cell disease, including DLBCL (Richter transformation, 2% to 8%), classic Hodgkin lymphoma (<1%), and PLL,[5,11] although there is rising concern that this complication is increasing, in association with rapidly expanding use of novel agents targeting the inhibition of the BCL2 and BCR signaling pathways.[116]

Copy number variations. Genetic aberrations are found in most cases of CLL. Conventional MC identifies abnormalities in only approximately 40% of cases.[117] However, FISH can detect cytogenetic changes in about 80% of CLL cases.[118] Unlike many other B-cell neoplasms, numerical changes, rather than translocations, predominate in CLL. Typical FISH panels interrogate four common chromosomal aberrancies: deletions of 13q14, 11q22-23, and 17p13 as well as trisomy of chromosome 12. Array CGH methods have the potential to identify even more aberrations, and some institutions routinely perform aCGH for CLL, although most of the published studies still use FISH as the gold standard for comparison.[119,120]

Deletions of 13q14 are the most common recurrent abnormality in CLL and account for 50% to 60% of cases.[118] Patients can show either homozygous or heterozygous losses of 13q14, both associated with favorable prognosis. The locus affected by this deletion appears to contain two miRNAs, *miR-15a* and *miR-16-1,* and deletion of these miRNAs are common in familial cases of CLL as well.[68,69] These miRNAs have been demonstrated to target and translationally repress a number of genes involved in apoptosis, including *BCL2, MCL1,* and *TP53.* Therefore, the loss of these miRNAs results in increased expression of the antiapoptotic genes *BCL2* and *MCL1* (Figure 89.11). Although *TP53* is proapoptotic, its role in CLL may be more complex than previously understood. The protein product of *TP53,* p53, also promotes transcription of two other miRNAs, *miR-34b* and *miR-34c,* both of which target the mRNA of *ZAP70.*[121] Thus in 13q14-deleted CLLs, there is increased p53 expression, increased *miR-34b* and *miR-34c,* and decreased ZAP70 protein. ZAP70 has independently been determined to portend a poor prognosis.[60]

Deletions of 11q22-23 are identified in approximately 17% of cases of CLL.[122] This locus contains a number of important genes

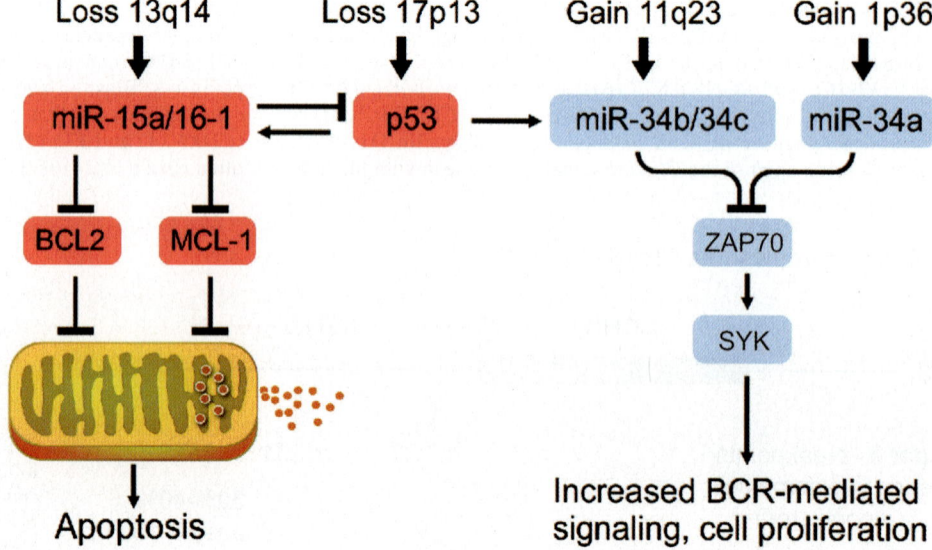

FIGURE 89.11 Chronic lymphocytic leukemia biology. Loss of 13q14 causes decreased miR15a/16-1, resulting in decreased apoptosis. Trisomy 11 results in increased miR-34b/34c, with resultant decreased ZAP 70 and decreased B-cell receptor (BCR) signaling. However, loss of 17q13 results in increased ZAP 70 and increased BCR-mediated signaling with decreased apoptosis.

in the pathogenesis of CLL, including *ATM* at 11q22.3. ATM phosphorylates p53, resulting in its protection from ubiquitination and degradation by MDM2. Therefore, loss of the *ATM* locus is tantamount to loss of p53. In addition, miRNAs, *miR-34b* and *miR-34c*, are located at 11q23.1 and are also deleted with *ATM*. The deletion of these miRNAs results in increased protein expression of the poor prognostic marker ZAP70.[60,121] Deletions of 11q22-23 are therefore consistent with a poor prognosis. Recent studies have suggested the importance of adding alkylating agents such as cyclophosphamide to regimens used to treat patients with deletion 11q22-23.[123] On the other hand, these patients have not shown worse response to targeted inhibitors of BCL2 (venetoclax) or Bruton tyrosine kinase (BTK) (ibrutinib) than patients lacking this alteration.[124,125]

Deletions of 17p13 involve the loss of the *TP53* locus and are found in approximately 8% of cases of CLL, also associated with a poor prognosis.[122] By itself, deletion of the tumor suppressor gene is typically associated across malignancies with negative prognosis. In CLL, it has been demonstrated that loss of p53 can also result in decreased *miR-34b* and *miR-34c* transcription and therefore increased ZAP70 expression.[121] The identification of del(17p) is a critical predictor of resistance to fludarabine, the backbone of most chemoimmunotherapy regimens for CLL, but patients may have a durable response to ibrutinib.[126]

Trisomy 12 is found in approximately 20% of cases of CLL and can be associated with more atypical morphologic features such as irregular nuclear contours and less condensed chromatin as well as increased CD11c expression.[5,122,127] Trisomy 12 is considered to be an intermediate risk factor in CLL but can be associated with specific other abnormalities that may modify its prognostic import.

Somatic hypermutation. CLL cases are nearly divided evenly in their immunoglobulin mutational status, approximately 40% to 50% SHM negative (called "*IGHV* unmutated") and 50% to 60% SHM positive (called "*IGHV* mutated").[5,41,42] The discovery of SHM in CLL caused a revolution in the thinking of the biologic origin of CLL. These same gene expression profiling studies also determined that CLL is a neoplasm of memory B cells, approximately 50% of which pass through the germinal center thereby acquiring SHM in an adaptive T-cell-dependent fashion, whereas the remaining memory B cells, part of our innate immune system, become memory B cells without SHM.[128,129] Prognostically, the IGH-mutated cases of CLL have longer overall survival (median 293 months for low-stage disease) and *IGHV*-unmutated cases portend a poor prognosis (median survival 95 months for low-stage disease).[41,130] Owing to the high 98% homology cutoff for determining SHM status, Ig gene rearrangement studies nonetheless have a universally high level of detection of clonal rearrangements using standard FR primers.[16-18]

The V_H repertoire utilized in CLL is biased, implying a common set of antigens or superantigens in the pathogenesis of CLL that have yet to be identified.[131-134] In some cases, certain Ig genes appear to be preferentially used in unmutated rearrangements (V_H1-69, V_K1-33, V_L3-21), whereas others are associated with *IGHV*-mutated cases (V_H4-34, V_K3-7, V_L3-23, V_L2-30, V_L2-8).[133,134] Within these gene regions even the specific amino acid changes that occur in these regions in those cases exhibiting SHM involve stereotyped changes, providing further evidence of selection for specific pathogenic antigens.[132] Certain of the stereotypes are associated with poor prognosis regardless of mutational status. The most well documented of these is V_H3-21, although V_H3-48 and V_H3-53 have been discussed in this context as well.[130,135,136] Other B-cell Ig gene stereotypes have been associated with better prognosis, including V_H4-34 and V_H2-30.[132] Monoclonal B-cell lymphocytosis appears to utilize V_H4-59/61 preferentially, although it has a similar array of cytogenetic changes as CLL.[137]

SLL, although derived from the same cell of origin as CLL, demonstrates slightly different prognostic markers. SLL is associated with a lower rate of SHM than CLL (26% of cases compared with 40% of cases).[138] The prevalence of trisomy 12 and V_H3-21 is also significantly increased in SLL compared with CLL.[139]

Somatic variants. The spectrum of somatic mutations in CLL has been characterized (*Figure 89.12*).[140-143] *SF3B1* was identified as one of the most common mutations in CLL, with its frequency rising from ~5% at diagnosis, up to 15% to 25% at time of treatment initiation and rising even higher with relapse following treatment.[144-146] The majority of the mutations are a single p.K700E mutation (mutational hotspots also include codons 662 and 666), which generates aberrant splicing in these patients.[147-149] This mutation is commonly associated with del(11q) or mutations in the *ATM* gene and found in predominantly unmutated cases of CLL.[150] *SF3B1* mutations have also been identified in the myeloid neoplasm, myelodysplastic syndrome, and clonal hematopoiesis.[151-155]

NOTCH1 mutations have been identified in 4% to 12% of CLLs, associated with decreased overall survival and the presence of trisomy 12.[142,156-158] The majority of these cases contain a two-nucleotide ΔCT deletion in the PEST domain, resulting in decreased ubiquitination. Additional modes by which Notch signaling is impacted include (i) activating recurrent noncoding mutations, occurring at a hotspot in the 3'-UTR or (ii) dysregulated splicing of downstream Notch pathway targets.[141,149] *NOTCH1* can directly stimulate *MYC* transcription, and *NOTCH1* mutation or *MYC* activation can coexist with decreased p53 function, especially in cases of fludarabine-refractory CLL or Richter transformation.[157,159,160]

MYD88 mutations, occurring stably at ~10% of cases across disease course, predominantly involve missense mutations occurring at only three sites within a 40-bp region of the gene.[156] These patients tend to be younger with disease presenting at a more advanced clinical state and are highly associated with SHM and del(13q). *FBXW7* mutations (4% of cases), as well as *NOTCH1* mutations, are associated with trisomy 12.[157,158,160]

TP53 mutations (present in 15% of cases at diagnosis and rising in frequency in the setting of chemotherapy treatment) often occur in conjunction with del(17p), to result in biallelic loss of function, although recent single cell studies also suggest that subclonal alterations in TP53 and del(17p) can also arise as separate lesions in distinct subpopulations.[149] Similarly, *ATM* (9%) mutations are also often found in conjunction with its corresponding gene deletion.

Progression. Disease progression, resistance to therapy, and transformation in CLL appears to be associated with an accumulation of genetic changes, particularly deletion of 6q21-q24.[118,161] Therefore, at relapse or progressive disease, the number and nature of cytogenetic aberrancies can differ from at the time of diagnosis. Acquisition of reciprocal translocations, even those commonly associated with other B-cell lymphomas such as rearrangements of *BCL2, MYC,* and *BCL3* often with IGH, can be seen at disease progression.[162-165] The accumulation of mutations during disease progression has been likewise documented by NGS studies, with mutations in *TP53, ATM, SF3B1, NOTCH1,* and *MYD88* commonly tested for associations with response in clinical trials in CLL.[143] Altogether, these studies have clearly confirmed *TP53* disruption as the most crucial and independent factor of resistance in the setting of cytotoxic chemotherapy,[140,145,166,167] while allogeneic transplantation remains a valid strategy for patients with *TP53* disruption, as well as the use of newer agents such as ibrutinib, idelalisib-rituximab, and venetoclax.[124,168-171] Importantly, small subclones with *TP53* mutations detected at diagnosis only by sensitive techniques are associated with the same adverse prognosis as macroscopic subclones and can anticipate fludarabine refractoriness.[143,172] *SF3B1* or *ATM* mutations appear to have variable evolution, with distinct clones rising or falling over time, suggesting that they likely do not bring the same advantage as *TP53* when considered individually. The prevalence of *NOTCH1* mutations increases with Richter transformation (from 8.3% to 31.0%) as well as with chemorefractoriness (20.8%).[157]

In contrast to the setting of chemotherapy, resistance to the targeted irreversible pathway inhibitor ibrutinib has been attributed to mutations directly affecting its target (BTK) or its downstream effector PLCγ2.[173] *BTK* mutations (p.C481S hotspot) are located in the ibrutinib-binding site, resulting in a protein that is only reversibly inhibited by ibrutinib.[174]

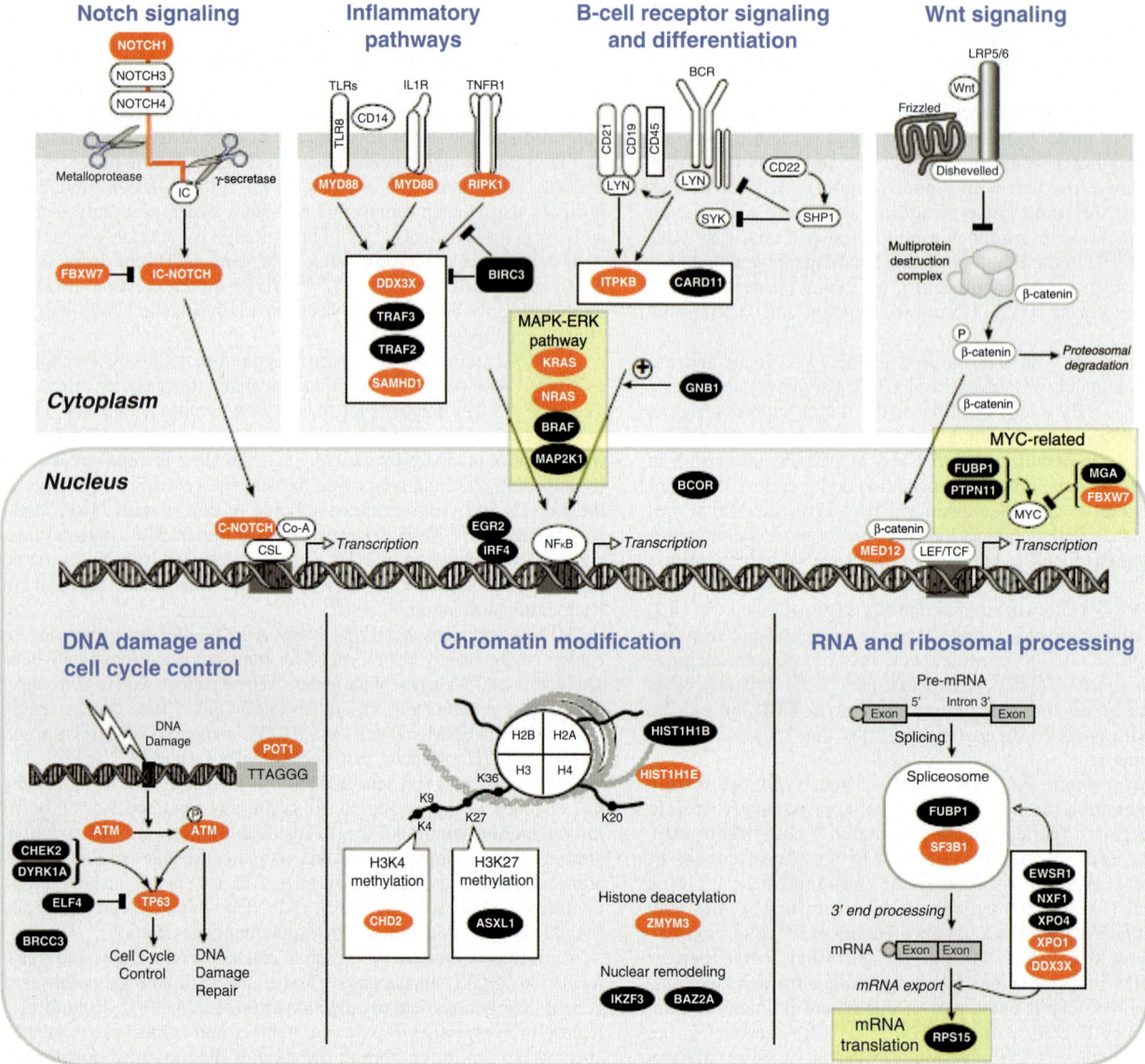

FIGURE 89.12 Pathways with genomic alterations in chronic lymphocytic leukemia. The Notch, inflammatory, B-cell receptor, Wnt signaling, DNA damage/cell cycle, chromatin modification, and RNA/ribosomal pathways are shown with their interactions. Key genes recurrently altered in CLL are shown in orange (note: not all the genes illustrated are specifically discussed in the text).

BTK mutations can be detected in patients on ibrutinib with residual clonal lymphocytosis, prior to overt relapse, and their presence is predictive of subsequent progression.[175] The same mutations appear to confer resistance to the second-generation BTK inhibitors acalabrutinib and zanubrutinib.[176-178] *PLCG2* mutations likewise provide gain of function and lead to activation of BCR signaling in a BTK-independent manner.[179] Resistance to ibrutinib has been also associated with marked clonal evolution.[180] Aside from *BTK* or *PLCG2* mutations, relapsing subclones have been shown to be progeny of parental del(8p) leukemic cells, present prior to therapy. Distinct modes of therapy thus may shape the CLL architecture differently.

Similarly, resistance to the targeted BCL2 inhibitor venetoclax has been associated with acquired mutations in BCL2. The most common such mutation, p.G101V, markedly reduces the affinity of BCL2 for venetoclax and has been identified in up to 50% of cases of CLL with acquired venetoclax resistance. Other mutations in BCL2 that confer venetoclax resistance include mutations at Asp103 (p.D103Y/G/V) and Val156 (p.V156D).[181-184]

Guidelines for Molecular Testing in Chronic Lymphocytic Leukemia

Diagnosis	MRD
FISH or aCGH recurrent numerical changes and SHM testing	Flow cytometry is the standard of care. Consider NGS for Ig gene rearrangement studies
Consider somatic mutation testing for *TP53, SF3B1, NOTCH1,* and *ATM* for prognostic and therapeutic purposes	
In the setting of disease resistant to ibrutinib or venetoclax, consider mutational testing of *BTK/PLCG2* or *BCL2*	

Extranodal Marginal Zone Lymphoma (Mucosa-Associated Lymphoid Tissue Lymphoma)

Mucosa-associated lymphoid tissue (MALT) lymphomas comprise 7% to 8% of all B-cell lymphomas and are the most common extranodal NHL.[5] MALT lymphoma is one of three subclasses of marginal zone lymphoma recognized by the World Health Organization (WHO) along with nodal marginal zone lymphoma (NMZL) and SMZL.[5] This neoplasm is not to be confused with NMZL or SMZL, as these entities lack the characteristic reciprocal translocations found in the MALT lymphomas. It is interesting that these MALT lymphomas are not traditionally found in normal physiologic sites of MALT, but rather in sites exposed to chronic inflammation that acquire a significant lymphoid infiltrate. This chronic inflammation is often associated with specific infectious agents or autoimmune disease, and these instigating etiologies segregate by the sites of the MALT lymphomas (Table 89.5).[185,186]

Rearrangements. Four recurrent reciprocal translocations are identified in MALT lymphomas: t(11;18)(q22;q21), t(1;14)(p22;q32), t(14;18)(q32;q21), and t(3;14)(p14.1;q32). The first three of these translocations all involve overexpression or fusion of components within the NF-κB pathway, resulting in overstimulation of the pathway and overexpression of NF-κB-dependent genes involved in antiapoptosis and cellular proliferation (Figure 89.13).[186] Typically, stimulation of the BCR (Ig complex) induces the interaction of BCL10 and MALT1, which promotes dimerization of MALT1. This complex in turn causes oligomerization of the TNF receptor–associated factor 6 (TRAF6). This activation of TRAF6 results in promotion of IKKγ-mediated phosphorylation of Ik-B. Phosphorylated Ik-B is then targeted for degradation, releasing NF-κB, which translocates to the nucleus and promotes transcription of genes involved in lymphocyte survival and proliferation. The various NF-κB pathway–related translocations cause induction of this pathway independent of stimulation through the BCR.

The t(11;18) (q22;q21) creates a fusion product between *BIRC3* (*API2*) on 11q22 and *MALT1* on 18q21 and is the most common recurrent translocation in MALT lymphomas.[187,188] All of the translocation sites in *BIRC3* (at least four known) are localized downstream from the BIR domains in the gene, resulting in full BIR domain activity in the fusion protein.[189] These domains mark BIRC3 as a member of the inhibitors of apoptosis (IAP) family of proteins that inhibit the caspases. However, these domains are also capable of homophilic interactions, causing dimerization. This fusion therefore results in MALT1 units that can dimerize independent of the BCR, thereby creating constitutive, antigen-independent stimulation of the NF-κB pathway. Over 90% of the translocation sites in *BIRC3* occur at a single site, just 5′ to its CARD domain, so designing primers against this most common breakpoint region is possible. Unfortunately, the *MALT1* breakpoint regions are spread over 300 bp throughout the middle portion of the gene, leaving the carboxyl terminus of the *MALT1* gene fused to *BIRC3*.[189] Nevertheless, PCR-based assays have been designed for this lesion, which, depending on the primers, have variable but overall moderate clinical sensitivity. FISH probes, which easily span the possible breakpoint sites, provide higher clinical sensitivity for this translocation, which has significant therapeutic relevance (vide infra).[190]

The t(1;14) (p22;q32) results in the overexpression of the *BCL10* gene on 1p22 through its relocation under the IGH enhancer. The resultant increased concentration of BCL10 in the cytoplasm results in its forced association with MALT1 and activation of the NF-κB pathway. Interestingly, the interaction of BCL10 with MALT1 appears to help localize BCL10 to the cytoplasm, and overexpression of BCL10 results in excess unbound BCL10 and consequent nuclear expression of BCL10 in cells with this translocation. The formation of *BIRC3::MALT1* fusion in cases harboring the t(11;18) likewise frees BCL10 from the cytoplasm and results in nuclear expression of BCL10. This can be seen immunohistochemically and may prove to be a good surrogate for these translocations.[189,191,192] Currently, there is limited offering of FISH or any molecular assay for this translocation, although IGH-break-apart probes can be used to identify the translocation, albeit not its partner.

The t(14;18)(q32;q21) seen in approximately 10% of MALT lymphomas contains the identical karyotypic breakpoints to those seen in FL.[193] However, the *BCL2* gene is in reality located 5 Mb telomeric to the *MALT1* gene.[194] This translocation juxtaposes the IGH partner, in this case *MALT1*, with the IGH enhancer to the J_H subunit of IGH.[193] The resultant overexpression of MALT1 protein results in elevated cytoplasmic concentrations of the protein, which stochastically force enough proximity to induce TRAF6 oligomerization and NF-κB activation. The majority of *MALT1* breakpoints appear to occur within an 87-bp region, which may permit the development of a PCR-based assay for this translocation. However, due to the relatively low frequency of this translocation in MALT lymphoma, FISH probes for these loci are commonly utilized.

Finally, the t(3;14)(p14.1;q32) involves the overexpression of the *FOXP1* gene on 3p14 due to its relocation to the IGH gene locus.[195] *FOXP1* encodes a transcriptional repressor in the Forkhead family, which is critical for B-cell development and whose overexpression is implicated in several B-cell lymphomas in addition to MALT lymphomas. Although FOXP1 can be interrogated by IHC, this antibody is not commonly used in clinical laboratories, and directed FISH probes or PCR-based assays are likewise not common. IGH-break-apart probes can be used to identify the translocation, albeit not its partner.

Table 89.5. Translocations in Extranodal Marginal Zone Lymphomas, Their Frequency by Site, and Their Association With Chronic Inflammatory Agents/Disorders

Translocation	t(11;18)(q22;q21)	t(1;14)(p22;q32)	t(14;18)(q32;q21)	t(3;14)(q14.1;q32)	Potential agent
Product	BIRC3::MALT1 Fusion (%)	Overexpression of BCL10 (%)	Overexpression of MALT1 (%)	Overexpression of FOXP1 (%)	
Locations:					
Stomach	22	3			*Helicobacter pylori*
Intestine	15	10			*Campylobacter jejuni*
Lung	42	7			*Chlamydia psittaci*
Ocular adnexa			13	20	*C. psittaci*
Salivary glands			5		Sjogren disease
Thyroid				50	Hashimoto disease
Skin			14	10	*Borrelia burgdorferi*

Abbreviations: BCL, B-cell lymphoma; MALT, mucosa-associated lymphoid tissue.
From Aigelsreiter A, Gerlza T, Deutsch AJA, et al. Chlamydia psittaci infection in nongastrointestinal extranodal MALT lymphomas and their precursor lesions. *Am J Clin Pathol.* 2011;135(1):70-75; Farinha P, Gascoyne RD. Molecular pathogenesis of mucosa-associated lymphoid tissue lymphoma. *J Clin Oncol.* 2005;23(26):6370-6378.

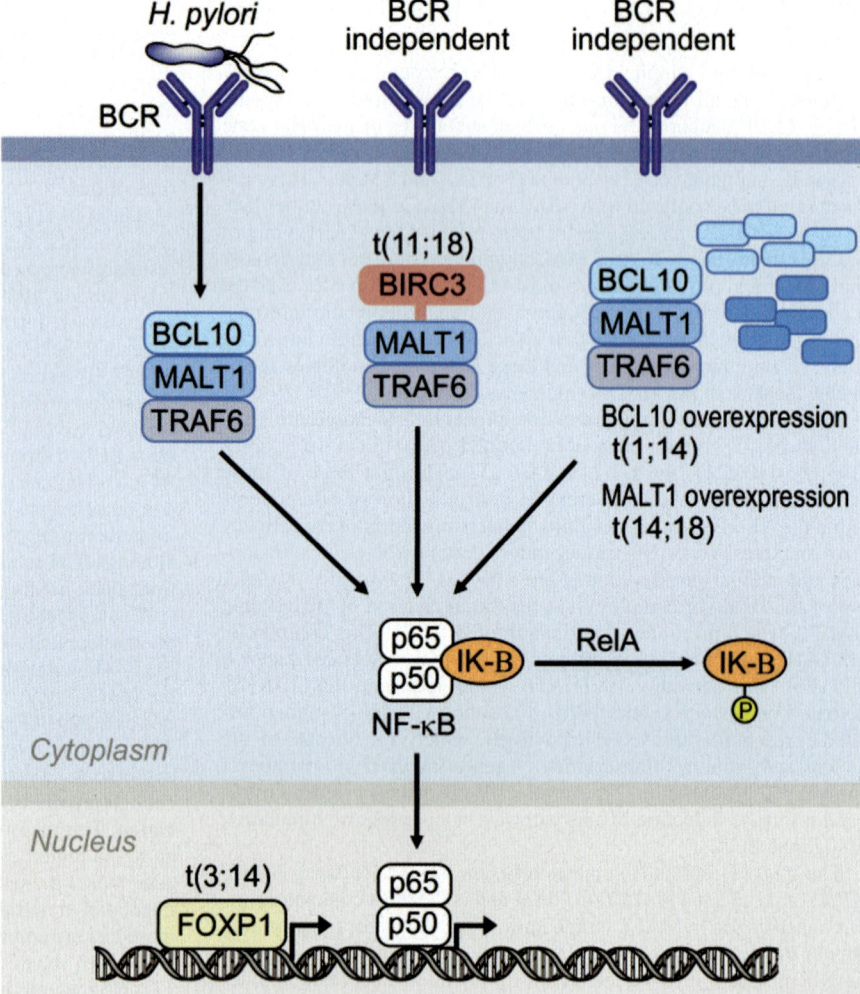

FIGURE 89.13 Biology of translocations common in extranodal marginal zone lymphomas. On the far left: *Helicobacter pylori* stimulation of the B-cell receptor (BCR) induces the interaction of BCL10 and MALT1, promoting dimerization of MALT1 and downstream oligomerization of TRAF6. This activation of TRAF6 results in promotion of IKKγ-mediated phosphorylation of Ik-B (IKKγ not shown). Phosphorylated Ik-B is then targeted for degradation, releasing NF-κB, which translocates to the nucleus and transcriptionally activates genes involved in lymphocyte survival and proliferation. The t(11;18) induces BCR-independent dimerization of MALT1 and activation of the pathway. The t(1;14) induces BCL10 overexpression and promotes dimerization of MALT1 as does overexpression of MALT1 itself via a t(14;18). Lastly, the t(3;14) induces a FOXP1 transcriptional program that must be related to the NF-κB program.

These translocations are associated with specific sites and etiologies of MALT lymphomas.[186] The t(11;18) and t(1;14) are most common in gastric, intestinal, and lung MALT lymphomas with the t(11;18) being especially prevalent in the gastric and lung neoplasms. By contrast, the t(14;18) and t(3;14) occur in the ocular adnexa and skin, with the t(14;18) also rarely found in the salivary gland lymphomas and the t(3;14) commonly found in the thyroid lesions. Each of these different sites has a distinct source of chronic inflammation that has been associated with MALT lymphomas in these sites, although exactly how the instigating agent causes specific reciprocal translocations remains to be understood. However, it is known that, although early gastric MALT lymphomas are dependent upon *Helicobacter pylori* stimulation of the B cell, once the neoplasm acquires a t(11;18), it becomes independent of the bacterium. Thus, whereas antibiotics successfully treat up to 75% of gastric MALT lymphomas, the cases with t(11;18) are refractory to antibiotic therapy.[196]

Inasmuch as MALT lymphomas are derived from post-germinal center marginal zone B cells, they tend to have significant SHM. Thus, immunoglobulin gene rearrangement studies identify clonal rearrangements in only 62% to 68% of cases using a single set of FR3 primers.[15-17] Distinguishing reactive lymphoid hyperplasia from MALT lymphoma in sites of chronic inflammation can be histologically challenging; in these cases, Ig gene rearrangement studies, when positive, can be helpful. However, these results must be interpreted with caution, as inflammatory lesions can demonstrate pseudoclonality due a limited repertoire of B cells responding to a given antigen.

Copy number variations and somatic variants. MALT lymphomas, as well as other marginal zone lymphomas, can demonstrate ancillary cytogenetic changes, in particular trisomies of 3, 7, 12, and 18.[197] In addition, with transformation to DLBCL, additional aberrations may accumulate in *TP53, CDKN2B (p15), CDKN2A (p16), RB1,* and *MYC*.[186] Recurrent somatic mutations are primarily found in the NF-κB pathway (*TNFAIP3* 25%, *MYD88* 10%) and epigenetic pathways (*KMT2D* 15%, *CREBBP* 17%, *TBL1XR1* 19%).[198-201]

Guidelines for Molecular Testing in Extranodal Marginal Zone Lymphoma

Diagnosis	MRD
Consider FISH for various translocations	Consider NGS for Ig gene rearrangement studies
Consider PCR or NGS for Ig gene rearrangement studies	

Nodal Marginal Zone Lymphoma

NMZL is one of three subclasses of marginal zone lymphoma recognized by the WHO, along with MALT lymphoma and SMZL.[5] However, while MALT lymphoma typically follows an indolent course with frequent protracted remission, NMZL is more aggressive, with 5-year survival of only 60% to 70%; therefore, it is critical to distinguish these entities.[202,203] NMZL accounts for 1.6% of all lymphoid neoplasms and approximately 30% of marginal zone lymphomas[204] and predominantly occurs in adults, with a median age of approximately 60 years, and males and females equally affected.[202,205] An association with specific infectious agents is not observed for NMZL, although epidemiologic data suggest an association with B-cell-activating autoimmune disease.[206] A pediatric variant has also been described, with histologic and immunophenotypic features similar to adult NMZL; however, unlike its adult counterpart, it has a marked male predominance and follows a more indolent clinical course.[207]

Rearrangements and cytogenetic alterations. NMZL lacks the recurrent chromosomal translocations seen in MALT lymphoma, as well as in other low-grade B-cell lymphomas, and the deletion of chromosome 7q31 characteristic of SMZL.[208] This absence may be critical in distinguishing NMZL from its histologic mimics. Trisomy of chromosomes 3, 12, and 18 and loss of 6q34 are frequently observed in NMZL; however, none of these findings are specific.[208] *IGHV* gene region usage is biased toward IGHV3 and IGHV4, with a particular bias toward IGHV4-34.[209,210]

Somatic variants. In the past several years, genomic analysis has helped to elucidate the pathogenesis of NMZL. Many of the genes that are most frequently mutated in NMZL (and SMZL) play central roles in marginal zone B-cell differentiation, implicating dysregulation of marginal zone development as the major pathophysiologic process in NMZL.[208]

NOTCH2 is the most frequently mutated gene in NMZL; mutations in this gene are observed in approximately 25% of cases of NMZL. Approximately 10% to 40% of cases of SMZL and monoclonal B-cell lymphocytosis of marginal zone phenotype also harbor *NOTCH2* mutations, suggesting some degree of overlap between these entities.[208,211] *NOTCH2* is essential for marginal zone B-cell differentiation in both mice and humans, and patients with Alagille syndrome, an inherited disorder caused by germline *NOTCH2* mutation, have reduced numbers of marginal zone B cells. Like the canonical *NOTCH1* mutations, the *NOTCH2* mutations seen in marginal zone lymphomas cluster in the C-terminal PEST domain and prevent its proteasomal degradation.[208] Mutations in other genes involved in NOTCH2 signaling, including *MAML2*, *SPEN*, and *DTX1*, are observed in an additional 15% of cases of NMZL and appear to be mutually exclusive with *NOTCH2* mutations. Overall, approximately 40% of NMZL harbor mutations that affect NOTCH2 signaling.[208,211]

NF-κB signaling is also required for marginal zone B-cell differentiation, and mutations involving the NF-κB signaling pathway have been identified in approximately 50% of NMZL. Like the NOTCH signaling pathway mutations in NMZL, the NF-κB pathway mutations observed in NMZL are mutually exclusive with one another and result in constitutive activation and pathologic gain of function; this is consistent with the observation that immunohistochemical markers of NF-κB activation, such as p50 and p52, are frequently positive in NMZL.[208] NF-κB signaling pathway components with observed aberrations in NMZL include *CARD11* of the canonical NF-κB pathway and *TRAF3*, *MAP3K14*, and *BIRC3* of the noncanonical NF-κB pathway.[208] Notably, the *MYD88* p.L265P mutation characteristic of lymphoplasmacytic lymphoma (LPL) is generally absent in NMZL, although it has been observed in rare cases.[212-214]

Nearly all the somatic variants described above show significant overlap between SMZL and NMZL; to date, few studies have identified aberrations that show a significant association with one relative to the other. A noteworthy exception is *PTPRD*, a protein tyrosine phosphatase expressed in naïve and marginal zone B cells, which is mutated in ~20% of NMZL but only rarely in SMZL. Mutations in *PTPRD* associated with NMZL are generally loss of function.[208,211,215]

Guidelines for Molecular Testing in Nodal Marginal Zone Lymphoma

The absence of characteristic cytogenetic abnormalities associated with MALT lymphoma (e.g., t(11;18)) and SMZL (e.g., 7q deletion) may be helpful in distinguishing NMZL from these entities, and in cases with plasmacytic differentiation, the absence of *MYD88* p.L265P mutation may assist in distinction from nodal LPL. In challenging cases, identification of the *NOTCH2* mutation or NF-κB pathway mutations may be helpful in distinguishing NMZL from other low-grade B-cell lymphomas.

Diagnosis	MRD
Consider FISH for various translocations	Consider NGS for Ig gene rearrangement studies
Consider PCR or NGS for Ig gene rearrangement studies	Consider PCR or NGS for mutational analysis
Consider PCR or NGS for mutational analysis	

Splenic Marginal Zone Lymphoma

SMZL is relatively rare, accounting for approximately 2% of all lymphoid neoplasms,[204] although this may be an underestimate due to frequent misdiagnosis as CD5-negative CLL/SLL.[5] It primarily affects adults, with a median age of 67 to 68 years and equal incidence among males and females and is not clearly associated with any infectious or immune-mediated pathology; an association with hepatitis C virus infection has been reported, but is controversial. While it is relatively indolent, with 10-year survival between 67% and 95%,[5] it is more aggressive than either MALT lymphoma or CLL/SLL and is poorly responsive to chemotherapy regimens effective against other low-grade B-cell neoplasms,[5,216-218] making distinction from these entities critical for appropriate therapy.

Rearrangements and cytogenetic alterations. Like NMZL, with which it shows significant overlap, SMZL lacks the chromosomal rearrangements characteristic of MALT lymphoma,[211] as well as other translocations characteristic of low-grade B-cell lymphomas.[5] Rarely, a translocation involving chromosomes 2 and 7 resulting in *IGK::CDK6* rearrangement may be observed[219]; however, this finding is rare and its specificity is uncertain.

The most frequent cytogenetic abnormality in SMZL is deletion of chromosome 7q, which is present in approximately 30% of SMZL and is highly specific for this entity.[5] The minimal deleted region has been mapped to cytoband 7q32,[220] although deletion of 7q22 has also been described.[221] However, the mechanistic basis for the link between 7q deletion and development of SMZL has not been determined despite extensive study. Proposed mechanisms include loss of *IRF5*[222] and underexpression of microRNAs encoded within the region.[223] Gain of 3q is also frequently seen in SMZL but is far less specific.[5] IGHV region usage in SMZL is highly biased, with usage of the IGHV1-2*04 allele in 30% of cases[224,225] and restricted CDR3 sequences, suggesting a role for antigen selection in lymphomagenesis.[226]

Somatic variants. As with NMZL, genomic analysis of SMZL has identified mutations in multiple genes and signaling pathways involved in marginal zone B-cell differentiation.[211] *NOTCH2* mutations, generally involving the C-terminal PEST domain, have been identified in 10% to 40% of cases.[227-232] Notably, *NOTCH2* mutation has been associated with reduced treatment-free survival in SMZL.[233] Mutations in *KLF2*, which, like *NOTCH2*, is involved in regulation of NF-κB signaling and marginal zone B-cell differentiation, are detected in a similar percentage of cases.[227,234]

MYD88 mutations, which are characteristic of LPL and frequently seen in CLL/SLL, are rare in SMZL.[213] Likewise, *PTPRD* mutations, which are seen in approximately 20% of cases of NMZL, are rare in SMZL, making this finding one of the few that can potentially distinguish NMZL and SMZL.[215]

Guidelines for Molecular Testing in Splenic Marginal Zone Lymphoma

Testing for the presence of 7q deletion is recommended to distinguish SMZL from other low-grade B-cell lymphomas with similar immunophenotype. In cases that lack 7q deletion, or are otherwise challenging, identification of a *NOTCH2* mutation, particularly in the absence of *PTPRD* or *MYD88* mutation, may be helpful in clarifying the diagnosis.

Diagnosis	MRD
Consider FISH for 7q deletion	Consider PCR or NGS for Ig gene rearrangement studies
Consider PCR or NGS for Ig gene rearrangement studies	Consider PCR or NGS for mutational analysis
Consider PCR or NGS for mutational analysis	

Lymphoplasmacytic Lymphoma/Waldenström Macroglobulinemia

LPL accounts for approximately 2% of NHLs. It occurs predominantly in older adults, with a median age in the 60s, and shows a slight male predominance.[5] In the vast majority of cases, LPL is associated with Waldenström macroglobulinemia (WM), which is formally defined as LPL with bone marrow involvement and IgM monoclonal gammopathy. While 18% of patients with LPL have a first-degree relative with a B-cell lymphoproliferative disorder, suggesting a familial component to the disease, no inherited germline mutations that predispose to LPL have yet been identified.[5] The clinical course of WM/LPL is typically indolent, with median survival of 5 to 10 years.[235,236]

The cell of origin in LPL is believed to be a post-germinal center B cell that has undergone some degree of plasmacytic differentiation and an unusually high degree of SHM.[237] Most patients with WM have a serum IgM paraprotein, implying that transformation occurs prior to class switch recombination (CSR), and functional studies have demonstrated impairment of CSR in WM cells, although mutations affecting CSR machinery have not been identified in LPL.[238] However, cases of LPL with secretion of IgG or IgA paraproteins are known to occur, indicating that impairment of CSR is not a causal or defining feature of the disease.[5]

Rearrangements and copy number variations. Although cytogenetic aberrations are frequently seen in LPL, none that are consistent or specific for the disease have been identified. The chromosomal translocation (9;14)(p13;q32), resulting in *PAX5::IGH* fusion, was previously reported to be present in as many as 50% of LPL based on karyotype data from small case series; however, larger studies largely debunked this association, demonstrating that this translocation is both rare and not particularly associated with LPL.[239,240] Deletions involving chromosome 6q are present in approximately 50% of LPL and are associated with poor prognosis.[241-243] However, this abnormality is not specific to LPL.[5] Trisomy 4 is seen in approximately 20% of LPL but is likewise nonspecific.[244] Other CNVs described in LPL include gains in chromosomes 3q, 8q, 18, and Xq and losses of 11q23, 13q14, and 17p.[245,246]

Somatic variants. The wide-scale application of NGS has led to the identification of point mutations that are highly sensitive and specific and likely causal in LPL. The key finding was the identification of the p.L265P point mutation in the *MYD88* gene on chromosome 3p22.2.[247] This mutation is present in greater than 90% of cases of LPL, as well as in approximately 30% of cases of non-germinal-center/activated type DLBCL, particularly those at immune-privileged sites, and in a small number of other low-grade B-cell lymphomas (e.g., MALT, CLL).[2] However, it appears to be absent in myeloma, (including IgM-expressing cases), and in gamma heavy chain disease, both of which can clinically mimic LPL.[2,212] The MYD88 protein functions as a signaling adaptor, interacting with toll-like receptor 4 (through BTK) and the IL-1 receptor expressed on B cells, resulting in upregulation of the NF-κB pathway. The p.L265P mutation induces constitutive association of BTK with the mutant MYD88 protein, resulting in constitutive activation of the NF-κB pathway, resistance to apoptosis, and enhanced cell survival.[247,248] The presence of the *MYD88* p.L265P mutation is predictive of response to the BTK inhibitor ibrutinib, which disrupts the interaction of BTK with *MYD88*.[249,250] Highly sensitive ASO-PCR assays have been developed to detect the *MYD88* p.L265P mutation, and the mutation is amenable to detection by NGS as well, although typically with lower analytical sensitivity.

Subsequent WGS studies of patients with LPL identified mutations in the *CXCR4* gene in a significant subset (27%-36%) of patients with LPL.[251,252] In the vast majority of *CXCR4*-mutant LPL cases (>98%), the *MYD88* p.L265P mutation is also present,[251,252] suggesting that the *MYD88* p.L265P mutation occurs first while *CXCR4* mutation is acquired later as a subclonal event.[253] *CXCR4* is a chemokine receptor that promotes adhesion to bone marrow stroma through interaction with its ligand, CXCL12.[254] Germline *CXCR4* mutations are associated with warts, hypogammaglobulinemia, infection, and myelokathexis (WHIM) syndrome, a rare congenital immunodeficiency disorder, but are otherwise somatically rare in other malignancies. The *CXCR4* mutations found in LPL are identical to those seen in the germline in association with WHIM syndrome and are divided into two classes that occur with approximately equal frequency in LPL: nonsense mutations that truncate the distal 15 to 20 amino acids of the protein and frameshift mutations occurring within a 40-amino-acid region of the distal C terminus. Both classes of mutation result in expression of a protein lacking the C-terminal regulatory domain and, consequently, blocked receptor internalization and gain of function resulting in enhanced cell survival and persistent cell adhesion to bone marrow stroma.[254-256] The presence of *CXCR4* mutation is associated with increased disease activity and more aggressive phenotype, including higher serum IgM, bone marrow disease burden, and increased likelihood of clinical symptoms requiring therapy,[252,256] as well as resistance to ibrutinib (although *MYD88/CXCR4* double mutated cases still respond to ibrutinib better than cases in which *MYD88* is wild type).[257,258] Nonsense *CXCR4* mutations are associated with a more severe phenotype than frameshift mutations.[256] Both ASO-PCR[253] and NGS-based assays have been developed to detect *CXCR4* mutation in LPL, although the latter may be preferable due to the heterogeneity of mutations.

Other genes with validated somatic mutations in LPL include *ARID1A* (present in 17% of LPL cases) and *CD79B*, *TP53*, *MYBBP1A*, *MUC16*, *TRAF2*, *TRAF3*, *RAG2*, and *NOTCH2* (all of which are present in less than 10% of LPL cases).[251] None of these mutations, however, are specific to LPL.

Gene expression profiling. Gene expression profiling in LPL has identified characteristic signatures, including upregulation of V(D)J-recombination related genes including *RAG1* and *RAG2*, upregulation of cell-adhesion molecules including both *CXCR4* and *CXCL12* as well as *VCAM1*, and upregulation of *IGF1*.[259] Notably, *CXCR4*-mutant and *CXCR4*-WT LPL cases showed distinct gene expression profiles, with the latter showing a gene expression pattern suggestive of an earlier stage of B-cell differentiation.[259]

Epigenetic analysis. Profiling of epigenetic modifications in LPL has identified a global pattern of aberrant histone hypoacetylation mediated, at least in part, by aberrant microRNA expression, particularly microRNA-206 and -209.[260] The histone deacetylase inhibitor panobinostat has shown clinical efficacy against LPL in clinical trials.[261]

Guidelines for Molecular Testing in Lymphoplasmacytic Lymphoma/Waldenström Macroglobulinemia

Upfront molecular testing for the *MYD88* p.L265P mutation is recommended.[262] *MYD88* mutation analysis may also be helpful in assessment of minimal residual disease.[263] Testing for *CXCR4* mutations should also be considered, particularly in patients who may receive ibrutinib therapy.[264]

Diagnosis	MRD
PCR or NGS for *MYD88* p.L265P mutation	PCR or NGS for *MYD88* p.L265P mutation
Consider NGS for *CXCR4* mutation	
Consider PCR or NGS for Ig gene rearrangement studies	Consider PCR or NGS for Ig gene rearrangement studies

Hairy Cell Leukemia

HCL is a rare leukemic mature B-cell neoplasm that affects middle-aged to older adults with a strong male:female bias (5:1) and unique presentation involving "hairy" morphology, cytopenias (especially monocytopenia), bone marrow fibrosis, and involvement of the splenic red pulp.[5] Up to 10% of cases of HCL show variant clinical presentation (typically leukocytosis rather than cytopenias), morphology (resembling PLL), and immunophenotype. These cases respond suboptimally to purine analogues (e.g., cladribine and pentostatin), the mainstay of therapy for HCL, and are provisionally classified as "hairy cell leukemia-variant" (HCLv) to distinguish them from classical HCL.[5]

Gene expression profiling demonstrates a molecular signature that matches the morphologic and clinical characteristics of the disease, with prominent signatures generated by adhesion molecules, homing molecules, and molecules involved in marrow fibrosis.[265] The cell of origin is believed to be a late post-germinal center memory B cell, since more than 85% of cases demonstrate significant SHM.[5,266] Reciprocal translocations are rare in HCL. Instead, many cases of HCL appear to have multiple clonally related Ig-isotypes, suggesting that the defect lies in the class switching process.[264]

Copy number variations. Until recently, no consistent or specific cytogenetic abnormalities had been identified in HCL, although gains in chromosome 5 (20%) and losses of the long arm of chromosome 7 (10%) had been identified.[267-269] Although HCL in general does not show biased IGHV region usage, a subset of HCL cases (10% of classical HCL and up to 40% of HCLv) have rearrangements involving IGHV4-34; these cases have a poor prognosis relative to IGHV4-34-negative HCL, independent of classification as classical vs variant HCL.[270]

Somatic variants. BRAF p.V600E mutation is 98% to 100% sensitive for classical HCL.[271] While frequently identified in solid tumors,[272] the mutation has not been identified in cases that can be morphologic mimics of HCL, such as SMZL, HCLv, and splenic diffuse red pulp small B-cell lymphoma.[273,274] This mutation that activates the MAPK pathway is most commonly found as a heterozygous somatic mutation, but in rare cases it can be homozygous. Dysregulation of the MAPK pathway results in constitutive transcription of cyclin D1 and downregulation of p27, both of which conspire to cause increased cellular proliferation and explain the expression of cyclin D1 by IHC in HCL without any evidence of the t(11;14). Highly sensitive PCR-based *BRAF* assays may be helpful in the diagnosis and almost certainly in the future monitoring of patients with applied to HCL.[275,276] The BRAF inhibitor vemurafenib has been demonstrated, in phase 2 clinical trials, to rapidly induce durable remission in HCL relapsed or refractory to purine analogues, with response rates of 96% to 100%.[277]

Clinical variants and related diseases. In contrast to classical HCL, no cases of HCLv with *BRAF* p.V600E mutation have been reported.[271] Instead, activating mutations of *MAP2K1*, encoding a kinase downstream of BRAF in the MAPK pathway, have been identified in 42% of cases of HCL-v.[278] *MAP2K1* mutations appear to be mutually exclusive with the *BRAF* p.V600E mutation. However, the rare cases of classical HCL lacking the *BRAF* p.V600E mutation are disproportionately likely to harbor *MAP2K1* mutations[278,279] and to show usage of IGHV4-34,[280] suggesting that *BRAF* and *MAP2K1* mutation status, in combination with IGHV usage, may be more predictive of disease biology and clinical behavior than conventional classification as classical vs variant HCL.

Guidelines for Molecular Testing in Hairy Cell Leukemia

The *BRAF* p.V600E mutation may be helpful in distinguishing HCL from some of its morphologic mimics. No studies to date have examined *BRAF* mutations in the MRD setting of HCL. Testing by NGS for *MAP2K1* mutations may be helpful in identifying cases of HCL that lack the *BRAF* p.V600E mutation, and NGS for IGHV4-34 usage may be a useful prognostic indicator.

Diagnosis	MRD
Consider *BRAF* p.V600E testing	Consider *BRAF* V600E testing
Consider PCR or NGS for Ig gene rearrangements	Consider PCR or NGS for Ig gene rearrangements
Consider NGS for *MAP2K1* mutations	Consider NGS for *MAP2K1* mutations
Consider NGS for IGHV4-34 usage	

Follicular Lymphoma

FL accounts for approximately 20% of all lymphomas and is the second most common B-cell lymphoma, especially prevalent in Western nations.[5] FL is predominantly a disease of adults, and morphologic subclassifications are based upon the histologic grade and degree of nodularity. Notable subtypes include primary cutaneous FL (PCFL), pediatric-type nodal FL (PTNFL), and FL of specific extranodal sites such as the duodenum or testes. Organized in follicles and expressing germinal center B-cell markers such as BCL6 and CD10, FL cells have the characteristic gene expression profile of centrocytes and centroblasts, consistent with their differentiation level. Approximately 25% to 35% of FL may transform to a more aggressive lymphoma, typically a DLBCL.[5]

Rearrangements. The longstanding hallmark of FL has been the IGH::*BCL2* translocation, t(14;18) (q32,q21), found in approximately 85% to 90% of cases of FL, including in situ follicular neoplasia and duodenal variants, and in 20% to 25% of de novo DLBCLs (not transformed from a known prior FL), occasional cases of CLL, and rarely in other lymphomas.[111,162,163,281-283] The translocation, occurring during VDJ rearrangement, results in the overexpression of BCL2, which can be determined by immunohistochemical staining (IHC) except in cases when a mutation in *BCL2*, superimposed on the rearrangement, prevents the antibody from binding.[284] The translocation itself is commonly identified by karyotype, FISH, or PCR-based assays. Overexpression of BCL2 results in the failure of apoptosis rather than a proliferative drive, explaining the typically indolent behavior of this lymphoma (*Figure 89.9*).

Within the *BCL2* locus there are several clusters of breakpoints spread out over the entire length of the coding gene and extending to more than 30 kb downstream from the final exon 3 (*Figure 89.14*).[94,285] The majority of the potential breakpoint

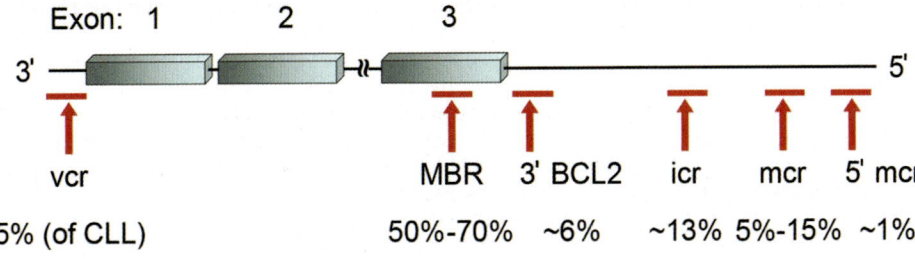

FIGURE 89.14 Location of breakpoint clusters in the *BCL2* gene and their relative frequencies in follicular lymphoma and other B-cell neoplasms. icr, intermediate cluster region; MBR, major breakpoint region; mcr, minor cluster region; vcr, variable cluster region.

clusters involve translocation of the full coding sequence of *BCL2* to chromosome 14. The major breakpoint region (MBR) is located within the 3′-UTR of exon 3 and accounts for 50% to 70% of potential breakpoints in *BCL2*. The minor cluster region (mcr) is located 20 to 30 kb farther downstream of exon 3, accounting for 5% to 15% of cases. These two sets of primers are able to detect approximately 70% to 85% of potential rearrangements.[281] However, there are several additional sites within the *BCL2* locus that can also be involved in rearrangements with immunoglobulin.[94,285] In addition, the intermediate cluster region (icr), accounting for 13% of translocations, is located between the MBR and the mcr as is the 3′ BCL2 cluster, which accounts for 6% of cases. The 5′ mcr is the farthest downstream breakpoint region but only accounts for approximately 1% of cases. Lastly, the variable cluster region (vcr) is located 5′ to the first exon but is found predominantly in the rare cases of CLL that harbor a t(14;18) as well as rare cases of FL and can be associated with translocations involving either IGK or IGL instead of IGH without prognostic differences.[285]

Given the only 70% to 85% clinical sensitivity of most clinical PCR-based assays for t(14;18)(q32;q21), FISH for the rearrangement plays a significant role in those cases where the diagnosis is not definitive or in lieu of molecular testing.[286] The clinical sensitivity of FISH is significantly higher (100% correlation with SB) due to the far longer probes used in this method, which are not dependent upon the specific site of the break. FISH is less useful in monitoring patients for MRD. For cases in which there is morphologic concern for a more high-grade process (foci of grade 3B or concomitant DLBCL), FISH for *MYC* and *BCL6* rearrangements may also be helpful to identify transformation to a double- or triple-hit lymphoma.[287,288]

Even with the more clinically sensitive FISH studies, still 10% to 15% of FLs will be negative for a t(14;18). These cases of FL may have translocations involving *BCL6* instead, often associated with more aggressive lesions with increased large cells.[289-292] In addition, the FL variants such as PCFL, PTNFL, testicular FL, and diffuse variants are also typically t(14;18)-negative.[2,5] Higher-grade FL is also associated with a higher incidence of t(14;18) negativity.[5] These t(14;18)-negative FLs have been associated with downregulation of miR-16, miR-26a, miR-101, miR-29c, and miR-138, supporting a later germinal center cell of origin.[293]

The use of molecular testing for *BCL2::IGH* rearrangements for MRD monitoring carries one significant caveat. Using highly sensitive nested PCR methods or RT-PCR, t(14;18) may be found in up to 50% of normal individuals, the incidence increasing with age.[294-296] At this time, there is no indication that these t(14;18)-positive individuals are at any higher risk of developing FL. This phenomenon may serve as the basis for those individuals who enjoy prolonged complete remission while remaining PCR positive.[297] Its presence in the majority of malignant cells within individuals with FL suggest that it is a founding lesion, but it is not itself sufficient or pathognomonic for pathogenesis of this entity.[298,299]

Because FL is a neoplasm of GCBs, ongoing SHM limits the utility of immunoglobulin gene rearrangement molecular assays. Indeed, these assays have a notoriously low clinical sensitivity for FL using a single set of IGH FR3 primers, ranging from 13% to 52%.[16-18] This corresponds to the extremely high average frequency of mutations in FL, of 11.6% for IgG clones, 9.9% for IgA clones, and 7.8% for IgM clones.[300] V_H contains an overall of 11.0% mutations in essentially 100% of cases of FL, where V_K contains a mean mutation rate of only 0.5% in only 33% of cases.[301] Therefore, the addition of IGK primers greatly enhances the clinical sensitivity of the assay for FLs. The IGK locus tends to harbor fewer mutations, 4.7% according to one study.[302] Therefore, by combining multiple immunoglobulin primers against both IGH and IGK, a clonal rearrangement can be identified.[16-18,301]

Copy number variations. In addition to translocations, nonrandom losses of chromosomes 1p36 and 6q, and gains of 7, 18, X have been detected in FL.[303] Cytogenetic abnormalities tend to accumulate with transformation of FL to DLBCL, and deletions or mutations of *TP53* located on 17p13 and deletions of 6q or 9p are particularly associated with poor prognosis.[303-305] Losses or copy number neutral LOH of 1p36, at which site *TP73* and *TNFRSF14* are located, have been associated predominantly with diffuse FL but can be seen in nodal FL, duodenal-type FL, PTNFL, and even in situ follicular neoplasia. In addition, acquisition of a *MYC* translocation may also be associated with transformation.[5]

Gene expression profiling. Gene expression profiling studies in FL have identified two separate prognostic groups distinguished by their tumor microenvironment. A prominent T-cell signature is associated with better prognosis, whereas a dominant macrophage signature is associated with poor outcomes.[306] Given the impracticality of diagnostic transcriptional profiling for all patients at this time, immunohistochemical surrogates have been sought including the quantitation of CD68+ macrophages, CD14+ follicular dendritic cells, and the histologic localization and number of FoxP3+ Treg cells, but the interpretation of these markers is technically challenging.[307-309]

Somatic variants. The rapidly evolving area of cancer molecular genetics has recently greatly expanded our understanding of the molecular subtypes of FL (*Figure 89.15*).[310-312] By deep sequencing, 97% of FLs have nonsilent mutations in epigenetic modifiers. Inactivating mutations of *KMT2D* have been discovered to be among the most commonly recurrent events, accounting for more than 80% of FLs. These mutations interfere with the ability of *KMT2D* to activate gene transcription through H3K4 methylation.[313] Other top recurrent lesions in the fully developed FL are typically detected in genes also involved in histone modification (i.e., *CREBBP*, *EZH2*, *MEF2B*, and *EP300* found in 33%, 27%, 15%, and 9% of FL, respectively).[312-314] Mutations in CREBBP, a histone acetyltransferase (HAT), are linked with loss of HAT activity, resulting in increased activity of the BCL6 oncogene. EZH2 is the catalytic unit of the polycomb repressive complex 2, with activating mutations (unlike the loss of function mutations in myeloid neoplasms) leading to increased H3K27 trimethylation and locking the transcriptional profile of GC B cells in a transcriptional profile that favors proliferation.[315-318] *MEF2B*, a gene that interacts with *CREBBP* and *EP300* to acetylate histones, is mutated in 13.4% of FL.[313]

Analyses of candidate genes within recurrent nonrandom losses of chromosomes 1p36 and 6q in FL have revealed inactivating mutations of *TNFRSF14* and loss of the tumor suppressors *TNFAIP3/A20* and *EPHA7*.[319] Mutations in *TNFRSF14* have been reported in 19% to 46% patients, with 57% of mutations predicted to result in a truncation of its transmembrane domain, thereby resulting in decreased surface expression. Mutations and chromosomal deletions affecting *TNFSF14* at 1p36 have been associated with high-risk clinical features and shorter overall survival.

Seven common recurrent molecular alterations (*EZH2*, *ARID1A*, *MEF2B*, *EP300*, *FOXP1*, *CREBBP*, *CARD11*) have been used to improve the predictability of Follicular Lymphoma International Prognostic Index (FLIPI) performance status.[320] This model, called m7-FLIPI, outperformed a model having only gene mutations, with a positive predictive value of 64% and negative predictive value for 5-year FS of 78% following frontline immunochemotherapy.

Progression and clinical variants. FL cases may transform into an aggressive lymphoma with poor prognosis.[303,314,321,322] There is currently no routine way to predict risk of transformation. The most frequently mutated genes in transformed FL are *KMT2D*, *CREBBP*, *EZH2*, *BCL2*, and *MEF2B*.[321,323] However, detailed evaluation of clonal phylogenies has demonstrated that transformed FL typically arises from clones that exist below the level of detection at diagnosis, hindering the identification of genetic biomarkers that predict aggressive transformation.[324]

At the opposite end of the clinical spectrum is PTNFL, which is clinically indolent and cured with surgical excision. Although it was originally identified in children, this entity is not defined by age, as

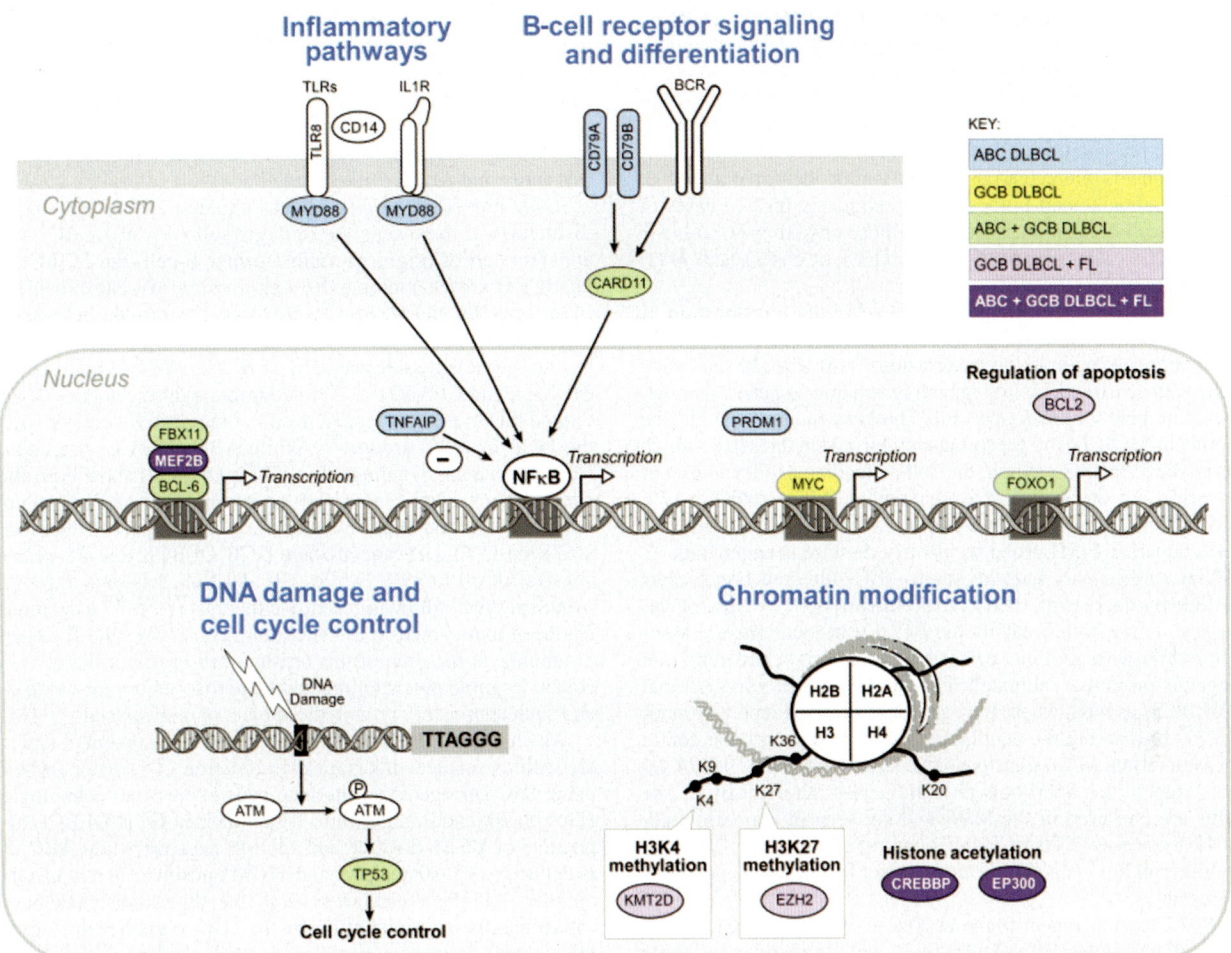

FIGURE 89.15 Pathways with genomic alterations in follicular lymphoma and diffuse large B-cell lymphoma. Mutations of membrane-proximal B-cell signaling components (e.g., *CD79A/B*), and those involving the proinflammatory NF-κB signaling pathway, are largely unique to ABC-type DLBCL (shown in blue). In contrast, genomic alterations involving regulation of apoptosis (e.g., *BCL2*) and regulation of the methylome (*KMT2D*, *EZH2*) are common to both follicular lymphoma and GCB-type DLBCL (shown in lavender), while mutation of *TP53* and of *BCL6* and its regulators occur in both ABC-type and GCB-type DLBCL (show in green). Other mutations, such as those of proteins that regulate histone acetylation, are found in all three entities (shown in dark purple).

there are biological and genetic similarities between pediatric and adult cases.[2] PTNFL is genomically bland and lacks recurrent mutations in epigenetic modifiers (*CREBBP* and *MLL2*) that otherwise characterize FL.[325-327] Copy number alterations affect only 0.5% PTNFL genomes, compared with 10% of limited-stage typical FL. On the other hand, the most common mutated gene is *MAP2K1* (encoding MEK1), at a mutational frequency of 43%. All *MAP2K1* mutations were activating mutations. Missense mutations in other ERK/MEK pathway genes such as *MAP1* and *RRAS* were identified in cases that lacked *MAP2K1* mutations. The second most common class of gene mutations in PTNFL was in *TNFSF14* (29%), like that seen in limited-stage typical FL.

Guidelines for Molecular Testing in Follicular Lymphoma

At diagnosis, many pathologists no longer performed PCR or FISH for confirmation of the t(14;18) if the lesional cells are immunohistochemically positive for BCL2. However, PCR or NGS for the t(14;18), if positive, can then be used to monitor MRD in this patient for prognostic import after maintenance therapy, even in cfDNA.[328] If there is morphologic evidence for a more high-grade process disease, then FISH for *MYC* and *BCL6* may also be appropriate. Owing to extensive SHM, only NGS for Ig gene rearrangements is appropriate for monitoring purposes.

Diagnosis	MRD
Consider PCR or FISH for *BCL2::IGH*	PCR for *BCL2::IGH* after maintenance
Consider FISH for *BCL6*, and *IRF4/MUM1* rearrangements for diagnostic clarity and prognostication as well as for deletion of 1p36	Consider NGS for Ig gene rearrangement studies
Consider FISH for *MYC* and *BCL6* if aggressive	
Consider NGS for Ig gene rearrangement studies	
Consider NGS for *TNFRSF14* and *MAP2K1* in young patients without t(14;18) or BCL2 expression to aid in distinction between FL and PTNFL	
Consider NGS if applying m7-FLIPI prior to R-CHOP or R-CVP	

Diffuse Large B-cell Lymphoma and Other High-Grade B-cell Lymphomas

The high-grade B-cell lymphomas discussed here include diffuse large B-cell lymphoma, not otherwise specified (DLBCL, NOS), and high-grade B-cell lymphoma with and without *MYC* and *BCL2* or *BCL6* translocations, that is, "double-hit" and "triple-hit" lymphomas.[2] DLBCL, NOS, is the most common adult lymphoma, comprising approximately 30% to 40% of cases of NHL.[5] Its nondescript appellation belies extensive biological heterogeneity and wide variation in clinical presentation and prognosis.

Rearrangements. Gene rearrangements can be identified by FISH, typically using break-apart probes, in approximately 65% of cases of high-grade B-cell lymphoma, split among those involving *BCL6* (45% of cases), *BCL2* (21% of cases), *BCL10* (18% of cases), and *MYC* (16% of cases).[329,330]

BCL6 gene rearrangements typically involve the translocation of the entire coding region of *BCL6* on chromosome 3q27 to its partner chromosome, resulting in its overexpression.[331] At least 20 such partners have been described, including both Ig and non-Ig genes, mandating the requirement for break-apart FISH probes against *BCL6*.[332] The breakpoints in the *BCL6* are predominantly located in the MBR, which consists of the 5′ flanking region, the first noncoding exon, and part of the first intron. An alternative breakpoint region (ABR), found in 17% of *BCL6* translocations, is located 240 to 280 kb 5′ to the MBR and requires a separate FISH probe to identify these rearrangements.[333] Most FISH studies only use the single MBR-directed break-apart probes, thereby decreasing their clinical sensitivity,[333-336] but newer FISH assays cover both breakpoints. *BCL6* translocations are associated primarily with germinal center histogenic origin and confer an advantageous prognosis, although they can be seen in non-germinal center DLBCLs as well, where they appear to be associated with poor outcome.[337] By locking the neoplastic B cells in the germinal center stage of maturation, *BCL6* translocations permit ongoing SHM. *BCL6* is itself a target of this SHM both physiologically and in DLBCL. The mutations are clustered in the MBR and are seen in approximately 25% to 45% of cases of DLBCL, often multiple or biallelic.[329,338-340] BCL6 inhibition has been explored as a target for the development of new therapeutics.[341,342]

The *BCL2* rearrangement found in 20% to 30% of DLBCLs is the identical hallmark t(14;18)(q32;q21) of FL.[5,282] In many cases these are de novo DLBCLs, without documented transformation from a preceding or concomitant FL. As in FL, this translocation is associated with a germinal center origin of the lymphomas. However, *BCL2* overexpression due to chromosomal gains at this locus can be associated with more ABC-type DLBCLs.[330]

BCL10 overexpression as a result of reciprocal translocations appear to be unrelated to any associated MALT lymphoma in most cases and are associated with a poor prognosis.[329]

MYC translocations are found in up to 15% of cases of high-grade B-cell lymphoma[5,329,330,343] and may be found in de novo DLBCL or as a secondarily acquired change during evolution from a low-grade B-cell lymphoma. It is associated with a poor prognosis, regardless of ontogeny of the lymphoma.[343,344] MYC alterations are frequently found in association with *BCL2* and, to a lesser extent, with *BCL6* gene rearrangements. The presence of *MYC* rearrangement in combination with *BCL2* and/or *BCL6* rearrangement (i.e., "double-hit" or "triple-hit" lymphoma) defines a distinct biological entity that carries a particularly dire prognosis, responding poorly to R-CHOP chemotherapy,[345] and showing inferior survival following hematopoietic stem cell transplantation.[346] Median overall survival ranges from 4.5 to 34 months, compared with a 2-year overall survival of 70% for conventional DLBCL.[347] More intensive induction regimens may prolong survival, although data are limited and conflicting.[347-349] "Single-hit" *MYC* rearranged lymphomas have a high association with overexpression of p53 and in those cases have a comparably poor prognosis to that of the double-hit lymphomas.[350]

Of note, MYC protein overexpression is detected in a significant proportion of DLBCLs that lack cytogenetic evidence of MYC gene rearrangement, frequently in association with BCL2 overexpression.[351] These cases, referred to as "double-expressor" lymphomas, have a worse outcome than DLBCLs lacking MYC/BCL2 overexpression but are not as aggressive as cases with cytogenetic evidence of *MYC* and *BCL2* and/or *BCL6* gene rearrangement.[352]

In ALK-positive large B-cell lymphomas, a recurrent translocation, t(2;17)(p23;q23), that results in a *CLTC::ALK* fusion is identified. These ALK-positive cases are uncommon but are considered their own category due to their characteristic behavior. Earlier studies suggest that these cases demonstrate hyperactivation of STAT3, reflecting overarching similarities in the predominant cellular pathways between this entity and ALCL (vide infra).[353]

Gene expression profiling. Gene expression profiling studies have distinguished three separate biologic subtypes of DLBCL based on apparent cell of origin. Germinal center B-cell-like DLBCLs (GCB DLBCLs) are characterized by expression of genes such as *MME* (*CD10*), *BCL6*, and *MYBL1* (A-MYB). By contrast, the activated B-cell-like (ABC-like) subtype of DLBCL expresses genes that are induced by mitogenic stimulation, such as *BCL2*, *IRF4* (which encodes for MUM1), and *CCND2*.[354,355] In addition, a third category of DLBCL, termed the "type 3" category, does not molecularly cluster with either the GCB or ABC groups.[355] While ABC DLBCLs are addicted to BCR-dependent signaling,[356,357] GCB DLBCLs show a profile more similar to germinal center–derived low-grade B-cell lymphomas and commonly harbor BCL2 translocations, e.g., t(14;18) IGH::BCL2, as also seen in FL. Advanced-stage GCB DLBCL has a 5-year overall survival of up to 75%, while ABC DLBCL has only a 50% 5-year overall survival following frontline therapy,[355,358-360] a decrement that has been maintained in the rituximab era.[361] Despite these different prognoses, at the time of this writing, cell of origin has proven inadequate to guide precision medicine approaches in real-world cohorts, and such approaches remain the subject of clinical trials.[362-369]

Much research has been devoted to the development of replacement algorithms for cell-of-origin classification of DLBCL, whether by using IHC surrogates or alternate gene expression technologies. The Hans classification algorithm, which defines GCB DLBCL as CD10 positive or BCL6 positive and MUM1 negative while ABC DLBCL is defined as CD10 negative and MUM1 positive,[370] remains the most popular.[2] Although there are several other algorithms, none has proven robust enough to supplant either the Hans classifier in routine practice or gene expression profiling as gold standard.[282,354,371-374] More recently, newer methods of gene expression profiling based on quantitation of RNA transcripts from FFPE tissue have been developed, some commercially available.[359,374-377] However, acknowledging the inaccessibility of even these assays to many laboratories, the most recent WHO classification permits use of either IHC or GEP for cell-of-origin assessment in DLBCL.[2] Additional gene expression profiling efforts have identified a molecular high-grade (MHG) group of GCB-type cell of origin and subset concordance with double hit cytogenetics. This MHG demonstrated worse progression-free survival while double-hit lymphomas without the MHG profile show no evidence of inferior outcomes to other GCB-type cases.[343]

Somatic variants. NGS has helped to further define the genomic landscape of high-grade B-cell lymphomas, identifying both somatic variants that are common to all types and others that are specific to the GCB and ABC subtypes (*Figure 89.15*).[378] Alterations common to both subtypes include inactivating mutations in *TP53*, mutation of genes involved in immunosurveillance (including *B2M* and *CD58*), mutation of epigenetic regulators (*CREBBP/EP300*, *KMT2C/2D*, *MEF2B*), and activating *BCL6* mutations.[378] Specific alterations found in GCB DLBCL include mutations in *EZH2* and *KMT2D*, and mutation of the *S1PR2* receptor and its downstream signal transduction protein *GNA13*,[311,378,379] while ABC-specific alterations include activating mutations in *CD79A*, *CARD11*, and *TNFAIP3*, all of which activate BCR/TLR signaling and NF-κB pathways.[378] In addition, ABC DLBCLs are far more likely to contain *MYD88* mutations, most frequently the same p.L265P mutation seen in LPL, than GCB DLBCLs. Other mutations identified by NGS in DLBCL include deletions of *CDKN2A* and *CDKN2B* and mutations in *PRDM1*.[311]

MicroRNA profiling. miRNA expression profiling studies have identified miRNA signatures that correlate with the cell of origin (GCB vs ABC), as well as a distinct set of miRNAs that correlate with outcome.[380] Two of the miRNAs overexpressed in the GCB DLBCLs, *miR-151* and *miR-28*, are predicted to downregulate FOXP1 (a marker expressed in the ABC subtype) whereas *miR-451*, an miRNA in the ABC signature is predicted to downregulate CD10 (a germinal center marker).[380] Some of these differentially expressed miRNAs may be independent predictors of survival in DLBCL.[381,382]

Molecular classification. Two groups from Harvard and the National Cancer Institute (NCI) independently identified reproducible signatures with biological relevance and clinical prognostic significance based not only on SNVs and small insertions/deletions but also on somatic copy number alterations and structural variants (*Table 89.6*).[383-385] For example, these systems revealed primary subgroups with the ABC-type DLBCLs with considerable prognostic divergence. The first is an adverse risk subgroup characterized by concurrent *MYD88* p.L265P and *CD79B* mutations and mutational inactivation of tumor suppressors including but not limited to *ETV6*, *BTG1*, and *TBL1XR1* and sharing features with primary extranodal lymphomas (Harvard Cluster 5 and the NCI MCD subgroups). The second is a favorable-risk subgroup harboring *BCL6* rearrangements and mutational activation of *NOTCH2*, NF-κB (including by *MYD88* non-L265P), and potential immune evasion pathways, sharing several key features with marginal zone lymphomas and raising the possibility of a common ontogeny (Harvard Cluster 1 and the NCI BN2 subgroups). Lastly, the NCI subsequently nominated a third subgroup of ABC-type DLBCLs, called N1, with mutations in *NOTCH1* and transcriptional regulators of B-lymphoid differentiation, such as *IRF4*, *ID3*, and *BCOR*, as well as transcriptional enrichment for T-cell activation.

The Harvard and NCI classification systems similarly resolve GC-type DLBCLs into prognostically divergent molecular subgroups. Favorable risk subgroups, termed Cluster 4 (Harvard) and ST2 (NCI), harbor recurrent mutations in genes influencing BCR/PI3K signaling including *SGK1* and *GNA13*, NF-κB modifiers including *NFKBIA*, and JAK/STAT signaling including *STAT3*. Harvard Cluster 4 is enriched in mutations of linker and core histone genes like those seen in FL, whereas the NCI ST2 mutational signature shares germinal center molecular features with nodular lymphocyte-predominant Hodgkin lymphoma and T-cell histiocyte-rich large B-cell lymphoma (THRLBCL). The Harvard and NCI systems similarly identify adverse molecular risk subgroups within GC-type DLBCL, termed Cluster 3 (Harvard) and EZB (NCI). Consensus features of these groups include activating *BCL2* structural and SNVs, mutations in epigenetic modifiers like *EZH2*, as well as B-cell transcriptional regulators, including *IRF8* and *MEF2B*.

Both the NCI and Harvard systems also resolved biological coherence across cell of origin classes with a molecular subgroup characterized by inactivation of *TP53* through copy loss and mutations, leading to increased DNA damage and chromosomal instability (Harvard Cluster 2, NCI group A53).

The prospective assessment of application of these subgroups with a broader array of treatment regimens is ongoing but requires inclusion of copy number and structural variant data.[386] The NCI group offers the use of the publicly available LymphGen algorithm (https://llmpp.nih.gov/lymphgen/index.php), which assigns probabilities that individual tumors belong to each of the seven NCI molecular subtypes based on available molecular inputs.[385]

Evaluation of response and MRD. Highly sensitive next-generation molecular technologies have enabled development of targeted molecular platforms for enumeration and characterization of MRD.[387] Immunoglobulin clonotype NGS has been tested for its ability to detect early relapse in patients with DLBCL. However, this method is limited by the requirement for clonotype identification on diagnostic tissue and adequate sensitivity for the clonotype in circulating disease. For example, interim analysis of a large multi-institution study in which patients underwent serial monitoring of peripheral blood mononuclear cells and plasma with clonotyping NGS revealed positive MRD in only 56% of patients prior to relapse.[388]

Additional efforts have utilized panel-based sequencing circulating tumor DNA (ctDNA) for MRD detection.[26] Retrospective analyses have demonstrated that panel-based ctDNA sequencing can identify ctDNA in nearly all patients with newly diagnosed DLBCL. Moreover, ctDNA dynamics have demonstrated independent prognostic value, with a 2-log reduction in ctDNA levels after one cycle (early molecular response) and a 2.5-log reduction after two cycles (major molecular response), both predicting event-free survival following various first-line immunochemotherapy regimens.[26] While this is promising, at the time of this writing, prospective trials remain needed to validate the ability of early ctDNA dynamics to guide individualized risk-adapted therapy.

Guidelines for Molecular Testing in High-Grade B-cell Lymphoma

Consensus guidelines recommend cytogenetic assessment of *MYC* rearrangement with reflex *BCL2* and *BCL6* testing as part of upfront diagnostic workup of all high-grade B-cell lymphomas.[2] In addition, upfront cell-of-origin classification is recommended, although either IHC or gene expression profiling may be used.[2] Clonotype, t(14;18), or somatic mutational panel NGS testing should be considered for MRD monitoring and prognostication purposes.

Diagnosis	MRD
FISH for *MYC* rearrangement	
FISH for *BCL2* and *BCL6* rearrangement (upfront or reflex if MYC rearrangement is present)	Consider PCR or NGS for *BCL2*::IGH
Gene expression profiling or IHC for cell of origin classification	Consider NGS for Ig gene rearrangement studies
Consider PCR or NGS for Ig gene rearrangement studies	Consider panel-based NGS for assessment of response dynamics within a clinical trial
Consider NGS for molecular cluster designation and assessment of novel mutations within a clinical trial	

Burkitt Lymphoma

BL is a highly aggressive B-cell neoplasm that can have a lymphomatous, leukemic, or combined presentation, although these forms are not biologically distinct. However, there are three subtypes of BL that appear to have different epidemiologic and molecular bases, while related by their common dependence upon *MYC* dysregulation.[5] The endemic variant of BL is prevalent in equatorial Africa, tending to occur in young children between the ages of 4 and 7 years, with involvement of the mandible, maxilla, other facial bones and abdomen.[6] Epstein-Barr virus (EBV) is endemic to that geographic region, and approximately 95% of endemic BL contains clonal EBV DNA. Sporadic BL is found predominantly in adolescents and young adults of Western countries and is the most common form of childhood lymphoma in the United States. In these cases, the disease is predominately abdominal with less frequent association with EBV in 5% to 30% of cases.[5,11,389] Immunodeficiency-associated BL is the third biologic subtype, where the most common association is with human immunodeficiency virus, although this form of BL can be seen secondary to other causes of immunodeficiency, both primary and secondary in nature. In approximately 25% to 40% of cases, there is an association with clonal EBV as well.[390,391]

Rearrangements. The most common translocation partner of *MYC*, located at 8q24, is the IGH locus on chromosome 14q32. This t(8;14)(q24;q32) can be identified in 80% of all BL and results in the overexpression of *MYC*.[392,393] The remaining cases of BL place *MYC* under the regulation, not of the heavy chain locus, but under one of the light chains, with a kappa light chain partner in a t(2;8)(p11;q24) and with lambda in t(8;22)(q24;q11).[394,395] The *MYC* gene is composed of three exons, the first noncoding and the remaining two coding. *MYC* encodes for a transcription factor involved in both cell proliferation as well as apoptosis (*Figure 89.9*). Dysregulated function of MYC results in increased cell cycling through its inhibition of p21 and p27 as well as its promotion of CDK2 and CDK4.[396] This is manifest pathologically by the numerous mitoses in BL as well as the extremely high proliferation rate, with Ki-67 expression typically >99%. In addition, MYC is proapoptotic, correlating with the numerous apoptotic bodies that create the classic "starry sky" histologic appearance of these tumors.

Table 89.6. Proposed Molecular Classification of DLBCL According to Two Independent, Large-Scale, Multiplatform Analyses at Harvard and the National Cancer Institute (NCI)

Cluster	COO	Enriched Molecular Features	Clinical Associations	Prognosis	Potential Therapeutic Targets
Cluster 1 (Harvard)	ABC	*BCL6* rearrangements; activating mutations in NOTCH2 pathway (*NOTCH2, SPEN*) and NF-κB pathway (*BCL10, TNFAIP3*); alterations implicated in immune evasion (mutations of *B2M, CD70, FAS* and SVs involving *PD-L1* and *PD-L2*); *MYD88*$^{non-L265P}$ mutations; low or absent cAID mutational signature	Mutational similarity to MZL	Favorable	Aberrant NOTCH2 signaling Immune evasion mechanisms
BN2 (NCI)	Any	***BCL6* rearrangements; mutations in NOTCH2 pathway** (*NOTCH2, SPEN, DTX1*), NF-κB regulators (*TNFAIP3, TNIP1*), and BCR-dependent NF-κB pathway (*PRKCB, TRAF6, BCL10* including amplifications); activating mutations in *CCND3* and *CXCR5*; loss of function mutations of *CD70* suggesting immune evasion	Mutational similarity to MZL raises possibility of occult MZL origin with transformation	Favorable	BCR-dependent NF-κB signaling (e.g., with BTK and PKCβ inhibitors) Aberrant NOTCH2 signaling, mTORC1, BCL2, PI3K signaling
Cluster 2 (Harvard)	Any	Biallelic TP53 inactivation through 17p copy loss and mutations; copy loss of 9p21.13 (*CDKN2A*) and 13q13.2 (*RB1*); copy gains of 1q23.3 (*MCL1*); 13q31.31 (miR-17-92) copy gain; 1q42.12 copy loss; genome doubling		Adverse	
A53 (NCI)	ABC> GCB	***TP53* inactivation through copy loss and mutations**; inactivating mutations or deletions of *TP53BP1* associated with DNA damage, **aneuploidy**; deletion of 6q (*TNFAIP3, PRDM1*); gain of 3q; amplification of *NFKBIZ, CNPY8, BCL2*; deletions of tumor suppressors *TP73* and *ING1*; *B2M* suggesting immune evasion	None	Adverse in ABC, more favorable in GCB	BCR-dependent NF-κB signaling
Cluster 3 (Harvard)	GCB	*BCL2* mutations and SVs; mutations in chromatin modifiers (*KMT2D, CREBBP, EZH2*), B-cell transcription factors (*MEF2B, IRF8*), BCR/PI3K signaling (*TNFSF14, HCNV1, GNA13*)	Mutational similarity to follicular lymphoma	Adverse	BCL2, PI3K, EZH2, and CREBBP
EZB (NCI)	GCB	**Mutations in *EZH2*; *BCL2* SVs**; *REL* amplification; inactivating mutations of epigenetic regulators *TNFRSF14, CREBBP, EP300, KMT2D, ARID1A, IRF8, MEF2B, EBF1*; mutations of genes involved in homing to GC (*S1PR2, GNA13*); mutational activation of JAK-STAT pathway (*SOCS1* mutations/deletions) and PI3K/mTOR pathway (inactivating *PTEN* mutations/deletion, *MTOR* mutations, *MIR17HG* amplification); mutations suggesting immune evasion (*CIITA, HLA-DMA*)	Mutational similarity to follicular lymphoma and DLBCL transformed from follicular lymphoma; MYC+ similar to BL	Adverse in MYC+, favorable in MYC−	BCL2
Cluster 4 (Harvard)	GCB	Mutations in linker and histone genes, mutations implicated in immune evasion (*CD83, CD58, CD70*), BCR/PI3K signaling (*RHOA, GNA13, SGK1*), NF-κB modifiers (*CARD11, NFKBIE, NFKBIA*) and RAS/JAK/STAT signaling (*BRAF, STAT3*); PTEN inactivation through focal 10q23.31 loss or truncating mutations; more frequent co-occurrence off *BCL2* and *MYC* SVs	Similar mutations in linker and core histone genes to follicular lymphoma	Favorable	JAK/STAT signaling BRAK/MEK1 signaling
ST2 (NCI)	GCB	**Truncating mutations in *SGK1* and *TET2***; mutational activation of JAK/STAT signaling (*STAT3, SOCS1, DUSP2*) and NF-κB (*NFKBIA*); mutational impairment of GC trafficking (*P2RY8, GNA13*)	Mutational similarity to NLPHL and THRLBCL	Favorable	PI3K, JAK2
Cluster 5 (Harvard)	ABC	*BCL2* gain; mutations of *MYD88*^{L265P}/*CD79B, ETV6, PIM1, GRHPR, TBL1XR1, BTG1*; cAID mutational signature	Extranodal tropism; mutational similarity to PCNSL and testicular lymphoma	Adverse	Proximal BCR/TLR signaling BCL2
MCD (NCI)	ABC	**Concurrent *MYD88*^{L265P}/*CD79B* mutations**; gains/amplifications of *SPIB*; inactivating mutations of *PRDM1*; mutations of known and potential tumor suppressors *CDKN2A, ETV6, BTG1, BTG2, TOX, SETD1B, FOXC1, TBL1XR1, KLHL14*; loss-of-function alterations in *HLA-A, HLA-B, HLA-C*, or *CD58* suggestive of immune evasion	Extranodal tropism; mutational similarity to primary extranodal lymphomas (e.g., PCNSL) as well as WM	Adverse	BCR signaling (e.g., with BTK, SYK, or PI3K inhibitors) BCR-dependent NF-κB signaling (e.g., with BTK and PKCβ inhibitors) mTORC1, JAK1, IRAK4, IRF4, and BCL2-BCLX$_L$-MCL1 axis
N1 (NCI)	ABC	**Mutations in *NOTCH1*** and B-cell transcriptional regulators (*IRF4, ID3, BCOR*); elevated T-cell gene expression signature	Plasmacytic phenotype; similarity to *NOTCH1*-mutated CLL	Adverse	Aberrant NOTCH1 signaling Immune checkpoint inhibition

Resolution of coordinate biological signatures incorporating single nucleotide variants, somatic copy number alterations, and structural variants reveals biological substructure with considerable overlap between the two systems. Clusters with similar biological and clinical features are shown adjacent to each another and visually demarcated by color.

Abbreviations: ABC, activated B cell–type DLBCL; Any, includes ABC subtype, GCB subtype, and unclassified type DLBCL; BL, Burkitt lymphoma; cAID, canonical activation-induced deaminase; COO, cell of origin; GCB, germinal center–type DLBCL; MYC−, negative for MYC rearrangements, amplifications, or activating mutations; MYC+, harboring MYC rearrangements, amplifications, or activating mutations; MZL, marginal zone lymphoma; NLPHL, nodular lymphocyte-predominant Hodgkin lymphoma; PCNSL, primary central nervous system lymphoma; SV, structural variant; THRLBCL, T-cell histiocyte-rich large B-cell lymphoma; WM, Waldenström macroglobulinemia.

Although all cases of BL contain a translocation of *MYC*, the different subtypes of BL are molecularly distinct as well.[397-400] All the translocations with immunoglobulin genes result in the transcription of the full *MYC* coding sequence. However, the breakpoints of *MYC* and immunoglobulin genes vary among the BL subtypes. In endemic BL, the *MYC* breakpoint is located approximately 300 kb upstream from exon 1. This breakpoint translocates the full *MYC* gene to the J_H region of IGH. By contrast, the *MYC* breakpoint in sporadic BL can occur 5′ to exon 1 or within intron 1, still translocating the full *MYC* coding region in either scenario to the one of the C regions of IGH (Cμ, Cγ, and Cα have all been documented). In the translocations involving either IGK or IGL, the *MYC* gene typically remains on chromosome 8, with the breakpoint 3′ to the third and final coding exon to which the IGK or IGL locus is affixed at either a V or J segment. These differing molecular breakpoints may be related to differences in the stages of B-cell development during which the oncogenic change occurs. The sporadic cases may develop during class switching, whereas endemic cases may occur during SHM.[5]

As a result of the wide range of potential breakpoints in both the *MYC* gene and the immunoglobulin genes, PCR-based assays for *MYC* translocations are not practical, although primers have been generated against specific *MYC* breakpoints.[401] Rather, FISH is the optimal means for detection of *MYC* translocations at diagnosis. Specific probes against both *MYC* and IGH can be used to assess for the t(8;14)(q24;q32). However, these probes will be less sensitive for the variant light chain rearrangements. Therefore, *MYC* break-apart probes provide greater sensitivity for any *MYC* rearrangement, regardless of the immunoglobulin partner.[402]

Clinical variants and related diseases. In addition to BL, *MYC* translocation is seen in a subset of high-grade B-cell lymphomas, including those that merit classification as DLBCL, NOS; high-grade B-cell lymphoma with *MYC* and *BCL2* and/or *BCL6* rearrangement (i.e., double- or triple-hit lymphoma); or high-grade B-cell lymphoma, NOS.[2] Therefore, the presence of an *MYC* translocation alone does not define BL in the absence of the appropriate morphologic and immunophenotypic features. In cases where either the morphology or the immunophenotype is not classic for BL, additional FISH studies are required for classification.[2,287,288] These include FISH assessment for the *BCL2::IGH* translocation t(14;18)(q32;q21) as well as for rearrangements of *BCL6* on chromosome 3q27. In addition, use of *MYC* break-apart probes is critical in these cases as the translocation partner in some cases may involve nonimmunoglobulin-related genes.[5]

The pathogenesis of non-Hodgkin B-cell lymphomas that resemble BL morphologically, but lack *MYC* rearrangement, remains an object of intensive study. A subset of such cases shows characteristic cytogenetic abnormalities involving chromosome 11q, with centromeric gains and telomeric losses. Notably, these cases appear to be clinically and biologically distinct from conventional BL, appearing more frequently in the posttransplant setting and displaying greater cytologic pleomorphism and karyotypic complexity and lower levels of MYC expression.[403,404] These cases are currently classified as "Burkitt-like lymphoma with 11q aberration."[2]

Gene expression profiling. Gene expression profiling studies have clearly supported the distinction of BL from DLBCL and the category formerly known as atypical BL (many of which are currently classified as high-grade B-cell lymphoma, NOS).[405,406] These studies have also highlighted the overexpression of T-cell leukemia 1 (TCL1) in BL, which appears to be dependent upon the presence of EBV.

Somatic variants. MYC dysregulation alone appears insufficient to drive BL, indicating that additional genomic changes are required for lymphomagenesis. Several recent studies applying whole-exome and genome sequencing have helped to define the genomic landscape of BL and identify somatic variants that may link MYC dysregulation to the development of lymphoma. These studies have notably identified the role of the transcription factor *TCF3*, a master regulator of germinal center B-cell differentiation, in the pathogenesis of BL. Activating mutations in *TCF3* are present in up to 23% of cases of BL, while inactivating mutations of *ID3* (68% of cases), a negative regulator of *TCF3*, and activating mutations in *CCND3* (38% of cases), a downstream target of *TCF3*, are even more frequently identified.[407-409] The TCF3 pathway functions primarily through upregulation of PI3 kinase signaling, highlighting the importance of this pathway in BL and drawing a distinction from other high-grade B-cell lymphomas, in which the NF-κB pathway, rather than PI3K, is constitutively activated.[410]

Guidelines for Molecular Testing in Burkitt Lymphoma

FISH confirmation of an *MYC* rearrangement is recommended at diagnosis of BL. However, FISH is not a sensitive marker of MRD. Owing to the extensive SHM of BL as a neoplasm of GCBs, PCR-based immunoglobulin gene rearrangement studies have very poor clinical sensitivity, and, in the absence of allele-specific primers, PCR for immunoglobulin gene rearrangements using consensus primers is not superior to FISH in terms of analytical sensitivity. PCR directed against the *MYC* rearrangement itself sees little practical use due to the low clinical sensitivity. NGS may provide a good means for MRD testing. Therefore, FISH remains the optimal diagnostic test, and there is a limited role for any testing for MRD other than potentially NGS. As mentioned earlier, in cases that do not have the classic morphologic or immunophenotypic profile of BL, additional FISH studies for *BCL2* and *BCL6* gene rearrangements are also recommended. In addition, FISH for aberration of chromosome 11q is recommended in cases that resemble BL morphologically but lack *MYC* translocation.

Diagnosis	MRD
FISH for *MYC*	Consider NGS for Ig gene rearrangement studies
Consider FISH for *BCL2*, *BCL6*, or 11q for cases without classic presentation	
Consider NGS for Ig gene rearrangement studies	

Mature Neoplasms of T Cells

There are several recurrent themes in the T-cell neoplasms with involvement of the TCR and costimulatory pathways, JAK/STAT pathway, epigenetic pathways (both DNA and chromatin modifying), and DNA damage repair and cell cycling pathways (*Figure 89.16*). Thus, although there are distinct clinicopathologic features in all these neoplasms, there are recurrent pathway utilization modes that group unexpected T-cell neoplasms into unique molecular groupings.

Anaplastic Large Cell Lymphoma, ALK Positive and ALK Negative

Anaplastic lymphoma kinase (ALK)-positive ALCLs comprise roughly 3% of all adult NHLs (12% of T-cell NHLs) and as much as 20% of childhood lymphomas.[4,5] Incidence peaks in the second decade of life, and cases in elderly adults are rare. These lymphomas are highly chemosensitive, although aggressive, and the overall 5-year survival approaches 80%, up to 90% in patients with low prognostic indices. By contrast, incidence of ALK-negative ALCLs peaks in the sixth decade of life, and survival is considerably less than in the ALK-positive cases (36% 5-year survival). For these reasons, these two forms of ALCL are classified separately, and, despite their similarities in morphology and CD30 expression that initially grouped them together as ALCLs, they have very different epidemiology and clinical outcomes.

Rearrangements. These two entities also differ significantly in what is known of their molecular underpinnings, although both have clonally rearranged T-cell genes: 76% of ALK-positive ALCLs, 89% of ALK-negative ALCLs. Together, 79% of all ALCLs can be detected by a combination of TRG and TRB sets of commercial primers.[32] The ALK-positive cases of ALCL have well-documented driving reciprocal translocations involving the *ALK* locus on chromosome 2p23 and a limited set of partner chromosomes. *ALK* encodes for a transmembrane tyrosine kinase protein, which is found in neural cells but has no appreciable expression in normal hematopoietic cells.[411] The breakpoints in *ALK* are located near this transmembrane domain and result in the full expression of the tyrosine kinase domain in the

Translocation	Fusion Partners	Staining Pattern	Frequency
t(2;5)(p23;q35)	NPM – ALK	Nuclear, diffuse cytoplasmic	84%
t(1;2)(q25;p23)	TPM3 – ALK	Diffuse cytoplasmic	13%
inv(2)(p23q35)	ATIC – ALK	Diffuse cytoplasmic	1%
t(2;3)(p23;q21)	TFG – ALK	Diffuse cytoplasmic	<1%
t(2;17)(p23;q23)	CLTC – ALK	Granular cytoplasmic	<1%
t(2;X)(p23;q11-12)	MSN – ALK	Membrane	<1%
t(2;22)(p23;q11.2)	MYH9 – ALK	Diffuse cytoplasmic	<1%
t(2;19)(p23;q13.1)	TPM4 – ALK	Diffuse cytoplasmic	<1%
t(2;17)(p23;q25)	ALO17 – ALK	Diffuse cytoplasmic	<1%

FIGURE 89.16 Anaplastic large cell lymphoma. The various translocations of *ALK* with its myriad partners is demonstrated with cytogenetic translocations and immunohistochemical pattern of AKT1 described. (Adapted with permission from Swerdlow SH; International Agency for Research on Cancer; World Health Organization. *WHO Classification of Tumours of Haematopoietic and Lymphoid Tissues*. 4th ed. International Agency for Research on Cancer; 2008.)

fusion product in all cases. The most common partner is the *NPM1* gene on chromosome 5q35.1, found in 84% of ALK-positive cases, resulting in a t(2;5)(p23;q35.1) (Figure 89.17).[5,412] *NPM1* encodes for nucleophosmin, a protein that shuttles ribonucleoproteins from the nucleus to the cytoplasm and is involved in preribosomal assembly.[413] As a result, the fusion protein is also found in both locations, and IHC stains targeting the normally cytoplasmic C terminus of ALK show both nuclear and cytoplasmic staining.[5] The fusion attaches the N terminus of NPM1 containing an oligomerization domain to ALK, resulting in constitutive activation of ALK kinase activity. This kinase activity activates numerous pathways involved in growth and cell survival, including AKT/PI3K/mTOR, JAK/STAT, JUN, and MYC

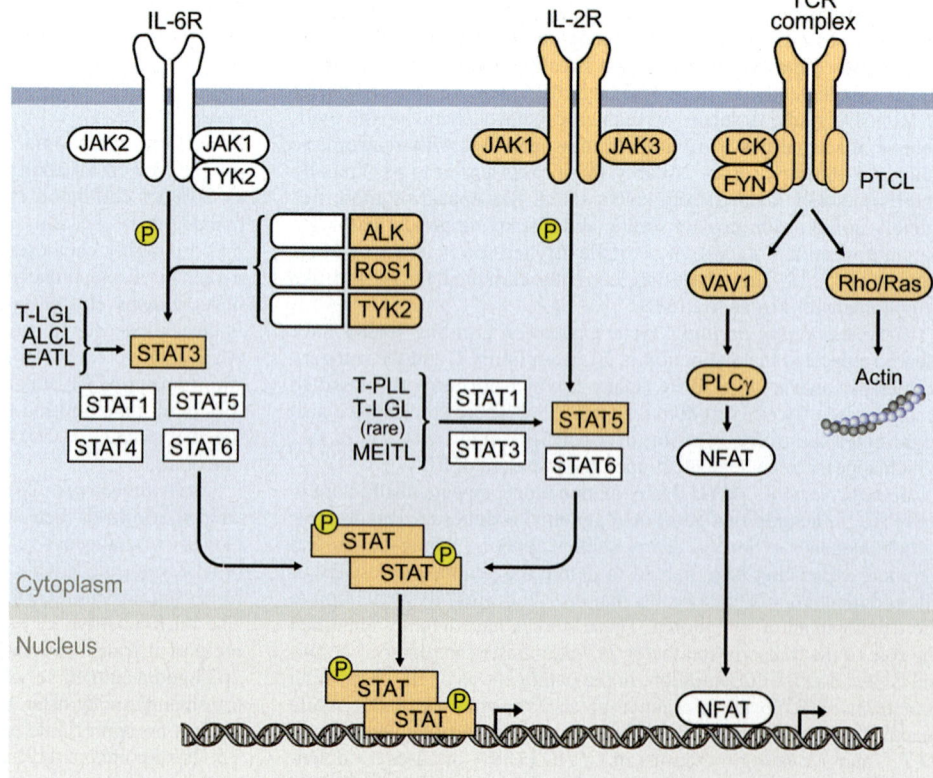

FIGURE 89.17 Pathways with genomic alterations in several T-cell lymphomas. The protein products of mutated or translocated genes are shown in orange. The STAT3 pathway is recurrently implicated in cases of T-LGL, ALCL (including those with translocations involving *ALK*, *ROS1*, and *TYK2*), EATL, ATLL, and ENKTCL. By contrast, the IL-2R-JAK(1/3)-STAT5 pathway is activated in T-PLL, a minority of cases of T-LGL, and in MEITL. In PTCL, there are a wide range of mutations involving the T-cell receptor and its signaling through actin reorganization and transcription while AITL signals frequently through RHOA. PTCL, AITL, ATLL, and ENKTCL have recurrent epigenetic mutations, and ATLL may have NOTCH signaling mutations.

pathways. The dependence of the ALCL cells upon the fusion protein has made the fusion and its downstream collaborators a target for the development of therapeutics.[414-416]

In addition to the t(2;5)(p23;q35.1), several other translocations of *ALK* are summarized in *Figure 89.17*.[5] In each case, the partner chromosome contains an oligomerization domain, and in most cases there is a single breakpoint region involved. The physiologic localization of the partner protein is mimicked in the fusion protein, resulting in characteristic patterns on ALK IHC. Although the t(2;5)(p23;q35.1) can be identified by a number of molecular techniques, including targeted PCR, anchored multiplex PCR, reverse transcription PCR, and FISH, the most prevalent method in clinical use is FISH, since it has the best clinical sensitivity for the variant rearrangements.[417-419]

In ALK-negative ALCLs, several recurrent translocations have also been identified. A recurrent t(6;7)(p25.3;q32.2) has recently been identified in ALK-negative ALCL via NGS methods.[420] This reciprocal translocation places the *DUSP22* phosphatase gene or the *IRF4* gene (encoding MUM1) on chromosome 6p25.3 adjacent to chromosome 7q32.3, near the *FRA7H* fragile genomic site and *miR-29*, and is the first balanced translocation identified in this diagnostic entity. Using FISH probes against these loci, 20% to 45% of cases of ALK-negative ALCL (both systemic and primary cutaneous) were shown to have this rearrangement, approximately two-thirds with *DUSP22*, whereas only rare PTCLs were positive and with no other cutaneous T-cell lymphomas.[416,420] *DUSP22* and *IRF4* are located within 40 kb of each other. In contrast to *DUSP22* rearrangements, which portend a favorable prognosis with 90% 5-year overall survival, rearrangements of the *TP53* homolog *TP63* located on 3q28, which are functionally homologous to the oncogenic ΔNp63 isoform, mark an adverse risk subgroup. *TP63* rearranged cases comprise 8% of ALK-negative ALCLs but have a 5-year overall survival of only 17%.[421] In the same report, cases lacking rearrangement of *ALK*, *DUSP22*, and *TP63*, so-called triple-negative ALCLs, had an intermediate prognosis, with a 5-year overall survival of 42%. Subsequent RNA-sequencing efforts have identified recurrent translocations of *VAV1* in 11% of cases as well as *ROS1* and *TYK2* in ALK-negative ALCL (*Figure 89.16*).[422,423] Most recently, RNA-based fusion analysis has identified cases of ALK-negative ALCL that can mimic classic Hodgkin lymphoma histologically and harbor potentially targetable rearrangements of *JAK2*, with a variety of fusion partners (*PCM1*, *TFG*, *PABPC1*, *ILF3*, *MAP7*).[10]

Copy number variations. CGH studies have determined that 58% of ALK-positive ALCLs may carry additional aberrations such as gains of 17p and 17q24-qter and losses of 4q13-q21 and 11q14.[424] These aberrations were not associated with any particular prognostic import. Here too, ALK-negative cases of ALCL demonstrate a different pattern of imbalances (gains of 1q, 6p21, 3p and losses of 16pter, 6q13q21 a15, and 17p13) in 65% of cases, which further supports their biologic separation.[424,425] Losses of 6p21 and 17p13 encompassing *PRDM1* and *TP53* have each been associated with poor prognosis.[420,426]

MicroRNA profiling. The *DUSP22*-containing rearrangements result not only in a decrease of DUSP22 expression, which has been shown to have tumor suppressor activity in some other T-cell neoplasms, but also in overexpression of miR-29.[420] By contrast, the *NPM1::ALK*-mediated downregulation of *miR-29a* may result in the downstream overexpression of MCL1 and inhibition of apoptosis.[427] In addition to *miR-29a*, ALK-positive ALCLs also upregulate *miR-135b*, resulting in blockage of IL-17 production by ALCL cells, suppressing a Th2 phenotype and inducing a Th17 phenotype.[428] These results are compatible with the gene expression profiling studies that also find a prominent Th17 signature.[429] Similarly, the *NPM1::ALK* fusion has also been implicated in the methylation of the *IL2RG* gene promoter directly through STAT3 regulation of DNA methyl transferases and indirectly through repression of *miR-21* expression.[430]

Gene expression profiling. Gene expression profiling studies of ALCLs have identified a profile of activated T cells involving the JAK3/STAT3 pathway (IL26, IL31RA, IL9), molecules that characterize Th17 cells (IL17A, IL17F, RORC), as well as overexpression of ALK, albeit with downregulation of a number of other molecules that typically characterize T cells.[431-433] In fact, the profiles of both ALK-positive and ALK-negative ALCLs resemble the signature obtained from cHL, with overexpression of members of the NF-κB pathway. Moreover, the cHL cell lines more closely resemble ALK-positive ALCL than other B-cell lymphomas, despite the differences in their cells of origin.[62,431,434] Both ALK-positive and ALK-negative cases also form a common ALCL signature that is distinct from that of other T-cell lymphomas, supporting their continued separation from peripheral T-cell lymphoma, not otherwise specified (PTCL, NOS).[433] However, distinct signatures separate the ALCLs by ALK status as well, with ALK-positive tumors overexpressing the cyclin, *CCND3*, as well other signal transduction molecules (SYK, LYN, CDC37) and ALK-negative lymphomas demonstrating decreased expression of p19INK4D, a cell cycle inhibitor, and underexpression of homeobox transcription factors, HOXC6 and HOXA4.[435]

Somatic variants. Recurrent somatic variants have been noted in ALCL and demonstrate a common recurrent theme in T-cell lymphomas of activation of the JAK/STAT pathways, consistent with the expression profiling phenotype (*Figure 89.16*). Variants in *STAT3* and/or *JAK1* are identified in up to 18% of systemic ALK-negative ALCLs and 5% of primary cutaneous ALCLs as well as in several cases of breast implant–associated ALCL.[422,436-438] While systemic ALK-negative ALCLs may carry mutations in both these genes, in the cutaneous ALCL these genetic lesions do not co-occur.[422] *STAT3* variants are typically located in the SH2 domain, resulting in activation, with an association with necrosis and high mitotic activity.[422,436] *JAK1* variants are activating mutations in the tyrosine kinase domain.[422] Although mutations of this pathway may be seen in other types of T-cell lymphomas, these variants were not identified in other diagnostic categories closely related to ALK-negative ALCL histologically, found neither in ALK-positive ALCL (where the pathway is instead activated by the ALK fusion) nor in PTCL, NOS, including CD30+ cases of the latter.[422]

Guidelines for Molecular Testing in Anaplastic Large Cell Lymphoma

FISH for the t(2;5) may be helpful for ALK-positive cases. FISH for *DUSP22/IRF4* and *FRA7H* can help discriminate ALK-negative ALCL and PTCL, NOS, permitting better prognostication.[439] In cases that are negative for *ALK* and *DUSP22* rearrangements, FISH for *TP63* using break-apart probes or dual-fusion probes for *TBL1XR1::TP63* can help identify patients with adverse clinical risk. Among those that remain, FISH or NGS for t(6;7) or *JAK2* rearrangements may inform prognosis and potential therapeutic targets.

Diagnosis	MRD
Consider PCR or NGS for TCR gene rearrangement studies	Consider NGS for TCR gene rearrangement studies
Consider FISH for t(2;5) (*NPM1::ALK*), the 6p25.3 region (*DUSP22-IRF4*), 3q28 (*TP63*), (and *TBL1XR1::TP63*)	
Consider FISH or NGS for t(6;7) (*DUSP22::FRA7H*) or *JAK2* rearrangements	

Peripheral T-cell Lymphoma, Not Otherwise Specified

Discrimination between ALK-positive ALCL, ALK-negative ALCL, and PTCL, NOS, has been the focus of much research in an attempt to define different cells of origin, aspiring to the success seen in the B-cell lymphomas. The diagnostic dilemma is particularly challenging between ALK-negative ALCL and PTCL, NOS, with high expression of CD30. The distinction between these two entities is clinically relevant since prognostically the ALK-negative ALCLs fare better than the PTCLs (74% 5-year overall survival for cases with a low international prognostic index, IPI 0-1, vs 52% to 56% for similar IPI PTCL groups, respectively).[439,440]

At the time of this writing, PTCL, NOS, remains a diagnosis of exclusion, accounting for approximately 26% of T-cell NHLs.[440] This category encompasses a wide range of neoplasms of T cells that fail to segregate clearly with other defined categories of T-cell lymphomas. Essentially all cases of PTCL, NOS, contain clonally rearranged TCR genes that can be detected by a combination of TRG and TRB commercial primers.[32] Yet, many of these lymphomas are defined by site, rather than by the biology of the cell of origin, resulting in a wide range of clinical, epidemiologic, and pathologic findings. There are, furthermore, few cytogenetic changes specifically associated with PTCL, but rather a panoply of nonspecific changes. However, recent efforts to define the molecular substructure of this heterogeneous class of disorders through comprehensive molecular profiling are now beginning to illuminate potential biological classifications with clinical relevance.[441]

Copy number variations. Cytogenetic studies have identified a wide spectrum of changes in PTCL, NOS, vs ALK-negative ALCL, which point to slightly different patterns of aberrations, albeit with some overlap. Both disease categories share common gains of 1q and 3p and losses of 13q.[425] As mentioned in the previous section, ALK-negative ALCL also demonstrate losses of 16pter, 6q13q21, 15, and 17p13, whereas PTCL, NOS, showed losses of 6q22q24, 9p21-pter, 10p13pter, 10q23-24, and 12q21-q22, as well as additional gains of 7q22q31, 5p, 11q13, and 12p13.[425,442,443] None of the specific aberrations appear to have discrete impacts on overall survival, although general cytogenetic complexity does correspond to poorer overall survival.

SNP arrays have identified candidate genes at the site of recurrent losses in PTCL at chromosome 9p21.3, encompassing *CDKN2A* and *CDKN2B*, loci that encode for key proteins in regulating cell cycling and apoptosis, p14/p16 and p15, respectively.[444] In addition, the recurrent gain at 7p22 contains the apoptosis-related gene *CARD11* (*CARMA1*), corresponding to overexpression of the corresponding mRNA. Other focal copy number alterations that have been reported by targeted capture and whole exome sequencing with a frequency of at least 5% include losses of the tumor suppressor *TP53*, the epigenetic regulator *ARID1A*, and MHC class I components *HLA-A* and *HLA-B*; inactivating structural variants and copy losses affect the epigenetic regulator *ARID2*, the lymphoid transcription factor *IKZF2*, and the TCR/NF-κB signaling mediator *TNFAIP3*.[441] Reported with similar frequencies are gains of *NOTCH1* and the stimulating TCR *CD28*, with activating structural variants supplementing copy gains of the immune inhibitory receptor ligand *CD274*.[441] Prognostically, gains at chromosomes 2 and 5 are associated with poor clinical outcomes in PTCL.[444]

Rearrangements. Recurrent translocations involving *VAV1* have been identified in 11% of cases of PTCL, NOS (as well as in ALK-negative ALCL), involving partners *GSS* or *MYO1F*, at least the former of which may be inhibited in vitro with RAC inhibition.[423,445] Several other novel fusions were noted in this same study, including an *IKZF2::ERBB4* fusion and an *ITK::FER* fusion analogous to the *ITK::SYK* translocation described under follicular helper (Tfh) T-cell lymphomas, below.[423] Rare cases of a *IRF4::TRA* fusion in PTCL have also been noted, resulting from a t(6;14)(p25;q11.2). These cases appear to be associated with a cytotoxic T-cell phenotype and involve the bone marrow and skin without concomitant lymphadenopathy.[446]

Gene expression profiling. Gene expression profiling has been perhaps the most useful in discerning differences in biology of different T-cell lymphomas. However, due to its heterogeneity, PTCL, NOS, not surprisingly has been difficult to associate with a clear defining transcriptional signature, often interspersed among the other subtypes of T-cell lymphomas.[447] The most successful profiling experiments have been able to assign profiles to PTCL, NOS, which most closely resemble activated CD4$^+$ or CD8$^+$ T cells.[448] Transcriptional profiling has identified one discrete subset of PTCL, NOS, which expresses a signature characteristic of cytotoxic T cells and is associated with a poor prognosis. Although not all these tumors are CD8$^+$ (in fact, 55% were CD4$^+$), they expressed two key transcription factors found in CD8$^+$ T cells, T-bet (*TBX21*) and eomesodermin, as well as their target genes (*CXCR3, IL2RB, CCL3, IFNG*). These cells also expressed typical cytotoxic molecules and even killer cell immunoglobulin-like receptor family members and other NK-cell markers.[432]

Although the *ITK::SYK* translocation is limited to follicular TCL (see below), approximately 95% of all PTCLs demonstrate overexpression of SYK by IHC, whereas nonneoplastic T cells are negative. The kinase in these lymphomas is phosphorylated and therefore in an activated state, suggesting the possibility of SYK inhibition in the treatment of PTCL.[449] Similarly, overexpression of *PDGFRA* has been identified in 85% to 90% of PTCLs by gene expression profiling studies and RT-PCR without any genomic imbalances involving the 4q11-q13 locus, providing another potential molecular target for treatment.[448,450]

Somatic variants. One of the largest recent series of PTCLs, with 133 cases, identified mutations in 12 genes at a frequency greater than 5%. These include epigenetic regulators *TET2, DNMT3A, CREBBP, KMT2C, SETD1B*, and *IDH2*; the tumor suppressor *TP53*; TCR/NK-κB signaling intermediates *RHOA, VAV1*, and *PLCG1*; the cytokine receptor–mediated signal transducer *JAK3*; and the MHC class I complex component *HLA-A* (*Figure 89.16*).[441] Mutations in *TET2* and *DNMT3A*, commonly associated with acute myeloid leukemias (AMLs), both involve epigenetic regulation of transcription through CpG methylation.[451,452] *TET2* is involved in the successive oxidation of the 5-methyl group of 5-methylcytosine, resulting ultimately in demethylation. *DNMT3A* is a DNA methyltransferase, and mutations demonstrate hypomorphic function. *TET2* mutations have been found in 12% of nodal and extranodal T-cell lymphomas (compared with only 2% of B-cell lymphomas), often in conjunction with *DNMT3A* mutations.[451,452] In addition to translocations, deletions and activating mutations of *VAV1* are also found in PTCL (*Figure 89.16*).[423,445,453] VAV1 acts downstream of CD28 and the TCR, activating the RHO and RAS families of GTPases, driving cytoskeletal reorganization, migration, and proliferation. Correspondingly, activating mutations in these GTPases as well as other members of this pathway (including *CD28, FYN, LCK*, and *PLCG1*) are also mutated in PTCL.[453]

Recent work has highlighted recurrent, mostly biallelic, inactivating mutations and copy number alterations in *TP53* and focal deletions of *CDKN2A* (*Figure 89.16*), associated with a striking increase in focal and arm-level copy number alterations.[441] These lesions, which reflect impaired DNA damage response, segregate with aberrations of the lymphoid transcription factor *IKZF2* and genes involved in immune presentation, including *HLA-A, HLA-B*, and *CD58*. Interestingly, these alterations appear mutually exclusive of *RHOA* p.G17V and, to a lesser extent, other features of Tfh TCLs. This divergence suggests a potential biological basis for resolving the molecular heterogeneity of PTCL, NOS. Indeed, in this same series, hierarchical clustering based on genomic driver lesions distinguished PTCLs with Tfh molecular features from those harboring *TP53* and *CDKN2A* alterations, as well as a third group lacking these genomic changes. Retrospective evaluation of a modest number of patients (n = 46) demonstrated an association between molecular subtype and survival, with *TP53/CDKN2A*-altered lymphomas, Tfh TCLs with *RHOA* p.G17V mutations, and those lacking these genomic drivers comprising adverse, intermediate, and favorable clinical risk strata, respectively. While these data are promising, replication in larger cohorts and clarification of how this potential molecular taxonomy relates to proposed transcriptional subgroups[429] are required before attempts at prospective clinical validation with clinically tractable molecular platforms are undertaken.

Guidelines for Molecular Testing in Peripheral T-cell Lymphoma, NOS

SYK and PDGFRα overexpression by IHC may become therapeutically relevant in the future as may molecular testing for mutations in *TET2* and *DNMT3A*.

Diagnosis	MRD
Consider PCR or NGS for TCR gene rearrangement studies	Consider NGS for TCR gene rearrangement studies
Consider IHC for SYK and PDGFRα	
Consider testing for somatic variants, particularly if necessary to distinguish from Tfh TCL	Consider testing for somatic variants

Follicular T-cell Lymphomas (Tfh Lymphomas)

The 2016 Revisions of the WHO[2] have created a broader category of follicular T-cell lymphomas that encompasses angioimmunoblastic T-cell lymphoma (AITL) as well as other cases of nodal PTCL with the Tfh phenotype. The below discussion will be focused on AITL; however, many of the findings may be extrapolated to other types of follicular T-cell lymphomas.

Angioimmunoblastic T-cell Lymphoma

AITL is an EBV-associated T-cell lymphoma associated with a wide range of systemic symptomatology. AITL is one of the more common subtypes of PTCLs, accounting for 15% to 20% of cases, although it comprises only 1% to 2% of all NHLs.[5] Patients typically present in their sixth or seventh decade. Systemic symptoms include hepatosplenomegaly, lymphadenopathy, polyclonal hypergammaglobulinemia, rash, pruritus, cold agglutinin disease associated with hemolytic anemia, positive rheumatoid factor, the presence of antismooth muscle antibodies, and immunodeficiency. Interestingly, although this lymphoma is associated with EBV, only the background B cells in this lymphoma are EBV positive. The EBV-driven B cells can undergo a resultant immunoblastic proliferation and often can demonstrate a clonal/pseudoclonal Ig gene rearrangement. The T cells, by contrast, are EBV negative. AITL is one of the few T-cell lymphomas for which the cell of origin is well established to be a CD4+ follicular helper T cell. Clonally rearranged TCR genes are identified in 95% of cases of AITL using commercial primers.[32]

Copy number variations. Until recently little was known about any recurrent genetic aberrations in AITL. aCGH studies identify gains of 22q, 19, and 11q11-q14 (11q13) and losses of 13q.[442] The gain of 11q13 is shared by both AITL and PTCL, NOS, and may involve either *CCND1* or *GSTP1*, a gene often coamplified with *CCND1* encoding for a glutathione transferase. aSNP studies show general copy number or LOH findings very similar to those of PTCL, NOS. Specifically in AITL, gains of 13q22.3 may involve *MYCBP2*, a gene that encodes an MYC binding protein with putative ubiquitin ligase activity that may regulate *MYC*-mediated transcription. These gains are associated with poor prognosis in these patients.[444]

Rearrangements. Recurrent translocations have been identified as well in AITL, including the *ITK::SYK* (18% of AITL), *CTLA4::CD28* (58% of AITL), and *ICOS::CD28* (6% of AITL) fusions (Figure 89.16). The *ITK::SYK* rearrangement was originally described in nodal PTCL with the Tfh phenotype, although recent studies appear to have identified this translocation in rare cases of AITL as well.[449,454-456] This rearrangement fuses the inducible T-cell kinase (*ITK*) with the spleen tyrosine kinase (*SYK*). *ITK* is activated through the TCR. *SYK* is integral in the function of both the BCR and the TCR, playing the predominant role in B cells, whereas ZAP-70 plays an analogous role in T cells.[457] The fusion results in loss of the *ITK* kinase domain and autoinhibitory SH2 and SH3 domains (with retention of the pleckstrin homology domain and proline-rich region) and their replacement by the kinase domain of *SYK*, which may prove to be a reasonable target for kinase inhibitors such as fostamatinib. These lymphomas demonstrate a characteristic histologic pattern of lymphoid follicles ("follicular pattern" PTCL), which immunophenotypically marks a neoplasm of Tfh cells. The *ICOS::CD28* rearrangement is not specific for AITL but may also be found in a range of PTCL, NOS, and extranodal NK/T-cell lymphomas.[458] Recurrent rearrangements involving the TCR costimulatory receptor CD28 are relatively rare in PTCLs as a whole but are enriched within TCLs with the Tfh phenotype, particularly AITL, where they are seen in up to 15% of cases.[322,459] Here, the cytoplasmic signal transducing portion of CD28 is fused to the transmembrane and extracellular domains of ICOS or CTLA4, with CD28 expression furthermore subject to the ICOS or CTLA4 promoter, providing two avenues for tonic TCR signaling through CD28.

Gene expression profiling. Early attempts at establishing a gene expression profile of AITL were plagued by the numerous contaminating B cells, dendritic cells, and endothelial cells in this lymphoma.[447,460,461] However, recent studies have confirmed a signature of follicular helper T cells in AITL, with expression of several members of the CD28 family of TCRs (the programmed death-1 [PD1 or CD279, gene name *PDCD1*] and inducible costimulator [ICOS]), as well as CD10, BCL6, CXCL13, CXCR5, CD40LG, SAP1 (gene name *PSAP*), CCRF, and NFATC1.[429,462] These studies have defined the characteristic protein profile of the neoplastic cells in AITL through the use of a range of IHC markers and in situ hybridization for EBV RNA. Current recommendations are to identify the expression of two or three of the corresponding antigens as sufficient to establish the follicular helper T-cell origin of these neoplastic cells.[2] In addition, a signature of immunosuppressive cytokines and their receptors was also notable (TNF-β1, TNF-βR2, IL-10Rα, IL-10-Rβ).[429] A prognostic signature was also obtained for AITL by gene expression profiling. Cases with a poor prognosis (1.05 years median overall survival vs 3.06 years, $P < .001$) demonstrate high expression levels of PDGFRa and PDGFRb, suggesting the potential for tyrosine kinase inhibitors in treating this disorder.[429]

Somatic variants. Recently, mutations in *RHOA*, *CD28*, *TET2*, *DNMT3A*, and *IDH2* have been identified at a high prevalence in AITL (Figure 89.16). *RHOA* is a GTPase molecular switch downstream of the TCR involved in signal transduction and actin nucleation that regulates cell shape, motility, and attachment. A hotspot missense p.G17V has been found in 53% to 68% of cases of AITL and is thought to be a driver mutation with dominant negative function.[463-465] By contrast, rare p.K18N mutations may show activating function in vitro of unclear significance.[465] Interestingly, these mutations appear to be commonly found in conjunction with *IDH2* and *TET2* mutations as well.[463,466] CD28 is a T cell–specific surface glycoprotein involved in proliferation, survival, cytokine production, and T-helper type 2 development. Hotspot missense mutations in *CD28* (p.D124 and p.T195) were found in 10% to 11% of cases of AITL, are nearly exclusive to this entity, and confer an adverse prognosis.[322,467] The latter three genes are involved in the DNA methylation. The roles of *TET2* and *DNMT3A* in the regulation of DNA methylation have been described above. *TET2* mutations have been found in up to 33% of cases of AITL, located throughout the gene on chromosome 10.[348] It is common for *TET2* mutations to occur in conjunction with *DNMT3A* mutations, implying some synergism.[451] *IDH2*, located on chromosome 15q21-qter, encodes for a mitochondrial NADP(+)-dependent isocitrate dehydrogenase, which physiologically plays a role in the citric acid cycle, converting isocitrate to α-ketoglutarate. The mutant enzyme is believed to catalyze the production of (R)-2-hydroxyglutarate, which may inhibit the function of TET2 and Jumonji histone demethylases, thereby affecting epigenetic regulation of the cell.[468,469] *IDH2* mutations (predominantly p.R172, with fewer p.R140) were identified in approximately 45% of all cases of AITL and are associated with the morphologic presence of clear cells.[466,470] Identical mutations are also seen in gliomas and AMLs. Unlike in these other disease types, mutations in *IDH1* are not identified and there is no suggestion of any prognostic import of the identification of this mutation at this time. Likewise, *TET2* and *DNMT3A* mutations are also common in AML and other myeloid neoplasms, pointing either to a common precursor or the relationship specifically between myeloid and T-cell lineages.[151,155,471] These mutations may also provide targets for novel therapeutics in AITL and MRD monitoring, although to date no studies have been conducted to investigate their use in MRD testing. *IDH2* provides the greatest potential for MRD testing inasmuch as a single mutation at R172 accounts for 15/16 cases examined, allowing for high clinical sensitivity and the development of highly sensitive allele-specific PCR assays. Additional non-*RHOA* mutations in the TCR pathway are mutually exclusive, including *PLCG1* (14%), *CTNNB1* (6%), *GTF2I* (6%), and infrequent mutations in the PI3K-AKT and JAK/STAT pathways. The consequent TCR pathway activation appears to be associated with poor response to anthracyclines.[465]

Guidelines for Molecular Testing in Angioimmunoblastic T-cell Lymphoma

FISH is not widely available for *ITK::SYK* or *CTLA4::CD28* currently. Testing for mutations in *TET2*, *DNMT3A*, *RHOA*, *IDH1*, and *IDH2* at diagnosis may help to discriminate AITL from other PTCLs. In addition, the identification of *CD28* hotspot mutations may inform prognosis. *IDH2* p.R172 or p.R140 mutations may be utilized in the monitoring of MRD for AITL.

Diagnosis	MRD
Consider PCR or NGS for TCR gene rearrangement studies	Consider NGS for TCR gene rearrangement studies
IHC for some set of PD-1, CD10, BCL6, CXCL13, CXCR5, CD40LG, SAP1	
Consider IHC for SYK	
Test for somatic variants, in particular *TET2, IDH1, IDH2, RHOA,* and *DNMT3A,* as well as possibly *CD28,* among others	Consider testing for somatic variants

T-prolymphocytic Leukemia

T-PLL is a rare aggressive T-cell neoplasm found in adults. Involvement is predominantly of the peripheral blood and bone marrow, with frequent infiltration of the lymph nodes and occasionally of the skin (20% of cases).[5] This neoplasm is not known to be virally driven, although it occurs with increased frequency in patients with ataxia-telangiectasia due to mutations in the *ATM* gene.[472] Clonal rearrangements of the TCR genes are detectable in essentially all cases of T-PLL using commercial primers against TRG and TRB.[32]

Rearrangements. Although the cell of origin is poorly understood, T-PLL is easily distinguished from other T-cell neoplasms by the presence of hallmark translocations and inversions involving the oncogenes *TCL1A, TCL1B,* or *MTCP1* with the TRA/D gene. These rearrangements are found in 80% to 90% of cases of T-PLL.[473,474] *TCL1A* and *TCL1B* are located on chromosome 14q32, resulting in inv(14)(q11;q32.1) or t(14;14)(q11;q32.1). Less frequently, translocations can involve the homologous *MTCP1* locus in chromosome Xq28 in a t(X;14)(q28;q11). Overexpression of the genes fused to the TRA/D locus at the J/D segment is the result in all these aberrations. This overexpression is independent of the orientation relative to the TRA/D enhancer, due to the presence of *TCL1A* and *TCL1B* in opposite orientations within a 120-kb region that separates the two breakpoint clusters common at 14q32.1.[472] Less commonly, rearrangements of *TCL1* can involve TRB as well.[475] A rare translocation has been anecdotally reported of a *SEPT9::ABL1* rearrangement, or t(9;17)(q34.12;q25.3), in a patient with T-PLL, resulting in insensitivity to ABL1 tyrosine kinase inhibitors.[476]

TCL1A and *TCL1B* encode for a cytoplasmic protein that is typically expressed in early double-negative T-cell progenitors and most B cells but not in mature T cells. However, its overexpression in T-PLL, a mature T-cell neoplasm, appears to be oncogenic, functioning through activation of the AKT pathway (*Figure 89.16*).[472] In addition, recently ATM has been identified as a TCL1-interaction protein, leading to activation of the NF-κB pathway.[477]

Copy number variations. Various profiling methods (aCGH, aSNP, and gene expression profiling) have identified other common secondary cytogenetic aberrations in T-PLL, which can lead to quite complex karyotypes with greater than three aberrations in the majority of cases.[474,478,479] These changes include large regions of gains in 6p and 8q, in particular i(8)(q10) that is observed in 61% to 77% of cases, often in association with translocations of TRA/D.[474,480] In addition, there are recurrent losses of 6q, 7q (involving the *EZH2* and *GIMAP* loci), 8p, 10p, 11q (involving the *ATM* locus), 17p (involving the *TP53* locus), and 22q (involving the *SMARCB1* locus).[474,478,481] In addition, aberrations involving the TRA/TRD locus on 14q11.2 at the site of the translocations were found in 86% of cases.[474]

Somatic variants. Recently, recurrent somatic mutations have been identified in T-PLL, including mutations in *ATM* (70%-73%), *STAT5B* (36%), *JAK3* (21%-34%), *TP53* (14%), *JAK1* (6%-8%), *EZH2* (13%), *BCOR* (8%), *FBWX10* (8%), *CHEK2* (5%), and *IL2RG* (2%).[474,480,482] *ATM* mutations are most commonly missense mutations, found throughout the gene (the majority in the C-terminal half) and typically co-occurring with deletion (LOH) of the second *ATM* allele. Cases with an *ATM* mutation tend to occur in conjunction with translocations of TRA/D while those with *TP53* mutations are more commonly found in cases without translocations of TRA/D.[474] *TP53*-mutated cases, typically missense mutations including the known hotspot p.R175, also tended to occur in the setting of LOH. Surprisingly, biallelic dysfunction of either *ATM* or *TP53* is not associated with particular prognostic import in T-PLL.[474,480]

Mutations of the *IL2RG-JAK1-JAK3-STAT5B* axis tend to be mutually exclusive, resulting in increased cytoplasmic and nuclear expression of pSTAT5 (*Figure 89.16*).[480] Somatic mutations in *JAK1, JAK3,* and *STAT5B* center on mutational hotspots that result in activation of the corresponding proteins. *JAK3* cases commonly involved the mutational hotspot p.M511I (over 50% of JAK3-positive cases), located in the region between the JH3 and pseudokinase (JH2) domains. This variant may occur in conjunction with a second variant in the pseudokinase domain.[482] The mutations in *STAT5B* are localized in the SH2 domain, in particular the p.N642H variant. Of all the mutations, only the *JAK3* variants are associated with poor overall survival in univariate analysis.[474,480]

Guidelines for Molecular Testing in T-prolymphocytic Leukemia

FISH for inv(14) or t(14;14) is diagnostically important. Mutational testing has the potential to provide enhanced sensitivity and may aid in the diagnosis of T-PLL if a typical pattern of cytogenetic and molecular findings is identified.

Diagnosis	MRD
Consider PCR or NGS for TCR gene rearrangement studies	Consider NGS for TCR gene rearrangement studies
FISH for inv(14) or t(14;14)	
Molecular testing for *ATM, JAK3, STAT5B,* and other common aberration in T-PLL	Consider NGS for somatic variants

T-cell Large Granular Lymphocytic Leukemia

T-cell large granular lymphocytic leukemia (T-LGL) is an uncommon, typically indolent disorder of clonal circulating cytotoxic T cells. T-LGL may be associated with neutropenia or even severe anemia due to red cell aplasia. An association with rheumatoid arthritis is also noted. Unfortunately, the differential diagnosis for an expanded population of large granular lymphocytes is broad and may include clonal expansions of T-LGLs without neoplasia, such as seen in the post–allogeneic stem cell transplantation setting. Therefore, although the TRG gene is rearranged in all cases (whether the cell of origin is αβ or γδ), the finding of clonality does not equate with neoplasia. Cases of LGL are more commonly associated with skewed TCR clonotypes.[483]

Somatic variants. Accordingly, recent findings of recurrent somatic mutations in T-LGL have been welcome supportive evidence of neoplasia. In particular, mutations of *STAT3* and *STAT5B* are recurrently found in T-LGL and not in normal controls and patients with circulating LGLs and concomitant neutropenia (*Figure 89.16*).[484,485] *STAT3* mutations are identified in 28% to 70% of these patients and are missense mutations located within exon 21, the src homology 2 (SH2) domain involved in dimerization, particularly the p.Y640F and p.D661 loci.[486-488] Less commonly, a recurrent hotspot missense mutation in the analogous domain of *STAT5B* has also been identified in approximately 2% of patients with T-LGL.[487,488] The mutational landscape is further complicated by the not uncommon finding of multiple *STAT3* clones and mutations in other genes within the *STAT3* pathway (*PTPRT*) as well as T-cell activation pathways (*BCL11B, SLIT2,* and *NRP1*).[489,490] *STAT3* variants are also found in patients with NK-LGL.[485,491] Although the presence of a *STAT3* mutation confers no particular prognostic significance, patients with were characterized by increased symptomatology, including pure red cell aplasia and the requirement for more lines of therapy.[485,491] Inhibition of STAT3 results in apoptosis of leukemic LGLs, demonstrating the oncogenic nature of these mutations.[485]

Guidelines for Molecular Testing in T-cell Large Granular Lymphocytic Leukemia

Activating *STAT3* mutations may assist in the differential between reactive and neoplastic LGLs and may be used to monitor disease.

Diagnosis	MRD
Consider PCR or NGS for TCR gene rearrangement studies	Consider NGS for TCR gene rearrangement studies
Molecular testing for *STAT3*	Consider PCR for *STAT3*

Enteropathy-Associated T-cell Lymphoma and Monomorphic Epitheliotropic Intestinal T-cell Lymphoma

Enteropathy-associated T-cell lymphoma (EATL) is a rare intestinal tumor of intraepithelial T cells, associated with celiac disease and the HLA-DQA1*0501, DBQ*0201 genotype, most commonly found in the patients of Northern European origin. This entity has now been formally separated from monomorphic epitheliotropic intestinal T-cell lymphoma (MEITL) that is found predominately in the Asian and Hispanic populations with no association with celiac disease (formerly known as EATL, type II). Combined, these two entities represent 10% to 25% of all lymphomas primary to the small intestine, predominantly the jejunum or ileum.[492] The neoplastic cell in EATL is a cytotoxic T cell, often negative for both CD4 and CD8, CD103, and TCRß, and is analogous to the intraepithelial T cell seen in celiac disease. MEITL may be either TCRαß or TCRγδ (or null in 40% of cases) and express CD8 with CD56 and cytotoxic markers. They have been found to express high levels of nuclear MATK.[493]

Copy number variations. Although there are no hallmark translocations found in either EATL or MEITL, both entities are associated with recurrent CNVs. Both demonstrate common gains of 9q34 or losses of 16q12.1 noted by FISH or aSNP analysis.[492,494] However, EATL is associated with gains of 1q32.2-q41 and 5q34-q35.2 while MEITL in the majority of cases is positive for gains of 8q24 (*MYC*).[5,495]

Somatic variants. MEITL cases harbor recurrent mutations of *SETD2* in nearly all cases (93% of cases), resulting in loss of H3K36 trimethylation that can be assessed by immunohistochemical stains.[496] In addition, there are frequent activating mutations in *STAT5B* (60% of cases) and *JAK3* (46% of cases, many co-occurring with *STAT5B* variants) as well as SH2B3 (20% of cases) (*Figure 89.16*).[494,496] In addition, recurrent mutations in *TP53*, *BRAF*, and *KRAS* are also found, although their therapeutic implications have not yet been explored. By contrast, neither *SETD2* nor *JAK3*/*STAT5B* mutations are common in EATL, although *JAK1* and *STAT3* mutations are recurrent, suggesting differential addiction to cytokine/T-cell subtypes (*Figure 89.16*).[496]

Guidelines for Molecular Testing in EATL and MEITL

Molecular assessment of various somatic variants can be considered both for diagnosis and monitoring, although their diagnostic and prognostic implications are less well characterized at this time. Although immunohistochemical studies for H3K36 trimethylation characterize MEITL and distinguish it from EATL, this stain is not widely available.

Diagnosis	MRD
Consider PCR or NGS for TCR gene rearrangement studies	Consider NGS for TCR gene rearrangement studies
Consider molecular (NGS) testing for *SETD2, STAT5B, JAK3, STAT3, JAK1*	Consider PCR for known variants

Adult T-cell Leukemia/Lymphoma

Adult T-cell leukemia/lymphoma (ATLL) is neoplasm of mature T cells characterized by monoclonal integration of the retrovirus, human T-cell leukemia virus type 1 (HTLV-1). HTLV-1 status can be confirmed by HTLV-1 serology or quantitative PCR of the proviral load.[497,498] Although the viral infection is acquired early in life, typically in individuals from southwest Japan, Caribbean basin, and central Africa, the disease has a long latency with low penetrance, with only 2.5% of HTLV-1 carriers in Japan developing the disease after 30 to 50 years (median age of diagnosis 58 years).[5] ATLL includes four distinct subtypes: acute, lymphomatous, chronic, and smoldering. The acute and lymphomatous subtypes are rapidly fatal, while the chronic and smoldering subtypes may progress to the acute variant in 25% of cases over the course of years. These clinical subtypes are characterized by different molecular genetic patterns, but all subtypes typically demonstrate clonal TCR gene rearrangements.

Rearrangements. In general, ATLL demonstrates genomic instability with numerous structural variants typically involving fragile sites of the genome. In addition, as with AITL, ATLL demonstrates recurrent activating translocation of *CD28*, including *CTLA4::CD28* (5% of cases) and *ICOS::CD28* (2% of cases).[499] WGS identified tandem duplications of 2q33.2, which result in these fusions. Since normally CD28 expression is downregulated after T-cell activation and replaced by expression of CTLA4 or ICOS, these fusions result in extension of the CD28-mediated signaling. This pathway may also be activated by recurrent mutations or amplification of CD28.

Copy number variations. Approximately 88% of cases of ATLL will demonstrate CNVs and/or CN-LOH, often co-occurring with mutations of affected genes to result in biallelic dysfunction.[499,500] Typically, loss-of-function mutations are accompanied by copy loss or CN-LOH, while gain-of-function mutations are associated with copy number gains or CN-LOH. More numerous CNVs are found in the more aggressive subtypes (acute and lymphomatous) with high association with deletions of *CDKN2A* (9p21, 20%-30%), *CCDC7* (10p11, 10%-30%), *ATXN1* (6p22, 10% to 20%), and *GPR183* (13q32, 20%-30%). Other frequent CNVs include amplification of *CD28* (2q33, 10%-20%), *IRF4* (6p25, 20%-30%), *BCL11B* (14q32, 20%-40%), and *CD274* (encoding PD-L1, 9p24, 10%-20%), as well as deletions of TRB (7q34, 40%-50%) and *TP53* (20%-40%, 17p13).

Somatic variants. Tax1, a viral oncogene, is encoded by HTLV-1, and its interactome involves both the TCR-NF-κB pathway and the p53 and p16 tumor suppressors. Not surprisingly, the recurrently mutated genes in ATLL, particularly in Japanese patients, reflect gain-of-function mutations in TCR signaling, such as *PLCG1* (36%), *VAV1* (18%), *FYN* (4%), and *CD28* (2%), as well as gain of function in NF-κB signaling, including *PRKCB* (33%), *CARD11* (24%), *IRF4* (14%), and *RHOA* (8%).[499-503] Negative regulators of these pathways are involved by loss-of-function mutations: *CBLB* (4%), *TRAF3* (2%), *TNFAIP3* (1%), *NFKB1A* (1%), *PTPRC* (2%), and *CSNK1A1* (5%). Genes involved in T-cell trafficking are also affected, including gain-of-function *CCR4* (29%) and *CCR7* (11%) mutations and loss-of-function *GPR183* (28%). Other pathways affected by somatic alterations in ATLL include the JAK/STAT pathways (*JAK3* [2%], *STAT3* [21%]) and NOTCH pathways (*NOTCH1* [15%], *ATXN1* [1%], *ZFP36L2* [1%]). In total 96% of cases of ATLL will have a somatic mutation, for a very high negative predictive value for the absence of any mutation. As with the CNVs, somatic mutational patterns correlate with prognosis, with *PRKCB*, *TP53*, and subclonal *IRF4* mutations significantly associated with aggressive subtypes and *STAT3* mutation associated with indolent subtypes. Interestingly, in North American cases of ATLL, the mutation signature is significantly skewed toward epigenetic genes with mutations in *EP300* found in 20% of cases along with mutations in *TET2*, *EZH2*, *MED12*, *PBRM1*, *DNMT3A*, *KMT2A*, *HIST1H1E*, *SPEN*, *IDH1*, *SMARCB1*, and *ASXL1* for an overall epigenetic aberration in 57% of cases.[504] By contrast, *CARD11* was found in only 7% of cases. The epigenetic signature was associated with poor prognosis but was sensitive in vitro to decitabine.

Guidelines for Molecular Testing in Adult T-Cell Leukemia/Lymphoma

HTLV-1 serology testing is critical for the diagnosis of ATLL, and *TCR* gene rearrangement studies should be positive. Importantly, quantitation of the HTLV-1 proviral load has been associated with response to therapy, although this methodology requires the complex mapping of the integration site and development of an oligoclonality score, which is too complex for routine clinical care at this time. Somatic variants (TCR-NF-κB pathway) may provide supportive evidence for the diagnosis of ATLL, and the number and type of somatic alterations can be prognostically relevant. The NOTCH pathway is seldom subject to somatic alteration in other mature T-cell neoplasms and, when positive, can be suggestive of ATLL.

Diagnosis	MRD
HTLV-1 serology	
Consider PCR or NGS for TCR gene rearrangement studies	Consider NGS for TCR gene rearrangement studies
Consider molecular (NGS) testing for prognostic purposes	Consider NGS for known variants

Extranodal NK/T-cell Lymphoma

Another virally driven lymphoma is extranodal NK/T-cell lymphoma (ENKTCL), a rare aggressive neoplasm typically characterized by ulcerative and angiocentric/angiodestructive lesions in extranodal sites, often in the nasopharynx and occasionally in the skin and other sites.[5] The disease is more prevalent in Asia and Central and South America in mature adults with a male predominance. Most cases show an NK-cell phenotype that is therefore negative for a clonal TCR gene rearrangement but may be clonal by KIR repertoire studies.[505,506] However, rare cases may exhibit a cytotoxic T-cell phenotype with clonal rearrangements.

Rearrangements. As with AILT and ATLL, ENKTCL demonstrates recurrent activating translocation *CTLA4-CD28* (23% of cases). Other structural rearrangements include i(6)(p10), which results in loss of 6q (see CNVs below).

Copy number variations. Deletion of 6q21-26 can be seen in up to 44% of cases of ENKTCL and is the most common cytogenetic change in this neoplasm, resulting in deletion of *PRDM1*, *ATG5*, and *HACE1*. Other CNVs include gain of 2q and loss of 1p36, 23-26.33, 4q12, 5q34-35.3, 7q21.3-22.1, 11a22.3-23.3, and 15q11.2-14. None of these changes is specific for ENKTCL.

Somatic variants. Recurrent somatic alterations in ENKTCL include mutations in an RNA helicase gene (*DDX3X*, 20%, associated with poor prognosis), the JAK/STAT pathway (*STAT3* [6%-27%], *JAK3*, [6%-35%], *STAT5B* [2%-6%]), the histone modification pathway (*BCOR* [21%], *KMT2D* [7%-18%], *ARID1A* [6%]), and *TP53* (12%-13%).[507-511]

Guidelines for Molecular Testing in ENKTCL

KIR repertoire studies may be helpful for the diagnosis of ENKTCL, but TCR gene rearrangement studies will only detect the minority of cases with cytotoxic T-cell origin. Molecular assessment of various somatic variants can be considered both for diagnosis and monitoring, and targeted therapies may become available in the future.

Diagnosis	MRD
Consider KIR repertoire testing	
Consider PCR or NGS for TCR gene rearrangement studies	Consider NGS for TCR gene rearrangement studies
Consider molecular (NGS) testing	Consider NGS for known variants

References

1. A clinical evaluation of the international lymphoma study group classification of non-Hodgkin's lymphoma. The non-Hodgkin's lymphoma classification project. *Blood*. 1997;89(11):3909-3918.
2. Swerdlow SH, Campo E, Pileri SA, et al. The 2016 revision of the World Health Organization classification of lymphoid neoplasms. *Blood*. 2016;127(20):2375-2390. doi:10.1182/blood-2016-01-643569
3. American Cancer Society (ACS. *Cancer Facts & Figures 2021*. American Cancer Society; 2021. https://seer.cancer.gov/explorer/
4. Howlader N, Noone AM, Krapcho M, et al, eds.*SEER Cancer Statistics Review, 1975-2013*. National Cancer Institute; 2016.
5. Swerdlow SH, Campo E, Harris NL, et al, eds. *WHO Classification of Tumours of Haematopoietic and Lymphoid Tissues*. Revised 4th ed. International Agency for Research on Cancer; 2017.
6. Burkitt DP. A sarcoma involving the jaws in African children. *Br J Surg*. 1958;46(197):218-223.
7. Tsujimoto Y, Finger LR, Yunis J, Nowell PC, Croce CM. Cloning of the chromosome breakpoint of neoplastic B cells with the t(14;18) chromosome translocation. *Science*. 1984;226(4678):1097-1099.
8. Klein U, Dalla-Favera R. Germinal centres: role in B-cell physiology and malignancy. *Nat Rev Immunol*. 2008;8(1):22-33. doi:10.1038/nri2217
9. Shaffer AL, Rosenwald A, Staudt LM. Lymphoid malignancies: the dark side of B-cell differentiation. *Nat Rev Immunol*. 2002;2(12):920-932. doi:10.1038/nri953nri953
10. Fitzpatrick MJ, Massoth LR, Marcus C, et al. JAK2 rearrangements are a recurrent alteration in CD30 + systemic T-cell lymphomas with anaplastic morphology. *Am J Surg Pathol*. 2021;45(7):895-904.
11. Roullet M, Bagg A. The basis and rational use of molecular genetic testing in mature B-cell lymphomas. *Adv Anat Pathol*. 2010;17(5):333-358. doi:10.1097/PAP.0b013e3181ec7466
12. HUGO Gene Nomenclature Committee website. Accessed September 8, 2021. www.genenames.org
13. Schroeder HW Jr, Cavacini L. Structure and function of immunoglobulins. *J Allergy Clin Immunol*. 2010;125(2 suppl):S41-S52. 10.1016/j.jaci.2009.09.046
14. Abbas AK, Lichtman AH, Pillai S. *Cellular and Molecular Immunology*. 7th ed. Elsevier/Saunders; 2012.
15. van Dongen JJM, Langerak AW, Bruggemann M, et al. Design and standardization of PCR primers and protocols for detection of clonal immunoglobulin and T-cell receptor gene recombinations in suspect lymphoproliferations: report of the BIOMED-2 Concerted Action BMH4-CT98-3936. *Leukemia*. 2003;17(12):2257-2317. doi:10.1038/sj.leu.24032022403202
16. Liu H, Bench AJ, Bacon CM, et al. A practical strategy for the routine use of BIOMED-2 PCR assays for detection of B- and T-cell clonality in diagnostic haematopathology. *Br J Haematol*. 2007;138(1):31-43. 10.1111/j.1365-2141.2007.06618.x
17. Evans PAS, Pott C, Groenen PJTA, et al. Significantly improved PCR-based clonality testing in B-cell malignancies by use of multiple immunoglobulin gene targets. Report of the BIOMED-2 Concerted Action BHM4-CT98-3936. *Leukemia*. 2007;21(2):207-214. 10.1038/sj.leu.2404479
18. van Krieken JHJM, Langerak AW, Macintyre EA, et al. Improved reliability of lymphoma diagnostics via PCR-based clonality testing: report of the BIOMED-2 Concerted Action BHM4-CT98-3936. *Leukemia*. 2007;21(2):201-206. doi:10.1038/sj.leu.2404467
19. Faham M, Zheng J, Moorhead M, et al. Deep-sequencing approach for minimal residual disease detection in acute lymphoblastic leukemia. *Blood*. 2012;120(26):5173-5180. doi:10.1182/blood-2012-07-444042
20. Logan AC, Vashi N, Faham M, et al. Immunoglobulin and t cell receptor gene high-throughput sequencing quantifies minimal residual disease in acute lymphoblastic leukemia and predicts post-transplantation relapse and survival. *Biol Blood Marrow Transplant*. 2014;20(9):1307-1313. doi:10.1016/j.bbmt.2014.04.018
21. Rosati E, Dowds CM, Liaskou E, Henriksen EKK, Karlsen TH, Franke A. Overview of methodologies for T-cell receptor repertoire analysis. *BMC Biotechnol*. 2017;17(1):61. doi:10.1186/s12896-017-0379-9
22. Arcila ME, Yu W, Syed M, et al. Establishment of immunoglobulin heavy (IGH) chain clonality testing by next-generation sequencing for routine characterization of B-cell and plasma cell neoplasms. *J Mol Diagn*. 2019;21(2):330-342. doi:10.1016/j.jmoldx.2018.10.008
23. Wu D, Emerson RO, Sherwood A, et al. Detection of minimal residual disease in B lymphoblastic leukemia by high-throughput sequencing of IGH. *Clin Cancer Res*. 2014;20(17):4540-4548. doi:10.1158/1078-0432.CCR-13-3231
24. Logan AC, Zhang B, Narasimhan B, et al. Minimal residual disease quantification using consensus primers and high-throughput IGH sequencing predicts post-transplant relapse in chronic lymphocytic leukemia. *Leukemia*. 2013;27(8):1659-1665. doi:10.1038/leu.2013.52
25. Martinez-Lopez J, Lahuerta JJ, Pepin F, et al. Prognostic value of deep sequencing method for minimal residual disease detection in multiple myeloma. *Blood*. 2014;123(20):3073-3079. doi:10.1182/blood-2014-01-550020
26. Kurtz DM, Scherer F, Jin MC, et al. Circulating tumor DNA measurements as early outcome predictors in diffuse large B-cell lymphoma. *J Clin Oncol*. 2018;36(28):2845-2853. doi:10.1200/JCO.2018.78.5246
27. Kurtz DM, Green MR, Bratman SV, et al. Noninvasive monitoring of diffuse large B-cell lymphoma by immunoglobulin high-throughput sequencing. *Blood*. 2015;125(24):3679-3687. doi:10.1182/blood-2015-03-635169
28. Rustad EH, Hultcrantz M, Yellapantula VD, et al. Baseline identification of clonal V(D)J sequences for DNA-based minimal residual disease detection in multiple myeloma. *PLoS One*. 2019;14(3):e0211600. doi:10.1371/journal.pone.0211600

29. van Dongen JJ, Comans-Bitter WM, Wolvers-Tettero IL, Borst J. Development of human T lymphocytes and their thymus-dependency. *Thymus*. 1990;16(3-4):207-234.
30. Winoto A, Baltimore D. Separate lineages of T cells expressing the alpha beta and gamma delta receptors. *Nature*. 1989;338(6214):430-432. doi:10.1038/338430a0
31. Lefranc MP. IMGT databases, web resources and tools for immunoglobulin and T cell receptor sequence analysis. *Leukemia*. 2003;17(1):260-266. doi:10.1038/sj.leu.24026372402637
32. Bruggemann M, White H, Gaulard P, et al. Powerful strategy for polymerase chain reaction-based clonality assessment in T-cell malignancies Report of the BIOMED-2 Concerted Action BHM4 CT98-3936. *Leukemia*. 2007;21(2):215-221. doi:10.1038/sj.leu.2404481
33. De Masson A, O'Malley JT, Elco CP, et al. High-throughput sequencing of the T cell receptor β gene identifies aggressive early-stage mycosis fungoides. *Sci Transl Med*. 2018;10(440):eaar5894. doi:10.1126/scitranslmed.aar5894
34. Sufficool KE, Lockwood CM, Abel HJ, et al. T-cell clonality assessment by next-generation sequencing improves detection sensitivity in mycosis fungoides. *J Am Acad Dermatol*. 2015;73(2):228-236.e2. doi:10.1016/j.jaad.2015.04.030
35. Wu D, Sherwood A, Fromm JR, et al. High-throughput sequencing detects minimal residual disease in acute T lymphoblastic leukemia. *Sci Transl Med*. 2012;4(134):134ra63. doi:10.1126/scitranslmed.3003656
36. Trask BJ. Fluorescence in situ hybridization: applications in cytogenetics and gene mapping. *Trends Genet*. 1991;7(5):149-154. doi:10.1016/0168-9525(91)90378-4
37. Gutierrez NC, Garcia JL, Hernandez JM, et al. Prognostic and biologic significance of chromosomal imbalances assessed by comparative genomic hybridization in multiple myeloma. *Blood*. 2004;104(9):2661-2666. doi:10.1182/blood-2004-04-13192004-04-1319
38. Schwaenen C, Nessling M, Wessendorf S, et al. Automated array-based genomic profiling in chronic lymphocytic leukemia: development of a clinical tool and discovery of recurrent genomic alterations. *Proc Natl Acad Sci U S A*. 2004;101(4):1039-1044. doi:10.1073/pnas.03047171010304717101
39. Maciejewski JP, Tiu RV, O'Keefe C. Application of array-based whole genome scanning technologies as a cytogenetic tool in haematological malignancies. *Br J Haematol*. 2009;146(5):479-488. doi:10.1111/j.1365-2141.2009.07757.x
40. ISCN rules for listing chromosomal rearrangements. *Curr Protoc Hum Genet*. 1998:Appendix 4:Appendix 4C.
41. Hamblin TJ, Davis Z, Gardiner A, Oscier DG, Stevenson FK. Unmutated Ig V(H) genes are associated with a more aggressive form of chronic lymphocytic leukemia. *Blood*. 1999;94(6):1848-1854.
42. Damle RN, Wasil T, Fais F, et al. Ig V gene mutation status and CD38 expression as novel prognostic indicators in chronic lymphocytic leukemia. *Blood*. 1999;94(6):1840-1847.
43. Rosenquist R, Ghia P, Hadzidimitriou A, et al. Immunoglobulin gene sequence analysis in chronic lymphocytic leukemia: Updated ERIC recommendations. *Leukemia*. 2017;31(7):1477-1481. doi:10.1038/leu.2017.125
44. Maciejewski JP, Mufti GJ. Whole genome scanning as a cytogenetic tool in hematologic malignancies. *Blood*. 2008;112(4):965-974. doi:10.1182/blood-2008-02-130435
45. de Ravel TJL, Devriendt K, Fryns JP, Vermeesch JR. What's new in karyotyping? The move towards array comparative genomic hybridisation (CGH). *Eur J Pediatr*. 2007;166(7):637-643. doi:10.1007/s00431-007-0463-6
46. Gunn SR, Mohammed MS, Gorre ME, et al. Whole-genome scanning by array comparative genomic hybridization as a clinical tool for risk assessment in chronic lymphocytic leukemia. *J Mol Diagn*. 2008;10(5):442-451. doi:10.2353/jmoldx.2008.080033
47. Balcárková J, Urbánková H, Scudla V, et al. Gain of chromosome arm 1q in patients in relapse and progression of multiple myeloma. *Cancer Genet Cytogenet*. 2009;192(2):68-72. doi:10.1016/j.cancergencyto.2009.02.020
48. Lennon PA, Zhuang Y, Pierson D, et al. Bacterial artificial chromosome array-Based comparative genomic hybridization using paired formalin-fixed, paraffin-embedded and fresh frozen tissue specimens in multiple myeloma. *Cancer*. 2009;115(2):345-354. doi:10.1002/cncr.24021
49. Sanger F, Nicklen S, Coulson AR. DNA sequencing with chain-terminating inhibitors. *Proc Natl Acad Sci U S A*. 1977;74(12):5463-5467.
50. Rizzo JM, Buck MJ. Key principles and clinical applications of "next-generation" DNA sequencing. *Cancer Prev Res*. 2012;5(7):887-900. doi:10.1158/1940-6207.CAPR-11-0432
51. Metzker ML. Sequencing technologies—the next generation. *Nat Rev Genet*. 2010;11(1):31-46. doi:10.1038/nrg2626
52. Kluk MJ, Lindsley RC, Aster JC, et al. Validation and implementation of a custom next-generation sequencing clinical assay for hematologic malignancies. *J Mol Diagn*. 2016;18(4):507-515. doi:10.1016/j.jmoldx.2016.02.003
53. Newman AM, Lovejoy AF, Klass DM, et al. Integrated digital error suppression for improved detection of circulating tumor DNA. *Nat Biotechnol*. 2016;34(5):547-555. doi:10.1038/nbt.3520
54. Zhang BM, Keegan A, Li P, et al. An overview of characteristics of clinical next-generation sequencing–based testing for hematologic malignancies. *Arch Pathol Lab Med*. 2021;145(9):1110-1116. doi:10.5858/arpa.2019-0661-cp
55. Nagarajan R, Bartley AN, Bridge JA, et al. A window into clinical next-generation sequencing-based oncology testing practices. *Arch Pathol Lab Med*. 2017;141(12):1679-1685. doi:10.5858/arpa.2016-0542-CP
56. Merker JD, Devereaux K, Iafrate AJ, et al. Proficiency testing of standardized samples shows very high interlaboratory agreement for clinical next-generation sequencing-based oncology assays. *Arch Pathol Lab Med*. 2019;143(4):463-471. doi:10.5858/arpa.2018-0336-CP
57. Surrey LF, Oakley FD, Merker JD, et al. Next-generation sequencing (NGS) methods show superior or equivalent performance to non-NGS methods on BRAF, EGFR, and KRAS proficiency testing samples. *Arch Pathol Lab Med*. 2019;143(8):980-984. doi:10.5858/arpa.2018-0394-CP
58. Keegan A, Bridge JA, Lindeman NI, et al. Proficiency testing of standardized samples shows high interlaboratory agreement for clinical next-generation sequencing-based hematologic malignancy assays with survey material-specific differences in variant frequencies. *Arch Pathol Lab Med*. 2020;144:959-966. doi:10.5858/arpa.2019-0352-CP
59. Mandruzzato S. Technological platforms for microarray gene expression profiling. *Adv Exp Med Biol*. 2007;593:12-18. doi:10.1007/978-0-387-39978-2-2
60. Crespo M, Bosch F, Villamor N, et al. ZAP-70 expression as a surrogate for immunoglobulin-variable-region mutations in chronic lymphocytic leukemia. *N Engl J Med*. 2003;348(18):1764-1775. doi:10.1056/NEJMoa023143348/18/1764
61. Rosenwald A, Staudt LM. Gene expression profiling of diffuse large B-cell lymphoma. *Leuk Lymphoma*. 2003;44(suppl 3):S41-S47.
62. Savage KJ, Monti S, Kutok JL, et al. The molecular signature of mediastinal large B-cell lymphoma differs from that of other diffuse large B-cell lymphomas and shares features with classical Hodgkin lymphoma. *Blood*. 2003;102(12):3871-3879. doi:10.1182/blood-2003-06-18412003-06-1841
63. Willenbrock K, Kuppers R, Renne C, et al. Common features and differences in the transcriptome of large cell anaplastic lymphoma and classical Hodgkin's lymphoma. *Haematologica*. 2006;91(5):596-604.
64. Lim LP, Lau NC, Garrett-Engele P, et al. Microarray analysis shows that some microRNAs downregulate large numbers of target mRNAs. *Nature*. 2005;433(7027):769-773. doi:10.1038/nature03315
65. Havelange V, Garzon R. MicroRNAs: emerging key regulators of hematopoiesis. *Am J Hematol*. 2010;85(12):935-942. doi:10.1002/ajh.21863
66. Garzon R, Croce CM. MicroRNAs in normal and malignant hematopoiesis. *Curr Opin Hematol*. 2008;15(4):352-358. doi:10.1097/MOH.0b013e328303e15d
67. Sevignani C, Calin GA, Siracusa LD, Croce CM. Mammalian microRNAs: a small world for fine-tuning gene expression. *Mamm Genome*. 2006;17(3):189-202. doi:10.1007/s00335-005-0066-3
68. Calin GA, Dumitru CD, Shimizu M, et al. Frequent deletions and down-regulation of micro- RNA genes miR15 and miR16 at 13q14 in chronic lymphocytic leukemia. *Proc Natl Acad Sci U S A*. 2002;99(24):15524-15529. doi:10.1073/pnas.242606799
69. Calin GA, Ferracin M, Cimmino A, et al. A MicroRNA signature associated with prognosis and progression in chronic lymphocytic leukemia. *N Engl J Med*. 2005;353(17):1793-1801. doi:10.1056/NEJMoa050995
70. Calin GA, Pekarsky Y, Croce CM. The role of microRNA and other non-coding RNA in the pathogenesis of chronic lymphocytic leukemia. *Best Pract Res Clin Haematol*. 2007;20(3):425-437. doi:10.1016/j.beha.2007.02.003
71. Metzler M, Wilda M, Busch K, Viehmann S, Borkhardt A. High expression of precursor microRNA-155/BIC RNA in children with Burkitt lymphoma. *Genes Chromosomes Cancer*. 2004;39(2):167-169. doi:10.1002/gcc.10316
72. Jiang J, Lee EJ, Schmittgen TD. Increased expression of microRNA-155 in Epstein-Barr virus transformed lymphoblastoid cell lines. *Genes Chromosomes Cancer*. 2006;45(1):103-106. doi:10.1002/gcc.20264
73. Eis PS, Tam W, Sun L, et al. Accumulation of miR-155 and BIC RNA in human B cell lymphomas. *Proc Natl Acad Sci U S A*. 2005;102(10):3627-3632. doi:10.1073/pnas.0500613102
74. He L, Thomson JM, Hemann MT, et al. A microRNA polycistron as a potential human oncogene. *Nature*. 2005;435(7043):828-833. doi:10.1038/nature03552
75. Gardiner-Garden M, Frommer M. CpG islands in vertebrate genomes. *J Mol Biol*. 1987;196(2):261-282. doi:10.1016/0022-2836(87)90689-9
76. Takai D, Jones PA. Comprehensive analysis of CpG islands in human chromosomes 21 and 22. *Proc Natl Acad Sci U S A*. 2002;99(6):3740-3745. doi:10.1073/pnas.052410099
77. Ammerpohl O, Martin-Subero JI, Richter J, Vater I, Siebert R. Hunting for the 5th base: techniques for analyzing DNA methylation. *Biochim Biophys Acta*. 2009;1790(9):847-862. doi:10.1016/j.bbagen.2009.02.001
78. Chang JW, Huang THM, Wang YC. Emerging methods for analysis of the cancer methylome. *Pharmacogenomics*. 2008;9(12):1869-1878. doi:10.2217/14622416.9.12.1869
79. Huang YW, Huang THM, Wang LS. Profiling DNA methylomes from microarray to genome-scale sequencing. *Technol Cancer Res Treat*. 2010;9(2):139-147. doi:10.1177/153303461000900203
80. Ondrejka SL, Lai R, Smith SD, Hsi ED. Indolent mantle cell leukemia: a clinicopathological variant characterized by isolated lymphocytosis, interstitial bone marrow involvement, kappa light chain restriction, and good prognosis. *Haematologica*. 2011;96(8):1121-1127. doi:10.3324/haematol.2010.036277.
81. Orchard J, Garand R, Davis Z, et al. A subset of t(11;14) lymphoma with mantle cell features displays mutated IgVH genes and includes patients with good prognosis, nonnodal disease. *Blood*. 2003;101(12):4975-4981. doi:10.1182/blood-2002-06-1864
82. Fu K, Weisenburger DD, Greiner TC, et al. Cyclin D1-negative mantle cell lymphoma: a clinicopathologic study based on gene expression profiling. *Blood*. 2005;106(13):4315-4321. doi:10.1182/blood-2005-04-1753
83. Royo C, Salaverria I, Hartmann EM, Rosenwald A, Campo E, Bea S. The complex landscape of genetic alterations in mantle cell lymphoma. *Semin Cancer Biol*. 2011;21(5):322-334. doi:10.1016/j.semcancer.2011.09.007
84. Matutes E, Brito-Babapulle V, Ellis J, et al. Translocation t(11;14)(q13;q32) in chronic lymphoid disorders. *Genes Chromosomes Cancer*. 1992;5(2):158-165.
85. Fiedler W, Weh HJ, Hossfeld DK. Comparison of chromosome analysis and BCL-1 rearrangement in a series of patients with multiple myeloma. *Br J Haematol*. 1992;81(1):58-61.
86. Ronchetti D, Finelli P, Richelda R, et al. Molecular analysis of 11q13 breakpoints in multiple myeloma. *Blood*. 1999;93(4):1330-1337.
87. Vandenberghe E, De Wolf Peeters C, Wlodarska I, et al. Chromosome 11q rearrangements in B non Hodgkin's lymphoma. *Br J Haematol*. 1992;81(2):212-217.
88. Belaud-Rotureau MA, Parrens M, Dubus P, Garroste JC, de Mascarel A, Merlio JP. A comparative analysis of FISH, RT-PCR, PCR, and immunohistochemistry for the diagnosis of mantle cell lymphomas. *Mod Pathol*. 2002;15(5):517-525. doi:10.1038/modpathol.3880556

89. Briggs RC, Miranda RN, Kinney MC, Veno PA, Hammer RD, Cousar JB. Immunohistochemical detection of cyclin D1 using optimized conditions is highly specific for mantle cell lymphoma and hairy cell leukemia. Mod Pathol. 2000;13(12):1308-1314. doi:10.1038/modpathol.3880239

90. Zukerberg LR, Yang WI, Arnold A, Harris NL. Cyclin D1 expression in non-Hodgkin's lymphomas. Detection by immunohistochemistry. Am J Clin Pathol. 1995;103(6):756-760.

91. Diehl JA. Cycling to cancer with cyclin D1. Cancer Biol Ther. 2002;1(3):226-231. doi:10.4161/cbt.72

92. Katzenberger T, Petzoldt C, Holler S, et al. The Ki67 proliferation index is a quantitative indicator of clinical risk in mantle cell lymphoma. Blood. 2006;107(8):3407. doi:10.1182/blood-2005-10-4079

93. Tiemann M, Schrader C, Klapper W, et al. Histopathology, cell proliferation indices and clinical outcome in 304 patients with mantle cell lymphoma (MCL): a clinicopathological study from the European MCL Network. Br J Haematol. 2005;131(1):29-38. doi:10.1111/j.1365-2141.2005.05716.x

94. Vega F, Medeiros JL. Chromosomal translocations involved in non-Hodgkin lymphomas. Arch Pathol Lab Med. 2003;127(9):1148-1160.

95. Wickham CL, Harries LW, Sarsfield P, Joyner MV, Ellard S. Large variation in t(11;14)(q13;q32) and t(14;18)(q32;q21) translocation product size is confirmed by sequence analysis of PCR products. Clin Lab Haematol. 2006;28(4):248-253. doi:10.1111/j.1365-2257.2006.00790.x

96. Chen RW, Bemis LT, Amato CM, et al. Truncation in CCND1 mRNA alters miR-16-1 regulation in mantle cell lymphoma. Blood. 2008;112(3):822-829. doi:10.1182/blood-2008-03-142182

97. Wiestner A, Tehrani M, Chiorazzi M, et al. Point mutations and genomic deletions in CCND1 create stable truncated cyclin D1 mRNAs that are associated with increased proliferation rate and shorter survival. Blood. 2007;109(11):4599-4606. doi:10.1182/blood-2006-08-039859

98. Schraders M, Oeschger S, Kluin PM, et al. Hypermutation in mantle cell lymphoma does not indicate a clinical or biological subentity. Mod Pathol. 2009;22(3):416-425. doi:10.1038/modpathol.2008.199

99. Gimenez E, Chauvet M, Rabin L, et al. Cloned IGH VDJ targets as tools for personalized minimal residual disease monitoring in mature lymphoid malignancies; a feasibility study in mantle cell lymphoma by the Groupe Ouest Est d'Etude des Leucemies et Autres Maladies du Sang. Br J Haematol. 2012;158(2):186-197. doi:10.1111/j.1365-2141.2012.09161.x

100. Mozos A, Royo C, Hartmann E, et al. SOX11 expression is highly specific for mantle cell lymphoma and identifies the cyclin D1-negative subtype. Haematologica. 2009;94(11):1555-1562. doi:10.3324/haematol.2009.010264

101. Chen YH, Gao J, Fan G, Peterson LC. Nuclear expression of sox11 is highly associated with mantle cell lymphoma but is independent of t(11;14)(q13;q32) in non-mantle cell B-cell neoplasms. Mod Pathol. 2010;23(1):105-112. doi:10.1038/modpathol.2009.140

102. Beà S, Valdés-Mas R, Navarro A, et al. Landscape of somatic mutations and clonal evolution in mantle cell lymphoma. Proc Natl Acad Sci U S A. 2013;110(45):18250-18255. doi:10.1073/pnas.1314608110

103. Dreyling MH, Bullinger L, Ott G, et al. Alterations of the cyclin D1/p16-pRB pathway in mantle cell lymphoma. Cancer Res. 1997;57(20):4608-4614.

104. Pinyol M, Cobo F, Bea S, et al. p16(INK4a) gene inactivation by deletions, mutations, and hypermethylation is associated with transformed and aggressive variants of non-Hodgkin's lymphomas. Blood. 1998;91(8):2977-2984.

105. Pinyol M, Hernandez L, Cazorla M, et al. Deletions and loss of expression of p16INK4a and p21Waf1 genes are associated with aggressive variants of mantle cell lymphomas. Blood. 1997;89(1):272-280.

106. Rosenwald A, Wright G, Wiestner A, et al. The proliferation gene expression signature is a quantitative integrator of oncogenic events that predicts survival in mantle cell lymphoma. Cancer Cell. 2003;3(2):185-197. doi:10.1016/s153561080300028-x

107. Greiner TC, Moynihan MJ, Chan WC, et al. p53 mutations in mantle cell lymphoma are associated with variant cytology and predict a poor prognosis. Blood. 1996;87(10):4302-4310.

108. Hernandez L, Fest T, Cazorla M, et al. p53 gene mutations and protein overexpression are associated with aggressive variants of mantle cell lymphomas. Blood. 1996;87(8):3351-3359.

109. Camacho E, Hernandez L, Hernandez S, et al. ATM gene inactivation in mantle cell lymphoma mainly occurs by truncating mutations and missense mutations involving the phosphatidylinositol-3 kinase domain and is associated with increasing numbers of chromosomal imbalances. Blood. 2002;99(1):238-244.

110. Tort F, Hernandez S, Bea S, et al. CHK2-decreased protein expression and infrequent genetic alterations mainly occur in aggressive types of non-Hodgkin lymphomas. Blood. 2002;100(13):4602-4608. doi:10.1182/blood-2002-04-1078

111. Kridel R, Meissner B, Rogic S, et al. Whole transcriptome sequencing reveals recurrent NOTCH1 mutations in mantle cell lymphoma. Blood. 2012;119(9):1963-1971. doi:10.1182/blood-2011-11-391474

112. Zhang J, Jima D, Moffitt AB, et al. The genomic landscape of mantle cell lymphoma is related to the epigenetically determined chromatin state of normal B cells. Blood. 2014;123(19):2988-2996. doi:10.1182/blood-2013-07-517177

113. Hartmann E, Fernandez V, Moreno V, et al. Five-gene model to predict survival in mantle-cell lymphoma using frozen or formalin-fixed, paraffin-embedded tissue. J Clin Oncol. 2008;26(30):4966-4972. doi:10.1200/JCO.2007.12.0410

114. Halldorsdottir AM, Kanduri M, Marincevic M, et al. Mantle cell lymphoma displays a homogenous methylation profile: a comparative analysis with chronic lymphocytic leukemia. Am J Hematol. 2012;87(4):361-367. doi:10.1002/ajh.23115

115. Leshchenko VV, Kuo PY, Shaknovich R, et al. Genomewide DNA methylation analysis reveals novel targets for drug development in mantle cell lymphoma. Blood. 2010;116(7):1025-1034. doi:10.1182/blood-2009-12-257485

116. Hillmen P. Richter's syndrome: CLL taking a turn for the worse. Oncology. 2012;26(12):1155-1156.

117. Dohner H, Stilgenbauer S, Dohner K, Bentz M, Lichter P. Chromosome aberrations in B-cell chronic lymphocytic leukemia: reassessment based on molecular cytogenetic analysis. J Mol Med. 1999;77(2):266-281.

118. Dohner H, Stilgenbauer S, Benner A, et al. Genomic aberrations and survival in chronic lymphocytic leukemia. N Engl J Med. 2000;343(26):1910-1916. doi:10.1056/NEJM200012283432602

119. O'Malley DP, Giudice C, Chang AS, et al. Comparison of array comparative genomic hybridization (aCGH) to FISH and cytogenetics in prognostic evaluation of chronic lymphocytic leukemia. Int J Lab Hematol. 2011;33(3):238-244. doi:10.1111/j.1751-553X.2010.01284.x

120. Sargent R, Jones D, Abruzzo LV, et al. Customized oligonucleotide array-based comparative genomic hybridization as a clinical assay for genomic profiling of chronic lymphocytic leukemia. J Mol Diagn. 2009;11(1):25-34. doi:10.2353/jmoldx.2009.080037

121. Fabbri M, Bottoni A, Shimizu M, et al. Association of a microRNA/TP53 feedback circuitry with pathogenesis and outcome of B-cell chronic lymphocytic leukemia. J Am Med Assoc. 2011;305(1):59-67. doi:10.1001/jama.2010.1919

122. Grever MR, Lucas DM, Dewald GW, et al. Comprehensive assessment of genetic and molecular features predicting outcome in patients with chronic lymphocytic leukemia: results from the US Intergroup Phase III Trial E2997. J Clin Oncol. 2007;25(7):799-804. doi:10.1200/JCO.2006.08.3089

123. Ding W, Ferrajoli A. Evidence-based mini-review: the role of alkylating agents in the initial treatment of chronic lymphocytic leukemia patients with the 11q deletion. Hematology Am Soc Hematol Educ Program. 2010;2010:90-92. doi:10.1182/asheducation-2010.1.90

124. Roberts AW, Davids MS, Pagel JM, et al. Targeting BCL2 with venetoclax in relapsed chronic lymphocytic leukemia. N Engl J Med. 2016;374(4):311-322. doi:10.1056/NEJMoa1513257

125. O'Brien S, Furman RR, Coutre SE, et al. Ibrutinib as initial therapy for elderly patients with chronic lymphocytic leukaemia or small lymphocytic lymphoma: an open-label, multicentre, phase 1b/2 trial. Lancet Oncol. 2014;15(1):48-58. doi:10.1016/S1470-2045(13)70513-8

126. Ahn IE, Tian X, Wiestner A. Ibrutinib for chronic lymphocytic leukemia with TP53 alterations. N Engl J Med. 2020;383(5):498-500. doi:10.1056/NEJMC2005943

127. Matutes E, Oscier D, Garcia-Marco J, et al. Trisomy 12 defines a group of CLL with atypical morphology: correlation between cytogenetic, clinical and laboratory features in 544 patients. Br J Haematol. 1996;92(2):382-388.

128. Klein U, Tu Y, Stolovitzky GA, et al. Gene expression profiling of B cell chronic lymphocytic leukemia reveals a homogeneous phenotype related to memory B cells. J Exp Med. 2001;194(11):1625-1638.

129. Chiorazzi N, Ferrarini M. Cellular origin(s) of chronic lymphocytic leukemia: cautionary notes and additional considerations and possibilities. Blood. 2011;117(6):1781-1791. doi:10.1182/blood-2010-07-155663

130. Lin KI, Tam CS, Keating MJ, et al. Relevance of the immunoglobulin VH somatic mutation status in patients with chronic lymphocytic leukemia treated with fludarabine, cyclophosphamide, and rituximab (FCR) or related chemoimmunotherapy regimens. Blood. 2009;113(14):3168-3171. doi:10.1182/blood-2008-10-184853

131. Ghia EM, Jain S, Widhopf GF II, et al. Use of IGHV3-21 in chronic lymphocytic leukemia is associated with high-risk disease and reflects antigen-driven, post-germinal center leukemogenic selection. Blood. 2008;111(10):5101-5108. doi:10.1182/blood-2007-12-130229

132. Maurerer K, Zahrieh D, Gorgun G, et al. Immunoglobulin gene segment usage, location and immunogenicity in mutated and unmutated chronic lymphocytic leukemia. Br J Haematol. 2005;129(4):499-510. doi:10.1111/j.1365-2141.2005.05480.x

133. Murray F, Darzentas N, Hadzidimitriou A, et al. Stereotyped patterns of somatic hypermutation in subsets of patients with chronic lymphocytic leukemia: implications for the role of antigen selection in leukemogenesis. Blood. 2008;111(3):1524-1533. doi:10.1182/blood-2007-07-099564

134. Stamatopoulos K, Belessi C, Moreno C, et al. Over 20% of patients with chronic lymphocytic leukemia carry stereotyped receptors: pathogenetic implications and clinical correlations. Blood. 2007;109(1):259-270. doi:10.1182/blood-2006-03-012948

135. Thorselius M, Krober A, Murray F, et al. Strikingly homologous immunoglobulin gene rearrangements and poor outcome in V H 3-21 – using chronic lymphocytic leukemia patients independent of geographic origin and mutational status. Blood. 2006;107(7):2889-2894. doi:10.1182/blood-2005-06-2227

136. Tobin G, Thunberg U, Johnson A, et al. Chronic lymphocytic leukemias utilizing the VH3-21 gene display highly restricted Vlambda2-14 gene use and homologous CDR3s: implicating recognition of a common antigen epitope. Blood. 2003;101(12):4952-4957. doi:10.1182/blood-2002-11-3485

137. Fazi C, Scarfo L, Pecciarini L, et al. General population low-count CLL-like MBL persists over time without clinical progression, although carrying the same cytogenetic abnormalities of CLL. Blood. 2011;118(25):6618-6625. doi:10.1182/blood-2011-05-357251

138. Yeung CCS, Powers MLE, Nguyen TD, et al. Relevance of IgVH gene somatic hypermutation and interphase cytogenetics in lymphomatous presentation of chronic lymphocytic leukemia/small lymphocytic lymphoma. Int J Surg Pathol. 2011;19(5):563-569. doi:10.1177/1066896911406918

139. Daudignon A, Poulain S, Morel P, et al. Increased trisomy 12 frequency and a biased IgVH 3-21 gene usage characterize small lymphocytic lymphoma. Leuk Res. 2010;34(5):580-584. doi:10.1016/j.leukres.2009.11.003

140. Landau DA, Carter SL, Stojanov P, et al. Evolution and impact of subclonal mutations in chronic lymphocytic leukemia. *Cell*. 2013;152(4):714-726. doi:10.1016/j.cell.2013.01.019
141. Puente XS, Beà S, Valdés-Mas R, et al. Non-coding recurrent mutations in chronic lymphocytic leukaemia. *Nature*. 2015;526(7574):519-524. doi:10.1038/nature14666
142. Puente XS, Pinyol M, Quesada V, et al. Whole-genome sequencing identifies recurrent mutations in chronic lymphocytic leukaemia. *Nature*. 2011;475(7354):101-105. doi:10.1038/nature10113
143. Lazarian G, Tausch E, Eclache V, et al. TP53 mutations are early events in chronic lymphocytic leukemia disease progression and precede evolution to complex karyotypes. *Int J Cancer*. 2016;139(8):1759-1763. doi:10.1002/ijc.30222
144. Rossi D, Bruscaggin A, Spina V, et al. Mutations of the SF3B1 splicing factor in chronic lymphocytic leukemia: association with progression and fludarabine-refractoriness. *Blood*. 2011;118(26):6904-6908. doi:10.1182/blood-2011-08-373159
145. Landau DA, Tausch E, Taylor-Weiner AN, et al. Mutations driving CLL and their evolution in progression and relapse. *Nature*. 2015;526(7574):525-530. doi:10.1038/nature15395
146. Guièze R, Wu CJ. Genomic and epigenomic heterogeneity in chronic lymphocytic leukemia. *Blood*. 2015;126(4):445-453. doi:10.1182/blood-2015-02-585042
147. Darman RB, Seiler M, Agrawal AA, et al. Cancer-associated SF3B1 hotspot mutations induce cryptic 3' splice site selection through use of a different branch point. *Cell Rep*. 2015;13(5):1033-1045. doi:10.1016/j.celrep.2015.09.053
148. DeBoever C, Ghia EM, Shepard PJ, et al. Transcriptome sequencing reveals potential mechanism of cryptic 3' splice site selection in SF3B1-mutated cancers. *PLoS Comput Biol*. 2015;11(3):e1004105. doi:10.1371/journal.pcbi.1004105
149. Wang L, Brooks AN, Fan J, et al. Transcriptomic characterization of SF3B1 mutation reveals its pleiotropic effects in chronic lymphocytic leukemia. *Cancer Cell*. 2016;30(5):750-763. doi:10.1016/j.ccell.2016.10.005
150. Wang L. *Genome-wide analysis of a novel murine model of chronic lymphocytic leukemia*. ASH Abstract *58th ASH Annual Meeting San Diego, CA*. 2016.
151. Bell JJ, Bhandoola A. The earliest thymic progenitors for T cells possess myeloid lineage potential. *Nature*. 2008;452(7188):764-767. doi:10.1038/nature06840
152. Malcovati L, Papaemmanuil E, Bowen DT, et al. Clinical significance of SF3B1 mutations in myelodysplastic syndromes and myelodysplastic/myeloproliferative neoplasms. *Blood*. 2011;118(24):6239-6246. doi:10.1182/blood-2011-09-377275
153. Papaemmanuil E, Cazzola M, Boultwood J, et al. Somatic SF3B1 mutation in myelodysplasia with ring sideroblasts. *N Engl J Med*. 2011;365(15):1384-1395. doi:10.1056/NEJMoa1103283
154. Patnaik MM, Lasho TL, Hodnefield JM, et al. SF3B1 mutations are prevalent in myelodysplastic syndromes with ring sideroblasts but do not hold independent prognostic value. *Blood*. 2012;119(2):569-572. doi:10.1182/blood-2011-09-377994
155. Wada H, Masuda K, Satoh R, et al. Adult T-cell progenitors retain myeloid potential. *Nature*. 2008;452(7188):768-772. doi:10.1038/nature06839
156. Wang L, Lawrence MS, Wan Y, et al. SF3B1 and other novel cancer genes in chronic lymphocytic leukemia. *N Engl J Med*. 2011;365(26):2497-2506. doi:10.1056/NEJMoa1109016
157. Fabbri G, Rasi S, Rossi D, et al. Analysis of the chronic lymphocytic leukemia coding genome: role of NOTCH1 mutational activation. *J Exp Med*. 2011;208(7):1389-1401. doi:10.1084/jem.20110921
158. Balatti V, Bottoni A, Palamarchuk A, et al. NOTCH1 mutations in CLL associated with trisomy 12. *Blood*. 2012;119(2):329-331. doi:10.1182/blood-2011-10-386144
159. Eischen CM, Weber JD, Roussel MF, Sherr CJ, Cleveland JL. Disruption of the ARF-Mdm2-p53 tumor suppressor pathway in Myc-induced lymphomagenesis. *Genes Dev*. 1999;13(20):2658-2669.
160. Rossi D, Rasi S, Fabbri G, et al. Mutations of NOTCH1 are an independent predictor of survival in chronic lymphocytic leukemia. *Blood*. 2012;119(2):521-529. doi:10.1182/blood-2011-09-379966
161. Finn WG, Kay NE, Kroft SH, Church S, Peterson LC. Secondary abnormalities of chromosome 6q in B-cell chronic lymphocytic leukemia: a sequential study of karyotypic instability in 51 patients. *Am J Hematol*. 1998;59(3):223-229. doi:10.1002/(sici)1096-8652(199811)59:3<223::aid-ajh7>3.0.co;2-y
162. Baseggio L, Geay MO, Gazzo S, et al. In non-follicular lymphoproliferative disorders, IGH/BCL2-fusion is not restricted to chronic lymphocytic leukaemia. *Br J Haematol*. 2012;158(4):489-498. doi:10.1111/j.1365-2141.2012.09178.x
163. Weiss LM, Warnke RA, Sklar J, Cleary ML. Molecular analysis of the t(14;18) chromosomal translocation in malignant lymphomas. *N Engl J Med*. 1987;317(19):1185-1189. doi:10.1056/NEJM198711053171904
164. Huh YO, Lin KIC, Vega F, et al. MYC translocation in chronic lymphocytic leukaemia is associated with increased prolymphocytes and a poor prognosis. *Br J Haematol*. 2008;142(1):36-44. doi:10.1111/j.1365-2141.2008.07152.x
165. Sen F, Lai R, Albitar M. Chronic lymphocytic leukemia with t(14;18) and trisomy 12. *Arch Pathol Lab Med*. 2002;126(12):1543-1546. doi:10.1043/0003-9985(2002)126<1543:CLLWTA>
166. Zenz T, Eichhorst B, Busch R, et al. TP53 mutation and survival in chronic lymphocytic leukemia. *J Clin Oncol*. 2010;28(29):4473-4479.
167. Zenz T, Kröber A, Scherer K, et al. Monoallelic TP53 inactivation is associated with poor prognosis in chronic lymphocytic leukemia: results from a detailed genetic characterization with long-term follow-up. *Blood*. 2008;112(8):3322-3329. doi:10.1182/blood-2008-04-154070
168. Hallek M. Chronic lymphocytic leukemia: 2015 Update on diagnosis, risk stratification, and treatment. *Am J Hematol*. 2015;90(5):446-460. doi:10.1002/ajh.23979
169. Dreger P, Corradini P, Kimby E, et al. Indications for allogeneic stem cell transplantation in chronic lymphocytic leukemia: the EBMT transplant consensus. *Leukemia*. 2007;21(1):12-17. doi:10.1038/sj.leu.2404441
170. Dreger P, Schnaiter A, Zenz T, et al. TP53, SF3B1, and NOTCH1 mutations and outcome of allotransplantation for chronic lymphocytic leukemia: six-year follow-up of the GCLLSG CLL3X trial. *Blood*. 2013;121(16):3284-3288. doi:10.1182/blood-2012-11-469627
171. Stilgenbauer S, Eichhorst B, Schetelig J, et al. Venetoclax in relapsed or refractory chronic lymphocytic leukaemia with 17p deletion: a multicentre, open-label, phase 2 study. *Lancet Oncol*. 2016;17(6):768-778. doi:10.1016/S1470-2045(16)30019-5
172. Rossi D, Khiabanian H, Spina V, et al. Clinical impact of small TP53 mutated subclones in chronic lymphocytic leukemia. *Blood*. 2014;123(14):2139-2147. doi:10.1182/blood-2013-11-539726
173. Woyach JA, Furman RR, Liu T-M, et al. Resistance mechanisms for the Bruton's tyrosine kinase inhibitor ibrutinib. *N Engl J Med*. 2014;370(24):2286-2294. doi:10.1056/NEJMoa1400029
174. Cheng S, Guo A, Lu P, Ma J, Coleman M, Wang YL. Functional characterization of BTK(C481S) mutation that confers ibrutinib resistance: exploration of alternative kinase inhibitors. *Leukemia*. 2015;29(4):895-900. doi:10.1038/leu.2014.263
175. Quinquenel A, Fornecker LM, Letestu R, et al. Prevalence of BTK and PLCG2 mutations in a real-life CLL cohort still on ibrutinib after 3 years: a FILO group study. *Blood*. 2019;134(7):641-644. doi:10.1182/blood.2019000854
176. Woyach J, Huang Y, Rogers K, et al. Resistance to acalabrutinib in CLL is mediated primarily by BTK mutations. *Blood*. 2019;134(suppl 1):504.
177. Handunnetti SM, Tang CPS, Nguyen T, et al. BTK Leu528Trp - a potential secondary resistance mechanism specific for patients with chronic lymphocytic leukemia treated with the next generation BTK inhibitor zanubrutinib. *Blood*. 2019;134(suppl 1):170.
178. Sedlarikova L, Petrackova A, Papajik T, Turcsanyi P, Kriegova E. Resistance-associated mutations in chronic lymphocytic leukemia patients treated with novel agents. *Front Oncol*. 2020;10:894-910. doi:10.3389/fonc.2020.00894
179. Liu T-M, Woyach JA, Zhong Y, et al. Hypermorphic mutation of phospholipase C, $\gamma 2$ acquired in ibrutinib-resistant CLL confers BTK independency upon B-cell receptor activation. *Blood*. 2015;126(1):61-68. doi:10.1182/blood-2015-02-626846
180. Burger JA, Landau DA, Taylor-Weiner A, et al. Clonal evolution in patients with chronic lymphocytic leukaemia developing resistance to BTK inhibition. *Nat Commun*. 2016;7:11589. doi:10.1038/ncomms11589
181. Blombery P, Anderson MA, Gong JN, et al. Acquisition of the recurrent Gly101Val mutation in BCL2 confers resistance to venetoclax in patients with progressive chronic lymphocytic leukemia. *Cancer Discov*. 2019;9(3):342-353. doi:10.1158/2159-8290.CD-18-1119
182. Blombery P, Thompson ER, Nguyen T, et al. Multiple BCL2 mutations cooccurring with Gly101Val emerge in chronic lymphocytic leukemia progression on venetoclax. *Blood*. 2020;135(10):773-777. doi:10.1182/blood.2019004205
183. Tausch E, Close W, Dolnik A, et al. Venetoclax resistance and acquired BCL2 mutations in chronic lymphocytic leukemia. *Haematologica*. 2019;104(9):e434-e437.
184. Lucas F, Larkin K, Gregory CT, et al. Novel BCL2 mutations in venetoclax-resistant, ibrutinib-resistant CLL patients with BTK/PLCG2 mutations. *Blood*. 2020;135(24):2192-2195. doi:10.1182/blood.2019003722
185. Aigelsreiter A, Gerlza T, Deutsch AJA, et al. Chlamydia psittaci infection in nongastrointestinal extranodal MALT lymphomas and their precursor lesions. *Am J Clin Pathol*. 2011;135(1):70-75. doi:10.1309/AJCPXMDRT1SY6KIV
186. Farinha P, Gascoyne RD. Molecular pathogenesis of mucosa-associated lymphoid tissue lymphoma. *J Clin Oncol*. 2005;23(26):6370-6378. doi:10.1200/JCO.2005.05.011
187. Auer IA, Gascoyne RD, Connors JM, et al. t(11;18)(q21;q21) is the most common translocation in MALT lymphomas. *Ann Oncol*. 1997;8(10):979-985.
188. Ott G, Katzenberger T, Greiner A, et al. The t(11;18)(q21;q21) chromosome translocation is a frequent and specific aberration in low-grade but not high-grade malignant non-Hodgkin's lymphomas of the Mucosa-Associated Lymphoid Tissue (MALT-) type. *Cancer Res*. 1997;57(18):3944-3948.
189. Liu H, Ye H, Dogan A, et al. T(11;18)(q21;q21) is associated with advanced mucosa-associated lymphoid tissue lymphoma that expresses nuclear BCL10. *Blood*. 2001;98(4):1182-1187.
190. Dierlamm J, Baens M, Stefanova-Ouzounova M, et al. Detection of t(11;18)(q21;q21) by interphase fluorescence in situ hybridization using API2 and MLT specific probes. *Blood*. 2000;96(6):2215-2218.
191. Nakagawa M, Seto M, Hosokawa Y. Molecular pathogenesis of MALT lymphoma: two signaling pathways underlying the antiapoptotic effect of API2-MALT1 fusion protein. *Leukemia*. 2006;20(6):929-936. doi:10.1038/sj.leu.2404192
192. Ye H, Dogan A, Karran L, et al. BCL10 expression in normal and neoplastic lymphoid tissue. Nuclear localization in MALT lymphoma. *Am J Pathol*. 2000;157(4):1147-1154. doi:10.1016/S0002-9440(10)64630-5
193. Murga Penas EM, Callet-Bauchu E, Ye H, et al. The t(14;18)(q32;q21)/IGH-MALT1 translocation in MALT lymphomas contains templated nucleotide insertions and a major breakpoint region similar to follicular and mantle cell lymphoma. *Blood*. 2010;115(11):2214-2219. doi:10.1182/blood-2009-08-236265
194. Sagaert X, De Wolf-Peeters C, Noels H, Baens M. The pathogenesis of MALT lymphomas: where do we stand? *Leukemia*. 2007;21(3):389-396. doi:10.1038/sj.leu.2404517
195. Streubel B, Vinatzer U, Lamprecht A, Raderer M, Chott A. T(3;14)(p14.1;q32) involving IGH and FOXP1 is a novel recurrent chromosomal aberration in MALT lymphoma. *Leukemia*. 2005;19(4):652-658. doi:10.1038/sj.leu.2403644
196. Liu H, Ye H, Ruskone-Fourmestraux A, et al. T(11;18) is a marker for all stage gastric MALT lymphomas that will not respond to *H. pylori* eradication. *Gastroenterology*. 2002;122(5):1286-1294. doi:10.1053/gast.2002.33047
197. Dierlamm J, Pittaluga S, Wlodarska I, et al. Marginal zone B-cell lymphomas of different sites share similar cytogenetic and morphologic features. *Blood*. 1996;87(1):299-307.

198. Jung H, Yoo HY, Lee SH, et al. The mutational landscape of ocular marginal zone lymphoma identifies frequent alterations in TNFAIP3 followed by mutations in TBL1XR1 and CREBBP. *Oncotarget.* 2017;8(10):17038-17049.
199. Johansson P, Klein-Hitpass L, Grabellus F, et al. Recurrent mutations in NF-κB pathway components, KMT2D, and NOTCH1/2 in ocular adnexal MALT-type marginal zone lymphomas. *Oncotarget.* 2016;7(38):62627-62639.
200. Gachard N, Parrens M, Soubeyran I, et al. IGHV gene features and MYD88 L265P mutation separate the three marginal zone lymphoma entities and Waldenström macroglobulinemia/lymphoplasmacytic lymphomas. *Leukemia.* 2013;27(1):183-189.
201. Novak U, Rinaldi A, Kwee I, et al. The NF-{kappa}B negative regulator TNFAIP3 (A20) is inactivated by somatic mutations and genomic deletions in marginal zone lymphomas. *Blood.* 2009;113(20):4918-4921. doi:10.1182/blood-2008-08-174110
202. Angelopoulou MK, Kalpadakis C, Pangalis GA, Kyrtsonis MC, Vassilakopoulos TP. Nodal marginal zone lymphoma. *Leuk Lymphoma.* 2014;55(6):1240-1250. doi:10.3109/10428194.2013.840888
203. Arcaini L, Lucioni M, Boveri E, Paulli M. Nodal marginal zone lymphoma: current knowledge and future directions of an heterogeneous disease. *Eur J Haematol.* 2009;83(3):165-174. doi:10.1111/j.1600-0609.2009.01301.x
204. Surveillance, Epidemiology and ER (SEER) Program. *SEER*Stat Database: Incidence - SEER Research Data*, 9 Registries. 2021.
205. van den Brand M, van Krieken JH, van Krieken JM. Recognizing nodal marginal zone lymphoma: recent advances and pitfalls. A systematic review. *Haematologica.* 2013;98(7):1003-1013. doi:10.3324/haematol.2012.083386
206. Bracci PM, Benavente Y, Turner JJ, et al. Medical history, lifestyle, family history, and occupational risk factors for marginal zone lymphoma: the InterLymph Non-Hodgkin Lymphoma Subtypes Project. *J Natl Cancer Inst Monogr.* 2014;2014(48):52-65. doi:10.1093/jncimonographs/lgu011
207. Taddesse-Heath L, Pittaluga S, Sorbara L, Bussey M, Raffeld M, Jaffe ES. Marginal zone B-cell lymphoma in children and young adults. *Am J Surg Pathol.* 2003;27(4):522-531.
208. Spina V, Khiabanian H, Messina M, et al. The genetics of nodal marginal zone lymphoma. *Blood.* 2016;128(10):1362-1373. doi:10.1182/blood-2016-02-696757
209. Camacho FI, Algara P, Mollejo M, et al. Nodal marginal zone lymphoma: a heterogeneous tumor. A comprehensive analysis of a series of 27 cases. *Am J Surg Pathol.* 2003;27(6):762-771.
210. Traverse-Glehen A, Davi F, Ben Simon E, et al. Analysis of VH genes in marginal zone lymphoma reveals marked heterogeneity between splenic and nodal tumors and suggests the existence of clonal selection. *Haematologica.* 2005;90(4):470-478.
211. Spina V, Rossi D. Molecular pathogenesis of splenic and nodal marginal zone lymphoma. *Best Pract Res Clin Haematol.* 2017;30(1-2):5-12. doi:10.1016/j.beha.2016.09.004
212. Hamadeh F, MacNamara SP, Aguilera NS, Swerdlow SH, Cook JR. MYD88 L265P mutation analysis helps define nodal lymphoplasmacytic lymphoma. *Mod Pathol.* 2015;28(4):564-574. doi:10.1038/modpathol.2014.120
213. Martinez-Lopez A, Curiel-Olmo S, Mollejo M, et al. MYD88 (L265P) somatic mutation in marginal zone B-cell lymphoma. *Am J Surg Pathol.* 2015;39(5):644-651. doi:10.1097/PAS.0000000000000411
214. Swerdlow SH, Kuzu I, Dogan A, et al. The many faces of small B cell lymphomas with plasmacytic differentiation and the contribution of MYD88 testing. *Virchows Arch.* 2016;468(3):259-275. doi:10.1007/s00428-015-1858-9
215. Piris MA. Nodal marginal zone mutational signature. *Blood.* 2016;128(10):1315-1316. doi:10.1182/blood-2016-07-724963
216. Berger F, Felman P, Thieblemont C, et al. Non-MALT marginal zone B-cell lymphomas: a description of clinical presentation and outcome in 124 patients. *Blood.* 2000;95(6):1950-1956. doi:10.1182/blood.v95.6.1950
217. Khalil MO, Morton LM, Devesa SS, et al. Incidence of marginal zone lymphoma in the United States, 2001-2009 with a focus on primary anatomic site. *Br J Haematol.* 2014;165(1):67-77. doi:10.1111/bjh.12730
218. Xing KH, Kahlon A, Skinnider BF, et al. Outcomes in splenic marginal zone lymphoma: analysis of 107 patients treated in British Columbia. *Br J Haematol.* 2015;169(4):520-527. doi:10.1111/bjh.13320
219. Corcoran MM, Mould SJ, Orchard JA, et al. Dysregulation of cyclin dependent kinase 6 expression in splenic marginal zone lymphoma through chromosome 7q translocations. *Oncogene.* 1999;18(46):6271-6277. doi:10.1038/sj.onc.1203033
220. Watkins AJ, Huang Y, Ye H, et al. Splenic marginal zone lymphoma: characterization of 7q deletion and its value in diagnosis. *J Pathol.* 2010;220(4):461-474.
221. Robledo C, García JL, Benito R, et al. Molecular characterization of the region 7q22.1 in splenic marginal zone lymphomas. *PLoS One.* 2011;6(9):e24939. doi:10.1371/journal.pone.0024939
222. Fresquet V, Robles EF, Parker A, et al. High-throughput sequencing analysis of the chromosome 7q32 deletion reveals IRF5 as a potential tumour suppressor in splenic marginal-zone lymphoma. *Br J Haematol.* 2012;158(6):712-726. doi:10.1111/j.1365-2141.2012.09226.x
223. Watkins AJ, Hamoudi RA, Zeng N, et al. An integrated genomic and expression analysis of 7q deletion in splenic marginal zone lymphoma. *PLoS One.* 2012;7(9):e44997-e44999. doi:10.1371/journal.pone.0044997
224. Algara P, Mateo MS, Sanchez-Beato M, et al. Analysis of the IgVH somatic mutations in splenic marginal zone lymphoma defines a group of unmutated cases with frequent 7q deletion and adverse clinical course. *Blood.* 2002;99(4):1299-1304. doi:10.1182/blood.v99.4.1299
225. Bikos V, Darzentas N, Hadzidimitriou A, et al. Over 30% of patients with splenic marginal zone lymphoma express the same immunoglobulin heavy variable gene: ontogenetic implications. *Leukemia.* 2012;26(7):1638-1646. doi:10.1038/leu.2012.3
226. Zibellini S, Capello D, Forconi F, et al. Stereotyped patterns of B-cell receptor in splenic marginal zone lymphoma. *Haematologica.* 2010;95(10):1792-1796. doi:10.3324/haematol.2010.025437
227. Clipson A, Wang M, De Leval L, et al. KLF2 mutation is the most frequent somatic change in splenic marginal zone lymphoma and identifies a subset with distinct genotype. *Leukemia.* 2015;29(5):1177-1185. doi:10.1038/leu.2014.330
228. Kiel MJ, Velusamy T, Betz BL, et al. Whole-genome sequencing identifies recurrent somatic NOTCH2 mutations in splenic marginal zone lymphoma. *J Exp Med.* 2012;209(9):1553-1565. doi:10.1084/jem.20120910
229. Martínez N, Almaraz C, Vaqué JP, et al. Whole-exome sequencing in splenic marginal zone lymphoma reveals mutations in genes involved in marginal zone differentiation. *Leukemia.* 2014;28(6):1334-1340. doi:10.1038/leu.2013.365
230. Parry M, Rose-Zerilli MJJ, Ljungström V, et al. Genetics and prognostication in splenic marginal zone lymphoma: revelations from deep sequencing. *Clin Cancer Res.* 2015;21(18):4174-4183. doi:10.1158/1078-0432.CCR-14-2759
231. Rossi D, Trifonov V, Fangazio M, et al. The coding genome of splenic marginal zone lymphoma: activation of *NOTCH2* and other pathways regulating marginal zone development. *J Exp Med.* 2012;209(9):1537-1551. doi:10.1084/jem.20120904
232. Shanmugam V, Craig JW, Hilton LK, et al. Notch activation is pervasive in SMZL and uncommon in DLBCL: implications for Notch signaling in B-cell tumors. *Blood Adv.* 2021;5(1):71-83. doi:10.1182/bloodadvances.2020002995
233. Campos-Martín Y, Martínez N, Martínez-López A, et al. Clinical and diagnostic relevance of NOTCH2 and KLF2 mutations in splenic marginal zone lymphoma. *Haematologica.* 2017;102(8):e310-e312.
234. Piva R, Deaglio S, Famà R, et al. The Krüppel-like factor 2 transcription factor gene is recurrently mutated in splenic marginal zone lymphoma. *Leukemia.* 2015;29(2):503-507. doi:10.1038/leu.2014.294
235. Vijay A, Gertz MA. Waldenstrom macroglobulinemia. *Blood.* 2007;109(12):5096-5103. doi:10.1182/blood-2006-11-055012
236. Dimopoulos MA, Kyle RA, Anagnostopoulos A, Treon SP. Diagnosis and management of Waldenstrom's macroglobulinemia. *J Clin Oncol.* 2005;23(7):1564-1577. doi:10.1200/JCO.2005.03.144
237. Wagner SD, Martinelli V, Luzzatto L. Similar patterns of V kappa gene usage but different degrees of somatic mutation in hairy cell leukemia, prolymphocytic leukemia, Waldenstrom's macroglobulinemia, and myeloma. *Blood.* 1994;83(12):3647-3653.
238. Kriangkum J, Taylor BJ, Treon SP, et al. Molecular characterization of Waldenstrom's macroglobulinemia reveals frequent occurrence of two B-cell clones having distinct IgH VDJ sequences. *Clin Cancer Res.* 2007;13(7):2005-2013. doi:10.1158/1078-0432.CCR-06-2788
239. Cook JR, Aguilera NI, Reshmi-Skarja S, et al. Lack of PAX5 rearrangements in lymphoplasmacytic lymphomas: reassessing the reported association with t(9;14). *Hum Pathol.* 2004;35(4):447-454. doi:10.1016/j.humpath.2003.10.014
240. George TI, Wrede JE, Bangs CD, Cherry AM, Warnke Ra, Arber Da. Low-grade B-cell lymphomas with plasmacytic differentiation lack PAX5 gene rearrangements. *J Mol Diagn.* 2005;7(3):346-351. doi:10.1016/S1525-1578(10)60563-6
241. Mansoor A, Medeiros LJ, Weber DM, et al. Cytogenetic findings in lymphoplasmacytic lymphoma/Waldenstrom macroglobulinemia: chromosomal abnormalities are associated with the polymorphous subtype and an aggressive clinical course. *Am J Clin Pathol.* 2001;116(4):543-549. doi:10.1309/6U88-357U-UKJ5-YPT3
242. Ocio EM, Schop RFJ, Gonzalez B, et al. 6q deletion in Waldenstrom macroglobulinemia is associated with features of adverse prognosis. *Br J Haematol.* 2007;136(1):80-86. doi:10.1111/j.1365-2141.2006.06389.x
243. Schop RFJ, Van Wier SA, Xu R, et al. 6q deletion discriminates Waldenstrom macroglobulinemia from IgM monoclonal gammopathy of undetermined significance. *Cancer Genet Cytogenet.* 2006;169(2):150-153. doi:10.1016/j.cancergencyto.2006.04.009
244. Terré C, Nguyen-Khac F, Barin C, et al. Trisomy 4, a new chromosomal abnormality in Waldenström's macroglobulinemia: a study of 39 cases. *Leukemia.* 2006;20(9):1634-1636. doi:10.1038/sj.leu.2404314
245. Braggio E, Keats JJ, Leleu X, et al. High-resolution genomic analysis in Waldenstrom's macroglobulinemia identifies disease-specific and common abnormalities with marginal zone lymphomas. *Clin Lymphoma Myeloma.* 2009;9(1):39-42. doi:10.3816/CLM.2009.n.009
246. Nguyen-Khac F, Lambert J, Chapiro E, et al. Chromosomal aberrations and their prognostic value in a series of 174 untreated patients with Waldenström's macroglobulinemia. *Haematologica.* 2013;98(4):649-654. doi:10.3324/haematol.2012.070458
247. Treon SP, Xu L, Yang G, et al. MYD88 L265P somatic mutation in waldenström's macroglobulinemia. *N Engl J Med.* 2012;367(9):826-833. doi:10.1056/NEJMoa1200710
248. Yang G, Zhou Y, Liu X, et al. A mutation in MYD88 (L265P) supports the survival of lymphoplasmacytic cells by activation of Bruton tyrosine kinase in Waldenstrom macroglobulinemia. *Blood.* 2013;122(7):1222-1232. doi:10.1182/blood-2012-12-475111
249. Treon SP, Xu L, Hunter Z. MYD88 mutations and response to ibrutinib in waldenström's macroglobulinemia. *N Engl J Med.* 2015;373(6):584-586. doi:10.1056/NEJMc1506192
250. Castillo JJ, Palomba ML, Advani RTS, Treon SP. Ibrutinib in Waldenström macroglobulinemia: latest evidence and clinical experience. *Ther Adv Hematol.* 2016;7(4):179-186. doi:10.1177/2040620716654102
251. Hunter ZR, Xu L, Yang G, et al. The genomic landscape of Waldenström macroglobulinemia is characterized by highly recurring MYD88 and WHIM-like CXCR4 mutations, and small somatic deletions associated with B-cell lymphomagenesis. *Blood.* 2014;123(11):1637-1646. doi:10.1182/blood-2013-09-525808
252. Schmidt J, Federmann B, Schindler N, et al. MYD88 L265P and CXCR4 mutations in lymphoplasmacytic lymphoma identify cases with high disease activity. *Br J Haematol.* 2015;169(6):795-803.
253. Xu L, Hunter ZR, Tsakmaklis N, et al. Clonal architecture of CXCR4 WHIM-like mutations in Waldenström macroglobulinaemia. *Br J Haematol.* 2016;172(5):735-744.

254. Ngo HT, Leleu X, Lee J, et al. SDF-1/CXCR4 and VLA-4 interaction regulates homing in Waldenstrom macroglobulinemia. *Blood*. 2008;112(1):150-158. doi:10.1182/blood-2007-12-129395
255. Lagane B, Chow KYC, Balabanian K, et al. CXCR4 dimerization and beta-arrestin-mediated signaling account for the enhanced chemotaxis to CXCL12 in WHIM syndrome. *Blood*. 2008;112(1):34-44. doi:10.1182/blood-2007-07-102103
256. Treon SP, Cao Y, Xu L, Yang G, Liu X, Hunter ZR. Somatic mutations in MYD88 and CXCR4 are determinants of clinical presentation and overall survival in Waldenström macroglobulinemia. *Blood*. 2014;123(18):2791-2796. doi:10.1182/blood-2014-01-550905
257. Treon SP, Tripsas CK, Meid K, et al. Ibrutinib in previously treated Waldenstrom's macroglobulinemia. *N Engl J Med*. 2015;372(15):1430-1440. doi:10.1056/NEJMoa1501548
258. Cao Y, Hunter ZR, Liu X, et al. The WHIM-like CXCR4(S338X) somatic mutation activates AKT and ERK, and promotes resistance to ibrutinib and other agents used in the treatment of Waldenstrom's Macroglobulinemia. *Leukemia*. 2015;29(1):169-176. doi:10.1038/leu.2014.187
259. Hunter ZR, Xu L, Yang G, et al. Transcriptome sequencing reveals a profile that corresponds to genomic variants in Waldenström macroglobulinemia. *Blood*. 2016;128(6):827-838. doi:10.1182/blood-2016-03-708263
260. Roccaro AM, Sacco A, Jia X, et al. microRNA-dependent modulation of histone acetylation in Waldenstrom macroglobulinemia. *Blood*. 2010;116(9):1506-1514. doi:10.1182/blood-2010-01-265686
261. Ghobrial IM, Campigotto F, Murphy TJ, et al. Results of a phase 2 trial of the single-agent histone deacetylase inhibitor panobinostat in patients with relapsed/refractory Waldenstrom macroglobulinemia. *Blood*. 2013;121(8):1296-1303. doi:10.1182/blood-2012-06-439307
262. Castillo JJ, Garcia-Sanz R, Hatjiharissi E, et al. Recommendations for the diagnosis and initial evaluation of patients with Waldenström macroglobulinaemia: a task force from the 8th international workshop on Waldenström macroglobulinaemia. *Br J Haematol*. 2016;175(1):77-86. doi:10.1111/bjh.14196
263. Drandi D, Genuardi E, Ghione P, et al. Highly sensitive Droplet digital PCR for MYD88L265P mutation detection and minimal residual disease monitoring in Waldenström macroglobulinemia. *Blood*. 2013;126(23):2645.
264. Forconi F, Sozzi E, Rossi D, et al. Selective influences in the expressed immunoglobulin heavy and light chain gene repertoire in hairy cell leukemia. *Haematologica*. 2008;93(5):697-705. doi:10.3324/haematol.12282
265. Basso K, Liso A, Tiacci E, et al. Gene expression profiling of hairy cell leukemia reveals a phenotype related to memory B cells with altered expression of chemokine and adhesion receptors. *J Exp Med*. 2004;199(1):59-68. doi:10.1084/jem.20031175199/1/59
266. Arons E, Roth L, Sapolsky J, Suntum T, Stetler-Stevenson M, Kreitman RJ. Evidence of canonical somatic hypermutation in hairy cell leukemia. *Blood*. 2011;117(18):4844-4851. doi:10.1182/blood-2010-11-316737
267. Wu X, Ivanova G, Merup M, et al. Molecular analysis of the human chromosome 5q13.3 region in patients with hairy cell leukemia and identification of tumor suppressor gene candidates. *Genomics*. 1999;60(2):161-171. doi:10.1006/geno.1999.5911
268. Andersen CL, Gruszka-Westwood A, Østergaard M, et al. A narrow deletion of 7q is common to HCL, and SMZL, but not CLL. *Eur J Haematol*. 2004;72(6):390-402. doi:10.1111/j.1600-0609.2004.00243.x
269. Cawley JC. The pathophysiology of the hairy cell. *Hematol Oncol Clin North Am*. 2006;20(5):1011-1021. doi:10.1016/j.hoc.2006.06.002
270. Arons E, Suntum T, Stetler-Stevenson M, Kreitman RJ. VH4-34+ hairy cell leukemia, a new variant with poor prognosis despite standard therapy. *Blood*. 2009;114(21):4687-4695. doi:10.1182/blood-2009-01-201731
271. Kreitman RJ. Hairy cell leukemia-new genes, new targets. *Curr Hematol Malig Rep*. 2013;8(3):184-195. doi:10.1007/s11899-013-0167-0
272. Davies H, Bignell GR, Cox C, et al. Mutations of the BRAF gene in human cancer. *Nature*. 2002;417(6892):949-954. doi:10.1038/nature00766
273. Blombery PA, Wong SQ, Hewitt CA, et al. Detection of BRAF mutations in patients with hairy cell leukemia and related lymphoproliferative disorders. *Haematologica*. 2012;97(5):780-783. doi:10.3324/haematol.2011.054874
274. Tiacci E, Trifonov V, Schiavoni G, et al. BRAF mutations in hairy-cell leukemia. *N Engl J Med*. 2011;364(24):2305-2315. doi:10.1056/NEJMoa1014209
275. Li WQ, Kawakami K, Ruszkiewicz A, Bennett G, Moore J, Iacopetta B. BRAF mutations are associated with distinctive clinical, pathological and molecular features of colorectal cancer independently of microsatellite instability status. *Mol Cancer*. 2006;5:2. doi:10.1186/1476-4598-5-2
276. Brose MS, Volpe P, Feldman M, et al. BRAF and RAS mutations in human lung cancer and melanoma. *Cancer Res*. 2002;62(23):6997-7000. doi:10.1093/jnci/93.14.1062
277. Tiacci E, Park JH, De Carolis L, et al. Targeting mutant BRAF in relapsed or refractory hairy-cell leukemia. *N Engl J Med*. 2015;373(18):1733-1747. doi:10.1056/NEJMoa1506583
278. Waterfall JJ, Arons E, Walker RL, et al. High prevalence of MAP2K1 mutations in variant and IGHV4-34-expressing hairy-cell leukemias. *Nat Genet*. 2014;46(1):8-10. doi:10.1038/ng.2828
279. Mason EF, Brown RD, Szeto DP, et al. Detection of activating MAP2K1 mutations in atypical hairy cell leukemia and hairy cell leukemia variant. *Leuk Lymphoma*. 2017;58(1):233-236. doi:10.1080/10428194.2016.1185786
280. Xi L, Arons E, Navarro W, et al. Both variant and IGHV4-34-expressing hairy cell leukemia lack the BRAF V600E mutation. *Blood*. 2012;119(14):3330-3332. doi:10.1182/blood-2011-09-379339
281. Aster JC, Longtine JA. Detection of BCL2 rearrangements in follicular lymphoma. *Am J Pathol*. 2002;160(3):759-763. doi:10.1016/S0002-9440(10)64897-3
282. Huang JZ, Sanger WG, Greiner TC, et al. The t(14;18) defines a unique subset of diffuse large B-cell lymphoma with a germinal center B-cell gene expression profile. *Blood*. 2002;99(7):2285-2290.
283. Kridel R, Sehn LH, Gascoyne RD. Pathogenesis of follicular lymphoma. *J Clin Invest*. 2012;122(10):3424-3431. doi:10.1172/JCI63186.3424
284. Tanaka S, Louie DC, Kant JA, Reed JC. Frequent incidence of somatic mutations in translocated BCL2 oncogenes of non-Hodgkin's lymphomas. *Blood*. 1992;79(1):229-237.
285. Weinberg OK, Ai WZ, Mariappan MR, Shum C, Levy R, Arber DA. "Minor" BCL2 breakpoints in follicular lymphoma: frequency and correlation with grade and disease presentation in 236 cases. *J Mol Diagn*. 2007;9(4):530-537. doi:10.2353/jmoldx.2007.070038
286. Vaandrager JW, Schuuring E, Raap T, Philippo K, Kleiverda K, Kluin P. Interphase FISH detection of BCL2 rearrangement in follicular lymphoma using breakpoint-flanking probes. *Genes Chromosomes Cancer*. 2000;27(1):85-94. doi:10.1002/(sici)1098-2264(200001)27:1<85::aid-gcc11>3.0.co;2-9
287. Aukema SM, Siebert R, Schuuring E, et al. Double-hit B-cell lymphomas. *Blood*. 2011;117(8):2319-2331. doi:10.1182/blood-2010-09-297879
288. Li S, Lin P, Fayad LE, et al. B-cell lymphomas with MYC/8q24 rearrangements and IGH@BCL2/t(14;18)(q32;q21): an aggressive disease with heterogeneous histology, germinal center B-cell immunophenotype and poor outcome. *Mod Pathol*. 2012;25(1):145-156. doi:10.1038/modpathol.2011.147
289. Guo Y, Karube K, Kawano R, et al. Bcl2-negative follicular lymphomas frequently have Bcl6 translocation and/or Bcl6 or p53 expression. *Pathol Int*. 2007;57(3):148-152. doi:10.1111/j.1440-1827.2006.02072.x
290. Guo Y, Karube K, Kawano R, et al. Low-grade follicular lymphoma with t(14;18) presents a homogeneous disease entity otherwise the rest comprises minor groups of heterogeneous disease entities with Bcl2 amplification, Bcl6 translocation or other gene aberrances. *Leukemia*. 2005;19(6):1058-1063. doi:10.1038/sj.leu.2403738
291. Katzenberger T, Ott G, Klein T, Kalla J, Müller-Hermelink HK, Ott MM. Cytogenetic alterations affecting BCL6 are predominantly found in follicular lymphomas grade 3B with a diffuse large B-cell component. *Am J Pathol*. 2004;165(2):481-490. doi:10.1016/S0002-9440(10)63313-5
292. Karube K, Guo Y, Suzumiya J, et al. CD10-MUM1+ follicular lymphoma lacks BCL2 gene translocation and shows characteristic biologic and clinical features. *Blood*. 2007;109(7):3076-3079. doi:10.1182/blood-2006-09-045989
293. Leich E, Zamo A, Horn H, et al. MicroRNA profiles of t(14;18)-negative follicular lymphoma support a late germinal center B-cell phenotype. *Blood*. 2011;118(20):5550-5558. doi:10.1182/blood-2011-06-361972
294. Schmitt C, Balogh B, Grundt A, et al. The bcl-2/IgH rearrangement in a population of 204 healthy individuals: occurrence, age and gender distribution, breakpoints, and detection method validity. *Leuk Res*. 2006;30(6):745-750. doi:10.1016/j.leukres.2005.10.001
295. Limpens J, Stad R, Vos C, et al. Lymphoma-associated translocation t(14;18) in blood B cells of normal individuals. *Blood*. 1995;85(9):2528-2536.
296. Dolken G, Illerhaus G, Hirt C, Mertelsmann R. BCL-2/JH rearrangements in circulating B cells of healthy blood Donors and patients with nonmalignant diseases. *J Clin Oncol*. 1996;14(4):1333-1344.
297. Finke J, Slanina J, Lange W, Dolken G. Persistence of circulating t(14;18)-positive cells in long-term remission after radiation therapy for localized-stage follicular lymphoma. *J Clin Oncol*. 1993;11(9):1668-1673.
298. McDonnell TJ, Korsmeyer SJ. Progression from lymphoid hyperplasia to high-grade malignant lymphoma in mice transgenic for the t(14; 18). *Nature*. 1991;349(6306):254-256. doi:10.1038/349254a0
299. Egle A, Harris AW, Bath ML, O'Reilly L, Cory S. VavP-Bcl2 transgenic mice develop follicular lymphoma preceded by germinal center hyperplasia. *Blood*. 2004;103(6):2276-2283. doi:10.1182/blood-2003-07-2469
300. Aarts WM, Bende RJ, Steenbergen EJ, et al. Variable heavy chain gene analysis of follicular lymphomas: correlation between heavy chain isotype expression and somatic mutation load. *Blood*. 2000;95(9):2922-2929.
301. Payne K, Wright P, Grant JW, et al. BIOMED-2 PCR assays for IGK gene rearrangements are essential for B-cell clonality analysis in follicular lymphoma. *Br J Haematol*. 2011;155(1):84-92. doi:10.1111/j.1365-2141.2011.08803.x
302. Stamatopoulos K, Kosmas C, Papadaki T, et al. Follicular lymphoma immunoglobulin kappa light chains are affected by the antigen selection process, but to a lesser degree than their partner heavy chains. *Br J Haematol*. 1997;96(1):132-146.
303. Bouska A, McKeithan TW, Deffenbacher KE, et al. Genome-wide copy-number analyses reveal genomic abnormalities involved in transformation of follicular lymphoma. *Blood*. 2014;123(11):1681-1690. doi:10.1182/blood-2013-05-500595
304. d'Amore F, Chan E, Iqbal J, et al. Clonal evolution in t(14;18)-positive follicular lymphoma, evidence for multiple common pathways, and frequent parallel clonal evolution. *Clin Cancer Res*. 2008;14(22):7180-7187. doi:10.1158/1078-0432.CCR-08-0752
305. Schwaenen C, Viardot A, Berger H, et al. Microarray-based genomic profiling reveals novel genomic aberrations in follicular lymphoma which associate with patient survival and gene expression status. *Genes Chromosomes Cancer*. 2009;48(1):39-54. doi:10.1002/gcc.20617
306. Dave SS, Wright G, Tan B, et al. Prediction of survival in follicular lymphoma based on molecular features of tumor-infiltrating immune cells. *N Engl J Med*. 2004;351(21):2159-2169. doi:10.1056/NEJMoa041869
307. Sander B, de Jong D, Rosenwald A, et al. The reliability of immunohistochemical analysis of the tumor microenvironment in follicular lymphoma: a validation study from the Lunenburg Lymphoma Biomarker Consortium. *Haematologica*. 2014;99(4):715-725. doi:10.3324/haematol.2013.095257
308. Blaker YN, Spetalen S, Brodtkorb M, et al. The tumour microenvironment influences survival and time to transformation in follicular lymphoma in the rituximab era. *Br J Haematol*. 2016;175(1):102-114. doi:10.1111/bjh.14201

309. Saifi M, Maran A, Raynaud P, et al. High ratio of interfollicular CD8/FOXP3-positive regulatory T cells is associated with a high FLIPI index and poor overall survival in follicular lymphoma. *Exp Ther Med.* 2010;1(6):933-938. doi:10.3892/etm.2010.146
310. Green MR, Kihira S, Liu CL, et al. Mutations in early follicular lymphoma progenitors are associated with suppressed antigen presentation. *Proc Natl Acad Sci U S A.* 2015;112(10):E1116-E1125. doi:10.1073/pnas.1501199112
311. Pasqualucci L, Trifonov V, Fabbri G, et al. Analysis of the coding genome of diffuse large B-cell lymphoma. *Nat Genet.* 2011;43(9):830-837. doi:10.1038/ng.892
312. Okosun J, Bodor C, Wang J, et al. Integrated genomic analysis identifies recurrent mutations and evolution patterns driving the initiation and progression of follicular lymphoma. *Nat Genet.* 2014;46(2):176-181. doi:10.1038/ng.2856
313. Morin RD, Mendez-Lago M, Mungall AJ, et al. Frequent mutation of histone-modifying genes in non-Hodgkin lymphoma. *Nature.* 2011;476(7360):298-303. doi:10.1038/nature10351
314. Pasqualucci L, Khiabanian H, Fangazio M, et al. Genetics of follicular lymphoma transformation. *Cell Rep.* 2014;6(1):130-140. doi:10.1016/j.celrep.2013.12.027
315. Velichutina I, Shaknovich R, Geng H, et al. EZH2-mediated epigenetic silencing in germinal center B cells contributes to proliferation and lymphomagenesis. *Blood.* 2010;116(24):5247-5255. doi:10.1182/blood-2010-04-280149
316. Bödör C, Grossmann V, Popov N, et al. EZH2 mutations are frequent and represent an early event in follicular lymphoma. *Blood.* 2013;122(18):3165-3168. doi:10.1182/blood-2013-04-496893
317. Morin RD, Johnson NA, Severson TM, et al. Somatic mutations altering EZH2 (Tyr641) in follicular and diffuse large B-cell lymphomas of germinal-center origin. *Nat Genet.* 2010;42(2):181-185. doi:10.1038/ng.518
318. Ryan RJH, Nitta M, Borger D, et al. EZH2 codon 641 mutations are common in BCL2-rearranged germinal center B cell lymphomas. *PLoS One.* 2011;6(12):e28585. doi:10.1371/journal.pone.0028585
319. Oricchio E, Nanjangud G, Wolfe AL, et al. The Eph-receptor A7 is a soluble tumor suppressor for follicular lymphoma. *Cell.* 2011;147(3):554-564. doi:10.1016/j.cell.2011.09.035
320. Pastore A, Jurinovic V, Kridel R, et al. Integration of gene mutations in risk prognostication for patients receiving first-line immunochemotherapy for follicular lymphoma: a retrospective analysis of a prospective clinical trial and validation in a population-based registry. *Lancet Oncol.* 2015;16(9):1111-1122. doi:10.1016/S1470-2045(15)00169-2
321. Bouska A, Zhang W, Gong Q, et al. Combined copy number and mutation analysis identifies oncogenic pathways associated with transformation of follicular lymphoma. *Leukemia.* 2017;31:83-91. doi:10.1038/leu.2016.175
322. Rohr J, Guo S, Huo J, et al. Recurrent activating mutations of CD28 in peripheral T-cell lymphomas. *Leukemia.* 2016;30(5):1062-1070. doi:10.1038/leu.2015.357
323. Casulo C, Burack WR, Friedberg JW. Transformed follicular non Hodgkin lymphoma. *Blood.* 2015;125(1):40-47. doi:10.1182/blood-2014-04-516815
324. Kridel R, Chan FC, Mottok A, et al. Histological transformation and progression in follicular lymphoma: a clonal evolution study. *PLoS Med.* 2016;13(12):e1002197. doi:10.1371/journal.pmed.1002197
325. Ozawa MG, Bhaduri A, Chisholm KM, et al. A study of the mutational landscape of pediatric-type follicular lymphoma and pediatric nodal marginal zone lymphoma. *Mod Pathol.* 2016;29(10):1212-1220. doi:10.1038/modpathol.2016.102
326. Louissaint A, Schafernak KT, Geyer JT, et al. Pediatric-type nodal follicular lymphoma: a biologically distinct lymphoma with frequent MAPK pathway mutations. *Blood.* 2016;128(8):1093-1100. doi:10.1182/blood-2015-12-682591
327. Schmidt J, Gong S, Marafioti T, et al. Genome-wide analysis of pediatric-type follicular lymphoma reveals low genetic complexity and recurrent alterations of TNFRSF14 gene. *Blood.* 2016;128(8):1101-1111. doi:10.1182/blood-2016-03-703819
328. Kurtz DM, Scherer F, Newman AM, et al. Noninvasive detection of BCL2, BCL6, and MYC translocations in diffuse large B-cell lymphoma. *Blood.* 2016;128(22):2930. doi:10.1182/blood.v128.22.2930.2930
329. Tibiletti MG, Martin V, Bernasconi B, et al. BCL2, BCL6, MYC, MALT 1, and BCL10 rearrangements in nodal diffuse large B-cell lymphomas: a multicenter evaluation of a new set of fluorescent in situ hybridization probes and correlation with clinical outcome. *Hum Pathol.* 2009;40(5):645-652. doi:10.1016/j.humpath.2008.06.032
330. Kramer MH, Hermans J, Wijburg E, et al. Clinical relevance of BCL2, BCL6, and MYC rearrangements in diffuse large B-cell lymphoma. *Blood.* 1998;92(9):3152-3162.
331. Ye BH, Chaganti S, Chang CC, et al. Chromosomal translocations cause deregulated BCL6 expression by promoter substitution in B cell lymphoma. *EMBO J.* 1995;14(24):6209-6217.
332. Akasaka H, Akasaka T, Kurata M, et al. Molecular anatomy of BCL6 translocations revealed by long-distance polymerase chain reaction-based assays. *Cancer Res.* 2000;60(9):2335-2341.
333. Iqbal J, Greiner TC, Patel K, et al. Distinctive patterns of BCL6 molecular alterations and their functional consequences in different subgroups of diffuse large B-cell lymphoma. *Leukemia.* 2007;21(11):2332-2343. doi:10.1038/sj.leu.2404856
334. Ueda C, Nishikori M, Kitawaki T, Uchiyama T, Ohno H. Coexistent rearrangements of c-MYC, BCL2, and BCL6 genes in a diffuse large B-cell lymphoma. *Int J Hematol.* 2004;79(1):52-54.
335. Gu K, Fu K, Jain S, et al. t(14;18)-negative follicular lymphomas are associated with a high frequency of BCL6 rearrangement at the alternative breakpoint region. *Mod Pathol.* 2009;22(9):1251-1257. doi:10.1038/modpathol.2009.81
336. Bosga-Bouwer AG, Haralambieva E, Booman M, et al. BCL6 alternative translocation breakpoint cluster region associated with follicular lymphoma grade 3B. *Genes Chromosomes Cancer.* 2005;44(3):301-304. doi:10.1002/gcc.20246
337. Barrans SL, O'Connor SJM, Evans PAS, et al. Rearrangement of the BCL6 locus at 3q27 is an independent poor prognostic factor in nodal diffuse large B-cell lymphoma. *Br J Haematol.* 2002;117(2):322-332. doi:10.1046/j.1365-2141.2002.03435.x
338. Shen HM, Peters A, Baron B, Zhu X, Storb U. Mutation of BCL-6 gene in normal B cells by the process of somatic hypermutation of Ig genes. *Science.* 1998;280(5370):1750-1752.
339. Pasqualucci L, Migliazza A, Fracchiolla N, et al. BCL-6 mutations in normal germinal center B cells: evidence of somatic hypermutation acting outside Ig loci. *Proc Natl Acad Sci U S A.* 1998;95(20):11816-11821. doi:10.1073/pnas.95.20.11816
340. Migliazza A, Martinotti S, Chen W, et al. Frequent somatic hypermutation of the 5′ noncoding region of the BCL6 gene in B-cell lymphoma. *Proc Natl Acad Sci U S A.* 1995;92(26):12520-12524. doi:10.1073/pnas.92.26.12520
341. Wagner SD, Ahearne M, Ko Ferrigno P. The role of BCL6 in lymphomas and routes to therapy. *Br J Haematol.* 2011;152(1):3-12. doi:10.1111/j.1365-2141.2010.08420.x
342. Tzankov A, Schneider A, Hoeller S, Dirnhofer S. Prognostic importance of BCL6 rearrangements in diffuse large B-cell lymphoma with respect to Bcl6 protein levels and primary lymphoma site. *Hum Pathol.* 2009;40(7):1055-1056, author reply 1056. doi:10.1016/j.humpath.2009.03.008
343. Sha C, Barrans S, Cucco F, et al. Molecular high-grade B-cell lymphoma: defining a poor-risk group that requires different approaches to therapy. *J Clin Oncol.* 2019;37(3):202-212. doi:10.1200/JCO.18.01314
344. Barrans S, Crouch S, Smith A, et al. Rearrangement of MYC is associated with poor prognosis in patients with diffuse large B-cell lymphoma treated in the era of rituximab. *J Clin Oncol.* 2010;28(20):3360-3365. doi:10.1200/JCO.2009.26.3947
345. Akyurek N, Uner A, Benekli M, Barista I. Prognostic significance of MYC, BCL2, and BCL6 rearrangements in patients with diffuse large B-cell lymphoma treated with cyclophosphamide, doxorubicin, vincristine, and prednisone plus rituximab. *Cancer.* 2012;118(17):4173-4183. doi:10.1002/cncr.27396
346. Herrera AF, Mei M, Low L, et al. Relapsed or refractory double-expressor and double-hit lymphomas have inferior progression-free survival after autologous stem-cell transplantation. *J Clin Oncol.* 2017;35(1):24-31.
347. Staton AD, Cohen JB. A clinician's approach to double-hit lymphoma: identification, evaluation, and management. *J Oncol Pract.* 2016;12(3):232-238. doi:10.1200/JOP.2015.009647
348. Petrich AM, Gandhi M, Jovanovic B, et al. Impact of induction regimen and stem cell transplantation on outcomes in double-hit lymphoma: a multicenter retrospective analysis. *Blood.* 2014;124(15):2354-2361. doi:10.1182/blood-2014-05-578963
349. Herrera AF. Double-hit lymphoma: practicing in a data-limited setting. *J Oncol Pract.* 2016;12(3):239-240. doi:10.1200/JOP.2015.010439
350. Li S, Weiss VL, Wang XJ, et al. High-grade B-cell lymphoma with MYC rearrangement and without BCL2 and BCL6 rearrangements is associated with high P53 expression and a poor prognosis. *Am J Surg Pathol.* 2016;40(2):253-261. doi:10.1097/PAS.0000000000000542
351. Karube K, Campo E. MYC alterations in diffuse large B-cell lymphomas. *Semin Hematol.* 2015;52(2):97-106. doi:10.1053/j.seminhematol.2015.01.009
352. Swerdlow SH. Diagnosis of "double hit" diffuse large B-cell lymphoma and B-cell lymphoma, unclassifiable, with features intermediate between DLBCL and Burkitt lymphoma: when and how, FISH versus IHC. *Hematology Am Soc Hematol Educ Program.* 2014;2014(1):90-99. doi:10.1182/asheducation-2014.1.90
353. Momose S, Tamaru Jichi, Kishi H, et al. Hyperactivated STAT3 in ALK-positive diffuse large B-cell lymphoma with clathrin-ALK fusion. *Hum Pathol.* 2009;40(1):75-82. doi:10.1016/j.humpath.2008.06.009
354. Shipp MA, Ross KN, Tamayo P, et al. Diffuse large B-cell lymphoma outcome prediction by gene-expression profiling and supervised machine learning. *Nat Med.* 2002;8(1):68-74. doi:10.1038/nm0102-68nm0102-68
355. Alizadeh AA, Eisen MB, Davis RE, et al. Distinct types of diffuse large B-cell lymphoma identified by gene expression profiling. *Nature.* 2000;403(6769):503-511. doi:10.1038/35000501
356. Davis RE, Ngo VN, Lenz G, et al. Chronic active B-cell-receptor signalling in diffuse large B-cell lymphoma. *Nature.* 2010;463(7277):88-92. doi:10.1038/nature08638
357. Young RM, Wu T, Schmitz R, et al. Survival of human lymphoma cells requires B-cell receptor engagement by self-antigens. *Proc Natl Acad Sci U S A.* 2015;112(44):13447-13454. doi:10.1073/pnas.1514944112
358. Rosenwald A, Wright G, Chan WC, et al. The use of molecular profiling to predict survival after chemotherapy for diffuse large-B-cell lymphoma. *N Engl J Med.* 2002;346(25):1937-1947. doi:10.1056/NEJMoa012914346/25/1937
359. Scott DW, Mottok A, Ennishi D, et al. Prognostic significance of diffuse large B-cell lymphoma cell of origin determined by digital gene expression in formalin-fixed paraffin-embedded tissue biopsies. *J Clin Oncol.* 2015;33(26):2848-2856. doi:10.1200/JCO.2014.60.2383
360. Mareschal S, Lanic H, Ruminy P, Bastard C, Tilly H, Jardin F. The proportion of activated B-cell like subtype among de novo diffuse large B-cell lymphoma increases with age. *Haematologica.* 2011;96(12):1888-1890. doi:10.3324/haematol.2011.050617
361. Thieblemont C, Briere J, Mounier N, et al. The germinal center/activated B-cell subclassification has a prognostic impact for response to salvage therapy in relapsed/refractory diffuse large B-cell lymphoma: a bio-CORAL study. *J Clin Oncol.* 2011;29(31):4079-4087. doi:10.1200/JCO.2011.35.4423
362. Delarue R, Tilly H, Mounier N, et al. Dose-dense rituximab-CHOP compared with standard rituximab-CHOP in elderly patients with diffuse large B-cell lymphoma (the LNH03-6B study): a randomised phase 3 trial. *Lancet Oncol.* 2013;14(6):525-533. doi:10.1016/S1470-2045(13)70122-0
363. Cunningham D, Hawkes EA, Jack A, et al. Rituximab plus cyclophosphamide, doxorubicin, vincristine, and prednisolone in patients with newly diagnosed diffuse large B-cell non-Hodgkin lymphoma: a phase 3 comparison of dose intensification with 14-day versus 21-day cycles. *Lancet.* 2013;381(9880):1817-1826. doi:10.1016/S0140-6736(13)60313-X

364. Bartlett NL, Wilson WH, Jung SH, et al. Dose-adjusted EPOCH-R compared with R-CHOP as frontline therapy for diffuse large B-cell lymphoma: clinical outcomes of the phase III intergroup trial alliance/CALGB 50303. *J Clin Oncol.* 2019;37(21):1790-1799. doi:10.1200/JCO.18.01994
365. Ruan J, Martin P, Furman RR, et al. Bortezomib plus CHOP-rituximab for previously untreated diffuse large B-cell lymphoma and mantle cell lymphoma. *J Clin Oncol.* 2011;29(6):690-697. doi:10.1200/JCO.2010.31.1142
366. Nowakowski GS, LaPlant B, Macon WR, et al. Lenalidomide combined with R-CHOP overcomes negative prognostic impact of non-germinal center B-cell phenotype in newly diagnosed diffuse large B-cell lymphoma: a phase II study. *J Clin Oncol.* 2015;33(3):251-257. doi:10.1200/JCO.2014.55.5714
367. Younes A, Sehn LH, Johnson P, et al. Randomized phase III trial of ibrutinib and rituximab plus cyclophosphamide, doxorubicin, vincristine, and prednisone in non–germinal center B-cell diffuse large B-cell lymphoma. *J Clin Oncol.* 2019;37(15):1285-1295. doi:10.1200/JCO.18.02403
368. Récher C, Coiffier B, Haioun C, et al. Intensified chemotherapy with ACVBP plus rituximab versus standard CHOP plus rituximab for the treatment of diffuse large B-cell lymphoma (LNH03-2B): an open-label randomised phase 3 trial. *Lancet.* 2011;378(9806):1858-1867. doi:10.1016/S0140-6736(11)61040-4
369. Molina TJ, Canioni D, Copie-Bergman C, et al. Young patients with non-germinal center B-cell-like diffuse large B-cell lymphoma benefit from intensified chemotherapy with ACVBP plus rituximab compared with CHOP plus rituximab: analysis of data from the Groupe d'Etudes des Lymphomes de l'Adulte/lymphoma study association phase III trial LNH 03-2B. *J Clin Oncol.* 2014;32(35):3996-4003. doi:10.1200/JCO.2013.54.9493
370. Hans CP, Weisenburger DD, Greiner TC, et al. Confirmation of the molecular classification of diffuse large B-cell lymphoma by immunohistochemistry using a tissue microarray. *Blood.* 2004;103(1):275-282. doi:10.1182/blood-2003-05-1545
371. Choi WWL, Weisenburger DD, Greiner TC, et al. A new immunostain algorithm classifies diffuse large B-cell lymphoma into molecular subtypes with high accuracy. *Clin Cancer Res.* 2009;15(17):5494-5502. 10.1158/1078-0432.CCR-09-0113
372. Meyer PN, Fu K, Greiner TC, et al. Immunohistochemical methods for predicting cell of origin and survival in patients with diffuse large B-cell lymphoma treated with rituximab. *J Clin Oncol.* 2011;29(2):200-207. 10.1200/JCO.2010.30.0368
373. Muris JJF, Meijer CJ, Vos W, et al. Immunohistochemical profiling based on Bcl-2, CD10 and MUM1 expression improves risk stratification in patients with primary nodal diffuse large B cell lymphoma. *J Pathol.* 2006;208(5):714-723. doi:10.1002/path.1924
374. Sujobert P, Salles G, Bachy E. Molecular classification of diffuse large B-cell lymphoma: what is clinically relevant? *Hematol Oncol Clin North Am.* 2016;30(6):1163-1177. doi:10.1016/j.hoc.2016.07.001
375. Scott DW, Wright GW, Williams PM, et al. Determining cell-of-origin subtypes of diffuse large B-cell lymphoma using gene expression in formalin-fixed paraffin-embedded tissue. *Blood.* 2014;123(8):1214-1217. doi:10.1182/blood-2013-11-536433
376. Masqué-Soler N, Szczepanowski M, Kohler CW, Spang R, Klapper W. Molecular classification of mature aggressive B-cell lymphoma using digital multiplexed gene expression on formalin-fixed paraffin-embedded biopsy specimens. *Blood.* 2013;122(11):1985-1986. doi:10.1182/blood-2013-06-508937
377. Mareschal S, Ruminy P, Bagacean C, et al. Accurate classification of germinal center B-cell-like/activated B-cell-like diffuse large B-cell lymphoma using a simple and rapid reverse transcriptase-multiplex ligation-dependent probe amplification assay: a CALYM study. *J Mol Diagn.* 2015;17(3):273-283. doi:10.1016/j.jmoldx.2015.01.007
378. Pasqualucci L, Dalla-Favera R. The genetic landscape of diffuse large B-cell lymphoma. *Semin Hematol.* 2015;52(2):67-76. doi:10.1053/j.seminhematol.2015.01.005
379. Muppidi JR, Schmitz R, Green JA, et al. Loss of signalling via Gα13 in germinal centre B-cell-derived lymphoma. *Nature.* 2014;516(7530):254-258. doi:10.1038/nature13765
380. Montes-Moreno S, Martinez N, Sanchez-Espiridion B, et al. miRNA expression in diffuse large B-cell lymphoma treated with chemoimmunotherapy. *Blood.* 2011;118(4):1034-1040. doi:10.1182/blood-2010-11-321554
381. Zheng Z, Li X, Zhu Y, Gu W, Xie X, Jiang J. Prognostic significance of MiRNA in patients with diffuse large B-cell lymphoma: a meta-analysis. *Cell Physiol Biochem.* 2016;39(5):1891-1904. doi:10.1159/000447887
382. Lim EL, Trinh DL, Scott DW, et al. Comprehensive miRNA sequence analysis reveals survival differences in diffuse large B-cell lymphoma patients. *Genome Biol.* 2015;16:18. doi:10.1186/s13059-014-0568-y
383. Chapuy B, Stewart C, Dunford AJ, et al. Molecular subtypes of diffuse large B cell lymphoma are associated with distinct pathogenic mechanisms and outcomes. *Nat Med.* 2018;24(5):679-690. doi:10.1038/s41591-018-0016-8
384. Schmitz R, Wright GW, Huang DW, et al. Genetics and pathogenesis of diffuse large B-cell lymphoma. *N Engl J Med.* 2018;378(15):1396-1407. doi:10.1056/NEJMoa1801445
385. Wright GW, Huang DW, Phelan JD, et al. A probabilistic classification tool for genetic subtypes of diffuse large B cell lymphoma with therapeutic implications. *Cancer Cell.* 2020;37(4):551.e14-568.e14. doi:10.1016/j.ccell.2020.03.015
386. Lacy SE, Barrans SL, Beer PA, et al. Targeted sequencing in DLBCL, molecular subtypes, and outcomes: a Haematological Malignancy Research Network report. *Blood.* 2020;135(20):1759-1771. doi:10.1182/blood.2019003535
387. Roschewski M, Dunleavy K, Pittaluga S, et al. Circulating tumour DNA and CT monitoring in patients with untreated diff use large B-cell lymphoma: a correlative biomarker study. *Lancet Oncol.* 2021;16(2015):541-549. doi:10.1016/S1470-2045(15)70106-3
388. Kumar A, Westin J, Schuster SJ, et al. Interim analysis from a prospective multicenter study of next-generation sequencing minimal residual disease assessment and CT monitoring for surveillance after frontline treatment in diffuse large B-cell lymphoma. *Blood.* 2020;136(suppl 1):46-47.
389. Jarrett RF. Viruses and lymphoma/leukaemia. *J Pathol.* 2006;208(2):176-186. doi:10.1002/path.1905
390. Hamilton-Dutoit SJ, Raphael M, Audouin J, et al. In situ demonstration of Epstein-Barr virus small RNAs (EBER 1) in acquired immunodeficiency syndrome-related lymphomas: correlation with tumor morphology and primary site. *Blood.* 1993;82(2):619-624.
391. Raphael M, Gentilhomme O, Tulliez M, Byron PA, Diebold J. Histopathologic features of high-grade non-Hodgkin's lymphomas in acquired immunodeficiency syndrome. The French Study Group of Pathology for Human Immunodeficiency Virus-Associated Tumors. *Arch Pathol Lab Med.* 1991;115(1):15-20.
392. Dalla-Favera R, Bregni M, Erikson J, Patterson D, Gallo RC, Croce CM. Human c-myc onc gene is located on the region of chromosome 8 that is translocated in Burkitt lymphoma cells. *Proc Natl Acad Sci U S A.* 1982;79(24):7824-7827.
393. Taub R, Kirsch I, Morton C, et al. Translocation of the c-myc gene into the immunoglobulin heavy chain locus in human Burkitt lymphoma and murine plasmacytoma cells. *Proc Natl Acad Sci U S A.* 1982;79(24):7837-7841.
394. Hollis GF, Mitchell KF, Battey J, et al. A variant translocation places the lambda immunoglobulin genes 3′ to the c-myc oncogene in Burkitt's lymphoma. *Nature.* 1984;307(5953):752-755. doi:10.1038/307752a0
395. Erikson J, Nishikura K, ar-Rushdi A, et al. Translocation of an immunoglobulin kappa locus to a region 3′ of an unrearranged c-myc oncogene enhances c-myc transcription. *Proc Natl Acad Sci U S A.* 1983;80(24):7581-7585.
396. Pelengaris S, Khan M, Evan G. c-MYC: more than just a matter of life and death. *Nat Rev Cancer.* 2002;2(10):764-776.
397. Barriga F, Kiwanuka J, Alvarez-Mon M, et al. Significance of chromosome 8 breakpoint location in Burkitt's lymphoma: correlation with geographical origin and association with Epstein-Barr virus. *Curr Top Microbiol Immunol.* 1988;141:128-137.
398. Pelicci PG, Knowles DM II, Magrath I, Dalla-Favera R. Chromosomal breakpoints and structural alterations of the c-myc locus differ in endemic and sporadic forms of Burkitt lymphoma. *Proc Natl Acad Sci U S A.* 1986;83(9):2984-2988.
399. Shiramizu B, Barriga F, Neequaye J, et al. Patterns of chromosomal breakpoint locations in Burkitt's lymphoma: relevance to geography and Epstein-Barr virus association. *Blood.* 1991;77(7):1516-1526.
400. Gutierrez MI, Bhatia K, Barriga F, et al. Molecular epidemiology of Burkitt's lymphoma from South America: differences in breakpoint location and Epstein-Barr virus association from tumors in other world regions. *Blood.* 1992;79(12):3261-3266.
401. Shiramizu B, Magrath I. Localization of breakpoints by polymerase chain reactions in Burkitt's lymphoma with 8;14 translocations. *Blood.* 1990;75(9):1848-1852.
402. Haralambieva E, Banham AH, Bastard C, et al. Detection by the fluorescence in situ hybridization technique of MYC translocations in paraffin-embedded lymphoma biopsy samples. *Br J Haematol.* 2003;121(1):49-56. doi:10.1046/j.1365-2141.2003.04238.x
403. Salaverria I, Martin-Guerrero I, Wagener R, et al. A recurrent 11q aberration pattern characterizes a subset of MYC-negative high-grade B-cell lymphomas resembling Burkitt lymphoma. *Blood.* 2014;123(8):1187-1198. doi:10.1182/blood-2013-06-507996
404. Ferreiro JF, Morscio J, Dierickx D, et al. Post-transplant molecularly defined Burkitt lymphomas are frequently MYC-negative and characterized by the 11q-gain/loss pattern. *Haematologica.* 2015;100(7):e275-e279. doi:10.3324/haematol.2015.124305
405. Dave SS, Fu K, Wright GW, et al. Molecular diagnosis of Burkitt's lymphoma. *N Engl J Med.* 2006;354(23):2431-2442. doi:10.1056/NEJMoa055759
406. Hummel M, Bentink S, Berger H, et al. A biologic definition of Burkitt's lymphoma from transcriptional and genomic profiling. *N Engl J Med.* 2006;354(23):2419-2430. doi:10.1056/NEJMoa055351
407. Richter J, Schlesner M, Hoffmann S, et al. Recurrent mutation of the ID3 gene in Burkitt lymphoma identified by integrated genome, exome and transcriptome sequencing. *Nat Genet.* 2012;44(12):1316-1320. doi:10.1038/ng.2469
408. Love C, Sun Z, Jima D, et al. The genetic landscape of mutations in Burkitt lymphoma. *Nat Genet.* 2012;44(12):1321-1325. doi:10.1038/ng.2468
409. Schmitz R, Young RM, Ceribelli M, et al. Burkitt lymphoma pathogenesis and therapeutic targets from structural and functional genomics. *Nature.* 2012;490(7418):116-120. doi:10.1038/nature11378
410. Sander S, Calado DP, Srinivasan L, et al. Synergy between PI3K signaling and MYC in Burkitt lymphomagenesis. *Cancer Cell.* 2012;22(2):167-179. doi:10.1016/j.ccr.2012.06.012
411. Falini B, Mason DY. Proteins encoded by genes involved in chromosomal alterations in lymphoma and leukemia: clinical value of their detection by immunocytochemistry. *Blood.* 2002;99(2):409-426. doi:10.1182/blood.V99.2.409
412. Morris SW, Kirstein MN, Valentine MB, et al. Fusion of a kinase gene, ALK, to a nucleolar protein gene, NPM, in non-Hodgkin's lymphoma. *Science.* 1994;263(5151):1281-1284.
413. Chan WY, Liu QR, Borjigin J, et al. Characterization of the cDNA encoding human nucleophosmin and studies of its role in normal and abnormal growth. *Biochemistry.* 1989;28(3):1033-1039.
414. Merkel O, Hamacher F, Sifft E, Kenner L, Greil R; European Research Initiative on Anaplastic Large Cell Lymphoma. Novel therapeutic options in anaplastic large cell lymphoma: molecular targets and immunological tools. *Mol Cancer Ther.* 2011;10(7):1127-1136. doi:10.1158/1535-7163.MCT-11-0042
415. Werner MT, Zhao C, Zhang Q, Wasik MA. Nucleophosmin-anaplastic lymphoma kinase: the ultimate oncogene and therapeutic target. *Blood.* 2017;129(7):823-831. doi:10.1182/blood-2016-05-717793
416. Bisig B, Gaulard P, de Leval L. New biomarkers in T-cell lymphomas. *Best Pract Res Clin Haematol.* 2012;25(1):13-28. doi:10.1016/j.beha.2012.01.004
417. Wellmann A, Otsuki T, Vogelbruch M, Clark HM, Jaffe ES, Raffeld M. Analysis of the t(2;5)(p23;q35) translocation by reverse transcription-polymerase chain reaction in CD30+ anaplastic large-cell lymphomas, in other non-Hodgkin's lymphomas of T-cell phenotype, and in Hodgkin's disease. *Blood.* 1995;86(6):2321-2328.

418. Sarris AH, Luthra R, Papadimitracopoulou V, et al. Amplification of genomic DNA demonstrates the presence of the t(2;5) (p23;q35) in anaplastic large cell lymphoma, but not in other non-Hodgkin's lymphomas, Hodgkin's disease, or lymphomatoid papulosis. *Blood.* 1996;88(5):1771-1779.
419. Mathew P, Sanger WG, Weisenburger DD, et al. Detection of the t(2;5)(p23;q35) and NPM-ALK fusion in non-Hodgkin's lymphoma by two-color fluorescence in situ hybridization. *Blood.* 1997;89(5):1678-1685.
420. Feldman AL, Dogan A, Smith DI, et al. Discovery of recurrent t(6;7)(p25.3;q32.3) translocations in ALK-negative anaplastic large cell lymphomas by massively parallel genomic sequencing. *Blood.* 2011;117(3):915-919. doi:10.1182/blood-2010-08-303305
421. Parrilla Castellar ER, Jaffe ES, Said JW, et al. ALK-negative anaplastic large cell lymphoma is a genetically heterogeneous disease with widely disparate clinical outcomes. *Blood.* 2014;124(9):1473-1480. doi:10.1182/blood-2014-04-571091
422. Crescenzo R, Abate F, Lasorsa E, et al. Convergent mutations and kinase fusions lead to oncogenic STAT3 activation in anaplastic large cell lymphoma. *Cancer Cell.* 2015;27(4):516-532. doi:10.1016/j.ccell.2015.03.006
423. Boddicker RL, Razidlo GL, Dasari S, et al. Integrated mate-pair and RNA sequencing identifies novel, targetable gene fusions in peripheral T-cell lymphoma. *Blood.* 2016;128(9):1234-1245. doi:10.1182/blood-2016-03-707141
424. Salaverria I, Bea S, Lopez-Guillermo A, et al. Genomic profiling reveals different genetic aberrations in systemic ALK-positive and ALK-negative anaplastic large cell lymphomas. *Br J Haematol.* 2008;140(5):516-526. doi:10.1111/j.1365-2141.2007.06924.x
425. Nelson M, Horsman DE, Weisenburger DD, et al. Cytogenetic abnormalities and clinical correlations in peripheral T-cell lymphoma. *Br J Haematol.* 2008;141(4):461-469. doi:10.1111/j.1365-2141.2008.07042.x
426. Boi M, Rinaldi A, Kwee I, et al. PRDM1/BLIMP1 is commonly inactivated in anaplastic large T-cell lymphoma. *Blood.* 2013;122(15):2683-2693. doi:10.1182/blood-2013-04-497933
427. Desjobert C, Renalier MH, Bergalet J, et al. MiR-29a down-regulation in ALK-positive anaplastic large cell lymphomas contributes to apoptosis blockade through MCL-1 overexpression. *Blood.* 2011;117(24):6627-6637. doi:10.1182/blood-2010-09-301994
428. Matsuyama H, Suzuki HI, Nishimori H, et al. miR-135b mediates NPM-ALK-driven oncogenicity and renders IL-17-producing immunophenotype to anaplastic large cell lymphoma. *Blood.* 2011;118(26):6881-6892. doi:10.1182/blood-2011-05-354654
429. Iqbal J, Wright G, Wang C, et al. Gene expression signatures delineate biological and prognostic subgroups in peripheral T-cell lymphoma. *Blood.* 2014;123(19):2915-2923. doi:10.1182/blood-2013-11-536359
430. Zhang Q, Wang HY, Liu X, Bhutani G, Kantekure K, Wasik M. IL-2R common gamma-chain is epigenetically silenced by nucleophosphin-anaplastic lymphoma kinase (NPM-ALK) and acts as a tumor suppressor by targeting NPM-ALK. *Proc Natl Acad Sci U S A.* 2011;108(29):11977-11982. doi:10.1073/pnas.1100319108
431. Eckerle S, Brune V, Doring C, et al. Gene expression profiling of isolated tumour cells from anaplastic large cell lymphomas: insights into its cellular origin, pathogenesis and relation to Hodgkin lymphoma. *Leukemia.* 2009;23(11):2129-2138. doi:10.1038/leu.2009.161
432. Iqbal J, Weisenburger DD, Greiner TC, et al. Molecular signatures to improve diagnosis in peripheral T-cell lymphoma and prognostication in angioimmunoblastic T-cell lymphoma. *Blood.* 2010;115(5):1026-1036. doi:10.1182/blood-2009-06-227579
433. Piva R, Agnelli L, Pellegrino E, et al. Gene expression profiling uncovers molecular classifiers for the recognition of anaplastic large-cell lymphoma within peripheral T-cell neoplasms. *J Clin Oncol.* 2010;28(9):1583-1590. doi:10.1200/JCO.2008.20.9759
434. Lamant L, de Reynies A, Duplantier MM, et al. Gene-expression profiling of systemic anaplastic large-cell lymphoma reveals differences based on ALK status and two distinct morphologic ALK+ subtypes. *Blood.* 2007;109(5):2156-2164. doi:10.1182/blood-2006-06-028969
435. Thompson MA, Stumph J, Henrickson SE, et al. Differential gene expression in anaplastic lymphoma kinase-positive and anaplastic lymphoma kinase-negative anaplastic large cell lymphomas. *Hum Pathol.* 2005;36(5):494-504. doi:10.1016/j.humpath.2005.03.004
436. Ohgami RS, Ma L, Merker JD, Martinez B, Zehnder JL, Arber DA. STAT3 mutations are frequent in CD30+ T-cell lymphomas and T-cell large granular lymphocytic leukemia. *Leukemia.* 2013;27(11):2244-2247. doi:10.1038/leu.2013.104
437. Blombery P, Thompson ER, Jones K, et al. Whole exome sequencing reveals activating JAK1 and STAT3 mutations in breast implant-associated anaplastic large cell lymphoma anaplastic large cell lymphoma. *Haematologica.* 2016;101(9):e387-e390. doi:10.3324/haematol.2016.146118
438. Di Napoli A, Jain P, Duranti E, et al. Targeted next generation sequencing of breast implant-associated anaplastic large cell lymphoma reveals mutations in JAK/STAT signalling pathway genes, TP53 and DNMT3A. *Br J Haematol.* 2018;180(5):741-744. doi:10.1111/bjh.14431
439. Savage KJ, Harris NL, Vose JM, et al. ALK- anaplastic large-cell lymphoma is clinically and immunophenotypically different from both ALK+ ALCL and peripheral T-cell lymphoma, not otherwise specified: report from the International Peripheral T-Cell Lymphoma Project. *Blood.* 2008;111(12):5496-5504. doi:10.1182/blood-2008-01-134270
440. Foss FM, Zinzani PL, Vose JM, Gascoyne RD, Rosen ST, Tobinai K. Peripheral T-cell lymphoma. *Blood.* 2011;117(25):6756-6767. doi:10.1182/blood-2010-05-231548
441. Watatani Y, Sato Y, Miyoshi H, et al. Molecular heterogeneity in peripheral T-cell lymphoma, not otherwise specified revealed by comprehensive genetic profiling. *Leukemia.* 2019;33(12):2867-2883. doi:10.1038/s41375-019-0473-1
442. Thorns C, Bastian B, Pinkel D, et al. Chromosomal aberrations in angioimmunoblastic T-cell lymphoma and peripheral T-cell lymphoma unspecified: a matrix-based CGH approach. *Genes Chromosomes Cancer.* 2007;46(1):37-44. doi:10.1002/gcc.20386
443. Zettl A, Rudiger T, Konrad MA, et al. Genomic profiling of peripheral T-cell lymphoma, unspecified, and anaplastic large T-cell lymphoma delineates novel recurrent chromosomal alterations. *Am J Pathol.* 2004;164(5):1837-1848. doi:10.1016/S0002-9440(10)63742-X
444. Fujiwara SI, Yamashita Y, Nakamura N, et al. High-resolution analysis of chromosome copy number alterations in angioimmunoblastic T-cell lymphoma and peripheral T-cell lymphoma, unspecified, with single nucleotide polymorphism-typing microarrays. *Leukemia.* 2008;22(10):1891-1898. doi:10.1038/leu.2008.191
445. Abate F, da Silva-Almeida AC, Zairis S, et al. Activating mutations and translocations in the guanine exchange factor VAV1 in peripheral T-cell lymphomas. *Proc Natl Acad Sci U S A.* 2017;114(4):764-769. doi:10.1073/pnas.1608839114
446. Feldman AL, Law M, Remstein ED, et al. Recurrent translocations involving the IRF4 oncogene locus in peripheral T-cell lymphoma. *Leukemia.* 2009;23(3):574-580. doi:10.1038/leu.2008.320
447. Ballester B, Ramuz O, Gisselbrecht C, et al. Gene expression profiling identifies molecular subgroups among nodal peripheral T-cell lymphomas. *Oncogene.* 2006;25(10):1560-1570. doi:10.1038/sj.onc.1209178
448. Piccaluga PP, Agostinelli C, Califano A, et al. Gene expression analysis of peripheral T cell lymphoma, unspecified, reveals distinct profiles and new potential therapeutic targets. *J Clin Invest.* 2007;117(3):823-834. doi:10.1172/JCI26833
449. Feldman AL, Sun DX, Law ME, et al. Overexpression of Syk tyrosine kinase in peripheral T-cell lymphoma. *Leukemia.* 2008;22(6):1139-1143. doi:10.1038/leu.2008.77
450. Piccaluga PP, Agostinelli C, Zinzani PL, Baccarani M, Dalla Favera R, Pileri SA. Expression of platelet-derived growth factor receptor alpha in peripheral T-cell lymphoma not otherwise specified. *Lancet Oncol.* 2005;6(6):440. doi:10.1016/S1470-2045(05)70213-8
451. Couronne L, Bastard C, Bernard OA. TET2 and DNMT3A mutations in human T-cell lymphoma. *N Engl J Med.* 2012;366(1):95-96. doi:10.1056/NEJMc1111708
452. Quivoron C, Couronne L, Della Valle V, et al. TET2 inactivation results in pleiotropic hematopoietic abnormalities in mouse and is a recurrent event during human lymphomagenesis. *Cancer Cell.* 2011;20(1):25-38. doi:10.1016/j.ccr.2011.06.003
453. Boddicker RL, Razidlo GL, FA. Genetic alterations affecting GTPases and T-cell receptor signaling in peripheral T-cell lymphoma. *Small GTPases.* 2016;29:1-7. doi:10.1080/21541248.2016.1263718
454. Attygalle AD, Feldman AL, Dogan A. ITK/SYK translocation in angioimmunoblastic T-cell lymphoma. *Am J Surg Pathol.* 2013;37(9):1456-1457.
455. Huang Y, Moreau A, Dupuis J, et al. Peripheral T-cell lymphomas with a follicular growth pattern are derived from follicular helper T cells (TFH) and may show overlapping features with angioimmunoblastic T-cell lymphomas. *Am J Surg Pathol.* 2009;33(5):682-690. doi:10.1097/PAS.0b013e3181971591
456. Streubel B, Vinatzer U, Willheim M, Raderer M, Chott A. Novel t(5;9)(q33;q22) fuses ITK to SYK in unspecified peripheral T-cell lymphoma. *Leukemia.* 2006;20(2):313-318. doi:10.1038/sj.leu.2404045
457. Mulloy JC. Peripheral T cell lymphoma: new model + new insight. *J Exp Med.* 2010;207(5):911-913. doi:10.1084/jem.20100608
458. Yoo HY, Kim P, Kim WS, et al. Frequent CTLA4-CD28 gene fusion in diverse types of T-cell lymphoma. *Haematologica.* 2016;101(6):757-763. doi:10.3324/haematol.2015.139253
459. Vallois D, Dupuy A, Lemonnier F, et al. RNA fusions involving CD28 are rare in peripheral T-cell lymphomas and concentrate mainly in those derived from follicular helper T cells. *Haematologica.* 2018;103(8):360-363.
460. Cuadros M, Dave SS, Jaffe ES, et al. Identification of a proliferation signature related to survival in nodal peripheral T-cell lymphomas. *J Clin Oncol.* 2007;25(22):3321-3329. doi:10.1200/JCO.2006.09.4474
461. Miyazaki K, Yamaguchi M, Imai H, et al. Gene expression profiling of peripheral T-cell lymphoma including gammadelta T-cell lymphoma. *Blood.* 2009;113(5):1071-1074. doi:10.1182/blood-2008-07-166363
462. de Leval L, Rickman DS, Thielen C, et al. The gene expression profile of nodal peripheral T-cell lymphoma demonstrates a molecular link between angioimmunoblastic T-cell lymphoma (AITL) and follicular helper T (TFH) cells. *Blood.* 2007;109(11):4952-4963. doi:10.1182/blood-2006-10-055145
463. Sakata-Yanagimoto M, Enami T, Yoshida K, et al. Somatic RHOA mutation in angioimmunoblastic T cell lymphoma. *Nat Genet.* 2014;46(2):171-175. doi:10.1038/ng.2872
464. Yoo HY, Sung MK, Lee SH, et al. A recurrent inactivating mutation in RHOA GTPase in angioimmunoblastic T cell lymphoma. *Nat Genet.* 2014;46(4):371-375. doi:10.1038/ng.2916
465. Vallois D, Dobay MPD, Morin RD, et al. Activating mutations in genes related to TCR signaling in angioimmunoblastic and other follicular helper T-cell-derived lymphomas. *Blood.* 2016;128(11):1490-1502. doi:10.1182/blood-2016-02-698977
466. Steinhilber J, Mederake M, Bonzheim I, et al. The pathological features of angioimmunoblastic T-cell lymphomas with IDH2 R172 mutations. *Mod Pathol.* 2019;32(8):1123-1134. doi:10.1038/s41379-019-0254-4
467. Lee SHL, Kim JS, Kim J, et al. A highly recurrent novel missense mutation in CD28 among angioimmunoblastic T-cell lymphoma patients. *Haematologica.* 2015;100(12):e505-e507.
468. Dang L, White DW, Gross S, et al. Cancer-associated IDH1 mutations produce 2-hydroxyglutarate. *Nature.* 2010;465(7300):966. doi:10.1038/nature09132
469. Ward PS, Cross JR, Lu C, et al. Identification of additional IDH mutations associated with oncometabolite R(-)-2-hydroxyglutarate production. *Oncogene.* 2012;31(19):2491-2498. doi:10.1038/onc.2011.416

470. Cairns RA, Iqbal J, Lemonnier F, et al. IDH2 mutations are frequent in angioimmunoblastic T-cell lymphoma. *Blood*. 2012;119(8):1901-1903. doi:10.1182/blood-2011-11-391748
471. Lewis NE, Petrova-Drus K, Huet S, et al. Clonal hematopoiesis in angioimmunoblastic T-cell lymphoma with divergent evolution to myeloid neoplasms. *Blood Adv*. 2020;4(10):2261-2271. doi:10.1182/bloodadvances.2020001636
472. Pekarsky Y, Hallas C, Croce CM. Molecular basis of mature T-cell leukemia. *J Am Med Assoc*. 2001;286(18):2308-2314. doi:10.1001/jama.286.18.2308
473. de Leval L, Gaulard P. Tricky and terrible T-cell tumors: these are thrilling times for testing. Molecular pathology of peripheral T-cell lymphomas. *Hematology Am Soc Hematol Educ Program*. 2011;2011:336-343. doi:10.1182/asheducation-2011.1.336
474. Stengel A, Kern W, Zenger M, et al. Genetic characterization of T-PLL reveals two major biologic subgroups and JAK3 mutations as prognostic marker. *Genes Chromosomes Cancer*. 2016;55(1):82-94.
475. Virgilio L, Isobe M, Narducci MG, et al. Chromosome walking on the TCL1 locus involved in T-cell neoplasia. *Proc Natl Acad Sci U S A*. 1993;90(20):9275-9279.
476. Suzuki R, Matsushita H, Kawai H, et al. Identification of a novel SEPT9-ABL1 fusion gene in a patient with T-cell prolymphocytic leukemia. *Leuk Res Rep*. 2014;3(2):54-57. doi:10.1016/j.lrr.2014.06.004
477. Gaudio E, Spizzo R, Paduano F, et al. Tcl1 interacts with Atm and enhances NF-κB activation in hematologic malignancies. *Blood*. 2012;119(1):180-187. doi:10.1182/blood-2011-08-374561
478. Durig J, Bug S, Klein-Hitpass L, et al. Combined single nucleotide polymorphism-based genomic mapping and global gene expression profiling identifies novel chromosomal imbalances, mechanisms and candidate genes important in the pathogenesis of T-cell prolymphocytic leukemia with inv(14)(q11q32). *Leukemia*. 2007;21(10):2153-2163. doi:10.1038/sj.leu.2404877
479. Urbankova H, Holzerova M, Balcarkova J, et al. Array comparative genomic hybridization in the detection of chromosomal abnormalities in T-cell prolymphocytic leukemia. *Cancer Genet Cytogenet*. 2010;202(1):58-62. doi:10.1016/j.cancergencyto.2010.06.006
480. Kiel MJ, Velusamy T, Rolland D, et al. Integrated genomic sequencing reveals mutational landscape of T-cell prolymphocytic leukemia. *Blood*. 2014;124(9):1460-1472. doi:10.1182/blood-2014-03-559542
481. Bug S, Durig J, Oyen F, et al. Recurrent loss, but lack of mutations, of the SMARCB1 tumor suppressor gene in T-cell prolymphocytic leukemia with TCL1A-TCRAD juxtaposition. *Cancer Genet Cytogenet*. 2009;192(1):44-47. doi:10.1016/j.cancergencyto.2009.03.001
482. Bergmann AK, Schneppenheim S, Seifert M, et al. Recurrent mutation of JAK3 in T-cell prolymphocytic leukemia. *Genes Chromosomes Cancer*. 2014;53(4):309-316. doi:10.1002/gcc.22141
483. Clemente MJ, Przychodzen B, Jerez A, et al. Deep sequencing of the T-cell receptor repertoire in CD8+ T-large granular lymphocyte leukemia identifies signature landscapes. *Blood*. 2013;122(25):4077-4085. doi:10.1182/blood-2013-05-506386
484. Kristensen T, Larsen M, Rewes A, Frederiksen H, Thomassen M, Møller MB. Clinical relevance of sensitive and quantitative STAT3 mutation analysis using next-generation sequencing in T-cell large granular lymphocyte leukemia. *J Mol Diagn*. 2014;16(4):382-392. doi:10.1016/j.jmoldx.2014.02.005
485. Jerez A, Clemente MJ, Makishima H, et al. STAT3 mutations unify the pathogenesis of chronic lymphoproliferative disorders of NK cells and T-cell large granular lymphocyte leukemia. *Blood*. 2012;120(15):3048-3057. doi:10.1182/blood-2012-06-435297
486. Koskela HLM, Eldfors S, Ellonen P, et al. Somatic STAT3 mutations in large granular lymphocytic leukemia. *N Engl J Med*. 2012;366(20):1905-1913. doi:10.1056/NEJMoa1114885
487. Rajala HLM, Eldfors S, Kuusanmaki H, et al. Discovery of somatic STAT5b mutations in large granular lymphocytic leukemia. *Blood*. 2013;121(22):4541-4550. doi:10.1182/blood-2012-12-474577
488. Rajala HLM, Porkka K, Maciejewski JP, Loughran TP, Mustjoki S. Uncovering the pathogenesis of large granular lymphocytic leukemia-novel STAT3 and STAT5b mutations. *Ann Med*. 2014;46(3):114-122. doi:10.3109/07853890.2014.882105
489. Rajala HLM, Olson T, Clemente MJ, et al. The analysis of clonal diversity and therapy responses using STAT3 mutations as a molecular marker in large granular lymphocytic leukemia. *Haematologica*. 2015;100(1):91-99. doi:10.3324/haematol.2014.113142
490. Andersson EI, Rajala HLM, Eldfors S, et al. Novel somatic mutations in large granular lymphocytic leukemia affecting the STAT-pathway and T-cell activation. *Blood Cancer J*. 2013;3(12):e168. doi:10.1038/bcj.2013.65
491. Ishida F, Matsuda K, Sekiguchi N, et al. STAT3 gene mutations and their association with pure red cell aplasia in large granular lymphocyte leukemia. *Cancer Sci*. 2014;105(3):342-346. doi:10.1111/cas.12341
492. Arps DP, Smith LB. Classic versus type II enteropathy-associated T-cell lymphoma: diagnostic considerations. *Arch Pathol Lab Med*. 2013;137(9):1227-1231. doi:10.5858/arpa.2013-0242-CR
493. Tan S-Y, Ooi A-S, Ang M-K, et al. Nuclear expression of MATK is a novel marker of type II enteropathy-associated T-cell lymphoma. *Leukemia*. 2011;25(3):555-557. doi:10.1038/leu.2010.295
494. Wilson AL, Swerdlow SH, Przybylski GK, et al. Intestinal γδ T-cell lymphomas are most frequently of type II enteropathy-associated T-cell type. *Hum Pathol*. 2013;44(6):1131-1145. doi:10.1016/j.humpath.2012.10.002
495. Tomita S, Kikuti YY, Carreras J, et al. Genomic and immunohistochemical profiles of enteropathy-associated T-cell lymphoma in Japan. *Mod Pathol*. 2015;28(10):1286-1296. doi:10.1038/modpathol.2015.85
496. Roberti A, Dobay MP, Bisig B, et al. Type II enteropathy-associated T-cell lymphoma features a unique genomic profile with highly recurrent SETD2 alterations. *Nat Commun*. 2016;7:12602. doi:10.1038/ncomms12602
497. Cook LBM, Demontis MA, Sagawe S, et al. Molecular remissions are observed in chronic adult T-cell leukemia/lymphoma in patients treated with mogamulizumab. *Haematologica*. 2019;104(12):E566-E569. doi:10.3324/haematol.2019.219253
498. Gillet NA, Malani N, Melamed A, et al. The host genomic environment of the provirus determines the abundance of HTLV-1-infected T-cell clones. *Blood*. 2011;117(11):3113-3122. doi:10.1182/blood-2010-10-312926
499. Kataoka K, Nagata Y, Kitanaka A, et al. Integrated molecular analysis of adult T cell leukemia/lymphoma. *Nat Genet*. 2015;47(11):1304-1315. doi:10.1038/ng.3415
500. Kataoka K, Iwanaga M, Yasunaga JI, et al. Prognostic relevance of integrated genetic profiling in adult T-cell leukemia/lymphoma. *Blood*. 2018;131(2):215-225. doi:10.1182/blood-2017-01-761874
501. Nagata Y, Kontani K, Enami T, et al. Variegated RHOA mutations in adult T-cell leukemia/lymphoma. *Blood*. 2016;127(5):596-604. doi:10.1182/blood-2015-06-644948
502. Pancewicz J, Taylor JM, Datta A, et al. Notch signaling contributes to proliferation and tumor formation of human T-cell leukemia virus type 1-associated adult T-cell leukemia. *Proc Natl Acad Sci U S A*. 2010;107(38):16619-16624. doi:10.1073/pnas.1010722107
503. Yeh C-H, Bellon M, Pancewicz-Wojtkiewicz J, Nicot C. Oncogenic mutations in the FBXW7 gene of adult T-cell leukemia patients. *Proc Natl Acad Sci U S A*. 2016;113(24):6731-6736. doi:10.1073/pnas.1601537113
504. Shah UA, Chung EY, Giricz O, et al. North American ATLL has a distinct mutational and transcriptional profile and responds to epigenetic therapies. *Blood*. 2018;132(14):1507-1518. doi:10.1182/blood-2018-01-824607
505. Can K, Xiaozhou H, Qiang G, et al. Diagnostic and biological significance of KIR expression profile determined by RNA-seq in natural killer/T-cell lymphoma. *Am J Pathol*. 2016;186:1435-1441. doi:10.1016/j.ajpath.2016.02.011
506. Lin CW, Chen YH, Chuang YC, Liu TY, Hsu SM. CD94 transcripts imply a better prognosis in nasal-type extranodal NK/T-cell lymphoma. *Blood*. 2003;102(7):2623-2631. doi:10.1182/blood-2003-01-0295
507. Lee S, Park HY, Kang SY, et al. Genetic alterations of JAK/STAT cascade and histone modification in extranodal NK/T-cell lymphoma nasal type. *Oncotarget*. 2015;6(19):17764-17776. doi:10.18632/oncotarget.3776
508. Küçük C, Jiang B, Hu X, et al. Activating mutations of STAT5B and STAT3 in lymphomas derived from γδ-T or NK cells. *Nat Commun*. 2015;6:6025. doi:10.1038/ncomms7025
509. Koo GC, Tan SY, Tang T, et al. Janus kinase 3-activating mutations identified in natural killer/T-cell lymphoma. *Cancer Discov*. 2012;2(7):591-597. doi:10.1158/2159-8290.CD-12-0028
510. Jiang L, Gu ZH, Yan ZX, et al. Exome sequencing identifies somatic mutations of DDX3X in natural killer/T-cell lymphoma. *Nat Genet*. 2015;47(9):1061-1066. doi:10.1038/ng.3358
511. Dobashi A, Tsuyama N, Asaka R, et al. Frequent BCOR aberrations in extranodal NK/T-Cell lymphoma, nasal type. *Genes Chromosomes Cancer*. 2016;55(5):460-471. doi:10.1002/gcc.22348

Chapter 90 ■ Non-Hodgkin Lymphoma in Adults

TARSHEEN K. SETHI • SHALIN KOTHARI • ERIN MULVEY • FRANCINE FOSS • JOHN P. LEONARD • JOHN P. GREER

HISTORICAL PERSPECTIVE

Since Thomas Hodgkin's initial recognition that lymphadenopathy could occur as a primary neoplasm, there have been four historical phases in the study of non-Hodgkin lymphoma (NHL): (1) clinical features, 1832 to 1900; (2) histopathology, 1900 to 1972; (3) immunopathology, 1972 to the present; and (4) molecular genetics, 1982 to the present. These phases (Table 90.1) naturally overlap and all contribute to the understanding of NHL. Immunotherapy with monoclonal antibodies and the development of targeted therapies, initially the tyrosine kinase inhibitors and subsequently the B-cell receptor inhibitors, have improved prognosis for hematopoietic neoplasms and have coincided with the expanded tools for diagnosis as outlined in the 2016 revision of the World Health Organization (WHO) classification of lymphoid malignancies.[1]

Therapy in NHL has improved with refinement of uniform diagnostic and classification criteria. In 1941, Gall and Mallory developed a classification scheme for NHL that had both clinical and histopathologic significance.[2] The histopathologic phase of NHL culminated in the 1956 classic work of Rappaport who developed a morphologic classification which stratified cases according to the pattern of growth with nodular replacing follicular and contrasting with diffuse.[3] Four categories of lymphoma were described: well differentiated lymphocytic, poorly differentiated lymphocytic, mixed lymphocytic and histiocytic, and histiocytic.

In 1967, Good and Finstad discussed the relationship of B and T cells to lymphoid neoplasia, and Dameshek introduced the concepts that lymphomas were aberrations of immunologically competent cells and that transformation of lymphocytes to "blast" forms (immunoblasts) could occur secondary to antigenic stimulation.[4] In 1972, the immunologic origin of lymphoid neoplasia was confirmed by the presence of monotypic immunoglobulin (Ig) on the cell surface (B cell) or by sheep erythrocyte rosette formation with neoplastic cells (T cell).[5,6] Lymphoblastic lymphoma (LBL) was determined to originate from thymocytes by Smith in 1973.[6] Barcos and Lukes described the clinicopathologic features of "convoluted lymphocytic lymphoma" of thymic origin and used the term LL, which was later preferred by Nathwani because of similarities to blasts of T-cell acute lymphoblastic leukemia (ALL).[7]

Table 90.1. History of Diagnosis and Classifications of Non-Hodgkin Lymphoma

Year	Investigator	Milestone
1832	Hodgkin	Wilks gave credit to Hodgkin in 1865 for recognizing cancer originating from lymph nodes
1863–1865	Virchow	Introduced term lymphosarcoma as distinct from leukemia
1871	Billroth	Used the term malignant lymphoma
1893	Kundrat	Lymphosarcoma should be reserved for sarcomatous tumors of lymph nodes
1898, 1902	Sternberg, Reed	Identified binucleated cells characteristic of Hodgkin lymphoma (HL)
1925, 1927	Brill, Symmers	Described follicular lymphoma as an indolent malignancy
1914, 1928, 1930	Ewing, Oberling, Roulet	Used the term reticulum cell sarcoma for large cell lymphoma
1942	Gall and Mallory	Classification of non-Hodgkin lymphoma (NHL)
1947	Robb-Smith; Jackson and Parker	Reviews of NHL and HL
1956	Rappaport	Classification of NHL: nodular replaced follicular and was distinguished from diffuse pattern. Four types were described (see text)
1958	Burkitt	Aggressive lymphoma in children across equatorial Africa
1964	Epstein, Barr, and Achong	Found viral particles in Burkitt lymphoma
1967	Cooper, Good, and Finstad	Recognized B and T cells
1967	Dameshek	Lymphomas were aberrations of immunologically competent cells and lymphocytes could transform to immunoblasts secondary to antigenic stimulation
1972	Aisenberg and Bloch; Preud'homme and Seligmann	B-cell origin of lymphoma was confirmed by the presence of monotypic immunoglobulin on the cell surface
1972	Smith	T-cell origin of lymphoblastic lymphoma was identified by sheep erythrocyte rosette formation with neoplastic cells
1973	Barcos and Lukes	Lymphoblastic lymphoma of thymic origin was described
1974	Lennert (Kiel); Lukes and Collins	Immunologic classifications for NHL, separating into B- and T-cell neoplasms
1976	Zech, Klein	Recurrent cytogenetic translocations involving the immunoglobulin gene on chromosome 14 were found in Burkitt lymphoma
1977	Takatsuki and Uchiyama	Clinical description of adult T-cell leukemia/lymphoma (ATL) in Japan
1978	Isaacson and Wright	Introduced the term of mucosa-associated lymphoid tissue (MALToma) for an indolent B-cell lymphoma arising in extranodal sites
1979	Fukuhara, Rowley	Recurrent translocations involving the immunoglobulin gene locus on chromosome 14 were found in follicular lymphoma

(Continued)

Table 90.1. History of Diagnosis and Classifications of Non-Hodgkin Lymphoma *(Continued)*

Year	Investigator	Milestone
1980-1982	Poiesz, Gallo; Yoshida, Hinuma	Discovered a retrovirus, HTLV-1, as the etiologic agent for ATL
1980-1982	Stein, Poppema, Warnke, and Mason	Lymphoid cells identified by immunohistochemistry on frozen and paraffin sections
1981	Korsmeyer	Rearrangement of immunoglobulin genes proved clonality of B-cell lymphomas
1982	Berard, Dorfman, DeVita, Rosenberg	Working Formulation separated lymphomas according to three histologic grades (see text)
1982	Doll, List	First case of lymphoma in a patient with acquired immunodeficiency syndrome (AIDS)
1982	Taub, Leder, Dalla-Favera, and Croce	*MYC* gene was translocated from chromosome 8 to immunoglobulin genes in Burkitt lymphoma
1984	Ziegler	NHL described in 90 homosexual patients; NHL recognized as a criterion for AIDS in 1987
1984-1985	Tsujimoto	Genetic translocations defined follicular lymphoma, *BCL2/IGH*, and mantle cell lymphoma, *CCND1/IGH*
1985	Waldmann, Minden, Aisenberg	Rearrangements of genes for the antigen receptors of T cells identified lineage and clonality in T-cell neoplasms
1985	Stein	Initial description of Ki-1+ (CD30) anaplastic large cell lymphoma (ALCL)
1989	Kaneko	A novel translocation, t(2:5) (p23;q35), was found in ALCL of T-cell origin
1991-1992	Isaacson and Stein	Founded the International Lymphoma Study Group (ILSG) and consensus report on the diagnosis of mantle cell lymphoma
1993-1994	Wotherspoon, Parsonett	*Helicobacter pylori* infection preceded gastric MALToma and antibiotics caused regression in two-thirds of cases
1994	Morris	The genes, *ALK/NPM*, were identified in t(2; 5) of ALCL
1994	Harris, Isaacson, and Stein	Revised European-American Lymphoma (REAL) classification developed a consensus for describing the B- and T-cell origins of NHL
1997	Armitage	Validation of the REAL classification by the ILSG
2000	Staudt	Gene expression profiling of lymphomas
2001	Hematopathology associations—Jaffe et al	World Health Organization (WHO) adopted the diagnostic principles of the REAL classification in a monograph: *Pathology and Genetics of Hematopoietic and Lymphoid Tissues* (Third edition)
2008	Hematopathology associations—Swerdlow et al	*WHO Classification of Tumors of Hematopoietic and Lymphoid Tissues* (Fourth edition)
2011	Tiacci	*BRAF* V600 E was found in most cases of hairy cell leukemia and in many histiocytic neoplasms
2012	Treon	*MYD88* L265P mutations were present in 90% of Waldenström macroglobulinemia
2016	Hematopathology associations—Swerdlow et al	Revisions of the WHO classifications for hematopoietic neoplasms *WHO Classification of Tumors of Hematopoietic and Lymphoid Tissues* (Revised Fourth edition)

In 1974, Lennert in Kiel, Germany, and Lukes and Collins in the United States classified NHL on the basis of the cell of origin within the immune system (*Figure 90.1*).[8] Monoclonal antibodies to lymphocyte differentiation antigens have been used to define sequential stages in the development of B and T cells and to identify subtypes of NHL. Recurrent cytogenetic translocations involving the Ig gene locus on chromosome 14 were identified in Burkitt lymphoma (BL) in 1976 and in follicular lymphoma (FL) in 1979.[9,10] In the 1980s, the lymphoid origin of NHL was confirmed at the molecular level with the identification of specific Ig gene and T-cell receptor (TCR) gene rearrangements in B-cell lymphoma and T-cell lymphoma (TCL), respectively.[11,12]

In 1982, a Working Formulation (WF) of NHL separated diseases according to histologic grade and made correlations with survival; however, the WF lumped disparate diseases together by basing the diagnosis on morphology without utilizing immunophenotyping or molecular genetic techniques. The laboratories of Leder and Croce in 1982 identified *MYC* as the gene translocated from chromosome 8 to the Ig locus in BL.[11,13] Subsequently, the genes defining FL, *BCL2/IGH*, and mantle cell lymphoma (MCL), *CCND1/IGH*, were described.[14,15] Although specific genetic changes are less common in TCLs, in 1989, a proportion of T-anaplastic large cell lymphomas (ALCLs) were found to have recurrent translocations involving t(2;5) (p23;q35)[16]; and in 1994, Morris identified the genes, *ALK/NPM*, involved in the translocation.[17]

Isaacson and Stein formed an international group of pathologists (International Lymphoma Study Group) to develop a consensus about diagnosis and terminology of lymphoid neoplasms.[18] In 1994, a Revised European-American Lymphoma (REAL) classification was proposed to identify specific types of lymphomas of B- and T-cell origin.[19] The REAL classification dropped the grading schema of lymphomas and developed a diagnosis by identifying clinical features, morphology, immunophenotype, and genetic data when available. An International Lymphoma Classification Project organized by Armitage affirmed the clinical utility and the reproducibility of the REAL classification.[20] The WHO adopted the diagnostic principles of the REAL classification and has periodically revised the diagnosis and classification of all hematopoietic neoplasms.[21]

EPIDEMIOLOGY

A worldwide epidemic of NHL, varying by gender, race, and geography, has occurred but reached a plateau at the end of the 20th century. Per the Surveillance, Epidemiology, and End Results (SEER) program, the age-adjusted incidence of NHL in the United States increased from 11.1 per 100,000 people in 1975 to 20.0 in 1995. Over

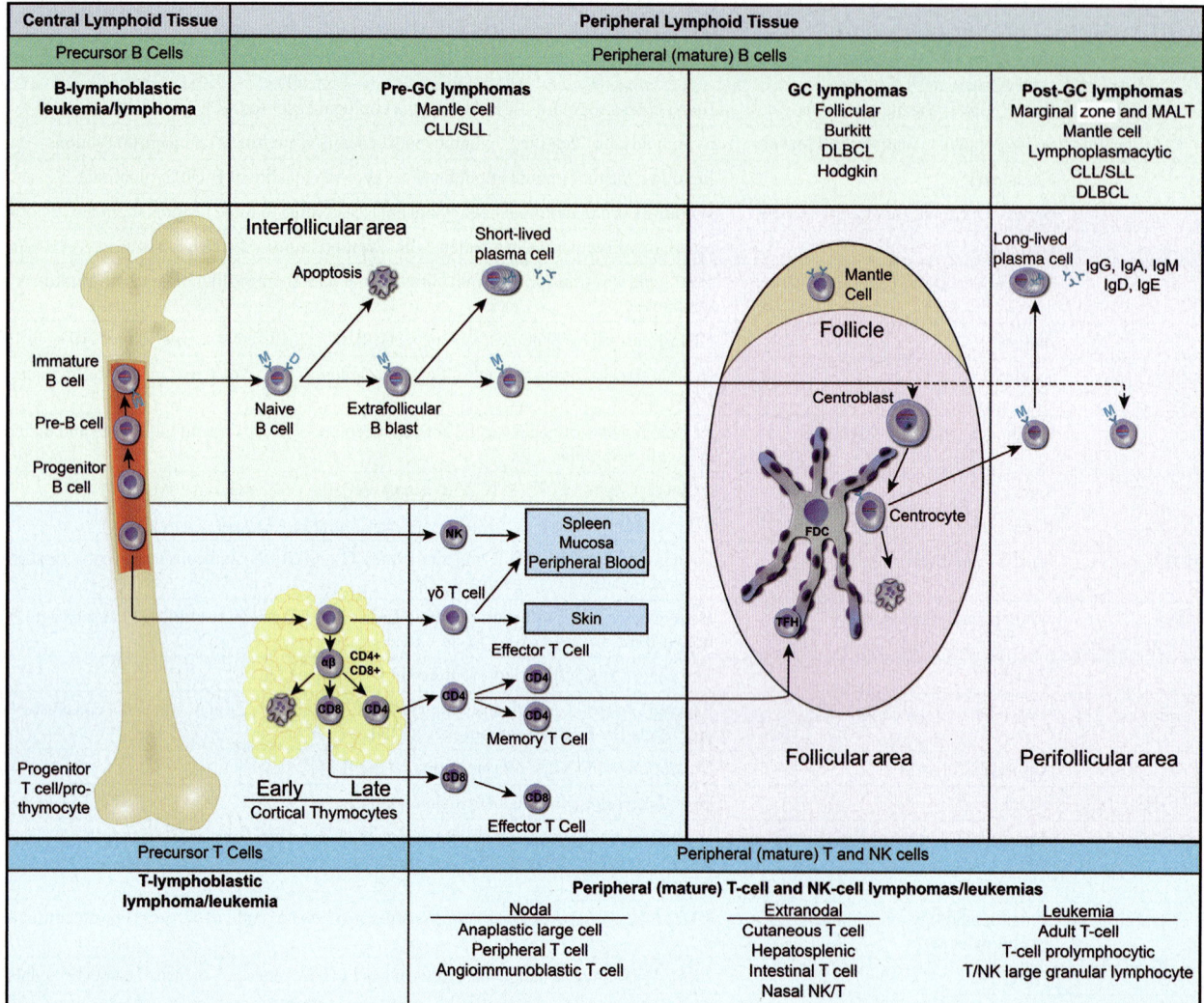

FIGURE 90.1 Cellular origins of non-Hodgkin lymphoma by B- and T-cell differentiation pathways: B and T cells originate in the marrow where they are antigen independent. In the germinal center (GC), B cells normally progress through stages in response to antigen exposure: (a) proliferation of centroblasts (large noncleaved cells), (b) selection of centrocytes (small cleaved cells) or cell death via apoptosis, (c) differentiation into postgerminal center memory B lymphocytes or plasma cells with increased antigen affinity and an Ig isotype switch. Early T-cell differentiation occurs in the thymus. The most immature T-cell precursors are negative for both CD4 and CD8. Thymocytes can become committed to either the γ-δ or α-β lineage. As thymocytes within the α-β lineage mature, they gain expression of both CD4 and CD8. Normal thymocytes downregulate the expression of CD4 or CD8 before moving into the periphery as naïve T cells, which are subdivided into helper (CD4$^+$) and suppressor/cytotoxic (CD8$^+$) subsets. Lymphomas arise with disordered or arrested development of malignant lymphocytes. Precursor B and T cells within the marrow or thymus are associated with acute lymphoblastic leukemia or lymphoblastic lymphoma. Mature lymphoid neoplasms correspond with stage of cellular differentiation and site(s) of nodal and/or extranodal origin. B-cell lymphomas include pre-GC, GC, and post-GC types. Mantle cell leukemia and chronic lymphocytic leukemia (CLL)/small B-cell lymphocytic lymphoma (SLL) have both pre- and post-GC variants. Diffuse large B-cell lymphoma (DLBCL) can be of a GC origin or an activated B cell, or post-GC, type. Marginal zone lymphomas are post-GC nodal type or extranodal mucosal–associated lymphoid type (MALT). Peripheral T/NK neoplasms may involve the interfollicular zone, the sinus (anaplastic large cell), specific extranodal sites, or bone marrow with leukemic presentation. (The figure was drawn by Kate Mittendorf, PhD, and is adapted from Jaffe ES, Harris NL, Stein H, Isaacson PG. Classification of lymphoid neoplasms: the microscope as a tool for disease discovery. *Blood*. 2008;112:4384-4399.)

the past 2 decades, the incidence has ranged between 19.4 and 21.4 (*Figure 90.2*). In 2021, the estimated number of new cases in the United States was 81,560 (4.3% of all cancers) and the deaths were 20,720 (3.4% of all cancer deaths). Death rates have dropped an average of 2.2% per year from 2010 to 2019, and the 5-year relative survival has improved from 51.9% in 1995 to 75.8% in 2013.

The increased incidence of NHL was partly attributed to opportunistic NHL in patients with the acquired immunodeficiency syndrome (AIDS); however, there are a myriad of other possible contributing factors to the epidemic (*Table 90.2*). Even before the AIDS crisis, there was a steady increase of 3% to 4% per year from the 1970s up until the mid-1990s, when there was a plateau and a decline in some subgroups of patients. Part of the drop-off was due to the introduction of antiretroviral therapy (ART) for AIDS patients.[22] Improved disease detection and cancer registration likely also inflated case number, but the consensus is that the initial increase in NHL remains unexplained by either the improvements in diagnosis or the AIDS epidemic. For similarly unclear reasons, age-adjusted rates subsequently fell 0.9% per year from 2009 to 2018.

Age, Race, Sex, and Familial Differences

The frequency of various lymphoid neoplasms is age dependent, has a variable worldwide distribution, and is more common in males than in females. Lymphomas represent approximately 10% of all childhood cancers in developed countries and are third in relative frequency behind acute leukemias and brain tumors. They are more common in adults than in children and have a steady increase in incidence from childhood through age 80 years (*Figure 90.3*). They are the seventh

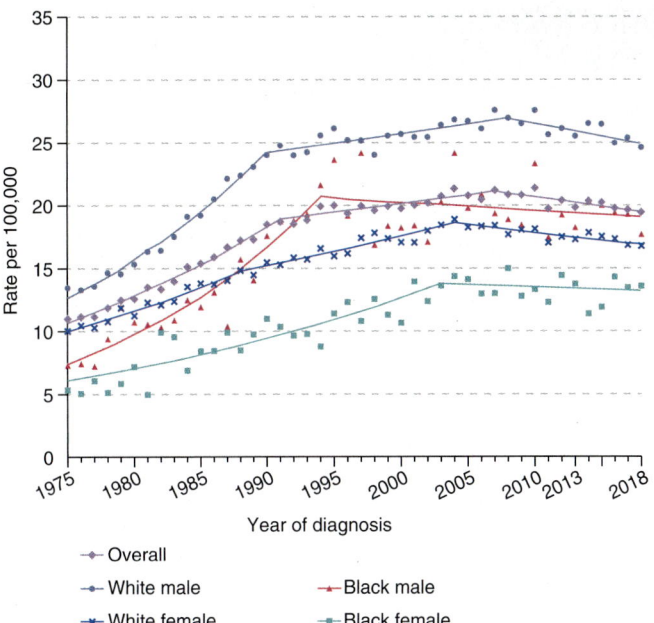

FIGURE 90.2 Temporal trends in the age-adjusted incidence rates of NHL in the United States (SEER data, 1975-2013).

Table 90.2. Epidemiologic Factors That Are Associated With an Increased Risk of Non-Hodgkin Lymphoma

Immunodeficiency
    Congenital
    Acquired

Infectious agents
Male gender
Increasing age
Family history of non-Hodgkin lymphoma
Prior cancer history

Drug Exposure:
    Immunosuppressive agents
    Antiepileptic medication

Occupational History
Exposure to: herbicides
    pesticides
    wood dust
    epoxy glue
    solvents

Other possible etiologic factors
    Hair dye use
    Nutritional factors
    Blood transfusion

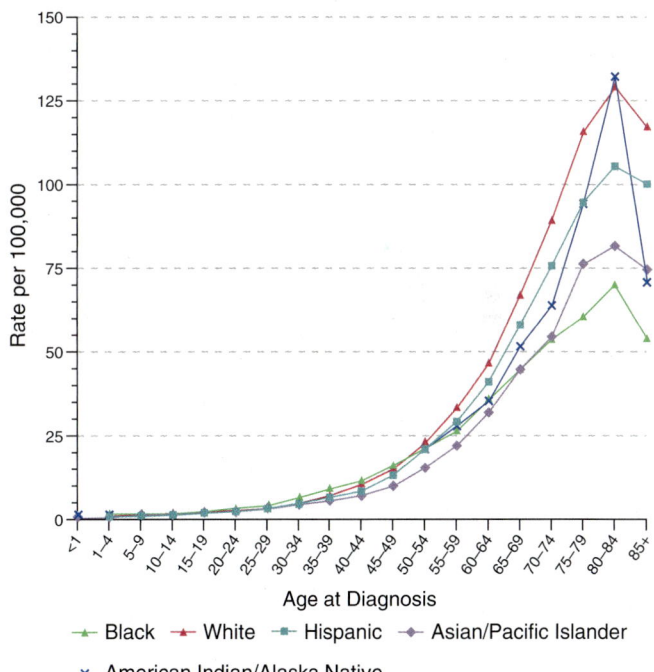

FIGURE 90.3 Age-specific incidence rates of NHL according to race (SEER data, 1975-2014).

most common cancer among males and the sixth most common among females in the United States. The median age at diagnosis was 67 years for 2014 to 2018. The annual incidence rate of NHL was 40% higher for males (23.7 per 100,000) than females (16.2 per 100,000). The median age of death was 76 years of age. The highest age-adjusted mortality is in white males (7.1 per 100,000) and the lowest mortality has been in Asian/Pacific Islander females (3.3 per 100,000). Per the Global Cancer Incidence, Mortality and Prevalence in 2020, there were 544,352 new cases worldwide and 259,793 deaths. The highest recorded incidence occurred in Australia and New Zealand, North America, and Europe (*Figure 90.4*).

A comparison of NHL in children and adults is outlined in *Table 90.3*. Lymphomas involving peripheral lymph nodes are usually of B-cell origin in North America and Europe and are more common in adults than in children who often present with gastrointestinal involvement (BL) or mediastinal widening (usually LBL of T-cell origin). The histologic appearance of NHL is more variable in adults, who frequently have low-grade follicular or diffuse patterns in which the majority of malignant cells are small, dormant lymphocytes; children predominantly have high-grade diffuse patterns in which the malignant cells have a "blastic" or transformed appearance and a high mitotic rate. Mature T-cell malignancies are more common in Asia due to viral associations, Epstein-Barr virus (EBV) in nasal natural killer (NK)/T-cell neoplasms and human T-lymphotropic virus type 1 (HTLV-1) in adult T-cell leukemia/lymphoma (ATL).

Extranodal presentation of NHL occurs in 15% to 25% of adult patients in the United States, is higher in Europe, and is 40% to 50% in Asia.[23] Clinicopathologic features of the epidemic of NHL included a faster rise in extranodal than nodal disease, an increase in diffuse pattern over nodular, and in aggressive over indolent disease.[24] NHL of the brain incidence rose four times as rapidly as other extranodal sites during the 1980s and early 1990s and was primarily due to AIDS in men, but the upward trend began before the AIDS crisis and was seen in immunocompetent hosts of all ages and in both genders.[25] After 1995, the overall incidence of central nervous system (CNS) lymphoma declined with a drop in cases in young and middle-aged men due to effective ART, but the rate continued to increase in men over 65 years of age and in women.[26]

Familial aggregation of NHL plays a small role in the epidemic and accounts for a 1.5- to 4-fold increased risk for NHL in close relatives of patients with lymphoma or other hematopoietic neoplasm.[27] The lifetime risk of NHL is 3.6% in first-degree relatives compared to 2.1% in the general population of the United States.[28] In a twin study, there was a 23-fold higher risk in monozygotic twins and a 14-fold higher risk in dizygotic twins, suggesting a genetic role in the former, but also an environmental factor in the latter.[29] Aggregation has been reported to be stronger for siblings and male relatives.[30] Anticipation (earlier age of onset in subsequent generation) has been reported in NHL[31]; however, others have disputed the finding by suggesting that the studies did not account for the increasing incidence of NHL.[32]

A family history of a specific subtype has been associated with higher risk of developing that same subtype, particularly for diffuse

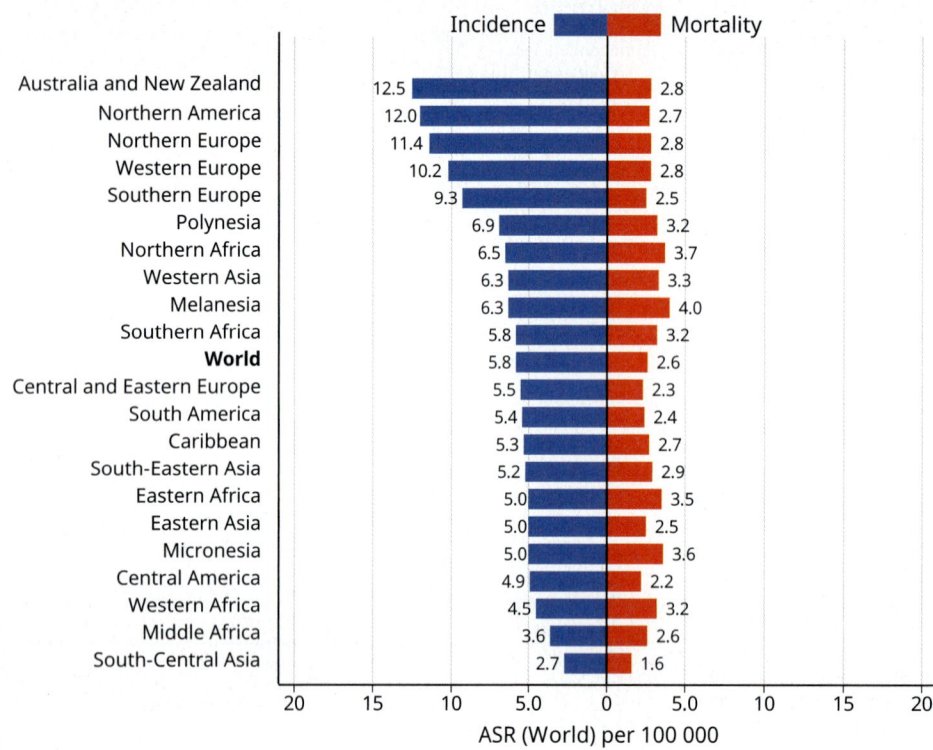

FIGURE 90.4 Age-adjusted incidence and mortality rates of NHL in selected world regions. ASR, age-standardized rate; NHL, non-Hodgkin lymphoma. (From International Agency for Research on Cancer. Globocan 2020: estimated cancer incidence, mortality and prevalence worldwide 2020.)

large B-cell lymphoma (DLBCL).[28] Genome-wide association studies have identified a locus at the human leukocyte class II region on chromosome 6p21.32 as a risk factor for both FL and DLBCL.[33] Other single nucleotide polymorphisms (SNPs; at 6p25.3 [*EXOC2*], 2p23.3 [*NCOA1*], and 8q24.21 [near *PVT1* and *MYC*]) have also been associated with DLBCL. There have been over 60 SNPs from 41 genetic loci associated with NHL; however, the modest familial risk and the relative low incidence of NHL, along with the lack of available interventions, presently argue against routine genomic screening for families affected by lymphomas.

Table 90.3. Clinicopathologic Differences Between Childhood and Adult Non-Hodgkin Lymphomas

	Children	Adults
Incidence	Rare	Common
Median Age	10-15 y	60-70 y
Presentation	Extranodal > nodal	Nodal > extranodal
Most common histologic diagnoses	B cell: Burkitt Diffuse large cell T cell: Lymphoblastic ALK+ Anaplastic large cell	B cell: Diffuse large cell Follicular T cell: Peripheral T cell, not otherwise specified Anaplastic large cell Angioimmunoblastic
Immunophenotype	60%-70% B cell	85%-90% B cell (United States, Europe); 20%-35% T/NK cell (Asia)
Paraprotein	None	Rare (<5%)
Clinical course	Aggressive	Variable-often indolent
Curability	70%-95%	<30%, except 50%-75% in aggressive subtypes, particularly diffuse large B-cell lymphoma

There is an increased risk for B-cell lymphomas in families with an autoimmune lymphoproliferative syndrome (ALPS, also known as the Canale-Smith syndrome) which is characterized by chronic lymphadenopathy, splenomegaly, autoimmune features, and defective lymphocyte apoptosis.[34,35] Expanded TCRαβ+ cells, double negative for CD4 and CD8, and elevated plasma levels of Fas ligand and interleukin (IL)-10 are diagnostic.[36] Both NHL and Hodgkin lymphoma (HL), particularly nodular lymphocyte predominant, may occur decades after recognition of the syndrome and are predominantly associated with germline and/or somatic mutations of the genes coding for FAS and its ligand.[37] Mutations in other subtypes of ALPS involve caspase 10 (*CASP10*), *CASP8*, *NRAS*, and *KRAS*; 20% to 30% of cases have an unidentified genetic defect.[35]

A prior history of cancer, Jewish ancestry, and small size families have been suggested as risk factors for lymphoma.[38] In families with a diagnosis of NHL, there are reports indicating an increased risk for other cancers, including melanoma, pancreatic, and gastric.[39] Patients who have both a family history of hematologic cancer and occupational exposures to certain substances (e.g., gasoline or benzene) may have an increased risk for NHL.[40] In a Swedish registry, there was a 40% higher rate of solid tumors and a fivefold increase in myelodysplastic syndrome (MDS)/acute myeloid leukemia (AML) in patients with NHL, with the latter likely related to chemotherapy.[41] The risk of MDS/AML has diminished in FL in the past decade likely due to a shift from chemotherapy to targeted and biologic agents.

Infectious Agents

Infectious diseases have contributed to understanding mechanisms of lymphomagenesis. The role infections play in specific lymphomas varies according to host factors, environment, and geography. There are at least two mechanisms in which infections contribute to lymphomagenesis. The best described is direct lymphocyte transformation by microbial agents. Lymphotropic viruses include EBV, HTLV-1, and human herpesvirus 8 (HHV-8). Other microorganisms, such as *Helicobacter pylori*, infect host tissues and elicit a lymphoproliferative response that remains dependent on the presence of the agent

Table 90.4. Infections and Associations With Lymphoma

Agent	Lymphoma Type(s)
Epstein-Barr virus	Burkitt lymphoma (Africa) Posttransplant lymphoproliferative disorders Acquired immunodeficiency syndrome–related lymphoma (central nervous system, others) Nasal natural killer/T-cell lymphoma Hodgkin lymphoma Diffuse large B-cell lymphoma Peripheral T-cell lymphoma, including angio-immunoblastic T-cell lymphoma
Human T-lymphotropic virus type 1	Adult T-cell leukemia/lymphoma
Human herpesvirus 8/ Kaposi sarcoma–associated herpesvirus	Primary effusion lymphoma Plasmablastic lymphoma
Helicobacter pylori	Gastric MALToma[a]
Hepatitis B virus	Diffuse large B-cell lymphoma
Hepatitis C virus	Splenic marginal zone lymphoma; other B-cell lymphomas
Campylobacter jejuni	Immunoproliferative small intestinal disease[a]
Borrelia burgdorferi	Primary cutaneous B-cell lymphoma[a]
Chlamydia psittaci	Ocular adnexal lymphoma[a]

[a]Extranodal marginal zone lymphoma, MALT type.

or an antigen. The former does not usually respond to antimicrobial therapy, whereas the latter does. There are an expanding number of infections associated with specific types of NHL (Table 90.4).

The complex interplay of environmental and host factors in the pathogenesis of lymphoma was recognized through Dennis Burkitt's description in 1958 of an aggressive tumor of young children that was characterized by frequent jaw and abdominal involvement (*Figure 90.5A*). Using careful epidemiologic surveys, Burkitt identified a tumor belt across equatorial Africa that was associated with temperature, rainfall, and elevation (*Figure 90.5B*).[42] Subsequently, the geographic distribution of this neoplasm was shown to correlate with that of endemic malaria. In 1964, Epstein, Achong, and Barr found viral particles in tumor cell lines derived from Burkitt's patients.[43] A direct causative role for the virus was subsequently questioned by its infrequency in BL occurring outside Africa; however, EBV was shown to be trophic for B cells, to induce B-cell proliferation and differentiation, and to be the etiologic agent for infectious mononucleosis. In 1965, Burkitt discovered that the lymphoma could be cured with chemotherapy.[44]

Following the discovery of the 8;14 translocation with endemic Burkitt NHL in the 1970s, lymphomagenesis was thought to arise in a state of EBV-induced polyclonal B-cell proliferation in the setting of immunodeficiency associated with chronic malaria.[45] Supporting this theory, EBV plays a role in lymphoproliferation in other immunodeficient conditions, such as post–organ transplant lymphomas, AIDS-related lymphomas (most CNS and variably with systemic), and plasmablastic lymphoma (PBL), often in the setting of AIDS. EBV has also been associated with some peripheral T/NK lymphomas, particularly nasal and angioimmunoblastic types, a proportion of HL, some DLBCL (formerly of the elderly type), hydroa vacciniforme (usually in childhood) that can evolve to lymphoma, and rare lymphomas that can occur after chronic infectious mononucleosis.

Shortly after immunologic classifications for NHL were proposed, adult T-cell leukemia/lymphoma was described in Japan by Takatsuki and Uchiyama in 1977.[46] The clinical course of ATL was variable, but the majority of patients presented with an acute leukemia or lymphoma forms, which were characterized by lymphadenopathy, organomegaly, skin lesions, hypercalcemia, and an elevated white count with multilobated lymphocytes (in the acute leukemia type), referred to as "cloverleaf" or "flower" cells, and a rapidly fatal course. In 1980 to 1982, Poiesz et al in Gallo's lab in the United States and Yoshida et al in Hinuma's lab in Japan independently discovered a unique retrovirus, HTLV-1, as the etiologic agent of ATL.[47,48] HTLV-1 was shown to be endemic to certain geographic areas: southwestern Japan, the Caribbean Islands, New Guinea, parts of Central and West equatorial Africa, parts of South America, the Middle East, and central Australia (*Figure 90.6*).[49] Epidemiologic data are incomplete from parts of the world such as India and China.

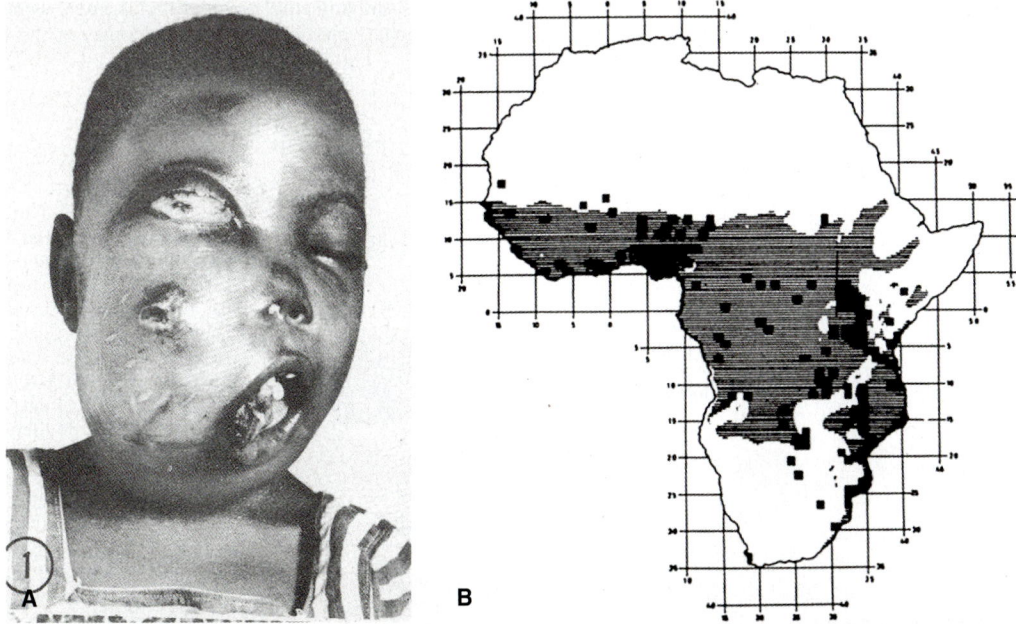

FIGURE 90.5 A, Burkitt lymphoma involving mandible, maxilla, and orbit. B, Lymphoma belt of Africa: Burkitt lymphoma occurred only in areas below 3000 ft (above sea level), with mean temperature above 15.6 °C, and with annual rainfall over 50 cm. Shaded area, where Burkitt lymphoma would be expected to occur; black squares, sites of cases identified by Burkitt. (A, From O'Conor GT. Significant aspects of childhood lymphoma in Africa. *Cancer Res*. 1963;23(9 Pt 1):1514-1527; Copyright ©1963 American Association for Cancer Research. With permission from AACR. B, From Haddow AJ. An improved map for study of Burkitt lymphoma syndrome in Africa. *East Afr Med J*. 1963;40:429-432. Reprinted by permission of Prof. Lukoye Atwoli.)

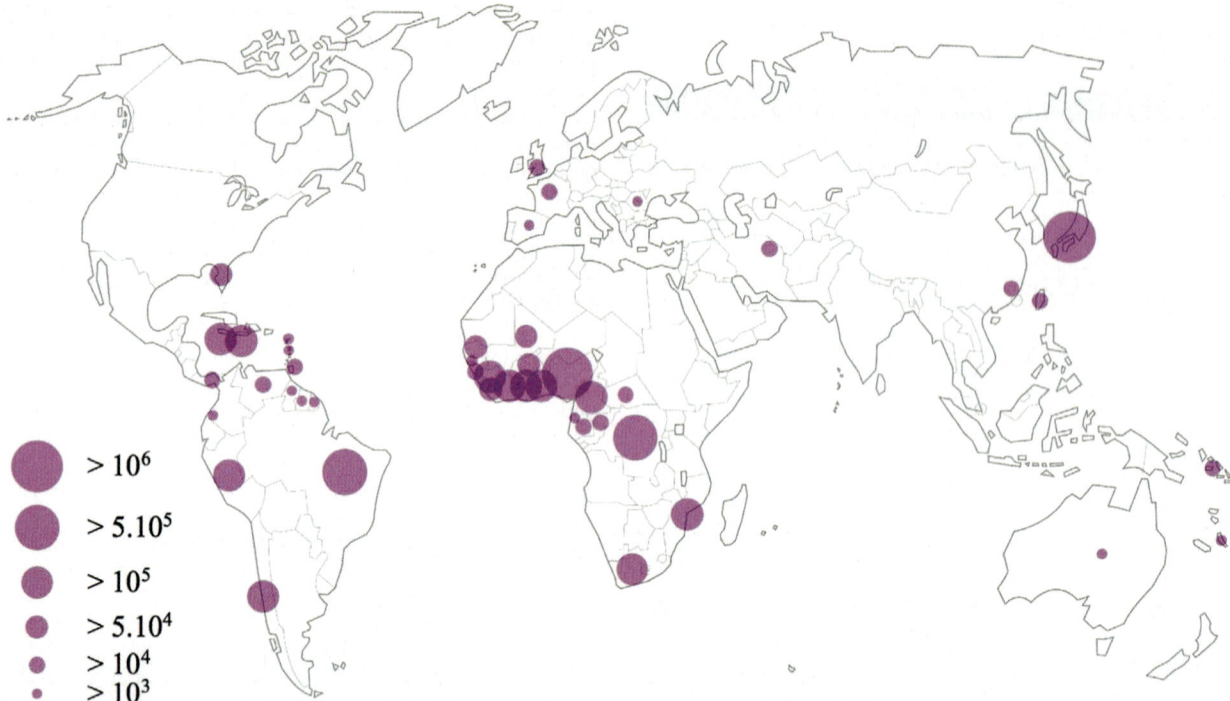

FIGURE 90.6 Geographic distribution of HTLV-1 infection. Estimates of the number of carriers based on approximately 1.5 billion individuals from known endemic areas and epidemiologic data. (From Gessain A, Cassar O. Epidemiological aspects and world distribution of HTLV-1 infection. *Front Microbiol.* 2012;3:388. https://creativecommons.org/licenses/by/3.0)

HTLV-1 is an RNA-containing delta retrovirus that infects a mature T cell, usually CD3+, CD4+, and HLA-DR+. The molecular pathogenesis revolves around Tax, a potent HTLV-1 transcription activator protein, and HTLV-1 basic ZIP factor, HBZ (*Figure 90.7*).[50] T-cell dysregulation may initially involve an autocrine IL-2 loop as well as paracrine effects from other cellular genes and cytokines. Tax is prominent during the initial infection by increasing the expression of viral genes through viral long terminal repeats (LTRs) and by stimulating the transcription of cellular genes through signaling pathways of nuclear factor kappa B (NFκB), serum response factor (SRF), cyclic AMP response element binding protein (CREB), and activated protein 1.[51] Tax induces proliferation and inhibits apoptosis of HTLV-1 cells through induction of IκB-α degradation, which activates the NFκB pathway, promoting expression of cell-cycle regulators (cyclin D2 and CDK6) and leads to increased activation of PI3-kinase signaling.[52] Tax deregulates the expression of cytokines (IL-2 and IL-15) and anti-apoptotic genes, upregulates vascular cell adhesion molecules, activates osteoclasts, and alters interferon (IFN) signaling, all of which contribute to the pathogenesis of ATL.

HBZ is transcribed from the 3′-LTR and is the only gene which is conserved and unmethylated in all ATL cases, whereas the *TAX* gene is often inactivated by epigenetic changes or the loss of 5′-LTR.[53]

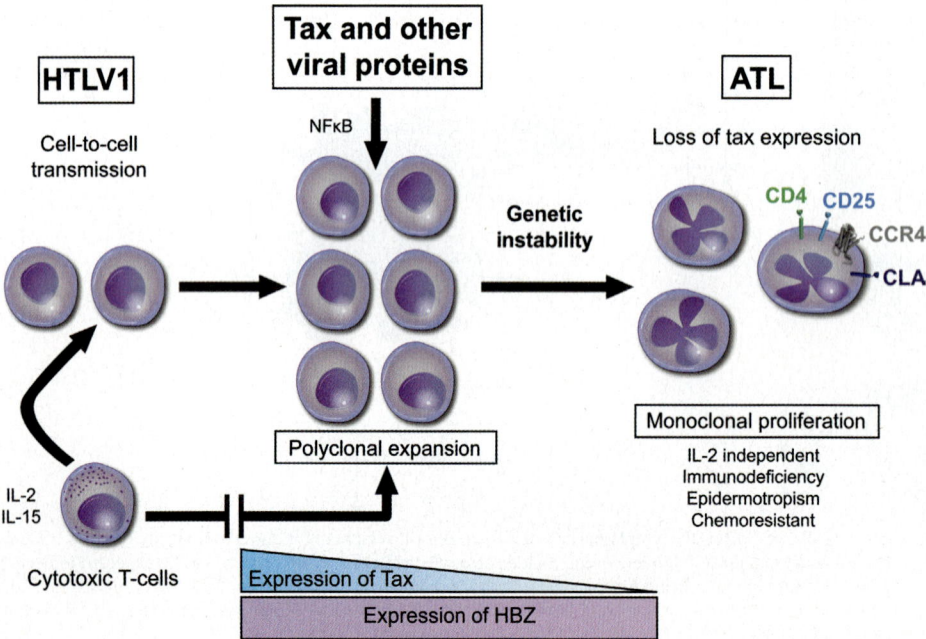

FIGURE 90.7 Course of human T-lymphotropic virus type 1 (HTLV-1) infection. After infection of a mature T_H cell, there is a long latency period (decades) which can be controlled by cytotoxic T cells and an autocrine IL-2 loop. Clonal proliferation is promoted by pleiotropic actions of Tax and other viral proteins that inhibit apoptosis and induce IκBα which activates the NFκB pathway. *HBZ* promotes T-cell proliferation and the HBZ protein suppresses *TAX*-mediated viral transcription. As TAX expression is lost, there is emergence of a monoclonal T-cell population that is independent of IL-2. CC chemokine receptor 4 (CCR4) and cutaneous lymphocyte antigen (CLA) on adult T-cell leukemia/lymphoma (ATL) cells interact with endothelial cells in the skin and contribute to epidermotropism. ATL follows a multistep process of worsening genetic instability and is subdivided into clinical syndromes characterized by immunodeficiency and chemoresistance. (The figure was drawn by Kate Mittendorf, PhD.)

HBZ promotes T-cell proliferation in its RNA form by the regulation of E2F transcription factor 1 pathway; the HBZ protein interacts with CREB-2 and suppresses Tax-mediated viral transcription. Initially, the T lymphoproliferation is polyclonal and controlled by host defense mechanisms; however, as Tax expression diminishes, an oligoclonal or monoclonal T-cell proliferation that is IL-2 independent emerges, resulting in the clinical manifestations of ATL. HTLV-1 contributes to a multistep process of worsening genetic instability characterized by mutation of *TP53*, deletion of tumor suppressor genes *CDKN2B/p15* and *CDKN2A/p16*, and DNA methylation.

HTLV-1 can be transmitted from mother to child through breast milk or the placenta and by blood transfusions, needle sharing, or sexual intercourse. Ten to 20 million people worldwide are estimated to be infected with HTLV-1, but over 90% will remain asymptomatic carriers.[54] The virus has a prolonged latency period of decades before clinical syndromes appear. Detecting driver mutations 2 to 10 years before a clinical syndrome occurs may enable early detection of individuals at risk and allow possible intervention.[55] There is a lifetime ATL risk of approximately 1% to 6% for those persons seropositive for HTLV-1 antibodies; males have had a risk of 6% to 7%, while females have been 2% to 3%.

In the 1980s, ATL had a male:female ratio in Japan of 1.4:1 and a peak age around 60 years but the ratio is now approaching one with a median age close to 70 years[56,57]; whereas in the Caribbean, there is no gender difference and the peak age is 40 to 50 years.[58,59] In Japan, there are approximately 1.1 million people infected; there are 1500 cases of ATL diagnosed yearly; and there has been steady rate of 1000 deaths from ATL for over 2 decades.[56] There are 4000 newly infected people with HTLV-1 found each year in Japan; however, the number is projected to decline due to HTLV-1 screening of pregnant women, limiting breast feeding for mothers who test positive, and antibody screening of blood donors since 1986. The majority of endemic areas do not have a policy about breastfeeding by HTLV-1 positive mothers.[59]

Other viruses have been implicated in lymphoid neoplasia and include HTLV-2, HHV-6, HHV-8 (also referred to as Kaposi sarcoma–associated herpesvirus), and hepatitis B virus (HBV) and hepatitis C virus (HCV). HTLV-2 was isolated in 1982 by Kalyanaraman et al from a patient with an unusual T-cell variant of hairy cell leukemia.[60] HTLV-2 is less common than HTLV-1 with less than 1 million people infected worldwide.[61] It has not been linked to lymphoproliferative disease and rarely has been found in HTLV-1-negative tropical spastic paraparesis. It is considered an ancestral virus that is prevalent in indigenous peoples of North, Central, and South America, particularly Brazil, and has been reported in intravenous drug users.[62] Two other related viruses, HTLV-3 and HTLV-4, were reported in 2005 in Central Africa but have not been linked to disease.[63] Salahuddin et al identified HHV-6 in B lymphocytes from six patients with various lymphoproliferative disorders[64]; it was subsequently found as the etiologic agent for exanthema subitum (roseola infantum) and as a cause for pneumonia in immunocompromised hosts.[65] HHV-8 has been identified in multicentric Castleman disease (CD) and AIDS-related body cavity–based B-cell lymphomas, where coinfection with EBV is common and absence of *MYC* gene rearrangements notable.[66,67]

There is a twofold to threefold and a twofold to fourfold risk of developing NHL in HBV- and HCV-infected patients, respectively. The risk of lymphoma in patients infected with HBV increases with increasing age so that there is a sixfold increase in patients 65 and older compared to those aged 25 to 44 years.[68] HBV is highly endemic in Asia, Africa, the Middle East, parts of Eastern Europe, and parts of South America. Although the data are limited in regard to the subtype of NHL, DLBCL appears to be associated with HBV more than other types with higher prevalence in endemic areas.[69] Besides the association of HBV with NHL, cytotoxic therapy, particularly when given with an anti-CD20 monoclonal antibody, can lead to HBV reactivation resulting in hepatitis and even liver failure.[70] Screening HBV serologies prior to therapy and prophylaxis with antiviral therapy for positive patients can decrease the rate of reactivation.[71]

The incubation time for lymphoma to occur in patients infected with HCV is estimated to be as long as 15 years.[72] The fraction of NHL caused by HCV varies widely according to country, but is estimated to be as high as 10% where HCV is endemic, such as Egypt, Italy, and South Korea. Chronic HCV infection is often (40%-90%) present in patients with type II mixed cryoglobulinemia (MC); and 5% to 10% of MC patients have or will develop a B-cell lymphoma.[73] The B-NHL subtypes most frequently associated with HCV are marginal zone lymphomas (MZL), particularly of the splenic type; DLBCL; and lymphoplasmacytic lymphoma (LPL).[74] HCV-infected NHL patients have more advanced stage disease, liver and spleen involvement, and adverse prognostic factors than NHL patients without HCV.[75] For MZL and other indolent lymphomas that may not require conventional chemotherapy, antiviral therapy, formerly with IFN and ribavirin and now with direct-acting antivirals (DAAs), may be used as frontline therapy due to reports of regression.[76] Due to higher antiviral response and better tolerability, there is a trend to use the DAA over IFN.[77] Although rituximab was previously omitted to avoid hepatic toxicity, there is emerging support for the concurrent administration of DAA with combination chemotherapy and anti-CD20 monoclonal antibody in hepatitis C patients with DLBCL.[78]

H. pylori is a gram-negative rod which was discovered by Warren and Marshall in 1983 and was shown to be associated with peptic ulcer disease, gastric carcinoma, and NHL.[79] Gastric lymphoma was found to have a high frequency in certain parts of Europe, such as the Veneto region of Italy, and was usually an indolent B-cell lymphoma of mucosa-associated lymphoid tissue (MALToma), a term proposed by Isaacson and Wright.[80] Parsonett recognized that *H. pylori* infection preceded the development of lymphoma,[81] and Wotherspoon reported in 1993 that antibiotic treatment for *H. pylori* caused regression of the lymphoma in over two-thirds of patients.[82] Over one-half of *H. pylori* large B-cell gastric lymphoma in an early stage will also respond to antibiotics.[83]

MALToma of the stomach serves as a model for lymphomagenesis secondary to antigenic stimulation (*Figure 90.8*). Both B and T cells are recruited to the gastric mucosa following *H. pylori* infection. Proliferation of B cells is dependent on reactive T cells. There is a continuous spectrum of pathologic lesions during the transition from gastritis to low-grade MALToma to the less frequent large B cell. Polymerase chain reaction (PCR) may be helpful in identifying a malignant B-cell clone that may persist after histologic regression following antibiotic therapy.[84] Somatic hypermutation is characteristic of the B-cell clone of MALToma and, along with the observation of plasmacytoid differentiation, indicates a post–germinal center origin. Translocation-positive gastric MALTomas lead to activation of the NFκB pathway that causes overexpression of BCL2, blocks apoptosis of B cells, and leads to antibiotic resistance, whereas translocation-negative cases involve inflammatory and immune responses which maintain B- and T-cell interaction and respond to *H. pylori* eradication.[85] The cytotoxin-associated gene A (CagA) protein has been shown to be directly delivered into B cells by *H. pylori* and likely contributes to lymphomagenesis.[86]

The most common genetic abnormality in gastric MALToma is the t(11;18) (q21;q21) which is present in one-quarter to one-third of cases, and up to one-half of *H. pylori*-negative cases.[87] The genes involved at t(11;18) are an apoptosis inhibitor-2 gene and a novel 18q gene, *MALT1*, and are more likely to result in disseminated disease but less likely to undergo histologic transformation (HT) than other genetic abnormalities.[88] The t(14;18) in MALToma involves *IGH/MALT1* and may coexist with trisomies 3, 12, or 18; occurs in 5% gastric MALTomas; and is more common in nongastrointestinal sites.[89] The t(1;14) (p22;q32) and t(1;2) (p22;q12) involve the *BCL10* gene and are present in 1% to 3% of gastric MALTomas. *BCL1* and *BCL2* gene rearrangements are usually not present in MALTomas, and *BCL-6* has rarely (1%-2%) been reported.[90] Loss of tumor suppressor genes and amplification of 3q27 have been associated with histologic progression and dissemination of MALTomas.[88]

Other infections associated with specific MALTomas include *Borrelia burgdorferi* with primary cutaneous B-cell lymphoma, *Chlamydia psittaci* with ocular adnexal MALTomas, *Campylobacter jejuni* with immunoproliferative small intestinal disease (also called

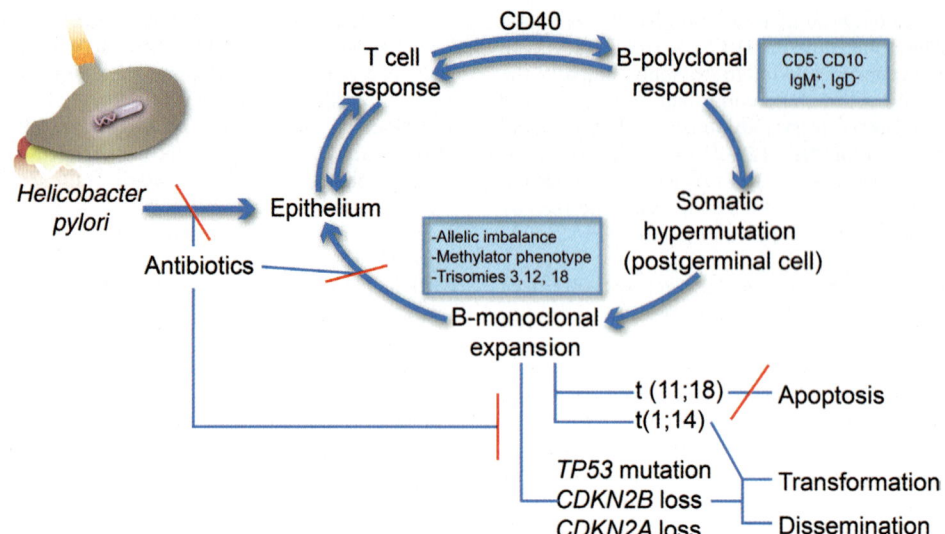

FIGURE 90.8 **MALToma of the stomach: model for lymphomagenesis.** *Helicobacter pylori* infects the epithelial cells and there is recruitment of both T and B cells. Contact-dependent T-cell help is mediated by CD40 and CD40 ligand interaction. B cells undergo a T-cell–dependent polyclonal response which can develop into a postgerminal center monoclonal B-cell lymphoma. Three-fourths of gastric MALTomas have allelic imbalance, methylator phenotype, and/or trisomies and respond to antibiotics that eradicate *H. pylori*. Alternatively, there can be clonal evolution that involves a specific translocation (i.e., t[11;18] or t[11;14]) and/or a loss of tumor suppressor genes (i.e., *TP53, CDKN2B/p15, CDKN2A/p16*), which are associated with dissemination of disease. t(11;18) rarely is associated with transformation, whereas t(11;14) may progress to a diffuse large B-cell lymphoma. (The figure was drawn by Kate Mittendorf, PhD.)

alpha heavy-chain disease or Mediterranean lymphoma), and possibly *Achromobacter xylosoxidans* with bronchial MALToma.[90] Their frequency varies according to endemic geography and has been found more commonly in Europe than in North America or Asia. The ability to diagnose the association depends on either immunohistochemistry using a monoclonal antibody detecting the agent or preferably, targeted PCR that detects the DNA of the infectious agent. Antibiotics for *H. pylori* and *C. psittaci*–related lymphomas are standard therapy, while treatment of the other infections linked to lymphoma is investigational.[90]

Environmental Factors

Environmental associations implicated in the pathogenesis of NHL include not only infections, but also drug exposure and toxic chemical exposure. InterLymph and EpiLymph, international consortia of NHL groups, are identifying associations of subtypes of NHL with medical and family histories, lifestyle, and occupations.[91,92] Immunosuppressive agents contribute to lymphomagenesis frequently through interaction with EBV, particularly in organ transplants. Phenytoin and carbamazepine have been associated with both pseudolymphoma and malignant lymphoma with the former condition presenting with fever, rash, and adenopathy that regress after drug withdrawal.[93] A large list of drugs, including anticonvulsants, antihypertensives, antihistamines, and statins, have been linked to skin rashes that can be confused with cutaneous lymphomas.[94]

Methotrexate and the tumor necrosis factor (TNF) alpha inhibitors have been associated with an increased risk of lymphoma in some, but not all, studies in rheumatoid arthritis (RA) which itself may have an increased risk.[95,96] Although epidemiologic studies are flawed by methodologic weaknesses, other drugs possibly associated with NHL include analgesics, antibiotics, steroids, digitalis, estrogen, and tranquilizers.[97] A Danish study found no increased risk of NHL in women using postmenopausal hormone replacement.[98] Statins have been reported to have a decreased risk.[99]

Occupational exposures have been reported as factors in the epidemic, but conclusions are inconsistent and are often flawed due to small numbers and to being retrospective. An increased risk of NHL has been reported among people employed in agriculture, forestry, fishing, construction, motor vehicles, telephone communication, leather industries, and education.[91,100] The strongest evidence has been for farmers and agricultural workers. Specific jobs reported to be at risk include plant and poultry farmers; butchers, gardeners; painters and plasterers; car repair and gasoline station workers; carpenters; brick and stone masons; plumbers; welders and solderers; roofers; hairdressers; and teachers. The latter has also been reported to have a reduced risk.[92] The associations tend to increase with longer duration of employment, and studies have correlated specific jobs with histologic types.[91]

Chemicals that have been implicated in the epidemic include organochlorines, organophosphates, and phenoxyacetic acids that are commonly found in pesticides and herbicides.[101] Recent studies are correlating exposures to specific subtypes of lymphoma.[102] A number of organochlorine compounds have been banned in the United States and include dichlorodiphenyltrichloroethane (used 1939-1972), polychlorinated biphenyls (1929-1977), and chlordane (1947-1988); however, studies have correlated the presence of these and similar chemicals in carpet dust and in adipose tissue with a higher risk of developing NHL. An excess risk for NHL has also been suggested for exposure to organic solvents, such as benzene, xylene, toluene, and trichloroethylene; fertilizers; epoxy glues; and leather or wood dust.[103,104]

Hair dyes have been associated with FL, small B lymphocytic lymphoma (SLL), and chronic lymphocytic leukemia (CLL) in early epidemiologic studies. There was an increased risk in women who used hair dyes before 1980, but not among women after 1980, probably related to removal of carcinogenic compounds, including aromatic amines.[105]

Ultraviolet (UV) light exposure and vitamin D have been investigated, but the findings have been inconsistent. An InterLymph study reported a protective effect of recreational sun exposure, but not total exposure.[106] A meta-analysis found a further decrease in NHL with increasing number of sunburns and sunbaths.[107] Another meta-analysis showed a protective effect of sunlight or UV exposure, while neither vitamin D intake nor 25-hydroxyvitamin D levels revealed an association with NHL.[108] Although studies linking vitamin D insufficiency to NHL have varied, there are reports showing an inferior survival in patients with NHL and low vitamin D levels compared to those with normal levels.[109] Supplementation of vitamin D3 (cholecalciferol) has been reported to improve survival with chemotherapy, and ongoing trials are evaluating its role in therapy.[110]

Nutritional factors, including milk, butter, liver, meat, coffee, and cola consumption, have been identified as possible risk factors, but the associations vary among studies.[111] A high intake of fat from animal sources has been linked to an increased risk of NHL in many, but not all, reports.[112,113] A Western diet with a high intake of red and processed meats, sweets, and refined grains has been considered proinflammatory and was found to have a modest association with B cell lymphomas.[114] Green leafy and cruciferous vegetables and fruit have been reported to have a lower risk of NHL.[115,116] A decreased risk for NHL has been found with higher intake of vegetables, lutein and zeaxanthin, and zinc.[117] Milk and dairy product consumption have had conflicting reports.[111,118] A dose-response of both was linked to an increase in DLBCL.[118] Obesity and lack of exercise have been suggested as contributing to the epidemic in some, but not all, studies.[119,120] Green tea has been associated with a reduced risk of NHL.[121]

Blood transfusion has been implicated as contributing to the increased incidence of NHL.[122] The use of blood products beginning in the 1950s coincided with the epidemic. Although cohort studies have supported the connection between blood transfusion and lymphoma, case-control studies have not consistently confirmed the association.[123] Transmission of infectious agents or suppression of cell-mediated immunity has been proposed as a possible mechanism. In a study of patients receiving transfusions in 2000 and beyond (after viral screening was standard), an increased risk of NHL was reported.[124] A meta-analysis found an increased overall risk for NHL and specifically for CLL/SLL,[122] but an InterLymph study reported no increased risk and even an inverse relationship for DLBCL and CLL/SLL in non-Hispanic white men.[123]

Other factors have been mentioned as contributing to the epidemic, including ionizing radiation, electromagnetic fields, alcohol, tobacco, and chronic fatigue syndrome, but the data are weak to support an association of any of these factors with an increased risk of NHL. Limited evidence suggests a mild increase in NHL following radiotherapy for NHL,[125] but there were no excess cases of NHL in atomic bomb survivors.[126] Precursor lymphoid leukemias were increased in a dose response relation in male survivors.[127] Investigation of NHL is now correlating exposures with genetics and specific subtypes.[92] There has been a reported increase of FL in female smokers.[128] Carefully designed studies with large cohorts and prolonged follow-up are required to determine the validity of an association between a factor and lymphomagenesis.

PRELYMPHOMATOUS CONDITIONS

The mechanism of developing lymphomas has been best studied in immunodeficiency states. These disorders can be subdivided into inborn errors of immunity, formerly known as congenital, or primary, immunodeficiencies and acquired, or secondary, immunodeficiencies (Table 90.5). Common components to all these disorders are defects in immunoregulation, particularly in T-cell immunity and uncontrolled B-cell growth in lymphoid tissue, often in association with EBV genome. Since 1973, cases of malignant disease in children with immunodeficiency have been recorded by immunodeficiency cancer registries, and NHL constitutes the majority of the cases.[129] The median age of onset is 7 years and there is a predominance of males over females due in part to the contribution of X-linked disorders.

The importance of EBV in the pathogenesis of lymphoproliferation in immunodeficiency was suggested by Purtilo et al in 1974 when they described an X-linked lymphoproliferative (XLP) disorder in which six boys in a single family died of infectious mononucleosis, agammaglobulinemia, or malignant lymphoma.[130] XLP type 1 is caused by mutations in the SH2 domain-containing 1A gene, which interacts with the lymphocyte activation molecule (SLAM)-associated protein, essential to T and NK cell development.[131] The role of EBV in lymphomas developing in patients with immunodeficiencies is addressed in Chapters 63 to 65.

Organ Transplants

In the early 1980s, a range of lymphoproliferative lesions, now known as post–transplant lymphoproliferative disease (PTLD), was described that occurred in patients receiving chronic immunosuppressive therapy after solid organ transplantation. The clinical and pathologic spectrum of diseases included primary infectious mononucleosis, polymorphic B-cell hyperplasia, and monomorphic B-cell lymphomas in which necrosis, cytologic atypia, monotypic Ig expression, and cytogenetic abnormalities are harbingers of neoplastic transformation and aggressive behavior. Serologic and molecular studies linked many of these lymphoproliferations to primary or secondary EBV infection. The risk of developing lymphoproliferation after transplantation is dependent on age, recipient EBV serostatus, type of transplant, and degree of immunosuppression. A lower chance occurs in older as opposed to younger age, sibling over cadaver donor, and single over multiple organ transplants. Early reports from Stanford University indicated that up to 40% of patients surviving cardiac transplantation developed a malignant lymphoma.[132] With less immunosuppression, the 5-year cumulative incidence of PTLD in the United States ranges from 0.7% to 9%, which is a 5- to 15-fold increase in lymphomas than occurs in the general population.[133] The diagnosis and management of PTLD is described in Chapter 63.

Acquired Immunodeficiency Syndrome

AIDS was recognized as a disease in 1981 and the first case of lymphoma in an AIDS patient was reported in 1982.[134] This was followed by a series of 90 homosexual patients with NHL reported by Ziegler et al in 1984.[135] In 1985, the diagnosis of NHL in association with positive serologic evidence for human immunodeficiency virus (HIV) became a criterion for the diagnosis of AIDS.[136] In Ziegler's series, presenting features included generalized adenopathy and opportunistic infections in one-third of patients.[135] Extranodal sites of disease and advanced stage disease, often with an aggressive course, tend to occur with AIDS-related lymphoma (ARL).[137] The most common extranodal sites are the meninges, gastrointestinal tract, bone marrow, liver, and lung/pleura; unusual sites include rectum, oral cavity, heart/pericardium, common bile duct, and skin. NHL in AIDS patients is usually of B-cell origin with the predominant types being DLBCL and BLs, but there are also increased rates of some peripheral T-cell lymphomas (PTCLs), MZL and LPL/Waldenström macroglobulinemia (WM). Unique presentations of ARL include PBL of the oral cavity and primary effusion lymphoma (PEL).[67,137]

The prevalence of NHL in AIDS is 3% to 6%, and before the era of ART there were projected increased risks over time.[138] The risk of lymphoma formerly was increased 60- to 650-fold among HIV-infected patients compared to the general population, but is now 9- to 23-fold higher in the ART era.[139] Severe immunodeficiency (defined by CD4 count and HIV viral load), prolonged HIV infection, older age, and transmission through sex between men are risk factors for NHL. In patients receiving ART, coinfection with HBV and HCV is associated with increased NHL.[140] Since the introduction of ART in 1996, epidemiologic studies in developed countries reported an increase in ARL as the first AIDS-defining illness but decreased overall incidence and improved survival in ARL.[141,142] Comparing pre-ART to late ART (2006-2015), there has been a downward shift in the United States in DLBCL from 63% to 35% to 37%, an increase in Burkitt from 3%

Table 90.5. Prelymphomatous Conditions

Congenital	Acquired
Ataxia telangiectasia	Immunodeficiency
Wiskott-Aldrich syndrome	Organ transplants
Severe combined immunodeficiency	Acquired immunodeficiency syndrome
Common variable immunodeficiency	Autoimmune disorders
	Sjögren syndrome
	Hashimoto thyroiditis
Hyper IgM syndrome	Rheumatoid arthritis
Hyper IgE syndrome	Systemic lupus erythematosus
X-linked hypogammaglobulinemia	Inflammatory bowel disease
	Castleman disease
X-linked lymphoproliferative syndrome	Hodgkin lymphoma
	Lymphomatoid granulomatosis
Autoimmune lymphoproliferative syndrome	Predisposition to T-cell lymphoma
	Nontropical sprue
	Angioimmunoblastic lymphadenopathy
	Lymphomatoid papulosis

to 16% to 20%, a recognition of HL (26%), and the presence of PBL (6%) and PEL (5%) in HIV+ patients.[138] Prognostic factors and therapy of ARL are addressed in Chapter 65.

Autoimmune and Other Immunologic Disorders

Chronic inflammation, immune hyperactivity, and/or immunosuppression are elements of autoimmune disorders (ADs) that predispose patients to lymphoma.[143,144] Shared genetic loci between AD and NHL have not been clearly identified.[145] Many of these lymphomas arise in extranodal sites where there is sparse lymphoid tissue; they are usually localized, low-grade B-cell lymphomas arising from MALToma. Isaacson and Wright initially recognized MALTomas in the gastrointestinal tract and indicated they were a subset of immunoproliferative small intestinal disease, or Mediterranean lymphoma; however, they subsequently identified similar lymphomas occurring in the lung and salivary gland.[146] Multiple other extranodal sites have been involved with MALTomas and include thyroid gland, thymus, breast, conjunctiva, gallbladder, skin, cervix, larynx, lung, and trachea. Although the term MALToma is misleading due to the fact that not all of the lesions arise in the mucosal tissue, two common features are chronic inflammation and the presence of glandular epithelium that is destroyed by progressive lymphocytic infiltration.

Lymphomas associated with Sjögren syndrome (SS) and Hashimoto thyroiditis are of B-cell origin and tend to occur in elderly females. The presumed pathogenesis of lymphomas in these patients is associated with chronic antigenic stimulation causing polyclonal B-cell growth with eventual development of a monoclonal B-cell lymphoma. Bunim and Talal reported the first association of lymphoma and SS in 1963,[147] and Kassan et al subsequently reported a 44-fold risk for NHL.[148] Five percent to 10% of patients with primary SS will develop lymphoma.[149]

The histologic lesion of SS is a myoepithelial sialoadenitis (MESA) characterized by lymphoid infiltration of the salivary gland along with acinar atrophy and proliferation of ductal cells to form myoepithelial islands.[150] Although the initial clinical course of SS usually is benign, clonally rearranged Ig genes can be detected in the biopsy of MESA.[151] The detection of germinal centers correlated with the development of lymphoma in some reports, but not in others.[152,153] The B-lymphocyte activator of the TNF-family (BAFF) is overexpressed in SS salivary glands, induces BCL-2 which impairs apoptosis, and likely contributes to lymphomagenesis.[154]

Overt lymphoma tends to occur in those lesions with extensive, confluent areas of monotypic B-cell proliferation. A risk factor model involves seven factors: salivary gland enlargement, lymphadenopathy, Raynaud phenomenon, anti-Sjögren antibodies, rheumatoid factor positivity, monoclonal gammopathy, and C4 hypocomplementemia.[155] Elevated chemokine levels, such as CXCL13, have also correlated with the development of lymphoma.[156] The most common type is MALToma and others include DLBCL and nodal marginal zone lymphoma.[157]

Lindsay and Dailey described an association between lymphoma and Hashimoto thyroiditis in 1957.[158] Subsequent studies indicate that over 75% of thyroid lymphomas are preceded by Hashimoto thyroiditis, made evident by thyroiditis in the nonlymphomatous portion of the pathologic specimens and by the presence of antithyroid antibodies.[159] There is a 40- to 80-fold increase in thyroid lymphoma and many occur 20 to 30 years after thyroiditis, but the lifetime risk is only 0.6% to 2%.[160] DLBCL is the most common type followed by MALToma, and there frequently is a mixture of the two pathologies.[161]

Lymphomas have been reported in patients with other ADs, including RA, systemic lupus erythematosus (SLE), scleroderma, inflammatory bowel disease, and dermatomyositis; however, the increased incidence in these disorders is complicated by the use of immunosuppressive therapy and by possible methodologic flaws of epidemiologic studies. The increased risk for lymphoma in RA varies from 2- to 15-fold and is higher in patients with more severe disease or with Felty syndrome.[162]

A large study reported an increased NHL risk (standardized incidence ratio 2.9 [1.7-4.9]) in RA patients treated with any biologic agent and a greater risk with anti-TNF agents than methotrexate[163]; however, other studies have reported no risk with either type of agent.[96] A meta-analysis of randomized clinical trials in RA reported no increased risk of malignancy with biologic therapy, but did find an increased risk for NHL (odds ratio 2.1 [0.55-8.4]) in patients receiving anti-TNF therapy compared with controls.[164] Despite conflicting reports, the Food and Drug Administration (FDA) in 2009 issued a Black Box warning of an increased risk of NHL with TNF inhibitors.[95]

A wide spectrum of lesions have been described in RA patients, ranging from lesions that resemble posttransplant polymorphous lymphoproliferation to DLBCL, the most common type, HL, and, rarely, PTCL.[165] EBV may be present in tumor cells, and the lymphoproliferations may regress with discontinuation of immunosuppression.[166] T-large granular lymphocyte leukemia is often associated with RA and neutropenia.[167] The risk of NHL in SLE is increased 2.7- to 4-fold, and MZL and DLBCL are the most common types.[143,168]

CD (giant lymph node hyperplasia, angiofollicular lymph node hyperplasia) was first recognized in the 1920s and was described by Castleman as a distinct entity in 1954.[169] It has two types of clinical presentations (unicentric [UCD] and multicentric [MCD]) and three types of histologic subtypes (hyaline vascular [HV], plasma cell [PC], and mixed).[170] The MCD is further subdivided into idiopathic (iMCD), HHV-8 associated, and POEMS (polyneuropathy, organomegaly, endocrinopathy, monoclonal PC disorder, and skin changes). Pathologists prefer describing a spectrum of pathologic changes not specific to a clinical type and use the term hypervascular rather than HV within iMCD.[171] Increased expression of the gene coding for IL-6 has been identified in CD, and retroviral transduction of the gene into mice has reproduced histology and symptoms.[172]

UCD tends to present as the HV type with localized adenopathy, often in the neck or mediastinum. It can be encapsulated and amenable to surgical resection. Although UCD was initially reported to be radioresistant, it has been successfully treated with radiation. The cell of origin of the HV variant is likely a stromal cell, the follicular dendritic cell.[173] If UCD is neither amenable to surgery or radiotherapy, embolization or neoadjuvant therapy with rituximab, anti-IL6 therapy or other agents can be tried.[174]

MCD usually has PC histology and is associated with systemic symptoms, anemia of chronic disease, hypergammaglobulinemia, and a variety of unusual syndromes, including myasthenia gravis, nephrotic syndrome, peripheral neuropathy, amyloidosis, and temporal arteritis. Another syndrome with thrombocytopenia, ascites, reticulin fibrosis, renal dysfunction, and organomegaly has been reported from Japan in multicentric form that has HV or mixed histology.[175] Siltuximab, an antibody to IL-6, the only FDA-approved treatment for MCD,[176] and tocilizumab, an anti-IL6 receptor antibody, approved in Japan, are effective in approximately one-half of patients with MCD.[177,178] Steroids can be added to the anti-IL6 agents.[178] Other agents that have been utilized include rituximab, IFN, imids, sirolimus, cyclosporine, antiviral therapy, and chemotherapy.[170]

The PC variant can present as UCD in a young adult, but more commonly occurs as iMCD in an older adult or as HHV8-associated MCD in an HIV-infected patient with diffuse adenopathy and an aggressive course with 20% to 30% of patients developing either a B-cell lymphoma or Kaposi sarcoma.[170,178] The lymphomas in CD have a variable histologic pattern, but they are usually of B-cell origin.[179] In HIV-negative patients, mantle cell is the most common type.[180] HL and follicular dendritic sarcoma have been reported in CD.[174] HIV-infected patients with HHV8-associated MCD have a 15-fold increase in NHL compared to HIV-positive patients without MCD.[170] Rituximab reduces the risk of lymphoma in HIV+ MCD.[181] In patients with MCD and KS, rituximab can worsen the KS, but adding liposomal doxorubicin can prevent KS progression.[182] The ARL in HHV8-associated MCD is predominantly PEL type that is often EBV+ or is PBL.[66]

NHL may follow HL, with prior therapy and the cell-mediated immune defect characteristic of HL serving as possible contributing factors. Krikorian et al reported six cases from Stanford University of aggressive lymphoma developing after HL.[183] There is a 5.5- to 11.5-fold higher incidence of NHL in patients with HL compared to the general population with the elevated risk occurring primarily in lymphocyte-predominant HL (LPHL) and lymphocyte-rich classical HL.[184] The risk is higher in advanced stage, older age (60-69 years), and usually occurs 5 to 9 years after the diagnosis of HL. The most common type of secondary NHL is DLBCL and is followed by FL and PTCL.[184,185] The LBLs associated with LPHL generally are regarded as progression of LPHL rather than as secondary neoplasms. The incidence has varied from 2% to 17%, including a 7.6% rate in a Mayo Clinic report.[186] There are rare patients with unclassifiable B-cell lymphoma and intermediate clinical and pathologic features between DLBCL and classical HL.[187] They were previously called mediastinal gray zone lymphoma (GZL) or LBL with Hodgkin-like features; there is also a nonmediastinal GZL.

PTCLs do not occur as commonly as B NHL in the setting of immunodeficiencies with the exception of ataxia telangiectasia; however, some immune disorders can occur prior to, during, or after a diagnosis of PTCL.[188] Up to one-tenth of lymphomas in organ transplants are of T-cell origin, tend to occur late, and have a poor prognosis.[189] Hepatosplenic γδ TCL can occur after solid organ transplantation and in patients with Crohn disease, the majority of whom were on anti-TNF therapy.[190] PTCL comprise up to 7% of all AIDS lymphoma with an increased risk for ALCL and PTCL-NOS (not otherwise specified) compared to the general population.[191] Patients with gluten-sensitive enteropathy, or celiac disease, have an increased incidence of enteropathy-associated T-cell lymphoma (EATL), formerly called type 1.[192] Autoimmune features are characteristic of angioimmunoblastic T-cell lymphoma (AITL). Cutaneous γδ TCL has been associated with SLE, SS, and hemophagocytosis.[188] The underlying etiology of secondary hemophagocytic lymphohistiocytosis is frequently PTCL.[193] Primary ALK-negative ALCL has been reported after breast implant surgery.[194]

Skin disorders, including psoriasis and pemphigus, may also evolve into a malignant cutaneous TCL (Chapter 94). Clonality, as evidenced by TCR gene rearrangements, has been detected in patients with lymphomatoid papulosis, as well as in those with other cutaneous T-cell processes of uncertain malignant potential, such as pityriasis lichenoides et varioliformis acuta, granulomatous slack skin disease, and pagetoid reticulosis.[195] The latter two disorders are considered variants of mycosis fungoides.

CLINICAL FEATURES AT PRESENTATION

The majority of patients with NHL present with painless adenopathy, more commonly in the cervical or supraclavicular regions[196]; however, extranodal disease can be detected at presentation in up to 40% of patients and varies depending on immune status and geographic differences. Systemic symptoms occur in less than 25% of patients in most large series. When present, however, they usually are associated with advanced stages of disease and often a poor prognosis. Significant cytopenias are rare unless marrow involvement is extensive or there are associated immune-mediated cytopenias, hypersplenism, or uncommonly, hemophagocytosis. Leukemia presentations in NHL are rare and variably impact prognosis.

The gastrointestinal tract is involved in 5% to 20% of adults with NHL and is the most common extranodal site at presentation, occurring in 20% to 40% of NHL.[197,198] The stomach is most frequently involved followed by the small intestine, the colon, and esophagus. Over 90% of primary gastrointestinal lymphomas are of B-cell origin, while T-cell origin occurs in 4% to 6% of cases.[198] Certain subtypes have a site predilection: MALToma and DLBCL in the stomach, Burkitt (non-African) in the terminal ileum; mantle cell in the terminal ileum, jejunum, and colon; EATL in the jejunum; and follicular in the duodenum.

Gastrointestinal symptoms are often nonspecific with vague abdominal pain the most common presenting symptom. Epigastric pain, dyspepsia, nausea, and, less often, early satiety suggest stomach involvement. Frank bleeding occurs in less than 30% of patients with gastrointestinal lymphomas, and usually is from either a gastric (melena) or large bowel source. Patients with rectal involvement can present with hematochezia or a change in bowel habits. Obstruction, specifically intussusception, or perforation is associated with aggressive small bowel lymphomas, particularly DLBCL, BL, and EATL.[199] MCL presents with gastrointestinal symptoms in 20% to 30% of patients, and multiple polyposis may be found on colonoscopy (*Figure 90.9*). Lymphomatous polyposis of the gastrointestinal tract is not restricted to MCL and has also been detected in FL and MALToma.[200] Although the mucosa may appear normal, abnormal histology in the gastrointestinal tract is found in over 80% of MCL patients.[201]

Dysphagia, airway obstruction, and eustachian tube blockage with or without cervical adenopathy are symptoms suggesting Waldeyer ring involvement. DLBCL is the most common pathology followed by FL and SLL. Epistaxis and nasal obstruction usually with facial edema are common signs of involvement of nasal lymphomas. Ulceration of the hard palate is seen in nasal NK/TCL.

Hepatosplenomegaly is a common feature of advanced indolent B-cell lymphoma, including SLL, and splenic marginal zone lymphoma (SMZL) and can be the predominant clinical feature of hepatosplenic TCL. Subclinical secondary involvement of the liver has been reported in 26% to 40% of NHL, whereas primary hepatic lymphoma is extremely rare, representing 0.05% of extranodal lymphoma.[202] Primary splenic lymphoma is similarly uncommon, and splenectomy may be considered for diagnosis and therapy in selected patients.[203,204]

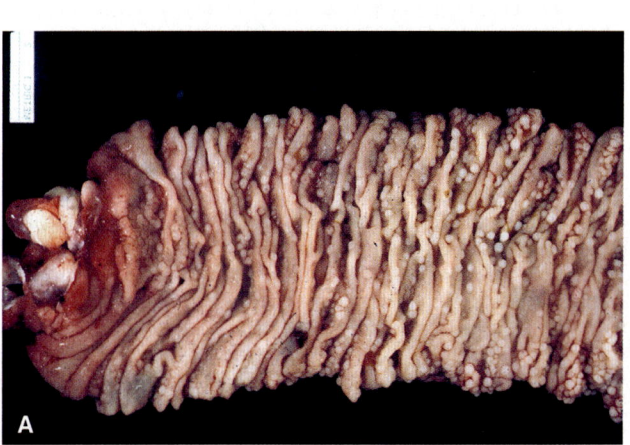 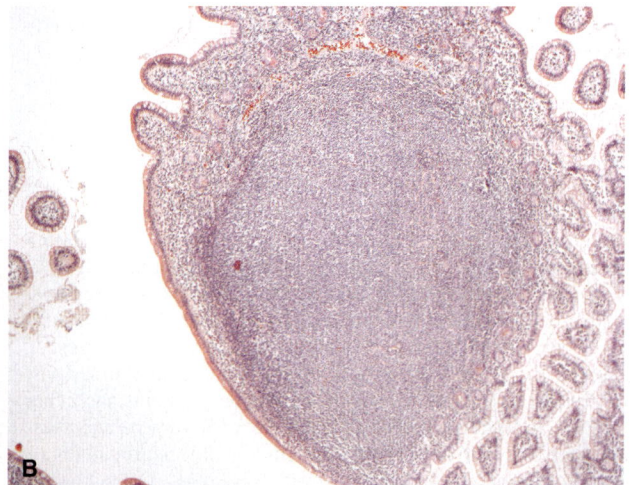

FIGURE 90.9 Mantle cell lymphoma. A, Intestine involved my multiple lymphomatous polyposis. Multiple small nodules extensively involve the bowel mucosa. B, Aggregates of small B cells from multiple nodules just beneath the mucosa express CD5 and cyclin D1. (A, Image provided by Dr Lawrence Weiss, City of Hope National Medical Center; B, Image provided by Dr Dan Arber, University of Chicago, Chicago, IL.)

Primary NHL of the liver is usually DLBCL, can be associated with HCV, and can arise in immunodeficient hosts.[205] Presenting features include right upper quadrant pain, anorexia, nausea, coagulopathy, and elevated liver enzymes without significant jaundice.[202] Hypodense, nonenhancing (possible rim enhancement) masses on CT imaging are characteristic of primary liver NHL. Solitary masses occur in approximately two-thirds; multiple masses, in one-third; and diffuse infiltration is unusual.[206] Obstructive jaundice can occur in NHL secondary to periportal lymphadenopathy or to primary lymphoma of the bile duct or pancreas. Rarely, liver involvement with NHL may present with hepatic failure.[207]

The skin is another common site of extranodal NHL, and the most common primary cutaneous type is the cerebriform T cell of mycosis fungoides/Sézary syndrome (Chapter 94). Mycosis fungoides tends to be confined to the skin with characteristic stages. B-cell lymphomas involving the skin only represent 20% to 30% of primary cutaneous lymphoma and usually present as nodules involving the head, neck, or trunk. The major types of primary cutaneous B-cell lymphoma and their distinguishing immunophenotype include marginal zone (MALT type) ($CD20^+$, $CD5^-$, $CD10^-$), primary cutaneous FL ($CD20^+$, $CD10^+$), and primary cutaneous LBL ($CD20^+$; usually $CD10^-$). Other TCLs with unique skin involvement include ALCL which can be a primary cutaneous type or a systemic disease, subcutaneous panniculitis–like PTCL, αβ subtype; cutaneous γδ TCL, aggressive epidermotropic $CD8^+$ cytotoxic TCL, primary cutaneous $CD4^+$ small/medium-sized pleomorphic TCL, and primary cutaneous acral $CD8^+$ TCL.

Neurologic symptoms and signs, including headache, confusion, lethargy, dysphasia, hemiparesis, seizures, and cranial nerve palsies, and rarely, multifocal leukoencephalopathy, may be presenting features of CNS involvement.[208,209] Focal neurologic deficits occur in 70% of primary CNS lymphoma (PCNSL) followed by cognitive and personality changes in 43% of patients due to a predilection for involvement in the frontal lobes, corpus callosum, and periventricular area.[208] Over 90% of PCNSL are DLBCL, predominantly of the activated B-cell–like (ABC)/nongerminal cell type[210]; the remainder are indolent B-cell lymphomas, BL, and PTCLs.

The detection of a single lesion on MRI favors PCNSL, but multifocal lesions can occur in approximately one-third of normal hosts and more frequently in AIDS patients (Figure 90.10). PCNSL is less common in HIV+ patients after the introduction of ART but has increased in patients over 60 (see Epidemiology). The differential in AIDS patients with intracranial mass lesions includes not only CNS lymphoma but also toxoplasmosis, progressive multifocal leukoencephalopathy, and other opportunistic infections. CT scanning of CNS lymphoma usually identifies a contrast-enhancing lesion or lesions with a mass effect and edema which may have ring enhancement, a common finding in toxoplasmosis. The definitive diagnostic procedure is CT-guided stereotactic biopsy. Positron emission tomography (PET) scanning may distinguish lymphoma and toxoplasmosis and obviate the need for biopsy in some AIDS patients.

Lymphomatous meningeal infiltration may be detected in up to 15% of patients with parenchymal PCNSL or may occur as an early or late complication in patients with specific sites of disease, including nasopharynx through local extension, testicular, or extensive marrow involvement.[211] The histologies involving the spinal fluid are usually aggressive and include DLBCL, BL, and T-lymphoblastic. Primary leptomeningeal lymphoma is when there is no systemic lymphoma or parenchymal disease and occurs in 7% of presentations with CNS disease.[211] Neurolymphomatosis is a rare syndrome characterized by a clinical neuropathy with variable pain and is due to lymphomatous infiltration of peripheral nerve(s), nerve root or plexus; or cranial nerves.[212] Intravascular B-cell lymphoma usually has subcutaneous skin lesions, but can present with a wide variety of neurologic symptoms, including neuropathies, myopathy, dementia, and stroke.[213] Rarely, paraneoplastic neurological syndromes, primarily sensorimotor neuropathies or dermatomyositis, have been associated with NHL.[214]

Because of the risk of leptomeningeal disease in PCNSL, ARL, Burkitt, LBL, and DLBCL with the specific sites noted above, the CSF should be examined by cytology and flow cytometry (FC), and

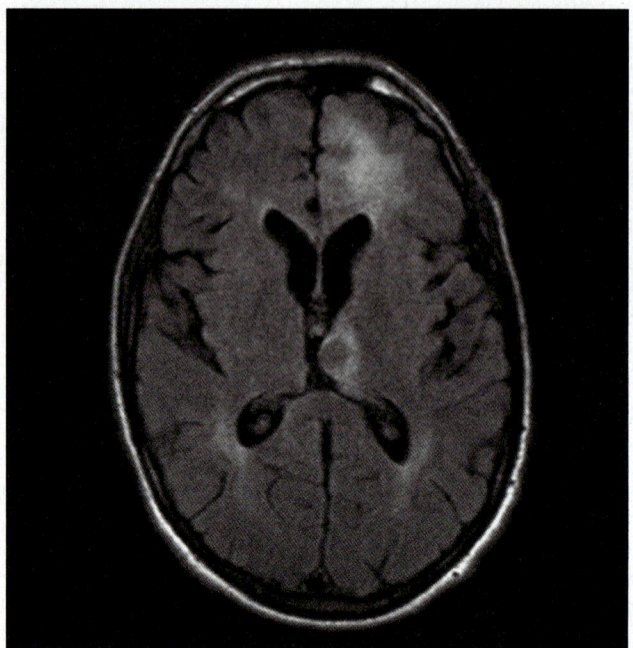

FIGURE 90.10 Primary central nervous system lymphoma. This FLAIR sequence MRI demonstrates a small periventricular mass lesion in the left thalamus. The lesion displays a signal intensity that is isointense compared with normal gray matter structures. This feature is consistent with a highly cellular lesion, a finding that suggests lymphoma but is not specific for that diagnosis. In addition, there are multiple areas of high signal intensity with ill-defined borders, most pronounced in the left frontal region. This appearance is also nonspecific, reflecting increased water content or decreased myelin in those regions, as may occur with any cause of inflammation. It is consistent with a multifocal, widely infiltrative process, and supportive of the diagnosis of lymphoma. Description provided by Dr Paul Moots, Vanderbilt University, Nashville, TN.

prophylaxis should be considered in these patients. In patients with DLBCL, elevated lactate dehydrogenase (LDH), and more than one extranodal site are among the factors predicting CNS relapse.[215]

Symptoms of spinal cord compression may include back pain, paresthesias, weakness, and incontinence and requires emergent recognition and therapy. Compression occurs through extension of a paravertebral mass or direct involvement of a vertebral body. MRI of the entire spine is recommended to exclude multiple sites of involvement. The thoracic spine is the most common area followed by lumbar and then cervical.[216]

Primary ocular lymphoma is part of the spectrum of CNS lymphoma, usually with DLBCL histology and is defined by infiltration by lymphoma cells in the visual tract, retina, vitreous, or optic nerve head. Approximately 5% to 20% of PCNSL have ocular involvement at diagnosis, whereas CNS involvement may follow isolated ocular lymphoma in 60% to 90% of patients.[217] Ocular symptoms include blurred vision, loss of visual acuity, or "floaters," but patients can be asymptomatic. Slit lamp examination is recommended for patients with CNS or ocular lymphoma. The external eye usually is normal, and the diagnosis can be confused with uveitis, vitritis, or glaucoma.

Lymphomas of the extraocular space are more common than ocular lymphomas and can arise in the superficial conjunctiva or eyelids or deeper in the lacrimal gland or retrobulbar tissues.[218] Blurred vision, ptosis, chemosis, epiphora, and proptosis can occur depending on the orbital site involved. Most orbital lymphomas are of low grade B-cell origin, predominantly of the marginal zone MALT type, occurring in the conjunctiva or eyelids, but can be a LBL in the lacrimal gland or retrobulbar area.[219] Bilateral involvement occurs in 10% to 15% of patients, mostly in conjunctival forms. CNS involvement rarely occurs, and the risk for distant spread is less with conjunctival lesions.

Other symptoms and signs depend on unusual extranodal presentations. Bone pain is uncommon unless the lymphoma has a leukemic component or the patient has extranodal bone lymphoma, which accounts for 3% to 5% of extranodal NHL.[220] The long bones are most commonly affected and there may be soft-tissue swelling. The lesions may be lytic, sclerotic, or mixed with periosteal erosion and are best evaluated by MRI (and differentiated from findings of bone marrow involvement). DLBCL accounts for 70% to 80% of all bone lymphomas.[220] Genitourinary presentations include renal mass, ureteral obstruction, testicular mass, ovarian mass, and vaginal bleeding. The most common cause of a testicular mass in an elderly male is NHL, usually DLBCL, ABC type.[221] Bilateral testicular involvement occurs in 6% to 10% of cases. Primary breast lymphoma accounts for less than 0.5% of all malignant breast tumors, 1% of NHL, and less than 3% of extranodal lymphoma.[222] DLBCL is the most common pathology, occurring in 56% to 84% of patients and is usually the ABC type, and is followed by MZL (9%-28%), FL (10%-19%), and BL (<6%).[222] Breast lymphoma in young women is associated with pregnancy and lactation and often has diffuse involvement of both breasts. Older women tend to have discrete masses with unilateral involvement.

Lung and heart are rarely involved in NHL but these patients commonly present with cardiopulmonary symptoms. Cough, dyspnea, and chest pain usually of a short duration may be the presenting symptoms of mediastinal nodal involvement. The superior vena cava syndrome can occur with either T-LBL or LBL of the mediastinum. Pleural effusions require cytology and immunophenotyping by FC to determine if there is lymphomatous involvement.

Primary pulmonary lymphoma represents less than 1% of NHL and 3%-4% of extranodal lymphoma. The most common pathology is a MALToma, a small B-cell bronchus–associated lymphoid tissue (BALT) lymphoma, which more commonly presents as localized opacities.[223] A subset of BALT with plasmacytic differentiation is seen in elderly women, often with autoimmune disease and localized but not systemic amyloidosis. Less common pathologies include indolent B-cell lymphomas, DLBCL, and lymphomatoid granulomatosis. Chest computerized tomography (CT) in BALT can detect single or multiple nodules or nonspecific findings, including ill-defined infiltrates; bilateral disease occurs in one-quarter of patients.[223] Bronchoscopy may reveal bronchial narrowing and biopsy can identify submucosal involvement.

Primary cardiac lymphoma is extremely rare, usually occurs as DLBCL in an immunocompromised host, and may present with heart failure, pericardial effusion, or arrhythmia, including heart block.[224]

NHL occasionally will present with metabolic and endocrine problems that tend to be more prominent following the introduction of therapy particularly in the setting of a large tumor volume or aggressive histologies. Hypercalcemia, hyperuricemic renal failure, and severe hypoglycemia are unusual metabolic presentations. Hypercalcemia is present in approximately one-fifth of patients with ATL at diagnosis and occurs in up to 70% during the course of the illness.[51] Cases of primary adrenal lymphoma have been reported and the initial presentation is usually due to the mass effect. Rarely, adrenal insufficiency may be the initial presentation of NHL and can be rapidly fatal if unrecognized.[225]

STAGING AND PROGNOSIS

The Ann Arbor staging classification (*Table 90.6*) developed for HL in 1971 has been the standard scheme for NHL[226]; however, it does not account for tumor burden and is only one of the factors contributing to prognosis. The Lugano classification devised in 2014 provided a universally applicable standard approach for patient evaluation both for staging and response assessment.[227] Other staging systems have been developed for NHL, particularly in children (Chapter 91), specific pathologies, and extranodal sites of disease, including gastrointestinal and CNS (*Table 90.6*).

As expected, prognosis and therapy depend not only on stage, but also on the pathologic features of the lymphoma and by a variety of clinical parameters which reflect tumor bulk and disease kinetics (e.g., size of mass, LDH level, number of extranodal sites). The international prognostic index (IPI) (*Table 90.6*) was developed to incorporate additional clinical parameters that correlate with prognosis which moved beyond the Ann Arbor staging system in predicting survival. There are NHLs for which the IPI may be less useful, such as primary mediastinal large B-cell lymphoma where prognosis depends on the extent of local disease. Modification in clinical prognostic indices has been made for different types of NHL and biologic parameters can further subdivide groups.

Table 90.7 outlines the clinical evaluation and staging studies to consider when evaluating patients with NHL. Bone marrow evaluation detects disease in 20% to 40% of all patients with NHL and from 50% to 70% of patients with indolent lymphomas. FC can increase the overall rate of detection, but morphology can be positive when FC is negative and vice versa. Immunohistochemistry is a mainstay of pathologic evaluation of tissue (Chapter 88). Molecular studies may be of diagnostic, prognostic, and predictive significance and are detailed further in Chapter 89.

Using ^{18}F-fluorodeoxyglucose ^{18}F-FDG, PET is commonly used to identify sites of disease and to assess response (see section "Functional Imaging"). ^{18}F-FDG uptake varies according to histology and proliferative activity with less uptake in the indolent lymphomas than in the aggressive lymphomas. Although there is increasing reliance on PET scans, there is no substitute for tissue diagnosis to confirm the presence of disease. The IPI score has utility in predicting survival for DLBCL based on readily available clinical and laboratory parameters. Revisions to the IPI have been based on the improved outcomes observed for patients treated with the R-CHOP immunochemotherapy regimen incorporating rituximab as opposed to earlier chemotherapy-only regimens.[228] The Revised IPI (R-IPI) stratifies patients into three risk groups, defined as very good (0 risk factors) (10% of patients, 4-year progression-free survival [PFS] 94% and overall survival [OS] 94%), good (1 or 2 factors) (45% of patients, 4-year PFS 80%, OS 79%), and poor (≥3 factors) (45% of patients, 4-year PFS 53%, OS 55%) (*Figure 90.11*). Another prognostic score derived from the National Comprehensive Cancer Network was able to better discriminate the high-risk group of patients by dividing age into three categories and LDH as >3 × ULN or 1 to 3 × ULN.[229]

The IPI is also predictive in FL, but its discriminatory value is limited, because most patients fall into low- or low-intermediate risk groups. A scoring system designated follicular lymphoma IPI (FLIPI) stratifies patients into low-, intermediate-, or high-risk groups based on the number of nodal groups involved, age, Ann Arbor stage, hemoglobin level, and LDH (*Table 90.6*).[230] The FLIPI has been validated as a useful prognostic tool and provides a means of comparing relative patient risk distribution among clinical trials. The FLIPI2 scoring system (*Table 90.6*) is more relevant to current patients, however, as it is based on initial therapy with rituximab-containing regimens (*Figure 90.12*). The acronym "BABA6" can be used for the five FLIPI2 markers: Beta-2 microglobulin >normal, Anemia with hemoglobin <120 g/L, Bone marrow positive for lymphoma, Age > 60 years, and one or more nodal masses ≥6 cm in diameter. Five- and 10-year OS rates had a strong inverse correlation with low-, intermediate-, and high-risk FLIPI2 scores.[230]

Pastore et al aimed to improve risk stratification by integrating genetic mutations into the clinical prognostic model. DNA deep sequencing of FL specimens led to the identification of genetically recurrent mutations that have been associated with prognosis (*EZH2, CARD11, ARID1A, MEF2B, EP300, FOXO1,* and *CREBBP*). The incorporation of these mutations in the clinical risk model, termed m7-FLIPI, outperformed FLIPI risk prognostication alone. This test, although not widely available, needs validation in prospective clinical trials.[231]

A mantle cell lymphoma IPI (MIPI) score has also been validated that incorporates age, LDH, white blood cell count, and performance status (PS), and has been further refined to include the proliferation marker Ki-67[231] Similarly, a prognostic index for PTCL (PIT) includes four variables: bone marrow involvement, age, PS, and LDH.[232]

Immunophenotypic and Molecular Markers

Advances in the molecular and cellular biology of lymphoma have contributed to better understanding of tumor biology that affect

Table 90.6. Staging and Prognostic Indexes of Non-Hodgkin Lymphoma

Ann Arbor Staging System

	I	Involvement of a single lymph node region or of a single extranodal organ or site (I_E)
	II	Involvement of two or more node regions on the same side of the diaphragm, or localized involvement of an extranodal site or organ (II_E) and one or more lymph node regions on the same side of the diaphragm
	III	Involvement of lymph node regions on both sides of the diaphragm which may also be accompanied by localized involvement of an extranodal organ or site (III_E) or spleen (III_S) or both (III_{SE})
	IV	Diffuse or disseminated involvement of one or more distant extranodal organs with or without associated lymph node involvement
	B symptoms	Fever >38 °C, night sweats, and/or weight loss >10% of body weight in the 6 mo preceding admission are defined as systemic symptoms.
Staging modification		The E designation is used when extranodal lymphoid malignancies arise in tissues separate from, but near, the major lymphatic aggregates. Stage IV refers to disease that is diffusely spread throughout an extranodal site, such as the liver. If pathologic proof of involvement of one or more extralymphatic sites has been documented, the symbol for the site of involvement, followed by a plus sign (+), is listed. Sites are identified by the following notation: H, liver; S, spleen; L, lung; P, pleura; M, bone marrow; O, bone; D, skin. Current practice assigns a clinical stage (CS) based on the findings of the clinical evaluation and a pathologic stage (PS) based on the findings made as a result of invasive procedures beyond the initial biopsy.

International Prognostic Index (IPI): Survival for Diffuse Large B Cell Lymphoma by IPI

Adverse Factor	Risk Group	Number of Factors	4 y Progression Free Survival[a] (%)
Performance status ≥2*	Low	0, 1	85
LDH > normal*	Low-intermediate	2	80
Extranodal sites ≥ 2 Stage III/IV disease*	High-intermediate	3	57
Age >60	High	4, 5	51

*Age-adjusted factors

Follicular Lymphoma International Prognostic Index (FLIPI)[b]

Adverse Factor		Risk Group	Number of Factors	10-y Overall Survival (%)
Age > 60 y		Low	0, 1	70
Stage III/IV		Intermediate	2	50
Hemoglobin < 120 g/L		High	≥3	35
Number of nodal areas > 4				
LDH > normal				

Adverse Factor	Risk Group	Number of Factors	5-y Progression-Free Survival (%)	5-y Overall Survival (%)
FLIPI2: (applies to time of first treatment)[c]	Low	0	79	98
β_2-Microglobulin elevated	Intermediate	1, 2	51	88
Age > 60 y	High	≥3	20	77
Positive bone marrow				
Hemoglobin < 120 g/L				
One or more nodes > 6 cm				

Staging System for Gastrointestinal Non-Hodgkin Lymphoma[d]

Stage	Description
Stage I	Tumor confined to gastrointestinal tract without serosal penetration Single primary site
Stage II	Tumor extending into abdomen from primary site—nodal involvement II_1 Local (gastric/mesenteric) II_2 Distant (para-aortic/paracaval)
Stage II_E	Penetration of serosa to involve adjacent "structures"; enumerate actual site of involvement, such as stage II_E (large intestine) Perforation/peritonitis
Stage IV	Disseminated extranodal involvement or a gastrointestinal tract lesion with supradiaphragmatic nodal involvement

(Continued)

Table 90.6. Staging and Prognostic Indexes of Non-Hodgkin Lymphoma (Continued)

Central Nervous System International Prognostic Index[e]

Adverse Factor	Risk Group	Number of Factors	Risk of CNS Disease at 2 y
Age > 60 y	Low	0, 1	0.6%
LDH > normal	Intermediate	2, 3	3.4%
PS > 1 Stage III/IV disease	High	4-6	10.2%
Extranodal site >1			
Kidney or adrenal			

[a]From Sehn LH, Berry B, Chhanabhai M, et al. The revised International Prognostic Index (R-IPI) is a better predictor of outcome than the standard IPI for patients with diffuse large B-cell lymphoma treated with R-CHOP. *Blood*. 2007;109:1857-1861.
[b]From Solal-Celigny P, Roy P, Colombat P, et al. Follicular lymphoma international prognostic index. *Blood*. 2004;104:1258-1265.
[c]From Federico M, Bellei M, Marcheselli L, et al. Follicular lymphoma international prognostic index 2: a new prognostic index for follicular lymphoma developed by the international follicular lymphoma prognostic factor project. *J Clin Oncol*. 2009;27:4555-4562.
[d]From Rohatiner A, d'Amore F, Coiffier B, et al. Report on a workshop convened to discuss the pathological and staging classifications of gastrointestinal tract lymphoma. *Ann Oncol*. 1994;5:397-400.
[e]From Schmitz N, Zeynalova S, Nickelsen M, et al. CNS international prognostic index: a risk model for CNS relapse in patients with diffuse large B-cell lymphoma treated with R-CHOP. *J Clin Oncol*. 2016;34:3150-3156.

clinical behavior and therapeutic response. In DLBCL and MCL, a high proliferative fraction as defined by expression of the nuclear proliferation antigen Ki-67 (MIB1; >30%-60% of malignant cells) has identified patients at risk for early relapse and short survival.[233]

Correlations between acquired molecular abnormalities and specific lymphoma entities are a central part of the WHO classification and the understanding of lymphomagenesis. Immunophenotyping further identifies protein expression patterns that correlate with specific cytogenetic abnormalities and with prognosis (*Table 90.8*). Examples include nuclear cyclin D1 expression with the t(11;14) (q13;q32) of MCL and anaplastic lymphoma kinase (ALK) expression with the t(2;5) and its variants in ALCL.[234,235] BCL-6 expression has been associated with an improved outcome in DLBCL, but its absence may be less deleterious in the rituximab era.[236]

Gene expression profiling (GEP) using cDNA microarrays has been a powerful tool for dissecting pathogenetically relevant mutations and therapeutically targetable pathways in lymphomas. For example, DLBCL may be stratified into prognostic subtypes based on molecular profile.[237,238] These include primary mediastinal B-cell lymphoma (PMBL), germinal center B-cell–like (GCB), ABC-like, and a fourth type with a microarray signature distinct from the other types. PMBL and GCB have better prognoses than the others in patients treated with CHOP-like chemotherapy (*Figure 90.13*).[239] As molecular profiling is not currently practical for routine clinical use, efforts have been made to use immunophenotypic expression patterns to stratify DLBCL into GCB or non-GCB subtypes. One of these systems, the Hans algorithm, uses immunostains for CD10, BCL-6, and MUM1, with good correlation with gene expression profile analysis.[240,241] A modification, the Choi algorithm, also uses these markers plus GCET1 and FOXP1 to stratify patients into GCB vs ABC DLBCL, again correlating with OS.[242]

About 5% to 8% of DLBCL carry translocations in the *MYC* oncogene, often with coexisting *BCL2* and/or *BCL6* translocations ("double-hit" or "triple-hit"). MYC protein expression identifies *MYC* deregulation not detected by fluorescent in situ hybridization (FISH); and coexpression with BCL-2 is present in 21% to 29% of DLBCL.[243,244] Double-hit DLBCL has a poor outcome with standard R-CHOP chemotherapy; as such, testing for these markers using immunohistochemistry or FISH analysis and applying alternative treatment strategies for these patients are now being assessed.[245,246]

It should be recognized that prognostic markers for treatment response and patient outcome are defined within the context of specific regimens and thus may become irrelevant when newer therapeutics are applied. As such, it is essential to revalidate these markers with new regimens and targeted therapies. Several agents such as *BCL6, SYK, BTK,* and *EZH2* inhibitors are currently under investigation.

Table 90.7. Staging Studies in Non-Hodgkin Lymphoma

Complete history and physical examination, inquiring about B symptoms, HIV risk, infections, autoimmune diseases, immunosuppressive therapy
Complete blood count, including leukocyte count with differential, platelet count
Chemistry profile, particularly lactate dehydrogenase: also alkaline phosphatase, uric acid, creatinine, calcium, and albumin
Positron emission tomography/CT of neck, chest, abdomen, and pelvis
Bone marrow aspiration and biopsy—cytogenetics (+ fluorescent in situ hybridization [FISH] in specific lymphomas: *BCL2, BCL1, MYC, ALK,* others) and consider molecular tests and gene rearrangement studies in selected patients
Lumbar puncture with cytology in selected patients: all patients with Burkitt and lymphoblastic lymphomas; patients with non-Hodgkin lymphoma (NHL) in certain sites: nasopharynx, epidural space, testes, and large cell with marrow involvement; HIV + patients
Gastrointestinal (GI) endoscopy for patients with Waldeyer ring involvement or abdominal symptoms, or in patients with specific pathologies that have a propensity to the GI tract (e.g., mantle cell NHL)
Immunophenotype and flow cytometry of pathology specimen
Cytogenetics and/or gene rearrangement data in selected patients
Cytologic assessment of third space fluids (pleura, peritoneum)
Selected radiologic procedures as clinically appropriate (e.g., MRI, ultrasound, bone scan)
Other blood evaluations: viral studies as indicated (HIV, hepatitis B, hepatitis C, Epstein-Barr virus by PCR, and HTLV-1); levels of β_2-microglobulin and cytokines if clinically relevant

Functional Imaging

The use of ^{18}F-FDG PET scans has improved the sensitivity for initial staging and posttreatment restaging of NHL.[247] Assessment of treatment response by anatomic staging with routine CT scans, especially in aggressive lymphomas, reveals that many patients have measurable residual abnormalities. The significance of such findings is often problematic as to whether they represent fibrous tissue only vs residual lymphoma, and biopsy of these residual masses may be inconclusive or falsely negative due to sampling error or necrosis. Properly performed and interpreted PET scans have a high discriminatory value in identifying residual lymphoma in patients with incomplete therapeutic response. Several studies have correlated posttreatment PET positivity with relapse and poor survival, and prospective clinical trials are ongoing to assess the use of PET imaging to stratify patients for early institution of dose-intensive therapy.[248]

The use of interim PET imaging following two cycles of chemotherapy has shown a strong correlation with outcome in HL; however, interim PET in DLBCL remains controversial. Interim 18-FDG-PET/

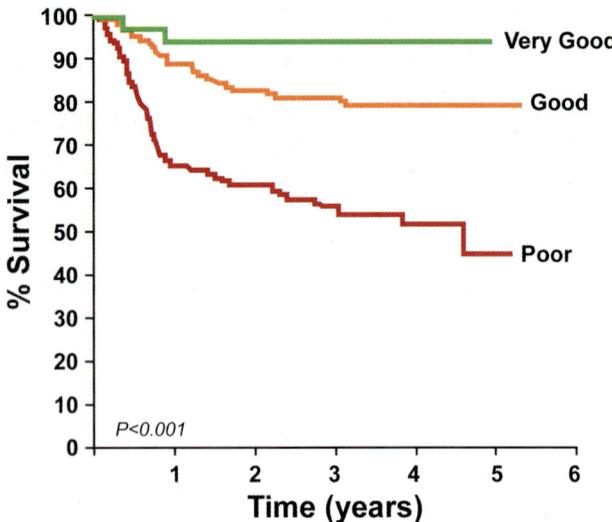

FIGURE 90.11 Progression-free survival according to the revised International Prognostic Index. (Reprinted from Sehn LH, Berry B, Chhanabhai M, et al. The revised International Prognostic Index (R-IPI) is a better predictor of outcome than the standard IPI for patients with diffuse large B-cell lymphoma treated with R-CHOP. *Blood*. 2007;109(5):1857-1861. Copyright © 2007 American Society of Hematology. With permission.)

CT failed to predict outcome in DLBCL patients treated at diagnosis with rituximab-CHOP.[249,250] Pre- and postinduction PET/CT imaging was performed in 122 patients with FL who took part in a prospective clinical trial of rituximab chemotherapy followed by maintenance rituximab (MR) vs observation.[251] Patients remaining PET-positive after induction therapy had significantly inferior PFS and increased risk of death compared to PET-negative individuals. Interestingly, response by traditional posttreatment restaging including CT scans did not correlate with outcome.

Response criteria for NHL include recommendations for incorporation of functional imaging by PET/CT scans (*Table 90.9*).[227] In addition, guidelines for standardization and interpretation of PET scans have been recommended for use in clinical trials and in prospective registries assessing treatment outcomes and prognosis.[252]

THERAPEUTIC PRINCIPLES

Therapy follows assessment of the patient, pathology, and stage of disease. Treatment tolerability is dependent on age, PS, and immune competence. How advanced age adversely affects outcome in therapy is controversial, but comorbid illnesses and biologic differences of lymphomas can contribute to higher mortality in the elderly. Treatment-related toxicities are greater in elderly patients, but deaths from unrelated causes are also increased.[253] Biologic differences of NHL between young and old patients are implicated by a greater

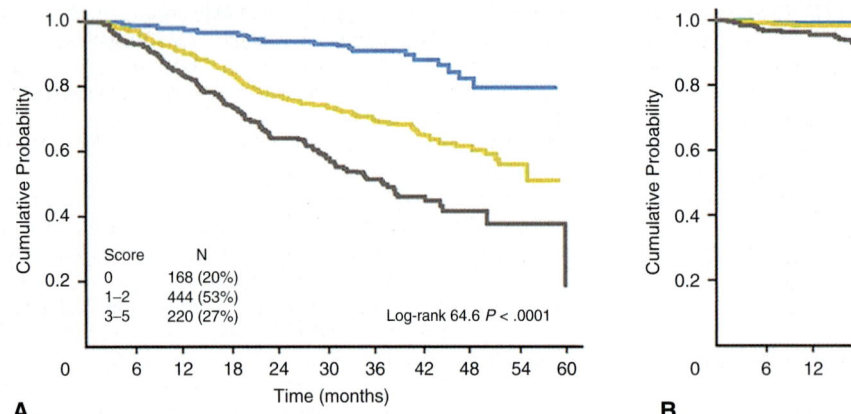
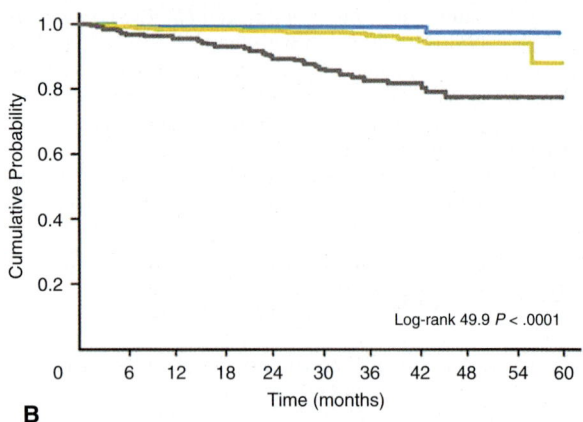

FIGURE 90.12 Progression-free survival (A) and overall survival (B) according to the Follicular Lymphoma International Prognostic Index 2. (Reprinted with permission from Federico M, Bellei M, Marcheselli L, et al. Follicular lymphoma international prognostic index 2: a new prognostic index for follicular lymphoma developed by the international follicular lymphoma prognostic factor project. *J Clin Oncol*. 2009;27(27):4555-4562. Copyright © 2009 by American Society of Clinical Oncology.)

Table 90.8. Prognostic Biomarkers by Immunohistochemistry in Aggressive Lymphoma

Biomarker	Pathway/Function	Correlation
ALK	Proliferation (tyrosine kinase)	Improved survival if positive in T-ALCL
BCL-2	Apoptosis	Decreased survival in ABC-like expressing BCL-2
Ki-67	Proliferation	Expression associated with increased proliferative rate and decreased survival in MCL, PTCL, and DLBCL
FOX P1	Transcription factor	Poor survival in cases with strong expression (DLBCL)
BCL-6	Transcriptional repressor, marker of germinal center origin	Improved response and survival in BCL-6–positive DLBCL
CD10$^+$; or CD10$^-$, BCL-6$^+$, MUM1$^-$	Markers for GCB-like subtype	Improved survival vs non-GCB (DLBCL)
CD10$^-$, BCL-6$^-$; or CD10$^-$, BCL-6$^+$, MUM1$^+$	Markers for non-GCB subtypes	Decreased survival vs GCB (DLBCL)
MYC plus BCL-2	Proliferation and apoptosis	Double expressor DLBCL, poor prognosis, but better than double hit
TP53$^+$, CDKN1A$^-$	Proliferation and apoptosis	*TP53* mutation, poor prognosis DLBCL and PTCL

Abbreviations: ABC, activated B cell; ALCL, anaplastic large cell lymphoma; DLBCL, diffuse large B-cell lymphoma; GCB, germinal center B; MCL, mantle cell lymphoma; PTCL, peripheral T-cell lymphoma.

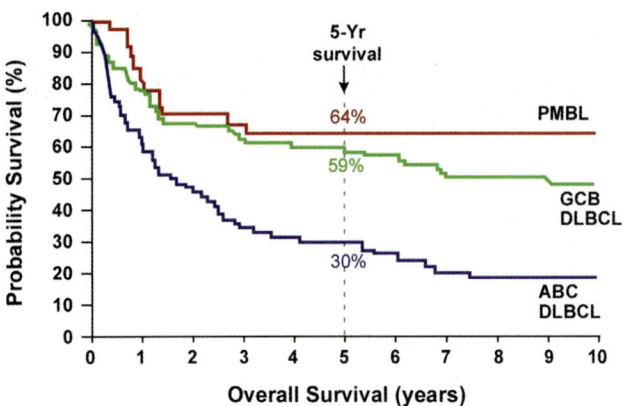

FIGURE 90.13 Gene expression arrays can stratify diffuse large B-cell lymphoma (DLBCL) into at least three subtypes, primary mediastinal B-cell lymphoma (PMBL), germinal center B-cell (GCB), and activated B-cell–like (ABC). This Kaplan-Meier curve indicates differing survival among the groups. (Reprinted with permission from Rosenwald A, Wright G, Leroy K, et al. Molecular diagnosis of primary mediastinal B-cell lymphoma identifies a clinically favorable subgroup of diffuse large B-cell lymphoma related to Hodgkin lymphoma. *J Exp Med*. 2003;198(6):851-862. Originally published in Journal of Experimental Medicine. https://doi.org/10.1084/jem.20031074. Copyright © 2003 by The Rockefeller University Press.)

lymphoma-related mortality in some series of elderly patients compared with younger cohorts[254] (see section "Therapy in the Elderly").

Treatment paradigms are based on pathology, disease biology, and risk stratification and will be discussed in the next several sections. *Table 90.10* outlines the current clinical schema based on the WHO classification.

INDOLENT B-CELL LYMPHOMAS

Indolent B-cell lymphomas include FL, LPL, small lymphocytic lymphoma, and MZL and are typically advanced at presentation but are still associated with long median survival. Most patients die with rather than from disease. There are many therapeutic options for indolent lymphomas based on symptoms, stage, and pathology (*Table 90.11*). Although they do respond to treatment, they tend to have a relapsing course. Immunotherapy, in particular anti-CD20 antibodies, has become a mainstay of treatment, often may be employed as frontline monotherapy with excellent outcomes, and has contributed to an improved survival in the past 2 decades. Newer chemotherapies and targeted agents have also contributed to an improved overall prognosis. However, a small proportion of indolent lymphomas will transform to more aggressive large cell phenotypes, typically with poorer outcomes. In these diseases, which are generally considered to be incurable, and where OS is often measured in decades, the goals of therapy prioritize minimizing symptoms and maximizing quality of life. As the treatment armamentarium continues to expand with the advent of novel therapies including CAR-T cell therapy and bispecific antibodies, long-lasting remissions are achievable and the potential for cure seems to be on the horizon for a proportion of patients.

Follicular Lymphoma

FL is the most common type of indolent lymphoma, accounting for approximately 60% of low-grade lymphomas and roughly 25% of all NHL.[20] FL commonly presents as asymptomatic lymphadenopathy, with a quarter of patients experiencing B symptoms.[223,255] Bone marrow involvement is common (30%-60%); only about one-third of patients will present with stage I/II disease.[224,256] Despite commonly advanced stage at presentation, median survival is approaching 20 years and has improved with the incorporation of anti-CD20 monoclonal antibodies and better supportive care into therapy.[257]

FL cells typically express CD10, CD19, CD20, CD22, CD79α, surface Ig, BCL-2, and BCL-6. Cytogenetic changes involving the *BCL2* gene locus, most commonly t(14;18) (q32;q21), result in overexpression of the anti–apoptotic BCL-2 protein. Evaluation for *BCL2* translocation may identify occult disease in the bone marrow or peripheral blood.[258] Cytologic examination by light microscopy classifies FL into grades based on the number of centrocytes per high power field. Grades 1, 2, and 3a are considered to be indolent disease, whereas grade 3b is felt to behave like aggressive lymphoma and is treated more aggressively with combination chemoimmunotherapy. In addition to clinical parameters incorporated into the FLIPI score, tumor intrinsic factors may predict outcomes. Immunohistochemical stains for Ki-67 measure the proliferation index and are correlated with cytologic grading.[259] Discordant low-grade, high Ki-67 occurred in 18% of cases in one study and had more aggressive clinical behavior as compared to low-grade, low Ki-67.[260] Thus, Ki-67 evaluation

Table 90.9. 2007 and 2014 Response Criteria for Non-Hodgkin Lymphoma

Response Category	Definition	Nodal and Extranodal Masses	Spleen/Liver	Bone Marrow
Complete response	Disappearance of all evidence of disease	a. FDG-avid or PET positive prior to therapy becomes negative (score of 1 or 2); a posttreatment mass of any size is permitted if PET negative b. If variably FDG-avid or PET positive prior to therapy, all lymph nodes should regress to normal size on CT	Not palpable; nodules disappear	Infiltrate cleared on repeat biopsy; if indeterminate by morphology, immunohistochemistry should be negative
Partial response	Regression of measurable disease and no new sites	a. ≥50% decrease in SPD of up to 6 largest masses; no increase in size of other nodes b. One or more persistently FDG-avid or PET-positive sites c. Regression on CT if variably FDG-avid or PET negative	≥50% decrease in SPD of nodules; no increase in size of liver or spleen	Irrelevant if positive prior to therapy and partial response at other sites
Stable disease	Failure to attain CR/PR, but does not meet criteria for progressive disease	a. FDG-avid or PET positive at prior sites of disease and no new sites on PET or CT b. Variably FDG-avid or PET negative; no change in size of previous lesions on CT		
Relapsed or progressive disease	Any new lesion or increase by ≥50% of previously involved sites from nadir	a. Appearance of a new lesion(s) >1.5 cm in any axis, ≥50% increase in SPD of more than one node, or ≥50% increase in longest diameter of a previously identified node >1 cm in short axis. Lesions PET positive if FDG-avid lymphoma or PET positive prior to therapy (score of 4 or 5)	>50% increase from nadir in the SPD of any previous lesions	New or recurrent involvement

Abbreviations: CT, computed tomography; FDG, [18]Ffluorodeoxyglucose; PET, positron emission tomography-using a 5-point scale; a score of 3 can indicate a good prognosis, particularly if an interim scan, but 3 may be called an inadequate response if de-escalation is considered (to avoid undertreatment); PR, partial remission; SPD, sum of the product of the diameters.
Adapted from Cheson BD, Pfistner B, Juweid ME, et al. Revised response criteria for malignant lymphoma. *J Clin Oncol*. 2007;25:579-586; Cheson BD, Fisher RI, Barrington SF, et al. Recommendations for initial evaluation, staging, and response assessment of Hodgkin and non-Hodgkin lymphoma: the Lugano classification. *J Clin Oncol*. 2014;32:3059-3067.

Table 90.10. Clinical Schema for Lymphoid Neoplasms

B-cell Lineage	T/NK-cell Lineage
Indolent	
Chronic lymphocytic leukemia/small lymphocytic lymphoma	Large granular lymphocytic leukemia, T- and NK-cell types
B-cell prolymphocytic leukemia	Mycosis fungoides/Sézary syndrome
Lymphoplasmacytic lymphoma/Waldenström macroglobulinemia Follicular lymphoma (grade I/II/IIIa)	Primary cutaneous CD30+ T-cell lymphoproliferative disorders Lymphomatoid papulosis
Duodenal-type follicular lymphoma	Primary cutaneous anaplastic large cell lymphoma
Primary cutaneous follicular lymphoma	Smoldering and chronic adult T-cell leukemia/lymphoma (HTLV-1+)
Marginal zone B-cell lymphoma	Subcutaneous panniculitis-like T-cell lymphoma (can be aggressive)
Splenic marginal zone lymphoma	*Indolent T-cell lymphoproliferative disorder of the GI tract*
Extranodal (MALT-B-cell lymphoma)	*Primary cutaneous acral CD8+ T-cell lymphoma*
Nodal (monocytoid)	*Primary cutaneous CD4+ small/medium T-cell lymphoproliferative disorder*
Splenic B-cell lymphoma/leukemia, unclassifiable	
Aggressive	
Mantle cell lymphoma (can be indolent)	T-cell prolymphocytic leukemia (can be indolent)
Follicular (large cell)-grade IIIb	Peripheral T cell lymphoma, not otherwise specified
Diffuse large B cell lymphoma (DLBCL)	Anaplastic large cell lymphoma, ALK+
Germinal center B-cell type	Anaplastic large cell lymphoma, ALK−
Activated B-cell type	Angioimmunoblastic T-cell lymphoma
T-cell/histiocyte-rich large B-cell lymphoma	*Follicular T-cell lymphoma*
Primary mediastinal (thymic) large B-cell lymphoma	*Nodal PTCL with T_{FH} phenotype*
Primary cutaneous DLBCL, leg type	Enteropathy-associated T-cell lymphoma
Intravascular B-cell lymphoma	Monomorphic epitheliotropic intestinal T-cell lymphoma Extranodal
Large B-cell lymphoma with IRF4 rearrangement	NK/T-cell lymphoma, nasal type
Primary DLBCL of the central nervous system	Hepatosplenic γδ T-cell lymphoma
EBV+ DLBCL, not otherwise specified	Primary cutaneous γδ T-cell lymphoma
ALK+ large B-cell lymphoma	*Primary cutaneous CD8+ aggressive epidermotropic cytotoxic T-cell lymphoma*
B-cell lymphoma, unclassifiable, with features intermediate between DLBCL and Hodgkin lymphoma	Breast implant–associated anaplastic large cell lymphoma
Highly Aggressive	
Precursor B-lymphoblastic lymphoma/leukemia	Precursor T-lymphoblastic lymphoma/leukemia
Burkitt lymphoma/B cell acute leukemia	Adult T-cell lymphoma/leukemia (HTLV-1+) (lymphoma and acute leukemia subtypes)
Burkitt-like lymphoma with 11q aberration	Aggressive NK-cell leukemia
High-grade B-cell lymphoma with intermediate features between DLBCL and Burkitt lymphoma with (*MYC, BCL2, BCL6*) and without gene rearrangements	

Provisional entities are listed in italics.
Abbreviations: ALK, anaplastic lymphoma kinase; EBV, Epstein-Barr virus; HTLV-1, human T-lymphotropic virus type 1; MALT, mucosa-associated lymphoid tissue; NK, natural killer.

Table 90.11. Therapeutic Options for Indolent Lymphoma

Watchful waiting
Local radiation for limited-stage disease
Chemotherapy with immunotherapy
    Bendamustine
    Combination chemotherapy
    Alkylating agent
Immunotherapy
    Unconjugated monoclonal antibodies
    Radioimmunotherapy
    CAR-T cell therapy
    Bispecific antibodies
Combined modality
    Chemotherapy and radiation
Transplantation
    Autologous ± purging
    Allogeneic
        Myeloablative
        Nonmyeloablative
Selected therapies
    Antibiotics in selected MALTomas
    Splenectomy
Novel agents
    BTK inhibitors
    EZH2 inhibitors
Immunomodulatory agents
    PI3K inhibitors

may have additional prognostic value and may be considered in treatment decisions. Elevation of serum β_2-microglobulin above the upper limit of normal has also been identified as a strong prognostic factor in FL, and has been incorporated into modern prognostic scoring systems developed in the rituximab era.[261] Translocations involving the minor cluster region 30 kb downstream of the *BCL2* gene occur in only 11% of cases but are associated with 95% failure-free survival (FFS) at 3 years, whereas translocations involving the major breakpoint region in the 3′ untranslated region of the *BCL2* gene occur in 71% of cases and are associated with 76% 3-year FFS.[262,263] Persistence of *BCL2* gene rearrangements has also been studied as a marker of residual disease after treatment and has been shown to predict shorter disease-free intervals but had no effect on OS.[258,264] Thus, its prognostic value remains controversial. The prognostic importance of the tumor microenvironment has also been investigated. Favorable and unfavorable gene expression signatures have been identified (respectively, "immune response 1" enriched for T-cell and macrophage-specific genes *CD7, CD8B1, ITK, LEF1, STAT4, ACTN1,* and *TNFSF3B,* and "immune response 2" reflecting macrophage/dendritic cell influence with high expression of *TLR5, FCGR1A, SEPT10, CCR1, LGMN,* and *C3AR1*) in nonmalignant tumor-infiltrating cells.[265] A clinicogenetic risk model (m7-FLIPI) has been developed which integrates the mutation status of seven genes (EZH2, ARID1A, MEF2B, EP300, FOXO1, CREBBP, and CARD11) and stratifies patients into risk groups predictive of failure of chemoimmunotherapy.[266] The most robust predictor of survival for patients with FL is the response to initial chemoimmunotherapy at 24 months. Work by Casulo et al from the National

LymphoCare Study demonstrated that 20% of patients initially treated with R-CHOP for FL had progression of disease at 2 years (POD24), and that the 5-year OS for this group of patients was 50%, as opposed to the non-POD24 group where it was 90%. In a multivariable model, male sex, impaired PS, elevated β-2-microglobulin, and high follicular FLIPI risk score were associated with an increased risk for POD24 and worse survival.[267,268]

Small B Lymphocytic Lymphoma

SLL comprises approximately 6% of all NHL.[20] SLL has extensive clinical overlap with CLL (Chapter 92). The WHO considers SLL and CLL different clinical presentations of the same disease,[1] and SLL accounts for 15% of cases within this spectrum.[269] SLL is characterized by prominent generalized lymphadenopathy without lymphocytosis, but over time, 10% to 20% of patients develop lymphocytosis.[270] Between 2% and 8% of CLL/SLL evolve into an aggressive large cell process known as *Richter syndrome*, which is characterized by bulky retroperitoneal adenopathy, rising LDH, and survival usually less than 1 year.[271,272]

Lymphoplasmacytic Lymphoma

LPL largely overlaps with WM (Chapter 102). LPL represents 1% of NHL and usually presents in the elderly (median age 60-70 years).[20,273] Patients may exhibit symptoms associated with lymphadenopathy, splenomegaly, or bone marrow involvement.[274] A paraprotein, most commonly IgM, is found in 29% to 50% of LPL cases and can contribute to hyperviscosity, neuropathy, and glomerular disease.[275] Plasmapheresis will reduce the paraprotein levels in the blood and improve hyperviscosity symptoms while definitive treatment is being initiated.[276] A positive Coombs test, cold agglutinin disease, cryoglobulinemia, autoimmune diseases, and positive HCV serology can be associated with LPL and WM.[277] Mutation analysis of the myeloid differentiation primary response gene-88 (*MYD88*) is now incorporated into the diagnostic workflow for WM, where *MYD88* L265P mutation occurs in nearly 90% of cases and predicts likelihood of response to the oral Bruton tyrosine kinase (BTK) inhibitor ibrutinib.[278,279] Median survivals prior to ibrutinib approval for first-line therapy in WM have been variable, usually in the 5- to 10-year range.[280] An International Prognostic Scoring System for WM was devised and incorporates the adverse risk factors of advanced age, cytopenias, elevated β$_2$-microglobulin, and paraprotein levels greater than 7.0 g/dL.

Marginal Zone Lymphoma

Marginal zone B-cell lymphomas account for between 5% and 7% of all NHL and include nodal based disease, extranodal lymphoma of MALToma, and SMZL.[20,273] Extranodal MALTomas are most common among them (50%-70%) and are discussed in the section "Management of Extranodal Lymphomas." Nodal MZL occurs in the elderly (median age 59-65 years) and preferentially in women (up to 2:1 female:male ratio).[273,281] It may present as localized lymphadenopathy.[281] Bone marrow involvement is less common than with other indolent lymphomas, and cytopenias and paraproteinemia are also rare. The most frequent cytogenetic abnormalities are gains in chromosomes 3 and 18q23.[282] Median OS is in the range of 9 to 12 years.[281,283]

Like nodal MZL, SMZL also occurs in the elderly (median age 61-70 years) and has a relatively long median survival (10.5 years).[284,285] In contrast, the clinical course is often more obtrusive, with symptoms related to splenomegaly, peripheral cytopenias, and marrow involvement.[284] Even with disseminated disease, splenectomy can alleviate symptoms and improve cytopenias.[286] A paraprotein may be present and is an adverse prognostic factor, as are elevated β$_2$-microglobulin and lymphocyte count >9 × 10^9/L.[287,288] In a simple prognostic scoring system, the 5-year cause-specific survival was correlated with the presence of no, one, or more than one adverse risk factor (hemoglobin <120 g/L, LDH greater than normal, and albumin <35 g/L) and corresponded to 88%, 73%, and 50%, respectively.[284] Multiple cytogenetic abnormalities have been identified in SMZL, although none is specific for the disease and the prognostic implications of any particular aberration are still debated.[282,289]

Special Clinicopathologic Features

Spontaneous regression has been reported in the indolent lymphomas. In a series of 83 untreated FL patients, Horning and Rosenberg reported spontaneous regression occurred in 23%, including complete regression in six patients.[290] Spontaneous regression occurs in approximately one-fourth of primary cutaneous ALCL (see section "Anaplastic Large Cell Lymphoma").

At the other end of the spectrum, indolent lymphomas may undergo HT, which is usually associated clinically with one or more rapidly growing lymph nodes and rising LDH levels. HT is the forerunner and counterpart of the Richter syndrome of CLL/SLL.[271,272] Although the actual incidence of HT is uncertain and historically has varied widely between studies, it is believed to be an infrequent event. Grade 1 FL is the most common lymphoma to undergo HT, but the risk of HT in FL is estimated at 2% to 4% per year.[291,292] Although the risk of transformation is generally accepted to increase over time, some series have suggested that the risk plateaus between 6 and 20 years after diagnosis.[292,293] Factors predictive of HT in FL have included failure to achieve complete response (CR) with prior treatments, hypoalbuminemia, elevated β$_2$-microglobulin (>3 mg/L), and a high FLIPI score at diagnosis.[293,294] Studies have confirmed that the majority of patients with POD24 after treatment with chemoimmunotherapy harbor transformed disease.[295] Transformation in low-grade FL is characterized by loss of a follicular pattern and an increase in the number of large noncleaved cells per high power field.[290,296] Some reports have implicated clonal evolution and accumulation of additional cytogenetic abnormalities.[297] HT carries a poor prognosis, with median survival historically reported as less than 1 year (range 2.5-22 months), although patients with limited-stage disease, low FLIPI, and no prior chemotherapy exposure at the time of HT have better outcomes than those with heavily pretreated and/or advanced stage disease.[291,292]

Treatment Options: Stages I and II Indolent B-cell Lymphoma

Indolent lymphomas are uncommonly diagnosed with limited-stage disease, ranging from 6% to 20% across multiple series, with pathologic staging providing the more conservative estimates. With more widespread use of sensitive imaging modalities, immunophenotyping, cyto- and molecular genetic testing, minor involvement in clinically unapparent sites may be identified; however, how to incorporate these findings into therapeutic decision-making remains unclear. In a prospective study in stage I FL, treatment strategies were highly variable (e.g., observation, chemoimmunotherapy, radiation therapy [XRT], single-agent rituximab, systemic therapy + XRT). No statistically significant differences were seen in OS at a median follow-up of 57 months.[298] For asymptomatic patients with minimal disease, treatment is not urgent and observation can be considered without adversely affecting prognosis.[299,300] However, reconciling a diagnosis of lymphoma with observation alone can be difficult and less intensive therapies may be employed. Radiation therapy may induce a durable remission, and possibly even cure a subset of patients, with the best results in patients <50 years of age with nonbulky (<2.5 cm) disease involving a single nodal group.[301,302] In limited-stage FL, radiation therapy achieved relapse-free survival at 10 and 20 years of 44% and 37%.[302,303] Efficacy of involved field or involved nodal radiation therapy was comparable with 10 years PFS and OS of 49 and 66%, respectively, and no difference in relapse rate.[304] Disease relapse outside of the radiation field is a common occurrence. An attractive therapeutic alternative, especially in light of the fact that many patients may have occult disease outside the radiation field, is single-agent anti-CD20 monoclonal antibody rituximab. CD20 is an ideal target in B-cell lymphoma, because it is expressed on the surface of B cells in all stages of maturation and virtually all B NHL cells, but is not expressed on hematopoietic stem cells or PCs.[305,306] Furthermore, CD20 does not shed or internalize after binding with antibody.[307,308] Rituximab, a chimeric monoclonal antibody that targets CD20, is the most widely used immunotherapy in the treatment of indolent NHL. When rituximab engages CD20 on the surface of a B lymphoma cell, it leads to antibody-dependent cellular cytotoxicity, via Ig heavy-chain receptors (FcR) on monocytes and T/NK cells, complement-mediated lysis, and induction of apoptosis.[309,310] Rituximab is both well tolerated and efficacious with first-line response rates ranging from 47% to 76%.[311,312]

Frontline Treatment Options: Stages III and IV Indolent B-cell Lymphoma

Among the most controversial decisions in the management of indolent lymphomas are when to initiate treatment and with what type of therapy (*Table 90.11*). Patient age, preference, PS, comorbid illnesses, histologic lymphoma grade, and physician training and bias influence therapeutic decisions. Indolent lymphomas have propensity to relapse and early chemotherapeutic intervention has not achieved improvement in OS in advanced stages compared to a delayed treatment approach.[290,313] Three trials randomized patients to watchful waiting or to some form of treatment upon diagnosis, and none showed improvement in OS with earlier therapy.[314-316] In one study, the median time to chemotherapy initiation in the observation group was 31 months. The actuarial chance of not requiring chemotherapy at 10 years was 19%.[316] In a trial comparing early employment of single-agent rituximab vs observation in advanced stage disease, PFS was significantly longer in patients treated with rituximab (not reached vs 24 months in the observation group).[317] However, there was again no difference in OS between the two groups. Thus, "watchful waiting" may be appropriate for asymptomatic patients despite advanced stage of disease.

Clinical features associated with more aggressive disease and which may warrant therapy include B symptoms, bulky lymphadenopathy, nodal encroachment on vital organs, massive organomegaly, cytopenias, and HT.[315,317] Frontline therapy for advanced indolent lymphoma, in particular FL, is evolving. As randomized trials with head-to-head comparison of different chemotherapeutic regimens are challenging due to long median survivals, requiring prolonged follow-up, therapeutic strategies are variable. There is, however, general consensus that incorporating anti-CD20 antibodies into the treatment plan optimizes the response of indolent B-cell NHL once the decision to treat has been made.

Rituximab is effective as a single agent[311,318] with response rates ranging from 47% to 76% (up to 20%-45% CR), depending on disease burden and B-cell lymphoma subtype. In a multicenter trial involving 166 patients with relapsed indolent NHL treated with single-agent rituximab given weekly for 4 weeks, McLaughlin et al reported a 48% response and a median time to progression of 13 months for responders.[319] This study led to rituximab's approval by the US FDA for relapsed indolent NHL in 1997. Subsequent studies of frontline rituximab have reported higher response rates of approximately 70% to 80%.[317] Rituximab has also improved response rates, duration of response, and OS when added to chemotherapy.[320,321] Randomized trials have almost uniformly favored the rituximab-plus-chemotherapy arms over chemotherapy alone for both indolent and more aggressive B-cell lymphomas. Regimens containing second-generation anti-CD20 antibodies, including obinutuzumab and ofatumumab, have also demonstrated efficacy in indolent NHL.[322-325]

The most commonly used frontline regimens in the United States in the multicenter, longitudinal National LymphoCare study published in 2009 were R-CHOP (rituximab, cyclophosphamide, adriamycin, vincristine, prednisone) (55%), followed by R-CVP (rituximab, cyclophosphamide, vincristine, prednisone) (23%), and R-fludarabine-based therapy (15.5%).[326] With the advent of newer and better-tolerated agents, such as bendamustine, the use of anthracyclines and fludarabine in initial therapy for advanced indolent lymphomas has become controversial. Two prospective studies comparing bendamustine + rituximab (BR) to R-CHOP and/or R-CVP have garnered support for the non–anthracycline-based therapy. In a randomized phase III trial of bendamustine plus rituximab (BR) vs R-CHOP by Rummel et al, the overall response rate (ORR) was equivalent, but BR achieved a higher CR rate (40% vs 30%, $P = .021$), longer PFS (69.5 vs 31.2 months, $P < .0001$), and was better tolerated (*Figure 90.14*).[327] Flinn et al also found that BR demonstrated better long-term disease control than R-CVP/R-CHOP in primarily advanced indolent lymphoma (PFS

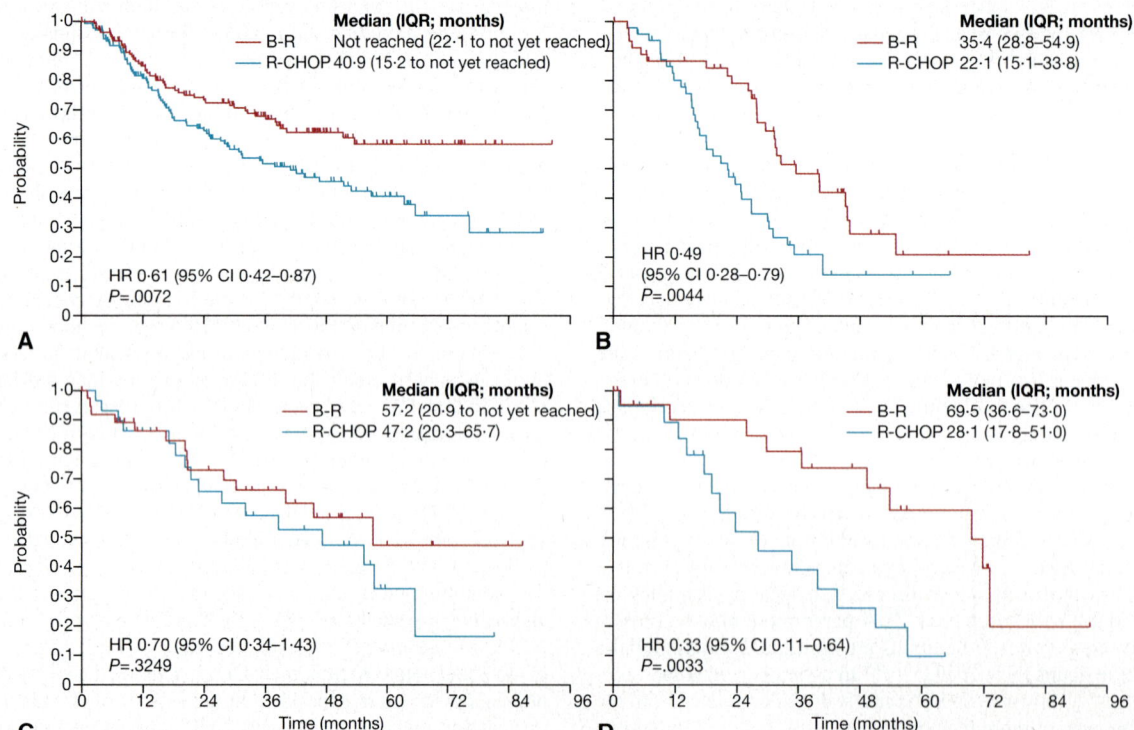

FIGURE 90.14 Median progression-free survival was longer in the bendamustine plus rituximab (BR) groups than in the CHOP plus rituximab (R-CHOP) groups except in marginal zone lymphoma: (A) follicular, (B) mantle cell, (C) marginal zone, and (D) Waldenström macroglobulinemia. (Reprinted from Rummel MJ, Niederle N, Maschmeyer G, et al. Bendamustine plus rituximab versus CHOP plus rituximab as first-line treatment for patients with indolent and mantle-cell lymphomas: an open-label, multicenter, randomized, phase 3 non-inferiority trial. *Lancet*. 2013;381(9873):1203-1210. Copyright © 2013 Elsevier. With permission.)

at 5 years 65.5% vs 55.8%, 95% CI, 0.45-0.85, P = .0025) and was associated with less peripheral neuropathy and alopecia.[328] Thus, BR has supplanted R-CHOP as first-line therapy for advanced indolent lymphoma in many centers, but R-CHOP is still favored in high-grade (especially grade 3b) FL and transformed indolent lymphomas. Obinutuzumab-based frontline chemoimmunotherapy has demonstrated prolonged PFS compared to rituximab-based regimens (5-year PFS: hazard ratio [HR] 0.76; 95% CI: 0.62-0.92; P = .0043; 70.5% [95% CI: 66.4-74.1] vs 63.2% [95% CI: 59.0-67.1]), with no improvement in OS but with an increased risk for high-grade adverse events, most commonly infections.[329]

Fludarabine has been shown to be efficacious in indolent NHL both as a single agent and in combination; however, modern regimens incorporating bendamustine are generally favored due to improved efficacy and tolerability.[330-333]

The roles of immunomodulatory and targeted agents in the treatment of indolent NHL are evolving, but in large part are reserved for the relapsed and refractory setting. In a multicenter phase II trial, the combination of lenalidomide with rituximab demonstrated efficacy in previously untreated FL with CR rates of over 70% and estimated 5-year PFS of nearly 70%.[334,335] The international, multicenter phase III RELEVANCE study compared the combination of lenalidomide and rituximab to rituximab plus chemotherapy in previously untreated FL. Rituximab plus lenalidomide (R^2) demonstrated comparable efficacy compared to rituximab plus chemotherapy (CR/CRu rate of 48% vs 53%, respectively (P = .13), and PFS of 77% vs 78% respectively). Fewer patients in the R^2 group experienced grade 3 or 4 neutropenia (32% vs 50% in the rituximab-chemotherapy group), or neutropenia of any grade (2% vs 7%), but had a higher occurrence of grade 3 or 4 cutaneous reactions (7% vs 1%).[336]

In combination with rituximab and/or dexamethasone, proteasome inhibitors (bortezomib and carfilzomib) produce rapid responses with low risk of IgM flare in treatment-naïve and relapsed LPL.[337-341] Ibrutinib and zanubrutinib have also demonstrated robust responses and are well tolerated when used as primary therapy for LPL. The treatment of LPL and Waldenström macroglobulinemia is reviewed in further detail in Chapter 102.

The treatment of SLL is analogous to CLL, where the BTK inhibitors ibrutinib, acalabrutinib, and zanubrutinib have demonstrated durable remissions and have emerged as preferred first-line therapy either as single agents or combined with the anti-CD20 agent obinutuzumab.[342,343] The BCL2 inhibitor venetoclax is FDA approved for use in CLL/SLL either as a single agent or in combination with obinutuzumab or rituximab. The treatment of SLL/CLL is reviewed in further detail in Chapter 92.

Beyond first-line therapy, maintenance therapy with anti-CD20 antibodies, mostly commonly MR, may be considered. In FL cases with high volume disease that were treated with and responded to cyclophosphamide-based chemoimmunotherapy, MR improved the PFS, but did not benefit OS and increased the risk of infectious complications.[344] The benefit of MR has not been defined following other frontline chemoimmunotherapy treatment options, such as BR. Obinutuzumab-chemotherapy induction and maintenance has also been shown to prolong PFS (compared to rituximab-chemotherapy induction and maintenance) without affecting OS.[345]

The Swiss Group for Clinical Cancer Research compared short-term (4 doses given 2 months apart) vs long-term rituximab maintenance (bimonthly doses for up to 5 years) in patients with previously untreated FL who achieved at least a PR after 4 weekly doses of rituximab induction. After a median follow-up for 10 years, the median event-free survival was 3.4 years (95% confidence interval [CI], 2.1-5.5) in the short-term MR arm and 5.3 years (95% CI, 3.5-7.5) in the long-term MR arm, which was not statistically significant.[346] Similarly, there was no statistically significant difference in OS, with median OS of 11.0 years (95% CI, 11.0-NA) in the short-term arm and was not reached in the long-term arm (P = .80), and long-term MR was associated with higher rates of toxicities, most commonly infections. The RESORT study compared MR (single dose every 3 months) to retreatment with rituximab (RR; 4 weekly doses given at disease progression) following frontline single-agent rituximab in patients with low tumor burden FL. Long-term follow-up has shown that retreatment with rituximab is effective for the majority of patients (ORR 61%) and that the OS of patients treated with MR vs RR is not statistically different (10-year OS of 84% for MR vs 83% for RR).[347,348]

Relapsed and Refractory Treatment Options

Conventional therapy for FL is not curative, and many patients will ultimately develop progressive disease following initial treatment. Following frontline therapy, patients are followed regularly with history, physical exam, and blood work to monitor for any signs or symptoms concerning for relapsed disease. Patients with asymptomatic relapses can often be monitored closely for symptomatic disease or other indications for treatment as in the frontline setting. Frequent imaging scans are not recommended in the absence of symptoms or signs of relapse. Patients who progress within 24 months of initial chemoimmunotherapy or within 12 months of single-agent rituximab have been shown to have significantly inferior outcomes and high rates of HT.[267,268] Repeat biopsy prior to retreatment is often indicated to rule out transformed disease, particularly in patients with early relapses. Multiple salvage therapies are available and include cytotoxic chemotherapy, immunomodulatory and targeted agents, and immunotherapy. For many patients, intermittent treatment over the course of decades is often required and the focus of second-line therapy and beyond is to alleviate symptoms, reverse cytopenias, and to improve quality of life. For patients experiencing early relapse, a more aggressive approach may be beneficial.

A main treatment option for patients with symptomatic relapsed FL is single-agent rituximab. Rituximab given weekly for 4 doses resulted in an ORR of 48% with a median time to progression of 13 months for responders in a multicenter trial in patients with relapsed FL.[319] In the Resort trial, patients who progressed after initial treatment with rituximab achieved an ORR of 67% with a median duration of response to second-line rituximab of 2.1 years.[348] Thus, this option is often utilized in patients with low tumor burden relapsed FL.

Chemoimmunotherapy also remains an option for relapsed FL, combining either rituximab or obinutuzumab with a chemotherapy backbone, typically differing from first-line therapy. BR demonstrated high response rates (ORR 90%, CR 55%) with median PFS of approximately 2 years in patients with FL who relapsed after rituximab or CHOP.[349,350] In patients who had a suboptimal response to rituximab, bendamustine plus obinutuzumab (BO), followed by 2 years of obinutuzumab maintenance, was studied in the GADOLIN trial, resulting in PFS of 25.8 months. This study demonstrated an OS benefit of BO compared to single-agent bendamustine (HR, 0.67; 95% CI, 0.47-0.96; P = .027) in patients with relapsed FL.[351] R-CHOP or O-CHOP can also be utilized in the relapsed setting. While BR has demonstrated improved PFS and tolerability vs R-CHOP in frontline FL, and similarly BO has demonstrated superior PFS compared to BR in previously untreated FL, such head-to-head comparisons have not been completed in the R/R setting. In patients who respond to salvage chemoimmunotherapy, consolidative autologous stem cell transplantation (auto-SCT) appears to improve long-term survival for patients who are eligible, based on retrospective analyses. The role of allogeneic transplantation has not been defined and is associated with high potential for toxicities, which must be carefully considered in indolent lymphoma where OS is often measured in decades even in the relapsed setting. Typically, allogeneic transplantation is reserved for patients who have had numerous prior regimens including some patients who receive an auto-SCT and relapsed.

The combination of rituximab and lenalidomide (R^2) is highly active in patients with R/R FL, with ORR of 80% including 35% CR, and is associated with improved PFS compared to rituximab monotherapy (39.4 vs 14.1 months, HR 0.46 95% CI, 0.34-0.62; P < .001). Infections (63% vs 49%), neutropenia (58% vs 23%), severe neutropenia (50% vs 13%), and cutaneous reactions (32% vs 12%) are more common with R^2 compared to single-agent rituximab; however, R^2 was not associated with any other serious grade 3 or 4 adverse events.[352]

The role of phosphoinositide-3-kinase (PI3K) inhibition in relapsed indolent lymphoma continues to evolve. Early data demonstrated promising activity in heavily pretreated patients, leading to the initial approval of four agents in R/R FL. Due to significant toxicities including neutropenia, diarrhea, transaminitis, and concerns for an increased risk of death in some trials, this enthusiasm has subsequently been tempered. Currently, copanlisib (pan-isoform inhibitor) is the only available PI3K inhibitor approved by the FDA for use in R/R FL where it has demonstrated an ORR of 59% including 12% CR and a median PFS of 11.2 months in patients previously treated with 2 or more prior therapies.[353] Idelalisib and duvelisib are approved for use in SLL/CLL and are discussed in further detail in Chapter 92.

EZH2 is an important epigenetic regulator of B-cell development, and approximately 25% of patients with FL possess EZH2 gain-of-function mutations.[354] Tazemetostat is an EZH2 inhibitor that has demonstrated an ORR of 70% in EZH2 mutated FL with DOR of 13.8 months and is a well-tolerated treatment option in patients with FL whose tumors are positive for EZH2 mutations who have received at least 2 prior systemic therapies.[355] Tazemetostat also demonstrated an ORR of 34% in EZH2 WT cases, and given its favorable toxicity profile, it is an option for patients with R/R FL who lack other treatment options, agnostic of EZH2 mutational status.

There is much fervor currently to harness the immune response to further improve on treatment strategies, and as these therapies evolve, the landscape of second-line treatment and beyond for indolent lymphomas remains dynamic. The optimal sequencing of these salvage therapies remains unknown.

Immunotherapy

Immunotherapy for indolent lymphoma includes a broad and expanding number of approaches. Historically, these have included nonspecific immunostimulation with IFNs, passive humoral therapy with antilymphoid monoclonal antibodies (such as rituximab), and radioimmunotherapy. Chimeric antigen receptor (CAR)–directed T cells are a recent addition to the treatment armamentarium and newer therapies including bispecific antibodies are also emerging in the relapsed/refractory setting.

The ability of an antibody to home to lymphoma cells has been co-opted to deliver radiation directly to tumor cells. The radioisotopes yttrium-90 (^{90}Y) or iodine-131 (^{131}I) have been conjugated to anti-CD20 antibodies. In a randomized trial comparing ^{90}Y-ibritumomab tiuxetan to rituximab in relapsed/refractory FL, radioimmunotherapy had a higher response rate (80% vs 56%, $P = .002$) with more durable responses of ≥6 months.[356] As compared to no further treatment, consolidation with a single dose of ^{90}Y-ibritumomab tiuxetan in FL patients, who achieved at least partial remission after first-line induction treatment, extended the PFS nearly threefold (36.5 vs 13.3 months).[357] ^{131}I-tositumomab (no longer available) also demonstrated improved response rates (65%) in chemorefractory indolent or transformed NHL[358] and 97% response rate (75% CR) with a median PFS of 6.1 years in treatment-naïve FL patients.[359] However, radioimmunotherapy is myelosuppressive with a trend toward increased incidence of treatment-related MDS. Thus, in current practice, radioimmunotherapy is typically reserved for very selected cases and is infrequently used given numerous other options.

Cellular immunotherapy for lymphomas is an important component of allogeneic stem cell transplantation efficacy, albeit with concomitant risk of graft-vs-host disease. A novel approach instead utilizes autologous T cells genetically engineered to express a CAR that directs the effector CAR-T cell to a B cell surface marker such as CD19. The intracellular portion of the CAR contains costimulatory elements that prime the T-cell response. After demonstrating impressive and durable responses in the phase II ZUMA-5 trial, the CD19 targeting axicabtagene ciloleucel, also called Yescarta, was granted FDA approval in R/R FL after two or more lines of therapy. Patients with FL had an ORR of 92% with 74% CRs, and a median PFS of nearly 40 months.[360] Based on the results of the phase II ELARA trial, a second CAR-T cell product tisagenlecleucel, also called Kymriah, has also been FDA approved as a third-line and beyond therapy for R/R FL. Following a median of four prior therapies, tisagenlecleucel produced an ORR of 86.2%, with a CRR of 66.0%.[361,362] CAR-T therapy is associated with unique and serious complications, including cytokine release syndrome (CRS), a severe systemic response to the activation of CAR-T cells, and neurologic toxicities (immune effector cell–associated neurotoxicity syndrome, or ICANS) which can be life threatening in extreme cases. In ZUMA-5, CRS of any grade was observed in 78% of patients, with grade 3 or worse CRS seen in 7% of patients and grade 3 or 4 neurological events in 19% of patients.[360] In ELARA, rates of CRS were 48.5% (grade ≥3, 0%), neurological events 37.1% (grade ≥3, 3%), and immune effector cell–associated neurotoxicity syndrome (ICANS) 4.1% (grade ≥3, 1%).[361] Given these toxicity concerns and the high associated cost of manufacturing, ideal patient selection remains a crucial challenge, and at present, this therapy is reserved for the third line and beyond in FL. CAR-T cell constructs have also showed dramatic efficacy and long remissions in patients with refractory CLL.[363]

As the understanding of host immune responses has evolved, new targets and strategies are being developed to optimize the antitumor immune response. Bispecific antibodies or bispecific T-cell engagers are novel protein constructs with separate B-cell and T-cell targeting domains that provide an off-the-shelf version of T-cell mediated therapy. Mosunetuzumab, which binds CD20 on the B lymphoma cell and simultaneously engages effector T cells via CD3, demonstrated deep and durable responses in heavily pretreated patients with FL. In a pivotal phase II trial, in patients with progressive disease after 2 or more prior therapies and 52% of patients with POD24, the CR rate to mosunetuzumab was 60% (ORR 80%). Among responders, the median duration of response was 22.8 months. Mosunetuzumab demonstrated a manageable safety profile, with CRS observed in 44% of patients, all of which were low grade apart from two cases. Neurotoxicity was seen in 4.4% of patients, with no grade ≥3 events.[364] Additional CD20 × CD3 bispecific antibodies including glofitamab (Genentech), epcoritamab (AbbVie), and odronextamab (Regeneron) are currently under investigation in indolent NHL. Bispecific antibodies are a promising new approach that will likely impact the future landscape of immunotherapy in indolent lymphoma.

A more detailed discussion of immunotherapy is reviewed in Chapter 71.

AGGRESSIVE LYMPHOMAS

Diffuse Large B-cell Lymphomas

LBLs are the most common type of adult NHL in North America and Europe, making up 30% to 40% of NHL. It represents a heterogeneous group of diseases and attempts to subdivide it have been based on morphology, cytogenetics, immunohistochemistry, predominant clinical presentations, associated viruses, and genomic profiles (*Table 90.12*).

DLBCL, NOS, is the most common clinicopathologic entity within the LBL classification. As noted in the Immunophenotypic and Molecular Markers section, DLBCL, NOS (henceforth referred to as DLBCL) has been subdivided by GEP using cDNA or oligonucleotide microarrays into four subgroups: GCB cell, activated B cells, and unclassified DLBCL.[365] The Hans algorithm staining for BCL-6, CD10, and MUM is 80% concordant with the DNA-expression analysis.[240] Comparative genomic hybridization has shown differences in genetic imbalances between GCB and ABC DLBCL. GCB is characterized by gain of 1q, 2p, 7q, and 12q; and ABC has gains of 3q, 18q, and 19q, and loss of 6q and 9p21, the latter of which includes the *CDKN2A* locus.[366]

More recently, the subclassification has become more complex. Molecular and cytogenetic profiling studies have independently identified 5 to 7 new genetic subgroups of DLBCL, validating the concept comprehensively.[367-370] The proposed subgroups are based on the underlying deregulated biologic pathways—BCR and NF-kB signaling (MCD/C5); NF-kB activation (N1); genetic instability and immune evasion (A53/C2); NOTCH2 signaling and immune evasion (BN2/C1); JAK/STAT signaling (ST2/C4); and epigenetic, PI3K

Table 90.12. Large B-cell Lymphomas

DLBCL, not otherwise specified (NOS)
Morphologic: centroblastic, immunoblastic, anaplastic, other
Immunophenotype/gene expression: germinal center-derived, activated B cell, other
Molecular/genetic: BCL6, BCL2, MYC, IRF4, 11q aberration
EBV-positive DLBCL, NOS
HHV8-positive DLBCL, NOS
Specified by site
Primary mediastinal large B-cell lymphoma
Mediastinal gray-zone lymphoma
Primary cutaneous large DLBCL, leg type
Intravascular B-cell lymphoma
HHV8 and EBV-negative primary effusion-based lymphoma
Other: CNS, testes, bone
Specified by histology or immunophenotype
T cell/histiocyte-rich large B-cell lymphoma
Nodular lymphocyte predominant B-cell lymphoma
Anaplastic lymphoma kinase-positive large B-cell lymphoma
DLBCL associated with chronic inflammation
Fibrin-associated DLBCL
Plasmablastic lymphoma
Primary effusion lymphoma (HHV8-associated)
High-grade B-cell lymphoma, NOS
High-grade B-cell lymphoma with MYC and BCL2 rearrangements
High-grade B-cell lymphoma with MYC and BCL6 rearrangements

Abbreviations: CNS, central nervous system; DLBCL, diffuse large B-cell lymphoma; EBV, Epstein-Barr virus; HHV8, human herpesvirus 8.

signaling, cell migration, and immune cell interactions (EZB/C3). At this time, the Hans algorithm remains the most employed method, but a combination of COO and molecular subclassification is expected to be used for designing future clinical trials in hopes of enhancing the therapeutic relevance of the categories.[371]

T-cell/histiocyte-rich large B-cell lymphoma (THRLBCL) represents 1% to 3% of DLBCL and is a subtype in which the malignant large B cell is the minority cell.[372] THRLBCL was first described in 1988 by Ramsay and may transform from an otherwise indolent nodular LPHL (both classical and nodular lymphocyte predominant types), PTCL, or an indolent lymphoma.[372,373] THRLBCL occurs at a younger median age than typical DLBCL with most series reporting fourth to fifth decade median ages compared to sixth decade.[374] Patients with THRLBCL have more B symptoms (26%-62%), splenomegaly (21%-60%), and marrow involvement (32%-53%) than traditional DLBCL. Although some series of THRLBCL have had inferior CR rates compared to DLBCL, there may have been a disproportionate number of patients with a high IPI; and case-controlled series have shown no differences in OS.[374] THRLBCL can be further defined by molecular profiling that identifies a unique cluster of genes involved in host response.[375]

EBV-positive DLBCL is a new entity which is clinically aggressive, has frequent extranodal presentation, and a poor prognosis.[376] This type of lymphoma is thought to be a result of immunosenescence with aging with a median age at presentation of 75 years. Another form of EBV-positive DLBCL is DLBCL associated with chronic inflammation involving joints or body cavities (pyothorax).[377]

There is no single cytogenetic abnormality which defines DLBCL, but there are a number of translocations commonly found with DLBCL, including t(3;14), t(14;18), and t(8;14), and related variants. These cytogenetic abnormalities are commonly found with other types of lymphomas; and when observed in DLBCL, there can be a clinical problem distinguishing transformation from a de novo presentation. BCL6 gene on 3q27 is associated with multiple chromosomal partners; and translocations involving 3q27 are found in 30% to 35% of DLBCL.[378] The prognostic implication of BCL6 abnormalities has been variable with data indicating a worse survival with non-Ig gene BCL6 rearrangements than with IGH/BCL6 translocations of t(3;14).[379]

t(14;18) is present in 20% to 25% of DLBCL and may represent transformation from a FL or a true de novo presentation. Although BCL2 genetic translocation has not been correlated with survival in de novo DLBCL, BCL2 protein expression has been associated with an inferior survival, specifically in the activated B-cell type of DLBCL.[380] t(8;14) is usually found in BL and is rare in DLBCL. "Double-hit lymphomas" (DHLs) now better known as either high-grade B-cell lymphoma (HGBCL) with MYC and BCL2 rearrangements or HGBCL with MYC and BCL6 rearrangements harbor dual translocations involving MYC, t(8;14); and BCL2, t(14;18) or MYC, t(8;14), and BCL6, t(3;14) are frequently refractory to standard chemotherapy regimens and have a poor prognosis.[381] The synergistic activity of antiapoptosis driven by BCL2 and proliferation by MYC is likely responsible for the poor outcome with traditional chemotherapy.[382-384] The presence of BCL2 and MYC by immunohistochemical staining, otherwise known as "double expressors," has an inferior prognosis compared with DLBCL that do not express the proteins; however, the double expressors are not considered as a separate entity in the 2022 WHO classification and the 2022 International Consensus Classification.[371]

LBL of the leg is seen in the elderly and has a poorer prognosis than other cutaneous B-cell lymphomas.[385,386] Intravascular B-cell lymphoma was recognized in 1959 and was known as malignant angioendotheliomatosis.[387] It occurs in the elderly (median age 65-70 years) and most commonly affects the skin and CNS. Symptoms are usually related to ischemia secondary to occlusion of blood vessels and approximately one-half of cases are first detected at autopsy.[388]

A newer provisional entity, LBL with IRF4 rearrangement, tends to be localized to Waldeyer ring and cervical nodes and primarily occurs in children and young adults.[389] It is usually of a germinal center origin, and BCL6 rearrangement may be present but BCL2 is always absent. It should be distinguished from a CD10⁻, IRF4/MUM1⁺ FL that can be associated with DLBCL, also lacks BCL2 rearrangement, and is seen in older patients.[390]

Unclassifiable B-cell lymphomas with morphologic and immunophenotypic features between classical HL and DLBCL are now called mediastinal gray-zone lymphomas and have tended to have a worse outcome than either HL or PMLBCL.[391] Unclassifiable B-cell lymphomas with features between DLBCL and BL (now included in HGBCL, NOS category) are aggressive and respond poorly to standard chemotherapy though the optimal treatment regimen is not defined; cases that are blastoid in appearance and lack MYC translocation are placed under the category HGBCL, NOS.

DLBCL can rarely involve the ALK gene, and most ALK⁺ DLBCLs have a single or complex t(2;17) (p23;q23) involving the ALK gene at chromosome band 2p23 and the clathrin gene at chromosome band 17q23.[392] ALK⁺ DLBCL lacks expression of pan-B cell antigens, CD20 and CD79a, but is positive for CD138 and epithelial membrane antigen (EMA). Although data are limited due to the rarity of the disease, ALK⁺ DLBCL is usually advanced stage and has a poor prognosis.[392]

Mutations in the TP53 gene have been detected in 20% of DLBCL and are associated with a poor prognosis. TP53 expression is detectable by immunohistochemistry in 30% to 40% of DLBCL, does not correlate with the presence of mutations, and has not consistently affected prognosis. However, evaluating expression of TP53 and its downstream target CDKN1A/P21 (acting as a cyclin-dependent kinase inhibitor) has shown that the TP53⁺/P21⁻ immunophenotype is a surrogate for TP53 mutations and is associated with poor survival in DLBCL, even with a low-risk IPI.[393]

Expression of individual antigens assessed by immunophenotyping may help define subsets of DLBCL and may have prognostic value (see Table 90.8). CD5, an antigen primarily expressed by T cells and a small subset of B cells (B-1 cells), is present on 5% to 10% of DLBCL. CD5+ DLBCL has been associated with a high IPI and poor survival in most, but not all, studies.[394]

Current therapy of DLBCL is directed by clinical features, pathology, and stage of disease. As DLBCL represents a group of potentially curable neoplasms, prognostic factors are important to recognize and can influence the type, intensity, and duration of therapy. Selecting the intensity of therapy based on prognostic factors is referred to as risk stratification and has been applied successfully in pediatrics in which the curability of all types and stages of NHL is over 80%. The IPI is currently the best prognosticator for survival in DLBCL. Immunohistochemistry can delineate different types of DLBCL, but there is no consensus about the best panel of markers to either subclassify or prognosticate DLBCL. In the rituximab era, the prognosis has improved and the impact of IPI and immunohistochemistry was reassessed and classifies patients into very good, good, or poor risk groups with 94%, 75%, and 55% 4-year OS, respectively.[395]

Frontline Therapy for DLBCL

In the early 1970s, DeVita introduced a combination chemotherapy regimen, C-MOPP (cyclophosphamide replacing mechlorethamine, vincristine, procarbazine, and prednisone), which produced a CR rate in excess of 40% in patients with diffuse "histiocytic" lymphoma, a neoplasm generally equivalent to DLBCL; approximately one-third of these patients were cured.[396] By the mid-1970s, doxorubicin had been added to cyclophosphamide, vincristine, and prednisone to produce the CHOP regimen, which produced CR rates of 50% to 60% and DFS of 30% to 40%.[397,398] CHOP is the most extensively studied and used regimen in the therapy of large cell lymphoma. The addition of rituximab has improved response and survival.[399] Clinical observations have been that rapid achievement of a CR was associated with a good prognosis[397,400] and that relapses after 2 years of DFS were rare. Further follow-up for large cell lymphoma, however, recorded relapses in 6% to 22% of patients after 2 years of CR.[400,401]

Subsequent regimens were developed in part on the concepts of Goldie and Coldman, who proposed that tumors develop drug resistance by spontaneous mutation soon after exposure to chemotherapy, and of Hryniuk and Bush, who proposed that increasing dose intensity could overcome drug resistance.[402,403] The CR rates of third-generation regimens were 78% to 88% with DFS of 58% to 69% in studies primarily at single institutions. Many of these newer regimens had considerable toxicity when used initially and were associated with mortality rates of 5% to 10%; however, the rate of toxic deaths decreased over time with more experience and with better patient selection.[401] Many of the series in which these regimens were used involved favorable prognostic groups, including patients with limited-stage disease and patients with a relatively young median age.

One of the most important clinical trials for lymphoma was performed by an intergroup (SWOG and ECOG) study which compared CHOP with three of the newer and reportedly more intensive regimens, m-BACOD (methotrexate, bleomycin, Adriamycin [doxorubicin], cyclophosphamide, Oncovin [vincristine], and dexamethasone), MACOP-B (methotrexate, bleomycin, Adriamycin, cyclophosphamide, Oncovin, and prednisone), and ProMACE-CytaBOM (prednisone, matulane, Adriamycin, cyclophosphamide, etoposide/cytarabine, bleomycin, Oncovin, and methotrexate).[404] There were no differences in CR, PFS, or OS.

Although the intergroup study re-established CHOP as standard therapy for large cell lymphoma, it did not address the issue of dose intensity, and it did not emphasize how poorly these regimens do in patients with adverse prognostic factors. Using these conventional regimens, CR rates of 55% and 44% and 5-year survivals of 43% and 26% were observed in the IPI high-intermediate and high-risk groups, respectively.[405,406]

The intergroup trial was met with praise as well as disappointment because it indicated no improvement in survival for nearly 2 decades after the establishment of CHOP as an effective regimen. The first study to show an improvement in survival was a randomized GELA comparison of CHOP to rituximab plus CHOP (R-CHOP) in elderly patients (age 60-80 years) with DLBCL.[407] The rate of CR/CRu was higher for R-CHOP compared to CHOP alone (75% vs 63%, $P = .005$). The 5-year EFS and OS were significantly higher in the R-CHOP arm: 47% vs 29%, $P < .001$ and 58% vs 45%, $P = .007$.[407,408] The results have held up at 10 years.[409] A similar intergroup trial reported a 3-year FFS of 53% for R-CHOP and 46% for CHOP ($P = .04$).[410] Randomized trials in young patients have confirmed the superiority of rituximab + chemotherapy: 79% vs 59% 3-year EFS ($P < .0001$).[411] The addition of rituximab to CHOP may partially overcome the adverse prognosis associated with the nongerminal center (ABC) DLBCL.[412] New prognostic models evaluating biologic markers and/or gene expression are under investigation in the rituximab era, although reproducibility remains a concern.[413,414]

Strategies to improve response and survival in aggressive lymphomas have included using alternating non–cross-resistant regimens, infusional therapy, additional drugs, shorter intervals, modifiers of multidrug-resistant genes, and dose intensification, including HCT. Phase II trials of non–cross-resistant regimens, such as alternating triple therapy from M. D. Anderson, appeared to overcome adverse prognostic factors, but they were not compared to CHOP in phase III trials.[415,416] Similarly, a continuous infusional regimen, EPOCH with dose adjustments (DA-EPOCH), based on an individual's drug clearance had a CR rate in large B-cell NHL of 92%, a 5-year PFS and OS of 70% and 73%, respectively and overcame the IPI.[417] An Alliance intergroup trial has compared DA-EPOCH-R to R-CHOP. The results indicated no improvement in PFS or OS with the infusional DA-EPOCH-R regimen. High-risk patients were underrepresented and on posthoc analysis, patients with IPI score of 3 to 5 had improved PFS with DA-EPOCH-R, although OS was similar. There was a higher incidence of febrile neutropenia and thrombocytopenia with DA-EPOCH-R as expected.[418] It is important to note that very few patients in this trial had "double-hit" lymphoma and strong conclusions cannot be made for this aggressive subtype from this trial. Numerous retrospective studies published over the past several years have highlighted the generally poor outcome of patients with DHL. In a multicenter meta-analysis of survival outcomes of 394 DHL patients receiving either R-CHOP (46%), R-EPOCH (23%), or one of R-hyper-CVAD or R-CODOX/M-IVAC (31%), the median PFS was 12.1, 22.2, and 18.9 months, respectively. Patients receiving R-EPOCH were found to have a 34% reduction in the likelihood of experiencing progression as compared to those receiving R-CHOP ($P = .032$). Median OS was 21.4, 31.4, and 25.2 months, respectively, and did not differ significantly by treatment received.[419] In spite of the lack of prospective studies of patients with *MYC*-altered lymphomas, it appears that these patients are at high risk of poor clinical outcomes and CNS relapse and may benefit from, intensified induction therapy, earlier CAR T-cell therapy, consolidation therapy, and/or novel/targeted therapies during their treatment course.[420]

Randomized trials in Germany, the United Kingdom, and France have compared R-CHOP-14 to R-CHOP-21 and addition of etoposide and have shown no differences in responses or survivals when rituximab is included in the regimen.[421-424]

Dose escalation has been advocated as a means to improve response and survival in aggressive lymphomas in phase II studies, but there are few phase III clinical trials that have shown the efficacy of dose intensity.

Some investigators advocate early autologous HCT for selected DLBCL patients with poor prognostic factors, but large randomized trials have failed to consistently show a survival benefit for early transplantation.[425,426] R-CHOP has been established over several years as the standard regimen for DLBCL for adults in the United States.

A second-generation monoclonal antibody, obinutuzumab (G), which reportedly has better cytotoxic cell death or direct cell killing, was added to CHOP and compared with R-CHOP in a phase III study. G-CHOP did not improve PFS, which was the primary endpoint compared with R-CHOP.[427]

Ibrutinib plus R-CHOP was studied in a randomized phase III clinical trial in non–GCB DLBCL based on strong preclinical data, but the study did not meet its primary endpoint of EFS. In subgroup analysis, patients younger than 60 years appeared to benefit from this combination with improved EFS, PFS, and OS but further investigation is ongoing to explore Bruton's tyrosine kinase inhibitor use in this population.[428] Lastly, polatuzumab vedotin, an antibody-drug conjugate composed of an anti-CD79b monoclonal antibody conjugated by a protease-cleavable linker to monomethyl auristatin E (a microtubule inhibitor), was studied in a randomized, double-blind, placebo-controlled, phase III clinical trial. Eligible de-novo DLBCL patients with IPI score of 2 to 5 received polatuzumab vedotin plus R-CHP (omitting vincristine from the R-CHOP regimen) for six 21-day cycles followed by two 21-day cycles of rituximab alone for a total of 8 cycles.[429] After a median follow-up of 28.2 months, there was statistically significant improvement in PFS, EFS, and DFS when compared to R-CHOP. There was no difference in OS between the two groups. Many consider this regimen to be superior to R-CHOP for eligible patients, but further guidance is awaited regarding the licensing of this regimen in the frontline setting.

Patients with limited-stage disease (commonly defined as stage I or II that is nonbulky and localized) have more favorable outcomes, though delayed relapses have been observed.[430] Efforts have been made to limit the number of chemotherapy cycles or omitting radiation therapy. Four cycles of R-CHOP plus two cycles of R were confirmed to be sufficient for patients <60 with limited stage disease and age-adjusted IPI of 0.[431] PET-CT–adapted approach has also been explored in limited-stage disease, wherein patients with IPI 0 who had a CR by PET-CT after four cycles of R-CHOP did not benefit from addition of RT.[432] Similarly, an intergroup study has shown that four cycles of R-CHOP alone is sufficient in patients with CR by PET-CT scan after three cycles of R-CHOP.[433]

Management of Relapsed/Refractory Disease

Approximately 15% of patients treated with R-CHOP have primary refractory disease (defined as incomplete response or a relapse within 6 months of treatment), and an additional 20% will have a relapse after initial response.[434,435] A repeat biopsy is generally required at relapse to confirm histology since relapses with underlying indolent lymphomas can occur.

Chemotherapy regimens at relapse usually involve agents that are noncross resistant with, or at least different from, drugs used in initial therapy. Rituximab is usually added to the regimen as long as the lymphoma remains CD20 positive. Multiple effective protocols have been developed: R-ICE (*i*fosfamide, *c*arboplatinum, *e*toposide) and R-DHAP (dexamethasone, high-dose cytarabine [ara-C], and cisplatin [Platinol]) are commonly used. Combination regimens have yielded response rates in the 49% to 69% range, but there are no obvious differences in outcome among the combinations. A phase III trial, CORAL, randomized patients with refractory or relapsed CD20+ DLBCL to R-ICE or R-DHAP and found similar response rates (63.5% vs 62.8%).[16] Only 50% of patients were able to undergo HCT. There was no difference in 3-year EFS (26% and 35%) or OS (47% and 51%) between the two regimens. EFS was adversely affected by initial relapse within 1 year from diagnosis, aaIPI of 2 to 3, and prior rituximab treatment.

In general, salvage chemotherapy regimens in DLBCL are utilized as a bridge to HCT because prolonged survivals without transplant are less than 15%. Single-agent therapy is rarely used in intermediate- to high-grade lymphoma except in phase I/II trials or as palliation. Because of significant activity in relapsed disease, some of the agents are being used in combination with other drugs earlier in the course of NHL.

Oxaliplatin, a third-generation platinum drug with no renal toxicity and minimal auditory damage, has a 40% response rate in refractory NHL and is used in salvage regimens.[436] Combining gemcitabine with oxaliplatin and rituximab (GEMOX-R) led to an ORR of 43% with 34% CR in refractory/relapsing DLBCL and is a regimen that is typically used in HCT ineligible patients.[437]

Nucleoside analogues have primarily been used in indolent lymphomas, but gemcitabine, a pyrimidine antimetabolite, has had activity in relapsed aggressive lymphomas. A response rate of 20% was observed in predominantly large B-cell NHL, and higher responses have been observed in PTCL (see section "Therapy for T/NK Neoplasms").[438] The ORRs in gemcitabine combination regimens with cisplatin and methylprednisolone and with vinorelbine have been 79% (21% CR) and 50% (14% CR), respectively.[439,440] The NCIC-CTG conducted a phase III study in relapsed aggressive lymphoma comparing gemcitabine, dexamethasone, and cisplatin (GDP) to DHAP prior to a plan to transplant.[441]

There were no differences in response, survival, and transplantation rates, but GDP was associated with less toxicity and better quality of life.

Availability of CAR T-cell therapy has provided alternatives with the potential of durable responses and even survival advantage. Axicabtagene ciloleucel, tisagenlecleucel, and lisocabtagene maraleucel have been associated with ORR in the range of 50% to 80% and CR around 50% among patients with relapsed/refractory DLBCL.[442-444] All 3 CAR T-cell products demonstrated capacity to induce durable remissions in approximately one-third of treated patients (including patients who had not had a durable remission with a prior HCT) and have been US Food and Drug Administration approved for patients with relapsed/refractory DLBCL after at least two lines of therapy. Real-world outcome analysis of patients treated in clinical care has confirmed this benefit,[445] although they show that trial outcomes are likely to be more optimistic because of patient selection and analyses criteria. As these products have never been compared head-to-head, their comparative effectiveness has not been determined. Given these encouraging pivotal phase 2 data, these three CAR T-cell products were studied directly against second-line therapy (salvage therapy followed by HCT) in three separate phase III trials for patients who had refractory disease or relapsed within 12 months from completion of first-line therapy.[446-448] Trials testing axicabtagene ciloleucel (ZUMA-7) and lisocabtagene maraleucel (TRANSFORM) met their primary endpoints of improved EFS, while tisagenlecleucel (BELINDA) did not. These results for axicabtagene ciloleucel and lisocabtagene maraleucel justify a significant shift to second-line CAR T-cell therapy in suitable patients and are now FDA approved in the United States for second-line use. It is argued that none of these trials shed any light on important issues of mechanism of resistance and the failure of persistent cells to expand at the time of relapse.[449] It is important to note that all three trials showed dismal outcomes in the standard of care arm in this otherwise high-risk population, underscoring the importance of studying new therapies for this high-risk group of patients.

Despite the advance of CAR T-cell therapy, off-the-shelf novel therapies are needed in the relapsed/refractory setting. Polatuzumab vedotin plus bendamustine and rituximab (PBR), tafasitamab plus lenalidomide, loncastuximab tesirine and selinexor are licensed agents for use in this setting. Tafasitamab, an anti-CD19 monoclonal antibody, plus lenalidomide combination was licensed based on the results of L-MIND study, a phase II trial enrolling 80 patients with relapsed/refractory DLBCL ineligible for HCT. The trial achieved ORR of 60% with CR of 43%, median DOR of 21.7 months, and median PFS of 12.1 months.[450] Long-term outcomes of this regimen confirmed durability of response.[451] Polatuzumab vedotin as part of the PBR (added to bendamustine-rituximab) regimen was the first FDA-licensed novel agent in this clinical setting. Approval was based on a randomized phase II trial enrolling 80 patients resulting in significant improvements in end-of-treatment and best ORR (45.0% vs 17.5%; 62.5% vs 25.0%) and CR (40.0% vs 17.5%; 50.0% vs 22.5%) compared with bendamustine/rituximab with a median duration of response, PFS, and OS of 12.6, 9.5, and 12.4 months, respectively, resulting in a survival benefit (12.4 vs 4.7; $P = .002$).[452] Loncastuximab tesirine, an antibody-drug conjugate comprising a humanized anti-CD19 antibody conjugated to a pyrrolobenzodiazepine dimer cytotoxin, SG3199, was studied in phase I and later a phase II study (LOTIS-1 and LOTIS-2, respectively) which led to its approval in this setting. LOTIS-2 enrolled 145 patients and observed ORR of 48.3% with CR of 24.1%.[453]

Long-term follow-up showed a median PFS of 4.9 months and median OS of 9.5 months.[454] Durable responses were observed in heavily pretreated patients with DLBCL.

In summary, tremendous progress has been made in DLBCL in the last 3 to 4 years with multiple approvals in various lines of therapy. In spite of the progress, much work continues to be required for high-risk population. Immunotherapeutic approaches such as macrophage immune checkpoint inhibitors and bispecific antibodies that induce T-cell activation leading to cell-mediated cytotoxicity hold promise and are currently being investigated.

Primary Mediastinal Large B-cell Lymphoma

The WHO and ICC classifications recognize a distinct LBL postulated to arise from a thymic B cell and that can be confused with LBL, HL, thymomas, and extragonadal germ cell neoplasms.[455] Older literature referred to this entity as primary sclerosing mediastinal large cell lymphoma. PMLBCL constitute 2% to 3% of NHL and occur predominantly in females (female:male ~ 2:1) and young adults; three-fourths of cases are less than 35 years old.[456] Gains in chromosome 9p24 or 2p15 have been recognized in up to 75% and 50% of patients, respectively.[455,457] BCL2 and BCL6 gene rearrangements rarely occur, whereas overexpression of the MAL gene is common.[458] Interestingly, gene expression analysis has revealed a molecular signature with similarities to classical HL, perhaps reflected in the shared clinical and pathologic features and dysregulation of c-REL/NFkB pathways.[459,460] Programmed death ligands 1 and 2 are also in the 9p region and are rearranged in 20% of PMLBCL, making them susceptible to PD1 inhibition similar to HL.[461] Exploiting this association, it was found that pembrolizumab, a PD-1 inhibitor, is associated with high response rate, durable activity, and a manageable safety profile in patients with relapsed or refractory PMLBCL.[462]

Presenting features are usually of recent onset, varying from a few weeks to several months, and include chest pain (73%), cough (60%), dyspnea (46%), and superior vena cava obstruction (30%-57%).[455] Over two-thirds of patients have large masses (>10 cm) (*Figure 90.15*). Local extension of the mass into the pericardium, chest wall, or lung is common, whereas distant involvement of peripheral nodes, marrow, or CNS is infrequent.[456,463] The stage of disease is I or II in 80% of patients at diagnosis, and the IPI has not correlated well with prognosis. Unusual extranodal sites of involvement include kidney, ovaries, and adrenal glands.

Although early reports indicated a poor prognosis despite combination chemotherapy in PMLBCL, recent studies have had a good prognosis similar to or better than other DLBCL.[464] Poor prognostic factors in PMLBCL have been the presence of pleural or pericardial effusion, multiple (≥2) extranodal sites of disease, bulk (≥10 cm), and high LDH (>3 × normal). Historically, therapy included involved field radiation therapy, but some series have had equally good outcomes without radiation, indicating that its need remains controversial. Some centers have favored regimens other than R-CHOP, including

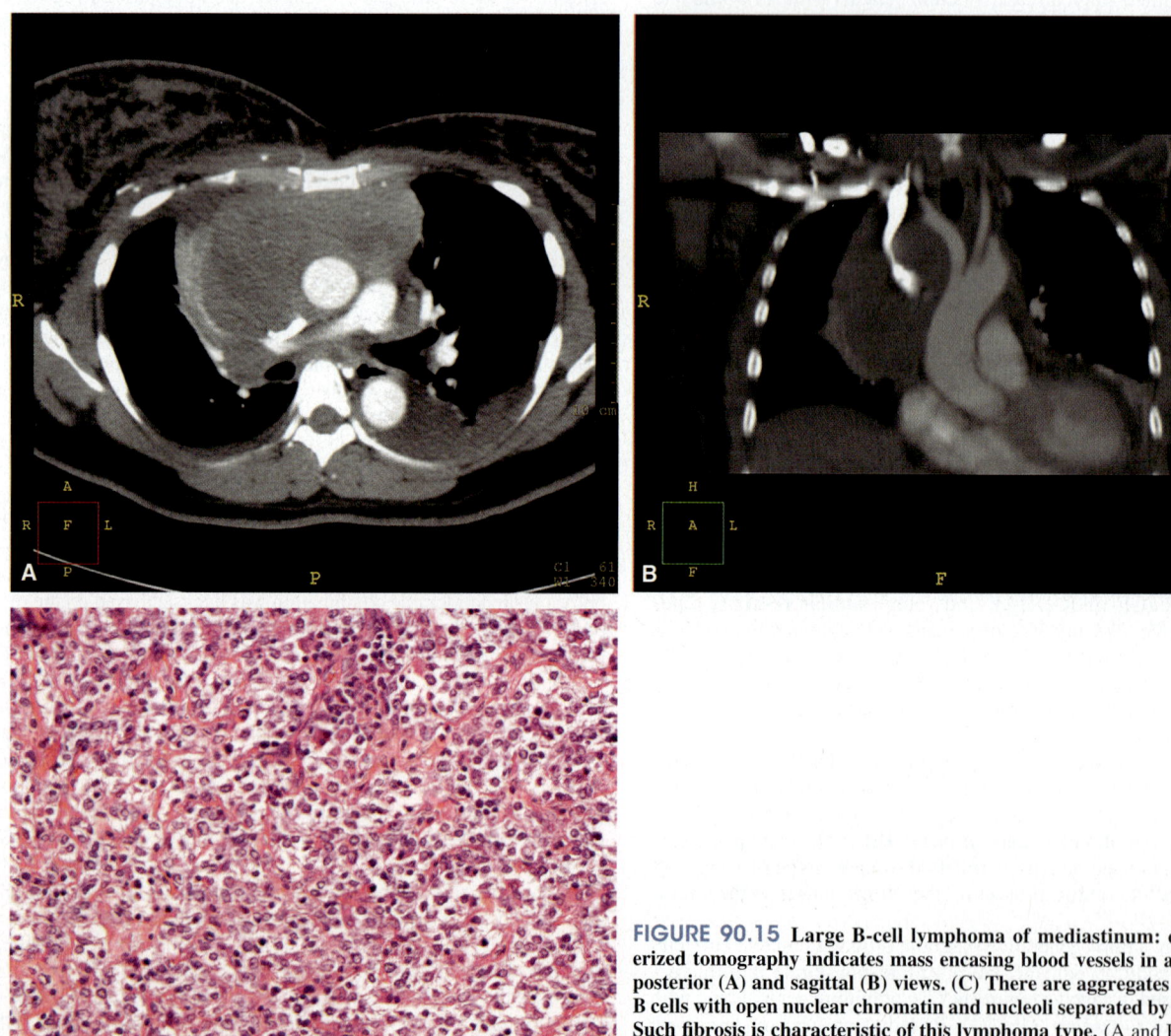

FIGURE 90.15 Large B-cell lymphoma of mediastinum: computerized tomography indicates mass encasing blood vessels in anterior-posterior (A) and sagittal (B) views. (C) There are aggregates of large B cells with open nuclear chromatin and nucleoli separated by fibrosis. Such fibrosis is characteristic of this lymphoma type. (A and B, Image provided by Dr Ron Arildsen, Vanderbilt University, Nashville, TN; C, Image provided by Dr Dan Arber, University of Chicago, Chicago, IL.)

R-MACOP-B/VACOP-B regimens, and DA-EPOCH-R.[465,466] The latter was reported to have EFS of 90% in a series of 26 patients, without the use of radiation therapy.[466] Others have advocated autologous HCT as consolidative therapy among patients with "high-risk" PMLBCL, but there are sparse phase II trials to commend this approach.[467] When deciding on an upfront treatment approach, the potential toxicity of more intensive regimens, such as DA-EPOCH-R, should be weighed against the potential toxicity of radiation therapy. For patients with primary refractory or relapsed disease, outcomes are poor. Immune checkpoint inhibitors such as pembrolizimab have activity in this setting, and combination trials with chemotherapy are underway.

MANTLE CELL LYMPHOMA

MCL was referred to as centrocytic, intermediate lymphocytic, and mantle zone lymphoma in earlier classifications and was given its present name in 1992.[468-470] MCL represents approximately 5% to 7% of NHL in Western populations. It occurs predominantly in the elderly (median age 68 years) and with a twofold to threefold male predominance.[471,472] Most patients present with diffuse lymphadenopathy and splenomegaly.[471,472] B symptoms are present in 25% to 50% of patients, and 15% to 30% have or will develop a unique gastrointestinal presentation with multiple lymphomatous polyposis (Figure 90.9).[471] Bone marrow involvement is detected in 60% to 90% of patients, and up to 25% will have an overt leukemic phase, although most patients have a small circulating clone detectable by FC.[471] CNS involvement has been documented in 9% of patients during the course of the illness, usually as a late event.[473]

MCL has a characteristic although not completely unique phenotype, with most expressing CD5 and negative for CD10 and CD23, which helps distinguish MCL from follicular and small lymphocytic lymphomas. Virtually all MCL demonstrate the classic cytogenetic marker t(11;14) (q13;q32) by conventional cytogenetic analysis and FISH.[473] Expression of nuclear cyclin D1 protein is found in >90% of cases and is considered the most reliable immunophenotypic marker in the diagnosis of MCL,[474] although variant MCL with cyclin D2 or cyclin D3 expression also occur.[475] A minimally deleted segment of 11q22-q23 affecting the *ATM* gene in 50% of MCL suggests that this is an early genetic event along with the *BCL-1/CCND1* (cyclin D1) translocation to chromosome 14.[476] Loss of tumor suppressor genes, including *TP53* and *CDKN2/p16*, appears to occur later and has been associated with an aggressive clinical course.[477]

Marked clinical and biologic heterogeneity of MCL is now well recognized, with about a quarter of patients having "indolent" disease that may not require immediate therapy. These patients often present with splenomegaly, bone marrow involvement, and lymphocytosis but without lymphadenopathy and systemic symptoms (also known as nonnodal MCL). Such MCL may be confused with CLL if proper FC and FISH markers are not obtained at diagnosis. Watchful waiting for the assessment of pace of disease has been proposed as initial management in these cases.[478] Biomarkers of clinically indolent cases include mutated Ig heavy-chain variable genes, lack of nuclear SOX11 expression, and lack of *TP53* aberration, few if any karyotypic changes aside from the t(11;14) and a characteristic molecular signature.[479] However, they can progress into an aggressive lymphoma with the acquisition of TP53 aberrations.

Clinically aggressive MCL typically has high tumor burden, blastoid morphology, complex cytogenetics in addition to t(11;14), and/or high Ki-67 expression. While several genes have been identified as commonly aberrated in MCL, the clinical significance for many of them is not fully clear.[480-482] Molecular markers that appear both pathogenically and prognostically relevant include TP53 aberrations,[483,484] *NOTCH1* mutation,[485] dysregulation of the Hippo tumor suppressor pathway,[486] and a unique microRNA signature and expression of miR-29.[487,488] The percentage of tumor cells expressing the proliferation marker Ki-67 has been incorporated into the MIPI score to enhance the discrimination of clinical outcomes among low-, intermediate-, and high-risk MCL patients treated with CHOP or R-CHOP regimens (Figure 90.16).[233,489]

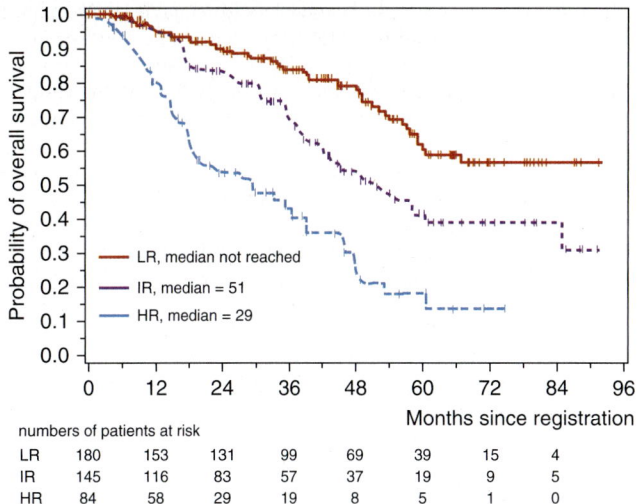

FIGURE 90.16 Overall survival in advanced stage patients according to the Mantle Cell International Prognostic Index (MIPI) and Ki67. Low risk (LR) score <5.7; intermediate risk (IR) ≥5.7 and <6.2; high risk (HR) ≥6.2. The combined biologic score is calculated as 0.03535 times age (years) plus 0.6978 (if ECOG >1) plus 1.367 times $\log_{10}$ (LDH/ULN) plus 0.9393 times $\log_{10}$ (WBC count) plus 0.02142 times Ki-67 (%). (Reprinted from Hoster E, Dreyling M, Klapper W, et al. A new prognostic index (MIPI) for patients with advanced-stage mantle cell lymphoma. *Blood*. 2008;111(2):558-565. Copyright © 2008 American Society of Hematology. With permission.)

Clinical outcomes and survival have improved in recent years as treatment options have expanded, although MCL remains incurable with standard approaches. The disease often responds initially to treatment, but relapses inevitably occur. Younger patients often receive an intensive regimen with or without auto-SCT in first remission, whereas older patients and those with significant comorbid disease are managed with less aggressive approaches. The OS benefits of aggressive approaches remain debated.

Currently, cytarabine-based chemoimmunotherapy regimen followed by autologous HCT and maintenance with an anti-CD20 antibody is the accepted standard of care approach in younger, fit patients in the frontline setting. Romaguera et al utilized rituximab-hyper-CVAD/MTX-AraC (fractionated cyclophosphamide plus vincristine, doxorubicin, dexamethasone alternating with high-dose methotrexate-cytarabine regimen) in a single-institution phase II trial.[490,491] Among 97 previously untreated patients, 87% achieved a CR. With a median 13.4-year follow-up, patients <65 years had a 5-, 10-, and 15-year FFS of 57% (95% CI, 44%-68%), 35% (95% CI, 23%-46%), and 30% (95% CI, 19%-41%) and a median OS of 13.4 years. A multicenter trial in 60 patients aged ≤70 years confirmed a high CR rate of 72% and a 5-year OS of 61%, and significant treatment-associated toxicity—only 37% of patients completed the planned course of therapy.[492] Patients with low- or intermediate-risk MIPI had much improved outcomes as compared to those with high-risk scores.

High-dose cytarabine has emerged as an important component of therapy in a large phase III trial by the European MCL Network comparing R-CHOP vs R-CHOP alternating with R-DHAP (dexamethasone, high-dose AraC, and cisplatin) followed by autologous HCT.[493] With a median follow-up of 11 years, TTF for the 420 patients was significantly improved with the addition of R-DHAP. Median OS was not reached in the R-DHAP arm vs 11.3 years in the R-CHOP arm (Figure right, $P = .12$), with 5/10-year OS probabilities of 76%/60% (R-DHAP) and 69%/55% (R-CHOP), respectively.[494] This study also showed that achievement of minimal residual disease (MRD) negativity in the peripheral blood and bone marrow was strongly associated with prolonged DFS.[495]

Bendamustine, a highly active chemotherapeutic in relapsed MCL, was studied as initial therapy in combination with rituximab (BR) and compared with R-CHOP in a phase III trial of non–transplant-eligible patients. PFS was improved in the BR arm, although with a similar continuous rate of relapse.

In a disease where relapse is considered inevitable, maintenance therapy is an attractive strategy to delay recurrence. The European MCL Network completed a phase III trial in 560 elderly, non–transplant-eligible patients comparing R-CHOP vs R-FC (fludarabine, cyclophosphamide) followed by a second randomization to IFN-alfa vs rituximab maintenance therapy.[496] The 4-year OS was significantly improved for R-CHOP followed by MR given once every 2 months until progression as compared with IFN (87% vs 63%, respectively, P = .005). Following autologous HCT, rituximab maintenance improved PFS and OS compared with no maintenance.[497] In young transplant-eligible patients, a randomized phase III study by the LYSA group showed that rituximab maintenance therapy for 3 years after auto-HCT prolonged EFS, PFS, and OS.[498] The utility for MR following bendamustine and rituximab induction is less clear and remains controversial.[499,500] A recently published randomized clinical trial studied the use of rituximab plus ibrutinib maintenance in patients treated with ibrutinib, bendamustine, and rituximab as the upfront regimen. At a median follow-up of 84.7 months, the median PFS was 80.6 months in the ibrutinib group and 52.9 months in the placebo group, while the OS was similar in the two groups.[501] The lack of OS benefit with this strategy suggests that the use of BTK inhibitor in the subsequent line rather than in frontline and maintenance setting may provide similar outcomes with potentially less additive toxicity.

A number of new treatment options are available for patients with MCL. The proteasome inhibitor bortezomib provides responses in 33% of relapsed or refractory MCL patients.[502] In a phase III trial, bortezomib was substituted for vincristine in frontline therapy with R-CHOP (VR-CAP) and compared with R-CHOP. At a median follow-up of 40 months, there was a significant improvement in PFS thus declaring the superiority of VR-CAP over R-CHOP.[503] Combination biologic therapy consisting of lenalidomide and rituximab was shown to be effective as initial therapy in elderly patients. The 7-year PFS rate was estimated at 60.3% (95% CI, 41.1%-75.0%) with 7-year OS rates at 73.2% (95% CI, 55.9%-84.6%).[504,505] Although lenalidomide-based treatment, BTK inhibitor–based treatment, BCL2 inhibitor-lenalidomide combinations, and BCL2 inhibitor-BTK inhibitor combinations all provide great promise as frontline treatment, none have been licensed to date.[506]

At relapse, patients should typically undergo another biopsy and restaging workup along with reassessment of prognostic markers. A pivotal randomized phase 3 clinical trial testing ibrutinib, a first-generation covalent BTK inhibitor, showed that the median PFS was 14.6 months for ibrutinib with an unparalleled ORR of 72%.[507] Pooled analysis provided further knowledge regarding the efficacy and depth of response in relation to the line of therapy. ORR, CR, median PFS, and median OS were superior for ibrutinib at first relapse rather than at subsequent relapses.[508] Ibrutinib, acalabrutinib, and zanubrutinib are licensed BTK inhibitors in relapsed/refractory MCL and dominate the space in recent years. Although no randomized data have been analyzed to determine toxicity differences between second-generation BTK inhibitors and ibrutinib in MCL, there are accumulating data to suggest their safety profile is superior. Where ibrutinib, zanubrutinib, and acalabrutinib are all available, therapeutic choice could be reasonably individualized based on the specific toxicity profiles of each agent.[506] BTK inhibitor–based combinations in relapsed/refractory MCL are currently being tested in various clinical trials. Lenalidomide, bortezomib, and temsirolimus are other options that are licensed for use in relapsed/refractory setting, though covalent BTK inhibitors dominate this space.

CAR-T cell therapy represents a significant advance in MCL. Brexucabtagene autoleucel is an anti-CD19 CAR-T cell therapy with a CD28 costimulatory domain approved by the FDA for all patients with R/R MCL. The ZUMA-2 trial enrolled patients with MCL after ≥3 prior lines including a prior covalent BTK inhibitor[509] and included a sizable number of patients with poor prognostic markers. With a recently reported follow-up of 35.6 months, ORR among all 68 treated patients was 91% with 68% CR with a median DOR, PFS, and OS of 28.2 months, 25.8 months, and 46.6 months, respectively.[510] Though numbers are small, preliminary data suggests that responses to CAR-T therapy may be agnostic to poor prognostic features such as aberrant TP53. It is presently unclear whether high-risk patients should receive BTK inhibitors before CAR-T therapy, or whether the effects of CAR-T therapy warrant earlier use in this population.

In younger, fit patients reinduction followed by related or unrelated allogeneic HCT has shown excellent response, with 50% to 60% of patients remaining event-free at 2 years, suggesting a possible graft-vs-lymphoma effect.[497,511] Treatment-associated morbidity and mortality remain high; hence, allogeneic transplant consolidation should be considered only for selected patients.

HIGHLY AGGRESSIVE LYMPHOMAS

BL and LBL, usually of immature T-cell origin, are rare NHL in adults, each representing less than 3% of NHL. As NHL is more common in adults, the absolute number of highly aggressive lymphoma exceeds that in children. Because children are treated primarily on clinical trials unlike adults at least in the United States, the main advances learned from pediatrics (Chapter 91) have been applied to the therapy of highly aggressive lymphoma in adults. In brief, short-course, dose-intensive cyclophosphamide therapy is utilized in BL, whereas therapy for ALL is the main approach to LBL. Both types of highly aggressive NHL require CNS prophylaxis, and have clinical overlap with adult ALL (Chapter 76).

Burkitt Lymphoma

Sporadic BL has a bimodal peak between 0 and 15 years and a later peak over 60 years.[512] SEER data indicate the median age is as high as 45 years with 30% over 60 years of age.[513] BL is characterized by a high proliferative rate (Ki-67 approaching 100%), a germinal center phenotype expressing CD10, BCL6, and weak BCL2, and a MYC/8q24 translocation.[514] A provisional entity that lacks MYC rearrangement is referred to as LBL with 11q aberration. This entity is frequently seen in children and young adults with good prognosis. These cases are genetically distinct from BL and closer to conventional DLBCL with GCB cell derivation harboring more complex karyotypes and absence of typical BL mutations.[371] HGBCL with features intermediate between DLBCL and BL has slightly deviant morphology and not as high a proliferative rate as BL; and are now known as HGBCL, NOS so long as there are no identified rearrangements of MYC and BCL2 or BCL6.

GEP is emerging as a technology to distinguish lymphomas with an intermediate morphology between DLBCL and BL. BL can be distinguished from DLBCL by a high level of MYC target genes, a subgroup of GCB genes, and a low level of expression of major histocompatibility complex class I genes and NF-κB target genes.[515] Until GEP becomes more available, detecting MYC translocations by FISH along with a high proliferative index can usually distinguish BL from DLBCL.[516]

In the United States, BL tends to occur in younger adults with frequent gastrointestinal presentations and have a risk for spontaneous tumor lysis. Intra-abdominal presentations usually involve the small bowel and intra-abdominal nodes and may mimic appendicitis or intussusception.[517] Surgery formerly played a role in staging and debulking disease, but now is reserved for the emergency acute abdomen. Early use of rasburicase and nephrology intervention should be considered in patients with elevated levels of LDH and uric acid. Bone marrow and CNS involvement have been reported in 30% to 38% and 13% to 17% of patients, respectively.[517]

Short-course, dose-intensive regimens have improved results in BL/mature B-ALL.[518-522] Results vary in part due to differences in age, stage, number of HIV-positive patients, and intensity of therapy. In general, the CR rates are greater than 80% and 5-year survival is 60% to 90% in young adults, 50% for adults, and 30% for the elderly.[513] CNS prophylaxis can be accomplished by a combination of intravenous and intrathecal drugs (methotrexate and/or cytarabine). Growth factors, either G- or GM-CSF, have decreased the length of myelosuppression and are a part of present-day regimens. Rituximab is incorporated into the therapy and appears to have improved outcome, but there are no comparative trials.[522] Relapses are usually confined to the first year after stopping therapy; there is no role for maintenance.

In pediatric and some adult trials, there is a prephase with low-dose cyclophosphamide, vincristine, and steroids to debulk and to lessen tumor lysis followed by intensive therapy stratified according to prognostic factors.[523] Prephase is probably unnecessary in most patients, particularly with the use of rasburicase. Patients with low-risk disease (defined as stage ≤2, ECOG PS ≤ 1, normal LDH, and tumor ≤7 cm) often require only two to three cycles of therapy delivered over 2.5 to 4 months.[524] In a retrospective review of adults treated with the pediatric LMB protocols, the CR rate was 89% with a 3-year OS of 74%.[523] The Magrath regimen of CODOX-M/IVAC has been administered to both children and adults and also utilizes risk stratification. The initial reports had a 4-year DFS of 84% but were in a young population with a median age of 25 years.[525] Selected older patients are now given the more intensive regimens but tend to have more treatment-related deaths unless modifications are made.[526]

The intensity of therapy in HIV patients with NHL was previously reduced due to the risk of infections and poor survival; however, in the era of ART and growth factor support, the CR rate with hyper-CVAD in HIV patients with BL/leukemia has reached 92% with a 2-year survival of 48%.[527] Myelosuppression can still be problematic in HIV patients and dose modifications may be required. There is a randomized trial indicating that rituximab did not improve survival if given with chemotherapy in HIV-related NHL.[528] The lack of improvement in the rituximab arm was attributed to increased infectious deaths in HIV patients with $CD4^+$ counts less than 50/mm^3. Rituximab with concurrent infusional DA-EPOCH achieved a high rate of CR in HIV patients and resulted in a 5-year PFS and OS of 84% and 68%, respectively.[529] DA-EPOCH-R is also used in non-HIV BL and may be particularly warranted in the elderly due to less toxicity.[518] A multicenter risk-adapted study of DA-EPOCH-R was recently conducted in which a total of 113 patients were enrolled.[518] Patients with low-risk disease received two cycles of DA-EPOCH-RR (rituximab on Days 1 and 5 of each cycle) followed by a PET-CT scan. Patients with a negative PET-CT went on to receive one additional cycle, while the ones with positive PET-CT scan received four cycles of DA-EPOCH-R with IT methotrexate. In contrast, high-risk patients (stage ≥3, ECOG PS ≥ 2, elevated LDH, or tumor ≥7 cm) received six cycles of DA-EPOCH-R with IT methotrexate. At median follow-up of 58.7 months, EFS and OS were 84.5% and 87.0%, respectively, and EFS was 100% and 82.1% in low- and high-risk patients, respectively.[518] Therapy was equally effective across age groups, HIV status, and IPI groups.

Advanced stage patients with CNS or marrow involvement previously had survival less than 30% and were considered candidates for early transplantation[530]; however, with the present-day regimens, DFS is in the 40% to 80% range for BL/B-ALL obviating the need for early transplantation in most adult patients. At relapse, there is no standard therapy, and there is no clear advantage of allogeneic HCT over autologous, even though many centers favor the former.[531] Transplantation is rarely successful for relapsed patients unless they are chemosensitive and in a second CR (see Chapter 106).

Lymphoblastic Lymphoma

T-cell LBL is more common than B-LBL in adults, accounting for up to 90% of cases. T-LBL is seen primarily in adolescents and young adults with a predominance of men (2-3:1) and a bimodal distribution (peaks at age 10-30 and 60-70 years).[532] T-LBL presents with a mediastinal mass in 60% to 70% of cases. Considerable overlap exists between T-LBL (<20% marrow involvement) and T-ALL; they are unified as precursor T-cell lymphoblastic/leukemia and are treated with regimens for ALL. B-cell LBL has a slight male predominance, a more even age distribution (median age ~39 years), and rarely has mediastinal or bone marrow involvement. Extranodal sites of disease are common in B-LBL and include skin, bone, and soft tissue.[533]

Multiple genes have been identified in the translocations associated with T-LBL/ALL (see Chapters 74 and 89). Approximately one-third of patients with T-LBL have translocations involving the loci of TCR genes, α and δ at 14q11.2, β at 7q35, and γ at 7p14-5, which produce high levels of transcription factor genes such as *HOX11/TLX1*, *TAL1/SCL*, *TAL2*, and *LYL*. GEP can subdivide T-LBL into subtypes with differing prognosis.[534] T-ALL is subdivided into early thymic precursor (ETP) and non-ETP subtypes, with the former having a worse prognosis. ETP ALL have mutations in genes associated with myeloid leukemias, including *RUNX1* and/or *ETV6*.[535] NOTCH1 is a transmembrane receptor and activating mutations occur in 50% to 60% of patients with non-ETP T-ALL.[536] FBXW7 is an ubiquitin ligase that triggers ubiquitination and degradation by the proteasome. Inactivating mutations *FBXW7* have been reported in 10% to 15% of patients. *NOTCH1* and *FBXW7* mutational status together identify a favorable group of T-ALL/LBL.[537] Loss of *CDKN2A/B* through chromosome 9 deletion is present in 50% to 60% of non-ETP ALL.

Rarely, T-LBL is associated with eosinophilia, myeloid malignancy, specific cytogenetic translocations t(8;13) (p11;q12), t(8;9) (p11;q32), or t(6;8) (q27;p11) and is known as 8p11 myeloproliferative disorder.[538] Unusual cases of T-cell LBL have been associated with prior epipodophyllotoxin chemotherapy and a cytogenetic translocation involving the *MLL* gene, t(11;19) (q23;p23).[539]

Controversial management issues for LBL include the types of induction, consolidation, and maintenance therapy; optimal type of CNS prophylaxis; the role of radiation to the mediastinum; and the role of transplantation.[540] With present-day ALL regimens, the CR rates are in the 75% to 95% range with prolonged DFS in 40% to 70% of responders[541-544] (see Chapter 76). For adolescents and young adults, pediatric-based protocols have had better EFS when compared with adult ALL protocols.[545] Pediatric protocols utilize more intrathecal doses of chemotherapy and have markedly reduced the role of radiation for CNS prophylaxis in ALL. In the era of intensive ALL regimens, mediastinal radiation is no rarely utilized. Because of poor survival with chemotherapy in high-risk patients, now primarily determined by the presence of MRD at the end of consolidation, there is a role for early allogeneic transplantation[546] (see Chapter 106).

Novel agents are being studied in relapsed T-LBL and for use in frontline therapy. Nelarabine, an analogue of AraG, had an ORR of 55% in pediatric patients with T-ALL/LBL in first relapse and 27% in second relapse.[547] An ORR of 46% (36% CR) was reported for adults with relapsed/refractory T-ALL/LBL[548]; it has also been incorporated into a salvage regimen with cyclophosphamide and etoposide in pediatric T-ALL/LBL[549] and with hyper-CVAD for upfront therapy of T-ALL.[550] Clofarabine, a nucleoside analog that inhibits ribonucleotide reductase, had an ORR of 30% (24% CR) in relapsed pediatric ALL and 17% in adult ALL.[551] Clofarabine combined with cyclophosphamide and/or etoposide had a 31% CR rate in adults with relapsed ALL/LBL, but had 23% treatment-related deaths.[552] The prevalent *NOTCH1* mutations in T-ALL are targets for inhibition, particularly with gamma secretase inhibitors that have activity but remain in phase I trials.[553] The proteasome inhibitor bortezomib has activity in both relapsed B and T-ALL, and is under investigation for upfront therapy.[554] Mutations of *NUP214-ABL1*, an activated tyrosine kinase in episomal DNA, present in 6% of T-ALL, may respond to tyrosine kinase inhibitors.[555]

Peripheral T- and NK-cell Lymphomas

T/NK-cell NHLs provide a unique therapeutic challenge due to the rarity, heterogeneity, and adverse disease biology and limited prospective studies evaluating treatment approaches.[556-558] PTCLs and NK-cell neoplasms represent 10% to 15% of all NHL in Western countries and 20% to 35% in Asia; there are multiple subtypes so that many represent less than 1% of NHL (*Table 90.13*). These diseases have a geographic variation with more nodal disease in North

Table 90.13. Mature T/NK Lymphoma/Leukemia

Nodal
Peripheral T-cell lymphoma, not otherwise specified
Anaplastic large cell lymphoma
ALK-positive
ALK-negative
Angioimmunoblastic T-cell lymphoma
Follicular T-cell lymphoma
Nodal PTCL with T_{FH} phenotype
Extranodal
Nasal NK/T-cell lymphoma
Localized
Disseminated (nasal type)
Enteropathy-associated T-cell lymphoma
Monomorphic epitheliotropic intestinal T-cell lymphoma
Indolent T-cell lymphoproliferative disorder of the GI tract
Hepatosplenic γδ T-cell lymphoma
Subcutaneous panniculitis-like T-cell lymphoma
Primary cutaneous γδ T-cell lymphoma
Leukemia
T-cell prolymphocytic leukemia
Adult T-cell lymphoma/leukemia
Large granular lymphocytic leukemia, T and NK types
Aggressive NK-cell leukemia

Abbreviations: ALK, anaplastic lymphoma kinase; NK, natural killer; PTCL, peripheral T-cell lymphoma; T_{FH}, T-follicular helper cell.

America and Europe, including PTCL, unspecified; ALCL and AITL; and more extranodal disease in Asia due to EBV-related nasal NK/T lymphoma and HTLV-1–associated ATL.[559] The prognosis in most peripheral T/NK neoplasms is poor with 5-year survival less than 35%.[559] PTCLs may be associated with paraneoplastic phenomena, including skin rashes, autoimmune hemolytic anemia, hypergammaglobulinemia, eosinophilia, hypercalcemia, vasculitis, hemophagocytosis, and fever of unknown origin, which may mask the initial diagnosis.[559]

Few characteristic translocations are noted in mature T/NK neoplasms; in fact, translocations involving the TCR genes at 14q11 (α/δ), 7q34 (β), and 7p14 (γ) are infrequent. One pathognomonic translocation is t(2;5) (p23;q35) associated with ALCL that produces a fusion gene encoding the cytoplasmic part of ALK, a receptor tyrosine kinase of the insulin receptor subfamily on chromosome 2, and the amino-terminal portion of nucleophosmin (NPM) on chromosome 5.[17] A t(5;9) translocation involving the IL-2-inducible T-cell kinase (ITK) gene on chromosome 5 and the spleen tyrosine kinase (SYK) on chromosome 9 is noted in a subset (17%) of PTCL-NOS cases.[560] Another translocation involving the multiple myeloma oncogene 1 (MUM1)/IFN-regulatory factor-4 (IRF4) gene locus with the TCRA gene, t(6;14) (p25;q11.2) was found in two cases of PTCL-NOS and led to the recognition by FISH screening of non-TCR-related IRF4 translocations in ALK-negative ALCLs.[561] A balanced translocation between DUSP22 phosphatase gene on 6p25.3 and FRA7H on 7q23 was subsequently found in both systemic and cutaneous ALCL.[562] Furthermore, gene expression signatures correspond to specific subtypes of PTCL, correlate with prognosis, and may identify potential targets for novel agents.[563]

The WHO classification separates mature T/NK neoplasms by site of involvement: nodal, extranodal, leukemic, and cutaneous. In the subsequent section, the focus is primarily on nodal and extranodal diseases followed by a description of the leukemias and therapeutic aspects unique to these malignancies. CTCLs are reviewed in Chapter 94.

Anaplastic Large Cell Lymphoma

ALCL pathology shows CD30 positive large cells in sheets. Based on the clinical presentation, ALCL is classified as systemic, cutaneous and breast implant–associated ALCL. Systemic ALCL predominantly involves lymph nodes, but extranodal involvement also occurs, especially skin involvement. Based on IHC for ALK protein expression, systemic ALCL is further classified as ALK+ and ALK− ALCL. ALK expression has both prognostic and predictive significance and impacts treatment decisions. In 1989, a proportion of ALCLs was associated with a specific chromosomal translocation,[16] and in 1994, Morris identified the genes involved in t(2;5).[17] ALK rearrangements are present in 50% to 70% of ALCL, and t(2;5) occurs in approximately three-fourths of these patients.[564] Additional variants have been described with t(1;2) (q25;p23) as the most common. IHC stain for the ALK protein is usually present in both cytoplasm and nuclei of classic t(2;5) (p23;q35) vs only in the cytoplasm of the variants.

ALK expression subdivides ALCL into at least four clinical subtypes: (1) ALK+ systemic ALCL, (2) ALK- systemic ALCL, (3) Breast implant–associated ALCL, and (4) primary cutaneous ALCL (also, ALK−). ALK+ ALCL occurs at a younger median age (15-30 years) than ALK- (45-65 years), has a male predominance (male:female = 2-6:1), and usually has advanced stage disease with frequent B symptoms (40%-75%) and extranodal involvement (50%-80%). Skin (21%-35%) (Figure 90.17), soft tissue (17%), and bone (8%-17%) are common extranodal sites, whereas gastrointestinal tract and CNS are rarely involved.[565] Bone marrow involvement in ALK-positive ALCL is identified in 10% to 15% with hematoxylin and eosin stains but up to 30% with immunohistochemistry stains.[565]

ALK+ ALCL is seen in younger patients with median age at diagnosis in 20s and is the most common lymphoma in children. Furthermore, ALK+ ALCL is more chemosensitive than ALK-negative ALCL with CR rates >75% for ALK+ and 50% to 75% in ALK+.[566,567] Better responses have resulted in a twofold or higher increase in survival for ALK+ ALCL (60%-93% at 5 years) compared with ALK-ALCL (15%-46%) in retrospective series.[558,567] Adverse prognostic factors in ALK+ patients include B symptoms, a high IPI, small cell variant histology, and expression of CD56 or survivin (a member of the inhibitor of apoptosis family).[568]

ALK− ALCL in itself is a heterogeneous group of diseases. Systemic ALK− may be primary or secondary to mycosis fungoides, lymphomatoid papulosis, or HL.[565] Based on cytogenetics, ALK− ALCL is classified into different prognostic groups. DUSP22 rearrangement (30% of cases) had similar outcome to ALK+ disease with a 90% 5-year OS, whereas TP63 (8%) had unfavorable OS at 17%; a triple negative (lacking ALK, DUSP22, and TP63) group (62%) had an intermediate prognosis (42% 5-year OS).[569] ALK− cases have more recurrent genetic losses than ALK+; losses at 6q21 (PRDM1) and at 17p (TP53) in ALK- disease have also been associated with a poor prognosis.[570] Although gene expression profiles overlap between the two groups, an overexpression of genes encoding signal transduction and downregulation of transcription factor genes has been reported in ALK+ vs ALK− ALCL.[571]

Primary cutaneous ALCL is ALK− and is a type of CD30+ cutaneous lymphoproliferative disease, which clinically overlaps with lymphomatoid papulosis (Chapter 94).[572] It usually presents with an isolated reddish violet skin tumor, ulcerated in a subset with a median age at diagnosis of 60 years. Less commonly, it may present as multiple nodules in a circumscribed area, or rarely with disseminated skin lesions. Localized lesions may be managed by watchful waiting as approximately one-quarter of patients regress, local excision ± radiation, or radiation alone.[565,572] Combination chemotherapy may be warranted with widespread skin disease or localized skin disease with adjacent nodal involvement, but these patients tend to relapse.[572]

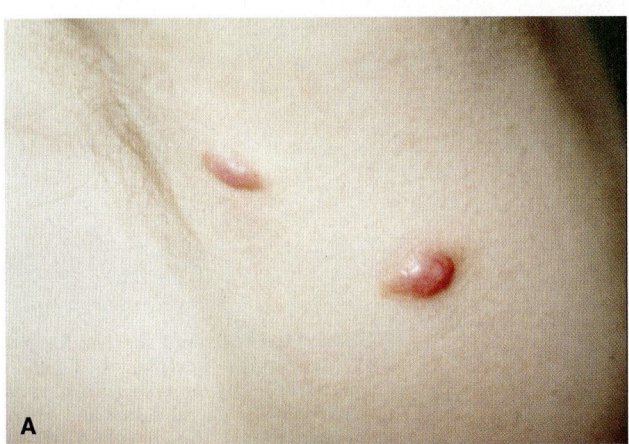 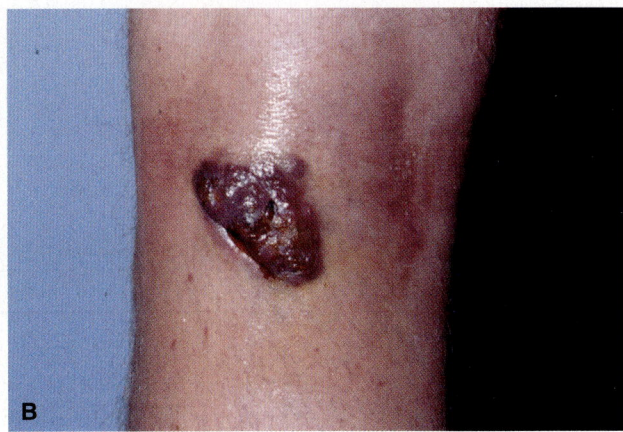

FIGURE 90.17 ALK-1–positive anaplastic large cell lymphoma: skin lesions can vary from nodules (A) in an axilla to ulcerations (B) in a popliteal fossa.

Another subtype, breast implant-associated ALCL was first reported in 1997 and is a rare disease with an estimated annual incidence of 0.1 to 0.3 per 100,000 women with implants, primarily of the textured type.[573] The median interval from implant to diagnosis was 8 years (range, 2-25 years); two-thirds of patients had an effusion, or seroma, with disease confined to a fibrous capsule.[574] Regional nodes were involved in 15% of patients. Although chemotherapy and/or radiation have been used, surgical excision of the lymphoma, capsule, and implant is the recommended therapy.

Two proteins, CD30 and ALK, provide unique therapeutic targets in ALCL. Brentuximab vedotin (BV) is an antibody-drug complex combining an anti-CD30 antibody with the antimicrotubule agent, monomethyl auristatin E. In a phase II trial in 58 patients with relapsed/refractory ALCL, the ORR was 86% (57% CR), and the median duration of response was 12.6 months for all patients.[575] A landmark phase 3 randomized controlled trial (ECHELON2) in CD30+ PTCL (CD30 expression 10% or more) found the combination of BV and cyclophosphamide, Adriamycin, and prednisone (BV-CHP) superior to CHOP in terms of PFS and OS.[576,577] The study included 452 patients, majority of patients with ALCL (70%), at a median follow-up of 5 months, the median PFS of BV-CHP vs CHOP were 63 vs 24 months. For the complete cohort, the estimated 5-year PFS rates were 51% and 43% and estimated 5-year OS rates of 69% and 60%, respectively. The estimated 5-year PFS rates for ALCL patients were 60% and 48%, respectively, for the BV-CHP vs CHOP (HR 0.55). The survival benefit for non-ALCL subtypes was less clear with HR for PFS of 0.75 and 1.4 for PTCL and AITL, respectively, and corresponding HR for OS of 0.83 and 0.87, respectively. The most common grade 3 or more side effects with BV-CHP were neutropenia, anemia, diarrhea, peripheral neuropathy, and nausea. Based on these data, BV-CHP is the preferred first-line treatment for patients with ALCL. Involved site radiation therapy may be considered in limited stage disease with more abbreviated chemotherapy similar to that in DLBCL.

Crizotinib is an oral small-molecule inhibitor of ALK tyrosine kinase that was first approved for use in the 2% of non–small cell lung cancers with a rearrangement involving *ALK*. It is FDA approved for children and young adults with R/R ALK+ ALCL and has also demonstrated activity in adults. A phase I trial reported seven CRs in nine relapsed pediatric ALK-positive ALCL.[578] A subsequent report confirmed CRs in adults.[579] Crizotinib has been associated with an ORR of 67% in R/R ALK+ ALCL, with all relapses/progressions occurring within 3 months.[580] This has been attributed to resistance to ALK inhibitor. A recent phase 2 study ($n = 12$), crizotinib at a dose of 250 mg BID, was associated with an ORR of 83% and CR rate of 58%. The 2-year PFS rate was 65% and OS rates of 66%.[581] Ceritinib is another ALK inhibitor that has induced CRs in xenograft models and in patients resistant to crizotinib.[582] Furthermore, alectinib, a second-generation ALK inhibitor with CNS penetration, is active in ALK+ R/R ALCL and a potential option in those with CNS involvement.[583,584]

Nodal Peripheral T-cell Lymphoma

PTCLs are a heterogeneous group of lymphoproliferative diseases that includes ALCL discussed above (13%). PTCL-NOS is the most common subtype (26%), others include AITL, 19%, EATLs in less than 5%. For years, therapy paradigms have been extrapolated from aggressive B-cell lymphomas, however, with inferior outcomes in PTCLs.[585,586]

PTCL-NOS represented the largest group (29.5%) in the International Peripheral T cell Lymphoma Project (IPTL) (*Figure 90.18*).[587] The median age was 60 years with a male predominance. Most patients presented with nodal (87%) disease and had advanced stage (69%); extranodal involvement occurred in 49%. The 5-year OS was 32% and FFS was 20%. GEP can further divide T/NK-cell lymphomas into different types and prognoses. Over one-third of morphologically diagnosed PTCL-NOS can be reclassified into other subtypes of PTCL according to molecular signatures.[588] High expression of GATA3 or TBX21 divides PTCL-NOS into two subtypes, with the former being associated with a poorer prognosis.[589] In addition to high IPI score, multivariable analysis showed PTCL-GATA 3 subtype based on IHC predicted a poorer OS.[590] In the large Swedish registry real world study ($n = 755$ PTCL cases), male sex was associated with an adverse outcome [(OS) (HR, 1.28; $P = .011$); PFS (HR, 1.26; $P = .014$)] in addition to IPI.[591] A smaller cohort from China reported Ki67 and thrombocytopenia (defined as count <100,000/μL) as potential adverse prognostic factors.[592]

Additional tumor-specific features prognostic evaluated include expression of cytotoxic molecules, Ki-67, TP53, chemokine receptors, and gene profiles.[593] Expression of the cytotoxic molecules TIA-1 and granzyme B is associated with the presence of B symptoms, a higher IPI, an inferior CR rate, and a worse OS.[594] Ki-67 positivity was additive to IPI factors (age, PS, LDH) in a series of PTCL-NOS.[595] TP53 overexpression was detected by immunohistochemistry in a minority (29%) of nodal PTCL cases; was associated with Ki-67, BCL-2, and P-glycoprotein; and was a better predictor of poor survival than IPI.[596]

AITL may be difficult to diagnose, because both B- and T-cell clones and EBV may be present and because it has a variable clinical course with autoimmune features.[597] AITL was the second most common type (18.5%) in the IPTL, usually occurring in the elderly (median age 57-68 years) as a systemic disease with diffuse adenopathy (84%-100%), B symptoms (52%-86%), maculopapular rash (38%-58%), arthritis (16%-18%), eosinophilia (32%-50%), and immunologic features (Coombs-positive hemolytic anemia [32%-75%], cold agglutinins, cryoglobulinemia, polyclonal hypergammaglobulinemia

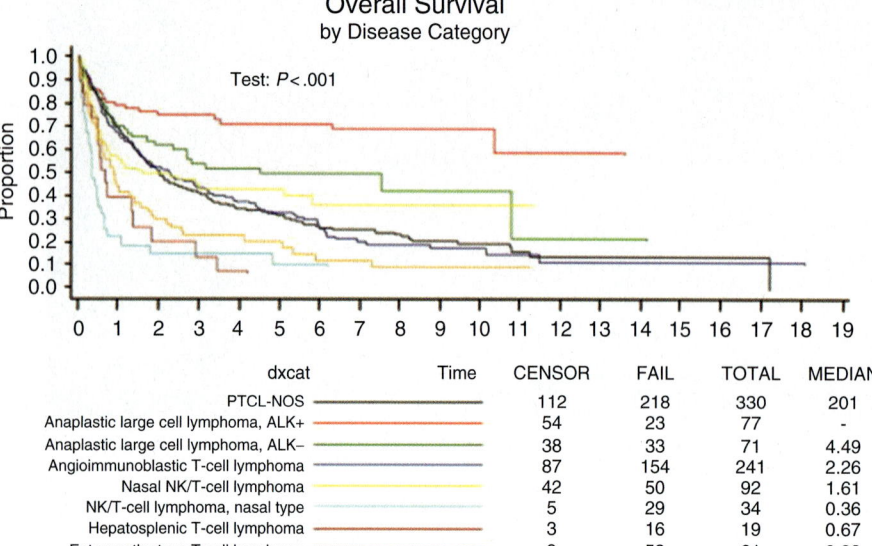

FIGURE 90.18 Overall survival for patients with aggressive peripheral T-cell lymphoma (PTCL) by subtype according to the International Peripheral T Cell and NK/T Cell Lymphoma Study. ALK, anaplastic lymphoma kinase. (From Armitage JO. The aggressive peripheral T-cell lymphomas: 2012 update on diagnosis, risk stratification, and management. *Am J Hematol.* 2012;87(5):511-519. Copyright © 2012 Wiley Periodicals, Inc. Reprinted by permission of John Wiley & Sons, Inc.)

[50%-83%], antinuclear antibodies, and rheumatoid factors). Most patients have extranodal disease and are in an advanced stage (68%-94%).

There is clonal evolution over time in AITL and EBV may participate in lymphomagenesis. The cell of origin is a T-follicular helper cell (T_{FH}); and there is cytoplasmic expression of the cytokine CXCL13.[598] Follicular T-cell lymphoma and PTCL of T_{FH} origin (T_{FH}-PTCL) are closely related to AITL and are now excluded from PTCL-NOS. TCR gene rearrangements occur early in the course of AITL indicating a clonal T-cell population, but one-third of patients will also have an Ig gene rearrangement. Similar to posttransplant lymphoproliferation but unlike other NHL, unrelated or oligoclonal cell populations are commonly found. The most common cytogenetic abnormalities are trisomy 3, trisomy 5, and an additional X chromosome, but patients who develop complex aberrant clones and structural abnormalities in the short arm of chromosome 1 progress rapidly.[599]

A model for AITL involves a premalignant lesion at *TET2* or *DNMT3A* followed by a secondary mutation in *RHOA* or *IDH2* that leads to malignant transformation of T_{FH} cells.[599] The *RHOA* gene encodes a small GTPase that regulates the actin cytoskeleton, cell adhesion, and TCR signaling, and is mutated in 60% to 70% of cases of AITL and T_{FH}-PTCL.[600] Epigenetic regulators, *TET2*, *IDH2*, and *DNMT3A*, are mutated in 50% to 75%, 20% to 30%, and 20% to 30% of AITL, respectively. The *IDH2* mutations are gain-of-function missense at the *R172* residue and have a distinct gene expression signature in AITL.

AITL may spontaneously regress in up to 10% of patients; and they may respond to single agents, including steroids, cyclosporine, methotrexate, IFN, nucleoside analogs, bortezomib, romidepsin, bendamustine, gemcitabine, and rituximab. Combination chemotherapy is usually warranted once a diagnosis is made with a CR rate of 50% to 70% following anthracycline-based therapy, but patients have frequent and early relapses or deaths due to infections with 5-year survival at 10% to 30%.[601] Due to the poor prognosis, early transplant has been advocated for selected AITL patients.[602]

Extranodal T-cell Lymphomas

Hepatosplenic γ/δ T-cell lymphoma (HSTL) was first described in 1990 as an aggressive illness with B symptoms and organomegaly in young adult males.[603] Up to 20% of HSTL arise in patients on immunosuppression agents, including anti-TNFα or thiopurines, for solid organ transplants or inflammatory bowel disease.[604] The median age is 25 to 35 years with a male:female ratio of 9:1. Patients have splenomegaly (98%), hepatomegaly (80%), minimal to no lymphadenopathy, anemia (84%), and severe thrombocytopenia (85%).[605] The bone marrow is involved in three-fourths of patients and erythrophagocytosis may occur. Isochrome 7q often associated with trisomy 8 is a common cytogenetic abnormality. Most patients have brief responses or are refractory to anthracycline-based therapy and have a median survival of 12 to 16 months.[605] There is an α/β variant with similar features and outcome.[606] Similar GEPs involving genes implicated in cytotoxic T and NK-cell function are present in both γ/δ and α/β variants.[607] Due to the poor prognosis, early allogeneic HCT has been advocated as a therapeutic strategy to improve survival.[608,609]

Subcutaneous panniculitis-like T-cell lymphoma (SPTCL) presents with subcutaneous nodules, usually on the extremities, and is an αβ subtype that should be distinguished from primary cutaneous γ/δ T-cell lymphoma (PCGDTCL).[610] SPTCL occurs at a younger median age (36 years) with a female predominance. The skin lesions tend to be self-healing subcutaneous plaques and nodules without ulceration. Disseminated disease and hemophagocytosis (17%) are rare. These patients may be controlled with single agent therapies, and have a 5-year OS of 82%.[438] PCGDTCL occurs in an older population (median age 59 years) with a roughly equal male:female ratio. Skin lesions may involve the epidermis and ulcerate. B symptoms, nodal disease, and hemophagocytosis are associated with a poor prognosis and a 5-year OS of 11% despite combination chemotherapy.[610]

EATLs account for 6% to 9% of PTCL, have a geographic variation, and may be associated with celiac disease.[611,612] EATL, formerly known as Type I, has a large cell or pleomorphic cytology, has chromosome 9q31.3 gain or 16q12.1 deletion, is associated with the HLA-DQ2 haplotype, is strongly associated with celiac disease, and is more common in Europe (*Table 90.14*). Monomorphic epitheliotropic intestinal TCL, formerly EATL Type II, is characterized by monomorphic cells often with CD56 expression; has chromosome 8q24 gain and less commonly, 1q and 5q gains; occurs sporadically; and is found primarily in Asia. The median age of EATLs is 50 to 64 years and males predominate in most series.[611,613] Abdominal pain and weight loss occur in over 80% of patients at presentation followed by diarrhea or vomiting in one-third of patients.[441,613] Small bowel obstruction or perforation is common, and the diagnosis of EATL is often made at laparotomy. Prognosis is poor with a median survival of 7.5 months and 1-year FFS less than 20%; the monomorphic type appears to have a worse prognosis.[611-614] Indolent T-cell lymphoproliferative disease of the gastrointestinal tract and NK enteropathy can be confused with EATLs.[615]

Extranodal T-cell and Natural Killer-cell Lymphomas

Extranodal NK/T-cell lymphoma (ENKTL), nasal and nasal-type, is characterized by angiocentric and angiodestructive proliferation;

Table 90.14. Management Issues for Extranodal Lymphomas

Site	Usual Pathology	Clinical Associations	Suggested Therapy[a]
Stomach	B-cell MALToma	*Helicobacter pylori*	Antibiotic trial, serial endoscopy; other therapy if t(11;18), t(1;14), transformation or progressive disease
Ileum	Burkitt	Obstruction	High-dose cyclophosphamide combination chemotherapy ± surgery
Immunoproliferative small intestinal disease	B-cell MALToma	Malabsorption, IgA heavy chain Middle East	Antibiotics, steroids, ±combination chemotherapy
Enteropathy-associated T-cell lymphoma	Peripheral T-cell lymphoma	Celiac disease, obstruction Western hemisphere	Combination chemotherapy ± surgery; nutrition
Waldeyer ring	Large B cell	Other gastrointestinal diseases	Combination chemotherapy or combined modality
Paranasal (sinus)	Large B cell	CNS disease	Combined modality, consider CNS prophylaxis
Nasal	Natural killer/T-cell lymphoma	Epstein-Barr virus; angiocentric features, Asia	Combined modality, consider CNS prophylaxis; radiation alone for small volume disease
Salivary gland	B-cell MALToma	Sjögren syndrome	Single agent, including monoclonal antibody; and/or radiation
Thyroid	Large B-cell, B-cell MALToma	Hashimoto thyroiditis	Radiation or combined modality, depending on histology and stage
Lung	Small B cell, B-cell MALToma		Single agent, including monoclonal antibody; surgery, or radiation
Orbital	Small B cell, B-cell MALTtoma Large B cell (rare)		Radiation and/or single agent, including monoclonal antibody; combination chemotherapy if large B cell
Primary CNS	Large B cell	Ocular involvement Leptomeningeal disease AIDS	Steroids, high-dose methotrexate ± radiation
Testis	Large B cell	Contralateral testicular disease, CNS disease, retroperitoneal spread	Orchiectomy, combination chemotherapy, radiation to contralateral testis, CNS prophylaxis
Breast	Large B cell	Pregnancy	Combination chemotherapy ± radiation
Ovary	Burkitt Large B cell	Bilateral disease	Combination chemotherapy
Bone	Large B cell		Combination chemotherapy ± radiation
Cutaneous	Mycosis fungoides B-cell MALToma Primary cutaneous follicular lymphoma Primary cutaneous large B-cell lymphoma		Skin-directed when limited stage Radiation if stage I$_E$ Single agents, including monoclonal antibody for indolent disease Combined modality, if large B cell (see Chapter 94)

[a]Combined modality refers to combination chemotherapy and radiation. Combination chemotherapy refers to doxorubicin-based therapy. Rituximab is added to therapy of most B cell (CD20+) lymphomas.
Abbreviations: AIDS, acquired immunodeficiency syndrome; CNS, central nervous system; MALToma, lymphoma of mucosa-associated lymphoid tissue.

large granular lymphocyte morphology; CD2+, CD3−, CD16−/+, CD56+, CD57− immunophenotype; and an aggressive course.[616] Only 10% express surface CD3 and have clonal TCR rearrangement with a similar course of disease.[617] ENKTL represents 3% to 5% of PTCL in North America and Europe, but 15% to 22% in Asia and Latin America. A diagnosis of hydroa vacciniforme-like lymphoproliferative disease may precede ENKTL, particularly in Latin America.[618] EBV is consistently detected in tumor cells and elevated levels of EBV DNA in tumor tissue or serum have correlated with a poor prognosis.[619,620]

Nasal NK/T cell lymphoma may present with facial swelling or midfacial destruction and was formerly called lethal midline granuloma or polymorphic reticulosis (*Figure 90.19*). The disease occurs more commonly in males with a median age of 50 to 55 years.[616,617] Nasal NK/T lymphoma is localized stage I/II in 80% of patients at diagnosis but can disseminate early to skin, gastrointestinal tract, testis, orbit, and CNS. Although radiation alone can achieve CR in two-thirds of localized, low volume disease, local relapse occurs in half the patients and disseminated disease develops in one-quarter.[616] Combined modality therapy with early radiation and chemotherapy with non–anthracycline-based regimens is recommended; the optimal sequencing of radiation (before, during, or after chemotherapy) is uncertain.[621,622] Patients with disease confined to the nasal cavity, larynx, pharynx, or oral cavity had 54% 5-year survival compared to 20% ($P = .0068$) with more advanced disease.[623] Patients with cutaneous-only involvement have a better survival than other disseminated ENKTL.[624]

L-Asparaginase was shown to be effective in relapsed/refractory ENKTL and has been incorporated into upfront chemotherapy.[625] Because of high expression of P-glycoprotein in the tumor, regimens containing multidrug-resistant independent agents, such as SMILE (steroids, methotrexate, ifosfamide, L-asparaginase, etoposide), GeLOX (gemcitabine, L-asparaginase, oxaliplatin), DeVIC (dexamethasone, etoposide, ifosfamide, carboplatin), and VIPD (etoposide, ifosfamide, cisplatin, dexamethasone), have been formulated to treat nasal-type NK/TCL.[626] PD-1 blockade with pembrolizumab has been effective in a limited number of patients with relapsed NK/T lymphoma.[627]

Mature T-cell and Natural Killer-cell Leukemias

Large granular lymphocytic (LGL) leukemia was first noted to be associated with chronic neutropenia in 1977, recognized as a clonal disorder in 1985, and classified into T (CD3+) and NK (CD3−) types

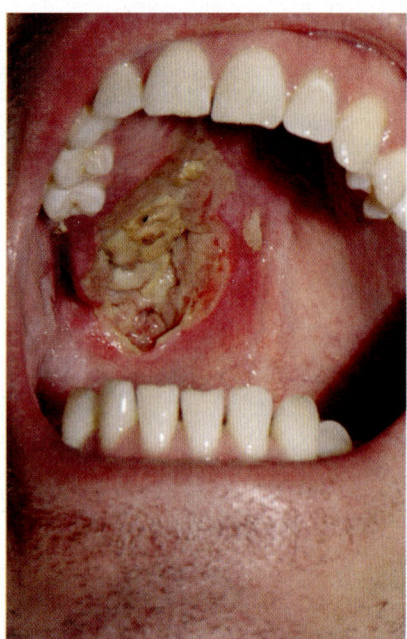

FIGURE 90.19 Nasal NK/T lymphoma: an ulcerated lesion in the hard palate.

in 1993 (*Figure 90.20A*).[628,629] Chronic NK lymphocytosis represents less than 10% of cases, but it shares the same clinical and biologic features of T-LGL leukemia. The median age is 60 years; there is no sex difference; and there is an association with RA (10%-20%) and autoimmune features.[628] Lymphocytosis is usually between 2 and 20×10^9/L and mild splenomegaly (25%-50%) may be present; one-third of patients are asymptomatic, but the typical clinical presentation is related to neutropenia or anemia. Severe neutropenia ($<0.5 \times 10^9$/L) occurs in 16% to 48% of cases. Recurrent infections (15%-39%) are usually respiratory or mucocutaneous.[629] Pure red cell aplasia (8%-19%), autoimmune hemolytic anemia, aplastic anemia, idiopathic thrombocytopenic purpura, B-cell lymphomas, and MDS (3%-10%) have been reported in patients with LGL leukemia.[629]

Constitutive activation of STAT3 plays a critical role in the pathogenesis of LGL leukemia.[629] LGL cells express high levels of both FAS and FAS ligand, but the cells are resistant to FAS-mediated death due to STAT3 activation which upregulates an antiapoptotic protein.[630] *STAT3* mutations are present in one-third of both T and NK types and are associated with symptomatic disease, but are not mandatory for LGL clonal expansion.[631] IL-6 and IL-15 are proinflammatory cytokines that are elevated in LGL patients and can promote LGL survival and activate the JAK/STAT3 pathway.[632]

LGL leukemia is an indolent disease with approximately 70% survival at 10 years.[629] Single-agent immunosuppressive agents, methotrexate, cyclophosphamide, or cyclosporine, are considered frontline therapy with no clear advantage of one agent over the other.[633] The ORR is broad (21%-85%) with a median of 50%.[629] Purine analogs (fludarabine, cladribine, deoxycoformycin, or bendamustine) are second line with response rates up to 79% in a limited number of patients.[629] Alemtuzumab (Campath) has had a response of 60% in refractory patients; it is recommended to use the lowest dose possible for this indication.[634] G-CSF can increase the neutrophils rapidly, but it is not effective in all patients and may exacerbate arthritis or splenomegaly; and erythropoietin is of little benefit. Therapy targeting activated pathways in LGL leukemia such as JAK and STAT is under investigation.[635]

Aggressive NK leukemia is a rare disorder that primarily occurs in Asia, is associated with EBV, and represents the leukemic phase of nasal-type NK lymphoma (*Figure 90.20B*). Patients are young (median age 30-40 years) with a slight male predominance and present with a fulminant illness characterized by B symptoms, diffuse adenopathy, organomegaly, and circulating LGL cells which can have a blastic appearance.[636] Patients are chemoresistant and have median survival less than 3 months.

T-prolymphocytic leukemia represents approximately 2% of small lymphocytic leukemia in adults (*Figure 90.20C*).[636] The median age is 57 to 69 years and the male:female ratio is 1.5:1. Patients usually have a marked lymphocytosis ($>100 \times 10^9$/L in 75% of patients), splenomegaly (73%), and lymphadenopathy (53%); and approximately 20% of patients have skin infiltration.[637] Cell morphology is variable; the nuclei are irregular, include a "knobby" variant, and usually have prominent nucleoli; cytoplasmic protrusions are characteristic. Sixty percent of patients are CD4+/CD8−; 25% coexpress CD4+/CD8+; and 15% are CD4−/CD8+.

The most common cytogenetic abnormality in T-PLL is an inversion of chromosome 14 occurring in 75% of patients.[637] Another 10% to 20% will have either t(X;14) (q28;q11) or a reciprocal translocation, t(14;14) (q11;q32). All three abnormalities juxtapose a gene at the *TCL1* family (*TCL1A* at 14q32 or *MTCP1* at Xq) with the *TCRA* locus at 14q11. Deletions at 11q23, the locus for the *ATM* gene, and abnormalities of chromosome 8 (isochromosome 8q or trisomy) are other common cytogenetic findings in T-PLL. 12p13 deletion occurs in up to one-half of cases, and may contribute to pathogenesis by causing haploinsufficiency of *CDKN1B*.[638] Three-quarters of cases have mutually exclusive activating mutations in the JAK-STAT pathway.[639]

The median survival in T-PLL is 12 to 20 months, although up to one-third can have an indolent phase.[640] The most active single agent is intravenous alemtuzumab (Campath) with 74% and 91% responses in previously treated and untreated patients, respectively.[640] Response rates in T-PLL with alkylating agents and anthracyclines are only 30% to 45% with few complete remissions and are slightly higher with purine nucleoside analogs, such as pentostatin and fludarabine, or with bendamustine.[641] Sequential chemotherapy (fludarabine, cyclophosphamide, mitoxantrone) followed by alemtuzumab had a 92% response rate, a PFS of 11.9 months, and an OS of 17.1 months in a series that included both treated and untreated patients.[642] Stem cell transplant, primarily allogeneic over autologous, has been utilized in select patients, but there has been a 30% to 40% transplant-related mortality (with allo), a high relapse rate of 30% to 50% (higher with auto than allo), and only a 20% to 30% 3- to 5-year survival.[643]

The clinical course of **ATL** follows four basic types per the 1991 Shimoyama classification: (1) acute (leukemic) (50%-60% of cases), (2) lymphoma (20%-25%), (3) chronic (10%-20%), and (4) smoldering (5%-19%). The male to female ratio is 1.3 to 2.2:1, and the median age varies from 47 to 65 years depending on the endemic region.[51] The median age at diagnosis in Central and South America is in the fifth decade, whereas it has increased in Japan from the sixth to the seventh decade due to a high prevalence in the elderly and a reduction in the young following universal screening of blood donors, prenatal testing, and avoidance of breastfeeding from infected mothers. In a Japanese study comparing patients diagnosed from 1983 to 1987 to those from 2000 to 2008, the median survivals modestly increased in three of the four types of ATL: 6.2 to 8.3 months for acute, 10.2 to 10.6 months for lymphoma, and 24.3 to 31.5 months for chronic.[644] The respective 4-year OS changes were 5% to 11%, 6% to 16%, and 27% to 36%. There was a worse survival for the smoldering type: a median not reached with 62% 4-year OS in the early group compared to 55 months and 52% OS.

The cutaneous lesions have a diverse appearance, including erythroderma, papules, nodules, plaques, tumors, and ulcers. Histologically, dermal invasion predominates although the lesions of ATL may resemble primary CTCL with epidermotropism and Pautrier microabscesses. Over one-quarter of patients have infections at diagnosis. Anemia and thrombocytopenia are infrequent findings because of a low degree of marrow infiltration. Eosinophilia may occur in up to 20% of patients. CNS involvement may develop in as many as 10% of patients with aggressive forms of ATL.[645]

The acute form is characterized by lymphadenopathy, organomegaly, skin lesions, elevated white count with multilobed lymphocytes, often referred to as "cloverleaf" or "flower" cells (*Figure 90.20D*);

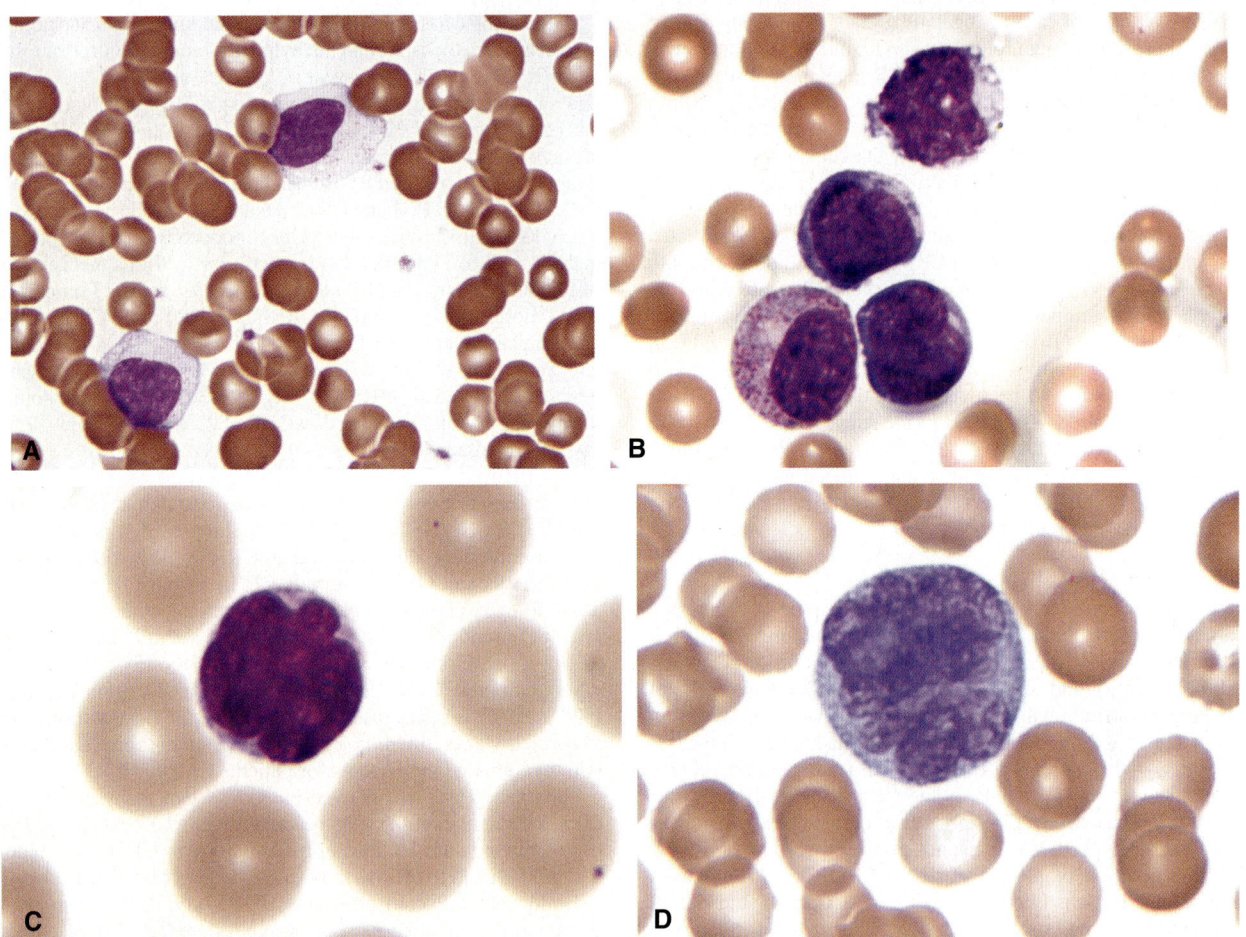

FIGURE 90.20 Mature T/NK leukemias. A, T-cell large granular lymphocytic leukemia. The lymphocytes are enlarged with dense nuclear chromatin and abundant cytoplasm with fine azurophilic granules. B, Natural killer/T-cell leukemia. Three leukemic cells and one myelocyte are present. The leukemia cells have blastic, fine nuclear chromatin with irregular nuclei and basophilic cytoplasm. Some cases may show cytoplasmic granules. C, T-cell prolymphocytic leukemia. The lymphocyte has clumped nuclear chromatin with irregular nuclear contours, sometimes referred to as "knobby cells." Nucleoli may be inconspicuous, in contrast to B-cell prolymphocytic leukemia which has prominent nucleoli. D, Abnormal T lymphocyte in the peripheral blood of a patient with adult T-cell leukemia. The cell is enlarged with a multilobated nucleus. These "flower cells" are usually easily found with this disorder. (Images provided by Dr Dan Arber, University of Chicago, Chicago, IL.)

hypercalcemia in 50% to 70% of patients (vs 15%-20% in the lymphomatous form), elevated LDH level, and usually a rapidly fatal course. Lymphoma is distinguished by prominent adenopathy without significant peripheral blood involvement. Primary extranodal lymphoma occurs in approximately 5% of lymphomatous presentations and has involved skin, Waldeyer ring, gastrointestinal tract, sinuses, and pleura.[646] A prognostic index for the aggressive subtypes has five factors: stage III/IV (2 points), ECOG score of 2 to 4 (1 point), age >70 years (1 point), serum albumin <3.5 g/dL (1 point), and soluble IL-2 receptor >20,000 U/mL (1 point).[647] A low score (0-2) had a median OS of 16.2 months; an intermediate score (3-4), 7 months; and a high score (5-6), 4.6 months.

The chronic type is associated with an increased leukocyte count (absolute T-lymphocytes > 4.0×10^9/L) and occasionally with slight adenopathy and organomegaly. Unfavorable factors include a low serum albumin, a high LDH, or elevated blood urea nitrogen. Patients with smoldering ATL have few ATL cells (0.5%-5%) in the peripheral blood and do not have lymphocytosis, adenopathy, or splenomegaly; they may have skin or lung infiltration. Chronic and smoldering ATL may evolve into an acute form after many years of indolent disease.

No consistent cytogenetic abnormality has been identified in ATL. The most common abnormalities are gains at chromosomes 14q, 7q, and 3p, and losses at 6q and 13q.[648] The acute type showed a gain of 3/3p, whereas the lymphoma type had more frequent gains at 1q, 2p, 4q, 7p, and 7q, and more losses of 10p, 13q, 16q, and 18p. Aneuploidy, multiple chromosomal breaks, and loss of tumor suppressor genes are associated with an aggressive course.[648,649]

ATL has been difficult to treat due to chemoresistance and lack of effective antiviral therapy. Options for therapy are based on presentation and prognostic subtype and include observation, chemotherapy, antiviral therapy, targeted therapies, and allogeneic stem cell transplantation. In a randomized trial, chemotherapy with a complex regimen, LSG15 protocol, was marginally superior (40% CR, 24% 3-year OS) to CHOP (25% CR, 13% 3-year OS); there was a higher response rate in the lymphoma form compared to acute.[650] Other combinations, including EPOCH and hyper-CVAD, and novel agents such as histone deacetylase inhibitors (HDACis), proteasome inhibitors, and nucleoside analogs have been used in ATL, but there is no consensus or data to support one regimen over another. Standard response criteria have been developed for ATL.[651]

IFN-α and zidovudine (AZT) has had a higher response rate than chemotherapy in the chronic, smoldering, and acute forms of ATL.[652] There may be a survival advantage for concurrent chemotherapy with low-dose IFN/AZT in acute and lymphoma subtypes compared to chemotherapy alone.[653] Arsenic trioxide synergizes with IFN and has been effective with or without AZT.[654] Lenalidomide has also shown responses as a single agent in phase II trials.[655]

Unconjugated and conjugated monoclonal antibodies directed at receptors on the malignant T cells have activity in ATL. Chemokine receptor 4 (CCR4), a chemokine involved in T_H2 regulation, is expressed in over 80% of cases. Mogamulizumab, an antibody against CCR4, was approved in Japan for relapsed ATL in 2012 and for newly diagnosed patients in 2014. It had a 50% ORR in relapsed disease with a median PFS and OS of 5.2 and 13.7 months, respectively.[656] In a randomized phase II trial, mogamulizumab with chemotherapy had a higher response rate (86% ORR, 52% CR) than chemotherapy alone (75% ORR, 33% CR).[657] Daclizumab, an antibody against CD25, the 55-kDa α chain of the IL-2 receptor, has had limited responses in chronic and smoldering forms.[658] Alemtuzumab (Campath) is directed at CD52 and had a 52% ORR (21% CR) of short duration (2-month PFS and 5.9-month OS).[659] There may be a role for the antibody-drug conjugate, BV, for the minority of ATL cases that are CD30 positive.

Allogeneic HCT was first reported as a curative option in ATL in 1996. Although the median survival of 9.9 to 10.5 months with allo HCT has not been shown to be superior to other therapy, the 3-year PFS of 20% to 30% and OS of 30% to 41% suggests HCT may offer the best chance for long-term survival.[660,661] There has been no difference in survival between myeloablative and reduced intensity conditioning regimens. GVHD and survival may be worse in patients who previously received mogamulizumab.[661]

Therapy for T/NK Neoplasms

Although CHOP has been the mainstay of therapy for aggressive lymphomas, its results have been poor for most mature T/NK neoplasms.[662] The response rates to CHOP have been inferior compared to B-cell lymphomas, and there has been no ubiquitous monoclonal antibody similar to rituximab to improve survival with the exception of BV in a subset. Adding etoposide to CHOP had modest improvement for only young patients, primarily with ALK-positive ALCL, in the combined analysis of trials by the German High-Grade Non-Hodgkin Lymphoma Study Group.[663] Escalating therapy, such as Mega-CHOEP or hyper-CVAD, has not improved responses or survival.[663] The addition of alemtuzumab to CHOP led to increased infections so that its use is likely limited.[664] Bevacizumab with CHOP was associated with congestive heart failure.[665] BV can be effective in CD30+ PTCL (see section "Anaplastic Large Cell Lymphoma").[576,577]

Despite the advances in the treatment of CD30+ aggressive TCLs with the incorporation of brentuximab, overall other attempts of incorporating newer agents in the frontline have not been successful. In phase II clinical trials of the HDACi romidepsin, response rates of 25% and 38% (CR 15% and 18%) were reported with 8% to 19% fatigue and 20% to 47% grade 3/4 neutropenia.[666,667] The updated data from the pivotal phase 2 study of romidepsin (n = 131) reported an ORR of 33% in the AITL cohort (n = 27), 6 patients achieved CR. Duration of response exceeded a year in 5 of the 9 patients with overall response. The rapidity, depth, and duration of response in AITL have led to its exploration in combinations for AITL and other TfH subtypes of TCL.[668] The pathophysiology of this increased sensitivity in these subtypes is thought to be related to frequent mutations involving *DNMT3A*, *TET2*, *IDH2*, and *RhoA* in AITL.[669,670] Leveraging the sensitivity of PTCLs to epigenetic modifiers, a combination of romidepsin with hypomethylating agent oral azacytidine was evaluated in R/R PTCL.[671] The ORR and CR rates across PTCL subtypes (n = 25) were 61% and 48%, respectively. The corresponding response rates in TfH subtypes were 80% and 67%, respectively. The most common grade 3/4 side effects were cytopenias (NCT01998035). Belinostat, a pan HDACi, had a 26% response (11% CR) and 6% to 11% cytopenias.[672] In a phase Ib/II study, romidepsin with CHOP (Ro-CHOP) had a 51% CR rate and a 30-month PFS of 41% and OS of 71%.[673] However, a recent phase III RCT evaluated Ro-CHOP vs CHOP in frontline therapy of PTCL. The addition of romidepsin to CHOP was associated with increased toxicity without an improvement of PFS, OS, or response rates.[674]

The response rate and toxicities in relapsed PTCL for the folate antagonist pralatrexate was 29% (11% CR) with 22% mucositis and 18% to 32% cytopenias.[675] A phase II trial of cyclophosphamide, etoposide, vincristine, and prednisone alternating with pralatrexate as initial therapy in PTCL had a 52% CR, a 2-year PFS of 39%, and OS of 60%, but the results were not considered superior to historical reports with CHOP.[676]

Gemcitabine has been combined with multiple agents, including a trial with cisplatin, etoposide, and methylprednisolone (PEGS) that resulted in an ORR of only 39% with 2-year PFS of 12% and OS of 30% for de novo and relapsed patients.[677] Another regimen with gemcitabine, ifosfamide, and oxaliplatin (GIFOX) for upfront patients had an 82% ORR (65% CR) and a 5-year PFS of 48% that included some patients who went to autologous HCT.[678] In relapsed PTCL, bendamustine had an ORR of 50% (28% CR) and a median PFS and OS of 3.6 and 6.2 months, respectively.[679] A recent large retrospective multicenter cohort study (n = 82) reported ORR and CR rates of 71% and 51%, respectively.[680] With a median follow-up of 9 months, the median PFS and OS were 8.3 and 26.3 months respectively. Bortezomib had a 67% ORR (17% CR) in CTCL and has been used in phase II trials for frontline PTCL with CHOP (76% ORR [65% CR] and 3-year PFS of 35% and OS of 47%) and with gemcitabine for relapsed PTCL (36% ORR [27% CR]).[681,682] The IMiD lenalidomide and the mTORi everolimus showed an ORR of 22% to 39% and 44%, respectively, in relapsed PTCL.[683,684]

Additional targets in PTCL include aurora A kinase, phosphoinositide-3-kinase (PI3K), isocitrate dehydrogenase (IDH2), NF-κB, JAK/STAT, and FYN tyrosine kinase.[685] Alisertib, an aurora A kinase inhibitor, demonstrated an ORR of 30% with a median PFS of 3 months and OS of 8 months.[686] In a phase III trial comparing alisertib to investigator's choice (pralatrexate, romidepsin, and gemcitabine) found no differences in response rates.[687] Duvelisib, an oral inhibitor of PI3 kinases, had an ORR of 47% (13% CR) and median OS of 9 months.[688] AG-221, an inhibitor of *IDH2*, is in a trial for AITL (NCT02273739). Because both *IDH2* and *TET2* mutations promote hypermethylation, there is a rationale for combining IDH2 inhibitors with hypomethylating agents for patients with AITL.

Because PTCLs are relatively chemoresistant, many centers advocate early transplantation for subtypes other than ALK+ ALCL. Prospective trials utilizing auto-HCT as upfront therapy in PTCL have reported a 5-year PFS and OS of 39% to 44% and 44% to 51%, respectively.[689,690] A randomized trial comparing auto-HCT to allo HCT was stopped early due to an interim analysis showing no difference; 38% of randomized patients did not proceed to HCT mainly due to progressive disease, again highlighting the problem of refractoriness in PTCL.[691]

References

1. Swerdlow SH, Campo E, Pileri SA, et al. The 2016 revision of the World Health Organization classification of lymphoid neoplasms. *Blood*. 2016;127(20):2375-2390.
2. Gall EA, Mallory TB. Malignant lymphoma: a clinico-pathologic survey of 618 cases. *Am J Pathol*. 1942;18(3):381-429.
3. Hicks EB, Rappaport H, Winter WJ. Follicular lymphoma; a re-evaluation of its position in the scheme of malignant lymphoma, based on a survey of 253 cases. *Cancer*. 1956;9(4):792-821.
4. Robb-Smith AHT, Taylor C. *Lymph Node Biopsy*. Oxford University Press; 1981.
5. Aisenberg AC, Bloch KJ. Immunoglobulins on the surface of neoplastic lymphocytes. *N Engl J Med*. 1972;287(6):272-276.
6. Smith JL, Clein GP, Barker CR, Collins RD. Characterisation of malignant mediastinal lymphoid neoplasm (Sternberg sarcoma) as thymic in origin. *Lancet*. 1973;1(7794):74-77.
7. Nathwani BN, Diamond LW, Winberg CD, et al. Lymphoblastic lymphoma: a clinicopathologic study of 95 patients. *Cancer*. 1981;48(11):2347-2357.
8. Lukes RJ, Collins RD. Immunologic characterization of human malignant lymphomas. *Cancer*. 1974;34(4 suppl):1488-1503.
9. Zech L, Haglund U, Nilsson K, Klein G. Characteristic chromosomal abnormalities in biopsies and lymphoid-cell lines from patients with Burkitt and non-Burkitt lymphomas. *Int J Cancer*. 1976;17(1):47-56.
10. Fukuhara S, Ueshima Y, Shirakawa S, Uchino H, Morikawa S. 14q translocations, having a break point at 14q13, in lymphoid malignancy. *Int J Cancer*. 1979;24(6):739-743.
11. Korsmeyer SJ, Hieter PA, Ravetch JV, Poplack DG, Waldmann TA, Leder P. Developmental hierarchy of immunoglobulin gene rearrangements in human leukemic pre-B-cells. *Proc Natl Acad Sci U S A*. 1981;78(11):7096-7100.
12. Waldmann TA, Davis MM, Bongiovanni KF, Korsmeyer SJ. Rearrangements of genes for the antigen receptor on T cells as markers of lineage and clonality in human lymphoid neoplasms. *N Engl J Med*. 1985;313(13):776-783.
13. Dalla-Favera R, Bregni M, Erikson J, Patterson D, Gallo RC, Croce CM. Human c-myc onc gene is located on the region of chromosome 8 that is translocated in Burkitt lymphoma cells. *Proc Natl Acad Sci U S A*. 1982;79(24):7824-7827.
14. Tsujimoto Y, Cossman J, Jaffe E, Croce CM. Involvement of the bcl-2 gene in human follicular lymphoma. *Science*. 1985;228(4706):1440-1443.
15. Tsujimoto Y, Yunis J, Onorato-Showe L, Erikson J, Nowell PC, Croce CM. Molecular cloning of the chromosomal breakpoint of B-cell lymphomas and leukemias with the t(11;14) chromosome translocation. *Science*. 1984;224(4656):1403-1406.

16. Kaneko Y, Frizzera G, Edamura S, et al. A novel translocation, t(2;5)(p23;q35), in childhood phagocytic large T-cell lymphoma mimicking malignant histiocytosis. *Blood.* 1989;73(3):806-813.
17. Morris SW, Kirstein MN, Valentine MB, et al. Fusion of a kinase gene, ALK, to a nucleolar protein gene, NPM, in non-Hodgkin's lymphoma. *Science.* 1994;263(5151):1281-1284.
18. Jaffe ES, Harris NL, Stein H, Isaacson PG. Classification of lymphoid neoplasms: the microscope as a tool for disease discovery. *Blood.* 2008;112(12):4384-4399.
19. Harris NL, Jaffe ES, Stein H, et al. A revised European-American classification of lymphoid neoplasms: a proposal from the International Lymphoma Study Group. *Blood.* 1994;84(5):1361-1392.
20. A clinical evaluation of the international lymphoma study group classification of non-hodgkin's lymphoma. The non-hodgkin's lymphoma classification project. *Blood.* 1997;89(11):3909-3918.
21. Swerdlow S, Campo E, Harris N, et al. *WHO Classification of Tumours of Haematopoietic and Lymphoid Tissues*. IARC Press; 2017.
22. Howlader N, Shiels MS, Mariotto AB, Engels EA. Contributions of HIV to non-Hodgkin lymphoma mortality trends in the United States. *Cancer Epidemiol Biomarkers Prev.* 2016;25(9):1289-1296.
23. Gurney KA, Cartwright RA. Increasing incidence and descriptive epidemiology of extranodal non-Hodgkin lymphoma in parts of England and Wales. *Hematol J.* 2002;3(2):95-104.
24. Groves FD, Linet MS, Travis LB, Devesa SS. Cancer surveillance series: non-Hodgkin's lymphoma incidence by histologic subtype in the United States from 1978 through 1995. *J Natl Cancer Inst.* 2000;92(15):1240-1251.
25. Olson JE, Janney CA, Rao RD, et al. The continuing increase in the incidence of primary central nervous system non-Hodgkin lymphoma: a surveillance, epidemiology, and end results analysis. *Cancer.* 2002;95(7):1504-1510.
26. O'Neill BP, Decker PA, Tieu C, Cerhan JR. The changing incidence of primary central nervous system lymphoma is driven primarily by the changing incidence in young and middle-aged men and differs from time trends in systemic diffuse large B-cell non-Hodgkin's lymphoma. *Am J Hematol.* 2013;88(12):997-1000.
27. Paltiel O, Schmit T, Adler B, et al. The incidence of lymphoma in first-degree relatives of patients with Hodgkin disease and non-Hodgkin lymphoma: results and limitations of a registry-linked study. *Cancer.* 2000;88(10):2357-2366.
28. Cerhan JR, Slager SL. Familial predisposition and genetic risk factors for lymphoma. *Blood.* 2015;126(20):2265-2273.
29. Mack TM, Cozen W, Shibata DK, et al. Concordance for Hodgkin's disease in identical twins suggesting genetic susceptibility to the young-adult form of the disease. *N Engl J Med.* 1995;332(7):413-418.
30. Wang SS, Slager SL, Brennan P, et al. Family history of hematopoietic malignancies and risk of non-Hodgkin lymphoma (NHL): a pooled analysis of 10211 cases and 11905 controls from the International Lymphoma Epidemiology Consortium (InterLymph). *Blood.* 2007;109(8):3479-3488.
31. Wiernik PH, Wang SQ, Hu XP, Marino P, Paietta E. Age of onset evidence for anticipation in familial non-Hodgkin's lymphoma. *Br J Haematol.* 2000;108(1):72-79.
32. Daugherty SE, Pfeiffer RM, Mellemkjaer L, Hemminki K, Goldin LR. No evidence for anticipation in lymphoproliferative tumors in population-based samples. *Cancer Epidemiol Biomarkers Prev.* 2005;14(5):1245-1250.
33. Smedby KE, Foo JN, Skibola CF, et al. GWAS of follicular lymphoma reveals allelic heterogeneity at 6p21.32 and suggests shared genetic susceptibility with diffuse large B-cell lymphoma. *PLoS Genet.* 2011;7(4):e1001378.
34. Matson DR, Yang DT. Autoimmune lymphoproliferative syndrome: an Overview. *Arch Pathol Lab Med.* 2020;144(2):245-251.
35. Li P, Huang P, Yang Y, Hao M, Peng H, Li F. Updated understanding of autoimmune lymphoproliferative syndrome (ALPS). *Clin Rev Allergy Immunol.* 2016;50(1):55-63.
36. Neven B, Magerus-Chatinet A, Florkin B, et al. A survey of 90 patients with autoimmune lymphoproliferative syndrome related to TNFRSF6 mutation. *Blood.* 2011;118(18):4798-4807.
37. Volkl S, Rensing-Ehl A, Allgauer A, et al. Hyperactive mTOR pathway promotes lymphoproliferation and abnormal differentiation in autoimmune lymphoproliferative syndrome. *Blood.* 2016;128(2):227-238.
38. Bernstein L, Ross RK. Prior medication use and health history as risk factors for non-Hodgkin's lymphoma: preliminary results from a case-control study in Los Angeles County. *Cancer Res.* 1992;52(19 Suppl):5510s-5515s.
39. Chatterjee N, Hartge P, Cerhan JR, et al. Risk of non-Hodgkin's lymphoma and family history of lymphatic, hematologic, and other cancers. *Cancer Epidemiol Biomarkers Prev.* 2004;13(9):1415-1421.
40. Linet MS, Pottern LM. Familial aggregation of hematopoietic malignancies and risk of non-Hodgkin's lymphoma. *Cancer Res.* 1992;52(19 Suppl):5468s-5473s.
41. Joelsson JK, Wasterlid T, Rosenquist R, et al. Incidence and time trends of second primary malignancies after non-Hodgkin lymphoma: a Swedish population-based study. *Blood Adv.* 2022;6(8):2657-2666.
42. Walusansa V, Okuku F, Orem J. Burkitt lymphoma in Uganda, the legacy of Denis Burkitt and an update on the disease status. *Br J Haematol.* 2012;156(6):757-760.
43. Epstein M, Achong B. *The Epstein-Barr Virus*. Springer; 1979:1-22. Introduction: discovery and general biology of the virus.
44. Burkitt D, Hutt MS, Wright DH. The African lymphoma: preliminary observations on response to therapy. *Cancer.* 1965;18:399-410.
45. Magrath I. Epidemiology: clues to the pathogenesis of Burkitt lymphoma. *Br J Haematol.* 2012;156(6):744-756.
46. Uchiyama T, Yodoi J, Sagawa K, Takatsuki K, Uchino H. Adult T-cell leukemia: clinical and hematologic features of 16 cases. *Blood.* 1977;50(3):481-492.
47. Poiesz BJ, Ruscetti FW, Gazdar AF, Bunn PA, Minna JD, Gallo RC. Detection and isolation of type C retrovirus particles from fresh and cultured lymphocytes of a patient with cutaneous T-cell lymphoma. *Proc Natl Acad Sci U S A.* 1980;77(12):7415-7419.
48. Yoshida M, Miyoshi I, Hinuma Y. Isolation and characterization of retrovirus from cell lines of human adult T-cell leukemia and its implication in the disease. *Proc Natl Acad Sci U S A.* 1982;79(6):2031-2035.
49. Gessain A, Cassar O. Epidemiological aspects and world distribution of HTLV-1 infection. *Front Microbiol.* 2012;3:388.
50. Panfil AR, Martinez MP, Ratner L, Green PL. Human T-cell leukemia virus-associated malignancy. *Curr Opin Virol.* 2016;20:40-46.
51. Taylor GP, Matsuoka M. Natural history of adult T-cell leukemia/lymphoma and approaches to therapy. *Oncogene.* 2005;24(39):6047-6057.
52. Fukuda RI, Tsuchiya K, Suzuki K, et al. HTLV-I Tax regulates the cellular proliferation through the down-regulation of PIP3-phosphatase expressions via the NF-κB pathway. *Int J Biochem Mol Biol.* 2012;3(1):95-104.
53. Zhao T, Matsuoka M. HBZ and its roles in HTLV-1 oncogenesis. *Front Microbiol.* 2012;3:247.
54. Goncalves DU, Proietti FA, Ribas JGR, et al. Epidemiology, treatment, and prevention of human T-cell leukemia virus type 1-associated diseases. *Clin Microbiol Rev.* 2010;23(3):577-589.
55. Rowan AG, Dillon R, Witkover A, et al. Evolution of retrovirus-infected premalignant T-cell clones prior to adult T-cell leukemia/lymphoma diagnosis. *Blood.* 2020;135(23):2023-2032.
56. Iwanaga M. Epidemiology of HTLV-1 infection and ATL in Japan: an update. *Front Microbiol.* 2020;11:1124.
57. Ito S, Iwanaga M, Nosaka K, et al. Epidemiology of adult T-cell leukemia-lymphoma in Japan: an updated analysis, 2012-2013. *Cancer Sci.* 2021;112(10):4346-4354.
58. Hisada M, Stuver SO, Okayama A, et al. Persistent paradox of natural history of human T lymphotropic virus type I: parallel analyses of Japanese and Jamaican carriers. *J Infect Dis.* 2004;190(9):1605-1609.
59. Oliveira PD, de Carvalho RF, Bittencourt AL. Adult T-cell leukemia/lymphoma in South and Central America and the Caribbean: systematic search and review. *Int J STD AIDS.* 2017;28(3):217-228.
60. Kalyanaraman VS, Sarngadharan MG, Robert-Guroff M, Miyoshi I, Golde D, Gallo RC. A new subtype of human T-cell leukemia virus (HTLV-II) associated with a T-cell variant of hairy cell leukemia. *Science.* 1982;218(4572):571-573.
61. Martinez MP, Al-Saleem J, Green PL. Comparative virology of HTLV-1 and HTLV-2. *Retrovirology.* 2019;16(1):21.
62. Paiva A, Casseb J. Origin and prevalence of human T-lymphotropic virus type 1 (HTLV-1) and type 2 (HTLV-2) among indigenous populations in the Americas. *Rev Inst Med Trop Sao Paulo.* 2015;57(1):1-13.
63. Mahieux R, Gessain A. The human HTLV-3 and HTLV-4 retroviruses: new members of the HTLV family. *Pathol Biol.* 2009;57(2):161-166.
64. Salahuddin SZ, Ablashi DV, Markham PD, et al. Isolation of a new virus, HBLV, in patients with lymphoproliferative disorders. *Science.* 1986;234(4776):596-601.
65. Yamanishi K, Okuno T, Shiraki K, et al. Identification of human herpesvirus-6 as a causal agent for exanthem subitum. *Lancet.* 1988;1(8594):1065-1067.
66. Oksenhendler E, Boulanger E, Galicier L, et al. High incidence of Kaposi sarcoma-associated herpesvirus-related non-Hodgkin lymphoma in patients with HIV infection and multicentric Castleman disease. *Blood.* 2002;99(7):2331-2336.
67. Cesarman E, Chang Y, Moore PS, Said JW, Knowles DM. Kaposi's sarcoma-associated herpesvirus-like DNA sequences in AIDS-related body-cavity-based lymphomas. *N Engl J Med.* 1995;332(18):1186-1191.
68. Lai YR, Chang YL, Lee CH, Tsai TH, Huang KH, Lee CY. Risk of non-hodgkin lymphoma among patients with hepatitis B virus and hepatitis C virus in Taiwan: a Nationwide Cohort Study. *Cancers.* 2022;14(3):583.
69. Dalia S, Chavez J, Castillo JJ, Sokol L. Hepatitis B infection increases the risk of non-Hodgkin lymphoma: a meta-analysis of observational studies. *Leuk Res.* 2013;37(9):1107-1115.
70. Kusumoto S, Arcaini L, Hong X, et al. Risk of HBV reactivation in patients with B-cell lymphomas receiving obinutuzumab or rituximab immunochemotherapy. *Blood.* 2019;133(2):137-146.
71. Cao X, Wang Y, Li P, Huang W, Lu X, Lu H. HBV reactivation during the treatment of non-Hodgkin lymphoma and management strategies. *Front Oncol.* 2021;11:685706.
72. Duberg AS, Nordstrom M, Torner A, et al. Non-Hodgkin's lymphoma and other nonhepatic malignancies in Swedish patients with hepatitis C virus infection. *Hepatology.* 2005;41(3):652-659.
73. Tasleem S, Sood GK. Hepatitis C associated B-cell non-Hodgkin lymphoma: clinical features and the role of antiviral therapy. *J Clin Transl Hepatol.* 2015;3(2):134-139.
74. Peveling-Oberhag J, Arcaini L, Hansmann ML, Zeuzem S. Hepatitis C-associated B-cell non-Hodgkin lymphomas. Epidemiology, molecular signature and clinical management. *J Hepatol.* 2013;59(1):169-177.
75. Zhang M, Gao F, Peng L, et al. Distinct clinical features and prognostic factors of hepatitis C virus-associated non-Hodgkin's lymphoma: a systematic review and meta-analysis. *Cancer Cell Int.* 2021;21(1):524.
76. Pellicelli A, Giannelli V, Zoli V, et al. Resolution of primary hepatic marginal zone lymphoma in a hepatitis C virus-infected patient treated with a direct-acting antiviral. *Oxf Med Case Reports.* 2021;2021(5):omab022.
77. Frigeni M, Besson C, Visco C, et al. Interferon-free compared to interferon-based antiviral regimens as first-line therapy for B-cell lymphoproliferative disorders associated with hepatitis C virus infection. *Leukemia.* 2020;34(5):1462-1466.
78. Merli M, Frigeni M, Alric L, et al. Direct-acting antivirals in hepatitis C virus-associated diffuse large B-cell lymphomas. *Oncol.* 2019;24(8):e720-e729.
79. Marshall BJ, Warren JR. Unidentified curved bacilli in the stomach of patients with gastritis and peptic ulceration. *Lancet.* 1984;1(8390):1311-1315.
80. Isaacson P, Wright DH. Malignant lymphoma of mucosa-associated lymphoid tissue. A distinctive type of B-cell lymphoma. *Cancer.* 1983;52(8):1410-1416.
81. Parsonnet J, Hansen S, Rodriguez L, et al. Helicobacter pylori infection and gastric lymphoma. *N Engl J Med.* 1994;330(18):1267-1271.

82. Wotherspoon AC, Doglioni C, Diss TC, et al. Regression of primary low-grade B-cell gastric lymphoma of mucosa-associated lymphoid tissue type after eradication of Helicobacter pylori. *Lancet.* 1993;342(8871):575-577.
83. Kuo SH, Yeh KH, Wu MS, et al. Helicobacter pylori eradication therapy is effective in the treatment of early-stage H pylori-positive gastric diffuse large B-cell lymphomas. *Blood.* 2012;119(21):4838-4844, quiz 5057.
84. Vladut C, Ciocirlan M, Costache RS, et al. Is mucosa-associated lymphoid tissue lymphoma an infectious disease? Role of *Helicobacter pylori* and eradication antibiotic therapy (Review). *Exp Ther Med.* 2020;20(4):3546-3553.
85. Hamoudi RA, Appert A, Ye H, et al. Differential expression of NF-kappaB target genes in MALT lymphoma with and without chromosome translocation: insights into molecular mechanism. *Leukemia.* 2010;24(8):1487-1497.
86. Wang HP, Zhu YL, Shao W. Role of Helicobacter pylori virulence factor cytotoxin-associated gene A in gastric mucosa-associated lymphoid tissue lymphoma. *World J Gastroenterol.* 2013;19(45):8219-8226.
87. Pereira MI, Medeiros JA. Role of *Helicobacter pylori* in gastric mucosa-associated lymphoid tissue lymphomas. *World J Gastroenterol.* 2014;20(3):684-698.
88. Starostik P, Patzner J, Greiner A, et al. Gastric marginal zone B-cell lymphomas of MALT type develop along 2 distinct pathogenetic pathways. *Blood.* 2002;99(1):3-9.
89. Owens SR, Smith LB. Molecular aspects of H. pylori-related MALT lymphoma. *Patholog Res Int.* 2011;2011:193149.
90. Zucca E, Bertoni F. The spectrum of MALT lymphoma at different sites: biological and therapeutic relevance. *Blood.* 2016;127(17):2082-2092.
91. Thandra KC, Barsouk A, Saginala K, Padala SA, Barsouk A, Rawla P. Epidemiology of non-Hodgkin's lymphoma. *Med Sci (Basel).* 2021;9(1):5.
92. Chihara D, Nastoupil LJ, Williams JN, Lee P, Koff JL, Flowers CR. New insights into the epidemiology of non-Hodgkin lymphoma and implications for therapy. *Expert Rev Anticancer Ther.* 2015;15(5):531-544.
93. Abbondazo SL, Irey NS, Frizzera G. Dilantin-associated lymphadenopathy. Spectrum of histopathologic patterns. *Am J Surg Pathol.* 1995;19(6):675-686.
94. Magro CM, Daniels BH, Crowson AN. Drug induced pseudolymphoma. *Semin Diagn Pathol.* 2018;35(4):247-259.
95. Calip GS, Patel PR, Adimadhyam S, et al. Tumor necrosis factor-alpha inhibitors and risk of non-Hodgkin lymphoma in a cohort of adults with rheumatologic conditions. *Int J Cancer.* 2018;143(5):1062-1071.
96. Hellgren K, Di Giuseppe D, Smedby KE, et al. Lymphoma risks in patients with rheumatoid arthritis treated with biological drugs-a Swedish cohort study of risks by time, drug and lymphoma subtype. *Rheumatology.* 2021;60(2):809-819.
97. Rasmussen MLH, Hjalgrim H, Molgaard-Nielsen D, Wohlfahrt J, Melbye M. Antibiotic use and risk of non-Hodgkin lymphomas. *Int J Cancer.* 2012;131(7):E1158-E1165.
98. Norgaard M, Poulsen AH, Pedersen L, et al. Use of postmenopausal hormone replacement therapy and risk of non-Hodgkin's lymphoma: a Danish Population-based Cohort Study. *Br J Cancer.* 2006;94(9):1339-1341.
99. Desai P, Wallace R, Anderson ML, et al. An analysis of the effect of statins on the risk of Non-Hodgkin's Lymphoma in the Women's Health Initiative cohort. *Cancer Med.* 2018;7(5):2121-2130.
100. Bassig BA, Lan Q, Rothman N, Zhang Y, Zheng T. Current understanding of lifestyle and environmental factors and risk of non-Hodgkin lymphoma: an epidemiological update. *J Cancer Epidemiol.* 2012;2012:978930.
101. Zhang L, Rana I, Shaffer RM, Taioli E, Sheppard L. Exposure to glyphosate-based herbicides and risk for non-Hodgkin lymphoma: a meta-analysis and supporting evidence. *Mutat Res Rev Mutat Res.* 2019;781:186-206.
102. Kachuri L, Beane Freeman LE, Spinelli JJ, et al. Insecticide use and risk of non-Hodgkin lymphoma subtypes: a subset meta-analysis of the North American Pooled Project. *Int J Cancer.* 2020;147(12):3370-3383.
103. Rêgo MAV, Sousa CSC, Kato M, de Carvalho AB, Loomis D, Carvalho FM. Non-Hodgkin's lymphomas and organic solvents. *J Occup Environ Med.* 2002;44(9):874-881.
104. Cocco P, Satta G, Meloni F, et al. Occupational exposure to organic dust and risk of lymphoma subtypes in the EPILYMPH case-control study. *Scand J Work Environ Health.* 2021;47(1):42-51.
105. Zhang Y, Birmann BM, Han J, et al. Personal use of permanent hair dyes and cancer risk and mortality in US women: prospective cohort study. *Br Med J.* 2020;370:m2942.
106. Kricker A, Armstrong BK, Hughes AM, et al. Personal sun exposure and risk of non Hodgkin lymphoma: a pooled analysis from the Interlymph Consortium. *Int J Cancer.* 2008;122(1):144-154.
107. Kim HB, Kim JH. Sunlight exposure in association with risk of lymphoid malignancy: a meta-analysis of observational studies. *Cancer Causes Control.* 2021;32(5):441-457.
108. Park HY, Hong YC, Lee K, Koh J. Vitamin D status and risk of non-Hodgkin lymphoma: an updated meta-analysis. *PLoS One.* 2019;14(4):e0216284.
109. Drake MT, Maurer MJ, Link BK, et al. Vitamin D insufficiency and prognosis in non-Hodgkin's lymphoma. *J Clin Oncol.* 2010;28(27):4191-4198.
110. Hohaus S, Tisi MC, Bellesi S, et al. Vitamin D deficiency and supplementation in patients with aggressive B-cell lymphomas treated with immunochemotherapy. *Cancer Med.* 2018;7(1):270-281.
111. Cross AJ, Lim U. The role of dietary factors in the epidemiology of non-Hodgkin's lymphoma. *Leuk Lymphoma.* 2006;47(12):2477-2487.
112. Han TJ, Li JS, Luan XT, Wang L, Xu HZ. Dietary fat consumption and non-Hodgkin's lymphoma risk: a meta-analysis. *Nutr Cancer.* 2017;69(2):221-228.
113. Bertrand KA, Giovannucci E, Rosner BA, Zhang SM, Laden F, Birmann BM. Dietary fat intake and risk of non-Hodgkin lymphoma in 2 large prospective cohorts. *Am J Clin Nutr.* 2017;106(2):650-656.
114. Solans M, Benavente Y, Saez M, et al. Inflammatory potential of diet and risk of lymphoma in the European Prospective Investigation into Cancer and Nutrition. *Eur J Nutr.* 2020;59(2):813-823.
115. Chiu BC, Cerhan JR, Folsom AR, et al. Diet and risk of non-Hodgkin lymphoma in older women. *J Am Med Assoc.* 1996;275(17):1315-1321.
116. Chiu BCH, Kwon S, Evens AM, Surawicz T, Smith SM, Weisenburger DD. Dietary intake of fruit and vegetables and risk of non-Hodgkin lymphoma. *Cancer Causes Control.* 2011;22(8):1183-1195.
117. Kelemen LE, Cerhan JR, Lim U, et al. Vegetables, fruit, and antioxidant-related nutrients and risk of non-Hodgkin lymphoma: a National Cancer Institute-Surveillance, Epidemiology, and End Results population-based case-control study. *Am J Clin Nutr.* 2006;83(6):1401-1410.
118. Wang J, Li X, Zhang D. Dairy product consumption and risk of non-Hodgkin lymphoma: a meta-analysis. *Nutrients.* 2016;8(3):120.
119. Abar L, Sobiecki JG, Cariolou M, et al. Body size and obesity during adulthood, and risk of lympho-haematopoietic cancers: an update of the WCRF-AICR systematic review of published prospective studies. *Ann Oncol.* 2019;30(4):528-541.
120. Etter JL, Cannioto R, Soh KT, et al. Lifetime physical inactivity is associated with increased risk for Hodgkin and non-Hodgkin lymphoma: a case-control study. *Leuk Res.* 2018;69:7-11.
121. Mirtavoos-Mahyari H, Salehipour P, Parohan M, Sadeghi A. Effects of coffee, black tea and green tea consumption on the risk of non-Hodgkin's lymphoma: a systematic review and dose-response meta-analysis of observational studies. *Nutr Cancer.* 2019;71(6):887-897.
122. Castillo JJ, Dalia S, Pascual SK. Association between red blood cell transfusions and development of non-Hodgkin lymphoma: a meta-analysis of observational studies. *Blood.* 2010;116(16):2897-2907.
123. Cerhan JR, Kane E, Vajdic CM, et al. Blood transfusion history and risk of non-Hodgkin lymphoma: an InterLymph pooled analysis. *Cancer Causes Control.* 2019;30(8):889-900.
124. Yang TO, Cairns BJ, Reeves GK, Green J, Beral V; Million Women Study collaborators. Cancer risk among 21st century blood transfusion recipients. *Ann Oncol.* 2017;28(2):393-399.
125. Kim CJ, Freedman DM, Curtis RE, Berrington de Gonzalez A, Morton LM. Risk of non-Hodgkin lymphoma after radiotherapy for solid cancers. *Leuk Lymphoma.* 2013;54(8):1691-1697.
126. Shimizu Y, Schull WJ, Kato H. Cancer risk among atomic bomb survivors. The RERF life span study. Radiation effects Research Foundation. *J Am Med Assoc.* 1990;264(5):601-604.
127. Fujihara M, Sakata R, Yoshida N, Ozasa K, Preston DL, Mabuchi K. Incidence of lymphoid neoplasms among atomic bomb survivors by histological subtype, 1950 to 1994. *Blood.* 2022;139(2):217-227.
128. Morton LM, Hartge P, Holford TR, et al. Cigarette smoking and risk of non-Hodgkin lymphoma: a pooled analysis from the International Lymphoma Epidemiology Consortium (interlymph). *Cancer Epidemiol Biomarkers Prev.* 2005;14(4):925-933.
129. Pai SY, Lurain K, Yarchoan R. How immunodeficiency can lead to malignancy. *Hematology Am Soc Hematol Educ Program.* 2021;2021(1):287-295.
130. Grierson H, Purtilo DT. Epstein-Barr virus infections in males with the X-linked lymphoproliferative syndrome. *Ann Intern Med.* 1987;106(4):538-545.
131. Panchal N, Booth C, Cannons JL, Schwartzberg PL. X-linked lymphoproliferative disease type 1: a clinical and molecular perspective. *Front Immunol.* 2018;9:666.
132. Krikorian JG, Anderson JL, Bieber CP, Penn I, Stinson EB. Malignant neoplasms following cardiac transplantation. *J Am Med Assoc.* 1978;240(7):639-643.
133. Dharnidharka VR. Comprehensive review of post-organ transplant hematologic cancers. *Am J Transplant.* 2018;18(3):537-549.
134. Doll DC, List AF. Burkitt's lymphoma in a homosexual. *Lancet.* 1982;1(8279):1026-1027.
135. Ziegler JL, Beckstead JA, Volberding PA, et al. Non-Hodgkin's lymphoma in 90 homosexual men. Relation to generalized lymphadenopathy and the acquired immunodeficiency syndrome. *N Engl J Med.* 1984;311(9):565-570.
136. Bilezikian JP. Surgery or no surgery for primary hyperparathyroidism. *Ann Intern Med.* 1985;102(3):402-403.
137. Noy A. Optimizing treatment of HIV-associated lymphoma. *Blood.* 2019;134(17):1385-1394.
138. Carbone A, Vaccher E, Gloghini A. Hematologic cancers in individuals infected by HIV. *Blood.* 2022;139(7):995-1012.
139. Achenbach CJ, Buchanan AL, Cole SR, et al. HIV viremia and incidence of non-Hodgkin lymphoma in patients successfully treated with antiretroviral therapy. *Clin Infect Dis.* 2014;58(11):1599-1606.
140. Wang Q, De Luca A, Smith C, et al. Chronic hepatitis B and C virus infection and risk for non-Hodgkin lymphoma in HIV-infected patients: a cohort study. *Ann Intern Med.* 2017;166(1):9-17.
141. Hernandez-Ramirez RU, Shiels MS, Dubrow R, Engels EA. Cancer risk in HIV-infected people in the USA from 1996 to 2012: a population-based, registry-linkage study. *Lancet HIV.* 2017;4(11):e495-e504.
142. Barta SK, Samuel MS, Xue X, et al. Changes in the influence of lymphoma- and HIV-specific factors on outcomes in AIDS-related non-Hodgkin lymphoma. *Ann Oncol.* 2015;26(5):958-966.
143. Ekstrom Smedby K, Vajdic CM, Falster M, et al. Autoimmune disorders and risk of non-Hodgkin lymphoma subtypes: a pooled analysis within the InterLymph Consortium. *Blood.* 2008;111(8):4029-4038.
144. Franks AL, Slansky JE. Multiple associations between a broad spectrum of autoimmune diseases, chronic inflammatory diseases and cancer. *Anticancer Res.* 2012;32(4):1119-1136.
145. Din L, Sheikh M, Kosaraju N, et al. Genetic overlap between autoimmune diseases and non-Hodgkin lymphoma subtypes. *Genet Epidemiol.* 2019;43(7):844-863.
146. Isaacson PG. Lymphomas of mucosa-associated lymphoid tissue (MALT). *Histopathology.* 1990;16(6):617-619.

147. Talal N, Bunim JJ. The development of malignant lymphoma in the course of Sjoegren's syndrome. *Am J Med*. 1964;36:529-540.
148. Kassan SS, Thomas TL, Moutsopoulos HM, et al. Increased risk of lymphoma in Sicca syndrome. *Ann Intern Med*. 1978;89(6):888-892.
149. Voulgarelis M, Ziakas PD, Papageorgiou A, Baimpa E, Tzioufas AG, Moutsopoulos HM. Prognosis and outcome of non-Hodgkin lymphoma in primary Sjogren syndrome. *Medicine (Baltimore)*. 2012;91(1):1-9.
150. Kroese FGM, Haacke EA, Bombardieri M. The role of salivary gland histopathology in primary Sjögren's syndrome: promises and pitfalls. *Clin Exp Rheumatol*. 2018;6(3):222-233.
151. Fishleder A, Tubbs R, Hesse B, Levine H. Uniform detection of immunoglobulin-gene rearrangement in benign lymphoepithelial lesions. *N Engl J Med*. 1987;316(18):1118-1121.
152. Theander E, Vasaitis L, Baecklund E, et al. Lymphoid organisation in labial salivary gland biopsies is a possible predictor for the development of malignant lymphoma in primary Sjögren's syndrome. *Ann Rheum Dis*. 2011;70(8):1363-1368.
153. Alunno A, Leone MC, Giacomelli R, Gerli R, Carubbi F. Lymphoma and lymphomagenesis in primary Sjögren's syndrome. *Front Med*. 2018;5:102.
154. Groom J, Kalled SL, Cutler AH, et al. Association of BAFF/BLyS overexpression and altered B cell differentiation with Sjogren's syndrome. *J Clin Invest*. 2002;109(1):59-68.
155. Fragkioudaki S, Mavragani CP, Moutsopoulos HM. Predicting the risk for lymphoma development in Sjogren syndrome: an easy tool for clinical use. *Medicine (Baltimore)*. 2016;95(25):e3766.
156. Traianos EY, Locke J, Lendrem D, et al. Serum CXCL13 levels are associated with lymphoma risk and lymphoma occurrence in primary Sjögren's syndrome. *Rheumatol Int*. 2020;40(4):541-548.
157. Chatzis LG, Stergiou IE, Goules AV, et al. Clinical picture, outcome, and predictive factors of lymphoma in primary Sjogren's syndrome. Results from a harmonized dataset (1981-2021). *Rheumatology*. 2022;61(9):3576-3585.
158. Lindsay S, Dailey ME. Malignant lymphoma of the thyroid gland and its relation to Hashimoto disease: a clinical and pathologic study of 8 patients. *J Clin Endocrinol Metab*. 1955;15(11):1332-1353.
159. Travaglino A, Pace M, Varricchio S, et al. Hashimoto thyroiditis in primary thyroid non-Hodgkin lymphoma. *Am J Clin Pathol*. 2020;153(2):156-164.
160. Walsh S, Lowery AJ, Evoy D, McDermott EW, Prichard RS. Thyroid lymphoma: recent advances in diagnosis and optimal management strategies. *Oncol*. 2013;18(9):994-1003.
161. Derringer GA, Thompson LD, Frommelt RA, Bijwaard KE, Heffess CS, Abbondanzo SL. Malignant lymphoma of the thyroid gland: a clinicopathologic study of 108 cases. *Am J Surg Pathol*. 2000;24(5):623-639.
162. Baecklund E, Backlin C, Iliadou A, et al. Characteristics of diffuse large B cell lymphomas in rheumatoid arthritis. *Arthritis Rheum*. 2006;54(12):3774-3781.
163. Wolfe F, Michaud K. Lymphoma in rheumatoid arthritis: the effect of methotrexate and anti-tumor necrosis factor therapy in 18,572 patients. *Arthritis Rheum*. 2004;50(6):1740-1751.
164. Lopez-Olivo MA, Tayar JH, Martinez-Lopez JA, et al. Risk of malignancies in patients with rheumatoid arthritis treated with biologic therapy: a meta-analysis. *J Am Med Assoc*. 2012;308(9):898-908.
165. Kedra J, Seror R, Dieudé P, et al. Lymphoma complicating rheumatoid arthritis: results from a French case-control study. *RMD Open*. 2021;7(3):e001698.
166. Hoshida Y, Xu JX, Fujita S, et al. Lymphoproliferative disorders in rheumatoid arthritis: clinicopathological analysis of 76 cases in relation to methotrexate medication. *J Rheumatol*. 2007;34(2):322-331.
167. Cheon H, Dziewulska KH, Moosic KB, et al. Advances in the diagnosis and treatment of large granular lymphocytic leukemia. *Curr Hematol Malig Rep*. 2020;15(2):103-112.
168. Song L, Wang Y, Zhang J, Song N, Xu X, Lu Y. The risks of cancer development in systemic lupus erythematosus (SLE) patients: a systematic review and meta-analysis. *Arthritis Res Ther*. 2018;20(1):270.
169. Castleman B, Iverson L, Menendez VP. Localized mediastinal lymphnode hyperplasia resembling thymoma. *Cancer*. 1956;9(4):822-830.
170. Dispenzieri A, Fajgenbaum DC. Overview of Castleman disease. *Blood*. 2020;135(16):1353-1364.
171. Wu D, Lim MS, Jaffe ES. Pathology of Castleman disease. *Hematol Oncol Clin North Am*. 2018;32(1):37-52.
172. Brandt SJ, Bodine DM, Dunbar CE, Nienhuis AW. Dysregulated interleukin 6 expression produces a syndrome resembling Castleman's disease in mice. *J Clin Invest*. 1990;86(2):592-599.
173. Chang KC, Wang YC, Hung LY, et al. Monoclonality and cytogenetic abnormalities in hyaline vascular Castleman disease. *Mod Pathol*. 2014;27(6):823-831.
174. van Rhee F, Oksenhendler E, Srkalovic G, et al. International evidence-based consensus diagnostic and treatment guidelines for unicentric Castleman disease. *Blood Adv*. 2020;4(23):6039-6050.
175. Kawabata H, Takai K, Kojima M, et al. Castleman-Kojima disease (TAFRO syndrome): a novel systemic inflammatory disease characterized by a constellation of symptoms, namely, thrombocytopenia, ascites (anasarca), microcytic anemia, myelofibrosis, renal dysfunction, and organomegaly. A status report and summary of Fukushima (6 June, 2012) and Nagoya meetings (22 September, 2012). *J Clin Exp Hematop*. 2013;53(1):57-61.
176. van Rhee F, Casper C, Voorhees PM, et al. Long-term safety of siltuximab in patients with idiopathic multicentric Castleman disease: a prespecified, open-label, extension analysis of two trials. *Lancet Haematol*. 2020;7(3):e209-e217.
177. Nishimoto N, Terao K, Mima T, Nakahara H, Takagi N, Kakehi T. Mechanisms and pathological significances in increase in serum interleukin-6 (IL-6) and soluble IL-6 receptor after administration of an anti-IL-6 receptor antibody, tocilizumab, in patients with rheumatoid arthritis and Castleman disease. *Blood*. 2008;112(10):3959-3964.
178. van Rhee F, Voorhees P, Dispenzieri A, et al. International, evidence-based consensus treatment guidelines for idiopathic multicentric Castleman disease. *Blood*. 2018;132(20):2115-2124.
179. Oksenhendler E, Boutboul D, Fajgenbaum D, et al. The full spectrum of Castleman disease: 273 patients studied over 20 years. *Br J Haematol*. 2018;180(2):206-216.
180. Larroche C, Cacoub P, Soulier J, et al. Castleman's disease and lymphoma: report of eight cases in HIV-negative patients and literature review. *Am J Hematol*. 2002;69(2):119-126.
181. Gerard L, Michot JM, Burcheri S, et al. Rituximab decreases the risk of lymphoma in patients with HIV-associated multicentric Castleman disease. *Blood*. 2012;119(10):2228-2233.
182. Uldrick TS, Polizzotto MN, Aleman K, et al. Rituximab plus liposomal doxorubicin in HIV-infected patients with KSHV-associated multicentric Castleman disease. *Blood*. 2014;124(24):3544-3552.
183. Krikorian JG, Burke JS, Rosenberg SA, Kaplan HS. Occurrence of non-Hodgkin's lymphoma after therapy for Hodgkin's disease. *N Engl J Med*. 1979;300(9):452-458.
184. Ali S, Olszewski AJ. Disparate survival and risk of secondary non-Hodgkin lymphoma in histologic subtypes of Hodgkin lymphoma: a population-based study. *Leuk Lymphoma*. 2014;55(7):1570-1577.
185. Xavier AC, Armeson KE, Hill EG, Costa LJ. Risk and outcome of non-Hodgkin lymphoma among classical Hodgkin lymphoma survivors. *Cancer*. 2013;119(18):3385-3392.
186. Kenderian SS, Habermann TM, Macon WR, et al. Large B-cell transformation in nodular lymphocyte-predominant Hodgkin lymphoma: 40-year experience from a single institution. *Blood*. 2016;127(16):1960-1966.
187. Bosch-Schips J, Granai M, Quintanilla-Martinez L, Fend F. The grey zones of classic Hodgkin lymphoma. *Cancers*. 2022;14(3):742.
188. Van den Bergh M, Alvarez-Argote J, Panwala AH, Dasanu CA. Autoimmune disorders in patients with T-cell lymphoma: a comprehensive review. *Curr Med Res Opin*. 2015;31(10):1861-1870.
189. Clarke CA, Morton LM, Lynch C, et al. Risk of lymphoma subtypes after solid organ transplantation in the United States. *Br J Cancer*. 2013;109(1):280-288.
190. Parakkal D, Sifuentes H, Semer R, Ehrenpreis ED. Hepatosplenic T-cell lymphoma in patients receiving TNF-α inhibitor therapy: expanding the groups at risk. *Eur J Gastroenterol Hepatol*. 2011;23(12):1150-1156.
191. Gibson TM, Morton LM, Shiels MS, Clarke CA, Engels EA. Risk of non-Hodgkin lymphoma subtypes in HIV-infected people during the HAART era: a population-based study. *AIDS*. 2014;28(15):2313-2318.
192. Ondrejka S, Jagadeesh D. Enteropathy-associated T-cell lymphoma. *Curr Hematol Malig Rep*. 2016;11(6):504-513.
193. Zoref-Lorenz A, Murakami J, Hofstetter L, et al. An improved index for diagnosis and mortality prediction in malignancy-associated hemophagocytic lymphohistiocytosis. *Blood*. 2022;139(7):1098-1110.
194. Mehta-Shah N, Ghione P. An updated approach and understanding of breast implant-associated anaplastic large cell lymphoma. *J Natl Compr Canc Netw*. 2022;20(3):309-315.
195. Chitgopeker P, Sahni D. T-cell receptor gene rearrangement detection in suspected cases of cutaneous T-cell lymphoma. *J Invest Dermatol*. 2014;134(4):1-5.
196. Rosenberg SA, Diamond HD, Jaslowitz B, Craver LF. Lymphosarcoma: a review of 1269 cases. *Medicine (Baltimore)*. 1961;40:31-84.
197. Ghimire P, Wu GY, Zhu L. Primary gastrointestinal lymphoma. *World J Gastroenterol*. 2011;17(6):697-707.
198. Alvarez-Lesmes J, Chapman JR, Cassidy D, et al. Gastrointestinal tract lymphomas. *Arch Pathol Lab Med*. 2021;145(12):1585-1596.
199. Vaidya R, Habermann TM, Donohue JH, et al. Bowel perforation in intestinal lymphoma: incidence and clinical features. *Ann Oncol*. 2013;24(9):2439-2443.
200. Kodama T, Ohshima K, Nomura K, et al. Lymphomatous polyposis of the gastrointestinal tract, including mantle cell lymphoma, follicular lymphoma and mucosa-associated lymphoid tissue lymphoma. *Histopathology*. 2005;47(5):467-478.
201. Romaguera JE, Medeiros LJ, Hagemeister FB, et al. Frequency of gastrointestinal involvement and its clinical significance in mantle cell lymphoma. *Cancer*. 2003;97(3):586-591.
202. Masood A, Kairouz S, Hudhud KH, Hegazi AZ, Banu A, Gupta NC. Primary non-Hodgkin lymphoma of liver. *Curr Oncol*. 2009;16(4):74-77.
203. Arcaini L, Rossi D, Paulli M. Splenic marginal zone lymphoma: from genetics to management. *Blood*. 2016;127(17):2072-2081.
204. Pan X, Ren D, Li Y, Zhao J. The effect of surgery on primary splenic lymphoma: a study based on SEER database. *Cancer Med*. 2021;10(20):7060-7070.
205. Qiu MJ, Fang XF, Huang ZZ, et al. Prognosis of primary hepatic lymphoma: a US population-based analysis. *Transl Oncol*. 2021;14(1):100931.
206. Salmon JS, Thompson MA, Arildsen RC, Greer JP. Non-Hodgkin's lymphoma involving the liver: clinical and therapeutic considerations. *Clin Lymphoma Myeloma*. 2006;6(4):273-280.
207. Thompson DR, Faust TW, Stone MJ, Polter DE. Hepatic failure as the presenting manifestation of malignant lymphoma. *Clin Lymphoma*. 2001;2(2):123-128.
208. Bataille B, Delwail V, Menet E, et al. Primary intracerebral malignant lymphoma: report of 248 cases. *J Neurosurg*. 2000;92(2):261-266.
209. Grommes C, Rubenstein JL, DeAngelis LM, Ferreri AJM, Batchelor TT. Comprehensive approach to diagnosis and treatment of newly diagnosed primary CNS lymphoma. *Neuro Oncol*. 2019;21(3):296-305.
210. Camilleri-Broet S, Criniere E, Broet P, et al. A uniform activated B-cell-like immunophenotype might explain the poor prognosis of primary central nervous system lymphomas: analysis of 83 cases. *Blood*. 2006;107(1):190-196.
211. Shenkier TN. Unusual variants of primary central nervous system lymphoma. *Hematol Oncol Clin North Am*. 2005;19(4):651-664, vi.

212. Bourque PR, Warman Chardon J, Bryanton M, Toupin M, Burns BF, Torres C. Neurolymphomatosis of the brachial plexus and its branches: case series and literature review. *Can J Neurol Sci*. 2018;45(2):137-143.
213. Ponzoni M, Campo E, Nakamura S. Intravascular large B-cell lymphoma: a chameleon with multiple faces and many masks. *Blood*. 2018;132(15):1561-1567.
214. Graus F, Arino H, Dalmau J. Paraneoplastic neurological syndromes in Hodgkin and non-Hodgkin lymphomas. *Blood*. 2014;123(21):3230-3238.
215. Savage KJ. Secondary CNS relapse in diffuse large B-cell lymphoma: defining high-risk patients and optimization of prophylaxis strategies. *Hematology Am Soc Hematol Educ Program*. 2017;2017(1):578-586.
216. Szekely G, Miltenyi Z, Mezey G, et al. Epidural malignant lymphomas of the spine: collected experiences with epidural malignant lymphomas of the spinal canal and their treatment. *Spinal Cord*. 2008;46(4):278-281.
217. Raval V, Binkley E, Aronow ME, Valenzuela J, Peereboom DM, Singh AD. Primary central nervous system lymphoma – ocular variant: an interdisciplinary review on management. *Surv Ophthalmol*. 2021;66(6):1009-1020.
218. Olsen TG, Heegaard S. Orbital lymphoma. *Surv Ophthalmol*. 2019;64(1):45-66.
219. Stefanovic A, Lossos IS. Extranodal marginal zone lymphoma of the ocular adnexa. *Blood*. 2009;114(3):501-510.
220. Messina C, Christie D, Zucca E, Gospodarowicz M, Ferreri AJM. Primary and secondary bone lymphomas. *Cancer Treat Rev*. 2015;41(3):235-246.
221. Cheah CY, Wirth A, Seymour JF. Primary testicular lymphoma. *Blood*. 2014;123(4):486-493.
222. Cheah CY, Campbell BA, Seymour JF. Primary breast lymphoma. *Cancer Treat Rev*. 2014;40(8):900-908.
223. Sanguedolce F, Zanelli M, Zizzo M, et al. Primary pulmonary B-cell lymphoma: a review and update. *Cancers*. 2021;13(3):415.
224. Petrich A, Cho SI, Billett H. Primary cardiac lymphoma: an analysis of presentation, treatment, and outcome patterns. *Cancer*. 2011;117(3):581-589.
225. Kuyama A, Takeuchi M, Munemasa M, et al. Successful treatment of primary adrenal non-Hodgkin's lymphoma associated with adrenal insufficiency. *Leuk Lymphoma*. 2000;38(1-2):203-205.
226. Carbone PP, Kaplan HS, Musshoff K, Smithers DW, Tubiana M. Report of the committee on Hodgkin's disease staging classification. *Cancer Res*. 1971;31:1860-1861.
227. Cheson BD, Fisher RI, Barrington SF, et al. Recommendations for initial evaluation, staging, and response assessment of Hodgkin and non-Hodgkin lymphoma: the Lugano classification. *J Clin Oncol*. 2014;32(27):3059-3068.
228. Sehn LH, Berry B, Chhanabhai M, et al. The revised International Prognostic Index (R-IPI) is a better predictor of outcome than the standard IPI for patients with diffuse large B-cell lymphoma treated with R-CHOP. *Blood*. 2007;109:1857-1861.
229. Zhou Z, Sehn LH, Rademaker AW, et al. An enhanced International Prognostic Index (NCCN-IPI) for patients with diffuse large B-cell lymphoma treated in the rituximab era. *Blood*. 2014;123(6):837-842.
230. Solal-Celigny P, Roy P, Colombat P, et al. Follicular lymphoma international prognosticindex. *Blood*. 2004;104:1258-1265.
231. Pastore A, Jurinovic V, Kridel R, et al. Integration of gene mutations in risk prognostication for patients receiving first-line immunochemotherapy for follicular lymphoma: a retrospective analysis of a prospective clinical trial and validation in a population-based registry. *Lancet Oncol*. 2015;16:1111-1122.
232. Gallamini A, Stelitano C, Calvi R, et al. Peripheral T-cell lymphoma unspecified (PTCL-U): a new prognostic model from a retrospective multicentric clinical study. *Blood*. 2004;103(7):2474-2479.
233. Determann O, Hoster E, Ott G, et al. Ki-67 predicts outcome in advanced-stage mantle cell lymphoma patients treated with anti-CD20 immunochemotherapy: results from randomized trials of the European MCL Network and the German Low Grade Lymphoma Study Group. *Blood*. 2008;111(4):2385-2387.
234. Miller TP, Grogan TM, Dahlberg S, et al. Prognostic significance of the Ki-67-associated proliferative antigen in aggressive non-Hodgkin's lymphomas: a prospective Southwest Oncology Group trial. *Blood*. 1994;83(6):1460-1466.
235. Kutok JL, Aster JC. Molecular biology of anaplastic lymphoma kinase-positive anaplastic large-cell lymphoma. *J Clin Oncol*. 2002;20(17):3691-3702.
236. Winter JN, Weller EA, Horning SJ, et al. Prognostic significance of Bcl-6 protein expression in DLBCL treated with CHOP or R-CHOP: a prospective correlative study. *Blood*. 2006;107(11):4207-4213.
237. Alizadeh AA, Eisen MB, Davis RE, et al. Distinct types of diffuse large B-cell lymphoma identified by gene expression profiling. *Nature*. 2000;403(6769):503-511.
238. Rosenwald A, Wright G, Chan WC, et al. The use of molecular profiling to predict survival after chemotherapy for diffuse large-B-cell lymphoma. *N Engl J Med*. 2002;346(25):1937-1947.
239. Rosenwald A, Wright G, Leroy K, et al. Molecular diagnosis of primary mediastinal B cell lymphoma identifies a clinically favorable subgroup of diffuse large B cell lymphoma related to Hodgkin lymphoma. *J Exp Med*. 2003;198(6):851-862.
240. Hans CP, Weisenburger DD, Greiner TC, et al. Confirmation of the molecular classification of diffuse large B-cell lymphoma by immunohistochemistry using a tissue microarray. *Blood*. 2004;103(1):275-282.
241. van Imhoff GW, Boerma EJG, van der Holt B, et al. Prognostic impact of germinal center-associated proteins and chromosomal breakpoints in poor-risk diffuse large B-cell lymphoma. *J Clin Oncol*. 2006;24(25):4135-4142.
242. Choi WWL, Weisenburger DD, Greiner TC, et al. A new immunostain algorithm classifies diffuse large B-cell lymphoma into molecular subtypes with high accuracy. *Clin Cancer Res*. 2009;15(17):5494-5502.
243. Johnson NA, Slack GW, Savage KJ, et al. Concurrent expression of MYC and BCL2 in diffuse large B-cell lymphoma treated with rituximab plus cyclophosphamide, doxorubicin, vincristine, and prednisone. *J Clin Oncol*. 2012;30(28):3452-3459.
244. Green TM, Young KH, Visco C, et al. Immunohistochemical double-hit score is a strong predictor of outcome in patients with diffuse large B-cell lymphoma treated with rituximab plus cyclophosphamide, doxorubicin, vincristine, and prednisone. *J Clin Oncol*. 2012;30(28):3460-3467.
245. Savage KJ, Johnson NA, Ben-Neriah S, et al. MYC gene rearrangements are associated with a poor prognosis in diffuse large B-cell lymphoma patients treated with R-CHOP chemotherapy. *Blood*. 2009;114(17):3533-3537.
246. Gascoyne RD, Rosenwald A, Poppema S, Lenz G. Prognostic biomarkers in malignant lymphomas. *Leuk Lymphoma*. 2010;51(suppl 1):11-19.
247. Cheson BD. Role of functional imaging in the management of lymphoma. *J Clin Oncol*. 2011;29(14):1844-1854.
248. Spaepen K, Stroobants S, Dupont P, et al. Prognostic value of pretransplantation positron emission tomography using fluorine 18-fluorodeoxyglucose in patients with aggressive lymphoma treated with high-dose chemotherapy and stem cell transplantation. *Blood*. 2003;102(1):53-59.
249. Pregno P, Chiappella A, Bellò M, et al. Interim 18-FDG-PET/CT failed to predict the outcome in diffuse large B-cell lymphoma patients treated at the diagnosis with rituximab-CHOP. *Blood*. 2012;119(9):2066-2073.
250. Safar V, Dupuis J, Itti E, et al. Interim [18F]fluorodeoxyglucose positron emission tomography scan in diffuse large B-cell lymphoma treated with anthracycline-based chemotherapy plus rituximab. *J Clin Oncol*. 2012;30(2):184-190.
251. Trotman J, Fournier M, Lamy T, et al. Positron emission tomography-computed tomography (PET-CT) after induction therapy is highly predictive of patient outcome in follicular lymphoma: analysis of PET-CT in a subset of PRIMA trial participants. *J Clin Oncol*. 2011;29(23):3194-3200.
252. Juweid ME, Stroobants S, Hoekstra OS, et al. Use of positron emission tomography for response assessment of lymphoma: consensus of the Imaging Subcommittee of International Harmonization Project in Lymphoma. *J Clin Oncol*. 2007;25(5):571-578.
253. Fields PA, Linch DC. Treatment of the elderly patient with diffuse large B cell lymphoma. *Br J Haematol*. 2012;157(2):159-170.
254. Effect of age on the characteristics and clinical behavior of non-Hodgkin's lymphoma patients. *Ann Oncol*. 1997;8(10):973-978.
255. Armitage JO, Weisenburger DD. New approach to classifying non-Hodgkin's lymphomas: clinical features of the major histologic subtypes. Non-Hodgkin's Lymphoma Classification Project. *J Clin Oncol*. 1998;16(8):2780-2795.
256. Johnson PW, Rohatiner AZ, Whelan JS, et al. Patterns of survival in patients with recurrent follicular lymphoma: a 20-year study from a single center. *J Clin Oncol*. 1995;13(1):140-147.
257. Junlén HR, Peterson S, Kimby E, et al. Follicular lymphoma in Sweden. Nationwide improved survival in the rituximab era, particularly in elderly women: a Swedish Lymphoma Registry study. *Leukemia*. 2015;29(3):668-676.
258. Arcaini L, Colombo N, Bernasconi P, et al. Role of the molecular staging and response in the management of follicular lymphoma patients. *Leuk Lymphoma*. 2006;47(6):1018-1022.
259. Broyde A, Boycov O, Strenov Y, Okon E, Shpilberg O, Bairey O. Role and prognostic significance of the Ki-67 index in non-Hodgkin's lymphoma. *Am J Hematol*. 2009;84(6):338-343.
260. Wang SA, Wang L, Hochberg EP, Muzikansky A, Harris NL, Hasserjian RP. Low histologic grade follicular lymphoma with high proliferation index: morphologic and clinical features. *Am J Surg Pathol*. 2005;29(11):1490-1496.
261. Federico M, Bellei M, Marcheselli L, et al. Follicular lymphoma international prognostic index 2: a new prognostic index for follicular lymphoma developed by the international follicular lymphoma prognostic factor project. *J Clin Oncol*. 2009;27(27):4555-4562.
262. Biagi JJ, Seymour JF. Insights into the molecular pathogenesis of follicular lymphoma arising from analysis of geographic variation. *Blood*. 2002;99(12):4265-4275.
263. López-Guillermo A, Cabanillas F, McDonnell TI, et al. Correlation of bcl-2 rearrangement with clinical characteristics and outcome in indolent follicular lymphoma. *Blood*. 1999;93(9):3081-3087.
264. Rambaldi A, Lazzari M, Manzoni C, et al. Monitoring of minimal residual disease after CHOP and rituximab in previously untreated patients with follicular lymphoma. *Blood*. 2002;99(3):856-862.
265. Dave SS, Wright G, Tan B, et al. Prediction of survival in follicular lymphoma based on molecular features of tumor-infiltrating immune cells. *N Engl J Med*. 2004;351(21):2159-2169.
266. Pastore A, Jurinovic V, Kridel R, et al. Integration of gene mutations in risk prognostication for patients receiving first-line immunochemotherapy for follicular lymphoma: a retrospective analysis of a prospective clinical trial and validation in a population-based registry. *Lancet Oncol*. 2015;16(9):1111-1122.
267. Casulo C, Byrtek M, Dawson KL, et al. Early relapse of follicular lymphoma after rituximab plus cyclophosphamide, doxorubicin, vincristine, and prednisone defines patients at high risk for death: an analysis from the National LymphoCare Study. *J Clin Oncol*. 2015;33(23):2516-2522.
268. Casulo C, Dixon JG, Le-Rademacher J, et al. Validation of POD24 as a robust early clinical end point of poor survival in FL from 5225 patients on 13 clinical trials. *Blood*. 2022;139(11):1684-1693.
269. Tsimberidou AM, Wen S, O'Brien S, et al. Assessment of chronic lymphocytic leukemia and small lymphocytic lymphoma by absolute lymphocyte counts in 2,126 patients: 20 years of experience at the University of Texas M.D. Anderson Cancer Center. *J Clin Oncol*. 2007;25(29):4648-4656.
270. Hallek M, Cheson BD, Catovsky D, et al. Guidelines for the diagnosis and treatment of chronic lymphocytic leukemia: a report from the International Workshop on Chronic Lymphocytic Leukemia Updating the National Cancer Institute-Working Group 1996 guidelines. *Blood*. 2008;111(12):5446-5456.
271. Richter MN. Generalized reticular cell sarcoma of lymph nodes associated with lymphatic leukemia. *Am J Pathol*. 1928;4(4):285-292.

272. Robertson LE, Pugh W, O'Brien S, et al. Richter's syndrome: a report on 39 patients. *J Clin Oncol*. 1993;11(10):1985-1989.
273. Armitage JO, Carbone PP, Connors JM, Levine A, Bennett JM, Kroll S. Treatment-related myelodysplasia and acute leukemia in non-Hodgkin's lymphoma patients. *J Clin Oncol*. 2003;21(5):897-906.
274. Lin P, Medeiros LJ. Lymphoplasmacytic lymphoma/waldenstrom macroglobulinemia: an evolving concept. *Adv Anat Pathol*. 2005;12(5):246-255.
275. Richards MA, Hall PA, Gregory WM, et al. Lymphoplasmacytoid and small cell centrocytic non-Hodgkin's lymphoma—a retrospective analysis from St Bartholomew's Hospital 1972-1986. *Hematol Oncol*. 1989;7(1):19-35.
276. Dimopoulos MA, Kastritis E, Owen RG, et al. Treatment recommendations for patients with Waldenström macroglobulinemia (WM) and related disorders: IWWM-7 consensus. *Blood*. 2014;124(9):1404-1411.
277. Kristinsson SY, Koshiol J, Björkholm M, et al. Immune-related and inflammatory conditions and risk of lymphoplasmacytic lymphoma or Waldenstrom macroglobulinemia. *J Natl Cancer Inst*. 2010;102(8):557-567.
278. Treon SP, Tripsas CK, Meid K, et al. Ibrutinib in previously treated Waldenström's macroglobulinemia. *N Engl J Med*. 2015;372(15):1430-1440.
279. Insuasti-Beltran G, Gale JM, Wilson CS, Foucar K, Czuchlewski DR. Significance of MYD88 L265P mutation status in the subclassification of low-grade B-cell lymphoma/leukemia. *Arch Pathol Lab Med*. 2015;139(8):1035-1041.
280. Dimopoulos MA, Kyle RA, Anagnostopoulos A, Treon SP. Diagnosis and management of Waldenstrom's macroglobulinemia. *J Clin Oncol*. 2005;23(7):1564-1577.
281. Arcaini L, Paulli M, Burcheri S, et al. Primary nodal marginal zone B-cell lymphoma: clinical features and prognostic assessment of a rare disease. *Br J Haematol*. 2007;136(2):301-304.
282. Rinaldi A, Mian M, Chigrinova E, et al. Genome-wide DNA profiling of marginal zone lymphomas identifies subtype-specific lesions with an impact on the clinical outcome. *Blood*. 2011;117(5):1595-1604.
283. Olszewski AJ, Castillo JJ. Survival of patients with marginal zone lymphoma: analysis of the Surveillance, Epidemiology, and End Results database. *Cancer*. 2013;119(3):629-638.
284. Arcaini L, Lazzarino M, Colombo N, et al. Splenic marginal zone lymphoma: a prognostic model for clinical use. *Blood*. 2006;107(12):4643-4649.
285. Liu L, Wang H, Chen Y, Rustveld L, Liu G, Du XL. Splenic marginal zone lymphoma: a population-based study on the 2001-2008 incidence and survival in the United States. *Leuk Lymphoma*. 2013;54(7):1380-1386.
286. Mollejo M, Camacho FI, Algara P, Ruiz-Ballesteros E, García JF, Piris MA. Nodal and splenic marginal zone B cell lymphomas. *Hematol Oncol*. 2005;23(3-4):108-118.
287. Franco V, Florena AM, Iannitto E. Splenic marginal zone lymphoma. *Blood*. 2003;101(7):2464-2472.
288. Thieblemont C, Felman P, Berger F, et al. Treatment of splenic marginal zone B-cell lymphoma: an analysis of 81 patients. *Clin Lymphoma*. 2002;3(1):41-47.
289. Salido M, Baró C, Oscier D, et al. Cytogenetic aberrations and their prognostic value in a series of 330 splenic marginal zone B-cell lymphomas: a multicenter study of the Splenic B-Cell Lymphoma Group. *Blood*. 2010;116(9):1479-1488.
290. Horning SJ, Rosenberg SA. The natural history of initially untreated low-grade non-Hodgkin's lymphomas. *N Engl J Med*. 1984;311(23):1471-1475.
291. Montoto S, Davies AJ, Matthews J, et al. Risk and clinical implications of transformation of follicular lymphoma to diffuse large B-cell lymphoma. *J Clin Oncol*. 2007;25(17):2426-2433.
292. Al-Tourah AJ, Gill KK, Chhanabhai M, et al. Population-based analysis of incidence and outcome of transformed non-Hodgkin's lymphoma. *J Clin Oncol*. 2008;26(32):5165-5169.
293. Bastion Y, Sebban C, Berger F, et al. Incidence, predictive factors, and outcome of lymphoma transformation in follicular lymphoma patients. *J Clin Oncol*. 1997;15(4):1587-1594.
294. Giné E, Montoto S, Bosch F, et al. The Follicular Lymphoma International Prognostic Index (FLIPI) and the histological subtype are the most important factors to predict histological transformation in follicular lymphoma. *Ann Oncol*. 2006;17(10):1539-1545.
295. Freeman CL, Kridel R, Moccia AA, et al. Early progression after bendamustine-rituximab is associated with high risk of transformation in advanced stage follicular lymphoma. *Blood*. 2019;134(9):761-764.
296. Freedman AS. Biology and management of histologic transformation of indolent lymphoma. *Hematology Am Soc Hematol Educ Program*. 2005:314-320.
297. Lossos IS, Alizadeh AA, Diehn M, et al. Transformation of follicular lymphoma to diffuse large-cell lymphoma: alternative patterns with increased or decreased expression of c-myc and its regulated genes. *Proc Natl Acad Sci U S A*. 2002;99(13):8886-8891.
298. Friedberg JW, Byrtek M, Link BK, et al. Effectiveness of first-line management strategies for stage I follicular lymphoma: analysis of the National LymphoCare Study. *J Clin Oncol*. 2012;30(27):3368-3375.
299. Advani R, Rosenberg SA, Horning SJ. Stage I and II follicular non-Hodgkin's lymphoma: long-term follow-up of no initial therapy. *J Clin Oncol*. 2004;22(8):1454-1459.
300. Solal-Céligny P, Bellei M, Marcheselli L, et al. Watchful waiting in low-tumor burden follicular lymphoma in the rituximab era: results of an F2-study database. *J Clin Oncol*. 2012;30(31):3848-3853.
301. Gallagher CJ, Gregory WM, Jones AE, et al. Follicular lymphoma: prognostic factors for response and survival. *J Clin Oncol*. 1986;4(10):1470-1480.
302. Guadagnolo BA, Li S, Neuberg D, et al. Long-term outcome and mortality trends in early-stage, Grade 1-2 follicular lymphoma treated with radiation therapy. *Int J Radiat Oncol Biol Phys*. 2006;64(3):928-934.
303. Mac Manus MP, Hoppe RT. Is radiotherapy curative for stage I and II low-grade follicular lymphoma? Results of a long-term follow-up study of patients treated at Stanford University. *J Clin Oncol*. 1996;14(4):1282-1290.
304. Campbell BA, Voss N, Woods R, et al. Long-term outcomes for patients with limited stage follicular lymphoma: involved regional radiotherapy versus involved node radiotherapy. *Cancer*. 2010;116(16):3797-3806.
305. Uckun FM. Regulation of human B-cell ontogeny. *Blood*. 1990;76(10):1908-1923.
306. Nadler LM, Ritz J, Hardy R, Pesando JM, Schlossman SF, Stashenko P. A unique cell surface antigen identifying lymphoid malignancies of B cell origin. *J Clin Invest*. 1981;67(1):134-140.
307. Press OW, Farr AG, Borroz KI, Anderson SK, Martin PJ. Endocytosis and degradation of monoclonal antibodies targeting human B-cell malignancies. *Cancer Res*. 1989;49(17):4906-4912.
308. Press OW, Howell-Clark J, Anderson S, Bernstein I. Retention of B-cell-specific monoclonal antibodies by human lymphoma cells. *Blood*. 1994;83(5):1390-1397.
309. Reff ME, Carner K, Chambers KS, et al. Depletion of B cells in vivo by a chimeric mouse human monoclonal antibody to CD20. *Blood*. 1994;83(2):435-445.
310. Golay J, Zaffaroni L, Vaccari T, et al. Biologic response of B lymphoma cells to anti-CD20 monoclonal antibody rituximab in vitro: CD55 and CD59 regulate complement-mediated cell lysis. *Blood*. 2000;95(12):3900-3908.
311. Hainsworth JD, Litchy S, Burris HA III, et al. Rituximab as first-line and maintenance therapy for patients with indolent non-Hodgkin's lymphoma. *J Clin Oncol*. 2002;20(20):4261-4267.
312. Ghielmini M, Schmitz SFH, Cogliatti SB, et al. Prolonged treatment with rituximab in patients with follicular lymphoma significantly increases event-free survival and response duration compared with the standard weekly × 4 schedule. *Blood*. 2004;103(12):4416-4423.
313. O'Brien ME, Easterbrook P, Powell J, et al. The natural history of low grade non-Hodgkin's lymphoma and the impact of a no initial treatment policy on survival. *Q J Med*. 1991;80(292):651-660.
314. Young RC, Longo DL, Glatstein E, Ihde DC, Jaffe ES, DeVita VT Jr. The treatment of indolent lymphomas: watchful waiting v aggressive combined modality treatment. *Semin Hematol*. 1988;25(suppl 2):11-16.
315. Brice P, Bastion Y, Lepage E, et al. Comparison in low-tumor-burden follicular lymphomas between an initial no-treatment policy, prednimustine, or interferon alfa: a randomized study from the Groupe d'Etude des Lymphomes Folliculaires. Groupe d'Etude des Lymphomes de l'Adulte. *J Clin Oncol*. 1997;15(3):1110-1117.
316. Ardeshna KM, Smith P, Norton A, et al. Long-term effect of a watch and wait policy versus immediate systemic treatment for asymptomatic advanced-stage non-Hodgkin lymphoma: a randomised controlled trial. *Lancet*. 2003;362(9383):516-522.
317. Ardeshna KM, Qian W, Smith P, et al. Rituximab versus a watch-and-wait approach in patients with advanced-stage, asymptomatic, non-bulky follicular lymphoma: an open-label randomised phase 3 trial. *Lancet Oncol*. 2014;15(4):424-435.
318. Colombat P, Salles G, Brousse N, et al. Rituximab (anti-CD20 monoclonal antibody) as single first-line therapy for patients with follicular lymphoma with a low tumor burden: clinical and molecular evaluation. *Blood*. 2001;97(1):101-106.
319. McLaughlin P, Grillo-López AJ, Link BK, et al. Rituximab chimeric anti-CD20 monoclonal antibody therapy for relapsed indolent lymphoma: half of patients respond to a four-dose treatment program. *J Clin Oncol*. 1998;16(8):2825-2833.
320. Herold M, Haas A, Srock S, et al. Rituximab added to first-line mitoxantrone, chlorambucil, and prednisolone chemotherapy followed by interferon maintenance prolongs survival in patients with advanced follicular lymphoma: an East German Study Group Hematology and Oncology Study. *J Clin Oncol*. 2007;25(15):1986-1992.
321. Salles G, Mounier N, de Guibert S, et al. Rituximab combined with chemotherapy and interferon in follicular lymphoma patients: results of the GELA-GOELAMS FL2000 study. *Blood*. 2008;112(13):4824-4831.
322. Sehn LH, Chua N, Mayer J, et al. Obinutuzumab plus bendamustine versus bendamustine monotherapy in patients with rituximab-refractory indolent non-Hodgkin lymphoma (GADOLIN): a randomised, controlled, open-label, multicentre, phase 3 trial. *Lancet Oncol*. 2016;17(8):1081-1093.
323. Sehn LH, Goy A, Offner FC, et al. Randomized phase II trial comparing obinutuzumab (GA101) with rituximab in patients with relapsed CD20+ indolent B-cell non-Hodgkin lymphoma: final analysis of the GAUSS study. *J Clin Oncol*. 2015;33(30):3467-3474.
324. Marcus R, Davies A, Ando K, et al. Obinutuzumab for the first-line treatment of follicular lymphoma. *N Engl J Med*. 2017;377(14):1331-1344.
325. Cheson BD. Ofatumumab, a novel anti-CD20 monoclonal antibody for the treatment of B-cell malignancies. *J Clin Oncol*. 2010;28(21):3525-3530.
326. Friedberg JW, Taylor MD, Cerhan JR, et al. Follicular lymphoma in the United States: first report of the National LymphoCare study. *J Clin Oncol*. 2009;27(8):1202-1208.
327. Rummel MJ, Niederle N, Maschmeyer G, et al. Bendamustine plus rituximab versus CHOP plus rituximab as first-line treatment for patients with indolent and mantle-cell lymphomas: an open-label, multicentre, randomised, phase 3 non-inferiority trial. *Lancet*. 2013;381(9873):1203-1210.
328. Flinn IW, van der Jagt R, Kahl B, et al. First-line treatment of patients with indolent non-hodgkin lymphoma or mantle-cell lymphoma with bendamustine plus rituximab versus R-CHOP or R-CVP: results of the BRIGHT 5-year follow-up study. *J Clin Oncol*. 2019;37(12):984-991.
329. Townsend W, Buske C, Cartron G, Cunningham D, Dyer MJ. Comparison of efficacy and safety with obinutuzumab plus chemotherapy versus rituximab plus chemotherapy in patients with previously untreated follicular lymphoma: updated results from the phase III Gallium Study. *J Clin Oncol*. 2020;35:8023.
330. Czuczman MS, Koryzna A, Mohr A, et al. Rituximab in combination with fludarabine chemotherapy in low-grade or follicular lymphoma. *J Clin Oncol*. 2005;23(4):694-704.
331. McLaughlin P, Hagemeister FB, Romaguera JE, et al. Fludarabine, mitoxantrone, and dexamethasone: an effective new regimen for indolent lymphoma. *J Clin Oncol*. 1996;14(4):1262-1268.
332. Zinzani PL, Magagnoli M, Bendandi M, et al. Efficacy of fludarabine and mitoxantrone (FN) combination regimen in untreated indolent non-Hodgkin's lymphomas. *Ann Oncol*. 2000;11(3):363-365.

333. Cheson BD, Pfistner B, Juweid ME, et al. Revised response criteria for malignant lymphoma. *J Clin Oncol*. 2007;25(5):579-586.
334. Fowler NH, Davis RE, Rawal S, et al. Safety and activity of lenalidomide and rituximab in untreated indolent lymphoma: an open-label, phase 2 trial. *Lancet Oncol*. 2014;15(12):1311-1318.
335. Martin P, Jung SH, Pitcher B, et al. A phase II trial of lenalidomide plus rituximab in previously untreated follicular non-Hodgkin's lymphoma (NHL): CALGB 50803 (Alliance). *Ann Oncol*. 2017;28(11):2806-2812.
336. Morschhauser F, Fowler NH, Feugier P, et al. Rituximab plus lenalidomide in advanced untreated follicular lymphoma. *N Engl J Med*. 2018;379(10):934-947.
337. Treon SP, Ioakimidis L, Soumerai JD, et al. Primary therapy of Waldenström macroglobulinemia with bortezomib, dexamethasone, and rituximab: WMCTG clinical trial 05-180. *J Clin Oncol*. 2009;27(23):3830-3835.
338. Dimopoulos MA, García-Sanz R, Gavriatopoulou M, et al. Primary therapy of Waldenstrom macroglobulinemia (WM) with weekly bortezomib, low-dose dexamethasone, and rituximab (BDR): long-term results of a phase 2 study of the European Myeloma Network (EMN). *Blood*. 2013;122(19):3276-3282.
339. Ghobrial IM, Xie W, Padmanabhan S, et al. Phase II trial of weekly bortezomib in combination with rituximab in untreated patients with Waldenström macroglobulinemia. *Am J Hematol*. 2010;85(9):670-674.
340. Treon SP, Tripsas CK, Meid K, et al. Carfilzomib, rituximab, and dexamethasone (CaRD) treatment offers a neuropathy-sparing approach for treating Waldenström's macroglobulinemia. *Blood*. 2014;124(4):503-510.
341. Chen CI, Kouroukis CT, White D, et al. Bortezomib is active in patients with untreated or relapsed Waldenstrom's macroglobulinemia: a phase II study of the National Cancer Institute of Canada Clinical Trials Group. *J Clin Oncol*. 2007;25(12):1570-1575.
342. Byrd JC, Woyach JA, Furman RR, et al. Acalabrutinib in treatment-naive chronic lymphocytic leukemia. *Blood*. 2021;137(24):3327-3338.
343. Tam CS, Giannopoulos K, Jurczak W, Šimkovič M. SEQUOIA: results of a phase 3 randomized study of zanubrutinib versus bendamustine + rituximab in patients with treatment-naïve chronic lymphocytic leukemia/small lymphocytic lymphoma (CLL/SLL). *Blood*. 2021;183:396.
344. Salles G, Seymour JF, Offner F, et al. Rituximab maintenance for 2 years in patients with high tumour burden follicular lymphoma responding to rituximab plus chemotherapy (PRIMA): a phase 3, randomised controlled trial. *Lancet*. 2011;377(9759):42-51.
345. Marcus RE, Davies AJ, Ando K, Klapper W. Obinutuzumab-based induction and maintenance prolongs progression-free survival (PFS) in patients with previously untreated follicular lymphoma: primary results of the randomized phase 3 GALLIUM study. *Blood*. 2016;128:6.
346. Moccia AA, Taverna C, Schär S, et al. Prolonged rituximab maintenance in follicular lymphoma patients: long-term results of the SAKK 35/03 randomized trial. *Blood Adv*. 2020;4(23):5951-5957.
347. Kahl BS, Hong F, Williams ME, et al. Rituximab extended schedule or re-treatment trial for low-tumor burden follicular lymphoma: eastern cooperative oncology group protocol e4402. *J Clin Oncol*. 2014;32(28):3096-3102.
348. Kahl BS, Hong F, Peterson C. Long term follow up of the Resort study (E4402): a randomized phase III study comparing two different rituximab dosing strategies for low tumor burden follicular lymphoma. *Blood*. 2021;138:815.
349. Rummel MJ, Al-Batran SE, Kim SZ, et al. Bendamustine plus rituximab is effective and has a favorable toxicity profile in the treatment of mantle cell and low-grade non-Hodgkin's lymphoma. *J Clin Oncol*. 2005;23(15):3383-3389.
350. Robinson KS, Williams ME, van der Jagt RH, et al. Phase II multicenter study of bendamustine plus rituximab in patients with relapsed indolent B-cell and mantle cell non-Hodgkin's lymphoma. *J Clin Oncol*. 2008;26(27):4473-4479.
351. Cheson BD, Chua N, Mayer J, et al. Overall survival benefit in patients with rituximab-refractory indolent non-Hodgkin lymphoma who received obinutuzumab plus bendamustine induction and obinutuzumab maintenance in the GADOLIN study. *J Clin Oncol*. 2018;36(22):2259-2266.
352. Leonard JP, Trneny M, Izutsu K, et al. AUGMENT: a phase III study of lenalidomide plus rituximab versus placebo plus rituximab in relapsed or refractory indolent lymphoma. *J Clin Oncol*. 2019;37(14):1188-1199.
353. Dreyling M, Santoro A, Mollica L, et al. Phosphatidylinositol 3-kinase inhibition by copanlisib in relapsed or refractory indolent lymphoma. *J Clin Oncol*. 2017;35(35):3898-3905.
354. Bodor C, Grossmann V, Popov N, et al. EZH2 mutations are frequent and represent an early event in follicular lymphoma. *Blood*. 2013;122(18):3165-3168.
355. Morschhauser F, Tilly H, Chaidos A, et al. Tazemetostat for patients with relapsed or refractory follicular lymphoma: an open-label, single-arm, multicentre, phase 2 trial. *Lancet Oncol*. 2020;21(11):1433-1442.
356. Witzig TE, Gordon LI, Cabanillas F, et al. Randomized controlled trial of yttrium-90-labeled ibritumomab tiuxetan radioimmunotherapy versus rituximab immunotherapy for patients with relapsed or refractory low-grade, follicular, or transformed B-cell non-Hodgkin's lymphoma. *J Clin Oncol*. 2002;20(10):2453-2463.
357. Morschhauser F, Radford J, Van Hoof A, et al. Phase III trial of consolidation therapy with yttrium-90-ibritumomab tiuxetan compared with no additional therapy after first remission in advanced follicular lymphoma. *J Clin Oncol*. 2008;26(32):5156-5164.
358. Kaminski MS, Zelenetz AD, Press OW, et al. Pivotal study of iodine I 131 tositumomab for chemotherapy-refractory low-grade or transformed low-grade B-cell non-Hodgkin's lymphomas. *J Clin Oncol*. 2001;19(19):3918-3928.
359. Kaminski MS, Tuck M, Estes J, et al. 131I-Tositumomab therapy as initial treatment for follicular lymphoma. *N Engl J Med*. 2005;352(5):441-449.
360. Jacobson CA, Chavez JC, Sehgal AR, et al. Axicabtagene ciloleucel in relapsed or refractory indolent non-Hodgkin lymphoma (ZUMA-5): a single-arm, multicentre, phase 2 trial. *Lancet Oncol*. 2022;23(1):91-103.
361. Schuster S, Dickinson M, Dreyling M, Martinez-Lopez J. Efficacy and safety of tisagenlecleucel (Tisa-cel) in adult patients (pts) with relapsed/refractory follicular lymphoma (r/r FL): primary analysis of the phase 2 Elara trial. *J Clin Oncol*. 2021;9(15):7508-7508.
362. Novartis. *FDA Approves Novartis Kymriah CAR-T Cell Therapy for Adult Patients With Relapsed or Refractory Follicular Lymphoma*. News Release. 2022. Accessed May 31, 2022. https://www.novartis.com/news/media-releases/fda-approves-novartis-kymriah-car-t-cell-therapy-adult-patients-relapsed-or-refractory-follicular-lymphoma
363. Porter DL, Levine BL, Kalos M, Bagg A, June CH. Chimeric antigen receptor-modified T cells in chronic lymphoid leukemia. *N Engl J Med*. 2011;365(8):725-733.
364. Budde L, Sehn L, Matasar M. Mosunetuzumab monotherapy is an effective and well-tolerated treatment option for patients with relapsed/refractory follicular lymphoma who have received ≥ 2 lines of therapy: pivotal results from a phase I/II study. *Blood*. 2021;138:127.
365. Sweetenham JW. Diffuse large B-cell lymphoma: risk stratification and management of relapsed disease. *Hematology Am Soc Hematol Educ Program*. 2005:252-259.
366. Tagawa H, Suguro M, Tsuzuki S, et al. Comparison of genome profiles for identification of distinct subgroups of diffuse large B-cell lymphoma. *Blood*. 2005;106(5):1770-1777.
367. Chapuy B, Stewart C, Dunford AJ, et al. Molecular subtypes of diffuse large B cell lymphoma are associated with distinct pathogenic mechanisms and outcomes. *Nat Med*. 2018;24(5):679-690.
368. Schmitz R, Wright GW, Huang DW, et al. Genetics and pathogenesis of diffuse large B-cell lymphoma. *N Engl J Med*. 2018;378(15):1396-1407.
369. Wright GW, Huang DW, Phelan JD, et al. A probabilistic classification tool for genetic subtypes of diffuse large B cell lymphoma with therapeutic implications. *Cancer Cell*. 2020;37(4):551.e14-568.e14.
370. Lacy SE, Barrans SL, Beer PA, et al. Targeted sequencing in DLBCL, molecular subtypes, and outcomes: a Haematological Malignancy Research Network report. *Blood*. 2020;135(20):1759-1771.
371. Campo E, Jaffe ES, Cook JR, et al. The international consensus classification of mature lymphoid neoplasms: a report from the Clinical Advisory Committee. *Blood*. 2022;140(11):1229-1253.
372. Tousseyn T, De Wolf-Peeters C. T cell/histiocyte-rich large B-cell lymphoma: an update on its biology and classification. *Virchows Arch*. 2011;459(6):557-563.
373. Ramsay AD, Smith WJ, Isaacson PG. T-cell-rich B-cell lymphoma. *Am J Surg Pathol*. 1988;12(6):433-443.
374. Abramson JS. T-cell/histiocyte-rich B-cell lymphoma: biology, diagnosis, and management. *Oncol*. 2006;11(4):384-392.
375. Van Loo P, Tousseyn T, Vanhentenrijk V, et al. T-cell/histiocyte-rich large B-cell lymphoma shows transcriptional features suggestive of a tolerogenic host immune response. *Haematologica*. 2010;95(3):440-448.
376. Oyama T, Yamamoto K, Asano N, et al. Age-related EBV-associated B-cell lymphoproliferative disorders constitute a distinct clinicopathologic group: a study of 96 patients. *Clin Cancer Res*. 2007;13(17):5124-5132.
377. Dojcinov SD, Venkataraman G, Pittaluga S, et al. Age-related EBV-associated lymphoproliferative disorders in the Western population: a spectrum of reactive lymphoid hyperplasia and lymphoma. *Blood*. 2011;117(18):4726-4735.
378. Lo Coco F, Ye BH, Lista F, et al. Rearrangements of the BCL6 gene in diffuse large cell non-Hodgkin's lymphoma. *Blood*. 1994;83(7):1757-1759.
379. Akasaka T, Ueda C, Kurata M, et al. Nonimmunoglobulin (non-Ig)/BCL6 gene fusion in diffuse large B-cell lymphoma results in worse prognosis than Ig/BCL6. *Blood*. 2000;96(8):2907-2909.
380. Iqbal J, Neppalli VT, Wright G, et al. BCL2 expression is a prognostic marker for the activated B-cell-like type of diffuse large B-cell lymphoma. *J Clin Oncol*. 2006;24(6):961-968.
381. Kanungo A, Medeiros LJ, Abruzzo LV, Lin P. Lymphoid neoplasms associated with concurrent t(14;18) and 8q24/c-MYC translocation generally have a poor prognosis. *Mod Pathol*. 2006;19(1):25-33.
382. Tomita N, Tokunaka M, Nakamura N, et al. Clinicopathological features of lymphoma/leukemia patients carrying both BCL2 and MYC translocations. *Haematologica*. 2009;94(7):935-943.
383. Johnson NA, Savage KJ, Ludkovski O, et al. Lymphomas with concurrent BCL2 and MYC translocations: the critical factors associated with survival. *Blood*. 2009;114(11):2273-2279.
384. Aukema SM, Siebert R, Schuuring E, et al. Double-hit B-cell lymphomas. *Blood*. 2011;117(8):2319-2331.
385. Pandolfino TL, Siegel RS, Kuzel TM, Rosen ST, Guitart J. Primary cutaneous B-cell lymphoma: review and current concepts. *J Clin Oncol*. 2000;18(10):2152-2168.
386. Senff NJ, Hoefnagel JJ, Jansen PM, et al. Reclassification of 300 primary cutaneous B-Cell lymphomas according to the new WHO-EORTC classification for cutaneous lymphomas: comparison with previous classifications and identification of prognostic markers. *J Clin Oncol*. 2007;25(12):1581-1587.
387. DiGiuseppe JA, Nelson WG, Seifter EJ, Boitnott JK, Mann RB. Intravascular lymphomatosis: a clinicopathologic study of 10 cases and assessment of response to chemotherapy. *J Clin Oncol*. 1994;12(12):2573-2579.
388. Miller DC, Hochberg FH, Harris NL, Gruber ML, Louis DN, Cohen H. Pathology with clinical correlations of primary central nervous system non-Hodgkin's lymphoma. The Massachusetts General Hospital experience 1958-1989. *Cancer*. 1994;74(4):1383-1397.
389. Salaverria I, Philipp C, Oschlies I, et al. Translocations activating IRF4 identify a subtype of germinal center-derived B-cell lymphoma affecting predominantly children and young adults. *Blood*. 2011;118(1):139-147.
390. Karube K, Guo Y, Suzumiya J, et al. CD10-MUM1+ follicular lymphoma lacks BCL2 gene translocation and shows characteristic biologic and clinical features. *Blood*. 2007;109(7):3076-3079.
391. Traverse-Glehen A, Pittaluga S, Gaulard P, et al. Mediastinal gray zone lymphoma: the missing link between classic Hodgkin's lymphoma and mediastinal large B-cell lymphoma. *Am J Surg Pathol*. 2005;29(11):1411-1421.

392. Gascoyne RD, Lamant L, Martin-Subero JI, et al. ALK-positive diffuse large B-cell lymphoma is associated with Clathrin-ALK rearrangements: report of 6 cases. *Blood*. 2003;102(7):2568-2573.
393. Leroy K, Haioun C, Lepage E, et al. p53 gene mutations are associated with poor survival in low and low-intermediate risk diffuse large B-cell lymphomas. *Ann Oncol*. 2002;13(7):1108-1115.
394. Lossos IS, Morgensztern D. Prognostic biomarkers in diffuse large B-cell lymphoma. *J Clin Oncol*. 2006;24(6):995-1007.
395. Sehn LH, Berry B, Chhanabhai M, et al. The revised International Prognostic Index (R-IPI) is a better predictor of outcome than the standard IPI for patients with diffuse large B-cell lymphoma treated with R-CHOP. *Blood*. 2007;109(5):1857-1861.
396. DeVita VT Jr, Canellos GP, Chabner B, Schein P, Hubbard SP, Young RC. Advanced diffuse histiocytic lymphoma, a potentially curable disease. *Lancet*. 1975;1(7901):248-250.
397. Armitage JO, Fyfe MA, Lewis J. Long-term remission durability and functional status of patients treated for diffuse histiocytic lymphoma with the CHOP regimen. *J Clin Oncol*. 1984;2(8):898-902.
398. Jones SE, Grozea PN, Metz EN, et al. Superiority of adriamycin-containing combination chemotherapy in the treatment of diffuse lymphoma: a Southwest Oncology Group study. *Cancer*. 1979;43(2):417-425.
399. Lee L, Crump M, Khor S, et al. Impact of rituximab on treatment outcomes of patients with diffuse large b-cell lymphoma: a population-based analysis. *Br J Haematol*. 2012;158(4):481-488.
400. Haw R, Sawka CA, Franssen E, Berinstein NL. Significance of a partial or slow response to front-line chemotherapy in the management of intermediate-grade or high-grade non-Hodgkin's lymphoma: a literature review. *J Clin Oncol*. 1994;12(5):1074-1084.
401. Armitage JO, Cheson BD. Interpretation of clinical trials in diffuse large-cell lymphoma. *J Clin Oncol*. 1988;6(8):1335-1347.
402. Longo DL, DeVita VT Jr, Duffey PL, et al. Superiority of ProMACE-CytaBOM over ProMACE-MOPP in the treatment of advanced diffuse aggressive lymphoma: results of a prospective randomized trial. *J Clin Oncol*. 1991;9(1):25-38.
403. Shipp MA, Yeap BY, Harrington DP, et al. The m-BACOD combination chemotherapy regimen in large-cell lymphoma: analysis of the completed trial and comparison with the M-BACOD regimen. *J Clin Oncol*. 1990;8(1):84-93.
404. Fisher RI, Gaynor ER, Dahlberg S, et al. Comparison of a standard regimen (CHOP) with three intensive chemotherapy regimens for advanced non-Hodgkin's lymphoma. *N Engl J Med*. 1993;328(14):1002-1006.
405. Shipp MA. Prognostic factors in aggressive non-Hodgkin's lymphoma: who has "high-risk" disease? *Blood*. 1994;83(5):1165-1173.
406. Waits TM, Greco FA, Greer JP, et al. Effective therapy for poor-prognosis non-Hodgkin's lymphoma with 8 weeks of high-dose-intensity combination chemotherapy. *J Clin Oncol*. 1993;11(5):943-949.
407. Coiffier B, Lepage E, Briere J, et al. CHOP chemotherapy plus rituximab compared with CHOP alone in elderly patients with diffuse large-B-cell lymphoma. *N Engl J Med*. 2002;346(4):235-242.
408. Feugier P, Van Hoof A, Sebban C, et al. Long-term results of the R-CHOP study in the treatment of elderly patients with diffuse large B-cell lymphoma: a study by the Groupe d'Etude des Lymphomes de l'Adulte. *J Clin Oncol*. 2005;23(18):4117-4126.
409. Coiffier B, Thieblemont C, Van Den Neste E, et al. Long-term outcome of patients in the LNH-98.5 trial, the first randomized study comparing rituximab-CHOP to standard CHOP chemotherapy in DLBCL patients: a study by the Groupe d'Etudes des Lymphomes de l'Adulte. *Blood*. 2010;116(12):2040-2045.
410. Habermann TM, Weller EA, Morrison VA, et al. Rituximab-CHOP versus CHOP alone or with maintenance rituximab in older patients with diffuse large B-cell lymphoma. *J Clin Oncol*. 2006;24(19):3121-3127.
411. Pfreundschuh M, Trümper L, Osterborg A, et al. CHOP-like chemotherapy plus rituximab versus CHOP-like chemotherapy alone in young patients with good-prognosis diffuse large-B-cell lymphoma: a randomised controlled trial by the MabThera International Trial (MInT) Group. *Lancet Oncol*. 2006;7(5):379-391.
412. Salles G, de Jong D, Xie W, et al. Prognostic significance of immunohistochemical biomarkers in diffuse large B-cell lymphoma: a study from the Lunenburg Lymphoma Biomarker Consortium. *Blood*. 2011;117(26):7070-7078.
413. Perry AM, Cardesa-Salzmann TM, Meyer PN, et al. A new biologic prognostic model based on immunohistochemistry predicts survival in patients with diffuse large B-cell lymphoma. *Blood*. 2012;120(11):2290-2296.
414. Alizadeh AA, Gentles AJ, Alencar AJ, et al. Prediction of survival in diffuse large B-cell lymphoma based on the expression of 2 genes reflecting tumor and microenvironment. *Blood*. 2011;118(5):1350-1358.
415. Cabanillas F, Rodriguez-Diaz Pavón J, Hagemeister FB, et al. Alternating triple therapy for the treatment of intermediate grade and immunoblastic lymphoma. *Ann Oncol*. 1998;9(5):511-518.
416. Fridrik MA, Hausmaninger H, Linkesch W, et al. CEOP-IMVP-Dexa in the treatment of aggressive lymphomas: an Austrian multicenter trial. *J Clin Oncol*. 1996;14(1):227-232.
417. Wilson WH, Grossbard ML, Pittaluga S, et al. Dose-adjusted EPOCH chemotherapy for untreated large B-cell lymphomas: a pharmacodynamic approach with high efficacy. *Blood*. 2002;99(8):2685-2693.
418. Bartlett NL, Wilson WH, Jung SH, et al. Dose-adjusted EPOCH-R compared with R-CHOP as frontline therapy for diffuse large B-cell lymphoma: clinical outcomes of the phase III intergroup trial Alliance/CALGB 50303. *J Clin Oncol*. 2019;37(21):1790-1799.
419. Howlett C, Snedecor SJ, Landsburg DJ, et al. Front-line, dose-escalated immunochemotherapy is associated with a significant progression-free survival advantage in patients with double-hit lymphomas: a systematic review and meta-analysis. *Br J Haematol*. 2015;170(4):504-514.
420. Landsburg DJ, Falkiewicz MK, Maly J, et al. Outcomes of patients with double-hit lymphoma who achieve first complete remission. *J Clin Oncol*. 2017;35(20):2260-2267.
421. Pfreundschuh M, Trümper L, Kloess M, et al. Two-weekly or 3-weekly CHOP chemotherapy with or without etoposide for the treatment of elderly patients with aggressive lymphomas: results of the NHL-B2 trial of the DSHNHL. *Blood*. 2004;104(3):634-641.
422. Pfreundschuh M, Trümper L, Kloess M, et al. Two-weekly or 3-weekly CHOP chemotherapy with or without etoposide for the treatment of young patients with good-prognosis (normal LDH) aggressive lymphomas: results of the NHL-B1 trial of the DSHNHL. *Blood*. 2004;104(3):626-633.
423. Cunningham D, Smith P, Mouncey P, et al. A phase III trial comparing R-CHOP 14 and R-CHOP 21 for the treatment of patients with newly diagnosed diffuse large B-cell non-Hodgkin's lymphoma. *J Clin Oncol*. 2009;27(15 suppl):8506.
424. Delarue R, Tilly H, Mounier N, et al. Dose-dense rituximab-CHOP compared with standard rituximab-CHOP in elderly patients with diffuse large B-cell lymphoma (the LNH03-6B study): a randomised phase 3 trial. *Lancet Oncol*. 2013;14(6):525-533.
425. Gisselbrecht C, Lepage E, Molina T, et al. Shortened first-line high-dose chemotherapy for patients with poor-prognosis aggressive lymphoma. *J Clin Oncol*. 2002;20(10):2472-2479.
426. Oliansky DM, Czuczman M, Fisher RI, et al. The role of cytotoxic therapy with hematopoietic stem cell transplantation in the treatment of diffuse large B cell lymphoma: update of the 2001 evidence-based review. *Biol Blood Marrow Transplant*. 2011;17(1):20.e30-47.e30.
427. Vitolo U, Trněný M, Belada D, et al. Obinutuzumab or rituximab plus cyclophosphamide, doxorubicin, vincristine, and prednisone in previously untreated diffuse large B-cell lymphoma. *J Clin Oncol*. 2017;35(31):3529-3537.
428. Younes A, Sehn LH, Johnson P, et al. Randomized phase III trial of ibrutinib and rituximab plus cyclophosphamide, doxorubicin, vincristine, and prednisone in non-germinal center B-cell diffuse large B-cell lymphoma. *J Clin Oncol*. 2019;37(15):1285-1295.
429. Tilly H, Morschhauser F, Sehn LH, et al. Polatuzumab vedotin in previously untreated diffuse large B-cell lymphoma. *N Engl J Med*. 2022;386(4):351-363.
430. Stephens DM, Li H, LeBlanc ML, et al. Continued risk of relapse independent of treatment modality in limited-stage diffuse large B-cell lymphoma: final and long-term analysis of southwest oncology group study S8736. *J Clin Oncol*. 2016;34(25):2997-3004.
431. Poeschel V, Held G, Ziepert M, et al. Four versus six cycles of CHOP chemotherapy in combination with six applications of rituximab in patients with aggressive B-cell lymphoma with favourable prognosis (FLYER): a randomised, phase 3, non-inferiority trial. *Lancet*. 2019;394(10216):2271-2281.
432. Lamy T, Damaj G, Soubeyran P, et al. R-CHOP 14 with or without radiotherapy in nonbulky limited-stage diffuse large B-cell lymphoma. *Blood*. 2018;131(2):174-181.
433. Persky DO, Li H, Stephens DM, et al. Positron emission tomography-directed therapy for patients with limited-stage diffuse large B-cell lymphoma: results of Intergroup National Clinical Trials Network study S1001. *J Clin Oncol*. 2020;38(26):3003-3011.
434. Maurer MJ, Ghesquieres H, Jais JP, et al. Event-free survival at 24 months is a robust end point for disease-related outcome in diffuse large B-cell lymphoma treated with immunochemotherapy. *J Clin Oncol*. 2014;32(10):1066-1073.
435. Crump M, Neelapu SS, Farooq U, et al. Outcomes in refractory diffuse large B-cell lymphoma: results from the international SCHOLAR-1 study. *Blood*. 2017;130(16):1800-1808.
436. Germann N, Brienza S, Rotarski M, et al. Preliminary results on the activity of oxaliplatin (L-OHP) in refractory/recurrent non-Hodgkin's lymphoma patients. *Ann Oncol*. 1999;10(3):351-354.
437. López A, Gutiérrez A, Palacios A, et al. GEMOX-R regimen is a highly effective salvage regimen in patients with refractory/relapsing diffuse large-cell lymphoma: a phase II study. *Eur J Haematol*. 2008;80(2):127-132.
438. Zinzani PL, Baliva G, Magagnoli M, et al. Gemcitabine treatment in pretreated cutaneous T-cell lymphoma: experience in 44 patients. *J Clin Oncol*. 2000;18(13):2603-2606.
439. Ng M, Waters J, Cunningham D, et al. Gemcitabine, cisplatin and methylprednisolone (GEM-P) is an effective salvage regimen in patients with relapsed and refractory lymphoma. *Br J Cancer*. 2005;92(8):1352-1357.
440. Papageorgiou ES, Tsirigotis P, Dimopoulos M, et al. Combination chemotherapy with gemcitabine and vinorelbine in the treatment of relapsed or refractory diffuse large B-cell lymphoma: a phase-II trial by the Hellenic Cooperative Oncology Group. *Eur J Haematol*. 2005;75(2):124-129.
441. Crump M, Kuruvilla J, Couban S, et al. Randomized comparison of gemcitabine, dexamethasone, and cisplatin versus dexamethasone, cytarabine, and cisplatin chemotherapy before autologous stem-cell transplantation for relapsed and refractory aggressive lymphomas: NCIC-CTG LY.12. *J Clin Oncol*. 2014;32(31):3490-3496.
442. Abramson JS, Palomba ML, Gordon LI, et al. Lisocabtagene maraleucel for patients with relapsed or refractory large B-cell lymphomas (TRANSCEND NHL 001): a multicentre seamless design study. *Lancet*. 2020;396(10254):839-852.
443. Neelapu SS, Locke FL, Bartlett NL, et al. Axicabtagene ciloleucel CAR T-cell therapy in refractory large B-cell lymphoma. *N Engl J Med*. 2017;377(26):2531-2544.
444. Schuster SJ, Bishop MR, Tam CS, et al. Tisagenlecleucel in adult relapsed or refractory diffuse large B-cell lymphoma. *N Engl J Med*. 2019;380(1):45-56.
445. Westin J, Sehn LH. CAR T cells as a second-line therapy for large B-cell lymphoma: a paradigm shift? *Blood*. 2022;139(18):2737-2746.
446. Bishop MR, Dickinson M, Purtill D, et al. Second-line tisagenlecleucel or standard care in aggressive B-cell lymphoma. *N Engl J Med*. 2022;386(7):629-639.

447. Kamdar M, Solomon SR, Arnason J, et al. Lisocabtagene maraleucel versus standard of care with salvage chemotherapy followed by autologous stem cell transplantation as second-line treatment in patients with relapsed or refractory large B-cell lymphoma (TRANSFORM): results from an interim analysis of an open-label, randomised, phase 3 trial. *Lancet.* 2022;399(10343):2294-2308.
448. Locke FL, Miklos DB, Jacobson CA, et al. Axicabtagene ciloleucel as second-line therapy for large B-cell lymphoma. *N Engl J Med.* 2022;386(7):640-654.
449. Roschewski M, Longo DL, Wilson WH. CAR T-cell therapy for large B-cell lymphoma – who, when, and how? *N Engl J Med.* 2022;386(7):692-696.
450. Salles G, Duell J, Gonzalez Barca E, et al. Tafasitamab plus lenalidomide in relapsed or refractory diffuse large B-cell lymphoma (L-MIND): a multicentre, prospective, single-arm, phase 2 study. *Lancet Oncol.* 2020;21(7):978-988.
451. Duell J, Maddocks KJ, Gonzalez-Barca E, et al. Long-term outcomes from the Phase II L-MIND study of tafasitamab (MOR208) plus lenalidomide in patients with relapsed or refractory diffuse large B-cell lymphoma. *Haematologica.* 2021;106(9):2417-2426.
452. Sehn LH, Herrera AF, Flowers CR, et al. Polatuzumab vedotin in relapsed or refractory diffuse large B-cell lymphoma. *J Clin Oncol.* 2020;38(2):155-165.
453. Caimi PF, Ai W, Alderuccio JP, et al. Loncastuximab tesirine in relapsed or refractory diffuse large B-cell lymphoma (LOTIS-2): a multicentre, open-label, single-arm, phase 2 trial. *Lancet Oncol.* 2021;22(6):790-800.
454. Zinzani PL, Quaglino P, Violetti SA, et al. Critical concepts and management recommendations for cutaneous T-cell lymphoma: a consensus-based position paper from the Italian Group of Cutaneous Lymphoma. *Hematol Oncol.* 2021;39(3):275-283.
455. Zinzani PL, Piccaluga PP. Primary mediastinal DLBCL: evolving biologic understanding and therapeutic strategies. *Curr Oncol Rep.* 2011;13(5):407-415.
456. Aisenberg AC. Primary large cell lymphoma of the mediastinum. *Semin Oncol.* 1999;26(3):251-258.
457. Joos S, Otaño-Joos MI, Ziegler S, et al. Primary mediastinal (thymic) B-cell lymphoma is characterized by gains of chromosomal material including 9p and amplification of the REL gene. *Blood.* 1996;87(4):1571-1578.
458. Copie-Bergman C, Gaulard P, Maouche-Chrétien L, et al. The MAL gene is expressed in primary mediastinal large B-cell lymphoma. *Blood.* 1999;94(10):3567-3575.
459. Savage KJ, Monti S, Kutok JL, et al. The molecular signature of mediastinal large B-cell lymphoma differs from that of other diffuse large B-cell lymphomas and shares features with classical Hodgkin lymphoma. *Blood.* 2003;102(12):3871-3879.
460. Feuerhake F, Kutok JL, Monti S, et al. NFkappaB activity, function, and target-gene signatures in primary mediastinal large B-cell lymphoma and diffuse large B-cell lymphoma subtypes. *Blood.* 2005;106(4):1392-1399.
461. Zinzani PL, Ribrag V, Moskowitz CH, et al. Safety and tolerability of pembrolizumab in patients with relapsed/refractory primary mediastinal large B-cell lymphoma. *Blood.* 2017;130(3):267-270.
462. Armand P, Rodig S, Melnichenko V, et al. Pembrolizumab in relapsed or refractory primary mediastinal large B-cell lymphoma. *J Clin Oncol.* 2019;37(34):3291-3299.
463. van Besien K, Kelta M, Bahaguna P. Primary mediastinal B-cell lymphoma: a review of pathology and management. *J Clin Oncol.* 2001;19(6):1855-1864.
464. Camus V, Rossi C, Sesques P, et al. Outcomes after first-line immunochemotherapy for primary mediastinal B-cell lymphoma: a LYSA study. *Blood Adv.* 2021;5(19):3862-3872.
465. Broccoli A, Casadei B, Stefoni V, et al. The treatment of primary mediastinal large B-cell lymphoma: a two decades monocentric experience with 98 patients. *BMC Cancer.* 2017;17(1):276.
466. Dunleavy K, Pittaluga S, Maeda LS, et al. Dose-adjusted EPOCH-rituximab therapy in primary mediastinal B-cell lymphoma. *N Engl J Med.* 2013;368(15):1408-1416.
467. Sehn LH, Antin JH, Shulman LN, et al. Primary diffuse large B-cell lymphoma of the mediastinum: outcome following high-dose chemotherapy and autologous hematopoietic cell transplantation. *Blood.* 1998;91(2):717-723.
468. Weisenburger DD, Armitage JO. Mantle cell lymphoma—an entity comes of age. *Blood.* 1996;87(11):4483-4494.
469. Banks PM, Chan J, Cleary ML, et al. Mantle cell lymphoma. A proposal for unification of morphologic, immunologic, and molecular data. *Am J Surg Pathol.* 1992;16(7):637-640.
470. Swerdlow SH, Williams ME. From centrocytic to mantle cell lymphoma: a clinicopathologic and molecular review of 3 decades. *Hum Pathol.* 2002;33(1):7-20.
471. Decaudin D. Mantle cell lymphoma: a biological and therapeutic paradigm. *Leuk Lymphoma.* 2002;43(4):773-781.
472. Andersen NS, Jensen MK, de Nully Brown P, Geisler CH. A Danish population-based analysis of 105 mantle cell lymphoma patients: incidences, clinical features, response, survival and prognostic factors. *Eur J Cancer.* 2002;38(3):401-408.
473. Gill S, Herbert KE, Prince HM, et al. Mantle cell lymphoma with central nervous system involvement: frequency and clinical features. *Br J Haematol.* 2009;147(1):83-88.
474. de Boer CJ, Schuuring E, Dreef E, et al. Cyclin D1 protein analysis in the diagnosis of mantle cell lymphoma. *Blood.* 1995;86(7):2715-2723.
475. Wlodarska I, Dierickx D, Vanhentenrijk V, et al. Translocations targeting CCND2, CCND3, and MYCN do occur in t(11;14)-negative mantle cell lymphomas. *Blood.* 2008;111(12):5683-5690.
476. Stilgenbauer S, Winkler D, Ott G, et al. Molecular characterization of 11q deletions points to a pathogenic role of the ATM gene in mantle cell lymphoma. *Blood.* 1999;94(9):3262-3264.
477. Martinez-Climent JA, Vizcarra E, Sanchez D, et al. Loss of a novel tumor suppressor gene locus at chromosome 8p is associated with leukemic mantle cell lymphoma. *Blood.* 2001;98(12):3479-3482.
478. Martin P, Chadburn A, Christos P, et al. Outcome of deferred initial therapy in mantle-cell lymphoma. *J Clin Oncol.* 2009;27(8):1209-1213.
479. Fernàndez V, Salamero O, Espinet B, et al. Genomic and gene expression profiling defines indolent forms of mantle cell lymphoma. *Cancer Res.* 2010;70(4):1408-1418.
480. Bea S, Valdes-Mas R, Navarro A, et al. Landscape of somatic mutations and clonal evolution in mantle cell lymphoma. *Proc Natl Acad Sci U S A.* 2013;110(45):18250-18255.
481. Zhang J, Jima D, Moffitt AB, et al. The genomic landscape of mantle cell lymphoma is related to the epigenetically determined chromatin state of normal B cells. *Blood.* 2014;123(19):2988-2996.
482. Silkenstedt E, Linton K, Dreyling M. Mantle cell lymphoma - advances in molecular biology, prognostication and treatment approaches. *Br J Haematol.* 2021;195(2):162-173.
483. Pararajalingam P, Coyle KM, Arthur SE, et al. Coding and noncoding drivers of mantle cell lymphoma identified through exome and genome sequencing. *Blood.* 2020;136(5):572-584.
484. Eskelund CW, Dahl C, Hansen JW, et al. TP53 mutations identify younger mantle cell lymphoma patients who do not benefit from intensive chemoimmunotherapy. *Blood.* 2017;130(17):1903-1910.
485. Kridel R, Meissner B, Rogic S, et al. Whole transcriptome sequencing reveals recurrent NOTCH1 mutations in mantle cell lymphoma. *Blood.* 2012;119(9):1963-1971.
486. Hartmann EM, Campo E, Wright G, et al. Pathway discovery in mantle cell lymphoma by integrated analysis of high-resolution gene expression and copy number profiling. *Blood.* 2010;116(6):953-961.
487. Zhao JJ, Lin J, Lwin T, et al. microRNA expression profile and identification of miR-29 as a prognostic marker and pathogenetic factor by targeting CDK6 in mantle cell lymphoma. *Blood.* 2010;115(13):2630-2639.
488. Iqbal J, Shen Y, Liu Y, et al. Genome-wide miRNA profiling of mantle cell lymphoma reveals a distinct subgroup with poor prognosis. *Blood.* 2012;119(21):4939-4948.
489. Hoster E, Dreyling M, Klapper W, et al. A new prognostic index (MIPI) for patients with advanced-stage mantle cell lymphoma. *Blood.* 2008;111(2):558-565.
490. Chihara D, Cheah CY, Westin JR, et al. Rituximab plus hyper-CVAD alternating with MTX/Ara-C in patients with newly diagnosed mantle cell lymphoma: 15-year follow-up of a phase II study from the MD Anderson Cancer Center. *Br J Haematol.* 2016;172(1):80-88.
491. Romaguera JE, Fayad LE, Feng L, et al. Ten-year follow-up after intense chemoimmunotherapy with Rituximab-HyperCVAD alternating with Rituximab-high dose methotrexate/cytarabine (R-MA) and without stem cell transplantation in patients with untreated aggressive mantle cell lymphoma. *Br J Haematol.* 2010;150(2):200-208.
492. Merli F, Luminari S, Ilariucci F, et al. Rituximab plus HyperCVAD alternating with high dose cytarabine and methotrexate for the initial treatment of patients with mantle cell lymphoma, a multicentre trial from Gruppo Italiano Studio Linfomi. *Br J Haematol.* 2012;156(3):346-353.
493. Hermine O, Hoster E, Walewski J, et al. Addition of high-dose cytarabine to immunochemotherapy before autologous stem-cell transplantation in patients aged 65 years or younger with mantle cell lymphoma (MCL Younger): a randomised, open-label, phase 3 trial of the European Mantle Cell Lymphoma Network. *Lancet.* 2016;388(10044):565-575.
494. Hermine O, Jiang L, Walewski J, et al. Addition of high-dose cytarabine to immunochemotherapy before autologous stem-cell transplantation in patients aged 65 years or younger with mantle cell lymphoma (MCL younger): a long-term follow-up of the randomized, open-label, phase 3 trial of the European Mantle Cell Lymphoma Network. *Blood.* 2021;138(suppl 1):380.
495. Pott C, Hoster E, Delfau-Larue MH, et al. Molecular remission is an independent predictor of clinical outcome in patients with mantle cell lymphoma after combined immunochemotherapy: a European MCL intergroup study. *Blood.* 2010;115(16):3215-3223.
496. Kluin-Nelemans HC, Hoster E, Hermine O, et al. Treatment of older patients with mantle cell lymphoma (MCL): long-term follow-up of the randomized European MCL elderly trial. *J Clin Oncol.* 2020;38(3):248-256.
497. Le Gouill S, Kröger N, Dhedin N, et al. Reduced-intensity conditioning allogeneic stem cell transplantation for relapsed/refractory mantle cell lymphoma: a multicenter experience. *Ann Oncol.* 2012;23(10):2695-2703.
498. Le Gouill S, Thieblemont C, Oberic L, et al. Rituximab after autologous stem-cell transplantation in mantle-cell lymphoma. *N Engl J Med.* 2017;377(13):1250-1260.
499. Rummel MJ, Knauf W, Goerner M, et al. Two years rituximab maintenance vs. observation after first-line treatment with bendamustine plus rituximab (B-R) in patients with mantle cell lymphoma: first results of a prospective, randomized, multicenter phase II study (a subgroup study of the StiL NHL7-2008 MAINTAIN trial). *J Clin Oncol.* 2016;34(15 suppl):7503.
500. Hill BT, Switchenko JM, Martin P, et al. Maintenance rituximab improves outcomes in mantle cell lymphoma patients who respond to induction therapy with bendamustine + rituximab without autologous transplant. *Blood.* 2019;134(suppl 1):1525.
501. Wang ML, Jurczak W, Jerkeman M, et al. Ibrutinib plus bendamustine and rituximab in untreated mantle-cell lymphoma. *N Engl J Med.* 2022;386(26):2482-2494.
502. Fisher RI, Bernstein SH, Kahl BS, et al. Multicenter phase II study of bortezomib in patients with relapsed or refractory mantle cell lymphoma. *J Clin Oncol.* 2006;24(30):4867-4874.
503. Robak T, Huang H, Jin J, et al. Bortezomib-based therapy for newly diagnosed mantle-cell lymphoma. *N Engl J Med.* 2015;372(10):944-953.
504. Yamshon S, Martin P, Shah B, et al. Initial treatment with lenalidomide plus rituximab for mantle cell lymphoma (MCL): 7-year analysis from a multi-center phase II study. *Blood.* 2020;136(supplement 1):45-46.
505. Ruan J, Martin P, Shah B, et al. Lenalidomide plus rituximab as initial treatment for mantle-cell lymphoma. *N Engl J Med.* 2015;373(19):1835-1844.
506. Eyre TA, Cheah CY, Wang ML. Therapeutic options for relapsed/refractory mantle cell lymphoma. *Blood.* 2022;139(5):666-677.
507. Dreyling M, Jurczak W, Jerkeman M, et al. Ibrutinib versus temsirolimus in patients with relapsed or refractory mantle-cell lymphoma: an international, randomised, open-label, phase 3 study. *Lancet.* 2016;387(10020):770-778.

508. Rule S, Dreyling M, Goy A, et al. Ibrutinib for the treatment of relapsed/refractory mantle cell lymphoma: extended 3.5-year follow up from a pooled analysis. *Haematologica*. 2019;104(5):e211-e214.
509. Wang M, Munoz J, Goy A, et al. KTE-X19 CAR T-cell therapy in relapsed or refractory mantle-cell lymphoma. *N Engl J Med*. 2020;382(14):1331-1342.
510. Wang M, Munoz J, Goy A, et al. Three-year follow-up of KTE-X19 in patients with relapsed/refractory mantle cell lymphoma, including high-risk subgroups, in the ZUMA-2 study. *J Clin Oncol*. 2023;41(3):555-567.
511. Maris MB, Sandmaier BM, Storer BE, et al. Allogeneic hematopoietic cell transplantation after fludarabine and 2 Gy total body irradiation for relapsed and refractory mantle cell lymphoma. *Blood*. 2004;104(12):3535-3542.
512. Boerma EG, van Imhoff GW, Appel IM, Veeger NJGM, Kluin PM, Kluin-Nelemans JC. Gender and age-related differences in Burkitt lymphoma – epidemiological and clinical data from the Netherlands. *Eur J Cancer*. 2004;40(18):2781-2787.
513. Mukhtar F, Boffetta P, Risch HA, et al. Survival predictors of Burkitt's lymphoma in children, adults and elderly in the United States during 2000-2013. *Int J Cancer*. 2017;140(7):1494-1502.
514. Linch DC. Burkitt lymphoma in adults. *Br J Haematol*. 2012;156(6):693-703.
515. Dave SS, Fu K, Wright GW, et al. Molecular diagnosis of Burkitt's lymphoma. *N Engl J Med*. 2006;354(23):2431-2442.
516. Hummel M, Bentink S, Berger H, et al. A biologic definition of Burkitt's lymphoma from transcriptional and genomic profiling. *N Engl J Med*. 2006;354(23):2419-2430.
517. Blum KA, Lozanski G, Byrd JC. Adult Burkitt leukemia and lymphoma. *Blood*. 2004;104(10):3009-3020.
518. Roschewski M, Dunleavy K, Abramson JS, et al. Multicenter study of risk-adapted therapy with dose-adjusted EPOCH-R in adults with untreated Burkitt lymphoma. *J Clin Oncol*. 2020;38(22):2519-2529.
519. Hoelzer D, Walewski J, Döhner H, et al. Improved outcome of adult Burkitt lymphoma/leukemia with rituximab and chemotherapy: report of a large prospective multicenter trial. *Blood*. 2014;124(26):3870-3879.
520. Corazzelli G, Frigeri F, Russo F, et al. RD-CODOX-M/IVAC with rituximab and intrathecal liposomal cytarabine in adult Burkitt lymphoma and 'unclassifiable' highly aggressive B-cell lymphoma. *Br J Haematol*. 2012;156(2):234-244.
521. Mead GM, Barrans SL, Qian W, et al. A prospective clinicopathologic study of dose-modified CODOX-M/IVAC in patients with sporadic Burkitt lymphoma defined using cytogenetic and immunophenotypic criteria (MRC/NCRI LY10 trial). *Blood*. 2008;112(6):2248-2260.
522. Thomas DA, Faderl S, O'Brien S, et al. Chemoimmunotherapy with hyper-CVAD plus rituximab for the treatment of adult Burkitt and Burkitt-type lymphoma or acute lymphoblastic leukemia. *Cancer*. 2006;106(7):1569-1580.
523. Soussain C, Patte C, Ostronoff M, et al. Small noncleaved cell lymphoma and leukemia in adults. A retrospective study of 65 adults treated with the LMB pediatric protocols. *Blood*. 1995;85(3):664-674.
524. Gerrard M, Cairo MS, Weston C, et al. Excellent survival following two courses of COPAD chemotherapy in children and adolescents with resected localized B-cell non-Hodgkin's lymphoma: results of the FAB/LMB 96 international study. *Br J Haematol*. 2008;141(6):840-847.
525. Magrath I, Adde M, Shad A, et al. Adults and children with small non-cleaved-cell lymphoma have a similar excellent outcome when treated with the same chemotherapy regimen. *J Clin Oncol*. 1996;14(3):925-934.
526. Lacasce A, Howard O, Lib S, et al. Modified magrath regimens for adults with Burkitt and Burkitt-like lymphomas: preserved efficacy with decreased toxicity. *Leuk Lymphoma*. 2004;45(4):761-767.
527. Cortes J, Thomas D, Rios A, et al. Hyperfractionated cyclophosphamide, vincristine, doxorubicin, and dexamethasone and highly active antiretroviral therapy for patients with acquired immunodeficiency syndrome-related Burkitt lymphoma/leukemia. *Cancer*. 2002;94(5):1492-1499.
528. Kaplan LD, Lee JY, Ambinder RF, et al. Rituximab does not improve clinical outcome in a randomized phase 3 trial of CHOP with or without rituximab in patients with HIV-associated non-Hodgkin lymphoma: AIDS-Malignancies Consortium Trial 010. *Blood*. 2005;106(5):1538-1543.
529. Dunleavy K, Little RF, Pittaluga S, et al. The role of tumor histogenesis, FDG-PET, and short-course EPOCH with dose-dense rituximab (SC-EPOCH-RR) in HIV-associated diffuse large B-cell lymphoma. *Blood*. 2010;115(15):3017-3024.
530. Sweetenham JW, Pearce R, Taghipour G, Blaise D, Gisselbrecht C, Goldstone AH. Adult Burkitt's and Burkitt-like non-Hodgkin's lymphoma – outcome for patients treated with high-dose therapy and autologous stem-cell transplantation in first remission or at relapse: results from the European Group for Blood and Marrow Transplantation. *J Clin Oncol*. 1996;14(9):2465-2472.
531. Ahmed SO, Sureda A, Aljurf M. The role of hematopoietic SCT in adult Burkitt lymphoma. *Bone Marrow Transplant*. 2013;48(5):617-629.
532. Portell CA, Sweetenham JW. Adult lymphoblastic lymphoma. *Cancer J*. 2012;18(5):432-438.
533. Lin P, Jones D, Dorfman DM, Medeiros LJ. Precursor B-cell lymphoblastic lymphoma: a predominantly extranodal tumor with low propensity for leukemic involvement. *Am J Surg Pathol*. 2000;24(11):1480-1490.
534. Baleydier F, Decouvelaere AV, Bergeron J, et al. T cell receptor genotyping and HOXA/TLX1 expression define three T lymphoblastic lymphoma subsets which might affect clinical outcome. *Clin Cancer Res*. 2008;14(3):692-700.
535. Taylor J, Xiao W, Abdel-Wahab O. Diagnosis and classification of hematologic malignancies on the basis of genetics. *Blood*. 2017;130(4):410-423.
536. Sulis ML, Williams O, Palomero T, et al. NOTCH1 extracellular juxtamembrane expansion mutations in T-ALL. *Blood*. 2008;112(3):733-740.
537. Callens C, Baleydier F, Lengline E, et al. Clinical impact of NOTCH1 and/or FBXW7 mutations, FLASH deletion, and TCR status in pediatric T-cell lymphoblastic lymphoma. *J Clin Oncol*. 2012;30(16):1966-1973.
538. Aguiar RC, Chase A, Coulthard S, et al. Abnormalities of chromosome band 8p11 in leukemia: two clinical syndromes can be distinguished on the basis of MOZ involvement. *Blood*. 1997;90(8):3130-3135.
539. Thandla S, Alashari M, Green DM, Aplan PD. Therapy-related T cell lymphoblastic lymphoma with t(11;19)(q23;p13) and MLL gene rearrangement. *Leukemia*. 1999;13(12):2116-2118.
540. Litzow MR, Ferrando AA. How I treat T-cell acute lymphoblastic leukemia in adults. *Blood*. 2015;126(7):833-841.
541. Hoelzer D, Gökbuget N, Digel W, et al. Outcome of adult patients with T-lymphoblastic lymphoma treated according to protocols for acute lymphoblastic leukemia. *Blood*. 2002;99(12):4379-4385.
542. DeAngelo DJ, Stevenson KE, Dahlberg SE, et al. Long-term outcome of a pediatric-inspired regimen used for adults aged 18-50 years with newly diagnosed acute lymphoblastic leukemia. *Leukemia*. 2015;29(3):526-534.
543. Hocking J, Schwarer AP, Gasiorowski R, et al. Excellent outcomes for adolescents and adults with acute lymphoblastic leukemia and lymphoma without allogeneic stem cell transplant: the FRALLE-93 pediatric protocol. *Leuk Lymphoma*. 2014;55(12):2801-2807.
544. Cortelazzo S, Intermesoli T, Oldani E, et al. Results of a lymphoblastic leukemia-like chemotherapy program with risk-adapted mediastinal irradiation and stem cell transplantation for adult patients with lymphoblastic lymphoma. *Ann Hematol*. 2012;91(1):73-82.
545. Stock W, La M, Sanford B, et al. What determines the outcomes for adolescents and young adults with acute lymphoblastic leukemia treated on cooperative group protocols? A comparison of Children's Cancer Group and Cancer and Leukemia Group B studies. *Blood*. 2008;112(5):1646-1654.
546. Hunault M, Truchan-Graczyk M, Caillot D, et al. Outcome of adult T-lymphoblastic lymphoma after acute lymphoblastic leukemia-type treatment: a GOELAMS trial. *Haematologica*. 2007;92(12):1623-1630.
547. Berg SL, Blaney SM, Devidas M, et al. Phase II study of nelarabine (compound 506U78) in children and young adults with refractory T-cell malignancies: a report from the Children's Oncology Group. *J Clin Oncol*. 2005;23(15):3376-3382.
548. Gökbuget N, Basara N, Baurmann H, et al. High single-drug activity of nelarabine in relapsed T-lymphoblastic leukemia/lymphoma offers curative option with subsequent stem cell transplantation. *Blood*. 2011;118(13):3504-3511.
549. Commander LA, Seif AE, Insogna IG, Rheingold SR. Salvage therapy with nelarabine, etoposide, and cyclophosphamide in relapsed/refractory paediatric T-cell lymphoblastic leukaemia and lymphoma. *Br J Haematol*. 2010;150(3):345-351.
550. Jain P, Kantarjian H, Ravandi F, et al. The combination of hyper-CVAD plus nelarabine as frontline therapy in adult T-cell acute lymphoblastic leukemia and T-lymphoblastic lymphoma: MD Anderson Cancer Center experience. *Leukemia*. 2014;28(4):973-975.
551. Jeha S, Gandhi V, Chan KW, et al. Clofarabine, a novel nucleoside analog, is active in pediatric patients with advanced leukemia. *Blood*. 2004;103(3):784-789.
552. Barba P, Sampol A, Calbacho M, et al. Clofarabine-based chemotherapy for relapsed/refractory adult acute lymphoblastic leukemia and lymphoblastic lymphoma. The Spanish experience. *Am J Hematol*. 2012;87(6):631-634.
553. Papayannidis C, DeAngelo DJ, Stock W, et al. A Phase 1 study of the novel gamma-secretase inhibitor PF-03084014 in patients with T-cell acute lymphoblastic leukemia and T-cell lymphoblastic lymphoma. *Blood Cancer J*. 2015;5(9):e350.
554. Bertaina A, Vinti L, Strocchio L, et al. The combination of bortezomib with chemotherapy to treat relapsed/refractory acute lymphoblastic leukaemia of childhood. *Br J Haematol*. 2017;176(4):629-636.
555. De Keersmaecker K, Lahortiga I, Mentens N, et al. In vitro validation of gamma-secretase inhibitors alone or in combination with other anti-cancer drugs for the treatment of T-cell acute lymphoblastic leukemia. *Haematologica*. 2008;93(4):533-542.
556. Foss FM, Zinzani PL, Vose JM, Gascoyne RD, Rosen ST, Tobinai K. Peripheral T-cell lymphoma. *Blood*. 2011;117(25):6756-6767.
557. Zain JM, Hanona P. Aggressive T-cell lymphomas: 2021 Updates on diagnosis, risk stratification and management. *Am J Hematol*. 2021;96(8):1027-1046.
558. Sethi TK, Montanari F, Foss F, Reddy N. How we treat advanced stage cutaneous T-cell lymphoma – mycosis fungoides and Sézary syndrome. *Br J Haematol*. 2021;195(3):352-364.
559. Vose J, Armitage J, Weisenburger D; International T-Cell Lymphoma Project. International peripheral T-cell and natural killer/T-cell lymphoma study: pathology findings and clinical outcomes. *J Clin Oncol*. 2008;26(25):4124-4130.
560. Schlegelberger B, Himmler A, Gödde E, Grote W, Feller AC, Lennert K. Cytogenetic findings in peripheral T-cell lymphomas as a basis for distinguishing low-grade and high-grade lymphomas. *Blood*. 1994;83(2):505-511.
561. Feldman AL, Law M, Remstein ED, et al. Recurrent translocations involving the IRF4 oncogene locus in peripheral T-cell lymphomas. *Leukemia*. 2009;23(3):574-580.
562. Feldman AL, Dogan A, Smith DI, et al. Discovery of recurrent t(6;7)(p25.3;q32.3) translocations in ALK-negative anaplastic large cell lymphomas by massively parallel genomic sequencing. *Blood*. 2011;117(3):915-919.
563. Iqbal J, Wright G, Wang C, et al. Gene expression signatures delineate biological and prognostic subgroups in peripheral T-cell lymphoma. *Blood*. 2014;123(19):2915-2923.
564. Duyster J, Bai RY, Morris SW. Translocations involving anaplastic lymphoma kinase (ALK). *Oncogene*. 2001;20(40):5623-5637.
565. Stein H, Foss HD, Dürkop H, et al. CD30(+) anaplastic large cell lymphoma: a review of its histopathologic, genetic, and clinical features. *Blood*. 2000;96(12):3681-3695.
566. Hapgood G, Savage KJ. The biology and management of systemic anaplastic large cell lymphoma. *Blood*. 2015;126(1):17-25.

567. Savage KJ, Harris NL, Vose JM, et al. ALK- anaplastic large-cell lymphoma is clinically and immunophenotypically different from both ALK+ ALCL and peripheral T-cell lymphoma, not otherwise specified: report from the International Peripheral T-Cell Lymphoma Project. *Blood*. 2008;111(12):5496-5504.

568. Schlette EJ, Medeiros LJ, Goy A, Lai R, Rassidakis GZ. Survivin expression predicts poorer prognosis in anaplastic large-cell lymphoma. *J Clin Oncol*. 2004;22(9):1682-1688.

569. Parrilla Castellar ER, Jaffe ES, Said JW, et al. ALK-negative anaplastic large cell lymphoma is a genetically heterogeneous disease with widely disparate clinical outcomes. *Blood*. 2014;124(9):1473-1480.

570. Boi M, Rinaldi A, Kwee I, et al. PRDM1/BLIMP1 is commonly inactivated in anaplastic large T-cell lymphoma. *Blood*. 2013;122(15):2683-2693.

571. Agnelli L, Mereu E, Pellegrino E, et al. Identification of a 3-gene model as a powerful diagnostic tool for the recognition of ALK-negative anaplastic large-cell lymphoma. *Blood*. 2012;120(6):1274-1281.

572. Rosen ST, Querfeld C. Primary cutaneous T-cell lymphomas. *Hematology Am Soc Hematol Educ Program*. 2006;2006:323-330.

573. de Jong D, Vasmel WLE, de Boer JP, et al. Anaplastic large-cell lymphoma in women with breast implants. *J Am Med Assoc*. 2008;300(17):2030-2035.

574. Clemens MW, Medeiros LJ, Butler CE, et al. Complete surgical excision is essential for the management of patients with breast implant-associated anaplastic large-cell lymphoma. *J Clin Oncol*. 2016;34(2):160-168.

575. Pro B, Advani R, Brice P, et al. Brentuximab vedotin (SGN-35) in patients with relapsed or refractory systemic anaplastic large-cell lymphoma: results of a phase II study. *J Clin Oncol*. 2012;30(18):2190-2196.

576. Horwitz S, O'Connor OA, Pro B, et al. The ECHELON-2 Trial: 5-year results of a randomized, phase III study of brentuximab vedotin with chemotherapy for CD30-positive peripheral T-cell lymphoma. *Ann Oncol*. 2022;33(3):288-298.

577. Horwitz S, O'Connor OA, Pro B, et al. Brentuximab vedotin with chemotherapy for CD30-positive peripheral T-cell lymphoma (ECHELON-2): a global, double-blind, randomised, phase 3 trial. *Lancet*. 2019;393(10168):229-240.

578. Mossé YP, Lim MS, Voss SD, et al. Safety and activity of crizotinib for paediatric patients with refractory solid tumours or anaplastic large-cell lymphoma: a Children's Oncology Group phase 1 consortium study. *Lancet Oncol*. 2013;14(6):472-480.

579. Gambacorti-Passerini C, Messa C, Pogliani EM. Crizotinib in anaplastic large-cell lymphoma. *N Engl J Med*. 2011;364(8):775-776.

580. Brugières L, Houot R, Cozic N, et al. Crizotinib in advanced ALK+ anaplastic large cell lymphoma in children and adults: results of the Acsé phase II trial. *Blood*. 2017;130:2831.

581. Bossi E, Aroldi A, Brioschi FA, et al. Phase two study of crizotinib in patients with anaplastic lymphoma kinase (ALK)-positive anaplastic large cell lymphoma relapsed/refractory to chemotherapy. *Am J Hematol*. 2020;95(12):E319-e321.

582. Richly H, Kim TM, Schuler M, et al. Ceritinib in patients with advanced anaplastic lymphoma kinase-rearranged anaplastic large-cell lymphoma. *Blood*. 2015;126(10):1257-1258.

583. Reed DR, Hall RD, Gentzler RD, Volodin L, Douvas MG, Portell CA. Treatment of refractory ALK rearranged anaplastic large cell lymphoma with Alectinib. *Clin Lymphoma Myeloma Leuk*. 2019;19(6):e247-e250.

584. Fukano R, Mori T, Sekimizu M, et al. Alectinib for relapsed or refractory anaplastic lymphoma kinase-positive anaplastic large cell lymphoma: an open-label phase II trial. *Cancer Sci*. 2020;111(12):4540-4547.

585. Gisselbrecht C, Gaulard P, Lepage E, et al. Prognostic significance of T-cell phenotype in aggressive non-Hodgkin's lymphomas. Groupe d'Etudes des Lymphomes de l'Adulte (GELA). *Blood*. 1998;92(1):76-82.

586. Savage KJ, Chhanabhai M, Gascoyne RD, Connors JM. Characterization of peripheral T-cell lymphomas in a single North American institution by the WHO classification. *Ann Oncol*. 2004;15(10):1467-1475.

587. Weisenburger DD, Savage KJ, Harris NL, et al. Peripheral T-cell lymphoma, not otherwise specified: a report of 340 cases from the International Peripheral T-cell Lymphoma Project. *Blood*. 2011;117(12):3402-3408.

588. Iqbal J, Wilcox R, Naushad H, et al. Genomic signatures in T-cell lymphoma: how can these improve precision in diagnosis and inform prognosis? *Blood Rev*. 2016;30(2):89-100.

589. Wang T, Feldman AL, Wada DA, et al. GATA-3 expression identifies a high-risk subset of PTCL, NOS with distinct molecular and clinical features. *Blood*. 2014;123(19):3007-3015.

590. Amador C, Greiner TC, Heavican TB, et al. Reproducing the molecular subclassification of peripheral T-cell lymphoma-NOS by immunohistochemistry. *Blood*. 2019;134(24):2159-2170.

591. Ellin F, Landström J, Jerkeman M, Relander T. Real-world data on prognostic factors and treatment in peripheral T-cell lymphomas: a study from the Swedish Lymphoma Registry. *Blood*. 2014;124(10):1570-1577.

592. Xu P, Yu D, Wang L, Shen Y, Shen Z, Zhao W. Analysis of prognostic factors and comparison of prognostic scores in peripheral T cell lymphoma, not otherwise specified: a single-institution study of 105 Chinese patients. *Ann Hematol*. 2015;94(2):239-247.

593. Piccaluga PP, Agostinelli C, Gazzola A, et al. Prognostic markers in peripheral T-cell lymphoma. *Curr Hematol Malig Rep*. 2010;5(4):222-228.

594. Asano N, Suzuki R, Kagami Y, et al. Clinicopathologic and prognostic significance of cytotoxic molecule expression in nodal peripheral T-cell lymphoma, unspecified. *Am J Surg Pathol*. 2005;29(10):1284-1293.

595. Went P, Agostinelli C, Gallamini A, et al. Marker expression in peripheral T-cell lymphoma: a proposed clinical-pathologic prognostic score. *J Clin Oncol*. 2006;24(16):2472-2479.

596. Pescarmona E, Pignoloni P, Puopolo M, et al. p53 over-expression identifies a subset of nodal peripheral T-cell lymphomas with a distinctive biological profile and poor clinical outcome. *J Pathol*. 2001;195(3):361-366.

597. Federico M, Rudiger T, Bellei M, et al. Clinicopathologic characteristics of angioimmunoblastic T-cell lymphoma: analysis of the international peripheral T-cell lymphoma project. *J Clin Oncol*. 2013;31(2):240-246.

598. Cortés JR, Palomero T. The curious origins of angioimmunoblastic T-cell lymphoma. *Curr Opin Hematol*. 2016;23(4):434-443.

599. Schlegelberger B, Zwingers T, Hohenadel K, et al. Significance of cytogenetic findings for the clinical outcome in patients with T-cell lymphoma of angioimmunoblastic lymphadenopathy type. *J Clin Oncol*. 1996;14(2):593-599.

600. Wang C, McKeithan TW, Gong Q, et al. IDH2R172 mutations define a unique subgroup of patients with angioimmunoblastic T-cell lymphoma. *Blood*. 2015;126(15):1741-1752.

601. Mourad N, Mounier N, Brière J, et al. Clinical, biologic, and pathologic features in 157 patients with angioimmunoblastic T-cell lymphoma treated within the Groupe d'Etude des Lymphomes de l'Adulte (GELA) trials. *Blood*. 2008;111(9):4463-4470.

602. El-Asmar J, Reljic T, Ayala E, et al. Efficacy of high-dose therapy and autologous hematopoietic cell transplantation in peripheral T cell lymphomas as front-line consolidation or in the relapsed/refractory setting: a systematic review/meta-analysis. *Biol Blood Marrow Transplant*. 2016;22(5):802-814.

603. Ferreri AJM, Govi S, Pileri SA. Hepatosplenic gamma-delta T-cell lymphoma. *Crit Rev Oncol Hematol*. 2012;83(2):283-292.

604. Jaffe ES. Pathobiology of peripheral T-cell lymphomas. *Hematology Am Soc Hematol Educ Program*. 2006:317-322.

605. Belhadj K, Reyes F, Farcet JP, et al. Hepatosplenic gammadelta T-cell lymphoma is a rare clinicopathologic entity with poor outcome: report on a series of 21 patients. *Blood*. 2003;102(13):4261-4269.

606. Macon WR, Levy NB, Kurtin PJ, et al. Hepatosplenic alphabeta T-cell lymphomas: a report of 14 cases and comparison with hepatosplenic gammadelta T-cell lymphomas. *Am J Surg Pathol*. 2001;25(3):285-296.

607. Travert M, Huang Y, de Leval L, et al. Molecular features of hepatosplenic T-cell lymphoma unravels potential novel therapeutic targets. *Blood*. 2012;119(24):5795-5806.

608. Tanase A, Schmitz N, Stein H, et al. Allogeneic and autologous stem cell transplantation for hepatosplenic T-cell lymphoma: a retrospective study of the EBMT Lymphoma Working Party. *Leukemia*. 2015;29(3):686-688.

609. Rashidi A, Cashen AF. Outcomes of allogeneic stem cell transplantation in hepatosplenic T-cell lymphoma. *Blood Cancer J*. 2015;5(6):e318.

610. Willemze R, Jansen PM, Cerroni L, et al. Subcutaneous panniculitis-like T-cell lymphoma: definition, classification, and prognostic factors. An EORTC Cutaneous Lymphoma Group Study of 83 cases. *Blood*. 2008;111(2):838-845.

611. Al-Toma A, Verbeek WHM, Hadithi M, von Blomberg BME, Mulder CJJ. Survival in refractory coeliac disease and enteropathy-associated T-cell lymphoma: retrospective evaluation of single-centre experience. *Gut*. 2007;56(10):1373-1378.

612. Delabie J, Holte H, Vose JM, et al. Enteropathy-associated T-cell lymphoma: clinical and histological findings from the International Peripheral T-cell Lymphoma Project. *Blood*. 2011;118(1):148-155.

613. Gale J, Simmonds PD, Mead GM, Sweetenham JW, Wright DH. Enteropathy-type intestinal T-cell lymphoma: clinical features and treatment of 31 patients in a single center. *J Clin Oncol*. 2000;18(4):795-803.

614. Tse E, Gill H, Loong F, et al. Type II enteropathy-associated T-cell lymphoma: a multicenter analysis from the Asia lymphoma Study Group. *Am J Hematol*. 2012;87(7):663-668.

615. Perry AM, Warnke RA, Hu Q, et al. Indolent T-cell lymphoproliferative disease of the gastrointestinal tract. *Blood*. 2013;122(22):3599-3606.

616. Kim GE, Cho JH, Yang WI, et al. Angiocentric lymphoma of the head and neck: patterns of systemic failure after radiation treatment. *J Clin Oncol*. 2000;18(1):54-63.

617. Liang R, Todd D, Chan TK, et al. Treatment outcome and prognostic factors for primary nasal lymphoma. *J Clin Oncol*. 1995;13(3):666-670.

618. Quintanilla-Martinez L, Ridaura C, Nagl F, et al. Hydroa vacciniforme-like lymphoma: a chronic EBV+ lymphoproliferative disorder with risk to develop a systemic lymphoma. *Blood*. 2013;122(18):3101-3110.

619. Ishii H, Ogino T, Berger C, et al. Clinical usefulness of serum EBV DNA levels of BamHI W and LMP1 for Nasal NK/T-cell lymphoma. *J Med Virol*. 2007;79(5):562-572.

620. Hsieh PP, Tung CL, Chan ABW, et al. EBV viral load in tumor tissue is an important prognostic indicator for nasal NK/T-cell lymphoma. *Am J Clin Pathol*. 2007;128(4):579-584.

621. Tse E, Zhao WL, Xiong J, Kwong YL. How we treat NK/T-cell lymphomas. *J Hematol Oncol*. 2022;15(1):74.

622. Tse E, Kwong YL. How I treat NK/T-cell lymphomas. *Blood*. 2013;121(25):4997-5005.

623. Lee J, Park YH, Kim WS, et al. Extranodal nasal type NK/T-cell lymphoma: elucidating clinical prognostic factors for risk-based stratification of therapy. *Eur J Cancer*. 2005;41(10):1402-1408.

624. Mraz-Gernhard S, Natkunam Y, Hoppe RT, LeBoit P, Kohler S, Kim YH. Natural killer/natural killer-like T-cell lymphoma, CD56+, presenting in the skin: an increasingly recognized entity with an aggressive course. *J Clin Oncol*. 2001;19(8):2179-2188.

625. Matsumoto Y, Nomura K, Kanda-Akano Y, et al. Successful treatment with Erwinia L-asparaginase for recurrent natural killer/T cell lymphoma. *Leuk Lymphoma*. 2003;44(5):879-882.

626. Yamaguchi M, Kwong YL, Kim WS, et al. Phase II study of SMILE chemotherapy for newly diagnosed stage IV, relapsed, or refractory extranodal natural killer (NK)/T-cell lymphoma, nasal type: the NK-Cell Tumor Study Group study. *J Clin Oncol.* 2011;29(33):4410-4416.
627. Kwong YL, Chan TSY, Tan D, et al. PD1 blockade with pembrolizumab is highly effective in relapsed or refractory NK/T-cell lymphoma failing l-asparaginase. *Blood.* 2017;129(17):2437-2442.
628. Lamy T, Loughran TP Jr. How I treat LGL leukemia. *Blood.* 2011;117(10):2764-2774.
629. Lamy T, Moignet A, Loughran TP Jr. LGL leukemia: from pathogenesis to treatment. *Blood.* 2017;129(9):1082-1094.
630. Epling-Burnette PK, Liu JH, Catlett-Falcone R, et al. Inhibition of STAT3 signaling leads to apoptosis of leukemic large granular lymphocytes and decreased Mcl-1 expression. *J Clin Invest.* 2001;107(3):351-362.
631. Jerez A, Clemente MJ, Makishima H, et al. STAT3 mutations unify the pathogenesis of chronic lymphoproliferative disorders of NK cells and T-cell large granular lymphocyte leukemia. *Blood.* 2012;120(15):3048-3057.
632. Teramo A, Gattazzo C, Passeri F, et al. Intrinsic and extrinsic mechanisms contribute to maintain the JAK/STAT pathway aberrantly activated in T-type large granular lymphocyte leukemia. *Blood.* 2013;121(19):3843-3854, S1.
633. Loughran TP, Jr, Zickl L, Olson TL, et al. Immunosuppressive therapy of LGL leukemia: prospective multicenter phase II study by the Eastern Cooperative Oncology Group (E5998). *Leukemia.* 2015;29(4):886-894.
634. Dumitriu B, Ito S, Feng X, et al. Alemtuzumab in T-cell large granular lymphocytic leukaemia: interim results from a single-arm, open-label, phase 2 study. *Lancet Haematol.* 2016;3(1):e22-e29.
635. Bilori B, Thota S, Clemente MJ, et al. Tofacitinib as a novel salvage therapy for refractory T-cell large granular lymphocytic leukemia. *Leukemia.* 2015;29(12):2427-2429.
636. Suzuki R, Suzumiya J, Nakamura S, et al. Aggressive natural killer-cell leukemia revisited: large granular lymphocyte leukemia of cytotoxic NK cells. *Leukemia.* 2004;18(4):763-770.
637. Dearden CE. T-cell prolymphocytic leukemia. *Med Oncol.* 2006;23(1):17-22.
638. Le Toriellec E, Despouy G, Pierron G, et al. Haploinsufficiency of CDKN1B contributes to leukemogenesis in T-cell prolymphocytic leukemia. *Blood.* 2008;111(4):2321-2328.
639. Kiel MJ, Velusamy T, Rolland D, et al. Integrated genomic sequencing reveals mutational landscape of T-cell prolymphocytic leukemia. *Blood.* 2014;124(9):1460-1472.
640. Dearden C. How I treat prolymphocytic leukemia. *Blood.* 2012;120(3):538-551.
641. Herbaux C, Genet P, Bouabdallah K, et al. Bendamustine is effective in T-cell prolymphocytic leukaemia. *Br J Haematol.* 2015;168(6):916-919.
642. Hopfinger G, Busch R, Pflug N, et al. Sequential chemoimmunotherapy of fludarabine, mitoxantrone, and cyclophosphamide induction followed by alemtuzumab consolidation is effective in T-cell prolymphocytic leukemia. *Cancer.* 2013;119(12):2258-2267.
643. Herling M. Are we improving the outcome for patients with T-cell prolymphocytic leukemia by allogeneic stem cell transplantation? *Eur J Haematol.* 2015;94(3):191-192.
644. Katsuya H, Ishitsuka K, Utsunomiya A, et al. Treatment and survival among 1594 patients with ATL. *Blood.* 2015;126(24):2570-2577.
645. Teshima T, Akashi K, Shibuya T, et al. Central nervous system involvement in adult T-cell leukemia/lymphoma. *Cancer.* 1990;65(2):327-332.
646. Shimamoto Y, Yamaguchi M. HTLV-I induced extranodal lymphomas. *Leuk Lymphoma.* 1992;7(1-2):37-45.
647. Katsuya H, Yamanaka T, Ishitsuka K, et al. Prognostic index for acute- and lymphoma-type adult T-cell leukemia/lymphoma. *J Clin Oncol.* 2012;30(14):1635-1640.
648. Tsukasaki K, Krebs J, Nagai K, et al. Comparative genomic hybridization analysis in adult T-cell leukemia/lymphoma: correlation with clinical course. *Blood.* 2001;97(12):3875-3881.
649. Itoyama T, Chaganti RS, Yamada Y, et al. Cytogenetic analysis and clinical significance in adult T-cell leukemia/lymphoma: a study of 50 cases from the human T-cell leukemia virus type-1 endemic area, Nagasaki. *Blood.* 2001;97(11):3612-3620.
650. Tsukasaki K, Utsunomiya A, Fukuda H, et al. VCAP-AMP-VECP compared with biweekly CHOP for adult T-cell leukemia-lymphoma: Japan Clinical Oncology Group Study JCOG9801. *J Clin Oncol.* 2007;25(34):5458-5464.
651. Tsukasaki K, Hermine O, Bazarbachi A, et al. Definition, prognostic factors, treatment, and response criteria of adult T-cell leukemia-lymphoma: a proposal from an International Consensus Meeting. *J Clin Oncol.* 2009;27(3):453-459.
652. Bazarbachi A, Plumelle Y, Carlos Ramos J, et al. Meta-analysis on the use of zidovudine and interferon-alfa in adult T-cell leukemia/lymphoma showing improved survival in the leukemic subtypes. *J Clin Oncol.* 2010;28(27):4177-4183.
653. Hodson A, Crichton S, Montoto S, et al. Use of zidovudine and interferon alfa with chemotherapy improves survival in both acute and lymphoma subtypes of adult T-cell leukemia/lymphoma. *J Clin Oncol.* 2011;29(35):4696-4701.
654. Kchour G, Tarhini M, Kooshyar MM, et al. Phase 2 study of the efficacy and safety of the combination of arsenic trioxide, interferon alpha, and zidovudine in newly diagnosed chronic adult T-cell leukemia/lymphoma (ATL). *Blood.* 2009;113(26):6528-6532.
655. Ishida T, Fujiwara H, Nosaka K, et al. Multicenter phase II study of lenalidomide in relapsed or recurrent adult T-cell leukemia/lymphoma: ATLL-002. *J Clin Oncol.* 2016;34(34):4086-4093.
656. Ishida T, Joh T, Uike N, et al. Defucosylated anti-CCR4 monoclonal antibody (KW-0761) for relapsed adult T-cell leukemia-lymphoma: a multicenter phase II study. *J Clin Oncol.* 2012;30(8):837-842.
657. Ishida T, Jo T, Takemoto S, et al. Dose-intensified chemotherapy alone or in combination with mogamulizumab in newly diagnosed aggressive adult T-cell leukaemia-lymphoma: a randomized phase II study. *Br J Haematol.* 2015;169(5):672-682.
658. Berkowitz JL, Janik JE, Stewart DM, et al. Safety, efficacy, and pharmacokinetics/pharmacodynamics of daclizumab (anti-CD25) in patients with adult T-cell leukemia/lymphoma. *Clin Immunol.* 2014;155(2):176-187.
659. Sharma K, Janik JE, O'Mahony D, et al. Phase II study of alemtuzumab (CAMPATH-1) in patients with HTLV-1-associated adult T-cell leukemia/lymphoma. *Clin Cancer Res.* 2017;23(1):35-42.
660. Ishida T, Hishizawa M, Kato K, et al. Allogeneic hematopoietic stem cell transplantation for adult T-cell leukemia-lymphoma with special emphasis on preconditioning regimen: a nationwide retrospective study. *Blood.* 2012;120(8):1734-1741.
661. Adrianzen Herrera D, Kornblum N, Acuna-Villaorduna A, et al. Barriers to allogeneic hematopoietic stem cell transplantation for human T cell lymphotropic virus 1-associated adult T cell lymphoma-leukemia in the United States: experience from a large cohort in a major tertiary center. *Biol Blood Marrow Transplant.* 2019;25(6):e199-e203.
662. Moskowitz AJ, Lunning MA, Horwitz SM. How I treat the peripheral T-cell lymphomas. *Blood.* 2014;123(17):2636-2644.
663. Schmitz N, Trümper L, Ziepert M, et al. Treatment and prognosis of mature T-cell and NK-cell lymphoma: an analysis of patients with T-cell lymphoma treated in studies of the German High-Grade Non-Hodgkin Lymphoma Study Group. *Blood.* 2010;116(18):3418-3425.
664. Gallamini A, Zaja F, Patti C, et al. Alemtuzumab (Campath-1H) and CHOP chemotherapy as first-line treatment of peripheral T-cell lymphoma: results of a GITIL (Gruppo Italiano Terapie Innovative nei Linfomi) prospective multicenter trial. *Blood.* 2007;110(7):2316-2323.
665. Advani RH, Hong F, Horning SJ, et al. Cardiac toxicity associated with bevacizumab (Avastin) in combination with CHOP chemotherapy for peripheral T cell lymphoma in ECOG 2404 trial. *Leuk Lymphoma.* 2012;53(4):718-720.
666. Piekarz RL, Frye R, Prince HM, et al. Phase 2 trial of romidepsin in patients with peripheral T-cell lymphoma. *Blood.* 2011;117(22):5827-5834.
667. Coiffier B, Pro B, Prince HM, et al. Results from a pivotal, open-label, phase II study of romidepsin in relapsed or refractory peripheral T-cell lymphoma after prior systemic therapy. *J Clin Oncol.* 2012;30(6):631-636.
668. Pro B, Horwitz SM, Prince HM, et al. Romidepsin induces durable responses in patients with relapsed or refractory angioimmunoblastic T-cell lymphoma. *Hematol Oncol.* 2017;35(4):914-917.
669. Odejide O, Weigert O, Lane AA, et al. A targeted mutational landscape of angioimmunoblastic T-cell lymphoma. *Blood.* 2014;123(9):1293-1296.
670. Sakata-Yanagimoto M, Enami T, Yoshida K, et al. Somatic RHOA mutation in angioimmunoblastic T cell lymphoma. *Nat Genet.* 2014;46(2):171-175.
671. Falchi L, Ma H, Klein S, et al. Combined oral 5-azacytidine and romidepsin are highly effective in patients with PTCL: a multicenter phase 2 study. *Blood.* 2021;137(16):2161-2170.
672. O'Connor OA, Horwitz S, Masszi T, et al. Belinostat in patients with relapsed or refractory peripheral T-cell lymphoma: results of the pivotal phase II BELIEF (CLN-19) study. *J Clin Oncol.* 2015;33(23):2492-2499.
673. Dupuis J, Morschhauser F, Ghesquières H, et al. Combination of romidepsin with cyclophosphamide, doxorubicin, vincristine, and prednisone in previously untreated patients with peripheral T-cell lymphoma: a non-randomised, phase 1b/2 study. *Lancet Haematol.* 2015;2(4):e160-e165.
674. Bachy E, Camus V, Thieblemont C, et al. Romidepsin plus CHOP versus CHOP in patients with previously untreated peripheral T-cell lymphoma: results of the Ro-CHOP phase III study (conducted by LYSA). *J Clin Oncol.* 2022;40(3):242-251.
675. O'Connor OA, Pro B, Pinter-Brown L, et al. Pralatrexate in patients with relapsed or refractory peripheral T-cell lymphoma: results from the pivotal PROPEL study. *J Clin Oncol.* 2011;29(9):1182-1189.
676. Advani RH, Ansell SM, Lechowicz MJ, et al. A phase II study of cyclophosphamide, etoposide, vincristine and prednisone (CEOP) Alternating with Pralatrexate (P) as front line therapy for patients with peripheral T-cell lymphoma (PTCL): final results from the T-cell consortium trial. *Br J Haematol.* 2016;172(4):535-544.
677. Mahadevan D, Unger JM, Spier CM, et al. Phase 2 trial of combined cisplatin, etoposide, gemcitabine, and methylprednisolone (PEGS) in peripheral T-cell non-Hodgkin lymphoma: Southwest Oncology Group Study S0350. *Cancer.* 2013;119(2):371-379.
678. Corazzelli G, Marcacci G, Frigeri F, et al. A phase II study of gemcitabine, ifosfamide, and oxaliplatin (GIFOX) as upfront treatment for high-risk, non-anaplastic large cell, peripheral T-cell lymphomas. *J Clin Oncol.* 2013;31(15 suppl):8564.
679. Damaj G, Gressin R, Bouabdallah K, et al. Results from a prospective, open-label, phase II trial of bendamustine in refractory or relapsed T-cell lymphomas: the BENTLY trial. *J Clin Oncol.* 2013;31(1):104-110.
680. Bouabdallah K, Aubrais R, Chartier L, et al. Salvage therapy with brentuximab-vedotin and bendamustine for patients with relapsed/refractory T cell lymphoma. A multicenter and retrospective study. *Blood.* 2021;138:620.
681. Kim SJ, Yoon DH, Kang HJ, et al. Bortezomib in combination with CHOP as first-line treatment for patients with stage III/IV peripheral T-cell lymphomas: a multicentre, single-arm, phase 2 trial. *Eur J Cancer.* 2012;48(17):3223-3231.
682. Evens AM, Rosen ST, Helenowski I, et al. A phase I/II trial of bortezomib combined concurrently with gemcitabine for relapsed or refractory DLBCL and peripheral T-cell lymphomas. *Br J Haematol.* 2013;163(1):55-61.
683. Toumishey E, Prasad A, Dueck G, et al. Final report of a phase 2 clinical trial of lenalidomide monotherapy for patients with T-cell lymphoma. *Cancer.* 2015;121(5):716-723.

684. Witzig TE, Reeder C, Han JJ, et al. The mTORC1 inhibitor everolimus has antitumor activity in vitro and produces tumor responses in patients with relapsed T-cell lymphoma. *Blood*. 2015;126(3):328-335.
685. Zhang Y, Xu W, Liu H, Li J. Therapeutic options in peripheral T cell lymphoma. *J Hematol Oncol*. 2016;9(1):37.
686. Barr PM, Li H, Spier C, et al. Phase II intergroup trial of alisertib in relapsed and refractory peripheral T-cell lymphoma and transformed mycosis fungoides: SWOG 1108. *J Clin Oncol*. 2015;33(21):2399-2404.
687. O'Connor OA, Özcan M, Jacobsen ED, et al. Randomized phase III study of alisertib or Investigator's choice (selected single agent) in patients with relapsed or refractory peripheral T-cell lymphoma. *J Clin Oncol*. 2019;37(8):613-623.
688. Horwitz SM, Porcu P, Flinn I, et al. Duvelisib (IPI-145), a phosphoinositide-3-kinase-δ, γ inhibitor, shows activity in patients with relapsed/refractory T-cell lymphoma. *Blood*. 2014;124(21):803.
689. d'Amore F, Relander T, Lauritzsen GF, et al. Up-front autologous stem-cell transplantation in peripheral T-cell lymphoma: NLG-T-01. *J Clin Oncol*. 2012;30(25):3093-3099.
690. Wilhelm M, Smetak M, Reimer P, et al. First-line therapy of peripheral T-cell lymphoma: extension and long-term follow-up of a study investigating the role of autologous stem cell transplantation. *Blood Cancer J*. 2016;6(7):e452.
691. Schmitz N, Nickelsen M, Altmann B, et al. Allogeneic or autologous transplantation as first-line therapy for younger patients with peripheral T-cell lymphoma: results of the interim analysis of the AATT trial. *J Clin Oncol*. 2015;33(15 suppl):8507.

Chapter 91 ■ Non-Hodgkin Lymphoma in Children

NITYA GULATI • LISA GIULINO ROTH

INTRODUCTION

There have been significant clinical and laboratory advances over the past 40 years in our understanding of the non-Hodgkin lymphomas (NHLs) of childhood. These include the refinement of diagnosis and classification of clinically relevant histologic subtypes, the elucidation of various pathogenic mechanisms, and, most importantly, improvements in therapy and supportive care that have resulted in improved event-free survival (EFS) and overall survival (OS) rates. Increased attention to reducing and eliminating late effects of therapy, such as infertility, cardiotoxicity, and second cancers, is another essential hallmark of clinical research over recent years.

Malignant lymphomas, which comprise both Hodgkin lymphoma (HL) and NHL, are the third most common type of childhood cancer after acute lymphoblastic leukemia (ALL) and brain tumors.[1-3] Among children < 18 years of age, there is a slight predominance of HL, whereas the reverse is true among those <15 years of age.[4,5]

It is important to note the distinction between the NHLs of adults and children.[2,3,6] Pediatric NHLs are typically high-grade tumors,[7] in contrast to the low- and intermediate-grade tumors, which are predominant among adults. In addition, specific lymphoma diagnoses and histological subtypes are more common in children (e.g., Burkitt lymphoma [BL]) than in older adults. While there is overlap in the underlying biology and pathophysiology between pediatric and adult lymphomas, molecular distinctions are increasingly identified, highlighting the need to focus on pediatric lymphoma-specific treatment strategies.[8,9]

EPIDEMIOLOGY

NHL accounts for approximately 7% of all cancer diagnoses under the age of 20 years, with an incidence of 10 to 15 cases per million children and adolescents in developed countries.[10] However, low- and middle-income countries are estimated to contribute to 90% of childhood NHL cases worldwide.[11] In general, five lymphoma subtypes account for over 90% of all pediatric NHL diagnoses worldwide: Burkitt lymphoma, which is the most common, followed by T-cell lymphoblastic lymphoma (T-LBL), diffuse large B-cell lymphoma (DLBCL), anaplastic large cell lymphoma (ALCL), and primary mediastinal B-cell lymphoma (PMBCL).[12,13] The incidence and spectrum of NHL subtypes varies by geographical regions. For example, endemic BL is the most common childhood cancer in regions of sub-Saharan Africa that are endemic for malaria. Here nearly 95% of cases are associated with Epstein-Barr virus (EBV). In contrast 20% to 30% of sporadic BL cases are EBV positive. EBV-associated T- and NK-cell lymphoproliferative disorders, which are rare in the United States and Europe, are more common in East Asia and Central and South America.[14]

Although there is no specific age peak for NHL within the pediatric population, there are differences among age groups. NHL is very rare among infants. The incidence of NHL, as a proportion of all cancers in the United States, increases from 3% in the 1- to 4-year age group to 8% to 9% in the 5- to 14-year age group and then stabilizes through adolescence.[15] NHL is more common among boys across all age groups and regions, with the gender difference most pronounced in children less than 15 years old.[15] PMBCL is an exception, which is more common among females. Similar to most other childhood cancers, the incidence of NHL is higher among white children than African Americans, the cause of which remains unknown.[15]

Although the majority of NHL cases arise in immunocompetent hosts, congenital and acquired immunodeficiency syndromes are well-established risk factors for the development of NHL. Congenital immunodeficiencies associated with increased risk for NHL include cell-mediated and humoral immunodeficiency syndromes, disorders of cell repair (e.g., ataxia telangiectasia, Wiskott-Aldrich syndrome), severe combined immunodeficiency, and X-linked lymphoproliferative disorder. Patients with acquired immunodeficiency who are at higher risk for developing NHL include those on immunosuppressives such as after bone marrow or solid organ transplant and patients with human immunodeficiency virus. The pathogenesis in these cases is often attributed to viral infections, with EBV being the most common.[16,17]

CLASSIFICATION

The most recent World Health Organization (WHO) Classifications of Tumors of Hematopoietic and Lymphoid Tissues designate NHLs according to their clinical, morphologic, immunophenotypic, and genetic features and also acknowledge difficulties in differentiating some of the clinically significant subtypes of B-cell lymphoma by introducing some borderline ("gray zone") categories to encompass these issues. Pediatric NHL, similar to adult NHL, is categorized based on the cell of origin as "B-" or "T/NK"-cell lymphoproliferative disorders/lymphomas. The vast majority of pediatric NHLs arise from mature lymphocytes, with mature B-cell lymphomas being the most common, including BL (35%-40% cases), DLBCL (10%-15% cases), and PMBL (1%-2%). ALCL is the most common mature T-cell lymphoma of childhood (10% of cases), with all other lymphomas falling into the rare category. Among the precursor lymphoblastic lymphomas T-LBL is more common than B-cell LBL (T-LBL 15%-20% cases).[16,18] *Table 91.1* summarizes the pediatric NHLs according to the 2016 WHO Classification.[19] *Table 91.2* summarizes the main diagnostic immunophenotypic, molecular, and genetic features of the most common subtypes of NHL encountered in this age group.

DIAGNOSTIC WORKUP, STAGING, AND INITIAL MANAGEMENT

Diagnostic workup: Therapy for the NHLs of childhood is determined by the histologic diagnosis, disease stage, and, in some cases, risk stratification. For histologic diagnosis an excisional biopsy is usually preferred; however, image-guided percutaneous core needle biopsy can also be considered if sufficient tissue can be obtained for histopathology, immunohistochemistry, fluorescence in situ hybridization, flow cytometry, and other molecular studies if needed.[20] Patients can present in severe tumor lysis and/or respiratory distress and may not be able to undergo tissue biopsy. In these situations it may be possible to obtain a diagnosis from pleural or pericardial effusions. Initial bloodwork should include a complete blood count with differential, chemistry panel, including serum lactate dehydrogenase (LDH), liver function tests, and uric acid to evaluate for tumor lysis.

Staging: A comprehensive staging workup should be performed once the diagnosis is established. This includes computerized tomography of the neck, chest, abdomen, and pelvis and typically fluorodeoxyglucose (FDG)-positron emission tomography (PET) imaging. In many cases bilateral bone marrow aspirate/biopsy and lumbar puncture for cerebrospinal fluid cytology should be performed.[21] The role for FDG-PET at diagnosis and interim imaging in pediatric NHL is not yet clearly established. Uniform criteria for interpreting FDG-PET findings in children are needed and are currently being evaluated in clinical trials. The St. Jude NHL staging classification is the most widely accepted staging approach in pediatric NHL (*Table 91.3*).[21]

Table 91.1. Subtypes of Non-Hodgkin Lymphoma Most Commonly Encountered in Children (Less Than 18 years) According to the 2016 World Health Organization (WHO) Classification

Precursor lymphoid neoplasms
B-lymphoblastic lymphoma/leukemia, NOS
B-lymphoblastic lymphoma/leukemia, NOS with recurrent genetic abnormalities
T-lymphoblastic lymphoma/leukemia
NK-lymphoblastic leukemia/lymphoma (provisional entity)
Mature B-Cell Lymphomas
Burkitt lymphoma
Burkitt-like lymphoma with 11q aberration (provisional entity)
Diffuse large B-cell lymphoma (DLBCL), NOS
Germinal center type
Activated B-cell type
T-cell/histiocyte-rich large B-cell lymphoma
Lymphomatoid granulomatosis
Primary mediastinal (thymic) large B-cell lymphoma
ALK+ large B-cell lymphoma
Plasmablastic lymphoma
B-cell lymphoma, unclassifiable, with features intermediate between DLBCL and classic Hodgkin lymphoma
Pediatric-type follicular lymphoma
Large B-cell lymphoma with *IRF4* rearrangement (provisional entity)
Pediatric nodal marginal zone lymphoma (provisional entity)
Mature T- and NK-Cell Neoplasms
Anaplastic large cell lymphoma, ALK+
Peripheral T-cell lymphoma, NOS
Hepatosplenic T-cell lymphoma
Extranodal NK/T-cell lymphoma, nasal type
Subcutaneous panniculitis-like T-cell lymphoma
Primary cutaneous CD30-positive T-cell lymphoproliferative disorders
Lymphomatoid papulosis
Mycosis fungoides
Systemic EBV-positive T-cell lymphoma of childhood
Chronic active EBV infection of T- and NK-cell type, systemic form
Hydroa vacciniforme–like lymphoproliferative disorder
Posttransplant lymphoproliferative disorders (PTLDs)
Plasmacytic hyperplasia PTLD
Infectious mononucleosis PTLD
Florid follicular hyperplasia PTLD
Polymorphic PTLD
Monomorphic PTLD (B- and T/NK-cell types)
Classical Hodgkin lymphoma PTLD

Abbreviations: ALK, anaplastic lymphoma kinase; EBV, Epstein-Barr virus; NK, natural killer; NOS, not otherwise specified.

A revised international pediatric NHL staging system (IPNHLSS) was proposed by an international multidisciplinary expert panel convened in Frankfurt, Germany, in 2009 at the Third International Childhood, Adolescent and Young Adult NHL symposium. The proposed IPNHLSS aims to define, in more detail, sites of involvement, including extranodal sites of disease, and to incorporate improved diagnostic methods and advanced imaging technologies in defining bone marrow and central nervous system (CNS) involvement (*Tables 91.3* and *91.4*).[22]

Initial management: Upon expeditious completion of the diagnostic and staging workup, appropriate therapeutic options can be implemented. Before chemotherapy is started, however, a number of issues must be considered. Some children are at high risk for tumor lysis syndrome (TLS). This primarily includes children with advanced-stage BL and some children with LBL who have a large tumor burden at diagnosis, which may be reflected by an elevated serum LDH. Some of these children will have metabolic abnormalities with some degree of renal dysfunction at diagnosis, which only worsens once chemotherapy is started (e.g., hyperkalemia, hyperuricemia, hyperphosphatemia). Therefore, these children should have excellent intravenous access and vigorous hydration before starting chemotherapy. Hyperuricemia has historically been managed using hyperhydration coupled with allopurinol, a xanthine oxidase inhibitor. Uricolytics, such as rasburicase, have been shown to be effective and well tolerated with a reduced risk of associated allergic reaction.[23] The advantage of these agents is the precipitous drop in serum uric acid, which negates the need for alkalinization, thus facilitating phosphorous excretion. Of note, a study of rasburicase in children at high risk for TLS demonstrated preservation of renal function with no significant associated hyperphosphatemia or hyperkalemia.[23] Chemotherapy approaches, which are tailored to NHL subtype, will be outlined below for each histologic subtype.

LYMPHOBLASTIC LYMPHOMAS (T- AND B-LYMPHOBLASTIC LYMPHOMA/LEUKEMIA)

ALL and LBL are neoplasms of precursor B cells or T cells, characterized by immature (blastic) morphology and immunophenotype. At the pathologic and clinical levels, both ALL and LBL appear to represent an overlapping continuum, with the distinction between these two processes being primarily quantitative and arbitrary: cases involving at least 25% of the marrow cellularity are managed as ALL, whereas cases with less or no marrow involvement are designated as LBL.[24-26] More recent studies have identified important differences in gene expression profiling, adhesion molecule expression, and T-ALL and T-LBL molecular pathways that explain at least partially their distinct dissemination patterns.[27-29] T-lymphoblastic lymphoma (T-LBL) is the more common subtype (70%-80% of LBL cases), presents with advanced stage III/IV disease, and involves most often the mediastinum, lymph nodes, skin, bone, or soft tissues, and, less commonly, kidney, lung, or orbit (*Figure 91.1*).[12,18] By contrast, the less common B-lymphoblastic lymphoma (B-LBL, 20%-25% cases) more often presents with localized stage I/II disease involving the lymph nodes, skin, bone, soft tissues, or breast, with mediastinal presentation being very uncommon. Bone marrow involvement is more common in B-LBL than in T-LBL, although CNS involvement is rare in both cases (≤5% cases).[30-32] The median age of diagnosis is 9 years for both T- and B-LBL. While T-LBL is 2.5 times more common in males, there is no difference in gender distribution for B-LBL.[32]

Histologically, B-LBL and T-LBL show a diffuse growth pattern, with extensive replacement of the underlying normal tissue architecture by sheets of blastic cells. The malignant lymphoblasts are small to intermediate in size, with scant to moderate amounts of basophilic cytoplasm, finely dispersed nuclear chromatin, and small indistinct nucleoli (*Figure 91.2*). In some cases, the nuclei may have markedly irregular or convoluted outlines, a feature more common in T-LBL. In addition, mitotic figures may be numerous in some cases, correlating with the presence of a "starry-sky" appearance imparted by scattered pale macrophages containing apoptotic nuclear debris. Therefore, BL should be considered in the differential diagnosis of such cases.

Most T-LBLs express cytoplasmic (cy) or membrane-bound CD3 and terminal deoxynucleotidyl transferase (TdT). They are variably positive for CD1a, CD2, CD4, CD5, CD7, and CD8, depending on the stage of differentiation of the T lymphoblast.[33] In addition to TdT,

Table 91.2. Immunophenotypic Features of the Most Common Pediatric Non-Hodgkin Lymphomas

	TdT	CD34	CD20	CD10	CD19	CD79a	Ig	CD5	CD7	CD3	CD4	CD8	CD30	ALK	CTA	MUM1[b]	BCL2	BCL6	Cytogenetic	Molecular Biology
T-LBL	+(−)	+	−	−/+	−	−(+)	−	+/−	+	+[a]	+/−	+/−	−	−	−	−/+	−	+/−	Translocations involving 14q11-13; few other data	NOTCH/FBXW7, PTEN, IGH/TCR rearrangements
B-LBL	+	+	+/−	+/−	+	+	−/+[b]	−	−	−	−	−	−	−	−	−	+/−	−	Few data	IGH/TCR rearrangements
Burkitt	−	−	+	+	+	+	+	−	−	−	−	−	−	−	−	−	−	+	t(8;14) (q24;q32) t(2;8) (p12;q24) t(8;22)(q24;q11)	MYC/IGH IGK/MYC MYC/IGL
DLBCL	−	−	+	+/−	+	+	+/−	− −/+	−	−	−	−	+/−	−/+[c]	−/+	+/−	+/−	+/−	Complex karyotype with structural and numerical abnormalities, see text for details	See text for details
PMBL	−	−	+	−/+	+	+	−	−	−	−	−	−	+/−	−	−	+/−	−/+	−/+	9p Amplifications	Nuclear factor-κB pathway dysregulation
ALCL, ALK+	−	−	−	−	−	−	−	+/−	−/+	−/+	−/+	−/+	++	+	+/−	+	−/+	+/−	T(2;5)(p23;q35) or other variants involving 2p23	NPM/ALK > 90% or variants
PTCL, NOS	−	−	−	−	−	−	−	−	−	+	+	−/+	−/+	−	−/+	+/−	−/+	−/+	t(5;9) (q33;q22) loss at 9p21.3 CTLA4-CD28 fusion VAV1 fusions	GATA3 and TBX21 subgroups based on GEP; mutations in TET2, DNMT3A, RHOA, FYN
HSL	−	−	−	−	−	−	−	−	−	+	−	−	−	−	+	−/+	−	+	Isochromosome 7q; trisomy 8; loss of sex chromosome	—
PTFL	−	−	+	+	+	+	−	−	−	−	−	−	−	−	−	−	−/+ (weak)	+	No BCL2, BCL2, IRF4, or aberrant IG rearrangement Gains/amplifications of 6pter-p24.3; del1p36	Del and mutations of TNFRSF14 MAP2K1 mutation
PMZL	−	−	+	−	+	+	+	−	−	−	−	−	−	−	−	−	+ (Variable)	−	Ig rearrangements trisomy 18 and 3 MYC, BCL2, BCL6, and IRF4 translocations usually absent	—

Abbreviations: +, positive; −, negative; (+), less than 15% of cases positive; +/−, commonly positive but may be negative; −/+, commonly negative but may be positive; ALCL, anaplastic large cell lymphoma; ALK, anaplastic lymphoma kinase; B-LBL, B-lymphoblastic lymphoma; CTA, cytotoxic antigen (e.g., TIA-1 and perforin); DLBCL, diffuse large B-cell lymphoma; GATA3, GATA-binding protein 3; GEP, gene expression profiling; HSL, hepatosplenic lymphoma; MUM1, interferon regulatory factor-4 (IRF4); PMBL, mediastinal large B-cell lymphoma; PMZL, pediatric marginal-zone lymphoma; PTCL, peripheral T-cell lymphoma; PTFL, pediatric-type follicular lymphoma; T-LBL, T-lymphoblastic lymphoma; TBX21, T-box 21.
[a]Cytoplasmic CD3.
[b]Cytoplasmic μ heavy chain only.
[c]ALK restricted to the ALK+ DLBCL subtype.

Table 91.3. Staging of Non-Hodgkin Lymphoma in Children[a]

Murphy Staging System	IPNHLSS
Stage I A single tumor (extranodal) or involvement of a single anatomic area (nodal), with the exclusion of the mediastinum and abdomen	**Stage I** Single tumor with exclusion of mediastinum and abdomen (N; EN; B or S: EN-B, EN-S)
Stage II A single tumor (extranodal) with regional node involvement Two or more nodal areas on the same side of the diaphragm Two single (extranodal) tumors, with or without regional node involvement on the same side of the diaphragm A primary gastrointestinal tract tumor (usually in the ileocecal area), with or without involvement of associated mesenteric nodes, that is completely resectable	**Stage II** Single EN tumor with regional node involvement Two nodal areas on same side of diaphragm Primary GI tract tumor (usually in ileocecal area), ± involvement of associated mesenteric nodes, that is completely resectable (if malignant ascites or extension of tumor to adjacent organs, it should be regarded as stage III)
Stage III Two single tumors (extranodal) on opposite sides of the diaphragm Two or more nodal areas above and below the diaphragm Any primary intrathoracic tumor (mediastinal, pleural, or thymic) Extensive primary intra-abdominal disease Any paraspinal or epidural tumor, regardless of whether other sites are involved	**Stage III** ≥ Two EN tumors (including EN-B or EN-S) above and/or below diaphragm ≥ Two nodal areas above and below the diaphragm Any intrathoracic tumor (mediastinal, hilar, pulmonary, pleural, or thymic) Intra-abdominal and retroperitoneal disease, including liver, spleen, kidney, and/or ovary localizations, regardless of degree of resection (except primary GI tract tumor [usually in ileocecal region] ±involvement of associated mesenteric nodes that is completely resectable) Any paraspinal or epidural tumor, regardless of whether other sites are involved Single B lesion with concomitant involvement of EN and/or nonregional N sites
Stage IV Any of the above findings with initial involvement of the central nervous system or bone marrow or both	**Stage IV** Any of the above findings with initial involvement of CNS (stage IV CNS), BM (stage IV BM), or both (stage IV combined) based on conventional methods

Abbreviations: B, bone; BM, bone marrow; EN, extranodal; N, nodal; S, skin.
[a]Based on the staging proposed by Murphy and proposed International Pediatric Non-Hodgkin Lymphoma Staging System (IPNHLSS).

Table 91.4. Staging Classification for BM and CNS Involvement From IPNHLSS

BM Involvement

Stage IV disease, resulting from BM involvement, is currently defined by morphologic evidence of ≥5% blasts or lymphoma cells by BM aspiration; this applies to any histologic subtype and will be maintained in IPNHLSS
For each stage, type and degree of BM involvement (by BM aspiration) should be specified, using the abbreviations below to identify involvement:
  BMm: BM positivity by morphology (specify % lymphoma cells)
  BMi: BM positivity by immunophenotypic methods (immunohistochemical or flow cytometric analysis; specify % lymphoma cells)
  BMc: BM positivity by cytogenetic or FISH analysis (specify % lymphoma cells)
  BMmol: BM positivity by molecular techniques (PCR based; specify level of involvement)
Same approach should be used for PB involvement (i.e., PBm, PBi, PBc, PBmol)

CNS involvement

Any CNS tumor mass (identified by imaging techniques [i.e., CT, MRI])
Cranial nerve palsy that cannot be explained by extradural lesions
Blasts morphologically identified in CSF. Condition that defines CNS positivity should be specified: CNS positive/mass, CNS positive/palsy, CNS positive/blasts
CSF status: CSF positivity is based on morphologic evidence of lymphoma cells
CSF should be considered positive when any number of blasts is detected
CSF unknown (not performed, technical difficulties)
Type of CSF involvement should be described whenever possible
  CSFm: CSF positivity by morphology (specify No. of blasts/µL)
  CSFi: CSF positivity by immunohistochemical or flow cytometric analysis; specify % lymphoma cells)
  CSFc: CSF positive by cytogenetic or FISH analysis (specify % lymphoma cells)
  CSFmol: CSF positivity by molecular techniques (PCR based; specify level of involvement)

Definition of BM involvement should be obtained from analysis of bilateral BM aspirates and BM biopsy.

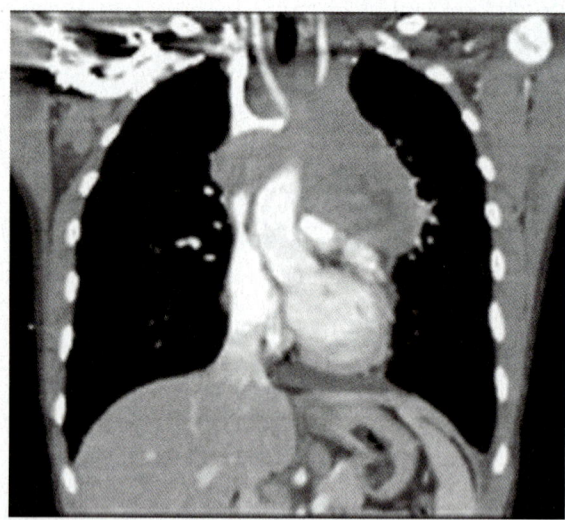

FIGURE 91.1 Sagittal CT of mediastinal LL. Computed tomography scan of child with mediastinal lymphoblastic lymphoma (LL).

CD99, CD34, and CD1a positivity are the most specific markers to point to the precursor nature of the T lymphoblasts. Cd79a may be weakly expressed, and myeloid antigens such as CD13 and CD33 may be coexpressed in some cases. A more frequent expression of T-cell receptor (TCR) αβ than γδ has been reported in T-LBL as compared with precursor T-ALL.[34,35] A rare form of T-ALL/T-LBL termed early T-cell precursor lymphoblastic leukemia (ETP) shows a characteristic immunophenotype with coexpression of CD7 and one or more stem cell markers such as CD34, CD117, HLA-DR, CD13, CD33, CD11, or CD65. These cells may be positive for cyCD3, CD2, and/or CD4 but are consistently negative for CD8 and CD1a as well as CD5 in most cases. ETP-ALL is associated with an increased incidence of AML-type mutations rather than the NOTCH mutations found more commonly in T-ALL/TLBL. ETP-ALL was associated with increased

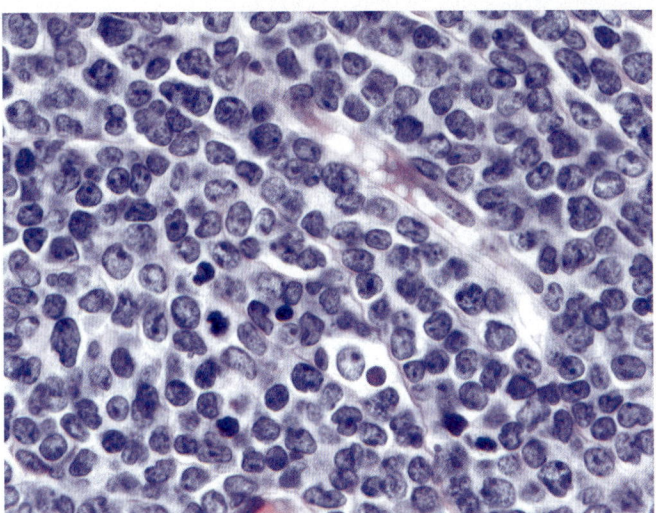

FIGURE 91.2 Histology LL. Lymphoblastic lymphoma (LL). Sheets of small lymphoid cells with fairly uniform chromatin without clearing and scant cytoplasm are present. They show little variation in size, and many show mitotic activity.

induction failures when it was first described; however, with current treatment protocols, there is no significant difference in overall prognosis.[36-39]

B-LBLs typically resemble normal progenitor B cells and express CD19, cyCD79a, and cyCD22 along with PAX5 and TdT, and may be negative or only weakly positive for the mature B-cell marker CD20.[33] Myeloid markers such as CD13 and CD33 may be positive, but MPO is usually absent.[19,33] The neoplastic cells most often lack expression of surface IG and light chain restriction. They often express cytoplasmic μ heavy chain without detectable κ or λ IG light chains (IGLs).[40-42]

While recurrent molecular alterations and their association with prognosis are well defined in B-ALL, less is known about the molecular makeup of B-LBL. Alterations in chromosome 21 (trisomy or duplication of 21q22) are the most commonly reported cytogenetic abnormalities in B-LBL.[43,44] A recent study comparing the copy number alterations between B-ALL and B-LBL using formalin-fixed tissue also identified significant differences between the two disease entities. The study reported a similar incidence of CDKN2A/B, IKZF1, and PAX5 deletions but a lower incidence of ETV6 and EBF1 deletions in patients with B-LBL. All cases where hyperdiploidy was found were in patients with limited-stage disease. Unlike B-ALL, where trisomies of chromosomes 4, 10, and 17 are associated with a favorable prognosis, none of the patients with B-LBL in this cohort harbored these favorable trisomies.[45]

T-LBL and T-ALL share similar chromosomal abnormalities; however, no characteristic translocations correlate with prognosis. Chromosomal abnormalities of the TCR are relatively common and include chromosomal abnormalities at 7q34-36, 7p15, and 14q11.[46,47] Other reported translocations include (9;17), t(8;13) (p11;q11-14), and t(10;11)(p13-14;q14-21).[48-53] B-LBLs and T-LBLs contain IG and *TCR* gene rearrangements at the molecular level, respectively, although there can be some overlap as well. The TCR rearrangement status appears to have prognostic significance in T-LBL, with the absence of biallelic *TRD* deletion, seen in approximately 7% of cases, associated with inferior outcome.[54] Additional genetic alterations associated with prognostic significance in patients treated with current therapy regimens include loss of heterozygosity for chromosome 6q (present in 12% of cases), activating mutations in *NOTCH1* and/or *FBXW7* gene (present in 50%-70% of cases), *PTEN* (loss-of-function mutations in 9%-23% of cases), *NRAS + KRAS* (5%-18% of cases), activating mutation in genes of the PI3K/AKT pathway (4%-15% of cases), and overexpression of *miR*-223.[54-65] These features appear to be useful for risk stratification in pediatric T-LBL and may be employed in the design of future therapy protocols. Along those lines, the role of minimal disseminated disease (MDD) in the diagnostic bone marrow (≥1% lymphoblasts) and minimal residual disease (MRD) as prognostic markers in T-LBL are yet to be unequivocally established.[36,66,67]

Stage at diagnosis is the only parameter consistently used for risk group stratification of children with LBL, dividing them into limited-stage (stages I and II) and advanced stage (stages III and IV) disease. Modern treatment regimens for LBL based on ALL-type regimens result in EFS rates between 75% and 90%. Current protocols used in the United States and Europe are derived from either the LSA2L2 regimen (Memorial Sloan Kettering Cancer Center) or the NHL–Berlin-Frankfurt-Munster (BFM) protocols modeled on the ALL-BFM strategy.[68-71] Limited data exist on pediatric LBL studies from the Asian subcontinent.[72-76] The various cooperative groups have tested several modifications of methotrexate administration to improve CNS-directed treatments. Overall, high-dose methotrexate has not shown to significantly affect EFS in patients with T-LBL, and CNS-directed therapy based on frequent intrathecal injections without the need for cranial radiation effectively prevents CNS relapses. The recent Children's Oncology Group (COG) ALL0434 trial evaluated the role of methotrexate and nelarabine, a nucleoside analogue, in T-ALL. Patients with T-LBL were also included in this trial. In this study patients were randomized between Capizzi dose MTX and high-dose MTX and with or without the addition of nelarabine. Patients with T-LBL did not participate in the methotrexate randomization, and all patients with T-LBL received augmented BFM regimen with Capizzi-style methotrexate and pegaspargase. Only patients with high-risk T-LBL (defined as having more than 1% T-lymphoblasts in the BM detected by MMD flow cytometry) were eligible for the nelarabine randomization. Patients with CNS3 disease were not eligible. For patients with T-ALL, the Capizzi methotrexate arm with the addition of nelarabine showed significantly improved 4-year disease-free survival (DFS). Among the 118 patients with high-risk T-LBL enrolled, there was no difference in DFS between those who received nelarabine ($n = 60$) and those who did not ($n = 58$, 4-year DFS $85.0 \pm 5.6\%$ vs $89.0 \pm 4.7\%$, respectively, $P = 0.2788$).[77] This trial, however, was not powered to evaluate nelarabine in T-LBL, leaving its role in T-LBL undefined.

In B-LBL in children there is no single standard of care. Patients are often treated with modified BMF therapy derived from ALL protocols. In the COG5791 study, these patients received a four-drug induction,[78] but the BFM and French groups have shown that dose reductions in cyclophosphamide and anthracyclines can be achieved for patients with localized LBL (stages I and II).[30,79] However, these studies combined patients with T- and B-LBL. Patients with localized B-LBL were included in the recently completed COG ALL trial AALL0932 to determine if we could decrease overall therapy for patients with localized LBL by using a three-drug induction that reduces the anthracycline dose to 75 mg/m^2 (compared with 175 mg/m^2 in past studies) and a standard consolidation that decreases cyclophosphamide exposure from 3 to 1 g/m^2. Patients with B-LBL on this trial were nonrandomly assigned to the standard-risk ALL arm. The results of this study are awaited.

The outcomes in children with relapsed LBL remains dismal, with survival rates of 10% to 30%. Available data indicate that high-dose therapy followed by hematopoietic stem cell transplant (HSCT) is the only option with a chance for cure. There is ongoing debate about whether auto- or allo-HSCT is superior in such circumstances. Published data seem to suggest that, while there may be higher treatment-related mortality with allo-HCTs, they may offer a higher probability of DFS. The numbers, however, remain too small to draw a definitive conclusion.[30,32,80,81]

BURKITT LYMPHOMA AND DIFFUSE LARGE B-CELL LYMPHOMA

BL and DLBCL are the most common mature B-NHLs of childhood and adolescence.[82,83] Although distinct histological, immunophenotypic, and genotypic characteristics are appreciated in typical cases, the two lymphomas share considerable histologic and clinical overlap and are treated on the same protocols in the pediatric population.

Pathology and Molecular Characteristics

BL resembles highly proliferative B cells present in the germinal center (GC). It accounts for 30% to 50% of all childhood lymphomas.[84] Three distinct epidemiological variants have been described; "endemic," "sporadic," and "immunodeficiency-associated BL." These variants differ in their geographical distribution, EBV association, biology, morphological and immunophenotypic features, and clinical features. For example, the endemic form is most commonly found in central Africa and presents with jaw involvement. The sporadic variant occurs worldwide and is the most common subtype in Western Europe and Africa and usually presents with abdominal masses involving the terminal ileum and ileocecal region.[85-90]

Histologically, BL is characterized by a diffuse growth pattern that extensively replaces the normal underlying tissue architecture. Frequent mitotic and apoptotic cells reflect this lymphoma's high proliferative rate and apoptotic index, respectively. Tingible body macrophages interspersed among the neoplastic cells impart a characteristic low-power microscopic starry-sky appearance. The proliferation index, measured by the immunohistochemical nuclear expression for Ki-67, typically approaches 100% of the tumor cells. In the classic BL variant, the neoplastic cells are monomorphous and medium-sized ("small noncleaved") with moderate amounts of basophilic cytoplasm (*Figure 91.3*).[19,91] The cells have round nuclei, clumped or condensed chromatin with clear parachromatin, and one to three nucleoli. When seen in Wright-stained cytologic preparations, BL cells have characteristically deeply basophilic cytoplasm with prominent, clear cytoplasmic vacuoles.

Immunophenotypically, BLs have a mature GC-like profile. They express CD10, CD19, strong uniform CD20, CD22, CD79a, PAX5, BCL-6, and surface IG (IgM or, less commonly, IgA or IgG), with κ or λ IGL restriction (*Table 91.2*).[92] They are typically negative for BCL2, CD34, and TdT. The latter two antigens are useful in the differential diagnosis with B-LBL, which is most often positive for these markers. CD21, the complement fragment Cd3 and the EBV receptor, is more frequently detected in the endemic than sporadic form.

BL is molecularly characterized by translocations of the *MYC* gene to either the immunoglobulin heavy or light chain and leading to its overexpression and the typical high proliferation rate. These translocations include t(8;14)(q24;q32)/*MYC-IGH* (80%-90% of the cases), t(2;8)(q11;q32)/*IGL-MYC*, and t(8;22)(q23;q11)/*MYC-IGK*.

The translocations associated with BL are relatively easily detected by classic cytogenetic methods and by fluorescent in situ hybridization.[91] In addition to these classic translocations, a significant proportion of pediatric BLs contain other nonspecific but recurrent cytogenetic abnormalities, such as chromosome 22 abnormalities, independent of t(8;22) and gains of chromosomes, typically +1q, +7q, +12, or losses of, for example, 17p, etc., some of which appear to increase in frequency with disease progression.[93-95] Some of these (e.g., abnormalities of 13q) may correlate with prognosis, at least in cases with high-stage presentation.[93] More recently, a subset of *MYC*-negative BL with abnormalities of 11q has been described and currently accepted as a provisional entity called "Burkitt-like lymphoma with 11q aberration" in the WHO Classification.[19] These lymphomas represent ~3% of BLs occurring in immunocompetent patients but are significantly enriched in the setting of immunosuppression following solid organ transplantation (SOT), where they represent 43% of all BLs. They have morphologic and clinical features and a gene expression signature similar to the *MYC*+ BL and harbor a recurrent pattern of 11q abnormalities, including interstitial gains at 11q23.2-q23.3 and telomeric losses at 11q24.1-qter.[96,97]

Gene expression profiling and comparative genome hybridization described a molecular signature for BL[98-100] with upregulation of MYC target genes and GC B-cell genes and decreased expression of nuclear factor (NF)-κB-associated genes and MHC class I.[98] miRNA profiling data showed only minor differences between sporadic and endemic BL.[101] High-throughput sequencing has revealed mutations in ID3, CCND3, ARID1A, and/or SMARCA4.[102-104] EBV-negative tumors are more likely to have additional mutations when compared with EBV-positive tumors.[102]

DLBCL accounts for ~20% of all pediatric NHLs.[1,105] It is composed predominantly of large cells (i.e., nuclear size equal to or exceeding that of macrophage nuclei), with a diffuse growth pattern and with a proliferation index typically less than that required for a diagnosis of BL (typically 90% or less). In addition, the neoplastic cells may have a predominantly centroblastic (>80% in children), immunoblastic (<10% in children), or anaplastic appearance, defining three morphologic variants with no known prognostic implications (*Figure 91.4*).[106,107] Tumors rich in T lymphocytes and histiocytes are defined as a distinct entity in the most recent WHO Classification as T-cell/histiocyte-rich large B-cell lymphoma.

Immunophenotypically, DLBCLs express one or more pan-B-cell-associated markers CD19, CD20, CD22, CD79a, and PAX5. Surface or cytoplasmic IG is expressed by 50% or more cases. Some cases may express CD5, CD10, BCL2, BCL6, IRF4/MUM1, and CD30

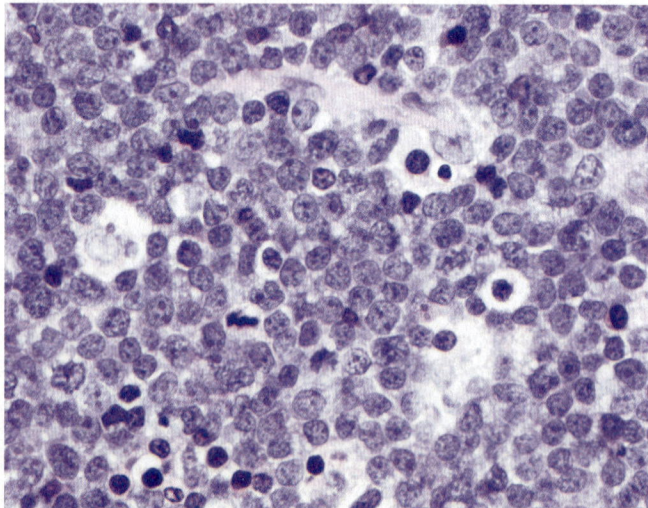

FIGURE 91.3 Histology BL. Burkitt lymphoma (BL). Sheets of medium-sized lymphocytes are present with fine chromatin and multiple nucleoli. In addition, there are scattered large histiocytes containing debris. These histiocytes give the "starry-sky" appearance to the histology of BL.

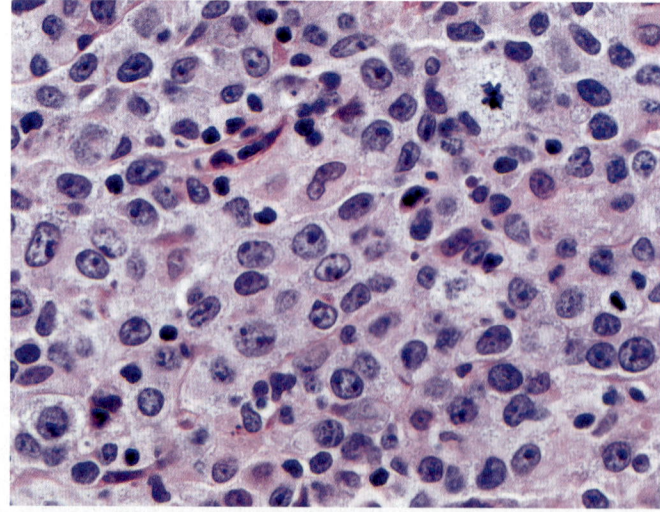

FIGURE 91.4 Histology DLBCL. Diffuse large B-cell lymphoma. Sheets of variably sized large cells with prominent nucleoli and chromatin clearing. There is variation in cell size, in contrast to the more uniform cells of Burkitt lymphoma.

(Table 91.2). Gene expression profiling and immunohistochemical studies have defined subgroups with distinct biology in DLBCL.[108] The gene expression profiles of the tumor cells when compared with signatures of their postulated physiologic counterparts were identified as either germinal center origin-like (GCB) or post–germinal center origin/activated B-cell-like (ABC) and type 3 subgroups traditionally. These three subgroups have shown fundamental survival differences in adult patients treated by chemotherapy; therefore, the distinction of the GCB from the non-GCB subtype is an important predictive factor in DLBCL. Currently, these subgroups do not currently determine therapy in children. The GC-like group, which is predominant in children,[106,109] is characterized by a $CD10^{+/-}$, $BCL6^{+/-}$, $IRF4/MUM1^-$ immunophenotype, whereas the non-GC subtype is characterized by $CD10^-$, $BCL6^{+/-}$, and $IRF4/MUM1^+$. In addition, cases classified pathologically as DLBCL in children appear to be associated with MYC overexpression.[109] Rare cases of anaplastic lymphoma kinase (ALK)-expressing DLBCL with plasmablastic features can be found among DLBCL of children.[110-112] These have been included under the designation of ALK-positive large B-cell lymphoma in the most recent WHO Classifications.

Cytogenetics of DLBCL often include complex karyotypes with recurrent, but nonspecific abnormalities. While, in adults, many of the GC-like cases contain the t(14;18) characteristic for follicular lymphoma (FL), this is not the case in pediatrics, perhaps because of the unique biology of FL, a potential precursor of DLBCL, in this age group. The rare ALK-positive cases may harbor the t(2;5) or t(2;17), resulting in *ALK* gene overexpression. Adult studies have shown recurrent somatic mutations depending on the cell of origin of DLBCL. For example, mutations within EZH2 and GNA13 are almost exclusively associated with the GCB subtype, while mutations for MYD88, CARD11, and CD79b are restricted to ABC-type lymphomas.[113] Alterations including translocations of BCL-6 at 3q27 and copy number alterations at 6q21 and 9p21 are more common in the ABC subgroup as compared with the BCL-2 rearrangements, which are more commonly found in GCB DLBCL.[114-117] MYC translocation, without a concurrent translocation of BCL-2 and/or BCL-6 ("single hit") is more common in pediatric cases of DLBCL as compared with adults.[118] BCL-2 translocations are very rarely seen in children.[106,118] However, in-depth genomic analysis in adult DLBCL has uncovered distinct functional profiles and genetic aberrations between the two groups (GCB vs ABC), but it has also uncovered genetic heterogeneity within these groups. Based on these findings new taxonomies for DLBCL have been proposed, designated as the LymphGen classification and the DLBCL clusters. The DLBCL cluster taxonomy subdivided GCB and ABC DLBCL into five clusters (C1-C5). The LymphGen classification on the other hand divides DLBCL into seven genetic subtypes, namely, BN2, MCD, N1,ST2,A53, $EZB-MYC^+$, and $EZB-MYC^-$. These are based on oncogenic pathway involvement, gene expression phenotype, tumor microenvironment, survival rates, and potential therapeutic targets.[119-121]

High-grade B-cell lymphoma is a heterogeneous category of mature B-cell lymphomas, often with morphologic features of both DLBCL and BL, but with intermediate biologic features. According to the most recent 2016 WHO Classification[19] these include (1) high-grade B-cell lymphoma with *MYC* and *BCL2* and/or *BCL6* rearrangements, to describe cases of DLBCL with a gene expression profiling similar to BL, many of which harbor dual translocations involving *MYC* and *BCL2* ("double-hit lymphomas"), correlating with a particularly poor outcome, and (2) high-grade B-cell lymphoma, not otherwise specified (NOS), referring to cases of DLBCL with a high proliferation rate and immunophenotype resembling BL, but lacking a detectable *MYC* translocation, or cases with morphology typical for BL but atypical immunophenotype or genetic features. Some of these cases would have been classified as "Burkitt-like lymphoma" in previous classification systems.

Clinical Features and Management

Sporadic BL and DLBCL commonly present with intra-abdominal disease involving the gastrointestinal (GI) tract. This can present as intussusception. Peripheral lymphadenopathy and involvement of the regions of the head and neck are more common in DLBCL. Bone marrow and CNS involvement is much more common in BL as compared with DLBCL.[122,123]

Risk Stratification: The French, American, British/Lymphoma malignancy group (FAB/LMB) and BFM risk group classifications elucidate characteristics specific to BL, Burkitt-like lymphoma, and DLBCL. Risk group stratification incorporates stage, disease site, surgical resectability, and LDH levels. Although the general principles are the same, there are subtle differences in the details of the risk group stratification between the two. The BFM risk stratification divides patients into four risk groups (R1-R4)[124] while the FAB/LMB protocols stratify patients into three risk groups(groups A, B, and C; Table 91.5).[128,130] In the most recent FAB/LMB international trial, group B patients were further subdivided into "lower" and "higher" risk based on baseline LDH levels with the intensification of therapy for the higher-risk group B patients (Table 91.5).[129]

Treatment: There have been significant improvements in outcome for children with newly diagnosed BL and DLBCL over the past 30 years.[1,12,131] This has been largely accomplished through incremental refinements in sequential multicenter trials that feature both a stage- and histology-directed approach as well as advances in supportive care to allow highly intensive therapy and control of tumor lysis. Compared with ALL-type therapy, shorter, more intensive therapy has been shown to improve survival for patients with B-NHL.[132] Advances in therapy were initially achieved by dose intensification of cyclophosphamide, methotrexate, and cytarabine and by the incorporation of etoposide. In the SFOP LMB-89 regimen,[122] group A treatment is restricted to those who have completely resected limited-stage disease, whereas group C, which is the most intensive arm, comprises those who have marrow or CNS disease. Group B is intermediate. Approximately 85% of children with advanced-stage B-cell lymphoma were cured with this approach. An international collaborative study (LMB-96) was conducted to determine whether the intensity of LMB-89 therapy could be safely reduced for patients with groups B and C therapies. Among group B patients, it was demonstrated that the avoidance of cyclophosphamide dose escalation in the second course of COPADM and deletion of a maintenance sequence could be safely implemented without compromising the outcome.[128] Among group C patients, however, reduction in therapy was associated with a poorer outcome.[130] The BFM cooperative group has also reported excellent results with a regimen that features high-dose methotrexate (5 g/m^2), ifosfamide, doxorubicin, etoposide, cytarabine, vincristine, and steroids.[133]

The monoclonal anti-CD20 antibody rituximab is known to improve outcomes when combined with chemotherapy in adults with DLBCL.[134] Rituximab has been studied in pediatric B-NHL in recent studies. The BFM group examined a rituximab window phase, and the toxicity profile was generally acceptable.[135] A recent international randomized clinical trial evaluated the efficacy of combining rituximab to the FAB/LMB96 chemotherapy backbone for patients with group C disease and group B with elevated LDH.[129] Patients on the rituximab arm had a superior 3-year EFS compared with standard chemotherapy (93.9% vs 82.3%, hazard ratio 0.32 P = .00096).[129] With this approach, EFS for all risk groups of BL/DLBCL in pediatrics is >90% (Table 91.5).

Outcomes for patients with relapsed or refractory disease, however, are dismal with the 5-year OS of <20%.[136-140] The treatment of relapsed disease is high-dose chemotherapy followed by HSCT. One of the most commonly used regimens for children with recurrent CD20 mature B-cell lymphoma (e.g., BL and DLBCL) is the R-ICE regimen, which includes rituximab, ifosfamide, carboplatin, and etoposide. A COG study demonstrated the activity of this regimen in patients with either BL or DLBCL with subsequent EFS following either auto-HSCT or allo-HSCT.[141] The role of autologous vs allogeneic HSCT remains controversial. Published studies featuring HSCT for pediatric B-NHL are relatively small in number and vary with respect to the type of HSCT, salvage therapy, preparative regimen, and histologic subtype, making direct comparisons difficult.[136-150]

Table 91.5. Mature B-NHL in Children: LMB/FAB Risk Stratification, Chemotherapy, and Outcome

Risk Strata	FAB/LMB Group	St. Jude/Murphy Staging	Chemotherapy	EFS, % (Year)	Trial	Reference
Low risk	Group A	Completely resected stage I or completely resected abdominal stage II	COPAD X 2 No intrathecal (IT) therapy	98 (4 y)	FAB/LMB 96	127
Intermediate risk[a]	Group B lower risk	Not in groups A or C, and stage I/II with any LDH, or stage III with LDH < twice the upper limit of normal	COP-RCOPADM1-RCOPADM1-RCYM-RCYM + IT chemotherapy[+]	95 (4 y)	FAB/LMB 96	128
	Group B higher risk	Not in groups A or C, and stage III with LDH > twice the upper limit of normal Non-CNS, non-leukemic stage IV with any LDH	COP-RCOPADM1-RCOPADM1-RCYM-RCYM + IT chemotherapy[+]	93.9 (3 y)	International B-NHL 2010	129
High risk	Group C1	Bone marrow involvement ≥25, and/or CNS positive with CSF cytology negative	COP-RCOPADM1-RCOPADM2-RCYVE-RCYVE-M1-M2 + IT chemotherapy[+]			
	Group C3	CSF cytology positive	COP-RCOPADM1-RCOPADM2-RCYVE-RCYVE-M1-M2 + IT chemotherapy[+]			

Abbreviations: COP (pre-phase), cyclophosphamide, vincristine, predniso(lo)ne; COPAD, cyclophosphamide, vincristine, predniso(lo)ne, doxorubicin; CPM, cyclophosphamide; M1, cyclophosphamide (250 mg/m^2/dose), vincristine, predniso(lo)ne, doxorubicin, methotrexate; M2, cytarabine, etoposide; RCOPADM1, rituximab, cyclophosphamide(250 mg/m^2/dose), vincristine, predniso(lo)ne, doxorubicin, methotrexate; RCOPADM2, rituximab, cyclophosphamide(500 mg/m^2/dose), vincristine, predniso(lo)ne, doxorubicin, methotrexate; RCYM, rituximab, cytarabine, methotrexate; RCYVE, rituximab, cytarabine, etoposide.
M-methotrexate, Group B patients receive 3 g/m^2/dose over 3 hours as a part of both RCOPADM1 and RCYM courses; group C1 patients receive 8 g/m^2/dose over 4 hours as a part of RCOPADM1, RCOPADM2, and M1. For CNS$^+$ group C1 patients an additional dose of 8 g/m^2/dose over 4 hours of methotrexate is given with the first CYVE cycle. Patients categorized as C3 are the highest risk for relapse, and therefore their therapy is further intensified via delivery of a 24-hour high-dose methotrexate infusion of 8 g/m^2/dose in RCOPADM2, first RCYVE, and M1.
R-Rituximab, a total of six doses of rituximab are administered as a part of group B and C therapy. Dose = 375 mg/m^2/dose.
[+]**IT (intrathecal) chemotherapy**: Group B—IT hydrocortisone and methotrexate on day 1 of pre-phase COP, days 2 and 6 of RCOPADM1 and day 2 of RCYM cycles. IT hydrocortisone and cytarabine on day 7 of RCYM cycles.
Group C1—IT hydrocortisone, methotrexate, and cytarabine on days 1, 3, and 5 of pre-phase COP, days 2, 4, and 6 of RCOPADM1 and 2, and day 2 of M1 cycles.
CNS$^+$ group C1 patients also receive additional IT hydrocortisone, methotrexate, and cytarabine on day 1 of both RYCVE cycles.
Group C3 IT chemotherapy schedule is identical to that of CNS$^+$ group C1 patients.
[a]The FAB/LMB96 trial did not include Rituximab. A subsequent single-arm pilot COG study demonstrated the safety of addition of six doses of rituximab to LMB therapy for children with group B and C disease. The intergroup B-NHL Rituximab 2010 trial was conducted based on these results.[125,126]

Several novel therapies including monoclonal antibodies (newer generations of anti-CD20 mAbs, BiTE or bispecific T-cell engager), chimeric antigen receptor (CAR) T-cell therapy, anti PD-1/PD-L1 or anti-CTLA4 antibodies, and small-molecule inhibitors are being studied alone and in combination with chemotherapy in adults with B-cell lymphomas. These have not yet been studied systematically in the pediatric population; however, they might help to advance outcomes in this very-high-risk group.[151]

PRIMARY MEDIASTINAL B-CELL LYMPHOMA

Primary mediastinal (thymic) large B-cell lymphoma (PMBCL) is an uncommon subtype of DLBCL (<10% of large cell lymphomas in children) thought to arise from thymic medullary B cells.[19] PMBCL has a peak incidence in the adolescent and young adult population. PMBCL is clinically and biologically closely related to nodular sclerosing Hodgkin lymphoma (NSHL).[152,153] In fact, PMBCL can be considered to lie on a pathological continuum of diseases with NSHL and PMBCL lying on either end, and in between mediastinal B-cell lymphomas with features intermediate between PMBCL and NSHL called mediastinal gray zone lymphoma (MGZL).[154]

Pathology and Molecular Characteristics

PMBCL is characterized by a diffuse growth pattern and is composed of tumor cells that may range from medium to large in size. They may have a centroblast-like appearance, may show lobated, "flower-like" nuclear outlines, or may have an anaplastic, Reed-Sternberg-like appearance. Often, they have abundant pale cytoplasm, with a "clear cell" appearance. The neoplastic cells are typically surrounded by thin to thick, dense fibrotic bands. Small benign-appearing lymphocytes and eosinophils may be present and add to the difficulty in differentiating PMBL from HL.

Immunophenotypically, PMBL cells express CD45 and B-cell-associated antigens PAX5, CD19, CD20, CD22, and CD79a (*Table 91.2*); characteristically lack IG; and very often show variable degrees of CD30 expression,[155] as well as CD23 and IRF4/MUM1 positivity. Expression of CD10, BCL-6, and BCL2 is less common. Although not unique to PMBL, the expression of the myelin and lymphocyte (MAL) protein may be useful in differentiating it from other mature B-cell and post-thymic T-cell lymphomas.[156] The transcription factors BOB-1 and OCT2, typically absent in HL, are strongly positive,[157] and similar to HL these tumors usually reveal a strong expression of PD-L1 and PD-L2.[158]

Immunoglobulin genes are rearranged in most cases even if IG expression is not demonstrable by immunologic techniques.[157,159] Gene expression profiling studies reveal a unique signature, similar to HL but distinct from DLBCL. Perturbations in the JAK-STAT and NF-kB pathways and acquired "immune privilege" are believed to act synergistically across the spectrum of these mediastinal lymphomas (HL, PMBCL, MGZL).[160] JAK-STAT signaling in PMBCL likely depends on both IL-13 receptor–mediated signaling as well as constitutive activation caused by somatic gene mutations-JAK2 amplifications, deletions or inactivation of negative regulators *SOCS1* and *PTPN1*, and mutations of *STAT6*.[161-165]

More than half the cases of PMBCL have genomic gains of chromosome 9p, which contains the locus for multiple genes including JAK2 and the programmed death ligands PDL1, PDL2, and JMJD2C.[158,160,166] Chromosomal gains at 2p16.1 are found in approximately 50% of cases, thereby associated with amplifications of REL and BCL11A.[163,167,168] "Immune privilege" in PMBCL likely results from downregulation of MHC class I and II molecules and the increased expression of the programmed death ligands resulting in reduced immunogenicity and T-cell anergy.[169-173]

Clinical Presentation and Management

PMBCL often presents as a large mediastinal mass and often infiltrates into adjacent organs such as the lung, pericardium, or walls of great vessels (Figure 91.5). Extrathoracic extension at diagnosis is uncommon but, with disease progression, can include the kidneys, brain, soft tissue, GI tract, skin, and adrenal glands; bone marrow and lymph node involvement is very rare.[174,175] The initial presentation often includes pleural and pericardial effusions, which can result in tamponade physiology.

The treatment of PMBCL in pediatrics has historically been included in trials/regimens designed for mature B-NHL including BL and DLBCL. However, this approach resulted in inferior outcomes in patients with PMBCL when compared with patients with DLBCL treated with the same approach (EFS 60%-70% for PMBCL vs ~85% for DLBCL).[128,176,177] Given the suboptimal outcomes with mature B-cell chemotherapy and in an effort to reduce the exposure to radiation in the young, predominantly female PMBCL population, infusional DA-EPOCH-R (dose-adjusted etoposide, prednisone, vincristine, cyclophosphamide, doxorubicin, and rituximab) is increasingly being used by the pediatric oncology community. Typically, 6 to 8 cycles of this chemoimmunotherapy is given without consolidative radiation therapy (RT). The success of this approach was first reported by the National Cancer Institute (NCI) in a phase II trial with 51 adult patients (5-year EFS OF 93%).[178] While the same exceptional outcomes have not recapitulated in other multicenter settings, the results remain encouraging. In a retrospective study with 118 adults and 38 pediatric patients (<21 years) across 24 centers the 3-year EFS was 87 and 81%, respectively.[179] In a retrospective registry conducted by the NHL-BFM study group, outcome among 67 pediatric patients treated with DA-EPOCH-R, the 60 month EFS was 84% (95% confidence interval [CI] 72%-91%).[180] The most recent international pediatric mature B-NHL trial studied the DA-EPOCH-R regimen for patients with PMBCL in a single arm phase II trial. Among the 46 patients treated on trial, the 4-year EFS was 69.6% (95% CI 55.2%-80.9%). This was disappointing compared with the single-center NCI adult data; however, it did not differ from the outcome among pediatric patients with PMBCL treated on historical trials (P = .59).[181] A recent prospective trial reported on the use of rituximab in combination with LMB-based chemotherapy for patients with mature B-NHL. Among 21 patients with PMBCL treated with this approach the 5-year EFS was 95.2% (95% CI 71%-97%).[182] Given the small numbers in each trial and the overlapping confidence intervals with different approaches, there remains no single standard of care for the initial management of PMBCL in children. An ongoing phase III NCTN-wide clinical trial is evaluating the role of the checkpoint inhibitor nivolumab in combination with chemoimmunotherapy for children and adults with previously untreated PMBCL (NCT04759586).

The role for RT in PMBCL is also not defined. RT is not routinely used in the upfront setting in DA-EPOCH-R or LMB-based therapy; however, it can be used to consolidate remission in those who fail to achieve complete remission with chemoimmunotherapy. Caution should be taken when using end of therapy FDG-PET to determine response to treatment and role for RT given the high rate of false positivity (likely due to posttreatment inflammatory mediastinal tissue).[178,179,183-187]

Relapses in PMBCL typically occur within 18 months of diagnosis. Disease can be localized to the mediastinum or spread to distant nodal or extranodal sites or the CNS.[188,189] No prospective trials exist to guide management of relapsed disease in children. In the adults treatment options include RT alone for relapse that is confined to the mediastinum[178,179]; high-dose chemotherapy, with or without RT, followed by autologous stem cell transplant (auto-SCT)[189-191]; and/or novel agents including CD-19 CAR-T.[192-194] Retrospective series of relapsed PMBCL in adults report PFS ranging from 57% to 61%.[188,189,195] Given the variable and suboptimal response to chemotherapy in the relapsed setting and recent advances in our understanding of the biology of PMBCL several novel agents have been identified and are being studied in clinical trials. The immune checkpoint inhibitor pembrolizumab is now US Food and Drug Administration approved in the relapsed setting based on activity in a phase II trial.[196] The combination of anti-CD30 antibody-drug conjugate brentuximab vedotin and nivolumab has also demonstrated activity in a phase II trial in relapsed PMBCL.[197,198] Other agents with activity include JAK2 inhibitors such as Ruxolitinib[199,200] and T cells engineered to express chimeric antigen receptors (CARs) directed at CD-19.[192-194]

ANAPLASTIC LARGE CELL LYMPHOMA

Pathology and Molecular Characteristics

ALCL is a CD30+ mature T-cell lymphoma that accounts for 10% to 15% of all childhood lymphomas.[1,201,202] In the revised 2016 WHO classification of lymphoid neoplasms ALCL is subdivided into ALK+ ALCL, ALK− ALCL, and primary cutaneous ALCL.[19] There are several morphologic patterns identified on histology in ALCL, but all morphologic variants harbor the large pleomorphic "hallmark cell," which is characterized by an eccentrically located, horseshoe- or

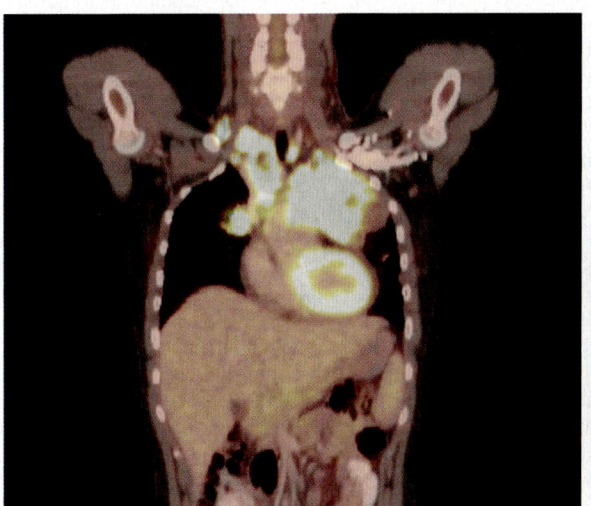
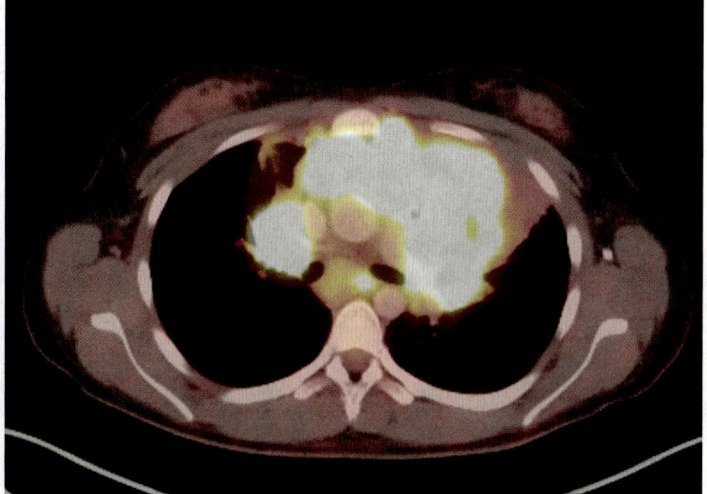

FIGURE 91.5 PET/CT primary mediastinal B-cell lymphoma. Positron emission tomography/computed tomography scan of an adolescent with primary mediastinal B-cell lymphoma, sagittal (L) and axial (R) views.

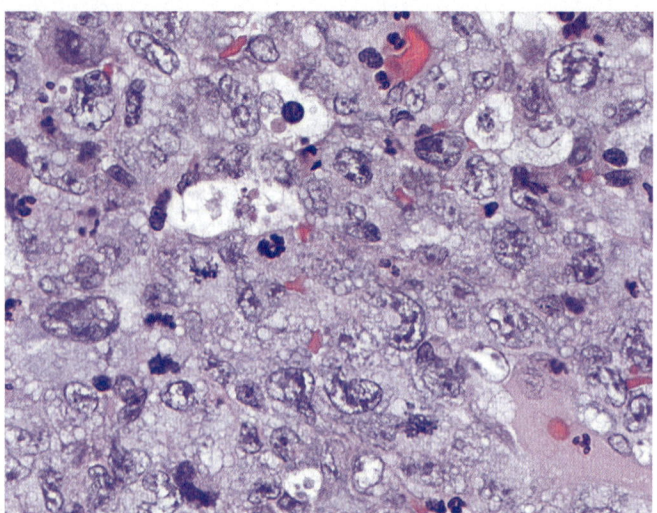

FIGURE 91.6 Histology ALCL. Anaplastic large cell lymphoma (ALCL). Heterogeneous population of large lymphocytes is present with clearing of the nuclear chromatin and moderately abundant *pink* cytoplasm. Some cells have *irregular* and *horseshoe*-shaped nuclei ("hallmark" cells).

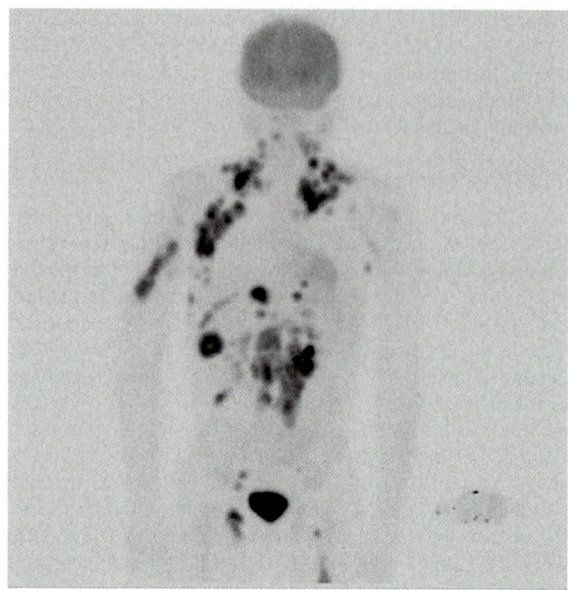

FIGURE 91.7 FDG-PET anaplastic large cell lymphoma. Positron emission computed tomography scan of child with disseminated anaplastic large cell lymphoma.

kidney-shaped nucleus with a paranuclear eosinophilic region (*Figure 91.6*). The morphologic subtypes are (i) common type (60% of cases), (ii) lymphohistiocytic type (10%), (iii) small cell variant (5%-10%), (iv) Hodgkin-like pattern (<5%), and (v) composite (20%-30%). Other poorly characterized, rare variants are sarcomatoid, signet-ring, neutrophil rich, and giant cell type.[19,203-205]

The tumor cells express CD30 in a membrane-bound foundation with dot-like enhancement of the Golgi zone. Most tumors show an aberrant T-cell phenotype with frequent T-cell antigen deletion (CD4+ CD45RO+ CD43+ CD3− CD8−, CD5−CD7−, EMA+ CD25+ TIA, Granzyme-B or Perforin +). Some cases without demonstration of any T-cell phenotype are called "null-type phenotype" (both these entities are clinicopathologically and genetically identical, thus considered the same entity). CD15 is usually absent or only weakly positive. Macrophage-associated antibodies PGM-1 or CD163 are usually negative, as is EBV staining.[203,206-214]

ALK+ ALCL expresses ALK proteins (nuclear/nucleolar and/or cytoplasmic staining). These tumors are characterized by the rearrangement of the *ALK* gene on chromosome 2q23 with several translocation partners, the most common being nucleophosmin (*NPM*) on chromosome 5q35 (t (2; 5)). Other common partners include genes such as *TPM3, ATIC, TFG, CLTC, MSN*, or *TPM4*. In adults, the prognosis of *ALK*-rearranged cases is superior to those without ALK alterations and is independent of the *ALK* fusion partner.[207,215-219]

ALK− ALCL is morphologically indistinguishable from ALK+ ALCL but lacks the *ALK* alterations. Alternative recurrent genetic alterations found include rearrangements of DUSP22 t(6;7), TP63 rearrangements, and other mutations/kinase fusions that lead to JAK/STAT3 pathway constitutive activation.[214,215,220-223]

Clinical Presentation and Management

ALK+ ALCL is most common in the first 3 decades (median age at diagnosis of approximately 12 years) with a slight male predominance (male to female ratio 1.5:1), while ALK- ALCL is primarily seen in older patients. Pediatric ALCL is frequently associated with B symptoms and advanced disease (stage III-IV disease). Greater than 90% of cases have nodal involvement both above and below the diaphragm (*Figure 91.7*). In addition, extranodal involvement such as skin (25%), bone (17%), lung (10%), and/or liver (8%) is also common. Bone marrow involvement is variable (<10% on basic morphologic analysis but 15%-30% if stained for CD30 and ALK and ~50% by polymerase chain reaction [PCR] detection).[207,224-229] A leukemic phase with the presence of leukocytosis and circulating lymphoma cells, although rare, has been reported, especially in the small cell variant ALCL.[230-232] CNS involvement occurs in <5% of cases.[233] Children with ALCL can present with hemophagocytic lymphohistiocytosis (HLH) or HLH-like symptoms, the association being more common when compared with any other kind of lymphoma.[226]

Pediatric ALCL is a chemosensitive tumor with EFS and OS range from 65%-75% and 70%-90%, respectively.[234] Over the past 2 decades variable therapeutic approaches have been used for children with CD30+ ALCL.[202,204,235] The APO regimen is one of the most active regimens and features an induction phase (doxorubicin, vincristine, prednisone, and intrathecal methotrexate) followed by sequential maintenance phases (doxorubicin, methotrexate, vincristine, prednisone, 6-mercaptopurine, and intrathecal methotrexate).[235-237] A Pediatric Oncology Group randomized trial that examined the potential benefit of adding intermediate-dose methotrexate and high-dose cytarabine to the APO regimen found no difference in outcome regardless of immunophenotype. Among the 86 patients with advanced-stage disease, a 4-year EFS and OS of 71.8% and 88.1%, respectively, were reported.[237]

More recent cooperative group trials in Europe and the United States have built on BFM B-cell and APO strategies. The international ALCL99 trial is now considered to be the standard of treatment in many centers worldwide. It is based on the BFM-NHL-90 protocol with a total duration of chemotherapy of 4 to 5 months. In the ALCL99 trial, the addition of vinblastine to the BFM backbone did not improve long-term EFS.[238] Another observation in this trial was that the infusion of methotrexate could be changed from 1 g/m^2 given over 24 hours with IT MTX to a 3-hour infusion of methotrexate at a dosage of 3 g/m^2 (without IT MTX), without compromising outcome.[239] The shorter infusion was also associated with less toxicity. In this trial, various prognostic factors were examined. Interestingly, stage was not associated with prognosis[240]; however, those with a small cell variant or lymphohistiocytic histologic component had a poorer outcome than those lacking this subtype.[208] The overall 2-year EFS was 73%.

Both CD30 and ALK are attractive therapeutic targets in ALCL. The antibody-drug conjugate brentuximab vedotin, which links monomethyl auristatin E to anti-CD30, has been shown to be active in relapsed ALCL in both phase I and phase II studies.[241-243] In addition, 80% complete response rates have been reported in phase I/II clinical trials using small molecule ALK inhibitors such as crizotinib in pediatric patients with relapsed ALCL.[244] Given activity for both agents in the relapsed setting, the COG recently completed the phase II ANHL12P1 trial, which randomized patients to receive either brentuximab vedotin or crizotinib in addition to the ALCL99 backbone chemotherapy. Each arm was compared with a historic ALCL99 cure model with a "cure" rate of 70%. The study was not designed to compare the two novel agents. The 2-year EFS in the brentuximab arm was 79.1% (95% CI 67.2%-87.1%) with an OS of 97% (95%CI 88.1%-99.2%). Therapy was overall well tolerated, and the addition of brentuximab prevented on-therapy relapses in comparison with historic controls.[234] The crizotinib arm was closed just prior to completing accrual due to an increased rate of thrombosis in this group. Results of outcome in the crizotinib arm are still awaited.

There is no standard frontline therapy for patients with CNS ALK+ ALCL or ALK- ALCL. At the current time many of the patients with CNS disease are treated with cranial irradiation and chemotherapy similar to CNS− cases. ALK− ALCL are also treated similarly to ALK+ patients. Adult studies indicate that patients with ALK− ALCL have a lower EFS and higher relapse rate than those with ALK+ ALCL, but this has not been systematically studied in children.

There have been focused efforts to identify factors predictive of failure for children with ALCL. The qualitative and quantitative measurement of *NPM-ALK* transcripts in the blood and bone marrow by PCR screening at the time of diagnosis (MDD) and persistent MRD after the first course of chemotherapy has been shown to predict outcome.[228,229,234,245,246] ALK antibody titers have also been shown to have prognostic significance. Specifically, those with high titers at the time of diagnosis and during treatment have an excellent prognosis compared with those with low titers.[247-249] Mussolin et al. have proposed a risk stratification model based on MDD and ALK antibody titers that may be useful in future trials.[250]

Relapse occurs in 25% to 30% of patients with ALCL. Most relapses occur soon after completion of chemotherapy with a median time to relapse of 1.7 months.[251] Treatment approaches for relapsed ALCL have included second-line chemotherapy followed by high-dose chemotherapy and autologous or allogeneic HSCT.[252-258] Weekly vinblastine monotherapy has shown high response rates and long-lasting remissions, especially in CD3-negative relapses that occurred >12 months after diagnosis as reported in one series.[251,259] In the same series patients with high-risk and very-high-risk disease defined as progression during frontline therapy and CD3+ relapse, respectively, were treated with allogeneic stem cell transplant after carmustine-etoposide-cytarabine-melphalan.[251] Five-year EFS was 41% and 62%, respectively, in the two groups. In the future, novel agents may benefit patients with high-risk relapse and/or replace ASCT in certain risk groups.

POSTTRANSPLANTATION LYMPHOPROLIFERATIVE DISORDERS

Posttransplantation lymphoproliferative disorders (PTLDs) encompass a heterogeneous group of pathologic and clinical entities that may develop in the setting of decreased T-cell function and altered immune surveillance following HSCT and SOT. It is the most common cancer following SOT during childhood and adolescence[260,261] and can range from uncomplicated, self-limited disease to widespread nodal and extranodal disease.

Risk factors include EBV status at the time of transplant (EBV-naïve recipients receiving a transplant from EBV-positive donors being at high risk),[262-264] host factors including younger age,[262,265] degree of immunosuppression as determined primarily by the organ transplanted (lung and intestinal transplants at highest risk),[266,267] donor source for HSCT (highest risk with mismatched unrelated donors and T-cell depletion), and cumulative exposure to immunosuppressive medications (increased incidence among recipients of SOT with history of rejection and among HSCT recipients with graft-versus-host disease).[268,269] However, the absolute risk associated with specific immunosuppression medications remains controversial.

Pathology and Molecular Characteristics

The 2016 revision of the WHO Classification divides PTLD into "early lesion," "polymorphic," "monomorphic," and "classical Hodgkin lymphoma (cHL)-like" PTLD (*Table 91.1*). PTLD is most commonly of B-cell origin and EBV associated, particularly among post-HSCT patients (typically within 3-4 months) or early after SOT (first 1-2 years post SOT). Late-onset disease (3-10 years post transplant) in the SOT population is increasingly described and is more likely to be EBV negative and of monomorphic pathology. EBV-negative PTLD appears to have more genomic alterations, including alterations in known genes in lymphoma genesis, that is, c-MYC, TP53, BCL6, and RAS.[263,270-272]

Clinical Presentation and Management

EBV viral load monitoring is a highly sensitive tool for surveillance and preemptive management of patients at risk for PTLD. However, it has several limitations including poor specificity for determining PTLD risk and a lack of standardization of the optimal sample type, reporting units, trigger points, and monitoring algorithms.[273-276] Treatment strategies for PTLD must consider several factors including disease presentation and pathology, organ graft function, risk of rejection, and immunosuppressive medications. The standard first-line approach to PTLD consists of reduction of immunosuppression to restore T-cell function; however, this leads to resolution in less than 50% of patients and is not always feasible because of increased risk of organ rejection. Other therapeutic approaches include rituximab as single agent ± chemotherapy or chemotherapy alone with reported EFS rates of approximately 70% for all approaches.[277-281] Preliminary studies have shown that adoptive cellular therapy with EBV-specific T lymphocytes (EBV-CTLs) are well tolerated and have efficacy in PTLD.[282] A recently completed COG pilot study, ANHL1522, studied the feasibility of using third-party EBV-CTLs at multiple pediatric centers for patients with incomplete response to three cycles of rituximab. The results are currently awaited.[283]

UNCOMMON PEDIATRIC LYMPHOMAS

Approximately 10% of childhood NHLs are subtypes of uncommon histologies of mature B-lineage such as pediatric-type follicular lymphoma (PTFL), marginal zone lymphoma (MZL), and primary CNS lymphoma or of mature T-lineage as peripheral T-cell lymphoma not otherwise specified (PTCL-NOS), hepatosplenic T-cell lymphoma (HSTCL), extranodal natural killer/T-cell lymphoma—nasal type, angioimmunoblastic T-cell lymphoma, subcutaneous panniculitis like T-cell lymphoma, and primary cutaneous γδ T-cell lymphoma.

Pediatric Follicular Lymphoma

Children may develop FL that is pathologically and clinically similar to the adult disease, as well as FLs with unique clinicopathologic features, designated by the most recent WHO Classification as PTFL.[284-289] More recent studies uncovered two distinct clinicopathologic entities with overlapping morphologic features and characteristic patterns of molecular alterations: nodal, PTFL, and FL/large B-cell lymphoma with interferon regulatory factor-4 (*IRF4*) gene rearrangement (LBCL with *IRF4* rearrangement).[290]

PTFL predominantly occurs in males and presents with limited stage, although advanced stage III/IV cases have been reported. Neoplastic cells of PTFL express a mature B-cell phenotype and are positive for pan B-cell markers. CD10 and BCL6 are persevered and cells may have weak BCL2 expression but are negative for MUM/IRF4.[19,286,289] In contrast to adult FL the malignant cells lack t(14;18)(q32;q21), *BCL2*, *BCL6*, and *IRF4* rearrangements and P53 overexpression, despite their apparent high histologic grade. Recent studies of PTFL have revealed a mutational landscape characterized by low genetic complexity, correlating with their indolent clinical behavior, with a limited number of gene mutations, uncommon mutations in histone-modifying genes and frequent mutations in the *TNFRSF14* gene and *MAP2K1* genes, gains or amplifications of 6p24.3, del1p36.[284,291-296] Optimal therapy for PTFL remains undefined and ranges from B-cell NHL-type chemotherapy or cyclophosphamide, doxorubicin, vincristine, prednisone-derived chemotherapy courses to a "watchful waiting" approach, which may be appropriate after complete resection of limited stage disease. In contrast to FL in adults, which is an incurable disease, outcomes in pediatric FL are excellent with long-term survival rates exceeding 95%.[284,293]

LBCL with *IRF4* rearrangements may have follicular (grade 3B), composite (follicular and diffuse), or exclusively diffuse growth patterns, the latter resembling GC-type DLBCL. This histologic subtype occurs predominantly in children and young adults and presents in the Waldeyer ring and/or cervical lymph nodes, typically at low stage. LBCLs are associated with rearrangements of *IRF4* to the *IGH* or *IGL* genes and, in a small percentage of cases, to an unknown partner gene. The tumor cells typically express IRF4/MUM1, BCL6, and BCL2, without *BCL2* gene rearrangements. Somatic BCL6 mutations and mutations in IRF4 and NF-κB pathway genes (*CARD*11, CD79b, and *MYD*88) are frequent. *IRF*-rearranged lymphomas appear to have an excellent prognosis when occurring in children and young adults.[290,293]

Marginal Zone B-Cell Lymphoma

MZL represents less than 2% of all pediatric NHLs.[289,297,298] As with adults, MZLs in children and young adults may be nodal or extranodal in their presentation. The extranodal MZLs of mucosa-associated tissue are also referred to as MALT lymphomas, and gastric forms are often associated with *Helicobacter pylori* infection. Extranodal sites of presentation include the salivary glands, lung, orbit, ocular adnexa, lip, breast, stomach, and sinonasal cavity. Both nodal and extranodal MZLs are reportedly more frequent in males and usually present with localized disease. MZLs in children demonstrate morphologic and immunophenotypic features similar to their adult counterparts. In addition, over two-thirds of pediatric nodal MZLs display disruption of residual normal follicles, resembling progressive transformation of GCs, a feature that appears to be unique to MZLs in this age group and that prompted their classification as a distinct provisional entity, pediatric nodal MZL.[19] Genetic abnormalities that can be observed in pediatric MZL cases are similar to those seen in MZL occurring in adult patients and include trisomy 18, trisomy 3, t(14;18)/*IGH*-*MALT1*, and, rarely, other *IGH* gene translocation to unknown partner genes.[299]

Therapeutic approaches to MZL in children vary considerably, and there are no defined treatment guidelines. Clinical data from international series currently support an approach of complete staging followed by wait and watch strategy with close clinical monitoring for completely resected, limited-stage disease. The approach may also be considered in cases with incomplete resection.[300,301] Radiation or systemic chemotherapy can be considered in advanced stage or relapsed disease, both of which are very rare. Overall outcomes in pediatric MZL are excellent with EFS and OS of 94% and 100% in a recent international series.[301]

Peripheral T-Cell Lymphoma Not Otherwise Specified

Nonanaplastic PTCLs are rare in children and comprise between 0.9% and 1.8% of childhood NHLs.[302,303] These are a heterogeneous group of diseases, divided in 28 subtypes[19] with PTCL-NOS being the most common subtype, followed by NK-/T-cell lymphoma, HSTCL, and subcutaneous panniculitis-like T-cell lymphoma.[302-307] Preexisting conditions are reported in 25% of children with PTCL.[304] PTCL-NOS is usually diagnosed at the end of the first decade of life, with a slight male predominance. These lymphomas are mainly nodal based, with infrequent involvement of the peripheral blood and bone marrow, as well as the skin and the GI tract. Patients usually present with advanced-stage disease, with most patients having an effusion in at least one location, pleural being the most common. CNS involvement at diagnosis is very rare.[302,304] Immunophenotypically, PTCL-NOS are composed of CD3$^+$/TCRbeta$^+$ and mostly CD4$^+$ T cells with frequent losses of antigens such as CD5 and CD7. Some cases may show CD30 expression, which is inhomogeneous and not as strong as in ALCL.[19,308] PTCL-NOS is a molecularly heterogeneous group. Gene expression profiling in adults has identified two major biological and clinical subgroups, the GATA-binding protein 3(GATA3) and the T-box 21(TBX21) and eomesodermin (EOMES) subtypes, with the GATA3 subgroup associated with poor OS.[309-311] Several recurrent mutations/chromosomal alterations have been identified in PTCL-NOS, such as mutations in the epigenetic modulator genes *TET2*, *DNMT3A*, *RHOA*, or the *FYN* gene; overexpression of spleen tyrosine kinase (SYK) characterized by a recurrent t(5;9)(q33;q22); loss at 9p21 associated with reduced expression of CDKN2A, CDKN2B, and MTAP; and fusion CTLA4-CD28 and fusions of VAV1.[312-317]

No standard of treatment for children with PTCL-NOS exists. B-cell/T-cell lymphoma and ALCL-like treatment regimens have been used with variable success with neither strategy showing a clear survival benefit over the other.[202,302-305] Allogenic HSCT seems to provide a clear survival benefit in first relapse. However, given suboptimal responses to first-line chemotherapy, it remains to be seen whether a high-risk group of patients who might benefit from an allogenic HSCT can be identified (such as those with induction failure or those who fail to achieve complete response with induction chemotherapy).[304,305]

Hepatosplenic T-Cell Lymphoma

HSTCL is an aggressive extranodal malignancy of cytotoxic T cells usually of γδ and, less commonly, αβ TCR types. This rare lymphoma has a peak incidence in adolescents and young adults, with male predominance,[19,293,304,318] although a female predisposition is reported for αβ hepatosplenic lymphomas. Cases of αβ hepatosplenic lymphoma are histologically, cytogenetically, and clinically similar to the γδ form.[319,320] A relatively high percentage of cases follow SOT or immunosuppressive therapies for other conditions.[293,302] Patients typically present with hepatosplenomegaly, B-symptoms, bone marrow involvement, and elevated LDH levels but no appreciable lymphadenopathy. Isolated thrombocytopenia is a common presentation. Circulating lymphoma cells are commonly present at diagnosis but may be difficult to distinguish from atypical lymphocytes. A more obvious leukemic phase may develop as the disease progresses.[319,320]

Histologically, the neoplastic cells are small to intermediate in size, with scant to moderate amounts of cytoplasm, and tend to infiltrate the splenic red pulp cords and sinuses, hepatic sinusoids, and bone marrow sinuses.[319,321] The lymphoma cells have a fairly consistent immunophenotypic expression pattern of CD2$^+$, CD3$^+$, CD4$^-$, CD8$^\pm$, CD5$^-$, CD7$^+$, CD16$^+$, and CD56$^\pm$ (*Table 91.2*).[19,320,322] Cytogenetically, an isochromosome 7q, often with trisomy 8, loss of Y chromosome, and other random chromosomal abnormalities, is found in the majority of reported cases.[293,304,322] Recent studies have better defined the genetic landscape of this lymphoma, which includes recurrent mutations in genes that activate signaling pathways critical for lymphoma survival (STAT5B, STAT3, and PIK3CD in 9%-30% of cases) and also represent potential targets for existing therapeutic agents. In addition, mutations in chromatin-modifying genes (*SETD2*, *INO80*, and *ARID1B*) are present in ~60% of cases.[323] Currently, there is no consensus on the standard of care. OS is dismal at 13± 12% at 5 years.[304] Chemotherapy alone (mature B-NHL or preferentially ALCL-derived therapy) is inadequate for the treatment of HSCTL. Allogenic HSCT appears to show survival benefit in cases in CR1 after induction or consolidation therapy.[324-327]

Primary CNS Lymphoma

Primary CNS lymphoma (PCNSL) is an extranodal subtype of NHL that is confined to the brain, leptomeninges, eyes, and/or spinal cord. It is rare in childhood and less than 150 cases have been reported in the literature. While most reported cases are in immunocompetent hosts, both acquired and congenital immunodeficiency increase the risk of PCNSL. The median age at diagnosis is 12 years. The most common histology of pediatric PCNSL is DLBCL; however, unlike adult PCNSL, this represents only 50% of all cases (>95% cases in adults are DLBCL). Other common histologies include ALCL (25% of cases) and BL (10% of cases).[328] The molecular biology of PCNSL in children remains largely undefined; however, a recent report characterized the genomic alterations in a cohort of 12 pediatric and young adult cases, identifying common alterations in *TP53*, *NFKBIE*, and *GNA13* with wild-type *MYD88* among younger patients.[329] The most common presenting symptoms include signs of increased intracranial pressure and/or cranial nerve palsies. Most of the patients (>90%) present with solid intracranial masses. Isolated intraspinal masses and/or isolated leptomeningeal disease are rare (<5%).[328]

A contrast-enhanced brain magnetic resonance imaging (MRI) is the imaging modality of choice for the detection of PCNSL. The diagnosis is typically made by a stereotactic brain biopsy. Additional diagnostic evaluation should include whole-body PET/computed tomography, bone marrow aspirate and biopsy, cerebrospinal fluid (CSF) analysis, and/or spinal MRI.

Complete surgical resection does not seem to confer any benefit to children with PCNSL given the multifocal and infiltrative nature of the disease. On the contrary, given the increased risk of toxicity and long-term neurological sequelae the role of surgery is restricted to obtaining a biopsy to establish the diagnosis. Similarly, whole-brain RT alone does not provide durable remissions (median OS of only 17 months).[330] Favorable outcomes have been reported with CNS-penetrating chemotherapy such as high-dose methotrexate and/or high-dose cytarabine containing chemotherapy regimens (5-yr EFS 74%, OS 85%).[328] Thus, most pediatric centers treat children with PCNSL without immunodeficiency with NHL-directed chemotherapy without RT as first-line therapy. Novel approaches are needed to improve outcomes in children with immunodeficiency who have inferior outcomes.

FUTURE DIRECTIONS

Although significant progress has been made in the treatment of children with NHL, 25% to 30% continue to have refractory or recurrent disease. Treatment-related late effects are of additional concern. Thus, the continued goal and challenge for the pediatric oncologist are to develop more effective treatment approaches that are not associated with significant late effects. This will require further refinement in risk-adapted treatment planning, which will be made possible by the identification of additional prognostic biologic and clinical factors. The continued molecular characterization associated with pediatric NHL may prove helpful in refining the classification of clinically relevant histologic subtypes, evaluating response to therapy, and developing novel therapeutic approaches that target the molecular lesion directly and reduce our reliance on chemotherapy.

References

1. Sandlund JT, Downing JR, Crist WM. Non-Hodgkin's lymphoma in childhood. *N Engl J Med.* 1996;334(19):1238-1248.
2. Wood WA, Lee SJ. Malignant hematologic diseases in adolescents and young adults. *Blood.* 2011;117(22):5803-5815.
3. Jaglowski SM, Linden E, Termuhlen AM, Flynn JM. Lymphoma in adolescents and young adults. *Semin Oncol.* 2009;36(5):381-418.
4. Young JL, Jr, Ries LG, Silverberg E, Horm JW, Miller RW. Cancer incidence, survival, and mortality for children younger than age 15 years. *Cancer.* 1986;58(2 suppl):598-602.
5. Percy CLSM, Linet M, et al. Lymphomas and reticuloendothelial, neoplasms. In: Ries LASM, Gurney JG, et al., eds. *Adolescents: eCiasaca, United States SEER Program 1975-1995 NPN, 99-4649.* National Cancer Institute SP; 1999:35-50.
6. Sandlund JT, Martin MG. Non-Hodgkin lymphoma across the pediatric and adolescent and young adult age spectrum. *Hematology Am Soc Hematol Educ Program.* 2016;2016(1):589-597.
7. National Cancer Institute sponsored study of classifications of non-Hodgkin's lymphomas: summary and description of a working formulation for clinical usage. The Non-Hodgkin's Lymphoma Pathologic Classification Project. *Cancer* 1982;49:2112-2135.
8. Hochberg J, El-Mallawany NK, Abla O. Adolescent and young adult non-Hodgkin lymphoma. *Br J Haematol.* 2016;173(4):637-650.
9. Miles RR, Shah RK, Frazer JK. Molecular genetics of childhood, adolescent and young adult non-Hodgkin lymphoma. *Br J Haematol.* 2016;173(4):582-596.
10. Linet MS, Brown LM, Mbulaiteye SM, et al. International long-term trends and recent patterns in the incidence of leukemias and lymphomas among children and adolescents ages 0-19 years. *Int J Cancer.* 2016;138(8):1862-1874.
11. Rodriguez-Galindo C, Friedrich P, Alcasabas P, et al. Toward the cure of all children with cancer through collaborative efforts: pediatric oncology as a global challenge. *J Clin Oncol.* 2015;33(27):3065-3073.
12. Minard-Colin V, Brugières L, Reiter A, et al. Non-Hodgkin lymphoma in children and adolescents: progress through effective collaboration, current knowledge, and challenges ahead. *J Clin Oncol.* 2015;33(27):2963-2974.
13. Ward E, DeSantis C, Robbins A, Kohler B, Jemal A. Childhood and adolescent cancer statistics, 2014. *CA Cancer J Clin.* 2014;64(2):83-103.
14. Ozuah NW, El-Mallawany NK. Childhood and adolescence non-Hodgkin lymphomas in low- and middle-income countries. In: Attarbaschi OAA, ed. *Non-Hodgkin's Lymphoma in Childhood and Adolescence.* Springer; 2019:337-351.
15. *SEER Cancer Statistics Review, 1975-2014.* National Cancer Institute. Based on November 2016 SEER data submission, posted to the SEER web site https://seer.cancer.gov/csr/1975_2014/. 2017.
16. Thacker N, Abla O. Epidemiology of non-Hodgkin lymphomas in childhood and adolescence. In: Abla O, Attarbaschi A, eds. *Non-Hodgkin's Lymphoma in Childhood and Adolescence.* Springer International Publishing; 2019:15-22.
17. Natkunam Y, Gratzinger D, Chadburn A, et al. Immunodeficiency-associated lymphoproliferative disorders: time for reappraisal? *Blood.* 2018;132(18):1871-1878.
18. Burkhardt B, Oschlies I, Klapper W, et al. Non-Hodgkin's lymphoma in adolescents: experiences in 378 adolescent NHL patients treated according to pediatric NHL-BFM protocols. *Leukemia.* 2011;25(1):153-160.
19. Swerdlow SH, Campo E, Pileri SA, et al. The 2016 revision of the World Health Organization classification of lymphoid neoplasms. *Blood.* 2016;127(20):2375-2390.
20. Blondiaux E, Laurent M, Audureau E, et al. Factors influencing the diagnostic yield and accuracy of image-guided percutaneous needle biopsy of pediatric tumors: single-center audit of a 26-year experience. *Pediatr Radiol.* 2016;46(3):372-382.
21. Murphy SB. Classification, staging and end results of treatment of childhood non-Hodgkin's lymphomas: dissimilarities from lymphomas in adults. *Semin Oncol.* 1980;7(3):332-339.
22. Rosolen A, Perkins SL, Pinkerton CR, et al. Revised international pediatric non-Hodgkin lymphoma staging system. *J Clin Oncol.* 2015;33(18):2112-2118.
23. Pui CH, Mahmoud HH, Wiley JM, et al. Recombinant urate oxidase for the prophylaxis or treatment of hyperuricemia in patients with leukemia or lymphoma. *J Clin Oncol.* 2001;19(3):697-704.
24. Head DR, Behm FG. Acute lymphoblastic leukemia and the lymphoblastic lymphomas of childhood. *Semin Diagn Pathol.* 1995;12(4):325-334.
25. Mitchell CD, Gordon I, Chessells JM. Clinical, haematological, and radiological features in T-cell lymphoblastic malignancy in childhood. *Clin Radiol.* 1986;37(3):257-261.
26. Williams AH, Taylor CR, Higgins GR, et al. Childhood lymphoma-leukemia. I. Correlation of morphology and immunological studies. *Cancer.* 1978;42(1):171-181.
27. Burkhardt B. Paediatric lymphoblastic T-cell leukaemia and lymphoma: one or two diseases? *Br J Haematol.* 2010;149(5):653-668.
28. Feng H, Stachura DL, White RM, et al. T-lymphoblastic lymphoma cells express high levels of BCL2, S1P1, and ICAM1, leading to a blockade of tumor cell intravasation. *Cancer Cell.* 2010;18(4):353-366.
29. Raetz EA, Perkins SL, Bhojwani D, et al. Gene expression profiling reveals intrinsic differences between T-cell acute lymphoblastic leukemia and T-cell lymphoblastic lymphoma. *Pediatr Blood Cancer.* 2006;47(2):130-140.
30. Ducassou S, Ferlay C, Bergeron C, et al. Clinical presentation, evolution, and prognosis of precursor B-cell lymphoblastic lymphoma in trials LMT96, EORTC 58881, and EORTC 58951. *Br J Haematol.* 2011;152(4):441-451.
31. Neth O, Seidemann K, Jansen P, et al. Precursor B-cell lymphoblastic lymphoma in childhood and adolescence: clinical features, treatment, and results in trials NHL-BFM 86 and 90. *Med Pediatr Oncol.* 2000;35(1):20-27.
32. Burkhardt B, Zimmermann M, Oschlies I, et al. The impact of age and gender on biology, clinical features and treatment outcome of non-Hodgkin lymphoma in childhood and adolescence. *Br J Haematol.* 2005;131(1):39-49.
33. Oschlies I, Burkhardt B, Chassagne-Clement C, et al. Diagnosis and immunophenotype of 188 pediatric lymphoblastic lymphomas treated within a randomized prospective trial: experiences and preliminary recommendations from the European childhood lymphoma pathology panel. *Am J Surg Pathol.* 2011;35(6):836-844.
34. Uckun FM, Sather HN, Gaynon PS, et al. Clinical features and treatment outcome of children with myeloid antigen positive acute lymphoblastic leukemia: a report from the Children's Cancer Group. *Blood.* 1997;90(1):28-35.
35. Pilozzi E, Pulford K, Jones M, et al. Co-expression of CD79a (JCB117) and CD3 by lymphoblastic lymphoma. *J Pathol.* 1998;186(2):140-143.
36. Coustan-Smith E, Mullighan CG, Onciu M, et al. Early T-cell precursor leukaemia: a subtype of very high-risk acute lymphoblastic leukaemia. *Lancet Oncol.* 2009;10(2):147-156.
37. Patel JL, Smith LM, Anderson J, et al. The immunophenotype of T-lymphoblastic lymphoma in children and adolescents: a Children's Oncology Group report. *Br J Haematol.* 2012;159(4):454-461.
38. Haydu JE, Ferrando AA. Early T-cell precursor acute lymphoblastic leukaemia. *Curr Opin Hematol.* 2013;20(4):369-373.
39. Patrick K, Wade R, Goulden N, et al. Outcome for children and young people with Early T-cell precursor acute lymphoblastic leukaemia treated on a contemporary protocol, UKALL 2003. *Br J Haematol.* 2014;166(3):421-424.
40. Link MP, Roper M, Dorfman RF, Crist WM, Cooper MD, Levy R. Cutaneous lymphoblastic lymphoma with pre-B markers. *Blood.* 1983;61(5):838-841.
41. Sheibani K, Nathwani BN, Winberg CD, et al. Antigenically defined subgroups of lymphoblastic lymphoma. Relationship to clinical presentation and biologic behavior. *Cancer.* 1987;60(2):183-190.
42. Borowitz MJ, Croker BP, Metzgar RS. Lymphoblastic lymphoma with the phenotype of common acute lymphoblastic leukemia. *Am J Clin Pathol.* 1983;79(3):387-391.
43. Maitra A, McKenna RW, Weinberg AG, Schneider NR, Kroft SH. Precursor B-cell lymphoblastic lymphoma. A study of nine cases lacking blood and bone marrow involvement and review of the literature. *Am J Clin Pathol.* 2001;115(6):868-875.
44. Geethakumari PR, Hoffmann MS, Pemmaraju N, et al. Extramedullary B lymphoblastic leukemia/lymphoma (B-ALL/B-LBL): a diagnostic challenge. *Clin Lymphoma Myeloma Leuk.* 2014;14(4):e115-e118.
45. Meyer JA, Zhou D, Mason CC, et al. Genomic characterization of pediatric B-lymphoblastic lymphoma and B-lymphoblastic leukemia using formalin-fixed tissues. *Pediatr Blood Cancer.* 2017;64(7). doi:10.1002/pbc.26363

46. Kaneko Y, Frizzera G, Shikano T, Kobayashi H, Maseki N, Sakurai M. Chromosomal and immunophenotypic patterns in T cell acute lymphoblastic leukemia (T ALL) and lymphoblastic lymphoma (LBL). *Leukemia.* 1989;3(12):886-892.
47. Shikano T, Ishikawa Y, Naito H, et al. Cytogenetic characteristics of childhood non-Hodgkin lymphoma. *Cancer.* 1992;70(3):714-719.
48. Naeem R, Singer S, Fletcher JA. Translocation t(8;13)(p11;q11-12) in stem cell leukemia/lymphoma of T-cell and myeloid lineages. *Genes Chromosomes Cancer.* 1995;12(2):148-151.
49. Inhorn RC, Aster JC, Roach SA, et al. A syndrome of lymphoblastic lymphoma, eosinophilia, and myeloid hyperplasia/malignancy associated with t(8;13)(p11;q11): description of a distinctive clinicopathologic entity. *Blood.* 1995;85:1881-1887.
50. Narita M, Shimizu K, Hayashi Y, et al. Consistent detection of CALM-AF10 chimaeric transcripts in haematological malignancies with t(10;11)(p13;q14) and identification of novel transcripts. *Br J Haematol.* 1999;105(4):928-937.
51. Xiao S, Nalabolu SR, Aster JC, et al. FGFR1 is fused with a novel zinc-finger gene, ZNF198, in the t(8;13) leukaemia/lymphoma syndrome. *Nat Genet.* 1998;18(1):84-87.
52. Ashihara E, Nakamura S, Inaba T, Taki T, Hayashi Y, Shimazaki C. A novel AF10-CALM fusion transcript in gamma/delta-T cell type lymphoblastic lymphoma. *Am J Hematol.* 2007;82(9):859-860.
53. Bohlander SK, Muschinsky V, Schrader K, et al. Molecular analysis of the CALM/AF10 fusion: identical rearrangements in acute myeloid leukemia, acute lymphoblastic leukemia and malignant lymphoma patients. *Leukemia.* 2000;14(1):93-99.
54. Callens C, Baleydier F, Lengline E, et al. Clinical impact of NOTCH1 and/or FBXW7 mutations, FLASH deletion, and TCR status in pediatric T-cell lymphoblastic lymphoma. *J Clin Oncol.* 2012;30:1966-1973.
55. Bonn BR, Rohde M, Zimmermann M, et al. Incidence and prognostic relevance of genetic variations in T-cell lymphoblastic lymphoma in childhood and adolescence. *Blood.* 2013;121(16):3153-3160.
56. Balbach ST, Makarova O, Bonn BR, et al. Proposal of a genetic classifier for risk group stratification in pediatric T-cell lymphoblastic lymphoma reveals differences from adult T-cell lymphoblastic leukemia. *Leukemia.* 2016;30(4):970-973.
57. Park MJ, Taki T, Oda M, et al. FBXW7 and NOTCH1 mutations in childhood T cell acute lymphoblastic leukaemia and T cell non-Hodgkin lymphoma. *Br J Haematol.* 2009;145(2):198-206.
58. Baleydier F, Decouvelaere AV, Bergeron J, et al. T cell receptor genotyping and HOXA/TLX1 expression define three T lymphoblastic lymphoma subsets which might affect clinical outcome. *Clin Cancer Res.* 2008;14(3):692-700.
59. Burkhardt B, Bruch J, Zimmermann M, et al. Loss of heterozygosity on chromosome 6q14-q24 is associated with poor outcome in children and adolescents with T-cell lymphoblastic lymphoma. *Leukemia.* 2006;20(8):1422-1429.
60. Burkhardt B, Moericke A, Klapper W, et al. Pediatric precursor T lymphoblastic leukemia and lymphoblastic lymphoma: differences in the common regions with loss of heterozygosity at chromosome 6q and their prognostic impact. *Leuk Lymphoma.* 2008;49(3):451-461.
61. Bandapalli OR, Zimmermann M, Kox C, et al. NOTCH1 activation clinically antagonizes the unfavorable effect of PTEN inactivation in BFM-treated children with precursor T-cell acute lymphoblastic leukemia. *Haematologica.* 2013;98(6):928-936.
62. Paganin M, Grillo MF, Silvestri D, et al. The presence of mutated and deleted PTEN is associated with an increased risk of relapse in childhood T cell acute lymphoblastic leukaemia treated with AIEOP-BFM ALL protocols. *Br J Haematol.* 2018;182(5):705-711.
63. Zuurbier L, Homminga I, Calvert V, et al. NOTCH1 and/or FBXW7 mutations predict for initial good prednisone response but not for improved outcome in pediatric T-cell acute lymphoblastic leukemia patients treated on DCOG or COALL protocols. *Leukemia.* 2010;24(12):2014-2022.
64. Basso K, Mussolin L, Lettieri A, et al. T-cell lymphoblastic lymphoma shows differences and similarities with T-cell acute lymphoblastic leukemia by genomic and gene expression analyses. *Genes Chromosomes Cancer.* 2011;50(12):1063-1075.
65. Pomari E, Lovisa F, Carraro E, et al. Clinical impact of miR-223 expression in pediatric T-Cell lymphoblastic lymphoma. *Oncotarget.* 2017;8(64):107886-107898.
66. Stark B, Avigad S, Luria D, et al. Bone marrow minimal disseminated disease (MDD) and minimal residual disease (MRD) in childhood T-cell lymphoblastic lymphoma stage III, detected by flow cytometry (FC) and real-time quantitative polymerase chain reaction (RQ-PCR). *Pediatr Blood Cancer.* 2009;52(1):20-25.
67. Mussolin L, Buldini B, Lovisa F, et al. Detection and role of minimal disseminated disease in children with lymphoblastic lymphoma: the AIEOP experience. *Pediatr Blood Cancer.* 2015;62(11):1906-1913.
68. Reiter A, Schrappe M, Ludwig WD, et al. Intensive ALL-type therapy without local radiotherapy provides a 90% event-free survival for children with T-cell lymphoblastic lymphoma: a BFM group report. *Blood.* 2000;95(2):416-421.
69. Reiter A, Schrappe M, Parwaresch R, et al. Non-Hodgkin's lymphomas of childhood and adolescence: results of a treatment stratified for biologic subtypes and stage—a report of the Berlin-Frankfurt-Münster Group. *J Clin Oncol.* 1995;13(2):359-372.
70. Wollner N, Burchenal JH, Lieberman PH, Exelby P, D'Angio G, Murphy ML. Non-Hodgkin's lymphoma in children. A comparative study of two modalities of therapy. *Cancer.* 1976;37(1):123-134.
71. Wollner N, Exelby PR, Lieberman PH. Non-Hodgkin's lymphoma in children: a progress report on the original patients treated with the LSA2-L2 protocol. *Cancer.* 1979;44(6):1990-1999.
72. Gao YJ, Pan C, Tang JY, et al. Clinical outcome of childhood lymphoblastic lymphoma in Shanghai China 2001-2010. *Pediatr Blood Cancer.* 2014;61(4):659-663.
73. Jin L, Zhang R, Huang S, Yang J, Duan YL, Zhang YH. Clinical features and prognosis of children with lymphoblastic lymphoma. [Article in Chinese]. *Zhonghua Zhong Liu Za Zhi.* 2012;34(2):138-142.
74. Kobayashi R, Takimoto T, Nakazawa A, et al. Inferior outcomes of stage III T lymphoblastic lymphoma relative to stage IV lymphoma and T-acute lymphoblastic leukemia: long-term comparison of outcomes in the JACLS NHL T-98 and ALL T-97 protocols. *Int J Hematol.* 2014;99(6):743-749.
75. Sun XF, Xia ZJ, Zhen ZJ, et al. Intensive chemotherapy improved treatment outcome for Chinese children and adolescents with lymphoblastic lymphoma. *Int J Clin Oncol.* 2008;13(5):436-441.
76. Sunami S, Sekimizu M, Takimoto T, et al. Prognostic impact of intensified maintenance therapy on children with advanced lymphoblastic lymphoma: a report from the Japanese pediatric leukemia/lymphoma study group ALB-NHL03 study. *Pediatr Blood Cancer.* 2016;63(3):451-457.
77. Dunsmore KP, Winter SS, Devidas M, et al. Children's oncology group AALL0434: a phase III randomized clinical trial testing nelarabine in newly diagnosed T-cell acute lymphoblastic leukemia. *J Clin Oncol.* 2020;38(28):3282-3293.
78. Termuhlen AM, Smith LM, Perkins SL, et al. Outcome of newly diagnosed children and adolescents with localized lymphoblastic lymphoma treated on Children's Oncology Group trial A5971: a report from the Children's Oncology Group. *Pediatr Blood Cancer.* 2012;59(7):1229-1233.
79. Burkhardt B, Reiter A, Landmann E, et al. Poor outcome for children and adolescents with progressive disease or relapse of lymphoblastic lymphoma: a report from the Berlin-Frankfurt-Muenster Group. *J Clin Oncol.* 2009;27(20):3363-3369.
80. Mitsui T, Mori T, Fujita N, Inada H, Horibe K, Tsurusawa M; Lymphoma Committee, Japanese Pediatric Leukemia/Lymphoma Study Group. Retrospective analysis of relapsed or primary refractory childhood lymphoblastic lymphoma in Japan. *Pediatr Blood Cancer.* 2009;52:591-595.
81. Gross TG, Hale GA, He W, et al. Hematopoietic stem cell transplantation for refractory or recurrent non-Hodgkin lymphoma in children and adolescents. *Biol Blood Marrow Transplant.* 2010;16(2):223-230.
82. Egan G, Goldman S, Alexander S. Mature B-NHL in children, adolescents and young adults: current therapeutic approach and emerging treatment strategies. *Br J Haematol.* 2019;185(6):1071-1085.
83. El-Mallawany NK, Cairo MS. Advances in the diagnosis and treatment of childhood and adolescent B-cell non-Hodgkin lymphoma. *Clin Adv Hematol Oncol.* 2015;13(2):113-123.
84. Magrath I. Epidemiology: clues to the pathogenesis of Burkitt lymphoma. *Br J Haematol.* 2012;156(6):744-756.
85. Magrath I. The pathogenesis of Burkitt's lymphoma. *Adv Cancer Res.* 1990;55:133-270.
86. Barth TFE, Müller S, Pawlita M, et al. Homogeneous immunophenotype and paucity of secondary genomic aberrations are distinctive features of endemic but not of sporadic Burkitt's lymphoma and diffuse large B-cell lymphoma with MYC rearrangement. *J Pathol.* 2004;203(4):940-945.
87. Burkitt D. A sarcoma involving the jaws in African children. *Br J Surg.* 1958;46(197):218-223.
88. Cairo MS, Sposto R, Perkins SL, et al. Burkitt's and Burkitt-like lymphoma in children and adolescents: a review of the Children's Cancer Group experience. *Br J Haematol.* 2003;120(4):660-670.
89. Chuang SS, Huang WT, Hsieh PP, et al. Sporadic paediatric and adult Burkitt lymphomas share similar phenotypic and genotypic features. *Histopathology.* 2008;52(4):427-435.
90. Hochberg J, Waxman IM, Kelly KM, Morris E, Cairo MS. Adolescent non-Hodgkin lymphoma and Hodgkin lymphoma: state of the science. *Br J Haematol.* 2009;144(1):24-40.
91. Jaffe ES, Harris NL, Stein H, Vardiman J. *World Health Organization classification of tumours, Pathology and Genetics of Tumours of Haematopoietic and Lymphoid Tissues.* IARC; 2001:10-302.
92. Behm FGCD. *Immunophenotyping.* In: C-H P eCLNY. Cambridge University Press; 1999:141-141.
93. Onciu M, Schlette E, Zhou Y, et al. Secondary chromosomal abnormalities predict outcome in pediatric and adult high-stage Burkitt lymphoma. *Cancer.* 2006;107(5):1084-1092.
94. Aukema SM, Theil L, Rohde M, et al. Sequential karyotyping in Burkitt lymphoma reveals a linear clonal evolution with increase in karyotype complexity and a high frequency of recurrent secondary aberrations. *Br J Haematol.* 2015;170(6):814-825.
95. Poirel HA, Cairo MS, Heerema NA, et al. Specific cytogenetic abnormalities are associated with a significantly inferior outcome in children and adolescents with mature B-cell non-Hodgkin's lymphoma: results of the FAB/LMB 96 international study. *Leukemia.* 2009;23(2):323-331.
96. Salaverria I, Martin-Guerrero I, Wagener R, et al. A recurrent 11q aberration pattern characterizes a subset of MYC-negative high-grade B-cell lymphomas resembling Burkitt lymphoma. *Blood.* 2014;123(8):1187-1198.
97. Ferreiro JF, Morscio J, Dierickx D, et al. Post-transplant molecularly defined Burkitt lymphomas are frequently MYC-negative and characterized by the 11q-gain/loss pattern. *Haematologica.* 2015;100(7):e275-e279.
98. Dave SS, Fu K, Wright GW, et al. Molecular diagnosis of Burkitt's lymphoma. *N Engl J Med.* 2006;354(23):2431-2442.
99. Hummel M, Bentink S, Berger H, et al. A biologic definition of Burkitt's lymphoma from transcriptional and genomic profiling. *N Engl J Med.* 2006;354(23):2419-2430.
100. Klapper W, Szczepanowski M, Burkhardt B, et al. Molecular profiling of pediatric mature B-cell lymphoma treated in population-based prospective clinical trials. *Blood.* 2008;112(4):1374-1381.
101. Lenze D, Leoncini L, Hummel M, et al. The different epidemiologic subtypes of Burkitt lymphoma share a homogenous micro RNA profile distinct from diffuse large B-cell lymphoma. *Leukemia.* 2011;25(12):1869-1876.

102. Giulino-Roth L, Wang K, MacDonald TY, et al. Targeted genomic sequencing of pediatric Burkitt lymphoma identifies recurrent alterations in antiapoptotic and chromatin-remodeling genes. *Blood.* 2012;120(26):5181-5184.
103. Schmitz R, Young RM, Ceribelli M, et al. Burkitt lymphoma pathogenesis and therapeutic targets from structural and functional genomics. *Nature.* 2012;490(7418):116-120.
104. Love C, Sun Z, Jima D, et al. The genetic landscape of mutations in Burkitt lymphoma. *Nat Genet.* 2012;44(12):1321-1325.
105. Cairo MS, Sposto R, Hoover-Regan M, et al. Childhood and adolescent large-cell lymphoma (LCL): a review of the Children's Cancer Group experience. *Am J Hematol.* 2003;72(1):53-63.
106. Oschlies I, Klapper W, Zimmermann M, et al. Diffuse large B-cell lymphoma in pediatric patients belongs predominantly to the germinal-center type B-cell lymphomas: a clinicopathologic analysis of cases included in the German BFM (Berlin-Frankfurt-Munster) Multicenter Trial. *Blood.* 2006;107(10):4047-4052.
107. Jaffe ES. Anaplastic large cell lymphoma: the shifting sands of diagnostic hematopathology. *Mod Pathol.* 2001;14(3):219-228.
108. Rosenwald A, Wright G, Chan WC, et al. The use of molecular profiling to predict survival after chemotherapy for diffuse large-B-cell lymphoma. *N Engl J Med.* 2002;346(25):1937-1947.
109. Miles RR, Raphael M, McCarthy K, et al. Pediatric diffuse large B-cell lymphoma demonstrates a high proliferation index, frequent c-Myc protein expression, and a high incidence of germinal center subtype: report of the French-American-British (FAB) international study group. *Pediatr Blood Cancer.* 2008;51(3):369-374.
110. Bubała H, Małdyk J, Włodarska I, Sońta-Jakimczyk D, Szczepański T. ALK-positive diffuse large B-cell lymphoma. *Pediatr Blood Cancer.* 2006;46(5):649-653.
111. Onciu M, Behm FG, Downing JR, et al. ALK-positive plasmablastic B-cell lymphoma with expression of the NPM-ALK fusion transcript: report of 2 cases. *Blood.* 2003;102(7):2642-2644.
112. Gesk S, Gascoyne RD, Schnitzer B, et al. ALK-positive diffuse large B-cell lymphoma with ALK-Clathrin fusion belongs to the spectrum of pediatric lymphomas. *Leukemia.* 2005;19(10):1839-1840.
113. Dobashi A. Molecular pathogenesis of diffuse large B-cell lymphoma. *J Clin Exp Hematop.* 2016;56(2):71-78.
114. Pasqualucci L, Bereshchenko O, Bereschenko O, et al. Molecular pathogenesis of non-Hodgkin's lymphoma: the role of Bcl-6. *Leuk Lymphoma.* 2003;44(suppl 3):S5-S12.
115. Visco C, Tzankov A, Xu-Monette ZY, et al. Patients with diffuse large B-cell lymphoma of germinal center origin with BCL2 translocations have poor outcome, irrespective of MYC status: a report from an International DLBCL rituximab-CHOP Consortium Program Study. *Haematologica.* 2013;98(2):255-263.
116. Huang JZ, Sanger WG, Greiner TC, et al. The t(14;18) defines a unique subset of diffuse large B-cell lymphoma with a germinal center B-cell gene expression profile. *Blood.* 2002;99(7):2285-2290.
117. Iqbal J, Greiner TC, Patel K, et al. Distinctive patterns of BCL6 molecular alterations and their functional consequences in different subgroups of diffuse large B-cell lymphoma. *Leukemia.* 2007;21(11):2332-2343.
118. Deffenbacher KE, Iqbal J, Sanger W, et al. Molecular distinctions between pediatric and adult mature B-cell non-Hodgkin lymphomas identified through genomic profiling. *Blood.* 2012;119(16):3757-3766.
119. Schmitz R, Wright GW, Huang DW, et al. Genetics and pathogenesis of diffuse large B-cell lymphoma. *N Engl J Med.* 2018;378(15):1396-1407.
120. Wright GW, Huang DW, Phelan JD, et al. A probabilistic classification tool for genetic subtypes of diffuse large B cell lymphoma with therapeutic implications. *Cancer Cell.* 2020;37(4):551-568.e14.
121. Sehn LH, Salles G. Diffuse large B-cell lymphoma. *N Engl J Med.* 2021;384(9):842-858.
122. Patte C, Auperin A, Michon J, et al. The Société Française d'Oncologie Pédiatrique LMB89 protocol: highly effective multiagent chemotherapy tailored to the tumor burden and initial response in 561 unselected children with B-cell lymphomas and L3 leukemia. *Blood.* 2001;97(11):3370-3379.
123. Salzburg J, Burkhardt B, Zimmermann M, et al. Prevalence, clinical pattern, and outcome of CNS involvement in childhood and adolescent non-Hodgkin's lymphoma differ by non-Hodgkin's lymphoma subtype: a Berlin-Frankfurt-Munster Group Report. *J Clin Oncol.* 2007;25:3915-3922.
124. Woessmann W, Seidemann K, Mann G, et al. The impact of the methotrexate administration schedule and dose in the treatment of children and adolescents with B-cell neoplasms: a report of the BFM Group Study NHL-BFM95. *Blood.* 2005;105(3):948-958.
125. Goldman S, Smith L, Anderson JR, et al. Rituximab and FAB/LMB 96 chemotherapy in children with Stage III/IV B-cell non-Hodgkin lymphoma: a Children's Oncology Group report. *Leukemia.* 2013;27(5):1174-1177.
126. Goldman S, Smith L, Galardy P, et al. Rituximab with chemotherapy in children and adolescents with central nervous system and/or bone marrow-positive Burkitt lymphoma/leukaemia: a Children's Oncology Group Report. *Br J Haematol.* 2014;167(3):394-401.
127. Gerrard M, Cairo MS, Weston C, et al. Excellent survival following two courses of COPAD chemotherapy in children and adolescents with resected localized B-cell non-Hodgkin's lymphoma: results of the FAB/LMB 96 international study. *Br J Haematol.* 2008;141(6):840-847.
128. Patte C, Auperin A, Gerrard M, et al. Results of the randomized international FAB/LMB96 trial for intermediate risk B-cell non-Hodgkin lymphoma in children and adolescents: it is possible to reduce treatment for the early responding patients. *Blood.* 2007;109(7):2773-2780.
129. Minard-Colin V, Aupérin A, Pillon M, et al. Rituximab for high-risk, mature B-cell non-Hodgkin's lymphoma in children. *N Engl J Med.* 2020;382(23):2207-2219.
130. Cairo MS, Gerrard M, Sposto R, et al. Results of a randomized international study of high-risk central nervous system B non-Hodgkin lymphoma and B acute lymphoblastic leukemia in children and adolescents. *Blood.* 2007;109(7):2736-2743.
131. Sandlund JT. Non-hodgkin lymphoma in children. *Curr Hematol Malig Rep.* 2015;10(3):237-243.
132. Gadner H, Müller-Weihrich S, Riehm H. Treatment strategies in malignant non-Hodgkin lymphomas in childhood. [Article in German]. *Onkologie.* 1986;9(2):126-130.
133. Reiter A, Schrappe M, Tiemann M, et al. Improved treatment results in childhood B-cell neoplasms with tailored intensification of therapy: a report of the Berlin-Frankfurt-Münster Group Trial NHL-BFM 90. *Blood.* 1999;94(10):3294-3306.
134. Coiffier B, Lepage E, Brière J, et al. CHOP chemotherapy plus rituximab compared with CHOP alone in elderly patients with diffuse large-B-cell lymphoma. *N Engl J Med.* 2002;346(4):235-242.
135. Meinhardt A, Burkhardt B, Zimmermann M, et al. Phase II window study on rituximab in newly diagnosed pediatric mature B-cell non-Hodgkin's lymphoma and Burkitt leukemia. *J Clin Oncol.* 2010;28(19):3115-3121.
136. Rigaud C, Auperin A, Jourdain A, et al. Outcome of relapse in children and adolescents with B-cell non-Hodgkin lymphoma and mature acute leukemia: a report from the French LMB study. *Pediatr Blood Cancer.* 2019;66(9):e27873.
137. Cairo M, Auperin A, Perkins SL, et al. Overall survival of children and adolescents with mature B cell non-Hodgkin lymphoma who had refractory or relapsed disease during or after treatment with FAB/LMB 96: a report from the FAB/LMB 96 study group. *Br J Haematol.* 2018;182(6):859-869.
138. Woessmann W, Zimmermann M, Meinhardt A, et al. Progressive or relapsed Burkitt lymphoma or leukemia in children and adolescents after BFM-type first-line therapy. *Blood.* 2020;135(14):1124-1132.
139. Burkhardt B, Taj M, Garnier N, et al. Treatment and outcome analysis of 639 relapsed non-Hodgkin lymphomas in children and adolescents and resulting treatment recommendations. *Cancers (Basel).* 2021;13(9):2075.
140. Jourdain A, Auperin A, Minard-Colin V, et al. Outcome of and prognostic factors for relapse in children and adolescents with mature B-cell lymphoma and leukemia treated in three consecutive prospective "Lymphomes Malins B" protocols. A Société Française des Cancers de l'Enfant study. *Haematologica.* 2015;100(6):810-817.
141. Griffin TC, Weitzman S, Weinstein H, et al. A study of rituximab and ifosfamide, carboplatin, and etoposide chemotherapy in children with recurrent/refractory B-cell (CD20+) non-Hodgkin lymphoma and mature B-cell acute lymphoblastic leukemia: a report from the Children's Oncology Group. *Pediatr Blood Cancer.* 2009;52(2):177-181.
142. Kobrinsky NL, Sposto R, Shah NR, et al. Outcomes of treatment of children and adolescents with recurrent non-Hodgkin's lymphoma and Hodgkin's disease with dexamethasone, etoposide, cisplatin, cytarabine, and l-asparaginase, maintenance chemotherapy, and transplantation: Children's Cancer Group Study CCG-5912. *J Clin Oncol.* 2001;19(9):2390-2396.
143. Ladenstein R, Pearce R, Hartmann O, Patte C, Goldstone T, Philip T. High-dose chemotherapy with autologous bone marrow rescue in children with poor-risk Burkitt's lymphoma: a report from the European Lymphoma Bone Marrow Transplantation Registry. *Blood.* 1997;90(8):2921-2930.
144. Appelbaum FR, Deisseroth AB, Graw RG, Jr, et al. Prolonged complete remission following high dose chemotherapy of Burkitt's lymphoma in relapse. *Cancer.* 1978;41(3):1059-1063.
145. Philip T, Biron P, Philip I, et al. Massive therapy and autologous bone marrow transplantation in pediatric and young adults Burkitt's lymphoma (30 courses on 28 patients: a 5-year experience). *Eur J Cancer Clin Oncol.* 1986;22(8):1015-1027.
146. Philip T, Hartmann O, Biron P, et al. High-dose therapy and autologous bone marrow transplantation in partial remission after first-line induction therapy for diffuse non-Hodgkin's lymphoma. *J Clin Oncol.* 1988;6(7):1118-1124.
147. Sandlund JT, Bowman L, Heslop HE, et al. Intensive chemotherapy with hematopoietic stem-cell support for children with recurrent or refractory NHL. *Cytotherapy.* 2002;4(3):253-258.
148. Loiseau HA, Hartmann O, Valteau D, et al. High-dose chemotherapy containing busulfan followed by bone marrow transplantation in 24 children with refractory or relapsed non-Hodgkin's lymphoma. *Bone Marrow Transplant.* 1991;8(6):465-472.
149. Philip T, Hartmann O, Pinkerton R, et al. Curability of relapsed childhood B-cell non-Hodgkin's lymphoma after intensive first line therapy: a report from the Société Française d'Oncologie Pédiatrique. *Blood.* 1993;81(8):2003-2006.
150. Satwani P, Jin Z, Martin PL, et al. Sequential myeloablative autologous stem cell transplantation and reduced intensity allogeneic hematopoietic cell transplantation is safe and feasible in children, adolescents and young adults with poor-risk refractory or recurrent Hodgkin and non-Hodgkin lymphoma. *Leukemia.* 2015;29(2):448-455.
151. Grace Egan SW, Alexander S. Epidemiology of non-Hodgkin lymphomas in childhood and adolescence. In: Abla O, Attarbaschi A, eds. *Non-Hodgkin's Lymphoma in Childhood and Adolescence.* Springer International Publishing; 2019:167-183.
152. Rosenwald A, Wright G, Leroy K, et al. Molecular diagnosis of primary mediastinal B cell lymphoma identifies a clinically favorable subgroup of diffuse large B cell lymphoma related to Hodgkin lymphoma. *J Exp Med.* 2003;198(6):851-862.
153. Gunawardana J, Chan FC, Telenius A, et al. Recurrent somatic mutations of PTPN1 in primary mediastinal B cell lymphoma and Hodgkin lymphoma. *Nat Genet.* 2014;46(4):329-335.
154. Grant C, Dunleavy K, Eberle FC, Pittaluga S, Wilson WH, Jaffe ES. Primary mediastinal large B-cell lymphoma, classic Hodgkin lymphoma presenting in the mediastinum, and mediastinal gray zone lymphoma: what is the oncologist to do? *Curr Hematol Malig Rep.* 2011;6(3):157-163.
155. Higgins JP, Warnke RA. CD30 expression is common in mediastinal large B-cell lymphoma. *Am J Clin Pathol.* 1999;112(2):241-247.

156. Copie-Bergman C, Plonquet A, Alonso MA, et al. MAL expression in lymphoid cells: further evidence for MAL as a distinct molecular marker of primary mediastinal large B-cell lymphomas. *Mod Pathol*. 2002;15(11):1172-1180.
157. Pileri SA, Gaidano G, Zinzani PL, et al. Primary mediastinal B-cell lymphoma: high frequency of BCL-6 mutations and consistent expression of the transcription factors OCT-2, BOB.1, and PU.1 in the absence of immunoglobulins. *Am J Pathol*. 2003;162(1):243-253.
158. Johnson PWM, Davies AJ. Primary mediastinal B-cell lymphoma. *Hematology Am Soc Hematol Educ Program*. 2008:349-358.
159. Küppers R, Rajewsky K, Hansmann ML. Diffuse large cell lymphomas are derived from mature B cells carrying V region genes with a high load of somatic mutation and evidence of selection for antibody expression. *Eur J Immunol*. 1997;27(6):1398-1405.
160. Steidl C, Gascoyne RD. The molecular pathogenesis of primary mediastinal large B-cell lymphoma. *Blood*. 2011;118(10):2659-2669.
161. Guiter C, Dusanter-Fourt I, Copie-Bergman C, et al. Constitutive STAT6 activation in primary mediastinal large B-cell lymphoma. *Blood*. 2004;104(2):543-549.
162. Melzner I, Bucur AJ, Brüderlein S, et al. Biallelic mutation of SOCS-1 impairs JAK2 degradation and sustains phospho-JAK2 action in the MedB-1 mediastinal lymphoma line. *Blood*. 2005;105(6):2535-2542.
163. Weniger MA, Melzner I, Menz CK, et al. Mutations of the tumor suppressor gene SOCS-1 in classical Hodgkin lymphoma are frequent and associated with nuclear phospho-STAT5 accumulation. *Oncogene*. 2006;25(18):2679-2684.
164. Mottok A, Renné C, Willenbrock K, Hansmann ML, Bräuninger A. Somatic hypermutation of SOCS1 in lymphocyte-predominant Hodgkin lymphoma is accompanied by high JAK2 expression and activation of STAT6. *Blood*. 2007;110(9):3387-3390.
165. Ritz O, Guiter C, Castellano F, et al. Recurrent mutations of the STAT6 DNA binding domain in primary mediastinal B-cell lymphoma. *Blood*. 2009;114(6):1236-1242.
166. Rui L, Emre NCT, Kruhlak MJ, et al. Cooperative epigenetic modulation by cancer amplicon genes. *Cancer Cell*. 2010;18(6):590-605.
167. Savage KJ, Monti S, Kutok JL, et al. The molecular signature of mediastinal large B-cell lymphoma differs from that of other diffuse large B-cell lymphomas and shares features with classical Hodgkin lymphoma. *Blood*. 2003;102(12):3871-3879.
168. Weniger MA, Gesk S, Ehrlich S, et al. Gains of REL in primary mediastinal B-cell lymphoma coincide with nuclear accumulation of REL protein. *Genes Chromosomes Cancer*. 2007;46(4):406-415.
169. Rigaud G, Moore PS, Taruscio D, et al. Alteration of chromosome arm 6p is characteristic of primary mediastinal B-cell lymphoma, as identified by genome-wide allelotyping. *Genes Chromosomes Cancer*. 2001;31(2):191-195.
170. Roberts RA, Wright G, Rosenwald AR, et al. Loss of major histocompatibility class II gene and protein expression in primary mediastinal large B-cell lymphoma is highly coordinated and related to poor patient survival. *Blood*. 2006;108(1):311-318.
171. Green MR, Monti S, Rodig SJ, et al. Integrative analysis reveals selective 9p24.1 amplification, increased PD-1 ligand expression, and further induction via JAK2 in nodular sclerosing Hodgkin lymphoma and primary mediastinal large B-cell lymphoma. *Blood*. 2010;116(17):3268-3277.
172. Twa DDW, Chan FC, Ben-Neriah S, et al. Genomic rearrangements involving programmed death ligands are recurrent in primary mediastinal large B-cell lymphoma. *Blood*. 2014;123(13):2062-2065.
173. Steidl C, Shah SP, Woolcock BW, et al. MHC class II transactivator CIITA is a recurrent gene fusion partner in lymphoid cancers. *Nature*. 2011;471(7338):377-381.
174. Lones MA, Perkins SL, Sposto R, et al. Large-cell lymphoma arising in the mediastinum in children and adolescents is associated with an excellent outcome: a Children's Cancer Group report. *J Clin Oncol*. 2000;18(22):3845-3853.
175. Dunleavy K, Steidl C. Emerging biological insights and novel treatment strategies in primary mediastinal large B-cell lymphoma. *Semin Hematol*. 2015;52(2):119-125.
176. Seidemann K, Tiemann M, Lauterbach I, et al. Primary mediastinal large B-cell lymphoma with sclerosis in pediatric and adolescent patients: treatment and results from three therapeutic studies of the Berlin-Frankfurt-Münster Group. *J Clin Oncol*. 2003;21:1782-1789.
177. Gerrard M, Waxman IM, Sposto R, et al. Outcome and pathologic classification of children and adolescents with mediastinal large B-cell lymphoma treated with FAB/LMB96 mature B-NHL therapy. *Blood*. 2013;121(2):278-285.
178. Dunleavy K, Pittaluga S, Maeda LS, et al. Dose-adjusted EPOCH-rituximab therapy in primary mediastinal B-cell lymphoma. *N Engl J Med*. 2013;368(15):1408-1416.
179. Giulino-Roth L, O'Donohue T, Chen Z, et al. Outcomes of adults and children with primary mediastinal B-cell lymphoma treated with dose-adjusted EPOCH-R. *Br J Haematol*. 2017;179(5):739-747.
180. Knorr F, Zimmermann M, Attarbaschi A, et al. Dose-adjusted EPOCH-rituximab or intensified B-NHL therapy for pediatric primary mediastinal large B-cell lymphoma. *Haematologica*. 2021;106(12):3232-3235.
181. Burke GAA, Minard-Colin V, Auperin A, et al. Dose-adjusted etoposide, doxorubicin, and cyclophosphamide with vincristine and prednisone plus rituximab therapy in children and adolescents with primary mediastinal B-cell lymphoma: a multicenter phase II trial. *J Clin Oncol*. 2021;39(33):3716-3724.
182. Dourthe ME, Phulpin A, Auperin A, et al. Rituximab in addition to LMB-based chemotherapy regimen in children and adolescents with primary mediastinal large B-cell lymphoma: results of the French LMB2001 prospective study. *Haematologica*. 2022;107(9):2173-2182.
183. Pinnix CC, Dabaja B, Ahmed MA, et al. Single-institution experience in the treatment of primary mediastinal B cell lymphoma treated with immunochemotherapy in the setting of response assessment by 18fluorodeoxyglucose positron emission tomography. *Int J Radiat Oncol Biol Phys*. 2015;92(1):113-121.
184. Filippi AR, Piva C, Giunta F, et al. Radiation therapy in primary mediastinal B-cell lymphoma with positron emission tomography positivity after rituximab chemotherapy. *Int J Radiat Oncol Biol Phys*. 2013;87(2):311-316.
185. Martelli M, Ceriani L, Zucca E, et al. [18F]fluorodeoxyglucose positron emission tomography predicts survival after chemoimmunotherapy for primary mediastinal large B-cell lymphoma: results of the International Extranodal Lymphoma Study Group IELSG-26 Study. *J Clin Oncol*. 2014;32(17):1769-1775.
186. Zinzani PL, Broccoli A, Casadei B, et al. The role of rituximab and positron emission tomography in the treatment of primary mediastinal large B-cell lymphoma: experience on 74 patients. *Hematol Oncol*. 2015;33(4):145-150.
187. Melani C, Advani R, Roschewski M, et al. End-of-treatment and serial PET imaging in primary mediastinal B-cell lymphoma following dose-adjusted EPOCH-R: a paradigm shift in clinical decision making. *Haematologica*. 2018;103(8):1337-1344.
188. Aoki T, Shimada K, Suzuki R, et al. High-dose chemotherapy followed by autologous stem cell transplantation for relapsed/refractory primary mediastinal large B-cell lymphoma. *Blood Cancer J*. 2015;5:e372.
189. Kuruvilla J, Pintilie M, Tsang R, Nagy T, Keating A, Crump M. Salvage chemotherapy and autologous stem cell transplantation are inferior for relapsed or refractory primary mediastinal large B-cell lymphoma compared with diffuse large B-cell lymphoma. *Leuk Lymphoma*. 2008;49(7):1329-1336.
190. Hamlin PA, Portlock CS, Straus DJ, et al. Primary mediastinal large B-cell lymphoma: optimal therapy and prognostic factor analysis in 141 consecutive patients treated at Memorial Sloan Kettering from 1980 to 1999. *Br J Haematol*. 2005;130(5):691-699.
191. Sehn LH, Antin JH, Shulman LN, et al. Primary diffuse large B-cell lymphoma of the mediastinum: outcome following high-dose chemotherapy and autologous hematopoietic cell transplantation. *Blood*. 1998;91(2):717-723.
192. Neelapu SS, Locke FL, Bartlett NL, et al. Axicabtagene ciloleucel CAR T-cell therapy in refractory large B-cell lymphoma. *N Engl J Med*. 2017;377(26):2531-2544.
193. Abramson JS, Palomba ML, Gordon LI, et al. CR rates in relapsed/refractory (R/R) aggressive B-NHL treated with the CD19-directed CAR T-cell product JCAR017 (TRANSCEND NHL 001). *Am Soc Clin Oncol*. 2017;35:7513
194. Kochenderfer JN, Dudley ME, Kassim SH, et al. Chemotherapy-refractory diffuse large B-cell lymphoma and indolent B-cell malignancies can be effectively treated with autologous T cells expressing an anti-CD19 chimeric antigen receptor. *J Clin Oncol*. 2015;33(6):540-549.
195. Vardhana S, Hamlin PA, Yang J, et al. Outcomes of relapsed and refractory primary mediastinal (thymic) large B cell lymphoma treated with second-line therapy and intent to transplant. *Biol Blood Marrow Transplant*. 2018;24(10):2133-2138.
196. Armand P, Rodig S, Melnichenko V, et al. Pembrolizumab in relapsed or refractory primary mediastinal large B-cell lymphoma. *J Clin Oncol*. 2019;37(34):3291-3299.
197. Zinzani PL, Pellegrini C, Chiappella A, et al. Brentuximab vedotin in relapsed primary mediastinal large B-cell lymphoma: results from a phase 2 clinical trial. *Blood*. 2017;129(16):2328-2330.
198. Zinzani PL, Santoro A, Gritti G, et al. Nivolumab combined with brentuximab vedotin for relapsed/refractory primary mediastinal large B-cell lymphoma: efficacy and safety from the phase II CheckMate 436 study. *J Clin Oncol*. 2019;37(33):3081-3089.
199. Kim SJ, Kang HJ, Dong-Yeop S, et al. The efficacy of JAK2 inhibitor in heavily pretreated classical Hodgkin lymphoma: a prospective pilot study of ruxolitinib in relapsed or refractory classical Hodgkin lymphoma and primary mediastinal large B-cell lymphoma. *Blood*. 2016;128:1820.
200. Younes A, Hilden P, Coiffier B, et al. International Working Group consensus response evaluation criteria in lymphoma (RECIL 2017). *Ann Oncol*. 2017;28(7):1436-1447.
201. Prokoph N, Larose H, Lim MS, Burke GAA, Turner SD. Treatment options for paediatric anaplastic large cell lymphoma (ALCL): current standard and beyond. *Cancers (Basel)*. 2018;10(4):E99.
202. Seidemann K, Tiemann M, Schrappe M, et al. Short-pulse B-non-Hodgkin lymphoma-type chemotherapy is efficacious treatment for pediatric anaplastic large cell lymphoma: a report of the Berlin-Frankfurt-Münster Group Trial NHL-BFM 90. *Blood*. 2001;97(12):3699-3706.
203. Benharroch D, Meguerian-Bedoyan Z, Lamant L, et al. ALK-positive lymphoma: a single disease with a broad spectrum of morphology. *Blood*. 1998;91(6):2076-2084.
204. Brugières L, Deley MC, Pacquement H, et al. CD30(+) anaplastic large-cell lymphoma in children: analysis of 82 patients enrolled in two consecutive studies of the French Society of Pediatric Oncology. *Blood*. 1998;92(10):3591-3598.
205. Pileri S, Sabattini E, Poggi S, Amini M, Falini B, Stein H. Lymphohistiocytic T-cell lymphoma. *Histopathology*. 1994;25(2):191-193.
206. Straus SE, Jaffe ES, Puck JM, et al. The development of lymphomas in families with autoimmune lymphoproliferative syndrome with germline Fas mutations and defective lymphocyte apoptosis. *Blood*. 2001;98(1):194-200.
207. Lowe EJ, Gross TG. Anaplastic large cell lymphoma in children and adolescents. *Pediatr Hematol Oncol*. 2013;30(6):509-519.
208. Lamant L, McCarthy K, d'Amore E, et al. Prognostic impact of morphologic and phenotypic features of childhood ALK-positive anaplastic large-cell lymphoma: results of the ALCL99 study. *J Clin Oncol*. 2011;29(35):4669-4676.
209. Mussolin L, Le Deley MC, Carraro E, et al. Prognostic factors in childhood anaplastic large cell lymphoma: long term results of the international ALCL99 trial. *Cancers (Basel)*. 2020;12(10):E2747.
210. Falini B, Pileri S, Zinzani PL, et al. ALK+ lymphoma: clinico-pathological findings and outcome. *Blood*. 1999;93(8):2697-2706.
211. Brousset P, Rochaix P, Chittal S, Rubie H, Robert A, Delsol G. High incidence of Epstein-Barr virus detection in Hodgkin's disease and absence of detection in anaplastic large-cell lymphoma in children. *Histopathology*. 1993;23(2):189-191.
212. Foss HD, Anagnostopoulos I, Araujo I, et al. Anaplastic large-cell lymphomas of T-cell and null-cell phenotype express cytotoxic molecules. *Blood*. 1996;88(10):4005-4011.

213. Penny RJ, Blaustein JC, Longtine JA, Pinkus GS. Ki-1-positive large cell lymphomas, a heterogenous group of neoplasms. Morphologic, immunophenotypic, genotypic, and clinical features of 24 cases. *Cancer*. 1991;68(2):362-373.
214. Stein H, Foss HD, Dürkop H, et al. CD30(+) anaplastic large cell lymphoma: a review of its histopathologic, genetic, and clinical features. *Blood*. 2000;96(12):3681-3695.
215. Falini B. Anaplastic large cell lymphoma: pathological, molecular and clinical features. *Br J Haematol*. 2001;114(4):741-760.
216. Pulford K, Morris SW, Turturro F. Anaplastic lymphoma kinase proteins in growth control and cancer. *J Cell Physiol*. 2004;199(3):330-358.
217. Pulford K, Lamant L, Espinos E, et al. The emerging normal and disease-related roles of anaplastic lymphoma kinase. *Cell Mol Life Sci*. 2004;61(23):2939-2953.
218. Morris SW, Xue L, Ma Z, Kinney MC. Alk+ CD30+ lymphomas: a distinct molecular genetic subtype of non-Hodgkin's lymphoma. *Br J Haematol*. 2001;113(2):275-295.
219. Duyster J, Bai RY, Morris SW. Translocations involving anaplastic lymphoma kinase (ALK). *Oncogene*. 2001;20(40):5623-5637.
220. Ferreri AJM, Govi S, Pileri SA, Savage KJ. Anaplastic large cell lymphoma, ALK-negative. *Crit Rev Oncol Hematol*. 2013;85(2):206-215.
221. Crescenzo R, Abate F, Lasorsa E, et al. Convergent mutations and kinase fusions lead to oncogenic STAT3 activation in anaplastic large cell lymphoma. *Cancer Cell*. 2015;27(4):516-532.
222. Parrilla Castellar ER, Jaffe ES, Said JW, et al. ALK-negative anaplastic large cell lymphoma is a genetically heterogeneous disease with widely disparate clinical outcomes. *Blood*. 2014;124(9):1473-1480.
223. King RL, Dao LN, McPhail ED, et al. Morphologic features of ALK-negative anaplastic large cell lymphomas with DUSP22 rearrangements. *Am J Surg Pathol*. 2016;40(1):36-43.
224. Sandlund JT, Pui CH, Santana VM, et al. Clinical features and treatment outcome for children with CD30+ large-cell non-Hodgkin's lymphoma. *J Clin Oncol*. 1994;12(5):895-898.
225. Fraga M, Brousset P, Schlaifer D, et al. Bone marrow involvement in anaplastic large cell lymphoma. Immunohistochemical detection of minimal disease and its prognostic significance. *Am J Clin Pathol*. 1995;103(1):82-89.
226. Le Deley MC, Reiter A, Williams D, et al. Prognostic factors in childhood anaplastic large cell lymphoma: results of a large European intergroup study. *Blood*. 2008;111(3):1560-1566.
227. Damm-Welk C, Schieferstein J, Schwalm S, Reiter A, Woessmann W. Flow cytometric detection of circulating tumour cells in nucleophosmin/anaplastic lymphoma kinase-positive anaplastic large cell lymphoma: comparison with quantitative polymerase chain reaction. *Br J Haematol*. 2007;138(4):459-466.
228. Damm-Welk C, Busch K, Burkhardt B, et al. Prognostic significance of circulating tumor cells in bone marrow or peripheral blood as detected by qualitative and quantitative PCR in pediatric NPM-ALK-positive anaplastic large-cell lymphoma. *Blood*. 2007;110(2):670-677.
229. Mussolin L, Pillon M, d'Amore ES, et al. Prevalence and clinical implications of bone marrow involvement in pediatric anaplastic large cell lymphoma. *Leukemia*. 2005;19(9):1643-1647.
230. Onciu M, Behm FG, Raimondi SC, et al. ALK-positive anaplastic large cell lymphoma with leukemic peripheral blood involvement is a clinicopathologic entity with an unfavorable prognosis. Report of three cases and review of the literature. *Am J Clin Pathol*. 2003;120(4):617-625.
231. Ok CY, Wang SA, Amin HM. Leukemic phase of ALK(+) anaplastic large-cell lymphoma, small-cell variant: clinicopathologic pitfalls of a rare entity. *Clin Lymphoma Myeloma Leuk*. 2014;14(4):e123-e126.
232. Bayle C, Charpentier A, Duchayne E, et al. Leukaemic presentation of small cell variant anaplastic large cell lymphoma: report of four cases. *Br J Haematol*. 1999;104(4):680-688.
233. Williams D, Mori T, Reiter A, et al. Central nervous system involvement in anaplastic large cell lymphoma in childhood: results from a multicentre European and Japanese study. *Pediatr Blood Cancer*. 2013;60(10):E118-E121.
234. Lowe EJ, Reilly AF, Lim MS, et al. Brentuximab vedotin in combination with chemotherapy for pediatric patients with ALK+ALCL: results of COG trial ANHL12P1. *Blood*. 2021;137(26):3595-3603.
235. Laver JH, Mahmoud H, Pick TE, et al. Results of a randomized phase III trial in children and adolescents with advanced stage diffuse large cell non-Hodgkin's lymphoma: a Pediatric Oncology Group study. *Leuk Lymphoma*. 2002;43(1):105-109.
236. Weinstein HJ, Lack EE, Cassady JR. APO therapy for malignant lymphoma of large cell "histiocytic" type of childhood: analysis of treatment results for 29 patients. *Blood*. 1984;64(2):422-426.
237. Laver JH, Kraveka JM, Hutchison RE, et al. Advanced-stage large-cell lymphoma in children and adolescents: results of a randomized trial incorporating intermediate-dose methotrexate and high-dose cytarabine in the maintenance phase of the APO regimen—a Pediatric Oncology Group phase III trial. *J Clin Oncol*. 2005;23(3):541-547.
238. Le Deley MC, Rosolen A, Williams DM, et al. Vinblastine in children and adolescents with high-risk anaplastic large-cell lymphoma: results of the randomized ALCL99-vinblastine trial. *J Clin Oncol*. 2010;28(25):3987-3993.
239. Brugières L, Le Deley MC, Rosolen A, et al. Impact of the methotrexate administration dose on the need for intrathecal treatment in children and adolescents with anaplastic large-cell lymphoma: results of a randomized trial of the EICNHL Group. *J Clin Oncol*. 2009;27(6):897-903.
240. Attarbaschi A, Mann G, Rosolen A, et al. Limited stage I disease is not necessarily indicative of an excellent prognosis in childhood anaplastic large cell lymphoma. *Blood*. 2011;117(21):5616-5619.
241. Pro B, Advani R, Brice P, et al. Five-year results of brentuximab vedotin in patients with relapsed or refractory systemic anaplastic large cell lymphoma. *Blood*. 2017;130(25):2709-2717.
242. Younes A, Bartlett NL, Leonard JP, et al. Brentuximab vedotin (SGN-35) for relapsed CD30-positive lymphomas. *N Engl J Med*. 2010;363(19):1812-1821.
243. Locatelli F, Mauz-Koerholz C, Neville K, et al. Brentuximab vedotin for paediatric relapsed or refractory Hodgkin's lymphoma and anaplastic large-cell lymphoma: a multicentre, open-label, phase 1/2 study. *Lancet Haematol*. 2018;5(10):e450-e461.
244. Mossé YP, Voss SD, Lim MS, et al. Targeting ALK with crizotinib in pediatric anaplastic large cell lymphoma and inflammatory myofibroblastic tumor: a Children's oncology group study. *J Clin Oncol*. 2017;35(28):3215-3221.
245. Damm-Welk C, Mussolin L, Zimmermann M, et al. Early assessment of minimal residual disease identifies patients at very high relapse risk in NPM-ALK-positive anaplastic large-cell lymphoma. *Blood*. 2014;123(3):334-337.
246. Damm-Welk C, Kutscher N, Zimmermann M, et al. Quantification of minimal disseminated disease by quantitative polymerase chain reaction and digital polymerase chain reaction for NPM-ALK as a prognostic factor in children with anaplastic large cell lymphoma. *Haematologica*. 2020;105(8):2141-2149.
247. Ait-Tahar K, Damm-Welk C, Burkhardt B, et al. Correlation of the autoantibody response to the ALK oncoantigen in pediatric anaplastic lymphoma kinase-positive anaplastic large cell lymphoma with tumor dissemination and relapse risk. *Blood*. 2010;115(16):3314-3319.
248. Mussolin L, Bonvini P, Ait-Tahar K, et al. Kinetics of humoral response to ALK and its relationship with minimal residual disease in pediatric ALCL. *Leukemia*. 2009;23:400-402.
249. Mussolin L, Pillon M, Zimmermann M, et al. Course of anti-ALK antibody titres during chemotherapy in children with anaplastic large cell lymphoma. *Br J Haematol*. 2018;182:733-735.
250. Mussolin L, Damm-Welk C, Pillon M, et al. Use of minimal disseminated disease and immunity to NPM-ALK antigen to stratify ALK-positive ALCL patients with different prognosis. *Leukemia*. 2013;27(2):416-422.
251. Knörr F, Brugières L, Pillon M, et al. Stem cell transplantation and vinblastine monotherapy for relapsed pediatric anaplastic large cell lymphoma: results of the international, prospective ALCL-relapse trial. *J Clin Oncol*. 2020;38(34):3999-4009.
252. Brugières L, Quartier P, Le Deley MC, et al. Relapses of childhood anaplastic large-cell lymphoma: treatment results in a series of 41 children--a report from the French Society of Pediatric Oncology. *Ann Oncol*. 2000;11(1):53-58.
253. Fukano R, Mori T, Kobayashi R, et al. Haematopoietic stem cell transplantation for relapsed or refractory anaplastic large cell lymphoma: a study of children and adolescents in Japan. *Br J Haematol*. 2015;168(4):557-563.
254. Smith SM, Burns LJ, van Besien K, et al. Hematopoietic cell transplantation for systemic mature T-cell non-Hodgkin lymphoma. *J Clin Oncol*. 2013;31(25):3100-3109.
255. Strullu M, Thomas C, Le Deley MC, et al. Hematopoietic stem cell transplantation in relapsed ALK+ anaplastic large cell lymphoma in children and adolescents: a study on behalf of the SFCE and SFGM-TC. *Bone Marrow Transplant*. 2015;50(6):795-801.
256. Woessmann W, Peters C, Lenhard M, et al. Allogeneic haematopoietic stem cell transplantation in relapsed or refractory anaplastic large cell lymphoma of children and adolescents—a Berlin-Frankfurt-Münster Group Report. *Br J Haematol*. 2006;133(2):176-182.
257. Woessmann W, Zimmermann M, Lenhard M, et al. Relapsed or refractory anaplastic large-cell lymphoma in children and adolescents after Berlin-Frankfurt-Muenster (BFM)-type first-line therapy: a BFM-group study. *J Clin Oncol*. 2011;29(22):3065-3071.
258. Mori T, Takimoto T, Katano N, et al. Recurrent childhood anaplastic large cell lymphoma: a retrospective analysis of registered cases in Japan. *Br J Haematol*. 2006;132(5):594-597.
259. Brugières L, Pacquement H, Le Deley MC, et al. Single-drug vinblastine as salvage treatment for refractory or relapsed anaplastic large cell lymphoma: a report from the French Society of Pediatric Oncology. *J Clin Oncol*. 2009;27(30):5056-5061.
260. Francis A, Johnson DW, Craig JC, Wong G. Incidence and predictors of cancer following kidney transplantation in childhood. *Am J Transplant*. 2017;17(10):2650-2658.
261. Smith JM, Dharnidharka VR. Viral surveillance and subclinical viral infection in pediatric kidney transplantation. *Pediatr Nephrol*. 2015;30(5):741-748.
262. Chinnock R, Webber SA, Dipchand AI, Brown RN, George JF; Pediatric Heart Transplant Study. A 16-year multi-institutional study of the role of age and EBV status on PTLD incidence among pediatric heart transplant recipients. *Am J Transplant*. 2012;12(11):3061-3068.
263. Dharnidharka VR, Webster AC, Martinez OM, Preiksaitis JK, Leblond V, Choquet S. Post-transplant lymphoproliferative disorders. *Nat Rev Dis Primers*. 2016;2:15088.
264. Höcker B, Fickenscher H, Delecluse HJ, et al. Epidemiology and morbidity of Epstein-Barr virus infection in pediatric renal transplant recipients: a multicenter, prospective study. *Clin Infect Dis*. 2013;56(1):84-92.
265. Weintraub L, Weiner C, Miloh T, et al. Identifying predictive factors for posttransplant lymphoproliferative disease in pediatric solid organ transplant recipients with Epstein-Barr virus viremia. *J Pediatr Hematol Oncol*. 2014;36(8):e481-e486.
266. Mynarek M, Schober T, Behrends U, Maecker-Kolhoff B. Posttransplant lymphoproliferative disease after pediatric solid organ transplantation. *Clin Dev Immunol*. 2013;2013:814973.
267. Nassif S, Kaufman S, Vahdat S, et al. Clinicopathologic features of post-transplant lymphoproliferative disorders arising after pediatric small bowel transplant. *Pediatr Transplant*. 2013;17(8):765-773.
268. Landgren O, Gilbert ES, Rizzo JD, et al. Risk factors for lymphoproliferative disorders after allogeneic hematopoietic cell transplantation. *Blood*. 2009;113(20):4992-5001.

269. Styczynski J, Gil L, Tridello G, et al. Response to rituximab-based therapy and risk factor analysis in Epstein Barr Virus-related lymphoproliferative disorder after hematopoietic stem cell transplant in children and adults: a study from the Infectious Diseases Working Party of the European Group for Blood and Marrow Transplantation. *Clin Infect Dis*. 2013;57(6):794-802.
270. Ferreiro JF, Morscio J, Dierickx D, et al. EBV-positive and EBV-negative posttransplant diffuse large B cell lymphomas have distinct genomic and transcriptomic features. *Am J Transplant*. 2016;16(2):414-425.
271. Luskin MR, Heil DS, Tan KS, et al. The impact of EBV status on characteristics and outcomes of posttransplantation lymphoproliferative disorder. *Am J Transplant*. 2015;15(10):2665-2673.
272. Morscio J, Dierickx D, Tousseyn T. Molecular pathogenesis of B-cell posttransplant lymphoproliferative disorder: what do we know so far? *Clin Dev Immunol*. 2013;2013:150835.
273. Fryer JF, Heath AB, Wilkinson DE, Minor PD; Collaborative Study Group. A collaborative study to establish the 1st WHO International Standard for Epstein-Barr virus for nucleic acid amplification techniques. *Biologicals*. 2016;44(5):423-433.
274. Parrish A, Fenchel M, Storch GA, et al. Epstein-Barr viral loads do not predict post-transplant lymphoproliferative disorder in pediatric lung transplant recipients: a multicenter prospective cohort study. *Pediatr Transplant*. 2017;21(6):10.1111/petr.13011.
275. Ruf S, Behnke-Hall K, Gruhn B, Reiter A, Wagner HJ. EBV load in whole blood correlates with LMP2 gene expression after pediatric heart transplantation or allogeneic hematopoietic stem cell transplantation. *Transplantation*. 2014;97(9):958-964.
276. Soriano-López DP, Alcántar-Fierros JM, Hernández-Plata JA, et al. A scheduled program of molecular screening for epstein-Barr virus decreases the incidence of post-transplantation lymphoproliferative disease in pediatric liver transplantation. *Transplant Proc*. 2016;48(2):654-657.
277. González-Barca E, Domingo-Domenech E, Capote FJ, et al. Prospective phase II trial of extended treatment with rituximab in patients with B-cell post-transplant lymphoproliferative disease. *Haematologica*. 2007;92(11):1489-1494.
278. Gross TG, Orjuela MA, Perkins SL, et al. Low-dose chemotherapy and rituximab for posttransplant lymphoproliferative disease (PTLD): a Children's Oncology Group Report. *Am J Transplant*. 2012;12(11):3069-3075.
279. Gross TG, Savoldo B, Punnett A. Posttransplant lymphoproliferative diseases. *Pediatr Clin North Am*. 2010;57(2):481-503. Table of Contents.
280. Messahel B, Taj MM, Hobson R, et al. Single agent efficacy of rituximab in childhood immunosuppression related lymphoproliferative disease: a United Kingdom Children's Cancer Study Group (UKCCSG) retrospective review. *Leuk Lymphoma*. 2006;47(12):2584-2589.
281. Wilsdorf N, Eiz-Vesper B, Henke-Gendo C, et al. EBV-specific T-cell immunity in pediatric solid organ graft recipients with posttransplantation lymphoproliferative disease. *Transplantation*. 2013;95(1):247-255.
282. Bollard CM, Rooney CM, Heslop HE. T-cell therapy in the treatment of post-transplant lymphoproliferative disease. *Nat Rev Clin Oncol*. 2012;9:510-519.
283. Bollard CM, Gottschalk S, Helen Huls M, Leen AM, Gee AP, Rooney CM. Good manufacturing practice-grade cytotoxic T lymphocytes specific for latent membrane proteins (LMP)-1 and LMP2 for patients with Epstein-Barr virus-associated lymphoma. *Cytotherapy*. 2011;13(5):518-522.
284. Attarbaschi A, Beishuizen A, Mann G, et al. Children and adolescents with follicular lymphoma have an excellent prognosis with either limited chemotherapy or a "Watch and wait" strategy after complete resection. *Ann Hematol*. 2013;92(11):1537-1541.
285. Heller KN, Teruya-Feldstein J, La Quaglia MP, Wexler LH. Primary follicular lymphoma of the testis: excellent outcome following surgical resection without adjuvant chemotherapy. *J Pediatr Hematol Oncol*. 2004;26(2):104-107.
286. Lorsbach RB, Shay-Seymore D, Moore J, et al. Clinicopathologic analysis of follicular lymphoma occurring in children. *Blood*. 2002;99(6):1959-1964.
287. Lu D, Medeiros LJ, Eskenazi AE, Abruzzo LV. Primary follicular large cell lymphoma of the testis in a child. *Arch Pathol Lab Med*. 2001;125:551-554.
288. Pakzad K, MacLennan GT, Elder JS, et al. Follicular large cell lymphoma localized to the testis in children. *J Urol*. 2002;168(1):225-228.
289. Swerdlow SH. Pediatric follicular lymphomas, marginal zone lymphomas, and marginal zone hyperplasia. *Am J Clin Pathol*. 2004;122(suppl):S98-S109.
290. Salaverria I, Philipp C, Oschlies I, et al. Translocations activating IRF4 identify a subtype of germinal center-derived B-cell lymphoma affecting predominantly children and young adults. *Blood*. 2011;118(1):139-147.
291. Jaffe ES, Harris NL, Siebert R. Paediatric-type follicular lymphoma. In: Swerdlow SH, Campo E, Harris NL, et al., eds. *WHO Classification of Tumours of Haematopoietic and Lymphoid Tissues WHO Classification of Tumours*, Revised. 4th ed, Vol 2. 2017.
292. Ferry JAdLL, Louissaint A, Jr, Harris NL. Follicular lymphoma. In: Jaffe ESAD, Campo E, Harris NL, Quintanilla-Martinez L, eds. *Hematopathology*. Elsevier; 2017:321-352.
293. Attarbaschi A, Abla O, Arias Padilla L, et al. Rare non-Hodgkin lymphoma of childhood and adolescence: a consensus diagnostic and therapeutic approach to pediatric-type follicular lymphoma, marginal zone lymphoma, and nonanaplastic peripheral T-cell lymphoma. *Pediatr Blood Cancer*. 2020;67(8):e28416.
294. Louissaint A, Jr, Schafernak KT, Geyer JT, et al. Pediatric-type nodal follicular lymphoma: a biologically distinct lymphoma with frequent MAPK pathway mutations. *Blood*. 2016;128(8):1093-1100.
295. Martin-Guerrero I, Salaverria I, Burkhardt B, et al. Recurrent loss of heterozygosity in 1p36 associated with TNFRSF14 mutations in IRF4 translocation negative pediatric follicular lymphomas. *Haematologica*. 2013;98(8):1237-1241.
296. Schmidt J, Gong S, Marafioti T, et al. Genome-wide analysis of pediatric-type follicular lymphoma reveals low genetic complexity and recurrent alterations of TNFRSF14 gene. *Blood*. 2016;128(8):1101-1111.
297. Mo JQ, Dimashkieh H, Mallery SR, Swerdlow SH, Bove KE. MALT lymphoma in children: case report and review of the literature. *Pediatr Dev Pathol*. 2004;7(4):407-413.
298. Taddesse-Heath L, Pittaluga S, Sorbara L, Bussey M, Raffeld M, Jaffe ES. Marginal zone B-cell lymphoma in children and young adults. *Am J Surg Pathol*. 2003;27(4):522-531.
299. Rizzo KA, Streubel B, Pittaluga S, et al. Marginal zone lymphomas in children and the young adult population; characterization of genetic aberrations by FISH and RT-PCR. *Mod Pathol*. 2010;23(6):866-873.
300. Makarova O, Oschlies I, Müller S, et al. Excellent outcome with limited treatment in paediatric patients with marginal zone lymphoma. *Br J Haematol*. 2018;182(5):735-739.
301. Ronceray L, Abla O, Barzilai-Birenboim S, et al. Children and adolescents with marginal zone lymphoma have an excellent prognosis with limited chemotherapy or a watch-and-wait strategy after complete resection. *Pediatr Blood Cancer*. 2018;65(4). doi:10.1002/pbc.26932
302. Kontny U, Oschlies I, Woessmann W, et al. Non-anaplastic peripheral T-cell lymphoma in children and adolescents—a retrospective analysis of the NHL-BFM study group. *Br J Haematol*. 2015;168(6):835-844.
303. Windsor R, Stiller C, Webb D. Peripheral T-cell lymphoma in childhood: population-based experience in the United Kingdom over 20 years. *Pediatr Blood Cancer*. 2008;50(4):784-787.
304. Mellgren K, Attarbaschi A, Abla O, et al. Non-anaplastic peripheral T cell lymphoma in children and adolescents-an international review of 143 cases. *Ann Hematol*. 2016;95(8):1295-1305.
305. Kobayashi R, Yamato K, Tanaka F, et al. Retrospective analysis of non-anaplastic peripheral T-cell lymphoma in pediatric patients in Japan. *Pediatr Blood Cancer*. 2010;54(2):212-215.
306. Hutchison RE, Laver JH, Chang M, et al. Non-anaplastic peripheral t-cell lymphoma in childhood and adolescence: a Children's Oncology Group study. *Pediatr Blood Cancer*. 2008;51(1):29-33.
307. Al Mahmoud R, Weitzman S, Schechter T, Ngan B, Abdelhaleem M, Alexander S. Peripheral T-cell lymphoma in children and adolescents: a single-institution experience. *J Pediatr Hematol Oncol*. 2012;34(8):611-616.
308. Jaffe ES. Pathobiology of peripheral T-cell lymphomas. *Hematology Am Soc Hematol Educ Program*. 2006:317-322.
309. Ballester B, Ramuz O, Gisselbrecht C, et al. Gene expression profiling identifies molecular subgroups among nodal peripheral T-cell lymphomas. *Oncogene*. 2006;25(10):1560-1570.
310. Sakata-Yanagimoto M, Chiba S. Molecular pathogenesis of peripheral T cell lymphoma. *Curr Hematol Malig Rep*. 2015;10(4):429-437.
311. Iqbal J, Wright G, Wang C, et al. Gene expression signatures delineate biological and prognostic subgroups in peripheral T-cell lymphoma. *Blood*. 2014;123(19):2915-2923.
312. Palomero T, Couronné L, Khiabanian H, et al. Recurrent mutations in epigenetic regulators, RHOA and FYN kinase in peripheral T cell lymphomas. *Nat Genet*. 2014;46(2):166-170.
313. Yoo HY, Sung MK, Lee SH, et al. A recurrent inactivating mutation in RHOA GTPase in angioimmunoblastic T cell lymphoma. *Nat Genet*. 2014;46(4):371-375.
314. Couronné L, Bastard C, Bernard OA. TET2 and DNMT3A mutations in human T-cell lymphoma. *N Engl J Med*. 2012;366(1):95-96.
315. Streubel B, Vinatzer U, Willheim M, Raderer M, Chott A. Novel t(5;9)(q33;q22) fuses ITK to SYK in unspecified peripheral T-cell lymphoma. *Leukemia*. 2006;20(2):313-318.
316. Fujiwara SI, Yamashita Y, Nakamura N, et al. High-resolution analysis of chromosome copy number alterations in angioimmunoblastic T-cell lymphoma and peripheral T-cell lymphoma, unspecified, with single nucleotide polymorphism-typing microarrays. *Leukemia*. 2008;22(10):1891-1898.
317. Sandell RF, Boddicker RL, Feldman AL. Genetic landscape and classification of peripheral T cell lymphomas. *Curr Oncol Rep*. 2017;19(4):28.
318. Weidmann E. Hepatosplenic T cell lymphoma. A review on 45 cases since the first report describing the disease as a distinct lymphoma entity in 1990. *Leukemia*. 2000;14(6):991-997.
319. Macon WR, Levy NB, Kurtin PJ, et al. Hepatosplenic alphabeta T-cell lymphomas: a report of 14 cases and comparison with hepatosplenic gammadelta T-cell lymphomas. *Am J Surg Pathol*. 2001;25(3):285-296.
320. Cooke CB, Krenacs L, Stetler-Stevenson M, et al. Hepatosplenic T-cell lymphoma: a distinct clinicopathologic entity of cytotoxic gamma delta T-cell origin. *Blood*. 1996;88(11):4265-4274.
321. Farcet JP, Gaulard P, Marolleau JP, et al. Hepatosplenic T-cell lymphoma: sinusal/sinusoidal localization of malignant cells expressing the T-cell receptor gamma delta. *Blood*. 1990;75(11):2213-2219.
322. Belhadj K, Reyes F, Farcet JP, et al. Hepatosplenic gammadelta T-cell lymphoma is a rare clinicopathologic entity with poor outcome: report on a series of 21 patients. *Blood*. 2003;102(13):4261-4269.
323. McKinney M, Moffitt AB, Gaulard P, et al. The genetic Basis of hepatosplenic T-cell lymphoma. *Cancer Discov*. 2017;7(4):369-379.
324. Voss MH, Lunning MA, Maragulia JC, et al. Intensive induction chemotherapy followed by early high-dose therapy and hematopoietic stem cell transplantation results in improved outcome for patients with hepatosplenic T-cell lymphoma: a single institution experience. *Clin Lymphoma Myeloma Leuk*. 2013;13(1):8-14.

325. Rashidi A, Cashen AF. Outcomes of allogeneic stem cell transplantation in hepatosplenic T-cell lymphoma. *Blood Cancer J*. 2015;5:e318.
326. Yabe M, Miranda RN, Medeiros LJ. Hepatosplenic T-cell Lymphoma: a review of clinicopathologic features, pathogenesis, and prognostic factors. *Hum Pathol*. 2018;74:5-16.
327. McThenia SS, Rawwas J, Oliveira JL, Khan SP, Rodriguez V. Hepatosplenic γδ T-cell lymphoma of two adolescents: case report and retrospective literature review in children, adolescents, and young adults. *Pediatr Transplant*. 2018;22(5):e13213.
328. Attarbaschi A, Abla O, Ronceray L, et al. Primary central nervous system lymphoma: initial features, outcome, and late effects in 75 children and adolescents. *Blood Adv*. 2019;3(24):4291-4297.
329. Guney E, Lucas C-HG, Qi Z, et al. A genetically distinct pediatric subtype of primary CNS large B-cell lymphoma is associated with favorable clinical outcome. *Blood Adv*. 2022;6(10):3189-3193.
330. Kai Y, Kuratsu J, Ushio Y. Primary malignant lymphoma of the brain in childhood. *Neurol Med Chir (Tokyo)*. 1998;38(4):232-237.

Chapter 92 ■ Chronic Lymphocytic Leukemia

SAMEER A. PARIKH • SAAD S. KENDERIAN • NEIL E. KAY • JAMES B. JOHNSTON

INTRODUCTION

Chronic lymphocytic leukemia (CLL) is characterized by the accumulation of mature-appearing malignant lymphocytes (CLL cells) in the blood, marrow, lymph nodes, and spleen.[1-3] Small lymphocytic lymphoma (SLL) is biologically the same disease, with primarily involvement of lymph nodes and spleen. Both CLL and SLL are antedated by monoclonal B-cell lymphocytosis (MBL) in which small numbers of CLL cells can be detected in the blood of asymptomatic individuals (Table 92.1).[5] The CLL cells are unique in being monoclonal B lymphocytes that express CD19, CD5, and CD23 with weak or no expression of surface immunoglobulin (Ig), CD20, CD79b, and FMC7.[1] Despite the fact that the CLL cells may look similar in different patients, there is heterogeneity in the biology, clinical features, and prognosis. In recent years remarkable advances have been made in our understanding of the biology of CLL and this has permitted the development of new prognostic/predictive markers and a variety of highly effective targeted therapies, including inhibitors of the B-cell receptor (BCR) pathway, for example, ibrutinib, and inhibitors of the antiapoptotic proteins, for example, venetoclax.[2,5]

In North America, CLL/SLL accounts for one-quarter of all leukemias, with the incidence reported by the Surveillance, Epidemiology and End Results (SEER) Program being 4.6 per 100,000 for the period 2014 to 2018.[6] However, the incidence is likely much higher, as many patients are diagnosed by flow cytometry and are not included in tumor registries.[7] By combining data from flow cytometry and the cancer registry, the incidence of CLL/SLL in the population of Manitoba, Canada, is 7.99 per 100,000, with the median age at diagnosis being 71.5 years.[7] The median age at diagnosis is younger for males (70 years) than for females (73 years), with the male:female ratio being 1.3:1[7] (Figure 92.1). One-third of patients are <65 years and 10% <50 years. However, because of referral bias, the median age of patients at diagnosis is lower in CLL clinics and in those entered onto clinical trials.[8]

In both population and clinic studies, relative survival (survival compared to sex- and age-matched population without CLL) has traditionally been poorest for men and those aged >70 to 80 years.[7,9,10] However, while the relative survival for all age groups has improved over the past 40 years, men have particularly benefited, diminishing the previously observed gender differences.[11]

Using SEER data, there has been a continued improvement in relative survival from 1985 to 2017, which was most striking after 2000, following the development of chemoimmunotherapy and ibrutinib.[11] As patients are now living longer with the addition of novel therapies, there is considerable interest in the long-term outcome of these patients.

PATHOPHYSIOLOGY

Cell of Origin

There has been controversy as to the normal counterpart of the CLL cell.[3,5] Based on the mutation status of the immunoglobulin heavy chain variable region (IGHV) gene, there are two forms of CLL, one in which there are >2% mutations from germline (mutated, 60% of cases) and one in which there are ≤2% mutations (unmutated, 40% of cases) (Figure 92.2). The IGHV gene is translated into one component of the immunoglobulin protein which, along with CD79, makes up the BCR. As mutations in the IGHV gene occur as the B cell is processed in the follicle centers in lymph nodes, these studies suggest that IGHV mutated CLL may arise from a memory B cell, whereas the unmutated form may be derived from a naïve B cell (Figure 92.3).[3,5] This hypothesis has been supported by DNA methylation studies. In normal B lymphocytes, there are progressive alterations in DNA methylation along the genome as naïve B cells develop into memory B cells.[12] Interestingly, the DNA methylation pattern in the IGHV unmutated form of CLL is similar to a CD5+ naïve B cell form, whereas the IGHV mutated form is most similar to a memory B cell.[13] A third intermediate form of CLL can also be identified by the methylation pattern, which has lower levels of mutations than the IGHV mutated form and an intermediate prognosis between the other two types.[13,14]

It has been suggested that the hematopoietic stem cell is abnormal in CLL, demonstrating increased expression of early lymphoid transcription factors, such as IKAROS.[15] When hematopoietic stem cells from CLL patients are transplanted into immunosuppressed

Table 92.1. Chronic Lymphocytic Leukemia and Variants

Marker	Monoclonal B-cell Lymphocytosis (MBL)[b]	Chronic Lymphocytic Leukemia (CLL)[b]	Small Lymphocytic Lymphoma (SLL)
Peripheral blood B-cell count	<5 × 10⁹/L	≥5 × 10⁹/L	<5 × 10⁹/L
Enlarged lymph nodes and/or spleen[a]	No	Maybe	Yes

[a]By physical examination.[1]
[b]Patients are considered to have CLL if they have a cytopenia or any disease-related symptom.[4]

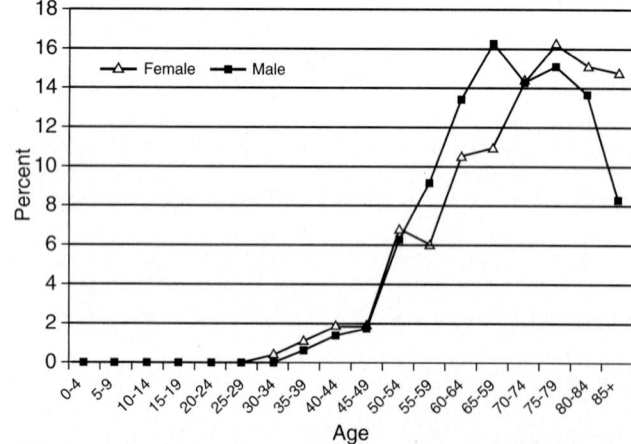

FIGURE 92.1 Age distribution of 351 males and 265 females diagnosed through the provincial cancer registry and a centralized flow cytometry facility in Manitoba over a 5-year period (1998-2003). The median age at diagnosis was 70 years for men and 73 years for women (P = .0281). Overall median age was 71.5 years. (Reprinted from Seftel MD, Demers AA, Banerji V, et al. High incidence of chronic lymphocytic leukemia (CLL) diagnosed by immunophenotyping: a population-based Canadian cohort. Leuk Res. 2009;33(11):1463-1468. Copyright © 2009 Elsevier. With permission.)

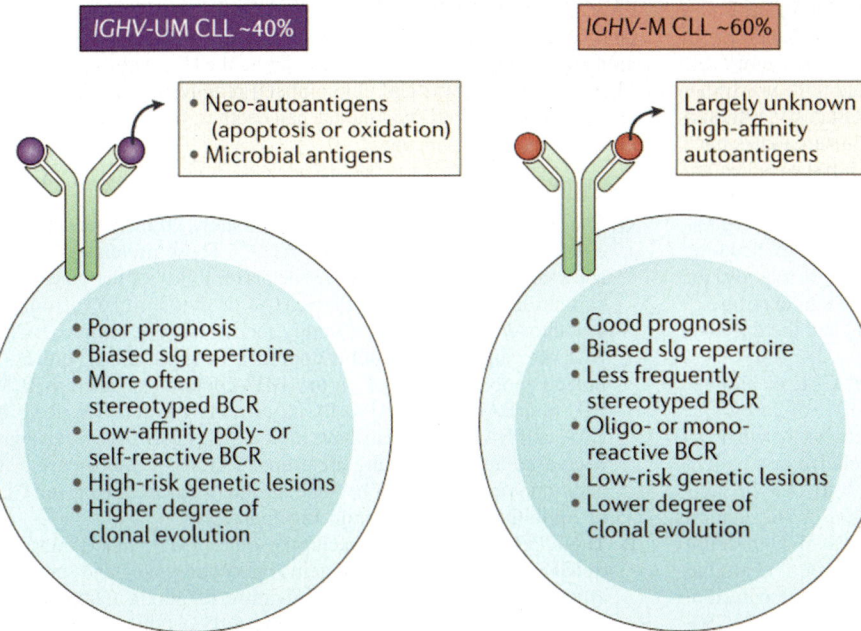

FIGURE 92.2 **Chronic lymphocytic leukemia (CLL) can be classified into two subgroups on the basis of the presence or absence of mutations in the immunoglobulin heavy chain variable region (*IGHV*) genes.** Stereotypy is seen in 30% of patients and is more common in unmutated patients. BCR, B-cell receptor. (Reprinted by permission from Nature: Fabbri G, Dalla-Favera R. The molecular pathogenesis of chronic lymphocytic leukaemia. *Nat Rev Cancer*. 2016;16(3):145-162. Copyright © 2016 Springer Nature.)

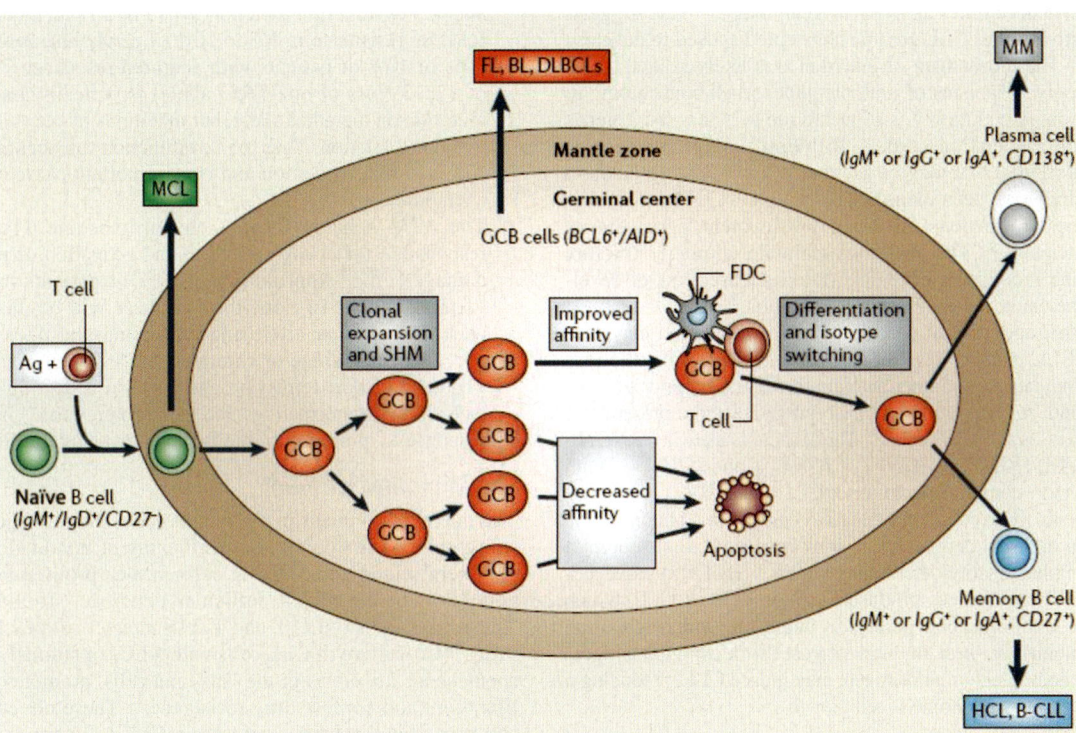

FIGURE 92.3 **The germinal center (GC) reaction is a key event in adaptive immunity to T-cell-dependent antigens.** In lymph nodes and the spleen, antigen (Ag)-activated naïve B cells (immunoglobulin [Ig] M+/IgD+) are driven into primary follicles where, aided by T cells, they undergo clonal expansion, form the GC, and displace nonproliferating naïve B cells to the periphery or mantle zone (shown in diagram). Within the GC, somatic hypermutation (SHM) mutates the Ig variable region of proliferating B cells to increase their affinity for the stimulating Ag. Although most GCB cells (GCB) acquire unfavorable mutations and die by apoptosis, a few improve their Ig affinity and are selected for further differentiation through interactions with T cells and follicular dendritic cells (FDC). A proportion of these selected B cells then undergo switch recombination of the Ig constant region, which changes the isotype and, consequently, the antibody-effector function. B cells of the GC express BCL6, which is required for GC formation, and activation-induced cytidine deaminase (AID), which is essential for SHM and switch recombination. Finally, selected B cells differentiate into memory B cells (CD27+) or antibody-secreting plasma cells (CD138+). Follicular lymphoma (FL), Burkitt lymphoma (BL), and some diffuse large B-cell lymphomas (DLBCLs) are thought to derive from B cells of the GC, mantle cell lymphoma (MCL) mainly from mantle-zone naïve B cells, B-cell chronic lymphocytic leukemia (B-CLL) and hairy-cell leukemia (HCL) from memory B cells, and multiple myeloma (MM) from plasma cells. The majority of cases of CLL and HCL have undergone SHM, but proportions have not and these cases have more aggressive disease. (Reprinted by permission from Nature: Tiacci E, Liso A, Piris M, et al. Evolving concepts in the pathogenesis of hairy-cell leukaemia. *Nature Rev*. 2006;6(6):437-448. Copyright © 2006 Springer Nature.)

mice, there is increased production of polyclonal and monoclonal (or oligoclonal) B cells that are either CD5+ or CD5−, and usually have mutated *IGHV*, similar to that seen with MBL.[15] The authors suggest that a "second hit" may then be required to develop CLL. However, further studies are required to confirm these findings.

Predisposing Factors Including Familial Chronic Lymphocytic Leukemia

There is a strong racial component to CLL/SLL (both will now be referred to as CLL), with the incidence being higher in North America and Europe than in Asia.[16] The incidence remains low in Asians living in North America suggesting genetic rather than environmental factors contribute to racial differences.[3,16] In addition, the incidence of CLL is 40% to 50% in Hispanics or American Indians and 65% in African Americans as compared to Caucasians in the United States.[17] It should be noted that most biological, genetic, and management studies have been carried out in the Caucasian population and further studies are required to determine whether findings from these studies hold true for all races. Other factors increasing the risk for CLL include a family history of a hematological cancer, farming, hairdressing, hepatitis C virus infections.[18] Factors decreasing risk include prior atopy, for example, hay fever, blood transfusions, smoking and sun exposure.[18] Agent Orange and insecticides also increase the risk, and there is controversy as to the role of irradiation.[3,19]

The strongest risk factor is a family history of CLL or another lymphoproliferative disorder, which is present in 10% of cases.[20-22] Concordance is more likely to occur in monozygotic twins than in dizygotic twins.[23] Moreover, the risk of a first-degree relative of a patient developing CLL is increased 8.5-fold,[21] while 13% to 18% of first-degree relatives have CD5+ MBL.[24,25] (As discussed in Differential Diagnosis, CLL is preceded by MBL, and about 1% of high-count MBL patients each year require treatment for progression.[26]) Familial CLL is similar to sporadic CLL in terms of age at presentation. However, familial CLL is more likely than sporadic CLL to be *IGHV* mutated, although *IGHV* gene family usage is similar in both and there is no concordance in families as to *IGHV* gene usage.[27] This suggests that patients with familial CLL are inherently predisposed to developing the disease. The mechanism of inheritance is likely related to the inheritance of polymorphisms of multiple genes, each contributing to the predisposition. A commonly used technique to assess these genes is genome-wide association studies, to identify single-nucleotide polymorphisms (SNPs) that may be associated with CLL. To date, 45 SNPs from 39 loci have been identified in familial CLL and a number of affected genes are involved in B-cell development, apoptosis, or telomere maintenance.[23] The shelterins maintain telomere structure and function, and individuals have a 3.6-fold increased risk of developing CLL if they have a germline *POT1* mutation.[28]

Evidence also suggests that chronic immune stimulation may lead to CLL. First, CLL patients have an increased incidence of infections or pernicious anemia (but not other autoimmune diseases) prior to diagnosis.[29,30] Second, surface immunophenotyping shows the presence of activation markers on the CLL cells.[31] Third, there is skewing in *IGHV* gene usage in CLL (*IGHV$_{1-69}$*, *IGHV$_{3-23}$*, *IGHV$_{3-7}$*, and *IGHV$_{4-34}$*) with *IGHV$_{1-69}$* being more common in unmutated CLL and *IGHV$_{3-23}$*, *IGHV$_{3-7}$*, and *IGHV$_{4-34}$* being more common in mutated cases.[32] In addition, ~30% of patients from different geographic regions have similar (stereotypic) heavy-chain complementarity-determining region 3 (HCDR3) sequences in their BCR.[33] These changes produce a unique BCR in CLL, which drives autonomous cell signaling, perhaps by interacting with neighboring BCRs.[34] In combination, these findings suggest that a common antigen, such as an infectious agent or autoantigen, may induce CLL, producing a unique BCR that drives autonomous cell growth.

Abnormalities in Apoptosis

Defects in apoptosis typify CLL, with the majority of cells being long-lived, noncycling, and in G0.[35,36] Apoptosis occurs through the activation of caspases, which are cysteine proteases that cleave other caspases at aspartate acid residues, converting the inactive proforms to active enzymes. The downstream caspases, caspases 3, 6, and 7, activate caspase-activated DNase, which cleaves DNA into 180 bp fragments.[35]

The *intrinsic apoptotic pathway* is typically initiated by chemotherapy, which causes activation of p53, an increase in the BAX:BCL2 ratio, and the release of cytochrome *c* from between the inner and outer mitochondrial membranes into the cytosol.

The *extrinsic apoptotic pathway* also plays a major role in CLL apoptosis. There are six death receptors (DRs), and these include the tumor necrosis factor (TNF) receptor, FAS (APO-1 or CD95), and DR4/DR5 (receptors for TNF-related apoptosis-inducing ligand [TRAIL]). Chemotherapeutic agents may upregulate receptors for FAS[37,38] or DR4/DR5,[39,40] which prime the cells to apoptosis by physiological levels of FAS ligand or TRAIL. p53 activation by chemotherapy increases DR4/DR5 sensitizing the CLL cells to TRAIL.[39] Thus, both fludarabine and chlorambucil require functional p53 activation to kill CLL cells and induce cell death through the intrinsic and extrinsic apoptotic pathways.

Modulators of the Apoptotic Pathway in CLL

a. The *BCL2 family* consists of approximately 20 members that can either promote or inhibit apoptosis.[35,41] These proteins can interact with each other to influence the permeability of the outer mitochondrial membrane and the release of cytochrome *c* from the mitochondria. Some BCL2 family members, for example, BCL2, BCL-xL, and MCL1 inhibit apoptosis whereas BAX and BAK induce apoptosis. A final group (BH3-containing), such as BIM, BID and BAD, can bind to BCL2 priming the cells for death by BAX and BAK. CLL cells have high BCL2 and MCL1 levels, with decreased apoptosis being a cardinal feature of the disease.[42] In addition, venetoclax has become an important treatment for CLL by inhibiting BCL-2 and inducing apoptosis.[2-4]

b. The *TP53 gene* is located on chromosome 17p13 and is a transcriptional activator.[43] The p53 protein is phosphorylated and stabilized after DNA damage through activation of ataxia telangiectasia mutation (ATM) kinase.[44] Activation of p53 is thus a key step for the activity of chemotherapy and chemoimmunotherapy in CLL, and p53 dysfunction (deletion 17p13 or a *TP53* mutation) accounts for drug resistance in 5% to 10% of newly diagnosed patients and 30% to 40% of patients with acquired resistance.[39,45,46] Deletion of 17p13 (loss of one *TP53* allele) is typically associated with a mutation on the other allele, but mutations of both alleles can occur without a deletion. Thus, p53 dysfunction can occur with a deletion 17p or a *TP53* mutation and is an important cause of resistance to chemotherapy.[5,47]

c. The *ATM gene* is located on chromosome 11q22-23 and is responsible for phosphorylation and activation of p53 after DNA damage.[44,48,49] Approximately 20% of patients have a deletion 11q22-23 (del 11q); one-third of these will be missing the *ATM* gene on the other allele and have abnormal phosphorylation of p53 with fludarabine or chlorambucil.[48,49] Thus, patients with del 11q have a short remission and survival following chemotherapy (see "FISH Abnormalities and Gene Expression") but an excellent response to inhibition of the BCR pathway by ibrutinib.[50]

The Microenvironment

The microenvironment in the lymph nodes play a major role in CLL cell growth with a continuous trafficking of nondividing cells in the peripheral blood and dividing cells in the "proliferation centers" in nodes.[2,3,5] In the nodes, follicular dendritic, stromal, fibroblasts, "nurse-like" cells (NLCs), and T cells interact with CLL cells (*Figure 92.4*).[51] Co-culture of CLL cells with NLCs or stromal cells decreases spontaneous apoptosis in the leukemia cells, promotes CLL cell proliferation, and confers drug resistance.[52] These effects require cell-cell contact and activation of certain CLL cell surface receptors. The BCR plays a central role in the microenvironment through maintenance and expansion of the CLL cell clone. BCR signaling is controlled by intracellular tyrosine kinases such as spleen tyrosine kinase (Syk), and Bruton tyrosine kinase (BTK).[53] In addition, aberrantly expressed CD40L on CLL cells can interact with CD40 on microvascular endothelial cells, which leads to the release of the TNF family members, BAFF (B-cell activating factor of the TNF family), and APRIL (a proliferation-inducing agent).[54] Receptors for BAFF and APRIL (BMCA, TAC1, and BAFF-R) are present on CLL cells and stimulation leads to increased survival and induction of the expression of CD40L, thus potentiating the cycle. This exemplifies the cross-talk between CLL and stromal cells in the microenvironment. Adhesion molecules are also important for CLL cell survival; β1 and β2 integrins on CLL cells bind to CD54 and CD106 on stromal cells and this promotes cell survival.[55] Moreover, neutralizing antibodies against various integrins induce CLL cells to undergo apoptosis.[55] Caveolin-1 expression by CLL cells in lymph nodes may stimulate

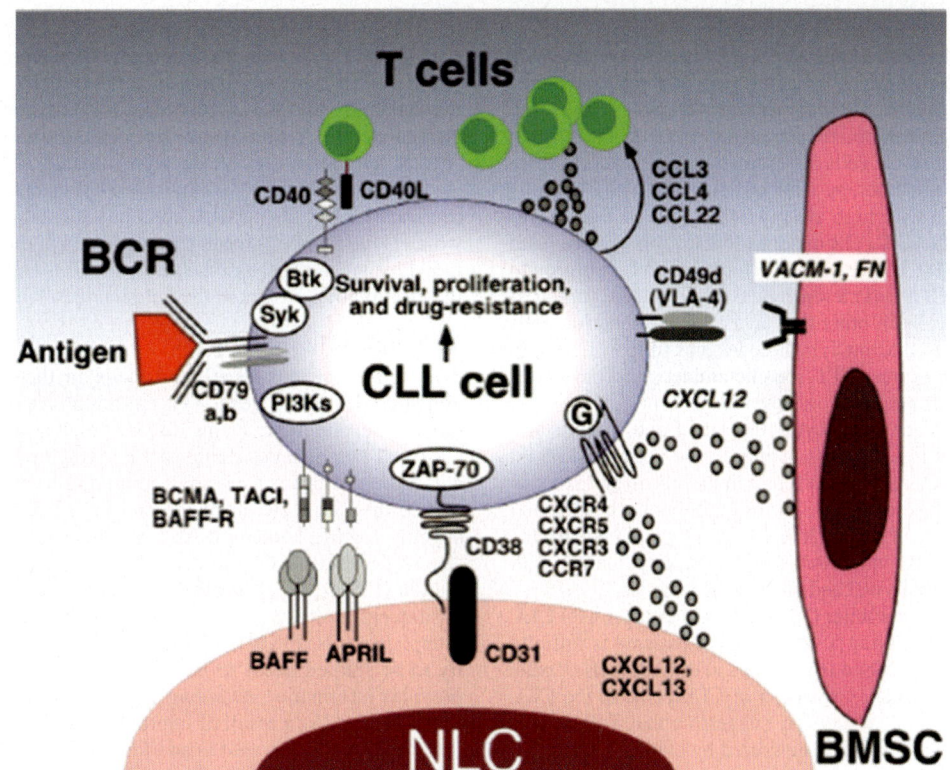

FIGURE 92.4 **Molecular interactions in the chronic lymphocytic leukemia (CLL) microenvironment.** Molecular interactions between CLL and stromal cells in the bone marrow and/or lymphoid tissue microenvironments that are considered important for CLL-cell survival and proliferation, CLL-cell homing, and tissue retention. Contact between CLL cells and nurse-like cells (NLCs) or bone marrow stromal cells (BMSCs) is established and maintained by chemokine receptors and adhesion molecules expressed on CLL cells. NLCs express the chemokines CXCL12 and CXCL13, whereas BMSCs predominantly express CXCL12. The chemokine receptors CXCR3 and CCR7 are additional chemokine receptors on CLL cells that are involved in lymphatic tissue homing. NLCs and BMSCs attract CLL cells via the G-protein–coupled chemokine receptors CXCR4 and CXCR5, which are expressed at high levels on CLL cells. Integrins, particularly VLA-4 integrins (CD49d), expressed on the surface of CLL cells cooperate with chemokine receptors in establishing cell-cell adhesion through respective ligands on the stromal cells (VCAM-1 and fibronectin). NLCs also express the TNF family members BAFF and APRIL, providing survival signals to CLL cells via corresponding receptors (BCMA, TACI, and BAFF-R). CD38 expression allows CLL cells to interact with CD31, the ligand for CD38 that is expressed by stromal and NLCs. Ligation of CD38 activates ZAP-70 and downstream survival pathways. Self- and/or environmental Ags are considered key factors in the activation and expansion of the CLL clone by activation of the B-cell receptor (BCR) and its downstream kinases. Stimulation of the BCR complex (BCR and CD79a,b) induces downstream signaling by recruitment and activation of Syk, Btk, and PI3Ks. Finally, BCR stimulation and co-culture with NLCs also induces CLL cells to secrete chemokines (CCL3, CCL4, and CCL22) for the recruitment of immune cells (T cells and monocytes) for cognate interactions. CD40L+ (CD154+) T cells are preferentially found in CLL-proliferation centers, and can interact with CLL cells via CD40. (Used with permission of American Society of Hematology from Burger JA.Nurture versus nature: the microenvironment in chronic lymphocytic leukemia. *Hematology Am Soc Hematol Educ Program.* 2011;2011:96-103; permission conveyed through Copyright Clearance Center, Inc.)

CLL proliferation and migration but also mediates CLL cell interactions with autologous T lymphocytes, which contributes to T cell inhibition leading to immune tolerance.[56] Finally, tyrosine kinase Lyn activated macrophages support CLL cell growth in a *Tcl-1* transgenic mouse model, indicating a role for macrophages in nurturing CLL growth in the microenvironment.

In addition to cell-cell contact, the extracellular milieu contains growth factors, proteins, and lipids that contribute to CLL survival and growth.[2,3,5,52] Stromal and CLL cells produce cytokines that may stimulate leukemia cell growth in an autocrine or paracrine fashion while inhibiting survival of normal lymphoid and marrow cells. This latter effect can lead to the immunosuppression and myelosuppression that typify this disease. In addition, the chemokine receptors, CXCR4 and CXCR5, on CLL cells regulate CLL cell trafficking to the stromal cells, which produce the receptor ligands CXCL12 (stromal-derived growth factor-1) and CXCL13, respectively.[3] There, the CLL cells produce IL-6 and IL-8, which enhance adhesion of the leukemia cells to the stromal cells and in turn provide signals for cell survival.[57] Upon BCR activation, CLL cells secrete cytokines, such as CCL3 and CCL4, that attract T and accessory cells to join the CLL and stromal cells.[58] In addition to signaling, stromal cells also supply essential nutrients to the CLL cells. For example, CLL cells have limited capacity to transport cysteine for glutathione synthesis due to low expression of Xc-transporter.[59] In contrast, stromal cells can effectively transport cysteine and convert it to cysteine, which can then be released into the microenvironment where the CLL cells take up the cysteine for glutathione synthesis. The CLL cell is thus believed to be in continuous transition between the lymph node and blood, with cells egressing from the node after division and being $CXCR4^{low}/CD5^{high}$.[3] After time in the circulation the cells become $CXCR4^{high}/CD5^{low}$ and are thus primed to respond to CXCL12 and return to the nodal microenvironment where cell division occurs again.[3]

CLL cells can also influence stromal cell signaling by the uptake of exosomes and microvesicles, which are different-sized extracellular vesicles released by CLL cells.[60-62] The exosomes contain proteins and microRNAs, which induce stromal cells to produce cytokines and angiogenic factors to promote CLL growth.[60] Microvesicles are larger than exosomes and are released by CLL cells modulating the activity of the bone marrow stromal cells (BMSCs).[61] The microvesicles can activate the AKT/mammalian target of rapamycin/p70S6K/hypoxia-inducible factor-1alpha axis in CLL-BMSCs with production of vascular endothelial growth factor, a survival factor for CLL cells.[63] They can also transfer various messages to target cells that may be critical to disease progression. BCR pathway kinase inhibitors (KIs), such as ibrutinib and idelalisib, act on the microenvironment causing direct death of the CLL cells (especially *IGHV* unmutated cases) and redistribution of leukemia cells into the peripheral bloodstream (especially *IGHV* mutated cases).[64]

Cellular Features of the Microenvironment

The lymph nodes and marrow and lymphatic tissue have intrinsic characteristics to support CLL cell functions.[51,65] Normal hematopoiesis depends upon BMSCs, which provide attachment sites and growth signals for the hematopoietic precursors. In CLL, the stromal cells create niches where CLL cells are nourished and protected from either spontaneous or chemotherapy-induced apoptosis. The CLL cells can bind to the BMSCs with high affinity, which allows tight adhesion and migration of the CLL cells underneath the stromal cells. Both murine and human BMSCs have similar effects on CLL cell growth and cell survival. BMSCs are of mesenchymal origin and are similar to mesenchymal stromal cells in other tissues. Follicular dendritic cells (FDCs) are also found in marrow/lymph nodes and support CLL cell survival.[66] These FDCs express CLL-specific antigens and have been investigated for the development of vaccines for CLL.

NLCs are differentiated monocytes that are large, round, and adherent cells that bind to CLL cells mainly in the peripheral blood system.[52] However, NLCs can also be found in the spleen and secondary lymphoid tissue.[52] There is diverse cross-talk between NLC and CLL cells. NLC express CXCL12, CXCL13, CD31, plexin B1, BAFF, APRIL, and vimentin.[67] All these cell-surface markers interact with CLL receptors providing survival and proliferative signals.

T lymphocytes and natural killer (NK) cells also interact with CLL cells. The number of circulating T cells in CLL patients is initially increased and this might be due to interactions with CLL cells. T cells can either suppress or stimulate expansion of CLL cells. In the CLL proliferation centers, T cells co-localize, suggesting that T cells support the CLL proliferation.[68] This is supported by evidence that CLL cells fail to grow in immunodeficient mice, demonstrating that activated CD4+ T cells are important for CLL proliferation.[69]

The interaction with these cells activates different receptors on the CLL cell surface, including interleukin receptors, CD40 and BCR (Figure 92.4).[65,70] However, based on the expression of downstream genes, activation of the BCR pathway appears to be most important as CLL cells in the lymph nodes, and to a lesser extent in marrow, have increased expression of genes related to BCR activation.[71] These changes include phosphorylated Syk and NF-κB. As expected, the changes are greater in unmutated IGHV cases than in mutated cases and correlate with the rate of cell proliferation and disease aggressiveness. Thus, inhibition of the BCR by ibrutinib inhibits CLL growth in the lymph nodes.[64,65]

Cell Proliferation

Although CLL cells in the peripheral blood are not dividing, the telomeres of CLL cells are shorter than in normal B cells, suggesting that the leukemic cells have undergone more frequent cell divisions than normal B cells.[72] Moreover, CLL cells with unmutated IGHV have shorter telomeres than those with mutated IGHV.[72] Using deuterated water to label DNA, it has been estimated that 0.11% to 1.76% (median 0.39%) of the CLL cells in patients are dividing each day, which is the same or greater than observed in the B cells from normal individuals.[73] As discussed above, the CLL cells divide primarily in the proliferation centers in the lymph nodes.[64]

Genomic Abnormalities

Tremendous strides have been made in the analysis of the CLL genome, identifying genes that are important in the pathogenesis of the disease, and in predicting disease progression and drug resistance. Classical cytogenetics demonstrates structural abnormalities in the chromosomes but is time consuming and it was initially difficult to induce the CLL cells to divide and to obtain metaphases that were specific for the leukemia. As a result, cytogenetics was generally superseded after 2000 for clinical use by fluorescent in situ hybridization (FISH). FISH has the advantage over cytogenetics in that it is simpler, faster, and can detect genetic abnormalities in nondividing interphase cells. FISH is highly sensitive, but the specific abnormality to be studied needs to be known in advance, while cytogenetics provides information regarding chromosome numbers and structural abnormalities. As a result of improved B-cell-specific mitogens, cytogenetics is now often used in addition to FISH as CLL metaphases can be obtained in over >90% of cases with abnormalities detected in 80% of cases.[74] Additionally, the changes identified by classical cytogenetics may provide additional prognostic information over FISH alone.[74] More recently, SNP analysis and DNA sequencing have dramatically improved our understanding of the molecular changes in CLL with disease progression and following therapy.

Analysis by FISH

The landmark study by Döhner et al[75] in 2000 demonstrated the importance of FISH in CLL. In 325 patients, 268 (82%) had abnormalities, with deletion 13q14.2-14.3 (del 13q) being most frequent (55%), followed by deletion 11q22.3-q23.1 (del 11q, 18%), trisomy 12q13 (trisomy 12q, 16%), deletion 17p13.1 (del 17p, 7%), and deletion 6q21

Table 92.2. Incidence of Genomic Abnormalities by the Döhner Hierarchical Classification

Genomic Abnormality	Hierarchical FISH[a]	Affected Genes	Clinical Features
Del 17p	7%-12% (increases to 30%-40% with drug resistance)	TP53 mutation	CLL/PLL morphology Drug resistance Short PFS and OS
Del 11q	11%-17%	ATM (mutated on other allele in one-third) SF3B1 (mutated in one-third)	Younger May have bulky disease Short TTFT and PFS
Trisomy 12q	14%	25% NOTCH mutations[76]	Atypical morphology Risk of Richter syndrome
Normal karyotype	18%-24%		
Del 13q	36%-39%	Rb MiR-15a/MiR-16-1	Good prognosis—worse if Rb deleted or >70%-85% cells affected[77-79]
Various	0%-8%	–	–

Abbreviations: ATM, ataxia telangiectasia mutation; CLL, chronic lymphocytic leukemia; FISH, fluorescent in situ hybridization; OS, overall survival; PFS, progression-free survival; PLL, prolymphocytic leukemia; TTFT, time to first treatment.
[a]The five major categories in the hierarchical model are del 17p, patients with a del 17p; del 11q, have a del 11q but not a del 17p; trisomy 12q, have a trisomy 12q but no del 17p or del 11q; normal karyotype; and del 13q as the only abnormality.
Obtained from Döhner H, Stilgenbauer S, Benner A, et al. Genomic aberrations and survival in chronic lymphocytic leukemia. N Engl J Med. 2000;343(26):1910-1916; Van Dyke DL, Werner L, Rassenti LZ, et al. The Dohner fluorescence in situ hybridization prognostic classification of chronic lymphocytic leukaemia (CLL): The CLL Research Consortium experience. Br J Haematol. 2016;173(1):105-113; Dal Bo M, Rossi FM, Rossi D, et al. 13q14 Deletion size and number of deleted cells both influence prognosis in chronic lymphocytic leukemia. Genes Chromosomes Cancer. 2011;50:633-643; Ouillette P, Collins R, Shakhan S, et al. The prognostic significance of various 13q14 deletions in chronic lymphocytic leukemia. ClinCancer Res. 2011;17(21):6778-6790.

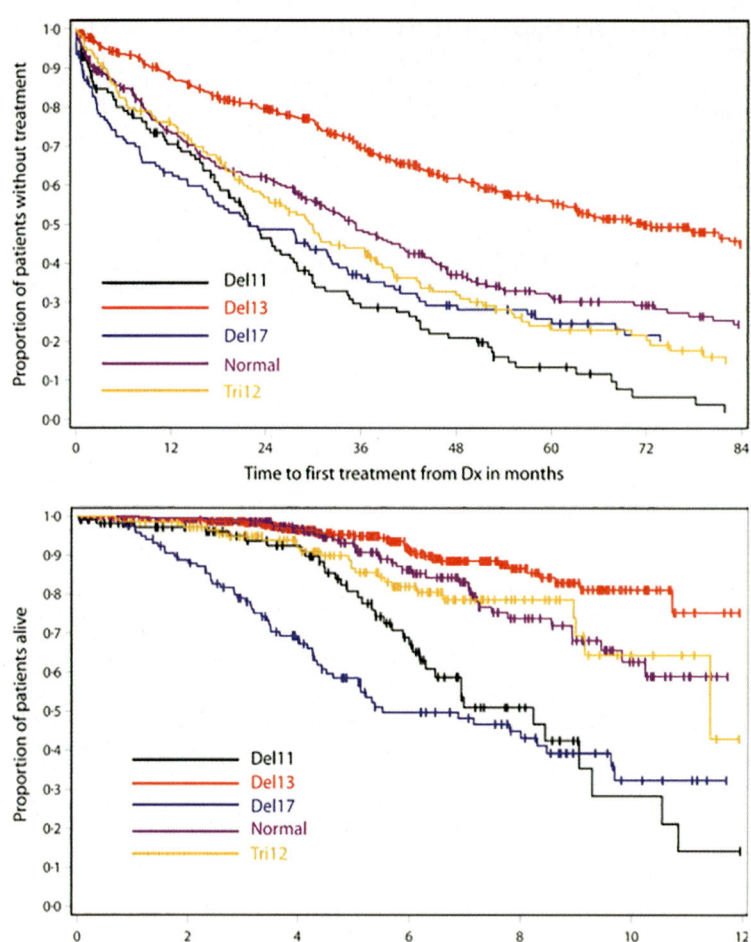

FIGURE 92.5 Time to first treatment and overall survival (OS) by FISH category from the date when FISH analysis was done. FISH, fluorescence in situ hybridization. (From, Van Dyke DL, Werner L, Rassenti LZ, et al. The Dohner fluorescence in situ hybridization prognostic classification of chronic lymphocytic leukaemia (CLL): the CLL Research Consortium experience. *Br J Haematol.* 2016;173(1):105-113. © 2016 The Authors. Reprinted by permission of John Wiley & Sons, Inc.)

(7%). There was one abnormality in 65% patients, two aberrations in 25%, and more than two aberrations in 10%. A hierarchical model categorized patients into five groups with different prognoses (*Table 92.2*). Using this model, the median survival times for patients with a del 17p, del 11q, trisomy 12q, normal karyotype, and a deletion 13q were 32, 79, 114, 111, and 133 months, respectively. Patients with unmutated *IGHV* were more likely to have del 17p or del 11q, whereas patients with mutated *IGHV* were more likely to have del 13q.[80] The incidence of trisomy 12q was the same in patients with mutated or unmutated *IGHV*.[80]

Very similar results in terms of hierarchy have been obtained in subsequent prospective studies.[77,81,82] An analysis by the CLL Research Consortium has demonstrated slight differences in the percentage of patients presenting with the different FISH hierarchies and in the survival of these patients (*Figure 92.5*; *Table 92.2*).[82] Of 1048 patients who had FISH within 4 years of diagnosis, the incidences of del 13q, normal FISH, trisomy 12, del 17p, and del 11q were 39%, 24%, 14%, 12% and 11%, respectively. The median time to first treatment (TTFT) was shortest for del 11q and del 17p (22 months), while it was longest for del 13q at 72 months; TTFT was 30 months for trisomy 12 patients and 35 months for those without an abnormality. The median overall survival (OS) was shortest for those with a del 17p or a del 11q, being 5 and 7 years, respectively. The median OS was 11 years for those with trisomy 12 and was not reached for those with a del 13q or no abnormalities. The OS data were derived primarily for patients treated with chemoimmunotherapy and will differ in patients receiving novel agents, which retain activity in patients with a del 17p or del 11q. An important additional finding was that the percentage of involved nuclei was important for prognosis. For del 17p patients, the TTFT was 44 months if the number of involved nuclei was ≤20%, but <8 months if >20%. For del 13q, the median TTFT was 24 months if >85% of the nuclei were affected, but 52 months to not reached if ≤85%. For trisomy 12, the median TTFT was 3 months if >75% of nuclei were affected, but 7 to 54 months as the number of involved nuclei decreased. For del 11q, the percentage of involved nuclei was not prognostically important when looking at all cases, but another study has demonstrated that the fraction is important in cases where del 11q is the only abnormality.[83]

It has been recommended that all CLL patients should also be routinely examined for an *IGH* translocation.[84,85] Of 1032 patients at the Mayo Clinic with a presumptive diagnosis of CLL, 76 (7%) were found to have an *IGH* translocation, with 34 involving a translocation with *cyclin D1*, consistent with a diagnosis of mantle cell lymphoma.[84] Eighteen had a translocation with *BCL2*, and six a translocation with *BCL3*.[84] Those with a *BCL3* translocation were associated with unmutated *IGHV* status, atypical morphology and aggressive disease, with short TTFT and OS.[85] In contrast, the presence of a *BCL2* translocation was associated with a benign clinical course.[85]

Conventional Cytogenetics

Metaphases may be obtained in >90% of patients with abnormalities being detected in >80% of patients.[74,86-90] Translocations occur in one-third of patients, with half of these being balanced, and complex karyotypes (CK; ≥3 abnormalities observed, either structural or numerical, in ≥2 metaphases in the same clone) occur in 10% to 20% of patients with CLL and 8% of patients with MBL.[74] Unsurprisingly, complex karyotyping occurs more frequently in *IGHV* unmutated cases and in those with *TP53* mutation, del 17p or del 11q.[74] Baliakas et al[91] have shown in a retrospective study of 5290 patients primarily treated with chemotherapy that those with ≥5 abnormalities (high-CK) had a very poor prognosis, regardless of p53 function (del 17p or *TP53* mutation), clinical stage, or *IGHV* status. In contrast those with three or four abnormalities only had a poor prognosis if there was p53 dysfunction. In addition, it has been shown that the presence of complex karyotyping adds additional information to del 17p in predicting relapse after ibrutinib.[90,92,93] Kittai et al[93] have shown in 456 patients receiving ibrutinib with or without rituximab, first line or in relapsed/resistant patients, that an increasing number of CK was an independent predictor for shorter progression-free survival (PFS) and OS. Moreover, the presence of clonal evolution was predictive of short survival. Further studies are required to standardize karyotyping in CLL and to confirm its role in CLL.

FISH Abnormalities and Gene Expression

Del 13q

The most frequent structural abnormality in CLL is del 13q (55% of cases) and is usually associated with *IGHV* mutated disease and good prognosis.[75,94] Of these cases 76% are monoallelic and 24% biallelic.[75,94] The deleted region involves the minimal deleted region, containing the *deleted in lymphocytic leukemia 2* (*DLEU2*) gene and microRNA (miR)-15a/16-1.[94] *DLEU2* encodes a noncoding RNA, but its function is unknown, whereas miR-15a/16-1 inhibits proliferation and apoptosis through upregulation of BCL-2.[94] Using transgenic mice, deletion of miR-15a/16-1 can lead to MBL and CLL.[78] Moreover, as in CLL patients, many of these mice have a very similar CDR3 structure (stereotypy), suggesting that a common antigen and/or autoantigen causes induction of the monoclonal population.

Del 11q

Del 11q occurs in 10% to 20% of cases, primarily in *IGHV* unmutated disease, and typically is seen in middle aged men who have rapid disease progression with earlier TTFT and reduced PFS with chemotherapy.[75,83,95-97] Original studies indicated that these patients had bulky lymphadenopathy at diagnosis, but this is not a universal finding.[83,98] The critical region for the deletion is a 3-Mb segment at 11q22.3-q23.1, and candidate genes in this region include radixin (*RDX*), which has homology to the neurofibromatosis-type 2 (*NF2*) tumor-suppressor gene, and the *ATM* gene.[95] The ATM protein is a protein kinase activated by DNA double-strand breaks and this leads to phosphorylation and activation of p53.

One-third of patients with a del 11q have a mutation on the remaining *ATM* allele and this subgroup has a defective response to DNA damage with radiation or chemotherapy and a poorer OS than the group of patients with a del 11q and wild-type *ATM* on the other allele.[48,49,99] The other two-thirds of patients must have an additional genetic defect leading to their poor prognosis. One candidate is *SF3B1*, which is involved in RNA slicing, as mutations of this gene are present in 36% of patients with del 11q.[100,101] CLL cells with a del 11q overexpress genes involved in cell signaling, cycling, and apoptosis and have reduced levels of a number of adhesion proteins, which may explain the marked lymphadenopathy observed in some cases.[95,96,102]

Del 17p

Del 17p is typically associated with loss of *TP53* on the deleted part of chromosome 17 with a mutation of *TP53* on the other allele.[45,103] This causes p53 dysfunction and cells are unable to undergo apoptosis with chemotherapy and exhibit genomic instability with complex karyotyping.[39,45] Thus, the likelihood of this abnormality increases following drug exposure and resistance.

Trisomy 12q

Trisomy 12q occurs because of duplication of one homologue and is seen in ~15% of patients. A *NOTCH1* mutation is seen in 24% of cases, typically occurring if trisomy 12q is the only abnormality and the cells are *IGHV* unmutated.[76] Trisomy 12q is frequently associated with "atypical" CLL. Patient survival is minimally affected when trisomy 12q is detected by FISH but may be shortened if detected by karyotyping.[80]

Translocations of 14q32

Translocations (t) of 14q32 involving *IGH* occurs in 7% of patients with CLL and many of these cases turn out to have a different malignancy disorder.[84] Most typically these patients have a t(11;14)(q13;q32), reflecting mantle cell lymphoma, or a t(14;18)(q32;q21), reflecting leukemic phase of a follicular lymphoma. More rarely, these patients may have a t(14;19)(q32;q13.1), where there is juxtapositioning of *BCL3* on chromosome 19 with the *Ig* gene on chromosome 14. BCL3 is a member of the IκB family, and this abnormality is associated with atypical morphology and progressive disease.[84,104]

Whole-Genome and Whole-Exome Sequencing

Important advances have recently been made in understanding the molecular genetic abnormalities in CLL.[19,94,105,106] Through whole-exome sequencing, 44 recurrently mutated genes and 11 recurrent copy number variations (where sections of a DNA sequence are repeated) were detected in 538 CLL patients including 278 untreated cases.[106] Mutations involving the MYC and MAPK-ERK pathways, RNA processing and DNA repair were commonly present. In a second landmark study, whole-genome sequencing was carried out in 452 CLL and 54 MBL pretreatment patients.[105] The mutation burden was similar in both MBL and CLL patients and both groups were thus studied together. Thirty-six genes were found to be recurrently mutated, with an additional 23 genes, which were preferentially mutated in either *IGHV* mutated or unmutated cases. Importantly the number of driver mutations (a gene mutation believed important in the causation of cancer) was greater in unmutated cases and the most commonly mutated genes in descending order were *NOTCH1* (12.6%), *ATM* (11%), *BIRC3* (8.8%), *SF3B1* (8.6%), *CHD2* (6%), *TP53* (5.3%), and *MYD88* (4%). Importantly because the whole genome was sequenced, a number of new mutations were detected in noncoding regions, which could influence gene expression and prognosis. Thus, mutations in the 3′ region of *NOTCH1* were observed, resulting in splicing and increased *NOTCH1* expression and activity. Mutations in *NOTCH1* typically occur in exon 34 and increase NOTCH1 activity by decreasing NOTCH1 protein clearance.[107] NOTCH1 is a transmembrane receptor and interaction with its ligands (Jagged or Delta families) leads to increased cell survival and drug resistance. Mutations within or outside the coding region were associated with more aggressive disease. Similarly, mutations in the PAX5 enhancer resulted in decreased activity of the transcription factor. This study showed that an increasing number of driver mutations correlated with shorter TTFT and OS, while patients without genomic mutations had an excellent prognosis. This area of research will increase our understanding of the heterogeneity in biology and clinical outcome in CLL.

Clonal Evolution in CLL

The clinical course in CLL is highly variable leading to studies evaluating the genetic changes that develop following diagnosis and how they influence the pattern of tumor growth and TTFT.[81,106,108,109] In general, stable CLL is associated with clonal equilibrium. With disease progression, the growth of CLL can be exponential (rapid and continued increase in white cell count), logistic (gradual increase in white cell count with plateauing), or indeterminate.[108] Those with unmutated *IGHV* have a tendency to have exponential growth with an increased risk of developing a del 17p or del 11q, while those with a logistic growth pattern are more likely to have mutated *IGHV* and del 13q. Clonal evolution over time can be linear or multibranching, with the latter being more commonly observed.[108,109] Linear is where the original single clone is maintained and additional mutations occur over time, while multibranching is where there are two or more subclones that continue to subdivide with the acquisition of new genetic abnormalities. The risk of developing new genetic abnormalities, particularly del 17p, is further increased by chemotherapy.[106] Indeed, 42% of patients who develop resistance to fludarabine have a *TP53* mutation or a del 17p.[110]

DIAGNOSIS

The International Workshop of Chronic Lymphocytic Leukemia (iwCLL) requires a peripheral blood B cell count of ≥5 × 10^9/L and the presence of monoclonal (kappa or lambda) B cells, which have the typical immunophenotype of CLL cells (CD19+, CD5+, CD23+, and decreased expression of surface Ig, CD20, and CD79b).[1] The CLL cells are mature-appearing lymphocytes admixed with larger or atypical cells, prolymphocytes (PL), and cleaved cells. Having more than 55% PL is consistent with prolymphocytic leukemia (PLL). Individuals with a peripheral blood B cell count of <5 × 10^9/L and CLL cells in the blood have either SLL or MBL. These two disorders can be distinguished as MBL lacks lymphadenopathy or splenomegaly (by physical examination or computed tomography [CT] scans, *Table 92.1*).[1]

DIFFERENTIAL DIAGNOSIS

In most patients, the diagnosis of CLL is easily made after a careful review of the peripheral smear and immunophenotyping, although other conditions must be considered (*Table 92.3*).

Benign Causes

T Cell–Associated Causes

Chronic infections, such as tuberculosis or syphilis, may produce a lymphocytosis. A transient lymphocytosis may also be seen in viral illnesses, for example, human immunodeficiency virus (HIV), hepatitis, or cytomegalovirus (CMV) infections, autoimmune diseases, hypersensitivity reactions, and stress.[26] However, these are easily distinguished from CLL by the clinical features and the lymphocytes are polyclonal by immunophenotyping.

B Cell–Associated Causes

Persistent polyclonal B-cell lymphocytosis is a rare and benign condition seen typically in middle-aged female smokers with a familial tendency.[111-113] The lymphocytes are binucleated and have abundant cytoplasm. There is a polyclonal increase in immunoglobulins and a strong association with HLA-DR7; an isochromosome 3q$^+$ (i3)(q10) is observed in some cases.[111,112] These cells are *IGHV* gene mutated, are immunophenotypically marginal zone lymphocytes, and contain multiple *BCL2/IGH* gene rearrangements.[112,113]

Tropical splenomegaly syndrome or hyperreactive malarial splenomegaly occurs in countries with endemic malaria and may mimic CLL.[114] This disease is believed to be a disordered response to malarial antigens leading to overproduction of B cells and is characterized by massive splenomegaly, an increase in IgM, and an increase in lymphocyte count in 10% of cases. The disorder responds to antimalarial therapy.

Malignant Causes

Before flow cytometry became a diagnostic requirement for CLL, many patients were diagnosed as having CLL based on abnormal blood counts, but likely had other disorders. The most common malignancies to be confused with CLL are PLL and the leukemic phase of non-Hodgkin lymphomas (NHLs, *Table 92.3*). Morphologically, these disorders may appear similar to CLL.

B Cell–Associated Causes

Monoclonal B-cell Lymphocytosis

MBL is defined as the persistent (>3 months) increase in the number of monoclonal B cells in the peripheral blood, without evidence of clinical lymphadenopathy/splenomegaly, normal blood counts (apart from a possible slight lymphocytosis), and no evidence of a coexisting active infection or autoimmune disorder.[115] The B-cell count is <5 × 10^9/L and there are three common variants: CLL-like MBL (CD5$^+$, CD20 dim), atypical MBL (CD5$^+$, CD20 bright), and CD5- MBL.[1,26,116,117] The majority are CLL-like. MBLs are found in 3.5% of adults older than 40 years with normal blood counts, being more common in males with the incidence increasing with age.[24] The incidence of MBL is even higher (13.5%) among healthy members of CLL families and in otherwise healthy people with a lymphocyte count >4 × 10^9/L.[24] Using eight-color flow cytometry, MBL has been detected in up to 12% of healthy individuals with normal blood counts.[118]

The number of clonal B cells detected in MBL depends on whether the study is evaluating patients in the population with normal blood counts (so-called population MBL or low-count MBL), or patients who present with slightly increased lymphocyte counts (clinical MBL or high-count MBL, *Figure 92.6*).[119] Thus, low-count MBL have <0.5 × 10^9/L clonal B cells and high-count MBL ≥0.5 × 10^9/L clonal B cells.[119] The B cell count is intimately related to risk of progression to CLL, with low count progressing to CLL at a rate of 1%/year, while the rate is 4% when all MBL patients are considered.[120,121] Compared to high-count MBL, low-count MBL patients are more likely to be *IGHV* mutated, to have good prognostic markers by FISH, and are unlikely to demonstrate *IGHV* stereotypy.[26,122]

The use of 5 × 10^9/L B cells to differentiate high-count MBL from Rai 0 CLL is an arbitrary number but, using these criteria 41% of patients previously diagnosed with Rai 0 CLL are now considered to have high-count MBL and have a survival no different to age- and sex-matched controls.[123,124] However, they do have an increased incidence of serious bacterial infections and second malignancies,[125-127] and 1% to 4% require treatment for progression to CLL each year.[119,128] Thus these patients need to be monitored and counseled annually.[128] Ig

Table 92.3. Differential Diagnosis of Chronic Lymphocytic Leukemia

Benign Causes
Bacterial (e.g., tuberculosis)
Viral (e.g., infectious mononucleosis)
Persistent polyclonal B-cell lymphocytosis
Hyperreactive malarial splenomegaly
Premalignant and Malignant Causes
B Cell
Monoclonal B-cell lymphocytosis (MBL)
Prolymphocytic leukemia (PLL)
Leukemic phase of non-Hodgkin lymphomas
    Mantle cell lymphoma
    Follicular lymphoma
    Marginal zone lymphoma
    Lymphoplasmacytic lymphoma
    Diffuse large-cell lymphoma
    Hairy cell leukemia (classical and variant)
T-cell
Prolymphocytic leukemia
Adult T-cell leukemia/lymphoma
Sézary syndrome
Large granular lymphocytic (LGL) leukemia

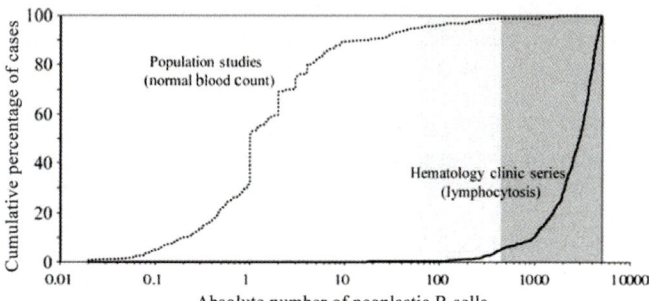

FIGURE 92.6 The cumulative percentage of cases according to the absolute number of clonal B cells for studies of individuals from the general population with a normal blood count (dotted line) and from series of individuals referred for clinical hematology investigations usually with a current or prior lymphocytosis (solid line). The clonal B-cell count in chronic lymphocytic leukemia–type monoclonal B-cell lymphocytosis shows a marked difference in cases from population studies (median 1 clonal B cell per µL with 95% of cases having less than 56 clonal B cells per µL highlighted by the white background) compared to clinical hematology series (median 2939 clonal B cells per µL with 95% of cases having more than 447 clonal B cells per µL highlighted by the dark gray background). Very few cases from either series have a clonal B-cell count within the same range as polyclonal B-cell levels in individuals with no detectable abnormal B cells (light gray background). (From Rawstron AC, Shanafelt T, Lanasa MC, et al. Different biology and clinical outcome according to the absolute numbers of clonal B-cells in monoclonal B-cell lymphocytosis (MBL). *Cytometry B Clin Cytom.* 2010;78(suppl 1):19-23. Copyright © 2010 International Clinical Cytometry Society. Reprinted by permission of John Wiley & Sons, Inc.)

levels are reduced in some patients (IgG 19%, IgA 9% and IgM, 45%) while 42% will have significant lymphadenopathy by CT scans.[129,130] However, CT scans are usually only performed if clinically indicated.

MBL has been detected in 7.1% of blood donors aged >45 years in Kansas City, raising the possibility that tumor cells could be inadvertently transmitted during transfusion.[131] While case reports have confirmed this concern, a recent large study from Scandinavia has indicated that the risk of transmission of CLL by blood transfusion is unlikely.[132,133]

Finally, there has been debate as to whether patients should be diagnosed as MBL or SLL based on the incidental involvement of lymph node or marrow with CLL cells, diagnosed when nodes are removed at surgery, for example, for prostate and breast cancer surgery, or when marrows are carried out for evaluation of other diseases.[26] Regardless of the extent of marrow or lymph node involvement by CLL, the patients should be considered as having MBL unless the blood counts are abnormal or the lymph nodes are clearly enlarged.[26]

B-cell Prolymphocytic Leukemia

B-cell prolymphocytic leukemia (B-PLL) is a rare disease, characterized by larger, less mature-appearing cells than are seen in CLL, and the nuclei have condensed chromatin with a prominent central nucleoli.[134,135] Patients with CLL/B-PLL have 11% to 54% PL, but in B-PLL ≥55% of the cells are PL.[136] B-PLL appearing de novo is an aggressive disease, and patients frequently are symptomatic with fever, weight loss, or abdominal discomfort and are found to have massive splenomegaly, minimal lymphadenopathy, and resistance to therapy. Leukocyte counts in excess of 150×10^9/L, consisting almost entirely of PL, are common, as are anemia and thrombocytopenia. The cells invariably have intense staining for surface membrane immunoglobulin, FMC7, CD20, and CD79b, and usually are CD5$^-$ and CD23$^-$.[134,135,137] The differential for B-PLL is CLL, mantle cell lymphoma, or splenic marginal zone lymphoma, and molecular studies can help differentiate these disorders as B-PLL tends to be *IGHV* mutated, half of the cases have a p53 dysfunction while two-thirds have MYC activation, usually by a t(8;14), and less frequently by an increase in gene copy number.[134,135,137] Chapiro et al[137] have recently classified B-PLL into three prognostic groups based on the presence of MYC activation or del 17p: indolent B-PLL (24%; no MYC aberration) intermediate-risk (MYC aberrations but no del 17p) and high-risk (MYC aberrations and del 17p).

Leukemic Phase of Non-Hodgkin Lymphoma

The leukemic phase of NHL used to be referred to as *lymphosarcoma cell leukemia* and includes the leukemic phase of mantle cell lymphoma, follicular lymphoma, splenic lymphoma with villous lymphocytes (splenic marginal zone lymphoma), other marginal zone lymphomas, and rarely large-cell lymphoma. These disorders may be suspected by cell morphology and clinical presentation, and diagnosis is made by immunophenotyping and molecular genetics (*Table 92.4*).

INVESTIGATIONS AND STAGING

Investigations

Physical examination, complete blood count, review of the peripheral smear, and immunophenotyping are required for diagnosis and staging in CLL. Additional recommended investigations have been published by the iwCLL and will be reviewed.[1] It should be emphasized that the extent of investigations will depend on whether a patient is being seen in general practice or for a clinical trial.

Standard Tests for General Practice

Physical Assessment

This includes measuring the bidimensional size of the largest nodes in the cervical, supraclavicular, axillary, inguinal, and femoral regions with measurement of the spleen and liver. The performance status should also be documented.

Laboratory Measurements

Complete blood count with white cell differential (including the percentage of PL) and reticulocyte count; direct antiglobulin test (DAT) routine plasma biochemistry (including renal/liver function tests and lactate dehydrogenase [LDH]), β2-microglobulin level, serum protein electrophoresis and/or immunoelectrophoresis, and immunoglobulin levels; the *IGHV* mutational status, FISH, and *TP53* sequencing may be carried out at diagnosis and provide useful prognostic information.[138]

Screening for hepatitis and HIV is usually carried out at diagnosis and repeated prior to treatment. Reactivation of hepatitis B, which can be fatal, typically occurs with the anti-CD20 monoclonal antibodies, but also can occur with novel agents.[139] Chronic carriers of hepatitis B virus (HBV) (positive for hepatitis B surface antigen, hepatitis B core antibody, and/or low HBV titers in serum) should receive prophylactic antiviral agent, such as lamivudine, while being treated for CLL.[1] Those with high titers of hepatitis C or hepatitis B DNA should be treated initially for the infection prior to receiving treatment for CLL.[1]

Table 92.4. Immunophenotypes of Chronic Lymphocytic Leukemia (CLL) and Other Chronic B-Cell Disorders

Diagnosis	smIg	CD5	CD10	CD11c	CD19	CD20	CD22	CD23	CD25	CD43	CD79b	CD103	CD200	FMC7
CLL	Dim	++	–	–/+	++	Dim	–/+	++	+/–	+	–/Dim	–	++	–/+
Mantle cell lymphoma	++	++	–/+	–	++	++	++	–	–	+	++	–	–	++
Prolymphocytic leukemia	+++	–/+	–/+	–/+	++	+++	++	++	–/+	+	++	–	Dim	+
Splenic marginal zone lymphoma	++	–/+	–/+	+/–	++	++	++	+/–	–/+	+	++	–/+	Dim	++
Marginal zone lymphoma	++	–	–	+/–	++	++	+/–	+/–	–	–/+	++	–	Dim	+
Follicular lymphoma	++	–/+	++	–	++	++	++	–/+	–	–	++	–	Dim	++
HCL	+++	–	–	++	+++	+++	+++	–	+++	+	++	+++	+++	+++
HCL variant	+++	–	–	++	+++	+++	+++	–	–	+	+	+++	–	+++
Lymphoplasmacytoid lymphoma	++	–	–	–/+	++	++	+	–	–/+	+/–	+	–	Dim	+

Abbreviations: –, not expressed; –/+, usually is not expressed; +/–, usually is expressed; + to +++, varying degrees of strength of expression; HCL, hairy cell leukemia; smIg, surface membrane Ig.
Adapted from Gascoyne RD. Differential diagnosis of the chronic B-cell lymphoid leukemias. In: Cheson BD, ed. *Chronic Lymphoid Leukemias*. 2nd ed. Marcel Dekker; 2001:209-230; Matutes E, Attygalle A, Wotherspoon A, Catovsky D. Diagnostic issues in chronic lymphocytic leukaemia (CLL). *Best Pract Res Clin Haematol*. 2010;23(1):3-20; Swerdlow SH, Campo E, Pileri SA, et al. The 2016 revision of the World Health Organization classification of lymphoid neoplasms. *Blood*. 2016;127(20):2375-2390; Rozman C, Montserrat E. Chronic lymphocytic leukemia. *N Engl J Med*. 1995;333(16):1052-1057.

Radiology

A baseline chest x-ray is useful to determine any preexisting lung disease.

Additional Tests for Clinical Trials and Specific Clinical Situations

Bone Marrow

A marrow aspirate/biopsy may be useful to (a) assess normal marrow reserve and establish the cause of anemia and thrombocytopenia for patients with Rai stage III or IV disease; (b) assess response and cause of persistent cytopenias following chemotherapy; and (c) determine the extent/pattern of marrow infiltration.[140]

Radiology

Baseline CT scans are not of value for routine management but are usually required for clinical trials.[141] Positron emission tomography (PET) scans are not useful for staging in CLL, as 2-deoxy-2-[fluorine-18] fluoro-D-glucose (18F-FDG) uptake in CLL is low. However, they are useful to identify a suitable node for biopsy when there is concern about disease transformation, or a second malignancy.[142,143]

Staging

Two staging systems are in general use and are based on physical examination and blood counts.[144,145] The Rai staging system is generally used in North America, and the original system divided patients into five groups, although a simplified three-stage version is sometimes used (Table 92.5).[1,144] The Binet staging system is most frequently used in Europe, and staging is based on the number of involved areas, the level of hemoglobin, and the platelet count (Table 92.6).

Several points should be emphasized about these staging systems: (a) Clinical staging is based on a physical examination and not on imaging methods; (b) although both staging systems provide useful prognostic information, they do not correlate well with each other. Thus, there are twofold more patients with Binet stage A as there are in the Rai stage 0 group; alternatively, there are twofold more patients with Rai I/II disease as those with Binet stage B disease[147]; (c) the cause of cytopenia was not defined in the original descriptions of staging. One-quarter of CLL patients develop cytopenia, with 54% due to marrow replacement, 18% to immune cytopenias, and 28% due to other causes, for example, uremia.[148,149] As survival depends on the cause of cytopenia, patients should be subclassified according to the cause of cytopenia; (d) the diagnosis of CLL in the original studies was based on lymphocyte count, the degree of marrow involvement by lymphocytes, and cell morphology but not on immunophenotyping (Tables 92.5 and 92.6). Thus, a number of patients in the original studies likely had other NHLs with leukemic involvement; (e) the lymphocyte threshold to diagnose CLL has changed since the original definitions (≥15 × 10^9/L for Rai classification and ≥4 × 10^9/L for Binet classification). Currently, we use a B-cell count of ≥5 × 10^9/L to diagnose CLL, as opposed to an absolute lymphocyte count, and (f) as a result of the above changes in diagnosis and new therapies, the survival of Rai stage III/IV patients has increased from 1.5 years to ≥5 years.[2,147]

CLINICAL FINDINGS

Most CLL patients in the general population are elderly at the time of diagnosis with a median age of 71.5 years.[7] However, the median age at diagnosis of patients in CLL clinics is younger, varying from 58 to 68 years, with 20% to 25% of patients being <55 years.[8,10,150-153]

The presenting symptoms are similar, regardless of age.[150] In addition, because of routine blood testing, most patients are diagnosed incidentally when they have a routine blood count and have early-stage disease (Rai 0/I). Alternatively, lymphadenopathy, splenomegaly, or both may be detected during a regular physical examination. The most frequent complaints are fatigue or a vague sense of being unwell. Less frequently, enlarged nodes or infections are the initial complaint. Fever and weight loss are uncommon at presentation but may occur with advanced and drug-resistant disease.

Most symptomatic patients have enlarged lymph nodes and/or splenomegaly. Enlargement of the cervical and supraclavicular nodes occurs more frequently than axillary or inguinal lymphadenopathy. The lymph nodes are usually discrete, soft, freely movable, and nontender. Painful enlarged nodes usually indicate a superimposed bacterial or viral infection, or possibly a Richter transformation (discussed later). Hard and fixed nodes are concerning for a carcinoma and should be investigated as secondary malignancies are frequent and an important cause of death in CLL (discussed in Second Malignancies). There is usually only mild to moderate enlargement of the spleen, and splenic infarction is uncommon. Less common manifestations are enlargement of the tonsils, abdominal masses due to mesenteric or retroperitoneal lymphadenopathy, and skin infiltration. Direct involvement of the skin by CLL typically affects the face and the features can be quite variable, varying from macules or papules (which may be vascular) to more extensive involvement that may simulate rhinophyma.[154,155]

Patients may also present with skin cancers, shingles, or recalcitrant warts secondary to immunosuppression.[155]

Symptomatic anemia can also be a presenting feature, which may be related to marrow replacement or, more rarely, to autoimmune hemolysis or red cell aplasia. Alternatively, patients may have bruising or bleeding, most commonly related to thrombocytopenia and infrequently to acquired von Willebrand disease. Rarely, patients present with a paraneoplastic syndrome, such as nephrotic syndrome, paraneoplastic pemphigus, or angioedema.

Peripheral Blood

The mean lymphocyte count at diagnosis is approximately 30 × 10^9/L, with 30% having a lymphocyte count of less than 10 × 10^9/L and one-quarter greater than 30 × 10^9/L.[10] As most patients present with early disease, it takes >12 months for the lymphocyte count to double in 90% of patients and the lymphocyte count can fluctuate in some patients.[156,157] The CLL cells are small to medium-sized lymphocytes with clumped chromatin, inconspicuous nucleoli, and a small ring of

Table 92.5. Rai Staging

Stage	Modified Stage	Description
0	Low-risk	Lymphocytosis[a]
I	Intermediate-risk	Lymphocytosis + lymphadenopathy[b]
II	Intermediate-risk	Lymphocytosis + splenomegaly[b] ± lymphadenopathy
III	High-risk	Lymphocytosis + anemia[a] ± lymphadenopathy or splenomegaly
IV	High-risk	Lymphocytosis + thrombocytopenia[a] ± anemia, splenomegaly or lymphadenopathy

[a]Lymphocytosis, originally lymphocytes ≥15 × 10^9/L for >4 weeks with ≥40% marrow involvement with lymphocytes; anemia, hemoglobin <110 g/L; and thrombocytopenia, platelets <100 × 10^9/L.[144]
[b]Enlarged nodes or spleen by physical examination.

Table 92.6. Binet Staging

Stage	Blood Counts	Involved Areas
A	Hgb >100 g/L and platelets >100 × 10^9/L	<3
B	Hgb >100 g/L and platelets >100 × 10^9/L	≥3
C	Hgb <100 g/L, or platelets <100 × 10^9/L, or both	Any number

Lymphocyte count of ≥4 × 10^9/L and ≥40% marrow involvement with lymphocytes. The five areas of involvement include palpable nodes in the head and neck, axillae, groins, palpable spleen, and clinically enlarged liver.[146]

cytoplasm. Crystalline, globular, tubular, or rod-shaped cytoplasmic inclusions may occasionally be observed.[158]

Smudge cells (basket cells or shadow cells of Gumprecht) are commonly seen in the peripheral blood smear in CLL, but not in other lymphoid disorders, and are caused by a decrease in the cellular content of vimentin, a cytoskeletal protein required for maintaining cell structure.[159,160] The number of smudge cells can vary from 1% to 75% (median 28%) and appears to be remarkably consistent in individual patients.[160]

There can be great variation in blood cell morphology in CLL, with mature-appearing lymphocytes being most prominent and a smaller number of cells having cleaved nuclei, abundant cytoplasm, or having prominent central nucleoli (PL).[136,161] In *classical CLL*, >90% of cells are small, and when 11% to 54% of the cells are PL, it is termed *CLL/PLL*.[161] When >15% of the lymphocytes are plasmoid or cleaved and <10% are PL, it is *atypical* or *mixed-cell type* CLL. Approximately 80% of patients have classical CLL, and 20% have CLL/PLL or atypical CLL. Although not routinely measured, as discussed in Prognostic and Predictive Markers, these morphologic variations may predict for more aggressive disease. If ≥55% of the cells are PL, the patient has PLL, a distinct disease to CLL.

Bone Marrow and Lymph Nodes

A bone marrow is not required for the diagnosis of CLL and is not usually carried out unless looking for an additional disorder. The marrow infiltration by CLL may be interstitial, nodular, mixed (nodular and interstitial), or diffuse, with mixed being the most common and nodular the least common.[140,162] Diffuse involvement, in which there is effacement of the fat spaces by tumor, carries the worst prognosis.[140] The marrow involvement is random and contrasts with follicular lymphomas, in which paratrabecular involvement is the rule. In contrast to marrow, involvement of the lymph node is diffuse. Proliferation centers are primarily observed in lymph nodes but can be seen in marrow.[163]

Immunophenotyping

CLL cells show clonal light chain restriction and are typically CD19+, CD20+ (low), CD23+, and CD5+ and their immunophenotypes compared with other chronic are shown in *Table 92.4*.[1,161,162] In addition the cells may also be CD27+, consistent with being memory B cells.[31] Alternatively, the presence of CD27, CD5, and CD23 could reflect the activated nature of the CLL cell.[31] The CD5 antigen is typically observed in T cells but normal B cells carrying the CD5 marker are located in the mantle zone of the lymph node, and small numbers of these cells are also present in the peripheral blood.[164] The overexpression of membrane CD23 is related to deregulation of NOTCH2 signaling and may play a role in decreasing apoptosis.[165] Cell surface CD23 undergoes spontaneous proteolysis, producing elevated serum levels of CD23, the level reflecting disease stage.[165] The presence of CD23 is useful to differentiate CLL from mantle cell lymphoma, which is also CD5+.[165] Similarly, CD200 is strongly expressed on CLL cells but not in mantle cell lymphoma.[166]

In contrast, the cells usually do not stain for FMC7, which identifies an epitope of CD20 that is usually not present in CLL as CD20 is weakly expressed.[167] Similarly, CLL cells lack CD79b, related to overexpression of an alternatively spliced form of the gene.[168]

Along with the diagnostic profile above, ZAP-70 and CD38 were previously measured by flow cytometry in CLL, as they were initially considered surrogate markers for *IGHV* mutational status and useful prognostic markers. However, they are less commonly used these days.

Immunoglobulin Production and Light Chain Ratio

By immunofixation and serum protein electrophoresis serum IgM or IgG paraproteins with the same light chain as the CLL cells have been detected in 18% and 17% of patients, respectively, and these patients have more advanced disease and a poorer prognosis than patients without a paraprotein.[169] However, standard serum protein electrophoresis detects a monoclonal protein in approximately 5% of CLL cases and an abnormal serum-free light chain ratio is observed in one-third of patients.[129,170-172] The presence of an abnormal ratio correlates with advanced and aggressive disease, with poor prognosis.[171,172]

IMMUNE DYSFUNCTION IN CHRONIC LYMPHOCYTIC LEUKEMIA

Abnormalities in the immune system are common and important in CLL leading to the infections, second malignancies, and autoimmune complications. These abnormalities will be discussed and their management reviewed later in the Treatment of CLL section.

Several factors lead to immunosuppression in CLL. Apart from hypogammaglobulinemia, there are alterations in T-cell function, abnormalities in complement activation, and dysfunction in the neutrophils/NK cells/monocytes.[173-175] While these complications are more prevalent with advanced disease, patients with MBL also have an increased risk of infections and second malignancies.[125-127] Moreover, immunosuppression can be potentiated by therapy of CLL, aging, and concomitant comorbidities, such as diabetes.[173,176] These abnormalities may lead to serious infections and second malignancies, important causes of death in CLL.[177,178] Whether the incidence of these complications will change in the future with the increasing use of targeted therapies is unknown.[179]

Infections in CLL typically involve the respiratory tract, urinary tract, and skin, with an increased incidence of bacterial, viral, and fungal infections.[173] An important cause of infections is a reduction in IgG and IgA levels, which is more pronounced with increasing disease burden and duration of disease (*Figure 92.7*). IgM levels are reduced in 50% of MBL, CLL, and SLL patients at diagnosis, but the decrease of this Ig does not appear to correlate with disease stage or risk of infections.[129] Reduced levels of IgG are seen in a quarter of all patients at diagnosis (especially IgG3 and IgG4), with the decrease correlating with disease burden and decreases in a further one-third at 10 years follow-up.[129,170,173] Interestingly, this decrease over time can occur without other evidence of tumor progression.[173] IgA differs from IgG in that it is produced at mucosal surfaces and reduced IgA levels at diagnosis have been associated with a short TTFT/OS and risk for subsequent infections.[129,180,181] This finding suggests that the CLL cells directly, or through factor(s) secreted by the CLL cells, suppress normal B and plasma cells.[182] CLL cells may have a direct effect on plasma cells through the surface expression of Fas ligand, CD27, and PDL1.[182] Additionally, TGF-β is secreted by CLL and marrow stromal cells in CLL and is a potent inhibitor of normal B and T cells.[183,184]

T cell abnormalities also occur in CLL, and likely play a role in the development of opportunistic infections, second malignancies, and red cell aplasia.[173] These changes are present very early in the disease course, being observed in MBL.[185] Described abnormalities include (a) an increase in the number of CD4 and CD8 cells in the peripheral blood in early-stage CLL, with inversion in the CD4:CD8 cell ratio.[173,174] In contrast, the CD4 cells are preferentially increased in the marrow and nodes[174]; (b) features of T cell exhaustion in the CD4+ and CD8+ cells, which is typically seen in chronic viral infections.[186] T cells express CD160, CD244, and PD1, key markers of T cell exhaustion, and the CD8+ cells show increased production of TNF-α and γ-IFN. It is speculated that these T cell changes are due to chronic stimulation by self-antigens or a response to interaction with CLL cells; (c) the gene expression profile of CD4+ and CD8+ cells differs in CLL patients as compared to normal individuals, and this abnormal expression can be induced in normal CD4+ and CD8+ cells by co-culturing them with CLL B cells.[187] This leads to altered production of filamentous actin polymerization and abnormal immunological synapse formation with antigen-presenting cells,[188] and (d) CLL cells might function as B regulatory (Breg) cells, suppressing CD4+ cells and inducing production of T regulatory (Treg) cells. Both CLL and Breg cells are CD5+/CD27+ B-cells with low sIgM and can secrete IL10. Treg cells are increased in CLL and are important in tumor immunesurveillance.[174] Similarly, CLL cells can induce the production of myeloid-derived suppressor cells (MDSCs) from

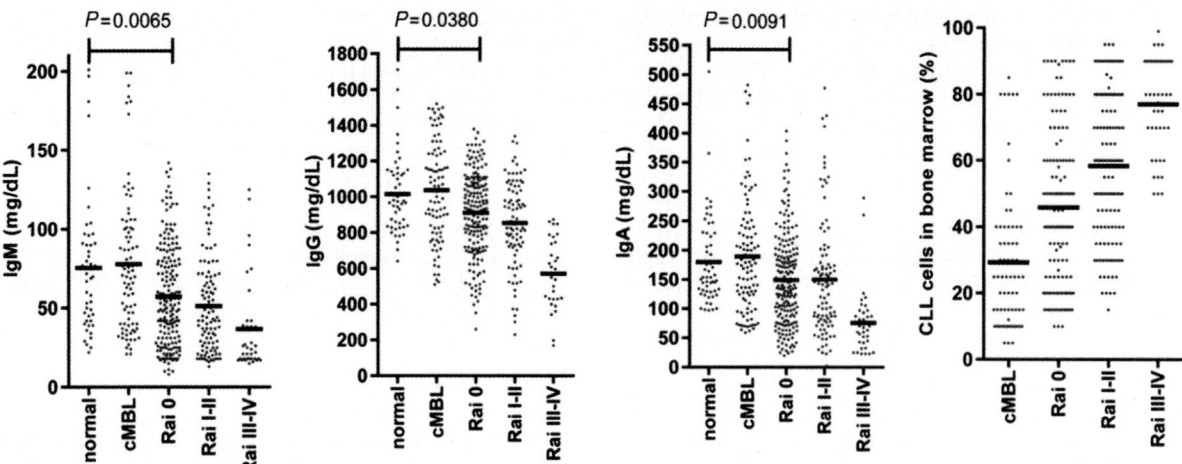

FIGURE 92.7 Early reduction of serum immunoglobulin levels in patients with chronic lymphocytic leukemia (CLL). Serum IgM, IgG, and IgA levels in high-count monoclonal B-cell lymphocytosis (MBL) and Rai stages 0, I-II, III-IV CLL at diagnosis are represented as dot plots. The normal age-matched donor cohort was used as internal reference values and for statistical comparison. The bone marrow infiltration by CLL cells at the early and late stage of disease according to Rai classification is also represented. (Reprinted from Forconi F, Moss P. Perturbation of the normal immune system in patients with CLL. *Blood.* 2015;126(5):573-581. Copyright © 2015 American Society of Hematology. With permission.)

polymorphonuclear cells or monocytes and MDSCs can increase Treg cell numbers.[189]

The levels of different serum complement components are also decreased in CLL, particularly in patients with advanced disease.[190] In addition, multiple defects in neutrophil, monocyte, and NK cell function have been described, and these are associated with an increased risk of infection.[175,191]

Infections, COVID-19, and Immunization
Infections

Infections are common in CLL, and patients with both MBL and CLL have a threefold increased likelihood of admission to hospital with infection compared to age- and sex-matched population with similar comorbidities.[192,193] In addition, even patients with low-count MBL have an increased risk of infection, although their risk of progression to CLL is very small.[127] Gram-positive bacterial infections tend to predominate in patients with early disease and can be related to reduced levels of IgG and IgA.[173] However, the correlation with immunoglobulin levels and risk of infection is not absolute and some patients with normal IgG will have repeated infections and others with hypogammaglobulinemia remain infection free.[175] While bacterial infections predominate, patients are also susceptible to opportunistic infections particularly if they have received steroids, purine nucleoside analogs, or anti-CD20 monoclonal antibodies. The nucleoside analogs are highly toxic to T lymphocytes, while the anti-CD20 monoclonal antibodies eliminate normal B cells increasing the risk of reactivation of hepatitis B and preventing a vigorous response to coronavirus disease 2019 (COVID-19) immunization for up to 12 months.[139,194] Ibrutinib also inhibits normal B cell activation and monocyte activity through inhibition of BTK while T-cell function is affected by ibrutinib through an off-target effect on inducible T-cell kinase (ITK); these effects can increase the risk for treated patients of infections initially, but the risk diminishes after 6 months.[195,196] IgA levels may increase over time with ibrutinib while IgG levels continue to decline.[195] Venetoclax does not affect normal B or T cells, but can cause infections by suppressing myelopoiesis.[197] As discussed below, the response of CLL patients to COVID-19 immunization is diminished in patients receiving ibrutinib.

Coronavirus Disease 2019

Severe acute respiratory syndrome coronavirus 2 (SARS-CoV-2) has caused the COVID-19 pandemic, producing significant morbidity and mortality in CLL patients.[198-200] This is likely multifactorial, related to immune-suppression, advanced age, and the multiple comorbidities in this patient population. In one multicenter study of 198 CLL patients with COVID-19, 90% required admission to hospital with one-third dying.[199] Importantly, both untreated and treated patients had a similar outcome to COVID infections with age ≥75 years and multiple comorbidities being poor prognostic features. Similar observations were made in a European study of 190 patients with COVID-19.[200] Results of this latter study suggested that treatment with ibrutinib may have been beneficial, perhaps by reducing the massive cytokine release from T/NK cells and monocytes, which causes the lung injury.[200,201] However, not all CLL patients become symptomatic when infected with SARS-CoV-2, but may be carriers of the disease. One carefully studied CLL patient with hypogammaglobulinemia demonstrated infectious virus by nasal swabs 70 days after the documented infection, suggesting that prolonged viral shedding may be a problem in immunosuppressed patients with CLL.[202] Finally, newer data with the Omicron variant of SARS-CoV-2 indicate that the mortality rates are much lower—whether this is due to a less virulent nature of the virus, vs a significant proportion of CLL patients having received vaccination, vs a combination of factors such as supportive/antiviral care remains unclear.[203]

Immunizations

There are two pathways for response to immunization, either a T-cell-independent pathway, which is typically seen with polysaccharide vaccines, or a T-cell-dependent pathway where examples include protein conjugate vaccines (PCV), protein vaccines, and viral vaccines.[193] Thus, patients with CLL have a reduced response to immunization, and while 58% of untreated early-stage patients responded to 13-valent pneumococcal vaccine, in comparison to 100% in the control group, this was considerably higher than seen with a pneumococcal polysaccharide vaccine.[204] As expected, the response was greatest in those with early-stage disease. Thus, it is recommended that the PCV13 vaccine (Prevnar 13; Wyeth/Pfizer) be given first followed 8 weeks later by the 23-valent pneumococcal polysaccharide vaccine (PPSV23) in CLL.[193] Because of their immune-compromised state, live vaccines should be avoided in CLL patients. Ibrutinib has been shown to inhibit response to influenza, hepatitis B, and SARS-CoV-2 vaccines, through its effects on the BCR pathway in normal B cells.[194,205-207] In contrast, ibrutinib does not affect the secondary response to recombinant herpes zoster vaccine (Shingrix; GlaxoSmithKline Biologicals) or the memory B cells generated by prior exposure to the virus through chickenpox.[205]

In keeping with these observations, either untreated or treated CLL patients may show a poor response to the BNT162b2 mRNA vaccine (Pfizer-BioNTech COVID-19 vaccine) or the mRNA-1273 vaccine (Moderna COVID-19 vaccine).[194,207,208] When tested 2 to 3 weeks after the second immunization BNT162b2 mRNA vaccine (given 21 days after the first immunization) only 39.5% of CLL patients had an antibody response to the vaccine; the responses in 52 patients and 52 age- and sex-matched controls were 52% and 100%, respectively.[207] Interestingly, there was no correlation between the development of local or systemic side effects with the vaccine and the development of antibodies. By multivariate analysis, the likelihood of responding to the vaccine was higher in females, if not actively receiving therapy, if ≤65 years, IgG ≥5.5 g/L, and IgM ≥0.4 g/L. In these studied patients, therapy was typically with a BTK inhibitor or venetoclax with or without an anti-CD20 antibody. Importantly, the highest response rate at 79.2% was seen in patients who had completed treatment and remained in remission at the time of immunization. Results of these studies and others have led to the recommendation that SARS-CoV-2 immunization be given prior to therapy.[194,208] Among the two most commonly used vaccinations in the United States against SARS-CoV-2, data indicate a more robust serological response with the use of the mRNA-1273 vaccine compared to the BNT162b2 vaccine. However, there are no data to suggest that specific levels of antibodies provide protection against clinical infection. In general, it is believed that evidence of seroconversion, if seen in CLL patients, can offer a degree of protection from coronavirus 2 infections and blunt the severity of the illness. Recent studies have also shown that CLL patients can generate T-cell-specific responses to SARS-CoV-2 vaccination, particularly among individuals who have not previously been treated for CLL.[209-211]

Second Malignancies

Second malignancies are common in CLL and are an important cause of death, particularly in the elderly.[177-179] Even patients with high-count MBL have an increased incidence of second malignancies.[126] Compared to the general population and patients with follicular lymphoma, the incidence of second malignancies is increased twofold, with the most common malignancies being squamous and basal cell carcinomas of the skin.[177,178,212] Immunosuppression is thought to be the primary cause of this complication, as a similar range of second malignancies is seen in immunosuppressed patients following organ transplantation.[178] In addition, these malignancies are more aggressive and an increased mortality has been seen with squamous cell carcinoma of the skin, melanomas, Merkel cell tumors, and solid tumors.[213-216] A recent publication has strongly suggested that treatment of CLL compared to untreated can greatly accelerate the incidence of second primary malignancies driven by increases in hematological malignancies.[217] This same study also determined that the increased incidence of second primary malignancies was not driven by increased surveillance.

The increased incidence of skin cancers is present at diagnosis and increases fourfold after diagnosis, with the main risk factors being male sex, age over 70 years, and a history of chemotherapy.[178] Thus, it is recommended that all patients have a careful skin examination at diagnosis with the frequency of follow-up depending on risk factors.[218] Careful skin surveillance with early detection has been reported in one study from Canada to reduce the expected mortality from skin cancers.[178,179] However, there does not appear to be a link between the incidence of skin cancers and the development of a solid tumor.[178]

The increased incidence of solid tumors appears to affect all types to a variable degree, and while prostate and breast cancers tend to predominate in most studies, because of their frequency, the predominant other types depend on the population studied.[212,213,219,220]

In contrast to the clear relationship between chemotherapy and risk of skin cancer, the relationship between therapy and the development of a solid tumor is less clear.[178,179] Moreover, a recent study on patients receiving first- or second-line ibrutinib or acalabrutinib showed a similar increase in skin cancers as observed with chemotherapy, and there was also an increased incidence of lung and bladder cancers in these patients.[220] Importantly, this study demonstrated that a history of smoking was a very strong risk factor. Thus, the increased risk of skin cancers and solid tumors in CLL may be a function of the disease itself, rather than the type of treatment, and is likely related to the combination of carcinogenic exposure combined with a global immunosuppression. As CLL patients are living longer with new therapies the incidence of second malignancies in CLL as a cause of death is expected to increase further in the future, highlighting the need for age-appropriate cancer screening.[179]

The risk of developing acute myeloid leukemia (AML) or myelodysplasia (MDS) appears to be closely linked to prior chemotherapy. The risk is low with alkylating agents or purine nucleoside analogs alone, but the risk increases if both are given together and the risk of developing AML/MDS with frontline fludarabine/cyclophosphamide/rituximab (FCR) chemotherapy is 5.1% after a median follow-up of 4.4 years.[221] Finally, CLL patients may develop other hematological malignancies, such as myeloma, lympho-, and myeloproliferative disorders.[222-224]

Autoimmune Disorders

Despite being immune deficient, CLL patients have an increased incidence of autoimmune cytopenias, with one-third being present before or at the time of diagnosis and two-thirds after the diagnosis.[148,225,226] Moreover, CLL is a commonly identified cause of autoimmune hemolytic anemia (AIHA) in adults (14% of cases) and patients with primary AIHA have an increased incidence of MBL and likelihood of developing CLL.[225,227] Overall, 4% to 10% of CLL patients develop AIHA and this is usually associated with a positive DAT.[148,226] Another 7% to 14% have a positive DAT without hemolysis. The incidence of AIHA is increased with male sex, older age, high lymphocyte count, advanced disease, and poor prognostic markers.[148,149,226,228] The diagnosis of AIHA can be difficult in CLL, as multiple factors can cause anemia, LDH may be increased from the disease itself, and the DAT may be negative. Zent et al[149] have developed stringent diagnostic criteria for the diagnosis of AIHA in CLL, which include (a) hemoglobin <100 g/L; (b) ≥1 marker of hemolysis, that is, reticulocytosis or increased marrow erythropoiesis (without bleeding), increased indirect bilirubin (without liver disease), or increased LDH (without another cause); and (c) evidence of an autoimmune mechanism, that is, positive DAT/cold agglutinins or ≥2 markers of hemolysis, without evidence of hypersplenism or bleeding.

AIHA may be triggered by chemotherapy, with an incidence around 10% for first-line chlorambucil or fludarabine as studied in the UK LRF CLL4 study.[229] However, the incidence was just 5% with fludarabine/cyclophosphamide, indicating that cyclophosphamide most likely has a protective effect. The incidence of DAT+ before treatment was 14% and one-third of DAT+ patients receiving single-agent chlorambucil or fludarabine developed AIHA. Conversely, 7% of the DAT− patients developed AIHA. The addition of rituximab to chemotherapy would be expected to reduce the incidence of AIHA further, and the incidence of AIHA was in fact <1% to 5.8% in patients receiving first-line FCR.[77,230] The development of an AIHA in CLL does not influence prognosis of CLL.[148,149] The risk of the targeted therapies triggering AIHA is still unclear, but a retrospective analysis suggests that it is low with ibrutinib and that patients receiving immune-suppressants for immune cytopenias can be weaned off these agents with control of the CLL by ibrutinib.[231]

Immune thrombocytopenia (ITP) occurs in <1% to 2% of patients and may be suspected if there is a sudden isolated fall in platelets in the absence of splenomegaly, as anemia usually precedes thrombocytopenia when cytopenia is caused by marrow replacement. The diagnosis is confirmed by an increase in platelet size in the peripheral blood and an increase in megakaryocytes in the marrow, although the latter is often difficult to ascertain as the marrow is usually infiltrated with CLL cells. Autoimmune neutropenia occurs rarely in CLL but should be considered if patients have an isolated neutropenia and the marrow will show myeloid arrest. Red cell aplasia is also rare and is suspected when a patient develops isolated anemia with reticulocytopenia and none of the usual signs of hemolysis.

The antibodies causing these cytopenias are produced by normal B cells and not CLL cells as the antibodies are polyclonal and usually IgG. In addition, the autoimmune disorders may occur while the patient's disease is responding to therapy. It has thus been suggested that CLL cells act as antigen-presenting cells for normal CD5+

or CD5⁻ antibody-producing B cells and that antibody production is increased after inhibition of T cells, either with advancement of disease or because of therapy.[225,232] Antigen presentation may occur in the spleen as it is the major site of removal of senescent red cells and may be potentiated by T cells through CD40L-CD40.[233] Moreover, there is an association between the likelihood of developing AIHA or ITP in CLL with certain BCR stereotypes.[233] In contrast to the other immune cytopenias, red cell aplasia is caused by T-cell dysfunction, rather than autoantibodies, and these patients usually respond well to cyclosporine.[232,233]

A number of other conditions may be caused by autoantibodies produced directly by the CLL cells and these include cold agglutinin disease, peripheral neuropathy, and paraneoplastic pemphigus.[232] Cold agglutinin disease is caused by a monoclonal antibody produced by the CLL cells against the red cell I antigen and the CLL cells are typically $IGHV_{4-21}$.[234] Polyneuropathy is caused by an antibody against myelin-associated glycoprotein.[233] Paraneoplastic pemphigus causes painful mouth ulcers, conjunctivitis, and pruritic blistering skin lesions.[235] It is diagnosed by typical histologic changes in the skin and the presence of autoantibodies in the blood directed against cutaneous epitopes. Acquired angioedema is associated with recurrent abdominal pain and is caused by consumption of the inhibitor of the first component complement by CLL cells.[232] Glomerulonephritis, frequently with nephrotic syndrome, may occur secondary to deposition of intact monoclonal antibody or light chains in the kidney and remits with treatment of the CLL.[232] As opposed to the immune cytopenias, all of the above occur with CLL disease progression and typically resolve with treatment of the leukemia.[236]

PROGNOSTIC AND PREDICTIVE MARKERS

Because of routine blood testing, most patients with CLL nowadays present with Rai stages 0/I disease. However, there is great variation in the rate of disease progression in these patients, and great efforts have been made to develop reliable prognostic markers to predict TTFT and OS, which are important when deciding which patients require close monitoring and to counsel patients regarding their prognosis (Table 92.7).[237] In addition, predictive markers are required to assess whether a patient will respond to therapy, which may influence survival. Several general points about these markers should be made: (a) these markers have generally been evaluated in patients less than 65 years of age and their value in older patients is less certain.[57,152] Thus, although *IGHV* status and FISH results are useful predictors of survival for younger patients, they are less useful in those ≥75 years[57,152]; (b) the markers have been studied at the time of diagnosis and their utility throughout the disease course is less clear. The exception here is for FISH and *TP53* sequencing, as abnormalities can evolve over time and these tests may be carried out at diagnosis and prior to each treatment. The results provide useful information regarding prognosis at diagnosis and influence treatment decisions[138,238]; (c) a prognostic marker may be able to predict one aspect of the disease course, for example TTFT, but may not be able to predict PFS or OS; (d) many prognostic markers are not independent markers and their usefulness diminishes when markers are examined using multivariate analysis[238]; and (e) existing prognostic and predictive markers have been evaluated with chemotherapy and their relevance in the era of novel agents is less clear.

Rai and Binet Staging

Clinical staging remains a simple and independent prognostic marker in CLL, but is limited since about 85% of patients now present with Rai stage 0/I. The rate of disease progression in this group of patients is highly variable, and biological markers are required to predict which patients will progress.

Age and Sex

Approximately 10% to 20% of CLL patients are ≤55 years at diagnosis, and these patients may have more aggressive disease than older patients.[150,153] The proportion of deaths directly attributed to CLL is greater than for older patients and they may be at increased risk of Richter syndrome (RS).[150] Epidemiological studies have shown that the relative survival of patients older than 75 years is reduced, likely related to inadequate treatment and lack of trial eligibility rather than to a difference in disease biology.[7,8,151]

The male-to-female ratio for CLL is 1.3:1, and women have a better prognosis than men. Women are more likely to have *IGHV* mutated disease, to present with earlier clinical stage, respond better to therapy, and have a better OS.[239] However, while women with unmutated *IGHV* disease have a better prognosis than men with unmutated disease, no difference in prognosis is seen for patients with mutated disease.[239]

Lymphocyte Characteristics
Morphology

Approximately 20% of patients have atypical CLL or CLL/PLL based on blood morphology, and these patients have a more advanced stage, a higher proliferative index, and a poorer prognosis.[161,240,241] These patients are more likely to have trisomy 12, mutated *NOTCH1*, be CD38⁺, and have unmutated *IGHV*.[161,240,241] In the UK LRF CLL4 study, 14% of patients had ≥10% PL in their peripheral blood and these patients had an increased risk of RS, and a shorter PFS and OS with chemotherapy compared to patients with <10% PL.[241] In contrast, the presence of smudge cells signifies a good prognosis, with patients having ≥30% smudge cells having a better OS than those with <30% smudge cells.[160]

Number

Survival decreases with increasing B-cell or lymphocyte count at diagnosis.[124] A B-cell count of >11 × 10⁹/L predicts a shorter treatment-free survival and OS independent of CD38, ZAP-70, and *IGHV* mutational status.[124]

Doubling Time

The lymphocyte doubling time (LDT) at diagnosis remains a simple and important prognostic measure.[157] In 848 patients, those with a LDT of <12 months required treatment at a median of 25 months vs not reached ($P < .001$) and the median OS was 95 vs 161 months ($P < .001$). As expected, short LDT was associated with unmutated *IGHV*, p53 dysfunction, del 11q, and high β2-microglobulin. However, LDT was an independent prognostic marker for TTFT, likely as it

Table 92.7. Prognostic Markers in CLL Including Those Used in CLL-IPI

Prognostic Marker	Better Prognosis	Worse Prognosis
Sex	Female	Male
Age[a]	<65 y	≥65 y
Stage[a] • Rai • Binet	 0 A	 I-IV B, C
Lymphocyte doubling time	>12 mo	<12 mo
β2-microglobulin level[a]	<3.5 mg/L	≥3.5
FISH/*TP53* mutations[a]	Del 13q	Del 17p and/or *TP53* mutation
IGHV mutation status[a]	Mutated	Unmutated

Abbreviations: CLL, chronic lymphocytic leukemia; CLL-IPI, International Prognostic Index for chronic lymphocytic leukemia; FISH, fluorescent in situ hybridization; IGHV, immunoglobulin heavy chain variable region.
[a]Five key independent prognostic markers used in the CLL-IPI. International CLL-IPI working group. An international prognostic index for patients with chronic lymphocytic leukaemia (CLL-IPI): a meta-analysis of individual patient data. *Lancet Oncology.* 2016;17(6):779-790. For scoring: age >65 years and Rai stages I-IV (or Binet B/C) each receive 1 point; β2-microglobulin concentration >3.5 mg/L and unmutated *IGHV* each receive 2 points; and del 17p and/or *TP53* mutation 4 points. Patients with scores of 0 to 1, 2 to 3, 4 to 6, and 7 to 10 are designated low-, intermediate-, high-, and very-high-risk.

reflects a number of genetic changes associated with cell proliferation/apoptosis. However, it did not predict response to chemoimmunotherapy but was an independent predictor of OS.

Flow Cytometry

i. **CD38** is a measure of cell proliferation but there has been controversy as to its value as levels can fluctuate over time.[242] However, positivity has been correlated with increasing Rai stage, lymphadenopathy, short doubling time, increased β_2-microglobulin levels, TTFT, PFS, and OS.[242-244] Moreover, the CD38 status may predict which early-stage patients will progress.[245]

ii. **ZAP-70** positivity enhances the BCR pathway but is difficult to measure reproducibly.[242] However, the CLL Research Consortium has demonstrated that ZAP-70+ patients had a median TTFT of 2.6 vs 8.4 years for ZAP-70– patients.[246] ZAP-70– patients and unmutated *IGHV* patients had a median OS of 6.3 vs 10 years for mutated *IGHV* patients.

iii. **CD49d** is the α chain of the $\alpha 4\beta 1$ integrin (VLA-4). VLA-4 is the ligand for the vascular cell adhesion molecule (VCAM1) receptor and fibronectin, which are present on stromal cells and matrix in the microenvironment, respectively. These interactions are important for CLL cell trafficking and survival, and the CD49d pathway is activated in peripheral blood CD49d+ cells but not CD49d– cells.[247] The overexpression of CD49d (>30% cells stained positive) is one of the best flow-based independent prognostic markers, alongside unmutated *IGHV* and p53 dysfunction, for predicting reduced TTFT and OS.[248-250] Approximately one-third of patients have increased CD49d, and these patients have more advanced disease, bulky lymphadenopathy, unmutated *IGHV*, and high β_2-microglobulin.[249] Importantly, the CD34d status may be used to separate *IGHV* mutated patients into two prognostic groups.[249]

Genetics

Fluorescence In Situ Hybridization

FISH is an important prognostic and predictive tool in CLL. Thus, FISH results can predict TTFT and OS, leading to suggestions that it be carried out at diagnosis.[120,138] The iwCLL 2018 guidelines recommended that FISH be carried out prior to each new line of therapy as new FISH abnormalities can develop over time and a del 17p is associated with resistance to chemoimmunotherapy and a shorter response to the novel agents.[1,75,82,251-253] A detailed description of FISH abnormalities was discussed in "Analysis by FISH" and the effects of the various abnormalities are shown in *Figure 92.5*. In brief, 80% of patients will have a FISH abnormality and using the hierarchical model, the incidences of del 13q, normal FISH, trisomy 12, del 17p, and del 11q have been reported by Van Dyke et al[82] as 39%, 24%, 14%, 12%, and 11%, respectively. Changes predicting TTFT, from shortest to longest, are del 11q, del 17p, trisomy 12, normal, and del 13q while changes associated with OS, from worst to best, are del 17p, del 11q, trisomy 12, normal, and del 13q.[75,82] In general, the prognosis is worse with increasing numbers of affected nuclei. However, it should be noted that these patients were treated with chemotherapy.

Del 17p is the most important predictive marker, as it reflects p53 dysfunction and resistance to chemotherapy and a decreased response to the novel agents.[251-253] It is typically seen with unmutated *IGHV* and in half the patients with CLL/PLL.[251,254] The incidence of this abnormality increases over time and with the development of resistance. Typically, 4% to 5% of patients at diagnosis have a del 17p; half require treatment in 3 years but one-third have stable disease.[255] At first-line therapy, 10% have del 17p while this increases to one-third with fludarabine resistance.[45,77,110] Most patients with del 17p have a *TP53* mutation on the other allele, but patients may have a del 17p or a *TP53* mutation alone.[45,251] Thus, fludarabine-resistant patients have del 17p alone (~7%), del 17p with a *TP53* mutation (~25%), or a *TP53* mutation alone (~5%).[45,251] Prognosis is equally poor in all groups and patients with either a del 17p or a *TP53* mutation are described as having p53 dysfunction. Thus, if possible, patients should thus have *TP53* sequencing in addition to FISH studies.

Del 11q is classically seen with unmutated *IGHV* disease, occurs in 10% to 20% patients, and is associated with short TTFT, PFS, and OS with chemotherapy.[75,83,95-97] While the number of nuclei in all patients with the del 11q does not influence prognosis, it may depend on whether the del 11q is the sole abnormality or coexists with a del 13q.[82,83] In a study of 196 patients studied at diagnosis, one-third had only del 11q while two-thirds had del 11q with del 13q.[83] Both groups had a short TTFT at ~6 months and similar OS (not reached). For the del 11q group alone the median TTFT was inversely related to the number of cells with the del (1.7 months if >58% and 19.1 months if ≤58%) as was OS (median 75 months if >58% and not reached if ≤58%).[83] Prognosis can be significantly improved with the addition of cyclophosphamide and rituximab to fludarabine (FC and FCR), with an improvement in the response rate and PFS.[77,146] In addition, while a del 11q predicted for shortened PFS for FCR in the CLL8 trial, it did not influence survival indicating that these patients can respond to further therapy.[97] In contrast to chemotherapy, patients with a del 11q do well with ibrutinib.[50]

Trisomy 12 can be associated with atypical immunophenotype, atypical morphology, and with CD38 positivity.[161,256] While atypical CLL or CLL/PLL are often associated with trisomy 12, not all the atypical cells contain trisomy 12, indicating that the chromosomal abnormality is not responsible for the morphology.[257] One-quarter of trisomy 12 cases have a *NOTCH1* mutation, and these patients have a worse prognosis than patients without a mutation.[76] In one study the primary causes of death for patients with trisomy 12 were RS and second malignancies, while these patients also had an increased incidence of ITP.[256]

Half of CLL patients have del 13q, which can affect one or both alleles, and generally these patients have a good prognosis. However, prognosis depends on the number of cells affected by the deletion, with the OS being poorer for those with a large deletion (including the retinoblastoma region) or those with >70% nuclei affected.[82,258,259] TTFT is also longer for those with <85% nuclei affected than those with a higher number.[82]

Classical Genetics

Complex karyotyping in CLL can independently predict TTFT and OS in patients receiving chemotherapy or ibrutinib.[74,91,93] Those with ≥5 abnormalities (high-CK) have a very poor prognosis with chemotherapy, regardless of p53 function (del 17p or *TP53* mutation), while those with 3 or 4 abnormalities only have a poor prognosis if there is p53 dysfunction.[93] For those receiving ibrutinib, an increasing number of CK is an independent predictor for shorter PFS and OS.[93] However, further studies are required before karyotyping becomes routine in CLL.

Mutations of *IGHV*, *IGHV*$_{3-21}$ Usage and Stereotypy

The *IGHV* mutational status is one of the most important biologic predictors of PFS and OS with chemoimmunotherapy, an effect that is not observed with the targeted therapies.[138,238,260,261] Approximately 40% of patients have unmutated *IGHV* and are more likely to develop del 17p and/or del 11q, progressive disease, drug resistance, and have shorter OS than mutated patients when treated with chemotherapy. Hamblin et al[261] showed that for Binet stage A patients, survival was 95 months for unmutated patients and 293 months for mutated patients. While a cut-off of 2% mutated is used to differentiate mutated from unmutated, caution should be taken with borderline mutation levels. The *IGHV*$_{3-21}$ mutational status is often borderline and these patients have a poor prognosis, regardless of mutation status.[262] Interestingly, over half of these cases show BCR stereotypy (subset #2) and these cases have a shorter TTFT than the nonsubset #2 cases, regardless of *IGVH* mutational status.[262] Stereotypy subsets refer to groups of patients who have similar HCDR3 sequences in their BCR immunoglobulin gene.

Telomere Length and Telomerase Activity

Short telomeres are associated with genomic instability, del 17p and/or del 11q, short OS, and an increased risk of developing RS.[263]

NOTCH, SF3B1, and Other Novel Mutations

The clinical significance of a number of novel molecular markers has been assessed in the CLL8 clinical trial.[77,264] Patients were characterized as having subclonal or clonal mutations, depending on the frequency of the mutation. A high number of clonal mutations were seen with a total frequency of *TP53* (10.6%), *ATM* (11.1%), *SF3B1* (12.6%), *NOTCH1* (21.8%), and *BIRC3* (4.2%). Mutations in *ATM*, clonal *SF3B1* mutations, and both clonal and subclonal *NOTCH1* mutations predicted for shorter TTFT while clonal and subclonal *TP53* mutations, and clonal *NOTCH1* mutations predicted for shortened OS. Thus, this study emphasized the importance of *TP53* in CLL, with even subclonal mutations carrying a poor prognosis. When CLL patients were examined following relapse or resistance to different treatments, 38% had ≥2 mutations while mutations in *TP53*, *NOTCH1*, and *SF3B1* were found in 22.8%, 14.9%, and 28.1% patients, respectively (*Figure 92.8*).[265] Interestingly these three gene mutations appeared to cluster together in 19% of patients (Cluster #3) and these patients had a poorer response to salvage therapy than others, with reduced PFS and OS.[265] When considered individually, the presence of a *TP53* mutation was the only genetic abnormality to predict for poor response to salvage therapy and a shorter PFS.[265]

NOTCH1 mutations are associated with unmutated *IGHV*, trisomy 12, advanced stage, and CD38/ZAP-70 positivity. In addition, the risk of developing RS for *NOTCH1* mutated patients is 45% compared to 4% in unmutated patients.[266] Mutations of *SF3B1* cause aberrations in splicing of a variety of mRNAs and have generated interest in CLL because of their frequency, interesting RNA regulatory function, and possible role in drug resistance.[267]

MicroRNA Expression

Low levels of MiR-181b at diagnosis can predict disease progression, and the level of the MiR decreases over time in patients with progressive disease.[268] This is likely related to the fact that both BCL2 and MCL1 are targets for MiR-181b and the levels of these antiapoptotic proteins increase as the level of MiR-181b falls.[268]

Marrow Histology

The bone marrow involvement in CLL can be interstitial, nodular, mixed (combination of interstitial and nodular), or diffuse, with the diffuse involvement primarily occurring in those with advanced stage and correlating with poor prognosis.[140,269] Similarly, ≥80% lymphocytes in the marrow aspirate usually indicates more rapid disease progression and shorter OS than an infiltrate of <80%.[269]

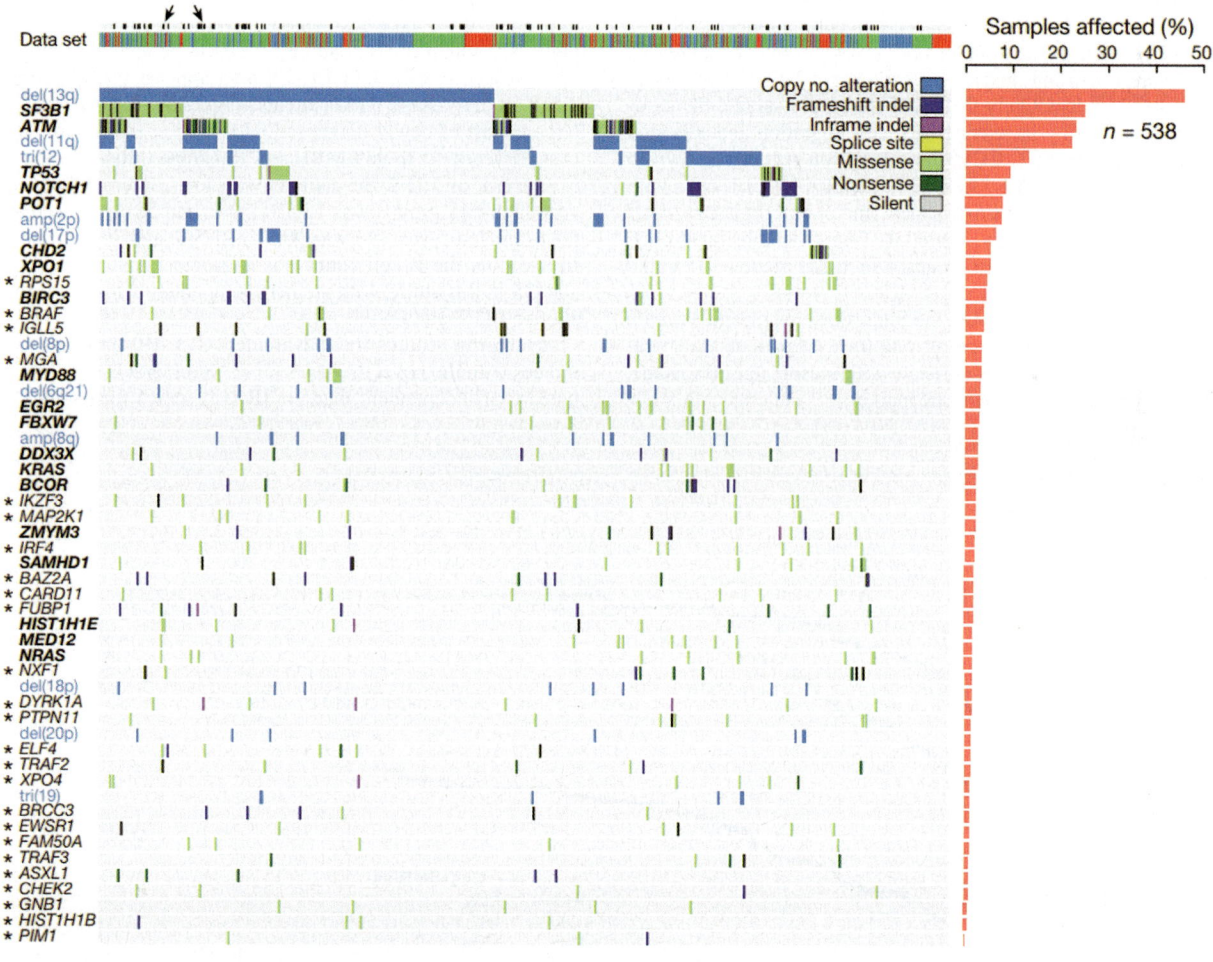

FIGURE 92.8 Clustering diagram of gene mutation distribution. Somatic mutation information is shown across the 55 putative driver genes and recurrent somatic copy number alterations (CNAs; rows) for 538 primary patient samples (from CLL8 [green], Spanish ICGC [red], and DFCI/Broad [blue]) that underwent whole-exome sequencing (columns). Blue labels, recurrent somatic CNAs; bold labels, putative chronic lymphocytic leukemia cancer genes; asterisked labels, additional cancer-associated genes identified in this study. Samples were annotated for IGHV (immunoglobulin heavy chain variable region) status (black, mutated; white, unmutated; red, unknown), and for exposure to therapy before sampling (black, previous therapy; white, no previous therapy; red, unknown previous treatment status). (Adapted by permission from Nature: Landau DA, Tausch E, Taylor-Weiner AN, et al. Mutations driving CLL and their evolution in progression and relapse. *Nature*. 2015;526(7574):525-530. Copyright © 2015 Springer Nature.)

Patients with persistent lymphoid nodules in the marrow after chemotherapy (nodular partial remission [nPR]) likely have persistent leukemia and have a shorter time to relapse compared to those in complete remission (CR).[1,270] Immunohistochemistry is important to ensure that residual nodules reflect CLL cells and not reactive T or normal B cells.[1]

Plasma Markers

Plasma *LDH* levels are a measure of cell turnover and increased levels are associated with the presence of other poor prognostic markers, such as high CD38 or ZAP-70, or the presence of del 17p.[271] A sudden and significant increase in LDH may indicate disease progression or the development of RS.

Plasma *β_2-microglobulin* is derived from the cell membrane of nucleated cells and is noncovalently linked to the α-chain of the class I major histocompatibility complex. An increased level of β_2-microglobulin predicts for short TTFT, PFS, and OS.[57,77,272-274] The β_2-microglobulin level may reflect tumor burden, but is still useful in Binet stage A disease to predict TTFT and PFS.[272,273] Thus, β_2-microglobulin levels also reflect the CLL biology. In this context the inflammatory cytokine (IL-6, IL-8, and TNF-α) levels reflect CLL disease activity and comorbidities.[57] While β-microglobulin is cleared by the kidneys, its prognostic value is increased by correcting for renal function.[274] Although β-microglobulin has been mainly evaluated with chemotherapy, the levels fall rapidly following initiation of ibrutinib, and normalization of levels at 6 months predicts for a longer PFS.[275]

The plasma levels of the inflammatory *cytokines* may be increased in CLL and are important prognostic markers for OS, particularly in the elderly.[57,276-278] It is likely that many cell types secrete the cytokines, which may act by increasing CLL cell migration and adhesion in the microenvironment.[57] CCL3 has also been recently shown to have prognostic value in CLL.[58] CCL3 is secreted by CLL cells with BCR stimulation in the microenvironment and elevated plasma levels predict a short TTFT.[58] Finally, Yan et al[279] have demonstrated clustering of 23 cytokines into three groups, which can predict TTFT and OS in CLL.

Two groups have demonstrated the importance of plasma *vitamin D* levels in CLL.[280,281] In one study, one-third of patients had vitamin D deficiency, which did not correlate with season, age, sex, stage, lymphocyte count, or other prognostic markers.[281] Patients with a low level had a shorter TTFT and OS and it has been suggested that vitamin D has a cytotoxic effect on CLL cells, which have high levels of the vitamin D receptor.[280,281]

Prognostic Index

With many markers having independent value for prognosis, there has been interest in combining these markers to generate a prognostic index. The MD Anderson[282] developed an index using six easily measured factors (age, sex, Rai stage, lymphocyte counts, number of lymph node regions involved, and β2-microglobulin level) to predict OS in previously untreated patients receiving chemotherapy and the value of this index was subsequently confirmed at the Mayo Clinic.[283]

More recently the International CLL-IPI Working Group has developed the CLL-IPI to predict OS (*Figure 92.9*), and this divides patients into four prognostic groups based on five independent prognostic markers, which are given different weights according to their prognostic significance.[238] 3472 patients were included from 8 phase III randomized clinical trials, and 27 prognostic markers were assessed. Although the initial score was based on relatively young (median age 62 years) patients being entered on clinical trials, the results were validated on newly diagnosed patients at the Mayo Clinic and Swedish CLL registry, many of whom did not require therapy. Age >65 years and Rai stages I-IV (or Binet B/C) each received 1 point; β2-microglobulin concentration >3.5 mg/L and unmutated *IGHV* 2 points, and del 17p and/or *TP53* mutation 4 points. Patients with scores of 0 to 1, 2 to 3, 4 to 6, and 7 to 10 were designated low-, intermediate-, high-, and very-high-risk; with a corresponding 5-year OS being 97%, 92%, 68%, and 21%, respectively. The CLL-IPI also appears useful for predicting TTFT in early-stage CLL patients; *Figure 92.8* shows the TTFT in a large cohort of newly diagnosed CLL seen at the Mayo Clinic in the past 15 years.[284] In 969 MBL and Rai stage 0 disease, the estimated 5-year risk of TTFT for patients with low-, intermediate-, and high/very-high-risk groups was 13.5%, 30%, and 58%, respectively, while the estimated 5-year OS was 96.3%, 91.5%, and 76%, respectively.[120] In addition, the B-cell count was an independent predictor of TTFT and OS in this study, with an increasing count being associated with a shorter TTFT and OS.[120]

Emerging studies have evaluated CLL-IPI and new prognostic indices with the novel therapies.[285-287] Soumerai et al[285] initially evaluated four independent markers (BALL score) for patients receiving

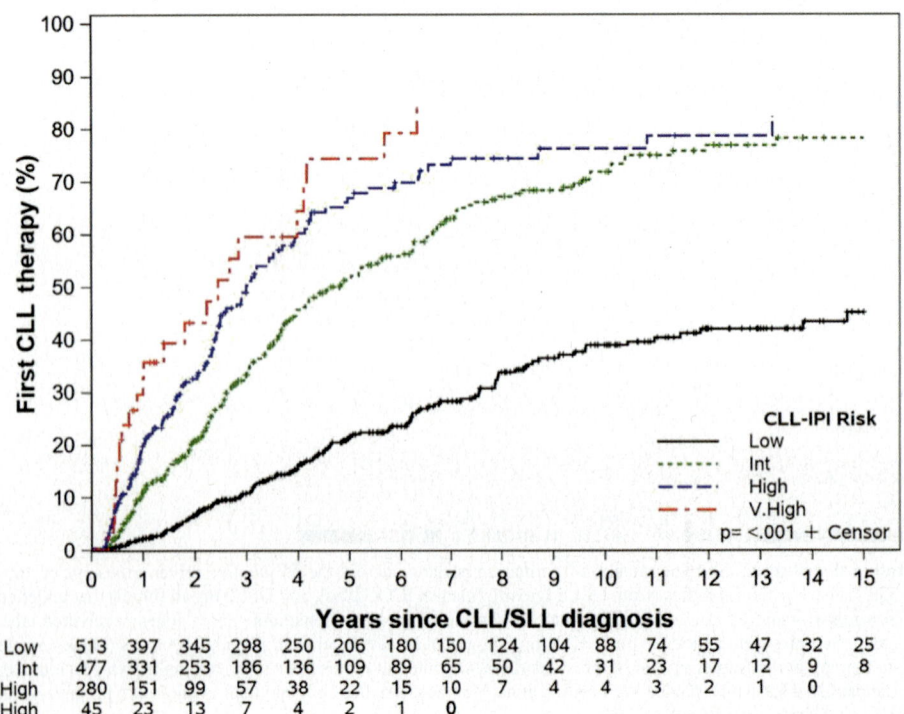

FIGURE 92.9 Time to first therapy according to the chronic lymphocytic leukemia—international prognostic index (CLL-IPI) in newly diagnosed CLL patients seen at the Mayo Clinic. SLL, small lymphocytic lymphoma. (Reprinted from Kay NE, Hampel PJ, Van Dyke DL, Parikh SA, CLL update 2022: A continuing evolution in care. *Blood Rev.* 2022;54:100930. Copyright © 2022 Elsevier. With permission.)

ibrutinib or venetoclax as second-line therapy using patients from six clinical trials and the Mayo Clinic CLL Database. One point was given for an increased serum β2-microglobulin (≥5 mg/dL), anemia (hemoglobin <110 g/L for women or <120 g/L for men), elevated LDH, and a short length of time from initiation of last therapy (<24 months). Patients were low- (score 0-1), intermediate- (score 2-3), or high-risk (score 4), which predicted for OS. A subsequent study of 541 patients receiving salvage ibrutinib in the real-world setting confirmed the importance of β$_2$-microglobulin, anemia, and LDH as independent prognostic markers.[286] In contrast to the above, Ahn et al[287] have shown that *TP53* dysfunction is an independent prognostic marker for ibrutinib resistance. Thus, in 804 patients, β$_2$-microglobulin ≥5 mg/dL, high LDH, prior treatment, and p53 dysfunction were each given 1 point and patients separated into low-risk (0,1 point), intermediate-risk (2 points), and high-risk (3,4 points). At 3 years the PFS for these groups was 87%, 74%, and 47%, respectively, whereas the OS was 93%, 83%, and 63%, respectively. These studies confirmed that *IGHV* mutation status did not influence response to the targeted agents and further studies are required to assess the importance of p53 dysfunction and other molecular markers for response to these agents, both in the first- and second-line settings.

TREATMENT OF CLL

Indications for Treatment

As all treatments can be toxic, it is important to only start therapy when indicated. Guidelines for initiation of therapy are as recommended by the iwCLL[1]: (a) Rai stage 0-II disease in patients who are symptomatic (weight loss of >10% body weight in previous 6 months, extreme fatigue, night sweats, or fevers of >100.5 °F or 38 °C for >2 weeks without evidence of infection) or have progressive anemia/thrombocytopenia or lymphocytosis (>50% increase over 2 months or LDT <6 months); (b) Rai stages III/IV to improve the hemoglobin level and/or platelet counts, although asymptomatic patients can be monitored and treatment initiated when there is clear evidence of disease progression; (c) bulky or progressive lymphadenopathy (masses >10 cm in diameter) or splenomegaly (>6 cm below left costal margin); and (d) immune cytopenias. Symptomatic or functional extranodal involvement (e.g., skin, kidney, spine, and lung) is also an indication for treatment.

Response Criteria, Resistance, and Minimal Residual Disease

To facilitate comparisons of results obtained in clinical trials, the iwCLL[1] has established criteria for clinical responses in CLL, as outlined in *Table 92.8*. The presence of organomegaly in clinical practice is based on clinical examination, but CT scans are required for clinical trials. The BCR inhibitors produce an initial lymphocytosis and this is reflected in response, for example, partial response with lymphocytosis (PR-L).

Complete responses (CRs)/partial responses (PRs) are routinely obtained with chemoimmunotherapy and venetoclax-containing regimens, while elimination of measurable residual disease (MRD) from blood and marrow can predict for longer PFS and improved OS.[288] This topic has recently been reviewed with consensus recommendations.[288] MRD assessments are primarily used following fixed-duration therapy, but whether marrow or peripheral blood should be assessed, which method should be used to assess MRD, and the assay sensitivity required are presently ill defined. Basic three-color flow cytometry (CD19/CD5 with evidence of cells being κ or λ) can detect 10^{-2} MRD (one CLL cell in 100 leukocytes [1%]) and is referred to as MRD2.[288,289] Subsequent four- to ten-color panels have increased sensitivity further. The minimum sensitivity is MRD4 (10^{-4}) developed in 2007 using four-color flow cytometry with CD5/CD19 with CD20/CD38, CD81/CD22, and CD79b/CD43, and concordance between peripheral blood and marrow MRD was ~90% when assessed >3 months after treatment.[289] This remains the gold standard and has been validated across different laboratories and in clinical trials. PCR assays on *IGHV* sequences or high-throughput next-generation sequencing are highly sensitive and can be done more easily on stored samples, but are more cumbersome and expensive.[288] In 2020, the clonoSEQ assay was approved by the FDA to assess MRD in CLL

Table 92.8. Criteria for Response in Chronic Lymphocytic Leukemia (CLL)

Group	Parameter	Complete Response (CR)	Partial Response (PR) and Partial Response With Lymphocytosis (PR-L)	Progressive Disease (PD)	Stable Disease (SD)
A	Lymph nodes	None ≥1.5 cm	Decrease ≥50% (from baseline)[a]	Increase ≥50% from baseline or from response	Change of –49% to +49%
	Liver and/or spleen size[b]	Spleen size, 13 cm; liver size normal	Decrease ≥50% from baseline	Increase ≥50% from baseline or from response	Change of –49% to +49%
	Constitutional symptoms	None	Any	Any	Any
	Circulating lymphocyte count	Normal	Decrease ≥50% from baseline	Increase ≥50% from baseline or from response	Change of –49% to +49%
B	Platelets	≥100 × 10^9/L	≥100 × 10^9/L or increase ≥50% over baseline	Decrease by ≥50% from baseline secondary to CLL	Change of –49% to +49%
	Hemoglobin	≥11.0 g/dL (untransfused and without erythropoietin)	≥11.0 g/dL or increase ≥50% over baseline	Decrease of ≥2 g/dL from baseline secondary to CLL	Increase, 11.0 g/dL or <50% over baseline, or decrease, 2 g/dL
	Marrow	Normocellular, no CLL cells, no B-lymphoid nodules	Presence of CLL cells, or of B-lymphoid nodules, or not done	Increase of CLL cells by ≥50% on successive biopsies	No change in marrow infiltrate

Abbreviations: CR, complete remission (all of the criteria have to be met); PD, progressive disease (at least one of the criteria of group A or group B has to be met); PR, partial remission (for a PR, at least two of the parameters of group A and one parameter of group B need to improve if previously abnormal; if only one parameter of both groups A and B is abnormal before therapy, only one needs to improve); SD, stable disease (all of the criteria have to be met; constitutional symptoms alone do not define PD).
[a]Sum of the products of six or fewer lymph nodes (as evaluated by CT scans and physical examination in clinical trials or by physical examination in general practice).
[b]Spleen size is considered normal if 13 cm. There is not firmly established international consensus of the size of a normal liver; therefore, liver size should be evaluated by imaging and manual palpation in clinical trials and be recorded according to the definition used in a study protocol.
Reprinted from Hallek M, Cheson BD, Catovsky D, et al. iwCLL guidelines for diagnosis, indications for treatment, response assessment and supportive management of chronic lymphocytic leukemia. *Blood.* 2018;131(25):2745-2760. Copyright © 2018 American Society of Hematology. With permission.

patient samples and using next-generation sequencing can detect one CLL cell in 1 million leukocytes (MRD6 [10^{-6}]).[290,291] While "undetectable-MRD" (U-MRD) is likely going to remain a therapeutic goal with chemoimmunotherapy, venetoclax, and following non-myeloablative allogeneic hematopoietic cell transplantation (HCT), whether those patients who do not achieve MRD negativity benefit from additional therapy requires further study. Prospective studies are necessary to determine if the current iwCLL standard of defining MRD negativity by flow cytometry (MRD4) needs to be replaced by more sensitive next-generation sequencing. Thus, at the present time MRD measurements remain a research tool and are not recommended in routine clinical practice.

Chemotherapy

While most chemotherapy is now combined with a monoclonal antibody (chemoimmunotherapy), for completeness we will initially discuss chemotherapy and immunotherapy separately, and then in combination.

Alkylating Agents

Chlorambucil was first used for CLL 60 years ago, and this simple and well-tolerated oral drug still plays a role in the treatment of CLL.[292] Its activity is likely through covalent binding to DNA, although it also binds to RNA and cellular proteins. Many treatment schedules have been used, with response depending on dose with intermittent dosing producing less myelosuppression.[293,294] The two most common regimens used today are the British (10 mg/m^2 daily × 7, repeated monthly for 6-12 months)[295] and German (0.5 mg/kg on days 1 and 15 for 6-12 months)[296] schedules, although daily low doses of chlorambucil, for example, 4 to 6 mg/d, may be used in elderly patients with dose-adjustments according to monthly blood counts. Approximately 50% of patients achieve a PR, and CRs are uncommon.

Cyclophosphamide is similar to chlorambucil and may be given orally using 2 to 3 mg/kg/d or 20 mg/kg once every 2 to 3 weeks.[297] Cyclophosphamide has the long-term risk of bladder cancer, but is advantageous over chlorambucil in being less myelosuppressive and less likely to cause immune cytopenias.[295,298]

To improve response rates, alkylating agents have been combined with steroids or other agents. Steroids cause a redistribution of the CLL cells and initially there is an increase in the peripheral lymphocyte count with shrinkage of nodes and spleen. In practice, prednisone may be combined with chlorambucil or used prior to chlorambucil to produce a rapid decrease in lymph node/spleen size and reduce pancytopenia related to marrow packing.[295] However, corticosteroids should be used carefully as they do not increase survival and may produce significant side effects.[293,299]

Bendamustine is a novel alkylating agent that produces more extensive DNA cross-linking and breaks than other alkylators and activates a base-excision DNA repair pathway rather than the O_6-alkylguanine-DNA alkyltransferase repair used by chlorambucil and cyclophosphamide.[300,301] As first-line therapy, bendamustine produces a higher CR rate than chlorambucil, a threefold increase in PFS and time to next treatment (31.7 vs 10.1 months) but no difference in OS.[302] The quality of life is similar with both drugs but adverse events are twofold more common with bendamustine, and include skin rashes, marrow suppression, and nausea/vomiting.

Nucleoside Analogs

The nucleoside analogs have demonstrated significant activity in the indolent lymphoproliferative disorders and their mechanisms of action has been reviewed.[303,304]

The adenosine deaminase inhibitor, *pentostatin*, produces CR and PR rates of 16% to 25% in previously treated CLL patients, with an additional 20% to 30% of patients exhibiting clinical improvement.[305,306] The standard dose is 4 mg/m^2 intravenously (IV) every other week.

Fludarabine is administered orally or IV, although a higher dose is required when given orally.[307] Using 25 to 30 mg/m^2 IV daily for 5 days, repeated monthly, the overall response rate (ORR) is ~45% in previously treated patients, with the CR rate being 3% to 20%.[308-310] In untreated patients, the response rate is ~70%, with the CR rate being 20% to 40%.[311-313] To reduce toxicity, fludarabine has been administered as 30 mg/m^2 IV daily for 3 days, repeated every 4 weeks.[314] Compared to the 5-day schedule, the response rate is lower at 46% (CR, 10%), but there are fewer infections and no difference in OS.

Toxicities: Neither cladribine nor fludarabine causes significant nausea/vomiting, but this occurs with pentostatin. Very rarely, these agents cause a peripheral neuropathy, which can be severe.[315] They are highly immunosuppressive, being both myelosuppressive and producing a marked fall in the $CD4^+$ cell count, which may persist for years.[316]

Combining Nucleoside Analogs With Alkylating Agents

Nucleoside analogs inhibit DNA repair, which explains the synergistic antitumor activity seen between these agents and irradiation or alkylating agents.[303] Enhanced clinical responses are observed on combining cyclophosphamide with fludarabine,[295] cladribine,[317] or pentostatin.[318] These combinations can be effective in fludarabine-resistant patients.[318]

Steroids

Although steroids alone are primarily used for immune cytopenias, they have been used for the treatment of CLL. Steroids can kill CLL cells with a *TP53* mutation[319] and are useful for palliation in patients resistant to alkylating agents and nucleoside analogs.[319] High-dose steroids, such as methylprednisolone at 1 g/m^2/d × 5 days, repeated monthly, can be helpful in advanced-stage patients, who are drug resistant and have bulky disease, marrow failure, or both.[319] The difficulty with this approach are the side effects with high-dose steroids.

Immunotherapy

Anti-CD20

The cell-surface antigen CD20 plays an important role in the activation, proliferation, and differentiation of B cells and antibodies to CD20 have transformed therapy of CLL.[320,321] The chimeric monoclonal antibody, *rituximab*, contains a human IgG1 Ig constant region and a murine variable region directed against CD20. Rituximab exerts its antitumor activity by complement-dependent cytotoxicity, antibody-dependent cell-mediated cytotoxicity, or by the direct induction of apoptosis. The anti-CD20 monoclonal antibodies are classified as type I or type II based on their ability to redistribute CD20 into lipid rafts.[320] Type I antibodies, exemplified by rituximab and ofatumumab, redistribute CD20 into lipid rafts and potently activate complement. Type II antibodies, for example, obinutuzumab, induce lysosome permeabilization with the release of cathepsin B into the cytoplasm.[322,323] This leads to increased free radical formation by NADPH oxidases, which results in loss of plasma cell membrane and cell death.[323] Biosimilar versions of rituximab are also now available in clinical practice.

Ofatumumab is a fully human type I monoclonal antibody directed against a different epitope on CD20 that results in tighter binding and increased complement activation.[320] The pivotal study by Wierda et al[324] showed a response rate of 58% in patients who were resistant to fludarabine and alemtuzumab and 47% in patients who were resistant to fludarabine with bulky (>5 cm) lymphadenopathy (BF). The median PFS/OS were 5.7/13.7 months for the fludarabine/alemtuzumab group and 5.9/15.4 months for the BF group.

Obinutuzumab (GA101) is a humanized type II antibody with a novel mechanism of action and has been evaluated in untreated CLL patients using either standard or escalated dosing.[325] Standard dosing involved 100 mg on day 1, 900 mg on day 2, 1000 mg on days 8 and 15, and 1000 mg on day 1 on cycles 2 to 6. The escalated dosing used 100 mg on day 1, 900 mg on day 2, 1000 mg on day 3, and then 2000 mg on days 8 and 15 and day 1 (cycles 2-6). With the standard and escalated doses the CR/PR were 5%/44% and 20%/47%, respectively.

Anti-CD52

The monoclonal antibody, **alemtuzumab (Campath-1H)**, is a humanized IgG1 antibody against CD52 and targets are B and T lymphocytes, NK cells, monocytes, and eosinophils with sparing of normal hematopoietic stem cells.[326] Before the novel agents, alemtuzumab was an important agent for treatment of patients who were fludarabine-resistant and those with *TP53* dysfunction. Unfortunately, the agent is no longer being marketed for CLL, but can be obtained on a compassionate basis.

Chemoimmunotherapy
Combinations With Anti-CD20 Antibodies
Fludarabine With Rituximab and Cyclophosphamide

Synergy has been demonstrated between rituximab and chemotherapy, possibly related to effects of rituximab on antiapoptotic proteins or through downregulation of CD55 on the cell surface.[327-329] The combination of fludarabine and rituximab (FR) is well tolerated, and more effective than fludarabine alone in CLL.[330-332] Byrd et al[330] compared concurrent vs sequential treatment with fludarabine and rituximab in untreated CLL patients (CALGB 9712). In the concurrent regimen, there were 47% CRs and 43% PRs, whereas the sequential regimen appeared less effective with 28% CR and 49% PR. However, a follow-up analysis showed that both groups had a similar outcome with the combined median PFS being 42 months and the median OS being 85 months.[331] A retrospective comparison to patients treated with fludarabine alone (CALGB 9011) demonstrated a survival advantage for patients receiving FR.[332] Similar results have been obtained with pentostatin and rituximab in untreated patients.[333]

The MD Anderson Cancer Center first combined FR with cyclophosphamide (FCR) which until recently became the standard first-line therapy for fit patients (*Table 92.9*). In 224 previously untreated patients the CR, nPR, and PR rates were 72%, 10%, and 13%, respectively.[337] At a median follow-up of 12.8 years the PFS was 30.9%, being 50.7% for *IGHV* mutated patients and 8.7% for unmutated patients.[291] Moreover, PFS appeared to plateau for mutated patients suggesting long-term remissions. Half the mutated patients had achieved an MRD negative marrow at the end of chemotherapy and for these patients the PFS at 12.8 years was 79.8%. In addition, a β2-microglobulin of ≥4 mg/L at diagnosis in mutated patients was associated with a shorter PFS at 12.8 years (38.8% vs 61.6%). OS at 12.8 years was 32.3% and 65.5% for *IGHV* unmutated and mutated patients, respectively. Deaths were due to progressive CLL (58.1%), followed by second malignancies (18.4%), RS (15.4%), and infections (6.6%). A concomitant study has shown that achieving an MRD negative marrow is more important for long-term outcome than the number of cycles of FCR.[338] The likelihood of achieving MRD negativity after 3 or 6 cycles of FCR was 17% and 43%, respectively. Patients who were *IGHV* mutated and did not have a del 17p were more likely to achieve MRD negativity.

A subsequent prospective randomized phase 3 study comparing FCR and FC (CLL8) from the German CLL Study Group confirmed these findings (*Table 92.9*).[77] Prophylaxis with antivirals was not given and prophylaxis against *Pneumocystis jirovecii* only recommended for severe leukopenia lasting >7 days. One-quarter of patients in both the FC and FCR groups were unable to tolerate the full 6 cycles of therapy and drug dosages had to be reduced by >10% in 47% of patients on FCR and 27% of patients on FC. The CR/PR for FCR were 44%/46% and for FC were 22%/58%. The median PFS was 51.8 months with FCR and 32.8 months with FC, whereas OS at 3 years was 87% with FCR and 83% with FC (*P* = .01). The marrows of patients in CR after FCR or FC were MRD negative in 44% and 28%, respectively, and this correlated with PFS.[339] The response of patients with a del 17p was equally poor for patients treated with FCR or FC, and although PFS was increased with FCR (11.3 vs 6.5 months, *P* = .019), there was no improvement in OS. However, FCR overcame the poor prognosis associated with FC in patients with a del 11q, with an improved CR rate (51% vs 15%, *P* = <.0001), prolonged PFS at 3 years (64% vs 32%, *P* = <.0001), and increased OS at 3 years (94% vs 83%). Long-term follow-up (median 5.9 years) has confirmed the better long-term survival with mutated *IGHV*.[97]

Toxicities: In the CLL8 study, FCR caused more neutropenia than FC, and neutropenia and infections occurred more commonly in those >65 years. Deaths related to both regimens only occurred in 2% to 3% of patients, but it should be emphasized that these patients were carefully chosen according to performance status, comorbidities, and renal function. In addition, the median age of patients was only 61 years. The MD Anderson studies have demonstrated that about 20% of patients can have cytopenias lasting longer than 3 months following FCR and that 28% of patients whose blood counts have recovered following treatment can have a late cytopenia that usually occurs in the first year of remission.[337] The incidence of immune cytopenias after first-line FCR was 6.5% in the MD Anderson series with AIHA typically occurring between cycles 3 and 6 and most patients responded to standard therapies.[230] In contrast, in the CLL8 study, only 1% of previously untreated patients developed immune cytopenias. The risk of serious or opportunistic infections in the MD Anderson study was 10% and 4% in the first and second years of remission, respectively, with a relatively high incidence of shingles at these times.[337] In addition, 5.1% developed AML/MDS and 9% RS at a median follow-up of 4.4 years.[221]

Bendamustine/Rituximab

In a follow-up to the CLL8 study, the German CLL10 study compared bendamustine/rituximab with FCR in fit patients.[340] This study demonstrated that FCR was more effective than bendamustine/

Table 92.9. Commonly Used First-Line Chemoimmunotherapy

Reference	Treatment[a]	Patient Number	CR (%)	nPR (%)	PR (%)	PFS	OS
Byrd et al, 2005[331]	F	178	20		43	67% at 2 y	2 y, 81%
	FR	104	38		46	45% at 2 y	2 y, 93%
Goede et al, 2018[334]	CLB	118	–		31.4	Median, 11.1 mo	Median, 66.7 mo
	CLB/Ob	238	22.3		55.0	Median, 31.1 mo	Median, NR
	CLB/R	233	7.3		58.4	Median, 15.7 mo	Median, 73.1 mo
Offner et al, 2020[335]	CLB	221	1		68	Median, 14.7 mo	Median, 84.7 mo
	CLB/Ofat	226	14		68	Median, 23.4 mo	Median, NR
Thompson et al, 2015[291]	FCR	224	72	10	13	Median, 6.4 y	Median, 12.7 y
Fischer et al, 2016[97]	FC	371	22		58	Median, 32.9	Median, 86 mo
	FCR	388	44		46	Median, 56.8	Median, NR
Kutsch et al, 2020[336]	FCR	282	40		55	Median 57.6 mo	5 y, 80.1%
	BR	279	31		65	Median, 42.3 mo	5 y, 80.9%

Abbreviations: CR, complete remission; nPR, nodular partial remission; OS, overall survival; PFS, progression-free survival; PR, partial remission.
[a]B, bendamustine; CLB, chlorambucil; C, cyclophosphamide; F, fludarabine; Ob, obinutuzumab; Ofat, ofatumumab; P, pentostatin; R, rituximab.

rituximab, both in obtaining a CR, obtaining marrow MRD negativity and PFS. The median observation time was 37.1 months and the CR/PR for FCR were 40%/55%, and for bendamustine/rituximab were 31%/65%. The PFS was 55.2 months for FCR and 41.7 months for bendamustine/rituximab ($P = .0003$) and to date there has been no difference in OS. Interestingly, patients with del 11q appeared to particularly benefit from FCR, with the CR rate being 38% and 19% for FCR and bendamustine/rituximab, respectively ($P = .016$), and the PFS being 37.8 and 25.3 months, respectively ($P = .0002$). However, FCR was more marrow toxic and produced a higher number of serious infections, which was seen primarily in those >65 years. Thus, while the PFS for FCR and bendamustine/rituximab for patients ≤65 years were 53.6 and 38.5 months, respectively ($P = .0004$), the PFS for those >65 years were similar being 48.5 months for bendamustine/rituximab and not reached for FCR ($P = .172$). Twenty-three percent of patients on FCR, but only 13% on bendamustine/rituximab, had to stop treatment because of toxicity ($P = .003$). Major toxicities included marrow suppression and infections; the difference in toxicities was most apparent in patients aged >65 years. In addition, 2% of patients on FCR developed MDS/AML, significantly higher than for bendamustine/rituximab. Thus, while FCR is the preferred treatment for fit patients ≤65 years, bendamustine/rituximab may be used for fit patients >65 years.

Chlorambucil With Obinutuzumab or Ofatumumab

In the German CLL11 phase III randomized study, the combination of chlorambucil/obinutuzumab was found to be significantly more effective than chlorambucil/rituximab, or chlorambucil alone, in patients with comorbidities or mild renal dysfunction.[341,342] The median age of patients was 73 years. The dose of chlorambucil was 0.5 mg/kg IV on days 1 and 15, monthly for 6 months with standard doses of obinutuzumab. The CR/PR rates for chlorambucil alone, chlorambucil/rituximab, and chlorambucil/obinutuzumab were 0/31.4%, 7.3%/58.4%, and 22.3%/55%, respectively, with the likelihood of a molecular remission being highest with the obinutuzumab arm (Table 92.9). Median PFS for chlorambucil/obinutuzumab, chlorambucil/rituximab, and chlorambucil were 26.7, 16.3, and 11.1 months, respectively. All these differences were significant. Remarkably, MRD-negative status was 19.5% in marrow and 37.5% in blood for patients receiving chlorambucil/obinutuzumab who achieved a CR. The OS was significantly longer with the addition of obinutuzumab, than for chlorambucil alone, and with longer follow-up OS was also increased with chlorambucil/rituximab over chlorambucil, although this was less significant than with chlorambucil/obinutuzumab.[342] The incidence of neutropenia was highest with chlorambucil/obinutuzumab and lowest with chlorambucil, although the incidence of infections was similar in all groups. Obinutuzumab caused a significant reaction with the first infusion and tumor lysis was observed. Because of the effectiveness in this group of elderly unfit patients, chlorambucil/obinutuzumab has become a standard treatment for this patient population.

Similar findings have been observed by Hillmen et al,[343] evaluating chlorambucil alone or with ofatumumab in the COMPLEMENT 1 trial. Patients who were not eligible for fludarabine were included; the median age was 69 years and the median follow-up time was 28.9 months. In general, the patients had renal dysfunction or at least two comorbidities. The dose of chlorambucil was 10 mg/m^2 orally daily × 7, repeated monthly until best response, or until 12 months. The CR/PR for chlorambucil/ofatumumab and chlorambucil were 14%/68% and 1%/68%, respectively. The PFS for chlorambucil/ofatumumab and chlorambucil were 22.4 months and 13.1 months, respectively ($P < .0001$) and it is too early to assess if there is a difference in survival. Neutropenia was more common in the combination group, but the incidence of infections was similar in both groups.

Novel Agents

A number of new agents are under development but only those agents already available for clinical use or that hold promise are discussed (Figure 92.10).[2,5]

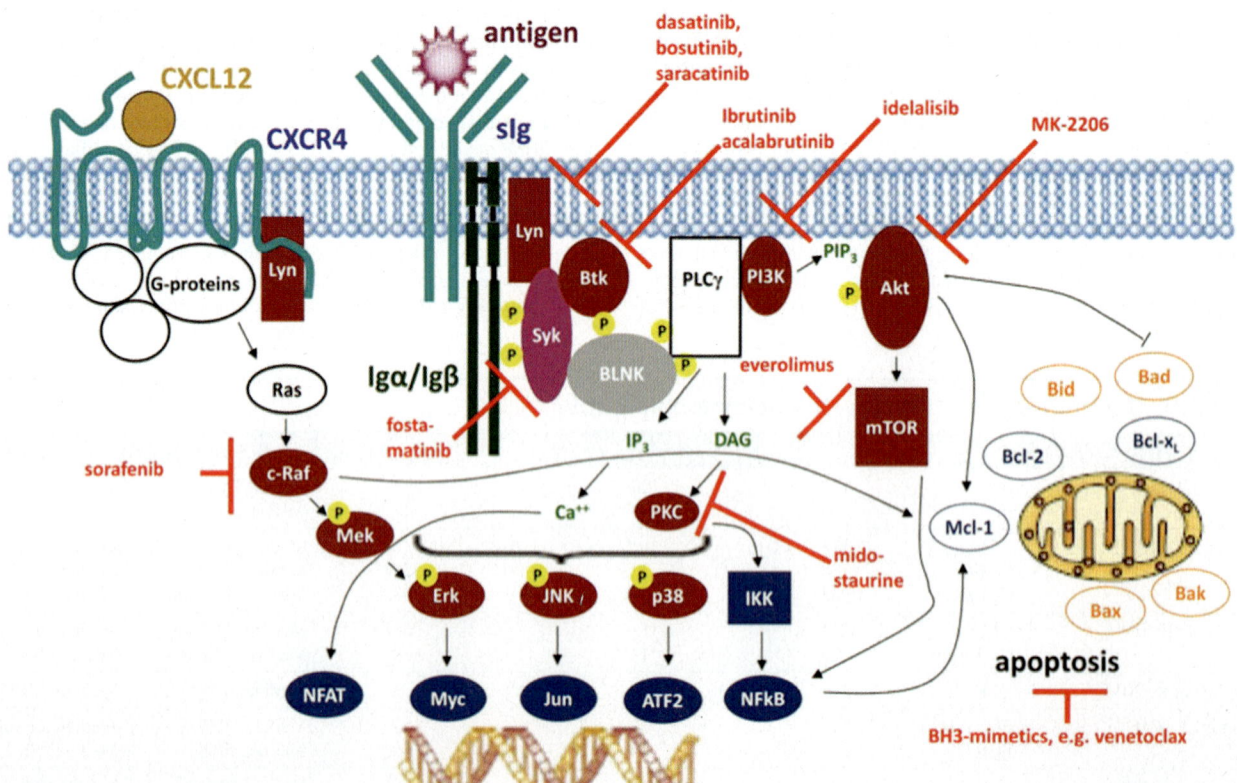

FIGURE 92.10 Targeting of signaling pathways in the chronic lymphocytic leukemia cell. Hallek, M. Targeting of BCR signaling in the treatment of CLL. (From Hallek M. Chronic lymphocytic leukemia: 2017 update on diagnosis, risk stratification, and treatment. *Am J Hematol.* 2017;92(9):946-965. Copyright © 2017 Wiley Periodicals, Inc. Reprinted by permission of John Wiley & Sons, Inc.)

Effectors of the BCR Pathway

With the understanding of the importance of the BCR pathway for cell survival and proliferation in CLL, a number of KIs have been developed to inhibit different stages in the pathway.[2,5] The most important of these are the BTK inhibitors and the phosphoinositide 3-kinase delta (PI3Kδ) inhibitors (idelalisib, duvelisib, and umbralisib). The activities of these agents are shown in Table 92.10. Next-generation noncovalent BTK inhibitors such as nemtabrutinib and pirtobrutinib have also shown promising activity in CLL.

Ibrutinib (PCI-32765)

Mutations in BTK result in Bruton agammaglobulinemia where there is a lack of peripheral blood B cells and hypogammaglobulinemia.[344] Ibrutinib is an oral covalent BTK inhibitor, which binds to CS481 and causes irreversible enzyme inhibition.[345] However, it inhibits many other kinases, including interleukin-2 inducible ITK and epidermal growth factor receptor.[344] It is administered as 420 mg once daily (3 × 140 mg capsules) until disease progression or toxicity. The drug has shown significant activity in both untreated CLL and in those with refractory and p53 dysfunctional disease and is now licensed by the FDA for both first- and second-line treatments.[2,5,345-349] Through inhibition of the BCR pathway CLL cells can no longer adhere to stromal cells in the nodes, spleen, and marrow; tumor cells can die at these sites while a proportion egress into the bloodstream where they gradual die over the ensuing months to years.[350] Thus in the first 4 to 6 weeks, there is a peripheral lymphocytosis with resolution of lymphadenopathy and splenomegaly; the lymphocytosis resolves in 1 year in 80% of patients but remains elevated in 20%.[351] Counterintuitively, patients with persistent lymphocytosis do as well as those whose lymphocyte counts normalize.[351]

The RESONATE R/R phase III trial was the pivotal study for ibrutinib in relapsed CLL, where ibrutinib was compared to ofatumumab in resistant/relapsed patients (Table 92.10).[347] Four percent of patients on ofatumumab had a PR, but 43% of the ibrutinib group (P= <.0001); the PR-L was 63% for ibrutinib. The PFS was 8.1 months with ofatumumab and was not reached at a median follow-up of 9.4 months with ibrutinib. In addition, ibrutinib significantly improved survival with 88% being alive at 6 months, compared to 65% with ofatumumab. With longer follow-up, patients

Table 92.10. Major Randomized Studies With Novel Agents in Frontline Therapy of Chronic Lymphocytic Leukemia (CLL)

Study	Treatment Regimen	Patient Population	N	ORR%	PFS	OS
BTK Inhibitor-Based Treatment						
Ibrutinib						
Resonate-2	Ibrutinib	Del 17p: excluded, unmutated IGHV: 44%	136	86	78-month: 61%	78-mo: 78%
	Chlorambucil		133	35	78-mo: 9%	NR
Alliance A041202	Ibrutinib	Del 17p: 6%, unmutated IGHV: 61%	182	93	48-mo: 76%	48-mo: 85%
	Ibrutinib + rituximab		182	94	48-mo: 76%	48-mo: 86%
	Bendamustine + rituximab		183	81	48-mo: 47%	48-mo: 84%
E1912	Ibrutinib + rituximab	Del 17p: excluded Unmutated IGHV: 71%	354	96	36-mo: 89%	36-mo: 99%
	FCR		175	81	36-mo: 71%	36-mo: 93%
ILLUMINATE	Ibrutinib + obinutuzumab	Del 17p: 14%, unmutated IGHV: 58%	113	88	30-mo: 79%	30-mo: 86%
	Chlorambucil + obinutuzumab		116	73	30-mo: 31%	30-mo: 85%
UK FLAIR	Ibrutinib + rituximab	Del 17p >20%: excluded, unmutated IGHV: 50%	386	91	48-mo: 85%	48-mo: 95%
	FCR		385	88	48-mo: 72%	48-mo: 95%
Acalabrutinib						
ELEVATE-TN	Acalabrutinib	Del 17p: 9%, unmutated IGHV: 61%	179	89	48-mo: 78%	48-mo: 88%
	Acalabrutinib + obinutuzumab		179	96	48-mo: 87%	48-mo: 93%
	Chlorambucil + obinutuzumab		177	82	48-mo: 48%	48-mo: 88%
Zanubrutinib						
SEQUOIA	Zanubrutinib	Del 17p: excluded, unmutated IGHV: 53%	241	95	24-mo: 86%	24-mo: 94%
	Bendamustine + rituximab		238	85	24-mo: 70%	24-mo: 95%
Venetoclax-Based Treatment						
CLL14	Venetoclax + obinutuzumab	Del 17p: 8%, unmutated IGHV: 60%	216	85	48-mo: 74%	48-mo: 85%
	Chlorambucil + obinutuzumab		216	71	48-mo: 35%	48-mo: 83%
GLOW	Ibrutinib + venetoclax	Del 17p: excluded, unmutated IGHV: 52%	106	NR	Median not reached after 27-mo follow-up	NR
	Chlorambucil + venetoclax		105	NR	Median = 21 mo	NR
PI3 Kinase Inhibitor-Based Treatment						
UNITY-CLL	Umbralisib + ublituximab	Del 17p: 10%, unmutated IGHV: 56%	210*	83.3%*	Median = 38.5 mo	NR
	Chlorambucil + obinutuzumab		211*	68.7%*	Median = 26.1 mo	NR

NR: not reported *includes patients with relapsed/refractory CLL.
Abbreviations: BTK, Bruton tyrosine kinase; FCR, fludarabine/cyclophosphamide/rituximab; IGHV, immunoglobulin heavy chain variable region; ORR, overall response rate; OS, overall survival; PFS, progression-free survival.

with del 17p who received ibrutinib were shown to have the shortest median PFS (40.6 months).[352] In contrast, patients with del 11q had a surprisingly longer median PFS (60.7 months) compared to patients with neither del 11q nor del 17p (42.5 months), suggesting that patients with del 11q preferentially benefit from ibrutinib therapy in the relapsed/refractory setting. The RESONATE-2 phase III pivotal trial for first-line ibrutinib in patients over 65 years demonstrated a significant advantage over chlorambucil alone.[348] Patients received 0.5 mg/kg chlorambucil every 14 days, increasing the dose to 0.75 mg/kg for up to 12 months, according to tolerance. Mean dose of chlorambucil was 0.6 mg/kg and 40% received 12 months of therapy. With a median follow-up of 18.4 months, the median PFS for ibrutinib and chlorambucil was not reached and 18.9 months, respectively, with the risk of death being reduced 84% by ibrutinib ($P < .001$). The overall response with lymphocytosis (OR-L) was 86% with ibrutinib and 35% for chlorambucil, with the ibrutinib group having a better improvement in normal blood counts. After a median follow-up of 75 months, a sustained benefit was seen with ibrutinib as compared to chlorambucil (61% progression free with ibrutinib compared to 9% with chlorambucil); this benefit was seen across all subgroups, including those with unmutated *IGHV*.[353]

The E1912 trial led by ECOG-ACRIN compared FCR to ibrutinib/rituximab (1:2 randomization) in 529 previously untreated CLL patients, ≤70 years of age, and without del 17p.[354] Therapy with FCR was administered in a standard fashion, whereas patients in the ibrutinib/rituximab arm received ibrutinib continuously at a dose of 420 mg daily and rituximab was given for 6 cycles (at standard doses) after one cycle of single-agent ibrutinib. After a median follow-up of 33.6 months, patients who received ibrutinib/rituximab experienced a significantly longer PFS (89.4% vs 72.9% at 3 years; $P < .001$) and longer OS (98.8% vs 91.5% at 3 years; hazard ratio for death, 0.17; 95% CI, 0.05-0.54; $P < .001$) compared to FCR. Although patients with unmutated *IGHV* experienced a longer PFS with the use of ibrutinib/rituximab compared to FCR (3-year PFS 90.7% vs 62.5%), there was no significant difference in PFS among those with mutated *IGHV* genes (3-year PFS 87.7% vs 88%, respectively).

The companion A041202 study randomized 547 previously untreated CLL patients ≥65 years of age to ibrutinib, ibrutinib/rituximab, or bendamustine/rituximab; cross-over to single-agent ibrutinib was allowed for patients progressing on bendamustine/rituximab.[355] Ibrutinib was given at a dose of 420 mg orally daily until disease progression or unacceptable toxicity. Bendamustine and rituximab were administered at standard doses. After a median follow-up of 38 months, patients in the ibrutinib-containing arms had a significantly improved PFS compared to those receiving bendamustine/rituximab (87% and 88% vs 74% at 2 years, respectively, $P < .001$), although there was no difference in OS. Surprisingly, there was no difference in outcomes between the single-agent ibrutinib and ibrutinib/rituximab arms suggesting that the addition of an anti-CD20 monoclonal antibody did not enhance the activity of ibrutinib.

The ILLUMINATE study compared ibrutinib/obinutuzumab to chlorambucil/obinutuzumab in 229 previously untreated CLL patients.[356] After a median follow-up of 31 months, PFS was significantly longer in the ibrutinib/obinutuzumab arm compared to chlorambucil/obinutuzumab arm (79% vs 31% at 30 months; $P < .001$).

Finally, the UK FLAIR study compared ibrutinib/rituximab to FCR (1:1 randomization) in 771 previously untreated CLL with a median age of 62 years.[357] Fludarabine was administered at a dose of 24 mg/m² orally daily for 5 days each month, cyclophosphamide at a dose of 150 mg/m² orally daily for 5 days each month, along with standard dosing for rituximab monthly for a total of 6 months. Patients in the ibrutinib/rituximab treatment arm received ibrutinib 420 mg/d and rituximab as in the FCR arm. After a median follow-up of 53 months, treatment with ibrutinib/rituximab was associated with a longer PFS (median PFS not reached for ibrutinib/rituximab vs 67 months for FCR; HR: 0.44; $P < .001$). In contrast to the E1912 study,[354] there was no difference in OS between the two arms with current follow-up (HR: 1.01; $P = .956$).

Collectively, the above studies have established the superiority of ibrutinib in the frontline management of CLL, regardless of the patient's age and comorbidities, compared to standard chemoimmunotherapy.

Ibrutinib monotherapy is also very effective in patients with del 17p, both in previously untreated and relapsed/refractory CLL patients. In a study conducted at the National Institutes of Health, among 34 previously untreated CLL patients who received single-agent ibrutinib, the 6-year PFS was 61%.[252] In a multicenter phase 2 study of single-agent ibrutinib in 144 patients with relapsed/refractory CLL with del 17p, the estimated 2-year PFS was 63% and the estimated 2-year OS was 75%.[358]

Acalabrutinib

Acalabrutinib, another covalent BTK inhibitor, is a derivative of ibrutinib with more specific inhibition of BTK and potentially less side effects.[359,360] In a single-arm phase 1b/2 study of acalabrutinib monotherapy given at a dose of 100 mg twice daily in 134 patients with relapsed/refractory CLL, the ORR was 94% (regardless of the presence of high-risk features such as unmutated *IGHV* genes or CK) and the estimated 45-month PFS was 62%.[360]

In the ACE-CL-001 study, acalabrutinib monotherapy was administered to 99 treatment naïve CLL patients, where the ORR was 97%, and the estimated 48-month PFS was 96%.[361] Two major phase 3 trials have led to the approval of acalabrutinib treatment in both frontline and relapsed CLL settings. The ASCEND study compared acalabrutinib monotherapy ($n = 155$) to investigators' choice of either bendamustine/rituximab ($n = 36$) or idelalisib/rituximab ($n = 119$) in patients with relapsed CLL.[362] After a median follow-up of 16 months, patients who received acalabrutinib had a significantly longer PFS compared to those who received either bendamustine/rituximab or idelalisib/rituximab (PFS not reached vs 16.5 months, $P < .0001$). In the ELEVATE-TN study, acalabrutinib monotherapy was compared to acalabrutinib/obinutuzumab and chlorambucil/obinutuzumab in 535 previously untreated CLL patients.[363] After a median follow-up of 28 months, the estimated PFS at 2 years was 93% with acalabrutinib/obinutuzumab vs 87% with acalabrutinib monotherapy vs 47% with chlorambucil/obinutuzumab ($P < .0001$ for comparison of acalabrutinib-containing regimens to chlorambucil/obinutuzumab).

Zanubrutinib

In a phase 1b/2 study of 98 patients with relapsed refractory CLL treated with zanubrutinib, a novel covalent BTK inhibitor, the ORR was 96%, and the estimated 2-year PFS was 88%.[364] The phase 3 SEQUOIA study has compared zanubrutinib at 160 mg orally twice daily ($n = 241$) to standard doses of bendamustine/rituximab ($n = 238$) in untreated CLL patients without del 17p. After a median follow-up of 26.2 months, PFS was significantly prolonged with zanubrutinib compared to bendamustine/rituximab (estimated 24 months PFS 85.5% vs 69.5%, $P < .0001$), although there was no difference in OS.[365]

Pirtobrutinib and Nemtabrutinib

Noncovalent BTK inhibitors, such as pirtobrutinib (formerly LOXO-305) and nemtabrutinib (formerly ARQ-531), differ to ibrutinib, acalabrutinib, or zanubrutinib in that they do not covalently bind to the C481 site on BTK and have thus the potential to retain activity in patients who have developed resistance due to a mutation at this site.[366-368] In addition, they potentially may have different toxicities. In a phase 1/2 study (BRUIN) in 323 patients with advanced B-cell malignancies who had received a median of three prior lines of therapy, treatment with oral pirtobrutinib was well-tolerated, with the most common toxicity being grade 3 or greater neutropenia at 10%.[367] Only 5 patients (1%) discontinued therapy due to adverse events. Of the 139 CLL patients who were evaluable for efficacy, the ORR was 63%; the response rate was similar in patients with or without the presence of the C481S BTK mutation. Similar results were also seen with the use of nemtabrutinib in a phase 2 single-arm study, where the ORR was 58% among 38 patients with CLL who were evaluated before response.[368] The most common adverse events included dysgeusia (15%), nausea (11%), fatigue (11%), and decreased neutrophil count (10%).

Toxicity With BTK Inhibitors

Although treatment with covalent BTK inhibitors is generally well-tolerated, there are several toxicities that need to be considered. Nausea, diarrhea, arthralgias, and skin rashes are common, but are usually mild and transient. Infections remain an important complication, particularly in patients who have previously received chemo-immunotherapy; however, the risk of infection diminishes with time. BTK and TEC are present in platelets and treatment with BTK inhibitors can interfere with collagen-mediated platelet aggregation.[369] The risk of bleeding is higher in patients who are on concomitant antiplatelet agents, other nonsteroidal anti-inflammatory agents, fish oil, or anticoagulants. Treatment with warfarin may be contraindicated in conjunction with covalent BTK inhibitors due to the risk of fatal hemorrhage. It is recommended that all covalent BTK inhibitors should be held for 3 days prior to and after any procedures with minor bleeding risk (e.g., colonoscopy), and for approximately 5 to 7 days prior to and after procedures with major bleeding risks such as surgeries requiring a skin incision. Nail splitting (onychoschizia) and brittleness (onychorrhexis) with breaking of the tips of the nails of the hands occurs in two-thirds of patients at a median of 6 months after starting therapy, while similar changes in the toe nails and alterations in hair texture each occur in a quarter of the patients at a median of 9 months.[370] The changes are thought related to the binding of ibrutinib to cysteine in the nails. Biotin 2.5 mg/d can improve the nail and skin changes.

Cardiovascular toxicities such as hypertension and atrial fibrillation are significant complications of therapy with covalent BTK inhibitors. In a head-to-head study (ELEVATE-RR) comparing acalabrutinib to ibrutinib in patients with relapsed CLL and high-risk features, such as del 11q and del 17p, both acalabrutinib and ibrutinib produced a median PFS of 38 months.[371] However, there was a significantly lower incidence of hypertension (9% vs 23%), bleeding (38% vs 51%), and atrial fibrillation (9% vs 16%) with acalabrutinib as compared to ibrutinib ($P < .05$ for all comparisons). The Phase III ALPINE study compared zanubrutinib to ibrutinib in 415 patients with relapsed CLL.[372] After a median follow-up of 15 months, the 12-month PFS was superior with the use of zanubrutinib compared to ibrutinib (95% vs 84%, respectively), and the risk of atrial fibrillation was also lower with zanubrutinib compared to ibrutinib (3% vs 10%, respectively). These results suggest that treatment with next-generation covalent BTK inhibitors such as acalabrutinib and zanubrutinib will likely be better tolerated with similar efficacy to ibrutinib in patients with CLL. However, these other agents have their own issues. Thus, acalabrutinib cannot be given with proton pump inhibitors, for example, rabeprazole, as they significantly reduce gastrointestinal absorption of acalabrutinib. In addition, zanubrutinib treatment is associated with significantly higher risk of neutropenia than seen with ibrutinib.

Outcome After Treatment With BTK Inhibitors

In a review of 308 patients receiving ibrutinib and followed for a median of 20 months in four clinical trials, 24% stopped the drug.[373] Of patients who discontinued ibrutinib, 41% had disease progression or RS, 37% infections, and 22% other causes. Importantly, transformation occurred in the first 2 years, while progression occurred after 1 year with the incidence increasing over time. Older age and prior therapies increased the risk of side effects and similar findings are observed in the "real-life" setting.[374] This latter study demonstrated that in the first year the ibrutinib dose was reduced in 26% of patients and there were >14-day treatment breaks in 13% of patients. One-year survival was reduced if drug treatment was interrupted but not if the drug dose was reduced. The most common reasons for dose reduction were gastrointestinal toxicity (mainly lower bowel), cytopenias, infections, and debility.

Resistance to Ibrutinib

Resistance to ibrutinib may involve a cysteine to serine mutation (C481S) in BTK preventing covalent binding and inhibition by ibrutinib while mutations in phospholipase C γ2 (PLCγ2) provides a gain-of-function activity for the BCR pathway, bypassing the need for BTK.[92,375] Other mechanisms also play a role and clones of resistant cells are present prior to treatment and grow out following ibrutinib.[376] Similar resistance mechanisms have also been described in patients treated with acalabrutinib. Resistance to the noncovalent BTK inhibitor, pirtobrutinib, has been associated with multiple mutations in BTK outside the C481 residue with activating mutations of PLCγ2.[377] These mutations can cause resistance to other noncovalent BTK inhibitors, which is associated with cross-resistance to covalent BTK inhibitors.[377]

Idelalisib

Idelalisib is a PI3Kδ inhibitor, and like ibrutinib blocks the BCR pathway. The landmark study used idelalisib plus rituximab compared to rituximab alone in refractory patients, and demonstrated a significant advantage for the former treatment.[378] Patients received intravenous rituximab 375 mg/m^2 followed by 500 mg/m^2 every 2 weeks × 4 doses, followed by a treatment every month × 3 (8 treatments total) with either idelalisib 150 mg orally twice daily or placebo indefinitely. The response rates for patients receiving idelalisib or placebo were 81% and 13%, respectively, with a median PFS of 93% and 46% at 24 months, respectively ($P = <.001$), and an OS of 92% vs 80% at 1 year, respectively ($P = .02$). While side effects, such as fatigue and nausea were common, they occurred with equal frequency in both groups. More serious side effects included marrow suppression and infections, which occurred in both study arms. Based on this study, idelalisib plus rituximab was licensed for relapsed CLL.

Idelalisib plus rituximab has been used as first-line treatment in elderly patients with a median age of 71 years.[379] The ORR was 97% with 19% CR, and a PFS of 83% at 36 months. All of the patients with dysfunctional *TP53* responded. However, 89% of patients had severe toxicities, with diarrhea/colitis (42%) and pneumonia (19%) being most common. The incidence of colitis and hepatitis was higher in this study than in previously treated patients and there was a lymphocyte infiltrate in the colon biopsies of affected patients. As the immune system is relatively intact in untreated patients, the authors suggested that the pneumonitis/pulmonary fibrosis, hepatitis, and colitis seen with idelalisib are likely autoimmune, perhaps caused by inhibition of PI3Kδ in regulatory T cells. The median time to diarrhea/colitis was 9.5 months and these autoimmune complications are treated by withdrawing drug and prescribing steroids.

Other BCR Pathway Inhibitors

Because of the success of the above agents, there has been considerable enthusiasm in evaluating other inhibitors of the BCR pathway.[380] For example, duvelisib inhibits both PI3K γ and δ, which are both expressed in CLL cells and has demonstrated significant activity in this disease. In a phase 3 study, duvelisib (25 mg orally twice daily) has been compared to ofatumumab (given in standard doses) in relapsed CLL. Compared to ofatumumab, duvelisib produced a significantly higher ORR (74% vs 45%; $P < .0001$) and a longer median PFS (13.3 vs 9.9 months; $P < .0001$), leading to the FDA approval of this agent in relapsed CLL.[381] Umbralisib is PI3K δ inhibitor that also inhibits C1ε. In the UNITY CLL phase III study, continuous umbralisib (800 mg orally daily) and the anti-CD20 monoclonal antibody, ublituximab (900 mg × 3 doses during cycle 1, then monthly with cycles 2-6, and then every 3 months) showed superior PFS compared to 6 cycles of obinutuzumab plus chlorambucil (19.5 vs 12.9 months) in 181 patients with relapsed CLL.[382] The rates of diarrhea (to 12.1% vs 2.5%), elevated liver function tests (8.3% vs 2%), colitis (3.4% vs 0%), and pneumonitis (2.9% vs 0%) were significantly higher with umbralisib and ublituximab compared to chlorambucil/obinutuzumab. Further toxicity data (including risk of death) led to the removal from the market of umbralisib in June 2022.

Inhibitors of Bcl-2

Venetoclax (ABT-199) is a BH-3 mimetic drug and a potent inhibitor of BCL-2, which has shown remarkable activity in CLL patients with refractory disease and those with p53 dysfunction.[383,384] In the initial study by Roberts et al,[383] there was a high incidence of tumor-lysis syndrome with the initiation of therapy and venetoclax was subsequently given in a ramped-up schedule (20 mg/d for 1 week, 50 mg/d for 1 week, 100 mg/d for 1 week, 200 mg/d for 1 week followed by 400 mg/d continuously). With the expansion cohort of 60 patients, the ORR was 82% with 10% CR (although the CR rate increased to 20% by including the dose-escalation cohort). The PFS in the expansion group was estimated to be 66% at 15 months. Remarkably, all patients, regardless of lymph node size and *TP53* status, responded equally well.

In a randomized phase II MURANO study, venetoclax and rituximab was compared to bendamustine/rituximab in patients with relapsed CLL.[385] Venetoclax was administered in the usual dose ramp-up for 5 weeks followed by daily 400 mg orally for a fixed duration of 2 years. Rituximab was administered starting week 6 monthly for a total of 6 cycles. Treatment with bendamustine/rituximab was administered in a standard fashion for 6 cycles. Treatment with venetoclax and rituximab was associated with a longer PFS compared to bendamustine/rituximab (2-year PFS rates were 84.9% and 36.3%, respectively, $P < .0001$). At the most recent update of these data, the venetoclax treated arm had a median PFS of 54 months and an estimated 5-year OS of 82%.[386] Three months after the end of therapy, 62% patients achieved undetectable MRD in the venetoclax/rituximab arm compared to 13% in the bendamustine/rituximab arm. Using landmark analyses, the investigators also showed that the patients with undetectable MRD had a longer PFS compared to those who had MRD.

The combination of venetoclax and obinutuzumab was compared to chlorambucil/obinutuzumab in 432 previously untreated patients with CLL in the CLL 14 study led by the German CLL study group.[387] Obinutuzumab was started on cycle 1 day 1 with standard dosing for 6 cycles. Patients received 1 year of venetoclax that started on cycle 1 day 22 with the weekly ramp-up, getting up to 400 mg after cycle 2 of obinutuzumab. Chlorambucil/obinutuzumab were given at the same dosing schedule as in the CLL 11 study, except that chlorambucil was given for a total of 12 months.[341] Patients with del 17p were included in the study. After a median follow-up of 28 months, the estimated 24-month PFS was significantly longer in the venetoclax/obinutuzumab group compared to patients receiving chlorambucil/obinutuzumab (88.2% vs 64.1%, $P < .0001$), but there was no difference in OS between the two groups. No clinical tumor lysis was seen and this fixed-duration venetoclax/obinutuzumab treatment regimen is now approved as first-line therapy in CLL.

Toxicity With BCL2 Inhibitors

Due to the risk of tumor lysis, CLL patients who start venetoclax undergo a weekly dose escalation at treatment initiation, with monitoring and prophylaxis including hydration, allopurinol, and/or rasburicase as indicated by their baseline risk for TLS outlined in the package insert.[388,389] The reported incidence of laboratory TLS in clinical trials ranges from 3% to 6%, compared to 8% to 13% among patients treated in routine practice outside the context of clinical trials.[389] In contrast, the rate of clinical tumor lysis is quite low (<3%) with weekly dose ramp-up. Other adverse events including ≥grade 3 neutropenia can occur in 57% patients treated with venetoclax/rituximab in relapsed CLL,[385] and in 52% patients treated with venetoclax/obinutuzumab for frontline CLL.[387] Despite the high rates of neutropenia, the risk of neutropenic fever remains low (<5%). The most frequent nonhematologic toxicity includes diarrhea, fatigue, and nausea, which typically decrease with dose reduction, and treatment discontinuation is usually not required.

Resistance to Venetoclax

Relapses do occur using time-limited therapy with venetoclax and an anti-CD20 monoclonal antibody, but 50% of patients will again respond to venetoclax. Several mechanisms of resistance have been identified for patients who do not respond to venetoclax and these include a novel Gly101Val mutation in *BCL2* gene.[390] This mutation reduces the affinity of BCL2 for venetoclax by approximately 180-fold, which prevents the drug from displacing pro-apoptotic mediators from BCL2, which leads to drug resistance. Multiple *BCL2* mutations (such as Asp103Tyr, Arg129Leu, or Ala113Gly) can occur (median 3 mutations per patient) in resistant patients suggesting an oligoclonal pattern of disease relapse.[391] Finally, overexpression of BCL-XL and amplification of the *MCL1* locus have also been described in patients progressing on venetoclax.[392] Testing for these mutations is not readily available in most clinics at the current time, but a more individualized treatment program may become available in the future. In this scenario, treatment with venetoclax or another type of treatment (such as a BTK inhibitor) may be recommended depending on the presence or absence of specific BCL2 or BTK mutations in resistant CLL patients.

Combination Therapy With Novel Agents

A number of clinical trials have examined the novel agents in combination, as preclinical studies have suggested complementary mechanisms of action and nonoverlapping toxicities. In a phase 2 study of 80 patients with previously untreated CLL, ibrutinib was combined with venetoclax for a total of 2 years of therapy.[393] Ibrutinib was started as a single agent in cycle 1 at a dose of 420 mg daily and venetoclax introduced at cycle 4 with standard ramp-up dosing. After a median follow-up of 33.8 months, 66% of patients achieved undetectable MRD in the marrow and the estimated 48-month PFS and OS exceeded 95%. These encouraging results led to the phase 3 randomized GLOW study in 211 previously untreated CLL patients.[394] Here, patients were randomly assigned to treatment with either a combination of ibrutinib and venetoclax (ibrutinib lead-in for 3 cycles, followed by a combination of ibrutinib and venetoclax for 12 cycles, for a total of 15 cycles of therapy) or standard chlorambucil/obinutuzumab. After a median follow-up of 27.7 months, the median PFS was not reached with the ibrutinib/venetoclax arm compared to 21 months for chlorambucil/obinutuzumab ($P < .0001$), although there was no difference in the OS between the two arms. It is likely that the combination of ibrutinib and venetoclax will be approved by the FDA for frontline treatment of CLL in 2022.

The phase II CLARITY trial evaluated the combination of ibrutinib and venetoclax in 50 patients with relapsed CLL, none of whom had received prior BTK inhibitor or venetoclax therapy.[395] After 12 months of combined therapy, undetectable MRD was achieved in 53% patients in the peripheral blood, and 36% patients in the bone marrow, suggesting that this combination is also very effective in patients with relapsed CLL.

Triplet therapies consisting of the combination of a BTK inhibitor, venetoclax, and an anti-CD20 monoclonal antibody have also been reported in previously untreated CLL patients.[396-398] Across these studies, a fixed duration of treatment has been utilized, varying between 8 and 16 months and a significant proportion of patients (ranging from 56% to 78%) achieved undetectable MRD in both the peripheral blood and bone marrow. It remains unclear whether these triplet combinations are better than therapy with a BTK inhibitor/venetoclax or a BTK inhibitor alone. Results of several ongoing large phase 3 studies (such as CLL17, EA9161, ALLIANCE A041702) will answer these questions in the coming years.

Hematopoietic Stem Cell Transplantation

HCT remains the only potentially curative therapy in CLL, particularly in younger patients with high-risk features, for example, p53 dysfunction. While this comes at the cost of increased mortality and morbidity, there is a clear graft-vs-leukemia effect and benefit in CLL. In a recent update from the European Bone Marrow Transplant (EBMT) registry, including 2589 patients who received HCT between 2000 and 2010 for CLL, the event-free survival, OS, and nonrelapse mortality (NRM) 10 years after HCT were 28%, 35%, and 40%, respectively.[399] Those patients who survived 5 years posttransplantation had a 79% probability of surviving 10 years, highlighting the potential curative nature of HCT. The potent graft-vs-leukemia effect in CLL is evidenced by the increased posttransplant relapse rates in the absence of chronic graft-vs-host disease (GVHD), increased relapses after T-cell-depleted transplantation and the favorable antitumor response after donor lymphocyte infusion in posttransplantation relapse.[400-402]

The prominent graft-vs-leukemia effect in CLL, along with the relatively high treatment-related mortality with myeloablative conditioning (MAC) raised considerable interest in reduced-intensity conditioning (RIC) transplantation, which has become the mainstay conditioning for HCT in the last decade. While there is no prospective comparison between RIC and MAC, RIC is associated with shorter duration of cytopenias, lower risk of opportunistic infections, and reduced NRM based on registry studies. A pivotal European registry-based study demonstrated that in 73 heavily pretreated patients receiving RIC-HCT, the cumulative transplant-related mortality (TRM) was relatively low at 19%.[403,404] With a median follow-up of 22 months, the cumulative event-free survival and OS were 58% and 70%, respectively.[403,404] A retrospective comparison of these 73 RIC cases with 82 matched MAC-HCT patients from the EBMT registry showed a significant reduction in TRM but an increased relapse incidence in the RIC conditioning population.[404] There was no significant difference between the two modalities in terms of event-free survival and OS. Moreover, in a recent report from the Center for International Blood and Marrow Transplant Research (CIBMTR) for patients who received a HCT for CLL, the 3-year survival was significantly higher for RIC compared to MAC (58% vs 50%, $P < .001$).[405,406] Based on this evidence, most current transplant guidelines continue to recommend RIC transplant for CLL.[406] In an updated analysis of 606 CLL patients who underwent RIC allogeneic HCT from the CIBMTR between 2008 and 2014 and had complete cytogenetic information available, a prognostic scoring system was developed that incorporated four variables identified on multivariable analysis—disease status, comorbidity index, lymphocyte count, and white blood cell count at HCT.[407] Using this prognostic score, patients were stratified into low-, intermediate-, high-, and very-high-risk (with corresponding 4-year PFS rates of 58%, 42%, 33%, and 25%, respectively, $P < .0001$; and 4-year OS rates of 70%, 57%, 54%, and 38%, respectively, $P < .0001$). In addition, the presence of del 17p or ≥5 karyotypic abnormalities were associated with shorter PFS. Finally, a composite risk index utilizing both the prognostic score and the karyotypic score was developed that helped predict outcomes following RIC allogeneic HCT. An important limitation of this model is that it does not include patients treated with novel agents.

Traditionally, related donors have been the preferred source of cells for HCT in CLL. However, there is concern over the high incidence of familial CLL and MBL. Anecdotal cases of MBL transmission from donor to recipient have been reported.[408-410] Therefore, it is prudent to screen all potential sibling donors for the presence of a clonal B cell population. If they have a monoclonal B cell clone, it is recommended to exclude them or discuss potential consequences, especially if no matched unrelated donor is identified.[406] It should also be noted that haploidentical HCT has been recently employed as an appropriate alternative in CLL patients with comparable outcomes to matched donors.[411]

The optimum timing for allogeneic HCT in CLL remains largely unknown. While transplantation was previously offered for patients with high-risk CLL in first remission following chemoimmunotherapy, recent guidelines recommend postponing transplantation until patients have received a BTK inhibitor and venetoclax.[406] It should be noted that these guidelines are based on expert opinion rather than evidence-based recommendations and therefore controlled trials are required to address optimal timing of transplantation in CLL in the era of highly active signal inhibitors. Roeker and colleagues[412] reported the outcomes of a large cohort of CLL patients ($n = 65$) who underwent RIC allogeneic HCT following the receipt of novel agents (median number of prior lines of therapy = 3; including ibrutinib in 82%, venetoclax in 40%, and idelalisib in 20% patients).[412] The estimated 12-month PFS was 63% at 24 months, and the estimated OS at 24 months was 81%. The cumulative incidence of grade III-IV acute GVHD at day 100 was 24%, and moderate-severe chronic GVHD occurred in 27% patients. An HCT comorbidity index score of greater than 1 (vs 0; HR, 3.3; $P = .035$) was the only pretransplant characteristic associated with shorter PFS. These data suggest that eligible CLL patients should be considered for a HCT if they are receiving a second-line novel agent, especially if they have p53 dysfunction or ≥5 chromosomal abnormalities (high-CK), given the potential for durable responses with HCT.

Chimeric Antigen Receptor T Cells in Chronic Lymphocytic Leukemia

Chimeric antigen receptor (CAR) T cell therapy has emerged as a potent and potentially curative therapy in hematological malignancies.[413] A CAR is a synthetic protein that comprises the antigen binding domain of an antibody, linked through a transmembrane domain to one or more T cell signaling domains.[414] Therefore, a CAR marries the specificity of an antibody with the effector functions of a T cell. To generate CAR-T cells, patients undergo leukapheresis, T cells are isolated, transduced with the transgene, stimulated *ex-vivo* where they expand several fold and are then re-infused back into patients. The most commonly used therapy in the clinic is CD19-directed CAR-T cells for B-cell malignancies. Several products have been FDA approved since 2017 for the treatment of acute lymphoblastic leukemia[415] and NHL,[416-419] based on unprecedented results in early-phase clinical trials of patients with refractory and relapsed disease. The application of CAR-T cell therapy in hematological malignancies has been associated with unique toxicities. The most notable and important toxicities include the development of cytokine release syndrome (CRS) and neurotoxicity.[420,421] CRS is characterized by fevers, capillary leak, and hypotension that can progress to multiorgan failure. It is associated with significant elevation of T cell cytokines and coincides with T cell proliferation in peripheral blood.[422] It is typically reversible with the use of tocilizumab (IL-6 receptor blocker), but refractory cases and deaths have been reported due to this syndrome. Neurotoxicity, on the other hand, is characterized by a range of neurological symptoms, ranging from somnolence to obtundation, seizure, and cerebral edema. The mechanism of development of neurotoxicity is poorly understood.[423]

The first report of CAR-T19 in CLL included three patients with relapsed refractory disease.[424,425] While it only included three patients, it showed that CAR-T cells were able to induce CRs in a heavily pretreated population, to proliferate and expand by several folds in vivo, to kill multiple tumor cells (up to 1000), to persist and in some cases differentiate into a memory phenotype.[425] In a follow-up of 14 patients with relapsed refractory CLL treated with CAR-T19 at the University of Pennsylvania, the ORR was 57% and the rate of CR was 29%.[426] There was a direct association between achieving CR and in vivo CAR-T cell expansion. Notably, no relapses were observed in patients achieving a CR, suggestive that durable remissions are possible with this approach. Turtle and colleagues[427] conducted an investigator-initiated phase 1/2 study of CAR-T19 cell therapy (41BB co-stimulated product that has equal proportion of CD8+ and CD4+ CAR-T cells), in 24 patients with relapsed CLL (median number of prior therapies was 5 and all patients had received ibrutinib previously). There were three dose-level cohorts: 2×10^5 CAR-T cells/kg, 2×10^6 CAR-T cells/kg, and 2×10^7 CAR-T cells/kg. All patients received lymphodepleting chemotherapy consisting of cyclophosphamide, fludarabine, or a combination of the two prior to receiving the CAR-T cell infusion. Twenty patients developed CRS (including one patient with grade 4 and one patient with grade 5 CRS) and 8 patients developed neurotoxicity. The ORR 4 weeks after the CAR-T cell infusion was 74% (including a CR in 21%), among 19 patients who were evaluable for response. Seven patients out of 18 who underwent assessment of MRD had no detectable CLL using *IGHV* sequencing, and these patients had a significantly longer PFS and OS compared to patients with detectable residual disease. Since preclinical studies demonstrated a potential improvement in the efficacy of CAR-T therapy with the concurrent use of ibrutinib,[428] a subsequent study used concurrent ibrutinib therapy with CAR-T19 in 19 patients (median number of prior CLL treatments was 5). Ibrutinib was started more than 2 weeks prior to leukapheresis and continued for ≥3 months following CAR-T cell infusion. The ORR at 4 weeks following CAR-T infusion was 81% (including CR in 22%) among 18 evaluable patients, and 61% patients achieved undetectable MRD in the bone marrow by *IGHV* sequencing. Notably, the risk of CRS was lower in this study compared to CAR-T cells alone (median CRS grade 1 in this study with concomitant ibrutinib compared to median CRS score of 2 in the prior study with CAR-T cells alone, $P = .04$, 19 patients in each study). The 1-year PFS and 1-year OS in this study were 59% and 86%, respectively.[429]

In a company-sponsored phase 1 dose escalation study of lisocabtagene maraleucel, an autologous CD19-directed CAR-T product that has equal proportion of $CD8^+$ and $CD4^+$ T cells, 24 patients with relapsed CLL (median prior lines of therapy was 4) were treated at two dose levels: 50×10^6 and 100×10^6 CAR-T cells.[430] No dose limiting toxicity was reported in the smaller dose-level cohort, whereas two dose-limiting toxicity events (1 patient with grade 4 hypertension, and 1 patient with grade 3 encephalopathy and grade 3 tumor lysis syndrome) were noted in the cohort that received 100×10^6 CAR-T cells. For all patients, the most commonly reported treatment-emergent adverse events of grade 3 or greater included anemia (74%), thrombocytopenia (70%), neutropenia (70%), febrile neutropenia (26%), and hypophosphatemia (22%). Two patients (9%, both in the higher dose-level cohort) developed grade 3 CRS; any grade CRS occurred in 74% patients. Among 22 patients who were evaluable for efficacy, the ORR was 82%, including a CR/CRi rate of 45%, after a median follow-up of 24 months. Overall, 15 (75%) patients achieved undetectable MRD in the peripheral blood, of whom 13 (65%) also achieved undetectable MRD in the bone marrow. Patients with undetectable MRD in the blood who also achieved a best response of CR or PR had a better median PFS compared to those who did not achieve undetectable MRD (median not reached for patients with undetectable MRD compared to 3 months for those with detectable MRD, $P = .006$). The median PFS for the entire study cohort was 18 months and was 13 months in a subset of patients who had disease progression on both prior BTK inhibitors and venetoclax. A phase 2 expansion cohort of this study is currently enrolling patients at the recommended phase 2 dose of 100×10^6 CAR-T cells.

The encouraging early results of CAR-T cell therapy in CLL and the durable remissions in some cases suggest a potentially important role for this modality in heavily pretreated patients. Active research is warranted to understand the mechanisms of the relatively lower response rates in CLL compared to other hematological malignancies, and combination strategies of CAR-T cells with other CLL-directed therapies or immune modulators are undergoing.

Radiotherapy

Irradiation of the spleen, mediastinum, extracorporeal irradiation of the blood, total body irradiation, and hemibody irradiation were all commonly used in the past for the treatment of CLL.[431] However, radiation is rarely used nowadays, because of the effectiveness of new therapies and chemoimmunotherapy-resistant patients are usually resistant to irradiation.[431] Occasionally, splenic irradiation may be considered to control immune cytopenias or to shrink bulky lymphadenopathy in patients considered unfit for other therapies.[432]

Splenectomy

Splenectomy is rarely carried out in CLL, but may have a role for refractory AIHA or ITP, or in resistant patients with massive painful splenomegaly where the leukemia is predominantly confined to the spleen.[433,434] Postoperative morbidity in CLL has been reported to be 25% to 50%, with a mortality rate of 5% to 7.5%.[433,434] Patients should be immunized with pneumococcal, meningococcal, and *Haemophilus influenzae* vaccines about a month before splenectomy.[173] Laparoscopic splenectomy may also on occasion be required for AIHA.[435]

HOW WE TREAT CLL OUTSIDE OF CLINICAL TRIALS

1. Despite advances in therapy for CLL, all treatments come at a cost and potential toxicity. Thus, treatment should only be initiated when indicated, as outlined in the 2018 iwCLL guidelines.[1,2,5]

2. Prior to initial therapy, patients should have *IGHV* mutational status analysis and be screened for HIV, hepatitis B, and hepatitis C. Before each line of therapy, patients should have a careful, thorough physical examination along with FISH analysis, and *TP53* sequencing. A baseline β2-microglobulin is also useful as a prognostic marker and will drop with effective therapy. In addition, we typically perform CT scans of the chest, abdomen, and pelvis to quantitate bulky lymphadenopathy and splenomegaly that may not be apparent on examination. Patients with Rai stages III/IV disease may require a bone marrow to ensure that the anemia/thrombocytopenia are related to marrow infiltration, and not to MDS, an immune mechanism or to another disease. These parameters will need to be reassessed at completion of therapy or at other intervals to truly monitor extent of remissions.

3. Given their excellent tolerability and high efficacy, we recommend a targeted therapy in the frontline management of CLL (Figure 92.11). Given the lack of prospective randomized data comparing BTK inhibitor or venetoclax in the frontline setting, the patient's comorbidities and treatment preferences play an important role in the selection of therapy. For patients who prefer a fixed duration of therapy or have a history of cardiovascular comorbidity, combination therapy with venetoclax and obinutuzumab according to the CLL14 protocol is recommended. Patients must be willing to come to the clinic frequently during the initial 2 months for the obinutuzumab infusions and venetoclax ramp-up. Other patients may prefer a long-term therapy with a BTK inhibitor. Among the presently available BTK inhibitors, acalabrutinib and zanubrutinib appear to have less cardiovascular toxicity compared to ibrutinib. We do not routinely combine an anti-CD20 monoclonal antibody with a BTK inhibitor in the frontline setting.

4. In the absence of novel agents, chemoimmunotherapy is an option and patients with good-risk cytogenetics (such as del 13q by FISH), mutated *IGHV*, and no *TP53* mutation can have a long PFS and OS. The choice of chemoimmunotherapy depends on the patient's age and fitness (often assessed by the CIRS score and renal function). Fit patients <65 years generally can receive FCR and those >65 bendamustine/rituximab if that is deemed the best upfront approach. For the unfit patient, a standard approach is chlorambucil/obinutuzumab. Elderly patients who are unable to receive novel agents or a standard chemoimmunotherapy regimen may benefit from chlorambucil alone, with or without prednisone.

5. Given the inferior PFS using fixed duration therapy with venetoclax and obinutuzumab in patients with p53 dysfunction, we recommend a single-agent BTK inhibitor for these patients.

6. For patients receiving second-line therapy after prior chemoimmunotherapy, and have not had a novel agent, we recommend venetoclax and rituximab for a fixed duration of 2 years according to the MURANO regimen, or indefinite treatment with a BTK inhibitor, using FDA-approved agents that include ibrutinib, acalabrutinib, or zanubrutinib (Figure 92.12). We do not recommend repeating chemoimmunotherapy in these individuals, given the excellent PFS and OS with the novel agents.

7. Among patients who have disease progression on a BTK inhibitor (and are naïve to venetoclax), treatment with venetoclax and an anti-CD20 monoclonal antibody should be considered (Figure 92.12). It is also important to ensure that patients are bridged with a BTK inhibitor during the venetoclax dose ramp-up, given the increased risk of ibrutinib withdrawal syndrome in such patients. For patients who have disease progression on venetoclax (and are naïve to BTK inhibitors), therapy with any of the BTK inhibitors is appropriate.

8. Patients described above (in 7) should be considered for an allogenic hematopoietic stem cell transplantation, particularly if they have p53 dysfunction. However, only young patients (<70 years), who are fit, and have a matched donor can proceed to a stem cell transplant. Therefore, other patients should be considered for enrollment on well-designed prospective clinical trials, including studies using novel CAR-T approaches.

Approach to Frontline CLL Therapy
Previously untreated CLL patient in need of therapy*
Clinical trial participation strongly encouraged
TP53 disrupted (either by del17p on FISH or TP53 mutation)
Yes
No
• BTKi +/- obinutuzumab
Ascertain IGHV mutation status and patient fitness
Mutated IGHV**
Unmutated IGHV
Fit
Unfit¶¶
• BTKi +/- obinutuzumab
• Venetoclax + obinutuzumab
• BTKi +/- obinutuzumab
• Venetoclax + obinutuzumab
• FCR¶
*In general, patient preference, side effect profile of individual therapies, comorbidities, and availability of treatments play an important role in choice of initial therapy. ** no VH 3-21 gene usage. ¶ maybe a reasonable treatment option where novel agents are not available; and should be used only when there is no del11q by FISH, may administer 3 cycles and stop if MRD-negative; may use obinutuzumab instead of rituximab. ¶¶ both bendamustine and rituximab or chlorambucil and obinutuzumab are reasonable treatment options if access to novel agents is limited

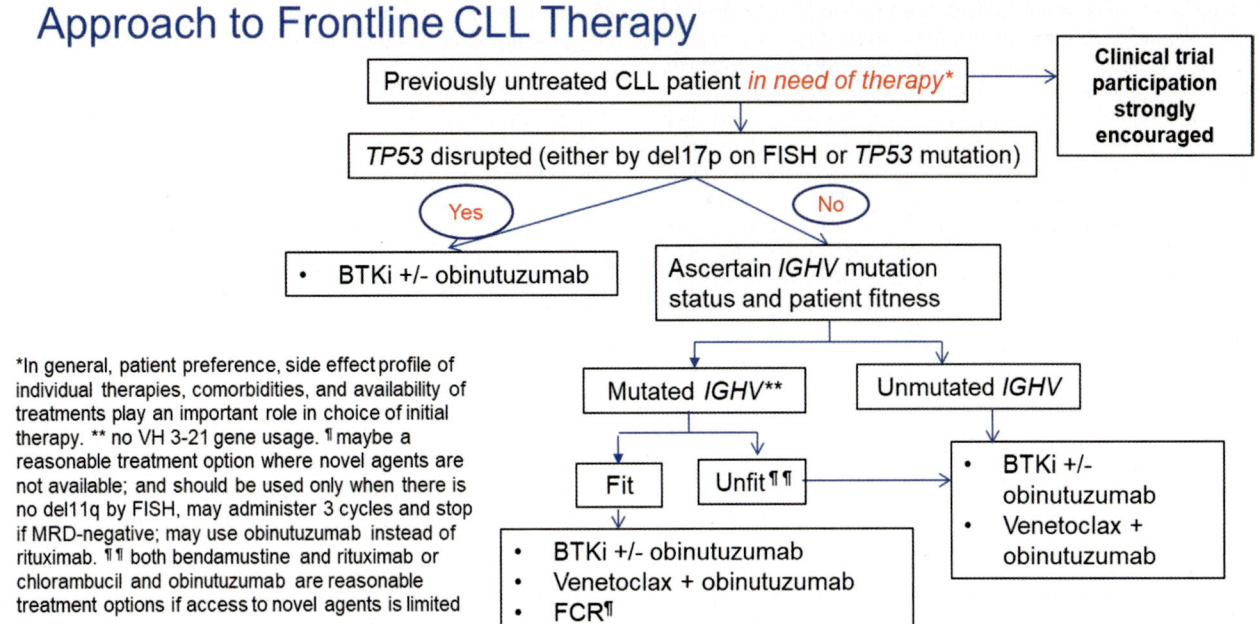

FIGURE 92.11 **Suggested algorithm for the management of frontline chronic lymphocytic leukemia (CLL). FCR, fludarabine/cyclophosphamide/rituximab; FISH, fluorescent in situ hybridization; IGHV, immunoglobulin heavy chain variable region.**

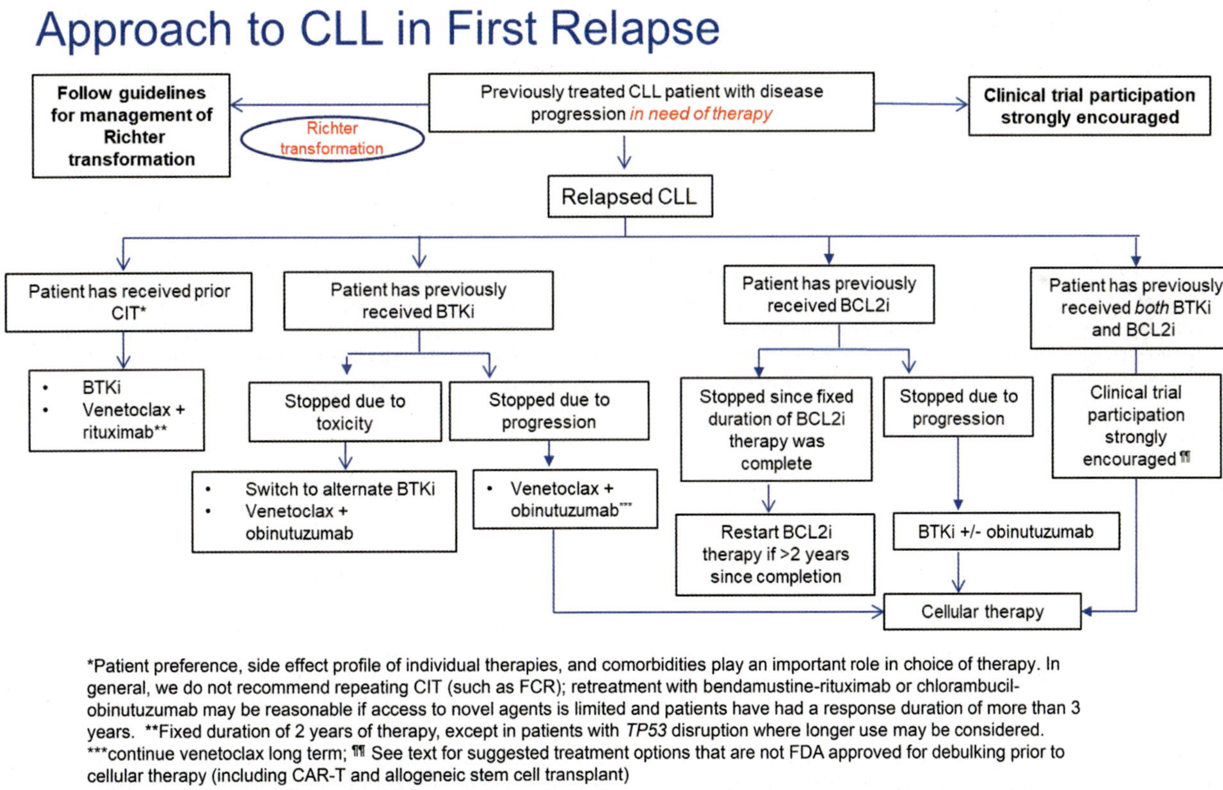

Approach to CLL in First Relapse
Follow guidelines for management of Richter transformation
Richter transformation
Previously treated CLL patient with disease progression in need of therapy
Clinical trial participation strongly encouraged
Relapsed CLL
Patient has received prior CIT*
Patient has previously received BTKi
Patient has previously received BCL2i
Patient has previously received both BTKi and BCL2i
• BTKi
• Venetoclax + rituximab**
Stopped due to toxicity
Stopped due to progression
Stopped since fixed duration of BCL2i therapy was complete
Stopped due to progression
Clinical trial participation strongly encouraged¶¶
• Switch to alternate BTKi
• Venetoclax + obinutuzumab
• Venetoclax + obinutuzumab***
Restart BCL2i therapy if >2 years since completion
BTKi +/- obinutuzumab
Cellular therapy
*Patient preference, side effect profile of individual therapies, and comorbidities play an important role in choice of therapy. In general, we do not recommend repeating CIT (such as FCR); retreatment with bendamustine-rituximab or chlorambucil-obinutuzumab may be reasonable if access to novel agents is limited and patients have had a response duration of more than 3 years. **Fixed duration of 2 years of therapy, except in patients with TP53 disruption where longer use may be considered. ***continue venetoclax long term; ¶¶ See text for suggested treatment options that are not FDA approved for debulking prior to cellular therapy (including CAR-T and allogeneic stem cell transplant)

FIGURE 92.12 **Suggested algorithm for the management of chronic lymphocytic leukemia (CLL) in first relapse. CAR-T, chimeric antigen receptor T cell; CIT, chemoimmunotherapy; FCR, fludarabine/cyclophosphamide/rituximab.**

MANAGEMENT OF IMMUNE DYSFUNCTION IN CLL

Infections

Strategies to reduce infections in patients with CLL include immunoglobulin replacement, prophylactic antibiotics, and vaccines.[193] In general, patients with markers of aggressive disease and prior treatment are at most risk of infections, with about 10% of patients developing significant infections.[129] Reductions in IgG and IgA in patients are major causes of infection and γ-globulin replacement can be effective in these patients, although these products are depleted of IgA. Original studies in the 1980s using high-dose γ-globulin, 400 mg/kg IV every 3 weeks, reduced the incidence of bacterial infections by 50%, particularly those caused by *Streptococcus pneumoniae* and *H. influenzae*; however, the total number of severe bacterial infections and nonbacterial infections was not reduced, and treatment did not prolong survival.[436] Moreover, this therapy was not cost-effective.[437] However, lower doses of γ-globulin were subsequently shown to be as effective, for example, 250 mg/kg every 4 weeks or 10 g every 3 weeks.[438,439] Molica et al[440] randomized CLL patients with an IgG of less than 6 g/L and a serious infection in the previous 6 months to 300 mg/kg γ-globulin every 4 weeks or to observation. Patients receiving γ-globulin had a reduced number of infections and effectiveness did not require restoration of the IgG levels. More recently, self-administration of low doses of subcutaneous γ-globulin (SCIG) on a weekly basis has been shown be highly effective in CLL, producing higher trough levels of IgG than intravenous γ-globulin.[441-443] This treatment produces sustained increased levels of IgG, decreases the infection rates, and compared to intravenous γ-globulin may improve patients' quality of life and be more cost-effective.[441-443]

Prophylactic antibiotics may be of benefit, particularly when patients are receiving nucleoside analogs, bendamustine, and steroids, and thus frequently antibiotics are incorporated into the newer and more immunosuppressive regimens. Accordingly, patients may be maintained on trimethoprim-sulfamethoxazole (cotrimoxazole) to prevent *P. jirovecii* pneumonia, acyclovir to prevent herpes viruses, valganciclovir to prevent both herpes and CMV, or fluconazole to prevent fungal infections. However, whether all patients should receive prophylactic antibiotics or only older patients or those with a history of infections is still unclear.[192,444]

While vaccines are less effective in CLL, it is still recommended to immunize these patients for pneumococcus (PCV13 followed by PPSV23) and influenza, the latter annually.[192,204,444,445] In addition, the shingle vaccine, Shingrix (GlaxoSmithKline Biologicals), is safe and effective in these patients.[205] As mentioned earlier in this chapter, these patients should not receive live vaccines, and these include, typhoid, yellow fever, measles, mumps, rubella, and BCG.[192,204,444,445]

Guidelines for the management of CLL patients were developed during the COVID-19 pandemic and will evolve over time depending on the effectiveness of herd immunity to new SARS-CoV-2 strains, which may necessitate ongoing immunization targeted to new variants.[198,446] Likewise, the impact of new variants will depend on their virulence and on the development of new antivirals and monoclonal antibodies to SARS-CoV-2. During the pandemic, recommendations were for patients to be immunized for COVID-19, preferably before starting therapy, and to reduce the risk of infection by social distancing, frequent hand washing, and wearing a facemask when in public.[198] Physicians reduced unnecessary patient visits, follow-ups were carried out remotely when possible, and treatment of CLL avoided, unless essential.[198] These recommendations have been modified recently as the incidence of COVID-19 fluctuates, but the infection will likely remain endemic with new variants emerging and CLL patients must remain vigilant as they may not respond to immunization, particularly if they have active disease or on therapy.[194,207,208] Moreover, CLL patients are typically elderly with comorbidities increasing the risk of complications if they do get infected.[199] Patients should continue to be immunized for COVID-19 as per validated recommendations and if they are infected, hospitalizations have been reduced by approximately 90% with the use of antivirals, for example, paxlovid (nirmatrelvir and ritonavir)[447] or molnupiravir,[448] with both treatments FDA approved and active against all SARS-CoV-2 variants, at present.[449] A number of monoclonal antibodies to SARS-CoV-2 are also available to treat infected patients, but have varying specificities, with decreased activity against the omicron variant.[449] For patients requiring hospitalization, improved outcomes have recently been reported, which may be related to the use of remdesivir, convalescent plasma, and the continuation of ibrutinib for patients admitted on this drug; in contrast, no benefit was seen with the addition of dexamethasone.[447,450]

More recently there has been interest in the use of long-acting monoclonal antibodies against SARS-CoV-2 to protect high-risk immunosuppressed patients from infection.[451] AZD7442 (tixagevimab-cilgavimab; Evusheld, AstraZeneca) has been licensed by the FDA for use in patients who cannot be immunized or on therapies that would reduce the efficacy of immunization. However, the effectiveness of these agents may be reduced with the ongoing appearance of more virulent omicron variants.

Second Malignancies

Patients should be educated about the twofold increased risk of secondary cancers in CLL, particularly skin cancers, and smokers should be encouraged to quit this habit because of the increased risk of squamous cell carcinomas of the skin, lung cancer, and other malignancies.[178,218,220] Patients should undergo regular skin self-examinations for skin and lip changes, have their skin assessed at their routine follow-up visits, and be seen by a dermatologist or physician with expertise in skin cancers at diagnosis and annually or more frequently for males aged >70 years particularly if there is a history of skin cancer or CLL treatment.[178,218] Patients should be educated about sun avoidance and use sun block and high-risk patients may benefit from retinoids or nicotinamide to prevent squamous cell carinomas.[218] Nicotinamide is well tolerated and 500 mg orally twice a day reduced the incidence of nonmelanotic skin cancers by 23% 1 year after starting the drug in non-CLL patients.[218] While therapy has not been linked to the development of solid tumors, patients should follow standard recommended screening recommendations.[178]

Immune Cytopenias

The immune cytopenias in CLL are treated initially with steroids, using prednisone 1 mg/kg/d, and 75% of patients respond to this therapy.[228,233] A response may be seen within days, although it may take several weeks in some patients and evidence of relapses are not uncommon. We recommend that patients with AIHA should also be maintained on folic acid, 1 mg/d and, after the hemoglobin and reticulocyte counts have normalized (usually in 1-2 weeks), the prednisone should be tapered slowly over a period of 2 to 3 months to help prevent a relapse. These patients should be advised of and monitored for prednisone side effects and maintained on prophylaxis against *P. jirovecii*.[452] They are also at risk of other infections, such as oral candidiasis or herpes simplex/zoster infections. Many of these patients are elderly, and the prolonged course of prednisone increases the risk of osteoporosis and vertebral collapse. Thus, patients should be maintained on vitamin D, calcium supplements, and a bisphosphonate. It is important that patients with AIHA and very low hemoglobin (<7 g/dL) are transfused, because, despite theoretical concerns, these patients rarely have severe transfusion reactions. In addition, any infection should be treated promptly, as sepsis may suppress marrow function and inhibit the compensatory reticulocytosis and worsen the anemia.

If a more rapid response is required, or if the patient does not respond to prednisone within 7 to 10 days, 1 gram of methylprednisolone IV or intravenous gamma-globulin (1 g/kg/d × 2 days) should be added.[228,453] This can produce a rapid but transient response and re-treatments are generally required every 3 to 4 weeks. There is no standard therapy for patients who do not respond to this therapy or who cannot be weaned off prednisone without a relapse. Cyclosporine is a reasonable option and produces a major response in two-thirds of CLL patients with ITP or AIHA and is highly effective in red cell aplasia.[454,455] Using 300 mg a day, the median time to response is 3 weeks with a median duration of response of 10 months.[454] Other immunosuppressives, such as 6-mercaptopurine or cyclophosphamide, can also be used.[228,233] Rituximab is also useful, either alone or in combination with a cyclophosphamide-containing regimen.[298,456,457] The response rate of 48 steroid-resistant CLL patients with immune cytopenias (AIHA 26, ITP 9, Evan syndrome 8, and red cell aplasia 5) receiving rituximab, cyclophosphamide, and dexamethasone (RCD) was 90% with the median duration of response being 24 months.[456] The immune cytopenia is often associated with active disease, and 40% of patients had progressive disease at the time of treatment and all patients who relapsed with immune cytopenias had progression of their CLL. Thus, maintaining remission of the immune cytopenias requires better control of the underlying CLL. Responses have also been observed with AIHA in CLL using alemtuzumab (an anti-CD52 monoclonal antibody), and this could be used in refractory cases if available.[458] Splenectomy is a helpful adjunct in AIHA, and the number of patients eligible for this procedure is increasing with the use of laparoscopic splenectomy.[435] Splenic irradiation may be carried out in those who are not surgical candidates, but it may take up to 2 months to see a response; the responses last for approximately 1 year.[432] The thrombopoietin analogs, romiplostim, and eltrombopag, are also effective for refractory thrombocytopenia, although the drugs need to be given indefinitely.[228,459]

MANAGEMENT OF RICHTER SYNDROME AND OTHER TRANSFORMATIONS

Patients with CLL often have hyperreactive lymph nodes, which can enlarge with an infection such as the flu, or sinusitis. In addition, painful enlargement of the axillary lymph nodes may occur after immunization. However, in the absence of infection, disease transformation should be considered if there is sudden enlargement of a lymph node(s), fevers, constitutional symptoms, and a high LDH.[266,460,461] RS occurs in ~2% to 8% patients.[461] The most common histology at the time of transformation is diffuse large B-cell lymphoma (DLBCL, 95%), followed by Hodgkin lymphoma (HL, <5%), and occasionally PLL or plasmablastic transformation (<1% each). The risk of RS is ~0.5% per year after CLL diagnosis; this risk increases to 1% per year among those patients on therapy.[460]

Richter Syndrome

Several risk factors for the development of RS in CLL patients have been described—these include clinical features (advanced Rai stage, lymph node size >3 cm), biological features (high expression of adverse prognostics including CD38, CD49d, or ZAP-70, and unmutated *IGHV*), and high-risk genetic factors (including del 17p and del 11q).[460,462] Other novel markers have been recently described including stereotyped BCRs ("subset 8"),[463] short telomere length[464] and $IGHV_{4-39}$ gene usage.[465] Next-generation sequencing has identified *NOTCH1* and *TP53* mutations as also being associated with an increased risk of RS. Rossi et al[465] have shown that the presence of both $IGHV_{4-39}$ gene usage and a *NOTCH1* mutation is associated with the highest risk of RS (~75% risk at 5 years) compared to <5% risk at 5 years in the absence of both these risk factors. Unfortunately, given the rarity of this condition, large cohorts of RS patients have not been studied systematically to perform adequate multivariable analyses to predict which of these factors are independently associated with an increased risk of transformation. Recent studies using whole-exome sequencing of DLBCL and CLL tissue have identified three major pathways involved in transformation: *TP53* disruption (del 17p or a *TP53* mutation) and *C-MYC* activation (~50% patients), *NOTCH1* mutations, which occur mostly in patients with trisomy 12 (~30% patients), and heterogenous genomic aberrations (~20% patients).[466]

In the era of targeted therapies, the presence of *TP53* dysfunction, a *BCL-6* abnormality, and a CK have been shown to predict an increased risk of transformation among ibrutinib-treated patients (occurs in ~5% of ibrutinib treated relapsed/refractory patients).[467] In contrast, the risk of transformation appears to be higher (12%) among relapsed/refractory CLL patients treated with venetoclax.[468] However, a direct comparison of the risk between these two novel agents is not possible given the heterogeneity of the patients studied and the varying lengths of follow-up. Among ibrutinib treated patients who experience progression of disease, the risk of RS appears to be highest in the first 12 to 18 months of therapy, whereas the risk of CLL progression is typically higher after 18 to 24 months on therapy.[467] This has important implications for the treating physician, who should make every effort to rule out RS in patients who progress during the first 12 to 18 months on novel agent therapy.

RS typically presents with rapidly enlarging discordant lymphadenopathy, with worsening B-type symptoms such as fever, night sweats, and weight loss. Laboratory studies typically show an increased LDH, although this is neither a sensitive nor a specific test for the diagnosis of transformation. All patients who are suspected of having RS should undergo PET with ^{18}F-FDG integrated with CT (^{18}F-FDG PET/CT) to determine if there is any evidence of increased FDG uptake in the enlarged lymph nodes. Additionally, all patients should also undergo a bone marrow biopsy. In the vast majority of patients who have undergone transformation, the standardized uptake value (SUV) in the lymph nodes generally exceeds 10, whereas in CLL the SUV is generally <5.[469] In 332 patients at the MD Anderson an SUV_{max} of ≥5 was found to be the useful to detect an optimum node to biopsy.[143] Patients with histologically aggressive CLL (large proliferation centers, increased proliferation index, and increased number of large cells) may also have increased LDH and constitutional symptoms but are less likely to have an SUV_{max} ≥5 (34% compared with 88% for RS) and have a better survival (27.6 vs 7.7 months).[143] Two studies on patients experiencing progression of disease in the novel agent era (mostly after BCR inhibitors) suggest using an SUV uptake of ≥5 as the optimal cut-off for determining if a biopsy is necessary to evaluate for RS.[470,471] Since infectious complications and other malignancies can mimic Richter transformation (both in terms of clinical presentation and imaging study findings),[472] an excisional lymph node biopsy is mandatory in establishing the diagnosis (typically performed on the most PET avid lymph node). In patients where the most PET avid lymph node is not accessible for an excisional biopsy, a core needle biopsy may be appropriate. A fine needle aspirate should not be performed, since it is unlikely to be diagnostic.

Many patients who are suspected of having transformed are on ibrutinib at the time of their evaluation. Since ibrutinib can increase the risk of bleeding during an excisional biopsy, it should be held for 3 to 5 days prior to and after the biopsy. In a subset of these patients, the disease "takes off rapidly" when ibrutinib is held resulting in significant enlargement in lymph nodes, increasing LDH and constitutional symptoms. If this occurs, it is reasonable to administer corticosteroids temporarily or to perform the biopsy while on ibrutinib, giving platelets to minimize bleeding.

Approximately 80% of cases of RS are clonally related to the underlying CLL, whereas the remaining 20% represents de novo DLBCL.[473] Clonal relationship may be simply determined by the surface light chain (κ or λ) expressions on the CLL and lymphoma cells; if different, then the RS is clonally unrelated. However, if similar the RS may be clonally related, but this can only be proven by comparing *IGHV* gene sequence between the DLBCL and the CLL cells.[461] Those patients with clonally related RS have a median OS of <1 year compared to patients with clonally unrelated de novo DLBCL where survival exceeds 5 years. There are no randomized phase 3 trials to guide treatment in patients with RS. Current therapy recommendations can be divided into the following categories:

Richter transformation occurring after chemoimmunotherapy and no past exposure of novel agents: Treatment of RS with traditional cytotoxic chemotherapy regimens (either anthracycline-containing regimens such as R-CHOP and R-EPOCH, or with platinum-containing regimens such as OFAR) is associated with CR rates of ~20%, ORRs of ~40% to 50%, and median survival of 1 to 2 years.[474-477] It is not surprising that these results are disappointing given that ~50% patients with RS have evidence of del 17p or a *TP53* mutation, where cytotoxic chemotherapy is less useful. Among patients who have a good response to therapy, an allogeneic HCT should be considered in first remission since it can lead to improved disease control and extend survival.[478] Unfortunately, given the advanced age of CLL patients with RS, their associated comorbidities and lack of response to standard therapy there are few patients to whom an allogeneic HCT can be offered. Therapy with ibrutinib (either as a single agent or in combination with corticosteroids) has shown some benefit in patients with RS. In a case series of 4 patients with relapsed/refractory RS, the median duration of response was ~6 months, with one patient achieving a CR.[479] Venetoclax has also been shown to offer modest benefit; in a phase 1 study of 7 patients with RS, 3 (43%) patients had a PR and 2 (29%) patients had stable disease.[480]

Richter transformation occurring while the patient is receiving novel targeted agents: Among patients who develop RS on ibrutinib, switching to a second-generation BTK inhibitor such as acalabrutinib may produce a transient response, with a median PFS of 2.1 months.[481]

Given these promising results, a randomized phase 2 study comparing acalabrutinib + R-CHOP to R-CHOP alone (STELLAR trial, NCT03899337) is currently enrolling patients. There are encouraging data demonstrating the utility of noncovalent BTK inhibitors, such as pirtobrutinib and nemtabrutinib, in patients where RS developed while patients were receiving covalent BTK inhibitors. Additional studies with larger numbers of patients are required to determine if these approaches will lead to durable responses.

Other novel approaches, such as pembrolizumab (a PD-1 inhibitor), have been studied. Ding and colleagues[482] reported an ORR of 44% among nine patients with RS who were treated with single-agent pembrolizumab (67% of whom had progressed on ibrutinib), with a median survival of ~11 months. Concurrent therapy with nivolumab and ibrutinib has also shown promising results. In a phase 2 study of 23 patients with RS, nivolumab was given 3 mg/kg IV every 2 weeks, starting cycle 1 day 1 for a total of 24 cycles, and ibrutinib was given 420 mg once daily starting cycle 2 day 1 until disease progression or unacceptable toxicity.[483] The ORR was 43%, with 8 patients (35%) achieving a complete metabolic response and the median OS for the entire cohort was 13.8 months.

A phase 2 trial of dose-adjusted R-EPOCH in combination with venetoclax among 26 patients with RS produced a CR rate of 50% with a median OS of 16.9 months.[484] Patients received one cycle of dose-adjusted R-EPOCH followed by rapid dose-escalation of venetoclax starting at the end of cycle 1 (days 22-27, with an initial dose of 20 mg daily and daily dose escalation to 50 mg, 100 mg, 200 mg, and finally 400 mg daily). Day 1, cycle 2, started the day following 400 mg venetoclax and patients received five further cycles of R-EPOCH at 3-week intervals, with 400 mg venetoclax given daily on days 1 to 10 of each cycle. At the end of cycle 6, patients could proceed to cellular therapy or continue venetoclax maintenance. Approximately 50% of eligible patients were eligible to proceed to cellular therapy (either HCT or CAR therapy) suggesting the feasibility of such an approach. In addition, among the 9 patients with clonally related RS who were evaluable for a response, the ORR was 80%, and the CR rate was 55%. However, this treatment was toxic, with a 38% risk of febrile neutropenia, and grade 3 or higher hematologic toxicities occurring in more than 50% patients. Therefore, an extension study is now being planned with the use of R-CHOP and venetoclax in these patients.

CAR-T therapy for patients with ibrutinib relapsed/refractory CLL has shown great promise and is now being tested in patients with RS.[427] In a study of 9 patients with RS who were treated with axicabtagene ciloleucel, 5 patients achieved CR, and 3 achieved a PR.[485] These patients were heavily pretreated with a median of four lines of prior CLL therapy, and all patients had previously received at least one novel agent, such as a BTK inhibitor or venetoclax.

HCT remains an important treatment modality in patients with RS, but most patients are unable to undergo HCT (either allogeneic or autologous HCT) due to inadequate response to initial therapy, poor performance status, advanced age, or lack of a matched donor. In a large retrospective study using the CIBMTR, Herrera and colleagues[486] reported on the outcomes of patients with RS who underwent an autologous HCT ($n = 53$) and an allogeneic HCT ($n = 118$). The 3-year relapse incidence, PFS, and OS were 37%, 48%, and 57%, respectively, among patients who underwent autologous HCT, whereas for those receiving an allogeneic HCT, the 3-year relapse incidence, PFS, and OS were 30%, 43%, and 52%, respectively. Receipt of more than three lines of prior therapy for RS was associated with an increased risk of NRM, and disease status prior to allogeneic HCT (PR vs resistant disease) was associated with a higher risk of disease relapse, and shorter PFS and OS following transplant. Other variables including del 17p status and receipt of novel agents prior to HCT did not predict for worse outcomes.

The natural history of RS is likely going to change with the use of novel therapies earlier in CLL treatment, and despite the introduction of such treatments, there remain a significant number of patients who develop transformation. The risk factors that contribute to the development of RS in CLL need to be evaluated in the context of these novel treatments, with the hope of ultimately developing strategies to reduce the incidence of this difficult complication. An improved participation of patients in properly designed clinical trials that target key aberrations in the pathogenesis of transformation will hopefully lead to more effective treatments for our patients.

Hodgkin Lymphoma

Occasionally, HL develops in CLL and is about 10% as common as RS.[487,488] HL typically occurs 4 to 6 years after CLL is diagnosed, with the mean age at diagnosis being 67 years vs a median age of 61 years for RS.[487,488] Histologically, there are two types of transformation. Type 1 transformation is characterized by scattered Reed-Sternberg cells in a field of CLL cells and type 2 transformation shows Reed-Sternberg cells in a field of inflammatory cells, separate from the CLL cells.[489] Most patients have advanced Rai stage disease at transformation and 70% of cases are mixed cellular or nodular sclerosing HL.[487] As with RS, patients present with fever, lymphadenopathy, and weight loss.[489] Previously treated patients have a much poorer survival than untreated patients. The cell of origin for the Reed-Sternberg cell in these patients is unclear, with some studies showing a clonal relationship to the underlying CLL cell, whereas others do not. In contrast to RS, Epstein-Barr viral infection is frequently seen in this transformation. Although initial studies suggested that the median survival of these patients is about 4 years (significantly worse compared to de novo HL),[488] more contemporary series suggest that the survival is significantly better than previously reported using ABVD-containing regimens.[490]

Prolymphocytic Transformation

Prolymphocytic transformation of CLL occurs slowly over several years with the gradual accumulation of increasing numbers of PLs (B-PLL/CLL).[161] In general, this type of transformation occurs more frequently in patients with unmutated *IGHV* and trisomy 12.[161] The underlying genetic cause for the transformation is presently unknown, but *MYC* rearrangements have been described.[491] Although most cases of PL in CLL represent a transformation of the CLL clone, cases of separate CLL and PL clones in the same patient have been described.[492]

References

1. Hallek M, Cheson BD, Catovsky D, et al. iwCLL guidelines for diagnosis, indications for treatment, response assessment and supportive management of chronic lymphocytic leukemia. *Blood*. 2018;131(25):2745-2760.
2. Burger JA. Treatment of chronic lymphocytic leukemia. *N Engl J Med*. 2020;383(5):460-473.
3. Chiorazzi N, Chen SS, Rai KR. Chronic lymphocytic leukemia. *Cold Spring Harb Perspect Med*. 2021;11(2):1-35.
4. Swerdlow SH, Campo E, Pileri SA, et al. The 2016 revision of the World Health Organization classification of lymphoid neoplasms. *Blood*. 2016;127(20):2375-2390.
5. Delgado J, Nadeu F, Colomer D, Campo E. Chronic lymphocytic leukemia: from molecular pathogenesis to novel therapeutic strategies. *Haematologica*. 2020;105(9):1-13.
6. Howlader N, Noone AM, Krapcho M, et al. *SEER Cancer Statistics Review, 1975-2014*. Posted to the SEER website. National Cancer Institute; 2017.
7. Seftel MD, Demers AA, Banerji V, et al. High incidence of chronic lymphocytic leukemia (CLL) diagnosed by immunophenotyping: a population-based Canadian cohort. *Leuk Res*. 2009;33(11):1463-1468.
8. Beiggi S, Banerji V, Deneka A, Griffith EJ, Gibson SB, Johnston JB. Comparison of outcome between referred and non-referred chronic lymphocytic leukemia patients to a specialized CLL clinic: a Canadian-based study. *Cancer Med*. 2016;5(6):971-979.
9. Brenner H, Gondos A, Pulte D. Trends in long-term survival of patients with chronic lymphocytic leukemia from the 1980s to the early 21st century. *Blood*. 2008;111:4916-4921.
10. Abrisqueta P, Pereira A, Rozman C, et al. Improving survival in patients with chronic lymphocytic leukemia (1980-2008): the Hospital Clínic of Barcelona experience. *Blood*. 2009;114(10):2044-2050.
11. Alrawashdh N, Sweasy J, Erstad B, McBride A, Persky DO, Abraham I. Survival trends in chronic lymphocytic leukemia across treatment eras: US SEER database analysis (1985-2017). *Ann Hematol*. 2021;100(10):2501-2512.
12. Kulis M, Merkel A, Heath S, et al. Whole-genome fingerprint of the DNA methylome during human B cell differentiation. *Nat Genet*. 2015;47(7):746-756.
13. Kulis M, Heath S, Bibikova M, et al. Epigenomic analysis detects widespread gene-body DNA hypomethylation in chronic lymphocytic leukemia. *Nat Genet*. 2012;44(11):1236-1242.
14. Queirós AC, Villamor N, Clot G, et al. A B-cell epigenetic signature defines three biological subgroups of chronic lymphocytic leukemia with clinical impact. *Leukemia*. 2015;29(3):598-605.

15. Kikushige Y, Ishikawa F, Miyamoto T, et al. Self-renewing hematopoietic stem cell is the primary target in pathogenesis of human chronic lymphocytic leukemia. *Cancer Cell*. 2011;20(2):246-259.
16. Yang S, Varghese AM, Sood N, et al. Ethnic and geographic diversity of chronic lymphocytic leukaemia. *Leukemia*. 2021;35(2):433-439.
17. National Cancer Insitiute: Surveillance, Epidemiology, and End Results Program. Cancer Stat Facts: NHL—Chronic Lymphocytic Leukemia/Small Lymphocytic Lymphoma (CLL/SLL). Accessed January 16, 2023. https://seer.cancer.gov/statfacts/html/cllsll.html
18. Slager SL, Benavente Y, Blair A, et al. Medical history, lifestyle, family history, and occupational risk factors for chronic lymphocytic leukemia/small lymphocytic lymphoma: the InterLymph non-Hodgkin lymphoma subtypes project. *J Natl Cancer Inst Monogr*. 2014;48:41-51.
19. Kipps TJ, Stevenson FK, Wu CJ, et al. Chronic lymphocytic leukaemia. *Nat Rev Dis Primers*. 2017;3:16096.
20. Goldin LR, Slager SL, Caporaso NE. Familial chronic lymphocytic leukemia. *Curr Opin Hematol*. 2010;17:350-355.
21. Speedy HE, Sava GS, Houlston RS. Inherited susceptibility to CLL. *Adv Exp Med Biol*. 2013;792:293-308.
22. Law PJ, Berndt SI, Speedy HE, et al. Genome-wide association analysis implicates dysregulation of immunity genes in chronic lymphocytic leukemia. *Nat Commun*. 2017;8:14175.
23. Cerhan JR, Slager SL. Familial predisposition and genetic risk factors for lymphoma. *Blood*. 2015;126(20):2265-2273.
24. Rawstron AC, Yuille MR, Fuller J, et al. Inherited predisposition to CLL is detectable as subclinical monoclonal B-lymphocyte expansion. *Blood*. 2002;100(7):2289-2291.
25. Marti GE, Carter P, Abbasi, et al. B-cell monoclonal lymphocytosis and B-cell abnormalities in the setting of familial B-cell chronic lymphocytic leukemia. *Cytometry B Clin Cytom*. 2003;52B:1-12.
26. Strati P, Shanafelt TD. Monoclonal B-cell lymphocytosis and early-stage chronic lymphocytic leukemia: diagnosis, natural history, and risk stratification. *Blood*. 2015;126(4):454-462.
27. Crowther-Swanepoel D, Wild R, Sellick G, et al. Insight into the pathogenesis of chronic lymphocytic leukemia (CLL) through analysis of IgVH gene usage and mutation status in familial CLL. *Blood*. 2008;111(12):5691-5693.
28. Speedy HE, Kinnersley B, Chubb D, et al. Germ line mutations in shelterin complex genes are associated with familial chronic lymphocytic leukemia. *Blood*. 2016;128(17):2319-2326.
29. Landgren O, Rapkin JSJ, Caporaso NE, et al. Respiratory tract infections and subsequent risk of chronic lymphocytic leukemia. *Blood*. 2007;109(5):2198-2201.
30. Landgren O, Engels E., Caporaso NE, et al. Patterns of autoimmunity and subsequent chronic lymphocytic leukemia in Nordic countries. *Blood*. 2006;108(1):292-296.
31. Damle RN, Ghiotto F, Valetto A, et al. B-cell chronic lymphocytic leukemia cells express a surface membrane phenotype of activated, antigen-experienced B lymphocytes. *Blood*. 2002;99(11):4087-4094.
32. Stevenson FK, Krysov S, Davies AJ, Steele AJ, Packham G. B-cell receptor signaling in chronic lymphocytic leukemia. *Blood*. 2011;118(16):4313-4320.
33. Agathangelidis A, Darzentas N, Hadzidimitriou A, et al. Stereotyped B-cell receptors in one third of chronic lymphocytic leukemia: towards a molecular classification with implications for targeted therapeutic interventions. *Blood*. 2012;119(19):4467-4476.
34. Minici C, Gounari M, Übelhart R, et al. Distinct homotypic B-cell receptor interactions shape the outcome of chronic lymphocytic leukaemia. *Nat Commun*. 2017;8(1):1-12.
35. Fegan C, Pepper C. Apoptosis deregulation in CLL. *Adv Exp Med Biol*. 2013;792:151-171.
36. Besbes S, Mirshahi M, Pocard M, Billard C. Strategies targeting apoptosis proteins to improve therapy of chronic lymphocytic leukemia. *Blood Rev*. 2015;29:345-350.
37. Friesen C, Herr I, Krammer PH, Debatin KM. Involvement of the CD95 (APO-1/FAS0 receptor/ligand system in drug-induced apoptosis in leukemia cells. *Nat Med*. 1996;2(5):574-577.
38. Jones DT, Ganeshaguru K, Virchis AE, et al. Caspase 8 activation independent of Fas (CD95/APO-1) signaling may mediate killing of B-chronic lymphocytic leukemia cells by cytotoxic drugs or gamma radiation. *Blood*. 2001;98(9):2800-2807.
39. Johnston JB, Kabore AF, Strutinsky J, et al. Role of the TRAIL/APO2-L death receptors in chlorambucil- and fludarabine-induced apoptosis in chronic lymphocytic leukemia. *Oncogene*. 2003;22(51):8356-8369.
40. Xiao W, Ishdorj G, Sun J, Johnston JB, Gibson SB. Death receptor 4 is preferentially recruited to lipid rafts in chronic lymphocytic leukemia cells contributing to tumor necrosis related apoptosis inducing ligand-induced synergistic apoptotic responses. *Leuk Lymphoma*. 2011;52(7):1290-1301.
41. Del Gaizo Moore V, Brown JR, Certo M, Love TM, Novina CD, Letai A. Chronic lymphocytic leukemia requires BCL2 to sequester prodeath BIM, explaining sensitivity to BCL2 antagonist ABT-737. *J Clin Invest*. 2007;117(1):112-121.
42. Pepper C, Lin TT, Pratt G, et al. Mcl-1 expression has in vitro and in vivo significance in chronic lymphocytic leukemia and is associated with other poor prognostic markers. *Blood*. 2008;112(9):3807-3817.
43. Yoshida K, Miki Y. The cell death machinery governed by the p53 tumor suppressor in response to DNA damage. *Cancer Sci*. 2010;101(4):831-835.
44. Shiloh Y, Ziv Y. The ATM protein kinase: regulating the cellular response to genotoxic stress, and more. *Nat Rev Mol Cell Biol*. 2013;14(4):197-210.
45. Zenz T, Häbe S, Denzel T, et al. Detailed analysis of p53 pathway defects in fludarabine-refractory chronic lymphocytic leukemia (CLL): dissecting the contribution of 17p deletion, TP53 mutation, p53-p21 dysfunction, and miR34a in a prospective clinical trial. *Blood*. 2009;114:2589-2597.
46. Zenz T, Eichhorst B, Busch R, et al. TP53 mutation and survival in chronic lymphocytic leukemia. *J Clin Oncol*. 2010;28(29):4473-4479.
47. te Raa GD, Malčiková J, Mraz M, et al. Assessment of TP53 functionality in chronic lymphocytic leukaemia by different assays; an ERIC-wide approach. *Br J Haematol*. 2014;167(4):565-569.
48. Austen B, Skowronska A, Baker C, et al. Mutation status of the residual ATM allele is an important determinant of the cellular response to chemotherapy and survival in patients with chronic lymphocytic leukemia containing an 11q deletion. *J Clin Oncol*. 2007;25(34):5448-5457.
49. Austen B, Powell JE, Alvi A, et al. Mutations in the ATM gene lead to impaired overall and treatment-free survival that is independent of IGVH mutation status in patients with B-CLL. *Blood*. 2005;106(9):3175-3182.
50. Kipps TJ, Fraser G, Coutre SE, et al. Long-term studies assessing outcomes of ibrutinib therapy in patients with del(11q) chronic lymphocytic leukemia. *Clin Lymphoma Myeloma Leuk*. 2019;19(11):715-722.e716.
51. Ten Hacken E, Burger JA. Molecular pathways: targeting the microenvironment in chronic lymphocytic leukemia—focus on the B-cell receptor. *Clin Cancer Res*. 2014;20(3):548-556.
52. Burger JA, Tsukada N, Burger M, Zvaifler NJ, Dell'Aquila M, Kipps TJ. Blood-derived nurse-like cells protect chronic lymphocytic leukemia B cells from spontaneous apoptosis through stromal cell-derived factor-1. *Blood*. 2000;96(8):2655-2663.
53. Davids MS, Brown JR. Targeting the B cell receptor pathway in chronic lymphocytic leukemia. *Leuk Lymphoma*. 2012;53(12):2362-2370.
54. Cols M, Barra CM, He B, et al. Stromal endothelial cells establish a bidirectional crosstalk with chronic lymphocytic leukemia cells through the TNF-related factors BAFF, APRIL, and CD40L. *J Immunol*. 2012;188(12):6071-6083.
55. Eble JA, Haier J. Integrins in cancer treatment. *Curr Cancer Drug Targets*. 2006;6(2):89-105.
56. Gilling CE, Mittal AK, Chaturvedi NK, et al. Lymph node-induced immune tolerance in chronic lymphocytic leukaemia: a role for caveolin-1. *Br J Haematol*. 2012;158(2):216-231.
57. Yoon JY, Lafarge S, Dawe D, et al. Association of interleukin-6 and interleukin-8 with poor prognosis in elderly patients with chronic lymphocytic leukemia. *Leuk Lymphoma*. 2012;53(9):1735-1742.
58. Sivina M, Hartmann E, Kipps TJ, et al. CCL3 (MIP-1α) plasma levels and the risk for disease progression in chronic lymphocytic leukemia. *Blood*. 2011;117(5):1662-1669.
59. Zhang W, Trachootham D, Liu J, et al. Stromal control of cystine metabolism promotes cancer cell survival in chronic lymphocytic leukemia. *Nat Cell Biol*. 2012;14(3):276-286.
60. Paggetti J, Haderk F, Seiffert M, et al. Exosomes released by chronic lymphocytic leukemia cells induce the transition of stromal cells into cancer-associated fibroblasts. *Blood*. 2015;126(9):1106-1117.
61. Boysen J, Nelson M, Magzoub G, et al. Dynamics of microvesicle generation in B-cell chronic lymphocytic leukemia: implication in disease progression. *Leukemia*. 2017;31(2):350-360.
62. Caivano A, Del Vecchio L, Musto P. Do we need to distinguish exosomes from microvesicles in hematological malignancies? *Leukemia*. 2017;31(9):2009-2010.
63. Ghosh AK, Secreto C, Boysen J, et al. The novel receptor tyrosine kinase Axl is constitutively active in B-cell chronic lymphocytic leukemia and acts as a docking site of nonreceptor kinases: implications for therapy. *Blood*. 2011;117(6):1928-1937.
64. Burger JA, Li KW, Keating MJ, et al. Leukemia cell proliferation and death in chronic lymphocytic leukemia patients on therapy with the BTK inhibitor ibrutinib. *JCI Insight*. 2017;2(2):1-11.
65. Woyach JA, Johnson AJ, Byrd JC. Review article the B-cell receptor signaling pathway as a therapeutic target in CLL. *Blood*. 2012;120(6):1175-1184.
66. Seke Etet PF, Vecchio L, Nwabo Kamdje AH. Interactions between bone marrow stromal microenvironment and B-chronic lymphocytic leukemia; any role for Notch, Wnt and Hh signaling pathways? *Cell Signal*. 2012;24:1433-1443.
67. Munk Pedersen I, Reed J. Microenvironmental interactions and survival of CLL B-cells. *Leuk Lymphoma*. 2004;45(12):2365-2372.
68. Burger J. Nurture versus nature: the microenvironment in chronic lymphocytic leukemia. *Hematology Am Soc Hematol Educ Program*. 2011;2011:96-103.
69. Christopoulos P, Pfeifer D, Bartholomé K, et al. Definition and characterization of the systemic T-cell dysregulation in untreated indolent B-cell lymphoma and very early CLL. *Blood*. 2011;117(14):3836-3846.
70. Crassini K, Shen Y, Mulligan S, et al. Modeling the chronic lymphocytic leukemia microenvironment in vitro. *Leuk Lymphoma*. 2017;58(2):266-279.
71. Herishanu Y, Pérez-Galán P, Liu D, et al. The lymph node microenvironment promotes B-cell receptor signaling, NF-κB activation, and tumor proliferation in chronic lymphocytic leukemia. *Blood*. 2011;117(2):563-574.
72. Damle RN, Batliwalla FM, Ghiotto F, et al. Telomere length and telomerase activity delineate distinctive replicative features of the B-CLL subgroups defined by immunoglobulin V gene mutations. *Blood*. 2004;103(2):375-382.
73. Messmer D, Kipps TJ. CD154 gene therapy for human B-cell malignancies. *Ann N Y Acad Sci*. 2005;1062:51-60.
74. Chatziakostantinou T, Demosthenous C, Baliakas P. Biology and treatment of high-risk CLL: significance of complex karyotype. *Front Oncol*. 2021;11:788761.
75. Döhner H, Stilgenbauer S, Benner A, et al. Genomic aberrations and survival in chronic lymphocytic leukemia. *N Engl J Med*. 2000;343(26):1910-1916.
76. Del Giudice I, Rossi D, Chiaretti S, et al. NOTCH1 mutations in +12 chronic lymphocytic leukemia (CLL) confer an unfavorable prognosis, induce a distinctive transcriptional profiling and refine the intermediate prognosis of +12 CLL. *Haematologica*. 2012;97(3):437-441.
77. Hallek M, Fischer K, Fingerle-Rowson G, et al. Addition of rituximab to fludarabine and cyclophosphamide in patients with chronic lymphocytic leukaemia: a randomised, open-label, phase 3 trial. *Lancet*. 2010;376(9747):1164-1174.

78. Klein U, Lia M, Crespo M, et al. The DLEU2/miR-15a/16-1 cluster controls B cell proliferation and its deletion leads to chronic lymphocytic leukemia. *Cancer Cell.* 2010;17(1):28-40.
79. Berndt SI, Skibola CF, Joseph V, et al. Genome-wide association study identifies multiple risk loci for chronic lymphocytic leukemia. *Nat Genet.* 2013;45(8):868-876.
80. Stilgenbauer S, Bullinger L, Lichter P, Do H. Genetics of chronic lymphocytic leukemia: genomic aberrations and V(H) gene mutation status in pathogenesis and clinical course. *Leukemia.* 2002;16:993-1007.
81. Shanafelt TD, Witzig TE, Fink SR, et al. Prospective evaluation of clonal evolution during long-term follow-up of patients with untreated early-stage chronic lymphocytic leukemia. *J Clin Oncol.* 2006;24(28):4634-4641.
82. Van Dyke DL, Werner L, Rassenti LZ, et al. The Dohner fluorescence in situ hybridization prognostic classification of chronic lymphocytic leukaemia (CLL): the CLL Research Consortium experience. *Br J Haematol.* 2016;173(1):105-113.
83. Jain P, Keating M, Thompson PA, et al. High fluorescence in situ hybridization percentage of deletion 11q in patients with chronic lymphocytic leukemia is an independent predictor of adverse outcome. *Am J Hematol.* 2015;90(6):471-477.
84. Nowakowski GS, Dewald GW, Hoyer JD, et al. Interphase fluorescence in situ hybridization with an IGH probe is important in the evaluation of patients with a clinical diagnosis of chronic lymphocytic leukaemia. *Br J Haematol.* 2005;130(1):36-42.
85. Fang H, Reichard KK, Rabe KG, et al. IGH translocations in chronic lymphocytic leukemia: clinicopathologic features and clinical outcomes. *Am J Hematol.* 2019;94(3):338-345.
86. Mayr C, Speicher MR, Kofler DM, et al. Chromosomal translocations are associated with poor prognosis in chronic lymphocytic leukemia. *Blood.* 2006;107:742-751.
87. Muthusamy N, Breidenbach H, Andritsos L, et al. Enhanced detection of chromosomal abnormalities in chronic lymphocytic leukemia by conventional cytogenetics using CpG oligonucleotide in combination with pokeweed mitogen and phorbol myristate acetate. *Cancer Genetics.* 2011;204:77-83.
88. Herling CD, Klaumunzer M, Krings Rocha C, et al. Complex karyotypes, KRAS and POT1 mutations impact outcome in CLL after chlorambucil based chemo- or chemoimmunotherapy. *Blood.* 2016;128(3):395-404.
89. Heerema NA, Byrd JC, Dal Cin PS, et al. Stimulation of chronic lymphocytic leukemia cells with CpG oligodeoxynucleotide gives consistent karyotypic results among laboratories: a CLL Research Consortium (CRC) Study. *Cancer Genet Cytogenet.* 2010;203:134-140.
90. Thompson PA, O'Brien SM, Wierda WG, et al. Complex karyotype is a stronger predictor than del(17p) for an inferior outcome in relapsed or refractory chronic lymphocytic leukemia patients treated with ibrutinib-based regimens. *Cancer.* 2015;121(20):3612-3621.
91. Baliakas P, Jeromin S, Iskas M, et al. Cytogenetic complexity in chronic lymphocytic leukemia: definitions, associations, and clinical impact. *Blood.* 2019;133(11):1205-1216.
92. Woyach JA, Furman RR, Liu TM, et al. Resistance mechanisms for the Bruton's tyrosine kinase inhibitor ibrutinib. *N Engl J Med.* 2014;370:2286-2294.
93. Kittai AS, Miller C, Goldstein D, et al. The impact of increasing karyotypic complexity and evolution on survival in patients with CLL treated with ibrutinib. *Blood.* 2021;138(23):2372-2382.
94. Fabbri G, Dalla-Favera R. The molecular pathogenesis of chronic lymphocytic leukaemia. *Nat Rev Cancer.* 2016;16(3):145-162.
95. Aalto Y, El-Rifa W, Vilpo L, et al. Distinct gene expression profiling in chronic lymphocytic leukemia with 11q23 deletion. *Leukemia.* 2001;15(11):1721-1728.
96. Herold T, Jurinovic V, Mulaw M, et al. Expression analysis of genes located in the minimally deleted regions of 13q14 and 11q22-23 in chronic lymphocytic leukemia - unexpected expression pattern of the RHO GTPase activator ARHGAP20. *Genes Chromosomes Cancer.* 2011;50:546-558.
97. Fischer K, Bahlo J, Fink AM, et al. Long-term remissions after FCR chemoimmunotherapy in previously untreated patients with CLL: updated results of the CLL8 trial. *Blood.* 2016;127(2):208-215.
98. Döhner H, Stilgenbauer S, James MR, et al. 11q deletions identify a new subset of B-cell chronic lymphocytic leukemia characterized by extensive nodal involvement and inferior prognosis. *Blood.* 1997;89(7):2516-2522.
99. Skowronska A, Austen B, Powell JE, et al. ATM germline heterozygosity does not play a role in chronic lymphocytic leukemia initiation but influences rapid disease progression through loss of the remaining ATM allele. *Haematologica.* 2012;97(1):142-146.
100. Wang L, Lawrence MS, Wan Y, et al. SF3B1 and other novel cancer genes in chronic lymphocytic leukemia. *N Engl J Med.* 2011;365(26):2497-2506.
101. Rossi D, Bruscaggin A, Spina V, et al. Mutations of the SF3B1 splicing factor in chronic lymphocytic leukemia: association with progression and fludarabine-refractoriness. *Blood.* 2011;118(26):6904-6908.
102. Dickinson JD, Smith LM, Sanger WG, et al. Unique gene expression and clinical characteristics are associated with the 11q23 deletion in chronic lymphocytic leukaemia. *Br J Haematol.* 2005;128:460-471.
103. Marinelli M, Peragine N, Di Maio V, et al. Identification of molecular and functional patterns of p53 alterations in chronic lymphocytic leukemia patients in different phases of the disease. *Haematologica.* 2013;98(3):371-375.
104. Au WY, Horsman DE, Ohno H, Klasa RJ, Gascoyne RD. Bcl-3/IgH translocation (14;19)(q32;q13) in non-Hodgkin's lymphomas. *Leuk Lymphoma.* 2002;43(4):813-816.
105. Puente XS, Beà S, Valdés-Mas R, et al. Non-coding recurrent mutations in chronic lymphocytic leukaemia. *Nature.* 2015;526:519-524.
106. Landau DA, Tausch E, Taylor-Weiner AN, et al. Mutations driving CLL and their evolution in progression and relapse. *Nature.* 2015;526(7574):525-530.
107. Arruga F, Gizdic B, Serra S, et al. Functional impact of NOTCH1 mutations in chronic lymphocytic leukemia. *Leukemia.* 2014;28(5):1060-1070.
108. Gutierrez C, Wu CJ. Clonal dynamics in chronic lymphocytic leukemia. *Blood Adv.* 2019;3(22):3759-3769.
109. Ojha J, Ayres J, Secreto C, et al. Deep sequencing identifies genetic heterogeneity and recurrent convergent evolution in chronic lymphocytic leukemia. *Blood.* 2015;125(3):492-498.
110. Lozanski G, Heerema NA, Flinn IW, et al. Alemtuzumab is an effective therapy for chronic lymphocytic leukemia with p53 mutations and deletions. *Blood.* 2004;103:3278-3281.
111. Mossafa H, Malaure H, Maynadie M, et al. Persistent polyclonal B lymphocytosis with binucleated lymphocytes: a study of 25 cases. Groupe Français d'Hématologie Cellulaire. *Br J Haematol.* 1999;104(3):486-493.
112. Delage R, Jacques L, Massinga-Loembe M, et al. Persistent polyclonal B-cell lymphocytosis: further evidence for a genetic disorder associated with B-cell abnormalities. *Br J Haematol.* 2001;114(3):666-670.
113. Salcedo I, Campos-Caro A, Sampalo A, Reales E, Brieva JA. Persistent polyclonal B lymphocytosis: an expansion of cells showing IgVH gene mutations and phenotypic features of normal lymphocytes from the CD27+ marginal zone B-cell compartment. *Br J Haematol.* 2002;116(3):662-666.
114. Bates I, Bedu-Addo G, Bevan DH, Rutherford TR. Use of immunoglobulin gene rearrangements to show clonal lymphoproliferation in hyper-reactive malarial splenomegaly. *Lancet.* 1991;337:505-507.
115. Marti GE, Rawstron AC, Ghia P, et al. Diagnostic criteria for monoclonal B-cell lymphocytosis. *Br J Haematol.* 2005;130(3):325-332.
116. Marti GE. MBL: mostly benign lymphocytes, but. *Blood.* 2011;118(25):6480-6481.
117. Shanafelt TD, Ghia P, Lanasa MC, Landgren O, Rawstron aC. Monoclonal B-cell lymphocytosis (MBL): biology, natural history and clinical management. *Leukemia.* 2010;24(3):512-520.
118. Nieto WG, Almeida J, Romero A, et al. Increased frequency (12%) of circulating chronic lymphocytic leukemia-like B-cell clones in healthy subjects using a highly sensitive multicolor flow cytometry approach. *Blood.* 2009;114(1):33-37.
119. Rawstron AC, Shanafelt T, Lanasa MC, et al. Different biology and clinical outcome according to the absolute numbers of clonal B-cells in monoclonal B-cell lymphocytosis (MBL). *Cytometry B Clin Cytometry.* 2010;78(suppl 1):19-23.
120. Parikh SA, Rabe KG, Kay NE, et al. The CLL-international prognostic index (CLL-IPI) predicts outcomes in monoclonal B-cell lymphocytosis and Rai 0 CLL. *Blood.* 2021;138(2):149-159.
121. Slager SL, Lanasa MC, Marti GE, et al. Natural history of monoclonal B-cell lymphocytosis among relatives in CLL families. *Blood.* 2021;137(15):2046-2056.
122. Vardi A, Dagklis A, Scar L, et al. Immunogenetics shows that not all MBL are equal: the larger the clone, the more similar to CLL. *Blood.* 2013;121(22):4521-4528.
123. Shanafelt TD, Kay NE, Rabe KG, et al. Survival of patients with clinically identified monoclonal B-cell lymphocytosis (MBL) relative to the age- and sex-matched general population. *Leukemia.* 2012;26(2):373-376.
124. Shanafelt TD, Kay NE, Jenkins G, et al. B-cell count and survival: differentiating chronic lymphocytic leukemia from monoclonal B-cell lymphocytosis based on clinical outcome. *Blood.* 2009;113(18):4188-4196.
125. Moreira J, Rabe KG, Cerhan JR, et al. Infectious complications among individuals with clinical monoclonal B-cell lymphocytosis (MBL): a cohort study of newly diagnosed cases compared to controls. *Leukemia.* 2012;27(1):136-141.
126. Solomon BM, Chaffee KG, Moreira J, et al. Risk of non-hematologic cancer in individuals with high-count monoclonal B-cell lymphocytosis. *Leukemia.* 2016;(30):331-336.
127. Shanafelt TD, Kay NE, Parikh SA, et al. Risk of serious infection among individuals with and without low count monoclonal B-cell lymphocytosis (MBL). *Leukemia.* 2021;35(1):239-244.
128. Rawstron AC, Bennett FL, O'Connor SJ, et al. Monoclonal B-cell lymphocytosis and chronic lymphocytic leukemia. *N Engl J Med.* 2008;359(6):575-583.
129. Ishdorj G, Streu E, Lambert P, et al. IgA levels at diagnosis predict for infections, time to treatment, and survival in chronic lymphocytic leukemia. *Blood Advances.* 2019;3(14):2188-2198.
130. Gentile M, Cutrona G, Fabris S, et al. Total body computed tomography scan in the initial work-up of Binet stage A chronic lymphocytic leukemia patients: results of the prospective, multicenter O-CLL1-GISL study. *Am J Hematol.* 2013;88(7):539-544.
131. Shim YK, Rachel JM, Ghia P, et al. Monoclonal B-cell lymphocytosis in healthy blood donors: an unexpectedly common finding. *Blood.* 2014;123(9):1319-1326.
132. Ferrand C, Garnache-Ottou F, Collonge-Rame MA, et al. Systematic donor blood qualification by flow cytometry would have been able to avoid CLL-type MBL transmission after unrelated hematopoietic stem cell transplantation. *Eur J Haematol.* 2012;88(3):269-272.
133. Hjalgrim H, Rostgaard K, Vasan SK, et al. No evidence of transmission of chronic lymphocytic leukemia through blood transfusion. *Blood.* 2015;126(17):2059-2061.
134. Dearden C. Management of prolymphocytic leukemia. *Hematology Am Soc Hematol Educ Program.* 2015;2015(1):361-367.
135. Kay NE, Hanson CA. B-cell prolymphocytic leukemia has 3 subsets. *Blood.* 2019;134(21):1777-1778.
136. Bennett JM, Catovsky D, Daniel MT, et al. Proposals for the classification of chronic (mature) B and T lymphoid leukaemias. French-American-British (FAB) Cooperative Group. *J Clin Pathol.* 1989;42(6):567-584.
137. Chapiro E, Pramil E, Diop MB, et al. Genetic characterization of B-cell prolymphocytic leukemia: a prognostic model involving MYC and TP53. *Blood.* 2019;134(21):1821-1831.
138. Parikh SA, Strati P, Tsang M, West CP, Shanafelt TD. Should IGHV status and FISH testing be performed in all CLL patients at diagnosis? A systematic review and meta-analysis. *Blood.* 2016;127(14):1752-1760.

139. Ozoya OO, Sokol L, Dalia S. Hepatitis B reactivation with novel agents in non-Hodgkin's lymphoma and prevention strategies. *J Clin Transl Hepatol.* 2016;4(2):143-150.
140. Rozman C, Montserrat E, Rodriguez-Fernandez JM, et al. Bone marrow histologic pattern - the best single prognostic parameter in chronic lymphocytic leukemia: a multivariate survival analysis of 329 cases. *Blood.* 1984;64(3):642-648.
141. Eichhorst BF, Fischer K, Fink AM, et al. Limited clinical relevance of imaging techniques in the follow-up of patients with advanced chronic lymphocytic leukemia: results of a meta-analysis. *Blood.* 2011;117(6):1817-1821.
142. Molica S. FDG/PET in CLL today. *Blood.* 2014;123(18):2749-2750.
143. Falchi L, Keating MJ, Marom EM, et al. Correlation between FDG/PET, histology, characteristics, and survival in 332 patients with chronic lymphoid leukemia. *Blood.* 2014;123(18):2783-2790.
144. Rai KR, Sawitsky A, Cronkite EP, Chanana AD, Levy RN, Pasternack BS. Clinical staging of chronic lymphocytic leukemia. *Blood.* 1975;46(2):219-234.
145. Binet JL, Leporrier M, Dighiero G, et al. Clinical staging system for chronic lymphocytic leukemia. *Cancer.* 1977;40:855-864.
146. Ding W, Ferrajoli A. Evidence-based mini-review: the role of alkylating agents in the initial treatment of chronic lymphocytic leukemia patients with the 11q deletion. *Hematology Am Soc Hematol Educ Program.* 2010;2010:90-92.
147. Dighiero G, Binet JL. When and how to treat chronic lymphocytic leukemia. *N Engl J Med.* 2000;343(24):1799-1801.
148. Moreno C, Hodgson K, Ferrer G, et al. Autoimmune cytopenia in chronic lymphocytic leukemia: prevalence, clinical associations, and prognostic significance. *Blood.* 2010;116(23):4771-4776.
149. Zent CS, Ding W, Schwager SM, et al. The prognostic significance of cytopenia in chronic lymphocytic leukaemia/small lymphocytic lymphoma. *Br J Haematol.* 2008;141(5):615-621.
150. Mauro FR, Foa R, Giannarelli D, et al. Clinical characteristics and outcome of young chronic lymphocytic leukemia patients: a single institution study of 204 cases. *Blood.* 1999;94(2):448-454.
151. Baumann T, Delgado J, Santacruz R, et al. Chronic lymphocytic leukemia in the elderly: clinico-biological features, outcomes, and proposal of a prognostic model. *Haematologica.* 2014;99(10):1599-1604.
152. Shanafelt TD, Rabe KG, Kay NE, et al. Age at diagnosis and the utility of prognostic testing in patients with chronic lymphocytic leukemia. *Cancer.* 2010;116(20):4777-4787.
153. Parikh S., Rabe KG, Kay NE, et al. Chronic lymphocytic leukemia in young (≤ 55 years) patients: a comprehensive analysis of prognostic factors and outcomes. *Haematologica.* 2014;99(1):140-147.
154. Barzilai A, Feuerman H, Quaglino P, et al. Cutaneous B-cell neoplasms mimicking granulomatous rosacea or rhinophyma. *Arch Dermatol.* 2012;148(7):824-831.
155. Agnew KL, Ruchlemer R, Catovsky D, Matutes E, Bunker CB. Cutaneous findings in chronic lymphocytic leukaemia. *Br J Dermatol.* 2004;150(6):1129-1135.
156. Galton DA. The pathogenesis of chronic lymphocytic leukemia. *Can Med Assoc J.* 1966;94:1005-1011.
157. Baumann T, Moia R, Gaidano G, et al. Lymphocyte doubling time in chronic lymphocytic leukemia modern era: a real-life study in 848 unselected patients. *Leukemia.* 2021;35(8):2325-2331.
158. Feliu E, Rozman C, Montserrat E, Gallart T, Marques-Pereira J. Cytoplasmic inclusions in lymphocytes of chronic lymphocytic leukaemia. *Scand J Haematol.* 1983;31(5):510-512.
159. Binet JL, Baudet S, Mentz F, et al. Basket cells or shadow cells of Gumprecht: a scanning electron microscopy study, and the correlation between percentages of basket cells, and cells with altered chromatin structure (dense cells) i chronic lymphocyic leukemia. *Blood Cell.* 1993;19:573-581.
160. Nowakowski GS, Hoyer JD, Shanafelt TD, et al. Percentage of smudge cells on routine blood smear predicts survival in chronic lymphocytic leukemia. *J Clin Oncol.* 2009;27(11):1844-1849.
161. Matutes E, Attygalle A, Wotherspoon A, Catovsky D. Diagnostic issues in chronic lymphocytic leukaemia (CLL). *Best Pract Res Clin Haematol.* 2010;23(1):3-20.
162. Swerdlow SH, Campo E, Harris NL, Al E. *WHO Classification of Tumours of Haematopoietic and Lymphoid Tissues.* 4th ed. International Agency for Research on Cancer; 2017.
163. Chang JC, Harrington AM, Olteanu H, VanTuinen P, Kroft SH. Proliferation centers in bone marrows involved by chronic lymphocytic leukemia/small lymphocytic lymphoma: a clinicopathologic analysis. *Ann Diagn Pathol.* 2016;25:15-19.
164. Kipps TJ, Carson DA. Autoantibodies in chronic lymphocytic leukemia and related systemic autoimmune diseases. *Blood.* 1993;81(10):2475-2487.
165. DiRaimondo F, Albitar M, Huh Y, et al. The clinical and diagnostic relevance of CD23 expression in the chronic lymphoproliferative disease. *Cancer.* 2002;94(6):1721-1730.
166. D'Arena G, De Feo V, Pietrantuono G, et al. CD200 and chronic lymphocytic leukemia: biological and clinical relevance. *Front Oncol.* 2020;10:584427.
167. Deans JP, Polyak MJ. FMC7 is an epitope of CD20. *Blood.* 2008;111(4):2492.
168. Alfarano a, Indraccolo S, Circosta P, et al. An alternatively spliced form of CD79b gene may account for altered B-cell receptor expression in B-chronic lymphocytic leukemia. *Blood.* 1999;93(7):2327-2335.
169. Rizzo D, Chauzeix J, Trimoreau F, et al. IgM peak independently predicts treatment-free survival in chronic lymphocytic leukemia and correlates with accumulation of adverse oncogenetic events. *Leukemia.* 2015;29:337-345.
170. Parikh SA, Leis JF, Chaffee KG, et al. Hypogammaglobulinemia in newly diagnosed chronic lymphocytic leukemia: natural history, clinical correlates, and outcomes. *Cancer.* 2015;121(17):2883-2891.
171. Pratt G, Harding S, Holder R, et al. Abnormal serum free light chain ratios are associated with poor survival and may reflect biological subgroups in patients with chronic lymphocytic leukaemia. *Br J Haematol.* 2009;144(2):217-222.
172. Morabito F, De Filippi R, Laurenti L, et al. The cumulative amount of serum-free light chain is a strong prognosticator in chronic lymphocytic leukemia. *Blood.* 2011;118(24):6353-6361.
173. Forconi F, Moss P. Perturbation of the normal immune system in patients with CLL. *Blood.* 2015;126(5):573-581.
174. Riches JC, Gribben JG. Understanding the immunodeficiency in chronic lymphocytic leukemia. Potential clinical implications. *Hematol Oncol Clin North Am.* 2013;27(2):207-235.
175. Ravandi F, O'Brien S. Immune defects in patients with chronic lymphocytic leukemia. *Cancer Immunol Immunother.* 2006;55(2):197-209.
176. Hilal T, Gea Banacloche JC, Leis JF. Chronic lymphocytic leukemia and infection risk in the era of targeted therapies: linking mechanisms with infections. *Blood Rev.* 2018;32(5):387-399.
177. Tsimberidou AM, Wen S, McLaughlin P, et al. Other malignancies in chronic lymphocytic leukemia/small lymphocytic lymphoma. *J Clin Oncol.* 2009;27(6):904-910.
178. Ishdorj G, Beiggi S, Nugent Z, et al. Risk factors for skin cancer and solid tumors in newly diagnosed patients with chronic lymphocytic leukemia and the impact of skin surveillance on survival. *Leuk Lymphoma.* 2019;60(13):3204-3213.
179. Mulligan SP, Shumack S, Guminski A. Chronic lymphocytic leukemia, skin and other second cancers. *Leuk Lymphoma.* 2019;60(13):3104-3106.
180. Andersen MA, Eriksen CT, Brieghel C, et al. Incidence and predictors of infection among patients prior to treatment of chronic lymphocytic leukemia: a Danish nationwide cohort study. *Haematologica.* 2018;103:e301-e303.
181. Reda G, Cassin R, Gentile M, et al. IgA hypogammaglobulinemia predicts outcome in chronic lymphocytic leukemia. *Leukemia.* 2019;33(6):1519-1522.
182. Mohr A, Renaudineau Y, Bagacean C, et al. Regulatory B lymphocyte functions should be considered in chronic lymphocytic leukemia. *Oncoimmunology.* 2016;5(5):e1132977.
183. Kremer JP, Reisbach G, Nerl C, Dormer P. B-cell chronic lymphocytic leukaemia cells express and release transforming growth factor-beta. *Br J Haematol.* 1992;80:480-487.
184. Lagneaux L, Delforge A, Dorval C, Bron D, Stryckans P. Excessive production of transforming growth factor-beta by bone marrow stromal cells in B-cell chronic lymphocytic leukemia inhibits growth of hematopoietic precursors and interleukin-6 production. *Blood.* 1993;82(8):2379-2385.
185. Purroy N, Tong YE, Lemvigh CK, et al. Single-cell analysis reveals immune dysfunction from the earliest stages of CLL that can be reversed by ibrutinib. *Blood.* 2022;139(14):2252-2256.
186. Riches JC, Davies JK, McClanahan F, et al. T cells from CLL patients exhibit features of T-cell exhaustion but retain capacity for cytokine production. *Blood.* 2013;121(9):1612-1621.
187. Görgün G, Holderried TW, Zahrieh D, Neuberg D, Gribben JG. Chronic lymphocytic leukemia cells induce changes in gene expression of CD4 and CD8 T cells. *J Clin Investig.* 2005;115(7):1797-1805.
188. Ramsay AG, Johnson AJ, Lee AM, et al. Chronic lymphocytic leukemia T cells show impaired immunological synapse formation that can be reversed with an immunomodulating drug. *J Clin Investig.* 2008;118(7):2427-2437.
189. Ferrer G, Jung B, Chiu PY, et al. Myeloid-derived suppressor cell subtypes differentially influence T-cell function, T-helper subset differentiation, and clinical course in CLL. *Leukemia.* 2021;35(11):3163-3175.
190. Middleton O, Cosimo E, Dobbin E, et al. Complement deficiencies limit CD20 monoclonal antibody treatment efficacy in CLL. *Leukemia.* 2015;29(1):107-114.
191. Itala M, Vainio O, Remes K. Functional abnormalities in granulocytes predict susceptibility to bacterial in chronic lymphocytic leukaemia. *Eur J Haematol.* 1996;57(1):46-53.
192. Morrison VA. Infectious complications of chronic lymphocytic leukaemia: pathogenesis, spectrum of infection, preventive approaches. *Best Pract Res Clin Haematol.* 2010;23(1):145-153.
193. Whitaker JA, Shanafelt TD, Poland GA, Kay NE. Room for improvement: immunizations for patients with monoclonal B-cell lymphocytosis or chronic lymphocytic leukemia. *Clin Adv Hematol Oncol.* 2014;12(7):440-450.
194. Roeker LE, Knorr DA, Thompson MC, et al. COVID-19 vaccine efficacy in patients with chronic lymphocytic leukemia. *Leukemia.* 2021;35(9):2703-2705.
195. Sun C, Tian X, Lee YS, et al. Partial reconstitution of humoral immunity and fewer infections in patients with chronic lymphocytic leukemia treated with ibrutinib. *Blood.* 2015;126(19):2213-2219.
196. Fiorcari S, Maffei R, Vallerini D, et al. BTK inhibition impairs the innate response against fungal infection in patients with chronic lymphocytic leukemia. *Front Immunol.* 2020;11:2158.
197. Maschmeyer G, De Greef J, Mellinghoff SC, et al. Infections associated with immunotherapeutic and molecular targeted agents in hematology and oncology. A position paper by the European Conference on Infections in Leukemia (ECIL). *Leukemia.* 2019;33(44):844-862.
198. Rossi D, Shadman M, Condoluci A, et al. How we manage patients with chronic lymphocytic leukemia during the SARS-CoV-2 pandemic. *HemaSphere.* 2020;4(4):e432-e432.
199. Mato AR, Roeker LE, Lamanna N, et al. Outcomes of COVID-19 in patients with CLL: a multicenter, international experience. *Blood.* 2020;136(10):1134-1143.
200. Scarfò L, Chatzikonstantinou T, Rigolin GM, et al. COVID-19 severity and mortality in patients with chronic lymphocytic leukemia: a joint study by ERIC, the European Research Initiative on CLL, and CLL Campus. *Leukemia.* 2020;34(9):2354-2363.

201. Fiorcari S, Atene CG, Maffei R, et al. Ibrutinib interferes with innate immunity in chronic lymphocytic leukemia patients during COVID-19 infection. *Haematologica.* 2021;106(8):2265-2268.
202. Avanzato VA, Matson MJ, Seifert SN, et al. Case study: prolonged infectious SARS-CoV-2 shedding from an asymptomatic immunocompromised individual with cancer. *Cell.* 2020;183(7):1901-1912.
203. Niemann CU, da Cunha-Bang C, Helleberg M, Ostrowski SR, Brieghel C. Patients with CLL have lower risk of death from COVID-19 in the Omicron era. *Blood.* 2022;140(5):445-450.
204. Pasiarski M, Rolinski J, Grywalska E, et al. Antibody and plasmablast response to 13-valent pneumococcal conjugate vaccine in chronic lymphocytic leukemia patients - preliminary report. *PLoS One.* 2014;9(12):1-14.
205. Pleyer C, Ali MA, Cohen JI, et al. Effect of Bruton tyrosine kinase inhibitor on efficacy of adjuvanted recombinant hepatitis B and zoster vaccines. *Blood.* 2021;137(2):185-189.
206. Douglas AP, Trubiano JA, Barr I, Leung V, Slavin MA, Tam CS. Ibrutinib may impair serological responses to influenza vaccination. *Haematologica.* 2017;102(10):e397-e399.
207. Herishanu Y, Avivi I, Aharon A, et al. Efficacy of the BNT162b2 mRNA COVID-19 vaccine in patients with chronic lymphocytic leukemia. *Blood.* 2021;137(23):3165-3173.
208. Roeker LE, Knorr DA, Pessin MS, et al. Anti-SARS-CoV-2 antibody response in patients with chronic lymphocytic leukemia. *Leukemia.* 2020;34(11):3047-3049.
209. Parry H, McIlroy G, Bruton R, et al. Impaired neutralisation of SARS-CoV-2 delta variant in vaccinated patients with B cell chronic lymphocytic leukaemia. *J Hematol Oncol.* 2022;15(1):3.
210. Mellinghoff SC, Robrecht S, Mayer L, et al. SARS-CoV-2 specific cellular response following COVID-19 vaccination in patients with chronic lymphocytic leukemia. *Leukemia.* 2022;36(2):562-565.
211. Haydu JE, Maron JS, Redd RA, et al. Humoral and cellular immunogenicity of SARS-CoV-2 vaccines in chronic lymphocytic leukemia: a prospective cohort study. *Blood Adv.* 2022;6(6):1671-1683.
212. Beiggi S, Johnston JB, Seftel MD, et al. Increased risk of second malignancies in chronic lymphocytic leukaemia patients as compared with follicular lymphoma patients: a Canadian population-based study. *Br J Cancer.* 2013;109(5):1287-1290.
213. Royle JA, Baade PD, Joske D, Girschik J, Fritschi L. Second cancer incidence and cancer mortality among chronic lymphocytic leukaemia patients: a population-based study. *Br J Cancer.* 2011;105(7):1076-1081.
214. Tadmor T, Aviv A, Polliack A. Merkel cell carcinoma, chronic lymphocytic leukemia and other lymphoproliferative disorders: an old bond with possible new viral ties. *Ann Oncol.* 2011;22(2):250-256.
215. Brewer JD, Shanafelt TD, Otley CC, et al. Chronic lymphocytic leukemia is associated with decreased survival of patients with malignant melanoma and merkel cell carcinoma in a SEER population-based study. *J Clin Oncol.* 2012;30(8):843-849.
216. Solomon BM, Rabe KG, Slager SL, Brewer JD, Cerhan JR, Shanafelt TD. Overall and cancer-specific survival of patients with breast, colon, kidney, and lung cancers with and without chronic lymphocytic leukemia: a SEER population-based study. *J Clin Oncol.* 2013;31(7):930-937.
217. Furstenau M, Giza A, Stumpf T, et al. Second primary malignancies in treated and untreated patients with chronic lymphocytic leukemia. *Am J Hematol.* 2021;96(12):E457-E460.
218. Mulcahy A, Mulligan SP, Shumack SP. Recommendations for skin cancer monitoring for patients with chronic lymphocytic leukemia. *Leuk Lymphoma.* 2018;59(3):578-582.
219. Falchi L, Vitale C, Keating MJ, et al. Incidence and prognostic impact of other cancers in a population of long-term survivors of chronic lymphocytic leukemia. *Ann Oncol.* 2016;27(6):1100-1106.
220. Bond DA, Huang Y, Fisher JL, et al. Second cancer incidence in CLL patients receiving BTK inhibitors. *Leukemia.* 2020;34(12):3197-3205.
221. Benjamini O, Jain P, Trinh L, et al. Second cancers in patients with chronic lymphocytic leukemia who received frontline fludarabine, cyclophosphamide and rituximab therapy: distribution and clinical outcomes. *Leuk Lymphoma.* 2015;56(6):1643-1650.
222. Maddocks-Christianson K, Slager SL, Zent CS, et al. Risk factors for development of a second lymphoid malignancy in patients with chronic lymphocytic leukaemia. *Br J Haematol.* 2007;139(3):398-404.
223. Kriangkum J, Motz SN, Debes Marun CS, et al. Frequent occurrence of highly expanded but unrelated B-cell clones in patients with multiple myeloma. *PLoS One.* 2013;8(5):e64927.
224. Todisco G, Manshouri T, Verstovsek S, et al. Chronic lymphocytic leukemia and myeloproliferative neoplasms concurrently diagnosed: clinical and biological characteristics. *Leuk Lymphoma.* 2016;57(5):1054-1059.
225. Hamblin TJ. Autoimmune complications of chronic lymphocytic leukemia. *Semin Oncol.* 2006;33:230-239.
226. Visco C, Cortelezzi A, Moretta F, et al. Autoimmune cytopenias in chronic lymphocytic leukemia at disease presentation in the modern treatment era: is stage C always stage C? *Leuk Lymphoma.* 2014;55(6):1261-1265.
227. Mittal S, Blaylock MG, Culligan DJ, Barker RN, Vickers MA. A high rate of CLL phenotype lymphocytes in autoimmune hemolytic anemia and immune thrombocytopenic purpura. *Haematologica.* 2008;93(1):151-152.
228. Hodgson K, Ferrer G, Pereira A, Moreno C, Montserrat E. Autoimmune cytopenia in chronic lymphocytic leukaemia: diagnosis and treatment. *Br J Haematol.* 2011;154(1):14-22.
229. Dearden C, Wade R, Else M, et al. The prognostic significance of a positive direct antiglobulin test in chronic lymphocytic leukemia: a beneficial effect of the combination of fludarabine and cyclophosphamide on the incidence of hemolytic anemia. *Blood.* 2008;111(4):1820-1826.
230. Borthakur G, O'Brien S, Wierda WG, et al. Immune anaemias in patients with chronic lymphocytic leukaemia treated with fludarabine, cyclophosphamide and rituximab - incidence and predictors. *Br J Haematol.* 2007;136(6):800-805.
231. Rogers KA, Ruppert AS, Bingman A, et al. Incidence and description of autoimmune cytopenias during treatment with ibrutinib for chronic lymphocytic leukemia. *Leukemia.* 2016;30(2):346-350.
232. Hodgson K, Ferrer G, Montserrat E, Moreno C. Chronic lymphocytic leukemia and autoimmunity: a systematic review. *Haematologica.* 2011;96(5):752-761.
233. Visco C, Barcellini W, Maura F, Neri A, Cortelezzi A, Rodeghiero F. Autoimmune cytopenias in chronic lymphocytic leukemia. *Am J Hematol.* 2014;89(11):1055-1062.
234. Ruzickova S, Pruss A, Odendahl M, et al. Chronic lymphocytic leukemia preceded by cold agglutinin disease: intraclonal immunoglobulin light-chain diversity in V H4-34 expressing single leukemic B cells. *Blood.* 2002;100(9):3419-3422.
235. Anhalt GJ, SooChan K, Stanley JR, et al. Paraneoplastic pemphigus. An autoimmune mucocutaneous disease associated with neoplasia. *N Engl J Med.* 1990;323(25):1729-1735.
236. Go RS, Winters JL, Kay NE. How I treat autoimmune hemolytic anemia. *Blood.* 2017;129(22):2971-2979.
237. Gaidano G, Rossi D. The mutational landscape of chronic lymphocytic leukemia and its impact on prognosis and treatment. *Hematology Am Soc Hematol Educ Program.* 2017;2017(1):329-337.
238. The International CLL-IPI Working Group. An international prognostic index for patients with chronic lymphocytic leukaemia (CLL-IPI): a meta-analysis of individual patient data. *Lancet Oncol.* 2016;17(6):779-790.
239. Catovsky D, Wade R, Else M. The clinical significance of patients' sex in chronic lymphocytic leukemia. *Haematologica.* 2014;99(6):1088-1094.
240. Matutes E, Oscier D, Garcia-Marco J, et al. Trisomy 12 defines a group of CLL with atypical morphology: correlation between cytogenetic, clinical and laboratory features in 544 patients. *Br J Haematol.* 1996;92(2):382-388.
241. Oscier D, Else M, Matutes E, Morilla R, Strefford JC, Catovsky D. The morphology of CLL revisited: the clinical significance of prolymphocytes and correlations with prognostic/molecular markers in the LRF CLL4 trial. *Br J Haematol.* 2016;174(5):767-775.
242. Rassenti LZ, Kipps TJ. Clinical utility of assessing ZAP-70 and CD38 in chronic lymphocytic leukemia. *Cytometry B Clin Cytometry.* 2006;70B:209-213.
243. Malavasi F, Deaglio S, Damle R, Cutrona G, Ferrarini M, Chiorazzi N. CD38 and chronic lymphocytic leukemia: a decade later. *Blood.* 2011;118(13):3470-3479.
244. Damle RN, Temburni S, Calissano C, et al. CD38 expression labels an activated subset within chronic lymphocytic leukemia clones enriched in proliferating B cells. *Blood.* 2007;110(9):3352-3359.
245. Pepper C, Majid A, Lin TT, et al. Defining the prognosis of early stage chronic lymphocytic leukaemia patients. *Br J Haematol.* 2012;156(4):499-507.
246. Rassenti LZ, Huynh L, Toy TL, et al. ZAP-70 compared with immunoglobulin heavy-chain gene mutation status as a predictor of disease progression in chronic lymphocytic leukemia. *N Engl J Med.* 2004;351(9):893-901.
247. Benedetti D, Tissino E, Caldana C, et al. Persistent CD49d engagement in circulating CLL cells: a role for blood-borne ligands?. *Leukemia.* 2016;30:513-517.
248. Dal Bo M, Bulian P, Bomben R, et al. CD49d prevails over the novel recurrent mutations as independent prognosticator of overall survival in chronic lymphocytic leukemia. *Leukemia.* 2016;30(10):2011-2018.
249. Baumann T, Delgado J, Santacruz R, et al. CD49d (ITGA4) expression is a predictor of time to first treatment in patients with chronic lymphocytic leukaemia and mutated IGHV status. *Br J Haematol.* 2016;172:48-55.
250. Bulian P, Shanafelt TD, Fegan C, et al. CD49d is the strongest flow cytometry-based predictor of overall survival in chronic lymphocytic leukemia. *J Clin Oncol.* 2014;32(9):897-904.
251. Zenz T, Kro A, Scherer K, et al. Monoallelic TP53 inactivation is associated with poor prognosis in chronic lymphocytic leukemia: results from a detailed genetic characterization with long-term follow-up. *Blood.* 2008;112(8):3322-3329.
252. Ahn IE, Tian X, Wiestner A. Ibrutinib for chronic lymphocytic leukemia with TP53 alterations. *N Engl J Med.* 2020;383(5):498-500.
253. Roberts AW, Ma S, Kipps TJ, et al. Efficacy of venetoclax in relapsed chronic lymphocytic leukemia is influenced by disease and response variables. *Blood.* 2019;134(2):111-122.
254. Lens D, Dyer MJ, Garcia-Marco JM, et al. p53 abnormalities in CLL are associated with excess of prolymphocytes and poor prognosis. *Br J Haematol.* 1997;99(4):848-857.
255. Tam CS, Shanafelt TD, Wierda WG, et al. De novo deletion 17p13.1 chronic lymphocytic leukemia shows significant clinical heterogeneity: the M. D. Anderson and Mayo Clinic experience. *Blood.* 2009;114(5):957-964.
256. Strati P, Abruzzo LV, Wierda WG, O'Brien S, Ferrajoli A, Keating MJ. Second cancers and Richter transformation are the leading causes of death in patients with trisomy 12 chronic lymphocytic leukemia. *Clin Lymphoma Myeloma Leuk.* 2015;15(7):420-427.
257. Hjalmar V, Kimby E, Matutes E, Sundstrom C, Wallvik J, Hast R. Atypical lymphocytes in B-cell chronic lymphocytic leukemia and trisomy 12 studied by conventional staining combined with fluorescence in situ hybridization. *Leuk Lymphoma.* 2000;37(5-6):571-576.
258. Dal Bo M, Rossi FM, Rossi D, et al. 13q14 Deletion size and number of deleted cells both influence prognosis in chronic lymphocytic leukemia. *Gene Chromosome Cancer.* 2011;50:633-643.
259. Ouillette P, Collins R, Shakhan S, et al. The prognostic significance of various 13q14 deletions in chronic lymphocytic leukemia. *Clin Cancer Res.* 2011;17(21):6778-6790.

260. Damle RN, Wasil T, Fais F, et al. Ig V gene mutation status and CD38 expression as novel prognostic indicators in chronic lymphocytic leukemia. *Blood.* 1999;94(6):1840-1847.
261. Hamblin BTJ, Davis Z, Gardiner A, Oscier DG, Stevenson FK. Unmutated Ig V(H) genes are associated with a more aggressive form of chronic lymphocytic leukemia. *Blood.* 1999;94(6):1848-1854.
262. Baliakas P, Agathangelidis A, Hadzidimitriou A, et al. Not all IGHV3-21 chronic lymphocytic leukemias are equal: prognostic considerations. *Blood.* 2015;125(5):856-859.
263. Jebaraj BMC, Stilgenbauer S. Telomere dysfunction in chronic lymphocytic leukemia. *Front Oncol.* 2021;10:612665.
264. Nadeu F, Delgado J, Royo C, et al. Clinical impact of clonal and subclonal TP53, SF3B1, BIRC3, NOTCH1, and ATM mutations in chronic lymphocytic leukemia. *Blood.* 2016;127(17):2122-2130.
265. Guieze R, Robbe P, Clifford R, et al. Presence of multiple recurrent mutations confers poor trial outcome of relapsed/refractory CLL. *Blood.* 2015;126(18):2110-2118.
266. Rossi D. Richter's syndrome: novel and promising therapeutic alternatives. *Best Pract Res Clin Haematol.* 2016;29(1):30-39.
267. Wan Y, Wu CJ. SF3B1 mutations in chronic lymphocytic leukemia. *Blood.* 2013;121(23):4627-4634.
268. Visone R, Veronese A, Rassenti LZ, et al. miR-181b is a biomarker of disease progression in chronic lymphocytic leukemia. *Blood.* 2011;118(11):3072-3079.
269. Montserrat E, Villamor N, Reverter JC, et al. Bone marrow assessment in B-cell chronic lymphocytic leukaemia: aspirate or biopsy? A comparative study in 258 patients. *Br J Haematol.* 1996;93(1):111-116.
270. Oudat R, Keating MJ, Lerner S, O'Brien S, Albitar M. Significance of the levels of bone marrow lymphoid infiltrate in chronic lymphocytic leukemia patients with nodular partial remission. *Leukemia.* 2002;16(4):632-635.
271. Van Bockstaele F, Verhasselt B, Philippé J. Prognostic markers in chronic lymphocytic leukemia: a comprehensive review. *Blood Rev.* 2009;23(1):25-47.
272. Letestu R, Lévy V, Eclache V, et al. Prognosis of Binet stage A chronic lymphocytic leukemia patients: the strength of routine parameters. *Blood.* 2010;116(22):4588-4590.
273. Gentile M, Cutrona G, Neri A, Molica S, Ferrarini M, Morabito F. Predictive value of β2-microgobulin (β2-m) levels in chronic lymphocytic leukemia since Binet A stages. *Haematologica.* 2009;94(6):887-888.
274. Delgado J, Pratt G, Phillips N, et al. Beta2-microglobulin is a better predictor of treatment-free survival in patients with chronic lymphocytic leukaemia if adjusted according to glomerular filtration rate. *Br J Haematol.* 2009;145(6):801-805.
275. Thompson PA, O'Brien SM, Xiao L, et al. β2-microglobulin normalization within 6 months of ibrutinib-based treatment is associated with superior progression-free survival in patients with chronic lymphocytic leukemia. *Cancer.* 2015;122(4):565-573.
276. Ferrajoli A, Keating MJ, Manshouri T, Giles FJ. The clinical significance of tumor necrosis factor-α plasma level in patients having chronic lymphocytic leukemia. *Blood.* 2002;100(4):1215-1220.
277. Fayad L, Keating MJ, Reuben JM, et al. Interleukin-6 and interleukin-10 levels in chronic lymphocytic leukemia: correlation with phenotypic characteristics and outcome. *Blood.* 2001;97(1):256-263.
278. Wierda WG, Johnson MM, Do KA, et al. Plasma interleukin 8 level predicts for survival in chronic lymphocytic leukaemia. *Br J Haematol.* 2003;120(3):452-456.
279. Yan XJ, Dozmorov I, Li W, et al. Identification of outcome-correlated cytokine clusters in chronic lymphocytic leukemia. *Blood.* 2011;118(19):5201-5210.
280. Molica S, Digiesi G, Antenucci A, et al. Vitamin D insufficiency predicts time to first treatment (TFT) in early chronic lymphocytic leukemia (CLL). *Leuk Res.* 2012;36(4):443-447.
281. Shanafelt TD, Drake MT, Maurer MJ, et al. Vitamin D insufficiency and prognosis in chronic lymphocytic leukemia. *Blood.* 2011;117(5):1492-1498.
282. Wierda WG, O'Brien S, Wang X, et al. Prognostic nomogram and index for overall survival in previously untreated patients with chronic lymphocytic leukemia. *Blood.* 2007;109(11):4679-4685.
283. Shanafelt TD, Jenkins G, Call TG, et al. Validation of a new prognostic index for patients with chronic lymphocytic leukemia. *Cancer.* 2009;115:363-372.
284. Molica S, Shanafelt TD, Giannarelli D, et al. The chronic lymphocytic leukemia international prognostic index predicts time to first treatment in early CLL: independent validation in a prospective cohort of early stage patients. *Am J Hematol.* 2016;91(11):1090-1095.
285. Soumerai JD, Ni A, Darif M, et al. Prognostic risk score for patients with relapsed or refractory chronic lymphocytic leukaemia treated with targeted therapies or chemoimmunotherapy: a retrospective, pooled cohort study with external validations. *Lancet Haematol.* 2019;6(7):e366-e374.
286. Gentile M, Morabito F, Del Poeta G, et al. Survival risk score for real-life relapsed/refractory chronic lymphocytic leukemia patients receiving ibrutinib. A campus CLL study. *Leukemia.* 2021;35:235-238.
287. Ahn IE, Tian X, Ipe D, et al. Prediction of outcome in patients with chronic lymphocytic leukemia treated with ibrutinib: development and validation of a four-factor prognostic model. *J Clin Oncol.* 2021;39(6):576-585.
288. Wierda WG, Rawstron A, Cymbalista F, et al. Measurable residual disease in chronic lymphocytic leukemia: expert review and consensus recommendations. *Leukemia.* 2021;35(11):3059-3072.
289. Rawstron AC, Villamor N, Ritgen M, et al. International standardized approach for flow cytometric residual disease monitoring in chronic lymphocytic leukaemia. *Leukemia.* 2007;21(5):956-964.
290. Thompson PA. MRD negativity as a surrogate for PFS in CLL? *Blood.* 2018;131(9):943-944.
291. Thompson PA, Tam CS, O'Brien SM, et al. Fludarabine, cyclophosphamide, and rituximab treatment achieves long-term disease-free survival in IGHV-mutated chronic lymphocytic leukemia. *Blood.* 2016;127(3):303-309.
292. Galton DAG, Israels LG, Nabarro JDN, Till M. Clinical trials of p-(di-2-chloroethylamino)-phenylbutyric acid (CB 1348) in malignant lymphoma. *Br Med J.* 1955;2(4949):1172-1176.
293. Sawitsky A, Rai KR, Glidewell O, Silver RT. Comparison of daily versus intermittent chlorambucil and prednisone therapy in the treatment of patients with chronic lymphocytic leukemia. *Blood.* 1977;50(6):1049-1059.
294. Knospe WH, Loeb V, Huculey CM. Bi-weekly chlorambucil treatment of chronic lymphocytic leukemia. *Cancer.* 1974;33(2):555-562.
295. Catovsky D, Richards S, Matutes E, et al. Assessment of fludarabine plus cyclophosphamide for patients with chronic lymphocytic leukaemia (the LRF CLL4 Trial): a randomised controlled trial. *Lancet.* 2007;370(9583):230-239.
296. Eichhorst BF, Busch R, Stilgenbauer S, et al. First-line therapy with fludarabine compared with chlorambucil does not result in a major benefit for elderly patients with advanced chronic lymphocytic leukemia. *Blood.* 2009;114:3382-3391.
297. Montserrat E, Rozman C, Ronan C. Chronic lymphocytic leukaemia treatment. *Blood Rev.* 1993;7(3):164-175.
298. Michallet AS, Rossignol J, Cazin B, Ysebaert L. Rituximab-cyclophosphamide-dexamethasone combination in management of autoimmune cytopenias associated with chronic lymphocytic leukemia. *Leuk Lymphoma.* 2011;52(7):1401-1403.
299. Han T, Ezdinli EZ, Shimaoka K, Desai DV. Chlorambucil vs. combined chlorambucil-corticosteroid therapy in chronic lymphocytic leukemia. *Cancer.* 1973;31(3):502-508.
300. Kost SEF, Bouchard EDJ, Labossière É, et al. Cross-resistance and synergy with bendamustine in chronic lymphocytic leukemia. *Leuk Res.* 2016;50:63-71.
301. Leoni LM, Bailey B, Reifert J, et al. Bendamustine (Treanda) displays a distinct pattern of cytotoxicity and unique mechanistic features compared with other alkylating agents. *Clin Cancer Res.* 2008;14(1):309-317.
302. Knauf WU, Lissitchkov T, Aldaoud A, et al. Bendamustine compared with chlorambucil in previously untreated patients with chronic lymphocytic leukaemia: updated results of a randomized phase III trial. *Br J Haematol.* 2012;159(1):67-77.
303. Johnston JB. Mechanism of action of pentostatin and cladribine in hairy cell leukemia. *Leuk Lymphoma.* 2011;52(suppl 2):43-45.
304. Genini D, Adachi S, Chao Q, et al. Deoxyadenosine analogs induce programmed cell death in chronic lymphocytic leukemia cells by damaging the DNA and by directly affecting the mitochondria. *Blood.* 2000;96(10):3537-3543.
305. Ho AD, Thaler J, Stryckmans P, et al. Pentostatin in refractory chronic lymphocytic leukemia: a phase II trial of the European organization for research and treatment of cancer. *J Natl Cancer Institute.* 1990;82(17):1416-1420.
306. Dillman RO, Mick R, McIntyre OR. Pentostatin in chronic lymphocytic leukemia: a phase II trial of Cancer and Leukemia Group B. *J Clin Oncol.* 1989;7(4):433-438.
307. Shustik C, Turner AR, Desjardins P, et al. Oral fludarabine in untreated patients with B-cell chronic lymphocytic leukemia. *Leukemia.* 2010;24(1):237-239.
308. Keating MJ, O'Brien S, Kantarjian H, et al. Long-term follow-up of patients with chronic lymphocytic leukemia treated with fludarabine as a single agent. *Blood.* 1993;81(11):2878-2884.
309. Sorensen JM, Vena DA, Allavollita A, Chun HG, Cheson BD. Treatment of refractory chronic lymphocytic leukemia with fludarabine phosphate via the group C protocol mechanism of the National Cancer Institute: five year follow-up report. *J Clin Oncol.* 1997;15(2):458-465.
310. Johnson S, Smith AG, Loffler H, et al. Multicentre prospective randomised trial of fludarabine versus cyclophosphamide, doxorubicin, and prednisone (CAP) for treatment of advanced-stage chronic lymphocytic leukaemia. The French Cooperative Group on CLL. *Lancet.* 1996;347(9013):1432-1438.
311. Rai KR, Peterson BL, Appelbaum FR, et al. Fludarabine compared with chlorambucil as primary therapy for chronic lymphocytic leukemia. *N Engl J Med.* 2000;343(24):1750-1757.
312. Leporrier M, Chevret S, Cazin B, et al. Randomized comparison of fludarabine CAP, ad CHOP in 938 untreated stage B and C chronic lymphocytic leukemia patients. *Blood.* 2001;98:2319-2325.
313. Keating MJ, O'Brien S, Lerner S, et al. Long-term follow-up of patients with chronic lymphocytic leukemia (CLL) receiving fludarabine regimens as initial therapy. *Blood.* 1998;92(4):1165-1171.
314. Robertson LE, O'Brien S, Kantarjian H, et al. A 3-day schedule of fludarabine in previously treated chronic lymphocytic leukemia. *Leukemia.* 1995;9:1444-1449.
315. Cheson BD, Vena DA, Foss FM, Sorensen JM. Neurotoxicity of purine analogs: a review. *J Clin Oncol.* 1994;12(10):2216-2228.
316. Tallman MS, Hakimian D. Purine nucleoside analogs: emerging roles in indolent lymphoproliferative disorders. *Blood.* 1995;86(7):2463-2474.
317. Robak T, Jamroziak K, Gora-Tybor J, et al. Comparison of cladribine plus cyclophosphamide with fludarabine plus cyclophosphamide as first-line therapy for chronic lymphocytic leukemia: a phase III randomized study by the Polish Adult Leukemia Group (PALG-CLL3 study). *J Clin Oncol.* 2010;28(11):1863-1869.
318. Weiss MA, Maslak PG, Jurcic JG, et al. Pentostatin and cyclophosphamide: an effective new regimen in previously treated patients with chronic lymphocytic leukemia. *J Clin Oncol.* 2003;21(7):1278-1284.
319. Thornton PD, Matutes E, Bosanquet AG, et al. High dose methylprednisolone can induce remissions in CLL patients with p53 abnormalities. *Ann Hematol.* 2003;82(12):759-765.
320. Alduaij W, Illidge TM. The future of anti-CD20 monoclonal antibodies: are we making progress? *Blood.* 2011;117(11):2993-3001.
321. Cartron G, Trappe RU, Solal-Céligny P, Hallek M. Interindividual variability of response to rituximab: from biological origins to individualized therapies. *Clin Cancer Res.* 2011;17(1):19-30.

322. Alduaij W, Ivanov A, Honeychurch J, et al. Novel type II anti-CD20 monoclonal antibody (GA101) evokes homotypic adhesion and actin-dependent, lysosome-mediated cell death in B-cell malignancies. *Blood.* 2011;117(17):4519-4529.
323. Honeychurch J, Alduaij W, Cheadle E, et al. Antibody-induced non-apoptotic cell death in human lymphoma and leukemia cells is mediated through NADPH oxidase-derived reactive oxygen species. *Blood.* 2012;119(15):3523-3533.
324. Wierda WG, Padmanabhan S, Chan GW, et al. Ofatumumab is active in patients with fludarabine-refractory CLL irrespective of prior rituximab: results from the phase 2 international study. *Blood.* 2011;118(19):5126-5129.
325. Byrd JC, Flynn JM, Kipps TJ, et al. Randomized phase 2 study of obinutuzumab monotherapy in symptomatic, Previously untreated chronic lymphocytic leukemia. *Blood.* 2016;127(1):79-86.
326. Gribben JG, Hallek M. Rediscovering alemtuzumab: current and emerging therapeutic roles. *Br J Haematol.* 2009;144(6):818-831.
327. Alas S, Emmanouilides C, Bonavida B. Inhibition of interleukin 10 by Rituximab results in down-regulation of Bcl-2 and sensitization of B-cell non-Hodgkin's lymphoma to apoptosis. *Clin Cancer Res.* 2001;7(3):709-723.
328. Byrd JC, Kitada S, Flinn IW, et al. The mechanism of tumor cell clearance by rituximab in vivo in patients with B-cell chronic lymphocytic leukemia: evidence of caspase activation and apoptosis induction. *Blood.* 2002;99(3):1038-1043.
329. Di Gaetano N, Xiao Y, Erba E, et al. Synergism between fludarabine and rituximab revealed in a follicular lymphoma cell line resistant to the cytotoxic activity of either drug alone. *Br J Haematol.* 2001;114(4):800-809.
330. Byrd JC, Peterson BL, Morrison Va, et al. Randomized phase 2 study of fludarabine with concurrent versus sequential treatment with rituximab in symptomatic, untreated patients with B-cell chronic lymphocytic leukemia: results from Cancer and Leukemia Group B 9712 (CALGB 9712). *Blood.* 2003;101(1):6-14.
331. Byrd JC, Rai K, Peterson BL, et al. Addition of rituximab to fludarabine may prolong progression-free survival and overall survival in patients with previously untreated chronic lymphocytic leukemia: an updated retrospective comparative analysis of CALGB 9712 and CALGB 9011. *Blood.* 2005;105(1):49-53.
332. Woyach JA, Ruppert AS, Heerema NA, et al. Chemoimmunotherapy with fludarabine and rituximab produces extended overall survival and progression-free survival in chronic lymphocytic leukemia: long-term follow-up of CALGB study 9712. *J Clin Oncol.* 2011;29(10):1349-1355.
333. Kay NE, Wu W, Kabat B, et al. Pentostatin and rituximab therapy for previously untreated patients with B-cell chronic lymphocytic leukemia. *Cancer.* 2010;116(9):2180-2187.
334. Goede VFK, Dyer M, Müller L, et al. Overall survival benefit ofobinutuzumab over rituximab when combined with chlorambucil inpatients with chronic lymphocytic leukemia and comorbidities: finalsurvival analysis of the CLL11 study. Presented at: the 2018 EHA Congress. 2018:S151.
335. Offner F, Robak T, Janssens A, et al. A five-year follow-up of untreated patients with chronic lymphocytic leukaemia treated with ofatumumab and chlorambucil: final analysis of the complement 1 phase 3 trial. *Br J Haematol.* 2020;190(5):736-740.
336. Kutsch N, Bahlo J, Robrecht S, et al. Long term follow-up data and health-related quality of life in frontline therapy of fit patients treated with FCR versus BR (CLL10 trial of the GCLLSG). *Hemasphere.* 2020;4(1):e336.
337. Tam CS, Brien SO, Wierda W, et al. Long-term results of the fludarabine, cyclophosphamide, and rituximab regimen as initial therapy of chronic lymphocytic leukemia. *Blood.* 2008;112(4):975-980.
338. Strati P, Keating MJ, O'Brien SM, et al. Eradication of bone marrow minimal residual disease may prompt early treatment discontinuation in CLL. *Blood.* 2014;123(24):3727-3732.
339. Böttcher S, Ritgen M, Fischer K, et al. Minimal residual disease quantification is an independent predictor of progression-free and overall survival in chronic lymphocytic leukemia: a Multivariate analysis from the randomized GCLLSG CLL8 trial. *J Clin Oncol.* 2012;30(9):980-988.
340. Eichhorst B, Fink AMM, Bahlo J, et al. First-line chemoimmunotherapy with bendamustine and rituximab versus fludarabine, cyclophosphamide, and rituximab in patients with advanced chronic lymphocytic leukaemia (CLL10): an international, open-label, randomised, phase 3, non-inferiority trial. *Lancet Oncol.* 2016;17(7):928-942.
341. Goede V, Fischer K, Busch R, et al. Obinutuzumab plus chlorambucil in patients with CLL and coexisting conditions. *N Engl J Med.* 2014;370(12):1101-1110.
342. Goede V, Fischer K, Engelke A, et al. Obinutuzumab as frontline treatment of chronic lymphocytic leukemia: updated results of the CLL11 study. *Leukemia.* 2015;29(7):1602-1604.
343. Hillmen P, Robak T, Janssens A, et al. Chlorambucil plus ofatumumab versus chlorambucil alone in previously untreated patients with chronic lymphocytic leukaemia (COMPLEMENT 1): a randomised, multicentre, open-label phase 3 trial. *Lancet.* 2015;385(9980):1873-1883.
344. Honigberg LA, Smith AM, Sirisawad M, et al. The Bruton tyrosine kinase inhibitor PCI-32765 blocks B-cell activation and is efficacious in models of autoimmune disease and B-cell malignancy. *Proc Natl Acad Sci U S A.* 2010;107(29):13075-13080.
345. Deeks ED. Ibrutinib: a review in chronic lymphocytic leukaemia. *Drugs.* 2017;77:225-236.
346. Byrd JC, Furman RR, Coutre SE, et al. Targeting BTK with ibrutinib in relapsed chronic lymphocytic leukemia. *N Engl J Med.* 2013;369(1):32-32.
347. Byrd JC, Brown JR, O'Brien S, et al. Ibrutinib versus ofatumumab in previously treated chronic lymphoid leukemia. *N Engl J Med.* 2014;371(3):213-223.
348. Burger J., Tedeschi A, Barr PM, et al. Ibrutinib as initial therapy for patients with chronic lymphocytic leukemia. *N Engl J Med.* 2015;373(25):2425-2437.
349. Farooqui MZH, Valdez J, Martyr S, et al. Ibrutinib for previously untreated and relapsed or refractory chronic lymphocytic leukaemia with TP53 aberrations: a phase 2, single-arm trial. *Lancet Oncol.* 2015;16(2):169-176.
350. Wodarz D, Garg N, Komarova NL, et al. Kinetics of CLL cells in tissues and blood during therapy with the BTK inhibitor ibrutinib. *Blood.* 2014;123(26):4132-4135.
351. Woyach JA, Smucker K, Smith LL, et al. Prolonged lymphocytosis during ibrutinib therapy is associated with distinct molecular characteristics and does not indicate a suboptimal response to therapy. *Blood.* 2014;123(12):1810-1817.
352. Munir T, Brown JR, O'Brien S, et al. Final analysis from RESONATE: up to 6 years of follow-up on ibrutinib in patients with previously treated chronic lymphocytic leukemia or small lymphocytic lymphoma. *Am J Hematol.* 2019;94:1353-1363.
353. Barr PM, Owen C, Robak T, et al. Up to seven years of follow-up in the RESONATE-2 study of first-line ibrutinib treatment for patients with chronic lymphocytic leukemia. *J Clin Oncol.* 2021;39(15 suppl):7523.
354. Shanafelt TD, Wang XV, Kay NE, et al. Ibrutinib–rituximab or chemoimmunotherapy for chronic lymphocytic leukemia. *N Engl J Med.* 2019;381(5):432-443.
355. Woyach JA, Ruppert AS, Heerema NA, et al. Ibrutinib regimens versus chemoimmunotherapy in older patients with untreated CLL. *N Engl J Med.* 2018;379(26):2517-2528.
356. Moreno C, Greil R, Demirkan F, et al. Ibrutinib plus obinutuzumab versus chlorambucil plus obinutuzumab in first-line treatment of chronic lymphocytic leukaemia (iLLUMINATE): a multicentre, randomised, open-label, phase 3 trial. *Lancet Oncol.* 2019;20(1):43-56.
357. Hillmen P, Pitchford A, Bloor A, et al. Ibrutinib plus rituximab is superior to FCR in previously untreated CLL: results of the phase III NCRI FLAIR trial. *Blood.* 2021;138(suppl 1):642.
358. O'Brien S, Jones JA, Coutre SE, et al. Ibrutinib for patients with relapsed or refractory chronic lymphocytic leukaemia with 17p deletion (RESONATE-17): a phase 2, open-label, multicentre study. *Lancet Oncol.* 2016;17(10):1409-1418.
359. Byrd JC, Harrington B, O'Brien S, et al. Acalabrutinib (ACP-196) in relapsed chronic lymphocytic leukemia. *N Engl J Med.* 2016;374(4):323-332.
360. Byrd JC, Wierda WG, Schuh A, et al. Acalabrutinib monotherapy in patients with relapsed/refractory chronic lymphocytic leukemia: updated phase 2 results. *Blood.* 2020;135(15):1204-1213.
361. Byrd JC, Woyach JA, Furman RR, et al. Acalabrutinib in treatment-naive chronic lymphocytic leukemia. *Blood.* 2021;137(24):3327-3338.
362. Ghia P, Pluta A, Wach M, et al. ASCEND: phase III, randomized trial of acalabrutinib versus idelalisib plus rituximab or bendamustine plus rituximab in relapsed or refractory chronic lymphocytic leukemia. *J Clin Oncol.* 2020;38(25):2849-2861.
363. Sharman JP, Egyed M, Jurczak W, et al. Acalabrutinib with or without obinutuzumab versus chlorambucil and obinutuzmab for treatment-naive chronic lymphocytic leukaemia (ELEVATE TN): a randomised, controlled, phase 3 trial. *Lancet.* 2020;395(10232):1278-1291.
364. Cull G, Simpson D, Opat S, et al. Treatment with the Bruton tyrosine kinase inhibitor zanubrutinib (BGB-3111) demonstrates high overall response rate and durable responses in patients with chronic lymphocytic leukemia/small lymphocytic lymphoma (CLL/SLL): updated results from a phase 1/2 trial. *Blood.* 2019;134(suppl 1):500.
365. Tam CS, Giannopoulos K, Jurczak W, et al. SEQUOIA: results of a phase 3 randomized study of zanubrutinib versus bendamustine + rituximab (BR) in patients with treatment-naïve (TN) chronic lymphocytic leukemia/small lymphocytic lymphoma (CLL/SLL). *Blood.* 2021;138(suppl 1):396.
366. Lewis KL, Cheah CY. Non-covalent BTK inhibitors-The new BTKids on the block for B-cell malignancies. *J Pers Med.* 2021;11(8):764.
367. Mato AR, Pagel JM, Coombs CC, et al. Pirtobrutinib, A next generation, highly selective, non-covalent BTK inhibitor in previously treated CLL/SLL: updated results from the phase 1/2 BRUIN study. *Blood.* 2021;138(suppl 1):391.
368. Woyach JA, Flinn IW, Awan FT, et al. Preliminary efficacy and safety of MK-1026, a non-covalent inhibitor of wild-type and C481S mutated Bruton tyrosine kinase, in B-cell malignancies: a phase 2 dose expansion study. *Blood.* 2021;138(suppl 1):392.
369. Kamel S, Horton L, Ysebaert L, et al. Ibrutinib inhibits collagen-mediated but not ADP-mediated platelet aggregation. *Leukemia.* 2015;29:783-787.
370. Bitar C, Farooqui MZH, Valdez J, et al. Hair and nail changes during long-term therapy with ibrutinib for chronic lymphocytic leukemia. *JAMA Dermatol.* 2016;152(6):698-701.
371. Byrd JC, Hillmen P, Ghia P, et al. First results of a head-to-head trial of acalabrutinib versus ibrutinib in previously treated chronic lymphocytic leukemia. *J Clin Oncol.* 2021;39(15 suppl):7500.
372. Hillmen P, Brown JR, Eichhorst BF, et al. ALPINE: zanubrutinib versus ibrutinib in relapsed/refractory chronic lymphocytic leukemia/small lymphocytic lymphoma. *Future Oncol.* 2020;16(10):517-523.
373. Maddocks KJ, Ruppert AS, Lozanski G, et al. Etiology of ibrutinib discontinuation and outcomes in chronic lymphocytic leukemia patients. *JAMA Oncol.* 2015;1(1):80-87.
374. Forum UC. Ibrutinib for relapsed/refractory chronic lymphocytic leukemia: a UK and Ireland analysis of outcomes in 315 patients. *Haematologica.* 2016;101(10112):1563-1572.
375. Liu TM, Woyach JA, Zhong Y, et al. Hypermorphic mutation of phospholipase C, γ2 acquired in ibrutinib-resistant CLL confers BTK independency upon B-cell receptor activation. *Blood.* 2015;126(1):61-68.
376. Burger JA, Landau DA, Taylor-Weiner A, et al. Clonal evolution in patients with chronic lymphocytic leukaemia developing resistance to BTK inhibition. *Nat Commun.* 2016;7:11589.
377. Wang E, Mi X, Thompson MC, et al. Mechanisms of resistance to noncovalent Bruton's tyrosine kinase inhibitors. *N Engl J Med.* 2022;386(8):735-743.
378. Furman RR, Sharman JP, Coutre SE, et al. Idelalisib and rituximab in relapsed chronic lymphocytic leukemia. *N Engl J Med.* 2014;370(11):997-1007.
379. O'Brien SM, Lamanna N, Kipps TJ, et al. A phase 2 study of idelalisib plus rituximab in treatment-naive older patients with chronic lymphocytic leukemia. *Blood.* 2015;126(25):2686-2694.

380. Brown JR, Hallek MJ, Pagel JM. Chemoimmunotherapy versus targeted treatment in chronic lymphocytic leukemia: when, how long, how much, and in which combination. *Am Soc Clin Oncol Educ Book*. 2016;35:387-398.
381. Flinn IW, Hillmen P, Montillo M, et al. The phase 3 DUO trial: duvelisib versus ofatumumab in relapsed and refractory CLL/SLL. *Blood*. 2018;132(23):2446-2455.
382. Gribben JG, Jurczak W, Jacobs RW, et al. Umbralisib plus ublituximab (U2) is superior to obinutuzumab plus chlorambucil (O+Chl) in patients with treatment naïve (TN) and relapsed/refractory (R/R) chronic lymphocytic leukemia (CLL): results from the phase 3 unity-CLL study. *Blood*. 2020;136(suppl 1):37-39.
383. Roberts AW, Davids MS, Pagel JM, et al. Targeting BCL2 with venetoclax in relapsed chronic lymphocytic leukemia. *N Engl J Med*. 2016;374(4):312-322.
384. Stilgenbauer S, Eichhorst B, Schetelig J, et al. Venetoclax in relapsed or refractory chronic lymphocytic leukaemia with 17p deletion: a multicentre, open-label, phase 2 study. *Lancet Oncol*. 2016;17(6):768-778.
385. Seymour JF, Kipps TJ, Eichhorst B, et al. Venetoclax-rituximab in relapsed or refractory chronic lymphocytic leukemia. *N Engl J Med*. 2018;378(12):1107-1120.
386. Kater AP, Kipps TJ, Eichhorst B, et al. Five-year analysis of murano study demonstrates enduring undetectable minimal residual disease (uMRD) in a subset of relapsed/refractory chronic lymphocytic leukemia (R/R CLL) patients (pts) following fixed-duration venetoclax-rituximab (VenR) therapy (tx). *Blood*. 2020;136(suppl 1):19-21.
387. Fischer K, Al-Sawaf O, Bahlo J, et al. Venetoclax and obinutuzumab in patients with CLL and coexisting conditions. *N Engl J Med*. 2019;380(23):2225-2236.
388. Davids MS, Hallek M, Wierda W, et al. Comprehensive safety analysis of venetoclax monotherapy for patients with relapsed/refractory chronic lymphocytic leukemia. *Clin Cancer Res*. 2018;24(18):4371-4379.
389. Koehler AB, Leung N, Call TG, et al. Incidence and risk of tumor lysis syndrome in patients with relapsed chronic lymphocytic leukemia (CLL) treated with venetoclax in routine clinical practice. *Leuk Lymphoma*. 2020;61(10):2383-2388.
390. Blombery P, Anderson MA, Gong JN, et al. Acquisition of the recurrent Gly101Val mutation in BCL2 confers resistance to venetoclax in patients with progressive chronic lymphocytic leukemia. *Cancer Discov*. 2019;9(3):342-353.
391. Blombery P, Thompson ER, Nguyen T, et al. Multiple BCL2 mutations cooccurring with Gly101Val emerge in chronic lymphocytic leukemia progression on venetoclax. *Blood*. 2020;135(10):773-777.
392. Guieze R, Liu VM, Rosebrock D, et al. Genetic determinants of venetoclax resistance in lymphoid malignancies. *Blood*. 2018;132(suppl 1):893.
393. Jain N, Keating M, Thompson P, et al. Ibrutinib and venetoclax for first-line treatment of CLL. *N Engl J Med*. 2019;380(22):2095-2103.
394. Kater A, Owen C, Moreno C, et al. Fixed-duration ibrutinib and venetoclax (I+V) versus chlorambucil plus obinutuzumab (CLB+O) for first-line (1L) chronic lymphocytic leukemia (CLL): primary analysis of the phase 3 GLOW study. 2021. European Hematology Association Meeting. 2021.
395. Hillmen P, Rawstron AC, Brock K, et al. Ibrutinib plus venetoclax in relapsed/refractory chronic lymphocytic leukemia: the CLARITY study. *J Clin Oncol*. 2019;37(30):2722-2729.
396. Rogers KA, Huang Y, Ruppert AS, et al. Phase II study of combination obinutuzumab, ibrutinib, and venetoclax in treatment-naïve and relapsed or refractory chronic lymphocytic leukemia. *J Clin Oncol*. 2020;38(31):3626-3637.
397. Davids MS, Lampson BL, Tyekucheva S, et al. Acalabrutinib, venetoclax, and obinutuzumab as frontline treatment for chronic lymphocytic leukaemia: a single-arm, open-label, phase 2 study. *Lancet Oncol*. 2021;22(10):1391-1402.
398. Soumerai JD, Mato AR, Dogan A, et al. Zanubrutinib, obinutuzumab, and venetoclax with minimal residual disease-driven discontinuation in previously untreated patients with chronic lymphocytic leukaemia or small lymphocytic lymphoma: a multicentre, single-arm, phase 2 trial. *Lancet Haematology*. 2021;8(12):e879-e890.
399. Van Gelder M, De Wreede L, Bornhäuser M, et al. Long-term survival of patients with CLL after allogeneic transplantation: a report from the European Society for Blood and Marrow Transplantation. *Bone Marrow Transplant*. 2017;52(10):372-380.
400. Rondon G, Giralt S, Huh Y, et al. Graft-versus-leukemia effect after allogenec bone marrow transplantation for chronic lymphocytic leukemia. *Bone Marrow Transplant*. 1996;18(3):669-672.
401. Khouri IF, Bassett R, Poindexter N, et al. Non-myeloablative allogeneic stem cell transplantation in relapsed/refractory chronic lymphocytic leukemia: long-term follow-up, prognostic factors, and effect of human leukocyte histocompatibility antigen subtype on outcome. *Cancer*. 2011;117(20):4679-4688.
402. Gribben JG, Zahrieh D, Stephans K, et al. Autologous and allogeneic stem cell transplantations for poor-risk chronic lymphocytic leukemia. *Blood*. 2005;106(13):4389-4396.
403. Dreger P, Corradini P, Kimby E, et al. Indications for allogeneic stem cell transplantation in chronic lymphocytic leukemia: the EBMT transplant consensus. *Leukemia*. 2007;21:12-17.
404. Dreger P, Brand R, Milligan D, et al. Reduced-intensity conditioning lowers treatment-related mortality of allogeneic stem cell transplantation for chronic lymphocytic leukemia: a population-matched analysis. *Leukemia*. 2005;19:1029-1033.
405. Auletta JJ, Kou J, Chen M, Shaw BE. Current use and outcome of hematopoietic stem cell transplantation: CIBMTR US summary slides. 2021. Accessed January 16, 2023. https://cibmtr.org/CIBMTR/Resources/Summary-Slides-Reports
406. Kharfan-Dabaja MA, Kumar A, Hamadani M, et al. Clinical practice recommendations for use of allogeneic hematopoietic cell transplantation in chronic lymphocytic leukemia on behalf of the guidelines committee of the American Society for Blood and Marrow Transplantation. *Biol Blood Marrow Transplant*. 2016;22(12):2119-2125.
407. Kim HT, Ahn KW, Hu ZH, et al. Prognostic score and cytogenetic risk classification for chronic lymphocytic leukemia patients: center for International Blood and Marrow Transplant Research report. *Clin Cancer Res*. 2019;25(16):5143-5155.
408. Aikawa V, Porter D, Luskin MR, Bagg A, Morrissette JJD. Transmission of an expanding donor-derived del(20q) clone through allogeneic hematopoietic stem cell transplantation without the development of a hematologic neoplasm. *Cancer Genetics*. 2015;208:625-629.
409. Perz JB, Ritgen M, Moos M, Ho AD, Kneba M, Dreger P. Occurrence of donor-derived CLL 8 years after sibling donor SCT for CML. *Bone Marrow Transplant*. 2008;42:687-688.
410. Pavletic SZ, Zhou G, Sobocinski K, et al. Genetically identical twin transplantation for chronic lymphocytic leukemia. *Leukemia*. 2007;21:2452-2455.
411. van Gorkom G, van Gelder M, Eikema DJ, et al. Outcomes of haploidentical stem cell transplantation for chronic lymphocytic leukemia: a retrospective study on behalf of the chronic malignancies working party of the EBMT. *Bone Marrow Transplant*. 2018;53(3):255-263.
412. Roeker LE, Dreger P, Brown JR, et al. Allogeneic stem cell transplantation for chronic lymphocytic leukemia in the era of novel agents. *Blood Adv*. 2020;4(16):3977-3989.
413. Kenderian SS, Porter DL, Gill S. Chimeric antigen receptor T cells and hematopoietic cell transplantation: how not to put the CART before the horse. *Biol Blood Marrow Transplant*. 2017;23:235-246.
414. Gill S, Maus MV, Porter DL. Chimeric antigen receptor T cell therapy: 25 years in the making. *Blood Rev*. 2016;30:157-167.
415. Maude SL, Frey N, Shaw PA, et al. Chimeric antigen receptor T cells for sustained remissions in leukemia. *N Engl J Med*. 2014;371(16):1507-1517.
416. Neelapu SS, Locke FL, Bartlett NL, et al. Axicabtagene ciloleucel CAR T-cell therapy in refractory large B-cell lymphoma. *N Engl J Med*. 2017;377(26):2531-2544.
417. Abramson JS, Palomba ML, Gordon LI, et al. Lisocabtagene maraleucel for patients with relapsed or refractory large B-cell lymphomas (TRANSCEND NHL 001): a multicentre seamless design study. *Lancet*. 2020;396(10254):839-852.
418. Schuster SJ, Bishop MR, Tam CS, et al. Tisagenlecleucel in adult relapsed or refractory diffuse large B-cell lymphoma. *N Engl J Med*. 2019;380(1):45-56.
419. Wang M, Munoz J, Goy A, et al. KTE-X19 CAR T-cell therapy in relapsed or refractory mantle-cell lymphoma. *N Engl J Med*. 2020;382(14):1331-1342.
420. Yang Q, Chen LS, Ha MJ, Do KA, Neelapu SS, Gandhi V. Idelalisib impacts cell growth through inhibiting translation-regulatory mechanisms in mantle cell lymphoma. *Clin Cancer Res*. 2017;23(1):181-192.
421. Grupp SA, Kalos M, Barrett D, et al. Chimeric antigen receptor–modified T cells for acute lymphoid leukemia. *N Engl J Med*. 2013;368:1509-1518.
422. Teachey DT, Lacey SF, Shaw PA, et al. Identification of predictive biomarkers for cytokine release syndrome after chimeric antigen receptor T-cell therapy for acute lymphoblastic leukemia. *Cancer Discov*. 2016;6(6):664-679.
423. Siegler EL, Kenderian SS. Neurotoxicity and cytokine release syndrome after chimeric antigen receptor T cell therapy: insights into mechanisms and novel therapies. *Front Immunol*. 2020;11:1973.
424. Porter DL, Levine BL, Kalos M, Bagg A, June CH. Chimeric antigen receptor–modified T cells in chronic lymphoid leukemia. *N Engl J Med*. 2011;365(8):725-733.
425. Kalos M, Levine BL, Porter DL, et al. T cells with chimeric antigen receptors have potent antitumor effects and can establish memory in patients with advanced leukemia. *Sci Transl Med*. 2011;3(95):95ra73.
426. Porter DL, Hwang WT, Frey NV, et al. Chimeric antigen receptor T cells persist and induce sustained remissions in relapsed refractory chronic lymphocytic leukemia. *Sci Transl Med*. 2015;7(303):303ra139.
427. Turtle CJ, Hay KA, Hanafi LA, et al. Durable molecular remissions in chronic lymphocytic leukemia treated with CD19-specific chimeric antigen receptor–modified T cells after failure of ibrutinib. *J Clin Oncol*. 2017;35:3010-3020.
428. Ruella M, Kenderian SS, Shestova O, et al. The addition of the BTK inhibitor ibrutinib to anti-CD19 chimeric antigen receptor T cells (CART19) improves responses against mantle cell lymphoma. *Clin Cancer Res*. 2016;22(11):2684-2696.
429. Gauthier J, Hirayama AV, Purushe J, et al. Feasibility and efficacy of CD19-targeted CAR T cells with concurrent ibrutinib for CLL after ibrutinib failure. *Blood*. 2020;135(19):1650-1660.
430. Siddiqi T, Soumerai JD, Dorritie KA, et al. Phase 1 TRANSCEND CLL 004 study of lisocabtagene maraleucel in patients with relapsed/refractory CLL or SLL. *Blood*. 2022;139(12):1794-1806.
431. Weinmann M, Becker G, Einsele H, Bamberg M. Clinical indications and biological mechanisms of splenic irradiation in chronic leukemias and myeloproliferative disorders. *Radiother Oncol*. 2001;58(2):235-246.
432. Guiney MJ, Liew KH, Quong GG, Cooper IA. A study of splenic irradiation in chronic lymphocytic leukemia. *Int J Radiat Oncol Biol Phys*. 1989;16:225-229.
433. Cusack JC, Seymour JF, Lerner S, Keating MJ, Pollock RE. Role of splenectomy in chronic lymphocytic leukemia. *J Am Coll Surg*. 1997;185(3):237-243.
434. Neil TF Jr, Tefferi A, Witzig TE, Su J, Phyliky RL, Nagorney DM. Splenectomy in advanced chronic lymphocytic leukemia: a single institution experience with 50 patients. *Am J Med*. 1992;93(4):435-440.
435. Hill J, Walsh RM, McHam S, Brody F, Kalaycio M. Laparoscopic splenectomy for autoimmune hemolytic anemia in patients with chronic lymphocytic leukemia: a case series and review of the literature. *Am J Hematol*. 2004;75(3):134-138.
436. Cooperative Group for the Study of Immunoglobulin in Chronic Lymphocytic Leukemia, Gale RP, Chapel HM, et al. Intravenous immunoglobulin for the prevention of infection in chronic lymphocytic leukemia. A randomized, controlled clinical trial. *N Engl J Med*. 1988;319:902-907.
437. Weeks JC, Tierney MR, Weinstein MC. Cost effectiveness of prophylactic intravenous immune globulin in chronic lymphocytic leukemia. *N Engl J Med*. 1991;325:81-86.
438. Chapel H, Dicato M, Gamm H, et al. Immunoglobulin replacement in patients with chronic lymphocytic leukaemia: a comparison of two dose regimes. *Br J Haematol*. 1994;88(1):209-212.

439. Jurlander J, Geisler CH, Hansen MM. Treatment of hypogammaglobulinaemia in chronic lymphocytic leukaemia by low-dose intravenous gammaglobulin. *Eur J Haematol.* 1994;53(2):114-118.
440. Molica S, Musto P, Chiurazzi F, et al. Prophylaxis against infections with low-dose intravenous immunoglobulins (IVIG) in chronic lymphocytic leukemia. Results of a crossover study. *Haematologica.* 1996;81(2):121-126.
441. Compagno N, Cinetto F, Semenzato G, Agostini C. Subcutaneous immunoglobulin in lymphoproliferative disorders and rituximab-related secondary hypogammaglobulinemia: a single-center experience in 61 patients. *Haematologica.* 2014;99(6):1101-1106.
442. Streu E, Bi J, De Sousa M, et al. The efficacy and cost effectiveness of subcutaneous immunoglobulin (SCIG) replacement in patients with immune deficiency secondary to chronic lymphocytic leukemia. *Blood.* 2016;128:4778.
443. Cinetto F, Neri R, Vianello F, et al. Subcutaneous immunoglobulins replacement therapy in secondary antibody deficiencies: real life evidence as compared to primary antibody deficiencies. *PLoS One.* 2021;16(3):e0247717.
444. Dearden C. Disease-specific complications of chronic lymphocytic leukemia. *Hematology Am Soc Hematol Educ Program.* 2008;2008:450-456.
445. Tsigrelis C, Ljungman P. Vaccinations in patients with hematological malignancies. *Blood Rev.* 2016;30(2):139-147.
446. Gavriatopoulou M, Ntanasis-Stathopoulos I, Korompoki E, et al. Emerging treatment strategies for COVID-19 infection. *Clin Exp Med.* 2021;21(2):167-179.
447. Hammond J, Leister-Tebbe H, Gardner A, et al. Oral nirmatrelvir for high-risk, nonhospitalized adults with Covid-19. *N Engl J Med.* 2022;386(15):1397-1408.
448. Jayk Bernal A, Gomes da Silva MM, Musungaie DB, et al. Molnupiravir for oral treatment of Covid-19 in nonhospitalized patients. *N Engl J Med.* 2022;386(6):509-520.
449. National Institutes of Health. *Coronavirus Disease 2019 (COVID-19) Treatment Guidelines.* 2022. https://www.covid19treatmentguidelines.nih.gov/
450. Roeker LE, Eyre TA, Thompson MC, et al. COVID-19 in patients with CLL: improved survival outcomes and update on management strategies. *Blood.* 2021;138(18):1768-1773.
451. Levin MJ, Ustianowski A, De Wit S, et al. Intramuscular AZD7442 (Tixagevimab-Cilgavimab) for prevention of covid-19. *N Engl J Med.* 2022;386(23):2188-2200.
452. Kovacs J, Gill VJ, Meshnick S, Masur H. New insights into transmission, diagnosis, and drug treatment of Pneumocystis carinii pneumonia. *J Am Med Assoc.* 2001;286(19):2450-2460.
453. Flores G, Cunningham-Rundels C, Newland AC, Bussel JB. Efficacy of intravenous immunoglobulin in the treatment of autoimmune hemolytic anemia: results in 73 patients. *Am J Hematol.* 1993;44(4):237-242.
454. Cortes J, Loscertales J, Kantarjian H, et al. Cyclosporin A for the treatment of cytopenia associated with chronic lymphocytic leukemia. *Cancer.* 2001;92(8):2016-2021.
455. Yamada O, Yun-Hua W, Motoji T, Mizoguchi H. Clonal T-cell proliferation causing pure red cell aplasia in chronic B-cell lymphocytic leukaemia: Successful treatment with cyclosporine following in vitro abrogation of erythroid colony-suppressing activity. *Br J Haematol.* 1998;101(2):335-337.
456. Kaufman M, Limaye S., Driscoll N, et al. A combination of rituximab, cyclophosphamide and dexamethasone effectively treats immune cytopenias of chronic lymphocytic leukemia. *Leuk Lymphoma.* 2009;50(6):892-899.
457. Bowen DA, Call TG, Shanafelt TD, et al. Treatment of autoimmune cytopenia complicating progressive chronic lymphocytic leukemia/small lymphocyticlymphoma with rituximab, cyclophosphamide, vincristine, and prednisone. *Leuk Lymphoma.* 2010;51(4):620-627.
458. Österborg A, Karlsson C, Lundin J. Alemtuzumab to treat refractory autoimmune hemolytic anemia or thrombocytopenia in chronic lymphocytic leukemia. *Current Hematologic Malignancy Reports.* 2009;4(1):47-53.
459. Koehrer S, Meating MJ, Wierda WG, Keating MJ, Wierda WG. Eltrombopag, a second-generation thrombopoietin receptor agonist, for chronic lymphocytic leukemia-associated ITP. *Leukemia.* 2010;24(5):1096-1098.
460. Parikh SA, Rabe KG, Call TG, et al. Diffuse large B-cell lymphoma (Richter syndrome) in patients with chronic lymphocytic leukaemia (CLL): a cohort study of newly diagnosed patients. *Br J Haematol.* 2013;162(6):774-782.
461. Parikh SA, Kay NE, Shanafelt TD. How we treat Richter syndrome. *Blood.* 2014;123(11):1647-1657.
462. Rossi D, Cerri M, Capello D, et al. Biological and clinical risk factors of chronic lymphocytic leukaemia transformation to Richter syndrome. *Br J Haematol.* 2008;142(2):202-215.
463. Parikh SA, Shanafelt TD. Risk factors for Richter syndrome in chronic lymphocytic leukemia. *Curr Hematol Malig Rep.* 2014;9(3):294-299.
464. Rossi D, Lobetti Bodoni C, Genuardi E, et al. Telomere length is an independent predictor of survival, treatment requirement and Richter's syndrome transformation in chronic lymphocytic leukemia. *Leukemia.* 2009;23(6):1062-1072.
465. Rossi D, Rasi S, Spina V, et al. Different impact of NOTCH1 and SF3B1 mutations on the risk of chronic lymphocytic leukemia transformation to Richter syndrome. *Br J Haematol.* 2012;158(3):426-429.
466. Fabbri G, Khiabanian H, Holmes AB, et al. Genetic lesions associated with chronic lymphocytic leukemia transformation to Richter syndrome. *J Exp Med.* 2013;210(11):2273-2288.
467. Woyach JA, Ruppert AS, Guinn D, et al. BTKC481S-Mediated resistance to ibrutinib in chronic lymphocytic leukemia. *J Clin Oncol.* 2017;35(13):1437-1443.
468. Anderson MA, Tam C, Lew TE, et al. Clinicopathological features and outcomes of progression of CLL on the BCL2 inhibitor venetoclax. *Blood.* 2017;129(25):3362-3370.
469. Bruzzi JF, Macapinlac H, Tsimberidou AM, et al. Detection of Richter's transformation of chronic lymphocytic leukemia by PET/CT. *J Nucl Med.* 2006;47(8):1267-1273.
470. Wang Y, Rabe KG, Bold MS, et al. The role of 18F-FDG-PET in detecting Richter's transformation of chronic lymphocytic leukemia in patients receiving therapy with a B-cell receptor inhibitor. *Haematologica.* 2020;105(11):2675-2678.
471. Mato AR, Wierda WG, Davids MS, et al. Analysis of PET-CT to identify Richter's transformation in 167 patients with disease progression following kinase inhibitor therapy. *Blood.* 2017;130(suppl 1):834.
472. Oppermann S, Ylanko J, Shi Y, et al. High-content screening identifies kinase inhibitors that overcome venetoclax resistance in activated CLL cells. *Blood.* 2016;128(7):934-947.
473. Rossi D, Spina V, Deambrogi C, et al. The genetics of Richter syndrome reveals disease heterogeneity and predicts survival after transformation. *Blood.* 2011;117(12):3391-3401.
474. Langerbeins P, Busch R, Anheier N, et al. Poor efficacy and tolerability of R-CHOP in relapsed/refractory chronic lymphocytic leukemia and Richter transformation. *Am J Hematol.* 2014;89:E239-E243.
475. Tsimberidou AM, Wierda WG, Plunkett W, et al. Phase I-II study of oxaliplatin, fludarabine, cytarabine, and rituximab combination therapy in patients with Richter's syndrome or fludarabine-refractory chronic lymphocytic leukemia. *J Clin Oncol.* 2008;26:196-203.
476. Tsimberidou AM, Wierda WG, Wen S, et al. Phase I-II clinical trial of oxaliplatin, fludarabine, cytarabine, and rituximab therapy in aggressive, relapsed/refractory chronic lymphocytic leukemia or Richter's syndrome. *Clin Lymphoma Myeloma Leuk.* 2013;13(5):568-574.
477. Rogers KA, Salem G, Stephens DM, et al. A single-institution retrspecctivecohort study of patients treated with R-EPOCH for Richter's transformation of chronic lymphocytic leukemia. *Blood.* 2015;126:2951.
478. Cwynarski K, van Biezen A, de Wreede L, et al. Autologous and allogeneic stem-cell transplantation for transformed chronic lymphocytic leukemia (Richter's Syndrome): a Retrospective Analysis From the Chronic Lymphocytic Leukemia Subcommittee of the Chronic Leukemia Working Party and Lymphoma Working Party of the European Group for Blood and Marrow Transplantation. *J Clin Oncol.* 2012;30(18):2211-2217.
479. Tsang M, Shanafelt TD, Call TG, et al. The efficacy of ibrutinib in the treatment of Richter syndrome. *Blood.* 2015;125(10):1676-1679.
480. Davids MS, Roberts AW, Seymour JF, et al. Phase I first-in-human study of venetoclax in patients with relapsed or refractory non-hodgkin lymphoma. *J Clin Oncol.* 2017;35:826-833.
481. Eyre T, Schuh A, Wierda WG, et al. Acalabrutinib monotherapy for treatment of chronic lymphocytic leukaemia (ACE-CL-001): analysis of the Richter transformation cohort of an open-label, single-arm, phase 1-2 study. *Lancet Haematol.* 2021;8(12):e912-e921.
482. Ding W, LaPlant BR, Call TG, et al. Pembrolizumab in patients with chronic lymphocytic leukemia with Richter's transformation and relapsed CLL. *Blood.* 2017;129:3419-3427.
483. Jain N, Ferrajoli A, Basu S, et al. A Phase II Trial of Nivolumab combined with Ibrutinib for patients with Richter transformation. *Blood.* 2018;132(suppl 1):296.
484. Davids MS, Rogers KA, Tyekucheva S, et al. Venetoclax plus dose-adjusted R-EPOCH (VR-EPOCH) for Richter's syndrome. *Blood.* 2021;139(5):686-689.
485. Kittai AS, Bond DA, William B, et al. Clinical activity of axicabtagene ciloleucel in adult patients with Richter syndrome. *Blood Adv.* 2020;4(19):4648-4652.
486. Herrera AF, Ahn KW, Litovich C, et al. Autologous and allogeneic hematopoietic cell transplantation for diffuse large B-cell lymphoma-type Richter syndrome. *Blood Adv.* 2021;5(18):3528-3539.
487. Bockorny B, Codreanu I, Dasanu CA. Hodgkin lymphoma as Richter transformation in chronic lymphocytic leukaemia: A retrospective analysis of world literature. *Br J Haematol.* 2012;156(1):50-66.
488. Parikh SA, Habermann TM, Chaffee KG, et al. Hodgkin transformation of chronic lymphocytic leukemia: Incidence, outcomes, and comparison to de novo Hodgkin lymphoma. *Am J Hematol.* 2015;90(4):334-338.
489. Tsimberidou AM, O'Brien S, Kantarjian HM, et al. Hodgkin transformation of chronic lymphocytic leukemia: the M. D. Anderson Cancer Center experience. *Cancer.* 2006;107(6):1294-1302.
490. Stephens DM, Boucher K, Kander E, et al. Hodgkin lymphoma arising in patients with chronic lymphocytic leukemia: outcomes from a large multi-center collaboration. *Haematologica.* 2021;106(11):2845-2852.
491. Huh YO, Lin KI, Vega F, et al. MYC translocation in chronic lymphocytic leukaemia is associated with increased prolymphocytes and a poor prognosis. *Br J Haematol.* 2008;142(1):36-44.
492. Cao F, Amato D, Wang C. Concurrent chronic lymphocytic leukemia and prolymphocytic leukemia derived from two separate B-cell clones. *Am J Hematol.* 2011;86(9):782.

Chapter 93 ■ Hairy Cell Leukemia

JAMES B. JOHNSTON • GRAEME R. QUEST • MICHAEL R. GREVER

INTRODUCTION

Hairy cell leukemia (HCL), or leukemic reticuloendotheliosis, is a chronic B-cell disorder that was initially described in detail by Bouroncle et al in 1958.[1] Consensus guidelines regarding the diagnosis and management of these patients have recently been published.[2] The disease is characterized by the presence of typical hairy cells in the peripheral blood and marrow, pancytopenia, and a variable degree of splenomegaly. The disease has always aroused special interest, initially over the unique morphologic and clinical features of this disorder, and later as the biology of the disease became better understood and effective therapies were developed. The tumor cells are B cells that typically express CD11c, CD25, CD103, and CD123, have usually mutations of the variable region of the immunoglobulin heavy chain gene (*IGHV*-mutated) and are unique memory B-cells in expressing multiple immunoglobulin (Ig) isotypes. More recently, it has been demonstrated that most hairy cells contain a mutated active form of the *BRAF* gene (V600E) which may be used as a diagnostic tool and a target for therapy. Most cases of HCL are very sensitive to interferon alpha (IFNα) and the purine nucleoside analogs, pentostatin (2′-deoxycoformycin dCF) and cladribine (2-chlorodeoxyadenosine CdA). Less responsive disease generally benefits from the addition of an anti-CD20 monoclonal antibody, such as rituximab, to the purine nucleoside analog, or to moxetumumab pasudotox (an immunotoxin-labeled antibodies to CD22). More recently, there has been great interest in the use of vemurafenib (an inhibitor of BRAF) and ibrutinib (an inhibitor of Bruton's tyrosine kinase (BTK)) for the treatment of HCL. Prior to the development of these treatments the median survival for HCL patients was 4 years whereas now the survival of most patients with HCL is similar to a control population. However, in order to achieve this improvement in survival, patients may require repeated treatments if relapses occur.

As will be discussed, the less-common variant form of HCL (HCLv) is quite distinct to classical HCL. For simplicity, we will refer to classical HCL as HCL and the variant form as HCLv.

INCIDENCE AND ETIOLOGY

HCL is a rare disorder, accounting for 2% of non-Hodgkin lymphomas (NHLs), and occurs more frequently in men, with an incidence in the United States of 2.9 per million per year for men and 0.6 per million per year for women.[3] The etiology of HCL is unknown, though case-controlled studies have identified possible relationships to farming (including exposure to farm animals, commercial herbicides and/or pesticides), and an inverse correlation with smoking.[4,5] A familial predisposition is suggested by reports of the disorder in 13 families where HCL occurred among first-degree relatives, appearing linked to HLA haplotypes within affected families, although no specific HLA markers appear disproportionately associated within familial occurences.[6] In addition, recent study using high-throughput sequencing of four families with at least two effected members with HCL was unable to identify a common genetic variant.[7]

PATHOGENESIS

The lineage of HCL has been a subject of much historical debate. Based on the unusual villous monocytoid appearance of the hairy cell, along with the phagocytic and cytochemical properties of these cells, early studies suggested a reticuloendothelial or monocytic origins.[1,8,9] However, subsequent identification of a clonal *IGH* rearrangement and immunoglobin production confirmed the mature B cell origin of this disease.[10] The gene expression profile of HCL is extremely homogeneous and distinct from other lymphoid neoplasms, while the increased expression of chemokine and adhesion genes explain many of the unique properties of this disease. These features include the unique cell structure, phagocytic function, marrow fibrosis, marrow suppression, and the tendency of tumor cells to home to spleen and marrow rather than to lymph nodes.[11]

Although hairy cells consistently do not express CD27, a classical marker of memory B cell status, gene expression profiling demonstrates that the hairy cell is most similar to a post-germinal center memory B cell origin (*Figure 93.1*), possibly arising from an obscure CD27-memory B subset.[11–13] Consistent with a memory B cell origin, the majority of cases with HCL demonstrate somatic hypermutations of the *IGHV* region, though 10% to 20% of cases are unmutated; these latter cases generally respond poorly to chemotherapy and have a poor prognosis.[14–16] Hairy cells are unique in their ability to express multiple immunoglobulin isotypes, and may concurrently express IgM, IgD, IgG, and/or IgA in approximately 40% of cases.[17,18] These studies suggest that the hairy cell is arrested at a memory-stage of maturation post somatic hypermutation, with differential splicing of IgH transcripts though incapable of excisional class-switch recombination. More recently, genome-wide DNA promoter methylation studies have demonstrated that HCL most closely aligns with low and intermediate-maturity post-germinal memory B cells, notably demonstrating significant similarities with splenic marginal zone B lymphoma.[19]

The *IGHV* gene usage is shown in *Figure 93.2* and demonstrates that in classical HCL *IGHV* 3-23 (17%), 3-30 (8%) and 4-34 (7%) are most commonly used, while *IGHV*1-69, 3-11, 3-48 and 4-39 are each used in 5% of cases.[15] The major difference between the HCL variant (HCL-V) and classical HCL, is the usage of *IGHV*4-34, which is present in 36% of variant cases but only 7% of classical cases, and the HCL-V is frequent unmutated (94%).[15] As expected, the *IGHV* is more likely to be unmutated in the HCL-V (54%) as compared to classical HCL (17%).[15] The patterns of *IGHV* gene family usage and somatic hypermutation status is different in HCL and chronic lymphocytic leukemia (CLL).[15] In CLL, approximately 60% of CLL cases have mutated *IGHV* and 40% are unmutated, while the most commonly used *IGHV* genes are *IGHV*1-69, 3-21, 3-30, 4-34 and 1-02.[20–22] Paradoxically, in CLL most *IGHV*1-69 cases are unmutated and most *IGHV*4-34 cases are mutated, while the opposite is seen in HCL; these findings suggest that disease-specific factors coordinately bias both *IGHV* allele-usage and somatic hypermutations.[15]

Molecular Genetics

It was demonstrated over a decade ago that the activities of mitogen-activated protein-ERK kinase (MEK) and extracellular signal-regulated kinase (ERK) are increased in HCL, and that inhibition of MEK causes loss of cell viability (*Figure 93.3*).[23,24] Activation of the pathway was subsequently demonstrated in 2011 to be due to increased activity of BRAF, a serine-threonine kinase upstream of MEK, as a result of the *BRAF* V600E mutation.[25] The *BRAF* proto-oncogene is located on chromosome 7q34, with a transversion mutation from GTG to GAG within codon 600 (c.1799T > A) resulting in substitution of glutamate (E) for valine (V). The variant BRAF protein (V600E) demonstrates constitutive kinase activity,[26] resulting in enhanced phosphorylation and activation of MEK and ERK, which promote cell survival and proliferation by increasing expression of cyclin D1 and decreasing expression of *CDKN1B* (encoding p27).[25,27] The functionality of the variant protein was demonstrated in primary hairy cells by confirming the presence of phosphorylated MEK and ERK in these cells (*Figure 93.3*). In addition, treatment of the cells

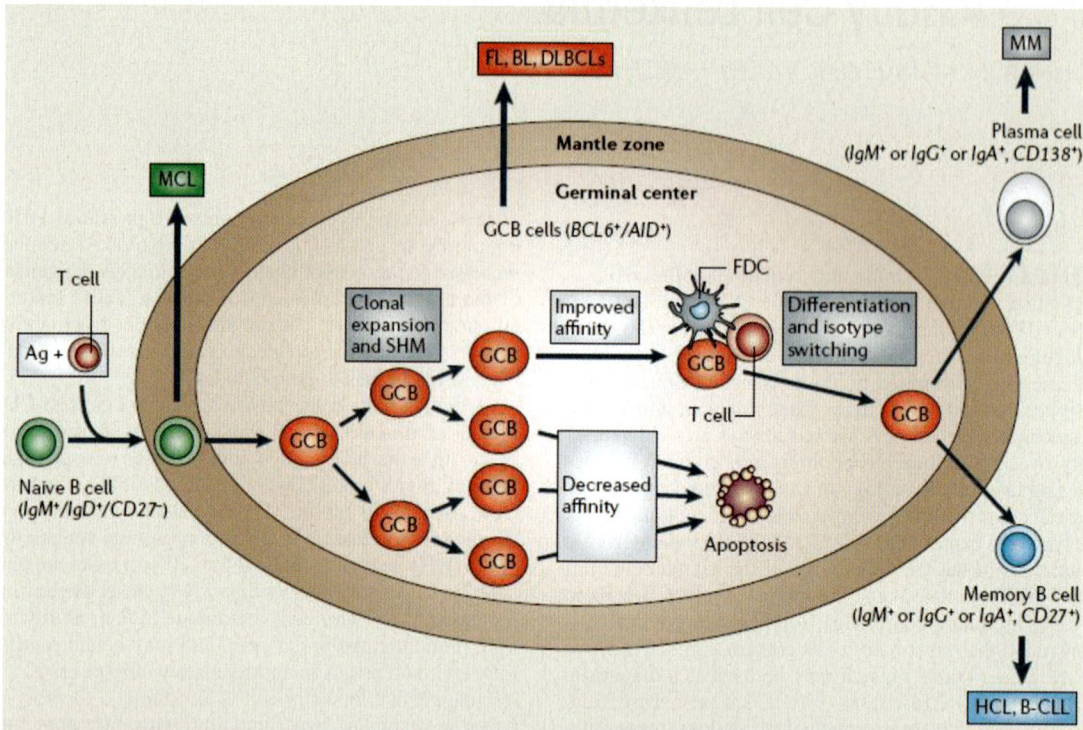

FIGURE 93.1 **The germinal center (GC) reaction is a key event in adaptive immunity to T-cell-dependent antigens.** In lymph nodes and the spleen, antigen (Ag)-activated naive B-cells (immunoglobulin [Ig] M+/IgD+) are driven into primary follicles where, aided by T-cells, they undergo clonal expansion, form the GC, and displace non-proliferating naive B-cells to the periphery or mantle zone (shown in diagram). Within the GC, somatic hypermutation (SHM) mutates the Ig variable region of proliferating B-cells to increase their affinity for the stimulating Ag. Although most GC B-cells (GCB) acquire unfavorable mutations and die by apoptosis, a few improve their Ig affinity and are selected for further differentiation through interactions with T-cells and follicular dendritic cells (FDC). A proportion of these selected B-cells then undergo switch recombination of the Ig constant region, which changes the isotype and, consequently, the antibody-effector function. B-cells of the GC express BCL6, which is required for GC formation, and activation-induced cytidine deaminase (AID) which is essential for SHM and switch recombination. Finally, selected B-cells differentiate into memory B-cells (CD27+) or antibody-secreting plasma cells (CD138+). Follicular lymphoma (FL), Burkitt lymphoma (BL), and some diffuse large B-cell lymphomas (DLBCLs) are thought to derive from B-cells of the GC, mantle cell lymphoma (MCL) mainly from mantle-zone naive B-cells, B-cell chronic lymphocytic leukemia (B-CLL) and hairy-cell leukemia (HCL) from memory B-cells, and multiple myeloma (MM) from plasma cells. The majority of cases of CLL and HCL have undergone SHM, but proportions have not and these cases have more aggressive disease. (Reprinted by permission from Nature: Tiacci E, Liso A, Piris M, et al. Evolving concepts in the pathogenesis of hairy-cell leukaemia. *Nat Rev Cancer*. 2006;6(6):437-448. Copyright © 2006 Springer Nature.)

with the BRAF inhibitor, PLX-4720 (vemurafenib), decreased MEK and ERK phosphorylation and caused loss of the characteristic "hairy" villous projections, with subsequent apoptosis.[25,27] In addition, whole exome sequencing has demonstrated that *CDKN1B* is mutated in 16% of patients with classical HCL, but not in the HCLv.[28] The gene product of *CDKN1B*, p27, prevents the activation of cyclin E-CDK2 and cyclin D-CDK4, thus inhibiting passage through G1. Missense mutations of *KLF2*, a transcription factor involved in B cell differentiation, is also found to be mutated in 16% of HCL cases.[29] It is likely that these additional abnormalities work cooperatively with BRAF mutations in the pathogenesis of HCL.

While initial studies suggested that all patients with classical HCL demonstrated the *BRAF* V600E mutation, subsequent studies have demonstrated very rare cases demonstrating an alternate activating *BRAF* mutation in exon 11,[30] as well as a subset cases lacking any *BRAF* mutation; this subset demonstrates a marked bias in utilization of *IGHV4-34* and is associated with an adverse prognosis.[31–34] Subsequent studies have demonstrated that cases of classical HCL lacking a *BRAF* mutation, HCL-V (which uniformly do not demonstrate *BRAF* mutations), and occasionally other mimics of HCL may alternately demonstrate mutations in *MAP2K1*, which encodes for MEK1, a kinase immediately downstream of BRAF.[32,33,35] Select *MAP2K1* mutations may be amenable to targeted MEK inhibitors, though many of the recurrent mutations described are reported to confer resistance.[32,36–39] Recently, Chung et al[40] have provided evidence that HCL may arise from early hematopoietic precursors, demonstrating that the *BRAF* mutation is also present in CD34+ hematopoietic stem cells in HCL. While the presence of a *BRAF* mutation appears

highly specific for HCL amongst its mimics, *BRAF* mutations may be seen in chronic lymphocytic leukemia,[41,42] multiple myeloma,[43] histiocytic malignancies,[44,45] as well as many solid tumor malignancies.[46] Rare case reports of synchronous HCL and histiocytic malignancies have been reported, raising the possibility of a common stem cell origin in these disorder or possible transdifferentiation between the mature malignant populations.[47–49]

Gene Expression in HCL

Gene expression profiling identifies a unique homogeneous signature for HCL distinct from other B-cell malignancies. In HCL samples, decreased expression was noted for *CXCR5*, *TNFRAF5*, *CD40*, *CD27*, and *CCR7*, whereas increased expression was noted for *GAS7*, *FGFR1*, *FGF2*, *FLT3*, *TIMP1*, *TIMP4*, *RECK*, *ANXA1*, *SDC3*, *CCND1*, *IGFBP*, and *NUDT6*.[11,27] The proposed effects of these changes on the pathophysiology of HCL are outlined in *Table 93.1*. The expression of several genes involved in monocytic differentiation, including the proto-oncogenic transcription factor *MAF* (which biases monocytic differentiation in granulocyte-monocytic progenitors), *ANXA1*, the monocyte-macrophage-specific isoform of CD68, and the macrophage colony stimulating factor receptor (CD115, *CSF1R*), are expressed in hairy cells and may explain the phagocytic ability and other features which suggested a monocytic-reticuloendothelial origin of HCL.[8,9,11] Inhibition of BRAF increased the expression of 30 genes and decreased expression of 105 genes (*Figure 93.4*), including decreased expression of TRAP, CD25 and cyclin D1 at the messenger and protein levels, and increased the expression of *CDKN1B* (p27) with the induction of apoptosis.

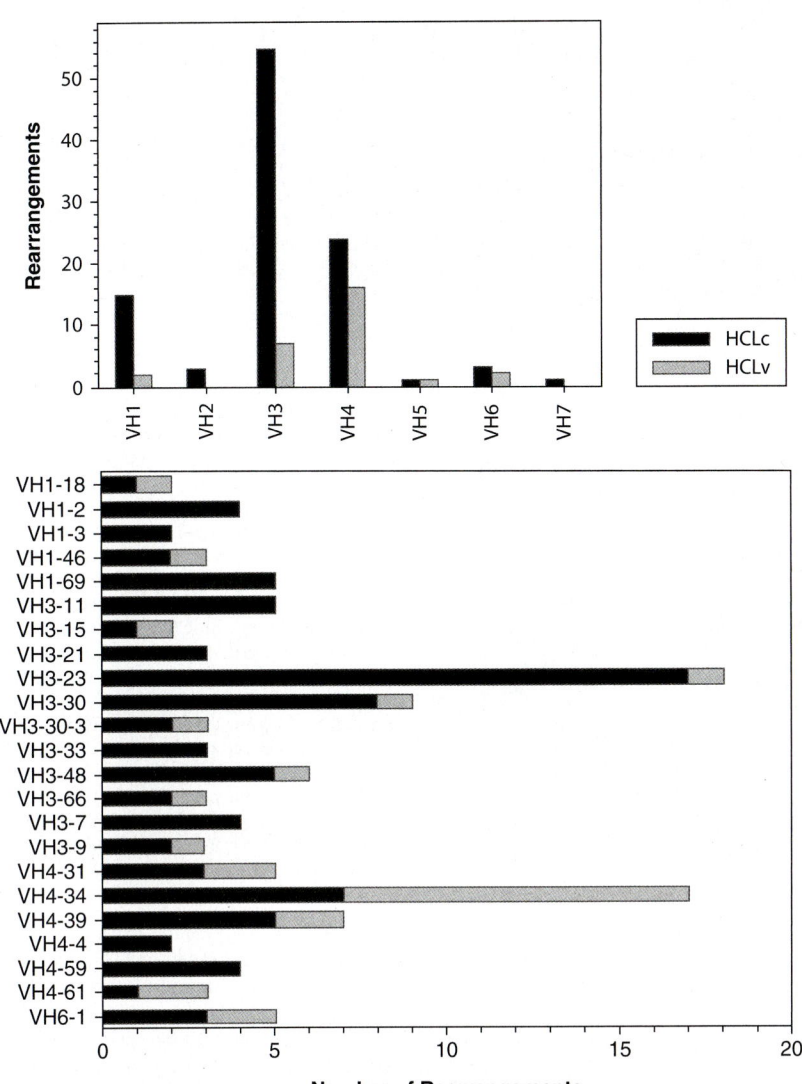

FIGURE 93.2 **Immunoglobulin (Ig) VH family and gene usage in hairy-cell leukemia (HCL).** Number of IGV_H rearrangements in each family (A) and for genes used by more than one patient (B) for HCLc (*black*) and HCL-V (*gray*). (Reprinted from Arons E, Roth L, Sapolsky J, et al. Evidence of canonical somatic hypermutation in hairy cell leukemia. *Blood*. 2011;117(18):4844-4851. Copyright © 2011 American Society of Hematology. With permission.)

Interestingly, apoptosis could be partially inhibited upon co-culture with stromal cells.[27] Prior to apoptosis, the cells showed a reduction in the filamentous projections which was ascribed to the reduction in expression of *ACTB* (β-actin) and *LST1* (leukocyte transcript 1).[27] ACTB is present in the cytoskeleton of the filamentous projections while LST1 is required for the formation of the projections. Studies of miRNA have demonstrated a distinctive expression profile in HCL, with the expression of miRNA which suppress CDKN1B, as well as the JNK and p38 MAPK pathways.[23,24,50] Thus, like mutant BRAF, overexpression of these miRNAs may cause hairy cells to be resistant to apoptosis.[50]

Cytogenetics

Cytogenetic studies have been difficult to carry out in HCL because the number of circulating hairy cells is small and attempts at marrow aspiration are frequently unsuccessful. In addition, it has been difficult to induce hairy cells to proliferate and to obtain hairy cells in metaphase until the recent identification of suitable stimulants to induce proliferation.[51–53] Clonal abnormalities involving chromosome 5q13 have been described by Haglund et al in 40% of cases (most commonly, trisomy 5, pericentric inversions, and interstitial deletions involving 5q13).[53] Subsequent studies of abnormalities in 5q13 in HCL have identified three expressed sequences as candidates for a putative tumor-suppressor gene at 5q13.3.[54] Cultures of HCL stimulated with anti-CD40 allowed cytogenetic analysis in 42 of 43 cases, demonstrating clonal abnormalities in 19% of cases, frequently involving numeric or structural abnormalities in chromosomes 5, 7 (frequently involving deletion of *BRAF*), and 14.[51] In contrast, abnormalities of chromosome 5 were not observed in the HCL-V, and translocations more frequently involved either chromosome 2 or 14.[55]

High-density genome-wide DNA profiling in HCL showed that, in contrast with CLL, HCL has a remarkably stable genome.[56–58] Using a high-density single nucleotide polymorphism (SNP)-array, only 25% of patients had gross copy number abnormalities.[57] Alterations in the genes for FGF12 and FGF receptor were observed, and increased expression of these genes is typically observed in HCL, which is responsible for the marrow fibrosis seen in this disease.[57] While a high incidence of *TP53* mutations was initially reported in HCL, subsequent studies have suggested that this is uncommon and occurs primarily in patients with unmutated *IGHV*.[14,59]

Cytokines

There has been great interest in the role of cytokines in the pathogenesis of HCL.[60–62] Identified factors that may be involved include interleukin-2 (IL-2), tumor necrosis factor (TNF)-α, IL-4, IL-6, B-cell growth factor, IFN-α, transforming growth factor-β (TGF-β), and basic fibroblast growth factor (bFGF, FGF2) (*Figure 93.5*).[63] Some of these factors may be produced by the hairy cells themselves or by normal T-cells.[63,64] T-cell clones have been shown to produce cytokines that stimulate the growth of hairy cells, but not normal B-cells, and this effect is prevented by the addition of IFN-α.[64]

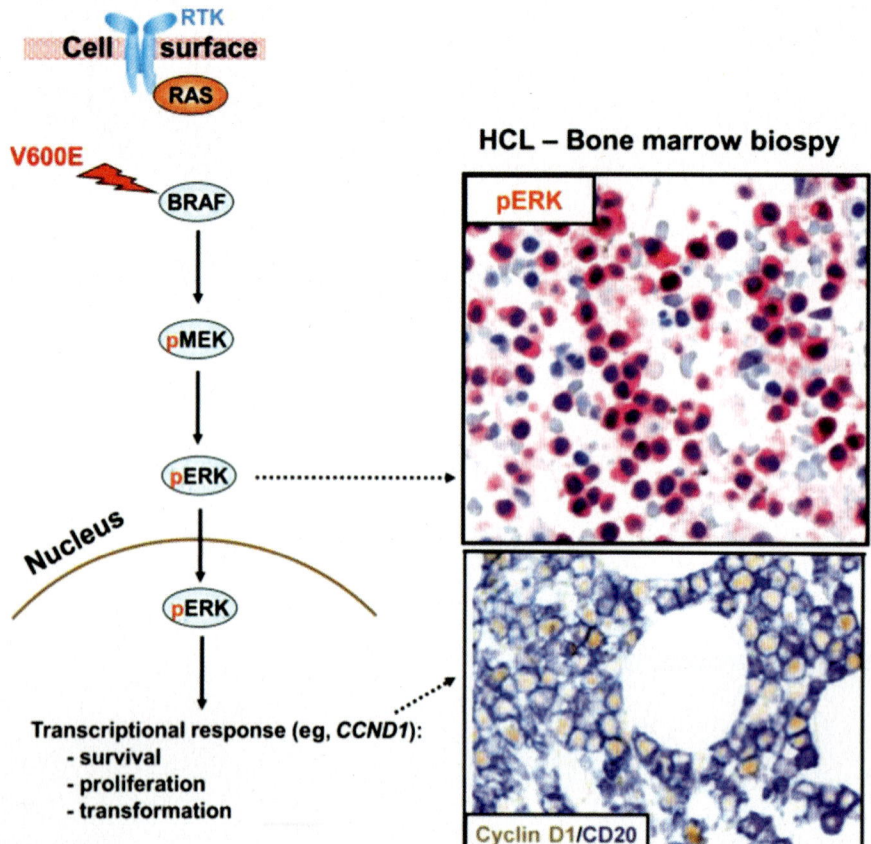

FIGURE 93.3 **The RAS-RAF-MEK-ERK signaling pathway.** The RAS–RAF–MAPK signaling pathway is physiologically triggered by the binding of surface receptor tyrosine kinases (RTKs) to their ligand. This activates RAS and, in turn, RAFs (BRAF and, not shown, CRAF). BRAF-CRAF heterodimers phosphorylate the MEK1 and MEK2 kinases (pMEK), which in turn phosphorylate extracellular signal-regulated kinases 1 and 2 (ERK1 and ERK2 - pERK). Active ERKs phosphorylate several substrates in the cytoplasm (not shown) as well as in the nucleus, where they initiate a transcriptional response (e.g., through the AP-1 transcription complex) that includes cyclin D1 upregulation and that promotes cell survival and proliferation, as well as feedback inhibitory mechanisms (not shown) to counter-regulate pathway activity. The latter, if uncontrolled, can result in neoplastic transformation. The BRAF V600E mutation renders BRAF constitutively active independent from upstream regulatory signals and from heterodimerization with CRAF. On the right, in vivo activation of the BRAF-MEK-ERK pathway in HCL patients is illustrated by the expression of pERK and cyclin-D1 by bone marrow leukemic hairy cells (counterstained with hematoxylin in the upper panel and with the surface B-cell marker CD20 in the lower panel). (Reprinted from Falini B, Martelli MP, Tiacci E. BRAF V600E mutation in hairy cell leukemia: from bench to bedside. *Blood*. 2016;128(15):1918-1927. Copyright © 2016 American Society of Hematology. With permission.)

Table 93.1. Mechanisms for Hairy Cell Leukemia Features

Hairy Cell Feature	Mechanism
Hairy cell projections	Alteration of F-actin structure through up-regulation of ACTB (β-actin) and LST1 (leukocyte transcript 1).
Prolonged survival of hairy cells	Autocrine stimulation by TNF-α, increased cellular levels of bcl-2.
Ability of hairy cell to phagocytose and expression of macrophage markers, for example, CD11c	Up-regulation of annexin1 mediates phagocytic function and c-Maf transcription factor for macrophage differentiation.
Marrow fibrosis and monocytopenia	Up-regulation of FGF2 which activates FGFR1 on the hairy cell producing fibronectin and TGF-β, which causes the adjacent fibroblasts to secrete collagen. TNF-α and TGF-β cause marrow suppression and monocytopenia.
Infiltration of red pulp of spleen by hairy cells with the formation of "pseudosinuses"	Up-regulation of TIMP1, TIMP4, RECK inhibitors of matrix metalloproteinases.
Lack of lymph node involvement by hairy cells	Hairy cells lack L-selectin which is required for binding to venule endothelium and chemokine receptor 7 (CCR7) which is required for transendothelial migration.

Abbreviations: GTPases, guanosine triphosphatases; TGF-β, transforming growth factor-β; TNF-α, tumor necrosis factor.
Adapted from Basso K, Liso A, Tiacci E, et al. Gene expression profiling of hairy cell leukemia reveals a phenotype related to memory B cells with altered expression of chemokine and adhesion receptors. *J Exp Med*. 2004;199:59-68; Pettirossi V, Santi A, Imperi E, et al. BRAF inhibitors reverse the unique molecular signature and phenotype of hairy cell leukemia and exert potent antileukemic activity. *Blood*. 2015;125:1207-1216; Cawley JC, Hawkins SF. The biology of hairy-cell leukemia. *Curr Opin Hematol*. 2010;17:341-349; Swerdlow SH, Campo E, Harris NL, et al. *WHO Classification of Tumors of Haematopoietic and Lymphoid Tissues*. Revised 4th ed. International Agency for Research on Cancer; 2017.

A feature of classical HCL is the reactivity of the hairy cells with CD25, which detects the α-chain of the IL-2 receptor.[65,66] Increased serum levels of the IL-2 receptor have been found in untreated HCL patients, and there is evidence that the leukemic cells release the receptor.[67] The serum levels of IL-2 receptor correlate with the extent of disease and decrease after effective therapy with IFN-α or purine nucleoside analogs.[68] Paradoxically, even though the IL-2 receptor is present on hairy cells, these cells do not respond to stimulation by IL-2, and IL-2 probably does not play a major role in the pathogenesis of HCL.[63]

It has been demonstrated that TNF-α, but not TNF-β, stimulates the growth of hairy cells, whereas in CLL, both forms of TNF stimulate leukemic cell growth (*Figure 93.5*).[69,70] Hairy cells can also produce TNF-α,[71,72] and the serum level of TNF-α is increased in HCL correlating with tumor burden.[72] The TNF-α receptor can also be detected in the serum of these patients, and the level of this receptor also decreases after treatment with IFN-α.[73,74] These findings suggest that TNF-α production by the hairy cells may play an important role in the pathogenesis of HCL by stimulating further growth of hairy cells, and producing pancytopenia through the inhibition of normal marrow function.[69,71,72]

Hairy cells secrete low levels of IL-6, and the serum level of this cytokine is increased in HCL.[63,75] The production of IL-6 messenger RNA and IL-6 secretion is markedly increased by incubating HCL cells with TNF.[75] IL-6 antisense oligonucleotide can inhibit the effect of TNF on IL-6 secretion and DNA synthesis, suggesting that IL-6 mediates the activity of TNF in HCL.[75] Hairy cells also produce bFGF, TGF-β, and express the bFGF receptor.[76,77] Adhesion of the hairy cells to hyaluronan via CD44 induces the secretion of bFGF, but not TGF-β.[76] The secreted bFGF then feeds back on the hairy cell to secrete fibronectin, which is a major component of the marrow fibrosis in this disease. As the spleen does not have hyaluronic acid, this explains the lack of bFGF and fibrosis in this organ despite abundant hairy cells.[76] TGF-β has been shown to be present in increased quantities in the plasma and marrow of patients with HCL, and this also contributes to the marrow fibrosis by inducing the production of collagen and reticulin by adjacent fibroblasts.[77]

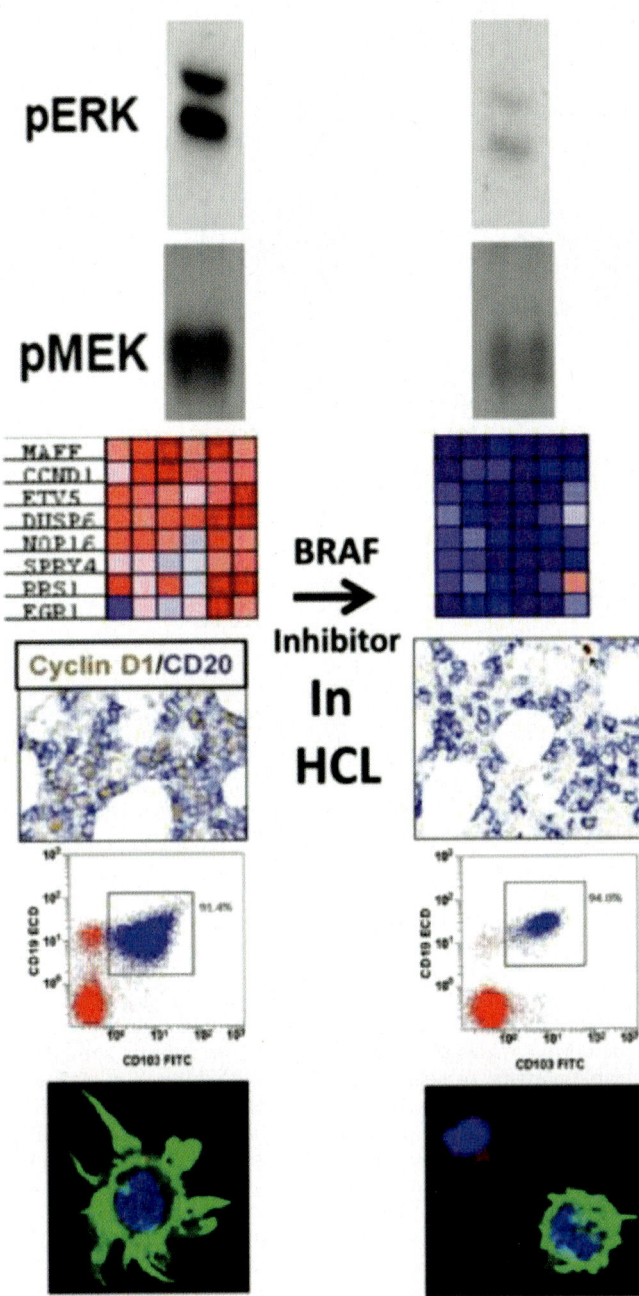

FIGURE 93.4 Studies performed by Pettirossi et al[27] to confirm the mechanism of BRAF inhibition in HCL. (Left) Before and (right) after BRAF inhibition with vemurafenib. From top to bottom: (A) phosphorylated ERK and MEK; (B) HCL-related genes with large differences in expression before and after vemurafenib (each column, 1 of 6 patients); (C) bone marrow immunohistochemistry for cyclin D1 and CD20; (D) flow cytometry of the bone marrow aspirate; and (E) confocal microscopy of HCL cells showing loss of hairy morphology. (Reprinted from Kreitman RJ. Removing a hair of doubt about BRAF targeting. Blood. 2015;125(8):1199-1200. Copyright © 2015 American Society of Hematology. With permission.)

CLINICAL FINDINGS

The diagnosis of HCL occurs at a median age of approximately 55 years (range, 18-95 years), with a significantly higher incidence in men and a male-to-female ratio of 4:1.[1,78–80] Classically, patients present with weakness, fatigue, and other symptoms related to pancytopenia and splenomegaly (Table 93.2). Early studies demonstrated splenomegaly in greater than 90% of patients, often massive, though presentations with marked splenomegaly appear to be declining, possibly due to earlier diagnosis through routine blood work.[79] Peripheral lymphadenopathy is uncommon in HCL, though abdominal adenopathy may be identified through imaging studies at diagnosis (17%), or more commonly at disease relapse (56%), and correlates with disease extent and progression.[81,82] The finding of significant abdominal adenopathy is associated with a decreased complete response rate to purine nucleoside analogs and consequent decreased overall survival.[83,84]

Patients commonly present with pancytopenia at presentation, which is multifactorial in nature and related to marrow infiltration, cytokine-induced myelosuppression and myelofibrosis, and splenic sequestration. Splenomegaly in HCL may produce pancytopenia by three mechanisms. First, the major factor responsible for the cytopenias is pooling of normal peripheral blood cells in the enlarged spleen.[85–90] As much as 90% of the peripheral platelet mass,[86] 30% of the red cell mass,[89] and 65% of the granulocytes[87] may pool in a massively enlarged spleen. In HCL, because of the formation of blood-filled pseudosinuses by hairy cells, a greater proportion of the peripheral red cell volume (as much as 48%) may be pooled in the spleen.[90] A second mechanism is the increased destruction of cells in the spleen. Finally, an expanded plasma volume contributes to the appearance of cytopenia, particularly anemia, with splenomegaly.[85,88] Finally, autoimmune thrombocytopenia or autoimmune hemolytic anemia have been rarely described in HCL.[91,92]

Infections

Fever is rarely a manifestation of the underlying HCL, and when present, it should prompt a careful search for an infectious process. Prior to the development of effective treatments for HCL, infections were a major problem and the leading cause of death in this disease.[93,94] Approximately one third of patients will develop an infection during the course of their disease, and two thirds of these will be serious.[93,95] Pyogenic infections account for ~50% of infectious episodes; Gram-negative and Gram-positive bacteria are identified with approximately equal frequency.[94,95] However, infections can occur with unusual organisms such as atypical mycobacteria, including *Mycobacterium kansasii*.[96,97] Other organisms include *Toxoplasma gondii*, *Legionella*, *Listeria monocytogenes*, and *Pneumocystis jirovecii*, as well as various fungi and viruses.[98–100]

The high risk of infections in untreated HCL is multifactorial. The high infection rate is partly related to neutropenia and monocytopenia, and functional abnormalities of these cells may occur.[99,101] The defects in monocyte production and function may account for the unusual susceptibility of these patients to atypical mycobacterial and fungal infections.[93,102] Lymphocyte functional studies reveal impaired delayed-type hypersensitivity to recall antigens, as well as near-absent antibody-dependent cellular cytotoxicity.[103] While the numbers of CD4+ and CD8+ cells are usually normal or slightly depressed in HCL,[104,105] poor antigen response has been described, thought to be related to the absence of CD28.[103,106] A clonogenic expansion of CD8+ cytotoxic lymphocytes has also been described, though the target or etiology of this expansion has not been identified.[107] These abnormalities can resolve with therapy, although it may take several years to see this effect.[108] Unlike chronic lymphocytic leukemia, the serum Ig levels are usually normal and any decline is usually restricted to IgM.[109]

Table 93.2. Hairy Cell Leukemia: Clinical Manifestations

Manifestation	Incidence (%)
Weakness, easy fatigue	80
Fever, sweats, weight loss, anorexia	20-35
Infection	20-30
Easy bruising, bleeding	20-30
Left upper quadrant abdominal discomfort	25
Autoimmune disorders	15-30
Splenomegaly	80-90
Hepatomegaly	30-40
Ecchymoses, petechiae	20-30

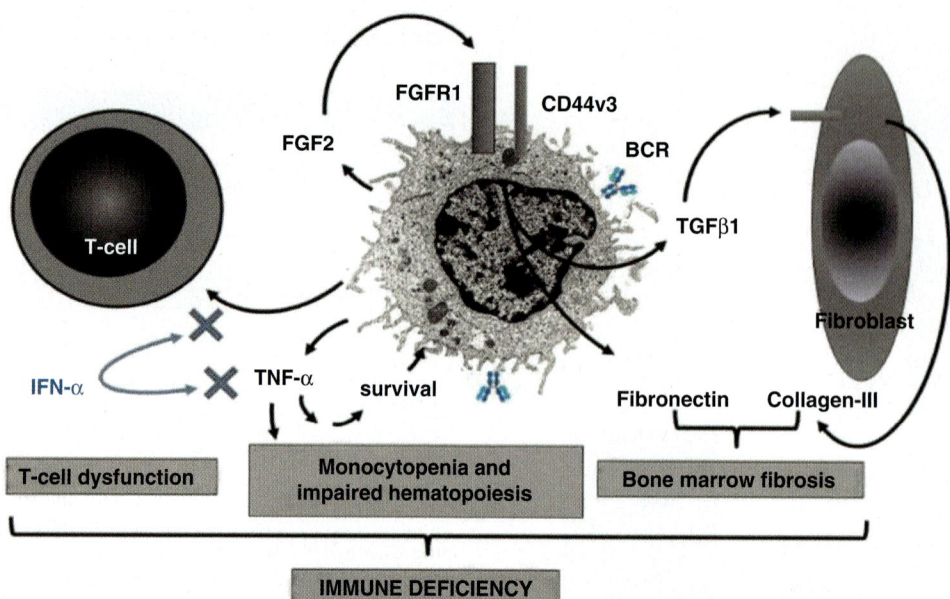

FIGURE 93.5 **Immune suppression in hairy-cell leukemia (HCL).** Immune suppression is a result of T-cell dysfunction and impaired hematopoiesis with pancytopenia, bone marrow fibrosis, and hypersplenism. T-cell activation, decreased numbers of memory T-cells, restricted T-cell repertoire, and opportunistic infections are the result of inappropriate activation and suppression of T-cell responses directly by cytokines produced by the neoplastic B-cells. Cytopenia with severe monocytopenia is caused by the secretion of tumor necrosis factor (TNF)-α by the hairy cells. TNF-α also has autocrine prosurvival effects on the tumor clone. Treatment of HCL with IFN-α is able to restore the abnormal T-cell repertoire and hematopoiesis by inhibiting cytokine (including TNF-α) mediated effects on the T-cells and tumor cell. Fibrosis is caused by production of fibroblast growth factor-2 (FGF-2) and overexpression of its receptor FGFR1. The FGF2-FGFR1 interaction increases with CD44v3 co-receptor and syndecan family members. FGFR1 signals secretion of autocrine fibronectin and of transforming growth factor-β (TGF-β) by hairy cells. TGF-β stimulates adjacent fibroblasts to produce fibronectin and collagen type III. (From Forconi F. Hairy cell leukaemia: biological and clinical overview from immunogenetic insights. *Hematol Oncol.* 2011;29(2):55-66. Copyright © 2010 John Wiley & Sons, Ltd. Reprinted by permission of John Wiley & Sons, Inc.)

Covid-19

In 2020, the emergence of the SARS CoV-2 pandemic (COVID-19) presented a new challenge in the management of patients with hematologic malignancies. While the risk of death was higher in general among those with a malignancy, patients with hematologic malignancy were at greater risk than that reported in those with solid tumors. In addition to an inherent increased risk related to impaired immunity from the underlying disease, many of the agents utilized in treating patients with HCL are associated with treatment-related immunosuppression. While reports in patients with leukemia and lymphoma have outlined the risks associated with COVID-19, specific data in patients with HCL has been limited to case reports.[110]

Recommendations based upon expert opinion in dealing with patients in the midst of the COVID-19 pandemic were recently published indicating that effective therapy for HCL should not be delayed in those presenting with severe pancytopenia.[111] If patients have active infection at presentation for therapy, every effort to control the infection should be pursued before treatment of the HCL. Because purine nucleoside analogs can produce profound and prolonged myelosuppression and immunosuppression, alternative strategies in the severely neutropenic patient with active infection may improve hematologic parameters enabling control of infection acting as a "bridge" to secure a remission. In classic HCL, the presence of the BRAFV600 E mutation has facilitated hematologic response to the "off-label" use of inhibitors (e.g., vemurafenib) of this mutation. The duration of the hematologic response to a BRAF mutation inhibitor alone is predicted by the quality of the response achieved. Patients with a complete response experience a longer duration of response compared to those achieving a partial response.

The addition of an anti-CD20 monoclonal antibody either to a purine analog or a BRAF inhibitor may improve the response of the leukemia but decrease the effectiveness of a potential vaccination against the COVID-19 infection. Therefore, if possible, immunizing patients with HCL should be pursued prior to the use of immunosuppressive anti-leukemia therapy. While the ability of patients with HCL to vigorously respond to vaccines is largely unknown, studies are needed to document the specific immune response in these patients. In the interim, patients are encouraged to pursue effective vaccination against influenza, pneumococcal infection, COVID-19 and other infections that could pose a threat.

Autoimmune Disorders

Clinical manifestations secondary to various autoimmune disorders are being recognized with increasing frequency in patients with HCL.[94,112–116] In one series of patients, these complications were second only to infection as a cause of morbidity.[112] The onset may occur at any time during the course of the disease and is not related to tumor burden. Most frequently, patients present with arthritis, arthralgias, palpable purpura, or nodular skin lesions resulting from cutaneous vasculitis, and low-grade fever.[112,114] Occasionally, patients may have involvement of the lung, liver, intestine, and kidney, with a clinical picture that resembles polyarteritis nodosa.[112,113,115] These patients often have fever, malaise, and weight loss, and a co-existent infection must be ruled out.[112] If skin lesions are present, the diagnosis can be confirmed by biopsy, which usually shows changes compatible with a diagnosis of polyarteritis nodosum or leukocytoclastic vasculitis; occasionally, a vasculitis related to the invasion of the vessel wall by hairy cells occurs and this may appear very similar to polyarteritis nodosa with the presence of aneurysms.[114] In some organs, such as the lung, a granulomatous vasculitis may be found.[112] Angiography may reveal peripheral aneurysms.[112] Antinuclear antibodies, rheumatoid factor, immune complexes, and hepatitis B antigen are variably positive.[117] Cryoglobulinemia has been detected in some patients.[118,119] It has been postulated that the increased incidence of vasculitis in HCL may be related to infections with hepatitis B and other viruses, cross-reactivity of antibodies against hairy cells with epitopes on endothelial cells, and decreased clearance of immune complexes by the impaired immune system.[114] These autoimmune manifestations may be self-limited, but if therapy is required, a short course of corticosteroids is usually effective.[114] Remissions have also been observed after splenectomy, IFN-α, and pentostatin.[112,114,115]

Unusual Manifestations
Bone Lesions

Bone lesions are unusual in HCL and are reported to occur in about 3% of cases, being most usually lytic although osteosclerosis or bone thinning can occur (*Table 93.3*).[120–124] In some patients HCL and multiple myeloma were thought to coexist,[125,126] but HCL alone

Table 93.3. Hairy Cell Leukemia: Unusual Clinical Manifestations

Manifestation	Incidence (%)
Peripheral lymphadenopathy	<5
Lytic bone lesions	3
Skin involvement	5
Splenic rupture	<5
Other organ dysfunction	<5

Table 93.4. Hairy Cell Leukemia: Laboratory Manifestations

Manifestation	Incidence (%)
Pancytopenia	70
Neutropenia	80
Thrombocytopenia	80
Anemia	75
Monocytopenia	98
Leukocytosis	15
Hairy cells in peripheral blood	85
Hairy cells in bone marrow	99

can cause this complication.[121–123] The proximal femurs and spine are typically involved and there is usually advanced disease with extensive marrow infiltration by hairy cells.[122–124] The lesions usually respond well to therapy of the HCL and prompt relief in bone pain can be obtained with steroids and radiotherapy.[18,120,124] F-FDG PET/CT can be useful to assess the extent of disease and response to therapy.[124]

Skin Involvement

Cutaneous lesions occur in about 10% of HCL patients and are usually related to thrombocytopenia (ecchymoses, petechiae), infection, drug reactions or vasculitis, but infiltration of the skin by hairy cells is unusual.[116,127] In a retrospective review of 600 cases, skin lesions thought to be due to infiltration by hairy cells were reported in 8.0% of cases, but histopathological verification was present in only 1.3%.[127] Infiltrative lesions usually are widely disseminated erythematous maculopapules and resolve promptly with cladribine.[116] Many different types of skin lesions can occur, including vasculitis, Sweet's syndrome and pyoderma gangrenosum, all resolving with therapy of the HCL.[116] Finally, the incidence of non-melanotic skin cancers, but not melanoma, may be increased in HCL when compared to an age- and sex-matched population without HCL.[116]

Splenic Rupture

Surprisingly, even with massive splenomegaly, spontaneous splenic rupture is rare in HCL, occurring in ~2% of cases.[1,128]

Other Organ Dysfunction

Although hairy cell infiltration of multiple organs and tissues is a frequent finding at autopsy, clinically significant organ dysfunction is unusual.[129] Infiltration of connective tissue and fat surrounding organs is common.[129] While infections of the central nervous system may occur, involvement of the brain or meninges is uncommon.[130] Infection is by far the most frequent cause for neurologic complications. Pleural effusions, ascites, protein-losing enteropathy, and spinal cord compression may occur rarely in HCL and result from tissue infiltration by hairy cells.[120]

LABORATORY FINDINGS

In line with the decreased clinical presentations of marked splenomegaly, adenopathy, and infection since the initial description of HCL, the degree of cytopenias noted on presentation also appear to be decreasing over time.[79] The relative incidence of the most characteristic laboratory findings is listed in *Table 93.4*. In a series of 725 cases studied by the Italian Cooperative Group, 80% of patients demonstrated significant cytopenias at presentation, with one third of all patients having a hemoglobin level <85 g/L, neutrophils <0.5 × 10^9/L, and platelets <50 × 10^9/L.[79] The authors' experience suggests that the prevalence of such marked cytopenias has further decreased over the past 20 years, with severe pancytopenia in less than 10% of initial presentations. Anemia frequently appears mild (>100 g/L in approximately 80%), while moderate-to-severe neutropenia and/or thrombocytopenia are seen in approximately 60% and 50% of cases, respectively. A careful inspection of the peripheral blood smear demonstrates the presence of typical hairy cells in >85% of patients, and in 13% of cases, there are >5 × 10^9/L hairy cells.[79] In Bouroncle's series of 82 patients, hairy cells accounted for ≥10% of the leukocytes in 80% of patients and ≥50% in 43% of patients.[130] The total leukocyte count was elevated in 20%, but in only 4% did the count exceed 50 × 10^9/L.[131] Monocytopenia also typically occurs in active HCL, though monocytes may be erroneously reported by automated hematology analyzers due to the increased size and light scatter of the hairy cells.[101,132,133]

An isolated elevation of serum alkaline phosphatase level is present in 10% to 19% of individuals with HCL.[134] Hypocholesterolemia is a frequent though non-specific finding in active HCL, which normalizes following purine nucleoside therapy.[135,136] The immunoglobulin levels are usually normal in HCL, although an increase in one or more immunoglobulins (most frequently IgG) occurs in 30% of cases.[109] Unlike chronic lymphocytic leukemia, hypogammaglobulinemia is uncommon in HCL (17%) and is usually restricted to IgM.[109] A low-level monoclonal immunoglobulin may be identified in serum (11.8%, usually IgGK) or urine (5.6%, and intriguingly may be of discordant light chain restriction in approximately 50% of cases.[109] A significant paraproteinemia should warrant consideration of a concomitant monoclonal gammopathy of unknown origin, myeloma, or another B-lymphoproliferative disorder.[122,125,126]

PATHOLOGIC DIAGNOSIS

Cytology

Hairy cells are frequently present on examination of a peripheral blood film and demonstrate a characteristic monocytoid appearance with pale blue-gray cytoplasm, circumferential fine villous projections and a cell diameter in the range of 10-25 μm (*Figure 93.6*). The development of the "hairy" villi in HCL has been related to up-regulation of the expression of ACTB (β-actin) and LST1 in the hairy cells, secondary to the increased activity of mutant BRAF.[27] The characteristic filamentous projections can be seen readily in living hairy cells; using supravital dyes and phase-contrast microscopy, one can observe the cytoplasmic projections protruding and then retracting constantly. While the leukemic cells of other B-cell disorders, such as B-cell prolymphocytic leukemia, HCLv, splenic marginal zone lymphoma, and splenic diffuse red pulp small B-cell lymphoma (SDRPL) may also demonstrate "hairy" villous projections, these are seldom circumferential in distribution but rather polar with broader villi. On both transmission and scanning electron microscopy, the cytoplasmic projections appear as elongated slender microvilli or broad-based ruffles or pseudopods (*Figure 93.6*). Ultrastructural features also include numerous mitochondria, polyribosomes, strands of rough endoplasmic reticulum, intermediate filaments, and some lysosomal granules, with ribosomal-lamellar complexes present in approximately 50% of cases (*Figure 93.6*).[137] The nuclei of hairy cells may be round, oval, or reniform, though dumbbell-shaped or other atypical nuclear forms occasionally present.[138] The chromatin pattern is homogeneous, less clumped and lighter staining than that of normal mature lymphocytes; nucleoli are small and inconspicuous, if seen at all.[139]

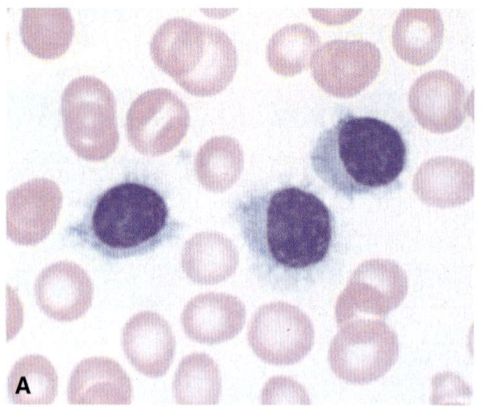
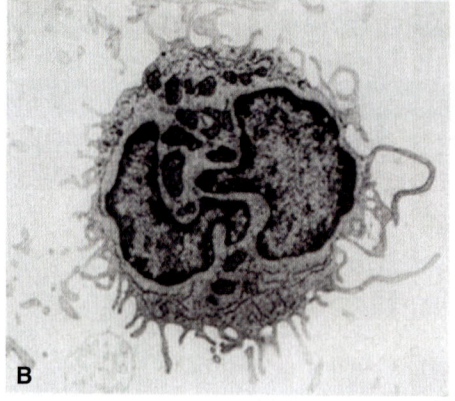

FIGURE 93.6 **Hairy cells from a peripheral blood smear.** Panel A: Light microscopy. Cells have abundant agranular cytoplasm with multiple cytoplasmic projections. Nucleus is round, oval, or reniform with light-staining homogeneous nuclear chromatin (May-Grunwald-Giemsa stain, 1,000×). Panel B: Transmission electron microscopy. The characteristic and delicate cytoplasmic projections are striking. Nucleus is irregular in shape with marginated chromatin (11,000×).

Bone Marrow Histology

Marrow infiltration is demonstrable in trephine biopsies of more than 99% of patients, though exceedingly rare cases with apparent isolated involvement of the spleen may be seen.[134] Overall marrow cellularity appears increased in 54% of patients, though may be hypoplastic to aplastic in 13% to 28% of cases.[139,140] The pattern of bone marrow involvement is typically an interstitial infiltration becoming diffuse, creating a "honeycomb" or "fried egg" appearance, with the nucleus of each hairy cell surrounded by a halo of cytoplasm (Figure 93.7A). The extravasation of red blood cells may be seen, forming "blood lake" pseudosinuses which may also be seen in the liver and spleen.[141] Areas of patchy, low-level infiltration may be difficult to appreciate using standard histologic stains alone, though become readily apparent upon immunohistochemical staining (Figure 93.7). The bone marrow cellularity frequently demonstrates relatively maintained erythropoiesis and megakaryocyte distribution, though a marked reduction in granulopoiesis is common; progressive infiltration eventually leads to suppression of all three lineages. Plasma cells, mast cells, and histiocytes may be seen in close relationship to the hairy cell infiltrate. Bone marrow aspiration may be difficult in HCL, with a "dry tap" or exceedingly hemodiluted aspirates obtained in approximately 50% of cases, secondary to a diffuse reticulin fibrosis produced by the hairy cell infiltrate through autocrine production and multimerization of fibronectin.[77,142] Notably, while extensive reticulin fibrosis may be present, collagenous fibrosis is not seen.

Spleen and Liver Involvement

The spleen is almost always involved in HCL, where the infiltrates are confined to the red pulp, and, unlike most other lymphoproliferative disorders, the white pulp is atrophic.[1,143–146] Blood-filled pseudosinuses lined by hairy cells may be present, and, despite monocytopenia, the number of histiocytes is increased in the red pulp.[141] Significant histologic overlap with splenic diffuse red pulp lymphoma (SDRPL) and HCLv exists, with the formation of pseudosinus "blood lakes" also shared between HCL and SDRPL.[141,143,144,147] Infiltration of the liver occurs in the portal areas, which may demonstrate angiomatous lesions, as well as in the sinuses, where hairy cells may mimic Kupffer cell hyperplasia.[1,137,145,146]

Immunophenotype and Molecular Pathology

Immunophenotyping has proved very useful in assisting in the diagnosis of HCL and in differentiating it from variants and other B-cell malignancies (Table 93.5 and Figure 93.7). Using flow cytometry, very small numbers of abnormal cells can be detected and the diagnosis of HCL can be made on the peripheral blood in the majority of patients. In HCL, the leukemic cells demonstrate exceptionally bright staining for CD19, CD20, and CD22, with pathognemonic coexpression of CD11c, CD25, CD103, and CD123 with homogenous intensity (Figure 93.7), and absence of staining for CD27.[13,139,148] HCL may also express bright CD160,[149,150] CD180,[151] CD200,[150,152] CD305,[153] ROR1,[154] while expression of CD79b is often dim.[155] Rare cases of classical HCL lacking CD25 or CD103 expression are recognized, as are cases with atypical expression of CD5, CD10, CD23, or CD38.[139,156,157]

A mutation-specific antibody for immunohistochemical detection of BRAF V600E has been developed, which appears concordant with molecular testing in both sensitivity and specificity for HCL amongst B cell lymphoproliferative disorders.[158,159] Immunohistochemistry for Annexin A1 is highly specific for HCL amongst B cell lymphoproliferative disorders[160] though it has been described in lymphoplasmacytic lymphoma[161] and a single case of SDRPL.[147] Notably, Annexin A1 staining also highlights myeloid cells and a subset of T lymphocytes, which may be difficult to interpret when involvement is sparse; double staining with PAX5 facilitates a definitive assessment in cases with minimal tissue involvement. Additional immunohistochemical markers commonly positive in HCL include CD11c, CD20, CD25, CD68, CD103, DBA.44, HBME-1, HC2, T-bet, TCL-1, TIA-1, PCA-1, and TRAP (acid phosphatase isoenzyme 5), as well as variable cyclin D1 in a subset of the population.[161–164] While these markers individually demonstrate limited specificity for HCL, they are of greater utility in combination.

Detection of Residual Disease and Minimal Residual Disease

The optimum time to assess for residual disease is not well defined, with evidence of a deepening response for up to 6 months following purine nucleoside analog therapy.[165] Detection of residual disease is defined by morphologically apparent residual hairy cells in the peripheral blood or bone marrow, while the detection of minimal residual disease (MRD) requires the use of ancillary methods. While attainment of a complete response (CR) correlates with an improved relapse-free survival,[80,166,167] the prognostic significance of MRD is less certain, as patients may demonstrate evidence of MRD without symptomatic progression for years, though increasing levels of MRD predicts relapse.[168] Immunohistochemistry for BRAF V600E, CD25,

Table 93.5. Hairy Cell Leukemia: Differential Diagnosis

Splenic diffuse red pulp small B-cell lymphoma
Hairy cell variant
Splenic marginal zone lymphomas/splenic lymphoma with villous lymphocytes
Lymphoplasmacytic lymphoma, including Waldenström macroglobulinemia
B-cell prolymphocytic leukemia
Chronic lymphocytic leukemia/small lymphocytic lymphoma
Mantle cell lymphoma
Other B cell lymphomas with primary splenic presentation
Large granular lymphocytic leukemia
Hepatosplenic T cell lymphoma
Primary myelofibrosis
Malignant histiocytosis
Systemic mast cell disease

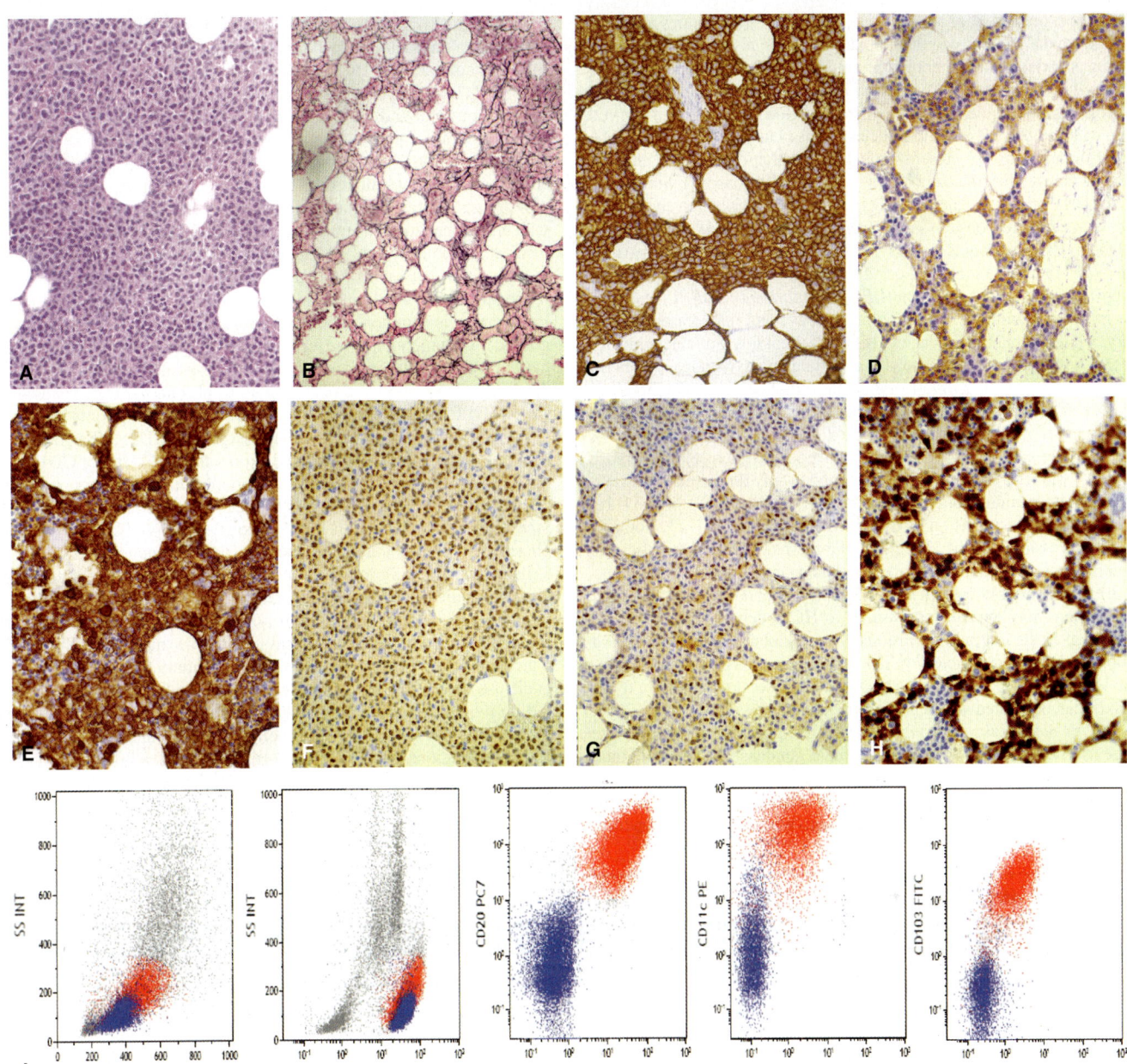

FIGURE 93.7 Bone marrow trephine biopsy (paraffin embedded). Panel A: Pattern of the infiltration gives a "honeycomb" appearance with the nucleus of each hairy cell surrounded by a generous halo of cytoplasm. Nuclei variably appear round, oval, or indented/reniform (hematoxylin and eosin, 400×). Panel B: Reticulin stain, highlighting increased reticulin deposition surrounding the hairy cell infiltrate. Panels C-H: Immunohistochemistry for CD20, CD25, Annexin A1, PAX5, Cyclin D1, and TCL1 may be of utility in highlighting the hairy cell population and confirming the diagnosis. Panel I: Flow cytometry (hemodilute marrow aspirate). The immunophenotype of hairy cell leukemia is distinctive (population in red), with bright and homogeneous coexpression of CD19, CD20, CD45, CD11c, CD25, CD103, and CD123, with monoclonal light chain restriction (not shown). Note is made of the increased light scatter characteristics of the hairy cell population, overlapping the typical "monocyte region." The T cell population (blue) is included as a light scatter and negative immunophenotypic reference.

CD103, cyclin D1, and/or DBA.44 (though scattered non-neoplastic B cell may be positive)[163] in conjunction with CD20 or PAX5, are useful for detection of MRD. It should be noted that loss of cyclin D1 and CD25 are commonly seen following treatment with BRAF inhibitors,[27] and CD20 may be lost or obscured upon treatment with anti-CD20 therapies. Immunohistochemistry for CD11c and annexin A1 are of limited utility in the assessment of small amounts residual disease, given their normal expression on myeloid, monocytic, and subsets of T cells, unless utilized with double staining for PAX5.

DIFFERENTIAL DIAGNOSIS

The differential diagnosis of HCL includes chiefly other hematological malignancies that present with cytopenias and splenomegaly in the absence of lymphadenopathy. These entities can usually be easily separated by their clinical features and histology, though some B cell lymphoproliferative disorders may demonstrate partially overlapping immunophenotypic features (*Table 93.6*).

Hairy cell leukemia-variant (HCLv) is typically seen at an older age of diagnosis (median age 71), and with a male:female ratio of 6:1.[169] HCLv does not demonstrate monocytopenia, while a significant lymphocytosis is common (often >50 × 10^9/L) associated with splenomegaly.

HCLv cells are medium sized lymphocytes with monocytoid features, though frequently demonstrate a prominent nucleolus with a more condensed chromatin, and HCLv has been referred to as the "prolymphocytic variant" of HCL. Villous projections are less commonly seen than in classical HCL and tend to be multi-polar but not circumferential. The immunophenotype includes common B cell markers as well as CD11c and CD103, though CD25 and annexin A1 are not present, and CD123 is weakly expressed, if at all. Marrow infiltration often features a prominent sinusoidal pattern, with interstitial infiltration also present; reticulin fibrosis is variable though commonly mild if present. As a result, unlike the "dry-tap" that occurs with classical HCL, marrow aspiration is usually possible. Splenic infiltration demonstrates diffuse infiltration of the red pulp, with atrophic white pulp follicles. Unlike classical HCL, the *BRAF* V600E mutation is not present, though a mutation of *MAP2K1* may be present—suggestive of a pathobiologic spectrum overlapping with classical *IGHV*4-34 HCL.[32] The clinical course of HCL-v is relatively aggressive, with a poor response to single-agent purine nucleoside analogs alone and the median survival is 9 years. Loss of TP53 function, either by deletion 17p13 or a TP53 mutation, occurs in one-third of cases.[169]

Splenic diffuse red pulp small B-cell lymphoma (SDRPL) presents at a median age range of 66 to 77 years of age and may closely mimic hairy cell leukemia in clinical and histologic features. Patients typically present with marked splenomegaly and cytopenias, without peripheral adenopathy, and with a mild-to-moderate lymphocytosis. The lymphocytes of SDRPL typically demonstrate a less abundant cytoplasm than HCL, with unevenly distributed polar villous projections (typically 1-4 poles) with broad bases.[144] The chromatin tends to be dense, with a more clumped character than the more finely and evenly dispersed chromatin of HCL. The immunophenotype notably may include DBA.44, CD11c, and weak/partial expression of CD25, CD103, and/or CD123. Notably, CD27 expression may be absent.[170] The marrow infiltration pattern is predominantly sinusoidal, though interstitial and nodular infiltration patterns may be variably present with minimal reticulin fibrosis.[144] Splenic involvement may appear very similar to HCL, demonstrating diffuse infiltration of the red pulp, occasionally with blood lake formation, and atrophic white pulp follicles.[144] The clinical course is frequently indolent, with overall survival of >15 years. Many cases do not require treatment or can be treated with splenectomy alone.[144]

Splenic marginal zone lymphoma (SMZL) presents at a similar age range as HCL, though with a mild female gender bias noted in some series. SMZL demonstrates splenomegaly though adenopathy may be seen at more advanced presentations, and a mild-to-moderate peripheral lymphocytosis is commonly present without monocytopenia. Circulating SMZL cells variably demonstrate broad based villi, typically with a unipolar or bipolar distribution, and less voluminous cytoplasm as compared to HCL.[171,172]

SMZL frequently expresses CD27, while DBA.44 and CD11c are variably present, and expression of CD25, CD103, and/or CD123 are typically weak, if present. Annexin A1 is not expressed.[160] Marrow infiltration demonstrates a sinusoidal pattern, which may be accompanied by interstitial or nodular elements without significant reticulin fibrosis. Splenic infiltration demonstrates expansion of the white pulp with a marginal zone pattern, with a variable degree of diffuse or nodular involvement of the red pulp. Median survival is approximately 10 years.[173]

Lymphoplasmacytic lymphoma may demonstrate marked splenomegaly with very limited adenopathy. Low-level peripheral blood involvement is common in both disorders, though monocytopenia is not a feature of lymphoplasmacytic lymphoma. The cytomorphologic features also bear little in common, with lymphoplasmacytic lymphoma demonstrating a spectrum of lymphoid to plasmacytoid morphologies, without villous projections. Lymphoplasmacytic lymphoma expresses typical B cell markers and frequently expresses CD25, though expression of CD11c is less common, and expression of CD103 or CD123 are not seen.[174] In contrast to HCL, lymphoplasmacytic lymphoma typically expresses IgM solely (rarely IgG), and may demonstrate markedly increased IgM resulting in hyperviscosity. Lymphoplasmacytic lymphoma may demonstrate paratrabecular, nodular, and/or interstitial patterns of marrow infiltration, with clear plasmacytic differentiation and Dutcher bodies (intranuclear inclusions of immunoglobulin) are commonly present. Interestingly, both lymphoplasmacytic lymphoma and HCL may induce a reactive increase in marrow mast cells. Significant marrow reticulin fibrosis is not a common feature. Splenic involvement is diffuse, involving the red and white pulp, with small nodules in the red pulp being occasionally present. Mutations in *BRAF* are not seen, though the *MYD88* L265P mutation is common and may occur with *CXCR4* mutations similar to those seen in WHIM (warts, hypogammaglobulinemia, immunodeficiency, and myelokathexis) syndrome.[175]

B-cell prolymphocytic leukemia presents at a median age of 69 years, often presenting with marked splenomegaly and B-symptoms, a marked

Table 93.6. Hairy Cell Leukemia (HCL) and Its Differential: Immunophenotypic Profile and Diagnostic Markers

Marker	HCL	HCL-V	SDRPL	SMZL	B-PLL	LPL
CD19, CD20, CD22	+BR	+	+	++	++	++
Surface Ig	+	+	+	+	++	+
CD11c	+BR	+BR	+	+/W	+	–/W
CD25	+BR	–	–/+	–/+	+	+/–
CD103	+BR	+	–/+	–/W	–	–
CD123	+BR	–/W	–/+	–/W	–	–
CD27	–	–	–	+/–	+	+
Annexin A1[a]	+	–	Rare	–	–	Rare
DBA.44	+	+	+	+/–	–	–
BRAF V600E	80%-100%	0%	Rare	0%	0%	0%
MAP2K1 mutation	5%	10%-50%	Rare	NR	NR	NR
KLF2 mutation	16%	NR	NR	20%-40%	NR	NR
Marrow Infiltration Patterns	IN	IS, IN	IS	IS, N, IN	D	IN, N, P

[a]Normally expressed in myeloid, monocytic, and T cells. MAP2K1 mutations occur in BRAF with HCL and are enriched in cases with IGHV4-34 use, estimated frequency.
Abbreviations: +BR, brightly expressed; +, predominantly positive; +/–, often positive; –/+, infrequently positive; –, negative; –/W, infrequent weak expression; +/W, rare case reports of positive findings; D, diffuse; IN, interstitial; IS, intrasinusoidal; N, nodular; NR, not reported; P, paratrabecular.
Adapted from Forconi F, Raspadori D, Lenoci M, Lauria F. Absence of surface CD27 distinguishes hairy cell leukemia from other leukemic B-cell malignancies. *Haematologica.* 2005;90:266-268; Tiacci E, Trifonov V, Schiavoni G, et al. BRAF mutations in hairy-cell leukemia. *N Engl J Med.* 2011;364:2305-2315; Waterfall JJ, Arons E, Walker RL, et al. High prevalence of MAP2K1 mutations in variant and IGHV4-34-expressing hairy-cell leukemias. *Nat Genet.* 2014;46:8-10; Mason EF, Brown RD, Szeto DP, et al. Detection of activating MAP2K1 mutations in atypical hairy cell leukemia and hairy cell leukemia variant. *Leuk Lymphoma.* 2017;58(1):233-236; Shao H, Calvo KR, Gronborg M, et al. Distinguishing hairy cell leukemia variant from hairy cell leukemia: development and validation of diagnostic criteria. *Leuk Res.* 2013;37:401-409; Del Giudice I, Matutes E, Morilla R, et al. The diagnostic value of CD123 in B-cell disorders with hairy or villous lymphocytes. *Haematologica.* 2004;89:303-308; Sherman MJ, Hanson CA, Hoyer JD. An assessment of the usefulness of immunohistochemical stains in the diagnosis of hairy cell leukemia. *Am J Clin Pathol.* 2011;136:390-399; Baseggio L, Traverse-Glehen A, Callet-Bauchu E, et al. Relevance of a scoring system including CD11c expression in the identification of splenic diffuse red pulp small B-cell lymphoma (SRPL). *Hematol Oncol.* 2011;29:47-51; Garcia-Sanz R, Jimenez C, Puig N, et al. Origin of Waldenstrom's macroglobulinaemia. *Best Pract Res Clin Haematol.* 2016;29:136-147.

lymphocytosis with intermediate-to-large circulating lymphocytes having a prominent central nucleolus and without villous cytoplasmic projections. The immunophenotype is similarly distinct; expressions of CD25, CD103, CD123, and annexin A1 are not seen in B-cell prolymphocytic leukemia. Marrow involvement typically demonstrates a marked diffuse infiltration, without significant reticulin fibrosis. Spleen involvement demonstrates diffuse expansion of the white pulp, although infiltration of the red pulp is also commonly present. This is an aggressive disease, and *TP53* mutations are common, with subsequent poor response to therapy and a survival typically less than 3 years.[176]

INDICATIONS FOR THERAPY AND TYPES OF TREATMENT

While most patients will require therapy when first seen, about 10% can be initially observed until there is disease progression. In general, patients are treated if they have symptoms referable to HCL, for example, uncomfortable splenomegaly, or if they have a progressive fall in their blood counts. Consensus guidelines are to start treatment are a hemoglobin of <110 g/L, platelets <100 × 10^9/L or a neutrophil count of <1 × 10^9/L.[2] Confirmation of these values is important with consideration of disease-related symptoms as a reason to begin therapy.

Although splenectomy was the previous standard treatment for HCL, therapy for this disease in the 1980s IFN-α became the standard first-line therapy but was rapidly replaced by the nucleoside analogs, pentostatin and cladribine. The purine analogs remain the initial standard treatments for HCL.[177–179] The anti-CD20 monoclonal antibody, rituximab, can enhance the activity of cladribine and under some circumstances may be used in combination. Over time, patients may become resistant to the nucleoside analogs and be considered for treatment with BRAF/ERK inhibitors, the Bruton's tyrosine kinase (BTK) inhibitor, ibrutinib, or the anti-CD22 monoclonal antibody, moxetumumab pasudotox.

Splenectomy

Until the mid-1980s, the standard therapy for HCL was splenectomy.[180–183] Occasionally, patients may achieve a CR with splenectomy, and these patients may have a pure "splenic" form of HCL. Approximately two thirds of patients have a hematologic response and the procedure may also alleviate early satiety, weight loss, and abdominal discomfort. While early studies demonstrated no improvement in survival after splenectomy,[180,181] a subsequent multicenter retrospective analysis of 391 patients demonstrated a highly significant survival advantage ($P < .0001$) for patients who underwent splenectomy.[182]

In 40% of patients a postsplenectomy hemoglobin of >110 g/L, neutrophils >1 × 10^9/L, and platelets >100 × 10^9/L, was achieved. Patients with larger spleens also responded better than those with smaller spleens. The duration of response after splenectomy is variable, but some patients remain asymptomatic for years. Approximately one third, however, achieve only a minimal response or relapse within a few months. Important prognostic markers are bone marrow cellularity and platelet count.[184] Thus, the time from splenectomy to death is shorter and the need for additional therapy more likely if the postoperative bone marrow cellularity is ≥85% and/or the platelet count is <60 × 10^9/L. Splenectomy is now rarely performed in HCL, but may be of value for patients with splenic rupture, patients with the pure "splenic" form of the disease, and patients with splenomegaly and profound thrombocytopenia due to hypersplenism.

Purine Nucleoside Analogs

The purine nucleoside analogs, pentostatin (deoxycoformycin, dCF) and cladribine (2-chlorodeoxyadenosine, CdA), have shown remarkable activity in HCL and have replaced IFN-α as first-line therapy for HCL. Their proposed mechanisms of action have been reviewed, although the exquisite sensitivity of HCL compared to other lymphoid malignancies is a unique feature of the disease.[185] After therapy with the adenosine deaminase inhibitor, pentostatin, deoxyadenosine and adenosine accumulate in the plasma and deoxyadenosine is preferentially phosphorylated in lymphocytes to deoxyadenosine triphosphate (dATP). The intracerebral accumulation of deoxyadenosine and adenosine likely causes the nausea and vomiting that are the major toxicities of this agent. Through the addition of a chlorine group to deoxyadenosine, cladribine is resistant to degradation by adenosine deaminase and is phosphorylated in lymphocytes to 2-CdATP. Through the intracellular accumulation of dATP or 2-CdATP, pentostatin and cladribine induce DNA breaks in lymphocytes, which leads to apoptosis. However, cladribine differs from deoxyadenosine in that it is also phosphorylated by deoxyguanosine kinase in the mitochondria to 2-CdATP, which is directly toxic to the mitochondria. This may explain the greater myelotoxicity of cladribine, as compared to pentostatin.

Pentostatin in HCL

Pentostatin is highly effective in HCL and produces a much higher rate of durable CR than is observed with IFN-α (*Table 93.7*).[187] Pentostatin has been administered in a variety of different doses and schedules for HCL, but regardless of the mode of administration, it produces responses in most patients. The CR rate ranges from 44% to 89% (median, 76%), and the PR rate varies from 0% to 52% (median, 16%).[84,187,189,190,195–198] Patients who relapse after splenectomy or who are resistant to IFN-α also respond to pentostatin, with a median CR rate of 42% and a PR rate of 45%.[198–200] In two large studies, the response rates to pentostatin were similar in untreated patients and in patients previously treated with IFN-α.[84,187] Moreover, these studies identified young age, initial high hemoglobin, high white cell count, and little or no splenomegaly as favorable prognostic features. The most commonly used treatment regimen is pentostatin 4 mg/m^2 intravenously (IV) every second week; the average number of treatments to CR is 8 (range, 4-15).[187,195] The peripheral blood lymphocyte count falls rapidly after the initiation of treatment, with the hairy cell count decreasing by 50% to 95% in the first week. The peripheral blood lymphocyte count falls rapidly after the initiation of treatment, with the hairy cell count decreasing by 50% to 95% in the first week.[133] Concomitantly, there is a rapid increase in platelets followed by recovery of neutrophils and hemoglobin; the median time to documented peripheral and marrow CR is 4 months.[133] In contrast to IFN-α, there is resolution of the marrow fibrosis after pentostatin.[133,201] Using immunophenotyping of peripheral blood or bone marrow, immunohistochemistry of the bone biopsy, or gene rearrangement studies, one can detect MRD in HCL patients who are in morphologic CR after pentostatin, suggesting that pentostatin cannot entirely eliminate the hairy cell population.[202,203] In addition, relapses are observed after discontinuation of treatment without evidence of a plateau, although the duration of remissions is considerably longer than for IFN-α.[166,187,204,205]

Several studies have evaluated the long-term outcome of patients treated with pentostatin (*Table 93.8*).[166,167,198,205,206] The longest follow-up is of 188 patients followed for a median of 14 years with the relapse rates at 5, 10, and 15 years being 24%, 42%, and 47%, respectively.[166,210] The likelihood of relapse depended on response and pre-treatment parameters with the longest remission being in those who achieved a CR and had a pre-treatment hemoglobin of >100 g/L and platelets >100 × 10^9/L, and the worst prognosis was in those who achieved a PR and were anemic and/or thrombocytopenic pre-treatment (*Figure 93.8*).[166] For patients who remained in CR at 5 years the likelihood of remaining in CR by 15 years was 75%. For patients requiring another treatment, the likelihood of achieving a CR decreased but for those who did achieve a CR the prognosis was similar as for those with a first-time CR.

In a Phase III intergroup study, patients were randomized to receive pentostatin, 4 mg/m^2 IV every 2 weeks, or IFN-α, 3 × 10^6 U SC three times per week.[167,187] Patients not responding to one treatment were switched to the other agent. There were 241 patients who received pentostatin and were followed for a median of 9.3 years; 154 received pentostatin as initial therapy, and 87 received pentostatin after failure with IFN-α. For all patients, the estimated 5- and 10-year survivals were 90% and 81%, similar to those predicted for the

Table 93.7. Response Rates Using Different Agents and Treatment Schedules for Hairy Cell Leukemia

Agent	Author[Ref] (Year)	Dose and Schedule	Number of Patients	CR (%)	PR (%)
Interferon-α					
	Spielberger[186] (1994)	2×10^6 U/m² SC; 3 ×/wk for 12 or 18 mo	69	13	62
	Grever[187] (1995)	3×10^6 U SC; 3 ×/wk for 12 mo	159	11	27
	Rai[188] (1995)	2×10^6 U SC; 3 ×/wk for 12 mo	55	24	49
Pentostatin					
	Spiers[189] (1987)[a]	5 mg/m² IV daily × 2; repeated every 14 d until CR	27	59	37
	Johnston[190] (1988)	Cycles (4 mg/m² IV/wk × 3); q8wk until CR + 2 further cycles	28	89	11
	Grever[187] (1995)	4 mg/m² IV q2wk; until CR + 2 to max 12 mo	154	76	3
	Maloisel[84] (2003)	4 mg/m² IV q2wk until max response or failure	238	79	17
	Else[166] (2009)	4 mg/m² IV q2wk; until CR + 2	188	82	14
Cladribine					
	Juliusson[191] (1995)	3.4 mg/m² SC daily × 7 d	73	81	14
	Saven[192] (1998)	0.1 mg/kg/d cont IV × 7 d	349	91	7
	Lauria[193] (1999)	0.15 mg/kg IV over 2 h weekly × 6	30	73	27
	Robak[194] (2007)	0.12 mg/kg/d IV over 2 h × 5 d	62	76	19
		0.12 mg/kg/wk IV × 6 wk	54	72	19
	Else[166] (2009)	0.1 mg/kg/d cont IV × 7 d	45	76	24

Abbreviations: cont, continuous; CR, complete remission; IV, intravenous; max, maximum; PR, partial remission; SC, subcutaneously.

general population. The survival was similar whether patients were treated initially with pentostatin or were crossed over to pentostatin after treatment with IFN-α (Figure 93.9A). Patients younger than 55 years of age did significantly better than patients 55 years of age or older, and the 10-year survivals for the two groups were 93% and 68%, respectively (Figure 93.9B). Similarly, in a large multicenter retrospective study from France, the estimated survivals at 5 and 10 years in 230 evaluable patients treated with pentostatin were both 89%.[84] In that study, a hemoglobin level <100 g/L, a white cell count $<2 \times 10^9$/L, and lymphadenopathy were associated with decreased survival.

Toxicity

Pentostatin is generally well tolerated, although nausea and vomiting and lethargy can occur. Drug-induced neutropenia with fever commonly occurs with initiation of treatment and deaths from infection have been observed. However, for patients receiving 4 mg/m² pentostatin every 2 weeks, infections can be avoided by delaying the treatments if the white blood count is $<1.5 \times 10^9$/L.[195] In addition, the dose of pentostatin can be delayed to every 3 weeks if the absolute neutrophil count falls below the baseline count as consequence of treatment. This delay of a week may permit improvement in blood counts, and then treatment may be resumed. Intermittent administration permits

Table 93.8. Long-Term Follow-Up of Patients With Hairy Cell Leukemia

Agent	Author[Ref] (year)	Number of Patients	CR (%)	Median Follow-Up Months (Range)	Relapse After CR (%)	Outcome for Patients in CR[e]
Interferon-α	Grever[187] (1995)	159	11	57 (19-82)	70	
Pentostatin	Johnston[206] (2000)	28	89	125 (61-137)	36	Median time to relapse 49 mo (15-122 mo)
	Flinn[167] (2000)	241	76	112 (19-139)	18	RFS 67% at 10 y
	Maloisel[84] (2003)	238[a]	79	63.5 (0.39-138.4)	14	DFS 68.8% at 10 y
	Else[166] (2009)	188	82	71 (6-139)	44	Relapse rate at 15 y, 47%
Cladribine	Saven[192] (1998)	358[b]	91	58 (1-134)	24	
	Jehn[207] (2004)	40		102 (1.2-146)	39	
	Goodman[208] (2003)	209[c]	95	108 (86-172)	34	Median time to relapse 44 mo (8-118 mo)
	Chadha[209] (2005)	86[d]	79	116 (4-165)	31	Median time to relapse 35 mo
	Else[166] (2009)	45	76	108 (5-192)	38	Relapse rate at 15 y, 48%

Abbreviation: NA, not available.
[a]Only 230 evaluable for response.
[b]Only 349 evaluable for response.
[c]Follow-up of at least 7 years. Only 207 evaluable for response.
[d]Only 85 evaluable for response.
[e]RFS, relapse-free survival.

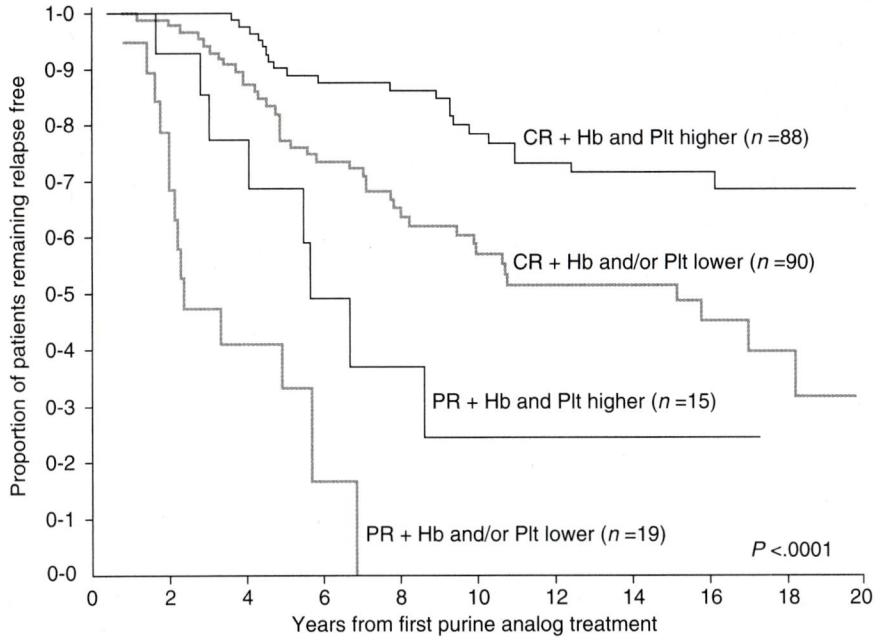

FIGURE 93.8 Relapse-free survival after first-line purine analog therapy. Patients were separated by pre-treatment blood counts and response to therapy. Relapse-free survival was longest in complete responders (CR) with hemoglobin (Hb) > 100 g/L and platelet count >100 × 10^9/L (CR + Hb and Plt higher) and shortest in partial responders with hemoglobin <10 g/dL and/or platelet count <100 × 10^9/L (PR + Hb and/or Plt lower). (From Else M, Dearden CE, Matutes E, et al. Long-term follow-up of 233 patients with hairy cell leukaemia, treated initially with pentostatin or cladribine, at a median of 16 years from diagnosis. *Br J Hematol.* 2009;145(6):733-740. Copyright © 2009 Blackwell Publishing Ltd. Reprinted by permission of John Wiley & Sons, Inc.)

titration of the dose of pentostatin depending on the neutropenia observed early in the course of therapy. Alternatively, low-dose pentostatin has been successfully administered to patients with infection when therapy was essential.[211] Pentostatin decreases the T-cells more than the B-cells, and CD4$^+$ cells are affected to a greater extent than CD8$^+$cells or NK-cells; in contrast, immunoglobulin levels are not affected.[105,202,212,213] The CD4$^+$ and CD8$^+$ cell counts both fall to <0.2 × 10^9/L during therapy, but the CD4$^+$ counts recover and normalize in 3.0 to 49.5 months (median, 14.5 months) after therapy.[202] The CD8$^+$ and B cells recover more rapidly, while NK cells increase during therapy.[105,202,212] Associated with the decrease in T-cells during therapy is an increase in the incidence of herpetic infections, and there is a gradual decrease in the incidence after discontinuation of therapy.[105,202,212] However, there is no increase in more unusual opportunistic infections, either during therapy or during long-term follow-up, and there is no evidence of a significant increase in second malignancies.[166,167]

Although neurotoxicity is a problem with high doses of pentostatin,[214] this is not observed with the doses used for HCL.

Cladribine in HCL

Cladribine has equivalent activity to pentostatin in HCL, with the advantage of rarely causing nausea and vomiting although it may be more myelosuppressive.[166,192,205,207–209,215–223] In initial studies, cladribine was administered as 0.1 mg/kg/d by continuous infusion for 7 days, because in vitro studies indicated that a prolonged exposure to cladribine was required for cytotoxic effect.[221] Response rates varied, with the CR ranging from 50% to 91% (median, 80%) and PR from 0% to 37% (median, 16%).[192,207–209,215–223] As with pentostatin, there was a rapid recovery in blood counts, with the platelet count increasing first, followed by an increase in neutrophils and hemoglobin. Some patients achieved a CR with normal blood counts, whereas the marrows remained hypocellular.[224] Technetium 99 m sulfur colloid scans have demonstrated increased uptake in the distal appendicular skeleton in some of these patients, suggesting abnormal areas of hematopoiesis.[224]

Although hairy cells may not be seen in the marrow 3 to 4 months after cladribine treatment, the leukemic cells can still be detected by immunostaining, using the monoclonal antibody, DBA.44,[225] or by

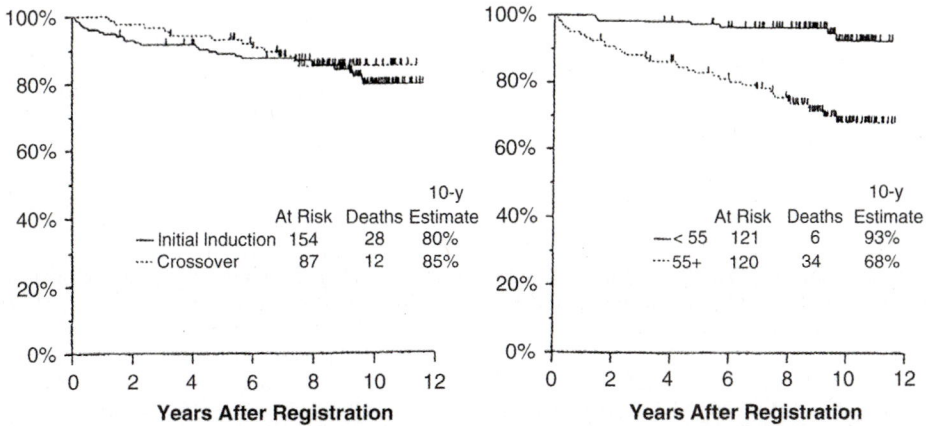

FIGURE 93.9 Long-term responses to treatment with the nucleoside analogs. A, Survival of patients treated initially with pentostatin or after crossover from interferon-α. Survival is similar in both groups (*P* = .59). Figure shows estimated distributions of overall survival (Kaplan-Meier estimates) from date of registration for 2′-deoxycoformycin (dCF) therapy, by phase of treatment. B, Overall survival by age of patients treated with dCF. Survival is significantly better for patients younger than 55 years of age (*P* < .0001). Figure shows estimated distributions of overall survival (Kaplan-Meier estimates) from date of registration for dCF therapy, by age at start of initial therapy. (Reprinted from Flinn IW, Kopecky KJ, Foucar MK, et al. Long-term follow-up of remission duration, mortality, and second malignancies in hairy cell leukemia patients treated with pentostatin. *Blood.* 2000;96:2981-2986. Copyright © 2000 American Society of Hematology. With permission.)

PCR with clone-specific probes for *IGH* genes.[226] When marrows were intermittently examined by DBA.44 for 25 months after treatment with cladribine, there was no increase in the number of hairy cells in the marrow in most cases, suggesting stabilization of residual disease.[225] However, others have suggested that the presence of residual disease is predictive of relapse.[227] Interestingly, 19 of 358 patients treated at Scripps have remained in long-term remission after a single cycle of cladribine. The median time from cladribine was 16 years and 9 had no evidence of MRD, 7 had MRD, and 3 had morphologic evidence of HCL.[223]

In a large, long-term study from the Scripps Clinic, 91% of patients achieved a CR with cladribine, and these 349 patients were followed for a median of 52 months (range, 1-134 months).[192] Of these patients, 24% relapsed at a median time of 30 months (range, 7-85 months). The overall survival at 48 months was 96%. The same group has evaluated 207 patients followed for at least 7 years, and 37% relapsed with patients achieving a CR relapsing later (median 44 months [8-118 months]) than those who achieved PR (median 31 months [10-108 months]). Of 60 patients who received a second cycle of cladribine, 75% achieved a CR and 17% a PR.[208] Two studies have evaluated the response of HCL patients ≤40 years of age treated with cladribine compared to older patients[78,80] Overall response of both age groups was similar, although the time to next treatment was shorter for younger patients and they needed more frequent treatments.

Because cladribine has not been compared with pentostatin in a randomized study, it is unknown whether one of these agents is superior in terms of toxicities and long-term outcomes (*Table 93.8*). However, in a retrospective analysis of patients treated either with pentostatin or cladribine at the Royal Marsden Hospital the overall response rates and survivals were the same for both drugs.[166,210] A number of patients who were resistant to pentostatin have obtained remissions with cladribine, suggesting a possible lack of cross-resistance between these agents.[228]

Toxicity

Cladribine was implicated as the cause of deaths in the National Cancer Institute group C Phase II study in 1.1% of 979 patients.[222] The major toxicity is marrow suppression; one-third to one-half of patients develop severe neutropenia with infections and often require prolonged blood support after therapy. This problem is not prevented by prophylactic antibiotics, and, although an infectious cause for the fever is not found in most cases, affected patients may require hospitalization for septic workup and antibiotics. The likelihood of this complication occurring increases with the severity of initial marrow involvement, and granulocyte colony-stimulating factor has been administered using 5 μg/kg/d SC on days −3, −2, and −1 before a standard 7-day course of cladribine, and then after cladribine until the neutrophil count was >2 × 10^9/L for 2 consecutive days.[229] However, although this increased the neutrophil count, there was no decrease in the number of febrile episodes and the number of hospitalizations for antibiotics. An identical phenomenon has been observed after treatment of HCL with standard doses of pentostatin,[190,204] suggesting that the fever following treatment can be partly related to the release of cytokines by tumor.[219]

It is important to realize that patients with active infection were not eligible to participate in the initial cladribine trials. Thus, a patient with hairy cell leukemia who requires therapy, but has an active infection, presents a challenging dilemma. In general, it is important to try to treat any infection before administering a purine analog and if there is urgency in treating the leukemia initial therapy with α-IFN, vemurafenib or low-dose pentostatin.[211,230–232]

Moreover, the incidence of febrile neutropenia may be less following biweekly pentostatin than seen with cladribine, as the intermittent schedule of drug administration following pentostatin affords an opportunity to titrate the drug administration depending upon the neutrophil count. It is clear that the optimal management of patients with HCL and concomitant active infection requires further investigation.

Cladribine also produces a profound fall in the $CD4^+$ and $CD8^+$ cell counts, and although $CD8^+$ cell counts may recover within 3 months, the $CD4^+$ count may take longer than 3 years to normalize.[104,233] Despite this, there have, to date, been no long-term problems with opportunistic infections after therapy with cladribine.[213,219] However, infections, sometimes opportunistic, do occur in some of these patients, and deaths have been reported.[218,234] More recently, Epstein-Barr virus, associated diffuse large B-cell non-Hodgkin lymphoma, have been described in two patients shortly after completion of cladribine therapy.[235,236] Significant neurotoxicity has also been observed with cladribine and may involve the legs or arms.[222] Transfusion-associated graft-vs-host disease has been observed with multiple cycles of cladribine in low-grade lymphomas but, to the authors' knowledge, this has not been observed in HCL.[237] However, we do recommend use of irradiated blood products for those requiring transfusions.[2]

There has been interest in investigating different modes of cladribine administration to simplify treatment and minimize toxicity. Liliemark et al 238 demonstrated an identical "area under the curve" for drug concentration vs time using the same cladribine concentration given by continuous infusion, as a 2-hour infusion, or given orally using twice the IV dose. Similar responses have been obtained with cladribine in HCL using 0.1 mg/kg IV over 2 hours daily × 5[239] or 0.1 mg/kg SC daily × 7[191,240] as when the drug was administered as 0.1 mg/kg/d by continuous infusion × 7. Weekly cladribine (e.g., 0.14-0.15 mg/kg/wk IV × 5-6 weeks) appears to be as effective as the other schedules.[193,194,241,242] While this regimen was initially felt to be associated with less marrow suppression and to be safer than conventional regimens, recent randomized studies demonstrated that the weekly regimen produced an equivalent incidence of infections and septic deaths as a standard regimen using 0.12 mg/kg over 2 hours daily × 5.[194,242] However, it should be noted that in these two studies cladribine was given weekly regardless of blood counts, rather than delaying treatment to allow recovery of the neutrophil count following each weekly treatment. Using biweekly pentostatin, the drug is frequently be held if the neutrophil count is <1.5 × 10^9/L.[195]

Fludarabine alone has not been evaluated extensively in HCL. However, complete and partial responses have been observed in the few patients treated thus far.[243,244]

Interferon-α

IFN-α is also useful in HCL,[187,188,245–251] due to its effects on TNF-α on hairy cells.[252] IFN-α induces apoptosis in nonadherent hairy cells by increasing the production of TNF-α by the hairy cells and increasing their sensitivity to TNF-α by reducing the levels of inhibitors of apoptosis (IAPs). However, IFN-α does not affect the IAPs or induce apoptosis in hairy cells adhering to vitronectin or fibronectin. These results may explain why IFN-α can clear hairy cells rapidly from the bloodstream, but not from the tissues, where the leukemic cells are adherent. Unfortunately, standard IFN-α is no longer available for clinical while the pegylated version of IFN-α is available the dosing of the pegylated form in HCL requires study. However, for completeness we will review prior studies with standard IFN-α.

The overall response rate with IFN-α is ~80%, with 13% having a CR and 69% having a PR (*Table 93.7*).[187,188,251] Responding patients have a reduced incidence of infections, even if they remain neutropenic.[249] The responses occur rapidly, regardless of whether the patients have previously had a splenectomy, with hairy cells disappearing from the peripheral blood within the first week; the platelet count returns to normal within 2 months, the hemoglobin level within 4 months, and the neutrophil count within 4 to 6 months.[249] The percentage of hairy cells in the bone marrow decreases, but they rarely disappear completely, and the reticulin fibrosis persists.[253,254]

In most series, the dose of IFN-α is 2 to 4 × 10^6 U/m^2 subcutaneously (SC) three to seven times weekly for 12 months. Higher doses do not appear to increase the response rate and are associated with more toxicity.[255] In addition, extending the treatment beyond 12 months does not improve the response rate, and the development of a chronic fatigue syndrome is more prevalent and severe.[256] Doses 1 log lower (2 × 10^5 U/m^2 three times weekly) show activity, but the response is inferior to that achieved with higher IFN-α doses.[257]

The relapse rate is high (33%-77%) after the discontinuation of IFN-α, usually 6 to 31 months after cessation of therapy.[186,250] Maintenance low-dose IFN-α (1×10^6 U, three times/week, or 3×10^6 U, once per week) can prolong remissions with minimal toxicity.[251,258,259] When patients relapse after IFN-α, a further remission can generally be obtained with IFN-α[258,259] or the nucleoside analogs.[187] In addition, patients who relapse after therapy with the nucleoside analogs may respond to IFN-α.[260]

Neutralizing anti-IFN antibodies appear in one third of patients treated with IFN-α2a but not with IFN-α2b.[261,262] However, the clinical significance of these antibodies and their role in the induction of resistance to therapy are controversial.[261] Generally these antibodies develop early in therapy and may disappear with ongoing therapy.[262]

Virtually all patients experience toxicity with IFN-α therapy, and the frequency and severity are dose- and age-related. Flu-like symptoms occur in most patients with the initiation of treatment; these symptoms can usually be controlled with acetaminophen or by reducing the IFN-α dosage, and symptoms usually resolve within 2 to 4 weeks. Less common symptoms include: nausea and vomiting; diarrhea; somnolence and confusion; cardiovascular disorders, including hypotension and tachycardia, and skin changes, such as rash and pruritus.[256]

With high doses, leukopenia, thrombocytopenia, and anemia may occur, but this is rare with the doses of IFN-α used for HCL. A worsening of pre-existing autoimmune disorders, or the emergence of new autoimmune problems, has also been reported with IFN-α.[263] In most reports, patients developed thyroiditis, autoimmune thrombocytopenia, or anemia.[264]

Rituximab

Monoclonal antibody therapy is an attractive option for HCL, because many patients have significant neutropenia at the time of diagnosis and the monoclonal antibodies should theoretically not worsen this problem. Rituximab is directed against CD20 and exerts its antitumor activity by complement-dependent cytotoxicity, antibody-dependent cell-mediated cytotoxicity, or the direct induction of apoptosis.[265]

Using rituximab, 375 mg/m² IV once per week for 4 weeks, response rates of 25% to 75% were observed with a variable number of CRs.[266–269] The poorest responses were observed in heavily pre-treated patients.[266] Prolonging therapy to 8 weeks may improve response, and a response rate of 80% with 53% CRs was observed in 15 patients with relapsed or refractory HCL.[268]

Enhancing Response by Repeating Treatment With the Purine Nucleoside Analog or Adding Rituximab

As patients who achieve a CR appear to have a much longer remission than those who achieve a PR, attempts have been made to convert PR to a CR. The group at the Royal Marsden Hospital have demonstrated in 8 patients who achieved a PR with cladribine that a second course of treatment at 4 to 7 months led to a CR in 6 patients and the relapse-free survival was the same whether one or two cycles of therapy was required to achieve the CR.[166,210]

An alternate approach has been to administer rituximab with or following chemotherapy to consolidate the remission.[269–272] Thus, rituximab given 3 to 6 months following cladribine can increase the number of CRs without additional toxicity.[268] In a phase II clinical trial, 59 previously untreated, 14 relapsed HCL and 7 HCLv patients received cladribine followed 1 month later by rituximab 375 mg/m² IV weekly for 8 weeks.[272] The CR rate was 100% for the HCL patients and 86% for the HCLv patients. The failure-free survivals at 5 years for the untreated HCL, relapsed HCL and HCLv patients were 95%, 100% and 86%, respectively. A subsequent phase II study has confirmed the benefit of adding rituximab to cladribine.[269] Sixty eight untreated HCL patients received cladribine and 8 weekly treatments with rituximab, either given concurrently or with rituximab given ≥6 months after cladribine, if the peripheral blood remained MRD positive. The marrow MRD negative CR rate at 6 months in cladribine alone vs cladribine with concurrent rituximab was 24% and 97%, respectively.

New Therapies

In the past 10 years, there has been the development of novel new therapies in HCL, partly based on our increased understanding about the biology of this disease.[177–179]

Moxetumomab Pasudotox

Moxetumumab pasudotox is an immunotoxin directed against CD22, and contains the modified light chains of the antibody bound to a truncated form of the Pseudomonas exotoxin.[273,274] The immunotoxin can kill the targeted cells through a variety of ways and the immune mechanisms utilized by rituximab are not required. A phase III global single-arm study in 80 relapsed/refractory patients received moxetumumab pasudotox 40 μg/kg intravenously on days 1, 3 and 5, repeated monthly.[275,276] Sixty-three percent patients completed 6 cycles and at a median of 24.6 months follow-up, 36% of patients had a durable CR (lasting >3 months) and the median duration of remission following the onset of CR was 62.8 months (range, 0.1+ to 62.8 months). In addition, another one-third of patients had a PR. Eighty five percent of patients achieving a CR had no marrow minimal residual disease (MRD negative), and these patients had a longer remission than those who were MRD positive. In contrast to the nucleoside analogs, moxetumumab pasudotox produced less myelotoxicity and immunosuppression. However, all patients had at least one toxicity, the most common being nausea, peripheral oedema, headaches and fevers. Unique toxicities included hemolytic uremic syndrome or a capillary leak syndrome, necessitating treatment discontinuation in 7.5% of patients.[276] Based on these results the US FDA has approved moxetumumab pasudotox for use in relapsed/refractory HCL after two or more prior therapies, including a purine nucleoside analog.

BRAF and MEK Inhibition

Several reports have documented the effectiveness of BRAF inhibition with vemurafenib for the treatment of refractory HCL.[231,232,277] Dietrich et al[277] provided the first description of a patient who had *BRAF* V600E mutated classical HCL and was resistant to nucleoside analogs and rituximab but had a rapid and complete response to a 56-day course of vemurafenib. Within 6 days of treatment ERK phosphorylation of hairy cells in the marrow was abolished, with the induction of apoptosis, and the marrow showed no evidence of minimal residual disease at 6 months. The author and his colleagues subsequently expanded on this study including 21 patients treated at multiple sites using various vemurafenib regimens. The median time on therapy was 90 days; 40% of patients achieved a CR with the median time to recovery of platelets, neutrophils and hemoglobin being 28, 43 and 55 days. 240 mg vemurafenib was sufficient to inhibit ERK phosphorylation by immunohistochemistry of marrow, and while the median time to next treatment or death was 17 months, the duration did not correlate with the dose of vemurafenib or duration of therapy. The authors concluded that 240 mg vemurafenib twice a day appeared to be effective for the treatment of HCL. Vemurafenib caused arthralgias, and skin changes, including photosensitivity, squamous carcinomas, squamous papillomas and keratoacanthomas, which occurred at all vemurafenib doses. Moreover, one patient developed acute myeloid leukemia on vemurafenib which regressed following withdrawal of the drug; whether the vemurafenib induced the AML or enhanced the growth of a previously undiagnosed AML was not known.

Tiacci et al[232] reported on two phase 2 studies in previously treated HCL patients, carried out in Italy (28 patients) and in the United States (26 patients), using vemurafenib 960 mg twice a day for a median of 16 or 18 weeks, respectively. Complete response rates of 35% to 42% and PR rates of 58% to 62% were seen by 8 to 12 weeks. However, immunohistochemical studies continued to show small numbers of hairy cells in the marrow after treatment. Interestingly, within several days of treatment there was loss of CD25 on the cell surface and loss of villi. The rate of hematological recovery was rapid, and in the Italian study the median time for recovery of platelets ($\geq 100 \times 10^9$/L) was 2 weeks, neutrophils ($\geq 1.5 \times 10^9$/L) was 4 weeks and hemoglobin (≥110 g/L) was 8 weeks. The remission duration was longer for patients who achieved a CR with the median treatment-free time being 25 months, as compared to 18 months for patients with a PR. Most frequent side effects requiring dose reductions were skin changes and arthralgias/arthritis. Skin changes included papillomas and hyperkeratosis of the palms of the hands or soles of feet. In addition, seven patients developed basal cell, squamous cell or superficial melanomas requiring surgical resection.

Tiacci and colleagues[278] have subsequently demonstrated that the activity of veumurafenib can be significant increased by the addition of rituximab. Patients received vemurafenib 960 mg twice a day for 8 weeks with rituximab 375 mg/m² intravenously on days 1 and 15 of each cycle. Two weeks following vemurafenib the patients received four more treatments with rituximab given every 2 weeks. In 30 refractory/relapsed patients, the CR rate was 87% (26 of 30 cases) with MRD negativity (as assessed by PCR for BRAF in bone marrow), being seen in 17 patients (65%). Normalization of blood counts was more rapid than seen with vemurafenib alone, with platelet recovery occurring at a median of 2 weeks and neutrophils/hemoglobin at 4 weeks. For all 30 patients, the progression-free survival from start of treatment was 78% at a median of 37 months. The treatment was generally well tolerated with the expected side-effects for vemurafenib and rituximab.

Dabrafenib is another oral reversible BRAF inhibitor and has been evaluated in 10 classical HCL patients with refractory/relapsed disease.[279] Patients received dabrafenib 150 mg orally twice a day for 8 to 12 weeks, and all patients responded. There were 3 CRs and 4 PRs, with the CR patients relapsing at 14, 15.5 and 21 months. Toxicities included arthralgias, an increase in lipase or liver function tests, and a prolongation in Q-T interval, resulting in drug dose tapering in 4 patients. Because of the short treatment duration no cutaneous malignancies were seen. A second study evaluated dabrafenib 150 mg orally twice a day with the MEK inhibitor, trametinib 2 mg/d, in 43 HCL patients with refractory/relapsed disease.[280] Preliminary results indicate that with a median follow-up of 17 months (range, 1-39 months), 20 (49%) had a CR and 12 (29%) a PR. Seventy percent of CR were MRD negative. However, side-effects were common necessitating dose-reductions or treatment interruptions in half the patients with permanent discontinuation in 5 patients.

Resistance to vemurafenib in melanoma frequently results in reactivation of the ERK pathway through a variety of mechanisms, leading to the use of combined BRAF/MEK inhibition in HCL.[281] In one HCL patient, new activating mutations in KRAS and *MAP2K* (encodes for MEK1) were detected with the development of vemurafenib resistance, and this was associated with recurrence of ERK phosphorylation.[281] With a combination of the MEK inhibitor, cobimetinib, and vemurafenib the patient had a rapid hematological response which has been maintained for over 12 months. Whether MEK inhibitors will be effective in all vemurafenib-resistant HCL patients requires further study.

While all of these approaches are exciting these agents are not yet officially approved for use in HCL and need to be used "off-label."[111]

Bruton Tyrosine Kinase (BTK) Inhibition

Total and phosphorylated Bruton tyrosine kinase (BTK) are present in hairy cells and inhibition of BTK phosphorylation by ibrutinib leads to reduced viability.[282] Thirty-seven patients with classical HCL (28/37) and variant HCL (9/37) were treated with 420 or 840 mg ibrutinib per day.[283] All patients had been heavily pretreated, except for 2 HCL variants who were untreated. The overall response was similar for both types of HCL, being 36% at 48 weeks and 54% overall. The best response at any time was CR for 7 patients, PR for 13 patients and stable disease for 10. The estimated progression-free survival at 36 months was 73%. Interestingly, ibrutinib did not cause a significant increase in hairy cells in the peripheral blood and a decrease in ERK phosphorylation did not correlate with response, suggesting a unique mechanism of action in this disease. Hematological toxicity occurred in 43% of patients with recovery of normal blood counts being relatively slow, occurring at median of 2 months for neutrophils and 5 months for hemoglobin and platelets.

Other Treatments of Historical Interest

Chemotherapy

Chlorambucil has been used when the disease progressed after splenectomy.[284,285] Although some patients improved, the course in others was often worse, with increased myelosuppression. The best results were reported by Golomb et al,[285] who administered chlorambucil 4 mg orally/day for at least 6 months to 24 post-splenectomy patients with progressive disease. A reduction in the number of circulating hairy cells and an increase in one or more of the normal peripheral blood cellular elements occurred in most patients. Six deaths occurred, and time to response was 6 months or longer. Other chemotherapeutic agents, either alone or in combination, have demonstrated some benefit, but the toxic effects were often severe.[286,287] Partial remissions have also been reported with androgens,[288] as well as with a combination of lithium carbonate and immunotherapy with Calmette-Guérin bacillus.[289] Steroids may provide a rapid improvement in pain when caused by lytic bone disease with HCL.[124]

Bone Marrow Transplantation

One case of successful bone marrow transplantation from an identical twin has been reported.[290]

Leukapheresis

Clinical and hematologic improvements have been reported by using leukapheresis to reduce the number of hairy cells in the peripheral blood.[291] However, others have found the responses less predictable and more transient.[292]

Radiation Therapy

Low-dose radiation to the spleen can produce transient clinical and hematologic improvements, but the response is slow and unpredictable.[293] However, radiation therapy can be effective for the treatment of massive retroperitoneal lymphadenopathy and lytic bone lesions.[294]

Treatment of Patients With Active Infections

While the purine nucleoside analogs have been the cornerstone of initial therapy in classical HCL, they produce significant myelo- and immune-suppression. Thus, an alternative approach is required for the 20% of patients presenting with active infection or where there is a risk of infection, such as with the COVID-19 pandemic.[111,295,296] Shenoi et al[295] described 3 patients with classical HCL who had neutropenia and active infections following initiation of purine nucleoside analog therapy. All three patients showed rapid recovery in the neutrophil counts following vemurafenib. A more recent retrospective analysis has described 22 HCL patients who presented with neutropenia and were treated with vemurafenib 240 mg once or twice a day.[296] Seventeen patients had infections and 7 were in intensive care. In 21 patients there was recovery of the neutrophil count with resolution of infections allowing subsequent definitive therapy with cladribine. Alternatively, moxetumumab or the pegylated version of α-interferon may be considered.[111] Further studies are thus required to determine the optimum approach for HCL patients who present with marked neutropenia and/or monocytopenia and for those who present with an active infection.

Minimal Residual Disease

Because of the ability of new therapies to eliminate MRD, there has been interest as to whether this should be the target for initial therapy.[178,297] Achieving the elimination of MRD in HCL is now possible with cladribine/rituximab,[269,272] moxetumumab,[275,276] and vemurafenib/rituximab,[278] with patients achieving MRD negativity having a longer time to relapse than those who remain MRD positive. Further studies are required to standardize MRD measurements and to determine which patients benefit most by achieving MRD negativity.

Treatment of Hairy Cell Leukemia Variant

In contrast to classical HCL, the HCL-V is notoriously difficult to treat.[169,298] Splenectomy has been reported to produce hematological remissions in three-quarters of patients with a median time to relapse of 48 months.[298] For patients unfit for splenectomy or chemotherapy, responses can be obtained with splenic irradiation.[169] Response to the nucleoside analogs alone is generally poor, but good results may be obtained with a rituximab-nucleoside analog combination.[272,299,300] Kreitman and colleagues have recently treated 10 patients with HCL variant using cladribine 0.15 mg/kg daily intravenously for 5 days with rituximab 375 mg/m² intravenously weekly for 8 weeks, starting on the same day as the cladribine.[299] Nine patients achieved a CR and these patients remained free of MRD at 12 to 48 (median 27) months. Small numbers of patients have also been reported to respond to bendamustine/rituximab, ibrutinib and the MEK inhibitor, trametinib.[169]

SUMMARY OF HCL TREATMENT

The following recommendations are based on the authors' experience and consensus guidelines.[2,111,300–302]

1. Asymptomatic patients with HCL may not require treatment; however, it is generally recommended to start therapy when the hemoglobin is <110 g/L, platelets <100 × 10⁹/L or neutrophils <1 × 10⁹/L or if there is evidence of disease progression.[2] Patients with active HCL are at risk of infection related to neutropenia, monocytopenia, and T cell dysfunction, and this will resolve after a remission is obtained. Persistent lymphopenia and lymphocyte dysfunction may persist for months to years following the use of a purine nucleoside analog. Concomitant use of rituximab may further deplete the lymphocytes. Although the value of prophylactic antibiotics in otherwise healthy patients is unclear, patients with prior infections may require prophylaxis for herpetic infections and *Pneumocystis jirovecii* for up to 6 months. As purine nucleoside analogs can increase the risk of reactions to other drug, it is recommended that the antibiotics be started after the analog.[301] Allopurinol is not usually required. In addition, it has been recommended that HCL patients who have been treated with a purine nucleoside analog should receive irradiated blood products for the rest of their lives, to prevent graft-vs-host disease.[2,301]

2. Our recommended approach to therapy is detailed in *Figure 93.10*. The standard therapy for HCL is with one of the purine nucleoside analogs, pentostatin or cladribine, which appear to have equal efficacy and produce CRs in the majority of patients. Cladribine appears to have similar efficacy as pentostatin, with equal activity whether administered as 0.1 mg/kg/d × 7, by continuous infusion, or as 0.14 mg/kg/d × 5, as a 2-hour infusion or SC, or on a weekly schedule using 0.15 mg/kg/wk × 6. Pentostatin is generally administered on a biweekly (4 mg/m² IV) basis. Because of the effectiveness of pentostatin and cladribine in HCL and the rarity of this disease, it is unlikely that there will be any prospective studies to compare the efficacy of these two agents and the different treatment regimens. The major toxicity with the nucleoside analogs is myelosuppression and the risk of infections with initiation of treatment. As a result, the authors prefer using pentostatin every other week or weekly cladribine with a blood count just prior to each treatment. For safety, the biweekly or weekly treatments are delayed until the neutrophil count is back to baseline or better. Both pentostatin and cladribine are excreted by the kidneys and the creatinine should be measured before each treatment and therapy only continued as long as renal function is not impaired. It has been suggested that 1.5l of IV fluid be given with each pentostatin treatment.

3. Achievement of a CR is associated with a longer remission than achieving a PR. Thus, for patients who remain in CR for 5 years, the likelihood of remaining in CR by 15 years is 75%.[166] However, as patients with classical HCL generally respond to subsequent therapies it is unclear whether survival is longer for patients who achieve a CR or a PR. Similarly, patients who achieve an MRD negative CR may have a longer remission than those with an MRD positive CR. However, the optimum technique to measure MRD and how this should be used in clinical practice requires further study.[297]

4. Prognosis for patients treated with pentostatin is worse for those older than 50 to 55 years of age at presentation and those with a hemoglobin level <100 g/L and white cell counts

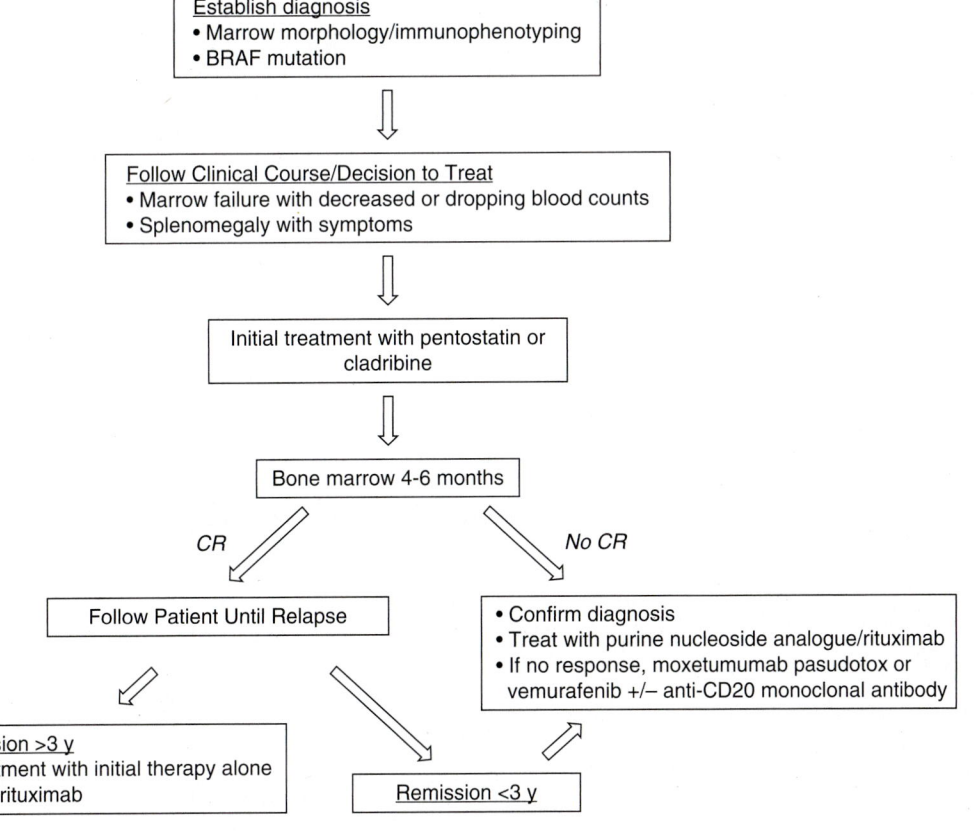

FIGURE 93.10 Recommended treatment schema for hairy cell leukemia (HCL). CR (complete response) is based on morphological appearance of marrow. The assessment of minimal residual disease is reserved for patients on clinical trials.

$<2 \times 10^9$/L.[84,166,167] In addition, patients with bulky abdominal lymphadenopathy have a poorer prognosis.[83]

5. Patients should have a marrow 4 to 6 months after starting cladribine or pentostatin and if there is residual disease, additional therapy with or without rituximab should be considered. The goal should be to strive for a CR, but to avoid excessive immunosuppressive and marrow toxicities remembering that consequences, for example, opportunistic infections, may result from excessive treatment.

6. Because of the COVID-19 pandemic, caution has to be used when using a purine nucleoside analog or rituximab, which will reduce the response to COVID-19 immunization and increase the risk of complications if the patient does get infected with the COVID-19 virus.[111,178] Thus, treatment should be deferred, if possible, until the patient has received COVID-19 immunization and any active infections treated prior to therapy. If therapy for HCL is required immediately and the risk of COVID-19 infection is high, or the patient has an active infection, treatment with a non-immunosuppressive therapy should be considered. Options include vemurafenib or moxetumumab pasudotox, as an interim measure prior to more definitive therapy with a purine nucleoside analog. In the past, IFN-α has also been been used in these patients, and the pegylated version of IFN-α should have similar efficacy.

7. Two-thirds of patients benefit from splenectomy, but a CR is rare. However, splenectomy is rarely considered now that effective therapies have been developed. Splenectomy is required for patients who have a splenic rupture and may be of value for patients with pure "splenic" HCL, as well as for patients who have severe thrombocytopenia with increased numbers of megakaryocytes in the marrow.

8. Treatment with rituximab and a nucleoside analog is highly effective and should be considered as initial therapy for HCLv.[272,299]

SECOND MALIGNANCIES

Some studies have shown an increased incidence of second malignancies in HCL, regardless of whether patients receive a nucleoside analog or α-interferon, and this has been related to immunosuppression secondary to HCL or therapy.[303–305] However, this increased incidence has not been observed by other investigators.[80,167,208,306]

PROGNOSIS

Before the availability of IFN-α and the nucleoside analogs, the median survival of HCL patients was 4.6 years for non-splenectomized patients and 6.9 years for splenectomized patients.[131] However, the prognosis has improved markedly with present therapies, and the survival rates for patients treated with the nucleoside analogs are now similar for most patients to those of the general population.[166,208,307] A recent population study from the Netherlands has confirmed an excellent relative survival for those less than 70 years while older individuals have a reduced relative survival, thought related to poorer tolerance to cladribine and the effects of additional comorbidities.[308] However, resistance to the nucleoside analogs is being seen with long-term follow up, and the outcome of these patients who receive salvage therapy requires further study.

References

1. Bouroncle BA, Wiseman BK, Doan CA. Leukemic reticuloendotheliosis. *Blood.* 1958;13:609-630. Accessed May 16, 2015. http://www.bloodjournal.org/content/bloodjournal/13/7/609.full.pdf
2. Grever MR, Abdel-Wahab O, Andritsos LA, et al. Consensus guidelines for the diagnosis and management of patients with classic hairy cell leukemia. *Blood.* 2017;129(1):553-561. doi:10.1182/blood-2016-01-689422
3. Teras LR, DeSantis CE, Cerhan JR, Morton LM, Jemal A, Flowers CR. 2016 US lymphoid malignancy statistics by World Health Organization subtypes. *CA Cancer J Clin.* 2016;66(6):443-459. doi:10.3322/caac.21357
4. Nordström M, Hardell L, Magnuson A, Hagberg H, Rask-Andersen A. Occupational exposures, animal exposure and smoking as risk factors for hairy cell leukaemia evaluated in a case-control study. *Br J Cancer.* 1998;77(11):2048-2052.
5. Monnereau A, Slager SL, Hughes AM, et al. Medical history, lifestyle, and occupational risk factors for hairy cell leukemia: the InterLymph Non-Hodgkin Lymphoma Subtypes Project. *J Natl Cancer Inst Monogr.* 2014;48:115-124. doi:10.1093/jncimonographs/lgu004
6. Villemagne B, Bay JO, Tournilhac O, Chaleteix C, Travade P. Two new cases of familial hairy cell leukemia associated with HLA haplotypes A2, B7, Bw4, Bw6. *Leuk Lymphoma.* 2005;46(2):243-245. doi:10.1080/10428190400013589
7. Pemov A, Pathak A, Jones SJ, et al. In search of genetic factors predisposing to familial hairy cell leukemia (HCL): exome-sequencing of four multiplex HCL pedigrees. *Leukemia.* 2020;34(7):1934-1938. doi:10.1038/s41375-019-0702-7
8. Rosner MC, Golomb HM. Phagocytic capacity of hairy cells from seventeen patients. *Virchows Arch B Cell Pathol Incl Mol Pathol.* 1982;40(3):327-337.
9. Hooper WC, Buss DH, Parker CL. Leukemic reticuloendotheliosis (hairy cell leukemia): a review of the evidence concerning the immunology and origin of the cell. *Leuk Res.* 1980;4(5):489-503.
10. Korsmeyer SJ, Greene WC, Cossman J, et al. Rearrangement and expression of immunoglobulin genes and expression of Tac antigen in hairy cell leukemia. *Proc Natl Acad Sci U S A.* 1983;80(14):4522-4526. doi:10.1073/pnas.80.14.4522
11. Basso K, Liso A, Tiacci E, et al. Gene expression profiling of hairy cell leukemia reveals a phenotype related to memory B cells with altered expression of chemokine and adhesion receptors. *J Exp Med.* 2004;199(1):59-68. doi:10.1084/jem.20031175
12. Weston-Bell N, Townsend M, Di Genova G, Forconi F, Sahota SS. Defining origins of malignant B cells: a new circulating normal human IgM(+)D(+) B-cell subset lacking CD27 expression and displaying somatically mutated IGHV genes as a relevant memory population. *Leukemia.* 2009;23(11):2075-2080. doi:10.1038/leu.2009.178
13. Forconi F, Raspadori D, Lenoci M, Lauria F. Absence of surface CD27 distinguishes hairy cell leukemia from other leukemic B-cell malignancies. *Haematologica.* 2005;90(2):266-268.
14. Forconi F, Sozzi E, Cencini E, et al. Hairy cell leukemias with unmutated IGHV genes define the minor subset refractory to single-agent cladribine and with more aggressive behavior. *Blood.* 2009;114(21):4696-4702. doi:10.1182/blood-2009-03-212449
15. Arons E, Roth L, Sapolsky J, Suntum T, Stetler-Stevenson M, Kreitman RJ. Evidence of canonical somatic hypermutation in hairy cell leukemia. *Blood.* 2011;117(18):4844-4851. doi:10.1182/blood-2010-11-316737
16. Arons E, Suntum T, Stetler-Stevenson M, Kreitman RJ. VH4-34+ hairy cell leukemia, a new variant with poor prognosis despite standard therapy. *Blood.* 2009;114(21):4687-4695. doi:10.1182/blood-2009-01-201731
17. Forconi F, Sahota SS, Raspadori D, et al. Hairy cell leukemia: at the crossroad of somatic mutation and isotype switch. *Blood.* 2004;104(10):3312-3317. doi:10.1182/blood-2004-03-0950
18. Forconi F, Sahota SS, Raspadori D, Mockridge CI, Lauria F, Stevenson FK. Tumor cells of hairy cell leukemia express multiple clonally related immunoglobulin isotypes via RNA splicing. *Blood.* 2001;98(4):1174-1181. doi:10.1182/blood.V98.4.1174
19. Arribas AJ, Rinaldi A, Chiodin G, et al. Genome-wide promoter methylation of hairy cell leukemia. *Blood Adv.* 2019;3(3):384-396. doi:10.1182/bloodadvances.2018024059
20. Tschumper RC, Geyer SM, Campbell ME, et al. Immunoglobulin diversity gene usage predicts unfavorable outcome in a subset of chronic lymphocytic leukemia patients. *J Clin Invest.* 2008;118(1):306-315. doi:10.1172/JCI32625
21. Messmer BT, Albesiano E, Efremov DG, et al. Multiple distinct sets of stereotyped antigen receptors indicate a role for antigen in promoting chronic lymphocytic leukemia. *J Exp Med.* 2004;200(4):519-525. doi:10.1084/jem.20040544
22. Murray F, Darzentas N, Hadzidimitriou A, et al. Stereotyped patterns of somatic hypermutation in subsets of patients with chronic lymphocytic leukemia: implications for the role of antigen selection in leukemogenesis. *Blood.* 2008;111(3):1524-1533. doi:10.1182/blood-2007-07-099564
23. Kamiguti AS, Harris RJ, Slupsky JR, Baker PK, Cawley JC, Zuzel M. Regulation of hairy-cell survival through constitutive activation of mitogen-activated protein kinase pathways. *Oncogene.* 2003;22(15):2272-2284. doi:10.1038/sj.onc.1206398
24. Slupsky JR, Kamiguti AS, Harris RJ, Cawley JC, Zuzel M. Central role of protein kinase Cepsilon in constitutive activation of ERK1/2 and Rac1 in the malignant cells of hairy cell leukemia. *Am J Pathol.* 2007;170(2):745-754. doi:10.2353/ajpath.2007.060557
25. Tiacci E, Trifonov V, Schiavoni G, et al. BRAF mutations in hairy-cell leukemia. *N Engl J Med.* 2011;364(24):2305-2315.
26. Wan PTC, Garnett MJ, Roe SM, et al. Mechanism of activation of the RAF-ERK signaling pathway by oncogenic mutations of B-RAF. *Cell.* 2004;116(6):855-867. doi:10.1016/S0092-8674(04)00215-6
27. Pettirossi V, Santi A, Imperi E, et al. BRAF inhibitors reverse the unique molecular signature and phenotype of hairy cell leukemia and exert potent antileukemic activity. *Blood.* 2015;125(8):1207-1216. doi:10.1182/blood-2014-10-603100
28. Dietrich S, Jennifer H, weiLee SC, et al. Recurrent CDKN1B (p27) mutations in hairy cell leukemia. *Blood.* 2015;125(8):1005-1008. doi:10.1182/blood-2015-04-643361
29. Piva R, Deaglio S, Famà R, et al. The Krüppel-like factor 2 transcription factor gene is recurrently mutated in splenic marginal zone lymphoma. *Leukemia.* 2014;29(2):503-507. doi:10.1038/leu.2014.294
30. Tschernitz S, Flossbach L, Bonengel M, Roth S, Rosenwald A, Geissinger E. Alternative BRAF mutations in BRAF V600E-negative hairy cell leukaemias. *Br J Haematol.* 2014;165(4):529-533. doi:10.1111/bjh.12735
31. Xi L, Arons E, Navarro W, et al. Both variant and IGHV4-34-expressing hairy cell leukemia lack the BRAF V600E mutation. *Blood.* 2012;119(14):3330-3332. doi:10.1182/blood-2011-09-379339
32. Waterfall JJ, Arons E, Walker RL, et al. High prevalence of MAP2K1 mutations in variant and IGHV4-34-expressing hairy-cell leukemias. *Nat Genet.* 2014;46(1):8-10. doi:10.1038/ng.2828
33. Mason EF, Brown RD, Szeto DP, et al. Detection of activating *MAP2K1* mutations in atypical hairy cell leukemia and hairy cell leukemia variant. *Leuk Lymphoma.* 2016;8194:1-4. doi:10.1080/10428194.2016.1185786

34. Verma S, Greaves WO, Ravandi F, et al. Rapid detection and quantitation of BRAF mutations in hairy cell leukemia using a sensitive pyrosequencing assay. *Am J Clin Pathol.* 2012;138(1):153-156. doi:10.1309/AJCPL0OPXI9LZITV
35. Martinez D, Navarro A, Martinez-Trillos A, et al. NOTCH1, TP53, and MAP2K1 mutations in splenic diffuse red pulp small B-cell lymphoma are associated with progressive disease. *Am J Surg Pathol.* 2016;40(2):192-201. doi:10.1097/PAS.0000000000000523
36. Andritsos LA, Anghelina M, Grieselhuber NR, et al. Trametinib for the treatment of IGHV4-34, MAP2K1 mutant variant hairy cell leukemia. *Blood.* 2016;128(22):5598.
37. Emery CM, Vijayendran KG, Zipser MC, et al. MEK1 mutations confer resistance to MEK and B-RAF inhibition. *Proc Natl Acad Sci U S A.* 2009;106(48):20411-20416. doi:10.1073/pnas.0905833106
38. Wagle N, Emery C, Berger MF, et al. Dissecting therapeutic resistance to RAF inhibition in melanoma by tumor genomic profiling. *J Clin Oncol.* 2011;29(22):3085-3096. doi:10.1200/JCO.2010.33.2312
39. Marks JL, Gong Y, Chitale D, et al. Novel MEK1 mutation identified by mutational analysis of epidermal growth factor receptor signaling pathway genes in lung adenocarcinoma. *Cancer Res.* 2009;68(14):5524-5528. doi:10.1158/0008-5472.CAN-08-0099
40. Chung SS, Kim E, Park JH, et al. Hematopoietic stem cell origin of BRAFV600E mutations in hairy cell leukemia. *Sci Transl Med.* 2014;6(238):238ra71. doi:10.1126/scitranslmed.3008004
41. Quesada V, Conde L, Villamor N, et al. Exome sequencing identifies recurrent mutations of the splicing factor SF3B1 gene in chronic lymphocytic leukemia. *Nat Genet.* 2012;44(1):47-52. doi:10.1038/ng.1032
42. Jebaraj BMC, Kienle D, Bühler A, et al. BRAF mutations in chronic lymphocytic leukemia. *Leuk Lymphoma.* 2013;54(6):1177-1182. doi:10.3109/10428194.2012.742525
43. Walker BA, Boyle EM, Wardell CP, et al. Mutational spectrum, copy number changes, and outcome: results of a sequencing study of patients with newly diagnosed myeloma. *J Clin Oncol.* 2015;33(33):3911-3920. doi:10.1200/JCO.2014.59.1503
44. Badalian-Very G, Vergilio JA, Degar BA, et al. Recurrent BRAF mutations in Langerhans cell histiocytosis. *Blood.* 2010;116(11):1919-1923. doi:10.1182/blood-2010-04-279083
45. Haroche J, Charlotte F, Arnaud L, et al. High prevalence of BRAF V600E mutations in Erdheim-Chester disease but not in other non-Langerhans cell histiocytoses. *Blood.* 2012;120(13):2700-2703. doi:10.1182/blood-2012-05-430140
46. Davies H, Bignell GR, Cox C, et al. Mutations of the BRAF gene in human cancer. *Nature.* 2002;417(6892):949-954. doi:10.1038/nature00766
47. Loghavi S, Khoury JD. Langerhans cell histiocytosis in a patient with hairy cell leukemia: a tale of divergence. *Blood.* 2017;129(11):1563. doi:10.1182/blood-2016-11-749374
48. Michonneau D, Kaltenbach S, Derrieux C, et al. BRAF(V600E) mutation in a histiocytic sarcoma arising from hairy cell leukemia. *J Clin Oncol.* 2014;32(35):e117-e121. doi:10.1200/JCO.2013.49.0078
49. Muslimani A, Chisti MM, Blenc AM, Boxwala M, Micale MA, Jaiyesimi I. Langerhans/dendritic cell sarcoma arising from hairy cell leukemia: a rare phenomenon. *Ann Hematol.* 2012;91(9):1485-1487. doi:10.1007/s00277-011-1399-5
50. Kitagawa Y, Brahmachary M, Tiacci E, Dalla-Favera R, Falini B, Basso K. A microRNA signature specific for hairy cell leukemia and associated with modulation of the MAPK-JNK pathways. *Leukemia.* 2012;26(12):2564-2567. doi:10.1038/leu.2012.149
51. Kluin-Nelemans HC, Beverstock GC, Mollevanger P, et al. Proliferation and cytogenetic analysis of hairy cell leukemia upon stimulation via the CD40 antigen. *Blood.* 1994;84(9):3134-3141.
52. Sambani C, Trafalis DTP, Mitsoulis-mentzikoff C, et al. Clonal chromosome rearrangements in hairy cell leukemia: personal experience and review of literature. *Cancer Genet Cytogenet.* 2001;129:138-144.
53. Haglund U, Juliusson G, Stellan B, Gahrton G. Hairy cell leukemia is characterized by clonal chromosome abnormalities clustered to specific regions. *Blood.* 1994;83(9):2637-2645.
54. Wu X, Ivanova G, Merup M, et al. Molecular analysis of the human chromosome 5q13.3 region in patients with hairy cell leukemia and identification of tumor suppressor gene candidates. *Genomics.* 1999;60(2):161-171. doi:10.1006/geno.1999.5911
55. Brito-Babapulle V, Matutes E, Oscier D, Mould S, Catovsky D. Chromosome abnormalities in hairy cell leukaemia variant. *Gene Chromosome Cancer.* 1994;10:197-202.
56. Nordgren A, Corcoran M, Sääf A, et al. Characterisation of hairy cell leukaemia by tiling resolution array-based comparative genome hybridisation: a series of 13 cases and review of the literature. *Eur J Haematol.* 2010;84(1):17-25. doi:10.1111/j.1600-0609.2009.01334.x
57. Forconi F, Poretti G, Kwee I, et al. High density genome-wide DNA profiling reveals a remarkably stable profile in hairy cell leukemia. *Br J Haematol.* 2008;141(5):622-630. doi:10.1111/j.1365-2141.2008.07106.x
58. Hockley SL, Morgan GJ, Leone PE, et al. High-resolution genomic profiling in hairy cell leukemia-variant compared with typical hairy cell leukemia. *Leukemia.* 2011;25(7):1189-1192. doi:10.1038/leu.2011.47
59. König Ea, Kusser WC, Day C, et al. P53 mutations in hairy cell leukemia. *Leukemia.* 2000;14(4):706-711.
60. Tiacci E, Liso A, Piris M, Falini B. Evolving concepts in the pathogenesis of hairy-cell leukaemia. *Nat Rev Cancer.* 2006;6(6):437-448. doi:10.1038/nrc1888
61. Cawley JC, Hawkins SF. The biology of hairy-cell leukaemia. *Curr Opin Hematol.* 2010;17(4):341-349. doi:10.1097/MOH.0b013e328338c417
62. Forconi F. Hairy cell leukemia: biological and clinical overview from immunogenetic insights. *Hematol Oncol.* 2011;29:55-66. doi:10.1002/hon.975
63. Schmid M, Porzsolt F. Autocrine and paracrine regulation of neoplastic cell growth in hairy cell leukemia. *Leuk Lymphoma.* 1995;17:401-410.
64. Schmid M, Schrezenmeier H, Staib G, Porzsolt F. Evidence for a paracrine pathway of B-cell stimulation in hairy cell leukaemia. *Br J Haematol.* 1995;90:156-162.
65. de Totero D, Tazzari PL, Lauria F, et al. Phenotypic analysis of hairy cell leukemia: "Variant" cases express the interleukin-2 receptor beta chain, but not the alpha chain (CD25). *Blood.* 1993;82(2):528-535. doi:10.1017/CBO9781107415324.004
66. Bulger K, Murphy J, Janckila A, Nichols J, McCaffrey R. Peripheral blood hairy cell leukemia cells express only low affinity IL-2 receptors. *Leuk Res.* 1994;18(2):101-104.
67. Semenzato G, Trentin L, Zambello R, et al. Origin of the soluble interleukin-2 receptor in the serum of patients with hairy cell leukemia. *Leukemia.* 1988;2:788-792.
68. Richards BJM, Mick R, Latta JM, et al. Serum soluble interleukin-2 receptor is associated with clinical and pathologic disease status in hairy cell leukemia. *Blood.* 1990;76(10):1941-1945.
69. Cordingley F, Bianchi A, Hoffbrand A, et al. Tumour necrosis factor as a autocrine tumour growth factor for chronic B-cell malignancies. *Lancet.* 1988;1(8592):969-971.
70. Buck C, Digel W, Schoniger W, et al. Tumor necrosis factor-alpha but not lymphotoxin, stimulated growth of tumor cells in hairy cell leukemia. *Leukemia.* 1990;4:431-434.
71. Foa R, Guarini A, Francia di Celle P, et al. Constitutive production of tumor necrosis factor-alpha in hairy cell leukemia: possible role in the pathogenesis of the cytopenia(s) and effect of treatment with interferon-alpha. *J Clin Oncol.* 1992;10:954-959.
72. Lindemann A, Ludwig W, Oster W, Mertelsmann R, Hermann F. High-level secretion of tumor necrosis factor-alpha contributes to hematopoietic failure in hairy cell leukemia. *Blood.* 1989;73(4):880-884.
73. Digel W, Porzsolt F, Schmid M, Hermann F, Lessiauer W, Brockhaus M. High levels of circulating soluble receptors for tumor necrosis factor in hairy cell leukemia and type B chronic lymphocytic leukemia. *J Clin Invest.* 1992;89:1690-1693.
74. Trentin L, Pizzolo G, Zambello R, et al. Leukemic cells in hairy cell leukemia and B cell chronic lymphocytic leukemia release soluble TNF receptors. *Leukemia.* 1995;9:1051-1055.
75. Barut B, Chauhan D, Uchiyama H, Anderson KC. Interleukin-6 functions as an intracellular growth factor in hairy cell leukemia in vitro. *J Clin Invest.* 1993;92(5):2346-2352. doi:10.1172/JCI116839
76. Aziz KA, Till KJ, Chen H, et al. The role of autocrine FGF-2 in the distinctive bone marrow fibrosis of hairy-cell leukemia (HCL). *Blood.* 2003;102(3):1051-1056. doi:10.1182/blood-2002-12-3737
77. Shehata M, Schwarzmeier JD, Hilgarth M, Hubmann R, Duechler M, Gisslinger H. TGF-1 induces bone marrow reticulin fibrosis in hairy cell leukemia. *J Clin Invest.* 2004;113(5):676-685. doi:10.1172/JCI200419540
78. Getta BM, Woo KM, Devlin S, et al. Treatment outcomes and secondary cancer incidence in young patients with hairy cell leukaemia. *Br J Haematol.* 2016;175(3):402-409. doi:10.1111/bjh.14207
79. Frassoldati A, Lamparelli T, Federico M, et al. Hairy cell leukemia: a clinical review based on 725 cases of the Italian cooperative group (ICGHCL). Italian cooperative group for hairy cell leukemia. *Leuk Lymphoma.* 1994;13(3-4):307-316. doi:10.3109/10428199409056295
80. Rosenberg J, Burian C, Waalen J, Saven A. Clinical characteristics and long-term outcome of young hairy cell leukemia patients treated with cladribine: a single-institution series. *Blood.* 2014;123(2):177-183. doi:10.1182/blood-2013-06-508754
81. Hakimian D, Tallman MS, Hogan DK, Rademaker AW, Rose E, Nemcek AA. Prospective evaluation of internal adenopathy in a cohort of 43 patients with hairy cell leukemia. *J Clin Oncol.* 1994;12(2):268-272. Accessed May 17, 2015. http://www.ncbi.nlm.nih.gov/pubmed/7906724
82. Mercieca J, Puga M, Matutes E, Moskovic E, Salim S, Catovsky D. Incidence and significance of abdominal lymphadenopathy in hairy cell leukaemia. *Leuk Lymphoma.* 1994;14(suppl 1):79-83. Accessed May 17, 2015. http://www.ncbi.nlm.nih.gov/pubmed/7820058
83. Mercieca J, Matutes E, Emmett E, Coles HC, Catovsky D. 2-Chlorodeoxyadenosine in the treatment of hairy cell leukaemia: differences in response in patients with and without abdominal lymphadenopathy. *Br J Haematol.* 1996;93(2):409-411.
84. Maloisel F, Benboubker L, Gardembas M, et al. Long-term outcome with pentostatin treatment in hairy cell leukemia patients. A French retrospective study of 238 patients. *Leukemia.* 2003;17(1):45-51. doi:10.1038/sj.leu.2402784
85. Castro-Malaspina H, Najean Y, Flandrin G. Erythrokinetic studies in hairy-cell leukaemia. *Br J Haematol.* 1979;42(2):189-197.
86. Aster R. Splenic platelet pooling as a cause of "hypersplenic" thrombocytopenia. *Trans Assoc Am Phys.* 1965;78:362-373.
87. Brubaker L, Johnson C. Correlation of splenomegaly and abnormal neutrophil pooling (margination). *J Lab Clin Med.* 1978;92:508-515.
88. Hess CE, Ayers CR, Sandusky WR, Carpenter MA, Wetzel RA, Mahler DN. Mechanism of dilutional anemia in massive splenomegaly. *Blood.* 1976;47(4):629-644.
89. Lewis SM, Catovsky D, Hows JM, Ardalan B. Splenic red cell pooling in hairy cell leukaemia. *Br J Haematol.* 1977;35:351-357.
90. Schaffner A, Augustiny N, Otto RC, Fehr J. The hypersplenic spleen. A contractile reservoir of granulocytes and platelets. *Arch Intern Med.* 1985;145:651-654.
91. Mainwaring CJ, Walewska R, Snowden J, et al. Fatal cold anti-i autoimmune haemolytic anaemia complicating hairy cell leukaemia. *Br J Haematol.* 2000;109(3):641-643.
92. Virchis AE, Jan-Mohamed R, Kaczmarski KS, Barker FG, Mehta AB. Primary splenic hairy cell leukaemia variant presenting as immune thrombocytopenic purpura. *Eur J Haematol.* 1998;61(4):288-291.

93. Damaj G, Kuhnowski F, Marolleau JP, Bauters F, Leleu X, Yakoub-Agha I. Risk factors for severe infection in patients with hairy cell leukemia: a long-term study of 73 patients. *Eur J Haematol.* 2009;83:246-250. doi:10.1111/j.1600-0609.2009.01259.x

94. Hoffman MA. Clinical presentations and complications of hairy cell leukemia. *Hematol Oncol Clin North Am.* 2006;20(5):1065-1073. doi:10.1016/j.hoc.2006.06.003

95. Golomb HM, Hanauer SB. Infectious complications associated with hairy cell leukemia. *J Infect Dis.* 1981;143(5):639-643. Accessed May 23, 2015. http://www.jstor.org.proxy2.lib.umanitoba.ca.proxy1.lib.umanitoba.ca/stable/30113282?seq=1#page_scan_tab_contents

96. Weinstein RA, Golomb HM, Grumet G, Gelmann E, Schechter GP. Hairy cell leukemia: association with disseminated atypical mycobacterial infection. *Cancer.* 1981;48:380-383.

97. Mackowiak PA, Demian SE, Sljtker WL, Smith JW, Tompsett R, Sheehan WW. Infections in hairy cell leukemia clinical evidence of a pronounced defect in cell-mediated immunity. *Am J Med.* 1980;68:718-724.

98. Knecht H, Rhyner K, Streuli RA. Toxoplasmosis in hairy-cell leukaemia. *Br J Haematol.* 1986;62:65-73.

99. Nielsen H, Bangsborg J, Rechnitzer C, Jacobsen N, Busk HE. Defective monocyte function in Legionnaires' disease complicating hairy cell leukaemia. *Acta Med Scand.* 1986;220(4):381-383.

100. Salata RA, King RE, Gose F, Pearson RD. Listeria monocytogenes cerebritis, bacteremia, and cutaneous lesions complicating hairy cell leukemia. *Am J Med.* 1986;81:1068-1072.

101. Janckila A, Wallace JH, Yam LT. Generalized monocyte deficiency in leukaemic reticuloendotheliosis. *Scand J Haematol.* 1982;29(2):153-160.

102. Stewart DJ, Bodey GP. Infections in hairy cell leukemia (leukemic reticuloendotheliosis). *Cancer.* 1981;47:801-805. doi:10.1002/1097-0142(19810215)47:4<801::AID-CNCR2820470428>3.0.CO;2-6

103. van de Corput L, Falkenburg J, Kluin-Nelemans J. T-Cell dysfunction in hairy cell leukemia: an updated review. *Leuk Lymphoma.* 1998;30(1-2):31-39. doi:10.3109/10428199809050927

104. Seymour JF, Kurzrock R, Freireich EJ, Estey EH. 2-chlorodeoxyadenosine Induces durable remissions and prolonged suppression of CD4+ lymphocyte counts in patients with hairy cell leukemia. *Blood.* 1994;83(10):2906-2911.

105. Urba WJ, Baseler MW, Kopp WC, et al. Deoxycoformycin-induced immunosuppression in patients with hairy cell leukemia. *Blood.* 1989;73(1):38-46.

106. van de Corput L, Falkenburg JH, Kester MG, Willemze R, Kluin-Nelemans JC. Impaired expression of CD28 on T cells in hairy cell leukemia. *Clin Immunol.* 1999;93(3):256-262. doi:10.1006/clim.1999.4794

107. Spaenij-Dekking EHA, Van der Meijden ED, Falkenburg JHF, Kluin-Nelemans JC. Clonally expanded T cells in hairy cell leukemia patients are not leukemia specific. *Leukemia.* 2004;18(1):176-178. doi:10.1038/sj.leu.2403149

108. Kluin-Nelemans HC, Kester MG, van deCorput L, et al. Correction of abnormal T-cell receptor repertoire during interferon-alpha therapy in patients with hairy cell leukemia. *Blood.* 1998;91(11):4224-4231.

109. Hansen DA, Robbins BA, Bylund DJ, Piro LD, Saven A, Ellison DJ. Identification of monoclonal immunoglobulins and quantitative immunoglobulin abnormalities in hairy cell leukemia and chronic lymphocytic leukemia. *Am J Clin Pathol.* 1994;102(5):580-585.

110. Kohla S, Ibrahim FA, Aldapt MB, Elsabah H, Mohamed S, Youssef R. A rare case of hairy cell leukemia with unusual loss of CD123 associated with COVID-19 at the time of presentation. *Case Rep Oncol.* 2020;94(12):1430-1440. doi:10.1159/000512830

111. Grever MR, Woermann B, Andritsos L, et al. Hairy cell leukemia and COVID-19 adaptation of treatment guidelines. *Leukemia.* 2021;35:1864-1872.

112. Westbrook C, Golde DW. Autoimmune disease in hairy cell leukaemia: clinical syndromes and treatment. *Br J Haematol.* 1985;61(2):349-356. doi:10.1111/j.1365-2141.1985.tb02835.x

113. Komadina KH, Houk RW. Polyarteritis nodosa presenting as recurrent pneumonia following splenectomy for hairy-cell leukemia. *Semin Arthritis Rheum.* 1989;18(4):252-257. doi:10.1007/s13398-014-0173-7.2

114. Hasler P, Kistler H, Gerber H. Vasculitides in hairy cell leukemia. *Semin Arthritis Rheum.* 1995;25(2):134-142. doi:10.1016/S0049-0172(95)80026-3

115. Carpenter MT, West SG. Polyarteritis nodosa in hairy cell leukemia: treatment with interferon-alpha. *J Rheumatol.* 1994;21(6):1150-1152.

116. Robak E, Jesionek-Kupnicka D, Robak T. Skin changes in hairy cell leukemia. *Ann Hematol.* 2020;100:615-625. doi:10.1007/s00277-020-04349-z

117. Dorsey JK, Penick GD. The association of hairy cell leukemia with unusual immunologic disorders. *Arch Intern Med.* 1982;142:902-903. doi:10.1001/archinte.1982.00340180060014

118. Douglas M, Schwartz M, Sharon Z. Cryoglobulinemia and immune-mediated glomerulonephritis in association with hairy cell leukemia. *Am J Kidney Dis.* 1985;6:181-184.

119. Raju SF, Chapman SW, Dreiling B, Tavassoli M. Hairy-cell leukemia with the appearance of mixed cryoglobulinemia and vasculitis. *Arch Intern Med.* 1984;144(6):1300-1302. doi:10.1001/archinte.1984.00350180248038

120. Bouroncle BA. Unusual presentations and complications of hairy cell leukemia. *Leukemia.* 1987;1(4):288-293. Accessed June 5, 2015. http://www.ncbi.nlm.nih.gov/pubmed/3669749

121. Arkel YS, Lake-Lewin D, Savopoulos AA, Berman E. Bone lesions in hairy cell leukemia. A case report and response of bone pains to steroids. *Cancer.* 1984;53:2401-2403.

122. Demanes DJ, Lane N, Beckstead JH. Bone involvement in hairy-cell leukemia. *Cancer.* 1982;49:1607-1701.

123. Lembersky BC, Ratain MJ, Golomb HM. Skeletal complications in hairy cell leukemia: diagnosis and therapy. *J Clin Oncol.* 1988;6(8):1280-1284. Accessed May 31, 2015. http://www.ncbi.nlm.nih.gov/pubmed/3411340

124. Robak P, Jesionek-Kupnicka D, Kupnicki P, Polliack A, Robak T. Bone lesions in hairy cell leukemia: diagnosis and treatment. *Eur J Haematol.* 2020;105(6):682-691. doi:10.1111/ejh.13505

125. Catovsky D, Costello C, Loukopoulos D, et al. Hairy cell leukemia and myelomatosis: chance association or clinical manifestations of the same B-cell disease spectrum. *Blood.* 1981;57(4):758-763.

126. Jansen J, Bolhuis RL, van Nieuwkoop JA, Schuit HR, Kroese WF. Paraproteinaemia plus osteolytic lesions in typical hairy-cell leukaemia. *Br J Haematol.* 1983;54(4):531-541.

127. Arai E, Ikeda S, Itoh S, Katayama I. Specific skin lesions as the presenting symptom of hairy cell leukemia. *Am J Clin Pathol.* 1988;90(4):459-464.

128. Yam LT, Crosby WH. Spontaneous rupture of spleen in leukemic reticuloendotheliosis. *Am J Surg.* 1979;137(2):270-273. doi:10.1016/0002-9610(79)90162-4

129. Vardiman J, Golomb H. Autopsy findings in hairy cell leukemia. *Semin Oncol.* 1984;11:370-380.

130. McDowell MM, Zhu X, Agarwal N, Nikiforova MN, Lieberman FS, Drappatz J. Response of relapsed central nervous system hairy cell leukemia to vemurafenib. *Leuk Lymphoma.* 2016;8194:1-3. doi:10.1080/10428194.2016.1177773

131. Bouroncle BA. Leukemic reticuloendotheliosis (hairy cell leukemia). *Blood.* 1979;53:412-436. http://www.bloodjournal.org/content/bloodjournal/53/3/412.full.pdf

132. Seshadri RS, Brown EJ, Zipursky A. Leukemic reticuloendotheliosis. A failure of monocyte production. *N Engl J Med.* 1976;295(4):181-184.

133. Dalal BI, Freier L, Johnston JB, Merry CC, Israels LG. Peripheral blood and bone marrow changes following 2′-deoxycoformycin therapy in hairy cell leukemia. Results of 200 weeks follow-up. *Cancer.* 1989;63(1):14-22.

134. Golomb HM, Catovsky D, Golde DW. Hairy cell leukemia: a clinical review based on 71 cases. *Ann Intern Med.* 1978;89(5_pt_1):677-683.

135. Juliusson G, Vitols S, Liliemark J. Disease-related hypocholesterolemia in patients with hairy cell leukemia. Positive correlation with spleen size but not with tumor cell burden or low density lipoprotein receptor activity. *Cancer.* 1995;76(3):423-428.

136. Pandolfino J, Hakimian D, Rademaker AW, Tallman MS. Hypocholesterolemia in hairy cell leukemia: a marker for proliferative activity. *Am J Hematol.* 1997;55(3):129-133.

137. Katayama I, Li CY, Yam LT. Histochemical study of acid phosphatase isoenzyme in leukemic reticuloendotheliosis. *Cancer.* 1972;29(1):157-164.

138. Lemez P, Kacirkova P. Variations of hairy cell nuclei shapes with regard to ring-shaped nuclei simulating dysplastic neutrophilic granulocytes and review of the literature. *Int J Lab Hematol.* 2014;36(5):580-586. doi:10.1111/ijlh.12195

139. Shao H, Calvo KR, Gronborg M, et al. Distinguishing hairy cell leukemia variant from hairy cell leukemia: development and validation of diagnostic criteria. *Leuk Res.* 2013;37(4):401-409. doi:10.1016/j.leukres.2012.11.021

140. Gillis S, Amir G, Bennett M, Polliack A. Unexpectedly high incidence of hypoplastic/aplastic foci in bone marrow biopsies of hairy cell leukemia patients in remission following 2-chlorodeoxyadenosine therapy. *Eur J Haematol.* 2001;66(1):7-10.

141. Nanba K, Soban EJ, Bowling MC, Berard CW. Splenic pseudosinuses and hepatic angiomatous lesions. Distinctive features of hairy cell leukemia. *Am J Clin Pathol.* 1977;67(5):415-426.

142. Burthem J, Cawley JC. The bone marrow fibrosis of hairy-cell leukemia is caused by the synthesis and assembly of a fibronectin matrix by the hairy cells. *Blood.* 1994;83(2):497-504.

143. Burke JS, Rappaport H. The diagnosis and differential diagnosis of hairy cell leukemia in bone marrow and spleen. *Semin Oncol.* 1984;11(4):334-346.

144. Traverse-Glehen A, Baseggio L, Salles G, Coiffier B, Felman P, Berger F. Splenic diffuse red pulp small-B cell lymphoma: toward the emergence of a new lymphoma entity. *Discov Med.* 2012;13(71):253-265.

145. Catovsky D, Pettit JE, Galton DAG, Spiers ASD, Harrison CV. Leukaemic reticuloendotheliosis ("Hairy" cell leukaemia): a distinct clinico-pathological entity. *Br J Haematol.* 1974;26(1):9-27. doi:10.1111/j.1365-2141.1974.tb00445.x

146. Burke JS, Byrne GE Jr, Rappaport H. Hairy cell leukemia (leukemic reticuloendotheliosis): I. A clinical pathologic study of 21 patients. *Cancer.* 1974;37(9):1929-1950.

147. Mendes LS, Attygalle A, Matutes E, Wotherspoon A. Annexin A1 expression in a splenic diffuse red pulp small B-cell lymphoma: report of the first case. *Histopathology.* 2013;63(4):590-593. doi:10.1111/his.12179

148. Del Giudice I, Matutes E, Morilla R, et al. The diagnostic value of CD123 in B-cell disorders with hairy or villous lymphocytes. *Haematologica.* 2004;89(3):303-308.

149. Farren TW, Giustiniani J, Liu FT, et al. Differential and tumor-specific expression of CD160 in B-cell malignancies. *Blood.* 2011;118(8):2174-2183. doi:10.1182/blood-2011-02-334326

150. Lesesve JF, Tardy S, Frotscher B, Latger-Cannard V, Feugier P, De Carvalho Bittencourt M. Combination of CD160 and CD200 as a useful tool for differential diagnosis between chronic lymphocytic leukemia and other mature B-cell neoplasms. *Int J Lit Humanit.* 2015;37(4):486-494. doi:10.1111/ijlh.12315

151. Mayeur-Rousse C, Guy J, Miguet L, et al. CD180 expression in B-cell lymphomas: a multicenter GEIL study. *Cytometry B Clin Cytometry.* 2016;90(5):462-466. doi:10.1002/cyto.b.21325

152. Brunetti L, di Noto R, Abate G, et al. CD200/OX2, a cell surface molecule with immunoregulatory function, is consistently expressed on hairy cell leukaemia neoplastic cells. *Br J Haematol.* 2009;145(5):665-667. doi:10.1111/j.1365-2141.2009.07644.x

153. van Dongen JJM, Lhermitte L, Böttcher S, et al. EuroFlow antibody panels for standardized n-dimensional flow cytometric immunophenotyping of normal, reactive and malignant leukocytes. *Leukemia.* 2012;26(9):1908-1975. doi:10.1038/leu.2012.120

154. Daneshmanesh AH, Porwit A, Hojjat-Farsangi M, et al. Orphan receptor tyrosine kinases ROR1 and ROR2 in hematological malignancies. *Leuk Lymphoma*. 2013;54(4):843-850. doi:10.3109/10428194.2012.731599
155. Olejniczak SH, Stewart CC, Donohue K, Czuczman MS. A quantitative exploration of surface antigen expression in common B-cell malignancies using flow cytometry. *Immunol Invest*. 2006;35(1):93-114. doi:10.1080/08820130500496878
156. Chen YH, Tallman MS, Goolsby C, Peterson L. Immunophenotypic variations in hairy cell leukemia. *Am J Clin Pathol*. 2006;125(2):251-259. doi:10.1309/PMQX-VY61-9Q8Y-43AR
157. Poret N, Fu Q, Guihard S, et al. CD38 in hairy cell leukemia is a marker of poor prognosis and a new target for therapy. *Cancer Res*. 2015;75(18):3902-3911. doi:10.1158/0008-5472.CAN-15-0893
158. Andrulis M, Penzel R, Weichert W, von Deimling A, Capper D. Application of a BRAF V600E mutation-specific antibody for the diagnosis of hairy cell leukemia. *Am J Surg Pathol*. 2012;36(12):1796-1800. doi:10.1097/PAS.0b013e3182549b50
159. Brown NA, Betz BL, Weigelin HC, Elenitoba-Johnson KSJ, Lim MS, Bailey NG. Evaluation of allele-specific PCR and immunohistochemistry for the detection of BRAF V600E mutations in hairy cell leukemia. *Am J Clin Pathol*. 2015;143(1):89-99. doi:10.1309/AJCPDN4Q1JTFGCFC
160. Falini B, Tiacci E, Liso A, et al. Simple diagnostic assay for hairy cell leukaemia by immunocytochemical detection of annexin A1 (ANXA1). *Lancet*. 2004;363:1869-1871. doi:10.1016/S0140-6736(04)16356-3
161. Sherman MJ, Hanson CA, Hoyer JD. An assessment of the usefulness of immunohistochemical stains in the diagnosis of hairy cell leukemia. *Am J Clin Pathol*. 2011;136(3):390-399. doi:10.1309/AJCP5GE1PSBMBZTW
162. Toth-Liptak J, Piukovics K, Borbenyi Z, Demeter J, Bagdi E, Krenacs L. A comprehensive immunophenotypic marker analysis of hairy cell leukemia in paraffin-embedded bone marrow trephine biopsies – a tissue microarray study. *Pathol Oncol Res*. 2015;21(1):203-211. doi:10.1007/s12253-014-9807-5
163. Went PT, Zimpfer A, Pehrs AC, et al. High specificity of combined TRAP and DBA.44 expression for hairy cell leukemia. *Am J Surg Pathol*. 2005;29(4):474-478.
164. Mori N, Murakami YI, Shimada S, et al. TIA-1 expression in hairy cell leukemia. *Mod Pathol*. 2004;17(7):840-846. doi:10.1038/modpathol.3800129
165. Bastie JN, Cazals-Hatem D, Daniel MT, et al. Five years follow-up after 2-chloro deoxyadenosine treatment in thirty patients with hairy cell leukemia: evaluation of minimal residual disease and CD4+ lymphocytopenia after treatment. *Leuk Lymphoma*. 1999;35(5-6):555-565. doi:10.1080/10428199909169620
166. Else M, Dearden CE, Matutes E, et al. Long-term follow-up of 233 patients with hairy cell leukaemia, treated initially with pentostatin or cladribine, at a median of 16 years from diagnosis. *Br J Haematol*. 2009;145(6):733-740. doi:10.1111/j.1365-2141.2009.07668.x
167. Flinn IW, Kopecky KJ, Foucar MK, et al. Long-term follow-up of remission duration, mortality, and second malignancies in hairy cell leukemia patients treated with pentostatin. *Blood*. 2000;96(9):2981-2986.
168. Mhawech-Fauceglia P, Oberholzer M, Aschenafi S, et al. Potential predictive patterns of minimal residual disease detected by immunohistochemistry on bone marrow biopsy specimens during a long-term follow-up in patients treated with cladribine for hairy cell leukemia. *Arch Pathol Lab Med*. 2006;130(3):374-377. doi:10.1043/1543-2165(2006)130[374:PPPOMR]2.0.CO;2
169. Liu Q, Harris N, Epperla N, Andritsos LA. Current and emerging therapeutic options for hairy cell leukemia variant. *OncoTargets Ther*. 2021;14:1797-1805.
170. Baseggio L, Traverse-Glehen A, Callet-Bauchu E, et al. Relevance of a scoring system including CD11c expression in the identification of splenic diffuse red pulp small B-cell lymphoma (SRPL). *Hematol Oncol*. 2011;29(1):47-51. doi:10.1002/hon.957
171. Sun T, Dittmar K, Koduru P, Susin M, Teichberg S, Brody J. Relationship between hairy cell leukemia variant and splenic lymphoma with villous lymphocytes: presentation of a new concept. *Am J Hematol*. 1996;51(4):282-288. doi:10.1002/(SICI)1096-8652(199604)51:4<282::AID-AJH6>3.0.CO;2-S
172. Matutes BE, Morilla R, Owusu-ankomah K, Houlihan A, Catovsky D. The Immunophenotype of splenic lymphoma with villous lymphocytes and its relevance to the differential diagnosis. *Blood*. 1994;83(6):1558-1562.
173. Kalpadakis C, Pangalis GA, Angelopoulou MK, Vassilakopoulos TP. Treatment of splenic marginal zone lymphoma. *Best Pract Res Clin Haematol*. 2017;30(1-2):139-148. doi:10.1016/j.beha.2016.07.004
174. Garcia-Sanz R, Jimenez C, Puig N, et al. Origin of Waldenstrom's macroglobulinaemia. *Best Pract Res Clin Haematol*. 2016;29(2):136-147. doi:10.1016/j.beha.2016.08.024
175. Hunter ZR, Xu L, Yang G, et al. The genomic landscape of Waldenström macroglobulinemia is characterized by highly recurring MYD88 and WHIM-like CXCR4 mutations, and small somatic deletions associated with B-cell lymphomagenesis. *Blood*. 2014;123(11):1637-1646. doi:10.1182/blood-2013-09-525808
176. Collignon A, Wanquet A, Maitre E, Cornet E, Troussard X, Aurran-Schleinitz T. Prolymphocytic leukemia: new insights in diagnosis and in treatment. *Curr Oncol Rep*. 2017;19(4):29. doi:10.1007/s11912-017-0581-x
177. Paillassa J, Troussard X. Biology and treatment of hairy cell leukemia. *Curr Treat Options Oncol*. 2020;21(6):44. doi:10.1007/s11864-020-00732-0
178. Kreitman RJ, Arons E. Diagnosis and treatment of hairy cell leukemia as the COVID-19 pandemic continues. *Blood Rev*. 2022;(51):100888.
179. Falini B, Tiacci E. New treatment options in hairy cell leukemia with focus on BRAF inhibitors. *Hematol Oncol*. 2019;37(S1):30-37. doi:10.1002/hon.2594
180. Jansen J, Hermans J, Remme J, den Ottolander G, Lopes Cardozo P. Hairy cell leukaemia. Clinical features and effect of splenectomy. *Scand J Haematol*. 1978;21:60-71.
181. Mintz U, Golomb HM. Splenectomy as initial therapy in twenty-six patients with leukemic reticuloendotheliosis (hairy cell leukemia). *Cancer Res*. 1979;39:2366-2370.
182. Jansen JAN, Hermans JO. Splenectomy in hairy cell leukemia: a retrospective muliticenter analysis. *Cancer*. 1981;47(8):2066-2076.
183. Golomb HM, Vardiman JW. Response to splenectomy in 65 patients with hairy cell leukemia an evaluation of spleen weight and bone marrow involvement. *Blood*. 1983;61(2):349-352.
184. Ratain MJ, Vardiman JW, Barker CM, Golomb HM. Prognostic variables in hairy cell leukemia after splenectomy as initial therapy. *Cancer*. 1988;62:2420-2424.
185. Johnston JB. Mechanism of action of pentostatin and cladribine in hairy cell leukemia. *Leuk Lymphoma*. 2011;52(suppl 2):43-45. doi:10.3109/10428194.2011.570394
186. Spielberger R, Mick R, Ratain M, Golomb H. Interferon treatment for hairycell leukemia. An update on a cohort of 69 patients treated from 1983-1986. *Leuk Lymphoma*. 1994;14(suppl 1):89-93.
187. Grever M, Kopecky K, Foucar M, et al. Randomized comparison of pentostatin versus interferon alfa-2a in previously untreated patients with hairy cell leukemia: an intergroup study. *J Clin Oncol*. 1995;13:974-982.
188. Rai K, Davey F, Peterson S, et al. Recombinant alpha-2b-interferon in therapy of previously untreated hairy cell leukemia: longterm results of study by cancer and leukemia group B. *Leukemia*. 1995;9:1116-1120.
189. Spiers AS, Moore D, Cassileth PA, et al. Remissions in hairy-cell leukemia with pentostatin (2′-deoxycoformycin). *N Engl J Med*. 1987;316:825-830.
190. Johnston JB, Eisenhauer E, Corbett WEN, Scott JG, Zaentz SD. Efficacy of 2′-deoxycoformycin in hairy-cell leukemia: a study of the National Cancer Institute of Canada Clinical Trials Group. *J Natl Cancer Inst* 1988;80(10):765-769. doi:10.1093/jnci/80.10.765
191. Juliusson G, Heldal D, Hippe E, et al. Subcutaneous injections of 2-chlorodeoxyadenosine for symptomatic hairy cell leukemia. *J Clin Oncol*. 1995;13:989-995.
192. Saven A, Burina C, Koziol JA, Piro LD. Long-term follow-up of patients with hairy cell leukemia after cladribine treatment. *Blood*. 1998;92(6):1918-1926. doi:10.1200/JCO.2003.05.093
193. Lauria F, Bocchia M, Marotta G, Raspadori D, Zinzani PL, Tondelli D. Weekly administration of 2-chlorodeoxyadenosine in patients with hairy-cell leukemia is effective and reduces infectious complications. *Haematologica*. 1999;84:22-25.
194. Robak T, Jamroziak K, Gora-Tybor J, et al. Cladribine in a weekly versus daily schedule for untreated active hairy cell leukemia: final report from the Polish Adult Leukemia Group (PALG) of a prospective, randomized, multicenter trial. *Blood*. 2007;109(9):3672-3675. doi:10.1182/blood-2006-08-042929
195. Kraut E, Bouroncle B, Grever M. Pentostatin in the treatment of advanced hairy ell leukemia. *J Clin Oncol*. 1989;7:168-172.
196. Catovsky D, Matutes E, Talavera J, et al. Long-term results with 2'deoxycoformcyin in hairy cell leukemia. *Leuk Lymphoma*. 1994;14(suppl 1):109-113.
197. Rafel M, Cervantes F, Beltrán JM, et al. Deoxycoformycin in the treatment of patients with hairy cell leukemia: results of a Spanish collaborative study of 80 patients. *Cancer*. 2000;88(2):352-357. doi:10.1002/(sici)1097-0142(20000115)88:2<352::aid-cncr15>3.0.co;2-8
198. Ribeiro P, Bouaffia F, Peaud Py, et al. Long term outcome of patients with hairy cell leukemia treated with pentostatin. *Cancer*. 1999;85(1):65-71.
199. Seymour JF, Talpaz M, Kurzrock R. Response duration and recovery of CD4+ lymphocytes following deoxycoformycin in interferon-alpha-resistant hairy cell leukemia: 7-year follow-up. *Leukemia*. 1997;11:42-47.
200. Ho A, Thaler J, Mandelli F, et al. Response to pentostatin in hairy-cell leukemia refractory to interferon alpha. *J Clin Oncol*. 1989;7:1533-1538.
201. Golomb H, Dodge R, Mick D, et al. Pentostatin treatment of hairy cell leukemia patients who failed initial therapy with recombinant alpha-interferon: a report of CALGB study 8515. *Leukemia*. 1994;8:2037-2040.
202. Thaler J, Grunewald K, Gattringer C, et al. Long-term follow-up of patients with hairy cell leukaemia treated with pentostatin: lymphocyte subpopulations and residual bone marrow infiltration. *Br J Haematol*. 1993;84:75-82.
203. Matutes E, Meeus P, McLennan K, Catovsky D. The significance of minimal residual disease in hairy cell leukaemia patients treated with deoxycoformcyin: a long-term follow-up study. *Br J Haematol*. 1997;98:375-383.
204. Cassileth P, Cheuvart B, Spiers A, et al. Pentostatin induces durable remissions in hairy cell leukemia. *J Clin Oncol*. 1991;9:243-246.
205. Zinzani PL, Pellegrini C, Stefoni V, et al. Hairy cell leukemia: evaluation of the long-term outcome in 121 patients. *Cancer*. 2010;116(20):4788-4792. doi:10.1002/cncr.25243
206. Johnston J, Eisenhauer E, Wainman N, Corbett W, Zaentz S, Daeninck P. Long-term outcome following treatment of hairy cell leukemia with pentostatin (Nipent): a National Cancer Institute of Canada study. *Semin Oncol*. 2000;27:32-36.
207. Jehn U, Bartl R, Dietzfelbinger H, Haferlach T, Heinemann V. An update: 12-year follow-up of patients with hairy cell leukemia following treatment with 2-chlorodeoxyadenosine. *Leukemia*. 2004;18(9):1476-1481. doi:10.1038/sj.leu.2403418
208. Goodman G, Burian C, Koziol J, Saven A. Extended follow-up of patients with hairy cell leukemia after treatment with cladribine. *J Clin Oncol*. 2003;21(5):891-896.
209. Chadha P, Rademaker Aw, Mendiratta P, et al. Treatment of hairy cell leukemia with 2-chlorodeoxyadenosine (2-CdA): long-term follow-up of the Northwestern University experience. *Blood*. 2005;106:241-246. doi:10.1182/blood-2005-01-0173
210. Dearden CE, Else M, Catovsky D. Long-term results of pentostatin and cladribine treatment of hairy cell leukemia. *Leuk Lymphoma*. 2011;52(suppl 2):21-24. doi:10.3109/10428194.2011.565093
211. Andritsos L, Dunavin N, Lozanski G, et al. Reduced dose pentostatin for initial management of hairy cell leukemia patients who have active infection or risk of hemorrhage is safe and effective. *Haematologica*. 2015;100:e18-e20. doi:10.3324/haematol.2014.108258

212. Kraut E, Neff J, Bouroncle B, Grever M. Immunosuppressive effects of pentostatin. *J Clin Oncol*. 1990;8:848-855.
213. Cheson B. Infectious and immunosuppressive effects of purine analog therapy. *J Clin Oncol*. 1995;13:2431-2448.
214. Cheson BD, Vena D, Foss F, Sorensen JM. Neurotoxicity of purine analogs: a review. *J Clin Oncol*. 1994;12(10):2216-2228.
215. Hoffman M, Janson D, Rose E, Rai K. Treatment of hairy-cell leukemia with cladribine: response, toxicity, and long-term follow-up. *J Clin Oncol*. 1997;15:1138-1142.
216. Estey EH, Kurzrock R, Kantarjian HM, et al. Treatment of hairy cell leukemia with 2-chlorodeoxyadenosine (2-CdA). *Blood*. 1992;79(4):882-887.
217. Tallman MS, Hakimian D, Variakojis D, et al. A single cycle of 2-chlorodeoxyadenosine results in complete remission in the majority of patients with hairy cell leukemia. *Blood*. 1992;80(9):2203-2209.
218. Juliusson BG, Liliemark J. Rapid recovery from cytopenia in hairy cell leukemia after treatment with 2-chloro-2'-deoxyadenosine (CdA): relation to opportunistic infections. *Blood*. 1992;79(4):888-894.
219. Piro L, Ellison D, Saven A. The Scripps Clinic experience with 2-chlorodeoxyadenosine in the treatment of hairy cell leukemia. *Leuk Lymphoma*. 1994;14 (S1):121-125.
220. Lauria F, Rondelli D, Zinzani PL, et al. Long-lasting complete remission in patients with hairy cell leukemia treated with 2-CdA: a 5-year survey. *Leukemia*. 1997;11(5):629-632. http://www.ncbi.nlm.nih.gov/entrez/query.fcgi?cmd=Retrieve&db=PubMed&dopt=Citation&list_uids=9180283
221. Piro LD, Carrera CJ, Beutler E, Carson DA. 2-Chlorodeoxyadenosine: an effective new agent for the treatment of chronic lymphocytic leukemia. *Blood*. 1988;72(3):1069-1073.
222. Cheson B, Sorensen J, Vena D, et al. Treatment of hairy cell leukemia with 2-chlorodeoxyadenosine via the Group C protocol mechanism of the National Cancer Institute: a report of 979 patients. *J Clin Oncol*. 1998;16:3007-3015.
223. Sigal DS, Sharpe R, Burian C, Saven A. Very long-term eradication of minimal residual disease in patients with hairy cell leukemia after a single course of cladribine. *Blood*. 2010;115(10):1893-1896.
224. Siegel RS, Hakimian D, Spies W, et al. Technetium-99M sulfur colloid scanning and correlative magnetic resonance imaging in patients with hairy cell leukemia and hypocellular bone marrow biopsies after 2-chlorodeoxyadenosine. *Leuk Lymphoma*. 1999;35(1-2):171-177.
225. Ellison BDJ, Sharpe R, Robbins BA, et al. Immunomorphologic analysis of bone marrow biopsies after treatment with 2-chlorodeoxyadenosine for hairy cell leukemia. *Blood*. 1994;84(12):4310-4315.
226. Filleul B, Delannoy A, Ferrant A, et al. A single corse of 2-chloro-deoxyadenosine does not eradicate leukemic cells in hairy cell leukemia patients in complete remission. *Leukemia*. 1994;8:1153-1156.
227. Wheaton S, Tallman MS, Hakimian D, Peterson L. Minimal residual disease may predict bone marrow relapse in patients with hairy cell leukemia treated with 2-chlorodeoxyadenosine. *Blood*. 1996;87(4):1556-1560. http://www.ncbi.nlm.nih.gov/pubmed/8608247
228. Saven A, Piro LD. Complete remissions in hairy cell leukemia with 2-chlorodeoxyadenosine after failure with 2'-deoxycoformycin. *Ann Intern Med*. 1993;119(4):278-283.
229. Saven A, Burian C, Adusumalli J, Koziol JA. Filgrastim for cladribine-induced neutropenic fever in patients with hairy cell leukemia. *Blood*. 1999;93(8):2471-2477. http://www.ncbi.nlm.nih.gov/pubmed/10194424
230. Legrand O, Vekhoff A, Marie JP, Zittoun R, Delmer A. Treatment of hairy cell leukaemia (HCL) with 2-chlorodeoxyadenosine (2-CdA): identification of parameters predictive of adverse effects. *Br J Haematol*. 1997;99(1):165-167. http://0-ovidsp.ovid.com.wam.city.ac.uk/ovidweb.cgi?T=JS&PAGE=reference&D=med4&NEWS=N&AN=9359518
231. Dietrich S, Pircher A, Endris V, et al. BRAF inhibition in hairy cell leukemia with low dose vemurafenib. *Blood*. 2016;127:2847-2855, doi:10.1182/blood-2015-11-680074
232. Tiacci E, Park JH, de Carolis L, et al. Targeting mutant BRAF in relapsed or refractory hairy-cell leukemia. *N Engl J Med*. 2015;373(18):1733-1747, doi:10.1056/NEJMoa1506583
233. Juliusson G, Lenkei R, Liliemark J. Flow cytometry of blood and bone marrow cells from patients with hairy cell leukemia: phenotype of hairy cells and lymphocyte subsets after treatment with 2-chlorodeoxyadenosine. *Blood*. 1994;83(12):3672-3681.
234. Juliusson G, Lenkei R, Tjonnford G, Heldal D, Liliemark J. Low-dose cladribine for symptomatic hairy cell leukaemia. *Br J Haematol*. 1995;89:637-639.
235. Lenz G, Golf A, Rudiger T, Hiddemann W, Haferlach T. Epstein-Barr virus-associated B-cell non-Hodgkin lymphoma following treatment of hairy cell leukemia with cladribine. *Blood*. 2003;102(9):3457-3458.
236. Bhargava R, Barbashina V, Filippa DA, Teruya-Feldstein J. Epstein-Barr virus positive large B-cell lymphoma arising in a patient previously treated with cladribine for hairy cell leukemia. *Leuk Lymphoma*. 2004;45(5):1043-1048. doi:10.1080/10428190310001625890
237. Zulian GB, Roux E, Tiercy JM, et al. Transfusion-associated graft-versus-host disease in a patient treated with Cladribine (2-chlorodeoxyadenosine): demonstration of exogenous DNA in various tissue extracts by PCR analysis. *Br J Haematol*. 1995;89(1):83-89, doi:10.1111/j.1365-2141.1995.tb08906.x
238. Liliemark J, Albertioni F, Hassan M, Juliusson G. On the bioavailability of oral and subcutaneous 2-chloro-2-deoxyadenosine in human; alternative routes of administration. *J Clin Oncol*. 1992;10:1514-1518.
239. Robak T, Blasinska-Morawiec M, Krykowski E, et al. 2-Chlorodeoxyadenosine (Cladribine) in a 2-hour versus 24-hour intravenous infusion in the treatment of patients with hairy cell leukemia. *Leuk Lymphoma*. 1996;22:107-111.
240. von Rohr A, Schmitz SFH, Tichelli A, et al. Treatment of hairy cell leukemia with cladribine (2-chlorodeoxyadenosine) by subcutaneous bolus injection: a phase II study. *Ann Oncol*. 2002;13(10):1641-1649. doi:10.1093/annonc/mdf272
241. Zenhäusern R, Schmitz SFH, Solenthaler M, et al. Randomized trial of daily versus weekly administration of 2-chlorodeoxyadenosine in patients with hairy cell leukemia: a multicenter phase III trial (SAKK 32/98). *Leuk Lymphoma*. 2009;50(9):1501-1511. doi:10.1080/10428190903131755
242. Chacko J, Murphy C, Duggan C, O'Briain D, Browne P, McCann S. Weekly intermittent 2-CdA is less toxic and equally efficacious when compared to continuous infusion in hairy cell leukaemia. *Br J Haematol*. 1999;105(4):1145-1146.
243. Kraut EH, Chun H. Fludarabine phosphate in refractory hairy cell leukemia. *Am J Hematol*. 1991;37(1):59-60.
244. Kantarjian HM, Schachner J, Keating MJ. Fludarabine therapy in hairy cell leukemia. *Cancer*. 1991;67:1291-1293. doi:10.1089/gen.32.20.21
245. Quesada JR, Reuben J, Maning JT, Hersh EM, Gutterman JU. Alpha interferon for induction of remission in hairy-cell leukemia. *N Engl J Med*. 1984;310:15-18.
246. Foon KA, Maluish AE, Abrams PG, et al. Recombinant leukocyte A interferon therapy for advanced hairy cell leukemia. Therapeutic and immunologic results. *Am J Med*. 1986;80(3):351-356. doi:10.1016/0002-9343(86)90705-9
247. Golomb H, Jacobs A, Fefer A, et al. Alpha2 interferon therapy of hairy-cell leukemia: a multicenter study of 64 patients. *J Clin Oncol*. 1986;4:900-905.
248. Golomb H, Fefer A, Golde D, et al. Sequential evaluation of alpha-2b-interferon in 128 patients with hairy cell leukemia. *Semin Oncol*. 1987;14 (2 suppl):13-17.
249. Quesada JR, Hersh EM, Manning J, et al. Treatment of hairy cell leukemia with recombinant alpha-interferon. *Blood*. 1986;68(2):493-497.
250. Ratain MJ, Golomb HM, Vardiman JW, Vokes EE, Jacobs RH, Daly K. Treatment of hairy cell leukemia with recombinant alpha2 interferon. *Blood*. 1985;65(3):644-648.
251. Benz R, Siciliano RD, Stussi G, Fehr J. Long-term follow-up of interferon-alpha induction and low-dose maintenance therapy in hairy cell leukemia. *Eur J Haematol*. 2009;82(3):194-200. doi:10.1111/j.1600-0609.2008.01190.x
252. Baker PK, Pettitt AR, Slupsky JR, et al. Response of hairy cells to IFN-alpha involves induction of apoptosis through autocrine TNF-alpha and protection by adhesion. *Blood*. 2002;100:647-653.
253. Bardawil R, Ratain M, Golomb H, Bitter M, Groves C, Vardiman J. Changes in peripheral blood and bone marrow specimens during and after alpha 2b-interferon therapy for hairy cell leukemia. *Leukemia*. 1987;1:340-343.
254. Naeim F, Jacobs AD. Bone marrow changes in patients with hairy cell leukemia treated by recombinant alpha2-interferon. *Hum Pathol*. 1985;16(12):1200-1205.
255. Weiss K. Safety profile of interferon-alpha therapy. *Semin Oncol*. 1998;25(suppl 1):9-13.
256. Golomb H, Ratain M, Fefer A, et al. Randomized Study of the Effect of the duration of treatment with interferon alfa-2B in patients with hairy cell leukemia. *J Natl Cancer Inst*. 1988;80(5):369-373.
257. Thompson JA, Kidd P, Rubin E, Fefer A. Very low dose alpha-2b interferon for the treatment of hairy cell leukemia. *Blood*. 1989;73(6):1440-1443.
258. Troussard X, Flandrin G. An update on a cohort of 93 patients treated in a single institution. Effects of interferon in patients relapsing after splenectomy and in patients with or without maintenance treatment. *Leuk Lymphoma*. 1994;14(suppl 1):99-105.
259. Capnist G, Federico M, Chisesi T, et al. Long-term results of interferon treatment in hairy cell leukemia. Italian Cooperative Group of Hairy Cell Leukemia (ICGHCL). *Leuk Lymphoma*. 1994;14:457-464.
260. Seymour J, Estey E, Keating M, Kurzrock R. Response to interferon-alpha in patients with hairy cell leukemia relapsing after treatment with 2-chlorodeoxyadenosine. *Leukemia*. 1995;(9):929-932.
261. Spiegel RJ, Spicehandler JR, Jacobs SL, Oden EM. Low incidence of serum neutralizing factors in patients receiving recombinant alfa-2b interferon (intron A). *Am J Med*. 1986;80:223-228.
262. Steis RG, Smith JW, Urba WJ, et al. Loss of interferon antibodies during prolonged continuous interferon-alpha 2a therapy in hairy cell leukemia. *Blood*. 1991;77(4):792-798. http://www.ncbi.nlm.nih.gov/pubmed/1704264
263. Conlon KC, Urba WJ, Smith JW, Steis RG, Longo DL, Clark JW. Exacerbation of symptoms of autoimmune disease in patients receiving alpha-interferon therapy. *Cancer*. 1990;65:2237-2242.
264. Akhard LP, Hoffman R, Elias L, Saiers J. Alpha-interferon and immune hemolytic anemia. *Ann Intern Med*. 1986;105(2):306.
265. Johnston JB. Enhancing monoclonal antibody activity in chronic lymphocytic leukemia. *Leuk Lymphoma*. 2015;56(8):2231-2232. doi:10.3109/10428194.2015.1080927
266. Nieva J, Bethel K, Saven A. Phase 2 study of rituximab in the treatment of cladribine-failed patients with hairy cell leukemia. *Blood*. 2003;102(3):810-813. doi:10.1182/blood-2003-01-0014
267. Thomas DA, O'Brien S, Bueso-Ramos C, et al. Rituximab in relapsed or refractory hairy cell leukemia. *Blood*. 2003;102(12):3906-3911. doi:10.1182/blood-2003-02-0630
268. Cervetti G, Galimberti S, Andreazzoli F, et al. Rituximab as treatment for minimal residual disease in hairy cell leukaemia. *Eur J Haematol*. 2004;73(6):412-417. doi:10.1111/j.1600-0609.2004.00325.x
269. Chihara D, Arons E, Stetler-Stevenson M, et al. Randomized phase II study of first-line cladribine with concurrent or delayed rituximab in patients with hairy cell leukemia. *J Clin Oncol*. 2020;38:1527-1538. doi:10.1200/JCO.19
270. Else M, Dearden CE, Matutes E, et al. Rituximab with pentostatin or cladribine: an effective combination treatment for hairy cell leukemia after disease recurrence. *Leuk Lymphoma*. 2011;52(suppl 2):75-78. doi:10.3109/10428194.2011.568650
271. Gerrie AS, Zypchen LN, Connors JM. Fludarabine and rituximab for relapsed or refractory hairy cell leukemia. *Blood*. 2012;119(9):1988-1991. doi:10.1182/blood-2011-08-371989

272. Chihara D, Kantarjian H, O'Brien S, et al. Long-term durable remission by cladribine followed by rituximab in patients with hairy cell leukaemia: update of a phase II trial. *Br J Haematol*. 2016;174(5):760-766. doi:10.1111/bjh.14129
273. Kreitman RJ, Arons E. Update on hairy cell leukemia. *Clin Adv Hematol Oncol*. 2018;16(3):205-215.
274. Kreitman RJ, Pastan I. Contextualizing the use of moxetumomab pasudotox in the treatment of relapsed or refractory hairy cell leukemia. *Oncol*. 2020;25(1):e170-e177. doi:10.1080/17474086.2019.1643231
275. Kreitman RJ, Dearden C, Zinzani PL, et al. Moxetumomab pasudotox in heavily pre-treated patients with relapsed/refractory hairy cell leukemia (HCL): long-term follow-up from the pivotal trial. *J Hematol Oncol*. 2021;14(35):1-11.
276. Kreitman RJ, Dearden C, Zinzani PL, et al. Moxetumomab pasudotox in relapsed/refractory hairy cell leukemia. *Leukemia*. 2018;32(8):1768-1777. doi:10.1038/s41375-018-0210-1
277. Dietrich S., Glimm H, Andrulis M, von Kalle C, Ho AD, Zenz T. BRAF inhibition in refractory hairy-cell leukemia. *N Engl J Med*. 2012;21(24):2038-2040.
278. Tiacci E, de Carolis L, Simonetti E, et al. Vemurafenib plus rituximab in refractory or relapsed hairy-cell leukemia. *N Engl J Med*. 2021;384:1810-1823, doi:10.1056/NEJMoa2031298
279. Tiacci E, de Carolis L, Simonetti E, et al. Safety and efficacy of the BRAF inhibitor dabrafenib in relapsed or refractory hairy cell leukemia: a pilot phase-2 clinical trial. *Leukemia*. 2021;35:3314-3318. doi:10.1038/s41375-021-01210-8
280. Kreitman RJ, Moreau P, Hutchings M, et al. Treatment with combination of dabrafenib and trametinib in patients with recurrent/refractory BRAF V600e-mutated hairy cell leukemia (HCL). *Blood*. 2018;132(suppl 1):391. doi:10.1182/blood-2018-99-113135
281. Caeser R, Collord G, Yao WQ, et al. Targeting MEK in vemurafenib-resistant hairy cell leukemia. *Leukemia*. 2018;33(2):541-545. doi:10.1038/s41375-018-0270-2
282. Sivina M, Kreitman RJ, Arons E, Ravandi F, Burger JA. The bruton tyrosine kinase inhibitor ibrutinib (PCI-32765) blocks hairy cell leukaemia survival, proliferation and B cell receptor signalling: a new therapeutic approach. *Br J Haematol*. 2014;166(2):177-188. doi:10.1111/bjh.12867
283. Rogers KA, Andritsos LA, Wei L, et al. Phase 2 study of ibrutinib in classic and variant hairy cell leukemia. *Blood*. 2021;137:3473-3483. doi:10.1182/blood.2020009688
284. Krigel R, Liebes LF, Pelle E, Silber R. Chlorambucil therapy in hairy cell leukemia: effects on lipid composition and lymphocyte subpopulations. *Blood*. 1982;60(1):272-275.
285. Golomb H, Schmidt K, Vardiman J. Chlorambucil therapy of twenty-four post-splenectomy patients with progressive hairy cell leukemia. *Semin Oncol*. 1984;11(4 suppl 2):502-508.
286. Calvo F, Castaigne S, Sigaux F, et al. Intensive Chemotherapy of hairy cell leukemia in patients with aggressive disease. *Blood*. 2016;65(1):115-119.
287. Cold S, Brincker H. Chemotherapy of progressive hairy-cell leukaemia. *Eur J Haematol*. 1987;38:251-255.
288. Magee MJ, McKenzie S, Filippa DA, Arlin ZA, Gee TS, Clarkson BD. Hairy Cell Leukemia. Durability of response to splenectomy in 26 patients and treatment of relapse with androgens in six patients. *Cancer*. 1985;56:2557-2562. doi:10.1016/B978-0-7216-0040-6.00015-0
289. Quesada JR, Hersh EM, Keating M, Zander A, Hester J. Hairy cell leukemia: clinical effects of the methanol extraction residue (MER) of BCG, lithium carbonate and mononuclear cell-enriched leukocyte transfusions. *Leuk Res*. 1981;5(6):463-476, doi:10.1017/CBO9781107415324.004
290. Cheever MA, Fefer A, Greeberg PD, et al. Treatment of hairy-cell leukemia with chemoradiotherapy and identical-twin bone-marrow transplantation. *Neoplasia*. 1982;307(8):479-481.
291. Mielke CH, Dobbs CE, Winkler CF, Yam LT. Therapeutic leukapheresis in hairy cell leukemia. *Arch Intern Med*. 1982;142:700-702.
292. Golomb HM, Kraut EH, Oviatt D, Prendergast E, Stein R, Sweet D. Absence of prolonged benefit of initial leukapheresis therapy for hairy cell leukemia. *Am J Hematol*. 1983;14:49-56.
293. Weinmann M, Becker G, Einsele H, Bamberg M. Clinical indications and biological mechanisms of splenic irradiation in chronic leukemias and myeloproliferative disorders. *Radiother Oncol*. 2001;58(2):235-246. doi:10.1007/PL00002384
294. Orringer EP, Varia MA. Role for radiation in the treatment of hairy cell leukemia complicated by massive lymphadenopathy. *Cancer*. 1980;45:2047-2050.
295. Shenoi DP, Andritsos LA, Blachly JS, et al. Classic hairy cell leukemia complicated by pancytopenia and severe infection: a report of 3 cases treated with vemurafenib. *Blood Adv*. 2019;3(2):116-118. doi:10.1182/bloodadvances.2018027466
296. Smirnova SY, Al-Radi LS, Moiseeva TN, et al. Inhibitor of BRAFV600E mutation as a treatment option for hairy cell leukemia with deep neutropenia and infectious complications. *Clin Lymphoma Myeloma Leuk*. 2021;21:427-430.
297. Ravandi F. MRD in HCL: does it matter? *Blood*. 2018;131(21):2277-2278. doi:10.1182/blood-2018-04-843128
298. Matutes E; Wotherspoon A, Brito-Babapulle V, Catovsky D. The natural history and clinico-pathological features of the variant form of hairy cell leukemia. *Leukemia*. 2001;15(1):184-186. http://www.ncbi.nlm.nih.gov/pubmed/11243388
299. Kreitman RJ, Wilson W, Calvo KR, et al. Cladribine with immediate rituximab for the treatment of patients with variant hairy cell leukemia. *Clin Cancer Res*. 2013;19(24):6873-6881. doi:10.1158/1078-0432.CCR-13-1752
300. Troussard X, Grever MR. The revised guidelines for the diagnosis and management of hairy cell leukaemia and the hairy cell leukaemia variant. *Br J Haematol*. 2021;193(1):11-14. doi:10.1111/bjh.17201
301. Parry-Jones N, Joshi A, Forconi F, Dearden C. Guideline for diagnosis and management of hairy cell leukaemia (HCL) and hairy cell variant (HCL-V). *Br J Haematol*. 2020;191(5):730-737. doi:10.1111/bjh.17055
302. Wierda WG, Byrd JC, Abramson JS, et al. Hairy cell Leukemia, Version 2.2018: clinical practice guidelines in oncology. *J Natl Compr Canc Netw*. 2017;15(11):1414-1427. doi:10.6004/jnccn.2017.0165
303. Cornet E, Tomowiak C, Tanguy-Schmidt A, et al. Long-term follow-up and second malignancies in 487 patients with hairy cell leukemia. *Br J Haematol*. 2014;166:390-400. doi:10.1111/bjh.12908
304. Hisada M, Chen BE, Jaffe ES, Travis LB. Second cancer incidence and cause-specific mortality among 3104 patients with hairy cell leukemia: a population-based study. *J Natl Cancer Inst*. 2007;99(3):215-222. doi:10.1093/jnci/djk030
305. Kampmeier BP, Spielberger R, Dickstein J, Mick R, Golomb H, Vardiman JW. Increased incidence of second neoplasms in patients treated with interferon alpha 2b for hairy cell leukemia: a clinicopathologic assessment. *Blood*. 1994;83:2931-2938.
306. Pawson R, A'Hern R, Catovsky D. Second malignancy in hairy cell leukaemia: no evidence of increased incidence after treatment with interferon alpha. *Leuk Lymphoma*. 1996;22:103-106.
307. Benz R, Arn K, Andres M, et al. Prospective long-term follow-up after first-line subcutaneous cladribine in hairy cell leukemia: a SAKK trial. *Blood Adv*. 2020;4(15):3699-3707. doi:10.1182/bloodadvances.2020002160
308. Dinmohamed AG, Posthuma EFM, Visser O, Kater AP, Raymakers RAP, Doorduijn JK. Relative survival reaches a plateau in hairy cell leukemia: a population-based analysis in The Netherlands. *Blood*. 2018;131(12):1380-1383. doi:10.1182/blood-2017-12-820381

Chapter 94 ■ Cutaneous T-Cell Lymphoma: Mycosis Fungoides and Sézary Syndrome

JOHN A. ZIC • FRANCINE FOSS • EVA NIKLINSKA • JEFF P. ZWERNER

Cutaneous lymphomas are a heterogeneous group of non-Hodgkin lymphomas (NHLs) of T- and B-cell origin in which the skin is the primary organ of involvement. Primary cutaneous lymphomas usually present without signs of extracutaneous malignancy at onset of symptoms; they represent an entity distinct from nodal lymphomas with secondary cutaneous involvement. In 1975, Lutzner, Edelson, and associates introduced the term cutaneous T-cell lymphoma (CTCL) to describe the spectrum of skin-based lymphomas of T-cell origin including classical mycosis fungoides (MF) and Sézary syndrome (SS).[1,2] This chapter is a review of the history, epidemiology, clinicopathologic features, and therapy of these lymphomas.

HISTORICAL PERSPECTIVE AND PATHOPHYSIOLOGY

Clinical Description

The first clinical description of MF was provided in 1806 by Alibert, a French physician, who identified a 56-year-old man presenting with skin tumors resembling mushrooms after having had a desquamating rash over several months; the lesions waxed and waned for 5 years before the patient died with a "hectic" fever.[3] In 1832, Alibert first used the term mycosis fungoïde in his treatise on diseases of the skin to describe the mushroom-like tumors.[4] Bazin described the three "classical" cutaneous stages in 1870: (a) the premycotic stage, which can be localized or diffuse with superficial eczematous or erythematous lesions; (b) the infiltrative plaque stage; and (c) the tumor stage.[5] The mycosis d'emblée variant, in which tumors develop rapidly without a preceding premycotic or plaque stage, was described by Vidal and Brocq in 1885.[6] In the early 1890s, Besnier and Hallopeau described the erythrodermic variant, which later became known as SS.[7,8]

Histopathology

By the end of the 19th century, most authorities agreed that the small round cells infiltrating the epidermis and forming tumors were lymphoid in origin.[9] Although the French authorities considered the disease lymphadenomatous in nature, the German, English, and American authorities were divided between sarcomatous and granulomatous (infectious) etiologies.[9,10]

The unique appearance of the cells involved in CTCL was identified in 1938 by Sézary and Bouvrain, who reported a triad of erythroderma, leukemia with circulating mononuclear cells that had convoluted nuclei, and adenopathy infiltrated with the same cells.[11] SS was recognized in the English literature by several groups in the 1950s, but it was not described in the US medical literature until Taswell and Winkelmann at the Mayo Clinic in 1961.[12] In 1968, Lutzner and Jordan extended the light microscopic description of the Sézary cell by using electron microscopy to visualize the "serpentine" or cerebriform cell nucleus.[13]

Immunology

The 1970s witnessed the introduction of cellular immunology into the study of hematopoietic neoplasms, and in 1971 Crossen et al confirmed the lymphocyte origin of SS.[14] In 1973, Broome et al[15] and Brouet et al[16] identified the neoplastic cell as a T cell, and Broder et al demonstrated in 1976 that the cells are usually of the helper phenotype (CD4+).[17]

Studies performed in the early 1990s further characterized the circulating malignant T cells in patients with SS as "memory" helper T cells because of the expression of CD45RO+.[18] In 1992, Vowels et al detected a cytokine profile similar to that produced by murine T_H2 cells from both stimulated peripheral blood mononuclear cells and serum from patients with SS.[19] Further studies identified a T_H2 cytokine profile (interleukin [IL]-4, IL-5, IL-6, IL-10) to be present in the skin of patients with MF and SS.[20-22] Increased levels of IL-4 and IL-5 produced by the malignant T-cell clone may account for the eosinophilia and increased levels of immunoglobulin-E (IgE) and IgA in the serum of patients with advanced CTCL.[23] In addition, T_H2 cytokines, IL-4 and IL-13, have been shown to increase periostin, which in turn stimulates the chemokine thymic stromal lymphopoietin (TSLP) expression, all of which have been shown to be upregulated in CTCL. Stimulation of CTCL cell lines with TSLP leads to further T_H2 cytokine expression as well and proliferative lymphocyte growth, demonstrating a T_H2-centric positive feedback loop in CTCL.[24] The T_H17-associated proinflammatory cytokine, IL-17, has also been found to be upregulated in MF skin lesions and appears to be activated through the Janus kinase and signal transducer and activator of transcription (JAK/STAT) pathway, although more recent data have been presented demonstrating instances of either increased or decreased T_H17 populations in CTCL.[25,26] The T-lymphocyte regulatory cells, typified by Forkhead box 3P (FOXP3), CD4, and CD25 expression, have also been found in increased numbers in CTCL, potentially leading to a dampening of the immune response against the tumor cells.[25]

Immunologic studies have addressed the pathogenesis of MF and SS by examining the tumor microenvironment and the complex interactions among malignant cerebriform T cells, keratinocytes, Langerhans cells, and other immunomodulating cells. Lymphocytes (malignant and inflammatory) that home to cutaneous sites differ from lymphocytes in noncutaneous infiltrates by expressing the cutaneous lymphocyte-associated antigen (CLA), which binds to the endothelial cell adhesion molecule E-selectin (ELAM-1), which is preferentially induced on cutaneous venules.[27,28] Both circulating and skin-based malignant T cells from patients with MF have been shown to express CLA, which may explain how the cells preferentially home into the skin (Figure 94.1A).[27,28] In addition, CLA+ T cells selectively express CC chemokine receptor 4 (CCR4) and CCR10, whose ligands CCL17 (TARC) and CCL27 (CTAK) are generated by the lesional keratinocytes and also on the luminal surface of postcapillary venules in the skin.[29,30] Narducci et al discovered that SS cells express a functionally active CXCR4 and that its ligand SDF-1 is abundantly produced in the skin, thus representing the main destination of SS cell spreading.[31] SDF-1 is normally inactivated by proteolytic cleavage by the CD26/dipeptidylpeptidase IV (DPPIV). The lack of CD26 from the cell surface is a hallmark of circulating SS cells (Figure 94.1B). In addition, it has been found that fibroblasts from lesional CTCL produce increased levels of the chemokine eotaxin, which is also expressed at increasingly higher levels as the disease advances.[32] The only receptor for eotaxin is CCR3, which is found on T_H2 lymphocytes and eosinophils and may further explain why we see an increase of T_H2 polarity as CTCL progresses.[32]

Within the skin, the specific epidermotropism of the malignant T cell is partially explained by the discovery of increased expression of intercellular adhesion molecule-1 (ICAM-1 or CD54) by epidermal keratinocytes in early MF lesions. The binding of ICAM-1 to lymphocyte function-associated protein 1 (LFA-1) or CD18 expressed by lymphocytes speaks to the histologic finding of atypical lymphocytes nesting within the epidermis.[33] Some authorities speculate that the expression of ICAM-1 by keratinocytes is induced by the release of interferon-γ (IFN-γ) from infiltrating CD8+ T cells or natural killer (NK) cells responding to the malignant T-cell population within the dermis (Figure 94.2).[23] Soluble chemotactic factors may also play a role in the epidermotropism of MF. The expression of the CXC

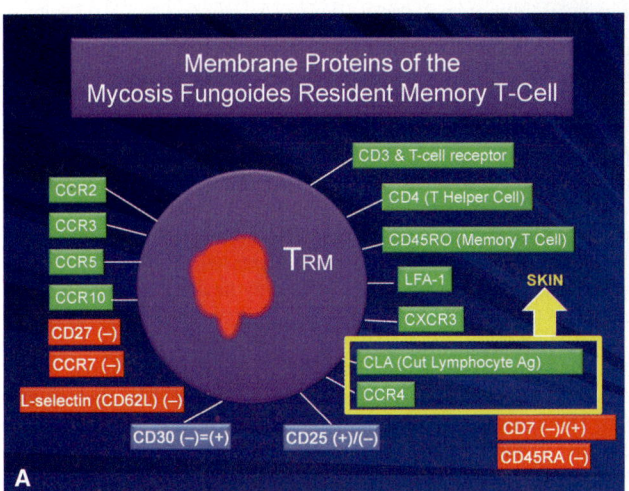
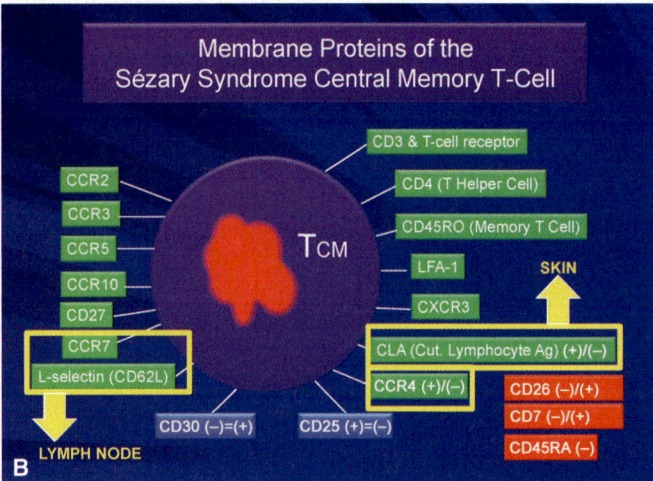

FIGURE 94.1 Membrane proteins of the malignant T cell. A, Mycosis fungoides is a malignancy of the resident memory T cell. B, Sézary syndrome is a malignancy of the central memory T cell. The cutaneous lymphoid antigen (CLA) and CCR4 are membrane proteins expressed by a vast majority of T cells found in inflamed skin including CTCL. Expression of CCR7 and L-selectin on the malignant T cell of Sézary syndrome allows the cell to traffic into lymph nodes. LFA-1 is a β_2 integrin expressed by all mature white blood cells. CCR, CC chemokine receptor; CTCL, cutaneous T-cell lymphoma; LFA-1, lymphocyte function-associated protein 1.

chemokine IP-10 (IFN-γ-inducible protein-10), which is chemotactic for CD4+ lymphocytes, has been shown to be markedly increased by basal and suprabasal keratinocytes in MF lesions.[34] Several studies suggest that, in early MF, epidermal Langerhans cells convert to hyperstimulatory antigen-presenting cells (CD1a+, CD1b+, CD36+) with a high expression of major histocompatibility complex MHC class II molecules and adhesion molecules capable of activating tumor-infiltrating lymphocytes.[23]

More advanced lesions of MF, characterized clinically as tumors or generalized erythroderma, often demonstrate a loss of epidermotropism, with malignant T cells infiltrating the deep dermis.[35] In 1989, Nickoloff et al found markedly diminished ICAM-1 expression by keratinocytes in a patient with SS,[36] and similar findings in tumor-stage patients were reported by Vejlsgaard et al.[37] Rook et al[38] hypothesized that, through evasion of the host immune response, an expansion of the malignant clonal population causes increased production of IL-4 and reduced IFN-γ. Through this mechanism, keratinocyte ICAM-1 expression is decreased along with reduced binding of malignant T cells within the epidermal compartment (*Figure 94.3*).[38] Others have suggested that the expression of CCR7 by some peripheral blood Sézary cells may enhance their ability to home into lymph nodes and extracutaneous spread.[39] Campbell et al revealed a disparate chemokine receptor expression profile in leukemic CTCL cells as compared with CTCL cells isolated from lesional skin. The leukemic cells had strong expression of CCR7, L-selectin, and CCR4, whereas the cells from CTCL skin expressed CCR4 and CLA.[40] The results of these investigators and others suggest that SS is a malignancy of central memory T cells and MF is a malignancy of skin-resident effector memory T cells (*Figure 94.1A and B*).[40,41]

The T cells in early-stage MF typically display a Th1 phenotype and produce immunostimulatory cytokines such as IFN-γ and IL-12 that help recruit the host's immune system to combat the malignant cells. As the disease progresses, however, there is a shift toward Th2 cytokine expression and cell-mediated immunity, critical for tumor cell recognition and destruction, is slowly dismantled.[42,43] The malignant cells also express immunosuppressive cell surface proteins, such

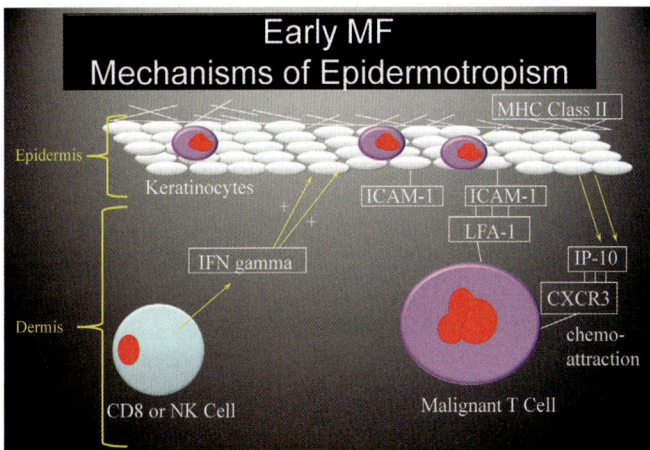

FIGURE 94.2 Early cutaneous T-cell lymphoma (CTCL): mechanisms of epidermotropism. The release of interferon (IFN)-γ by early, reactive CD8-cytotoxic T cells or NK cells leads to increased keratinocyte expression of intercellular adhesion molecule-1 (ICAM-1) and release of the C-X-C chemokine IP-10, which binds to the CXCR3 receptor, and may lead to nesting of CTCL cells within the epidermis. MF, mycosis fungoides; NK, natural killer.

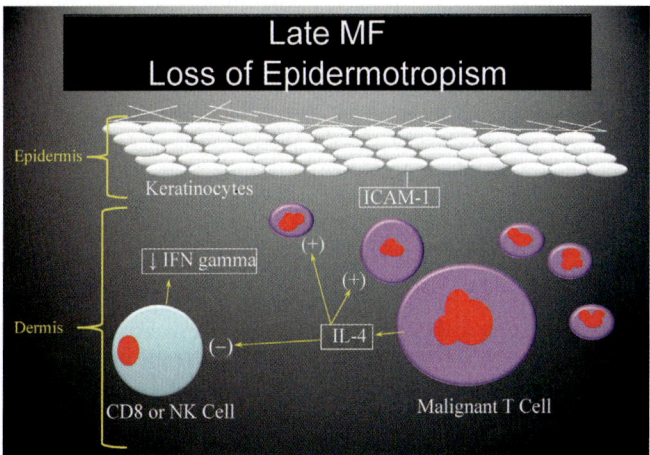

FIGURE 94.3 Late cutaneous T-cell lymphoma (CTCL): loss of epidermotropism. As the clonal population of CTCL cells expands, more IL-4 is released, which drives autocrine-induced proliferation of the CTCL cells and inhibition of CD8-cytotoxic T cells and NK cells. The impaired release of interferon (IFN)-γ may lead to less intercellular adhesion molecule-1 (ICAM-1) expression and decreased keratinocyte-CTCL cell adhesion. IL, interleukin; MF, mycosis fungoides; NK, natural killer.

as PD-1, PD-L1, and CTLA-4, that prevent the host's immune system from mounting a response.[44,45] The Th2-driven expression of CD47 on Sézary cells inhibits macrophage-mediated phagocytosis of tumor cells and is associated with worse overall survival (OS).[46] In addition, late-stage disease is characterized by diminished complexity of the T-cell receptor (TCR) repertoire that could limit the number of antigens the immune system is able to recognize.[47] All of these changes lead to unchecked proliferation of the malignant clone and generalized immunosuppression leading to life-threatening opportunistic infections.

Molecular Genetics

Clonality in T-cell lymphoma was difficult to establish before the development of molecular genotyping methods in the 1980s. Initial evidence of clonality in MF/SS was provided by cytogenetic analysis.[48,49] Several of these early studies demonstrated the same abnormal clone in separate lesions from skin, peripheral blood, lymph nodes, and bone marrow.[48,49]

The identification of a defined cytogenetic abnormality would be a major advance in the diagnosis and our understanding of the pathogenesis of MF/SS. Unfortunately, to date, no such abnormality has been identified consistently in MF, with most reported findings being largely of a random nature.[50] Some of the specific chromosomal deletions and amplifications that have been identified in CTCL include 8q gains, 10q and 17p deletions, and 17q gains (isochromosome 17).[51-54] Abnormalities in chromosome 10 have been correlated with progression to tumor stage, including loss of heterozygosity on 10q and microsatellite instability.[55] Salgado et al demonstrated through comparative genomic hybridization oligonucleotide array that, in tumor stage MF, loss of 9p21.3 (encodes *CDKN2A* and *CDKN2B*) and 10q26qter, and gain of 8q.24.21, was associated with decreased survival.[56] In addition, p16^{INK4a}, a protein coded at the 9p21 locus, has been shown to be silenced in tumor-stage MF.[57] Microsatellite instability was detected in 16 of 56 patients with CTCL that may be a consequence of *hMLH1* promoter hypermethylation and may prevent transcription in a subset of patients.[58] van Doorn and colleagues reported that the malignant T cells of patients with CTCL display widespread promoter hypermethylation associated with inactivation of several tumor-suppressor genes involved in DNA repair (*MGMT*, *MLH1*), cell cycle (*CHFR*), and apoptosis signaling pathways.[59] Rindler et al recently identified several biomarkers of disease progression using single-cell RNA sequencing.[60]

Comparative transcriptome analysis was performed on tissue from patients with early-stage MF and benign dermatoses, which identified increased expression of the TOX protein in MF. TOX is strongly expressed in thymic tissue but is normally silenced in mature CD4$^+$ T cells.[61] This finding was recapitulated in a number of follow-up studies, and efforts were made to identify a role in pathogenesis. Recently it was shown that cyclin-dependent kinase inhibitors p27 and p57 are upregulated with knockdown of TOX, whereas increased TOX expression was associated with AKT phosphorylation and CTCL proliferation.[62,63] Inhibition of the GATA-binding protein 3 (GATA3) is integral in T-cell development and can be upregulated in lymphoma cells leading to reduced levels of TOX in CTCL cells.[64] All of these data speak to a possible pathogenic role of TOX overexpression in CTCL.

Overexpression of the tumor-suppressor gene *TP53* has been detected in some cases of high-grade CTCL such as cutaneous anaplastic large cell lymphoma (LCL), but rarely in low-grade CTCL.[65] Infrequent *FAS* mutations, but no *BAX* or *TP53* mutations, were discovered in a study of 44 patients with early MF.[65] Aberrant expression of the *BCL-2* gene, which normally codes for an inner mitochondrial membrane protein, can suppress apoptosis, an important pathogenic mechanism in lymphomas. Although Dummer and colleagues detected *BCL-2* expression in 22 of 26 MF cases, it was also present in 5 of 6 cases of benign inflammatory dermatoses.[66] A cDNA microarray study of 29 cases of MF and 11 cases of inflammatory dermatoses revealed a signature of 27 genes implicated in the tumorigenesis of MF, including tumor necrosis factor receptor (TNFR)-dependent apoptosis regulators, *STAT4*, *CD40L*, and other oncogenes and apoptosis inhibitors.[67] Loss of SHP-1 tyrosine phosphatase expression appears to correlate with the advanced stages of CTCL.[68] The epigenetic silencing of *SHP-1* is induced by an activated phosphorylated (p)-STAT3 transcription factor in cooperation with DNA methyltransferase 1 (DNMT1), the key member of the epigenetic gene silencing machinery.[68] *JUNB* amplification leads to enhanced T$_H$2 cell function, a hallmark of the malignant T cell in CTCL. Mao and colleagues reported the amplification and overexpression of JUNB in tissue from patients with CTCL.[69] In addition, mutations involving the RAS pathway have been identified in a minority of CTCL.[70]

More recently, there has been a veritable explosion of data generated through next-generation sequencing, allowing for rapid whole genome sequencing and analysis of individual patient tumors and blood. The number of "nonsynonymous" and "premature stop" single nucleotide variants ranged from around 60 to 100, as has been found with other malignancies.[71-73] Interestingly, one study demonstrated that somatic copy number variants were found to play a significant role in CTCL, with copy number alteration, specifically focal deletions, accounting for up to 92% of oncogenic mutations, often affecting genes including *TP53* and *FAS*, among others.[74]

Although these next-generation sequencing studies failed to identify a single "founder" mutation, there were numerous aberrations found affecting similar pathways, as summarized by Damsky et al.[71] The JAK-STAT pathway, integral to IL-2 signaling and cellular proliferation, is known to be deregulated in MF and CTCL.[73,75] Mutations of the *JAK1*, *JAK3*, *STAT3*, and *STAT5B* genes were also discovered within a small percentage of CTCL patient samples, and *STAT5B* has also been found to have copy number gain in up to 63% of late-stage MF.[71,72] The nuclear factor kappa B (NF-κB) pathway also bears significant dysregulation in CTCL/MF along with constitutive activation downstream of TCR signaling. Mutations have been identified with genes integral to the NF-κB pathway, including caspase recruitment domain family member 11 (*CARD11*) and TNF receptor superfamily member 1B (*TNFRSF1B*), which encodes the tumor necrosis factor receptor 2 (*TNFR2*).[76,77] TCR signaling has been shown to harbor significant alteration in CTCL. Phospholipase C gamma 1 (PLGC1), a TCR-associated enzyme integral to transduction of tyrosine kinase signaling, has been reported within CTCL to have activating mutations leading to nuclear factor of activated T-cells (NFAT) activation and potential lymphomagenesis or exacerbation of disease.[76,78] Zinc finger E-box-binding homeobox 1 (*ZEB1*), an inhibitor of the T-lymphocyte stimulatory cytokine IL-2, was found to have both mutations (presumably inactivating) and loss of expression.[72,79] Lastly, gain-of-function or activating mutations have also been reported in the CD28 TCR costimulatory molecule, which would cause continued stimulation of the T lymphocytes.[74] Over the coming years, we will continue to learn and benefit from the data generated through these and future studies.

The small, single-stranded, noncoding RNAs, known as microRNAs (miRNAs), have been found to be differentially expressed in MF/CTCL.[80,81] A CTCL miRNA signature (miR-155, miR-203, and miR-205) was found to be capable of distinguishing between CTCL and benign inflammatory dermatoses with 95% accuracy.[81] It has also been demonstrated that there is a loss of miR-223 and miR-342 in SS vs normal CD4$^+$ T cells.[82] Numerous studies have continued to demonstrate aberrant miRNA expression in MF/CTCL, and efforts were then turned toward better understanding the role of these dysregulated miRNAs. It was first shown that reduced miR-342 leads to inhibition of apoptosis in CTCL cells.[82] Narducci et al also reported that knockdown of the overexpressed miR-21 in a CTCL cell line led to increased apoptosis.[83] A further study revealed that miR-21 is under positive transcriptional control of STAT3, known to be constitutively activated in SS.[84] McGirt et al demonstrated that TOX is a target gene of miR-223, and overexpression of miR-223 led to decreased TOX expression with associated reduction in CTCL proliferation.[85] It was hypothesized that the low levels of miR-223 found in CTCL may allow increased transcription of TOX and therefore increased cell growth.[85]

In 1985, Aisenberg et al and Weiss et al independently described Southern blot analysis techniques using probes for the β chain of the *TCR* to establish clonality in T-cell lymphoproliferative disorders (LPDs).[86,87] Because earlier cytogenetic studies suggested that CTCL arises from a single malignant clone of mature T cells,[48] the presence of *TCR* β-chain rearrangement in pathologically suspicious tissue has been considered strong evidence for the diagnosis of CTCL. More sensitive techniques involving polymerase chain reaction (PCR) were then developed to evaluate clonality in CTCL and related skin diseases.[88] Although the vast majority of CTCL express the α/β *TCR* heterodimer, most laboratories using the PCR technique take advantage of the fact that all α/β *TCR*-positive T cells also contain at least one rearranged allele of the *TCR* γ-chain gene. The γ gene contains a very limited number of clinically significant V segments (eight) and C regions (two), making it possible to use specific primers for all known *TCR* γ V segments. It is important to note that clonality does not indicate malignancy, as suggested by one study in which 25% of tissue from patients with lichen planus, a benign dermatosis, were found to have *TCR* gene rearrangements using the PCR technique.[89]

In the late 1990s, a European consortium of 45 laboratories (BIOMED-2 Concerted Action BMH4-CT98-3936) was initiated with the aim of establishing a highly reliable standard in PCR-based clonality testing, for B-cell as well as for T-cell malignancies.[90] Because of the higher speed, efficiency, and sensitivity of the BIOMED-2 multiplex PCR protocol, it can reliably replace Southern blot analysis in clonality diagnostics in routine laboratory settings.[91] Expertise with clonality diagnostics and knowledge about the biology of *TCR* gene recombination are essential for correct interpretation of *TCR* clonality data. Patel and colleagues showed that combining *TCR*-γ primers with *TCR*-β primers significantly improved the sensitivity of *TCR* gene analysis, to 94%.[92] Yang et al used the strategy of multiple PCR/heteroduplex analysis for *TCR*-γ gene rearrangement combined with a laser-capture microdissection–proteinase K approach to increase the detection rate of clonal *TCR*-γ gene rearrangement in early MF cases.[93] This approach could provide strong evidence to confirm the diagnosis of early MF when the diagnosis can be most challenging.

Recently, with the technologic advancements, high-throughput sequencing of the TCR has also been utilized to aid in diagnosis of CTCL as well as monitoring for minimal residual disease (MRD).[94,95]

EPIDEMIOLOGY

The incidence of the primary CTCLs has risen dramatically and consistently since 1973.[96] Based on data from the Surveillance, Epidemiology, and End Results (SEER) Program of cancer registries, the incidence of CTCL in the United States increased from 3.0 (1973-1979) to 4.7 (1980-1989), to 5.3 (1990-1999), to 5.9 (2000-2009) per one million person-years.[97] The most recent SEER data analysis from 2010 to 2016 by Kaufman et al demonstrates an incidence of 5.8 per one million person-years.[97] Because the number of patients with early-stage MF often is not reported to tumor registries, the actual incidence may be higher. In one study, missed cases were estimated to constitute 17% of MF.[98] The incidence of MF increases with advancing age, with median age usually between 60 and 70 years.[96,99]

In a review of cutaneous lymphoma incidence patterns between 2001 and 2005, Bradford et al found that patients who self-identified as black/African American or non-Hispanic white had the highest incidence rates (11.5/1,000,000 person-years), compared with Hispanic white (7.9/1,000,000 person-years), and Asian/Pacific-Islander (7.1/1,000,000 person-years).[99] In a review of SEER data from the 1970s to 2010s, Kaufman et al found that there was a decrease in the percentage of patients of European ancestry with light skin (79% vs 60%, respectively) and a concurrent increase in the percentage of patients of Hispanic ancestry (4% vs 11%, respectively).[97] The percentage of patients of African ancestry with dark skin remained stable (13% vs 15%). Men are more likely to develop CTCL; however, the ratio of male to female has decreased over time from 1.9 in the 1970s to 1.4 after 1990.[97,99] The epidemiologic study by Criscione and Weinstock found the incidence rates of CTCL to be correlated with high physician density, high family income, high percentage of population with a bachelor's degree or higher, and high home values, suggesting that socioeconomic factors and increased detection of CTCL may play a role in the increased incidence rates since 1973.[96]

MF is rare in patients <30 years of age. However, in the 1990s there emerged several reports of children and adolescents affected with MF and SS.[100] Recent epidemiologic studies showed about 1% to 2% of cases of CTCL to be in the <20 years age group.[96,101] A study from the International Childhood Registry of Cutaneous Lymphoma found the mean age of onset and diagnosis of pediatric cutaneous lymphoma to be 7.5 years (±3.8 years) and 9.9 years (±3.4 years), respectively.[102] In the United States, pediatric MF is rare with an incidence of 0.5 per 1,000,000 person-years before 20 years of age and 1.2 per 1,000,000 person-years for 20 to 29 years of age.[103] The prevalence of pediatric MF compared with adult-reported cases varies geographically with pediatric MF composing 4% to 5% of total MF cases in the United States, 16.6% of total MF cases in Kuwait, and 11% of total MF cases in Singapore.[104-107] As in adults, pediatric MF is more prevalent in populations of color. In those under 30 years of age, MF has the highest prevalence in individuals of Asian, Pacific Islander, or African descent.[96,103]

The etiology of MF/SS remains unknown, but genetic, environmental, and infectious agents have been implicated as possible factors in triggering lymphocyte activation and/or lymphocyte transformation. One study found that not only did the antioxidative effects of wine consumption fail to protect against the development of MF but also patients who consume >24 g of alcohol daily demonstrated a higher incidence of MF than matched controls regardless of beverage type (adjusted odds ratio [OR] 3.02, 95% confidence interval [CI] 1.34-6.79).[108] Tobacco use has also been evaluated, and although mostly inconclusive, more recently, it was shown that people with a greater than 40-year history of cigarette smoking have a significant increase in risk of developing CTCL.[109]

Despite the rarity of MF, there have been geographic clusters reported of patients with MF in Sweden,[110] the United States (Texas,[111] Pennsylvania[112]), and Canada.[113] These groupings may suggest contributing and cumulative environmental exposures.[114] In fact, the study in Canada found CTCL clustering in heavy industrial areas, with relative sparing in areas of limited industrial presence.[113] Early reports implicated an increased risk of developing CTCL in people employed in a manufacturing occupation, particularly those related to petrochemicals, textiles, or metals, or in farming, with exposure to pesticides or herbicides.[115] Although two case-control studies failed to confirm these observations, a 2014 study again demonstrated the highest risk of CTCL was in general carpenters (OR 4.07) and painters (OR 3.71), with vegetable/crop farmers and wood workers also having increased risk. The authors suggested that a potential increase in exposure to halogenated hydrocarbon-containing solvents and pesticides led to the increase of CTCL in these populations.[109,116,117] Results of other studies have suggested that patients with MF have increased contact allergies, but Whittemore et al were unable to substantiate the association in a case-control clinical study.[117] Cumulatively, while data suggest that exposure to chemicals (including pesticides), air pollution, and certain detergents may increase the risk of MF, SS, and NHL development, further investigation is required.[118,119]

Exploration of familial clusters, in addition to geographic clusters, offers insight into the combination of environmental and genetic exposures. In addition to multiple cases involving first-degree relatives that were reported,[115,120-122] Hodak et al reported a cluster of 6 Jewish families (12 patients with MF total).[123] Human leukocyte antigen (HLA) analysis of the families revealed no specific haplotype, HLA class I antigen, or HLA-DR allele predominant. However, the DQB1*03 allele was found to be significantly increased compared with control. In this cohort, 2 of 12 patients were pediatric (<18 years). In addition, a case report was published on two pediatric siblings (14, 10 years), diagnosed with MF.[124] These reports suggest that there may be a genetic predisposition or susceptibility for developing MF in some families.

Human retroviruses have been suggested as possible etiologic agents in CTCL. Human T-cell lymphotropic virus (HTLV)-I was described initially in a patient with CTCL who had an aggressive clinical course; however, this disease was later identified as adult T-cell leukemia/lymphoma (ATL), which is endemic to Japan, the Caribbean, and other areas of the world but can have cutaneous lesions similar to CTCL (see ATL in Chapter 90).[125] Serologic findings for HTLV-I/II in patients with CTCL are negative in the vast majority of patients.[126-128] Seven series found no proviral HTLV-I sequences in 332 patients with CTCL,[127,129-133] and four studies detected the proviral sequences in 10% of 176 patients.[134-137] Recent molecular biology studies have found critical differences between HTLV-1$^+$ leukemia cell and SS/leukemic MF cell behavior.[138] There have been studies evaluating for the presence of human herpesvirus-8 and the polyoma Merkel cell virus, but neither of these infectious agents have been significantly identified.[139,140] More recent efforts have identified low levels of polyoma Merkel cell virus in folliculotropic MF (FMF; 89%, $n = 9$), but it is not clear what role the virus actually plays.[141] A separate group evaluated MF skin samples for the presence of multiple infectious agents (HTLV, Epstein-Barr virus [EBV], and *Borrelia burgdorferi*) and found that 21 of 83 MF samples had 2 or more infectious agents identified as compared with 1 of 83 healthy controls.[142] EBV-associated conditions such as extranodal NK/T-cell lymphoma, nasal type, and chronic active EBV infection are conditions recognized as CTCL entities via the WHO-EORTC 2018 classification and will be discussed in detail in the chapter.

CLINICAL PRESENTATION

MF usually evolves over a long period, so patients often have a long premycotic or premalignant phase with eczematous skin eruptions between 4 and 10 years before a histologic diagnosis is established.[143] The differential diagnosis during this period includes chronic eczematous dermatitis, atopic dermatitis, or contact dermatitis, which may evolve slowly into eruptions clinically suggestive of benign papulosquamous skin diseases such as eczema or psoriasis or less commonly parapsoriasis en plaque, poikiloderma atrophicans vasculare, or others.[144] Failure of the lesions to respond to standard topical therapy may be an early clue of a different diagnosis. However, initial lesions occasionally appear to improve following topical steroid application, which masks early recognition of the underlying malignancy. Because of the difficulty in diagnosis in the premycotic phase of MF, careful follow-up with serial skin biopsies is warranted in patients with suspect lesions (see "Diagnostic Evaluation").[145]

The earliest diagnostic phase of MF is the patch phase, characterized by persistent scaly macules and patches that vary in size, shape, and color; tend to involve sun-protected sites; and are occasionally associated with pruritus (*Figure 94.4A*).[5,144,146] Early MF patches and plaques, unlike other eczematous eruptions, are usually asymptomatic. Other, less common early skin findings in MF include poikiloderma,[147] hypopigmentation,[148] hyperpigmentation (*Figure 94.4B*), alopecia, pruritus alone,[149-151] dermatomal,[152] pityriasis lichenoides-like lesions,[153,154] purpura,[155] and porokeratosis-like lesions.[156] Several cases of "invisible MF" have been described. Afflicted patients present only with persistent, generalized pruritus and no clinical eruption.[149-151] Random biopsies of "normal" skin confirmed the diagnosis of MF.

Plaques are sharply demarcated, scaly, elevated lesions that may have annular, arcuate, or serpiginous borders (*Figure 94.4C*). Plaques with thick scale can mimic psoriasis or nummular eczema, whereas annular lesions with central clearing may be confused with tinea corporis.[144] Ultraviolet radiation occasionally induces regression of patches and plaques, further delaying correct diagnosis. Prominent involvement of the palms and/or soles may result in hyperkeratosis, fissuring, or frank keratoderma (*Figure 94.4D*).[157]

The tumor phase is heralded by the onset of dome-shaped, deep red to violaceous nodules emerging in areas of uninvolved skin or in preexisting plaques.[158] The tumors may ulcerate and become secondarily infected (*Figure 94.4E*), and there is a predilection for the body folds and face, where dermal thickening, coalescing plaques, and tumors may result in characteristic "leonine facies" (*Figure 94.4F*). The tumor stage is more clinically aggressive than the patch and plaque stages and may be associated with histologic transformation to a large cell process with a vertical growth phase (see "Histopathology" and "Prognosis").[158] Rarely, patients with MF will present initially with tumors without the preceding patch and plaque phases (the MF d'emblée variant).[6,159] It is very common for more advanced patients to have patches, plaques, and/or tumors present simultaneously on different areas of their skin.[143]

Generalized erythroderma may develop as the initial presenting sign of MF/SS or may accompany plaques and tumors.[143] In SS, the leukemic variant of CTCL, erythroderma and circulating tumor cells (Sézary cells) in the peripheral blood may be accompanied by generalized lymphadenopathy, splenomegaly, keratoderma, vitiligo-like hypopigmented patches,[160] alopecia, ectropion, nail dystrophy,[161] and ankle edema.[162] The first cutaneous sign of SS is usually a nonspecific dermatitis leading to a mean diagnostic delay of about 4 years.[163] Intense pruritus and cutaneous pain are common in SS, and when the palms and soles are affected with scaling and fissuring, walking and manual dexterity become difficult.[162]

CLASSIFICATION OF CUTANEOUS T-CELL LYMPHOMAS

The term cutaneous T-cell lymphoma (CTCL) is a general term that encompasses a variety of diseases, including MF and SS. In addition, there are other cutaneous T-cell LPDs that appear to be specific entities with unique clinical, histologic, and prognostic features. In an effort to recognize the separate disease processes, the World Health Organization (WHO) and the European Organisation for Research and Treatment of Cancer (EORTC) jointly formulated a new classification of primary cutaneous lymphomas in 2005, with modifications in 2018 mirroring the original system, save for minor revisions.[164-166] The 2018 fourth edition WHO classification of Skin Tumors monograph incorporated the definitions and terminology of the most recent 2017 WHO classification of tumors of hematopoietic and lymphoid tissue with a few exceptions and modifications (*Table 94.1*).[165,167,168] MF is the most common subtype, accounting for almost 60% of all CTCL,[166] and this term should be used only for patients with the classic presentation of patches and plaques with slow progression as described by Alibert and Bazin. The following sections will focus on the histopathology and immunopathology of MF, SS, and the other types of primary CTCLs.

DIAGNOSTIC EVALUATION

Tissue Handling

Skin biopsies for diagnosis of MF/SS must be properly handled to maximize the diagnostic information obtained. These studies include routine histology, immunophenotyping, and molecular genotyping. Communication between the clinical staff, dermatologists, and pathologists is essential to ensure that the appropriate types of biopsies are done and are properly handled. In general, 6-mm punch skin biopsies are recommended. Multiple biopsies from different skin lesions may be necessary to establish a definitive diagnosis of MF/SS, particularly in early-patch-stage lesions. Topical steroids may blunt many of the histologic features of MF/SS and should be discontinued for 2 to 3 weeks prior to biopsy. A careful drug history should be taken prior to biopsy, because certain drug eruptions can closely mimic early MF, particularly phenytoin and other anticonvulsants.[169] Although advancements in immunohistochemical protocols and molecular diagnostics allow most studies to be performed on formalin-fixed paraffin-embedded tissue, skin biopsies for possible CTCL may be sent to the pathology or dermatopathology laboratory fresh, on saline-soaked gauze or in tissue culture media such as RPMI. These biopsies can then be divided for the various diagnostic studies. Punch biopsies can be divided into halves, one half for routine histology and the other half for immunophenotyping (flow cytometry) and/or molecular diagnostic studies. Sections for routine histology should be fixed in a good

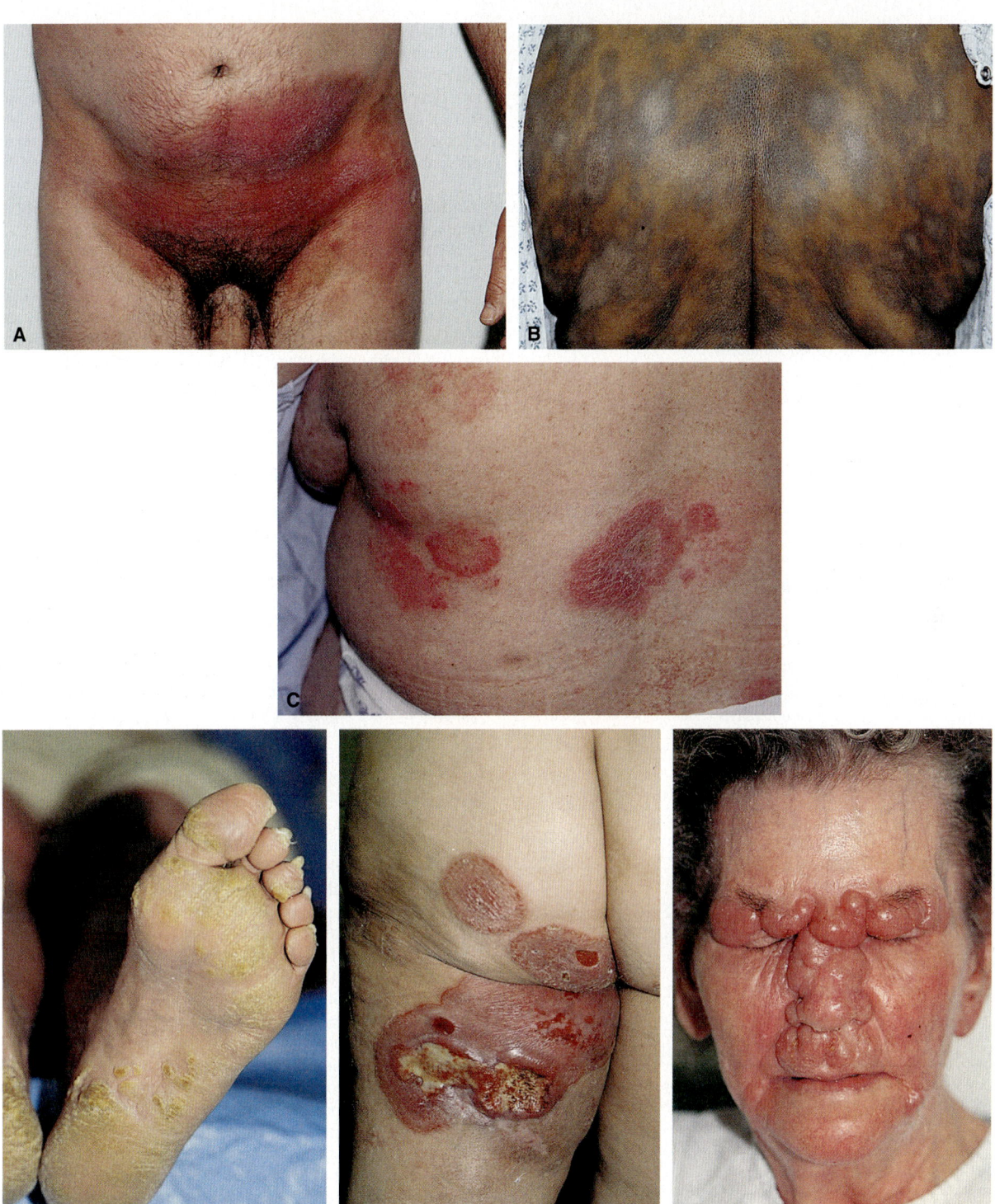

FIGURE 94.4 A–F, The cutaneous phases of mycosis fungoides. A, Early patch-stage lesions in a sun-protected region. B, Hyperpigmented diffuse patches on the back of a dark-skinned patient. C, Scattered thin and thick plaques on the back. D, Early keratoderma of the sole. E, Ulcerated tumor within a plaque on the posterior leg. F, Coalescing nodules and tumors with dermal thickening forming "leonine facies" in this patient with transformed cutaneous T-cell lymphoma. See text for full description.

nuclear fixative, such as B-Plus, to facilitate evaluation of nuclear morphology and recognition of the characteristic complex nuclear folding yielding cerebriform cells. If the biopsy is sufficiently cellular, flow cytometry can be performed allowing for simultaneous assessment of multiple antigens. The tissue for flow cytometry should be promptly delivered to the appropriate laboratory in cell culture media. Lymph nodes should be worked up as previously described.[170]

Histopathology
Cutaneous Features of MF/SS

In general, the histologic diagnosis of MF/SS in skin biopsies is based on criteria similar to those used for the diagnosis of other lymphoid neoplasms, including the presence of an infiltrative or destructive growth pattern and cytologic atypia. The distribution of the infiltrate

Table 94.1. Survival for Subtypes of Cutaneous Lymphoma

WHO-EORTC Classification of Cutaneous Lymphoma	5-Year Disease Specific Survival
Cutaneous T-cell Lymphomas	
Mycosis fungoides	88%
MF variants:	
Folliculotropic mycosis fungoides	75%
Pagetoid reticulosis	100%
Granulomatous slack skin	100%
Sézary syndrome	36%
Primary cutaneous CD30+ lymphoproliferative disorders	
Lymphomatoid papulosis	99%
Primary cutaneous anaplastic large cell lymphoma	95%
Subcutaneous panniculitis-like T-cell lymphoma	87%
Chronic active EBV infection *includes hydroa vacciniforme-like LPD	NDA
Primary cutaneous γδ T-cell lymphoma	11%
Primary cutaneous peripheral T-cell lymphoma, NOS	15%
Provisional entities	
Primary cutaneous CD8+ aggressive epidermotropic cytotoxic T-cell lymphoma	31%
Primary cutaneous CD4+ small/medium-sized pleomorphic T-cell lymphoproliferative disorder	100%
Primary cutaneous acral CD8+ T-cell lymphoma	100%
Adult T-cell leukemia/lymphoma[a]	NDA
Extranodal NK/T-cell lymphoma, nasal type[a]	16%
Cutaneous B-cell Lymphomas	
Primary cutaneous marginal zone lymphoma	99%
Primary cutaneous follicle center lymphoma	95%
Primary cutaneous diffuse large B-cell lymphoma, leg type	56%
Intravascular large B-cell lymphoma[a]	72%
Provisional entities:	
EBV+ mucocutaneous ulcer	100%

Abbreviations: EORTC, European Organization for Research and Treatment of Cancer; MF, mycosis fungoides; NDA, no data available; NOS, not otherwise specified; WHO, World Health Organization.
[a]Typically, an extracutaneous lymphoma with skin as a secondary site.
Adapted from Willemze R, Cerroni L, Kempf W, et al. The 2018 update of the WHO-EORTC classification for primary cutaneous lymphomas. *Blood.* 2019;133(16):1703-1714. Copyright © 2019 American Society of Hematology. With permission.

lesions by Massone et al, the histologic features most helpful for diagnosing MF were (a) epidermotropism, particularly with a basilar lymphocytosis (23%) or with "haloed" lymphocytes (40%); (b) a dermal lymphocytic infiltrate that is bandlike (30%) or patchy-lichenoid (66%); and (c) interface dermatitis (59%).[172] Large convoluted lymphocytes in the epidermis were found only in 9% of cases, and Pautrier microabscesses were found in 19%. The authors noted that, although these cytologic changes are highly specific, the architectural abnormalities (pattern of infiltrate, epidermotropism) were more sensitive in diagnosing MF.

Spongiosis should be minimal in relationship to epidermotropism in MF and SS. Biopsies with prominent spongiosis must be differentiated from eczematous or spongiotic dermatitis. Microvesiculation and Langerhans cell microabscesses are rarely present in MF/SS and would point toward a spongiotic process. Eosinophils and plasma cells are rarely present in early-patch-stage MF but are more common in plaque- and tumor-stage disease. Caution is advised, however, as spongiotic variants of MF have been described.[173] The presence of mild spongiosis should not exclude a diagnosis of MF if other classic features are present.[174]

It is important to understand that a definitive diagnosis of MF may not be possible in some early-patch-stage lesions. Multiple biopsies of separate skin lesions, immunophenotyping, and clonality studies may help confirm the diagnosis in difficult cases. Even these ancillary studies may be inconclusive in early lesions. The reported range of sensitivity of T-cell clonality detection is large, with some studies reporting as few as 20% of early-patch-stage lesions being clonal[175] to as many as 71%.[176] Likely, this variability reflects variability in density of infiltrate in early lesions, variability in source material for DNA extraction (frozen vs paraffin), and variability of the clonality assay (Southern blot vs PCR vs denaturing gel electrophoresis vs capillary electrophoresis). Newer detection methods, such as high-throughput TCR sequencing, are improving the ability to detect clonality even in the earliest disease.[95] In later plaque- and tumor-stage lesions, T-cell clonality can typically be detected in >90% of cases.[176,177] Several techniques have been advocated, such as comparing clonality studies from disparate clinical lesions and using complementary clonality studies (*TCR ß* and *TCR γ*), that may increase the specificity and sensitivity of the molecular studies.[178,179] Despite these advancements, however, a lack of demonstrated clonality in a histologically or clinically suspicious lesion should not prevent a diagnosis of CTCL. Likewise, the presence of a clonal population does not equate with malignancy as many benign dermatoses may demonstrate clonality.[180]

Tumor-stage MF is characterized histologically by a dense dermal infiltrate involving the papillary and reticular dermis, often with extension into the subcutis. In contrast to patch- and plaque-stage lesions, MF tumors often lack epidermotropism. Furthermore, the malignant T cells in tumor-stage MF often display various degrees of histologic transformation. The diagnosis of malignancy in the tumor stage is rarely in question, but recognition of MF origin for tumors with large cell transformation may be obscured by their resemblance to other NHLs. A careful search for dysplastic cerebriform T cells and residual foci of epidermal infiltration near the edges of tumors often provides histologic evidence of MF origin in difficult cases.[181] Previous or concurrent biopsies of earlier-stage MF lesions may also help confirm the diagnosis in these cases.

Generalized exfoliative erythroderma is characteristic of SS, but it may also occur in MF. Cutaneous biopsies of erythroderma in MF/SS often lack many of the hallmark features found in patch/plaque MF, as they generally demonstrate spongiosis and often lack epidermotropism. In fact, in one study, up to 17% of skin biopsies of patients with established SS were considered nondiagnostic because of insufficient epidermotropism.[182] Evaluation of the peripheral blood for circulating tumor cells and/or molecular analysis of the skin and peripheral blood for a clonal rearrangement of the TCR may help establish the diagnosis of MF/SS in cases for which skin biopsies are histologically suspicious but nondiagnostic. In addition, the finding of identical clonal populations in the skin and peripheral blood is very supportive of a lymphoma diagnosis.[183] Finally, immunohistochemical stains can be helpful, as the presence of PD-1, CD7, Ki-67, and TOX staining and a

within the skin biopsy is also important (Figure 94.5A). The characteristic atypical lymphocytes in MF and SS are intermediate-sized dysplastic cerebriform T cells with enlarged hyperchromatic nuclei. Demonstration of cerebriform nuclear folding requires good fixation (such as B5 fixation), thin (4-μm) sections, and examination under 100× oil immersion. Diagnostic criteria for cutaneous involvement by MF are best illustrated in plaque-stage lesions (Figure 94.5B and C). The essential criteria for diagnosis are (a) a bandlike lymphocytic infiltrate in the superficial papillary dermis, (b) epidermotropism, and (c) atypical intermediate-sized cerebriform T cells in the dermal and epidermal infiltrates.[171] Pautrier microabscesses (Figure 94.5D) are characteristic of MF but are often absent in early-patch-stage lesions, erythroderma, and tumors. Diagnosing early-patch-stage lesions is often difficult. In a morphologic study of >700 early-patch-stage

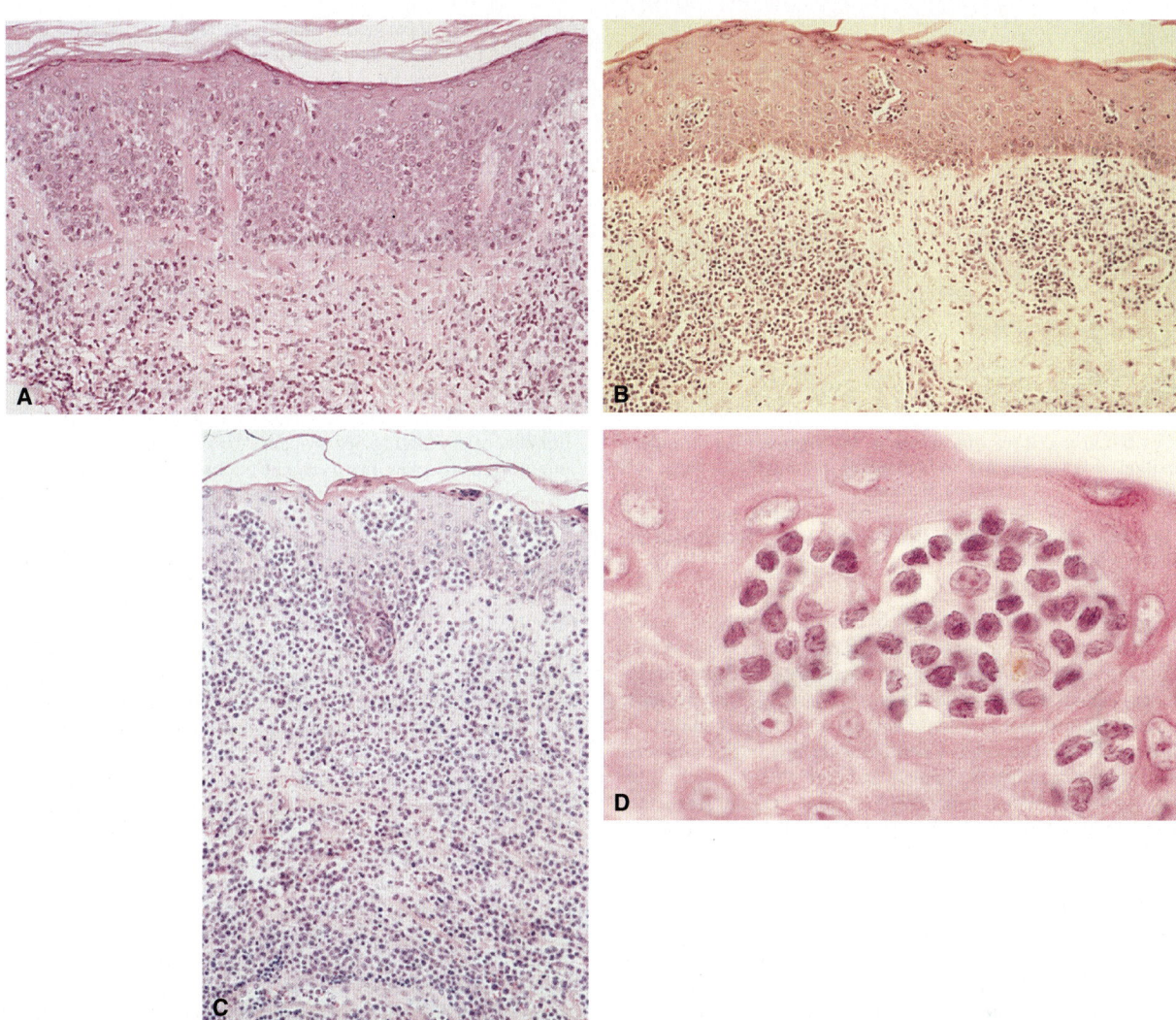

FIGURE 94.5 A, MF, patch stage. A band-like lymphocytic infiltrate occupies the superficial papillary dermis with single cell epidermotropism by atypical, "haloed" cerebriform T cells, preferentially involving the basal layer (H&E, ×50). B, MF, plaque stage. A band-like lymphocytic infiltrate occupies the papillary dermis with epidermotropism by atypical cerebriform T cells, focally forming small Pautrier microabscesses (H&E, ×25). C, MF, thick plaque. A dense band-like lymphocytic infiltrate fills the papillary dermis and extends into the reticular dermis. Prominent epidermotropism by atypical, enlarged cerebriform T cells creates large Pautrier microabscesses (H&E, ×25). D, MF, Pautrier microabscess. High magnification of a Pautrier microabscess shows characteristic small to medium cerebriform T cells with highly convoluted nuclear folding. The Pautrier microabscess recapitulates normal interactions between components of the skin-associated lymphoid tissue, that is, cutaneous T cells, Langerhans' histiocytes (2 cells with large pale nuclei in the center), and keratinocytes (H&E, ×500). H&E, hematoxylin and eosin; MF, mycosis fungoides.

decreased numbers of CD8+ cells have been shown to support a diagnosis of SS over benign erythroderma.[184-186]

Large Cell Transformation of MF/SS

Approximately 20% of low-grade MF and SS undergo secondary transformation to high-grade LCL with a predominance (>25%) of large (>4 times the size of a small lymphocyte) transformed lymphocytes (*Figure 94.6*).[181] The transformed lymphocytes can be CD30+ or CD30−. Cutaneous LCT usually occurs in tumor-stage lesions, but it can occasionally be seen in plaques or erythrodermic MF. Lymph nodes are the most common site of extracutaneous LCT, but it may also occur in other extracutaneous sites. In patients with MF with LCT the absence of CD30 expression has been associated with a reduced disease-specific survival (DSS).[187] MF/SS with LCT must be distinguished from primary cutaneous ALCL (PCALCL), lymphomatoid papulosis (LyP), and secondary cutaneous involvement by systemic ALCL because of prognostic differences.[188] This is particularly true with CD30-expressing transformed MF/SS, which has a poor prognosis, in contrast to PCALCL and LyP, both of which have a favorable prognosis.[189,190] Absence of perforin expression, a dermal infiltrate comprising less than 75% large cells, and the presence of folliculotropism all favor MF with LCT over PCALCL.[191] Unfortunately, differentiating these entities is often impossible on histologic grounds alone and requires close collaboration between the clinician and pathologist.

Extracutaneous MF/SS

Extracutaneous dissemination is a late occurrence in MF/SS because the disease is clinically limited to the skin for prolonged periods of time in most patients. There is evidence that nodal involvement as detected with highly sensitive molecular techniques can segregate otherwise low-stage patients into high-risk and low-risk groups[192]; however, assessment of regional lymph nodes is not standard practice in patients with early-stage MF. Although autopsy studies have histologically documented widespread extracutaneous disease in most patients,[193] most series were performed several decades ago, when detection of early disease was difficult.

Extracutaneous MF/SS has morphologic features that are usually similar to those seen in the skin. Dysplastic cerebriform T cells are the most helpful diagnostic feature for recognition as extracutaneous disease. Almost every organ has been involved by MF/SS in autopsy series, but the

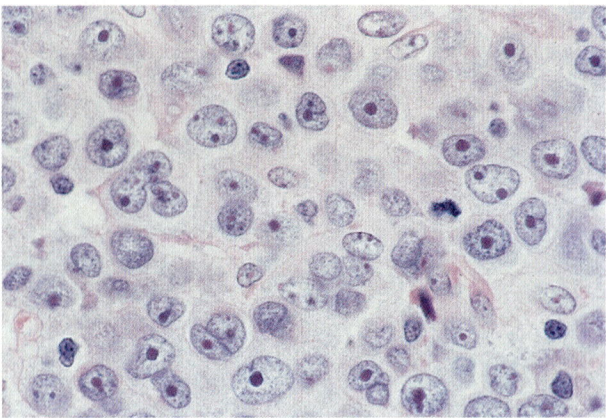

FIGURE 94.6 **Large cell transformation of MF representing secondary transformation of low-grade MF to high-grade immunoblastic large cell lymphoma.** This tumor is composed of sheets of large transformed cells or immunoblasts with round to oval nuclei, dispersed chromatin, and prominent nucleoli. Several mitoses are present (H&E, ×500). H&E, hematoxylin and eosin; MF, mycosis fungoides.

most frequent sites are the lymph nodes, liver, spleen, and lungs, which may be involved in >50% of more advanced cases.[193] Other less common sites include kidney, bone marrow, thyroid, heart, pancreas, gastrointestinal tract, and central nervous system. Lymph nodes represent the most frequent site of extracutaneous disease in pathologic staging studies.[194] Extracutaneous CTCL, particularly visceral disease, is strongly associated with advanced-stage skin disease (tumors and erythroderma) and SS.[195] Because tumor-stage MF and generalized erythroderma are frequently nonepidermotropic, it has been suggested that loss of epidermotropism may play an important role in systemic dissemination.

Lymph Node Pathology

With up to 50% of staging lymph node biopsies being microscopically involved by MF/SS, lymph nodes are the earliest and most common site of extracutaneous dissemination.[194] The International Society for Cutaneous Lymphomas (ISCL), the United States Cutaneous Lymphoma Consortium (USCLC), and the Cutaneous Lymphoma Task Force of the European Organization for the Research and Treatment of Cancer (EORTC) have proposed updated staging guidelines and recommend biopsy of lymph nodes if they are >1.5 cm in the longest diameter confirmed by imaging, especially if accompanied by other features of concern (firm, rubbery, and/or fixed).[196] Nodal involvement is typically staged using the ISCL/EORTC staging system that is based on the National Cancer Institute Veterans Affairs (NCI-VA) guidelines (Table 94.2). N1 nodes in the ISCL/EORTC staging system show either LN1 (rare single atypical cells in paracortical area) or LN2 (LN1 with some small clusters with fewer than 10 cells per cluster and dermatopathic change) morphology. LN3 (LN2 with increased paracortical clusters containing at least 10 and often >15 atypical cells per cluster) do not show nodal effacement and are classified as N2 stage in the ISCL/EORTC staging system. Lymph nodes with effacement of nodal architecture by atypical cells or large immunoblastic cells are NCI-VA classification system LN4 and ISCL/EORTC stage N2. As lymph nodes become progressively infiltrated, the cerebriform T cells tend to become larger and more pleomorphic, with increased numbers of large transformed cells.[197] Over 35% of positive nodes will show complete large cell transformation with pleomorphic, immunoblastic, or anaplastic large cell morphology.[181,197,198] In contrast to MF, lymph nodes from patients with SS tend to be effaced by more monomorphic infiltrates of small to medium cerebriform T cells[199] and may also undergo large cell transformation in some cases.[181,200]

Bone Marrow Involvement

The bone marrow in MF and SS is generally thought to be spared until late in the course of the disease, including in patients with large numbers of circulating Sézary cells.[143,201] Early studies suggested that antemortem marrow involvement occurred in <3% of patients with MF/SS,[201] yet the marrow was involved in nearly 50% of patients at autopsy in several series from the 1970s.[193,202] Marrow involvement typically manifests as nonparatrabecular lymphoid aggregates with cerebriform lymphocytes. Molecular studies have shown that, in patients with a defined clonal T-cell rearrangement in the skin, approximately 20% will have an identical T-cell clone detected in their blood or bone marrow. Moreover, all patients with bone marrow involvement by molecular studies had blood involvement as well, but only 76% of patients with blood involvement had bone marrow involvement.[203] This suggests that marrow examination should not be performed with a confirmed circulating clone or evidence of marrow dysfunction. Sibaud et al were unable to demonstrate that bone marrow involvement was associated with a worse prognosis in a multivariate analysis of their data; however, blood involvement was an independent variable for disease progression. In patients with SS, subtle small interstitial clusters of Sézary cells have been identified in up to 90% of cases, suggesting that most patients with circulating Sézary cells have early systemic dissemination of disease.[195] Detection of these subtle interstitial infiltrates of Sézary cells requires careful examination under oil immersion (100×) to identify the cells with abnormal cerebriform nuclear folds. Identification can be facilitated with immunoperoxidase studies for T-cell markers such as CD3, CD4, and CD7. Flow cytometry using a broad array of T-cell markers including CD3, CD4, CD8, CD7, and CD26 is also useful for detecting marrow involvement.

Other Extracutaneous Sites

Splenic and hepatic involvement by MF and SS is common and can be staged using imaging criteria rather than by invasive methods.[204] Liver involvement in initial staging procedures has been found in 8% to 16% of cases.[194] Disseminated MF and SS tends to form nodular infiltrates of atypical cerebriform T cells within the portal tracts or hepatic lobules. Cerebriform T cells within the hepatic sinusoids without formation of focal aggregates are not considered diagnostic of liver involvement in the presence of peripheral blood involvement. Splenic infiltration was documented in 31% of staging laparotomies in one series.[205] The atypical cerebriform T cells usually infiltrate the red pulp diffusely, but they may home to the periarteriolar lymphocyte sheath.[202] Splenic rupture has been reported in a rare case with massive splenic involvement by CTCL.[206]

All other suspected sites of visceral involvement should be confirmed by biopsy if possible. Antemortem pulmonary manifestations of MF and SS are generally uncommon but may occasionally present clinically as interstitial or nodular pulmonary infiltrates.[207] However, the lungs are frequently involved by MF/SS at autopsy.[193] Infiltrates of atypical cerebriform T cells usually spread along the alveolar septae with preservation of the alveolar architecture. In some cases, the infiltrates may also fill alveolar spaces.

Blood Involvement

The ISCL defined three stages of blood involvement for MF/SS.[208] Patients with B2 peripheral blood involvement have >1000 Sézary

Table 94.2. NCI-VA Grading Scheme for Lymph Node Histology in CTCL

Grade	Histopathologic Features
LN-1	DL with occasional CTC
LN-2	DL with CTC singly or in small clusters (<6 cells)
LN-3	DL with numerous CTC, singly or in large clusters (>15 cells)
LN-4	Partial or complete effacement by MF/SS ± DL

Abbreviations: CTC, cerebriform T cells; DL, dermatopathic lymphadenopathy; LN, lymph node; MF, mycosis fungoides; NCI, National Cancer Institute; SS, Sézary syndrome; VA, Veterans Affairs.
Modified from: Sausville EA, Eddy JL, Makuch RW, et al. Histopathologic staging at initial diagnosis of mycosis fungoides and the Sézary syndrome. Definition of three distinctive prognostic groups. *Ann Intern Med*. 1988;109:372-382.

cells/mm³, where the Sézary cells are distinguished by their large nuclear size (>15 µm) and high nuclear contour index (Figure 94.7).[209] All B2-stage blood samples require evidence of clonality by PCR or Southern blot analysis of the TCR gene.[208] In one study, increased large Sézary cells correlated significantly with poorer survival.[210] However, size criteria alone would fail to recognize the small Sézary cell variant, which is similar in size to a normal resting lymphocyte. Because of the inherent difficulties in diagnosing peripheral blood involvement by MF/SS on peripheral smear review, additional technologies are used including flow cytometry and molecular studies such as PCR. The ISCL considered a positive clonal TCR rearrangement in the blood coupled with either a CD4 to CD8 ratio >10:1 in the presence of >1000/µL of CD4⁺ or CD3⁺ cells or an elevated CD4 count and abnormal immunophenotype by flow cytometry (>40% lymphocytes CD4⁺CD7⁻ or >30% lymphocytes CD4⁺CD26⁻) as adequate evidence to constitute a positive peripheral blood for B2 staging purposes.[208]

Blood staging by ISCL/EORTC criteria also requires assessment of clonality using either PCR or Southern blot analysis of the TCR gene. As noted earlier, all B2-stage patients must not only reach morphologic criteria of >1000 Sézary cells per microliter but also be shown to be clonal.[208] ISCL B0 is defined as no increase in Sézary cells (<5% of peripheral blood lymphocytes). B0 cases with molecular detection of T-cell clonality (B0b) have a worse prognosis than molecularly negative (B0a) cases even when the histologic criteria for blood involvement have not been met.[183,211,212] In fact, T-cell clonality in the peripheral blood even in the absence of increased lymphocytes by morphology or flow cytometry (B0b) conveys a worse OS, DSS, and risk of disease progression.[213]

In 2021 the ISCL, USCLC, and EORTC published modified staging guidelines for blood involvement.[196] The simplified guidelines use absolute abnormal circulating lymphocyte count to assess blood involvement.[214] Absolute counts should be determined by the percentage of aberrant lymphocytes (CD4⁺CD7⁻ or CD4⁺CD26⁻ or another aberrant lymphocyte population) identified by flow cytometry, multiplied by the total lymphocyte count of a complete blood count. Alternatively, the percentage of aberrant CD45⁺ leukocytes multiplied by the white blood count may be used.[196,214] B0 is defined as absolute count <250/µL; B1, absolute count 250 to <1000/µL; and B2, absolute count ≥1000/µL. In addition, each B stage is subdivided into substage A if T-cell clone is absent or equivocal and substage B if T-cell clone is present and identical to skin (e.g., B_{2A} or B_{2B}).

Recently, reliable detection of T-cell clonality by flow cytometry has been reported with the use of antibodies to T-cell receptor constant β chain-1 (TRBC1).[215-219] The α/β TCR rearranges one of two constant β genes in its formation. Abnormal ratios of TRBC1⁺ to TRBC1⁻ (a mimic for TRBC2) in T-cell populations imply clonality in a similar way to kappa and lambda light chain ratios in B-cell populations. This approach may be more cost-effective than PCR-based TCR gene rearrangement techniques.[219]

Immunophenotyping Studies

T-cell origin of the neoplastic cells in MF and SS is well established as a memory T cell that expresses CLA, the cutaneous lymphoid antigen homing receptor.[220] The vast majority are derived from T-helper cells that express CD4 and other T cell–associated antigens including CD2, CD3, CD5, CD45RO, and αβ TCRs (Figure 94.8).[221] Of the less common CD8⁺ CTCL, clinical presentation and behavior are crucial in distinguishing the more indolent CD8⁺ MF variant[222] from the more aggressive primary cutaneous aggressive epidermotropic CD8⁺-cytotoxic T-cell lymphoma (PC8TCL) described in the updated WHO-EORTC nomenclature as a provisional subtype of peripheral CTCL.[167] Activation-associated (HLA-DR, CD25, CD30, CD38) and proliferation-associated (CD71, Ki-67) antigens are also frequently expressed in MF/SS, particularly in advanced stages.[181]

Aberrant T-antigen expression is often seen in MF and SS, particularly advanced plaque- or tumor-stage lesions, and can be used to help differentiate reactive dermatitis from MF/SS.[223] Flow cytometry is used to assess antigen expression on the T cells present in circulation or, less commonly, directly from involved skin biopsies. Aberrant T-cell phenotypes are defined as diminished or absent expression of pan–T-cell antigens (CD2, CD3, or CD5), absent T-cell subset antigen expression (CD4⁻CD8⁻), or coexpression of T-cell subset antigens (CD4⁺CD8⁺). Diminished or absent CD7 expression is one of the most common aberrant T-cell phenotypes in tissue sections of MF and SS.[223] However, the isolated findings of loss of CD7 expression must be considered in the context of other clinical, histologic, and immunophenotypic findings in that expanded populations of CD7-negative T cells can also be seen in benign dermatoses.[221] Several studies have shown that the loss of CD26 (dipeptidyl-aminopeptidase IV) expression is a characteristic feature of circulating Sézary cells that is likely more sensitive than loss of CD7 expression.[224-226] Killer Ig-like receptor (KIR) 3DL2 expression in MF and SS has been discovered and may represent a new marker for diagnosis and a new target for therapy.[227,228] For histologic diagnosis of cutaneous lymphomas, immunohistochemistry can reliably differentiate between T-cell lymphomas, B-cell lymphomas, and Hodgkin lymphoma. The most widely used paraffin-reactive T-cell antibodies include CD2, CD3, CD4, CD5, CD7, CD8, CD30, CD43, CD45RO, PD-1, and βF1. Although immunohistochemistry for CD7 can be helpful in evaluating early MF biopsies, loss of CD7 can be seen in a wide variety of reactive, benign conditions requiring correlation with clinical, histologic, other immunophenotypic and molecular findings.[229,230] An elevated CD4 to CD8 ratio favors MF over benign inflammatory cutaneous disorders.[231] NK-cell or cytotoxic lymphocyte markers (CD56, granzyme

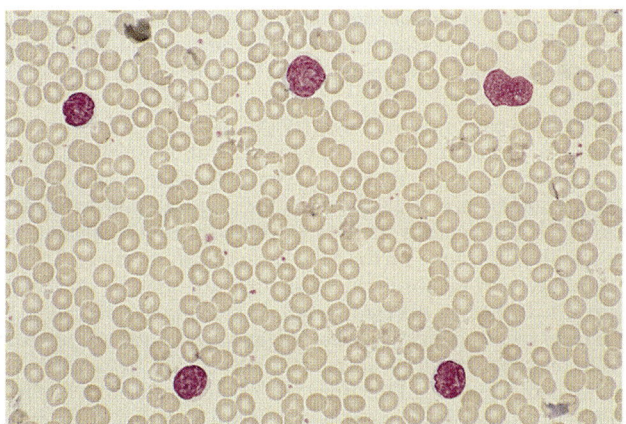

FIGURE 94.7 Sézary syndrome. The peripheral blood shows lymphocytosis. Most lymphocytes are Sézary cells with enlarged, highly convoluted nuclei and scant cytoplasm (H&E, ×250). H&E, hematoxylin and eosin.

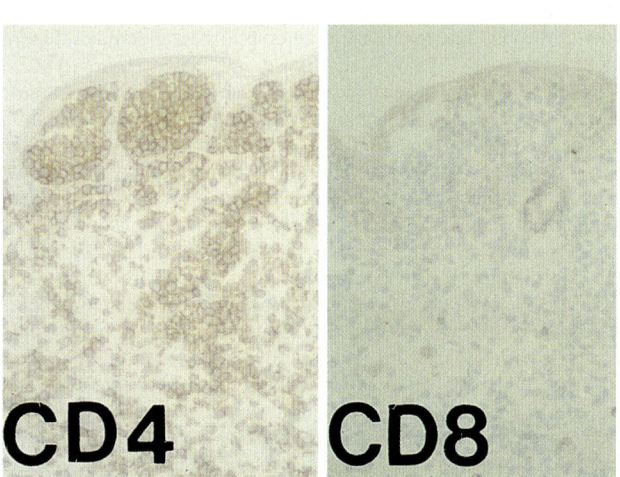

FIGURE 94.8 Frozen section immunohistochemistry of a cutaneous plaque in a patient with MF shows a marked predominance of CD4⁺ T-helper cells within Pautrier microabscesses and within the dermis. CD8 is essentially negative (diaminobenzidine-hematoxylin, ×50). MF, mycosis fungoides.

B, perforin, and T-cell intracellular antigen-1 [TIA-1]) can be used as well if non-MF NK/T cell lymphomas are in the differential. CD20, CD79a, CD5, CD10, BCL-6, BCL-2, κ, λ, MUM1, and CD138 are the most widely used B-cell paraffin-reactive antibodies. When used in panels, these antibodies allow subclassification of most cutaneous lymphomas when combined with clinical history and examination, which are vital to correct classification.

DIFFERENTIAL DIAGNOSIS

The clinicopathologic differential diagnosis for MF/SS includes several forms of benign dermatitis, other primary low-grade CTCLs, and secondary cutaneous involvement by disseminated lymphomas or leukemias. Differentiation of these mimickers from CTCL often requires careful correlation of clinical, histopathologic, immunophenotypic, and genotypic characteristics and may require multiple or serial biopsies. The following discussion describes methods to differentiate MF/SS from similar benign conditions, indolent CTCL, and other primary CTCLs.

To assist clinicians with the diagnosis of early MF, Pimpinelli et al proposed an algorithm using clinical, histopathologic, molecular biologic, and immunopathologic criteria in which a total of four points from any of the four categories was necessary to make the diagnosis of early MF.[146] The scoring system would allow, for example, a patient with persistent patches in non-sun-exposed areas with size/shape variation (2 points) and histologic findings of a superficial lymphocytic infiltrate, epidermotropism without spongiosis, and lymphocyte atypia (2 points) to meet criteria for early MF diagnosis without any immunostains or *TCR* gene rearrangement analysis of the skin tissue. Recently, the sensitivity 87.5% and specificity 60% of the algorithm were validated in a cohort of 34 cases.[232] Modifications have recently been suggested.[174]

Benign Conditions

Benign inflammatory skin lesions are most likely to be confused with early-patch-stage MF. In general, these conditions have clinical presentations and courses that are different from MF, lack enlarged atypical cerebriform T cells, and lack epidermotropism that is disproportionately increased in relationship to spongiosis. However, in difficult cases, immunophenotypic analysis and gene rearrangement studies may be necessary to look for aberrant T-cell phenotypes or clonal *TCR* gene rearrangements. The benign inflammatory dermatoses that most closely resemble CTCL include small plaque parapsoriasis and large plaque parapsoriasis (LPP), psoriasis vulgaris, poikiloderma vasculare atrophicans (PVA), pityriasis lichenoides, pigmented purpuric eruption, lichenoid keratosis, benign erythroderma, contact dermatitis, persistent arthropod bite reactions, drug eruptions, and actinic reticuloid (AR).[233,234]

Despite the name, the chronic skin diseases under the term parapsoriasis are unrelated to the much more common skin disease psoriasis.[235] Most dermatologists separate parapsoriasis into one of two types. The benign subtype is known as small plaque parapsoriasis, digitate dermatosis, or chronic superficial dermatitis. The other type is considered premalignant and is most often called large plaque parapsoriasis (LPP) or parapsoriasis en plaques (having in the past been called prereticulotic poikiloderma). LPP is clinically indistinguishable from patch-stage MF.[146] However, the patches of MF tend to be fixed, whereas the patches of LPP tend to wane in the summer and flare in the winter. Because of clinical and histologic overlap, some authorities consider LPP to be an early stage of MF.[236] Others consider LPP to be a latent form of MF because ~10% of patients eventually develop overt MF.[237] A retrospective review documented a higher rate of evolution to MF in 12 of 36 (33%) patients with LPP.[238] A recent Danish population-based registry study of 582 patients with parapsoriasis found a significant increased risk of subsequent cancers of all types and increased mortality (standardized incidence ratio, 1.3 [95% CI, 1.1-1.5]).[239]

In support of the close relationship of LPP and early MF is the demonstration of clonal *TCR* gene rearrangement in 50% of LPP biopsies.[240] Furthermore, demonstration of clonal *TCR* gene rearrangements in small plaque or digitate parapsoriasis has suggested that this may be an abortive form of MF.[241,242] Gug and Solovan reported the similarity between LPP and MF in terms of genetic copy number alterations is striking, emphasizing once again the difficulty of differentiating the two entities.[243] A recent study found TOX expression to be helpful in distinguishing MF from benign inflammatory dermatoses but not from LPP, suggesting an unappreciated role in the development of MF.[64]

Histologically, the lymphoid infiltrate of LPP is perivascular and epidermotropism is generally less than is seen in MF. The presence of Pautrier microabscesses would strongly argue against LPP in favor of MF. Furthermore, cytologically atypical cerebriform T cells with highly convoluted nuclei are inconspicuous or absent in LPP. However, immunophenotypic analysis is usually not helpful for differentiating LPP from patch-stage MF as both have a predominance of CD4+ helper cells with absent CD7.[244]

PVA can also present similarly to early MF, so much so, that most experts believe PVA to be a rare variant of MF,[245-248] whereas others separate PVA from poikilodermatous MF.[248-251] The macules and patches of PVA show the poikilodermatous features of hypopigmentation, hyperpigmentation, atrophy, and telangiectasias. PVA macules/patches tend to also be localized to sun-protected sites, most commonly appearing on the buttocks, breasts, and flexural areas. And, like LPP, some clinicians believe that PVA may potentially precede or coexist with MF. Histologically, PVA is characterized by an atrophic epidermis; chronic, ill-defined inflammatory changes; and dilated capillaries. Often, lymphoid cells form a bandlike pattern in the superficial dermis, with only rare epidermotropism.[245,246]

Pityriasis lichenoides is considered a spectrum of diseases including an acute and a chronic form: pityriasis lichenoides et varioliformis acuta (PLEVA) and pityriasis lichenoides chronica (PLC), respectively.[252] Many patients demonstrate lesions of both forms during their disease course. PLEVA, also known as Mucha-Habermann disease, is a benign cutaneous disorder characterized by recurrent, self-healing papulonecrotic lesions that may resemble LyP, which is discussed later.[253] PLC, which is a benign eruption with lymphocytic infiltrates of the skin, presents as a persistent, erythematous, papular eruption with scale.[254] PLC must be distinguished from pityriasis lichenoides–like MF.[153,255] Biopsies may show slightly atypical cerebriform T cells with some epidermotropism, but vacuolar degeneration of the epidermal basilar layer, necrotic keratinocytes, and dermal hemorrhage in PLEVA distinguish it from MF. The lymphoid infiltrate is composed predominantly of CD8+ cells as opposed to the typical CD4+ phenotype of MF.[256] The histology of PLC is similar to PLEVA, although the findings are muted with only focal basal vacuolar change and limited lymphocytic exocytosis. The intraepidermal lymphocytes tend to be CD4+, which further complicates the distinction from early MF. As in PLEVA, the lymphocytes lack significant cytologic atypia. Some consider pityriasis lichenoides to be a T-cell LPD or a form of indolent cutaneous T-cell dyscrasia related to LyP, and clonal *TCR* gene rearrangement has been demonstrated.[257-259] While cases of patients with pityriasis lichenoides progressing to MF have been described, this is definitely a rare event.[258,260-262]

Pigmented purpuric dermatoses (PPDs) are a group of chronic and benign skin disorders categorized by rupture of the small capillaries in the superficial papillary dermis. Clinically, patients present with petechiae and bronze discoloration of the skin on the lower extremities.[263,264] Histologically, there is a primarily chronic inflammation that may be superficial perivascular or lichenoid in nature. Dermal hemorrhage and hemosiderin deposition are present to varying degrees. Lymphocytic exocytosis may be present, whereas cytologic atypia and intraepidermal lymphocytic microabscesses are generally absent. Immunohistochemical and molecular studies are typically not helpful in differentiating PPD from MF.[155] Lichen aureus, a rare type of PPD, can mimic the purpuric variant of MF both clinically and histologically and progress to MF in very rare cases.[155,265] One study showed that, of 43 cases of PPD, 21 showed a clonal population of T cells. Only 40% of the cases with demonstrated clonality, however, had clinical and pathologic features consistent with MF. In addition, loss of CD7 was frequently observed in both the polyclonal and monoclonal groups.[266] Other studies have documented the frequent occurrence of T-cell clonality in cases of PPD that fail to develop disease typical of MF.[267] The presence of extensive PPD-like skin disease, especially when present outside of the lower extremities, should raise the suspicion of MF regardless of the histologic features.

Lymphomatoid keratosis is a benign epithelial skin neoplasm related to an inflamed seborrheic keratosis or lichenoid keratosis. Patients generally demonstrate one or a few scattered small hyperkeratotic plaques on the trunk and are biopsied to rule out the possibility of a nonmelanoma skin cancer.[268] The histologic features can be indistinguishable from MF with a lichenoid infiltrate and extensive lymphocytic exocytosis. Unilesional MF may be misdiagnosed.[269,270] In addition, clonal populations of T cells have been detected.[271] The presence of epidermotropic CD20+ B cells is suggestive of a lymphomatoid keratosis; however, clinicopathologic correlation is paramount in arriving at the correct diagnosis.[272]

Erythroderma may occur in a variety of benign dermatologic disorders including psoriasis, pityriasis rubra pilaris, eczematous dermatitis, seborrheic dermatitis, severe contact dermatitis, crusted scabies, and drug eruptions.[273-276] These patients may also have circulating cerebriform cells and lymphadenopathy, further complicating the diagnosis. Erythroderma secondary to drug reactions, especially anticonvulsants as part of drug reaction with eosinophilia and systemic symptoms (DRESS), can be particularly difficult to distinguish from MF/SS because of the presence of convoluted cerebriform T cells and the formation of Pautrier microabscesses.[169,277] In addition, patients with DRESS may have atypical lymphocytes detected in blood.[278] Several studies have compared the histologic features of erythrodermic MF/SS with other causes of reactive erythroderma. Although not present in all cases, Pautrier microabscesses and a dense, often lichenoid, dermal lymphocytic infiltrate were more commonly associated with erythrodermic MF/SS.[279,280] As mentioned previously, when compared with benign erythroderma SS biopsies more commonly show expression of PD-1, a higher proliferative index as detected by Ki-67 staining, loss of CD7 expression, and a decreased number of associated CD8+ lymphocytes.[186] Differentiation of benign erythroderma from erythrodermic CTCL can usually be accomplished through careful evaluation of the history, skin biopsy of the more typical lesions of the underlying disease, molecular genetic analysis of both skin and blood, and flow cytometry of peripheral blood.[279,280]

Subacute or chronic spongiotic dermatitis and interface dermatitis resulting from contact dermatitis,[281,282] drug eruption, and persistent arthropod bite reaction may have atypical cerebriform T cells with epidermotropism and Pautrier-like microabscesses mimicking MF.[283] Caution should be exercised in interpretation of epidermotropism associated with significant spongiosis, especially microvesiculation, which is only rarely observed in MF.[284] The Pautrier-like microabscesses seen in spongiotic processes typically have a flask shape and are composed of Langerhans cells and keratinocytes. Immunophenotyping may be helpful in this differential diagnosis because cutaneous T-cell pseudolymphomas rarely show aberrant loss of CD2, CD3, or CD5 expression, especially a combination of these markers.[283] In addition, TOX staining has been shown to help differentiate early MF from benign inflammatory dermatitides.[61,64] CD7 is not as helpful as its expression is commonly lost in both MF and reactive dermatoses.[283] Typically, T cell–predominant pseudolymphomas are characterized by perivascular, "sleevelike" infiltrates around vessels in the dermis, with accompanying plasma cells, eosinophils, and macrophages. The T cells are typically a mixture of CD4+ and CD8+ cells as opposed to the CD4+-predominant population characteristic of most cases of MF. The utility of gene rearrangement studies in this setting is unclear as clonal TCR gene rearrangements have been reported in some cutaneous T-cell pseudolymphomas.[285] Next-generation sequencing may hold promise as the exact clone can be followed over time.[286] B cell–predominant pseudolymphomas often present as pink to purple papules or nodules and may be triggered by a wide range of causative agents (e.g., Borrelia, tattoos, arthropod bites).[287] They are notable for reactive follicle formation with tangible-body macrophages, centroblasts, and centrocytes in the germinal centers surrounded by distinct marginal and mantle zones. There are polyclonal plasma cells, a mix of CD4+ and CD8+ T cells, and often eosinophils in the accompanying inflammatory infiltrate.[288,289]

AR is a severe form of photosensitive dermatitis that may closely mimic MF or SS clinically and histologically when fully developed.[290,291] AR is a chronic, persistent eruption that can be induced by a broad spectrum of light wavelengths (ultraviolet A [UVA], ultraviolet B [UVB], and visible wavelengths of light).[290] The skin lesions are typically plaques and papules on the sun-exposed areas of the face and hands but may extend to covered areas or even become generalized erythroderma.[292] There is typically spongiosis and mixed dermal inflammation with scattered eosinophils and multinucleated cells. CD8+ lymphocytes predominate and often demonstrate mild cytologic atypia and subtle exocytosis. Severe cases of erythrodermic AR may have generalized lymphadenopathy and circulating Sézary cells mimicking SS. Positive photo testing and patch testing, as well as a lack of clonality, all would support a diagnosis of AR over MF/SS.[293]

CD30+ Lymphoproliferative Diseases

The differential diagnosis for suspected MF also includes a variety of related conditions, which are equally concerning for their malignant or premalignant clinical course. LyP and PCALCL are both characterized by the presence of CD30+ T cells; together, they represent the poles of a continuous disease spectrum (Table 94.3). Both LyP and PCALCL are subtypes of the CTCLs.[164,295] There is no clear-cut boundary between the diseases, however, and many patients fall into a borderline category when definitive diagnosis is not possible based on the current clinicopathologic features. CD30+ lymphomatoid drug reactions may resemble LyP and PCALCL both clinically and histologically; therefore, drugs should be identified with a temporal association with the onset of the cutaneous eruption.[296-298]

Lymphomatoid Papulosis

LyP is a CD30-positive T-cell LPD characterized by chronically recurring, self-healing crops of mildly pruritic papulonodular lesions that are clinically benign but histologically malignant.[299] LyP initially presents with crops of erythematous, often pruritic papules on the trunk and limbs that wax and wane. Individual lesions range from 2 mm to 2 cm in diameter (usually <1 cm). In their clinical course, the papules become hemorrhagic and necrotic before undergoing spontaneous regression over an average duration of 5 weeks, ranging from 2 weeks to 6 months, with subsequent postinflammatory hyperpigmentation and eventual atrophic varioliform scar formation. Rare cases have presented with acral or facial involvement, and uncommon variants include mucosal, follicular, bullous, and pustular.[300]

LyP is classically divided into three histologic types, type A, type B, and type C. More recently, type D, type E, 6p25.3-associated and follicular variants, have been described and added to the 2018 WHO-EORT classification update.[165,168,301-304] Any of the histologic types may occur simultaneously in the same patient or during the course of their disease, and the individual histologic type provides no prognostic significance.[305] LyP type A, the most common type (>80%),[166] is characterized by a polymorphous infiltrate of eosinophils, neutrophils, and scattered anaplastic large transformed lymphocytes and binucleate Reed-Sternberg-like cells (Figure 94.9). LyP type B (<5%)[166] is characterized by small to medium cerebriform T cells resembling MF. CD30 expression may not be present in LyP type B, and clinical correlation is paramount to differentiate it from MF. LyP type C (10%)[166] is characterized by sheets of large, anaplastic CD30+ cells and can be histologically identical to PCALCL but follows a waxing-and-waning clinical course. The atypical cells in LyP types A, B, and C are typically CD4+. LyP type D is characterized by an extensively epidermotropic population of cytologically atypical CD8+ lymphocytes in a pattern that is nearly identical to that observed in PC8TCL (see "Other Primary Cutaneous T-cell Lymphomas").[301,306,307] LyP type E (<%5) presents with large, necrotic ulcers with eschars. Histologically, LyP type E shows an angioinvasive infiltrate of atypical cells in a similar

Table 94.3. Primary Cutaneous CD30+ Lymphoproliferative Disorders

	Lymphomatoid Papulosis (LyP)	Primary Cutaneous Anaplastic Large-Cell Lymphoma (PCALCL)
Definition	• Lymphoproliferative disorder with histologic features suggestive of a CD30+ lymphoma; 5 main types (A-E)	• Lymphoma characterized by large, anaplastic cells where >75% are CD30+
Clinical features	• Chronic, recurring crops of erythematous, pruritic papules/nodules affecting trunk/limbs with spontaneous resolution over 1-2 mo • No extracutaneous dissemination	• Most commonly affects adult males[164] • Isolated nodule(s) ± ulceration with uncommon spontaneous resolution
Prognosis	• Excellent • 99% 5 y DSS[166] • Patients with LyP do not die from their disease[312] • Up to 20% of patients with LyP will go on to develop another lymphoma (PCALCL, MF, other lymphomas)[294] • Patients with LyP may be at increased risk for nonhematologic malignancies (squamous cell carcinoma, melanoma)[294]	• 95% 5 y DSS[166] • Owing to prognostic differences, needs to be differentiated from secondary CD30+ LCL resulting from MF/SS large cell transformation
Treatment	• No curative therapies • Chronic management with low-dose weekly methotrexate or phototherapy[164] • Severe disease may respond to brentuximab	• Radiotherapy and surgical excision are preferred • Patients may respond to low-dose methotrexate[164] • Patients with refractory or extracutaneous disease should be treated with brentuximab

Abbreviations: DSS, disease-specific survival; LCL, large cell lymphoma; MF, mycosis fungoides; SS, Sézary syndrome.

pattern to NK/T-cell lymphomas. The 6p25.3 variant of LyP is the first subtype to be defined by a consistent chromosomal abnormality and typically shows a biphasic pattern of inflammation with small to medium-sized epidermotropic cells and a dermal infiltrate of large atypical cells.[303] Finally, the follicular variant is characterized by a folliculocentric infiltrate of atypical cells. Eosinophils are often present, and associated follicular mucinosis (FM) has been described.[304] The atypical cells in all of the types often have clonal rearrangement of the *TCR* gene and absent or diminished expression of pan-T-cell antigens.

The incidence of LyP is 1.2 to 1.9 cases per 1 million person-years, and it is more common in males.[308] Although LyP is diagnosed more frequently in adults, over 250 cases of LyP in children and adolescents have been reported.[259] The etiology of LyP is unknown, although cases have been associated with hepatitis E[309] and the drug fingolimod.[310-312] Clinical behavior of LyP is usually benign; however, development of overt lymphoma, usually MF, PCALCL, or Hodgkin lymphoma, has been documented.[313] The incidence of LyP-associated hematologic malignancies (HMs) in the literature varies widely, ranging from 10% to 60%.[313-315] In a recent review of 504 Dutch patients with LyP, associated HM was observed in 15.5% of patients (median follow-up time 120 months), with rates not exceeding 20% after a 25-year follow-up period.[294] Compared with the general population, patients with LyP may be at increased risk for nonhematologic malignancies such as cutaneous squamous cell carcinoma, melanoma, and intestinal/lung/bladder cancers.[294] No clinical, histologic, immunophenotypic, or molecular genetic features have been identified that can predict which patients will develop lymphoma. However, onset of LyP at a younger age is associated with a 13% cumulative risk for overt lymphoma, and therefore, all patients with LyP should be closely monitored throughout their lives.[259] The benign or malignant nature of LyP is controversial, but the WHO-EORTC considers LyP to be a latent or low-grade stage of the primary cutaneous CD30+ LPDs that are considered to be malignancies.[164,316] Its clinical, histologic, and immunophenotypic similarities to PCALCL; aberrant T-cell antigen expression; clonal *TCR* gene rearrangements; and increased risk for transformation to malignant lymphoma support this view.

Primary Cutaneous Anaplastic Large Cell Lymphoma

Distinguishing PCALCL from LyP type C may be challenging. Clinically, PCALCL presents as larger solitary or localized nodules/tumors (>1 cm) ± ulceration instead of crops of papules. PCALCL has a higher frequency of persistent or progressive cutaneous lesions with less frequent or incomplete spontaneous regression.[317,318] PCALCL is differentiated from LyP type C by cohesive sheets or >75% CD30+ large transformed cells, fewer admixed neutrophils and eosinophils, a diffuse infiltrate that extends into the deep dermis vs a more superficial wedge-shaped infiltrate.[317,318]

Differentiation of PCALCL from LyP and secondary CD30+ LCL resulting from large cell transformation of MF/SS is important because of differences in prognosis and therapy.[164,319] PCALCL has a good prognosis and can be effectively managed with local excision and/or radiation therapy,[320,321] whereas secondary CD30+ LCL due to large cell transformation of MF/SS has a very poor prognosis requiring systemic therapy that often includes aggressive combination chemotherapy.[188,322] LyP also has an excellent prognosis with >98% 5-year survival and >90% 10-year survival.[313,314] LyP can often be managed with no therapy, topical steroids, phototherapy, and low-dose methotrexate[323,324] without the need for aggressive therapy.[325] More refractory, severe cases of LyP may be managed with bexarotene capsules[326] or brentuximab vedotin infusions.[327] Furthermore, PCALCL must be differentiated from secondary cutaneous involvement by extracutaneous ALCL.[328] Primary nodal ALCL and secondary cutaneous involvement by extracutaneous ALCL are more aggressive than PCALCL.[328] In malignant cells, the presence of anaplastic lymphoma kinase-1 protein (ALK-1) from the t(2;5) (p23;q35) chromosomal translocation favors primary nodal ALCL.[317] A thorough dermatologic

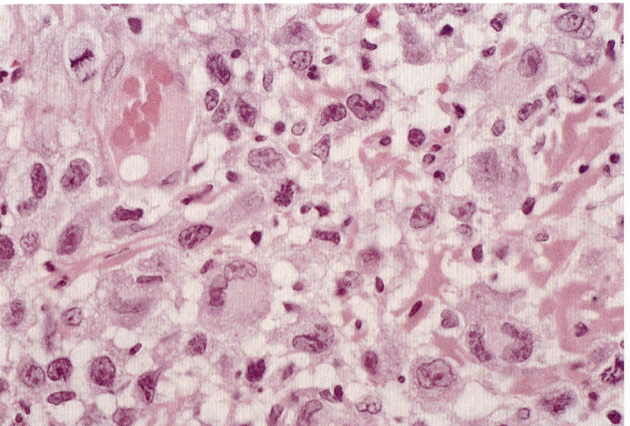

FIGURE 94.9 Lymphomatoid papulosis, type A. Anaplastic large cells with abundant cytoplasm, reniform nuclei, and prominent nucleoli are scattered among small lymphocytes and eosinophils. Note occasional binucleate Reed-Sternberg-like cells (H&E, ×250). The large cells were strongly positive for CD30 (not shown). H&E, hematoxylin and eosin.

examination, history, and staging for extracutaneous disease are necessary to exclude secondary large cell transformation of low-grade MF or secondary cutaneous involvement by extracutaneous lymphoma before a case is accepted as PCALCL. Other aspects of ALCL are discussed in more detail in Chapter 90.

Other Primary Cutaneous T-cell Lymphomas

Using the WHO-EORTC classification for cutaneous lymphomas as a guide, other primary CTCLs need to be considered in patients with atypical lymphocytic infiltrates of the skin.[164,329,330] These lymphomas include three variants of MF (pagetoid reticulosis, FMF, and granulomatous slack skin [GSS] disease); subcutaneous panniculitis-like T-cell lymphoma (SPTL); PCGDTCL, chronic EBV infection; and three provisional entities (PC8TL, primary cutaneous CD4+ small/medium-sized pleomorphic T-cell lymphoproliferative disorder [PCSMPTCLPD], and primary cutaneous acral CD8+ T-cell lymphoma [PCATCL]). See *Tables 94.4* and *94.5*.

Pagetoid reticulosis and FMF are variants of MF implying minor clinicopathologic differences from classical MF, whereas GSS is a subtype of MF with more significant differences from classical MF.[341] Like classical MF, these diseases are low-grade clonal T-cell lymphomas that generally follow a benign course but may behave aggressively over time.

Pagetoid Reticulosis

Pagetoid reticulosis is a rare epidermotropic variant of MF that usually presents as localized, hyperkeratotic, verrucous plaques on the hands or feet (Woringer-Kolopp disease)[342,343] but may also present with disseminated cutaneous plaques (Ketron-Goodman disease).[344] Given its more aggressive clinical course, Ketron-Goodman disease would currently be better classified as tumor-stage MF, PCGDTCL, or PC8TL.[164,345,346] Pagetoid reticulosis may mimic a more unusual variant of MF localized to the palms and soles known as MF palmaris et plantaris.[347] Skin biopsies of pagetoid reticulosis show pagetoid epidermotropism by enlarged, atypical cerebriform T cells, with relative sparing of the dermis (*Figure 94.10*). The malignant cells in pagetoid reticulosis may be CD8+ or, less commonly, CD4+ and, rarely, CD4−CD8−.[348,349] Pagetoid reticulosis has a clinically benign course, with only rare reports of cutaneous dissemination of localized pagetoid reticulosis.[346] Local excision or radiation therapy is generally adequate treatment for pagetoid reticulosis, especially the localized form.

Folliculotropic Mycosis Fungoides

FMF is another variant of CTCL first reported in 1985 with a folliculotropic infiltration by atypical cerebriform T cells with minimal or absent epidermotropism[350] (*Figure 94.11*). While patients often present with patches and plaques similar to classic MF, FMF is typified by more involvement of sun-exposed areas such as the head and neck and patches devoid of hair.[351] Less commonly, patients with FMF present with acne-like comedones, facial papules, milia, and rarely spiky follicular papules.[352,353] The follicles may show plugging, cystic dilatation, and mucinous degeneration, as seen with mucin stains such as Alcian blue. The folliculotropic cerebriform T cells are typically CD4+[354] and may express an aberrant T-cell phenotype with loss of CD7 and other T-cell antigens.[355] Other less frequent histologic features that have been described include eosinophilic folliculitis, basaloid follicular hyperplasia, and granulomatous inflammation.[354,356] Differential upregulation of ICAM-1 (CD54) on follicular epithelium instead of epidermal keratinocytes has been implicated in the folliculotropic homing pattern of folliculotropic MF.[355] Lymph node involvement and large cell transformation have also been described.[355]

FMF is the most common MF subtype in adults and the second most common form of pediatric MF.[357,358] FMF, whether or not exhibiting FM, was initially reported to show a more aggressive course than classic MF.[213,359] Approximately 7% of reported cases have demonstrated rapid lymph node involvement.[360,361] Patients with extracutaneous spread at first presentation have poor 5-year and 10-year DSSs of 23% and 2%.[353] Agar and colleagues completed an outcome analysis on 1502 patients with MF/SS concluding that folliculotropic MF was one of several independent predictors of poor survival and increased risk of disease progression.[213]

More recently, indolent (early-stage FMF) and more aggressive (advanced-stage FMF) subgroups have been identified based on clinicohistologic presentation.[331,353,357] The indolent subgroup with 5- and 10-year DSSs of 96% and 93% to 96%, respectively, presents with follicular papules, acneiform or keratosis pilaris-like lesions, and/or "early-stage" patches and thin plaques with sparse small-cell neoplastic infiltrates. The more aggressive subgroup with 5- and 10-year DSSs of 65% to 70% and 40% to 70%, respectively, presents with "advanced-stage" thick plaques with dense medium- to large-cell neoplastic infiltrates, tumors, nodules, or erythroderma.[331,353,357] In a single-center study, the estimated 5-year survival for early-stage FMF was similar to that of early-stage MF, while advanced-stage FMF was similar to classic tumor-stage MF.[357] The indolent subgroup may respond to skin-directed therapy, whereas the more aggressive group often requires systemic therapy.[351,353]

FM is frequently associated with FMF and less commonly with classical MF. FM is a rare cutaneous disease with unknown etiology, which has been described in two forms. The first is a primary benign idiopathic form, also known as alopecia mucinosa, which is characterized histologically by follicular mucin deposition.[362] The secondary form is closely connected with cutaneous lymphomas. FM is characterized by an eruption of hypopigmented or flesh-colored, eczematous or edematous plaques or follicular papules on the head/neck devoid of hair.[363] The concurrence of FM associated with MF and FMF varies widely among studies (9.4%-60%).[363] Controversy exists whether FM is a clonal inflammatory process or a neoplastic process serving as an MF precursor. However, recent data comparing the two prognostic

Table 94.4. MF Variants

	Pagetoid Reticulosis	Folliculotropic MF	Granulomatous Slack Skin
Clinical features	• Slowly progressing, isolated psoriasiform, hyperkeratotic patch/plaque • Usually affects the hands and feet • No extracutaneous dissemination	• Classic finding: indurated patches and plaques with alopecia and follicular prominence • More commonly affects adult males & children • Preferential involvement of the sun-exposed areas (head and neck) • Occasional intense pruritus	• Initial patches/plaques that progress to pendulous, lax skin preferentially in folds of axillae and groin
Prognosis	• 100% 5 y DSS[166] • Indolent course, rarely aggressive local involvement	• Patches, papules, thin plaques: indolent form, good prognosis (96% 5 y DSS)[331] • Thick plaques, tumors: aggressive, guarded prognosis (<70% 5 y DSS)[331]	• Indolent course • 100% 5 y DSS[166] • Increased risk of Hodgkin lymphoma[332]
Treatment	• Radiotherapy is preferred • Surgical excision is uncommon[164]	• Owing to perifollicular dermal infiltrates, patients are less responsive to topical therapies • Combination treatments including PUVA are more effective	• Radiotherapy • Systemic retinoids • Methotrexate

Abbreviations: DSS, disease-specific survival; MF, mycosis fungoides; PUVA, psoralen + ultraviolet A phototherapy.

Table 94.5. Rare CTCL Variants

	PC CD4+ Small/Medium T-cell LPD	PC Acral CD8+ T-cell Lymphoma	Hydroa Vacciniforme-Like LPD	Subcutaneous Panniculitis-Like TCL	PC CD8+ Aggressive Epidermotropic Cytotoxic TCL	PC Gamma-Delta TCL
Clinical features	• Typically presents as a solitary plaque or tumor on the head, neck, or trunk without preceding erythematous patches or plaques[333]	• Slow-growing, isolated nodule on the ear, nose, hands, or feet, without other or prior patches/plaques[8] • Indolent clinical course in older adults (>50 y old)	• EBV-associated • Primarily affects Asian and Latin-American children • 10-15 y clinical course[334] • Early-stage papulovesicular eruptions on sun-exposed areas, such as the face, upper extremities, and chest, which develop into pox-like scars • Late-stage ulceration, necrosis, and systemic symptoms • Carries risk of development into systemic lymphoma	• Isolated or multiple subcutaneous nodules often on the extremities • Rarely complicated by a hemophagocytic syndrome, causing more rapid disease progression	• Rapid development of large plaques/tumors marked with ulceration and necrosis • Involvement of oral/genital mucosa, and extracutaneous spread is common[335]	• Disseminated plaques/ulceronecrotic nodules w/frequent mucosal involvement • Varied appearance of patches and plaques, even within the same patient • Predilection of the extremities and relative sparing of the trunk[336] • Hemophagocytic syndrome can also develop in panniculitis-like presentations, contributing to worse prognosis[336]
Prognosis	• Favorable (especially for localized skin lesions) with 5 y DSS of 100%[166]	• Favorable, 5 y DSS 100%[166]	• Variable	• 5 y DSS 87%[166]	• Poor, with 5 y DSS 31%[166]	• Poor with median survival of 15 mo and 5 y survival of approximately 10%[166,336]
Treatment	• Lesions often spontaneously resolve post biopsy • Surgical excision or radiotherapy are preferred treatment for local, isolated skin lesions • Multiple, relapsing lesions may require radiotherapy + topical steroids • Generalized skin spread may require cyclophosphamide or interferon alpha chemotherapy[337]	• Conservative treatment varying from simple observation to surgical excision, radiotherapy[338]	• Early stages: lesions responsive to topical steroids, retinoic acid and interferon • Later stage: more aggressive measures such as radiotherapy and chemotherapy may be required[334]	• Common initial treatment with oral steroids alone ± low-dose methotrexate/cyclosporine • Additional therapies include radiotherapy, doxorubicin-based chemotherapy, and, rarely, hematopoietic stem cell transplantation[339]	• Doxorubicin-based multiagent chemotherapy	• Varied tumor response to doxorubicin-based multiagent chemotherapy, radiation, and even stem cell transplant[340]

Worsening Prognosis →

Abbreviations: CTCL, cutaneous T-cell lymphoma; DSS, disease-specific survival; LPD, lymphoproliferative disorder; PC, primary cutaneous; TCL, T-cell lymphoma.

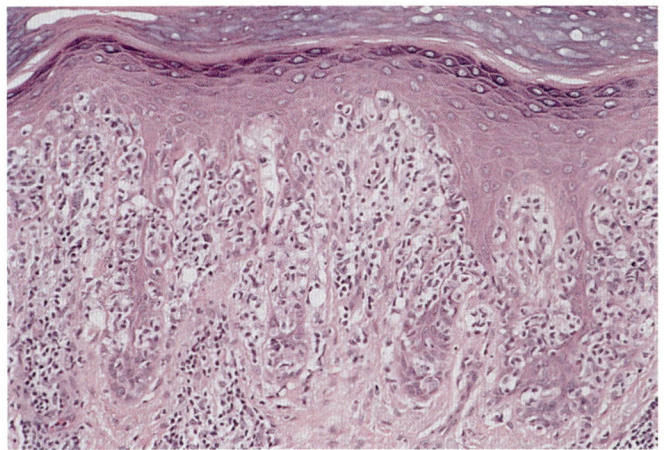

FIGURE 94.10 Pagetoid reticulosis. Note the pronounced pagetoid pattern of epidermotropism by enlarged, atypical cerebriform T cells (H&E, ×50). H&E, hematoxylin and eosin.

Granulomatous Slack Skin Disease

GSS disease is a rare but distinctive subtype of MF that begins with patches and plaques that steadily progress to characteristic pendulous, erythematous skin folds in the axilla and groin. Several authors stress the importance of distinguishing the mature lesions of GSS from the histologic variant of granulomatous MF, which can be differentiated quantitatively, not qualitatively.[332] GSS has histologic features of MF including superficial papillary dermal and epidermotropic infiltrates of atypical cerebriform T cells, but it also exhibits expansive infiltration into the deep dermis and subcutis with extensive elastolysis, a prominent granulomatous reaction with Langhans-type multinucleated giant cells, and uncommon infiltration of vessel walls (*Figure 94.12*).[368,369] These multinucleated giant cells are histiocytic in origin with 20 to 30 nuclei, frequently show emperipolesis and elastophagocytosis, and express CD68 and CD1a.[332] Similar to MF, GSS is a clonal proliferation of CD4+ T-helper cells that frequently lack expression of CD7. GSS has a slow, progressive course and usually remains localized to the skin, although hypercalcemia, lymph node involvement, and fatal systemic dissemination have been reported.[368,370-374] Importantly, in contrast to other CTCL variants, patients with GSS have an increased incidence of Hodgkin lymphoma at a frequency between 25% and 50%.[332,375]

Subcutaneous Panniculitis-Like T-cell Lymphoma

SPTL presents as tender, erythematous nodules or subcutaneous palpable masses, mostly on the legs, trunk, arms, or face. Histologically, this lesion is confined to the subcutis and does not typically extend to the dermis or epidermis.[376,377] Classically, T cells ranging from small and inconspicuous to large and transformed cells with hyperchromatic nuclei rim individual fat cells.[378,379] As the name implies, this lymphoma is similar in histology to a lobular panniculitis and, in fact, many patients present with a history of previously biopsied panniculitis. In addition, there is some clinical and histologic overlap with lupus panniculitis and many patients with SPTL will present with or develop evidence of concomitant systemic lupus erythematosus.[380-382] In addition, patients with SPTL may show the histologic features of SPTL and lupus panniculitis in the same biopsy specimen.[383] By immunohistochemistry, the neoplastic T cells express αβ TCR, CD3, CD8, and

subtypes of FMF (as described above) did not show a difference in FM presence between the groups.[363] In general, no single clinicopathologic feature can differentiate FM associated with MF from alopecia mucinosa.[362,364,365] Alopecia mucinosa tends to occur in younger patients with fewer lesions localized to the head and neck as opposed to the more general distribution commonly seen in MF-associated cases. Histologically, alopecia mucinosa tends to have fewer atypical cerebriform T cells, less epidermotropism and/or lymphocytic infiltration of follicular epithelium, and a normal CD4 to CD8 ratio. In FM associated with MF the infiltrate tends to be more dense and cytologically atypical with a CD4+-predominant immunophenotype.[362] Clonal *TCR* gene rearrangement can be detected in many cases of alopecia mucinosa, thus limiting its usefulness in the differentiation from MF.[366] In support of this, a long-term follow-up study of seven patients with FM concluded that, despite the presence of a clonal *TCR* gene rearrangement, there was no evidence of progression to CTCL in any patient.[367]

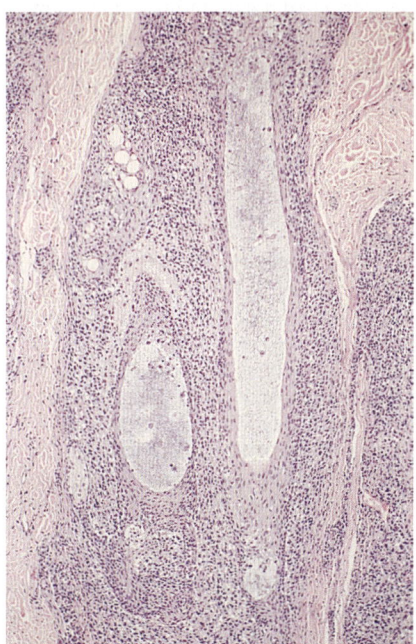

FIGURE 94.11 Folliculotropic MF with follicular mucinosis. Note the preferential pattern of perifollicular infiltration by atypical cerebriform T cells with prominent folliculotropism forming small Pautrier microabscesses. Also note the bluish pools of mucin within the hair follicles (H&E, ×25). H&E, hematoxylin and eosin; MF, mycosis fungoides.

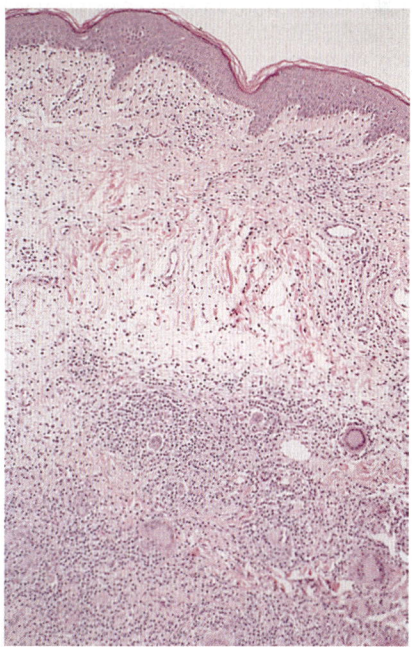

FIGURE 94.12 Granulomatous slack skin. This variant of mycosis fungoides shows a deep lymphocytic infiltrate with dermal edema, disruption of elastic fibers, and numerous foreign body giant cells (H&E, ×10). H&E, hematoxylin and eosin.

cytotoxic granule proteins, although CD56 and CD30 are rarely detected.[376,378,379,384] The CD8+ lymphocytes that rim the adipocytes typically have an elevated Ki-67 proliferative index, a finding that can be used to differentiate SPTL from lupus panniculitis.[385] Historically, SPTL had been associated with a poor prognosis often secondary to an aggressive hemophagocytic syndrome (HPS). The present WHO-EORTC classification separates cases into SPTL with an αβ phenotype and PCGDTCL based both on immunohistologic features and clinical behavior. SPTL with an αβ phenotype are CD4−, CD8+, CD56−, ßF1+; are limited to the subcutaneous fat and are uncommonly associated with an HPS[386]; and have a favorable prognosis (5-year OS 82%).[387] PCGDTCL is generally CD4−, CD8−, CD56±, ßF1−; tends to involve the epidermis with resulting ulceration; is commonly associated with HPS; and has a dire prognosis (5-year OS 11%).[339,340] Repeat biopsies may be necessary to confirm the diagnosis of SPTL.

Primary Cutaneous γδ T-cell Lymphoma

PCGDTCL is characterized clinically by disseminated plaques and ulceronecrotic nodules that frequently also involve mucosal sites. The different clinicopathologic presentations may resemble MF, pagetoid reticulosis, psoriasis, peripheral T-cell lymphoma (PTCL) unspecified, and SPTL.[336,340,379,388] Patients presenting with nodules/tumors/plaques localized predominantly to the extremities should alert the clinician to PCGDTCL. One series found all 23 of their patients with PCGDTCL to have nodules or tumors on the extremities, with less than half exhibiting concurrent truncal lesions.[336] While PCGDTCL may appear as solitary lesions or generalized disease, the skin tumor burden does not correlate with prognosis.[340] Whether these lesions are primary to the mucosa or the skin, most reports suggest that PCGDTCL is aggressive and poorly responsive to therapy,[389] except in rare cases.[390] Five-year DSS is estimated at 11%, with poor median survival of 15 months.[166,336] As mentioned previously, PCGDTCL includes subcutaneous lesions previously considered to be γδ variants of SPTL associated with a potentially very aggressive HPS.[336,340] There are reports of a more indolent subcutaneous form of PCGDTCL associated with atypical lymphocytic lobular panniculitis,[390] which may be difficult to distinguish without clinical correlation. Histologically, the neoplastic clone of PCGDTCL is a mature, activated γδ T cell with a cytotoxic phenotype. The subcutis, dermis, or epidermis may be involved by medium- to large-sized cells with irregular nuclei and clumped chromatin. Cases with extensive epidermotropism have been described and can be difficult to distinguish from MF and pagetoid reticulosis solely on histologic grounds.[391] Interestingly, this epidermotropic variant may have a slightly better prognosis than classic PCGDTCL. Basal vacuolar interface change and interface dermatitis is common. The background tissue shows apoptosis and necrosis with occasional angioinvasion. Often, one patient may show different histologic patterns at different sites. In contrast to αβ+ MF and SS, the neoplastic γδ+ T cells are typically negative for both CD4 and CD8, with rare CD8+ cases.[336,340,388] The cells stain with a TCR γ stain and are TCR ßF1 negative. In addition, the neoplastic γδ T cells express CD3, CD2, CD43, and CD45RO.[392] The T cells also express cytotoxic granule proteins such as TIA-1, perforin, and granzyme B.[376]

EBV+ Lymphoproliferative Disorders

Chronic active EBV infection is a new section in the updated WHO-EORTC classifications. This group contains EBV+ LPDs such as hydroa vacciniforme-like LPD (HV-like LPD) and hypersensitivity reactions to mosquito bites. HV-like LPD primarily affects Asian and Latin American children with a clinical course of 10 to 15 years.[334] In the early stage, papulovesicular eruptions arise on sun-exposed areas, such as the face, upper extremities, and chest, and develop into pox-like scars over several weeks. In later stages, ulceration, necrosis, and facial edema are common, with potential systemic symptom development (such as fever, wasting, lymphadenopathy, hepatosplenomegaly). Patients with mosquito bite hypersensitivity may develop ulceronecrotic lesions at bite sites with systemic symptom development. While the clinical course is variable, both HV-like LPD and mosquito bite hypersensitivity carry the risk of progression to systemic EBV+ T/NK-cell lymphoma.[334] The histologic features of HV-like LPD can be somewhat variable. Spongiosis, epidermal necrosis, intraepidermal vesiculation, and epidermotropsim are frequently seen. The dermal infiltrate typically comprises small to medium-sized hyperchromatic cytotoxic T cells (CD3+/CD8+/cytotoxic marker+ [TIA-1, perforin, granzyme B]) or NK cells (CD56+). The number of EBV-infected cells varies and must be detected by EBV-encoded small RNA in situ hybridization as LMP-1 staining is negative. Extension into the subcutaneous fat and angiotropism can be seen. Mosquito bite hypersensitivity is characterized histologically by epidermal necrosis and ulceration. There is marked papillary dermal edema and dense mixed dermal inflammation with CD4+ T cells, CD8+ T cells, and NK cells. Vasculitis may be present. EBV-positive cells are often rare.[393]

Primary Cutaneous Aggressive Epidermotropic CD8+ Cytotoxic T-cell Lymphoma

PC8TCL is a provisional entity comprising epidermotropic CD8+ T cells with an aggressive clinical course.[335,394] Patients with this aggressive variant usually present with widespread eruptive ulcerative plaques with necrotic eschars. Mucosal and genital involvement is common. The disease course is often complicated by spread to the central nervous system, lung, and testis.[335] Of note, the lymph nodes are rarely involved. Histologically, there is a pagetoid pattern or occasionally a linear distribution of T cells in an atrophic or acanthotic epidermis. Spongiosis may accompany the intraepidermal lymphocytes.[335] Angioinvasion and adnexal destruction are common findings. Immunohistochemically, the neoplastic cells express CD3, CD8, CD45RA, and cytotoxic granule proteins such as perforin, granzyme B, and TIA-1.[395] CD2 and CD5 expressions are often lost, while CD7 expression is retained, a pattern that is generally the inverse of what is typically observed in MF.[396] PC8TCL must clinically and histologically be differentiated from CD8+ MF, pagetoid reticulosis, and type D LyP, all of which tend to follow an indolent course.[307,397-399] Nofal and colleagues have proposed diagnostic criteria for PC8TCL that must include these constant features[335]: (1) clinical—a history of onset within weeks to months of an aggressively behaving eruption of widespread papules, plaques, and tumors that often ulcerate, without any precursor lesions; (2) histopathological—epidermotropism, often prominent with a nodular or diffuse infiltrates of pleomorphic T cells; (3) immunohistochemical—CD8+, CD4− staining pleomorphic T cells. Patients with PC8TCL have a poor prognosis with a median survival of 32 months.[335,396] This is further exemplified by an average 5-year DSS of 31% as compared with 88% in the more indolent MF.[166]

Primary Cutaneous CD4+ Small/Medium-Sized Pleomorphic T-cell Lymphoproliferative Disorder

The second provisional entity is PCSMPTCLPD, formerly a lymphoma. PCSMPTCLPD typically presents as a solitary plaque or tumor on the head and neck or trunk without preceding erythematous patches or plaques more typical of MF.[333,337] Spontaneous regression has been reported.[400] Uncommonly, the papulonodules, tumors, or deep plaques can be multiple.[401] Histologically, there is a nodular or diffuse infiltrate of small or medium-sized pleomorphic lymphocytes in the dermis, with minimal or no epidermotropism and without cerebriform nuclei. The infiltrate can extend deeply into the dermis and subcutis and can include histiocytes, plasma cells, and eosinophils. Large, atypical lymphocytes should comprise <30% of total cellularity. There have been rare cases with granulomatous features that may be confusing for GSS, yet GSS typically presents with more epidermotropism and shows some cerebriform cells.[333,402] The neoplastic T cells are by definition CD4+ and also express CD3, αβ TCR, but they are negative for CD8, CD30, and cytotoxic proteins. Pan-T-cell markers may be lost. The neoplastic cells consistently express PD-1, CXCL13, and BCL-6 indicating derivation from follicular T-helper cells.[403-405] The CD4+/PD-1+ atypical cells are often seen in clusters and in "pseudorosettes" around B cells.[406] Nuclear staining with NFATc1 may be helpful to differentiate PCSMPTCLPD from MF and pseudolymphomas, which show a predominant cytoplasmic staining pattern.[407] The prognosis is usually excellent with recently reported 5-year DSS of 100%.[166] In typical cases, staging is not required or recommended. If involved lesions do not spontaneously resolve post biopsy, they can be treated with intralesional steroids, surgical excision or, rarely, radiotherapy.[166] Rare cases of generalized lesions and large, rapidly growing tumors with >30% large pleomorphic T cells do not belong in this category and should be classified as PTCL, not otherwise specified (NOS).[408]

Primary Cutaneous Acral CD8+ T-cell Lymphoma

The third provisional entry is PCATCL, a rare, indolent lymphoma typified by a slowly progressive papule/nodule on the ear or less common acral sites, such as the nose and foot. The entity was identified by Petrella et al in 2007,[409] with approximately 60 reported cases in the literature since that time.[338,410] The disease largely affects those >50 years in age. While solitary lesions are predominant at presentation, bilateral symmetric and multifocal cutaneous disease has been described.[338] PCATCL is characterized histologically by a dense and diffuse dermal infiltrate of medium-sized CD3+/CD8+ blast cells. The dermal infiltrate is separated from the epidermis by a clear grenz zone and expresses TIA-1 but not the other cytotoxic proteins (granzyme B and perforin), findings that contrast with many of the other CD8+ CTCLs. The proliferation rate is typically low (<10%).[411] The prognosis for this condition is excellent, with 5-year DSS of 100%. Therefore, in typical cases staging is not recommended and conservative management is preferred with surgical excision or radiotherapy.

Other Hematopoietic Neoplasms With Similar Cutaneous Presentations

Other lymphomas and hematopoietic tumors that may involve the skin include HTLV-1+ ATL, extranodal NK/T-cell lymphoma, Hodgkin lymphoma, cutaneous B-cell lymphomas, leukemia cutis, and extramedullary myeloid tumor (EMT; including granulocytic sarcoma and monoblastic sarcoma). PTCL and NK/T-cell lymphomas are discussed in Chapters 90 and 91. Hodgkin lymphoma is discussed in Chapters 95. Cutaneous B-cell lymphoma, leukemia cutis, and EMTs are discussed in the following section.

Primary cutaneous B-cell lymphomas are uncommon (incidence of 3.1 per million person-years) and must be differentiated from secondary cutaneous involvement by systemic B-cell lymphoma and cutaneous lymphoid hyperplasia of B-cell type.[99,412] The primary cutaneous B-cell lymphomas include primary cutaneous follicle center lymphoma (PCFCL); primary cutaneous marginal zone B-cell lymphoma (PCMZL); primary cutaneous diffuse large B-cell lymphoma (PCDLBCL), leg type; and primary cutaneous large B-cell lymphoma, other.[164,413,414] Other systemic B-cell lymphomas may involve the skin, including intravascular large B-cell lymphoma, lymphomatoid granulomatosis, chronic lymphocytic leukemia/small cell lymphoid neoplasm, mantle cell lymphoma, and Burkitt lymphoma.[164,316] Cutaneous B-cell lymphomas usually present as single or multiple violaceous nodules on the head and neck or trunk and tend to infiltrate the deeper portions of the dermis, sparing the epidermis ("bottom-heavy"). PCFCLs are the most common cutaneous B-cell lymphomas. PCFCLs may have a nodular or a nodular and diffuse growth pattern and more frequently have a predominance of large noncleaved cells[415] than their nodal counterparts (*Figure 94.13*). The Mann-Berard grading system used for nodal follicular lymphomas is not predictive in PCFCL. In fact, in contrast to the aggressive behavior of nodal large cell follicular lymphomas, PCFCL tend to be localized, follow an indolent course, and can often be managed with local excision, radiation therapy, and uncommonly rituximab.[412,413,416-419] However, careful staging must be performed to exclude extracutaneous lymphoma before a case is classified as primary cutaneous B-cell lymphoma. Typically, nodal follicular lymphomas express BCL-2 and are characterized by the chromosomal translocation t(14;18). PCFCLs, on the other hand, rarely show characteristic chromosomal translocations, and BCL-2 is uncommonly expressed.[420,421]

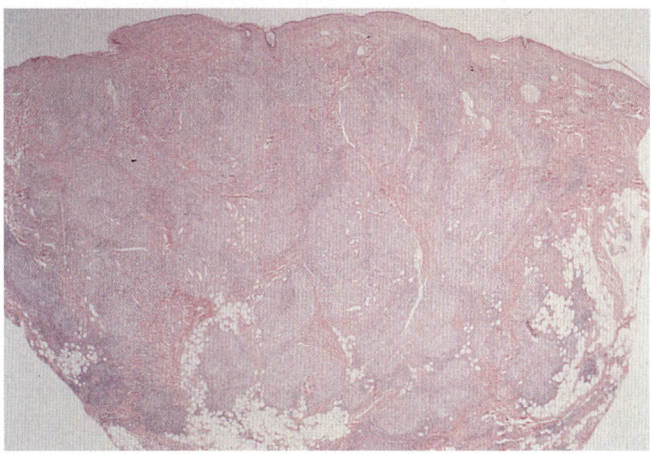

FIGURE 94.13 Primary cutaneous follicle center lymphoma. Note the back-to-back nodular pattern. The infiltrate extends from the superficial reticular dermis to the superficial subcutis in a "bottom-heavy" pattern sparing the papillary dermis and epidermis (H&E, ×2). H&E, hematoxylin and eosin.

PCMZL is an indolent lymphoma characterized clinically by small purple-pink irregular plaques on the trunk, in contrast to PCFCL, in which the violaceous nodules are usually confined to the head and neck.[422,423] Histologically, PCMZL is generally characterized by small, monocytoid, or lymphoplasmacytoid B cells. The infiltrate may be predominantly plasmacytic, and in instances where there is no evidence of systemic disease, these lesions are still considered part of the spectrum of primary cutaneous marginal zone B-cell lymphomas.

The neoplastic cells typically express CD20, CD79, and BCL-2 but are negative for CD5, CD10, and BCL-6, the last two markers helping to distinguish it from PCFCL (Table 94.6).[423,424] The presence of large clusters of CD123+ plasmacytoid dendritic cells has also been proposed as a differentiating feature of PCMZL from the other primary cutaneous B-cell lymphomas.[425] There are now thought to be two subtypes of PCMZL. The more common variant expresses class switched immunoglobulins, IgG in approximately 72% to 95% and IgA in approximately 5% to 17%.[422] There is a predominance of T cells and only a small population of neoplastic B cells. Monotypic plasma cells are usually present at the periphery of the infiltrate. The second, less common type of PCMZL is characterized by a diffuse proliferation or large nodules of neoplastic B cells that express IgM. This subtype is more frequently associated with extracutaneous disease.[166]

PCLBCL, leg type, typically presents in the elderly (average age of onset, 78 years) with rapidly growing reddish to violaceous nodules and tumors on the lower legs, but they can occur at any cutaneous site.[426-428] Histologically, the lesion is composed of sheets of immunoblasts and centroblasts without the admixed centrocytes that are more often seen in PCFCL. The infiltrate rarely involves the epidermis but can extend into the deep dermis and subcutaneous tissue. Because PCLBCL has a poor prognosis compared with the more indolent course of PCFCL, it is important to be able to distinguish these two entities.[427-430] As noted earlier, PCFCL and also PCLBCL can have a purely diffuse infiltrate with many centroblasts and immunoblasts, yet PCFCL will also contain centrocytes, whereas PCLBCL, leg type, will not. By immunohistochemistry, PCFCL expresses CD10 and BCL-6 and only expresses BCL-2 or MUM1/IRF4 in a minority population, whereas PCLBCL diffusely expresses BCL-2, MUM1/IRF4, and IgM but does not express CD10 and only rarely expresses BCL-6 (Table 94.6).[424,427,428,431,432] Gene chip expression profiling has shown that PCLBCL has an activated B-cell genotype, whereas PCFCL has more of a germinal center B-cell genotype.[433] A further study evaluating apoptosis-related genes identified a strong cellular cytotoxic immune response in PCFCL, whereas PCLBCL, leg type, had constitutive activation of the intrinsic-mediated apoptosis pathway and downstream inhibition of apoptosis.[434] In addition, miR20a and miR20b have been shown to be upregulated in PCLBCL as compared with PCFCL. One

Table 94.6. Immunohistochemistry Pattern of the Primary Cutaneous B-cell Lymphomas

CBCL Type	BCL-2	BCL-6	CD10	CD20	Ig	MUM1/IRF4
PCFCL	−(10% +)	+	+ Follicular pattern; − diffuse pattern	+	−	−(10% +)
Secondary FCCL	+	+	+	+	+	−
PCMZL	+	−	−	+	+	+ On associated plasma cells
PCLBL, leg type	++	rarely	−	+	+ IgM	++

Abbreviations: FCCL, follicle center cell lymphoma; PCFCL, primary cutaneous follicle center lymphoma; PCLBL, primary cutaneous large B-cell lymphoma; PCMZL, primary cutaneous marginal zone lymphoma.

of the miRNA target genes, PTEN, was found to be downregulated in PCLBCL and was associated with decreased disease-free survival (DFS).[435]

PCDLBCL, other, is a WHO-EORTC classification that includes those B-cell lymphomas that do not conform to the PCFCL or PLBCL, leg type, criteria. This category includes large B-cell lymphoma subtypes such as anaplastic, plasmablastic, T-cell/histiocyte-rich, and intravascular large B-cell lymphoma.[436-442] Although these entities can present initially as cutaneous lesions, they often represent cutaneous involvement by a systemic lymphoma. Of note, some cases of intravascular large B-cell lymphoma appear to be confined exclusively to the venules, capillaries, and arterioles of the skin, without systemic involvement.[442] These rare cases have a better prognosis (3-year OS: 56% vs 22%) than their systemic counterparts.[442] More detailed discussion of the other systemic B-cell lymphomas is in Chapter 90.

Leukemia cutis and EMT are cutaneous infiltrates of myeloblasts and immature myeloid precursors that are often difficult to differentiate from cutaneous lymphoma. EMT, also known as granulocytic sarcoma or chloroma, is an extramedullary tumor composed of immature granulocytic precursor cells. The most common sites of presentation are bone, periosteum, soft tissue, lymph node, skin, and, infrequently, small intestine. The tumor may develop during the course of acute myeloid leukemia, chronic myeloid leukemia, or other myelodysplastic disorders.[443-445] EMT usually presents as nodules or tumors that are often solitary, whereas leukemia cutis presents with multiple skin lesions with a varied clinical appearance, including papules, nodules, plaques, palpable purpura, or ulcers.[445] Histologically, EMT and leukemia cutis tend to infiltrate between collagen bundles and fat spaces in an interstitial pattern (*Figure 94.14*). Cytologically, the myeloblasts of EMT and leukemia cutis are medium-sized cells with finely dispersed chromatin, small or inconspicuous nucleoli, and scant cytoplasm. Occasionally, eosinophilic or neutrophilic granules may point to the cells' myeloid lineage. In difficult cases, immunohistochemistry, flow cytometry, and cytochemical stains will usually confirm the diagnosis and exclude lymphoma.[446] CD68, CD43, and lysozyme, while not lineage specific for monocytes or macrophages, have been shown to be the most sensitive markers for detecting myeloid leukemia cutis.[447,448] Although nearly half of the cases of may be myeloperoxidase (MPO) negative, a study looking at 173 skin biopsies of myeloid leukemia cutis demonstrated a 100% diagnostic accuracy utilizing CD68, CD33, and MPO.[449] If the patient has systemic leukemia, comparing the immunohistochemical profile of the cutaneous infiltrate with that from the peripheral blood or bone marrow can be helpful. It must be kept in mind, however, that many of the immunophenotypic markers used in defining blastic cells in the blood or bone marrow (CD117 and CD34) are often negative in the cutaneous infiltrates.[432,443] MPO, Sudan black B, and chloroacetate esterase cytochemical stains can be used to confirm myeloid differentiation if air-dried touch imprints are available.

STAGING

In 1979, a staging system for CTCL was proposed by an international panel of experts who devised a tumor-node-metastasis (TNM) system.[450] In the original TNM staging system, peripheral blood involvement with >5% atypical circulating cells was indicated by a separate peripheral blood stage B1 (vs B0) and did not affect the clinical stage designation. Two large series have shown that blood involvement is more commonly seen in higher-stage disease, with 0% to 12% of patients with plaques only, 16% to 27% of patients with tumors, and >90% with erythroderma, demonstrating peripheral blood involvement.[194,451] Vonderheid et al have shown that blood involvement has distinct prognostic implications.[452]

In 2007, the ISCL/EORTC recommended revisions to the Mycosis Fungoides Cooperative Group classification and staging system for CTCL.[208] These revisions were made to incorporate advances related to tumor cell biology, diagnostic techniques, and prognostic variables pertaining exclusively to MF and SS as opposed to non-MF/SS CTCLs (*Table 94.7*). Stage I refers to patients with patches and plaques without adenopathy and is divided into stage IA for patients with <10% body surface area involvement (T1) and stage IB for more generalized patches and plaques (T2). Stage II has two unique categories: stage IIA patients have patches/plaques with palpable adenopathy (histology negative), whereas stage IIB patients have tumors (nodules > 1 cm in size) with or without palpable adenopathy (histology negative). Patients with erythroderma are placed into stage III with or without palpable adenopathy (histology negative). Stage IV patients have evidence of CTCL beyond the skin. Stage IVA$_1$ reflects significant blood involvement. Patients with stage IVA$_2$ have nodal involvement without visceral disease, and stage IVB reflects patients with visceral disease. The lymph node staging includes N1 for dermatopathic lymph nodes (NCI grades 0-2), N2 for NCI grade 3 lymph nodes, and N3 for NCI grade 4 lymph nodes (*Table 94.2*). New modifications to blood staging have been recently proposed by the ISCL/USCLC/EORTC.[196] See "Blood Involvement" under "Histopathology" and *Table 94.7*. B0 is defined as absolute abnormal T-cell count <250/μL; B1, absolute count 250 to <1000/μL; and B2, absolute count ≥1000/μL. The blood stage is factored into the clinical stage to create a TNMB matrix. Changes also included the creation of clinical stages

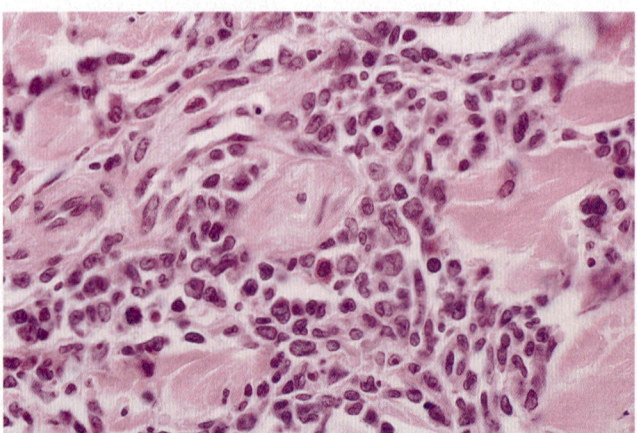

FIGURE 94.14 Leukemia cutis. Clusters of myeloblasts with fine chromatin and scant cytoplasm infiltrate between collagen bundles in the reticular dermis (H&E, ×250). H&E, hematoxylin and eosin.

Table 94.7. ISCL/EORTC Staging of Mycosis FUNGOIDES/Sézary Syndrome

Stage	Clinical-pathologic features
T Skin Stage	
T1	Patches/plaques <10% BSA
T2	Patches/plaques >10% BSA
T3	At least one tumor nodule >1 cm in diameter
T4	Confluence of erythema (erythroderma) covering >80% BSA
N Lymph Node Stage	
N0	No clinically abnormal peripheral lymph nodes (pLNs)
N1	Clinically abnormal pLNs with NCI grade 1 or 2 pathology
N2	Clinically abnormal pLNs with NCI grade 3 pathology
N3	Clinically abnormal pLNs with NCI grade 4 pathology
Nx	Clinically abnormal pLNs with no histologic confirmation
M Visceral Stage	
M0	No visceral involvement
M1	Visceral involvement
B Blood Stage	
B0	Abnormal lymphocyte count* <250/μL
B1	Abnormal lymphocyte count 250 to <1000/μL
B2	Abnormal lymphocyte count ≥1000/μL * Absolute counts should be determined by the percentage of aberrant lymphocytes (CD4$^+$CD7$^-$ or CD4$^+$CD26$^-$ or another aberrant lymphocyte population) identified by flow cytometry, multiplied by the total lymphocyte count of a complete blood count. - In addition, each B stage is subdivided into substage A if T-cell clone is absent or equivocal and substage B if T-cell clone is present and identical to skin (e.g., B_{2A} or B_{2B}).
Clinical Stage	**TNMB Stages**
Early-Stage Disease	
IA	T1 N0 M0 B0-1
IB	T2 N0 M0 B0-1
IIA	T1-2 N1-2 M0 B0-1
Late-Stage Disease	
IIB	T3 N0-2 M0 B0-1
IIIA	T4 N0-2 M0 B0
IIIB	T4 N0-2 M0 B1
IVA$_1$	T1-4 N0-2 M0 B2
IVA$_2$	T1-4 N3 M0 B0-2
IVB	T1-4 N0-3 M1 B0-2
Sézary Syndrome	
IVA$_{1\ or\ 2}$ or IVB	T4 N0-3 M0-1 B2

Abbreviations: BSA, body surface area; EORTC, European Organization for the Research and Treatment of Cancer; ISCL, International Society of Cutaneous Lymphomas; pLNs, peripheral lymph nodes.
Modified from: Olsen EA, Whittaker S, Willemze R, et al. Primary cutaneous lymphoma: recommendations for clinical trial design and staging update from the ISCL, USCLC, and EORTC. *Blood*. 2021;140(5):419-437. doi:10.1182/blood.2021012057

IIIA (T4N0-2M0B0), IIIB (T4N0-2M0B1), IVA$_1$ (T1–4N0-2M0B2), and IVA$_2$ (T1–4N3M0B0–2).[208]

Lymph node biopsy of a nonpalpable lymph node in patients without adenopathy and liver and bone marrow biopsies are rarely helpful in those patients with limited skin disease and no lymphadenopathy.[204] Table 94.8 outlines staging procedures for MF/SS adapted from the ISCL/USCLC/EORTC guidelines.[196] All patients should have a complete physical examination with special attention to skin and lymph nodes. Careful mapping of skin involvement and/or total-body photographs are recommended to document the initial extent of disease at diagnosis and to assess response to treatment. Laboratory studies should include serum comprehensive metabolic panel, lactate dehydrogenase (LDH), and complete blood count with manual differential.

In addition, peripheral blood should be examined for abnormal lymphocytes by flow cytometry with attention to CD4$^+$/CD7$^-$ or CD4$^+$/CD26$^-$ gated populations. A manual Sézary cell count (number per microliter) is less accurate than flow cytometry. *TCR* gene rearrangement of peripheral blood is also recommended, including an attempt to correlate a positive finding with any clone in the skin. Although there is no significant benefit to performing bone marrow biopsies for staging purposes,[196,203] they may be helpful in working up unexplained hematologic abnormalities.

Imaging

The role of diagnostic imaging in the initial staging of CTCL has been examined by several authors.[453,454] A study of 63 patients with CTCL

Table 94.8. Recommended Initial Staging Evaluation of Mycosis Fungoides/Sézary Syndrome

	Evaluation and Studies
Skin	
Physical examination	Identify primary skin lesion (patches, plaques, tumors, erythroderma) and % BSA involved
Skin biopsy	Punch biopsy of thickest or oldest skin lesions (>1 skin biopsy)
Immunophenotyping	CD2, CD3, CD4, CD5, CD7, CD8, CD20, CD30
Molecular genetics	T-cell receptor rearrangement analysis if needed
Lymph Nodes	
Physical examination	Identify abnormal peripheral lymph nodes ≥1.5 cm or irregular
Radiologic tests	CT scans of chest, abdomen, pelvis except in stage IA or limited IB. PET scans may be helpful to identify which LN to biopsy
LN biopsy	Complete LN biopsy or several core LN biopsies favored over FNA
Immunophenotyping	CD2, CD3, CD4, CD5, CD7, CD8, CD20, CD30
Molecular genetics	T-cell receptor rearrangement analysis if needed
Viscera	
Physical examination	Identify abnormal liver, spleen, or other organs
Radiologic tests	CT scans of chest, abdomen, pelvis except in stage IA or limited IB. PET scans may be helpful to identify visceral abnormalities
Liver biopsy	Not indicated, unless involvement would change management
Spleen biopsy	Not indicated, unless involvement would change management
Bone marrow biopsy	Not indicated, unless abnormalities would change management
Other biopsies	Not indicated, unless involvement would change management
Immunophenotyping	CD2, CD3, CD4, CD5, CD7, CD8, CD20, CD30
Molecular genetics	T-cell receptor rearrangement analysis if needed
Blood	
Chemistries	Comprehensive panel including liver enzymes, lactate dehydrogenase, HTLV-1 serology if indicated
Blood cells	Complete blood count and differential, manual Sézary cell count (if flow cytometry not available)
Immunophenotyping	Flow cytometry for absolute count and %: CD2, CD3, CD4, CD5, CD7, CD8, CD20, CD26, CD30. Also include CD4/CD8 ratio, CD4+CD7−, CD4+ CD26−, TRBC1 (if available)
Molecular genetics	T-cell receptor rearrangement analysis

Abbreviations: BSA, body surface area; CT, computed tomography; FNA, fine-needle aspiration; HTLV-1, human T-lymphotropic virus-1; LN, lymph node; PET, positron emission tomography; TRBC1, T-cell receptor constant β chain-1.
Modified from: Olsen EA, Whittaker S, Willemze R, et al. Primary cutaneous lymphoma: recommendations for clinical trial design and staging update from the ISCL, USCLC, and EORTC. Blood. 2021;140(5):419-437. doi:10.1182/blood.2021012057

(78% with stage I or II disease) who had staging body computed tomography (CT) scans found positive findings in 18 (29%) patients, half of whom had clinically unsuspected advanced-stage disease.[455] Of these 18 patients, 8 had biopsies, with 5 of 8 confirming extracutaneous CTCL. Of the 38 patients with stage I disease, however, only 2 had positive findings on CT scan.[455] Another retrospective study of 33 patients with CTCL (70% with stage I or II disease) who had CT scans found that 3 of the 20 patients with initial clinical stage I disease were staged higher on the basis of CT findings as stage II.[456] Subsequent lymph node biopsies confirmed extracutaneous disease in all three patients (stage IVA). In summary, pelvic, abdominal, and thoracic CT scans have a low yield in patients without palpable adenopathy (stage I) and are not necessary for staging these patients.[454] The highest yield of CT scans appears to be in cases of non-MF/SS CTCL (nonepidermotropic, transformed CTCL, PCALCL) and stage III disease (erythroderma), in contrast to stage II and IV patients, in whom CT findings often do not change treatment or stage.[455] Therefore, staging CT scans of the chest, abdomen, and pelvis are recommended for patients with generalized plaques, erythroderma, tumors, palpable lymph nodes, or blood involvement.[196]

Positron emission tomography (PET) may provide an alternative staging and response-assessment tool for patients with CTCL. Thirteen patients with MF and SS at risk for secondary lymph node involvement were evaluated using integrated PET/CT followed by excisional biopsy of the lymph nodes.[457] Two of seven patients with LN4 effaced lymph nodes had nodes <1.5 cm on CT scan and would have been assigned an N0 classification without the use of integrated PET/CT. The intensity of PET activity correlated roughly with lymph node histologic grade but did not reach statistical significance because of the small sample size. Feeney and colleagues evaluated the fluorodeoxyglucose PET/CT findings in patients with a variety of T-cell lymphomas noting a significant difference in the mean maximum standardized uptake value (SUV) in patients with MF with transformation (SUV, 11.3) compared with patients with MF without transformation (SUV, 3.82; $P < .05$).[458] Other studies suggest a beneficial role of CT/PET in the staging of patients with MF/SS.[459-461] The recently proposed updated staging guidelines of the ISCL, USCLC, and EORTC recommend using the Lugano classification of PET/CT imaging in the staging and assessment of extracutaneous disease in CTCL.[196,462]

Lymph Nodes

Although the presence of palpable nodes has prognostic value, lymph node histology is even more important in staging and assessing prognosis, not only at diagnosis but also later in the course of the disease. Enlarged lymph nodes from patients with MF/SS show either dermatopathic lymphadenopathy or involvement by MF/SS. Sausville et al described a system of grading lymph nodes in patients with CTCL (NCI VA classification) that correlated well with prognosis: LN1, a few atypical cerebriform T cells; LN2, dermatopathic lymphadenopathy with small clusters (<6 cells) of atypical cerebriform T cells; LN3, dermatopathic lymphadenopathy with large clusters (>6 cells) of atypical cerebriform T cells; and LN4, partial or complete effacement of lymph node architecture (Table 94.5).[194] Although clusters of atypical cerebriform T cells are present in grades LN2 and LN3, lymph node architecture is preserved. Only LN4 lymph nodes are considered involved with CTCL (histology positive) for purposes of the TNM staging system (Table 94.4). The NCI VA classification has been criticized because of the nonspecificity of grades LN1-3 and because lymph nodes from patients with unrelated diseases can show similar findings, and many consider LN3 lymph nodes to be histologically borderline.[463,464]

The ISCL/EORTC consensus staging system for lymph nodes distinguishes stage N3 lymph nodes that show effacement of nodal architecture (grade LN4) from stage N2 lymph nodes that contain clusters of atypical lymphocytes (>6 cells) that do not efface architecture (grade LN3). ISCL/EORTC stage N1 lymph nodes may show dermatopathic lymphadenopathy, or small clusters of atypical lymphocytes (3-6 cells) that do not distort nodal architecture (grade LN1-2). In general, there is good correlation between histologic and molecular evaluation of lymph nodes for involvement by MF/SS. Three studies have shown that most histologically negative lymph nodes (LN1-2) do not show *TCR* gene rearrangements, whereas ~90% or more histologically involved LNs (LN4) do show clonal *TCR* gene rearrangements by Southern blot analysis.[465,466] All three studies also showed a mixture of clonal and polyclonal populations in histologically borderline cases (LN3 or histologically equivalent to LN3). Although not statistically significant in all studies, histologically borderline cases that have a positive *TCR* gene rearrangement tend to have a poorer prognosis, similar to cases with histologically involved lymph nodes (LN4).[465]

Fine-needle aspiration of lymph nodes to assess for involvement by MF/SS has been evaluated in a limited number of patients, with good correlation between cytologic grade of the FNA specimen and histologic classification of the lymph node biopsy.[464,467] However, as with other types of lymphomas, there is an inherent risk of sampling only low-grade involvement and missing a focal area of transformation to a LCL. Therefore, excisional biopsy of peripheral lymph nodes >1.5 cm in the longest diameter is recommended, with preference for the largest lymph node draining the involved skin area or, if available, the lymph node with the highest SUV from PET scan data.[196] A core needle biopsy (CNB) of a representative abnormal lymph node may suffice in certain circumstances, and suggestions to enhance the diagnostic yield of CNB have been published.[196,468]

Bone Marrow

Studies of bone marrow involvement in patients with MF at initial staging found disease in 2% to 22% of patients.[195] Histologic findings in involved marrows include clusters of $CD3^+$ atypical lymphocytes with cerebriform nuclei and occasional large dysplastic cells.[195] Bone marrow involvement by MF is more common in higher-stage disease and correlates with a poorer prognosis; however, when other factors such as skin stage and visceral involvement were considered, bone marrow involvement was not shown to be an adverse prognostic factor.[469] These findings were supported by a study that evaluated the prognostic significance of histologic and molecular evidence of bone marrow involvement at the time of diagnosis. This study also showed a correlation between histologic or molecular bone marrow involvement and clinical stage of disease, but bone marrow involvement failed to be an independent prognostic indicator.[203] Therefore, despite being considered in initial staging of non-MF/SS lymphoma patients, routine staging bone marrow biopsies in patients with MF are not currently recommended. The ISCL/USCLC/EORTC consensus publication recommends performing bone marrow biopsies only in patients with unexplained hematologic abnormalities.[196]

PROGNOSIS

Prognosis correlates with the extent of skin disease and status of the lymph nodes, blood, and visceral involvement. MF behaves in a manner similar to other low-grade or indolent NHL, with prolonged survival despite recurrent relapses (see Chapter 90). Zackheim et al assessed relative (observed/expected) long-term survival among the four skin stages. Stage and survival data for 489 patients with CTCL were extracted from a University of California, San Francisco, CTCL registry dated 1957 to 1994 and compared with a control group matched for age, sex, race, and geographic variables. Using the control group to generate expected survival values, researchers found a relative survival at 10 years for each group as follows: 100% for T1, 67% for T2, 40% for T3, and 41% for T4.[470]

Utilizing the newest staging criteria from the ISCL/EORTC, the 5-year survival rates are similar: 94% for stage IA, 84% for stage IB, 78% for stage IIA, 47% for stage IIB, 47% for stage IIIA, 40% for stage IIIB, 37% for stage IVA$_1$, 18% for stage IVA$_2$, and 18% for stage IVB.[213] Data from a retrospective cohort analysis suggest that the long-term (30-year) survival of patients with stage IA (limited patch/plaque) MF is similar to the expected survival of a matched control population.[470,471] Therefore, it is unlikely that stage IA MF will affect the life expectancy of afflicted patients.

Kim et al performed a retrospective cohort analysis of 525 patients with MF/SS at Stanford University from 1958 to 1999.[471] In the multivariate analysis, patient age, T classification, and the presence of extracutaneous disease were the most important independent factors. The risk for disease progression to a more advanced TNM or B classification, worse clinical stage, the development of extracutaneous disease, or death due to MF correlated with the severity of the initial T classification. None of the patients had T1 disease when their extracutaneous disease was detected.[471]

Several reports suggest that patients with dermatopathic or early lymph node involvement with *TCR* gene rearrangement have a worse prognosis than similar patients without evidence of gene rearrangement.[192,472]

A retrospective analysis of 1502 patients with MF/SS using the revised ISCL/EORTC staging for CTCL found a significant difference in survival between those with patch-only disease (T1a/T2a) vs patch and plaque disease (T1b/T2b).[213] Multivariate analysis revealed that advanced T stage, the presence of a peripheral blood tumor clone without Sézary cells (B0b), increased LDH, and folliculotropic MF were associated with both decreased survival and increased risk of disease progression.[213] The same analysis showed that large cell transformation was predictive only of increased risk of disease progression, and male sex, increasing age, and poikilodermatous MF were associated with decreased survival.[213]

Young patients <20 years have an overall favorable prognosis in contrast to progressive disease associated with age >20 years, individuals of African ancestry, poikilodermatous variant, and advanced-stage disease.[473] Hypopigmented patches are the most common presentation in young patients and children and portends a favorable prognosis.[101,473]

In a retrospective analysis of 100 patients with transformed MF, Benner et al identified decreased overall and DSS in those with folliculotropic MF and those lacking CD30.[187] They developed a "prognostic index" for those with transformed MF based upon the following four negative prognostic factors: CD30 negativity, generalized skin lesions, extracutaneous transformation, and folliculotropic MF. There was a significant decrease in survival in those with 2+ negative prognostic factors vs those with 0 to 1.[187]

Patients with SS have a relatively poor prognosis, with a median survival of ~3 to 4 years.[162,471,474] In a series of 29 patients with SS, features linked with a bad prognosis included fast evolution of the disease (from symptoms onset up to diagnosis) ($P = .0274$), raised levels of serum LDH ($P = .0379$), and β_2-microglobulin ($P = .0151$), the last being the most important prognostic factor.[474] Some of these findings were confirmed in another series of 28 patients with SS in whom the detrimental prognostic value of increasing age and LDH level and the identification of the EBV genome in the skin were reported.[475]

The prognosis for patients with extracutaneous disease is poor, with median survivals between 1 and 2.5 years.[476] Virtually all patients with extracutaneous disease die of CTCL, compared with nearly one-third of patients with generalized plaques and a majority of patients with tumors or erythroderma without visceral involvement.[477,478] Very few patients with limited plaques (T1) actually die of MF, with most deaths due to cardiovascular events or other malignancies.[470,471,477] Agar et al found that 26% died due to their cutaneous lymphoma.[213] Overall, the bulk of patients with CTCL do not die from their malignancy.[476,479] Second malignancies other than skin cancers include NHL, Hodgkin lymphoma, colon cancer, and lung cancer.[480] Infection remains the most common cause of death in patients who succumb to CTCL, with *Staphylococcus aureus* and *Pseudomonas aeruginosa* being the most common pathogens infecting the skin, leading to bacteremia and sepsis.[478,479] Visceral involvement with CTCL may lead to organ failure and ultimately death.

An international collaboration has led to the most recent data for prognosis in advanced MF/SS. A total of 1275 patients (29 international sites) were evaluated, and the median OS was 63 months. The 2- and 5-year survival rates were 77% and 52%, respectively. Stage IIB had a slightly worse OS as compared with stage III (5-year OS: 57.4 vs 58.2 months). The 5-year OS for both stages IVA and IVB continues to be poor (42.9 and 39 months, respectively). Similar to previous studies the only independent prognostic factors for reduced survival included advanced stage (stage IV), greater than 60 years of age, elevated LDH, and large-cell transformation.[481]

THERAPY

The mainstay of treatment of CTCL has been control of the cutaneous manifestations of disease with topical therapies in the hope of preventing spread to extracutaneous sites. However, because of the risk of progression to extracutaneous sites and worsening cutaneous symptoms, systemic agents alone or in combination with topical therapies have been studied to control more advanced disease. Therapy in MF/SS is based on the extent of disease, age, performance status, potential for remission, availability of treatments, efficacy, and treatment toxicity.[482,483] Because MF usually behaves as a low-grade or indolent lymphoma, controversial issues have involved the timing, selection, and intensity of systemic therapy. Unfortunately, there are few randomized clinical trials comparing the efficacy of the numerous therapeutic options available for patients with MF/SS. The following discussion summarizes the efficacy and toxicity of each therapy and relates these parameters to disease stage (*Figure 94.15*).

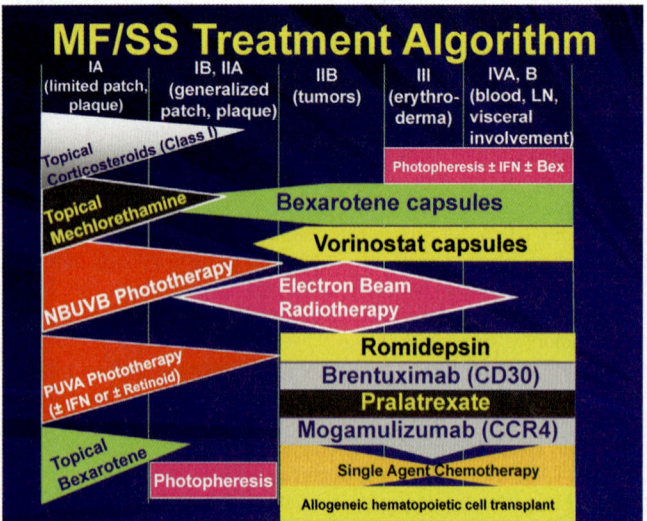

FIGURE 94.15 MF/SS treatment algorithm. Note that single-agent chemotherapeutic agents with impressive benefit/risk ratios include pegylated liposomal doxorubicin, gemcitabine, and pralatrexate. Bex, bexarotene capsules; IFN, interferon; MF, mycosis fungoides; NBUVB, narrow beam ultraviolet B phototherapy; PUVA, psoralen + ultraviolet A phototherapy; SS, Sézary syndrome.

Topical Chemotherapy

Mechlorethamine hydrochloride, or nitrogen mustard (HN2), was introduced in 1947 as the first topical agent to demonstrate activity in treating MF[484] and remains one of the major therapies of choice for early-stage MF. In 1942, HN2 became the first chemotherapy agent to be infused into a human being for the treatment of cancer.[485] HN2 is an alkylating agent that undergoes rapid degradation to an active ethyleniminium ion that has high antimitotic activity and a brief half-life.[476] Several studies have suggested that the mode of action of HN2 may involve induction of G_2 arrest, gene-specific DNA cross-links, and blockage of transcription factor–binding sites.[486] Some investigators have suggested that immunogenic properties of HN2 demonstrated by its propensity to induce delayed-type hypersensitivity contribute to its antineoplastic activity.[487] Topical HN2 may be prepared in a variety of ways. Initial studies dissolved HN2 in water to reach a concentration of 10 to 20 mg/dL,[488] whereas more recently HN2 has been suspended in an emollient such as Aquaphor (0.01%, 0.02%) or a gel (0.016%).[489,490] Topical HN2 is usually applied once daily to the active regions or entire skin surface with relative sparing of the eyelids, genitalia, rectum, lips, and intertriginous areas. The length of treatment is variable but usually involves daily applications until the patient achieves a complete or significant clearing of skin lesions, followed by a maintenance regimen of daily or every-other-day applications for a period of 6 months to 2 years. No author has advocated a maintenance regimen of indefinite HN2 applications. Kim et al found that longer maintenance regimens had no impact on the relapse rate in patients treated with topical HN2.[489] Treatment may be intensified for localized lesions by increasing either the concentration or frequency of application.

The response rate of topical HN2 is related to the morphology (patch/plaque vs tumor) and extent of disease (T1 vs T2). Several large series with >100 patients have been reported.[489,491,492] It is difficult to compare overall response rates among these studies because of differences in the clinical stages treated, adjunctive therapies, and staging systems. The percentage of patients with early-stage MF achieving an initial complete response (CR) ranged from 64%[491] to 75%[492] in stage I disease. The newer gel formulation was found to have a 58.5% response rate, and about 20% of subjects withdrew from the study due to skin irritation.[490] Including more advanced stages, the CR ranged from 37% in stage I/IIA disease to 50% in stage I-III disease.[489] The median time to achieve CR is shorter for stage I patients than for those with more advanced stages.[489] Vonderheid et al found a durable CR to HN2 lasting more than 8 years occurring in 34 of 324 (10%) patients with early-stage MF,[492] and Kim et al demonstrated that freedom-from-progression rates at 10 years were 85% and 83% for T1 and T2 patients, respectively.[489] Relapse is common, as Kim et al observed relapses in 42% of 107 patients after an initial CR, all of which occurred within 5 years, and disease progression to a higher skin stage has been reported in 12% and 17% of T1 and T2 patients, respectively.[489] However, among patients who had an initial response to HN2 and relapsed, 67% achieved a CR after receiving HN2 salvage therapy. In summary, HN2 is effective in achieving an initial response in early-stage disease. Relapse occurs frequently but can often be treated with a second course of therapy.

The side effects of topical HN2 include local allergic reactions, xerosis, hyperpigmentation, and secondary cutaneous cancers. Immediate hypersensitivity reactions manifesting as urticaria are rare but do occur in ~5% of patients using topical HN2 and necessitate discontinuing treatment to avoid a potentially life-threatening anaphylactic reaction.[487] Delayed-type hypersensitivity reactions (allergic contact dermatitis) manifesting as erythematous eczematous patches occur in up to 64% of patients treated with aqueous HN2[493] but occur less frequently (<10%) with the ointment-based preparation[489] and gel formulations.[494] Some investigators have suggested that the delayed-type hypersensitivity reaction to topical HN2 may have a beneficial effect in clearing MF lesions[487] and advocate topical desensitization rather than discontinuation of the HN2 when delayed-type hypersensitivity reactions occur.[487] Despite this, discontinuation of the medication occurs in about 20% of patients.[490,493] Hyperpigmentation of the skin, especially in sites of MF involvement, occur commonly in patients using topical HN2, and patients should be reassured that the hyperpigmentation will resolve spontaneously within several months.

In their study of 331 patients treated with HN2, Vonderheid et al calculated an 8.6-fold ($n = 31$, 9%) and 1.8-fold ($n = 27$, 8%) increased risk for the development of squamous cell carcinoma (SCC) and basal cell carcinoma (BCC) of the skin, respectively, when compared with the general US population.[492] In contrast, Kim et al found BCC or SCC skin neoplasms in only 8 of 203 (4%) patients with CTCL treated initially with HN2.[489] Melanoma occurred in one patient in the Kim et al cohort. This patient had Fitzpatrick skin type 1 and had had a previous BCC.[489] Because HN2 is a known radiomimetic agent, its carcinogenic potential may be amplified with the simultaneous use of other agents, most notably ultraviolet therapy.[487] To help minimize this risk, patients using HN2 should adhere to strict protection from sun exposure. The risk of environmental contamination from topical HN2 appears to be minimal, as there are no epidemiologic data of increased malignancy in family members of treated patients; however, treatment assistants should wear latex gloves and wash accidently exposed skin thoroughly.

Topical carmustine (BCNU), a nitrosourea compound that causes DNA damage through alkylation at an O^6 site of guanine and interstrand cross-linkage, is also used to treat early-stage MF, although experience is more limited than with topical HN2.[495] The use of topical nitrosoureas for the treatment of MF was first reported in 1972.[496] Patients mix a 5-mL (10-mg) aliquot of a 0.2% alcoholic stock solution with 60 mL of tap water and apply the solution to only the involved areas of MF. Applications are repeated daily for no more than 8 to 10 weeks at a time. Zackheim et al reported a CR in 86% of T1 stage patients and 48% of T2 patients treated with BCNU solution.[497] In their follow-up report of 188 early-stage MF patients treated with topical BCNU, 91% of stage T1 patients and 62% of stage T2 patients had not failed treatment after 36 months, and 5-year survivals were 97% and 80%, respectively.[487] A phase 1 to 2 clinical trial evaluating the use of topical carmustine and intravenous O^6-benzylguanine was reported.[498] The therapeutic combination was initiated in 17 patients with refractory early stage MF (IA-IIA). The objective response rate (ORR) was 88% (CR 41%), with a mean (standard deviation) duration of CR of 14.43 (6.6) months. The maximally tolerated dose was 20 mg of carmustine applied once in combination with two daily doses of 120 mg/m^2 of O^6-benzylguanine. Most adverse events (112 [67%]) were grade I. Of 15 patients with dermatitis, 5 individuals (33%) demonstrated grade II dermatitis that was unresponsive to topical corticosteroid therapy.[498]

Phototherapy

Psoralen photochemotherapy was introduced in 1974 for refractory psoriasis and has been used extensively in the early stages of CTCL. Psoralen and ultraviolet A light therapy (PUVA) involves the ingestion of 8-methoxypsoralen (8-MOP), a photosensitizing compound, which is activated after exposure to ultraviolet A light (320- to 400-nm wavelength). 5-Methoxy-psoralen has been used as the photosensitizing agent in PUVA, and early studies indicated similar efficacy.[499] Because of the similar efficacy of narrow band ultraviolet B (NBUVB) phototherapy as compared with PUVA phototherapy in the treatment of psoriasis, the availability of UVA light boxes in dermatology offices is diminishing. Psoralen intercalates with DNA and, after UVA exposure, forms mono- or bifunctional adducts to pyrimidine bases and cross-links between strands of DNA. In addition to interfering with DNA synthesis and the subsequent death of neoplastic T cells,[500] PUVA may have other effects, including a direct cytotoxic effect, immunomodulation,[501] and the induction of apoptosis in peripheral blood lymphocytes.[502]

Approximately 1 to 2 hours after ingesting 8-MOP, patients are exposed to increasing doses of UVA light, initially in the range of 1.5 to 3.0 J/cm^2 based on the patient's skin type (I-VI) determined from skin color and sun sensitivity or, less commonly, based on the direct measurement of a patient's minimal phototoxic dose.[500] Treatments are given at a frequency of two to three times per week until complete clearing occurs, followed by a maintenance regimen with increasing intervals between treatments over 2 to 7 months.[500,503] In a small study, the number of patients in the relapse vs the nonrelapse group receiving maintenance therapy was the same.[504] Therefore, the risk of increased cumulative UVA dose in patients treated with maintenance therapy must be balanced against the potential side effects.

In their combined analysis of five studies reflecting the response of 244 patients with CTCL to PUVA, Herrmann et al reported the following CR rates for each stage: IA, 54/60 (90%); IB, 88/116 (76%); IIA, 7/9 (78%); IIB, 16/27 (59%); III, 11/18 (61%); IVA, 4/10 (40%); IVB, 0/4 (0%).[500] Median time to CR was 3 months in the study of Herrmann et al.[503] Patients with early-stage disease readily respond to PUVA, but relapse among complete responders is common, affecting ~31%, 56%, and 71% of stage IA, IB, and IIA patients, respectively.[503] In a retrospective review of 104 patients with early-stage MF treated with PUVA, Querfeld et al reported a 63% CR rate, although 50% relapsed on maintenance PUVA therapy.[504] Even higher relapse rates were seen in erythrodermic patients treated with PUVA alone. Tumor-stage (IIB) patients usually require localized radiation therapy or systemic chemotherapy to achieve a significant response and PUVA should play only an adjunctive role. Approximately one-third of relapsing stage IA patients will achieve a second long-lasting disease-free remission with reinitiation of PUVA, whereas ~22% of stage IB patients can be expected to do the same.[500,503] Hermann et al reported the same 5- and 10-year survival rates of 89%, 78%, and 100% for stages IA ($n = 19$), IB ($n = 49$), and IIA ($n = 6$) patients, respectively, and a 5-year survival rate of 80% for stage III ($n = 6$) patients.[503] A recent systemic review of phototherapy for MF found PUVA to be safe, effective, and well tolerated for the management of early-stage MF.[505] In an attempt to minimize side effects, Weber et al evaluated 16 patients who received bath PUVA. Patients were treated with 30 mL of 0.5% alcoholic 8-MOP in 150 L of water; all 16 patients achieved a CR.[506]

Acute side effects of PUVA include delayed (24 hours) burning and erythema (10%), pruritus (7%), nausea due to psoralen (4%), and reactivation of herpes simplex (2%).[500] The photosensitivity due to psoralen may last up to 24 hours, and patients should wear protective clothing and sunscreens to prevent sunburn. Potential complications to long-term PUVA therapy include cataract formation, nonmelanoma skin cancer (8%-10%), benign solar lentigos (4%), actinic keratoses, keratoacanthomas (3%), and vitiligo (2%).[500,503] Because of the potential of PUVA to induce cataracts, patients are instructed to wear ultraviolet light–blocking eyeglasses for 24 hours. BCC and SCC of the skin can be expected to occur in 8% to 10% of patients receiving PUVA after several years, with a clear predominance of SCC, unlike the general population.[500,503] More importantly, the risk of invasive and noninvasive melanoma skin cancer increases substantially after 250 PUVA treatments and appears to increase with the passage of time.[507]

Wide-band ultraviolet B phototherapy (WBUVB) (280-320 nm wavelength) has also been used effectively to treat patients with stage I CTCL[508] but has largely been replaced by NBUVB phototherapy.[509]

Studies have established the effectiveness of NBUVB phototherapy (311-312 nm wavelength) in the management of early MF.[510] NBUVB was first introduced in 1984 with the Philip TL-01 lamp as the optimal wavelength for antipsoriatic activity.[511] NBUVB treatment has a lower carcinogenic potential and is associated with less erythema than PUVA and WBUVB, respectively.[512-515] One in vitro study, however, reported cyclobutane pyrimidine dimer (CPD) formation, a sign of carcinogenicity, following a minimum erythema dose by NBUVB was significantly higher than that following 1 MED by WBUVB, whereas the formation of (6-4) photoproducts and 8-oxoG following WBUVB was significantly higher than those following NBUVB exposure. These results suggest that CPD formation is closely related to higher carcinogenic characteristics of NBUVB.[516]

In the initial clinical report, Clark et al reported a CR in six of eight patients with MF treated with NBUVB.[517] Since that time, several larger studies have emerged. Gathers et al evaluated 24 patients with stage IA/IB disease; 13 (54%) achieved a CR, 7 (29%) achieved a partial response (PR), and 4 (17%) had no response. In the four patients who achieved a CR and discontinued therapy, the average time to relapse was 12.5 weeks.[518] In two comparative studies of NBUVB and PUVA in stage IA/IB disease, no difference in CR rates were observed in patients receiving NBUVB or PUVA.[519,520] Pavlotsky et al conducted a retrospective analysis of patients with stage IA/IB disease receiving NBUVB and WBUVB. CR was seen in 84% and 89% of stage IA patients receiving NBUVB and WBUVB, respectively. The CR dropped to 78% and 44% in patients with stage IB disease. Once maintenance therapy was stopped, 65% were relapse free at 27 weeks. The study found no difference in relapse rates regardless of use of maintenance therapy.[521] Other small series of patients with early-stage MF treated with NBUVB therapy have been reported, with CR rates of 57% to 100% (for patch-stage disease) and relapse rates of ~50%.[513,522-524] Side effects of NBUVB therapy were minor and did not require discontinuation of therapy. Gathers et al report erythema in 42% of patients and pruritus in 29% of patients.[518] Permanent tan freckles (lentigines) and white macules (idiopathic guttate hypomelanosis) have also been reported recently as side effects of NBUVB.[525-527] In early MF, there is no statistically significant difference between the response to oral PUVA and NBUVB.[528] NBUVB is a safe and effective treatment of stage IA/IB MF, especially patch-stage disease. In addition, several studies have confirmed the safety of NBUVB in children as opposed to PUVA phototherapy, which should be avoided.[529,530]

Retinoids

Retinoids are a class of pharmaceuticals whose structure and function resemble vitamin A and its metabolites. Vitamin A and its analogues, the retinoids, have antiproliferative activity, may induce cellular maturation, and probably modulate immune response.[531,532] Isotretinoin (13-cis-retinoic acid) and etretinate, a monoaromatic retinoid compound no longer available, have demonstrated similar efficacy in the treatment of CTCL.[533] Three clinical trials have demonstrated overall objective clinical responses in 66 of 113 patients (58%) treated with isotretinoin or etretinate and a CR in 19%.[533-535] Median duration of response, however, has ranged from 3 to >8 months.[535] Etretinate is no longer available and has largely been replaced with its metabolite, acitretin, because of its superior safety profile. Acitretin may reduce the thick palmoplantar keratoderma of advanced MF or SS.[531]

In 1999 the US Food and Drug Administration (FDA) approved the use of bexarotene capsules, a novel retinoid, for the treatment of CTCL. Unlike isotretinoin and acitretin, which bind to nuclear retinoic acid receptor (RAR), bexarotene binds to and activates the nuclear retinoid X receptor (RXR) and is therefore referred to as a "rexinoid." RXRs are unique in that they form heterodimers with a vast array of nuclear receptors including the RARs, liver X receptors (LXRs), and peroxisome proliferator activator receptors.[536,537] The ultimate antiproliferative effect is mediated, in part, by the induction of apoptosis and expression of adhesion molecules.[538] Two multicenter clinical trials established the optimal dose of 300 mg/m^2/d, with an ORR of 45%.[539,540] Higher response rates were seen in patients with higher initial doses (up to 650 mg/m^2), but side effects of hypertriglyceridemia were dose limiting. Subsequent pancreatitis occurred in 4 of the 152 patients enrolled in the two clinical trials.[539,540] The advanced-stage CTCL trial showed a relapse rate of 36% but an impressive median duration of response of 299 days.[539]

Talpur et al summarized the experience of treating 70 patients with CTCL using bexarotene capsules as monotherapy and combined with other modalities.[541] Many of the patients participated in the two pivotal clinical trials. The overall response rate seen in the monotherapy group (n = 54) was 48%, in contrast to the 69% response rate in the combination-therapy group. Bexarotene was safely added to photopheresis (extracorporeal photochemotherapy [ECP]), ECP/IFN, IFN/PUVA, and ECP/IFN/PUVA. Adverse effects were similar between the clinical trials and included hypertriglyceridemia (87%), central hypothyroidism requiring thyroid supplementation (80%),[542,543] neutropenia (41%),[544] skin peeling (43%), hypercholesterolemia (20%), and pancreatitis (3%). Seventy-eight percent of the monotherapy group (n = 54) and 100% of the combination-therapy group (n = 16) required at least one lipid-lowering agent (LLA). Of the 10 patients with diabetes, 3 had hypertriglyceridemia that could not be controlled with an LLA.[541] In this series, atorvastatin and fenofibrate were the LLAs of choice. Interestingly, 9 of 10 (90%) patients on bexarotene monotherapy taking two LLAs responded, which was significantly higher than those groups on one or no LLA (P = .0001). The explanation for this finding is not clear, but using two LLAs may allow patients to maintain maximum doses of bexarotene.[541] The utility of bexarotene in managing patients with CTCL has been summarized more recently.[544,545]

Vigilance for rhabdomyolysis should be exercised when combining atorvastatin and fenofibrate. In contrast, omega-3 fatty acids may be combined with other LLAs to effectively manage hypertriglyceridemia in patients receiving bexarotene.[546] Gemfibrozil and drugs that inhibit the CYP 3A4 enzyme are contraindicated with bexarotene, to avoid elevated drug levels and worsened side effects. Although patients taking bexarotene are at increased risk for elevated triglycerides, elevated low-density lipoprotein, and decreased high-density lipoprotein, there are very few reports to date indicating an increased risk of cardiac events.[547] Several animal studies have shown that bexarotene may have a favorable pharmacological effect on atherosclerosis despite the induction of hypertriglyceridemia via LXR,[548] via a beneficial action on intestinal absorption and macrophage efflux,[549] inhibition of the initial inflammatory response that precedes the atherogenic process by targeting different steps of the mononuclear recruitment cascade,[536] and protective effects against H_2O_2-induced apoptosis in H9c2 rat ventricular cells through antioxidant and mitochondria-protective mechanisms.[550]

Bexarotene is also available as a 1% gel. The gel formulation is most helpful in early-stage patients (IA) without prior therapies. In a phase 1/2 multicenter trial, bexarotene 1% gel was applied to lesional skin with increasing frequency, once daily the first week and twice daily the second week, with a goal of four times daily if tolerated.[551] Patients achieved an ORR of 63% and a clinical CR of 21%. Median projected time to onset of response was 20.1 weeks (range, 4.0-86.0 weeks), and the estimated median response duration from the start of therapy was 99 weeks.[551] The most common side effect was irritation (retinoid "paint splatter" dermatitis) at the sites of application, which might make it difficult to assess response to the drug. The study was followed by a phase 3 study that included patients with stages IA/B and IIA disease. The ORR was 44% according to the Physicians Global Assessment. Similar to the previous study, the median time to response was 142 days (range, 28-505 days) and the relapse rate in responding patients was 26%. The most frequent adverse response was irritant dermatitis, which occurred more frequently in patients applying the drug more frequently.[552] Overall, topical bexarotene is a moderately effective and well-tolerated treatment of early-stage MF most often used for refractory patches or thin plaques. The retinoid dermatitis may obscure evaluation of the patches of MF so patients should be instructed to avoid enlarging the original treatment area and to stop applying the gel 1 to 2 weeks before clinical evaluation.

Interferon

Interferons (IFNs) are glycoproteins, naturally occurring or synthesized by recombinant DNA technology. These agents act as immunomodulators with both cytostatic and antiviral activity.[553] Although three classes, IFN-α, IFN-β, and IFN-γ, are described, the IFN-α class has been most extensively studied in MF and SS, and their efficacy was first reported by Bunn et al in 1984.[554] The exact mechanism of action of IFN in MF and SS is unknown. Interferon may act to inhibit IL-4 and IL-5 production by normal and aberrant T cells in patients with SS, induce myelomonocytic My7 antigen (CD13) in epidermal basal cells,[555] induce the ds-RNA-dependent enzyme 2'5'-oligoadenylate synthetase leading to cleavage of cellular RNAs, and phosphorylate eIF-2, a peptide elongation initiation factor that blocks protein synthesis.[553] The pharmacokinetics of IFN delivered via the intramuscular and subcutaneous routes are equivalent, allowing patients the opportunity to self-administer the drug subcutaneously.

Treatment of MF and SS with IFN-α has been reported in >200 patients, and the results have been summarized.[553] The ORR for IFN-α alone was 52%, with a 17% CR among 207 patients with MF and SS, summarized by Bunn et al.[556] Over three-quarters of the patients received IFN-α2a, which is no longer available in the United States, although there were no apparent differences in clinical efficacy between IFN-α2a and IFN-α2b (Intron-A, Schering-Plough Research Institute).[553,556] However, interpretation of pooled data is complicated by variations in initial dose, target dose, frequency, and length of therapy among study centers.[553]

In an attempt to define the optimal dose of IFN-α in CTCL, a randomized study from Duke and Northwestern Universities was designed comparing low dose (3 MU/d) to escalating doses (up to 36 MU/d); however, because of slow patient accrual, the proposed study was terminated.[557] For the 22 patients evaluated, the objective response rate was 64% and was greater, although not statistically significant, for those receiving high doses (11 of 14) than for those receiving low doses (3 of 8), in part because of late responses in unresponsive patients who crossed over into the higher-dose arm.[556,557] Of interest, two of the three CR patients were induced by the low-dose regimen, suggesting that patients could achieve a CR with 3 million units (MU) daily of IFN-α2a.[553,557]

Daily dosing of IFN-α2a for an induction period of several months was used by all of the larger studies of IFN-treated CTCL patients,[558,559] whereas many fewer patients have been studied using an initial three times-a-week schedule.[560-562] Nonetheless, some authorities[556] recommend an optimal dose of 3 MU of IFN-α2a three times a week, based in part on randomized dose studies in B-cell indolent NHL showing no benefit of higher-dose interferon with respect to response rate or duration.[563] Maximum daily dosing is dependent on several patient factors but, in general, should not exceed 15 MU.[564] About 2 to 5 months is generally necessary to obtain an objective response with IFN, but a CR or maximal response can take much longer.[553,558] Treatment is generally continued for ~1 year after a CR to prevent the high potential for relapse when treatment is discontinued before clearing.[553] Three studies have reported a median duration of response to IFN-α as follows: 6 months,[565] 8 months,[559] and 14 months.[558] Olsen et al noted a mean duration of PR while on therapy of 7.9 months (range, 2.1-26.5 months) and durations of CR off therapy ranging from 4 to 28 months.[553] The numerous side effects associated with IFN have led to dose reductions in 50% to 86% of patients in some studies.[557,566] A more recent study in 377 patients with relapsed/refractory CTCL demonstrated that IFN-α2b (5 MU three times a week) combined with either all-trans retinoic acid or methotrexate 15 mg twice a week both led to 80% response rates.[567]

Recombinant IFN-γ and IFN-β have been studied in many fewer patients with CTCL, as they appear to offer no major advantage over IFN-α.[568-570] IFN-β has reportedly shown little effectiveness in treating CTCL,[568] and IFN-γ has been linked with more intense and frequent side effects than IFN-α.[553] Interestingly, it has been demonstrated in vitro that the combination of IFN-γ and a Toll-like receptor (TLR) 7/8 agonist increases NK-cell cytotoxic activity against CTCL cell lines.[571] This combination of the two therapies led to an increase in IL-12 and IFN-α levels, which was regulated through IFN regulating factor 8.[571]

Electron Beam Radiotherapy and Photon Beam Irradiation

Radiation was one of the earliest effective treatments for MF, first reported in 1902.[572] In 1953, Trump et al were first to suggest using accelerated electrons for treatment.[573] Modern total-skin electron beam radiotherapy (TSEBRT) is among the most effective and well-studied therapies for MF.[574] The total skin surface can be treated by linear accelerator–generated electron beams that are scattered by a penetrable plate at the collimator site.[574] The usual depth of penetration is <10 mm and is proportional to the energy of the electrons generated, allowing effective dosing to the skin and adnexal structures without internal organ toxicity.[574] The most common technique uses a dual fixed-angle six-field or rotation methods with 4- to 9-MeV electrons, with total doses in the range of 2400 to 3600 cGy over an 8- to 10-week period.[574] With this technique, relatively lower doses are delivered to the scalp, soles, and areas of self-shielding such as the ventral penis, perineum, upper medial thighs, perianal skin, inframammary folds, and folds under any pannus.[574] Only the eyes are routinely shielded, and unless there is involvement of the head and neck, a scalp shield is used after a dose of 2500 to 2600 cGy has been delivered, to decrease the degree of alopecia. The hands, forearms, ankles, and dorsal penis may receive doses >100%, and shielding all of these structures for part of TSEBRT is not uncommon.[574] Recently, low-dose regimens of TSEBRT (10-12 Gy in 8-12 fractions) approach the response rates of the high-dose therapy and allow repeat therapy to be given more safely.[575,576]

The long-term results of 561 patients with MF treated at Stanford University and Hamilton Regional Cancer Centre from the mid-1950s to 1993 with TSEBRT alone were summarized by Jones et al.[577] Over 80% of stage IA patients can be expected to achieve a CR after TSEBRT, with 40% to 60% remaining relapse-free at 5 years.[577] Two other studies showed similar CR rates, ranging from 80% to 90% for IA and IB disease.[578,579] Less encouraging were the relapse-free rates, at 2.5 years for stages IB (35%-40%), IIA (21%-37%), IIB (7%-26%), and III (10%-23%).[577] However, most patients who relapse with what is usually minimal disease will reenter remission with other topical therapies.[577] In these studies, a new diagnosis of MF, low stage, lack of blood involvement, and intensity of TSEBRT were independently associated with progression-free survival (PFS).[577,578] TSEBRT was less effective in advanced-stage disease (II–IV), with a CR rate of 60%.[578] Another report suggests that prognosis for tumor-stage patients with <10% skin involvement treated with TSEBRT is significantly better than for patients with >10% involvement.[580]

Acute cutaneous side effects, peaking 1 to 2 weeks after TSEBRT, include erythema, edema, dry or moist desquamation, tenderness, and rare blister formation that is most severe at sites of disease.[574] Total-body alopecia and loss of nails will occur in all unshielded patients, but the skin appendages will normally regrow within 6 months.[574] During the first year, heat intolerance may develop as a result of the suppression of sweat gland production, which may be permanent.[581] Patients with erythroderma (T4) may experience more severe acute side effects from TSEBRT; however, radiation may be effective in stage III, especially with no blood involvement.[582] When there is blood, lymph node, or visceral involvement in patients with erythroderma, combined-modality therapies, in particular photopheresis, should be explored.[583] Chronic cutaneous side effects most commonly include xerosis, superficial atrophy, telangiectasia, and dyspigmentation.[581] The role of TSEBRT in the development of secondary cutaneous malignancies has not been clearly established, as most patients have received a variety of therapies that could contribute to the development of skin cancer.[574]

Several studies have evaluated the response and toxicity of multiple courses of TSEBRT for CTCL, with similar results.[579,584] Wilson et al[585] reported on 14 patients with CTCL, 5 receiving three courses of TSEBRT and 9 receiving two courses. The total median dose was 5700 cGy (range, 4500-8200 cGy) with 86% (n = 12) achieving a CR after the second course of therapy (median relapse-free interval, 11.5 months) and three of five (60%) achieving a CR after a third course (limited follow-up).[585]

Because of the toxicities of TSEBRT and the effectiveness of topical therapies, most authorities recommend using TSEBRT for patients with progressive disease, those failing topical therapies, or patients with extensive, deeply infiltrated plaques and tumors.[578,586] Because of the high relapse rates after TSEBRT, posttreatment with nitrogen mustard, PUVA, photopheresis, or oral bexarotene have been studied to maintain remissions.[578,583,587] A recent retrospective study of patients with MF who received TSEBRT (n = 180, T2 and T3 skin stage) from Stanford University found no difference in outcomes between those who received adjunctive topical nitrogen mustard to prevent relapse and those patients who did not.[584]

Small-field megavoltage photon beam irradiation can be applied as palliation to either deep-seated cutaneous lesions in the tumor phase or for extracutaneous disease.[588] A single dose of 1.0 Gy can lead to a PR and a single dose of 8.0 Gy can achieve a CR of 94.4%.[589] Nearly all cutaneous lesions respond completely, with the risk of relapse (up to 45%) being inversely proportional to the dose, and with recurrence usually developing within 2 years of treatment.

Photopheresis or Extracorporeal Photochemotherapy

Because of the development of resistance to conventional chemotherapy and radiation and the high potential for relapse in advanced-stage patients, new modalities to treat CTCL have been developed. Leukapheresis, which had been used in patients with high Sézary cell counts, was the forerunner for a new adaptation of PUVA called extracorporeal photochemotherapy (ECP) or photopheresis. In the original protocol, patients ingested 8-MOP prior to undergoing fractionation of their blood. A leukocyte-enriched blood fraction was then isolated and exposed to UVA in an extracorporeal system, which photoactivated the psoralen.[590] The photopheresis procedure currently performed uses liquid 8-MOP injected directly into the collection bag containing the enriched white blood cell fraction to achieve a concentration of 340 ng/mL within the collection bag. All treated and untreated blood products are then returned to the patient.

In 1987, Edelson et al were the first to report responses in 27 of 37 patients (64%) with resistant CTCL treated with ECP, including 8 of 10 patients with lymph node involvement and 24 of 29 patients with erythroderma. However, patients with extensive plaques or tumors did not respond as well (three of eight patients).[590]

The immunomodulatory mechanism underlying patient response to ECP is still under debate. However, evidence currently supports the following two simultaneous and synergistic processes occurring during ECP: induction of apoptosis in malignant T cells and a mass conversion of blood monocytes to dendritic cells (DCs).[591,592] Animal studies demonstrate that ECP induces a CD8+ T-cell response against expanded clones of pathogenic T cells,[593] as well as an increased synthesis of class I MHC molecules on murine T-cell lymphoma cells.[594] In vitro studies using family-specific monoclonal antibodies and magnetic bead technology demonstrated a tumor-specific cytolytic CD8+ T-cell response to distinctive class I surface peptides on CTCL tumor cells of four patients with advanced disease. These results suggest that reduced class I expression of relevant tumor antigen epitopes may limit the extent of CD8+ T cell–mediated cytolysis.[595] In support of this hypothesis, investigators have found a favorable response to correlate with the following two scenarios at the onset of ECP: normal or near-normal numbers of CD8+ peripheral blood T cells[596] and a lower CD4 to CD8 ratio in the peripheral blood.[597]

Other investigators have found that ECP and in vitro PUVA induce apoptosis in peripheral blood lymphocytes but not in monocytes.[502] The apoptosis induction mechanism remains unknown but may be explained by the observation that a significant amount of TNF-α, which mediates various antitumor effects, is produced by macrophages following ECP.[598] Berger et al identified monocytes transitioning to immature DCs during overnight incubation in gas-permeable bags of ECP-treated white blood cells from five patients with intractable CTCL.[599] Both the initial leukapheresis step as well as the subsequent passage through the narrow photoactivation plate initiated and contributed to monocytes-to-DC differentiation.[599,600] Edelson proposed that the innumerable encounters of monocytes with the plastic surface of the photoactivation plate activated the cells to begin differentiation to immature DCs.[591] An immature DC can engulf an apoptotic T cell and present tumor antigen via MHC class I molecules, which stimulates a potent antitumor CD8 T-cell response.[591,592,600-602]

Treatment of CTCL with ECP has been reported in >400 patients and summarized.[603-606] The majority of patients with CTCL treated with ECP have generalized erythroderma (skin stage T4), a finding most likely due to the encouraging preliminary study results of Edelson et al.[603] A combined analysis of >400 patients treated with ECP and adjunctive therapies showed an ORR for all stages of CTCL of 55.7% (244 of 438), with 17.6% (77 of 438) achieving a CR.[603] Efficacy in treating certain clinical stages (IB, IIA, III, and IVA) and skin stages (T2 and T4) of MF and SS is favorable, although randomized trials comparing ECP with other standard therapies are needed. Combined analysis of five North American series[590,607-611] of ECP-treated CTCL patients ($N = 157$) demonstrates an objective response (>25% improvement of skin lesions) in 67 of 111 stage T4 patients (60%), with ~20% achieving a CR. A long-term follow-up study of the original 29 erythrodermic patients with CTCL in the report of Edelson et al[590] demonstrated a median survival of 60 months, which compared favorably with historical controls.[597] Many authorities recommend that ECP be considered the first line of treatment of erythrodermic-stage patients.[612-614] However, other authorities differ in their opinions regarding the role of ECP in the treatment of CTCL, stating that the data have been inconsistent and the need for prospective randomized studies.[615-617]

Preliminary and long-term follow-up studies by Zic et al on 20 patients with refractory CTCL treated with ECP and adjunctive therapies demonstrated an objective response (>50% clearing of skin lesions) in 9 of 14 (64%) early-stage T2 patients, with CR in 4.[607,618] Talpur and colleagues reported the results of a prospective study of 19 patients with MF stages IA, IB, and IIA who were treated with photopheresis administered 2 days every 4 weeks for 6 months.[619] Patients with PRs by skin-weighted assessment continued for an additional 6 months while nonresponders added oral bexarotene and/or IFN-α. The overall response rate was 42%, and the authors concluded that ECP is effective for patients with early-stage MF alone or in combination with biologic response modifiers with low toxicity and improved quality of life.[619] Other studies support a trial of ECP in early-stage patients with refractory disease.[620,621] Observations by other investigators, however, question the use of ECP to treat stage IB patients when less expensive and more widely accessible therapies are available.[622-624]

ECP is well tolerated, with few complications or adverse effects.[603,614] Uncommon adverse reactions are usually vascular related and include the fluid-responsive hypotension and venipuncture-site hematomas.[618] Rarely, adverse reactions have included exacerbation of congestive heart failure or arrhythmias,[612] superficial thrombophlebitis,[612] catheter-related sepsis,[625] herpes infections,[612] disseminated fungal infection,[612] and a single episode of hemolysis.[607]

Several studies have focused on the effects of combining ECP with systemic chemotherapy, PUVA, IFN and other cytokines,[626-628] radiation therapy, oral bexarotene with and without IFN,[629,630] and HN2. Raphael and colleagues summarized their experience treating 98 patients with SS with at least 3 months of photopheresis and 1 or more systemic immunostimulatory agents (INF-α, oral retinoids, IFN-γ, granulocyte-macrophage colony-stimulating factor).[631] A total of 73 patients (75%) responded (30% CR, 45% PR), and a lower CD4 to CD8 ratio, a higher percentage of monocytes, and lower numbers of circulating abnormal T cells at baseline were the strongest predictive factors for CR compared with nonresponse.[631] A much smaller cohort of patients with SS ($n = 12$) showed a lower response rate of 42%, and the parameters that correlated best with response were number of Sézary cells, CD4 to CD8 ratio, and white blood cell count.[632] McGirt and colleagues found that increased eosinophils and decreased percentages of Sézary cells were associated with a favorable clinical response to ECP, but they were not able to identify the predictors of ECP response within the first 3 months of treatment.[633]

Systemic Chemotherapy

Single-agent and combination chemotherapy are reserved for patients who have advanced-stage (IIb-IVb), REL or refractory disease or are part of a clinical trial.[634,635] Treatments that maintain or augment the immune response, such as IFN, bexarotene, and ECP, may be preferable over chemotherapy, which is immunosuppressive. Sequential use of single agents should be considered over combinations since CTCL is chronic and the clinical goals are control of the disease, amelioration of pruritus, and prevention of skin breakdown; however, combination chemotherapy may be warranted if the disease is progressive, extensive, or advanced stage.[635-638] There is no consensus about the optimal order of single agents or combination regimens.[634] In a retrospective series of MF (53% with advanced stage), IFN had the longest time to next treatment at 8.7 months ($P < .00001$) and histone deacetylase (HDAC) inhibitors (HDIs) had a slight advantage over other chemotherapy agents (4.5 vs 3.9 months, $P = .01$).[639]

Previously, single agents used for MF/SS were the same as those used in all types of NHL and included oral corticosteroids, alkylating agents, and methotrexate, but median response durations were short.[629,640] Daily or pulse chlorambucil with a steroid has been used to successfully treat SS.[641,642] In two retrospective series using weekly low-dose oral methotrexate, Zackheim et al reported a 33% response rate (12% CR) in T2 skin disease and a 55% response rate (41% CR) in erythrodermic CTCL with time to progression and OS of 15 and 31 months, respectively.[643,644] Etoposide has shown activity in a small reported series, where the ORR was 69% but response durations were short (43 weeks).[645]

A number of novel agents have shown activity in CTCL, including nucleoside analogues, HDIs, the antifolate pralatrexate, CD25- and CD30-targeted recombinant toxins, and pathway-directed agents.

HDIs were shown to have activity in T-cell lymphomas in phase 1 trials by Piekarz et al at the National Cancer Institute (NCI).[646,647] HDIs cause histone hyperacetylation, alter chromatin structure, and modulate gene expression.[648] They also acetylate nonhistone proteins such as p53 and downmodulate cytokines such as IL-10, both of which contribute to apoptosis of cancer cells.[648-650] HDI can be divided into six groups based on their chemical structures, and it is unknown whether pan-HDAC inhibition (HDACi) or more selective HDACi is better in treating malignancies.[651] Two HDIs have been approved for therapy in REL CTCL, vorinostat (Zolinza, Merck & Co, Whitehouse Station, NJ; suberoylanilide hydroxamic acid), a relatively nonselective inhibitor of HDAC, and romidepsin (Istodax, formerly depsipeptide; Bristol Myers Squib, Summit, NJ), a specific inhibitor of class I HDAC enzymes.[649]

Vorinostat was approved for the treatment of REL CTCL in October 2006. The maximum tolerated daily oral dose of vorinostat was 400 mg given orally on a daily basis. In a phase 2 trial of 33 patients with heavily treated CTCL (median number of prior systemic therapy = 5), Duvic et al reported an ORR of 24% (all PR) and an additional 33% had stable disease (SD) or pruritus relief, or both.[652] In a multicenter phase 2 trial in 74 patients treated with at least two previous systemic therapies, the ORR was similar at 29.7%.[653] The median time to progression was 4.9 and 9.8 months for responders with stage IIB-IVB disease. The adverse effects for the two phase 2 trials were diarrhea (49%-60%), fatigue (46%-78%), nausea (43%-60%), thrombocytopenia (22%-54%), and dysgeusia (24%-51%). Grade 3/4 adverse events were thrombocytopenia (5%-19%), dehydration (1%-8%), and pulmonary embolism (5%).[652,653] Cardiac complications have been reported including QT prolongation.[654] Vorinostat has been evaluated in combinations with bexarotene, bortezomib, and lenalidomide.[648,655] A recent randomized trial comparing vorinostat with mogamulizumab, a novel CCR4-directed monoclonal antibody, demonstrated a lower overall response rate for vorinostat, with an overall response rate of 5% and a PFS of 3.1 months when a global assessment scoring was used.[656] In that study, 16% of patients had response (CR or PR) in the skin and 14% had response in the blood compartment of the disease.

Romidepsin was approved for the treatment of relapsed CTCL in November 2009.[657,658] In two phase 2 trials in REL CTCL patients ($n = 71$ and 96), the ORRs were 34% in both, including 6% CR in both, and the median durations were 13.7 and 15.4 months.[659,660] Both studies used a dose of 14 mg/m^2 as a 4-hour infusion weekly times 3 every 4 weeks.

Adverse events (all grades) for romidepsin were nausea (52%-54%), fatigue (41%-42%), emesis (19%-26%), anorexia (20%-21%), diarrhea (8%-14%), and ageusia (13%-19%). There was concern that HDI, including romidepsin, would have significant prolongation of the QT interval and risk of arrhythmia, but the studies found minimal risk; however, antiemetics that prolong QT should be limited and the potassium and magnesium levels should be normalized before romidepsin infusion.[661]

Other isoform-specific HDIs have been developed and are in clinical trials for T-cell lymphomas. Belinostat is a hydroxamic acid type of HDI that reported an ORR of 14% in CTCL and 25% in PTCL.[662-665] Panobinostat is also a hydroxamic acid HDI with both intravenous and oral formulations and had a 60% ORR in a study of 10 patients with CTCL[666]; however, a larger study of 95 patients reported only 16% ORR.[667]

Pralatrexate (Folotyn; Allos Therapeutics Inc) is a novel antifolate with a high affinity for the reduced folate carrier 1, which is overexpressed in neoplastic cells. Pralatrexate inhibits dihydrofolate reductase, an enzyme involved in the synthesis of deoxythymidine and the purine DNA nucleotides, and promotes apoptosis. Pralatrexate received approval in September 2009 for relapsed or refractory PTCL at a dose of 30 mg/m^2 weekly for 6 or 7 weeks.[668] A de-escalation trial identified an effective dose of 15 mg/m^2 weekly for 3 or 4 weeks in patients with REL CTCL.[669] The ORR was 45% (13/29: 1 CR, 12 PR); 73% of responses were continuing at 6 months by Kaplan-Meier estimate. The main toxicities were mild except for mucositis (48% all grades, 17% grade 3). To reduce mucositis, vitamin B12 and folate supplementation are started before therapy with pralatrexate. A recent study demonstrated that the addition of leucovorin given the day following each dose of pralatrexate significantly ameliorated mucositis.[670] Skin flare after pralatrexate occurs in up to 21% of patients and responds to topical or oral corticosteroids.[669] Ongoing trials are investigating combination therapies that incorporate pralatrexate. A combination of pralatrexate with bexarotene reported a response rate of 60% (4 CR, 14 PR) with a response duration of 29 months. The major toxicity was mucositis.[671] A number of nucleoside analogues have demonstrated activity in T-cell lymphomas and in CTCL. Gemcitabine at a dose of 1200 mg/m^2 on days 1, 8, and 15 of a 28-day cycle had a 70% ORR, including 10% CR and a median response duration of 8 months, and 83% of patients with tumor-stage MF had a response in the first two cycles.[672] Side effects with gemcitabine included neutropenia (34%), thrombocytopenia (25%), cutaneous hyperpigmentation (17%), and elevated liver enzymes (13%).[672] Another phase 2 trial with lower doses (1000 mg/m^2 on days 1, 8, and 15 for six cycles) demonstrated a similar response rate (68%) and side-effect profile.[673] Marchi et al reported a high ORR of 78% including 22% CR, when gemcitabine was administered to patients who had no prior systemic therapy.[674] The combination of gemcitabine, liposomal doxorubicin (Doxil), and vinorelbine was also found to be effective in a small number of patients with advanced disease.[675] The purine nucleoside analogues 2-deoxycoformycin (DCF or pentostatin) and fludarabine monophosphate (FAMP) have activity in CTCL.[676,677] Dosing of DCF has varied among studies and yields an ORR of 33% to 71% with approximately one-third of the responses being CR.[678] The median time to progression ranges from 1.3 to 8.3 months, and there appears to be a better response in SS than in MF.[678,679] The most common side effects are granulocytopenia, renal insufficiency, and prolonged CD4 lymphopenia. A combination study of DCF with high-dose IFN resulted in an ORR of 41% with a median PFS of 13.1 months.[680]

Fludarabine as a single agent has demonstrated response rates of 19% to 29.5%[681]; however, response rates improved in small series when FAMP was combined with IFN (51%), cyclophosphamide (42%), or ECP (63%).[681-683] The median PFS for IFN and ECP were 5.9 and 13 months, respectively.[681,682]

Forodesine is a selective purine nucleoside phosphorylase inhibitor and causes increased levels of deoxyguanosine and deoxyguanosine triphosphate, which inhibit T-cell proliferation.[684,685] In a phase 1 intravenous trial of 13 patients with CTCL, there were 4 responses (3 CR, 1 PR) and 6 with SD. In a phase 1/2 trial using an oral formulation at 80 mg/m^2 once daily, the objective response rate was 53.6% (2 CR, 13 PR, and 22 SD).[686] However, in a large phase 2 trial in patients who had received three or more treatments, forodesine had limited activity with an ORR of 11% (no CR; 50% with SD) and a median time to progression of 6.3 months.[687] In addition, one-third of patients had serious adverse events and there were increased infections (49%), a few of which were fatal.

Pegylated liposomal doxorubicin,[688] Doxil, has shown activity as a single agent in patients with relapsed/refractory MF/SS. At a dose of 20 mg/m^2 once a month, 60% of patients experienced a CR, 10%

PR, and 10% SD.[689] In a retrospective review of 34 patients using doses of 20 to 40 mg/m^2 every 2 to 4 weeks, the ORR was 88% (44% CR + CRu [patients who achieved a CR defined by clinical criteria only with no biopsy] and 44% PR) with an OS of 17.8 months and event-free survival of 12 months.[690] Adverse events were reported in 41% of patients with 17% grade 3/4, including only one with palmar-plantar erythrodysesthesias. The ORR in a phase 2 trial was lower at 41% (6% CR), but Doxil is considered to be one of the more effective single agents for CTCL.[691]

Bortezomib (Velcade; Millennium Pharmaceuticals, Boston, MA), a proteasome inhibitor, downregulates NF-κB activation and causes apoptosis of CTCL cell lines.[692] In a phase 2 trial of 12 REL patients (10 MF, 2 PTCL with skin involvement), the ORR was 67% (2CR, 6PR) and all responses were durable, lasting from 7 to > 14 months.[693] There were no grade 4 toxicities, and the grade 3 toxicities were neutropenia ($n = 2$), thrombocytopenia ($n = 2$), and sensory neuropathy ($n = 2$). A phase 1 trial of bortezomib, gemcitabine, and liposomal doxorubicin reported a PR in six of seven REL CTCL patients.[694] The combination of bortezomib with the HDI vorinostat induced apoptosis in CTCL and was associated with an upregulation of cell cycle regulating proteins p21 and p27, an increased expression of phosphorylated p38, and a suppression of vascular endothelial growth factor by tumor cells.[695] It has also been combined with romidepsin in a phase 1 trial since it prevents romidepsin-induced NF-κB activation.[696]

Temozolomide, an oral derivative of dacarbazine that causes DNA damage by methylating nucleotide bases, has demonstrated some efficacy in the treatment of CTCL. This alkylating agent produces O^6-alkylguanine adducts, which are deactivated by O^6-alkylguanine-DNA alkyltransferase (AGT), a DNA repair enzyme often found in tumor cells. Dolan et al found that patients with MF demonstrated lower-than-expected levels of AGT in tumor cells, thus emphasizing temozolomide's potential therapeutic efficacy in this specific malignancy.[697] In a phase 2 trial, nine patients were treated with 150 mg/m^2 of temozolomide orally for 5 days for the first 4-week cycle and then 200 mg/m^2 of temozolomide for 5 days for the second and third 4-week cycle. A total response rate of 33% was observed with two patients developing grade 3 hematopoietic toxicities.[698] In a larger trial of 26 REL patients using the 200 mg/m^2 dosing schedule, the ORR was 27% (2 CR, 5 PR); the median DFS and OS were 4 and 24 months, respectively.[699] The response did not correlate with levels of AGT. The most common grade 1/2 toxicities were gastrointestinal, and treatment was stopped in three patients due to grade 3 thrombocytopenia, lymphopenia, and skin reaction.

Owing to its immunomodulatory effects such as NK- and T-cell activation and induction of T$_H$1 cytokine production, lenalidomide has been investigated in CTCL. In a phase 2 trial of refractory patients, the ORR was 28% (no CR) with a median OS of 43 months and PFS of 8 months.[700] In a small phase 3 trial comparing maintenance lenalidomide with observation following debulking chemotherapy in advanced-stage patients, lenalidomide had a slight advantage with a PFS of 5.3 vs 2 months with observation.[701]

Combination chemotherapy regimens tend to be reserved for REL, aggressive, and advanced-stage MF/SS. Responses occur in the 40% to 89% range but are brief with PFS in the 5- to 9-month range.[702-704] In a phase 2 trial of etoposide, prednisone, vincristine, cyclophosphamide, doxorubicin (EPOCH) in 15 refractory patients with CTCL, including 4 ALCL, the ORR was 80% (4 CR, 8 PR); the median PFS was 8.0 months and the median OS was 13.5 months.[704] Infectious complications, including staphylococcal bacteremia related to open skin lesions, are a significant problem for patients receiving combination chemotherapy.

Combined-Modality Therapy

Because there is no single therapy for CTCL that can consistently induce long-lasting remissions, various combinations of therapeutic modalities have been studied.

Following TSEBRT, subsequent PUVA therapy appears to aid in maintaining remission status in patients with CTCL. A significant benefit in DFS but no statistically significant improvement in OS was observed. However, prospective, randomized data are needed to confirm these results. Incidentally, PUVA has also demonstrated effectiveness as a salvage therapy after TSEBT in early-stage patients with recurrence, with acceptable toxicity.[705] Elsayed et al showed significant increased median PFS for 27 patients with CTCL who received oral bexarotene after TSEBRT compared with 19 patients who received TSEBRT alone.[587]

The most significant study to evaluate the role of combined modality therapy was that of Kaye et al at the NCI in the 1980s comparing TSEBRT and combination chemotherapy (cyclophosphamide, doxorubicin, etoposide, and vincristine) with conservative topical therapy (beginning with topical HN2 followed sequentially, if needed, by PUVA, TSEBRT, and combination chemotherapy) in a randomized trial of 103 patients with MF.[706] Although the rate of CR was significantly increased in the combined modality arm (38% vs 10%, $P = .032$), toxicity was greater and no significant difference was noted between the groups in DFS or OS. Thus, this study indicated that, similar to other low-grade lymphomas, early aggressive therapy in MF does not have a major impact on survival.

A nonrandomized study from Yale University compared relapse-free survival (RFS) and OS between patients with CTCL who achieved a CR following TSEBRT, with subsequent treatment consisting of adjuvant chemotherapy (cyclophosphamide and doxorubicin; $n = 77$), photopheresis ($n = 11$), or no adjuvant therapy ($n = 43$).[707] Adjunctive therapy was also offered to 32 patients who achieved a "good PR" to TSEBRT. The statistical analysis found no appreciable impact on RFS among the patients receiving adjuvant chemotherapy or photopheresis when compared with patients receiving no adjuvant therapy. However, a marginally significant ($P < .06$) improvement on OS was demonstrated when stage T3/T4 patients treated with adjuvant photopheresis ($n = 7$) were compared with stage T3/T4 patients receiving no adjuvant therapy ($n = 22$).[707]

Retinoids and IFN-α have been combined to treat CTCL in several open studies.[708-710] Combined analysis of the results of 102 reported patients treated with retinoids and IFN-α showed that approximately 60% of patients respond and 10% achieve a CR, which is similar to the response for IFN-α alone.[556] PUVA phototherapy has been combined with systemic retinoids to treat CTCL demonstrating response rates similar to PUVA alone.[711] Bexarotene has been combined with ECP, PUVA phototherapy,[712] and IFN-α in several patients with potential beneficial effects, as well as no increased toxicity.[541,713]

The combination of PUVA and IFN-α is well tolerated and generates impressive CR rates.[714-716] In the combined analysis of the phase 1 and phase 2 trials of IFN-α and PUVA for CTCL at Northwestern University, 39 patients with CTCL (stage IB, $n = 14$; IIA, $n = 5$; IIB, $n = 6$; III, $n = 8$; IVA, $n = 5$; IVB, $n = 1$) received intramuscular or subcutaneous IFN-α2a three times a week at initial intermediate doses (6 MU, $n = 3$; 12 to 18 MU, $n = 13$; 21 to 30 MU, $n = 23$) with subsequent dose reduction in 19 patients due to apparent toxicity.[714] IFN-α was continued for the planned 2-year period in only 10 of 39 patients (26%) with 8 patients receiving four or less months of IFN-α due to tumor progression, toxic effects, or patient request. PUVA was initiated three times per week and tapered to one monthly treatment indefinitely for patients achieving a CR. The objective ORR was 90% with 24 patients (62%) achieving a pathologically confirmed CR, 15 of whom had early-stage disease (stage IB/IIA). Nineteen patients (54%) relapsed demonstrating a median duration of response of 28 months (range, 1-64 months). Median survival for the entire cohort was 62 months with mean survivals for stage I/II and stage III/IV patients of 55 and 35 months, respectively.[714] Thus, although patients respond impressively, a majority of patients will relapse despite maintenance PUVA and experience nontrivial toxicities at higher doses of interferon. The overall impact on survival of combined PUVA and IFN-α has yet to be determined.

A prospective phase 2 trial examined escalating doses of IFN-α2a combined with PUVA in 63 symptomatic patients representing all stages of MF and SS.[716] Fifty-one patients achieved a CR (74.6%) or PR (6%), with a median response duration of 32 months. The 5-year OS rate was 91% and included 17 patients with advanced disease.[716]

Rupoli et al completed a multicenter prospective phase 2 clinical study on 89 patients with early-stage IA to IIA MF treated for 14 months with low-dose IFN-α2b (6-18 MU/wk) and PUVA.[717] Complete remission was achieved in 84% and an ORR in 98% of cases. Long-term CR was associated with high epidermal CD1a+ dendritic-cell density ($P = .030$), and high CD8+ lymphoid T-cell density was associated with a lower relapse rate ($P = .002$).[717]

Stadler and colleagues completed a prospective randomized multicenter trial to compare IFN plus PUVA and IFN plus acitretin in stage I and II patients with CTCL (n = 82 evaluable patients).[718] Interferon-α2a was administered subcutaneously at 9 MU three times weekly and combined with either PUVA at an initial interval of five times weekly, or with acitretin up to 50 mg daily. Interferon-α + PUVA (n = 40) was significantly superior to the IFN + acitretin (n= 42), as marked by a 70% complete remission rate in the former, vs a 38.1% complete remission rate in the latter.[718] A recent report appeared to suggest that elevated levels of the cutaneous T-cell attracting chemokine CTACK/CCL27 in skin and sera after combined PUVA and IFNα-2b therapy might be correlated with risk of recurrence.[30] Reports have emerged of the successful combination of low-dose bexarotene and phototherapy. Narrow-band UVB phototherapy has been combined with oral bexarotene with success in one recent case.[719] The successful combination of oral bexarotene with PUVA phototherapy has also been reported.[541,712,713,720-726] Recently, a randomized, open-label, two-parallel-group, active-control specified clinical study in patients diagnosed with CTCL compared 22 patients treated with bexarotene monotherapy with 24 patients treated with bexarotene and with bath-PUVA or narrowband UVB.[727] The ORR was similar in both groups, but the combined therapy arm showed a higher skin resolution rate.

Immunotherapy

Over the past decade, researchers have developed immunotherapies to correct abnormalities and also directly stimulate the immune response in patients with CTCL. As described in previous sections, recombinant forms of natural cytokines such as interferons and immunomodulation with photopheresis and more recently the blockade of inhibitor pathways in the host immune response have all shown promise in the treatment of CTCL, with tolerable toxicity profiles and reasonable efficacy. This section focuses on other cytokines and monoclonal antibody–based therapies for the treatment of CTCL.

Denileukin diftitox (DD) was the first immunotherapy approved for T-cell lymphoma. DD is a recombinant fusion protein consisting of the full-length sequence of interleukin-2 and the toxin and membrane translocating domains of diphtheria toxin. DD targets the intermediate- and high-affinity isoforms of the interleukin receptor and is internalized via receptor-mediated endocytosis and translocated into the cytosol where the toxin moiety induces cell death by inhibition of protein synthesis.[728] The interleukin-2 receptor (IL-2R) is present in low-, medium-, and high-affinity isoforms on normal and neoplastic T cells. The high-affinity IL-2R has been a specific target that is commonly present on cells in ATLL.[729] Approximately 60% of patients with CTCL demonstrate expression of IL-2R on their tumor cells.[730,731]

A pivotal phase 3 trial evaluated the safety, efficacy, and pharmacokinetics of two dose levels of DD (9 and 18 μg/kg/d for 5 days on a 21-day cycle) in REL/refractory CTCL stage IB-IV.[732] For study inclusion, patients had to have detectible CD25 on ≥25% of their tissue biopsy lymphocytes via immunoperoxidase assay. The overall response rate was 30% (20% PR and 10% CR), and there was no difference in efficacy or tolerability between the doses. The median response duration was 6.9 months, range 2.7-46.1+ months.[732] Upon stratification with respect to disease stage, 18 μg/kg/d of DD proved more effective in treating stage IIB patients (36% OR) than the lower dose (23% OR).[732] A phase 3, placebo-controlled trial, again evaluating the two dosing regimens of 9- and 18-μg/kg/d, was performed with 144 patients with CD25+ earlier-stage CTCL.[733] The ORR was higher in the 18-μg/kg/d group as compared with the 9-μg/kg/d group (49.1% vs 37.8%), and both were higher than placebo (15.9%).[733] There was also increased estimated PFS in the 18-μg/kg/d group vs the 9-μg/kg/d group (32.4 vs 26.5 months), but the adverse events were similar for both dosing arms.[733] This study, importantly, reported results from placebo treatment of CTCL and, not surprisingly, the placebo group had significantly fewer adverse events and reduced PFS. Side effects of DD have included reversible elevated hepatic transaminases (15% with grade 3 or 4) and constitutional symptoms (fever/chills, nausea/vomiting, and arthralgias/myalgias) seen in 92% of patients in the pivotal trial. A delayed vascular leak syndrome (hypoalbuminemia, edema, and hypotension) was seen in 25% of patients in the same patient population. Acutely, hypersensitivity reactions during infusion may show as dyspnea, back pain, chest pain, and hypotension. As noted above, pretreatment of these patients with steroids make acute hypersensitivity reactions less likely. Bone marrow suppression or secondary immunosuppressive effects have not been noted as significant adverse events related to denileukin diftitox.[728,732] Infections were seen in 56% of subjects. However, 80% of these infections were typical in patients with advanced-stage or heavily pretreated CTCL and were thus not attributed to therapy.[732] Currently, a new formulation of DD, E7777, has been manufactured with improved purity and more active protein monomer species. A phase 1/2 study has been completed and shows similar efficacy.[734,735]

Resimmune, a second-generation recombinant immunotoxin (composed of catalytic and translocation domains of diphtheria toxin fused to two single chain antibody fragments reactive with the extracellular domain of CD3ε), had a 36% ORR (16% CR) in 25 patients with CTCL.[736] Similar to DD, vascular leak syndrome occurred in 40% of patients with 7% grade 4/5. Reactivation of cytomegalovirus or EBV was seen in 23% and elevated transaminases in 20%.

Alemtuzumab (CAMPATH-1H), a monoclonal antibody directed against CD52, has been studied in the treatment of advanced, low-grade NHLs, including CTCL. This humanized antibody targets T and B lymphocytes, and it appears to have a predilection for circulating cells, relatively sparing those localized within lymph nodes.[41,737] Two small phase 2 studies evaluated the safety and efficacy of alemtuzumab in stage IIB to IV disease. Kennedy et al reported a 38% ORR, whereas Lundin reported a 55% ORR. Both studies used 30 mg twice-weekly dosing. The time to progression and the time to treatment failure were short in both studies, at <4 and 12 months, respectively.[738,739] A more recent open-label trial from Querfeld et al treated 19 patients with erythrodermic CTCL with escalating IV doses of alemtuzumab up to a maximum of 30 mg, three times weekly, for 4 weeks, followed by 8 weeks of subcutaneous administration.[740] The ORR was 84%, with 47% having a CR. Similar to previous studies, the median PFS was 6 months. Significant side effects occurred, including grade 3 to 4 cytopenias, cardiac events, and severe infections.[740,741]; however, Lundin et al did not experience any adverse cardiac events in their study patients.[742] The side-effect profile for alemtuzumab includes significant neutropenia with subsequent increased susceptibility to opportunistic infections and bacterial septicemia, thus limiting its utility in the treatment of advanced-stage patients with compromised immune systems.[738,739,743,744] Although subcutaneous low-dose alemtuzumab shows promise in the setting of SS, larger clinical trials are needed to clarify the role of alemtuzumab in the treatment of CTCL.[162,744-748] In a multicenter retrospective analysis examining the long-term efficacy, 39 patients (SS; n = 23, MF; n = 16) received alemtuzumab 30 mg two to three times per week for a median duration of 12 weeks (range 1-35). There was a 51% ORR with better response found in SS as compared with MF (70% vs 25%). The median time to progression was 3 to 4 months, and six patients (SS, n = 5; MF, n = 1) remained progression free for >2 years.[749]

Brentuximab vedotin ([BV]; Adcetris, Seattle Genetics) is an antibody-drug conjugate targeting the CD30 receptor. BV contains a chimeric IgG1 mAb CAC10 specific for human CD30; the microtubule disrupting agent MMAE; and a protease cleavable covalent linker that attaches the antibody to MMAE.[750] A phase 2 trial of BV in 58 patients with REL ALCL (72% ALK negative) reported an objective response in 86% of patients including 57% CR and 29% PR.[751] The median durations of OR and CR were 12.6 and 13.2 months, respectively. Grade 3 or 4 adverse events were neutropenia (21%), thrombocytopenia (14%), and peripheral sensory neuropathy (12%). In a phase 2 open-label trial of 48 patients with CD30+ LPDs including LyP and primary cutaneous pc-ALCL (pc-ALCL) or CD30+ MF, brentuximab demonstrated an ORR of 71% (34/48) with 35% of patients achieving a complete remission.[752] Interestingly, there was no correlation between the degree of CD30 expression and response as reported subsequently.[753]

A phase 3 open label randomized trial was conducted to evaluate the efficacy of BV in patients with CD30-expressing CTCL. The study (ALCANZA) enrolled 97 patients with CD30+ MF and 21 with PCALCL.[754] Patients were randomized to receive brentuximab vedotin 1.8 mg/kg once every 3 weeks up to 16 cycles or physician's choice (methotrexate 5-50 mg once weekly or bexarotene capsules 300 mg/m^2 once daily) for up to 48 weeks. Patients with CD30+ MF achieved an objective response lasting at least 4 months in 50% (brentuximab arm) and 10% (physician's choice arm). Of note, 63% of patients receiving brentuximab with tumor-stage CD30+ MF achieved an objective response lasting at least 4 months vs 5% in the physician's choice arm. Patients with PCALCL achieved an objective response lasting at least 4 months in 75% (brentuximab arm) and 20% (physician's choice arm). Peripheral neuropathy was diagnosed in 67% (n = 44) of patients receiving brentuximab (9% grade 3). At last follow-up (median 22.9 months) 36 (82%) of 44 patients had improvement (≥1 grade) or resolution of the peripheral neuropathy.[754,755]

Mogamulizumab (Poteligeo, Kyowa Kirin, Tokyo, Japan) is another FDA-approved immunotherapy for CTCL. Mogamulizumab is a humanized defucosylated anti-CCR4 monoclonal antibody with enhanced antibody-dependent cellular cytotoxicity, which targets the CCR4 chemokine receptor, expressed on CTCL as well as Tregs and other populations of normal T-lymphocytes. The drug demonstrated an overall response rate of 50%, including 31% CR in patients with HTLVL-1-associated adult T-cell leukemia, which demonstrates a high level of expression of CCR4.[756] Adverse events included infusion reactions (89%) and skin rashes (63%). In a phase 1/2 study of 41 pretreated patients with CTCL, there was no dose-limiting toxicity and the dose in the phase 2 part was 1.0 mg/kg weekly for 4 weeks followed by every 2 weeks until progression.[757] The ORR rate was 36.8, higher in SS (47.1%) compared with MF (28.6%). A randomized phase 3 trial (MAVORIC trial) of mogamulizumab compared with vorinostat was conducted in patients with CTCL irrespective of the level of CCR4 expression. The study enrolled 372 patients with REL or refractory stage IB-IVB MF or SS to receive mogamulizumab 1 mg/kg weekly (n = 186) for the first 28-day cycle, followed by every other week for subsequent cycles or vorinostat 400 mg daily (n = 186), with a crossover for patients who progressed in the vorinostat arm.[656] The median PFS was 7.7 months in the mogamulizumab arm vs 3.1 months in the vorinostat arm, and the ORR in the mogamulizumab arm was 28%, with a higher response rate in SS (37% ORR) than in patients with predominantly skin involvement (ORR 21%). Compartment responses were 68% in blood, 42% in skin, and 17% in lymph nodes. Infusion reactions and drug-mediated immune skin rash were the most common adverse events.[758,759] Mogamulizumab has now become a preferred treatment of patients with SS.[760,761]

IPH4012 is a novel humanized monoclonal antibody targeting the KIR3DL2 receptor, which is expressed on NK cells and on Sézary leukemia cells.[762,763] In a phase 1 study of 44 patients with advanced CTCL of which 35 had SS, the maximum dose was 75 mg IV and toxicities included lymphopenia and fatigue.[228] The ORR was 36%, and the response in patients with SS was 43%. Like mogamulizumab, this novel antibody holds promise as an effective therapy for patients with circulating Sézary cells, and a larger confirmatory trial is underway.

In addition to monoclonal antibodies, there have been efforts to harness the patients' own immune system to enhance the cytotoxic antitumor response. Utilizing TLRs and additional cytokines to stimulate NK cells, in vitro studies have shown increased cellular death in CTCL lines.[571] A phase 1 trial initially evaluated the use of a TLR9 agonist in patients with treatment-refractory CTCL (stage IB-IVA), using a dose escalation ranging from 0.08 to 0.36 mg/kg in 24 weekly subcutaneous injections.[764] Common side effects included rigors, cytopenias, and pyrexia. Although the trial was not designed to evaluate for efficacy, they did identify a 32% overall response rate, of which most lasted for the duration of the study (24 weeks).[764] More recently, a phase 1/2 study combined an intratumoral injection of a TLR9 agonist with radiation (to enhance tumor immunogenicity) in a cohort of 15 patients with MF (stage IA-IVA) who had failed at least one standard therapy.[765] They again found a 33% ORR, and the therapy was well tolerated with mild injection site reaction or flu-like symptoms.[765]

Checkpoint inhibitors target the inhibitory pathways of the immune response and include the cytotoxic T lymphocyte–associated protein 4 (CTLA-4) inhibitor, ipilimumab, as well the inhibitors of programmed death-1 (PD-1) and programmed death-ligand 1 (PD-L1), nivolumab, pembrolizumab, atezolizumab, and others. In a study of patients with relapsed lymphoma, nivolumab 13 patients with MF were treated with nivolumab. Two (15%) had a PR, whereas the majority of patients (69%) had stable disease.[766] Pembrolizumab was evaluated in a multicenter phase 2 trial that enrolled 24 patients with MF and SS.[767] The ORR was 38% (1 CR and 8 PR). An additional nine patients (38%) had stable disease. The median time to response was 11 weeks; median duration of response was 14 months, and 2-year PFS was 69%. Skin flare occurred in patients with SS, especially with Sézary cells showing high PD-1 expression. Pembrolizumab is now being studied in combination with radiation therapy and other biological agents.[768,769]

Hematopoietic Cell Transplantation

Hematopoietic stem cell transplantation (HCT) has been increasingly explored using various donor sources, donor sites, and therapeutic conditioning regimens as an option for patients with advanced and refractory CTCL. See Chapter 90 for a full discussion of HCT. Earlier data with autologous stem cell transplant showed no benefit, with a high relapse rate, and thus autologous stem cell transplant is not considered an acceptable treatment of MF/SS.[770-772]

Allogeneic stem cell transplantation is an immunotherapy that relies on a graft-vs lymphoma effect from minor HLA-mismatched antigen recognition by donor cells toward malignant lymphoma cells. Early studies demonstrated a graft-vs-lymphoma effect in six of eight patients treated with ablative conditioning.[773] Retrospective transplant registry reviews from the Center for International Blood and Marrow Transplant Research (CIBMTR) and the European Group for Blood and Marrow Transplantation (EBMT) described outcomes for 129 and 137 patients with MF/SS, respectively, who underwent allogeneic stem cell transplant.[774,775] All patients had relapsed or refractory disease, and about 60% received reduced-intensity conditioning. The PFS at 1 year were 31% and 34%, respectively, and at 5 years were 17% and 26%, respectively. A more recent US multicenter review of 66 patients with MF/SS undergoing allo-BMT reported a 5-year PFS of 18% and OS of 44%.[776]

The use of TSEBRT as part of allogeneic conditioning for allotransplant in patients with MF/SS has been pioneered at MD Anderson Cancer Center, who reported results in 42 patients.[777] The ORR was 58% with 79% response in SS. Of those patients who had total skin radiation prior to transplant, 58% achieved a CR.[778] Another study reported results using total skin radiation prior to conditioning with a reduced-intensity pentostatin/TBI regimen. Of 16 patients with MF/SS, there were 8 CR and OS and DFS were 75% and 62%, respectively.[779]

Another novel regimen reported by Weng et al incorporated total skin radiation followed by total lymphoid irradiation and antithymocyte globulin as a conditioning regimen.[780] In this study, 35 patients with MF/SS were enrolled and MRD status was determined by TCR sequencing before and after transplant. Forty-three percent of patients achieved MRD in blood and skin at a median time to MRD of 146 days. The risk of progression was much lower (13%) for MRD-negative CR patients compared with MRD-positive patients (75%). Donor lymphocyte infusions and a second allo-BMT resulted in long-term survival in some of the patients who had progression. These results suggest that allogeneic stem cell transplant has the capacity to induce long-term remissions and potential cure in a subset of patients with MF/SS and should be considered as a potentially curative modality in transplant eligible patients.

SUMMARY AND FUTURE INVESTIGATIONS

Molecular studies are unraveling the complex interactions of cytokines, adhesion molecules, and the immune system responsible for the pathogenesis of CTCL and are continuing to provide insight for novel approaches to treatment. As with other indolent lymphomas, an array of therapies can produce responses in CTCL but are generally not curative. In contrast to other lymphomas, however, there is a high degree of efficacy with topical treatments (HN2, TSEBRT, NBUVB, and PUVA phototherapies) for patients with early-stage MF/SS. Because CTCL is not cured by systemic chemotherapy, initial management of early-stage disease should include skin-directed therapy. Ongoing clinical trials may define the roles of systemic therapy in managing more advanced-stage patients including combinations of skin-directed therapies, photopheresis, retinoids, monoclonal antibodies, chemotherapy agents, and HCT.

References

1. Lutzner M, Edelson R, Schein P, Green I, Kirkpatrick C, Ahmed A. Cutaneous T-cell lymphomas: the Sezary syndrome, mycosis fungoides, and related disorders. *Ann Intern Med.* 1975;83(4):534-552.
2. Edelson RL. Cutaneous T-cell lymphomas: clues of a skin-thymus interaction. *J Invest Dermatol.* 1976;67(3):419-424.
3. Alibert JL. *Description des Maladies de la Peau: Observees a l'Hospital St. louis et Exposition des Meilleurs Methodes Suivies pour leur Traitement.* Barrois l'aine et Fil; 1806.
4. Alibert MLB. *Monographie des Dermatoses*, Vol Tome Second. Daynac; 1832.
5. Bazin E. *Lecons sur le Traitement des Maldies Chroniques en General affections de la Peau en Particular par l'Emploi Compare des Eaux Minerales de l'Hydrotherapie et des Moyens Pharmaceutiques.* Adrien Delahaye; 1870.
6. Vidal E, Brocq L. Etude sur le mycosis fongoide. *La France Me'dical.* 1885;2:946-1019.
7. Hallopeau H. Sur une e'rythrodermie chronique a' pousse'es aigue; de'but probable d'un mycosis fongoide. *Bull Soc Franc de Dermat et Syph.* 1890;1:220.
8. Besnier E, Hallopeau H. On the erythroderma of mycosis fungoides. *J Cutan Genitourin Dis.* 1892;10:453.
9. Stelwagon HW, Hatch JL. A study of mycosis fungoides with a report of two cases. *J Cutan Genitourin Dis.* 1892;10(1):57-64.
10. Tilden GH. So-called mycosis fongoide. *Boston Med Surg J.* 1885;2:386-392.
11. Sezary A, Bouvrain Y. Erythrodermia avec presence de cellules monstreuses dans le derme et le sang circulant. *Bull Soc Fr Dermatol Syphil.* 1938;45:254.
12. Taswell HF, Winkelmann RK. Sezary syndrome—a malignant reticulemic erythroderma. *J Am Med Assoc.* 1961;177:465-472.
13. Lutzner MA, Jordan HW. The ultrastructure of an abnormal cell in Sezary's syndrome. *Blood.* 1968;31(6):719-726.
14. Crossen PE, Mellor JE, Finley AG, Ravich RB, Vincent PC, Gunz FW. The Sezary syndrome: cytogenetic studies and identification of the Sezary cell as an abnormal lymphocyte. *Am J Med.* 1971;50(1):24-34.
15. Broome JD, Zucker-Franklin D, Weiner MS, Bianco C, Nussenzweig V. Leukemic cells with membrane properties of thymus-derived (T) lymphocytes in a case of Sezary's syndrome: morphologic and immunologic studies. *Clin Immunol Immunopathol.* 1973;1(3):319-329.
16. Brouet JC, Flandrin G, Seligmann M. Indications of the thymus-derived nature of the proliferating cells in six patients with Sezary's syndrome. *N Engl J Med.* 1973;289(7):341-344.
17. Broder S, Edelson RL, Lutzner MA, et al. The Sezary syndrome: a malignant proliferation of helper T cells. *J Clin Invest.* 1976;58(6):1297-1306.
18. Heald PW, Yan SL, Edelson RL, Tigelaar R, Picker LJ. Skin-selective lymphocyte homing mechanisms in the pathogenesis of leukemic cutaneous T-cell lymphoma. *J Invest Dermatol.* 1993;101(2):222-226.
19. Vowels BR, Cassin M, Vonderheid EC, Rook AH. Aberrant cytokine production by Sezary syndrome patients: cytokine secretion pattern resembles murine Th2 cells. *J Invest Dermatol.* 1992;99(1):90-94.
20. Saed G, Fivenson DP, Naidu Y, Nickoloff BJ. Mycosis fungoides exhibits a Th1-type cell-mediated cytokine profile whereas Sezary syndrome expresses a Th2-type profile. *J Invest Dermatol.* 1994;103(1):29-33.
21. Vowels BR, Lessin SR, Cassin M, et al. Th2 cytokine mRNA expression in skin in cutaneous T-cell lymphoma. *J Invest Dermatol.* 1994;103(5):669-673.
22. Lessin SR, Vowels BR, Rook AH. Th2 cytokine profile in cutaneous T-cell lymphoma. *J Invest Dermatol.* 1995;105(6):855-856.
23. Hansen ER. Immunoregulatory events in the skin of patients with cutaneous T-cell lymphoma. *Arch Dermatol.* 1996;132(5):554-561.
24. Takahashi N, Sugaya M, Suga H, et al. Thymic stromal chemokine TSLP acts through Th2 cytokine production to induce cutaneous T-cell lymphoma. *Cancer Res.* 2016;76(21):6241-6252.
25. Rubio Gonzalez B, Zain J, Rosen ST, Querfeld C. Tumor microenvironment in mycosis fungoides and Sezary syndrome. *Curr Opin Oncol.* 2016;28(1):88-96.
26. Wolk K, Mitsui H, Witte K, et al. Deficient cutaneous antibacterial competence in cutaneous T-cell lymphomas: role of Th2-mediated biased Th17 function. *Clin Cancer Res.* 2014;20(21):5507-5516.
27. Ransohoff RM, Kivisakk P, Kidd G. Three or more routes for leukocyte migration into the central nervous system. *Nat Rev Immunol.* 2003;3(7):569-581.
28. Kim EJ, Hess S, Richardson SK, et al. Immunopathogenesis and therapy of cutaneous T cell lymphoma. *J Clin Invest.* 2005;115(4):798-812.
29. Saeki H, Tamaki K. Thymus and activation regulated chemokine (TARC)/CCL17 and skin diseases. *J Dermatol Sci.* 2006;43(2):75-84.
30. Goteri G, Rupoli S, Campanati A, et al. Serum and tissue CTACK/CCL27 chemokine levels in early mycosis fungoides may be correlated with disease-free survival following treatment with interferon alfa and psoralen plus ultraviolet A therapy. *Br J Dermatol.* 2012;166(5):948-952.
31. Narducci MG, Scala E, Bresin A, et al. Skin homing of Sezary cells involves SDF-1-CXCR4 signaling and down-regulation of CD26/dipeptidylpeptidase IV. *Blood.* 2006;107(3):1108-1115.
32. Miyagaki T, Sugaya M, Fujita H, et al. Eotaxins and CCR3 interaction regulates the Th2 environment of cutaneous T-cell lymphoma. *J Invest Dermatol.* 2010;130(9):2304-2311.
33. Uccini S, Ruco LP, Monardo F, La Parola IL, Cerimele D, Baroni CD. Molecular mechanisms involved in intraepithelial lymphocyte migration: a comparative study in skin and tonsil. *J Pathol.* 1993;169(4):413-419.
34. Sarris AH, Esgleyes-Ribot T, Crow M, et al. Cytokine loops involving interferon-gamma and IP-10, a cytokine chemotactic for CD4+ lymphocytes: an explanation for the epidermotropism of cutaneous T-cell lymphoma? *Blood.* 1995;86(2):651-658.
35. Pals ST, de Gorter DJJ, Spaargaren M. Lymphoma dissemination: the other face of lymphocyte homing. *Blood.* 2007;110(9):3102-3111.
36. Nickoloff BJ, Griffiths CE, Baadsgaard O, Voorhees JJ, Hanson CA, Cooper KD. Markedly diminished epidermal keratinocyte expression of intercellular adhesion molecule-1 (ICAM-1) in Sezary syndrome. *J Am Med Assoc.* 1989;261(15):2217-2221.
37. Vejlsgaard GL, Ralfkiaer E, Avnstorp C, Czajkowski M, Marlin SD, Rothlein R. Kinetics and characterization of intercellular adhesion molecule-1 (ICAM-1) expression on keratinocytes in various inflammatory skin lesions and malignant cutaneous lymphomas. *J Am Acad Dermatol.* 1989;20(5 pt 1):782-790.
38. Rook AH, Heald P. The immunopathogenesis of cutaneous T-cell lymphoma. *Hematol Oncol Clin North Am.* 1995;9(5):997-1010.
39. Sokolowska-Wojdylo M, Wenzel J, Gaffal E, et al. Circulating clonal CLA(+) and CD4(+) T cells in Sezary syndrome express the skin-homing chemokine receptors CCR4 and CCR10 as well as the lymph node-homing chemokine receptor CCR7. *Br J Dermatol.* 2005;152(2):258-264.
40. Campbell JJ, Clark RA, Watanabe R, Kupper TS. Sezary syndrome and mycosis fungoides arise from distinct T-cell subsets: a biologic rationale for their distinct clinical behaviors. *Blood.* 2010;116(5):767-771.
41. Clark RA, Watanabe R, Teague JE, et al. Skin effector memory T cells do not recirculate and provide immune protection in alemtuzumab-treated CTCL patients. *Sci Transl Med.* 2012;4(117):117ra117.
42. Girardi M, Heald PW, Wilson LD. The pathogenesis of mycosis fungoides. *N Engl J Med.* 2004;350(19):1978-1988.
43. Dummer R, Cozzio A, Urosevic M. Pathogenesis and therapy of cutaneous lymphomas—progress or impasse? *Exp Dermatol.* 2006;15(5):392-400.
44. Kantekure K, Yang Y, Raghunath P, et al. Expression patterns of the immunosuppressive proteins PD-1/CD279 and PD-L1/CD274 at different stages of cutaneous T-cell lymphoma/mycosis fungoides. *Am J Dermatopathol.* 2012;34(1):126-128.
45. Wong RM, Scotland RR, Lau RL, et al. Programmed death-1 blockade enhances expansion and functional capacity of human melanoma antigen-specific CTLs. *Int Immunol.* 2007;19(10):1223-1234.
46. Johnson LDS, Banerjee S, Kruglov O, et al. Targeting CD47 in Sézary syndrome with SIRPαFc. *Blood Adv.* 2019;3(7):1145-1153.
47. Yawalkar N, Ferenczi K, Jones DA, et al. Profound loss of T-cell receptor repertoire complexity in cutaneous T-cell lymphoma. *Blood.* 2003;102(12):4059-4066.
48. Edelson RL, Berger CL, Raafat J, Warburton D. Karyotype studies of cutaneous T cell lymphoma: evidence for clonal origin. *J Invest Dermatol.* 1979;73(6):548-550.
49. Nowell PC, Finan JB, Vonderheid EC. Clonal characteristics of cutaneous T cell lymphomas: cytogenetic evidence from blood, lymph nodes, and skin. *J Invest Dermatol.* 1982;78(1):69-75.
50. Mao X, Lillington DM, Czepulkowski B, Russell-Jones R, Young BD, Whittaker S. Molecular cytogenetic characterization of Sezary syndrome. *Genes Chromosomes Cancer.* 2003;36(3):250-260.
51. Karenko L, Sarna S, Kahkonen M, Ranki A. Chromosomal abnormalities in relation to clinical disease in patients with cutaneous T-cell lymphoma: a 5-year follow-up study. *Br J Dermatol.* 2003;148(1):55-64.
52. Mao X, Lillington D, Scarisbrick JJ, et al. Molecular cytogenetic analysis of cutaneous T-cell lymphomas: identification of common genetic alterations in Sezary syndrome and mycosis fungoides. *Br J Dermatol.* 2002;147(3):464-475.
53. Wain EM, Mitchell TJ, Russell-Jones R, Whittaker SJ. Fine mapping of chromosome 10q deletions in mycosis fungoides and Sezary syndrome: identification of two discrete regions of deletion at 10q23.33-24.1 and 10q24.33-25.1. *Genes Chromosomes Cancer.* 2005;42(2):184-192.
54. Lin WM, Lewis JM, Filler RB, et al. Characterization of the DNA copy-number genome in the blood of cutaneous T-cell lymphoma patients. *J Invest Dermatol.* 2012;132(1):188-197.
55. Scarisbrick JJ, Woolford AJ, Russell-Jones R, Whittaker SJ. Loss of heterozygosity on 10q and microsatellite instability in advanced stages of primary cutaneous T-cell lymphoma and possible association with homozygous deletion of PTEN. *Blood.* 2000;95(9):2937-2942.
56. Salgado R, Servitje O, Gallardo F, et al. Oligonucleotide array-CGH identifies genomic subgroups and prognostic markers for tumor stage mycosis fungoides. *J Invest Dermatol.* 2010;130(4):1126-1135.
57. Navas IC, Algara P, Mateo M, et al. p16(INK4a) is selectively silenced in the tumoral progression of mycosis fungoides. *Lab Invest.* 2002;82(2):123-132.

58. Scarisbrick JJ, Mitchell TJ, Calonje E, Orchard G, Russell-Jones R, Whittaker SJ. Microsatellite instability is associated with hypermethylation of the hMLH1 gene and reduced gene expression in mycosis fungoides. *J Invest Dermatol.* 2003;121(4):894-901.
59. van Doorn R, Zoutman WH, Dijkman R, et al. Epigenetic profiling of cutaneous T-cell lymphoma: promoter hypermethylation of multiple tumor suppressor genes including BCL7a, PTPRG, and p73. *J Clin Oncol.* 2005;23(17):3886-3896.
60. Rindler K, Jonak C, Alkon N, et al. Single-cell RNA sequencing reveals markers of disease progression in primary cutaneous T-cell lymphoma. *Mol Cancer.* 2021;20(1):124.
61. Zhang Y, Wang Y, Yu R, et al. Molecular markers of early-stage mycosis fungoides. *J Invest Dermatol.* 2012;132(6):1698-1706.
62. Huang Y, Su MW, Jiang X, Zhou Y. Evidence of an oncogenic role of aberrant TOX activation in cutaneous T-cell lymphoma. *Blood.* 2015;125(9):1435-1443.
63. Yu X, Luo Y, Liu J, Liu Y, Sun Q. TOX acts an oncological role in mycosis fungoides. *PLoS One.* 2015;10(3):e0117479.
64. McGirt LY, Degesys CA, Johnson VE, Zic JA, Zwerner JP, Eischen CM. TOX expression and role in CTCL. *J Eur Acad Dermatol Venereol.* 2016;30(9):1497-1502.
65. Dereure O, Levi E, Vonderheid EC, Kadin ME. Infrequent Fas mutations but no Bax or p53 mutations in early mycosis fungoides: a possible mechanism for the accumulation of malignant T lymphocytes in the skin. *J Invest Dermatol.* 2002;118(6):949-956.
66. Dummer R, Michie SA, Kell D, et al. Expression of bcl-2 protein and Ki-67 nuclear proliferation antigen in benign and malignant cutaneous T-cell infiltrates. *J Cutan Pathol.* 1995;22(1):11-17.
67. Tracey L, Villuendas R, Dotor AM, et al. Mycosis fungoides shows concurrent deregulation of multiple genes involved in the TNF signaling pathway: an expression profile study. *Blood.* 2003;102(3):1042-1050.
68. Witkiewicz A, Raghunath P, Wasik A, et al. Loss of SHP-1 tyrosine phosphatase expression correlates with the advanced stages of cutaneous T-cell lymphoma. *Hum Pathol.* 2007;38(3):462-467.
69. Mao X, Orchard G, Lillington DM, Russell-Jones R, Young BD, Whittaker SJ. Amplification and overexpression of JUNB is associated with primary cutaneous T-cell lymphomas. *Blood.* 2003;101(4):1513-1519.
70. Kiessling MK, Oberholzer PA, Mondal C, et al. High-throughput mutation profiling of CTCL samples reveals KRAS and NRAS mutations sensitizing tumors toward inhibition of the RAS/RAF/MEK signaling cascade. *Blood.* 2011;117(8):2433-2440.
71. Damsky WE, Choi J. Genetics of cutaneous T cell lymphoma: from Bench to Bedside. *Curr Treat Options Oncol.* 2016;17(7):33.
72. McGirt LY, Jia P, Baerenwald DA, et al. Whole-genome sequencing reveals oncogenic mutations in mycosis fungoides. *Blood.* 2015;126(4):508-519.
73. Tensen CP, Quint KD, Vermeer MH. Genetic and epigenetic insights into cutaneous T-cell lymphoma. *Blood.* 2022;139(1):15-33.
74. Choi J, Goh G, Walradt T, et al. Genomic landscape of cutaneous T cell lymphoma. *Nat Genet.* 2015;47(9):1011-1019.
75. Abraham RM, Zhang Q, Odum N, Wasik MA. The role of cytokine signaling in the pathogenesis of cutaneous T-cell lymphoma. *Cancer Biol Ther.* 2011;12(12):1019-1022.
76. Ungewickell A, Bhaduri A, Rios E, et al. Genomic analysis of mycosis fungoides and Sezary syndrome identifies recurrent alterations in TNFR2. *Nat Genet.* 2015;47(9):1056-1060.
77. Wang L, Ni X, Covington KR, et al. Genomic profiling of Sezary syndrome identifies alterations of key T cell signaling and differentiation genes. *Nat Genet.* 2015;47(12):1426-1434.
78. Vaque JP, Gomez-Lopez G, Monsalvez V, et al. PLCG1 mutations in cutaneous T-cell lymphomas. *Blood.* 2014;123(13):2034-2043.
79. Yasui DH, Genetta T, Kadesch T, et al. Transcriptional repression of the IL-2 gene in Th cells by ZEB. *J Immunol.* 1998;160(9):4433-4440.
80. Valencak J, Schmid K, Trautinger F, et al. High expression of Dicer reveals a negative prognostic influence in certain subtypes of primary cutaneous T cell lymphomas. *J Dermatol Sci.* 2011;64(3):185-190.
81. Ralfkiaer U, Hagedorn PH, Bangsgaard N, et al. Diagnostic microRNA profiling in cutaneous T-cell lymphoma (CTCL). *Blood.* 2011;118(22):5891-5900.
82. Ballabio E, Mitchell T, van Kester MS, et al. MicroRNA expression in Sezary syndrome: identification, function, and diagnostic potential. *Blood.* 2010;116(7):1105-1113.
83. Narducci MG, Arcelli D, Picchio MC, et al. MicroRNA profiling reveals that miR-21, miR486 and miR-214 are upregulated and involved in cell survival in Sezary syndrome. *Cell Death Dis.* 2011;2(4):e151.
84. van der Fits L, van Kester MS, Qin Y, et al. MicroRNA-21 expression in CD4+ T cells is regulated by STAT3 and is pathologically involved in Sezary syndrome. *J Invest Dermatol.* 2011;131(3):762-768.
85. McGirt LY, Adams CM, Baerenwald DA, Zwerner JP, Zic JA, Eischen CM. miR-223 regulates cell growth and targets proto-oncogenes in mycosis fungoides/cutaneous T-cell lymphoma. *J Invest Dermatol.* 2014;134(4):1101-1107.
86. Weiss LM, Hu E, Wood GS, et al. Clonal rearrangements of T-cell receptor genes in mycosis fungoides and dermatopathic lymphadenopathy. *N Engl J Med.* 1985;313(9):539-544.
87. Aisenberg AC, Krontiris TG, Mak TW, Wilkes BM. Rearrangement of the gene for the beta chain of the T-cell receptor in T-cell chronic lymphocytic leukemia and related disorders. *N Engl J Med.* 1985;313(9):529-533.
88. Wood GS, Haeffner A, Dummer R, Crooks CF. Molecular biology techniques for the diagnosis of cutaneous T-cell lymphoma. *Dermatol Clin.* 1994;12(2):231-241.
89. Holm N, Flaig MJ, Yazdi AS, Sander CA. The value of molecular analysis by PCR in the diagnosis of cutaneous lymphocytic infiltrates. *J Cutan Pathol.* 2002;29(8):447-452.
90. Groenen PJ, Langerak AW, van Dongen JJ, van Krieken JH. Pitfalls in TCR gene clonality testing: teaching cases. *J Hematop.* 2008;1(2):97-109.
91. Sandberg Y, van Gastel-Mol EJ, Verhaaf B, Lam KH, van Dongen JJM, Langerak AW. BIOMED-2 multiplex immunoglobulin/T-cell receptor polymerase chain reaction protocols can reliably replace Southern blot analysis in routine clonality diagnostics. *J Mol Diagn.* 2005;7(4):495-503.
92. Patel KP, Pan Q, Wang Y, et al. Comparison of BIOMED-2 versus laboratory-developed polymerase chain reaction assays for detecting T-cell receptor-gamma gene rearrangements. *J Mol Diagn.* 2010;12(2):226-237.
93. Yang H, Xu C, Tang Y, Wan C, Liu W, Wang L. The significance of multiplex PCR/heteroduplex analysis-based TCR-gamma gene rearrangement combined with laser-capture microdissection in the diagnosis of early mycosis fungoides. *J Cutan Pathol.* 2012;39(3):337-346.
94. Weng WK, Armstrong R, Arai S, Desmarais C, Hoppe R, Kim YH. Minimal residual disease monitoring with high-throughput sequencing of T cell receptors in cutaneous T cell lymphoma. *Sci Transl Med.* 2013;5(214):214ra171.
95. Kirsch IR, Watanabe R, O'Malley JT, et al. TCR sequencing facilitates diagnosis and identifies mature T cells as the cell of origin in CTCL. *Sci Transl Med.* 2015;7(308):308ra158.
96. Criscione VD, Weinstock MA. Incidence of cutaneous T-cell lymphoma in the United States, 1973-2002. *Arch Dermatol.* 2007;143(7):854-859.
97. Kaufman AE, Patel K, Goyal K, et al. Mycosis fungoides: developments in incidence, treatment and survival. *J Eur Acad Dermatol Venereol.* 2020;34(10):2288-2294.
98. Weinstock MA, Gardstein B. Twenty-year trends in the reported incidence of mycosis fungoides and associated mortality. *Am J Public Health.* 1999;89(8):1240-1244.
99. Bradford PT, Devesa SS, Anderson WF, Toro JR. Cutaneous lymphoma incidence patterns in the United States: a population-based study of 3884 cases. *Blood.* 2009;113(21):5064-5073.
100. Zackheim HS, McCalmont TH, Deanovic FW, Odom RB. Mycosis fungoides with onset before 20 years of age. *J Am Acad Dermatol.* 1997;36(4):557-562.
101. Boulos S, Vaid R, Aladily TN, Ivan DS, Talpur R, Duvic M. Clinical presentation, immunopathology, and treatment of juvenile-onset mycosis fungoides: a case series of 34 patients. *J Am Acad Dermatol.* 2014;71(6):1117-1126.
102. Pope E, Weitzman S, Ngan B, et al. Mycosis fungoides in the pediatric population: report from an international Childhood Registry of Cutaneous Lymphoma. *J Cutan Med Surg.* 2010;14(1):1-6.
103. Ai WZ, Keegan TH, Press DJ, et al. Outcomes after diagnosis of mycosis fungoides and Sezary syndrome before 30 years of age: a population-based study. *JAMA Dermatol.* 2014;150(7):709-715.
104. Tan E, Tay YK, Giam YC. Profile and outcome of childhood mycosis fungoides in Singapore. *Pediatr Dermatol.* 2000;17(5):352-356.
105. Fink-Puches R, Chott A, Ardigo M, et al. The spectrum of cutaneous lymphomas in patients less than 20 years of age. *Pediatr Dermatol.* 2004;21(5):525-533.
106. Nanda A, AlSaleh QA, Al-Ajmi H, et al. Mycosis fungoides in Arab children and adolescents: a report of 36 patients from Kuwait. *Pediatr Dermatol.* 2010;27(6):607-613.
107. Wu JH, Cohen BA, Sweren RJ. Mycosis fungoides in pediatric patients: clinical features, diagnostic challenges, and advances in therapeutic management. *Pediatr Dermatol.* 2020;37(1):18-28.
108. Morales Suarez-Varela MM, Olsen J, Kaerlev L, et al. Are alcohol intake and smoking associated with mycosis fungoides? A European multicentre case-control study. *Eur J Cancer.* 2001;37(3):392-397.
109. Aschebrook-Kilfoy B, Cocco P, La Vecchia C, et al. Medical history, lifestyle, family history, and occupational risk factors for mycosis fungoides and Sezary syndrome: the InterLymph Non-Hodgkin Lymphoma Subtypes Project. *J Natl Cancer Inst Monogr.* 2014;2014(48):98-105.
110. Gip L, Nilsson E. Clustering of mycosis fungoides in the county of Vasternorrland. *Lakartidningen.* 1977;74(12):1174-1176.
111. Litvinov IV, Tetzlaff MT, Rahme E, et al. Identification of geographic clustering and regions spared by cutaneous T-cell lymphoma in Texas using 2 distinct cancer registries. *Cancer.* 2015;121(12):1993-2003.
112. Moreau JF, Buchanich JM, Geskin JZ, Akilov OE, Geskin LJ. Non-random geographic distribution of patients with cutaneous T-cell lymphoma in the Greater Pittsburgh Area. *Dermatol Online J.* 2014;20(7):13030/qt4nw7592w.
113. Ghazawi FM, Netchiporouk E, Rahme E, et al. Comprehensive analysis of cutaneous T-cell lymphoma (CTCL) incidence and mortality in Canada reveals changing trends and geographic clustering for this malignancy. *Cancer.* 2017;123(18):3550-3567.
114. Ghazawi FM, Alghazawi N, Le M, et al. Environmental and other extrinsic risk factors contributing to the pathogenesis of cutaneous T cell lymphoma (CTCL). *Front Oncol.* 2019;9:300.
115. Cohen SR, Stenn KS, Braverman IM, Beck GJ. Clinicopathologic relationships, survival, and therapy in 59 patients with observations on occupation as a new prognostic factor. *Cancer.* 1980;46(12):2654-2666.
116. Tuyp E, Burgoyne A, Aitchison T, MacKie R. A case-control study of possible causative factors in mycosis fungoides. *Arch Dermatol.* 1987;123(2):196-200.
117. Whittemore AS, Holly EA, Lee IM, et al. Mycosis fungoides in relation to environmental exposures and immune response: a case-control study. *J Natl Cancer Inst.* 1989;81(20):1560-1567.
118. Fischmann AB, Bunn PA Jr, Guccion JG, Matthews MJ, Minna JD. Exposure to chemicals, physical agents, and biologic agents in mycosis fungoides and the Sezary syndrome. *Cancer Treat Rep.* 1979;63(4):591-596.
119. Chang ET, Delzell E. Systematic review and meta-analysis of glyphosate exposure and risk of lymphohematopoietic cancers. *J Environ Sci Health B.* 2016;51(6):402-434.
120. Sandbank M, Katzenellenbogen I. Mycosis fungoides of prolonged duration in siblings. *Arch Dermatol.* 1968;98(6):620-627.

121. Naji AA, Waiz MM, Sharquie KE. Mycosis fungoides in identical twins. *J Am Acad Dermatol.* 2001;44(3):532-533.
122. Hodak E, Friedman E. Familial mycosis fungoides: model of genetic susceptibility. *Clin Lymphoma Myeloma Leuk.* 2010;10(suppl 2):S67-S69.
123. Hodak E, Klein T, Gabay B, et al. Familial mycosis fungoides: report of 6 kindreds and a study of the HLA system. *J Am Acad Dermatol.* 2005;52(3 pt 1):393-402.
124. Vassallo C, Brazzelli V, Cestone E, et al. Mycosis fungoides in childhood: description and study of two siblings. *Acta Derm Venereol.* 2007;87(6):529-532.
125. Poiesz BJ, Ruscetti FW, Gazdar AF, Bunn PA, Minna JD, Gallo RC. Detection and isolation of type C retrovirus particles from fresh and cultured lymphocytes of a patient with cutaneous T-cell lymphoma. *Proc Natl Acad Sci U S A.* 1980;77(12):7415-7419.
126. Zucker-Franklin D, Pancake BA. The role of human T-cell lymphotropic viruses (HTLV-I and II) in cutaneous T-cell lymphomas. *Semin Dermatol.* 1994;13(3):160-165.
127. Bazarbachi A, Soriano V, Pawson R, et al. Mycosis fungoides and Sezary syndrome are not associated with HTLV-I infection: an international study. *Br J Haematol.* 1997;98(4):927-933.
128. Shohat M, Shohat B, Mimouni D, et al. Human T-cell lymphotropic virus type 1 provirus and phylogenetic analysis in patients with mycosis fungoides and their family relatives. *Br J Dermatol.* 2006;155(2):372-378.
129. Li G, Vowels BR, Benoit BM, Rook AH, Lessin SR. Failure to detect human T-lymphotropic virus type-I proviral DNA in cell lines and tissues from patients with cutaneous T-cell lymphoma. *J Invest Dermatol.* 1996;107(3):308-313.
130. Wood GS, Salvekar A, Schaffer J, et al. Evidence against a role for human T-cell lymphotrophic virus type I (HTLV-I) in the pathogenesis of American cutaneous T-cell lymphoma. *J Invest Dermatol.* 1996;107(3):301-307.
131. Capesius C, Saal F, Maero E, et al. No evidence for HTLV-I infection in 24 cases of French and Portuguese mycosis fungoides and Sezary syndrome (as seen in France). *Leukemia.* 1991;5(5):416-419.
132. Lisby G, Reitz MS Jr, Vejlsgaard GL. No detection of HTLV-I DNA in punch skin biopsies from patients with cutaneous T-cell lymphoma by the polymerase chain reaction. *J Invest Dermatol.* 1992;98(4):417-420.
133. Boni R, Davis-Daneshfar A, Burg G, Fuchs D, Wood GS. No detection of HTLV-I proviral DNA in lesional skin biopsies from Swiss and German patients with cutaneous T-cell lymphoma. *Br J Dermatol.* 1996;134(2):282-284.
134. D'Incan M, Southteyrand P, Bignon Y, Dastugue B, Claudy A, Desgranges C. Retroviral sequences related to HTLV-I endemic areas. *Eur J Dermatol.* 1992;2:363-371.
135. Srivastava BI, Banki K, Perl A. Human T-cell leukemia virus type I or a related retrovirus in patients with mycosis fungoides/Sezary syndrome and Kaposi's sarcoma. *Cancer Res.* 1992;52(16):4391-4395.
136. Whittaker SJ, Luzzatto L. HTLV-1 provirus and mycosis fungoides. *Science.* 1993;259(5100):1470, discussion 1471.
137. Chan WC, Hooper C, Wickert R, et al. HTLV-I sequence in lymphoproliferative disorders. *Diagn Mol Pathol.* 1993;2(3):192-199.
138. Netchiporouk E, Gantchev J, Tsang M, et al. Analysis of CTCL cell lines reveals important differences between mycosis fungoides/Sézary syndrome *vs. HTLV-1*$^{+}$ leukemic cell lines. *Oncotarget.* 2017;8(56):95981-95998.
139. Amitay-Laish I, Sarid R, Ben-Amitai D, et al. Human herpesvirus 8 is not detectable in lesions of large plaque parapsoriasis, and in early-stage sporadic, familial, and juvenile cases of mycosis fungoides. *J Am Acad Dermatol.* 2012;66(1):46-50.
140. Mirvish ED, Pomerantz RG, Geskin LJ. Infectious agents in cutaneous T-cell lymphoma. *J Am Acad Dermatol.* 2011;64(2):423-431.
141. Gormley RH, Kim EJ, Rook AH, et al. Merkel cell polyomavirus in low levels in folliculotropic mycosis fungoides represents a passenger, not a driver. *Int J Dermatol.* 2015;54(5):e182-e183.
142. Bonin S, Tothova SM, Barbazza R, Brunetti D, Stanta G, Trevisan G. Evidence of multiple infectious agents in mycosis fungoides lesions. *Exp Mol Pathol.* 2010;89(1):46-50.
143. Diamandidou E, Cohen PR, Kurzrock R. Mycosis fungoides and Sezary syndrome. *Blood.* 1996;88(7):2385-2409.
144. Koh HK, Charif M, Weinstock MA. Epidemiology and clinical manifestations of cutaneous T-cell lymphoma. *Hematol Oncol Clin North Am.* 1995;9(5):943-960.
145. Foo SH, Shah F, Chaganti S, Stevens A, Scarisbrick JJ. Unmasking mycosis fungoides/Sezary syndrome from preceding or co-existing benign inflammatory dermatoses requiring systemic therapies: patients frequently present with advanced disease and have an aggressive clinical course. *Br J Dermatol.* 2016;174(4):901-904.
146. Pimpinelli N, Olsen EA, Santucci M, et al. Defining early mycosis fungoides. *J Am Acad Dermatol.* 2005;53(6):1053-1063.
147. Pankratov O, Gradova S, Tarasevich S, Pankratov V. Poikilodermatous mycosis fungoides: clinical and histopathological analysis of a case and literature review. *Acta Dermatovenerol Alp Pannonica Adriat.* 2015;24(2):37-41.
148. Lambroza E, Cohen SR, Phelps R, Lebwohl M, Braverman IM, DiCostanzo D. Hypopigmented variant of mycosis fungoides: demography, histopathology, and treatment of seven cases. *J Am Acad Dermatol.* 1995;32(6):987-993.
149. Pujol RM, Gallardo F, Llistosella E, et al. Invisible mycosis fungoides: a diagnostic challenge. *J Am Acad Dermatol.* 2002;47(2 suppl):S168-S171.
150. Hwong H, Nichols T, Duvic M. "Invisible" mycosis fungoides? *J Am Acad Dermatol.* 2001;45(2):318.
151. Dereure O, Guilhou JJ. Invisible mycosis fungoides: a new case. *J Am Acad Dermatol.* 2001;45(2):318-319.
152. Rieger KE, Kim J, Kim YH. Zosteriform mycosis fungoides: a new clinical presentation with a dermatomal distribution. *Am J Dermatopathol.* 2017;39(2):e17-e18.
153. Jang MS, Kang DY, Park JB, et al. Pityriasis lichenoides-like mycosis fungoides: clinical and histologic features and response to phototherapy. *Ann Dermatol.* 2016;28(5):540-547.
154. de Unamuno Bustos B, Ferriols AP, Sanchez RB, et al. Adult pityriasis lichenoides-like mycosis fungoides: a clinical variant of mycosis fungoides. *Int J Dermatol.* 2014;53(11):1331-1338.
155. Nasimi M, Bonabiyan M, Lajevardi V, et al. Pigmented purpuric dermatoses versus purpuric mycosis fungoides: clinicopathologic similarities and new insights into dermoscopic features. *Australas J Dermatol.* 2022;63(1):81-85.
156. Hsu WT, Toporcer MB, Kantor GR, Vonderheid EC, Kadin ME. Cutaneous T-cell lymphoma with porokeratosis-like lesions. *J Am Acad Dermatol.* 1992;27(2 pt 2):327-330.
157. Stasko T, Vander Ploeg DE, De Villez RL. Hyperkeratotic mycosis fungoides restricted to the palms. *J Am Acad Dermatol.* 1982;7(6):792-796.
158. Patrawala SA, Broussard KC, Wang L, Zic JA. Tumor stage mycosis fungoides: a single-center study on clinicopathologic features, treatments, and patient outcome. *Dermatol Online J.* 2016;22(5):13030/qt1q15b903.
159. O'Quinn RP, Zic JA, Boyd AS. Mycosis fungoides d'emblee: CD30-negative cutaneous large T-cell lymphoma. *J Am Acad Dermatol.* 2000;43(5 pt 1):861-863.
160. Bouloc A, Grange F, Delfau-Larue MH, et al. Leucoderma associated with flares of erythrodermic cutaneous T-cell lymphomas: four cases. The French Study Group of Cutaneous Lymphomas. *Br J Dermatol.* 2000;143(4):832-836.
161. Bishop BE, Wulkan A, Kerdel F, El-Shabrawi-Caelen L, Tosti A. Nail alterations in cutaneous T-cell lymphoma: a case series and review of nail manifestations. *Skin Appendage Disord.* 2015;1(2):82-86.
162. Olsen EA, Rook AH, Zic J, et al. Sezary syndrome: immunopathogenesis, literature review of therapeutic options, and recommendations for therapy by the United States Cutaneous Lymphoma Consortium (USCLC). *J Am Acad Dermatol.* 2011;64(2):352-404.
163. Mangold AR, Thompson AK, Davis MD, et al. Early clinical manifestations of Sezary syndrome: a multicenter retrospective cohort study. *J Am Acad Dermatol.* 2017;77(4):719-727.
164. Willemze R, Jaffe ES, Burg G, et al. WHO-EORTC classification for cutaneous lymphomas. *Blood.* 2005;105(10):3768-3785.
165. Kempf W, Zimmermann AK, Mitteldorf C. Cutaneous lymphomas-An update 2019. *Hematol Oncol.* 2019;37(suppl 1):43-47.
166. Willemze R, Cerroni L, Kempf W, et al. The 2018 update of the WHO-EORTC classification for primary cutaneous lymphomas. *Blood.* 2019;133(16):1703-1714.
167. Swerdlow SH, Campo E, Pileri SA, et al. The 2016 revision of the World Health Organization classification of lymphoid neoplasms. *Blood.* 2016;127(20):2375-2390.
168. Willemze R. *WHO Classification of Skin Tumours.* 4th ed. Vol 11. World Health Organization; 2018.
169. Rijlaarsdam JU, Scheffer E, Meijer CJ, Willemze R. Cutaneous pseudo-T-cell lymphomas. A clinicopathologic study of 20 patients. *Cancer.* 1992;69(3):717-724.
170. Collins RD. Lymph node examination. What is an adequate workup? *Arch Pathol Lab Med.* 1985;109(9):797-799.
171. Guitart J, Kennedy J, Ronan S, Chmiel JS, Hsiegh YC, Variakojis D. Histologic criteria for the diagnosis of mycosis fungoides: proposal for a grading system to standardize pathology reporting. *J Cutan Pathol.* 2001;28(4):174-183.
172. Massone C, Kodama K, Kerl H, Cerroni L. Histopathologic features of early (patch) lesions of mycosis fungoides: a morphologic study on 745 biopsy specimens from 427 patients. *Am J Surg Pathol.* 2005;29(4):550-560.
173. Shamim H, Johnson EF, Gibson LE, Comfere N. Mycosis fungoides with spongiosis: a potential diagnostic pitfall. *J Cutan Pathol.* 2019;46(9):645-652.
174. Krishnasamy S, Correia E, Kartan S, et al. Application of the current diagnostic algorithm for early mycosis fungoides to a single center cohort: identification of challenges and suggestions for modification. *J Cutan Pathol.* 2022;49(9):772-779.
175. Alessi E, Coggi A, Venegoni L, Merlo V, Gianotti R. The usefulness of clonality for the detection of cases clinically and/or histopathologically not recognized as cutaneous T-cell lymphoma. *Br J Dermatol.* 2005;153(2):368-371.
176. Ponti R, Quaglino P, Novelli M, et al. T-cell receptor gamma gene rearrangement by multiplex polymerase chain reaction/heteroduplex analysis in patients with cutaneous T-cell lymphoma (mycosis fungoides/Sezary syndrome) and benign inflammatory disease: correlation with clinical, histological and immunophenotypical findings. *Br J Dermatol.* 2005;153(3):565-573.
177. Cordel N, Lenormand B, Courville P, Helot MF, Benichou J, Joly P; French Study Group on Cutaneous Lymphomas. Usefulness of cutaneous T-cell clonality analysis for the diagnosis of cutaneous T-cell lymphoma in patients with erythroderma. *Arch Pathol Lab Med.* 2005;129(3):372-376.
178. Thurber SE, Zhang B, Kim YH, Schrijver I, Zehnder J, Kohler S. T-cell clonality analysis in biopsy specimens from two different skin sites shows high specificity in the diagnosis of patients with suggested mycosis fungoides. *J Am Acad Dermatol.* 2007;57(5):782-790.
179. Zhang B, Beck AH, Taube JM, et al. Combined use of PCR-based TCRG and TCRB clonality tests on paraffin-embedded skin tissue in the differential diagnosis of mycosis fungoides and inflammatory dermatoses. *J Mol Diagn.* 2010;12(3):320-327.
180. Plaza JA, Morrison C, Magro CM. Assessment of TCR-beta clonality in a diverse group of cutaneous T-Cell infiltrates. *J Cutan Pathol.* 2008;35(4):358-365.
181. Salhany KE, Cousar JB, Greer JP, Casey TT, Fields JP, Collins RD. Transformation of cutaneous T cell lymphoma to large cell lymphoma. A clinicopathologic and immunologic study. *Am J Pathol.* 1988;132(2):265-277.
182. Buechner SA, Winkelmann RK. Sezary syndrome. A clinicopathologic study of 39 cases. *Arch Dermatol.* 1983;119(12):979-986.
183. Delfau-Larue MH, Laroche L, Wechsler J, et al. Diagnostic value of dominant T-cell clones in peripheral blood in 363 patients presenting consecutively with a clinical suspicion of cutaneous lymphoma. *Blood.* 2000;96(9):2987-2992.
184. Cetinozman F, Jansen PM, Willemze R. Expression of programmed death-1 in skin biopsies of benign inflammatory vs. lymphomatous erythroderma. *Br J Dermatol.* 2014;171(3):499-504.

185. Boonk SE, Cetinozman F, Vermeer MH, Jansen PM, Willemze R. Differential expression of TOX by skin-infiltrating T cells in Sezary syndrome and erythrodermic dermatitis. *J Cutan Pathol*. 2015;42(9):604-609.
186. Klemke CD, Booken N, Weiss C, et al. Histopathological and immunophenotypical criteria for the diagnosis of sezary syndrome in differentiation from other erythrodermic skin diseases: a European Organisation for Research and Treatment of Cancer (EORTC) cutaneous lymphoma task force study of 97 cases. *Br J Dermatol*. 2015;173(1):93-105.
187. Benner MF, Jansen PM, Vermeer MH, Willemze R. Prognostic factors in transformed mycosis fungoides: a retrospective analysis of 100 cases. *Blood*. 2012;119(7):1643-1649.
188. Greer JP, Salhany KE, Cousar JB, et al. Clinical features associated with transformation of cerebriform T-cell lymphoma to a large cell process. *Hematol Oncol*. 1990;8(4):215-227.
189. Greer JP, Kinney MC, Collins RD, et al. Clinical features of 31 patients with Ki-1 anaplastic large-cell lymphoma. *J Clin Oncol*. 1991;9(4):539-547.
190. Willemze R. New concepts in the classification of cutaneous lymphomas. *Arch Dermatol*. 1995;131(9):1077-1080.
191. Fauconneau A, Pham-Ledard A, Cappellen D, et al. Assessment of diagnostic criteria between primary cutaneous anaplastic large-cell lymphoma and CD30-rich transformed mycosis fungoides; a study of 66 cases. *Br J Dermatol*. 2015;172(6):1547-1554.
192. Fraser-Andrews EA, Mitchell T, Ferreira S, et al. Molecular staging of lymph nodes from 60 patients with mycosis fungoides and Sezary syndrome: correlation with histopathology and outcome suggests prognostic relevance in mycosis fungoides. *Br J Dermatol*. 2006;155(4):756-762.
193. Arai E, Katayama I, Ishihara K. Mycosis fungoides and Sezary syndrome in Japan. Clinicopathologic study of 107 autopsy cases. *Pathol Res Pract*. 1991;187(4):451-457.
194. Sausville EA, Eddy JL, Makuch RW, et al. Histopathologic staging at initial diagnosis of mycosis fungoides and the Sezary syndrome. Definition of three distinctive prognostic groups. *Ann Intern Med*. 1988;109(5):372-382.
195. Salhany KE, Greer JP, Cousar JB, Collins RD. Marrow involvement in cutaneous T-cell lymphoma. A clinicopathologic study of 60 cases. *Am J Clin Pathol*. 1989;92(6):747-754.
196. Olsen EA, Whittaker S, Willemze R, et al. Primary cutaneous lymphoma: recommendations for clinical trial Design and staging update from the ISCL, USCLC, and EORTC. *Blood*. 2022;140(5):419-437. doi:10.1182/blood.2021012057
197. Vonderheid EC, Diamond LW, Lai SM, Au F, Dellavecchia MA. Lymph node histopathologic findings in cutaneous T-cell lymphoma. A prognostic classification system based on morphologic assessment. *Am J Clin Pathol*. 1992;97(1):121-129.
198. Scheffer E, Meijer CJ, Van Vloten WA. Dermatopathic lymphadenopathy and lymph node involvement in mycosis fungoides. *Cancer*. 1980;45(1):137-148.
199. Scheffer E, Meijer CJ, van Vloten WA, Willemze R. A histologic study of lymph nodes from patients with the Sezary syndrome. *Cancer*. 1986;57(12):2375-2380.
200. Li G, Salhany KE, Rook AH, Lessin SR. The pathogenesis of large cell transformation in cutaneous T-cell lymphoma is not associated with t(2;5)(p23;q35) chromosomal translocation. *J Cutan Pathol*. 1997;24(7):403-408.
201. Bunn PA Jr, Huberman MS, Whang-Peng J, et al. Prospective staging evaluation of patients with cutaneous T-cell lymphomas. Demonstration of a high frequency of extracutaneous dissemination. *Ann Intern Med*. 1980;93(2):223-230.
202. Rappaport H, Thomas LB. Mycosis fungoides: the pathology of extracutaneous involvement. *Cancer*. 1974;34(4):1198-1229.
203. Sibaud V, Beylot-Barry M, Thiebaut R, et al. Bone marrow histopathologic and molecular staging in epidermotropic T-cell lymphomas. *Am J Clin Pathol*. 2003;119(3):414-423.
204. Olsen EA, Whittaker S, Kim YH, et al. Clinical end points and response criteria in mycosis fungoides and Sezary syndrome: a consensus statement of the International Society for Cutaneous Lymphomas, the United States Cutaneous Lymphoma Consortium, and the Cutaneous Lymphoma Task Force of the European Organisation for Research and Treatment of Cancer. *J Clin Oncol*. 2011;29(18):2598-2607.
205. Variakojis D, Rosas-Uribe A, Rappaport H. Mycosis fungoides: pathologic findings in staging laparotomies. *Cancer*. 1974;33(6):1589-1600.
206. Bennett SR, Greer JP, Stein RS, Glick AD, Cousar JB, Collins RD. Death due to splenic rupture in suppressor cell mycosis fungoides: a case report. *Am J Clin Pathol*. 1984;82(1):104-109.
207. Wolfe JD, Trevor ED, Kjeldsberg CR. Pulmonary manifestations of mycosis fungoides. *Cancer*. 1980;46(12):2648-2653.
208. Olsen E, Vonderheid E, Pimpinelli N, et al. Revisions to the staging and classification of mycosis fungoides and Sezary syndrome: a proposal of the International Society for Cutaneous Lymphomas (ISCL) and the Cutaneous Lymphoma Task Force of the European Organization of Research and Treatment of Cancer (EORTC). *Blood*. 2007;110(6):1713-1722.
209. Vonderheid EC, Bernengo MG, Burg G, et al. Update on erythrodermic cutaneous T-cell lymphoma: report of the International Society for Cutaneous Lymphomas. *J Am Acad Dermatol*. 2002;46(1):95-106.
210. Vonderheid EC, Sobel EL, Nowell PC, Finan JB, Helfrich MK, Whipple DS. Diagnostic and prognostic significance of Sezary cells in peripheral blood smears from patients with cutaneous T cell lymphoma. *Blood*. 1985;66(2):358-366.
211. Fraser-Andrews EA, Woolford AJ, Russell-Jones R, Seed PT, Whittaker SJ. Detection of a peripheral blood T cell clone is an independent prognostic marker in mycosis fungoides. *J Invest Dermatol*. 2000;114(1):117-121.
212. Beylot-Barry M, Sibaud V, Thiebaut R, et al. Evidence that an identical T cell clone in skin and peripheral blood lymphocytes is an independent prognostic factor in primary cutaneous T cell lymphomas. *J Invest Dermatol*. 2001;117(4):920-926.
213. Agar NS, Wedgeworth E, Crichton S, et al. Survival outcomes and prognostic factors in mycosis fungoides/Sezary syndrome: validation of the revised International Society for Cutaneous Lymphomas/European Organisation for Research and Treatment of Cancer staging proposal. *J Clin Oncol*. 2010;28(31):4730-4739.
214. Vermeer MH, Moins-Teisserenc H, Bagot M, Quaglino P, Whittaker S. Flow cytometry for the assessment of blood tumour burden in cutaneous T-cell lymphoma: towards a standardised approach. *Br J Dermatol*. 2022;187(1):21-28.
215. Berg H, Otteson GE, Corley H, et al. Flow cytometric evaluation of TRBC1 expression in tissue specimens and body fluids is a novel and specific method for assessment of T-cell clonality and diagnosis of T-cell neoplasms. *Cytometry B Clin Cytom*. 2021;100(3):361-369.
216. Chen M, Wang A, Liu S, et al. Analysis of the Expression of the TRBC1 in T lymphocyte tumors. *Indian J Hematol Blood Transfus*. 2021;37(2):271-279.
217. Horna P, Shi M, Jevremovic D, Craig FE, Comfere NI, Olteanu H. Utility of TRBC1 expression in the diagnosis of peripheral blood involvement by cutaneous T-cell lymphoma. *J Invest Dermatol*. 2021;141(4):821-829.e2.
218. Munoz-Garcia N, Lima M, Villamor N, et al. Anti-TRBC1 antibody-based flow cytometric detection of T-cell clonality: standardization of sample preparation and diagnostic implementation. *Cancers (Basel)*. 2021;13(17):4379. doi:10.3390/cancers13174379
219. Waldron D, O'Brien D, Smyth L, Quinn F, Vandenberghe E. Reliable detection of T-cell clonality by flow cytometry in mature T-cell neoplasms using TRBC1: implementation as a reflex test and comparison with PCR-based clonality testing. *Lab Med*. 2022;53(4):417-425. https://www.ncbi.nlm.nih.gov/pubmed/25046454
220. Picker LJ, Michie SA, Rott LS, Butcher EC. A unique phenotype of skin-associated lymphocytes in humans. Preferential expression of the HECA-452 epitope by benign and malignant T cells at cutaneous sites. *Am J Pathol*. 1990;136(5):1053-1068.
221. Ralfkiaer E. Immunohistological markers for the diagnosis of cutaneous lymphomas. *Semin Diagn Pathol*. 1991;8(2):62-72.
222. Martinez-Escala ME, Kantor RW, Cices A, et al. CD8+ mycosis fungoides: a low-grade lymphoproliferative disorder. *J Am Acad Dermatol*. 2017;77(3):489-496.
223. Bogen SA, Pelley D, Charif M, et al. Immunophenotypic identification of Sezary cells in peripheral blood. *Am J Clin Pathol*. 1996;106(6):739-748.
224. Bernengo MG, Novelli M, Quaglino P, et al. The relevance of the CD4+ CD26− subset in the identification of circulating Sezary cells. *Br J Dermatol*. 2001;144(1):125-135.
225. Sokolowska-Wojdylo M, Wenzel J, Gaffal E, et al. Absence of CD26 expression on skin-homing CLA+ CD4+ T lymphocytes in peripheral blood is a highly sensitive marker for early diagnosis and therapeutic monitoring of patients with Sezary syndrome. *Clin Exp Dermatol*. 2005;30(6):702-706.
226. Vonderheid EC, Hou JS. CD4(+)CD26(−) lymphocytes are useful to assess blood involvement and define B ratings in cutaneous T cell lymphoma. *Leuk Lymphoma*. 2018;59(2):330-339.
227. Bagot M, Moretta A, Sivori S, et al. CD4(+) cutaneous T-cell lymphoma cells express the p140-killer cell immunoglobulin-like receptor. *Blood*. 2001;97(5):1388-1391.
228. Bagot M, Porcu P, Marie-Cardine A, et al. IPH4102, a first-in-class anti-KIR3DL2 monoclonal antibody, in patients with relapsed or refractory cutaneous T-cell lymphoma: an international, first-in-human, open-label, phase 1 trial. *Lancet Oncol*. 2019;20(8):1160-1170.
229. Ormsby A, Bergfeld WF, Tubbs RR, Hsi ED. Evaluation of a new paraffin-reactive CD7 T-cell deletion marker and a polymerase chain reaction-based T-cell receptor gene rearrangement assay: implications for diagnosis of mycosis fungoides in community clinical practice. *J Am Acad Dermatol*. 2001;45(3):405-413.
230. Murphy M, Fullen D, Carlson JA. Low CD7 expression in benign and malignant cutaneous lymphocytic infiltrates: experience with an antibody reactive with paraffin-embedded tissue. *Am J Dermatopathol*. 2002;24(1):6-16.
231. Tirumalae R, Panjwani PK. Origin use of CD4, CD8, and CD1a immunostains in distinguishing mycosis fungoides from its inflammatory mimics: a pilot study. *Indian J Dermatol*. 2012;57(6):424-427.
232. Vandergriff T, Nezafati KA, Susa J, et al. Defining early mycosis fungoides: validation of a diagnostic algorithm proposed by the International Society for Cutaneous Lymphomas. *J Cutan Pathol*. 2015;42(5):318-328.
233. Kelati A, Gallouj S, Tahiri L, Harmouche T, Mernissi FZ. Defining the mimics and clinico-histological diagnosis criteria for mycosis fungoides to minimize misdiagnosis. *Int J Womens Dermatol*. 2017;3(2):100-106.
234. Arps DP, Chen S, Fullen DR, Hristov AC. Selected inflammatory imitators of mycosis fungoides: histologic features and utility of ancillary studies. *Arch Pathol Lab Med*. 2014;138(10):1319-1327.
235. Chairatchaneeboon M, Thanomkitti K, Kim EJ. Parapsoriasis-A diagnosis with an identity crisis: a narrative review. *Dermatol Ther*. 2022;12(5):1091-1102. doi:10.1007/s13555-022-00716-y
236. Kikuchi A, Naka W, Harada T, Sakuraoka K, Harada R, Nishikawa T. Parapsoriasis en plaques: its potential for progression to malignant lymphoma. *J Am Acad Dermatol*. 1993;29(3):419-422.
237. Bordignon M, Belloni Fortina A, Pigozzi B, Alaibac M. γδ T cells as potential contributors to the progression of parapsoriasis to mycosis fungoides. *Mol Med Rep*. 2008;1(4):485-488.
238. Vakeva L, Sarna S, Vaalasti A, Pukkala E, Kariniemi AL, Ranki A. A retrospective study of the probability of the evolution of parapsoriasis en plaques into mycosis fungoides. *Acta Derm Venereol*. 2005;85(4):318-323.
239. Lindahl LM, Fenger-Gron M, Iversen L. Subsequent cancers, mortality, and causes of death in patients with mycosis fungoides and parapsoriasis: a Danish nationwide, population-based cohort study. *J Am Acad Dermatol*. 2014;71(3):529-535.
240. Staib G, Sterry W. Use of polymerase chain reaction in the detection of clones in lymphoproliferative diseases of the skin. *Recent Results Cancer Res*. 1995;139:239-247.
241. Burg G, Dummer R. Small plaque (digitate) parapsoriasis is an 'abortive cutaneous T-cell lymphoma' and is not mycosis fungoides. *Arch Dermatol*. 1995;131(3):336-338.

242. Ackerman AB, Schiff TA. If small plaque (digitate) parapsoriasis is a cutaneous t-cell lymphoma, even an abortive one, it must be mycosis fungoides. *Arch Dermatol*. 1996;132(5):562-566.
243. Gug G, Solovan C. From benign inflammatory dermatosis to cutaneous lymphoma. DNA copy number Imbalances in mycosis fungoides versus large plaque parapsoriasis. *Medicina (Kaunas)*. 2021;57(5):502.
244. Lindae ML, Abel EA, Hoppe RT, Wood GS. Poikilodermatous mycosis fungoides and atrophic large-plaque parapsoriasis exhibit similar abnormalities of T-cell antigen expression. *Arch Dermatol*. 1988;124(3):366-372.
245. Kreuter A, Hoffmamm K, Altmeyer P. A case of poikiloderma vasculare atrophicans, a rare variant of cutaneous T-cell lymphoma, responding to extracorporeal photopheresis. *J Am Acad Dermatol*. 2005;52(4):706-708.
246. Nakai K, Yoneda K, Moriue T, et al. Narrow-band ultraviolet B decreases serum interleukin-2 receptor levels in patients with poikiloderma vasculare atrophicans. *J Eur Acad Dermatol Venereol*. 2009;23(7):844-846.
247. Mahajan VK, Chauhan PS, Mehta KS, Sharma AL. Poikiloderma vasculare atrophicans: a distinct clinical entity? *Indian J Dermatol*. 2015;60(2):216.
248. Vasconcelos Berg R, Valente NYS, Fanelli C, et al. Poikilodermatous mycosis fungoides: comparative study of clinical, histopathological and immunohistochemical features. *Dermatology*. 2020;236(2):117-122.
249. Nofal A, Salah E. Acquired poikiloderma: proposed classification and diagnostic approach. *J Am Acad Dermatol*. 2013;69(3):e129-e140.
250. Syrnioti A, Aikaterini P, Georgiou E, Avgeros C, Koletsa T. FOXP3+ atypical cells in poikilodermatous mycosis fungoides may implicate in treatment resistance. *Acta Derm Venereol*. 2022;102:adv00701. doi:10.2340/actadv.v102.2037
251. Rohmer E, Mitcov M, Cribier B, Lipsker D, Lenormand C. Clinical heterogeneity of poikilodermatous mycosis fungoides: a retrospective study of 12 cases. *Ann Dermatol Venereol*. 2020;147(6-7):418-428.
252. Lupu J, Chosidow O, Wolkenstein P, Bergqvist C, Ortonne N, Ingen-Housz-Oro S. Pityriasis lichenoides: a clinical and pathological case series of 49 patients with an emphasis on follow-up. *Clin Exp Dermatol*. 2021;46(8):1561-1566.
253. Pereira N, Brinca A, Manuel Brites M, Jose Juliao M, Tellechea O, Goncalo M. Pityriasis lichenoides et varioliformis acuta: case report and review of the literature. *Case Rep Dermatol*. 2012;4(1):61-65.
254. Henning JS. Pityriasis lichenoides chronica *Dermatol Online J*. 2004;10(3):8. http://dermatology-s10.cdlib.org/103/NYU/case_presentations/111803n3.html
255. Mohd Amin SN, Muhamad R, Wan Abdullah WNH, Mohd Zulkifli M, Bakrin IH, Tangam T. A case report of pityriasis lichenoides-like mycosis fungoides in children: a challenging diagnosis. *Korean J Fam Med*. 2021;42(4):334-338. doi:10.4082/kjfm.20.0036
256. Willemze R, Scheffer E. Clinical and histologic differentiation between lymphomatoid papulosis and pityriasis lichenoides. *J Am Acad Dermatol*. 1985;13(3):418-428.
257. Martorell-Calatayud A, Hernandez-Martin A, Colmenero I, et al. Lymphomatoid papulosis in children: report of 9 cases and review of the literature. *Actas Dermosifiliogr*. 2010;101(8):693-701.
258. Magro CM, Crowson AN, Morrison C, Li J. Pityriasis lichenoides chronica: stratification by molecular and phenotypic profile. *Hum Pathol*. 2007;38(3):479-490.
259. Wieser I, Wohlmuth C, Nunez CA, Duvic M. Lymphomatoid papulosis in children and adolescents: a systematic review. *Am J Clin Dermatol*. 2016;17(4):319-327.
260. Tomasini D, Zampatti C, Palmedo G, Bonfacini V, Sangalli G, Kutzner H. Cytotoxic mycosis fungoides evolving from pityriasis lichenoides chronica in a seventeen-year-old girl. Report of a case. *Dermatology*. 2002;205(2):176-179.
261. Sibbald C, Pope E. Systematic review of cases of cutaneous T-cell lymphoma transformation in pityriasis lichenoides and small plaque parapsoriasis. *Br J Dermatol*. 2016;175(4):807-809.
262. Sidiropoulou P, Nikolaou V, Marinos L, et al. A case of lymphomatoid papulosis, pityriasis lichenoides acuta, and mycosis fungoides coexistence. *Australas J Dermatol*. 2019;60(2):e154-e156.
263. Kaplan J, Burgin S, Sepehr A. Granulomatous pigmented purpura: report of a case and review of the literature. *J Cutan Pathol*. 2011;38(12):984-989.
264. Caytemel C, Baykut B, Agirgol S, et al. Pigmented purpuric dermatosis: ten years of experience in a tertiary hospital and awareness of mycosis fungoides in differential diagnosis. *J Cutan Pathol*. 2020;48(5):611-616.
265. Yazdi AS, Mayser P, Sander CA. Lichen aureus with clonal T cells in a child possibly induced by regular consumption of an energy drink. *J Cutan Pathol*. 2008;35(10):960-962.
266. Magro CM, Schaefer JT, Crowson AN, Li J, Morrison C. Pigmented purpuric dermatosis: classification by phenotypic and molecular profiles. *Am J Clin Pathol*. 2007;128(2):218-229.
267. Solomon GJ, Magro CM. Foxp3 expression in cutaneous T-cell lymphocytic infiltrates. *J Cutan Pathol*. 2008;35(11):1032-1039.
268. Maor D, Ondhia C, Yu LL, Chan JJ. Lichenoid keratosis is frequently misdiagnosed as basal cell carcinoma. *Clin Exp Dermatol*. 2017;42(6):663-666.
269. Al-Hoqail IA, Crawford RI. Benign lichenoid keratoses with histologic features of mycosis fungoides: clinicopathologic description of a clinically significant histologic pattern. *J Cutan Pathol*. 2002;29(5):291-294.
270. Kossard S. Unilesional mycosis fungoides or lymphomatoid keratosis? *Arch Dermatol*. 1997;133(10):1312-1313.
271. Arai E, Shimizu M, Tsuchida T, Izaki S, Ogawa F, Hirose T. Lymphomatoid keratosis. An epidermotropic type of cutaneous lymphoid hyperplasia: clinicopathological, immunohistochemical, and molecular biological study of 6 cases. *Arch Dermatol*. 2007;143(1):53-59.
272. Choi MJ, Kim HS, Kim HO, Song KY, Park YM. A case of lymphomatoid keratosis. *Ann Dermatol*. 2010;22(2):219-222.
273. Zhang P, Chen HX, Xing JJ, et al. Clinical analysis of 84 cases of erythrodermic psoriasis and 121 cases of other types of erythroderma from 2010-2015. *J Huazhong Univ Sci Technolog Med Sci*. 2017;37(4):563-567.
274. Cesar A, Cruz M, Mota A, Azevedo F. Erythroderma. A clinical and etiological study of 103 patients. *J Dermatol Case Rep*. 2016;10(1):1-9.
275. Miyashiro D, Sanches JA. Erythroderma: a prospective study of 309 patients followed for 12 years in a tertiary center. *Sci Rep*. 2020;10(1):9774.
276. Devi GC, Hazarika N. Erythroderma secondary to crusted scabies. *BMJ Case Rep*. 2021;14(12):e248000.
277. Tashiro Y, Azukizawa H, Asada H, et al. Drug-induced hypersensitivity syndrome/drug reaction with eosinophilia and systemic symptoms due to lamotrigine differs from that due to other drugs. *J Dermatol*. 2019;46(3):226-233.
278. Pukhalskaya T, El Hussein S. Hematologic findings in drug reaction with eosinophilia and systemic symptoms (DRESS). *Am J Hematol*. 2021;96(11):1548-1550.
279. Vonderheid EC. On the diagnosis of erythrodermic cutaneous T-cell lymphoma. *J Cutan Pathol*. 2006;33(suppl 1):27-42.
280. Ram-Wolff C, Martin-Garcia N, Bensussan A, Bagot M, Ortonne N. Histopathologic diagnosis of lymphomatous versus inflammatory erythroderma: a morphologic and phenotypic study on 47 skin biopsies. *Am J Dermatopathol*. 2010;32(8):755-763.
281. Uzuncakmak TK, Akdeniz N, Özkanlı Ş, Türkoğlu Z, Zemheri EI, Ka Radağ AS. Lymphomatoid contact dermatitis associated with textile dye at an unusual location. *Indian Dermatol Online J*. 2015;6(suppl 1):S24-S26.
282. Knackstedt TJ, Zug KA. T cell lymphomatoid contact dermatitis: a challenging case and review of the literature. *Contact Dermatitis*. 2015;72(2):65-74.
283. Rijlaarsdam JU, Willemze R. Cutaneous pseudolymphomas: classification and differential diagnosis. *Semin Dermatol*. 1994;13(3):187-196.
284. Smoller BR, Bishop K, Glusac E, Kim YH, Hendrickson M. Reassessment of histologic parameters in the diagnosis of mycosis fungoides. *Am J Surg Pathol*. 1995;19(12):1423-1430.
285. Magro CM, Schaefer JT. T- and B-cell clonally restricted pseudolymphoma in the setting of phytoestrogen therapy. *J Eur Acad Dermatol Venereol*. 2008;22(5):642-643.
286. Phyo ZH, Shanbhag S, Rozati S. Update on biology of cutaneous T-cell lymphoma. *Front Oncol*. 2020;10:765.
287. Mitteldorf C, Kempf W. Cutaneous pseudolymphoma. *Surg Pathol Clin*. 2017;10(2):455-476.
288. Bergman R, Khamaysi K, Khamaysi Z, Ben Arie Y. A study of histologic and immunophenotypical staining patterns in cutaneous lymphoid hyperplasia. *J Am Acad Dermatol*. 2011;65(1):112-124.
289. Hasan M, Shahid M, Varshney M, Mubeen A, Gaur K. Idiopathic lymphocytoma cutis: a diagnostic dilemma. *BMJ Case Rep*. 2011;2011:bcr1220103662. doi:10.1136/bcr.12.2010.3662
290. Lugović-Mihić L, Duvancić T, Situm M, Mihić J, Krolo I. Actinic reticuloid – photosensitivity or pseudolymphoma?—A review. *Coll Antropol*. 2011;35(suppl 2):325-329.
291. De Silva BD, McLaren K, Kavanagh GM. Photosensitive mycosis fungoides or actinic reticuloid? *Br J Dermatol*. 2000;142(6):1221-1227.
292. Byrne M, Stefanato CM, Sarkany R. A photosensitive pseudolymphomatous eruption. Actinic reticuloid (AR). *Clin Exp Dermatol*. 2012;37(2):203-204.
293. Sidiropoulos M, Deonizio J, Martinez-Escala ME, Gerami P, Guitart J. Chronic actinic dermatitis/actinic reticuloid: a clinicopathologic and immunohistochemical analysis of 37 cases. *Am J Dermatopathol*. 2014;36(11):875-881.
294. Melchers RC, Willemze R, Bekkenk MW, et al. Frequency and prognosis of associated malignancies in 504 patients with lymphomatoid papulosis. *J Eur Acad Dermatol Venereol*. 2020;34(2):260-266.
295. Sauder MB, O'Malley JT, LeBoeuf NR. CD30+ lymphoproliferative disorders of the skin. *Hematol Oncol Clin North Am*. 2017;31(2):317-334.
296. Chen YC, Wu YH. Linear folliculotropic CD30-positive lymphomatoid drug reaction. *Am J Dermatopathol*. 2017;39(5):e62-e65.
297. Magro CM, Olson LC, Nguyen GH, de Feraudy SM. CD30 positive lymphomatoid angiocentric drug reactions: characterization of a series of 20 cases. *Am J Dermatopathol*. 2017;39(7):508-517.
298. Pulitzer MP, Nolan KA, Oshman RG, Phelps RG. CD30+ lymphomatoid drug reactions. *Am J Dermatopathol*. 2013;35(3):343-350.
299. Macaulay WL. Lymphomatoid papulosis. A continuing self-healing eruption, clinically benign—histologically malignant. *Arch Dermatol*. 1968;97(1):23-30.
300. Wagner G, Rose C, Klapper W, Sachse MM. Lymphomatoid papulosis. *J Dtsch Dermatol Ges*. 2020;18(3):199-205.
301. Saggini A, Gulia A, Argenyi Z, et al. A variant of lymphomatoid papulosis simulating primary cutaneous aggressive epidermotropic CD8+ cytotoxic T-cell lymphoma. Description of 9 cases. *Am J Surg Pathol*. 2010;34(8):1168-1175.
302. Kempf W, Mitteldorf C, Karai LJ, Robson A. Lymphomatoid papulosis – making sense of the alphabet soup: a proposal to simplify terminology. *J Dtsch Dermatol Ges*. 2017;15(4):390-394.
303. Karai LJ, Kadin ME, Hsi ED, et al. Chromosomal rearrangements of 6p25.3 define a new subtype of lymphomatoid papulosis. *Am J Surg Pathol*. 2013;37(8):1173-1181.
304. Ross NA, Truong H, Keller MS, Mulholland JK, Lee JB, Sahu J. Follicular lymphomatoid papulosis: an eosinophilic-rich follicular subtype masquerading as folliculitis clinically and histologically. *Am J Dermatopathol*. 2016;38(1):e1-e10.
305. El Shabrawi-Caelen L, Kerl H, Cerroni L. Lymphomatoid papulosis: reappraisal of clinicopathologic presentation and classification into subtypes A, B, and C. *Arch Dermatol*. 2004;140(4):441-447.
306. Cardoso J, Duhra P, Thway Y, Calonje E. Lymphomatoid papulosis type D: a newly described variant easily confused with cutaneous aggressive CD8-positive cytotoxic T-cell lymphoma. *Am J Dermatopathol*. 2012;34(7):762-765.
307. Magro CM, Crowson AN, Morrison C, Merati K, Porcu P, Wright ED. CD8+ lymphomatoid papulosis and its differential diagnosis. *Am J Clin Pathol*. 2006;125(4):490-501.
308. Martinez-Cabriales SA, Walsh S, Sade S, Shear NH. Lymphomatoid papulosis: an update and review. *J Eur Acad Dermatol Venereol*. 2020;34(1):59-73.

309. Mallet V, Bruneau J, Zuber J, et al. Hepatitis E virus-induced primary cutaneous CD30(+) T cell lymphoproliferative disorder. *J Hepatol*. 2017;67(6):1334-1339.
310. Matoula T, Nikolaou V, Marinos L, et al. Lymphomatoid papulosis type D in a fingolimod-treated multiple sclerosis patient. *Mult Scler*. 2016;22(12):1630-1631.
311. Cohen V, Saber M, Provost N, Friedmann D. Lymphomatoid papulosis and fingolimod-A new connection? *Mult Scler*. 2016;22(12):1629-1630.
312. Samaraweera APR, Cohen SN, Akay EM, Evangelou N. Lymphomatoid papulosis: a cutaneous lymphoproliferative disorder in a patient on fingolimod for multiple sclerosis. *Mult Scler*. 2016;22(1):122-124.
313. Liu HL, Hoppe RT, Kohler S, Harvell JD, Reddy S, Kim YH. CD30+ cutaneous lymphoproliferative disorders: the Stanford experience in lymphomatoid papulosis and primary cutaneous anaplastic large cell lymphoma. *J Am Acad Dermatol*. 2003;49(6):1049-1058.
314. Cordel N, Tressieres B, D'Incan M, et al. Frequency and risk factors for associated lymphomas in patients with lymphomatoid papulosis. *Oncol*. 2016;21(1):76-83.
315. Wieser I, Oh CW, Talpur R, Duvic M. Lymphomatoid papulosis: treatment response and associated lymphomas in a study of 180 patients. *J Am Acad Dermatol*. 2016;74(1):59-67.
316. Burg G, Kempf W, Cozzio A, et al. WHO/EORTC classification of cutaneous lymphomas 2005: histological and molecular aspects. *J Cutan Pathol*. 2005;32(10):647-674.
317. Kinney MC, Kadin ME. The pathologic and clinical spectrum of anaplastic large cell lymphoma and correlation with ALK gene dysregulation. *Am J Clin Pathol*. 1999;111(suppl 1):S56-S67.
318. Massone C, El-Shabrawi-Caelen L, Kerl H, Cerroni L. The morphologic spectrum of primary cutaneous anaplastic large T-cell lymphoma: a histopathologic study on 66 biopsy specimens from 47 patients with report of rare variants. *J Cutan Pathol*. 2008;35(1):46-53.
319. Kempf W. A new era for cutaneous CD30-positive T-cell lymphoproliferative disorders. *Semin Diagn Pathol*. 2017;34(1):22-35.
320. Brown RA, Fernandez-Pol S, Kim J. Primary cutaneous anaplastic large cell lymphoma. *J Cutan Pathol*. 2017;44(6):570-577.
321. Hapgood G, Pickles T, Sehn LH, et al. Outcome of primary cutaneous anaplastic large cell lymphoma: a 20-year British Columbia Cancer Agency experience. *Br J Haematol*. 2017;176(2):234-240.
322. Demierre M-F, Goldberg LJ, Kadin ME, Koh HK. Is it lymphoma or lymphomatoid papulosis. *J Am Acad Dermatol*. 1997;36(5 pt 1):765-772.
323. Bruijn MS, Horvath B, van Voorst Vader PC, Willemze R, Vermeer MH. Recommendations for treatment of lymphomatoid papulosis with methotrexate: a report from the Dutch Cutaneous Lymphoma Group. *Br J Dermatol*. 2015;173(5):1319-1322.
324. Newland KM, McCormack CJ, Twigger R, et al. The efficacy of methotrexate for lymphomatoid papulosis. *J Am Acad Dermatol*. 2015;72(6):1088-1090.
325. Tan AWH, Giam YC. Lymphomatoid papulosis associated with recurrent cutaneous T-cell lymphoma. *Ann Acad Med Singap*. 2004;33(1):110-112.
326. Fujimura T, Furudate S, Tanita K, et al. Successful control of phototherapy-resistant lymphomatoid papulosis with oral bexarotene. *J Dermatol*. 2018;45(2):e37-e38.
327. Lewis DJ, Talpur R, Huen AO, Tetzlaff MT, Duvic M. Brentuximab vedotin for patients with refractory lymphomatoid papulosis: an analysis of phase 2 results. *JAMA Dermatol*. 2017;153(12):1302-1306.
328. Querfeld C, Khan I, Mahon B, Nelson BP, Rosen ST, Evens AM. Primary cutaneous and systemic anaplastic large cell lymphoma: clinicopathologic aspects and therapeutic options. *Oncology (Williston Park)*. 2010;24(7):574-587.
329. Vardiman JW, Thiele J, Arber DA, et al. The 2008 revision of the World Health Organization (WHO) classification of myeloid neoplasms and acute leukemia: rationale and important changes. *Blood*. 2009;114(5):937-951.
330. Swerdlow SH, Campo E, Harris NL, et al. *WHO Classification of Tumours of Haematopoietic and Lymphoid Tissues*. 4th ed. World Health Organization Press; 2008.
331. Charli-Joseph Y, Kashani-Sabet M, McCalmont TH, et al. Association of a proposed new staging system for folliculotropic mycosis fungoides with prognostic variables in a US cohort. *JAMA Dermatol*. 2021;157(2):157-165.
332. Shah A, Safaya A. Granulomatous slack skin disease: a review, in comparison with mycosis fungoides. *J Eur Acad Dermatol Venereol*. 2012;26(12):1472-1478.
333. Keeling BH, Gavino ACP, Admirand J, Soldano AC. Primary cutaneous CD4-positive small/medium-sized pleomorphic T-cell lymphoproliferative disorder: report of a case and review of the literature. *J Cutan Pathol*. 2017;44(11):944-947.
334. Guo N, Chen Y, Wang Y, et al. Clinicopathological categorization of hydroa vacciniforme-like lymphoproliferative disorder: an analysis of prognostic implications and treatment based on 19 cases. *Diagn Pathol*. 2019;14(1):82-11.
335. Nofal A, Abdel-Mawla MY, Assaf M, Salah E. Primary cutaneous aggressive epidermotropic CD8+ T-cell lymphoma: proposed diagnostic criteria and therapeutic evaluation. *J Am Acad Dermatol*. 2012;67(4):748-759.
336. Toro JR, Liewehr DJ, Pabby N, et al. Gamma-delta T-cell phenotype is associated with significantly decreased survival in cutaneous T-cell lymphoma. *Blood*. 2003;101(9):3407-3412.
337. Surmanowicz P, Doherty S, Sivanand A, et al. The clinical spectrum of primary cutaneous CD4+ small/medium-sized pleomorphic T-cell lymphoproliferative disorder: an updated systematic literature review and case series. *Dermatology*. 2021;237(4):618-628.
338. Kluk J, Kai A, Koch D, et al. Indolent CD8-positive lymphoid proliferation of acral sites: three further cases of a rare entity and an update on a unique patient. *J Cutan Pathol*. 2016;43(2):125-136.
339. Willemze R, Jansen PM, Cerroni L, et al. Subcutaneous panniculitis-like T-cell lymphoma: definition, classification, and prognostic factors. An EORTC Cutaneous Lymphoma Group Study of 83 cases. *Blood*. 2008;111(2):838-845.
340. Guitart J, Weisenburger DD, Subtil A, et al. Cutaneous γδ T-cell lymphomas: a spectrum of presentations with overlap with other cytotoxic lymphomas. *Am J Surg Pathol*. 2012;36(11):1656-1665.
341. Bagot M. Epitheliotropic lymphomas: better identification for improved treatment. *Bull Acad Natl Med*. 2010;194(7):1365-1372.
342. Woringer F, Kolopp P. Lesion erythemato-squameuse polycyclique de l'avant-bras evoluant depuis 6 ans chez un garconnet de 13 ans: histologiquement infiltrat intra epidermique d'apparence tumorale. *Ann Dermatol Syphil*. 1939;10:945.
343. Wang SC, Mistry N. Woringer-Kolopp disease mimicking psoriasis. *Can Med Assoc J*. 2015;187(17):1310.
344. Nakada T, Sueki H, Iijima M. Disseminated pagetoid reticulosis (Ketron-Goodman disease): six-year follow-up. *J Am Acad Dermatol*. 2002;47(2 suppl):S183-S186.
345. Pagnanelli G, Bianchi L, Cantonetti M, et al. Disseminated pagetoid reticulosis presenting as cytotoxic CD4/CD8 double negative cutaneous T-cell lymphoma. *Acta Derm Venereol*. 2002;82(4):314-316.
346. Shiozawa E, Shiokawa A, Shibata M, et al. Autopsy case of CD4/CD8 cutaneous T-cell lymphoma presenting disseminated pagetoid reticulosis with aggressive granulomatous invasion to the lungs and pancreas. *Pathol Int*. 2005;55(1):32-39.
347. Kaufmann F, Kettelhack N, Hilty N, Kempf W. Unilesional plantar mycosis fungoides treated with topical photodynamic therapy - case report and review of the literature. *J Eur Acad Dermatol Venereol*. 2017;31(10):1633-1637.
348. Mourtzinos N, Puri PK, Wang G, Liu ML. CD4/CD8 double negative pagetoid reticulosis: a case report and literature review. *J Cutan Pathol*. 2010;37(4):491-496.
349. Larson K, Wick MR. Pagetoid reticulosis: report of two cases and review of the literature. *Dermatopathology (Basel)*. 2016;3(1):8-12.
350. Kim SY. Follicular mycosis fungoides. *Am J Dermatopathol*. 1985;7(3):300-301.
351. Bagot M. Folliculotropic mycosis fungoides is a heterogenous group. *Br J Dermatol*. 2017;177(1):17-18.
352. Tomasini C, Kempf W, Novelli M, et al. Spiky follicular mycosis fungoides: a clinicopathologic study of 8 cases. *J Cutan Pathol*. 2015;42(3):164-172.
353. van Santen S, van Doorn R, Neelis KJ, et al. Recommendations for treatment in folliculotropic mycosis fungoides: report of the Dutch Cutaneous Lymphoma Group. *Br J Dermatol*. 2017;177(1):223-228.
354. Gerami P, Guitart J. The spectrum of histopathologic and immunohistochemical findings in folliculotropic mycosis fungoides. *Am J Surg Pathol*. 2007;31(9):1430-1438.
355. Gilliam AC, Lessin SR, Wilson DM, Salhany KE. Folliculotropic mycosis fungoides with large-cell transformation presenting as dissecting cellulitis of the scalp. *J Cutan Pathol*. 1997;24(3):169-175.
356. Demirkesen C, Esirgen G, Engin B, Songur A, Oğuz O. The clinical features and histopathologic patterns of folliculotropic mycosis fungoides in a series of 38 cases. *J Cutan Pathol*. 2015;42(1):22-31.
357. Hodak E, Amitay-Laish I, Atzmony L, et al. New insights into folliculotropic mycosis fungoides (FMF): a single-center experience. *J Am Acad Dermatol*. 2016;75(2):347-355.
358. Hodak E, Amitay-Laish I, Feinmesser M, et al. Juvenile mycosis fungoides: cutaneous T-cell lymphoma with frequent follicular involvement. *J Am Acad Dermatol*. 2014;70(6):993-1001.
359. Ke MS, Kamath NV, Nihal M, et al. Folliculotropic mycosis fungoides with central nervous system involvement: demonstration of tumor clonality in intrafollicular T cells using laser capture microdissection. *J Am Acad Dermatol*. 2003;48(2):238-243.
360. Bonta MD, Tannous ZS, Demierre MF, Gonzalez E, Harris NL, Duncan LM. Rapidly progressing mycosis fungoides presenting as follicular mucinosis. *J Am Acad Dermatol*. 2000;43(4):635-640.
361. van Doorn R, Scheffer E, Willemze R. Follicular mycosis fungoides, a distinct disease entity with or without associated follicular mucinosis: a clinicopathologic and follow-up study of 51 patients. *Arch Dermatol*. 2002;138(2):191-198.
362. Rongioletti F, De Lucchi S, Meyes D, et al. Follicular mucinosis: a clinicopathologic, histochemical, immunohistochemical and molecular study comparing the primary benign form and the mycosis fungoides-associated follicular mucinosis. *J Cutan Pathol*. 2010;37(1):15-19.
363. Khalil J, Kurban M, Abbas O. Follicular mucinosis: a review. *Int J Dermatol*. 2021;60(2):159-165.
364. Cerroni L, Fink-Puches R, Back B, Kerl H. Follicular mucinosis: a critical reappraisal of clinicopathologic features and association with mycosis fungoides and Sezary syndrome. *Arch Dermatol*. 2002;138(2):182-189.
365. Hooper KK, Smoller BR, Brown JA. Idiopathic follicular mucinosis or mycosis fungoides? classification and diagnostic challenges. *Cutis*. 2015;95(6):E9-E14.
366. Cerroni L, Kerl H. Primary follicular mucinosis and association with mycosis fungoides and other cutaneous T-cell lymphomas. *J Am Acad Dermatol*. 2004;51(1):146-147.
367. Brown HA, Gibson LE, Pujol RM, Lust JA, Pittelkow MR. Primary follicular mucinosis: long-term follow-up of patients younger than 40 years with and without clonal T-cell receptor gene rearrangement. *J Am Acad Dermatol*. 2002;47(6):856-862.
368. Swoboda R, Kaminska-Winciorek G, Wesolowski M, Dulik K, Giebel S. Granulomatous slack skin variant of mycosis fungoides: clinical and dermoscopic follow-up of a very rare entity. *Dermatol Ther*. 2021;34(2):e14822.
369. Tronnier M, Akarawita J, Sirimanna G, De Silva C, Kempf W. Granulomatous slack skin with vascular involvement. *J Dtsch Dermatol Ges*. 2017;15(10):1029-1030.
370. Gadzia J, Kestenbaum T. Granulomatous slack skin without evidence of a clonal T-cell proliferation. *J Am Acad Dermatol*. 2004;50(2 suppl):S4-S8.
371. Karakelides H, Geller JL, Schroeter AL, et al. Vitamin D-mediated hypercalcemia in slack skin disease: evidence for involvement of extrarenal 25-hydroxyvitamin D 1α-hydroxylase. *J Bone Miner Res*. 2006;21(9):1496-1499.
372. Liu J, Jin H, Liu Y, Zheng H, Fang K, Wang B. Granulomatous slack skin with extracutaneous involvement. *Arch Dermatol*. 2005;141(9):1178-1179.
373. Osuji N, Fearfield L, Matutes E, Wotherspoon AC, Bunker C, Catovsky D. Granulomatous slack skin disease—disease features and response to pentostatin. *Br J Haematol*. 2003;123(2):297-304.

374. Wollina U, Graefe T, Fuller J. Granulomatous slack skin or granulomatous mycosis fungoides—a case report. Complete response to percutaneous radiation and interferon alpha. *J Cancer Res Clin Oncol.* 2002;128(1):50-54.
375. Noto G, Pravata G, Miceli S, Arico M. Granulomatous slack skin: report of a case associated with Hodgkin's disease and a review of the literature. *Br J Dermatol.* 1994;131(2):275-279.
376. Santucci M, Pimpinelli N, Massi D, et al. Cytotoxic/natural killer cell cutaneous lymphomas. Report of EORTC cutaneous lymphoma task force workshop. *Cancer.* 2003;97(3):610-627.
377. Takeshita M, Okamura S, Oshiro Y, et al. Clinicopathologic differences between 22 cases of CD56-negative and CD56-positive subcutaneous panniculitis-like lymphoma in Japan. *Hum Pathol.* 2004;35(2):231-239.
378. Massone C, Chott A, Metze D, et al. Subcutaneous, blastic natural killer (NK), NK/T-cell, and other cytotoxic lymphomas of the skin: a morphologic, immunophenotypic, and molecular study of 50 patients. *Am J Surg Pathol.* 2004;28(6):719-735.
379. Massone C, Lozzi GP, Egberts F, et al. The protean spectrum of non-Hodgkin lymphomas with prominent involvement of subcutaneous fat. *J Cutan Pathol.* 2006;33(6):418-425.
380. Rose C, Leverkus M, Fleischer M, Shimanovich I. Histopathology of panniculitis – aspects of biopsy techniques and difficulties in diagnosis. *J Dtsch Dermatol Ges.* 2012;10(6):421-425.
381. Weingartner JS, Zedek DC, Burkhart CN, Morrell DS. Lupus erythematosus panniculitis in children: report of three cases and review of previously reported cases. *Pediatr Dermatol.* 2012;29(2):169-176.
382. Fernandez-Pol S, Costa HA, Steiner DF, et al. High-throughput sequencing of subcutaneous panniculitis-like T-cell lymphoma reveals Candidate pathogenic mutations. *Appl Immunohistochem Mol Morphol.* 2019;27(10):740-748.
383. Bosisio F, Boi S, Caputo V, et al. Lobular panniculitic infiltrates with overlapping histopathologic features of lupus panniculitis (lupus profundus) and subcutaneous T-cell lymphoma: a conceptual and practical dilemma. *Am J Surg Pathol.* 2015;39(2):206-211.
384. Hoque SR, Child FJ, Whittaker SJ, et al. Subcutaneous panniculitis-like T-cell lymphoma: a clinicopathological, immunophenotypic and molecular analysis of six patients. *Br J Dermatol.* 2003;148(3):516-525.
385. Sitthinamsuwan P, Pattanaprichakul P, Treetipsatit J, et al. Subcutaneous panniculitis-like T-cell lymphoma versus lupus erythematosus panniculitis: distinction by means of the periadipocytic cell proliferation index. *Am J Dermatopathol.* 2018;40(8):567-574.
386. Rudolph N, Klemke CD, Ziemer M, Simon JC, Treudler R. Hemophagocytic lymphohistiocytosis associated with subcutaneous panniculitis-like T-cell lymphoma. *J Dtsch Dermatol Ges.* 2016;14(11):1140-1142.
387. Musick SR, Lynch DT. *Subcutaneous panniculitis like T-cell lymphoma.* In: StatPearls. 2021.
388. Toro JR, Beaty M, Sorbara L, et al. Gamma delta T-cell lymphoma of the skin: a clinical, microscopic, and molecular study. *Arch Dermatol.* 2000;136(8):1024-1032.
389. Munn SE, McGregor JM, Jones A, et al. Clinical and pathological heterogeneity in cutaneous gamma-delta T-cell lymphoma: a report of three cases and a review of the literature. *Br J Dermatol.* 1996;135(6):976-981.
390. Magro CM, Wang X. Indolent primary cutaneous γ/δ T-cell lymphoma localized to the subcutaneous panniculus and its association with atypical lymphocytic lobular panniculitis. *Am J Clin Pathol.* 2012;138(1):50-56.
391. Merrill ED, Agbay R, Miranda RN, et al. Primary cutaneous T-cell lymphomas showing gamma-delta (γδ) phenotype and predominantly epidermotropic pattern are clinicopathologically distinct from classic primary cutaneous γδ T-cell lymphomas. *Am J Surg Pathol.* 2017;41(2):204-215.
392. Ahmad E, Kingma DW, Jaffe ES, et al. Flow cytometric immunophenotypic profiles of mature gamma delta T-cell malignancies involving peripheral blood and bone marrow. *Cytometry B Clin Cytom.* 2005;67(1):6-12.
393. Gru AA, Jaffe ES. Cutaneous EBV-related lymphoproliferative disorders. *Semin Diagn Pathol.* 2017;34(1):60-75.
394. Gormley RH, Hess SD, Anand D, Junkins-Hopkins J, Rook AH, Kim EJ. Primary cutaneous aggressive epidermotropic CD8+ T-cell lymphoma. *J Am Acad Dermatol.* 2010;62(2):300-307.
395. Agnarsson BA, Vonderheid EC, Kadin ME. Cutaneous T cell lymphoma with suppressor/cytotoxic (CD8) phenotype: identification of rapidly progressive and chronic subtypes. *J Am Acad Dermatol.* 1990;22(4):569-577.
396. Berti E, Tomasini D, Vermeer MH, Meijer CJ, Alessi E, Willemze R. Primary cutaneous CD8-positive epidermotropic cytotoxic T cell lymphomas. A distinct clinicopathological entity with an aggressive clinical behavior. *Am J Pathol.* 1999;155(2):483-492.
397. Onsun N, Dizman D, Emiroğlu N, et al. Challenges in early diagnosis of primary cutaneous CD8+ aggressive epidermotropic cytotoxic T-cell lymphoma: a case series of four patients. *Eur J Dermatol.* 2020;30(4):358-361.
398. Tomasini C, Novelli M, Fanoni D, Berti EF. Erythema multiforme-like lesions in primary cutaneous aggressive cytotoxic epidermotropic CD8+ T-cell lymphoma: a diagnostic and therapeutic challenge. *J Cutan Pathol.* 2017;44(10):867-873.
399. Poszepczynska-Guigne E, Jagou M, Wechsler J, Dieng MT, Revuz J, Bagot M. Cutaneous CD8+ epidermotropic cytotoxic T-cell lymphoma with aggressive course. *Ann Dermatol Venereol.* 2006;133(3):253-256.
400. Ayala D, Ramon MD, Cabezas M, Jorda E. Primary cutaneous CD4+ small/medium-sized pleomorphic T-cell lymphoma with expression of follicular T-helper cell markers and spontaneous remission. *Actas Dermosifiliogr.* 2016;107(4):357-359.
401. von den Driesch P, Coors EA. Localized cutaneous small to medium-sized pleomorphic T-cell lymphoma: a report of 3 cases stable for years. *J Am Acad Dermatol.* 2002;46(4):531-535.
402. Scarabello A, Leinweber B, Ardigo M, et al. Cutaneous lymphomas with prominent granulomatous reaction: a potential pitfall in the histopathologic diagnosis of cutaneous T- and B-cell lymphomas. *Am J Surg Pathol.* 2002;26(10):1259-1268.
403. Rodriguez Pinilla SM, Roncador G, Rodriguez-Peralto JL, et al. Primary cutaneous CD4+ small/medium-sized pleomorphic T-cell lymphoma expresses follicular T-cell markers. *Am J Surg Pathol.* 2009;33(1):81-90.
404. Cetinozman F, Jansen PM, Willemze R. Expression of programmed death-1 in primary cutaneous CD4-positive small/medium-sized pleomorphic T-cell lymphoma, cutaneous pseudo-T-cell lymphoma, and other types of cutaneous T-cell lymphoma. *Am J Surg Pathol.* 2012;36(1):109-116.
405. Battistella M, Beylot-Barry M, Bachelez H, Rivet J, Vergier B, Bagot M. Primary cutaneous follicular helper T-cell lymphoma: a new subtype of cutaneous T-cell lymphoma reported in a series of 5 cases. *Arch Dermatol.* 2012;148(7):832-839.
406. Alberti-Violetti S, Torres-Cabala CA, Talpur R, et al. Clinicopathological and molecular study of primary cutaneous CD4+ small/medium-sized pleomorphic T-cell lymphoma. *J Cutan Pathol.* 2016;43(12):1121-1130.
407. Magro CM, Momtahen S. Differential NFATc1 expression in primary cutaneous CD4+ small/medium-sized pleomorphic T-cell lymphoma and other forms of cutaneous T-cell lymphoma and pseudolymphoma. *Am J Dermatopathol.* 2017;39(2):95-103.
408. Kempf W, Mitteldorf C, Battistella M, et al. Primary cutaneous peripheral T-cell lymphoma, not otherwise specified: results of a multicentre European Organization for Research and Treatment of Cancer (EORTC) cutaneous lymphoma taskforce study on the clinico-pathological and prognostic features. *J Eur Acad Dermatol Venereol.* 2021;35(3):658-668.
409. Petrella T, Maubec E, Cornillet-Lefebvre P, et al. Indolent CD8-positive lymphoid proliferation of the ear: a distinct primary cutaneous T-cell lymphoma? *Am J Surg Pathol.* 2007;31(12):1887-1892.
410. Tjahjono LA, Davis MDP, Witzig TE, Comfere NI. Primary cutaneous acral CD8+ T-cell lymphoma-A single center review of 3 cases and recent literature review. *Am J Dermatopathol.* 2019;41(9):644-648.
411. Li JY, Guitart J, Pulitzer MP, et al. Multicenter case series of indolent small/medium-sized CD8+ lymphoid proliferations with predilection for the ear and face. *Am J Dermatopathol.* 2014;36(5):402-408.
412. Goyal A, LeBlanc RE, Carter JB. Cutaneous B-cell lymphoma. *Hematol Oncol Clin North Am.* 2019;33(1):149-161.
413. Sokol L, Naghashpour M, Glass LF. Primary cutaneous B-cell lymphomas: recent advances in diagnosis and management. *Cancer Control.* 2012;19(3):236-244.
414. Wilcox RA. Cutaneous B-cell lymphomas: 2016 update on diagnosis, risk-stratification, and management. *Am J Hematol.* 2016;91(10):1052-1055.
415. Gulia A, Saggini A, Wiesner T, et al. Clinicopathologic features of early lesions of primary cutaneous follicle center lymphoma, diffuse type: implications for early diagnosis and treatment. *J Am Acad Dermatol.* 2011;65(5):991-1000.
416. Pandolfino TL, Siegel RS, Kuzel TM, Rosen ST, Guitart J. Primary cutaneous B-cell lymphoma: review and current concepts. *J Clin Oncol.* 2000;18(10):2152-2168.
417. Kerl H, Kodama K, Cerroni L. Diagnostic principles and new developments in primary cutaneous B-cell lymphomas. *J Dermatol Sci.* 2004;34(3):167-175.
418. Anghel G, Pulsoni A, De Rosa L. Primary cutaneous follicle center cell lymphoma and limited stage follicular non-Hodgkin's lymphoma: a comparison of clinical and biological features. *Leuk Lymphoma.* 2002;43(11):2109-2115.
419. Quereux G, Brocard A, Peuvrel L, Nguyen JM, Knol AC, Dreno B. Systemic rituximab in multifocal primary cutaneous follicle centre lymphoma. *Acta Derm Venereol.* 2011;91(5):562-567.
420. Pileri A, Agostinelli C, Bertuzzi C, et al. BCL-2 expression in primary cutaneous follicle center B-cell lymphoma and its prognostic role. *Front Oncol.* 2020;10:662.
421. Jelic TM, Berry PK, Jubelirer SJ, et al. Primary cutaneous follicle center lymphoma of the arm with a novel chromosomal translocation t(12;21)(q13;q22): a case report. *Am J Hematol.* 2006;81(6):448-453.
422. Gibson SE, Swerdlow SH. How I diagnose primary cutaneous marginal zone lymphoma. *Am J Clin Pathol.* 2020;154(4):428-449.
423. Hoefnagel JJ, Vermeer MH, Jansen PM, et al. Primary cutaneous marginal zone B-cell lymphoma: clinical and therapeutic features in 50 cases. *Arch Dermatol.* 2005;141(9):1139-1145.
424. Willemze R. Primary cutaneous B-cell lymphoma: classification and treatment. *Curr Opin Oncol.* 2006;18(5):425-431.
425. Kempf W, Kerl H, Kutzner H. CD123-positive plasmacytoid dendritic cells in primary cutaneous marginal zone B-cell lymphoma: a crucial role and a new lymphoma paradigm. *Am J Dermatopathol.* 2010;32(2):194-196.
426. Fujita N, Ono Y, Sano A, Tanaka Y. Primary cutaneous diffuse large B-cell lymphoma, leg type. *Intern Med.* 2020;59(14):1785.
427. Grange F, Beylot-Barry M, Courville P, et al. Primary cutaneous diffuse large B-cell lymphoma, leg type: clinicopathologic features and prognostic analysis in 60 cases. *Arch Dermatol.* 2007;143(9):1144-1150.
428. Brogan BL, Zic JA, Kinney MC, Hu JY, Hamilton KS, Greer JP. Large B-cell lymphoma of the leg: clinical and pathologic characteristics in a North American series. *J Am Acad Dermatol.* 2003;49(2):223-228.
429. Massone C, Fink-Puches R, Wolf I, Zalaudek I, Cerroni L. Atypical clinicopathologic presentation of primary cutaneous diffuse large B-cell lymphoma, leg type. *J Am Acad Dermatol.* 2015;72(6):1016-1020.
430. Gellrich S, Rutz S, Golembowski S, et al. Primary cutaneous follicle center cell lymphomas and large B cell lymphomas of the leg descend from germinal center cells. A single cell polymerase chain reaction analysis. *J Invest Dermatol.* 2001;117(6):1512-1520.
431. Koens L, Vermeer MH, Willemze R, Jansen PM. IgM expression on paraffin sections distinguishes primary cutaneous large B-cell lymphoma, leg type from primary cutaneous follicle center lymphoma. *Am J Surg Pathol.* 2010;34(7):1043-1048.

432. Sundram U, Kim Y, Mraz-Gernhard S, Hoppe R, Natkunam Y, Kohler S. Expression of the bcl-6 and MUM1/IRF4 proteins correlate with overall and disease-specific survival in patients with primary cutaneous large B-cell lymphoma: a tissue microarray study. *J Cutan Pathol.* 2005;32(3):227-234.
433. Hoefnagel JJ, Dijkman R, Basso K, et al. Distinct types of primary cutaneous large B-cell lymphoma identified by gene expression profiling. *Blood.* 2005;105(9):3671-3678.
434. van Galen JC, Hoefnagel JJ, Vermeer MH, et al. Profiling of apoptosis genes identifies distinct types of primary cutaneous large B cell lymphoma. *J Pathol.* 2008;215(3):340-346.
435. Battistella M, Romero M, Castro-Vega LJ, et al. The high expression of the microRNA 17-92 cluster and its pralogs, and the downregulation of the target gene PTEN, is associated with primary cutaneous B-cell lymphoma progression. *J Invest Dermatol.* 2015;135(6):1659-1667.
436. Ponzoni M, Ferreri AJM. Intravascular lymphoma: a neoplasm of "homeless" lymphocytes? *Hematol Oncol.* 2006;24(3):105-112.
437. Terrier B, Aouba A, Vasiliu V, et al. Intravascular lymphoma associated with haemophagocytic syndrome: a very rare entity in western countries. *Eur J Haematol.* 2005;75(4):341-345.
438. Nixon BK, Kussick SJ, Carlon MJ, Rubin BP. Intravascular large B-cell lymphoma involving hemangiomas: an unusual presentation of a rare neoplasm. *Mod Pathol.* 2005;18(8):1121-1126.
439. Cerroni L, Zalaudek I, Kerl H. Intravascular large B-cell lymphoma colonizing cutaneous hemangiomas. *Dermatology.* 2004;209(2):132-134.
440. Dědic K, Belada D, Zak P, Nozicka Z. Intravascular large B-cell lymphoma presenting as cutaneous panniculitis. *Acta Med.* 2003;46(3):121-123.
441. Eros N, Karolyi Z, Kovacs A, Takacs I, Radvanyi G, Kelenyi G. Intravascular B-cell lymphoma. *J Am Acad Dermatol.* 2002;47(5 suppl):S260-S262.
442. Ferreri AJM, Campo E, Seymour JF, et al. Intravascular lymphoma: clinical presentation, natural history, management and prognostic factors in a series of 38 cases, with special emphasis on the 'cutaneous variant. *Br J Haematol.* 2004;127(2):173-183.
443. Rochate D, Pavao C, Amaral R, et al. Extramedullary acute leukemia-still an unforeseen presentation. *Hematol Rep.* 2022;14(2):143-148.
444. Kurata H, Okukubo M, Fukuda E, Ichihashi M, Ueda M. Myeloid markers should be undertaken in cases of CD56 positivity to exclude granulocytic sarcoma. *Br J Dermatol.* 2002;147(3):609-611.
445. Khalid S, Adil SN, Vaziri IA. Granulocytic sarcoma in the absence of acute myeloid leukemia: a case report. *Indian J Pathol Microbiol.* 2007;50(1):88-90.
446. Beswick SJ, Jones EL, Mahendra P, Marsden JR. Chloroma (aleukaemic leukaemia cutis) initially diagnosed as cutaneous lymphoma. *Clin Exp Dermatol.* 2002;27(4):272-274.
447. Cronin DMP, George TI, Sundram UN. An updated approach to the diagnosis of myeloid leukemia cutis. *Am J Clin Pathol.* 2009;132(1):101-110.
448. Cibull TL, Thomas AB, O'Malley DP, Billings SD. Myeloid leukemia cutis: a histologic and immunohistochemical review. *J Cutan Pathol.* 2008;35(2):180-185.
449. Benet C, Gomez A, Aguilar C, et al. Histologic and immunohistologic characterization of skin localization of myeloid disorders: a study of 173 cases. *Am J Clin Pathol.* 2011;135(2):278-290.
450. Lamberg SI, Bunn PA Jr. Cutaneous T-cell lymphomas. Summary of the mycosis fungoides cooperative group-national cancer institute workshop. *Arch Dermatol.* 1979;115(9):1103-1105.
451. Schechter GP, Sausville EA, Fischmann AB, et al. Evaluation of circulating malignant cells provides prognostic information in cutaneous T cell lymphoma. *Blood.* 1987;69(3):841-849.
452. Vonderheid EC, Pena J, Nowell P. Sezary cell counts in erythrodermic cutaneous T-cell lymphoma: implications for prognosis and staging. *Leuk Lymphoma.* 2006;47(9):1841-1856.
453. Shapiro M, Yun M, Junkins-Hopkins JM, et al. Assessment of tumor burden and treatment response by 18F-fluorodeoxyglucose injection and positron emission tomography in patients with cutaneous T- and B-cell lymphomas. *J Am Acad Dermatol.* 2002;47(4):623-628.
454. Spencer A, Gazzani P, Gadvi R, et al. Computed tomography scanning in mycosis fungoides: optimizing the balance between benefit and harm. *Br J Dermatol.* 2018;178(2):563-564.
455. Bass JC, Korobkin MT, Cooper KD, Kane NM, Platt JF. Cutaneous T-cell lymphoma: CT in evaluation and staging. *Radiology.* 1993;186(1):273-278.
456. Miketic LM, Chambers TP, Lembersky BC. Cutaneous T-cell lymphoma: value of CT in staging and determining prognosis. *AJR Am J Roentgenol.* 1993;160(5):1129-1132.
457. Tsai EY, Taur A, Espinosa L, et al. Staging accuracy in mycosis fungoides and Sezary syndrome using integrated positron emission tomography and computed tomography. *Arch Dermatol.* 2006;142(5):577-584.
458. Feeney J, Horwitz S, Gonen M, Schoder H. Characterization of T-cell lymphomas by FDG PET/CT. *AJR Am J Roentgenol.* 2010;195(2):333-340.
459. Xu L, Pang H, Zhu J, et al. Mycosis fungoides staged by 18F-flurodeoxyglucose positron emission tomography/computed tomography: case report and review of literature. *Medicine (Baltimore).* 2016;95(45):e5044.
460. Alanteri E, Usmani S, Marafi F, et al. The role of fluorine-18 fluorodeoxyglucose positron emission tomography in patients with mycosis fungoides. *Indian J Nucl Med.* 2015;30(3):199-203.
461. Besson FL, Galateau-Salle F, Comoz F, Troussard X, Agostini D, Dompmartin A. Folliculotropic mycosis fungoides with rare secondary pulmonary extension: potential role of FDG PET/CT in the assessment of epidermotropic T cell lymphoma. *Eur J Dermatol.* 2013;23(3):398-399.
462. Cheson BD, Fisher RI, Barrington SF, et al. Recommendations for initial evaluation, staging, and response assessment of Hodgkin and non-Hodgkin lymphoma: the Lugano classification. *J Clin Oncol.* 2014;32(27):3059-3068.
463. Vonderheid EC, Diamond LW, van Vloten WA, et al. Lymph node classification systems in cutaneous T-cell lymphoma. Evidence for the utility of the Working Formulation of Non-Hodgkin's Lymphomas for Clinical Usage. *Cancer.* 1994;73(1):207-218.
464. Galindo LM, Garcia FU, Hanau CA, et al. Fine-needle aspiration biopsy in the evaluation of lymphadenopathy associated with cutaneous T-cell lymphoma (mycosis fungoides/Sezary syndrome). *Am J Clin Pathol.* 2000;113(6):865-871.
465. Bakels V, Van Oostveen JW, Geerts ML, et al. Diagnostic and prognostic significance of clonal T-cell receptor beta gene rearrangements in lymph nodes of patients with mycosis fungoides. *J Pathol.* 1993;170(3):249-255.
466. Kern DE, Kidd PG, Moe R, Hanke D, Olerud JE. Analysis of T-cell receptor gene rearrangement in lymph nodes of patients with mycosis fungoides. Prognostic implications. *Arch Dermatol.* 1998;134(2):158-164.
467. Laforga JB, Chorda D, Sevilla F. Intramammary lymph node involvement by mycosis fungoides diagnosed by fine-needle aspiration biopsy. *Diagn Cytopathol.* 1998;19(2):124-126.
468. Calvani J, de Masson A, de Margerie-Mellon C, et al. Image-guided lymph node core-needle biopsy predicts survival in mycosis fungoides and Sezary syndrome. *Br J Dermatol.* 2021;185(2):419-427.
469. Graham SJ, Sharpe RW, Steinberg SM, Cotelingam JD, Sausville EA, Foss FM. Prognostic implications of a bone marrow histopathologic classification system in mycosis fungoides and the Sezary syndrome. *Cancer.* 1993;72(3):726-734.
470. Zackheim HS, Amin S, Kashani-Sabet M, McMillan A. Prognosis in cutaneous T-cell lymphoma by skin stage: long-term survival in 489 patients. *J Am Acad Dermatol.* 1999;40(3):418-425.
471. Kim YH, Liu HL, Mraz-Gernhard S, Varghese A, Hoppe RT. Long-term outcome of 525 patients with mycosis fungoides and Sezary syndrome: clinical prognostic factors and risk for disease progression. *Arch Dermatol.* 2003;139(7):857-866.
472. Assaf C, Hummel M, Steinhoff M, et al. Early TCR-beta and TCR-gamma PCR detection of T-cell clonality indicates minimal tumor disease in lymph nodes of cutaneous T-cell lymphoma: diagnostic and prognostic implications. *Blood.* 2005;105(2):503-510.
473. Virmani P, Levin L, Myskowski PL, et al. Clinical outcome and prognosis of young patients with mycosis fungoides. *Pediatr Dermatol.* 2017;34(5):547-553.
474. Marti RM, Pujol RM, Servitje O, et al. Sezary syndrome and related variants of classic cutaneous T-cell lymphoma. A descriptive and prognostic clinicopathologic study of 29 cases. *Leuk Lymphoma.* 2003;44(1):59-69.
475. Foulc P, N'Guyen JM, Dreno B. Prognostic factors in Sezary syndrome: a study of 28 patients. *Br J Dermatol.* 2003;149(6):1152-1158.
476. Hoppe RT, Wood GS, Abel EA. Mycosis fungoides and the Sezary syndrome: pathology, staging, and treatment. *Curr Probl Cancer.* 1990;14(6):293-371.
477. Abel EA, Wood GS, Hoppe RT. Mycosis fungoides: clinical and histologic features, staging, evaluation, and approach to treatment. *CA Cancer J Clin.* 1993;43(2):93-115.
478. Axelrod PI, Lorber B, Vonderheid EC. Infections complicating mycosis fungoides and Sezary syndrome. *J Am Med Assoc.* 1992;267(10):1354-1358.
479. Kuzel TM, Roenigk HH Jr, Rosen ST. Mycosis fungoides and the Sezary syndrome: a review of pathogenesis, diagnosis, and therapy. *J Clin Oncol.* 1991;9(7):1298-1313.
480. Kantor AF, Curtis RE, Vonderheid EC, van Scott EJ, Fraumeni JF Jr. Risk of second malignancy after cutaneous T-cell lymphoma. *Cancer.* 1989;63(8):1612-1615.
481. Scarisbrick JJ, Prince HM, Vermeer MH, et al. Cutaneous lymphoma international consortium study of outcome in advanced stages of mycosis fungoides and Sezary syndrome: effect of specific prognostic markers on survival and development of a prognostic model. *J Clin Oncol.* 2015;33(32):3766-3773.
482. Trautinger F, Knobler R, Willemze R, et al. EORTC consensus recommendations for the treatment of mycosis fungoides/Sezary syndrome. *Eur J Cancer.* 2006;42(8):1014-1030.
483. Bloom T, Kuzel TM, Querfeld C, Guitart J, Rosen ST. Cutaneous T-cell lymphomas: a review of new discoveries and treatments. *Curr Treat Options Oncol.* 2012;13(1):102-121.
484. Kierland RR, Watkins CH, Shullenberger CC. The use of nitrogen mustard in the treatment of mycosis fungoides. *J Invest Dermatol.* 1947;9(4):195-201.
485. Fenn JE, Udelsman R. First use of intravenous chemotherapy cancer treatment: rectifying the record. *J Am Coll Surg.* 2011;212(3):413-417.
486. Brulikova L, Hlavac J, Hradil P. DNA interstrand cross-linking agents and their chemotherapeutic potential. *Curr Med Chem.* 2012;19(3):364-385.
487. Ramsay DL, Meller JA, Zackheim HS. Topical treatment of early cutaneous T-cell lymphoma. *Hematol Oncol Clin North Am.* 1995;9(5):1031-1056.
488. Van Scott EJ, Kalmanson JD. Complete remissions of mycosis fungoides lymphoma induced by topical nitrogen mustard (HN2). Control of delayed hypersensitivity to HN2 by desensitization and by induction of specific immunologic tolerance. *Cancer.* 1973;32(1):18-30.
489. Kim YH, Martinez G, Varghese A, Hoppe RT. Topical nitrogen mustard in the management of mycosis fungoides: update of the stanford experience. *Arch Dermatol.* 2003;139(2):165-173.
490. Lessin SR, Duvic M, Guitart J, et al. Topical chemotherapy in cutaneous T-cell lymphoma: positive results of a randomized, controlled, multicenter trial testing the efficacy and safety of a novel mechlorethamine, 0.02%, gel in mycosis fungoides. *JAMA Dermatol.* 2013;149(1):25-32.
491. Ramsay DL, Halperin PS, Zeleniuch-Jacquotte A. Topical mechlorethamine therapy for early stage mycosis fungoides. *J Am Acad Dermatol.* 1988;19(4):684-691.
492. Vonderheid EC, Tan ET, Kantor AF, Shrager L, Micaily B, Van Scott EJ. Long-term efficacy, curative potential, and carcinogenicity of topical mechlorethamine chemotherapy in cutaneous T cell lymphoma. *J Am Acad Dermatol.* 1989;20(3):416-428.
493. Lindahl LM, Fenger-Gron M, Iversen L. Topical nitrogen mustard therapy in patients with Langerhans cell histiocytosis. *Br J Dermatol.* 2012;166(3):642-645.

494. Liner K, Brown C, McGirt LY. Clinical potential of mechlorethamine gel for the topical treatment of mycosis fungoides-type cutaneous T-cell lymphoma: a review on current efficacy and safety data. *Drug Des Devel Ther*. 2018;12:241-254.
495. Apisarnthanarax N, Wood GS, Stevens SR, et al. Phase I clinical trial of O6-benzylguanine and topical carmustine in the treatment of cutaneous T-cell lymphoma, mycosis fungoides type. *Arch Dermatol*. 2012;148(5):613-620.
496. Zackheim HS. Treatment of mycosis fungoides with topical nitrosourea compounds. *Arch Dermatol*. 1972;106(2):177-182.
497. Zackheim HS, Epstein EH Jr, Crain WR. Topical carmustine (BCNU) for cutaneous T cell lymphoma: a 15-year experience in 143 patients. *J Am Acad Dermatol*. 1990;22(5 pt 1):802-810.
498. Tacastacas JD, Chan DV, Carlson S, et al. Evaluation of O6-benzylguanine-potentiated topical carmustine for mycosis fungoides: a phase 1-2 clinical trial. *JAMA Dermatol*. 2017;153(5):413-420.
499. Wackernagel A, Hofer A, Legat F, Kerl H, Wolf P. Efficacy of 8-methoxypsoralen vs. 5-methoxypsoralen plus ultraviolet A therapy in patients with mycosis fungoides. *Br J Dermatol*. 2006;154(3):519-523.
500. Herrmann JJ, Roenigk HH Jr, Honigsmann H. Ultraviolet radiation for treatment of cutaneous T-cell lymphoma. *Hematol Oncol Clin North Am*. 1995;9(5):1077-1088.
501. Okamoto H, Takigawa M, Horio T. Alteration of lymphocyte functions by 8-methoxypsoralen and longwave ultraviolet radiation. I. Suppressive effects of PUVA on T-lymphocyte migration in vitro. *J Invest Dermatol*. 1985;84(3):203-205.
502. Yoo EK, Rook AH, Elenitsas R, Gasparro FP, Vowels BR. Apoptosis induction of ultraviolet light A and photochemotherapy in cutaneous T-cell Lymphoma: relevance to mechanism of therapeutic action. *J Invest Dermatol*. 1996;107(2):235-242.
503. Herrmann JJ, Roenigk HH Jr, Hurria A, et al. Treatment of mycosis fungoides with photochemotherapy (PUVA): long-term follow-up. *J Am Acad Dermatol*. 1995;33(2 pt 1):234-242.
504. Querfeld C, Rosen ST, Kuzel TM, et al. Long-term follow-up of patients with early-stage cutaneous T-cell lymphoma who achieved complete remission with psoralen plus UV-A monotherapy. *Arch Dermatol*. 2005;141(3):305-311.
505. Dogra S, Mahajan R. Phototherapy for mycosis fungoides. *Indian J Dermatol Venereol Leprol*. 2015;81(2):124-135.
506. Weber F, Schmuth M, Sepp N, Fritsch P. Bath-water PUVA therapy with 8-methoxypsoralen in mycosis fungoides. *Acta Derm Venereol*. 2005;85(4):329-332.
507. Stern RS; PUVA Follow Up Study. The risk of melanoma in association with long-term exposure to PUVA. *J Am Acad Dermatol*. 2001;44(5):755-761.
508. Ramsay DL, Lish KM, Yalowitz CB, Soter NA. Ultraviolet-B phototherapy for early-stage cutaneous T-cell lymphoma. *Arch Dermatol*. 1992;128(7):931-933.
509. Coven TR, Burack LH, Gilleaudeau R, Keogh M, Ozawa M, Krueger JG. Narrowband UV-B produces superior clinical and histopathological resolution of moderate-to-severe psoriasis in patients compared with broadband UV-B. *Arch Dermatol*. 1997;133(12):1514-1522.
510. Olsen EA, Hodak E, Anderson T, et al. Guidelines for phototherapy of mycosis fungoides and Sezary syndrome: a consensus statement of the United States Cutaneous Lymphoma Consortium. *J Am Acad Dermatol*. 2016;74(1):27-58.
511. el-Ghorr AA, Norval M. Biological effects of narrow-band (311 nm TL01) UVB irradiation: a review. *J Photochem Photobiol B*. 1997;38(2-3):99-106.
512. Grandi V, Baldo A, Berti E, et al. Italian expert-based recommendations on the use of photo(chemo)therapy in the management of mycosis fungoides: results of an e-Delphi consensus. *Photodermatol Photoimmunol Photomed*. 2021;37(4):334-342.
513. Ghodsi SZ, Hallaji Z, Balighi K, Safar F, Chams-Davatchi C. Narrow-band UVB in the treatment of early stage mycosis fungoides: report of 16 patients. *Clin Exp Dermatol*. 2005;30(4):376-378.
514. Hearn RMR, Kerr AC, Rahim KF, Ferguson J, Dawe RS. Incidence of skin cancers in 3867 patients treated with narrow-band ultraviolet B phototherapy. *Br J Dermatol*. 2008;159(4):931-935.
515. Lee E, Koo J, Berger T. UVB phototherapy and skin cancer risk: a review of the literature. *Int J Dermatol*. 2005;44(5):355-360.
516. Kunisada M, Kumimoto H, Ishizaki K, Sakumi K, Nakabeppu Y, Nishigori C. Narrow-band UVB induces more carcinogenic skin tumors than broad-band UVB through the formation of cyclobutane pyrimidine dimer. *J Invest Dermatol*. 2007;127(12):2865-2871.
517. Clark C, Dawe RS, Evans AT, Lowe G, Ferguson J. Narrowband TL-01 phototherapy for patch-stage mycosis fungoides. *Arch Dermatol*. 2000;136(6):748-752.
518. Gathers RC, Scherschun L, Malick F, Fivenson DP, Lim HW. Narrowband UVB phototherapy for early-stage mycosis fungoides. *J Am Acad Dermatol*. 2002;47(2):191-197.
519. El-Mofty M, El-Darouty M, Salonas M, et al. Narrow band UVB (311 nm), psoralen UVB (311 nm) and PUVA therapy in the treatment of early-stage mycosis fungoides: a right-left comparative study. *Photodermatol Photoimmunol Photomed*. 2005;21(6):281-286.
520. Diederen PV, van Weelden H, Sanders CJG, Toonstra J, van Vloten WA. Narrowband UVB and psoralen-UVA in the treatment of early-stage mycosis fungoides: a retrospective study. *J Am Acad Dermatol*. 2003;48(2):215-219.
521. Pavlotsky F, Barzilai A, Kasem R, Shpiro D, Trau H. UVB in the management of early stage mycosis fungoides. *J Eur Acad Dermatol Venereol*. 2006;20(5):565-572.
522. Ahmad K, Rogers S, McNicholas PD, Collins P. Narrowband UVB and PUVA in the treatment of mycosis fungoides: a retrospective study. *Acta Derm Venereol*. 2007;87(5):413-417.
523. Coronel-Perez IM, Carrizosa-Esquivel AM, Camacho-Martinez F. Narrow band UVB therapy in early stage mycosis fungoides. A study of 23 patients. *Actas Dermosifiliogr*. 2007;98(4):259-264.
524. Gokdemir G, Barutcuoglu B, Sakiz D, Köşlü A. Narrowband UVB phototherapy for early-stage mycosis fungoides: evaluation of clinical and histopathological changes. *J Eur Acad Dermatol Venereol*. 2006;20(7):804-809.
525. Friedland R, David M, Feinmesser M, Barzilai A, Hodak E. NB-UVB (311-312 nm)-induced lentigines in patients with mycosis fungoides: a new adverse effect of phototherapy. *J Eur Acad Dermatol Venereol*. 2012;26(9):1158-1162.
526. Xu HH, Xiao T, Chen HD. Lentigines following narrow-band ultraviolet B phototherapy for mycosis fungoides. *Clin Exp Dermatol*. 2010;35(3):326-328.
527. Friedland R, David M, Feinmesser M, Fenig-Nakar S, Hodak E. Idiopathic guttate hypomelanosis-like lesions in patients with mycosis fungoides: a new adverse effect of phototherapy. *J Eur Acad Dermatol Venereol*. 2010;24(9):1026-1030.
528. El-Mofty M, Mostafa WZ, Bosseila M, et al. A large scale analytical study on efficacy of different photo(chemo)therapeutic modalities in the treatment of psoriasis, vitiligo and mycosis fungoides. *Dermatol Ther*. 2010;23(4):428-434.
529. Pavlovsky M, Baum S, Shpiro D, Pavlovsky L, Pavlotsky F. Narrow band UVB: is it effective and safe for paediatric psoriasis and atopic dermatitis? *J Eur Acad Dermatol Venereol*. 2011;25(6):727-729.
530. Veith W, Deleo V, Silverberg N. Medical phototherapy in childhood skin diseases. *Minerva Pediatr*. 2011;63(4):327-333.
531. Burg G, Dummer R. Historical perspective on the use of retinoids in cutaneous T-cell lymphoma (CTCL). *Clin Lymphoma*. 2000;1(suppl 1):S41-S44.
532. Huen AO, Kim EJ. The role of systemic retinoids in the treatment of cutaneous T-cell lymphoma. *Dermatol Clin*. 2015;33(4):715-729.
533. Molin L, Thomsen K, Volden G, et al. Oral retinoids in mycosis fungoides and Sezary syndrome: a comparison of isotretinoin and etretinate. A study from the Scandinavian Mycosis Fungoides Group. *Acta Derm Venereol*. 1987;67(3):232-236.
534. Thomsen K, Molin L, Volden G, Lange Wantzin G, Hellbe L. 13-cis-retinoic acid effective in mycosis fungoides. A report from the Scandinavian Mycosis Fungoides Group. *Acta Derm Venereol*. 1984;64(6):563-566.
535. Kessler JF, Jones SE, Levine N, Lynch PJ, Booth AR, Meyskens FL Jr. Isotretinoin and cutaneous helper T-cell lymphoma (mycosis fungoides). *Arch Dermatol*. 1987;123(2):201-204.
536. Sanz MJ, Albertos F, Otero E, Juez M, Morcillo EJ, Piqueras L. Retinoid X receptor agonists Impair arterial mononuclear cell recruitment through peroxisome proliferator-activated receptor-gamma activation. *J Immunol*. 2012;189(1):411-424.
537. Boergesen M, Pedersen TA, Gross B, et al. Genome-wide profiling of liver X receptor, retinoid X receptor, and peroxisome proliferator-activated receptor alpha in mouse liver reveals extensive sharing of binding sites. *Mol Cell Biol*. 2012;32(4):852-867.
538. Zhang C, Hazarika P, Ni X, Weidner DA, Duvic M. Induction of apoptosis by bexarotene in cutaneous T-cell lymphoma cells: relevance to mechanism of therapeutic action. *Clin Cancer Res*. 2002;8(5):1234-1240.
539. Duvic M, Hymes K, Heald P, et al. Bexarotene is effective and safe for treatment of refractory advanced-stage cutaneous T-cell lymphoma: multinational phase II-III trial results. *J Clin Oncol*. 2001;19(9):2456-2471.
540. Duvic M, Martin AG, Kim Y, et al. Phase 2 and 3 clinical trial of oral bexarotene (Targretin capsules) for the treatment of refractory or persistent early-stage cutaneous T-cell lymphoma. *Arch Dermatol*. 2001;137(5):581-593.
541. Talpur R, Ward S, Apisarnthanarax N, Breuer-Mcham J, Duvic M. Optimizing bexarotene therapy for cutaneous T-cell lymphoma. *J Am Acad Dermatol*. 2002;47(5):672-684.
542. Makita N, Manaka K, Sato J, Mitani K, Nangaku M, Iiri T. Bexarotene-induced hypothyroidism: characteristics and therapeutic strategies. *Clin Endocrinol*. 2019;91(1):195-200.
543. Sherman SI. Etiology, diagnosis, and treatment recommendations for central hypothyroidism associated with bexarotene therapy for cutaneous T-cell lymphoma. *Clin Lymphoma*. 2003;3(4):249-252.
544. Hamada T, Morita A, Suga H, et al. Safety and efficacy of bexarotene for Japanese patients with cutaneous T-cell lymphoma: real-world experience from post-marketing surveillance. *J Dermatol*. 2022;49(2):253-262.
545. Panchal MR, Scarisbrick JJ. The utility of bexarotene in mycosis fungoides and Sezary syndrome. *OncoTargets Ther*. 2015;8:367-373.
546. Cabello I, Servitje O, Corbella X, Bardes I, Pinto X. Omega-3 fatty acids as adjunctive treatment for bexarotene-induced hypertriglyceridaemia in patients with cutaneous T-cell lymphoma. *Clin Exp Dermatol*. 2017;42(3):276-281.
547. DeAngelo S, Mann KI, Abdulbasit M, Ahnert A, Sundlof DW. A case report: rapid progression of coronary atherosclerosis in a patient taking Targretin (Bexarotene). *Cardiooncology*. 2020;6(1):31.
548. Lalloyer F, Pedersen TA, Gross B, et al. Rexinoid bexarotene modulates triglyceride but not cholesterol metabolism via gene-specific permissivity of the RXR/LXR heterodimer in the liver. *Arterioscler Thromb Vasc Biol*. 2009;29(10):1488-1495.
549. Lalloyer F, Fievet C, Lestavel S, et al. The RXR agonist bexarotene improves cholesterol homeostasis and inhibits atherosclerosis progression in a mouse model of mixed dyslipidemia. *Arterioscler Thromb Vasc Biol*. 2006;26(12):2731-2737.
550. Shan P, Pu J, Yuan A, et al. RXR agonists inhibit oxidative stress-induced apoptosis in H9c2 rat ventricular cells. *Biochem Biophys Res Commun*. 2008;375(4):628-633.
551. Breneman D, Duvic M, Kuzel T, Yocum R, Truglia J, Stevens VJ. Phase 1 and 2 trial of bexarotene gel for skin-directed treatment of patients with cutaneous T-cell lymphoma. *Arch Dermatol*. 2002;138(3):325-332.
552. Heald P, Mehlmauer M, Martin AG, Crowley CA, Yocum RC, Reich SD; Worldwide Bexarotene Study Group. Topical bexarotene therapy for patients with refractory or persistent early-stage cutaneous T-cell lymphoma: results of the phase III clinical trial. *J Am Acad Dermatol*. 2003;49(5):801-815.
553. Olsen EA, Bunn PA. Interferon in the treatment of cutaneous T-cell lymphoma. *Hematol Oncol Clin North Am*. 1995;9(5):1089-1107.
554. Bunn PA Jr, Foon KA. Therapeutic options in advanced cutaneous T cell lymphomas: a role for interferon alfa-2a (Roferon-A). *Semin Oncol*. 1985;12(4 suppl 5):18-24.
555. Dreno B, Fleischmann M, Valard S, et al. Induction of myelo-monocytic My7 antigen (CD13) expression by interferon-alpha in basal cells of cutaneous T-cell lymphomas. *Br J Dermatol*. 1992;126(4):320-323.

556. Bunn PA Jr, Hoffman SJ, Norris D, Golitz LE, Aeling JL. Systemic therapy of cutaneous T-cell lymphomas (mycosis fungoides and the Sezary syndrome). *Ann Intern Med.* 1994;121(8):592-602.
557. Olsen EA, Rosen ST, Vollmer RT, et al. Interferon alfa-2a in the treatment of cutaneous T cell lymphoma. *J Am Acad Dermatol.* 1989;20(3):395-407.
558. Papa G, Tura S, Mandelli F, et al. Is interferon alpha in cutaneous T-cell lymphoma a treatment of choice? *Br J Haematol.* 1991;79(suppl 1):48-51.
559. Kohn EC, Steis RG, Sausville EA, et al. Phase II trial of intermittent high-dose recombinant interferon alfa-2a in mycosis fungoides and the Sezary syndrome. *J Clin Oncol.* 1990;8(1):155-160.
560. Dreno B, Godefroy WY, Fleischmann M, Bureau B, Litoux P. Low-dose recombinant interferon-alpha in the treatment of cutaneous T-cell lymphomas. *Br J Dermatol.* 1989;121(4):543-544.
561. Mughal TI. Role of interferon alfa-2b in the management of patients with advanced cutaneous T-cell lymphoma. *Eur J Cancer.* 1991;27(suppl 4):S39-S40.
562. Estrach T, Marti R, Lecha M, Mascaro JM. Treatment of cutaneous T cell lymphoma with recombinant alfa 2b interferon [abstract]. *J Invest Dermatol.* 1989;93(4):549.
563. VanderMolen LA, Steis RG, Duffey PL, et al. Low- versus high-dose interferon alfa-2a in relapsed indolent non-Hodgkin's lymphoma. *J Natl Cancer Inst.* 1990;82(3):235-238.
564. Siegel RS, Kuzel TM. Cutaneous T-cell lymphoma/leukemia. *Curr Treat Options Oncol.* 2000;1(1):43-50.
565. Bunn PA Jr, Foon KA, Ihde DC, et al. Recombinant leukocyte A interferon: an active agent in advanced cutaneous T-cell lymphomas. *Ann Intern Med.* 1984;101(4):484-487.
566. Tura S, Mazza P, Zinzani PL, et al. Alpha recombinant interferon in the treatment of mycosis fungoides (MF). *Haematologica.* 1987;72(4):337-340.
567. Aviles A, Neri N, Fernandez-Diez J, Silva L, Nambo MJ. Interferon and low doses of methotrexate versus interferon and retinoids in the treatment of refractory/relapsed cutaneous T-cell lymphoma. *Hematology.* 2015;20(9):538-542.
568. Zinzani PL, Mazza P, Gherlinzoni F. Beta interferon in the treatment of mycosis fungoides. *Haematologica.* 1988;73(6):547-548.
569. Jimbow K, Yamana K, Ishida O, Kawamura M, Ito Y, Maeda K. Evaluation of rIFN-gamma in the treatment of lymphoma and melanoma of the skin by systemic and intralesional administration. *Gan To Kagaku Ryoho.* 1987;14(1):152-158.
570. Kaplan EH, Rosen ST, Norris DB, Roenigk HH Jr, Saks SR, Bunn PA Jr. Phase II study of recombinant human interferon gamma for treatment of cutaneous T-cell lymphoma. *J Natl Cancer Inst.* 1990;82(3):208-212.
571. Wysocka M, Dawany N, Benoit B, et al. Synergistic enhancement of cellular immune responses by the novel Toll receptor 7/8 agonist 3M-007 and interferon-γ: implications for therapy of cutaneous T-cell lymphoma. *Leuk Lymphoma.* 2011;52(10):1970-1979.
572. Scholtz W. Ueber den Einfluss der Rontgenstrahlen auf die Haut in gesundem und krankem Zustande. *Arch Dermatol Syph.* 1902;59:421-449.
573. Trump JG, Wright KA, Evans WW, et al. High energy electrons for the treatment of extensive superficial malignant lesions. *Am J Roentgenol Radium Ther Nucl Med.* 1953;69(4):623-629.
574. Whittaker S, Hoppe R, Prince HM. How I treat mycosis fungoides and Sezary syndrome. *Blood.* 2016;127(25):3142-3153.
575. Hoppe RT, Harrison C, Tavallaee M, et al. Low-dose total skin electron beam therapy as an effective modality to reduce disease burden in patients with mycosis fungoides: results of a pooled analysis from 3 phase-II clinical trials. *J Am Acad Dermatol.* 2015;72(2):286-292.
576. Newman NB, Patel CG, Ding GX, et al. Prospective observational trial of low-dose skin electron beam therapy in mycosis fungoides using a rotational technique. *J Am Acad Dermatol.* 2021;85(1):121-127.
577. Jones GW, Hoppe RT, Glatstein E. Electron beam treatment for cutaneous T-cell lymphoma. *Hematol Oncol Clin North Am.* 1995;9(5):1057-1076.
578. Jones G, Wilson LD, Fox-Goguen L. Total skin electron beam radiotherapy for patients who have mycosis fungoides. *Hematol Oncol Clin North Am.* 2003;17(6):1421-1434.
579. Ysebaert L, Truc G, Dalac S, et al. Ultimate results of radiation therapy for T1-T2 mycosis fungoides (including reirradiation). *Int J Radiat Oncol Biol Phys.* 2004;58(4):1128-1134.
580. Quiros PA, Kacinski BM, Wilson LD. Extent of skin involvement as a prognostic indicator of disease free and overall survival of patients with T3 cutaneous t-cell lymphoma treated with total skin electron beam radiation therapy. *Cancer.* 1996;77(9):1912-1917.
581. Hauswald H, Zwicker F, Rochet N, et al. Total skin electron beam therapy as palliative treatment for cutaneous manifestations of advanced, therapy-refractory cutaneous lymphoma and leukemia. *Radiat Oncol.* 2012;7(1):118.
582. Jones GW, Rosenthal D, Wilson LD. Total skin electron radiation for patients with erythrodermic cutaneous T-cell lymphoma (mycosis fungoides and the Sezary syndrome). *Cancer.* 1999;85(9):1985-1995.
583. Wilson LD, Jones GW, Kim D, et al. Experience with total skin electron beam therapy in combination with extracorporeal photopheresis in the management of patients with erythrodermic (T4) mycosis fungoides. *J Am Acad Dermatol.* 2000;43(1 pt 1):54-60.
584. Navi D, Riaz N, Levin YS, Sullivan NC, Kim YH, Hoppe RT. The Stanford University experience with conventional-dose, total skin electron-beam therapy in the treatment of generalized patch or plaque (T2) and tumor (T3) mycosis fungoides. *Arch Dermatol.* 2011;147(5):561-567.
585. Wilson LD, Quiros PA, Kolenik SA, et al. Additional courses of total skin electron beam therapy in the treatment of patients with recurrent cutaneous T-cell lymphoma. *J Am Acad Dermatol.* 1996;35(1):69-73.
586. Panizzon RG. Irradiation therapy: from UV light to electron beam. *J Cutan Pathol.* 2006;33(suppl 1):43-46.
587. Elsayad K, Rolf D, Sunderkotter C, et al. Low-dose total skin electron beam therapy plus oral bexarotene maintenance therapy for cutaneous T-cell lymphoma. *J Dtsch Dermatol Ges.* 2022;20(3):279-285.
588. Maingon P, Truc G, Dalac S, et al. Radiotherapy of advanced mycosis fungoides: indications and results of total skin electron beam and photon beam irradiation. *Radiother Oncol.* 2000;54(1):73-78.
589. Thomas TO, Agrawal P, Guitart J, et al. Outcome of patients treated with a single-fraction dose of palliative radiation for cutaneous T-cell lymphoma. *Int J Radiat Oncol Biol Phys.* 2013;85(3):747-753.
590. Edelson R, Berger C, Gasparro F, et al. Treatment of cutaneous T-cell lymphoma by extracorporeal photochemotherapy. Preliminary results. *N Engl J Med.* 1987;316(6):297-303.
591. Edelson RL. Cutaneous T cell lymphoma: the helping hand of dendritic cells. *Ann N Y Acad Sci.* 2001;941:1-11.
592. Berger CL, Hanlon D, Kanada D, Girardi M, Edelson RL. Transimmunization, a novel approach for tumor immunotherapy. *Transfus Apher Sci.* 2002;26(3):205-216.
593. Perez M, Edelson R, Laroche L, Berger C. Inhibition of antiskin allograft immunity by infusions with syngeneic photoinactivated effector lymphocytes. *J Invest Dermatol.* 1989;92(5):669-676.
594. Moor AC, Schmitt IM, Beijersbergen van Henegouwen GM, Chimenti S, Edelson RL, Gasparro FP. Treatment with 8-MOP and UVA enhances MHC class I synthesis in RMA cells: preliminary results. *J Photochem Photobiol B.* 1995;29(2-3):193-198.
595. Berger CL, Wang N, Christensen I, Longley J, Heald P, Edelson RL. The immune response to Class I-associated tumor-specific cutaneous T-cell lymphoma antigens. *J Invest Dermatol.* 1996;107(3):392-397.
596. Wolfe JT, Lessin SR, Singh AH, Rook AH. Review of immunomodulation by photopheresis: treatment of cutaneous T-cell lymphoma, autoimmune disease, and allograft rejection. *Artif Organs.* 1994;18(12):888-897.
597. Heald P, Rook A, Perez M, et al. Treatment of erythrodermic cutaneous T-cell lymphoma with extracorporeal photochemotherapy. *J Am Acad Dermatol.* 1992;27(3):427-433.
598. Vowels BR, Cassin M, Boufal MH, Walsh LJ, Rook AH. Extracorporeal photochemotherapy induces the production of tumor necrosis factor-alpha by monocytes: implications for the treatment of cutaneous T-cell lymphoma and systemic sclerosis. *J Invest Dermatol.* 1992;98(5):686-692.
599. Berger CL, Xu AL, Hanlon D, et al. Induction of human tumor-loaded dendritic cells. *Int J Cancer.* 2001;91(4):438-447.
600. Berger C, Hoffmann K, Vasquez JG, et al. Rapid generation of maturationally synchronized human dendritic cells: contribution to the clinical efficacy of extracorporeal photochemotherapy. *Blood.* 2010;116(23):4838-4847.
601. Ni X, Duvic M. Dendritic cells and cutaneous T-cell lymphomas. *G Ital Dermatol Venereol.* 2011;146(2):103-113.
602. Kibbi N, Sobolev O, Girardi M, Edelson RL. Induction of anti-tumor CD8 T cell responses by experimental ECP-induced human dendritic antigen presenting cells. *Transfus Apher Sci.* 2016;55(1):146-152.
603. Zic JA. The treatment of cutaneous T-cell lymphoma with photopheresis. *Dermatol Ther.* 2003;16(4):337-346.
604. Zic JA. Extracorporeal photopheresis in the treatment of mycosis fungoides and sezary syndrome. *Dermatol Clin.* 2015;33(4):765-776.
605. Alfred A, Taylor PC, Dignan F, et al. The role of extracorporeal photopheresis in the management of cutaneous T-cell lymphoma, graft-versus-host disease and organ transplant rejection: a consensus statement update from the UK Photopheresis Society. *Br J Haematol.* 2017;177(2):287-310.
606. Sanyal S, Child F, Alfred A, et al. U.K. national audit of extracorporeal photopheresis in cutaneous T-cell lymphoma. *Br J Dermatol.* 2018;178(2):569-570.
607. Zic J, Arzubiaga C, Salhany KE, et al. Extracorporeal photopheresis for the treatment of cutaneous T-cell lymphoma. *J Am Acad Dermatol.* 1992;27(5 pt 1):729-736.
608. Heald PW, Perez MI, Christensen I, Dobbs N, McKiernan G, Edelson R. Photopheresis therapy of cutaneous T-cell lymphoma: the Yale-New Haven Hospital experience. *Yale J Biol Med.* 1989;62(6):629-638.
609. Koh HK, Davis BE, Meola T, Lim HW. Extracorporeal photopheresis for the treatment of 34 patients with cutaneous T cell lymphoma (CTCL). *J Invest Dermatol.* 1994;102:567.
610. Duvic M, Hester JP, Lemak NA. Photopheresis therapy for cutaneous T-cell lymphoma. *J Am Acad Dermatol.* 1996;35(4):573-579.
611. Zic JA, Miller JL, Stricklin GP, King LE Jr. The North American experience with photopheresis. *Ther Apher.* 1999;3(1):50-62.
612. Lim HW, Edelson RL. Photopheresis for the treatment of cutaneous T-cell lymphoma. *Hematol Oncol Clin North Am.* 1995;9(5):1117-1126.
613. Scarisbrick JJ, Taylor P, Holtick U, et al. U.K. consensus statement on the use of extracorporeal photopheresis for treatment of cutaneous T-cell lymphoma and chronic graft-versus-host disease. *Br J Dermatol.* 2008;158(4):659-678.
614. Zic JA. Photopheresis in the treatment of cutaneous T-cell lymphoma: current status. *Curr Opin Oncol.* 2012;24(suppl 1):S1-S10.
615. Russell-Jones R. Extracorporeal photopheresis in cutaneous T-cell lymphoma. Inconsistent data underline the need for randomized studies. *Br J Dermatol.* 2000;142(1):16-21.
616. Martino M, Fedele R, Cornelio G, et al. Extracorporeal photopheresis, a therapeutic option for cutaneous T-cell lymphoma and immunological diseases: state of the art. *Expert Opin Biol Ther.* 2012;12(8):1017-1030.
617. Atta M, Papanicolaou N, Tsirigotis P. The role of extracorporeal photopheresis in the treatment of cutaneous T-cell lymphomas. *Transfus Apher Sci.* 2012;46(2):195-202.
618. Zic JA, Stricklin GP, Greer JP, et al. Long-term follow-up of patients with cutaneous T-cell lymphoma treated with extracorporeal photochemotherapy. *J Am Acad Dermatol.* 1996;35(6):935-945.
619. Talpur R, Demierre MF, Geskin L, et al. Multicenter photopheresis intervention trial in early-stage mycosis fungoides. *Clin Lymphoma Myeloma Leuk.* 2011;11(2):219-227.

620. Lewis DJ, Duvic M. Extracorporeal photopheresis for the treatment of early-stage mycosis fungoides. *Dermatol Ther.* 2017;30(3).
621. Seremet S, Abhyankar S, Herd TJ, Aires D. 75% complete response and 15% partial response to extracorporeal photopheresis combined with other therapies in resistant early stage cutaneous T-cell lymphoma. *J Drugs Dermatol.* 2016;15(10):1212-1216.
622. Rubegni P, De Aloe G, Fimiani M. Extracorporeal photochemotherapy in long-term treatment of early stage cutaneous T-cell lymphoma. *Br J Dermatol.* 2000;143(4):894-896.
623. Child FJ, Mitchell TJ, Whittaker SJ, Scarisbrick JJ, Seed PT, Russell-Jones R. A randomized cross-over study to compare PUVA and extracorporeal photopheresis in the treatment of plaque stage (T2) mycosis fungoides. *Clin Exp Dermatol.* 2004;29(3):231-236.
624. Miller JD, Kirkland EB, Domingo DS, et al. Review of extracorporeal photopheresis in early-stage (IA, IB, and IIA) cutaneous T-cell lymphoma. *Photodermatol Photoimmunol Photomed.* 2007;23(5):163-171.
625. Duvic M, Hagemeister F, Hester J. Accelerated delivery of extracorporeal photopheresis in patients with cutaneous T-cell lymphoma. *J Invest Dermatol.* 1989;92:423.
626. Suchin KR, Cucchiara AJ, Gottleib SL, et al. Treatment of cutaneous T-cell lymphoma with combined immunomodulatory therapy: a 14-year experience at a single institution. *Arch Dermatol.* 2002;138(8):1054-1060.
627. Rook AH, Gottlieb SL, Wolfe JT, et al. Pathogenesis of cutaneous T-cell lymphoma: implications for the use of recombinant cytokines and photopheresis. *Clin Exp Immunol.* 1997;107(suppl 1):16-20.
628. McGinnis KS, Ubriani R, Newton S, et al. The addition of interferon gamma to oral bexarotene therapy with photopheresis for Sezary syndrome. *Arch Dermatol.* 2005;141(9):1176-1178.
629. Apisarnthanarax N, Talpur R, Duvic M. Treatment of cutaneous T cell lymphoma: current status and future directions. *Am J Clin Dermatol.* 2002;3(3):193-215.
630. Siakantaris MP, Tsirigotis P, Stavroyianni N, et al. Management of cutaneous T-Cell lymphoma patients with extracorporeal photopheresis. The Hellenic experience. *Transfus Apher Sci.* 2012;46(2):189-193.
631. Raphael BA, Shin DB, Suchin KR, et al. High clinical response rate of Sezary syndrome to immunomodulatory therapies: prognostic markers of response. *Arch Dermatol.* 2011;147(12):1410-1415.
632. Booken N, Weiss C, Utikal J, Felcht M, Goerdt S, Klemke CD. Combination therapy with extracorporeal photopheresis, interferon-alpha, PUVA and topical corticosteroids in the management of Sezary syndrome. *J Dtsch Dermatol Ges.* 2010;8(6):428-438.
633. McGirt LY, Thoburn C, Hess A, Vonderheid EC. Predictors of response to extracorporeal photopheresis in advanced mycosis fungoides and Sezary syndrome. *Photodermatol Photoimmunol Photomed.* 2010;26(4):182-191.
634. Prince HM, Whittaker S, Hoppe RT. How I treat mycosis fungoides and Sezary syndrome. *Blood.* 2009;114(20):4337-4353.
635. Virmani P, Hwang SH, Hastings JG, et al. Systemic therapy for cutaneous T-cell lymphoma: who, when, what, and why? *Expert Rev Hematol.* 2017;10(2):111-121.
636. Duvic M. Systemic monotherapy vs combination therapy for CTCL: rationale and future strategies. *Oncology (Williston Park).* 2007;21(2 suppl 1):33-40.
637. Lansigan F, Foss FM. Current and emerging treatment strategies for cutaneous T-cell lymphoma. *Drugs.* 2010;70(3):273-286.
638. Sethi TK, Montanari F, Foss F, Reddy N. How we treat advanced stage cutaneous T-cell lymphoma - mycosis fungoides and Sezary syndrome. *Br J Haematol.* 2021;195(3):352-364.
639. Hughes CFM, Khot A, McCormack C, et al. Lack of durable disease control with chemotherapy for mycosis fungoides and Sezary syndrome: a comparative study of systemic therapy. *Blood.* 2015;125(1):71-81.
640. Rosen ST, Foss FM. Chemotherapy for mycosis fungoides and the Sezary syndrome. *Hematol Oncol Clin North Am.* 1995;9(5):1109-1116.
641. Winkelmann RK, Diaz-Perez JL, Buechner SA. The treatment of Sezary syndrome. *J Am Acad Dermatol.* 1984;10(6):1000-1004.
642. Coors EA, von den Driesch P. Treatment of erythrodermic cutaneous T-cell lymphoma with intermittent chlorambucil and fluocortolone therapy. *Br J Dermatol.* 2000;143(1):127-131.
643. Zackheim HS, Kashani-Sabet M, McMillan A. Low-dose methotrexate to treat mycosis fungoides: a retrospective study in 69 patients. *J Am Acad Dermatol.* 2003;49(5):873-878.
644. Zackheim HS, Kashani-Sabet M, Hwang ST. Low-dose methotrexate to treat erythrodermic cutaneous T-cell lymphoma: results in twenty-nine patients. *J Am Acad Dermatol.* 1996;34(4):626-631.
645. Purnak S, Azar J, Mark LA. Etoposide as a single agent in the treatment of mycosis fungoides: a retrospective analysis. *Dermatol Ther.* 2018;31(2):e12586.
646. Piekarz RL, Robey R, Sandor V, et al. Inhibitor of histone deacetylation, depsipeptide (FR901228), in the treatment of peripheral and cutaneous T-cell lymphoma: a case report. *Blood.* 2001;98(9):2865-2868.
647. O'Connor OA, Heaney ML, Schwartz L, et al. Clinical experience with intravenous and oral formulations of the novel histone deacetylase inhibitor suberoylanilide hydroxamic acid in patients with advanced hematologic malignancies. *J Clin Oncol.* 2006;24(1):166-173.
648. Horwitz SM. The emerging role of histone deacetylase inhibitors in treating T-cell lymphomas. *Curr Hematol Malig Rep.* 2011;6(1):67-72.
649. Tiffon C, Adams J, van der Fits L, et al. The histone deacetylase inhibitors vorinostat and romidepsin downmodulate IL-10 expression in cutaneous T-cell lymphoma cells. *Br J Pharmacol.* 2011;162(7):1590-1602.
650. Glaser KB. HDAC inhibitors: clinical update and mechanism-based potential. *Biochem Pharmacol.* 2007;74(5):659-671.
651. Marks PA, Richon VM, Rifkind RA. Histone deacetylase inhibitors: inducers of differentiation or apoptosis of transformed cells. *J Natl Cancer Inst.* 2000;92(15):1210-1216.
652. Duvic M, Talpur R, Ni X, et al. Phase 2 trial of oral vorinostat (suberoylanilide hydroxamic acid, SAHA) for refractory cutaneous T-cell lymphoma (CTCL). *Blood.* 2007;109(1):31-39.
653. Olsen EA, Kim YH, Kuzel TM, et al. Phase IIb multicenter trial of vorinostat in patients with persistent, progressive, or treatment refractory cutaneous T-cell lymphoma. *J Clin Oncol.* 2007;25(21):3109-3115.
654. Jr DR, Washam JB, Newby LK. QT interval prolongation and torsades de pointes in a patient undergoing treatment with vorinostat: a case report and review of the literature. *Cardiol J.* 2012;19(4):434-438.
655. Dummer R, Beyer M, Hymes K, et al. Vorinostat combined with bexarotene for treatment of cutaneous T-cell lymphoma: in vitro and phase I clinical evidence supporting augmentation of retinoic acid receptor/retinoid X receptor activation by histone deacetylase inhibition. *Leuk Lymphoma.* 2012;53(8):1501-1508.
656. Kim YH, Bagot M, Pinter-Brown L, et al. Mogamulizumab versus vorinostat in previously treated cutaneous T-cell lymphoma (MAVORIC): an international, open-label, randomised, controlled phase 3 trial. *Lancet Oncol.* 2018;19(9):1192-1204.
657. Lyseng-Williamson KA, Yang LPH. Romidepsin: a guide to its clinical use in cutaneous T-cell lymphoma. *Am J Clin Dermatol.* 2012;13(1):67-71.
658. Jain S, Zain J. Romidepsin in the treatment of cutaneous T-cell lymphoma. *J Blood Med.* 2011;2:37-47.
659. Piekarz RL, Frye R, Turner M, et al. Phase II multi-institutional trial of the histone deacetylase inhibitor romidepsin as monotherapy for patients with cutaneous T-cell lymphoma. *J Clin Oncol.* 2009;27(32):5410-5417.
660. Whittaker SJ, Demierre MF, Kim EJ, et al. Final results from a multicenter, international, pivotal study of romidepsin in refractory cutaneous T-cell lymphoma. *J Clin Oncol.* 2010;28(29):4485-4491.
661. Afifi S, Mohamed S, Zhao J, Foss F. A drug safety evaluation of mogamulizumab for the treatment of cutaneous T-Cell lymphoma. *Expert Opin Drug Saf.* 2019;18(9):769-776.
662. Pohlman B, Advani R, Duvic M, et al. Final results of a phase II trial of Belinostat (PXD101) in patients with recurrent or refractory peripheral or cutaneous T-cell lymphoma. *Blood.* 2009;114:920.
663. Gimsing P. Belinostat: a new broad acting antineoplastic histone deacetylase inhibitor. *Expert Opin Investig Drugs.* 2009;18(4):501-508.
664. Molife LR, de Bono JS. Belinostat: clinical applications in solid tumors and lymphoma. *Expert Opin Investig Drugs.* 2011;20(12):1723-1732.
665. Steele NL, Plumb JA, Vidal L, et al. Pharmacokinetic and pharmacodynamic properties of an oral formulation of the histone deacetylase inhibitor Belinostat (PXD101). *Cancer Chemother Pharmacol.* 2011;67(6):1273-1279.
666. Ellis L, Pan Y, Smyth GK, et al. Histone deacetylase inhibitor panobinostat induces clinical responses with associated alterations in gene expression profiles in cutaneous T-cell lymphoma. *Clin Cancer Res.* 2008;14(14):4500-4510.
667. Duvic M, Becker JC, Dalle S, et al. Phase II trial of oral panobinostat (LBH589) in patients with refractory cutaneous T-cell lymphoma (CTCL). *Blood.* 2008;112:1005.
668. O'Connor OA, Pro B, Pinter-Brown L, et al. Pralatrexate in patients with relapsed or refractory peripheral T-cell lymphoma: results from the pivotal PROPEL study. *J Clin Oncol.* 2011;29(9):1182-1189.
669. Horwitz SM, Kim YH, Foss F, et al. Identification of an active, well-tolerated dose of pralatrexate in patients with relapsed or refractory cutaneous T-cell lymphoma. *Blood.* 2012;119(18):4115-4122.
670. Foss FM, Parker TL, Girardi M, Li A. Effect of leucovorin administration on mucositis and skin reactions in patients with peripheral T-cell lymphoma or cutaneous T-cell lymphoma treated with pralatrexate. *Leuk Lymphoma.* 2019;60(12):2927-2930.
671. Duvic M, Kim YH, Zinzani PL, Horwitz SM. Results from a phase I/II open-label, dose-finding study of pralatrexate and oral bexarotene in patients with relapsed/refractory cutaneous T-cell lymphoma. *Clin Cancer Res.* 2017;23(14):3552-3556.
672. Zinzani PL, Baliva G, Magagnoli M, et al. Gemcitabine treatment in pretreated cutaneous T-cell lymphoma: experience in 44 patients. *J Clin Oncol.* 2000;18(13):2603-2606.
673. Duvic M, Talpur R, Wen S, Kurzrock R, David CL, Apisarnthanarax N. Phase II evaluation of gemcitabine monotherapy for cutaneous T-cell lymphoma. *Clin Lymphoma Myeloma.* 2006;7(1):51-58.
674. Marchi E, Alinari L, Tani M, et al. Gemcitabine as frontline treatment for cutaneous T-cell lymphoma: phase II study of 32 patients. *Cancer.* 2005;104(11):2437-2441.
675. Affandi AM, Blumetti TP, Wells J, Hertzberg M, Fernandez-Penas P. Gemcitabine and vinorelbine treatment in cutaneous T-cell lymphoma in four patients. *Australas J Dermatol.* 2015;56(4):294-297.
676. Grever MR, Bisaccia E, Scarborough DA, Metz EN, Neidhart JA. An investigation of 2'-deoxycoformycin in the treatment of cutaneous T-cell lymphoma. *Blood.* 1983;61(2):279-282.
677. Saven A, Carrera CJ, Carson DA, Beutler E, Piro LD. 2-Chlorodeoxyadenosine: an active agent in the treatment of cutaneous T-cell lymphoma. *Blood.* 1992;80(3):587-592.
678. Kurzrock R, Ravandi F. Purine analogues in advanced T-cell lymphoid malignancies. *Semin Hematol.* 2006;43(2 suppl 2):S27-S34.
679. Foss FM. Activity of pentostatin (Nipent) in cutaneous T-cell lymphoma: single-agent and combination studies. *Semin Oncol.* 2000;27(2 suppl 5):58-63.
680. Foss FM, Ihde DC, Breneman DL, et al. Phase II study of pentostatin and intermittent high-dose recombinant interferon alfa-2a in advanced mycosis fungoides/Sezary syndrome. *J Clin Oncol.* 1992;10(12):1907-1913.
681. Quaglino P, Fierro MT, Rossotto GL, Savoia P, Bernengo MG. Treatment of advanced mycosis fungoides/Sezary syndrome with fludarabine and potential adjunctive benefit to subsequent extracorporeal photochemotherapy. *Br J Dermatol.* 2004;150(2):327-336.
682. Foss FM, Ihde DC, Linnoila IR, et al. Phase II trial of fludarabine phosphate and interferon alfa-2a in advanced mycosis fungoides/Sezary syndrome. *J Clin Oncol.* 1994;12(10):2051-2059.

683. Scarisbrick JJ, Child FJ, Clift A, et al. A trial of fludarabine and cyclophosphamide combination chemotherapy in the treatment of advanced refractory primary cutaneous T-cell lymphoma. *Br J Dermatol.* 2001;144(5):1010-1015.
684. Galmarini CM. Drug evaluation: forodesine—PNP inhibitor for the treatment of leukemia, lymphoma and solid tumor. *IDrugs.* 2006;9(10):712-722.
685. Balakrishnan K, Verma D, O'Brien S, et al. Phase 2 and pharmacodynamic study of oral forodesine in patients with advanced, fludarabine-treated chronic lymphocytic leukemia. *Blood.* 2010;116(6):886-892.
686. Duvic M, Forero A, Foss F, Olsen E, Kim Y. Oral Forodesine (Bcx-1777) is clinically active in refractory cutaneous T-cell lymphoma: results of a phase I/II study. *Blood.* 2006;108:2467.
687. Dummer R, Duvic M, Scarisbrick J, et al. Final results of a multicenter phase II study of the purine nucleoside phosphorylase (PNP) inhibitor forodesine in patients with advanced cutaneous T-cell lymphomas (CTCL) (Mycosis fungoides and Sezary syndrome). *Ann Oncol.* 2014;25(9):1807-1812.
688. Gabizon AA. Selective tumor localization and improved therapeutic index of anthracyclines encapsulated in long-circulating liposomes. *Cancer Res.* 1992;52(4):891-896.
689. Wollina U, Graefe T, Kaatz M. Pegylated doxorubicin for primary cutaneous T-cell lymphoma: a report on ten patients with follow-up. *J Cancer Res Clin Oncol.* 2001;127(2):128-134.
690. Wollina U, Dummer R, Brockmeyer NH, et al. Multicenter study of pegylated liposomal doxorubicin in patients with cutaneous T-cell lymphoma. *Cancer.* 2003;98(5):993-1001.
691. Straus DJ, Duvic M, Horwitz SM, et al. Final results of phase II trial of doxorubicin HCl liposome injection followed by bexarotene in advanced cutaneous T-cell lymphoma. *Ann Oncol.* 2014;25(1):206-210.
692. Sors A, Jean-Louis F, Pellet C, et al. Down-regulating constitutive activation of the NF-kappaB canonical pathway overcomes the resistance of cutaneous T-cell lymphoma to apoptosis. *Blood.* 2006;107(6):2354-2363.
693. Zinzani PL, Musuraca G, Tani M, et al. Phase II trial of proteasome inhibitor bortezomib in patients with relapsed or refractory cutaneous T-cell lymphoma. *J Clin Oncol.* 2007;25(27):4293-4297.
694. Falchook GS, Duvic M, Hong DS, et al. Age-stratified phase I trial of a combination of bortezomib, gemcitabine, and liposomal doxorubicin in patients with advanced malignancies. *Cancer Chemother Pharmacol.* 2012;69(5):1117-1126.
695. Heider U, Rademacher J, Lamottke B, et al. Synergistic interaction of the histone deacetylase inhibitor SAHA with the proteasome inhibitor bortezomib in cutaneous T cell lymphoma. *Eur J Haematol.* 2009;82(6):440-449.
696. Holkova B, Yazbeck V, Kmieciak M, et al. A phase 1 study of bortezomib and romidepsin in patients with chronic lymphocytic leukemia/small lymphocytic lymphoma, indolent B-cell lymphoma, peripheral T-cell lymphoma, or cutaneous T-cell lymphoma. *Leuk Lymphoma.* 2017;58(6):1349-1357.
697. Dolan ME, McRae BL, Ferries-Rowe E, et al. O6-alkylguanine-DNA alkyltransferase in cutaneous T-cell lymphoma: implications for treatment with alkylating agents. *Clin Cancer Res.* 1999;5(8):2059-2064.
698. Tani M, Fina M, Alinari L, Stefoni V, Baccarani M, Zinzani PL. Phase II trial of temozolomide in patients with pretreated cutaneous T-cell lymphoma. *Haematologica.* 2005;90(9):1283-1284.
699. Querfeld C, Rosen ST, Guitart J, et al. Multicenter phase II trial of temozolomide in mycosis fungoides/Sezary syndrome: correlation with O6-methylguanine-DNA methyltransferase and mismatch repair proteins. *Clin Cancer Res.* 2011;17(17):5748-5754.
700. Querfeld C, Rosen ST, Guitart J, et al. Results of an open-label multicenter phase 2 trial of lenalidomide monotherapy in refractory mycosis fungoides and Sezary syndrome. *Blood.* 2014;123(8):1159-1166.
701. Bagot M, Hasan B, Whittaker S, et al. A phase III study of lenalidomide maintenance after debulking therapy in patients with advanced cutaneous T-cell lymphoma - EORTC 21081 (NCT01098656): results and lessons learned for future trial designs. *Eur J Dermatol.* 2017;27(3):286-294.
702. Molin L, Thomsen K, Volden G, et al. Combination chemotherapy in the tumour stage of mycosis fungoides with cyclophosphamide, vincristine, vp-16, adriamycin and prednisolone (cop, chop, cavop): a report from the Scandinavian mycosis fungoides study group. *Acta Derm Venereol.* 1980;60(6):542-544.
703. Duvic M, Apisarnthanarax N, Cohen DS, Smith TL, Ha CS, Kurzrock R. Analysis of long-term outcomes of combined modality therapy for cutaneous T-cell lymphoma. *J Am Acad Dermatol.* 2003;49(1):35-49.
704. Akpek G, Koh HK, Bogen S, O'Hara C, Foss FM. Chemotherapy with etoposide, vincristine, doxorubicin, bolus cyclophosphamide, and oral prednisone in patients with refractory cutaneous T-cell lymphoma. *Cancer.* 1999;86(7):1368-1376.
705. Quiros PA, Jones GW, Kacinski BM, et al. Total skin electron beam therapy followed by adjuvant psoralen/ultraviolet-A light in the management of patients with T1 and T2 cutaneous T-cell lymphoma (mycosis fungoides). *Int J Radiat Oncol Biol Phys.* 1997;38(5):1027-1035.
706. Kaye FJ, Bunn PA Jr, Steinberg SM, et al. A randomized trial comparing combination electron-beam radiation and chemotherapy with topical therapy in the initial treatment of mycosis fungoides. *N Engl J Med.* 1989;321(26):1784-1790.
707. Wilson LD, Licata AL, Braverman IM, et al. Systemic chemotherapy and extracorporeal photochemotherapy for T3 and T4 cutaneous T-cell lymphoma patients who have achieved a complete response to total skin electron beam therapy. *Int J Radiat Oncol Biol Phys.* 1995;32(4):987-995.
708. Aviles A, Guzman R, Garcia EL, Diazmaqueo JC. Biological modifiers (etretinate (changed from etretinate) and alfa 2a) in the treatment of refractory cutaneous T-cell lymphoma. *Cancer Biother Radiopharm.* 1996;11(1):21-24.
709. Altomare GF, Capella GL, Pigatto PD, Finzi AF. Intramuscular low dose alpha-2B interferon and etretinate for treatment of mycosis fungoides. *Int J Dermatol.* 1993;32(2):138-141.
710. Knobler RM, Trautinger F, Radaszkiewicz T, Kokoschka EM, Micksche M. Treatment of cutaneous T cell lymphoma with a combination of low-dose interferon alfa-2b and retinoids. *J Am Acad Dermatol.* 1991;24(2 pt 1):247-252.
711. Serri F, De Simone C, Venier A, Rusciani L, Marchetti F. Combination of retinoids and PUVA (Re-PUVA) in the treatment of cutaneous T cell lymphoma. *Curr Probl Dermatol.* 1990;19:252-257.
712. Rupoli S, Canafoglia L, Goteri G, et al. Results of a prospective phase II trial with oral low-dose bexarotene plus photochemotherapy (PUVA) in refractory and/or relapsed patients with mycosis fungoides. *Eur J Dermatol.* 2016;26(1):13-20.
713. Singh F, Lebwohl MG. Cutaneous T-cell lymphoma treatment using bexarotene and PUVA: a case series. *J Am Acad Dermatol.* 2004;51(4):570-573.
714. Kuzel TM, Roenigk HH Jr, Samuelson E, et al. Effectiveness of interferon alfa-2a combined with phototherapy for mycosis fungoides and the Sezary syndrome. *J Clin Oncol.* 1995;13(1):257-263.
715. Stadler R, Otte HG. Combination therapy of cutaneous T cell lymphoma with interferon alpha-2a and photochemotherapy. *Recent Results Cancer Res.* 1995;139:391-401.
716. Chiarion-Sileni V, Bononi A, Fornasa CV, et al. Phase II trial of interferon-alpha-2a plus psolaren with ultraviolet light A in patients with cutaneous T-cell lymphoma. *Cancer.* 2002;95(3):569-575.
717. Rupoli S, Goteri G, Pulini S, et al. Long-term experience with low-dose interferon-alpha and PUVA in the management of early mycosis fungoides. *Eur J Haematol.* 2005;75(2):136-145.
718. Stadler R, Otte HG, Luger T, et al. Prospective randomized multicenter clinical trial on the use of interferon -2a plus acitretin versus interferon -2a plus PUVA in patients with cutaneous T-cell lymphoma stages I and II. *Blood.* 1998;92(10):3578-3581.
719. D'Acunto C, Gurioli C, Neri I. Plaque stage mycosis fungoides treated with bexarotene at low dosage and UVB-NB. *J Dermatolog Treat.* 2010;21(1):45-48.
720. Morita A, Tateishi C, Muramatsu S, et al. Efficacy and safety of bexarotene combined with photo(chemo)therapy for cutaneous T-cell lymphoma. *J Dermatol.* 2020;47(5):443-451.
721. Coors EA, Von den Driesch P. Treatment of mycosis fungoides with bexarotene and psoralen plus ultraviolet A. *Br J Dermatol.* 2005;152(6):1379-1381.
722. Kronke A, Schlaak M, Arin M, Mauch C, Kurschat P. Successful treatment of a folliculotropic mycosis fungoides with bexarotene and PUVA. *Eur J Dermatol.* 2012;22(2):259-260.
723. Stern DK, Lebwohl M. Treatment of mycosis fungoides with oral bexarotene combined with PUVA. *J Drugs Dermatol.* 2002;1(2):134-136.
724. Papadavid E, Antoniou C, Nikolaou V, et al. Safety and efficacy of low-dose bexarotene and PUVA in the treatment of patients with mycosis fungoides. *Am J Clin Dermatol.* 2008;9(3):169-173.
725. Ortiz-Romero PL, Sanchez-Largo ME, Sanz H, et al. Treatment of mycosis fungoides with PUVA and bexarotene. *Actas Dermosifiliogr.* 2006;97(5):311-318.
726. Guitart J. Combination treatment modalities in cutaneous T-cell lymphoma (CTCL). *Semin Oncol.* 2006;33(1 suppl 3):S17-S20.
727. Morita A, Tateishi C, Ikumi K, et al. Comparison of the efficacy and safety of bexarotene and photo(Chemo)Therapy combination therapy and bexarotene monotherapy for cutaneous T-cell lymphoma. *Dermatol Ther (Heidelb).* 2022;12(3):615-629.
728. Foss FM, Kuzel TM. Experimental therapies in the treatment of cutaneous T-cell lymphoma. *Hematol Oncol Clin North Am.* 1995;9(5):1127-1137.
729. Waldmann TA. The IL-2/IL-2 receptor system: a target for rational immune intervention. *Immunol Today.* 1993;14(6):264-270.
730. LeMaistre CF, Kuzel T, Foss F, et al. DAB389IL2 is well tolerated at doses inducing responses in IL-2R expressing lymphomas. *Blood.* 1993;82(suppl 1):137a.
731. Foss FM, Borkowski TA, Gilliom M, et al. Chimeric fusion protein toxin DAB486IL-2 in advanced mycosis fungoides and the Sezary syndrome: correlation of activity and interleukin-2 receptor expression in a phase II study. *Blood.* 1994;84(6):1765-1774.
732. Olsen E, Duvic M, Frankel A, et al. Pivotal phase III trial of two dose levels of denileukin diftitox for the treatment of cutaneous T-cell lymphoma. *J Clin Oncol.* 2001;19(2):376-388.
733. Prince HM, Duvic M, Martin A, et al. Phase III placebo-controlled trial of denileukin diftitox for patients with cutaneous T-cell lymphoma. *J Clin Oncol.* 2010;28(11):1870-1877.
734. Kawai H, Ando K, Maruyama D, et al. Phase II study of E7777 in Japanese patients with relapsed/refractory peripheral and cutaneous T-cell lymphoma. *Cancer Sci.* 2021;112(6):2426-2435.
735. Ohmachi K, Ando K, Ogura M, et al. E7777 in Japanese patients with relapsed/refractory peripheral and cutaneous T-cell lymphoma: A phase I study. *Cancer Sci.* 2018;109(3):794-802.
736. Frankel AE, Woo JH, Ahn C, et al. Resimmune, an anti-CD3ε recombinant immunotoxin, induces durable remissions in patients with cutaneous T-cell lymphoma. *Haematologica.* 2015;100(6):794-800.
737. Pangalis GA, Dimopoulou MN, Angelopoulou MK, et al. Campath-1H (anti-CD52) monoclonal antibody therapy in lymphoproliferative disorders. *Med Oncol.* 2001;18(2):99-107.
738. Kennedy GA, Seymour JF, Wolf M, et al. Treatment of patients with advanced mycosis fungoides and Sezary syndrome with alemtuzumab. *Eur J Haematol.* 2003;71(4):250-256.
739. Lundin J, Hagberg H, Repp R, et al. Phase 2 study of alemtuzumab (anti-CD52 monoclonal antibody) in patients with advanced mycosis fungoides/Sezary syndrome. *Blood.* 2003;101(11):4267-4272.
740. Querfeld C, Mehta N, Rosen ST, et al. Alemtuzumab for relapsed and refractory erythrodermic cutaneous T-cell lymphoma: a single institution experience from the Robert H. Lurie Comprehensive Cancer Center. *Leuk Lymphoma.* 2009;50(12):1969-1976.

741. Lenihan DJ, Alencar AJ, Yang D, Kurzrock R, Keating MJ, Duvic M. Cardiac toxicity of alemtuzumab in patients with mycosis fungoides/Sezary syndrome. *Blood.* 2004;104(3):655-658.
742. Lundin J, Kennedy B, Dearden C, Dyer MJS, Osterborg A. No cardiac toxicity associated with alemtuzumab therapy for mycosis fungoides/Sezary syndrome. *Blood.* 2005;105(10):4148-4149.
743. Hotz C, Ingen-Housz-Oro S, Tran Van Nhieu J, et al. Pulmonary cryptococcoma in a patient with Sezary syndrome treated with alemtuzumab. *Eur J Dermatol.* 2011;21(6):1018-1020.
744. Ure UB, Ar MC, Salihoglu A, et al. Alemtuzumab in Sezary syndrome: efficient but not innocent. *Eur J Dermatol.* 2007;17(6):525-529.
745. Stewart JR, Desai N, Rizvi S, Zhu H, Goff HW. Alemtuzumab is an effective third-line treatment versus single-agent gemcitabine or pralatrexate for refractory Sezary syndrome: a systematic review. *Eur J Dermatol.* 2018;28(6):764-774.
746. Oliveira A, Lobo I, Alves R, Lima M, Selores M. Sezary syndrome presenting with leonine facies and treated with low-dose subcutaneous alemtuzumab. *Dermatol Online J.* 2011;17(11):6.
747. Alinari L, Geskin L, Grady T, Baiocchi RA, Bechtel MA, Porcu P. Subcutaneous alemtuzumab for Sezary Syndrome in the very elderly. *Leuk Res.* 2008;32(8):1299-1303.
748. Bernengo MG, Quaglino P, Comessatti A, et al. Low-dose intermittent alemtuzumab in the treatment of Sezary syndrome: clinical and immunologic findings in 14 patients. *Haematologica.* 2007;92(6):784-794.
749. de Masson A, Guitera P, Brice P, et al. Long-term efficacy and safety of alemtuzumab in advanced primary cutaneous T-cell lymphomas. *Br J Dermatol.* 2014;170(3):720-724.
750. Younes A, Yasothan U, Kirkpatrick P. Brentuximab vedotin. *Nat Rev Drug Discov.* 2012;11(1):19-20.
751. Pro B, Advani R, Brice P, et al. Brentuximab vedotin (SGN-35) in patients with relapsed or refractory systemic anaplastic large-cell lymphoma: results of a phase II study. *J Clin Oncol.* 2012;30(18):2190-2196.
752. Duvic M, Tetzlaff MT, Gangar P, Clos AL, Sui D, Talpur R. Results of a phase II trial of brentuximab vedotin for CD30+ cutaneous T-cell lymphoma and lymphomatoid papulosis. *J Clin Oncol.* 2015;33(32):3759-3765.
753. Hofer V, Maurus K, Houben R, et al. Treatment of mycosis fungoides with brentuximab vedotin: assessing CD30 expression by immunohistochemistry and quantitative real-time polymerase chain reaction. *J Cutan Pathol.* 2022;49(3):314-317.
754. Prince HM, Kim YH, Horwitz SM, et al. Brentuximab vedotin or physician's choice in CD30-positive cutaneous T-cell lymphoma (ALCANZA): an international, open-label, randomised, phase 3, multicentre trial. *Lancet.* 2017;390(10094):555-566.
755. Corbin ZA, Nguyen-Lin A, Li S, et al. Characterization of the peripheral neuropathy associated with brentuximab vedotin treatment of Mycosis Fungoides and Sezary Syndrome. *J Neuro Oncol.* 2017;132(3):439-446.
756. Ishida T, Joh T, Uike N, et al. Defucosylated anti-CCR4 monoclonal antibody (KW-0761) for relapsed adult T-cell leukemia-lymphoma: a multicenter phase II study. *J Clin Oncol.* 2012;30(8):837-842.
757. Duvic M, Pinter-Brown LC, Foss FM, et al. Phase 1/2 study of mogamulizumab, a defucosylated anti-CCR4 antibody, in previously treated patients with cutaneous T-cell lymphoma. *Blood.* 2015;125(12):1883-1889.
758. Trum NA, Zain J, Martinez XU, et al. Mogamulizumab efficacy is underscored by its associated rash that mimics cutaneous T-cell lymphoma: a retrospective single-centre case series. *Br J Dermatol.* 2022;186(1):153-166.
759. Wang JY, Hirotsu KE, Neal TM, et al. Histopathologic characterization of mogamulizumab-associated rash. *Am J Surg Pathol.* 2020;44(12):1666-1676.
760. Roelens M, de Masson A, Andrillon A, et al. Mogamulizumab induces long-term immune restoration and reshapes tumour heterogeneity in Sézary syndrome. *Br J Dermatol.* 2022;186(6):1010-1025. doi:10.1111/bjd.21018
761. Xu S, Foss F. New nonchemotherapy treatment options for cutaneous T-cell lymphomas. *Expert Rev Anticancer Ther.* 2021;21(9):1017-1028.
762. Van Der Weyden C, Bagot M, Neeson P, Darcy PK, Prince HM. IPH4102, a monoclonal antibody directed against the immune receptor molecule KIR3DL2, for the treatment of cutaneous T-cell lymphoma. *Expert Opin Investig Drugs.* 2018;27(8):691-697.
763. Ortonne N, Le Gouvello S, Tabak R, et al. CD158k/KIR3DL2 and NKp46 are frequently expressed in transformed mycosis fungoides. *Exp Dermatol.* 2012;21(6):461-463.
764. Kim YH, Girardi M, Duvic M, et al. Phase I trial of a Toll-like receptor 9 agonist, PF-3512676 (CPG 7909), in patients with treatment-refractory, cutaneous T-cell lymphoma. *J Am Acad Dermatol.* 2010;63(6):975-983.
765. Kim YH, Gratzinger D, Harrison C, et al. In situ vaccination against mycosis fungoides by intratumoral injection of a TLR9 agonist combined with radiation: a phase 1/2 study. *Blood.* 2012;119(2):355-363.
766. Lesokhin AM, Ansell SM, Armand P, et al. Nivolumab in patients with relapsed or refractory hematologic malignancy: preliminary results of a phase Ib study. *J Clin Oncol.* 2016;34(23):2698-2704.
767. Khodadoust MS, Rook AH, Porcu P, et al. Pembrolizumab in relapsed and refractory mycosis fungoides and sezary syndrome: a multicenter phase II study. *J Clin Oncol.* 2020;38(1):20-28.
768. Beygi S, Fernandez-Pol S, Duran G, et al. Pembrolizumab in mycosis fungoides with PD-L1 structural variants. *Blood Adv.* 2021;5(3):771-774.
769. Walker CJ, Donnelly ED, Moreira J, et al. Pembrolizumab and palliative radiotherapy in 2 cases of refractory mycosis fungoides. *JAAD Case Rep.* 2021;7:87-90.
770. Bigler RD, Crilley P, Micaily B, et al. Autologous bone marrow transplantation for advanced stage mycosis fungoides. *Bone Marrow Transplant.* 1991;7(2):133-137.
771. Sterling JC, Marcus R, Burrows NP, Roberts SO. Erythrodermic mycosis fungoides treated with total body irradiation and autologous bone marrow transplantation. *Clin Exp Dermatol.* 1995;20(1):73-75.
772. Olavarria E, Child F, Woolford A, et al. T-cell depletion and autologous stem cell transplantation in the management of tumour stage mycosis fungoides with peripheral blood involvement. *Br J Haematol.* 2001;114(3):624-631.
773. Molina A, Zain J, Arber DA, et al. Durable clinical, cytogenetic, and molecular remissions after allogeneic hematopoietic cell transplantation for refractory Sezary syndrome and mycosis fungoides. *J Clin Oncol.* 2005;23(25):6163-6171.
774. Lechowicz MJ, Lazarus HM, Carreras J, et al. Allogeneic hematopoietic cell transplantation for mycosis fungoides and Sezary syndrome. *Bone Marrow Transplant.* 2014;49(11):1360-1365.
775. Domingo-Domenech E, Duarte RF, Boumedil A, et al. Allogeneic hematopoietic stem cell transplantation for advanced mycosis fungoides and Sezary syndrome. An updated experience of the Lymphoma Working Party of the European Society for Blood and Marrow Transplantation. *Bone Marrow Transplant.* 2021;56(6):1391-1401.
776. Mehta-Shah N, Kommalapati A, Teja S, et al. Successful treatment of mature T-cell lymphoma with allogeneic stem cell transplantation: the largest multicenter retrospective analysis [Abstract]. *Blood.* 2020;136(suppl 1):35-36.
777. Hosing C, Bassett R, Dabaja B, et al. Allogeneic stem-cell transplantation in patients with cutaneous lymphoma: updated results from a single institution. *Ann Oncol.* 2015;26(12):2490-2495.
778. Duvic M, Donato M, Dabaja B, et al. Total skin electron beam and non-myeloablative allogeneic hematopoietic stem-cell transplantation in advanced mycosis fungoides and Sezary syndrome. *J Clin Oncol.* 2010;28(14):2365-2372.
779. Isufi I, Seropian S, Gowda L, et al. Outcomes for allogeneic stem cell transplantation in refractory mycosis fungoides and primary cutaneous gamma Delta T cell lymphomas. *Leuk Lymphoma.* 2020;61(12):2955-2961.
780. Weng WK, Arai S, Rezvani A, et al. Nonmyeloablative allogeneic transplantation achieves clinical and molecular remission in cutaneous T-cell lymphoma. *Blood Adv.* 2020;4(18):4474-4482.

Chapter 95 ■ Hodgkin Lymphoma in Adults

REID W. MERRYMAN • ANN LACASCE

INTRODUCTION

Hodgkin lymphoma (*HL*) is a lymphoproliferative malignancy accounting for 10% of all lymphomas, and 0.5% of newly diagnosed malignancies in the United States. 95% of cases are classic Hodgkin lymphoma (cHL) with nodular lymphocyte predominant HL (NLPHL) accounting for the remaining 5%. From a historical perspective, HL was the first cancer treated with curative intent using combination chemotherapy.

HL has a bimodal age distribution with the majority of patients diagnosed between the ages of 20 to 34, although patients in all age groups may be affected. The disease typically presents with lymphadenopathy that spreads in a contiguous fashion, and most patients have disease limited to lymph nodes and/or the spleen. Overall, durable remission can be achieved in approximately 85% of patients with HL with first-line treatment in the early stages of the disease and 75% in the later stages. Available therapies for relapsed disease are also highly effective resulting in no difference in overall survival (OS) in the vast majority of randomized clinical trials. Given the long life expectancy of patients with HL, particularly in young adults, balancing disease control with the risk of therapy associated late toxicities is crucial.

HISTORY

In 1832, Thomas Hodgkin described the autopsy findings of seven patients, outlining a *primary* process involving the lymph glands and spleen in a paper titled, "On Some Morbid Appearances of the Absorbent Glands and Spleen." In 1856, Samuel Wilks published a series of cases involving enlargement of the lymph glands and noted Hodgkin's original description. In 1865, Wilks wrote, "Cases of Enlargement of the Lymphatic Glands and Spleen (or Hodgkin Disease) with Remarks," updating and extending his findings. After these gross pathologic descriptions, the first microscopic description of HL was reported by Langhans in 1872. This report was followed by independent reports by Sternberg in 1898 and Reed in 1902 describing the characteristic giant cells subsequently termed Reed-Sternberg (*RS*) *cells*. These early authors were divided over the pathophysiology of HL and whether it represented an infectious disease, an inflammatory disorder, or a malignancy involving the lymph glands.

EPIDEMIOLOGY

It is estimated that 8830 new cases of HL will be diagnosed in 2021 in the United States.[1] The male-to-female ratio is 1.3:1. In most economically developed countries, the majority of cases occur in patients between the ages of 15 and 35 with small peaks in patients under 15 and over 50.[2] The occurrence of HL in patients between the ages of 15 and 39 has been positively associated with increased maternal education, decreased numbers of siblings, and single-family dwellings in childhood.[3] In less economically developed countries, HL is less common but affects children, particularly boys. The Epstein-Barr virus (EBV)-associated subtypes, mixed cellularity HL (MCHL), and lymphocyte-depleted HL are more commonly seen in this population.[2] These data have been interpreted as supporting the hypothesis that HL is associated with delayed exposure of a common childhood infectious agents.[4] Race also influences the incidence patterns and may impact outcome, with population-based studies reporting inferior OS in African Americans and Hispanics in the United States.[5,6] In the United States and Europe, the proportions of different subtypes are nodular sclerosis HL (NSHL), 70%; MCHL, 20% to 25%; lymphocyte-rich HL, 5%; and lymphocyte-depleted HL, 1%.[7] Human immunodeficiency virus (HIV) infection is associated with 10% of new cases of MCHL in the United States.[8]

RISK FACTORS

Close relatives of patients with HL have a three- to fivefold higher risk of HL than the general population,[9,10] which may be due to a genetic predisposition or common environmental factors. The risk in monozygotic twins is 50- to 100-fold higher. There is an association with certain HLA haplotypes, most notably, HLA-A1.[11]

Infections including EBV and HIV have been associated with an increased risk of HL. Epidemiologic evidence points to an association of EBV with cHL. In developed countries, infectious mononucleosis is associated with an increased risk of subsequent cHL.[12] Using in situ hybridization, EBV genome fragments have been found in RS cells from approximately 40% of patients with HL, more commonly in cases of MCHL and lymphocyte-depleted HL.[13,14] In addition, the EBV DNA associated with RS cells in cHL has been shown to be monoclonal, establishing that EBV preceded the development of cHL. Although a causal role of EBV in cHL pathogenesis is not established, the proposed mechanisms of EBV contributing to disease pathogenesis include increased expression of EBV genes, latent membrane protein 1 (LMP1), LMP2a, and EBV nuclear antigen 1 (EBNA1). LMP1 and LMP2a are associated with an antiapoptotic effect.[15-19] Immunosuppression related to autoimmune disease, solid organ or hematopoietic cell transplantation (HCT), underlying chronic lymphocytic leukemia, or HIV infection is associated with an increased risk of HL. Most of these cases are EBV-associated and are often of the mixed cellularity subtype.

PATHOGENESIS

In the 1990s, clonal immunoglobulin rearrangements were found in RS cells, establishing the cell of origin of HL as a germinal center or postgerminal center B cell.[20] RS cells do not express the common B-cell transcription factors and thus its B-cell phenotype (including the B-cell receptor) because of downregulation and epigenetic silencing.[21,22] Normally, such nonfunctional B cells would undergo apoptosis, and activation of several antiapoptotic pathways, including the nuclear factor NF-κB pathway, the Janus kinase-signal transducer, and the transcription signaling (JAK-STAT) pathways, has been proposed as a mechanism for the molecular pathogenesis of HL.[23]

The role of the tumor microenvironment in the pathogenesis of HL has been extensively studied in recent years. The malignant RS cells comprise a small percentage of the tumor bulk with T cells, nonmalignant B cells, granulocytes, eosinophils, and stromal cells occupying the majority of the involved tissue. Through a complex interplay of cytokines and chemokines, these cells contribute to the pathogenesis and maintenance of HL.[24] One of the mechanisms of immune evasion is the amplification of the 9p24.1 locus, which results in upregulation of both programmed death ligands (PD-L1 and PD-L2) and JAK2.[25,26] EBV infections also result in increased PD-L1 expression.[27] The PD-L1 ligand on the RS cells engages PD-1 on T cells in the tumor microenvironment blocking the immune response against the malignant RS cells.[28]

HISTOPATHOLOGY

The malignant RS cells constitute a minority of the overall cellularity in a background of a robust inflammatory infiltrate consisting of lymphocytes, histiocytes, granulocytes, eosinophils, and plasma cells. The

RS cells are large bilobed cells with two or more nuclei and eosinophilic nucleoli. Ideally, the diagnosis of HL requires an excisional or incisional biopsy of an involved lymph node. In some cases, the diagnosis can be established from a core needle biopsy of a lymph node or extranodal site, though subclassification may be difficult with limited tissue specimens. A fine-needle aspiration is not adequate for making a diagnosis. It is important to note that inflammatory nodes may be interspersed among nodes harboring HL. In general, a larger node with more abnormal features on imaging is a better target for biopsy. Almost all RS cells in cHL express CD30, and about 85% express CD15. CD45 is typically absent. CD20 is positive in a small proportion of cases. PAX-5 is dimly expressed in up to 95% of cases and is useful in distinguishing HL from anaplastic large-cell lymphoma. HL may also be confused with primary mediastinal B cell lymphoma, or T-cell-rich B-cell lymphoma (TCRBCL). Correct classification can usually be achieved using immunohistochemistry and cytogenetic techniques. The World Health Organization classification recognizes mediastinal gray zone lymphoma, which has features between diffuse large B-cell lymphoma (DLBCL) and cHL as a separate entity, which is typically treated with therapy based on the treatment for DLBCL.[29,30]

Variant forms of RS cells exist, especially in the nodular sclerosis subtype of cHL and the nodular form of lymphocyte-predominant HL (NLPHL). The RS cells in NLPHL are CD30 and CD15 negative as detailed later. RS cells are not specific for HL and have been noted in cases of infectious mononucleosis and other malignancies including non-Hodgkin lymphoma (NHL), carcinomas, and sarcomas.[31] Therefore, RS cells alone are not sufficient to establish the diagnosis of HL. Instead, the diagnosis depends on the presence of both the characteristic RS cells and the characteristic cellular environment. Supportive immunohistochemistry includes staining for CD30, CD15, and PAX-5 on RS cells in cHL, as mentioned above.

The subclassification of HL depends in large part on the ratio of neoplastic to reactive cells and their orientation. The subclassification stems from the classification of Lukes and Butler, as modified at the Rye Conference in 1966.[32] These investigators recognized a distinct subcategory of HL, NLPHL, characterized by what was thought to be an RS cell variant, previously known as the "L and H cell" ("lymphocytic and histiocytic" because of the associated background) or "popcorn cell" variants and now as lymphocyte predominant (LP) cell. Based on clinical, immunophenotyping, and gene expression profiling grounds, NLPHL is a clinicopathologic entity distinct from other types of HL.[33] Thus, the current WHO classification distinguishes cHL from NLPHL.

Classic HL has four subtypes, namely, NSHL, MCHL, lymphocyte-rich classic HL (LRCHL), and lymphocyte-depleted HL (see Chapter 88). In the past, the subtype of HL was felt to give the clinician valuable prognostic information; however, it is now recognized that the histologic subtype covaries with stage, which is likely the major driver of prognosis. When patients are stratified by stage and receive equivalent modern therapy, differences attributable to histologic subtype are small. The incidence of each histologic subtype is shown in *Table 95.1*.

In NSHL, nodularity is produced by dense collagenous bands that divide the cellular portion of the node into sections (*Figure 95.1*). RS cell variants, rather than classic RS cells, are common. These lacunar

Table 95.1. Relative Incidence of Histopathologic Subtypes of Hodgkin Lymphoma

Author	Lymphocyte Predominant (%)	Nodular Sclerosis (%)	Mixed Cellularity (%)	Lymphocyte Depleted (%)
Dorfman[34]	7	74	17	2
Jones et al[35]	2	65	26	6
Bernhards et al[36]	3	74	22	1
Medeiros et al[37]	7	63	26	4

Percentages refer to "classified" cases, as some studies contain cases of unclassified Hodgkin disease.

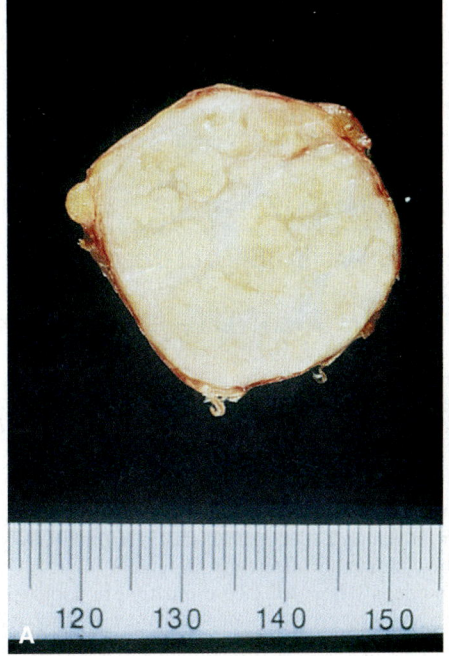
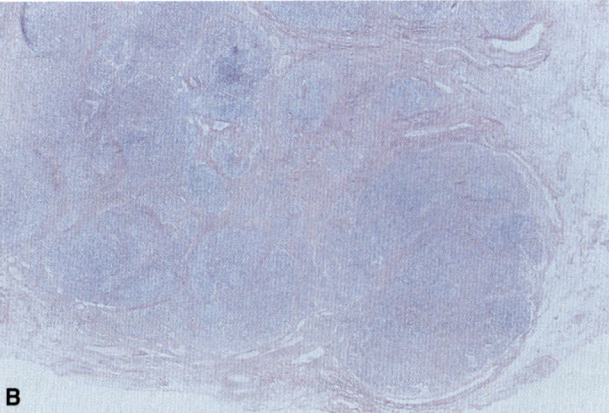

FIGURE 95.1 **Nodular sclerosing Hodgkin lymphoma.** A, Gross appearance of the cut surface of a resected node shows a thickened capsule, white fibrous bands, and yellow parenchymal nodules. B, Low magnification shows a fibrous capsule and bands of sclerosis circumscribing abnormal lymphoid nodules.

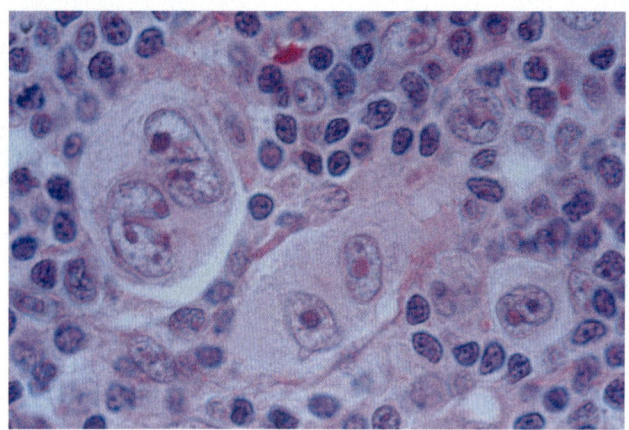

FIGURE 95.2 Nodular sclerosing Hodgkin lymphoma. High magnification shows Reed-Sternberg cells and lacunar variants in B5 fixed material.

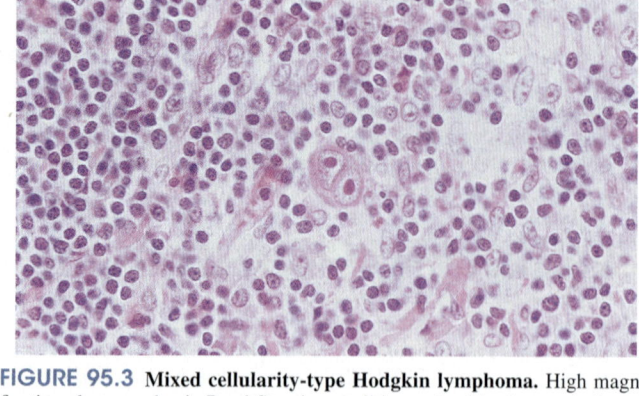

FIGURE 95.3 Mixed cellularity-type Hodgkin lymphoma. High magnification shows a classic Reed-Sternberg cell in a mixed background of small lymphocytes, plasma cells, and eosinophils.

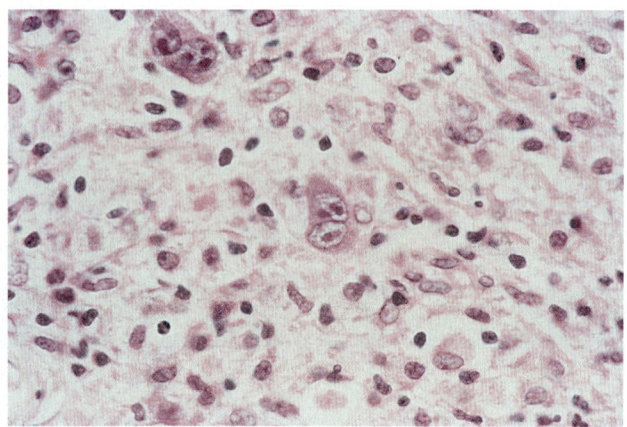

FIGURE 95.4 Lymphocyte-depleted type Hodgkin lymphoma, diffuse fibrosis subtype. Reed-Sternberg cells are easily found, and the background is depleted of cellularity and composed of amorphous eosinophilic connective tissue.

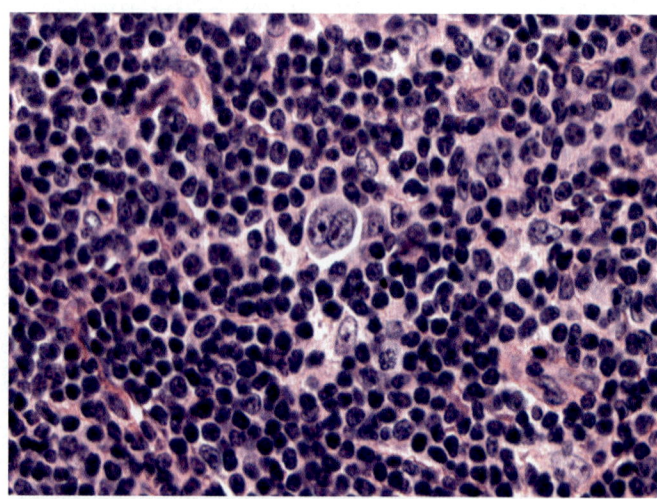

FIGURE 95.5 Lymphocyte-rich "classic" Hodgkin lymphoma. The background is primarily lymphocytes, and the Reed–Sternberg cells are usually CD15+ and CD30+ and negative for the B-cell marker CD20.

RS cells have faintly stained cytoplasm and appear separated from adjacent cells by empty space, an artifact of formalin fixation (*Figure 95.2*). NSHL is the most distinctive form of HL. NSHL commonly presents in young adults with stage I or II disease involving the cervical and mediastinal nodes, although more advanced stages of disease are not uncommon.

A "syncytial variant" of NSHL has been recognized in which numerous RS cell variants are observed in sheets and clusters. This variant of HL may be confused with NHL, thymoma, or metastatic cancer.[38] Studies suggest that this variant may be associated with a worse prognosis than the typical NSHL cases.[39]

MCHL is a diffuse lymphoma composed of a mixture of cells including RS cells (*Figure 95.3*). Distinguishing MCHL from diffuse mixed forms of NHL may be difficult on the basis of histologic features alone but should be resolved with immunohistochemical stains. This subtype of HL has a greater tendency than NSHL to be advanced at the time of presentation and to be associated with systemic symptoms. MCHL and NSHL make up the majority of HL cases.

Lymphocyte-depleted HL is composed predominantly of histiocytes and lymphocytes with varying numbers of eosinophils and RS cells (*Figure 95.4*). The host reaction is often scant relative to the number of malignant RS cells, and a varying amount of fibrosis is generally present. The disease is the least common type of HL, is associated with immunocompromised states (including HIV), and tends to be advanced at diagnosis (i.e., stage III or IV). B symptoms are common.[40] Many older case series include cases that would now be classified as peripheral T-cell lymphomas or anaplastic large-cell lymphomas. Therefore, the older literature regarding this entity must be interpreted cautiously.

LRCHL is characterized by rare RS cells or variants dispersed in a background of predominantly small lymphocytes[33] (*Figure 95.5*).

CLINICAL EVALUATION

Physical Examination: Sites of Disease and Pattern of Spread

Staging begins with physical examination. HL almost always presents with lymphadenopathy, and the involved nodes are often mobile with a rubbery consistency. Cases in which the microscopic appearance reveals fibrosis or sclerosis can be associated with hard or firm nodes. Although any lymph node group can be involved, cervical and supraclavicular adenopathy are the most common.

Mediastinal disease is common and usually occurs in conjunction with cervical or supraclavicular disease. HL can present with iliac, inguinal, or femoral adenopathy, and in approximately 3% of cases, only subdiaphragmatic disease is present.[41]

Splenomegaly is noted at presentation in approximately 10% of cases of cHL. However, splenomegaly may be a nonspecific manifestation of the cHL, and in only one-half of patients with splenomegaly was splenic involvement confirmed at laparotomy in a study from the era of staging laparotomies.[42] Additionally, splenic involvement

Table 95.2. Lugano Classification for Hodgkin Lymphoma[45]

Stage I	
Involvement of a single lymph node region or lymphoid structure (e.g., spleen, thymus, and Waldeyer ring)	
Stage II	
Involvement of two or more lymph node regions on the same side of the diaphragm (the mediastinum is a single site; hilar lymph nodes are lateralized); number of anatomic sites should be indicated by a suffix (e.g., II$_3$)	
Stage III	
Involvement of lymph node regions of structures on both sides of the diaphragm	
III$_1$	With or without splenic hilar, celiac, or portal nodes
III$_2$	With paraaortic, iliac, or mesenteric nodes
Stage IV	
Involvement of extranodal site(s) beyond that designated E	
A	No symptoms
B	Fever, drenching sweats, and weight loss
X	Bulky disease, greater than one-third widening of the mediastinum, >10 cm maximum dimension of nodal mass
E	Involvement of a single extranodal site, contiguous, or proximal to a known nodal site
CS	Clinical stage
PS	Pathologic stage

may occur in 20% to 30% of patients in the absence of splenomegaly and may be limited to a few microscopic nodules. Extranodal disease can occur at any site. At presentation, lung, liver, bone, and bone marrow are the most common extranodal sites of disease, with each of these sites seen in approximately 5% to 10% of cases. The central nervous system and the testis are exceptionally rare sites for cHL. Of note, marrow-only cHL is a common presentation in HIV-infected patients.[43,44] Classic HL tends to spread in a contiguous nodal fashion except in mixed cellularity type in which there may be skip lesions, likely due to hematogenous spread of disease.

Initial Evaluation of the Hodgkin Lymphoma Patient
Clinical History

A thorough clinical history is key to the management of HL patients and can guide staging and baseline testing. The presence of certain symptoms is associated with a less favorable prognosis and may be a clue to more advanced disease. The constitutional symptoms that are known to have prognostic value are unexplained fever greater than 100.4 °F, drenching night sweats, and weight loss greater than or equal to 10% of the patient's weight in the preceding 6 months. These symptoms are accounted for in the Lugano staging system (denoted by B appended on the numerical stage). Fever in HL can have any pattern, including continuous low-grade fever or occasional fever spikes. The pattern of recurrent episodes of daily high fevers separated by days without fever, known as Pel-Ebstein fever, was first associated with HL in 1885. However, in the modern era, it is a rare manifestation of HL. Rarely, fever may be the only clinical manifestation of HL, as in the case of patients with lymphocyte-depleted HL who present with fever and disease limited to retroperitoneal nodes or the bone marrow, or both. The night sweats of HL are frequently drenching and not simply associated with increased ambient temperature. Generalized fatigue and weakness may also be initial symptoms. Pain at the site of HL in association with the ingestion of alcohol is well described, but the mechanism of this phenomenon is unknown, and it does not have prognostic significance. Generalized pruritus can also be a prominent symptom of HL for up to 15% of patients. Improvement in the above symptoms can be an early marker of treatment response and their recurrence can be the first hint of a relapse.

The Lugano Staging System

The stage of the patient is the main determinant of therapy and prognosis in HL. The current classification system is the Lugano classification, which was derived from older staging symptoms, like the Cotswold system[45] (*Table 95.2*). The modalities used to stage patients have changed since the Cotswold conference in 1990 with positron emission tomography with integrated computed tomography (PET/CT), now a key component of the staging workup.

Stage I disease is the involvement of a single lymph node region (or a single lymphoid structure). Stage II disease is the involvement of multiple lymph node regions (e.g., cervical nodes and supraclavicular nodes) on only one side of the diaphragm. Stage III disease is the involvement of lymph node regions on both sides of the diaphragm. Stage IV disease is involvement of extranodal structures (e.g., lung, liver, or bone marrow) that is not due to direct extension from a nodal site. The subscript E represents extension from a nodal site, such as extension of a mediastinal mass directly into the lung, for example, II$_E$. The designations *A* and *B* are used to represent the absence and presence of symptoms (i.e., unexplained fever, drenching night sweats, and weight loss of 10% of body weight), respectively. The presence of bulky disease is defined as a mediastinal mass with a diameter greater than one-third the diameter of the chest at any level of the thoracic vertebrae as determined by CT, or any nodal mass with the greatest diameter of more than 10 cm.

Required and Suggested Studies for Initial Evaluation

Evaluation begins with a clinical history and physical examination as described earlier. PET/CT is the imaging modality of choice for initial assessment of patients with HL due to its high sensitivity and specificity. With its introduction, PET/CT (as compared to CT alone) altered the stage in up to 20% to 40% of cases and changed the recommended treatment in 5% to 15%.[46] If a PET/CT is unavailable, patients should have contrast-enhanced CT scans of the chest, abdomen, and pelvis. A neck CT should be included if there is any clinical suspicion of involvement of neck nodes. Based on data suggesting that PET/CT accurately identifies or rules out marrow involvement, the NCCN Guidelines recommend bone marrow biopsy only if there are cytopenias in the absence of PET evidence of bone marrow involvement.

Low-level bone marrow uptake is common in patients with HL, which is likely related to inflammation. In general, if the PET/CT shows homogeneous marrow uptake, a bone marrow biopsy is not required, and if there are multifocal (three or more) skeletal PET/CT lesions, marrow may be assumed to be involved.[46] Standard PET criteria used for response assessment are known as the Deauville Criteria on a 5-point scale. A score of 1 (no uptake), 2 (slight uptake but lower than uptake in the normal mediastinal blood pool), or 3 (uptake equal to or slightly above uptake in the blood pool but less than uptake in the liver) is regarded as indicating negative findings, and a score of 4 (uptake moderately higher than uptake in the liver) or 5 (uptake markedly higher than uptake in the liver) is regarded as positive.[45]

Blood tests should include a complete blood count; erythrocyte sedimentation rate (ESR); liver function tests including alkaline phosphatase, lactate dehydrogenase, albumin, and bilirubin; BUN and creatinine; and thyroid function tests as a baseline (if neck radiotherapy is contemplated). Serology for HIV is appropriate in selected cases. A pregnancy test should be performed for all women of childbearing potential, and patients should be counseled about fertility preservation. An assessment of ejection fraction by echocardiogram or radionuclide study is necessary for all patients receiving anthracycline chemotherapy. Pulmonary function tests with diffusing capacity should be ordered if bleomycin-containing chemotherapy is used.

A summary list of suggested initial procedures and tests is presented in *Table 95.3*.

Table 95.3. Recommended Initial Evaluation for Patients With Hodgkin Lymphoma

History and Physical Examination, Including
- Past medical history: including B symptoms (fever, night sweats, and weight loss of >10% in past 6 mo), alcohol intolerance, itching, HIV risks, cardiac, renal, and liver impairment
- Family history: including lung cancer, coronary disease, and breast cancer
- Personal history: smoking
- Examination of all peripheral lymph node regions (including epitrochlear, popliteal, and Waldeyer ring), liver, and spleen

Radiologic Studies
- Chest radiograph
- PET/CT
- Assessment of EF
- Pulmonary function tests

Laboratory Studies
- Hematocrit, white blood cell count, differential, and platelet count
- Erythrocyte sedimentation rate and lactic dehydrogenase
- Liver function tests including albumin, alkaline phosphatase transaminases, and bilirubin
- Bilirubin, alkaline phosphatase, and liver function tests
- Thyroid function tests if radiation to neck is contemplated
- Bone scan (selected patients)
- HIV serology

Bone Marrow Aspiration and Biopsy (consider if PET negative; not essential if bone marrow is PET positive)

Discuss fertility preservation measures

Abbreviations: CT, computed tomography; EF, ejection fraction; HIV, human immunodeficiency virus; PET, positron emission tomography.

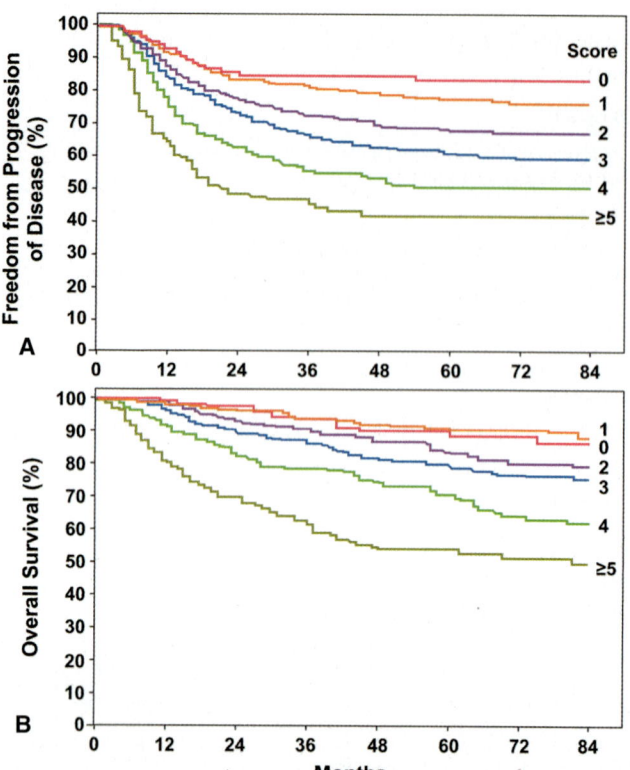

FIGURE 95.6 Progression-free survival (A) and survival (B) as related to number of risk factors. (From Hasenclever D, Diehl V, Armitage JO, et al. A prognostic score for advanced Hodgkin's disease. *N Engl J Med.* 1998;339(21):1506-1514. Copyright © 1998 Massachusetts Medical Society. Reprinted with permission from Massachusetts Medical Society.)

Prognostic Indicators

Stage is the major prognostic factor in HL, but patients can be further risk stratified based on additional prognostic factors. In a study of 5141 patients with "advanced" HL, primarily stage III and IV diseases, Hasenclever and Diehl performed a multivariate analysis of risk factors (*Figure 95.6*).[47] Seven independent factors that predicted freedom from progression (FFP) were identified: albumin <4.0 g/dL; hemoglobin <10.5 g/dL; male sex; 45 years of age or more; stage IV disease; leukocytosis at or above 15,000/mm³; and lymphocytopenia (lymphocytes ≤600/mm³ and/or lymphocytes <8% of total white count). For patients with no risk factors (7% of all patients), 5-year FFP was 84%; 1 risk factor (22% of patients), 5-year FFP was 77%; 2 risk factors (29% of patients), 5-year FFP was 67%; 3 risk factors (23% of patients), 5-year FFP was 60%; 4 risk factors (12% of patients), 5-year FFP was 51%; and 5 or more risk factors (7% of patients), 5-year FFP was 42%.

Of note, B symptoms did not have independent prognostic value in this model. This model, referred to as the "International Prognostic Score (IPS)," is validated only for advanced-stage patients.

A number of prognostic classifications have been used for (1) to identify early-stage HL patients with unfavorable clinical characteristics and (2) to tailor therapy further in clinical trials (*Table 95.4*). These commonly employ a combination of age, ESR, mediastinal bulk, and the number of involved nodal sites.

TREATMENT OF CLASSIC HODGKIN LYMPHOMA

Over time, the management of HL has evolved from the use of extensive radiation fields to the use of combination chemotherapy with or without more focal radiation. For patients younger than 65 to 75 years

Table 95.4. Unfavorable Characteristics for Stage I and II HL

Risk Factor	GHSG	EORTC
Age		≥50
ESR and B symptoms	>50 if A; >30 if B	>50 if A; >30 if B
Mediastinal mass	MMR ≥0.33	MTR ≥0.33
# Nodal sites	>2[a]	>3
E lesions	Any	

[a]Uses alternate definition of nodal sites.
Abbreviations: EORTC, European Organisation for the Research and Treatment of Cancer; GSHG, German Hodgkin Study Group; MMR, mediastinal mass ratio: maximal width of mass/maximal intrathoracic width; MTR, mass to thoracic width at T5-T6 interspace on standing PA chest radiograph.

who relapse and have chemotherapy-sensitive disease, consolidation with high-dose chemotherapy followed by autologous stem cell transplant (auto-HCT) remains the standard of care with curative intent. Novel agents including the anti-CD30 antibody drug conjugate, brentuximab vedotin (BV), and PD-1 inhibitors demonstrated significant efficacy in the relapsed and refractory setting. BV was subsequently approved in combination with chemotherapy in previously untreated patients with advanced-stage disease. Multiple clinical trials are studying the incorporation of novel agents in the upfront setting in stage III/IV patients as well as those with localized disease.

Radiotherapy

The modern radiotherapy era began with the Swiss radiotherapist Gilbert in 1925. Based on observed patterns of spread in patients with HL, Gilbert advocated treatment of both involved areas and adjacent, apparently uninvolved, areas. Over the next 2 decades, the curability of HL with radiation therapy was confirmed by Peters, Easson and Russell, and Kaplan, the latter investigator establishing the critical relationship between radiation dose and the risk of recurrence in the treatment field.

Since the demonstration that advanced HL was curable with combination chemotherapy, the incorporation of radiotherapy in initial treatment algorithms for HL has fallen over time given the risk of radiation-induced late toxicities as well as improvements in systemic therapy.[48] The dose of RT and the size of fields have both decreased, in concert with the development of new techniques and improved machinery. The impact of these changes, however, will take time to assess.

Chemotherapy

The development of cancer chemotherapy arose from the observation of lymph node and bone marrow necrosis in soldiers exposed to nitrogen mustard gas during World War I. HL and NHL were among the first disorders treated with nitrogen mustard.[49] During the 1960s, efforts were made to combine effective agents to reduce the emergence of resistance, culminating in the landmark demonstration by DeVita et al that MOPP (Mustargen [mechlorethamine], Oncovin [vincristine], procarbazine, and prednisone) combination chemotherapy could cure advanced HL.[50] In the initial publication reporting results achieved with the MOPP regimen, 81% of patients with advanced HL achieved a complete remission, and by actuarial analysis, 47% were projected to be long-term disease-free survivors.[51] Follow-up studies confirmed a long-term disease-free survival (DFS) rate of 56%.[52]

Studies of MOPP established combination chemotherapy as the treatment of choice for advanced HL. Subsequent trials, as detailed later in the section on frontline therapy of advanced disease, led to the use of alternative regimens given superior efficacy and toxicity compared to MOPP.

THERAPY OF EARLY-STAGE CLASSIC HODGKIN LYMPHOMA

Management of HL starts with determining the stage of disease and assessing risk factors. Early-stage disease refers to stage I or II. Risk factors are used to define *favorable early-stage HL* (defined as stage I or II HL without unfavorable risk factors) and *unfavorable early-stage HL* (defined as stage I or II with one or more risk factors). Risk factors have been variously defined by different groups (*Table 95.4*) but generally include (1) a greater number of nodal sites, (2) elevated ESR, (3) B symptoms, (4) a large mediastinal mass or other bulky disease, and (5) age over 50 years. Unfavorable early-stage HL may also be thought of as comprising two further groups: those unfavorable on the basis of bulky disease, and those unfavorable on the basis of another risk factor.

Treatment of Favorable Early-Stage Hodgkin Lymphoma

Historically, favorable early-stage HL was treated with extended-field radiotherapy, with cure rates as high as 80%. Given the risk of late toxicity including secondary cancers and cardiovascular disease, chemotherapy with limited fields and doses of radiotherapy or chemotherapy alone is standardly employed.[53-59]

A number of studies in stage I/II HL demonstrate the superiority of combined modality therapy compared with radiation alone. The European Organisation for Research and Treatment of Cancer (EORTC) H8F trial compared three cycles of MOPP/ABV (mechlorethamine, vincristine, procarbazine, prednisone, doxorubicin, bleomycin, and vinblastine) hybrid ($n = 270$) and involved field radiotherapy (IFRT) to subtotal nodal irradiation (STNRT) ($n = 272$). Event-free survival (EFS) at 5 years (98% vs 74%) and OS at 10 years (97% vs 92%) favored the combined modality arm.[53] The German Hodgkin Study Group (GHSG) subsequently examined the role of fewer cycles of chemotherapy and lower dose radiation in the HD10 study: 1370 patients without risk factors (fewer than three nodal sites, nonbulky disease without extranodal extension, ESR < 30 without B symptoms, or ESR < 50 with B symptoms) were randomized in a two-by-two design to four vs two cycles of ABVD and 30 vs 20 Gy of IFRT. With a median follow-up of 7.5 years, there was no difference between any of the arms, with freedom from treatment failure (FFTF) ranging from 91% to 93% at 5 years and 86% to 90% at 8 years, respectively.[60]

The HD6 trial of the National Cancer Institute of Canada randomized nonbulky early-stage patients to either ABVD alone (four to six cycles) or a strategy in which favorable (<40 years, ESR <50, no MCHL or lymphocyte-depleted histology, <4 sites of disease) patients received extended field radiation alone and unfavorable patients received ABVD × 2 followed by STNRT.[61] The study closed early after the emergence data supporting the use of IFRT in place of extended fields. At a median follow-up of 11.3 years, there was a lower rate of OS in the radiotherapy arm, with or without two cycles of ABVD, compared to ABVD alone (HR: 0.50). Although the trial was criticized for being underpowered and a number of the deaths in the radiotherapy arm were unrelated to treatment, this study led to the use of chemotherapy alone as a therapeutic option in early-stage disease. Straus et al subsequently randomized 152 nonbulky stage I, II, and IIIA patients to ABVD × 6 vs ABVD × 6 and 36 Gy of extended or involved field radiation therapy.[62] At 60 months, FFP was 81% vs 86% (NS) and OS was 90% vs 97% (NS).[63] The authors point out that the trial, which closed early due to slow accrual, was not powered to detect difference smaller than 20%.

Clinicians recognized early in the chemotherapy era that an early clinical response to therapy in HL predicted a good outcome. After several studies demonstrated the remarkable prognostic value of PET/CT done after one, two, or three cycles of chemotherapy in advanced-stage HL, trials were designed to test the omission of radiotherapy in interim PET negative patients.[64] The randomized EORTC/LYSA/FIL H10 trial included 444 favorable stage I/II HL patients who were randomized to a standard treatment vs experimental treatment arms.[65] PET/CT was performed after two cycles, and those with a negative PET/CT on the standard arm received a total of three cycles of ABVD followed by INRT (involved-node radiotherapy) 30 Gy. Those with a negative PET/CT, defined as a Deauville 1 or 2, on the experimental arm received two more cycles of ABVD for a total of four cycles without INRT. Interim PET was negative in 83%. PFS rates at 5 years were 99% and 87% in the standard and experimental arms, respectively. Those with a positive PET received escalated BEACOPP (bleomycin, etoposide, adriamycin, cyclophosphamide, vincristine, procarbazine, and prednisone; BEACOPP-esc) × 2 followed by INRT. The study combined the results of unfavorable and favorable patients with a positive PET; those in the standard arm (ABVD × 3 + INRT) who had a positive PET had a 5-year PFS of 77% and those on the experimental arm (ABVD × 2 + BEACOPP-esc × 2 + INRT) had a 5-year PFS of 91%.

The UK (Randomized Phase III Trial to Determine the Role of FDG-PET Imaging in Clinical Stages IA/IIA Hodgkin Disease [RAPID]) trial also evaluated the role of PET-adapted therapy in favorable early-stage HL.[66] Patients received three cycles of ABVD and then underwent PET scanning. Patients with negative PET (Deauville 1-2) were randomly assigned to receive IFRT or no further treatment; patients with positive PET findings received a fourth cycle of ABVD followed by radiotherapy. The trial was designed as a noninferiority study to exclude a difference in the 3-year PFS rate of 7% or more points from the assumed 95% PFS rate in the combined modality group. A total of 420 patients with negative interim PET/CT underwent randomization, 209 to the radiotherapy group, and 211 to no further therapy. At a median follow-up of 60 months, the 3-year PFS rate was 95% in the radiotherapy group and 91% in the group that received no further therapy, with an absolute risk difference of −3.8% points. The trial did not meet its noninferiority endpoint as the lower limit of CI exceeded the noninferiority cutoff, though both the chemotherapy and combined modality arms had excellent 3-year PFS.

The GHSG HD16 study randomized early favorable patients to a standard treatment of ABVD × 2 followed by 20 Gy IFRT or an experimental PET-adapted arm where those with a negative PET (Deauville

1-2) after two cycles of ABVD receive no further therapy.[67] The 5-year PFS in PET negative patients was 93% in the standard arm and 86% in the group receiving ABVD × 2 only. Five-year OS was similar in both groups at approximately 98%. PET2 positive patients experienced a 5-year PFS of 88%.

In the PET-directed phase 2 US cooperative group study, Alliance 50,604, patients with nonbulky stage II patients (both favorable and unfavorable) received two cycles of ABVD.[68] PET2 negative patients (Deauville 1-3) received an additional two cycles of ABVD, and PET2 positive patients were treated with BEACOPP-esc × 2 followed by RT. The 3-year PFS in the PET negative and PET positive groups was 91% and 66%, respectively.

Summary of Treatment for Early-Stage Favorable Classic Hodgkin Lymphoma

Therapeutic options for patients with early-stage, favorable HL include combined modality therapy vs chemotherapy alone. The incorporation of RT yields improved progression-free but not overall survival at the expense of risk of late toxicities including second cancers and cardiovascular disease. Balancing the risk/benefits of both options at the individual patient level is important. For women under 30, in particular, the risk of radiation-associated breast cancer is high and chemotherapy alone is typically preferred in patients who are interim PET negative. Radiotherapy, however, in PET2 positive patients almost certainly reduces the risk of disease recurrence as does intensification of chemotherapy. In addition, the incorporation of newer agents, including BV and/or a PD-1 inhibitor, in early-stage patients is being tested and could lead to further reductions in the use of radiotherapy and improvements in DFS.

Treatment of Unfavorable Early-Stage Hodgkin Lymphoma

Many patients who are classified as having unfavorable early-stage HL present with bulky mediastinal disease, whereas others are unfavorable on the basis of a high ESR or multiple nodal sites (>2 in the GHSG or >3 in the EORTC). Combined modality therapy has long been the recommended approach for this group of patients. The EORTC/GELA (Groupe d'Etude des Lymphoma de l'Adulte) H8U study randomized patients to one of three treatment strategies, two of which were MOPP/ABV × 6 followed by involved field radiation and MOPP/ABV × 4 followed by involved field radiation.[53] There was no statistical difference in the 5-year FFTF (84% vs 88%) or the 10-year OS (88% vs 85%). The same group's H9U study randomized patients to ABVD × 6, ABVD × 4, or baseline BEACOPP, each followed by involved field radiation.[69] The ABVD arms were equivalent, with a 4-year FFTF of 94% and 89%, respectively, and a 4-year OS of 96% and 95%. BEACOPP was not more effective (4-year FFTF of 91%) and was more toxic. These studies established ABVD × 4 followed by 30 Gy involved field radiation as a standard for unfavorable early-stage HL.

After the HD11 study of the GHSG showed no benefit to baseline BEACOPP over ABVD, HD14 trial compared ABVD × 4 to BEACOPP-esc × 2 followed by ABVD × 2 ("2 + 2"), each followed by 30 Gy involved field radiation; a total of 1528 patients entered the study.[70,71] The 2 + 2 arm was superior in PFS at 5 years (95% vs 89%) but OS was not significantly different. Toxicity was higher in the 2 + 2 arm as compared to the ABVD arm (at least one grade 3 or 4 toxicity of 87% vs 51%) and four patients died from toxicity in the 2 + 2 arm.[72] Despite the higher efficacy of the 2 + 2 arm, many would question the utility of the small increase in PFS without an increase in OS in this relatively short follow-up.

The EORTC H10 trial and UK RATHL trials also included patients with unfavorable disease. In the EORTC trial, the standard arm received ABVD × 4 + INRT 30 Gy. The experimental arm received ABVD × 6 if PET after two cycles was negative, and ABVD × 2 + BEACOPP-esc × 2 + INRT if the PET was positive.[65] Among the PET negative group, the 5-year PFS for ABVD alone and ABVD followed by INRT was 90% and 92%, respectively. Again, the study combines the results of unfavorable and favorable patients with a positive PET. Those in the standard arm (ABVD × 3 + INRT) who had a positive PET had a 5-year PFS of 77%, and those on the experimental arm (ABVD × 2 + BEACOPP-esc × 2 + INRT) had a 5-year PFS of 91%. In addition, the UK RATHL study also included 500 patients with early unfavorable cHL (defined as IIB with bulky disease or ≥3 nodal sites of involvement). PET2 negative (Deauville 1-3) patients after two cycles of ABVD were randomly assigned to four additional cycles of ABVD vs AVD.[73] PET2 positive patients were randomized to BEACOPP-esc vs BEACOPP-14. In the PET2 negative group with stage II disease, the 3-year PFS was 90% and was 92% in the 119 patients with bulky disease.

The recently published GHSG HD17 randomized 1100 early unfavorable patients to a standard treatment of BEACOPP-esc × 2 + ABVD × 2 followed by 30 Gy IFRT or an experimental PET-adapted arm where those with a negative PET after BEACOPP-esc × 2 cycles + ABVD × 2 of ABVD receive no further therapy. The 5-year PFS in the standard arm was 97% vs 95% in the PET-directed group and excluded the noninferiority, which was set at 8%.

A recent phase 2 study of 117 patients with early-stage unfavorable disease treated with BV plus four cycles of AVD in four cohorts with three radiotherapy doses/techniques (30 Gy ISRT, 20 Gy ISRT 30 Gy consolidation volume RT) and no RT.[74] The 2-year PFS in the cohorts was 93%, 97%, 90%, and 97%, respectively, supporting the omission of radiotherapy.

Summary of Treatment for Early-Stage Unfavorable Classic Hodgkin Lymphoma

In summary, ABVD × 4 to 6 followed by 30 Gy involved field radiation has been considered a standard for unfavorable early-stage HL. Recent data suggest that even for patients with bulky disease, the omission of radiotherapy after six cycles of ABVD is associated with favorable PFS. Moving forward, the use of intensified regimens and/or the incorporation of novel agents may further decrease the need for radiotherapy.

INITIAL THERAPY FOR ADVANCED-STAGE HODGKIN LYMPHOMA

Adriamycin (Doxorubicin), Bleomycin, Vinblastine, and Dacarbazine

HL was the first advanced adult malignancy cured with combination chemotherapy. Investigators at the NCI tested the MOPP regimen (mechlorethamine, vincristine, procarbazine, and prednisone),[50] which yielded a 4-year PFS rate of 47% in complete responders. Long-term toxicities, however, included secondary myelodysplasia/acute leukemia, and infertility, which is particularly relevant for patients with HL given the young median age of onset. The ABVD regimen was developed by Bonadonna and colleagues in 1975 as an effective, non–cross-resistant chemotherapy option for patients with relapsed HL.[75] ABVD was not associated with gonadotoxicity or secondary myelodysplasia/acute myeloid leukemia (AML).[76,77] A series of randomized clinical trials in the 1980s compared MOPP, ABVD, alternating MOPP/ABVD, and MOPP/ABV hybrid regimens demonstrated that ABVD was more effective and better tolerated than MOPP.[78-82] Thus, ABVD became the preferred regimen for the initial treatment of HL. With supportive care and other advances (such as treating patients without delays despite leukopenia), the PFS at 5 years is in the 70% to 75% range for an unselected academic center population.[83-85]

Bleomycin, Etoposide, Doxorubicin, Cyclophosphamide, Vincristine, Procarbazine, and Prednisone

Intensification of initial therapy is one approach to improve outcomes in patients with advanced-stage HL. However, this approach can lead to increased short- and long-term toxicity, which may ultimately have a negative impact on OS, particularly in lower-risk patients. The GHSG HD9 trial randomized patients aged 15 to 65 years with stage IIB, III, and IV HL to one of three arms: eight cycles of COPP/ABVD (cyclophosphamide, vincristine, procarbazine, and prednisone alternating with ABVD), BEACOPP-baseline, or BEACOPP-esc.[86] With 10 years of follow-up, FFTF was 64%, 70%, and 82% with OS of 75%, 80%, and 86% in the COPP/ABVD, BEACOPP-baseline, and BEACOPP-esc arms, respectively.[87] By IPS, FFTF at 5 years was 92%, 87%, and 82% with BEACOPP-esc for patients with 0 to 1, 2 to 3, and 4 to 7 risk factors, respectively. However, it is important to note that only 13% of patients receiving BEACOPP-esc had 4 to 7 risk factors on this trial, and although differences in FFTF were significantly in favor of BEACOPP-esc among all three risk groups, statistically significant improvements in OS were only observed in patients with IPS scores of 2 to 3. When analyzed by age, there was not a significant improvement in FFTF and OS for patients aged 60 to 65 years and increased toxicity occurred with BEACOPP-esc. Therefore, BEACOPP-esc is not recommended in patients beyond 60 years of age.

In an attempt to reduce toxicity, the HD12 trial examined eight cycles of BEACOPP-esc vs four cycles of BEACOPP-esc plus four cycles of BEACOPP-baseline.[88] Five-year FFTF and OS were 86% and 92%, respectively with eight BEACOPP-esc compared to 85% and 90% with 4 + 4 arm, and toxicities were not significantly reduced with the 4 + 4 approach.

In a randomized Italian study comparing six cycles of ABVD with four cycles of BEACOPP-esc plus two cycles BEACOPP-baseline, 5-year PFS was superior for BEACOPP (81%) compared to ABVD (68%), although there were no differences in OS perhaps because of the smaller numbers of patients on this trial compared to the 1201 patients on the HD9 trial.[63,87] In a second Italian cooperative group study, the 7-year rate of FFP was 85% in patients receiving four cycles of BEACOPP-esc plus four cycles BEACOPP-baseline compared to 73% in patients receiving six to eight cycles of ABVD.[89] In this same trial, the 7-year rate of freedom from second progression was 88% in the BEACOPP group compared to 82% in the ABVD group, suggesting that long-term outcomes may not differ between the two regimens when one factors in the efficacy of salvage chemotherapy and auto-HCT following ABVD.

Despite the success of the BEACOPP-esc regimen compared to hybrid regimens and ABVD in patients less than or equal to 60 years of age, this regimen is associated with infertility and a 6.0% second malignancy rate, including a 3.2% incidence of secondary AML/myelodysplastic syndrome (MDS).[63,87-90] In addition, BEACOPP-esc is associated with more acute toxicities including hematologic and infectious complications than observed with ABVD. Therefore, although several studies demonstrate the superiority of BEACOPP-esc with respect to PFS in patients with advanced-stage HL, it remains unclear if the risks of second malignancies, infertility, and acute infections associated with BEACOPP-esc are justified to improve patient outcomes in all patients with advanced-stage HL, especially if relapsing patients after ABVD can be effectively salvaged with high-dose therapy and HCT.

Brentuximab Vedotin, Doxorubicin, Vinblastine, and Dacarbazine

The ECHELON-1 study compared ABVD ($n = 670$) with brentuximab (Adcetris, A) + AVD ($n = 664$) in patients with stage III and IV cHL.[91] Patients were stratified according to geographic region and IPS risk group. The primary endpoint was modified PFS defined as time to disease progression, death from any cause, or modified progression (evidence of incomplete response after completion of frontline therapy according to review by an independent committee, followed by subsequent anticancer therapy). Secondary endpoints included OS. At a median follow-up of 24.6 months, the 2-year modified PFS rates were 82% and 77% in the A+AVD and ABVD groups, respectively. There were 28 and 39 deaths in A+AVD and ABVD, respectively, which was not statistically significant with respect to OS. The incidence of neutropenia (58% vs 45%) and neuropathy was more common (67% vs 43%) in A+AVD compared with ABVD groups. In contrast, the pulmonary toxicity rate was 1% in the A+AVD group and 3% in the ABVD group. A+AVD was associated with more neutropenia and neuropathy; and required growth factor support, adding to cost for a small difference in outcome. There was not a statistically significant difference between the 2 arms in patients over 60. Updated results after 5 years of follow-up showed a persistent PFS benefit for treatment with A+AVD (5-year PFS 82% vs 75%), but no difference in OS.[92]

Risk-Adapted Treatment Strategies in Advanced Hodgkin Lymphoma

Similar to early-stage HL, studies have examined the feasibility of response-adapted treatment strategies in the hope of avoiding excessive treatment in those with good prognosis or escalating treatment in those without response. Gallamini et al evaluated 260 patients mostly treated with ABVD with or without radiation and with stage IIB-IV HL.[93] A PET/CT was performed after two cycles of therapy. The 2-year PFS in the PET-negative patients was 95% compared to 12.8% in those with PET positive disease at a median follow-up of 2 years. The RATHL study randomized patients with a negative PET scan (Deauville 1-3) after two cycles of ABVD to either complete six cycles of ABVD or continue AVD for the last four cycles without radiation consolidation.[73] The primary outcome was the difference in the 3-year PFS and noninferiority margin was set at 5% or more. The absolute difference in the 3-year progression-free survival rate (ABVD vs AVD) was 1.6% (95% CI, −3.2-5.3) and did not meet the noninferiority margin. The omission of bleomycin with a negative interim PET-CT did not significantly increase the risk of recurrence and was associated with fewer respiratory adverse events. Those with positive PET findings after two cycles received BEACOPP. The 3-year progression-free survival rate was 67.5%, and the OS rate was 87.8%. Although this dose intensification strategy has not been studied extensively, these results did show improved outcome compared with continuation of ABVD after a positive PET in other studies.

The LYSA group studied using interim PET to de-escalate therapy in PET2 negative patients with advanced-stage HL.[72] In this noninferiority, phase 3 study patients, 823 patients were randomized to standard therapy with BEACOPP-esc for 6 cycles vs a PET-directed approach. In the experimental arm, PET2 negative patients (87%) received two cycles of ABVD followed by another PET scan. If PET4 was negative (96%), the patients completed two additional cycles of ABVD (six total cycles of ABVD). The 5-year PFS was 86.2 in the standard arm vs 85.4% in the PET-directed group.

Radiation Therapy as Consolidation in Stage III-IV Classic Hodgkin Lymphoma

With the incorporation of PET, it is no longer common to use radiation as consolidation for the majority of advanced-stage patients with bulky disease. In the RATHL study, 32.1% patients had bulky disease, radiation was not recommended for patients with a negative interim PET.[73] The omission of consolidative radiation did not change the outcome of patients with bulky disease. In addition, the more common approach for residual masses at the end of treatment is to determine PET avidity. Those that are PET negative generally do not need further intervention, whereas those with PET positive disease will usually need confirmatory biopsy to proceed to salvage chemotherapy.

Autologous Transplant as Consolidation in Stage III-IV Hodgkin Lymphoma

Several trials have examined the role of auto-HCT to improve outcomes in patients with high-risk, advanced-stage HL, and to date none have demonstrated a role for this following standard ABVD chemotherapy. A European intergroup trial enrolled patients with stage III-IV HL and two risk factors (elevated lactate dehydrogenase, bulky disease, stage IV with two or more extranodal sites, anemia, or inguinal involvement) who achieved a complete response (CR) or partial response (PR) after four cycles of ABVD or another doxorubicin containing induction (MOPP/ABVD, MOPP/ABV, CVPP/ABV). In the trial, 163 patients were randomized to either four additional cycles of the same induction chemotherapy or auto-HCT after BEAM (carmustine, etoposide, cytarabine, and melphalan) or CBV (cyclophosphamide, carmustine, and etoposide) conditioning.[94] The 5-year FFS with continued chemotherapy was 82% compared to 75% with consolidative auto-HCT, and the 5-year OS were 88% and 88%, demonstrating no clear benefit from early high-dose consolidation in high-risk advanced-stage HL. Two other studies using hybrid induction chemotherapy regimens vs chemotherapy followed by myeloablative transplant in 126 and 158 high-risk patients also demonstrated no difference in OS with frontline auto-HCT.[95,96]

Summary for Therapy of Classic Hodgkin Lymphoma

Overall, rates of long-term disease control in HL are high. Particularly in young patients, the efficacy of upfront therapeutic options must be balanced with the risk of late toxicity, particularly with regard to radiotherapy. Newer agents, such as BV and the PD-1 inhibitors, are being studied as part of frontline treatment in multiple ongoing trials and may result in additional changes to standard treatment approaches. Identifying which patients may require novel approaches and those who will have excellent outcomes with standard chemotherapy is critical, as is evaluating late toxicity and cost effectiveness of newer regimens. Assessing interim PET response using more quantitative approaches and the use of circulating tumor DNA have promise to improve risk adapted approaches.

THERAPY FOR RELAPSED OR REFRACTORY HODGKIN LYMPHOMA

Salvage Therapy and Autologous Hematopoietic Cell Transplant

The standard treatment for relapsed or refractory HL is salvage chemotherapy, which has historically consisted of a combination of chemotherapy agents not used in first-line therapy. For fit patients who demonstrate a response to treatment, consolidation with high-dose chemotherapy and auto-HCT is the standard of care based on two randomized trials from the 1990s that showed an improvement in EFS with this approach.[97,98] There are no randomized data to guide selection of second-line treatment and numerous options exist. Regimens such as ICE (ifosfamide, carboplatin, etoposide), GVD (gemcitabine, vinorelbine, liposomal doxorubicin), DHAP (dexamethasone, cytarabine, cisplatin), ESHAP (etoposide, methylprednisolone, cytarabine, cisplatin), GDP (gemcitabine, dexamethasone, and cisplatin), IGEV (ifosfamide, gemcitabine, vinorelbine, prednisolone), mini-BEAM (carmustine, etoposide, cytarabine, melphalan), and Dexa-BEAM (dexamethasone, carmustine, etoposide, cytarabine, melphalan; Table 95.5) have been used with similar results.[97,99-105] Multiple phase II trials have studied second-line treatment regimens that incorporate BV, including single agent BV, BV followed by multiagent chemotherapy, such as ICE,[104,106] or BV in combination with traditional chemotherapy regimens like ESHAP,[107] DHAP,[108] and bendamustine.[109,110] Most recently, combination regimens that include PD-1 blockade have shown encouraging results. These include nivolumab in combination with BV[111] and pembrolizumab plus GVD,[112] among others. In the absence of randomized trials, a salvage chemotherapy regimen should be selected based on patient factors and institutional experience. Ideally, the salvage regimen chosen should result in a high complete response rate with acceptable toxicity and not impair stem cell mobilization if auto-HCT is planned.

The MSKCC group prospectively evaluated prognostic factors in 153 patients undergoing ICE-based salvage therapy followed by auto-HCT.[113] In the multivariate analysis, pre-HCT PET scan positivity emerged as the most important factor that predicted both EFS and OS; the 5-year EFS was 31% and 75% for PET positive vs PET negative patients. Despite high-dose chemotherapy and auto-HCT, many patients will relapse. The double-blind, placebo-controlled, phase III AETHERA trial studied the role of BV consolidation after auto-HCT in patients at high risk of relapse, defined as patients who had at least one of the following: primary refractory disease, an initial remission duration of less than 12 months, or extranodal disease at the start of pretransplantation salvage chemotherapy.[114] Patients were treated with a dose of 1.8 mg/kg of BV every 3 weeks up to 16 cycles. Median PFS in the brentuximab arm was 42.9 months compared with 24.1 months in the placebo group. After 5 years of follow-up, BV continued to provide a sustained PFS benefit, but there was not yet an improvement in OS.[114]

Toxicity of Autologous Hematopoietic Cell Transplant

Patients who undergo auto-HCT should be monitored for risks of secondary leukemia, other secondary malignancies, hypogonadism, and its complications including declines in bone mineral density. Patients should also undergo revaccination to reduce the risk of infectious complications. In a retrospective study of 153 patients treated with autologous HCT for relapsed HL, the relative risk of second malignancies was 6.5 compared to the general population and 2.4 compared to nontransplanted patients with HL.[115] Second malignancies occurred in 15 patients, at a median of 9 years after auto-HCT and consisted of AML/MDS ($n = 6$), NHL ($n = 3$), non–small cell lung cancer ($n = 2$), colon cancer ($n = 2$), gastric cancer ($n = 1$), and adenocarcinoma of unknown primary ($n = 1$). All patients with AML/MDS had MOPP as part of their initial treatment regimen. In 100 patients treated with autologous HCT in Vancouver, second malignancies occurred in 7 patients at a median time of 4.2 years from transplantation and consisted of AML/MDS, glioblastoma, renal cell carcinoma, colon carcinoma, NHL, and breast cancer.[116] In this series, five patients developed cardiovascular disease including myocardial infarctions (MIs) 4 to 11 years posttransplant, arrhythmia, and aortic stenosis. In a large retrospective series of outcomes post-auto-HCT, 16 of 494 patients who underwent autologous HCT for relapsed or refractory disease developed second malignancies, and the risk of secondary malignancy was associated with use of total body irradiation as part of conditioning, age greater than or equal to 40, or use of radiation prior to transplantation.[117] Therefore, all survivors of HL who are transplanted should be have lifelong monitoring for second malignancies, with close attention to those treated with radiation either pre- or posttransplant or with TBI during transplant conditioning.

Because of the high risk of hypogonadism after auto-HCT, it is important to monitor for consequences of hormonal deficiency, including bone mineral density reduction using DEXA scanning. Lastly, immunity typically wanes post–autologous transplantation, and it is recommended that patients receive pneumococcal, tetanus, *Haemophilus influenza* type B, hepatitis B, and annual influenza vaccinations. Measles, mumps, rubella, and varicella vaccinations can be considered in immunocompetent patients 24 months after auto-HCT.

Therapeutic Options for Patients Relapsing After Autologous Hematopoietic Cell Transplantation

A significant number of patients experience disease relapse after auto-HCT. Fortunately, there are several options for treatment of relapsed HL in the post-HCT setting including single agent and combination chemotherapies. Many of the previously discussed combination salvage regimens including ICE, GVD, DHAP, ESHAP, GDP, and IGEV have activity in patients with HL that have progressed after autologous HCT; however, BV and the PD-1 inhibitors, nivolumab and pembrolizumab, have emerged as preferred options in this setting for patients who have not yet received these agents.[26,92]

Brentuximab Vedotin

BV is comprised of a CD30 antibody conjugated by a plasma-stable linker to the antimicrotubule agent, monomethyl auristatin E. In a pivotal phase II study with 102 patients with relapsed (29%) or refractory (71%) HL who had previously received a median of 3.5 prior therapies (range 1-13), the ORR was 75% with a 34% CR rate.[118] The median duration of response was 20.5 months in this trial, and grade 3 to 4 toxicity consisted of sensory neuropathy (8%), fatigue (2%), neutropenia (20%), and thrombocytopenia (8%). After 5 years of follow-up, 9 complete responders (9% of trial population) remained in remission without consolidative transplantation,

Table 95.5. Salvage Combination Chemotherapy Regimens Utilized for Relapsed or Refractory Hodgkin Lymphoma

Regimen	Drugs	Route	Schedule	Cycle Length
GVD (not previously transplanted)	Gemcitabine 1000 mg/m^2 Vinorelbine 20 mg/m^2 Liposomal doxorubicin 15 mg/m^2	IV IV IV	Days 1 and 8 Days 1 and 8 Days 1 and 8	Q21d
GVD (previously transplanted)	Gemcitabine 800 mg/m^2 Vinorelbine 15 mg/m^2 Liposomal doxorubicin 10 mg/m^2	IV IV IV	Days 1 and 8 Days 1 and 8 Days 1 and 8	Q21d
Gem-Ox	Gemcitabine 1000 mg/m^2 Oxaliplatin 100 mg/m^2	IV IV	Days 1 and 15 Days 1 and 15	Q28d
ICE	Ifosfamide 5000 mg/m^2 Mesna 5000 mg/m^2 Etoposide 100 mg/m^2 Carboplatin AUC = 5 (maximum dose of 800 mg)	IV over 24 h IV over 24 h IV IV	Day 2 Day 2 Days 1-3 Day 2	Q14d
DHAP	Dexamethasone 40 mg Cisplatin 100 mg/m^2 Cytarabine 2000 mg/m^2	IV/PO IV over 24 h IV every 12 h	Days 1-4 Day 1 Day 2	Q21d
ESHAP	Etoposide 40 mg/m^2 Methylprednisolone 500 mg Cytarabine 2000 mg/m^2 Cisplatin 25 mg/m^2	IV IV IV CIV	Days 1-4 Days 1-5 Day 5 Days 1-4	Q21d
Mini-BEAM	BCNU (carmustine) 60 mg/m^2 Etoposide 75 mg/m^2 Cytarabine 100 mg/m^2 Melphalan 30 mg/m^2 (maximum of 50 mg)	IV IV IV every 12 h IV	Day 1 Days 2-5 Days 2-5 Day 5	Q21-28d
Dexa-BEAM	Dexamethasone 24 mg BCNU (carmustine) 60 mg/m^2 Melphalan 20 mg/m^2 Etoposide 200 mg/m^2 Cytarabine 100 mg/m^2 G-CSF 300-480 µg	PO IV IV IV every 12 h IV every 12 h SQ	Days 1-10 Day 2 Day 3 Days 4-7 Days 4-7 Day 9 until WBC >2500/µL	Q28d
IGEV	Ifosfamide 2000 mg/m^2 Gemcitabine 800 mg/m^2 Vinorelbine 20 mg/m^2 Prednisolone 100 mg	IV IV IV PO	Days 1-4 Days 1 and 4 Day 1 Days 1-4	Q21d
GDP	Gemcitabine 1000 mg/m^2 Cisplatin 75 mg/m^2 Dexamethasone 40 mg	IV IV PO	Days 1 and 8 Days 1 and 8 Days 1-4	Q21d
ChlVPP	Chlorambucil 6 mg/m^2 Vinblastine 6 mg/m^2 Procarbazine 100 mg/m^2 Prednisone 40 mg	PO IV PO PO	Days 1-14 Days 1 and 8 Days 1-14 Days 1-14	Q28d
Brentuximab vedotin	1.8 mg/kg (capped at maximum of 100 kg)	IV	Day 1	Q21d
Brentuximab vedotin + Bendamustine	1.8 mg/kg (capped at maximum of 100 kg) 90 mg/m^2	IV IV	Day 1 Days 1, 2	Q21d
Brentuximab vedotin + Nivolumab	1.8 mg/kg (capped at maximum of 100 kg) 240 mg (flat dose) (study used 3 mg/kg)	IV IV	Day 1 Day 8 (cycle 1) Day 1 (cycles 2-4)	Q21d
Nivolumab	240 mg (flat dose) 480 mg (flat dose)	IV IV	Day 1 Day 1	Q14d Q28d
Pembrolizumab	200 mg (flat dose)	IV	Day 1	Q21d
Pembrolizumab + GVD	Pembrolizumab 200 mg (flat dose) Gemcitabine 1000 mg/m^2 Vinorelbine 20 mg/m^2 Liposomal doxorubicin 15 mg/m^2	IV IV IV IV	Day 1 Days 1 and 8 Days 1 and 8 Days 1 and 8	Q21d

suggesting that BV alone may be curative in a small percentage of patients.[119] BV may be administered for up to 16 cycles, with dose reductions or delays if needed for myelosuppression or neuropathy. In recent years, brentuximab has been approved for maintenance therapy in high-risk patients following auto-HCT and as part of first-line therapy (BV-AVD). As a result, most patients who relapse after auto-HCT will have already received BV.

PD-1 Inhibitors

Based on nearly universal alterations in PD-1 signaling in HL, expansion cohorts of HL patients were included in phase 1 trials of both nivolumab and pembrolizumab. These trials showed very high response rates among heavily pretreated patients.[120] Subsequent pivotal phase II trials of PD-1 blockade confirmed high ORRs (69% for nivolumab, 72% for pembrolizumab) among much larger cohorts of patients who had relapsed after auto-HCT or were ineligible for auto-HCT because of chemorefractory disease. Notably, response rates were similar for high-risk patients, including those with primary refractory disease or those refractory to BV. Median PFS was 14.7 months for nivolumab and 13.7 months for pembrolizumab.[121,122] As with BV, a subset of patients who achieve a complete response to PD-1 blockade may experience long-term PFS without consolidative transplantation. Based on these results, both nivolumab and pembrolizumab were FDA approved for relapsed/refractory disease post HCT. The toxicity of PD-1 blockade for patients with HL appears similar to that seen in other malignancies.

Other Treatment Options

There is not a standard approach for patients with R/R cHL who have progressed after both BV and PD-1 blockade. In most cases, the best option for these patients is a clinical trial. Retrospective series have suggested that response rates to traditional chemotherapy regimens may be higher following PD-1 blockade, leading some to hypothesize that PD-1 blockade may have a chemosensitization effect. Options after BV and PD-1 blockade include IFRT, single-agent chemotherapy, combination chemotherapy, or immunomodulatory therapy. Studies have also shown the efficacy of lenalidomide in this setting with an ORR of 14% to 50%.[123,124] Furthermore, prolonged therapy over several months rather than two to three cycles may be necessary to control disease.

Radiotherapy may also be considered in the setting of relapsed HL. In a retrospective analysis of salvage radiotherapy used in 100 patients at first-treatment failure, typically after COPP/ABVD initial therapy, 5-year FFTF and OS were 28% and 51% with radiotherapy alone.[125] Advanced stage at relapse and B-symptoms adversely affected OS in multivariate analysis. Therefore, in highly selected patients with limited-stage disease at relapse who may not be eligible for autologous HCT because of age and comorbid conditions, IFRT may lead to prolonged remissions. For younger patients with relapsed HL, owing to potential risks of second malignancies within the radiation field and improved survival with auto-HCT, radiotherapy alone is not recommended at first relapse. However, IFRT should be considered in these patients as consolidation post-auto-HCT to bulky, nonirradiated sites or to sites of relapsed limited-stage disease in previously nonirradiated fields. For those patients with limited-stage relapse posttransplantation, radiotherapy may lead to prolonged remissions and delay the need for palliative chemotherapy or allogeneic transplantation.

Allogeneic Transplant

Allogeneic hematopoietic stem cell transplantation (allo-HCT) can be curative in relapsed/refractory cHL, but there is a high risk of relapse (Chapter 106), as high as 40% even with alternate donor sources.[126] In recent years, outcomes with allo-HCT appear to be improving with advances in supportive care and the use reduced intensity conditioning (RIC).

RIC regimens use lower doses of chemoradiotherapy, have lower early posttransplantation morbidity and mortality, and rely more on the graft vs lymphoma effect, which does not depend on the intensity of conditioning. A retrospective study evaluated groups of HL patients receiving RIC vs myeloablative conditioning prior to allo-HCT. RIC was associated with improvements in both nonrelapse mortality.[127] Another other challenge in the use of allo-HCT was the lack of or delay in donor availability. The use of alternate donor sources such as haploidentical and cord blood donors has provided possible solutions in this regard. In a retrospective study evaluating RIC, allo-HCT found comparable outcomes with cord blood and matched sibling donors.[128] The use of double cord blood transplantation has shown a 5-year PFS of 31% in HL patients.[129]

Finally, the availability of novel agents for pretransplant salvage treatment may also be improving outcomes of allo-HCT. Data show that treatment with BV before RIC allo-HCT for relapsed cHL may improve outcome. BV was administered prior to RIC allogeneic HCT and resulted in an improvement in a 2-year PFS compared to historical control (59.3% vs 26.1%); however, there was no difference in OS.[130]

Treatment with nivolumab or pembrolizumab before allo-HCT also impacts post-allo-HCT outcomes. PD-1 blockade before allo-HCT has been associated with increased rates of severe acute graft-vs-host disease (GVHD), particularly for patients with a short interval from last dose of PD-1 to allo-HCT.[131,132] Even so, outcomes for allo-HCT after PD-1 blockade also appear to be better than historical controls, which may be driven in part by lower rates of relapse. In one large retrospective series, the 2-year PFS and OS were 69% and 82%, respectively. In this study, use of posttransplant cyclophosphamide for GVHD prophylaxis was associated with significant improvements in both PFS and GVHD and relapse-free survival.[132]

Adoptive T-cell Therapy

Adoptive T-cell therapy options are also under investigation for cHL. For patients with EBV-associated cHL, autologous cytotoxic T lymphocytes directed against EBV latent membrane proteins have shown efficacy.[133] A recent proof-of-concept study has shown early safety and efficacy of a modified T-cell product, which is resistant to the immune inhibitory cytokine, transforming growth factor β.[134] The application of CD19-directed chimeric antigen receptor (CAR) T cells to cHL has been limited by the lack of B-cell antigens including CD19 on RS cells; however, early studies with CD30-directed CAR-T cells have shown high overall response rates.[135-138] Additional studies and longer follow-up are needed to determine if CAR-T cell therapy can be curative in HL as it appears to be for several NHL subtypes.

NODULAR LYMPHOCYTE-PREDOMINANT HODGKIN LYMPHOMA

Epidemiology and Pathobiology

NLPHL is a rare subtype of HL, representing about 5% of all HL cases, with unique pathologic features distinguishing it from cHL.[139,140] The neoplastic cell is a large cell, which is the LP cell. This is also known as a popcorn cell because of its single, large, folded, or multilobulated nucleus that is typically smaller than observed in RS cells (*Figure 95.7*). Unlike the RS cell, these cells are typically CD30 and CD15 negative, and CD19, CD20, CD45, and CD79a positive. These cells also express transcription factors PAX-5 and OCT-2a. The background lymphocytes are predominantly small CD20 B-cells, with rare eosinophils, neutrophils, or plasma cells. Surrounding the LP cells, CD4+, CD57+, and PD1+ T-cell rosettes are found, and CD21-positive follicular dendritic cells are present, consistent with the germinal center derivation of this malignancy.[140] At least one nodule with a mixture of LP cells and small B cells is required for diagnosis.

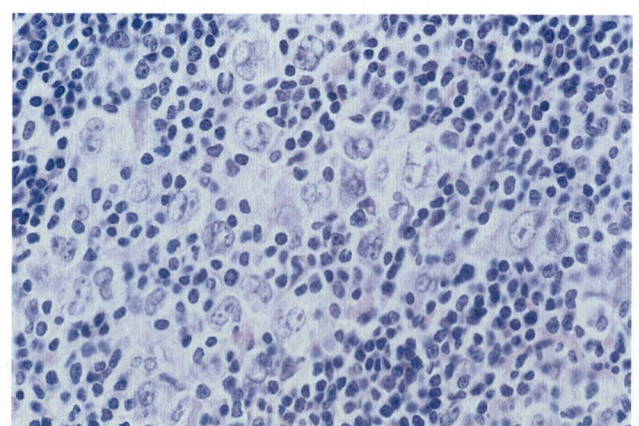

FIGURE 95.7 Lymphocyte-predominant Hodgkin lymphoma. High magnification shows variant lymphocytic and histiocytic cells (L and H cells), which have "popcorn" nuclei. A background of small lymphocytes and histiocytes is present.

Clinical Features

Owing to the rarity of NLPHL, the presentation, treatment, and patient outcomes are less well described than those of cHL. In a retrospective analysis of 8298 patients enrolled on clinical trials for HL through the GHSG, 394 patients had NLPHL.[139] In this series, the median age at diagnosis was 37 years, 75% patients were male, and 79% of patients had early-stage disease. Clinically, there appear to be two age peaks, one in children and the other in patients aged 30 to 50 years. The presence of B-symptoms or bulky disease is unusual, observed in fewer than 10% of patients. Patients with NLPHL typically have peripheral adenopathy (axillary or inguinal) at diagnosis rather than predominance of cervical and mediastinal adenopathy seen in cHL. Late relapses are more common in NLPHL.

Associated Conditions

Patients with NLPHL may have other lymph node disorders, including progressive transformation of germinal centers (PTGC) and NHL. PTGC is described as lymph nodes with large, well-defined nodules with an excess of B-cells, or germinal centers overrun by lymphocytes.[139] This entity may be observed prior to, simultaneously with, or following a diagnosis of NLPHL. Likewise, a subtype of NHL, TCRBCL, and NLPHL can occur simultaneously or in succession, and frequently TCRBCL can be pathologically confused with NLPHL. TCRBCL is characterized by large atypical B-cells that are CD20 positive, surrounded by an abundant background of T-cells and histiocytes. About 5% to 10% of NLPHL patients eventually develop NHL. Recurrent lymphadenopathy requires biopsy to distinguish among recurrent NLPHL, PTGC, and NHL patients. Relapses and transformation may occur late. In a French registry of 164 patients, 66 presented with recurrent disease and 19 of these had histologic transformation to DLBCL at a median of 4.7 years.[141] In a report of long-term follow-up of 95 cases of NLPHL, 13 patients had transformation at a median of 8.1 years.[142] Several risk factors for transformation have been described including advanced stage at diagnosis, splenic involvement, and abdominal involvement.

Therapy for Nodular Lymphocyte-Predominant Hodgkin Lymphoma

There is not a standard approach for treatment of newly diagnosed or relapsed NLPHL, but good outcomes have been observed with multiple different treatment approaches. In the large GHSG series, outcomes for NLPHL patients were excellent, with an ORR of 85% to 91% in patients with early-stage NLPHL compared to an ORR of 83% to 86% in patients with early-stage cHL treated with the same regimens.[139] For advanced-stage patients, outcomes were similarly good with ORR of 78% in patients with NLPHL compared to 78% in patients with stage III-IV cHL. FFTF at 50 months was 88% in patients with NLPHL and 82% for patients with cHL. Interestingly, relapses occurring more than 1 year after therapy completion were observed more commonly in patients with NLPHL (7%) compared to cHL (5%). Adverse prognostic factors in NLPHL include advanced stage, hemoglobin less than 10.5 g/dL, age greater than or equal to 45 years, and lymphopenia (<8% of total white cell count).[139] Patients with NLPHL are also at risk for transformation to an aggressive NHL, a phenomenon that is not typically observed with other HL subtypes. One study of 95 patients estimated the risk of transformation as 7% at 10 years and 30% at 20 years.[142] For patients who fail to respond to initial therapy or who develop recurrent disease, a tumor biopsy is recommended to confirm diagnosis and exclude transformation.

Initial treatment depends upon the presence of symptoms and staging. Given the good prognosis of NLPHL, limiting acute and long-term toxicity should be a priority whenever possible. For early-stage NLPHL, typically IFRT alone is recommended. A large multicenter study analyzed outcomes of patients with stage I-II NLPHL who were treated with various approaches between 1995 and 2018. For the entire cohort the 5-year PFS and OS were 87% and 98%, respectively. 5-year PFS was similar for patients who received RT alone (91%) and combined modality treatment (91%), while PFS was lower for patient receiving chemotherapy (78%) or rituximab alone (39%).[143] The GHSG evaluated 131 patients with stage IA NLPHL treated with extended field (n = 45), involved field (n = 45), and combined modality treatment (n = 41), and found an FFTF rate of 95% and OS of 99% at 43 months, with no differences with respect to FFTF or OS among the three treatment arms.[139] Based on these results, combined modality therapy is not recommended for most patients. Owing to the risks of second malignancies and the excellent long-term outcomes observed in patients with NLPHL, in selected patients where the disease is completely resected, observation may also be a suitable alternative to IFRT.[144]

Chemotherapy is typically reserved for those patients with advanced-stage disease or early-stage disease where the risks of late complications of radiotherapy are increased because of field or dose of radiotherapy required. Initial management of such patients depends upon extent of lymphoma involvement and the presence of symptoms. There are growing data to support active surveillance as an initial treatment strategy for asymptomatic patients with NLPHL. A single-center retrospective study of 163 consecutive patients with NLPHL demonstrated similar OS for patients managed with active surveillance compared to RT alone, combined modality therapy, or chemotherapy alone. Patients managed with active surveillance had a 5-year PFS of 77%, which was only slightly inferior to that seen with active treatment (87%).[145]

When patients require systemic therapy, multiple options are available including ABVD, alkylator regimens, like CVP or CHOP (with or without rituximab), or rituximab alone. Owing to the CD20 expression on LP cells, rituximab is increasingly utilized in the frontline treatment of NLPHL. In a study of single-agent rituximab as frontline therapy in 28 patients with stage IA NLPHL, the ORR was 100% and at 36 months the PFS was 81%.[146] Based on these results, rituximab is frequently combined with ABVD or alkylator-based (CHOP or CVP) therapy as part of initial treatment with those for stage III-IV disease. Limited data exist comparing ABVD to alkylator therapy either alone or in combination with rituximab, and therefore, these regimens are all frequently utilized as frontline and salvage therapy for relapsed stage III-IV NLPHL.

SPECIAL CONSIDERATIONS IN MANAGEMENT OF HODGKIN LYMPHOMA

Hodgkin Lymphoma in the Elderly

Older patients with HL have inferior outcomes compared to younger patients. In part, this is related to poor tolerance of intensified regimens but differences in disease biology may also be important. BEACOPP-esc is poorly tolerated in patients over 60 and is not recommended. In addition, subset analysis of the ECHELON-1 study demonstrated that patients over 60 did not experience improved PFS in the BV-AVD compared to ABVD. Added toxicity may lead to dose reduction and compromise in efficacy. Evens and colleagues tested a sequential approach in older patients. After two doses of BV, patients received six cycles of AVD followed by four additional doses of BV. 77% of patients completed six cycles of AVD and 73% received at least on dose on BV consolidation. Outcomes were excellent with this approach with 2-year PFS and OS of 84% and 93%, respectively.[147]

Friedberg et al studied the combination of brentuximab with dacarbazine or bendamustine in patients aged greater than or equal to 60 years in the frontline setting.[148] Both regimens had good efficacy with an ORR of 100%, and CR rates of 62% and 88% with the dacarbazine and bendamustine combinations, respectively. The bendamustine combination had unacceptable toxicity with 90% patients having grade 3 toxicity. The most common adverse event was diarrhea and the most common grade 3 or higher adverse events were fatigue, peripheral sensory neuropathy, and infection.

Classic Hodgkin Lymphoma and Human Immunodeficiency Virus

Although cHL is not considered an AIDS-defining illness, the incidence of cHL is increased as much as 10-fold among patients with HIV infection.[149,150] In contrast to patients without HIV infection, HL in patients with HIV infection is most commonly of the mixed cellularity subtype, and is associated with B symptoms and with advanced stage, commonly because of bone marrow involvement.[151] Despite the excellent results seen in patients with advanced-stage HL in the absence of HIV infection, early in the AIDS epidemic, median survival in HIV-positive patients with HL was poor, generally less than 2 years. With the advent of immune reconstitution with highly active antiretroviral therapy, outcomes approach those in the HIV-negative population using standard chemotherapy.[152-154] As in the general population, an interim PET scan is highly predictive of good outcome though there are likely more false positives.[155]

Hodgkin Lymphoma and Pregnancy

Because HL is commonly seen in women of childbearing years, it is not surprising that HL may occur in women who are pregnant. This problem has been reviewed.[156] Although agreement regarding optimal management of these patients does not exist, several key observations have been made, and guidelines for therapy have been advocated. Pregnancy does not affect the course of HL as compared to age-adjusted controls in patients with Hodgkin disease who are not pregnant.[157] CT and PET/CT are contraindicated during pregnancy but MRI may be used to stage patients and assess disease burden.

The risk of fetal malformations is approximately 15% when chemotherapy is given in the first trimester, but there is no evidence of an increase in fetal malformations when chemotherapy is given in the second and third trimester.[158] For patients with low burden, asymptomatic disease, delaying therapy until after delivery may be feasible. In those with higher volume of disease or progression during pregnancy, necessitating therapy, ABVD is safe and effective with the goal of getting patients to full term with the assistance of maternal fetal medicine physicians.

Chemotherapy Toxicity

Chemotherapy-associated toxicity is regimen specific, though neutropenia is common in all. With ABVD, patients are often neutropenic on the day of treatment. Despite this, the risk of febrile neutropenia is less than 1% per cycle in the absence of growth factors, likely due to the lack of mucositis with risk of bacterial translocation.[159] In addition, data suggest a possible increased risk of bleomycin lung toxicity with the use of granulocyte colony-stimulating factor (G-CSF). Therefore, particularly in younger patients, the prophylactic use of G-CSF can be safely avoided and incorporated only if patients develop febrile neutropenia. Dose intensity and schedule should be maintained to maximize outcome and delaying therapy for neutropenia is not necessary. BV, when combined with AVD, however, is associated with higher risk of febrile neutropenia, necessitating the prophylactic use of growth factors. BEACOPP-esc also requires the use of G-CSF. Thrombocytopenia is uncommon with ABVD but frequently occurs with BEACOPP.

Peripheral neuropathy, predominantly sensory in nature, is associated with both vinblastine and vincristine and commonly improves over time after the completion of therapy but numbness and tingling can be persistent in particularly older patients. Painful neuropathy is uncommon. BV, particularly when given in combination with vinblastine, also causes high rates of peripheral neuropathy, that can be higher grade and include motor symptoms may also occur. Long-term follow-up of the ECHELON-1 trial suggests that this also typically improves or resolves over time.

Gastrointestinal toxicity is common in patients treated for HL. Nausea should be preventable in the majority of patients with the use of highly effective anti-emetics including ondansetron and the more potent intravenous formulation palonosetron, as well as the NK1 receptor antagonists aprepitant and fosaprepitant. Anticipatory nausea is also common, particularly in younger patients, and benzodiazepines are typically effective. In addition, constipation is a common toxicity of vinca alkaloids, necessitating the use of bowel regimens.

Doxorubicin is associated with dose-dependent cardiotoxicity, which may be exacerbated with chest irradiation. Baseline echocardiograms are typically recommended, though young patients are rarely found to have asymptomatic cardiac dysfunction at baseline. The risk of lung toxicity from bleomycin requires careful clinical monitoring of patients. The drug is renally cleared and caution is indicated in patients over 60. For those over 70 or with baseline renal insufficiency, the bleomycin should be avoided.

MDS or secondary leukemia is rarely associated with ABVD chemotherapy but can be observed in up to 3.2% of patients treated with eight cycles of BEACOPP-esc.[87] Patients treated with BEACOPP or who have received MOPP should have a complete blood count monitored annually for this risk.

Infertility

The risk of infertility after ABVD chemotherapy is low with rates of amenorrhea in women younger than 40 years between 3% and 7%, though the rates with BEACOPP-esc are high at 40% to 67%.[160] For men, azoospermia is extremely rare after ABVD and >60% after BEACOPP-esc. Early data from the randomized trial comparing BV-AVD to ABVD suggest no increased risk with the addition of brentuximab. Salvage chemotherapy and high-dose chemotherapy with autologous stem rescue is associated with high rates of both male and female infertility. Given the ease of sperm cryopreservation, this is generally recommended for all men undergoing therapy for HL, though azoospermia may be present in prior to the initiation of therapy, particularly in patients with symptomatic or advanced-stage disease and may improve with therapy. For women oocyte retrieval, in vitro fertilization and embryo cryopreservation, or ovarian tissue freezing are not necessary with low-risk regimens but should be considered in patients who require second-line therapy/auto-HCT or BEACOPP-esc. Gonadotropin-releasing hormone analogues have been used as ovarian protection during therapy. The efficacy of this approach has not been clearly demonstrated but is generally well tolerated, particularly if progesterone is coadministered to prevent hot flashes.[161]

LONG-TERM TREATMENT-RELATED TOXICITY

Radiation Toxicity

Cardiac toxicity of radiation therapy can include myocarditis, cardiomyopathy, conduction abnormalities, pericardial disease, and accelerated coronary artery disease predominantly after mediastinal radiation.[162-164] The risk of cardiac morbidity is increased in patients treated with both doxorubicin and mediastinal radiation.[165] In a Dutch study of 1474 HL survivors greater than 41 years of age, at a median follow-up of 18.7 years, there was an increased risk of MI and congestive heart failure with standardized incidence ratios of 3.6 and 4.9, respectively.[166] The risk of MI significantly increased after 10 years and remained elevated for at least 25 years after treatment. In a Harvard study of 1279 HL survivors who had received mediastinal radiation, the 10- and 15-year cumulative incidence rates of cardiac events were 4.5% and 9.6%, respectively. Male sex and age were important risk factors for cardiac events.[167]

Long-term cardiac toxicity is therefore an important consideration in HL survivorship and is the most common nonmalignant cause of mortality in HL survivors. Several groups including Children's Oncology Group, National Comprehensive Cancer Network (NCCN), the Radiology Appropriateness Criteria Expert Panel on HL, and European Society for Medical Oncology have released consensus guidelines for screening and surveillance in high-risk patients.[168] The NCCN survivorship panel recommends consideration of an echocardiogram within 1 year of completion of anthracyclines, addressing underlying risk factors, including lipids, hypertension, tobacco use and obesity, and following a healthy diet with regular exercise. The HL guidelines also suggest echocardiogram or stress testing, as well as carotid ultrasonography for patients receiving neck radiation, every 10 years.

Hypothyroidism is a common complication of radiation therapy with actuarial analysis indicating that 52% of patients develop hypothyroidism 20 years after radiation. Thyroid cancer is an uncommon complication.[169] Annual thyroid function tests are recommended for patients with radiation to the neck or upper mediastinum and evaluation for pulmonary fibrosis should be considered in symptomatic patients.

An increased risk of second malignancies, including lung cancer, stomach cancer, melanoma, and breast cancer, has been noted in patients receiving radiation therapy for HL.[170,171] These malignancies generally occur 10 to 20 years after radiation therapy, with the risk of second malignancies being increased in patients who have also received chemotherapy. In a cohort of 3905 patients treated in the Netherlands from 1965 to 2000, 27% received radiotherapy only and 61% combined modality therapy and 12% were treated with chemotherapy only.[172] With median follow-up of 19.1 years, 1055 cancers were diagnosed in 908 patients. The standard incidence ratio was 4.6 compared to the general population with cumulative incidence of second cancer of 48.5% at 40 years. When comparing study periods, the risk did not differ between those treated between 1965 to 1976, 1977 to 1988, or 1989 to 2000.

Patient receiving previous radiotherapy should be monitored for second malignancy. The relative risk of breast cancer secondary to radiation is age related. The relative risk of developing breast cancer is 38 for patients radiated before age 20; 17 for patients radiated between the ages of 20 and 29; 4 for patients radiated after the age of 30 (not significantly different from 1).[164,170,173] Fortunately, the baseline risk of breast cancer in patients younger than age 30 is low, muting the quantitative impact of this increase in relative risk. Nevertheless, it has been recommended that women who receive radiation therapy for HL prior to age 30 should undergo annual mammography starting 8 to 10 years after completion of therapy or at the age of 40, whichever comes first because 95% of such tumors occur more than 10 years after radiation.[170,174,175] In addition, recent NCCN guidelines have also recommended breast MRI in addition to mammograms for this patient population also starting at 8 years after radiation. Lung cancer risk has also increased in patients receiving mediastinal radiation, particularly patients with a smoking history, and chest imaging annually should be considered for these patients at greatest risk.[174]

FOLLOW-UP OF PATIENTS WITH HODGKIN LYMPHOMA

Follow-up of patients with HL must address both the risk of relapse as well as potential late complications of therapy. The value of surveillance imaging in survivors of HL is controversial and has not been evaluated in randomized trials. The majority of recurrences are diagnosed in the setting of patient symptoms. In a retrospective analysis of 2071 patients who underwent 5352 CT scans, only 125 patients were treated with salvage therapy.[176] Routine surveillance imaging has not been associated with survival benefit and is not cost effective.[174,177-179] NCCN guidelines suggest clinical follow-up every 3 to 6 months for years 1 to 2, every 6 to 12 months until year 3 and then annually with CT scans no more often that every 6 months following the completion of therapy unless clinically indicated. PET scans should not be performed as surveillance in patients who demonstrated remission at the completion of therapy given high rates of subsequent false positives with a study demonstrating a positive predictive value if only 28%.[175] In this study, 161 patients had 299 routine or clinically indicated follow-up of PET/CTs (inferred as PET/CT was performed based on clinical suspicion), and in this setting the true-positive rates were only 5% and 13%, respectively. Biopsies should be performed to confirm suspected relapse.

Secondary late therapy-related effects in HL survivors include hypothyroidism, fertility issues, secondary cancers, and cardiovascular disease. The risks of second malignancies and cardiovascular disease continue even beyond 30 years from diagnosis, and therefore, monitoring of late complications is a lifelong endeavor for HL survivors.[170,172] The details of radiation, chemotherapy, and transplant-related toxicity and their long-term surveillance are detailed earlier.

SUMMARY

More than 80% of patients with HL achieve long term remission with current therapies. Individualizing treatment approaches to balance risk of recurrence as well as short and long term toxicity is key, particularly in young and geriatric patients. Novel agents including antibody drug conjugates and immunotherapy have an increasing role in the management of patients with relapsed and newly diagnosed HL.

References

1. Siegel RL, Miller KD, Fuchs HE, Jemal A. Cancer Statistics, 2021. *CA Cancer J Clin.* 2021;71(1):7-33.
2. Correa P, O'Conor GT. Epidemiologic patterns of Hodgkin's disease. *Int J Cancer.* 1971;8(2):192-201.
3. Gutensohn N, Cole P. Childhood social environment and Hodgkin's disease. *N Engl J Med.* 1981;304(3):135-140.
4. Mueller N, Evans A, Harris NL, et al. Hodgkin's disease and Epstein-Barr virus. Altered antibody pattern before diagnosis. *N Engl J Med.* 1989;320(11):689-695.
5. Evens AM, Antillón M, Aschebrook-Kilfoy B, Chiu BC. Racial disparities in Hodgkin's lymphoma: a comprehensive population-based analysis. *Ann Oncol.* 2012;23(8):2128-2137.
6. Kahn JM, Keegan THM, Tao L, Abrahao R, Bleyer A, Viny AD. Racial disparities in the survival of American children, adolescents, and young adults with acute lymphoblastic leukemia, acute myelogenous leukemia, and Hodgkin lymphoma. *Cancer.* 2016;122(17):2723-2730.
7. Swerdlow SH, Campo E, Harris NL, et al. *WHO Classification of Tumours of Haematopoietic and Lymphoid Tissues.* IARC Press; 2008.
8. Shiels MS, Koritzinsky EH, Clarke CA, Suneja G, Morton LM, Engels EA. Prevalence of HIV Infection among U.S. Hodgkin lymphoma cases. *Cancer Epidemiol Biomarkers Prev.* 2014;23(2):274-281.
9. Goldin LR, Pfeiffer RM, Gridley G, et al. Familial aggregation of Hodgkin lymphoma and related tumors. *Cancer.* 2004;100(9):1902-1908.
10. Kharazmi E, Fallah M, Pukkala E, et al. Risk of familial classical Hodgkin lymphoma by relationship, histology, age, and sex: a joint study from five Nordic countries. *Blood.* 2015;126(17):1990-1995.
11. Diepstra A, Niens M, Vellenga E, et al. Association with HLA class I in Epstein-Barr-virus-positive and with HLA class III in Epstein-Barr-virus-negative Hodgkin's lymphoma. *Lancet.* 2005;365(9478):2216-2224.
12. Rosdahl N, Larsen SO, Clemmesen J. Hodgkin's disease in patients with previous infectious mononucleosis: 30 years' experience. *Br Med J.* 1974;2(5913):253-256.
13. Weiss LM, Movahed LA, Warnke RA, Sklar J. Detection of Epstein-Barr viral genomes in Reed-Sternberg cells of Hodgkin's disease. *N Engl J Med.* 1989;320(8):502-506.
14. Gulley ML, Eagan P, Quintanilla-Martinez L, et al. Epstein-Barr virus DNA is abundant and monoclonal in the Reed-Sternberg cells of Hodgkin's disease: association with mixed cellularity subtype and Hispanic American ethnicity. *Blood.* 1994;83(6):1595-1602.
15. Jarrett RF, MacKenzie J. Epstein-Barr virus and other candidate viruses in the pathogenesis of Hodgkin's disease. *Semin Hematol.* 1999;36(3):260-269.
16. Kulwichit W, Edwards RH, Davenport EM, Baskar JF, Godfrey V, Raab-Traub N. Expression of the Epstein-Barr virus latent membrane protein 1 induces B cell lymphoma in transgenic mice. *Proc Natl Acad Sci U S A.* 1998;95(20):11963-11968.
17. Sylla BS, Hung SC, Davidson DM, et al. Epstein-Barr virus-transforming protein latent infection membrane protein 1 activates transcription factor NF-kappaB through a pathway that includes the NF-kappaB-inducing kinase and the IkappaB kinases IKKalpha and IKKbeta. *Proc Natl Acad Sci U S A.* 1998;95(17):10106-10111.
18. Cader FZ, Vockerodt M, Bose S, et al. The EBV oncogene LMP1 protects lymphoma cells from cell death through the collagen-mediated activation of DDR1. *Blood.* 2013;122(26):4237-4245.
19. Mancao C, Hammerschmidt W. Epstein-Barr virus latent membrane protein 2A is a B-cell receptor mimic and essential for B-cell survival. *Blood.* 2007;110(10):3715-3721.
20. Kuppers R, Rajewsky K, Zhao M, et al. Hodgkin disease: Hodgkin and Reed-Sternberg cells picked from histological sections show clonal immunoglobulin gene rearrangements and appear to be derived from B cells at various stages of development. *Proc Natl Acad Sci U S A.* 1994;91(23):10962-10966.
21. Schwering I, Brauninger A, Klein U, et al. Loss of the B-lineage-specific gene expression program in Hodgkin and Reed-Sternberg cells of Hodgkin lymphoma. *Blood.* 2003;101(4):1505-1512.
22. Ushmorov A, Ritz O, Hummel M, et al. Epigenetic silencing of the immunoglobulin heavy-chain gene in classical Hodgkin lymphoma-derived cell lines contributes to the loss of immunoglobulin expression. *Blood.* 2004;104(10):3326-3334.
23. Garcia JF, Camacho FI, Morente M, et al. Hodgkin and Reed-Sternberg cells harbor alterations in the major tumor suppressor pathways and cell-cycle checkpoints: analyses using tissue microarrays. *Blood.* 2003;101(2):681-689.

24. Re D, Kuppers R, Diehl V. Molecular pathogenesis of Hodgkin's lymphoma. *J Clin Oncol*. 2005;23(26):6379-6386.
25. Green MR, Monti S, Rodig SJ, et al. Integrative analysis reveals selective 9p24.1 amplification, increased PD-1 ligand expression, and further induction via JAK2 in nodular sclerosing Hodgkin lymphoma and primary mediastinal large B-cell lymphoma. *Blood*. 2010;116(17):3268-3277.
26. Ansell SM, Lesokhin AM, Borrello I, et al. PD-1 blockade with nivolumab in relapsed or refractory Hodgkin's lymphoma. *N Engl J Med*. 2015;372(4):311-319.
27. Chen BJ, Chapuy B, Ouyang J, et al. PD-L1 expression is characteristic of a subset of aggressive B-cell lymphomas and virus-associated malignancies. *Clin Cancer Res*. 2013;19(13):3462-3473.
28. Vardhana S, Younes A. The immune microenvironment in Hodgkin lymphoma: T cells, B cells, and immune checkpoints. *Haematologica*. 2016;101(7):794-802.
29. Swerdlow SH, Campo E, Pileri SA, et al. The 2016 revision of the World Health Organization classification of lymphoid neoplasms. *Blood*. 2016;127(20):2375-2390.
30. Hoeller S, Copie-Bergman C. Grey zone lymphomas: lymphomas with intermediate features. *Adv Hematol*. 2012;2012:460801.
31. Strum SB, Park JK, Rappaport H. Observation of cells resembling Sternberg-Reed cells in conditions other than Hodgkin's disease. *Cancer*. 1970;26(1):176-190.
32. Lukes RJ, Butler JJ. The pathology and nomenclature of Hodgkin's disease. *Cancer Res*. 1966;26(6):1063-1083.
33. Anagnostopoulos I, Hansmann ML, Franssila K, et al. European Task Force on Lymphoma project on lymphocyte predominance Hodgkin disease: histologic and immunohistologic analysis of submitted cases reveals 2 types of Hodgkin disease with a nodular growth pattern and abundant lymphocytes. *Blood*. 2000;96(5):1889-1899.
34. Dorfman RF. Relationship of histology to site in Hodgkin's disease. *Cancer Res*. 1971;31(11):1786-1793.
35. Jones SE, Byrne GE, Jr, Coltman CA, Jr, Moon TE. Histopathologic review of lymphoma cases from the Southwest Oncology Group. *Cancer*. 1977;39(3):1071-1076.
36. Bernhards J, Fischer R, Hubner K, Schwarze EW, Georgii A. Histopathological classification of Hodgkin's lymphomas. Results from the reference pathology of the German Hodgkin Trial. *Ann Oncol*. 1992;3(suppl 4):31-33.
37. Medeiros LJ, Greiner TC. Hodgkin's disease. *Cancer*. 1995;75(1 suppl):357-369.
38. Strickler JG, Michie SA, Warnke RA, Dorfman RF. The "syncytial variant" of nodular sclerosing Hodgkin's disease. *Am J Surg Pathol*. 1986;10(7):470-477.
39. Sethi T, Nguyen V, Li S, Morgan D, Greer J, Reddy N. Differences in outcome of patients with syncytial variant Hodgkin lymphoma compared with typical nodular sclerosis Hodgkin lymphoma. *Ther Adv Hematol*. 2017;8(1):13-20.
40. Bearman RM, Pangalis GA, Rappaport H. Hodgkin's disease, lymphocyte depletion type: a clinicopathologic study of 39 patients. *Cancer*. 1978;41(1):293-302.
41. Kaplan HS. Contiguity and progression in Hodgkin's disease. *Cancer Res*. 1971;31(11):1811-1813.
42. Kaplan HS, Dorfman RF, Nelsen TS, Rosenberg SA. Staging laparotomy and splenectomy in Hodgkin's disease: analysis of indications and patterns of involvement in 285 consecutive, unselected patients. *Natl Cancer Inst Monogr*. 1973;36:291-301.
43. Shah BK, Subramaniam S, Peace D, Garcia C. HIV-associated primary bone marrow Hodgkin's lymphoma: a distinct entity? *J Clin Oncol*. 2010;28(27):e459-e460.
44. Ponzoni M, Fumagalli L, Rossi G, et al. Isolated bone marrow manifestation of HIV-associated Hodgkin lymphoma. *Mod Pathol*. 2002;15(12):1273-1278.
45. Cheson BD, Fisher RI, Barrington SF, et al. Recommendations for initial evaluation, staging, and response assessment of Hodgkin and non-Hodgkin lymphoma: the Lugano classification. *J Clin Oncol*. 2014;32(27):3059-3068.
46. Connors JM. Positron emission tomography in the management of Hodgkin lymphoma. *Hematology Am Soc Hematol Educ Program*. 2011;2011:317-322.
47. Hasenclever D, Diehl V. A prognostic score for advanced Hodgkin's disease. International prognostic factors project on advanced Hodgkin's disease. *N Engl J Med*. 1998;339(21):1506-1514.
48. DeVita VT, Jr, Canellos GP, Moxley JH III. A decade of combination chemotherapy of advanced Hodgkin's disease. *Cancer*. 1972;30(6):1495-1504.
49. Gilman A. The initial clinical trial of nitrogen mustard. *Am J Surg*. 1963;105:574-578.
50. Devita VT, Jr, Serpick AA, Carbone PP. Combination chemotherapy in the treatment of advanced Hodgkin's disease. *Ann Intern Med*. 1970;73(6):881-895.
51. Longo DL. The use of chemotherapy in the treatment of Hodgkin's disease. *Semin Oncol*. 1990;17(6):716-735.
52. DeVita VT, Jr, Simon RM, Jr, Hubbard SM, et al. Curability of advanced Hodgkin's disease with chemotherapy. Long-term follow-up of MOPP-treated patients at the National Cancer Institute. *Ann Intern Med*. 1980;92(5):587-595.
53. Ferme C, Eghbali H, Meerwaldt JH, et al. Chemotherapy plus involved-field radiation in early-stage Hodgkin's disease. *N Engl J Med*. 2007;357(19):1916-1927.
54. Press OW, LeBlanc M, Lichter AS, et al. Phase III randomized intergroup trial of subtotal lymphoid irradiation versus doxorubicin, vinblastine, and subtotal lymphoid irradiation for stage IA to IIA Hodgkin's disease. *J Clin Oncol*. 2001;19(22):4238-4244.
55. Engert A, Franklin J, Eich HT, et al. Two cycles of doxorubicin, bleomycin, vinblastine, and dacarbazine plus extended-field radiotherapy is superior to radiotherapy alone in early favorable Hodgkin's lymphoma: final results of the GHSG HD7 trial. *J Clin Oncol*. 2007;25(23):3495-3502.
56. Bonadonna G, Bonfante V, Viviani S, Di Russo A, Villani F, Valagussa P. ABVD plus subtotal nodal versus involved-field radiotherapy in early-stage Hodgkin's disease: long-term results. *J Clin Oncol*. 2004;22(14):2835-2841.
57. De Bruin ML, Sparidans J, van't Veer MB, et al. Breast cancer risk in female survivors of Hodgkin's lymphoma: lower risk after smaller radiation volumes. *J Clin Oncol*. 2009;27(26):4239-4246.
58. Hancock SL, Tucker MA, Hoppe RT. Factors affecting late mortality from heart disease after treatment of Hodgkin's disease. *J Am Med Assoc*. 1993;270(16):1949-1955.
59. Maraldo MV, Brodin NP, Vogelius IR, et al. Risk of developing cardiovascular disease after involved node radiotherapy versus mantle field for Hodgkin lymphoma. *Int J Radiat Oncol Biol Phys*. 2012;83(4):1232-1237.
60. Engert A, Plutschow A, Eich HT, et al. Reduced treatment intensity in patients with early-stage Hodgkin's lymphoma. *N Engl J Med*. 2010;363(7):640-652.
61. Meyer RM, Gospodarowicz MK, Connors JM, et al. ABVD alone versus radiation-based therapy in limited-stage Hodgkin's lymphoma. *N Engl J Med*. 2012;366(5):399-408.
62. Straus DJ, Portlock CS, Qin J, et al. Results of a prospective randomized clinical trial of doxorubicin, bleomycin, vinblastine, and dacarbazine (ABVD) followed by radiation therapy (RT) versus ABVD alone for stages I, II, and IIIA nonbulky Hodgkin disease. *Blood*. 2004;104(12):3483-3489.
63. Federico M, Luminari S, Iannitto E, et al. ABVD compared with BEACOPP compared with CEC for the initial treatment of patients with advanced Hodgkin's lymphoma: results from the HD2000 Gruppo Italiano per lo Studio dei Linfomi Trial. *J Clin Oncol*. 2009;27(5):805-811.
64. Hutchings M, Loft A, Hansen M, et al. FDG-PET after two cycles of chemotherapy predicts treatment failure and progression-free survival in Hodgkin lymphoma. *Blood*. 2006;107(1):52-59.
65. Andre MPE, Girinsky T, Federico M, et al. Early positron emission tomography response-adapted treatment in stage I and II Hodgkin lymphoma: final results of the randomized EORTC/LYSA/FIL H10 trial. *J Clin Oncol*. 2017;35(16):1786-1794.
66. Radford J, Illidge T, Counsell N, et al. Results of a trial of PET-directed therapy for early-stage Hodgkin's lymphoma. *N Engl J Med*. 2015;372(17):1598-1607.
67. Fuchs M, Goergen H, Kobe C, et al. Positron emission tomography-guided treatment in early-stage favorable Hodgkin lymphoma: final results of the international, randomized phase III HD16 trial by the German Hodgkin study group. *J Clin Oncol*. 2019;37(31):2835-2845.
68. Straus DJ, Jung SH, Pitcher B, et al. CALGB 50604: risk-adapted treatment of nonbulky early-stage Hodgkin lymphoma based on interim PET. *Blood*. 2018;132(10):1013-1021.
69. Ferme C, Thomas J, Brice P, et al. ABVD or BEACOPP$_{baseline}$ along with involved-field radiotherapy in early-stage Hodgkin Lymphoma with risk factors: results of the European Organisation for Research and Treatment of Cancer (EORTC)-Groupe d'Etude des Lymphomes de l'Adulte (GELA) H9-U intergroup randomised trial. *Eur J Cancer*. 2017;81:45-55.
70. Eich HT, Diehl V, Gorgen H, et al. Intensified chemotherapy and dose-reduced involved-field radiotherapy in patients with early unfavorable Hodgkin's lymphoma: final analysis of the German Hodgkin Study Group HD11 trial. *J Clin Oncol*. 2010;28(27):4199-4206.
71. von Tresckow B, Plutschow A, Fuchs M, et al. Dose-intensification in early unfavorable Hodgkin's lymphoma: final analysis of the German Hodgkin Study Group HD14 trial. *J Clin Oncol*. 2012;30(9):907-913.
72. Casasnovas RO, Bouabdallah R, Brice P, et al. PET-adapted treatment for newly diagnosed advanced Hodgkin lymphoma (AHL2011): a randomised, multicentre, non-inferiority, phase 3 study. *Lancet Oncol*. 2019;20(2):202-215.
73. Johnson P, Federico M, Kirkwood A, et al. Adapted treatment guided by interim PET-CT scan in advanced Hodgkin's lymphoma. *N Engl J Med*. 2016;374(25):2419-2429.
74. Borchmann P, Plutschow A, Kobe C, et al. PET-guided omission of radiotherapy in early-stage unfavourable Hodgkin lymphoma (GHSG HD17): a multicentre, open-label, randomised, phase 3 trial. *Lancet Oncol*. 2021;22(2):223-234.
75. Bonadonna G, Zucali R, Monfardini S, De Lena M, Uslenghi C. Combination chemotherapy of Hodgkin's disease with adriamycin, bleomycin, vinblastine, and imidazole carboxamide versus MOPP. *Cancer*. 1975;36(1):252-259.
76. Viviani S, Santoro A, Ragni G, Bonfante V, Bestetti O, Bonadonna G. Gonadal toxicity after combination chemotherapy for Hodgkin's disease. Comparative results of MOPP vs ABVD. *Eur J Cancer Clin Oncol*. 1985;21(5):601-605.
77. Valagussa P, Santoro A, Fossati-Bellani F, Banfi A, Bonadonna G. Second acute leukemia and other malignancies following treatment for Hodgkin's disease. *J Clin Oncol*. 1986;4(6):830-837.
78. Canellos GP, Anderson JR, Propert KJ, et al. Chemotherapy of advanced Hodgkin's disease with MOPP, ABVD, or MOPP alternating with ABVD. *N Engl J Med*. 1992;327(21):1478-1484.
79. Santoro A, Bonadonna G, Bonfante V, Valagussa P. Alternating drug combinations in the treatment of advanced Hodgkin's disease. *N Engl J Med*. 1982;306(13):770-775.
80. Glick JH, Young ML, Harrington D, et al. MOPP/ABV hybrid chemotherapy for advanced Hodgkin's disease significantly improves failure-free and overall survival: the 8-year results of the intergroup trial. *J Clin Oncol*. 1998;16(1):19-26.
81. Somers R, Carde P, Henry-Amar M, et al. A randomized study in stage IIIB and IV Hodgkin's disease comparing eight courses of MOPP versus an alteration of MOPP with ABVD: a European Organization for Research and Treatment of Cancer Lymphoma Cooperative Group and Groupe Pierre-et-Marie-Curie controlled clinical trial. *J Clin Oncol*. 1994;12(2):279-287.
82. Duggan DB, Petroni GR, Johnson JL, et al. Randomized comparison of ABVD and MOPP/ABV hybrid for the treatment of advanced Hodgkin's disease: report of an intergroup trial. *J Clin Oncol*. 2003;21(4):607-614.
83. Boleti E, Mead GM. ABVD for Hodgkin's lymphoma: full-dose chemotherapy without dose reductions or growth factors. *Ann Oncol*. 2007;18(2):376-380.
84. Gordon LI, Hong F, Fisher RI, et al. Randomized phase III trial of ABVD versus Stanford V with or without radiation therapy in locally extensive and advanced-stage Hodgkin lymphoma: an intergroup study coordinated by the Eastern Cooperative Oncology Group (E2496). *J Clin Oncol*. 2013;31(6):684-691.
85. Hoskin PJ, Lowry L, Horwich A, et al. Randomized comparison of the stanford V regimen and ABVD in the treatment of advanced Hodgkin's lymphoma: United

Kingdom National Cancer Research Institute lymphoma group study ISRCTN 64141244. *J Clin Oncol*. 2009;27(32):5390-5396.
86. Diehl V, Franklin J, Pfreundschuh M, et al. Standard and increased-dose BEACOPP chemotherapy compared with COPP-ABVD for advanced Hodgkin's disease. *N Engl J Med*. 2003;348(24):2386-2395.
87. Engert A, Diehl V, Franklin J, et al. Escalated-dose BEACOPP in the treatment of patients with advanced-stage Hodgkin's lymphoma: 10 years of follow-up of the GHSG HD9 study. *J Clin Oncol*. 2009;27(27):4548-4554.
88. Borchmann P, Haverkamp H, Diehl V, et al. Eight cycles of escalated-dose BEACOPP compared with four cycles of escalated-dose BEACOPP followed by four cycles of baseline-dose BEACOPP with or without radiotherapy in patients with advanced-stage Hodgkin's lymphoma: final analysis of the HD12 trial of the German Hodgkin Study Group. *J Clin Oncol*. 2011;29(32):4234-4242.
89. Viviani S, Zinzani PL, Rambaldi A, et al. ABVD versus BEACOPP for Hodgkin's lymphoma when high-dose salvage is planned. *N Engl J Med*. 2011;365(3):203-212.
90. Sieniawski M, Reineke T, Nogova L, et al. Fertility in male patients with advanced Hodgkin lymphoma treated with BEACOPP: a report of the German Hodgkin Study Group (GHSG). *Blood*. 2008;111(1):71-76.
91. Connors JM, Jurczak W, Straus DJ, et al. Brentuximab vedotin with chemotherapy for stage III or IV Hodgkin's lymphoma. *N Engl J Med*. 2018;378(4):331-344.
92. Straus DJ, Długosz-Danecka M, Connors JM, et al. Brentuximab vedotin with chemotherapy for stage III or IV classical Hodgkin lymphoma (ECHELON-1): 5-year update of an international, open-label, randomised, phase 3 trial. *Lancet Haematol*. 2021;8(6):e410-e421.
93. Gallamini A, Hutchings M, Rigacci L, et al. Early interim 2-[18F]fluoro-2-deoxy-D-glucose positron emission tomography is prognostically superior to international prognostic score in advanced-stage Hodgkin's lymphoma: a report from a joint Italian-Danish study. *J Clin Oncol*. 2007;25(24):3746-3752.
94. Federico M, Bellei M, Brice P, et al. High-dose therapy and autologous stem-cell transplantation versus conventional therapy for patients with advanced Hodgkin's lymphoma responding to front-line therapy. *J Clin Oncol*. 2003;21(12):2320-2325.
95. Proctor SJ, Mackie M, Dawson A, et al. A population-based study of intensive multi-agent chemotherapy with or without autotransplant for the highest risk Hodgkin's disease patients identified by the Scotland and Newcastle Lymphoma Group (SNLG) prognostic index. A Scotland and Newcastle Lymphoma Group study (SNLG HD III). *Eur J Cancer*. 2002;38(6):795-806.
96. Arakelyan N, Berthou C, Desablens B, et al. Early versus late intensification for patients with high-risk Hodgkin lymphoma-3 cycles of intensive chemotherapy plus low-dose lymph node radiation therapy versus 4 cycles of combined doxorubicin, bleomycin, vinblastine, and dacarbazine plus myeloablative chemotherapy with autologous stem cell transplantation: five-year results of a randomized trial on behalf of the GOELAMS Group. *Cancer*. 2008;113(12):3323-3330.
97. Schmitz N, Pfistner B, Sextro M, et al. Aggressive conventional chemotherapy compared with high-dose chemotherapy with autologous haemopoietic stem-cell transplantation for relapsed chemosensitive Hodgkin's disease: a randomised trial. *Lancet*. 2002;359(9323):2065-2071.
98. Linch DC, Winfield D, Goldstone AH, et al. Dose intensification with autologous bone-marrow transplantation in relapsed and resistant Hodgkin's disease: results of a BNLI randomised trial. *Lancet*. 1993;341(8852):1051-1054.
99. Bartlett NL, Niedzwiecki D, Johnson JL, et al. Gemcitabine, vinorelbine, and pegylated liposomal doxorubicin (GVD), a salvage regimen in relapsed Hodgkin's lymphoma: CALGB 59804. *Ann Oncol*. 2007;18(6):1071-1079.
100. Colwill R, Crump M, Couture F, et al. Mini-BEAM as salvage therapy for relapsed or refractory Hodgkin's disease before intensive therapy and autologous bone marrow transplantation. *J Clin Oncol*. 1995;13(2):396-402.
101. Crump M, Smith AM, Brandwein J, et al. High-dose etoposide and melphalan, and autologous bone marrow transplantation for patients with advanced Hodgkin's disease: importance of disease status at transplant. *J Clin Oncol*. 1993;11(4):704-711.
102. Josting A, Rudolph C, Reiser M, et al. Time-intensified dexamethasone/cisplatin/cytarabine: an effective salvage therapy with low toxicity in patients with relapsed and refractory Hodgkin's disease. *Ann Oncol*. 2002;13(10):1628-1635.
103. Kuruvilla J, Nagy T, Pintilie M, Tsang R, Keating A, Crump M. Similar response rates and superior early progression-free survival with gemcitabine, dexamethasone, and cisplatin salvage therapy compared with carmustine, etoposide, cytarabine, and melphalan salvage therapy prior to autologous stem cell transplantation for recurrent or refractory Hodgkin lymphoma. *Cancer*. 2006;106(2):353-360.
104. Moskowitz CH, Nimer SD, Zelenetz AD, et al. A 2-step comprehensive high-dose chemoradiotherapy second-line program for relapsed and refractory Hodgkin disease: analysis by intent to treat and development of a prognostic model. *Blood*. 2001;97(3):616-623.
105. Santoro A, Magagnoli M, Spina M, et al. Ifosfamide, gemcitabine, and vinorelbine: a new induction regimen for refractory and relapsed Hodgkin's lymphoma. *Haematologica*. 2007;92(1):35-41.
106. Chen R, Palmer JM, Martin P, et al. Results of a multicenter phase II trial of brentuximab vedotin as second-line therapy before autologous transplantation in relapsed/refractory Hodgkin lymphoma. *Biol Blood Marrow Transplant*. 2015;21(12):2136-2140.
107. Garcia-Sanz R, Sureda A, de la Cruz F, et al. Brentuximab vedotin and ESHAP is highly effective as second-line therapy for Hodgkin lymphoma patients (long-term results of a trial by the Spanish GELTAMO Group). *Ann Oncol*. 2019;30(4):612-620.
108. Shah GL, Moskowitz CH. Transplant strategies in relapsed/refractory Hodgkin lymphoma. *Blood*. 2018;131(15):1689-1697.
109. LaCasce AS, Bociek RG, Sawas A, et al. Brentuximab vedotin plus bendamustine: a highly active first salvage regimen for relapsed or refractory Hodgkin lymphoma. *Blood*. 2018;132(1):40-48.
110. O'Connor OA, Lue JK, Sawas A, et al. Brentuximab vedotin plus bendamustine in relapsed or refractory Hodgkin's lymphoma: an international, multicentre, single-arm, phase 1-2 trial. *Lancet Oncol*. 2018;19(2):257-266.
111. Advani R, Skrypets T, Civallero M, et al. Brentuximab vedotin in combination with nivolumab in relapsed or refractory Hodgkin lymphoma: 3-year study results. *Blood*. 2021;138(6):427-438.
112. Moskowitz AJ, Shah G, Schöder H, et al. Phase II trial of pembrolizumab plus gemcitabine, vinorelbine, and liposomal doxorubicin as second-line therapy for relapsed or refractory classical Hodgkin lymphoma. *J Clin Oncol*. 2021;39(28):3109-3117.
113. Moskowitz AJ, Yahalom J, Kewalramani T, et al. Pretransplantation functional imaging predicts outcome following autologous stem cell transplantation for relapsed and refractory Hodgkin lymphoma. *Blood*. 2010;116(23):4934-4937.
114. Moskowitz CH, Walewski J, Nademanee A, et al. Five-year PFS from the AETHERA trial of brentuximab vedotin for Hodgkin lymphoma at high risk of progression or relapse. *Blood*. 2018;132(25):2639-2642.
115. Goodman KA, Riedel E, Serrano V, Gulati S, Moskowitz CH, Yahalom J. Long-term effects of high-dose chemotherapy and radiation for relapsed and refractory Hodgkin's lymphoma. *J Clin Oncol*. 2008;26(32):5240-5247.
116. Lavoie JC, Connors JM, Phillips GL, et al. High-dose chemotherapy and autologous stem cell transplantation for primary refractory or relapsed Hodgkin lymphoma: long-term outcome in the first 100 patients treated in Vancouver. *Blood*. 2005;106(4):1473-1478.
117. Sureda A, Arranz R, Iriondo A, et al. Autologous stem-cell transplantation for Hodgkin's disease: results and prognostic factors in 494 patients from the Grupo Espanol de Linfomas/Transplante Autologo de Medula Osea Spanish Cooperative Group. *J Clin Oncol*. 2001;19(5):1395-1404.
118. Younes A, Gopal AK, Smith SE, et al. Results of a pivotal phase II study of brentuximab vedotin for patients with relapsed or refractory Hodgkin's lymphoma. *J Clin Oncol*. 2012;30(18):2183-2189.
119. Chen R, Gopal AK, Smith SE, et al. Five-year survival and durability results of brentuximab vedotin in patients with relapsed or refractory Hodgkin lymphoma. *Blood*. 2016;128(12):1562-1566.
120. Armand P, Shipp MA, Ribrag V, et al. Programmed death-1 blockade with pembrolizumab in patients with classical Hodgkin lymphoma after brentuximab vedotin failure. *J Clin Oncol*. 2016;34(31):3733-3739.
121. Ansell SM, Minnema MC, Johnson P, et al. Nivolumab for relapsed/refractory diffuse large B-cell lymphoma in patients ineligible for or having failed autologous transplantation: a single-arm, phase II study. *J Clin Oncol*. 2019;37(6):481-489.
122. Chen R, Zinzani PL, Lee HJ, et al. Pembrolizumab in relapsed or refractory Hodgkin lymphoma: 2-year follow-up of KEYNOTE-087. *Blood*. 2019;134(14):1144-1153.
123. Fehniger TA, Larson S, Trinkaus K, et al. A phase 2 multicenter study of lenalidomide in relapsed or refractory classical Hodgkin lymphoma. *Blood*. 2011;118(19):5119-5125.
124. Boll B, Borchmann P, Topp MS, et al. Lenalidomide in patients with refractory or multiple relapsed Hodgkin lymphoma. *Br J Haematol*. 2010;148(3):480-482.
125. Josting A, Nogova L, Franklin J, et al. Salvage radiotherapy in patients with relapsed and refractory Hodgkin's lymphoma: a retrospective analysis from the German Hodgkin Lymphoma Study Group. *J Clin Oncol*. 2005;23(7):1522-1529.
126. Burroughs LM, O'Donnell PV, Sandmaier BM, et al. Comparison of outcomes of HLA-matched related, unrelated, or HLA-haploidentical related hematopoietic cell transplantation following nonmyeloablative conditioning for relapsed or refractory Hodgkin lymphoma. *Biol Blood Marrow Transplant*. 2008;14(11):1279-1287.
127. Sureda A, Robinson S, Canals C, et al. Reduced-intensity conditioning compared with conventional allogeneic stem-cell transplantation in relapsed or refractory Hodgkin's lymphoma: an analysis from the Lymphoma Working Party of the European Group for Blood and Marrow Transplantation. *J Clin Oncol*. 2008;26(3):455-462.
128. Majhail NS, Weisdorf DJ, Wagner JE, Defor TE, Brunstein CG, Burns LJ. Comparable results of umbilical cord blood and HLA-matched sibling donor hematopoietic stem cell transplantation after reduced-intensity preparative regimen for advanced Hodgkin lymphoma. *Blood*. 2006;107(9):3804-3807.
129. Thompson PA, Perera T, Marin D, et al. Double umbilical cord blood transplant is effective therapy for relapsed or refractory Hodgkin lymphoma. *Leuk Lymphoma*. 2016;57(7):1607-1615.
130. Chen R, Palmer JM, Tsai NC, et al. Brentuximab vedotin is associated with improved progression-free survival after allogeneic transplantation for Hodgkin lymphoma. *Biol Blood Marrow Transplant*. 2014;20(11):1864-1868.
131. Merryman RW, Kim HT, Zinzani PL, et al. Safety and efficacy of allogeneic hematopoietic stem cell transplant after PD-1 blockade in relapsed/refractory lymphoma. *Blood*. 2017;129(10):1380-1388.
132. Merryman RW, Castagna L, Giordano L, et al. Allogeneic transplantation after PD-1 blockade for classic Hodgkin lymphoma. *Leukemia*. 2021;35(9):2672-2683.
133. Bollard CM, Gottschalk S, Torrano V, et al. Sustained complete responses in patients with lymphoma receiving autologous cytotoxic T lymphocytes targeting Epstein-Barr virus latent membrane proteins. *J Clin Oncol*. 2014;32(8):798-808.
134. Bollard CM, Tripic T, Cruz CR, et al. Tumor-specific T-cells engineered to overcome tumor immune evasion induce clinical responses in patients with relapsed Hodgkin lymphoma. *J Clin Oncol*. 2018;36(11):1128-1139.
135. Ramos CA, Heslop HE, Brenner MK. CAR-T cell therapy for lymphoma. *Annu Rev Med*. 2016;67:165-183.
136. Wang CM, Wu ZQ, Wang Y, et al. Autologous T cells expressing CD30 chimeric antigen receptors for relapsed or refractory Hodgkin lymphoma: an open-label phase I trial. *Clin Cancer Res*. 2017;23(5):1156-1166.
137. Ramos CA, Ballard B, Zhang H, et al. Clinical and immunological responses after CD30-specific chimeric antigen receptor-redirected lymphocytes. *J Clin Invest*. 2017;127(9):3462-3471.

138. Ramos CA, Grover NS, Beaven AW, et al. Anti-CD30 CAR-T Cell therapy in relapsed and refractory Hodgkin lymphoma. *J Clin Oncol.* 2020;38(32):3794-3804.
139. Nogova L, Reineke T, Brillant C, et al. Lymphocyte-predominant and classical Hodgkin's lymphoma: a comprehensive analysis from the German Hodgkin Study Group. *J Clin Oncol.* 2008;26(3):434-439.
140. Nogova L, Reineke T, Eich HT, et al. Extended field radiotherapy, combined modality treatment or involved field radiotherapy for patients with stage IA lymphocyte-predominant Hodgkin's lymphoma: a retrospective analysis from the German Hodgkin Study Group (GHSG). *Ann Oncol.* 2005;16(10):1683-1687.
141. Biasoli I, Stamatoullas A, Meignin V, et al. Nodular, lymphocyte-predominant Hodgkin lymphoma: a long-term study and analysis of transformation to diffuse large B-cell lymphoma in a cohort of 164 patients from the Adult Lymphoma Study Group. *Cancer.* 2010;116(3):631-639.
142. Al-Mansour M, Connors JM, Gascoyne RD, Skinnider B, Savage KJ. Transformation to aggressive lymphoma in nodular lymphocyte-predominant Hodgkin's lymphoma. *J Clin Oncol.* 2010;28(5):793-799.
143. Binkley MS, Rauf MS, Milgrom SA, et al. Stage I-II nodular lymphocyte-predominant Hodgkin lymphoma: a multi-institutional study of adult patients by ILROG. *Blood.* 2020;135(26):2365-2374.
144. Pellegrino B, Terrier-Lacombe MJ, Oberlin O, et al. Lymphocyte-predominant Hodgkin's lymphoma in children: therapeutic abstention after initial lymph node resection – a study of the French Society of Pediatric Oncology. *J Clin Oncol.* 2003;21(15):2948-2952.
145. Borchmann S, Joffe E, Moskowitz CH, et al. Active surveillance for nodular lymphocyte-predominant Hodgkin lymphoma. *Blood.* 2019;133(20):2121-2129.
146. Eichenauer DA, Fuchs M, Pluetschow A, et al. Phase 2 study of rituximab in newly diagnosed stage IA nodular lymphocyte-predominant Hodgkin lymphoma: a report from the German Hodgkin Study Group. *Blood.* 2011;118(16):4363-4365.
147. Evens AM, Advani RH, Helenowski IB, et al. Multicenter phase II study of sequential brentuximab vedotin and doxorubicin, vinblastine, and dacarbazine chemotherapy for older patients with untreated classical Hodgkin lymphoma. *J Clin Oncol.* 2018;36(30):3015-3022.
148. Friedberg JW, Forero-Torres A, Bordoni RE, et al. Frontline brentuximab vedotin in combination with dacarbazine or bendamustine in patients aged ≥60 years with HL. *Blood.* 2017;130(26):2829-2837.
149. Lyter DW, Bryant J, Thackeray R, Rinaldo CR, Kingsley LA. Incidence of human immunodeficiency virus-related and nonrelated malignancies in a large cohort of homosexual men. *J Clin Oncol.* 1995;13(10):2540-2546.
150. Engels EA, Pfeiffer RM, Goedert JJ, et al. Trends in cancer risk among people with AIDS in the United States 1980-2002. *AIDS.* 2006;20(12):1645-1654.
151. Levine AM. Hodgkin's disease in the setting of human immunodeficiency virus infection. *J Natl Cancer Inst Monogr.* 1998;(23):37-42.
152. Spina M, Gabarre J, Rossi G, et al. Stanford V regimen and concomitant HAART in 59 patients with Hodgkin disease and HIV infection. *Blood.* 2002;100(6):1984-1988.
153. Xicoy B, Ribera JM, Miralles P, et al. Results of treatment with doxorubicin, bleomycin, vinblastine and dacarbazine and highly active antiretroviral therapy in advanced stage, human immunodeficiency virus-related Hodgkin's lymphoma. *Haematologica.* 2007;92(2):191-198.
154. Hartmann P, Rehwald U, Salzberger B, et al. BEACOPP therapeutic regimen for patients with Hodgkin's disease and HIV infection. *Ann Oncol.* 2003;14(10):1562-1569.
155. Okosun J, Warbey V, Shaw K, et al. Interim fluoro-2-deoxy-D-glucose-PET predicts response and progression-free survival in patients with Hodgkin lymphoma and HIV infection. *AIDS.* 2012;26(7):861-865.
156. Bachanova V, Connors JM. How is Hodgkin lymphoma in pregnancy best treated? ASH evidence-based review 2008. *Hematology Am Soc Hematol Educ Program.* 2008:33-34.
157. Barry RM, Diamond HD, Craver LF. Influence of pregnancy on the course of Hodgkin's disease. *Am J Obstet Gynecol.* 1962;84:445-454.
158. Doll DC, Ringenberg QS, Yarbro JW. Antineoplastic agents and pregnancy. *Semin Oncol.* 1989;16(5):337-346.
159. Evens AM, Cilley J, Ortiz T, et al. G-CSF is not necessary to maintain over 99% dose-intensity with ABVD in the treatment of Hodgkin lymphoma: low toxicity and excellent outcomes in a 10-year analysis. *Br J Haematol.* 2007;137(6):545-552.
160. Poorvu PD, Frazier AL, Feraco AM, et al. Cancer treatment-related infertility: a critical review of the evidence. *JNCI Cancer Spectr.* 2019;3(1):pkz008.
161. Lambertini M, Falcone T, Unger JM, Phillips KA, Del Mastro L, Moore HCF. Debated role of ovarian protection with gonadotropin-releasing Hormone agonists during chemotherapy for preservation of ovarian function and fertility in women with Cancer. *J Clin Oncol.* 2017;35(7):804-805.
162. Hancock SL, Donaldson SS, Hoppe RT. Cardiac disease following treatment of Hodgkin's disease in children and adolescents. *J Clin Oncol.* 1993;11(7):1208-1215.
163. Gottdiener JS, Katin MJ, Borer JS, Bacharach SL, Green MV. Late cardiac effects of therapeutic mediastinal irradiation. Assessment by echocardiography and radionuclide angiography. *N Engl J Med.* 1983;308(10):569-572.
164. Aleman BM, van den Belt-Dusebout AW, Klokman WJ, Van't Veer MB, Bartelink H, van Leeuwen FE. Long-term cause-specific mortality of patients treated for Hodgkin's disease. *J Clin Oncol.* 2003;21(18):3431-3439.
165. Myrehaug S, Pintilie M, Tsang R, et al. Cardiac morbidity following modern treatment for Hodgkin lymphoma: supra-additive cardiotoxicity of doxorubicin and radiation therapy. *Leuk Lymphoma.* 2008;49(8):1486-1493.
166. Aleman BM, van den Belt-Dusebout AW, De Bruin ML, et al. Late cardiotoxicity after treatment for Hodgkin lymphoma. *Blood.* 2007;109(5):1878-1886.
167. Galper SL, Yu JB, Mauch PM, et al. Clinically significant cardiac disease in patients with Hodgkin lymphoma treated with mediastinal irradiation. *Blood.* 2011;117(2):412-418.
168. Ng AK. Review of the cardiac long-term effects of therapy for Hodgkin lymphoma. *Br J Haematol.* 2011;154(1):23-31.
169. Hancock SL, Cox RS, McDougall IR. Thyroid diseases after treatment of Hodgkin's disease. *N Engl J Med.* 1991;325(9):599-605.
170. Ng AK, Bernardo MVP, Weller E, et al. Second malignancy after Hodgkin disease treated with radiation therapy with or without chemotherapy: long-term risks and risk factors. *Blood.* 2002;100(6):1989-1996.
171. Yahalom J, Petrek JA, Biddinger PW, et al. Breast cancer in patients irradiated for Hodgkin's disease: a clinical and pathologic analysis of 45 events in 37 patients. *J Clin Oncol.* 1992;10(11):1674-1681.
172. Schaapveld M, Aleman BMP, van Eggermond AM, et al. Second cancer risk up to 40 years after treatment for Hodgkin's lymphoma. *N Engl J Med.* 2015;373(26):2499-2511.
173. Hancock SL, Tucker MA, Hoppe RT. Breast cancer after treatment of Hodgkin's disease. *J Natl Cancer Inst.* 1993;85(1):25-31.
174. Ng A, Constine LS, Advani R, et al. ACR appropriateness criteria: follow-up of Hodgkin's lymphoma. *Curr Probl Cancer.* 2010;34(3):211-227.
175. El-Galaly TC, Mylam KJ, Brown P, et al. Positron emission tomography/computed tomography surveillance in patients with Hodgkin lymphoma in first remission has a low positive predictive value and high costs. *Haematologica.* 2012;97(6):931-936.
176. Hodgson DC, Grunfeld E, Gunraj N, Del Giudice L. A population-based study of follow-up care for Hodgkin lymphoma survivors: opportunities to improve surveillance for relapse and late effects. *Cancer.* 2010;116(14):3417-3425.
177. Torrey MJ, Poen JC, Hoppe RT. Detection of relapse in early-stage Hodgkin's disease: role of routine follow-up studies. *J Clin Oncol.* 1997;15(3):1123-1130.
178. Dryver ET, Jernström H, Tompkins K, Buckstein R, Imrie KR. Follow-up of patients with Hodgkin's disease following curative treatment: the routine CT scan is of little value. *Br J Cancer.* 2003;89(3):482-486.
179. Guadagnolo BA, Punglia RS, Kuntz KM, Mauch PM, Ng AK. Cost-effectiveness analysis of computerized tomography in the routine follow-up of patients after primary treatment for Hodgkin's disease. *J Clin Oncol.* 2006;24(25):4116-4122.

Chapter 96 ■ Hodgkin Lymphoma in Children

CHRISTINE MOORE SMITH • DEBRA L. FRIEDMAN

INTRODUCTION

The first description of Hodgkin lymphoma (HL) was in 1832 when Thomas Hodgkin described seven patients with enlarged lymph glands and spleen. This was followed by histologic descriptions of multinucleated giant cells, by Sternberg[1] in 1898 and Reed in 1902.[2] In the 1960s, the clonality of the Reed-Sternberg (RS) cell was established.[3] More recently, work has focused on the molecular biology of the disease, including the role of immunoglobulin genes, transcription factors, apoptotic pathways, and Epstein-Barr virus (EBV) incorporation.[4-7]

Therapeutic advances in HL began in 1902 when Pusey reported on the use of radiotherapy,[8] followed by the use of single-agent chemotherapy, mechlorethamine (nitrogen mustard) in 1946,[9] then combination chemotherapy with MOPP (mechlorethamine [nitrogen mustard], vincristine, procarbazine, and prednisone) in 1964[10] and ABVD (doxorubicin, bleomycin, vinblastine, and dacarbazine) in the 1970s.[11] Donaldson and colleagues at Stanford introduced the concept of combined modality therapy for pediatric patients using the MOPP backbone and low-dose radiation therapy (RT)[12] (for acronyms of treatment protocols, see Table 96.1). Multimodality, risk-adapted therapies are now the standard of care for pediatric and adolescent HL, with more recent advances in targeted antibody conjugates and immunotherapies tested in clinical trials and being brought to standard of care. The goals of contemporary clinical trials and treatment regimens are to balance short- and long-term toxicity with efficacy to maximize cure and minimize adverse sequelae of treatment, simultaneously.

EPIDEMIOLOGY

Incidence

Supported by data from U.S. Surveillance, Epidemiology End Results,[13,14] HL makes up 6.4% of all childhood cancer under the age of 20 years, but 13.2% of cancer in children between ages 15 and 19 years. The overall annual incidence rate in the United States is 12.2 per million for children under 20 years and increases to 32 per million when limiting the analysis to adolescents between ages 15 and 19 years. Overall, there is a slight female predominance when considering all children less than 20 years (M:F = 0.9). The Caucasian to African American ratio is 1.3:1.[13,14]

Adolescent and young adults are most likely to have disease of the nodular sclerosing subtype. Although among children <20 years of age, the nodular sclerosing subtype accounts for 70% of cases, this subtype accounts for 74% of cases in those 15 to 19 years of age. The mixed cellularity subtype accounts for 16% of cases under the age of 20 years but it represents 32% of cases under the age of 10 years; across the pediatric age group, it is more common in males.[13,14]

Risk Factors

There are several factors that are known to increase the risk of HL, which include family history of HL, EBV infections, socioeconomic status, and social contacts. For young adult disease (ages 16–44 years), there is a 99-fold increased risk among monozygotic twins and a 7-fold increased risk among other siblings.[15-17] There is a fascinating interaction between EBV and HL epidemiology and biology. EBV-associated HL, with incorporation of the EBV in the genome, is most commonly reported with the mixed cellularity histologic subtype in children from underdeveloped and developing nations and in young adult males. Conversely, in young adult HL, incorporation of EBV in the tumor genome is unusual, but a history of infectious mononucleosis and high-titer antibodies to EBV are associated.[7,18-21] Interestingly, the association between HL and socioeconomic status also differs by age. In children under 10 years, the disease is associated with lower socioeconomic status and large sibship.[22,23] In contrast, risk in young adult patients increases with socioeconomic status and with the related characteristics of a small nuclear family, single-family housing, and fewer siblings or childhood playmates. These findings may be related to an association with infections, where increased infections in early childhood may reduce risk of young adult HL.[24,25] There are inconsistent data regarding clustering of young adult cases.[26,27]

Biology

The hallmark of classic Hodgkin lymphoma (CHL) is the RS cell which most commonly derives from a neoplastic clone originating from B lymphocytes in lymph node germinal centers but is then embedded within a reactive infiltrate of lymphocytes, macrophages, granulocytes, and eosinophils.[28] The RS cell is a binucleated or multinucleated giant cell that is often characterized with a bilobed nucleus, with two large nucleoli, described commonly as an owl's eye appearance.[29] Sequence analyses of RS cell clones reveal rearrangements of immunoglobulin variable region genes, resulting in deficient immunoglobulin production. RS cells then evade the apoptotic pathway, leading to the genesis of HL, and perhaps the paraneoplastic immune-mediated phenomena that sometimes accompany the disease.[4,5] The B-lymphoid cells from which RS arise have high levels of constitutive nuclear factor (NF)-κB, a transcription factor known to mediate gene expression related to inflammatory and immune responses, and deregulation of NF-κB has been postulated as a mechanism by which RS cells evade apoptosis.[6,30] NF-κB dimers are held in an inactive cytoplasmic complex with inhibitory proteins, the IκBs.[30] B-cell stimulation by diverse signals results in rapid activation of the IκB kinase (IKK). The IKK complex phosphorylates two critical serine residues of IκBs,[31-33] thereby targeting them for rapid ubiquitin-mediated proteasomal degradation. Active NF-κB dimers are then released and translocated to the nucleus, where they activate gene transcription. Activation of NF-κB appears to be a final common effect of costimulatory interactions, genetic aberrations, or viral proteins that operate in HL.[34]

RS cell survival is dependent on several downstream pathways. RS cells express CD40, and CD40 ligand (CD40L) is expressed on inflammatory T and dendritic cells that surround them. CD40/CD40L interactions normally provide a second signal from activated helper T cells to normal B cells, resulting in activation of NF-κB. NF-κB, in turn, causes proliferation and induces expression of BCL-x_L, which protects B cells from apoptosis.[35] Tumor necrosis factor receptor–associated factor-1 (TRAF1) is overexpressed in EBV-transformed lymphoid cells and RS cells[36] and is associated with activation of NF-κB and protection of lymphoid cells from antigen-induced apoptosis. Activation of NF-κB, in turn, leads to expression of TRAF1, thereby establishing a positive feedback loop that maximizes NF-κB–dependent gene expression.[37] EBV latent membrane protein-1 (LMP1) interacts with TRAF1, tumors with TRAF1-LMP1 aggregates exhibit high NF-κB activity,[38,39] and LMP1 activates NF-κB by promoting IκBa turnover.[40] RS cells express CD30, and CD30 ligation promotes proliferation of HL-derived cells with constitutive activation of NF-κB.[41]

EBV genome fragments can be found in approximately 30% to 50% of HL specimens, and may play a role in the rescue and repair of RS cells, further aiding in their evasion of apoptosis and enhanced survival.[7,42-44] Three latent viral antigens are expressed in EBV-positive HL in RS cells: Epstein-Barr nuclear antigen-1, required for viral episome maintenance, LMP1 with transforming properties, and LMP2, which is nontransforming.[45,46]

Malignant cells of CHL are characterized by genetic alterations at the 9p24.1 locus that affects the immune checkpoint pathway.[47]

Table 96.1. Common First-Line Chemotherapy Protocols and Acronyms

Acronym	Chemotherapy Agents
ABV	Doxorubicin, bleomycin, and vinblastine
ABVD	Doxorubicin, bleomycin, vinblastine, and dacarbazine
AEPA	Brentuximab vedotin, etoposide, prednisone, and doxorubicin
ABvVE-PC	Doxorubicin, brentuximab vedotin, vincristine, and etoposide-prednisone and cyclophosphamide
ABvD	Doxorubicin, brentuximab vedotin, and dacarbazine
A-AVD	Brentuximab vedotin, doxorubicin, vinblastine, dacarbazine
BEACOPP	Bleomycin, etoposide, doxorubicin, cyclophosphamide, vincristine, procarbazine, and prednisone
CAPDac	Cyclophosphamide, brentuximab vedotin, prednisone, and dacarbazine
CHOP	Cyclophosphamide, doxorubicin, vincristine, and prednisone
COP (P)	Cyclophosphamide, vincristine, and procarbazine (prednisone)
COPDAC	Cyclophosphamide, vincristine, prednisone, and dacarbazine
D(A)BVE (PC)	Doxorubicin, bleomycin, vincristine, and etoposide (prednisone and cyclophosphamide)
MOPP	Mechlorethamine (nitrogen mustard), vincristine, procarbazine, and prednisone
VAMP	Vincristine, doxorubicin, methotrexate, and prednisone
VEPA	Vinblastine, etoposide, prednisone, and doxorubicin
OEPA	Vincristine, etoposide, prednisone, and doxorubicin

Programmed cell death protein-1 (PD-1) is an inhibitory checkpoint molecule expressed in activated T cells. PD-1 on the T cell interacts with PD-1 ligands (PD-L1), which induce inhibitory signals to the T-cell receptor pathway.[47,48] In HL, the background inflammatory cells and tumor-infiltrating lymphocytes express PD-L1 at a higher rate than healthy controls, with expression rate as high as 70% to 87% by immunohistochemistry on both the RS cells and background cells.[47] This expression by the malignant cells decreases lymphoid proliferation and activation subsequently decreasing the immune response and allowing escape from the immune system antitumor response.[47,48]

Histology

HL can broadly be divided into two pathologic classes: CHL and nodular lymphocyte predominant Hodgkin lymphoma (NLPHL).[49,50] In turn, CHL can be further divided into four subtypes: lymphocyte-rich CHL, nodular sclerosis HL, mixed cellularity HL, and lymphocyte-depleted HL (for descriptions of the subtypes, see Chapter 88).

In CHL, the RS cells do not express B-cell antigens, such as CD45, CD19, and CD79A, but virtually all express CD30 and approximately 70% express CD15, with only 20% to 30% expressing CD20.[51] In comparison, in NLPHL, the tumor cells do express B-cell antigens such as CD19, CD20, CD22, and CD79A, may or may not express CD30, and do not express CD15.[52] In addition, the OCT.2 and BOB.1 oncogenes are downregulated in CHL but not in NLPHL, correlating with immunoglobulin transcription.[53]

CLINICAL CONSIDERATIONS

Presentation and Staging

The most common presentation of HL, occurring in 80% of patients, is painless adenopathy. Mediastinal involvement is present in approximately 76% of adolescents, but only in 33% of children aged 10 years and younger. A large mediastinal mass with a maximum diameter that is greater than one-third of the chest diameter and/or a node or nodal aggregate greater than 10 cm occurs in about 20% of patients.[54,55] B symptoms, defined as (1) unexplained loss of >10% of body weight in the 6 months preceding the diagnosis; (2) unexplained fever with temperatures >38 °C for more than 3 days; or (3) drenching night sweats, are seen in 20% of patients at the time of initial disease presentation.[55-57] Staging is performed clinically, based on the Ann Arbor staging system[58] as revised in 1989.[56] Approximately 80% to 85% of children and adolescents with HL have involvement limited to or with direct extension from the lymph nodes and/or the spleen (stages I-III), whereas 15% to 20% of patients are stage IV with involvement of the lung, bone marrow, bone, or liver.[58] Although staging definitions by nodal region, B symptoms, and definition of extranodal involvement are well defined, bulk disease and substaging have not been consistent across studies (Table 96.2).

Diagnostic Evaluation

A detailed history is required to elucidate B symptoms for risk stratification. A thorough physical evaluation should be performed, documenting the location of adenopathy, the presence of splenomegaly, and any evidence of organ dysfunction. This should be complemented by cross-sectional imaging with computed tomography (CT) scan of chest and CT or magnetic resonance imaging scans of the neck, abdomen, and pelvis.[59,60] Fluorodeoxyglucose (FDG)-positron emission tomography (PET) imaging is the standard of care in HL, and response to disease is now judged by FDG-PET alone or in combination with CT. With the advent of combined CT-PET scans, areas of disease can be evaluated simultaneously with both modalities in an overlapping manner.[61,62] In addition, an upright chest radiograph (CXR) with posteroanterior (PA) and lateral views had traditionally been required for documentation of a large mediastinal mass (bulk mediastinal disease) for clinical trials, defined as tumor diameter > one-third the thoracic diameter (measured transversely at the level of the dome of the diaphragm on a 6-ft upright PA CXR).[61] However, with CT and PET imaging, the need for this is now largely obsolete. Bone marrow biopsy had been recommended in the past for stage III and IV patients or patients with B symptoms, but PET imaging can evaluate for bone marrow involvement, and PET avidity in the marrow can be accepted as evidence of disease, without a bone marrow biopsy.[62] Laboratory studies include a complete blood count, blood chemistries to evaluate hepatic and renal function, and may include acute-phase reactants, such as ferritin, erythrocyte sedimentation rate, and serum copper, which may be seen as nonspecific markers of tumor activity but may correlate with prognosis or response.

Prognostic Factors

Adverse prognostic markers established from clinical trials often form the basis for risk stratification and subsequent modification of therapeutic algorithms. In sequential trials, because treatment is then risk based, these adverse factors are abrogated by the changes in therapy. Pretreatment factors that have been shown to be associated with adverse outcomes include advanced stage, B symptoms, bulk disease, extranodal extension, male sex, and elevated erythrocyte sedimentation rate and, in some studies, hemoglobin < 110 g/dL or white blood cell count > 11.5×10^9/L, age 5 to 10 years, and increased numbers of sites of disease.[63-69] A predictive model for event-free survival (EFS), the Childhood Hodgkin International Prognostic Score (CHIPS), was developed as part of the Children's Oncology Group (COG) study AHOD0031 and is being validated in AHOD1331. Using the ABVE-PC study, stage IV disease, large mediastinal mass, albumin (<3.5), and fever were independent predictors of EFS that were each assigned one point in the CHIPS. The four-year EFS was 93.1% for patients with CHIPS = 0, 88.5% for patients with CHIPS = 1, 77.6% for patients with CHIPS = 2, and 69.2% for patients with CHIPS = 3.[70]

Patients with NLPHL appear to have an overall better prognosis than those with CHL, and among those with CHL, histologic subtype is not consistently associated with prognosis.[67] Serum markers that may confer adverse prognostic risk include soluble vascular adhesion molecule-1, tumor necrosis factor, soluble CD30, β-2 microglobulin,

Table 96.2. Clinical and Staging Criteria for Hodgkin Lymphoma

A. Stage

Stage I:
- Involvement of single lymph node region (I)
- OR localized contiguous involvement of a single extralymphatic organ or site (IE).

Stage II:
- Involvement of two or more lymph node regions on the same side of the diaphragm (II)
- OR localized contiguous involvement of a single extralymphatic organ or site with locoregional lymph node(s) and involvement of one or more additional lymph node regions on the same side of the diaphragm (IIE).

Stage III:
- Involvement of lymph node regions on both sides of the diaphragm (III)
- Can include localized contiguous involvement of an extralymphatic organ or site (IIIE), splenic involvement (IIIS), or both (IIIE + S)

Stage IV:
- Disseminated (multifocal) involvement of one or more extralymphatic organs or tissues including bone marrow, with or without associated lymph node involvement
- OR isolated extralymphatic organ involvement with distant (nonregional) nodal involvement

B. Symptoms and Presentations

"A" Symptoms: "B" symptoms not present.

"B" Symptoms: Presence of at least one of the following:
- Unexplained weight loss > 10% in the preceding 6 mo
- Unexplained recurrent fever > 38 °C
- Drenching night sweats

X: Bulk disease (see "C. Bulk Disease")

E: Involvement of a single extranodal site, i.e., contiguous or proximal to the known nodal site.

S: Splenic involvement

C. Bulk Disease

One or both of the following is consistent with "bulk" disease:
- *Large mediastinal mass:* Mass diameter > one-third the thoracic diameter (measured transversely at the level of the dome of the diaphragm on a 6-ft upright PA CXR). In the presence of hilar nodal disease, the maximal mediastinal tumor measurement may be taken at the level of the hilus. This should be measured as the maximum mediastinal width (at a level containing the tumor and any normal mediastinal structures at the level) over the maximum thoracic ratio.
- *Large extramediastinal nodal aggregate:* A conglomerate of nodal tissue that measures >6 cm[a] in the longest transverse diameter.

[a]Some studies use 10 cm for definition of extramediastinal bulk disease.

---

transferrin, serum interleukin-10, and serum CD8 antigen.[71-76] High RS cell levels of caspase 3 may be associated with a more favorable outcome.[77] Early response to treatment, which may be a correlate for biology, may also be an important prognostic factor, allowing titration of therapy to the individual.[68,78-80]

INITIAL TREATMENT FOR PEDIATRIC HODGKIN LYMPHOMA

Contemporary standard approaches to adolescent and young adult HL may include multiagent chemotherapy, targeted or immunotherapies with or without low-dose involved-field radiotherapy (IFRT). The overriding principles of pediatric treatment regimens are to balance efficacy with both acute and, perhaps, more importantly, long-term toxicities.[81-83] Treatment recommendations are based on staging and risk group stratification. While staging is consistent, risk groups may vary by clinical trial and cooperative group. A summary of common risk group stratifications from the NCCN Clinical Practice Guidelines in Oncology (NCCN Guidelines®) for Pediatric Hodgkin Lymphoma is found in *Table 96.3*.[84] *Figure 96.1* shows the timeline of evolution of therapy for pediatric HL.

Statistics from 2010 to 2016 show great response in this era of risk-adapted therapies with survival rates for children and adolescents with HL ages birth to 19 years of 97% to 99% relative survival rates compared with 87% to 89% of all age groups when combined. This represents a continued decline in death rates for HL across the age spectrum, continuing a trend started around 1975 but with impressive 4% per year decreases from 2008 to 2017 for HL.[85-87]

Initial chemotherapy regimens through the Pediatric Oncology Group (POG) and Children's Cancer Group (CCG), which merged into the COG, were largely built upon the MOPP and ABVD backbones and evaluated in part the ability to avoid radiation in certain populations. CCG 521, POG 8725, and CCG 5942 evaluated chemotherapy backbones with or without radiation.[88-90] POG 8725 used a backbone of MOPP/ABVD and showed that EFS was strongly associated with early response to chemotherapy.[89] In CCG 5942, randomization to IFRT or no further therapy after chemo including cyclophosphamide, vincristine, procarbazine, and prednisone (COPP)/ABV, cytarabine/etoposide, and CHOP resulted in overall EFS of 91% at 3 and 10 years for the group who received IFRT and 86% at 3 years and 83% at 10 years for those who did not receive IFRT.[63,90] A pilot study of 99 patients in CCG 59704 utilized the German Hodgkin Disease Group's BEACOPP backbone for patients with B symptoms or advanced stage disease. The study's five-year EFS was 94% with patients receiving six to eight cycles of chemotherapy with or without radiotherapy based on a gender-stratified, response-based therapeutic algorithm.[91]

To decrease late effects from alkylator therapy and potential cardiotoxicity, in the mid-1990s, the POG developed a series of studies with changes to the ABVD backbone, substituting dacarbazine with etoposide and vinblastine with vincristine allowing for escalation of doxorubicin and etoposide. POG 9226 piloted therapy with ABVE followed by low-dose IFRT lower risk patient with five-year EFS of 89% and POG 9426 used a similar backbone with reduction of therapy for early responders with EFS of 88.3%.[92,93] For advanced stage disease, POG 9425 added prednisone and cyclophosphamide to the ABVE backbone with response assessment determining number of cycles and all receiving RT with three-year EFS of 87%.[79]

Building on these findings, a series of studies in the COG have evaluated the principles of response-based risk-adapted therapy, where therapy is decreased for those at lowest risk and with favorable early

Table 96.3. Risk Stratification for Pediatric Classical Hodgkin Lymphoma

Clinical Stage	Bulk	E-Lesions	Risk Group
IA, IIA	No	No	Low risk (per EuroNet-PHL-C1)
	Yes	No	Low risk (per EuroNet-PHL-C1) if ESR<30 or Intermediate risk (per EuroNet-PHL-C1 or AHOD0031) if ESR >30
	Yes	Yes	Intermediate risk (per EuroNet-PHL-C1 or AHOD0031)
IB	Any	No	Low risk (per EuroNet-PHL-C1) if ESR<30 or Intermediate risk (per EuroNet-PHL-C1) if ESR >30
	Any	Any	Intermediate risk (per AHOD0031)
IIB[a]	No	No	Intermediate risk (per EuroNet-PHL-C1 or AHOD0031)
	No	Yes	Intermediate risk (per AHOD0031) or High risk (per EuroNet-PHL-C1)
	Yes	Any	High risk (per AHOD1331)
	Yes	Yes	High risk (per EuroNet-PHL-C1)
IIIA	Any	No	Intermediate risk (per EuroNet-PHL-C1 or AHOD0031)
	Any	Yes	Intermediate risk (per AHOD0031) or High risk (per EuroNet-PHL-C1)
IIIB, IV	Any	Any	High risk (per EuroNet-PHL-C1 or AHOD1331)

[a]Only IIB with bulk was upstaged to high risk in the most recent series of COG clinical trials. The panel acknowledges that current trials have modified these groupings.

Adapted with permission from the NCCN Clinical Practice Guidelines in Oncology (NCCN Guidelines) for Pediatric Hodgkin Lymphoma V.1.2022. © 2022 National Comprehensive Cancer Network, Inc. All rights reserved. The NCCN Guidelines and illustrations herein may not be reproduced in any form for any purpose without the express written permission of NCCN. To view the most recent and complete version of the NCCN Guidelines, go online to NCCN.org. The NCCN Guidelines are a work in progress that may be refined as often as new significant data become available.

responses to chemotherapy and augmented for those with more advanced disease or a slow response to initial chemotherapy. These studies have utilized the ABVE-PC backbone. COG AHOD0031 enrolled 1712 patients with intermediate risk disease and used early response assessment to determine the need for radiation or chemotherapy intensification. Overall EFS was 85.0%, and overall survival (OS) rate was 97.8%. For patients with rapid early response and complete response (CR), EFS did not differ significantly among those who were randomly assigned to IFRT (87.9%) versus no IFRT (84.3%). There was also no difference in EFS (79.3% vs 75.2%) for slow early responders (SERs) who were randomly assigned to dexamethasone, etoposide, cisplatin, and cytarabine (DECA) versus no DECA. In those SERs, those PET-positive results at response assessment had worse EFS than those PET-2 negative (70.7% vs 54.6%).[94]

For low-stage disease, COG AHOD0431 treated 278 patients with stage IA/IIA CHL without bulk with three cycles of adriamycin, prednisone, vincristine, cyclophosphamide. Patients achieving a CR after three cycles received no further therapy, while those with a partial response received IFRT. Overall EFS was 79.8% and OS rate was 99.6%. Patients with a negative PET after one cycle of chemotherapy had a four-year EFS of 88.2% vs 68.5% for those positive. Patients with mixed cellularity histology also had excellent EFS of 95.2% compared with 75.8% for those with nodular sclerosis histology.[95]

For advanced-stage disease, in COG AHOD0831, patients with stages IIIB and IVB received four cycles of ABVE-PC with a higher cyclophosphamide dose than in AHOD0031 and SERs received additional therapy with IV. Radiotherapy was given in a targeted manner. EFS was 80.2% (73%-85.6%), and OS rate was 95.9%.[96]

The Dana Farber-Stanford-St. Jude pediatric Hodgkin lymphoma consortium studies have similarly focused efforts on reduction in alkylating agent, anthracycline, and radiotherapy doses. Past studies for low-risk patients included four cycles of an alkylator-free chemotherapy protocol, vincristine, doxorubicin, methotrexate, and prednisone (VAMP), with radiotherapy doses of 15 Gy or 25.5 Gy based upon response to the first two cycles of chemotherapy. This approach resulted in a five-year EFS of 93% and 10-year EFS of 89%.[97] For patients with higher risk disease, two protocols have been evaluated, VAMP/COP and vinblastine, etoposide, prednisone, and doxorubicin, both with IFRT. Results have shown a five-year EFS of 74% and 68%, respectively.[98,99]

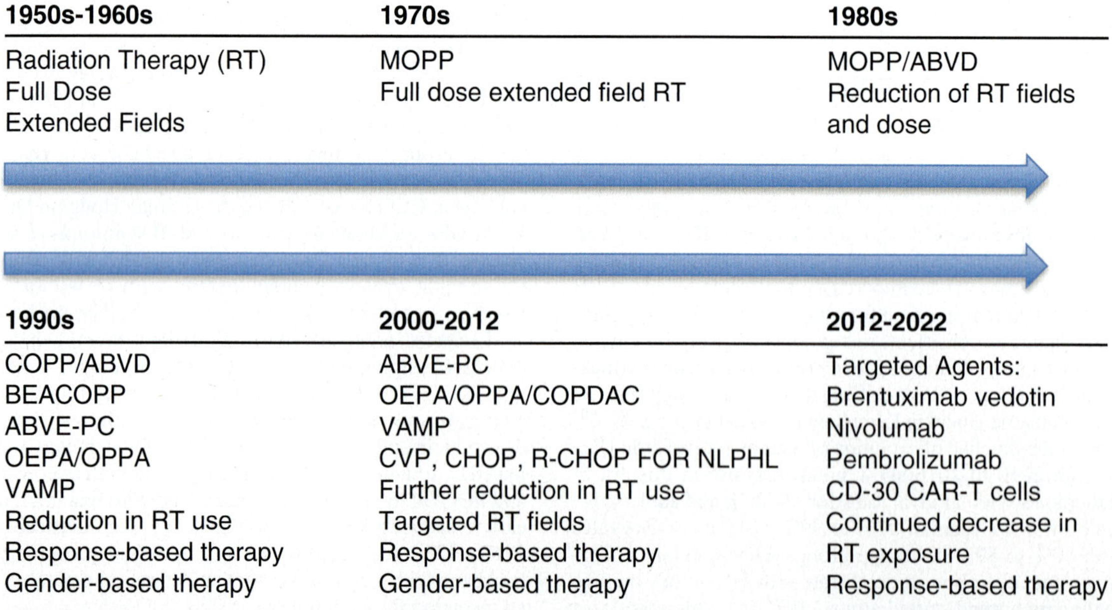

1950s-1960s	1970s	1980s
Radiation Therapy (RT) Full Dose Extended Fields	MOPP Full dose extended field RT	MOPP/ABVD Reduction of RT fields and dose

1990s	2000-2012	2012-2022
COPP/ABVD BEACOPP ABVE-PC OEPA/OPPA VAMP Reduction in RT use Response-based therapy Gender-based therapy	ABVE-PC OEPA/OPPA/COPDAC VAMP CVP, CHOP, R-CHOP FOR NLPHL Further reduction in RT use Targeted RT fields Response-based therapy Gender-based therapy	Targeted Agents: Brentuximab vedotin Nivolumab Pembrolizumab CD-30 CAR-T cells Continued decrease in RT exposure Response-based therapy

FIGURE 96.1 Timeline of Hodgkin lymphoma upfront therapy. ABVD, doxorubicin, bleomycin, vinblastine, dacarbazine; BEACOPP, bleomycin, etoposide, doxorubicin, cyclophosphamide, vincristine, procarbazine, prednisone; CHOP, cyclophosphamide, doxorubicin, vincristine, prednisone; COPDAC, cyclophosphamide, vincristine, prednisone, dacarbazine; COPP, cyclophosphamide, vincristine, procarbazine (prednisone); CVP, cyclophosphamide, vincristine, prednisone; MOPP, mechlorethamine (nitrogen mustard), vincristine, procarbazine, and prednisone; NLPHL, nodular lymphocyte predominant Hodgkin lymphoma; OEPA, vincristine, etoposide, prednisone, doxorubicin; OPPA, vincristine, procarbazine, prednisone, doxorubicin; VAMP, vincristine, doxorubicin, methotrexate, prednisone.

In the same era, the German cooperative groups have built upon COPP chemotherapy in both pediatric and adult HL. To decrease gonadotoxicity, which is more prevalent in males exposed to alkylating agents, some of these therapies were gender based. The DAL-HL-90 study used OEPA/COPP for males and vincristine and vincristine, etoposide, prednisone, doxorubicin (OPPA)/COPP for females, both followed by IFRT. EFS for stages II, III, and IV was 92%, 86%, and 90%, respectively.[100] The German Pediatric Oncology Group (GPOH)-95 study was designed to assess elimination of radiotherapy for those with a CR which was defined as complete resolution of all disease, which only 22% of patients achieved. It was built on the OPPA/OEPA backbones by adding cycles of COPP for patients with more advanced disease. Radiotherapy dose was determined by the post–chemotherapy disease reduction. Overall, the EFS was 92% for those receiving radiotherapy, compared with 88% in those treated with chemotherapy alone, but for patients with stages IA, IB, and IIA disease, EFS was not different among those with a CR to chemotherapy with no subsequent therapy (97%) and in those with a partial response subsequently treated with radiotherapy (94%). However, for all other patients, the EFS was 79% for those treated with chemotherapy alone compared with 91% for those treated with combined modality therapy.[101] This was followed by the GPOH-HD-2002 study, where OEPA-cyclophosphamide, vincristine, prednisone, and dacarbazine (COPDAC) chemotherapy was tested in males compared with OPPA-COPP in females for intermediate and advanced HL. The five-year EFS was 89.0%, without significant difference between males and females and so following studies have used OEPA instead of OPPA to reduce late effects.[102,103]

The European Network Pediatric Hodgkin Lymphoma (EURONET-PHL) collaborative network continued this work with two additional trials with final results yet to be published. EuroNet-PHL-C1 evaluated two cycles of OEPA with an early response assessment to determine further therapy ranging from no additional therapy for low-risk patients with good responses to radiation and/or additional chemotherapy randomized between two and four cycles of COPP vs COPDAC. Interim analysis revealed similar efficacy between COPP and COPDAC, so amendments led to treatment with COPDAC for all patients in those treatment groups. EuroNet-PHL-C2 is evaluating two cycles of OEPA followed by response assessment and one cycle COPDAC-28 or involved site radiation for TL-1 patients, and randomization between two and four cycles of COPDAC-28 versus an intensified regimen of doxorubicin, etoposide, cyclophosphamide, vincristine, prednisone, and dacarbazine (DECOPDAC-21).[103]

For low-risk patients with NLPHL, some patients may be treated with surgery alone. There are multiple small reports in both adult and pediatric HL of patients in the successful treatment of completely resected stage I disease. For those who did relapse, salvage rates were encouraging and death from disease very low.[104-106] Although adults with NLPHL may be treated with radiotherapy alone, the dose required without adjuvant chemotherapy exceeds that optimal in children and adolescents, and thus, this strategy is not used in pediatric NLPHL. In COG AHOD03P1, among patients who underwent complete resection of a single node with observation, EFS was 77%, and all were salvaged with chemotherapy. Of those treated either primarily with doxorubicin, vincristine, prednisone, cyclophosphamide or following recurrence postobservation, EFS was 88.8%. The EFS for the entire cohort was 85.5%, and OS rate was 100%.[107]

The optimal treatment of patients with more advanced stages of NLPHL remains undetermined. These patients are traditionally treated with regimens that are used for patients with advanced stage CHL with outcomes equivalent to or better than those with CHL. For intermediate risk patients, a subanalysis of COG AHOD0031 showed that patients with NLPHL had better outcomes than patients with CHL treated on the same chemotherapy backbone of ABVE-PC with EFS of 92.2% vs 83.5% but similar OS.[108] With an exceptional OS and low incidence of the NLPHL subtype, it is unlikely that prospective multicenter randomized studies for pediatrics will be conducted, but retrospective analyses are ongoing and the GPOH-HD Study Group and adult groups have published recommendations for treatment of NLPHL.[109,110]

Given such overall success in the treatment of HL in pediatrics, attention to immunotherapy and targeted agents has become important to either augment or replace conventional chemotherapy. The first of these to evaluate brentuximab vedotin (Bv) was the ECHELON-1 trial for patients aged 18 years and older with stage III and IV CHL. This showed improved outcomes for patients who received A-AVD (A- is Bv) compared with the standard ABVD backbone with five-year PFS of 82.2% with A-AVD versus 75.3% with ABVD. The benefit held regardless of PET2 status. PET2-negative patients had PFS of 84.9% vs 78.9% with ABVD. For PET2-positive patients, A-AVD had PFS of 60.6% vs 45.9%, showing benefit even in this harder to treat population.[111]

In pediatric upfront studies, two recent trials incorporated Bv. A recently completed multicenter clinical trial led by St. Jude Children's Research Hospital evaluated the safety of A-EPA/CAPDac in patients with stages IIB, IIIB, IVA, and IVB. Results showed Bv was tolerable in combination with chemotherapy and with outcomes of three-year EFS of 97.4% with OS rate of 98.7%.[112] The COG has completed accrual to a study where the ABVE-PC backbone compared to ABvVE-PC in the same patient population with results expected in the near future.

Ongoing studies include the COG evaluation of the PD-1 inhibitors pembrolizumab for slow responding disease in low-risk patients getting an ABVD backbone. The COG is also collaborating with the National Clinical Trials Network to investigate the substitution of Bv or nivolumab for bleomycin in the ABVD backbone in high-risk patients. An upcoming study by the COG aims to compare immunotherapy and standard chemotherapy with evaluation of patient reported outcomes to help determine the most effective and most tolerable therapy. A phase I/II study at St. Jude Children's Research Hospital is evaluating substitution of bendamustine for mechlorethamine in the Stanford V backbone for low and intermediate-risk patients.

Radiotherapy for Hodgkin Lymphoma

It has been recognized since the 1950s that HL is an extremely radiosensitive disease. Currently, for children and adolescents with HL, radiotherapy is exclusively delivered in the context of multimodality therapy. Doses of 15 to 30 Gy are commonly used, and as noted earlier, clinical trials have been and continue to be conducted to identify groups of patients for whom the exclusion of radiotherapy is possible, without affecting disease-free survival.

Delivery of radiotherapy, particularly in children and adolescents, requires careful considerations of the age, tumor burden and location, response to chemotherapy, and an assessment of both short- and long-term potential toxicity.

RT for HL started as fields including subtotal or total lymphoid irradiation then decreased to more regional fields such as mantle, abdominal, or pelvic based on disease involvement. Subsequent trials have narrowed the field, and thus, the total exposure of healthy tissue.[113] The COG's AHOD0031 used involved field radiation (IFRT).[94] Current studies are using involved site radiation that excludes tissues and nodes that are in the same nodal region but not involved with HL. In addition, as described previously, fewer patients are receiving radiation if they have early complete metabolic responses with chemotherapy. A recent St. Jude study and the current EuroNet-PHL-C2 trial are evaluating involved node radiation, which even further reduced the target volumes.[103,112-114]

Proton beam radiotherapy is being used to decrease dose delivered to surrounding structures including higher risk organs with the goal of decreased long-term risks and side effects while maintaining disease control.[113,115-119] In addition, more targeted doses to involved site or involved node as opposed to IFRT have been investigated with promising results in both early stage and higher stage disease.[115,116,119,120]

TREATMENT FOR RELAPSED HODGKIN LYMPHOMA

While upfront therapies have reduced relapses for HL, there are many curative options even in the relapsed or refractory setting including chemotherapy, radiotherapy, autologous stem cell transplant, targeted antibodies, and immunotherapies.[121,122] Some common chemotherapy retrieval regimens are presented in *Table 96.4*, and the choice of regimen is dependent on previous treatment and patterns of relapse. Combinations of vinorelbine, gemcitabine, ifosfamide, and bendamustine have been used with successful outcomes.[123-126]

Although not in trials all restricted to pediatric and adolescent patients, Bv has now been evaluated as a single agent in a number of trials and is now being testing in combination therapy both in the relapsed and upfront setting.[127-129] In the phase III AETHERA trial, post-autologous stem cell transplantation (ASCT) treatment with Bv for 16 cycles for those at with unfavorable risk relapsed or primary refractory CHL demonstrated that progression-free survival was significantly improved in patients in the Bv group compared with those in the placebo group.[130] Bv is also now being combined with other agents in the relapse setting. A phase I/II study of Bv and bendamustine had a promising 93% overall response rate and other similar trials or institutional reviews had similar response rates including one that included children and young adults.[131-134] A phase II study combining Bv with gemcitabine and vinorelbine was conducted in the COG, with results showing 57% of patients with a CR with four cycles and 31% with a partial response.[135]

Another class of drugs being utilized for relapsed or refractory HL are the PD-1 inhibitors, nivolumab, and pembrolizumab. Because of overexpression of PD-1 ligands and evasion of immune surveillance, a phase Ib study of nivolumab showed significant promise as single-agent therapy.[136] In a single-arm phase II study of nivolumab among patients failing a median of four prior therapies, including Bv and autologous transplantation, objective response rate was 66%.[137] In a phase Ib study of another PD-1 inhibitor, pembrolizumab, with a similar population, overall response rate was 65%.[138] In the phase II study, overall response rates ranged from 65% to 68%.[139]

Chemotherapy regimens in combination with PD-1 inhibition are also showing promise, with a recent trial showing 95% response with a combination of pembrolizumab with gemcitabine, vinorelbine, and liposomal doxorubicin.[140] In a study by the COG evaluating a backbone of Bv and nivolumab, followed by Bv and bendamustine if CMR not achieved at end of four cycles, interim results showed high overall response rates.[141] PD-1 inhibition is also being used in the setting of relapse after ASCT and is being investigated as a maintenance therapy after ASCT with or without Bv.[142,143] Ongoing retrieval trials in the COG include combinations of PD-1 inhibition, Bv, and cytotoxic T lymphocyte-associated antigen (CTLA-4) immunotherapies such as ipilimumab that showed favorable response rates in the adult population and are being extended to the pediatric population.[144]

Chimeric antigen receptor (CAR) T-cells directed at CD30 have been studied with a phase I trial showing some clinical efficacy and overall safety but no CR.[145] When proceeded by lymphodepletion with either fludarabine and bendamustine, cyclophosphamide and fludarabine, or bendamustine alone in phase I/II studies, CD30-directed CAR T-cells had an overall response rate of 72% with 59% with a complete response CR.[146] Other CAR T-cell products with coexpression are also under investigation.[147,148] For the majority of cases, salvage therapies are utilized as a bridge to definitive consolidative therapy for relapsed HL with stem cell transplant, although there is ongoing work to determine if there is a low-risk population who may not require HSCT. Autologous HSCT is most commonly used for recurrent or refractory HL, but full and reduced intensity allogeneic approaches as well as immune modulation and induction of autologous graft-versus-host disease have been explored to enhance the allogeneic effect.[149-154]

ADVERSE LONG-TERM OUTCOMES OF THERAPY

In pediatrics, a significant consideration when deciding therapy is the risk of adverse long-term risks of therapy including organ dysfunction and second malignancies. The era of treatment must be taken into account when assessing risk for an individual patient given the significant changes in therapy for HL in the past 4 decades.[155,156] The common potential long-term effects of radiotherapy and chemotherapy for HL are summarized together with general monitoring recommendations in *Table 96.5*.

In a review from the Childhood Cancer Survivor Study (CCSS), among 2633 HL 5-year survivors, initially treated between 1970 and 1986, there were 500 deaths with the highest attributable causes being HL, 35%; second malignancies, 23%; cardiovascular disease, 14%; and pulmonary disease, 4%. Adjusting for demographics and medical conditions, treatment with radiotherapy or alkylating agents was an independent risk factor for overall mortality. Radiotherapy, alkylating agents, and anthracyclines treatment increased risk of second malignancies with a 30-year cumulative incidence of 18.7%. Based on self-report, the 30-year incidences of chronic health conditions in the cohort were primarily cardiovascular, 11%; pulmonary, 5%; and thyroid, 51%.[157] The expanded CCSS cohort, treated from 1987 to 1999, showed a marked reduction in early mortality from causes other than primary malignancy, including for survivors of HL.[158] A retrospective review of the expanded CCSS cohort revealed risk-adapted therapy, primarily reduction of RT exposure, decreased treatment-related morbidity with cumulative incidence of endocrinopathy, 13.3%; cardiovascular disease, 10.1%; and second malignancy, 9.4% by age 35 years.[159] With changes in therapy over the past 2 decades, these adverse long-term outcomes are likely to be lower.

Other studies of subsequent malignancy cite female gender, radiotherapy field and dose, and follow-up time since diagnosis as risk factors. The most significant risk is for secondary breast cancer in female survivors treated with thoracic radiotherapy, where even lower doses of radiotherapy are still associated with increased risk.[160-162] With ongoing aging of the HL survivor population, increased risk for skin cancer and head and neck cancers, both related to radiotherapy, has

Table 96.4. Common Treatment Options for Recurrent Hodgkin Lymphoma

Multiagent Chemotherapy Regimens (in Alphabetical Order):
APE (cytosine arabinoside, cisplatin, and etoposide)
DECA (dexamethasone, etoposide, cisplatin, and cytarabine)
DHAP (dexamethasone, cytarabine, cisplatin)
EPIC (etoposide, prednisolone, ifosfamide, cisplatin)
GV (gemcitabine and vinorelbine)
GDP (gemcitabine, dexamethasone, cisplatin)
ICE (ifosfamide, carboplatin, etoposide)
IEP-ABVD (ifosfamide, etoposide, and prednisone-doxorubicin, bleomycin, vinblastine, and dacarbazine)
IGEV (ifosfamide, gemcitabine, vinorelbine)
IV (ifosfamide and vinorelbine)
Immunotherapy and Targeted Agents (in alphabetical order):
Brentuximab vedotin antibody-drug conjugate targeting CD30
Nivolumab
Pembrolizumab
Combination Chemotherapy and/or Targeted Agents (in alphabetical order):
Brentuximab vedotin + bendamustine
Brentuximab vedotin + nivolumab
Chimeric antigen receptor (CAR) T-cell therapy directed at CD30
GBv (gemcitabine and brentuximab vedotin)
Pembrolizumab + GVD (gemcitabine, vinorelbine, liposomal doxorubicin)

These therapies can be used as standalone therapy or as reinduction prior to planned stem cell transplant depending on risk stratification. Ongoing clinical trials should be considered. Radiotherapy can be considered together with this therapy.

Table 96.5. General Guidelines for Risk and Surveillance for Adverse Long-Term Outcomes

Routine Follow-Up Should Include History and Physical to Monitor for Relapse as Well as Secondary Effects of Therapy, Some of which are Highlight Below:			
System	Therapeutic Exposure	Potential Effects	Monitoring Recommendations[a]
Cardiac	Thoracic RT Doxorubicin	Arrhythmia Cardiomyopathy Congestive heart failure Pericarditis Coronary artery disease Valvular disease	Electrocardiogram and echocardiogram (frequency depending on doxorubicin isotoxic dose equivalents and/or radiation dose in Gy)
Pulmonary	Thoracic RT Bleomycin	Pulmonary fibrosis Interstitial pneumonitis	Pulmonary function tests (including DLCO and spirometry)
Thyroid	Neck RT	Hypothyroidism Hyperthyroidism Thyroid nodules or cancer	Free T4; TSH
Gonadal (female)	Pelvic RT Alkylating agents	Delayed/arrested puberty Early menopause Ovarian failure	Monitoring for pubertal progression with Tanner staging until mature and menstrual history; other studies include FSH, LH, estradiol
Gonadal (male)	Pelvic RT Alkylating agents	Germ cell failure Infertility/azoospermia Leydig cell dysfunction Hypogonadism Delayed/arrested puberty	Monitoring for pubertal progression with Tanner staging until mature; Other studies include FSH, LH, testosterone Semen analysis
Bone	Corticosteroids	Decreased bone mineral density	Bone density evaluation (DEXA)
Second malignancies	Radiotherapy Doxorubicin Etoposide Mechlorethamine Cyclophosphamide	Sarcomas CNS tumors Breast cancer Melanoma Nonmelanoma skin cancer Thyroid cancer Other solid tumors Therapy-related myelodysplasia and acute leukemia	Routine cancer screening per general population guidelines Mammography or Breast MRI to screen for female breast cancer at age 25 y or 8 y post-RT exposure, whichever is later Annual CBC with differential for 10-y postexposure

Abbreviations: CBC, complete blood count; CNS, central nervous system; DEXA, dual-energy X-ray absorptiometry; DLCO, diffusing capacity of the lung for carbon monoxide; FSH, follicle-stimulating hormone; LH, luteinizing hormone; RT, radiation therapy; TSH, thyroid-stimulating hormone.
[a]Monitoring recommendations all include a risk-adapted health history and physical examination. The frequency with which diagnostic studies should be performed is dependent on many factors, including radiotherapy dose, chemotherapy exposures, age at exposure, and other clinical parameters. See Children's Oncology Group guidelines for more details (www.survivorshipguidelines.org).

been noted.[163,164] With ongoing follow-up, however, of more contemporary populations treated with lower doses and fields of radiotherapy, one would expect this risk to decline in subsequent decades. This principle is illustrated by the decrease in therapy-related leukemia among HL survivors treated at Stanford over successive decades, where decreases in alkylating agent exposure were deliberately brought into therapeutic regimens.[165] An analysis of the COG AHOD0031 population revealed a 10-year cumulative incidence of 1.3% of subsequent malignancies, with leukemias, lymphomas, and solid tumors occurring but at relatively low rates with only 17 secondary malignancies out of 1711 patients.[166]

Thyroid dysfunction and thyroid cancer are also of concern in this population. In the CCSS, self-report thyroid status was assessed in 1791 HL survivors treated from 1970 to 1986. Of the entire cohort, 34% have been diagnosed with at least one thyroid abnormality. Hypothyroidism was the most common disturbance, with a relative risk of 17.1 compared to sibling controls. Hyperthyroidism was reported by 5% of survivors, which was eightfold greater than the incidence reported by the controls. The risk of thyroid nodules was 27 times that observed in sibling controls. Female gender and higher radiation dose increased risk for thyroid abnormalities including thyroid cancers related to radiation dose.[167-169] Data from more recent years of treatment with protocols that decreased radiation exposure suggest a decreased risk with chemotherapy alone and lower doses of radiation (<30 Gy) to the supradiaphragmatic regions.[170] Continued monitoring for thyroid dysfunction will be needed with increasing use of immunotherapies and checkpoint inhibitors that can cause autoimmune toxicities including thyroid disease though long-term findings with these newer agents are still being evaluated.[171]

Cardiac toxicity following anthracycline therapy and mediastinal radiotherapy is well recognized among survivors. In a cohort of five-year survivors diagnosed between 1966 and 1996 cumulative incidence of anthracycline (dose), cardiac irradiation (dose), combination of these treatments, and congenital heart disease were significantly associated with developing a cardiac event.[172] The St. Jude Lifetime Cohort Study (SJLIFE) found that by age 50, 45.5% of pediatric HL survivors had a cardiovascular complication in comparison to a community control cohort with 15.7% experiencing a cardiovascular condition.[173] Cardiac risk varies by treatment regimen, but anthracycline exposure with or without mediastinal radiation continues to elevate the risk of late cardiovascular effects.[174] The concurrent use of dexrazoxane showed a decreased overall risk, but this must be balanced with the regimen and some concern for increased secondary malignancies with dexrazoxane, when used in regimens with both doxorubicin and etoposide.[175,176] Modern radiation techniques can significantly reduce the cardiac dose to less than 15 Gy in many cases which is the dose associated in other studies with higher risk of adverse outcomes.[175] A structured program of exercise should be considered for those at risk for cardiac disease as SJLIFE study showed HL survivors are more likely to have impaired fitness and quality of life compared with community controls.[177] A study from the CCSS demonstrated that adherence to vigorous intensity exercise was associated with a 51% reduction in the risk of any cardiovascular event in comparison with not meeting the guidelines.[178]

Both alkylating agent chemotherapy and gonadal radiation increase the risk of premature ovarian failure in females[179,180] though more recent data show resumption of menstrual cycles in more than 90% and pregnancy rates equivalent to age-matched controls of 75% to 80% in females treated with ABVD.[175] Sterility in males was common with more alkylator-based regimens,[181] but with ABVD and more recent regimens, there is preservation of sperm counts and follicle-stimulating hormone levels in 50% to 75% of males.[175]

Various pediatric cooperative groups have developed long-term follow-up guidelines, which provide a foundation for the type of follow-up care that should be delivered. However, the recommendations are not completely consistent with one another and are consensus based, and thus, the optimal follow-up strategy is yet to be fully elucidated. Efforts are underway for international harmonization among large childhood cancer groups to develop more universal guidelines despite different treatment strategies among groups.[174,182-185]

CONCLUSIONS

Cure rates for HL are one of the highest in pediatric oncology, but the very therapies that have afforded such cure rates share the etiologic limelight for adverse long-term health outcomes. Ongoing clinical trials thus seek to balance efficacy with both short- and long-term toxicity and are examining reductions in or avoidance of cytotoxic chemotherapy and RT. For a meaningful minority of patients with higher risk initial disease, refractory, and recurrent disease, the challenge remains maintaining and even increasing the cure rate and incorporating novel agents that may better target the underlying biology and pathophysiology. And lastly, additional study is required to understand the complex biology and epidemiology of HL to understand better how they interface with one another, affect disease presentation, response to therapy, and long-term toxicity.

References

1. Sternberg C. Uber eind Eigenartige unter dem Bilde der Pseudoleuk mie verlaufende Turberculose des lymphatischen. *Apparates Z Heldk*. 1898;19:21.
2. Reed D. On the pathological changes in Hodgkin's disease, with special reference to its relation to tuberculosis. *Johns Hopkins Hosp Rep*. 1902;10:133.
3. Seif GS, Spriggs AI. Chromosome changes in Hodgkin's disease. *J Natl Cancer Inst*. 1967;39(3):557-570.
4. Jox A, Zander T, Diehl V, Wolf J. Clonal relapse in Hodgkin's disease. *N Engl J Med*. 1997;337(7):499.
5. Kanzler H, Kuppers R, Helmes S, et al. Hodgkin and Reed-Sternberg-like cells in B-cell chronic lymphocytic leukemia represent the outgrowth of single germinal-center B-cell-derived clones: potential precursors of Hodgkin and Reed-Sternberg cells in Hodgkin's disease. *Blood*. 2000;95(3):1023-1031.
6. Fiumara P, Snell V, Li Y, et al. Functional expression of receptor activator of nuclear factor kappaB in Hodgkin disease cell lines. *Blood*. 2001;98(9):2784-2790.
7. Ambinder RF, Browning PJ, Lorenzana I, et al. Epstein-Barr virus and childhood Hodgkin's disease in Honduras and the United States. *Blood*. 1993;81(2):462-467.
8. Pusey WA. Cases of sarcoma and Hodgkin's disease treated with exposures to x-rays: a preliminary report. *JAMA*. 1902;132:166.
9. Goodman LS, Wintrobe MM, Dameshek W, Goodman MJ, Gilman AZ, McLennan MT. Nitrogen mustard therapy: use of methyl-bis (beta-chloroethyl)amine hydrochloride for Hodgkin's disease, lymphosarcoma, leukemia and certain allied and miscellaneous disorders. *J Am Med Assoc*. 1946;132:126-132.
10. DeVita VT, Jr, Canellos GP, Moxley JH, III. A decade of combination chemotherapy of advanced Hodgkin's disease. *Cancer*. 1972;30(6):1495-1504.
11. Santoro A, Bonadonna G, Valagussa P, et al. Long-term results of combined chemotherapy-radiotherapy approach in Hodgkin's disease: superiority of ABVD plus radiotherapy versus MOPP plus radiotherapy. *J Clin Oncol*. 1987;5(1):27-37.
12. Donaldson SS, Link MP. Combined modality treatment with low-dose radiation and MOPP chemotherapy for children with Hodgkin's disease. *J Clin Oncol*. 1987;5:742-749.
13. Howlader N, Noone AM, Krapcho M, et al. SEER Cancer Statistics Review, 1975-2017. National Cancer Institute; 2020. based on November 2019 SEER data submission, posted to the SEER web sitehttps://seer.cancer.gov/csr/1975_2017/.
14. Percy CL, Smith MA, Linet M, et al. Lymphomas and reticuloendothelial neoplasms. In: Ries LAG, Smith MA, Gurney JG, et al, eds. *Cancer Incidence and Survival Among Children and Adolescents: United States SEER Program 1975-1995*. National Cancer Institute, SEER program; 1999.
15. Mack TM, Cozen W, Shibata DK, et al. Concordance for Hodgkin's disease in identical twins suggesting genetic susceptibility to the young-adult form of the disease. *N Engl J Med*. 1995;332(7):413-418.
16. Devesa SS, Blot WJ, Stone BJ, Miller BA, Tarone RE, Fraumeni JF, Jr. Recent cancer trends in the Henited States. *J Natl Cancer Inst*. 1995;87:175-182.
17. Kersey JH, Shapiro RS, Filipovich AH. Relationship of immunodeficiency to lymphoid malignancy. *Pediatr Infect Dis J*. 1988;7(5 suppl):S10-S12.
18. Kusuda M, Toriyama K, Kamidigo NO, Itakura H. A comparison of epidemiologic, histologic, and virologic studies on Hodgkin's disease in western Kenya and Nagasaki, Japan. *Am J Trop Med Hyg*. 1998;59(5):801-807.
19. Armstrong AA, Alexander FE, Cartwright R, et al. Epstein-Barr virus and Hodgkin's disease: further evidence for the three disease hypothesis. *Leukemia*. 1998;12(8):1272-1276.
20. Glaser SL, Lin RJ, Stewart SL, et al. Epstein-Barr virus-associated Hodgkin's disease: epidemiologic characteristics in international data. *Int J Cancer*. 1997;70(4):375-382.
21. Sleckman BG, Mauch PM, Ambinder RF, et al. Epstein-Barr virus in Hodgkin's disease: correlation of risk factors and disease characteristics with molecular evidence of viral infection. *Cancer Epidemiol Biomarkers Prev*. 1998;7(12):1117-1121.
22. Gruffferman S, Delzell E. Epidemiology of Hodgkin's disease. *Epidemiol Rev*. 1984;6:76-106.
23. Stiller CA. What causes Hodgkin's disease in children? *Eur J Cancer*. 1998;34(4):523-528.
24. Gutensohn NM. Social class and age at diagnosis of Hodgkin's disease: new epidemiologic evidence for the "two-disease hypothesis." *Cancer Treat Rep*. 1982;66(4):689-695.
25. Gruffferman S, Cole P, Smith PG, Lukes RJ. Hodgkin's disease in siblings. *N Engl J Med*. 1977;296(5):248-250.
26. Gruffferman S, Cole P, Levitan TR. Evidence against transmission of Hodgkin's disease in high schools. *N Engl J Med*. 1979;300(18):1006-1011.
27. Gruffferman S. Is Hodgkin's disease infectious? *Eur J Cancer*. 1995;31A:1388-1389.
28. Staudt LM. The molecular and cellular origins of Hodgkin's disease. *J Exp Med*. 2000;191(2):207-212.
29. Brauninger A, Schmitz R, Bechtel D, Renné C, Hansmann ML, Küppers R. Molecular biology of Hodgkin's and Reed/Sternberg cells in Hodgkin's lymphoma. *Int J Cancer*. 2006;118(8):1853-1861.
30. Baeuerle PA, Baltimore D. NF-κB: ten years after. *Cell*. 1996;87(1):13-20.
31. Karin M, Delhase M. The IκB kinase (IKK) and NF-κB: key elements of proinflammatory signalling. *Semin Immunol*. 2000;12(1):85-98.
32. Delhase M, Hayakawa M, Chen Y, Karin M. Positive and negative regulation of IkappaB kinase activity through IKKbeta subunit phosphorylation. *Science*. 1999;284(5412):309-313.
33. Li ZW, Chu W, Hu Y, et al. The IKKβ subunit of IκB kinase (IKK) is essential for nuclear factor κB activation and prevention of apoptosis. *J Exp Med*. 1999;189:1839-1845.
34. Bargou RC, Leng C, Krappmann D, et al. High-level nuclear NF-kappa B and Oct-2 is a common feature of cultured Hodgkin/Reed-Sternberg cells. *Blood*. 1996;87(10):4340-4347.
35. Ravi R, Bedi GC, Engstrom LW, et al. Regulation of death receptor expression and TRAIL/Apo2L-induced apoptosis by NF-kappaB. *Nat Cell Biol*. 2001;3(4):409-416.
36. Durkop H, Foss HD, Demel G, Klotzbach H, Hahn C, Stein H. Tumor necrosis factor receptor-associated factor 1 is overexpressed in Reed-Sternberg cells of Hodgkin's disease and Epstein-Barr virus-transformed lymphoid cells. *Blood*. 1999;93(2):617-623.
37. Wang CY, Mayo MW, Korneluk RG, Goeddel DV, Baldwin AS, Jr. NF-kappaB anti-apoptosis: induction of TRAF1 and TRAF2 and c-IAP1 and c-IAP2 to suppress caspase-8 activation. *Science*. 1998;281(5383):1680-1683.
38. Mosialos G, Birkenbach M, Yalamanchili R, VanArsdale T, Ware C, Kieff E. The Epstein-Barr virus transforming protein LMP1 engages signaling proteins for the tumor necrosis factor receptor family. *Cell*. 1995;80(3):389-399.
39. Devergne O, Hatzivassiliou E, Izumi KM, et al. Association of TRAF1, TRAF2, and TRAF3 with an Epstein-Barr virus LMP1 domain important for B-lymphocyte transformation: role in NF-kappaB activation. *Mol Cell Biol*. 1996;16(12):7098-7108.
40. Sylla BS, Hung SC, Davidson DM, et al. Epstein-Barr virus-transforming protein latent infection membrane protein 1 activates transcription factor NF-kappaB through a pathway that includes the NF-kappaB-inducing kinase and the IkappaB kinases IKKalpha and IKKbeta. *Proc Natl Acad Sci U S A*. 1998;95(17):10106-10111.
41. Mir SS, Richter BW, Duckett CS. Differential effects of CD30 activation in anaplastic large cell lymphoma and Hodgkin disease cells. *Blood*. 2000;96(13):4307-4312.
42. Klein G. Epstein-Barr virus-carrying cells in Hodgkin's disease. *Blood*. 1992;80(2):299-301.
43. Weiss LM, Movahed LA, Warnke RA, Sklar J. Detection of Epstein-Barr viral genomes in Reed-Sternberg cells of Hodgkin's disease. *N Engl J Med*. 1989;320(8):502-506.
44. Weiss LM, Strickler JG, Warnke RA, Purtilo DT, Sklar J. Epstein-Barr viral DNA in tissues of Hodgkin's disease. *Am J Pathol*. 1987;129(1):86-91.
45. Khanna R, Burrows SR. Role of cytotoxic T lymphocytes in Epstein-Barr virus-associated diseases. *Annu Rev Microbiol*. 2000;54:19-48.
46. Yang Y, Lemas VM, Flinn IW, Krone C, Ambinder RF. Application of the ELISPOT assay to the characterization of CD8(+) responses to Epstein-Barr virus antigens. *Blood*. 2000;95(1):241-248.
47. Xie W, Medeiros LJ, Li S, Yin CC, Khoury JD, Xu J. PD-1/PD-L1 pathway and its blockade in patients with classic Hodgkin lymphoma and non-Hodgkin large-cell lymphomas. *Curr Hematol Malig Rep*. 2020;15(4):372-381.
48. Xu-Monette ZY, Zhou J, Young KH. PD-1 expression and clinical PD-1 blockade in B-cell lymphomas. *Blood*. 2018;131(1):68-83.
49. Harris NL. Hodgkin's lymphomas: classification, diagnosis, and grading. *Semin Hematol*. 1999;36(3):220-232.
50. Pileri SA, Ascani S, Leoncini L, et al. Hodgkin's lymphoma: the pathologist's viewpoint. *J Clin Pathol*. 2002;55(3):162-176.
51. Tzankov A, Zimpfer A, Pehrs AC, et al. Expression of B-cell markers in classical Hodgkin lymphoma: a tissue microarray analysis of 330 cases. *Mod Pathol*. 2003;16(11):1141-1147.

52. Anagnostopoulos I, Hansmann ML, Franssila K, et al. European Task Force on Lymphoma project on lymphocyte predominance Hodgkin disease: histologic and immunohistologic analysis of submitted cases reveals 2 types of Hodgkin disease with a nodular growth pattern and abundant lymphocytes. *Blood.* 2000;96(5):1889-1899.
53. Stein H, Marafioti T, Foss HD, et al. Down-regulation of BOB.1/OBF.1 and Oct2 in classical Hodgkin disease but not in lymphocyte predominant Hodgkin disease correlates with immunoglobulin transcription. *Blood.* 2001;97(2):496-501.
54. Mauch PM, Kalish LA, Kadin M, Coleman CN, Osteen R, Hellman S. Patterns of presentation of Hodgkin disease. Implications for etiology and pathogenesis. *Cancer.* 1993;71(6):2062-2071.
55. Kaplan H. *Hodgkin's Disease*. Harvard University Press; 1980.
56. Lister TA, Crowther D, Sutcliffe SB, et al. Report of a committee convened to discuss the evaluation and staging of patients with Hodgkin's disease: Cotswolds meeting. *J Clin Oncol.* 1989;7(11):1630-1636.
57. Lister TA, Crowther D. Staging for Hodgkin's disease. *Semin Oncol.* 1990;17(6):696-703.
58. Carbone PP, Kaplan HS, Musshoff K, Smithers DW, Tubiana M. Report of the Committee on Hodgkin's disease staging classification. *Cancer Res.* 1971;31(11):1860-1861.
59. Castellino RA, Blank N, Hoppe RT, Cho C. Hodgkin disease: contributions of chest CT in the initial staging evaluation. *Radiology.* 1986;160(3):603-605.
60. Hanna SL, Fletcher BD, Boulden TF, Hudson MM, Greenwald CA, Kun LE. MR imaging of infradiaphragmatic lymphadenopathy in children and adolescents with Hodgkin disease: comparison with lymphography and CT. *J Magn Reson Imaging.* 1993;3:461-470.
61. Castellani MR, Cefalo G, Terenziani M, et al. Gallium scan in adolescents and children with Hodgkin's disease (HD). Treatment response assessment and prognostic value. *Q J Nucl Med.* 2003;47(1):22-30.
62. El Galaly TC, Gormsen LC, Hutchings M. PET/CT for staging; past, present, and future. *Semin Nucl Med.* 2018;48(1):4-16.
63. Nachman JB, Sposto R, Herzog P, et al. Randomized comparison of low-dose involved-field radiotherapy and no radiotherapy for children with Hodgkin's disease who achieve a complete response to chemotherapy. *J Clin Oncol.* 2002;20(18):3765-3771.
64. Ruhl U, Albrecht M, Dieckmann K, et al. Response-adapted radiotherapy in the treatment of pediatric Hodgkin's disease: an interim report at 5 years of the German GPOH-HD 95 trial. *Int J Radiat Oncol Biol Phys.* 2001;51:1209-1218.
65. Krasin MJ, Raj SN, Kun LE, et al. Patterns of treatment failure in pediatric and young adult patients with Hodgkin's disease: local disease control with combined-modality therapy. *J Clin Oncol.* 2005;23(33):8406-8413.
66. Smith RS, Chen Q, Hudson MM, et al. Prognostic factors for children with Hodgkin's disease treated with combined-modality therapy. *J Clin Oncol.* 2003;21(10):2026-2033.
67. Shankar AG, Ashley S, Radford M, Barrett A, Wright D, Pinkerton CR. Does histology influence outcome in childhood Hodgkin's disease? Results from the United Kingdom Children's Cancer Study Group. *J Clin Oncol.* 1997;15(7):2622-2630.
68. Landman-Parker J, Pacquement H, Leblanc T, et al. Localized childhood Hodgkin's disease: response-adapted chemotherapy with etoposide, bleomycin, vinblastine, and prednisone before low-dose radiation therapy – results of the French Society of Pediatric Oncology Study MDH90. *J Clin Oncol.* 2000;18(7):1500-1507.
69. Schwartz CL. Prognostic factors in pediatric Hodgkin disease. *Curr Oncol Rep.* 2003;5(6):498-504.
70. Schwartz CL, Chen L, McCarten K, et al. Childhood Hodgkin international prognostic Score (CHIPS) predicts event-free survival in Hodgkin lymphoma: a report from the Children's Oncology Group. *Pediatr Blood Cancer.* 2017;64(4):e26278.
71. Bohlen H, Kessler M, Sextro M, Diehl V, Tesch H. Poor clinical outcome of patients with Hodgkin's disease and elevated interleukin-10 serum levels. Clinical significance of interleukin-10 serum levels for Hodgkin's disease. *Ann Hematol.* 2000;79(3):110-113.
72. Hann HW, Lange B, Stahlhut MW, McGlynn KA. Prognostic importance of serum transferrin and ferritin in childhood Hodgkin's disease. *Cancer.* 1990;66(2):313-316.
73. Chronowski GM, Wilder RB, Tucker SL, et al. An elevated serum beta-2-microglobulin level is an adverse prognostic factor for overall survival in patients with early-stage Hodgkin disease. *Cancer.* 2002;95(12):2534-2538.
74. Nadali G, Tavecchia L, Zanolin E, et al. Serum level of the soluble form of the CD30 molecule identifies patients with Hodgkin's disease at high risk of unfavorable outcome. *Blood.* 1998;91(8):3011-3016.
75. Warzocha K, Bienvenu J, Ribeiro P, et al. Plasma levels of tumour necrosis factor and its soluble receptors correlate with clinical features and outcome of Hodgkin's disease patients. *Br J Cancer.* 1998;77(12):2357-2362.
76. Christiansen I, Sundstrom C, Enblad G, Tötterman TH. Soluble vascular cell adhesion molecule-1 (sVCAM-1) is an independent prognostic marker in Hodgkin's disease. *Br J Haematol.* 1998;102(3):701-709.
77. Dukers DF, Meijer CJLM, ten Berge RL, Vos W, Ossenkoppele GJ, Oudejans JJ. High numbers of active caspase 3-positive Reed-Sternberg cells in pretreatment biopsy specimens of patients with Hodgkin disease predict favorable clinical outcome. *Blood.* 2002;100(1):36-42.
78. Carde P, Koscielny S, Franklin J, et al. Early response to chemotherapy: a surrogate for final outcome of Hodgkin's disease patients that should influence initial treatment length and intensity? *Ann Oncol.* 2002;13(suppl 1):86-91.
79. Schwartz CL, Constine LS, Villaluna D, et al. A risk-adapted, response-based approach using ABVE-PC for children and adolescents with intermediate- and high-risk Hodgkin lymphoma: the results of P9425. *Blood.* 2009;114(10):2051-2059.
80. Weiner MA, Leventhal BG, Marcus R, et al. Intensive chemotherapy and low-dose radiotherapy for the treatment of advanced-stage Hodgkin's disease in pediatric patients: a Pediatric Oncology Group study. *J Clin Oncol.* 1991;9:1591-1598.
81. Donaldson SS. Pediatric Hodgkin's disease—up, up, and beyond. *Int J Radiat Oncol Biol Phys.* 2002;54:1-8.
82. Hudson MM. Pediatric Hodgkin's therapy: time for a paradigm shift. *J Clin Oncol.* 2002;20(18):3755-3757.
83. Schwartz CL. Special issues in pediatric Hodgkin's disease. *Eur J Haematol Suppl.* 2005;(66):55-62.
84. Referenced with permission from the NCCN Guidelines® for Pediatric Hodgkin Lymphoma V.1.2022 © National Comprehensive Cancer Network, Inc. 2022. All rights reserved. NCCN makes no warranties of any kind whatsoever regarding their content, use or application and disclaims any responsibility for their application or use in any way. Accessed April 18, 2022. www.NCCN.org.
85. Siegel RL, Miller KD, Fuchs HE, Jemal A. Cancer Statistics, 2021. *CA Cancer J Clin.* 2021;71(1):7-33.
86. American Cancer Society. *Cancer Facts & Figures 2020*. American Cancer Society; 2020. Accessed November 2021.
87. American Cancer Society. *Cancer Facts & Figures 2021*. American Cancer Society; 2021. Accessed November 2021.
88. Hutchinson RJ, Fryer CJ, Davis PC, et al. MOPP or radiation in addition to ABVD in the treatment of pathologically staged advanced Hodgkin's disease in children: results of the Children's Cancer Group Phase III Trial. *J Clin Oncol.* 1998;16(3):897-906.
89. Weiner MA, Leventhal B, Brecher ML, et al. Randomized study of intensive MOPP-ABVD with or without low-dose total-nodal radiation therapy in the treatment of stages IIB, IIIA2, IIIB, and IV Hodgkin's disease in pediatric patients: a Pediatric Oncology Group study. *J Clin Oncol.* 1997;15(8):2769-2779.
90. Wolden SL, Chen L, Kelly KM, et al. Long-term results of CCG 5942: a randomized comparison of chemotherapy with and without radiotherapy for children with Hodgkin's lymphoma—a report from the Children's Oncology Group. *J Clin Oncol.* 2012;30(26):3174-3180.
91. Kelly KM, Sposto R, Hutchinson R, et al. BEACOPP chemotherapy is a highly effective regimen in children and adolescents with high-risk Hodgkin lymphoma: a report from the Children's Oncology Group. *Blood.* 2011;117(9):2596-2603.
92. Tebbi CK, Mendenhall N, London WB, Williams JL, de Alarcon PA, Chauvenet AR; Children's Oncology Group. Treatment of stage I, IIA, IIIA$_1$ pediatric Hodgkin disease with doxorubicin, bleomycin, vincristine and etoposide (DBVE) and radiation: a Pediatric Oncology Group (POG) study. *Pediatr Blood Cancer.* 2006;46(2):198-202.
93. Tebbi CK, Mendenhall NP, London WB, et al. Response-dependent and reduced treatment in lower risk Hodgkin lymphoma in children and adolescents, results of P9426: a report from the Children's Oncology Group. *Pediatr Blood Cancer.* 2012;59(7):1259-1265.
94. Friedman DL, Chen L, Wolden S, et al. Dose-intensive response-based chemotherapy and radiation therapy for children and adolescents with newly diagnosed intermediate-risk Hodgkin lymphoma: a report from the Children's Oncology Group Study AHOD0031. *J Clin Oncol.* 2014;32(32):3651-3658.
95. Keller FG, Castellino SM, Chen L, et al. Results of the AHOD0431 trial of response adapted therapy and a salvage strategy for limited stage, classical Hodgkin lymphoma: a report from the Children's Oncology Group. *Cancer.* 2018;124(15):3210-3219.
96. Kelly KM, Cole PD, Chen L, et al. Phase III study of response adapted therapy for the treatment of children with newly diagnosed very high risk Hodgkin lymphoma (stages IIIB/IVB) (AHOD0831): a report from the Children's Oncology Group. *Blood.* 2015;126:3927.
97. Donaldson SS, Link MP, Weinstein HJ, et al. Final results of a prospective clinical trial with VAMP and low-dose involved-field radiation for children with low-risk Hodgkin's disease. *J Clin Oncol.* 2007;25(3):332-337.
98. Hudson MM, Krasin M, Link MP, et al. Risk-adapted, combined-modality therapy with VAMP/COP and response-based, involved-field radiation for unfavorable pediatric Hodgkin's disease. *J Clin Oncol.* 2004;22:4541-4550.
99. Friedmann AM, Hudson MM, Weinstein HJ, et al. Treatment of unfavorable childhood Hodgkin's disease with VEPA and low-dose, involved-field radiation. *J Clin Oncol.* 2002;20(14):3088-3094.
100. Schellong G, Potter R, Bramswig J, et al. High cure rates and reduced long-term toxicity in pediatric Hodgkin's disease: the German-Austrian multicenter trial DAL-HD-90. The German-Austrian Pediatric Hodgkin's Disease Study Group. *J Clin Oncol.* 1999;17(12):3736-3744.
101. Dorffel W, Luders H, Ruhl U, et al. Preliminary results of the multicenter trial GPOH-HD 95 for the treatment of Hodgkin's disease in children and adolescents: analysis and outlook. *Klin Pädiatr.* 2003;215(3):139-145.
102. Mauz-Korholz C, Hasenclever D, Dorffel W, et al. Procarbazine-free OEPA-COPDAC chemotherapy in boys and standard OPPA-COPP in girls have comparable effectiveness in pediatric Hodgkin's lymphoma: the GPOH-HD-2002 study. *J Clin Oncol.* 2010;28(23):3680-3686.
103. Lo AC, Dieckmann K, Pelz T, et al. Pediatric classical Hodgkin lymphoma. *Pediatr Blood Cancer.* 2021;68(suppl 2):e28562.
104. Shankar A, Daw S. Nodular lymphocyte predominant Hodgkin lymphoma in children and adolescents—a comprehensive review of biology, clinical course and treatment options. *Br J Haematol.* 2012;159(3):288-298.
105. Pellegrino B, Terrier-Lacombe MJ, Oberlin O, et al. Lymphocyte-predominant Hodgkin's lymphoma in children: therapeutic abstention after initial lymph node resection—a study of the French Society of Pediatric Oncology. *J Clin Oncol.* 2003;21(15):2948-2952.
106. Murphy SB, Morgan ER, Katzenstein HM, Kletzel M. Results of little or no treatment for lymphocyte-predominant Hodgkin disease in children and adolescents. *J Pediatr Hematol Oncol.* 2003;25(9):684-687.
107. Appel BE, Chen L, Buxton AB, et al. Minimal treatment of low-risk pediatric lymphocyte-predominant Hodgkin lymphoma: a report from the Children's Oncology Group. *J Clin Oncol.* 2016;34(20):2372-2379.

108. Milgrom SA, Kim J, Chirindel A, et al. Prognostic value of baseline metabolic tumor volume in children and adolescents with intermediate-risk Hodgkin lymphoma treated with chemo-radiation therapy: FDG-PET parameter analysis in a subgroup from COG AHOD0031. *Pediatr Blood Cancer*. 2021;68(9):e29212.
109. Eichenauer DA, Engert A. How I treat nodular lymphocyte-predominant Hodgkin lymphoma. *Blood*. 2020;136(26):2987-2993.
110. Mauz-Körholz C, Lange T, Hasenclever D, et al. Pediatric nodular lymphocyte-predominant Hodgkin lymphoma: treatment recommendations of the GPOH-HD study group. *Klin Pädiatr*. 2015;227(6-7):314-321.
111. Straus DJ, Długosz-Danecka M, Connors JM, et al. Brentuximab vedotin with chemotherapy for stage III or IV classical Hodgkin lymphoma (ECHELON-1): 5-year update of an international, open-label, randomised, phase 3 trial. *Lancet Haematol*. 2021;8(6):e410-e421.
112. Metzger ML, Link MP, Billett AL, et al. Excellent outcome for pediatric patients with high-risk Hodgkin lymphoma treated with brentuximab vedotin and risk-adapted residual node radiation. *J Clin Oncol*. 2021;39(20):2276-2283.
113. Hoppe RT. Evolution of the techniques of radiation therapy in the management of lymphoma. *Int J Clin Oncol*. 2013;18(3):359-363.
114. Hodgson DC. Late effects in the era of modern therapy for Hodgkin lymphoma. *Hematology Am Soc Hematol Educ Program*. 2011;2011(1):323-329.
115. Lautenschlaeger S, Iancu G, Flatten V, et al. Advantage of proton-radiotherapy for pediatric patients and adolescents with Hodgkin's disease. *Radiat Oncol*. 2019;14(1):157.
116. Li J, Dabaja B, Reed V, et al. Rationale for and preliminary results of proton beam therapy for mediastinal lymphoma. *Int J Radiat Oncol Biol Phys*. 2011;81(1):167-174.
117. Wilson VC, McDonough J, Tochner Z. Proton beam irradiation in pediatric oncology: an overview. *J Pediatr Hematol Oncol*. 2005;27(8):444-448.
118. Wray J, Flampouri S, Slayton W, et al. Proton therapy for pediatric Hodgkin lymphoma. *Pediatr Blood Cancer*. 2016;63(9):1522-1526.
119. Nielsen K, Maraldo MV, Berthelsen AK, et al. Involved node radiation therapy in the combined modality treatment for early-stage Hodgkin lymphoma: analysis of relapse location and long-term outcome. *Radiother Oncol*. 2020;150:236-244.
120. Maraldo MV, Aznar MC, Vogelius IR, Petersen PM, Specht L. Involved node radiation therapy: an effective alternative in early-stage Hodgkin lymphoma. *Int J Radiat Oncol Biol Phys*. 2013;85(4):1057-1065.
121. Moskowitz AJ, Herrera AF, Beaven AW. Relapsed and refractory classical Hodgkin lymphoma: keeping pace with novel agents and new options for salvage therapy. *Am Soc Clin Oncol Educ Book*. 2019;39:477-486.
122. Daw S, Wynn R, Wallace H. Management of relapsed and refractory classical Hodgkin lymphoma in children and adolescents. *Br J Haematol*. 2011;152(3):249-260.
123. Cole PD, Schwartz CL, Drachtman RA, de Alarcon PA, Chen L, Trippett TM. Phase II study of weekly gemcitabine and vinorelbine for children with recurrent or refractory Hodgkin's disease: a Children's Oncology Group report. *J Clin Oncol*. 2009;27(9):1456-1461.
124. Horton TM, Drachtman RA, Chen L, et al. A phase 2 study of bortezomib in combination with ifosfamide/vinorelbine in paediatric patients and young adults with refractory/recurrent Hodgkin lymphoma: a Children's Oncology Group study. *Br J Haematol*. 2015;170(1):118-122.
125. Trippett TM, Schwartz CL, Guillerman RP, et al. Ifosfamide and vinorelbine is an effective reinduction regimen in children with refractory/relapsed Hodgkin lymphoma, AHOD00P1: a Children's Oncology Group report. *Pediatr Blood Cancer*. 2015;62(1):60-64.
126. Santoro A, Mazza R, Pulsoni A, et al. Bendamustine in combination with gemcitabine and vinorelbine is an effective regimen as induction chemotherapy before autologous stem-cell transplantation for relapsed or refractory Hodgkin lymphoma: final results of a multicenter phase II study. *J Clin Oncol*. 2016;34(27):3293-3299.
127. Scott LJ. Brentuximab vedotin: a review in CD30-positive Hodgkin lymphoma. *Drugs*. 2017;77(4):435-445.
128. Senter PD, Sievers EL. The discovery and development of brentuximab vedotin for use in relapsed Hodgkin lymphoma and systemic anaplastic large cell lymphoma. *Nat Biotechnol*. 2012;30(7):631-637.
129. Michallet AS, Guillermin Y, Deau B, et al. Sequential combination of gemcitabine, vinorelbine, pegylated liposomal doxorubicin and brentuximab as a bridge regimen to transplant in relapsed or refractory Hodgkin lymphoma. *Haematologica*. 2015;100(7):e269-e271.
130. Moskowitz CH, Nademanee A, Masszi T, et al; AETHERA Study Group. Brentuximab vedotin as consolidation therapy after autologous stem-cell transplantation in patients with Hodgkin's lymphoma at risk of relapse or progression (AETHERA): a randomised, double-blind, placebo-controlled, phase 3 trial. *Lancet*. 2015;385(9980):1853-1862.
131. LaCasce AS, Bociek RG, Sawas A, et al. Brentuximab vedotin plus bendamustine: a highly active first salvage regimen for relapsed or refractory Hodgkin lymphoma. *Blood*. 2018;132(1):40-48.
132. Broccoli A, Argnani L, Botto B, et al. First salvage treatment with bendamustine and brentuximab vedotin in Hodgkin lymphoma: a phase 2 study of the Fondazione Italiana Linfomi. *Blood Cancer J*. 2019;9(12):100.
133. McMillan A, O'Neill AT, Townsend W, et al. The addition of bendamustine to brentuximab vedotin leads to improved rates of complete metabolic remission in children, adolescents and young adults with relapsed and refractory classical Hodgkin lymphoma: a retrospective single-centre series. *Br J Haematol*. 2021;192(3):e84-e87. Web.
134. Forlenza CJ, Gulati N, Mauguen A, et al. Combination brentuximab vedotin and bendamustine for pediatric patients with relapsed/refractory Hodgkin lymphoma. *Blood Adv*. 2021;5(24):5519-5524. [published online ahead of print, 2021 Sep 24] bloodadvances.2021005268.
135. Cole PD, McCarten KM, Pei Q, et al. Brentuximab vedotin with gemcitabine for paediatric and young adult patients with relapsed or refractory Hodgkin's lymphoma (AHOD1221): a Children's Oncology Group, multicentre single-arm, phase 1-2 trial. *Lancet Oncol*. 2081;19(9):1229-1238.
136. Ansell SM, Lesokhin AM, Borrello I, et al. PD-1 blockade with nivolumab in relapsed or refractory Hodgkin's lymphoma. *N Engl J Med*. 2015;372(4):311-319.
137. Younes A, Santoro A, Shipp M, et al. Nivolumab for classical Hodgkin's lymphoma after failure of both autologous stem-cell transplantation and brentuximab vedotin: a multicentre, multicohort, single-arm phase 2 trial. *Lancet Oncol*. 2016;17(9):1283-1294.
138. Armand P, Shipp MA, Ribrag V, et al. Programmed death-1 blockade with pembrolizumab in patients with classical Hodgkin lymphoma after brentuximab vedotin failure. *J Clin Oncol*. 2016;34(31):3733-3739.
139. Chen R, Zinzani PL, Fanale MA, et al. Phase II study of the efficacy and safety of pembrolizumab for relapsed/refractory classic Hodgkin lymphoma. *J Clin Oncol*. 2017;35(19):2125-2132.
140. Moskowitz AJ, Shah G, Schöder H, et al. Phase II trial of pembrolizumab plus gemcitabine, vinorelbine, and liposomal doxorubicin as second-line therapy for relapsed or refractory classical Hodgkin lymphoma. *J Clin Oncol*. 2021;39(28):3109-3117.
141. Harker-Murray P, Leblanc T, Mascarin M, et al. Response-adapated therapy with nivolumab and brentuximab vedotin (BV), followed by BV and bendamustine for suboptimal response, in children, adolescents, and young adults with standard-risk relapsed/refractory classical Hodgkin lymphoma. *Blood*. 2018;132(suppl 1):927.
142. Armand P, Chen YB, Redd RA, et al. PD-1 blockade with pembrolizumab for classical Hodgkin lymphoma after autologous stem cell transplantation. *Blood*. 2019;134(1):22-29.
143. Herrera AF, Chen L, Nieto Y, et al. Consolidation with nivolumab and brentuximab vedotin after autologous hematopoietic cell transplantation in patients with high-risk Hodgkin lymphoma. *Blood*. 2020;136(suppl 1):19-20.
144. Diefenbach CS, Hong F, Ambinder RF, et al. Ipilimumab, nivolumab, and brentuximab vedotin combination therapies in patients with relapsed or refractory Hodgkin lymphoma: phase 1 results of an open-label, multicentre, phase 1/2 trial. *Lancet Haematol*. 2020;7(9):e660-e670.
145. Wang CM, Wu ZQ, Wang Y, et al. Autologous T cells expressing CD30 chimeric antigen receptors for relapsed or refractory Hodgkin lymphoma: an open-label phase I trial. *Clin Cancer Res*. 2017;23(5):1156-1166.
146. Ramos CA, Grover NS, Beaven AW, et al. Anti-CD30 CAR-T cell therapy in relapsed and refractory Hodgkin lymphoma. *J Clin Oncol*. 2020;38(32):3794-3804.
147. Voorhees TJ, Beaven AW. Therapeutic updates for relapsed and refractory classical Hodgkin lymphoma. *Cancers*. 2020;12(10):2887.
148. Othman T, Herrera A, Mei M. Emerging therapies in relapsed and refractory Hodgkin lymphoma: what comes next after Brentuximab vedotin and PD-1 inhibition? *Curr Hematol Malig Rep*. 2021;16:1-7.
149. Perales MA, Ceberio I, Armand P, et al. Role of cytotoxic therapy with hematopoietic cell transplantation in the treatment of Hodgkin lymphoma: guidelines from the American Society for Blood and Marrow Transplantation. *Biol Blood Marrow Transplant*. 2015;21(6):971-983.
150. Harris RE, Termuhlen AM, Smith LM, et al. Autologous peripheral blood stem cell transplantation in children with refractory or relapsed lymphoma: results of Children's Oncology Group study A5962. *Biol Blood Marrow Transplant*. 2011;17(2):249-258.
151. Holmberg L, Maloney DG. The role of autologous and allogeneic hematopoietic stem cell transplantation for Hodgkin lymphoma. *J Natl Compr Canc Netw*. 2011;9:1060-1071.
152. Gauthier J, Castagna L, Garnier F, et al. Reduced-intensity and non-myeloablative allogeneic stem cell transplantation from alternative HLA-mismatched donors for Hodgkin lymphoma: a study by the French Society of Bone Marrow Transplantation and Cellular Therapy. *Bone Marrow Transplant*. 2017;52(5):689-696.
153. Genadieva-Stavrik S, Boumendil A, Dreger P, et al. Myeloablative versus reduced intensity allogeneic stem cell transplantation for relapsed/refractory Hodgkin's lymphoma in recent years: a retrospective analysis of the lymphoma working party of the European Group for Blood and Marrow Transplantation. *Ann Oncol*. 2016;27(12):2251-2257.
154. Claviez A, Canals C, Dierickx D, et al. Allogeneic hematopoietic stem cell transplantation in children and adolescents with recurrent and refractory Hodgkin lymphoma: an analysis of the European Group for Blood and Marrow Transplantation. *Blood*. 2009;114(10):2060-2067.
155. Ng AK, van Leeuwen FE. Hodgkin lymphoma: late effects of treatment and guidelines for surveillance. *Semin Hematol*. 2016;53(3):209-215.
156. Friedman DL, Constine LS. Late effects of treatment for Hodgkin lymphoma. *J Natl Compr Canc Netw*. 2006;4(3):249-257.
157. Castellino SM, Geiger AM, Mertens AC, et al. Morbidity and mortality in long-term survivors of Hodgkin lymphoma: a report from the childhood cancer survivor study. *Blood*. 2011;117(6):1806-1816.
158. Armstrong GT, Chen Y, Yasui Y, et al. Reduction in late mortality among 5-year survivors of childhood cancer. *N Engl J Med*. 2016;374(9):833-842.
159. Oeffinger KC, Stratton KL, Hudson MM, et al. Impact of risk-adapted therapy for pediatric Hodgkin lymphoma on risk of long-term morbidity: a report from the Childhood Cancer Survivor Study. *J Clin Oncol*. 2021;39(20):2266-2275.
160. Constine LS, Tarbell N, Hudson MM, et al. Subsequent malignancies in children treated for Hodgkin's disease: associations with gender and radiation dose. *Int J Radiat Oncol Biol Phys*. 2008;72(1):24-33.
161. Inskip PD, Robison LL, Stovall M, et al. Radiation dose and breast cancer risk in the childhood cancer survivor study. *J Clin Oncol*. 2009;27(24):3901-3907.
162. Moskowitz CS, Chou JF, Wolden SL, et al. Breast cancer after chest radiation therapy for childhood cancer. *J Clin Oncol*. 2014;32(21):2217-2223.

163. Chowdhry AK, McHugh C, Fung C, Dhakal S, Constine LS, Milano MT. Second primary head and neck cancer after Hodgkin lymphoma: a population-based study of 44, 879 survivors of Hodgkin lymphoma. *Cancer*. 2015;121(9):1436-1445.
164. Daniëls LA, Krol ADG, Schaapveld M, et al. Long-term risk of secondary skin cancers after radiation therapy for Hodgkin's lymphoma. *Radiother Oncol*. 2013;109(1):140-145.
165. Koontz MZ, Horning SJ, Balise R, et al. Risk of therapy-related secondary leukemia in Hodgkin lymphoma: the Stanford University experience over three generations of clinical trials. *J Clin Oncol*. 2013;31(5):592-598.
166. Giulino-Roth L, Pei Q, Buxton A, et al. Subsequent malignant neoplasms among children with Hodgkin lymphoma: a report from the Children's Oncology Group. *Blood*. 2021;137(11):1449-1456.
167. Sklar C, Whitton J, Mertens A, et al. Abnormalities of the thyroid in survivors of Hodgkin's disease: data from the childhood cancer survivor study. *J Clin Endocrinol Metab*. 2000;85(9):3227-3232.
168. Kovalchik SA, Ronckers CM, Veiga LHS, et al. Absolute risk prediction of second primary thyroid cancer among 5-year survivors of childhood cancer. *J Clin Oncol*. 2013;31(1):119-127.
169. Veiga LHS, Lubin JH, Anderson H, et al. A pooled analysis of thyroid cancer incidence following radiotherapy for childhood cancer. *Radiat Res*. 2012;178(4):365-376.
170. Macklin-Doherty A, Jones M, Coulson P, et al. Risk of thyroid disorders in adult and childhood Hodgkin lymphoma survivors 40 years after treatment. *Leuk Lymphoma*. 2021;63(3):1-11. [published online ahead of print, 2021 Nov 5].
171. Illouz F, Drui D, Caron P, Do Cao C. Expert opinion on thyroid complications in immunotherapy. *Ann Endocrinol*. 2018;79(5):555-561.
172. van der Pal HJ, van Dalen EC, van Delden E, et al. High risk of symptomatic cardiac events in childhood cancer survivors. *J Clin Oncol*. 2012;30(13):1429-1437.
173. Bhakta N, Liu Q, Yeo F, et al. Cumulative burden of cardiovascular morbidity in paediatric, adolescent, and young adult survivors of Hodgkin's lymphoma: an analysis from the St Jude Lifetime Cohort Study. *Lancet Oncol*. 2016;17(9):1325-1334.
174. Ehrhardt MJ, Flerlage JE, Armenian SH, Castellino SM, Hodgson DC, Hudson MM. Integration of pediatric Hodgkin lymphoma treatment and late effects guidelines: Seeing the forest beyond the trees. *J Natl Compr Canc Netw*. 2021;19(6):755-764.
175. Hodgson DC. Long-term toxicity of chemotherapy and radiotherapy in lymphoma survivors: optimizing treatment for individual patients. *Clin Adv Hematol Oncol*. 2015;13(2):103-112.
176. Tebbi CK, London WB, Friedman D, et al. Dexrazoxane-associated risk for acute myeloid leukemia/myelodysplastic syndrome and other secondary malignancies in pediatric Hodgkin's disease. *J Clin Oncol*. 2007;25(5):493-500.
177. Wogksch MD, Howell CR, Wilson CL, et al. Physical fitness in survivors of childhood Hodgkin lymphoma: a report from the St. Jude Lifetime Cohort. *Pediatr Blood Cancer*. 2019;66(3):e27506.
178. Jones LW, Liu Q, Armstrong GT, et al. Exercise and risk of major cardiovascular events in adult survivors of childhood Hodgkin lymphoma: a report from the childhood cancer survivor study. *J Clin Oncol*. 2014;32(32):3643-3650.
179. Sklar CA, Mertens AC, Mitby P, et al. Premature menopause in survivors of childhood cancer: a report from the childhood cancer survivor study. *J Natl Cancer Inst*. 2006;98(13):890-896.
180. van der Kaaij MAE, Heutte N, Meijnders P, et al. Premature ovarian failure and fertility in long-term survivors of Hodgkin's lymphoma: a European Organisation for Research and Treatment of Cancer Lymphoma Group and Groupe d'Etude des Lymphomes de l'Adulte Cohort Study. *J Clin Oncol*. 2012;30(3):291-299.
181. Green DM, Kawashima T, Stovall M, et al. Fertility of male survivors of childhood cancer: a report from the Childhood Cancer Survivor Study. *J Clin Oncol*. 2010;28(2):332-339.
182. Landier W, Bhatia S, Eshelman DA, et al. Development of risk-based guidelines for pediatric cancer survivors: the Children's oncology group long-term follow-up guidelines from the Children's oncology group late effects committee and nursing discipline. *J Clin Oncol*. 2004;22(24):4979-4990.
183. Landier W, Armenian SH, Lee J, et al. Yield of screening for long-term complications using the Children's oncology group long-term follow-up guidelines. *J Clin Oncol*. 2012;30(35):4401-4408.
184. Kenney LB, Bradeen H, Kadan-Lottick NS, Diller L, Homans A, Schwartz CL. The current status of follow-up services for childhood cancer survivors, are we meeting goals and expectations: a report from the consortium for New England childhood cancer survivors. *Pediatr Blood Cancer*. 2011;57(6):1062-1066.
185. Kremer LCM, Mulder RL, Oeffinger KC, et al. A worldwide collaboration to harmonize guidelines for the long-term follow-up of childhood and young adult cancer survivors: a report from the International Late Effects of Childhood Cancer Guideline Harmonization Group. *Pediatr Blood Cancer*. 2013;60(4):543-549.

Section 5 ■ PLASMA CELL DYSCRASIAS

Chapter 97 ■ Practical Approach to the Evaluation of Monoclonal Gammopathies

TAXIARCHIS KOURELIS • FRANCIS K. BUADI

INTRODUCTION

The real incidence of monoclonal gammopathy is unknown; it however increases with age, with most cases being identified in the seventh or eighth decade of life.[1] Monoclonal gammopathy simply implies the presence of a monoclonal protein in the serum or urine. Monoclonal proteins are immunoglobulins or components of immunoglobulins that can be detected by protein electrophoresis with immunofixation. The presence of a monoclonal protein is indicative of an underlying clonal plasma cell or B-cell disorder. These disorders encompass a spectrum of disease entities ranging from clinically benign monoclonal gammopathy of undetermined significance (MGUS) to clinically significant plasma cell disorders such as multiple myeloma, AL amyloidosis, POEMS syndrome, and also including B-cell disorders such as Waldenström macroglobulinemia and chronic lymphocytic leukemia.[2–5] Various neurologic, renal, and cutaneous conditions have also been associated with monoclonal gammopathy.[6–10] Among 60,568 monoclonal gammopathies evaluated at Mayo Clinic from 1960 to 2020, most had MGUS (55%), multiple myeloma (20%), and immunoglobulin light chain (AL) amyloidosis (10%) (*Figure 97.1*). However, about 4% of these monoclonal gammopathies were associated with other conditions such as POEMS syndrome, cryoglobulinemia, Castleman disease, and monoclonal gammopathy of renal significance (MGRS), which do require therapy and should not be missed during evaluation (Chapter 103). Mayo clinic is a tertiary referral center, and this distribution may not reflect the actual distribution in the general population. A systematic approach to the patient with a monoclonal gammopathy is required both to prevent unnecessary testing in the majority, who will not need treatment for the underlying condition, and to ensure that those with a clinically significant condition will be appropriately diagnosed. The initial indication for obtaining the testing for a monoclonal protein should guide the extent of evaluation.

This chapter addresses the initial approach to an individual with a monoclonal gammopathy or suspected disorder usually associated with monoclonal gammopathy. The basic principles on the use of the various tests, their interpretation, and limitations are also reviewed. Subsequent chapters in this book will deal with the detailed evaluation of specific diseases, associated with a monoclonal gammopathy.

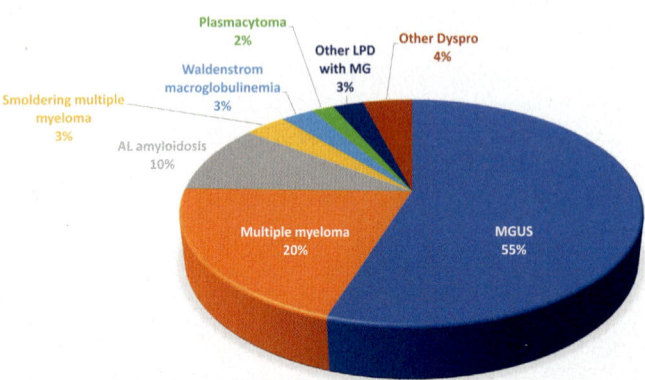

FIGURE 97.1 Distribution of Monoclonal Gammopathies seen at Mayo Clinic between 1960 and 2020. MGUS, monoclonal gammopathy of undetermined significance. LPD, lymphoproliferative disorder.

CLASSIFICATION OF MONOCLONAL IMMUNOGLOBULIN DISORDERS

A prior understanding of the various conditions associated with the production of monoclonal immunoglobulins (monoclonal protein) is essential. The clinical presentation may be due to the magnitude of the underlying tumor burden or the direct toxic effect of the monoclonal protein. However, a simple way of approaching the evaluation of these cases is to start with the type of monoclonal protein. Although the various diseases can be broadly classified based on the type of monoclonal protein, there is overlap in the underlying conditions. The type of monoclonal protein may give a clue about the underlying clonal cell disorder. For example, an IgM monoclonal protein is usually associated with lymphoproliferative diseases such as Waldenström macroglobulinemia and some lymphomas, but is rarely seen in a plasma cell disorder such as multiple myeloma.[11] IgG is the most common monoclonal protein in MGUS and myeloma, followed by IgM and IgA. Lambda light chain restriction is much more common in AL amyloidosis and POEMS syndrome as compared to kappa light chain restriction, which is more common in MGUS, myeloma, Waldenström macroglobulinemia, and light chain deposition disease.

DIAGNOSTIC ALGORITHM

In a patient suspected to have an underling gammopathy, one should first define the isotype and then quantity of the monoclonal protein (*Figure 97.2*). This will help in identifying and defining the underling clonal cell disorder. In the majority of cases, appropriate tissue biopsy and histopathologic evaluation should aid in providing a definitive diagnosis. In most cases, a bone marrow biopsy will help identify the underlying clonal cell. In certain cases, directed biopsy of a single bone lesion, lymph node, or soft tissue mass may be needed. In certain cases, appropriate tissue biopsy and histopathologic evaluation is required to define the associated clinical diagnosis.

Once the type of monoclonal protein and underling clonal cell disorder has been established, the clinician then needs to review the patients' history, physical examination, and laboratory data to determine whether this clonal disorder is the cause of the patient's symptoms or laboratory abnormality. The typical issues are usually with the hematopoietic (anemia, thrombocytopenia, bulky lymphadenopathy), skeletal (lytic lesion, pathologic fracture, and sclerotic lesions), renal (decrease in the glomerular filtration rate and/or nephrotic range proteinuria), nervous system (peripheral neuropathy, autonomic dysfunction), and cardiovascular (restrictive cardiomyopathy) systems. There may be overlap of symptoms, but understanding the various syndromes is important in helping to arrive at the correct diagnosis.

DIFFERENTIAL DIAGNOSIS OF MONOCLONAL GAMMOPATHY

The majority of non-IgM monoclonal gammopathies are classified as MGUS.[3] In most MGUS patients, the M-protein is a complete immunoglobulin molecule; however, some may only have a light chain component and are classified as light chain MGUS.[12] MGUS patients do not have any symptoms or laboratory abnormalities attributable to the

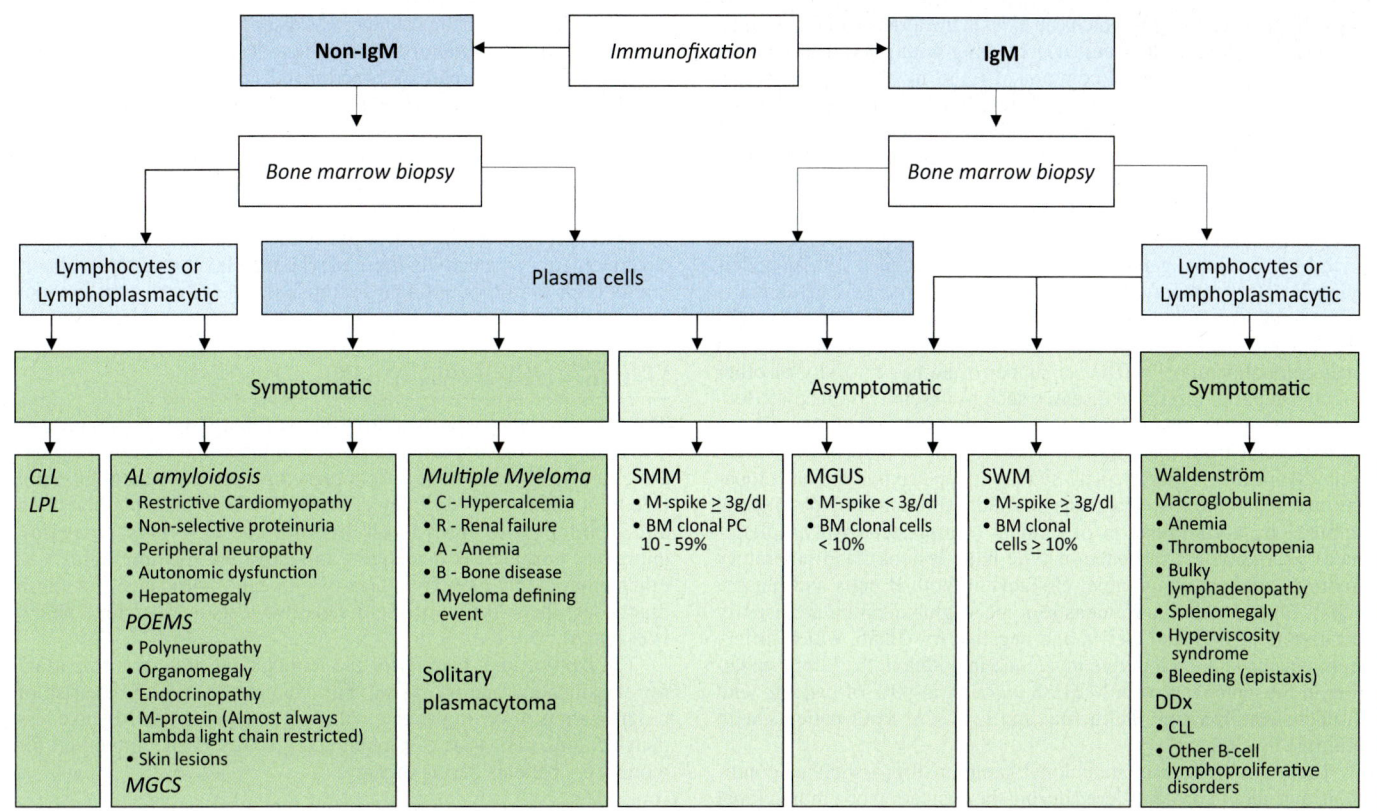

FIGURE 97.2 Simple diagnostic algorithm for patients with a monoclonal gammopathy. BM, bone marrow; CLL, chronic lymphocytic leukemia; LPL, lymphoplasmacytic lymphoma; MGCS, monoclonal gammopathy of clinical significance; MGUS, monoclonal gammopathy of undetermined significance; SMM, smoldering multiple myeloma; SWM, smoldering Waldenstrom macroglobulinemia.

underlying plasma cell clone. They should have less than 3 g/dL of monoclonal protein and bone marrow plasma cell less than 10%.

Asymptomatic patients with an M-protein > 3 g/dL or > 10% but <60% clonal bone marrow plasma cell are classified as smoldering multiple myeloma (SMM).[13] As will be discussed in Chapter 98, distinguishing between MGUS and SMM has prognostic significance and will determine frequency of follow-up. As bone marrow examination may be the only factor that will upstage an MGUS to SMM, this must be strongly considered in the evaluation of all monoclonal gammopathies, especially those with low-intermediate-risk or higher risk MGUS.[14] It is unlikely, one will miss significant pathology in patients with a blood panel consistent with low-risk MGUS if a bone marrow is omitted. In one retrospective study,[15] 79% of SMM patients required a bone marrow to distinguish their MGUS from SMM, but fewer than 1% would have been classified as "low risk MGUS" had the bone marrow been omitted; nearly 50% would have been considered intermediate or high-risk MGUS.

Patients with multiple myeloma should meet the CRAB criteria defined as hypercalcemia, renal insufficiency, anemia, or bone disease and/or have myeloma defining events (MDEs).[13] It is necessary to confirm that these complications are due to the underlying clonal plasma cell disorder. This is particularly important, especially considering the older age of patients with monoclonal gammopathies, who may have several other reasons to present with CRAB-like features. MDEs that required therapy include (a) bone marrow clonal plasma cells of 60% or more; (b) serum involved/uninvolved free light chain ratio of 100 or greater, provided the absolute level of the involved free light chain is at least 100 mg/L; and (c) more than one focal lesion on magnetic resonance imaging (MRI) that is at least 5 mm or greater in size.

Solitary plasmacytomas or solitary plasmacytoma with minimal bone marrow involvement should also be recognized, since these require only limited therapy.[16] These patients have a single bone or soft-tissue mass, a negative or <10% plasma cells on a bone marrow biopsy and do not meet the CRAB or MDE criteria.[13]

A significant number of patients with monoclonal gammopathy develop complications because of the toxic effect of the monoclonal protein in the absence of overt multiple myeloma. In AL amyloidosis, misfolding of the monoclonal protein, usually the light chain component, results in the formation of insoluble amyloid deposits in major organs of the body.[5] This deposition results in structural and physiologic dysfunction of the affected organ. An amyloid diagnosis (Chapter 100) is easy to make when presenting with macroglossia in association with periorbital purpura. Most, however, will present with symptoms secondary to the organ involvement, such as chest pain and shortness of breath due to restrictive cardiomyopathy in cardiac cases, and peripheral neuropathy and autonomic dysfunction in nervous system disease. Nonselective proteinuria with hypoalbuminemia is seen in kidney involvement. Hepatomegaly with elevated alkaline phosphatase will be seen in those with liver disease, and those with gastrointestinal involvement will have constipation or diarrhea. Patients may present with multiple organ involvement causing a protean constellation of findings; in such cases a strong suspicion for amyloidosis is required in order not to miss the diagnosis.

Nonamyloidotic immunoglobulin deposition diseases such as light chain deposition diseases are a group of conditions that should be considered during the evaluation of monoclonal gammopathy.[17] This involves the deposition of light chains usually in the kidney and less often in the heart, lungs, and liver. More rarely other organs can be also involved such as the cornea in the case of paraproteinemic crystalline keratopathy,[18] which can exist in the absence of other organ involvement. Renal involvement presenting with renal insufficiency and proteinuria is the most common.[19] Heart involvement, although not common, usually presents with restrictive cardiomyopathy and should be differentiated from amyloidosis.[20] There are a number of other monoclonal gammopathy–related diseases that are due to immunoglobulin deposition or humoral effects, which are currently designated monoclonal gammopathies of clinical significance (Chapter 102).

IgM monoclonal gammopathy is usually associated with an underlying B-cell lymphoproliferative disorder, and true IgM myeloma is exceedingly rare (Chapter 99). A large percentage of these IgM monoclonal gammopathy patients will have an IgM MGUS or Waldenström macroglobulinemia.[21,22] The remainder often has a variety of other B-cell lymphoproliferative diseases such as chronic lymphocytic leukemia, marginal zone lymphoma, and large cell lymphoma. Those with Waldenström macroglobulinemia (Chapter 101) may present with cytopenias, hyperviscosity syndrome, epistaxis, lymphadenopathy, and splenomegaly. Diagnosis of Waldenström macroglobulinemia is made by a combination of clinical (lymphadenopathy, splenomegaly), radiologic (absence of lytic bone lesions), and laboratory findings (macroglobulinemia, clonality in both B cells and plasma cells). Plasma cells in Waldenström macroglobulinemia are usually positive for CD45 and CD19, and negative for CD56, which differs from plasma cells in multiple myeloma. In addition, the L265P mutation in the adaptor protein MYD88 is found in 90% of patients with Waldenström macroglobulinemia and is absent from patients with multiple myeloma.[23]

There are other rare monoclonal gammopathy–associated conditions that should be considered during the evaluation of a monoclonal protein and these are discussed in detail in Chapter 102. The evaluation in these cases is usually dictated by the clinical presentation; for example, those with neuromuscular complications should be evaluated for conditions such as POEMS syndrome, IgM-associated neuropathy, or sporadic late-onset nemaline myopathy (SLONM).[4,24,25] POEMS patients, in addition to the neuropathy, have organomegaly (lymphadenopathy, splenomegaly, cardiomegaly, or hepatomegaly), multiple endocrinopathies, and skin changes (glomeruloid hemangiomata, hyperpigmentation). Almost all POEMS patients do have a lambda light chain restricted monoclonal protein, and most commonly non-IgM. If a patient has a kappa light chain or IgM heavy chain monoclonal protein, they most probably do not have POEMS syndrome.

Skin conditions such as scleromyxedema, necrobiotic xanthogranuloma, Schnitzler syndrome, and cryoglobulinemia should be considered in the differential diagnosis when patients present with cutaneous lesions.[6,8,9,26,27] TEMPI syndrome should be considered in patients presenting with telangiectasias, erythrocytosis, and intrapulmonary shunt.[28,29]

More recently, 20% of patients with VEXAS syndrome were found to have a coexisting monoclonal gammopathy or multiple myeloma. VEXAS is an adult-onset autoinflammatory disease affecting males, caused by a mutation in the UBA1 gene. The name derives from Vacuoles, E1 enzyme, X-linked, Autoinflammatory, Somatic. The causal association between the monoclonal gammopathy and VEXAS is unknown but this should be considered in all males with unexplained autoimmune symptoms that are refractory to management who present with anemia with or without a monoclonal protein.[30,31]

INITIAL EVALUATION

The usual test that will detect a monoclonal protein is not part of the typical healthy adult physical evaluation. It is therefore usually detected during the evaluation of a clinical symptom or during further evaluation of an abnormal laboratory test. Abnormalities in laboratory tests that suggest the possibility of a monoclonal protein disorder include rouleaux formation in a peripheral blood smear, elevated total serum protein, proteinuria, anemia, renal dysfunction, or hypercalcemia. Clinical situations that may require evaluation for a monoclonal protein include back pain, osteoporosis disproportionate to age, pathologic fracture, osteolytic or sclerotic bone lesions, recurrent sinopulmonary infections, progressive peripheral neuropathy, infiltrative or restrictive cardiomyopathy, skin changes, Raynaud phenomenon, or acrocyanosis. It must however be noted that in these conditions a monoclonal protein may not always be detected by standard testing and further evaluation may be needed to confirm or exclude an underlying plasma cell or lymphoproliferative disorder, particularly if the index of suspicion is high. Most patients with monoclonal protein are asymptomatic, especially in those in whom an incidental blood abnormality leads to further testing resulting in the identification of a monoclonal protein.

LABORATORY EVALUATION

The following are important tests that will help in the evaluation of a patient with or suspected to have a monoclonal protein. In general, the use of protein electrophoresis with serum immunoglobulin free light chain assay will detect nearly 100% of multiple myeloma and Waldenström macroglobulinemia cases.[32] This screening approach, however, is inadequate to screen for AL amyloidosis or other monoclonal gammopathies of clinical significance; for these diagnoses, the addition of more sensitive tests as described below is essential.

The isotype and quantity of the monoclonal protein is important for classification and prognosis. For example, in MGUS, the risk of progression is lower in patients with IgG isotype and an M-spike less than 1.5 g/dL. The type of protein and quantity is also important for monitoring patients during therapy.

Protein Electrophoresis

Serum and urine should both be evaluated for the presence of a monoclonal protein. High-resolution agarose gel electrophoresis or capillary zone electrophoresis is the preferred method for screening for a monoclonal protein.[32-34] These tests will separate serum or urine proteins into their various components in an electric field based primarily on their physical properties such as size and charge; the proteins are detected either by staining a solid matrix or their electrical impedance as they exit the column. There are usually five components seen on electrophoresis: albumin, alpha-1 and alpha-2, beta and gamma globulin (Figure 97.3A).

Monoclonal proteins will usually migrate into the gamma regions (Figure 97.3B); however, they may be seen in the beta or alpha-2 region, especially in the case of IgA and IgM monoclonal proteins. These bands are referred to as the M-protein or M-spike with the "M" referring to monoclonal. It must also be stressed that the gamma region contains all immunoglobulin isotypes (IgM, IgA, IgD, and IgE) and not only IgG. A monoclonal protein spike should not be confused with a polyclonal increase in immunoglobulin, which usually will be seen as a broad-based band in the gamma region in inflammatory conditions[35] (Figure 97.3C).

Protein electrophoresis may occasionally fail to identify the presence of a monoclonal protein, especially in cases where there is only minimal production of the monoclonal protein or if the protein migrates in the beta region. In such cases performing immunofixation despite a negative protein electrophoresis and using the serum free light chain analysis may be the only way to confirm the presence of an underlying clonal disorder. For this reason, when a monoclonal gammopathy is suspected all five tests should be performed: protein electrophoresis with immunofixation of both serum and urine and serum (not urine) free light chain levels. Of note, a 24-hour urine collection is preferred since random urine samples have lower sensitivity to identify a monoclonal protein.

The protein electrophoresis can be used to determine the amount of monoclonal protein present using the densitometer tracing (Figure 97.3B) or peak size by capillary zone electrophoresis. In the case of very high M-protein levels, the measured M-protein by densitometry tracing is typically lower than the total involved immunoglobulin measured by nephelometry.[33]

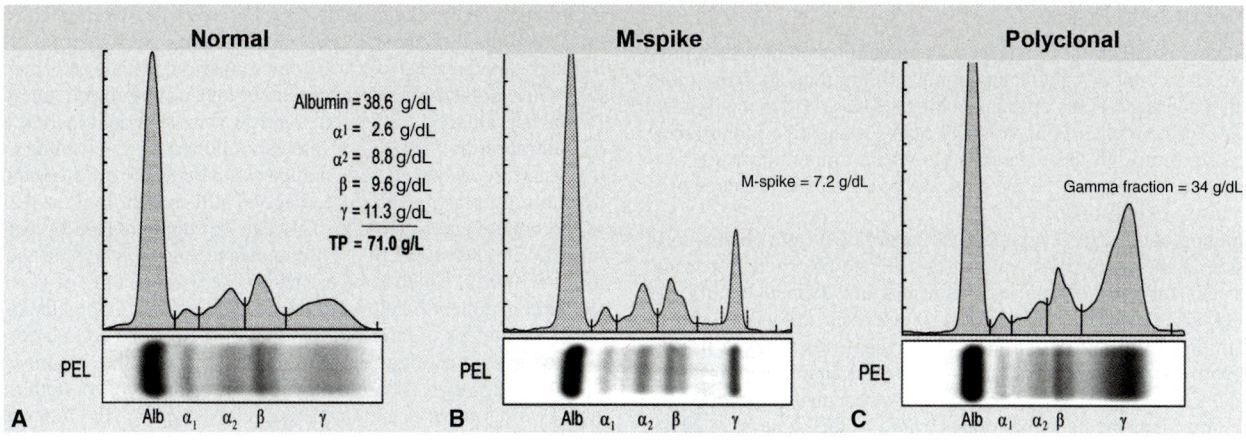

FIGURE 97.3 Serum protein electrophoresis. A, Normal serum electrophoresis, showing the five electrophoretic regions. B, Serum protein electrophoresis with a small monoclonal protein. C, Polyclonal hypergammaglobulenemia. PEL, protein electrophoresis.

Identification of the Type of the Monoclonal Protein

Immunofixation electrophoresis, immunosubtraction, or mass spectrometry should be used to type the M-protein (Figure 97.4) and to confirm the disappearance of an M-protein after therapy.[32,33,36,37] These methods are about ten-fold more sensitive than protein electrophoresis or capillary zone electrophoresis alone. Patients may have more than one type of M-protein, migrating together or separately, and this should not be missed.[38] Each of these methods employs antibodies directed against the heavy (IgG, IgA, and IgM) and light (kappa and lambda) chain isotypes.[32,33] Most laboratories do not initially perform immunofixation for IgD and IgE. If initial immunofixation studies detect only a monoclonal light chain, immunofixation for IgD and IgE should be performed.

The newest approach to detect monoclonal proteins is that of matrix-assisted laser desorption/ionization (MALDI) mass spectroscopy. This method is the standard practice at the Mayo Clinic, and other academic centers are eager to adopt this assay. This method exploits the biophysical properties of immunoglobulins, specifically the light chain. Each immunoglobulin light and heavy chain has unique amino acid sequences and thus a unique molecular mass. The unique molecular mass signatures of a given patient's monoclonal light chain generates allows for consistent identification.[37,39,40] This method is both more sensitive and specific than immunofixation and is less laborious than immunofixation. It can easily resolve false positives caused by therapeutic monoclonal antibodies, which are now commonly used in clinical practice, especially in rheumatologic diseases and other lymphoproliferative disorders. In multiple myeloma where response to therapy is largely based on monitoring of serum monoclonal proteins, this assay helps to differentiate persistent disease from therapeutic monoclonal antibodies used in the management of multiple myeloma.

Quantitation of Immunoglobulins

Immunoglobulin (IgG, IgA, IgM) levels should always be measured at diagnosis and monitored regularly during therapy, especially the involved immunoglobulin. If immunofixation showed an IgD or IgE M-protein, then the appropriate immunoglobulin level should also be determined. In most clonal plasma cell disorders the levels of the uninvolved immunoglobulins are suppressed or reduced.

Furthermore, the response to therapy among patients with IgA or IgM plasma cell disorders is better determined by quantification of the involved immunoglobulin rather than quantitation of the M-spike when the M-protein migrates outside of the gamma region.[41] In addition, a quantitative IgG level is used to document the level of gammaglobulins among patients with severe hypogammaglobulinemia and recurrent sinopulmonary infections to guide immunoglobulin replacement.

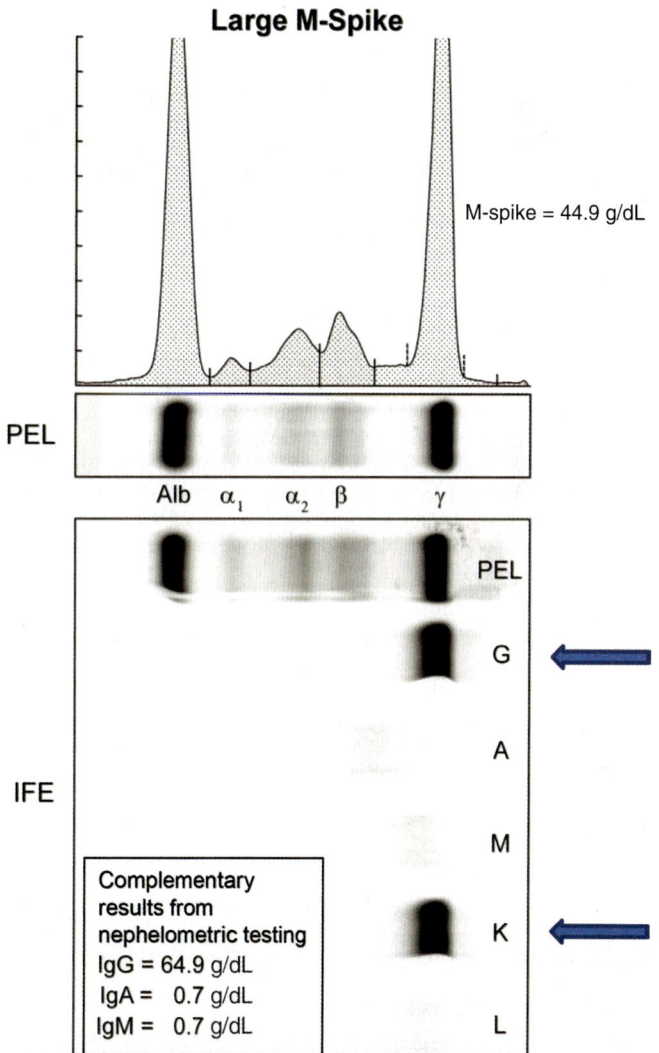

FIGURE 97.4 Serum protein electrophoresis and immunofixation electrophoresis. A monoclonal IgG kappa protein. The arrows indicate the lanes that show reactivity with the specific antibodies. Also illustrated is the discordance that may be seen between nephelometry and electrophoresis when M-protein is very large and narrow. IFE, immunofixation electrophoresis; PEL, protein electrophoresis.

Free Light Chain Assay

A significant population of patients with clonal plasma disorders produce excess amount of light chain but not a full immunoglobulin molecule, that is, Bence Jones proteins.[42] Most of these patients will have a negative protein electrophoresis and many, a negative immunofixation of the serum. In these patients the serum immunoglobulin free light chain assay test may be the only way to detect the presence of a clonal plasma cell disorder.[43,44]

Immunoglobulin free kappa (κ) and lambda (λ) light chains concentration in the serum is dependent on the rate of production from plasma cells and renal clearance. This results in a defined serum concentration and ratio. In clonal plasma cell disorders, there is an excess production of only one of the light chain types, resulting in higher levels, with suppression of the uninvolved light chain, leading to an abnormal κ/λ ratio. The levels and ratio however may be affected by renal failure, since the light chains are cleared by the kidneys. In 2014, the International Myeloma Working Group (IMWG) has defined the presence of the serum involved/uninvolved free light chain ratio of 100 or greater in patients with monoclonal gammopathies as an MDE warranting therapy, provided the absolute level of the involved free light chain is at least 100 mg/L.[13] Furthermore, the serum-free light chain test has become very important in the evaluation and monitoring of patients with amyloidosis, since this is the major protein involved in the formation of AL-type amyloid deposits.

The serum FLC assay can be used in place of urine protein electrophoresis and immunofixation in the initial screening algorithm for M-proteins. In a study of 428 patients, Katzmann et al found that urine studies can be eliminated by using the serum FLC assay in combination with the SPEP and immunofixation.[45] However, if a monoclonal plasma cell disorder is identified on screening, a 24-hour urine collection followed by electrophoresis and immunofixation should be considered to aid in the assessment of disease progression and response to therapy over time and to rule out nephrotic range albuminuria, such as is seen in AL amyloidosis. In addition to its role as a substitute for urine studies in the screening of plasma cell disorders, the FLC assay is used to predict prognosis in MGUS, SMM, AL, and solitary plasmacytoma.[46-48] In addition, it is also used to monitor oligosecretory MM, light-chain only form of MM, and AL amyloidosis.[43,49-51] An important caveat regarding the free light chain assay is that all of the original diagnostic and prognostic systems were developed using the free light chain assay developed by the Binding Site, LTD; subsequently, other manufacturers have developed different versions of the assay. These assays are not interchangeable since they have different performance characteristics and normal intervals.[52]

Urine Evaluation

In all patients with a serum M-protein or suspected to have a clonal plasma cell or lymphoplasmacytic disorder, a 24-hour urine collection should be examined for the presence of a monoclonal protein using protein electrophoresis and immunofixation electrophoresis. Although free light chains in the urine can be measured by nephelometry, the electrophoretic tests are favored. The excretion of immunoglobulin free light chain in the urine is referred to as Bence Jones proteinuria.[42] The pattern of protein excretion seen on electrophoresis, as to whether the urine protein is solely albumin or Bence Jones protein, is of diagnostic importance. For example, nonselective proteinuria (albumin predominance) is associated with glomerular diseases such as AL amyloidosis caused by the presence of a monoclonal protein.[53]

Bone Marrow and Tissue Evaluation

Bone marrow aspiration and biopsy should be performed in all patients except in a selected group of completely asymptomatic patients with a very small monoclonal protein if a diagnosis of MGUS is favored.[54,55] Studies have shown that the yield in an elderly patient with low-risk MGUS is very low and such patients can be spared the discomfort of a bone marrow biopsy.[3,15,46] However, most hematologists will recommend this test in patients with higher risk MGUS, since apart from giving information on the type of clonal cell disorder, it also provides information on the extent of disease. For example, the presence of less than 10% marrow plasma cells distinguishes MGUS from SMM.[3] Similarly, the presence of 60% or more marrow plasma cells meets the IMWG criteria for an MDE warranting myeloma-directed therapy.[13]

Basic evaluation of the bone marrow sample should include extent of infiltration by the cells of interest, reported as a percentage of the total marrow nucleated cells and/or cellularity. The gold standard for determining plasma cell percentage is still morphologic assessment of the bone marrow aspirate. This can be supplemented by performing CD138 and/or MUM-1 immunohistochemical stains on the bone marrow biopsy, which is of particular use if the quality of aspirate is suboptimal. Quantification of plasma cells by flow cytometry in diagnostic specimens usually underestimates the plasma cell percentages, as specimen processing tends to exclude lipid-adhesive plasma cells.[56]

Flow cytometric or immunophenotyping can confirm both the cell type (lymphoid vs plasma cell) and clonality.[57,58] Myeloma plasma cells are light chain restricted (kappa or lambda) and usually show aberrant expression of CD19, CD45, CD56, and/or CD117 (Figure 97.5). Flow cytometry is particularly useful when following patients on therapy as it is more sensitive in assessing the depth of response. Recent studies have also shown that minimal residual disease negative status using flow cytometry after treatment for newly diagnosed multiple myeloma is associated with better long-term survival.[59-63] Plasma cell DNA content can also be measured by flow cytometry allowing measurement of ploidy status and proliferation rate, which along with the proportion of normal plasma cells provides important prognostic information.[64] In addition, flow cytometry immunophenotyping of the peripheral blood can detect circulating plasma cells, which are associated with a more aggressive clinical course in patients with multiple myeloma.[65,66]

Assessing the genetic status of plasma cells is important for prognosis in plasma cell disorders. Fluorescent in situ hybridization (FISH) assessing break-apart of chromosome 14 along with potential partners of chromosome 4, 11, and 20; deletion of chromosome 13 or its long arm; deletion of the long arm of chromosome 17; additions of chromosome 1q; deletion of chromosome 1p; and trisomies of the odd chromosomes are a standard plasma cell disorder FISH set.[67,68] Metaphase cytogenetics in general is less relevant although they do give a proliferation signal. Gene expression profile analysis of the malignant plasma cells in multiple myeloma is of prognostic value.[69,70]

Congo Red Stain

In certain cases, a Congo red stain of subcutaneous fat aspirate or the bone marrow biopsy should be performed looking for amyloid deposition[5,71] (Chapter 101). In 70% to 85% of cases of AL amyloidosis, Congo red staining of bone marrow and subcutaneous fat aspirate will be sufficient to make the diagnosis. The remaining cases will require biopsy of the involved organ. All patients with peripheral neuropathy, significant albuminuria, or infiltrative cardiomyopathy in the setting of a monoclonal protein should have this test done. It should also be considered in patients in whom there is a high clinical suspicion of amyloidosis. If Congo red is positive, then liquid chromatography tandem mass spectrometry of peptide extracts from the congophilic material should be done for subtyping of the amyloid deposits.[72,73]

IMAGING

The imaging required for the evaluation of a patient with monoclonal protein depends on the clinical syndrome and type of monoclonal protein. In patients with non-IgM monoclonal protein who do not meet criteria for low or low-intermediate risk MGUS, bone imaging should be performed to look for lytic bone lesions. Cross-sectional imaging is preferred over plain radiographs for the detection of bone involvement in patients being evaluated for suspected MM.[74] Whole-body low-dose computed tomography (CT) has been considered as a better alternative to standard metastatic skeletal survey since it increases the sensitivity of detecting lytic bone lesions (Figure 97.6A and B).[75-79]

MRI or PET-CT may provide further information.[80] MRI is particularly useful for the assessment of the extent and nature of soft-tissue

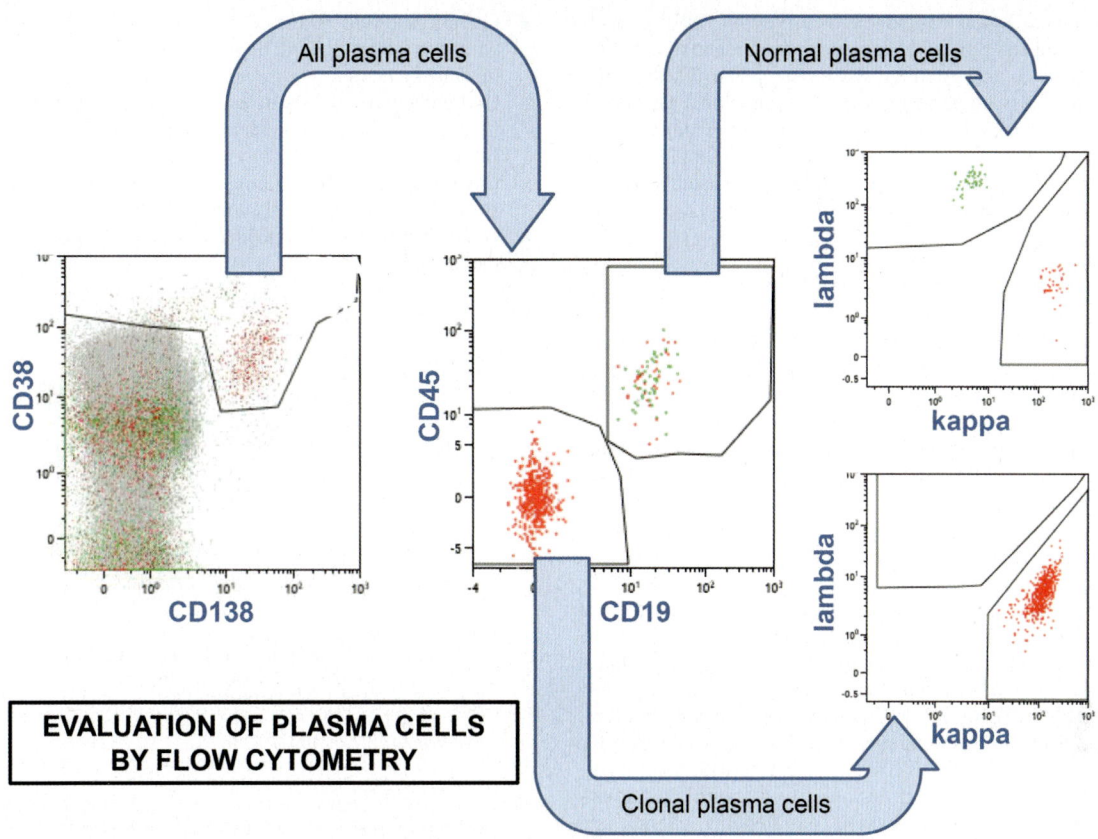

FIGURE 97.5 Identification of abnormal and normal plasma cells by flow cytometry. All plasma cells are CD38 and CD138 positive. The abnormal plasma cells are CD19 and CD45 negative and lambda immunoglobulin light chain restricted.

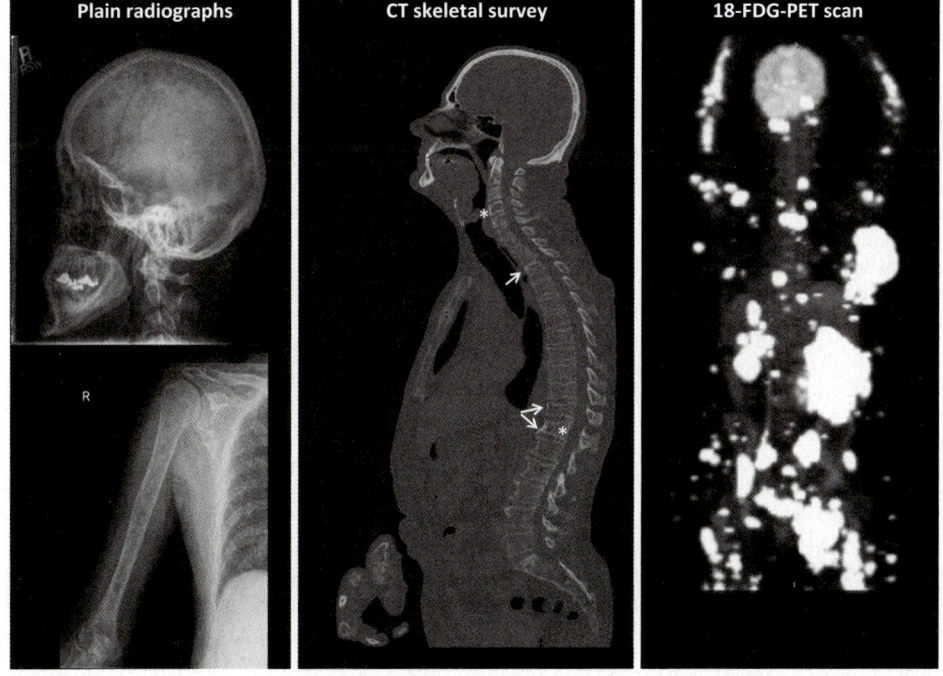

FIGURE 97.6 Radiographic imaging in plasma cell disorders. A, Skeletal bone survey showing lytic lesions typically seen in multiple myeloma. B, Low-dose CT-skeletal survey showing lytic lesions (*) and compression fractures (→). C, PET-CT scan showing multiple soft-tissue fluorodeoxyglucose avid plasmacytomas.

disease arising from bone lesions, especially those in the spine, which may cause neurologic compromise. The IMWG has included the use of whole-body MRI to identify patients with monoclonal gammopathies with more than one focal lesion that is at least 5 mm or greater in size as an MDE warranting myeloma-directed therapy. PET-CT is usually helpful in the evaluation of bone and extramedullary plasmacytomas and cases of nonsecretory multiple myeloma[16,81] (*Figure 97.6C*). In our experience, this modality has been helpful in the evaluation of patients with POEMS syndrome, by helping identify hypermetabolic osteosclerotic bone lesions. All three modalities are more sensitive than plain radiographic-based skeletal surveys, which are now considered a suboptimal standard of care. However, if advanced imaging not available, standard metastatic skeletal survey may still provide valuable information since all of these methods help identify vertebrae compression fractures, and osteoporosis or osteopenia. These radiologic studies should also be performed in IgM monoclonal gammopathies if there is the strong clinical suspicion for IgM myeloma.

CT scanning of the chest, abdomen, and pelvis should be performed in cases of IgM gammopathy, since they are usually associated with lymphoproliferative disorders, which may involve the lymph nodes and spleen.

HISTORY AND PHYSICAL EVALUATION

A detailed history and physical examination should be obtained any time a monoclonal protein is identified. Certain signs and symptoms may help guide the evaluation and ultimately result in the appropriate diagnosis. For instance, patients presenting with bone pain, pathologic fractures, weight loss, and symptoms of hypercalcemia or acute renal failure are more likely to have multiple myeloma.[2] Alternatively, those with night sweats, epistaxis, and lymphadenopathy are more likely to have lymphoproliferative disorders such as Waldenström macroglobulinemia, marginal zone lymphoma, or chronic lymphocytic leukemia/small lymphocytic lymphoma.[22,57,82]

Other less common conditions may also be revealed by patient assessment. A diagnosis of AL amyloidosis may be indicated by the presence of edema, shortness of breath, hepatomegaly, peripheral neuropathy, carpal tunnel syndrome, autonomic dysfunction, periorbital purpura, and macroglossia[5,83] (Chapter 101). Skin rash, purpura, neuropathy, and Raynaud phenomenon should prompt evaluation for cryoglobulinemia (Chapter 102).[26] Those presenting with polyradiculoneuropathy, endocrinopathy, skin lesions like glomeruloid hemangiomatas, organomegaly, thrombocytosis, papilledema, edema, and sclerotic bone lesions may have POEMS syndrome.[4]

Importantly, one should never overlook the initial reason that led to the identification of the monoclonal protein. Most patients in whom a monoclonal protein is identified are asymptomatic. For these patients, the key to a correct diagnosis may be the reason for the initial testing for the monoclonal protein. In a case where a mildly elevated serum creatinine was the key factor, a nephrology evaluation with possible kidney biopsy may be the only way to diagnose MGRS such as immunoglobulin deposition disease of the kidney.[10,19,84] Monoclonal gammopathies are common in the elderly, who are also at risk for other pathologic conditions and are usually on multiple medications with their side effects. For example, mild hypercalcemia in association with a monoclonal protein may be due to parathyroid disease or medication in a patient with benign MGUS rather than myeloma. Renal failure or proteinuria in a hypertensive or diabetic patient with monoclonal protein should be investigated thoroughly before attributing it to the monoclonal protein. Such cases may require a kidney biopsy.

SUMMARY AND RECOMMENDATIONS

The diagnostic approach to monoclonal gammopathy should be thorough and involve a detailed history, physical examination, appropriate laboratory testing, and imaging. This should distinguish benign from clinically relevant conditions that need immediate intervention. A good understanding of conditions associated with monoclonal gammopathy is essential. Testing and evaluation should include:

- Serum and urine protein electrophoresis followed by immunofixation will confirm the presence of the monoclonal protein, identify and classify the isotype, and provide an estimation of the amount. Immunoglobulin free light assay will help identify cases with only free light chain production, but negative protein electrophoresis.
- Quantitative immunoglobulin of the involved isotype is helpful for monitoring.
- A bone marrow evaluation will determine the nature of the underlying B-lineage disorder (plasma cell or lymphoproliferative), the extent of marrow infiltration, and prognostic stratification by immunophenotypic, cytogenetic, and molecular findings.
- Complete blood count analysis is used to identify cytopenias, which may be due to bone marrow replacement or immune-mediated causes.
- Comprehensive metabolic panel looking at serum calcium, creatinine, bilirubin, lactate dehydrogenase, and liver transaminases is essential.
- Bone and soft-tissue imaging looking for bony lesions and soft tissue masses such as lymphadenopathy or plasmacytoma is required.
- A detailed history and physical evaluation should help direct further testing.

References

1. Kyle RA, Therneau TM, Rajkumar SV, et al. Prevalence of monoclonal gammopathy of undetermined significance. *N Engl J Med*. 2006;354(13):1362-1369.
2. Kyle RA, Rajkumar SV. Multiple myeloma. *N Engl J Med*. 2004;351(18):1860-1873.
3. Kyle RA, Rajkumar SV, Rajkumar SV. Management of monoclonal gammopathy of undetermined significance (MGUS) and smoldering multiple myeloma (SMM). *Oncology (Williston Park)*. 2011;25(7):578-586.
4. Dispenzieri A. POEMS syndrome: 2021 update on diagnosis, risk-stratification, and management. *Am J Hematol*. 2021;96(7):872-888.
5. Kyle RA, Linos A, Beard CM, et al. Incidence and natural history of primary systemic amyloidosis in Olmsted County, Minnesota, 1950 through 1989. *Blood*. 1992;79(7):1817-1822.
6. Wood AJ, Wagner MVU, Abbott JJ, Gibson LE. Necrobiotic xanthogranuloma: a review of 17 cases with emphasis on clinical and pathologic correlation. *Arch Dermatol*. 2009;145(3):279-284.
7. Sethi S, Fervenza FC. Membranoproliferative glomerulonephritis—a new look at an old entity. *N Engl J Med*. 2012;366(12):1119-1131.
8. Pomann JJ, Rudner EJ. Scleromyxedema revisited. *Int J Dermatol*. 2003;42(1):31-35.
9. Cokonis Georgakis CD, Falasca G, Georgakis A, Heymann WR. Scleromyxedema. *Clin Dermatol*. 2006;24(6):493-497.
10. Leung N, Bridoux F, Nasr SH. Monoclonal gammopathy of renal significance. *N Engl J Med*. 2021;384(20):1931-1941.
11. Schuster SR, Rajkumar SV, Dispenzieri A, et al. IgM multiple myeloma: disease definition, prognosis, and differentiation from Waldenstrom's macroglobulinemia. *Am J Hematol*. 2010;85(11):853-855.
12. Dispenzieri A, Katzmann JA, Kyle RA, et al. Prevalence and risk of progression of light-chain monoclonal gammopathy of undetermined significance: a retrospective population-based cohort study. *Lancet*. 2010;375(9727):1721-1728.
13. Rajkumar SV, Dimopoulos MA, Palumbo A, et al. International Myeloma Working Group updated criteria for the diagnosis of multiple myeloma. *Lancet Oncol*. 2014;15(12):e538-e548.
14. Kyle RA, Rajkumar SV. Monoclonal gammopathy of undetermined significance. *Br J Haematol*. 2006;134(6):573-589.
15. Sidiqi MH, Aljama M, Kumar SK, et al. The role of bone marrow biopsy in patients with plasma cell disorders: should all patients with a monoclonal protein be biopsied? *Blood Cancer J*. 2020;10(5):52.
16. Dagan R, Morris CG, Kirwan J, Mendenhall WM. Solitary plasmacytoma. *Am J Clin Oncol*. 2009;32(6):612-617.
17. Buxbaum J, Gallo G. Nonamyloidotic monoclonal immunoglobulin deposition disease. Light-chain, heavy-chain, and light- and heavy-chain deposition diseases. *Hematol Oncol Clin North Am*. 1999;13(6):1235-1248.
18. Skalicka P, Dudakova L, Palos M, et al. Paraproteinemic keratopathy associated with monoclonal gammopathy of undetermined significance (MGUS): clinical findings in twelve patients including recurrence after keratoplasty. *Acta Ophthalmol*. 2019;97(7):e987-e992.
19. Bridoux F, Leung N, Hutchison CA, et al. Diagnosis of monoclonal gammopathy of renal significance. *Kidney Int*. 2015;87(4):698-711.
20. Gallo G, Goni F, Boctor F, et al. Light chain cardiomyopathy. Structural analysis of the light chain tissue deposits. *Am J Pathol*. 1996;148(5):1397-1406.
21. Kyle RA, Garton JP. The spectrum of IgM monoclonal gammopathy in 430 cases. *Mayo Clin Proc*. 1987;62(8):719-731.
22. Owen RG, Treon SP, Al-Katib A, et al. Clinicopathological definition of Waldenstrom's macroglobulinemia: consensus panel recommendations from the Second International Workshop on Waldenstrom's Macroglobulinemia. *Semin Oncol*. 2003;30(2):110-115.
23. Treon SP, Xu L, Yang G, et al. MYD88 L265P somatic mutation in Waldenstrom's macroglobulinemia. *N Engl J Med*. 2012;367(9):826-833.
24. Chahin N, Selcen D, Engel AG. Sporadic late onset nemaline myopathy. *Neurology*. 2005;65(8):1158-1164.
25. Kyle RA. Monoclonal proteins in neuropathy. *Neurol Clin*. 1992;10(3):713-734.
26. Cuellar ML, Garcia C, Molina JF. Cryoglobulinemia and other dysproteinemias, familial Mediterranean fever, and POEMS syndrome. *Curr Opin Rheumatol*. 1995;7(1):58-64.
27. Jain T, Offord CP, Kyle RA, Dingli D. Schnitzler syndrome: an under-diagnosed clinical entity. *Haematologica*. 2013;98(10):1581-1585.
28. Sykes DB, Schroyens W, O'Connell C. The TEMPI syndrome—a novel multisystem disease. *N Engl J Med*. 2011;365(5):475-477.
29. Sykes DB, O'Connell C, Schroyens W. The TEMPI syndrome. *Blood*. 2020;135(15):1199-1203.
30. Beck DB, Ferrada MA, Sikora KA, et al. Somatic mutations in UBA1 and severe adult-onset autoinflammatory disease. *N Engl J Med*. 2020;383(27):2628-2638.

31. Grayson PC, Patel BA, Young NS. VEXAS syndrome. *Blood.* 2021;137(26):3591-3594.
32. Katzmann JA, Kyle RA, Benson J, et al. Screening panels for detection of monoclonal gammopathies. *Clin Chem.* 2009;55(8):1517-1522.
33. Katzmann JA, Clark R, Wiegert E, et al. Identification of monoclonal proteins in serum: a quantitative comparison of acetate, agarose gel, and capillary electrophoresis. *Electrophoresis.* 1997;18(10):1775-1780.
34. Jenkins MA, Guerin MD. Capillary electrophoresis procedures for serum protein analysis: comparison with established techniques. *J Chromatogr B Biomed Sci Appl.* 1997;699(1-2):257-268.
35. Dispenzieri A, Gertz MA, Therneau TM, Kyle RA. Retrospective cohort study of 148 patients with polyclonal gammopathy. *Mayo Clin Proc.* 2001;76(5):476-487.
36. Litwin CM, Anderson SK, Philipps G, Martins TB, Jaskowski TD, Hill HR. Comparison of capillary zone and immunosubtraction with agarose gel and immunofixation electrophoresis for detecting and identifying monoclonal gammopathies. *Am J Clin Pathol.* 1999;112(3):411-417.
37. Mills JR, Kohlhagen MC, Dasari S, et al. Comprehensive assessment of M-proteins using nanobody enrichment coupled to MALDI-TOF mass spectrometry. *Clin Chem.* 2016;62(10):1334-1344.
38. Kyle RA, Robinson RA, Katzmann JA. The clinical aspects of biclonal gammopathies. Review of 57 cases. *Am J Med.* 1981;71(6):999-1008.
39. Barnidge DR, Dasari S, Botz CM, et al. Using mass spectrometry to monitor monoclonal immunoglobulins in patients with a monoclonal gammopathy. *J Proteome Res.* 2014;13(3):1419-1427.
40. Kohlhagen MC, Barnidge DR, Mills JR, et al. Screening method for M-proteins in serum using nanobody enrichment coupled to MALDI-TOF mass spectrometry. *Clin Chem.* 2016;62(10):1345-1352.
41. Visram A, Vaxman I, S Al Saleh A, et al. Disease monitoring with quantitative serum IgA levels provides a more reliable response assessment in multiple myeloma patients. *Leukemia.* 2021;35(5):1428-1437.
42. Pascali E, Pezzoli A. The clinical spectrum of pure Bence Jones proteinuria. A study of 66 patients. *Cancer.* 1988;62(11):2408-2415.
43. Drayson M, Tang LX, Drew R, Mead GP, Carr-Smith H, Bradwell AR. Serum free light-chain measurements for identifying and monitoring patients with nonsecretory multiple myeloma. *Blood.* 2001;97(9):2900-2902.
44. Katzmann JA, Abraham RS, Dispenzieri A, Lust JA, Kyle RA. Diagnostic performance of quantitative kappa and lambda free light chain assays in clinical practice. *Clin Chem.* 2005;51(5):878-881.
45. Katzmann JA, Dispenzieri A, Kyle RA, et al. Elimination of the need for urine studies in the screening algorithm for monoclonal gammopathies by using serum immunofixation and free light chain assays. *Mayo Clin Proc.* 2006;81(12):1575-1578.
46. Rajkumar SV, Kyle RA, Therneau TM, et al. Serum free light chain ratio is an independent risk factor for progression in monoclonal gammopathy of undetermined significance. *Blood.* 2005;106(3):812-817.
47. Lakshman A, Rajkumar SV, Buadi FK, et al. Risk stratification of smoldering multiple myeloma incorporating revised IMWG diagnostic criteria. *Blood Cancer J.* 2018;8(6):59.
48. Dingli D, Kyle RA, Rajkumar SV, et al. Immunoglobulin-free light chains and solitary plasmacytoma of bone. *Blood.* 2006;108(6):1979-1983.
49. Bradwell AR, Carr-Smith HD, Mead GP, Harvey TC, Drayson MT. Serum test for assessment of patients with Bence Jones myeloma. *Lancet.* 2003;361(9356):489-491.
50. Lachmann HJ, Gallimore R, Gillmore JD, et al. Outcome in systemic AL amyloidosis in relation to changes in concentration of circulating free immunoglobulin light chains following chemotherapy. *Br J Haematol.* 2003;122(1):78-84.
51. Dispenzieri A, Kyle R, Merlini G, et al. International Myeloma Working Group guidelines for serum-free light chain analysis in multiple myeloma and related disorders. *Leukemia.* 2009;23(2):215-224.
52. Lock RJ, Saleem R, Roberts EG, et al. A multicentre study comparing two methods for serum free light chain analysis. *Ann Clin Biochem.* 2013;50(pt 3):255-261.
53. Leung N, Gertz M, Kyle RA, et al. Urinary albumin excretion patterns of patients with cast nephropathy and other monoclonal gammopathy-related kidney diseases. *Clin J Am Soc Nephrol.* 2012;7(12):1964-1968.
54. Bartl R, Frisch B, Burkhardt R, et al. Bone marrow histology in myeloma: its importance in diagnosis, prognosis, classification and staging. *Br J Haematol.* 1982;51(3):361-375.
55. Rajkumar SV, Harousseau JL, Durie B, et al. Consensus recommendations for the uniform reporting of clinical trials: report of the International Myeloma Workshop Consensus Panel 1. *Blood.* 2011;117(18):4691-4695.
56. Nadav L, Katz BZ, Baron S, et al. Diverse niches within multiple myeloma bone marrow aspirates affect plasma cell enumeration. *Br J Haematol.* 2006;133(5):530-532.
57. Ansell SM, Kyle RA, Reeder CB, et al. Diagnosis and management of Waldenstrom macroglobulinemia: Mayo stratification of macroglobulinemia and risk-adapted therapy (mSMART) guidelines. *Mayo Clin Proc.* 2010;85(9):824-833.
58. Lin P, Owens R, Tricot G, Wilson CS. Flow cytometric immunophenotypic analysis of 306 cases of multiple myeloma. *Am J Clin Pathol.* 2004;121(4):482-488.
59. Landgren O, Devlin S, Boulad M, Mailankody S. Role of MRD status in relation to clinical outcomes in newly diagnosed multiple myeloma patients: a meta-analysis. *Bone Marrow Transplant.* 2016;51(12):1565-1568.
60. Munshi NC, Avet-Loiseau H, Rawstron AC, et al. Association of minimal residual disease with superior survival outcomes in patients with multiple myeloma: a meta-analysis. *JAMA Oncol.* 2017;3(1):28-35.
61. Munshi NC, Avet-Loiseau H, Anderson KC, et al. A large meta-analysis establishes the role of MRD negativity in long-term survival outcomes in patients with multiple myeloma. *Blood Adv.* 2020;4(23):5988-5999.
62. Goicoechea I, Puig N, Cedena MT, et al. Deep MRD profiling defines outcome and unveils different modes of treatment resistance in standard- and high-risk myeloma. *Blood.* 2021;137(1):49-60.
63. Perrot A, Lauwers-Cances V, Corre J, et al. Minimal residual disease negativity using deep sequencing is a major prognostic factor in multiple myeloma. *Blood.* 2018;132(23):2456-2464.
64. Paiva B, Vidriales MB, Mateo G, et al. The persistence of immunophenotypically normal residual bone marrow plasma cells at diagnosis identifies a good prognostic subgroup of symptomatic multiple myeloma patients. *Blood.* 2009;114(20):4369-4372.
65. Chakraborty R, Muchtar E, Kumar SK, et al. Risk stratification in myeloma by detection of circulating plasma cells prior to autologous stem cell transplantation in the novel agent era. *Blood Cancer J.* 2016;6(12):e512.
66. Gonsalves WI, Rajkumar SV, Gupta V, et al. Quantification of clonal circulating plasma cells in newly diagnosed multiple myeloma: implications for redefining high-risk myeloma. *Leukemia.* 2014;28(10):2060-2065.
67. Avet-Loiseau H. Role of genetics in prognostication in myeloma. *Best Pract Res Clin Haematol.* 2007;20(4):625-635.
68. Fonseca R, Blood E, Rue M, et al. Clinical and biologic implications of recurrent genomic aberrations in myeloma. *Blood.* 2003;101(11):4569-4575.
69. Nair B, Shaughnessy JD Jr, Zhou Y, et al. Gene expression profiling of plasma cells at myeloma relapse from tandem transplantation trial Total Therapy 2 predicts subsequent survival. *Blood.* 2009;113(26):6572-6575.
70. Waheed S, Shaughnessy JD, van Rhee F, et al. International staging system and metaphase cytogenetic abnormalities in the era of gene expression profiling data in multiple myeloma treated with total therapy 2 and 3 protocols. *Cancer.* 2011;117(5):1001-1009.
71. Magy-Bertrand N, Dupond JL, Mauny F, et al. Incidence of amyloidosis over 3 years: the AMYPRO study. *Clin Exp Rheumatol.* 2008;26(6):1074-1078.
72. Klein CJ, Vrana JA, Theis JD, et al. Mass spectrometric-based proteomic analysis of amyloid neuropathy type in nerve tissue. *Arch Neurol.* 2011;68(2):195-199.
73. Vrana JA, Gamez JD, Madden BJ, Theis JD, Bergen HR III, Dogan A. Classification of amyloidosis by laser microdissection and mass spectrometry based proteomic analysis in clinical biopsy specimens. *Blood.* 2009;114(24):4957-4959.
74. Hillengass J, Usmani S, Rajkumar SV, et al. International myeloma working group consensus recommendations on imaging in monoclonal plasma cell disorders. *Lancet Oncol.* 2019;20(6):e302-e312.
75. Dimopoulos MA, Moulopoulos LA, Datseris I, et al. Imaging of myeloma bone disease—implications for staging, prognosis and follow-up. *Acta Oncol.* 2000;39(7):823-827.
76. Roodman GD. Skeletal imaging and management of bone disease. *Hematology Am Soc Hematol Educ Program.* 2008;2008:313-319.
77. Dimopoulos M, Terpos E, Comenzo RL, et al. International myeloma working group consensus statement and guidelines regarding the current role of imaging techniques in the diagnosis and monitoring of multiple Myeloma. *Leukemia.* 2009;23(9):1545-1556.
78. Pianko MJ, Terpos E, Roodman GD, et al. Whole-body low-dose computed tomography and advanced imaging techniques for multiple myeloma bone disease. *Clin Cancer Res.* 2014;20(23):5888-5897.
79. Princewill K, Kyere S, Awan O, Mulligan M. Multiple myeloma lesion detection with whole body CT versus radiographic skeletal survey. *Cancer Invest.* 2013;31(3):206-211.
80. Zamagni E, Nanni C, Patriarca F, et al. A prospective comparison of 18F-fluorodeoxyglucose positron emission tomography-computed tomography, magnetic resonance imaging and whole-body planar radiographs in the assessment of bone disease in newly diagnosed multiple myeloma. *Haematologica.* 2007;92(1):50-55.
81. Salaun PY, Gastinne T, Frampas E, Bodet-Milin C, Moreau P, Bodere-Kraeber F. FDG-positron-emission tomography for staging and therapeutic assessment in patients with plasmacytoma. *Haematologica.* 2008;93(8):1269-1271.
82. Pangalis GA, Angelopoulou MK, Vassilakopoulos TP, Siakantaris MP, Kittas C. B-chronic lymphocytic leukemia, small lymphocytic lymphoma, and lymphoplasmacytic lymphoma, including Waldenstrom's macroglobulinemia: a clinical, morphologic, and biologic spectrum of similar disorders. *Semin Hematol.* 1999;36(2):104-114.
83. Gertz MA, Rajkumar SV. Primary systemic amyloidosis. *Curr Treat Options Oncol.* 2002;3(3):261-271.
84. Nasr SH, Valeri AM, Cornell LD, et al. Renal monoclonal immunoglobulin deposition disease: a report of 64 patients from a single institution. *Clin J Am Soc Nephrol.* 2012;7(2):231-239.

Chapter 98 ■ Molecular Genetic Aspects of Plasma Cell Disorders

PETER LEIF BERGSAGEL • LINDA B. BAUGHN • DRAGAN JEVREMOVIC • YAN ASMANN

INTRODUCTION

Multiple myeloma (MM) is an age-dependent monoclonal tumor of the bone marrow (BM) plasma cells (PCs), often with significant end-organ damage that can include lytic bone lesions, anemia, loss of kidney function, immunodeficiency, and amyloid deposits in various tissues. It has an estimated incidence of 34,920 in 2021, with 12,410 deaths in the United States.[1] Despite recent therapeutic advances, MM continues to be a mostly incurable disease but with a five-year survival rate reported in the surveillance, epidemiology, and end results program (SEER) database that has nearly doubled over the last 20 years, going from 27% (1987-1989) to 56% (2011-2017).[2] In fact, a subset of younger patients initially treated in 1999 can be identified with a 10-year survival rate of 75%,[3] with presumably even better results possible for patients starting treatment today. The incidence of both MM and MGUS is ~2-3-fold higher in Blacks compared to Whites, and in men than women.[2,4,5] In addition, the onset of MGUS and MM in Blacks occurs ~4 years prior to the onset in Whites.[6-8] It is evident from the SEER registry data that although the incidence of MM continues to rise with an annual percentage change of close to 1%, since 1994, the mortality rate has generally been decreasing likely due to the use of novel modern treatments and transplantation.

PLASMA CELL DEVELOPMENT

PCs are terminally differentiated B lymphocytes, each carrying a unique immunoglobulin (Ig) heavy and light chain sequence. The uniqueness of Igs is achieved by a combination of two temporally separated mutagenic processes (*Figure 98.1*):

1. VDJ rearrangement of the Ig heavy chains and VJ rearrangement of Ig light chains during the B-cell development. Ig loci at 14q32.33 (heavy chain, IgH), 2p11.2 (kappa, IgK), and 22q11.22 (lambda, IgL) are composed of multiple segments. In the initial stages of B-cell development in the BM, recombination-activating genes (RAG1/2) DNA recombinase introduces double-stranded DNA breaks in the Ig genes. These breaks result in hairpin formation of the DNA chain and juxtaposition of a single V, (D), and J segments with excision of the interposed DNA. Subsequently, DNA breaks are repaired by a nonhomologous end-joining mechanism, thus contributing to diversity in the DNA sequence.

2. Somatic hypermutation (SHM) and class switch recombination (CSR) upon antigen encounter, that is, germinal center (GC) reaction. When a B cell encounters an antigen, which binds to its unique Ig surface receptor, it migrates to the T-cell–rich areas of the lymphoid follicles and initiates formation of germinal centers. This reaction is characterized by marked proliferation of the B-cell clone. On the subcellular level, there occurs the second round of DNA modifications mediated by activation-induced cytidine deaminase (AID). CSR juxtaposes the unique VDJ sequence of the heavy chain away from the Ig mu constant region and instead joins it with Ig gamma, alpha, or epsilon constant regions. This results in Igs with different effector functions, an important feature of the adaptive immune system. At the same time, VDJ segments of the IgH locus are targets of AID that converts cytidine into uracil. This triggers an error-prone DNA repair mechanism and results in SHM, with multiple new but closely related DNA sequences. As multiple related clones move from the dark to the light zone of the germinal center, they are surrounded with follicular dendritic cells (FDCs) expressing antigens on the surface. Only clones with sufficiently high avidity to the antigen found on FDCs survive this process and differentiate into memory B cells or migrate to the BM, where stromal cells facilitate terminal differentiation into long-lived PC.[9]

MULTIPLE MYELOMA IS A PLASMA CELL TUMOR OF POSTGERMINAL CENTER B CELLS

MM cells and their precursors are similar to postgerminal center (GC) long-lived PCs, characterized by strong BM dependence, extensive SHM of Ig genes, and absence of IgM expression in all but 1% of tumors.[10] However, MM cells differ from healthy PCs because they retain the potential for a low rate of proliferation (1%-3% of cycling cells). Further, the two processes described above, mainly SHM and CSR, mediated by AID create the potential to generate oncogenic events that will be further described below.[10] In addition, these two processes produce PCs with unique Ig sequence, which can be followed during the process of malignant transformation resulting in a PC disorder. Secreted Igs by PCs can be detected in serum, and its protein sequence is identical to that of the Ig receptor on PCs, as both are encoded by the same unique DNA sequence. This uniqueness enables

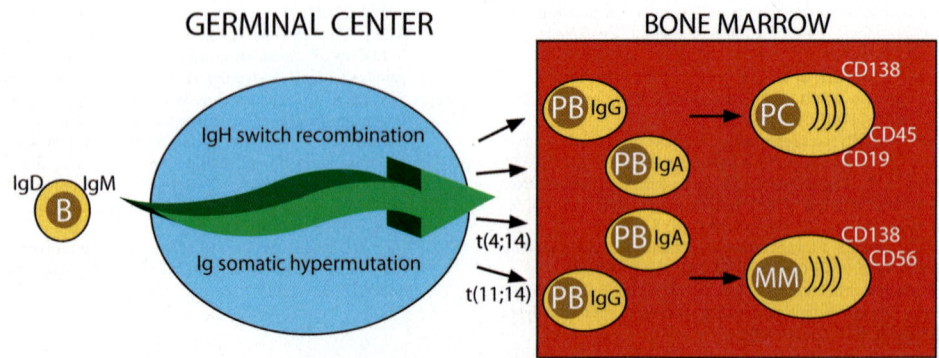

FIGURE 98.1 Normal and malignant plasma cell development. Pregerminal center (GC) B cells expressing surface immunoglobulin can enter germinal centers where the immunoglobulin genes undergo repeated rounds of somatic hypermutation followed by IgH isotype switch recombination. In multiple myeloma (MM), IgH translocations occur as a result of errors in these two physiologic DNA modification processes (10% and 90%, respectively). Post-GC B cells can generate plasmablast that homes to the bone marrow where stromal cells facilitate differentiation into long-lived PC. Normal plasma cell (PC) expresses surface CD138, CD19, and CD45, whereas MM cells express CD138, only 10% express CD19, 99% are CD45⁻ or dim, and 70% express CD56. Ig, immunoglobulin; PB, plasmablasts.

close follow-up of the evolution of a PC disorder and is also used in mass spectrometry assessment of the Ig in the serum, as well as minimal residual disease detection by sequencing methods.

As is the case with other malignancies, genetic changes observed in PC disorders are complex. In fact, the more sophisticated genetic tools are used such as whole genome sequencing (WGS), the more it becomes obvious how complex they are. However, there are still major limitations for the use of high-resolution technologies in routine clinical practice. As new clinical trials assess the role of particular genetic changes as prognostic (survival) and predictive (therapy specific) markers, the more of the "research" genetic markers are moving into clinical practice. Much of the data we have about the clinical impact of genetic changes in PC disorders have been derived from low-resolution techniques, namely chromosome and fluorescence in situ hybridization (FISH) studies.

EARLY GENETIC ABNORMALITIES IN MULTIPLE MYELOMA

Seven Primary IgH Translocations Are an Early Oncogenic Event in Multiple Myeloma and Its Precursor Conditions

Like other B-cell tumors, translocations involving the IgH locus are common in PC disorders and represent early primary genetic events. It seems likely that these events are mediated by errors in IgH CSR or SHM, since >90% of breakpoints in PC disorders are located near or within IgH switch regions characterizing them as postgerminal center cells, but sometimes near VDJ sequences.[11,12] Since there is no evidence that IgH CSR or SHM mechanisms mediated by AID are active in normal PC or PC tumors, it is presumed that these translocations usually represent primary—perhaps initiating—oncogenic events as normal B cells pass through GCs on their path toward affinity maturation.[13] The translocations result in dysregulated or increased expression of an oncogene that is positioned near one or more of the strong Ig enhancers. However, translocations involving an IgH switch region uniquely dissociate the intronic from one or both 3′ IgH enhancers, so that an oncogene might be juxtaposed to an IgH enhancer on either or both of the derivative chromosomes, as first demonstrated for *FGFR3* on der(14) and *NSD2* (*MMSET*) on der(4) in MM. Rarely, tumors can have translocations involving two of the primary translocation groups, such as both t(4;14) and t(14;16) within the same cell, suggesting that there can be some complementation.[14]

There are three recurrent primary IgH translocation groups that target oncogenes with an approximate prevalence in MM (~40% prevalence for all three groups) as follows: *CYCLIN D* (11q13-*CYCLIN D1*-15%; 12p13-*CYCLIN D2*- < 1%; 6p25-*CYCLIN D3*-2%); *MAF* (16q23-*MAF*-5%; 20q12-*MAFB*-2%; 8q24.3-*MAFA*-< 1%; and *NSD2/(FGFR3)*-4p16-(*NSD2* in all but also *FGFR3* in 80% of these tumors)-15%.[10,15] (Table 98.1). These recurrent IgH translocations are efficiently detected by dual-color, dual-fusion FISH probes. Large studies from several groups show that the prevalence of IgH translocations increases with disease stage: about 50% in MGUS or SMM, 55% to 70% for intramedullary MM, 85% in PCL, and >90% in human myeloma cell lines (HMCLs).[10] In addition, single-nucleotide polymorphism, rs9344 within the *CCND1* gene, has been identified as a germline risk factor associated with increased risk of t(11;14) MM.[16] Further, an increased prevalence of the rs9344 risk allele along with t(11;14) and *MAF* translocations has been found in association with African ancestry.[8,17,18]

Chromosome Content Is Associated With at Least Two Different Oncogenic Pathways

Chromosome content reflects at least two pathways of pathogenesis[15] (Figure 98.2). Nearly half of MGUS and MM tumors are hyperdiploid (HRD), with 48 to 75 (mostly 49-56) chromosomes, usually with extra copies of three or more specific "odd-numbered" chromosomes (3,5,7,9,11,15,19,21). The other half of MGUS and MM tumors are nonhyperdiploid (NHRD) with <48 and/or >75 chromosomes when their chromosome content has doubled representing a tetraploidy.[19] Strikingly, HRD tumors rarely (<10%) have a primary IgH translocation, whereas NHRD tumors usually (>70%) have an IgH translocation.[20] Tumors with a t(11;14) may represent a distinct category of NHRD tumors as they often are diploid or tetraploid. Curiously, extramedullary tumors and MM cell lines nearly always have a NHRD genotype, suggesting that HRD tumors are more stromal cell dependent than NHRD tumors. Although it has been proposed that NHRD and HRD tumors represent different pathways of pathogenesis, the timing, mechanism, and molecular consequences of hyperdiploidy is unknown. Interestingly, in patients with t(4;14) or t(14;16) or t(14;20) or del(17p), the presence of one or more trisomies is associated with a substantially better prognosis than with the absence of trisomies. This suggests that the phenotype associated with trisomies may be dominant.[21] Hyperdiploidy is usually detected by FISH using probes directed toward the centromere regions of certain odd-numbered chromosomes or in some instances, by flow cytometry.[22] In rare instances, MM tumors can be hyperhaploid with 24 to 34 chromosomes, and usually also lack a primary IgH translocation. This high-risk subtype is also often characterized by *TP53* mutations.[23-26]

SECONDARY ONCOGENIC EVENTS ASSOCIATED WITH PROGRESSION OF MGUS TO MULTIPLE MYELOMA

MYC Dysregulation

Increased expression of c-*MYC* has been observed in most newly diagnosed MM tumors compared to MGUS cells.[27] Sporadic activation of a *MYC* transgene in GC B cells in the C57Bl/6 MGUS prone, but not the Balb/c, mouse strain led to the universal development of MM tumors.[28,29] Hence, increased *MYC* expression seems to be responsible for progression from MGUS to MM.[30] Complex rearrangements involving *MYC* (c-*MYC* >> N-*MYC* > L-*MYC*) appear to be secondary progression events that involve Ig loci in about 40% of cases with the remaining 60% involving non-Ig enhancer sequences.[31-34] *MYC* rearrangements are rare or absent in MGUS, but occur in 30% to 45% of newly diagnosed MM and 90% of MM cell lines and have been reported in the progression from SMM to MM.[30,31,33,35,36] There are numerous types of *MYC* rearrangements in MM and most (50%-70%) are cryptic and not detected by interphase FISH using the *MYC* break apart probe, with the remainder only detected by higher resolution studies included targeted or WGS.[32,37] The frequency of *MYC* rearrangements varies considerably across different primary genetic subtypes, with a low frequency (22%) in t(11;14) and a high frequency (63%) in the HRD TC D1 subtype (see Table 98.2).[34]

About 60% of the *MYC* rearrangements involve a promiscuous array of loci characterized by the presence of superenhancers, many PC specific (the most common include *NSMCE2*, *TXNDC5*,

Table 98.1. Frequency of Cytogenetic Categories in Multiple Myeloma

Primary Cytogenetic Category	
Hyperdiploid	50%
Nonhyperdiploid	40%
Cyclin D translocations	
t(11;14) (q13;q32) *CCND1/IGH*	16%
t(6;14) (p25;q32) *CCND3/IGH*	3%
t(12;14) (p13;q32) *CCND2/IGH*	<1%
NSD2 translocations	15%
t(4;14) (p16;q32) NSD2 ± FGFR3/IGH	
MAF translocations	
t(14;16) (q32;q23) *IGH/MAF*	5%
t(14;20) (q32;q11) *IGH/MAFB*	2%
t(8;14) (q24;q32) *MAFA/IGH*	<1%
Unclassified (other)	10%

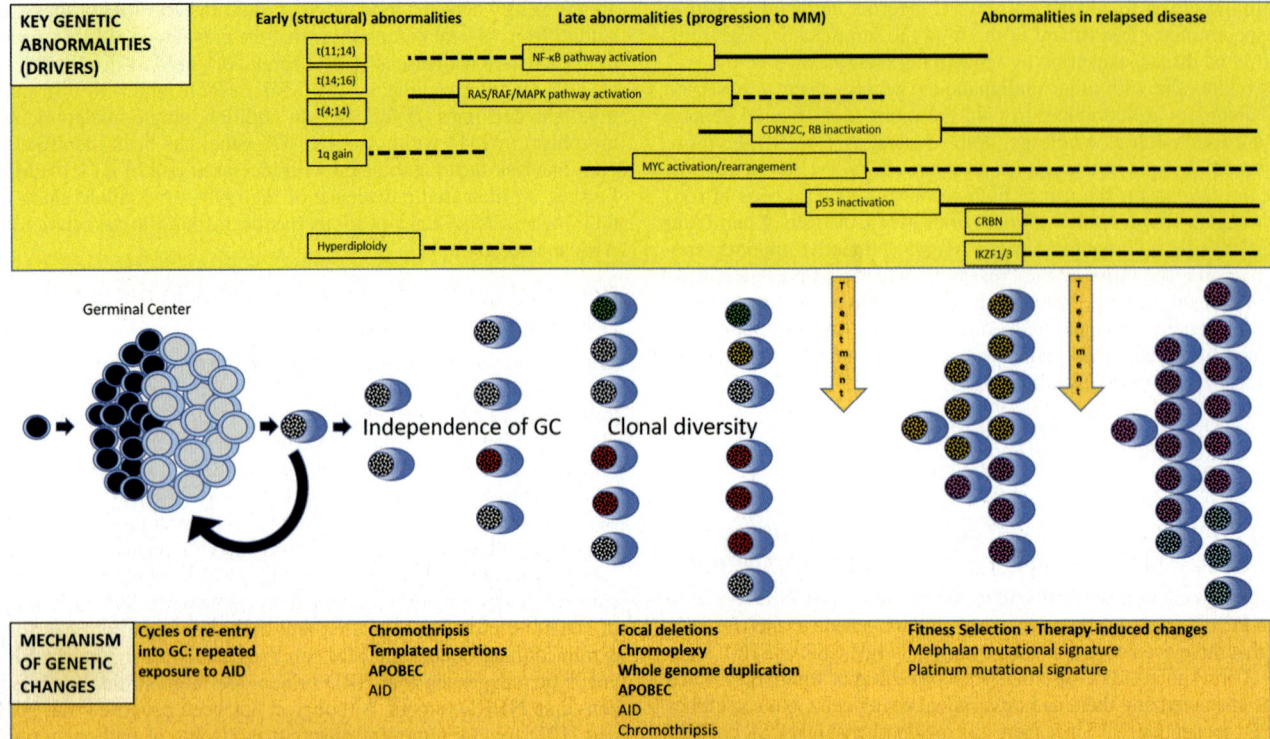

FIGURE 98.2 A model for the multistep molecular pathogenesis of multiple myeloma. Initiating events in the development of MGUS include immunoglobulin [Ig] translocations and multiple trisomies; these are likely driven by re-entry of plasma cells into germinal centers (GCs) and their repeated exposure to mutagenic activities of activation–induced cytidine deaminase (AID). Clonal plasma cells establish their residence in the bone marrow microenvironment and retain a low proliferative activity. As the clone slowly grows, it accumulates additional genetic changes, both point mutations and larger structural changes, including catastrophic events such as chromothripsis. These genetic changes activate important driver genes/pathways (cyclin D, NFκB, RAS/MAPK, MYC) adding to the proliferative and/or survival advantage of the clone. At this stage multiple different subclones emerge, some of which may become dominant at a later stage (post-therapy). A combination of genetic and epigenetic changes within clonal plasma cells, and interaction with the bone microenvironment and the immune system, eventually results in a clinically evident progression of MGUS to MM. Additional genetic changes can be introduced by chemotherapy (melphalan). Under selective pressure from proteasome inhibitors and immune modulators, resistant clones emerge late in the disease.

Table 98.2. Comparison of Different Molecular Classifications in Multiple Myeloma

Group	TC	Gene	%	CYCLIN D[38]	UAMS[39]	HOVON-GMMG[40]
Cyclin D translocation	11q13	*CCND1*	16	CYCLIN D1	CD-1 CD-2	CD-1 CD-2
	12p13	*CCND2*	<1	CYCLIN D2		
	6p25	*CCND3*	3	CYCLIN D3		
MAF translocation	16q23	*MAF*	5	CYCLIN D2	MF	MF
	20q12	*MAFB*	2	CYCLIN D2		
	8q24	*MAFA*	<1	CYCLIN D2		
NSD2 translocation	4p16	*NSD2/FGFR3*	15	CYCLIN D2	MS	MS
Hyperdiploid with trisomy 11	D1	*CCND1*	33	CYCLIN D1	HY	HY CD-1 NFκB CTA PRL3
	D1 + D2	*CCND1, CCND2*	7	CYCLIN D1 and D2	PR	PR, CTA
Hyperdiploid without trisomy 11 and others	D2	*CCND2*	18	CYCLIN D2	LB	LB, CTA, PRL3
Other	None	*RB1* biallelic deletion	2	No CYCLIN D	PR	PR, CTA

FAM46C (TENT5C), CSMD3, FOXO3, PRDM1). These superenhancers are characterized by long stretches of acetylated H3K27 that bind the acetyl-reader BRD4. Small molecule acetyl-mimic bromo-domain inhibitors can displace BRD4 from superenhancers leading to downregulation of *MYC* RNA expression and show therapeutic efficacy in preclinical models of MM.[41] In addition, lenalidomide and pomalidomide have been shown to degrade Ikaros and Aiolos in a cereblon-dependent fashion, leading to downregulation of MYC and IRF4.[42,43] This likely represents an important mechanism of action of immunomodulatory drugs (IMiDs) in MM and likely underlies their relatively greater efficacy in HRD MM.[44] Somatic mutations of *MYC* are rare,[32] but mutations in *MYC* pathway members *IRF4* and *MAX*, each in about 3% of patients, have characteristics of oncogenes (no loss of heterozygosity, recurrent hotspots) and may potentially substitute for MYC dysregulation in some patients.[45] Certain *MYC* subtypes appear to be associated with improved survival outcomes, while *MYC*/IgL translocations have been associated with poorer survival outcomes.[30-32,46] The poor outcome associated with IgL rearrangements is likely associated with the strong association of Ikaros to the IgL locus rendering cases with IgL rearrangements less sensitive to IMiD treatment.[46]

Chromosome 17p Loss and Abnormalities of TP53

Deletions that include the TP53 locus at 17p occur in ~7% of untreated MM tumors, and the prevalence increases with disease stage and is associated with extramedullary disease.[12,47] Overall, TP53 mutations are found in about 5% of newly diagnosed MM. Importantly, TP53 mutations are found in a higher frequency (37%) of untreated MM tumors with del(17p).[48] Thus, the poor prognosis associated with del(17p) appears to be a result of inactivation of TP53, as poor prognosis was found in patients with biallelic deletion of 17p, or monoallelic deletion together with a TP53 mutation, but not in those with only a heterozygous del(17p) or TP53 mutation.[47,49]

Gain of Chromosome 1q and Loss of Chromosome 1p

The prevalence of gain (three total copies) or amplification (four or more total copies) of 1q is about 30% of patients with SMM and 40% in untreated MM.[3,50] Gain or amplification of 1q appears to be an independent risk factor for progression from SMM to MM. Although the relevant gene(s) on 1q are not fully understood, some potential candidates include CKS1B (a cell cycle regulator), MCL-1 (an antiapoptosis BCL2 family member), and ADAR1 (an RNA editing protein).[50] Amplification of 1q is considered a high-risk cytogenetic abnormality associated with poor survival, while gain of 1q does not appear to be as detrimental as 1q amplification.[50-53]

Deletion 1p occurs in 20% to 25% of MM and has been associated with poor outcome.[54] There are potential targets on two regions of 1p that are associated with a poor prognosis: CDKN2C (p18INK4c) at 1p32.3 in 11%, and FAM46C at 1p12 in 19% of cases. Homozygous deletion of CDKN2C, which is present in about 30% of HMCL and about 4% of untreated and 6% of relapsed MM tumors, is associated with increased proliferation and a poor prognosis, whereas monoallelic deletion is not.[55] Mutations of FAM46C—often with hemizygous deletion—were identified in 5% of MM tumors, and in 25% of 16 HMCLs.[45,55]

Chromosome 13 Deletion

Deletion of chromosome 13, presenting as either monosomy 13 or deletion of a portion of the long arm of chromosome 13 (13q del) occurs in about half of MM tumors.[12,56] Deletion of chromosome 13 can be an early event in MGUS (e.g., in MAF, NSD2 tumors) or a progression event (for example, in t(11;14) tumors).[57] It is much more frequent in t(4;14) (90%) and MAF (68%) than in t(11;14) (28%) or HRD with trisomy 11 (20%). The pathogenic effect of this chromosome deletion is unknown, although important genes on chromosome 13 implicated in MM pathogenesis include RB1, DLEU2/miR-15a/16-1 locus, and DIS3. Mostly missense (>90%) and presumably hypomorphic mutations of the exoribonuclease DIS3, only about half of which are associated with loss of heterozygosity, have been identified in about 10% patients.[45,58] These characteristics suggest that the mutation is a dominant one and that DIS3 is an oncogene and not a tumor suppressor gene in MM. Abnormalities of chromosome 13 appeared to have prognostic significance independent of high-risk cytogenetics although monosomy 13 and deletion 13q appear to have opposite effects on outcome.[59] The poor outcome associated with chromosome 13 deletion may be overcome by the use of proteasome inhibitors (PIs)[12]; therefore, deletion of chromosome 13 is considered a neutral prognostic marker.

Light Chain Rearrangements

Secondary Ig translocations, including most IgK and IgL (kappa, 2p11.2 or lambda, 22q11.2) and IgH translocations not involving one of the seven primary partners, can occur at all stages of disease, and with a similar frequency in HRD and NHRD tumors. IgL translocations are present in about 10% of MGUS, SMM, or newly diagnosed MM tumors, about 15% to 20% of intramedullary MM tumors, and about 20% of relapsed/refractory MM and HMCL.[12,46,60] Translocations involving an IgK locus are rare, occurring in only 1% to 2% of MM tumors and HMCL.[46,60] IgL translocations, not IgK, have been shown to be prognostic of poor outcome.[46]

Activating Mutations of RAS/MAPK Pathway

Activating mutations of KRAS (21%), NRAS (19%), BRAF (7%), and FGFR3 (2% of all patients, but 17% of t(4;14) MM) make the RAS/MAPK pathway the most frequent target of mutations in untreated MM.[45] NRAS mutations are more common in HRD MM and KRAS mutations in t(11;14) MM. Mutations of NRAS, but not KRAS, are associated with resistance to bortezomib.[61] Mutations of NRAS and KRAS are much less common in MGUS, identified in 3/33 patients in a recent study,[62] suggesting a role in tumor progression from MGUS to MM. MM tumors depend on the continued expression of activated but not wild-type RAS[63] and tumors with RAS mutations sometimes respond to treatment with the MEK inhibitor trametinib.[64] Similarly, there are anecdotal cases of responses to the BRAF inhibitor vemurafenib in MM with BRAF mutations.[9,65]

Activating Mutations of NFκB Pathway

Extrinsic ligands (APRIL and BAFF) produced by BM stromal cells provide critical survival signals to long-lived PCs by stimulating transmembrane activator and CAML interactor (TACI), B cell maturation antigen (BCMA), and B-cell activating factor (BAFF) receptors to activate the nuclear factor kappa B (NFκB) pathways. Most MGUS and MM tumors highly express NFκB target genes, suggesting a continued role of extrinsic signaling in PC tumors.[66,67] Activating mutations in positive regulators (MAP3K14, NFKB1, NFKB2, CD40, TACI, LTBR) and inactivating mutations in negative regulators (TRAF3, TRAF2, cIAP1/2, CYLD, NFKBIA) of the NFκB pathway have been identified in at least 20% of untreated MM tumors and 50% of HMCLs, rendering the cells less dependent on ligand-mediated NFκB activation (Figure 98.3). Small molecules that inhibit extrinsic signaling (IKKβ, and NIK [MAP3K14]) are being developed as potential therapeutic agents.[68] In addition, several reagents are being developed that block TACI signaling (Atacicept) or that target BCMA expression (chimeric antigen receptorT cells, bispecific and conjugated anti-BCMA antibodies).[69-71] A theoretical concern is that these approaches may select for MM cells that have acquired activating mutations of NFκB, where continued expression of TACI or BCMA may be dispensable.

Mutations in Other Significant Pathways

Mutations in MYC pathway genes IRF4 and MAX each are found in about 3% of cases, and mutations in DNA repair genes ATM, ATR and EGR1 each are found in about 1% to 4% of MM. Other mutations in CDKN2C, RB1, FAM46C, and DIS3 have also been reported.[45,72,73] Mutations in ATM and ATR have been associated with a poor prognosis, while mutations in EGR1 have been associated with a good prognosis.[45]

HIGH-RESOLUTION SEQUENCING STUDIES AND ADDITIONAL COMPLEXITY OF MM GENOMES

Mechanisms of Mutagenesis in Plasma Cell Neoplasms

Comprehensive genomic analysis of MM has been significantly improved with the use of longer read WGS techniques, which has the ability to reveal most genome wide structural variants, single-nucleotide variants (point mutations) and copy number variants. Using these data, it has been discovered that there are three main complex chromosomal structural events in MM: (1) chromoplexy due to multiple translocations leading to numerous copy number losses, (2) templated insertions associated with focal copy number gains, and (3) chromothripsis involving shattering and random assembly of chromosomes leading to oscillating copy number abnormalities.[74] Complex genetic abnormalities including chromothripsis are found in 20% to 30% of MM and chromothripsis is an independent marker of adverse prognostic marker.[75] Thus, for newly diagnosed MM, integration of genome wide chromothripsis can significantly enhance current risk prediction.[74]

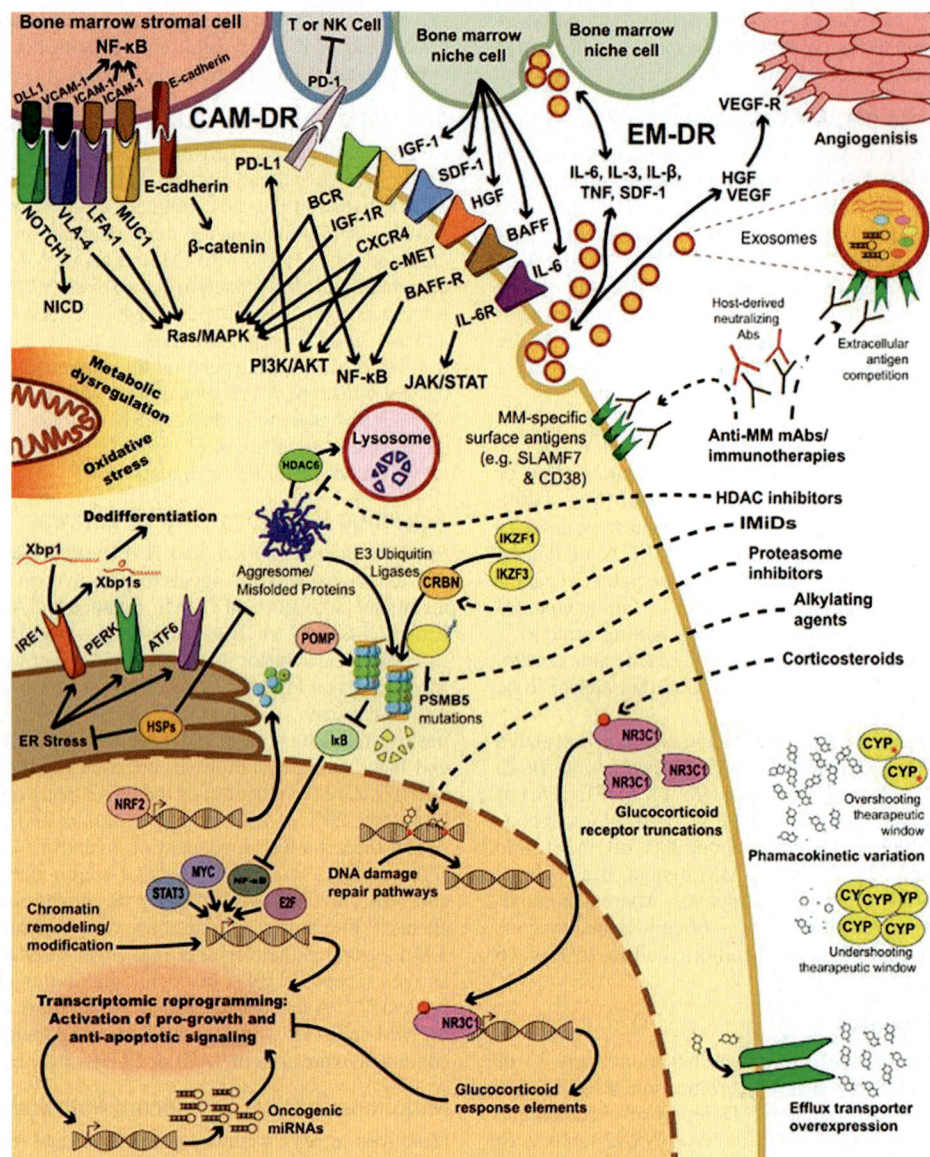

FIGURE 98.3 A schematic of mechanisms of resistance to MM therapies. Mechanisms of resistance depicted in the figure include variations in pharmacokinetics, efflux transporter aberrations, mutations of drug targets, epigenetic dysregulation, DNA damage repair, alterations in the ubiquitin proteasome system, and others mechanisms. (Reprinted by permission from Nature: Harding T, Baughn L, Kumar S, et al. The future of myeloma precision medicine: integrating the compendium of known drug resistance mechanisms with emerging tumor profiling technologies. *Leukemia*. 2019;33(4):863-883. Copyright © 2019 Springer Nature.)

In addition to detecting structural changes, high-resolution studies have also been able to detect specific mutagenic signatures (patterns of base changes) in MM cells. It appears that in most types of MM, earliest genetic changes (clonal, present in all cells) are driven by AID activity, likely as a result of aberrant re-entry of PCs into the germinal center. These early changes occur several decades prior to the onset of symptoms, underlying slow growth of PCs within the BM microenvironment. In contrast, the most important late signature (subclonal/progression driving) appears to be that of APOBEC activity.[76-79] Melphalan exposure signature is seen only in patients who have undergone autologous stem cell transplant with melphalan conditioning.[79]

Intraclonal Tumor Heterogeneity Associated With High-Risk Multiple Myeloma

Although the evidence is still emerging, it appears that many of the genetic events in MM are secondary and often present only in subclones of the tumor population.[72,80] A high level of intraclonal tumor heterogeneity has been described in some patients with high-risk MM associated in one case with alternating clonal dominance under therapeutic selective pressure, observations with important clinical implications. The findings suggest a competition between subclones for limited resources and raise the possibility that early, suboptimal treatment may eradicate the "good" drug-sensitive clone, making room for the "bad" drug-resistant clone to expand. They support the use of aggressive multidrug combination approaches for high-risk disease with unstable genomes and clonal heterogeneity, and sequential one- or two-drug approaches for low-risk disease with stable genomes and lacking clonal heterogeneity.

Bulk and single cell studies using various DNA sequencing methodologies, FISH, or genomic microarrays have revealed extensive intratumor clonal genetic heterogeneity in MM.[72,80-91] MM subclones with characteristic genetic signatures can dynamically evolve over time, within different locations of the BM resulting in spatial heterogeneity and in response to various chemotherapeutic agents.[92] The predominate mechanism driving clonal evolution appears to be a result of branching evolutionary patterns,[83,85,87,89-91] although evidence of neutral evolution in MM has also been reported.[93] Branching evolution enhances the fitness of select clones and is thought to be the cause of increased mutation burden resulting in chemotherapeutic resistance and disease relapse in comparison to patients with stable evolutionary patterns demonstrating fewer genetic changes over time.[85]

Genetic Changes in Myeloma as a Result of Therapy

Over the past 20 years, two classes of myeloma-directed therapies have become ubiquitous in the frontline therapy: IMIDs and PIs. The sensitivity of cells to IMIDs is regulated by several pathways, but the most important one appears to be binding of IMIDs to CRBN, a component of CLR4 E3 ubiquitin ligase, resulting in recruitment, ubiquitination, and degradation of multiple E3 neosubstrates, including transcription factors IKZF1/3. As a consequence of the cellular loss of IKZF1/3, multiple genes involved in myeloma cell survival are downregulated, including IRF4 and MYC. Due to branching evolution of myeloma cells, clones with genetic alterations (point mutations and structural alterations) of CRBN, CRL4, and IKZF1/3 are positively selected in patients undergoing IMID therapy, resulting in decreased expression of the corresponding proteins and IMID resistance[86,94-97] (Figure 98.3).

PIs are short peptide-like molecules that bind directly to catalytic sites of proteasome 20S catalytic particle. As PC translational machinery is highly active and prone to mistakes, the inhibition of proteasome activity leads to extreme accumulation of misfolded proteins and resulting endoplasmic reticulin stress and PCs death.[98] Resistance to PIs occurs through several mechanisms, including mutations in proteasome catalytic subunits[99] and dysregulation of proteasome subunit expression[100,101] (Figure 98.3).

BEYOND DNA: LESSONS FROM RNA EXPRESSION STUDIES

Almost all cases of PC neoplasms starting from the MGUS stage express one or more of the CYCLIN D genes in an aberrant fashion, despite a low proliferation index.[38,102] Therefore, it has been proposed that dysregulation of a CYCLIN D gene provides a unifying, early oncogenic event in MGUS and MM. MGUS and MM appear closer to normal, nonproliferating PCs than to normal proliferating plasmablasts, for which 30% or more of the cells can be in S phase; yet, the expression level of CYCLIN D1, CYCLIN D2, or CYCLIN D3 mRNA in MM and MGUS is distinctly higher than in normal PCs. This can be due to direct dysregulation in MM tumors with a CYCLIN D gene translocation or indirectly in tumors with a translocation of MAF, encoding a transcription factor that markedly upregulates CYCLIN D2. Although NSD2/FGFR3 tumors express moderately high levels of CYCLIN D2, the cause of increased CYCLIN D2 expression remains unknown. While normal BM PC express little or no detectable CYCLIN D1, the majority of HRD tumors express CYCLIN D1 biallelically, whereas most other tumors express increased levels of CYCLIN D2 compared to normal BM PC, both by unknown mechanisms. Only a few percent of MM tumors do not express increased levels of a CYCLIN D gene compared to normal PC, but many of these tumors appear to represent samples that are substantially contaminated by normal cells and another large fraction of these tumors often have inactivated RB1, the inhibitor downstream of CYCLIN D, eliminating the necessity of overexpressing a CYCLIN D gene. Mutations of CCND1 are seen in 12% of t(11;14) and are associated with a worse prognosis.[45]

The Role of Genes Dysregulated by Primary IgH Translocations

It is thought that CYCLIN D translocations only dysregulate expression of a CYCLIN D gene. By contrast, MAF translocations dysregulate expression of a MAF transcription factor that causes increased expression of many genes, including CYCLIN D2 and adhesion molecules that are thought to enhance the ability of the tumor cell to interact with the BM microenvironment.[103] The contributions of the two genes dysregulated by t(4;14) remain controversial. NSD2 is a chromatin-remodeling factor that is overexpressed in all tumors with a t(4;14), whereas about 20% of tumors lack der(14) and FGFR3 expression. The acquisition of FGFR3 activating mutations during progression confirms a role for FGFR3 in MM pathogenesis. Although an activated mutant FGFR3 can be oncogenic, a wild-type FGFR3 (as is found in most t[4;14]) has been shown to contribute to B-cell oncogenesis.[104] It remains to be determined if FGFR3 is critical early in pathogenesis but becomes dispensable during progression of t(4;14) MM. Preclinical studies suggest that tyrosine kinase inhibitors are active only against t(4;14) with activating mutations of FGFR3, whereas anti-FGFR3 monoclonal antibodies that inhibit FGFR3 signaling but also elicit antibody-dependent cell-mediated cytotoxicity are active against MM expressing wild-type FGFR3.[105,106] Despite an apparently indispensable role in t(4;14) MM, it remains to be determined how NSD2, which sometimes has amino-terminal truncations caused by the translocation, contributes to MM pathogenesis. There are some clues. It is a histone methyltransferase for H3K36me2, and when overexpressed, it results in a global increase in H3K36 methylation, and a decrease in H3K27 methylation, which might explain some of the many changes in gene expression associated with t(4;14) tumors.[107,108] In addition, it has been determined that NSD2 has a role in DNA repair and isotype CSR.[109,110] In particular, it has been shown to enhance DNA damage repair leading to an increase resistance to chemotherapeutic agents.[111] Importantly, loss of NSD2 expression alters adhesion, suppresses growth, and results in apoptosis of HMCLs, suggesting that it is an attractive therapeutic target.[107]

Molecular Classification of Multiple Myeloma

The patterns of spiked expression of genes deregulated by primary IGH translocations and the universal overexpression of CCND genes either by these translocations or other mechanisms led to the translocations and cyclin D (TC) classification that includes eight groups: those with primary translocations (designated 4p16, 11q13, 6p21, MAF), those that overexpressed CCND1 and CCND2 either alone or in combination (D1, D1 and D2, D2), and the rare cases that do not overexpress any CCND genes ("none") (Table 98.1).[38] Greater than 95% of the D1 group are HRD. In addition, most of the patients with HRD MM and trisomy 11 fall within the D1 and D1 and D2 groups, while those without trisomy 11 fall within the D2 group, although a majority of the D2 group are NHRD. This classification system therefore focuses on the different kinds of mechanisms that dysregulate a CCND gene as an early and unifying event in pathogenesis.

A MM classification based on an unsupervised analysis of microarray gene expression profiling from the University of Arkansas for Medical Sciences (UAMS) identified seven tumor groups characterized by the coexpression of unique gene clusters.[39] This classification was partially replicated in an independent unsupervised analysis of a combined HOVON-GMMG dataset that identified 10 tumor groups with considerable overlap with the UAMS groups.[40] Interestingly, these clusters also identify subgroups corresponding to the different primary translocations and hyperdiploidy. Importantly, however, they also highlight other important secondary events that can occur in each subtype of MM: proliferation (PR), expression of NFκB target genes (NFκB), cancer-testis antigens, and the phosphatase PTP4A3/PRL3 (PRL3). The CD-1 and CD-2 groups represent subgroups of patients with t(11;14) and t(6;14), with the former characterized by argininosuccinate synthetase 1 expression, and the latter by expression of B-cell antigens (CD20, VPREB, CD79A). Interestingly, they identify patients with markedly different clinical outcomes. Of all the molecular subgroups, CD-1 has the quickest onset and highest frequency of complete response (90%), whereas CD-2 has the slowest onset and lowest frequency of complete response (45%), when treated with total therapy 3. However, after the MF, the CD-1 has the shortest complete response duration (77% at 2 years), whereas the CD-2 has the longest (100% at 2 years).[112,113] A recent study using RNAseq data identified 12 different RNA subtypes of MM, significantly overlapping with previously identified subtypes.[114]

CONCLUSION

Significant progress has been made in understanding the molecular pathogenesis and biology of MM (Figure 98.3). Oncogenic pathways can be activated through cell intrinsic or extrinsic mechanisms. The use of whole genome and exome sequencing with powerful bioinformatics has allowed the comprehensive analysis of MM tumor genomes and the introduction of novel prognostic markers including chromothripsis and identification of mutation signatures. Similar to other cancers, MM is characterized by multistage accumulation of genetic abnormalities deregulating different pathways. Much of this knowledge is already being utilized for diagnosis, prognosis, and risk stratification of patients. Importantly, from a clinical standpoint, this knowledge has led to development of novel therapeutic strategies, some of which are already in clinical use and many others showing promise in preclinical and early clinical studies.

References

1. Siegel RL, Miller KD, Fuchs HE, Jemal A. Cancer statistics, 2021. *CA A Cancer J Clin*. 2021;71(1):7-33.
2. *SEER Cancer Statistics Review, 1975-2014*. National Cancer Institute; 2017.
3. Avet-Loiseau H, Attal M, Campion L, et al. Long-term analysis of the IFM 99 trials for myeloma: cytogenetic abnormalities [t(4;14), del(17p), 1q gains] play a major role in defining long-term survival. *J Clin Oncol*. 2012;30(16):1949-1952.
4. Weiss BM, Abadie J, Verma P, Howard RS, Kuehl WM. A monoclonal gammopathy precedes multiple myeloma in most patients. *Blood*. 2009;113(22):5418-5422.
5. Landgren O, Kyle RA, Pfeiffer RM, et al. Monoclonal gammopathy of undetermined significance (MGUS) consistently precedes multiple myeloma: a prospective study. *Blood*. 2009;113(22):5412-5417.
6. Landgren O, Katzmann JA, Hsing AW, et al. Prevalence of monoclonal gammopathy of undetermined significance among men in Ghana. *Mayo Clin Proc*. 2007;82(12):1468-1473.
7. Waxman AJ, Mink PJ, Devesa SS, et al. Racial disparities in incidence and outcome in multiple myeloma: a population-based study. *Blood*. 2010;116(25):5501-5506.
8. Baughn LB, Pearce K, Larson D, et al. Differences in genomic abnormalities among African individuals with monoclonal gammopathies using calculated ancestry. *Blood Cancer J*. 2018;8(10):96.
9. Jourdan M, Cren M, Robert N, et al. IL-6 supports the generation of human long-lived plasma cells in combination with either APRIL or stromal cell-soluble factors. *Leukemia*. 2014;28(8):1647-1656.
10. Kuehl WM, Bergsagel PL. Molecular pathogenesis of multiple myeloma and its pre-malignant precursor. *J Clin Invest*. 2012;122(10):3456-3463.
11. Walker BA, Wardell CP, Johnson DC, et al. Characterization of IGH locus breakpoints in multiple myeloma indicates a subset of translocations appear to occur in pregerminal center B cells. *Blood*. 2013;121(17):3413-3419.
12. Barwick BG, Gupta VA, Vertino PM, Boise LH. Cell of origin and genetic alterations in the pathogenesis of multiple myeloma. *Front Immunol*. 2019;10:1121.
13. Maura F, Rustad EH, Yellapantula V, et al. Role of AID in the temporal pattern of acquisition of driver mutations in multiple myeloma. *Leukemia*. 2020;34(5):1476-1480.
14. Ravindran A, Greipp PT, Wongchaowart N, et al. Dual primary IGH translocations in multiple myeloma: a novel finding. *Clin Lymphoma Myeloma Leuk*. 2021;21(9):e710-e713.
15. Kumar SK, Rajkumar SV. The multiple myelomas—current concepts in cytogenetic classification and therapy. *Nat Rev Clin Oncol*. 2018;15(7):409-421.
16. Weinhold N, Johnson DC, Chubb D, et al. The CCND1 c.870G>A polymorphism is a risk factor for t(11;14)(q13;q32) multiple myeloma. *Nat Genet*. 2013;45(5):522-525.
17. Baughn LB, Li Z, Pearce K, et al. The CCND1 c.870G risk allele is enriched in individuals of African ancestry with plasma cell dyscrasias. *Blood Cancer J*. 2020;10(3):39.
18. Kazandjian D, Hill E, Hultcrantz M, et al. Molecular underpinnings of clinical disparity patterns in African American vs. Caucasian American multiple myeloma patients. *Blood Cancer J*. 2019;9(2):15.
19. Sidana S, Jevremovic D, Ketterling RP, et al. Tetraploidy is associated with poor prognosis at diagnosis in multiple myeloma. *Am J Hematol*. 2019;94(5):E117-E120.
20. Fonseca R, Debes-Marun CS, Picken EB, et al. The recurrent IgH translocations are highly associated with nonhyperdiploid variant multiple myeloma. *Blood*. 2003;102(7):2562-2567.
21. Kumar S, Fonseca R, Ketterling RP, et al. Trisomies in multiple myeloma: impact on survival in patients with high-risk cytogenetics. *Blood*. 2012;119(9):2100-2105.
22. Sidana S, Jevremovic D, Ketterling RP, et al. Rapid assessment of hyperdiploidy in plasma cell disorders using a novel multi-parametric flow cytometry method. *Am J Hematol*. 2019;94(4):424-430.
23. Ashby C, Tytarenko RG, Wang Y, et al. Poor overall survival in hyperhaploid multiple myeloma is defined by double-hit bi-allelic inactivation of TP53. *Oncotarget*. 2019;10(7):732-737.
24. Peterson JF, Rowsey RA, Marcou CA, et al. Hyperhaploid plasma cell myeloma characterized by poor outcome and monosomy 17 with frequently co-occurring TP53 mutations. *Blood Cancer J*. 2019;9(3):20.
25. Sawyer JR, Morgan GJ. Hyperhaploid karyotypes in multiple myeloma. *Oncotarget*. 2017;8(45):78259-78260.
26. Sawyer JR, Tian E, Shaughnessy JD, Jr, et al. Hyperhaploidy is a novel high-risk cytogenetic subgroup in multiple myeloma. *Leukemia*. 2017;31(3):637-644.
27. Chng WJ, Huang GF, Chung TH, et al. Clinical and biological implications of MYC activation: a common difference between MGUS and newly diagnosed multiple myeloma. *Leukemia*. 2011;25(6):1026-1035.
28. Chesi M, Robbiani DF, Sebag M, et al. AID-dependent activation of a MYC transgene induces multiple myeloma in a conditional mouse model of post-germinal center malignancies. *Cancer Cell*. 2008;13(2):167-180.
29. Chesi M, Matthews GM, Garbitt VM, et al. Drug response in a genetically engineered mouse model of multiple myeloma is predictive of clinical efficacy. *Blood*. 2012;120(2):376-385.
30. Misund K, Keane N, Stein CK, et al. MYC dysregulation in the progression of multiple myeloma. *Leukemia*. 2019;34(1):322-326.
31. Mikulasova A, Ashby C, Tytarenko RG, et al. Microhomology-mediated end joining drives complex rearrangements and overexpression of MYC and PVT1 in multiple myeloma. *Haematologica*. 2020;105(4):1055-1066.
32. Sharma N, Smadbeck JB, Abdallah N, et al. The prognostic role of MYC structural variants identified by NGS and FISH in multiple myeloma. *Clin Cancer Res*. 2021;27(19):5430-5439.
33. Shou Y, Martelli ML, Gabrea A, et al. Diverse karyotypic abnormalities of the c-myc locus associated with c-myc dysregulation and tumor progression in multiple myeloma. *Proc Natl Acad Sci U S A*. 2000;97(1):228-233.
34. Affer M, Chesi M, Chen WD, et al. Promiscuous MYC locus rearrangements hijack enhancers but mostly super-enhancers to dysregulate MYC expression in multiple myeloma. *Leukemia*. 2014;28(8):1725-1735.
35. Chiecchio L, Dagrada GP, Protheroe RK, et al. Loss of 1p and rearrangement of MYC are associated with progression of smouldering myeloma to myeloma: sequential analysis of a single case. *Haematologica*. 2009;94(7):1024-1028.
36. Dib A, Gabrea A, Glebov OK, Bergsagel PL, Kuehl WM. Characterization of MYC translocations in multiple myeloma cell lines. *J Natl Cancer Inst*. 2008;39:25-31.
37. Smadbeck J, Peterson JF, Pearce KE, et al. Mate pair sequencing outperforms fluorescence in situ hybridization in the genomic characterization of multiple myeloma. *Blood Cancer J*. 2019;9(12):103.
38. Bergsagel PL, Kuehl WM, Zhan F, Sawyer J, Barlogie B, Shaughnessy J, Jr. Cyclin D dysregulation: an early and unifying pathogenic event in multiple myeloma. *Blood*. 2005;106(1):296-303.
39. Zhan F, Huang Y, Colla S, et al. The molecular classification of multiple myeloma. *Blood*. 2006;108(6):2020-2028.
40. Broyl A, Hose D, Lokhorst H, et al. Gene expression profiling for molecular classification of multiple myeloma in newly diagnosed patients. *Blood*. 2010;116(14):2543-2553.
41. Delmore JE, Issa GC, Lemieux ME, et al. BET bromodomain inhibition as a therapeutic strategy to target c-Myc. *Cell*. 2011;146(6):904-917.
42. Bjorklund CC, Lu L, Kang J, et al. Rate of CRL4(CRBN) substrate Ikaros and Aiolos degradation underlies differential activity of lenalidomide and pomalidomide in multiple myeloma cells by regulation of c-Myc and IRF4. *Blood Cancer J*. 2015;5:e354.
43. Zhu YX, Shi CX, Bruins LA, et al. Identification of lenalidomide resistance pathways in myeloma and targeted resensitization using cereblon replacement, inhibition of STAT3 or targeting of IRF4. *Blood Cancer J*. 2019;9(2):19.
44. Brioli A, Kaiser MF, Pawlyn C, et al. Biologically defined risk groups can be used to define the impact of thalidomide maintenance therapy in newly diagnosed multiple myeloma. *Leuk Lymphoma*. 2013;54(9):1975-1981.
45. Walker BA, Boyle EM, Wardell CP, et al. Mutational spectrum, copy number changes, and outcome: results of a sequencing study of patients with newly diagnosed myeloma. *J Clin Oncol*. 2015;33(33):3911-3920.
46. Barwick BG, Neri P, Bahlis NJ, et al. Multiple myeloma immunoglobulin lambda translocations portend poor prognosis. *Nat Commun*. 2019;10(1):1911.
47. Thanendrarajan S, Tian E, Qu P, et al. The level of deletion 17p and bi-allelic inactivation of TP53 has a significant impact on clinical outcome in multiple myeloma. *Haematologica*. 2017;102(9):e364-e367.
48. Lode L, Eveillard M, Trichet V, et al. Mutations in TP53 are exclusively associated with del(17p) in multiple myeloma. *Haematologica*. 2010;95(11):1973-1976.
49. Walker BA, Mavrommatis K, Wardell CP, et al. A high-risk, Double-Hit, group of newly diagnosed myeloma identified by genomic analysis. *Leukemia*. 2019;33(1):159-170.
50. Schmidt TM, Fonseca R, Usmani SZ. Chromosome 1q21 abnormalities in multiple myeloma. *Blood Cancer J*. 2021;11(4):83.
51. Weinhold N, Kirn D, Seckinger A, et al. Concomitant gain of 1q21 and MYC translocation define a poor prognostic subgroup of hyperdiploid multiple myeloma. *Haematologica*. 2016;101(3):e116-e119.
52. Weinhold N, Salwender HJ, Cairns DA, et al. Chromosome 1q21 abnormalities refine outcome prediction in patients with multiple myeloma—a meta-analysis of 2,596 trial patients. *Haematologica*. 2021;106(10):2754-2758.
53. Abdallah N, Greipp P, Kapoor P, et al. Clinical characteristics and treatment outcomes of newly diagnosed multiple myeloma with chromosome 1q abnormalities. *Blood Adv*. 2020;4(15):3509-3519.
54. Hebraud B, Leleu X, Lauwers-Cances V, et al. Deletion of the 1p32 region is a major independent prognostic factor in young patients with myeloma: the IFM experience on 1195 patients. *Leukemia*. 2014;28(3):675-679.
55. Boyd KD, Ross FM, Walker BA, et al. Mapping of chromosome 1p deletions in myeloma identifies FAM46C at 1p12 and CDKN2C at 1p32.3 as being genes in regions associated with adverse survival. *Clin Cancer Res*. 2011;17(24):7776-7784.
56. Fonseca R, Oken MM, Harrington D, et al. Deletions of chromosome 13 in multiple myeloma identified by interphase FISH usually denote large deletions of the q arm or monosomy. *Leukemia*. 2001;15(6):981-986.
57. Chiecchio L, Dagrada GP, Ibrahim AH, et al. Timing of acquisition of deletion 13 in plasma cell dyscrasias is dependent on genetic context. *Haematologica*. 2009;94(12):1708-1713.
58. Lohr JG, Stojanov P, Carter SL, et al. Widespread genetic heterogeneity in multiple myeloma: implications for targeted therapy. *Cancer Cell*. 2014;25(1):91-101.
59. Binder M, Rajkumar SV, Ketterling RP, et al. Prognostic implications of abnormalities of chromosome 13 and the presence of multiple cytogenetic

60. Gabrea A, Martelli ML, Qi Y, et al. Secondary genomic rearrangements involving immunoglobulin or MYC loci show similar prevalences in hyperdiploid and nonhyperdiploid myeloma tumors. *Genes Chromosomes Cancer.* 2008;47(7):573-590.
61. Mulligan G, Lichter DI, Di Bacco A, et al. Mutation of NRAS but not KRAS significantly reduces myeloma sensitivity to single-agent bortezomib therapy. *Blood.* 2014;123(5):632-639.
62. Mikulasova A, Wardell CP, Murison A, et al. The spectrum of somatic mutations in monoclonal gammopathy of undetermined significance indicates a less complex genomic landscape than that in multiple myeloma. *Haematologica.* 2017;102(9):1617-1625.
63. Steinbrunn T, Stuhmer T, Gattenlohner S, et al. Mutated RAS and constitutively activated Akt delineate distinct oncogenic pathways, which independently contribute to multiple myeloma cell survival. *Blood.* 2011;117(6):1998-2004.
64. Heuck CJ, Jethava Y, Khan R, et al. Inhibiting MEK in MAPK pathway-activated myeloma. *Leukemia.* 2016;30(4):976-980.
65. Andrulis M, Lehners N, Capper D, et al. Targeting the BRAF V600E mutation in multiple myeloma. *Cancer Discov.* 2013;3(8):862-869.
66. Keats JJ, Fonseca R, Chesi M, et al. Promiscuous mutations activate the noncanonical NF-kappaB pathway in multiple myeloma. *Cancer Cell.* 2007;12(2):131-144.
67. Annunziata CM, Davis RE, Demchenko Y, et al. Frequent engagement of the classical and alternative NF-kappaB pathways by diverse genetic abnormalities in multiple myeloma. *Cancer Cell.* 2007;12(2):115-130.
68. Demchenko YN, Brents LA, Li Z, Bergsagel LP, McGee LR, Kuehl MW. Novel inhibitors are cytotoxic for myeloma cells with NFkB inducing kinase-dependent activation of NFkB. *Oncotarget.* 2014;5(12):4554-4566.
69. Seckinger A, Delgado JA, Moser S, et al. Target expression, generation, preclinical activity, and pharmacokinetics of the BCMA-T cell bispecific antibody EM801 for multiple myeloma treatment. *Cancer Cell.* 2017;31(3):396-410.
70. Tai YT, Mayes PA, Acharya C, et al. Novel anti-B-cell maturation antigen antibody-drug conjugate (GSK2857916) selectively induces killing of multiple myeloma. *Blood.* 2014;123(20):3128-3138.
71. Lee L, Draper B, Chaplin N, et al. An APRIL based chimeric antigen receptor for dual targeting of BCMA and TACI in Multiple Myeloma. *Blood.* 2018;131(7):746-758.
72. Bolli N, Avet-Loiseau H, Wedge DC, et al. Heterogeneity of genomic evolution and mutational profiles in multiple myeloma. *Nat Commun.* 2014;5:2997.
73. Walker BA, Mavrommatis K, Wardell CP, et al. Identification of novel mutational drivers reveals oncogene dependencies in multiple myeloma. *Blood.* 2018;132(6):587-597.
74. Maura F, Boyle EM, Rustad EH, et al. Chromothripsis as a pathogenic driver of multiple myeloma. *Semin Cell Dev Biol.* 2022;123:115-123.
75. Maclachlan KH, Rustad EH, Derkach A, et al. Copy number signatures predict chromothripsis and clinical outcomes in newly diagnosed multiple myeloma. *Nat Commun.* 2021;12(1):5172.
76. Maura F, Petljak M, Lionetti M, et al. Biological and prognostic impact of APOBEC-induced mutations in the spectrum of plasma cell dyscrasias and multiple myeloma cell lines. *Leukemia.* 2018;32(4):1044-1048.
77. Rustad EH, Yellapantula V, Leongamornlert D, et al. Timing the initiation of multiple myeloma. *Nat Commun.* 2020;11(1):1917.
78. Maura F, Degasperi A, Nadeu F, et al. A practical guide for mutational signature analysis in hematological malignancies. *Nat Commun.* 2019;10(1):2969.
79. Maura F, Weinhold N, Diamond B, et al. The mutagenic impact of melphalan in multiple myeloma. *Leukemia.* 2021;35(8):2145-2150.
80. Keats JJ, Chesi M, Egan JB, et al. Clonal competition with alternating dominance in multiple myeloma. *Blood.* 2012;120(5):1067-1076.
81. Quinn JG, Sadek I. Clonal heterogeneity in plasma cell myeloma. *Lancet.* 2016;387(10022):e22.
82. Egan JB, Shi CX, Tembe W, et al. Whole-genome sequencing of multiple myeloma from diagnosis to plasma cell leukemia reveals genomic initiating events, evolution, and clonal tides. *Blood.* 2012;120(5):1060-1066.
83. Melchor L, Brioli A, Wardell CP, et al. Single-cell genetic analysis reveals the composition of initiating clones and phylogenetic patterns of branching and parallel evolution in myeloma. *Leukemia.* 2014;28(8):1705-1715.
84. Hoang PH, Cornish AJ, Sherborne AL, et al. An enhanced genetic model of relapsed IGH-translocated multiple myeloma evolutionary dynamics. *Blood Cancer J.* 2020;10(10):101.
85. Jones JR, Weinhold N, Ashby C, et al. Clonal evolution in myeloma: the impact of maintenance lenalidomide and depth of response on the genetics and subclonal structure of relapsed disease in uniformly treated newly diagnosed patients. *Haematologica.* 2019;104(7):1440-1450.
86. Kortum KM, Mai EK, Hanafiah NH, et al. Targeted sequencing of refractory myeloma reveals a high incidence of mutations in CRBN and Ras pathway genes. *Blood.* 2016;128(9):1226-1233.
87. Weinhold N, Ashby C, Rasche L, et al. Clonal selection and double-hit events involving tumor suppressor genes underlie relapse in myeloma. *Blood.* 2016;128(13):1735-1744.
88. Walker BA, Wardell CP, Melchor L, et al. Intraclonal heterogeneity and distinct molecular mechanisms characterize the development of t(4;14) and t(11;14) myeloma. *Blood.* 2012;120(5):1077-1086.
89. Corre J, Cleynen A, Robiou du Pont S, et al. Multiple myeloma clonal evolution in homogeneously treated patients. *Leukemia.* 2018;32(12):2636-2647.
90. Diamond B, Yellapantula V, Rustad EH, et al. Positive selection as the unifying force for clonal evolution in multiple myeloma. *Leukemia.* 2021;35(5):1511-1515.
91. Landau HJ, Yellapantula V, Diamond BT, et al. Accelerated single cell seeding in relapsed multiple myeloma. *Nat Commun.* 2020;11(1):3617.
92. Pawlyn C, Morgan GJ. Evolutionary biology of high-risk multiple myeloma. *Nat Rev Cancer.* 2017;17(9):543-556.
93. Johnson DC, Lenive O, Mitchell J, et al. Neutral tumor evolution in myeloma is associated with poor prognosis. *Blood.* 2017;130(14):1639-1643.
94. Gooding S, Ansari-Pour N, Towfic F, et al. Multiple cereblon genetic changes are associated with acquired resistance to lenalidomide or pomalidomide in multiple myeloma. *Blood.* 2021;137(2):232-237.
95. Lu G, Middleton RE, Sun H, et al. The myeloma drug lenalidomide promotes the cereblon-dependent destruction of Ikaros proteins. *Science.* 2014;343(6168):305-309.
96. Kronke J, Udeshi ND, Narla A, et al. Lenalidomide causes selective degradation of IKZF1 and IKZF3 in multiple myeloma cells. *Science.* 2014;343(6168):301-305.
97. Barrio S, Munawar U, Zhu YX, et al. IKZF1/3 and CRL4(CRBN) E3 ubiquitin ligase mutations and resistance to immunomodulatory drugs in multiple myeloma. *Haematologica.* 2020;105(5):e237-e241.
98. Lee AH, Iwakoshi NN, Anderson KC, Glimcher LH. Proteasome inhibitors disrupt the unfolded protein response in myeloma cells. *Proc Natl Acad Sci U S A.* 2003;100(17):9946-9951.
99. Barrio S, Stuhmer T, Da-Via M, et al. Spectrum and functional validation of PSMB5 mutations in multiple myeloma. *Leukemia.* 2019;33(2):447-456.
100. Acosta-Alvear D, Cho MY, Wild T, et al. Paradoxical resistance of multiple myeloma to proteasome inhibitors by decreased levels of 19S proteasomal subunits. *Elife.* 2015;4:e08153.
101. Tsvetkov P, Sokol E, Jin D, et al. Suppression of 19S proteasome subunits marks emergence of an altered cell state in diverse cancers. *Proc Natl Acad Sci U S A.* 2017;114(2):382-387.
102. Ely S, Di Liberto M, Niesvizky R, et al. Mutually exclusive cyclin-dependent kinase 4/cyclin D1 and cyclin-dependent kinase 6/cyclin D2 pairing inactivates retinoblastoma protein and promotes cell cycle dysregulation in multiple myeloma. *Cancer Res.* 2005;65(24):11345-11353.
103. Hurt EM, Wiestner A, Rosenwald A, et al. Overexpression of c-maf is a frequent oncogenic event in multiple myeloma that promotes proliferation and pathological interactions with bone marrow stroma. *Cancer Cell.* 2004;5(2):191-199.
104. Zingone A, Cultraro CM, Shin D-M, et al. Ectopic expression of wild-type FGFR3 cooperates with MYC to accelerate development of B-cell lineage neoplasms. *Leukemia.* 2010;24(6):1171-1178.
105. Qing J, Du X, Chen Y, et al. Antibody-based targeting of FGFR3 in bladder carcinoma and t(4;14)-positive multiple myeloma in mice. *J Clin Invest.* 2009;119(5):1216-1229.
106. Trudel S, Li ZH, Wei E, et al. CHIR-258, a novel, multitargeted tyrosine kinase inhibitor for the potential treatment of t(4;14) multiple myeloma. *Blood.* 2005;105(7):2941-2948.
107. Martinez-Garcia E, Popovic R, Min D-J, et al. The MMSET histone methyl transferase switches global histone methylation and alters gene expression in t(4;14) multiple myeloma cells. *Blood.* 2011;117(1):211-220.
108. Kuo AJ, Cheung P, Chen K, et al. NSD2 links dimethylation of histone H3 at lysine 36 to oncogenic programming. *Mol Cell.* 2011;44(4):609-620.
109. Pei H, Wu X, Liu T, Yu K, Jelinek DF, Lou Z. The histone methyltransferase MMSET regulates class switch recombination. *J Immunol.* 2013;190(2):756-763.
110. Pei H, Zhang L, Luo K, et al. MMSET regulates histone H4K20 methylation and 53BP1 accumulation at DNA damage sites. *Nature.* 2011;470(7332):124-128.
111. Shah MY, Martinez-Garcia E, Phillip JM, et al. MMSET/WHSC1 enhances DNA damage repair leading to an increase in resistance to chemotherapeutic agents. *Oncogene.* 2016;35(45):5905-5915.
112. Nair B, van Rhee F, Shaughnessy JD, et al. Superior results of Total Therapy 3 (2003-33) in gene expression profiling-defined low-risk multiple myeloma confirmed in subsequent trial 2006-66 with VRD maintenance. *Blood.* 2010;115(21):4168-4173.
113. Weinhold N, Heuck CJ, Rosenthal A, et al. Clinical value of molecular subtyping multiple myeloma using gene expression profiling. *Leukemia.* 2016;30(2):423-430.
114. Skerget S, Penaherrera D, Chari A, et al. Genomic basis of multiple myeloma subtypes from the MMRF CoMMpass study. Preprint. Posted online 2021. *medRxiv.* 2021.2008.2002.21261211.

Chapter 99 ■ Monoclonal Gammopathy of Undetermined Significance and Smoldering Multiple Myeloma

S. VINCENT RAJKUMAR • ROBERT A. KYLE • RONALD S. GO

INTRODUCTION

Definition

Monoclonal gammopathy of undetermined significance (MGUS) is an asymptomatic, pre–malignant clonal plasma cell proliferative disorder.[1] It is characterized by the presence of a monoclonal immunoglobulin in the blood and/or urine, referred to commonly as a monoclonal (M) protein. MGUS was initially referred to as *essential hyperglobulinemia* by Jan Waldenström, as well as several other terms such as benign, idiopathic, asymptomatic, nonmyelomatous, discrete, cryptogenic, and rudimentary monoclonal gammopathy; dysimmunoglobulinemia; lanthanic monoclonal gammopathy; idiopathic paraproteinemia; and asymptomatic paraimmunoglobul.[2,3] However, since there is an indefinite risk of progression to multiple myeloma (MM) or related disorder such as Waldenström macroglobulinemia (WM) or immunoglobulin light chain (AL) amyloidosis, the term MGUS is now the accepted nomenclature.[4] Smoldering multiple myeloma (SMM) is a clinically defined premalignant stage between MGUS and MM.[5,6] MGUS and SMM must be differentiated from MM, and from a number of related plasma cell disorders using the criteria listed on *Table 99.1*.[4]

Detection of Monoclonal Proteins

Immunoglobulins consist of two heavy polypeptide chains of the same class and subclass and two light polypeptide chains of the same type. The various types of immunoglobulins are designated by capital letters that correspond to the isotype of their heavy chains, which are designated by Greek letters: gamma constitutes immunoglobulin G (IgG), alpha (α) is found in IgA, mu is present in IgM, delta occurs in IgD, and IgE is characterized by epsilon. IgG1, IgG2, IgG3, and IgG4 are the subclasses of IgG; the subclasses of IgA are IgA1 and IgA2. Kappa (κ) and lambda (λ) are the two types of light chains. An intact immunoglobulin consists of two heavy chains of the same class and two light chains of the same type. A monoclonal increase in immunoglobulins results from a clonal process such as MGUS or MM, and a polyclonal increase in immunoglobulins is caused by a reactive or inflammatory process. The monoclonal immunoglobulin secreted by clonal plasma cells in MGUS, SMM, MM, and related monoclonal gammopathies is referred to as a monoclonal protein or M protein.

As described in Chapter 97, monoclonal proteins are detected using agarose gel or capillary electrophoresis of the serum and urine.[7] In addition, immunofixation or mass spectrometry is done when MM, WM, AL amyloidosis, or a related disorder is suspected, because small M proteins may not be detected with electrophoresis alone. Rate nephelometry and measurement of serum immunoglobulin free light chains (FLCs) are also important measurements in patients with monoclonal gammopathies.

The serum FLC assay is an automated nephelometric assay that measures free κ and λ light chains that are not bound to intact immunoglobulin.[8,9] Patients with a κ/λ FLC ratio below the normal range are considered to have a monoclonal λ FLC and those with ratios above the normal range are defined as having a monoclonal κ FLC. The normal reference range varies based on the manufacturer of the assay.

MONOCLONAL GAMMOPATHY OF UNDETERMINED SIGNIFICANCE

Definition and Terminology

MGUS is defined by the presence of a serum monoclonal (M) protein of <3 g/dL (or increased serum FLC level with abnormal FLC ratio), <10% clonal bone marrow plasma cells (BMPCs) with no evidence of SMM, end-organ damage or other myeloma defining event (MDE) (*Table 99.1*).[4] MGUS is classified into three major subtypes: IgM MGUS, non-IgM MGUS, and light chain MGUS (LC-MGUS) based on the predominant mode of clinical progression.[4,10] IgM MGUS carries a risk of progression to WM, although rarely patients can develop IgM MM.[11] Non-IgM MGUS is associated with a risk of progression to MM, and LC-MGUS is a precursor of light chain MM. All forms of MGUS can lead to AL amyloidosis. MGUS with a κ light chain type can predispose to light chain deposition disease.

MGUS is a disease of exclusion, and progression of MGUS to more serious plasma cell proliferative disorders such as MM, SMM, WM, solitary plasmacytoma, AL amyloidosis, and light chain deposition disease must be considered and excluded. In addition, to these disorders that are well established clear progression events, MGUS can also be seen in conjunction with a wide variety of malignant and nonmalignant disorders such as peripheral neuropathy,[12] proliferative glomerulonephritis,[13] and several skin disorders (Chapter 103). However, the causal relationship between the M protein and many of these disorders cannot often be established. Further these disorders typically also have other well-established etiologies unrelated to the presence or absence of an M protein. Thus, it is a matter of semantics as to whether, for instance, peripheral neuropathy presumed to be causally related to M protein (in the absence of MM, AL amyloidosis, WM, etc) should be referred to as "MGUS-associated peripheral neuropathy" or "monoclonal gammopathy associated peripheral neuropathy." Technically, the words "undetermined significance" in MGUS were coined to highlight the fact that despite all available testing and years of follow-up, one can never be certain as to whether malignant progression to MM, WM will or will not occur in a given patient with MGUS. It was never meant to suggest that the M protein in MGUS by itself cannot cause other tissue damage prior to clonal progression. To highlight the concept that monoclonal proteins can be the cause of specific end-organ damage that is distinct from malignant progression, terms such as monoclonal gammopathy of renal significance (MGRS) have been proposed to indicate renal damage and disease caused by M proteins in patients who do not have MM (Chapter 103).

Epidemiology

Prevalence

MGUS is the most common plasma cell proliferative disorder. The prevalence of MGUS has been estimated in a large population-based study that included 21,463 of the 28,038 enumerated residents (77%) of Olmsted County, Minnesota, who were 50 years or older.[14] MGUS was identified in 694 (3.2%) of these subjects. Age-adjusted rates were greater in men than in women, 4.0% vs 2.7% ($P < .001$) (*Figure 99.1*). The prevalence of MGUS was 5.3% among persons 70 years or older and 7.5% among those 85 years or older. Several other studies have reported similar prevalence estimates.[15] In addition, approximately 1% of the general population over the age of 50 has LC-MGUS.[10]

The incidence of M proteins is higher in Blacks than in whites.[16,17] A large population-based study ($n = 12,482$) of persons 50 years of age and older, using samples from the National Health and Nutrition Examination Survey (NHANES), confirmed that MGUS is twice as common in African-Americans compared to whites; adjusted prevalence of MGUS was significantly higher in Blacks (3.7%) compared with whites (2.3%) or Hispanics (1.8%) ($P < .001$).[18] A follow-up NHANES study revealed that racial disparity in prevalence occurs even at younger ages, with MGUS having an onset approximately a decade earlier in Blacks compared with whites.[19] *Table 99.2* gives the estimated prevalence of MGUS by race and age based on the MGUS studies.[18,19]

Table 99.1. International Myeloma Working Group Diagnostic Criteria for MGUS, Multiple Myeloma, and Related Disorders

Disorder	Disease Definition
IgM Monoclonal gammopathy of undetermined significance (IgM MGUS)	All three criteria must be met: • Serum IgM monoclonal protein < 3 g/dL • Bone marrow lymphoplasmacytic infiltration < 10% • No evidence of anemia, constitutional symptoms, hyperviscosity, lymphadenopathy, or hepatosplenomegaly that can be attributed to the underlying lymphoproliferative disorder.
Non-IgM monoclonal gammopathy of undetermined significance (MGUS)	All three criteria must be met: • Serum monoclonal protein (non-IgM type) < 3 g/dL • Clonal bone marrow plasma cells < 10%[a] • Absence of end-organ damage such as hypercalcemia, renal insufficiency, anemia, and bone lesions (CRAB) that can be attributed to the plasma cell proliferative disorder
Light Chain MGUS	All criteria must be met: • Abnormal free light chain (FLC) ratio (<0.26 or >1.65) • Increased level of the appropriate involved light chain (increased kappa FLC in patients with ratio >1.65 and increased lambda FLC in patients with ratio <0.26) • No immunoglobulin heavy chain expression on immunofixation • Absence of end-organ damage that can be attributed to the plasma cell proliferative disorder • Clonal bone marrow plasma cells < 10% • Urinary monoclonal protein < 500 mg/24 h
Smoldering multiple myeloma	Both criteria must be met: • Serum monoclonal protein (IgG or IgA) ≥ 3 g/dL or urinary monoclonal protein ≥ 500 mg/24 h and/or clonal bone marrow plasma cells 10%–60% • Absence of myeloma defining events or amyloidosis

Multiple Myeloma	Both criteria must be met:
	• Clonal bone marrow plasma cells ≥ 10% or biopsy-proven bony or extramedullary plasmacytoma
	• Any one or more of the following myeloma defining events:
	  • Evidence of end-organ damage that can be attributed to the underlying plasma cell proliferative disorder, specifically:
	    • Hypercalcemia: serum calcium > 0·25 mmol/L (>1 mg/dL) higher than the upper limit of normal or >2·75 mmol/L (>11 mg/dL)
	    • Renal insufficiency: creatinine clearance <40 mL per minute or serum creatinine > 177 μmol/L (>2 mg/dL)
	    • Anemia: hemoglobin value of >2 g/dL below the lower limit of normal, or a hemoglobin value < 10 g/dL
	    • Bone lesions: one or more osteolytic lesions on skeletal radiography, computed tomography (CT), or positron emission tomography-CT (PET-CT)
	  • Clonal bone marrow plasma cell percentage ≥60%
	  • Involved:uninvolved serum FLC ratio ≥100 (involved FLC level must be ≥100 mg/L)
	  • >1 focal lesions on magnetic resonance imaging (MRI) studies (at least 5 mm in size)

Smoldering Waldenström macroglobulinemia (also referred to as indolent or asymptomatic Waldenström macroglobulinemia)	Both criteria must be met: • Serum IgM monoclonal protein ≥ 3 g/dL and/or bone marrow lymphoplasmacytic infiltration ≥10% • No evidence of anemia, constitutional symptoms, hyperviscosity, lymphadenopathy, or hepatosplenomegaly that can be attributed to the underlying lymphoproliferative disorder.
Waldenström macroglobulinemia	All criteria must be met: • IgM monoclonal gammopathy (regardless of the size of the M protein) • ≥10% bone marrow lymphoplasmacytic infiltration (usually intertrabecular) by small lymphocytes that exhibit plasmacytoid or plasma cell differentiation and a typical immunophenotype (e.g., surface IgM+, CD5+/−, CD10−, CD19+, CD20+, CD23−) that satisfactorily excludes other lymphoproliferative disorders including chronic lymphocytic leukemia and mantle cell lymphoma • Evidence of anemia, constitutional symptoms, hyperviscosity, lymphadenopathy, or hepatosplenomegaly that can be attributed to the underlying lymphoproliferative disorder
Solitary Plasmacytoma	All four criteria must be met • Biopsy-proven solitary lesion of bone or soft tissue with evidence of clonal plasma cells • Normal bone marrow with no evidence of clonal plasma cells • Normal skeletal survey and MRI (or CT) of the spine and pelvis (except for the primary solitary lesion) • Absence of end-organ damage such as CRAB that can be attributed to a lympho-plasma cell proliferative disorder
Solitary Plasmacytoma with minimal marrow involvement[b]	All four criteria must be met • Biopsy-proven solitary lesion of bone or soft tissue with evidence of clonal plasma cells • Clonal bone marrow plasma cells < 10% • Normal skeletal survey and MRI (or CT) of the spine and pelvis (except for the primary solitary lesion) • Absence of end-organ damage such as CRAB that can be attributed to a lympho-plasma cell proliferative disorder
Systemic AL Amyloidosis	All four criteria must be met: • Presence of an amyloid-related systemic syndrome (such as renal, liver, heart, gastrointestinal tract, or peripheral nerve involvement) • Positive amyloid staining by Congo red in any tissue (e.g., fat aspirate, bone marrow, or organ biopsy) • Evidence that amyloid is light chain related established by direct examination of the amyloid using Mass Spectrometry–based proteomic analysis, or immuno-electron microscopy • Evidence of a monoclonal plasma cell proliferative disorder (serum or urine M protein, abnormal FLC ratio, or clonal plasma cells in the bone marrow) Note: Approximately 2% to 3% of patients with AL amyloidosis will not meet the requirement for evidence of a monoclonal plasma cell disorder listed above; the diagnosis of AL amyloidosis must be made with caution in these patients. Patients with AL amyloidosis who also meet criteria for multiple myeloma are considered to have both diseases.

Table 99.1. International Myeloma Working Group Diagnostic Criteria for MGUS, Multiple Myeloma, and Related Disorders (Continued)

Disorder	Disease Definition

POEMS syndrome	All four criteria must be met
	• Polyneuropathy
	• Monoclonal plasma cell proliferative disorder (almost always lambda)
	• Any one of the following three other <u>Major</u> criteria:
	  1. Sclerotic bone lesions
	  2. Castleman disease
	  3. Elevated levels of vascular endothelial growth factor (VEGF)[c]
	• Any one of the following six Minor Criteria
	  1. Organomegaly (splenomegaly, hepatomegaly, or lymphadenopathy)
	  2. Extravascular volume overload (edema, pleural effusion, or ascites)
	  3. Endocrinopathy (adrenal, thyroid, pituitary, gonadal, parathyroid, pancreatic)[d]
	  4. Skin changes (hyperpigmentation, hypertrichosis, glomeruloid hemangiomata, plethora, acrocyanosis, flushing, white nails)
	  5. Papilledema
	  6. Thrombocytosis/polycythemia
	Note: Not every patient meeting the above criteria will have POEMS syndrome; the features should have a temporal relationship to each other and no other attributable cause. Anemia and/or thrombocytopenia are distinctively unusual in this syndrome unless Castleman disease is present.

Abbreviations: POEMS, polyneuropathy, organomegaly, endocrinopathy, monoclonal plasma cell disorder, and skin changes; MGUS, monoclonal gammopathy of undetermined significance.
Modified from Rajkumar SV, Dimopoulos MA, Palumbo A, et al. International Myeloma Working Group updated criteria for the diagnosis of multiple myeloma. *Lancet Oncol.* 2014;15(12):e538-e548. Copyright © 2014 Elsevier. With permission.
[a]A bone marrow can be deferred in patients with low-risk MGUS (IgG type, M protein <15 g/L, normal free light chain ratio) in whom there are no clinical features concerning for myeloma.
[b]Solitary plasmacytoma with 10% or more clonal plasma cells is considered as multiple myeloma.
[c]The source data do not define an optimal cut off value for considering elevated VEGF level as a major criterion. We suggest that VEGF measured in the serum or plasma should be at least three to fourfold higher than the normal reference range for the laboratory, i.e., doing the testing to be considered a major criteria.
[d]In order to consider endocrinopathy as a minor criterion, an endocrine disorder other than diabetes or hypothyroidism is required since these two disorders are common in the general population.

The higher incidence of MGUS in Blacks may be related to genetic or environmental factors. A population-based study found that the increased risk of MGUS seen in African Americans was also seen in Blacks in Ghana, suggesting that the racial disparity may be due more to genetic factors.[20] Furthermore, a study of women in the southern part of the United States found that the racial disparity between Blacks and whites persisted even after adjusting for socio-economic status, again suggesting that the differences were more likely genetic rather than environmental.[21]

One study found that only 2.7% of elderly Japanese patients had a monoclonal gammopathy.[22] A subsequent population-based study in Japan found that the risk of MGUS was lower compared with the white population of Olmsted County.[23]

Incidence

The annual incidence of MGUS in males is estimated to be 120/100,000 at age 50, and rises to 530/100,000 at age 90 years.[24] The rates for women are 60/100,000 at age 50 and 370/100,000 at age 90. The fact that the increased prevalence of MGUS with rising age is not just related to accumulation of new cases but due to an actual increase in incidence suggests that an age-related cumulative damage model is at play in the pathogenesis of MGUS.

Risk Factors

The incidence and prevalence of MGUS rises with age.[14,24] MGUS is also more common in males. Blacks have a higher risk of MGUS than whites as discussed above.[18] Besides age, race, and gender, there are other risk factors that have been identified, both genetic and environmental. First-degree relatives of patients with MGUS and MM have a two to threefold higher risk of MGUS compared to those with no known affected relatives.[25-27] Obesity and immunosuppression are also known risk factors for MGUS.[21,28,29] An increased risk of MGUS has been noted with exposure to certain pesticides.[30]

Pathophysiology

MM is almost always preceded by the asymptomatic premalignant MGUS stage.[31,32] As part of the screening arm of the nationwide population-based prospective prostate, lung, colon, ovarian cancer screening trial, annual blood samples were collected on 77,469 healthy adults. From this cohort, a joint study by the National Cancer Institute and the Mayo Clinic identified 71 individuals who developed MM during the course of the study. Serial serum samples (up to six) obtained 2 to 9.8 years prior to MM diagnosis were then studied. The study found that an asymptomatic MGUS phase always preceded MM and was found in 100% of cases 6 years prior to MM.[31]

The specific alterations that lead to the establishment of the MGUS clone and subsequent malignant transformation of MGUS to MM or a

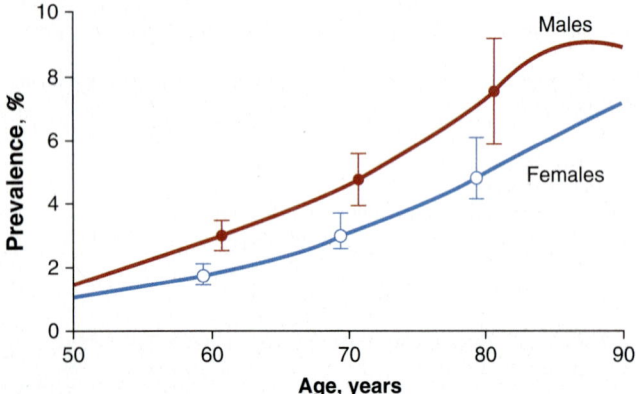

FIGURE 99.1 Prevalence of monoclonal gammopathy of undetermined significance, according to age. Of 21,463 residents 50 years of age or older, 694 had a monoclonal protein. The I bars represent 95% confidence interval. Years of age older than 90 have been condensed to 90 years of age (x-axis). (From Kyle RA, Therneau TM, Rajkumar SV, et al. Prevalence of monoclonal gammopathy of undetermined significance. *N Engl J Med.* 2006;354(13):1362-1369. Copyright © 2006 Massachusetts Medical Society. Reprinted with permission from Massachusetts Medical Society.)

Table 99.2. Prevalence of Monoclonal Gammopathy of Undetermined Significance (MGUS) (%), by Race/ethnicity and age

Age Group (Years)	Blacks % (95% CI)	Whites % (95% CI)	Hispanic American % (95% CI)	Total[a] % (95% CI)
10-19	0.00 (NA)	0.00 (NA)	0.11 (0.02-0.84)	0.01 (0.00-0.07)
20-29	0.26 (0.08-0.84)	0.00 (NA)	0.00 (NA)	0.03 (0.01-0.11)
30-39	0.81 (0.43-1.53)	0.32 (0.11-0.99)	0.23 (0.06-0.79)	0.49 (0.27-0.91)
40-49	3.26 (2.04-5.18)	0.53 (0.20-1.37)	2.20 (1.22-3.95)	0.88 (0.53-1.47)
50-59	2.19 (1.32-3.60)	1.01 (0.62-1.66)	0.85 (0.33-2.23)	1.20 (0.83-1.72)
60-69	3.48 (2.26-5.33)	2.43 (1.72-3.43)	2.41 (1.69-3.44)	2.45 (1.85-3.23)
70-79	5.67 (3.66-8.70)	3.44 (2.55-4.63)	2.51 (1.36-4.58)	3.43 (2.64-4.47)
80+	8.56 (4.92-14.47)	4.42 (3.31-5.87)	3.97 (1.33-11.22)	4.58 (3.54-5.90)

[a]Includes "Other" race/ethnicity group.
Modified from Landgren O, Graubard BI, Kumar S, et al. Prevalence of myeloma precursor state monoclonal gammopathy of undetermined significance in 12372 individuals 10-49 old: a population-based study from the National Health and Nutrition Examination Survey. *Blood Cancer J.* 2017;7(10):e618. http://creativecommons.org/licenses/by/4.0/

related plasma cell proliferative disorder are not fully known.[33,34] The pathogenesis of MGUS and MM is described in Chapter 98. Briefly, approximately 50% of patients with MGUS have primary translocations on chromosome 14q32 (IgH translocated MGUS/SMM).[35,36] The most common partner chromosome loci are: 11q13, 4p16.3, 6p21, 16q23, and 20q11.[37-39] These translocations lead to the dysregulation of oncogenes such as *CCND1* (cyclin D1) (11q13), *FGFR3/WHSC1* (fibroblastic growth factor receptor 3/Wolf-Hirschhorn syndrome candidate) (4p16.3), *CCND3* (cyclin D3) (6p21), *MAF* (16q23), and *MAFB* (20q11). The dysregulation of these oncogenes is thought to be critical for the initiation of the MGUS clone rather than progression of MGUS to MM. Approximately 40% of patients (40%) with MGUS have trisomies of odd-numbered chromosomes leading to hyperdiploidy (hyperdiploid MGUS). In a small subset, there are likely both IgH translocations and trisomies, and in some neither abnormality can be detected.

The rate of progression of MGUS to MM or related malignancy occurs at a fixed rate of 1% per year regardless of the known duration of antecedent MGUS, suggesting that the second hit (or series of hits) is a random event.[40] Recent studies using gene sequencing indicate that there are two main paths by which the progression event occurs, *MYC* translocations and mutations in the MAP kinase pathway.[41,42] In addition to these changes, there are also additional genetic abnormalities that occur in subpopulations resulting in clonal heterogeneity.[43]

Changes in Bone Marrow Microenvironment

Bone marrow angiogenesis is increased in MM and has prognostic value.[44,45] Using a chick embryo chorioallantoic membrane angiogenesis assay, Vacca et al found that 76% of MM bone marrow samples had increased angiogenic potential compared with 20% of MGUS samples.[46] Collectively these findings suggest that induction of angiogenesis may play a role in progression of MGUS to MM.

Changes in the bone marrow microenvironment may be triggered by cell-cell contact of clonal plasma cells with surrounding bone marrow stroma and endothelial cells. However, autocrine and paracrine secretion of various cytokines is thought to play an important role as well. There is overexpression of CD126 (interleukin-6 [IL-6] receptor α-chain) in MGUS compared to normal plasma cells.[47,48] IL-6 and interleukin-1β may play a role in the clonal proliferation of plasma cells in MGUS.[49]

One consequence of alteration in bone marrow microenvironment is the gradual disappearance of normal BMPCs that occurs with the transformation of MGUS to MM.[50] This is accompanied by an increase in the population of aberrant clonal plasma cells, and a reduction in B-cell precursors and CD34+ hematopoietic stem cells.

Alterations in Bone Turnover and New Bone Formation

As the MGUS clone evolves with additional cytogenetic abnormalities and changes in the microenvironment, there is overexpression of receptor activator of nuclear factor-κB ligand (RANKL) by osteoblasts (and possible plasma cells) and macrophage inflammatory protein 1-α by plasma cells.[51,52] Further there is a reduction in osteoprotegerin, the decoy receptor for RANKL. This leads to osteoclast activation and bone resorption. In addition, increased dickkopf 1 expression by MM cells is felt to play a major role in simultaneous suppression of osteoblasts and new bone formation.[53] This combination of factors is thought to be critical for development of lytic bone lesions in MM.

Clinical Features

MGUS is an asymptomatic condition. It is typically detected as an incidental finding when electrophoresis and immunofixation of the serum and/or urine or the serum FLC assay are performed during the work-up of suspected MM, AL amyloidosis, or WM. Thus, MGUS is usually detected during the work-up of unexplained weakness or fatigue, increased erythrocyte sedimentation rate, anemia, unexplained back pain, osteoporosis, osteolytic lesions or fractures, hypercalcemia, proteinuria, renal insufficiency, or recurrent infections. MGUS is also detected during work-up of patients with symptoms suggestive of AL amyloidosis such as unexplained sensorimotor peripheral neuropathy, carpal tunnel syndrome, refractory congestive heart failure, nephrotic syndrome, orthostatic hypotension, malabsorption, weight loss, change in the tongue or voice, paresthesias, numbness, increased bruising, bleeding, and steatorrhea.

Most cases of MGUS remain undiagnosed due to the asymptomatic nature of the condition. At age 60, the proportion of prevalent cases that are clinically recognized is only 13%.[24] This rate rises to 33% at age 80. When MGUS is first diagnosed, it is estimated that the condition has already been present in an undiagnosed form for a median duration of over 10 years.[24] For example, it is estimated that 56% of women age 70 diagnosed with MGUS have had the condition for over 10 years, including 28% for over 20 years. Corresponding values for men are 55% and 31%, respectively.

The risk and mode of progression of MGUS varies based on the subtype of MGUS as shown in *Table 99.3*.[4,10,11,54]

Prognosis

The prognosis of MGUS was first established in a study of 241 patients seen at the Mayo Clinic from 1956 through 1970.[55] The actuarial rate of progression to MM or related disorder at 10 years was 17%; at 20 years, 34%; and at 25 years, 39%.[56]

A subsequent larger population-based study of 1384 persons with MGUS from Southeastern Minnesota found that the risk of progression of MGUS to MM or related disorder is 1% per year (*Figure 99.2* and *Table 99.4*).[40] The risk of progression with MGUS persists even after over 30 years of follow-up.[1] Although the risk of progression is 1% per year, it must be emphasized that this does not take into account other competing causes of death in elderly patients. After adjusting for

Table 99.3. Risk and Pattern of Progression Monoclonal Gammopathy of Undetermined Significance (MGUS)

Type	Risk of Progression
Non-IgM MGUS[a]	1% per year risk of progression to multiple myeloma, AL amyloidosis, or related disorder
IgM MGUS[b]	1.5% per year risk of progression to Waldenström macroglobulinemia; rare patients can progress to IgM multiple myeloma
Light chain MGUS[c]	Risk of progression to light chain myeloma and AL amyloidosis. Rate of progression not defined.

[a]Almost all patients are IgG or IgA type. Occasional patients may have IgD or IgE monoclonal proteins.
[b]Note that conventionally IgM MGUS is considered a subtype of MGUS. Thus, when the term MGUS is used, in general, it includes IgM MGUS.
[c]Since light chain MGUS was only defined in 2010, studies pertaining to MGUS prior to that time do not include patients with this entity; unless otherwise specified studies since then may also not include patients with light chain MGUS.
Adapted from Rajkumar SV. Preventive strategies in monoclonal gammopathy of undetermined significance and smoldering multiple myeloma. Am J Hematol. 2012;87(5):453-454. Copyright © 2012 Wiley Periodicals, Inc. Reprinted by permission of John Wiley & Sons, Inc.

Table 99.4. Risk of Progression Among 1384 Residents of Southeastern Minnesota in Whom Monoclonal Gammopathy of Undetermined Significance Was Diagnosed, 1960-1994

Type of Progression	No. of Patients Observed	No. of Patients Expected[a]	Relative Risk (95% CI)
Multiple myeloma	75	3.0	25.0 (20-32)
Lymphoma[b]	19	7.8	2.4 (2-4)
AL amyloidosis	10	1.2	8.4 (4-16)
Macroglobulinemia	7	0.2	46.0 (19-95)
Chronic lymphocytic leukemia[c]	3	3.5	0.9 (0.2-3)
Plasmacytoma	1	0.1	8.5 (0.2-47)
Total	115	15.8	7.3 (6-9)

Abbreviation: AL, immunoglobulin light chain; CI, confidence interval.
From Kyle RA, Therneau TM, Rajkumar SV, et al. A long-term study of prognosis in monoclonal gammopathy of undetermined significance. N Engl J Med. 2002;346(8):564-569. Copyright © 2002 Massachusetts Medical Society. Reprinted with permission from Massachusetts Medical Society.
[a]Expected numbers of cases were derived from the age- and sex-matched white population of the Surveillance, Epidemiology, and End Results program in Iowa,[57] except for primary amyloidosis for which data are from Kyle et al.[58]
[b]All 19 patients had serum IgM monoclonal protein. If the 30 patients with IgM, IgA, or IgG monoclonal protein and lymphoma were included, the relative risk would be 3.9 (95% CI, 2.6-5.5).
[c]All three patients had serum IgM monoclonal protein. If all six patients with IgM, IgA, or IgG monoclonal protein and chronic lymphocytic leukemia were included, the relative risk would be 1.7 (95% CI, 0.6-3.7).

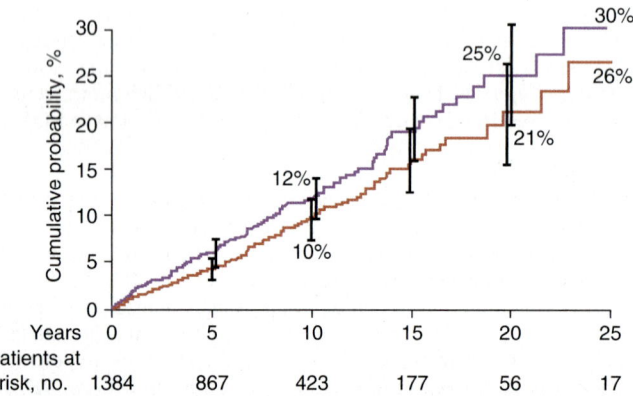

FIGURE 99.2 Probability of disease progression among 1384 residents of southeastern Minnesota in whom monoclonal gammopathy of undetermined significance (MGUS) was diagnosed from 1960 through 1994. The top curve shows the probability of progression to a plasma cell cancer (115 patients) or of an increase in the monoclonal protein concentration to more than 3 g/dL or in the proportion of plasma cells in the bone marrow to more than 10% (32 patients). The bottom curve shows only the probability of progression of MGUS to multiple myeloma, IgM lymphoma, primary amyloidosis, macroglobulinemia, chronic lymphocytic leukemia, or plasmacytoma (115 patients). The error bars indicate 95% confidence intervals. (From Kyle RA, Therneau TM, Rajkumar SV, et al. A long-term study of prognosis of monoclonal gammopathy of undetermined significance. N Engl J Med. 2002;346(8):564-569. Copyright © 2002 Massachusetts Medical Society. Reprinted with permission from Massachusetts Medical Society.)

competing causes of death, the true lifetime probability of progression of MGUS for the average patient is only approximately 10% (Figure 99.3).

In addition to progression to MM or related malignancy, patients with MGUS are at risk for several associated syndromes that are caused not due to malignant transformation, but rather due to the specific chemical or physical properties of the secreted M protein. These include disorders such as AL amyloidosis, light chain deposition disease, and proliferative glomerulonephritis.[13]

Spontaneous disappearance of M protein after the diagnosis of MGUS is uncommon.[40] In the Southeastern Minnesota study, the M protein disappeared without an apparent cause in 27 patients (2%), and only 6 of these 27 patients (0.4% of all patients) had a discrete spike on the densitometer tracing of the initial electrophoresis (median, 1.2 g/dL); the rest had small M proteins detected on immunofixation only.

Follow-Up in Other Series

The risk of progression of MGUS has been estimated in several other studies, and the results mirror those seen in the Southeastern Minnesota study. For example, Baldini et al noted that 6.8% of 335 patients with MGUS had progression during a median follow-up of 70 months.[59] In the Danish Cancer Registry, 64 new cases of malignancy (5 expected; relative risk, 12.9) were found among 1229 patients with MGUS.[60]

Prognostic Factors

No findings at diagnosis of MGUS can reliably distinguish patients whose condition will remain stable indefinitely from those in whom MM or related malignancy develops. However, there are several known prognostic factors that assist in estimation of the risk of progression for appropriate counseling and management.

Size of Monoclonal Protein

The size of the M protein at recognition of MGUS is one of the most important predictors for the risk of progression. In the study of 1384 patients from Southeastern Minnesota, the risk of progression to MM or a related disorder 10 years after diagnosis of MGUS was 6% for patients with an initial M protein level of 0.5 g/dL or less, 7% for 1 g/dL, 11% for 1.5 g/dL, 20% for 2 g/dL, 24% for 2.5 g/dL, and 34% for 3.0 g/dL.[40] Corresponding rates for progression at 20 years were 14%, 16%, 25%, 41%, 49%, and 64%, respectively.

Type of Monoclonal Protein

Patients with an IgM or IgA M protein have a higher risk of progression (1.5% per year) compared with those with an IgG or IgA M protein (1% per year).[40] IgM MGUS is a unique subtype of MGUS in which patients are mainly at risk of progression to WM rather than MM.[61] Rarely patients with IgM MGUS evolve into IgM MM.[11] The risk of progression of LC-MGUS relative to IgA, IgG, or IgM MGUS is not known.

Abnormal Serum-FLC Ratio

An abnormal FLC ratio is an independent risk factor for progression of MGUS. In a study of 1148 patients with MGUS, 379 (33%) had

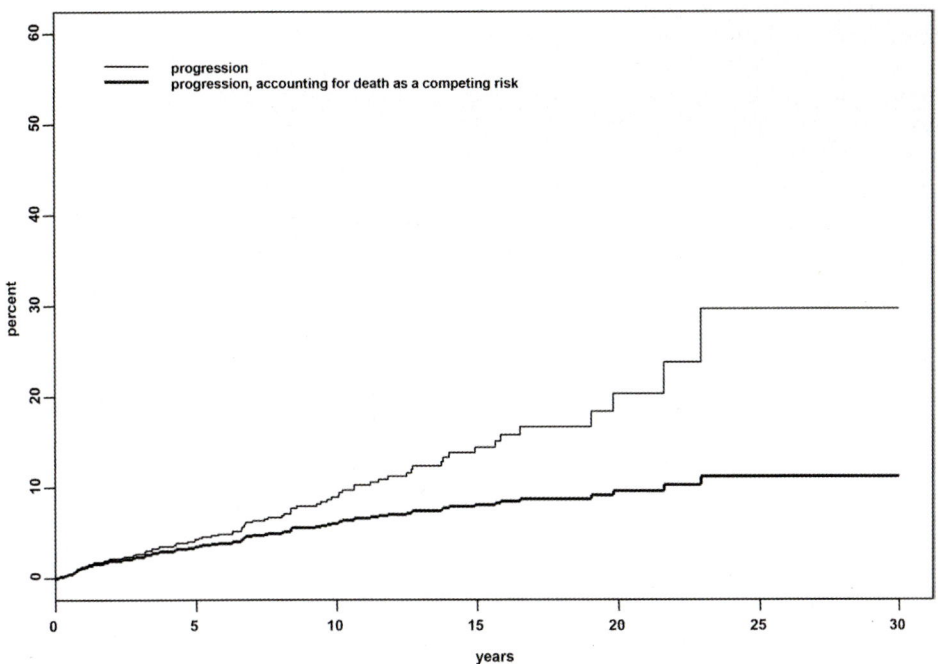

FIGURE 99.3 The risk of Progression to Myeloma or Related Disorder in 1148 patients with Monoclonal Gammopathy of Undetermined Significance. The upper curve illustrates risk of progression of all patients without taking into account competing causes of death. The lower curve illustrates risk of progression after accounting for other competing causes of death. (Reprinted from Rajkumar SV, Kyle RA, Therneau TM, et al. Serum free light chain ratio is an independent risk factor for progression in monoclonal gammopathy of undetermined significance. *Blood*. 2005;106(3):812-817. Copyright © 2005 American Society of Hematology. With permission.)

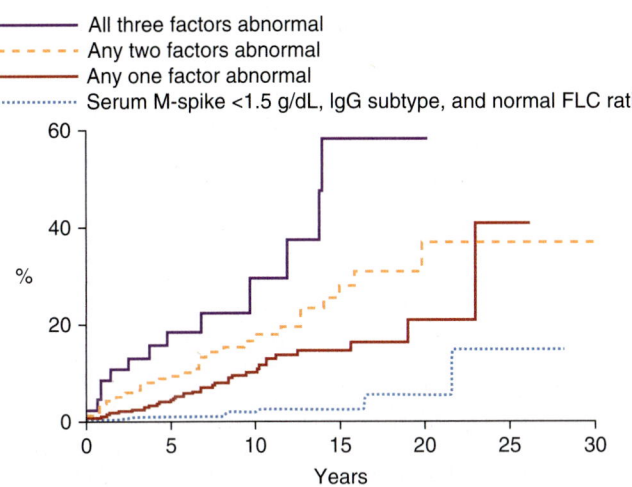

FIGURE 99.4 Risk of progression of monoclonal gammopathy of undetermined significance (MGUS) to myeloma or related disorder. The top curve illustrates the risk of progression with time in patients with three risk factors: abnormal serum κ:λ free light chain (FLC) ratio (<0.26 or >1.65), a high serum monoclonal (M) protein level (≥1.5 g/dL), and non-immunoglobulin G (IgG) MGUS. The second curve is the risk of progression in patients with any two of these risk factors. The third curve illustrates the risk of progression with one of these risk factors. The bottom curve is the risk of progression for patients with none of the risk factors. (Reprinted from Rajkumar SV, Kyle RA, Therneau TM, et al. Serum free light chain ratio is an independent risk factor for progression in monoclonal gammopathy of undetermined significance. *Blood*. 2005;106(3):812-817. Copyright © 2005 American Society of Hematology. With permission.)

an abnormal FLC ratio.[62] The risk of progression in patients with an abnormal FLC ratio was significantly higher than that in patients with a normal ratio (hazard ratio 3.5; $P < .001$) and was independent of the size and type of serum M protein (*Figure 99.4*). The production of excess monoclonal FLC in MGUS may be a biomarker for plasma cells bearing a higher degree of cytogenetic abnormalities thereby serving as a biomarker for a higher risk of progression.

Bone Marrow Plasma Cells

Cesana et al have found that patients with MGUS who have 5% to 9% BMPCs have a higher risk of progression compared with those with <5% BMPCs.[63] Of 1104 patients with MGUS in this study, patients with greater than 5% marrow plasmacytosis had a significantly higher risk of progression compared to those with 5% or fewer plasma cells, 1.35 vs 0.64 per 100 person years, respectively, $P = .004$.

Suppression of Uninvolved Immunoglobulins

Studies suggest that the risk of progression of MGUS may be increased if there is associated suppression of the other uninvolved immunoglobulins.[40]

Risk-Stratification

A risk-stratification model can be used to predict risk of progression in MGUS, and is useful for management.[62] The model is based on the size and type of the M protein and the FLC ratio (*Table 99.5*). Patients with all three risk factors consisting of an abnormal serum FLC ratio, IgA or IgM MGUS, and an increased serum M protein value (≥1.5 g/dL) have a risk of progression at 20 years of 58%, whereas the risk is 37% with any two risk factors present, 21% with one risk factor present, and 5% when none of the risk factors are present. When competing causes of death were taken into account, the risk of progression in the low risk group is only 2% at 20 years.

Life Expectancy and Cause of Death

In the Mayo Clinic study of 241 patients with MGUS, survival was shorter compared with an age- and sex-adjusted 1980 US population (13.7 vs 15.7 years).[64] Patients with MGUS had a shorter median survival compared to an age- and gender-matched control population, 8.1 vs. 12.4 years, $P < .001$.[1] In the study by van de Poel et al,[65] the long-term survival of 334 patients with MGUS was slightly shorter than the expected survival of an age- and sex-adjusted population. However, it is not clear from these studies if there is an excess risk of death from MGUS once the deaths due to malignant progression are accounted for.

Management

The differentiation between MGUS and MM and other related disorders is based on the criteria listed on *Table 99.1*.[4] At the time of initial diagnosis all patients need a complete blood count (CBC), serum calcium, and serum creatinine. If available, peripheral blood flow cytometry for circulating plasma cells should also be done. Radiographic studies of the bones can be omitted in asymptomatic patients with IgM MGUS or low-risk MGUS (*Table 99.5*). All other patients require

Table 99.5. Risk-Stratification Model to Predict Progression of Monoclonal Gammopathy of Undetermined Significance to Myeloma or Related Disorders

Risk Group	No. of Patients	Relative Risk	Absolute Risk of Progression at 20 Years (%)	Absolute Risk of Progression at 20 Years Accounting for Death as a Competing Risk (%)
Low risk (Serum M protein < 1.5 g/dL, IgG subtype, normal FLC ratio (0.26-1.65)	449	1	5	2
Low-Intermediate risk (Any one factor abnormal)	420	5.4	21	10
High-Intermediate risk (Any two factors abnormal)	226	10.1	37	18
High risk (All three factors abnormal)	53	20.8	58	27

Abbreviations: FLC, free light chain; IgG, immunoglobulin G; M, monoclonal.
Adapted from Rajkumar SV, Kyle RA, Therneau TM, et al. Serum free light chain ratio is an independent risk factor for progression in monoclonal gammopathy of undetermined significance. *Blood.* 2005;106(3):812-817. Copyright © 2005 American Society of Hematology. With permission.

examination of the skeleton preferably by low-dose whole body computed tomography to rule out osteolytic bone lesions. Similarly, although a bone marrow biopsy is required for the disease definition of MGUS, not all patients need to have such an examination if the clinical picture is otherwise entirely consistent with MGUS and the patient is considered to be at low risk (*Figure 99.5*).[66] If a bone marrow aspiration and biopsy is done, cytogenetic studies should be done at baseline. The recommendation to defer bone imaging and bone marrow examination is based on a study that found that the yield of these studies in such patients is extremely low.[67]

Once the diagnosis is made, the CBC, serum calcium, creatinine and serum protein electrophoresis, and serum FLC must be repeated in 6 months.[68] If stable, then in patients with low-risk MGUS, an assessment of the M protein level is needed only if symptoms worrisome for progression develop. This recommendation is based on the fact that the progression risk is very low in these patients, and that there are no data that monitoring can prevent complications in a timely manner.[69] In all other patients with MGUS, annual follow-up of the M protein is recommended lifelong.

Screening of the general population for MGUS is not recommended. A large randomized trial in Iceland (iStopMM) is testing the role of screening and early intervention. However, screening can be considered clinically in selected high-risk populations, namely Black people with one or more first-degree relatives with MM, and in all others who have two or more affected first-degree relatives.[70]

SMOLDERING MULTIPLE MYELOMA

Definition

SMM is defined by the presence of a serum monoclonal (M) protein of ≥ 3 g/dL (or urine M protein ≥500 mg/24 h) and/or 10% to 60% clonal BMPCs with no evidence of end-organ damage (i.e., CRAB criteria) or other MDE (*Table 99.1*).[4] It is distinguished from MGUS based on the level of serum M protein and the percentage of clonal BMPCs (*Table 99.1*).[71] The diagnostic criteria for SMM were revised in 2014 to exclude patients with clonal BMPC ≥60%, serum involved/uninvolved FLC ratio of ≥100, and those with two or more focal lesions on magnetic resonance imaging (MRI).[4] Such patients have an approximately 40% per year risk of progression and are now considered as MM.[72-77] Light chain SMM is a unique subtype of SMM in which there is monoclonal FLC excess with no expression of immunoglobulin heavy chain (IgH).[78] This entity is characterized by excess secretion (≥500 mg/24 h) of monoclonal FLC in the urine (Bence Jones proteinuria).

Epidemiology

SMM accounts for approximately 15% of all cases of newly diagnosed MM.[79,80] Other investigators have found a higher proportion of patients with SMM, but the sample size in these studies is small.[81,82] The prevalence estimates for SMM are distorted because many reports include asymptomatic patients with lytic bone lesions on skeletal survey or focal lesions on MRI. A Swedish Myeloma Registry, a prospective observational registry, study found that 14% of MM patients can be considered to have SMM.[83] Calculation of the true prevalence of SMM on the basis of updated criteria is not available.

Pathophysiology

SMM is not a unique biologic entity.[33,34] It is heterogeneous entity created primarily for clinical purposes to identify a group of patients with asymptomatic plasma cell dyscrasia that have a much higher risk of progression than MGUS (10% per year) so that these patients can be monitored more closely.[6,33,84] From a biologic standpoint, SMM includes patients with premalignancy (biological MGUS) and patients with early asymptomatic malignancy (MM).[34,85] Unfortunately, at present, histopathologic and other laboratory methods cannot distinguish SMM patients with premalignant MGUS from those who have early MM since there is no clear marker of malignancy that can distinguish a clonal premalignant plasma cell from a clonal malignant MM cell.

Clinical Features

As with MGUS, SMM is asymptomatic and is diagnosed during the routine work-up for a variety of symptoms and signs.[66,84] SMM should be differentiated from related plasma cell disorders using the criteria listed on *Table 99.1*.[4]

Prognosis

The risk of progression of SMM is much higher compared with MGUS, 10% per year compared with 1% per year. In a study of 276 patients with SMM, the risk of progression was 10% per year for the first 5 years, 5% per year for the next 3 years, and then 1% to 2% per year thereafter.[6] This pattern of progression in which there is a plateau after 10 years is consistent with the heterogeneous nature of SMM; in the first 10 years, the subset of patients with early MM

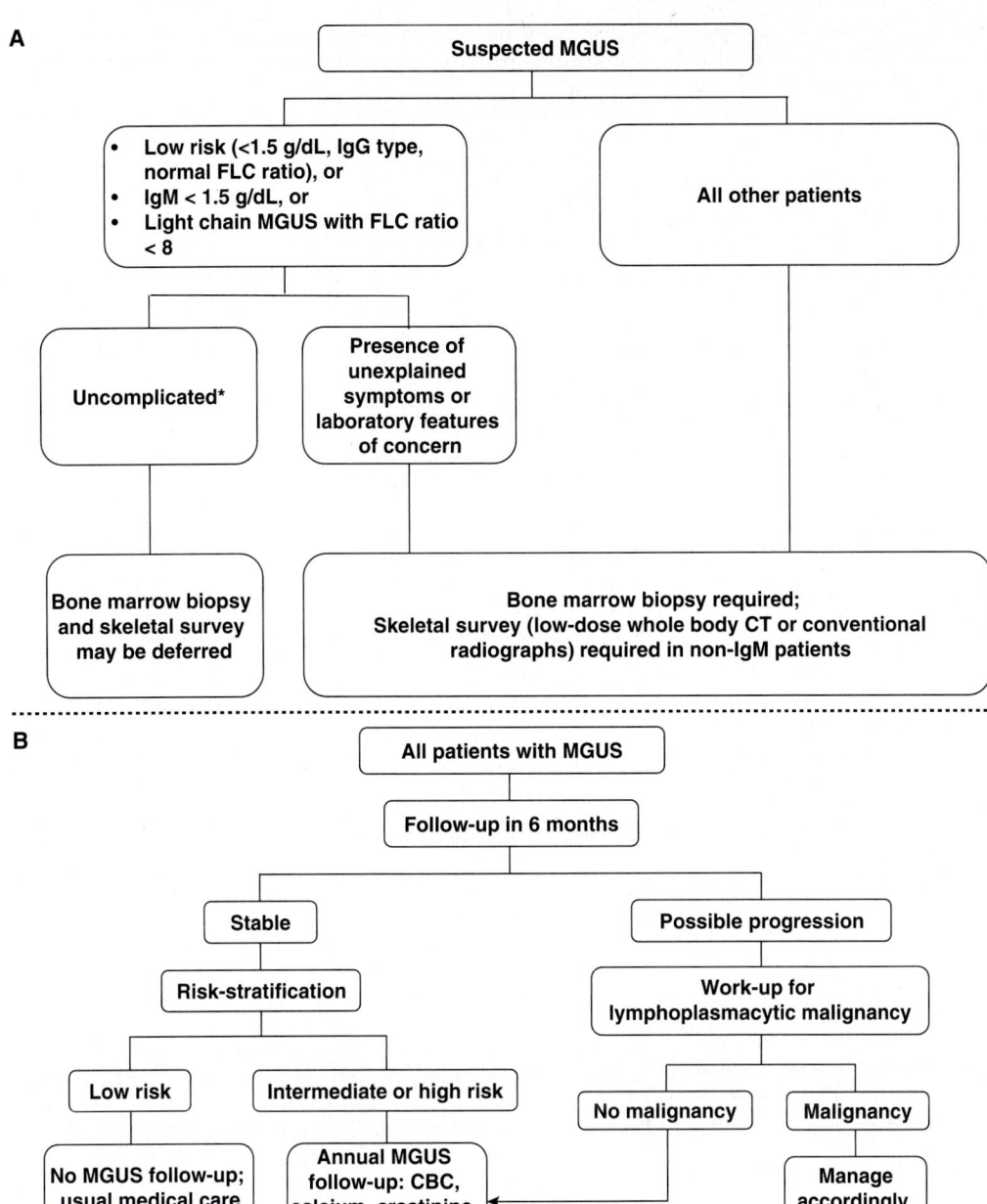

FIGURE 99.5 Approach to monoclonal gammopathy of undetermined significance (MGUS). Approach to diagnostic work-up (A) and approach to follow-up (B) FLC, free light chain; CBC, complete blood count; CT, computed tomography; SPEP, serum protein electrophoresis. (Reprinted from Go RS, Rajkumar SV. How I manage monoclonal gammopathy of undetermined significance. *Blood*. 2018;131(2):163-173. Copyright © 2018 American Society of Hematology. With permission.)

declare themselves with symptomatic disease, while after 10 years, the remaining cohort of patients is identical to MGUS in biology and clinical behavior.

Prognostic Factors

The assessment of prognostic factors for SMM is hampered by varying diagnostic criteria used to define the cohort. Although the prognostic factors listed below were studied prior to recent changes to the definition of SMM, the effect is likely to be minimal since the proportion of patients upstaged from SMM to MM on the basis of the new diagnostic criteria are relatively small (10%-15%).[4]

Size and Type of Monoclonal Protein

The size of the serum M protein is a significant risk factor for progression in SMM.[6] Similarly, in light chain SMM, the risk of progression is higher based on the level of the urinary M protein.[6] The risk of progression in light chain SMM may be lower than the risk of progression in SMM with presence of an intact immunoglobulin M protein with median time to progression (TTP) of 159 months in one study.[78]

Extent of Bone Marrow Involvement

Even after excluding patients with ≥60% clonal BMPC, the risk of progression in SMM is still affected by extent of bone marrow involvement. In the Mayo Clinic study, median TTP was 117 months for patients with <20% BMPC vs 26 months for patients with BMPC of 20% to 50%, $P < .001$.[6] BMPC estimates should be done on either the bone marrow aspirate or biopsy examination, and in the event of a discrepancy, the higher of the two values should be used.[4]

Suppression of Uninvolved Immunoglobulins

Suppression of one or more uninvolved immunoglobulins (immunoparesis) is seen in most patients with SMM; approximately 50% of patients have suppression of two or more uninvolved immunoglobulin isotypes.[6] In one study, median TTP was 159 months in patients with normal levels of uninvolved immunoglobulins, 89 months in those with a reduction in one isotype, and 32 months in patients with reduction in two isotypes of uninvolved immunoglobulins, $P = .001$.[6] Similar results have been reported in a Spanish study of SMM, where a decrease in one or two of the uninvolved immunoglobulins was a significant prognostic parameter in SMM; median TTP not reached with normal immunoglobulins vs 31 months with reduction in one or more uninvolved immunoglobulins, $P < .01$.[86]

Circulating Plasma Cells

The ability of plasma cells to escape from the bone marrow microenvironment and circulate in the peripheral blood ("marrow emancipation") is a likely hallmark of aggressive disease as well as malignant transformation. Patients with a high level of circulating plasma cells are at higher risk of progression to active disease.[87]

Abnormalities on Magnetic Resonance Imaging

Patients who undergo MRI often have abnormalities detected even when the skeletal survey shows no lytic lesions.[79,88] Patients with one focal lesion and those with solely diffuse (nonfocal) abnormalities on MRI are at increased risk of progression to MM, but not at the magnitude required to classify them as having MM.[76] These patients are still classified as SMM, but are at a high risk of progression and require more close follow-up and repeat imaging in 3 to 6 months.

Abnormalities on Positron Emission Tomography-Computed Tomography

There are emerging data on the value of (18) F-fluorodeoxyglucose positron emission tomography-computed tomography (PET-CT) in SMM.[89] Zamagni and colleagues studied 120 SMM patients who had undergone PET/CT imaging, to assess the impact of increased uptake without underlying osteolysis.[90] They found increased PET-CT uptake without osteolysis in 16% of patients. The median TTP was significantly shorter for patients with increased PET-CT uptake compared with patients with negative PET-CT, median TTP 1.1 vs 4.5 years, $P = .001$. The probability of progression within 2 years was 58% for PET-CT positive vs 33% for PET-CT negative patients. Thus, the presence of increased uptake on PET-CT without underlying osteolysis is a risk factor for progression of SMM, and should be considered as a high risk factor.

Serum Free Light Chain Assay

The serum FLC ratio can predict risk of progression in MGUS.[62] Similarly, among 116 patients with solitary plasmacytoma, an abnormal FLC ratio was associated with higher risk of progression to MM ($P = .039$).[91] In a study of 273 patients with SMM, an FLC ratio of ≤0.125 or ≥8 was an independent risk factor for progression (hazard ratio, 2.3; 95% confidence interval [CI], 1.6-3.2). Patients identified as high risk based on this assay had a 25% per year risk of progression in the first 2 years.[92]

Absence of Normal Plasma Cells on Multiparametric Flow Cytometry

Immunophenotyping with multiparametric flow cytometry is useful in determining prognosis in SMM by accurately distinguishing and quantitating BMPCs with malignant potential from normal plasma cells.[93] Certain immunophenotypic markers distinguish MM cells from normal plasma cells with a high degree of accuracy.[94] A Spanish study defines abnormal (MM-type) plasma cell immunophenotype as lack of expression of CD19 and/or CD45, expression of CD56, or weak expression of CD38. In MGUS, a substantial proportion of plasma cells are polyclonal and exhibit normal immunophenotype, whereas in MM almost all plasma cells seen (>95%) are clonal and have an aberrant immunophenotype.[86,94,95] Perez-Persona and colleagues have found that approximately 60% of patients with SMM have an aberrant immunophenotype similar to MM (>95% plasma cells aberrancy; <5% of the detected plasma cells are normal).[86,95] The risk of progression in SMM when >95% plasma cells in the bone marrow had an abnormal immunophenotype is significantly higher compared to those who had a lower rate of aberrancy in the detected BMPC population.[86]

Cytogenetic Abnormalities

A Mayo Clinic series of 351 patients with SMM found that patients with t(4;14) and/or del(17p) were at high risk of progression.[96] These patients had a significantly shorter median TTP (24 months) compared with patients with trisomies (intermediate risk), other cytogenetic abnormalities including t(11;14) (standard risk), and no cytogenetic abnormalities (low risk). Similar results have also been reported by Neben and colleagues in a study of 249 patients with SMM.[97]

Dhodapkar and colleagues have assessed the value of gene expression profiling (GEP) signatures in 331 patients with MGUS and SMM.[98] An increased risk score (≥0.26) based on a 70-gene signature (GEP70) was an independent predictor of the risk of progression to MM.

Change in Monoclonal Protein Level

A key variable that can identify patients with a high risk of progression is change in M protein levels over time. In one study of 53 patients with SMM, patients with a progressive rise in M protein (evolving type) had a higher risk of progression compared to those with stable M protein levels.[99] A Southwest Oncology Group study found that patients with an M protein of <3 g/dL that increased to an M protein level of ≥3 g/dL over 3 months were associated with a risk of progression of approximately 50% at 2 years.[98] Ravi and colleagues studied 190 patients with SMM seen at the Mayo Clinic between 1973 and 2014.[100] An evolving change in monoclonal protein level was defined as 10% increase in M protein within the first 6 months of diagnosis (if M protein 3 g/dL) and/or 25% increase in M protein within the first 12 months, with a minimum required increase of 0.5 g/dL in M protein. Evolving change in hemoglobin was defined as 0.5 g/dL decrease within 12 months of diagnosis. A total of 134 patients (70.5%) progressed to MM over a median follow-up of 10.4 years. On multivariable analysis adjusting for factors known to predict for progression to MM, BMPCs ≥ 20%, evolving M protein, and evolving hemoglobin were independent predictors of progression within 2 years of SMM diagnosis. A risk model comprising these variables found median TTP of 12.3, 5.1, 2.0, and 1.0 years among patients with 0, 1, 2, or 3 risk factors, respectively. The two-year progression rate was 81.5% in persons with evolving M protein and evolving hemoglobin and 90.5% in those with all 3 risk factors.

Risk-Stratification of SMM

Multiple risk-stratification models have been proposed by combining prognostic factors discussed above. Recently, the Mayo 2018 criteria have simplified the identification of patients with high-risk SMM using three variables: serum FLC ratio > 20, serum M protein level > 2 g/dL, and bone marrow clonal plasma cells > 20% (Table 99.6).[101] Presence of two or three of these factors is associated with a median TTP to MM of approximately 2 years, and is considered high-risk SMM. These criteria have subsequently been validated in a separate cohort by the International Myeloma Working Group (IMWG).[102] In addition, the IMWG validation study provides a scoring system for more accurate estimation of prognosis incorporating cytogenetic abnormalities and the Mayo 2018 criteria parameters.

Management

Initial diagnostic studies should include CBC, serum creatinine, serum calcium, skeletal survey (preferably whole body low-dose computed tomography), serum protein electrophoresis with immunofixation, 24-hour urine protein electrophoresis with immunofixation, and serum FLC assay.[68] Specialized imaging with either MRI (whole body or of the spine and pelvis) or PET-CT is recommended to exclude MM.[103] Bone marrow examination is required and should include fluorescent in situ hybridization studies to detect high-risk cytogenetic abnormalities, as well as plasma cell immunophenotyping by multiparametric flow cytometry to enable accurate risk-stratification.

Patients with high risk SMM are candidates for early intervention with lenalidomide or lenalidomide plus dexamethasone after a careful consideration of risks and benefits (Figure 99.6). These patients are also candidates for clinical trials. Patients with SMM who have an evolving M protein, evolving hemoglobin, or imaging changes should also be considered for early intervention similar to MM. In contrast, SMM patients without high-risk factors (low-risk SMM) likely have a risk of progression of 5% per year or less and should be observed without therapy.

Table 99.6. Definition of High-Risk Smoldering Multiple Myeloma[a]

Mayo 2018 Criteria (20-2-20 Criteria)
Any 2-3 of the following:
Serum free light chain ratio (involved/uninvolved) >20
Serum M protein > 2 g/dL
Bone marrow plasma cells >20%
Cytogenetic Risk Factors
t(4;14) translocation
Deletion 17p
Gain or Amp 1q
Other High-Risk Factors
Progressive increase in M protein level (Evolving type of SMM)[b]
Increased circulating plasma cells
MRI with diffuse abnormalities or with one focal lesion
PET-CT with focal lesion with increased uptake but without underlying osteolytic bone destruction

Abbreviations: M, monoclonal; MRI, magnetic resonance imaging; SMM, smoldering multiple myeloma; PET-CT, positron emission tomography-computed tomography.
Modified from Rajkumar SV. Multiple myeloma: 2020 update on diagnosis, risk-stratification, and management. *Am J Hematol.* 2020;95(5):548-567. Copyright © 2020 Wiley Periodicals, Inc. Reprinted by permission of John Wiley & Sons, Inc.

[a]Note that the term smoldering multiple myeloma excludes patients without end-organ damage who meet revised definition of multiple myeloma, namely clonal bone marrow plasma cells ≥60% or serum free light chain (FLC) ratio ≥100 (plus measurable involved FLC level ≥100 mg/L), or more than one focal lesion on magnetic resonance imaging. The risk factors listed in this Table variables associated with a higher risk of progression of SMM and identified patients who need consideration for early therapy and clinical trials. Patients who are high risk by Mayo 2018 criteria are candidates for prophylactic therapy with lenalidomide or lenalidomide plus dexamethasone in the absence of clinical trials.
[b]Increase in serum monoclonal protein by ≥25% on two successive evaluations within a 6-month period.

In patients being observed, the M protein, serum FLC levels, CBC, calcium, and creatinine should be monitored. In high-risk patients, follow-up should continue indefinitely and should include periodic imaging studies to rule out asymptomatic progression. In patients with MRI showing diffuse infiltration, solitary focal lesion, or equivocal lesions, follow-up examinations in 3 to 6 months are strongly recommended.[104] In low-risk patients, follow-up can be reduced to once every 6 months after the first 5 years.[71]

Drug Therapy

Early studies in SMM with melphalan and prednisone found no significant benefit.[105-107] Thalidomide was shown to delay time to progression, but there are long-term side effects associated with this treatment that make it unsuitable for intervention in an asymptomatic population.[108]

More recent randomized trials have focused on the subset of patients with high-risk SMM and have found benefit with early therapy. In a randomized trial conducted in Spain, TTP was significantly longer in patients treated with Rd compared with observation, median TTP not reached vs 21 months, $P < .001$.[93,109] Overall survival (OS) was also longer with Rd compared with observation, three-year survival rate 94% vs 80%, respectively, $P = .03$. A subsequent randomized trial conducted in the United States found that early therapy with lenalidomide as a single agent prolongs time to end-organ damage in patients with high-risk SMM.[110] Based on these two trials, patients with newly diagnosed high-risk SMM patients can be considered for early intervention with lenalidomide or Rd (*Figure 99.6*). An ongoing randomized trial is testing whether a standard myeloma therapeutic triplet (daratumumab, lenalidomide, dexamethasone) will be superior to prophylactic doublet therapy with lenalidomide plus dexamethasone (NCT03937635).

The role of bisphosphonates to delay bony events has also been studied. In one randomized trial, a reduction in skeletal-related events (SRE) was noted with pamidronate (60-90 mg once a month for 12 months) compared with observation.[111] However, no improvement in TTP or OS was noted. In another randomized trial, 163 patients with SMM were randomized to zoledronic acid (4 mg once a month for 12 months) vs observation.[112] A reduction in the rate of SREs was noted, 56% vs 78%, respectively, $P = .041$. Once-yearly bisphosphonate used for the treatment of osteoporosis is appropriate for most patients, but based on these data, more frequent dosing every 3 to 4 months can be considered for selected high-risk SMM patients.

Patients with high-risk SMM who are treated with lenalidomide or Rd should have peripheral blood stem cells collected for cryopreservation after approximately 4 to 6 cycles of therapy.[113,114]

VARIANTS OF MGUS

Secondary MGUS

During the course of MM, new M proteins of an isotype distinct from the original clone can arise and are referred to as secondary MGUS. In a study of 1942 patients with MM, 128 (6.6%) developed a secondary MGUS, at a median time of 12 months from the diagnosis of MM.[115] The median duration of secondary MGUS was 6 months. In 34 (27%)

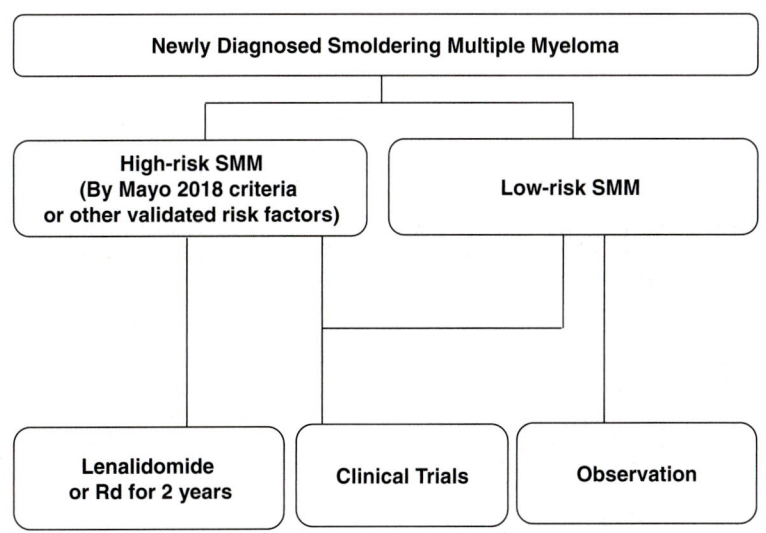

FIGURE 99.6 Approach to the management of smoldering multiple myeloma. Rd, lenalidomide plus dexamethasone; SMM, smoldering multiple myeloma.

of the 128 patients with secondary MGUS, there were multiple secondary MGUSs of varying isotypes. Secondary MGUS was more common in patients who had undergone stem cell transplant (SCT) compared to those who had not undergone such a procedure; 23% vs 2%, respectively, $P < .001$. Most secondary MGUS M proteins were small and detectable by immunofixation only in 84 patients (66%). OS was significantly superior among patients who developed secondary MGUS compared with those who did not develop a secondary MGUS, 73 vs 38 months respectively, $P < .001$. Other studies on secondary MGUS have also found a survival benefit with secondary MGUS that appears in MM patients following SCT.[20] Among patients with secondary MGUS, there is a trend to better OS in those in whom the MGUS resolved compared to those with persistent MGUS.

Biclonal and Triclonal Gammopathy

Biclonal gammopathies are characterized by the presence of two different M proteins and occur in 3% to 6% of patients with monoclonal gammopathies. Riddell et al reported that 2.5% of 1135 patients with monoclonal gammopathy had biclonal gammopathy.[116] They postulated that in some patients complete class switching in a single plasma cell clone resulted in the production of two M proteins, but in others the M proteins arose from two separate plasma cell clones. Triclonal gammopathy is rare. Most reported cases have been associated with immunodeficiency syndromes or lymphoproliferative disorders.

Idiopathic Bence Jones Proteinuria (Benign Monoclonal Light Chain Proteinuria)

Idiopathic Bence Jones proteinuria represents a more advanced stage of LC-MGUS, in which there is excretion of monoclonal light chains in the urine without any evidence of end-organ damage to suggest MM or related disorder.[117,118] Patients with idiopathic Bence Jones proteinuria who have urinary M protein ≥500 mg/24 h and/or ≥10% clonal BMPC are considered to have light chain SMM.[4,78] Kyle and colleagues studied all patients seen at the Mayo Clinic within 30 days of diagnosis of idiopathic Bence Jones proteinuria between January 1, 1960, and June 30, 2004.[78] Of 101 patients followed for 901 total person-years, 27 (27%) patients developed MM and 7 (7%) developed light chain amyloidosis. There was a higher risk of progression in patients with monoclonal light chain excretion ≥500 mg/24 h, ≥10% clonal BMPC, or both compared to the remaining patients and was used to establish the disease definition of light chain SMM. The risk of progression of patients defined as having light chain SMM was 27.8% at 5 years, 44.6% at 10 years, and 56.5% at 15 years.

IgD MGUS

In most studies of MGUS, there are few if any patients with IgD MGUS making it hard to ascertain the natural history of this entity. In general, since IgD is not usually secreted, the presence of a serum IgD M protein almost always indicates MM, AL amyloidosis, or plasma cell leukemia. However, IgD MGUS has been reported occasionally.[119]

ASSOCIATION OF MONOCLONAL GAMMOPATHY WITH OTHER DISEASES

Serum protein electrophoresis is commonly done in patients presenting with a wide variety of clinical symptoms. This results in the incidental diagnosis of MGUS in a wide variety of clinical settings. Since MGUS is common in the general population, and since the prevalence increases with age, "associations" with various diseases can occur just coincidentally. Thus, over the years, over a hundred different medical conditions have been reported to be associated with MGUS, and most such reported associations are not likely causally related. The only method to definitively ascertain true disease associations with MGUS that are etiologically related is to screen all persons in a geographic population for the presence or absence of MGUS, and then determine the diseases that are significantly associated in patients with and without MGUS. Only one such systematic study has been conducted so far. Bida and colleagues studied the association of MGUS with all diseases in a population-based cohort of 17,398 patients, all uniformly tested for the presence or absence of MGUS.[120] Among 17,398 persons, 605 MGUS cases and 16,793 negative controls were identified. The computerized Mayo Medical Index was used to obtain information on all diagnoses entered between January 1, 1975 and May 31, 2006 totaling 422,663 person-years of observations. The study studied all prior reported associations in detail and also looked for new associations not hitherto described. Data were analyzed using stratified Poisson regression, adjusting for age, gender, and total person-years of observation. The study confirmed a significant association in 14 (18.7%) of 75 previously reported disease associations with MGUS, including vertebral and hip fractures and osteoporosis (*Table 99.7*). Several of these associations were known progression events of MGUS such as MM and WM. A systematic analysis of all 16,062 diagnostic disease codes found additional previously unreported associations, including hyperlipidemia, mycobacterium infection, and superficial thrombophlebitis.

Some commonly reported disease associations are briefly discussed below. In some of these cases, the association with a monoclonal protein is undoubtedly causal and has great clinical relevance such as monoclonal gammopathy–associated neuropathy and monoclonal gammopathy–associated proliferative glomerulonephritis (Chapter 103). In others, the association is real, but carries limited clinical consequences such as M proteins that arise with immunosuppression. In others, such as the association with connective tissue disorders and neurologic disorders, it is impossible to determine whether the reported associations are coincidental, and they have limited clinical or etiologic significance. Most such associations are reported from studies in which not all patients were screened for the presence or absence of MGUS. Thus, the reported associations may merely reflect the type of diseases and clinical settings in which a serum protein electrophoresis is ordered rather than a true association with the result of the test.

Monoclonal Gammopathy–Associated Neuropathy

Monoclonal gammopathy associated neuropathy is a well-described entity[12,121,122] (Chapter 103). Approximately 3% to 5% of patients with monoclonal gammopathy have a peripheral neuropathy, and approximately 3% to 5% of patients with a peripheral neuropathy have evidence of an M protein on testing.[123-126] Since 3% to 4% of the general population over the age of 50 has MGUS, it is very common to encounter patients with peripheral neuropathy in whom further work-up reveals an M protein. Distinguishing patients in whom the M protein is causally related to the peripheral neuropathy from patients in whom the presence of an M protein is incidental and unrelated to the neuropathy is difficult. Clearly, the need to differentiate causal associations from coincidental is less important in patients with MM or WM, since these patients need therapy to eradicate the plasma cell clone anyway, and so the decision on whether or not therapy targeting the clone is needed does not arise. Similarly, monoclonal gammopathy–associated peripheral neuropathy must be differentiated from two other plasma cell disorders that cause neuropathy that have been well characterized and have strict diagnostic criteria, namely immunoglobulin light chain (AL) amyloidosis (Chapter 101) and neuropathy associated with POEMS (polyneuropathy, organomegaly, endocrinopathy, monoclonal plasma cell disorder, and skin changes) syndrome (Chapter 103). In AL amyloidosis neuropathy and in POEMS syndrome, the causal relationship between the neurologic process and the underlying M protein is not in question, and therapy is needed targeting at the underlying disorder. The main therapeutic dilemma is in patients with MGUS who have an associated progressive neuropathy in the absence of other causes that may explain the neuropathy.

Monoclonal Gammopathy of Renal Significance

The expression MGRS is gaining popularity as an important descriptor of the group of patients with renal disorders caused by a monoclonal immunoglobulin secreted by a nonmalignant B-cell clone (Chapter 103).[127,128] The same histologic lesions can be seen in cases of B-cell malignancy. MGRS encompasses nearly a dozen histologic entities, the most common of which are AL amyloidosis, monoclonal

Table 99.7. Disease Associations Previously Reported in the Literature in which a Significant Disease Association With Monoclonal Gammopathy of Undetermined Significance (MGUS) Could Be Confirmed Among Residents of Olmsted County, Minnesota.

Description[ref]	Positive MGUS Cases	Age- and Sex-Adjusted Case Rate per 100,000 Person-Years[a]	Positive Controls	Age- and Sex-Adjusted Control Rate per 100,000 Person-Years[a]	Risk Ratio (95% CI)	P-Value
Macroglobulinemia	5	55.1	1	0.6	96.2(11.0-836.5)	<0.001
Multiple myeloma	29	257.4	19	7.9	32.6(18.1-58.7)	<0.001
Plasma cell proliferative disorder	11	87.1	9	3.1	28.0(11.4-68.7)	<0.001
Amyloidosis	7	85.2	18	11.8	7.2(3.0-17.4)	<0.001
CIDP	2	14.9	8	2.5	5.9(1.2-28.4)	0.03
Liver transplant	2	13.9	10	2.6	5.4(1.2-25.3)	0.03
Kidney transplant	5	34.6	38	9.8	3.5(1.4-9.1)	0.01
Lymphoproliferative Disease	17	161.2	105	48.0	3.4(2.0-5.6)	<0.001
Autonomic neuropathy	5	35.8	39	11.0	3.2(1.3-8.3)	0.01
Vertebral Fracture	46	511.1	478	263.9	1.9(1.4-2.6)	<0.001
Hip fracture	36	581.6	388	377.1	1.5(1.1-2.2)	0.01
Hypercalcemia	40	297.5	736	214.9	1.4(1.0-1.9)	0.05
Osteoporosis	153	1701.1	3013	1407.7	1.2(1.0-1.4)	0.02
Urticaria	20	144.8	1003	242.9	0.6(0.4-0.9)	0.02

Abbreviations: CI, confidence interval; CIDP, chronic inflammatory demyelinating polyradiculoneuropathy; MGUS, monoclonal gammopathy of undetermined significance.
Reprinted from Bida JP, Kyle RA, Therneau TM, et al. Disease associations with monoclonal gammopathy of undetermined significance: a population-based study of 17,398 patients. Mayo Clin Proc. 2009;84(8):685-693. Copyright © 2009 Mayo Foundation for Medical Education and Research. With permission.
[a]Rates age and sex adjusted.

immunoglobulin deposition disease, and proliferative glomerulonephritis with monoclonal immunoglobulin deposits. A substantial proportion of cases with "idiopathic" immune-complex–mediated membranoproliferative glomerulonephritis (MPGN) are now felt to be related to monoclonal gammopathies.[13,129,130] In a study of 126 patients with MPGN conducted at the Mayo Clinic, 22% were associated with a monoclonal gammopathy.[129] Excluding other known causes such as hepatitis B and hepatitis C, approximately 40% of cases of idiopathic MPGN could be attributed to a monoclonal gammopathy separate from cryoglobulinemia which has long been associated.

Monoclonal gammopathies can lead to proliferative glomerulonephritis through direct and indirect mechanisms.[13] The direct mechanism involves deposition of M protein in the mesangium and along capillary walls resulting in an immune complex-mediated proliferative glomerulonephritis. The M protein activates the classical and terminal pathway of complement resulting in glomerular accumulation of complement factors of the classical and terminal complement pathway along with the M protein. On renal biopsy, the most common pattern of injury is MPGN, but less commonly other patterns of proliferative glomerulonephritis can be seen including mesangial proliferative glomerulonephritis, diffuse proliferative glomerulonephritis, crescentic and necrotizing glomerulonephritis, and sclerosing glomerulonephritis. Immunofluorescence microscopy will reveal M protein deposits in the mesangium and along capillary walls with evidence of light chain restriction (either κ or λ light chain staining but not both) indicating the clonal nature of the process.

The indirect mechanism involves activation of the alternative pathway of complement by the M protein resulting in accumulation of complement factors of alternative and classical pathway in the absence of significant M protein deposition resulting in C3 glomerulopathy. The term C3 glomerulopathy is used to define conditions associated with abnormalities of the alternative pathway abnormalities and includes C3 glomerulonephritis and dense deposit disease.[13] The renal biopsy will show bright mesangial and capillary wall staining for C3 with no significant M protein deposits on immunofluorescence microscopy.

The diagnosis of monoclonal gammopathy–associated proliferative glomerulonephritis should be suspected in any patient in whom there are no other identifiable causes such as infections (especially hepatitis C) or autoimmune disease. Immunofluorescence examination of the kidney biopsy is essential. The optimal treatment of monoclonal gammopathy–associated proliferative glomerulonephritis has not been well defined, but depending on the clinical symptoms, therapy targeted against the M protein is reasonable.[13,130]

Since the kidney is often involved in plasma cell disorders such as light chain cast nephropathy, light chain deposition disease, AL amyloidosis, and proliferative glomerulonephritis, renal involvement in patients with M proteins requires a careful evaluation and differential diagnosis.

Dermatologic Diseases

A variety of dermatologic diseases have been associated with MGUS (Chapter 103).[131] Lichen myxedematosus (papular mucinosis, scleromyxedema) is a rare dermatologic condition frequently associated with an IgG λ monoclonal protein. Scleredema (Buschke disease) has been noted with an M protein, but the role of the M protein is unknown. Other known associations include pyoderma gangrenosum, diffuse plane xanthomatosis, and subcorneal pustular dermatosis.[132,133] Necrobiotic xanthogranuloma is frequently found with an IgG M protein, while Schnitzler syndrome is a rare disorder characterized by the presence of chronic urticaria and an IgM monoclonal gammopathy.[134]

Immunosuppression

M proteins have been reported in patients with the acquired human immunodeficiency syndrome, but do not appear to have any prognostic significance. M proteins can be detected in approximately 5% to 10% of patients following renal transplantation. Approximately 25% of patients following heart transplantation[135,136] and approximately 30% of patients following liver transplantation have been reported to develop M proteins.[137,138]

The effect of organ transplantation on patients with MGUS is unclear. In one study, 3518 patients who underwent renal transplantation at Mayo Clinic were analyzed.[139] MGUS was identified in 42 patients: 23 prior to transplantation and 19 after transplantation. Two of the patients who had MGUS prior to renal transplantation developed progression of the plasma cell disorder, both to SMM. None of the 19 patients who developed an MGUS after transplant progressed to MM or related disorder. Thus, progression of MGUS following renal transplantation is rare.

Other Hematologic Disorders

MGUS has also been linked to a variety of coagulation disorders including acquired von Willebrand disease and lupus anticoagulant syndrome. A bleeding diathesis may also occur in MGUS from binding of an M protein to thrombin. Thromboembolic disease has also been noted to be more frequent in patients with MGUS. Other rare associations that have been reported include Gaucher disease, pernicious anemia, and pure red cell aplasia caused by a block in the maturation of the erythroid burst forming unit.

Connective Tissue Disorders

Rheumatoid arthritis, seronegative erosive arthritis, systemic lupus erythematosus, and other connective tissue disorders have been reported with MGUS. Polymyalgia rheumatica and polymyositis have also been reported with monoclonal gammopathy. Although there may be a higher prevalence of MGUS with these disorders, a causal or clinically significant relationship has not been established.

Other Neurologic Disorders

Several instances of monoclonal gammopathy and amyotrophic lateral sclerosis have been reported. However, a causal relationship has not been established. Other neurologic disorders that been reported in association with MGUS include myasthenia gravis, ataxia-telangiectasia, and sporadic late onset nemaline myopathy.

Miscellaneous Conditions

Systemic Capillary Leak Syndrome

This disorder is characterized by sudden onset shock and anasarca caused by plasma extravasation and is associated with at monoclonal protein in the majority of cases (Chapter 103).

Hepatitis C

Most cases of type II cryoglobulinemia are related to hepatitis C and are associated with an IgM monoclonal protein. The incidence of hepatitis C virus infection was 69% in 94 patients with mixed cryoglobulinemia and 14% in 107 patients without cryoglobulinemia[140] (Chapter 103). In another series of 102 cases of MM, WM, or MGUS, hepatitis C virus infection was found in 16% of patients but in only 5% of controls.[141] An M protein was found in 11% of 239 hepatitis C virus–positive patients but in only 1% of 98 hepatitis C virus–negative patients. Thus, the prevalence of M proteins in patients with hepatitis C virus–related chronic liver diseases is high.

Other Disorders

M proteins have been noted in numerous other disorders such as chronic active hepatitis, primary biliary cirrhosis, Henoch-Schönlein purpura, bacterial endocarditis, Hashimoto thyroiditis, idiopathic pulmonary fibrosis, pulmonary alveolar proteinosis, idiopathic pulmonary hemosiderosis, sarcoidosis, thymoma, hereditary spherocytosis, Doyne macular heredodystrophy, and eosinophilic fibrohistiocytic lesions of the bone marrow, but these associations are likely coincidental.[120] M proteins have also been associated with corneal crystalline deposits.[142]

M Proteins With Antibody Activity

M proteins may have autoantibody activity, and there have been numerous reported associations. Of 612 patients in whom M proteins were studied for their antibody activity against actin, tubulin, thyroglobulin, myosin, myoglobin, fetuin, albumin, transferrin, and double-stranded DNA, 36 (5.9%) had antibody activity.[143] In some patients with MGUS, MM, or WM, the M protein has exhibited unusual specificities to dextran, antistreptolysin O, platelet glycoprotein IIIa, smooth muscle, platelets, calcium, riboflavin, thyroglobulin, insulin, double-stranded DNA, apolipoprotein, thyroxine, cephalin, lactate dehydrogenase, anti–human immunodeficiency virus, and antibiotics. Of note, yellow discoloration of the skin and hair can be caused by an M protein with antiriboflavin antibody activity. Similarly, an M protein directed against platelet glycoprotein IIIa can lead to a thrombasthenia-like state. An IgM κ M protein that agglutinated platelets and produced a pseudothrombocytopenia has been reported. The binding of calcium by M protein may produce hypercalcemia without symptomatic or pathologic consequences. Binding of an M protein with transferrin can result in a high serum iron level, while binding to phosphate can result in a spurious elevation of the serum phosphorus level.[144]

References

1. Kyle RA, Larson DR, Therneau TM, et al. Long-term follow-up of monoclonal gammopathy of undetermined significance. *N Engl J Med*. 2018;378:241-249.
2. Waldenstrom J. Studies on conditions associated with disturbed gamma globulin formation (gammopathies). *Harvey Lect*. 1960-1961;56:211-231.
3. Axelsson U, Bachmann R, Hallen J. Frequency of pathological proteins (M-components) om 6,995 sera from an adult population. *Acta Med Scand*. 1966;179:235-247.
4. Rajkumar SV, Dimopoulos MA, Palumbo A, et al. International myeloma working group updated criteria for the diagnosis of multiple myeloma. *Lancet Oncol*. 2014;15:e538-e548.
5. Kyle RA, Greipp PR. Smoldering multiple myeloma. *N Engl J Med*. 1980;302:1347-1349.
6. Kyle RA, Remstein ED, Therneau TM, et al. Clinical course and prognosis of smoldering (asymptomatic) multiple myeloma. *N Engl J Med*. 2007;356:2582-2590.
7. Katzmann JA, Kyle RA, Benson J, et al. Screening panels for detection of monoclonal gammopathies. *Clin Chem*. 2009;55:1517-1522.
8. Katzmann JA, Clark RJ, Abraham RS, et al. Serum reference intervals and diagnostic ranges for free kappa and free lambda immunoglobulin light chains: relative sensitivity for detection of monoclonal light chains. *Clin Chem*. 2002;48:1437-1444.
9. Bradwell AR, Carr-Smith HD, Mead GP, Harvey TC, Drayson MT. Serum test for assessment of patients with Bence Jones myeloma. *Lancet*. 2003;361:489-491.
10. Dispenzieri A, Katzmann JA, Kyle RA, et al. Prevalence and risk of progression of light-chain monoclonal gammopathy of undetermined significance: a retrospective population-based cohort study. *Lancet*. 2010;375:1721-1728.
11. Schuster S, Rajkumar SV, Dispenzieri A, et al. IgM multiple myeloma: disease definition, prognosis, and differentiation from Waldenstrom's macroglobulinemia. *Am J Hematol*. 2010;85:853-855.
12. Chaudhry HM, Mauermann ML, Rajkumar SV. Monoclonal gammopathy-associated peripheral neuropathy: diagnosis and management. *Mayo Clin Proc*. 2017;92:838-850.
13. Sethi S, Rajkumar SV. Monoclonal gammopathy-associated proliferative glomerulonephritis. *Mayo Clin Proc*. 2013;88:1284-1293.
14. Kyle RA, Therneau TM, Rajkumar SV, et al. Prevalence of monoclonal gammopathy of undetermined significance. *N Engl J Med*. 2006;354:1362-1369.
15. Wadhera RK, Rajkumar SV. Prevalence of monoclonal gammopathy of undetermined significance: a systematic review. *Mayo Clinic Proc*. 2010;85:933-942.
16. Cohen HJ, Crawford J, Rao MK, Pieper CF, Currie MS. Racial differences in the prevalence of monoclonal gammopathy in a community-based sample of the elderly. *Am J Med*. 1998;104:439-444. erratum appears in Am J Med. 1998;105(4):362.
17. Landgren O, Gridley G, Turesson I, et al. Risk of monoclonal gammopathy of undetermined significance (MGUS) and subsequent multiple myeloma among African American and white veterans in the United States. *Blood*. 2006;107:904-906.
18. Landgren O, Graubard BI, Katzmann JA, et al. Racial disparities in the prevalence of monoclonal gammopathies: a population-based study of 12 482 persons from the national health and nutritional examination survey. *Leukemia*. 2014;28:1537-1542.
19. Landgren O, Graubard BI, Kumar S, et al. Prevalence of myeloma precursor state monoclonal gammopathy of undetermined significance (MGUS) in 12,309 individuals 10 to 49 years old: a population-based study from the National Health and Nutritional Examination Survey. *Blood Cancer J*. 2017;7:e618.
20. Landgren O, Katzmann JA, Hsing AW, et al. Prevalence of monoclonal gammopathy of undetermined significance among men in Ghana. *Mayo Clin Proc*. 2007;82:1468-1473.
21. Landgren O, Rajkumar SV, Pfeiffer RM, et al. Obesity is associated with an increased risk of monoclonal gammopathy of undetermined significance (MGUS) among African-American and Caucasian women. *Blood*. 2010;116:1056-1059.

22. Bowden M, Crawford J, Cohen HJ, Noyama O. A comparative study of monoclonal gammopathies and immunoglobulin levels in Japanese and United States elderly. *J Am Geriatr Soc.* 1993;41:11-14.
23. Iwanaga M, Tagawa M, Tsukasaki K, Kamihira S, Tomonaga M. Prevalence of monoclonal gammopathy of undetermined significance: study of 52,802 persons in Nagasaki city, Japan. *Mayo Clin Proc.* 2007;82:1474-1479.
24. Therneau TM, Kyle RA, Melton LJ, III, et al. Incidence of monoclonal gammopathy of undetermined significance and estimation of duration before first clinical recognition. *Mayo Clin Proc.* 2012;87:1071-1079.
25. Greenberg AJ, Rajkumar SV, Vachon CM. Familial monoclonal gammopathy of undetermined significance and multiple myeloma: epidemiology, risk factors, and biological characteristics. *Blood.* 2012;119:4771-4779.
26. Vachon CM, Kyle RA, Therneau TM, et al. Increased risk of monoclonal gammopathy in first-degree relatives of patients with multiple myeloma or monoclonal gammopathy of undetermined significance. *Blood.* 2009;114:785-790.
27. Greenberg AJ, Rajkumar SV, Larson DR, et al. Increased prevalence of light chain monoclonal gammopathy of undetermined significance (LC-MGUS) in first-degree relatives of individuals with multiple myeloma. *Br J Haematol.* 2012;157:472-475.
28. Zemble RM, Takach PA, Levinson AI. The relationship between hypogammaglobulinemia, monoclonal gammopathy of undetermined significance and humoral immunodeficiency: a case series. *J Clin Immunol.* 2011;31:737-743.
29. Passweg J, Thiel G, Bock HA. Monoclonal gammopathy after intense induction immunosuppression in renal transplant patients. *Nephrol Dial Transplant.* 1996;11:2461-2465.
30. Landgren O, Kyle RA, Hoppin JA, et al. Pesticide exposure and risk of monoclonal gammopathy of undetermined significance (MGUS) in the Agricultural Health Study. *Blood.* 2009;25:6386-6391.
31. Landgren O, Kyle RA, Pfeiffer RM, et al. Monoclonal gammopathy of undetermined significance (MGUS) consistently precedes multiple myeloma: a prospective study. *Blood.* 2009;113:5412-5417.
32. Weiss BM, Abadie J, Verma P, Howard RS, Kuehl WM. A monoclonal gammopathy precedes multiple myeloma in most patients. *Blood.* 2009;113:5418-5422.
33. Rajkumar SV. Prevention of progression in monoclonal gammopathy of undetermined significance. *Clin Cancer Res.* 2009;15:5606-5608.
34. Rajkumar SV. Preventive strategies in monoclonal gammopathy of undetermined significance and smoldering multiple myeloma. *Am J Hematol.* 2012;87:453-454.
35. Fonseca R, Barlogie B, Bataille R, et al. Genetics and cytogenetics of multiple myeloma: a workshop report. *Cancer Res.* 2004;64:1546-1558.
36. Kyle RA, Rajkumar SV. Multiple myeloma. *N Engl J Med.* 2004;351:1860-1873.
37. Kuehl WM, Bergsagel PL. Multiple myeloma: evolving genetic events and host interactions. *Nat Rev Cancer.* 2002;2:175-187.
38. Bergsagel PL, Kuehl WM. Chromosome translocations in multiple myeloma. *Oncogene.* 2001;20:5611-5622.
39. Fonseca R, Bailey RJ, Ahmann GJ, et al. Genomic abnormalities in monoclonal gammopathy of undetermined significance. *Blood.* 2002;100:1417-1424.
40. Kyle RA, Therneau TM, Rajkumar SV, et al. A long-term study of prognosis of monoclonal gammopathy of undetermined significance. *N Engl J Med.* 2002;346:564-569.
41. Misund K, Keane N, Stein CK, et al. MYC dysregulation in the progression of multiple myeloma. *Leukemia.* 2020;34:322-326.
42. Hanamura I, Stewart JP, Huang Y, et al. Frequent gain of chromosome band 1q21 in plasma-cell dyscrasias detected by fluorescence in situ hybridization: incidence increases from MGUS to relapsed myeloma and is related to prognosis and disease progression following tandem stem-cell transplantation. *Blood.* 2006;108:1724-1732.
43. Keats JJ, Chesi M, Egan JB, et al. Clonal competition with alternating dominance in multiple myeloma. *Blood.* 2012;120:1067-1076.
44. Rajkumar SV, Leong T, Roche PC, et al. Prognostic value of bone marrow angiogenesis in multiple myeloma. *Clin Cancer Res.* 2000;6:3111-3116.
45. Rajkumar SV, Mesa RA, Fonseca R, et al. Bone marrow angiogenesis in 400 patients with monoclonal gammopathy of undetermined significance, multiple myeloma, and primary amyloidosis. *Clin Cancer Res.* 2002;8:2210-2216.
46. Vacca A, Ribatti D, Presta M, et al. Bone marrow neovascularization, plasma cell angiogenic potential, and matrix metalloproteinase-2 secretion parallel progression of human multiple myeloma. *Blood.* 1999;93:3064-3073.
47. Perez-Andres M, Almeida J, Martin-Ayuso M, et al. Clonal plasma cells from monoclonal gammopathy of undetermined significance, multiple myeloma and plasma cell leukemia show different expression profiles of molecules involved in the interaction with the immunological bone marrow microenvironment. *Leukemia.* 2005;19:449-455.
48. Rawstron AC, Fenton JA, Ashcroft J, et al. The interleukin-6 receptor alpha-chain (CD126) is expressed by neoplastic but not normal plasma cells. *Blood.* 2000;96:3880-3886.
49. Donovan KA, Lacy MQ, Kline MP, et al. Contrast in cytokine expression between patients with monoclonal gammopathy of undetermined significance or multiple myeloma. *Leukemia.* 1998;12:593-600.
50. Paiva B, Perez-Andres M, Vidriales MB, et al. Competition between clonal plasma cells and normal cells for potentially overlapping bone marrow niches is associated with a progressively altered cellular distribution in MGUS vs myeloma. *Leukemia.* 2011;25:697-706.
51. Sezer O. Myeloma bone disease: recent advances in biology, diagnosis, and treatment. *Oncologist.* 2009;14:276-283.
52. Roodman GD. Pathogenesis of myeloma bone disease. *Leukemia.* 2009;23:435-441.
53. Tian E, Zhan F, Walker R, et al. The role of the Wnt-signaling antagonist DKK1 in the development of osteolytic lesions in multiple myeloma. *N Engl J Med.* 2003;349:2483-2494. [see comment].
54. Rajkumar SV, Kyle RA, Buadi FK. Advances in the diagnosis, classification, risk stratification, and management of monoclonal gammopathy of undetermined significance: implications for recategorizing disease entities in the presence of evolving scientific evidence. *Mayo Clinic Proc.* 2010;85:945-948.
55. Kyle RA. Monoclonal gammopathy of undetermined significance. Natural history in 241 cases. *Am J Med.* 1978;64:814-826.
56. Kyle RA, Therneau TM, Rajkumar SV, Larson DR, Plevak MF, Melton LJ, IIIrd. Long-term follow-up of 241 patients with monoclonal gammopathy of undetermined significance: the original Mayo Clinic series 25 years later. *Mayo Clin Proc.* 2004;79:859-866. [see comment].
57. Surveillance, Epidemiology, and End Results (SEER) Program public use data (1973-1998). National Cancer Institute, Cancer Statistics Branch; April 2001.
58. Kyle RA, Linos A, Beard CM, et al. Incidence and natural history of primary systemic amyloidosis in Olmsted County, Minnesota, 1950 through 1989. *Blood.* 1992;79:1817-1822.
59. Baldini L, Guffanti A, Cesana BM, et al. Role of different hematologic variables in defining the risk of malignant transformation in monoclonal gammopathy. *Blood.* 1996;87:912-918.
60. Gregersen H, Mellemkjaer L, Salling Ibsen J, et al. Cancer risk in patients with monoclonal gammopathy of undetermined significance. *Am J Hematol.* 2000;63:1-6.
61. Kyle RA, Therneau TM, Rajkumar SV, et al. Long-term follow-up of IgM monoclonal gammopathy of undetermined significance. *Blood.* 2003;102:3759-3764.
62. Rajkumar SV, Kyle RA, Therneau TM, et al. Serum free light chain ratio is an independent risk factor for progression in monoclonal gammopathy of undetermined significance (MGUS). *Blood.* 2005;106:812-817.
63. Cesana C, Klersy C, Barbarano L, et al. Prognostic factors for malignant transformation in monoclonal gammopathy of undetermined significance and smoldering multiple myeloma. *J Clin Oncol.* 2002;20:1625-1634.
64. Kyle RA. "Benign" monoclonal gammopathy--after 20 to 35 years of follow-up. *Mayo Clin Proc.* 1993;68:26-36.
65. van de Poel MH, Coebergh JW, Hillen HF. Malignant transformation of monoclonal gammopathy of undetermined significance among out-patients of a community hospital in southeastern Netherlands. *Br J Haematol.* 1995;91:121-125.
66. Go RS, Rajkumar SV. How I manage monoclonal gammopathy of undetermined significance. *Blood.* 2017;131(2):163-173.
67. Mangiacavalli S, Cocito F, Pochintesta L, et al. Monoclonal gammopathy of undetermined significance: a new proposal of work up. *Eur J Haematol.* 2013;91:356-360.
68. Kyle RA, Durie BGM, Rajkumar SV, et al. Monoclonal gammopathy of undetermined significance (MGUS) and smoldering (asymptomatic) multiple myeloma: IMWG consensus perspectives risk factors for progression and guidelines for monitoring and management. *Leukemia.* 2010;24:1121-1127.
69. Bianchi G, Kyle RA, Colby CL, et al. Impact of optimal follow-up of Monoclonal Gammopathy of Undetermined Significance (MGUS) on early diagnosis and prevention of myeloma-related complications. *Blood.* 2010;116:2019-2025.
70. Rajkumar SV. The screening imperative for multiple myeloma. *Nature.* 2020;587:S63.
71. Rajkumar SV, Landgren O, Mateos MV. Smoldering multiple myeloma. *Blood.* 2015;125:3069-3075.
72. Rajkumar SV, Larson D, Kyle RA. Diagnosis of smoldering multiple myeloma. *N Engl J Med.* 2011;365:474-475.
73. Kastritis E, Terpos E, Moulopoulos L, et al. Extensive bone marrow infiltration and abnormal free light chain ratio identifies patients with asymptomatic myeloma at high risk for progression to symptomatic disease. *Leukemia.* 2012;27:947-953.
74. Larsen JT, Kumar SK, Dispenzieri A, Kyle RA, Katzmann JA, Rajkumar SV. Serum free light chain ratio as a biomarker for high-risk smoldering multiple myeloma. *Leukemia.* 2013;27:941-946.
75. Waxman AJ, Mick R, Garfall AL, et al. Modeling the risk of progression in smoldering multiple myeloma. *J Clin Oncol.* 2014;32:A8607.
76. Hillengass J, Fechtner K, Weber MA, et al. Prognostic significance of focal lesions in whole-body magnetic resonance imaging in patients with asymptomatic multiple myeloma. *J Clin Oncol.* 2010;28:1606-1610.
77. Kastritis E, Moulopoulos LA, Terpos E, Koutoulidis V, Dimopoulos MA. The prognostic importance of the presence of more than one focal lesion in spine MRI of patients with asymptomatic (smoldering) multiple myeloma. *Leukemia.* 2014;28:2402-2403.
78. Kyle RA, Larson DR, Therneau TM, et al. Clinical course of light-chain smoldering multiple myeloma (idiopathic Bence Jones proteinuria): a retrospective cohort study. *Lancet Haematol.* 2014;1:e28-e36.
79. Dimopoulos MA, Moulopoulos LA, Maniatis A, Alexanian R. Solitary plasmacytoma of bone and asymptomatic multiple myeloma. *Blood.* 2000;96:2037-2044.
80. Dimopoulos MA, Moulopoulos A, Smith T, Delasalle KB, Alexanian R. Risk of disease progression in asymptomatic multiple myeloma. *Am J Med.* 1993;94:57-61.
81. Riccardi A, Gobbi PG, Ucci G, et al. Changing clinical presentation of multiple myeloma. *Eur J Cancer.* 1991;27:1401-1405.
82. Wisloff F, Andersen P, Andersson TR, et al. Incidence and follow-up of asymptomatic multiple myeloma. The myeloma project of health region I in Norway. II. *Eur J Haematol.* 1991;47:338-341.
83. Kristinsson SY, Holmberg E, Blimark C. Treatment for high-risk smoldering myeloma. *N Engl J Med.* 2013;369:1762-1763.
84. Blade J, Dimopoulos M, Rosinol L, Rajkumar SV, Kyle RA. Smoldering (asymptomatic) multiple myeloma: current diagnostic criteria, new predictors of outcome, and follow-up recommendations. *J Clin Oncol.* 2010;28:690-697.
85. Rajkumar SV, Merlini G, San Miguel JF. Redefining myeloma. *Nat Rev Clin Oncol.* 2012;9:494-496.
86. Perez-Persona E, Vidriales MB, Mateo G, et al. New criteria to identify risk of progression in monoclonal gammopathy of uncertain significance and smoldering multiple myeloma based on multiparameter flow cytometry analysis of bone marrow plasma cells. *Blood.* 2007;110:2586-2592.

87. Bianchi G, Kyle RA, Larson DR, et al. High levels of peripheral blood circulating plasma cells as a specific risk factor for progression of smoldering multiple myeloma. *Leukemia.* 2013;27:680-685.
88. Mouloupoulos LA, Dimopoulos MA, Smith TL, et al. Prognostic significance of magnetic resonance imaging in patients with asymptomatic multiple myeloma. *J Clin Oncol.* 1995;13:251-256.
89. Cavo M, Terpos E, Nanni C, et al. Role of 18F-FDG PET/CT in the diagnosis and management of multiple myeloma and other plasma cell disorders: a consensus statement by the International Myeloma Working Group. *Lancet Oncol.* 2017;18:e206-e217.
90. Zamagni E, Nanni C, Gay F, et al. 18F-FDG PET/CT focal, but not osteolytic, lesions predict the progression of smoldering myeloma to active disease. *Leukemia.* 2016;30:417-422.
91. Dingli D, Kyle RA, Rajkumar SV, et al. Immunoglobulin free light chains and solitary plasmacytoma of bone. *Blood.* 2006;108:1979-1983.
92. Dispenzieri A, Kyle RA, Katzmann JA, et al. Immunoglobulin free light chain ratio is an independent risk factor for progression of smoldering (asymptomatic) multiple myeloma. *Blood.* 2008;111:785-789.
93. Mateos M-V, Hernández M-T, Giraldo P, et al. Lenalidomide plus dexamethasone for high-risk smoldering multiple myeloma. *N Engl J Med.* 2013;369:438-447.
94. Rawstron AC, Orfao A, Beksac M, et al. Report of the European Myeloma Network on multiparametric flow cytometry in multiple myeloma and related disorders. *Haematologica.* 2008;93:431-438.
95. Pérez-Persona E, Mateo G, García-Sanz R, et al. Risk of progression in smouldering myeloma and monoclonal gammopathies of unknown significance: comparative analysis of the evolution of monoclonal component and multiparameter flow cytometry of bone marrow plasma cells. *Br J Haematol.* 2009;148:110-114.
96. Rajkumar SV, Gupta V, Fonseca R, et al. Impact of primary molecular cytogenetic abnormalities and risk of progression in smoldering multiple myeloma. *Leukemia.* 2013;27:1738-1744.
97. Neben K, Jauch A, Hielscher T, et al. Progression in smoldering myeloma is independently determined by the chromosomal abnormalities del(17p), t(4;14), gain 1q, hyperdiploidy, and tumor load. *J Clin Oncol.* 2013;31:4325-4332.
98. Dhodapkar MV, Sexton R, Waheed S, et al. Clinical, genomic, and imaging predictors of myeloma progression from asymptomatic monoclonal gammopathies (SWOG S0120). *Blood.* 2014;123:78-85.
99. Rosinol L, Blade J, Esteve J, et al. Smoldering multiple myeloma: natural history and recognition of an evolving type. *Br J Haematol.* 2003;123:631-636.
100. Ravi P, Kumar S, Larsen JT, et al. Evolving changes in disease biomarkers and risk of early progression in smoldering multiple myeloma. *Blood Cancer J.* 2016;6:e454.
101. Lakshman A, Rajkumar SV, Buadi FK, et al. Risk stratification of smoldering multiple myeloma incorporating revised IMWG diagnostic criteria. *Blood Cancer J.* 2018;8:59.
102. Mateos MV, Kumar S, Dimopoulos MA, et al. International Myeloma Working Group risk stratification model for smoldering multiple myeloma (SMM). *Blood Cancer J.* 2020;10:102.
103. Hillengass J, Usmani S, Rajkumar SV, et al. International myeloma working group consensus recommendations on imaging in monoclonal plasma cell disorders. *Lancet Oncol.* 2019;20:e302-e312.
104. Merz M, Hielscher T, Wagner B, et al. Predictive value of longitudinal whole-body magnetic resonance imaging in patients with smoldering multiple myeloma. *Leukemia.* 2014;28:1902-1908.
105. Hjorth M, Hellquist L, Holmberg E, Magnusson B, Rodjer S, Westin J. Initial versus deferred melphalan-prednisone therapy for asymptomatic multiple myeloma stage I--a randomized study. Myeloma Group of Western Sweden. *Eur J Haematol.* 1993;50:95-102.
106. Grignani G, Gobbi PG, Formisano R, et al. A prognostic index for multiple myeloma. *Br J Cancer.* 1996;73:1101-1107.
107. Riccardi A, Mora O, Tinelli C, et al. Long-term survival of stage I multiple myeloma given chemotherapy just after diagnosis or at progression of the disease: a multicentre randomized study. Cooperative Group of Study and Treatment of Multiple Myeloma. *Br J Cancer.* 2000;82:1254-1260.
108. Witzig TE, Laumann KM, Lacy MQ, et al. A phase III randomized trial of thalidomide plus zoledronic acid versus zoledronic acid alone in patients with asymptomatic multiple myeloma. *Leukemia.* 2013;27:220-225.
109. Mateos MV, Hernandez MT, Giraldo P, et al. Lenalidomide plus dexamethasone versus observation in patients with high-risk smouldering multiple myeloma (QuiRedex): long-term follow-up of a randomised, controlled, phase 3 trial. *Lancet Oncol.* 2016;17:1127-1136.
110. Lonial S, Jacobus SJ, Weiss M, et al. E3A06: randomized phase III trial of lenalidomide versus observation alone in patients with asymptomatic high-risk smoldering multiple myeloma. *J Clin Oncol.* 2020;38(11):1126-1137.
111. D'Arena G, Gobbi PG, Broglia C, et al. Pamidronate versus observation in asymptomatic myeloma: final results with long-term follow-up of a randomized study. *Leuk Lymphoma.* 2011;52:771-775.
112. Musto P, Petrucci MT, Bringhen S, et al. A multicenter, randomized clinical trial comparing zoledronic acid versus observation in patients with asymptomatic myeloma. *Cancer.* 2008;113:1588-1595.
113. Tsuda K, Tanimoto T, Komatsu T. Treatment for high-risk smoldering myeloma. *N Engl J Med.* 2013;369:1763.
114. Mateos MV, San Miguel JF. Treatment for high-risk smoldering myeloma. *N Engl J Med.* 2013;369:1764-1765.
115. Wadhera RK, Kyle RA, Larson DR, et al. Incidence, clinical course, and prognosis of secondary monoclonal gammopathy of undetermined significance in patients with multiple myeloma. *Blood.* 2011;118:2985-2987.
116. Riddell S, Traczyk Z, Paraskevas F, Israels LG. The double gammopathies. Clinical and immunological studies. *Medicine (Baltimore).* 1986;65:135-142.
117. Kyle RA, Maldonado JE, Bayrd ED. Idiopathic Bence Jones proteinuria–a distinct entity? *Am J Med.* 1973;55:222-226.
118. Kyle R, Therneau T, Dispenzieri A, et al. Idiopathic bence Jones proteinuria: clinical course and prognosis. *ASH Annual Meeting Abstracts.* 2006;108:3493.
119. Blade J, Kyle RA. IgD monoclonal gammopathy with long-term follow-up. *Br J Haematol.* 1994;88:395-396.
120. Bida JP, Kyle RA, Therneau TM, et al. Disease associations with monoclonal gammopathy of undetermined significance: a population-based study of 17,398 patients. *Mayo Clin Proc.* 2009;84:685-693.
121. Kyle RA, Dyck PJ. Neuropathy associated with the monoclonal gammopathies. In: Dyck PJ, Thomas PK, Griffin JW, Low PA, Poduslo JF, eds. *Peripheral Neuropathy.* 3rd ed. W. B. Saunders; 1993:1275-1287.
122. Kelly JJ, Jr. Polyneuropathies associated with plasma cell dyscrasias. *Semin Neurol.* 1987;7:30-39.
123. Kelly JJ, Kyle RA, Obrien PC, Dyck PJ. The prevalence of monoclonal gammopathy in peripheral neuropathy - a prospective survey. *Neurology.* 1981;31:155.
124. Kahn SN, Riches PG, Kohn J. Paraproteinaemia in neurological disease: incidence, associations, and classification of monoclonal immunoglobulins. *J Clin Pathol.* 1980;33:617-621.
125. Baldini L, Nobile-Orazio E, Guffanti A, et al. Peripheral neuropathy in IgM monoclonal gammopathy and Waldenstrom's macroglobulinemia: a frequent complication in elderly males with low MAG-reactive serum monoclonal component. *Am J Hematol.* 1994;45:25-31.
126. Nobile-Orazio E, Barbieri S, Baldini L, et al. Peripheral neuropathy in monoclonal gammopathy of undetermined significance: prevalence and immunopathogenetic studies. *Acta Neurol Scand.* 1992;85:383-390.
127. Leung N, Bridoux F, Hutchison CA, et al. Monoclonal gammopathy of renal significance: when MGUS is no longer undetermined or insignificant. *Blood.* 2012;120:4292-4295.
128. Bridoux F, Leung N, Hutchison CA, et al. Diagnosis of monoclonal gammopathy of renal significance. *Kidney Int.* 2015;87:698-711.
129. Sethi S, Zand L, Leung N, et al. Membranoproliferative glomerulonephritis secondary to monoclonal gammopathy. *Clin J Am Soc Nephrol.* 2010;5:770-782.
130. Sethi S, Fervenza FC. Membranoproliferative glomerulonephritis--a new look at an old entity. *N Engl J Med.* 2012;366:1119-1131.
131. Daoud MS, Lust JA, Kyle RA, Pittelkow MR. Monoclonal gammopathies and associated skin disorders. *J Am Acad Dermatol.* 1999;40:507-535. quiz 36-8.
132. Ryatt KS, Dodman BA, Cotterill JA. Subcorneal pustular dermatosis and IgA gammopathy. *Acta Derm Venereol.* 1981;61:560-562.
133. Lutz ME, Daoud MS, McEvoy MT, Gibson LE. Subcorneal pustular dermatosis: a clinical study of ten patients. *Cutis.* 1998;61:203-208.
134. Jain T, Offord CP, Kyle RA, Dingli D. Schnitzler syndrome: an under-diagnosed clinical entity. *Haematologica.* 2013;98:1581-1585.
135. Caforio AL, Gambino A, Belloni Fortina A, et al. Monoclonal gammopathy in heart transplantation: risk factor analysis and relevance of immunosuppressive load. *Transplant Proc.* 2001;33:1583-1584.
136. Caforio AL, Gambino A, Fortina AB, et al. Monoclonal gammopathy in heart transplantation: clinical significance and risk factors. *J Heart Lung Transplant.* 2001;20:237.
137. Badley AD, Portela DF, Patel R, et al. Development of monoclonal gammopathy precedes the development of Epstein-Barr virus-induced posttransplant lymphoproliferative disorder. *Liver Transpl Surg.* 1996;2:375-382.
138. Pageaux GP, Bonnardet A, Picot MC, et al. Prevalence of monoclonal immunoglobulins after liver transplantation - relationship with posttransplant lymphoproliferative disorders. *Transplantation.* 1998;65:397-400.
139. Naina HV, Harris S, Dispenzieri A, et al. Long-term follow-up of patients with monoclonal gammopathy of undetermined significance after kidney transplantation. *Am J Nephrol.* 2012;35:365-371.
140. Mussini C, Ghini M, Mascia MT, et al. HCV and monoclonal gammopathies. *Clin Exp Rheumatol.* 1995;13(suppl 13):S45-S49.
141. Mangia A, Clemente R, Musto P, et al. Hepatitis C virus infection and monoclonal gammopathies not associated with cryoglobulinemia. *Leukemia.* 1996;10:1209-1213.
142. Paladini I, Pieretti G, Giuntoli M, Abbruzzese G, Menchini U, Mencucci R. Crystalline corneal deposits in monoclonal gammopathy: in-vivo confocal microscopy. *Semin Ophthalmol.* 2013;28:37-40.
143. Dighiero G, Guilbert B, Fermand JP, Lymberi P, Danon F, Avrameas S. Thirty-six human monoclonal immunoglobulins with antibody activity against cytoskeleton proteins, thyroglobulin, and native DNA: immunologic studies and clinical correlations. *Blood.* 1983;62:264-270.
144. Pettersson T, Hortling L, Teppo AM, Totterman KJ, Fyhrquist F. Phosphate binding by a myeloma protein. *Acta Med Scand.* 1987;222:89-91.

Chapter 100 ■ Multiple Myeloma

WILSON I. GONSALVES • PRASHANT KAPOOR • SHAJI K. KUMAR

INTRODUCTION

Multiple myeloma (MM) is a neoplastic plasma cell dyscrasia (PCD). With the exception of monoclonal gammopathy of undetermined significance (MGUS; see Chapter 99), it is the most common PCD, with an incidence of about 1 per 10,000 per year in the United States.[1] Smoldering myeloma, solitary plasmacytoma, and plasma cell leukemia (PCL) are recognized as separate entities and are much less prevalent. The underlying pathogenesis of the plasma cell malignancies is not well understood but is an area of active investigation. At present, according to the World Health Organization classification system, there is only one category for MM.[2] Results of clinical trials are confounded by this under classification. Emerging information about the genetic underpinning of the disease, however, will likely rectify this deficiency.

The interactions among the plasma cells, their antibody product, the local bone and bone marrow environment, and other organs are complex. MM is not yet considered a curable disease, but there are many effective treatments that prolong and improve the quality of life in patients with the disease.

HISTORY

Samuel Solley reported the first well-documented case of MM (mollities ossium) in Sarah Newbury in 1844.[3] Several years later, William MacIntyre described and recorded the properties of the disease we now called MM in Thomas Alexander McBean. Both Drs MacIntyre and Bence Jones noted and described some of the peculiar urine properties of this same patient. On heating, the urine was found to be "abound in animal matter," which dissolved on the addition of nitric acid but reappeared after cooling. These urinary proteins became known as Bence Jones proteins. MacIntyre and Dalrymple described the postmortem examination of Mr McBean's bones. The term "multiple myeloma" was coined in 1873 by von Rustizky, who independently described a similar patient to emphasize the multiple bone tumors that were present. In 1889, Professor Otto Kahler described a case and published a major review in which he described the skeletal pain, albuminuria, pallor, anemia, a precipitable urinary protein, and the findings on necropsy linking these findings as part of a clinical syndrome, which was known as Kahler disease, another name for MM.

Serum electrophoresis, described by Tiselius in 1937, made it possible to separate serum proteins. Longsworth et al applied electrophoresis to the study of MM and described the tall narrow-based "church spire" peak. The use of filter paper as a support for protein electrophoresis permitted the separation of protein into distinct zones that could be stained with various dyes. Paper electrophoresis was supplanted by filter paper in 1957 and later by high-resolution electrophoresis on agarose gel. Kunkel hypothesized that monoclonal proteins were the product of malignant plasma cells and were the equivalent of normal antibodies produced by normal plasma cells. Immunoelectrophoresis and immunofixation or direct immunoelectrophoresis made it possible to detect small monoclonal light chains not recognizable by electrophoresis. The immunoglobulin free light-chain assay made it possible to detect circulating free light chains in the majority of patients previously designated nonsecretory.

Prior to the discovery in 1950[4] of salutary effects of adrenocorticotropic hormones on MM (*Figure 100.1*), medications used to that point included stibidine and urethane, neither of which had activity upon critical testing.[3] Corticosteroids decreased bone pain, improved hypercalcemia, increased hemoglobin values, and decreased abnormal serum and urine globulin concentrations. However, it was not until 1967 that high-dose corticosteroids were recognized as effective antineoplastic agents against MM.

Blokhin et al[5] reported benefits in three of six patients with MM who were treated with sarcolysin (a racemic mixture of the D- and L-isomers of phenylalanine mustard). Subsequently, the D- and L-isomers were tested separately, and the anti-MM activity was found to reside in the L-isomer, melphalan. Bergsagel et al[6] reported significant improvement in 14 of 24 patients with MM with the use of melphalan; this activity was quickly substantiated by others.[7] Similar effectiveness was noted with cyclophosphamide.[8] Subsequently, interferon (IFN)-α, anthracyclines, etoposide, cisplatin, carmustine, thalidomide, bortezomib, lenalidomide, bendamustine, carfilzomib, pomalidomide, ixazomib, and daratumumab[9-21] each were shown to have activity as a single agent in MM. The only Food and Drug Administration (FDA)–approved drugs for MM that do not have single-agent activity are elotuzumab and panobinostat.[22,23]

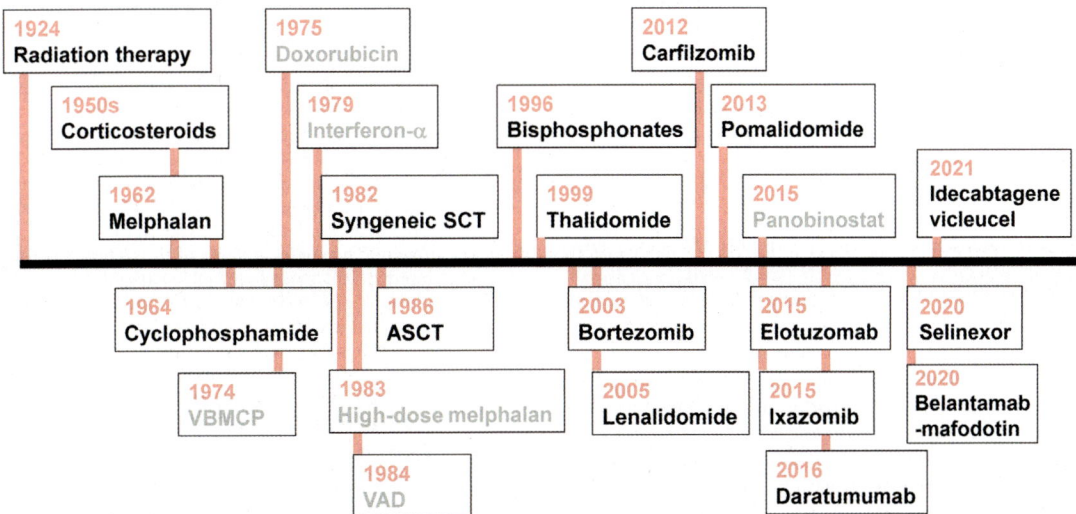

FIGURE 100.1 Landmark therapeutic innovations. ASCT, autologous stem cell transplant; CCT, conventional chemotherapy; VAD, vincristine, doxorubicin, and dexamethasone; VBMCP, vincristine.

INCIDENCE AND EPIDEMIOLOGY

As described in Chapters 98 and 99, recent evidence supports the theory that all MM arises from a preceding MGUS.[24] Increasingly, it is becoming apparent that there is increased risk of developing MM or MGUS among first-degree relatives of both MGUS and MM patients.[25,26] Whether this family linkage is caused by either genetic susceptibility factors or shared environmental risk factors (or both) is yet to be determined.

The 2021 annual estimate in the United States for new cases of MM is 30,770 and for deaths is 12,770.[1] Surveillance, Epidemiology, and End Results data incidence age-adjusted rates from 2010 to 2014 show an incidence among blacks of about twofold higher than whites, the incidence in men is about 1.6-fold that of women. The median age at diagnosis of MM is 69 years. Since the turn of the century, the 5-year survival rates in blacks and whites have equalized. MM accounts for 1.8% of all malignancies. International mortality data reveal that the highest rates of MM occur in Northern Europe, North America, Australia, and New Zealand, and the lowest rates are in Japan, Yugoslavia, and Greece.[27] Geographic clusters[28] and familial clusters of MM among first-degree relatives have been documented.[29,30]

Radiation Exposure

Reports of increased MM incidence and mortality among Japanese atomic bomb survivors have suggested an association between ionizing radiation and MM. Initial evaluations of cancer incidence[31] and mortality[32] among Japanese atomic bomb survivors suggested an increased risk of MM with increasing radiation dose, an observation that was no longer seen with additional years of follow-up.[33] Subsequent data would suggest that the prevalence of MGUS is higher among those younger patients exposed to higher doses of radiation.[34]

An excess of MM deaths among American radiologists was reported in the 1960s.[35] MM risk was considered to be two times higher among radiologists exposed to low doses of radiation than among physicians not exposed to radiation.[36] However, among 27,000 Chinese diagnostic radiography workers, no excess incidence of MM was observed in a 30-year period.[37] An analysis of 115,000 workers from the combined roster of four different nuclear plants showed a positive association between MM and radiation exposure in older age groups.[38] No increases in MM incidence and mortality have been observed among British[39] or New Zealand[40] military men who participated in atmospheric nuclear weapons testing.

Diagnostic x-ray exposure has not been linked with the development of MM in most epidemiologic studies.[41,42] A large multicenter population-based case-control study showed no evidence of excess risk of MM among individuals who reported exposure for 10 or more diagnostic radiographs.[43] One study reported that the overall risk for MM was not high (relative risk, 1.14), but that there was evidence of increasing risk with exposure to increasing numbers of radiographic procedures.[44] Studies of the effects of therapeutic irradiation on MM risk have shown conflicting results, but a study of 180,000 women treated for cervical cancer demonstrated no overall excess risk of developing MM.[45] Similarly, a study of 14,000 patients suffering from ankylosing spondylitis and treated with radiation revealed no significant increase in the risk of developing MM.[45,46]

Workplace Exposures

Several epidemiologic studies have evaluated the risk of MM among agricultural workers, with positive associations reported by many[47-50] but not all of the studies.[51-53] Khuder and Mutgi[54] found a relative risk of 1.23 in a meta-analysis of several studies. Workers in various metal occupations and industries have been reported to have an increased MM risk.[55-57]

Benzene has been suggested as a possible etiologic agent for MM, but several comprehensive reviews and meta-analyses found no evidence of a link between benzene exposure and MM.[58-60]

Recently, it has been found that white, male firefighters with environmental exposure to known and suspected carcinogens at the site of the World Trade Center attacks on September 11, 2001 had an increased age-standardized prevalence of MGUS and light chain MGUS compared to a reference population in Olmsted County, Minnesota.[61] This increased prevalence may be a risk factor for the development of MM.

Cigarette Smoking, Alcohol Consumption, and Diet

Multiple studies to date have found no etiologic role for cigarette smoking or alcohol consumption in the development of MM.[62-65] In contrast, Tavani et al[66] suggested a dietary link for MM and found a higher risk among people consuming large quantities of liver (odds ratio [OR], 2.0) and butter (OR, 2.8) and a lower risk among people consuming large amounts of vegetables (OR, 0.4). No association of MM and consumption of coffee or red meat has been found.[66] Brown and colleagues[67] looked at diet and nutrition as risk factors for MM among blacks and whites in the United States. Only obesity was associated with increased risk, and obesity was more frequent in black than in white controls. Frequent consumption of cruciferous vegetables, fish, and vitamin C supplements was associated with decreased risk of MM.

Personal use of hair dyes was evaluated as a risk factor for MM,[64] but subsequent studies have showed no increased risk.

Socioeconomic Status

Some investigators have reported that there is an inverse relationship between the risk of MM and socioeconomic status[68] and that this inverse correlation may account for a substantial amount of the black and white differential of MM incidence.[69]

Chronic Antigenic Stimulation

Repeated or chronic antigenic stimulation of the immune system may lead to MM. Several case-controlled studies have suggested that MM risk is associated with past history of infections, inflammatory conditions, connective tissue disorders, autoimmune illnesses, and allergy-related disorders.[63,70,71] Patients with the human immunodeficiency virus may have an increased likelihood of developing MM.[72] In addition, MM and hepatitis C may be associated.[73] The data are mixed regarding associations between rheumatoid arthritis and MM.[29] Recently, long-term immune activation by lysolipids has been demonstrated to be the likely explanation for the increased risk of monoclonal gammopathies in Gaucher disease.[74]

DIAGNOSIS

The diagnosis of MM has not been subject to static norms. In 1973, the Chronic Leukemia-Myeloma Task Force[75] set forth guidelines for the diagnosis of MM. These criteria, which by today's standards are not stringent enough, were replaced in 2003[76] and further revised in 2015 (Table 100.1).[77] In the past 3 decades, the terms and definitions of MGUS,

Table 100.1. Criteria for Diagnosis of Multiple Myeloma

Both Criteria Must Be Met[a]:
1. Clonal bone marrow plasma cells ≥10% or biopsy-proven bony or extramedullary plasmacytoma

2. Any one or more of the following myeloma defining events:
• *CRAB*: Evidence of end-organ damage that can be attributed to the underlying plasma cell proliferative disorder, specifically:
   • *Hypercalcemia*: serum calcium >0.25 mmol/L (>1 mg/dL) higher than the upper limit of normal or >2.75 mmol/L (>11 mg/dL)
   • *Renal insufficiency*: creatinine clearance <40 mL/min or serum creatinine >177 µmol/L (>2 mg/dL)
   • *Anemia*: hemoglobin value of >2 g/dL below the lower limit of normal, or a hemoglobin value <10 g/dL
   • *Bone lesions*: one or more osteolytic lesions on skeletal radiography, computed tomography, or positron emission tomography-CT
• Other myeloma defining event (new 2014):
   • Clonal bone marrow plasma cell percentage ≥60%
   • Involved: uninvolved serum free light chain (FLC) ratio ≥100 (involved FLC level must be ≥100 mg/L)
   • >1 focal lesions on magnetic resonance imaging studies (at least 5 mm in size)

[a]If both criteria are not met, then diagnosis is likely monoclonal gammopathy of undetermined significance, smoldering multiple myeloma, or immunoglobulin light-chain amyloidosis.
Reprinted from Rajkumar SV, Dimopoulos MA, Palumbo A, et al. International Myeloma Working Group updated criteria for the diagnosis of multiple myeloma. *Lancet Oncol.* 2014;15(12):e538-e548. Copyright © 2014 Elsevier. With permission.

smoldering MM, indolent MM, and symptomatic MM[78-81] have evolved and are now to be replaced by the following designations: MGUS, smoldering (asymptomatic) MM, and MM (see Chapter 99).[76,77]

Because MM includes a spectrum of biologic features, physicians should not feel compelled to start treatment as a result of a single threshold value. The diagnosis of active MM is not a straightforward pathologic one; rather, it is a clinical diagnosis that requires thoughtful synthesis of multiple variables. Patients with Durie-Salmon stage I disease, who also meet the criteria for smoldering MM without myeloma defining events, should be managed expectantly.

DIFFERENTIAL DIAGNOSIS

The diagnosis of MM is made from a constellation of findings, including anemia, monoclonal proteins, bone lesions, renal complications, hypercalcemia, and bone marrow plasmacytosis. Often the diagnosis is straightforward, but other disease entities associated with hypergammaglobulinemia or monoclonal bone marrow plasma cells must also be considered. These include reactive plasmacytosis, MGUS (see Chapters 97 and 99), immunoglobulin light-chain amyloidosis (see Chapter 101), Waldenström macroglobulinemia (see Chapter 102), osteosclerotic myeloma or POEMS (polyneuropathy, organomegaly, endocrinopathy, M-protein, and skin changes) syndrome (see Chapter 103), light-chain deposition disease (LCDD), acquired Fanconi syndrome (see Chapter 103), solitary plasmacytoma with or without marrow involvement, and PCL (see section "Special Cases of Myeloma").

CLINICAL MANIFESTATIONS

The symptoms and signs of MM may be nonspecific and include fatigue, bone pain, easy bruisability and bleeding, recurrent infections, manifestations of anemia, hypercalcemia, renal insufficiency, lytic bone lesions, hyperviscosity, thrombocytopenia, and hyper- or hypogammaglobulinemia (*Figure 100.2*). Weakness, infection, bleeding, and weight loss are reported in as many as 82%, 13%, 13%, and 24% of patients, respectively.[82-84] Hypercalcemia is present in 18% to 30% of patients.[82,83] One- to two-thirds of patients present with spontaneous bone pain.[82,83] "Tumor fever" is present in less than 1% of presenting patients.

Monoclonal Proteins

The M-protein (M-component, myeloma protein, or M spike) is a hallmark of the disease; 97% of MM patients have either an intact immunoglobulin or a free light chain that can be detected by protein electrophoresis, immunoelectrophoresis, or immunofixation studies of the serum or urine (*Figure 100.3A* and *B*).[83] Those cases without a detectable monoclonal protein have been referred to as nonsecretory MM, which had accounted for approximately 1% to 3% of MM cases. With the advent of the immunoglobulin free light-chain assay, small free light-chain monoclonal proteins hereto forth not seen by aforementioned methods are seen in approximately two-thirds of the cases that had been referred to as nonsecretory.[85]

In a series of 1027 newly diagnosed cases of MM (NDMM), the immunoglobulin type was IgG, IgA, IgD, and free light chain only (Bence Jones MM) in 52%, 20%, 2%, and 16% of cases, respectively.[83] Fewer than 1% of MM cases are IgM; most IgM monoclonal proteins are associated with diagnoses of MGUS, lymphoma, Waldenström macroglobulinemia, or immunoglobulin light-chain amyloidosis.[86] Higher proportion of patients with IgD MM have been reported in from Chinese studies. About 90% of MM patients have reduction in at least one of their uninvolved immunoglobulins. About 70% have a monoclonal protein—or fragment thereof—detected in the urine.

Anemia

The most common clinical feature of MM is anemia; hemoglobin <10 g/dL or less than 2 g/dL below lower limit is part of the diagnostic criteria. A hemoglobin concentration of less than 120 g/L occurs in 40% to 73% of patients at presentation[82,83] and contributes to the weakness and fatigue observed in as many as 82% of patients.[82,83] The anemia is normochromic, normocytic in most patients, but macrocytosis may be observed as well. When there are high concentrations of serum immunoglobulin, rouleaux formation may be observed (*Figure 100.3C*). The combination of anemia and hyperproteinemia leads to a marked increase in the erythrocyte sedimentation rate.

The anemia is related partially to direct infiltration and replacement of the bone marrow. Hemoglobin concentration is also correlated directly with the percentage of MM cells in S phase,[87] suggesting that the bone marrow cytokine milieu, permissive for MM cell proliferation, is not conducive to efficient erythropoiesis. Cytokines, like tumor necrosis factor-α and interleukin (IL)-1, may inhibit erythropoiesis.[88] Fas ligand–mediated erythroid apoptosis is also increased in patients with MM.[89] Finally, relative erythropoietin deficiency from MM-induced renal insufficiency also contributes to the observed anemia.

Histopathology

The bone marrow microenvironment is hospitable to malignant plasma cells that circulate through the blood. There is a complex interaction among the malignant clone, its surrounding stromal cells, and the remaining immune cells. The morphologic and immunologic phenotypes of MM cells can vary, and they often resemble normal plasma cells. (For information on immunophenotype, see "Immunophenotype of Myeloma Cells" in "Prognosis" section.) Plasma cells are at least two to three times the size of peripheral lymphocytes and are round to oval, with one or more eccentrically placed nuclei (*Figure 100.3D*). The nucleus, which contains either diffuse or clumped chromatin, is displaced from the center by an abundance of rough-surfaced endoplasmic reticulum—the site of specialized immunoglobulin synthesis. Intranuclear and cytoplasmic inclusions are not uncommon.[90] There

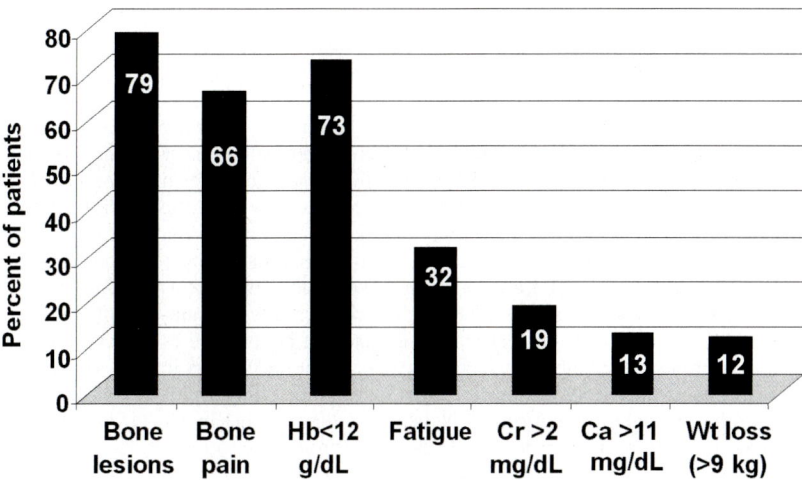

FIGURE 100.2 Signs and symptoms of 1027 newly diagnosed myeloma patients seen at the Mayo Clinic from 1985 to 1998.

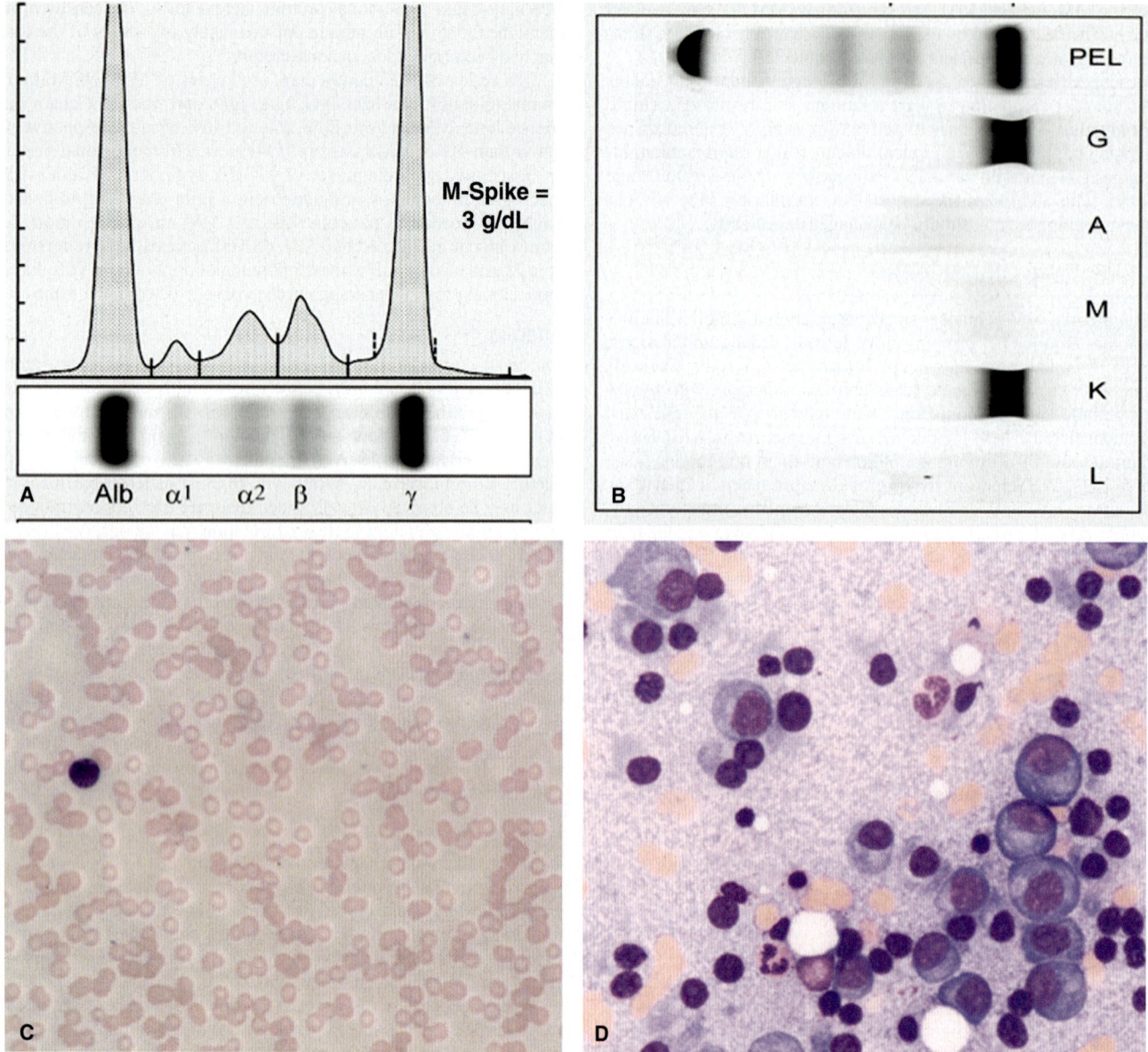

FIGURE 100.3 Laboratory findings in patients with multiple myeloma. A, Serum protein electrophoresis illustrating a 3 g/dL monoclonal protein spike. B, Immunofixation electrophoresis illustrating a monoclonal IgGλ monoclonal protein. C, Rouleaux. D, Bone marrow: myeloma cells on aspirate specimen.

is a perinuclear clear zone that is the site of the Golgi apparatus, the machinery used for immunoglobulin packaging and glycosylation for secretion. Derangements of immunoglobulin secretion are responsible for an assortment of cytologic aberrations, including flaming cells, Mott cells, Russell bodies, and Gaucher-like cells. Flaming cells are plasma cells that have intensely eosinophilic cytoplasm with a magenta or carmine coloring of their margins, which is because of plugging of peripheral secretory channels by precipitated immunoglobulin or immunoglobulin fragments. These cells are most commonly seen in IgA MM. Thesaurocytes are large flaming cells with a pyknotic nucleus that is pushed to the side. Mott cells (grape cells or morula forms) are plasma cells filled with dense spherical immunoglobulin inclusions; these inclusions are colorless, pink, or blue. Other inclusions are Russell bodies and their intranuclear counterparts (intranuclear dense bodies); these appear cherry red and can be as large as several microns in diameter. Gaucher-like cells are not uncommon in MM infiltrates; these cells are macrophages laden with sphingolipids released by the dying plasma cells.[91] None of these interesting inclusions are specific for malignancy nor do they have prognostic value.

In MM, there is often discordance between the nucleus and cytoplasm, the former appearing immature and the latter highly differentiated. About 20% of MM cases have plasmablastic morphology: a diffuse chromatin pattern, nucleus greater than 10 μm or nucleolus greater than 2 μm, relatively less abundant cytoplasm, and a concentrically placed nucleus with little or no hof.[92,93] Both diffuse and nodular infiltration patterns can be observed, although the former is more common. A minority of patients have plasma cells that have a lymphoplasmacytic appearance. MM cells are commonly present in cords around bone marrow microvessels. There is a high correlation between the extent of bone marrow angiogenesis, evaluated as microvessel area, and the proliferating fraction of marrow plasma cells in patients with MM.[94,95] Mild marrow fibrosis may be observed in as many as 27% of cases; extensive fibrosis is rare.[96] Less than 1% of cases have an extensive idiopathic granulomatous reaction.[90]

No individual bone marrow finding, however, is pathognomonic for a malignant plasma cell process other than plasmacytosis of 60% or greater; the bone marrow diagnosis of MM relies on the percentage of clonal bone marrow plasma cells, with 10% accepted as a cutoff to move a patient from MGUS to smoldering MM or MM. A clinical diagnosis of MM, however, can be made with fewer bone marrow plasma cells if CRAB (calcium elevated, renal failure, anemia, lytic bone lesions) feature(s) attributable to MM are present.

Bone Disease

Approximately one- to two-thirds of patients present with bone pain,[82-84] and bone disease is a major source of morbidity. There is an uncoupling of the balance between osteoclastic and osteoblastic activity. Even before the development of bone lesions, enhanced osteoblastic recruitment with an increased generation of new osteoclasts is observed in early MM and even in MGUS. Regardless of the initiating signal, whether IL-1β, IL-6, and sIL-6R, tumor necrosis factor-α, macrophage inflammatory protein 1α, receptor activator of NF-κβ (RANK) ligand, or parathyroid hormone–related protein,[97] the eventual outcome is bone destruction.[98]

Imaging Bone Disease

A myelomatous lesion may extend through the cortex of a vertebral body and cause either nerve root or spinal cord compression in less than 2% of patients.[82] Alternatively, the MM can disturb the mechanical integrity of a vertebral body, resulting in compression fracture with retropulsion of either plasmacytoma or bony fragments into the spinal canal, again causing neurologic deficit. Approximately 75% of patients have punched-out lytic lesions, osteoporosis, or fractures on conventional radiography (*Figure 100.4A* and *B*). The vertebrae, skull, ribs, sternum, proximal humeri, and femora are involved most frequently.[83,84] A small subset of patients have de novo osteosclerotic lesions,[99] and in a few patients, osteosclerosis is seen after therapy and may serve as a marker of healing.

Advanced imaging such as whole-body low-dose computed tomography (CT), [18]fluorodeoxyglucose positron emitting tomography/CT (FDG-PET/CT), or magnetic resonance imaging (MRI) is necessary in patients who are thought to have smoldering myeloma or solitary plasmacytoma of bone because finding additional bone lesions will upstage patients to active myeloma and affect treatment approaches.

Because myelomatous bone lesions are characteristically lytic, conventional radiography is superior to technetium-99m bone scanning.[100] About twice as many myelomatous bone lesions are detected by radiograph as by bone scan; an exception to this general finding is at the lumbar spine and the rib cage, where the two methods are equally reliable.[100] Whole-body CT skeletal surveys are considered to be preferred over plain radiographs.[101] In one series of 212 patients with MM, no lytic bone disease was detected with either technique in 49% of patients, and lesions were detected by both methods in 20%. Whole-body CT skeletal survey detected lesions where conventional radiography did not in 25% and conventional radiography detected lesions (most often in appendicular skeleton) in 6%.

Both whole-body CT skeletal surveys and MRI reveal specific lesions in 40% of stage I MM patients.[102] The presence of lacunae larger than 5 mm with trabecular disruption on CT appears to be sensitive and specific for MM. This information may be useful in distinguishing between senile and myelomatous osteoporosis and compression fractures.[103] Among asymptomatic myeloma patients with normal radiographs, 50% have tumor-related abnormalities on MRI of the lower spine (*Figure 100.4C*).[104] In patients with Durie-Salmon stage I MM, MRI can distinguish patients at higher and lower risks of progression.[105] According to modern definitions of MM, the presence of more than one lesion greater than 0.5 cm now satisfies the criteria for MM requiring therapy.[77] One-third of patients with an apparent solitary plasmacytoma of bone have evidence of other plasma cell tumors on MRI.[106]

MRI is superior to radiographs for the detection of lesions in the pelvis and the spine, but overall it is inferior to radiographs for detecting bone involvement in MM (79% vs 87%, respectively).[107] On MRI, vertebral fractures due to spinal infiltration or osteoporosis are seen in 48% of patients with symptomatic MM, and spinal canal narrowing with impingement occurs in 20%.[104] In one study of 28 NDMM, in 25% of patients, FDG-PET/CT detected more lytic bone lesions, all of which were out of the field-of-view of MRI, and in 25% of patients, MRI detected an infiltrative pattern in the spine that was not discerned on FDG-PET/CT.[108] In subsequent studies, whole-body MRI has been reported to have a higher sensitivity and specificity than FDG-PET/CT[109] and multidetector-row CT.[110] Detection of marrow infiltration on MRI does not translate into a deficit of cortical bone integrity. MRI can also be used as a prognostic factor and for identifying minimal residual disease (MRD).[111]

FDG-PET/CT has sensitivity and specificity rates of 84% to 92% and 83% to 100%, respectively[112,113] (*Figure 100.4D* and *E*). FDG-PET/CT can be considered a valuable tool for the workup of patients with both NDMM and relapsed or refractory MM because it assesses bone damage with relatively high sensitivity and specificity and detects extramedullary sites of clonal plasma cells while providing important prognostic information. A drawback of PET scan is its inability to detect very small lesions (<1 cm). Radiation-induced inflammatory changes can lead to false-positive PET, which should, therefore, only be performed at least 2 months after the therapy, if repeated.[114] Finally, approximately 10% of patients with MM who have extensive disease burden may be reported to be disease-free on FDG-PET that is PET false negative.[115] This has been attributed to the low expression of the gene coding for the hexokinase-2 enzyme which is responsible for catalyzing the first step of glycolysis and thus impairing the routine intracellular metabolism of the FDG tracer.

The use of FDG-PET/CT or that of whole-body MRI is mandatory to confirm a suspected diagnosis of presumed solitary plasmacytoma or smoldering myeloma.[116] Changes in FDG avidity can provide an earlier evaluation of response to therapy compared to MRI scans. It can also be used to identify MRD.[111]

Hypercalcemia

Hypercalcemia occurs in 18% to 30% of patients. About 13% have concentrations greater than 11 mg/dL. Rates of hypercalcemia at presentation have been decreasing in the past few decades, perhaps because of the earlier diagnosis of patients.[82-84] Hypercalcemic patients may complain of fatigue, constipation, nausea, or confusion. Calcium can precipitate in the kidneys and aggravate renal insufficiency.

Renal Insufficiency

Approximately 25% of MM patients have a serum creatinine value greater than 2 mg/dL at diagnosis. Another 25% have mildly elevated creatinine values.[82-84,117-120] Patients with Bence Jones or IgD MM have the highest rates of renal insufficiency.[118,120] Free light-chain proteinuria is a risk factor for renal failure.[121] Contributing factors to the renal insufficiency associated with MM kidney include hypercalcemia, dehydration, hyperuricemia, and the use of nephrotoxic drugs. If the renal insufficiency reverses with therapy as it does in the majority of cases,[122,123] survival is fourfold to sevenfold higher than in those in whom it does not,[117] but still inferior to those who never developed renal failure.[124] Factors predicting for renal function recovery include a serum creatinine less than 4 mg/dL, serum calcium value greater than 11.5 mg/dL, proteinuria less than 1 g/24 hour, adequate rehydration,[117] and highly effective MM-directed therapy.[125] Achieving at least a 60% reduction in free light chain by 21 days was associated with recovery of renal function for 80% of the population.[126]

The pathologic lesion of MM kidney consists of monoclonal light chains in the tubules in the form of dense, often laminated, tubular casts. These casts contain albumin and Tamm-Horsfall protein. Light chains are normally filtered by the glomeruli and reabsorbed and catabolized in the nephron's proximal tubules. It is postulated that these systems become overwhelmed, and casts result. When other causes contributing to renal insufficiency are excluded, there is a good correlation between the extent of MM cast formation and the severity of renal insufficiency.[127,128] The most common findings on autopsy include tubular atrophy and fibrosis (77%), tubular hyaline casts (62%), tubular epithelial giant cell reaction (48%), and nephrocalcinosis (42%). Evidence of acute and chronic pyelonephritis was observed in 20% and 23% of cases, respectively. Plasma cell infiltrates and amyloid may be observed in 10% and 5% of cases, respectively.[84] Rarely, MM may be associated with the acquired Fanconi syndrome.

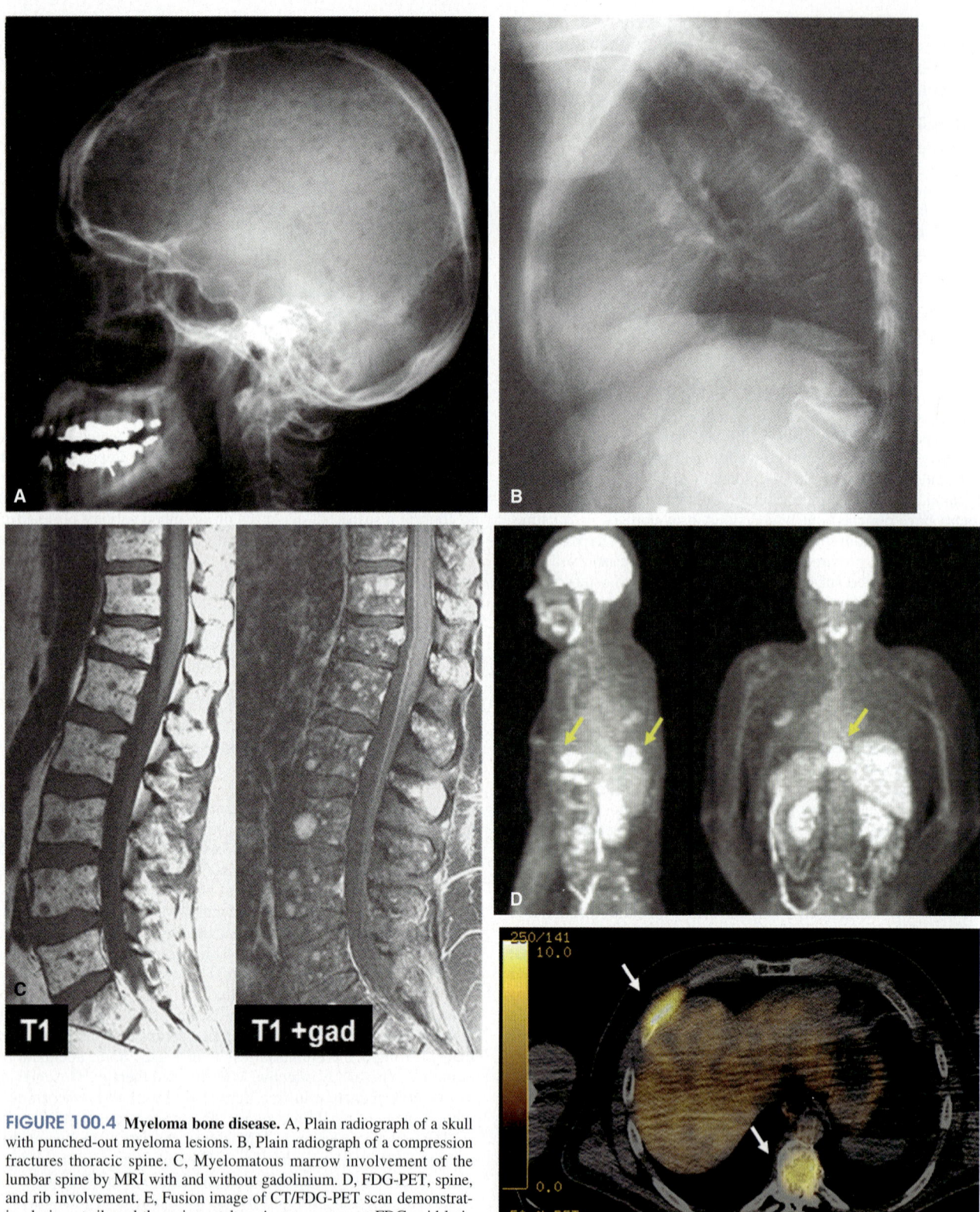

FIGURE 100.4 **Myeloma bone disease.** A, Plain radiograph of a skull with punched-out myeloma lesions. B, Plain radiograph of a compression fractures thoracic spine. C, Myelomatous marrow involvement of the lumbar spine by MRI with and without gadolinium. D, FDG-PET, spine, and rib involvement. E, Fusion image of CT/FDG-PET scan demonstrating lesion at rib and thoracic vertebra. Arrows represent FDG avid lytic bone lesions. CT, computed imaging; FDG-PET, [18]fluorodeoxyglucose positron emitting tomography; MRI, magnetic resonance imaging.

An important feature of myeloma kidney is that it is primarily a tubular, rather than a glomerular, disease.[129] Glomerular function is preserved initially, and there is a predominance of immunoglobulin light-chain protein in the urine instead of the nonspecific protein loss observed in glomerular disease. This feature helps predict the renal lesion. Nonspecific protein loss (i.e., mostly albumin) is more compatible with immunoglobulin light-chain amyloidosis, LCDD of the kidney, pamidronate use or proteinuria unrelated to the PCD[127]; a light-chain predominance is consistent with myeloma kidney.

Infection

Patients with MM are at high risk for bacterial infections and for dying of overwhelming bacteremia (see Infection Management in section "Treatment of Complications and Supportive Care").

Hemostasis in Multiple Myeloma

Bleeding as a complication of MM may be present in as many as one-third of patients[130] and is related to thrombocytopenia, uremia, hyperviscosity, and interference with the function of coagulation factors. Rarely, MM proteins may also interact with coagulation proteins.[130,131] Fewer than 7% of MM patients have a viscosity greater than 4 cP.[83] Symptoms of hyperviscosity include bleeding (particularly of the oronasal areas), purpura, decrease in visual acuity, retinopathy, neurologic symptoms, dyspnea, expanded plasma volume, and congestive heart failure. Most patients become symptomatic when the serum viscosity is 6 or 7 cP (normal is ≤1.8 cP).

The association with thrombosis is less clear because of coexisting factors such as old age and immobility that confound the interpretation of available data; however, the risk of thrombosis may be increased in MM patients. Monoclonal proteins have been shown to be responsible for lupus anticoagulants, acquired protein S deficiency, acquired activated protein C resistance, and inhibition of tissue plasminogen activator.

"Acute Terminal Phase of Plasma Cell Myeloma" and Cause of Death

Bergsagel and Pruzanski[132] described the "acute terminal phase" of patients with MM, which they observed in about one-third of their preterminal patients. They defined the syndrome as rapidly progressive disease with an unexplained fever and pancytopenia and a hypercellular marrow. Extramedullary plasmacytomas are also not uncommon preterminally.[133] As the disease progresses, and at autopsy, cutaneous, visceral, and even meningeal involvement is possible. Besides "progressive disease," the most frequent causes of death are infection in 24% to 52% and renal failure in about 20%.[84,134] Acute leukemia, myelodysplastic syndromes, and hemorrhage are the causes of death in a minority of patients,[84] and in an autopsy series, 85% of patients had evidence of either bacterial or fungal infection, and myelomatous involvement was found in the spleen, liver, lymph nodes, and kidneys in 45%, 28%, 27%, and 10% of patients, respectively.

PROGNOSIS

Prognosis is dependent on patient (age, performance status, renal function, and frailty), tumor-related factors, and the interaction between these factors. Survival of MM patients varies from months to more than a decade varying significantly among the different studies.[135,136] Given the disease heterogeneity and differing outcomes, it is important to understand the prognostic factors and develop adequate risk stratification systems, in order to compare different group of patients from different studies or clinical trials. However, prognostication is a dynamic process changing within a given patient during the disease course as dictated by the response to therapies and acquisition of new genetic changes. It is also constantly changing for the disease with incorporation of newer therapeutic strategies for the disease.

Staging is one form of prognostic modeling. The Durie-Salmon system, which until 1995 had been the most widely accepted MM staging system, separates patients predominantly by tumor burden and renal function.[137] Because the biology of MM is better understood, novel markers reflecting MM cell kinetics, signaling, genetic aberrations, and apoptosis have eclipsed the prognostic significance of tumor burden as a predictor of survival.[138-144] The Durie-Salmon staging system was an elegant system that incorporated information about immunoglobulin production and half-life, hemoglobin, calcium, creatinine, and extent of bone disease to derive mathematically the total MM cell burden.[137] Quantification of bone lesions used in this staging system, however, was not always reliable as a prognostic factor[140] in that patients classified as stage III solely on the basis of bone lesion criteria do not have a poorer prognosis.

Other variables, including patient age, performance status, serum albumin, immunoglobulin isotype, and bone marrow plasma cell infiltration, have long been recognized to predict survival,[145,146] and subsequent models have incorporated these factors,[143] whereas others have shown the prognostic value of serum β_2-microglobulin (β_2M), C-reactive protein, lactate dehydrogenase (LDH), elevations in serum immunoglobulin free light chains, the presence and quantity of circulating plasma cells,[147-149] bone marrow plasma cell proliferative rate, plasmablastic morphology, bone marrow angiogenesis, and chromosomal abnormalities.[94,139,141-144,150-155] MRI and PET-CT imaging has been shown to have prognostic importance.[114,156-159]

A staging system's relevance is based not only on its ability to predict outcome but also on its availability and cost.[160] An international consensus panel addressed this issue and developed the International Staging System (ISS) for MM (Table 100.2); it incorporates serum albumin levels and β_2M.[161] Though this staging system is inexpensive and readily available, it does not get to the heart of MM cell biology as do genetic changes, as will be discussed later. However, it does rely heavily on β_2M concentration, which is the strongest and most reliable prognostic factor for MM that is routinely available. β_2M concentration is influenced by both tumor burden and renal function. Formulas to correct the β_2M concentrations for the effects of renal insufficiency have not improved its predictive value,[162] and the β_2M value is still prognostic in MM patients with normal renal function.[138] As will be discussed, investigators have tried to enhance the performance of the ISS by adding other soluble markers or genetic risk features. The most important modification is the addition of LDH and fluorescence in situ hybridization (FISH), which is the Revised International Staging System (R-ISS; see below).

Cytogenetics, Fluorescence In Situ Hybridization, and Other Genetic Abnormalities

The first cytogenetic abnormalities in MM were documented nearly 30 years ago. Cytogenetic testing is an integral element of establishing prognosis and a treatment plan for all NDMM patients. Nearly all MM patients have abnormal chromosomes by FISH, including deletions, aneuploidy, and translocations[163,164] (Figure 100.5A and B), although abnormal karyotypes are seen in only 18% to 30% of cases. This apparent discrepancy is explained by the generally low proliferative rate of MM cells and the requirement of obtaining plasma cells (and not just the rapidly dividing normal myeloid precursors) in metaphase to generate conventional cytogenetics. Therefore, any abnormality in conventional cytogenetics identifies a group with a higher proliferative

Table 100.2. International Staging System and Revised International Staging System

Stage	Criterion	Overall Survival
ISS		Median, mo
Stage I	β_2M < 3.5 mg/L and alb ≥3.5 g/dL	62
Stage II	Not stage I or III	45
Stage III	β_2M ≥ 5.5 mg/L	29
R-ISS		**5-y, %**
R-ISS I	ISS I and normal LDH and no high-risk FISH	81
R-ISS II	Not R-ISS I or R-ISS III	60
R-ISS III	ISS III and either high LDH or high-risk FISH	40

High-risk FISH include t(4;14), t(14;16), or deletion 17p.
Abbreviations: β_2M, β_2-microgloulin; FISH, fluorescence in situ hybridization; ISS, International Staging System; LDH, lactate dehydrogenase; R-ISS, Revised International Staging System.
From Greipp PR, San Miguel J, Durie BG, et al. International staging system for multiple myeloma. *J Clin Oncol.* 2005;23(15):3412-3420; Palumbo A, Avet-Loiseau H, Oliva S, et al. Revised international staging system for multiple myeloma: a report from international myeloma working group. *J Clin Oncol.* 2015;33(26):2863-2869.

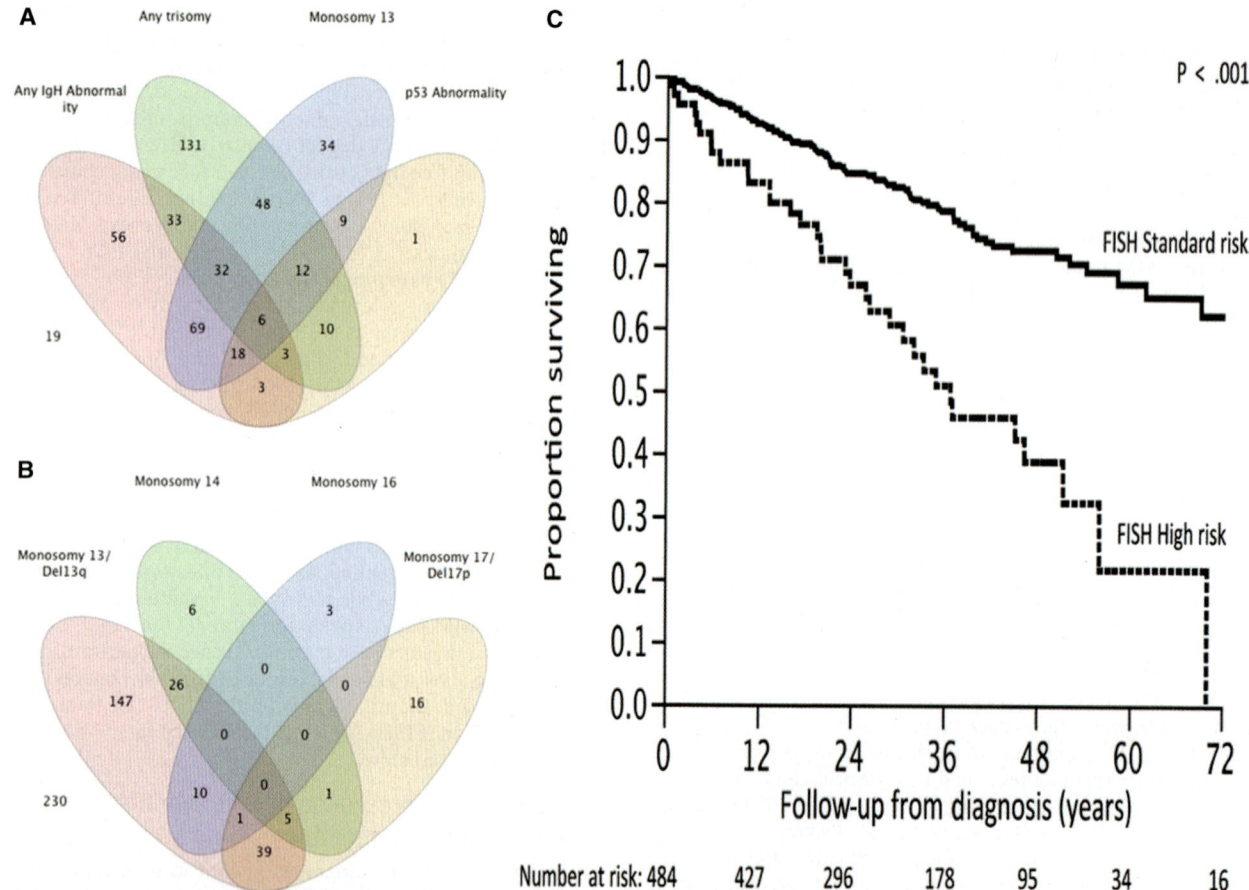

FIGURE 100.5 The relationship between genetic abnormalities among patients with multiple myeloma (MM). A, Venn diagram demonstrating the overlapping nature between the common abnormalities seen with fluorescence in situ hybridization (FISH) in patients with newly diagnosed MM. The actual number of patients with different abnormalities is presented from among 484 patients. The remaining 19 patients either had a normal FISH (n = 15) or another abnormality (n = 4). B, Distribution of various monosomies/deletions and their overlap. C, Modification of genetic risk system, using a hierarchical approach. High-risk includes deletion 17p, t(14;16), t(14;20), but with this new system, patients were reclassified into a new high-risk group, moving those patients previously classified as high-risk but with a trisomy into the standard-risk group. The survival of patients reclassified as high-risk (n = 66; 14%) was 3 years compared with not reached for the standard-risk group (P < .001). (Reprinted from Kumar S, Fonseca R, Ketterling RP, et al. Trisomies in multiple myeloma: impact on survival in patients with high-risk cytogenetics. *Blood*. 2012;119(9):2100-2105. Copyright © 2012 American Society of Hematology. With permission.)

rate[165] and poorer prognosis. With interphase FISH, several chromosomal abnormalities, such as immunoglobulin heavy-chain translocations and deletion of chromosome 13, are observed at equal frequencies among the spectrum of plasma cell proliferative disorders from MGUS to MM to PCL.[166,167]

Details of the molecular genetics of MM are detailed in Chapter 98, but from a practical prognostic standpoint, the most important aberrations observed with FISH are deletion 17p, t(4;14), t(14;16), t(14;20), additions of chromosome 1q, and deletions of chromosome 1p.[168] t(6;14) and t(11;14) are considered prognostically neutral translocations. The R-ISS incorporates "high-risk FISH" (t[4;14], t[14;16] or deletion 17p), the ISS, and LDH. R-ISS I is defined as ISS I, normal LDH, and no high-risk FISH; R-ISS III is present if ISS III and either high-risk FISH or abnormal LDH. R-ISS II includes the remaining patients.[169] The 5-year overall survival (OS) rate was 82% in the R-ISS I, 62% in the R-ISS II, and 40% in the R-ISS III groups; the 5-year progression-free survival (PFS) rates were 55%, 36%, and 24%, respectively (*Figure 100.6*).

Hypodiploid MM has a worse prognosis than diploid or hyperdiploid MM. This has been demonstrated by flow cytometric methods[170] and metaphase cytogenetics.[171,172] Controversy exists about whether the deletion 13q adds any additional prognostic information to a hypodiploid karyotype.[171-173]

Trisomy is common by FISH and most often includes chromosomes 3, 6, 9, 11, and 15.[174] In another study, trisomy of chromosomes 3, 7, and 11 accounted for over 50% of the hyperdiploid cases.[163] Trisomies of chromosomes 6, 9, and 17 were associated with prolonged survival.[175] The presence of trisomies is associated with better outcomes even among patients with high-risk cytogenetic markers, such as t(4;14), t(14;16), and 17p deletion (*Figure 100.5C*).[164]

Monoallelic loss of chromosome 13 (del 13) or its long arm (del 13q), when determined by metaphase cytogenetics, is a powerful adverse prognostic factor in patients treated with standard chemotherapy[142,170] or with autologous stem cell transplantation (ASCT).[151,176] Approximately 50% of NDMM patients have del 13 or del 13q by FISH,[167,177] and when detected by FISH is a much less potent risk factor.

Gene Expression Profiling

Many hematologic malignancies have witnessed the development of prognostically relevant disease subclassification through microarray profiling. MM is no exception, and considerable progress has been made to accurately predict individual patient's clinical course and survival outcomes using a molecular classification. Zhan and colleagues have comprehensively studied the gene expression on purified plasma cells of 414 NDMM patients who underwent high-dose therapy (HDT) with tandem transplants.[178] They introduced seven molecular subtypes of MM: PR (proliferation), LB (low bone disease), MS (*MMSET*), HY (hyperdiploid), CD-1 (*CCND1*), CD-2 (*CCND3*), and MF (*MAF/MAFB*). HY, CD1, CD2, and LB comprised the low-risk group with

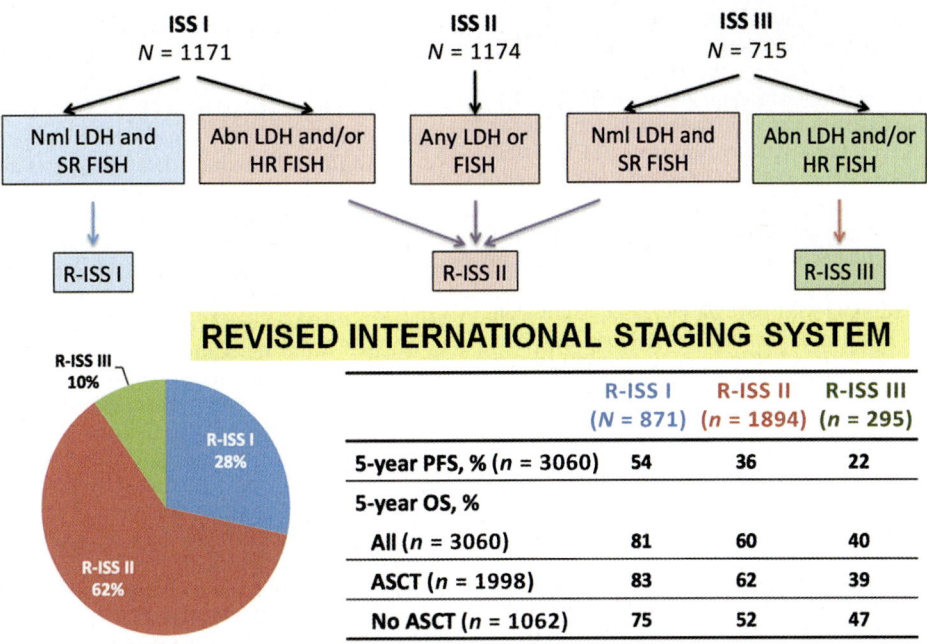

FIGURE 100.6 Revised International Staging System (R-ISS). ASCT, autologous hematopoietic stem cell transplantation; FISH, fluorescence in situ hybridization; HR, high-risk (t(4;14), t(14;16) or del(17p)); LDH, lactate dehydrogenase; OS, overall survival; PFS, progression-free survival; SR, not high risk. (Based on reference Palumbo A, Avet-Loiseau H, Oliva S, et al. Revised International Staging System for multiple myeloma: a report from International Myeloma Working Group. J Clin Oncol. 2015;33(26):2863-2869.)

3-year actuarial probabilities of 81% to 88%. The two high-risk groups, MS and PR, did not achieve a therapeutic benefit on total therapy 2 (TT2).[178] The same group of investigators identified 70 genes linked to shortened survival, with 30% of 51 overexpressed and 50% of 19 underexpressed genes mapping to chromosome 1, in a cohort of 532 newly diagnosed patients who received tandem transplants. This model was supplanted by an extremely powerful 17-gene prognostic model to detect the high-risk disease. In addition, this model could successfully prognosticate the patients with relapsed disease on either single-agent bortezomib or high-dose dexamethasone.[179] It has been validated using Mayo Clinic data set of 71 NDMM patients treated with ASCT, but practical impediments remain in the routine clinical utilization of this model. The GEP70 signature has also been validated in the nontransplant setting among a group of patients with NDMM receiving initial therapy with lenalidomide and dexamethasone (Rd).[180]

Several risk stratification systems have been proposed on the basis of gene expression profiling (GEP) results in addition to the ones from the University of Arkansas, including those from the French and Dutch groups.[181] These studies have helped us develop insights into the disease biology. However, the minimal overlap between different signatures raises questions as to the independence of these signatures from the type of therapy utilized as well as the potential influence of the sample preparation on the results and the ability to uniformly apply the method in real-life clinical setting.

Genetic evolution occurs in MM. Keats et al showed that tumors can follow several evolutionary paths over a patient's disease course.[182] With the use of serial genomic analysis of samples collected at different points during the disease course of 28 patients with MM, they showed that the genomes of standard-risk patients show few changes over time, whereas those of cytogenetically high-risk patients show significantly more changes over time. The results indicated that the pattern of genetic evolution over time can follow either a quiescent pathway with little changes, incremental changes with addition of new abnormalities over time (clonal evolution), or consist of a mixture of clones that wax and wane over time based on treatment selection pressure (clonal selection).

Plasma Cell Proliferative Rate

That the rate of clonal plasma cell expansion determines the disease outcome has been known for a long time, and several methodologies have been used to assess the degree of proliferation. One such test, the plasma cell labeling index (PCLI), is a slide-based method that measures the percentage of bone marrow MM cells in the S phase of the cell cycle,[92] which is a powerful prognostic factor in MM.[183,184] An increased PCLI predicts a short remission and survival but does not predict response to therapy. All large studies published to date have confirmed the independent prognostic value of the PCLI for survival after treatment with conventional chemotherapy or HDT.[184] A study highlighted the prognostic relevance of PCLI in the patients treated with immunomodulatory agents, thalidomide and lenalidomide, with high PCLI (≥1) at the time of initiation of therapy predicting a poorer PFS. However, lenalidomide appears to negate the adverse impact of high PCLI on OS, an effect not seen in the thalidomide arm. Undoubtedly, a longer follow-up of patients is required to determine the true impact of the PCLI in patients on lenalidomide therapy.[185]

Determination of S phase by flow cytometry using a DNA/CD38 double-staining technique is also possible and is prognostic but may not perfectly correlate with the slide-based method.

Immunophenotype of Myeloma Cells

The immunophenotype of MM cells is complex and potentially dynamic.[186,187] In general, MM cells are CD45 negative and CD38 and CD138 positive.[143,188] However, there is increasing evidence that a subset of MM cells is CD45 positive,[188,189] with an increasing proportion of CD45-positive MM cells in less advanced disease.[190,191] CD19 and CD20 are earlier B-cell antigens that are variably expressed on MM cells; surface immunoglobulin is seen in up to one-third of patients. CD56 is strongly positive in about 55% to 78% of MM cases.[188,192] CD56-negative MM cells tend to be present in more aggressive disease, such as end-stage MM or PCL.

The value of immunophenotyping NDMM by multiparametric flow cytometry was clearly established by the Spanish group in a prospective analysis of 685 patients treated with ASCT.[193] A prognostic model, risk-stratifying the NDMM patients into three categories, the poor risk (CD28+/CD117−; 23%), the intermediate risk (CD28−/CD117− or CD28+/CD117+; 56%), and the good risk (CD28−/CD117+, 21%), with OS 45 months, 68 months, and not reached (NR), respectively, was promulgated by this group. Patients with the t(11;14) translocation are more likely to have surface expression of CD56 and CD117. The extramedullary extension of the neoplastic plasma cells has been associated with a reduced expression or total absence of the adhesion molecule, CD56,[192] and upregulation of CD44 on the plasma cells. CD28 expression correlates with disease progression and is associated with t(14;16) and del(17p).

Patients with nonhyperdiploid MM have an increased expression of both CD20 and CD28 in the absence of reactivity for CD56 and CD117—all poor prognostic findings.[189] The absence of CD45 and CD27 portends a worse outcome. In a multivariate analysis of 95 NDMM patients who underwent ASCT, the lack of CD45 expression was the only significant variable that affected the outcome (median OS of 42 months for CD45− vs NR at 4 years for CD45+ MM, $P = .004$).[190] A small subset of CD45+ plasma cells constitutes the proliferative compartment of the bone marrow, and the expression of this antigen is required for IL-6 signaling, but prevents insulin growth factor 1 (IGF-1)–mediated AKT pathway activation. Furthermore, a lower degree of angiogenesis, likely because of reduced vascular endothelial growth factor production, was observed with CD45+ expression.

Other surface antigens like CD10 (CALLA), CD28, CD117 (c-KIT), CD13, CD33, and CD20 are present on a minority of patients' MM cells.[143,188,189] CD27 expression is associated with a better OS (92% at 3 years for CD27+ MM vs 50% in CD27− MM).[194] CD221 (IGF-1 receptor) overexpression is linked with t(4;14) or t(14;16), whereas CD20 expression is tightly associated with the more favorable t(11;14) and small lymphoplasmacytic morphology. CD200 is a membrane glycoprotein that imparts an immunoregulatory signal through CD200R, leading to the suppression of T-cell–mediated immune responses; downregulation of CD200 is associated with better prognosis.[195]

SYSTEMIC THERAPY FOR NEWLY DIAGNOSED MULTIPLE MYELOMA

Before starting therapy for MM, a distinction must be made between smoldering MM and MM requiring therapy (Chapters 97 and 99). Approximately 20% of patients with MM are recognized by chance without significant symptoms and may not meet the criteria for symptomatic myeloma; such patients can be carefully monitored without instituting therapy. Once the decision has been made to treat, a long-term plan for managing the disease should be formulated before instituting therapy. Because HDT with ASCT is an important treatment modality for patients younger than 70 years and even fit patients in their 70s, alkylator-based therapy should be limited or avoided prior to the collection of hematopoietic stem cells in patients considered candidates for HDT.

Prior to 1999, the bifunctional alkylators (melphalan and cyclophosphamide), nitrosoureas, doxorubicin, vincristine, and glucocorticoids were the mainstay of chemotherapy for MM. Until the advent of immunomodulatory drugs (IMiDs) and proteasome inhibitors, the higher response rates seen with combination therapies had not resulted in improved OS rates.[196] Both autologous and, to lesser extent, allogeneic stem cell transplantation (allo-SCT) have become important therapeutic options since McElwain and Powles' description in 1983[197] of the benefit of dose intensification of melphalan in patients with MM. With the recognition of thalidomide's activity against MM in 1999[12] and the subsequent development of bortezomib,[13] lenalidomide,[14] carfilzomib,[198] pomalidomide,[199] ixazomib,[200] daratumumab,[21] elotuzumab,[201] panobinostat,[202] isatuximab,[203] selinexor,[204] and idecabtagene vicleucel,[205] there is hope that the next 2 decades of MM treatment will be even more promising than the last.

Interpreting Treatment Response

Several points are emphasized regarding the interpretation and comparisons of the MM treatment literature. First, historically definitions of response have varied.[75,111,206-209] Second, definitions of evaluable patients may be different. Finally, patient population risk and prognosis may differ substantially. Lead-time bias and inappropriate treatment of MGUS or smoldering MM can confound survival estimates, as can effective salvage regimens.

The measurement of MM disease burden is complex, and investigators have used different methods to define response. The four most common response criteria that had been used until acceptance of the International Myeloma Working Group (IMWG) Response Criteria in 2006[210] were the Chronic Leukemia-Myeloma Task Force,[75] Southwest Oncology Group (SWOG),[206,207] Eastern Cooperative Oncology Group,[208] and Autologous Blood and Marrow Transplant Registry and the International Bone Marrow Transplant Registry (IBMTR/ABMTR).[209] In 2016, there were a further updates of response to allow for codification of deeper responses (*Table 100.3*).[111] In terms of the response criteria prior to the IMWG criteria, the main distinction among them was how the changes in serum and urine M components were classified.

The first iteration of an international consensus definition of MM response was the IBMTR/ABMTR response criteria.[209] After nearly 8 years of use, several deficiencies were noted, and the IMWG issued new consensus response definitions that included the Intergroupe Français du Myélome (IFM) very good partial response (VGPR) category,[211] the ability to measure response using the serum immunoglobulin free light chain, and a new category of "stringent complete response (CR)," which required documentation of the absence of clonality in the bone marrow and a normal serum immunoglobulin free light-chain ratio.[210] Most recently, molecular and high-sensitivity flow cytometry responses have been incorporated into response categories along with imaging-defined CR.[111] These latter criteria are most relevant for assessing deep responses in the context of clinical trials and are not considered necessary for routine clinical practice.

Combination Therapy for Induction

The last 3 decades of the 20th century were spent combining alkylators, anthracyclines, corticosteroids, and IFN. Thirty years of study indicated that the higher response rates afforded by these combinations as initial therapy did not translate into longer OS rates than standard melphalan and prednisone (MP) therapy,[196] and the data were conflicting as to whether patients with more advanced disease benefited from combined alkylator chemotherapy.

Clinical research in MM began to move at breakneck speed starting in the first decade of the 21st century. Once IMiDs and proteasome inhibitors were shown to have activity, clinical investigators began using these drugs in combination. Quadruplets incorporating daratumumab are also under investigation and showing promise.[212] Consideration of risk-adapted therapy became more prevalent in the 21st century, including host risk (age, performance status, frailty, and renal function) and tumor risk (GEP, cytogenetics, and FISH).[213,214] There have been increasing publications about frailty measures and scores[215-217] and important hints that bortezomib partially abrogates the risk of t(4;14) especially when used over extended periods of time[218-224] and that tandem transplant may abrogate risk of t(4;14) and deletion 17p.[219,220]

Because of the abundance of induction data and the absence of definitive "best options," the Mayo Clinic group has published a treatment algorithm for patients with NDMM called mSMART.[213,225,226] This is an online algorithm that is updated as new data emerge (*Figure 100.7*), https://www.msmart.org/. For patients, not considered to be ASCT candidates, the most commonly used regimens are bortezomib, lenalidomide, and dexamethasone (VRd), Rd, daratumumab-Rd, or bortezomib, melphalan, and prednisone (VMP). There have been no trials comparing Rd to VMP though modeling has been done by two separate groups, one favoring Rd[227] and the other favoring VMP.[228] As a

Table 100.3. IMWG Response Criteria

	MRD Criteria (All MRD States Also Require Minimal Criteria for a CR)
Sustained MRD-negative	MRD negativity in the marrow (NGF or NGS or both) and by imaging as defined below, confirmed minimum of 1 y apart
Flow MRD-negative	Absence of phenotypically aberrant clonal BMPC by NGF assay with a minimum sensitivity of 1 in 10^5 nucleated cells or higher (EuroFlow or validated equivalent method)
Sequencing MRD-negative	Absence of clonal BMPC by NGS using the LymphoSIGHT platform (or validated equivalent method) with a minimum sensitivity of 1 in 10^5 nucleated cells or higher
Imaging plus MRD-negative	MRD negativity as defined by NGF or NGS plus negative PET/CT (or decrease to less mediastinal blood pool SUV).
Standard IMWG Criteria	
Stringent CR	CR as defined below and normal FLC ratio and absence of clonal BMPC biopsy by immunohistochemistry (κ/λ ratio ≤4:1 or ≥1:2 for κ and λ patients, respectively, after counting ≥100 plasma cells)
Complete response	Negative immunofixation[a] on the serum and urine and disappearance of any soft-tissue plasmacytomas and <5% plasma cells in bone marrow aspirates
Very good partial response	Serum and urine M-protein detectable by immunofixation but not on electrophoresis or ≥90% reduction in serum M-protein plus urine M-protein level <100 mg/24 h
Partial response	• ≥50% reduction of serum M-protein and reduction in urinary M-protein by ≥90% or to <200 mg/24 h; • If the serum and urine M-protein are unmeasurable, a ≥50% decrease in the difference between involved and uninvolved FLC levels is required in place of the M-protein criteria; • If serum and urine M-protein are unmeasurable, and serum free light assay is also unmeasurable, ≥50% reduction in plasma cells is required in place of M-protein, provided baseline BMPC percentage was ≥30%. In addition to these criteria, if present at baseline, a ≥50% reduction in the SPD of soft-tissue plasmacytomas is also required
Minimum response	≥25% but ≤49% reduction of serum M-protein and reduction in 24-h urine M-protein by 50%-89%. In addition, if present at baseline, a ≥50% reduction in the SPD of soft-tissue plasmacytomas is also required
Stable	Not meeting criteria for complete response, very good partial response, partial response, minimal response, or progressive disease

Progressive disease	Any one or more of the following criteria:
	• Increase in 25% from lowest confirmed response value in one or more of the following criteria:
	  • Serum M-protein (absolute increase must be ≥0.5 g/dL);
	  • Serum M-protein increase ≥1 g/dL, if the lowest M-component was ≥5 g/dL;
	  • Urine M-protein (absolute increase must be ≥200 mg/24 h);
	  • In patients without measurable serum and urine M-protein levels, the difference between involved and uninvolved FLC levels (absolute increase must be >10 mg/dL);
	  • In patients without measurable serum and urine M-protein levels and without measurable involved FLC levels, BMPC percentage irrespective of baseline status (absolute increase must be ≥10%);
	• Appearance of a new lesion(s), ≥50% increase from nadir in SPD of >1 lesion, or ≥50% increase in the longest diameter of a previous lesion >1 cm in short axis;
	• ≥50% increase in circulating plasma cells (minimum of 200 cells/μL) if this is the only measure of disease

Clinical relapse	One or more of the following criteria: • Direct indicators of increasing disease and/or end-organ dysfunction (CRAB features) related to the MM; • Development of new soft-tissue plasmacytomas or bone lesions (osteoporotic fractures do not constitute progression); • Definite increase in the size of existing plasmacytomas or bone lesions. A definite increase is defined as a 50% (and ≥1 cm) increase as measured serially by the SPD of the measurable lesion; • Hypercalcemia (>11 mg/dL); • Decrease in hemoglobin of ≥2 g/dL not related to therapy or other non–myeloma-related conditions; • Rise in serum creatinine by 2 mg/dL or more from the start of the therapy and attributable to myeloma; • Hyperviscosity related to serum paraprotein
Relapse from CR	Any one or more of the following criteria: • Reappearance of serum or urine M-protein by immunofixation[a] or electrophoresis; • Development of ≥5% plasma cells in the bone marrow; • Appearance of any other sign of progression (i.e., new plasmacytoma, lytic bone lesion, or hypercalcemia, see above)
Relapse from MRD negative	Meeting criteria for relapse from CR or loss of MRD-negative state

All response categories require two consecutive assessments made any time before starting any new therapy; for MRD, there is no need for two consecutive assessments, but information on MRD after each treatment stage is recommended (e.g., after induction, high-dose therapy/ASCT, consolidation, maintenance). MRD tests should be initiated only at the time of suspected complete response.

Abbreviations: ^{18}F-FDG-PET, ^{18}F-fluorodeoxyglucose PET; ASCT, autologous stem cell transplantation; BMPC, bone marrow plasma cell; CR, complete response; CRAB features, calcium elevated, renal failure, anemia, lytic bone lesions; FCM, flow cytometry; FLC, free light chain; IMWG, International Myeloma Working Group; MFC, multiparameter flow cytometry; M-protein, myeloma protein; MRD, minimal residual disease; NGF, next-generation flow; NGS, next-generation sequencing; SPD, sum of the products of the maximal perpendicular diameters of measured lesions; SUV_{max}, maximum standardized uptake value.

[a]Special attention should be given to the emergence of a different monoclonal protein following treatment, especially in the setting of patients having achieved a conventional complete response, often related to oligoclonal reconstitution of the immune system. Also, appearance of monoclonal IgGκ in patients receiving monoclonal antibodies should be differentiated from the therapeutic antibody.

Reprinted from Kumar S, Paiva B, Anderson KC, et al. International Myeloma Working Group consensus criteria for response and minimal residual disease assessment in multiple myeloma. *Lancet Oncol.* 2016;17(8):e328-e346. Copyright © 2016 Elsevier. With permission.

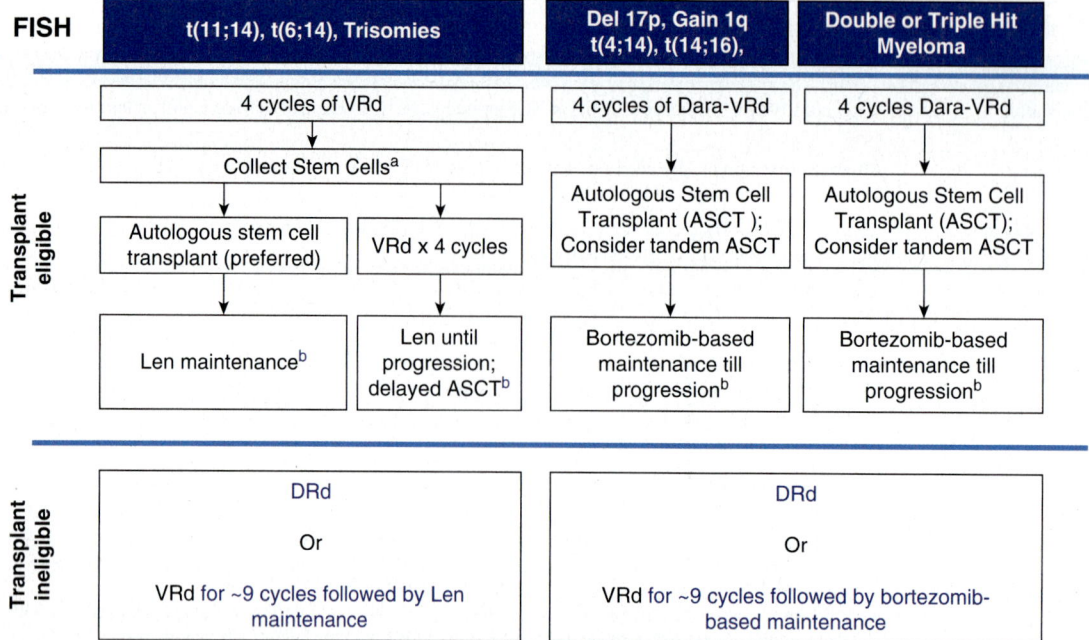

FIGURE 100.7 Mayo stratification for myeloma and risk-adapted therapy (mSMART).[213,225,226] Possible treatment algorithm for patients with newly diagnosed myeloma not being treated on a clinical trial. ASCT, autologous stem cell transplant; FISH, fluorescence in situ hybridization; KRd, carfilzomib, lenalidomide, and dexamethasone; VRd, bortezomib, lenalidomide, and dexamethasone. [a]If age >65 or >4 cycles of VRd, consider mobilization with G-CSF plus cytoxan or plerixafor. [b]Duration based on tolerance; consider risks and benefits for treatment beyond 3 years. [c]DVMP is also a reasonable option. [d]Dex is usually discontinued after first year.

general rule, patients who are being considered for stem cell collection and SCT receive VRd for 4 to 6 months in countries where this combination is available; otherwise, the lenalidomide is replaced with thalidomide, doxorubicin, or cyclophosphamide. For patients who are in renal failure, many prefer holding the lenalidomide and using either a dose-intensified dexamethasone along with the bortezomib or one of the other nonrenally metabolized drugs. If alkylator containing regimens are used, the number of cycles is restricted to four prior to stem cell mobilization. For expediency, the section on induction regimens will be separated into those specifically for transplant-ineligible patients and those for transplant-eligible patients. Table 100.4 lists the dosing and schedules of some of the most commonly used or discussed regimens.

Transplant-Ineligible Patients

MP was the standard for those not eligible for ASCT for decades.[206,252] Response rates are 40% to 60%, and anticipated median survival was 18 to 42 months. Because of the variable gastrointestinal tract absorption of melphalan, intravenous (IV) regimens of 15 to 25 mg/m² every 4 weeks along with oral prednisone or dexamethasone had been tried and resulted in response rates of 50% to 82%.[253,254] An important phase III trial (IFM 95-01) directed at the elderly (age 65-75 years) was a four arm study comparing MP to melphalan-dexamethasone (MD), dexamethasone, or dexamethasone-IFN.[251] Four hundred eighty-eight patients were randomized, and follow-up was 83 months. Response rates were significantly higher among patients receiving MD, and PFS was significantly better among patients receiving melphalan (22 vs 13 months), but there was no difference in OS between the four treatment groups. The median survival for the whole series was 35 months. The morbidity associated with dexamethasone-based regimens was significantly higher than with MP. The 1970s and 1980s were a testing ground for various combinations of alkylators, corticosteroids, and doxorubicin, but no regimen was shown to consistently be superior to MP. It was not until the 2000s with the advent of the IMiD and proteasome inhibitor classes of drugs that MP was shown to be inferior.[218,235,255-264]

Doublets

Lenalidomide and Dexamethasone. An important regimen for elderly patients with NDMM is lenalidomide and dexamethasone. This combination yields ORRs of 91% to 95%, with CR/VGPR rates of 32% to 38%.[265,266] The first report was that of Rajkumar et al [265] who treated 34 patients with lenalidomide 25 mg orally days 1-21 and dexamethasone 40 mg days 1 to 4, 9 to 12, and 17 to 20 in a 28 day cycle. Aspirin (ASA) was given as deep venous thrombosis (DVT) prophylaxis. The ORR was 91%, with 6% achieving CR and 32% VGPR.[267] This study was followed by a randomized controlled trial (E4A03) comparing lenalidomide with standard dexamethasone (12 d/mo schedule)—RD—to lenalidomide with reduced-intensity dexamethasone (weekly dexamethasone)—Rd.[230] After 4 months of therapy, 79% of the RD patients and 68% of the Rd patients had achieved a PR or better; however, at 1 year, OS was superior in the Rd arm as compared to the RD arm (92% vs 87%, $P = .0002$), making Rd the preferred doublet over RD. Among patients aged less than 65, the 1-year OS was 91% with RD and 98% with Rd; among those older than 65, the 1-year OS was 83% with RD and 94% with Rd. The trial was stopped because of this safety concern, and patients receiving high-intensity dexamethasone (RD) were crossed over to the low-intensity arm (Rd). Grade 3 to 4 AEs and early deaths were higher in the RD group (52% vs 35%, $P = .0001$; and 5.4% vs 0.5%, $P = .003$), respectively. The most common grade 3 or higher toxicities were DVT (26% vs 12%, $P = .0003$), infections (16% vs 9%, $P = .04$), and fatigue (15% vs 9%, $P = .08$).

Larocca and colleagues in a recent multicenter, phase 3 Italian trial (NCT02215980) involving 199 patients showed that Rd related toxicities could be further reduced by dose and schedule modification, without compromising efficacy.[268] The study population comprised a select group of vulnerable elderly patients with newly diagnosed MM who were categorized as intermediate-fit based on the IMWG frailty index. Therapy was deintensified after 9 months of the Rd doublet such that patients in the steroid-sparing investigational arm discontinued dexamethasone and deintensified the lenalidomide dose from 25 to 10 mg. The control arm received continuous full dose Rd, and the primary end point was event-free survival (EFS), a composite of both

Table 100.4. Commonly Cited Regimens and Their Dosage Schedules

Regimen	Proteasome Inhibitor	IMiD	Alkylator	Glucocorticoid	Other
VRD[229,c]	B: 1.3 mg/m² IV days 1, 4, 8, 11	L: 25 mg days 1-14	–	D: 20 mg days 1, 2, 4, 5, 8, 9, 11, 12	
L-dex[230,a]	–	L: 25 mg days 1-21	–	D: 40 mg/wk	–
VMP[231,d]	B: 1.3 mg/m²,d	–	M: 9 mg/m² days 1-4	P: 60 mg/m² days 1-4	
CyBorD[232,233,a]	B: 1.5 mg/m²/wk	–	C: 300 mg/m²/wk	D: 40 mg/wk[f]	
CTD[234,c]	–	T: 100-200 mg/d	C: 500 mg/wk	D: 40 mg days 1-4 and 12-15	–
MPT[235,b]	–	T: 200 mg/d	M: 0.25 mg/kg days 1-4	P: 2 mg/kg days 1-4	–
Carfilzomib (twice weekly dosing)[192,236]	Car: 20 mg/m² days 1, 2, in cycle 1; increase to 27 or 56 mg/m² on days 8, 9, 15, and 16. Cycle 2 and thereafter—27 or 56 mg/m² on days 1, 2, 8, 9, 15, and 16.	–		Premedicate with 4 mg on days 1, 2 8, 9 15,16, 22, and 23 of each cycle.	–
Carfilzomib (once weekly dosing)-Dex[237]	Car: Cycle 1—20 mg/m² on day 1, increase to 70 mg/m² on days 8 and 15. Cycle 2 and thereafter—70 mg/m² on days 1, 8, and 15.			D: 40 mg on days 1, 8, 15, and 22 of each cycle.	
Car-Len-Dex[238]	Car: 20/36 mg/m²/d days 1, 2, 8, 9, 15, 16 (cycle 1 uses lower dose days 1 and 2)	L: 25 mg/d days 1-21	–	D: 20-40 mg weekly	–
Daratumumab[21]	–	–	–	–	Dara: 16 mg/m²/wk if IV or 1800 mg SubQ × 2 cycles → QOW × 4 cycles → q 4 wk
Dara-Len-dex[239]	–	L: 25 mg/d days 1-21	–	D: 40 mg weekly (split dose on daratumumab weeks)	As single-agent daratumumab
Dara-Pom-dex[240]	–	P: 4 mg/d days 1-21	–	D: 40 mg weekly	As single-agent daratumumab
Dara-Bor-dex[241]	B: 1.3 mg/m² SQ days 1, 4, 8, 11			D: 20 mg day of and day after bortezomib	As single-agent daratumumab
Dara-Car-dex[242]	Car: 20/56 mg/m²/d days 1, 2, 8, 9, 15, 16 (cycle 1 uses lower dose days 1 and 2)Car: 20/70 mg/m²/d days 1, 8, 15 (cycle 1 uses lower dose of 20 mg/m² on days 1 and 2)			D: 20 mg day on carfilzomib infusion days in the twice-weekly schedule or 40 mg on the day of once weekly Car infusion.	As single-agent daratumumab
Dara-VMP[212,b]	B: 1.3 mg/m² days 1, 4, 8, 11, 22, 25, 29, 32 cycle 1cycles 2-9, day 1, 8, 22, 29	–	M: 9 mg/m² days 1-4	P: 60 mg/m² days 1-4	As single-agent daratumumab
Isa-Car-dex[243]	Car: 20/56 mg/m²/d days 1, 2, 8, 9, 15, 16 (cycle 1 uses lower dose days 1 and 2)			D: 20 mg day on carfilzomib infusion days in the twice-weekly schedule.	I: 10 mg/kg IV weekly for cycle → QOW for subsequent cycles.
Isa-Pom-dex[203]		P: 4 mg/d days 1-21		D: 40 mg day on days 1, 8, 15, and 22 of each cycle.	I: 10 mg/kg IV weekly for cycle → QOW for subsequent cycles.
Elo-Len-dex[244]		L: 25 mg/d days 1-21		D: 36 mg/wk C 1, 2 → 36 mg/wk alternating with 40 mg/wk	E: 10 mg/kg IV weekly for 2 cycles → QOW
Elo-Pom-dex[245]		P: 4 mg/d days 1-21		D: 28 mg oral and 8 mg IV on Elo infusion days and 40 mg/wk on non-Elo infusion days.	E: 10 mg/kg IV weekly for 2 cycles → 20 mg/kg q4 weeks
Belantamab-mafodotin[246]					Bel: 2.5 mg/kg IV every 3 wk.
Selinexor[204]				D: 20 mg on days 1 and 3 each week.	S: 80 mg on days 1 and 3 each week.

(Continued)

Table 100.4. Commonly Cited Regimens and Their Dosage Schedules (Continued)

Regimen	Proteasome Inhibitor	IMiD	Alkylator	Glucocorticoid	Other
Selinexor-bort-dex[247]	B: 1.3 mg/m² days 1, 8, 15, and 22 of 35 d cycle.			D: 20 mg on days 1 and 2 of each week.	S: 100 mg weekly on 35-d cycle.
CPa	—	—	C: 300 mg/m² weekly or 50-100 mg qd	P: 100 mg/d days 1-4 or P: 50-100 mg qod	—
T-Dex[248,a]		T: 50-200 mg daily		D: 40 mg days 1-4, 9-12 or D: 40 mg weekly	—
PAD[249]	V: 1.3 mg/m² SQ days 1, 4, 8, 11			D: 40 mg days 1-4	Dox: 9 mg/m² CI days 1-4
VDTPACE[250,e]	V: 1.0 mg/m² SQ days 1, 4, 8, 11	T: 200 mg daily	C: 400 mg/m²/d CI days 1-4 CDDP: 10 mg/m²/d CI days 1-4 Etop: 40 mg/m²/d CI days 1-4	D: 40 mg days 1-4	V, Dox as above

Abbreviations: B, bortezomib; BCNU, carmustine; C, cyclophosphamide; Car, carfilzomib; CDDP, cisplatin; CI, continuous infusion; CP, cyclophosphamide and prednisone; CTX, cyclophosphamide; C-VAMP, cyclophosphamide, vincristine, doxorubicin, and methylprednisolone; D, dexamethasone; Dex, dexamethasone; Dox, doxorubicin; IMiD, immunomodulatory drug; IV, intravenous; L, lenalidomide; M, melphalan; M-2, VBMCP; MP, melphalan and prednisone; MPT, MP and thalidomide; P, prednisone; PAD, bortezomib, doxorubicin, and dexamethasone; q, every; qod, every other day; T, thalidomide; VAD, vincristine, doxorubicin, and dexamethasone; VAMP, vincristine, doxorubicin, and methylprednisolone; VCR, vincristine; VDT-PACE, bortezomib, dex, thalidomide, cisplatin, doxorubicin, cyclophosphamide, etoposide; gluco, corticosteroid; VMCP, vincristine, melphalan, cyclophosphamide, and prednisone; VMP, MP and bortezomib.

[a]Repeated at 4-week intervals.
[b]Repeated at 6-week intervals.
[c]Repeated at 3-week intervals.
[d]Initial treatment strategy for VISTA trial was bortezomib 1.3 mg/m² on days 1, 4, 8, 11, 22, 25, 29, and 32, repeated every 6 weeks for four cycles, and then repeated every 5 weeks, with bortezomib schedule changing to weekly administration for 4 weeks followed by 1 week rest. Owing to high rates of neuropathy, recommended modification is to start with weekly administration and 5-week cycles.[251]
[e]Repeated every 5 weeks.
[f]Dexamethasone 40 mg days 1 to 4, 9 to 12, and 17 to 20 for cycle 1; then days 1, 8, 15, and 22.

efficacy and toxicity, and defined as progression/death from any cause, lenalidomide discontinuation, or hematologic grade 4 or nonhematologic grade 3 to 4 adverse events (AEs). Surprisingly, a divergence in the PFS curves was evident in the initial 9 months of treatment itself when both the arms had received similar therapy, highlighting the limitation of a non–placebo-controlled design. After a median follow-up of 37 months, the EFS was prolonged (median 10.4 vs 6.9 months, HR, 0.70; 95% confidence interval [CI], 0.51-0.95; $P = .02$), with comparable PFS (median 20.2 vs 18.3 months, HR, 0.78; 95% CI, 0.55-1.10; $P = .16$) and a trend toward OS benefit (3-year OS, 74% vs 63%; HR, 0.62; 95% CI, 0.37-1.03; $P = .06$) with reduced dose intensity Rd treatment vs full-dose Rd, respectively. The omission of dexamethasone not only reduced dexamethasone-related AEs, but also favorably impacted lenalidomide AE–related discontinuation rates. Lenalidomide was discontinued for AEs in 24% vs 30% and reduced in 45% vs 62% of patients receiving reduced dose intensity Rd treatment vs full-dose Rd, respectively.

At the same time Rd regimens were being explored, MP was being challenged by other triplets incorporating thalidomide or bortezomib. The results with MP and thalidomide (MPT) (see section "Melphalan, Prednisone, and Thalidomide") and those with Rd were the basis of the FIRST trial (also known as MM-020). Sixteen hundred twenty patients were randomized in 1:1:1 ratio to receive either lenalidomide and dexamethasone 21 days of 28-day cycles until progression (Rd-continuous) or lenalidomide and dexamethasone same schedule but for a limited duration of 18 cycles (Rd18) or MPT.[269] MPT was given in 42 days cycles for 72 weeks (12 cycles). Patient's risk stratified according to age (≤75 vs >75 years) or ISS stage (I or II vs III). All patients received protocol-specific antithrombotic prophylaxis.

ORRs are shown in *Table 100.5*. PR or better was achieved in 75% of patients, including 18% with CR and 42% with VGPR or better. Median time to first response was less than 2 months.[288] For those patients who achieved CR, median time to first CR was 10, 8, and 11 months in the Rd-continuous, Rd18, and MPT arms, respectively. In the first report, follow-up among surviving patients was 37 months.[269] The median PFS was 25 months with Rd-continuous, 21 months with 18 cycles of Rd, and 21 months with MPT. The 3-year OS rates were 70%, 66%, and 62%, respectively. Estimated 4-year OS rates at 4 years were 59%, 56%, and 51%, respectively. There was no difference in OS between the Rd-continuous arm and the Rd18 arm. There was, however, a difference in OS between and MPT and the pooled Rd populations (HR, 0.78; 95% CI: 0.64-0.96; $P = .02$).

Subsequent analyses comparing outcomes by regimen and by depth of response showed superior PFS in the Rd-continuous arm as compared to the other two arms regardless of depth of response with a median follow-up of 45 months.[288] For those achieving CR, the PFS rates were 60, 41, and 37 months, respectively. Although OS was best in those patients achieving CR, when patients were separated by depth of response and further by regimen, there was still no difference in OS between the Rd18 and the Rd-continuous arms, though trends were seen favoring Rd-continuous among those achieving a VGPR or stable disease. What was quite striking was the 4-year OS of approximately 80% for those patients achieving CR with Rd induction.

Rates of grade 3 or 4 neutropenia were lower in the Rd arms than in the MPT arm (26%-28% vs 45%). Grade 3 or 4 infections occurred in 29% of patients receiving Rd-continuous, 22% of lenalidomide-dexamethasone 18 cycles, and in 17% of those who received MPT. Rates of DVT or pulmonary embolism (PE) or both were 8% in the Rd-continuous group, 6% in the Rd18 group, and 5% in the MPT group. Respective rates of cardiac events of grade 3 or 4 were 12%, 7%, and 9%. Grade 3 or higher peripheral sensory neuropathy was rare in the lenalidomide-dexamethasone arms in 1% or less vs 9% in those treated with an MPT. Rates of invasive second primary cancers were reported in up to 6% of patients, with no difference between the arms. Specifically, hematologic cancers were slightly more frequent with MPT (2% of patients) and then with Rd (<1%).

Thalidomide and Dexamethasone. Thalidomide and dexamethasone (TD) was compared to single-agent high-dose dexamethasone in the early 2000s. Although it was an advance at the time, it is not used as an induction regimen in the modern era. In the TD arm, time to progression (TTP) was significantly better (17.4 months, 95% CI: 8.1 months to NR vs 6.4 months, 95% CI: 5.6-7.4 months), but grade 3 to 4 AEs were also higher: DVT/PE 15.4% vs 4.3%, cerebral ischemia 3.4% vs 1.3%, myocardial infarction 4.7% vs 1.3%, and peripheral neuropathy 3.8% vs 0.4%.[248,287] This was done prior to the recognition that ASA should be included when IMiDs are combined with corticosteroids.

TD has also been compared to MP.[286] In these 282 elderly patients, while there were higher response rates using TD (68% vs 52%,

Table 100.5. Randomized Trials of Induction Regimens for Elderly Patients/Patients Not Destined for ASCT

Study	Regimen	N	CR, %	P	≥PR, %	P	Median PFS/EFS, mo	P	Median OS, mo	P
MAIA[270]	DRd	368	48	<0.001	93	<0.001	NR	<0.001	5-y 66%	0.013
	Rd	369	25		81		32		5-y 53%	
TOURMALINE[271]	IRd	351	26	<0.001	82	0.436	35	0.073	54	0.495
	Rd	354	14		80		22		57	
S0777[272]	VRD-R	264	16	NS	81	0.02	43	0.004	75	0.02
	Rd-R	261	8		71		30		64	
MM-020 (FIRST trial)[269]	Rd Cont.	535	15	NS	75	<0.001	25	<0.001 Rd cont vs other	4-y 59%	NS
	Rd 18-mo	541	14		73	Rd vs MPT	21		4-y 56%	
	MPT	547	9		62		21		4-y 51%	
E4A03 ≥ 70[230,273]	Rd	71	NA	NA	74	NS	22	0.1	2-y 90%	0.03
	RD	76			75		16		2-y 69%	
VISTA(209)[261,274]	VMP	344	30	<0.001	71	<0.001	24	<0.001	56	<0.001
	MP	338	4		35		17		43	
PETHEMA/GEM05[275,276]	VMP[d]	130	20	NS	80	NS	32	NS	63	0.01
	VTP	130	28		81		23		43	
VMPT + VT[262,277]	VMP	257	24	<0.001	81	NS	24	<0.001	5-y 51%	0.01
	VMPT + VT	254	38		89		35		5-y 61%	
UPFRONT[278]	VD	168	3	NS	73	NS	15	NS	50	NS
	VTD	167	4		90		15		51	
	VMP	167	4		70		17		53	
Clarion[279]	KMP	478	26	NS	84	NS	22	NS	NA	NA
	VMP	477	23		79		22			
ALCYONE[212]	D-VMP	350	43	<0.001	91	<0.001	NA	<0.001	2-y 79%	NS
	VMP	356	24		74		18		2-y 79%	
IFM99-06[235,a]	MPT	125	13	<0.001	76	<0.001	28	<0.001	52	0.0006
	MP	196	2		35		18		33	
	MEL100 × 2	126	18		65		19		38	
IFM01-01[257]	MPT	113	7	<0.001	62	<0.001	24	0.001	45	0.03
	MP	116	1		31		19		28	
GIMEMA[255,256]	MPT[b]	129	15	<0.001	60	NA	22	0.004	45	NS
	MP	126	2		45		14		48	
NMSG #12[258]	MPT[b]	182	13	<0.001	57	<0.001	15	NS	29	NS
	MP	175	4		40		14		32	
HOVON 49[259]	MPT[b]	165	23[c]	<0.001	66	<0.001	13	<0.001	40	0.05
	MP	168	8[c]		45		9		31	
TMSG[260]	MPT	57	9	NS	58	0.03	21	NS	26	NS
	MP	57	9		37		14		28	
Meta-analysis[280]	MPT	809	25[c]	NA	59	<0.0001	20	<0.0001	39	0.004
	MP	876	9[d]		37		15		33	
MRC IX—nonintensive[264,281]	CTDa	419	13	NA	64	<0.001	13	0.01	34	NS
	MP	418	2		33		12		32	
MM-015[282]	MPR-R	152	33[c]	NA	77	0.002	31	<0.001	3-y 70%	NS
	MPR	153	33[c]		68		14		3-y 62%	
	MP	154	12[c]		50		13		3-y 66%	
E1A06[283]	MPT-T	154	5	NS	75	NS	21	NS	53	NS
	MPR-R	152	11		70		19		48	
HOVON87/NMSG18 trial[284]	MPR-T	318	10	NS	81	NS	20	NS	4-y 52%	NS
	MPT-R	319	13		84		23		4-y 56%	
Magarotto et al, 2016[285]	MPR + R ± P	211	3	NS	71	NS	24	NS	4-y 65%	NS
	CPR + R ± P	220	0.5		66		20		4-y 68%	
	Rd + R ± P	217	3		74		21		4-y 58%	
Ludwig et al, 2005[286]	Thal-Dex	142	2	NS	68	0.002	17	NS	2-y 61%	NS
	MP	141	2		52		21		2-y 70%	
THAL-MM-003[287]	TD	240	8	NS	63	<0.001	15	<0.001	2-y 69%	NS
	D	235	3		46		6		2-y 63%	
Facon (IFM 95-01)[251]	Dex	127	1	NS	42	<0.001	12	With M vs no M, P < .001	33	NS
	Dex-IFN	121	1		43		15		32	
	MP	122	1		41		21		34	
	MD	118	3		70		23		40	

Abbreviations: ASCT, autologous hematopoietic stem cell transplantation; CR, complete response; MD, melphalan-dexamethasone; MP, melphalan and prednisone; MPR-R, MPR with lenalidomide maintenance; MPT, melphalan, prednisone, and thalidomide; NA, not available; OS, overall survival; PFS/EFS, progression-free survival or event-free survival; TD, thalidomide and dexamethasone; VMP, bortezomib, melphalan, and prednisone; VMPT, bortezomib, melphalan, prednisone, and thalidomide.

[a]Third arm of this study that treated patients with two sequential mini-ASCTs is not included.
[b]Thalidomide was continued as maintenance in MPT arm.
[c]CR + very good partial response.
[d]Secondary randomization to either VT or VP.

$P = .002$), there was also higher rates AEs: neuropathy (72% vs 33%), psychological toxicity (36% vs 18%, $P < .001$), constipation (33% vs 13%, $P < .001$), and a trend toward more DVTs (10% vs 4%). The only toxicity more commonly seen in the MP arm was myelosuppression. With a median follow-up of 28 months, there was no difference in PFS, but there was a trend toward shorter OS among TD-treated patients, which was more notable in patients older than 75 years.

Triplets

Bortezomib, Lenalidomide, and Dexamethasone. Even before randomized data were available, VRd became one of the most commonly used induction regimes, even in the elderly. The justification for its use was the very impressive response rates seen in a small phase I/II study performed by Richardson and colleagues.[229] They treated 66 previously untreated patients with the combination of VRd. Patients received eight 3-week cycles and either proceeded to transplantation or maintenance. All patients responded, and 67% achieved a VGPR or better. Forty-two percent proceeded to ASCT. With median follow-up of 21 months, estimated 18-month PFS and OS for the combination treatment with/without transplantation were 75% and 97%, respectively. Sensory neuropathy occurred in 80% of patients, and 32% reported neuropathic pain (grade 2/3 in 14%). Grade 3 to 4 neutropenia and thrombocytopenia occurred in 9% and 6% of patients, respectively.

In 2017, a randomized trial comparing VRd vs Rd was reported (*Table 100.5*). The population was not restricted to transplant-ineligible patients.[272] In fact, 69% of patients had an intent to transplant, making this study an atypical "transplant-ineligible trial." This S0777 trial was an open-label, phase III trial that randomized 525 patients between two arms: 264 to VRd and 261 to Rd. Forty-three percent of patients were 65 years or older. The VRd regimen was given as eight 21-day cycles, and the Rd regimen was given as six 28-day cycles. All patients received 325 mg of oral ASA a day to reduce the risk of thromboembolic complications. Patients on the VRd arm received herpes simplex virus prophylaxis. After induction, all patients received ongoing maintenance with lenalidomide 25 mg/d for 21 days plus dexamethasone 40 mg once weekly. Stem cell collection was allowed for those patients considering future transplant. One hundred thirty-five VRd arm and 143 Rd patients proceeded to maintenance therapy. At the time of primary analysis, the median overall follow-up was 56 months. The median duration of maintenance was 385 days.

The primary endpoint of PFS was met: VRd at 43 months (95% CI: 39-52) vs Rd at 30 months (95% CI: 25-39 months). The respective median OS rates were 75 and 64 months, stratified hazard ratio (HR) 0.71 (95% CI: 0.52-0.96). The median duration of response (DOR) was 52 months in the VRd group vs 38 months for the Rd group ($P = .01$). Significant differences in PFS were observed only among patients younger than 65 years and in OS among patients older than 75 years.

Although overall response rates (ORRs) were improved in the VRd group as compared to the Rd group, confirmed CR rates were lower than expected.[289] Overall AEs were balanced between the two arms with the exception of a higher rate of grade 3 or higher neuropathy in the VRd group as compared to the Rd group (33% vs 11%; $P < .0001$).[272] Note that the bortezomib was given twice-weekly IV rather than subcutaneously (SQ), which is known to be associated with significantly higher peripheral nerve toxicity.[290]

A reduced intensity bortezomib-lenalidomide-dexamethasone (VRd lite) regimen was evaluated in transplant ineligible myeloma patients in a small single arm, phase 2 study involving 50 patients.[291] It utilized a modified schedule in which bortezomib was given 1·3 mg/m^2 weekly subcutaneously on days 1, 8, 15, and 22, lenalidomide at 15 mg orally on days 1 to 21; and dexamethasone 20 mg orally on the day of and day after bortezomib for nine 35-day cycles followed by 6 cycles of consolidation with lenalidomide and bortezomib. The ORR after 4 cycles of VRd lite was impressive at 86%, with 66% of patients achieving a VGPR or better. The estimated median PFS was 35·1 months (95% CI 30.9—NR) and median OS was not reached at a median follow-up of 30 months. The toxicities were quite manageable as well, with hypophosphatemia being the only grade 3 toxicity evident in more 10% of the study population. Although nearly 60% of the patients reported peripheral neuropathy, the subcutaneous route well as weekly administration resulted in grade 3 symptoms in only one patient. Although the global health status improved, it did not meet statistical significance.

Daratumumab, Lenalidomide, and Dexamethasone. The MAIA trial investigators evaluated the impact of adding daratumumab to the Rd backbone until disease progression or unacceptable toxicity in a randomized controlled trial involving 737 patients with newly diagnosed multiple myeloma who were ineligible for ASCT, with lenalidomide and dexamethasone doublet as the control group.[270] In a recently updated report, after a median follow-up of 56 months, not only was the PFS difference maintained in favor of the triplet (5 year-PFS rate was 52.5% (95% CI 46.7-58.0) in the daratumumab group establishing a new benchmark for the transplant ineligible patients; HR, 0.53), but importantly OS difference also emerged (median OS had not reached in either group; HR 0.68, $P = .0013$) in favor of the daratumumab group. Although there were no new safety concerns with extended follow-up, the triplet resulted in higher rates of neutropenia, pneumonia, and serious AEs. Among patients in the lenalidomide and dexamethasone group who underwent subsequent treatment, only 21% had received a daratumumab-based regimen as the first salvage therapy, hampering analysis for OS which may have been adversely impacted by the limited access to daratumumab by the control group. The MAIA trialists did not seek answers to key the questions regarding the consequences of sequencing a daratumumab-based regimen following progression on lenalidomide and dexamethasone, nor was the impact of a finite duration of daratumumab instead of continuous use of a third agent in the frontline setting examined.

The ELOQUENT 1 study (NCT01335399) is a phase 3, randomized, open labeled trial of continuous lenalidomide/dexamethasone ± elotuzumab administered in subjects with previously untreated MM who were deemed ineligible for ASCT because of age or coexisting conditions. The topline results from the final analysis of ELOQUENT1 [NCT01335399] data showed a lack of PFS benefit with the addition of elotuzumab in this patient population, indicating the failure of the study to meet its primary endpoint; a full publication is awaited.

Melphalan, Prednisone, and Thalidomide. There have been six randomized controlled trials comparing MP to MPT (*Table 100.5*).[235,255-260] All have favored MPT with regard to higher CR rates. Four of six have been positive with regard to PFS, again in favor of three drugs over two drugs, but only three of six have been positive with regard to OS. An individual patient meta-analysis demonstrated in aggregate that MPT was superior to MP in terms of ORR (59% vs 37%), median PFS (20 vs 15 months), and median OS (39 vs 33 months).[280] In a side meta-analysis examining serious AEs of individual patient data of these same six trials,[263] a higher cumulative incidence of grade 3 to 4 nonhematologic (39% vs 17%, HR 2.78, 95% CI: 2.21-3.50) and hematologic (28% vs 22%, HR 1.32, 95% CI: 1.05-1.66) toxicities was documented with MPT. Nonhematologic toxicities were more likely to occur in patients with a baseline poorer performance status (HR 1.18, 95% CI: 1.06-1.32). The specific serious AEs that were more common in patients receiving MPT were peripheral neuropathy, neurologic other than peripheral neuropathy, thrombosis, and dermatologic toxicity. The experience of a nonhematologic grade 3 to 4 AE had a negative impact on both PFS (HR 1.24, 95% CI: 1.07-1.45, $P = .006$) and OS (HR 1.23, 95% CI: 1.03-1.47, $P = .006$).

Cyclophosphamide, Thalidomide, and Dexamethasone. CTDa (cyclophosphamide, thalidomide, and dexamethasone) is a variation on the theme of MPT. The Medical Research Council (MRC) IX trial[264,281] randomized elderly patients to either MP or CTDa (*Table 100.5*) to maximum response, with a minimum of six cycles to a maximum of nine cycles. There was a secondary randomization to thalidomide or no thalidomide maintenance. PFS was marginally better in the CTDa arm, but OS was not different between the two arms even with a median follow-up of 71 months. Patients in the CTDa group had a higher rate of sensory and motor neuropathy, thromboembolic events, constipation, infection, rash, and elevated alkaline phosphatase levels than did those in the MP group, but lower incidence of cytopenias.

Bortezomib, Melphalan, and Prednisone. The VISTA trial[261] is the one large trial comparing MP to VMP (*Tables 100.4* and *100.5*) and is the one that established VMP as a standard for elderly myeloma patients. Patients received nine 6-week cycles of MP either alone or in combination with bortezomib (1.3 mg/m^2, on days 1, 4, 8, 11, 22, 25, 29, and 32 during cycles 1 to 4 and on days 1, 8, 22, and 29 during cycles 5 to 9). All response and survival outcomes were superior with the VMP, most notably CR rates of 30% vs 4%. Median PFS was 24 months as compared to 17 months, and 3-year OS was 68% as compared to 54%.[218] Time to response was also quicker with VMP 1.4 vs 4.2 months. Grade 3 to 4 AEs, however, were more frequent in patients receiving VMP (46% vs 36%). Thirty-three percent of patients discontinued bortezomib because of toxicity. Peripheral sensory neuropathy occurred in 44% of patients with grade 3 to 4 in 13%. Neuralgia was also reported in 36% of patients.

There are three phase III trials for the elderly that compare VMP to other regimens.[275,292] A major finding of two of these trials was the feasibility and efficacy of changing the bortezomib scheduled from days 1, 4, 8, and 11 every 21 days to a once-weekly schedule. This alteration dramatically reduced rates of peripheral neuropathy as did SQ instead of IV administration.

In the GEM2005 study, patients were randomized to VMP or VTP.[275,276] There was a secondary randomization, to VT or VP maintenance. In the initial report with a follow-up of less than 3 years, response rates, PFS, and OS were comparable, but grade 3 to 4 AEs were significantly higher in the VTP arm; however, with additional follow-up (median of 6 years), patients randomized to VMP had a significantly prolonged OS as compared to VTP cohort (median 63 and 43 months, $P = .01$). There was a trend for better PFS with VMP as compared to VTP (32 vs 23 months). There was no difference in outcome between patients receiving VT or VP as maintenance. Achieving a CR translated into a median OS of 80 months (81 months for VMP and 76 months for VTP, $P = .05$). Not only was immunophenotypic CR (by four-color flow cytometry) more common after VMP than VTP, patients achieving immunophenotypic CR after VMP had a significantly longer median OS than those achieving same level of response after VTP (NR vs 73 months). Among patients with high-risk cytogenetics, median PFS was comparable for VMP and VTP (18 and 20 months, respectively); however, OS was shorter in patients treated with VTP as compared to the VMP (29 vs 51 months). On multivariate analysis, factors independently associated with longer OS included a VMP as induction, standard-risk cytogenetics, and attainment of CR. More patients in the VTP arm discontinued therapy prematurely, and they had higher rates of cardiac events (8% vs 0%) but lower rates of infection (1% vs 7%).

In a pooled trial analysis of elderly NDMM patient, Mateos and colleagues have demonstrated that higher cumulative doses of bortezomib appeared to be associated with better OS.[293] Results of this posthoc analysis need to be balanced with the reality of side effects in this potentially frail population.

The UPFRONT Trial. The multicenter, phase IIIb UPFRONT study compared the efficacy and safety in 502 NDMM patients ineligible for HDT-SCT of three bortezomib-based induction regimens (24 weeks) followed by weekly bortezomib (1.6 mg/m^2 4 weeks out of 5) maintenance (25 weeks): VCD (bortezomib-dexamethasone), VTD, and VMP.[278] The median age of this population was 73 years. Owing to difficulties with tolerability, the mean bortezomib dose intensities for the respective three arms were 72%, 63%, and 68% during induction and 75%, 81%, and 87% during maintenance, respectively. Best confirmed ORR was 73%, 80%, and 70%, respectively, including CR rates of 3%, 4%, and 4%. Despite the highest rates of VGPR or better in the VTD arm (37% vs 51% and 41%), with a median follow-up of 43 months, there was no difference in PFS (15, 15, and 17 months) or OS (50, 51, and 53 months) among the groups. Peripheral neuropathy was the most common AE across arms: 50%, 60%, and 47%, respectively. Grade 3 or higher infections were seen in approximately 18% of all patients. EORCTC QLQ-C30 assessments were done. In all arms, there was a trend for worsening function in symptoms during induction followed by improvement/stabilization during maintenance except for cognitive functioning, nausea, vomiting, and diarrhea. In a multivariable regression analysis, only ISS stage I and Karnofsky performance status of 90% or better were associated with a longer PFS. This trial is a striking example of how good response rates do not always correlate with better outcomes. This phenomenon is exaggerated in the elderly, a population especially susceptible to toxicity.

Carfilzomib, Melphalan, and Prednisone. In the relapsed setting, there are studies that would suggest that carfilzomib is a more potent proteasome inhibitor than bortezomib. This assumption prompted the CLARION trial, which compared KMP with VMP in transplant-ineligible NDMM patients.[294] This was an open-label, multicenter randomized trial. Patients received 42-day cycles for nine cycles, that is, 54 weeks of therapy. The primary endpoint was PFS. Median PFS was 22.3 vs 22.1 months in the KMP and VMP arms, respectively. With fewer than 20% death events, OS data were immature, but no difference in OS was evident. Rates of treatment discontinuation because of AEs and fatal treatment-emergent AEs were comparable. In terms of notable AEs, for KMP and VMP, respectively, any grade AE included renal failure (6% vs 2%), cardiac failure (7% vs 2%), dyspnea (16% vs 8%), and hypertension (22% vs 7%). Any grade sensory peripheral neuropathy rate was lower in KMP as compared to the VMP arm (2% vs 14%).

Carfilzomib, Lenalidomide, and Dexamethasone. The combination of carfilzomib, lenalidomide, and dexamethasone (KRd) has been explored both in the nontransplant setting and in the transplant setting as part of a phase I/II trial.[295] Rd was given as described in *Table 100.5* for eight 28-day cycles; for cycles 9 to 25, the carfilzomib was given on days 1, 2, 15, and 16 along with the Rd; after 24 cycles, patients were maintained on lenalidomide off-study. All patients responded to this regimen, with 79% of the 24 elderly patients (median age 72) achieving a CR or better. Of 14 patients tested for MRD, 12 were MRD negative. Treatment was maintained throughout 24 cycles for all but four patients, albeit with dose modifications of KRd in 74%, 83%, and 70% of patients during induction and in more than 50% of each drug during maintenance. The results of the ENDURANCE trial (E1A11, NCT01863550) clarified that this regimen is not superior to VRd for the traditionally defined standard-risk myeloma patients.[296] This phase 3 trial randomly assigned patients with standard-risk or t(4;14) newly diagnosed multiple myeloma, without immediate intent for ASCT, to 36 weeks of induction with the standard of care, to VRd, or KRd, followed by a secondary randomization to lenalidomide maintenance for 2 years vs indefinite maintenance. The trial did not account for chromosome 1 abnormalities in risk stratification. At the planned interim analysis, the median PFS was comparable between the 2 arms (34.4 months in VRd arm vs 34.6 in the KRd arm, HR 1.04, $P = .74$). However, more patients in the VRd group had discontinued treatment early due to adverse effects or preference for an alternative therapy. Among the most common grade 3 to 4 nonhematologic toxicities, the treatment emergent peripheral neuropathy was more common in the VRd arm (8% vs 1%), while a composite of treatment-related cardiopulmonary and renal toxicities at grades 3 to 5 was higher in the KRd group (16% vs 5%). Treatment-related deaths were reported in 2 patients in the VRd group in contrast to 11 patients in the KRd group. A more recent update in abstract form after a median of 29 months of follow-up again failed to show any PFS or OS advantage of KRd over VRd in the entire cohort, although in an unplanned, posthoc analysis, the patients with chromosome 1 abnormalities (+1q and del 1p) showed inferior outcomes with both regimens compared to the outcomes of those without chromosome 1 abnormalities. Interestingly, the OS of patients with gain 1q (3 copies) and deletion 1p who were randomly assigned to the KRd arm was comparable to their respective counterparts without such abnormalities. By contrast, patients in the VRd group with gain 1q or deletion 1p had inferior OS compared to those without such abnormalities. However, among patients with amplification 1q (≥4 copies), the OS with KRd was remarkably short. The study was limited by the absence of data on the subsequent salvage therapies that could have potentially impacted the survival outcomes.

Ixazomib, Lenalidomide, and Dexamethasone. Ixazomib, a second-generation oral proteasome inhibitor, was perceived as a convenient replacement to its more neurotoxic predecessor, bortezomib for exploiting the proteasome inhibitor-immuno modulatory drug synergy. The TOURMALINE-MM2 trial (NCT01850524) randomly assigned 705 transplant ineligible newly diagnosed patients with MM to weekly ixazomib 4 mg or placebo plus lenalidomide dexamethasone doublet, with discontinuation of dexamethasone after 18 cycles and reduction of ixazomib and lenalidomide dose.[271] Although the odds of achieving complete (26% vs 14%; OR, 2.10; $P < .001$) and ≥ VGPR (63% vs 48%; OR, 1.87; $P < .001$) rates were greater with ixazomib-based triplet and despite achieving what appeared to be a clinically meaningful 13.5 months median PFS difference (median PFS 35.3 vs 21.8 months with ixazomib-Rd vs placebo-Rd, respectively, HR, 0.830; 95% CI, 0.676-1.018), the study failed to meet its primary endpoint of superior PFS ($P = .073$). Additionally, PFS advantage was not evident in the patients who were 75 year or older, patients age 75 years or older. Furthermore, after a median follow-up of 50 months, no OS benefit was observed with strikingly superimposable survival curves. However, a prespecified subgroup analysis demonstrated a significant PFS benefit (median PFS 23.8 vs 18.0 months, HR, 0.690; $P = .019$) among the patients with high-risk cytogenetics. Mean global health status scores over time suggested similar patient-reported health-related quality of life in the two arms. On-study deaths were deemed treatment-related in 5 of 27 patients in the ixazomib-Rd arm and 4 of 22 patients in the control arm.

Melphalan, Prednisone, and Lenalidomide. As it became clear that lenalidomide was both a more potent and better-tolerated IMiD than thalidomide, the melphalan, prednisone, and lenalidomide (MPR) regimen was studied.[282] Palumbo and colleagues performed a three-arm phase III trial: MP vs MPR vs MPR with lenalidomide maintenance (MPR-R). Four hundred fifty-nine patients were randomized to either MP (nine 4-week cycles of melphalan 0.18 mg/kg/d and prednisone 2 mg/kg/d days 1-4), MPR (nine 4-week cycles of MP plus lenalidomide 10 mg days 1-21), or nine cycles of MPR with indefinite lenalidomide maintenance (10 mg days 1-21 every 4 weeks). ORRs were lowest in the MP (50%) arm with progressively better rates for MPR (68%) and MPR-R (77%). With a median follow-up period of 30 months, however, neither PFS nor OS was better among patients treated with MPR as compared to MP. MPR-R patients had better PFS (31 vs 14 and 13 months) but not 3-year OS (70%) as compared to the other two groups (62% vs 66%). Toxicity was substantially higher in the lenalidomide arms.

Head-to-head comparisons of the combination of MPR-R to MPT with thalidomide maintenance (MPT-T) followed in two trials E1A06 and HOVON87/NMSG18.[283,284] The median age of participants on E1A06 was 76 years, and one-third of patients on HOVON87/NMSG18 were 76 years or older. The results of the two trials were quite similar with comparable response rates, PFS, and OS observed between the arms and between the trials. Overall, MPT-T caused more peripheral neuropathy, and MPR-R caused more myelosuppression. More patients discontinued MPT-T owing to toxicity than MPR-R. In the HOVON87/NMSG18 trial, rates of non–melanoma skin cancers were higher in the MPR-R arm (20 vs 5 patients).

MPR, CPR, and Rd were compared in a phase III study of patients ineligible for ASCT.[285] The MPR and the Rd were given as previously described. The CPR was administered as lenalidomide 10 mg days 1 to 21 every 38 days, cyclophosphamide 50 mg every other day for either 28 or 21 days depending on patient age, and prednisone was given as 50 or 25 mg every other day, again depending on age. Part way through the protocol, the CPR induction was changed to lenalidomide 25 mg days 1 to 21 and cyclophosphamide 50 mg daily for the younger cohort. After nine cycles of induction, patients were randomly assigned to receive maintenance treatment with lenalidomide either alone at 10 mg on days 1 to 21 every 28 days or in combination with prednisone at 25 mg every other day continuously.

Nearly 60% of MPR patients, one-quarter of CPR patients, and 20% of Rd patients required Neupogen, reducing the duration of neutropenia. The addition of alkylator did not appear to add anything to response rate, PFS, or OS for the overall group. In a posthoc analysis including fit patients only, the MPR group had a better median PFS (30 months) as compared to the other two groups (22 months), and the 4-year OS was better in the MPR and CPR groups than the Rd group (77% vs 57%).

Quadruplets

Daratumumab, Bortezomib, Melphalan, and Prednisone. Mateos and colleagues combined daratumumab with VMP and compared that to VMP as part of an open-label, randomized controlled trial.[212] Standard VMP was administered to all patients for nine cycles (*Tables 100.4* and *100.5*). In the experimental arm, daratumumab was given according to usual schedule and continued indefinitely. Oral dexamethasone at a dose of 20 mg was given with each dose of daratumumab along with premedications. A total of 700 patients received the assigned intervention.

The median age of the cohort was 71 years. During the first nine cycles, 19% of the daratumumab, bortezomib, melphalan, and prednisone (DVMP) and 33% of the VMP group discontinued therapy. With a median follow-up of 16.5 months, the median duration of treatment was 14.7 months in the DVMP group and 12 months in the VMP group. Dose intensity of bortezomib and melphalan was comparable between two arms, though there was a slightly higher prednisone dose equivalent given in the DVMP arm: 252 vs 237 mg/cycle. The 12-month PFS was 72% vs 50% for the respective arms (HR 0.5, 95% CI: 0.38-0.65, $P < .001$). Both ORRs and CR rates were superior in the DVMP arm. Rates of MRD negativity (at a threshold of 1 tumor cell per 10^5 white cells) were superior for DVMP as well (22% vs 6%, $P < .001$). Time to first response was 0.8 months for both groups, and time to best response was 4.9 and 4.1 months for DVMP and VMP. Side effects were relatively comparable between arms, including grade 3 or 4 neutropenia in nearly 40% both arms, thrombocytopenia in just over one-third of patients, and anemia in just under 20% of patients. Grade 3 or 4 infections were more common in the daratumumab group than the control group (23% vs 15%).

Bortezomib, Lenalidomide, Dexamethasone, and Elotuzumab. A companion phase 2 trial for the high-risk patient, SWOG-1211, assessed the value of adding elotuzumab, an anti-SLAMF7 (CS1) monoclonal antibody to VRd induction for eight 21-day cycles followed by its incorporation to 28-day cycles of dose-attenuated VRd maintenance until progression in a non–transplant-based approach.[297] Elotuzumab was administered at 10 mg/kg intravenously on days 1, 8, and 15 for cycles 1 to 2, on days 1 and 11 for cycles 3 to 8, and on days 1 and 15 during the maintenance phase. High-risk disease was defined by the presence of one or more of the following: GEP high risk, t(14;16), t(14;20), del(17p), or gain/amp1q21, primary plasma cell leukemia, and elevated serum LDH. The study did not meet the primary endpoint of improved PFS with the addition of elotuzumab. After a median follow-up of 53 months, PFS rates were similar in both groups (VRd median 33.6 months [95% CI 19.55—NR], VRd-elotuzumab 31.5 months [18.56-53.98]; HR 0.968 [80% CI 0.697-1.344]; one-sided $P = .45$]). Although comparable, the PFS rates for both arms exceeded the original statistical assumptions made based on the Total Therapy protocols, underscoring the value of continuous proteasome inhibitors and IMiD combination maintenance therapies for high-risk MM. The safety profile was largely comparable as well, although higher rates of grade 3 to 5 infections (4 [8%] of 52 in the VRd group, 8 [17%] of 48 in the VRd-elotuzumab group), sensory neuropathy (4 [8%] of 52 in the VRd group, 6 [13%] of 48 in the VRd-elotuzumab group), and motor neuropathy (1 [2%] of 52 in the VRd group, 4 [8%] of 48 in the VRd-elotuzumab group) were observed. One treatment-related death occurred in the VRd-elotuzumab group vs none in the VRd group.

A smaller open label phase 2a study (NCT02375555) used the elotuzumab VRd quadruplet as induction treatment for 4 cycles in transplant-eligible MM patients. Following cycle 4, pts could proceed with either ASCT or defer transplant and receive four additional cycles followed by risk-adapted maintenance with dose-attenuated quadruplet for both ASCT and nontransplant. Of 41 patients who were enrolled, all responded, but two died due to sepsis or respiratory failure–associated complications.

Bortezomib, Melphalan, Prednisone, and Thalidomide. Palumbo and colleagues randomized patients to receive either nine 5-week cycles of VMP (*Table 100.5*) or nine 5-week cycles of bortezomib, melphalan, prednisone, and thalidomide (VMPT), which also added thalidomide 50 mg continuously and continued with maintenance thalidomide along with alternate-week bortezomib. Median follow-up at the time of the initial publication was 23 months. Response rates and PFS were higher in the four-drug combination with maintenance as compared to the three-drug combination with no maintenance, but OS was not different. In a subsequent update with longer follow-up, for the VMP arm, the 5-year OS was 51%, and for the VMPT + VT, OS was 61%.[277] This benefit was mainly evident in patients aged 65 to 75 years. Toxicity was significantly higher using the four-drug regimen: grade 3 to 4 neutropenia (38% vs 28%; $P < .02$), cardiologic events (10% vs 5%; $P < .04$), and thromboembolic events (5% vs 2%, $P < .08$). A higher frequency of treatment discontinuation was reported in the VMPT + VT arm. Younger patients were able to receive 81% of the planned cumulative dose intensity of bortezomib, but older patients could only tolerate 58% of the planned dose. The VMPT + VT regimen became more tolerable when the once per week administration of bortezomib began in lieu of the twice-weekly administration. Severe sensory peripheral neuropathy was reduced from 16% to 3%. It is difficult to know whether the improvement seen in the VMPT + VT arm was because of the use of a quadruplet as induction or because of the use of maintenance treatment with VT. Another limitation of this study is the absence of any prespecified salvage therapy.

Alkylator Combinations

The 1970s and 1980s were a testing ground for various combinations of alkylators, corticosteroids, and doxorubicin. Melphalan-cyclophosphamide-prednisone,[298] carmustine-cyclophosphamide-prednisone,[299,300] melphalan-cyclophosphamide-carmustine-prednisone (MCBP),[298,301] and vincristine-melphalan-cyclophosphamide-prednisone (VMCP)[298] resulted in response rates of 47%, 37% to 50%, 49% to 68%, and 62%, respectively. Median survivals with these regimens were 25 to 36 months.[298-301] Lee and Case[302] introduced the five-drug regimen of vincristine-carmustine-melphalan-cyclophosphamide-prednisone (VBMCP or the M-2 regimen), which included the same four drugs as MCBP plus vincristine; dose intensities, however, were different in these two regimens. Response rate for VBMCP was about 85% in previously untreated patients with a median survival of 38 months.[302,303] The success of the VBMCP regimen supported the value of vincristine. However, the MRC IV trial, which randomized 530 previously untreated patients with MM to MP vs melphalan-vincristine-prednisone, revealed no difference in either response rate or OS between the two arms.[304] VMCP did not produce a response or survival advantage over MP.[305,306]

Although subsequent randomized trials substantiated the superior response rates of VBMCP over standard MP, they did not demonstrate superior survival. In fact, the meta-analysis performed by the Myeloma Trialists' Collaborative Group[196] involving 6633 patients in 27 randomized trials revealed a superior response rate (60.2% vs 53.2%, $P < .000001$, two-tailed), but no survival benefit for combination chemotherapy over standard MP. A prior meta-analysis of 18 published trials (3814 patients) also demonstrated no benefit for combination chemotherapy in terms of survival. There was a suggestion of a survival advantage in the subgroup of patients with more aggressive disease,[307] but this was not substantiated in the larger meta-analysis.[196]

The use of alkylator doxorubicin-based combination chemotherapy was stimulated by a report on the benefits of a combination of doxorubicin and BCNU in patients who had become resistant to melphalan.[308] Regimens such as MAP (melphalan-doxorubicin-prednisone), CAP (cyclophosphamide-doxorubicin-prednisone), VCAP (vincristine and CAP), and VBAP (vincristine-BCNU-doxorubicin-prednisone) were tried; by SWOG response criteria, objective response rates were 41%, 46%, 64%, and 61%, respectively.[298,309] Median survival ranged from 30 to 32 months; subsequent analysis demonstrated a superior median survival for the VBAP arm of 37 months.[144] Enthusiasm for alternating VMCP and VBAP (or VCAP) was generated by the SWOG study of 237 patients randomized to MP or the above regimens.[310,311] Response rates and OS were superior in the alternating combination chemotherapy arms compared to the MP arm,[144,309] but the survival benefits of this initial study were not reproducible by others. The MRC MM V trial randomized patients to ABCM (VBAP-VMCP without the vincristine or prednisone) or melphalan as a single agent on the basis of findings emanating from the MRC IV trial, which demonstrated a lack of benefit attributable to the addition of vincristine. Median survival in the ABCM group was superior to that of the melphalan-only arm (32 vs 24 months, $P = .0003$).[312,313]

Combination Chemotherapy With Interferon-α for Induction

IFN and dexamethasone were combined as an induction regimen in patients with NDMM and a low tumor mass. A multitude of trials adding IFN to MP and numerous alkylator corticosteroid combinations with or without anthracycline as part of an induction regimen were performed, but results were mixed. Two meta-analyses were performed in an attempt to reconcile these conflicting results.[314,315] The first, reported in 2000,[314] used published data and included 17 induction trials with 2333 evaluable patients; the second, reported by the Myeloma Trialists' Collaborative Group in 2001,[314] used primary data from 12 induction trials involving 2469 patients. PFS and OS were better with IFN by approximately 5 to 6 and 3 months, respectively; quality of life, however, suffered significantly.[316]

Transplant-Eligible Patients

The most commonly used induction regimen for patients who are considered ASCT candidates is VRd in the United States. In Europe and other parts of the world, VTD or VCD is preferred owing to cost constraints. There are ongoing studies evaluating other triplets and even quadruplets, including therapeutic monoclonal antibodies. Other induction regimens have been tested (e.g., VAD, single-agent dexamethasone, TD, Rd), but are now considered inferior. By the end of the 20th century, it was accepted that the strategies of early vs delayed transplant were equally effective in terms of OS if alkylator, anthracycline, and steroid combinations were used as induction and as part of the comparator arm. With the advent of IMiDs and proteasome inhibitors, the question of whether early ASCT is the best approach is being reconsidered. Preliminary data would suggest that there is a definite improvement in PFS with early ASCT, but more time will be required to determine whether this translates into better OS and better quality of life. It is generally accepted that lenalidomide maintenance is preferred over no maintenance, but other maintenance strategies are currently being studied, as will be discussed.

Doublets

Lenalidomide and Dexamethasone (Rd). This combination has been used as induction prior to transplantation,[230,273,317,318] but data have emerged from the S0777 trial, demonstrating inferiority in terms of both PFS and OS among patients receiving Rd.[273]

Bortezomib and Dexamethasone. The IFM 2005-1 randomized 482 patients to either four cycles of VAD or bortezomib-dexamethasone (BD)[319] followed by DCEP (dexamethasone-cyclophosphamide-etoposide-cisplatin) for two cycles vs no DCEP. Patients were to have a single ASCT, and those without a VGPR or better were to receive a second ASCT. An undefined number of patients received maintenance lenalidomide as part of a different trial of lenalidomide vs placebo (IFM 2005-2 trial). Pretransplant CR, VGPR, and PR were superior with BD. By protocol, fewer patients who received BD were deemed candidates for second ASCT compared to those who had VAD induction, but only 21% and 27%, respectively, actually received a second ASCT. The improvement in response in the BD arm persisted after transplant, but with a median follow-up of 32 months, there was no difference in PFS or OS. The incidence of grade 3 to 4 AEs appeared similar between groups, but hematologic toxicity and deaths related to toxicity (0 vs 7) were more frequent with VAD. In contrast, rates of grade 2 (20.5% vs 10.5%) and grades 3 to 4 (9.2% vs 2.5%) peripheral neuropathy during induction through first transplantation were significantly higher with BD.

Four phase II studies used either single-agent bortezomib or bortezomib in combination with dexamethasone. One study is notable because all patients on that study (E2A02) were high risk as defined by β_2M and/or cytogenetic abnormalities, and none of the patients had early transplantation. Median PFS was 8 months, and 2-year OS was 76%.[320]

Other Doublets. E1A00,[248] E4A03,[230] and S0232[321] (Table 100.6) were conducted with response endpoints rather than PFS or OS and have been discussed earlier. The two trials comparing variants of VAD using pegylated doxorubicin (PLD) had response and toxicity as major endpoints.[335,336] E1A00 compared single-agent dexamethasone to thalidomide-dexamethasone (TD). Its premise was to validate whether the addition of thalidomide to dexamethasone increased response rates as reported in phase II studies. The ORR of TD was significantly higher than dexamethasone alone (63% vs 41%); however, toxicity was greater using the combination with grade 4 to 5 toxicities being 45% vs 21% ($P < .001$).[248] For nearly a decade, TD was used as induction in the months before stem cell collection because of its high response rates and its ease of administration, but with the introduction lenalidomide and bortezomib, the TD doublet is not commonly used in the United States as induction.

Triplets

Bortezomib, Lenalidomide, and Dexamethasone. The IFM 2009 is one of the most important modern trials in that it delineates the response rates of VRd as induction in patients destined for transplant with a longer term goal of clarify the role of early vs delayed ASCT in the modern era (Table 100.7).[289] It builds on knowledge about VRd induction from other trials.[229,272] Attal and colleagues conducted an open-label, multicenter randomized trial that included 700 patients with NDMM.[289] All patients were given induction with three cycles of VRd. Patients were then randomized to consolidation either with VRd for five additional cycles or with high-dose melphalan with ASCT followed by two additional cycles of VRd. Both groups received maintenance therapy with lenalidomide for 1 year. The bortezomib was given IV according to the standard days 1, 4, 8, and 11 schedule. The consolidation regimen of VRd included a reduction of the dose of dexamethasone to 10 mg/dose rather than 20 mg/dose; the starting dose of the maintenance lenalidomide was 10 mg for the first 3 months with a possible dose escalation to 15 mg thereafter. Patients were stratified according to the ISS and by cytogenetic risk profile as determined by FISH. Without ASCT as consolidation, the ORR was 97%. In all, 48% of patients achieved CR and 49% were MRD negative by 7-color flow cytometry (sensitivity of 10^{-4}). Similar findings have been reported in abstract form from the STAMiNA (NCT01109004) and DETERMINATION (NCT01208662) trials.[350]

Bortezomib, Thalidomide, and Dexamethasone. Based on the promising phase II results using VTD in previously untreated MM,[349] the Gruppo Italiano Malattie Ematologiche dell'Adulto (GIMEMA) group randomly allocated 480 patients to either three 21-day cycles of thalidomide (100 mg daily for the first 14 days and 200 mg daily thereafter) plus dexamethasone (40 mg daily on 8 of the first 12 days), either alone or with bortezomib (1.3 mg/m² on days 1, 4, 8, and 11).[339] After double ASCT, patients received two 35-day cycles of their assigned

Table 100.6. Selected Phase II Induction Regimens

Reference	Regimen	Phase	N	CR, %	VGPR, %	PR, %	OR, %	PFS	OS
Voorhees et al, 2020[322]	D-VRd	II	104	19	53	26	98	2-y 96%	NR
Costa et al, 2021[323]	D-KRd	II	123	42	N/A	N/A	N/A	2-y 87%	2-y 94%
Niesvizky et al, 2008[267]	BiRD	II	40	25	18	53	95	2-y 75%	NA
Gosh et al, 2011[324]	VT	II	27	10	20	43	73	17 mo	3-y 74%
Reeder et al, 2009[234]	CyBorD	II	33	39[a]	22	17	88	NA	NA
Reeder et al, 2010[235]	mCyBorD	II	30	43[a]	17	33	93	NA	NA
Kumar et al, 2012[325]	VCD	II	33	22	19	34	75	1-y 93%	1-y 100%
Kumar et al, 2012[325]	mVCD	II	17	47	6	47	100	1-y 100%	1-y 100%
Bensiger et al, 2010[326]	VCD + VTD	II	42	45	12	38	95	1-y 81%	1-y 91%
Kumar et al, 2011[327]	CRD	II	53	13	34	38	85	28 mo	2-y 87%
Jakubowiak et al, 2012[238]	KRd	I/II	53	42	39	17	98	1-y 97%	NA
Dytfeld et al, 2014[295]	KRd	I/II	24	79	8	13	100	3-y 80%	3-y 100%
Sonneveld et al, 2015[328]	KTd	II	91	25	43	NA	NA	3-y 72%	NA
Kumar et al, 2012[325]	VDRC	II	48	25	33	30	88	1-y 86%	1-y 92%
Mikhael et al, 2015[329]	CYKLONE	Ib/II	64	8	51	22	91	2-y 76%	2-y 96%
Berenson et al, 2011[330]	VDD	II	35	20	9	43	72	NA	NA
Hussein et al, 2006[331]	DVd-T	II	55	36	13	34	83	28 mo	NA
Offidani et al, 2006[332]	ThaDD	II	50	34	24	30	88	3-y 57%	3-y 74%
Zervas et al, 2004[333]	T-DVD	II	39	10	0	64	74	1-y 70%	1-y 80%
Jaubowiak et al, 2011[334]	RVDD	I/II	72	44	23	29	96	2-y 70%	2-y 75%

Abbreviations: BiRD, biaxin, lenalidomide, and dexamethasone; bortez, bortezomib; CarRd, carfilzomib, lenalidomide, and dexamethasone; CRD, cyclophosphamide, lenalidomide, and dexamethasone; CR, complete response; CyBorD, cyclophosphamide, bortezomib, and dexamethasone; CYKLONE, cyclophosphamide, carfilzomib, thalidomide, dexamethasone; Dex, dexamethasone; EFS, event-free survival; KTd, carfilzomib, thalidomide, dexamethasone; KRd, carfilzomib, lenalidomide, and dexamethasone; LD-PAD, low-dose PAD; mCyBorD, modified CyBoD; MDT, MD and thalidomide; MPR, melphalan, prednisone, and lenalidomide; mVCD, modified VCD; N, number of patients; NA, not available; ORR, overall response rate; OS, overall survival; PAD, bortezomib, doxorubicin, and dexamethasone; PFS, progression-free survival; PR, partial response; RVDD, lenalidomide, bortezomib, doxorubicin, and dexamethasone; T-DVd, thalidomide, pegylated doxorubicin, vincristine, and dexamethasone; ThaDD, thalidomide, pegylated doxorubicin, and dexamethasone; thal, thalidomide; VCD, bortezomib, cyclophosphamide, and dexamethasone; VDD, bortezomib, doxorubicin, and dexamethasone; VDRC, bortezomib, dexamethasone, lenalidomide, and cyclophosphamide; VDT, bortezomib, pegylated liposomal doxorubicin, and thalidomide; VGPR, very good partial response; VMP, MP and bortezomib; VRD, bortezomib, lenalidomide, and dexamethasone; VT, bortezomib and thalidomide.
[a]Includes nCR as well as CR.

Table 100.7. Outcomes for Induction Regimens Among Patients Destined for ASCT, Randomized Controlled Trial

Reference	Regimen[a]	N	Postinduction Response, % Overall	Postinduction Response, % VGPR (CR)	Post-ASCT/Maintenance Response, % Overall	Post-ASCT/Maintenance Response, % VGPR (CR)	Median PFS/EFS	OS
CASSIOPEIA[337]	DVTd	543	93	65 (14)	93	83 (54)	18-mo 93%	Median: NR
	VTd	542	90	56 (9)	90	78 (39)	18-mo 85%	Median: NR
FORTE[338]	KRd	158	93[f]	70 (8)	97	82 (54)	4-y: 69%	Median: NR
	KCd	159	85	53 (6)	87	66 (42)	4-y: 51%	Median: NR
GRIFFIN[322]	DVRd	104	98	72 (19)	98	77 (70)	24-mo 96%	Median: NR
	VRd	103	92	57 (13)	92	66 (61)	24-mo 90%	Median: NR
IFM 2009[289]	VRD-ASCT-VRD -R	350	NA	47	97	88 (59)[c]	50 mo[c]	4-y 81%
	VRD-R	350	NA	45	97	77 (48)[c]	36 mo[c]	4-y 82%
GIMEMA-MMY-3006[339]	VTD + VTD/	236	93[c]	62 (19)[c]	96	89 (58)[c]	3-y 68%[c]	3-y 86%
	DTD + TD/D	238	79[c]	28 (5)[c]	89	74 (4)[c]	3-y 56%[c]	3-y 84%
HOVON-65/GMMG-HD4[340]	VAD + IFN	414	54[c]	14 (2)[c]	83[c]	56 (24)[c]	28 mo	5-y 55%[c]
	PAD + Velcade	413	78[c]	42 (7)[c]	90[c]	76 (36)[c]	35 mo	5-y 61%[c]
PETHEMA/GEM05MEN0S65[341]	VTD	130	85	60 (35)[c]	NA	NA (46)[c]	56 mo[c]	4-y 74%
	TD	127	62	29 (14)[c]	NA	NA (24)[c]	28 mo[c]	4-y 65%
	VBMCP/BVAD/B	129	75	36 (21)[c]	NA	NA (38)[c]	35 mo[c]	4-y 70%
IFM 2007-02[342]	VD	99	81	36[c] (12)	86	58[c] (31)	30 mo	No Difference
	vtD	100	88	49[c] (13)	89	74[c] (29)	26 mo	
IFM2013-04 (2016)[343]	VTD	170	92[c]	66[c] (13)	NA	NA	NA	NA
	VCD	170	83[c]	56[c] (9)	NA	NA	NA	NA
Mai et al, 2015[250]	PAD	251	72	34 (4)	NA	NA	NA	NA
	VCD	251	78	37 (8)	NA	NA	NA	NA
MRC IX[234,281]	CVAD + Thal or P	556	71	27 (8)	90[d]	62 (37)[d]	25 mo	81 mo
	CTD + Thal or P	555	82	43 (13)	92[d]	74 (50)[d]	27 mo	98 mo
Ludwig[346,345]	VTDC	49	100	69 (24)	NA	NA	5-y 48%	5-y 69%
	VTD	49	96	69 (23)	NA	NA	5-y 29%	5-y 65%
HOVON-50[346]	VAD + IFN	268	57[c]	18[c] (2)	79[c]	54 (23)[c]	25 mo[c]	60 mo
	TAD + Thal	268	71[c]	37[c] (3)	88[c]	66 (31)[c]	34 mo[c]	73 mo
E1A00[248,e]	TD	99	63[c]	NA (4)	NA	NA	NA	1-y 82%
	D	104	41[c]	NA (0)	NA	NA	NA	1-y 82%
E4A03[230,e]	Rd	208	70[c]	26[c] (4)	NA	NA	25 mo[c]	2-y 87%
	RD	214	81[c]	33[c] (5)	NA	NA	19 mo[c]	2-y 75%
S0232[321,e]	RD	97	78[c]	63 (26)[c]	NA	NA	3-y 52%[c]	3-y 79%
	D	95	48[c]	16 (4)[c]	NA	NA	3-y 32%[c]	3-y 73%
IFM 2005-1[319]	VAD + DCEP	121	63[c]	15 (6)[c]	79	37 (18)[c]	30 mo	3-y 77%
	BD + DCEP	121	79[c]	38 (15)[c]	84	54 (35)[c]	36 mo	3 y 81%
MAG/Macro[347]	VAD	104	NA	7 (NA)	NA	42 (NA)	NA	NA
	Thal-Dex	100	NA	25 (NA)	NA	44 (NA)	NA	NA
Rifkin et al, 2006[336,e]	DVd	97	44	NA (3)	NA	NA	2-y 53%	2-y 79%
	VAd	95	41	NA (0)	NA	NA	2-y 56%	2-y 72%
Dimopoulos et al, 2003[335,e]	DVD	132	61	NA (13)	NA	NA	2-y 49%	2-y 60%
	VAD	127	62	NA (13)	NA	NA	2-y 49%	2-y 68%
German MM study Group[347]	None	213	30	NA (1)	79	NA (9)	20 mo	56 mo
	VAD	207	48	NA (0)	78	NA (6)	21 mo	53 mo
Barlogie et al, 2006[348]	TT2 no thal[b]	323	40	(10)	78	(43)[c]	5-y[c] 44%	5-y 63%
	TT2 + thal[b]	345	60	(19)	86	(62)[c]	5-y[c] 56%	5-y 64%

Abbreviations: ASCT, autologous hematopoietic stem cell transplantation; BD, bortezomib-dexamethasone; CVAD, cyclophosphamide, vincristine, doxorubicin, and dexamethasone; DVd, daratumumab, bortezomib, and dexamethasone; DVD, doxil-vincristine-dexamethasone; OS, overall survival; PAD, bortezomib, doxorubicin, and dexamethasone; PFS/OFS, progression-free survival or event-free survival; Rd, lenalidomide and dexamethasone; TAD, thalidomide, adriamycin, and dexamethasone; TT2, total therapy 2; VAD, vincristine, doxorubicin, dexamethasone; VBMCP, vincristine-carmustine-melphalan-cyclophosphamide-prednisone; VCD, bortezomib, cyclophosphamide, and dexamethasone; VRD, bortezomib, lenalidomide, and dexamethasone; VTD, bortezomib-thalidomide-dexamethasone.

[a]Regimens listed as "induction" + "consolidation/maintenance."
[b]The basis of TT2 is a complex 6- or 7-drug induction followed by two autologous stem cell transplants, followed by two cycles of 5-drug consolidation, indefinite interferon maintenance, and 1 year of dexamethasone.
[c]Statistically significant difference between arms.
[d]Maintenance not included in response, though patients were randomized to thalidomide or prednisone.
[e]ASCT was not a predetermined part of these trials, so data include both patients who did and did not undergo ASCT.
[f]Includes an additional 157 patients who received KRd induction without ASCT.

drug regimen, VTD or TD, as consolidation therapy. All patients were subsequently maintained on dexamethasone 40 mg days 1 to 4 every 28 days. After induction therapy, higher rates of CR or near-complete response (nCR) were observed in the VTD arm as compared to TD (31% vs 11%, $P < .0001$). These improved response rates persisted after first and second ASCT and after two cycles of consolidation. A 3-year PFS was better in the VTD group (68% vs 56%, $P = .006$), but with a median follow-up of 36 months, the estimated 3-year OS rates were no different. Grade 3 or 4 AEs postinduction were recorded in a significantly higher number of patients on VTD than in those on TD (56% vs 33%, $P < .0001$), with a higher occurrence of grade 3 to 4 peripheral neuropathy in patients on VTD (10% vs 2%, $P = .0004$). A subsequent per protocol analysis, which included only those patients who made it to consolidation (68%), showed a better 3-year PFS from consolidation using the triplet (60% vs 48%).[219] A subanalysis was performed to characterize treatment-emergent peripheral neuropathy.[352] The incidence of grade ≥2 peripheral neuropathy was 35% in the VTD arm and 10% in the TD arm ($P < .001$). Peripheral neuropathy resolved in 88% and 95% of patients in VTD and TD groups, respectively. GEP analysis suggested an interaction between MM genetic profiles and development of VTD-induced peripheral neuropathy.

The Spanish Myeloma Group conducted a trial to compare VTD vs TD vs vincristine-BCNU-melphalan-cyclophosphamide-prednisone alternating with vincristine-BCNU-doxorubicin-dexamethasone plus bortezomib (VBMCP/VBAD/B) in patients aged 65 years or younger with MM destined for ASCT.[341] Three hundred eighty-six patients were allocated. The CR rate was significantly higher with VTD than with TD (35% vs 14%, $P = .001$) or with VBMCP/VBAD/B (35% vs 21%, $P = .01$). The median PFS was significantly longer with VTD (56 vs 28 vs 35 months, $P = .01$). With a median follow-up of 35 months, the 4-year OS was 74% for VTD, 65% for TD, and 70% for VBMCP/VBAD/B ($P =$ nonsignificant).

The IFM 2007-2 trial[342] was a randomized trial to compare bortezomib-dexamethasone (VD) as induction ASCT to a combination consisting of reduced doses of bortezomib and thalidomide plus dexamethasone (vtD), the latter of which was comprised of four 3-week cycles of IV bortezomib 1 mg/m²/m² days 1, 4, 8, and 11 along with thalidomide 100 mg/d orally, and dexamethasone 40 mg days 1 to 4 (all cycles) and days 9 to 12 (cycles 1 and 2). In the case of less than PR after cycle 2, the dose of bortezomib was increased to 1.3 mg/m² and the dose of thalidomide to 200 mg/d. The VD patients received two drugs as the same schedule as vtD, but the dose of bortezomib was 1.3 mg. Patients receiving the three-drug regimen had similar ORRs and CR rates, but VGPR or better was more frequent in the vtD group. This same pattern was observed after a single ASCT. Of note, the number of stem cells collected was less in patients receiving the three-drug regimen. Subsequent post-ASCT consolidation and/or maintenance was at treating physician's discretion; more patients receiving VD received maintenance therapy. Despite these differences, there was no significant difference in PFS or OS with a median follow-up of 32 months. There were significantly higher rates of peripheral neuropathy among patients on the VD arm—overall 70% vs 53%, $P = .01$; and grade 3 in 11% vs 3%, $P = .03$. The authors concluded that vtD, including reduced doses of bortezomib and thalidomide, yields higher VGPR rates compared with VD and can be considered a new effective triplet combination before HDT/ASCT.

Cyclophosphamide, Bortezomib, and Dexamethasone. Another popular regimen that worked its way into use initially without any phase III data is the cyclophosphamide, bortezomib, and dexamethasone (CyBorD or VCD) regimen (*Table 100.6*).[232,233,325,326] It is a variation of VMP—that is bortezomib with an alkylator and a corticosteroid. More recently, two randomized trials using VCD have been conducted, the first showing lower CR rates as compared to VTD[343] and the second showing noninferiority and better tolerability as compared to bortezomib, doxorubicin, and dexamethasone (PAD).[340]

The IFM randomized 340 patients with NDMM to either VTD or VCD as induction before HDT and ASCT.[343] VTD treatment consisted of four 3-week cycles of 1.3 mg/m² bortezomib administered SQ on days 1, 4, 8, and 11; 40 mg dexamethasone on days 1 to 4 and 9 to 12; plus 100 mg/d thalidomide administered orally. Therapy with VCD was composed of four 3-week cycles of bortezomib and dexamethasone (Bd) at the same doses and schedules as for the VTD regimen plus 500 mg/m² cyclophosphamide administered orally on days 1, 8, and 15. After four cycles, 66% of the patients in the VTD arm achieved VGPR or better vs 56% in the VCD arm ($P = .05$) and PR or better 92% vs 83% ($P = .01$). Overall, more dose reductions were required of the thalidomide than of the cyclophosphamide. Hematologic toxicity was higher in the VCD arm, with significantly increased rates of grade 3 and 4 anemia, thrombocytopenia, and neutropenia, but the rate of peripheral neuropathy was significantly higher in the VTD arm (grades 2-4, 22% vs 13%, $P = .008$). The median number of CD34+ cells collected was also higher in the VTD arm (10.7 vs 9.2 × 10⁶ cells/kg).

As part of the German speaking myeloma Multicenter Group (GMMG) MM5 trial, either VCD or PAD was administered in a randomized fashion for three cycles to 504 transplant-eligible NDMM patients.[249] Response rates and VGPR rates were comparable (72% vs 78% and 34% vs 37%), but PAD was more toxic; there were significantly more grade 3 to 4 events in general (33% vs 24%), more myelosuppression (35% vs 11%), and thromboembolic events (2.8% vs 0.4%), and more grade 2 to 4 neuropathy (15% vs 8%). In patients with high-risk cytogenetics as defined by deletion 17p and/or translocation (4;14) and/or gain of 1q21, there was a higher rate of progressive disease in the PAD arm. Additionally, the trial evaluated an approach involving ASCT followed by a recommendation for a second (tandem) ASCT if not in a nCR, followed by two cycles of lenalidomide as consolidation, and then finally another randomization to either lenalidomide maintenance for 2 years or until achievement of a CR. In the latter group, lenalidomide maintenance was not started if the subjects had already achieved a CR post-ASCT consolidation.[353]

A randomized phase II study comparing bortezomib, dexamethasone, cyclophosphamide, and lenalidomide (VDCR), VRd, and two VCD regimens in 140 previously untreated patients was reported.[325] A maximum of eight 21-day cycles followed by maintenance bortezomib (1.3 mg/m² every other week for 24 weeks) was administered. The VCD patients received cyclophosphamide 500 mg/m² days 1 and 8, whereas the VCD-mod patients received cyclophosphamide 500 mg/m² days 1, 8, and 15. The VGPR or better (and CR) rates were 58% (25%), 51% (24%), 41% (22%), and 53% (47%) for patients on VDCR, VDR, VCD, and VCD-mod, respectively. The corresponding 1-year PFS was 86%, 83%, 93%, and 100%. Grade 3 or higher AEs were seen in 76% to 88% of patients, with the highest rate of AE resulting in discontinuation in the VDCR arm. The highest rate of grade 3/4 hematologic AEs was in the VDCR and the VCD arms. Grade 3/4 peripheral neuropathy rates ranged from 9% to 18%. The two regimens recommended by the authors were VCD-mod and VRD.

Carfilzomib, Lenalidomide, and Dexamethasone. KRd has been used in the upfront setting with excellent response rates.[238] Most patients did not require dose modifications. Thirty-five patients underwent stem cell collection after cycle 4, and seven proceeded to early transplant. After a median of 12 cycles (range, 1-25), 62% achieved at least nCR and 42% stringent CR. With a median follow-up of 13 months, 24-month PFS estimate was 92%. Grade 3/4 toxicities included hypophosphatemia (25%), hyperglycemia (23%), anemia (21%), thrombocytopenia (17%), and neutropenia (17%); peripheral neuropathy was limited to grade 1/2 (23%). As discussed before, KRd did not emerge as a superior regimen to VRd in the ENDURANCE phase III trial (NCT01863550) that enrolled patients with standard risk disease or t(4;14).[270]

The FORTE trial involved the comparison of three approaches using the carfilzomib and dexamethasone (Kd) backbone in the frontline setting ($n = 474$).[338] This two-part, three-arm, phase 2 trial evaluated the comparative safety and efficacy of the combination of carfilzomib, cyclophosphamide, and dexamethasone (KCd, $n = 159$) induction therapy (four cycles), followed by ASCT, followed by four additional cycles of KCd consolidation (KCd-ASCT-KCd), KRd ($n = 158$), four-cycle induction therapy, followed by ASCT, followed by four additional cycles of KRd consolidation (KRd-ASCT-KRd) vs 12 cycles of KRd induction without ASCT (KRd12, $n = 157$). After a median follow-up of 51 months, 222 (70%) of 315 patients in the KRd (+/−ASCT) group and 84 (53%) of 159 patients in the KCd group had achieved the study coprimary endpoint of postinduction VGPR or better response rate (OR 2.14, 95% CI 1.44-3.19, P = .0002), indicating the superior efficacy of PI-IMid combination over PI-alkylator, albeit at a cost of higher nonhematologic toxicity. The median PFS was also superior for KRd-ASCT vs KCd-ASCT (NR vs 53 months; HR, 0.53; P < .001) and significantly longer for KRd-ASCT vs KRd12 (NR vs 57 months; HR, 0.64; P = .023) underscoring the additive value of ASCT even when utilized in the context of novel IMiD-PI–based induction/consolidation therapies. An additional important observation was the lack of any significant PFS difference between KRd12 and KCd-ASCT (HR, 0.82; P = .262). The 3-year OS rates for both KRd-ASCT and KRd12 were similar so far at 90% vs 83% for KCd. Although the postconsolidation (premaintenance) MRD-negative (sensitivity 10^{-5}) rates were similar to KRd plus ASCT (62%) and KRd12 (56%) but higher than with KCd plus ASCT (43%), the rate of sustained MRD negativity at 1 year was superior with KRd plus ASCT vs KRd12 (47% vs 35%, respectively; HR 1.69 [1.07-2.66], P = .024). The rate of sustained MRD negativity at 1 year for KCd plus ASCT was only 25%.

For the second part of the trial, 356 patients were randomly assigned to carfilzomib plus lenalidomide (n = 178) or lenalidomide alone (n = 178) as maintenance therapy following consolidation. While lenalidomide was given until progression or intolerable toxicity in both the arms, carfilzomib was administered every 2 weeks for up to 2 years. After a median follow-up interval of 37 months from the second randomization, the 3-year PFS rates were 75% with carfilzomib plus lenalidomide vs 65% with lenalidomide alone (HR 0.64 [95% CI 0.44-0.94], P = .023). Maintenance with the doublet appeared to be advantageous across both the high-risk and the standard-risk subsets. However, the 3-year OS is similar (94% with carfilzomib plus lenalidomide vs 90% with lenalidomide alone) thus far and the quality-of-life data are lacking.

In a subsequent analysis, among patients in the high-risk group, defined as the presence of del17p, t(4;14), t(14;16), del1p, and 1q gain (3 copies) or amp1q (≥4 copies), KRd-ASCT resulted in improved PFS rates in comparison to KRd12 (HR 0.6; P = .04) as well as KCd-SCT (HR, 0.57; P = .01) with corresponding to 4-year PFS rates of 62%, 45%, and 45%.[354] By contrast, the respective 4-year PFS rates among the standard risk patients were 80%, 67%, and 57%, respectively. Although the analyses by single cytogenetic abnormalities were hindered by the small sample sizes of the subgroups, a trend toward a PFS benefit from observed with KRd-ASCT vs KRd12 among groups with del17p (HR 0.61, P = .3), t(4;14) (HR 0.59, P = .2), and 1q gain (HR 0.45, P = .02). Patients with amp1q had the worst outcome, irrespective of the treatment assigned, suggesting that even KRd plus ASCT approach was inadequate in overcoming the poor prognostic impact of amp1q.

Ixazomib, Lenalidomide, and Dexamethasone. Ixazomib is the first oral proteasome inhibitor to enter the clinic and has been combined with lenalidomide.[353] In a phase II trial, 66 patients with NDMM were treated with oral ixazomib (escalation doses of 1.68-3.95 mg/m² days 1, 8, and 15) plus lenalidomide 25 mg (days 1-21) and dexamethasone 40 mg (days 1, 8, 15, and 22) for up to 12 28-day cycles, followed by maintenance therapy with ixazomib alone. The recommended phase II dose was 2.23 mg/m², which was converted to 4.0 mg fixed dose based on population pharmacokinetic results. In four response-evaluable patients, the ORR was 92%, including a VGPR or better in 58%. Common grade 3 or higher AEs were reported in 63%, including skin and SQ tissue disorders, neutropenia, and thrombocytopenia; grade 3 or higher drug-related peripheral neuropathy occurred in 6%.

Carfilzomib, Thalidomide, and Dexamethasone. Carfilzomib, thalidomide, and dexamethasone (KTd) is an interesting regimen that has only phase II data at present. The European Myeloma Network investigated the KTd combination as induction/consolidation therapy in 91 transplant-eligible patients with previously untreated MM as part of a phase II trial.[328] During KTd induction therapy, patients received four cycles of carfilzomib 20/27 mg/m² (n = 50), 20/36 mg/m² (n = 20), 20/45 mg/m² (n = 21), or 20/56 mg/m² (n = 20) on days 1, 2, 8, 9, 15, and 16 of a 28-day cycle; thalidomide 200 mg on days 1 to 28; and dexamethasone 20 mg on days 1, 2, 8, 9, 15, and 16. After ASCT, patients proceeded to KTd consolidation therapy, where the target doses of carfilzomib were 27, 36, 45, or 56 mg/m², respectively, and thalidomide 50 mg. Common grade 3/4 AEs included respiratory (15%), gastrointestinal (12%), and skin disorders (10%); polyneuropathy was infrequent (1%). CR rates after induction and consolidation treatment were 25% and 63%, respectively; rates of VGPR or better after induction and consolidation were 68% and 89%, respectively. At a median follow-up of 23 months, the 36-month PFS rate was 72%.

Bortezomib, Doxorubicin, and Dexamethasone. The Dutch-Belgian Hemato-Oncology Cooperative Group (HOVON-65) trial randomized 827 patients to 3 weeks of initial therapy with either VAD or PAD, followed by one or two ASCT.[340] Post-ASCT maintenance for the VAD group was thalidomide 50 mg daily and for the PAD group bortezomib 1.3 mg/m² once every 2 weeks. Maintenance was continued for 2 years. After completing induction therapy with PAD, 31% of patients had achieved a CR in contrast to 15% of VAD patients. This improved CR rate persisted even after one or two ASCTs. PFS was superior in the PAD-bortezomib maintenance arm as compared to the VAD-thalidomide arm (35 vs 28 months). After a median follow-up of 66 months, OS was also better in the PAD arm, 5-year OS of 61% vs 55% (P = .05), when adjusted for risk factors (age, performance status, ISS, double ASCT, and FISH abnormalities). In an update with follow-up of 8 years, the 5-year OS were 65% and 59% with an 8-year OS of 48% and 45%.[224] At second line, more VAD patients received bortezomib (60% vs 33%), and fewer of the VAD patients received lenalidomide (51% vs 71%). Peripheral neuropathy grades 2 to 4 were reported in 18% of VAD patients vs 40% of PAD patients (P < .001).[340] The discontinuation rate of thalidomide maintenance was higher than that with bortezomib maintenance (30% vs 11%, P < .001). An important observation made in this trial is that the use of bortezomib both pre- and post-ASCT appeared to attenuate the poor prognostic impact of deletion 17p, and this advantage persisted over time.[220,224] A challenge in interpreting this trial is knowing whether the induction, the maintenance, or merely access to bortezomib was the value-added step, in terms of the PFS and OS benefits seen in this trial.

Cyclophosphamide, Thalidomide, and Dexamethasone. In the MRC IX trial (transplant pathway), 1111 patients were randomized either to oral cyclophosphamide-thalidomide-dexamethasone (CTD) or to infusional cyclophosphamide, vincristine, doxorubicin, and dexamethasone (CVAD).[234,281] As many as six cycles were given prior to ASCT. The postinduction ORR was significantly higher with CTD than with CVAD (82.5% vs 71.2%, P < .0001), including superior CR rates (13.0% vs 8.1%, P = .008). This response advantage persisted post-ASCT (CR, 50.0% vs 37.2%, respectively; P = .00052). Patients had a secondary randomization to either maintenance thalidomide or prednisone. With a median follow-up of 71 months, there was no difference in either PFS or OS. FISH risk had no impact on outcome.

Thalidomide, Doxorubicin, and Dexamethasone. The HOVON 50/GMMG-HD3 trial is a phase III study randomized 536 patients up to 65 years[346] to either three cycles of TAD (thalidomide, 200 mg for HOVON and 400 mg for GMMG; adriamycin 9 mg/m², days 1-4; and dexamethasone 40 mg, days 1-4, 9-12, and 17-21) or VAD. TAD resulted in more grade 2 to 4 AEs as compared with the VAD arm (31% vs 21%, P = .008). The TAD had superior ORRs pre- and post-ASCT, but with a median follow-up of 52 months, there was no significant difference in median OS (73 vs 60 months, P = .77). Patients who had been randomized to thalidomide arm had a markedly shorter survival post relapse.

Quadruplets

Daratumumab, Bortezomib, Lenalidomide, and Dexamethasone. The GRIFFIN trial was a randomized phase 2 study conducted in transplant-eligible patients with MM ages 18 to 70 years.[324] It comprised of an initial safety run-in phase that demonstrated both safety and tolerability of adding subcutaneous daratumumab to bortezomib, lenalidomide and dexamethasone (D-RVd). The phase 2 portion of the study randomized patients to receive four pretransplant induction and two posttransplant consolidation cycles of lenalidomide, bortezomib, and dexamethasone (RVd) alone, or in combination with daratumumab (D-RVd) in a 1:1 ratio. All patients received subsequent lenalidomide maintenance after posttransplant consolidation until disease progression, but the D-RVd group also received daratumumab every 4 weeks as part of maintenance therapy.

In updated results after 24 months of maintenance therapy, among the intent-to-treat population, MRD-negativity (10^{-5}) rates were higher for D-RVd (64% vs 30%, $P < .0001$).[356] With 38.6 months follow-up, median PFS was not reached in either arm but trended toward favoring D-RVd vs RVd (HR, 0.46; 95% CI, 0.21-1.01). The estimated 36-month PFS rate was 88.9% for D-RVd and 81.2% for RVd. There was more grade 3 or higher cytopenias with D-RVd than with RVd. While there were more infections of any grade in the D-RVd group (91% vs 62%), these were due to more grade 1/2 upper respiratory tract infections in the D-RVd group since the incidence of grade 3/4 infections was similar between the two groups (23% vs 22%). A phase III trial comparing these two regimens is ongoing currently in Europe and Australia.

Daratumumab, Bortezomib, Thalidomide, and Dexamethasone. The CASSIOPEIA trial is a two-part, phase 3 study conducted in the transplant-eligible patients. In Part 1 of the study, 1085 patients with newly diagnosed MM were randomly assigned to receive four pretransplant induction and two posttransplant consolidation cycles of bortezomib, thalidomide, and dexamethasone (VTd) alone (considered a standard of care in Europe), or in combination with daratumumab (D-VTd).[337] Both the response depth and PFS improved with the frontline quadruplet, culminating in its regulatory approval.

With an extended follow-up, the favorable impact of using an upfront quadruplet was evident on OS as well (*Table 100.7*), supporting the use of daratumumab as induction and consolidation for patients undergoing ASCT. However, whether the use of daratumumab as primary therapy translates to improved OS in comparison to reserving it for use as the first salvage therapy on disease progression remains unknown. Besides the infusion reactions, the DVTd group most frequently encountered the adverse effects of neutropenia, lymphopenia, thrombocytopenia, sensory neuropathy, constipation, asthenia, nausea, pyrexia, stomatitis, and peripheral edema. The applicability of these results to current practice in the United States appears to be limited because thalidomide use has declined considerably, yielding to more effective and better-tolerated lenalidomide regimens.

The Part 2 evaluated the impact of daratumumab maintenance following consolidation and is discussed separately.

Elotuzumab, Bortezomib, Lenalidomide, and Dexamethasone. The GMMG trial, HD6 (NCT02495922), a randomized phase 3, four-arm trial investigated the effect of adding elotuzumab to VRD induction/post-ASCT consolidation and lenalidomide maintenance, specifically to examine whether there is advantage to using elotuzumab for the transplant-eligible patients with newly diagnosed myeloma. Like the preceding ELOQUENT 1 and SWOG1211 studies that examined the impact of integrating elotuzumab in the nontransplant and high-risk newly diagnosed patient populations, respectively, the HD6 trial could not show a benefit of a monoclonal antibody targeting SLAMF7 in the frontline setting.[357]

Carfilzomib, Thalidomide, Cyclophosphamide, and Dexamethasone. Investigators from the Mayo Clinic tested KTd plus cyclophosphamide, which they called CYKLONE, as part of a phase Ib/II trial.[329] They treated 64 transplant-eligible patients with NDMM with carfilzomib (days 1, 2, 8, 9, 15, and 16), 300 mg/m^2 cyclophosphamide (days 1, 8, and 15), 100 mg thalidomide (days 1-28), and 40 mg dexamethasone (days 1, 8, 15, and 22) in 28-day cycles. Carfilzomib was dose escalated to 15/20, 20/27, 20/36, and 20/45 mg/m^2 to determine the maximum tolerated dose (MTD), which was 20/36 mg/m^2. Regardless of attribution, common grade 3 or higher AEs were lymphopenia (38%), neutropenia (23%), and anemia (20%). All peripheral neuropathy (31%) was grade 1 and considered most likely to be thalidomide related. Common cardiac or pulmonary events of any grade in ≥5% of patients included dyspnea (20%) and cough (6%). Overall ($N = 64$), 91% of patients achieved a best response of PR or better across all cycles of treatment, including five patients with CRs. At the MTD, 59% of patients achieved a VGPR or better after four cycles. Stem cell collection was successful in all 42 patients in whom it was attempted. With a median follow-up of 17 months, the PFS and OS at 24 months were 76% and 96%, respectively.

VAD-like Regimens. Incorporating different corticosteroids[358-360] and C-VAMP (cyclophosphamide-vincristine-doxorubicin-methylprednisolone)[360] had commonly been used as induction therapy before stem cell collection and transplantation, but have been largely replaced by regimens incorporating IMiDs and/or proteasome inhibitors. These VAD-like regimens had initially been piloted with salutary effect in relapsed disease and were subsequently applied in previously untreated patients with response rates 50% to 84%. Median survival for patients treated initially with VAD and no transplant was about 36 months.[361] The CR rate of C-VAMP was higher than that of VAMP alone, but survival was not different.[362] Response rates of 80% have also been achieved using the CAD (cyclophosphamide-doxorubicin-dexamethasone) regimen.[363] The addition of etoposide to CVAD appears to contribute only toxicity.[364]

By the late 1990s and early 2000s, single-agent high-dose dexamethasone was used by some experts in lieu of VAD for induction in those patients destined for stem cell collection based on a nearly comparable response rate of single-agent high-dose dexamethasone of 43%[365] and the advantage of an oral, noninfusional therapy. This strategy was used successfully, resulting in adequate collections of peripheral blood stem cells without any apparent adverse effects on complete remission rates or PFS in several single-arm studies.[366,367] With the advent of additional therapies, single-agent dexamethasone is no longer a standard induction option.

In an attempt to avoid the continuous infusion required to administer VAD, the use of the pegylated liposomal doxorubicin has been explored in two randomized trials. Doxil-vincristine-dexamethasone (DVD)—using either standard high-dose dexamethasone[335] or attenuated doses of dexamethasone[336]—was compared to VAD. Results were comparable between arms with regard to response rates, 42% in the attenuated dexamethasone trial[336] and 61% with the standard-dose dexamethasone trial.[335] PFS and OS were comparable, but there was more alopecia, grade 3/4 neutropenia in the nonliposomal doxorubicin arms and more palmar-plantar erythrodysesthesia in liposomal doxorubicin arms.

Other Induction Regimens of Interest

Table 100.7 includes a number of regimens that have been reported in the upfront setting.[232,233,238,266,295,324-326,329-334]

Two regimens exclude corticosteroids, VT (bortezomib and thalidomide)[324] and VDT (bortezomib, pegylated liposomal doxorubicin, and thalidomide).[368] The VT study treated 27 patients with bortezomib 1.3 mg/m^2 on days 1, 4, 8, and 11 every 21 days and thalidomide 150 mg/d for a maximum of eight cycles.[324] The ORR was 81.5% with 25.8% nCR or greater. The most common grade 3 toxicities were peripheral neuropathy (22%), pneumonia (15%), fatigue (7%), and anemia (7%). No venous thromboembolic events were observed even in the absence of prophylactic anticoagulation. Forty-three NDMM patients were enrolled on to the VDT study.[368] The ORR and CR + nCR rates were 78% and 35%, respectively. Median TTP was 29.5 months. Fatigue, rash, neuropathy, constipation, and infections were the most common side effects.[368]

Kumar et al built on the Rd experience by adding cyclophosphamide.[327] Eighty-five percent of patients responded, and the toxicities were manageable with over 80% of planned doses delivered; six patients went off-study for toxicity. The median PFS for the entire group was 28 months (95% CI: 22.7-32.6), and the OS at 2 years was 87% (95% CI: 78-96). Importantly, 14 patients with high-risk MM had similar PFS and OS as the standard-risk patients ($n = 39$).

Lenalidomide, bortezomib, pegylated doxorubicin, and dexamethasone was tested in a phase I/II trial including 72 patients.[334]

The MTD was 3-week cycles of lenalidomide 25 mg/m² days 1 to 14, bortezomib 1.3 mg/m² days 1, 4, 8, and 11, PLD 30 mg/m² day 4, and dexamethasone 20 mg days 1, 2, 4, 5, 8, 9, 11, and 12 (cycles 1-4, but 10 mg for cycles 5-8). The maximum number of treatment cycles was eight, and patients who did not go to ASCT were to receive maintenance, which included lenalidomide, bortezomib, and dexamethasone indefinitely. The median treatment duration was 4.5 cycles, and 15% of patients achieved stringent CR. Grade 3/4 AEs included neutropenia (19.4%), infections (14%), thrombocytopenia (11%), sensory peripheral neuropathy (6%), and thromboembolism in 3%. All grade fatigue, constipation, sensory neuropathy, and infection occurred in 83%, 69%, 65%, and 57%, respectively. The 18-month PFS for patients proceeding and not proceeding to ASCT was 93% and 64%, respectively. Although the decision of proceeding to ASCT was nonrandomized, there was a significant difference in PFS between the groups. With a median follow-up of 15 months, the 2-year OS for all patients was approximately 75%.

There are three phase II reports of adding thalidomide to PLD and dexamethasone with[331,369] or without vincristine.[370] Response rates were comparable. In the ThaDD trial that did not include vincristine, grade 3 to 4 infections and thromboembolic accidents were observed in 22% and 14% of patients, respectively.[332] In the DVd-T and T-DVD trials, grade 3 to 4 toxicities included neutropenia (14%-15%), thrombosis (10%-25%), pneumonia (12%), constipation (10%), rash (5%-8%), and peripheral neuropathy (5%-22%). It is notable that although the ThaDD cohort[370] was older and received lower doses of the thalidomide and no vincristine, similar response rates and less toxicity were seen.

Hematopoietic Stem Cell Transplantation
Autologous Transplant

To overcome resistance of the MM cells to conventional-dose chemotherapy, McElwain and Powles[197] pioneered the use of high-dose melphalan to treat MM and PCL. The treatment was complicated by prolonged myelosuppression. Barlogie et al[371] subsequently used a regimen combining high-dose melphalan with total body irradiation (TBI) supported by autologous bone marrow transplantation in MM patients refractory to VAD. Ten years hence, Attal et al published the first prospective randomized controlled trial, demonstrating an improved OS for patients undergoing HDT with autologous stem cell support compared to conventional chemotherapy.[211]

By the end of the 20th century, it was accepted that a strategy of early vs delayed transplant was equally effective in terms of OS if alkylator, anthracycline, and steroid combinations were used as induction and as part of the comparator arm, but with the advent of IMiDs and proteasome inhibitors, this question is being readdressed. Data are emerging that ASCT is especially important among patients with high-risk FISH.[371]

In contrast to the experience with malignant lymphoma, SCT appears to be useful for patients with primary resistant disease in the case of induction with alkylator-based regimens, VAD, thalidomide/dexamethasone, or lenalidomide/dexamethasone.[372-376] Indeed, patients who have refractory disease do worse than their highly responsive counterparts in terms of PFS (22.1 vs 13.1 months) and OS (73.5 vs 30.4 months).[376] In a creative retrospective study performed by the Center for International Blood and Marrow Transplant Registry (CIBMTR), it was shown that there was no apparent survival benefit if induction strategies were changed prior to ASCT.[377] In contrast, the Myeloma XI trial addressed this question in a prospective randomized fashion after cyclophosphamide, lenalidomide, and dexamethasone (CRd) induction by providing additional cycles of therapy consisting of bortezomib, cyclophosphamide, and dexamethasone to half of the patients achieving only an MR or PR after induction therapy, and found that while additional PI-based therapy deepened hematological response to a VGPR or better in 41% of evaluable patients as well as improved PFS (55 vs 30 months, $P = .0003$), this did not translate to an improved OS compared to patients who received no further therapy prior to proceeding to an ASCT.[378]

Hematopoietic Stem Cell Collection

Autologous peripheral blood SCT has replaced autologous bone marrow transplantation because engraftment is more rapid and there is less contamination with MM cells.[379-381] Prolonged melphalan exposure leads to an impaired harvest of peripheral blood stem cells when stem cells are mobilized with chemotherapy plus growth factors[382] or growth factors alone.[383] Data also suggest lenalidomide exposure may have adverse effects on the ability to collect stem cells.[384] This appears to be related to the duration of lenalidomide therapy as well as the age of the patient. For this reason, early mobilization of stem cells, preferably within the first four cycles of initial therapy, is now recommended.[385] Stem cell mobilization for MM patients is primarily performed using filgrastim granulocyte colony–stimulating factor alone or after cyclophosphamide chemotherapy. The target CD34+ cell dose to be collected as well as the number of apheresis performed vary by center, but a minimum of two million CD34+ cells/kg has been traditionally used for the support of one cycle of HDT.[386] In the setting of ASCT, CD34+ cell doses greater than three million/kg have been associated with better outcomes, primarily due to faster hematologic recovery and lower incidence of infectious and bleeding complications.[387,388] The use of plerixafor in conjunction with filgrastim has enhanced the ability to successfully mobilize the majority of patients undergoing ASCT. Plerixafor is a novel stem cell–mobilizing agent. It is a bicyclam molecule that inhibits the SDF-1α/CXCR4 binding that occurs between CD34+ stem cells and the marrow stroma. The inhibition of this interaction results in the release of CD34+ stem cells into the bloodstream, facilitating their collection through apheresis methods.[389]

Historically, all peripheral blood cell products have been shown to be contaminated with malignant cells.[390,391] Purging marrow with cyclophosphamide derivatives[390] or with monoclonal antibodies[393-395] is feasible although associated with prolonged myelosuppression after transplantation. Two phase III randomized trials have shown no clinical benefit to using CD34+ selected autologous peripheral blood stem cells.[396,397] Moreover, the risk of infection was higher in the CD34 selected group.[397]

Single Autologous Stem Cell Transplantation

Prior to the advent of IMiDs and proteasome inhibitor therapy, HDT followed by ASCT improved EFS and OS in three[211,398,399] of the seven published randomized controlled trials[400-404] (Table 100.8). Three of the four "negative" studies are largely "early" vs "delayed" transplant trials,[400-402] and the fourth "negative" study (the PETHEMA trial) excluded from their randomization those patients who did not respond to induction therapy.[403] In this era, response rates after ASCT were 75% to 90%, and CR rates were 20% to 40%.[211,398-403] In the positive studies, PFS was improved by approximately 10 to 12 months, median OS by approximately 12 months, and 7-year OS was doubled (Figure 100.8). There are now three published trials comparing ASCT to regimens including novel agents,[289,317,318] but only one—the IFM 2009 trial—that uses a proteasome, IMiD, corticosteroid triplet.[289]

As previously discussed, the IFM 2009 is one of the most important modern trials in that it addresses the question of early vs delayed ASCT in the VRd induction era.[289] As previously discussed, all patients were given induction with three cycles of VRD. Patients were then randomized to consolidation either with VRd for five additional cycles or with high-dose melphalan with ASCT followed by two additional cycles of VRD. Both groups received maintenance therapy with lenalidomide for 1 year. Nearly all patients responded to therapy. In all, 65% and 79% attained MRD-negative status (7-color flow cytometry; sensitivity of 10^{-4}). With a median follow-up of 44 months, the median PFS is 36 and 50 months, thus favoring ASCT consolidation ($P < .001$). A 4-year OS is 82% in both the arms. Seventy-nine percent of patients who progressed in the VRd-only consolidation arm (or 39% of all patients on that arm) had ASCT as salvage. There were significantly more early grade 3 to 4 AEs in the ASCT-only consolidation arm (95% vs 64%), most notably hematologic AEs (95% vs 64%), gastrointestinal AEs (28% vs 7%), and infections (20% vs 9%). There was no difference in the

Table 100.8. Nontransplant Approach vs Autologous Hematopoietic Stem Cell Transplantation as First-Line Therapy, Randomized Trials

		N	CR/VGPR, %	ORR, %	PFS, mo	OS, mo	SCT, %
IFM90[211,403]	CCT	200	13	57	18[a]	44[a]	9
	ASCT		38[a]	81[a]	28[a]	57[a]	74
MRC7[396]	CCT	401	8	46	20[a]	42[a]	15
	ASCT		44[a]	86[a]	32[a]	54[a]	75
MAG91[398]	CCT	190	4	56	19[a]	48	22
	ASCT		6	59	25[a]	48	75
MAG90[399]	CCT	185	57	58	13	64	78
	ASCT		20	78	39	65	98
PEETHMA[401]	CCT	164	11	83	33	61	18
	ASCT		30[a]	82	42	66	90
S921[400]	CCT	516	17	90	7-y 14%	7-y 38%	34
	ASCT		15	93	7-y 17%	7-y 38%	82
MMSG97[397,b]	CCT	194	6	66	16	42[a]	39
	ASCT		25[a]	72	28[a]	58+[a]	92
HOVON-24[402,b]	CCT	303	13	86	23[a]	50	NA
	ASCT		28[a]	90	24[a]	55	
Palumbo et al, 2014[315]	Rd + MPR ± R	273	18/45	91	22[a]	4-y 65%[a]	74
	Rd + ASCT × 2 ± R		23/36	93	43[a]	4-y 82%[a]	100
Gay et al, 2015[316]	Rd + CRD + R ± P	356	20/22	70	29[b,d]	73[b,d]	41
	Rd + ASCT × 2 + R ± P		32/40	87	43[b,d]	86[b,d]	100
IFM 2009[287]	VRD + R	700	48/29	97	36[c]	4-y 82%	92
	VRD + ASCT + R		59[a]/29	99[a]	50[a]	4-y 81%	39

Abbreviations: CR/VGPR, complete response or very good partial response; ORR, overall response rate; OS, overall survival; P, prednisone; PFS, progression-free survival; SCT, stem cell transplant.
[a]Significant.
[b]Transplant arm is two low-dose melphalan 100 mg/m² autologous stem cell transplants.
[c]Often included in "double-transplant" tables because both arms received melphalan 70 mg/m² × 2 without stem cell support as induction therapy.
[d]Includes only those patients eligible for consolidation—not intention-to-treat analysis.

incidence of second primary cancers between the groups (1.1 vs 1.5 cases per 100 patient-years, respectively). Five cases of acute myeloid leukemia occurred: four in the ASCT group and one in the VRd-only group. In the long-term analysis after a median follow-up of 93 months, the median PFS was 47.3 months after ASCT and 35 months with VRd alone (HR = 0.70; 95% CI = 0.59-0.83), with evidence of benefit across all subgroups benefited from transplant, including patients with high-risk cytogenetics. No discernible PFS2 or OS differences were observed so far, although the second PFS, defined as the time from date of first progression to progression on next line therapy or death, was markedly longer in the VRd group (36 vs 25 months in ASCT group (HR [95CI] 1.41 [1.11-1.79] $P = .003$). The undetectable MRD rate was 29.8% with transplant vs 20% with VRd ($P = .01$). Notably, nearly 23% of patients who had relapsed after VRd and required the first salvage regimen did not undergo delayed ASCT. After 8 years, comparable rates of second primary malignancies (SPMs) were noted, without any differences in the rates of second hematologic malignancies as well.[404]

In another study, Palumbo and colleagues[276] randomly assigned 273 patients aged 65 years or younger to high-dose melphalan plus ASCT for two cycles or MPR consolidation therapy after induction with four cycles of Rd followed by cyclophosphamide stem cell mobilization. A secondary randomization of 251 patients to lenalidomide maintenance therapy or no maintenance therapy was subsequently performed. The primary endpoint was PFS. The median follow-up period was 51.2 months. Both PFS and OS were significantly longer with high-dose melphalan plus SCT than with MPR (median PFS, 43.0 vs 22.4 months; HR for progression or death, 0.44; 95% CI: 0.32-0.61; $P < .001$; and 4-year OS, 81.6% vs 65.3%; HR for death, 0.55; 95% CI: 0.32-0.93; $P = .02$). The CR rate improved from 16% to 36% from after consolidation to after maintenance in the ASCT group and from 20% to 34% in the MPR group. Median PFS was significantly longer with lenalidomide maintenance than with no maintenance (41.9 vs 21.6 months; HR for progression or death, 0.47; 95% CI: 0.33-0.65; $P < .001$), but a 3-year OS was not significantly prolonged (88.0% vs 79.2%; HR for death, 0.64; 95% CI: 0.36-1.15; $P = .14$). Grade 3 or 4 neutropenia was significantly more frequent with high-dose melphalan than with MPR (94.3% vs 51.5%), as were gastrointestinal AEs (18.4% vs 0%) and infections (16.3% vs 0.8%); neutropenia and dermatologic toxic effects were more frequent with lenalidomide maintenance than with no maintenance (23.3% vs 0% and 4.3% vs 0%, respectively).

Gay et al[316] compared consolidation with high-dose melphalan plus ASCT vs CRd and maintenance with lenalidomide plus prednisone vs lenalidomide alone in 389 patients. In an open-label, multicenter phase III study, they enrolled transplant-eligible patients with NDMM aged 65 years or younger. Patients received a common induction with four 28-day cycles of Rd. All patients had chemotherapy mobilization attempted and were randomized patients to consolidation with either six cycles of CRd or two courses of high-dose melphalan and ASCT. A secondary randomization for maintenance was done: lenalidomide (10 mg, days 1-21) plus prednisone (50 mg, every other day) or lenalidomide alone. Median follow-up was 52.0 months. PFS during consolidation was significantly shorter with CRd than with high-dose melphalan and ASCT (median 28.6 vs 43.3 months; $P < .0001$). PFS did not differ between maintenance treatments (median 37.5 months with lenalidomide plus prednisone vs 28.5 months with lenalidomide alone; $P = .34$). Fewer grade 3 or 4 AEs were recorded with CRd than with high-dose melphalan and ASCT.

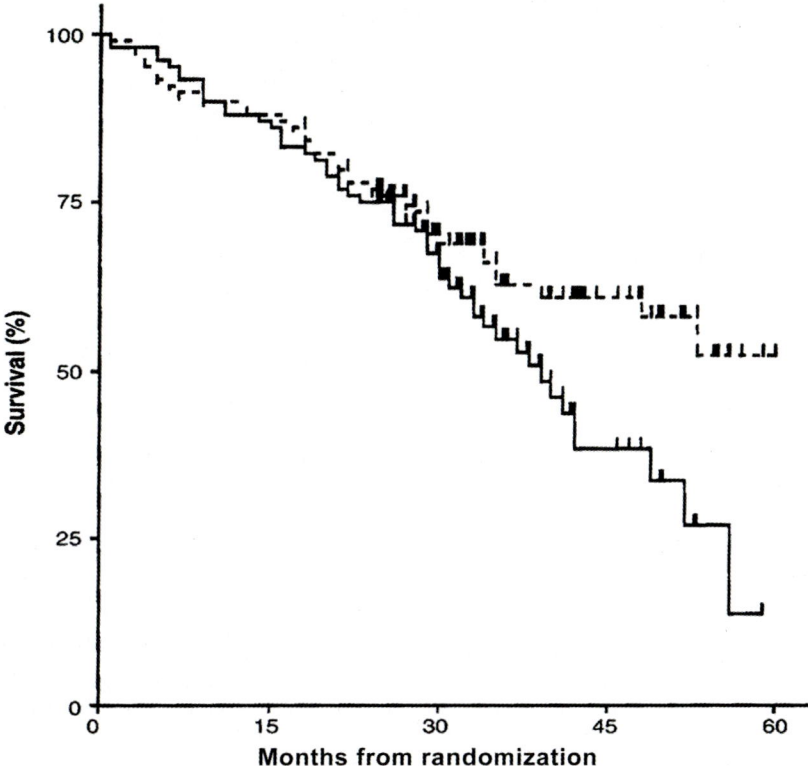

FIGURE 100.8 Conventional chemotherapy vs autologous hematopoietic stem cell transplantation (IFM 90 trial). (From Attal M, Harousseau JL, Stoppa AM, et al. A prospective, randomized trial of autologous bone marrow transplantation and chemotherapy in multiple myeloma. Intergroupe Français du Myélome. N Engl J Med. 1996;335(2):91-97. Copyright © 1996 Massachusetts Medical Society. Reprinted with permission from Massachusetts Medical Society.)

Single vs Double Transplantation

Because the evidence was mounting that one course of dose-intensified chemotherapy with ASCT was superior to conventional chemotherapy, investigators began experimenting with applying two consecutive ASCTs. The concept of double or tandem transplant was promulgated by Dr Barlogie and colleagues at the University of Arkansas.[249,347,405-409] These investigators reported high CR rates and survival. In the first report of "total therapy 1 (TT1)" that included 231 patients with NDMM, the OS with this approach was 68 months.[408] Their concept was not only to use two back-to-back ASCTs but also to use all therapies with activity against malignant plasma cells as early as possible with prolonged treatment courses. With successive tandem transplant trials—TT1, TT2, and total therapy 3 (TT3)—there were improvements in outcomes, including CR, PFS, and OS.[408] CR rates increased from 38% to 62% of patients, and 5-year OS rates have increased from 57% to 73%. Although other investigators had not previously reported duration of CR rates that approach those of TT3, since the 21st century, 5-year OS rates of 50% to 80% among transplant-eligible patients are increasingly common using less intensive and less toxic treatment strategies.[410,411]

It was the IFM group who were the first to perform a randomized controlled trial comparing a single upfront ASCT to a tandem ASCT approach in the IFM 94 study (Table 100.9). They found no difference in EFS or OS between double and single ASCTs after 2 years of follow-up[211]; however, by 4 years and beyond, an OS benefit was detected.[403] Though the response rate was not significantly different between the two groups (greater than a VGPR 42% in the single-transplant arm vs 50% in the double-transplant group, $P = .15$), both EFS (25 vs 30 months) and OS (48 vs 58 months) were improved in the double-ASCT arm. The respective 7-year OS (21% vs 42%) and EFS rates (10% vs 20%) also significantly favored the double-ASCT group[412] (Figure 100.9). In this trial, four factors were associated with a longer survival: low $\beta_2 M$ levels at diagnosis ($P < .01$), young age ($P < .05$), low LDH at diagnosis ($P < .01$), and the treatment arm to which the patient was assigned ($P < .05$). When the authors did an unplanned subgroup analysis, they found that patients who benefited most from the tandem ASCT were those who did not achieve a VGPR or better after their first ASCT. Cavo et al have made similar observations, including the benefit of a second ASCT being limited to those patients who do not achieve an nCR or better after their first ASCT.[413]

Table 100.9. Single vs Double Hematopoietic Stem Cell Transplantation, Randomized Trials

			Progression-Free Survival, mo			Overall Survival, %		
Study	N	FU, mo	Single	Double	P	Single	Double	P
IFM, 94[412]	403	75	25	30	0.03	48	58	0.01
Bologna, 96[413]	228	~48	21	31	0.001	44% at 6 y	63% at 6 y	NS
MAG, 95[399]	193	27	41 events	43 events	NS	27 deaths	22 deaths	NS
GMMG-HD2[414]	358	132	25	29	NS	73	75	NS

Abbreviations: FU, follow-up; IFM, Intergroupe Français du Myélome; MAG, Myelome Auto Greffe; NS, not significant.

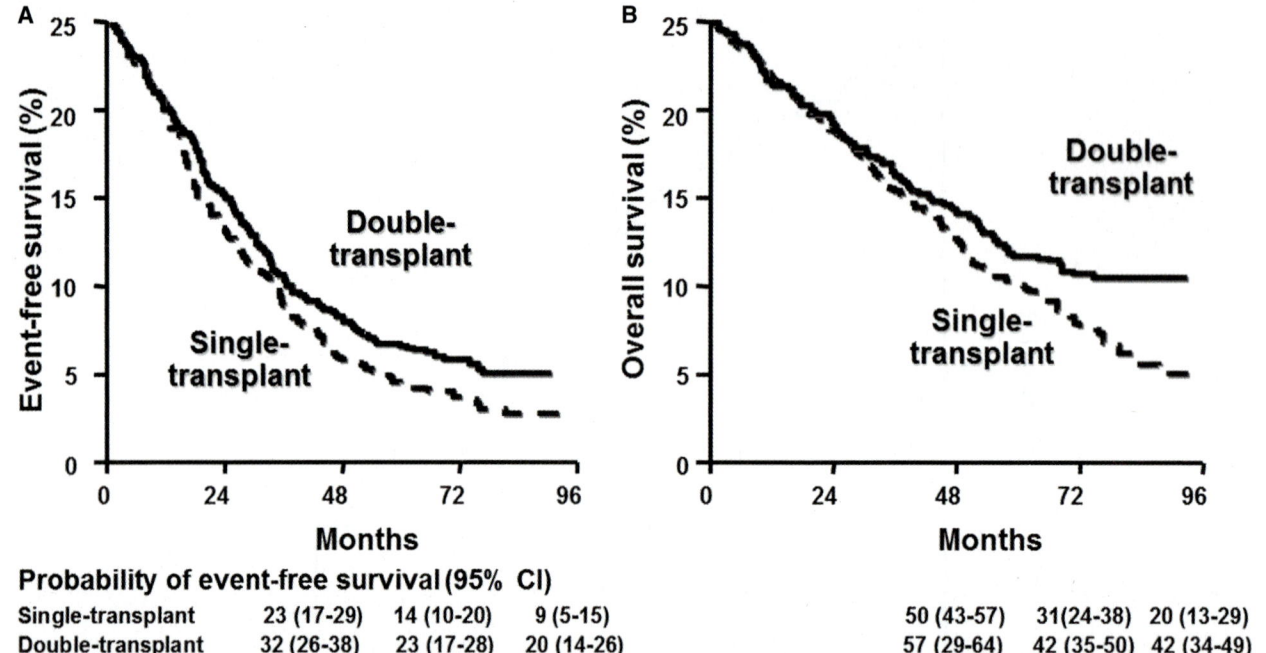

FIGURE 100.9 Single autologous vs double hematopoietic stem cell transplantation (IFM 94 trial). A, Event-free survival. B, Overall survival. (From Attal M, Harousseau JL, Facon T, et al. Single vs double autologous stem-cell transplantation for multiple myeloma. *N Engl J Med*. 2003;349(26):2495-2502. Copyright © 2003 Massachusetts Medical Society. Reprinted with permission from Massachusetts Medical Society.)

A meta-analysis was done comparing single ASCT to tandem ASCT for patients with MM.[337,399,412,414,415] Patients treated with tandem ASCT did not have a better OS or EFS than patients treated with a single ASCT. Some of this difference may be in part related to patients receiving a second ASCT at relapse.

With the advent of highly effective induction regimens, it appeared that a majority of patients would achieve VGPR or better with a proteasome inhibitor, IMiD, steroid combination leaving very few patients as candidates for their early second transplant. What has been emerging, however, is that the tandem ASCT strategy may be especially effective in the context of patients with high-risk FISH, especially those with deletion 17p.[370]

THE EMN02/HO95 study is a randomized, phase 3 study that compared ASCT (or single or double HSCT in centers with a double HSCT policy) to VMP as intensification therapy (first randomization, $n = 1197$) and VRd as consolidation therapy to no consolidation (second randomization, $n = 877$).[416] It supported intensification with ASCT because at a median follow-up of 60 months, ASCT significantly prolonged PFS compared with VMP (56.7 months [95% CI 49.3-64.5] vs 41.9 months [37.5-46.9]; HR 0.73, 0.62-0.85; $P = .0001$), although no OS benefit was evident (HR 0.90, 0.71-1.13, adjusted $P = .35$). However, in the high-risk subgroup, OS improvement was noticeable with ASCT (HR 0.66, 0.45-0.99; $P = .042$, in particular, in the del(17p) subpopulation (HR 0.48, 0.27-0.86; $P = .014$).

At the interim analysis, with a median follow-up of 42.1 months from the second randomization, VRd consolidation appeared to substantially improve the PFS compared with no consolidation (58.9 months [54.0—not estimable] vs 45.5 months [39.5-58.4]; HR 0.77, 0.63 to 0.95; $P = .014$).

Double HSCT in comparison to single ASCT significantly improved 5-year PFS (53.5%, 95% CI 46.6-61.3 vs 44.9%, 38.0-53.0; HR 0.74, 95% CI 0.56-0.98; $P = .036$) as well as 5-year OS (80.3% [74.5-86.4] vs 72.6% [66.5-79.3]; HR 0.62, 95% CI 0.41 to 0.93; $P = .022$). However, the standard-risk patients did not derive the same degree of benefit from double transplant as was observed among the patients carrying one or more of the following three adverse cytogenetic abnormalities on FISH analysis: translocation (4;14), translocation (14;16), or deletion (17p). Interestingly, the median PFS for the patients with a high-risk cytogenetic profile was 46.0 months (38.7—not estimable) with double HSCT vs 26.7 months (19.9-49.6) with single ASCT (HR 0.59, 0.34-1.03; $P = .062$), although the 5-year OS superiority is not yet evident [61.3% (45.8-82.1) vs 54.7% (41.1-72.7); HR 0.70, 0.35 to 1.42; $P = .32$]. Notably, among the patients with del(17p), a trend for the improvement in the OS rate is beginning to emerge [5-year 80.2% (62.4-100) with double ASCT vs 57.1% (39.2-83.2) with single ASCT (HR 0.30, 0.08-1.08; $P = .066$)]. The del(17p)- subset of patients that underwent double ASCT showed comparable survival rates with the standard-risk cytogenetics subgroup (HR 1.48, 0.43-5.04; $P = .53$). Moreover, the random allocation to double ASCT emerged as an independent variable for improved outcomes.

After an extended median follow-up, the OS was significantly superior for patients randomized to ASCT vs VMP. At the final analysis from the second randomization, the median follow-up time from was 75 months, VRd consolidation compared with no consolidation continued to improve ORR, CR rates and prolong PFS (HR 0.81; 95% CI, 0.68-0.96; $P = .016$), but consolidation-associated OS advantage from the second randomization was not discernible.

Salvage Hematopoietic Stem Cell Transplant

Table 100.10 illustrates that a second ASCT can performed in the salvage setting, providing patients with median OS rates ranging from 19 to 53 months following second ASCT.[417-427] Factors affecting OS included TTP after first ASCT, number of prior lines of therapy, and chemosensitivity at time of second ASCT. Cook and colleagues performed a randomized controlled trial in which they treated patient with PAD followed by ASCT or PAD followed by cyclophosphamide. Both PFS and OS favored a second ASCT at relapse.

Autologous Hematopoietic Stem Cell Transplantation in Special Populations

The mortality rate from ASCT is currently less than 5%. Age older than 65 years alone is not a contraindication for transplantation, although there are no randomized data proving or disproving its utility in this age group. Such patients are candidates for transplantation if they have good functional status and limited comorbidities.[428-431] Patients with renal failure, including dialysis patients, can successfully

Table 100.10. Second ASCT as Salvage

Study	Number of Pts	TRM, %	ORR, %	Median PFS, mo	Median OS, mo
Randomized					
BSBMT/UKMF					
Myeloma X[417]					
PAd-ASCT	89	1	83	67	67
PAd-CTX	85	0	75	35	52
Case Series					
Gonsvales et al, 2013[418]	98	4	86	10[a,b,c]	33[a]
Alveres et al, 2006[419]	83	–	–	16	35
Jimenez-Zepeda et al, 2012[420]	81	3	97	16	53[a,c]
Silva Rondon et al, 2012[421]	60	–	77	11	24
Fenk et al, 2011[422]	55	5	75	14[a]	52[a]
Shah et al, 2012[423]	44	2	90	12	32[a,b]
Mehta et al, 1998[424]	42	10[d]	81	12[d]	32[d]
Olin et al, 2009[425]	41	7	55	8[b]	21[a,b]
Elice et al, 2006[426]	26	0	69	15	38
Burzynski et al, 2009[427]	25	8	64	12	19
Summary		0-8	55-97	8-67	19-67

Abbreviations: ASCT, autologous hematopoietic stem cell transplantation; CR, complete response; ORR, overall response rate; OS, overall survival; PFS, progression-free survival; TRM, treatment-related mortality; VGPR, very good partial response.
[a]TTP after initial ASCT affected OS.
[b]Number of lines of therapy affected OS.
[c]VGPR or CR after salvage affected OS.
[d]Included allogeneic transplant patients.

undergo ASCT with melphalan 140 mg/m^2, with similar response rates and PFS, and a proportion will even have reversal of their renal failure. Treatment-related morbidity is higher,[432] and their OS is inferior to their dialysis-independent counterparts.[433,434]

Conditioning Therapy for Stem Cell Transplantation

In an effort to improve ASCT, various preparative regimens have been used. There has been only one positive prospective randomized controlled trial published in full comparing conditioning regimens in patients with MM.[435] Moreau et al[435] randomized 282 patients to receive either melphalan (140 mg/m^2) plus TBI or melphalan alone (200 mg/m^2). There was no difference in response rates or EFS. Survival at 45 months favored the melphalan alone arm (65.8% vs 45.5%, $P = .05$). Toxicity with melphalan alone was significantly less. Most investigators have now discontinued the use of TBI and give only melphalan (200 mg/m^2) as the preparative regimen.

The PETHEMA/GEM (Spanish myeloma) groups reported on their experience using busulfan/melphalan (Bu-Mel) combination that was associated with high rates of VOD, prompting them to switch to melphalan 200 mg/m^2 as conditioning.[436] Response rates were comparable, but rates of veno-occlusive disease and death were higher in the Bu-Mel arm; however, PFS was significantly longer with the Bu-Mel (41 vs 31 months, $P = .009$), with comparable OS. This experience led the randomized trial from MD Anderson comparing AUC targeted busulfan with melphalan vs melphalan.[437] Two hundred and five patients with newly diagnosed multiple myeloma who were 70 years or younger, with at least stable disease, were randomly assigned (1:1) to one of the two conditioning regimens. With a median follow-up of 28 months, treatment-related mortality (TRM), CR, and OS rates were comparable (90% at 3 years), but a 3-year PFS was better in the experimental arm (72% vs 50%). This PFS difference was most striking for patients with high-risk MM (median PFS was 44.7 and 25.7 months in the Bu-Mel and Mel arms, respectively (HR 0.48, $P = .044$).

Toxicities between the two arms were different with more grade 2 to 3 mucositis (74% vs 14%), constipation, rises in alanine aminotransferase, and neutropenic fever in the Bu-Mel arm, without any increase in treatment related deaths in either arm (0% day-100 mortality in both groups).

Bensinger et al compared melphalan 200 mg/m^2 to melphalan 280 mg/m^2 with amifostine support.[438] They found that hospitalization rates were more frequent in the mel280 group, but overall with a nonsignificant difference in grade 3 to 4 toxicities. Respective nCR rates were 22% and 39% ($P = .03$). With a median follow-up of approximately 3 years, there was no difference in either PFS or OS between the two groups. PFS at 3 years were 46% and 54%.

Other regimens including various combinations of melphalan, cyclophosphamide, idarubicin, etoposide, and/or thiotepa have been used,[439-444] without any evidence of superiority of these regimens over melphalan 200 mg/m^2 and several with significantly more toxicity[440,444] and morbidity.[439] Innovative trials supplementing melphalan with skeletal-targeted radiation (samarium-153-ethylenediamine tetramethylene phosphonate[445] and holmium-166 to 1,4,7,10-tetraazocyclodo-decane-1,4,7,10-tetramethylenephosphonic acid)[446] have been reported. Others have been studying bortezomib and carfilzomib as chemosensitizers for melphalan.[447-450]

Desikan et al retrospectively compared the impact of different conditioning regimens used for the second ASCT.[451] Outcomes of patients treated with melphalan 200 mg/m^2 were better than those conditioned with melphalan 200 mg/m^2 plus cyclophosphamide 120 mg/m^2 and melphalan 140 mg/m^2 plus TBI (1125 cGy).

Allogeneic Stem Cell Transplantation

Given the toxicity of allo-SCT approaches—rates of chronic graft-vs-host disease (GVHD) of 50%—and the lack of suitable donors, allogeneic transplant, whether myeloablative or reduced-intensity conditioning (RIC), should be considered experimental in patients with MM. Considering allo-SCT in patients with high-risk cytogenetics is reasonable, but data supporting this strategy are quite limited. Allo-SCT includes both myeloablative and nonmyeloablative or RIC transplants. Allo-SCT is appealing in theory because it avoids infusion of stem cells contaminated with MM cells and because there can be a beneficial graft-vs-myeloma effect. The use of myeloablative SCT fell out of favor by the end of the 20th century because of its high TRM in patients with MM. The RIC approach had lower TRM, but much higher rates of relapse and not insignificant rates of chronic GVHD. In fact, the lack of progression appeared to be tightly linked to the presence of chronic GVHD.[452]

Myeloablative Allogeneic Stem Cell Transplantation

CR rates of 22% to 67%, including molecular remissions in about one-third, can be achieved (Table 100.11).[453-455,457-460] Prolonged PFS is observed in approximately one-quarter to one-third of patients. The high TRM (10%-63%) and significant toxicity from GVHD have limited the role of this procedure in the treatment of MM.

There are no prospective randomized controlled trials that examine the role of myeloablative allo-SCT in MM. The US intergroup trial S9321 was an attempt at such a trial.[400] Patients with NDMM were treated with four cycles of VAD. Patients were randomly assigned to either HDT with melphalan plus TBI or to standard-dose therapy with VBMCP. Patients who were ≤55 years of age with an HLA-compatible sibling donor were offered the option of allogeneic transplantation with melphalan 140 mg/m^2 plus TBI. However, this arm was closed when an excessive first-year TRM rate of 53% was observed after enrollment of 36 eligible patients. With a median follow-up of 7 years, the OS of the conventional chemotherapy, autologous, and allogeneic transplant groups were identical at 39%. It was intriguing that allo-SCT group showed a survival plateau, whereas the other two groups did not, suggesting long-term benefit.

There have been eight case-control or cohort-control studies comparing ASCT to myeloablative allo-SCTs.[453-455,457-460] The largest of these was by Bjorkstrand et al.[453] In their retrospective analysis of data compiled by the European Blood and Marrow Transplantation Group, there was inferior OS for MM patients treated with allo-SCT compared to case-matched controls treated with ASCT (18 vs 36 months). The other smaller studies, which had relatively short follow-up, showed mixed results with regard to PFS and OS; TRM, however, was consistently higher in the allogeneic groups (19%-25%). Only one report favored allogeneic transplantation.[456] However, patients in the allo-SCT group were better prognosis patients in that they were significantly younger and less likely to have IgA MM. Though not reaching statistical significance, there were more ASCT patients having their transplant as salvage (37% vs 23%). In addition, cyclophosphamide and TBI were used to condition both the ASCT and allo-SCT patients. With follow-up times for the two groups of 24 and 43 months, respectively, the 1-year OS was 86% and 64%, and the 4-year OS was 50% and 64%.

Reduced-Intensity Conditioning Allo-SCT as Part of First-Line Therapy

Another strategy is to use ASCT to cytoreduce the MM followed by a reduced-intensity conditioning allo-SCT (allo-RIC). After two large series reported encouraging results,[462,463] five prospective trials have looked at this approach (Table 100.12). Only two of the five trials noted improved OS in patients undergoing tandem auto/allo-transplants, and in these two positive trials, the tandem ASCT patients did worse than expected. Graft-vs-myeloma effect appears to be tightly linked to GVHD (Figure 100.10),[452] which has the potential to significantly affect the quality of life.

In the first of the positive randomized trials, Bruno and colleagues enrolled 162 consecutive patients with NDMM who were ≤65 years of age.[466-468] All patients were initially treated with VAD, followed by high-dose melphalan and ASCT. Patients without an HLA-identical sibling received a second ASCT. Patients with an HLA-identical sibling then received nonmyeloablative TBI and stem cells from the sibling. With a median follow-up of 13 years, the median OS was longer in the 80 patients with HLA-identical siblings than in the 82 patients without HLA-identical siblings (8.7 vs 4.2 years, $P < .001$). Median EFS was 2.9 vs 2.4 years favoring the allo-SCT group. A 2-year

Table 100.11. Nonrandomized Comparisons of Autologous and Allogeneic Hematopoietic Stem Cell Transplantation for Multiple Myeloma

Study		N	TRM, %	PFS, mo	P	OS, mo	P
Bjorkstrand et al, 1996[453]	Auto	189	13	~22	NS	34	0.001
	Allo	189	41	~12		18	
Varterasian et al, 1997[454]	Auto	24	12	17	NS	33	NS
	Allo	24	25	31		39	
Couban et al, 1997[455]	Auto	40	5	14	–	>48	<0.001
	Allo	22	27	~11		7	
Reynolds et al, 2001[456]	Auto	35	6	2-y 30%	NS	2-y 42%	NS
	Allo	21	19	2-y 60%		2-y 60%	
Lokhorst et al, 1999[457]	Auto	50[a]	6	3-y 67%	NS	3-y 82%	NS
	Allo	11[a,b]	18	3-y 67%		3-y 82%	
Alyea et al, 2003[458]	Auto	166	13	4-y 28%	NS	4-y 41%	NS
	Allo[b]	66	24	4-y 18%		4-y 39%	
Arora et al, 2005[459]	Auto[c]	70	6	4-y 18%	NS	4-y 50%	NS
	Allo	17	31	4-y 32%		4 y 64%	
Kruvilla et al, 2007[460]	Auto	86	14	5-y 32%	NS	5-y 46%	NS
	Allo	72	22	5-y 33%		5-y 48%	
Freyetes et al, 2014[461]	Auto[d]	137	2	3-y 12%	0.03	3-y 46%	<0.001
	Allo[d]	152	13	3-y 6%		3-y 20%	

Abbreviations: MS, median survival; NS, not significant; OS, overall survival; PFS, progression-free survival; TRM, treatment-related mortality.
[a]Chemotherapy-sensitive patients only.
[b]T-cell–depleted allogeneic stem cells.
[c]Cyclophosphamide and total body irradiation conditioning.
[d]Salvage (second) transplant; this is the only study in this table in which the allo group received reduced-intensity conditioning regimens instead of myeloablative regimens.

Table 100.12. Prospective Randomized Trials Comparing Tandem Autologous SCT to Tandem Autologous Followed by HLA-Identical Reduced-Intensity Allogeneic SCT

Study	N	Regimen	Completed Both SCT, %	Median FU, mo	TRM, %	CR, %	PFS	OS
IFM99-03/4[464,465]	219[a]	Auto mel 200/220 ± IL-6 Ab	76	24	5	33	5-y 0%	6-y 40%
	65	Auto mel/Allo Bu/Flu/ATG	71	28	8	43	5-y 0%	6-y 28%
Bruno et al[466-468]	59	Auto mel 200/200	78	156	4	16	8-y 10%[b]	Median 4.3 y[b]
	60	Auto mel 200/Allo TBI	97	154	11	46	8-y 20%[b]	Median 8.7 y[b]
PeTHEMA[469]	85	Auto mel 200/mel 200 or CVB	85	>62	5	11	4-y 40%	4-y 65%
	25	Auto mel 200/Allo Flu/mel	25	>62	16	40	4-y 60%	4-y 65%
EBMT[470,471]	251	Auto mel 200/200	41	61	3	41	8-y 18%[b]	8-y 36%[b]
	107	Auto mel 200/Allo Flu/TBI	85	61	12	51	8-y 33%[b]	8-y 49%[b]
CTN 0102[472]	484	Auto mel 200/200	91	40	4	40	3-y 46%	3-y 80%
	226	Auto mel 200/Allo Flu/TBI	84	40	11	50	3-y 43%	3-y 77%

Abbreviations: CR, complete response; FU, follow-up; OS, overall survival; PFS, progression-free survival; SCT, stem cell transplantation; TRM, treatment-related mortality.
[a]High-risk patients as defined by the presence of deletion 13 by FISH and β_2 microglobulin of >3 mg/L.
[b]Significant difference between arms.

cumulative incidence of chronic GVHD was 67%. Fourteen patients received donor lymphocyte infusion (DLI) and two received a second allo-SCT from original donor. Three of the ASCT patients received an allo-SCT from unrelated donors.

The IFM enrolled 503 patients with high-risk MM (β_2M level greater than 3 mg/L and chromosome 13 deletion at diagnosis) in two clinical trials.[464,465] In both protocols, the induction regimen consisted of VAD followed by first ASCT prepared by melphalan 200 mg/m². Patients with an HLA-identical sibling donor were subsequently treated with allo-RIC (IFM99-03 trial), and patients without an HLA-identical sibling donor were randomly assigned to undergo second ASCT prepared by melphalan 220 mg/m² and 160 mg dexamethasone with or without anti–IL-6 monoclonal antibody (IFM99-04 protocol). In all, 284 patients in the IFM99-03 trial and 219 in the IFM99-04 trial were enrolled. There were no differences in OS or EFS.

The PETHEMA group enrolled 110 patients with MM who had failed to achieve at least near-complete remission after a first ASCT.[469] They received a second ASCT (85 patients) or an allo-RIC (25 patients), depending on the availability of an HLA-identical sibling donor. Those who received the allo-RIC had higher rates of complete remission (40% vs 11%, $P = .001$), but no difference in EFS and OS. They noted a 66% incidence of chronic GVHD.

The European Bone Marrow Transplant MM subcommittee enrolled 357 patients up to age 69.[470,471] Patients with an HLA-identical sibling were allocated to the ASCT-allo-RIC arm and the remaining to a tandem ASCT arm. CR rates were higher in the ASCT-allo-RIC group as was PFS, but there was no difference in OS with a median follow-up of 61 months, but with 96-month follow-up, the 8-year OS was 49% vs 36% ($P = .03$). Only 41% of patients in the tandem ASCT arm actually got a second ASCT, whereas 85% of patients in the ASCT-allo-RIC group received their second transplant.

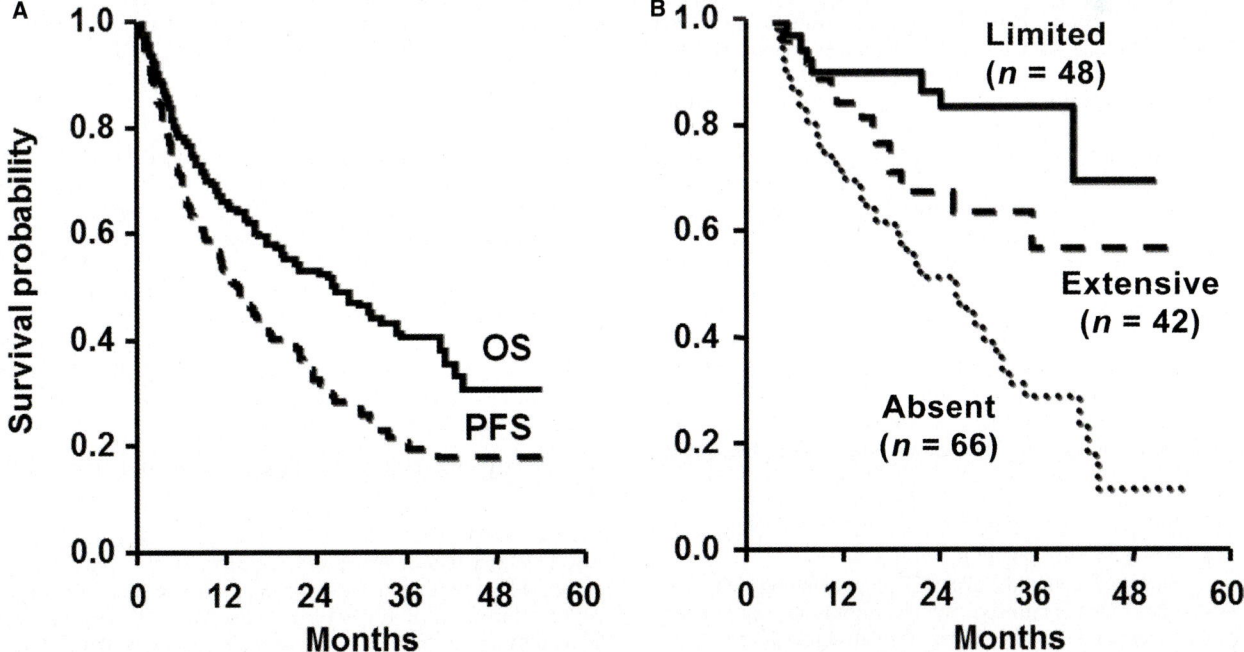

FIGURE 100.10 European Blood and Marrow Transplantation registry data on the role of reduced-intensity conditioning allogeneic transplantation regimens. A, Overall and progression-free survival. B, Overall survival relative to the presence or absence of graft-vs-host disease. (Reprinted from Crawley C, Lalancette M, Szydlo R, et al. Outcomes for reduced-intensity allogeneic transplantation for multiple myeloma: an analysis of prognostic factors from the Chronic Leukemia Working Party of the EBMT. *Blood*. 2005;105(11):4532-4539. Copyright © 2005 American Society of Hematology. With permission.)

The Blood Marrow Transplant Clinical Trials Network enrolled 710 patients[472] and biologically randomized them to tandem ASCT or ASCT-allo-RIC. They, too, noted no difference in OS or PFS.

A meta-analysis was performed combining results of four of the six trials listed earlier. The conclusion was that over the first 3 years, the auto-auto strategy was favored for TRM, PFS, and OS, but after 3 years, the HR for OS favored the auto-allo strategy.[473]

Reduced-Intensity Conditioning Allo-SCT in the Relapsed Setting

Kroger and colleagues reported on their experience using matched unrelated donor (MUD) RIC in 48 patients who relapsed after ASCT. The 5-year PFS and OS were 20% and 26%, respectively, and the rate of chronic GVHD was 35%.[474] Freytes on behalf of the CIBMTR compared outcomes of 289 patients who relapsed post-ASCT and went onto either a second ASCT or to an allo-RIC.[461] All parameters favored the ASCT over the allo-RIC. A major limitation of this study is that no cytogenetic data were available to balance patient biologic risk. There was no difference in outcomes between those patients who had related or those patients who had unrelated donors. Results from the Netherlands in 89 relapsed/refractory patients[475] did quite poorly, especially in the subgroup of patients relapsing within 18 months after ASCT.

An innovative strategy employing CD34-selected stem cells followed by planned DLI in an effort to reduce TRM has been applied, with some interesting results reported in 44 MM patients with relapsed and high-risk MM.[476] These patients had a 1-year TRM of 18%; a 2-year PFS and OS of 31% and 54%, respectively; and no chronic GVHD.

Haploidentical SCT with posttransplantation cyclophosphamide for heavily pretreated MM patients has been reported by groups from Italy and the United States.[477,478] Among 30 patients (8 myeloablative and 22 RIC) reported by Castagna, the 18-month nonrelapse mortality was 10%, and the incidence of relapse or progression was 42%. The incidence of chronic GVHD was 7%. With a median follow-up of 25 months, the 18-month PFS and OS were 33% and 63%, respectively. Chemorefractory disease at transplantation was associated with a lower/reduced 18-month PFS (9% vs 47%, $P = .01$) and OS (45% vs 74%, $P = .03$). Similar results were reported by Ghosh et al who reported on 39 patients (9 myeloablative and 30 RIC) with MM who received post–allo-SCT cyclophosphamide for GVHD prophylaxis for relapsed disease ($n = 26$) or as part of first-line therapy ($n = 13$).[478] Seven of these patients were haploidentical; the remainder were HLA matched. After allo-SCT, the CR was 26%. Eighteen patients received DLI. With a median follow-up of 10 years, 23% of patients remain without evidence of disease. Median OS was 4.4 years, and 5- and 10-year OS rates were 49% and 43%, respectively.

The European Group for Blood and Marrow Transplant Chronic Malignancies Working Party reported on their experience with salvage RIC using unrelated donors in 570 MM patients between 2001 and 2013.[479] Their sample included 419 10/10 HLA-MUD, 93 9/10 HLA MUD, and 58 cord blood patients. All patients had at least one prior ASCT. Only a small minority of patients had information about cytogenetics. Allo-SCT was performed after a median time of one ($n = 336$) or two ($n = 234$) ASCTs. The 2-year TRM for the three respective donor groups were 22%, 33%, and 27%, respectively. Respective 3-year relapse rates were 50%, 35%, and 54%, resulting in 3-year PFS of 25%, 31%, and 19%, and 3-year OS of 47%, 45%, and 38%. No information was provided about chronic GVHD or quality of life.

Allogeneic Stem Cell Transplantation in Patients With High-Risk Fluorescence In Situ Hybridization

There are limited data on the role allo-SCT plays among patients with high-risk disease. Much is retrospective, and most is based on tandem auto-allo approach, rather than a full myeloablative transplant.

Kroger and colleagues studied the incidence and impact of achievement of molecular remission and high-risk cytogenetics within a prospective protocol including 73 patients with MM.[480] After induction chemotherapy, patients received melphalan 200 mg/m^2 before undergoing ASCT, followed 3 months later by melphalan 140 mg/m^2 and fludarabine 180 mg/m^2 before allo-SCT. Sixteen patients had high-risk cytogenetic features, defined by positive FISH for del(17p13) and/or t(4;14). After a median follow-up of 6 years, overall 5-year PFS was 29%, with no significant difference between del(17p)13/t(4;14)-harboring patients and others (24% vs 30%; $P = .70$). Only depth of response influenced the 5-year PFS. These results suggest that auto-allo tandem SCT may overcome the negative prognostic effect of del(17p13) and/or t(4;14) and that achievement of molecular remission resulted in long-term freedom from disease.

The Societe Francaise de Greffe de Moelle et de Therapie Cellulaire reviewed 143 MM patients transplanted between 1999 and 2008, 53 of whom had del(17p), t(4;14), or t(14;16) and 32 who were tested for at least two of these three abnormalities and were negative for them.[481] Forty-eight patients received allo-SCT as part of first-line therapy; 32 patients had a myeloablative-conditioning regimen as part of their allo-SCT. For the entire heterogeneous population, there was no difference observed between the HR-FISH and SR-FISH patients in terms of 3-year PFS (30% vs 17%) or OS (45% vs 39%).

Schilling et al studied 101 patients with cytogenetic studies performed who underwent allo-RIC, more than half of whom had match unrelated donors.[482] Only four patients received allo-SCT without a preceding autograft. Fifty-one patients were treated as part of an ASCT-allo-SCT approach; 50 patients had experienced a relapse to a prior ASCT. There was a trend toward inferior EFS and OS for patients with del(17p), but no difference in either for patients with t(4;14).

Donor Lymphocyte Infusions

A graft-vs-myeloma effect has been noted after the administration of donor peripheral blood mononuclear cells for relapse after allogeneic transplantation.[483,484] DLI has been used in two ways in MM patients. Initially, it was used to treat relapsed or residual disease after full myeloablative allo-SCT.[483,484] Subsequently, it was used to reintroduce T cells into patients receiving allogeneic T-cell–depleted grafts.[485,486] Most recently, it has been implemented in the context of allo-RIC programs to treat mixed chimerism, as well as for the older indications.[487-489] In the largest DLI series for relapsed MM ($n = 54$), 52% of patients responded (35% with a PR and 17% with a CR). The majority of patients received some chemotherapy before DLI. PFS and OS were 19 and 23 months, respectively. Rates of overall acute GVHD and grade 3 to 4 acute GVHD were 57% and 20%, respectively. Rates of overall chronic GVHD and extensive GVHD were 47% and 30%, respectively. Acute and chronic GVHD following DLI were the strongest predictors for response.[490]

Maintenance Therapy

Strategies for maintenance therapy can be divided into two broad categories: (1) continued induction therapy and infinitum and (2) addition of a novel therapy after induction therapy. The former strategy was prevalent with alkylators until recognition of the risk of developing alkylator-induced myelodysplastic syndromes and leukemia.[491-496] Both strategies are used in the context of immune modulators, including prednisone, IFN, cellular therapies, thalidomide and lenalidomide, and, most recently, proteasome inhibitors. The standard is now considered lenalidomide maintenance for a minimum of 18 to 24 months, as will be discussed later. The role of maintenance proteasome inhibitors and antibodies is currently the areas of study.

Maintenance Lenalidomide Post–Autologous Stem Cell Transplantation

All of the randomize trials addressing lenalidomide maintenance after ASCT demonstrate improved PFS (*Table 100.13*) and a higher rate of secondary malignancies with maintenance lenalidomide,[501,502] but only the CALGB 100404 trial had a better OS (3-year OS 88 vs 80 months, $P = .03$)[502]; however, a meta-analysis, combining the three published trials, showed improved OS when lenalidomide was used as maintenance.[504] In the meta-analysis, the pooled PFS for maintenance vs no maintenance was 53 vs 23 months, an HR of 0.48 (95% CI: 0.41-0.55), and median OS was not reached vs 86 months (HR 0.75,

95% CI: 0.63-0.90). On subgroup analysis, the most benefit was seen among those under 60, males, ISS stage I/II, and ≥VGPR post-ASCT. Fewer than half of placebo patients in the IFM and GIMEMA trials received lenalidomide as part of their second-line therapy. Cumulative incidence rate of secondary malignancies was 23% in the lenalidomide groups as compared to 8.6% in the placebo/observation groups.

There were differences between the IFM 2005-02 trial and the CALGB 100404 trial. In the CALGB 100404 trial, patients were unblinded and crossed over early when a planned interim analysis revealed a superior PFS in the lenalidomide arm. In the IFM 2005-02 study,[501] all patients received two cycles of lenalidomide upon post-ASCT registration prior to getting either placebo or lenalidomide.[501] In addition, the duration of maintenance was limited to 2 years once their data safety monitoring board noted a higher cumulative incidence of secondary malignancies in the lenalidomide arm; their 4-year OS rates were 73% and 75%.

The GIMEMA RV-MM-PI-209 was an open-label, randomized, phase III study that compared ASCT with MPR as well as lenalidomide maintenance therapy with no maintenance therapy in patients with NDMM.[276] This study included 273 patients for the double randomization. With a median follow-up period of 51.2 months, PFS was significantly longer with lenalidomide maintenance than with no maintenance (41.9 vs 21.6 months; $P < .001$), but a 3-year OS was not significantly prolonged (88.0% vs 79.2%; $P = .14$) for the group at large or the ASCT group when considered separately. Neutropenia and dermatologic toxic effects were more frequent with lenalidomide maintenance than with no maintenance.

Maintenance lenalidomide was also tested in the Myeloma XI trial[505] and the PFS was once again markedly improved with lenalidomide maintenance (20 vs 39 months, $P < .001$), but the 3-year OS was similar.

In the GMMG-MM5 trial evaluating response-adapted lenalidomide maintenance following induction and consolidation therapy, there was a second randomization to either lenalidomide maintenance for a fixed duration of 2 years (LEN-2y) or lenalidomide maintenance that was stopped either due to achieving a subsequent CR or not started due to achieving a CR immediately after ASCT (LEN-CR).[351] In a pooled comparison of lenalidomide maintenance strategies, it was observed that there was no difference in PFS between LEN-2y and LEN-CR; however, OS was significantly prolonged with the LEN-2y vs LEN-CR maintenance strategy (HR = 1.42, 95% CI: 1.04-1.93, $P = .03$).[351] Furthermore, patients who had any high-risk cytogenetic abnormalities (defined by the presence of deletion 17p13 in >10% of nucleated, CD138-purified cells and/or translocation t(4;14), and/or amplification of 1q21) had a worse PFS and OS if they received the LEN-CR maintenance strategy compared to the LEN-2y strategy (PFS: HR = 1.93, 95% CI: 1.34-2.77, $P < .001$; OS: HR = 2.96, 95% CI: 1.91-4.61, $P < .001$). As such, this study suggests the need for utilizing lenalidomide maintenance for at least 2 years irrespective of CR status.

Maintenance Lenalidomide Post-Allogeneic Stem Cell Transplantation

In the post-allogeneic stem cell setting, lenalidomide appears to increase GVHD.[506,507] To improve the outcome of allo-SCT in MM as part of first-line treatment, the HOVON group prospectively investigated the feasibility and efficacy of lenalidomide maintenance. Lenalidomide was dosed 10 mg on days 1 to 21 of a 28-day schedule for a total of 24 cycles. In all, 30 patients started lenalidomide, but 13 patients (43%) stopped treatment because of development of GVHD, 5 patients (17%) because of other AEs, and 5 patients (17%) because of progression. Responses improved in 37% of patients, and the estimated 1-year PFS from start of maintenance was 69% (90% CI: 53%-81%). In a similar study, 30 allo-SCT patients received escalating doses of lenalidomide as part of a phase IIa clinical trial.[507] Eleven patients completed the planned maintenance of 12 months; 10 mg daily was the most commonly delivered dose. The incidence of acute GVHD was 38%. Five patients had their hematologic response upgraded with the maintenance. Cumulative incidence of MM relapse or progression at 18 months was 27%.

Maintenance Lenalidomide in the Non-Stem Cell Transplantation Setting

Of the three studies addressing this question, the findings are consistent: Maintenance lenalidomide provides a PFS advantage, but not an OS benefit. The most experience with lenalidomide maintenance is the continuous use of lenalidomide plus dexamethasone as primary induction therapy without early transplant as in the MM-020 trial.[503] The two arms of this trial that relate to the question at hand were lenalidomide and dexamethasone at diagnosis to be continued indefinitely, and lenalidomide and dexamethasone from diagnosis to be continued for only 18 months. An improved PFS was seen (4-year PFS 33% vs 14%), but OS between the two groups was identical (4-year OS 59% vs 58%).[503] The MM-015 trial, which randomized patients between three arms (MP, MPR, and MPR-R maintenance), also revealed superior PFS in the maintenance arm (31 vs 14 months, HR 0.49, $P < .001$), but no difference in OS between MPR with or without maintenance lenalidomide (45 months vs NR, $P = .25$).[280] The authors noted that the greatest benefit was observed in those patients aged 65 to 75 years. Slightly more than twice as many secondary malignancies were seen in the lenalidomide maintenance arm. In the Myeloma XI trial, among the transplant-ineligible cohorts, PFS from randomization was 26 months in the maintenance group and only 11 months in the observation arm (HR 0.44, 95% CI: 0.37-0.53); OS from randomization was 50.8 months for the maintenance group and 57.2 months in the observation group.[508]

Maintenance Thalidomide

In terms of randomized controlled trials evaluating the role of thalidomide maintenance as compared to placebo or prednisone, there have been seven performed in the post-ASCT setting[344,347,472,497-500] and another three in the setting of low-dose alkylator-based therapy.[255,257,258,499] (Table 100.13) In all the post-ASCT trials, there was a PFS benefit among patients receiving maintenance thalidomide, but there was an OS benefit in only two of these trials.[497,498] Quality of life was significantly worse among patients receiving thalidomide in the NCIC CTG-MY.10 trial.[500]

Among the four nontransplant trials,[255,257,258,499] there was improvement in PFS in three of the trials, but an OS benefit in only one.[258] Three of these four nontransplant trials not only tested the value of maintenance thalidomide but also using it as part of an induction triplet of MPT.[255,257,258] Owing to this design limitation, it is impossible to state whether the induction component or the maintenance component contributed to any differences in outcomes. The MRC IX trial,[499] which compared attenuated CTD to MP, had a double randomization, so the effect of induction vs maintenance could be more easily separated. Although there was a modest improvement in PFS in this study (11 vs 9 months), there was no difference in OS between the maintained and the nonmaintained groups.

Maintenance Strategies Incorporating Proteasome Inhibitors

There are four randomized clinical trials that incorporate bortezomib into a maintenance strategy.[261,274,339,338] Owing to the complexity of these trials, however, it is difficult to isolate the actual clinical benefit of the bortezomib maintenance. The first of the two ASCT trials was the HOVON-65/GMMG-HD4 trial,[338] which randomized patients to either PAD induction followed by one or two ASCT followed by maintenance bortezomib every other week for 2 years vs VAD induction followed by one or two ASCT followed by thalidomide maintenance for 2 years. Although OS was superior (5-year OS 61% vs 55%) in the bortezomib containing arm, it is impossible to isolate the effect of induction vs maintenance. Moreover, there was no information regarding the availability of salvage bortezomib in the VAD plus thalidomide arm.

The other post-ASCT trial is the PETHEMA/GEM05MEN0S65 trial,[339] which is a complicated study of 387 patients who were

Table 100.13. Randomized Clinical Trials Incorporating Immunomodulatory Drugs or Bortezomib for Maintenance vs No Maintenance or Comparing Maintenance Options, Transplant Eligible and Ineligible

Study	Trial Design[a]	N	Intended Months of Maintenance	FU, mo	EFS or PFS or Median	OS or Median	Percent Getting Maintenance Drug as Salvage
TT2[347]	TT2 ± T	668	Indefinite	72	5-y 56% vs 44%	8-y 57% vs 44%	
TT2 Abn Cytogenetics subgroup					5-y 56% vs 43%[b]		83
IFM99-02[497]	ASCT × 2 ± T	597	Indefinite	36	3-y 52% vs 36%	4-y 87% vs 77%	62
ALLG MM6[498]	ASCT × 1 + P ± T	243	1 y	24	3-y 42% vs 23%[b]	3-y 86% vs 75%[b]	54
MRC IX intensive path[499]	ASCT × 1 ± T[d]	492	Indefinite	38	30 vs 23 mo[b]	3-y 75% vs 80%[c]	62
NCIC CTG-MY.10[500]	ASCT × 1 ± TP	332	Indefinite	48	28 vs 17 mo[b]	4-y 68% vs 60%	NA
HOVON-50[344]	TAD vs VAD → ASCT × 1 or 2 ± T (vs IFN)[d]	536	Indefinite	52	34 vs 25 mo[b]	73 vs 60 mo	NA
BMT CTN 0102[472]	ASCT × 2 ± T	366	Indefinite	36	3-y 49% vs 43%	3-y 80% vs 81%	NA
IFM 2005-2[501]	ASCT × 1 or 2 ± L	614	2 y	45	4-y 43% vs 22%[b]	4-y 73% vs 75%[b]	45
CALGB 100104[502]	ASCT × 1 ± L	460	Indefinite	34	46 vs 27 mo[b]	3-y 88% vs 80%[b]	NA
HOVON-65/GMMG-HD4[338]	PAD vs VAD ASCT × 1 or 2 ± B (vs T)[d]	827	2 y	66	35 vs 28 mo[b]	5-y 61% vs 55%[b]	NA
PETHEMA/GEM05MEN0S65[339]	ASCT × 1 → VT vs T vs IFN	<387	3 y	24	2-y 78% vs 63% vs 49%[b]	Not different	NA
GIMEMA[255]	MPT vs MP	355	Indefinite	38	22 vs 14 mo[b]	45 vs 48 mo	42[e]
Nordic[257]	MPT vs MP	357	Indefinite	42	15 vs 14 mo	29 vs 32 mo	45
HOVON 49[258]	MPT vs MP	333	Indefinite	39	13 vs 9 mo[b]	40 vs 31 mo[b]	80
MRC IX nonintensive path	CTDa ± T vs MP ± T	326	Indefinite	38	11 vs 9 mo[b]	38 vs 39 mo	NA
MM-015[280]	MPR-R vs MPR/MP	459	Indefinite	30	31 vs 13 mo[b]	3-y 70% vs 64%	40-50
VMPT + VT[261]	VMPT + VT vs VMP	511	2 y	23	3-y 56% vs 41%[b]	3-y 89% vs 87%	NA
PETHEMA/GEM[274]	VTP vs VMP, 2° random to VT vs VP	260	3 y	32	32 vs 24 mo[b]	HR 1.2 (0.6-2.4)	NA
MM-020/FIRST[503]	Rd-R vs Rd 18	1076	Indefinite vs 18 mo	67	25 vs 21 mo	59 vs 62 mo	22
HOVON87/NMSG18 trial[282]	MPR-TMPT-R	318319	Indefinite	36	20 vs 23 mo	4-y 52% vs 56%	NA

Abbreviations: ASCT, autologous stem cell transplantation; f/u, follow-up; MP, melphalan and prednisone; MPT, MP and thalidomide; MS, median survival; NA, not available; OS, overall survival; Thal, thalidomide; VMP, bortezomib, melphalan, and prednisone; VMPT, bortezomib, melphalan, prednisone, and thalidomide.
[a]Induction regimens for trial design not specified if same in both arms. If no comparator maintenance drug listed, the comparator is either nothing or placebo.
[b]Statistically significant difference between arms.
[c]Risk of death × 1.8 higher in patients with adverse cytogenetics if thalidomide arm.
[d]Other details of this study included in *Table 100.6*.
[e]Received thalidomide or bortezomib—number of patients in control arm receiving thalidomide as salvage not specified.

randomized to one of three induction regimens followed by an ASCT followed by a secondary randomization to bortezomib (1.3 mg/m² days 1, 4, 8, and 11 every 3 months) plus thalidomide (100 mg/d), to single-agent thalidomide, or to thrice-weekly IFN. PFS was superior with the VT as compared to the T or the IFN, but with 24 months follow-up, there was no difference in OS.

The other two bortezomib maintenance trials were among elderly patients, who did not undergo ASCT. The first is the PETHEMA/GEM trial,[218] which randomized newly diagnosed elderly patients to either VMP or VTP with a secondary randomization to either VT or VP. After a median follow-up of 22 months from second randomization, PFS from this time point was 32 months for patients receiving VT and 24 months for those receiving VP (HR 1.4, 95% CI: 0.8-2.1; $P = .1$). No difference in OS was observed. In the Italian study comparing VMP with no maintenance to VMPT plus VT maintenance,[261] PFS was superior with the four-drug combination with two-drug maintenance compared to the three-drug regimen without maintenance (32 vs 24 months), but there was no difference in OS.

Based on these data, no recommendation regarding the utility of bortezomib maintenance in the general MM population can be provided; however, it—or another proteasome inhibitor—is commonly used as part of a maintenance strategy in patients with high-risk cytogenetics.

The TOURMALINE-MM03 (NCT02181413) reported that post-ASCT ixazomib maintenance for a fixed duration is well tolerated and prolongs PFS in comparison to placebo (median PFS 26.5 months [95% CI 23.7-33.8] vs 21.3 months [18.0-24.7]; HR 0.72, 95% CI 0.58-0.89; $P = 0.0023$).[509] However, cross study comparisons do not suggest similar degree of benefit as observed in the posttransplant lenalidomide maintenance trials for patients with newly diagnosed multiple myeloma. OS benefit has also not been observed so far. It is reasonable to consider using ixazomib in patients who are intolerant of lenalidomide in the maintenance setting, although it should be emphasized that ixazomib has not been studied specifically in this patient population.

In the FORTE trial, following consolidation therapy with KCd or KRd, 356 patients underwent a second randomization (R2), with assignment to either carfilzomib plus lenalidomide (KR) or lenalidomide (R) monotherapy as maintenance.[336] After a median follow-up of 31 months and a median duration of maintenance of 27 months, substantially more patients who were MRD positive at second randomization attained MRD negative state with KR doublet vs lenalidomide monotherapy (46% vs 32%; $P = .04$). Three-year PFS was significantly longer after R2 in the KR arm vs lenalidomide alone (75% vs 66%; HR 0.63; $P = .026$), albeit at the cost of higher grade 3 to 4 nonhematologic toxicities. KR maintenance appeared to improve PFS in comparison lenalidomide monotherapy among the standard risk patients (3-year PFS 90% vs 73%, HR 0.42, $P = .06$), high-risk patient (3-year PFS 69% vs 56%, HR 0.6, $P = .04$), and patients with double hit MM characterized by the presence of two or more high-risk cytogenetic abnormalities (3-year PFS 67% vs 42%, HR 0.53, $P = .1$). Three-year OS was similar: 90% with both KR and R, and a longer follow-up will shed more light on this endpoint.

Maintenance Daratumumab

In Part 2 of the CASSIOPEIA trial, 886 patients were randomly reassigned after consolidation therapy to IV daratumumab, 16 mg/kg every 8 weeks for up to 2 years or observation because they had achieved at least a partial response following peri-ASCT induction and consolidation with VTd,+/− daratumumab.[510] Barring a notable exception of patients receiving daratumumab during induction/consolidation (DVTd arm) all pre-specified subgroups advantage of incorporating daratumumab during maintenance. The daratumumab-naïve patient-population that received VTd induction/consolidation appeared to reap all the benefits of daratumumab maintenance (PFS-HR 0.32), and incontrovertibly drove the PFS improvement. However, this advantage of daratumumab maintenance was not observed in the DVTd induction/consolidation group. These findings suggest that incorporation of daratumumab in the frontline regimen is important, be it during the induction/consolidation phases, or the maintenance phase for the patients in whom it was not used during induction-consolidation. Daratumumab maintenance was well tolerated, with toxicity-related discontinuation rate of 3%. However, the SPM rate was twice as much in the IV daratumumab maintenance arm, with a shorter time to onset of SPM.

Oral agents, including ixazomib and lenalidomide, offer advantages over daratumumab therapy, but the new, subcutaneous route of administration, proven to be equally effective in the relapsed refractory setting in comparison to the IV route, as well as the low frequency of administration (once every 8 weeks), could in part overcome the burden associated with using this parenteral agent in the maintenance setting.

Maintenance With Alkylators, Steroids, or Interferon

Through the 1970s and 1980s, several randomized studies established that alkylator-based maintenance therapy does not produce a survival benefit.[304,511-515] Induction was commonly discontinued after plateau was reached.[515] There are four studies that address the utility of corticosteroids as maintenance therapy.[359,516-518] None justifies a recommendation of prednisone as a standard maintenance regimen for all patients. IFN has been studied both after conventional chemotherapy and after ASCT. Meta-analyses clarified divergent results observed in over 1500 patients in 13 maintenance trials[312,313]; IFN maintenance provided a 4.4-month prolongation of relapse-free survival ($P < .01$) and a 7.0-month increase in OS ($P < .01$),[312] but its toxicity profile and alternate available therapies at relapse have moved this from standard practice.

Management of Relapsed or Refractory Disease

The median survival of patients with MM has significantly increased over the past decade and is currently estimated to be 8 to 10 years. The median PFS after initial therapy, even with ASCT and maintenance, is estimated to be around 4 years. Given this scenario, patients will live with relapsed disease for at least half of their MM course if not more, making the management of relapsed disease an important component for the care of the MM patient. Significant changes have occurred in the management of relapsed MM during this time, as a result of increasing availability of new drugs and drug classes with significant efficacy. In fact, the median PFS from the start of new therapy for initial relapse with modern triplet regimens is 2 to 3 years, surpassing the result seen with initial therapy in the past decade.

At the same time, the increasing number of initial treatment approaches employed for MM has led to a significant heterogeneity among patients with relapsed MM. This combined with the underlying biologic heterogeneity intrinsic to the disease has precluded development of uniform approaches to the management of relapsed disease. Recent studies using advanced genomic analyses have clearly shown that significant clonal evolution as well as clonal selection occurs as the disease suffer multiple relapses over time. However, the deep response achieved with initial therapy also allows patients to recover from the complications of disease present at the time of initial diagnosis, thus allowing the patients to be in a much better performance status at the time of initial relapse. This, in turn, allows these patients to tolerate multidrug combination regimens that are highly effective.

Definitions

Despite the significant heterogeneity, uniform definitions have been developed for defining relapsed and refractory disease, which is critical for comparison of patient groups from a clinical trial standpoint. In general, relapses can be classified as biochemical relapses where the increase in the monoclonal protein component, bone marrow plasmacytosis, or size of plasmacytoma(s) meets the definitions of relapse as per the International IMWG Response Criteria.[210] However, a significant proportion of patients who meet this criteria do not require therapy right away, a concept similar to how we manage early-stage asymptomatic myeloma also known as smoldering myeloma. However, patients can have clinical evidence of progression that may or may not satisfy the biochemical criteria, but clearly require therapeutic intervention. These typically include development of one or more components of the CRAB criteria that is used at the time of diagnosis. Several additional qualifying criteria need to be included in the defining the patient with relapsed disease. This is not only important from a clinical trial perspective, allowing us to better compare results across different trials, but also helps us in deciding the future course of therapy.

The most important aspect is the differentiation between relapses occurring on therapy and off therapy, with the former often having a poorer prognosis. An accepted definition for refractory disease, currently used in most of the clinical trials, is relapse occurring while on a particular therapy or relapse within 60 days of stopping the therapy. A subset of these patients may have never responded to the initial therapy or may have progressed within 60 days of stopping the initial therapy, a group referred to as having primary refractory disease.[519] These definitions should be further qualified by the class of agents or the treatment modality to which the patient is refractory. Another disease characteristic that is critically important when comparing different patient groups is the number of lines of therapy that the patient has received. Criteria have been developed to better define a line of therapy. For example, induction therapy followed by 1 to 2 ASCT, posttransplant consolidation, and posttransplant maintenance are all considered as part of one line of therapy. More recently, with the advent of multiple drugs from within the same class, disease characteristics have been defined more in terms of the drug classes that an individual patient is refractory to rather using lines of therapy or refractoriness to specific drugs.

Prognostic Factors in Relapsed Disease

Many of the prognostic factors that are relevant at the time of initial diagnosis continue to be important at the time of relapse. These include the ISS, serum LDH, performance status, refractory status with respect to various drugs or drug classes, cytogenetics and/or FISH findings, and in particular development of new abnormalities, the plasma cell proliferation rate, and the presence of circulating cells or extramedullary disease. Two key factors that become evident at the time of relapse are particularly relevant to the prognosis of patients with relapsed disease. The DOR to the initial therapy is one of the most important prognostic factors at the time of relapse. Patients with a short-lasting response to initial therapy or are primary refractory to the newer drugs have very poor OS. In fact, in a retrospective study, the OS from relapse among a cohort of patients relapsing within 12 months of an ASCT was less than a year. Similar findings have been seen in nontransplant therapy settings as well. The second critical factor is the acquisition of new genetic abnormalities with disease evolution. The two most common abnormalities seen with increasing frequency among relapsed disease are loss of the *TP53* gene and chromosome 1 abnormalities (most commonly 1q amplification), both of which portends a poor outcome.

Treatment of Relapsed Disease: General Approach

Before the era of high-dose chemotherapy with stem cell support, IMiDs, proteasome inhibitors, and monoclonal antibodies, treatment guidelines were simpler. The approach to treatment can be quite varied, and there is a lack of consensus as to how best to treat disease relapse. There are a few broad principles that should be kept in mind while deciding the management approach to relapsed disease in any given patient. Many patients have an indolent disease relapse, marked by biochemical progression and no worsening or new end-organ damage despite extensive evaluation. It is not clear whether patients benefit from early intervention at the time of biochemical relapse, and it is reasonable to observe these patients for some time until a firm trend can be established. In patients with high-risk disease and those who presented with life-threatening complications of disease, treatment should be restarted early. Regimens that have been effective previously, and to which the patient is not refractory to, can and should be considered again. Combinations of two drugs, where the individual drugs have not been very effective, may be able to capitalize on the synergy and produce meaningful responses. In fact, a series of large phase III trials have shown improved OS among patients receiving a triplet regimen. Given the clonal selection process that occurs in the MM cells as has been shown through elegant genomic studies,[182] drugs that have previously become ineffective can be of benefit later on, alone or as part of combinations. While deep responses typically translate into prolonged disease control, minor responses can be quite meaningful in those patient populations from the point of clinical benefit. Therapeutic selection should take into account residual toxicities from earlier therapies in order not to exacerbate the ongoing symptoms and must be tailored to the patient's performance status. Care should be taken in terms of the use of drugs with cumulative toxicity, particularly hematologic toxicity, that will preclude subsequent use of some of the newer drugs.

The typical approach would be to use a combination of two active drugs and a corticosteroid, a strategy that has been born out from phase III trials. If possible, there should be at least one drug class that the patient has not been previously exposed to or at least one new drug. The specific drugs in the combination could depend on a variety of factors, including the drug classes the patient has most recently been exposed to, the residual toxicity from prior therapy, age, patient performance status, comorbidities, logistics of clinic visits for parenteral drugs vs oral therapies, and patient preference with respect to quality-of-life issues.

The approach to treatment for relapsed or refractory disease will be divided into two sections: activity of individual drugs with or without steroids (*Table 100.14*) and combinations of newer drugs or of new drugs with traditional chemotherapy agents. The latter is broadly divided into four groups based on the resistance to bortezomib and lenalidomide, given that they are the most commonly used initial therapies, as described in previous sections.

Immunomodulatory Drugs

Thalidomide

Single-agent thalidomide can induce a response in 25% to 58% of relapsed/refractory patients[12,520] and higher response rates of 41% to 55% when combined with dexamethasone[521,534-537] (*Table 100.14*). Thalidomide doses have ranged between 100 and 400 mg/d in the different regimens, without any clear dose-response effect.

Lenalidomide

As a single agent, approximately 18% to 25% of relapsed or refractory patients have achieved a PR with lenalidomide, and the median DOR for responding patients is 20 months[522] (*Table 100.14*). In the randomized phase II trial of lenalidomide, the addition of dexamethasone (40 mg days 1-4 and 15-18) to patients not responding to 2 months of lenalidomide resulted in PR rates in an additional 22% of patients.[522]

The combination of lenalidomide and dexamethasone was studied in two large phase III trials.[523,524] The results of both were comparable, with 59% of patients responding to the combination, including a 14% CR rate. This was significantly better than what was observed with single-agent dexamethasone (PR 22.5% and CR 2%). In addition, both TTP (11-13 vs ~5 months) and OS (NR vs 24 months) were superior in the lenalidomide/dexamethasone arm. The benefit with lenalidomide was independent of prior exposure to thalidomide.[538] Significant number of patients who initially had a PR improved the response to a CR or VGPR with continued treatment, especially among those obtaining a PR within the first four cycles.[317] As with other therapies, patients who achieved a CR/VGPR as their best response had significantly longer median DOR, TTP, and OS compared with those with only a PR.[539] Continuation of lenalidomide treatment until disease progression in patients achieving a PR was associated with a significant survival advantage.[540]

Pomalidomide

Pomalidomide (CC-4047) is another thalidomide-based IMiD used for relapsed MM[541,542] (*Table 100.14*). The initial trials with pomalidomide established the MTD of pomalidomide as 2 mg daily or 5 mg on alternate days.[19,543] These studies used pomalidomide as monotherapy and showed excellent activity with an ORR of 52%.[19] In the initial phase II trial from Mayo Clinic, pomalidomide 2 mg daily in combination with dexamethasone 40 mg weekly was given to cohort of 60 patients with relapsed MM, who had two to three prior regimens.[199] Thirty-eight patients (63%) achieved confirmed response, including CR in 3 patients (5%), VGPR in 17 patients (28%), and PR in 18 patients (30%). Responses were seen irrespective of their prior drug exposures, with 40% of lenalidomide-refractory patients, 37% of thalidomide-refractory patients, and 60% of bortezomib-refractory patients achieving a response. Subsequent cohorts of patients were enrolled studying different doses and schedules in different groups with respect to their refractoriness to bortezomib or lenalidomide.[544,545] Long-term outcomes of the 345 patients enrolled into the various cohorts showed response rate of ~35% (range, 23%-65%) with higher responses in cohorts with fewer prior lines of therapy.[546] The longest PFS and OS seen in any cohort were 13.1 and 47.9 months, respectively.

Pomalidomide and dexamethasone (Pd) were also studied in an open-label, randomized multicenter phase III trial comparing it with pulsed dose dexamethasone.[528] Patients with refractory MM or relapsed/refractory MM (RRMM), who had failed at least two previous treatments containing bortezomib and lenalidomide, were enrolled. Three hundred two patients were assigned in a 2:1 ratio to either 28-day cycles of pomalidomide (4 mg/d on days 1-21, orally) plus low-dose dexamethasone (40 mg/d on days 1, 8, 15, and 22, orally) or high-dose dexamethasone (40 mg/d on days 1-4, 9-12, and

Table 100.14. Single Agent and Dexamethasone Doublets for Relapsed or Refractory Disease

Author	Regimen	Phase	N	ORR, %	VGPR/CR, %	PFS/EFS, mo	OS, mo
Singhal[12,520]	Thalidomide	2	169	30	–	2 y 20%	2 y 48%
Dimopoulos et al, 2001[521]	Thal-Dex	2	44	55	–	4.2	12.6
Richardson et al, 2006[522]	Len (30 mg QD)	2	67	17		8	28
	Len (15 mg BID)	2	35	17	0	4	27
Dimopoulos et al, 2007[523]	Len/Dex	3	176	60	16	TTP 11.3	NR
	Dex	3	175	24	3.4	TTP 4.7	20.6
Weber et al, 2007[524]	Len/Dex	3	177	61	14	TTP 11	29.6
	Dex	3	177	20	1	TTP 4.7	20.2
Richardson et al, 2006[522]	Len	2	222	25	0	4.9	23.2
Richardson et al, 2006[525]	Bortezomib	2	193	28	10	7	17
Jagannath et al, 2004[526]	Bortez-Dex (1.0 mg/m²)	2	27	37	19	TTP 10.9	26.7
	Bortez-Dex (1.3 mg/m²)	2	26	50	4	TTP 7.0	NR
Richardson et al, 2005[527]	Bortezomib	3	315	38	13	6	1 y 80%
	Dex	3	312	18	2	3	1 y 66%
Moreau et al, 2011[288]	Bortez-Dex SQ	3	148	52	25	10.4	1 y 72.6
	Bortez-Dex IV	3	74	52	25	9.4	1 y 76.7
San Miguel et al, 2013[528]	Pom-Dex	3	302	31	6	4.0	12.7
	Dex	3	153	10	<1	1.9	8.1
Dimopoulos et al, 2016[529]	Pom-Dex	3b	682	33	8	4.6	11.9
Seigel et al, 2012[530]	Carfilzomib	2	266	23.7	5.4	3.7	15.6
Dimopoulos et al, 2016[531]	Carfilzomib Dex	3	464	77	54	18.7	47.6
	Bortezomib Dex	3	465	63	29	9.4	40
Kumar et al, 2014[200]	Ixazomib weekly	2	66	27	0	NA	NA
Richardson et al, 2014[20]	Ixazomib twice weekly	2	60	15	0	NA	NA
Kumar et al, 2016[532]	Ixazomib (4 mg)—Dex	2	35	31	23	EFS 8.4	NA
	Ixazomib (5.5 mg)—Dex	2	35	54	31	EFS 7.8	NA
Lonial et al, 2016[533]	Daratumumab	2	106	29	12	3.7	1 y 65%
Lokhorst et al, 2015[21]	Daratumumab	2	72	36	8	5.6	NA
Vogl et al, 2018[204]	Selinexor	2	79	21	5	2.3	9.3

Abbreviations: CR, complete response; ORR, overall response rate; OS, overall survival; PFS/EFS, progression-free survival/event-free survival; TTP, time to progression; VGPR, very good partial response.

17-20, orally) until disease progression or unacceptable toxicity. The median PFS with Pd was 4.0 vs 1.9 months with Dex. The most common grade 3 to 4 hematologic AEs were neutropenia, anemia, and thrombocytopenia. Grade 3 to 4 nonhematologic AEs included pneumonia, bone pain, and fatigue. The STRATUS study assessed safety and efficacy of Pd in RRMM.[529] Overall, 682 patients were enrolled with median number of prior regimens of 5. Most frequent grade 3/4 treatment-emergent AEs were hematologic. Most common grade 3/4 nonhematologic toxicities were pneumonia and fatigue. The ORR was 32.6%, and the median PFS and OS were 4.6 and 11.9 months, respectively.

The optimal dose and schedule for pomalidomide remains an issue of debate. The studies done so far have examined either 2 or 4 mg, and given either continuously or for 3 out of every 4 weeks. Richardson and colleagues in a phase I/II dose-escalation study showed that 4 mg pomalidomide daily given for 3 of 4 weeks is the MTD for that particular schedule.[547] The IFM group performed a randomized phase II trial looking at two dosing schedules, 21/28 days or 28/28 days with pomalidomide administered at 4 mg daily with weekly dexamethasone. The ORR and the DOR were comparable with the two strategies as was the overall toxicity.[548]

Proteasome Inhibitors

Bortezomib

Single-agent response rates in RRMM for bortezomib range from 28% to 38% with a median DOR of 8 months[525-527,549] (Table 100.14). In a phase III study, Richardson et al randomly assigned 669 patients with relapsed MM to receive either an IV bortezomib or high-dose dexamethasone.[527] The ORR was significantly higher with bortezomib (38%) compared with dexamethasone (18%), and the median TTPs in the Bd groups were 6.2 and 3.5 months, respectively. Although the original studies using this drug included only eight cycles of therapy, 63 patients were treated on an extension study without significantly more serious AEs than were seen on the parent studies of eight cycles alone.[550]

After the initial studies, peripheral neuropathy remained one of the major issues with use of bortezomib, and attempts were made to reduce the toxicity while maintaining efficacy. Subcutaneous administration of bortezomib was evaluated in a phase III trial comparing the SQ approach with IV administration. Two hundred twenty-two patients were randomized to SQ or IV bortezomib.[288] ORR after four cycles was 42% in both groups, with comparable PFS and OS, showing comparable efficacy. Grade 3 or worse AEs were reported in 57% patients in the SQ group vs 70% in the IV group; the most common were thrombocytopenia, neutropenia, and anemia. Peripheral neuropathy of any grade (38% vs 53%) was significantly less common with SQ than with IV administration. Subcutaneous administration was locally well tolerated.

Bd has been used as the control arm of several large phase III trials in relapsed MM with one to three prior line of therapy and have shown consistent results with a median PFS of 8 to 10 months.[202,240,531]

As with other MM drugs, retreatment with bortezomib is effective, and this strategy has been studied in a phase II trial.[276] In the RETRIVE study, 130 patients with median of two prior lines of therapy were enrolled. At retreatment, 28% and 72% of patients received bortezomib and VD, respectively. ORR was 40%. In patients who achieved PR, median DOR and TTP were 6.5 and 8.4 months, respectively. Thrombocytopenia was the most common grade 3 AE.

Carfilzomib

Carfilzomib is a next-generation, selective proteasome inhibitor that has been approved for treatment of relapsed MM (*Table 100.14*).[198,530,551] In an open-label, single-arm phase II study (PX-171-003-A1), patients received single-agent carfilzomib 20 mg/m^2 IV twice weekly for 3 of 4 weeks in cycle 1, followed by 27 mg/m^2 at the same schedule.[530] Among the enrolled patients, 95% were refractory to their last therapy, and 80% were refractory or intolerant to both bortezomib and lenalidomide. ORR was 24% with a median DOR of 7.8 months and OS of 15.6 months. Common toxicities encountered were fatigue, anemia, nausea, and thrombocytopenia. Neutropenia was limited to grades 1 and 2, occurring in 10% to 15% of the patients.

In another phase II trial, 35 patients with relapsed and/or refractory MM who have received at least one bortezomib-based regimen received carfilzomib 20 mg/m^2 in a twice-weekly, consecutive-day dosing schedule.[198] The best ORR was 17.1%, and the clinical benefit response rate (ORR + minor response) was 31.4%. The median DOR was ~10 months, and the median TTP was 4.6 months. In a similar phase II study, 129 bortezomib-naive patients with RRMM received IV carfilzomib either at 20 mg/m^2 for all treatment cycles, or 20 mg/m^2 for cycle 1 and then 27 mg/m^2 for all subsequent cycles.[551] The ORR was 42.4% in former group and 52.2% in the latter. The clinical benefit response was 59.3% and 64.2%; median DOR was 13.1 months and NR, and median TTP was 8.3 months and NR, respectively.

Carfilzomib at a higher dose of 56 mg/m^2 has been studied in combination with dexamethasone in a large phase III trial, where it was compared with Bd given at standard doses (*Table 100.15*).[531] Overall, 929 patients were randomized to carfilzomib group and 465 to the bortezomib group. At a median follow-up of 11.9 months, the median PFS was 18.7 months in the carfilzomib group vs 9.4 months in the bortezomib group at a preplanned interim analysis. Serious AEs were reported in 224 (48%) of 463 patients in the carfilzomib group and in 162 (36%) of 456 patients in the bortezomib group.

Ixazomib

Ixazomib is the first oral proteasome inhibitor to enter the clinic. Given the success of bortezomib in MM, it was studied extensively in phase I and III trials as single agent as well as in various combinations (*Table 100.14*). Sixty patients with relapsed and/or refractory MM were enrolled on this phase I trial of single-agent ixazomib, given weekly for 3 of 4 weeks, and the MTD was determined to be 2.97 mg/m^2.[200] Common drug-related AEs were thrombocytopenia (43%), diarrhea (38%), nausea (38%), fatigue (37%), and vomiting (35%). The observed rate of peripheral neuropathy was 20%, with only one grade 3 AE. PR or better was seen in 18% patients. In a parallel study, 60 patients received increasing doses of single-agent ixazomib on days 1, 4, 8, and 11 of a 21-day cycle; MTD was 2.0 mg/m^2.[20] The toxicity profile was similar to the once-weekly dosing. Among 55 response-evaluable patients, 15% achieved PR or better.

Ixazomib has been studied in combination with dexamethasone in several phase II trials. Thirty-three patients with relapsed MM were treated with ixazomib, with dexamethasone added for lack of an adequate response.[561] Dexamethasone was initiated in two-thirds of patients, 17 for not reaching the desired response and 5 for progression with an ORR of 34%. Different doses of ixazomib have also been explored in combination with dexamethasone. Seventy patients with relapsed MM were randomized to ixazomib at 4 or 5.5 mg weekly, given for 3 of 4 weeks.[532] Overall, 31% had a response with 4 mg and 54% with 5.5 mg of ixazomib. The median EFS for the entire study population was 8.4 months; 1-year OS was 96%. A grade 3 or 4 AEs considered at least possibly related to treatment were seen in 32% patients at 4 mg and in 60% at 5.5 mg.

Monoclonal Antibodies

Monoclonal antibody therapy has seen resounding success in B-cell malignancies, but has had minimal success with plasma cell disorders until the introduction of elotuzumab and daratumumab.

Elotuzumab

Elotuzumab is a humanized monoclonal IgG1 antibody targeting human CS1, a cell surface glycoprotein. CS1 is highly and uniformly expressed on MM cells, with limited expression on natural killer (NK) cells and CD8$^+$ cells and little to no expression in normal tissues. It was studied as a single agent in 35 patients with RRMM at escalating doses given every 2 weeks. No MTD was identified up to the maximum planned dose of 20 mg/kg. The most common AEs, regardless of attribution, were cough, headache, back pain, fever, and chills. The ORR was disappointing as a single agent, with 9 patients (26.5%) with stable disease.

Daratumumab

Daratumumab is a humanized monoclonal antibody targeted against CD38, which is typically expressed brightly on MM cells. In the GEN502 trial, a dose-escalation phase was followed by a dose-expansion phase with 30 patients treated at 8 mg/kg and 42 at 16 mg/kg.[21] The drug was well tolerated, with no MTD identified and infusion-related reactions easily managed with supportive care. The most common grade 3 or 4 AEs were pneumonia and thrombocytopenia. The ORR was 36% at 16 mg/kg and 10% at 8 mg/kg. In another parallel study, SIRIUS, daratumumab was studied as a single agent in a similar group of patients with relapsed disease.[533] Overall, 106 patients have a median of five previous lines of therapy DOR of 7.4 months and PFS of 3.7 months (*Table 100.14*).

Belantamab-Mafodotin

Belantamab-mafodotin is a monoclonal antibody with a drug conjugate that has been studied in RRMM.[562] The initial recommended dose of the drug based on phase I trials is 3.4 mg/kg dosed once every 3 weeks as a 1-hour IV infusion. The study enrolled 35 patients with multidrug refractory MM; the ORR was 60%. The most frequent AEs included corneal events, thrombocytopenia, anemia, increased aspartate aminotransferase, and cough. A subsequent open-label phase II study evaluated 196 patients (97 in the 2.5 mg/kg cohort and 99 in the 3.4 mg/kg cohort).[245] Thirty (31%) patients in the 2.5 mg/kg cohort and 34 (34%) patients in the 3.4 mg/kg cohort achieved an overall response. The most common grade 3-4 AEs were keratopathy in 27% of patients in the 2.5 mg/kg cohort and 21% of patients in the 3.4 mg/kg cohort in addition to thrombocytopenia and anemia. The current approved dosing for belantamab-mafodotin is at 2.5 mg/kg once every 3 weeks.

Anti-CD20 Antibodies

The human anti-CD20 antibody has demonstrated some effect in patients with MM. About 20% of patients with MM have CD20 expression on their plasma cells. In one study, 1 of 19 patients had a PR to therapy; an additional 5 had stable disease.[563]

Histone Deacetylase Inhibitors

Acetylation and deacetylation of histone proteins play an important role in the regulation of gene expression. Deacetylated histones by binding tightly to the DNA limit access to transcription factors, leading to inhibition of transcription. Acetylation, on the other hand, neutralizes the charge of histones and opens up the DNA conformation, allowing expression of the corresponding genes. The opposing activities of two sets of enzymes, histone acetyltransferase and histone deacetylase (HDAC), control the acetylation status, with normal cells existing in a state of balance. Existing evidence suggest that aberrant recruitment of HDAC may play a role in the changes in gene expression in cancer cells. HDAC inhibitors are thought to affect multiple pathways in MM reversing the abnormalities of cell apoptosis and cell cycle, potentially sensitizing MM cells to apoptosis.[564,565] Several HDAC inhibitors have been studied in the context of MM, including suberoylanilide hydroxamic acid (vorinostat),[566] ITF2357,[567] LBH589 (panobinostat),[23] and romidepsin.[568] Results so far suggest modest single-agent activity in patients with MM.[565]

A phase I trial studied escalating doses of oral vorinostat 200, 250, or 300 mg twice daily for 5 days every week or 200, 300, or 400 mg twice daily for 2 of 3 weeks in patients with RRMM.[569] Thirteen patients were enrolled, and MTD was not reached. Drug-related adverse experiences included fatigue, anorexia, dehydration, diarrhea, and nausea. Of 10 evaluable patients, 1 had a minimal response and 9 had stable disease. Romidepsin is an IV-administered HDAC inhibitor that was studied in a phase II trial, in which patients with MM who were refractory to standard therapy were treated with romidepsin (13 mg/m^2) given as a 4-hour IV infusion on days 1, 8, and 15 every 4 weeks.[568] No objective responses were seen among the 123 patients treated.

Patients ($n = 38$) with relapsed MM and at least two prior lines of chemotherapy and refractory to their most recent line of therapy were enrolled on a trial of single-agent panobinostat.[23] Panobinostat was administered at a dose of 20 mg thrice weekly in a 21-day treatment cycle. There was one PR and one minimal response observed; however, these responses were maintained for 19 and 28 months, respectively.

Other Targeted Therapies With Promising Single-Agent Activity

Venetoclax
Venetoclax is a small molecule inhibitor of bcl2 that has shown considerable activity in chronic lymphocytic leukemia. Sixty-six patients with relapsed MM were placed on escalating doses of venetoclax at 300 to 1200 mg daily after a 2-week lead-in with weekly dose escalation.[570] Patients had received a median of five prior therapies (range, 1-15); 61% were bortezomib and lenalidomide double refractory, and 46% had t(11;14). Most common AEs included nausea, vomiting and diarrhea with thrombocytopenia, neutropenia, anemia, and leukopenia reported in one-quarter of patients. The ORR was 21%, including 15% VGPR or better. Most responses (12/14) were in patients with t(11;14), translating to 40% ORR.

Selinexor
Selinexor is a selective inhibitor of the nuclear export protein XPO1. In a dose-escalation study, 22 patients with heavily pretreated MM and 3 patients with Waldenström macroglobulinemia were treated with selinexor (3-60 mg/m^2) in 8 or 10 doses per 28-day cycle.[571] An additional 59 patients were treated at 45 or 60 mg/m^2 with 20 mg dexamethasone, twice weekly in 28-day cycles, or selinexor (40 or 60 mg flat dose) without corticosteroids in 21-day cycles. The most common nonhematologic AEs were nausea, fatigue, anorexia, vomiting, weight loss, and diarrhea. The most common grade 3 or 4 AEs were hematologic, particularly thrombocytopenia. There was a modest antimyeloma activity with an objective response rate of 4%. However, when it was given with dexamethasone, the ORR was 50% with all responses of greater than or equal to PR occurring in the 45 mg/m^2 selinexor plus 20 mg dexamethasone twice-weekly cohort. In another phase II trial, selinexor 80 mg with dexamethasone 20 mg was administered twice weekly to 79 patients with MM refractory to bortezomib, carfilzomib, lenalidomide, and pomalidomide (quad-refractory disease $n = 48$), with a subset also refractory to an anti-CD38 antibody (penta-refractory disease $n = 31$).[204] The ORR was 21% and was similar for patients with quad-refractory (21%) and penta-refractory (20%) disease; median DOR was 5 months. AEs were similar to the previous study.

Combinations of Novel Agents

The newer drug classes (proteasome inhibitors, IMiDs, monoclonal antibodies, and HDAC inhibitors) have been studied in various combinations, predominantly two drugs with corticosteroids, in several phase III trials (*Table 100.15*).

Carfilzomib, Lenalidomide, and Dexamethasone
Carfilzomib was studied in combination in the ASPIRE phase III trial, where 792 patients with relapsed MM were randomized to lenalidomide and dexamethasone with or without carfilzomib.[553] The PFS was significantly higher in the carfilzomib group (median, 26.3 vs 17.6 months in the control group; $P < .001$). Recent update of the data also demonstrated an OS advantage to the triplet combination. The overall response (PR or better) rates were 87.1% and 66.7% in the carfilzomib and control groups, respectively.

Ixazomib, Lenalidomide, and Dexamethasone
Ixazomib, lenalidomide, and dexamethasone was compared with Rd in a double-blind, placebo-controlled, phase III trial that enrolled 722 patients with relapsed and/or refractory MM.[555] Addition of ixazomib to lenalidomide and dexamethasone led to significantly longer PFS (20.6 vs 14.7 months; $P = .01$). The ORR was 78% in the ixazomib group and 72% in the placebo group. The rates of serious AEs were similar in the two study groups. Thrombocytopenia, skin rash, and gastrointestinal side effects were more common with ixazomib. The incidence of peripheral neuropathy was 27% in the ixazomib group and 22% in the placebo group.

Daratumumab, Lenalidomide, and Dexamethasone
The combination of daratumumab, lenalidomide, and dexamethasone was studied in a large phase III trial, where it was compared with lenalidomide and dexamethasone in 569 patients with relapsed MM who had received one or more previous lines of therapy.[239] The PFS at 12 months was 83.2% in the daratumumab group, compared with 60.1% in the control group. With longer follow-up (44 months) in these lenalidomide nonrefractory patients, median PFS was 44.5 vs 17.5 months.[572] The ORR was higher with addition of daratumumab (92.9% vs 76.4%), as was CR or better (43.1% vs 19.2%), and MRD negativity rates were 30.4% and 5.3% respectively.[572] The most common AEs were neutropenia, thrombocytopenia, and anemia. Daratumumab-associated infusion-related reactions occurred in 47.7% of the patients and were mostly of grade 1 or 2.

Daratumumab, Bortezomib, and Dexamethasone
This combination was compared with Bd in a phase III trial of patients with relapsed MM.[519] Bd was given for only 6 months in both arms, and the daratumumab was continued indefinitely in the experimental arm. The 12-month rates of PFS were 60.7% and 26.9%, respectively. ORR was higher with daratumumab (82.9% vs 63.2%), as were the rates of CR or better (19.2% vs 9.0%). With 40-month follow-up, median PFS was greater with the addition of daratumumab (16.7 vs 7.1 months) as was the MRD-negativity rates (10^{-5}) (14% vs 2%).[573] Common AEs included thrombocytopenia, anemia, and neutropenia. Infusion-related reactions were seen in half of the patients receiving daratumumab.

Elotuzumab, Lenalidomide, and Dexamethasone
This regimen was compared with lenalidomide and dexamethasone in 646 patients in a phase III trial.[556] Elotuzumab, lenalidomide, and dexamethasone had a significantly higher median PFS (19.4 vs 14.9 months); PFS at 1 year (68% vs 57%) and at 2 years (41% vs 27%), respectively. The ORR was higher with elotuzumab at 79% vs 66%. Common grade 3 or 4 AEs in the two groups were lymphocytopenia, neutropenia, fatigue, and pneumonia. Infusion-related reactions

Table 100.15. Randomized Phase II/III Trials of Novel Combinations for Relapsed and/or Refractory Disease

Trial	Regimen	N	ORR, %	VGPR/CR, %	EFS/PFS, mo	Median OS, mo
ENDEAVOR[531]	Kd vs Vd	929	86 vs 82	54 vs 24	18.7 vs 9.4	46.7 vs 40.0
MMVAR/IFM 2005-04[552]	VTD vs TD	269	87 vs 72	56 vs 35	19.5 vs 13.8	2-y 71% vs 65%
ASPIRE[553,554]	KRd vs Rd	792	87 vs 67	70 vs 40	26.3 vs 17.6	73.3% and 65% at 24 mo
TOURMALINE MM1[555]	IRd vs Rd	722	78 vs 72	48 vs 39	20.6 vs 14.7	NR
POLLUX[239]	DRd vs Rd	569	93 vs 76	76 vs 44	NR vs 18.4 mo	1-y 92% vs 87%
CASTOR[240]	DVd vs Vd	498	83 vs 63	59 vs 29	NR vs 7.2	NR
ELOQUENT-2[556]	ERd vs Rd	321	79 vs 66	33 vs 28	19.4 vs 14.9	3-y 60% vs 53%
PANORAMA1[202]	Pano-Vd vs Vd	768	61 vs 55	28 vs 16	12.0 vs 8.1	40.3 vs 35.8
VANTAGE 088[557]	V + Vorinostat vs V	317	56 vs 41	NA	7.6 vs 6.8	NR vs 28
BELLINI[558]	VenVd vs Vd	291	82 vs 68	59 vs 36	22.4 vs 11.5	NR vs NR
OPTIMISMM[559]	PVd vs Vd	559	82 vs 50	53 vs 18	11.2 vs 7.1	N/A
BOSTON[246]	SVd vs Vd	402	76 vs 62	45 vs 32	13.9 vs 9.5	NR vs 25
CANDOR[241]	DKd vs Kd	466	84 vs 75	69 vs 49	NR vs 15.8	18 mo: 80% vs 74%
ELOQUENT-3[244]	EPd vs Pd	117	53 vs 26	20 vs 9	10 vs 5	N/A
APOLLO[560]	DPd vs Pd	304	69 vs 46	51 vs 20	12.4 vs 6.9	N/A
ICARIA-MM[203]	IPd vs Pd	307	60 vs 35	32 vs 9	11.5 vs 6.5	1 y: 72% vs 63%
IKEMA[242]	IKd vs Kd	302	87 vs 83	73 vs 56	NR vs 19.2	N/A

Abbreviations: CR, complete response; Dex, dexamethasone; DKd, daratumumab, carfilzomib, and dexamethasone; DPd, daratumumab, pomalidomide, and dexamethasone; DRd, daratumumab, lenalidomide, and dexamethasone; DVd, daratumumab, bortezomib, and dexamethasone; EFS/PFS, event-free survival/progression-free survival; EPd, elotuzumab, pomalidomide, and dexamethasone; ERd, elotuzumab, lenalidomide, and dexamethasone; IRd, ixazomib, lenalidomide, and dexamethasone; KRd, carfilzomib, lenalidomide, and dexamethasone; NR, not reached; ORR, overall response rate; OS, overall survival; Pano, panobinostat; Pd, pomalidomide and dexamethasone; PVd, pomalidomide, bortezomib, and dexamethasone; SVd, selinexor, bortezomib, and dexamethasone; TD, thalidomide; Vd, bortezomib and dexamethasone; VenVd, venetoclax, bortezomib and dexamethasone; VGPR, very good partial response; VTD, bortezomib, thalidomide, and dexamethasone.

occurred in 10% in the elotuzumab group. With nearly 71-month follow-up, the median OS was 48.3 months for the triplet and 39.6 for the doublet ($P = .048$). The magnitude of the benefit was greatest among patients with adverse prognostic factors such as older age, ISS stage III, IMWG high-risk disease, and 2 to 3 prior lines of therapy.[574]

Panobinostat, Bortezomib, and Dexamethasone

Based on promising results from phase II trial, panobinostat was studied in a phase III trial in combination with Bd.[196] Patients ($n = 768$) received 21-day cycles of placebo or panobinostat (20 mg, 3 days a week for 2 weeks), in combination with bortezomib (1.3 mg/m^2 on days 1, 4, 8, and 11) and dexamethasone (20 mg on days 1, 2, 4, 5, 8, 9, 11, and 12). Median PFS was significantly longer in the panobinostat group (12 vs 8 months; $P < .0001$). The proportion of patients achieving an overall response did not differ between treatment groups 60.7% vs 54.6%, even though the panobinostat group had higher VGPR rate. Common grade 3 to 4 laboratory abnormalities and AEs included thrombocytopenia, lymphopenia, diarrhea, asthenia or fatigue, and peripheral neuropathy.

A similar study assessing the value of vorinostat was negative.[557] Panobinostat had received accelerated FDA approval for its PFS benefit observed when used in combination with Bd and compared to Bd alone. However, the post–approval confirmatory clinical trials were not completed as required and hence its indication for use in the treatment of MM was withdrawn in 2021.

Thalidomide Combinations

In addition to corticosteroids, thalidomide has been combined with a variety of drugs, both old and new.[552] Investigators have combined thalidomide with alkylators either with or without corticosteroids achieving ORRs as high as 79%, including CR rates as high as 26% (Table 100.16). These have included combinations of thalidomide with melphalan, cyclophosphamide or bendamustine, doxorubicin, and corticosteroids.[329-331,575-584]

Pomalidomide, Bortezomib, and Dexamethasone

This combination was evaluated in a phase I/II trial of 50 patients treated with standard dose of Pd with 1 or 1.3 mg/m^2 of bortezomib given weekly SQ.[590] Objective response rate was 86% among all evaluable patients including VGPR or better in 50%. With a median follow-up of 42 months, median PFS was 13.7 months. The most common toxicities were neutropenia, thrombocytopenia, anemia, and fatigue.

Carfilzomib, Pomalidomide, and Dexamethasone

In a phase I dose-escalation study, 32 patients were treated with carfilzomib on days 1, 2, 8, 9, 15, and 16 of 28-day cycles, starting at 20/27 mg/m^2, along with Pd at standard doses.[591] The MTD of the regimen was dose level 1 (carfilzomib 20/27 mg/m^2, pomalidomide 4 mg, and dexamethasone 40 mg). Hematologic AEs were common, but rates of neuropathy were low. The ORR was 50% with a median PFS of 7.2 months. Similar results have also been observed with once-weekly carfilzomib given at similar dose with Pd.[592]

Daratumumab, Pomalidomide, and Dexamethasone

This combination was studied in 103 patients with RRMM who had at least two prior lines of therapy and was refractory to their last treatment.[593] Treatment consisted of standard dose and schedule of the three agents. Daratumumab was associated with infusion-related reactions in half of the patients. ORR was 60%, including 29% who were MRD negative. The median PFS was 8.8 months, and median OS was 17.5 months.

Daratumumab, Carfilzomib, and Dexamethasone

A phase III, open-label, multicenter trial included 466 patients randomized RRMM patients with 1 to 3 prior lines of therapy in 2:1 fashion to carfilzomib, dexamethasone, and daratumumab (KdD) or Kd.[241] After median follow-up of approximately 17 months, median PFS was not reached in the KdD group vs 15.8 months in the Kd group.

Table 100.16. Combinations of Immunomodulatory Drugs With Traditional Chemotherapy for Relapsed/Refractory Disease

Author	Regimen	Phase	N	ORR, %	VGPR/CR, %	PFS/EFS, mo	OS, mo
Offidani et al, 2003[575]	Mel-Thal	2	27	60	12	2-y PFS 61%	2-y OS 61%
Hovenga et al, 2005[576]	CTX Thal	2	38	75	11	30	20
Garcia-Sanz et al, 2004[577]	CTX-Dex-Thal	2	71	55	2	2-y EFS 57%	2-y OS 66%
Dimopoulos et al, 2004[578]	CTX-Dex-Thal	2	53	60	5	TTP 8.2	17.5
Kropff et al, 2003[579]	CTX-Dex-Thal	2	60	68	3	11	19
Kyriakou et al, 2005[580]	LD CTX-Dex-Thal	2	52	79	17	—	—
Sidra et al, 2006[581]	CTX-Dex-Thal	2	47	83	19	—	—
Palumbo et al, 2006[582]	Mel-Pred-Thal IV	2	24	42	13	9	—
Suvannasankha et al, 2007[583]	CTX-Thal-Pred	2	35	63	26	—	—
Ponisch et al, 2008[584]	Benda-Thal-Pred	1/2	28	85	35	11	19
Offidani et al, 2006[330]	Thal-PLD-Dex	2	50	76	38	17	NR
Zervas et al, 2004[331]	Thal-PLD-Vcr-Dex	2	39	74	10	—	—
Hussein et al, 2006[329]	Thal-PLD-Vcr-Dex	2	49	75	44	15.5	39.9
Knop et al, 2015[585]	Len-Dox-Dex	1/2	69	77	—	—	—
Schey et al, 2010[586]	Cyclo-Len-Dex	1/2	31	81	36	56% at 2 y	80% at 2.5 y
Lentzsch et al, 2012[587]	Len-Benda-Dex	1/2	36	52	24	4.4	NR
Palumbo et al, 2010[588]	Len-Mel-Pred-Thal	1/2	44	75	34	51% at 1 y	72% at 1 y
Baz et al, 2006[589]	PLD-Vcr-Dex-Len	1/2	62	75	29	12	NR

Abbreviations: Benda, bendamustine; Bortez, bortezomib; CR, complete response; CTX, cyclophosphamide; Dex, dexamethasone; Dox, doxorubicin; EFS, event-free survival; Len, lenalidomide; LD, low-dose; Mel, melphalan; N, number of patients; NR, not reached; ORR, overall response rate; OS, overall survival; PFS, progression-free survival; PLD, pegylated doxorubicin; PR, partial response; Pred, prednisone; Thal, thalidomide; TTP, time to progression; Vcr, vincristine; VGPR, very good partial response.

MRD-negative CR at 12 months was 13% in the KdD group compared to 1% in the Kd group. Grade 3 or higher AEs were reported in 82% of patients in the KdD group and 74% patients in the Kd group. The frequency of AEs leading to treatment discontinuation was similar in both groups.

Isatuximab, Pomalidomide, and Dexamethasone

A phase III, open-label, multicenter trial included 307 patients randomized RRMM patients with 1 to 3 prior lines of therapy in 1:1 fashion to isatuximab, pomalidomide, and dexamethasone (IPd) or Pd.[203] At a median follow-up of 11.6 months, median PFS was 11.5 months in the IPd group vs 6.5 months in the Pd group. MRD-negativity (in the intention-to-treat population) was observed in 5% of patients at 10^{-5} in the IPd group, but none in the Pd group. The most frequent any grade treatment emergent AEs for IPd vs Pd were infusion reactions (38% vs 0%), upper respiratory tract infections (28% vs 17%), and diarrhea (26% vs 20%).

Isatuximab, Carfilzomib, and Dexamethasone

A phase III, open-label, multicenter trial included 466 patients randomized RRMM patients with 1 to 3 prior lines of therapy in 3:2 fashion to isatuximab, carfilzomib, and dexamethasone (IKd) or Kd.[242] Median PFS was not reached in the IKd group compared with 19 months in the Kd group. Twenty percent of patients in the IPd group and 11% in the Pd group had a CR and MRD-negative response. Grade 3 or higher TEAEs was observed in 77% of patients in the IPd group vs 67% in the Pd group.

Elotuzumab, Bortezomib, and Dexamethasone

In a randomized phase II study, patients with RRMM were treated with elotuzumab with bortezomib and dexamethasone (EBd) or Bd.[594] Overall, 152 patients were randomized (77 EBd and 75 Bd): Median PFS was longer with EBd (9.7 months) vs Bd (6.9 months). ORR was 66% (EBd) vs 63% (Bd), including VGPR or better occurred in 36% of patients (EBd) vs 27% (Bd). In general, infusion reaction rate was low and easily managed with premedication.

Elotuzumab, Pomalidomide, and Dexamethasone

In a randomized phase II study, patients with RRMM who were refractory to lenalidomide and a proteasome inhibitor were treated with elotuzumab with pomalidomide and dexamethasone (EPd) or Pd.[244] The ORR was 53% in the elotuzumab group as compared with 26% in the control group. The median PFS among these patients was 10.3 months in the EPd group compared to 4.7 months in the Pd group. The most common grade 3 or higher AEs were cytopenias of neutropenia and anemia.

Venetoclax and Its Combinations

Preclinical studies demonstrating synergy when venetoclax was combined with bortezomib formed the basis for a dose-escalation study of the combination in patients with RRMM.[595] Treatment consisted of daily venetoclax (50-1200 mg per designated dose cohort; 800 mg in safety expansion) in combination with Bd. Overall, 66 patients with a median of three prior therapies were enrolled. The most common AEs included diarrhea, constipation, nausea, and cytopenias (thrombocytopenia and anemia). The ORR was 67%; 42% achieved VGPR or better. Median TTP was 9.5 months. Patients with high BCL2 expression had a higher ORR (17/18) than those with low BCL2 expression (16/27). This combination of venetoclax, bortezomib, and dexamethasone was compared in a phase III randomized and double-blind trial to Bd and yielded a superior PFS (22.4 vs 11.5 months).[558] The benefit was confined to those with t(11;14) and high *BCL-2* expression; however, there were more deaths in the venetoclax arm early on after randomization. Infectious causes of death were higher with venetoclax, but given the imbalance of deaths being predominant in the non t(11;14) and low *BCL-2* expression cohort, possibilities of venetoclax selecting out a more aggressive and resistant clone leading to rapid disease progression have been hypothesized but not proven.

The safety and tolerability as well as efficacy of venetoclax was also evaluated in combination with carfilzomib and dexamethasone (VenKd) in adults with RRMM were investigated in this phase 2 dose-escalation study.[596] Oral venetoclax (400 or 800 mg) was administered daily in combination with IV carfilzomib (27, 56, or 70 mg/m^2) and oral dexamethasone (20 or 40 mg). The expansion cohort received venetoclax 800 mg, carfilzomib 70 mg/m^2, and dexamethasone 40 mg. The ORR was 80% in all patients, 92% in patients with t(11;14) (n = 13), and 75% in patients without (n = 36). The rate of CR or better was 41%. Median PFS was 22.8 months. The most common treatment-emergent AEs were diarrhea (65%), fatigue (47%), nausea (47%), and lymphopenia (35%).

Finally, the safety and efficacy of venetoclax was also evaluated in combination with daratumumab and dexamethasone without bortezomib (VenDd) or with bortezomib (VenDVd) in a phase 1 dose escalation and expansion trial.[597] The expansion phase dose of venetoclax in both regimens was 800 mg. The ORR was 96% with VenDd all of which were ≥ VGPR and 92% with VenDVd of which 79% were ≥ VGPR. The 18-month PFS rate was 91% with VenDd and 67% with VenDVd. Common AEs with VenDd and VenDVd included diarrhea (63% and 54%) and nausea (50% and 50%).

Combinations of Novel Agents With Conventional Agents

The newer drugs can also be combined the traditional antimyeloma agent to develop effective drug combinations. These include the alkylating agents such as melphalan, cyclophosphamide and bendamustine, anthracyclines, and platinum drugs (Table 100.17). A myriad of combinations have been studied in smaller trials, and the discussion here regimens listed in Tables 100.16 and 100.18 are limited to the regimens that have shown promising activity.[13,586-589,606-619]

Bortezomib, Pegylated Doxorubicin, and Dexamethasone

In an international phase III study, 646 patients were randomly assigned to receive either IV bortezomib with or without PLD.[620] The ORR was similar between bortezomib (41%) and PLD + bortezomib (44%). Median TTP was increased from 6.5 to 9.3 months with the combination, and the 15-month survival rate for the combination was 76% compared with 65% for bortezomib alone.

Bortezomib, Cyclophosphamide, and Dexamethasone

This combination has been used extensively in the setting of NDMM, but also may have a role in the management of relapsed disease.[621,622] In phase I to II trials evaluating escalating doses of bortezomib, 1.3 mg/m^2 on days 1, 4, 8, and 11 and 1.5 mg/m^2 on days 1, 8, and 15, each on a 28-day cycle, was safely combined with cyclophosphamide 300 mg/m^2/wk and prednisone.[608] The ORR was 95% with CR observed in more than 50% of patients. The weekly bortezomib regimen resulted in lower rates of thrombocytopenia and peripheral neuropathy. The 1-year PFS and OS were 83% and 100%, respectively. Studies combining the newer proteasome inhibitors such as carfilzomib and bortezomib with cyclophosphamide are ongoing.

Lenalidomide, Adriamycin, and Dexamethasone

In a phase II trial, Knop et al studied 69 patients with relapsed MM; MTD was not reached at lenalidomide (R), 25 mg on days 1 to 21; adriamycin (A), 9 mg/m^2 IV on days 1 to 4; and dexamethasone (D), 40 mg on days 1 to 4 and 17 to 20.[585] Hematologic toxicity was the main finding, thromboembolic events occurred in 4.5% and severe infections in 10.5% of patients. The ORR was 73% for the whole study.

Cyclophosphamide, Lenalidomide, Dexamethasone/Prednisone

Reece et al studied the combination of cyclophosphamide 300 mg/m^2 on days 1, 8, and 15, lenalidomide 25 mg on days 1 to 21, and prednisone 100 mg every other day in a 28-day cycle.[623] The regimen resulted in no dose-limiting toxicity with an ORR of 94%. The median PFS was 16.1 months, and median OS was 27.6 months. β_2M level at protocol entry correlated with a better survival (P = .047).

Pomalidomide, Cyclophosphamide, and Dexamethasone

Baz et al studied the combination in a multicenter randomized phase II study in patients with lenalidomide-refractory MM.[624] Patients were randomized to receive pomalidomide-dexamethasone or pomalidomide, dexamethasone, and cyclophosphamide (PCd) 400 mg orally on days 1, 8, and 15. The ORR was 38.9% for Pd and 64.7% for PCd; median PFS was 4.4 and 9.5 months, respectively. Hematologic toxicity was the most common AE and was higher with cyclophosphamide. Other studies have shown comparable results.[625]

Table 100.17. Ongoing Single Arm Studies Evaluating Bispecific Antibodies Targeting Various MM Antigens and CD3

	Teclistamab[598]	Elranatamab[599,a]	TNB-383B[600,a]	AMG-701[601,a]	CC-93269[602,a]	REGN-5458[603,a]	Talquetamab[604,a]	Cevostamab[605,a]
Target	BCMA	BCMA	BCMA	BCMA	BCMA	BCMA	GPRC5D	FCRh5
Frequency	Weekly	Weekly	Q3 weeks	Weekly	Weekly	Weekly	Weekly	Weekly
Administration	SubQ	SubQ	IV	IV	IV	IV	SubQ	IV
No of Pts	40 pts treated at phase 2 dosing (1500 µg/kg after 60 and 300 µg/kg step up doses)	30	44 pts treated at dose of 40 mg or higher (RP2D is 60 mg)	75	30	45	72 (RP2D is SC 405 µg/kg)	51 (Arm A: Dose escalation)
Median Prior[a] therapies	5	8	5	6	6	5	6	6
Triple class refractory	83%	87%	55%	62%	90%	100%	100%	67%
ORR%	65% (≥VGPR 58%)	83% (≥VGPR 67%)	79% (≥VGPR 63%)	83% (≥VGPR 50%)	89%	36% (60% at highest dose level)	63% (≥VGPR 50%) at RP2D	52% (dose level of 3.6/20 mg or higher)
Duration of response	Median is NR	NR at 13 mo	N/A	NR at 7 mo	NR	6 mo	NR at 7 mo	NR at 7 mo
Grade 3+ CRS	None	None	None	N/A	N/A	N/A	1%	2%

Abbreviations: BCMA, B-cell maturation antigen; CRS, cytokine release syndrome; NR, not reached; ORR, overall response rate; VGPR, very good partial response.
[a]Reported only in abstract form and presented at national meetings but has not been presented in a peer-reviewed publication.

Table 100.18. Multidrug Combinations of Proteasome Inhibitors and Traditional Drugs for Relapsed, Refractory Disease

Author	Regimen	Phase	N	Or, %	VGPR, %	PFS/EFS, mo	OS, mo
Berenson et al, 2008[606]	Bortez-Mel-Pred	1/2	46	70	35	9	32
Popat et al, 2009[607]	Bortez-IV Mel	2	53	68	23	10	28
Reece et al, 2008[608]	CTX-Bortez-Pred	1/2	37	95	50	83% at 1 y	100% at 1 y
Kropff et al, 2007[609]	CTX-Bortez-Dex	2	54	90	16	12	22
Ciolli et al, 2006[610]	Low-dose Bortez-Thal-Dex	2	18	44	11	–	–
Pineda-Roman et al, 2005[611]	Bortez-Thal-Dex	2	85	55	–	9	22
Palumbo et al, 2007[612]	Bortez-MP-Thal	1/2	30	67	43	61% at 1 y	84% at 1 y
Terpos et al, 2008[613]	Bortez-MD-Thal	2	25	66	43	9.3	–
Kim et al, 2010[614]	Bortez-CTX-Thal-Dex	2	70	88	55	14.6	31.6
Berenson et al, 2012[615]	Bortez-PLD-Dex	2	40	48	31	–	–
Orlowski[13,616]	Bortez-PLD	3		44		9.3	76%
	Bortez			41		6.5	65%
Chanan-Khan et al, 2010[617]	Bortez-PLD-Dex-Thal	2	23	56	–	10.9	15.7
Ciolli et al, 2008[618]	Bortez-Thal-Dex	2	28	50	–	8	–
	Bortez-Thal-Dex-PLD	2	42	81	–	15	–
Richardson et al, 2010[619]	Bortez-Len-Dex	1/2	38	39	–	6.9	37

Abbreviations: Bortez, bortezomib; CR, complete response; CTX, cyclophosphamide; Dex, dexamethasone; EFS, event-free survival; Len, lenalidomide; Mel, melphalan; N, number of patients; NR, not-reached; OR, overall response; OS, overall survival; PFS, progression-free survival; PLD, pegylated doxorubicin; PR, partial response; Pred, prednisone; Thal, thalidomide; TTP, time to progression; VGPR, very good partial response.

Bendamustine, Lenalidomide, and Dexamethasone

In a phase II trial in patients with relapsed MM, bendamustine 75 mg/m² was given on days 1 and 2, with lenalidomide 25 mg on days 1 to 21 and dexamethasone 40 mg on days 1, 8, 15, and 22.[626] Seventy-one patients were accrued with median of three prior lines of therapy. ORR was 49%, including 29% with a VGPR or better; median PFS was 11.8 months. Grade 3 or higher hematologic toxicity was seen in 94% and nonhematologic toxicities in 50%.

Bendamustine, Bortezomib, and Dexamethasone

This combination has been studied in several trials. In one study, 79 patients with RRMM were treated with bendamustine 70 mg/m² days 1 and 4; bortezomib 1.3 mg/m² IV days 1, 4, 8, and 11; and dexamethasone 20 mg days 1, 4, 8, and 11 once every 28 days was given for up to eight cycles.[627] The ORR was 60.8%, PFS was 9.7, and OS was 25.6 months. Hematologic toxicity and neuropathy were the most common toxicities.

VDTPACE

In a retrospective analysis of outcomes of 141 patients with RRMM who received VDTPACE and similar regimens, a minimal response was seen in 68.4%, PR in 54.4%, and ≥VGPR in 10.3% patients.[628] Median PFS was 3.1 months, and median OS was 8.1 months. In heavily pretreated patients, these regimens can provide meaningful responses that can be the bridge to additional therapies, such as transplant.

Conventional Drug Combinations for Relapsed or Refractory Disease

With the increasing use of the novel drug combinations in the frontline and early relapse settings, patients are often not exposed to the traditional chemotherapy agents, such as alkylators and anthracyclines (Table 100.19). The drugs, especially the alkylating agents, can often be combined with steroids or a multidrug regimen with remarkable efficacy and benefit even in the late stages of disease.[18,562,629–636,638] Although there is cross-resistance among the alkylators, it is not absolute and may be circumvented by increasing dose intensity. Without extreme dose intensification, response rates as high as 30% to 38% can be obtained if prednisone is administered with cyclophosphamide.[629,639,640] Higher doses of cyclophosphamide (e.g., 600 mg/m² IV for 4 consecutive days) result in response rates of 29% to 43%.[631,641] Both DOR and OS tend to be short, approximately 3 and 9 months, respectively.

Dose intensification of melphalan can also be quite effective and is the basis for HDT with stem cell support.[197] Selby et al[642] reported that 66% of patients with resistant disease treated with 140 mg/m² without stem cell support responded, but median DOR was 6 months, with all patients relapsing within a year. Median times to leukocyte and platelet recovery were 42 and 37 days, respectively, and the regimen-related toxicity was 13%. Doses of 50 to 70 mg/m² result in a 50% response rate and leukocyte and platelet recovery time of 20 and 16 days, respectively.[633,643] Further reducing the intensity to 30 mg/m² every 2 months results in response rate of 38% and PFS of 10 months.[644]

VBMCP (the M-2 regimen) or MOCCA (melphalan, vincristine, cyclophosphamide, lomustine, doxorubicin) provided responses in 20% to 30% of refractory patients with a median survival of about 11 months.[635] After studying high-dose cytosine arabinoside, cisplatin, and etoposide as single agents, Barlogie et al[408] did preliminary studies of DAP (dexamethasone, cytosine arabinoside, and cisplatin) and later EDAP (etoposide and DAP). In patients with refractory disease, response rates with these treatments were 7%, 14%, 17%, 0%, and 40%, respectively. Median survival in patients treated with EDAP was 4.5 months. This regimen is myelosuppressive, with more than half of treated patients requiring platelet transfusions and 80% requiring hospitalization for neutropenic fever. In the first month, TRM was 15%.

Cellular Therapies

Recent advances in the manufacturing of cellular therapies such as the chimeric antigen receptor (CAR)-T cells have led to a novel modality of therapy for MM. CARs are fusion proteins in which an antigen recognition moiety is coupled via an extracellular spacer region

Table 100.19. Conventional Drug Combinations for Relapsed, Refractory Disease

Author	Regimen	N	ORR, %	DOR, mo	OS, mo
de Weerdt et al, 2001[629]	Continuous low-dose CTX; Pred	42	38	—	—
Trieui et al, 2005[630]	Weekly CTX; Pred	66	41	—	28.6
Lenhard et al, 1994[631]	CTX IV; Pred	48	29	—	8.6
Petrucci et al, 1989[632]	IV Mel25/m^2	34	34	16	8
Tsakanikas et al, 1991[633]	IV Mel50-70/m^2	18	50	—	11.5
Barlogie et al, 1984[357]	VAD	29	59	>12	—
Dimopoulos et al, 1996[634]	HyperCVAD	58	40	8	15
Finnish Leukaemia Group, 1992[635]	MOCCA	80	49	22	31
Lee et al, 2003[636]	DTPACE	148	32	—	—
Barlogie et al, 1989[18]	EDAP	20	40	—	4.5
Bonnet et al, 1982[637]	VBAP	151	25	—	7.6

Abbreviations: CTX, cyclophosphamide; DOR, duration of response; DTPACE, dexamethasone, thalidomide, cisplatin, doxorubicin, cyclophosphamide, etoposide; EDAP, etoposide, dexamethasone, doxorubicin, cisplatin; HyperCVAD, cyclophosphamide, vincristine, doxorubicin, dexamethasone; mel, melphalan; MOCCA, melphalan, vincristine, cyclophosphamide, lomustine, doxorubicin; N, number of patients; ORR, overall response rate; OS, overall survival; Pred, prednisone; VAD, vincristine, doxorubicin, dexamethasone; VBAP, vincristine, carmustine, doxorubicin.

(hinge) and a transmembrane-spanning element to a T-cell activation domain, which has typically been CD3ζ. Furthermore, incorporation of a costimulatory domain (CD28, 4-1BB or others) into the CAR endodomain has resulted in improved antitumor activity of these modified T cells. After a short course of lymphodepleting chemotherapy, CAR-T cells are infused into patients intravenously where they subsequently expand in number upon recognition of tumor cells. The tumor cells are then destroyed by the CAR-T cells in a non–major histocompatibility complex-restricted manner. While the antigen recognition moiety can be modified to target various unique antigens expressed on the target tumor cell, CAR-T cells targeting the B-cell maturation antigen (BCMA) protein are farthest along in clinical development. BCMA is consistently expressed on the surface of normal and malignant plasma cells and by mature B cells. It has a crucial role in the survival of long-lived plasma cells in the bone marrow.

Idecabtagene Vicleucel

Idecabtagene vicleucel is an FDA-approved CAR T-cell product expressing a murine BCMA-targeting single-chain variable fragment with a 4-1BB costimulatory motif. In the phase 1 CRB-401 study, an overall response was observed in 85% of patients who were heavily pretreated, including a CR or better in 42% of patients.[645] Median PFS was 11.8 months with improved PFS in patients receiving doses equal to or higher than 150 × 10^6 CAR T cells. A total of 25 patients (76%) had cytokine release syndrome (CRS), which was of grade 1 or 2 in 23 patients (70%) and grade 3 in 2 patients (6%). Neurologic toxic effects occurred in 14 patients (42%) and were of grade 1 or 2 in 13 patients (39%). As a result, the subsequent phase 2 KarMMa study used idecabtagene vicleucel with a target dose of 450 × 10^6 CAR T cells; range 150 × 10^6 to 450 × 10^6 in a group of 128 patients with triple-class exposed MM.[205] Across all administered doses, a PR or better response was observed in 94 (73%) of 128 patients with 42 (33%) having a CR or better. MRD-negative status (<10^{-5} nucleated cells) was confirmed in 33 (26%) patients. The median PFS was 8.8 months. CRS was reported in 107 patients (84%), including 7 (5%) who had events of grade 3 or higher. Neurotoxic effects developed in 23 patients (18%) and were of grade 3 in 4 patients (3%); no neurotoxic effects higher than grade 3 occurred.

Ciltacabtagene Autoleucel

Ciltacabtagene autoleucel is a 4-1BB–based CAR T-cell therapy with two BCMA-targeting domains.[646] The activity of ciltacabtagene autoleucel was explored in a phase 1b/2 study (CARTITUDE-1) in triple-class exposed patients with MM. A single cilta-cel infusion (target dose 0.75 × 10^6 CAR-positive viable T cells per kg) was administered 5 to 7 days after start of lymphodepletion. Of 97 patients treated with ciltacabtagene autoleucel at the phase II target dose of 0.75 × 10^6 CAR T cells per kg, there was a 97% response rate, and 65 (67%) patients had a CR. Of 57 evaluable patients for MRD status, 53 (93%) achieved MRD negativity. The 12-month PFS and OS was 77% and 89% respectively. Finally, AEs such as CRS occurred in 92 (95%) patients (4% were grade 3 or 4), whereas CAR T-cell neurotoxicity occurred in 20 (21%) patients (9% were grade 3 or 4).

Bispecific Antibodies

Bispecific antibodies are designed to bind both a target on the malignant plasma cells as well as a target on cytotoxic immune effector cells [T cells (CD3)/NK (CD16) cells] to create an immunologic synapse, leading to T/NK-cell activation and destruction of malignant plasma cells. To maximize efficacy and minimize toxicity, bispecific antibodies are designed to target an antigen that is unique and specific to MM cells, with minimal expression in other healthy tissues. Although there are numerous potential myeloma cell targets, four targets have been used in current phase I trials: BCMA, CD38, GPRC5D, and FcRH5 and are described in Table 100.17.[598-600,602-605] Given the off-the-shelf nature of these products and the absence for a lead time needed to manufacture T-cells, this modality is an attractive immunotherapy option for patients with MM and has significant potential to move into earlier lines of therapy.

RADIATION THERAPY

As early as the mid-1920s, there was recognition that external beam radiation therapy could promote immediate relief of pain, healing of pathologic fractures, and resolution of extramedullary plasmacytomas.[647-649] Until the 1950s, radiation therapy was the only effective treatment available for the management of plasma cell tumors. With the advent of systemic chemotherapy, indications for irradiation were primarily palliation of bone pain and solitary plasmacytomas. Concern for maintaining bone marrow reserve also constrains the use of radiation in patients with MM. Sykes et al[650] showed that radiation has long-term effects on the bone marrow; the majority of patients receiving concentrated local doses of 3500 cGy or more showed persistent localized marrow aplasia. One must administer enough radiation to provide palliation, without jeopardizing opportunities for further systemic therapy. In a retrospective review, Norin[651] has found that objective improvement was lacking when the tumor dose was below a cumulative dose (single-dose equivalent) of 1000 cGy. For palliation, the recommendation is, therefore, a cumulative dose of 1500 cGy, corresponding to a tumor dose of 3400 cGy in 10 to 15 fractions.[651,652] Leigh et al[653] recommended a total cumulative dose of 1000 cGy in these same patients. There is controversy as to whether the DOR correlates with the radiation dose in MM patients.[653,654]

In contrast, the conventional wisdom has been that patients with solitary plasmacytoma of bone should receive higher doses in an attempt at cure. Although the optimal dose has not been established by randomized controlled trials, 4000 to 5000 cGy encompassing all disease with a margin of normal tissue is recommended by most experts.[655-657] A study of 203 patients with solitary plasmacytoma of bone has brought this principle into question.[658] These authors found that therapeutic doses above 3000 cGy had no bearing on local control.

Radiation can often spare patients from undergoing surgery.[659] In a retrospective analysis of 35 cases of patients with cervical lesions and spinal instability, it was found that 19 of the 20 patients experience resolution of pain, 15 of whom received radiation alone. Of the 10 patients with sufficient follow-up data, none showed clinical progression of instability.

The first report of using whole-body irradiation to treat MM was by Medinger and Craver[660] in 1942. Partial or complete relief of pain was noted in the majority of patients. Once effective systemic chemotherapy came into wide use, this approach became less popular until 1971 when Bergsagel[661] postulated that sequential hemibody radiation could be a means of debulking tumor. He suggested that if a dose of approximately 725 cGy were given to the upper half of the body and 1000 cGy to the lower half, a theoretical 3-log kill could be achieved and survival prolonged. After a series of retrospective studies and a randomized study[518,662] evaluating its role in the earlier phases of MM, hemibody irradiation has once again fallen out of favor. In patients who have end-stage disease, with poor pain control, this treatment may still be important.

The majority of series involving hemibody or sequential hemibody radiation are retrospective and include patients who were either resistant to or relapsing from alkylator-based therapy. Significant relief of bone pain occurred in 80% to 90% of patients, and the median duration of survival was 5 to 11 months.[652,663] Objective biochemical response occurred in 25% to 50% of patients.[663] Pain relief typically occurred 1 to 2 days after institution of therapy, with a maximal response in 1 to 2 weeks.[664] The most common side effects were moderate myelosuppression, pneumonitis, nausea, vomiting, diarrhea, and stomatitis.[652] If an oral lead shield was not used, mucositis also occurred. Nadirs occurred within 3 weeks,[663] and white cell count and platelet count recovery occurred by about 6 weeks. Decrements in pulmonary function occurred in about half of the treated patients.[652] The most serious complication was radiation-induced pneumonitis, which was seen in 14% of patients.[663]

TREATMENT OF COMPLICATIONS AND SUPPORTIVE CARE

Complications Specific to Immunomodulatory Drugs

Thrombosis is an important complication in patients undergoing treatment with IMiDs. As a single agents, there does not appear to be any heightened risk; however, concomitant chemotherapy[612]—especially anthracyclines[665,666]—high-dose corticosteroids,[247,264,667] and erythropoietin[668] appear to increase the risk of thrombosis to as high 58%. A phase III trial[669] compared ASA (100 mg/d), low-dose warfarin (1.25 mg/d), and enoxaparin (40 mg/d) in 667 patients with previously untreated MM receiving a thalidomide-based regimen. The primary endpoint was a composite that included serious thromboembolic events, acute cardiovascular events, or sudden deaths during the first 6 months of treatment. The most frequent complications were thromboembolic events that occurred in 5.9% in the ASA group, 8.2% in the warfarin group, and 3.2% in the low–molecular-weight heparin (LMWH) group. Symptomatic PE episodes occurred only in the ASA and warfarin groups. The absolute differences for serious thromboembolic events were +2.7% ($P = .173$) between ASA and LMWH groups and +5.0% ($P = .024$) between warfarin and LMWH groups. These results did not reach a statistical significance. The same group conducted a prospective trial compared ASA to LMWH in 342 newly diagnosed patients[670] who were treated with lenalidomide and dexamethasone or MPR. Patients were randomly assigned to receive ASA 100 mg/d ($n = 176$) or LMWH enoxaparin 40 mg/d ($n = 166$). The incidence of VTE was 2.27% in the ASA group and 1.20% in the LMWH group, a difference that was not significant. Based on this, ASA can be an effective and less-expensive alternative to LMWH thromboprophylaxis. Of note, however, patients considered high risk for VTE were excluded from both these studies. Those patients with advanced age, inherited thrombophilic abnormalities, recent surgery, or a history of VTE should be considered for full-dose anticoagulation.

Pharmacologic Therapy of Myeloma Bone Disease

Myeloma bone disease is a significant contributor to morbidity, and relationships between bone turnover and plasma cell growth and survival are described. Bisphosphonate therapy has been the standard since the late 1990s. A randomized trial has demonstrated that treating with bisphosphonates not only helps prevent secondary bony events in patients with existing bone lesions, but that the use of monthly zoledronic acid (ZA) as compared to clodronate increases median OS of all patients (whether they have bone lesions or not) by 6 months.[671] In a double-blind, randomized phase III trial, denosumab has been shown to be noninferior to ZA.[672] Adequate calcium and vitamin D supplementation are also essential.

A meta-analysis was not able to confirm superiority of ZA over pamidronate, but remarkably revealed a survival advantage of ZA vs placebo.[673] This analysis also showed that in order to prevent one SRE, we need to treat 6 to 15 MM patients with BP. Bisphosphonates inhibit dissolution of the hydroxyapatite crystals and downregulate the major osteoclast functions. After internalization, the nitrogen-containing bisphosphonates interfere with the biosynthetic mevalonate pathway by inhibiting farnesyl diphosphonate synthase with resultant inability of osteoclasts to form the ruffled borders of their membrane needed to activate bone resorption.

The first study showing a reduction of almost 50% of secondary skeletal events among MM patients who received monthly IV administration of pamidronate was published in 1996.[674] At 12 months, there were fewer skeletal-related events in the pamidronate group than in placebo-treated patients (28% vs 44%; $P < .001$). With longer follow-up of 21 months, the difference between groups persisted but narrowed slightly to 28% in the pamidronate group vs 51% in the placebo group ($P < .015$).[675] This prospective study subsequently led the FDA to approve the use of the drug in this setting. In February 2002, the FDA approved an expanded indication for ZA for the treatment of patients with bone metastases that included its use in MM.

Despite the fact that the longest follow-up of patient in these studies was 24 months, the recommendation by the American Society of Clinical Oncology was to continue these agents indefinitely at monthly intervals.[676] In the short-term, the drugs were well tolerated—occasional episodes of mild pyrexia, renal function impairment, myalgias, and hypocalcemia. However, by 2003, avascular osteonecrosis of the jaw (ONJ) was described as a complication associated with their use. Bisphosphonate-associated ONJ has been described in various malignancies. Although most patients who develop ONJ had recent dental or oral surgical procedures (70%), the remainder developed spontaneous ONJ.[677] Proposed mechanisms include that inhibition of osteoclast activity reduces bone turnover and remodeling and that bisphosphonates prevent release of bone-specific factors that promote bone formation.[678] In addition, bisphosphonates, particularly ZA, may have antiangiogenic effects, which have been implicated in the development of ONJ. Finally, healing of an open bony oral wound may be challenged by bacterial insult from oral microflora. The true incidence of this complication is hard to estimate, but is somewhere around 6.8% to 9.9%.[679,680] Risk factors for ONJ are longer duration of treatment, ZA (as compared to pamidronate). In one study,[679] patients who developed ONJ received a median number of 35 infusions (range, 13-68) compared to 15 infusions (range, 6-74) for patients with no ONJ. The optimal dosing schedule and duration of therapy have not been adequately defined by randomized clinical trials. One retrospective study suggested quarterly infusions of ZA are as effective as monthly infusions with less risk of ONJ.[681] A randomized trial comparing 12-weekly vs 4-weekly ZA among breast cancer patients showed equivalency between the two schedules.[682]

Most would agree that 1 to 2 years of IV bisphosphonate is standard after a dental checkup. The role of these drugs after this time point is uncertain, especially if patients are in CR. Many opt to reduce the frequency of administration after 2 years, especially if disease is in remission. Once on these drugs, invasive dental procedures should be limited if possible.

Denosumab (a fully human monoclonal antireceptor activator of nuclear factor-κB ligand antibody) was compared to ZA for delaying or preventing skeletal-related events.[672] Denosumab was noninferior to ZA in delaying first skeletal event. Hypocalcemia was more commonly seen in the denosumab-treated patients. Care should be taken with discontinuing denosumab because in patients with osteoporosis, there may be a rebound in osteoporotic fractures among patients who had not previously received bisphosphonates. Although denosumab does not adversely affect renal function, patients with severe renal dysfunction are more sensitive to the development of hypocalcemia.

The standard method of following patients is with periodic (every 12-24 months) skeletal imaging—CT skeletal radiography is the preferred standard.

Nonpharmacologic Treatment of Myeloma Bone Disease

When a lytic bone lesion is present, significant risk factors for fracture of a long bone include increased pain with use and the involvement of more than the diameter of the bone. These lesions should be treated prophylactically with surgery if they are situated in weight-bearing bones. Endosteal resorption of one-half the cortical width of the femur weakens the bone by 70%. Surgical treatment should be considered for these lesions as well.[683] Once a bone has fractured, healing can occur, especially if proper internal fixation is performed and if patients have an anticipated survival of >6 months. Much of the data regarding malignant bone disease are derived from patients with carcinoma rather than MM. In patients with carcinoma metastatic to bone, modest postoperative radiation doses (≤3000 cGy) as adjuvant therapy are associated with better healing,[684] but the role of adjuvant radiation therapy in MM patients is less clear. MM is often chemotherapy sensitive; adjuvant systemic chemotherapy in MM patients may be more appropriate than adjuvant radiation therapy. In general, radiation therapy should be used for pain relief in chemotherapy-refractory disease because it relieves pain in 80% to 90% of patients with bony metastases,[685] long term in 55% to 70%.[686]

Percutaneous vertebroplasty is occasionally an option for patients with vertebral body compression fracture. Pain relief is generally apparent within 1 to 2 days after injection and persists for at least several months up to several years.[687] Complications are relatively rare, although some studies reported a high incidence of clinically insignificant leakage of bone cement into the paravertebral tissues. Compression of spinal nerve roots or neuralgia as a result of the leakage of polymer and PE has also been reported. Percutaneous kyphoplasty is also an option.[688] There is one published trial in patients with MM that randomized patients in an unblinded fashion to kyphoplasty or nonsurgical management.[689] At 1 month, the back-specific disability score was significantly better in the kyphoplasty group. Because patients in the control group had the option of crossing over to the kyphoplasty arm, there are no long-term data on outcomes.

Spinal Cord Compression

In a paper published in 1979, it was estimated that nearly 10% of patients with MM either present with spinal cord compression or that it develops during the course of the disease[690]; with higher awareness of MM and better imaging technology, the incidence is likely lower now. Cord compression, however, remains an important and emergent subject. The usual standard treatment is high-dose corticosteroids and radiation therapy. On rare occasions, surgical decompression may be considered. Because most myelomatous lesions arise from the vertebral body, an anterior surgical approach is generally used, which may contribute additional morbidity. One small randomized trial addressing the question of radiation vs laminectomy and radiation showed no benefit attributable to laminectomy[691]; similarly, a larger retrospective series found no benefit.[692] If the deficit is caused by compression by the plasma cell tumor (rather than a bone fragment retropulsed by a pathologic compression fracture), outcomes with radiation therapy are probably equal to (or superior to) surgical intervention in a radiosensitive tumor-like MM.[691,692]

High-dose corticosteroids may provide immediate pain relief and improvement in neurologic function. The optimal corticosteroid dose has not been established, but common dose schedules for metastatic disease include dexamethasone in an initial bolus of 10 mg IV or 100 mg IV followed by 4 mg orally four times daily, or a 100 mg IV bolus followed by 96 mg in four divided doses for 3 days followed by tapering doses.

Hypercalcemia

Patients with MM are at risk of severe hypercalcemia that can precipitate acute renal failure, hypertension, nausea, vomiting, pancreatitis, cardiac arrhythmia, coma, and death. The extracellular volume depletion associated with hypercalcemia should be corrected by vigorous hydration[663,693] followed by an antiresorptive agent such as IV bisphosphonate or subcutaneous denosumab. Serum calcium values usually declines rapidly, reaching the normal range within 2 to 3 days in more than 80% of cases. It occasionally goes below normal at the nadir. Corticosteroids can also reduce serum calcium concentration in about 60% of patients with hypercalcemia.[694]

Secondary Myelodysplasia and Acute Leukemia

The most ominous cause of anemia in the setting of previously treated MM is a secondary myelodysplastic syndrome or acute leukemia. Kyle et al were among the first to recognize that cytotoxic agents can induce myelodysplasia and acute myeloid leukemia.[491-494] With alkylator-based therapy, the risk of a secondary myelodysplastic syndrome or acute leukemia is approximately 3% at 5 years and 10% at 8 to 9 years,[695,696] with estimates as high as 25% at 10 years.[697] Some authors have suggested that higher cumulative doses of melphalan are implicated as a risk for acute leukemia.[695] Others have shown no difference in incidence based on the number of courses of chemotherapy or the cumulative melphalan dose between the patients who did and did not develop acute leukemia.[696] Although cyclophosphamide has been shown to be leukemogenic, data suggest that it is less so than melphalan.

The occurrence of concurrent acute leukemia in MM suggests that there may be a proclivity for acute leukemia to develop in patients with MM. After SCT for MM, the risk of myelodysplastic syndrome appears to be related to prior chemotherapy rather than to the transplant itself, at least in one retrospective series. Lenalidomide maintenance also has been shown to increase the risk of myelodysplastic syndromes and secondary malignancies.

Cryoglobulinemia and Hyperviscosity

Approximately 5% of MM gamma globulins exhibit reversible precipitation in the cold, so-called cryoglobulins, forming either a flocculent precipitate or a gel-like coagulum when the serum is cooled.[698] Plasmapheresis relieves the symptoms of hyperviscosity, but the benefit of this treatment in the absence of concurrent chemotherapy is short-lived.[699]

Renal Failure

Normal creatinine values are present in approximately 50% of MM patients at diagnosis,[83,117] and only 15% to 25% have a creatinine value above 2 mg/dL.[83,700] Patients in whom the renal failure is reversed have a better OS than those without improvement.[121,701] Factors that increase renal tubular cast formation include dehydration, infection, and hypercalcemia. There is some controversy around best management of patients with renal failure in terms of plasmapheresis and the relative importance of alkalinizing urine, but there are four points that are incontrovertible: (1) achieve a deep hematologic response as soon as possible, (2) avoid nephrotoxic drugs, (3) correct hypercalcemia, and (4) correct dehydration (maintaining a 24-hour fluid intake of at least 3 L can improve renal function).[121]

In terms of best chemotherapeutic regimens to achieve rapid hematologic response, several have already been discussed. A bortezomib-based regimen, such as CyBorD, VTD, or PAD, is often favored in the setting of renal failure. In a recent trial in which patients were randomized to VAD or PAD followed by ASCT, the subset of patients presenting with creatinine above 2 mg/dL and who were randomized to PAD had a markedly improved median survival as compared to the VAD patients (54 vs 21 months, $P < .001$). Because light chains with the lowest isoelectric points tend to be more nephrotoxic in animal models, avoidance of a low or acidic urinary pH is recommended. Oral or IV bicarbonate is useful in the setting of acute renal failure. The third MRC MM trial randomized MM patients with significant renal failure to oral sodium bicarbonate to neutralize urine pH (or not), and there was a trend toward better survival in the bicarbonate recipients.[121]

The use of plasmapheresis in the setting of renal failure remains controversial. There are three randomized trials addressing this question, with conflicting results. One small randomized study of patients with active MM and progressive renal failure suggested benefit in a subset of patients.[702] Twenty-one patients were randomized to either forced diuresis and chemotherapy (10 patients) or forced diuresis, chemotherapy, and plasmapheresis (11 patients). There was a trend toward better outcome in the plasmapheresis group, but the difference was not statistically significant. It is unclear whether the lack of significance is either because of the small sample size or because of an equivalence of the two therapeutic strategies. The study did demonstrate that the severity of MM cast formation directly correlated with lack of improvement regardless of treatment strategy.

Another randomized study in MM patients with severe renal compromise compared plasma exchange (and hemodialysis when needed) with peritoneal dialysis.[703] All patients received chemotherapy and corticosteroids. Of the 29 patients in the study, 24 received dialysis and 5 maintained serum creatinine concentrations of greater than 5 mg/dL without dialysis. Of the 15 patients in the plasmapheresis ± hemodialysis group, 13 recovered renal function, reaching serum creatinine values of less than or equal to 2.5 mg/dL in most cases, whereas only 2 patients in the peritoneal dialysis group had enough improvement to stop dialysis. The 1-year survival rates were 66% and 28%, respectively ($P < .01$). The study's design was flawed in that one group received peritoneal dialysis and the other hemodialysis; the question about the role of plasmapheresis is not adequately settled.

The largest trial was a negative study.[704] One hundred four patients with NDMM and a creatinine of 2.3 mg/dL were randomized to conventional chemotherapy with or without five to seven sessions of plasma exchange over 10 days. The primary outcome was a composite measure of death, dialysis dependence, or glomerular filtration rate of less than 30 mL/min/1.73 m^2. At 6 months, the endpoint was reached in 58% of the plasma exchange group and 69% of the control group. At 6 months, 7 of the 39 control patients (18%) and 5 of 58 plasma exchange patients (9%) were on dialysis. At 6 months, 33% of each group had died. Criticisms of this study included the patient selection, including the absence of renal biopsy, the use of relatively ineffective conventional chemotherapy, and small sample size. Patients were eligible if the serum creatinine level was 2.3 mg/dL with an increase greater than 0.6 mg/dL in the preceding 2 weeks despite correction of hypercalcemia, hypovolemia, and metabolic acidosis. This would imply that institution of plasma exchange was delayed and that there could have been other underlying pathologic renal lesions other than cast nephropathy, which would not be responsive to plasma exchange. More than twice as many patients on the plasma exchange group had MP as in the control group, which could have confounded the results because both ORRs are lower and time to response is longer with MP than with VAD.

Infection Management

Infections are a major cause of morbidity in MM patients.[705,706] Pneumonias and urinary tract infections caused by *Streptococcus pneumoniae*, *Haemophilus influenzae*, and *Escherichia coli* are most frequent.[273,707-709] The susceptibility to infection varies with the phase of illness. In one prospective study, the overall serious infection rate was 0.92 infections per patient-year and was four times higher during periods of active disease (1.90) than in plateau-phase MM (0.49).[710] A recent trial randomized 959 newly diagnosed ASCT-eligible patients to either levofloxacin 500 mg daily for 12 weeks or placebo and found that significantly fewer of the levofloxacin-treated patients than placebo-treated patients had events (febrile episode or death) during these 12 weeks: 19% vs 27%.[711] Other studies have not consistently demonstrated benefit from antibiotic prophylaxis.[712,713] Infections late in the course of MM may be an inevitable result of long-standing immunosuppression and overwhelming tumor burden. Prevention of infection is a critical goal for improving survival.

Prevention of infections by use of vaccines is an attractive strategy. Unfortunately, responses to vaccines are poor among MM patients. In one study, specific antibody titers to pneumococcal capsular polysaccharides and tetanus and diphtheria toxoids were significantly reduced in MM patients compared with the control population.[710] In addition, among 41 immunized patients, responses to pneumococcus vaccine and tetanus and diphtheria toxoids were poor.

A randomized, double-blind placebo-controlled trial demonstrated that intravenous immunoglobulin (IVIg) significantly reduced the number of infections in high-risk patients with plateau-phase MM.[714] Eighty-two such patients received either IVIg (0.4 g/kg/mo) or an equal volume of placebo for 1 year. There were no episodes of septicemia or pneumonia in patients receiving IVIg compared with 10 in placebo patients ($P = .002$). There were 38 serious infections in 470 patient-months for the placebo group, compared with 19 in 449 patient-months for the IVIg group ($P = .019$). A poor antibody response to pneumococcal vaccination (<twofold increase) identified patients who had maximum benefit from IVIg. However, IVIg is expensive and inconvenient and can be associated with toxicity. Therefore, use of this agent is recommended only for patients with a significant history of severe infections.

SPECIAL CASES OF MYELOMA

Concurrent AL Amyloidosis

AL (immunoglobulin light chain) amyloidosis is a plasma proliferative disorder associated with the overproduction of monoclonal light chains. Rarely, patients with MM may be diagnosed with AL amyloidosis before or around the time of the MM diagnosis. MM that develops more than 6 months after the diagnosis of AL amyloidosis is even less common.[715] The concurrent diagnoses occur when the monoclonal light chains are also amyloidogenic in nature. These AL-amyloidosis patients that have a coexisting MM have a worse OS prognosis than patients with AL-amyloidosis alone.[716] While anti–plasma cell therapies used in MM remain the cornerstone for the treatment of this variant, management of this entity is discussed in more detail in Chapter 101.

Plasma Cell Leukemia

PCL is a rare form of PCD. Between 2% and 4%[174,717,718] of malignant PCD cases are PCL. By definition, there are more than 20% plasma cells in the peripheral blood with an absolute plasma cell count of more than 2×10^9/L. Some authors accept the diagnosis with only one of these criteria.[719] The presentation may be primary, de novo, or secondary, evolving from an existing case of MM as part of the terminal phase of the disease. About 60% to 70% of cases are primary.[717] Recently, the IMWG[720] has redefined the cutoff of plasma cells in the peripheral blood to 5% or more rather than 20% based on similar poor survival outcomes observed in patients with 5% to 19% circulating plasma cells.[721-723]

PCL plasma cells more frequently express the CD20 antigen[174] than those of MM (50% vs 17%), and they often lack CD56 antigen,[174,192] which is present on the majority of MM cells.[174] CD56 is considered important in anchoring plasma cells to bone marrow stroma and is associated with a poor prognosis.[724,725] CD28 is more frequently expressed on malignant plasma cells in secondary than in primary PCL, which is consistent with an observation made in MM, that is, that acquisition of the CD28 antigen on plasma cells appears to correlate with an increased proliferative rate and disease progression.[726]

PCL plasma cells have higher proliferative rates[174] and more complex karyotypes than MM plasma cells.[718] By comparative genomic hybridization and FISH techniques, losses on 13q[727,728] and monosomy 13[174] exist in more than 80% of PCL patients.[727,728] Losses on chromosome 16 also occur in about 80% of cases.[728] Gains in 1q are present in about half of the patients by FISH,[174] but in all by comparative genomic hybridization.[728] In addition, PCL patients have unique losses of 2q and 6p. Overexpression of PRAD1/cyclin D1 and t(11;14) is commonly observed in PCL.[729] The gene expression profile of PCL is different from that of MM.[730]

The clinical presentation of primary PCL is more aggressive than that of MM, with a higher presenting tumor burden and higher frequencies of extramedullary involvement, anemia, thrombocytopenia, hypercalcemia, renal impairment,[174,717,718,731] increased levels of serum LDH and β_2M, and plasma cell proliferative activity.[174] The incidence of lytic bone lesions is slightly lower than that usually observed in MM.

Though the clinical and laboratory features of primary and secondary PCL are similar,[732,733] the response to therapy and OS in primary and secondary PCL go from poor to worse.[734,735] Higher response rates can be achieved with multiagent chemotherapy rather than single alkylator programs (47%-66% vs 8%-13%). Novel agent-based therapy that includes proteasome inhibitors, immunomodulators, and monoclonal antibodies followed by ASCT is a preferred approach.[736-738] However, at times with highly proliferative disease and significant disease burden, older regimens such as VTD-PACE, HyperCVAD-VTD, PAD, etc, can be helpful in acutely debulking the amount of disease burden before proceeding to a consolidation and maintenance strategy. Some patients derive excellent responses and 2- to 3-year disease-free survival after ASCT.[739-743] In a prospective phase II trial, patients with primary PCL were treated with a regimen that combined standard chemotherapy, a proteasome inhibitor, and high-dose melphalan and ASCT followed by either allogeneic transplantation or bortezomib/lenalidomide maintenance. In the intention-to-treat analysis, the median PFS and OS were 15.1 (95% CI: 8.4; -) and 36.3 (95% CI: 25.6; -) months, respectively.[744]

Saccaro et al[745] reported on the cumulative outcomes of the literature of PCL patients undergoing hematopoietic SCT. Median survival post-ASCT was 36 months, whereas it was only 12 months after allo-SCT. Registry studies have shown that OS with primary PCL approaches that of MM, and upfront ASCT appears to outperform allo-SCT even when reduced-intensity protocols are used.[746] Response and survival rates with secondary PCL remain low.

Osteosclerotic Myeloma (POEMS Syndrome)

Osteosclerotic myeloma is a rare variant of MM (≤3.3% of cases).[747] There is an osteosclerotic variant that is similar to MM in that anemia, significant bone marrow plasmacytosis, hypercalcemia, and renal insufficiency occur.[99] Survival in these patients is comparable to that of classic MM patients. There is, however, a more interesting form, which is known as Crow-Fukase syndrome, PEP (PCD, endocrinopathy, polyneuropathy) syndrome, Takatsuki syndrome, and POEMS syndrome. This variant is discussed in Chapter 103.

Light-Chain Deposition Disease

The nonamyloidogenic LCDDs are caused by pathologic protein deposition in various tissues and organs. Unlike the light-chain deposits observed in patients with immunoglobulin light-chain amyloidosis, these infiltrates are not congophilic by light microscopy, and by electron microscopy, nonbranching fibrils are not observed. Instead, amorphous nodular deposits are seen. LCDD may occur with or without coexistent MM. For more information, see Chapter 102.

Nonsecretory Multiple Myeloma

Nonsecretory MM accounts for 1% to 5% of MM cases. With more sensitive testing like immunofixation[748] and free light-chain assays,[85] a majority of these "nonsecretory" patients are found to be low secretors or oligosecretory. More than 85% of cases have a cytoplasmic monoclonal protein; in the remainder, no monoclonal protein can be detected in the cytoplasm.[749-751] Individuals in this latter group are referred to as "nonproducers." From a clinical standpoint, both are termed "nonsecretory." Median survival of these patients is at least as good as for those with secretory MM. Response is difficult to document, but with the new serum assays, quantitation of free light chains is possible in about two-thirds of these patients.[85]

Immunoglobulin M, D, and E Multiple Myeloma

IgM MM, which comprises only about 1% of MM cases, should not be confused with Waldenström macroglobulinemia.[83] IgD MM accounts for about 2% of all cases of MM.[752] The presence of a monoclonal IgD in the serum usually indicates MM, but three cases of IgD MGUS have been documented.[719] Patients with IgD MM generally present with a small band or no evident M spike on serum protein electrophoresis. Their clinical presentation is similar to that of patients with Bence Jones MM (light-chain MM) in that both have a higher incidence of renal insufficiency and coincident amyloidosis as well as a higher degree of proteinuria than in IgG or IgA MM.[752] IgD MM patients, however, appear to have a higher frequency of monoclonal λ light chain than κ light chains. With an incidence of 19% to 27%, extramedullary involvement is more prevalent in patients with IgD MM.

IgE MM is a rare form of MM. A disproportionate number of cases are PCL, although the sample size is small, with only about 40 cases of IgE MM reported in the literature.

Solitary Plasmacytoma of Bone

Solitary plasmacytoma of bone is a rare form of plasma cell proliferative disease. It accounts for about 2% to 5% of malignant PCDs treated at large referral centers. In most series, the definition has required the following characteristics: (1) histologic proof that the solitary lesion is a plasmacytoma; (2) no other bone lesions on metastatic bone survey; (3) less than 5% plasma cells from a random bone marrow biopsy site; and (4) the absence of anemia, hypercalcemia, or renal insufficiency that had no attributable cause. Some definitions allow for <10% bone marrow plasma cells, and others have restricted the quantity of the serum or urine M spike. Others have excluded patients who developed disseminated MM within a year after diagnosis of the solitary plasmacytoma.[753] The IMWG has adopted the above definition, but adds that if done, MRI should not demonstrate any other areas of marrow involvement.[76] Monoclonal proteins are present in about 50% of patients.

There is a clear male preponderance, and the median age is 55 years. Plasmacytomas most commonly arise from the axial skeleton, particularly the vertebral bodies. Pain is the usual presentation. Spinal cord or nerve root compression may also be present. If the patient also has evidence of a peripheral neuropathy, and especially if the bone lesion is sclerotic, one should consider the diagnosis of POEMS syndrome (see Chapter 103).

Careful staging should be done in all patients, including a complete blood cell count, protein electrophoresis and immunofixation of the serum and urine, serum immunoglobulin–free light chains, a complete radiographic skeletal survey, and random bone marrow aspiration and biopsy. At a minimum, immunohistochemical stains should be done on the bone marrow to identify a clone apart from the solitary plasmacytoma. MRI of the entire spine and pelvis should also be done to determine whether the lesion is solitary. Using MRI, Moulopoulos et al[106] found unexpected bone marrow involvement in 4 of 12 patients with apparently solitary plasmacytomas of bone. FDG-PET may also provide useful information.

From an historical perspective, solitary plasmacytomas of bone were treated surgically with or without adjuvant radiation. Present-day, single-modality, definitive radiation therapy is the treatment of choice. Although the optimal dose has not been established by randomized controlled trials, 4000 to 5000 cGy encompassing all disease with a margin of normal tissue is recommended by most experts on the basis of retrospective local relapse rate data.[655] This principle, however, has been challenged by recent data, which show no difference in local control as long as the therapeutic dose is over 3000 cGy.[658]

Median 10-year disease-free survival is about 25% to 40%.[655,754] Median time to failure, that is, local relapse, appearance of another plasmacytoma, or disseminated MM, is about 2 years,[655,658] but these figures are contaminated by inadequate staging of patients. In a retrospective study at a major academic institution, fewer than 5% of patients referred for a diagnosis solitary plasmacytoma of bone had adequate baseline staging.[755] The majority of patients with a solitary "plasmacytoma of bone" had a low burden of clonal plasma cells in their marrow. Because these patients are typically not offered immediate chemotherapy, a novel term was used to label these patients, "plasmacytoma plus." The 21-month disease-free survival of patients that did not satisfy criteria for "plasmacytoma plus" was 100%. Furthermore, detection of even very low numbers of clonal plasma cells in the bone marrow by adopting advanced multiparametric flow cytometry technologies is a risk factor for shorter TTP to MM.[756]

Risk factors for evolution to MM include the absence of a monoclonal protein at presentation (nonsecretory disease), depression of immunoglobulin values at presentation, persistence of the monoclonal protein after treatment,[754] abnormal immunoglobulin free light chain ratio at presentation,[757] tumor size of more than 5 cm, and a nonvertebral presentation.[658] The persistence of a monoclonal protein after radiation therapy does not guarantee relapse,[655] even after more than 10 years of follow-up.[754] In rare instances, the maximum reduction of myeloma protein may take several years after completion of the radiation therapy.[655] Median survival for all patients presenting with solitary plasmacytoma of bone—based on data from patients staged before routine use of MRI and bone marrow clonality studies—was approximately 10 years.[655,658,754] Adjuvant chemotherapy has not been shown to produce a survival advantage and carries the risk of treatment-related myelodysplastic syndromes or acute leukemia; it cannot be recommended.

Solitary Extramedullary Plasmacytoma

Solitary extramedullary plasmacytomas represent about 3% of all plasma cell neoplasms.[758] They most commonly affect men in their early 60s and occur in the upper respiratory tract (paranasal sinuses, nose, nasopharynx, and tonsils). They also occur in lymph nodes, lung, thyroid, gastrointestinal tract, liver, spleen, pancreas, testes, breast, or skin.[759] Amyloid involvement of the plasmacytoma occurs on occasion. Although extramedullary plasmacytomas are not common in NDMM, classic MM must be excluded by thorough staging. A monoclonal protein in the serum and urine, lytic bone lesions, anemia, renal insufficiency, and hypercalcemia should be excluded. Histologically, an extramedullary plasmacytoma should be differentiated from reactive plasmacytosis, plasma cell granuloma, poorly differentiated neoplasms, and immunoblastic lymphoma. Some extramedullary plasmacytomas may represent marginal zone B-cell lymphomas that have undergone plasmacytic differentiation.[760] Dimopoulos et al[758] compiled 128 extramedullary plasmacytoma patients from eight published series and summarized their clinical course. The local failure rate was 7%, multifocal extramedullary relapse occurred in 13%, and classic MM developed in 15%. Local radiation therapy is the treatment of choice, and adjuvant chemotherapy is not recommended. The 10-year disease-free survival is 70% to 80%. Ozsahin et al[761] compiled 52 patients through a Rare Cancer Network study. Their findings were similar with a 5-year progression rate of about 25% and a 5-year survival approaching 90%. Finally, a rare but distinct form of extramedullary plasmacytomas that express IgA has been identified and is characterized by frequent lymph node involvement and an indolent clinical course as reflected by a lower risk of progression to MM.[762]

Websites

Helpful websites for patients and doctors may include the following:
  http://myeloma.org/
  http://www.themmrf.org/
  msmart.org
  clinicaltrials.gov

References

1. Siegel RL, Miller KD, Fuchs HE, Jemal A. Cancer statistics, 2021. *CA Cancer J Clin.* 2021;71(1):7-33.
2. Harris NL, Jaffe ES, Stein H, et al. A revised European-American classification of lymphoid neoplasms: a proposal from the International Lymphoma Study Group. *Blood.* 1994;84(5):1361-1392.
3. Kyle RA. Multiple myeloma: an odyssey of discovery. *Br J Haematol.* 2000;111(4):1035-1044.
4. Thorn GW, Forsham PH, Frawley RF, et al. The clinical usefulness of ACTH and cortisone. *N Engl J Med.* 1950;242:824.
5. Blokhin N, Larionov L, Perevodchikova N, Chebotareva L, Merkulova N. Clinical experiences with sarcolysin in neoplastic diseases. *Ann N Y Acad Sci.* 1958;68(3):1128-1132.
6. Bergsagel DE, Sprague CC, Austin C, Griffith KM. Evaluation of new chemotherapeutic agents in the treatment of multiple myeloma. IV. L-Phenylalanine mustard (NSC-8806). *Cancer Chemother Rep.* 1962;21:87-99.
7. Bergsagel DE, Griffith KM, Haut A, Stuckey WJ Jr. The treatment of plasma cell myeloma. *Adv Cancer Res.* 1967;10:311-359.
8. Korst DR, Clifford GO, Fowler WM, Lewis J, Will J, Wilson HE. Multiple myeloma. II. Analysis of cyclophosphamide therapy in 165 patients. *J Am Med Assoc.* 1964;189:758-762.
9. Mellstedt H, Aahre A, Bjorkholm M, et al. Interferon therapy in myelomatosis. *Lancet.* 1979;2(8144):697.
10. Alberts DS, Salmon SE. Adriamycin (NSC-123127) in the treatment of alkylator-resistant multiple myeloma: a pilot study. *Cancer Chemother Rep.* 1975;59(2 pt 1):345-350.
11. Salmon SE. Nitrosoureas in multiple myeloma. *Cancer Treat Rep.* 1976;60(6):789-794.
12. Singhal S, Mehta J, Desikan R, et al. Antitumor activity of thalidomide in refractory multiple myeloma. *N Engl J Med.* 1999;341(21):1565-1571.
13. Orlowski RZ, Stinchcombe TE, Mitchell BS, et al. Phase I trial of the proteasome inhibitor PS-341 in patients with refractory hematologic malignancies. *J Clin Oncol.* 2002;20(22):4420-4427.
14. Richardson PG, Schlossman RL, Weller E, et al. Immunomodulatory drug CC-5013 overcomes drug resistance and is well tolerated in patients with relapsed multiple myeloma. *Blood.* 2002;100(9):3063-3067.
15. Alberts DS, Balcerzak SP, Bonnet JD, Stephens RL. Phase II trial of mitoxantrone in multiple myeloma: a Southwest Oncology Group Study. *Cancer Treat Rep.* 1985;69(11):1321-1323.
16. Sumpter K, Powles RL, Raje N, et al. Oral idarubicin as a single agent therapy in patients with relapsed or resistant multiple myeloma. *Leuk Lymphoma.* 1999;35(5-6):593-597.
17. Chisesi T, Capnist G, de Dominicis E, Dini E. A phase II study of idarubicin (4-demethoxydaunorubicin) in advanced myeloma. *Eur J Cancer Clin Oncol.* 1988;24(4):681-684.
18. Barlogie B, Velasquez WS, Alexanian R, Cabanillas F. Etoposide, dexamethasone, cytarabine, and cisplatin in vincristine, doxorubicin, and dexamethasone-refractory myeloma. *J Clin Oncol.* 1989;7(10):1514-1517.
19. Streetly MJ, Gyertson K, Daniel Y, Zeldis JB, Kazmi M, Schey SA. Alternate day pomalidomide retains anti-myeloma effect with reduced adverse events and evidence of in vivo immunomodulation. *Br J Haematol.* 2008;141(1):41-51.
20. Richardson PG, Baz R, Wang M, et al. Phase 1 study of twice-weekly ixazomib, an oral proteasome inhibitor, in relapsed/refractory multiple myeloma patients. *Blood.* 2014;124(7):1038-1046.
21. Lokhorst HM, Plesner T, Laubach JP, et al. Targeting CD38 with daratumumab monotherapy in multiple myeloma. *N Engl J Med.* 2015;373(13):1207-1219.
22. Zonder JA, Mohrbacher AF, Singhal S, et al. A phase 1, multicenter, open-label, dose escalation study of elotuzumab in patients with advanced multiple myeloma. *Blood.* 2012;120(3):552-559.
23. Wolf JL, Siegel D, Goldschmidt H, et al. Phase II trial of the pan-deacetylase inhibitor panobinostat as a single agent in advanced relapsed/refractory multiple myeloma. *Leuk Lymphoma.* 2012;53(9):1820-1823.
24. Landgren O, Kyle RA, Pfeiffer RM, et al. Monoclonal gammopathy of undetermined significance (MGUS) consistently precedes multiple myeloma: a prospective study. *Blood.* 2009;113(22):5412-5417.
25. Greenberg AJ, Rajkumar SV, Larson DR, et al. Increased prevalence of light chain monoclonal gammopathy of undetermined significance (LC-MGUS) in first-degree relatives of individuals with multiple myeloma. *Br J Haematol.* 2012;157(4):472-475.
26. Vachon CM, Kyle RA, Therneau TM, et al. Increased risk of monoclonal gammopathy in first-degree relatives of patients with multiple myeloma or monoclonal gammopathy of undetermined significance. *Blood.* 2009;114(4):785-790.
27. Cuzick J. Multiple myeloma. *Cancer Surv.* 1994;19-20:455-474.
28. Schwartz GG. Multiple myeloma: clusters, clues, and dioxins. *Cancer Epidemiol Biomarkers Prev.* 1997;6(1):49-56.
29. Landgren O, Linet MS, McMaster ML, Gridley G, Hemminki K, Goldin LR. Familial characteristics of autoimmune and hematologic disorders in 8,406 multiple myeloma patients: a population-based case-control study. *Int J Cancer.* 2006;118(12):3095-3098.

30. Altieri A, Chen B, Bermejo JL, Castro F, Hemminki K. Familial risks and temporal incidence trends of multiple myeloma. *Eur J Cancer.* 2006;42(11):1661-1670.
31. Ichimaru M, Ishimaru T, Mikami M, Matsunaga M. Multiple myeloma among atomic bomb survivors in Hiroshima and Nagasaki, 1950-76: relationship to radiation dose absorbed by marrow. *J Natl Cancer Inst.* 1982;69(2):323-328.
32. Shimizu Y, Kato H, Schull WJ. Studies of the mortality of A-bomb survivors. 9. Mortality, 1950-1985: Part 2. Cancer mortality based on the recently revised doses (DS86). *Radiat Res.* 1990;121(2):120-141.
33. Preston DL, Kusumi S, Tomonaga M, et al. Cancer incidence in atomic bomb survivors. Part III. Leukemia, lymphoma and multiple myeloma, 1950-1987. *Radiat Res.* 1994;137(2 suppl):S68-S97.
34. Iwanaga M, Tagawa M, Tsukasaki K, et al. Relationship between monoclonal gammopathy of undetermined significance and radiation exposure in Nagasaki atomic bomb survivors. *Blood.* 2009;113(8):1639-1650.
35. Lewis EB. Leukemia, multiple myeloma, and aplastic anemia in American radiologists. *Science.* 1963;142(3598):1492-1494.
36. Matanoski GM, Seltser R, Sartwell PE, Diamond EL, Elliott EA. The current mortality rates of radiologists and other physician specialists: specific causes of death. *Am J Epidemiol.* 1975;101(3):199-210.
37. Wang JX, Boice JD Jr, Li BX, Zhang JY, Fraumeni JF Jr. Cancer among medical diagnostic x-ray workers in China. *J Natl Cancer Inst.* 1988;80(5):344-350.
38. Wing S, Richardson D, Wolf S, Mihlan G, Crawford-Brown D, Wood J. A case control study of multiple myeloma at four nuclear facilities. *Ann Epidemiol.* 2000;10(3):144-153.
39. Muirhead CR, Bingham D, Haylock RGE, et al. Follow up of mortality and incidence of cancer 1952-98 in men from the UK who participated in the UK's atmospheric nuclear weapon tests and experimental programmes. *Occup Environ Med.* 2003;60(3):165-172.
40. Pearce N, Prior I, Methven D, et al. Follow up of New Zealand participants in British atmospheric nuclear weapons tests in the Pacific. *Br Med J.* 1990;300(6733):1161-1166.
41. Friedman GD. Multiple myeloma: relation to propoxyphene and other drugs, radiation and occupation. *Int J Epidemiol.* 1986;15(3):424-426.
42. Andersson M, Storm HH. Cancer incidence among Danish Thorotrast-exposed patients. *J Natl Cancer Inst.* 1992;84(17):1318-1325.
43. Hatcher JL, Baris D, Olshan AF, et al. Diagnostic radiation and the risk of multiple myeloma (United States). *Cancer Causes Control.* 2001;12(8):755-761.
44. Boice JD Jr, Morin MM, Glass AG, et al. Diagnostic x-ray procedures and risk of leukemia, lymphoma, and multiple myeloma. *J Am Med Assoc.* 1991;265(10):1290-1294.
45. Boice JD Jr, Day NE, Andersen A, et al. Second cancers following radiation treatment for cervical cancer. An international collaboration among cancer registries. *J Natl Cancer Inst.* 1985;74(5):955-975.
46. Darby SC, Doll R, Gill SK, Smith PG. Long term mortality after a single treatment course with X-rays in patients treated for ankylosing spondylitis. *Br J Cancer.* 1987;55(2):179-190.
47. Wiklund K, Dich J. Cancer risks among male farmers in Sweden. *Eur J Cancer Prev.* 1995;4(1):81-90.
48. Ronco G, Costa G, Lynge E. Cancer risk among Danish and Italian farmers. *Br J Ind Med.* 1992;49(4):220-225.
49. Kristensen P, Andersen A, Irgens LM, Laake P, Bye AS. Incidence and risk factors of cancer among men and women in Norwegian agriculture. *Scand J Work Environ Health.* 1996;22(1):14-26.
50. Sonoda T, Ishida T, Mori M, et al. A case-control study of multiple myeloma in Japan: association with occupational factors. *Asian Pac J Cancer Prev.* 2005;6(1):33-36.
51. Cerhan JR, Cantor KP, Williamson K, Lynch CF, Torner JC, Burmeister LF. Cancer mortality among Iowa farmers: recent results, time trends, and lifestyle factors (United States). *Cancer Causes Control.* 1998;9(3):311-319.
52. Nanni O, Falcini F, Buiatti E, et al. Multiple myeloma and work in agriculture: results of a case-control study in Forli, Italy. *Cancer Causes Control.* 1998;9(3):277-283.
53. Pahwa P, McDuffie HH, Dosman JA, et al. Exposure to animals and selected risk factors among Canadian farm residents with Hodgkin's disease, multiple myeloma, or soft tissue sarcoma. *J Occup Environ Med.* 2003;45(8):857-868.
54. Khuder SA, Mutgi AB. Meta-analyses of multiple myeloma and farming. *Am J Ind Med.* 1997;32(5):510-516.
55. Gallagher RP, Threlfall WJ. Cancer mortality in metal workers. *Can Med Assoc J.* 1983;129(11):1191-1194.
56. Fritschi L, Siemiatycki J. Lymphoma, myeloma and occupation: results of a case-control study. *Int J Cancer.* 1996;67(4):498-503.
57. McLaughlin JK, Malker HS, Linet MS, et al. Multiple myeloma and occupation in Sweden. *Arch Environ Health.* 1988;43(1):7-10.
58. Bergsagel DE, Wong O, Bergsagel PL, et al. Benzene and multiple myeloma: appraisal of the scientific evidence. *Blood.* 1999;94(4):1174-1182.
59. Sonoda T, Nagata Y, Mori M, Ishida T, Imai K. Meta-analysis of multiple myeloma and benzene exposure. *J Epidemiol.* 2001;11(6):249-254.
60. Wong O, Raabe GK. A critical review of cancer epidemiology in the petroleum industry, with a meta-analysis of a combined database of more than 350,000 workers. *Regul Toxicol Pharmacol.* 2000;32(1):78-98.
61. Landgren O, Zeig-Owens R, Giricz O, et al. Multiple myeloma and its precursor disease among firefighters exposed to the World Trade Center disaster. *JAMA Oncol.* 2018;4(6):821-827.
62. Thompson MA, Kyle RA, Melton LJ III, Plevak MF, Rajkumar SV. Effect of statins, smoking and obesity on progression of monoclonal gammopathy of undetermined significance: a case-control study. *Haematologica.* 2004;89(5):626-628.
63. Gramenzi A, Buttino I, D'Avanzo B, Negri E, Franceschi S, La Vecchia C. Medical history and the risk of multiple myeloma. *Br J Cancer.* 1991;63(5):769-772.
64. Brown LM, Everett GD, Burmeister LF, Blair A. Hair dye use and multiple myeloma in white men. *Am J Public Health.* 1992;82(12):1673-1674.
65. Brownson RC. Cigarette smoking and risk of myeloma. *J Natl Cancer Inst.* 1991;83(14):1036-1037.
66. Tavani A, La Vecchia C, Gallus S, et al. Red meat intake and cancer risk: a study in Italy. *Int J Cancer.* 2000;86(3):425-428.
67. Brown LM, Gridley G, Pottern LM, et al. Diet and nutrition as risk factors for multiple myeloma among blacks and whites in the United States. *Cancer Causes Control.* 2001;12(2):117-125.
68. Koessel SL, Theis MK, Vaughan TL, et al. Socioeconomic status and the incidence of multiple myeloma. *Epidemiology.* 1996;7(1):4-8.
69. Baris D, Brown LM, Silverman DT, et al. Socioeconomic status and multiple myeloma among US blacks and whites. *Am J Public Health.* 2000;90(8):1277-1281.
70. Gregersen H, Pedersen G, Svendsen N, Thulstrup AM, Sorensen HT, Schonheyder HC. Multiple myeloma following an episode of community-acquired pneumococcal bacteraemia or meningitis. *APMIS.* 2001;109(11):797-800.
71. Bourguet CC, Logue EE. Antigenic stimulation and multiple myeloma. A prospective study. *Cancer.* 1993;72(7):2148-2154.
72. Grulich AE, Wan X, Law MG, Coates M, Kaldor JM. Risk of cancer in people with AIDS. *AIDS.* 1999;13(7):839-843.
73. Yoshikawa M, Imazu H, Ueda S, et al. Prevalence of hepatitis C virus infection in patients with non-Hodgkin's lymphoma and multiple myeloma. A report from Japan. *J Clin Gastroenterol.* 1997;25(4):713-714.
74. Nair S, Branagan AR, Liu J, Boddupalli CS, Mistry PK, Dhodapkar MV. Clonal immunoglobulin against lysolipids in the origin of myeloma. *N Engl J Med.* 2016;374(6):555-561.
75. Proposed guidelines for protocol studies. I. Introduction. II. Plasma cell myeloma. 3. Chronic lymphocytic leukemia. IV. Chronic granulocytic leukemia. *Cancer Chemother Rep.* 1973;4(1):141-173.
76. International Myeloma Working Group. Criteria for the classification of monoclonal gammopathies, multiple myeloma and related disorders: a report of the International Myeloma Working Group. *Br J Haematol.* 2003;121(5):749-757.
77. Rajkumar SV, Dimopoulos MA, Palumbo A, et al. International Myeloma Working Group updated criteria for the diagnosis of multiple myeloma. *Lancet Oncol.* 2014;15(12):e538-e548.
78. Kyle RA. Monoclonal gammopathy of undetermined significance. Natural history in 241 cases. *Am J Med.* 1978;64(5):814-826.
79. Kyle RA. Multiple myeloma: review of 869 cases. *Mayo Clin Proc.* 1975;50(1):29-40.
80. Kyle RA, Greipp PR. Smoldering multiple myeloma. *N Engl J Med.* 1980;302(24):1347-1349.
81. Alexanian R. Localized and indolent myeloma. *Blood.* 1980;56(3):521-525.
82. Riccardi A, Gobbi PG, Ucci G, et al. Changing clinical presentation of multiple myeloma. *Eur J Cancer.* 1991;27(11):1401-1405.
83. Kyle RA, Gertz MA, Witzig TE, et al. Review of 1027 patients with newly diagnosed multiple myeloma. *Mayo Clin Proc.* 2003;78(1):21-33.
84. Kapadia SB. Multiple myeloma: a clinicopathologic study of 62 consecutively autopsied cases. *Medicine (Baltimore).* 1980;59(5):380-392.
85. Drayson M, Tang LX, Drew R, Mead GP, Carr-Smith H, Bradwell AR. Serum free light-chain measurements for identifying and monitoring patients with nonsecretory multiple myeloma. *Blood.* 2001;97(9):2900-2902.
86. Kyle RA, Garton JP. The spectrum of IgM monoclonal gammopathy in 430 cases. *Mayo Clin Proc.* 1987;62(8):719-731.
87. Fossa A, Brandhorst D, Myklebust JH, Seeber S, Nowrousian MR. Relation between S-phase fraction of myeloma cells and anemia in patients with multiple myeloma. *Exp Hematol.* 1999;27(11):1621-1626.
88. Musto P, Falcone A, D'Arena G, et al. Clinical results of recombinant erythropoietin in transfusion-dependent patients with refractory multiple myeloma: role of cytokines and monitoring of erythropoiesis. *Eur J Haematol.* 1997;58(5):314-319.
89. Silvestris F, Cafforio P, Tucci M, Dammacco F. Negative regulation of erythroblast maturation by Fas-L(+)/TRAIL(+) highly malignant plasma cells: a major pathogenetic mechanism of anemia in multiple myeloma. *Blood.* 2002;99(4):1305-1313.
90. Larson RS, Sukpanichnant S, Greer JP, Cousar JB, Collins RD. The spectrum of multiple myeloma: diagnostic and biological implications. *Hum Pathol.* 1997;28(12):1336-1347.
91. Kapff CT, Jandl JH. *Blood: Altas and Sourcebook of Hematology.* 2nd ed. Little, Brown, and Company; 1991.
92. Greipp PR, Raymond NM, Kyle RA, O'Fallon WM. Multiple myeloma: significance of plasmablastic subtype in morphological classification. *Blood.* 1985;65(2):305-310.
93. Bayrd ED. The bone marrow on sternal aspiration in multiple myeloma. *Blood.* 1948;3(9):987-1018.
94. Vacca A, Ribatti D, Roncali L, et al. Bone marrow angiogenesis and progression in multiple myeloma. *Br J Haematol.* 1994;87(3):503-508.
95. Rajkumar SV, Fonseca R, Witzig TE, Gertz MA, Greipp PR. Bone marrow angiogenesis in patients achieving complete response after stem cell transplantation for multiple myeloma. *Leukemia.* 1999;13(3):469-472.
96. Abildgaard N, Bendix-Hansen K, Kristensen JE, et al. Bone marrow fibrosis and disease activity in multiple myeloma monitored by the aminoterminal propeptide of procollagen III in serum. *Br J Haematol.* 1997;99(3):641-648.
97. Roodman GD. Role of the bone marrow microenvironment in multiple myeloma. *J Bone Miner Res.* 2002;17(11):1921-1925.
98. Silvestris F, Lombardi L, De Matteo M, Bruno A, Dammacco F. Myeloma bone disease: pathogenetic mechanisms and clinical assessment. *Leuk Res.* 2007;31(2):129-138.
99. Lacy MQ, Gertz MA, Hanson CA, Inwards DJ, Kyle RA. Multiple myeloma associated with diffuse osteosclerotic bone lesions: a clinical entity distinct from osteosclerotic myeloma (POEMS syndrome). *Am J Hematol.* 1997;56(4):288-293.

100. Lindstrom E, Lindstrom FD. Skeletal scintigraphy with technetium diphosphonate in multiple myeloma—a comparison with skeletal x-ray. *Acta Med Scand*. 1980;208(4):289-291.
101. Hillengass J, Moulopoulos LA, Delorme S, et al. Whole-body computed tomography versus conventional skeletal survey in patients with multiple myeloma: a study of the International Myeloma Working Group. *Blood Cancer J*. 2017;7(8):e599.
102. Laroche M, Assoun J, Sixou L, Attal M. Comparison of MRI and computed tomography in the various stages of plasma cell disorders: correlations with biological and histological findings. Myelome-Midi-Pyrenees Group. *Clin Exp Rheumatol*. 1996;14(2):171-176.
103. Lecouvet FE, Vande Berg BC, Malghem J, Maldague BE. Magnetic resonance and computed tomography imaging in multiple myeloma. *Semin Musculoskelet Radiol*. 2001;5(1):43-55.
104. Pertuiset E, Bellaiche L, Liote F, Laredo JD. Magnetic resonance imaging of the spine in plasma cell dyscrasias. A review. *Rev Rhum Engl Ed*. 1996;63(11):837-845.
105. Mariette X, Zagdanski AM, Guermazi A, et al. Prognostic value of vertebral lesions detected by magnetic resonance imaging in patients with stage I multiple myeloma. *Br J Haematol*. 1999;104(4):723-729.
106. Moulopoulos LA, Dimopoulos MA, Weber D, Fuller L, Libshitz HI, Alexanian R. Magnetic resonance imaging in the staging of solitary plasmacytoma of bone. *J Clin Oncol*. 1993;11(7):1311-1315.
107. Lecouvet FE, Malghem J, Michaux L, et al. Skeletal survey in advanced multiple myeloma: radiographic versus MR imaging survey. *Br J Haematol*. 1999;106(1):35-39.
108. Nanni C, Zamagni E, Farsad M, et al. Role of (18)F-FDG PET/CT in the assessment of bone involvement in newly diagnosed multiple myeloma: preliminary results. *Eur J Nucl Med Mol Imaging*. 2006;33(5):525-531.
109. Shortt CP, Gleeson TG, Breen KA, et al. Whole-Body MRI versus PET in assessment of multiple myeloma disease activity. *AJR Am J Roentgenol*. 2009;192(4):980-986.
110. Baur-Melnyk A, Buhmann S, Becker C, et al. Whole-body MRI versus whole-body MDCT for staging of multiple myeloma. *AJR Am J Roentgenol*. 2008;190(4):1097-1104.
111. Kumar S, Paiva B, Anderson KC, et al. International Myeloma Working Group consensus criteria for response and minimal residual disease assessment in multiple myeloma. *Lancet Oncol*. 2016;17(8):e328-e346.
112. Schirrmeister H, Bommer M, Buck AK, et al. Initial results in the assessment of multiple myeloma using (18)F-FDG PET. *Eur J Nucl Med Mol Imaging*. 2002;29(3):361-366.
113. Cavo M, Terpos E, Nanni C, et al. Role of 18F-FDG PET/CT in the diagnosis and management of multiple myeloma and other plasma cell disorders: a consensus statement by the International Myeloma Working Group. *Lancet Oncol*. 2017;18(4):e206-e217.
114. Bredella MA, Steinbach L, Caputo G, Segall G, Hawkins R. Value of FDG PET in the assessment of patients with multiple myeloma. *AJR Am J Roentgenol*. 2005;184(4):1199-1204.
115. Rasche L, Angtuaco E, McDonald JE, et al. Low expression of hexokinase-2 is associated with false-negative FDG-positron emission tomography in multiple myeloma. *Blood*. 2017;130(1):30-34.
116. Dimopoulos MA, Hillengass J, Usmani S, et al. Role of magnetic resonance imaging in the management of patients with multiple myeloma: a consensus statement. *J Clin Oncol*. 2015;33(6):657-664.
117. Blade J, Fernandez-Llama P, Bosch F, et al. Renal failure in multiple myeloma: presenting features and predictors of outcome in 94 patients from a single institution. *Arch Intern Med*. 1998;158(17):1889-1893.
118. Knudsen LM, Hippe E, Hjorth M, Holmberg E, Westin J. Renal function in newly diagnosed multiple myeloma—a demographic study of 1353 patients. The Nordic Myeloma Study Group. *Eur J Haematol*. 1994;53(4):207-212.
119. Prognostic features in the third MRC myelomatosis trial. Medical research Council's working party on leukaemia in adults. *Br J Cancer*. 1980;42(6):831-840.
120. Irish AB, Winearls CG, Littlewood T. Presentation and survival of patients with severe renal failure and myeloma. *QJM*. 1997;90(12):773-780.
121. MRC Working Party on Leukaemia in Adults. Analysis and management of renal failure in fourth MRC myelomatosis trial. *Br Med J*. 1984;288(6428):1411-1416.
122. Roussou M, Kastritis E, Christoulas D, et al. Reversibility of renal failure in newly diagnosed patients with multiple myeloma and the role of novel agents. *Leuk Res*. 2010;34(10):1395-1397.
123. Dimopoulos MA, Terpos E, Chanan-Khan A, et al. Renal impairment in patients with multiple myeloma: a consensus statement on behalf of the International Myeloma Working Group. *J Clin Oncol*. 2011;28(33):4976-4984.
124. Gonsalves WI, Leung N, Rajkumar SV, et al. Improvement in renal function and its impact on survival in patients with newly diagnosed multiple myeloma. *Blood Cancer J*. 2015;5:e296.
125. Dimopoulos MA, Sonneveld P, Leung N, et al. International myeloma working group recommendations for the diagnosis and management of myeloma-related renal impairment. *J Clin Oncol*. 2016;34(13):1544-1557.
126. Hutchison CA, Cockwell P, Stringer S, et al. Early reduction of serum-free light chains associates with renal recovery in myeloma kidney. *J Am Soc Nephrol*. 2011;22(6):1129-1136.
127. Hill GS, Morel-Maroger L, Mery JP, Brouet JC, Mignon F. Renal lesions in multiple myeloma: their relationship to associated protein abnormalities. *Am J Kidney Dis*. 1983;2(4):423-438.
128. Montseny JJ, Kleinknecht D, Meyrier A, et al. Long-term outcome according to renal histological lesions in 118 patients with monoclonal gammopathies. *Nephrol Dial Transplant*. 1998;13(6):1438-1445.
129. DeFronzo RA, Cooke CR, Wright JR, Humphrey RL. Renal function in patients with multiple myeloma. *Medicine (Baltimore)*. 1978;57(2):151-166.
130. Lackner H. Hemostatic abnormalities associated with dysproteinemias. *Semin Hematol*. 1973;10(2):125-133.
131. Saif MW, Allegra CJ, Greenberg B. Bleeding diathesis in multiple myeloma. *J Hematother Stem Cell Res*. 2001;10(5):657-660.
132. Bergsagel DE, Pruzanski W. Treatment of plasma cell myeloma with cytotoxic agents. *Arch Intern Med*. 1975;135(1):172-176.
133. McArthur JR, Athens JW, Wintrobe MM, Cartwright GE. Melphalan and myeloma. Experience with a low-dose continuous regimen. *Ann Intern Med*. 1970;72(5):665-670.
134. MacLennan IC, Cooper EH, Chapman CE, Kelly KA, Crockson RA. Renal failure in myelomatosis. *Eur J Haematol Suppl*. 1989;51:60-65.
135. Kyle RA. Long-term survival in multiple myeloma. *N Engl J Med*. 1983;308(6):314-316.
136. Anonymous. Long-term survival in multiple myeloma: a Finnish Leukaemia Group study. *Br J Haematol*. 1999;105(4):942-947.
137. Durie BG, Salmon SE. A clinical staging system for multiple myeloma. Correlation of measured myeloma cell mass with presenting clinical features, response to treatment, and survival. *Cancer*. 1975;36(3):842-854.
138. Greipp PR, Katzmann JA, O'Fallon WM, Kyle RA. Value of beta 2-microglobulin level and plasma cell labeling indices as prognostic factors in patients with newly diagnosed myeloma. *Blood*. 1988;72(1):219-223.
139. Greipp PR, Leong T, Bennett JM, et al. Plasmablastic morphology – an independent prognostic factor with clinical and laboratory correlates: Eastern Cooperative Oncology Group (ECOG) myeloma trial E9486 report by the ECOG Myeloma Laboratory Group. *Blood*. 1998;91(7):2501-2507.
140. Rapoport BL, Falkson HC, Falkson G. Prognostic factors affecting the survival of patients with multiple myeloma. A retrospective analysis of 86 patients. *S Afr Med J*. 1991;79(2):65-67.
141. Bataille R, Boccadoro M, Klein B, Durie B, Pileri A. C-reactive protein and beta-2 microglobulin produce a simple and powerful myeloma staging system. *Blood*. 1992;80(3):733-737.
142. Konigsberg R, Zojer N, Ackermann J, et al. Predictive role of interphase cytogenetics for survival of patients with multiple myeloma. *J Clin Oncol*. 2000;18(4):804-812.
143. San Miguel JF, Garcia-Sanz R, Gonzalez M, Orfao A. Immunophenotype and DNA cell content in multiple myeloma. *Baillieres Clin Haematol*. 1995;8(4):735-759.
144. Crowley J, Jacobson J, Alexanian R. Standard-dose therapy for multiple myeloma: the Southwest Oncology Group experience. *Semin Hematol*. 2001;38(3):203-208.
145. Ludwig H, Bolejack V, Crowley J, et al. Survival and years of life lost in different age cohorts of patients with multiple myeloma. *J Clin Oncol*. 2010;28(9):1599-1605.
146. Ludwig H, Durie BGM, Bolejack V, et al. Myeloma in patients younger than age 50 years presents with more favorable features and shows better survival: an analysis of 10549 patients from the International Myeloma Working Group. *Blood*. 2008;111(8):4039-4047.
147. Gonsalves WI, Jevremovic D, Nandakumar B, et al. Enhancing the R-ISS classification of newly diagnosed multiple myeloma by quantifying circulating clonal plasma cells. *Am J Hematol*. 2020;95(3):310-315.
148. Gonsalves WI, Morice WG, Rajkumar V, et al. Quantification of clonal circulating plasma cells in relapsed multiple myeloma. *Br J Haematol*. 2014;167(4):500-505.
149. Gonsalves WI, Rajkumar SV, Gupta V, et al. Quantification of clonal circulating plasma cells in newly diagnosed multiple myeloma: implications for redefining high-risk myeloma. *Leukemia*. 2014;28(10):2060-2065.
150. Snozek CLH, Katzmann JA, Kyle RA, et al. Prognostic value of the serum free light chain ratio in newly diagnosed myeloma: proposed incorporation into the international staging system. *Leukemia*. 2008;22(10):1933-1937.
151. Tricot G, Barlogie B, Jagannath S, et al. Poor prognosis in multiple myeloma is associated only with partial or complete deletions of chromosome 13 or abnormalities involving 11q and not with other karyotype abnormalities. *Blood*. 1995;86(11):4250-4256.
152. Rajkumar SV, Leong T, Roche PC, et al. Prognostic value of bone marrow angiogenesis in multiple myeloma. *Clin Cancer Res*. 2000;6(8):3111-3116.
153. Goasguen JE, Zandecki M, Mathiot C, et al. Mature plasma cells as indicator of better prognosis in multiple myeloma. New methodology for the assessment of plasma cell morphology. *Leuk Res*. 1999;23(12):1133-1140.
154. Dimopoulos MA, Barlogie B, Smith TL, Alexanian R. High serum lactate dehydrogenase level as a marker for drug resistance and short survival in multiple myeloma. *Ann Intern Med*. 1991;115(12):931-935.
155. Simonsson B, Brenning G, Kallander C, Ahre A. Prognostic value of serum lactic dehydrogenase (S-LDH) in multiple myeloma. *Eur J Clin Invest*. 1987;17(4):336-339.
156. D'Sa S, Abildgaard N, Tighe J, Shaw P, Hall-Craggs M. Guidelines for the use of imaging in the management of myeloma. *Br J Haematol*. 2007;137(1):49-63.
157. Nosas-Garcia S, Moehler T, Wasser K, et al. Dynamic contrast-enhanced MRI for assessing the disease activity of multiple myeloma: a comparative study with histology and clinical markers. *J Magn Reson Imaging*. 2005;22(1):154-162.
158. Moulopoulos LA, Dimopoulos MA, Christoulas D, et al. Diffuse MRI marrow pattern correlates with increased angiogenesis, advanced disease features and poor prognosis in newly diagnosed myeloma treated with novel agents. *Leukemia*. 2010;24(6):1206-1212.
159. Zamagni E, Patriarca F, Nanni C, et al. Prognostic relevance of 18-F FDG PET/CT in newly diagnosed multiple myeloma patients treated with up-front autologous transplantation. *Blood*. 2011;118(23):5989-5995.
160. Munshi NC, Anderson KC, Bergsagel PL, et al; International Myeloma Workshop Consensus Panel 2. Consensus recommendations for risk stratification in multiple myeloma: report of the International Myeloma Workshop Consensus Panel 2. *Blood*. 2011;117(18):4696-4700.
161. Greipp PR, San Miguel J, Durie BGM, et al. International staging system for multiple myeloma. *J Clin Oncol*. 2005;23(15):3412-3420.

162. Ortega F, Gonzalez M, Moro MJ, et al. Prognostic effect of beta 2-microglobulin in multiple myeloma. *Med Clin.* 1992;99(17):645-648.
163. Drach J, Schuster J, Nowotny H, et al. Multiple myeloma: high incidence of chromosomal aneuploidy as detected by interphase fluorescence in situ hybridization. *Cancer Res.* 1995;55(17):3854-3859.
164. Kumar S, Fonseca R, Ketterling RP, et al. Trisomies in multiple myeloma: impact on survival in patients with high-risk cytogenetics. *Blood.* 2012;119(9):2100-2105.
165. Rajkumar SV, Fonseca R, Dewald GW, et al. Cytogenetic abnormalities correlate with the plasma cell labeling index and extent of bone marrow involvement in myeloma. *Cancer Genet Cytogenet.* 1999;113(1):73-77.
166. Avet-Loiseau H, Li JY, Morineau N, et al. Monosomy 13 is associated with the transition of monoclonal gammopathy of undetermined significance to multiple myeloma. Intergroupe Francophone du Myélome. *Blood.* 1999;94(8):2583-2589.
167. Fonseca R, Oken MM, Harrington D, et al. Deletions of chromosome 13 in multiple myeloma identified by interphase FISH usually denote large deletions of the q arm or monosomy. *Leukemia.* 2001;15(6):981-986.
168. Boyd KD, Ross FM, Chiecchio L, et al; NCRI Haematology Oncology Studies Group. A novel prognostic model in myeloma based on co-segregating adverse FISH lesions and the ISS: analysis of patients treated in the MRC Myeloma IX trial. *Leukemia.* 2012;26(2):349-355.
169. Palumbo A, Avet-Loiseau H, Oliva S, et al. Revised international staging system for multiple myeloma: a report from International Myeloma Working Group. *J Clin Oncol.* 2015;33(26):2863-2869.
170. Chng WJ, Santana-Davila R, Van Wier SA, et al. Prognostic factors for hyperdiploid-myeloma: effects of chromosome 13 deletions and IgH translocations. *Leukemia.* 2006;20(5):807-813.
171. Smadja NV, Bastard C, Brigaudeau C, Leroux D, Fruchart C; Groupe Français de Cytogénétique Hématologique. Hypodiploidy is a major prognostic factor in multiple myeloma. *Blood.* 2001;98(7):2229-2238.
172. Shaughnessy J Jr, Tian E, Sawyer J, et al. Prognostic impact of cytogenetic and interphase fluorescence in situ hybridization-defined chromosome 13 deletion in multiple myeloma: early results of total therapy II. *Br J Haematol.* 2003;120(1):44-52.
173. Fonseca R, Debes-Marun CS, Picken EB, et al. The recurrent IgH translocations are highly associated with nonhyperdiploid variant multiple myeloma. *Blood.* 2003;102(7):2562-2567.
174. Garcia-Sanz R, Orfao A, Gonzalez M, et al. Primary plasma cell leukemia: clinical, immunophenotypic, DNA ploidy, and cytogenetic characteristics. *Blood.* 1999;93(3):1032-1037.
175. Perez-Simon JA, Garcia-Sanz R, Tabernero MD, et al. Prognostic value of numerical chromosome aberrations in multiple myeloma: a FISH analysis of 15 different chromosomes. *Blood.* 1998;91(9):3366-3371.
176. Tricot G, Sawyer JR, Jagannath S, et al. Unique role of cytogenetics in the prognosis of patients with myeloma receiving high-dose therapy and autotransplants. *J Clin Oncol.* 1997;15(7):2659-2666.
177. Facon T, Avet-Loiseau H, Guillerm G, et al; Intergroupe Francophone du Myelome. Chromosome 13 abnormalities identified by FISH analysis and serum beta2- microglobulin produce a powerful myeloma staging system for patients receiving high-dose therapy. *Blood.* 2001;97(6):1566-1571.
178. Zhan F, Huang Y, Colla S, et al. The molecular classification of multiple myeloma. *Blood.* 2006;108(6):2020-2028.
179. Zhan F, Barlogie B, Mulligan G, Shaughnessy JD Jr, Bryant B. High-risk myeloma: a gene expression based risk-stratification model for newly diagnosed multiple myeloma treated with high-dose therapy is predictive of outcome in relapsed disease treated with single-agent bortezomib or high-dose dexamethasone. *Blood.* 2008;111(2):968-969.
180. Kumar SK, Uno H, Jacobus SJ, et al. Impact of gene expression profiling-based risk stratification in patients with myeloma receiving initial therapy with lenalidomide and dexamethasone. *Blood.* 2011;118(16):4359-4362.
181. Decaux O, Lode L, Magrangeas F, et al; Intergroupe Francophone du Myelome. Prediction of survival in multiple myeloma based on gene expression profiles reveals cell cycle and chromosomal instability signatures in high-risk patients and hyperdiploid signatures in low-risk patients: a study of the Intergroupe Francophone du Myelome. *J Clin Oncol.* 2008;26(29):4798-4805.
182. Keats JJ, Chesi M, Egan JB, et al. Clonal competition with alternating dominance in multiple myeloma. *Blood.* 2012;120(5):1067-1076.
183. Greipp PR, Lust JA, O'Fallon WM, Katzmann JA, Witzig TE, Kyle RA. Plasma cell labeling index and beta 2-microglobulin predict survival independent of thymidine kinase and C-reactive protein in multiple myeloma. *Blood.* 1993;81(12):3382-3387.
184. Rajkumar SV, Greipp PR. Prognostic factors in multiple myeloma. *Hematol Oncol Clin North Am.* 1999;13(6):1295-1314, xi.
185. Kapoor P, Kumar S, Mandrekar SJ, et al. Efficacy of thalidomide- or lenalidomide-based therapy in proliferative multiple myeloma. *Leukemia.* 2011;25(7):1195-1197.
186. Nadav L, Katz BZ, Baron S, Cohen N, Naparstek E, Geiger B. The generation and regulation of functional diversity of malignant plasma cells. *Cancer Res.* 2006;66(17):8608-8616.
187. Yaccoby S. The phenotypic plasticity of myeloma plasma cells as expressed by dedifferentiation into an immature, resilient, and apoptosis-resistant phenotype. *Clin Cancer Res.* 2005;11(21):7599-7606.
188. Lin P, Owens R, Tricot G, Wilson CS. Flow cytometric immunophenotypic analysis of 306 cases of multiple myeloma. *Am J Clin Pathol.* 2004;121(4):482-488.
189. Mateo G, Castellanos M, Rasillo A, et al. Genetic abnormalities and patterns of antigenic expression in multiple myeloma. *Clin Cancer Res.* 2005;11(10):3661-3667.
190. Moreau P, Robillard N, Avet-Loiseau H, et al. Patients with CD45 negative multiple myeloma receiving high-dose therapy have a shorter survival than those with CD45 positive multiple myeloma. *Haematologica.* 2004;89(5):547-551.
191. Kumar S, Rajkumar SV, Kimlinger T, Greipp PR, Witzig TE. CD45 expression by bone marrow plasma cells in multiple myeloma: clinical and biological correlations. *Leukemia.* 2005;19(8):1466-1470.
192. Pellat-Deceunynck C, Barille S, Jego G, et al. The absence of CD56 (NCAM) on malignant plasma cells is a hallmark of plasma cell leukemia and of a special subset of multiple myeloma. *Leukemia.* 1998;12(12):1977-1982.
193. Mateo G, Montalban MA, Vidriales MB, et al; PETHEMA Study Group; GEM Study Group. Prognostic value of immunophenotyping in multiple myeloma: a study by the PETHEMA/GEM cooperative study groups on patients uniformly treated with high-dose therapy. *J Clin Oncol.* 2008;26(16):2737-2744.
194. Moreau P, Robillard N, Jego G, et al. Lack of CD27 in myeloma delineates different presentation and outcome. *Br J Haematol.* 2006;132(2):168-170.
195. Moreaux J, Hose D, Reme T, et al. CD200 is a new prognostic factor in multiple myeloma. *Blood.* 2006;108(13):4194-4197.
196. Myeloma Trialists' Collaborative Group. Combination chemotherapy versus melphalan plus prednisone as treatment for multiple myeloma: an overview of 6, 633 patients from 27 randomized trials. *J Clin Oncol.* 1998;16(12):3832-3842.
197. McElwain TJ, Powles RL. High-dose intravenous melphalan for plasma-cell leukaemia and myeloma. *Lancet.* 1983;2(8354):822-824.
198. Vij R, Wang M, Kaufman JL, et al. An open-label, single-arm, phase 2 (PX-171-004) study of single-agent carfilzomib in bortezomib-naive patients with relapsed and/or refractory multiple myeloma. *Blood.* 2012;119(24):5661-5670.
199. Lacy MQ, Hayman SR, Gertz MA, et al. Pomalidomide (CC4047) plus low-dose dexamethasone as therapy for relapsed multiple myeloma. *J Clin Oncol.* 2009;27(30):5008-5014.
200. Kumar SK, Bensinger WI, Zimmerman TM, et al. Phase 1 study of weekly dosing with the investigational oral proteasome inhibitor ixazomib in relapsed/refractory multiple myeloma. *Blood.* 2014;124(7):1047-1055.
201. van Rhee F, Szmania SM, Dillon M, et al. Combinatorial efficacy of anti-CS1 monoclonal antibody elotuzumab (HuLuc63) and bortezomib against multiple myeloma. *Mol Cancer Ther.* 2009;8(9):2616-2624.
202. San-Miguel JF, Hungria VTM, Yoon SS, et al. Panobinostat plus bortezomib and dexamethasone versus placebo plus bortezomib and dexamethasone in patients with relapsed or relapsed and refractory multiple myeloma: a multicentre, randomised, double-blind phase 3 trial. *Lancet Oncol.* 2014;15(11):1195-1206.
203. Attal M, Richardson PG, Rajkumar SV, et al; ICARIA-MM study group. Isatuximab plus pomalidomide and low-dose dexamethasone versus pomalidomide and low-dose dexamethasone in patients with relapsed and refractory multiple myeloma (ICARIA-MM): a randomised, multicentre, open-label, phase 3 study. *Lancet.* 2019;394(10214):2096-2107.
204. Vogl DT, Dingli D, Cornell RF, et al. Selective inhibition of nuclear export with oral selinexor for treatment of relapsed or refractory multiple myeloma. *J Clin Oncol.* 2018;36(9):859-866.
205. Munshi NC, Anderson LD Jr, Shah N, et al. Idecabtagene vicleucel in relapsed and refractory multiple myeloma. *N Engl J Med.* 2021;384(8):705-716.
206. Alexanian R, Bonnet J, Gehan E, et al. Combination chemotherapy for multiple myeloma. *Cancer.* 1972;30(2):382-389.
207. McLaughlin P, Alexanian R. Myeloma protein kinetics following chemotherapy. *Blood.* 1982;60(4):851-855.
208. Oken MM, Kyle RA, Greipp PR, et al. Complete remission induction with combined VBMCP chemotherapy and interferon (rIFN alpha 2b) in patients with multiple myeloma. *Leuk Lymphoma.* 1996;20(5-6):447-452.
209. Blade J, Samson D, Reece D, et al. Criteria for evaluating disease response and progression in patients with multiple myeloma treated by high-dose therapy and haemopoietic stem cell transplantation. Myeloma Subcommittee of the EBMT. European Group for Blood and Marrow Transplant. *Br J Haematol.* 1998;102(5):1115-1123.
210. Durie BGM, Harousseau JL, Miguel JS, et al; International Myeloma Working Group. International uniform response criteria for multiple myeloma. *Leukemia.* 2006;20(9):1467-1473.
211. Attal M, Harousseau JL, Stoppa AM, et al. A prospective, randomized trial of autologous bone marrow transplantation and chemotherapy in multiple myeloma. Intergroupe Français du Myélome. *N Engl J Med.* 1996;335(2):91-97.
212. Mateos MV, Dimopoulos MA, Cavo M, et al; ALCYONE Trial Investigators. Daratumumab plus bortezomib, melphalan, and prednisone for untreated myeloma. *N Engl J Med.* 2018;378(6):518-528.
213. Dispenzieri A, Rajkumar SV, Gertz MA, et al. Treatment of newly diagnosed multiple myeloma based on Mayo Stratification of Myeloma and Risk-adapted Therapy (mSMART): consensus statement. *Mayo Clin Proc.* 2007;82(3):323-341.
214. Dispenzieri A. Myeloma: management of the newly diagnosed high-risk patient. *Hematology Am Soc Hematol Educ Program.* 2016;2016(1):485-494.
215. Engelhardt M, Domm AS, Dold SM, et al. A concise revised Myeloma Comorbidity Index as a valid prognostic instrument in a large cohort of 801 multiple myeloma patients. *Haematologica.* 2017;102(5):910-921.
216. Milani P, Vincent Rajkumar S, Merlini G, et al. N-terminal fragment of the type-B natriuretic peptide (NT-proBNP) contributes to a simple new frailty score in patients with newly diagnosed multiple myeloma. *Am J Hematol.* 2016;91(11):1129-1134.
217. Palumbo A, Bringhen S, Mateos MV, et al. Geriatric assessment predicts survival and toxicities in elderly myeloma patients: an International Myeloma Working Group report. *Blood.* 2015;125(13):2068-2074.
218. Mateos MV, Richardson PG, Schlag R, et al. Bortezomib plus melphalan and prednisone compared with melphalan and prednisone in previously untreated multiple myeloma: updated follow-up and impact of subsequent therapy in the phase III VISTA trial. *J Clin Oncol.* 2010;28(13):2259-2266.
219. Cavo M, Pantani L, Petrucci MT, et al; GIMEMA Gruppo Italiano Malattie Ematologiche dell'Adulto Italian Myeloma Network. Bortezomib-thalidomide-dexamethasone is superior to thalidomide-dexamethasone as consolidation therapy after autologous hematopoietic stem cell transplantation in patients with newly diagnosed multiple myeloma. *Blood.* 2012;120(1):9-19.

220. Neben K, Lokhorst HM, Jauch A, et al. Administration of bortezomib before and after autologous stem cell transplantation improves outcome in multiple myeloma patients with deletion 17p. *Blood.* 2012;119(4):940-948.
221. Sonneveld P, Salwender HJ, Van Der Holt B, et al. Bortezomib induction and maintenance in patients with newly diagnosed multiple myeloma: long-term follow-up of the HOVON-65/GMMG-HD4 trial. *Blood.* 2015;126(23):27.
222. Weinhold N, Heuck CJ, Rosenthal A, et al. Clinical value of molecular subtyping multiple myeloma using gene expression profiling. *Leukemia.* 2016;30(2):423-430.
223. Nooka AK, Kaufman JL, Muppidi S, et al. Consolidation and maintenance therapy with lenalidomide, bortezomib and dexamethasone (RVD) in high-risk myeloma patients. *Leukemia.* 2014;28(3):690-693.
224. Goldschmidt H, Lokhorst HM, Mai EK, et al. Bortezomib before and after high-dose therapy in myeloma: long-term results from the phase III HOVON-65/GMMG-HD4 trial. *Leukemia.* 2018;32(2):383-390.
225. Kumar SK, Mikhael JR, Buadi FK, et al. Management of newly diagnosed symptomatic multiple myeloma: updated Mayo Stratification of Myeloma and Risk-Adapted Therapy (mSMART) consensus guidelines. *Mayo Clin Proc.* 2009;84(12):1095-1110.
226. Mikhael JR, Dingli D, Roy V, et al; Mayo Clinic. Management of newly diagnosed symptomatic multiple myeloma: updated Mayo Stratification of Myeloma and Risk-Adapted Therapy (mSMART) consensus guidelines 2013. *Mayo Clin Proc.* 2013;88(4):360-376.
227. Weisel K, Doyen C, Dimopoulos M, et al. A systematic literature review and network meta-analysis of treatments for patients with untreated multiple myeloma not eligible for stem cell transplantation. *Leuk Lymphoma.* 2017;58(1):153-161.
228. Gentile M, Magarotto V, Offidani M, et al. Lenalidomide and low-dose dexamethasone (Rd) versus bortezomib, melphalan, prednisone (VMP) in elderly newly diagnosed multiple myeloma patients: a comparison of two prospective trials. *Am J Hematol.* 2017;92(3):244-250.
229. Richardson PG, Weller E, Lonial S, et al. Lenalidomide, bortezomib, and dexamethasone combination therapy in patients with newly diagnosed multiple myeloma. *Blood.* 2010;116(5):679-686.
230. Rajkumar SV, Jacobus S, Callander NS, et al; Eastern Cooperative Oncology Group. Lenalidomide plus high-dose dexamethasone versus lenalidomide plus low-dose dexamethasone as initial therapy for newly diagnosed multiple myeloma: an open-label randomised controlled trial. *Lancet Oncol.* 2010;11(1):29-37.
231. Mateos MV, Hernandez JM, Hernandez MT, et al. Bortezomib plus melphalan and prednisone in elderly untreated patients with multiple myeloma: results of a multicenter phase 1/2 study. *Blood.* 2006;108(7):2165-2172.
232. Reeder CB, Reece DE, Kukreti V, et al. Cyclophosphamide, bortezomib and dexamethasone induction for newly diagnosed multiple myeloma: high response rates in a phase II clinical trial. *Leukemia.* 2009;23(7):1337-1341.
233. Reeder CB, Reece DE, Kukreti V, et al. Once- versus twice-weekly bortezomib induction therapy with CyBorD in newly diagnosed multiple myeloma. *Blood.* 2010;115(16):3416-3417.
234. Morgan GJ, Davies FE, Gregory WM, et al; National Cancer Research Institute Haematological Oncology Clinical Studies Group. Cyclophosphamide, thalidomide, and dexamethasone as induction therapy for newly diagnosed multiple myeloma patients destined for autologous stem-cell transplantation: MRC Myeloma IX randomized trial results. *Haematologica.* 2012;97(3):442-450.
235. Facon T, Mary JY, Hulin C, et al; Intergroupe Francophone du Myelome. Melphalan and prednisone plus thalidomide versus melphalan and prednisone alone or reduced-intensity autologous stem cell transplantation in elderly patients with multiple myeloma (IFM 99-06): a randomised trial. *Lancet.* 2007;370(9594):1209-1218.
236. Ailawadhi S, Sexton R, Lentzsch S, et al. Low-dose versus high-dose carfilzomib with dexamethasone (S1304) in patients with relapsed-refractory multiple myeloma. *Clin Cancer Res.* 2020;26(15):3969-3978.
237. Moreau P, Mateos MV, Berenson JR, et al. Once weekly versus twice weekly carfilzomib dosing in patients with relapsed and refractory multiple myeloma (A.R.R.O.W.): interim analysis results of a randomised, phase 3 study. *Lancet Oncol.* 2018;19(7):953-964.
238. Jakubowiak AJ, Dytfeld D, Griffith KA, et al. A phase 1/2 study of carfilzomib in combination with lenalidomide and low-dose dexamethasone as a frontline treatment for multiple myeloma. *Blood.* 2012;120(9):1801-1809.
239. Dimopoulos MA, Oriol A, Nahi H, et al; POLLUX Investigators. Daratumumab, lenalidomide, and dexamethasone for multiple myeloma. *N Engl J Med.* 2016;375(14):1319-1331.
240. Dimopoulos MA, Terpos E, Boccadoro M, et al. Daratumumab plus pomalidomide and dexamethasone versus pomalidomide and dexamethasone alone in previously treated multiple myeloma (APOLLO): an open-label, randomised, phase 3 trial. *Lancet Oncol.* 2021;22(6):801-812.
241. Palumbo A, Chanan-Khan A, Weisel K, et al. Daratumumab, bortezomib, and dexamethasone for multiple myeloma. *N Engl J Med.* 2016;375(8):754-766.
242. Dimopoulos M, Quach H, Mateos MV, et al. Carfilzomib, dexamethasone, and daratumumab versus carfilzomib and dexamethasone for patients with relapsed or refractory multiple myeloma (CANDOR): results from a randomised, multicentre, open-label, phase 3 study. *Lancet.* 2020;396(10245):186-197.
243. Moreau P, Dimopoulos MA, Mikhael J, et al; IKEMA study group. Isatuximab, carfilzomib, and dexamethasone in relapsed multiple myeloma (IKEMA): a multicentre, open-label, randomised phase 3 trial. *Lancet.* 2021;397(10292):2361-2371.
244. Dimopoulos MA, Lonial S, White D, et al. Elotuzumab plus lenalidomide/dexamethasone for relapsed or refractory multiple myeloma: ELOQUENT-2 follow-up and post-hoc analyses on progression-free survival and tumour growth. *Br J Haematol.* 2017;178(6):896-905.
245. Dimopoulos MA, Dytfeld D, Grosicki S, et al. Elotuzumab plus pomalidomide and dexamethasone for multiple myeloma. *N Engl J Med.* 2018;379(19):1811-1822.
246. Lonial S, Lee HC, Badros A, et al. Belantamab mafodotin for relapsed or refractory multiple myeloma (DREAMM-2): a two-arm, randomised, open-label, phase 2 study. *Lancet Oncol.* 2020;21(2):207-221.
247. Grosicki S, Simonova M, Spicka I, et al. Once-per-week selinexor, bortezomib, and dexamethasone versus twice-per-week bortezomib and dexamethasone in patients with multiple myeloma (BOSTON): a randomised, open-label, phase 3 trial. *Lancet.* 2020;396(10262):1563-1573.
248. Rajkumar SV, Blood E, Vesole D, Fonseca R, Greipp PR; Eastern Cooperative Oncology Group. Phase III clinical trial of thalidomide plus dexamethasone compared with dexamethasone alone in newly diagnosed multiple myeloma: a clinical trial coordinated by the Eastern Cooperative Oncology Group. *J Clin Oncol.* 2006;24(3):431-436.
249. Mai EK, Bertsch U, Durig J, et al. Phase III trial of bortezomib, cyclophosphamide and dexamethasone (VCD) versus bortezomib, doxorubicin and dexamethasone (PAd) in newly diagnosed myeloma. *Leukemia.* 2015;29(8):1721-1729.
250. Barlogie B, Anaissie E, van Rhee F, et al. Incorporating bortezomib into upfront treatment for multiple myeloma: early results of total therapy 3. *Br J Haematol.* 2007;138(2):176-185.
251. Facon T, Mary JY, Pegourie B, et al; Intergroupe Francophone du Myelome IFM group. Dexamethasone-based regimens versus melphalan-prednisone for elderly multiple myeloma patients ineligible for high-dose therapy. *Blood.* 2006;107(4):1292-1298.
252. Costa G, Engle RL, Schilling A, et al. Melpahlan and prednisone: an effective combination for the treatment of multiple myeloma. *Am J Med.* 1973;54:589-599.
253. Peest D, Deicher H, Coldewey R, et al. A comparison of polychemotherapy and melphalan/prednisone for primary remission induction, and interferon-alpha for maintenance treatment, in multiple myeloma. A prospective trial of the German Myeloma Treatment Group. *Eur J Cancer.* 1995;31A:146-151.
254. Schey SA, Kazmi M, Ireland R, Lakhani A. The use of intravenous intermediate dose melphalan and dexamethasone as induction treatment in the management of de novo multiple myeloma. *Eur J Haematol.* 1998;61(5):306-310.
255. Palumbo A, Bringhen S, Caravita T, et al; Italian Multiple Myeloma Network, GIMEMA. Oral melphalan and prednisone chemotherapy plus thalidomide compared with melphalan and prednisone alone in elderly patients with multiple myeloma: randomised controlled trial. *Lancet.* 2006;367(9513):825-831.
256. Palumbo A, Bringhen S, Liberati AM, et al. Oral melphalan, prednisone, and thalidomide in elderly patients with multiple myeloma: updated results of a randomized, controlled trial. *Blood.* 2008;112(8):3107-3114.
257. Hulin C, Facon T, Rodon P, et al. Efficacy of melphalan and prednisone plus thalidomide in patients older than 75 years with newly diagnosed multiple myeloma: IFM 01/01 trial. *J Clin Oncol.* 2009;27(22):3664-3670.
258. Waage A, Gimsing P, Fayers P, et al; Nordic Myeloma Study Group. Melphalan and prednisone plus thalidomide or placebo in elderly patients with multiple myeloma. *Blood.* 2010;116(9):1405-1412.
259. Wijermans P, Schaafsma M, Termorshuizen F, et al; Dutch-Belgium Cooperative Group HOVON. Phase III study of the value of thalidomide added to melphalan plus prednisone in elderly patients with newly diagnosed multiple myeloma: the HOVON 49 Study. *J Clin Oncol.* 2010;28(19):3160-3166.
260. Beksac M, Haznedar R, Firatli-Tuglular T, et al. Addition of thalidomide to oral melphalan/prednisone in patients with multiple myeloma not eligible for transplantation: results of a randomized trial from the Turkish Myeloma Study Group. *Eur J Haematol.* 2011;86(1):16-22.
261. San Miguel JF, Schlag R, Khuageva NK, et al; VISTA Trial Investigators. Bortezomib plus melphalan and prednisone for initial treatment of multiple myeloma. *N Engl J Med.* 2008;359(9):906-917.
262. Palumbo A, Bringhen S, Rossi D, et al. Bortezomib-melphalan-prednisone-thalidomide followed by maintenance with bortezomib-thalidomide compared with bortezomib-melphalan-prednisone for initial treatment of multiple myeloma: a randomized controlled trial. *J Clin Oncol.* 2010;28(34):5101-5109.
263. Palumbo A, Waage A, Hulin C, et al. Safety of thalidomide in newly diagnosed elderly myeloma patients: a meta-analysis of data from individual patients in six randomized trials. *Haematologica.* 2013;98(1):87-94.
264. Morgan GJ, Davies FE, Gregory WM, et al; NCRI Haematological Oncology Study Group. Cyclophosphamide, thalidomide, and dexamethasone (CTD) as initial therapy for patients with multiple myeloma unsuitable for autologous transplantation. *Blood.* 2011;118(5):1231-1238.
265. Rajkumar SV, Hayman SR, Lacy MQ, et al. Combination therapy with lenalidomide plus dexamethasone (Rev/Dex) for newly diagnosed myeloma. *Blood.* 2005;106(13):4050-4053.
266. Niesvizky R, Jayabalan DS, Christos PJ, et al. BiRD (Biaxin [clarithromycin]/Revlimid [lenalidomide]/dexamethasone) combination therapy results in high complete- and overall-response rates in treatment-naive symptomatic multiple myeloma. *Blood.* 2008;111(3):1101-1109.
267. Lacy MQ, Gertz MA, Dispenzieri A, et al. Long-term results of response to therapy, time to progression, and survival with lenalidomide plus dexamethasone in newly diagnosed myeloma. *Mayo Clin Proc.* 2007;82(10):1179-1184.
268. Larocca A, Bonello F, Gaidano G, et al. Dose/schedule-adjusted Rd-R vs continuous Rd for elderly, intermediate-fit patients with newly diagnosed multiple myeloma. *Blood.* 2021;137(22):3027-3036.
269. Benboubker L, Dimopoulos MA, Dispenzieri A, et al; FIRST Trial Team. Lenalidomide and dexamethasone in transplant-ineligible patients with myeloma. *N Engl J Med.* 2014;371(10):906-917.

270. Facon T, Kumar S, Plesner T, et al; MAIA Trial Investigators. Daratumumab plus lenalidomide and dexamethasone for untreated myeloma. *N Engl J Med.* 2019;380(22):2104-2115.
271. Facon T, Venner CP, Bahlis NJ, et al. Oral ixazomib, lenalidomide, and dexamethasone for transplant-ineligible patients with newly diagnosed multiple myeloma. *Blood.* 2021;137(26):3616-3628.
272. Durie BGM, Hoering A, Abidi MH, et al. Bortezomib with lenalidomide and dexamethasone versus lenalidomide and dexamethasone alone in patients with newly diagnosed myeloma without intent for immediate autologous stem-cell transplant (SWOG S0777): a randomised, open-label, phase 3 trial. *Lancet.* 2017;389(10068):519-527.
273. Vesole DH, Jacobus S, Rajkumar SV, et al. Lenalidomide plus low-dose dexamethasone (Ld): superior one and two year survival regardless of age compared to lenalidomide plus high-dose dexamethasone (LD). *Blood.* 2010;116(21):308.
274. Meyers BR, Hirschman SZ, Axelrod JA. Current patterns of infection in multiple myeloma. *Am J Med.* 1972;52(1):87-92.
275. Mateos MV, Oriol A, Martinez-Lopez J, et al. Bortezomib, melphalan, and prednisone versus bortezomib, thalidomide, and prednisone as induction therapy followed by maintenance treatment with bortezomib and thalidomide versus bortezomib and prednisone in elderly patients with untreated multiple myeloma: a randomised trial. *Lancet Oncol.* 2010;11(10):934-941.
276. Mateos MV, Oriol A, Martinez-Lopez J, et al. GEM2005 trial update comparing VMP/VTP as induction in elderly multiple myeloma patients: do we still need alkylators? *Blood.* 2014;124(12):1887-1893.
277. Palumbo A, Bringhen S, Larocca A, et al. Bortezomib-melphalan-prednisone-thalidomide followed by maintenance with bortezomib-thalidomide compared with bortezomib-melphalan-prednisone for initial treatment of multiple myeloma: updated follow-up and improved survival. *J Clin Oncol.* 2014;32(7):634-640.
278. Niesvizky R, Flinn IW, Rifkin R, et al. Community-based phase IIIB trial of three UPFRONT bortezomib-based myeloma regimens. *J Clin Oncol.* 2015;33(33):3921-3929.
279. Facon T, Lee GH, Moreau P, et al. Phase 3 Study (CLARION) of carfilzomib, melphalan, prednisone (KMP) vs bortezomib, melphalan, prednisone (VMP) in newly diagnosed multiple myeloma (NDMM). *Clin Lymphoma Myeloma Leuk.* 2017;17(1):e26-e27.
280. Fayers PM, Palumbo A, Hulin C, et al; Nordic Myeloma Study Group; Italian Multiple Myeloma Network, Turkish Myeloma Study Group; Hemato-Oncologie voor Volwassenen Nederland; Intergroupe Francophone du Myelom; European Myeloma Network. Thalidomide for previously untreated elderly patients with multiple myeloma: meta-analysis of 1685 individual patient data from 6 randomized clinical trials. *Blood.* 2011;118(5):1239-1247.
281. Morgan GJ, Davies FE, Gregory WM, et al. Long-term follow-up of MRC Myeloma IX trial: survival outcomes with bisphosphonate and thalidomide treatment. *Clin Cancer Res.* 2013;19(21):6030-6038.
282. Palumbo A, Hajek R, Delforge M, et al; MM-015 Investigators. Continuous lenalidomide treatment for newly diagnosed multiple myeloma. *N Engl J Med.* 2012;366(19):1759-1769.
283. Stewart AK, Jacobus S, Fonseca R, et al. Melphalan, prednisone, and thalidomide vs melphalan, prednisone, and lenalidomide (ECOG E1A06) in untreated multiple myeloma. *Blood.* 2015;126(11):1294-1301.
284. Zweegman S, van der Holt B, Mellqvist UH, et al. Melphalan, prednisone, and lenalidomide versus melphalan, prednisone, and thalidomide in untreated multiple myeloma. *Blood.* 2016;127(9):1109-1116.
285. Magarotto V, Bringhen S, Offidani M, et al. Triplet vs doublet lenalidomide-containing regimens for the treatment of elderly patients with newly diagnosed multiple myeloma. *Blood.* 2016;127(9):1102-1108.
286. Ludwig H, Hajek R, Tothova E, et al. Thalidomide-dexamethasone compared with melphalan-prednisolone in elderly patients with multiple myeloma. *Blood.* 2009;113(15):3435-3442.
287. Rajkumar SV, Rosinol L, Hussein M, et al. Multicenter, randomized, double-blind, placebo-controlled study of thalidomide plus dexamethasone compared with dexamethasone as initial therapy for newly diagnosed multiple myeloma. *J Clin Oncol.* 2008;26(13):2171-2177.
288. Bahlis NJ, Corso A, Mugge LO, et al. Benefit of continuous treatment for responders with newly diagnosed multiple myeloma in the randomized FIRST trial. *Leukemia.* 2017;31(11):2435-2442.
289. Attal M, Lauwers-Cances V, Hulin C, et al; IFM 2009 Study. Lenalidomide, bortezomib, and dexamethasone with transplantation for myeloma. *N Engl J Med.* 2017;376(14):1311-1320.
290. Moreau P, Pylypenko H, Grosicki S, et al. Subcutaneous versus intravenous administration of bortezomib in patients with relapsed multiple myeloma: a randomised, phase 3, non-inferiority study. *Lancet Oncol.* 2011;12(5):431-440.
291. O'Donnell EK, Laubach JP, Yee AJ, et al. A phase 2 study of modified lenalidomide, bortezomib and dexamethasone in transplant-ineligible multiple myeloma. *Br J Haematol.* 2018;182(2):222-230.
292. Niesvizky R, Flinn IW, Rifkin RM, et al. Impact of baseline characteristics on efficacy and safety after bortezomib-based induction and maintenance in newly diagnosed multiple myeloma (MM) patients ineligible for transplant in the phase IIIb UPFRONT study. *J Clin Oncol.* 2011;29(15 suppl):8072.
293. Mateos MV, Richardson PG, Dimopoulos MA, et al. Effect of cumulative bortezomib dose on survival in multiple myeloma patients receiving bortezomib-melphalan-prednisone in the phase III VISTA study. *Am J Hematol.* 2015;90(4):314-319.
294. Facon T, Lee JH, Moreau P, et al. Carfilzomib or bortezomib with melphalan-prednisone for transplant-ineligible patients with newly diagnosed multiple myeloma. *Blood.* 2019;133(18):1953-1963.
295. Dytfeld D, Jasielec J, Griffith KA, et al. Carfilzomib, lenalidomide, and low-dose dexamethasone in elderly patients with newly diagnosed multiple myeloma. *Haematologica.* 2014;99(9):e162-e164.
296. Kumar SK, Jacobus SJ, Cohen AD, et al. Carfilzomib or bortezomib in combination with lenalidomide and dexamethasone for patients with newly diagnosed multiple myeloma without intention for immediate autologous stem-cell transplantation (ENDURANCE): a multicentre, open-label, phase 3, randomised, controlled trial. *Lancet Oncol.* 2020;21(10):1317-1330.
297. Usmani SZ, Hoering A, Ailawadhi S, et al; SWOG1211 Trial Investigators. Bortezomib, lenalidomide, and dexamethasone with or without elotuzumab in patients with untreated, high-risk multiple myeloma (SWOG-1211): primary analysis of a randomised, phase 2 trial. *Lancet Haematol.* 2021;8(1):e45-e54.
298. Alexanian R, Salmon S, Bonnet J, Gehan E, Haut A, Weick J. Combination therapy for multiple myeloma. *Cancer.* 1977;40(6):2765-2771.
299. Cohen HJ, Silberman HR, Tornyos K, Bartolucci AA. Comparison of two long-term chemotherapy regimens, with or without agents to modify skeletal repair, in multiple myeloma. *Blood.* 1984;63(3):639-648.
300. Abramson N, Lurie P, Mietlowski WL, Schilling A, Bennett JM, Horton J. Phase III study of intermittent carmustine (BCNU), cyclophosphamide, and prednisone versus intermittent melphalan and prednisone in myeloma. *Cancer Treat Rep.* 1982;66(6):1273-1277.
301. Harley JB, Pajak TF, McIntyre OR, et al. Improved survival of increased-risk myeloma patients on combined triple- alkylating-agent therapy: a study of the CALGB. *Blood.* 1979;54(1):13-22.
302. Case DC Jr, Lee DJ III, Clarkson BD. Improved survival times in multiple myeloma treated with melphalan, prednisone, cyclophosphamide, vincristine and BCNU: M-2 protocol. *Am J Med.* 1977;63(6):897-903.
303. Case DC Jr, Sonneborn HL, Paul SD, et al. Combination chemotherapy for multiple myeloma with BCNU, cyclophosphamide, vincristine, melphalan, and prednisone (M-2 protocol). *Oncology.* 1985;42(3):137-140.
304. MacLennan IC, Cusick J. Objective evaluation of the role of vincristine in induction and maintenance therapy for myelomatosis. Medical Research Council Working Party on Leukaemia in Adults. *Br J Cancer.* 1985;52(2):153-158.
305. Peest D, Coldewey R, Deicher H. Overall vs. tumor-related survival in multiple myeloma. German Myeloma Treatment Group. *Eur J Cancer.* 1991;27(5):672.
306. Peest D, Deicher H, Coldewey R, Schmoll HJ, Schedel I. Induction and maintenance therapy in multiple myeloma: a multicenter trial of MP versus VCMP. *Eur J Cancer Clin Oncol.* 1988;24(6):1061-1067.
307. Gregory WM, Richards MA, Malpas JS. Combination chemotherapy versus melphalan and prednisolone in the treatment of multiple myeloma: an overview of published trials. *J Clin Oncol.* 1992;10(2):334-342.
308. Alberts DS, Durie BG, Salmon SE. Doxorubicin/B.C.N.U. chemotherapy for multiple myeloma in relapse. *Lancet.* 1976;1(7966):926-928.
309. Alexanian R, Salmon S, Gutterman J, Dixon D, Bonnet J, Haut A. Chemoimmunotherapy for multiple myeloma. *Cancer.* 1981;47(8):1923-1929.
310. Salmon SE, Haut A, Bonnet JD, et al. Alternating combination chemotherapy and levamisole improves survival in multiple myeloma: a Southwest Oncology Group Study. *J Clin Oncol.* 1983;1(8):453-461.
311. Durie BG, Dixon DO, Carter S, et al. Improved survival duration with combination chemotherapy induction for multiple myeloma: a Southwest Oncology Group Study. *J Clin Oncol.* 1986;4(8):1227-1237.
312. MacLennan IC, Chapman C, Dunn J, Kelly K. Combined chemotherapy with ABCM versus melphalan for treatment of myelomatosis. The Medical Research Council Working Party for Leukaemia in Adults. *Lancet.* 1992;339(8787):200-205.
313. MacLennan IC, Kelly K, Crockson RA, Cooper EH, Cuzick J, Chapman C. Results of the MRC myelomatosis trials for patients entered since 1980. *Hematol Oncol.* 1988;6(2):145-158.
314. Ludwig H, Fritz E. Interferon in multiple myeloma--summary of treatment results and clinical implications. *Acta Oncol.* 2000;39(7):815-821.
315. Myeloma Trialists' Collaborative Group. Interferon as therapy for multiple myeloma: an individual patient data overview of 24 randomized trials and 4012 patients. *Br J Haematol.* 2001;113(4):1020-1034.
316. Wisloff F, Hjorth M, Kaasa S, Westin J. Effect of interferon on the health-related quality of life of multiple myeloma patients: results of a Nordic randomized trial comparing melphalan-prednisone to melphalan-prednisone + alpha-interferon. The Nordic Myeloma Study Group. *Br J Haematol.* 1996;94(2):324-332.
317. Palumbo A, Cavallo F, Gay F, et al. Autologous transplantation and maintenance therapy in multiple myeloma. *N Engl J Med.* 2014;371(10):895-905.
318. Gay F, Oliva S, Petrucci MT, et al. Chemotherapy plus lenalidomide versus autologous transplantation, followed by lenalidomide plus prednisone versus lenalidomide maintenance, in patients with multiple myeloma: a randomised, multicentre, phase 3 trial. *Lancet Oncol.* 2015;16(16):1617-1629.
319. Harousseau JL, Attal M, Avet-Loiseau H, et al. Bortezomib plus dexamethasone is superior to vincristine plus doxorubicin plus dexamethasone as induction treatment prior to autologous stem-cell transplantation in newly diagnosed multiple myeloma: results of the IFM 2005-01 phase III trial. *J Clin Oncol.* 2010;28(30):4621-4629.
320. Dispenzieri A, Jacobus S, Vesole DH, Callandar N, Fonseca R, Greipp PR. Primary therapy with single agent bortezomib as induction, maintenance and re-induction in patients with high-risk myeloma: results of the ECOG E2A02 trial. *Leukemia.* 2010;24(8):1406-1411.
321. Zonder JA, Crowley J, Hussein MA, et al. Lenalidomide and high-dose dexamethasone compared with dexamethasone as initial therapy for multiple myeloma: a randomized Southwest Oncology Group trial (S0232). *Blood.* 2010;116(26):5838-5841.
322. Voorhees PM, Kaufman JL, Laubach J, et al. Daratumumab, lenalidomide, bortezomib, and dexamethasone for transplant-eligible newly diagnosed multiple myeloma: the GRIFFIN trial. *Blood.* 2020;136(8):936-945.
323. Costa LJ, Chhabra S, Callander NS, et al. Daratumumab, carfilzomib, lenalidomide and dexamethasone (Dara-KRd), autologous transplantation and MRD

response-adapted consolidation and treatment cessation. Final primary endpoint analysis of the master trial. *Blood.* 2021;138(suppl 1):481.
324. Ghosh N, Ye X, Ferguson A, Huff CA, Borrello I. Bortezomib and thalidomide, a steroid free regimen in newly diagnosed patients with multiple myeloma. *Br J Haematol.* 2011;152(5):593-599.
325. Kumar S, Flinn I, Richardson PG, et al. Randomized, multicenter, phase 2 study (EVOLUTION) of combinations of bortezomib, dexamethasone, cyclophosphamide, and lenalidomide in previously untreated multiple myeloma. *Blood.* 2012;119(19):4375-4382.
326. Bensinger WI, Jagannath S, Vescio R, et al. Phase 2 study of two sequential three-drug combinations containing bortezomib, cyclophosphamide and dexamethasone, followed by bortezomib, thalidomide and dexamethasone as frontline therapy for multiple myeloma. *Br J Haematol.* 2010;148(4):562-568.
327. Kumar SK, Lacy MQ, Hayman SR, et al. Lenalidomide, cyclophosphamide and dexamethasone (CRd) for newly diagnosed multiple myeloma: results from a phase 2 trial. *Am J Hematol.* 2011;86(8):640-645.
328. Sonneveld P, Asselbergs E, Zweegman S, et al. Phase 2 study of carfilzomib, thalidomide, and dexamethasone as induction/consolidation therapy for newly diagnosed multiple myeloma. *Blood.* 2015;125(3):449-456.
329. Mikhael JR, Reeder CB, Libby EN, et al. Phase Ib/II trial of CYKLONE (cyclophosphamide, carfilzomib, thalidomide and dexamethasone) for newly diagnosed myeloma. *Br J Haematol.* 2015;169(2):219-227.
330. Berenson JR, Yellin O, Chen CS, et al. A modified regimen of pegylated liposomal doxorubicin, bortezomib and dexamethasone (DVD) is effective and well tolerated for previously untreated multiple myeloma patients. *Br J Haematol.* 2011;155(5):580-587.
331. Hussein MA, Baz R, Srkalovic G, et al. Phase 2 study of pegylated liposomal doxorubicin, vincristine, decreased-frequency dexamethasone, and thalidomide in newly diagnosed and relapsed-refractory multiple myeloma. *Mayo Clin Proc.* 2006;81(7):889-895.
332. Offidani M, Corvatta L, Piersantelli MN, et al. Thalidomide, dexamethasone, and pegylated liposomal doxorubicin (ThaDD) for patients older than 65 years with newly diagnosed multiple myeloma. *Blood.* 2006;108(7):2159-2164.
333. Zervas K, Dimopoulos MA, Hatzicharissi E, et al; Greek Myeloma Study Group. Primary treatment of multiple myeloma with thalidomide, vincristine, liposomal doxorubicin and dexamethasone (T-VAD doxil): a phase II multicenter study. *Ann Oncol.* 2004;15(1):134-138.
334. Jakubowiak AJ, Griffith KA, Reece DE, et al. Lenalidomide, bortezomib, pegylated liposomal doxorubicin, and dexamethasone in newly diagnosed multiple myeloma: a phase 1/2 Multiple Myeloma Research Consortium trial. *Blood.* 2011;118(3):535-543.
335. Dimopoulos MA, Pouli A, Zervas K, et al; Greek Myeloma Study Group. Prospective randomized comparison of vincristine, doxorubicin and dexamethasone (VAD) administered as intravenous bolus injection and VAD with liposomal doxorubicin as first-line treatment in multiple myeloma. *Ann Oncol.* 2003;14(7):1039-1044.
336. Rifkin RM, Gregory SA, Mohrbacher A, Hussein MA. Pegylated liposomal doxorubicin, vincristine, and dexamethasone provide significant reduction in toxicity compared with doxorubicin, vincristine, and dexamethasone in patients with newly diagnosed multiple myeloma: a phase III multicenter randomized trial. *Cancer.* 2006;106(4):848-858.
337. Moreau P, Attal M, Hulin C, et al. Bortezomib, thalidomide, and dexamethasone with or without daratumumab before and after autologous stem-cell transplantation for newly diagnosed multiple myeloma (CASSIOPEIA): a randomised, open-label, phase 3 study. *Lancet.* 2019;394(10192):29-38.
338. Gay F, Musto P, Rota-Scalabrini D, et al. Carfilzomib with cyclophosphamide and dexamethasone or lenalidomide and dexamethasone plus autologous transplantation or carfilzomib plus lenalidomide and dexamethasone, followed by maintenance with carfilzomib plus lenalidomide or lenalidomide alone for patients with newly diagnosed multiple myeloma (FORTE): a randomised, open-label, phase 2 trial. *Lancet Oncol.* 2021;22(12):1705-1720.
339. Cavo M, Tacchetti P, Patriarca F, et al; GIMEMA Italian Myeloma Network. Bortezomib with thalidomide plus dexamethasone compared with thalidomide plus dexamethasone as induction therapy before, and consolidation therapy after, double autologous stem-cell transplantation in newly diagnosed multiple myeloma: a randomised phase 3 study. *Lancet.* 2010;376(9758):2075-2085.
340. Sonneveld P, Schmidt-Wolf IGH, van der Holt B, et al. Bortezomib induction and maintenance treatment in patients with newly diagnosed multiple myeloma: results of the randomized phase III HOVON-65/GMMG-HD4 trial. *J Clin Oncol.* 2012;30(24):2946-2955.
341. Rosinol L, Oriol A, Teruel AI, et al; Programa para el Estudio y la Terapeutica de las Hemopatias Malignas/Grupo Espanol de Mieloma PETHEMA/GEM group. Superiority of bortezomib, thalidomide, and dexamethasone (VTD) as induction pretransplantation therapy in multiple myeloma: a randomized phase 3 PETHEMA/GEM study. *Blood.* 2012;120(8):1589-1596.
342. Moreau P, Avet-Loiseau H, Facon T, et al. Bortezomib plus dexamethasone versus reduced-dose bortezomib, thalidomide plus dexamethasone as induction treatment before autologous stem cell transplantation in newly diagnosed multiple myeloma. *Blood.* 2011;118(22):5752-5758, quiz 982.
343. Moreau P, Hulin C, Macro M, et al. VTD is superior to VCD prior to intensive therapy in multiple myeloma: results of the prospective IFM2013-04 trial. *Blood.* 2016;127(21):2569-2574.
344. Ludwig H, Viterbo L, Greil R, et al. Randomized phase II study of bortezomib, thalidomide, and dexamethasone with or without cyclophosphamide as induction therapy in previously untreated multiple myeloma. *J Clin Oncol.* 2013;31(2):247-255.
345. Ludwig H, Greil R, Masszi T, et al. Bortezomib, thalidomide and dexamethasone, with or without cyclophosphamide, for patients with previously untreated multiple myeloma: 5-year follow-up. *Br J Haematol.* 2015;171(3):344-354.
346. Lokhorst HM, van der Holt B, Zweegman S, et al; Dutch-Belgian Hemato-Oncology Group HOVON. A randomized phase 3 study on the effect of thalidomide combined with adriamycin, dexamethasone, and high-dose melphalan, followed by thalidomide maintenance in patients with multiple myeloma. *Blood.* 2010;115(6):1113-1120.
347. Macro M, Divine M, Uzunhan Y, et al. Dexamethasone+Thalidomide (Dex/Thal) compared to VAD as a pre-transplant treatment in newly diagnosed multiple myeloma (mm): a randomized trial. *Blood.* 2006;108(11):57.
348. Straka C, Liebisch P, Salwender H, et al. Autotransplant with and without induction chemotherapy in older multiple myeloma patients: long-term outcome of a randomized trial. *Haematologica.* 2016;101(11):1398-1406.
349. Barlogie B, Tricot G, Anaissie E, et al. Thalidomide and hematopoietic-cell transplantation for multiple myeloma. *N Engl J Med.* 2006;354(10):1021-1030.
350. Stadtmauer EA, Pasquini MC, Blackwell B, et al. Comparison of autologous hematopoietic cell transplant (autoHCT), bortezomib, lenalidomide (len) and dexamethasone (RVD) consolidation with len maintenance (ACM), tandem autohct with len maintenance (TAM) and autohct with len maintenance (AM) for up-front treatment of patients with multiple myeloma (MM): primary results from the randomized phase III trial of the blood and marrow transplant clinical trials network (BMT CTN 0702 - StaMINA trial). *Blood Adv.* 2016;128(22):LBA-1.
351. Wang M, Delasalle K, Giralt S, Alexanian R. Rapid control of previously untreated multiple myeloma with bortezomib-thalidomide-dexamethasone followed by early intensive therapy. *Blood.* 2005;106:231a.
352. Tacchetti P, Terragna C, Galli M, et al. Bortezomib- and thalidomide-induced peripheral neuropathy in multiple myeloma: clinical and molecular analyses of a phase 3 study. *Am J Hematol.* 2014;89(12):1085-1091.
353. Goldschmidt H, Mai EK, Durig J, et al; German-speaking Myeloma Multicenter Group GMMG. Response-adapted lenalidomide maintenance in newly diagnosed myeloma: results from the phase III GMMG-MM5 trial. *Leukemia.* 2020;34(7):1853-1865.
354. Gay F, Mina R, Rota-Scalabrini D, et al. Carfilzomib-based induction/consolidation with or without autologous transplant (ASCT) followed by lenalidomide (R) or carfilzomib-lenalidomide (KR) maintenance: efficacy in high-risk patients. *J Clin Oncol.* 2021;39(15 suppl):8002.
355. Kumar SK, Berdeja JG, Niesvizky R, et al. Safety and tolerability of ixazomib, an oral proteasome inhibitor, in combination with lenalidomide and dexamethasone in patients with previously untreated multiple myeloma: an open-label phase 1/2 study. *Lancet Oncol.* 2014;15(13):1503-1512.
356. Laubach JP, Kaufman JL, Sborov DW, et al. Daratumumab (DARA) plus lenalidomide, bortezomib, and dexamethasone (RVd) in patients (pts) with transplant-eligible newly diagnosed multiple myeloma (NDMM): updated analysis of Griffin after 24 months of maintenance. *Blood.* 2021;138(suppl 1):79.
357. Goldschmidt H, Mai EK, Bertsch U, et al. Elotuzumab in combination with lenalidomide, bortezomib, dexamethasone and autologous transplantation for newly-diagnosed multiple myeloma: results from the randomized phase III GMMG-HD6 trial. *Blood.* 2021;138(suppl 1):486.
358. Alexanian R, Yap BS, Bodey GP. Prednisone pulse therapy for refractory myeloma. *Blood.* 1983;62(3):572-577.
359. Barlogie B, Smith L, Alexanian R. Effective treatment of advanced multiple myeloma refractory to alkylating agents. *N Engl J Med.* 1984;310(21):1353-1356.
360. Forgeson GV, Selby P, Lakhani S, et al. Infused vincristine and adriamycin with high dose methylprednisolone (VAMP) in advanced previously treated multiple myeloma patients. *Br J Cancer.* 1988;58(4):469-473.
361. Salmon SE, Crowley JJ, Grogan TM, Finley P, Pugh RP, Barlogie B. Combination chemotherapy, glucocorticoids, and interferon alfa in the treatment of multiple myeloma: a Southwest Oncology Group study. *J Clin Oncol.* 1994;12(11):2405-2414.
362. Raje N, Powles R, Kulkarni S, et al. A comparison of vincristine and doxorubicin infusional chemotherapy with methylprednisolone (VAMP) with the addition of weekly cyclophosphamide (C-VAMP) as induction treatment followed by autografting in previously untreated myeloma. *Br J Haematol.* 1997;97(1):153-160.
363. Szelenyi H, Kreuser ED, Keilholz U, et al. Cyclophosphamide, adriamycin and dexamethasone (CAD) is a highly effective therapy for patients with advanced multiple myeloma. *Ann Oncol.* 2001;12(1):105-108.
364. Giles FJ, Wickham NR, Rapoport BL, et al. Cyclophosphamide, etoposide, vincristine, adriamycin, and dexamethasone (CEVAD) regimen in refractory multiple myeloma: an International Oncology Study Group (IOSG) phase II protocol. *Am J Hematol.* 2000;63(3):125-130.
365. Alexanian R, Dimopoulos MA, Delasalle K, Barlogie B. Primary dexamethasone treatment of multiple myeloma. *Blood.* 1992;80(4):887-890.
366. Anagnostopoulos A, Aleman A, Williams P, et al. Autologous stem cell transplantation (ASCT) after nonmyelosuppressive induction therapy with dexamethasone alone is safe and effective for newly diagnosed multiple myeloma (MM) pts who receive high dose chemotherapy (HDC). *Blood.* 2001;98:2858a.
367. Kumar S, Lacy MQ, Dispenzieri A, et al. Single agent dexamethasone for pre-stem cell transplant induction therapy for multiple myeloma. *Bone Marrow Transplant.* 2004;34(6):485-490.
368. Sher T, Ailawadhi S, Miller KC, et al. A steroid-independent regimen of bortezomib, liposomal doxorubicin and thalidomide demonstrate high response rates in newly diagnosed multiple myeloma patients. *Br J Haematol.* 2011;154(1):104-110.
369. Hassoun H, Reich L, Klimek VM, et al. Doxorubicin and dexamethasone followed by thalidomide and dexamethasone is an effective well tolerated initial therapy for multiple myeloma. *Br J Haematol.* 2006;132(2):155-161.

370. Offidani M, Corvatta L, Marconi M, et al. Low-dose thalidomide with pegylated liposomal doxorubicin and high-dose dexamethasone for relapsed/refractory multiple myeloma: a prospective, multicenter, phase II study. *Haematologica.* 2006;91(1):133-136.
371. Barlogie B, Hall R, Zander A, Dicke K, Alexanian R. High-dose melphalan with autologous bone marrow transplantation for multiple myeloma. *Blood.* 1986;67(5):1298-1301.
372. Cavo M, Gay FM, Patriarca F, et al. Double autologous stem cell transplantation significantly prolongs progression-free survival and overall survival in comparison with single autotransplantation in newly diagnosed multiple myeloma: an analysis of phase 3 EMN02/HO95 study. *Blood.* 2017;130(suppl 1):401.
373. Alexanian R, Dimopoulos MA, Delasalle KB, Hester J, Champlin R. Myeloablative therapy for primary resistant multiple myeloma. *Stem Cell.* 1995;13(suppl 2):118-121.
374. Rajkumar SV, Fonseca R, Lacy MQ, et al. Autologous stem cell transplantation for relapsed and primary refractory myeloma. *Bone Marrow Transplant.* 1999;23(12):1267-1272.
375. Kumar S, Lacy MQ, Dispenzieri A, et al. High-dose therapy and autologous stem cell transplantation for multiple myeloma poorly responsive to initial therapy. *Bone Marrow Transplant.* 2004;34(2):161-167.
376. Gertz MA, Kumar S, Lacy MQ, et al. Stem cell transplantation in multiple myeloma: impact of response failure with thalidomide or lenalidomide induction. *Blood.* 2010;115(12):2348-2353, quiz 2560.
377. Vij R, Kumar S, Zhang MJ, et al. Impact of pretransplant therapy and depth of disease response before autologous transplantation for multiple myeloma. *Biol Blood Marrow Transplant.* 2015;21(2):335-341.
378. Jackson GH, Davies FE, Pawlyn C, et al. Response adapted induction treatment improves outcomes for myeloma patients; results of the phase III myeloma XI study. *Blood.* 2016;128(22):244.
379. Bensinger WI, Buckner CD, Anasetti C, et al. Allogeneic marrow transplantation for multiple myeloma: an analysis of risk factors on outcome. *Blood.* 1996;88(7):2787-2793.
380. Harousseau JL, Attal M, Divine M, et al. Comparison of autologous bone marrow transplantation and peripheral blood stem cell transplantation after first remission induction treatment in multiple myeloma. *Bone Marrow Transplant.* 1995;15(6):963-969.
381. Larsson K, Bjorkstrand B, Ljungman P. Faster engraftment but no reduction in infectious complications after peripheral blood stem cell transplantation compared to autologous bone marrow transplantation. *Support Care Cancer.* 1998;6(4):378-383.
382. Goldschmidt H, Hegenbart U, Wallmeier M, Hohaus S, Haas R. Factors influencing collection of peripheral blood progenitor cells following high-dose cyclophosphamide and granulocyte colony-stimulating factor in patients with multiple myeloma. *Br J Haematol.* 1997;98(3):736-744.
383. Kroger N, Zeller W, Hassan HT, et al. Successful mobilization of peripheral blood stem cells in heavily pretreated myeloma patients with G-CSF alone. *Ann Hematol.* 1998;76(6):257-262.
384. Kumar S, Dispenzieri A, Lacy MQ, et al. Impact of lenalidomide therapy on stem cell mobilization and engraftment post-peripheral blood stem cell transplantation in patients with newly diagnosed myeloma. *Leukemia.* 2007;21(9):2035-2042.
385. Kumar S, Giralt S, Stadtmauer EA, et al; International Myeloma Working Group. Mobilization in myeloma revisited: IMWG consensus perspectives on stem cell collection following initial therapy with thalidomide-lenalidomide-or bortezomib-containing regimens. *Blood.* 2009;114(9):1729-1735.
386. Giralt S, Stadtmauer EA, Harousseau JL, et al; IMWG. International myeloma working group (IMWG) consensus statement and guidelines regarding the current status of stem cell collection and high-dose therapy for multiple myeloma and the role of plerixafor (AMD 3100). *Leukemia.* 2009;23(10):1904-1912.
387. Bensinger W, Appelbaum F, Rowley S, et al. Factors that influence collection and engraftment of autologous peripheral-blood stem cells. *J Clin Oncol.* 1995;13(10):2547-2555.
388. Desikan KR, Tricot G, Munshi NC, et al. Preceding chemotherapy, tumour load and age influence engraftment in multiple myeloma patients mobilized with granulocyte colony-stimulating factor alone. *Br J Haematol.* 2001;112(1):242-247.
389. Devine SM, Flomenberg N, Vesole DH, et al. Rapid mobilization of CD34+ cells following administration of the CXCR4 antagonist AMD3100 to patients with multiple myeloma and non-Hodgkin's lymphoma. *J Clin Oncol.* 2004;22(6):1095-1102. doi:10.1200/JCO.2004.07.131
390. Galimberti S, Morabito F, Guerrini F, et al. Peripheral blood stem cell contamination evaluated by a highly sensitive molecular method fails to predict outcome of autotransplanted multiple myeloma patients. *Br J Haematol.* 2003;120(3):405-412.
391. Gertz MA, Witzig TE, Pineda AA, Greipp PR, Kyle RA, Litzow MR. Monoclonal plasma cells in the blood stem cell harvest from patients with multiple myeloma are associated with shortened relapse-free survival after transplantation. *Bone Marrow Transplant.* 1997;19(4):337-342.
392. Reece DE, Barnett MJ, Connors JM, et al. Treatment of multiple myeloma with intensive chemotherapy followed by autologous BMT using marrow purged with 4-hydroperoxycyclophosphamide. *Bone Marrow Transplant.* 1993;11(2):139-146.
393. Seiden MV, Schlossman R, Andersen J, et al. Monoclonal antibody-purged bone marrow transplantation therapy for multiple myeloma. *Leuk Lymphoma.* 1995;17(1-2):87-93.
394. Anderson KC, Andersen J, Soiffer R, et al. Monoclonal antibody-purged bone marrow transplantation therapy for multiple myeloma. *Blood.* 1993;82(8):2568-2576.
395. Tricot G, Gazitt Y, Leemhuis T, et al. Collection, tumor contamination, and engraftment kinetics of highly purified hematopoietic progenitor cells to support high dose therapy in multiple myeloma. *Blood.* 1998;91(12):4489-4495.
396. Stewart AK, Vescio R, Schiller G, et al. Purging of autologous peripheral-blood stem cells using CD34 selection does not improve overall or progression-free survival after high-dose chemotherapy for multiple myeloma: results of a multicenter randomized controlled trial. *J Clin Oncol.* 2001;19(17):3771-3779.
397. Bourhis JH, Bouko Y, Koscielny S, et al; European Group for Blood and Marrow Transplantation. Relapse risk after autologous transplantation in patients with newly diagnosed myeloma is not related with infused tumor cell load and the outcome is not improved by CD34+ cell selection: long term follow-up of an EBMT phase III randomized study. *Haematologica.* 2007;92(8):1083-1090.
398. Child JA, Morgan GJ, Davies FE, et al; Medical Research Council Adult Leukaemia Working Party. High-dose chemotherapy with hematopoietic stem-cell rescue for multiple myeloma. *N Engl J Med.* 2003;348(19):1875-1883.
399. Palumbo A, Bringhen S, Petrucci MT, et al. Intermediate-dose melphalan improves survival of myeloma patients aged 50 to 70: results of a randomized controlled trial. *Blood.* 2004;104(10):3052-3057.
400. Fermand JP, Katsahian S, Divine M, et al; Group Myelome-Autogreffe. High-dose therapy and autologous blood stem-cell transplantation compared with conventional treatment in myeloma patients aged 55 to 65 years: long-term results of a randomized control trial from the Group Myelome-Autogreffe. *J Clin Oncol.* 2005;23(36):9227-9233.
401. Fermand JP, Ravaud P, Chevret S, et al. High-dose therapy and autologous peripheral blood stem cell transplantation in multiple myeloma: up-front or rescue treatment? Results of a multicenter sequential randomized clinical trial. *Blood.* 1998;92(9):3131-3136.
402. Barlogie B, Kyle RA, Anderson KC, et al. Standard chemotherapy compared with high-dose chemoradiotherapy for multiple myeloma: final results of phase III US Intergroup Trial S9321. *J Clin Oncol.* 2006;24(6):929-936.
403. Blade J, Rosinol L, Sureda A, et al; Programa para el Estudio de la Terapeutica en Hemopatia Maligna PETHEMA. High-dose therapy intensification compared with continued standard chemotherapy in multiple myeloma patients responding to the initial chemotherapy: long-term results from a prospective randomized trial from the Spanish Cooperative Group PETHEMA. *Blood.* 2005;106(12):3755-3759.
404. Sonneveld P, van der Holt B, Segeren CM, et al; Dutch-Belgian Hemato-Oncology Cooperative Group HOVON. Intermediate-dose melphalan compared with myeloablative treatment in multiple myeloma: long-term follow-up of the Dutch Cooperative Group HOVON 24 trial. *Haematologica.* 2007;92(7):928-935.
405. Harousseau JL, Attal M. The role of stem cell transplantation in multiple myeloma. *Blood Rev.* 2002;16(4):245-253.
406. Perrot A, Lauwers-Cances V, Cazaubiel T, et al. Early versus late autologous stem cell transplant in newly diagnosed multiple myeloma: long-term follow-up analysis of the IFM 2009 trial. *Blood.* 2020;136(suppl 1):39.
407. Vesole DH, Barlogie B, Jagannath S, et al. High-dose therapy for refractory multiple myeloma: improved prognosis with better supportive care and double transplants. *Blood.* 1994;84(3):950-956.
408. Barlogie B, Jagannath S, Vesole DH, et al. Superiority of tandem autologous transplantation over standard therapy for previously untreated multiple myeloma. *Blood.* 1997;89(3):789-793.
409. Desikan R, Barlogie B, Sawyer J, et al. Results of high-dose therapy for 1000 patients with multiple myeloma: durable complete remissions and superior survival in the absence of chromosome 13 abnormalities. *Blood.* 2000;95(12):4008-4010.
410. Barlogie B, Jagannath S, Desikan KR, et al. Total therapy with tandem transplants for newly diagnosed multiple myeloma. *Blood.* 1999;93(1):55-65.
411. Usmani SZ, Crowley J, Hoering A, et al. Improvement in long-term outcomes with successive Total Therapy trials for multiple myeloma: are patients now being cured? *Leukemia.* 2013;27(1):226-232.
412. Khan ML, Reeder CB, Kumar SK, et al. A comparison of lenalidomide/dexamethasone versus cyclophosphamide/lenalidomide/dexamethasone versus cyclophosphamide/bortezomib/dexamethasone in newly diagnosed multiple myeloma. *Br J Haematol.* 2012;156(3):326-333.
413. Kumar SK, Lacy MQ, Dispenzieri A, et al. Early versus delayed autologous transplantation after immunomodulatory agents-based induction therapy in patients with newly diagnosed multiple myeloma. *Cancer.* 2012;118(6):1585-1592.
414. Attal M, Harousseau JL, Facon T, et al; InterGroupe Francophone du Myelome. Single versus double autologous stem-cell transplantation for multiple myeloma. *N Engl J Med.* 2003;349(26):2495-2502.
415. Cavo M, Tosi P, Zamagni E, et al. Prospective, randomized study of single compared with double autologous stem-cell transplantation for multiple myeloma: Bologna 96 clinical study. *J Clin Oncol.* 2007;25(17):2434-2441.
416. Mai EK, Benner A, Bertsch U, et al. Single versus tandem high-dose melphalan followed by autologous blood stem cell transplantation in multiple myeloma: long-term results from the phase III GMMG-HD2 trial. *Br J Haematol.* 2016;173(5):731-741.
417. Kumar A, Kharfan-Dabaja MA, Glasmacher A, Djulbegovic B. Tandem versus single autologous hematopoietic cell transplantation for the treatment of multiple myeloma: a systematic review and meta-analysis. *J Natl Cancer Inst.* 2009;101(2):100-106.
418. Cavo M, Gay F, Beksac M, et al. Autologous haematopoietic stem-cell transplantation versus bortezomib-melphalan-prednisone, with or without bortezomib-lenalidomide-dexamethasone consolidation therapy, and lenalidomide maintenance for newly diagnosed multiple myeloma (EMN02/HO95): a multicentre, randomised, open-label, phase 3 study. *Lancet Haematol.* 2020;7(6):e456-e468.
419. Cook G, Ashcroft AJ, Cairns DA, et al; National Cancer Research Institute Haemato-oncology Clinical Studies Group. The effect of salvage autologous stem-cell transplantation on overall survival in patients with relapsed multiple myeloma (final results from BSBMT/UKMF Myeloma X Relapse [Intensive]): a randomised, open-label, phase 3 trial. *Lancet Haematol.* 2016;3(7):e340-e351.
420. Gonsalves WI, Gertz MA, Lacy MQ, et al. Second auto-SCT for treatment of relapsed multiple myeloma. *Bone Marrow Transplant.* 2013;48(4):568-573.

421. Alvares CL, Davies FE, Horton C, Patel G, Powles R, Morgan GJ. The role of second autografts in the management of myeloma at first relapse. *Haematologica*. 2006;91(1):141-142.
422. Jimenez-Zepeda VH, Mikhael J, Winter A, et al. Second autologous stem cell transplantation as salvage therapy for multiple myeloma: impact on progression-free and overall survival. *Biol Blood Marrow Transplant*. 2012;18(5):773-779.
423. Silva Ronden C, Hassoun H, Chimento D, Jia X, Giralt S, Landau HJ. Outcomes following salvage autologous stem cell transplant (Sct) for multiple myeloma. *Biol Blood Marrow Transplant*. 2012;18(2 suppl):S254.
424. Fenk R, Liese V, Neubauer F, et al. Predictive factors for successful salvage high-dose therapy in patients with multiple myeloma relapsing after autologous blood stem cell transplantation. *Leuk Lymphoma*. 2011;52(8):1455-1462.
425. Shah N, Ahmed F, Bashir Q, et al. Durable remission with salvage second autotransplants in patients with multiple myeloma. *Cancer*. 2012;118(14):3549-3555.
426. Mehta J, Tricot G, Jagannath S, et al. Salvage autologous or allogeneic transplantation for multiple myeloma refractory to or relapsing after a first-line autograft? *Bone Marrow Transplant*. 1998;21(9):887-892.
427. Olin RL, Vogl DT, Porter DL, et al. Second auto-SCT is safe and effective salvage therapy for relapsed multiple myeloma. *Bone Marrow Transplant*. 2009;43(5):417-422.
428. Elice F, Raimondi R, Tosetto A, et al. Prolonged overall survival with second on-demand autologous transplant in multiple myeloma. *Am J Hematol*. 2006;81(6):426-431.
429. Burzynski JA, Toro JJ, Patel RC, et al. Toxicity of a second autologous peripheral blood stem cell transplant in patients with relapsed or recurrent multiple myeloma. *Leuk Lymphoma*. 2009;50(9):1442-1447.
430. Siegel DS, Desikan KR, Mehta J, et al. Age is not a prognostic variable with autotransplants for multiple myeloma. *Blood*. 1999;93(1):51-54.
431. Badros A, Barlogie B, Morris C, et al. High response rate in refractory and poor-risk multiple myeloma after allotransplantation using a nonmyeloablative conditioning regimen and donor lymphocyte infusions. *Blood*. 2001;97(9):2574-2579.
432. Muchtar E, Dingli D, Kumar S, et al. Autologous stem cell transplant for multiple myeloma patients 70 years or older. *Bone Marrow Transplant*. 2016;51(11):1449-1455.
433. Dhakal B, Nelson A, Guru Murthy GS, et al. Autologous hematopoietic cell transplantation in patients with multiple myeloma: effect of age. *Clin Lymphoma Myeloma Leuk*. 2017;17(3):165-172.
434. San Miguel JF, Lahuerta JJ, Garcia-Sanz R, et al. Are myeloma patients with renal failure candidates for autologous stem cell transplantation? *Hematol J*. 2000;1(1):28-36.
435. Lee CK, Zangari M, Barlogie B, et al. Dialysis-dependent renal failure in patients with myeloma can be reversed by high-dose myeloablative therapy and autotransplant. *Bone Marrow Transplant*. 2004;33(8):823-828.
436. Knudsen LM, Nielsen B, Gimsing P, Geisler C. Autologous stem cell transplantation in multiple myeloma: outcome in patients with renal failure. *Eur J Haematol*. 2005;75(1):27-33.
437. Moreau P, Facon T, Attal M, et al; Intergroupe Francophone du Myelome. Comparison of 200 mg/m^2 melphalan and 8 Gy total body irradiation plus 140 mg/m^2 melphalan as conditioning regimens for peripheral blood stem cell transplantation in patients with newly diagnosed multiple myeloma: final analysis of the Intergroupe Francophone du Myelome 9502 randomized trial. *Blood*. 2002;99(3):731-735.
438. Lahuerta JJ, Mateos MV, Martinez-Lopez J, et al; Grupo Espanol de MM and Programa para el Estudio de la Terapeutica en Hemopatia Maligna Cooperative Study Groups. Busulfan 12 mg/kg plus melphalan 140 mg/m^2 versus melphalan 200 mg/m^2 as conditioning regimens for autologous transplantation in newly diagnosed multiple myeloma patients included in the PETHEMA/GEM2000 study. *Haematologica*. 2010;95(11):1913-1920.
439. Bashir Q, Thall PF, Milton DR, et al. Conditioning with busulfan plus melphalan versus melphalan alone before autologous haemopoietic cell transplantation for multiple myeloma: an open-label, randomised, phase 3 trial. *Lancet Haematol*. 2019;6(5):e266-e275.
440. Bensinger WI, Becker PS, Gooley TA, et al. A randomized study of melphalan 200 mg/m^2 vs 280 mg/m^2 as a preparative regimen for patients with multiple myeloma undergoing auto-SCT. *Bone Marrow Transplant*. 2016;51(1):67-71.
441. Fenk R, Schneider P, Kropff M, et al; West German Myeloma Study Group. High-dose idarubicin, cyclophosphamide and melphalan as conditioning for autologous stem cell transplantation increases treatment-related mortality in patients with multiple myeloma: results of a randomised study. *Br J Haematol*. 2005;130(4):588-594.
442. Huijgens PC, Dekker-Van Roessel HM, Jonkhoff AR, et al. High-dose melphalan with G-CSF-stimulated whole blood rescue followed by stem cell harvesting and busulphan/cyclophosphamide with autologous stem cell transplantation in multiple myeloma. *Bone Marrow Transplant*. 2001;27(9):925-931.
443. Schiller G, Nimer S, Vescio R, et al. Phase I-II study of busulfan and cyclophosphamide conditioning for transplantation in advanced multiple myeloma. *Bone Marrow Transplant*. 1994;14(1):131-136.
444. Lahuerta JJ, Grande C, Blade J, et al; Spanish Multiple Myeloma Group. Myeloablative treatments for multiple myeloma: update of a comparative study of different regimens used in patients from the Spanish registry for transplantation in multiple myeloma. *Leuk Lymphoma*. 2002;43(1):67-74.
445. Capria S, Petrucci MT, Pulsoni A, et al. High-dose idarubicin, busulphan and melphalan for autologous stem cell transplantation in multiple myeloma responsive to DAV chemotherapy: comparison with a historical control. *Acta Haematol*. 2006;115(1-2):9-14.
446. Carrion Galindo R Sr, Serrano D, Perez-Corral A, et al. High-dose chemotherapy and autologous peripheral blood stem cell rescue (Auto-SCT) in multiple myeloma (MM) patients: busulfan + melphalan-140 (BuMel) versus (vs) melphalan-200 (Mel-200) as conditioning regimens. *J Clin Oncol*. 2006;24(18 suppl):7612.
447. Dispenzieri A, Wiseman GA, Lacy MQ, et al. A phase I study of 153Sm-EDTMP with fixed high dose melphalan as a peripheral blood stem cell conditioning regimen in patients with multiple myeloma. *Leukemia*. 2005;19(1):118-125.
448. Giralt S, Bensinger W, Goodman M, et al. 166Ho-DOTMP plus melphalan followed by peripheral blood stem cell transplantation in patients with multiple myeloma: results of two phase 1/2 trials. *Blood*. 2003;102(7):2684-2691.
449. Hollmig K, Stover T, Talamo G, et al. Addition of bortezomib (Velcade™) to high dose melphalan (Vel-Mel) as an effective conditioning regimen with autologous stem cell support in multiple myeloma (MM). *Blood*. 2004;104(11):929.
450. Palumbo A, Avonto I, Bruno B, et al. Intermediate-dose melphalan (100 mg/m^2)/bortezomib/thalidomide/dexamethasone and stem cell support in patients with refractory or relapsed myeloma. *Clin Lymphoma Myeloma*. 2006;6(6):475-477.
451. Lonial S, Kaufman J, Tighiouart M, et al. A phase I/II trial combining high-dose melphalan and autologous transplant with bortezomib for multiple myeloma: a dose- and schedule-finding study. *Clin Cancer Res*. 2010;16(20):5079-5086.
452. Roussel M, Moreau P, Huynh A, et al; Intergroupe Francophone du Myelome IFM. Bortezomib and high-dose melphalan as conditioning regimen before autologous stem cell transplantation in patients with de novo multiple myeloma: a phase 2 study of the Intergroupe Francophone du Myelome (IFM). *Blood*. 2010;115(1):32-37.
453. Desikan KR, Tricot G, Dhodapkar M, et al. Melphalan plus total body irradiation (MEL-TBI) or cyclophosphamide (MEL-CY) as a conditioning regimen with second autotransplant in responding patients with myeloma is inferior compared to historical controls receiving tandem transplants with melphalan alone. *Bone Marrow Transplant*. 2000;25(5):483-487.
454. Crawley C, Lalancette M, Szydlo R, et al; Chromic Leukaemia Working Party of the EBMT. Outcomes for reduced-intensity allogeneic transplantation for multiple myeloma: an analysis of prognostic factors from the Chronic Leukaemia Working Party of the EBMT. *Blood*. 2005;105(11):4532-4539.
455. Bjorkstrand BB, Ljungman P, Svensson H, et al. Allogeneic bone marrow transplantation versus autologous stem cell transplantation in multiple myeloma: a retrospective case-matched study from the European Group for Blood and Marrow Transplantation. *Blood*. 1996;88(12):4711-4718.
456. Varterasian M, Janakiraman N, Karanes C, et al. Transplantation in patients with multiple myeloma: a multicenter comparative analysis of peripheral blood stem cell and allogeneic transplant. *Am J Clin Oncol*. 1997;20(5):462-466.
457. Couban S, Stewart AK, Loach D, Panzarella T, Meharchand J. Autologous and allogeneic transplantation for multiple myeloma at a single centre. *Bone Marrow Transplant*. 1997;19(8):783-789.
458. Reynolds C, Ratanatharathorn V, Adams P, et al. Allogeneic stem cell transplantation reduces disease progression compared to autologous transplantation in patients with multiple myeloma. *Bone Marrow Transplant*. 2001;27(8):801-807.
459. Lokhorst HM, Sonneveld P, Cornelissen JJ, et al. Induction therapy with vincristine, adriamycin, dexamethasone (VAD) and intermediate-dose melphalan (IDM) followed by autologous or allogeneic stem cell transplantation in newly diagnosed multiple myeloma. *Bone Marrow Transplant*. 1999;23(4):317-322.
460. Alyea E, Weller E, Schlossman R, et al. Outcome after autologous and allogeneic stem cell transplantation for patients with multiple myeloma: impact of graft-versus-myeloma effect. *Bone Marrow Transplant*. 2003;32(12):1145-1151.
461. Arora M, McGlave PB, Burns LJ, et al. Results of autologous and allogeneic hematopoietic cell transplant therapy for multiple myeloma. *Bone Marrow Transplant*. 2005;35(12):1133-1140.
462. Kuruvilla J, Shepherd JD, Sutherland HJ, et al. Long-term outcome of myeloablative allogeneic stem cell transplantation for multiple myeloma. *Biol Blood Marrow Transplant*. 2007;13(8):925-931.
463. Freytes CO, Vesole DH, LeRademacher J, et al. Second transplants for multiple myeloma relapsing after a previous autotransplant-reduced-intensity allogeneic vs autologous transplantation. *Bone Marrow Transplant*. 2014;49(3):416-421.
464. Kroger N, Schwerdtfeger R, Kiehl M, et al. Autologous stem cell transplantation followed by a dose-reduced allograft induces high complete remission rate in multiple myeloma. *Blood*. 2002;100(3):755-760.
465. Maloney DG, Molina AJ, Sahebi F, et al. Allografting with nonmyeloablative conditioning following cytoreductive autografts for the treatment of patients with multiple myeloma. *Blood*. 2003;102(9):3447-3454.
466. Garban F, Attal M, Michallet M, et al. Prospective comparison of autologous stem cell transplantation followed by dose-reduced allograft (IFM99-03 trial) with tandem autologous stem cell transplantation (IFM99-04 trial) in high-risk de novo multiple myeloma. *Blood*. 2006;107(9):3474-3480.
467. Moreau P, Hullin C, Garban F, et al; Intergroupe Francophone du Myelome group. Tandem autologous stem cell transplantation in high-risk de novo multiple myeloma: final results of the prospective and randomized IFM 99-04 protocol. *Blood*. 2006;107(1):397-403.
468. Bruno B, Rotta M, Patriarca F, et al. A comparison of allografting with autografting for newly diagnosed myeloma. *N Engl J Med*. 2007;356(11):1110-1120.
469. Giaccone L, Storer B, Patriarca F, et al. Long-term follow-up of a comparison of nonmyeloablative allografting with autografting for newly diagnosed myeloma. *Blood*. 2011;117(24):6721-6727.
470. Giaccone L, Evangelista A, Patriarca F, et al. Impact of new drugs on the long-term follow-up of upfront tandem autograft-allograft in multiple myeloma. *Biol Blood Marrow Transplant*. 2018;24(1):189-193.
471. Rosinol L, Perez-Simon JA, Sureda A, et al; Programa para el Estudio y la Terapeutica de las Hemopatias Malignas y Grupo Espanol de Mieloma PETHEMA/GEM. A prospective PETHEMA study of tandem autologous transplantation versus autograft followed by reduced-intensity conditioning allogeneic transplantation in newly diagnosed multiple myeloma. *Blood*. 2008;112(9):3591-3593.

472. Bjorkstrand B, Iacobelli S, Hegenbart U, et al. Tandem autologous/reduced-intensity conditioning allogeneic stem-cell transplantation versus autologous transplantation in myeloma: long-term follow-up. *J Clin Oncol*. 2011;29(22):3016-3022.
473. Gahrton G, Iacobelli S, Bjorkstrand B, et al; EBMT Chronic Malignancies Working Party Plasma Cell Disorders Subcommittee. Autologous/reduced-intensity allogeneic stem cell transplantation vs autologous transplantation in multiple myeloma: long-term results of the EBMT-NMAM2000 study. *Blood*. 2013;121(25):5055-5063.
474. Krishnan A, Pasquini MC, Logan B, et al; Blood Marrow Transplant Clinical Trials Network BMT CTN. Autologous haemopoietic stem-cell transplantation followed by allogeneic or autologous haemopoietic stem-cell transplantation in patients with multiple myeloma (BMT CTN 0102): a phase 3 biological assignment trial. *Lancet Oncol*. 2011;12(13):1195-1203.
475. Armeson KE, Hill EG, Costa LJ. Tandem autologous vs autologous plus reduced intensity allogeneic transplantation in the upfront management of multiple myeloma: meta-analysis of trials with biological assignment. *Bone Marrow Transplant*. 2013;48(4):562-567.
476. Kroger N, Einsele H, Derigs G, Wandt H, Krull A, Zander A. Long-term follow-up of an intensified myeloablative conditioning regimen with in vivo T cell depletion followed by allografting in patients with advanced multiple myeloma. *Biol Blood Marrow Transplant*. 2010;16(6):861-864.
477. Franssen LE, Raymakers RAP, Buijs A, et al. Outcome of allogeneic transplantation in newly diagnosed and relapsed/refractory multiple myeloma: long-term follow-up in a single institution. *Eur J Haematol*. 2016;97(5):479-488.
478. Smith E, Devlin SM, Kosuri S, et al. CD34-Selected allogeneic hematopoietic stem cell transplantation for patients with relapsed, high-risk multiple myeloma. *Biol Blood Marrow Transplant*. 2016;22(2):258-267.
479. Castagna L, Mussetti A, Devillier R, et al. Haploidentical allogeneic hematopoietic cell transplantation for multiple myeloma using post-transplantation cyclophosphamide graft-versus-host disease prophylaxis. *Biol Blood Marrow Transplant*. 2017;23(9):1549-1554.
480. Ghosh N, Ye X, Tsai HL, et al. Allogeneic blood or marrow transplantation with post-transplantation cyclophosphamide as graft-versus-host disease prophylaxis in multiple myeloma. *Biol Blood Marrow Transplant*. 2017;23(11):1903-1909.
481. Sobh M, Michallet M, Dubois V, et al. Salvage use of allogeneic hematopoietic stem cell transplantation after reduced intensity conditioning from unrelated donors in multiple myeloma. A study by the Plasma Cell Disorders subcommittee of the European Group for Blood and Marrow Transplant Chronic Malignancies Working Party. *Haematologica*. 2017;102(7):e271-e274.
482. Kroger N, Badbaran A, Zabelina T, et al. Impact of high-risk cytogenetics and achievement of molecular remission on long-term freedom from disease after autologous-allogeneic tandem transplantation in patients with multiple myeloma. *Biol Blood Marrow Transplant*. 2013;19(3):398-404.
483. Roos-Weil D, Moreau P, Avet-Loiseau H, et al; Societe Francaise de Greffe de Moelle et de Therapie Cellulaire SFGM-TC. Impact of genetic abnormalities after allogeneic stem cell transplantation in multiple myeloma: a report of the Societe Francaise de Greffe de Moelle et de Therapie Cellulaire. *Haematologica*. 2011;96(10):1504-1511.
484. Schilling G, Hansen T, Shimoni A, et al. Impact of genetic abnormalities on survival after allogeneic hematopoietic stem cell transplantation in multiple myeloma. *Leukemia*. 2008;22(6):1250-1255.
485. Tricot G, Vesole DH, Jagannath S, Hilton J, Munshi N, Barlogie B. Graft-versus-myeloma effect: proof of principle. *Blood*. 1996;87(3):1196-1198.
486. Lokhorst HM, Schattenberg A, Cornelissen JJ, Thomas LL, Verdonck LF. Donor leukocyte infusions are effective in relapsed multiple myeloma after allogeneic bone marrow transplantation. *Blood*. 1997;90(10):4206-4211.
487. Alyea E, Weller E, Schlossman R, et al. T-cell – depleted allogeneic bone marrow transplantation followed by donor lymphocyte infusion in patients with multiple myeloma: induction of graft-versus-myeloma effect. *Blood*. 2001;98(4):934-939.
488. Peggs KS, Mackinnon S, Williams CD, et al. Reduced-intensity transplantation with in vivo T-cell depletion and adjuvant dose-escalating donor lymphocyte infusions for chemotherapy-sensitive myeloma: limited efficacy of graft-versus-tumor activity. *Biol Blood Marrow Transplant*. 2003;9(4):257-265.
489. Peggs KS, Thomson K, Hart DP, et al. Dose-escalated donor lymphocyte infusions following reduced intensity transplantation: toxicity, chimerism, and disease responses. *Blood*. 2004;103(4):1548-1556.
490. Ayuk F, Shimoni A, Nagler A, et al. Efficacy and toxicity of low-dose escalating donor lymphocyte infusion given after reduced intensity conditioning allograft for multiple myeloma. *Leukemia*. 2004;18(3):659-662.
491. van de Donk NWCJ, Kroger N, Hegenbart U, et al. Prognostic factors for donor lymphocyte infusions following non-myeloablative allogeneic stem cell transplantation in multiple myeloma. *Bone Marrow Transplant*. 2006;37(12):1135-1141.
492. Lokhorst HM, Wu K, Verdonck LF, et al. The occurrence of graft-versus-host disease is the major predictive factor for response to donor lymphocyte infusions in multiple myeloma. *Blood*. 2004;103(11):4362-4364.
493. Kyle RA, Pierre RV, Bayrd ED. Multiple myeloma and acute myelomonocytic leukemia. *N Engl J Med*. 1970;283(21):1121-1125.
494. Nordenson NG. Myelomatosis: a clinical review of 310 cases. *Acta Med Scand Suppl*. 1966;(suppl 445):178-186.
495. Osserman EF, Takatsuki K, Talal N. The pathogenesis of "amyloidosis". *Semin Hematol*. 1964;1:3-85.
496. Edwards GA, Zawadzki ZA. Extraosseous lesions in plasma cell myeloma: a report of six cases. *Am J Med*. 1967;43(2):194-205.
497. Gonzalez F, Trujillo JM, Alexanian R. Acute leukemia in multiple myeloma. *Ann Intern Med*. 1977;86(4):440-443.
498. Bergsagel DE, Bailey AJ, Langley GR, MacDonald RN, White DF, Miller AB. The chemotherapy on plasma-cell myeloma and the incidence of acute leukemia. *N Engl J Med*. 1979;301(14):743-748.
499. Attal M, Harousseau JL, Leyvraz S, et al; Inter-Groupe Francophone du Myelome IFM. Maintenance therapy with thalidomide improves survival in patients with multiple myeloma. *Blood*. 2006;108(10):3289-3294.
500. Spencer A, Prince HM, Roberts AW, et al. Consolidation therapy with low-dose thalidomide and prednisolone prolongs the survival of multiple myeloma patients undergoing a single autologous stem-cell transplantation procedure. *J Clin Oncol*. 2009;27(11):1788-1793.
501. Morgan GJ, Gregory WM, Davies FE, et al; National Cancer Research Institute Haematological Oncology Clinical Studies Group. The role of maintenance thalidomide therapy in multiple myeloma: MRC Myeloma IX results and meta-analysis. *Blood*. 2012;119(1):7-15.
502. Stewart AK, Trudel S, Bahlis NJ, et al. A randomized phase III trial of thalidomide and prednisone as maintenance therapy following autologous stem cell transplantation (ASCT) in patients with multiple myeloma (MM): the NCIC CTG MY.10 trial. *Blood*. 2010;116(21):39.
503. Attal M, Lauwers-Cances V, Marit G, et al; IFM Investigators. Lenalidomide maintenance after stem-cell transplantation for multiple myeloma. *N Engl J Med*. 2012;366(19):1782-1791.
504. McCarthy PL, Owzar K, Hofmeister CC, et al. Lenalidomide after stem-cell transplantation for multiple myeloma. *N Engl J Med*. 2012;366(19):1770-1781.
505. Facon T, Dimopoulos MA, Dispenzieri A, et al. Final analysis of survival outcomes in the phase 3 FIRST trial of up-front treatment for multiple myeloma. *Blood*. 2018;131(3):301-310.
506. McCarthy PL, Holstein SA, Petrucci MT, et al. Lenalidomide maintenance after autologous stem-cell transplantation in newly diagnosed multiple myeloma: a meta-analysis. *J Clin Oncol*. 2017;35(29):3279-3289.
507. Jackson GH, Davies FE, Pawlyn C, et al; UK NCRI Haemato-oncology Clinical Studies Group. Lenalidomide maintenance versus observation for patients with newly diagnosed multiple myeloma (Myeloma XI): a multicentre, open-label, randomised, phase 3 trial. *Lancet Oncol*. 2019;20(1):57-73.
508. Kneppers E, van der Holt B, Kersten MJ, et al. Lenalidomide maintenance after nonmyeloablative allogeneic stem cell transplantation in multiple myeloma is not feasible: results of the HOVON 76 Trial. *Blood*. 2011;118(9):2413-2419.
509. Alsina M, Becker PS, Zhong X, et al; Resource for Clinical Investigation in Blood and Marrow Transplantation. Lenalidomide maintenance for high-risk multiple myeloma after allogeneic hematopoietic cell transplantation. *Biol Blood Marrow Transplant*. 2014;20(8):1183-1189.
510. Jackson G, Davies FE, Pawlyn C, et al. Lenalidomide maintenance significantly improves outcomes compared to observation irrespective of cytogenetic risk: results of the myeloma XI trial. *Blood*. 2017;130(suppl 1):436.
511. Dimopoulos MA, Gay F, Schjesvold F, et al; TOURMALINE-MM3 study group. Oral ixazomib maintenance following autologous stem cell transplantation (TOURMALINE-MM3): a double-blind, randomised, placebo-controlled phase 3 trial. *Lancet*. 2019;393(10168):253-264.
512. Moreau P, Hulin C, Perrot A, et al. Maintenance with daratumumab or observation following treatment with bortezomib, thalidomide, and dexamethasone with or without daratumumab and autologous stem-cell transplant in patients with newly diagnosed multiple myeloma (CASSIOPEIA): an open-label, randomised, phase 3 trial. *Lancet Oncol*. 2021;22(10):1378-1390.
513. Alexanian R, Gehan E, Haut A, Saiki J, Weick J. Unmaintained remissions in multiple myeloma. *Blood*. 1978;51(6):1005-1011.
514. Cohen HJ, Bartolucci AA, Forman WB, Silberman HR. Consolidation and maintenance therapy in multiple myeloma: randomized comparison of a new approach to therapy after initial response to treatment. *J Clin Oncol*. 1986;4(6):888-899.
515. Kildahl-Andersen O, Bjark P, Bondevik A, et al. Multiple myeloma in central and northern Norway 1981-1982: a follow-up study of a randomized clinical trial of 5-drug combination therapy versus standard therapy. *Eur J Haematol*. 1988;41(1):47-51.
516. Belch A, Shelley W, Bergsagel D, et al. A randomized trial of maintenance versus no maintenance melphalan and prednisone in responding multiple myeloma patients. *Br J Cancer*. 1988;57(1):94-99.
517. Riccardi A, Ucci G, Luoni R, et al. Treatment of multiple myeloma according to the extension of the disease: a prospective, randomised study comparing a less with a more aggressive cystostatic policy. Cooperative Group of Study and Treatment of Multiple Myeloma. *Br J Cancer*. 1994;70(6):1203-1210.
518. Berenson JR, Crowley JJ, Grogan TM, et al. Maintenance therapy with alternate-day prednisone improves survival in multiple myeloma patients. *Blood*. 2002;99(9):3163-3168.
519. Alexanian R, Weber D, Dimopoulos M, Delasalle K, Smith TL. Randomized trial of alpha-interferon or dexamethasone as maintenance treatment for multiple myeloma. *Am J Hematol*. 2000;65(3):204-209.
520. Cornwell GG III, Pajak TF, Kochwa S, et al. Vincristine and prednisone prolong the survival of patients receiving intravenous or oral melphalan for multiple myeloma: Cancer and Leukemia Group B experience. *J Clin Oncol*. 1988;6(9):1481-1490.
521. Anderson KC, Kyle RA, Rajkumar SV, Stewart AK, Weber D, Richardson P; ASH/FDA Panel on Clinical Endpoints in Multiple Myeloma. Clinically relevant end points and new drug approvals for myeloma. *Leukemia*. 2008;22(2):231-239.
522. Barlogie B, Desikan R, Eddlemon P, et al. Extended survival in advanced and refractory multiple myeloma after single-agent thalidomide: identification of prognostic factors in a phase 2 study of 169 patients. *Blood*. 2001;98(2):492-494.
523. Dimopoulos MA, Zervas K, Kouvatseas G, et al. Thalidomide and dexamethasone combination for refractory multiple myeloma. *Ann Oncol*. 2001;12(7):991-995.

524. Richardson PG, Blood E, Mitsiades CS, et al. A randomized phase 2 study of lenalidomide therapy for patients with relapsed or relapsed and refractory multiple myeloma. *Blood.* 2006;108(10):3458-3464.
525. Dimopoulos M, Spencer A, Attal M, et al; Multiple Myeloma 010 Study Investigators. Lenalidomide plus dexamethasone for relapsed or refractory multiple myeloma. *N Engl J Med.* 2007;357(21):2123-2132.
526. Weber DM, Chen C, Niesvizky R, et al; Multiple Myeloma 009 Study Investigators. Lenalidomide plus dexamethasone for relapsed multiple myeloma in North America. *N Engl J Med.* 2007;357(21):2133-2142.
527. Richardson PG, Barlogie B, Berenson J, et al. Extended follow-up of a phase II trial in relapsed, refractory multiple myeloma:: final time-to-event results from the SUMMIT trial. *Cancer.* 2006;106(6):1316-1319.
528. Jagannath S, Barlogie B, Berenson J, et al. A phase 2 study of two doses of bortezomib in relapsed or refractory myeloma. *Br J Haematol.* 2004;127(2):165-172.
529. Richardson PG, Sonneveld P, Schuster MW, et al; Assessment of Proteasome Inhibition for Extending Remissions APEX Investigators. Bortezomib or high-dose dexamethasone for relapsed multiple myeloma. *N Engl J Med.* 2005;352(24):2487-2498.
530. Miguel JS, Weisel K, Moreau P, et al. Pomalidomide plus low-dose dexamethasone versus high-dose dexamethasone alone for patients with relapsed and refractory multiple myeloma (MM-003): a randomised, open-label, phase 3 trial. *Lancet Oncol.* 2013;14(11):1055-1066.
531. Dimopoulos MA, Palumbo A, Corradini P, et al. Safety and efficacy of pomalidomide plus low-dose dexamethasone in STRATUS (MM-010): a phase 3b study in refractory multiple myeloma. *Blood.* 2016;128(4):497-503.
532. Siegel DS, Martin T, Wang M, et al. A phase 2 study of single-agent carfilzomib (PX-171-003-A1) in patients with relapsed and refractory multiple myeloma. *Blood.* 2012;120(14):2817-2825.
533. Dimopoulos MA, Moreau P, Palumbo A, et al; ENDEAVOR Investigators. Carfilzomib and dexamethasone versus bortezomib and dexamethasone for patients with relapsed or refractory multiple myeloma (ENDEAVOR): a randomised, phase 3, open-label, multicentre study. *Lancet Oncol.* 2016;17(1):27-38.
534. Kumar SK, LaPlant BR, Reeder CB, et al. Randomized phase 2 trial of ixazomib and dexamethasone in relapsed multiple myeloma not refractory to bortezomib. *Blood.* 2016;128(20):2415-2422.
535. Lonial S, Weiss BM, Usmani SZ, et al. Daratumumab monotherapy in patients with treatment-refractory multiple myeloma (SIRIUS): an open-label, randomised, phase 2 trial. *Lancet.* 2016;387(10027):1551-1560.
536. Anagnostopoulos A, Weber D, Rankin K, Delasalle K, Alexanian R. Thalidomide and dexamethasone for resistant multiple myeloma. *Br J Haematol.* 2003;121(5):768-771.
537. Palumbo A, Giaccone L, Bertola A, et al. Low-dose thalidomide plus dexamethasone is an effective salvage therapy for advanced myeloma. *Haematologica.* 2001;86(4):399-403.
538. Myers B, Grimley C, Dolan G. Thalidomide and low-dose dexamethasone in myeloma treatment. *Br J Haematol.* 2001;114(1):245.
539. Weber D, Rankin K, Gavino M, Delasalle K, Alexanian R. Thalidomide alone or with dexamethasone for previously untreated multiple myeloma. *J Clin Oncol.* 2003;21(1):16-19.
540. Wang M, Knight R, Dimopoulos M, et al. Comparison of lenalidomide in combination with dexamethasone to dexamethasone alone in patients who have received prior thalidomide in relapsed or refractory multiple myeloma. *J Clin Oncol.* 2006;24(18 suppl):7522.
541. Harousseau JL, Dimopoulos MA, Wang M, et al. Better quality of response to lenalidomide plus dexamethasone is associated with improved clinical outcomes in patients with relapsed or refractory multiple myeloma. *Haematologica.* 2010;95(10):1738-1744.
542. San-Miguel JF, Dimopoulos MA, Stadtmauer EA, et al. Effects of lenalidomide and dexamethasone treatment duration on survival in patients with relapsed or refractory multiple myeloma treated with lenalidomide and dexamethasone. *Clin Lymphoma Myeloma Leuk.* 2010;11(1):38-43.
543. Verhelle D, Corral LG, Wong K, et al. Lenalidomide and CC-4047 inhibit the proliferation of malignant B cells while expanding normal CD34+ progenitor cells. *Cancer Res.* 2007;67(2):746-755.
544. Galustian C, Meyer B, Labarthe MC, et al. The anti-cancer agents lenalidomide and pomalidomide inhibit the proliferation and function of T regulatory cells. *Cancer Immunol Immunother.* 2009;58(7):1033-1045.
545. Schey SA, Fields P, Bartlett JB, et al. Phase I study of an immunomodulatory thalidomide analog, CC-4047, in relapsed or refractory multiple myeloma. *J Clin Oncol.* 2004;22(16):3269-3276.
546. Lacy MQ, Hayman SR, Gertz MA, et al. Pomalidomide (CC4047) plus low dose dexamethasone (Pom/dex) is active and well tolerated in lenalidomide refractory multiple myeloma (MM). *Leukemia.* 2010;24(11):1934-1939.
547. Lacy MQ, Allred JB, Gertz MA, et al. Pomalidomide plus low-dose dexamethasone in myeloma refractory to both bortezomib and lenalidomide: comparison of 2 dosing strategies in dual-refractory disease. *Blood.* 2011;118(11):2970-2975.
548. Ailawadhi S, Mikhael JR, LaPlant BR, et al. Pomalidomide-dexamethasone in refractory multiple myeloma: long-term follow-up of a multi-cohort phase II clinical trial. *Leukemia.* 2018;32(3):719-728.
549. Richardson PG, Siegel D, Baz R, et al. A phase 1/2 multi-center, randomized, open label dose escalation study to determine the maximum tolerated dose, safety, and efficacy of pomalidomide alone or in combination with low-dose dexamethasone in patients with relapsed and refractory multiple myeloma who have received prior treatment that includes lenalidomide and bortezomib. *Blood.* 2010;116(21):864.
550. Leleu X, Attal M, Moreau P, et al. Phase 2 study of 2 modalities of pomalidomide (CC4047) plus low-dose dexamethasone as therapy for relapsed multiple myeloma. IFM 2009-02. *Blood.* 2010;116(21):859.
551. Richardson PG, Barlogie B, Berenson J, et al. A phase 2 study of bortezomib in relapsed, refractory myeloma. *N Engl J Med.* 2003;348(26):2609-2617.
552. Berenson JR, Jagannath S, Barlogie B, et al. Safety of prolonged therapy with bortezomib in relapsed or refractory multiple myeloma. *Cancer.* 2005;104(10):2141-2148.
553. Vij R, Siegel DS, Jagannath S, et al. An open-label, single-arm, phase 2 study of single-agent carfilzomib in patients with relapsed and/or refractory multiple myeloma who have been previously treated with bortezomib. *Br J Haematol.* 2012;158(6):739-748.
554. Garderet L, Iacobelli S, Moreau P, et al. Superiority of the triple combination of bortezomib-thalidomide-dexamethasone over the dual combination of thalidomide-dexamethasone in patients with multiple myeloma progressing or relapsing after autologous transplantation: the MMVAR/IFM 2005-04 Randomized Phase III Trial from the Chronic Leukemia Working Party of the European Group for Blood and Marrow Transplantation. *J Clin Oncol.* 2012;30(20):2475-2482.
555. Stewart AK, Rajkumar SV, Dimopoulos MA, et al; ASPIRE Investigators. Carfilzomib, lenalidomide, and dexamethasone for relapsed multiple myeloma. *N Engl J Med.* 2015;372(2):142-152.
556. Dimopoulos MA, Stewart AK, Masszi T, et al. Carfilzomib-lenalidomide-dexamethasone vs lenalidomide-dexamethasone in relapsed multiple myeloma by previous treatment. *Blood Cancer J.* 2017;7(4):e554.
557. Moreau P, Masszi T, Grzasko N, et al; TOURMALINE-MM1 Study Group. Oral ixazomib, lenalidomide, and dexamethasone for multiple myeloma. *N Engl J Med.* 2016;374(17):1621-1634.
558. Lonial S, Dimopoulos M, Palumbo A, et al; ELOQUENT-2 Investigators. Elotuzumab therapy for relapsed or refractory multiple myeloma. *N Engl J Med.* 2015;373(7):621-631.
559. Dimopoulos M, Siegel DS, Lonial S, et al. Vorinostat or placebo in combination with bortezomib in patients with multiple myeloma (VANTAGE 088): a multicentre, randomised, double-blind study. *Lancet Oncol.* 2013;14(11):1129-1140.
560. Kumar SK, Harrison SJ, Cavo M, et al. Venetoclax or placebo in combination with bortezomib and dexamethasone in patients with relapsed or refractory multiple myeloma (BELLINI): a randomised, double-blind, multicentre, phase 3 trial. *Lancet Oncol.* 2020;21(12):1630-1642.
561. Richardson PG, Oriol A, Beksac M, et al; OPTIMISMM Trial Investigators. Pomalidomide, bortezomib, and dexamethasone for patients with relapsed or refractory multiple myeloma previously treated with lenalidomide (OPTIMISMM): a randomised, open-label, phase 3 trial. *Lancet Oncol.* 2019;20(6):781-794.
562. Dimopoulos MA, Terpos E, Boccadoro M, et al; APOLLO Trial Investigators. Daratumumab plus pomalidomide and dexamethasone versus pomalidomide and dexamethasone alone in previously treated multiple myeloma (APOLLO): an open-label, randomised, phase 3 trial. *Lancet Oncol.* 2021;22(6):801-812.
563. Kumar SK, LaPlant B, Roy V, et al. Phase 2 trial of ixazomib in patients with relapsed multiple myeloma not refractory to bortezomib. *Blood Cancer J.* 2015;5:e338.
564. Trudel S, Lendvai N, Popat R, et al. Deep and durable responses in patients (pts) with relapsed/refractory multiple myeloma (MM) treated with monotherapy GSK2857916, an antibody drug conjugate against B-cell maturation antigen (BCMA): preliminary results from part 2 of study BMA117159. *Blood.* 2017;2017(suppl 1):741.
565. Treon SP, Pilarski LM, Belch AR, et al. CD20-directed serotherapy in patients with multiple myeloma: biologic considerations and therapeutic applications. *J Immunother.* 2002;25(1):72-81.
566. Ocio EM, Mateos MV, Maiso P, Pandiella A, San-Miguel JF. New drugs in multiple myeloma: mechanisms of action and phase I/II clinical findings. *Lancet Oncol.* 2008;9(12):1157-1165.
567. Mahindra A, Cirstea D, Raje N. Novel therapeutic targets for multiple myeloma. *Future Oncol.* 2010;6(3):407-418.
568. Richardson PG, Sonneveld P, Schuster M, et al. Extended follow-up of a phase 3 trial in relapsed multiple myeloma: final time-to-event results of the APEX trial. *Blood.* 2007;110(10):3557-3560.
569. Galli M, Salmoiraghi S, Golay J, et al. A phase II multiple dose clinical trial of histone deactylase inhibitor5 ITF2357 in patients with relapsed or progressive multiple myeloma: preliminary results. *Blood.* 2007;2007(110):1175.
570. Niesvizky R, Ely S, Mark T, et al. Phase 2 trial of the histone deacetylase inhibitor romidepsin for the treatment of refractory multiple myeloma. *Cancer.* 2011;117:336-342.
571. Richardson P, Mitsiades C, Colson K, et al. Phase I trial of oral vorinostat (suberoylanilide hydroxamic acid, SAHA) in patients with advanced multiple myeloma. *Leuk Lymphoma.* 2008;49(3):502-507.
572. Kumar S, Kaufman JL, Gasparetto C, et al. Efficacy of venetoclax as targeted therapy for relapsed/refractory t(11;14) multiple myeloma. *Blood.* 2017;130(22):2401-2409.
573. Chen C, Siegel D, Gutierrez M, et al. Safety and efficacy of selinexor in relapsed or refractory multiple myeloma and Waldenstrom macroglobulinemia. *Blood.* 2018;131(8):855-863.
574. Bahlis NJ, Dimopoulos MA, White DJ, et al. Daratumumab plus lenalidomide and dexamethasone in relapsed/refractory multiple myeloma: extended follow-up of POLLUX, a randomized, open-label, phase 3 study. *Leukemia.* 2020;34(7):1875-1884.
575. Mateos MV, Sonneveld P, Hungria V, et al. Daratumumab, bortezomib, and dexamethasone versus bortezomib and dexamethasone in patients with previously treated multiple myeloma: three-year follow-up of CASTOR. *Clin Lymphoma Myeloma Leuk.* 2020;20(8):509-518.

576. Dimopoulos MA, Lonial S, White D, et al. Elotuzumab, lenalidomide, and dexamethasone in RRMM: final overall survival results from the phase 3 randomized ELOQUENT-2 study. *Blood Cancer J.* 2020;10(9):91.
577. Offidani M, Marconi M, Corvatta L, Olivieri A, Catarini M, Leoni P. Thalidomide plus oral melphalan for advanced multiple myeloma: a phase II study. *Haematologica.* 2003;88(12):1432-1433.
578. Hovenga S, Daenen SM, de Wolf JTM, et al. Combined thalidomide and cyclophosphamide treatment for refractory or relapsed multiple myeloma patients: a prospective phase II study. *Ann Hematol.* 2005;84(5):311-316.
579. Garcia-Sanz R, Gonzalez-Porras JR, Hernandez JM, et al. The oral combination of thalidomide, cyclophosphamide and dexamethasone (ThaCyDex) is effective in relapsed/refractory multiple myeloma. *Leukemia.* 2004;18(4):856-863.
580. Dimopoulos MA, Hamilos G, Zomas A, et al. Pulsed cyclophosphamide, thalidomide and dexamethasone: an oral regimen for previously treated patients with multiple myeloma. *Hematol J.* 2004;5(2):112-117.
581. Kropff MH, Lang N, Bisping G, et al. Hyperfractionated cyclophosphamide in combination with pulsed dexamethasone and thalidomide (HyperCDT) in primary refractory or relapsed multiple myeloma. *Br J Haematol.* 2003;122(4):607-616.
582. Kyriakou C, Thomson K, D'Sa S, et al. Low-dose thalidomide in combination with oral weekly cyclophosphamide and pulsed dexamethasone is a well tolerated and effective regimen in patients with relapsed and refractory multiple myeloma. *Br J Haematol.* 2005;129(6):763-770.
583. Sidra G, Williams CD, Russell NH, Zaman S, Myers B, Byrne JL. Combination chemotherapy with cyclophosphamide, thalidomide and dexamethasone for patients with refractory, newly diagnosed or relapsed myeloma. *Haematologica.* 2006;91(6):862-863.
584. Palumbo A, Avonto I, Bruno B, et al. Intravenous melphalan, thalidomide and prednisone in refractory and relapsed multiple myeloma. *Eur J Haematol.* 2006;76(4):273-277.
585. Suvannasankha A, Fausel C, Juliar BE, et al. Final report of toxicity and efficacy of a phase II study of oral cyclophosphamide, thalidomide, and prednisone for patients with relapsed or refractory multiple myeloma: a Hoosier Oncology Group Trial, HEM01-21. *Oncol.* 2007;12(1):99-106.
586. Ponisch W, Rozanski M, Goldschmidt H, et al; East German Study Group of Haematology and Oncology OSHO. Combined bendamustine, prednisolone and thalidomide for refractory or relapsed multiple myeloma after autologous stem-cell transplantation or conventional chemotherapy: results of a Phase I clinical trial. *Br J Haematol.* 2008;143(2):191-200.
587. Knop S, Gerecke C, Liebisch P, et al. Lenalidomide, adriamycin, and dexamethasone (RAD) in patients with relapsed and refractory multiple myeloma: a report from the German Myeloma Study Group DSMM (Deutsche Studiengruppe Multiples Myelom). *Blood.* 2009;113(18):4137-4143.
588. Schey SA, Morgan GJ, Ramasamy K, et al. The addition of cyclophosphamide to lenalidomide and dexamethasone in multiply relapsed/refractory myeloma patients; a phase I/II study. *Br J Haematol.* 2010;150(3):326-333.
589. Lentzsch S, O'Sullivan A, Kennedy RC, et al. Combination of bendamustine, lenalidomide, and dexamethasone (BLD) in patients with relapsed or refractory multiple myeloma is feasible and highly effective: results of phase 1/2 open-label, dose escalation study. *Blood.* 2012;119(20):4608-4613.
590. Palumbo A, Larocca A, Falco P, et al. Lenalidomide, melphalan, prednisone and thalidomide (RMPT) for relapsed/refractory multiple myeloma. *Leukemia.* 2010;24(5):1037-1042.
591. Baz R, Walker E, Karam MA, et al. Lenalidomide and pegylated liposomal doxorubicin-based chemotherapy for relapsed or refractory multiple myeloma: safety and efficacy. *Ann Oncol.* 2006;17(12):1766-1771.
592. Paludo J, Mikhael JR, LaPlant BR, et al. Pomalidomide, bortezomib, and dexamethasone for patients with relapsed lenalidomide-refractory multiple myeloma. *Blood.* 2017;130(10):1198-1204.
593. Shah JJ, Stadtmauer EA, Abonour R, et al. Carfilzomib, pomalidomide, and dexamethasone for relapsed or refractory myeloma. *Blood.* 2015;126(20):2284-2290.
594. Bringhen S, Mina R, Cafro AM, et al. Once-weekly carfilzomib, pomalidomide, and low-dose dexamethasone for relapsed/refractory myeloma: a phase I/II study. *Leukemia.* 2018;32(8):1803-1807.
595. Chari A, Suvannasankha A, Fay JW, et al. Daratumumab plus pomalidomide and dexamethasone in relapsed and/or refractory multiple myeloma. *Blood.* 2017;130(8):974-981.
596. Jakubowiak A, Offidani M, Pegourie B, et al. Randomized phase 2 study: elotuzumab plus bortezomib/dexamethasone vs bortezomib/dexamethasone for relapsed/refractory MM. *Blood.* 2016;127(23):2833-2840.
597. Moreau P, Chanan-Khan A, Roberts AW, et al. Promising efficacy and acceptable safety of venetoclax plus bortezomib and dexamethasone in relapsed/refractory MM. *Blood.* 2017;130(22):2392-2400.
598. Costa LJ, Davies FE, Monohan GP, et al. Phase 2 study of venetoclax plus carfilzomib and dexamethasone in patients with relapsed/refractory multiple myeloma. *Blood Adv.* 2021;5(19):3748-3759.
599. Bahlis NJ, Baz R, Harrison SJ, et al. Phase I study of venetoclax plus daratumumab and dexamethasone, with or without bortezomib, in patients with relapsed or refractory multiple myeloma with and without t(11;14). *J Clin Oncol.* 2021;39(32):3602-3612.
600. Berenson JR, Yang HH, Vescio RA, et al. Safety and efficacy of bortezomib and melphalan combination in patients with relapsed or refractory multiple myeloma: updated results of a phase 1/2 study after longer follow-up. *Ann Hematol.* 2008;87(8):623-631.
601. Popat R, Oakervee H, Williams C, et al. Bortezomib, low-dose intravenous melphalan, and dexamethasone for patients with relapsed multiple myeloma. *Br J Haematol.* 2009;144(6):887-894.
602. Reece DE, Rodriguez GP, Chen C, et al. Phase I-II trial of bortezomib plus oral cyclophosphamide and prednisone in relapsed and refractory multiple myeloma. *J Clin Oncol.* 2008;26(29):4777-4783.
603. Kropff M, Bisping G, Schuck E, et al; Deutsche Studiengruppe Multiples Myelom. Bortezomib in combination with intermediate-dose dexamethasone and continuous low-dose oral cyclophosphamide for relapsed multiple myeloma. *Br J Haematol.* 2007;138(3):330-337.
604. Ciolli S, Leoni F, Gigli F, Rigacci L, Bosi A. Low dose Velcade, thalidomide and dexamethasone (LD-VTD): an effective regimen for relapsed and refractory multiple myeloma patients. *Leuk Lymphoma.* 2006;47(1):171-173.
605. Pineda-Roman M, Zangari M, van Rhee F, et al. VTD combination therapy with bortezomib-thalidomide-dexamethasone is highly effective in advanced and refractory multiple myeloma. *Leukemia.* 2008;22(7):1419-1427.
606. Palumbo A, Ambrosini MT, Benevolo G, et al; Italian Multiple Myeloma Network; Gruppo Italiano Malattie Ematologicche dell'Adulto. Bortezomib, melphalan, prednisone, and thalidomide for relapsed multiple myeloma. *Blood.* 2007;109(7):2767-2772.
607. Terpos E, Kastritis E, Roussou M, et al. The combination of bortezomib, melphalan, dexamethasone and intermittent thalidomide is an effective regimen for relapsed/refractory myeloma and is associated with improvement of abnormal bone metabolism and angiogenesis. *Leukemia.* 2008;22(12):2247-2256.
608. Kim YK, Sohn SK, Lee JH, et al; Korean Multiple Myeloma Working Party KMMWP. Clinical efficacy of a bortezomib, cyclophosphamide, thalidomide, and dexamethasone (Vel-CTD) regimen in patients with relapsed or refractory multiple myeloma: a phase II study. *Ann Hematol.* 2010;89(5):475-482.
609. Berenson JR, Yellin O, Kazamel T, et al. A phase 2 study of pegylated liposomal doxorubicin, bortezomib, dexamethasone and lenalidomide for patients with relapsed/refractory multiple myeloma. *Leukemia.* 2012;26(7):1675-1680.
610. Orlowski RZ, Voorhees PM, Garcia RA, et al. Phase 1 trial of the proteasome inhibitor bortezomib and pegylated liposomal doxorubicin in patients with advanced hematologic malignancies. *Blood.* 2005;105(8):3058-3065.
611. Chanan-Khan AA, Giralt S. Importance of achieving a complete response in multiple myeloma, and the impact of novel agents. *J Clin Oncol.* 2010;28(15):2612-2624.
612. Ciolli S, Leoni F, Casini C, Breschi C, Santini V, Bosi A. The addition of liposomal doxorubicin to bortezomib, thalidomide and dexamethasone significantly improves clinical outcome of advanced multiple myeloma. *Br J Haematol.* 2008;141(6):814-819.
613. Richardson PG, Weller E, Jagannath S, et al. Multicenter, phase I, dose-escalation trial of lenalidomide plus bortezomib for relapsed and relapsed/refractory multiple myeloma. *J Clin Oncol.* 2009;27(34):5713-5719.
614. de Weerdt O, van de Donk NW, Veth G, Bloem AC, Hagenbeek A, Lokhorst HM. Continuous low-dose cyclophosphamide-prednisone is effective and well tolerated in patients with advanced multiple myeloma. *Neth J Med.* 2001;59(2):50-56.
615. Trieu Y, Trudel S, Pond GR, et al. Weekly cyclophosphamide and alternate-day prednisone: an effective, convenient, and well-tolerated oral treatment for relapsed multiple myeloma after autologous stem cell transplantation. *Mayo Clin Proc.* 2005;80(12):1578-1582.
616. Lenhard RE, Daniels MJ, Oken MM, et al. An aggressive high dose cyclophosphamide and prednisone regimen for advanced multiple myeloma. *Leuk Lymphoma.* 1994;13(5-6):485-489.
617. Petrucci MT, Avvisati G, Tribalto M, Cantonetti M, Giovangrossi P, Mandelli F. Intermediate-dose (25 mg/m^2) intravenous melphalan for patients with multiple myeloma in relapse or refractory to standard treatment. *Eur J Haematol.* 1989;42(3):233-237.
618. Tsakanikas S, Papanastasiou K, Stamatelou M, Maniatis A. Intermediate dose of intravenous melphalan in advanced multiple myeloma. *Oncology.* 1991;48(5):369-371.
619. Dimopoulos MA, Weber D, Kantarjian H, Delasalle KB, Alexanian R. HyperCVAD for VAD-resistant multiple myeloma. *Am J Hematol.* 1996;52(2):77-81.
620. Finnish Leukaemia Group. Combination chemotherapy MOCCA in resistant and relapsing multiple myeloma. *Eur J Haematol.* 1992;48(1):37-40.
621. Lee CK, Barlogie B, Munshi N, et al. DTPACE: an effective, novel combination chemotherapy with thalidomide for previously treated patients with myeloma. *J Clin Oncol.* 2003;21(14):2732-2739.
622. Bonnet JD, Alexanian R, Salmon SE, Haut A, Dixon DO. Addition of cisplatin and bleomycin to vincristine-carmustine-doxorubicin-prednisone (VBAP) combination in the treatment of relapsing or resistant multiple myeloma: a Southwest Oncology Group study. *Cancer Treat Rep.* 1984;68(3):481-485.
623. Orlowski RZ, Nagler A, Sonneveld P, et al. Randomized phase III study of pegylated liposomal doxorubicin plus bortezomib compared with bortezomib alone in relapsed or refractory multiple myeloma: combination therapy improves time to progression. *J Clin Oncol.* 2007;25(25):3892-3901.
624. de Waal EGM, de Munck L, Hoogendoorn M, et al. Combination therapy with bortezomib, continuous low-dose cyclophosphamide and dexamethasone followed by one year of maintenance treatment for relapsed multiple myeloma patients. *Br J Haematol.* 2015;171(5):720-725.
625. Kropff M, Vogel M, Bisping G, et al. Bortezomib and low-dose dexamethasone with or without continuous low-dose oral cyclophosphamide for primary refractory or relapsed multiple myeloma: a randomized phase III study. *Ann Hematol.* 2017;96(11):1857-1866.
626. Reece DE, Masih-Khan E, Atenafu EG, et al. Phase I-II trial of oral cyclophosphamide, prednisone and lenalidomide for the treatment of patients with relapsed and refractory multiple myeloma. *Br J Haematol.* 2015;168(1):46-54.
627. Baz RC, Martin TG III, Lin HY, et al. Randomized multicenter phase 2 study of pomalidomide, cyclophosphamide, and dexamethasone in relapsed refractory myeloma. *Blood.* 2016;127(21):2561-2568.

628. Larocca A, Montefusco V, Bringhen S, et al. Pomalidomide, cyclophosphamide, and prednisone for relapsed/refractory multiple myeloma: a multicenter phase 1/2 open-label study. *Blood.* 2013;122(16):2799-2806.
629. Kumar SK, Krishnan A, LaPlant B, et al. Bendamustine, lenalidomide, and dexamethasone (BRD) is highly effective with durable responses in relapsed multiple myeloma. *Am J Hematol.* 2015;90(12):1106-1110.
630. Ludwig H, Kasparu H, Leitgeb C, et al. Bendamustine-bortezomib-dexamethasone is an active and well-tolerated regimen in patients with relapsed or refractory multiple myeloma. *Blood.* 2014;123(7):985-991.
631. Lakshman A, Singh PP, Rajkumar SV, et al. Efficacy of VDT PACE-like regimens in treatment of relapsed/refractory multiple myeloma. *Am J Hematol.* 2018;93(2):179-186.
632. Usmani SZ, Garfall AL, van de Donk NW, et al. Teclistamab, a B-cell maturation antigen × CD3 bispecific antibody, in patients with relapsed or refractory multiple myeloma (MajesTEC-1): a multicentre, open-label, single-arm, phase 1 study. *Lancet.* 2021;398(10301):665-674.
633. Bahlis NJ, Raje NS, Costello C, et al. Efficacy and safety of elranatamab (PF-06863135), a B-cell maturation antigen (BCMA)-CD3 bispecific antibody, in patients with relapsed or refractory multiple myeloma (MM). *J Clin Oncol.* 2021;39(15 suppl):8006.
634. Kumar S, D'Souza A, Shah N, et al. A phase 1 first-in-human study of Tnb-383B, a BCMA x CD3 bispecific T-cell redirecting antibody, in patients with relapsed/refractory multiple myeloma. *Blood.* 2021;138(suppl 1):900.
635. Harrison SJ, Minnema MC, Lee HC, et al. A phase 1 first in human (FIH) study of AMG 701, an anti-B-cell maturation antigen (BCMA) half-life extended (HLE) BiTE® (bispecific T-cell engager) molecule, in relapsed/refractory (RR) multiple myeloma (MM). *Blood.* 2020;136(suppl 1):28-29.
636. Costa LJ, Wong SW, Bermúdez A., et al. *Interim Results From the First Phase 1 Clinical Study of the B-cell Maturation Antigen (BCMA) 2+1 T Cell Engager (TCE) CC-93269 in Patients (pts) With Relapsed/Refractory Multiple Myeloma (RRMM).* European Hematoloy Association; 2020.
637. Madduri D, Rosko A, Brayer J, et al. REGN5458, a BCMA x CD3 bispecific monoclonal antibody, induces deep and durable responses in patients with relapsed/refractory multiple myeloma (RRMM). *Blood.* 2020;136(suppl 1):41-42.
638. Berdeja JG, Krishnan AY, Oriol A, et al. Updated results of a phase 1, first-in-human study of talquetamab, a G protein-coupled receptor family C group 5 member D (GPRC5D) × CD3 bispecific antibody, in relapsed/refractory multiple myeloma (MM). *J Clin Oncol.* 2021;39(15 suppl):8008.
639. Cohen AD, Harrison SJ, Krishnan A, et al. Initial clinical activity and safety of BFCR4350A, a FcRH5/CD3 T-cell-engaging bispecific antibody, in relapsed/refractory multiple myeloma. *Blood.* 2020;136(suppl 1):42-43.
640. Bonnet J, Alexanian R, Salmon S, et al. Vincristine, BCNU, doxorubicin, and prednisone (VBAP) combination in the treatment of relapsing or resistant multiple myeloma: a Southwest Oncology Group study. *Cancer Treat Rep.* 1982;66(6):1267-1271.
641. Brandes LJ, Israels LG. Treatment of advanced plasma cell myeloma with weekly cyclophosphamide and alternate-day prednisone. *Cancer Treat Rep.* 1982;66(6):1413-1415.
642. Wilson K, Shelley W, Belch A, et al. Weekly cyclophosphamide and alternate-day prednisone: an effective secondary therapy in multiple myeloma. *Cancer Treat Rep.* 1987;71(10):981-982.
643. Lenhard RE Jr, Oken MM, Barnes JM, Humphrey RL, Glick JH, Silverstein MN. High-dose cyclophosphamide. An effective treatment for advanced refractory multiple myeloma. *Cancer.* 1984;53(7):1456-1460.
644. Selby PJ, McElwain TJ, Nandi AC, et al. Multiple myeloma treated with high dose intravenous melphalan. *Br J Haematol.* 1987;66(1):55-62.
645. Lokhorst HM, Sonneveld P, Wijermans PW, et al. Intermediate-dose melphalan (IDM) combined with G-CSF (filgrastim) is an effective and safe induction therapy for autologous stem cell transplantation in multiple myeloma. *Br J Haematol.* 1996;92(1):44-48.
646. Palumbo A, Pileri A, Triolo S, et al. Multicyclic, dose-intensive chemotherapy supported by hemopoietic progenitors in refractory myeloma patients. *Bone Marrow Transplant.* 1997;19(1):23-29.
647. Raje N, Berdeja J, Lin Y, et al. Anti-BCMA CAR T-cell therapy bb2121 in relapsed or refractory multiple myeloma. *N Engl J Med.* 2019;380(18):1726-1737.
648. Berdeja JG, Madduri D, Usmani SZ, et al. Ciltacabtagene autoleucel, a B-cell maturation antigen-directed chimeric antigen receptor T-cell therapy in patients with relapsed or refractory multiple myeloma (CARTITUDE-1): a phase 1b/2 open-label study. *Lancet.* 2021;398(10297):314-324.
649. Stone WJ. Multiple myelomata. *Am J Roentgenol.* 1924;12:543-545.
650. Jacox JW, Kahn EA. Multiple myeloma with spinal cord involvement. *Am J Roentgenol.* 1933;30:201-205.
651. Geschickter CF, Copeland MM. Multiple myeloma. *Arch Surg.* 1928;16:807-863.
652. Sykes MP, Chu FCH, Savel H, Bonadonna G, Mathis H. The effects of varying dosages of irradiation upon sternal-marrow regeneration. *Radiology.* 1964;83:1084-1088.
653. Norin T. Roentgen treatment of myeloma with special consideration to the dosage. *Acta radiol.* 1957;47(1):46-54.
654. Rostom AY, O'Cathail SM, Folkes A. Systemic irradiation in multiple myeloma: a report on nineteen cases. *Br J Haematol.* 1984;58(3):423-431.
655. Leigh BR, Kurtts TA, Mack CF, Matzner MB, Shimm DS. Radiation therapy for the palliation of multiple myeloma. *Int J Radiat Oncol Biol Phys.* 1993;25(5):801-804.
656. Adamietz IA, Schober C, Schulte RW, Peest D, Renner K. Palliative radiotherapy in plasma cell myeloma. *Radiother Oncol.* 1991;20(2):111-116.
657. Frassica DA, Frassica FJ, Schray MF, Sim FH, Kyle RA. Solitary plasmacytoma of bone: Mayo Clinic experience. *Int J Radiat Oncol Biol Phys.* 1989;16(1):43-48.
658. Mendenhall CM, Thar TL, Million RR. Solitary plasmacytoma of bone and soft tissue. *Int J Radiat Oncol Biol Phys.* 1980;6(11):1497-1501.
659. Mill WB. Radiation therapy in multiple myeloma. *Radiology.* 1975;115(1):175-178.
660. Knobel D, Zouhair A, Tsang RW, et al; Rare Cancer Network. Prognostic factors in solitary plasmacytoma of the bone: a Multicenter Rare Cancer Network study. *BMC Cancer.* 2006;6:118.
661. Rao G, Ha CS, Chakrabarti I, Feiz-Erfan I, Mendel E, Rhines LD. Multiple myeloma of the cervical spine: treatment strategies for pain and spinal instability. *J Neurosurg Spine.* 2006;5(2):140-145.
662. Medinger FG, Craver LF. Total body irradiation with review of cases. *Am J Roentgenol.* 1942;48:651-671.
663. Bergsagel DE. Total body irradiation for myelomatosis. *Br Med J.* 1971;2(5757):325.
664. Salmon SE, Tesh D, Crowley J, et al. Chemotherapy is superior to sequential hemibody irradiation for remission consolidation in multiple myeloma: a Southwest Oncology Group study. *J Clin Oncol.* 1990;8(9):1575-1584.
665. Singer FR, Ritch PS, Lad TE, et al. Treatment of hypercalcemia of malignancy with intravenous etidronate. A controlled, multicenter study. The Hypercalcemia Study Group. *Arch Intern Med.* 1991;151(3):471-476.
666. Jaffe JP, Bosch A, Raich PC. Sequential hemi-body radiotherapy in advanced multiple myeloma. *Cancer.* 1979;43(1):124-128.
667. Zangari M, Barlogie B, Anaissie E, et al. Deep vein thrombosis in patients with multiple myeloma treated with thalidomide and chemotherapy: effects of prophylactic and therapeutic anticoagulation. *Br J Haematol.* 2004;126(5):715-721.
668. Baz R, Li L, Kottke-Marchant K, et al. The role of aspirin in the prevention of thrombotic complications of thalidomide and anthracycline-based chemotherapy for multiple myeloma. *Mayo Clin Proc.* 2005;80(12):1568-1574.
669. Rajkumar SV, Blood E. Lenalidomide and venous thrombosis in multiple myeloma. *N Engl J Med.* 2006;354(19):2079-2080.
670. Knight R, DeLap RJ, Zeldis JB. Lenalidomide and venous thrombosis in multiple myeloma. *N Engl J Med.* 2006;354(19):2079-2080.
671. Palumbo A, Cavo M, Bringhen S, et al. Aspirin, warfarin, or enoxaparin thromboprophylaxis in patients with multiple myeloma treated with thalidomide: a phase III, open-label, randomized trial. *J Clin Oncol.* 2011;29(8):986-993.
672. Larocca A, Cavallo F, Bringhen S, et al. Aspirin or enoxaparin thromboprophylaxis for patients with newly diagnosed multiple myeloma treated with lenalidomide. *Blood.* 2012;119(4):933-939, quiz 1093.
673. Morgan GJ, Davies FE, Gregory WM, et al; National Cancer Research Institute Haematological Oncology Clinical Study Group. First-line treatment with zoledronic acid as compared with clodronic acid in multiple myeloma (MRC Myeloma IX): a randomised controlled trial. *Lancet.* 2010;376(9757):1989-1999.
674. Raje N, Terpos E, Willenbacher W, et al. Denosumab versus zoledronic acid in bone disease treatment of newly diagnosed multiple myeloma: an international, double-blind, double-dummy, randomised, controlled, phase 3 study. *Lancet Oncol.* 2018;19(3):370-381.
675. Mhaskar R, Redzepovic J, Wheatley K, et al. Bisphosphonates in multiple myeloma: a network meta-analysis. *Cochrane Database Syst Rev.* 2012;(5):CD003188.
676. Berenson JR, Lichtenstein A, Porter L, et al. Efficacy of pamidronate in reducing skeletal events in patients with advanced multiple myeloma. Myeloma Aredia Study Group. *N Engl J Med.* 1996;334(8):488-493.
677. Berenson JR, Rosen LS, Howell A, et al. Zoledronic acid reduces skeletal-related events in patients with osteolytic metastases. *Cancer.* 2001;91(7):1191-1200.
678. Berenson JR, Hillner BE, Kyle RA, et al; American Society of Clinical Oncology Bisphosphonates Expert Panel. American Society of Clinical Oncology clinical practice guidelines: the role of bisphosphonates in multiple myeloma. *J Clin Oncol.* 2002;20(17):3719-3736.
679. Ruggiero SL, Mehrotra B, Rosenberg TJ, Engroff SL. Osteonecrosis of the jaws associated with the use of bisphosphonates: a review of 63 cases. *J Oral Maxillofac Surg.* 2004;62(5):527-534.
680. Lacy MQ, Dispenzieri A, Gertz MA, et al. Mayo clinic consensus statement for the use of bisphosphonates in multiple myeloma. *Mayo Clin Proc.* 2006;81(8):1047-1053.
681. Bamias A, Kastritis E, Bamia C, et al. Osteonecrosis of the jaw in cancer after treatment with bisphosphonates: incidence and risk factors. *J Clin Oncol.* 2005;23(34):8580-8587.
682. Durie BGM, Katz M, Crowley J. Osteonecrosis of the jaw and bisphosphonates. *N Engl J Med.* 2005;353(1):99-102, discussion 99-102.
683. Corso A, Varettoni M, Zappasodi P, et al. A different schedule of zoledronic acid can reduce the risk of the osteonecrosis of the jaw in patients with multiple myeloma. *Leukemia.* 2007;21(7):1545-1548.
684. Amadori D, Aglietta M, Alessi B, et al. Efficacy and safety of 12-weekly versus 4-weekly zoledronic acid for prolonged treatment of patients with bone metastases from breast cancer (ZOOM): a phase 3, open-label, randomised, non-inferiority trial. *Lancet Oncol.* 2013;14(7):663-670.
685. McBroom RJ, Cheal EJ, Hayes WC. Strength reductions from metastatic cortical defects in long bones. *J Orthop Res.* 1988;6(3):369-378.
686. Gainor BJ, Buchert P. Fracture healing in metastatic bone disease. *Clin Orthop Relat Res.* 1983;178:297-302.
687. Allen KL, Johnson TW, Hibbs GG. Effective bone palliation as related to various treatment regimens. *Cancer.* 1976;37(2):984-987.
688. Tong D, Gillick L, Hendrickson FR. The palliation of symptomatic osseous metastases: final results of the study by the Radiation Therapy Oncology Group. *Cancer.* 1982;50(5):893-899.
689. Levine SA, Perin LA, Hayes D, Hayes WS. An evidence-based evaluation of percutaneous vertebroplasty. *Manag Care.* 2000;9(3):56-60.
690. Pflugmacher R, Kandziora F, Schroeder RJ, Melcher I, Haas NP, Klostermann CK. Percutaneous balloon kyphoplasty in the treatment of pathological vertebral body fracture and deformity in multiple myeloma: a one-year follow-up. *Acta Radiol.* 2006;47(4):369-376.

691. Berenson J, Pflugmacher R, Jarzem P, et al. Balloon kyphoplasty versus non-surgical fracture management for treatment of painful vertebral body compression fractures in patients with cancer: a multicentre, randomised controlled trial. *Lancet Oncol.* 2011;12(3):225-235.
692. Benson WJ, Scarffe JH, Todd ID, Palmer M, Crowther D. Spinal-cord compression in myeloma. *Br Med J.* 1979;1(6177):1541-1544.
693. Young RF, Post EM, King GA. Treatment of spinal epidural metastases. Randomized prospective comparison of laminectomy and radiotherapy. *J Neurosurg.* 1980;53(6):741-748.
694. Gilbert RW, Kim JH, Posner JB. Epidural spinal cord compression from metastatic tumor: diagnosis and treatment. *Ann Neurol.* 1978;3(1):40-51.
695. Gucalp R, Theriault R, Gill I, et al. Treatment of cancer-associated hypercalcemia. Double-blind comparison of rapid and slow intravenous infusion regimens of pamidronate disodium and saline alone. *Arch Intern Med.* 1994;154(17):1935-1944.
696. Mundy GR, Wilkinson R, Heath DA. Comparative study of available medical therapy for hypercalcemia of malignancy. *Am J Med.* 1983;74(3):421-432.
697. Cuzick J, Erskine S, Edelman D, Galton DA. A comparison of the incidence of the myelodysplastic syndrome and acute myeloid leukaemia following melphalan and cyclophosphamide treatment for myelomatosis. A report to the Medical Research Council's working party on leukaemia in adults. *Br J Cancer.* 1987;55(5):523-529.
698. Finnish Leukaemia Group Study. Acute leukaemia and other secondary neoplasms in patients treated with conventional chemotherapy for multiple myeloma: a Finnish Leukaemia Group study. *Eur J Haematol.* 2000;65(2):123-127.
699. Bergsagel DE. Chemotherapy of myeloma: drug combinations versus single agents, an overview, and comments on acute leukemia in myeloma. *Hematol Oncol.* 1988;6(2):159-166.
700. Wintrobe M, Buell M. Hyperproteinemia associated with multiple myeloma. *Bull Johns Hopkins Hosp.* 1933;52:156-165.
701. Siami GA, Siami FS. Plasmapheresis and paraproteinemia: cryoprotein-induced diseases, monoclonal gammopathy, Waldenstrom's macroglobulinemia, hyperviscosity syndrome, multiple myeloma, light chain disease, and amyloidosis. *Ther Apher.* 1999;3(1):8-19.
702. Knudsen LM, Hjorth M, Hippe E. Renal failure in multiple myeloma: reversibility and impact on the prognosis. Nordic Myeloma Study Group. *Eur J Haematol.* 2000;65(3):175-181.
703. Bernstein SP, Humes HD. Reversible renal insufficiency in multiple myeloma. *Arch Intern Med.* 1982;142(12):2083-2086.
704. Johnson WJ, Kyle RA, Pineda AA, O'Brien PC, Holley KE. Treatment of renal failure associated with multiple myeloma. Plasmapheresis, hemodialysis, and chemotherapy. *Arch Intern Med.* 1990;150(4):863-869.
705. Zucchelli P, Pasquali S, Cagnoli L, Ferrari G. Controlled plasma exchange trial in acute renal failure due to multiple myeloma. *Kidney Int.* 1988;33(6):1175-1180.
706. Clark AD, Shetty A, Soutar R. Renal failure and multiple myeloma: pathogenesis and treatment of renal failure and management of underlying myeloma. *Blood Rev.* 1999;13(2):79-90.
707. Jacobson DR, Zolla-Pazner S. Immunosuppression and infection in multiple myeloma. *Semin Oncol.* 1986;13(3):282-290.
708. Paradisi F, Corti G, Cinelli R. Infections in multiple myeloma. *Infect Dis Clin North Am.* 2001;15(2):373-384, vii-viii.
709. Savage DG, Lindenbaum J, Garrett TJ. Biphasic pattern of bacterial infection in multiple myeloma. *Ann Intern Med.* 1982;96(1):47-50.
710. Shaikh BS, Lombard RM, Appelbaum PC, Bentz MS. Changing patterns of infections in patients with multiple myeloma. *Oncology.* 1982;39(2):78-82.
711. Doughney KB, Williams DM, Penn RL. Multiple myeloma: infectious complications. *South Med J.* 1988;81(7):855-858.
712. Hargreaves RM, Lea JR, Griffiths H, et al. Immunological factors and risk of infection in plateau phase myeloma. *J Clin Pathol.* 1995;48(3):260-266.
713. Drayson MT, Bowcock S, Planche T, et al; TEAMM Trial Management Group and Trial Investigators. Levofloxacin prophylaxis in patients with newly diagnosed myeloma (TEAMM): a multicentre, double-blind, placebo-controlled, randomised, phase 3 trial. *Lancet Oncol.* 2019;20(12):1760-1772.
714. Oken MM, Pomeroy C, Weisdorf D, Bennett JM. Prophylactic antibiotics for the prevention of early infection in multiple myeloma. *Am J Med.* 1996;100(6):624-628.
715. Vesole DH, Oken MM, Heckler C, et al; University of Rochester Cancer Center and the Eastern Cooperative Oncology Group. Oral antibiotic prophylaxis of early infection in multiple myeloma: a URCC/ECOG randomized phase III study. *Leukemia.* 2012;26(12):2517-2520.
716. Chapel HM, Lee M, Hargreaves R, Pamphilon DH, Prentice AG. Randomised trial of intravenous immunoglobulin as prophylaxis against infection in plateau-phase multiple myeloma. The UK Group for Immunoglobulin Replacement Therapy in Multiple Myeloma. *Lancet.* 1994;343(8905):1059-1063.
717. Rajkumar SV, Gertz MA, Kyle RA. Primary systemic amyloidosis with delayed progression to multiple myeloma. *Cancer.* 1998;82(8):1501-1505.
718. Kourelis TV, Kumar SK, Gertz MA, et al. Coexistent multiple myeloma or increased bone marrow plasma cells define equally high-risk populations in patients with immunoglobulin light chain amyloidosis. *J Clin Oncol.* 2013;31(34):4319-4324.
719. Kyle RA, Maldonado JE, Bayrd ED. Plasma cell leukemia. Report on 17 cases. *Arch Intern Med.* 1974;133(5):813-818.
720. Dimopoulos MA, Palumbo A, Delasalle KB, Alexanian R. Primary plasma cell leukaemia. *Br J Haematol.* 1994;88(4):754-759.
721. Blade J, Kyle RA. Nonsecretory myeloma, immunoglobulin D myeloma, and plasma cell leukemia. *Hematol Oncol Clin North Am.* 1999;13(6):1259-1272.
722. Fernandez de Larrea C, Kyle R, Rosinol L, et al. Primary plasma cell leukemia: consensus definition by the International Myeloma Working Group according to peripheral blood plasma cell percentage. *Blood Cancer J.* 2021;11(12):192.
723. Ravi P, Kumar SK, Roeker L, et al. Revised diagnostic criteria for plasma cell leukemia: results of a Mayo Clinic study with comparison of outcomes to multiple myeloma. *Blood Cancer J.* 2018;8(12):116.
724. Granell M, Calvo X, Garcia-Guinon A, et al; GEMMAC (Grup per l'estudi del mieloma i l'amiloidosi de Catalunya). Prognostic impact of circulating plasma cells in patients with multiple myeloma: implications for plasma cell leukemia definition. *Haematologica.* 2017;102(6):1099-1104.
725. An G, Qin X, Acharya C, et al. Multiple myeloma patients with low proportion of circulating plasma cells had similar survival with primary plasma cell leukemia patients. *Ann Hematol.* 2015;94(2):257-264.
726. Van Riet I, De Waele M, Remels L, Lacor P, Schots R, Van Camp B. Expression of cytoadhesion molecules (CD56, CD54, CD18 and CD29) by myeloma plasma cells. *Br J Haematol.* 1991;79(3):421-427.
727. Barker HF, Hamilton MS, Ball J, Drew M, Franklin IM. Expression of adhesion molecules LFA-3 and N-CAM on normal and malignant human plasma cells. *Br J Haematol.* 1992;81(3):331-335.
728. Robillard N, Jego G, Pellat-Deceunynck C, et al. CD28, a marker associated with tumoral expansion in multiple myeloma. *Clin Cancer Res.* 1998;4(6):1521-1526.
729. Avet-Loiseau H, Andree-Ashley LE, Moore D II, et al. Molecular cytogenetic abnormalities in multiple myeloma and plasma cell leukemia measured using comparative genomic hybridization. *Genes Chromosomes Cancer.* 1997;19(2):124-133.
730. Gutierrez NC, Hernandez JM, Garcia JL, et al. Differences in genetic changes between multiple myeloma and plasma cell leukemia demonstrated by comparative genomic hybridization. *Leukemia.* 2001;15(5):840-845.
731. Shimazaki C, Goto H, Araki S, et al. Overexpression of PRAD1/cyclin D1 in plasma cell leukemia with t(11;14)(q13;q32). *Int J Hematol.* 1997;66(1):111-115.
732. Usmani SZ, Nair B, Qu P, et al. Primary plasma cell leukemia: clinical and laboratory presentation, gene-expression profiling and clinical outcome with Total Therapy protocols. *Leukemia.* 2012;26(11):2398-2405.
733. Pruzanski W, Platts ME, Ogryzlo MA. Leukemic form of immunocytic dyscrasia (plasma cell leukemia). A study of ten cases and a review of the literature. *Am J Med.* 1969;47(1):60-74.
734. Noel P, Kyle RA. Plasma cell leukemia: an evaluation of response to therapy. *Am J Med.* 1987;83(6):1062-1068.
735. Pasqualetti P, Festuccia V, Collacciani A, Aciteli P, Casale R. Plasma cell leukemia. A report on 11 patients and review of the literature. *Panminerva Med.* 1996;38(3):179-184.
736. Fernandez de Larrea C, Kyle RA, Durie BGM, et al; International Myeloma Working Group. Plasma cell leukemia: consensus statement on diagnostic requirements, response criteria and treatment recommendations by the International Myeloma Working Group. *Leukemia.* 2013;27(4):780-791.
737. Gonsalves WI, Rajkumar SV, Go RS, et al. Trends in survival of patients with primary plasma cell leukemia: a population-based analysis. *Blood.* 2014;124(6):907-912.
738. Musto P, Simeon V, Martorelli MC, et al. Lenalidomide and low-dose dexamethasone for newly diagnosed primary plasma cell leukemia. *Leukemia.* 2014;28(1):222-225.
739. Dhakal B, Patel S, Girnius S, et al. Hematopoietic cell transplantation utilization and outcomes for primary plasma cell leukemia in the current era. *Leukemia.* 2020;34(12):3338-3347.
740. Nandakumar B, Kumar SK, Dispenzieri A, et al. Clinical characteristics and outcomes of patients with primary plasma cell leukemia in the era of novel agent therapy. *Mayo Clin Proc.* 2021;96(3):677-687.
741. Panizo C, Rifon J, Rodriguez-Wilhelmi P, Cuesta B, Rocha E. Long-term survival in primary plasma cell leukemia after therapy with VAD, autologous blood stem cell transplantation and interferon-alpha. *Acta Haematol.* 1999;101(4):193-196.
742. Sica S, Chiusolo P, Salutari P, et al. Long-lasting complete remission in plasma cell leukemia after aggressive chemotherapy and CD34-selected autologous peripheral blood progenitor cell transplant: molecular follow-up of minimal residual disease. *Bone Marrow Transplant.* 1998;22(8):823-825.
743. Hovenga S, de Wolf JT, Klip H, Vellenga E. Consolidation therapy with autologous stem cell transplantation in plasma cell leukemia after VAD, high-dose cyclophosphamide and EDAP courses: a report of three cases and a review of the literature. *Bone Marrow Transplant.* 1997;20(10):901-904.
744. Yeh KH, Lin MT, Tang JL, Yang CH, Tsay W, Chen YC. Long-term disease-free survival after autologous bone marrow transplantation in a primary plasma cell leukaemia: detection of minimal residual disease in the transplant marrow by third-complementarity-determining region-specific probes. *Br J Haematol.* 1995;89(4):914-916.
745. Yang CH, Lin MT, Tsay W, Liu LT, Wang CH, Chen YC. Autologous bone marrow transplantation for plasma cell leukemia: report of a case. *Transplant Proc.* 1992;24(4):1531-1532.
746. Royer B, Minvielle S, Diouf M, et al. Bortezomib, doxorubicin, cyclophosphamide, dexamethasone induction followed by stem cell transplantation for primary plasma cell leukemia: a prospective phase II study of the Intergroupe Francophone du Myelome. *J Clin Oncol.* 2016;34(18):2125-2132.
747. Saccaro S, Fonseca R, Veillon DM, et al. Primary plasma cell leukemia: report of 17 new cases treated with autologous or allogeneic stem-cell transplantation and review of the literature. *Am J Hematol.* 2005;78(4):288-294.
748. Mahindra A, Kalaycio ME, Vela-Ojeda J, et al. Hematopoietic cell transplantation for primary plasma cell leukemia: results from the Center for International Blood and Marrow Transplant Research. *Leukemia.* 2012;26(5):1091-1097.
749. Evison G, Evans KT. Sclerotic bone deposits in multiple myeloma. *Br J Radiol.* 1983;56(662):145.
750. Tormey WP. Low concentration monoclonal and oligoclonal bands in serum and urine using the Sebia Hydragel Protein Electrophoresis System. *Clin Chem Lab Med.* 1998;36(4):253-254.

751. Rubio-Felix D, Giralt M, Giraldo MP, et al. Nonsecretory multiple myeloma. *Cancer*. 1987;59(10):1847-1852.
752. Cavo M, Galieni P, Gobbi M, et al. Nonsecretory multiple myeloma. Presenting findings, clinical course and prognosis. *Acta Haematol*. 1985;74(1):27-30.
753. Turesson I, Grubb A. Non-secretory or low-secretory myeloma with intracellular kappa chains. Report of six cases and review of the literature. *Acta Med Scand*. 1978;204(6):445-451.
754. Blade J, Kyle RA. IgD monoclonal gammopathy with long-term follow-up. *Br J Haematol*. 1994;88(2):395-396.
755. Dimopoulos MA, Moulopoulos LA, Maniatis A, Alexanian R. Solitary plasmacytoma of bone and asymptomatic multiple myeloma. *Blood*. 2000;96(6):2037-2044.
756. Liebross RH, Ha CS, Cox JD, Weber D, Delasalle K, Alexanian R. Solitary bone plasmacytoma: outcome and prognostic factors following radiotherapy. *Int J Radiat Oncol Biol Phys*. 1998;41(5):1063-1067.
757. Warsame R, Gertz MA, Lacy MQ, et al. Trends and outcomes of modern staging of solitary plasmacytoma of bone. *Am J Hematol*. 2012;87(7):647-651.
758. Paiva B, Chandia M, Vidriales MB, et al. Multiparameter flow cytometry for staging of solitary bone plasmacytoma: new criteria for risk of progression to myeloma. *Blood*. 2014;124(8):1300-1303.
759. Dingli D, Kyle RA, Rajkumar SV, et al. Immunoglobulin free light chains and solitary plasmacytoma of bone. *Blood*. 2006;108(6):1979-1983.
760. Dimopoulos MA, Kiamouris C, Moulopoulos LA. Solitary plasmacytoma of bone and extramedullary plasmacytoma. *Hematol Oncol Clin North Am*. 1999;13(6):1249-1257.
761. Galieni P, Cavo M, Pulsoni A, et al. Clinical outcome of extramedullary plasmacytoma. *Haematologica*. 2000;85(1):47-51.
762. Hussong JW, Perkins SL, Schnitzer B, Hargreaves H, Frizzera G. Extramedullary plasmacytoma. A form of marginal zone cell lymphoma? *Am J Clin Pathol*. 1999;111(1):111-116.
763. Ozsahin M, Tsang RW, Poortmans P, et al. Outcomes and patterns of failure in solitary plasmacytoma: a Multicenter Rare Cancer Network study of 258 patients. *Int J Radiat Oncol Biol Phys*. 2006;64(1):210-217.
764. Shao H, Xi L, Raffeld M, et al. Nodal and extranodal plasmacytomas expressing immunoglobulin a: an indolent lymphoproliferative disorder with a low risk of clinical progression. *Am J Surg Pathol*. 2010;34(10):1425-1435.

Chapter 101 ■ Immunoglobulin Light Chain Amyloidosis

MORIE A. GERTZ • ELI MUCHTAR • ANGELA DISPENZIERI

HISTORY

"The term lardaceous change has ... come more into use chiefly through the instrumentality of the Vienna School.... The term, lardaceous changes ... has but very little to do with these tumours, and rather refers to things, upon which the old writers ... who were better connoisseurs in bacon than our friends in Vienna, would hardly have bestowed such a name.... The appearance of such organs ... are said to look like bacon, bears ... a much greater resemblance to wax, and I have therefore now for a long time ... made use of the term waxy change.... These structures ... by the simple action of iodine ... assume just as blue a colour as vegetable starch...."[1]

Schleiden, a German botanist, first used the term *amyloid* in 1838 to describe a normal constituent of plants.[2] In 1858, Virchow, head of the pathology department in Berlin, gave a lecture entitled "Amyloid Degeneration" and described amyloid deposits that stained blue with iodine and sulfuric acid, similar to the chemical reaction markers of starch. Virchow concluded that the substance was composed of starch and used the word *amyloid* to describe it. During the lecture, Virchow also criticized his chief competitor in Vienna, Rokitansky, who believed that amyloid was a lardlike substance, perhaps because amyloid deposits were white and glistening, found in patients with syphilis, tuberculosis, or malaria. In 1859, Friedreich, Nikolau, and Kekule recognized that the waxy spleen described by Virchow did not contain any starch-like substances and that the deposits probably were derived from modified proteins. Budd analyzed the liver of a patient with amyloidosis and found that it was not lardaceous. Wilks identified what is likely the first reported case of immunoglobulin light chain amyloidosis (AL) (described as "idiopathic" at the time), a 52-year-old patient with lardaceous change unrelated to an obvious cause.

The amino acid composition of amyloid deposits was first described by Schmiedeberg in 1920.[2] Amyloid proteins strongly resembled serum globulin and therefore were neither fat nor carbohydrate. The first use of Congo red as the specific stain for detection of amyloid was reported in 1922 by Bennhold. In 1927, Divry and Florkin reported green birefringence under polarized light when amyloid-laden material from the brain of a patient with Alzheimer disease was stained with Congo red; the association between the neurodegeneration of Alzheimer disease and amyloid was forgotten for nearly 50 years. Magnus-Levy postulated that Bence Jones proteins were a precursor of amyloid and noted a relationship among amyloid deposits, Bence Jones proteins, and multiple myeloma.

The finding that amyloid proteins consisted of organized fibrils was credited to Cohen and Calkins in 1959.[2] They determined that all forms of amyloid were nonbranching and fibrillar. The fibril length varied, but the width was 9.5 nm. Apitz claimed that amyloid in the tissues was analogous to the excretion of immunoglobulin light chain proteins by the kidneys; he coined the term *paraprotein* to describe monoclonal immunoglobulins. Isobe and Osserman reported in 1974 that Bence Jones proteins had a direct role in the pathogenesis of AL. Physiologically normal proteins primarily have an α-helix configuration. In 1968, Eanes and Glenner reported that they used x-ray diffraction to determine that amyloid proteins formed an alternate configuration of β-pleated sheets, similar to the configuration of silk proteins.

As with silk, amyloid proteins are highly resistant to solvents, and this resistance is a feature of the purification process.[2] Amyloid-laden tissue is homogenized repeatedly in saline and centrifuged. The supernatant, which contains soluble components, is discarded, and the residual pelletized material contains amyloid proteins. After the pellet is resuspended in distilled water, a relatively pure preparation of amyloid fibrils is obtained. Pras et al first described the purification of amyloid in 1968.

Levin et al were the first to sequence an amyloid protein, and they designated it as *amyloid A* (the precursor protein responsible for AA amyloidosis, historically known as secondary amyloidosis).[2] Benditt et al independently sequenced amyloid A at the same time. The first sequence of an immunoglobulin light chain form of amyloid was reported in 1970 by Glenner et al and was recognized as an N-terminal fragment of an immunoglobulin light chain. All forms of AL amyloid were subsequently thought to be derived from misfolded fragments of immunoglobulin light chains, but heavy-chain fragments have also been shown to produce amyloid (designated as *AH*). Studies of recombinant-derived variable region fragments of immunoglobulins have shown a relationship between thermodynamic instability and fibrillogenic potential. Structural parameters and overall thermodynamic stability contribute to the fibril-forming propensity. Human monoclonal immunoglobulin light chains can be converted to amyloid fibrils in vitro by digestion with pepsin. Synthetically, amyloid fibrils can be produced by breaking the disulfide bonds of intact immunoglobulins.

CLASSIFICATION

The diagnosis of amyloidosis requires biopsy of tissue specimen with deposits that are positively stained by Congo red. With hematoxylin and eosin staining, amyloid deposits resemble hyalin. Deposits are always extracellular and appear amorphous. Apple-green birefringence is seen when Congo red stained material is viewed under polarized light. The Congo red stain can be technically difficult to use and can form precipitates, yielding false-positive results.[3] Pathologists need to perform diagnostic assays regularly to be experts in the interpretation of these stains. All forms of amyloid have a fibrillar appearance when viewed with electron microscopy, and the fibrils are rigid and nonbranching. Not all fibrils identified with electron microscopy are amyloid proteins; in the absence of a positive result on Congo red stain and apple-green birefringence, the diagnosis remains unconfirmed.

The classification scheme of amyloidosis has undergone revision as understanding of the pathophysiology of the disease has improved. In the 19th century, involvement of the liver, spleen, and kidneys was incorrectly thought to represent secondary amyloidosis (AA); amyloid that involved the heart, tongue, and peripheral nerves was classified as *AL or idiopathic or primary amyloidosis*. Familial amyloidosis was recognized generally by the presentation of progressive peripheral neuropathy with an autosomal dominant inheritance pattern. Families with inherited renal amyloidosis were also described. Mutations in transthyretin (TTR), apolipoprotein A1, apolipoprotein A2, apolipoprotein CII, apolipoprotein CIII, fibrinogen A-α chain, gelsolin, and lysozyme are also types of hereditary amyloidosis. More recently, another form of acquired amyloidosis, leukocyte chemotactic factor 2 (LECT2)[4] has been described. Although it is more prevalent in certain ethnic populations, no gene mutation has been identified. For more information on other forms of systemic amyloidosis, see section "Other types of systemic amyloidosis." A classification of the various forms of amyloidosis is shown in *Table 101.1*.

In AL, the tertiary structure and amino acid sequence of immunoglobulin light chains are abnormal. For patients with AL, 75% of immunoglobulin light chains are of the λ type. In contrast, for patients with multiple myeloma and monoclonal gammopathy of undetermined significance (MGUS) approximately 60% are of κ type (*Figure 101.1*).

Table 101.1. Nomenclature of the Most Common Forms of Amyloidosis

Amyloid Type	Precursor Protein	Clinical
AL or AH	Immunoglobulin (light or heavy chain), acquired	Formerly known as primary amyloidosis. Can be systemic or localized amyloidosis; associated with clonal plasma cell disorder
AA	Serum amyloid A, acquired	Formerly known as secondary amyloidosis. Caused by long-standing inflammation or infection and in periodic fever syndromes, such as familial Mediterranean fever; familial periodic fever syndromes associated with mutated tumor necrosis factor receptor
$ATTR_{mut}$	Transthyretin, inherited	Familial amyloidosis; most often heart and/or nerve
$ATTR_{wt}$	Transthyretin, acquired	Age-related (formerly known as senile) amyloidosis; heart and ligaments, CTS
AFib	Inherited	Familial renal amyloidosis (Ostertag amyloidosis)
$A\beta_2M$	β_2-Microglobulin, acquired	Dialysis associated; CTS, painful arthropathy
AApoAI, AApoAII	Apolipoprotein AI/AII, inherited	Heart (AApoAI only), kidney
AApoAIV	Apolipoprotein AIV, acquired	Kidney or heart
AGel	Gelsolin, inherited	Hereditary amyloidosis, common in Finnish descents. Triad of cutis laxa, corneal lattice dystrophy, and facial paralysis
ALys	Lysozyme, inherited	Renal
ALECT2	Leukocyte chemotactic factor 2, inherited	Renal and/or liver amyloidosis

Abbreviations: AA, secondary amyloid; AF, inherited amyloid proteins; AH, immunoglobulin heavy-chain amyloid; AL, primary amyloid; Apo1, apolipoprotein A1 amyloid; Apo2, apolipoprotein A2 amyloid; ATTR, amyloid transthyretin; $A\beta_2M$, amyloid β_2-microglobulin; AβPP, amyloid β protein precursor; CTS, carpal tunnel syndrome; LECT, leukocyte chemotactic factor; SAA, serum amyloid A.

The implication is that λ immunoglobulin light chains have a greater tendency to form a β-pleated sheet.

Certain immunoglobulins have "amyloidogenic" properties. Human amyloid deposits develop in the kidneys of mice after injection of light chains purified from the urine of patients with AL; this does not occur with similar samples from patients with multiple myeloma who do not have AL. There is preferential germline gene usage in AL. Of systemic AL cases, the IGVL-6-57 and the IGVL3-1 genes account for 23% and 15% of all lambda cases in which a lambda variable gene can be found.[5] The IGVL-6-57 seems to always be associated with amyloid proteins, which suggests that unique amino acid sequences may result in formation of amyloidogenic proteins (*Table 101.2*).

In AL, the plasma cell process is clonal but typically is not proliferative, and the unrestrained growth associated with malignancy is absent. AL with 10% or greater clonal marrow plasma cells is referred to as myeloma-associated AL. The distinction between AL and myeloma-associated AL is somewhat arbitrary. Even in the presence of greater than 10% plasma cells in the bone marrow, the clinical course is still dominated by organ involvement rather than by the features related to the plasma cell clone, although the higher the marrow plasma cell burden, the worse the outcome and more of a myeloma phenotype including less λ-skewed isotype, more intact immunoglobulin secretion, higher S-phase, higher rate of high-risk fluorescent in situ hybridization (FISH), and higher likelihood of lytic bone disease.[9,10] Regardless, lytic bone disease or spinal compression fractures are uncommon in patients with AL. Renal insufficiency in AL is almost never a consequence of the formation of light chain cast nephropathy, as is the case in multiple myeloma. For patients with AL, renal failure is attributable to glomerular and tubular atrophy, a consequence of long-term albuminuria, and time to dialysis in AL is predicted by the level of urinary albumin excretion.

DIAGNOSIS OF AMYLOIDOSIS

When should a clinician initiate a diagnostic algorithm to confirm the presence of AL? The symptoms and physical findings of AL generally are nonspecific and unhelpful to the clinician. Nevertheless, eight critical clinical syndromes commonly associated with amyloidosis should trigger screening: (1) infiltrative cardiomyopathy with restrictive hemodynamics (heart failure with preserved ejection fraction), (2) nephrotic-range proteinuria, (3) hepatomegaly, (4) peripheral neuropathy, (5) carpal tunnel syndrome, (6) gastrointestinal tract symptoms of pseudo-obstruction or malabsorption, (7) tongue enlargement, and (8) "atypical" MGUS or smoldering multiple myeloma. The diagnosis of AL must be considered when any one of these presentations is seen (*Table 101.3*), most notably in any patient with a plasma cell disorder who has unexplained weight loss, fatigue, or any of the above presentations.

For any patient with a compatible clinical syndrome, tests to confirm the diagnosis of AL should be pursued rigorously with immunofixation of the serum and urine as well as serum immunoglobulin free light chain (FLC) measurement.[11] Serum electrophoresis alone is inadequate because the light chains in AL frequently do not produce a spike on an electrophoretic pattern. More than 50% of patients have no detectable heavy chain by serum immunofixation (*Figure 101.2*).[12] As stand-alone tests, serum protein electrophoresis, serum immunofixation, and serum immunoglobulin FLC assay are positive in 66%, 77%, and 88% of patients with AL.[13] The urine should be evaluated because it adds to the sensitivity of the monoclonal protein testing and provides insight into the possibility of nephrotic syndrome. The combination

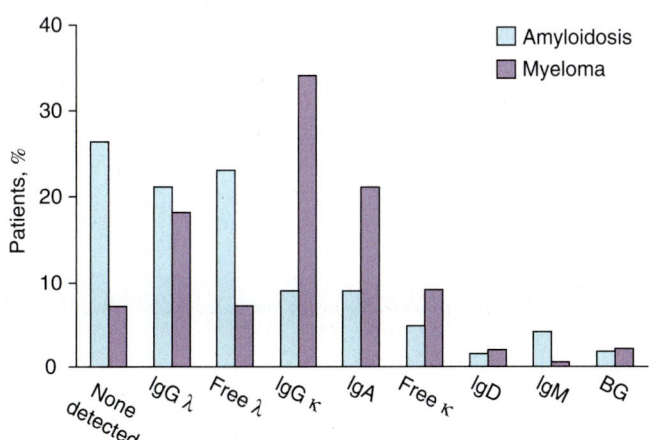

FIGURE 101.1 Distribution of serum monoclonal protein in patients with amyloidosis ($N = 270$) or myeloma ($N = 1000$) before the era of the immunoglobulin free light chain assay. BG, biclonal gammopathy. Ig, immunoglobulin. (Reprinted with permission from Gertz MA, Lacy MQ, Dispenzieri A, et al. Transplantation for amyloidosis. *Curr Opin Oncol.* 2007;19(2):136-141)

Table 101.2. Light Chain Class Usage in Amyloidosis

Light Chain Family	Study			
	Comenzo et al[6] (%)	Perfetti et al[7] (%)[a]	Abraham et al[8] (%)	Kourelis et al[5] (%)
IGVL1	31	15	22	20
IGVL2	14	16	34	17
IGVL3	17	47	28	19
IGVL6	38	20	16	23

Abbreviation: IGVL, immunoglobulin lambda variable.
[a]For polyclonal conditions, IGVL1 usage is 25%, IGVL2 usage is 24%, and IGVL3 usage is 43%.

of serum protein electrophoresis, serum immunofixation, and serum immunoglobulin FLC assay brings the sensitivity to 98%, and adding urine immunofixation brings the sensitivity to greater than 99%. The presence of a monoclonal protein does not assure a diagnosis of AL.

All patients with AL should have a bone marrow biopsy along with a FISH panel. A clonal population of plasma cells is detectable in virtually all patients with AL, even those with very low tumor burden, especially if high-sensitivity multiparametric flow cytometry is used in conjunction with marrow aspirate and trephine biopsy especially. If the patient does not have monoclonal protein in the serum or urine, has a normal FLC ratio, and has no detection of a clonal population of plasma cells in the bone marrow, the diagnosis of systemic AL is very unlikely; however, if amyloidosis is present, further evaluation for other types of systemic or localized amyloidosis should be performed.

The diagnosis of AL must always be confirmed by tissue biopsy. For patients who have neuropathy, nephrotic syndrome, cardiac failure, or hepatomegaly, the diagnosis could be established by direct biopsy of the involved organs, but an invasive visceral biopsy usually is not required to confirm AL. Because amyloid deposits typically are widespread at diagnosis and have involved the vasculature extensively, biopsy procedures that are less invasive, at a lower risk, and at a lower cost may be used to establish the diagnosis (*Table 101.4*). For a patient with a syndrome consistent with AL and confirmed presence of a monoclonal protein, we begin the diagnostic evaluation with a subcutaneous fat aspirate and bone marrow biopsy. The subcutaneous fat aspirate is a 75%-sensitive, risk-free procedure that is performed by registered nurses. Results are available within 24 hours (*Figure 101.3*).[14] A YouTube video on performance of a fat aspiration can be found at https://www.youtube.com/watch?v=tctYTmxd9gQ. Punch biopsy of fat is an alternative as is surgical incisional biopsy with a higher yield albeit more invasive. Amyloid deposits are seen in 69% of the bone marrow biopsy specimens of patients with AL and generally are identified in blood vessels.[14] With Congo red studies of fat and bone marrow, the diagnosis is established in 89% of patients. For the other 11%, the diagnosis may be established by a biopsy of the affected organ.

Table 101.3. Syndromes in patients with AL Amyloidosis Typed by Mass Spectrometry, Mayo Clinic 2008-2015 (n = 591)

Syndrome	Patients (%)
Cardiac	76
Renal	53
Neurologic	24
Hepatic	18
Gastrointestinal	17
>2 organs involved	25

Based on the data from Muchtar E, Gertz MA, Kyle RA, et al. A modern primer on light chain amyloidosis in 592 patients with mass spectrometry-verified typing. *Mayo Clin Proc*. 2019;94(3):472-483.

Other minimally invasive biopsy procedures may be used to establish a diagnosis of AL. Xerostomia in amyloidosis is attributable to salivary gland infiltration, and lip biopsy findings have high sensitivity (up to 87%).[15] Subcutaneous blood vessels may be accessed through a skin biopsy and may show AL deposits. Amyloid deposits regularly were confirmed by rectal biopsy in the 1970s and 1980s. Rectal biopsy is an outpatient procedure, although occasionally it results in bleeding. Endoscopic biopsy specimens have been used to establish a tissue diagnosis of amyloidosis.

Congo red may precipitate in tissue, and overstaining, particularly in subcutaneous fat, may produce a false-positive result.[16] Skin and subcutaneous fat have a high content of elastin and collagen; both bind Congo red and may also be interpreted as a false-positive result.[17] Rectal biopsy specimens containing amyloid may be misinterpreted as collagenous colitis if stained only with hematoxylin and eosin.[18] To recognize amyloid in the myocardium, our cardiac pathologists prefer to use the sulfated alcian blue stain. The Peripheral Nerve Laboratory at Mayo Clinic stains sural nerve biopsy specimens with crystal violet during screening and confirms the diagnosis subsequently with Congo red.

Once a diagnosis of amyloidosis is made, the amyloid must be typed. When the referral diagnosis was AL, 34 of 350 patients (9.7%) were reported to have a hereditary form of amyloidosis, the majority of which were AFib and ATTRv[19]; a low-grade monoclonal gammopathy was detectable in 8 patients. In another series of 54 patients who underwent screening with polymerase chain reaction assays to detect hereditary variants,[20] 3 patients had monoclonal gammopathy and concomitant hereditary amyloidosis variant. Approximately 25% of patients with ATTR cardiac amyloidosis have a monoclonal gammopathy so the finding of amyloid with a monoclonal protein should not be considered AL without specific identification of the protein subunit in the tissue specimen. These studies highlight the importance of accurate typing, a crucial part in the diagnostic evaluation of amyloidosis. We believe the gold standard for typing is mass spectroscopic analysis of the tissue and direct sequencing to identify the amyloid protein; this evaluation is now standard for all pathologic specimens that test Congo red positive seen at Mayo. The procedure can be performed on subcutaneous fat and any paraffin-embedded tissue.[21,22] The presence of serum amyloid P (SAP), apolipoprotein E, and apolipoprotein AIV are useful positive controls confirming the presence of amyloid. Immunohistochemistry yields equivocal results in over 20% of specimens, while mass spectroscopy fails to appropriately identify the subunit in only 7% most often due to scant amyloid deposits in the submitted specimen.

All forms of amyloid deposits contain a SAP component, a pentagonal glycoprotein structurally similar to C-reactive protein and present in all vertebrates. SAP may represent as much as 10% of the amyloid fibril by weight. Healthy adults have 50 to 100 mg of amyloid P component in the extravascular and intravascular compartments, whereas patients with amyloidosis may have up to 20,000 mg. The concentration of SAP in plasma is relatively stable, and it maintains a dynamic circulating equilibrium between the serum and tissue amyloid deposits. This dynamic equilibrium is exploited for imaging purposes using an I^{131}-labeled SAP scan.[24] The diagnostic sensitivity of SAP scintigraphy for systemic AA, AL, and amyloid TTR origin amyloidosis is 90%, 90%, and 48%, respectively; specificity is 93%, although the

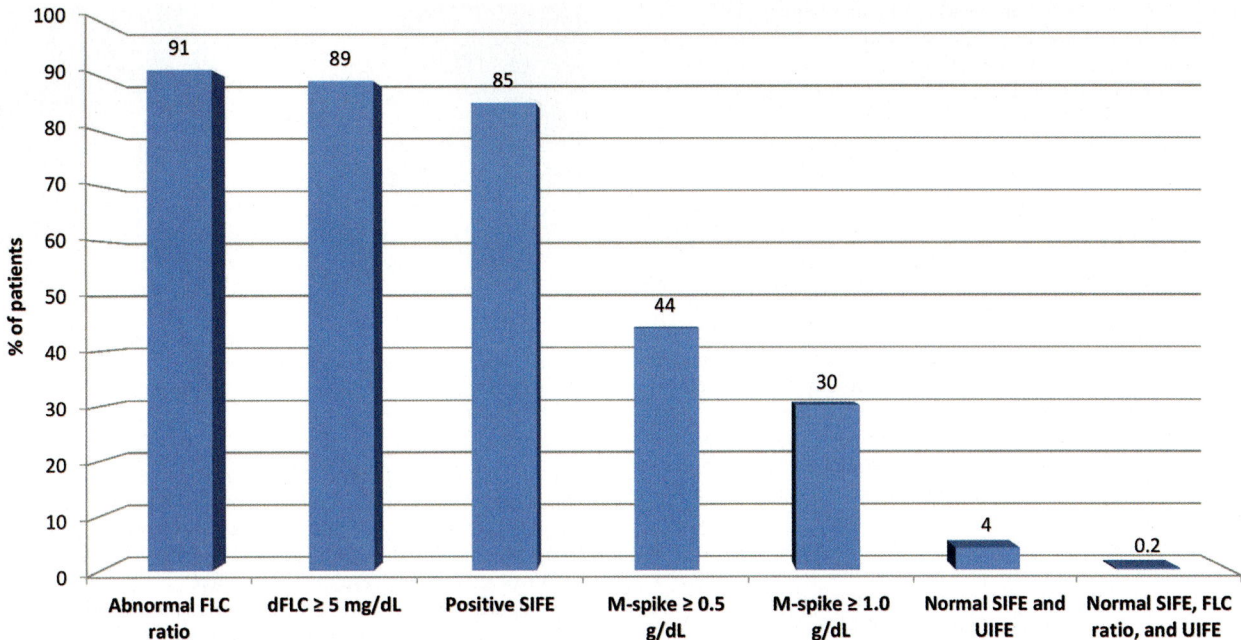

FIGURE 101.2 **Frequency of positive special protein results in patients with newly diagnosed AL.** A total of 1009 patients were seen at the Mayo Clinic between 2000 and 2014 who had serum protein electrophoresis, serum immunoelectrophoresis (IFE), and serum immunoglobulin free light chains measured. dFLC, difference between involved and uninvolved serum immunoglobulin free light chain. (From Muchtar E, Gertz MA, Kyle RA, et al. *Mayo Clin Proc.* (Submitted)).

Table 101.4. Findings of Biopsies Among Patients With AL With More Than One Biopsy for AL

Affected organ	Sensitivity of direct organ biopsy		Sensitivity of CR Performed on Either Bone Marrow or Fat Aspirate	
	N	CR+, N (%)	N	CR+ Bone Marrow or Fat, N (%)
Heart	96	96 (100)	93	67 (72)
Kidneys	207	205 (97)	198	148 (75)
Liver	34	33 (97)	33	26 (79)
Nerve	7	4 (57)	4	2 (50)

Abbreviation: CR, Congo red.
Based on data from Muchtar E, Dispenzieri A, Lacy MQ, et al. Overuse of organ biopsies in immunoglobulin light chain amyloidosis (AL): the consequence of failure of early recognition. *Ann Med.* 2017;49(7):1-7.

technique cannot distinguish between types. The clearance rate of radiolabeled SAP components from the plasma may be used to assess the total-body burden of amyloid and to evaluate the effect of therapy. Patients with large burdens of amyloid have rapid clearance, which is associated with shorter survival, but those with trace amounts of systemic amyloid deposits have plasma clearance rates similar to those of healthy individuals. Cardiac amyloid deposits cannot be detected using SAP scans, but uptake of I^{131}-labeled amyloid P component is seen in the spleen, liver, and kidneys in 87%, 60%, and 25% of patients, respectively. The correlation is poor between imaging and the extent of organ dysfunction assessed clinically. More widespread organ involvement is identified with a scan than with clinical examination. Iodine-labeled SAP scanning is not available in the United States. Although not clinically available for this indication, whole-body (18) F-Florbetapir positron emission tomography (PET)/computed tomography (CT) identifies amyloid deposits in a high percentage of subjects for several organ systems including tongue, lung, kidney, and abdominal wall fat.[25] Imaging using 124I-p5 + 14 PET is under active investigation for the detection of amyloid deposits in vivo.[26]

PRESENTATION AND CLINICAL FEATURES

The incidence of AL is 10 per million per year and has been stable for more than 50 years[27]; its incidence is similar to that of nodular sclerosing Hodgkin lymphoma, chronic myeloid leukemia, and polycythemia rubra vera. Multiple myeloma is five times more prevalent than AL. Sixty-four percent of AL cases occur in men. Although we have seen patients with AL who were as young as 23 years, the median age of patients with AL at our referral center is 64 years (range, 39-89 years).[28] The median age of patients who present with AL in Olmsted County, Minnesota, is 73 years.

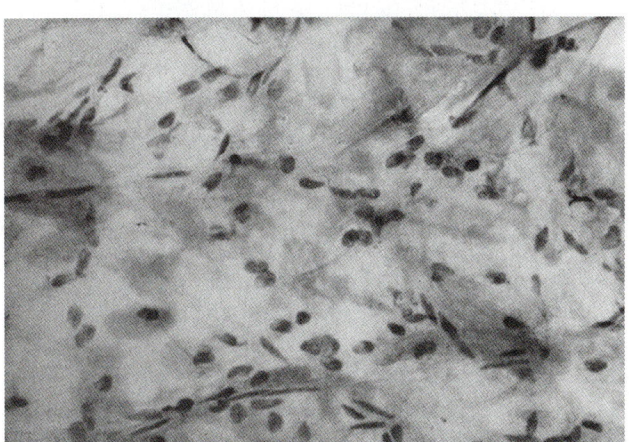

FIGURE 101.3 **Subcutaneous fat aspirate showing amyloid deposits (Congo red, original magnification ×100).** (Courtesy of Paul J. Kurtin, MD, Mayo Clinic, Rochester, Minnesota.)

The organs most affected are heart (76%) and kidney (53%), followed by nerve (24%) and liver (21%) (Table 101.3).[28] Fewer than 10% of patients have amyloid deposits that were identified in only the tongue, lung, joints, or soft tissues. Amyloid arthropathy occasionally occurs in amyloidosis. Synovial fluid aspiration and/or synovial biopsy may establish the diagnosis, and chemotherapy may effectively alleviate the joint manifestations.[29] At Mayo Clinic, 25% of patients with AL have more than two organs affected.

Symptoms and Signs

Weight loss, paresthesia, edema, dyspnea, and fatigue are the most common symptoms of AL (Figure 101.4). These nonspecific complaints provide little help to a clinician evaluating patients. Patients with extreme weight loss frequently undergo evaluation for an occult malignancy. The fatigue may be diagnosed incorrectly as stress-related or functional fatigue. We have seen many patients undergo coronary angiography because of fatigue and breathlessness, only to have the evaluation end when angiogram findings are normal. Over one-third of patients have a delay of over 1 year from symptom onset to diagnosis. Patients see a median of three physicians to establish a diagnosis.[30]

Lightheadedness occurs frequently in amyloidosis, but this is a common and nonspecific complaint in the primary care setting. In AL, the cause of light-headedness is multifactorial. Patients with nephrotic syndrome have dizziness because of hypoalbuminemia and marked intravascular volume contraction, which leads to orthostatic hypotension. Patients with cardiac AL have a low end-diastolic volume (because of restriction to filling during diastole) and low cardiac output, but a normal ejection fraction is maintained until late in the course of the disease. The echocardiographic finding of a normal ejection fraction may be highly misleading and may hinder recognition of cardiac involvement in AL. Patients may have orthostatic hypotension because of autonomic neuropathy. Syncope is not unusual.

Some of the physical findings of AL are specific and diagnostic; however, they are present in only 15% of patients and may easily be overlooked. Amyloid purpura is seen in only one of every six patients with AL (Figure 101.5). Purpura may be periorbital and also may occur in the face, webbing of the neck, and upper chest. Purpura on the arms is not characteristic of AL, but petechial lesions on the eyelids should not be overlooked. The liver is palpable 5 cm below the right costal margin in only 10% of patients. Splenomegaly, if present, is usually of modest degree. Overall, any degree of hepatomegaly is present in one-fifth of patients. Edema occurs in approximately 45% of patients.

Macroglossia is the most specific finding of AL (Figure 101.6). In our experience, enlargement of the tongue is never found in AA or hereditary, age-related (ATTR$_{WT}$) amyloidosis. Tongue enlargement is seen in 1 of 11 patients with AL and may be overlooked easily unless the physician knows to look for dental indentations on the underside of the tongue. However, presentation with fatigue, edema, breathlessness, or paresthesias would not immediately lead the physician to examine the patient's tongue. Tongue enlargement is almost always accompanied by concomitant enlargement of the submandibular salivary glands, but salivary gland involvement should not be misinterpreted as submandibular lymphadenopathy. Major and minor salivary gland involvement may result in xerostomia.

Vascular involvement without visceral organ dysfunction produces occlusion and ischemic symptoms, such as jaw claudication, when the temporal arteries are involved; calf and limb claudication may occur when the microvasculature that supplies the extremities is involved; and acute coronary syndrome is reported due to involvement of intramural coronary arteries. A monoclonal protein in the serum may increase the sedimentation rate, and it is not unusual for AL and jaw claudication to be misdiagnosed as temporal arteritis.[31] Amyloid deposits may be found if a temporal artery biopsy is performed, but Congo red staining typically is not performed on such specimens.

Carpal tunnel syndrome is observed in 21% of patients with systemic AL. The presence of carpal tunnel syndrome with cardiac failure or infiltrative cardiomyopathy can be a clue to the presence of amyloidosis. The shoulder-pad sign is a consequence of periarticular infiltration with amyloid and may produce pseudohypertrophy. Despite enlargement of the musculature of the shoulder and hip girdle, these patients present with diffuse muscular weakness and may have muscular atrophy because of chronic vascular occlusion.[32]

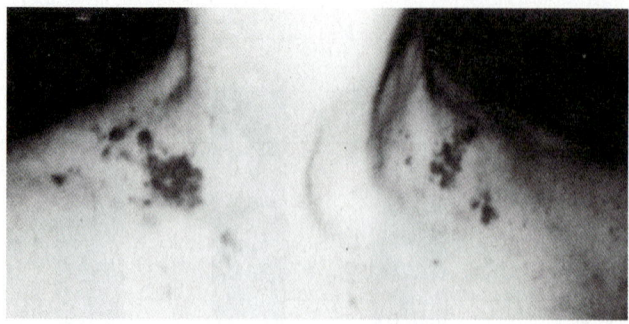

FIGURE 101.5 Classic truncal purpura in primary amyloidosis. (Reprinted from Gertz MA, Lacy MQ, Dispenzieri A. Amyloidosis. *Hematol Oncol Clin North Am.* 1999;13(6):1211-1233. Copyright © 1999 Elsevier. With permission.)

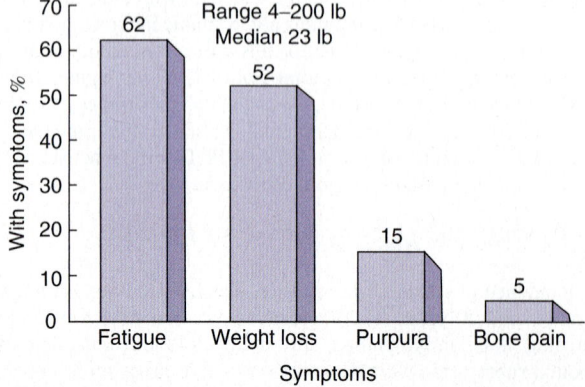

FIGURE 101.4 Prevalence of symptoms for patients with primary amyloidosis evaluated 1 month before or after diagnosis at Mayo Clinic, 1981 to 1992. (Reprinted from Kyle RA, Gertz MA. Primary systemic amyloidosis. Clinical and laboratory features in 474 cases. *Semin Hematol.* 1995;32(1):45-59. Copyright © 1995 Elsevier. With permission.)

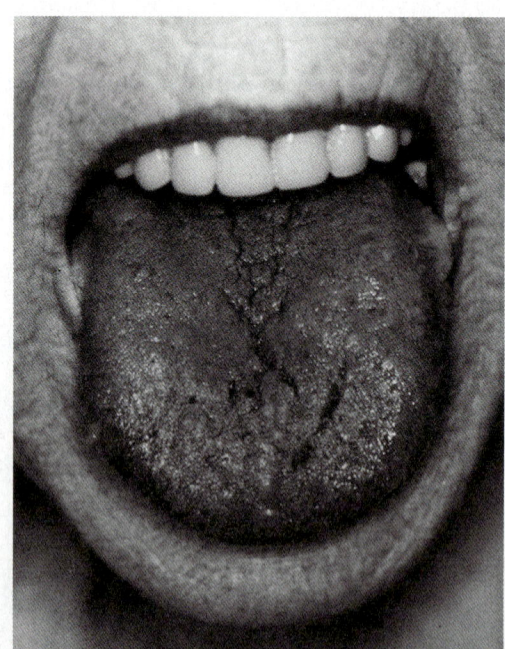

FIGURE 101.6 Tongue enlargement in primary amyloidosis. (Reprinted from Gertz MA, Lacy MQ, Dispenzieri A. Amyloidosis. *Hematol Oncol Clin North Am.* 1999;13(6):1211-1233. Copyright © 1999 Elsevier. With permission.)

AL is rarely associated with anemia. The hemoglobin level was greater than 100 g/L for 90% of patients and greater than 120 g/L for 71%.[12] Only 1.6% had hemoglobin levels less than 90 g/L, and the cause was usually active gastrointestinal tract bleeding or renal failure. The median platelet count of patients with AL was 257×10^9/L (range, 46×10^9/L to 809×10^9/L). A platelet count greater than 500×10^9/L was seen in 5.5% of patients. The most common cause of thrombocytosis in AL is hepatic involvement with associated hyposplenism.[33,34] The median number of bone marrow plasma cells at diagnosis is 10%. A serum creatinine value of 2 mg/dL or greater was present for 13.1% of patients, and 6.7% had alkaline phosphatase levels greater than twice the maximum normal value.

By immunofixation, monoclonal λ and κ light chains (in the serum and urine) were found in 77% and 16% of patients, respectively, with none detected in 7%. The serum heavy chain isotype frequency was no heavy chain, IgG, IgA, IgM, and IgD for 53%, 33%, 7%, 2%, and 1% of patients, respectively.[28] The presence of an IgM monoclonal protein is important for two reasons: first, we have seen many referred patients with a diagnosis of Waldenström macroglobulinemia, for whom the amyloid syndrome was overlooked.[35] Second, the management of IgM-related AL is more challenging and may require special considerations.

Heart

The heart is the organ that determines the patient outcome most (see section "Prognostic Features"), and it is affected in 76% of AL cases.[36] Amyloid is deposited extracellularly and results in a noncompliant and thickened left ventricle (*Figure 101.7*).[37] The echocardiogram has been the diagnostic standard for recognizing amyloid cardiomyopathy, but magnetic resonance imaging (MRI) may aid reaching a diagnosis. Occasionally, a patient has nondiagnostic imaging, and such that an endomyocardial biopsy is required.[38] Endomyocardial biopsy will provide the correct diagnosis for all patients when at least three endomyocardial specimens are obtained. For those not in overt heart failure but with cardiac involvement, presenting symptoms are fatigue, weight loss, and dyspnea on exertion. Syncope and arrhythmias may also occur. In one study, syncope with exercise was associated with a median survival time of 2 months.[39,40]

The electrocardiogram shows low voltage, but this also may be easily overlooked. The pseudoinfarction pattern of amyloidosis, with nearly two-thirds of patients showing loss of anterior forces in V_1 through V_3, may be misinterpreted as ischemic heart disease.[41] Electrocardiographic findings are clinically suspicious of silent ischemic disease, and patients invariably undergo coronary arteriography. Coronary angiogram findings are generally normal.[42] Failure to do an endomyocardial biopsy at the time of catheterization when high filling pressures are found is a major source of misdiagnosis. Soluble cardiac biomarkers troponin and NT-proBNP are also typically elevated in patients with cardiac AL and can be useful in the diagnosis and prognostication of AL.[43-45]

Early cardiac AL produces diastolic dysfunction without systolic dysfunction,[46] and chest radiographs do not show evidence of pulmonary vascular congestion or cardiomegaly. All patients being assessed for AL should have an echocardiographic evaluation that includes Doppler studies of diastolic performance, LV longitudinal strain, ejection fraction, and mitral deceleration time. A characteristic echocardiogram shows thickening of the left ventricular septum and free wall, thickening of the right ventricular wall, valve thickening, diastolic dysfunction with poor diastolic filling, reduced end-diastolic volume, and low cardiac output (*Figure 101.8*). Global longitudinal strain is frequently abnormal in the presence of cardiac amyloidosis with typical bull's-eye pattern of base to apex gradient (apical sparing).[47] The size of the left ventricular cavity is often reduced. Because of a low stroke volume, a hyperdynamic myocardium may develop with an elevated ejection fraction. This constellation of findings is frequently misinterpreted, and the presence of amyloid may be overlooked. The median septal thickness for patients with AL is 14 mm. Wall thickening frequently is misinterpreted as concentric left ventricular hypertrophy or asymmetrical septal hypertrophy, rather than infiltrative cardiomyopathy,[48,49] but the electrocardiogram typically shows low voltage and not hypertrophy. For patients who are assumed to have hypertrophy because of thickened ventricular walls, the finding of thickened mitral and tricuspid valves is a common and important clue; thickened valves are not found in hypertensive cardiomyopathy.

Doppler studies are best for accurate assessment of myocardial function for patients with AL and help in facilitating early diagnosis even in the absence of morphological echocardiographic abnormalities, especially when combined with strain imaging.[50] The Doppler filling patterns accurately indicate the extent of amyloid infiltration.[51] Valvular regurgitation is commonly seen by Doppler echocardiography, but it does not appear to have a clinically significant effect on myocardial performance. An important functional measurement is the deceleration time; a short deceleration time is indicative of restrictive physiologic characteristics, and a deceleration time shorter than 150 milliseconds is associated with worse outcomes. Decreased fractional shortening and increased ventricular wall thickness are the best predictors of outcome in AL.

Atrial or ventricular thrombi may develop in patients with AL because of stasis of blood within the cardiac chambers even in patients in sinus rhythm.[52] Systemic embolism may result, and the first manifestation of AL may be a stroke.[53] Anticoagulation therapy is indicated for patients with AL with atrial standstill. Distinguishing pericardial

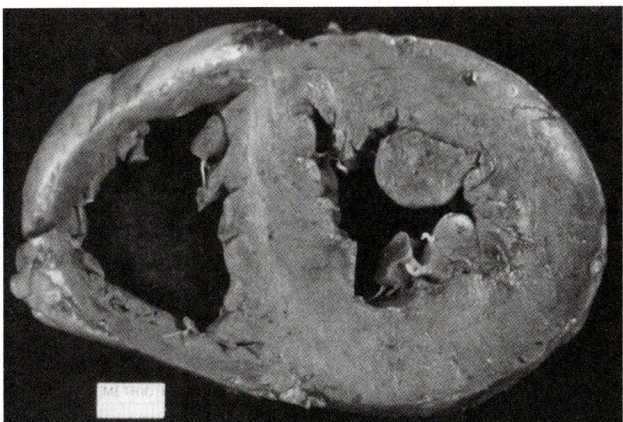

FIGURE 101.7 Myocardial wall diffusely thickened with amyloid. The whitish deposits represent the amyloid and are the lardaceous changes first recognized by Rokitansky. (From Gertz MA, Kyle RA. Amyloidosis [AL]. In: Wiernik PH, Goldman JM, Dutcher JP, et al., eds. *Neoplastic Diseases of the Blood.* 4th ed. Cambridge University Press; 2003:595-618. Used with permission of Mayo Foundation for Medical Education and Research. All rights reserved.)

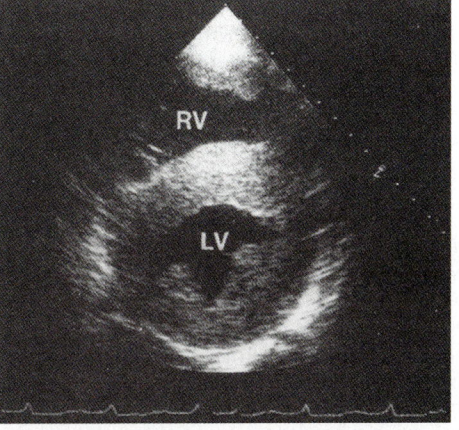

FIGURE 101.8 Echocardiographic image of concentric thickening of the wall of the left ventricle (LV) due to amyloid. RV, right ventricle. (From Gertz MA, Kyle RA. Amyloidosis [AL]. In: Wiernik PH, Goldman JM, Dutcher JP, et al., eds. *Neoplastic Diseases of the Blood.* 4th ed. Cambridge University Press; 2003:595-618. Used with permission of Mayo Foundation for Medical Education and Research. All rights reserved.)

disease from restrictive cardiomyopathy may be difficult.[54] It is rare for surgical pericardiectomy to provide clinical benefits to patients with AL. The hazards of surgery for patients with cardiac amyloidosis are well established.[55]

MRI may be a useful diagnostic technique. The combination of subtle, widespread heterogeneous myocardial enhancement on delayed postcontrast inversion recovery in T1-weighted images (also known as late gadolinium enhancement), with ancillary features of restrictive cardiac disease, may be highly suggestive of cardiac amyloidosis.[56] The presence of a positive cardiac MRI in AL was associated with a significantly increased risk of death, in particular of cardiac origin, but was not independent of clinical congestive heart failure.

Patients rarely present with symptoms of myocardial infarction due to amyloid deposition in the coronary arteries.[57] Angiographic findings are normal because epicardial coronary arteries are spared. In one pathology study 56/58 (97%) had amyloid *involvement* of the epicardial coronary arteries, but none had *obstruction* with amyloid of the epicardial vessels; in contrast, 63 of 96 patients (66%) had severe intramural coronary amyloidosis.[58] Myocardial ischemia affected 25% of patients with obstructive intramural coronary amyloidosis. For patients presenting with exertional angina, standard exercise tests show ischemia, but the diagnosis of intracoronary amyloid is difficult to establish before death. Right ventricular myocardial biopsy may show amyloid deposits in small intramural vessels. In a series of 11 patients with AL who presented with angina or an unstable coronary syndrome, a classic low-voltage electrocardiogram was seen in only two patients. Virtually all patients were assigned the diagnosis of cardiac amyloidosis at autopsy, which reflects the difficulty of recognizing small-vessel coronary arteriolar amyloidosis.

Kidney

AL affects the kidneys in 50% to 60% of patients. Kidneys are typically normal looking on ultrasound. When a patient has free monoclonal light chains in the urine, the differential diagnosis is cryoglobulinemia, amyloidosis, Randall-type light chain deposition disease and myeloma cast nephropathy. The presence of proteinuria does not always indicate albuminuria. The urine of patients with AL contains fat or fatty acid crystals but no casts or red blood cells. Of 118 patients with monoclonal gammopathy undergoing renal biopsy, 30% had AL. For nondiabetic adults with nephrotic syndrome, amyloidosis is observed in 12% of renal biopsy specimens; 2.5% to 2.8% of all kidney biopsy specimens contain amyloid deposits. In a series of 131 renal biopsies in patients aged 75 years or greater amyloidosis accounted for 9.1%.

AL most commonly affects the glomerulus with amyloid penetrating the glomerular basement membrane and resulting in proteinuria (predominantly albuminuria) with preserved estimated glomerular filtration rate (eGFR). Severe hypoalbuminemia is the result of nephrotic-range proteinuria. In one series, only 14% of patients had a presenting serum creatinine value that exceeded 2 mg/dL. The median urinary protein excretion for all patients with AL was 0.75 g in 24 hours (*Figure 101.9*),[7] but 30% had greater than 3 g of urinary protein in 24 hours. Only 5% of patients with AL had urinary protein loss in the reference range. The λ light chain may predispose patients to a higher level of renal involvement (5-fold higher rate of nephrotic range proteinuria in patients with λ clones as compared with κ clones); median urinary protein loss for patients with κ or λ amyloidosis is 3.6 or 4.6 g/d, respectively.

Continuous urinary protein loss results in tubular damage, and the long-term complication is end-stage renal disease.[59] The amount of protein in the urine and the extent of amyloid deposits in a kidney biopsy specimen correlate poorly.[6] Severe nephrotic syndrome may occur, even with low levels of amyloid deposits. Prognostic factors for development of end-stage renal disease are serum creatinine value at presentation and 24-hour urinary protein loss. These risk factors have been formalized in a renal staging system, which uses 24-hour urine protein greater than or equal to 5 g and eGFR < 50 mL/min as risk factors. They estimated the 2-year risk of dialysis of <3%, 11% to 25%, and 60% to 75% based on whether patients were stage I, II, or III, respectively.[8] Although the λ light chain may predispose patients to a

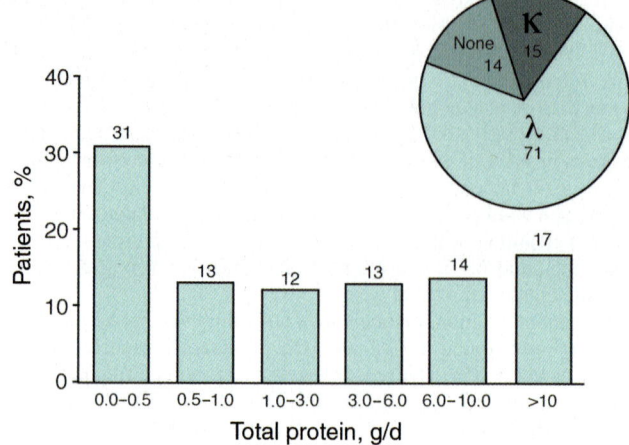

FIGURE 101.9 **Total protein excreted in the urine of patients with primary amyloidosis (24-hour period).** Inset, identification of immunoglobulin light chains, %. (From Gertz MA, Lacy MQ, Dispenzieri A. Amyloidosis. In: Mehta J, Singhal S, eds. *Myeloma*. Martin Dunitz; 2002:445-463. Copyright © 2002 by Martin Dunitz Ltd. Reproduced by permission of Taylor & Francis Group.)

higher level of proteinuria, there is no difference in the frequency of renal failure in κ or λ amyloidosis. Among patients presenting with renal AL, 42% received renal replacement therapy compared with 5% of patients who did not present with renal involvement.[60]

There are other conditions in the differential diagnosis for renal AL.[61] Fibrillary (immunotactoid) glomerulopathy refers to the deposition of fibrils in the kidney that initially may be confused with AL, but the fibrils are negative for Congo red stain and monoclonal protein typically is not detected in the serum or urine. Examination by electron microscopy shows that the fibrils of fibrillary glomerulopathy are twice the width of amyloid fibrils, and extrarenal disease does not develop in patients with fibrillary glomerulopathy. Randall-type light chain deposition disease indicates granular deposition of nonamyloid immunoglobulin light chain along the glomerular basement membrane. Light chain deposition disease and amyloidosis in the same patient has been reported. Electron microscopy studies of tissues affected by light chain deposition disease do not show fibrils.

Liver

Nearly three-quarters of patients with liver involvement experience involuntary weight loss.[62] Palpable hepatomegaly is present in 18% to 25% of patients with AL, but a dominant hepatic syndrome was seen in only 5% to 17%, although SAP scans show that hepatic amyloid is present in virtually all patients with AL.[63] Hepatomegaly is not synonymous with hepatic involvement because right-sided heart failure may produce congestive hepatomegaly. A symptomatic hepatic amyloid syndrome is defined as an increased serum alkaline phosphatase or γ-glutamyltransferase level and unexplained hepatomegaly. On physical examination of patients with a confirmed diagnosis of hepatic AL, the median measurement of the liver edge extending below the right costal margin was 7 cm. Hepatomegaly was not present in one-tenth of patients with biopsy-proven liver AL involvement. In patients with hepatic AL, splenomegaly is present in 11%. It is common to see ascites in patients with hepatic AL, but most of these patients also have nephrotic-range proteinuria, hypoalbuminemia, or congestive heart failure, all of which can contribute to ascites.[62]

At diagnosis, the median increase of the serum alkaline phosphatase level was 2.3 times the maximum normal value among patients with liver involvement. The serum alkaline phosphatase value was the most important screen for determining whether a patient had clinically significant hepatic involvement. Hyperbilirubinemia, when present, is usually a preterminal finding. The finding of Howell-Jolly bodies is highly specific for splenic involvement, but their absence does not exclude it.

Portal hypertension with varices and bleeding is rare. Presumably, patients succumb to hepatic or extrahepatic complications of AL before portal hypertension develops.[64] Homogeneous patterns are seen on radionuclide imaging, CT, and MRI. Scintigraphy generally is not useful for establishing the diagnosis of hepatic AL. The findings are nonspecific and include irregular distribution of the radionuclide and, occasionally, splenic uptake is absent.[65] Sinusoidal amyloid deposits may compress branches of the hepatic artery, which results in the angiographic appearance of luminal irregularity and abrupt changes in vascular caliber. CT is good for seeing hepatic rupture or subcapsular hematoma. Scanning of the spleen also does not correlate well with the presence of Howell-Jolly bodies observed on a peripheral blood smear. Splenic rupture is a recognized complication in patients with hepatic amyloid.[66] Fibroelastography is being explored as a tool to diagnose hepatic amyloidosis based on increased liver stiffness as well as a potential monitoring tool for response or progression over time.[67]

Amyloidosis is not a contraindication for liver biopsy. Although spontaneous hepatic rupture has been described, rupture after a percutaneous liver biopsy has not been reported. The risk of complications after liver biopsy ranges from 0.31% to 3%. In our experience, 4% of patients with amyloidosis had bleeding after liver biopsy, and none died of the bleeding. Despite the relative safety of liver biopsy, liver biopsy usually is not required if the diagnosis is suspected and alternate biopsy sites, like fat and/or bone marrow, are tested. Amyloid deposits are found in liver biopsy specimens distributed in the portal tract and perisinusoidally.[68] At autopsy, involvement of the portal triad vasculature frequently is seen, but the effect of amyloid deposits in the vasculature is not clinically significant.

Eighty-nine percent of patients with hepatic involvement have renal amyloid, half excreting greater than 1 g protein per day and a third excreting more than 3 g of protein per day.[62] Patients with hepatic AL also have higher levels of C-reactive protein than those without hepatic involvement.[69] In one series, predictors of a poor prognosis were heart failure, elevated bilirubin levels, and thrombocytosis.[62]

In summary, key clues that may be helpful in establishing the diagnosis of hepatic amyloidosis: (1) hepatomegaly out of proportion to the degree of liver function abnormality; (2) increase of the alkaline phosphatase value with minimal increase in transaminase values; (3) presence of Howell-Jolly bodies in a peripheral blood film (suggestive of reduced splenic function, a consequence of splenic replacement with amyloid deposits); (4) monoclonal protein (detectable by immunofixation) in the serum or urine or abnormal serum FLCs; and (5) proteinuria.

Gastrointestinal Tract

Symptomatic gastrointestinal tract amyloidosis occurred in 7.1% of patients with AL, and they presented with intestinal bleeding, pseudo-obstruction, or diarrhea. No correlation exists between the presence of gastrointestinal tract amyloid deposits and liver amyloid deposits. Only 15% of our patients with gastrointestinal tract amyloidosis had hepatomegaly and less than one-third had increased alkaline phosphatase values.[70] When routine screening biopsies are performed on the rectum or intestinal tract, amyloid deposits are found in most patients with AL.[71] Generally, deposits are vascular, but occasionally, they are in the submucosa of the bowel; amyloid deposits in the gastrointestinal tract can produce symptoms (e.g., steatorrhea, nausea, vomiting, abdominal pain, hematemesis, and hematochezia), but only for a minority of patients. Bowel dysfunction in AL may result from direct infiltration of the bowel lining or from a motility disturbance attributable to damaged regulatory nerves of the intestinal tract.[72] The high prevalence of anorexia and weight loss does not correlate with the presence of gastrointestinal tract amyloid deposits. Typically, patients had a median delay of 7 months between the onset of gastrointestinal symptoms and the histologic recognition of AL, although one patient had a delay of 4 years. Four of our 19 patients with gastrointestinal tract AL underwent laparotomy for evaluation of intestinal symptoms. For three of these four patients, diagnosis was delayed because the surgical specimens were not stained with Congo red.

Steatorrhea was seen in less than 5% of patients with gastrointestinal tract amyloidosis. These patients were not distinguishable clinically from those with celiac sprue, Whipple disease, or bacterial overgrowth. Small-bowel biopsy findings showed amyloid deposits for 19 of our patients with AL.[70] This number constitutes only 1% of the AL population at our institution, and it does not include patients who had clinical evidence of malabsorption, for whom a small-bowel biopsy was not performed (widespread amyloidosis was evident in other organs). Diarrhea, anorexia, dizziness, and abdominal pain were the most common symptoms. All patients had weight loss (median loss, 30 lb). Half the patients had orthostatic hypotension. A prolongation of prothrombin time, primarily from malabsorption of vitamin K, was present in one-fourth of patients. Factor X deficiency also was seen in one-fourth, but only one patient had factor X activity below 30%. A multivariate analysis showed that the degree of weight loss and the hemoglobin value at diagnosis affected survival. For patients presenting with a weight loss of 20 lb or more, the median survival was 10 months. Ten patients died due to nutritional failure, and five died of heart failure. Severe diarrhea may be due to neuropathy, which is rapid gastrointestinal tract transit.[73]

Esophageal dysmotility and gastroesophageal reflux may also occur. Multiple reports describe patients who had surgical intervention for bowel obstruction, only to have amyloid deposits identified histologically.[74] The most frequent symptoms of pseudo-obstruction are nausea (even during fasting) and emesis. Abdominal distention and pain are common.[75] For patients with pseudo-obstruction, extensive replacement of the muscularis propria by amyloid is prominent.[76] Dilatation of small-bowel loops is rare. The typical radiographic findings of a patient with intestinal amyloid deposits include increased fluid accumulation in the small bowel, loop dilatation with delayed transit, and thickening or nodularity. Computed tomography may show mild splenomegaly or lymphadenopathy, but it generally does not help establish the diagnosis. Esophagitis, duodenitis, and gastritis are commonly found during endoscopic procedures.[77] It is rare for these changes to cause symptomatic bleeding outside of the setting of high-dose chemotherapy with autologous stem cell transplantation (ASCT).

Vascular obstruction from AL has been reported to cause duodenal perforation. Ischemic colitis rarely is the presenting feature of AL.[78] The amyloid deposits obstruct vessels of the muscularis mucosa and lamina propria. The obstructed blood supply leads to mucosal ischemia, sloughing of the bowel lining, and hemorrhage. Barium studies show luminal narrowing, mucosal fold thickening, and ulcers. The most common location of ischemia is the rectosigmoid and descending colon.[79] Finding deposits of amyloid on endoscopic or colonoscopy biopsies of polyps or the margins of ulcers may reflect a localized form of amyloidosis with no risk of becoming systemic. Seeing a patient with a positive bowel biopsy for amyloid and normal light chain levels should raise the possibility that the amyloidosis is localized not requiring therapy.[80]

Nervous System

In 1938, the first description of peripheral nerve amyloidosis was published.[81] Among patients with AL, 15% to 20% have paresthesias and neuropathy symptoms.[82] Paresthesias, pain, numbness, muscle weakness, impotence, urinary retention, and orthostatic symptomatology are the most frequent symptoms of amyloid neuropathy.[83] Twelve percent of the patients had syncope. Dysesthesia that manifests as distal burning is present in one-fourth of the patients. Lower-extremity involvement precedes upper-extremity involvement for nearly 90%. Of those with peripheral neuropathy, autonomic neuropathy is seen in two-thirds. Involvement of the cranial nerves in AL is rare.[84] Half the patients with amyloid peripheral neuropathy also have carpal tunnel syndrome, a soft-tissue manifestation of amyloidosis. Weight loss was recognized in one-third of patients.

The clinical picture is often dominated by cardiac or renal involvement, and the peripheral neuropathy is minimally symptomatic. Echocardiographic abnormalities are found in 44% of patients who present with AL neuropathy. When a predominant neuropathy is seen in a patient with biopsy-proven amyloidosis, the possibility of hereditary amyloidosis should be considered.

An important diagnostic clue for amyloid neuropathy is its association with autonomic neuropathy.[85] Voiding difficulties are often due to detrusor weakness and impaired bladder sensation. The underlying mechanism of urinary dysfunction seems to involve postganglionic, cholinergic, and afferent somatic nerves. However, when patients present with peripheral neuropathy, amyloidosis usually is not considered in the differential diagnosis. The median delay between onset of paresthesias and biopsy proof of amyloidosis is 29 months.[86]

Amyloidosis typically causes loss of small myelinated and unmyelinated fibers. Electromyography does not easily detect changes in small unmyelinated fibers. Consequently, patients may have symptoms of amyloid neuropathy and have normal electromyographic findings. As it progresses, the neuropathy of amyloidosis is more axonal than demyelinating. The loss of myelin results in an elevation of cerebrospinal fluid protein value in one-third of patients. Axonal degeneration is detected in 96% of patients with amyloid myopathy. Typical electromyographic changes consist of reduced amplitude of compound muscle action potentials, decreased or absent sensory responses, mild slowing of nerve conduction velocity and fibrillation potentials on needle examination.

Although sural nerve biopsy is the standard method of diagnosing amyloid neuropathy, less invasive fat or bone marrow biopsies may also confirm the diagnosis. With sural nerve biopsy, amyloid deposits are found in the endoneurial capillaries or in the epineurium.[87] Teased fibers show axonal degeneration and a marked decrease in myelin fiber density. A sural nerve biopsy is not 100% sensitive. Nine patients were reported to have amyloid neuropathy, but six had negative sural nerve biopsy findings, despite being diagnosed subsequently with amyloidosis. Amyloid proteins may have been deposited at the nerve root, which resulted in distal demyelination without recognizable deposits in the sural nerve. Amyloid is deposited focally in the nerve, and multiple sections of the sural nerve need to be examined to confirm the diagnosis. Other methods to detect nerve involvement, especially small fiber nerve involvement include quantitative sensory testing and epidermal nerve fiber density. Testing for autonomic nerve involvement in the appropriate clinical setting should include testing for sweating, cardiovagal, and adrenergic function as well as gastric motility and bladder emptying.

All patients who present with a peripheral neuropathy should be screened with immunofixation assays of serum and urine and with immunoglobulin free light chain measurements. A patient with peripheral neuropathy and monoclonal light chains has a restricted differential diagnosis that includes (1) amyloidosis; (2) cryoglobulinemia; (3) polyneuropathy, organomegaly, endocrinopathy, M protein, and skin change syndrome (POEMS syndrome, osteosclerotic myeloma); and (4) neuropathy associated with monoclonal gammopathy (typically IgM isotype).

Respiratory Tract

Pulmonary deposition of amyloid is uncommon. Most patients who present with amyloidosis involving the respiratory tract have only localized tracheobronchial or nodular pulmonary amyloid deposits (see section "Localized Amyloidosis"). However, patients who present with systemic AL may have diffuse, interstitial pulmonary involvement and concomitant cardiac involvement that usually overshadow any respiratory symptoms.[88] Patients whose AL is associated with an IgM monoclonal protein or Waldenström macroglobulinemia have a higher prevalence of pulmonary amyloid deposits. Gas exchange is preserved until amyloid deposition in the alveolar interstitial space is advanced. Symptoms and involvement do not always align. In an autopsy study of pulmonary amyloidosis, histologic specimens from 11 of 12 patients had deposits in the lung (blood vessel walls and the alveolar septum), but only 4 of the 12 had clinical dyspnea. Diffuse alveolar septal amyloid deposits rarely cause hemoptysis. Radiographic findings are a nonspecific interstitial or reticulonodular pattern.[89] The diagnosis is easily obtained by a transbronchial lung biopsy, which is not associated with excessive bleeding. Rarely, pleural deposits of amyloid cause pleural effusions.[90] Occlusive amyloid deposits in the pulmonary circulation system may occasionally cause pulmonary hypertension with resultant right-sided cardiac failure.[91]

Thus, patients with unexplained dyspnea or fluid overload who have normal left ventricular diastolic and systolic function should be evaluated for pulmonary hypertension attributable to AL.

Coagulation System

Amyloidosis increases the fragility of blood vessels because of infiltration of the vessel wall,[92] and complications may include clinically significant hemorrhage or thrombosis. The most common manifestation of hemorrhage is eyelid purpura. Prolonged thrombin time is a frequently observed abnormality of amyloidosis,[93] and it is attributed to the presence of an inhibitor of fibrin polymerization in the plasma or the effects of prolonged nephrotic-range proteinuria with urinary loss of coagulation factors. Acquired hemostatic abnormalities include coagulation factor deficiencies, hyperfibrinolysis, and platelet dysfunction.

Acquired factor X deficiency is an uncommon, but well-documented, complication of AL[94,95]; nevertheless, bleeding is unlikely if factor X levels are higher than 25%. Fewer than 5% of patients have a serious deficiency of factor X with plasma levels less than 10% of the reference level for factor X, and patients with cardiac and renal involvement in the absence of hepatic involvement do not show clinically significant reductions in factor X levels. However, clinically significant bleeding complications may occur, especially for patients with ischemic colitis attributable to vascular occlusions. For one patient, factor X deficiency was treated with recombinant human factor VIIa during preparation for surgical splenectomy.[96] A factor X concentrate, a plasma-derived product, has been developed for inherited factor X deficiency. Its role in the acquired factor X deficiency of amyloidosis has not been defined. Bleeding disorders resulting from low levels of α_2 plasmin inhibitors, increased levels of plasminogen activators, and abnormal platelet aggregation also have been reported. Life-threatening bleeding from acquired factor V deficiency has been reported.[97]

Black et al described patients with amyloidosis who had documented episodes of thromboembolism. Similarly, Halligan et al[98] described patients with documented thromboembolism. Of 2132 patients, those with myocardial infarction, peripheral vascular disease, and stroke were excluded, and records of 40 patients (median age, 65 years) with documented thromboembolism were examined. In 11 of the 40 patients, thromboembolism preceded the diagnosis of amyloidosis, and for 9 of these 11 patients, the thromboembolic event occurred 1 month or more before the diagnosis of amyloidosis was established. In 20 of the 40 patients, the thromboembolism occurred 1 month or more after the diagnosis of AL was established. The thrombosis was venous for 29 patients and arterial in 11. Of the 40 patients, 37 had additional risk factors for thrombosis, the most common of which was nephrotic syndrome in 20 patients. Five patients had activated protein C resistance.

PROGNOSTIC FEATURES

Survival for patients with AL has been improving over time (*Figure 101.10*), but early death rates remain high.[12] The 4-year overall survival (OS) after AL diagnosis has improved over time: 1977 through 1986, 21%; 1987 through 1996, 24%; 1997 through 2006, 33%[99]; 2005 through 2009, 42%; and 2010 through 2014, 54% ($P < .001$).[12] At another institution, the median survival was 18 months in patients diagnosed before 2005 and was 5 years in patients diagnosed 2010 to 2019.

Congestive heart failure (caused by progressive cardiomyopathy) and sudden death (caused by pulseless electrical activity, asystole or ventricular tachycardia/fibrillation) are the most common causes of death for patients with AL. The two most important determinants of clinical outcome are the extent of cardiac involvement and depth of hematologic response to chemotherapy.[100-102] Twenty-two percent of patients with AL diagnosed between 2000 and 2008 survived for 10 or more years after diagnosis.[103] The most prognostic baseline tests

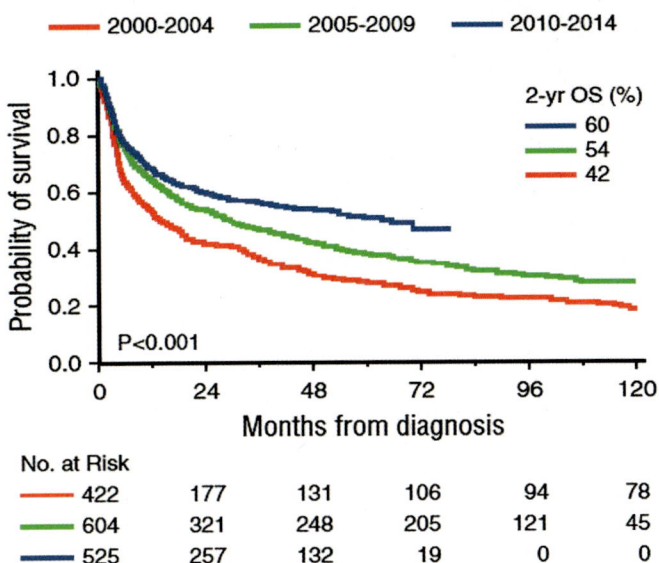

FIGURE 101.10 Improving overall survival over three time periods. (Reprinted from Muchtar E, Gertz MA, Kumar SK, et al. Improved outcomes for newly diagnosed AL amyloidosis between 2000 and 2014: cracking the glass ceiling of early death. *Blood*. 2017;129(15):2111-2119. Copyright © 2017 American Society of Hematology. With permission.)

include cardiac troponin, N-terminal probrain natriuretic peptide (NT-proBNP) or brain natriuretic peptide (BNP), dFLC, and resting systolic blood pressure.[100]

In 2004, a staging system that included serum cardiac troponin levels and NT-proBNP levels was developed at the Mayo Clinic for patients with AL. Depending on whether troponin and NT-proBNP levels were both low, both high, or high for only one component, three stages were defined with approximately a 2-fold risk of death for each increasing stage (*Figure 101.11*).[45,104] This system was later modified by the Europeans, where stage III was further subdivided based on whether NT-proBNP was ultrahigh cutoff (greater 8500 pg/mL) to stage IIIA and IIIB. A four-stage system adding dFLC to cardiac biomarkers was published by Mayo authors in 2012 and widely adopted[105]; for stages I, II, III, and IV, median survival rates were not reached, 96.5, 58.2, and 22.2 months, respectively.[105] The addition of the dFLC into the staging system was based on the observation that patients with higher baseline levels of free light chains had an increased risk of death (hazard ratio, 2.6).[106] These staging systems have withstood the test of time differentiating the healthiest patients from the sickest patients even among more contemporary patients who have access to even better therapies. These systems are widely used as stratification factors in clinical trials. Ultrahigh NT-proBNP is not part of the Mayo 2012 staging system. The exclusion of patients with ultrahigh NT-proBNP from most clinical trials skews the anticipated results (*Figure 101.12*) since nearly half of stage IV patients have ultrahigh values.[107] Stage IV patients' expected OS at 1 year was 18% vs 57% depending on whether or not the NT-proBNP was greater than 8500 pg/mL.

There are other important prognostic markers in AL including exertional syncope,[39,40] overt congestive heart failure, echocardiographic features[36,108,109] including interventricular wall thickness (>15 mm), right ventricular dilatation and wall thickness, restrictive filling (deceleration time < 150 ms), time to tertiary center,[110] year of diagnosis,[12,99] hyposplenic peripheral blood film,[111] elevated serum creatinine level, bone marrow plasmacytosis greater than 20%, chromosomal abnormalities, circulating plasma cells in the peripheral blood, elevated bone marrow plasma cell labeling index, increased β_2-microglobulin levels,[112] and the numbers of viscera clinically involved by AL.

If patients have over 10% plasma cells even in the absence of myeloma symptoms, their survival is comparable with patients with amyloidosis with overt myeloma and inferior to patients with AL with <10% marrow plasma cells.[9] When outcomes were reported in 1574 patients with AL with 20% or greater plasma cells poorer outcomes were seen independent of cardiac risk; median survival was only 12 months compared with 81 months with <5% plasma cells.[10] Translocation t(11;14), which is present in nearly half of all patients with AL, is associated with an adverse impact on progression-free

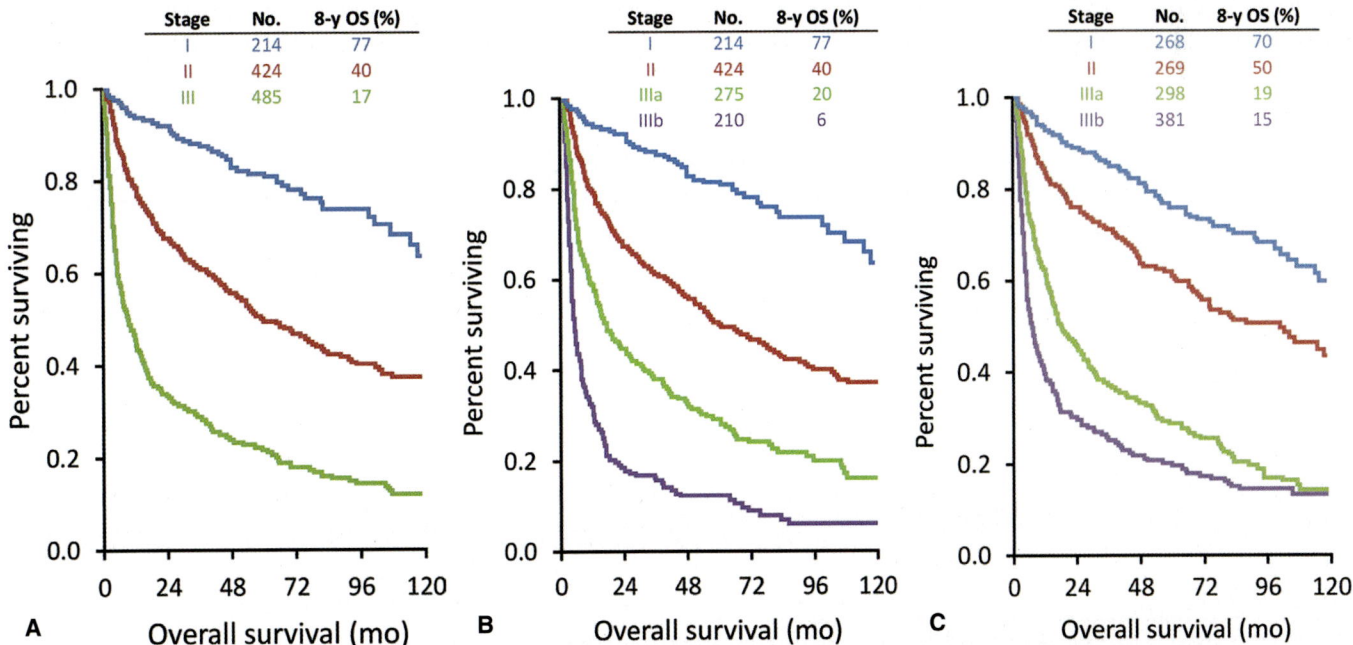

FIGURE 101.11 Overall survival of patients with AL seen at the Mayo Clinic 2000 to 2014 according to three staging systems. A, According to Mayo 2004 staging system: stage I, both troponin T < 0.035 μg/L and NT-proBNP < 332 ng/L; stage II, one value equal to or above threshold; stage III, both values equal to or above thresholds. B, According to European modification of Mayo 2004 staging system: as above for stages I and II, but stage III divided by NT-proBNP greater than or equal to 8500 ng/L; C, According to Mayo 2012 staging system: stage I, troponin T < 0.025 μg/L, NT-proBNP < 1800 ng/L, and dFLC < 180 mg/L; stage II, one marker above cut-point; stage III, two markers above cut-point; and stage IV, all three markers above cut-point. (Based on data from Muchtar E, Gertz MA, Kyle RA, et al. A modern primer on light chain amyloidosis in 592 patients with mass spectrometry-verified typing. *Mayo Clin Proc*. 2019;94(3):472-483.)

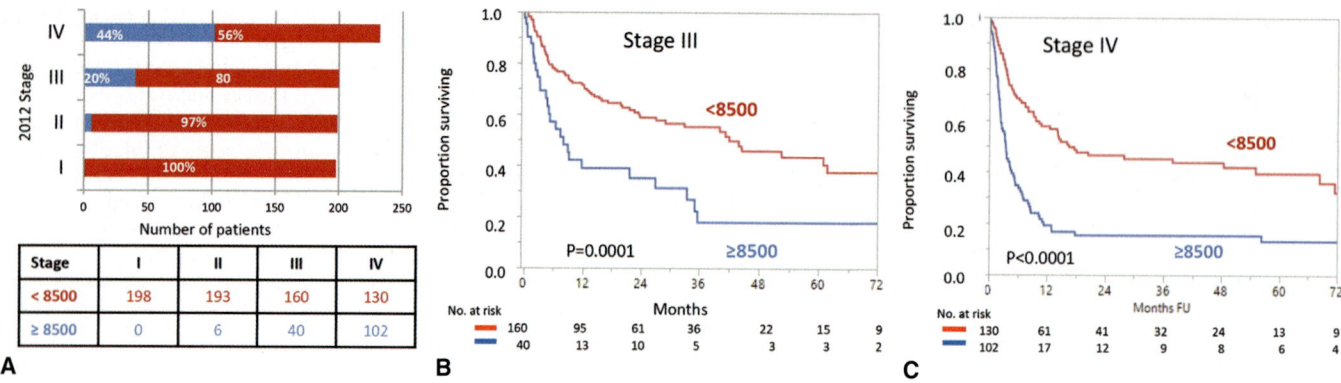

FIGURE 101.12 Interaction between biomarker stage and ultrahigh levels of NT-proBNP. A, Proportion of patients with ultrahigh NT-proBNP by Mayo 2012 stage; B, overall survival of the Mayo 2012 stage III parsed by ultrahigh NT-proBNP; C, overall survival of the Mayo 2012 stage III parsed by ultrahigh NT-proBNP. (Modified from Vaxman I, Kumar SK, Buadi F, et al. Outcomes among newly diagnosed AL amyloidosis patients with a very high NT-proBNP: implications for trial design. *Leukemia*. 2021;35(12):3604-3607. https://creativecommons.org/licenses/by/4.0/)

survival (PFS).[113,114] It appears that patients with t(11;14) do better with alkylator-based therapy than proteasome inhibitor–based therapy.[115] The presence of gain of chromosome 1q, which is present in 23% of patients, is an adverse prognostic factor among patients treated with melphalan and dexamethasone.[116] The presence of deletion 13/13q and trisomies, which are present in one-third and one-fourth of patients, respectively, have apparent prognostic impact.[114,116-118]

TREATMENT

Measuring Responses in Systemic AL Amyloidosis

Response measurement for patients with AL is divided into hematologic and organ responses (*Table 101.5*). Hematologic response involves measuring the monoclonal protein and free light chain component (the precursor protein) and applying criteria akin to those established for patients with multiple myeloma. Surrogate measurements typically are used to assess organ responses. Of note, even when patients show an organ response, follow-up tissue biopsy specimens show persistent deposits of amyloid. Because follow-up biopsies are performed infrequently, it is unclear whether clinical improvement is regularly associated with histologic regression. SAP scans suggest, however, that these deposits may be mobilized and that the total amyloid body burden is reduced. Although amyloid deposition in fat tissue has been reported to undergo substantial histologic regression only after normalization of the level of serum free light chain,[120] amyloid deposition in fat is not a standard measure.

As mentioned in the section "Prognostic Features," achieving a deep hematologic response is one of the most important prognostic factors in AL. Serum FLCs are typically measured every therapy cycle. The measure typically used is the dFLC, which is the difference of the involved minus the uninvolved FLC. Reducing the level of amyloidogenic FLC (iFLC) or the dFLC by more than 50% has been associated with substantial survival benefit, regardless of the type of chemotherapy used. The dFLC level used as a response criterion is a more useful measure than M protein response. When FLCs are not reduced after therapy, patients have a high risk of early death.[121] In a multinational study comparing outcomes based on hematologic response, at a 3-month landmark analysis the respective 3-year OS rates were approximately 90%, 80%, 50%, and 30% for patients who

Table 101.5. AL Response Criteria[17,119]

Response Type	Criteria
Hematologic	
Complete response (CR)	Negative serum and urine IFE and normal serum immunoglobulin κ/λ FLC ratio[a]
Very good partial response (VGPR)	dFLC < 40 mg/L[b]
Partial response (PR)	dFLC decrease of greater than or equal to 50%[c]
No response (NR)	Less than a partial response
Organ Response	
Cardiac response[d]	Decrease of NT-proBNP by >30% and 300 ng/L (if baseline NT-proBNP > 650 ng/L), or at least a 2 point decrease of NYHA class (if baseline NYHA class is III or IV)
Renal response	2005 criteria[119]: 50% increase in urinary protein loss (at least 1 g/24 h), or 25% worsening of creatinine or creatinine clearance 2014 criteria[58]: At least 30% decrease in proteinuria or drop below 0.5 g/24 h, in the absence of renal progression defined as a >25% decrease in eGFR[e]
Hepatic response	50% decrease in abnormal alkaline phosphatase value or decrease in radiographic liver size by at least 2 cm

dFLC, difference between involved and uninvolved serum immunoglobulin free light chain; a value adequate to measure response was deemed to be 50 mg/dL.
Reprinted from Dispenzieri A, Buadi F, Kumar SK, et al. Treatment of immunoglobulin light chain amyloidosis: mayo stratification of myeloma and risk-adapted Therapy (mSMART) consensus statement. *Mayo Clin Proc*. 2015;90(8):1054-1081. Copyright © 2015 Mayo Foundation for Medical Education and Research. With permission.
[a]Mandatory bone marrow removed from response criteria in 2012[17] as compared with 2005[119] response criteria.
[b]New response criterion in 2012.[17]
[c]Serum M-spike relegated to secondary status and used only if no measurable involved serum free light chain in 2012 criteria.
[d]Echocardiographic response replaced by NT-proBNP response in 2012.[17]
[e]New criteria proposed by European amyloid community, suggesting replacement of the 50% reduction of proteinuria used in 2005 criteria.[8]

achieved complete response (CR), very good partial response (VGPR), partial response (PR), and no response (see Table 101.5 for response criteria definitions).[17] For most patients the serum protein electrophoresis and immunofixation are not necessary testing each cycle unless the patient is a rare case in which the FLCs are normal and the patient has a measurable M protein by electrophoresis or a qualitatively positive immunofixation only. The immunofixation is still necessary to document a complete hematologic response.

Among 373 newly diagnosed patients assessed for response, we found that attainment of an iFLC less than 20 mg/L and dFLC of less than 10 mg/L were additive in survival discrimination. The serum FLC ratio did not add to these measures questioning its significance for response assessment.[122,123] Future directions in hematologic response may include the use of blood mass spectrometry. In one study, 12% of patients with AL were found to have residual disease by blood mass spectrometry that was missed by serum and urine immunofixation and serum FLC.[124]

According to current amyloid CR definitions, the bone marrow need not be done to document response. In the future, this criterion may be revised since patients with a negative bone marrow for clonal cells by multicolor flow cytometry have superior PFS than those who do not. In addition, bone marrow minimal residual disease (MRD) status is associated with higher organ response rates and better PFS, but no difference in OS has yet been observed.[125-127]

Organ response criteria have been defined. Cardiac response had been based largely on echocardiographic findings, but in 2012, consensus criteria for cardiac improvement changed to an improvement in NT-proBNP.[17] NT-proBNP values can be labile related to medications and or illness, and confirmatory measures may be necessary. A major advantage to NT-proBNP response over echocardiographic response is that the former occurs more quickly than the latter. The standard renal response was a 50% reduction in proteinuria, based on the criteria defined at the Tenth International Symposium on Amyloid and Amyloidosis.[119] In 2014, it was proposed that a 30% reduction in the amount of protein excreted in the urine within 24 hours, with no increase in serum creatinine levels and no decrease in serum albumin concentration be the revised renal amyloid response criteria. The purpose of relaxing the criteria for response is to document organ response in a timely fashion. A 50% reduction in serum alkaline phosphatase with no increase in transaminase or bilirubin levels is considered an organ response for hepatic AL. Reduction in liver size is less common. There are no consensus criteria for nerve, lung, gastrointestinal, or soft tissue amyloidosis. Trials use the neuroimpairment (NIS-LL) score to assess neuropathy between treatment groups. Currently organ responses are binary: response yes or no. Recently there is an initiative to qualify organ responses by depth clustering organ response into complete, very good partial, partial, and no response. It appears that deeper responses have improved survival and relapse rates are lower when responses are deeper.[128]

An advantage to hematologic response is that one can judge response (or progression) on a month-to-month basis; in contrast organ responses can be quite delayed.[102,106] In a retrospective analysis of 313 patients who achieved normalization of their serum FLC ratios, approximately two-thirds of patients had achieved an organ response by 6 months of normalization of the FLC ratio, but by 12 months, an additional 10% to 15% of patients had documented organ response.[129]

Nontransplant Systemic Therapies for Systemic AL Amyloidosis

To date, therapies for AL have been directed toward killing the underlying plasma cell clone, which in turn reduces the precursor protein (immunoglobulin FLC) and hopefully leads to regression of AL in tissues.[100] Successful cytotoxic chemotherapy to induce regression of AL was reported in 1972.[23] The backbone of therapy for nearly 5 decades had been steroids and alkylator, initially low-dose intermittent and later, for selected patients, high-dose alkylator with ASCT. The subsequent conversion from melphalan and prednisone (MP) to melphalan and dexamethasone (MDex) was transformative in terms of response rates and OS. Until recently the best non-ASCT outcomes were achieved with the combination of an alkylator, bortezomib, and dexamethasone. Most recently, the CD38 antibody, daratumumab, in combination with bortezomib, cyclophosphamide, and dexamethasone has become the new standard for the treatment of previously untreated AL.[130] The authors decision pathway to treat patients with AL is shown in Figure 101.13 and Table 101.6.

Alkylator-Based Therapy

The earliest reports of MP therapy showed responses and prolongation of survival for a minority of patients.[131-135] Patients with renal, cardiac, or liver AL appeared to benefit, but elevated β_2-microglobulin levels and cardiac involvement were predictors of failure of response. Although therapy with MP had been shown repeatedly to benefit a subgroup of patients with AL, most patients did not respond. Even with subset analysis, no cohort had a response rate that exceeded 40%, including patients with single-organ renal involvement and normal serum creatinine values (Table 101.7).

Two prospective, randomized noncrossover studies were performed to evaluate MP therapy for patients with AL. In one study, 220 patients were enrolled. Patients were stratified by age, sex, and clinical manifestation.[132] Half of the patients had nephrotic-range proteinuria, and 20% had heart failure. The median survival was significantly longer in the groups treated with MP (17 months) than in patients treated with single agent colchicine group (8.5 months). The second study randomly assigned 100 patients to receive colchicine therapy or a combination of MP and colchicine.[133] The OS of the patient group was 6.7 months in the colchicine-only group and 12.2 months in the melphalan group. With multivariate analysis, melphalan had a significant impact on survival when heart failure was not present.

Despite the relatively low response rates with alkylator-based therapy, long-term survival was possible for patients with AL. One report described 841 patients with AL who were studied over a 21-year period.[153] The actuarial survival rate for the patients at 1, 5, and 10 years was 51%, 16%, and 4.7%, respectively. The thirty 10-year survivors had received treatment with melphalan and prednisone; 14 had a documented hematologic response with eradication of M protein from the serum and urine. Ten patients had nephrotic-range proteinuria, and four had a reduction in urinary protein excretion of greater than 50%.

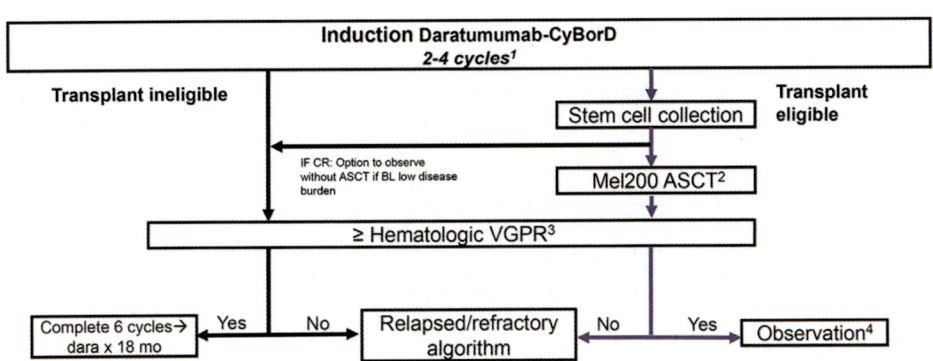

FIGURE 101.13 Initial treatment for newly diagnosed AL. [1]If daratumumab is not accessible, CyBorD is an acceptable alternative regimen (weekly bortezomib only). [2]For CrCl < 30, use Mel 140 mg/m². [3]Decision to change therapy if in VGPR but < CR is based on a number clinical factors. Re-refer to amyloid center of excellence. [4]For patients with overt multiple, use myeloma-type maintenance; consider for bone marrow plasma cells ≥ 20% and high-risk FISH (del 17p, t(4;14), t(14;16) and t(14;20)). (Based on Mayo Clinic mSMART treatment algorithm. http://msmart.org version October 2020.)

Based on hematologic response rates of 33% to 50% and organ responses in 12% to 35% of patients treated with dexamethasone plus or minus interferon,[136-139] Palladini and colleagues studied the combination of melphalan with dexamethasone (MDex) for the management of AL.[145,146] Patients were selected on the basis of ineligibility for stem cell transplantation. Of 46 patients, a hematologic response was seen in 31 (67%); of these, a hematologic CR was seen in 15 (33%). Improvement in organ dysfunction was observed in 22 patients (48%). A strong correlation was noted between hematologic response and organ response. Of the patients who achieved a hematologic CR, 87% had organ improvement. Among the patients who achieved a hematologic response, organ function improved in 56% of patients. The 15 who had no hematologic response also had no improvement in organ function. Advantages of this regimen included a 4% mortality rate on day 100 and resolution of cardiac failure for 6 of 32 patients. The median time to hematologic response was 4.5 months, and only 11% had adverse effects. Comparable response rates have been reported by some,[149,154] but not by others.[147,148,150,151] Response is dependent on how many patients have severe cardiac involvement; among patients with significant cardiac involvement, there is a race between hematologic response and early cardiac death.

Melphalan is potentially leukemogenic, especially with long-term use. Of 153 patients receiving melphalan, cytogenetic abnormalities were recognized in 10.[155] All cytogenetic changes were consistent with damage to hematopoietic stem cells. Morphologically, four patients had acute leukemia and five had myelodysplasia. The actuarial risk was 21% for myelodysplasia or acute leukemia developing 42 months after initiation of therapy. The median survival period was 8 months after receiving the diagnosis of leukemia or myelodysplasia. Of the 10 patients, 8 died of pancytopenia, 1 died of progressive renal amyloidosis, and 1 was alive at the time of publication.

Although not a classic alkylating agent, bendamustine has activity in previously treated AL. In a phase 2 trial of 31 patients treated with bendamustine 100 mg/m squared intravenously on 2 consecutive days every 4 weeks with 40 mg of dexamethasone weekly, 57% of patients achieved a PR or better. In addition, there were 11% CRs and 18% VGPR. The overall organ response rate was 29%. Adverse events included myelosuppression, fatigue, and nausea. The median PFS was 11.3 months.[152] Bendamustine may be particularly well suited for the 7% of patients with AL that is associated with an IgM immunoglobulin protein.[156]

The continuous infusion vincristine, doxorubicin, and dexamethasone regimen was borrowed from the treatment armamentarium of myeloma and was in many cases incorporated into induction regimens pre-ASCT.[102,140-144] As a stand-alone, however, response rates were seen in 42% to 50% of patients, overall.

Immune Modulatory Drug–Based Therapy

There are a few cautionary notes when using immune modulatory drugs (IMiDs) like thalidomide, lenalidomide, or pomalidomide in patients with AL. First, patients typically cannot tolerate the same doses that patients with myeloma can. Second, the NT-proBNP level increases not infrequently after the initiation of therapy.[157] Recognition of potential IMiD-induced toxicity including bradycardia, hypotension, and worsening congestive heart failure is important when these agents are used. High levels of NT-proBNP are predictive of an inability to tolerate IMiDs for amyloidosis, although there are patients whose NT-proBNP levels rise, without associated clinical stigmata (Table 101.8).

Table 101.6. mSMART Eligibility Criteria for Autologous Stem Cell Transplant for Patients With AL

"Physiologic" age ≤ 70 y
Performance score ≤ 2
Troponin T < 0.06 ng/mL (or high-sensitivity Troponin T < 75 ng/mL)
Systolic BP ≥ -90 mm Hg
Creatinine clearance ≥ 30 mL/min (unless on chronic dialysis)
NYHA class I/II

Modified from Dispenzieri A, Buadi F, Kumar SK, et al. Treatment of immunoglobulin light chain amyloidosis: mayo stratification of myeloma and risk-adapted therapy (mSMART) consensus statement. *Mayo Clin Proc.* 2015;90(8):1054-1081.

Table 101.7. Alkylator-Based Chemotherapy for AL

	N	No Prior Rx, %	OHR/CR, %	Organ Response, %	Median f/u, mo	Median Survival, m
MP[131-135]	~200[a]	Majority	28	20-30	NA	18-29
VBMCP[135]	49	100	29/NR	30	35	29
Melphalan IV[102]	20[b]		50	...		~50
Dex[136]	19	26	53/31	16	27	11
Dex[137]	25	100	40/12	12	18	13.8
Dex[138]	23	43	NR	35	33	24
Dex-IFN[139]	93	84	31/14	35	41	31
VAD[102,140-144]	32[b]	NR	42-50	...	NR	...
Mel-Dex[145,146]	46	100	67/33	48	60	61
Mel-Dex[147]	50	100	72/24	39	36	60
Mel-Dex[148]	140[b]	100	51/12	>20	60	20
Mel-Dex[149]	40[b]	100	58/13	NR	NR	10.5
Mel-IV-Dex[150]	61[b]	100	44/11	25	27	17.5
Mel-Dex[151]	70[b]	0	26/8	NR	17	66% at 2 y
Bendamustine[152]	31	0	57/11	29	14.9	18.2

Abbreviations: AL, light chain-associated amyloidosis; CR, complete response; Dex, dexamethasone; f/u, follow-up; IFN, interferon-alpha; IV, intravenous; Mel-Dex, melphalan and dexamethasone; MP, melphalan and prednisone; NA, not applicable; NR, not reported; OHR, overall hematologic response; Rx, treatment; VAD, vincristine, doxorubicin, and dexamethasone; VBMCP, vincristine, carmustine, melphalan, cyclophosphamide, prednisone.

Taken with permission from Dispenzieri A, Buadi F, Kumar SK, et al. Treatment of immunoglobulin light chain amyloidosis: mayo stratification of myeloma and risk-adapted therapy (mSMART) consensus statement. *Mayo Clin Proc.* 2015;90(8):1054-1081.
[a]Conglomeration of multiple trials.
[b]Case series/reports.

Table 101.8. Immune Modulatory Derivatives in Patients With AL

Regimen	N	No Prior Rx, %	OHR/CR, %	Organ Response, %	Median f/u, mo	OS
Thal 200-800 mg[158]	16	6	25/0	0	NR	NR
ThalDex[159]	31	0	48/0	26	32	NR
Thal 200-800[160]	12	58	0	11	2[a]	NR
Thal 50-200[161]	18	28	0	11	6[a]	NR
Cy-Thal-Dex[162]	65[c]	41	74/21	33	18	2-y 77%
MDex-thal[163]	22	86	36/5	18	28	1-y 20%
Len ±Dex[163]	22	43	43/5	26	17	2-y 50%
Len ± Dex[164]	69	6	47[c]/16	21	NR	NR[b]
Len ± Dex[165]	24	0	38/0	4	23	1-y 50%
Len-MDex[166]	26	100	58/23	50	19	2-y 81%
Len-MDex[167]	25	92	58/8	8	17	1-y 58%
Len-MDex[168]	16	69	43/7	6	34	2-y 70% PFS 24 mo
Len-Cy-Dex[169]	21	0	62/5	15	38	3-y 50% PFS 13 mo
Len-CyDex[170]	35	69	60/11	29	32	38 mo PFS 28 mo
Len-Cy- Dex[171]	37	65	55/8	22	29	2-y 41% PFS 10 mo
Len-Cy- Dex[172]	24	100	46/25	46	24	2-y 59% 2-y PFS 53%
Pom-Dex[173]	33	0	48/3	15	28	28 mo PFS 14 mo
Pom-Dex[174]	27	0	44/30	4	17	2-y 51 mo EFS 17 mo
Pom Dex[175]	153	0	44/28	H: 11; K: 20	32	29 mo
Len Bor-Dex[176]	34	100	89/82	H: 41; K: 22	12.5	1-y-87%

Abbreviations: AE, adverse events; Bor, bortezomib; Cy, cyclophosphamide; Dex, dexamethasone; f/u, follow-up; mo, months; H, heart; IFN, interferon; K, kidney; Len, lenalidomide; Pom, pomalidomide; Rx, treatment; Thal, thalidomide.

Taken with permission from Dispenzieri A, Buadi F, Kumar SK, et al. Treatment of immunoglobulin light chain amyloidosis: mayo stratification of myeloma and risk-adapted therapy (mSMART) consensus statement. *Mayo Clin Proc*. 2015;90(8):1054-1081.

[a]Median time on treatment.
[b]Case series, not a clinical trial.
[c]Partial response rate based on first 34 patients treated. No information on the additional 35.

Use of thalidomide has been explored in the treatment of AL as a single agent,[158,160,161] with dexamethasone,[159] and in combination with dexamethasone and alkylator.[162,163] As a single agent, there were no hematologic responses; with dexamethasone, the hematologic response rate was 48% with no CRs and an organ response rate of 26%. The median maximum tolerated dose was 300 mg, a dose that is never used in practice today. Patients with AL had poor tolerance of thalidomide. Exacerbation of peripheral neuropathy and pulmonary edema occurred frequently, and 50% of patients had grade 3 or 4 toxicity. Also seen were cognitive difficulty, edema, constipation, deep vein thrombosis, and syncope.[160] The median time receiving thalidomide therapy was only 72 days. In doses of up to 400 mg/d combined with dexamethasone treatment-related toxicity occurred for 65%. Thalidomide, dexamethasone, and cyclophosphamide have been reported to produce a hematologic response rate of 74%,[162] but with further study they were found to be relatively toxic. In another study, 22 newly diagnosed patients with cardiac involvement were treated with the combination of melphalan, thalidomide, and dexamethasone.[163] Despite a hematologic response rate of 36%, only 20% of patients were alive at 1 year, and toxicity was significant. Thalidomide is rarely used in our practice today, but when it is used, the dose will be from 50 to 100 mg daily with careful monitoring of patient's cardiac symptomatology and NT-proBNP levels.

Lenalidomide has also been studied as a single agent with on-demand dexamethasone[163-165] and in combination with alkylator and dexamethasone.[166-171] Hematologic response rates for single agent is only about 11%, but with dexamethasone, between 38% to 47% including CRs in 5% to 16% of patients. Lenalidomide was fairly well tolerated, but patients were prone to hypotension, worsening of heart failure,[157,177] and reduced renal function. PFS in patients achieving CR was 50 months.[178] The maximum tolerated dose of lenalidomide is 15 mg. If this agent is to be used, initiating a 10-mg dose and then increasing or decreasing based on symptoms is reasonable.

Lenalidomide also has been combined with MDex in the upfront setting in patients with a performance score of 0 to 1.[166] This three-drug oral combination produced hematologic responses in 58% and CRs in 42%, organ responses in 50%, and 2-year event-free survival and OS rates of 54% and 81%, respectively. Less selected patients did not fare as well in a subsequent study of predominantly previously untreated patients.[167] In another cohort of previously untreated and previously treated patients, hematologic response rate was 43% and organ response rate was 6% with a 2-year PFS of 70%.[168]

Similar studies using the combination of lenalidomide, cyclophosphamide, and dexamethasone have been conducted.[169-172] Overall hematologic response rates were about 60% with CRs in 5% to 11% of patients. Organ responses occurred in 15% to 29%, median PFS ranged from 13 to 28 months, and median OS was close to 3 years in most of the studies.

Lenalidomide bortezomib and dexamethasone (VRD) was given to 34 patients with newly diagnosed AL. The starting lenalidomide dose was 5 to 15 mg in 86% of patients. About 37.5% of patients required lenalidomide dose reduction, 27% discontinued lenalidomide, and 12% discontinued bortezomib. For patients with stage IIIb cardiac disease, 80% died by 6 months. When VRD was matched to 68 CyBorD-treated patients, there was a trend for deeper hematologic responses with VRD.[176]

Pomalidomide, a derivative of thalidomide with structural similarity to thalidomide and lenalidomide, was given to 33 evaluable patients in one study.[173] It was administered at a dose of 2 mg daily continuously along with dexamethasone 40 mg once weekly. All patients had received prior therapy including ASCT in 48%, other immune modulators in 21%, and proteasome inhibitors in 42%. On an intention to treat analysis, 48% had a confirmed hematologic response. Median duration of response was 19 months. Organ response was documented in 15% of patients. Median OS and PFS was 28 and 14 months, respectively. The authors retrospectively looked for "NT-proBNP progressions" according to the revised cardiac response criteria, although this response criterion was not part of the trial; of the 29 patients alive at 3 months from registration with NT-proBNP baseline and subsequent measures, 18 patients (62%) satisfied criteria for NT-proBNP progression. There was no difference between "NT-proBNP progressors" in terms of hematologic response rates, but there was a difference in OS. The three most common grade 3 to 5 adverse events regardless of attribution were hematologic (45%), cardiovascular (30%), and infections (27%). In another study, the pomalidomide and dexamethasone combination was studied in 27 previously treated patients with AL.[174] The MTD was 4 mg days 1 to 21 every 28 days with dexamethasone 20 mg weekly. With a median follow-up of 17 months, the median event-free survival was 18 months. A European retrospective of 153 previously treated patients with AL who received pomalidomide and dexamethasone reported 44% of patients achieving a hematologic response with a VGPR or better rate of 28%. OS for the entire cohort was 29 months, but those achieving at least a partial hematologic response enjoyed a median OS of 50 months.[175] Pomalidomide is probably the best tolerated of the immunomodulatory drugs. We would recommend a starting dose of 2 mg with plans to increase to 4 mg if clearly tolerated.

Proteasome Inhibitor–Based Therapy

Most of the data about bortezomib use in patients with AL had come not from clinical trials[179-183] but from case series (Table 101.9).[148,186,187,189-193] These data suggested high hematologic response rates, including CR rates as high as 33% as a single agent or when combined with dexamethasone[186,187] and 71% when combined with alkylator and dexamethasone.[148,189-193] The Heidelberg group demonstrated that patients with t(11;14), which is approximately 50% of patients with AL, have lower response rates and lower EFS and OS when treated with bortezomib than patients not harboring that abnormality.[115] This observation was subsequently confirmed in other retrospective studies. In contrast, t(11;14) did not appear to be a risk factor for patients treated with either standard-dose melphalan or high-dose melphalan as part of an ASCT. Risk-adapted bortezomib has been reported to produce a hematologic response in 67% with less toxicity and lower early mortality.[195]

Table 101.9. Proteasome Inhibitors in Patients With AL

Regimen	N	No Prior Rx, %	OHR/CR, %	Organ Response, %	Median f/u, mo	OS
Bor[179]	70	0	63 (33)[b]	24[c]	52	4-y 67%
BMDex[184] v. MDex	53 56	100	81/23 52/20	H: 38/K: 44 H: 28/K: 43	50	3-y 72% 3-y 48%
CyBorD[130]	193	100	77/18	22-44	11.4	1-y 85%
Ixa-Dex[185]	85	0	53/26	36	45	4-y 50%
Bor ± Dex[186]	94[a]	19	72/25	30	12	1-y 76%
Bor + Dex[187]	26[a]	69	54/31	12	15	Med 19 mo
Bor-MDex[182]	17	100	94/56	NR	11	NR
Bor-MDex[148] v. MDex	87[a,d] 87[a,d]	100	69/42 51/19	NR	26	3-y 58% 3-y 45%
Bor-MP[188]	19[a]	100	84/37	47	8	2-y 39%
Cy-Bor-Dex[189] v. Thal-Cy-Dex	69[a,d] 69[a,d]	100	71/40 80/25	NR	13 25	1-y 65% 1-y 67%
Cy-Bor-Dex[190]	17[a]	58	94/71	NR	21	21-mo 71%
Cy-Bor-Dex[191]	20[a]	100	90/65	46	14	2-y 98%
Cy-Bor-Dex[191]	23[a]	0	74/22			
Cy-Bor-Dex[192]	60[a,e]	100	68/17	32	12	1-y 57%
Cy-Bor-Dex[193]	230[a]	100	62/21	NR	NR	2-y 67%
Bor-Ritux Dex[181]	10[a]	60	78/0	0	13	1-y 90%
Ixa-Len-Dex[194]	40[a]	0	66/26	H: 6; K: 13	10	29

Abbreviations: AE, adverse events; BMDex, bortezomib, melphalan, and dexamethasone; bor, bortezomib; Cy, cyclophosphamide; CyBorD, cyclophosphamide, bortezomib, and dexamethasone; Dex, dexamethasone; f/u, follow-up; mo, months; H, heart; K, kidney; NR, not reported; Rx, treatment.

Taken with permission from Dispenzieri A, Buadi F, Kumar SK, et al. Treatment of immunoglobulin light chain amyloidosis: mayo stratification of myeloma and risk-adapted therapy (mSMART) consensus statement. Mayo Clin Proc. 2015;90(8):1054-1081.

[a]Case series, not a clinical trial.
[b]Excluding the phase 1 patients.
[c]The denominator (n = 62) for this calculation includes some of the 18 dose escalation patients since that group contained 5 of the 15 organ responses.
[d]Matched case control studies.
[e]Retrospective look at patients with stage III (Mayo 2004) disease.

A phase 1 dose-escalation study of bortezomib given either twice weekly on days 1, 4, 8, and 11 every 21 days or on days 1, 8, 15, and 22 every 35 days reported hematologic responses in 50% of patients.[179] The weekly regimen was associated with decreased neurotoxicity. Paradoxically, the once weekly group had at least as good or better outcomes than the twice weekly group, presumably due to better tolerability. Hematologic response (including CR) was documented in 67% (24%) and 69% (37%) for the twice weekly and once weekly schedules, respectively. There was a 1-year hematologic progression-free rate of 72% and 77% and a 4-year survival rate of 63% and 75%, respectively, for the twice-weekly and once-weekly dose groups. Among 70 patients, 29% had renal responses and 13% had cardiac responses. Bortezomib has been used as pre-ASCT induction[183,196] and post-ASCT consolidation,[197] but this will be discussed in the section on ASCT.

A multicenter randomized phase 3 trial comparing MDex, a prior standard of care, and BMDex in newly diagnosed AL was performed in Europe and Australia.[184] Patients with Mayo 2004 stage IIIb or significant peripheral neuropathy were ineligible. One hundred and nine patients were randomized to receive either MDex (melphalan at 0.22 mg/kg and dexamethasone at 40 mg daily for 4 consecutive days every 28 days) or BMDex (MDex plus bortezomib added at 1.3 mg/m^2, on days 1, 4, 8, and 11 in cycles 1 and 2, and on days 1, 8, 15, and 22 in the following cycles). Treatment was planned for 8 or 9 cycles, or achievement of CR or of at least PR plus organ response after cycle 6 and was discontinued in case PR was not achieved by cycle 3. The primary endpoint was overall hematologic response at 3 months. Respective hematologic PR or better rates (including CR) at 3 months were 52% (4%) and 79% (8%), $P = .002$, in the MDex and BMDex arms. At the end of treatment overall hematologic PR rates (including CR) were 57% (20%) and 81% (20%), respectively. No difference in organ responses were noted between the treatment arms. Cardiac response at 9 months was reached in 28% of evaluable patients treated with MDex and in 38% who received BMDex ($P = .195$). Renal response at 9 months was attained in 43% and 44% of evaluable patients, respectively. After a median follow-up of living patients of 50 months, there was a survival advantage for the BMDex arm over MDex arm (median not reached vs 34 months; $P = .02$). The proportion of patients experiencing grade 3 to 4 severe adverse events was significantly higher in the BMDex than in the MDex arm (occurring in 20% vs 10% of cycles performed, respectively). Most common grade 3 to 4 adverse events (MDex vs BMDex) were cytopenias (2%-5% vs 4%-10%), fluid retention (4% vs 10%), and neuropathy (1% vs 7%). The response rates seen with MDex in other series have been comparable.[148,182] A series of 17 patients treated with bortezomib, melphalan, and prednisone seemed to fare less well.[188]

Until the ANDROMEMA trial, all reports of the combination of CyBorD had been case series (see section on antibodies).[189-193] Although no direct comparisons are possible with BMDex, it appears that cyclophosphamide-containing regimens perform equally well. CyBorD has been used as pre-ASCT induction,[190,198] but this will be discussed in the section on ASCT.

Bortezomib, rituximab, and dexamethasone have been used in 10 patients with IgM-associated AL with monoclonal protein in a prospective clinical trial.[181] Overall hematologic response was seen in 78% of patients with no CRs.

In relapsed, refractory patients, ixazomib and dexamethasone produced a 53% hematologic response rate and a 26% CR rate, which was no higher than physicians' choice in a randomized phase 3 trial.[185] There was a trend toward higher CR rates with ixazomib dexamethasone than physicians' choice (26% vs 19%), and there was a superior time to vital organ deterioration or mortality (35 vs 26 months) with this proteasome inhibitor. Among patients who were proteasome inhibitor naïve, ixazomib and dexamethasone yielded response rates of 63% PR or better and 33% CR as compared with proteasome inhibitor-exposed patients who had PR of 41% and CR of 18%.

Ixazomib, lenalidomide, and dexamethasone in relapsed AL resulted in 41% VGPR or better. The median PFS was 17 months but was 28.8 months in those achieving a VGPR or better. This is an all oral treatment option for amyloidosis.[194]

Carfilzomib, a second-generation proteasome inhibitor, was administered to five patients with AL.[199] All had cardiac peripheral and autonomic neuropathy. All achieved at least a very good partial hematologic response with no worsening in cardiac function. Carfilzomib could be considered in patients with peripheral or autonomic neuropathy were bortezomib might be considered excessively toxic. Among patients with cardiac involvement, there is significant concern for cardiac toxicity based on data in patients with multiple myeloma.

Antibodies

Daratumumab is an anti-CD38 monoclonal antibody developed for the treatment of multiple myeloma. Daratumumab is exceptionally successful in the management of AL given its high efficacy and low toxicity profile. As such, its use in patients with newly diagnosed AL represents a major step forward in the management of this disease.

The design of the ANDROMEDA trial was an unblinded 1:1 randomization of 388 newly diagnosed patients to either CyBorD alone or with daratumumab.[130] The triplet was planned to be administered to all patients for 6 months. Patients on the daratumumab arm also received daratumumab from the time of therapy initiation for as long as 24 cycles of therapy. Patients were ineligible if they had an NT-proBNP of 8500 pg/mL or greater or an eGFR less than 20 mL/minute. The primary endpoint, which was hematologic CR rate, was met: 53% for the daratumumab-containing arm compared with 18% in the CyBorD only arm. Organ responses were significantly higher in the daratumumab arm: cardiac response rates of 42% vs 22%, respectively, and renal response rates of 54% vs 27%, respectively. These results prompted accelerated approval of the quadruplet as first-line therapy for newly diagnosed patients with AL.

In the relapsed setting, there have been two phase 2 studies and a plethora of case series (Table 101.10). Roussel et al treated 40 patients with relapsed or refractory AL with daratumumab for a planned duration of 24 weeks as part of a prospective phase 2 study.[200] Complete hematologic responses were seen in 15% of patients and VGPRs in

Table 101.10. Trials and Case Series of Daratumumab to Treat Immunoglobulin Light Chain Amyloidosis

Regimen	N	No Prior Rx, %	OHR/CR, %	Organ Response, %	Median f/u, mo	OS
Dara-VCD[130]	195	100	92/53	42-53	11	1-y 85%
Dara[200]	40	0	70/15	H: 29; K: 31	26	Not reached
Dara[201]	22	0	90/41	H: 50; K:67	20	Not reached
Dara-Dex[a,202]	106	0	64/8	H: 22; K: 24	21	26
Dara[a,203]	72[b]	0	77/40	H: 55; K: 52	27	2-y 87%
Dara-Bor-Dex[a,202]	62	0	66/28	H: 26; K: 24	17	Not reached

Abbreviations: bor, bortezomib; Dex, dexamethasone; f/u, follow-up; H, heart; K, kidney; mo, months; NR, not reported; Rx, treatment; VCD, bortezomib, cyclophosphamide, and dexamethasone.
[a]Case series, not a clinical trial.
[b]Only 52 had "measurable disease" with a dFLC greater than or equal to 2 mg/dL.

42%. The hematologic PFS was 25 months, and OS was not reached with a median follow-up of 26 months. Organ responses were observed in 31% and 29% of renal and cardiac patients, respectively.

In another phase 2 study, Sanchorawala et al treated 22 relapsed or refractory patients with daratumumab (and high-dose methylprednisolone as a premedication) for a planned duration of 24 months.[201] The hematologic CR rate was 41% with a VGPR rate of 45%. The hematologic PFS was 28 months, and OS was not reached at median follow-up of 20 months. The hematologic CR rate and organ response rates of this study are the highest seen and may relate to the fact that the median dFLC at on-study was only 81 mg/L.

In case series, VGPR or better occurred in approximately 70% of patients and CR in 8% to 40%, with the highest responses among those with the lowest clonal burden at institution of therapy. PFS/time to next therapy rates varied considerably ranging from 1 to 2 years.[202-205] Duration of therapy also varied considerably ranging from six cycles to indefinite. Nephrotic range albuminuria was deemed to be an adverse factor for hematologic event-free survival.[202] Response with combinations including bortezomib or lenalidomide or pomalidomide appear to be comparable with just daratumumab and dexamethasone, but these cases series are underpowered to detect a difference. Randomized trials will be required to better clarify the relative roles of combinations vs single agent among patients with relapsed refractory AL.

Trials of anti-SAP antibodies have been abandoned in AL. Birtamimab is an antibody to a cryptic epitope of the fibril, which has been reported to produce both renal and cardiac responses in patients following anti–plasma cell chemotherapy.[206] A trial of the antibody in treatment-naïve cardiac amyloidosis was abandoned for futility. A trial for stage IV (Mayo 2012) is planned. The fibril-reactive mAb 11-1F4, when labeled with iodine-124 was shown to bind AL amyloid in patients by using PET/CT imaging and is being studied. This antibody now called CAEL-101 has an established recommended dose,[207] and phase 3 trials are underway.

BCL2 Inhibitors

Venetoclax appears to be highly active in patients with AL who carry t(11;14). In a retrospective report of 43 patients from 14 centers, 32 harbored t(11;14).[208] Regimens and dosage varied. Fifty-eight percent received venetoclax plus or minus corticosteroid; 23% received venetoclax in combination with proteasome inhibitor plus or minus glucocorticoid. Other combinations were used in the remaining 19%. In the 30 evaluable patients harboring t(11;14), the hematologic response rate was 82% of whom 37% achieved VGPR and 41% achieved CR; their 24-month PFS and OS were approximately 80% and 100%, respectively.

Stem Cell Transplantation

Hematopoietic stem cell transplantation for AL is inherently different from that for other hematologic cancers. Patients with lymphoma, multiple myeloma, or leukemia typically have considerable bone marrow abnormalities that manifest as multiple cytopenias, but these patients generally have excellent cardiac, hepatic, and renal function and a performance status of 0 or 1. In contrast, patients with AL often have clinically significant visceral organ dysfunction, which puts them at a high risk for complications after high-dose chemotherapy.

Autologous Stem Cell Transplantation

Most reported experiences with myeloablative chemotherapy involve progenitor cell replacement with autologous peripheral blood stem cells. The blood stem cells are used because they are easy to collect and have relatively rapid engraftment kinetics. Clinicians at Boston University first reported five patients with AL receiving ASCT, and all showed a clinical response. When the cohort was expanded to 25 patients, a hematologic response was reported for 62% and an organ response for 65% of surviving patients.[209]

The role ASCT plays in the treatment of AL remains controversial, although the authors would advocate that it is an important therapeutic modality in selected patients. There is only one small prospective randomized controlled trial to address the role of ASCT in AL. One hundred patients were randomized to either low-dose oral MDex or ASCT.[147] In the ASCT arm, dose-modified melphalan was used based on the risk factors of the period, rather than the current cardiac biomarker staging systems. The trial demonstrated that there was no difference in hematologic response between the MDex and the ASCT arms (64% and 65%, respectively), and the landmark analysis performed to correct for the unexpectedly high treatment-related mortality from ASCT (24%) also showed no difference in OS (49 and 57 months, respectively). Among the 50 patients randomized to receive ASCT, only 37 received the planned ASCT, and 9 of those died within 100 days; in contrast, of the 50 patients randomized to MDex, 43 patients received 3 or more cycles of therapy.

As shown in *Table 101.11*, the results with ASCT are excellent, although patients are highly selected.[147,197,210-221] To demonstrate this bias, 1288 patients with AL seen at Mayo Clinic between 1983 and 1997 were retrospectively screened for eligibility for ASCT using the following criteria: symptomatic amyloidosis without multiple myeloma, an age less than 70 years, serum creatinine less than 2 mg/dL, direct bilirubin less than 2 mg/dL, an interventricular septal thickness no more than 15 mm, and an ejection fraction greater than 55%.[222] Only 229 patients (18%) would have been eligible for ASCT. The median survival of this ASCT-eligible, but conventionally treated, cohort was 42 months, and the 5- and 10-year survival rates were 36% and 15%. The expected median survival of the ASCT-ineligible patients during that period was 12 to 18 months. This study was followed by a case-control study that demonstrated superior OS among patients who received ASCT as compared with standard-dose chemotherapy.[101]

Currently, ASCT at the Mayo Clinic yields a 10-year survival of 43% and day 100 therapy-related mortality of 2% (*Figure 101.14*).[223] Registry data show reduced day 100 therapy-related mortality from 20% to 5% and improvement in 5-year survival from 55% to 77%.[221] In more modern series, hematologic responses occur in 50% to 92%, hematologic CR in 24% to 42%, and organ responses in 34% to 64% of patients. Organ response is a time-dependent variable, and organ responses may be delayed up to 36 months after ASCT. Fifty percent of patients who have received ASCT at our institution survived 10 years, and the 10-year survival rate for complete responders was approximate 80%.[223] Finally, there is a study demonstrating an improvement in the quality of life of patients who underwent stem cell transplantation.[224]

Given excellent long-term survival rates in patients undergoing ASCT,[219,220] it is our approach to carefully select patients using the criteria shown in *Table 101.6*.[100] The best outcomes are with patients with renal involvement, but patients with early cardiac or liver involvement also derive benefit as well. The two most important risk factors for death among patients undergoing ASCT are cardiac status and low systolic blood pressure (<90 mm Hg). In the modern era, a troponin T level of 0.06 μg/L (or high sensitivity troponin T higher than 75 ng/L) is a very powerful predictor of early death (*Figure 101.15*).[225] Other reported risk factors for death among patients with AL undergoing ASCT include[226,227]: weight gain of greater than 2% during stem cell mobilization, an absolute lymphocyte count at day 15 of less than 500 cells/μL, serum creatinine, NT-proBNP, left ventricular septal thickness, left ventricular ejection fraction, and transplant center experience. Data from the Center for International Blood and Marrow Transplant Research demonstrated that centers performing fewer than four ASCT for AL per year had inferior outcomes.[221]

A propensity score matching approach was applied to 136 patients with AL treated in the United Kingdom, 68 receiving bortezomib-based therapy and 68 receiving ASCT. The authors concluded that outcomes were not significantly different between the two groups, yet for every measure, there were trends favoring ASCT.[228] There were trends for better hematologic CR rates (41% vs 30%), cardiac response (70% vs 54%), and renal response (74% vs 24%) among patients treated with ASCT. With a median follow-up of 38 months for the ASCT group and 26 months for the bortezomib group, the OS curves were superimposable; however, there was a trend for better PFS among ASCT-treated patients (50 vs 42 months, $P = .058$), and time to next treatment was longer among patients who had at least a VGPR and received ASCT as

Table 101.11. Trials and Case Series of ASCT for Immunoglobulin Light Chain Amyloidosis[a]

Regimen	N	Mel Dose, Mg/m^2	TRM, %	OHR/CR, %	Median FU, mo	Overall Survival
Moreau[210]	21	140-200[b]	43	NR/14	14	4-y 57%
Goodman[211]	92	80-200[b]	23	37/20	NR	Med 5.3 y
Vesole[212]	107	>130[b]	27	32/16	NR	2-y 56%
Gertz[c,213]	28	200	14	NR/NR	30	3-y 62%
Jaccard[c,147]	50	140-200	24	52/24	36	2-y 48
Mollee[214]	20	140-200[b]	35	50/25	18	3-y 56%
Perz[c,215]	24	100-200	13	54/46	31	3-y 83%
Perfetti[216]	22	100-200	14	55/36	73	5-y 56%
Cohen[c,217]	42	100-200	4	60/20[d]	31	2-y 81%
Landau[c,197]	40	100-200	10	55/27[d]	45	3-y 82%
Kim[218]	24	100-200	0	92/42[e]	NR	2-y 90%
Cibeira[219]	421	100-200	11	NR/34	48	Med 6.3 y
Dispenzieri[220]	454	100-200[b]	9	80/40	60	5-y 66%
D'Souza[221]	1536[f]	140-200	5-20	61/33	61	5-y 55%-77%

Abbreviations: CR, complete hematologic response; FU, follow-up; med, median; Mel, melphalan; OHR, overall hematologic response; TRM, transplant-related mortality.
Reprinted from Dispenzieri A, Buadi F, Kumar SK, et al. treatment of immunoglobulin light chain amyloidosis: mayo stratification of myeloma and risk-adapted therapy (mSMART) consensus statement. *Mayo Clin Proc.* 2015;90(8):1054-1081. Copyright © 2015 Mayo Foundation for Medical Education and Research. With permission.
[a]All responses in table are ITT.
[b]Alternate regimens including Mel/TBI and/or BEAM some patients.
[c]Clinical trial.
[d]Response rates before consolidation. For Cohen study[217] post-dexamethasone ± thalidomide OHR and CR increased to 60 and 21; for Landau study[197] after bortezomib and dexamethasone consolidation, OR and CR increased to 79% and 58%.
[e]All but one received induction treatment.
[f]Registry data that may include patients from other series; the range of TRM and OS are period based, with the more recent period (2007-2012) having the lower TRM and higher OS and the oldest time period (1995-2000) having the higher TRM and lower OS.

compared with those who received bortezomib-based therapy without ASCT 66 vs 45 months (not significant). More patients required treatment in the bortezomib group at 24 and 48 months, $P = .004$.

Not all experts agree that patients should be so stringently selected for ASCT. There is the philosophy that sicker patients can undergo ASCT with attenuated doses of conditioning melphalan with reasonable levels of toxicity (*Table 101.12*).[197,217,219] The data are clear that attenuated doses of melphalan are associated with lower rates of TRM, but they are also associated with lower response rates and shorter PFS and OS.[219,229] An approach of consolidating patients with thalidomide, dexamethasone, or bortezomib post-ASCT has been employed by investigators at MSKCC in the context of small phase 2 trials in order to recoup response in patients treated with attenuated doses of melphalan conditioning. Rates of CR are increased, but it has yet to be shown whether this strategy is better than nonintensive chemotherapy strategies for these higher risk patients.[197,217] Tandem stem cell transplantations are feasible and have been performed infrequently in patients with amyloidosis, but the ultimate effect on outcome is unknown.[230,231]

In an early study that did not impose strict selection criteria and used dose-attenuated melphalan, 11% of patients who initiated stem cell collection did not undergo ASCT because of death or mobilization toxicities that precluded safe transplantation.[232] Gastrointestinal

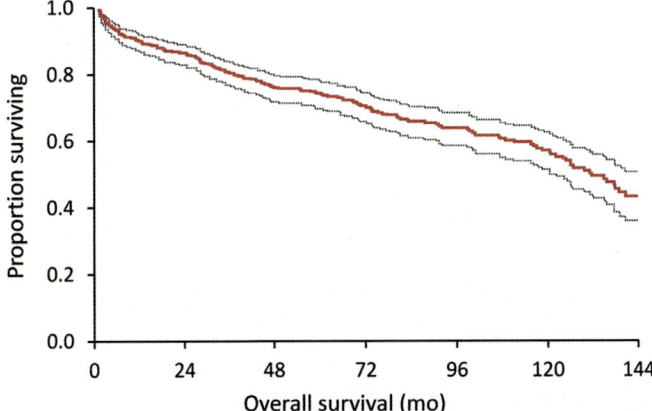

FIGURE 101.14 Overall survival of patients with AL who underwent autologous stem cell transplantation at Mayo Clinic as first-line therapy, years 1996 through 2016 (N = 672). The median survival time was 122 months. Hundred-day mortality rate reduced from 14.5% to 8.6% to 2.4% over the three time periods, 1996 to 2002, 2003 to 2009, and 2010 to 206, respectively.

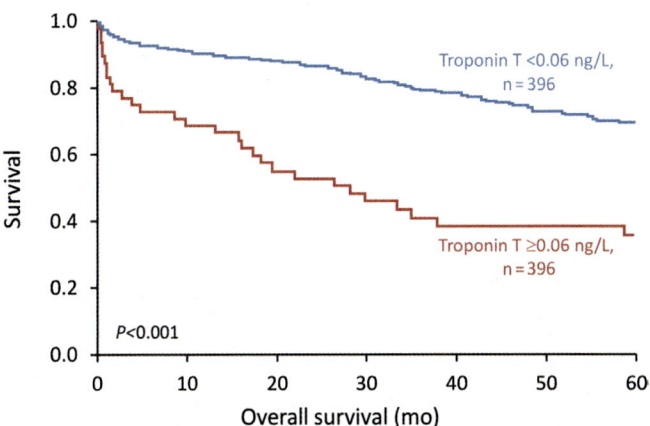

FIGURE 101.15 Effect of troponin T on transplant-related mortality. (Reprinted by permission from Nature: Gertz MA, Lacy MQ, Dispenzieri A, et al. Refinement in patient selection to reduce treatment-related mortality from autologous stem cell transplantation in amyloidosis. *Bone Marrow Transplantation.* 2013;48(4):557-561. Copyright © 2012 Springer Nature.)

Table 101.12. Toxic Responses Post Autologous Stem Cell Transplantation (Southwest Oncology Group Grade, ≥2)

Toxic Response	Frequency, % (n) 200 mg/m²	Frequency, % (n) 100 mg/m²
Nausea or vomiting	83 (19)	52 (14)
Diarrhea	65 (15)	48 (13)
Mucositis	91 (21)	37 (10)
Pulmonary edema	35 (8)	26 (7)
Peripheral edema	48 (11)	15 (4)
Non-GI tract bleeding	17 (4)	0 (0)
GI tract bleeding	22 (5)	7 (2)
Hepatic	13 (3)	22 (6)
Renal	35 (8)	19 (5)
Metabolic	35 (8)	7 (2)
Sepsis	26 (6)	11 (3)

Abbreviation: GI, gastrointestinal.

hemorrhage, progressive renal failure that required dialysis, and splenic rupture occurred in 7%, 5%, and 0.7% of patients. Rates of gastrointestinal tract bleeding appear to be much higher when total body irradiation was part of the conditioning regimen.[233] It is noteworthy that since the introduction of plerixafor on demand, mobilization failures are virtually nonexistent, and weight gain is less.[234]

Induction Before ASCT

There are limited data on the role of induction chemotherapy prior to ASCT.[183,196,215,235-238] Most of the reports of ASCT have been without application of induction therapy given the fact that AL tends to be a disease of low tumor burden. We and others have shown that patients undergoing ASCT who achieve CR without induction have exceedingly good outcomes, that is, 10-year OS of more than 70%.[239] With the recent introduction of daratumumab-CyBorD as the regimen of choice for AL, we recommend administration of induction therapy to all patients, and the decision to proceed to ASCT is based on several clinical factors including whether the patient attained or not CR to induction. Table 101.13 lists trials that incorporated induction prior to ASCT. One small phase 3 was positive,[183] another phase 3 was negative,[235] and the remaining are phase 2 reports.[196,215,236-238] Several case series also support the use of induction, especially bortezomib-containing induction regimens.[154,241]

Bortezomib-Based Induction Prior to ASCT

A phase 3 trial included 56 patients and compared bortezomib and dexamethasone for two cycles followed by ASCT vs direct ASCT.[183] The primary endpoint was achieved with 65% of bortezomib, dexamethasone, and ASCT patients and 36% of the ASCT only achieving a CR by 1 year. More importantly, however, the respective 2-year OS rates were 95% and 69% and the respective 2-year PFS rates were 81% and 51%. Two-year renal survival rates among the ASCT only group were surprisingly low at 62%. However, on multivariate analysis, only troponin-I, and not induction, was predictive of OS. There was only a trend toward benefit with bortezomib and dexamethasone induction, potentially due to small sample size.

In the HOVON 104 trial, 50 patients were designated to receive 4 cycles of bortezomib and dexamethasone prior to ASCT.[237] Thirty percent did not make it to ASCT due to death (n = 2), worsening functional status or bortezomib toxicity (n = 8), and patient refusal (n = 1). On an intention to treat basis, overall hematologic PR rate was 60% and CR was 32%; respective response rates were higher (86% and 46%) if only the patients who reached ASCT were included. Organ responses were observed in 72% of the cardiac patients, 61% of the renal patients, and 62% of the liver patients. With a median follow-up of 37 months, the 3-year PFS and OS were 63% and 86%.

Table 101.13. Induction and Consolidation Pre- and Post-ASCT Overall Outcomes

	N	No Prior Rx, %	OHR/CR, %	Median f/u, mo	Overall Survival
INDUCTION					
B-Dex × 2 + ASCT[183]	28	100	86/68 vs	NR	2-y 95% vs
vs ASCT[183]	28		48/36		2-y 69%
Oral MEL + ASCT[235]	48	100	NR/17	45	5-y 39%
vs ASCT	52		NR/21		5-y 51%
B-Dex × 4 + ASCT[237]	50	100	60/32	37	4-y 88%
B-Dex × 2 + ASCT[196]	35	97	77ª/57	36	5-y 84%
VAD[215]	28	89	43/39	31	3-y 71%
VAD[236]	69	90	46/13	115	5-y 54% 10-y 34%
INDUCTION and CONSOLIDATION					
B-dex × 2 + B-ASCT + B × 4[238]	21	100	86/48	53	5-y 100%
B-Dex ASCT – B-Dex[240]	19	100	95/37	61	2-y 68%
CONSOLIDATION					
Tandem ASCT[230]	53	85	NR/60	43	4-y 80%ᵇ
Tandem ASCT[231]	68	87	6/NR	47-51	Med 68 mo
ASCT → thal-dex[217]	42	100	72/36	31	2-y 81%
ASCT → B[197]	40	100	75/55	45	3-y 82%

Abbreviations: ASCT, autologous stem cell transplant; B, bortezomib; dex, dexamethasone; VAD, vincristine, doxorubicin, and dexamethasone.
Taken with permission from Dispenzieri A, Buadi F, Kumar SK, et al. Treatment of immunoglobulin light chain amyloidosis: Mayo stratification of myeloma and risk-adapted therapy (mSMART) consensus statement. Mayo Clin Proc. 2015;90(8):1054-1081.
ªVGPR or better.
ᵇThis figure also includes the 9 patients who never received any ASCT due to inadequate stem cell collection; all other figures are based on the 53 who received at least 1 ASCT.

In another phase 2 study of bortezomib induction prior to ASCT, 35 patients were treated with biweekly bortezomib and dexamethasone for two cycles.[196] Five patients who were transplant eligible at enrollment had clinical deterioration during induction necessitating withdrawal prior to ASCT. Those who underwent ASCT had bortezomib included as part of their conditioning regimen as well. By intention to treat CR and VGPR rates were 55% and 16%, respectively.

In a case series, ASCT-ineligible patients were treated with either bortezomib and dexamethasone (years 2006-2009, n = 14) or cyclophosphamide, bortezomib, and dexamethasone (after 2009, n = 14).[198] The rates of PR (including CR) were 93% (29%) and 93% (43%), respectively. Improved organ function and performance status permitted three and five patients to subsequently undergo ASCT. The median PFS for the bortezomib and dexamethasone and the CyBorD cohorts were 24 and 29 months, respectively, and the 3-year OS was 50% and 64%. In another retrospective review of 31 patients undergoing ASCT, 13 proceeded directly to ASCT after diagnosis and 12 received a bortezomib-containing regimen, while 6 received other induction regimens.[242] Overall hematologic response rates and organ response rates were 92% and 75% for the bortezomib-pretreated group and only 69% and 54% in the group that received no pretreatment.

Non-Bortezomib Induction Prior to ASCT

A phase 3 trial employing oral MP for 2 cycles prior to ASCT (experimental arm) did not show any benefit with 45-month follow-up.[235] Fewer patients in the experimental arm received ASCT.

A phase 2 trial by the HOVON group employed vincristine, doxorubicin, and dexamethasone (VAD) as induction followed by ASCT.[236] Of the 69 patients 55% had two or more organs involved, including 46% of patients with cardiac involvement. Twelve died during induction with VAD, and 46 proceeded to ASCT. Two patients died within 100 days of ASCT. On intent to treat, median OS from registration was 90 months, and if the analysis is limited to those patients who underwent ASCT, the median OS from ASCT was approximately 10 years.

Consolidation Post ASCT

There are even fewer trial data on consolidation therapy post ASCT. It, however, is not uncommon to start consolidation chemotherapy for those patients who have not achieved at least VGPR post ASCT.[243,244] Some would even recommend consolidation if less than a hematologic CR,[245] but this too is controversial. It is important to realize that approximately one-quarter of patents who achieve hematologic CR may not do that until 9 months after completion of therapy.[246]

In an open-label prospective trial Huang et al treated 21 patients with two standard 21-day cycles of bortezomib and dexamethasone induction, followed by ASCT using melphalan 140 mg/m² or 200 mg/m², depending on patient risk. Bortezomib was also used as part of the conditioning at a dose of 1 mg/m² on days −6, −3, +1, and +4, and then starting 60 to 90 days after ASCT additional bortezomib was used for an additional four 21-day cycle. The proportion of patients with Mayo 2004 stages I, II, and III were 52%, 24%, and 24%, respectively. Forty-eight percent achieved CR. At 3 years, the renal response rate was 67% and the cardiac response rate was 62%. The 5-year OS and PFS were 100% and 80%, respectively (see *Table 101.13*).

A prospective pilot analysis using bortezomib and dexamethasone before and after risk-adapted melphalan conditioning ASCT was performed in 19 patients.[240] There were three cycles of induction therapy and six cycles of posttransplant consolidation. The overall hematologic response rate was 95% including 37% MRD negativity. The 2-year PFS and OS were 68% and 84%, respectively.

Tandem ASCT has been used as consolidation in a limited number of patients as part of phase 2 studies.[230,231] This is not a therapy that has gained significant traction in the treatment of AL.

Allogeneic Stem Cell Transplantation

Syngeneic transplantation was reported in the treatment of a patient with AL in 1995. An SAP scan showed a reduction in amyloid deposits. In one report, two patients with AL had ablative allogeneic bone marrow transplantation.[247] The first had a hematologic response and underwent an allogeneic transplantation after melphalan treatment (110 mg/m²) and total body irradiation (1200 cGy). The patient achieved a complete hematologic response and was alive 29 months after transplantation. The second patient received a stem cell transplant from a human leukocyte antigen-identical sibling after treatment with melphalan (140 mg/m²) and total body irradiation (800 cGy). The urinary protein loss decreased from 9.15 to 1.3 g/d. The patient had chronic graft-vs-host disease of the skin and liver but was alive 18 months after transplantation.

The mortality rate of allogeneic stem cell transplant is high in patients with AL. The European Group for Blood and Marrow Transplantation reported 15 patients with AL, who underwent allogeneic transplantation: seven had full-intensity conditioning and eight had reduced-intensity conditioning.[248] OS and PFS at 1 year were 60% and 53%, respectively. The treatment-related mortality rate was 40%. Eight patients had a CR and two had a PR. For five of seven evaluable patients who had a CR, chronic graft-vs-host disease was observed, which implied existence of a graft-vs-plasma cell effect. Cardiac failure was a clinically significant problem. Mayo Clinic does not offer allogeneic stem cell transplantation to patients with AL.

Supportive Therapy for Amyloidosis
Cardiac Amyloidosis

Diuretic agents are the mainstay of therapy for patients with cardiac AL. Diuretic therapy is complicated because many patients have orthostatic hypotension and intravascular volume contraction, which are consequences of concomitant nephrotic syndrome. Diuretic therapy may precipitate a decrease in renal blood flow resulting in both an increase in serum creatinine concentration and syncope. Loop diuretics like torsemide, furosemide, or bumetanide are typically used to control edema. Our cardiologists use torsemide in preference to furosemide based on its superior bioavailability. Spironolactone is often beneficial. If loop diuretics fail to control edema, the addition of metolazone may be beneficial.

The role defibrillators and pacemakers play in these patients is unclear. In a recent study, implantable loop recorders were inserted within 24 hours of baseline evaluation into 20 consecutive patients with newly diagnosed severe cardiac AL and symptoms of syncope or presyncope. With a median follow-up of 308 days, 13 patients died, and median survival in the whole cohort was 61 days from device insertion. In each of eight evaluable cases, death was heralded by bradycardia, usually associated with complete atrioventricular block, followed shortly thereafter by pulseless electrical activity. Four patients received pacemakers after development of symptomatic complete atrioventricular block, but these did not prevent rapid cardiac decompensation and death in three cases. The discovery that bradyarrhythmia heralded terminal cardiac decompensation in most patients with severe cardiac AL prompts the question of whether pacemakers should be implanted in patients with severe cardiomyopathy.[249] Anecdotal reports of implantable defibrillators have yielded mixed results.[250-252] In a comparison between 472 patients with cardiac amyloidosis and 2360 propensity-matched nonischemic cardiomyopathies, the 1-year mortality following implantable cardioverter-defibrillator implantation was 27% in patients with AL, which was significantly higher than that seen for the controls.[253] Among 15 patients with defibrillators who underwent ASCT, one died.[254] The median OS was 40.8 months.

Left ventricular assist devices are commonly used in the support of chronic heart failure. Case reports have demonstrated that this therapy can be beneficial with a low complication rate. Many patients with amyloid have small left ventricles due to infiltration of the myocardium making placement of a cannula technically very difficult.[255]

The standard treatment of patients with ischemia-induced heart failure includes orally administered angiotensin-converting enzyme inhibitors and beta blockers. Their use is problematic for patients with AL because of the high incidence of associated hypotension and reduced stroke volume. Congestive heart failure may be precipitated by use of calcium channel blockers, such as nifedipine and diltiazem. Amyloid fibrils selectively bind nifedipine, which could result in high intracellular levels of the medication.[256] We avoid use of beta blockers, as many patients require sinus tachycardia to maintain cardiac output, and we avoid angiotensin-converting enzyme inhibitors due to the lack of published evidence of benefit. For atrial fibrillation the use of digoxin for rate control is safe with appropriate serum monitoring of drug levels. Attempts to manage atrial fibrillation by cardioversion have been reported. A transesophageal echocardiogram is mandatory prior to proceeding, since in one study 28% had an atrial thrombus as compared with 2.5% of controls.[257] Among those proceeding to direct current cardioversion of atrial arrhythmias, patients with cardiac amyloidosis experienced a higher procedural complication rate than control patients (14% vs 2%), but immediate success rates of the cardioversion was no different from controls (90% vs 94%), nor was arrhythmia recurrence at 1 year.

The results of orthotopic cardiac transplant are mixed (Table 101.14).[258-265] Five-year OS is reported to be as high as 77% in modern series. Key determinants for the best outcomes include limiting candidates to those who have lower tumor burden and clinical organ involvement limited to the heart and administering chemotherapy that is effective against the clone. Most patients do not satisfy these criteria, and even those who are placed on a transplant list do not survive long enough to receive an orthotopic heart.[263] Some of the best results have been in patients who have ASCT after their cardiac transplant.[264] Historically, the greatest risk of death post cardiac transplant was reoccurrence in the heart and/or progression in other organs, but now with highly effective plasma cell–directed therapies, infection and graft failure are competing factors. There is no clear guidance on how to and whether to incorporate ASCT after the cardiac transplant. There is a suggestion that IMiDs like lenalidomide and pomalidomide may contribute to acute cardiac rejection, so close surveillance is recommended if these drugs are used in cardiac recipients.[269]

Renal Amyloidosis

Effective chemotherapy slows progression to end-stage renal disease.[8] Diuretics, compressive support hose, low-sodium diet, and selective use of albumin diuresis are the mainstays of renal therapy for amyloidosis. Although diuretics typically are required to control edema, they may further aggravate intravascular volume contraction, increase hypotension, and decrease renal blood flow. Bilateral catheter embolization of renal arteries reduces the loss of urinary protein and increases the serum total protein of patients with advanced anasarca. Angiotensin-converting enzyme inhibitors are often not tolerated in these patients due to concomitant hypotension due to autonomic dysfunction.

The results of hemodialysis for patients with AL are inferior to those for patients with primary kidney disorders. Heart failure, cardiac arrhythmias, and refractory hypotension are the most common extrarenal complications of renal AL. Cardiac amyloidosis with renal failure regularly results in dialysis that is complicated by severe hypotension (a difficult clinical condition to manage). Hemodialysis and chronic ambulatory peritoneal dialysis had identical long-term survival rates.[270] In a review of 61 patients with AL receiving dialysis, 18 died within a month after initiating dialysis.[271] Of the 43 other patients, the median survival time was 61 months. In the Mayo Clinic experience, two-thirds of the deaths of dialysis patients with AL resulted from extrarenal progression (mostly cardiac amyloidosis).

Renal transplantation is an option for some patients with AL (Table 101.13), but the development of amyloidosis in a transplanted kidney is well recognized.[259,267,268] Many of the reports of renal transplantation for amyloidosis combine AL with AA amyloidosis making outcomes for the former condition difficult to discern. The three largest series are from the United Kingdom, Boston, and the Mayo Clinic. Among the 22 patients receiving a renal transplant over 25 years in the United Kingdom, there were no renal graft failures at 4.8 years. The 1- and 5-year OS rates were 95% and 67%, respectively. Seventeen patients received chemotherapy without ASCT either before or after renal transplantation; 4 patients had ASCT prior to kidney transplantation. The Boston group has reported outcomes among 49 patients showing a median OS from renal transplantation of 10.5 years, longer for patients in hematological VGPR or CR. In addition, the 1-year and 5-year renal survival was 94% and 81%, respectively.[267] The Mayo series, the largest to date, with 60 patients, showed superior outcomes for CR/VGPR patients, with time to amyloid recurrence significantly longer in CR compared with VGPR patients.[268]

Fifteen patients with systemic amyloidosis who underwent renal transplantation had SAP scintigraphy studies.[272] Abnormal uptake of radioactive iodine in the transplanted kidney was observed in 4 of 10 patients, and none had a reduction in the level of fibril precursor protein. Of 22 patients with renal amyloidosis, poor cortisol reserves were identified for 7, and hypoadrenalism resulted in the death of 4. Amyloid deposits are regularly found in the adrenal glands at autopsy. One set of recommendations that appears reasonable is to consider renal transplantation for those patients with AL who developed end-stage renal disease and achieve a hematologic CR or VGPR to plasma cell–directed chemotherapy. Organ involvement should not be present outside the kidney to be eligible.[267]

Amyloidosis Involving the Peripheral Nervous System

For patients with AL who present with a dominant neuropathy, survival is better than observed with other dominant systems involved.[86] Clinical improvement in peripheral neuropathy is rare with traditional chemotherapy, and it is infrequent even with high-dose therapy. One-third of patients with significant peripheral nerve and autonomic nerve involvement are ultimately bedridden, and three-fourths have marked restriction in their mobility and a reduced ability to perform the activities of daily living. Management with drugs like gabapentin, pregabalin, and duloxetine may help if neuropathy is painful. Topical compounds containing lidocaine, amitriptyline, and ketamine may also be beneficial. Collaborative symptom management with physiotherapists and/or palliative medicine teams may also be of value.[18] F-florbetapir PRT/MRI imaging reveals abnormal low-level uptake in tibial and peroneal nerves and can identify a target for nerve biopsy in patients where nerve and muscle biopsies miss the pathology.[273]

Amyloidosis Involving the Autonomic Nervous System

Midodrine is commonly used to treat hypotension in patients with AL. Midodrine dosage starts at 2.5 mg three times per day at 4-hour

Table 101.14. Solid Organ Transplant in Patients With AL

Reference	N	Organ	Outcomes
Registry of ISHT 1990, 1991[258]	10*	Heart	1-y 88% 4-y 38%
UK 2010[259]	14	Heart	1-y OS 86% 5-y OS 45%
French registry 2008[260]	8	Heart	1-y 89%
Heidelberg 2009[261]	12	Heart	1-y OS 83% 3-y OS 83%
Spanish registry 2009[262]	13	Heart	1-y OS 43% 5-y OS 16%
Boston 2014[263]	18	Heart	5-y 60%
Stanford 2015[264]	9	Heart	1-y 100%
Mayo 2016[265]	23	Heart	1-y OS 77% 5-y OS 43%
Houston 2018[266]	16	Heart	1-y OS 87% 5-y OS 77%
UK 2010[259]	22	Kidney	1-y OS 95% 5-y OS 67%
Boston 2019[267]	49	Kidney	1-y OS 96% 5-y OS 86%
Mayo 2021[268]	60	Kidney	1-y OS 93% 5-y OS 87%

Abbreviation: ISHT, International Society for Heart Transplant.
^aAt least eight were AL; unclear what the other two were.

intervals. Supine hypertension is an adverse effect of midodrine, and the drug is normally given only during waking hours. The drug is absorbed rapidly from the intestinal tract, and peak serum levels are attained within 30 minutes. The initial dose may be increased as needed to achieve therapeutic endpoints. The maximum recommended daily dose for midodrine is 40 mg. Active metabolites of midodrine are excreted by the kidney, and patients with renal insufficiency should begin with a reduced dose. Evidence of midodrine toxicity includes restlessness, supine hypertension, urinary retention, and reflex bradycardia. Fludrocortisone acetate (0.1 mg orally daily) may be used to treat AL orthostatic hypotension, but adverse effects include supine hypertension, increased fluid retention with aggravation of heart failure, severe hypokalemia, and edema. Fludrocortisone is not well tolerated in elderly patients with AL or those with significant heart failure or hypoalbuminuria. Severe orthostatic hypotension that was not affected by midodrine and fludrocortisone may be treated successfully with erythropoietin, but success is not correlated with the correction of anemia. Droxidopa is approved for the treatment of symptomatic neurogenic orthostatic hypotension in patients with Parkinson disease, multiple system atrophy, dopamine beta-hydroxylase deficiency, and nondiabetic autonomic neuropathy and in patients with pure autonomic failure. It has been attempted in amyloid autonomic failure with orthostatic syncope. Among six patients with light chain amyloidosis standing blood pressure improved from a mean of 82 to 98 mm Hg; although these patients required higher doses of droxidopa, the average dose was 837 mg daily.[274]

Hepatic Amyloidosis

No specific supportive care measures are available for hepatic amyloidosis. Ascites seen in these patients is more commonly associated with concurrent right-sided heart failure or nephrotic syndrome because portal hypertension is not common. Diuresis and, on occasion, paracentesis are the mainstays of support. Patients with hepatic AL have been treated with transjugular intrahepatic portal systemic shunting, which results in resolution of ascites and hydrothorax. For a patient with renal and hepatic amyloidosis, bilateral nephrectomy resulted in markedly improved liver function and normalization of a previously elevated bilirubin value. The median survival of 98 patients with amyloidosis (histologically proven with liver biopsy specimens) was 8.5 months. Stem cell transplantation performed in tandem at 10 and 14 months after liver transplantation resulted in a good clinical outcome 28 months after liver transplantation.

Gastrointestinal Tract Amyloidosis

Therapy for diarrhea includes diphenoxylate, tincture of opium, and loperamide, but results vary. Treating bacterial overgrowth may help, and occasionally the addition of pancreatic enzymes and/or bile acid binders may also provide some benefit. Octreotide (a somatostatin analog) has been reported to reduce diarrhea. In the short-acting form, the dose is 200 to 300 μg/d, divided into two or three doses. A long-acting form of octreotide, which comes in 10-, 20-, and 30-mg doses, may be used. A dose may be given on a monthly basis for 2 months, and it may then be adjusted according to the patient's response. Patients who are disabled because of diarrhea and fecal incontinence may undergo a diverting colostomy, which may result in high patient satisfaction. Patients with intestinal AL sometimes have such severe nutritional failure that long-term total parenteral nutrition is required. We have not found metoclopramide or cholinergic agents to be effective. A colon biopsy showing amyloid deposits may indicate localized form of amyloidosis and not systemic disease.

Respiratory Amyloidosis

For patients with localized tracheobronchial or laryngeal amyloidosis or with nodular pulmonary amyloidosis, see "Localized Amyloidosis" section. For patients with diffuse interstitial pulmonary amyloidosis and true disruption of the alveolar arterial gradient, low doses of prednisone produce symptomatic benefits, although radiographic changes are not evident. The therapy for pulmonary hypertension includes vasodilators and calcium channel blockers. Many patients with amyloidosis are intolerant of these medications because of the associated orthostatic hypotension.

Factor X Deficiency

Therapy for factor X deficiency has included anti-plasma cell–directed therapy.[275] For a patient who is an appropriate candidate, splenectomy results in improvement of factor X levels[276] and infusion of activated factor VII can temporarily normalize coagulation factors and permit safe splenectomy. The management of factor X deficiency with recombinant human factor VII and splenectomy has resolved intractable hematuria. Prothrombin complex concentrates containing high levels of factor X have also been used before performing a hemicolectomy in AL.[277] Factor X concentrate has been introduced for the management of congenital factor X deficiency. Its role in the management of factor X deficiency and AL remains undefined.

Localized Amyloidosis

Localized AL syndrome, which usually involves the skin, larynx, tracheobronchial tree and lungs, eyes, gastrointestinal tract, or urogenital tract, virtually does not progress to become systemic. The fibrils of localized amyloidosis light chain type are immunoglobulin light chain derived, but clonal plasma cells are not seen in the bone marrow; rather there are plasma cells and/or lymphoid cells in these local tissues depositing the amyloid in situ. A circulating monoclonal protein is not seen in localized AL (although coexisting MGUS can happen, which may complicate the diagnosis process, unless the light chain restriction differs between the amyloid deposits and the circulating monoclonal protein). Depending on the site of the localized amyloidosis, these patients may present with hematuria,[278] respiratory difficulties,[279] or visual disturbances; such symptoms may easily be confused with those of systemic amyloidosis, but the site of amyloid deposition provides an important clue for recognizing localized amyloidosis.

Localized Laryngeal Amyloidosis

Laryngeal amyloidosis can involve the true vocal cords, but it more commonly affects the false vocal cords and causes traction on the structures, leading to hoarseness; this form of laryngeal amyloidosis is always localized,[280] and it is diagnosed by laryngoscopy. A patient with laryngeal amyloidosis was treated with adjuvant external beam radiation to a dose of 45 Gy. At 11 months, the patient's voice, breathing, and swallowing had improved substantially.[281]

Localized Pulmonary Amyloidosis

Pulmonary amyloid may be subdivided into nodular, tracheobronchial, or diffuse interstitial deposits (the latter being systemic). Neither localized tracheobronchial nor nodular pulmonary amyloid deposits are associated with systemic disease, and generally have good prognosis, with prognosis less favorable for localized tracheobronchial amyloidosis due to respiratory complications.[282] The diagnosis of tracheobronchial amyloidosis is made by bronchoscopy during evaluation of a patient with obstruction, cough, dyspnea, wheezing, or hemoptysis. The usual treatment is resection of the tissue with an yttrium-aluminum-garnet laser[283,284] or radiation therapy.[285] Nodular pulmonary amyloidosis presents as a solitary pulmonary nodule or multiple nodules, and the nodules do not indicate systemic AL. The nodules, which can reach large size owing to their slow growth, are often resected to exclude a diagnosis of malignancy. The diagnosis is established during a thoracotomy or a video-assisted thoracoscopic surgical procedure. Traces of amyloid are often found in the nodules of pulmonary MALT lymphoma. Nodular pulmonary amyloidosis, if recognized, does not always require intervention. It frequently may be nonprogressive for 5 years or longer.[286]

Localized Ureterovesicular Amyloidosis

Obstructive ureterovesicular amyloidosis is always localized. Patients present with hematuria and have an incorrect prebiopsy diagnosis of cancer. Amyloid deposits are found when cystoscopic biopsies are performed. Eighty-five percent of patients with this type of amyloidosis present with hematuria. Patients may undergo partial cystectomy, fulguration, or transurethral resection. Dimethyl sulfoxide instillation in the bladder has been reported to reduce these deposits.[287,288] These patients present with renal colic because of obstruction or hematuria, and deposits are found during surgery. Nephrectomy can erroneously be performed because the ureteral mass preoperatively is thought to represent a transitional cell malignancy, but the recognition of amyloidosis avoids nephrectomy. Patients may present with dysuria and hematuria when amyloidosis involves the urethra.[289] Resection is the treatment of choice.

Localized Cutaneous Amyloidosis

Three forms of cutaneous amyloidosis are recognized. The lichen and macular forms are localized, innocuous conditions that usually are associated with a history of local skin trauma or inflammation. Nodular amyloidosis is associated with either systemic or localized AL, and evidence of nodular deposits may be an important clinical clue to an underlying life-threatening process. Degraded keratin molecules are the source of macular and papular amyloid deposits. Dermabrasion and other forms of local therapy adequately control localized cutaneous amyloidosis.

Localized Ocular Amyloidosis

Localized amyloidosis is seen in the conjunctiva and orbits. The best treatment is surgical excision. Amyloid has also been localized to breasts,[290] mesenteric lymph nodes, colonic polyps, thyroid, retroperitoneum, and ovaries. Localized deposits of amyloid commonly are observed in trace amounts within the cartilage on the hip surface after a total hip arthroplasty.[291] Similarly, localized deposits are found in resected knee arthroplasty specimens. These deposits are not associated with systemic disease and are usually of the TTR type.

Other Types of Systemic Amyloidosis

Amyloid neuropathy, cardiomyopathy, or nephropathy without monoclonal protein or clonal plasma cell disorder should raise clinical suspicion for other forms of amyloidosis.

AA Amyloidosis (Formerly Known as Secondary Amyloidosis)

AA is a consequence of poorly controlled, long-term systemic inflammation. From a simple syndrome standpoint, its presentation is similar to that of AL. AA is more common than AL in underdeveloped countries because of the persistence of tuberculosis, syphilis, malaria, and leprosy, but in the United States, AA is not easily distinguished from AL. At Mayo Clinic, AA accounts for only 2% of all patients with amyloidosis.[292] AA is not associated with a monoclonal protein or clonal marrow plasma cells. Patients with AA most commonly present with nephrotic-range proteinuria.

In the 19th century, when tuberculosis, leprosy, syphilis, and chronic infections were more prevalent, patients with these infections often had concomitant AA. In the postantibiotic era, the underlying cause of AA most commonly includes ankylosing spondylitis,[293] juvenile rheumatoid arthritis, psoriatic arthritis,[294] and rheumatoid arthritis.[295] For most patients with AA, the cause is clear because the arthritis is disabling and develops a median of 15 years before the development of AA.[296] In patients with rheumatoid arthritis, AA develops in 3.1%. With the introduction of anti-TNF therapies for inflammatory arthropathy, the prevalence of AA in industrialized nations continues to decrease as these disorders are better controlled. AA is also seen in patients with decades of Crohn disease, bronchiectasis[297] (including long-term survivors of cystic fibrosis), and chronic osteomyelitis in which the infected tissue is not amenable to surgical excision and antibiotic therapy results in poor control.[298] AA has been described in patients with Hodgkin lymphoma, Castleman disease, or hypernephroma; surgical excision leads to remission.[299] It has also been described in individuals who subcutaneously inject contaminated illegal substances (i.e., "skin poppers") and paraplegic patients with chronic infected decubitus ulcers or chronic urinary tract infection.[300] Amyloid deposits are identified during autopsy for half of all patients who sustained a spinal cord injury 10 years or more before death.

Hereditary periodic fever syndromes, such as familial Mediterranean fever (FMF), hyperimmunoglobulinemia-D syndrome, and tumor necrosis factor (TNF) receptor-associated periodic syndrome (TRAPS), can give rise to AA amyloidosis as a complication. Anti-cytokine-based therapies like etanercept, adalimumab, infliximab, anakinra, and canakinumab are new treatment options for the TRAPS, and they potentially may prevent amyloidosis.

FMF is the most common of the periodic fever syndromes, and it is caused by mutations in the *MEFV* gene. Clinical features of FMF are pleuritis, peritonitis, synovitis, and migratory skin rash.[301] This disorder is rarely seen in the Western hemisphere, and it primarily affects individuals of Sephardic Jewish, Armenian, Arabic, and Turkish ethnicity. Recurrent attacks of polyserositis are not required for development of amyloidosis, as one-fourth of patients in whom AA develops do not have any history of arthritis or polyserositis. Colchicine has been shown to prevent attacks of polyserositis effectively in two double-blind placebo-controlled studies; the frequency of attacks was reduced by 82% and 78%, and the development of amyloidosis was rare.[302] Occasionally, colchicine in FMF reversed the proteinuria associated with established renal amyloidosis, and after renal failure develops from AA in FMF, colchicine prevents recurrent amyloid deposition in the grafted kidney. Colchicine can be administered safely to children and pregnant women. Colchicine is not effective in the other periodic fever syndromes. Anti-TNF and anti Il-6 therapy has been used to treat AA amyloidosis that is inherited but not related to FMF.

ATTR Amyloidosis

There are two forms of systemic ATTR amyloidosis: the wild type or unmutated form ($ATTR_{wt}$) and the mutated or hereditary form ($ATTR_v$). $ATTR_{wt}$ is currently called age-related ATTR amyloidosis (formerly known as senile systemic amyloidosis) because the prevalence rises with increasing age. Over 80% of patients with $ATTR_{wt}$ amyloidosis are men. In autopsy studies, as much as a quarter of patients older than 90 years (general patient population) have cardiac $ATTR_{wt}$ amyloidosis. Patients present with heart failure symptoms, atrial fibrillation/flutter, conduction abnormalities, and carpal tunnel syndrome. Other clues to diagnosis include lumbar spinal stenosis and biceps tendon rupture. Proteinuria is typically not present. The severity of heart failure is less, and the median survival time is longer than that of patients with cardiac AL.[303] Approximately one-fourth of these patients may have mild length-dependent peripheral neuropathy. Upward of 25% are found to have MGUS, which increases the risk of missed diagnosis as AL when in reality this is TTR amyloidosis with an incidental MGUS.

The use of radionuclide imaging of the heart with Tc99m-PYP or Tc99m-DPD is useful in the diagnostic evaluation, but as uptake can also be seen in patient with AL, this study can be used to confirm the diagnosis of ATTR amyloidosis only in the absence of monoclonal protein.

Presentation of patients with $ATTR_v$ is clinically indistinguishable from that of AL; patients most commonly present with cardiomyopathy,[304] neuropathy, or both.[305] More than 130 different mutations in the *TTR* gene have been described with these clinical phenotypes.[306] Nearly half of the patients with hereditary forms of amyloidosis seen at Mayo Clinic do not have a family history of the disease, so absence of a family history is a poor screening method to exclude hereditary forms of amyloidosis.[296] The most common TTR mutation seen at Mayo Clinic is TTRT60A, caused by a nucleotide substitution in *TTR* DNA of 238A > G.

Patients with hereditary amyloidosis involving only the heart (without peripheral neuropathy) present with heart failure or arrhythmias, and the clinical picture is virtually indistinguishable from that of age-related cardiac amyloidosis ($ATTR_{wt}$) or AL. The TTRV122I mutation is a major cause of inherited cardiac amyloidosis for African Americans. The first report of the mutation described an African American man aged 68 years. The TTRV122I allele is carried by 3.9% of African Americans, which translates to 1.3 million people in the United States; therefore, a finding of cardiac amyloidosis without monoclonal gammopathy could represent $ATTR_v$ cardiomyopathy (even without a family history), and clinicians should not assume that the patient is affected by AL.

The treatment of ATTR$_v$ includes silencing RNA drugs, TTR stabilizers, and liver transplantation, which makes the distinction between it and AL critical for treatment decisions. TTR is produced in the choroid plexus and the liver. Regression of amyloid deposits has been reported when liver transplantation is performed before the development of disabling peripheral neuropathy, autonomic neuropathy, or advanced cardiomyopathy. Patients with the Val30Met mutation in the TTR gene appear to have the best outcome after liver transplantation.[307] Progressive cardiac amyloidosis has been reported after liver transplantation for patients with other TTR mutations.[308] After mutant TTR is deposited in the myocardium, it may serve as a nidus for further deposition of native TTR produced by the transplanted liver. Autopsy findings show cardiac amyloid fibrils with mutant and wild-type TTR.[309] Trials of siRNA against TTR and anti-sense mRNA to stop TTR production have demonstrated stabilization of neurological impairment and improved quality of life.[310,311] The use of these gene silencing therapies have sharply reduced utilization of liver transplantation and are now first-line therapies for TTR mutant peripheral neuropathy. These agents are also being investigated for use in TTR mutant cardiomyopathy. Diflunisal has been shown to slow the progression of TTR neuropathy, and Tafamidis is approved for ATTR$_{wt}$ based on a large phase 3 placebo-controlled study.[312] In that study Tafamidis has been shown to reduce all-cause mortality and cardiac hospitalization in TTR cardiomyopathy, both ATTR$_{wt}$ and ATTR$_v$. It is an oral medication that is well tolerated and has been approved for this use.

Other Rare Forms of Amyloidosis

Among more than 16,000 mass spectrometry typed cases of amyloidosis, AL/AH, ATTR, ALECT2, and AA amyloidosis accounted for 95.72% of all specimens.[313] Rare hereditary forms of amyloidosis include mutated fibrinogen,[314] lysozyme,[315] apolipoprotein A1, and apolipoprotein A2.[316,317] The amyloidosis associated with these mutations has a much better prognosis than that of renal AL. We have regularly seen patients who have proteinuria for more than a decade without renal failure. The absence of a monoclonal immunoglobulin disorder or the absence of free light chains in the serum/urine is an important distinguishing feature. However, only immunohistochemical staining or sequencing of the amyloid by mass spectrometry can differentiate these entities definitively.[21,22] Mass spectrometry often can detect mutations in both TTR and apolipoprotein amyloid.

ALECT2 was discovered by tandem mass spectrometry.[318] Isolation of genomic DNA and polymerase chain reaction amplification of LECT2-encoding exons showed no mutations; however, all were homozygous for the G allele encoding valine at position 40 in the mature protein. ALECT2-associated renal amyloidosis represents a unique form of renal amyloidosis, especially in Mexican Americans and Punjabi Indians. To date, it has not been classified as a hereditary form of amyloidosis. At Mayo Clinic it is currently the 3rd most recognized form of systemic amyloidosis.

CONCLUSION

Amyloidosis should be considered in the differential diagnosis of any patient with nephrotic-range proteinuria, heart failure with preserved fraction, neuropathy, or hepatomegaly as well as those with MGUS with atypical clinical features. The symptoms of amyloidosis are vague and not useful for establishing a diagnosis. The pathognomonic physical findings are seen in less than one-fifth of patients and therefore are not reliable for disease detection. When a patient has a compatible clinical syndrome, the best screening tests include immunofixation of the serum and urine and a serum free light chain assay. Monoclonal light chains may be detected in the serum or urine (or both) of nearly 90% of patients with AL, and 99% of those who have free light chain assays of the serum have abnormal findings. Noninvasive studies, such as fat aspiration and bone marrow biopsy, confirm the diagnosis for 85% to 90% of patients with AL. For patients with biopsy-proven amyloidosis who do not have detectable monoclonal protein in the serum or urine, a nonimmunoglobulin form of amyloidosis should be considered. The prognosis should be assessed by two-dimensional Doppler echocardiography, and levels of NT-proBNP and troponin T should be measured.

Systemic therapy is appropriate for most patients. Bortezomib has significant activity as a single agent and is widely used for transplant-ineligible patients and as part of multidrug induction strategies including alkylators and corticosteroids. Thalidomide, lenalidomide, and pomalidomide are often used in the relapsed or refractory settings. The development of daratumumab has been very important in the management of AL and combinations of daratumumab with bortezomib should be the basis for intervention in newly diagnosed patients. The more aggressive approach of stem cell transplantation may have long-term benefits. Very good partial or better response rates with stem cell transplantation approach 80%, and responders have the potential for long-term survival. However, firm evidence-based data that prove the survival benefit of stem cell transplantation do not exist. Currently, patients who receive a daratumumab bortezomib-based induction therapy who do not achieve MRD negative stringent CRs are candidates for ASCT at Mayo Clinic if they meet ASCT eligibility.

References

1. Virchow R. Cellular pathology (translation by chance F.). In: De Witt RM, ed. *Cellular Pathology*. 2nd ed. 1860:409-413.
2. Kyle RA. Amyloidosis: a convoluted story. *Br J Haematol*. 2001;114(3):529-538.
3. Blumenfeld W, Hildebrandt RH. Fine needle aspiration of abdominal fat for the diagnosis of amyloidosis. *Acta Cytol*. 1993;37(2):170-174.
4. Murphy C, Wang S, Kestler D, et al. Leukocyte chemotactic factor 2 (LECT2)-associated renal amyloidosis. *Amyloid*. 2011;18(suppl 1):223-225.
5. Kourelis TV, Dasari S, Theis JD, et al. Clarifying immunoglobulin gene usage in systemic and localized immunoglobulin light chain amyloidosis by mass spectrometry. *Blood*. 2017;129(3):299-306.
6. Sasatomi Y, Kiyoshi Y, Uesugi N, Hisano S, Takebayashi S. Prognosis of renal amyloidosis: a clinicopathological study using cluster analysis. *Nephron*. 2001;87(1):42-49.
7. Gertz MA, Kyle RA. Prognostic value of urinary protein in primary systemic amyloidosis (AL). *Am J Clin Pathol*. 1990;94(3):313-317.
8. Palladini G, Hegenbart U, Milani P, et al. A staging system for renal outcome and early markers of renal response to chemotherapy in AL amyloidosis. *Blood*. 2014;124(15):2325-2332.
9. Kourelis TV, Kumar SK, Gertz MA, et al. Coexistent multiple myeloma or increased bone marrow plasma cells define equally high-risk populations in patients with immunoglobulin light chain amyloidosis. *J Clin Oncol*. 2013;31(34):4319-4324.
10. Muchtar E, Gertz MA, Kourelis TV, et al. Bone marrow plasma cells 20% or greater discriminate presentation, response, and survival in AL amyloidosis. *Leukemia*. 2020;34(4):1135-1143.
11. Abraham RS, Katzmann JA, Clark RJ, Bradwell AR, Kyle RA, Gertz MA. Quantitative analysis of serum free light chains. A new marker for the diagnostic evaluation of primary systemic amyloidosis. *Am J Clin Pathol*. 2003;119(2):274-278.
12. Muchtar E, Gertz MA, Kumar SK, et al. Improved outcomes for newly diagnosed AL amyloidosis between 2000 and 2014: cracking the glass ceiling of early death. *Blood*. 2017;129(15):2111-2119.
13. Katzmann JA, Kyle RA, Benson J, et al. Screening panels for detection of monoclonal gammopathies. *Clin Chem*. 2009;55(8):1517-1522.
14. Muchtar E, Dispenzieri A, Lacy MQ, et al. Overuse of organ biopsies in immunoglobulin light chain amyloidosis (AL): the consequence of failure of early recognition. *Ann Med*. 2017;49(7):1-7.
15. Lechapt-Zalcman E, Authier FJ, Creange A, Voisin MC, Gherardi RK. Labial salivary gland biopsy for diagnosis of amyloid polyneuropathy. *Muscle Nerve*. 1999;22(1):105-107.
16. Guy CD, Jones CK. Abdominal fat pad aspiration biopsy for tissue confirmation of systemic amyloidosis: specificity, positive predictive value, and diagnostic pitfalls. *Diagn Cytopathol*. 2001;24(3):181-185.
17. Palladini G, Dispenzieri A, Gertz MA, et al. New criteria for response to treatment in immunoglobulin light chain amyloidosis based on free light chain measurement and cardiac biomarkers: impact on survival outcomes. *J Clin Oncol*. 2012;30(36):4541-4549.
18. Gradwell E. Amyloid colitis mimicking collagenous colitis. *Histopathology*. 1998;32(4):383.
19. Lachmann HJ, Booth DR, Booth SE, et al. Misdiagnosis of hereditary amyloidosis as AL (primary) amyloidosis. *N Engl J Med*. 2002;346(23):1786-1791.
20. Comenzo RL, Zhou P, Fleisher M, Clark B, Teruya-Feldstein J. Seeking confidence in the diagnosis of systemic AL (Ig light-chain) amyloidosis: patients can have both monoclonal gammopathies and hereditary amyloid proteins. *Blood*. 2006;107(9):3489-3491.
21. Klein CJ, Vrana JA, Theis JD, et al. Mass spectrometric-based proteomic analysis of amyloid neuropathy type in nerve issue. *Arch Neurol*. 2011;68(2):195-199.
22. Vrana JA, Gamez JD, Madden BJ, Theis JD, Bergen HR, IIIrd, Dogan A. Classification of amyloidosis by laser microdissection and mass spectrometry-based proteomic analysis in clinical biopsy specimens. *Blood*. 2009;114(24):4957-4959.

23. Jones NF, Hilton PJ, Tighe JR, Hobbs JR. Treatment of "primary" renal amyloidosis with melphalan. *Lancet*. 1972;2(7778):616-619.
24. Hawkins PN, Lavender JP, Pepys MB. Evaluation of systemic amyloidosis by scintigraphy with 123I-labeled serum amyloid P component. *N Engl J Med*. 1990;323(8):508-513.
25. Ehman EC, El-Sady MS, Kijewski MF, et al. Early detection of multiorgan light-chain amyloidosis by whole-body (18)F-florbetapir PET/CT. *J Nucl Med*. 2019;60(9):1234-1239.
26. Wall JS, Heidel RE, Stuckey AC, et al. Detection of systemic AL amyloidosis and differentiation of AL from Attr using 124I-p5+14 PET imaging. *Blood*. 2020;136:17-18.
27. Kyle RA, Linos A, Beard CM, et al. Incidence and natural history of primary systemic amyloidosis in Olmsted County, Minnesota, 1950 through 1989. *Blood*. 1992;79(7):1817-1822.
28. Muchtar E, Gertz MA, Kyle RA, et al. A modern primer on light chain amyloidosis in 592 patients with mass spectrometry-verified typing. *Mayo Clin Proc*. 2019;94(3):472-483.
29. Gisserot O, Landais C, Cremades S, et al. Amyloid arthropathy and Waldenstrom macroglobulinemia. *Joint Bone Spine*. 2006;73(4):456-458.
30. Lousada I, Comenzo RL, Landau H, Guthrie S, Merlini G. Light chain amyloidosis: patient experience survey from the amyloidosis Research consortium. *Adv Ther*. 2015;32(10):920-928.
31. Salvarani C, Gabriel SE, Gertz MA, Bjornsson J, Li CY, Hunder GG. Primary systemic amyloidosis presenting as giant cell arteritis and polymyalgia rheumatica. *Arthritis Rheum*. 1994;37(11):1621-1626.
32. Roke ME, Brown WF, Boughner D, Ang LC, Rice GP. Myopathy in primary systemic amyloidosis. *Can J Neurol Sci*. 1988;15(3):314-316.
33. Jacobson IM, Isselbacher KJ. Amyloidosis and hyposplenism with leukocytosis and thrombocytosis. *Ann Intern Med*. 1983;99(4):573.
34. Selroos O, Pettersson T. Platelet values in amyloidosis. *Scand J Rheumatol*. 1973;2(3):97-100.
35. Gertz MA, Kyle RA, Noel P. Primary systemic amyloidosis: a rare complication of immunoglobulin M monoclonal gammopathies and Waldenstrom's macroglobulinemia. *J Clin Oncol*. 1993;11(5):914-920.
36. Klein AL, Hatle LK, Taliercio CP, et al. Prognostic significance of Doppler measures of diastolic function in cardiac amyloidosis. A Doppler echocardiography study. *Circulation*. 1991;83(3):808-816.
37. Chew C, Ziady GM, Raphael MJ, Oakley CM. Proceedings: functional defect in amyloid heart disease "the stiff heart syndrome." *Br Heart J*. 1976;38(5):537.
38. Gertz MA, Grogan M, Kyle RA, Tajik AJ. Endomyocardial biopsy-proven light chain amyloidosis (AL) without echocardiographic features of infiltrative cardiomyopathy. *Am J Cardiol*. 1997;80(1):93-95.
39. Chamarthi B, Dubrey SW, Cha K, Skinner M, Falk RH. Features and prognosis of exertional syncope in light-chain associated AL cardiac amyloidosis. *Am J Cardiol*. 1997;80(9):1242-1245.
40. Fujii B, Matsuda Y, Ohno H, et al. A case of cardiac amyloidosis presenting with symptoms of exertional syncope. *Clin Cardiol*. 1991;14(3):267-268.
41. Hongo M, Yamamoto H, Kohda T, et al. Comparison of electrocardiographic findings in patients with AL (primary) amyloidosis and in familial amyloid polyneuropathy and anginal pain and their relation to histopathologic findings. *Am J Cardiol*. 2000;85(7):849-853.
42. Ogawa H, Mizuno Y, Ohkawara S, et al. Cardiac amyloidosis presenting as microvascular angina—a case report. *Angiology*. 2001;52(4):273-278.
43. Dispenzieri A, Kyle RA, Gertz MA, et al. Survival in patients with primary systemic amyloidosis and raised serum cardiac troponins. *Lancet*. 2003;361(9371):1787-1789.
44. Palladini G, Campana C, Klersy C, et al. Serum N-terminal pro-brain natriuretic peptide is a sensitive marker of myocardial dysfunction in AL amyloidosis. *Circulation*. 2003;107(19):2440-2445.
45. Dispenzieri A, Gertz MA, Kyle RA, et al. Serum cardiac troponins and N-terminal pro-brain natriuretic peptide: a staging system for primary systemic amyloidosis. *J Clin Oncol*. 2004;22(18):3751-3757.
46. Klein AL, Canale MP, Rajagopalan N, et al. Role of transesophageal echocardiography in assessing diastolic dysfunction in a large clinical practice: a 9-year experience. *Am Heart J*. 1999;138(5 pt 1):880-889.
47. Kim D, Choi JO, Kim K, Kim SJ, Kim JS, Jeon ES. Association of left ventricular global longitudinal strain with cardiac amyloid load in light chain amyloidosis. *JACC Cardiovasc Imaging*. 2021;14(6):1283-1285.
48. Hemmingson LO, Eriksson P. Cardiac amyloidosis mimicking hypertrophic cardiomyopathy. *Acta Med Scand*. 1986;219(4):421-423.
49. Sedlis SP, Saffitz JE, Schwob VS, Jaffe AS. Cardiac amyloidosis simulating hypertrophic cardiomyopathy. *Am J Cardiol*. 1984;53(7):969-970.
50. Bellavia D, Pellikka PA, Dispenzieri A, et al. Comparison of right ventricular longitudinal strain imaging, tricuspid annular plane systolic excursion, and cardiac biomarkers for early diagnosis of cardiac involvement and risk stratification in primary systematic (AL) amyloidosis: a 5-year cohort study. *Eur Heart J Cardiovasc Imaging*. 2012;13(8):680-689.
51. Elliott PM, Mahon NG, Matsumura Y, Hawkins PN, Gillmore JD, McKenna WJ. Tissue Doppler features of cardiac amyloidosis. *Clin Cardiol*. 2000;23(9):701.
52. Dubrey S, Pollak A, Skinner M, Falk RH. Atrial thrombi occurring during sinus rhythm in cardiac amyloidosis: evidence for atrial electromechanical dissociation. *Br Heart J*. 1995;74(5):541-544.
53. Browne RS, Schneiderman H, Kayani N, Radford MJ, Hager WD. Amyloid heart disease manifested by systemic arterial thromboemboli. *Chest*. 1992;102(1):304-307.
54. Kornberg A, Rapoport M, Yona R, Kaufman S. Amyloidosis of the pericardium in multiple myeloma: an unusual cause of bloody pericardial effusion. *Isr J Med Sci*. 1993;29(12):794-797.
55. Navarro JF, Rivera M, Ortuno J. Cardiac tamponade as presentation of systemic amyloidosis. *Int J Cardiol*. 1992;36(1):107-108.
56. vanden Driesen RI, Slaughter RE, Strugnell WE. MR findings in cardiac amyloidosis. *AJR Am J Roentgenol*. 2006;186(6):1682-1685.
57. Mueller PS, Edwards WD, Gertz MA. Symptomatic ischemic heart disease resulting from obstructive intramural coronary amyloidosis. *Am J Med*. 2000;109(3):181-188.
58. Neben-Wittich MA, Wittich CM, Mueller PS, Larson DR, Gertz MA, Edwards WD. Obstructive intramural coronary amyloidosis and myocardial ischemia are common in primary amyloidosis. *Am J Med*. 2005;118(11):1287.
59. Montseny JJ, Kleinknecht D, Meyrier A, et al. Long-term outcome according to renal histological lesions in 118 patients with monoclonal gammopathies. *Nephrol Dial Transplant*. 1998;13(6):1438-1445.
60. Gertz MA, Leung N, Lacy MQ, et al. Clinical outcome of immunoglobulin light chain amyloidosis affecting the kidney. *Nephrol Dial Transplant*. 2009;24(10):3132-3137.
61. Bridoux F, Leung N, Hutchison CA, et al. Diagnosis of monoclonal gammopathy of renal significance. *Kidney Int*. 2015;87(4):698-711.
62. Park MA, Mueller PS, Kyle RA, Larson DR, Plevak MF, Gertz MA. Primary (AL) hepatic amyloidosis: clinical features and natural history in 98 patients. *Medicine (Baltimore)*. 2003;82(5):291-298.
63. Lovat LB, Persey MR, Madhoo S, Pepys MB, Hawkins PN. The liver in systemic amyloidosis: insights from 123I serum amyloid P component scintigraphy in 484 patients. *Gut*. 1998;42(5):727-734.
64. Serra L, Poppi MC, Criscuolo M, Zandomeneghi R. Primary systemic amyloidosis with giant hepatomegaly and portal hypertension: a case report and a review of the literature. *Ital J Gastroenterol*. 1993;25(8):435-438.
65. Powsner RA, Simms RW, Chudnovsky A, Lee VW, Skinner M. Scintigraphic functional hyposplenism in amyloidosis. *J Nucl Med*. 1998;39(2):221-223.
66. Okazaki K, Moriyasu F, Shiomura T, et al. Spontaneous rupture of the spleen and liver in amyloidosis–a case report and review of the literature. *Gastroenterol Jpn*. 1986;21(5):518-524.
67. Venkatesh SK, Hoodeshenas S, Venkatesh SH, et al. Magnetic resonance elastography of liver in light chain amyloidosis. *J Clin Med*. 2019;8(5):739.
68. Iwai M, Ishii Y, Mori T, et al. Cholestatic jaundice in two patients with primary amyloidosis: ultrastructural findings of the liver. *J Clin Gastroenterol*. 1999;28(2):162-166.
69. Gertz MA, Kyle RA. Hepatic amyloidosis: clinical appraisal in 77 patients. *Hepatology*. 1997;25(1):118-121.
70. Hayman SR, Lacy MQ, Kyle RA, Gertz MA. Primary systemic amyloidosis: a cause of malabsorption syndrome. *Am J Med*. 2001;111(7):535-540.
71. Gilat T, Spiro HM. Amyloidosis and the gut. *Am J Dig Dis*. 1968;13(7):619-633.
72. Tada S, Iida M, Yao T, Kitamoto T, Yao T, Fujishima M. Intestinal pseudo-obstruction in patients with amyloidosis: clinicopathologic differences between chemical types of amyloid protein. *Gut*. 1993;34(10):1412-1417.
73. Guirl MJ, Hogenauer C, Santa Ana CA, et al. Rapid intestinal transit as a primary cause of severe chronic diarrhea in patients with amyloidosis. *Am J Gastroenterol*. 2003;98(10):2219-2225.
74. Lau CF, Fok KO, Hui PK, et al. Intestinal obstruction and gastrointestinal bleeding due to systemic amyloidosis in a woman with occult plasma cell dyscrasia. *Eur J Gastroenterol Hepatol*. 1999;11(6):681-685.
75. Friedman S, Janowitz HD. Systemic amyloidosis and the gastrointestinal tract. *Gastroenterol Clin North Am*. 1998;27(3):595-614. vi.
76. Koppelman RN, Stollman NH, Baigorri F, Rogers AI. Acute small bowel pseudo-obstruction due to AL amyloidosis: a case report and literature review. *Am J Gastroenterol*. 2000;95(1):294-296.
77. Tada S, Iida M, Yao T, et al. Endoscopic features in amyloidosis of the small intestine: clinical and morphologic differences between chemical types of amyloid protein. *Gastrointest Endosc*. 1994;40(1):45-50.
78. Vernon SE. Amyloid colitis. *Dis Colon Rectum*. 1982;25(7):728-730.
79. Racanelli V, D'Amore FP. Localized AL amyloidosis of the colon and clinical features of intestinal obstruction. A case report. *Ann Ital Med Int*. 1999;14(1):58-60.
80. Alshehri SA, Hussein MRA. Primary localized amyloidosis of the intestine: a pathologist viewpoint. *Gastroenterology Res*. 2020;13(4):129-137.
81. De Navasquez S, Treble HA. Case of primary generalized amyloid disease with involvement of nerves. *Brain*. 1938;61:116-128.
82. Yamada M, Hatakeyama S, Tsukagoshi H. Peripheral and autonomic nerve lesions in systemic amyloidosis. Three pathological types of amyloid polyneuropathy. *Acta Pathol Jpn*. 1984;34(6):1251-1266.
83. Rinaldi R, Azzimondi G, Preda P, Ricci P, D'Alessandro R, Pazzaglia P. Primary systemic amyloidosis presenting with polyneuropathy characterized by very long survival. *Acta Neurol Scand*. 1995;91(6):511-513.
84. Braganza RA, Tien R, Hoffman HT, Haghighi PH. Amyloid of the facial nerve. *Laryngoscope*. 1992;102(12 pt 1):1372-1376.
85. Lingenfelser T, Linke RP, Dette S, Roggendorf W, Wietholter H. AL amyloidosis mimicking a preferentially autonomic chronic Guillain-Barre syndrome. *Clin Investig*. 1992;70(2):159-162.
86. Rajkumar SV, Gertz MA, Kyle RA. Prognosis of patients with primary systemic amyloidosis who present with dominant neuropathy. *Am J Med*. 1998;104(3):232-237.
87. Sommer C, Schroder JM. Amyloid neuropathy: immunocytochemical localization of intra- and extracellular immunoglobulin light chains. *Acta Neuropathol*. 1989;79(2):190-199.
88. Howard ME, Ireton J, Daniels F, et al. Pulmonary presentations of amyloidosis. *Respirology*. 2001;6(1):61-64.
89. Matsumoto K, Ueno M, Matsuo Y, Kudo S, Horita K, Sakao Y. Primary solitary amyloidoma of the lung: findings on CT and MRI. *Eur Radiol*. 1997;7(4):586-588.
90. Bontemps F, Tillie-Leblond I, Coppin MC, et al. Pleural amyloidosis: thoracoscopic aspects. *Eur Respir J*. 1995;8(6):1025-1027.

91. Dingli D, Utz JP, Gertz MA. Pulmonary hypertension in patients with amyloidosis. *Chest.* 2001;120(5):1735-1738.
92. Sucker C, Hetzel GR, Grabensee B, Stockschlaeder M, Scharf RE. Amyloidosis and bleeding: pathophysiology, diagnosis, and therapy. *Am J Kidney Dis.* 2006;47(6):947-955.
93. Gastineau DA, Gertz MA, Daniels TM, Kyle RA, Bowie EJ. Inhibitor of the thrombin time in systemic amyloidosis: a common coagulation abnormality. *Blood.* 1991;77(12):2637-2640.
94. Greipp PR, Kyle RA, Bowie EJ. Factor-X deficiency in amyloidosis: a critical review. *Am J Hematol.* 1981;11(4):443-450.
95. Hoshino Y, Hatake K, Muroi K, et al. Bleeding tendency caused by the deposit of amyloid substance in the perivascular region. *Intern Med.* 1993;32(11):879-881.
96. Boggio L, Green D. Recombinant human factor VIIa in the management of amyloid-associated factor X deficiency. *Br J Haematol.* 2001;112(4):1074-1075.
97. Emori Y, Sakugawa M, Niiya K, et al. Life-threatening bleeding and acquired factor V deficiency associated with primary systemic amyloidosis. *Blood Coagul Fibrinolysis.* 2002;13(6):555-559.
98. Halligan CS, Lacy MQ, Vincent Rajkumar S, et al. Natural history of thromboembolism in AL amyloidosis. *Amyloid.* 2006;13(1):31-36.
99. Kumar SK, Gertz MA, Lacy MQ, et al. Recent improvements in survival in primary systemic amyloidosis and the importance of an early mortality risk score. *Mayo Clin Proc.* 2011;86(1):12-18.
100. Dispenzieri A, Buadi F, Kumar SK, et al. Treatment of immunoglobulin light chain amyloidosis: mayo stratification of myeloma and risk-adapted therapy (mSMART) consensus statement. *Mayo Clin Proc.* 2015;90(8):1054-1081.
101. Dispenzieri A, Kyle RA, Lacy MQ, et al. Superior survival in primary systemic amyloidosis patients undergoing peripheral blood stem cell transplantation: a case-control study. *Blood.* 2004;103(10):3960-3963.
102. Lachmann HJ, Gallimore R, Gillmore JD, et al. Outcome in systemic AL amyloidosis in relation to changes in concentration of circulating free immunoglobulin light chains following chemotherapy. *Br J Haematol.* 2003;122(1):78-84.
103. Muchtar E, Gertz MA, Lacy MQ, et al. Ten-year survivors in AL amyloidosis: characteristics and treatment pattern. *Br J Haematol.* 2019;187(5):588-594.
104. Dispenzieri A, Gertz MA, Kyle RA, et al. Prognostication of survival using cardiac troponins and N-terminal pro-brain natriuretic peptide in patients with primary systemic amyloidosis undergoing peripheral blood stem cell transplantation. *Blood.* 2004;104(6):1881-1887.
105. Kumar S, Dispenzieri A, Lacy MQ, et al. Revised prognostic staging system for light chain amyloidosis incorporating cardiac biomarkers and serum free light chain measurements. *J Clin Oncol.* 2012;30(9):989-995.
106. Dispenzieri A, Lacy MQ, Katzmann JA, et al. Absolute values of immunoglobulin free light chains are prognostic in patients with primary systemic amyloidosis undergoing peripheral blood stem cell transplantation. *Blood.* 2006;107(8):3378-3383.
107. Vaxman I, Kumar SK, Buadi F, et al. Outcomes among newly diagnosed AL amyloidosis patients with a very high NT-proBNP: implications for trial design. *Leukemia.* 2021;35(12):3604-3607.
108. Tei C, Dujardin KS, Hodge DO, Kyle RA, Tajik AJ, Seward JB. Doppler index combining systolic and diastolic myocardial performance: clinical value in cardiac amyloidosis. *J Am Coll Cardiol.* 1996;28(3):658-664.
109. Patel AR, Dubrey SW, Mendes LA, et al. Right ventricular dilation in primary amyloidosis: an independent predictor of survival. *Am J Cardiol.* 1997;80(4):486-492.
110. Kyle RA, Greipp PR, O'Fallon WM. Primary systemic amyloidosis: multivariate analysis for prognostic factors in 168 cases. *Blood.* 1986;68(1):220-224.
111. Gertz MA, Kyle RA, Greipp PR. Hyposplenism in primary systemic amyloidosis. *Ann Intern Med.* 1983;98(4):475-477.
112. Pardanani A, Witzig TE, Schroeder G, et al. Circulating peripheral blood plasma cells as a prognostic indicator in patients with primary systemic amyloidosis. *Blood.* 2003;101(3):827-830.
113. Bryce AH, Ketterling RP, Gertz MA, et al. Translocation t(11;14) and survival of patients with light chain (AL) amyloidosis. *Haematologica.* 2009;94(3):380-386.
114. Warsame R, Kumar SK, Gertz MA, et al. Abnormal FISH in patients with immunoglobulin light chain amyloidosis is a risk factor for cardiac involvement and for death. *Blood Cancer J.* 2015;5:e310.
115. Bochtler T, Hegenbart U, Kunz C, et al. Translocation t(11;14) is associated with adverse outcome in patients with newly diagnosed AL amyloidosis when treated with bortezomib-based regimens. *J Clin Oncol.* 2015;33(12):1371-1378.
116. Bochtler T, Hegenbart U, Kunz C, et al. Gain of chromosome 1q21 is an independent adverse prognostic factor in light chain amyloidosis patients treated with melphalan/dexamethasone. *Amyloid.* 2014;21(1):9-17.
117. Hayman SR, Bailey RJ, Jalal SM, et al. Translocations involving the immunoglobulin heavy-chain locus are possible early genetic events in patients with primary systemic amyloidosis. *Blood.* 2001;98(7):2266-2268.
118. Muchtar E, Dispenzieri A, Kumar SK, et al. Interphase fluorescence in situ hybridization in untreated AL amyloidosis has an independent prognostic impact by abnormality type and treatment category. *Leukemia.* 2017;31(7):1562-1569.
119. Gertz MA, Comenzo R, Falk RH, et al. Definition of organ involvement and treatment response in immunoglobulin light chain amyloidosis (AL): a consensus opinion from the 10th International Symposium on Amyloid and Amyloidosis, Tours, France, 18-22 April 2004. *Am J Hematol.* 2005;79(4):319-328.
120. van G, II, van Rijswijk MH, Bijzet J, Vellenga E, Hazenberg BP. Histological regression of amyloid in AL amyloidosis is exclusively seen after normalization of serum free light chain. *Haematologica.* 2009;94(8):1094-1100.
121. Palladini G, Lavatelli F, Russo P, et al. Circulating amyloidogenic free light chains and serum N-terminal natriuretic peptide type B decrease simultaneously in association with improvement of survival in AL. *Blood.* 2006;107(10):3854-3858.
122. Muchtar E, Gertz MA, Lacy MQ, et al. Refining amyloid complete hematological response: quantitative serum free light chains superior to ratio. *Am J Hematol.* 2020;95(11):1280-1287.
123. Palladini G, Schonland SO, Sanchorawala V, et al. Clarification on the definition of complete haematologic response in light-chain (AL) amyloidosis. *Amyloid.* 2021;28(1):1-2.
124. Dispenzieri A, Arendt B, Dasari S, et al. Blood mass spectrometry detects residual disease better than standard techniques in light-chain amyloidosis. *Blood Cancer J.* 2020;10(2):20.
125. Palladini G, Paiva B, Wechalekar A, et al. Minimal residual disease negativity by next-generation flow cytometry is associated with improved organ response in AL amyloidosis. *Blood Cancer J.* 2021;11(2):34.
126. Sidana S, Muchtar E, Sidiqi MH, et al. Impact of minimal residual negativity using next generation flow cytometry on outcomes in light chain amyloidosis. *Am J Hematol.* 2020;95(5):497-502.
127. Staron A, Burks EJ, Lee JC, Sarosiek S, Sloan JM, Sanchorawala V. Assessment of minimal residual disease using multiparametric flow cytometry in patients with AL amyloidosis. *Blood Adv.* 2020;4(5):880-884.
128. Muchtar E, Dispenzieri A, Leung N, et al. Depth of organ response in AL amyloidosis is associated with improved survival: grading the organ response criteria. *Leukemia.* 2018;32(10):2240-2249.
129. Kaufman GP, Dispenzieri A, Gertz MA, et al. Kinetics of organ response and survival following normalization of the serum free light chain ratio in AL amyloidosis. *Am J Hematol.* 2015;90(3):181-186.
130. Kastritis E, Palladini G, Minnema MC, et al. Daratumumab-based treatment for immunoglobulin light-chain amyloidosis. *N Engl J Med.* 2021;385(1):46-58.
131. Kyle RA, Greipp PR. Primary systemic amyloidosis: comparison of melphalan and prednisone versus placebo. *Blood.* 1978;52(4):818-827.
132. Kyle RA, Gertz MA, Greipp PR, et al. A trial of three regimens for primary amyloidosis: colchicine alone, melphalan and prednisone, and melphalan, prednisone, and colchicine. *N Engl J Med.* 1997;336(17):1202-1207.
133. Skinner M, Anderson J, Simms R, et al. Treatment of 100 patients with primary amyloidosis: a randomized trial of melphalan, prednisone, and colchicine versus colchicine only. *Am J Med.* 1996;100(3):290-298.
134. Kyle RA, Greipp PR, Garton JP, Gertz MA. Primary systemic amyloidosis. Comparison of melphalan/prednisone versus colchicine. *Am J Med.* 1985;79(6):708-716.
135. Gertz MA, Lacy MQ, Lust JA, Greipp PR, Witzig TE, Kyle RA. Prospective randomized trial of melphalan and prednisone versus vincristine, carmustine, melphalan, cyclophosphamide, and prednisone in the treatment of primary systemic amyloidosis. *J Clin Oncol.* 1999;17(1):262-267.
136. Gertz MA, Lacy MQ, Lust JA, Greipp PR, Witzig TE, Kyle RA. Phase II trial of high-dose dexamethasone for previously treated immunoglobulin light-chain amyloidosis. *Am J Hematol.* 1999;61(2):115-119.
137. Gertz MA, Lacy MQ, Lust JA, Greipp PR, Witzig TE, Kyle RA. Phase II trial of high-dose dexamethasone for untreated patients with primary systemic amyloidosis. *Med Oncol.* 1999;16(2):104-109.
138. Palladini G, Anesi E, Perfetti V, et al. A modified high-dose dexamethasone regimen for primary systemic (AL) amyloidosis. *Br J Haematol.* 2001;113(4):1044-1046.
139. Dhodapkar MV, Hussein MA, Rasmussen E, et al. Clinical efficacy of high-dose dexamethasone with maintenance dexamethasone/alpha interferon in patients with primary systemic amyloidosis: results of United States Intergroup Trial Southwest Oncology Group (SWOG) S9628. *Blood.* 2004;104(12):3520-3526.
140. Levy Y, Belghiti-Deprez D, Sobel A. Treatment of AL amyloidosis without myeloma. [Article in French]. *Ann Med Interne.* 1988;139(3):190-193.
141. Wardley AM, Jayson GC, Goldsmith DJ, Venning MC, Ackrill P, Scarffe JH. The treatment of nephrotic syndrome caused by primary (light chain) amyloid with vincristine, doxorubicin and dexamethasone. *Br J Cancer.* 1998;78(6):774-776.
142. van Gameren I, Hazenberg BP, Jager PL, Smit JW, Vellenga E. AL amyloidosis treated with induction chemotherapy with VAD followed by high dose melphalan and autologous stem cell transplantation. *Amyloid.* 2002;9(3):165-174.
143. Ichida M, Imagawa S, Ohmine K, et al. Successful treatment of multiple myeloma—associated amyloidosis by interferon-alpha, dimethyl sulfoxide, and VAD (vincristine, adriamycin, and dexamethasone). *Int J Hematol.* 2000;72(4):491-493.
144. Gono T, Matsuda M, Shimojima Y, et al. VAD with or without subsequent high-dose melphalan followed by autologous stem cell support in AL amyloidosis: Japanese experience and criteria for patient selection. *Amyloid.* 2004;11(4):245-256.
145. Palladini G, Perfetti V, Obici L, et al. Association of melphalan and high-dose dexamethasone is effective and well tolerated in patients with AL (primary) amyloidosis who are ineligible for stem cell transplantation. *Blood.* 2004;103(8):2936-2938.
146. Palladini G, Russo P, Nuvolone M, et al. Treatment with oral melphalan plus dexamethasone produces long-term remissions in AL amyloidosis. *Blood.* 2007;110(2):787-788.
147. Jaccard A, Moreau P, Leblond V, et al. High-dose melphalan versus melphalan plus dexamethasone for AL amyloidosis. *N Engl J Med.* 2007;357(11):1083-1093.
148. Palladini G, Milani P, Foli A, et al. Melphalan and dexamethasone with or without bortezomib in newly diagnosed AL amyloidosis: a matched case-control study on 174 patients. *Leukemia.* 2014;28(12):2311-2316.
149. Lebovic D, Hoffman J, Levine BM, et al. Predictors of survival in patients with systemic light-chain amyloidosis and cardiac involvement initially ineligible for stem cell transplantation and treated with oral melphalan and dexamethasone. *Br J Haematol.* 2008;143(3):369-373.
150. Dietrich S, Schonland SO, Benner A, et al. Treatment with intravenous melphalan and dexamethasone is not able to overcome the poor prognosis of patients with newly diagnosed systemic light chain amyloidosis and severe cardiac involvement. *Blood.* 2010;116(4):522-528.

151. Sanchorawala V, Seldin DC, Berk JL, Sloan JM, Doros G, Skinner M. Oral cyclic melphalan and dexamethasone for patients with AL amyloidosis. *Clin Lymphoma Myeloma Leuk.* 2010;10(6):469-472.
152. Lentzsch S, Lagos GG, Comenzo RL, et al. Bendamustine with dexamethasone in relapsed/refractory systemic light-chain amyloidosis: results of a phase II study. *J Clin Oncol.* 2020;38(13):1455-1462.
153. Kyle RA, Gertz MA, Greipp PR, et al. Long-term survival (10 years or more) in 30 patients with primary amyloidosis. *Blood.* 1999;93(3):1062-1066.
154. Afrough A, Saliba RM, Hamdi A, et al. Impact of induction therapy on the outcome of immunoglobulin light chain amyloidosis after autologous hematopoietic stem cell transplantation. *Biol Blood Marrow Transplant.* 2018;24(11):2197-2203.
155. Gertz MA, Kyle RA. Acute leukemia and cytogenetic abnormalities complicating melphalan treatment of primary systemic amyloidosis. *Arch Intern Med.* 1990;150(3):629-633.
156. Manwani R, Sachchithanantham S, Mahmood S, et al. Treatment of IgM-associated immunoglobulin light-chain amyloidosis with rituximab-bendamustine. *Blood.* 2018;132(7):761-764.
157. Dispenzieri A, Dingli D, Kumar SK, et al. Discordance between serum cardiac biomarker and immunoglobulin-free light-chain response in patients with immunoglobulin light-chain amyloidosis treated with immune modulatory drugs. *Am J Hematol.* 2010;85(10):757-759.
158. Seldin DC, Choufani EB, Dember LM, et al. Tolerability and efficacy of thalidomide for the treatment of patients with light cahin-associated (AL) amyloidosis. *Clin Lymphoma.* 2003;3(4):241-246.
159. Palladini G, Perfetti V, Perlini S, et al. The combination of thalidomide and intermediate-dose dexamethasone is an effective but toxic treatment for patients with primary amyloidosis (AL). *Blood.* 2005;105(7):2949-2951.
160. Dispenzieri A, Lacy MQ, Rajkumar SV, et al. Poor tolerance to high doses of thalidomide in patients with primary systemic amyloidosis. *Amyloid.* 2003;10(4):257-261.
161. Dispenzieri A, Lacy MQ, Geyer SM, et al. Low dose single agent thalidomide is tolerated in patients with primary systemic amyloidosis, but responses are limited. [ASH Annual Meeting Abstracts]. *Blood.* 2004;104(11):312b Abstract 4920.
162. Wechalekar AD, Goodman HJ, Lachmann HJ, Offer M, Hawkins PN, Gillmore JD. Safety and efficacy of risk-adapted cyclophosphamide, thalidomide, and dexamethasone in systemic AL amyloidosis. *Blood.* 2007;109(2):457-464.
163. Palladini G, Russo P, Lavatelli F, et al. Treatment of patients with advanced cardiac AL amyloidosis with oral melphalan, dexamethasone, and thalidomide. *Ann Hematol.* 2009;88(4):347-350.
164. Sanchorawala V, Wright DG, Rosenzweig M, et al. Lenalidomide and dexamethasone in the treatment of AL amyloidosis: results of a phase 2 trial. *Blood.* 2007;109(2):492-496.
165. Palladini G, Russo P, Foli A, et al. Salvage therapy with lenalidomide and dexamethasone in patients with advanced AL amyloidosis refractory to melphalan, bortezomib, and thalidomide. *Ann Hematol.* 2012;91(1):89-92.
166. Moreau P, Jaccard A, Benboubker L, et al. Lenalidomide in combination with melphalan and dexamethasone in patients with newly diagnosed AL amyloidosis: a multicenter phase 1/2 dose-escalation study. *Blood.* 2010;116(23):4777-4782.
167. Dinner S, Witteles W, Afghahi A, et al. Lenalidomide, melphalan and dexamethasone in an immunoglobulin light chain amyloidosis patient population with high rates of advanced cardiac involvement. *Haematologica.* 2013;98(10):1593-1599.
168. Sanchorawala V, Patel JM, Sloan JM, Shelton AC, Zeldis JB, Seldin DC. Melphalan, lenalidomide and dexamethasone for the treatment of immunoglobulin light chain amyloidosis: results of a phase II trial. *Haematologica.* 2013;98(5):789-792.
169. Palladini G, Russo P, Milani P, et al. A phase II trial of cyclophosphamide, lenalidomide and dexamethasone in previously treated patients with AL amyloidosis. *Haematologica.* 2013;98(3):433-436.
170. Kumar SK, Hayman SR, Buadi FK, et al. Lenalidomide, cyclophosphamide, and dexamethasone (CRd) for light-chain amyloidosis: long-term results from a phase 2 trial. *Blood.* 2012;119(21):4860-4867.
171. Kastritis E, Terpos E, Roussou M, et al. A phase 1/2 study of lenalidomide with low-dose oral cyclophosphamide and low-dose dexamethasone (RdC) in AL amyloidosis. *Blood.* 2012;119(23):5384-5390.
172. Cibeira MT, Oriol A, Lahuerta JJ, et al. A phase II trial of lenalidomide, dexamethasone and cyclophosphamide for newly diagnosed patients with systemic immunoglobulin light chain amyloidosis. *Br J Haematol.* 2015;170(6):804-813.
173. Dispenzieri A, Buadi F, Laumann K, et al. Activity of pomalidomide in patients with immunoglobulin light-chain amyloidosis. *Blood.* 2012;119(23):5397-5404.
174. Sanchorawala V, Shelton AC, Lo S, Varga C, Sloan JM, Seldin DC. Pomalidomide and dexamethasone in the treatment of AL amyloidosis: results of a phase 1 and 2 trial. *Blood.* 2016;128(8):1059-1062.
175. Milani P, Sharpley F, Schonland SO, et al. Pomalidomide and dexamethasone grant rapid haematologic responses in patients with relapsed and refractory AL amyloidosis: a European retrospective series of 153 patients. *Amyloid.* 2020;27(4):231-236.
176. Kastritis E, Dialoupi I, Gavriatopoulou M, et al. Primary treatment of light-chain amyloidosis with bortezomib, lenalidomide, and dexamethasone. *Blood Adv.* 2019;3(20):3002-3009.
177. Tapan U, Seldin DC, Finn KT, et al. Increases in B-type natriuretic peptide (BNP) during treatment with lenalidomide in AL amyloidosis. *Blood.* 2010;116(23):5071-5072.
178. Sanchorawala V, Finn KT, Fennessey S, et al. Durable hematologic complete responses can be achieved with lenalidomide in AL amyloidosis. *Blood.* 2010;116(11):1990-1991.
179. Reece DE, Hegenbart U, Sanchorawala V, et al. Long-term follow-up from a phase 1/2 study of single-agent bortezomib in relapsed systemic AL amyloidosis. *Blood.* 2014;124(16):2498-2506.
180. Kastritis E, Leleu X, Arnulf B, et al. A randomized phase III trial of melphalan and dexamethasone (MDex) versus bortezomib, melphalan and dexamethasone (BMDex) for untreated patients with AL amyloidosis. *Blood.* 2016;128(22):646.
181. Palladini G, Foli A, Russo P, et al. Treatment of IgM-associated AL amyloidosis with the combination of rituximab, bortezomib, and dexamethasone. *Clin Lymphoma Myeloma Leuk.* 2011;11(1):143-145.
182. Gasparetto C, Sanchorawala V, Snyder RM, et al. Use of melphalan (M)/dexamethasone (D)/bortezomib in AL amyloidosis. *J Clin Oncol.* 2010;28(15_suppl):8024.
183. Huang X, Wang Q, Chen W, et al. Induction therapy with bortezomib and dexamethasone followed by autologous stem cell transplantation versus autologous stem cell transplantation alone in the treatment of renal AL amyloidosis: a randomized controlled trial. *BMC Med.* 2014;12:2.
184. Kastritis E, Leleu X, Arnulf B, et al. Bortezomib, melphalan, and dexamethasone for light-chain amyloidosis. *J Clin Oncol.* 2020;38(28):3252-3260.
185. Dispenzieri A, Kastritis E, Wechalekar AD, et al. A randomized phase 3 study of ixazomib-dexamethasone versus physician's choice in relapsed or refractory AL amyloidosis. *Leukemia.* 2022;36(1):225-235.
186. Kastritis E, Wechalekar AD, Dimopoulos MA, et al. Bortezomib with or without dexamethasone in primary systemic (light chain) amyloidosis. *J Clin Oncol.* 2010;28(6):1031-1037.
187. Lamm W, Willenbacher W, Lang A, et al. Efficacy of the combination of bortezomib and dexamethasone in systemic AL amyloidosis. *Ann Hematol.* 2011;90(2):201-206.
188. Lee JY, Lim SH, Kim SJ, et al. Bortezomib, melphalan, and prednisolone combination chemotherapy for newly diagnosed light chain (AL) amyloidosis. *Amyloid.* 2014;21(4):261-266.
189. Venner CP, Gillmore JD, Sachchithanantham S, et al. A matched comparison of cyclophosphamide, bortezomib and dexamethasone (CVD) versus risk-adapted cyclophosphamide, thalidomide and dexamethasone (CTD) in AL amyloidosis. *Leukemia.* 2014;28(12):2304-2310.
190. Mikhael JR, Schuster SR, Jimenez-Zepeda VH, et al. Cyclophosphamide-bortezomib-dexamethasone (CyBorD) produces rapid and complete hematologic response in patients with AL amyloidosis. *Blood.* 2012;119(19):4391-4394.
191. Venner CP, Lane T, Foard D, et al. Cyclophosphamide, bortezomib, and dexamethasone therapy in AL amyloidosis is associated with high clonal response rates and prolonged progression-free survival. *Blood.* 2012;119(19):4387-4390.
192. Jaccard A, Comenzo RL, Hari P, et al. Efficacy of bortezomib, cyclophosphamide and dexamethasone in treatment-naive patients with high-risk cardiac AL amyloidosis (Mayo Clinic stage III). *Haematologica.* 2014;99(9):1479-1485.
193. Palladini G, Sachchithanantham S, Milani P, et al. A European collaborative study of cyclophosphamide, bortezomib, and dexamethasone in upfront treatment of systemic AL amyloidosis. *Blood.* 2015;126(5):612-615.
194. Cohen OC, Sharpley F, Gillmore JD, et al. Use of ixazomib, lenalidomide and dexamethasone in patients with relapsed amyloid light-chain amyloidosis. *Br J Haematol.* 2020;189(4):643-649.
195. Kastritis E, Roussou M, Gavriatopoulou M, et al. Long-term outcomes of primary systemic light chain (AL) amyloidosis in patients treated upfront with bortezomib or lenalidomide and the importance of risk adapted strategies. *Am J Hematol.* 2015;90(4):E60-E65.
196. Sanchorawala V, Brauneis D, Shelton AC, et al. Induction therapy with bortezomib followed by bortezomib-high dose melphalan and stem cell transplantation for light chain amyloidosis: results of a prospective clinical trial. *Biol Blood Marrow Transplant.* 2015;21(8):1445-1451.
197. Landau H, Hassoun H, Rosenzweig MA, et al. Bortezomib and dexamethasone consolidation following risk-adapted melphalan and stem cell transplantation for patients with newly diagnosed light-chain amyloidosis. *Leukemia.* 2013;27(4):823-828.
198. Cornell RF, Zhong X, Arce-Lara C, et al. Bortezomib-based induction for transplant ineligible AL amyloidosis and feasibility of later transplantation. *Bone Marrow Transplant.* 2015;50(7):914-917.
199. Manwani R, Mahmood S, Sachchithanantham S, et al. Carfilzomib is an effective upfront treatment in AL amyloidosis patients with peripheral and autonomic neuropathy. *Br J Haematol.* 2019;187(5):638-641.
200. Roussel M, Merlini G, Chevret S, et al. A prospective phase 2 trial of daratumumab in patients with previously treated systemic light-chain amyloidosis. *Blood.* 2020;135(18):1531-1540.
201. Sanchorawala V, Sarosiek S, Schulman A, et al. Safety, tolerability, and response rates of daratumumab in relapsed AL amyloidosis: results of a phase 2 study. *Blood.* 2020;135(18):1541-1547.
202. Kimmich CR, Terzer T, Benner A, et al. Daratumumab for systemic AL amyloidosis: prognostic factors and adverse outcome with nephrotic range albuminuria. *Blood.* 2020;135(18):1517-1530.
203. Chung A, Kaufman GP, Sidana S, et al. Organ responses with daratumumab therapy in previously treated AL amyloidosis. *Blood Adv.* 2020;4(3):458-466.
204. Dispenzieri A. AL patients don't dare go without dara. *Blood.* 2020;135(18):1509-1510.
205. Lecumberri R, Krsnik I, Askari E, et al. Treatment with daratumumab in patients with relapsed/refractory AL amyloidosis: a multicentric retrospective study and review of the literature. *Amyloid.* 2020;27(3):163-167.
206. Gertz MA, Landau H, Comenzo RL, et al. First-in-Human phase I/II study of NEOD001 in patients with light chain amyloidosis and persistent organ dysfunction. *J Clin Oncol.* 2016;34(10):1097-1103.
207. Edwards CV, Rao N, Bhutani D, et al. Phase 1a/b study of monoclonal antibody CAEL-101 (11-1F4) in patients with AL amyloidosis. *Blood.* 2021;138(25):2632-2641.
208. Premkumar VJ, Lentzsch S, Pan S, et al. Venetoclax induces deep hematologic remissions in t(11;14) relapsed/refractory AL amyloidosis. *Blood Cancer J.* 2021;11(1):10.

209. Comenzo RL, Vosburgh E, Falk RH, et al. Dose-intensive melphalan with blood stem-cell support for the treatment of AL (amyloid light-chain) amyloidosis: survival and responses in 25 patients. *Blood*. 1998;91(10):3662-3670.
210. Moreau P, Leblond V, Bourquelot P, et al. Prognostic factors for survival and response after high-dose therapy and autologous stem cell transplantation in systemic AL amyloidosis: a report on 21 patients. *Br J Haematol*. 1998;101(4):766-769.
211. Goodman HJ, Gillmore JD, Lachmann HJ, Wechalekar AD, Bradwell AR, Hawkins PN. Outcome of autologous stem cell transplantation for AL amyloidosis in the UK. *Br J Haematol*. 2006;134(4):417-425.
212. Vesole DH, Perez WS, Akasheh M, Boudreau C, Reece DE, Bredeson CN. High-dose therapy and autologous hematopoietic stem cell transplantation for patients with primary systemic amyloidosis: a Center for International Blood and Marrow Transplant Research Study. *Mayo Clin Proc*. 2006;81(7):880-888.
213. Gertz MA, Blood E, Vesole DH, Abonour R, Lazarus HM, Greipp PR. A multicenter phase 2 trial of stem cell transplantation for immunoglobulin light-chain amyloidosis (E4A97): an Eastern Cooperative Oncology Group Study. *Bone Marrow Transplant*. 2004;34(2):149-154.
214. Mollee PN, Wechalekar AD, Pereira DL, et al. Autologous stem cell transplantation in primary systemic amyloidosis: the impact of selection criteria on outcome. *Bone Marrow Transplant*. 2004;33(3):271-277.
215. Perz JB, Schonland SO, Hundemer M, et al. High-dose melphalan with autologous stem cell transplantation after VAD induction chemotherapy for treatment of amyloid light chain amyloidosis: a single centre prospective phase II study. *Br J Haematol*. 2004;127(5):543-551.
216. Perfetti V, Siena S, Palladini G, et al. Long-term results of a risk-adapted approach to melphalan conditioning in autologous peripheral blood stem cell transplantation for primary (AL) amyloidosis. *Haematologica*. 2006;91(12):1635-1643.
217. Cohen AD, Zhou P, Chou J, et al. Risk-adapted autologous stem cell transplantation with adjuvant dexamethasone +/- thalidomide for systemic light-chain amyloidosis: results of a phase II trial. *Br J Haematol*. 2007;139(2):224-233.
218. Kim SJ, Lee GY, Jang HR, et al. Autologous stem cell transplantation in light-chain amyloidosis patients: a single-center experience in Korea. *Amyloid*. 2013;20(4):204-211.
219. Cibeira MT, Sanchorawala V, Seldin DC, et al. Outcome of AL amyloidosis after high-dose melphalan and autologous stem cell transplantation: long-term results in a series of 421 patients. *Blood*. 2011;118(16):4346-4352.
220. Dispenzieri A, Seenithamby K, Lacy MQ, et al. Patients with immunoglobulin light chain amyloidosis undergoing autologous stem cell transplantation have superior outcomes compared with patients with multiple myeloma: a retrospective review from a tertiary referral center. *Bone Marrow Transplant*. 2013;48(10):1302-1307.
221. D'Souza A, Dispenzieri A, Wirk B, et al. Improved outcomes after autologous hematopoietic cell transplantation for light chain amyloidosis: a center for international blood and marrow transplant Research study. *J Clin Oncol*. 2015;33(32):3741-3749.
222. Dispenzieri A, Lacy MQ, Kyle RA, et al. Eligibility for hematopoietic stem-cell transplantation for primary systemic amyloidosis is a favorable prognostic factor for survival. *J Clin Oncol*. 2001;19(14):3350-3356.
223. Sidiqi MH, Aljama MA, Buadi FK, et al. Stem cell transplantation for light chain amyloidosis: decreased early mortality over time. *J Clin Oncol*. 2018;36(13):1323-1329.
224. Seldin DC, Anderson JJ, Sanchorawala V, et al. Improvement in quality of life of patients with AL amyloidosis treated with high-dose melphalan and autologous stem cell transplantation. *Blood*. 2004;104(6):1888-1893.
225. Gertz MA, Lacy MQ, Dispenzieri A, et al. Trends in day 100 and 2-year survival after auto-SCT for AL amyloidosis: outcomes before and after 2006. *Bone Marrow Transplant*. 2011;46(7):970-975.
226. Gertz MA, Lacy MQ, Dispenzieri A, et al. Autologous stem cell transplant for immunoglobulin light chain amyloidosis: a status report. *Leuk Lymphoma*. 2010;51(12):2181-2187.
227. Leung N, Leung TR, Cha SS, Dispenzieri A, Lacy MQ, Gertz MA. Excessive fluid accumulation during stem cell mobilization: a novel prognostic factor of first-year survival after stem cell transplantation in AL amyloidosis patients. *Blood*. 2005;106(10):3353-3357.
228. Sharpley FA, Manwani R, Petrie A, et al. Autologous stem cell transplantation vs bortezomib based chemotheraphy for the first-line treatment of systemic light chain amyloidosis in the UK. *Eur J Haematol*. 2021;106(4):537-545.
229. Gertz MA, Lacy MQ, Dispenzieri A, et al. Risk-adjusted manipulation of melphalan dose before stem cell transplantation in patients with amyloidosis is associated with a lower response rate. *Bone Marrow Transplant*. 2004;34(12):1025-1031.
230. Sanchorawala V, Wright DG, Quillen K, et al. Tandem cycles of high-dose melphalan and autologous stem cell transplantation increases the response rate in AL amyloidosis. *Bone Marrow Transplant*. 2007;40(6):557-562.
231. Sanchorawala V, Hoering A, Seldin DC, et al. Modified high-dose melphalan and autologous SCT for AL amyloidosis or high-risk myeloma: analysis of SWOG trial S0115. *Bone Marrow Transplant*. 2013;48(12):1537-1542.
232. Skinner M, Sanchorawala V, Seldin DC, et al. High-dose melphalan and autologous stem-cell transplantation in patients with AL amyloidosis: an 8-year study. *Ann Intern Med*. 2004;140(2):85-93.
233. Gertz MA, Lacy MQ, Dispenzieri A, et al. Stem cell transplantation for the management of primary systemic amyloidosis. *Am J Med*. 2002;113(7):549-555.
234. Dhakal B, Strouse C, D'Souza A, et al. Plerixafor and abbreviated-course granulocyte colony-stimulating factor for mobilizing hematopoietic progenitor cells in light chain amyloidosis. *Biol Blood Marrow Transplant*. 2014;20(12):1926-1931.
235. Sanchorawala V, Wright DG, Seldin DC, et al. High-dose intravenous melphalan and autologous stem cell transplantation as initial therapy or following two cycles of oral chemotherapy for the treatment of AL amyloidosis: results of a prospective randomized trial. *Bone Marrow Transplant*. 2004;33(4):381-388.
236. Hazenberg BP, Croockewit A, van der Holt B, et al. Extended follow up of high-dose melphalan and autologous stem cell transplantation after vincristine, doxorubicin, dexamethasone induction in amyloid light chain amyloidosis of the prospective phase II HOVON-41 study by the Dutch-Belgian Co-operative Trial Group for Hematology Oncology. *Haematologica*. 2015;100(5):677-682.
237. Minnema MC, Nasserinejad K, Hazenberg B, et al. Bortezomib based induction followed by stem cell transplantation in light chain amyloidosis: results of the multicenter HOVON 104 trial. *Haematologica*. 2019;104(11):2274-2282.
238. Huang X, Fu C, Chen L, et al. Combination of bortezomib in the induction, conditioning and consolidation with autologous hematopoietic stem cell transplantation in patients with immunoglobulin light chain amyloidosis. *Am J Hematol*. 2019;94(4):E101-E104.
239. Hwa YL, Kumar SK, Gertz MA, et al. Induction therapy pre-autologous stem cell transplantation in immunoglobulin light chain amyloidosis: a retrospective evaluation. *Am J Hematol*. 2016;91(10):984-988.
240. Landau H, Lahoud O, Devlin S, et al. Pilot study of bortezomib and dexamethasone pre- and post-risk-adapted autologous stem cell transplantation in AL amyloidosis. *Biol Blood Marrow Transplant*. 2020;26(1):204-208.
241. Vaxman I, Sidiqi MH, Al Saleh AS, et al. Depth of response prior to autologous stem cell transplantation predicts survival in light chain amyloidosis. *Bone Marrow Transplant*. 2021;56(4):928-935.
242. Scott EC, Heitner SB, Dibb W, et al. Induction bortezomib in Al amyloidosis followed by high dose melphalan and autologous stem cell transplantation: a single institution retrospective study. *Clin Lymphoma Myeloma Leuk*. 2014;14(5):424-430 e421.
243. Muchtar E, Dispenzieri A, Gertz MA, et al. Treatment of AL amyloidosis: mayo stratification of myeloma and risk-adapted therapy (mSMART) consensus statement 2020 update. *Mayo Clin Proc*. 2021;96(6):1546-1577.
244. Al Saleh AS, Sidiqi MH, Sidana S, et al. Impact of consolidation therapy post autologous stem cell transplant in patients with light chain amyloidosis. *Am J Hematol*. 2019;94(10):1066-1071.
245. Landau H, Smith M, Landry C, et al. Long-term event-free and overall survival after risk-adapted melphalan and SCT for systemic light chain amyloidosis. *Leukemia*. 2017;31(1):136-142.
246. Muchtar E, Gertz MA, Kumar SK, et al. Characterization and prognostic implication of delayed complete response in AL amyloidosis. *Eur J Haematol*. 2021;106(3):354-361.
247. Gertz MA, Lacy MQ, Dispenzieri A. Amyloidosis: recognition, confirmation, prognosis, and therapy. *Mayo Clin Proc*. 1999;74(5):490-494.
248. Schonland SO, Lokhorst H, Buzyn A, et al. Allogeneic and syngeneic hematopoietic cell transplantation in patients with amyloid light-chain amyloidosis: a report from the European Group for Blood and Marrow Transplantation. *Blood*. 2006;107(6):2578-2584.
249. Sayed RH, Rogers D, Khan F, et al. A study of implanted cardiac rhythm recorders in advanced cardiac AL amyloidosis. *Eur Heart J*. 2015;36(18):1098-1105.
250. Itoh M, Ohmori K, Yata K, et al. Implantable cardioverter defibrillator therapy in a patient with cardiac amyloidosis. *Am J Hematol*. 2006;81(7):560-561.
251. Lin G, Dispenzieri A, Kyle R, Grogan M, Brady PA. Implantable cardioverter defibrillators in patients with cardiac amyloidosis. *J Cardiovasc Electrophysiol*. 2013;24(7):793-798.
252. Wright BL, Grace AA, Goodman HJ. Implantation of a cardioverter-defibrillator in a patient with cardiac amyloidosis. *Nat Clin Pract Cardiovasc Med*. 2006;3(2):110-114. quiz 115.
253. Higgins AY, Annapureddy AR, Wang Y, et al. Survival following implantable cardioverter-defibrillator implantation in patients with amyloid cardiomyopathy. *J Am Heart Assoc*. 2020;9(18):e016038.
254. Phull P, Sanchorawala V, Brauneis D, et al. High-dose melphalan and autologous peripheral blood stem cell transplantation in patients with AL amyloidosis and cardiac defibrillators. *Bone Marrow Transplant*. 2019;54(8):1304-1309.
255. Lim CP, Lim YP, Lim CH, et al. Ventricular assist device support in end-stage heart failure from cardiac amyloidosis. *Ann Acad Med Singap*. 2019;48(12):435-438.
256. Gertz MA, Falk RH, Skinner M, Cohen AS, Kyle RA. Worsening of congestive heart failure in amyloid heart disease treated by calcium channel-blocking agents. *Am J Cardiol*. 1985;55(13 pt 1):1645.
257. El-Am EA, Dispenzieri A, Melduni RM, et al. Direct current cardioversion of atrial arrhythmias in adults with cardiac amyloidosis. *J Am Coll Cardiol*. 2019;73(5):589-597.
258. Hosenpud JD, DeMarco T, Frazier OH, et al. Progression of systemic disease and reduced long-term survival in patients with cardiac amyloidosis undergoing heart transplantation. Follow-up results of a multicenter survey. *Circulation*. 1991;84(5 suppl):III338-III343.
259. Sattianayagam PT, Gibbs SD, Pinney JH, et al. Solid organ transplantation in AL amyloidosis. *Am J Transplant*. 2010;10(9):2124-2131.
260. Mignot A, Varnous S, Redonnet M, et al. Heart transplantation in systemic (AL) amyloidosis: a retrospective study of eight French patients. *Arch Cardiovasc Dis*. 2008;101(9):523-532.
261. Kristen AV, Sack F-U, Schonland SO, et al. Staged heart transplantation and chemotherapy as a treatment option in patients with severe cardiac light-chain amyloidosis. *Eur J Heart Fail*. 2009;11(10):1014-1020.
262. Roig E, Almenar L, Gonzalez-Vilchez F, et al. Outcomes of heart transplantation for cardiac amyloidosis: subanalysis of the Spanish registry for heart transplantation. *Am J Transplant*. 2009;9(6):1414-1419.
263. Gray Gilstrap L, Niehaus E, Malhotra R, et al. Predictors of survival to orthotopic heart transplant in patients with light chain amyloidosis. *J Heart Lung Transplant*. 2014;33(2):149-156.
264. Davis MK, Kale P, Liedtke M, et al. Outcomes after heart transplantation for amyloid cardiomyopathy in the modern era. *Am J Transplant*. 2015;15(3):650-658.

265. Grogan M, Gertz M, McCurdy A, et al. Long term outcomes of cardiac transplant for immunoglobulin light chain amyloidosis: the Mayo Clinic experience. *World J Transplant*. 2016;6(2):380-388.
266. Trachtenberg BH, Kamble RT, Rice L, et al. Delayed autologous stem cell transplantation following cardiac transplantation experience in patients with cardiac amyloidosis. *Am J Transplant*. 2019;19(10):2900-2909.
267. Angel-Korman A, Stern L, Sarosiek S, et al. Long-term outcome of kidney transplantation in AL amyloidosis. *Kidney Int*. 2019;95(2):405-411.
268. Heybeli C, Bentall A, Wen J, et al. A study from the Mayo Clinic evaluated long-term outcomes of kidney transplantation in patients with immunoglobulin light chain amyloidosis. *Kidney Int*. 2021;99(3):707-715.
269. Qualls DA, Lewis GD, Sanchorawala V, Staron A. Orthotopic heart transplant rejection in association with immunomodulatory therapy for AL amyloidosis: a case series and review of the literature. *Am J Transplant*. 2019;19(11):3185-3190.
270. Browning M, Banks R, Tribe C, et al. Renal involvement in systemic amyloidosis. *Proc Eur Dial Transplant Assoc*. 1983;20:595-602.
271. Gertz MA, Kyle RA, O'Fallon WM. Dialysis support of patients with primary systemic amyloidosis. A study of 211 patients. *Arch Intern Med*. 1992;152(11):2245-2250.
272. Gillmore JD, Madhoo S, Pepys MB, Hawkins PN. Renal transplantation for amyloid end-stage renal failure-insights from serial serum amyloid P component scintigraphy. *Nucl Med Commun*. 2000;21(8):735-740.
273. Shouman K, Broski SM, Muchtar E, et al. Novel imaging techniques using (18) F-florbetapir PET/MRI can guide fascicular nerve biopsy in amyloid multiple mononeuropathy. *Muscle Nerve*. 2021;63(1):104-108.
274. McDonell KE, Preheim BA, Diedrich A, et al. Initiation of droxidopa during hospital admission for management of refractory neurogenic orthostatic hypotension in severely ill patients. *J Clin Hypertens (Greenwich)*. 2019;21(9):1308-1314.
275. Choufani EB, Sanchorawala V, Ernst T, et al. Acquired factor X deficiency in patients with amyloid light-chain amyloidosis: incidence, bleeding manifestations, and response to high-dose chemotherapy. *Blood*. 2001;97(6):1885-1887.
276. Rosenstein ED, Itzkowitz SH, Penziner AS, Cohen JI, Mornaghi RA. Resolution of factor X deficiency in primary amyloidosis following splenectomy. *Arch Intern Med*. 1983;143(3):597-599.
277. Takabe K, Holman PR, Herbst KD, Glass CA, Bouvet M. Successful perioperative management of factor X deficiency associated with primary amyloidosis. *J Gastrointest Surg*. 2004;8(3):358-362.
278. Tirzaman O, Wahner-Roedler DL, Malek RS, Sebo TJ, Li CY, Kyle RA. Primary localized amyloidosis of the urinary bladder: a case series of 31 patients. *Mayo Clin Proc*. 2000;75(12):1264-1268.
279. O'Regan A, Fenlon HM, Beamis JF, Jr, Steele MP, Skinner M, Berk JL. Tracheobronchial amyloidosis. The Boston university experience from 1984 to 1999. *Medicine (Baltimore)*. 2000;79(2):69-79.
280. Hocevar-Boltezar I, Zidar N, Zargi M, Zupevc A, Lestan B, Andoljsek D. Amyloidosis of the larynx. *Wien Klin Wochenschr*. 2000;112(15-16):732-734.
281. Neuner GA, Badros AA, Meyer TK, Nanaji NM, Regine WF. Complete resolution of laryngeal amyloidosis with radiation treatment. *Head Neck*. 2012;34(5):748-752.
282. Srinivas P, Liam CK, Jayaram G. Localised nodular pulmonary amyloidosis in a patient with sicca syndrome. *Med J Malaysia*. 2000;55(3):385-387.
283. Madden BP, Lee M, Paruchuru P. Successful treatment of endobronchial amyloidosis using Nd:YAG laser therapy as an alternative to lobectomy. *Monaldi Arch Chest Dis*. 2001;56(1):27-29.
284. Cordier JF. Pulmonary amyloidosis in hematological disorders. *Semin Respir Crit Care Med*. 2005;26(5):502-513.
285. Utz JP, Gertz MA, Kalra S. External-beam radiation therapy in the treatment of diffuse tracheobronchial amyloidosis. *Chest*. 2001;120(5):1735-1738.
286. Suzuki H, Matsui K, Hirashima T, et al. Three cases of the nodular pulmonary amyloidosis with a longterm observation. *Intern Med*. 2006;45(5):283-286.
287. Nurmi MJ, Ekfors TO, Rajala PO, Puntala PV. Intravesical dimethyl sulfoxide instillations in the treatment of secondary amyloidosis of the bladder. *J Urol*. 1990;143(4):808-810.
288. Hayashi T, Kojima S, Sekine H, Mizuguchi K. Primary localized amyloidosis of the ureter. *Int J Urol*. 1998;5(4):383-385.
289. Dias R, Fernandes M, Patel RC, de Shadarevian JJ, Lavengood RW. Amyloidosis of renal pelvis and urinary bladder. *Urology*. 1979;14(4):401-404.
290. Gluck BS, Cabrera J, Strauss B, Ricca R, Brancaccio W, Tamsen A. Amyloid deposition of the breast. *AJR Am J Roentgenol*. 2000;175(6):1590.
291. Athanasou NA, Sallie B. Localized deposition of amyloid in articular cartilage. *Histopathology*. 1992;20(1):41-46.
292. Hazenberg BP, van Rijswijk MH. Where has secondary amyloid gone? *Ann Rheum Dis*. 2000;59(8):577-579.
293. Kovacsovics-Bankowski M, Zufferey P, So AK, Gerster JC. Secondary amyloidosis: a severe complication of ankylosing spondylitis. Two case-reports. *Joint Bone Spine*. 2000;67(2):129-133.
294. Ahmed Q, Chung-Park M, Mustafa K, Khan MA. Psoriatic spondyloarthropathy with secondary amyloidosis. *J Rheumatol*. 1996;23(6):1107-1110.
295. Chevrel G, Jenvrin C, McGregor B, Miossec P. Renal type AA amyloidosis associated with rheumatoid arthritis: a cohort study showing improved survival on treatment with pulse cyclophosphamide. *Rheumatology (Oxford)*. 2001;40(7):821-825.
296. Gertz MA. Secondary amyloidosis (AA). *J Intern Med*. 1992;232(6):517-518.
297. Goldsmith DJ, Roberts IS, Short CD, Mallick NP. Complete clinical remission and subsequent relapse of bronchiectasis-related (AA) amyloid induced nephrotic syndrome. *Nephron*. 1996;74(3):572-576.
298. Alabi ZO, Ojo OS, Odesanmi WO. Secondary amyloidosis in chronic osteomyelitis. *Int Orthop*. 1991;15(1):21-22.
299. Moon WK, Kim SH, Im JG, Yeon KM, Han MC. Castleman disease with renal amyloidosis: imaging findings and clinical significance. *Abdom Imaging*. 1995;20(4):376-378.
300. Silver JR. Pressure ulcer and amyloidosis. *Spinal Cord*. 1998;36(4):293.
301. Grateau G. The relation between familial Mediterranean fever and amyloidosis. *Curr Opin Rheumatol*. 2000;12(1):61-64.
302. Livneh A, Langevitz P. Diagnostic and treatment concerns in familial Mediterranean fever. *Baillieres Best Pract Res Clin Rheumatol*. 2000;14(3):477-498.
303. Ng B, Connors LH, Davidoff R, Skinner M, Falk RH. Senile systemic amyloidosis presenting with heart failure: a comparison with light chain-associated amyloidosis. *Arch Intern Med*. 2005;165(12):1425-1429.
304. Svendsen IH, Steensgaard-Hansen F, Nordvag BY. A clinical, echocardiographic and genetic characterization of a Danish kindred with familial amyloid transthyretin methionine 111 linked cardiomyopathy. *Eur Heart J*. 1998;19(5):782-789.
305. Plante-Bordeneuve V, Said G. Transthyretin related familial amyloid polyneuropathy. *Curr Opin Neurol*. 2000;13(5):569-573.
306. Connors LH, Richardson AM, Theberge R, Costello CE. Tabulation of transthyretin (TTR) variants as of 1/1/2000. *Amyloid*. 2000;7(1):54-69.
307. Nishino M, Tagaya N, Lynch SV, Steadman C, Balderson GA, Strong RW. Liver transplantation for familial amyloidotic polyneuropathy in Australia. *J Hepatobiliary Pancreat Surg*. 2000;7(3):312-315.
308. Garcia-Herola A, Prieto M, Pascual S, et al. Progression of cardiomyopathy and neuropathy after liver transplantation in a patient with familial amyloidotic polyneuropathy caused by tyrosine-77 transthyretin variant. *Liver Transpl Surg*. 1999;5(3):246-248.
309. Yazaki M, Mitsuhashi S, Tokuda T, et al. Progressive wild-type transthyretin deposition after liver transplantation preferentially occurs onto myocardium in FAP patients. *Am J Transplant*. 2007;7(1):235-242.
310. Adams D, Gonzalez-Duarte A, O'Riordan WD, et al. Patisiran, an RNAi therapeutic, for hereditary transthyretin amyloidosis. *N Engl J Med*. 2018;379(1):11-21.
311. Benson MD, Waddington-Cruz M, Berk JL, et al. Inotersen treatment for patients with hereditary transthyretin amyloidosis. *N Engl J Med*. 2018;379(1):22-31.
312. Maurer MS, Schwartz JH, Gundapaneni B, et al. Tafamidis treatment for patients with transthyretin amyloid cardiomyopathy. *N Engl J Med*. 2018;379(11):1007-1016.
313. Dasari S, Theis JD, Vrana JA, et al. Amyloid typing by mass spectrometry in clinical practice: a comprehensive review of 16,175 samples. *Mayo Clin Proc*. 2020;95(9):1852-1864.
314. Hamidi Asl L, Fournier V, Billerey C, et al. Fibrinogen A alpha chain mutation (Arg554 Leu) associated with hereditary renal amyloidosis in a French family. *Amyloid*. 1998;5(4):279-284.
315. Pepys MB, Hawkins PN, Booth DR, et al. Human lysozyme gene mutations cause hereditary systemic amyloidosis. *Nature*. 1993;362(6420):553-557.
316. Benson MD, Liepnieks JJ, Yazaki M, et al. A new human hereditary amyloidosis: the result of a stop-codon mutation in the apolipoprotein AII gene. *Genomics*. 2001;72(3):272-277.
317. Caballeria J, Bruguera M, Sole M, Campistol JM, Rodes J. Hepatic familial amyloidosis caused by a new mutation in the apolipoprotein AI gene: clinical and pathological features. *Am J Gastroenterol*. 2001;96(6):1872-1876.
318. Murphy CL, Wang S, Kestler D, et al. Leukocyte chemotactic factor 2 (LECT2)-associated renal amyloidosis: a case series. *Am J Kidney Dis*. 2010;56(6):1100-1107.

Chapter 102 ▪ Waldenström Macroglobulinemia

STEPHEN M. ANSELL • RAFAEL FONSECA

INTRODUCTION

Waldenström macroglobulinemia (WM) is an indolent B-cell malignancy characterized by low-grade proliferation of lymphoplasmacytic (LP) cells that primarily inhabit the bone marrow (BM), but it can involve other organs, such as the lymph nodes, liver, and spleen.[1,2] It is unique among B-cell malignancies in that it usually produces a large amount of monoclonal immunoglobulin M (IgM).[1,2] Both the proliferation of LP cells and the increased production of IgM can lead to the characteristic symptoms associated with the disease. These symptoms arise because of the infiltrative nature of these cells, causing enlargement of tissues (lymphadenopathy, hepatomegaly, or splenomegaly) or displacement of the normal BM function, leading to impaired hematopoiesis. The rheologic properties of the monoclonal IgM protein can also lead to characteristics symptoms, including hyperviscosity, immune deposits, or other antibody-mediated disorders.[3-5]

The extent of clonal growth and the rapidity of the expansion of these clonal cells will lead to a spectrum of clinical presentations. Some patients will present with extensive organ involvement and are highly symptomatic, whereas others are only incidentally discovered. Likewise, patients can have a long indolent course without evolution to a more aggressive stage, whereas others quickly declare a need for treatment. Logically, patients with more modest degrees of clonal expansion will be less likely to be symptomatic; however, sometimes the attributes of the monoclonal IgM can result in a clinical phenotype (e.g., IgM-associated amyloid deposits) even when the serum concentration of such protein is low. Because of this heterogeneity, and to mimic what has been a canonical description of the plasma cell neoplasms, IgM LP neoplasms that harbor MYD88 mutations can be categorized as IgM monoclonal gammopathy of undetermined significance (IgM MGUS), smoldering WM, and symptomatic WM.[6]

Even though WM has an indolent course, for most patients, the disease remains incurable, and depending on the age at diagnosis, the disease remains a likely life-ending diagnosis. The median survival for newly diagnosed symptomatic patients is approximately 8 years. However, because the disease is indolent and it primarily afflicts the elderly, it is estimated that about one-half of patients will die from other reasons and not WM. Because of the aforementioned considerations, decisions on when to start therapy remain the cornerstone of optimal clinical management of WM. Treatment planning for asymptomatic elderly patients is quite different from that of symptomatic younger individuals. To this effect, several meetings of international experts have aimed to provide guidance on when to start treatment.[7-9] As always, the individuality of every situation makes the complexity of such decisions at the bedside be unique.

EPIDEMIOLOGY

WM is rare among the hematologic malignancies, accounting for only about 1% of these diagnoses, and has an annual incidence of about 5 cases per million persons in the United States, leading to a total of about 1500 new cases per year.[10-14] Given the rarity of the disease, it is difficult to be precise about the relative incidence of WM across various populations—it is perceived to be more common among Caucasians although this could include bias in diagnostic capabilities.[15] There is a greater proportion of men versus women with WM, and most patients are diagnosed in their mid-60s.[3] Patients with IgM-type MGUS are at greater risk of progression to WM because this state is a precursor to WM.[16] Population-based studies have shown that the rate of progression from IgM MGUS to WM is approximately 2% per year.[16-18]

Although the majority of cases of WM are likely sporadic, several studies have shown situations where a familial predisposition can be identified.[19-22] This increased propensity is also noted for IgM MGUS, which, in turn, suggests a greater propensity for this precursor state.[21] Genetic susceptibility linkage has been identified for loci in chromosomes 1q, 3q, and 4q.[17] How this susceptibility increases the risk for WM and IgM MGUS remains to be determined, although a long-standing process of antigenic stimulation has been proposed.[22-25] The specific antigenic recognition sites that may be driven by chronic stimulation are not known to be unique, although, just like for myeloma, a subset of patients shows reactivity to the protein of unknown function paratarg-7 (P-7).[26] A hyperphosphorylated state of this protein (pP7), inherited as a dominant trait, can be detected in family members of individuals with IgM monoclonal processes. Although hyperphosphorylation of P-7 may be the culprit in some cases, other potential mechanisms remain to be discovered and could include defects in other regulatory elements of the natural immune function that fail to control proper reactivity of terminally differentiated B cells.

DIAGNOSIS

Although multiple diagnostic criteria have been proposed, the diagnosis of WM is usually not difficult and is based on the combination of clinical and pathologic features. Three groups, the World Health Organization (WHO) Lymphoma Classification,[27] a consensus statement by the Second International Workshop on Waldenström Macroglobulinemia,[1] and our group, have proposed criteria that are largely overlapping but not identical.[28] These groups all incorporate the combination of the pathologic presence of LP lymphoma and the consequent IgM monoclonal protein. One key divergence for these criteria is that the WHO broadens its definition by including other lymphoma entities as well as cases with a monoclonal IgA and IgG. In contrast, the Second International Workshop on Waldenström Macroglobulinemia restricts the diagnosis of WM exclusively to cases with LP lymphoma and an IgM monoclonal protein. Both the Mayo classification and the classification from the Second International Workshop on Waldenström Macroglobulinemia include the need for LP lymphoma and a monoclonal IgM, but the Mayo classification requires an involvement of at least 10% of the BM in asymptomatic patients. Another key difference is that the WHO criteria place added importance to nodal pathology, whereas the Mayo classification places greater emphasis on the BM pathology.

A key aspect of the LP lymphoma morphology[29] is that it is rather pleomorphic with some cases having a small lymphocytic morphology with condensed chromatin at one end of the spectrum to cells that have plasma cell morphology at the other end.[1,30] Some cases also have a variant described as "plasmacytoid lymphocytes," also known as "plymphs," with intermediate morphologic features. The architectural pattern of involvement of lymph nodes by WM is typically characterized by paracortical and hilar infiltration but sparing of subscapular and marginal sinuses. The infiltration of the BM space can also be heterogeneous with patterns that can range from nodular, to paratrabecular, to interstitial. Light microscopy can often identify Dutcher bodies–containing plasma cells.

The expression of cell surface markers is quite consistent with the state of B-cell maturation corresponding to the clonal expansions of these cells. The cells display high levels of surface CD19, CD20, and immunoglobulin light chain expression.[30] In contrast to follicular lymphoma, WM cells lack expression of CD10.[30] It is important to recognize that the malignant cells of WM can, like chronic lymphocytic leukemia and mantle cell lymphoma, show expression of CD5 (in about one-half of cases), although its level of expression is not strong. Consistent with some maturation that is retained by these clonal cells, one can see that plasmacytic cells will have the same immunoglobulin light chain restriction and are also positive for CD138 and lose expression of PAX5, CD19, and CD20. In classic WM, cells express surface IgM, although other isotypes would be acceptable by the WHO classification. LP cells of WM can also express CD25, CD27, FMC7, and Bcl-2, and lack expression of Bcl-6 and CD75.

The most common cytogenetic findings in WM are deletions of chromosome 6q. Karyotype analyses initially identified this genetic abnormality in up to one-half of patients studied.[31] We identified that 23% of patients with detectable karyotypic abnormalities, a rarity in WM because of its indolent nature, had 6q deletion. This study is limited because it requires proliferating cells to yield abnormal metaphases.[32] Using interphase fluorescent in situ hybridization, we could detect deletions in 42% of patients,[32] with a minimal area of deletion located at 6q23-24.3.[33] Although deletions of 6q are the most common genetic aberration in WM, their finding is not specific, and their detection alone is not pathognomonic because these deletions can be identified in many other B-cell neoplasias.[34-37] Although no specific gene mutations have been associated with 6q deletions, the consistency at which these deletions are seen in WM suggests that there is an important role, yet to be defined, for this chromosomal deletion. Notably, genes in the commonly deleted region include modulators of NF-kappa-B, Bcl-2, apoptosis, and plasma cell differentiation.

The key finding, now identified as nearly universal in WM, is a mutation of the gene *MYD88*. In the seminal study by the group of Treon and colleagues, *MYD88* was detected in 90% of cases (46/51). The specific mutation leads to a leucine to proline substitution in codon 265 (L265P).[38] Detection of this mutation is commonly used to support the diagnosis of WM because its presence is rare in similar lymphoma subtypes. One unresolved issue is whether the mutation is an initiating or a progression event because it is detectable in some cases of IgM MGUS, but not all.[39,40] Furthermore, mutations of CXCR4 have also been described in patients with WM, and activate Akt and extracellular-regulated kinase.[41-43] The presence of these mutations seems to be associated with resistance to ibrutinib, particularly when they occur in the absence of MYD88 mutations.[41-44]

The transcriptional profile of WM studied by gene expression profiling is unique and dissimilar from what is seen in myeloma. We and others have studied, in a comparative manner, the clonal cells of WM and contrasted them with the transcriptional profile of cells from chronic lymphocytic lymphoma (CLL) and multiple myeloma.[45,46] We concluded that there are more similarities between the profiles of WM cells and CLL cells than those of myeloma.[45] These profiling results align with some of the clinicopathologic similarities between WM and CLL, including expression of similar B-cell markers, low proliferative rates, and a lack of somatic hypermutation.[46] Gene expression profiling also revealed a high level of expression of interleukin 6 (IL-6), clinically correlating with the elevated C-reactive protein levels seen in some WM patients.[45,46] This finding is of great interest because IL-6 participates in the normal inflammatory response and plays a key role by activating the mitogen-activated protein kinase pathway.[47] This overexpression is also likely a culprit in the anemia seen in some cases, where the hemoglobin levels may be more suppressed than would be dictated by the level of BM involvement and likely mediated via hepcidin, as seen in anemia of inflammation.[48] IL-6 expression in WM probably results in an autocrine loop where IL-6 binds to the tyrosine kinase receptor Janus kinases 1 and 2, activating Stat3, and consequent IgM increased production.[49,50]

CLINICAL PRESENTATION

The clinical presentation is dictated both by the infiltration of the BM and other organs by the WM cells and by the rheologic properties of the monoclonal IgM. Given that WM is part of a spectrum, some patients are detected earlier in the course of clonal evolution and may be completely asymptomatic, whereas others will be symptomatic. Common symptomatology may include fatigue due to anemia, bleeding, or neurologic complaints.[51] The monoclonal protein can cause a phenotype because of its large size and discordant dimensions (pentameric molecule), leading to hyperviscosity, or because of its ability to deposit or recognize autoantigens.[3] Although hyperviscosity is quite characteristic for WM, it is not common and is only reported in about one-third of patients. Symptoms of hyperviscosity include mucosal bleeding, retinopathy including venous occlusion leading to visual disturbances, neurocognitive dysfunction, headache, and cold sensitivity.[5,51,52] A large retrospective analysis identified a cutoff value for the IgM of about 6000 mg/dL as a high risk for the development of hyperviscosity, suggesting that these patients should be considered for initiating therapy.[5] Hyperviscosity is not associated with prognosis, but with mutations of CXCR4.[5,44]

Approximately twenty percent of patients may present with neuropathy at diagnosis. The most frequent neurologic abnormality is a distal, symmetric, and slowly progressive sensorimotor peripheral neuropathy.[53-55] Anti–myelin-associated glycoprotein antibodies are found in approximately 50% of patients, but there is no correlation between antibody titers and the patient symptoms.[53] Additional neurologic manifestations include cranial nerve palsies, mononeuritis multiplex, multifocal leukoencephalopathy, and infiltration of the central nervous system (Bing-Neel syndrome).[55-57] Other possible associated syndromes or symptoms include renal involvement,[58] cryoglobulinemia,[59] and systemic amyloidosis.[60]

Deciding when to start treatment is one of the most important decisions in the disease course of patients with WM. Because currently available therapies are not considered curative, decisions to treat will be mostly based on the need to improve symptoms thought to be emanating from excessive proliferation of cells or IgM-related complications. Central to the decision as to when to start therapy is the correct diagnostic allocation of patients who present with monoclonal IgM proteins. To facilitate this staging allocation, we have developed criteria that can aid in differentiating the various IgM gammopathies and providing a framework on when to start treatment (*Table 102.1*).[28]

Table 102.1. Diagnostic Criteria for Waldenström Macroglobulinemia

	Serum IgM Monoclonal Protein	Bone Marrow Infiltrate[a]	End-Organ Damage[b]
Waldenström macroglobulinemia	Any size, and →	>10% bone marrow, and →	Present and attributable to the lymphoplasmacytic disorder
Smoldering Waldenström macroglobulinemia (indolent or asymptomatic)	≥3 g/dL, and/or →	Lymphoplasmacytic infiltration ≥10%, and →	None that can be attributed to the lymphoplasmacytic disorder[c]
IgM MGUS	<3 g/dL and →	Lymphoplasmacytic infiltration <10%, and →	None that can be attributed to the lymphoplasmacytic disorder[c]

Abbreviation: IgM MGUS, immunoglobulin M monoclonal gammopathy of undetermined significance.
[a]Lymphoplasmacytic infiltration by small lymphocytes that exhibit plasmacytoid or plasma cell differentiation and a typical immunophenotype surface IgM+, CD5−, CD10−, CD19+, CD20+, CD23−. This phenotype satisfactorily excludes other lymphoproliferative disorders, including chronic lymphocytic leukemia, and mantle cell lymphoma.
[b]Anemia, constitutional symptoms, hyperviscosity, lymphadenopathy, or hepatosplenomegaly.
[c]As appropriate, exclude hemoglobulin light chain amyloidosis and other monoclonal gammopathies of clinical significance.
Modified from Kapoor P, Ansell SM, Fonseca R, et al. Diagnosis and management of Waldenström macroglobulinemia: Mayo Stratification of Macroglobulinemia and Risk-Adapted Therapy (mSMART) guidelines 2016. *JAMA Oncol*. 2017;3(9):1257-1265.

PROGNOSTIC FACTORS

Although many patients will ultimately succumb to the disease, the prognosis is usually good, and many patients can complete a normal life expectancy, if diagnosed later in life. To better understand the individual prognostic implications, several prognostic indexes have been developed. An international collaborative project, the International Prognostic Staging System for Waldenström Macroglobulinemia (IPSSWM), has defined five prognostic factors associated with a shorter survival and that can segregate patients into three groups.[61] The negative prognostic factors are age >65 years, hemoglobin <11.5 g/dL, platelet count <100,000, β2-microglobulin >3 mg/L, and a monoclonal IgM >7 g/dL.[61] Patients are divided according to the presence of these five variables into those that have 0 to 1, 2, or >2 factors and have a 5-year survival probability of 87%, 68%, and 37%. Even though ultimately every case is unique, the IPSSWM can be used for patient counseling, consideration of inclusion in clinical trials, and is a reminder of criteria usually associated with need for therapy. As previously stated and based on the lack of simple curative therapies, asymptomatic patients should not be treated.[51]

WHEN TO START TREATMENT

While the decision on when to start therapy remains highly individualized and to some degree subjective, there is a desire to create standardized criteria that would allow inclusion patients to clinical trials and would serve as a guide to practicing clinicians. The consensus panel of the Second International Workshop on Waldenström Macroglobulinemia agreed on principles to be used such that therapy initiation should be considered, and these principles were affirmed by the Eighth International Workshop Consensus Panel.[9,62] The panel recommended treatment initiation in the presence of constitutional symptoms, such as fever, night sweats, or weight loss; lymphadenopathy or splenomegaly; hemoglobin <10 g/dL or a platelet count lower than 100×10^9/L (if believed to be as a result of BM infiltration), as well as protein-related complications, such as hyperviscosity or amyloid deposits. The panel affirmed the recommendation not to treat patients with IgM MGUS or asymptomatic WM.

Patients at higher risk of hyperviscosity (unusual with IgM < 4000 mg/dL and nearly universal when the IgM is >8000 mg/dL) should be evaluated for visual impairments, neurologic symptoms, or mucosal bleeding. If hyperviscosity is documented, immediate removal of the monoclonal IgM with plasmapheresis is recommended, even prior to initiation of systemic therapy.[28]

RISK STRATIFICATION

Based on the variety of agents that are clinically active in this disease, a risk-adapted approach to the management of WM is necessary (*Figure 102.1*). Three groups of patients have previously been identified.[28] First, patients with IgM MGUS or smoldering (asymptomatic) WM and normal hematologic function constitute a low-risk group. Second, symptomatic WM patients with modest hematologic compromise, IgM-related neuropathy, or hemolytic anemia are at intermediate risk of disease progression and subsequent morbidity or mortality. Third, WM patients who have constitutional symptoms, significant hematologic compromise, bulky disease, or hyperviscosity have a high risk of disease progression and early mortality. Utilizing these risk groups, we recommend the following: (1) patients with IgM MGUS or smoldering (asymptomatic) WM and preserved hematologic function should be observed without initial therapy. (2) Symptomatic WM patients with IgM-related neuropathy, hemolytic anemia unresponsive to corticosteroids, or symptomatic cryoglobulinemia should receive four standard doses of rituximab alone without maintenance therapy.

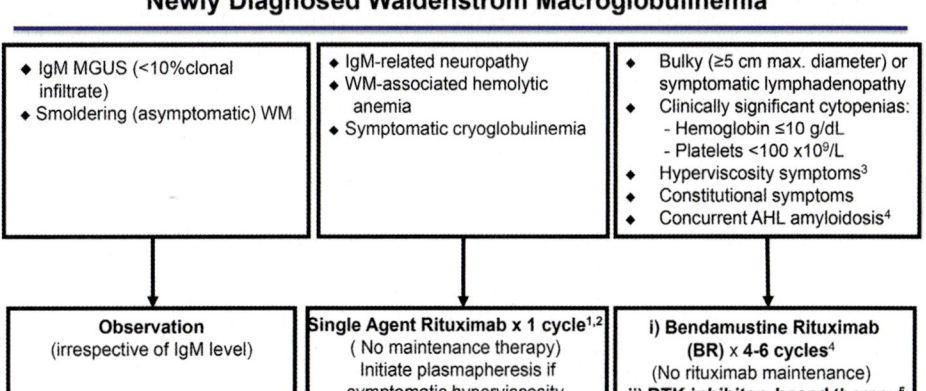

FIGURE 102.1 Mayo Clinic (Mayo Stratification of Macroglobulinemia and Risk-Adapted Therapy [mSMART]) consensus for the management of newly diagnosed Waldenström macroglobulinemia.

(3) WM patients who have constitutional symptoms, clinically significant hematologic compromise, bulky disease, systemic amyloidosis, or hyperviscosity should be treated with chemoimmunotherapy or a Bruton tyrosine kinase (BTK) inhibitor. Younger patients with systemic amyloidosis and adequate cardio-renal function may be considered for an autologous stem cell transplant in first remission. Any patient with symptoms of hyperviscosity should first be treated with plasmapheresis.[28]

THERAPEUTIC OPTIONS

There is now a large array of agents available for the initial treatment of WM. However, once a decision is made to start treatment, several principles should be considered. The intensity of the regimen should be weighed against the severity of symptoms. The delivery route, frequency of administration, and length of therapy vary between agents and may impact treatment choices. It may be important to choose between a fixed duration of therapy compared to long-term treatment administration, as well as whether the treatment is administered intravenously, subcutaneously, or orally. The plan for subsequent therapy should be considered, as patients who are candidates for autologous stem cell transplantation (SCT) should avoid treatment with agents that might interfere with stem cell collection. It is also important to be aware that rituximab administration is frequently associated with a transient increase in serum IgM, which may result in hyperviscosity.

Goals of Therapy

Because WM is not considered to be a curable disease and because it often occurs in elderly patients, complete response (CR) is not typically a primary goal. Response criteria have been defined by the IWWM and are akin to those for multiple myeloma with categories of CR, very good partial response (VGPR), partial response (PR), and minor response, which largely depend on changes in the monoclonal IgM protein.[63] Respectively, these require disappearance by immunofixation, 90% reduction, a 50%-90% reduction, and a 25% to 50% reduction. Additional features of response rely on lymphadenopathy and splenomegaly in the case of CR and VGPR. For all categories, there should also be no new signs of active disease.

Rituximab as a Single Agent

Rituximab is broadly used in the treatment of WM. The rates of response reported vary substantially and likely reflect the patient population used for the various clinical trials. The single-agent response rate varies from a low 29% to up to 65%. Under some circumstances, mainly in patients with neuropathy, hemolytic anemia, or cryoglobulinemia, single-agent rituximab represents a reasonable therapeutic option.[28] An Eastern Cooperative Oncology Group study of 69 WM patients reported an overall response rate of 52% for single-agent rituximab.[64] An important practical aspect for the proper management of rituximab as a treatment for WM is the awareness of a flare phenomenon that can be seen in up to one-half of cases.[28,65] This paradoxical increase in the serum IgM levels can be misinterpreted as evidence of disease progression and may last for up to 4 months. It is also important to anticipate this possibility in patients who have a very high IgM (anyone with an IgM > 4000 mg/dL) who may be treated with rituximab. Although the addition of other agents may abrogate the increase, careful monitoring is necessary to intervene as necessary with plasmapheresis to prevent or treat hyperviscosity.[66] It may also be prudent to withhold rituximab during the first cycle of chemoimmunotherapy in patients with high serum IgM levels.

Nucleoside Analogs

Historically, regimens that contain nucleoside analogs, such as cladribine and fludarabine, have been used with great success, including when used in combination with other drugs such as cyclophosphamide/rituximab (FCR) and rituximab alone (FR). The FCR regimen has a reported overall response rate of 79%, including 12% complete remission and 21% very good partial remission.[67] However, myelosuppression and immunosuppression are known immediate- and long-term toxicities of these combinations. In one study, grade 3-4 neutropenia was seen in 45% of cases and often led to treatment abandonment. A simpler approach has been to merely combine fludarabine with rituximab (FR).[68] Of 43 patients enrolled, the overall response rate was 81%, including some cases that achieved a complete remission and very good partial remission. The toxicities reported in this study are similar to those seen in the FCR study, including myelosuppression and infections.

The interest in the use of purine nucleoside analogs as frontline therapy has waned after reports were made of an increased rate of transformation to aggressive lymphoma and myelodysplasia.[69] One longitudinal study of 439 WM patients, 193 of whom were previously treated with nucleoside analogs, addressed this issue. With a median follow-up of 5 years, among those treated with purine nucleoside analogs, 5% of patients developed large cell lymphoma and 2% evolved to myelodysplasia, whereas only one patient transformed within the other groups.[69] Because of these findings, purine nucleoside analogs are uncommonly used as frontline therapy.

Alkylators and Bendamustine

For many years, alkylating agents were the mainstay of treatment for WM. Although other cytotoxic medications have been used, classic alkylators, predominantly chlorambucil and cyclophosphamide, had been the treatment of choice.[70-72] Over time, these alkylators have been combined with rituximab resulting in improved outcomes. A comparison of rituximab, cyclophosphamide, vincristine, and prednisone (R-CHOP) to CHOP showed a significantly higher response rate for R-CHOP (94% vs 67%, $P = .008$) and similar toxicity.[73] The increased level of response also translated into a longer duration of disease control (63 vs 22 months, $P = .003$). Alkylators are generally well tolerated at the doses used in WM and have gained acceptance as part of the initial combinations to be used in the treatment of WM. The combination of rituximab, dexamethasone, and cyclophosphamide, for example, has been tested in newly diagnosed WM and produced an overall response rate of 83%, with 7% of patients achieving a CR.[74]

Similar to results in other indolent lymphoma patients, bendamustine has proven to be active against WM and has been tested in combination with rituximab. The use of this combination in previously treated patients has resulted in an overall response rate of 80%.[75] The combination is well tolerated but can cause substantial myelosuppression in patients with prior exposure to purine nucleoside analogs. The combination of bendamustine and rituximab has now become a standard frontline therapy for WM. It has been directly compared with R-CHOP in a larger cohort of indolent lymphomas, where it was shown to be better tolerated and associated with a lower risk of relapse, including a longer progression-free survival (PFS).[76] In a subset analysis of the 41 patients with WM, BR was better tolerated than R-CHOP, resulted in a similar overall response rate, and patients had an improved median PFS (70 vs 28 months). Similar response rates and PFS were subsequently reported in a larger multicenter retrospective study.[77]

Proteasome Inhibitors

Proteasome inhibitors have also been used for the treatment of WM. Their use in WM stems from the similarity that WM has to multiple myeloma, where protein homeostasis is essential to assure cell survival. Bortezomib has been used in similar combinations to those used in myeloma, including corticosteroids and alkylators. Bortezomib has also been combined with rituximab in WM. The combination of bortezomib, dexamethasone, and rituximab (BDR) was tested as a primary therapy for newly diagnosed WM and yielded responses in nearly all cases (96%), with a median time to response of 1.4 months.[78] Peripheral neuropathy was common and led to treatment discontinuation in most patients (61%), but these patients received bortezomib in a schedule that is now known to cause a higher rate of peripheral neuropathy. The results with BDR were confirmed in a multicenter phase II trial of 59 patients with symptomatic, previously untreated WM. This study reported an overall response rate of 85% with most patients demonstrating an initial response at 3 months.[79] In a subsequent study by Ghobrial et al, the combination of bortezomib and rituximab was tested with dexamethasone omitted and was found to be active in WM when bortezomib was administered once weekly. Fifty-four percent of patients developed peripheral neuropathy, although none of them were grade 3 or 4.[80] Somewhat unexpectedly, 12% of patients developed neutropenia. Carfilzomib and dexamethasone have also been tested in combination against WM with similar activity to what was seen with bortezomib. In a study by Treon and colleagues, there was an overall response rate of 90% in a cohort of 31 patients.[81] Although some patients experienced asymptomatic hyperlipasemia, and there is a risk of cardiotoxicity and hypogammaglobulinemia, this regimen is attractive in that it has very low risk of inducing peripheral neuropathy. Also, ixazomib, an oral proteosome inhibitor, has been tested in combination with dexamethasone and rituximab (IDR) in 26 treatment-naive patients with WM.[82] The overall response rate was 96% and the median PFS was 40 months. The safety profile was excellent with no grade 4 adverse events. It is concluded that IDR provides a safe and effective frontline treatment option for symptomatic patients with WM.

Bruton Tyrosine Kinase Inhibitors

The identification of *MYD88* mutations by Treon and colleagues in the majority of patients with WM paved the way for the development of BTK inhibitors as therapeutic tools for this disease.[38] *MYD88* L265P is present in >90% of patients with WM, and inhibition of the downstream signaling emanating from the constitutive activation state dictated by these mutations presented an opportunity for a small molecule inhibitor (*Table 102.2*). Ibrutinib is the canonical inhibitor of BTK signaling and induces apoptosis of malignant cells with *MYD88* mutations. A seminal clinical trial of ibrutinib in patients with relapsed or refractory WM showed an impressive overall response rate of 90%, a major response (PR or better) rate of 73%, and a median time to response of 1 month.[83] More importantly, the responses were durable, and a 2-year PFS of 69% was reported. Furthermore, response rates were higher in patients with mutated *MYD88* compared to wild type. The study confirmed that ibrutinib is highly active and well tolerated in patients with relapsed or refractory WM, and this agent is now an approved therapy in this disease. With long-term follow-up of this trial, the median 5-year PFS rate for all patients was not reached, and the 5-year overall survival rate was 87%.[84]

The efficacy of ibrutinib has been confirmed in additional studies of both relapsed and treatment-naïve patients. An international, multicenter study tested ibrutinib as a single agent as therapy for WM ($n = 31$). At a median follow-up of 18.1 months, the proportion of patients with an overall response was 28 (90%) of 31, including 22 (71%) patients who had a major response; the estimated 18-month PFS rate was 86%, and the estimated 18-month overall survival rate was 97%.[85] As previously mentioned, mutations of CXCR4 correlate with resistance to ibrutinib.[90] However, in the international study, the depth of the response was greater than those with wild-type CXCR4, but subsequent studies have shown an association between CXCR4 mutations and BTK mutations.[91] A prospective study of ibrutinib monotherapy in 30 symptomatic, untreated patients with WM tested the effect of CXCR4 mutational status on outcome.[91] The overall response rate for all patients was 100% but the rates of major (94% vs 71%) and very good partial (31 vs 7%) responses were higher in patients with wild-type CXCR4 versus those with CXCR4 mutations, respectively. It was concluded that ibrutinib produces durable responses, is safe as a primary therapy in patients with symptomatic WM, but CXCR4 mutational status does affect responses to ibrutinib.

The combination of ibrutinib plus rituximab has been compared to placebo plus rituximab in a randomized trial of WM patients with symptomatic disease.[86] The addition of ibrutinib to rituximab resulted in higher rates of major response (72% vs 32%) and improved PFS (30-month PFS 82% vs 28%). While ibrutinib plus rituximab resulted in higher rates of atrial fibrillation and hypertension, the rates of anemia, infusion reactions, and IgM flare were lower. These results confirmed that the addition of ibrutinib to rituximab improved patient

Table 102.2. BTK Inhibitors in Symptomatic Waldenström Macroglobulinemia

Agent(s)	Patients, N	Treatment Naïve (%)	Overall Response (%)	PFS	Safety
Ibrutinib[83,84]	63	0	90	69% at 24 mo	Bleeding, atrial fibrillation, mild hematologic toxicity
Ibrutinib[85]	31	0	90	86% at 18-mo	10 patients had serious AEs, mostly infection. Four patients discontinued: two because of AEs.
Ibrutinib plus rituximab (IR) vs placebo plus rituximab[86]	75 75	45	72 32	82% vs 28% at 30 mo	AEs grade 3 or higher: more frequent with IR were atrial fibrillation and hypertension; less frequent: with IR were infusion reactions and IgM flare. Major hemorrhage rate was 4% both arms.
Zanubrutinib vs ibrutinib (ASPEN)[87]	102 99	18	94 vs 94	85% vs 84% at 18 mo	Atrial fibrillation, contusion, diarrhea, edema, Hemorrhage, muscle spasms, and pneumonia, were more common with ibrutinib. Neutropenia more common with zanubrutinib
Zanubrutinib[88]	77	31	96	80.5% at 36 mo	AEs of interest included contusion, neutropenia, major hemorrhage, atrial fibrillation/flutter, and grade 3 diarrhea.
Acalabrutinib[89]	122	13	93	TN: 90% at 24-moRelapsed: 82% at 24 mo	Grade 3-4 AEs occurring in more than 5% of patients were neutropenia and pneumonia.

Abbreviations: AEs, adverse events; BTK, Bruton tyrosine kinase; IgM, immunoglobulin M; PFS, progression-free survival; TN, treatment naive.

outcome; however, it is unknown how this combination compares with ibrutinib as a single agent or with other rituximab-based combinations.

Other BTK inhibitors have also been tested in WM and have been found to be highly effective. Acalabrutinib has been evaluated in a multicenter phase II trial of 122 patients with WM. In this study, the overall response rate was 93% in both treatment-naïve ($n = 14$) and relapsed ($n = 92$) patients.[89] After a median follow-up of 27.4 months, the median duration of response had not been reached in either cohort, with a 24-month duration of response of 90% for treatment-naïve patients and 82% for relapsed or refractory patients. Similar results have been seen with another BTK inhibitor, zanubrutinib, in WM patients.[87,88] In this phase 1/2 study of 77 patients, the overall response rate was 96%, the estimated 3-year PFS rate was 80%, and overall survival rate was 85%.[88] Zanubrutinib has been compared to ibrutinib in a randomized phase III trial (ASPEN).[87] In this study of 201 patients, both arms demonstrated similar efficacy with regards to response rates (28% vs 19%) and PFS (18-month PFS 85% vs 84%). Zanubrutinib was associated with lower rates of hemorrhage, peripheral edema, hypertension, and atrial fibrillation, but there was a higher rate of neutropenia in that treatment arm.

OTHER THERAPEUTIC ALTERNATIVES

Novel Agents

Venetoclax is a Bcl-2 inhibitor that has been used in a series of other late B-cell malignancies. In an open-label phase 2 study, it was tested in a large cohort of patients with indolent B-cell malignancies, including four patients with WM. All four patients with WM had a PR with duration of responses at the time of the report between 12 and 42 months.[92] With longer term follow-up, the median PFS for WM patients was 30.4 months and the median duration of response was 25.3 months, suggesting that venetoclax achieves durable responses in patients with WM.[93] Additional studies of this drug are warranted given this promising preliminary data.

The phosphatidylinositol-3-kinase (PI3K)/Akt/ mammalian target of rapamycin (mTOR) pathway has been identified as important for the survival of WM cells. Accordingly, everolimus, an inhibitor of the mTOR, has been studied in WM with evidence of disease response.[94] Single-agent treatment with everolimus achieved an overall response rate of 72% in previously treated WM and yielded a 12-month PFS of 62%. Clinical trials have tested this agent in newly diagnosed patients as well. In a study by Treon and colleagues, 33 patients with WM, not previously treated, received single-agent everolimus and achieved an overall response of 73%, with major responses occurring in 67% of patients.[95] The median time to progression was 21 months, and responses occurred fast, usually within the first month. However, toxicity was significant and led to treatment discontinuation in 27% of cases, with an 18% incidence of pneumonitis. A randomized trial of the PI3K inhibitor, copanlisib, in combination with rituximab included a subgroup of WM patients and showed that copanlisib plus rituximab improved PFS in patients with relapsed indolent non-Hodgkin lymphoma including WM when compared with placebo plus rituximab.[96]

Other monoclonal antibodies that target CD20 and CXCR4 have been being explored as treatment for WM. Ofatumumab is a monoclonal antibody that targets CD20, but with a different antigenic site of recognition than rituximab. Ofatumumab targets both the large and small extracellular loops of CD20, as opposed to rituximab that only targets the large loop.[97] Single-agent activity of ofatumumab as treatment for WM patients ($n = 37$) showed an overall response rate of 59%, and a lower prevalence of flare reactions was reported.[98] The CXCR4-antagonist antibody, ulocuplumab, has been combined with ibrutinib in a phase 1 study.[99] The major response rate was 100% in 12 evaluable WM patients. With a median follow-up of 22.4 months, the estimated 2-year PFS was 90%.

Stem Cell Transplant

SCT is effective in controlling the disease and has been described as being underutilized.[100] Autologous SCT is the most common modality used and can produce durable remissions in suitable candidates. With improved medical and nursing care, SCT can be said to be relatively well tolerated and capable of inducing durable responses.[28] Kyriakou and colleagues reported a series of 158 patients with WM who had been extensively treated and were experiencing relapse that went on to be treated with autologous SCT.[101] Five years from treatment, nearly one-half remained in remission, with a mortality of 3.8%. The PFS and overall survival rates at 5 years were 40% and 68%, respectively.[101]

This group subsequently published an updated registry report on 615 patients. At a median follow-up of 53 months, the 5-year PFS and overall survival rate were 46% and 65%, respectively. The nonrelapse mortality rate was 7% at 5 years. Patients receiving transplant in first response had a significantly superior 5-year PFS (50% vs 40%) and overall survival (71% vs 63%) rates compared to those transplanted in later response or with refractory/progressive disease. Although the PFS was superior in patients transplanted in the rituximab era, the overall survival was not significantly different, likely because of availability of novel salvage regimens upon relapse.[102] Although additional studies are needed, these results provide a strong rationale to consider SCT in selected WM patients.

Allogeneic SCT has also been studied by Kyriakou and colleagues although its utilization is not common in standard clinical practice and should not be routinely recommended. They reported on 86 patients with WM who were treated with myeloablative or reduced-intensity conditioning (RIC) regimens. Not surprisingly, both regimens were associated with higher risks of nonrelapse mortality at 3 years (33% and 23%, respectively).[103] In a similar series using data from the Center for International Blood and Marrow Transplant Research database (2001-2013), patients who received myeloablative ($n = 67$) or RIC ($n = 67$) transplants were evaluated.[104] The rates of PFS, overall survival, relapse, and nonrelapse mortality at 5 years were 46%, 52%, 24%, and 30%, respectively. There were no significant differences in PFS based on conditioning (myeloablative, 50%, vs RIC, 41%) or graft source and the most common causes of death were primary disease and graft-versus-host disease. These results confirm that allogeneic SCT yielded durable survival in select patients with WM.

Overall Approach for Relapsed and Refractory Waldenström Macroglobulinemia

Because there is currently no standard approach to the management of patients with relapsed WM, the approach of our group (*Figure 102.2*) is to consider all patients for participation in a clinical trial either as definitive therapy for their disease or as preparative therapy prior to considering an autologous SCT.[28] For patients who are ineligible or unwilling to go on a clinical trial, the choice of therapy is determined by their response to frontline treatment. Because response rates to initial therapies are often high and clinical benefit is typically quite durable, we recommend using a 4-year cutoff to determine treatment. For patients with a durable response that lasted >4 years, the original therapy can be repeated. For patients who have an inadequate response to initial therapy or a response lasting <4 years, an alternative approach should be used. Our group will commonly use ibrutinib in these patients if not previously used. An autologous SCT can also be considered in eligible patients with relapsed disease.

CONCLUSIONS

WM is a rare condition for which a plethora of effective treatments exist. Given the complexity of the decision process of when to start treatment and what agents to choose, referral to comanage patients with experts in the field is recommended. We have worked to create guidelines that provide guidance of the various management options.[28] We update these recommendations on a regularly basis as new data become available and are available at www.mSMART.org.

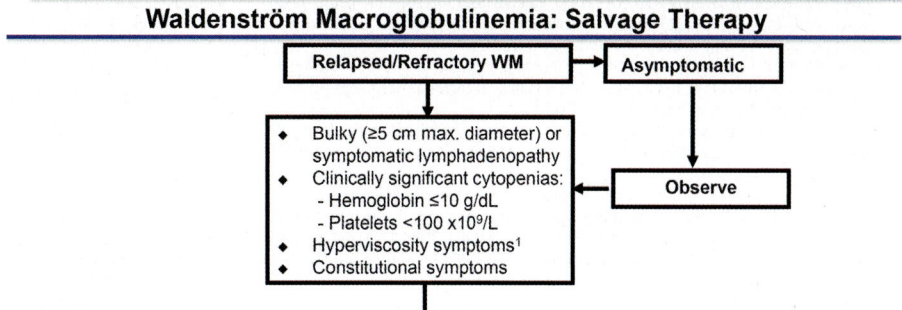

FIGURE 102.2 Mayo Clinic (Mayo Stratification of Macroglobulinemia and Risk-Adapted Therapy [mSMART]) consensus for the management of relapsed Waldenström macroglobulinemia.

References

1. Owen RG, Treon SP, Al-Katib A, et al. Clinicopathological definition of Waldenström's macroglobulinemia: consensus panel recommendations from the Second International Workshop on Waldenström's Macroglobulinemia. *Semin Oncol*. 2003;30(2):110-115.
2. Dimopoulos MA, Kyle RA, Anagnostopoulos A, Treon SP. Diagnosis and management of Waldenström's macroglobulinemia. *J Clin Oncol*. 2005;23(7):1564-1577.
3. Dimopoulos MA, Panayiotidis P, Moulopoulos LA, Sfikakis P, Dalakas M. Waldenström's macroglobulinemia: clinical features, complications, and management. *J Clin Oncol*. 2000;18(1):214-226.
4. Gertz MA. Waldenström macroglobulinemia: 2021 update on diagnosis, risk stratification, and management. *Am J Hematol*. 2021;96(2):258-269.
5. Gustine JN, Meid K, Dubeau T, et al. Serum IgM level as predictor of symptomatic hyperviscosity in patients with Waldenström macroglobulinaemia. *Br J Haematol*. 2017;177(5):717-725.
6. Kyle RA, Rajkumar SV. Criteria for diagnosis, staging, risk stratification and response assessment of multiple myeloma. *Leukemia*. 2009;23(1):3-9.
7. Gertz MA, Anagnostopoulos A, Anderson K, et al. Treatment recommendations in Waldenström's macroglobulinemia: consensus panel recommendations from the Second International Workshop on Waldenström's Macroglobulinemia. *Semin Oncol*. 2003;30(2):121-126.
8. Dimopoulos MA, Gertz MA, Kastritis E, et al. Update on treatment recommendations from the Fourth International Workshop on Waldenström's macroglobulinemia. *J Clin Oncol*. 2009;27(1):120-126.
9. Castillo JJ, Advani RH, Branagan AR, et al. Consensus treatment recommendations from the tenth International Workshop for Waldenström macroglobulinaemia. *Lancet Haematol*. 2020;7(11):e827-e837.
10. Ailawadhi S, Kardosh A, Yang D, et al. Outcome disparities among ethnic subgroups of Waldenström's macroglobulinemia: a population-based study. *Oncology*. 2014;86(5-6):253-262.
11. Kyle RA, Larson DR, McPhail ED, et al. Fifty-year Incidence of Waldenström macroglobulinemia in Olmsted county, Minnesota, from 1961 through 2010: a population-based study with complete case capture and hematopathologic review. *Mayo Clin Proc*. 2018;93(6):739-746.
12. Castillo JJ, Olszewski AJ, Kanan S, Meid K, Hunter ZR, Treon SP. Overall survival and competing risks of death in patients with Waldenström macroglobulinaemia: an analysis of the Surveillance, Epidemiology and End Results database. *Br J Haematol*. 2015;169(1):81-89.
13. Wang H, Chen Y, Li F, et al. Temporal and geographic variations of Waldenström macroglobulinemia incidence: a large population-based study. *Cancer*. 2012;118(15):3793-3800.
14. Weiss BM, Minter A, Abadie J, et al. Patterns of monoclonal immunoglobulins and serum free light chains are significantly different in black compared to white monoclonal gammopathy of undetermined significance (MGUS) patients. *Am J Hematol*. 2011;86(6):475-478.
15. Benjamin M, Reddy S, Brawley OW. Myeloma and race: a review of the literature. *Cancer Metastasis Rev*. 2003;22(1):87-93.
16. Kyle RA, Therneau TM, Rajkumar SV, et al. Long-term follow-up of IgM monoclonal gammopathy of undetermined significance. *Semin Oncol*. 2003;30(2):169-171.
17. McMaster ML, Goldin LR, Bai Y, et al. Genomewide linkage screen for Waldenström macroglobulinemia susceptibility loci in high-risk families. *Am J Hum Genet*. 2006;79(4):695-701.
18. Bustoros M, Sklavenitis-Pistofidis R, Kapoor P, et al. Progression risk stratification of asymptomatic Waldenström macroglobulinemia. *J Clin Oncol*. 2019;37(16):1403-1411.
19. Steingrimsson V, Lund SH, Turesson I, et al. Population-based study on the impact of the familial form of Waldenström macroglobulinemia on overall survival. *Blood*. 2015;125(13):2174-2175.
20. Treon SP, Hunter ZR, Aggarwal A, et al. Characterization of familial Waldenström's macroglobulinemia. *Ann Oncol*. 2006;17(3):488-494.
21. McMaster ML. Familial Waldenström's macroglobulinemia. *Semin Oncol*. 2003;30(2):146-152.
22. Sud A, Chattopadhyay S, Thomsen H, et al. Analysis of 153115 patients with hematological malignancies refines the spectrum of familial risk. *Blood*. 2019;134(12):960-969.
23. Aoki H, Takishita M, Kosaka M, Saito S. Frequent somatic mutations in D and/or JH segments of Ig gene in Waldenström's macroglobulinemia and chronic lymphocytic leukemia (CLL) with Richter's syndrome but not in common CLL. *Blood*. 1995;85(7):1913-1919.
24. Kristinsson SY, Koshiol J, Björkholm M, et al. Immune-related and inflammatory conditions and risk of lymphoplasmacytic lymphoma or Waldenström macroglobulinemia. *J Natl Cancer Inst*. 2010;102(8):557-567.
25. Martin-Jimenez P, Garcia-Sanz R, Balanzategui A, et al. Molecular characterization of heavy chain immunoglobulin gene rearrangements in Waldenström's macroglobulinemia and IgM monoclonal gammopathy of undetermined significance. *Haematologica*. 2007;92(5):635-642.
26. Grass S, Preuss KD, Wikowicz A, et al. Hyperphosphorylated paratarg-7: a new molecularly defined risk factor for monoclonal gammopathy of undetermined significance of the IgM type and Waldenström macroglobulinemia. *Blood*. 2011;117(10):2918-2923.
27. Swerdlow SH, Campo E, Pileri SA, et al. The 2016 revision of the World Health Organization classification of lymphoid neoplasms. *Blood*. 2016;127(20):2375-2390.
28. Kapoor P, Ansell SM, Fonseca R, et al. Diagnosis and management of Waldenström macroglobulinemia: Mayo stratification of macroglobulinemia and risk-adapted therapy (mSMART) guidelines 2016. *JAMA Oncol*. 2017;3(9):1257-1265.
29. Paiva B, Corchete LA, Vidriales MB, et al. The cellular origin and malignant transformation of Waldenström macroglobulinemia. *Blood*. 2015;125(15):2370-2380.
30. Morice WG, Chen D, Kurtin PJ, Hanson CA, McPhail ED. Novel immunophenotypic features of marrow lymphoplasmacytic lymphoma and correlation with Waldenström's macroglobulinemia. *Mod Pathol*. 2009;22(6):807-816.
31. Mansoor A, Medeiros LJ, Weber DM, et al. Cytogenetic findings in lymphoplasmacytic lymphoma/Waldenström macroglobulinemia. Chromosomal abnormalities are associated with the polymorphous subtype and an aggressive clinical course. *Am J Clin Pathol*. 2001;116(4):543-549.

32. Schop RF, Kuehl WM, Van Wier SA, et al. Waldenström macroglobulinemia neoplastic cells lack immunoglobulin heavy chain locus translocations but have frequent 6q deletions. *Blood*. 2002;100(8):2996-3001.
33. Schop RF, Van Wier SA, Xu R, et al. 6q deletion discriminates Waldenström macroglobulinemia from IgM monoclonal gammopathy of undetermined significance. *Cancer Genet Cytogenet*. 2006;169(2):150-153.
34. Braggio E, Dogan A, Keats JJ, et al. Genomic analysis of marginal zone and lymphoplasmacytic lymphomas identified common and disease-specific abnormalities. *Mod Pathol*. 2012;25(5):651-660.
35. Ferreira BI, Garcia JF, Suela J, et al. Comparative genome profiling across subtypes of low-grade B-cell lymphoma identifies type-specific and common aberrations that target genes with a role in B-cell neoplasia. *Haematologica*. 2008;93(5):670-679.
36. Rinaldi A, Mian M, Chigrinova E, et al. Genome-wide DNA profiling of marginal zone lymphomas identifies subtype-specific lesions with an impact on the clinical outcome. *Blood*. 2011;117(5):1595-1604.
37. Dohner H, Stilgenbauer S, Benner A, et al. Genomic aberrations and survival in chronic lymphocytic leukemia. *N Engl J Med*. 2000;343(26):1910-1916.
38. Treon SP, Xu L, Yang G, et al. MYD88 L265P somatic mutation in Waldenström's macroglobulinemia. *N Engl J Med*. 2012;367(9):826-833.
39. Landgren O, Staudt L. MYD88 L265P somatic mutation in IgM MGUS. *N Engl J Med*. 2012;367(23):2255-2256. author reply 6-7.
40. Xu L, Hunter ZR, Yang G, et al. Detection of MYD88 L265P in peripheral blood of patients with Waldenström's Macroglobulinemia and IgM monoclonal gammopathy of undetermined significance. *Leukemia*. 2014;28(8):1698-1704.
41. Cao Y, Hunter ZR, Liu X, et al. The WHIM-like CXCR4(S338X) somatic mutation activates AKT and ERK, and promotes resistance to ibrutinib and other agents used in the treatment of Waldenström's Macroglobulinemia. *Leukemia*. 2015;29(1):169-176.
42. Roccaro AM, Sacco A, Jimenez C, et al. C1013G/CXCR4 acts as a driver mutation of tumor progression and modulator of drug resistance in lymphoplasmacytic lymphoma. *Blood*. 2014;123(26):4120-4131.
43. Treon SP, Cao Y, Xu L, Yang G, Liu X, Hunter ZR. Somatic mutations in MYD88 and CXCR4 are determinants of clinical presentation and overall survival in Waldenström macroglobulinemia. *Blood*. 2014;123(18):2791-2796.
44. Treon SP, Xu L, Guerrera ML, et al. Genomic landscape of Waldenström macroglobulinemia and Its Impact on treatment strategies. *J Clin Oncol*. 2020;38(11):1198-1208.
45. Chng WJ, Schop RF, Price-Troska T, et al. Gene-expression profiling of Waldenström macroglobulinemia reveals a phenotype more similar to chronic lymphocytic leukemia than multiple myeloma. *Blood*. 2006;108(8):2755-2763.
46. Gutierrez NC, Ocio EM, de Las Rivas J, et al. Gene expression profiling of B lymphocytes and plasma cells from Waldenström's macroglobulinemia: comparison with expression patterns of the same cell counterparts from chronic lymphocytic leukemia, multiple myeloma and normal individuals. *Leukemia*. 2007;21(3):541-549.
47. Hodge DR, Hurt EM, Farrar WL. The role of IL-6 and STAT3 in inflammation and cancer. *Eur J Cancer*. 2005;41(16):2502-2512.
48. Ciccarelli BT, Patterson CJ, Hunter ZR, et al. Hepcidin is produced by lymphoplasmacytic cells and is associated with anemia in Waldenström's macroglobulinemia. *Clin Lymphoma Myeloma Leuk*. 2011;11(1):160-163.
49. Elsawa SF, Novak AJ, Ziesmer SC, et al. Comprehensive analysis of tumor microenvironment cytokines in Waldenström macroglobulinemia identifies CCL5 as a novel modulator of IL-6 activity. *Blood*. 2011;118(20):5540-5549.
50. Hodge LS, Ansell SM. Jak/Stat pathway in Waldenström's macroglobulinemia. *Clin Lymphoma Myeloma Leuk*. 2011;11(1):112-114.
51. Garcia-Sanz R, Montoto S, Torrequebrada A. Spanish Group for the Study of Waldenström Macroglobulinaemia and PETHEMA, et al. Waldenström macroglobulinaemia: presenting features and outcome in a series with 217 cases. *Br J Haematol*. 2001;115(3):575-582.
52. Stone MJ, Pascual V. Pathophysiology of Waldenström's macroglobulinemia. *Haematologica*. 2010;95(3):359-364.
53. Nobile-Orazio E, Marmiroli P, Baldini L, et al. Peripheral neuropathy in macroglobulinemia: incidence and antigen-specificity of M proteins. *Neurology*. 1987;37(9):1506-1514.
54. Rudnicki SA, Harik SI, Dhodapkar M, et al. Nervous system dysfunction in Waldenström's macroglobulinemia: response to treatment. *Neurology*. 1998;51(4):1210-1213.
55. Baehring JM, Hochberg EP, Raje N, Ulrickson M, Hochberg FH. Neurological manifestations of Waldenström macroglobulinemia. *Nat Clin Pract Neurol*. 2008;4(10):547-556.
56. Simon L, Fitsiori A, Lemal R, et al. Bing-Neel syndrome, a rare complication of Waldenström macroglobulinemia: analysis of 44 cases and review of the literature. A study on behalf of the French Innovative Leukemia Organization (FILO). *Haematologica*. 2015;100(12):1587-1594.
57. Minnema MC, Kimby E, D'Sa S, et al. Guideline for the diagnosis, treatment and response criteria for Bing-Neel syndrome. *Haematologica*. 2017;102(1):43-51.
58. Higgins L, Nasr SH, Said SM, et al. Kidney Involvement of patients with Waldenström macroglobulinemia and other IgM-producing B cell lymphoproliferative disorders. *Clin J Am Soc Nephrol*. 2018;13(7):1037-1046.
59. Michael AB, Lawes M, Kamalarajan M, Huissoon A, Pratt G. Cryoglobulinaemia as an acute presentation of Waldenström's macroglobulinaemia. *Br J Haematol*. 2004;124(5):565.
60. Gertz MA, Kyle RA, Noel P. Primary systemic amyloidosis: a rare complication of immunoglobulin M monoclonal gammopathies and Waldenström's macroglobulinemia. *J Clin Oncol*. 1993;11(5):914-920.
61. Morel P, Duhamel A, Gobbi P, et al. International prognostic scoring system for Waldenström macroglobulinemia. *Blood*. 2009;113(18):4163-4170.
62. Kyle RA, Treon SP, Alexanian R, et al. Prognostic markers and criteria to initiate therapy in Waldenström's macroglobulinemia: consensus panel recommendations from the Second International Workshop on Waldenström's Macroglobulinemia. *Semin Oncol*. 2003;30(2):116-120.
63. Owen RG, Kyle RA, Stone MJ, et al. Response assessment in Waldenström macroglobulinaemia: update from the VIth International Workshop. *Br J Haematol*. 2013;160(2):171-176.
64. Gertz MA, Rue M, Blood E, Kaminer LS, Vesole DH, Greipp PR. Multicenter phase 2 trial of rituximab for Waldenström macroglobulinemia (WM): an Eastern Cooperative Oncology Group Study (E3A98). *Leuk Lymphoma*. 2004;45(10):2047-2055.
65. Ghobrial IM, Fonseca R, Greipp PR, et al. Initial immunoglobulin M 'flare' after rituximab therapy in patients diagnosed with Waldenström macroglobulinemia: an Eastern Cooperative Oncology Group Study. *Cancer*. 2004;101(11):2593-2598.
66. Schwartz J, Padmanabhan A, Aqui N, et al. Guidelines on the use of therapeutic apheresis in clinical practice-evidence-based approach from the Writing committee of the American society for apheresis: the seventh special Issue. *J Clin Apher*. 2016;31(3):149-162.
67. Tedeschi A, Benevolo G, Varettoni M, et al. Fludarabine plus cyclophosphamide and rituximab in Waldenström macroglobulinemia: an effective but myelosuppressive regimen to be offered to patients with advanced disease. *Cancer*. 2012;118(2):434-443.
68. Treon SP, Branagan AR, Ioakimidis L, et al. Long-term outcomes to fludarabine and rituximab in Waldenström macroglobulinemia. *Blood*. 2009;113(16):3673-3678.
69. Leleu X, Soumerai J, Roccaro A, et al. Increased incidence of transformation and myelodysplasia/acute leukemia in patients with Waldenström macroglobulinemia treated with nucleoside analogs. *J Clin Oncol*. 2009;27(2):250-255.
70. Annibali O, Petrucci MT, Martini V, et al. Treatment of 72 newly diagnosed Waldenström macroglobulinemia cases with oral melphalan, cyclophosphamide, and prednisone: and cost analysis. *Cancer*. 2005;103(3):582-587.
71. Petrucci MT, Avvisati G, Tribalto M, Giovangrossi P, Mandelli F. Waldenström's macroglobulinaemia: results of a combined oral treatment in 34 newly diagnosed patients. *J Intern Med*. 1989;226(6):443-447.
72. Leblond V, Levy V, Maloisel F; French Cooperative Group on Chronic Lymphocytic Leukemia and Macroglobulinemia, et al. Multicenter, randomized comparative trial of fludarabine and the combination of cyclophosphamide-doxorubicin-prednisone in 92 patients with Waldenström macroglobulinemia in first relapse or with primary refractory disease. *Blood*. 2001;98(9):2640-2644.
73. Buske C, Hoster E, Dreyling M; German Low-Grade Lymphoma Study Group, et al. The addition of rituximab to front-line therapy with CHOP (R-CHOP) results in a higher response rate and longer time to treatment failure in patients with lymphoplasmacytic lymphoma: results of a randomized trial of the German Low-Grade Lymphoma Study Group (GLSG). *Leukemia*. 2009;23(1):153-161.
74. Dimopoulos MA, Anagnostopoulos A, Kyrtsonis MC, et al. Primary treatment of Waldenström macroglobulinemia with dexamethasone, rituximab, and cyclophosphamide. *J Clin Oncol*. 2007;25(22):3344-3349.
75. Tedeschi A, Picardi P, Ferrero S, et al. Bendamustine and rituximab combination is safe and effective as salvage regimen in Waldenström macroglobulinemia. *Leuk Lymphoma*. 2015;56(9):2637-2642.
76. Rummel MJ, Niederle N, Maschmeyer G; Study Group Indolent Lymphomas, et al. Bendamustine plus rituximab versus CHOP plus rituximab as first-line treatment for patients with indolent and mantle-cell lymphomas: an open-label, multicentre, randomised, phase 3 non-inferiority trial. *Lancet*. 2013;381(9873):1203-1210.
77. Laribi K, Poulain S, Willems L, et al. Bendamustine plus rituximab in newly-diagnosed Waldenström macroglobulinaemia patients. A study on behalf of the French Innovative Leukaemia Organization (FILO). *Br J Haematol*. 2019;186(1):146-149.
78. Treon SP, Ioakimidis L, Soumerai JD, et al. Primary therapy of Waldenström macroglobulinemia with bortezomib, dexamethasone, and rituximab: WMCTG clinical trial 05-180. *J Clin Oncol*. 2009;27(23):3830-3835.
79. Dimopoulos MA, García-Sanz R, Gavriatopoulou M, et al. Primary therapy of Waldenström macroglobulinemia (WM) with weekly bortezomib, low-dose dexamethasone, and rituximab (BDR): long-term results of a phase 2 study of the European Myeloma Network (EMN). *Blood*. 2013;122(19):3276-3282.
80. Ghobrial IM, Xie W, Padmanabhan S, et al. Phase II trial of weekly bortezomib in combination with rituximab in untreated patients with Waldenström Macroglobulinemia. *Am J Hematol*. 2010;85(9):670-674.
81. Leblebjian H, Noonan K, Paba-Prada C, Treon SP, Castillo JJ, Ghobrial IM. Cyclophosphamide, bortezomib, and dexamethasone combination in Waldenström macroglobulinemia. *Am J Hematol*. 2015;90(6):E122-E123.
82. Treon SP, Tripsas CK, Meid K, et al. Carfilzomib, rituximab, and dexamethasone (CaRD) treatment offers a neuropathy-sparing approach for treating Waldenström's macroglobulinemia. *Blood*. 2014;124(4):503-510.
83. Castillo JJ, Meid K, Flynn CA, et al. Ixazomib, dexamethasone, and rituximab in treatment-naive patients with Waldenström macroglobulinemia: long-term follow-up. *Blood Adv*. 2020;4(16):3952-3959.
84. Treon SP, Tripsas CK, Meid K, et al. Ibrutinib in previously treated Waldenström's macroglobulinemia. *N Engl J Med*. 2015;372(15):1430-1440.
85. Dimopoulos MA, Trotman J, Tedeschi A; iNNOVATE Study Group and the European Consortium for Waldenström's Macroglobulinemia, et al. Ibrutinib for patients with rituximab-refractory Waldenström's macroglobulinaemia (iNNOVATE): an open-label substudy of an international, multicentre, phase 3 trial. *Lancet Oncol*. 2017;18(2):241-250.
86. Dimopoulos MA, Tedeschi A, Trotman J, et al. Phase 3 trial of Ibrutinib plus rituximab in Waldenström's macroglobulinemia. *N Engl J Med*. 2018;378(25):2399-2410.
87. Tam CS, Opat S, D'Sa S, et al. A randomized phase 3 trial of zanubrutinib vs ibrutinib in symptomatic Waldenström macroglobulinemia: the ASPEN study. *Blood*. 2020;136(18):2038-2050.

88. Trotman J, Opat S, Gottlieb D, et al. Zanubrutinib for the treatment of patients with Waldenström macroglobulinemia: 3 years of follow-up. *Blood*. 2020;136(18):2027-2037.
89. Owen RG, McCarthy H, Rule S, et al. Acalabrutinib monotherapy in patients with Waldenström macroglobulinemia: a single-arm, multicentre, phase 2 study. *Lancet Haematol*. 2020;7(2):e112-e121.
90. Xu L, Tsakmaklis N, Yang G, et al. Acquired mutations associated with ibrutinib resistance in Waldenström macroglobulinemia. *Blood*. 2017;129(18):2519-2525.
91. Treon SP, Gustine J, Meid K, et al. Ibrutinib monotherapy in symptomatic, treatment-naïve patients with Waldenström macroglobulinemia. *J Clin Oncol*. 2018;36(27):2755-2761.
92. Davids MS, Roberts AW, Seymour JF, et al. Phase I first-in-human study of venetoclax in patients with relapsed or refractory non-hodgkin lymphoma. *J Clin Oncol*. 2017;35(8):826-833.
93. Davids MS, Roberts AW, Kenkre VP, et al. Long-term follow-up of patients with relapsed or refractory non-hodgkin lymphoma treated with venetoclax in a phase I, first-in-human study. *Clin Cancer Res*. 2021;27(17):4690-4695. doi:10.1158/1078-0432.CCR-20-4842
94. Ghobrial IM, Gertz M, Laplant B, et al. Phase II trial of the oral mammalian target of rapamycin inhibitor everolimus in relapsed or refractory Waldenström macroglobulinemia. *J Clin Oncol*. 2010;28(8):1408-1414.
95. Treon SP, Meid K, Tripsas C, et al. Prospective, multicenter clinical trial of everolimus as primary therapy in Waldenström macroglobulinemia (WMCTG 09-214). *Clin Cancer Res*. 2017;23(10):2400-2404.
96. Matasar MJ, Capra M, Özcan M, et al. Copanlisib plus rituximab versus placebo plus rituximab in patients with relapsed indolent non-Hodgkin lymphoma (CHRONOS-3): a double-blind, randomised, placebo-controlled, phase 3 trial. *Lancet Oncol*. 2021;22(5):678-689.
97. Cheson BD. Ofatumumab, a novel anti-CD20 monoclonal antibody for the treatment of B-cell malignancies. *J Clin Oncol*. 2010;28(21):3525-3530.
98. Furman RR, Eradat HA, DiRienzo CG, et al. Once-weekly ofatumumab in untreated or relapsed Waldenström macroglobulinaemia: an open-label, single-arm, phase 2 study. *Lancet Haematol*. 2017;4(1):e24-e34.
99. Treon SP, Meid K, Hunter ZR, et al. Phase I study of Ibrutinib and the CXCR4 antagonist ulocuplumab in CXCR4 mutated Waldenström macroglobulinemia. *Blood*. 2021;138(17):1535-1539. doi:10.1182/blood.2021012953
100. Gertz MA, Reeder CB, Kyle RA, Ansell SM. Stem cell transplant for Waldenström macroglobulinemia: an underutilized technique. *Bone Marrow Transplant*. 2012;47(9):1147-1153.
101. Kyriakou C, Canals C, Sibon D, et al. High-dose therapy and autologous stem-cell transplantation in Waldenström macroglobulinemia: the lymphoma working party of the European group for blood and marrow transplantation. *J Clin Oncol*. 2010;28(13):2227-2232.
102. Kyriakou C, Boumendil A, Finel H, et al. Autologous stem cell transplantation (ASCT) for the treatment of patients with Waldenström's macroglobulinemia/ lymphoplasmacytic lymphoma (WM/LPL). A risk factor analysis by the European Society for Blood and Marrow Transplantation (EBMT) lymphoma work. *Blood*. 2014;124:678.
103. Kyriakou C, Canals C, Cornelissen JJ, et al. Allogeneic stem-cell transplantation in patients with Waldenström macroglobulinemia: report from the lymphoma working party of the European group for blood and marrow transplantation. *J Clin Oncol*. 2010;28(33):4926-4934.
104. Cornell RF, Bachanova V, D'Souza A, et al. Allogeneic transplantation for relapsed Waldenström macroglobulinemia and lymphoplasmacytic lymphoma. *Biol Blood Marrow Transplant*. 2017;23(1):60-66.

Chapter 103 ■ Monoclonal Gammopathies of Clinical Significance

ANGELA DISPENZIERI • DAVID DINGLI • RAHMA WARSAM

INTRODUCTION

This chapter addresses plasma cell disorders that are not "malignant" but that cause significant morbidity and mortality. These entities are known as monoclonal gammopathies of clinical significance (MGCS). Typically, the bone marrows and monoclonal proteins of patients with MGCS when observed in isolation of the clinical scenario would be classified as monoclonal gammopathy of undetermined significance (MGUS); however, this label could be construed as a misnomer for patients with MGCS since their plasma cell disorder has determined significance—albeit not malignant significance. These entities can be broken down into three large categories based on their dominant pathological presentation: neurologic, dermatologic, and renal (*Figure 103.1*).

MONOCLONAL GAMMOPATHIES OF NEUROLOGICAL SIGNIFICANCE

The first step in a diagnostic evaluation should be to consider and exclude other causes of neuropathy. Since intervention often involves administering anticancer therapy in patients without malignancy, a diagnosis of monoclonal gammopathy–associated neuropathy should not be made lightly. The major MGCS considerations for a patient with neuropathy include amyloid light-chain (AL) amyloidosis (Chapter 101), POEMS syndrome, cryoglobulinemia, CANOMAD (chronic ataxic neuropathy, ophthalmoplegia, IgM paraprotein, cold agglutinins, and disialosyl antibodies), and DADS-M (distal, acquired, demyelinating, symmetric neuropathy with M-protein; formerly known as MGUS-associated peripheral neuropathy). The first three are diseases with multiple systemic manifestations, whereas the last two are primarily nerve related.

POEMS Syndrome

POEMS syndrome is a rare paraneoplastic syndrome due to an underlying plasma cell disorder. The acronym, which was coined by Bardwick in 1980,[1] refers to several, but not all, of the features of the syndrome: polyradiculoneuropathy, organomegaly, endocrinopathy, monoclonal plasma cell disorder, and skin changes. There are three important points that relate to this memorable acronym: (1) not all of the features within the acronym are required to make the diagnosis; (2) there are other important features not included in the

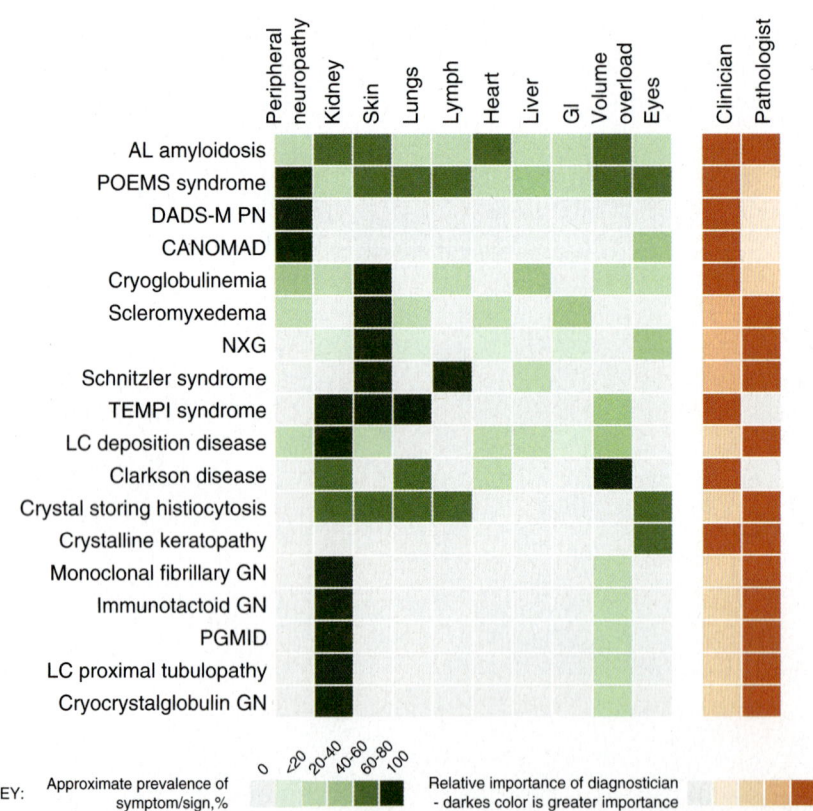

FIGURE 103.1 Organ involvement and diseases. CANOMAD, chronic ataxic neuropathy, ophthalmoplegia, IgM paraprotein, cold agglutinins, and disialosyl antibodies; DADS-M-PN, distal, acquired, demyelinating, symmetric neuropathy with M-protein; GN, glomerulonephritis; LC, light chain; NXG necrobiotic xanthogranuloma; PGNMID, proliferative glomerulonephritis with monoclonal immune deposition; POEMS, polyradiculoneuropathy, organomegaly, endocrinopathy, monoclonal protein, skin changes. (Used with permission of American Society of Hematology from Dispenzieri A. Monoclonal gammopathies of clinical significance. *Hematology Am Soc Hematol Educ Program.* 2020;2020(1):380-388; permission conveyed through Copyright Clearance Center, Inc.)

POEMS acronym, including *p*apilledema, *e*xtravascular volume overload, *s*clerotic bone lesions, *t*hrombocytosis/erythrocytosis (P.E.S.T.), elevated vascular endothelial growth factor (VEGF) levels, a predisposition toward thrombosis, and abnormal pulmonary function tests; and (3) there is a Castleman disease variant of POEMS syndrome that me be associated with a clonal plasma cell disorder. Other names of the POEMS syndrome that are less frequently used are osteosclerotic myeloma, Takatsuki syndrome, Crow-Fukase syndrome, and PEP (plasma cell dyscrasia, endocrinopathy, polyneuropathy) syndrome.[2,3]

The disease was initially thought to be more common in patients of Japanese descent given the largest initial reports from Japan.[2,3] However, over the years, large series have also been reported from other countries.[4] A national survey conducted in Japan in 2003 showed a prevalence of approximately 0.3 per 100,000.[5]

Etiology of POEMS Syndrome

The pathogenesis of the syndrome is not understood. Distinctive presenting characteristics of the syndrome that differentiate POEMS syndrome from standard multiple myeloma (MM) include the following: (1) dominant symptoms have little to nothing to do with bone pain, extremes of bone marrow infiltration by plasma cells, or renal failure; (2) dominant symptoms are typically neuropathy, endocrine dysfunction, and volume overload; (3) VEGF levels are high; (4) sclerotic bone lesions are present in the majority of cases; (5) overall survival is typically superior; and (6) lambda clones predominate.[6]

To date, VEGF is the cytokine that correlates best with disease activity, although it is likely not the driving force of the disease based on the mixed results seen with anti-VEGF therapy.[4] VEGF is known to target endothelial cells, induce a rapid and reversible increase in vascular permeability, and be important in angiogenesis. It is expressed by osteoblasts, in bone tissue, macrophages, malignant plasma cells,[7-9] and megakaryocytes/platelets.[10] Both interleukin (IL)-1ß and IL-6 have been shown to stimulate VEGF production.[7] Little is known about the plasma cells in POEMS syndrome except that more than 95% of the time they are lambda light chain restricted with restricted immunoglobulin light chain variable gene usage (*IGLV1*).[11,12] Lambda V domain usage is restricted to IGLV1-40, IGLV1-4, and IGVL1-36 variable gene, and stereotypic substitutions have also been observed including the H40→N in the FR2 region of IGV1-40 and T38→P/A substitution in the CDR1 of IGLV1-44.[13] Aneuploidy and deletion of chromosome 13 have been described, but hyperdiploidy is not seen.[14]

Diagnosis of POEMS Syndrome

The diagnosis is made based on a composite of clinical and laboratory features. The most notable symptoms include the constellation of neuropathy and any of the following: monoclonal protein (especially lambda light chain); thrombocytosis; anasarca; or papilledema. The requirements set forth in *Table 103.1* are designed to retain both sensitivity and specificity, potentially erring on the side of specificity. Making the diagnosis can be a challenge, but a good history and physical examination followed by appropriate testing—most notably radiographic assessment of bones,[19] measurement of VEGF,[20-24] and careful analysis of a bone marrow biopsy[25]—can differentiate this syndrome from other conditions like chronic inflammatory polyradiculoneuropathy (CIDP), MGUS neuropathy, and immunoglobulin light chain amyloid neuropathy. *Figure 103.2* demonstrates several classic findings among patients with POEMS syndrome.

Table 103.1. Diagnostic Criteria for Five Selected Syndromes

POEMS Syndrome[4,a]	Schnitzler Syndrome[15,e,f]	Necrobiotic Xanthogranuloma[16,k]
Mandatory major criteria 1. Polyneuropathy (typically demyelinating) 2. Monoclonal plasma cell-proliferative disorder (almost always lambda) *Major criteria* 3. Castleman disease[b] 4. Sclerotic bone lesions 5. Vascular endothelial growth factor elevation *Minor criteria* 6. Organomegaly (splenomegaly, hepatomegaly, or lymphadenopathy) 7. Extravascular volume overload (edema, pleural effusion, or ascites) 8. Endocrinopathy[c] (adrenal, thyroid, pituitary, gonadal, parathyroid, pancreatic) 9. Skin changes (hyperpigmentation, hypertrichosis, glomeruloid hemangiomata, plethora, lipodystrophy, acrocyanosis, flushing, white nails) 10. Papilledema 11. Thrombocytosis/polycythemia[d] **Other**: Clubbing, weight loss, hyperhidrosis, pulmonary hypertension/restrictive lung disease, thrombotic diatheses, diarrhea, low vitamin B_{12}	*Obligate criteria* 1. Chronic urticarial rash 2. Monoclonal IgM or IgG *Minor criteria* 3. Recurrent fever[g] 4. Objective findings of abnormal bone remodeling with or without bone pain[h] 5. A neutrophilic dermal infiltrate on skin biopsy[i] 6. Leukocytosis and/or elevated CRP[j] **Scleromyxedema**[17] 1. Generalized papular and sclerodermoid eruption 2. Evidence of monoclonal gammopathy 3. Microscopic triad associating dermal mucin deposition, thickened collagen, and fibroblast proliferation or an interstitial granuloma annulare-like pattern 4. Absence of thyroid disease	*Major criteria* 1. Cutaneous papules, plaques, and/or nodules, most often yellow or orange in color 2. Histopathological features demonstrating palisading granulomas with lympho-plasmacytic infiltrate and zones of necrobiosis. Variably present cholesterol clefts and/or giant cells *Minor criteria* 3. Periorbital distribution of cutaneous lesions 4. Paraproteinemia, most often IgG-κ, plasma-cell dyscrasia, and/or other associated lymphoproliferative disorder **TEMPI Syndrome**[18] **Major** 1. Telangiectasias 2. Monoclonal gammopathy 3. Elevated erythropoietin and erythrocytosis **Minor** 4. Perinephric fluid 5. Intrapulmonary shunting **Other**: Venous thrombosis

[a]POEMS syndrome diagnosis is confirmed when both of the mandatory major criteria, 1 of the 3 other major criteria, and 1 of the 6 minor criteria are present.
[b]There is a Castleman disease variant of POEMS syndrome that occurs without evidence of a clonal plasma cell disorder that is not accounted for in this table. This entity should be considered separately.
[c]Because of the high prevalence of diabetes mellitus and thyroid abnormalities, this diagnosis alone is not sufficient to meet this minor criterion.
[d]Approximately 50% of patients will have bone marrow changes that distinguish it from a typical MGUS or myeloma bone marrow. Anemia and/or thrombocytopenia are distinctively unusual in this syndrome unless Castleman disease is present.
[e]Definite diagnosis of Schnitzler syndrome. If IgM: both obligate criteria AND at least 2 minor criteria; if IgG: both obligate criteria AND 3 minor criteria.
[f]Probable diagnosis Schnitzler syndrome. If IgM: both obligate criteria AND 1 minor criteria; if IgG: both obligate criteria AND 2 minor criteria.
[g]Must be >38 °C, and otherwise unexplained. Occurs usually—but not obligatory—together with the skin rash.
[h]As assessed by bone scintigraphy, MRI or elevation of bone alkaline phosphatase.
[i]Corresponds usually to the entity described as "neutrophilic urticarial dermatosis"; absence of fibrinoid necrosis; and significant dermal edema.
[j]Neutrophils >10 000/mm^3 and/or CRP >30 mg/L.
[k]For necrobiotic xanthogranuloma diagnosis, both major criteria and at least 1 minor criterion, applicable only in the absence of foreign body, infection, or other identifiable cause.
Abbreviations: POEMS, polyneuropathy, organomegaly, endocrinopathy, M protein, skin changes; TEMPI, telangiectasias, elevated erythropoietin and erythropoiesis, monoclonal gammopathy, perinephric fluid, intrapulmonary shunting.

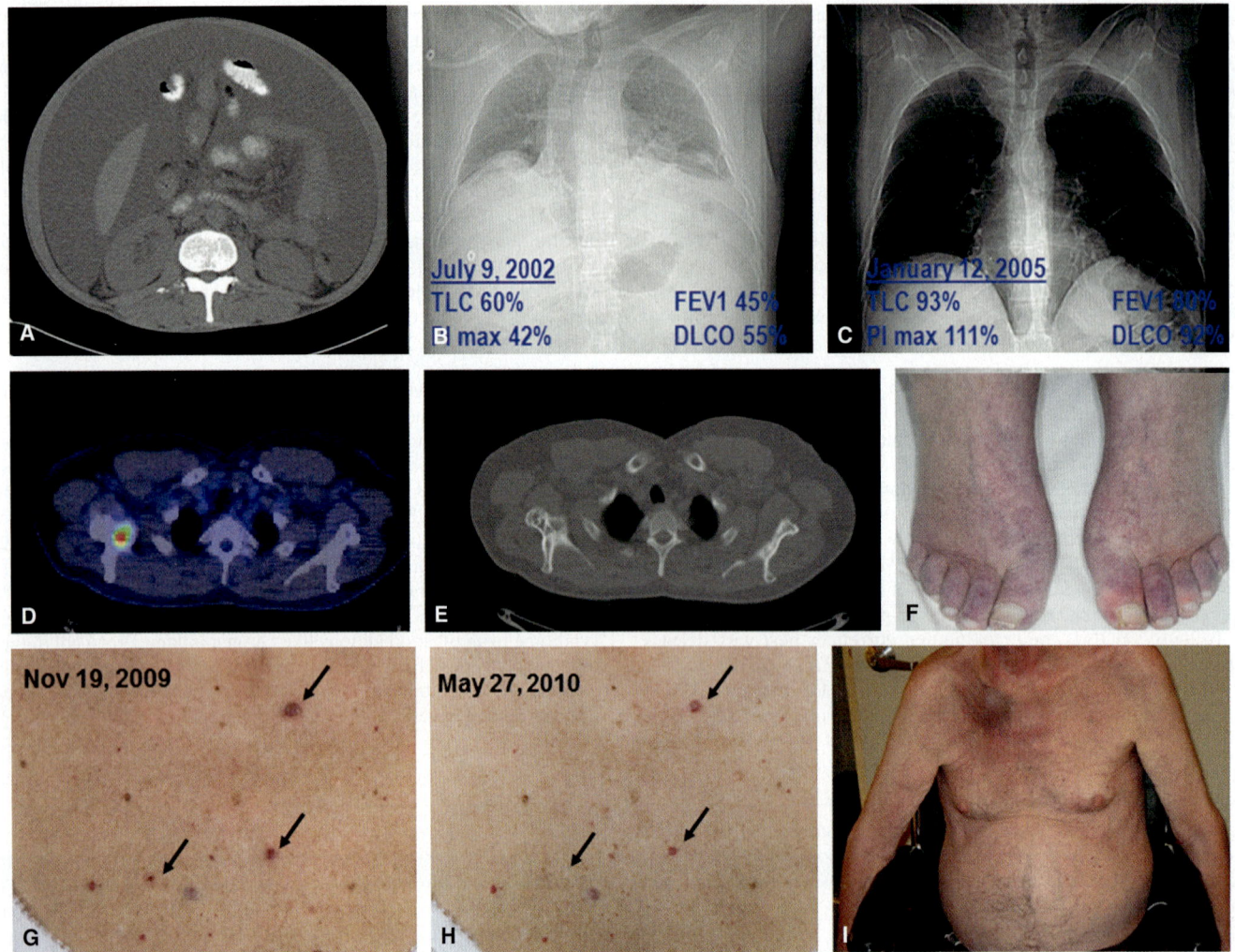

FIGURE 103.2 **Classic findings of POEMS syndromes.** A, Massive ascites and lipodystrophy. B, Chest radiograph and pulmonary function test results demonstrating reduced lung volumes due to neuromuscular weakness, small effusions, and reduced diffusing capacity of carbon monoxide. C, Improved chest radiograph and pulmonary function tests 2.5 years after autologous stem cell transplantation (same patient as H). D, Fusion CT PET of mixed lytic/sclerotic lesion in right scapula. E, Bone windows of CT of mixed lytic/sclerotic lesion in right scapula. F, Hyperemia of extremities and white nails. G, Outcropping of cherry angiomata at diagnosis. H, Shrinkage and disappearance of cherry angiomata after radiation to solitary osteosclerotic lesion right femur. I, Plasmacytoma right scapula with overlying erythema as well as gynecomastia, muscle wasting, and ascites. Also present but unrelated is florid tinea corporis due to chronic steroid used for the incorrect diagnosis of chronic inflammatory polyradiculoneuropathy. (Reprinted from Dispenzieri A. How I treat POEMS syndrome. *Blood.* 2012;119(24):5650-5658. Copyright © 2012 American Society of Hematology. With permission.)

Clinical Presentation of POEMS Syndrome

Polyradiculoneuropathy

The peripheral neuropathy is the dominant characteristic.[2,3,26-28] It is ascending, symmetrical, and affecting both sensation and motor function.[29] In our experience, pain may be a dominant feature in about 10% to 15% of patients, though in one report as many as 76% of patients had painful neuropathy.[5,30] Nerve conduction studies in patients with POEMS syndrome show slowing of nerve conduction that is more predominant in the intermediate than distal nerve segments as compared to CIDP, and there is more severe attenuation of compound muscle action potentials in the lower than upper limbs.[5,31,32] In contrast to CIDP, conduction block is rare.[5,32] The conduction findings suggest that demyelination is predominant in the nerve trunk rather than the distal nerve terminals, and axonal loss is predominant in the lower limb nerves.[5] Axonal loss is greater in POEMS syndrome than it is in CIDP.[32] The nerve biopsy is not specific, but uncompacted myelin lamellae, endothelial cytoplasmic enlargement, opening of the tight junctions between endothelial cells and presence of many pinocytic vesicles adjacent to the cell membranes, absence of macrophage-associated demyelination have been described.[33,34] As compared to CIDP, POEMS syndrome demonstrates more axonal degeneration and epineurial neovascularization but less endoneurial inflammation and onion-bulb formation.[35]

Organomegaly, Endocrinopathy, Skin Changes, Papilledema, and Extravascular Overload

Depending on the series, 45% to 85% of patients will have any combination of splenomegaly, hepatomegaly, and/or lymphadenopathy. The histology of the liver and spleen tends to be nonspecific. Lymph nodes may appear reactive or reveal frank Castleman disease or merely "Castleman disease-like" changes. Historically, it was estimated that 11% to 30% of POEMS patients with documented clonal plasma cell disorder also have documented Castleman disease or Castleman-like histology.[4] Among individuals with POEMS who undergo lymph node biopsy, about 50% show angiofollicular hyperplasia typical of Castleman disease,[3,28] and 84% of these are hyaline vascular type.[28] Only those with peripheral neuropathy AND a plasma cell clone should classified as standard POEMS syndrome; without both, patients can be classified as Castleman disease variant of POEMS if they have other POEMS features.[4]

Endocrinopathy is a central but poorly understood feature of POEMS. In one series,[36] approximately 84% of patients had a recognized endocrinopathy, with hypogonadism as the most common endocrine abnormality, followed by thyroid abnormalities, glucose metabolism abnormalities, and lastly by adrenal insufficiency. The majority of patients have evidence of multiple endocrinopathies in the four major endocrine axes (gonadal, thyroid, glucose, and adrenal). Gynecomastia may be present on physical examination.

The characteristic skin changes include hyperpigmentation, a recent outcropping of hemangioma, hypertrichosis, dependent rubor and acrocyanosis, white nails, sclerodermoid changes, facial lipodystrophy, flushing, or clubbing.[4] Rarely calciphylaxis is also seen. The histologic findings of the dermis have been reported to range from nonspecific to glomeruloid hemangiomata to vascular abnormalities in apparently normal dermis.[37-39]

Papilledema is present in at least one-third of patients[40]; the majority of these patients do not have specific symptoms relating to this finding but a minority will report blurred vision, diplopia, or ocular pain.

Peripheral edema, ascites, and effusions are the symptoms and signs that cause the next most morbidity after the peripheral neuropathy. The manifestations of extravascular overload occur in 29% to 87% of patients with POEMS syndrome and are not typically associated with severe hypoalbuminemia. Severe third spacing can lead to worsening renal function. Serum creatinine levels are normal in most cases, but serum cystatin C, which is a surrogate marker for renal function, is high in 71% of patients.[41] In our experience, at presentation, fewer than 10% of patients have proteinuria exceeding 0.5 g/24 hours, and only 6% have a serum creatinine greater than or equal to 1.5 mg/dL. Four percent of patients developed renal failure as preterminal events.[27] In a series from China, 22% of patients had a creatinine clearance (CrCl) of less than 60 mL/min including 8% with a CrCl of less than 30 mL/min; 10% had microhematuria.[42] The renal histologic findings are diverse with membranoproliferative features and evidence of endothelial injury being most common.[43] On both light and electron microscopy, mesangial expansion, narrowing of capillary lumina, basement membrane thickening, subendothelial deposits, widening of the sub-endothelial space, swelling and vacuolization of endothelial cells, and mesangiolysis predominate.[44] Standard immunofluorescence is negative, which differentiates it from primary membranoproliferative glomerulitis.[43] Rarely infiltration by plasma cells nests or Castleman-like lymphoma has been described.[44]

Monoclonal Plasma Cell Disorder, Sclerotic Bone Lesions, and Myeloproliferation

Finding the monoclonal plasma cell disorder can sometimes be a challenge. In one series, only 53% percent of patients had a positive protein electrophoresis, with another 31% being immunoelectrophoresis positively only, and 16% had their clone discovered only by either bone marrow biopsy or biopsy of a plasmacytoma, that is bone lesion.[27]

Among patients with POEMS syndrome, the complete blood count is notable for an absence of cytopenias. In fact, nearly half of patients will have thrombocytosis or erythrocytosis.[27] In a series from China, 26% of patients had anemia, which the authors attributed to impaired renal function.[28] Their series was enriched with Castleman disease cases (25%), which may have also contributed to this unprecedentedly high rate of anemia.

The bone marrow biopsy reveals megakaryocyte hyperplasia and megakaryocyte clustering in 54% and 93% of cases, respectively.[25] These megakaryocyte findings are reminiscent of a myeloproliferative disorder, but *JAK2* V617F mutation is uniformly absent. One-third of patients do not have clonal plasma cells on their iliac crest biopsy. These are the patients who present with a solitary or "multiple solitary plasmacytomas." The median percent of plasma cells observed is less than 5%. Immunohistochemical staining is more sensitive than is six-color flow since the former provides information on bone marrow architecture, which is key in making the diagnosis in nearly half of cases. In our study of 67 pretreatment bone marrow biopsies from patients with POEMS syndrome, lymphoid aggregates were found in 49% of cases. Of these, there was plasma cell rimming in all but one; and of these 32 cases, 31 were clonal lambda and 1 was kappa. This finding was not seen in bone marrows from normal controls or from patients with MGUS, MM, or amyloidosis. Overall, only 8/67 (12%) of POEMS cases had normal iliac crest bone marrow biopsies, that is no detectable clonal plasma cells, no plasma cell rimmed lymphoid aggregates, and no megakaryocyte hyperplasia.

Osteosclerotic lesions occur in approximately 95% of patients, and can be confused with benign bone islands, aneurysmal bone cysts, nonossifying fibromas, and fibrous dysplasia.[3,27] Some lesions are densely sclerotic, while others are lytic with a sclerotic rim, while still others have a mixed soap-bubble appearance. Occasionally patients with have a lytic lesion without any evident sclerosis. Bone windows of CT body images are often very informative,[45] often even more so than FDG-uptake, which can be variable and most useful when there is an obvious lytic component to the bone lesion.

Elevated VEGF and Other Cytokines

Plasma and serum levels of VEGF are markedly elevated in patients with POEMS[7,24,46] and correlate with the activity of the disease.[7,20,21,24] The principal isoform of VEGF expressed is VEGF165.[20] VEGF levels are independent of M-protein size.[20] IL-1ß, TNF-α, IL-6, and IL-12 levels are often also increased.[47] Serum VEGF levels are 10 to 50 times higher than plasma levels of VEGF,[48] making it unclear which test is preferred. In patients with POEMS, VEGF is found in both plasma cells[8,9] and platelets.[49] The higher level observed in serum is attributable to the release of VEGF from platelets in vitro during serum processing. Our group has demonstrated that a plasma VEGF level of 200 pg/mL had a specificity of 95% with a sensitivity of 68% in support of a diagnosis of POEMS syndrome. Other diseases with high VEGF include connective tissue disease and vasculitis.[24]

Pulmonary and Coagulation Abnormalities

Respiratory complaints are usually limited given patients' neurologic status impairing their ability to induce cardiovascular challenges.[50] The pulmonary manifestations are protean, including pulmonary hypertension, restrictive lung disease, impaired neuromuscular respiratory function, and impaired diffusion capacity of carbon monoxide, but improve with effective therapy.[28,50,51] Pulmonary hypertension has been reported to occur in 27% of unselected patients with POEMS syndrome.[52] Finger-nail clubbing is seen in about 4% to 49% of cases.[3,50]

Patients are at increased risk for arterial and/or venous thromboses during their course, with nearly 20% of patients experiencing one of these complications.[6,53,54] Ten percent of patients present with a cerebrovascular event, most commonly embolic or vessel dissection and stenosis.[55] Thrombocytosis, erythrocytosis, and increased bone marrow infiltration are associated with risk for cerebrovascular accidents.[54,55] Aberrations in the coagulation cascade have been implicated in POEMS syndrome, but are not usually clinically apparent.[34]

Treatment of POEMS Syndrome

Despite the relationship between disease response and dropping levels of VEGF, the most experience with successful outcomes has been associated with directing therapy at the underlying clonal plasma cell disorder rather than solely targeting VEGF with anti-VEGF antibodies. The treatment algorithm is based on the extent of the plasma cell infiltration (*Figure 103.3*). The approach to therapy differs based on whether there is bone marrow involvement as determined by blind iliac crest sampling.[56]

The course of POEMS syndrome is usually chronic with an estimated 10-year survivorship rate of 77% to 79%[57,58] and of more than 90% for those who undergo autologous stem cell transplantation (ASCT).[27,50,59] Baseline risk factors for inferior survival have included fingernail clubbing, extravascular volume overload,[27] low serum albumin,[58] coexistent Castleman disease,[28] and respiratory symptoms.[50] In a publication from China of 362 patients, factors associated with inferior survival were age, pulmonary hypertension, pleural effusion, and estimated glomerular filtration rate < 30 mL/min/1.73 m^2. The

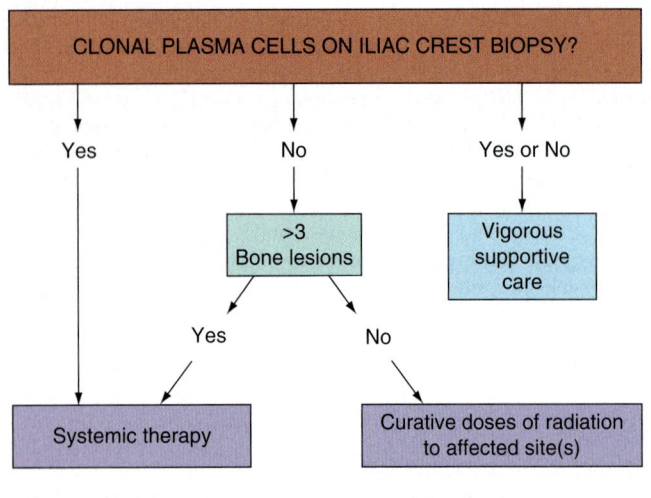

FIGURE 103.3 Algorithm for the treatment of POEMS Syndrome. (Reprinted from Dispenzieri A. How I treat POEMS syndrome. *Blood.* 2012;119(24):5650-5658. Copyright © 2012 American Society of Hematology. With permission.)

number of POEMS features does not affect survival.[6,26] Factors contributing to a shorter progression-free survival include low albumin and lack of achieving a complete hematologic response.[59]

Management of POEMS Syndrome Without Disseminated Bone Marrow Involvement

In the case of patients with an isolated bone lesion without clonal plasma cells found on iliac crest biopsy, radiation is the recommended therapy as it is in the case of a more straightforward solitary plasmacytoma of bone. Not only does radiation to an isolated (or even two or three isolated) lesion(s) improve the symptoms of POEMS syndrome over the course of 3 to 36 months, but it can be curative.

Management of POEMS Syndrome With Disseminated Bone Marrow Involvement

Typically, once there is disseminated disease identified, systemic therapy is recommended with the caveat that large bony lesions with a significant lytic component may require adjuvant radiation therapy.[56] Decisions about adjuvant radiation should be made on a case-by-case basis, and typically not until a minimal of 6 months after completing chemotherapy. It is important to remember that the there is a lag between completion of successful therapy and neurologic response, often with no discernible improvement until 6 months after completion of therapy. Maximal response is not seen until 2 to 3 years hence. Other features like anasarca, papilledema, and skin changes may improve sooner. Optimal FDG-PET response may also lag by 6 to 12 months.

Since there is a paucity of clinical trials among patients with POEMS syndrome,[60-64] treatment recommendations are largely based on case series and anecdote. The treatment armamentarium is borrowed from other plasma cell disorders. *Table 103.2* summarizes regimens and observed outcomes. Corticosteroids may provide symptomatic improvement, but response duration is limited. The most experience has been with alkylator-based therapy, either low dose or high dose with peripheral blood stem cell transplant. The first prospective clinical trial to treat POEMS syndrome was reported from China.[65] Thirty-one patients were treated with 12 cycles of melphalan and dexamethasone and 81% of patients achieved hematologic response, 100% had VEGF response, and 100% had at least some improvement in neurologic status. At 21 months, 100% were progression free and alive. Personal experience and retrospective reports of the use of cyclophosphamide-based therapy are also promising.[56]

High-dose alkylator with peripheral blood stem cell transplant can also be quite effective, but selection basis may confound these reports.[60] Case series suggest 100% of patients achieve at least some neurologic improvement. Doses of melphalan ranging from 140 to 200 mg/m^2 have been used, with the lower doses used for sicker patients. In addition, tandem transplant has been applied in one patient, but again, no information is available regarding any added value of the second transplant. In one series, progression-free survival was 98%, 94%, and 75% at 1, 2, and 5 years, respectively.[66] Symptomatic progressions were rare, whereas radiographic and VEGF progressions were most common. Treatment-related morbidity and mortality can be minimized by recognizing and treating an engraftment-type syndrome characterized by fevers, rash, diarrhea, weight gain, and respiratory symptoms and signs that occur anytime between days 7 and 15 post–stem cell infusion.[67] In an EBMT series, engraftment syndrome was reported in 23% of patients. Survival figures were comparable to that seen in the Mayo series.[68]

Misawa and colleagues conducted a randomized, double-blind, placebo-controlled phase 2/3 trial for patients with POEMS syndrome who were not candidates for ASCT.[63] Twenty-five patients were randomized to either daily thalidomide plus 4 days of dexamethasone every 4 weeks or placebo and 4 days of dexamethasone for 24 weeks; thereafter all patients received open-label, single-agent thalidomide for 48 weeks. Patients treated with thalidomide had higher rates of VEGF reduction, greater change in summated muscle test scores, and smaller changes in SF-36 QoL physical function and physical scores. Not surprisingly, side effects including sinus bradycardia, constipation, and mild sensory neuropathy were more frequent in patients treated with thalidomide.

Table 103.2. Activity of Therapy for the Treatment of POEMS Syndrome

Regimen	Outcome
Radiation	50%-70% of patients have significant clinical improvement
Melphalan-dexamethasone	81% hematologic response rate; 100% with some neurologic improvement
Corticosteroids	50% of patients have significant clinical improvement
Cyclophosphamide-dexamethasone	At least 50% of patients have significant improvement
ASCT	100% of surviving patients have significant clinical improvement
Thalidomide-dexamethasone	Reported responses in 12 patients, but not recommended as first line due to risk of neuropathy. Additional 25 patients treated in randomized trial with cross-over revealed improved VEGF and motor function.[63]
Lenalidomide-dexamethasone	75%-95% patients have significant clinical improvement and VEGF improvement
Bortezomib	Nearly 100% in combination with cyclophosphamide and dexamethasone. Caution regarding risk of worsening neuropathy. Usually used after first line.
Bevacizumab	No consistent benefit

Modified from Dispenzieri A. POEMS syndrome: 2021 Update on diagnosis, risk-stratification, and management. *Am J Hematol.* 2021;96(7):872-888. Copyright © 2021 Wiley Periodicals LLC. Reprinted by permission of John Wiley & Sons, Inc.

Lenalidomide has also yielded favorable results, seemingly with fewer side effects. As part of a phase II study, Li et al treated 41 patients with 12 cycles of lenalidomide and dexamethasone. The hematologic complete response rate was 46%, neurologic response 95%, and VEGF response rate was 83%. With a median follow-up of 34 months, 3-year PFS was 75% and 3-year survival was 90%.[69] The French have reported in abstract form their results of a phase 2 study of lenalidomide and dexamethasone for 2 cycles as neoadjuvant therapy preceding radiation or high-dose therapy or as primary therapy as 9 cycles followed by 12 cycles of single agent lenalidomide.[70] They treated 27 patients: 10 preradiation therapy; 8 pre-ASCT; and 9 as primary therapy. Although follow-up is short, the authors report that several patients had rapid neurological response, no patient has died, and 1 patient has progressed. These results are similar to case reports and case series.[71-73] In the largest case series of 20 patients,[73] all patients responded, but 4 patients relapsed 3 to 10 months after the end of treatment. Another retrospective case series of 12 patients with relapsed or refractory POEMS syndrome treated with lenalidomide and dexamethasone reported a 2-year PFS and overall survival of 92%.[74] A systematic review of lenalidomide use in patients with POEMS has been published,[75] which estimates a 1- and 2-year PFS of 92% and 42% using lenalidomide. Given the intrinsic risk patients with POEMS syndrome have for thrombosis, it is imperative that at least an aspirin be used for prophylaxis. The use of low molecular weight heparin or warfarin should be balanced against fall risk.

Like thalidomide and lenalidomide, bortezomib can have anti-VEGF and anti-TNF effects. Enthusiasm for thalidomide and bortezomib should be tempered by the high rate of peripheral neuropathy induced by these drugs. Bortezomib use has been reported in a limited number of patients, with favorable results, especially those with severe ascites.[60] Although an anti-VEGF strategy is appealing, the results with bevacizumab have been mixed. Most of the reports include patients who had also received either radiation or alkylator during and/or predating the bevacizumab had benefit.[56] Both our experience and the literature would support that single agent intravenous gammaglobulin (IVIG) or plasmapheresis is not helpful.

Managing Symptoms of Disease
Attention to supportive care is imperative. Orthotics, physical therapy, and CPAP all play an important role in patients' recovery. Ankle foot orthotics can increase mobility and reduce falls. Physical therapy reduces the risk for permanent contractures and leads to improved function both in the long and short term. For those with severe neuromuscular weakness, CPAP and/or biBAP provides better oxygenation and potentially reduces the risk complications associated with hypoventilation like pulmonary infection and pulmonary hypertension.

Monitoring Response
Patients must be followed carefully on a quarterly basis tracking the status of deficits comparing these to baseline.[66] VEGF responses may occur as soon as 3 months,[76] but they can be delayed. VEGF is an imperfect marker since discordance between disease activity and response have been reported,[77] so trends rather than absolute values should direct therapeutic decisions. Serum M-protein responses by protein electrophoresis, immunofixation electrophoresis, or serum immunoglobulin free light chains also pose a challenge. The size of the M-protein is typically small making standard MM response criteria inapplicable in most cases. In addition, patients can derive very significant clinical benefit in the absence of an M-protein response.[65,67] Finally, although the immunoglobulin free light chains are elevated in 90% of POEMS patients, the ratio is normal in all but 18%,[41] making the test of limited value for patients with POEMS syndrome.

Measuring organ response is complex since there are more than two-dozen parameters that can be assessed in a given patient with POEMS syndrome given the multisystem nature of the disease.[66,78] Response criteria for POEMS syndrome could be abridged as follows: (1) hematologic response using a modified amyloid response criteria; (2) VEGF response; and (3) a simplified organ response, which is limited to those systems causing the most morbidity, like peripheral neuropathy assessment, pulmonary function testing (diffusion capacity of carbon monoxide), and extravascular overload (grading ascites and pleural effusion as absent, mild, moderate, or severe).[4]

Distal, Acquired Demyelinating, Symmetric Neuropathy With M-protein
DADS-M was previously known as MGUS-associated peripheral neuropathy. Patients are most often male and in their 50 to 80s. They present with a distal, demyelinating symmetric neuropathy. Sensory ataxia is the most common sign. The IgM monoclonal gammopathy accounts for approximate 60% of neuropathies associated with monoclonal gammopathy.[79] Even in the presence of a monoclonal gammopathy, other explanations like inherited neuropathies, diabetes, alcoholism, and drugs should be ruled out.

Pathologic studies have identified demyelination and IgM deposits in the widened lamellae of myelin fibers and myelin debris contained in Schwann cells and macrophages. Even though these M-proteins may bind to myelin-associated glycoprotein (MAG) or other gangliosides, anti-MAG antibodies are not specific for peripheral neuropathy, and reduction in anti-MAG antibody titers with rituximab or other anti-CD20 antibodies has not correlated with clinical improvement. Treatments include IVIG and rituximab.

Two small, randomized trials have investigated the role of rituximab in IgM MGUS, MAG neuropathy, 80 patients total.[80,81] An improvement in neuropathy was noted in approximately 25% of patients.

Chronic Ataxic Neuropathy, Ophthalmoplegia, IgM Paraprotein, Cold Agglutinins, and Disialosyl Antibodies
CANOMAD is a rare condition characterized by a chronic neuropathy with sensory ataxia and IgM disialosyl antibodies.[82] Patients may or may not have motor weakness involving oculomotor and bulbar muscles or cold agglutinins. The most frequently targeted gangliosides are CD1b, GD3, GT1b, and GQ1b. Both axonal and demyelinating patterns have been recognized. The most effective therapies are IVIG, rituximab, and plasmapheresis.

Sporadic Late-Onset Nemaline Myopathy
Sporadic late-onset nemaline myopathy is a rare muscle disease that can be associated with a monoclonal protein or HIV infection.[83] It is not a neuropathy, but it does cause significant motor dysfunction. On biopsy, muscle fibers accumulate nemaline rods, and there is no associated inflammation. Patients present with predominantly proximal or axial muscle weakness, including respiratory muscle weakness. Treatment strategies include IVIG and plasma cell directed therapies, including ASCT.

MONOCLONAL GAMMOPATHIES OF DERMATOLOGIC SIGNIFICANCE

Schnitzler Syndrome
In the early 1970s, Liliane Schnitzler, described a clinical syndrome characterized by chronic urticaria in association with a monoclonal IgM.[84] Subsequent work by Lipsker[85] and de Koning[86] as well as the Schnitzler syndrome study group[15] led to a standardized definition of the syndrome and the Strasbourg criteria for diagnosis (Table 103.1). Most patients are in their sixth decade at diagnosis (range 30-76 in one series) and men are affected more than females (1.2:1).[87] The syndrome is almost certainly underrecognized and consequently there is considerable delay between the symptom onset and diagnosis.[15,87] Apart from the urticarial rash, other clinical features that are often present include malaise, fever, myalgia, arthralgia or bone pain, and enlarged lymph nodes. Symptoms of peripheral neuropathy may also be present (Figure 103.1).

Clinical Features
The urticarial eruption is typically recurrent and generally difficult to treat since it is either resistant to therapy or relapses fairly quickly once therapy is stopped. It presents as a macular eruption that is pale

rose in appearance and may develop into raised papules and plaques and be associated with mild to moderate pruritus. The urticaria generally resolves spontaneously within 24 hours without any scarring only to appear somewhere else. The trunk and proximal extremities are the main areas affected.[88] It is uncommon for a patient to be free of any skin lesions for more than a few weeks at a time. The eruption can be exacerbated by exposure to cold or heat, alcohol consumption, or even stress.[85] Angioedema is unusual and seen in less than 10% of patients.[85,87]

In one series, 75% of patients developed fever,[87] may reach 40 °C.[89] There is no direct relationship between the fever and the skin rash and in time, patients seem to get used to the recurrent pyrexia, perhaps due to the relative lack of associated chills, sweats (25%), and rigors.

Musculoskeletal symptoms are seen in at least two-thirds of patients, if not more.[86,87] In one series, arthralgias were reported in 68% of patients while bone pain has been reported in 63%. Lipsker initially reported a low frequency of peripheral neuropathy in this syndrome (1 patient)[90] but a larger series from a single institution found a frequency of 56% although in most cases this was mild.[87]

On physical examination, apart from the rash, other notable findings can include pallor due to anemia. Lymphadenopathy in found in approximately 45% of patients while enlargement of the liver and spleen are found in a third of patients.[15,85-87] The lymph nodes are mainly in the axillae and groin, can vary in size, and be up to several centimeters in diameter.

Laboratory Features

The presence of a monoclonal protein in the serum is required for diagnosis. The first reported patients had a monoclonal IgM in the serum,[84] but there are anecdotal reports of monoclonal IgA and IgG that otherwise fit the clinical syndrome.[89,91] The IgM is kappa light chain restricted in over 90% of patients. In one series the ratio of kappa to lambda light chain restriction was 15:1,[87] which is quite different from patients with IgM MGUS where the ratio is generally 56:44. The serum M-protein is generally below 1 g/dL. It is essential that serum immunofixation is performed to detect very small monoclonal proteins. In most patients, the uninvolved immunoglobulins (IgA and IgG) are normal. A monoclonal protein in the urine may be found in up to a third of patients. In the bone marrow the plasma cells constitute less than 10% (median of 4%) of the bone marrow cellularity and may even be polyclonal.[15,85-87]

At diagnosis, most patients will be anemic while leukocytosis and thrombocytosis (both reactive) are very common. The leukocytosis is invariably due to neutrophilia and resolves promptly with initiation of therapy. The sedimentation rate is generally quite high as is the C-reactive protein while serum ferritin is normal.[15,85-87] Complement levels are normal; if they are abnormal, one should suspect other diagnoses such as cryoglobulinemia, hypocomplementemic urticarial vasculitis, systemic lupus erythematosus, or perhaps a congenital deficiency of a complement component such as C4a.[15,85,86] C1 esterase inhibitor levels are generally normal.

Imaging Abnormalities

Early reports included plain imaging of the skeleton but techniques such as nuclear bone scanning, magnetic resonance imaging, and CT or PET/CT provide more sensitive. A radiologic abnormality may be found in 40% to 64% of patients.[92,93] A systematic radiologic analysis of a cohort of 22 patients suggested that the most commonly affected bones are the distal femur and the proximal tibia followed by the innominate bone.[92] Other bones that may be affected include the spine, humerus, talus, and fibula. The most common finding is bone sclerosis around the knee with the femur somewhat more likely to be affected compared to the tibia.[93] The pattern of sclerosis varies from trabecular thickening to patchy or confluent osteosclerosis. The sclerotic process always extends to involve the endosteum. Sometimes, the bone abnormality may be mixed with both sclerosis and lytic lesions. Isolated diaphysial involvement should suggest another diagnosis since in one series of Schnitzler syndrome, this was never observed.[92]

When the innominate bone is involved, the process tends to affect the medial and anterolateral aspects of the bone while the mid-superior iliac wing is spared, leading to a "V" shaped area of osteosclerosis on frontal views of the pelvis.

Radionuclide bone scans are more sensitive that plain radiographs and show focal radiotracer uptake at the sites of bone sclerosis. Imaging findings may be symmetric. Nuclear imaging can be positive when planar skeletal imaging is normal. MRI typically shows cortical thickening as well as medullary bone involvement in the absence of a tumor.[93] Sometimes, the abnormality is restricted to the medulla with T2 hyperintensity. PET/CT imaging is the most sensitive for radiologic evaluation of Schnitzler syndrome since organomegaly, periosteal bone thickening, and abnormal glucose uptake in the bone marrow. PET/CT is also helpful in evaluating other potential diagnostic considerations such as lymphoma.[92]

Differential Diagnosis

While the differential diagnosis of Schnitzler syndrome is broad, other diagnoses can be easily excluded based on laboratory studies as well as an informative skin biopsy. Diagnostic considerations include Waldenstrom macroglobulinemia (WM), hypocomplementemic urticarial vasculitis, adult-onset Still disease (AOSD), systemic lupus erythematosus, cryoglobulinemic vasculitis, C1 esterase inhibitor deficiency, chronic idiopathic urticaria, and several familial fever syndromes such as cryopyrin-associated periodic syndromes (CAPS), Muckel-Wells syndrome or familial cold auto-inflammatory syndrome, TRAPS (TNF-receptor associated periodic syndrome), and mevalonate kinase deficiency syndrome (also known as hyper-IgD syndrome).

Although AOSD may mimic Schnitzler syndrome, the very high ferritin and elevated hepatic transaminases are not features of Schnitzler syndrome. In WM, the monoclonal protein is generally high, the lymphoplasmacytic component in the bone marrow is also considerable, and most patients do not have a leukocytosis, thrombocytosis, or joint pains. Patients with systemic lupus erythematosus will have positive serologies for antibodies against DNA, extractable nuclear antigens, and other diagnostic criteria. Patients with cryoglobulinemia generally have Raynaud phenomenon and low complement levels that are absent in Schnitzler syndrome.

The familial fever syndromes generally present at an earlier age and are not associated with a serum monoclonal protein. One also has to note that an IgM monoclonal protein is not as common as IgG or IgA, and the combination of an IgM monoclonal protein and chronic, resistant urticaria along with fever and systemic manifestations and evidence of inflammation should be highly suggestive of Schnitzler syndrome.[85,87] Diagnosis of Schnitzler syndrome has been placed on a more secure footing by the publication of the "Strasbourg criteria"[15] These guidelines should be followed to establish the diagnosis in the absence of a specific diagnostic test for the syndrome.

Pathophysiology

The underlying pathogenesis of this syndrome is unclear. A unifying link between the monoclonal protein, rash, and the systemic inflammatory process has not been established.

Cytokines such as IL-1 and perhaps IL-18 are important mediators of the syndrome. Although serum IL-1 levels are normal in patients with Schnitzler syndrome, isolated mononuclear cells from such patients secrete large amounts of IL-1 and IL-6 in response to lipopolysaccharide stimulation.[94] Moreover, the rapid and often complete response to IL-1 directed agents such as anakinra,[15] canakinumab,[95] and rilonacept[96] point to the central role of IL-1 in this disease. IL-1 has protean manifestations including stimulation of chondrocytes that may explain the joint symptoms that often afflict these patients.

The skin rash is similar to that observed in several inherited periodic fever syndromes especially the auto-inflammatory CAPS. In CAPS, a mutation in the NLRP3 is often found.[97] Recent deep sequencing studies make the tantalizing suggestion that perhaps an acquired mutation in NLRP3 may in part be responsible for Schnitzler syndrome in some patients,[98,99] but not the majority.[99]

Histopathology

The histologic evaluation of a typical skin lesion would show a neutrophilic infiltrate within the dermis and usually in a perivascular pattern.[88,100] The neutrophils may be dispersed interstitially between the collagen bundles together with leukocytoclasia. Eosinophils may also form a minor component of the infiltrate. Less common is a mononuclear cell infiltrate with perivascular inflammation.[100] Features of vasculitis should not be present. In addition, the lack of dermal edema distinguishes this syndrome from Sweet syndrome.[85] Fibrinoid necrosis within blood vessels or dermal hemorrhage should not be present.[89] Sometimes, the neutrophils can cluster around the sweat ducts with a pattern of eccrine hidradenitis.[100]

When performed, immunofluorescence studies will reveal vascular deposition of IgM in a minority of patients, typically around the superficial dermal vessels.[89,100] Even less commonly C3 deposits may also be found. Deposition of IgM and C3 within the granular basement membrane can also be seen.[100] Sometimes, the IgM is deposited at the junction between the dermis and epidermis and there is evidence that these antibodies may target antigens present in the skin[101] and possibly induce an inflammatory response leading to the skin lesions and symptoms. Sometimes, patients with the syndrome undergo lymph node biopsy but in the absence of lymphoma but the findings tend to be nonspecific.

Therapy

While patients often respond to high doses of steroids, the disease often flares once they are tapered or discontinued. The introduction of the IL-1 receptor antagonist anakinra, which is given subcutaneously daily, was a breakthrough for this disease. The initial report[102] was soon followed by many others as well as small cohorts of patients.[99] Anakinra provides rapid, sustained, and complete resolution of symptoms as well as normalization of the inflammatory markers. The anemia resolves and the reactive leukocytosis and thrombocytosis normalize, but the monoclonal IgM persists. Anakinra has a short half-life (~6 hours) and has to be taken daily; if patients skip dose(s) they will rapidly experience resurgence of symptoms but will respond again if regular therapy is reinstituted.[85] In patients who are unresponsive to the drug, the diagnosis of Schnitzler syndrome should be revisited. Sometimes, patients may respond to higher doses of anakinra. The drug is generally well tolerated apart from local injection site reactions.[103] Patients should be monitored regularly for neutropenia, especially soon after the introduction of the drug. In women who are contemplating pregnancy, the drug should be withheld. Some patients have also responded to therapy with canakinumab (anti IL-1β)[95] or the IL-1 trap rilonacept[96] although the experience with the latter agents is more limited. The monoclonal protein should be followed up as per standard guidelines for MGUS for the development of WM, non-Hodgkin lymphoma, IgM MM, or amyloidosis.

Immunosuppressive agents such as cyclophosphamide, azathioprine, and methotrexate are ineffective.[85] IVIG and tumor necrosis factor alpha blocking agents are ineffective.[85] Colchicine and dapsone can provide relief in mild cases and may help the cutaneous manifestations of the disease.[89] Joint symptoms may sometimes respond to hydroxychloroquine. Pefloxacin, which is unavailable in many countries, has been used with success in some patients.

Prognosis and Long-term Complications

Schnitzler syndrome is a chronic condition and spontaneous and sustained remission is rare.[85,104] It may be reasonable to stop therapy and observe patients if they achieve a complete remission and were on therapy for at least 2 years.[15] In one cohort of patients from a single institution, the median overall survival was 12.8 years from the time of diagnosis.[87]

The initial reports suggested that perhaps 20% of patients may develop a lymphoproliferative disorder within 10 years of diagnosis.[86,89] However, in a more recent series the incidence of lymphoma was 12% with a median follow-up of 13 years from diagnosis.[87] It is unknown whether therapy with anakinra and good control of the inflammatory process is associated with a reduction in the risk of development of a lymphoproliferative disorder.

There are anecdotal reports of patients who developed reactive (AA) amyloidosis with nephrotic syndrome,[86] pseudoxanthoma elasticum, nodular hyperplasia of the liver, antiphospholipid antibody syndrome, and hearing loss. The link between Schnitzler syndrome and these uncommon conditions is difficult to establish except the hearing loss that is a feature of Muckle-Wells and CINCA (chronic infantile neurological cutaneous and articular) syndromes that share features with Schnitzler syndrome. The incidence of AA amyloidosis due to a longstanding acute phase response in the untreated patient will hopefully be a thing of the past with faster recognition and prompt institution of therapy that rapidly controls the inflammation characteristic of this syndrome.

Scleromyxedema

Scleromyxedema is a rare, chronic disorder characterized by a papular lichenoid eruption with sclerosis and deposition in the skin of glycosaminoglycans within the dermis. Diagnosis requires the presence of four criteria as defined by Rongioletti and Rebora (Table 103.1).[17,105] The disease appears to affect females and males equally and generally presents in the sixth decade, although patients may be in their third decade at diagnosis.[106]

Cutaneous Manifestations

The skin manifestations include small (2-3 mm) dome- or flat-shaped waxy papules typically in sun-exposed areas of the skin such as the face, neck, upper trunk, forearms, and thighs. Involvement of the skin of the face with deep furrows leads to the leonine facies while similar involvement of the skin of the upper back causes the "shar pei" sign.[107] Pruritus may be present in half of the patients.[106]

Extracutaneous Features

Scleromyxedema can affect several organ systems including the central nervous system, the heart, gastrointestinal tract, joints, lungs, and the kidneys. In one large series, neurologic involvement occurred in 54% of patients with the most common being carpal tunnel syndrome.[106] Central nervous system involvement with the so-called dermato-neuro syndrome occurs in 18%. The latter can have protean manifestations and is often preceded by a flu-like illness. Symptoms include dysarthria, seizures, ataxia, hemiparesis, extrapyramidal syndrome, and even coma.[106,108] Rheumatologic complications are found in up to 27% and include arthralgia or arthritis involving peripheral joints. An inflammatory myopathy is less common. Patients may present with heart block, myocardial ischemia, or even congestive heart failure although these are uncommon.[109] Gastrointestinal involvement may present with dysphagia due to involvement of the upper esophagus. The lungs may be affected relating in either obstructive or restrictive pattern leading to dyspnea on exertion. All patients will have a circulating monoclonal protein, invariably an IgG and more likely to be lambda light chain restricted. The size of the monoclonal protein is typically small and around 4.5 g/L.[106]

Differential Diagnosis

The main differential diagnosis is with systemic sclerosis (SS). Several features can distinguish between the two including the presence of Raynaud phenomenon and calcinosis in SS, which are absent in scleromyxedema. Moreover, the skin behind the ears and upper back are often spared in SS and characteristic of scleromyxedema. Nailfold capillaroscopy will not show the abnormal capillaries that are present in SS. Nephrogenic fibrosing dermopathy, also known as nephrogenic systemic fibrosus, also shares features with scleromyxedema, but patients with the former typically have significant renal dysfunction and do not have monoclonal proteins or facial involvement.

Pathogenesis

The pathogenesis of the disease is unknown. The histologic features include diffuse deposition of glycosaminoglycans (mucin) in the upper dermis with collagen deposition and the presence of irregularly arranged fibroblasts. The elastic fibers tend to be reduced in number and fragmented. Sometimes, a lymphoplasmacytic infiltrate may be present. Biopsies of other involved organ systems also demonstrate mucin deposition and increased collagen. The serum of patients with scleroderma may have high levels of IL-4, a profibrotic cytokine,[110] while elevated levels of mRNA coding for TGF-β, collagen 1a, IL8, and IL-10 have been reported based on skin transcriptomic analysis.[106] The role of the monoclonal protein in the causation of the disease is unclear. While the serum from patients with the disease can stimulate fibroblast proliferation, the monoclonal protein itself does not stimulate fibroblast growth.[111]

Therapy

Data on therapy for scleromyxedema is based on small case series and no randomized controlled trials exist. Patients with limited cutaneous disease can be treated with topical steroids, dimethyl sulfoxide or oral retinoids or ultraviolet A1 therapy. Recent studies suggest that compared to historical controls, the current interventions for systemic disease improve outcomes and survival.[106] With the advent of novel therapies, 97% of patients are alive at 3 years.[106]

The goal of therapy is not only to control the disease and reverse the cutaneous and systemic manifestations but also to reduce the risk of the dermato-neuro syndrome that can be life threatening. The current agent of choice is IVIG given at 2 g/kg over at least 2 days every 4 weeks. Therapy is associated with a relatively rapid improvement in the skin and rheumatologic manifestations of the disease. In one series, 42% of patients achieved a complete clinical improvement compared to their baseline. If remission is achieved, maintenance therapy with intermittent IVIG is recommended since the risk of relapse is quite high and may occur within 1 to 24 months of holding therapy.

For patients who cannot tolerate IVIG or patients who progress on this therapy, glucocorticosteroids alone or in combination with immunomodulatory agents such as thalidomide or lenalidomide are a reasonable option. Both thalidomide and lenalidomide are effective but in our experience lenalidomide is preferred due to its superior side effect profile.[112,113] Once a response is achieved, the medication dose should be reduced to the lowest level compatible with maintaining the response. There are anecdotal reports of efficacy with bortezomib or melphalan, but the latter agent is not recommended due to its risk of leukemogenesis. ASCT has been reported as an effective therapy by several groups with complete resolution of disease manifestations in up to 59% of patients although the duration of response is limited.[114,115] The role of maintenance therapy after ASCT is not known.

Therapy for dermato-neuro syndrome requires a multimodality approach including IVIG, dexamethasone, and sometimes plasmapheresis. The patient should be cared for in intensive care and given anticonvulsants due to the high risk/frequency of seizures. Dexamethasone and bortezomib have also been used to treat this syndrome.[106,116]

Necrobiotic Xanthogranuloma

In 1980, Kossard and Winkelmann described a syndrome where patients had multiple violaceous atrophic plaques and nodules that affected the face in a periorbital distribution, the skin flexures, and trunk in association with a monoclonal protein.[117] The condition was named necrobiotic xanthogranuloma (NXG) due to the presence of histiocytic granulomas with necrobiosis and the presence of Touton giant cells or foreign body giant cells.[118] The condition is rare, and a series from a single institution reported 35 patients over a 15-year interval.[119] The average age at diagnosis is 62 and some studies suggest that females are affected more frequently.[16] The pathogenesis of this condition is unknown. Hypotheses include a foreign body reaction to deposition of immunoglobulin/lipid complexes, complement activation and accumulation of lipids in monocytes or impaired lipid hemostasis with an inflammatory response.

Clinical Features

The typical cutaneous features of NXG are yellowish to red-orange or violaceous plaques, nodules, or papules with areas of ulceration, telangiectasia, and atrophy. The most commonly affected areas are the periorbital region of the face (60%-80%),[118,120] sites of prior scars, or the trunk, arms, thighs, and legs. Extracutaneous involvement can occur including in the orbit and eye, liver, lungs, gastrointestinal tract, brain, and other organ systems.[16,119] Ocular involvement is common, and almost half of the patients with NXG may have ocular symptoms including uveitis or scleritis.[118,121]

Most patients with NXG will have a monoclonal protein, with IgG kappa being significantly more common than IgG lambda.[119] In one series, 23% of patients progressed to MM after a median follow-up of 67 months. Three of these patients had smoldering MM at the time of NXG diagnosis.[119] Some patients may also have antecedent, concomitant, or subsequent low-grade B cell lymphoproliferative disorders.[16,119]

Diagnosis requires the presence of typical cutaneous lesions that on biopsy show the palisading granulomas with a lymphoplasmacytic infiltrate and zones of necrobiosis, often with the presence of giant cells (Touton or foreign body) together with the presence of a monoclonal protein or a plasma cell or lymphoproliferative disorder (Table 103.1). The periorbital distribution of the lesions helps with the diagnostic evaluation. A punch biopsy showing the typical histologic features is required for diagnosis. Complement C4 levels are often low[16,119] and may help with the diagnosis since low C4 would be unusual in conditions such as xanthelasma palpebrarum or necrobiotic lipoidica. A concomitant cryoglobulin may be present in about 25% of patients[16,119] while a substantial number may have low high-density cholesterol levels.[16]

Therapy

There are no randomized controlled trials exploring therapies in NXG, and recommendations are based on case series. In the past, patients with an associated plasma cell or lymphoproliferative disorder were treated with chlorambucil or melphalan. IVIG is considered the most effective therapy.[16,119,122,123] There are anecdotal reports of responses to more modern therapies including IMIDs, proteasome inhibitors, and ASCT.[119] Intralesional triamcinolone may also work.

Cryoglobulinemia

In 1933, Wintrobe and Buell originally reported observing cryoglobulins in a serum sample from a patient with MM.[124] These cold precipitable immunoglobulins were observed in some patients with vasculitis, viral infection, or lymphoproliferative disorders and were found to be byproducts of lymphoid dysfunction—unchecked and misdirected stimulation and proliferation that cause dysfunction and pathological changes.

The term "cryoglobulin" was coined by Lerner and Watson in 1947.[125] Precipitation of cryoglobulins is dependent on temperature, pH, cryoglobulin concentration, and weak noncovalent factors.[126] Meltzer and others described a distinct syndrome of purpura, arthralgias, asthenia, renal disease, and neuropathy—often occurring with immune complex deposition or vasculitis, or both.[127,128] Brouet et al popularized a system of classifying cryoglobulinemia based on the components of the cryoprecipitate[129]: type I, isolated monoclonal immunoglobulins; type II, a monoclonal component, usually IgM that binds to the Fc component of polyclonal IgG (i.e., has rheumatoid factor activity); and type III, polyclonal immunoglobulins of more than one isotype.[129] This classification provided a framework by which clinical correlations could be made. Associated conditions, such as lymphoproliferative disorders, connective tissue disorders, infection, and liver disease were observed in some patients.[130,131] Early studies did not identify an underlying condition in 34% to 71% of cryoglobulinemia cases, and such patients were considered to have *essential* or *primary* cryoglobulinemia.[129,130,132] However, with the discovery of hepatitis C virus (HCV) in 1990 and 1991 came the recognition that the majority of these cases were related to HCV.[133,134] Therefore, essential cryoglobulinemia represents less than 10% of cases of cryoglobulinemia.[135]

Epidemiology

It is difficult to determine the prevalence of cryoglobulinemia since the syndrome is clinically heterogenous, and it may be difficult to distinguish incidental laboratory findings from symptomatic

Table 103.3. Clinical Features of Cryoglobulinemia at Diagnosis

Reference[a]	N	F:M	Essential[b]	Type I	Type II	Type III	LPD	Liver[c]	Sicca	Skin	Raynaud	Renal	Arthralgia	Neuro
126	29	3:1	41	59	41[d]	41[d]	31	72[e]	17[e]	92[e]	–	25[e]	92[e]	17[e]
127	86	–	34	25	25	50	44	–	9	55	50	21	35	17
	40	1.7:1	100	0	32	68	–	70	15	100	25	55	72	12
143 f	44	1:7	82	–	–	–	0[g]	14	2	59	7	100	57	7
144	16	–	–	12	63	25	6	–	–	94	–	63	63	56
145	891	2:1	72	6	62	32	6	39	5	76	19	20	–	21
146	231	3:1	<8%	–	62	38	10	77	53	98	48	30	98	80
133	206[h]	–	–	–	–	–	10	–	–	51	11	39	40	14
147	49	1.7:1	12	6[i]	49	33	0	43	35	82	35	24	51	55
136	66	45:55	15	–	100	–	9	50	2	55	12	26	21	18

[a]Publications are listed chronologically, from oldest to most recent.
[b]Cryoglobulinemia without any identified predisposing condition. These values do not represent actual incidence but rather the make-up of the population analyzed for symptoms.
[c]Patients with abnormal liver function tests or hepatomegaly, or both.
[d]Value is for types II and III combined.
[e]Symptoms of the essential mixed cryoglobulinemia (types II and III) population only.
[f]Series restricted to patients with renal involvement.
[g]Patients with multiple myeloma, Waldenström macroglobulinemia, and infection were excluded from this study by design.
[h]Only patients with a cryocrit ≥1% were included. The percentages were calculated on the basis of the 206 symptomatic patients described by the authors.
[i]In this study, 12% of the patients were not typed.
Abbreviations: Abd, abdominal; cryo, cryoglobulinemia; LPD, lymphoproliferative disorder; neuro, neurologic disease.
Modified from Dispenzieri A, Gorevic PD. Cryoglobulinemia. *Hematol Oncol Clin North Am.* 1999;13(6):1315-1349. Copyright © 1999 Elsevier. With permission.

disease states. Cryoglobulins may be found in patients with cirrhosis (up to 45%), alcoholic hepatitis (32%), autoimmune hepatitis (40%), subacute bacterial endocarditis (90%), rheumatoid arthritis (47%), Sjogren syndrome, IgG myeloma (10%), and WM (19%).[129-131,136-138] The presence of cryoglobulins should alert the physician to the possibility of undiagnosed chronic infections such as bacterial endocarditis, Lyme disease, and Q fever.[131] Case reports describe cryoglobulinemia in association with hepatitis A virus, hepatitis B virus, Hantavirus, cytomegalovirus, Epstein-Barr virus, human T-cell lymphotropic virus type I, hepatitis G virus, human immunodeficiency virus, and parvovirus B19. The majority (42%-100%) of cases of mixed cryoglobulinemia are due to infection with HCV.[134,139-144] The median age at diagnosis is the sixth decade with a female predominance that may be greater than 2:1 (Table 103.3).[138,150,151] Although no racial differences are reported, the incidence is higher in regions with a high prevalence of HCV (for example, southern Europe).[152]

Etiology

Cryoglobulinemia is driven or associated primarily with four groups of diseases: liver disease (predominantly HCV), infection (again, predominantly HCV), connective tissue disorders, and lymphoproliferative disorders (Figure 103.4). Type I and II cryoglobulins are associated with monoclonal expansion of B cells or plasma cells while type III cryoglobulins result from polyclonal B cell expansion. Infection and/or inflammation ostensibly induce a nonspecific stimulation of B cells, leading to polyclonal hypergammaglobulinemia. Immune activation can lead to formation of antibodies to auto-antigens. In animal models, a strong B-cell stimulus disrupts the sequential order of idiotype–anti-idiotype interactions, resulting in both immunosuppression and idiotype–anti-idiotype immune complexes.[153] Furthermore, poorly regulated production and clearance of IgM rheumatoid factor contributes to immune complex formation.[126,130] Deposition of these antibody complexes on the walls of blood vessels leads to a variety of pathologic conditions, including vasculitis, thrombosis, and glomerulonephritis.

Complement components, fibronectin, and lipoproteins can be found along with antigen-antibody complexes within cryoprecipitates. Although hepatitis B virus, Epstein-Barr virus, and bacterial products may be present, the most common pathogen within cryoprecipitates is HCV.[154] HCV RNA, HCV-specific proteins, and antibodies against HCV are found in the supernatant and within the cryoprecipitate itself in 42% to 98% of patients with type II cryoglobulinemia.[140-144] Cryoprecipitates contain 20 to 1000 times more HCV RNA than what is detectable in the supernatant.[155] The IgG component to which the IgM-rheumatoid factor fraction binds is directed against the HCV proteins.[156]

The biochemical basis for the temperature-dependent precipitation of these proteins is not completely understood. Cryoglobulins may precipitate at temperatures substantially higher than the 4 °C that is used to determine their presence in the laboratory. Precipitation also depends on temperature, pH, the ionic strength, and the structure (sequence) of the immunoglobulin components.

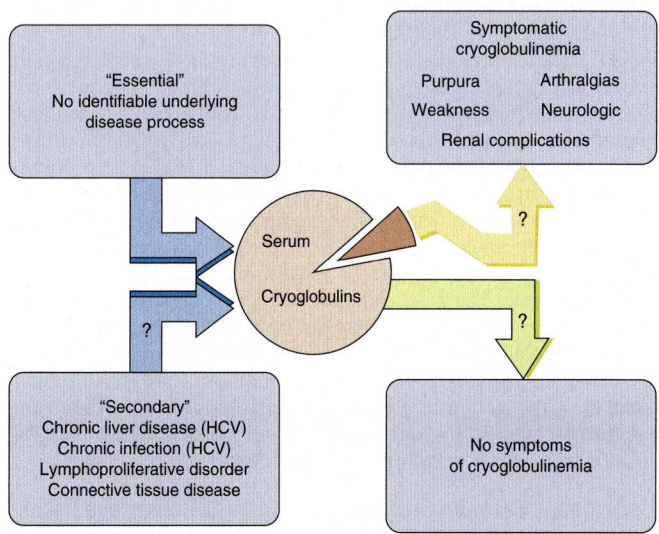

FIGURE 103.4 Relationship among underlying diseases, cryoglobulins, and symptoms of cryoglobulinemia. Question marks represent unknown contributing factors. HCV, hepatitis C virus. (From Dispenzieri A, Gertz MA. Cryoglobulinemia. In: Gertz MA, Greipp PA, eds. *Hematologic Malignancies: Multiple Myeloma and Related Plasma Cell Disorders*. Springer-Verlag; 2003:227-256. Used with permission of Mayo Foundation for Medical Education and Research. All rights reserved.)

Hepatitis C Virus

HCV can infect B-lymphocytes through CD81 or the LDL receptor.[157,158] There is considerable evidence that: (1) HCV can serve as a chronic immune stimulus; (2) cryoglobulins are present in up to 50% of HCV-infected patients[159-161]; (3) HCV is associated with autoimmune phenomena even in the absence of cryoglobulinemia; and (4) HCV may predispose patients to lymphoma.[131,162] Predisposing factors for cryoglobulinemia in HCV patients are female gender, alcohol consumption, detectable serum HCV-RNA, longer duration of hepatitis, higher serum gamma globulin levels, higher rheumatoid factor levels, steatosis, and extensive liver fibrosis or cirrhosis.[144,159,163-165]

The major envelope protein of HCV (HCV-E2) binds with high affinity to CD81, a tetraspanin expressed on several cell types, including B and T lymphocytes.[157] CD81 expression on CD19+ B lymphocytes is significantly higher in patients with mixed cryoglobulinemia compared to those without mixed cryoglobulinemia, patients chronically infected with hepatitis B virus, and healthy controls.[166] Engagement of CD81 on human B cells by a combination of HCV-E2 and an anti-CD81 monoclonal antibody triggers the JNK pathway and leads to the preferential proliferation of naive (CD27−) B cells.[167] The interaction between CD19/CD21 and CD81 provides a strong activation signal for B cells that drives the polyclonal proliferation of naive B lymphocytes and may be an important initial step in the development of HCV-associated B lymphocyte disorders.[167] These B cells have a biased usage of rheumatoid factor encoding V_H1-69 and $V_\kappa 3$-20 gene segments, similar to what is observed in patients with HCV-related lymphoma.[168] Interestingly, these cells express low levels of CD21 and are associated with an anergic phenotype.[169] Eradication of HCV infection by interferon therapy leads to normalization of the activation markers expression on B lymphocytes[167] as well as restoration of immune homeostasis, especially after therapy with rituximab.[170,171]

Connective Tissue Disease

The incidence of cryoglobulinemia, most commonly type II or III, in relation to specific connective tissue diseases is quite variable.[128,131] Among patients with systemic lupus erythematosus, 25% have detectable cryoglobulins and cryoglobulins have been detected in 12.5% of patients with SS.[136,172] Measurable amounts of cryoglobulins, usually polyclonal, can be found in up to 46% of patients with active rheumatoid arthritis. Among patients with Sjögren syndrome, 16% to 37% have serum cryoglobulins[131]; conversely, 5% to 15% of patients with mixed cryoglobulinemia have Sjögren syndrome.[129,130,132]

Lymphoproliferative Disorders

Type I cryoglobulinemia occurs in the setting of clonal B cell and plasma cell expansion such as MGUS, MM, WM, and chronic lymphocytic leukemia (CLL). Up to 31% of all patients with secondary symptomatic cryoglobulinemia have a diagnosed lymphoproliferative disorder when cryoglobulinemia is found.[132] Higher percentages are reported in series when bone marrow biopsies, flow cytometry, Southern blot analysis, and polymerase chain reaction are performed routinely.[131] In another 6% to 28% of patients, symptomatic lymphoma develops at follow-up, 50% of these are intermediate- or high-grade lymphoma. The most common histologic diagnoses among the remaining low-grade lymphomas are immunocytoma followed by mucosa-associated lymphoid tissue (MALT) and centrocytic follicular lymphoma. Among patients whose conditions transform to overt lymphoma, the malignant clone is derived from one of the dominant baseline B-cell clones in only a minority of patients, implying a predisposition for the development of mutant clones and evolution.

Associations Between Cryoglobulinemia, HCV, Connective Tissue Disease, and Lymphoma

A recognized model for progression from chronic antigenic stimulation to benign or malignant lymphoproliferation is *Helicobacter pylori* and MALT lymphoma.[173] HCV, Sjögren syndrome, cryoglobulinemia, and immunocytoma may follow a similar model.[131] Similar degrees of homology are seen between the immunoglobulin receptors in the lymphoproliferation of patients with Sjögren syndrome and those in the lymphomas of HCV-infected patients with or without type II cryoglobulinemia.

In a series of 1255 patients in Italy with HCV and symptomatic mixed cryoglobulinemia, the risk of aggressive non-Hodgkin lymphoma was 35-fold higher compared with the general population with 224.1 new cases per 100,000 patient-years.[174] The median time from the diagnosis of cryoglobulinemia to the clinical onset of NHL was 6.3 years (range, 0.81-24 years). The clinical course and response to chemotherapy in the patients with cryoglobulinemia and NHL were similar to those usually described for patients with NHL without cryoglobulinemia.

Productive t(14;18) translocations with resultant BCL-2 overexpression occur in about 12% to 38% of HCV-positive patients without symptomatic cryoglobulinemia and in 39% to 85% of their cryoglobulin-positive counterparts.[175]

Clinical Presentation of Cryoglobulinemia

Involvement of the skin, peripheral nerves, kidneys, and liver is common (*Table 103.3*). Lymphadenopathy is present in approximately 17% of patients.[128,130] On autopsy, widespread vasculitis involving small and medium vessels in the heart, gastrointestinal tract, central nervous system, muscles, lungs, and adrenal glands may also be seen.[130] The interval between the onset of symptoms and the time of diagnosis varies considerably (range, 0-10 years). Type I cryoglobulinemia is usually asymptomatic. When symptomatic, it most commonly causes occlusive symptoms such as Raynaud phenomenon rather than the vasculitis of types II and III.[128-130] Symptoms of hyperviscosity may occur (*Figure 103.5*). Type II cryoglobulinemia is more frequently symptomatic (61% of patients) than type III (21% of patients). The most common causes of death include renal failure, infection, lymphoproliferative disorders, liver failure, cardiovascular complications, and hemorrhage.[129,130,132,146,149]

In a series of 231 patients seen between 1972 and 2001, the mixed cryoglobulinemia syndrome followed a relatively benign clinical course in more than 50% of cases, whereas a moderate-severe clinical course was observed in one-third of patients whose prognosis was severely affected by renal or liver failure. For 15% of individuals the disease was complicated by malignancy: B-cell NHL was more common than hepatocellular and thyroid malignancies. Ten-year overall survival was 56%. Lower survival rates were seen in males and in individuals with renal involvement.[148]

Dermatologic and Joint Manifestations of Cryoglobulinemia

Purpura is the most frequent cutaneous symptom, being present in 55% to 100% of patients with mixed cryoglobulinemia (*Table 103.3* and *Figure 103.5*).[129,130,132,146] The incidence varies from 15% to 33% in type I, from 60% to 93% in type II, and from 70% to 83% in type III.[176] Petechiae and palpable purpura are the most common lesions, although ecchymoses, erythematous spots, and dermal nodules occur in up to 20% of patients. Bullous or vesicular lesions are distinctly uncommon.[129] Successive purpuric rashes, which may be preceded by a burning or itching sensation, occur most commonly on the lower extremities, gradually extending to the thighs and lower abdomen. Occasionally the arms are involved, but the face and trunk are generally spared.[129] Head and mucosal involvement, livedoid vasculitis, and cold-induced acrocyanosis of the helices of the ears are more frequently observed in type I; infarction, hemorrhagic crusts, or ulcers occur in 10% to 25% of all patients with mixed cryoglobulinemia.[177] Showers of purpura last for 1 to 2 weeks and occur once or twice a month. Cold precipitates these types of lesions in only 10% to 30% of patients.[129,177] Raynaud phenomenon occurs in between 19% and 50% of patients[129,130,132,146]; in a quarter of these, the symptoms may be severe, including necrosis of fingertips.[129] Skin necrosis, urticaria, and livedo, which are all rare, are more commonly associated with exposure to cold.

Arthralgias are common, affecting 35% to 92% of patients, with the highest incidence in type III cryoglobulinemia (*Table 103.3*). The small distal joints are affected more frequently than larger proximal joints. Symmetrical polyarthralgia is often exacerbated by cold temperatures. Frank arthritis is rare.[129,130,132,135,146]

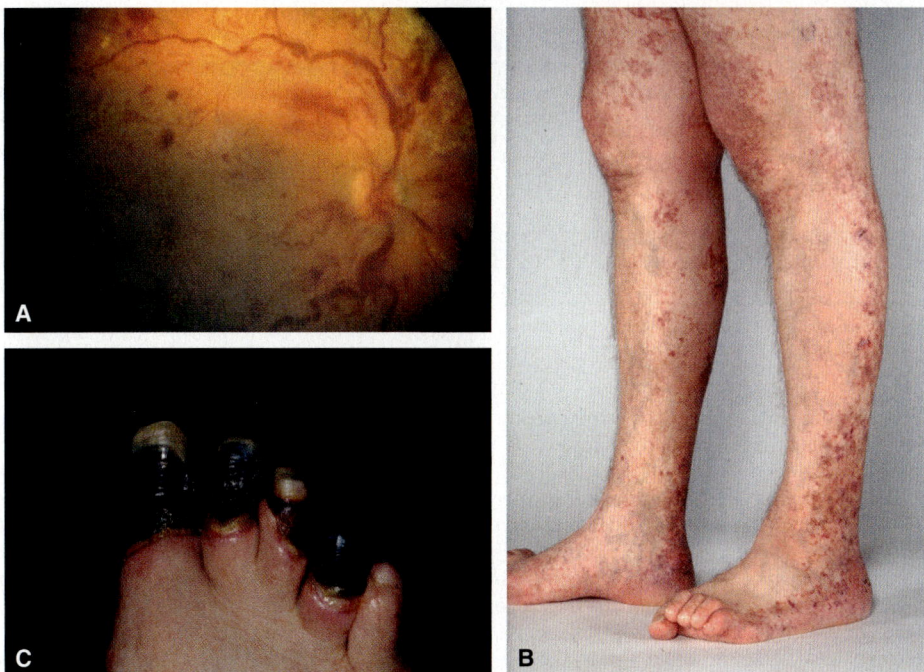

FIGURE 103.5 Cryoglobulin-associated physical findings. A, Hyperviscosity manifested as retinopathy with venous engorgement and hemorrhage. B, Purpura. C, Gangrene.

Nervous System Manifestations of Cryoglobulinemia

Peripheral neuropathy is the more common presentation, although central nervous system involvement may occur. Peripheral nerve involvement is described in 12% to 56% of patients (Table 103.3).[129,130,132,135,146] Signs and symptoms of sensory neuropathy usually precede those of motor neuropathy.[129,178] The presentation may be an acute or subacute distal symmetric polyneuropathy or a mononeuritis multiplex with a chronic or chronic-relapsing evolution.[179] The neuropathy is most often characterized by axonal degeneration. Epineurial vasculitis is a common finding on sural nerve biopsy. Even when other manifestations of mixed cryoglobulinemia are stable over time, there is typically worsening of the peripheral neuropathy.[180]

Central nervous system abnormalities are not uncommon in patients with mixed cryoglobulinemia. Casato et al compared 40 patients with mixed cryoglobulinemic vasculitis and chronic active HCV infection with normal controls and HCV patients without mixed cryoglobulinemia. Twenty-four of the 27 (89%) patients with HCV-mixed cryoglobulinemia had a deficiency in one or more of 10 cognitive domains examined.[181] Cappellari et al have also found central nervous system abnormalities in a majority of patients studied.[182]

Renal Manifestations of Cryoglobulinemia

Approximately 21% to 39% of patients with mixed cryoglobulinemia have renal involvement.[129,135] The incidence of renal injury is highest in patients with type II cryoglobulins.[132] Although renal and extrarenal manifestations may occur concurrently, renal involvement usually follows the onset of purpura by approximately 4 years.[130,183] Proteinuria greater than 0.5 g/d and hematuria are the most common features of renal disease at diagnosis (present in 50% of patients); nephrotic syndrome affects approximately 20% of patients and acute nephritic syndrome affects approximately 25% of patients.[183,184] Although cryopathic membranoproliferative glomerulonephritis portends a poor prognosis progression to end-stage renal failure due to sclerosing nephritis is uncommon.[130,136,184,185] Among patients with mixed cryoglobulinemia-associated membranoproliferative glomerulonephritis followed up for a median of 11 years, 15% had disease progression to end-stage renal failure, and 43% died of cardiovascular, hepatic, or infectious causes.[184]

Liver Manifestations of Cryoglobulinemia

Approximately 39% of patients with symptomatic cryoglobulinemia[132] and as many as 77% with mixed cryoglobulinemia[130,186] have documented liver abnormalities at the time of diagnosis (Table 103.3). Hepatomegaly is present in up to 70% of patients, and splenomegaly is observed in 52%.[127,130,145] Among patients with symptomatic cryoglobulinemia, liver failure is the cause of death in 2.5% to 7.6% of patients and in 5.6% to 29% of all reported deaths.[130,147,184]

Histologic findings include portal fibrosis, chronic persistent hepatitis, chronic active hepatitis, chronic active hepatitis with cirrhosis, and postnecrotic cirrhosis. Most specimens are characterized by a diffuse lymphocytic infiltrate ranging from minimal periportal to extensive infiltration with nodule formation. These changes correlate with the severity of other pathologic findings. Plasma-cell infiltration has also been noted in several specimens.[186,187] The lymphoid population in the liver may form pseudo-follicular structures with morphologic features similar to those previously reported in chronic HCV without cryoglobulinemia.[188] These hepatic lymphoid nodules contain B cells predominantly with a $CD5^+/Bcl-2^+/Ki67^-$ phenotype—that is, low apoptotic and proliferative rates.[189]

Other Manifestations of Cryoglobulinemia

Given the propensity of immune complexes to deposit in blood vessels and activate complement, in principle, cryoglobulinemic vasculitis can affect any vascular distribution including the mesenteric vessels,[135] leading to intestinal ischemia, cholecystitis, and pancreatitis. Pulmonary vascular involvement, in severe cases, may lead to acute alveolar hemorrhage and diffuse pulmonary infiltrates. Rarely, coronary vasculitis may lead to myocardial infarction.

Diagnosis of Cryoglobulinemia

By definition, all patients with cryoglobulinemia have a detectable serum cryoglobulin. The collection and processing of the specimens are critical because the cold-induced reversible precipitates can be lost with improper handling.[131] A minimum of 10 mL of blood is required, and the specimen must be allowed to clot at 37 °C for 30 to 60 minutes before centrifugation. The serum supernatant is stored at 4 °C for up to 7 days and inspected daily for cryoprecipitate. Methods to evaluate

Table 103.4. Treatments for Symptomatic Mixed Cryoglobulinemia

Most Effective	Probably Effective	Possibly Effective	Variable Efficacy	Probably Not Effective
Sofosbuvir	Plasmapheresis	Azathioprine	IV immunoglobulin[a]	Anti-TNF-α antibody
Interferon/PEG-interferon	Corticosteroids	Cyclosporin	Splenectomy	Colchicine
Ribavirin	Alkylators			Chloroquine
Rituximab	Thalidomide			H_1 and H_2 blockers
Low-antigen diet (mild disease)			Purine nucleoside analogs	Penicillamine

[a]One case report of precipitating acute renal failure and another of systemic vasculitis.
Abbreviations: IV, intravenous; PEG, pegylated; TNF, tumor necrosis factor.

the composition of the cryoglobulin include immunoelectrophoresis, immunofixation, immunoblotting, and capillary electrophoresis.

Concentrations of cryoglobulins tend to vary by type: type III, less than 1 mg/mL; type II, 1 mg/mL or greater; and type I, greater than 5 mg/mL.[129,190] The type or quantity does not reliably predict the presence or nature of symptoms. On serum protein electrophoresis, polyclonal hypergammaglobulinemia is the most common finding, although normal patterns or hypogammaglobulinemia may also be seen.[128,130,138] Even among patients with type II cryoglobulinemia, only 15% have a visible monoclonal spike on serum protein electrophoresis. Frequently, serum IgM levels are elevated; cryoprecipitable IgM may comprise up to one-third of the total serum IgM concentration[130] but hyperviscosity occurs only occasionally.[127] Marked depression of complement CH50, C1q, and C4 in the presence of relatively normal C3 levels is usual.[130,135] Neither C4 concentrations nor cryoglobulin levels correlate with overall clinical severity, although for individual patients the cryoglobulin level can sometimes serve as a marker for disease activity.[130,191] Rheumatoid factor activity—that is, anti-Fc activity—is detectable in the sera of 87% to 100% of patients with mixed cryoglobulinemia, and levels may decrease with response to therapy.[128,129,147] An elevated erythrocyte sedimentation rate and a mild normochromic, normocytic anemia are fairly common.[130] Cytopenias have been described, as have pseudoleukocytosis and pseudothrombocytosis.[127] Among patients with cryoglobulinemia, the antinuclear antibody results may be positive in as many as two-thirds of patients and in as many as one-third of the HCV-positive patients.[135] Because HCV is frequently concentrated in cryoglobulins,[140] serial measurements of plasma or serum HCV RNA levels in these patients are not reliable.[164]

Treatment of Cryoglobulinemia

Since cryoglobulinemia has a fluctuating course with spontaneous exacerbations and remissions, controlled clinical trials are important to evaluate therapeutic efficacy. Although there are several "accepted" or "standard" treatments there are limited data from randomized trials to support their practice (Table 103.4).[131] Although therapies such as the use of histamine (H) H_1 and H_2 blockers and penicillamine have sound scientific basis for consideration, they have shown no clear clinical benefit.[130,131] Figure 103.6 outlines a strategy for managing symptomatic cryoglobulinemia.

The standard treatment of mild symptomatic cryoglobulinemia (purpura, asthenia, arthralgia, and mild sensory neuropathy) has included bed rest, analgesics, low-dose glucocorticosteroid therapy, low-antigen content diet, and protective measures against cold exposure; the treatment of severe disease (glomerulonephritis, motor neuropathy, and systemic vasculitis) has included plasmapheresis, high-dose glucocorticosteroid therapy, and cytotoxic therapy. With the recognition of the association between HCV and mixed cryoglobulinemia, immunosuppressive therapy has been viewed less favorably, and now antiviral therapy is considered the preferred treatment approach for patients without a medical emergency.[192-199] The availability of highly active direct acting antiviral agent combinations based on sofosbuvir has resulted in sustained remissions and viral clearance in a large number of patients with HCV. Antiviral therapy is associated with a concomitant reduction in the cryoglobulins and resolution of symptoms of cryoglobulinemia.[198,199]

Patients with symptomatic type 1 cryoglobulinemia should receive therapy directed at the underlying lymphoproliferative disorder. Although rituximab is effective in patients with WM, care has to be taken to avoid the risk of precipitating hyperviscosity syndrome when rituximab is used alone since it can lead to a transient increase in the monoclonal IgM ("Rituximab flare"). In such circumstances, apart from the use of plasma exchange, bortezomib can be added to rapidly reduce the B cell or plasma cell burden responsible for production of the monoclonal immunoglobulin (cryoglobulin). Ibrutinib is now an approved therapy for WM, and this may be a potential therapeutic approach. The authors have anecdotal evidence for its efficacy in this setting. Similarly, treatment of an underlying connective tissue disease or infection would be first-line therapy in patients with type II or III cryoglobulinemia. The importance of not overtreating patients must be emphasized.

Treatment of Life-Threatening Disease

For clinical emergency situations (acute nephritis or severe vasculitis), initial measures are aimed at reducing the inflammatory activity of the renal lesions (corticosteroids), removing circulating cryoglobulins (plasmapheresis), and reducing the formation of new antibodies (e.g., cyclophosphamide). Plasma exchange or plasmapheresis alone can reverse serious complications, but these procedures are typically used in combination with cytotoxic agents or corticosteroids for more durable responses.[191] According to case reports, responses may be seen in 60% to 100% of patients.[131] Skin manifestations and arthralgias usually respond the fastest, whereas the degree of neural and renal response depends on the acuity of their occurrence, with poorer

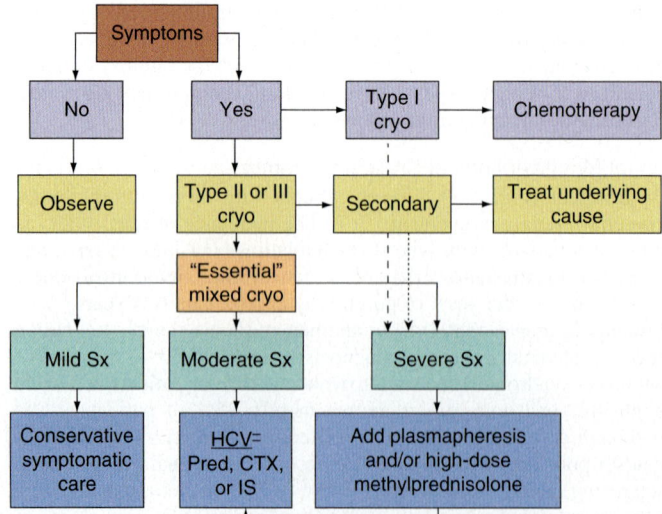

FIGURE 103.6 Treatment schema for cryoglobulinemia. Cryo, cryoglobulin; CTX, cyclophosphamide; HCV, hepatitis C virus; IS, immunosuppressant; pred, low-dose therapy with prednisone; Sx, symptoms.

responses observed in chronic cases.[200] With combination immunosuppressive therapy and plasma exchange, reversal of catastrophic complications such as encephalopathy and acute glomerulonephritis has been documented. High-dose pulse therapy with methylprednisolone is also a favored therapeutic intervention for acute events, with 90% response rates in rapidly progressive glomerulonephritis.[183,201] Once the acute exacerbation has been mitigated, antiviral strategies are implemented in HCV positive patients to consolidate and maintain the response and potentially cure the cryoglobulinemia.

Antiviral Therapy

Historically, interferon (IFN) alpha monotherapy, followed by combination with ribavirin was the standard of care for HCV-related cryoglobulinemia.[192-197,202-207] Several randomized trials evaluated the efficacy of IFN therapy in HCV-positive patients with symptomatic type II mixed cryoglobulinemia. These studies documented clinical responses in 60% to 89% of patients.[192-196] However, when compared with HCV-related chronic hepatitis, treatment of mixed cryoglobulinemia with IFN monotherapy was associated with a relatively poorer response and a high relapse rate, especially in severe cases. A majority of patients relapsed within 6 months of discontinuation.[193-197] Purpuric lesions and liver function abnormalities are the features that tend to respond rapidly (within weeks), but neuropathy and nephropathy respond more slowly.[197,202] There have been reports of peripheral neuropathy, nephritis, vasculitis, and ischemic manifestations being exacerbated by IFN-α.

The availability of direct-acting antiviral agents has transformed therapy for HCV. As a result, sofosbuvir-based therapy has emerged as a highly effective treatment for HCV-related cryoglobulinemia with the advantage of fewer side effects, high rates of viral eradication, and a shorter course of therapy. Gragnani et al reported on a cohort of 44 patients treated with direct antiviral agents and showed that all the patients had cleared HCV at 12 and 24 weeks post therapy. Concomitantly, the cryocrit fell from a mean of 7.2 (±15.4)% to 1.5 (±5.1)% at 24 weeks and this was associated with significant improvement in the Birmingham vasculitis activity scores. This approach opens the possibility of curing such patients of their disease.[198] Bonacci et al recently reported their experience with 64 patients who had HCV-related cryoglobulinemia.[199] After a standard course of direct-acting antivirals, 94% of the patients had sustained clearance of the virus 12 weeks after therapy. 71% of the patients achieved a complete clinical response while 48% of the patients achieved a complete immunologic response, defined as no detectable cryoglobulin and normalization of serum complement levels and/or rheumatoid factor.[199] The Birmingham vasculitis activity score also improved significantly. The latter study had rather short follow-up and further updates on this cohort should inform the field about the longer-term outcomes of this therapy.

Rituximab Therapy

Anti-CD20 therapy with rituximab has been shown to produce responses in patients with all types of cryoglobulinemia[208-211]; however, those patients with HCV are at risk for increased HCV replication.[208,209] Initial studies reported responses in the majority of patients, including improvements in the manifestations of cutaneous vasculitis (ulcers, purpura, or urticaria), subjective symptoms of peripheral neuropathy, low-grade B-cell lymphoma, arthralgias, fever, nephritis, levels of rheumatoid factor, cryoglobulins, and C4. In a randomized trial including 59 patients with cryoglobulinemic vasculitis, the patients were randomized to either rituximab or conventional therapy, which included glucocorticoids, azathioprine, cyclophosphamide, or plasmapheresis. Time to treatment failure at 1 year was superior in the rituximab group (64% vs 3%). The vasculitis activity also improved significantly on rituximab, whereas it did not for the other treatment arm. The median duration of response to rituximab was 18 months.[150]

The combination of pegylated IFN-α, ribavirin, and rituximab has been reported to hasten symptomatic improvement, organ (renal) response, cryoglobulin clearance, and elimination of HCV viremia.[171,212] Responses are generally more durable with a median duration of response in excess of 3 years.[171] Two trials used a similar regimen for the IFN-α and ribavirin but differed in the use of rituximab. While Saadoun et al started therapy with rituximab alone (weekly for 4 doses),[212] Dammacco et al started the triple combination simultaneously and subsequently gave additional single doses of rituximab at 6 and 11 months after the initiation of therapy.[171] The addition of rituximab to the combination of antiviral agents did not lead to an increase in the HCV burden as measured by quantitative PCR and therapy was associated with a significant reduction or elimination of clonal B cells from the circulation.

Other Therapies for Cryoglobulinemia

Although not formally studied, high-dose therapy with autologous stem-cell transplantation may be considered for patients with symptomatic, refractory type I cryoglobulinemia that results from a plasma cell proliferative disorder.

MONOCLONAL GAMMOPATHIES OF RENAL SIGNIFICANCE

Monoclonal gammopathy of renal significance, a term coined in 2012 by the International Kidney and Monoclonal Gammopathy Research Group (IKMG), refers to small B cell clones that lack criteria for a symptomatic disease, but secrete monoclonal proteins that are pathogenic and responsible for disease in the kidney.[213] In 2017, the term was updated to include all clonal proliferative disorders that do not meet criteria for a specific hematologic malignancy but produce a nephrotoxic immunoglobulin.[214] The renal disease is not associated with the degree of clonal burden but rather the pathogenic properties of the monoclonal protein secreted. This group of conditions includes monoclonal immunoglobulin deposition disease (MIDD), proliferative glomerulonephritis and monoclonal immunoglobulin deposits (PGNMID), crystal storing histiocytosis, and light chain proximal tubulopathy (LCPT). Light chain or heavy amyloidosis and cryoglobulinemia are considered MGRS but are discussed elsewhere (Chapter 101 and previously, respectively). Some of these renal manifestations have been documented in patients with CLL, MM, or WM. However, these conditions have also been seen in low clonal burden disorders that do not meet diagnostic criteria for other malignancies. Distinct from other non-monoclonal-related diseases like IgA nephropathy, MGRS disorders do not respond to standard immunosuppression nor spontaneously regress but require clone directed treatment to prevent further damage to kidney or end-stage renal disease.[213,215-218] If the underlying hematological condition progresses to overt MM, WM, CLL, or lymphoma, then the patient no longer has MGRS and should be managed according to the disease directed procedures.

Classification of MGRS Disorders

The renal lesions are defined by the structural characteristics and properties of the monoclonal protein rather than the underlying cell that produced it.[219] The IKMG classification is based on findings of immunofluorescence and structural appearance of the deposits on electron microscopy, but notably electron microscopy is not widely available. Therefore, light microscopy and immunofluorescence studies are also accepted.[214] The classification is first defined as diseases with or without monoclonal deposits. Monoclonal deposits are then further subdivided into organized and nonorganized. Organized deposits are then further divided into fibrillar, microtubular, and inclusion/crystalline deposits (*Figure 103.7*).

Organized Monoclonal Deposits

There are three categories of organized monoclonal deposits: fibrillar, microtubular, and inclusions or crystalline deposits. Among the fibrillar includes light chain or heavy chain amyloidosis (Chapter 101) and monoclonal fibrillary glomerulonephritis (FGN). FGN deposits are glomerular, nonbranching fibrils lacking a hollow center by electron microscopy; Congo Red stains are negative. Glomerular staining of DNJ homologue subfamily B member 9 (DNAJB9) is a reliable

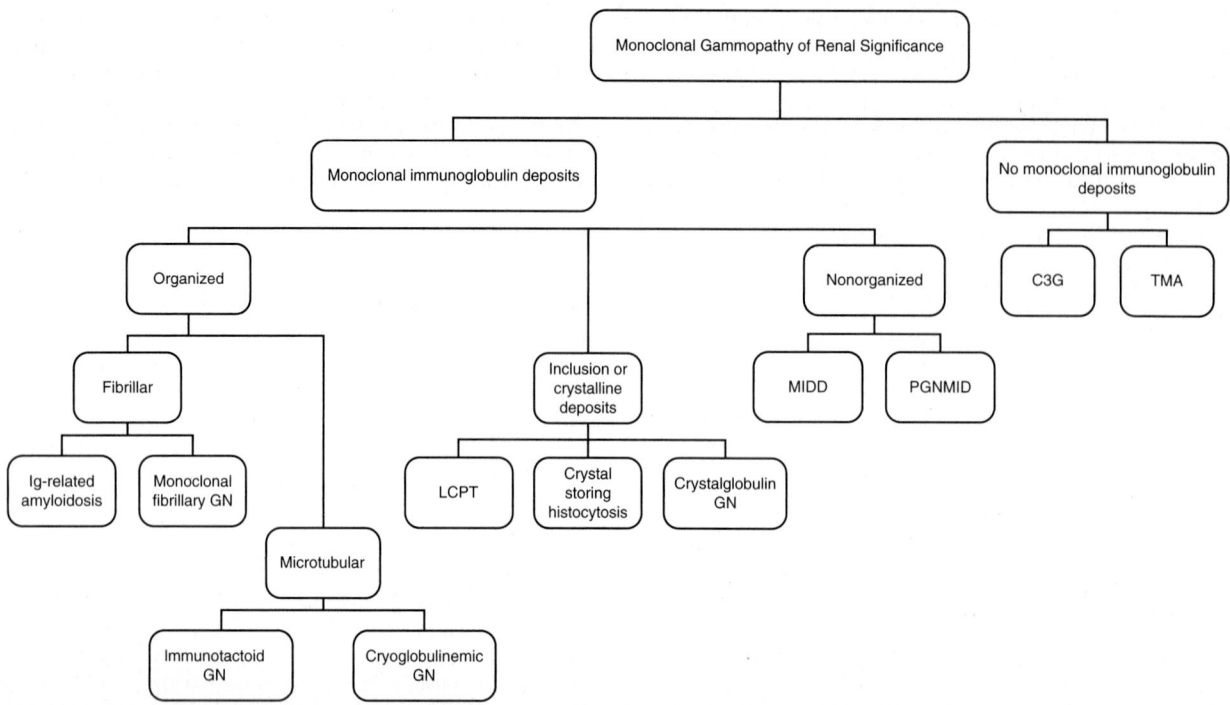

FIGURE 103.7 Classification of monoclonal gammopathy of renal significance. C3G, C3 glomerulopathy with monoclonal gammopathy; Ig, immunoglobulin; GN, glomerulonephritis; LCPT, light chain proximal tubulopathy; MIDD, monoclonal immunoglobulin deposit disease; PGNMID, proliferative glomerulonephritis with monoclonal immunoglobulin deposits; TMA, thrombomicroangiopathy with monoclonal gammopathy. (Modified from Leung N, Bridoux F, Batuman V, et al. The evaluation of monoclonal gammopathy of renal significance: a consensus report of the International Kidney and Monoclonal Gammopathy Research Group. *Nat Rev Nephrol.* 2019;15(1):45-59.)

marker to distinguish for FGN,[220] but when a case is DNAJB9 positive, it almost never is associated with a monoclonal gammopathy. Rarely, there are patients with DNAJB9 negative FGN that are associated with a monoclonal gammopathy.[214] Monoclonal FGN is a rare disorder found in 0.4% to 1.4% of kidney biopsies.[221]

Microtubular deposits have hollow centers with large diameters and include immunotactoid glomerulonephritis and cryoglobulinemic glomerulonephritis.[222] Cryoglobulinemia is discussed in depth elsewhere. Immunotactoid glomerulonephritis is a renal limited disease in which deposits are uniform microtubules in parallel located within the subepithelium and/or subendothelium.

The crystalline or inclusion group consists of LCPT, crystal storing histiocytosis, and crystalglobulin glomerulonephritis.[223] LCPT is characterized by light chain inclusions of monoclonal light chains (κ more commonly than λ) in proximal tubules; the inclusions can be crystalline or noncrystalline. The crystalline subtype is frequently associated with acquired Fanconi syndrome, and has light chain (virtually all κ) crystal deposits in various areas in proximal tubules, both free in cytoplasm and inside lysosomes.[224] A clue to acquired Fanconi syndrome includes evidence of failure of reabsorption at the proximal tubule, which can result in hypophosphatemia, low serum uric acid, glycosuria, aminoaciduria, secondary hyperparathyroidism, and renal tubular acidosis. The noncrystalline subtype results in injury to proximal tubules due to accumulation of noncrystalline light chains in lysosomes.[225] For both crystalline or noncrystalline acute tubular injury is observed with essentially normal glomeruli.[226] In crystal-storing histiocytosis, there can be renal and extra renal depositions such as bone marrow, lymph nodes, lungs, thyroid, parotid gland, cornea, skin, subcutaneous fat, liver, intestines, and brain.[227] Lastly, crystalglobulinemic glomerulonephritis is a rare disorder marked by immunoglobulin thrombi in arterioles and capillaries of the glomerulus.[228] Occasionally this deposition is prompted by cold exposure and termed cryocrystalglobulinemia.[229] Similar to cryoglobulinemia, small thrombi result in small vessel occlusions and inflammatory vasculitis.

Nonorganized Monoclonal Deposits

MIDD and PGNMID are both part of the nonorganized classification of MGRS. MIDD represents a group of conditions; heavy chain deposition disease (HCDD), light chain deposition disease (LCDD), or both (LHCDD) that deposit on the basement membranes of the kidney.[230] Among those three subtypes, HCDD is the rarest with the first description in 1992 case report.[231] Diagnosis is based on immunofluorescence of kidney biopsies demonstrating linear deposits of the involved monoclonal immunoglobulin along glomerular or tubular basement membranes and granular deposits on electron microscopy.[232] MIDD usually lacks the first constant domain of the immunoglobulin.[233] MIDD usually is a truncated IgG1 that is deposited, while PGNMID is commonly IgG3, and rarely IgA or IgM.[234] Whereas PGNMID deposits are limited to glomeruli and in the mesangium and subendothelium and usually contain completely intact immunoglobulins.[235]

MGRS With Nonimmunoglobulin Deposits

There are conditions where no immunoglobulin is deposited that are still considered MGRS and include C3 glomerulopathy (C3G) with monoclonal gammopathy and thrombotic microangiopathy.

In C3G with monoclonal gammopathy, complement component C3 fragments are deposited in the glomeruli without immunoglobulin deposits[236]; it is considered a MGRS because 60% to 80% of patients over age 50 with C3G have a detectable circulating monoclonal gammopathy.[237,238] There are two patterns seen: glomerulonephritis with isolated C3 deposits and dense deposit disease. The dense deposit disease appears as electron dense intramembranous deposit and mesangial rounded nodular deposits, whereas the isolated C3 deposits appear large hump shaped subepithelial deposits.[214,215] Both patterns are associated with dysregulation of the complement alternative pathway from autoantibodies directed at complement proteins.[239,240] There is a small proportion of cases that appears to be C3G except in actuality possess membranoproliferative glomerulonephritis with masked monoclonal deposits which require additional immunofluorescence studies to be recognized.[241]

Thrombotic microangiopathy has provisional status as MGRS. It is frequently seen with microangiopathy with hemolytic anemia and can occur in patients with MGUS, MM, and WM. The mechanism is not well understood and instead hypothesized to be related to the monoclonal antibody behaving as an autoantibody against complement proteins.[242,243] There is also a glomerular angiopathy associated with POEMS syndrome. Histologically, subacute to chronic glomerular thrombotic microangiopathy described as mesangial and endothelial proliferation and widening of the subendothelial zone and double contouring are seen.[42] The presumption is that these lesions observed in some POEMS syndrome patients are related to cytokine-mediated endothelial cell injury.[244]

Workup of MGRS

Diagnosis should be suspected of MGRS when patients with a monoclonal gammopathy or B cell disorder have unexplained kidney dysfunction or proteinuria. In patients with a monoclonal gammopathy who had a kidney biopsy, 40% were found to have a MGRS lesion.[245] The workup is a combined hematologic and renal evaluation and requires a kidney biopsy. Simply having MGUS or B cell lymphocytosis and kidney impairment is not sufficient for the diagnosis. It is critical to distinguish MGRS from other renal disorders since treatment of MGRS is usually aimed at the underlying hematologic condition for kidney preservation.[214] Risk of bleeding is 4% for a kidney biopsy and is no worse in patients with MGRS vs those without MGRS.[246] The biopsy requires review via light microscopy, immunofluorescence, and electron microscopy, and can be sent to specialized renal pathologists if there is question of the diagnosis. Renal biopsy can be avoided for those MGRS conditions that are part of a systemic illness (e.g., AL amyloidosis or cryoglobulinemia), which has been confirmed in another organ.

Once a MGRS lesion is determined, confirmation of the source of the monoclonal protein is also required (if not already identified) and could include serum and urine protein electrophoresis and immunofixation, serum free light chains, and frequently blood flow cytometry and a bone marrow biopsy to identify clone. If there is no clone found in bone marrow, imaging can be done to look for a plasmacytoma or lymphadenopathy that could be biopsied. Unfortunately, a clone is not always identified during evaluation particularly with PGMID with only 20% to 30% having detectable monoclonal proteins.[234]

Treatment of MGRS

The IKMG recommends treatment, even without the existence of malignant conditions.[237] There are limited studies on some of the rarer MGRS disorders, and clear treatment guidelines have not been developed. Most evidence is from case reports, case series, and retrospective studies. The goal of therapy is to preserve function of the kidney and avoid progression of extra-renal manifestations of disease for those conditions that do not limit themselves to the kidney. There are no therapies specifically designed to remove deposited monoclonal proteins from the kidney or any other affected organ. Typical immunosuppressing medications are not successful in managing MGRS. Treatment is directed at the clone (plasma cell, lymphoplasmacytic, or B cell) that is producing the toxic monoclonal immunoglobulin.[215] Typically, the better the hematologic response, the better the renal survival is.[232,238] The treatment of AL amyloidosis and cryoglobulinemia are covered in Chapter 101 and previous text, respectively.

Clone Directed therapy

For the most part MIDD is treated like AL amyloidosis, with excellent outcomes documented with bortezomib monotherapy and combination therapy as well as ASCT.[232,238] Impaired glomerular filtration rates are more common with MIDD than AL amyloidosis, but otherwise MIDD patients are less likely to have cardiac involvement. This has implications in terms of the treatment choices. Retrospective studies reveal 5-year renal survival rates approaching 60%.[238]

Immunotactoid glomerulopathy has a CLL clone underlying in as many as 50% of cases. For that reason, rituximab therapy can be effective in those cases. For cases with a plasma cell clone, bortezomib and/or alkylator can be effective.[222,247]

For LCPT—specifically acquired Fanconi syndrome—benefit has been reported using classic myeloma therapies.[218] The deeper the hematologic response, the more likely the chance of having preserved renal function.

Despite finding a monotypic protein in the kidney, a clone is not found in the bone marrow in a majority of PGMID patients. In one series, 10/16 cases did not have a detectable bone marrow clone and were thus treated empirically: 8 received rituximab-based therapy; the other 2 received alkylator or bortezomib.[248] Renal complete and partial responses were seen in 3 and 5 of these 10 empirically treated patients.

A cohort of 50 patients with C3G with monoclonal gammopathy was reported.[215] Twenty-nine received chemotherapy, 8 immunosuppressive agents, and 13 symptomatic management. Patients who received chemotherapy and achieved a hematologic response had higher renal response rates ($P = .0001$) and median renal survival (HR 0.22; 95% CI 0.05-0.92; $P = .009$). Several studies have shown that hematologic response and kidney response are closely related.[249]

Kidney Transplantation

Consideration for kidney transplantation is appropriate in MGRS but risk of relapse in the allograft must be considered. A recent case series of 28 patients between 1987 and 2016 who received renal transplant LCDD (n = 10), C3 glomerulopathy with monoclonal gammopathy (n = 5) and LCPT (n = 4) revealed that there was a high risk of recurrence in the allograft if hematologic response was not achieved (57.8% of LCDD, 100% of C3G, and 75% of LCPT).[250]

Six patients with MIDD underwent kidney transplantation.[251] The median survival was 19.8 years from diagnosis (range 13.7-27.8 years). Three patients died; the time from the first kidney transplantation to death was 7.4, 18.8, and 20.4 years. Two patients lost their graft due to disease recurrence at 4 months and 3.8 years after kidney transplantation. Neither had achieved hematologic response.

Among 19 patients with ESRD due to PGNMID who underwent renal transplant due to end-stage renal disease, 17 recurred in the allograft. Sixteen patients with documented reoccurrence received some combination of chemotherapy, corticosteroid and/or antibody therapy, and more than half had improvement in proteinuria and in glomerular pathology.

In summary, each case undergoing consideration for a kidney transplant should be weighed against avoiding dialysis/stopping dialysis and the risk of recurrence in the allograft, the speed of recurrence, and overall mortality. It is consistent with the evidence that patients who can receive systemic therapy and achieve a hematologic response do better long term.

OTHER MONOCLONAL GAMMOPATHIES OF CLINICAL SIGNIFICANCE

TEMPI Syndrome

TEMPI syndrome is a rare acquired disorder characterized by the features that comprise the acronym: telangiectasias; elevated erythropoietin and erythrocytosis; monoclonal gammopathy; perinephric fluid collections; and intrapulmonary shunting.[18] The underlying pathophysiology is not understood, but it is clear that plasma cell directed therapy reverses the clinical manifestations.

Telangiectasias involving the face and upper body and erythrocytosis is the most common presentation. Unlike the erythrocytosis of polycythemia rubra vera and of POEMS syndrome, patients with TEMPI syndrome have a high erythropoietin.[252] Patients develop progressive hypoxia. The pulmonary shunting is not evident on high resolution computed tomography of the chest and is best demonstrated by ^{101}mTc macro-aggregated albumin scintigraphy. The perinephric fluid collections have the same electrolyte composition of serum. Unlike

POEMS syndrome, there is no bias in clonality for lambda restricted clones and there are no features of a myeloproliferative neoplasm.

Plasma cell directed therapy appears to be useful, specifically bortezomib, daratumumab, lenalidomide, and high-dose melphalan. All of the features can improve upon achievement of complete hematologic response.

Idiopathic Systemic Capillary Leak Syndrome (Clarkson Disease)

This devastating disease was described in 1960. Systemic capillary leak syndrome (SCLS) is characterized by capillary leak resulting in sudden-onset shock and anasarca caused by plasma extravasation (up to 70% of total plasma volume). The diagnostic triad is composed of the "3 Hs," which occur in the absence of secondary causes for these findings: hypotension; hemoconcentration, and hypoalbuminemia. Sixty-eight percent of adult cases SCLS have monoclonal proteins, most commonly IgG kappa. Details for the limited understanding of disease mechanism for the vascular endothelial hyperpermeability for SCLS can be found in review.[253]

The differential diagnosis for an acute attack includes sepsis, anaphylaxis, and hereditary angioedema. Treatment at the time of an acute attack is supportive with fluid resuscitation until flare subsides, which typically occurs over the course of a few days. Empiric prophylaxis with IVIG is recommended as it has been demonstrated that there are fewer attacks for those managed as such.[254]

References

1. Bardwick PA, Zvaifler NJ, Gill GN, Newman D, Greenway GD, Resnick DL. Plasma cell dyscrasia with polyneuropathy, organomegaly, endocrinopathy, M protein, and skin changes: the POEMS syndrome. Report on two cases and a review of the literature. *Medicine*. 1980;59(4):311-322.
2. Takatsuki K, Sanada I. Plasma cell dyscrasia with polyneuropathy and endocrine disorder: clinical and laboratory features of 109 reported cases. *Jpn J Clin Oncol*. 1983;13(3):543-555.
3. Nakanishi T, Sobue I, Toyokura Y, et al. The Crow-Fukase syndrome: a study of 102 cases in Japan. *Neurology*. 1984;34(6):712-720.
4. Dispenzieri A. POEMS syndrome: 2021 update on diagnosis, risk-stratification, and management. *Am J Hematol*. 2021;96(7):872-888.
5. Nasu S, Misawa S, Sekiguchi Y, et al. Different neurological and physiological profiles in POEMS syndrome and chronic inflammatory demyelinating polyneuropathy. *J Neurol Neurosurg Psychiatry*. 2012;83(5):476-479.
6. Dispenzieri A. POEMS syndrome. *Blood Rev*. 2007;21(6):285-299.
7. Soubrier M, Dubost JJ, Serre AF, et al. Growth factors in POEMS syndrome: evidence for a marked increase in circulating vascular endothelial growth factor. *Arthritis Rheum*. 1997;40(4):786-787.
8. Endo I, Mitsui T, Nishino M, Oshima Y, Matsumoto T. Diurnal fluctuation of edema synchronized with plasma VEGF concentration in a patient with POEMS syndrome. *Intern Med*. 2002;41(12):1196-1198.
9. Nakano A, Mitsui T, Endo I, Takeda Y, Ozaki S, Matsumoto T. Solitary plasmacytoma with VEGF overproduction: report of a patient with polyneuropathy. *Neurology*. 2001;56(6):818-819.
10. Koga H, Tokunaga Y, Hisamoto T, et al. Ratio of serum vascular endothelial growth factor to platelet count correlates with disease activity in a patient with POEMS syndrome. *Eur J Intern Med*. 2002;13(1):70-74.
11. Martin S, Labauge P, Jouanel P, Viallard JL, Piette JC, Sauvezie B. Restricted use of Vλ genes in POEMS syndrome. *Haematologica*. 2004;89(4):ECR02.
12. Nakaseko C, Abe D, Takeuchi M, et al. Restricted Oligo-clonal usage of monoclonal immunoglobulin {lambda} light chain germline in POEMS syndrome. *ASH Annual Meeting Abstracts*. 2007;110(11):2483.
13. Bender R, Javaugue V, Saintamand A, et al. Immunoglobulin variable domain high-throughput sequencing reveals specific novel mutational patterns in POEMS syndrome. *Blood*. 2020;135(20):1750-1758.
14. Bryce AH, Ketterling RP, Gertz MA, et al. A novel report of cig-FISH and cytogenetics in POEMS syndrome. *Am J Hematol*. 2008;83(11):840-841.
15. Simon A, Asli B, Braun-Falco M, et al. Schnitzler's syndrome: diagnosis, treatment, and follow-up. *Allergy*. 2013;68(5):562-568.
16. Nelson CA, Zhong CS, Hashemi DA, et al. A multicenter cross-sectional study and systematic review of necrobiotic xanthogranuloma with proposed diagnostic criteria. *JAMA Dermatol*. 2020;156(3):270-279.
17. Rongioletti F, Merlo G, Carli C, et al. Histopathologic characteristics of scleromyxedema: a study of a series of 34 cases. *J Am Acad Dermatol*. 2016;74(6):1194-1200.
18. Sykes DB, O'Connell C, Schroyens W. The TEMPI syndrome. *Blood*. 2020;135(15):1199-1203.
19. Alberti MA, Martinez-Yelamos S, Fernandez A, et al. 18F-FDG PET/CT in the evaluation of POEMS syndrome. *Eur J Radiol*. 2010;76(2):180-182.
20. Watanabe O, Maruyama I, Arimura K, et al. Overproduction of vascular endothelial growth factor/vascular permeability factor is causative in Crow-Fukase (POEMS) syndrome. *Muscle Nerve*. 1998;21(11):1390-1397.
21. Scarlato M, Previtali SC, Carpo M, et al. Polyneuropathy in POEMS syndrome: role of angiogenic factors in the pathogenesis. *Brain*. 2005;128(pt 8):1911-1920.
22. Nobile-Orazio E, Terenghi F, Giannotta C, Gallia F, Nozza A. Serum VEGF levels in POEMS syndrome and in immune-mediated neuropathies. *Neurology*. 2009;72(11):1024-1026.
23. Briani C, Fabrizi GM, Ruggero S, et al. Vascular endothelial growth factor helps differentiate neuropathies in rare plasma cell dyscrasias. *Muscle Nerve*. 2011;43(2):164-167.
24. D'Souza A, Hayman SR, Buadi F, et al. The utility of plasma vascular endothelial growth factor levels in the diagnosis and follow-up of patients with POEMS syndrome. *Blood*. 2011;118(17):4663-4665.
25. Dao LN, Hanson CA, Dispenzieri A, Morice WG, Kurtin PJ, Hoyer JD. Bone marrow histopathology in POEMS syndrome: a distinctive combination of plasma cell, lymphoid and myeloid findings in 87 patients. *Blood*. 2011;117(24):6438-6444.
26. Soubrier MJ, Dubost JJ, Sauvezie BJ. POEMS syndrome: a study of 25 cases and a review of the literature. French Study Group on POEMS Syndrome. *Am J Med*. 1994;97(6):543-553.
27. Dispenzieri A, Kyle RA, Lacy MQ, et al. POEMS syndrome: definitions and long-term outcome. *Blood*. 2003;101(7):2496-2506.
28. Li J, Zhou DB, Huang Z, et al. Clinical characteristics and long-term outcome of patients with POEMS syndrome in China. *Ann Hematol*. 2011;90(7):819-826.
29. Kelly JJ Jr, Kyle RA, Miles JM, Dyck PJ. Osteosclerotic myeloma and peripheral neuropathy. *Neurology*. 1983;33(2):202-210.
30. Koike H, Iijima M, Mori K, et al. Neuropathic pain correlates with myelinated fibre loss and cytokine profile in POEMS syndrome. *J Neurol Neurosurg Psychiatry*. 2008;79(10):1171-1179.
31. Kelly JJ Jr. The electrodiagnostic findings in peripheral neuropathy associated with monoclonal gammopathy. *Muscle Nerve*. 1983;6(7):504-509.
32. Mauermann ML, Sorenson EJ, Dispenzieri A, et al. Uniform demyelination and more severe axonal loss distinguish POEMS syndrome from CIDP. *J Neurol Neurosurg Psychiatry*. 2012;83(5):480-486.
33. Arimura K. Increased vascular endothelial growth factor (VEGF) is causative in Crow-Fukase syndrome. Article in Japanese. *Rinsho Shinkeigaku Clinical Neurology*. 1999;39(1):84-85.
34. Saida K, Kawakami H, Ohta M, Iwamura K. Coagulation and vascular abnormalities in Crow-Fukase syndrome. *Muscle Nerve*. 1997;20(4):486-492.
35. Piccione EA, Engelstad J, Dyck PJB, Mauermann ML, Dispenzieri A, Dyck PJ. Nerve pathologic features differentiate POEMS syndrome from CIDP. *Acta Neuropathol Commun*. 2016;4(1):116.
36. Gandhi GY, Basu R, Dispenzieri A, Basu A, Montori VM, Brennan MD. Endocrinopathy in POEMS syndrome: the Mayo clinic experience. *Mayo Clin Proc*. 2007;82(7):836-842.
37. Ishikawa O, Nihei Y, Ishikawa H. The skin changes of POEMS syndrome. *Br J Dermatol*. 1987;117(4):523-526.
38. Jitsukawa K, Hayashi Y, Sato S, Anzai T. Cutaneous angioma in Crow-Fukase syndrome: the nature of globules within the endothelial cells. *J Dermatol*. 1988;15(6):513-522.
39. Rongioletti F, Gambini C, Lerza R. Glomeruloid hemangioma. A cutaneous marker of POEMS syndrome. *Am J Dermatopathol*. 1994;16(2):175-178.
40. Kaushik M, Pulido JS, Abreu R, Amselem L, Dispenzieri A. Ocular findings in patients with polyneuropathy, organomegaly, endocrinopathy, monoclonal gammopathy, and skin changes syndrome. *Ophthalmology*. 2011;118(4):778-782.
41. Stankowski-Drengler T, Gertz MA, Katzmann JA, et al. Serum immunoglobulin free light chain measurements and heavy chain isotype usage provide insight into disease biology in patients with POEMS syndrome. *Am J Hematol*. 2010;85(6):431-434.
42. Ye W, Wang C, Cai QQ, et al. Renal impairment in patients with polyneuropathy, organomegaly, endocrinopathy, monoclonal gammopathy and skin changes syndrome: incidence, treatment and outcome. *Nephrol Dial Transplant*. 2016;31(2):275-283.
43. Sanada S, Ookawara S, Karube H, et al. Marked recovery of severe renal lesions in POEMS syndrome with high-dose melphalan therapy supported by autologous blood stem cell transplantation. *Am J Kidney Dis*. 2006;47(4):672-679.
44. Nakamoto Y, Imai H, Yasuda T, Wakui H, Miura AB. A spectrum of clinicopathological features of nephropathy associated with POEMS syndrome. *Nephrol Dial Transplant*. 1999;14(10):2370-2378.
45. Glazebrook K, Guerra Bonilla FL, Johnson A, Leng S, Dispenzieri A. Computed tomography assessment of bone lesions in patients with POEMS syndrome. *Eur Radiol*. 2015;25(2):497-504.
46. Watanabe O, Arimura K, Kitajima I, Osame M, Maruyama I. Greatly raised vascular endothelial growth factor (VEGF) in POEMS syndrome. *Lancet*. 1996;347(9002):702.
47. Kanai K, Sawai S, Sogawa K, et al. Markedly upregulated serum interleukin-12 as a novel biomarker in POEMS syndrome. *Neurology*. 2012;79(6):575-582.
48. Tokashiki T, Hashiguchi T, Arimura K, Eiraku N, Maruyama I, Osame M. Predictive value of serial platelet count and VEGF determination for the management of DIC in the Crow-Fukase (POEMS) syndrome. *Intern Med*. 2003;42(12):1240-1243.
49. Hashiguchi T, Arimura K, Matsumuro K, et al. Highly concentrated vascular endothelial growth factor in platelets in Crow-Fukase syndrome. *Muscle Nerve*. 2000;23(7):1051-1056.
50. Allam JS, Kennedy CC, Aksamit TR, Dispenzieri A. Pulmonary manifestations in patients with POEMS syndrome: a retrospective review of 137 patients. *Chest*. 2008;133(4):969-974.
51. Lesprit P, Godeau B, Authier FJ, et al. Pulmonary hypertension in POEMS syndrome: a new feature mediated by cytokines. *Am J Respir Crit Care Med*. 1998;157(3 pt 1):907-911.
52. Li J, Tian Z, Zheng HY, et al. Pulmonary hypertension in POEMS syndrome. *Haematologica*. 2013;98(3):393-398.
53. Lesprit P, Authier FJ, Gherardi R, et al. Acute arterial obliteration: a new feature of the POEMS syndrome? *Medicine*. 1996;75(4):226-232.

54. Mellors PW, Kourelis T, Go RS, et al. Characteristics and risk factors for thrombosis in POEMS syndrome: a retrospective evaluation of 230 patients. *Am J Hematol.* 2022;97(2):209-215.
55. Dupont SA, Dispenzieri A, Mauermann ML, Rabinstein AA, Brown RD Jr. Cerebral infarction in POEMS syndrome: incidence, risk factors, and imaging characteristics. *Neurology.* 2009;73(16):1308-1312.
56. Dispenzieri A. How I treat POEMS syndrome. *Blood.* 2012;119(24):5650-5658.
57. Wang C, Huang XF, Cai QQ, et al. Prognostic study for overall survival in patients with newly diagnosed POEMS syndrome. *Leukemia.* 2017;31(1):100-106.
58. Kourelis TV, Buadi FK, Kumar SK, et al. Long-term outcome of patients with POEMS syndrome: an update of the Mayo Clinic experience. *Am J Hematol.* 2016;91(6):585-589.
59. Kourelis TV, Buadi FK, Gertz MA, et al. Risk factors for and outcomes of patients with POEMS syndrome who experience progression after first-line treatment. *Leukemia.* 2016;30(5):1079-1085.
60. Dispenzieri A. POEMS syndrome: update on diagnosis, risk-stratification, and management. *Am J Hematol.* 2015;90(10):951-962.
61. Suichi T, Misawa S, Nagashima K, et al. Lenalidomide treatment for thalidomide-refractory POEMS syndrome: a prospective single-arm clinical trial. *Intern Med.* 2020;59(9):1149-1153.
62. Nozza A, Terenghi F, Gallia F, et al. Lenalidomide and dexamethasone in patients with POEMS syndrome: results of a prospective, open-label trial. *Br J Haematol.* 2017;179(5):748-755.
63. Misawa S, Sato Y, Katayama K, et al. Safety and efficacy of thalidomide in patients with POEMS syndrome: a multicentre, randomised, double-blind, placebo-controlled trial. *Lancet Neurol.* 2016;15(11):1129-1137.
64. Katayama K, Misawa S, Sato Y, et al. Japanese POEMS syndrome with Thalidomide (J-POST) Trial: study protocol for a phase II/III multicentre, randomised, double-blind, placebo-controlled trial. *BMJ Open.* 2015;5(1):e007330.
65. Li J, Zhang W, Jiao L, et al. Combination of melphalan and dexamethasone for patients with newly diagnosed POEMS syndrome. *Blood.* 2011;117(24):6445-6449.
66. D'Souza A, Lacy M, Gertz M, et al. Long-term outcomes after autologous stem cell transplantation for patients with POEMS syndrome (osteosclerotic myeloma): a single-center experience. *Blood.* 2012;120(1):56-62.
67. Dispenzieri A, Lacy MQ, Hayman SR, et al. Peripheral blood stem cell transplant for POEMS syndrome is associated with high rates of engraftment syndrome. *Eur J Haematol.* 2008;80(5):397-406.
68. Cook G, Iacobelli S, van Biezen A, et al. High-dose therapy and autologous stem cell transplantation in patients with POEMS syndrome: a retrospective study of the Plasma Cell Disorder sub-committee of the Chronic Malignancy Working Party of the European Society for Blood & Marrow Transplantation. *Haematologica.* 2017;102(1):160-167.
69. Li J, Huang XF, Cai QQ, et al. A prospective phase II study of low dose lenalidomide plus dexamethasone in patients with newly diagnosed polyneuropathy, organomegaly, endocrinopathy, monoclonal gammopathy, and skin changes (POEMS) syndrome. *Am J Hematol.* 2018;93(6):803-809.
70. Jaccard A, Lazareth A, Karlin L, et al. A prospective phase II trial of lenalidomide and dexamethasone (LEN-DEX) in POEMS syndrome. *Blood.* 2014;124(21):36.
71. Vannata B, Laurenti L, Chiusolo P, et al. Efficacy of lenalidomide plus dexamethasone for POEMS syndrome relapsed after autologous peripheral stem-cell transplantation. *Am J Hematol.* 2012;87(6):641-642.
72. Dispenzieri A, Klein CJ, Mauermann ML. Lenalidomide therapy in a patient with POEMS syndrome. *Blood.* 2007;110(3):1075-1076.
73. Royer B, Merlusca L, Abraham J, et al. Efficacy of lenalidomide in POEMS syndrome: a retrospective study of 20 patients. *Am J Hematol.* 2013;88(3):207-212.
74. Cai QQ, Wang C, Cao XX, Cai H, Zhou DB, Li J. Efficacy and safety of low-dose lenalidomide plus dexamethasone in patients with relapsed or refractory POEMS syndrome. *Eur J Haematol.* 2015;95(4):325-330.
75. Zagouri F, Kastritis E, Gavriatopoulou M, et al. Lenalidomide in patients with POEMS syndrome: a systematic review and pooled analysis. *Leuk Lymphoma.* 2014;55(9):2018-2023.
76. Kuwabara S, Misawa S, Kanai K, et al. Neurologic improvement after peripheral blood stem cell transplantation in POEMS syndrome. *Neurology.* 2008;71(21):1691-1695.
77. Goto H, Nishio M, Kumano K, Fujimoto K, Yamaguchi K, Koike T. Discrepancy between disease activity and levels of vascular endothelial growth factor in a patient with POEMS syndrome successfully treated with autologous stem-cell transplantation. *Bone Marrow Transplant.* 2008;42(9):627-629.
78. Dispenzieri A. Ushering in a new era for POEMS. *Blood.* 2011;117(24):6405-6406.
79. Chaudhry HM, Mauermann ML, Rajkumar SV. Monoclonal gammopathy-associated peripheral neuropathy: diagnosis and management. *Mayo Clin Proc.* 2017;92(5):838-850.
80. Leger JM, Viala K, Nicolas G, et al. Placebo-controlled trial of rituximab in IgM anti-myelin-associated glycoprotein neuropathy. *Neurology.* 2013;80(24):2217-2225.
81. Dalakas MC, Rakocevic G, Salajegheh M, et al. Placebo-controlled trial of rituximab in IgM anti-myelin-associated glycoprotein antibody demyelinating neuropathy. *Ann Neurol.* 2009;65(3):286-293.
82. Yuki N, Uncini A. Acute and chronic ataxic neuropathies with disialosyl antibodies: a continuous clinical spectrum and a common pathophysiological mechanism. *Muscle Nerve.* 2014;49(5):629-635.
83. Naddaf E, Milone M, Kansagra A, Buadi F, Kourelis T. Sporadic late-onset nemaline myopathy: clinical spectrum, survival, and treatment outcomes. *Neurology.* 2019;93(3):e298-e305.
84. Schnitzler L, Schubert B, Boasson M, Gardais J, Tourmen A. Urticaire chronique, lesions osseuses, macroglobulinemie IgM: maladie de Waldenstrom-IIe presentation. *Bull Soc Fr Dermatol Syphiligr.* 1974;81:363.
85. Lipsker D. The Schnitzler syndrome. *Orphanet J Rare Dis.* 2010;5:38.
86. de Koning HD, Bodar EJ, van der Meer JWM, Simon A; Schnitzler Syndrome Study Group. Schnitzler syndrome: beyond the case reports. Review and follow-up of 94 patients with an emphasis on prognosis and treatment. *Semin Arthritis Rheum.* 2007;37(3):137-148.
87. Jain T, Offord CP, Kyle RA, Dingli D. Schnitzler syndrome: an under-diagnosed clinical entity. *Haematologica.* 2013;98(10):1581-1585.
88. Kieffer C, Cribier B, Lipsker D. Neutrophilic urticarial dermatosis: a variant of neutrophilic urticaria strongly associated with systemic disease. Report of 9 new cases and review of the literature. *Medicine (Baltimore).* 2009;88(1):23-31.
89. Lipsker D, Veran Y, Grunenberger F, Cribier B, Heid E, Grosshans E. The Schnitzler syndrome. Four new cases and review of the literature. *Medicine (Baltimore).* 2001;80(1):37-44.
90. Lebbe C, Rybojad M, Klein F, et al. Schnitzler's syndrome associated with sensorimotor neuropathy. *J Am Acad Dermatol.* 1994;30(2 pt 2):316-318.
91. Nashan D, Sunderkotter C, Bonsmann G, Luger T, Goerdt S. Chronic urticaria, arthralgia, raised erythrocyte sedimentation rate and IgG paraproteinaemia: a variant of Schnitzler's syndrome? *Br J Dermatol.* 1995;133(1):132-134.
92. Niederhauser BD, Dingli D, Kyle RA, Ringler MD. Imaging findings in 22 cases of Schnitzler syndrome: characteristic para-articular osteosclerosis, and the "hot knees" sign differential diagnosis. *Skeletal Radiol.* 2014;43(7):905-915.
93. Lecompte M, Blais G, Bisson G, Maynard B. Schnitzler's syndrome. *Skeletal Radiol.* 1998;27(5):294-296.
94. Launay D, Dutoit-Lefevre V, Faure E, et al. Effect of in vitro and in vivo anakinra on cytokines production in Schnitzler syndrome. *PLoS One.* 2013;8(3):e59327.
95. de Koning HD, Schalkwijk J, van der Meer JWM, Simon A. Successful canakinumab treatment identifies IL-1β as a pivotal mediator in Schnitzler syndrome. *J Allergy Clin Immunol.* 2011;128(6):1352-1354.
96. Krause K, Weller K, Stefaniak R, et al. Efficacy and safety of the interleukin-1 antagonist rilonacept in Schnitzler syndrome: an open-label study. *Allergy.* 2012;67(7):943-950.
97. Hoffman HM, Mueller JL, Broide DH, Wanderer AA, Kolodner RD. Mutation of a new gene encoding a putative pyrin-like protein causes familial cold autoinflammatory syndrome and Muckle-Wells syndrome. *Nat Genet.* 2001;29(3):301-305.
98. de Koning HD, van Gijn ME, Stoffels M, et al. Myeloid lineage-restricted somatic mosaicism of NLRP3 mutations in patients with variant Schnitzler syndrome. *J Allergy Clin Immunol.* 2015;135(2):561-564.
99. Rowczenio DM, Pathak S, Arostegui JI, et al. Molecular genetic investigation, clinical features, and response to treatment in 21 patients with Schnitzler syndrome. *Blood.* 2018;131(9):974-981.
100. Sokumbi O, Drage LA, Peters MS. Clinical and histopathologic review of Schnitzler syndrome: the Mayo Clinic experience (1972-2011). *J Am Acad Dermatol.* 2012;67(6):1289-1295.
101. Janier M, Bonvalet D, Blanc MF, et al. Chronic urticaria and macroglobulinemia (Schnitzler's syndrome): report of two cases. *J Am Acad Dermatol.* 1989;20(2 pt 1):206-211.
102. Martinez-Taboada VM, Fontalba A, Blanco R, Fernandez-Luna JL. Successful treatment of refractory Schnitzler syndrome with anakinra: comment on the article by Hawkins et al. *Arthritis Rheum.* 2005;52(7):2226-2227.
103. Gusdorf L, Asli B, Barbarot S, et al. Schnitzler syndrome: validation and applicability of diagnostic criteria in real-life patients. *Allergy.* 2017;72(2):177-182.
104. Asli B, Brouet JC, Fermand JP. Spontaneous remission of Schnitzler syndrome. *Ann Allergy Asthma Immunol.* 2011;107(1):87-88.
105. Rongioletti F, Rebora A. Updated classification of papular mucinosis, lichen myxedematosus, and scleromyxedema. *J Am Acad Dermatol.* 2001;44(2):273-281.
106. Mahevas T, Arnulf B, Bouaziz JD, et al. Plasma cell-directed therapies in monoclonal gammopathy-associated scleromyxedema. *Blood.* 2020;135(14):1101-1110.
107. Kapoor P, Gonsalves WI. Of lions, shar-pei, and doughnuts: a tale retold. *Blood.* 2020;135(14):1074-1076.
108. Fleming KE, Virmani D, Sutton E, et al. Scleromyxedema and the dermato-neuro syndrome: case report and review of the literature. *J Cutan Pathol.* 2012;39(5):508-517.
109. De Simone C, Castriota M, Carbone A, Marini Bettolo P, Pieroni M, Rongioletti F. Cardiomyopathy in scleromyxedema: report of a fatal case. *Eur J Dermatol.* 2010;20(6):852-853.
110. Kalli F, Cioni M, Parodi A, et al. Increased frequency of interleukin-4 and reduced frequency of interferon-gamma and IL-17-producing CD4+ and CD8+ cells in scleromyxedema. *J Eur Acad Dermatol Venereol.* 2020;34(5):1092-1097.
111. Ferrarini M, Helfrich DJ, Walker ER, Medsger TA Jr, Whiteside TL. Scleromyxedema serum increases proliferation but not the glycosaminoglycan synthesis of dermal fibroblasts. *J Rheumatol.* 1989;16(6):837-841.
112. Sansbury JC, Cocuroccia B, Jorizzo JL, Gubinelli E, Gisondi P, Girolomoni G. Treatment of recalcitrant scleromyxedema with thalidomide in 3 patients. *J Am Acad Dermatol.* 2004;51(1):126-131.
113. Brunet-Possenti F, Hermine O, Marinho E, Crickx B, Descamps V. Combination of intravenous immunoglobulins and lenalidomide in the treatment of scleromyxedema. *J Am Acad Dermatol.* 2013;69(2):319-320.
114. Feasel AM, Donato ML, Duvic M. Complete remission of scleromyxedema following autologous stem cell transplantation. *Arch Dermatol.* 2001;137(8):1071-1072.
115. Lacy MQ, Hogan WJ, Gertz MA, et al. Successful treatment of scleromyxedema with autologous peripheral blood stem cell transplantation. *Arch Dermatol.* 2005;141(10):1277-1282.
116. Fett NM, Toporcer MB, Dalmau J, Shinohara MM, Vogl DT. Scleromyxedema and dermato-neuro syndrome in a patient with multiple myeloma effectively treated with dexamethasone and bortezomib. *Am J Hematol.* 2011;86(10):893-896.
117. Kossard S, Winkelmann RK. Necrobiotic xanthogranuloma with paraproteinemia. *J Am Acad Dermatol.* 1980;3(3):257-270.

118. Mehregan DA, Winkelmann RK. Necrobiotic xanthogranuloma. *Arch Dermatol.* 1992;128(1):94-100.
119. Higgins LS, Go RS, Dingli D, et al. Clinical features and treatment outcomes of patients with necrobiotic xanthogranuloma associated with monoclonal gammopathies. *Clin Lymphoma Myeloma Leuk.* 2016;16(8):447-452.
120. Szalat R, Pirault J, Fermand JP, et al. Physiopathology of necrobiotic xanthogranuloma with monoclonal gammopathy. *J Intern Med.* 2014;276(3):269-284.
121. Peyman A, Walsh N, Green P, Dorey MW, Seamone C, Pasternak S. Necrobiotic xanthogranuloma associated with necrotizing scleritis. *Am J Dermatopathol.* 2012;34(6):644-647.
122. Hallermann C, Tittelbach J, Norgauer J, Ziemer M. Successful treatment of necrobiotic xanthogranuloma with intravenous immunoglobulin. *Arch Dermatol.* 2010;146(9):957-960.
123. Rubinstein A, Wolf DJ, Granstein RD. Successful treatment of necrobiotic xanthogranuloma with intravenous immunoglobulin. *J Cutan Med Surg.* 2013;17(5):347-350.
124. Wintrobe M, Buell M. Hyperproteinemia associated with multiple myeloma. *Bull Johns Hopkins Hosp.* 1933;52:156-165.
125. Lerner A, Watson C. Studies of cryoglobulins. Unusual purpura associated with the presence of a high concentration of cryoglobulin (cold precipitable serum globulin). *Am J Med Sci.* 1947;214(4):410-415.
126. Grey HM, Kohler PF. Cryoimmunoglobulins. *Semin Hematol.* 1973;10(2):87-112.
127. Meltzer M, Franklin EC. Cryoglobulinemia – a study of twenty-nine patients. I. IgG and IgM cryoglobulins and factors affecting cryoprecipitability. *Am J Med.* 1966;40(6):828-836.
128. Meltzer M, Franklin EC, Elias K, McCluskey RT, Cooper N. Cryoglobulinemia – a clinical and laboratory study. II. Cryoglobulins with rheumatoid factor activity. *Am J Med.* 1966;40(6):837-856.
129. Brouet JC, Clauvel JP, Danon F, Klein M, Seligmann M. Biologic and clinical significance of cryoglobulins. A report of 86 cases. *Am J Med.* 1974;57(5):775-788.
130. Gorevic PD, Kassab HJ, Levo Y, et al. Mixed cryoglobulinemia: clinical aspects and long-term follow-up of 40 patients. *Am J Med.* 1980;69(2):287-308.
131. Dispenzieri A, Gorevic PD. Cryoglobulinemia. *Hematol Oncol Clin North Am.* 1999;13(6):1315-1349.
132. Monti G, Galli M, Invernizzi F, et al. Cryoglobulinaemias: a multi-centre study of the early clinical and laboratory manifestations of primary and secondary disease. GISC. Italian Group for the Study of Cryoglobulinaemias. *Q J Med.* 1995;88(2):115-126.
133. Pascual M, Perrin L, Giostra E, Schifferli JA. Hepatitis C virus in patients with cryoglobulinemia type II. *J Infect Dis.* 1990;162(2):569-570.
134. Ferri C, Greco F, Longombardo G, et al. Antibodies to hepatitis C virus in patients with mixed cryoglobulinemia. *Arthritis Rheum.* 1991;34(12):1606-1610.
135. Trejo O, Ramos-Casals M, Garcia-Carrasco M, et al. Cryoglobulinemia: study of etiologic factors and clinical and immunologic features in 443 patients from a single center. *Medicine (Baltimore).* 2001;80(4):252-262.
136. Invernizzi F, Galli M, Serino G, et al. Secondary and essential cryoglobulinemias. Frequency, nosological classification, and long-term follow-up. *Acta Haematol.* 1983;70(2):73-82.
137. Osserman E. Plasma-cell myeloma. II. Clinical aspects. *N Engl J Med.* 1959;261:952-960.
138. Bryce AH, Kyle RA, Dispenzieri A, Gertz MA. Natural history and therapy of 66 patients with mixed cryoglobulinemia. *Am J Hematol.* 2006;81(7):511-518.
139. Disdier P, Harle JR, Weiller PJ. Cryoglobulinaemia and hepatitis C infection. *Lancet.* 1991;338(8775):1151-1152.
140. Agnello V, Chung RT, Kaplan LM. A role for hepatitis C virus infection in type II cryoglobulinemia. *N Engl J Med.* 1992;327(21):1490-1495.
141. Misiani R, Bellavita P, Fenili D, et al. Hepatitis C virus infection in patients with essential mixed cryoglobulinemia. *Ann Intern Med.* 1992;117(7):573-577.
142. Pechere-Bertschi A, Perrin L, de Saussure P, Widmann JJ, Giostra E, Schifferli JA. Hepatitis C: a possible etiology for cryoglobulinaemia type II. *Clin Exp Immunol.* 1992;89(3):419-422.
143. Cacoub P, Fabiani FL, Musset L, et al. Mixed cryoglobulinemia and hepatitis C virus. *Am J Med.* 1994;96(2):124-132.
144. Tanaka K, Aiyama T, Imai J, Morishita Y, Fukatsu T, Kakumu S. Serum cryoglobulin and chronic hepatitis C virus disease among Japanese patients. *Am J Gastroenterol.* 1995;90(10):1847-1852.
145. Tarantino A, De Vecchi A, Montagnino G, et al. Renal disease in essential mixed cryoglobulinaemia. Long-term follow-up of 44 patients. *Q J Med.* 1981;50(197):1-30.
146. Singer DR, Venning MC, Lockwood CM, Pusey CD. Cryoglobulinaemia: clinical features and response to treatment. *Q J Med.* 1986;137(3):251-253.
147. Monti G, Saccardo F, Pioltelli P, Rinaldi G. The natural history of cryoglobulinemia: symptoms at onset and during follow-up. A report by the Italian Group for the Study of Cryoglobulinemias (GISC). *Clin Exp Rheumatol.* 1995;13(suppl 13):S129-S133.
148. Ferri C, Sebastiani M, Giuggioli D, et al. Mixed cryoglobulinemia: demographic, clinical, and serologic features and survival in 231 patients. *Semin Arthritis Rheum.* 2004;33(6):355-374.
149. Rieu V, Cohen P, Andre MH, et al. Characteristics and outcome of 49 patients with symptomatic cryoglobulinaemia. *Rheumatology.* 2002;41(3):290-300.
150. De Vita S, Quartuccio L, Isola M, et al. A randomized controlled trial of rituximab for the treatment of severe cryoglobulinemic vasculitis. *Arthritis Rheum.* 2012;64(3):843-853.
151. Foessel L, Besancenot JF, Blaison G, et al. Clinical spectrum, treatment, and outcome of patients with type II mixed cryoglobulinemia without evidence of hepatitis C infection. *J Rheumatol.* 2011;38(4):716-722.
152. Monti G, Saccardo F, Castelnovo L, et al. Prevalence of mixed cryoglobulinaemia syndrome and circulating cryoglobulins in a population-based survey: the Origgio study. *Autoimmun Rev.* 2014;13(6):609-614.
153. Goldman M, Renversez JC, Lambert PH. Pathological expression of idiotypic interactions: immune complexes and cryoglobulins. *Springer Semin Immunopathol.* 1983;6(1):33-49.
154. Wilson MR, Arroyave CM, Miles L, Tan EM. Immune reactants in cryoproteins. Relationship to complement activation. *Ann Rheum Dis.* 1977;36(6):540-548.
155. Lunel F, Musset L, Cacoub P, et al. Cryoglobulinemia in chronic liver diseases: role of hepatitis C virus and liver damage. *Gastroenterology.* 1994;106(5):1291-1300.
156. Sansonno D, Iacobelli AR, Cornacchiulo V, et al. Immunochemical and biomolecular studies of circulating immune complexes isolated from patients with acute and chronic hepatitis C virus infection. *Eur J Clin Invest.* 1996;26(6):465-475.
157. Pileri P, Uematsu Y, Campagnoli S, et al. Binding of hepatitis C virus to CD81. *Science.* 1998;282(5390):938-941.
158. Agnello V, Abel G, Elfahal M, Knight GB, Zhang QX. Hepatitis C virus and other flaviviridae viruses enter cells via low density lipoprotein receptor. *Proc Natl Acad Sci U S A.* 1999;96(22):12766-12771.
159. Hartmann H, Schott P, Polzien F, et al. Cryoglobulinemia in chronic hepatitis C virus infection: prevalence, clinical manifestations, response to interferon treatment and analysis of cryoprecipitates. *Z Gastroenterol.* 1995;33(11):643-650.
160. Galli M, Monti G, Monteverde A, et al. Hepatitis C virus and mixed cryoglobulinaemias. *Lancet.* 1992;339(8799):989.
161. Cacoub P, Lunel F, Musset L, Opolon P, Piette JC. Hepatitis C virus and cryoglobulinemia. *N Engl J Med.* 1993;328(15):1121-1122; author reply 1123-1124.
162. Zignego AL, Ferri C, Giannini C, et al. Hepatitis C virus infection in mixed cryoglobulinemia and B-cell non-Hodgkin's lymphoma: evidence for a pathogenetic role. *Arch Virol.* 1997;142(3):545-555.
163. Lunel F. Hepatitis C virus and autoimmunity: fortuitous association or reality? *Gastroenterology.* 1994;107(5):1550-1555.
164. Schmidt WN, Stapleton JT, LaBrecque DR, et al. Hepatitis C virus (HCV) infection and cryoglobulinemia: analysis of whole blood and plasma HCV-RNA concentrations and correlation with liver histology. *Hepatology.* 2000;31(3):737-744.
165. Saadoun D, Asselah T, Resche-Rigon M, et al. Cryoglobulinemia is associated with steatosis and fibrosis in chronic hepatitis C. *Hepatology.* 2006;43(6):1337-1345.
166. Hofmann WP, Herrmann E, Kronenberger B, et al. Association of HCV-related mixed cryoglobulinemia with specific mutational pattern of the HCV E2 protein and CD81 expression on peripheral B lymphocytes. *Blood.* 2004;104(4):1228-1229.
167. Rosa D, Saletti G, De Gregorio E, et al. Activation of naive B lymphocytes via CD81, a pathogenetic mechanism for hepatitis C virus-associated B lymphocyte disorders. *Proc Natl Acad Sci U S A.* 2005;102(51):18544-18549.
168. Charles ED, Green RM, Marukian S, et al. Clonal expansion of immunoglobulin M+CD27+ B cells in HCV-associated mixed cryoglobulinemia. *Blood.* 2008;111(3):1344-1356.
169. Charles ED, Brunetti C, Marukian S, et al. Clonal B cells in patients with hepatitis C virus-associated mixed cryoglobulinemia contain an expanded anergic CD21low B-cell subset. *Blood.* 2011;117(20):5425-5437.
170. Saadoun D, Rosenzwajg M, Landau D, Piette JC, Klatzmann D, Cacoub P. Restoration of peripheral immune homeostasis after rituximab in mixed cryoglobulinemia vasculitis. *Blood.* 2008;111(5):5334-5341.
171. Dammacco F, Tucci FA, Lauletta G, et al. Pegylated interferon-alpha, ribavirin, and rituximab combined therapy of hepatitis C virus-related mixed cryoglobulinemia: a long-term study. *Blood.* 2010;116(3):343-353.
172. Husson JM, Druet P, Contet A, Fiessinger JN, Camilleri JP. Systemic sclerosis and cryoglobulinemia. *Clin Immunol Immunopathol.* 1976;6(1):77-82.
173. Wotherspoon AC, Ortiz-Hidalgo C, Falzon MR, Isaacson PG. Helicobacter pylori-associated gastritis and primary B-cell gastric lymphoma. *Lancet.* 1991;338(8776):1175-1176.
174. Monti G, Pioltelli P, Saccardo F, et al. Incidence and characteristics of non-Hodgkin lymphomas in a multicenter case file of patients with hepatitis C virus-related symptomatic mixed cryoglobulinemias. *Arch Intern Med.* 2005;165(1):101-105.
175. Zignego AL, Ferri C, Giannelli F, et al. Prevalence of bcl-2 rearrangement in patients with hepatitis C virus-related mixed cryoglobulinemia with or without B-cell lymphomas. *Ann Intern Med.* 2002;137(7):571-580.
176. Montagnino G. Reappraisal of the clinical expression of mixed cryoglobulinemia. *Springer Semin Immunopathol.* 1988;10(1):1-19.
177. Cohen SJ, Pittelkow MR, Su WP. Cutaneous manifestations of cryoglobulinemia: clinical and histopathologic study of seventy-two patients. *J Am Acad Dermatol.* 1991;25(1 pt 1):21-27.
178. Gemignani F, Brindani F, Alfieri S, et al. Clinical spectrum of cryoglobulinaemic neuropathy. *J Neurol Neurosurg Psychiatry.* 2005;76(10):1410-1414.
179. Gemignani F, Melli G, Inglese C, Marbini A. Cryoglobulinemia is a frequent cause of peripheral neuropathy in undiagnosed referral patients. *J Peripher Nerv Syst.* 2002;7(1):59-64.
180. Ammendola A, Sampaolo S, Ambrosone L, et al. Peripheral neuropathy in hepatitis-related mixed cryoglobulinemia: electrophysiologic follow-up study. *Muscle Nerve.* 2005;31(3):382-385.
181. Casato M, Saadoun D, Marchetti A, et al. Central nervous system involvement in hepatitis C virus cryoglobulinemia vasculitis: a multicenter case-control study using magnetic resonance imaging and neuropsychological tests. *J Rheumatol.* 2005;32(3):484-488.
182. Cappellari A, Origgi L, Spina MF, et al. Central nervous system involvement in HCV-related mixed cryoglobulinemia. *Electromyogr Clin Neurophysiol.* 2006;46(3):149-158.
183. D' Amico G. Renal involvement in hepatitis C infection: cryoglobulinemic glomerulonephritis. *Kidney Int.* 1998;54(2):650-671.

184. Tarantino A, Campise M, Banfi G, et al. Long-term predictors of survival in essential mixed cryoglobulinemic glomerulonephritis. *Kidney Int.* 1995;47(2):618-623.
185. Gorevic PD, Frangione B. Mixed cryoglobulinemia cross-reactive idiotypes: implications for the relationship of MC to rheumatic and lymphoproliferative diseases. *Semin Hematol.* 1991;28(2):79-94.
186. Levo Y, Gorevic PD, Kassab HJ, Tobias H, Franklin EC. Liver involvement in the syndrome of mixed cryoglobulinemia. *Ann Intern Med.* 1977;87(3):287-292.
187. Donada C, Crucitti A, Donadon V, et al. Systemic manifestations and liver disease in patients with chronic hepatitis C and type II or III mixed cryoglobulinaemia. *J Viral Hepat.* 1998;5(3):179-185.
188. Monteverde A, Ballare M, Bertoncelli MC, et al. Lymphoproliferation in type II mixed cryoglobulinemia. *Clin Exp Rheumatol.* 1995;13(suppl 13):S141-S147.
189. Monteverde A, Ballare M, Pileri S. Hepatic lymphoid aggregates in chronic hepatitis C and mixed cryoglobulinemia. *Springer Semin Immunopathol.* 1997;19(1):99-110.
190. Cream JJ. Clinical and immunological aspects of cutaneous vasculitis. *Q J Med.* 1976;45(178):255-276.
191. Ferri C, Moriconi L, Gremignai G, et al. Treatment of the renal involvement in mixed cryoglobulinemia with prolonged plasma exchange. *Nephron.* 1986;43(4):246-253.
192. Ferri C, Marzo E, Longombardo G, et al. Interferon alfa-2b in mixed cryoglobulinaemia: a controlled crossover trial. *Gut.* 1993;34(2 suppl):S144-S145.
193. Misiani R, Bellavita P, Fenili D, et al. Interferon alfa-2a therapy in cryoglobulinemia associated with hepatitis C virus. *N Engl J Med.* 1994;330(11):751-756.
194. Dammacco F, Sansonno D, Han JH, et al. Natural interferon-alpha versus its combination with 6-methyl-prednisolone in the therapy of type II mixed cryoglobulinemia: a long-term, randomized, controlled study. *Blood.* 1994;84(10):3336-3343.
195. Lauta VM, De Sangro MA. Long-term results regarding the use of recombinant interferon alpha-2b in the treatment of II type mixed essential cryoglobulinemia. *Med Oncol.* 1995;12(4):223-230.
196. Mazzaro C, Lacchin T, Moretti M, et al. Effects of two different alpha-interferon regimens on clinical and virological findings in mixed cryoglobulinemia. *Clin Exp Rheumatol.* 1995;13(suppl 13):S181-S185.
197. Migliaresi S, Tirri G. Interferon in the treatment of mixed cryoglobulinemia. *Clin Exp Rheumatol.* 1995;13(suppl 13):S175-S180.
198. Gragnani L, Visentini M, Fognani E, et al. Prospective study of guideline-tailored therapy with direct-acting antivirals for hepatitis C virus-associated mixed cryoglobulinemia. *Hepatology.* 2016;64(5):1473-1482.
199. Bonacci M, Lens S, Londoño MC, et al. Virologic, clinical, and immune response outcomes of patients with hepatitis C virus-associated cryoglobulinemia treated with direct-acting antivirals. *Clin Gastroenterol Hepatol.* 2017;15(4):575.e1-583.e1.
200. Valbonesi M, Montani F, Mosconi L, Florio G, Vecchi C. Plasmapheresis and cytotoxic drugs for mixed cryoglobulinemia. *Haematologia.* 1984;17(3):341-351.
201. De Vecchi A, Montagnino G, Pozzi C, Tarantino A, Locatelli F, Ponticelli C. Intravenous methylprednisolone pulse therapy in essential mixed cryoglobulinemia nephropathy. *Clin Nephrol.* 1983;19(5):221-227.
202. Casato M, Lagana B, Antonelli A, Dianzani F, Bonomo L. Long-term results of therapy with interferon-alpha for type II essential mixed cryoglobulinemia. *Blood.* 1991;78(12):3142-3147.
203. Calleja JL, Albillos A, Moreno-Otero R, et al. Sustained response to interferon-alpha or to interferon-alpha plus ribavirin in hepatitis C virus-associated symptomatic mixed cryoglobulinaemia. *Aliment Pharmacol Ther.* 1999;13(9):1179-1186.
204. Donada C, Crucitti A, Donadon V, Chemello L, Alberti A. Interferon and ribavirin combination therapy in patients with chronic hepatitis C and mixed cryoglobulinemia. *Blood.* 1998;92(8):2983-2984.
205. Mazzaro C, Zorat F, Comar C, et al. Interferon plus ribavirin in patients with hepatitis C virus positive mixed cryoglobulinemia resistant to interferon. *J Rheumatol.* 2003;30(8):1775-1781.
206. Mazzaro C, Zorat F, Caizzi M, et al. Treatment with peg-interferon alfa-2b and ribavirin of hepatitis C virus-associated mixed cryoglobulinemia: a pilot study. *J Hepatol.* 2005;42(5):632-638.
207. Saadoun D, Resche-Rigon M, Thibault V, Piette JC, Cacoub P. Antiviral therapy for hepatitis C virus-associated mixed cryoglobulinemia vasculitis: a long-term followup study. *Arthritis Rheum.* 2006;54(11):3696-3706.
208. Zaja F, De Vita S, Mazzaro C, et al. Efficacy and safety of rituximab in type II mixed cryoglobulinemia. *Blood.* 2003;101(10):3827-3834.
209. Sansonno D, De Re V, Lauletta G, Tucci FA, Boiocchi M, Dammacco F. Monoclonal antibody treatment of mixed cryoglobulinemia resistant to interferon alpha with an anti-CD20. *Blood.* 2003;101(10):3818-3826.
210. Bryce AH, Dispenzieri A, Kyle RA, et al. Response to rituximab in patients with type II cryoglobulinemia. *Clin Lymphoma Myeloma.* 2006;7(2):140-144.
211. Roccatello D, Baldovino S, Rossi D, et al. Long-term effects of anti-CD20 monoclonal antibody treatment of cryoglobulinaemic glomerulonephritis. *Nephrol Dial Transplant.* 2004;19(12):3054-3061.
212. Saadoun D, Resche Rigon M, Sene D, et al. Rituximab plus Peg-interferon-alpha/ribavirin compared with Peg-interferon-alpha/ribavirin in hepatitis C-related mixed cryoglobulinemia. *Blood.* 2010;116(3):326-334; quiz 504-505.
213. Leung N, Bridoux F, Hutchison CA, et al. Monoclonal gammopathy of renal significance: when MGUS is no longer undetermined or insignificant. *Blood.* 2012;120(22):4292-4295.
214. Leung N, Bridoux F, Batuman V, et al. The evaluation of monoclonal gammopathy of renal significance: a consensus report of the International Kidney and Monoclonal Gammopathy Research Group. *Nat Rev Nephrol.* 2019;15(1):45-59.
215. Chauvet S, Fremeaux-Bacchi V, Petitprez F, et al. Treatment of B-cell disorder improves renal outcome of patients with monoclonal gammopathy-associated C3 glomerulopathy. *Blood.* 2017;129(11):1437-1447.
216. Cohen C, El-Karoui K, Alyanakian MA, Noel LH, Bridoux F, Knebelmann B. Light and heavy chain deposition disease associated with CH1 deletion. *Clin Kidney J.* 2015;8(2):237-239.
217. Cohen C, Joly F, Sibille A, et al. Randall-type monoclonal immunoglobulin deposition disease: new insights into the pathogenesis, diagnosis and management. *Diagnostics.* 2021;11(3):420.
218. Vignon M, Javaugue V, Alexander MP, et al. Current anti-myeloma therapies in renal manifestations of monoclonal light chain-associated Fanconi syndrome: a retrospective series of 49 patients. *Leukemia.* 2017;31(1):123-129.
219. Solomon A, Weiss DT, Kattine AA. Nephrotoxic potential of bence Jones proteins. *N Engl J Med.* 1991;324(26):1845-1851.
220. Nasr SH, Vrana JA, Dasari S, et al. DNAJB9 is a specific immunohistochemical marker for fibrillary glomerulonephritis. *Kidney Int Rep.* 2018;3(1):56-64.
221. Nasr SH, Valeri AM, Cornell LD, et al. Fibrillary glomerulonephritis: a report of 66 cases from a single institution. *Clin J Am Soc Nephrol.* 2011;6(4):775-784.
222. Nasr SH, Fidler ME, Cornell LD, et al. Immunotactoid glomerulopathy: clinicopathologic and proteomic study. *Nephrol Dial Transplant.* 2012;27(11):4137-4146.
223. Stokes MB, Valeri AM, Herlitz L, et al. Light chain proximal tubulopathy: clinical and pathologic characteristics in the modern treatment era. *J Am Soc Nephrol.* 2016;27(5):1555-1565.
224. Larsen CP, Bell JM, Harris AA, Messias NC, Wang YH, Walker PD. The morphologic spectrum and clinical significance of light chain proximal tubulopathy with and without crystal formation. *Mod Pathol.* 2011;24(11):1462-1469.
225. Herrera GA. Proximal tubulopathies associated with monoclonal light chains: the spectrum of clinicopathologic manifestations and molecular pathogenesis. *Arch Pathol Lab Med.* 2014;138(10):1365-1380.
226. Sethi S, Rajkumar SV, D'Agati VD. The complexity and heterogeneity of monoclonal immunoglobulin-associated renal diseases. *J Am Soc Nephrol.* 2018;29(7):1810-1823.
227. Dogan S, Barnes L, Cruz-Vetrano WP. Crystal-storing histiocytosis: report of a case, review of the literature (80 cases) and a proposed classification. *Head Neck Pathol.* 2012;6(1):111-120.
228. Leung N, Buadi FK, Song KW, Magil AB, Cornell LD. A case of bilateral renal arterial thrombosis associated with cryocrystalglobulinaemia. *NDT Plus.* 2010;3(1):74-77.
229. Ball NJ, Wickert W, Marx LH, Thaell JF. Crystalglobulinemia syndrome. A manifestation of multiple myeloma. *Cancer.* 1993;71(4):1231-1234.
230. Bridoux F, Leung N, Hutchison CA, et al. Diagnosis of monoclonal gammopathy of renal significance. *Kidney Int.* 2015;87(4):698-711.
231. Katsuno T, Mizuno S, Mabuchi M, Tsuboi N, Komatsuda A, Maruyama S. Long-term renal survival of γ3-heavy chain deposition disease: a case report. *BMC Nephrol.* 2017;18(1):239.
232. Joly F, Cohen C, Javaugue V, et al. Randall-type monoclonal immunoglobulin deposition disease: novel insights from a nationwide cohort study. *Blood.* 2019;133(6):576-587.
233. Bridoux F, Javaugue V, Bender S, et al. Unravelling the immunopathological mechanisms of heavy chain deposition disease with implications for clinical management. *Kidney Int.* 2017;91(2):423-434.
234. Bhutani G, Nasr SH, Said SM, et al. Hematologic characteristics of proliferative glomerulonephritides with nonorganized monoclonal immunoglobulin deposits. *Mayo Clin Proc.* 2015;90(5):587-596.
235. Nasr SH, Markowitz GS, Stokes MB, et al. Proliferative glomerulonephritis with monoclonal IgG deposits: a distinct entity mimicking immune-complex glomerulonephritis. *Kidney Int.* 2004;65(1):85-96.
236. Fakhouri F, Fremeaux-Bacchi V, Noel LH, Cook HT, Pickering MC. C3 glomerulopathy: a new classification. *Nat Rev Nephrol.* 2010;6(8):494-499.
237. Fermand JP, Bridoux F, Kyle RA, et al. How I treat monoclonal gammopathy of renal significance (MGRS). *Blood.* 2013;122(22):3583-3590.
238. Kourelis TV, Nasr SH, Dispenzieri A, et al. Outcomes of patients with renal monoclonal immunoglobulin deposition disease. *Am J Hematol.* 2016;91(11):1123-1128.
239. Sethi S, Fervenza FC, Zhang Y, et al. Proliferative glomerulonephritis secondary to dysfunction of the alternative pathway of complement. *Clin J Am Soc Nephrol.* 2011;6(5):1009-1017.
240. Smith RJH, Harris CL, Pickering MC. Dense deposit disease. *Mol Immunol.* 2011;48(14):1604-1610.
241. Larsen CP, Messias NC, Walker PD, et al. Membranoproliferative glomerulonephritis with masked monotypic immunoglobulin deposits. *Kidney Int.* 2015;88(4):867-873.
242. Blanc C, Togarsimalemath SK, Chauvet S, et al. Anti-factor H autoantibodies in C3 glomerulopathies and in atypical hemolytic uremic syndrome: one target, two diseases. *J Immunol.* 2015;194(11):5129-5138.
243. Leung N, Drosou ME, Nasr SH. Dysproteinemias and glomerular disease. *Clin J Am Soc Nephrol.* 2018;13(1):128-139.
244. Pulivarthi S, Gurram MK. An atypical presentation of POEMS syndrome with IgG kappa type M protein and normal VEGF level: case report and review of literature. *J Cancer Res Therapeut.* 2018;14(3):679-681.
245. Klomjit N, Leung N, Fervenza F, Sethi S, Zand L. Rate and predictors of finding monoclonal gammopathy of renal significance (MGRS) lesions on kidney biopsy in patients with monoclonal gammopathy. *J Am Soc Nephrol.* 2020;31(10):2400-2411.
246. Fish R, Pinney J, Jain P, et al. The incidence of major hemorrhagic complications after renal biopsies in patients with monoclonal gammopathies. *Clin J Am Soc Nephrol.* 2010;5(11):1977-1980.
247. Javaugue V, Dufour-Nourigat L, Desport E, et al. Results of a nation-wide cohort study suggest favorable long-term outcomes of clone-targeted chemotherapy in immunotactoid glomerulopathy. *Kidney Int.* 2021;99(2):421-430.

248. Gumber R, Cohen JB, Palmer MB, et al. A clone-directed approach may improve diagnosis and treatment of proliferative glomerulonephritis with monoclonal immunoglobulin deposits. *Kidney Int.* 2018;94(1):199-205.
249. Contejean A, Larousserie F, Bouscary D, et al. A colonic mass revealing a disseminated crystal storing histiocytosis secondary to indolent multiple myeloma: a case report with literature review. *BMC Gastroenterol.* 2020;20(1):239.
250. Heybeli C, Alexander MP, Bentall AJ, et al. Kidney transplantation in patients with monoclonal gammopathy of renal significance (MGRS)-associated lesions: a case series. *Am J Kidney Dis.* 2022;79(2):202-216.
251. Angel-Korman A, Stern L, Angel Y, et al. The role of kidney transplantation in monoclonal Ig deposition disease. *Kidney Int Rep.* 2020;5(4):485-493.
252. Rosado FG, Oliveira JL, Sohani AR, et al. Bone marrow findings of the newly described TEMPI syndrome: when erythrocytosis and plasma cell dyscrasia coexist. *Mod Pathol.* 2015;28(3):367-372.
253. Druey KM, Parikh SM. Idiopathic systemic capillary leak syndrome (Clarkson disease). *J Allergy Clin Immunol.* 2017;140(3):663-670.
254. Xie Z, Chan EC, Long LM, Nelson C, Druey KM. High-dose intravenous immunoglobulin therapy for systemic capillary leak syndrome (Clarkson disease). *Am J Med.* 2015;128(1):91-95.

Part 8

HEMATOPOIETIC CELLULAR THERAPY

Chapter 104 ▪ Hematopoietic Cell Transplantation

RACHEL B. SALIT • FREDERICK R. APPELBAUM

HISTORY OF HEMATOPOIETIC CELL TRANSPLANTATION

In 1949, Leon Jacobsen demonstrated for the first time that mice could be protected from the otherwise lethal effects of total body irradiation (TBI) by shielding the spleen or hind limb (Figure 104.1).[1] Subsequent experiments found that radiation-induced marrow aplasia could be reversed with the infusion of bone marrow (BM) from a mouse of the same strain.[2] E. Donnall Thomas and others then hypothesized that it should therefore be possible to eradicate an abnormal marrow and replace it with one from a normal healthy donor. In 1960, Thomas performed the first successful bone marrow transplant (BMT) when he cured a 7-year-old girl of aplastic anemia by infusing marrow from an identical twin. Efforts in patients without twin donors uniformly failed. Using an outbred canine model, Thomas and associates determined the dose of TBI needed to prevent the host from rejecting nontwin donor marrow, the need for histocompatibility matching, and the utility of posttransplant methotrexate (MTX) to prevent otherwise lethal graft-vs-host disease (GVHD).[3,4] With those measures, long-term stable engraftment of donor marrow could be achieved in almost all matched littermates.

Bone marrow from human leukocyte antigen (HLA)-identical sibling donors was first successfully used to treat patients with immune deficiencies in 1968.[5,6] In 1970, Thomas and colleagues performed the first successful allogeneic transplants for patients with end-stage leukemia, and a year later for patients with aplastic anemia.[7] In 1975, the Seattle group reported their experience with marrow transplantation for 110 patients with either aplastic anemia or end-stage leukemia, showing that cures could be achieved in both settings.[8] In 1979, Hansen and colleagues performed the first successful marrow graft from an unrelated donor for a patient with leukemia.[9]

Since the initial clinical trials, more than 1 million hematopoietic cell transplants (HCTs) have been performed around the world using BM, peripheral blood, or cord blood (CB) following myeloablative and reduced-intensity conditioning (RIC) regimens for a variety of malignant and nonmalignant indications. In the last edition of this book, the most significant advance was the ability of the transplant community to find donors for almost all patients in need. Since then, there has been a substantial increase in the number of patients receiving mismatched related donor transplants (haploidentical) with overall survival (OS) approaching that of matched unrelated donor transplants and in some cases HLA-matched sibling transplantation. The biggest advances in the past several years pertain to the prevention and treatment of acute and chronic GVHD. For the first time in 30 years, a drug (ruxolitinib) was United States Federal Drug Administration

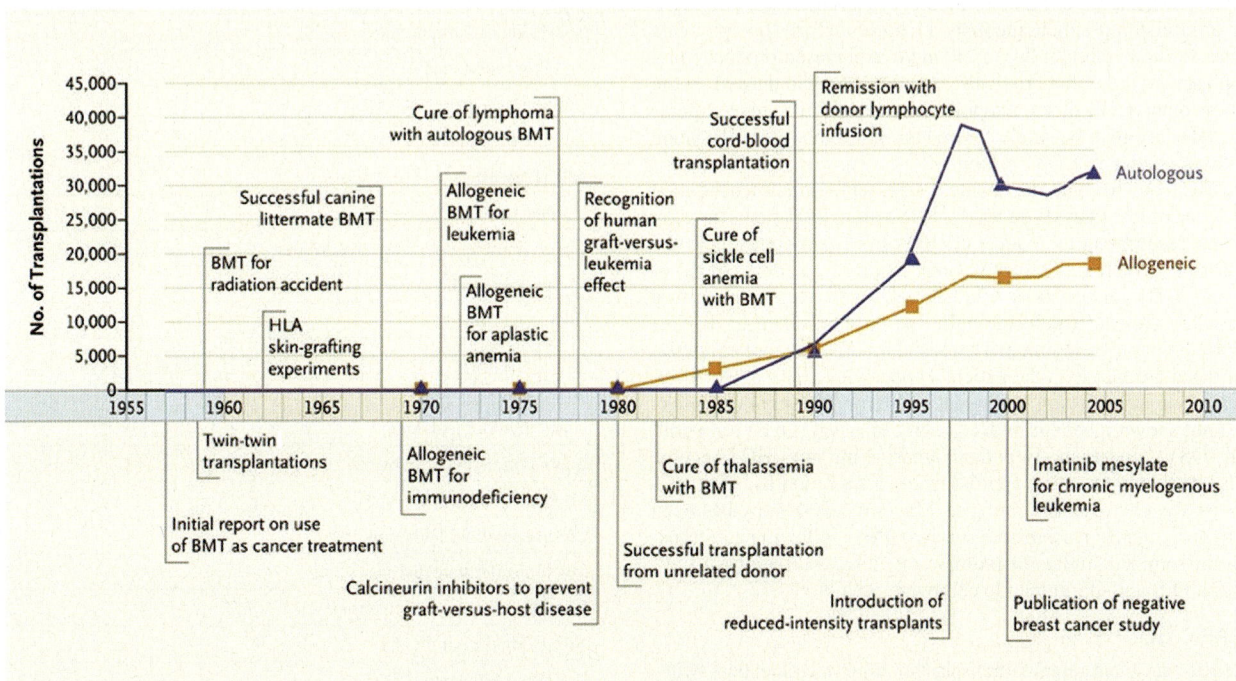

FIGURE 104.1 Historical Timeline. (From Appelbaum FR. Hematopoietic-cell transplantation at 50. *N Engl J Med.* 2007;357(15):1472-1475. Copyright © 2007 Massachusetts Medical Society. Reprinted with permission from Massachusetts Medical Society.)

(FDA) approved for the treatment of steroid refractory acute GVHD by showing superiority to best available therapy. Furthermore, for the first time ever, we have three FDA-approved medications specifically for the treatment of chronic GVHD (ibrutinib, ruxolitinib, and belumosudil). In another first, the drug abatacept, a costimulation modulator, was recently FDA approved in combination with tacrolimus (TAC) and MTX for the prevention of acute GVHD. Posttransplant cyclophosphamide (PTCy), initially used only in haplo-HCT, has now been explored in most donor sources with a significant decrease in the incidence of chronic GVHD. Last but certainly not least, cytomegalovirus (CMV), which used to be a deadly virus in transplant patients, is now almost completely preventable with the early post-HCT use of letermovir, a drug that has shown substantial effects even in patients receiving CB or T-cell-depleted transplants.

This chapter will focus on general principles of HCT including stem cell sources, conditioning regimens, and methods to prevent or treat complications. The role of HCT in the treatment of specific diseases will be mentioned briefly but discussed in greater detail in the chapters dedicated to those diseases.

DONOR SOURCES

Autologous HCT

The goal of an autologous (auto) HCT is to be able to give a patient disease targeted myeloablative chemotherapy and then rescue them with their own previously saved stem cells. Auto-HCT is used most frequently in patients with multiple myeloma and lymphoma. Auto–stem cells are usually collected either from granulocyte colony stimulating factor (G-CSF) or from chemo-mobilized peripheral blood and much less frequently collected from BM. Prior to mobilization, peripheral blood flow cytometry is sent to ensure only a minimal disease burden is present. Mobilization strategies for autologous stem cell transplant in patients with malignancy vary. One approach is to treat patients with chemotherapy followed by (G-CSF) at 6 μg/kg/d. After chemotherapy, patients are apheresed when the total white blood cell count has recovered to 1000/μL and the CD34$^+$ cell count in the peripheral blood is at >20/μL, with the goal of collecting 5 million CD34$^+$ stem cells or 10 million in the case of multiple myeloma (enough for two transplants).[10] For patients not requiring chemotherapy, mobilization is with G-CSF alone (5-16 μg/kg) by daily subcutaneous injection for 5 to 8 days.[11] If the patient fails to mobilize, plerixafor 0.24 mg/kg/d may be administered subcutaneously 11 hours before the apheresis procedure.[12] The maximum dose is 40 mg/d. Apheresed products may be cryopreserved in 5% dimethylsulfoxide (DMSO) and thawed on the day of transplant. Cells that are kept frozen at liquid nitrogen temperatures for later use may be safely thawed and used more than 10 years later without change in CD34$^+$ viability.[13]

Auto-HCT has become increasingly safe, with a treatment-related mortality rate of less than 1% to 3%.[14,15] Occasionally patients develop a syndrome resembling mild acute GVHD of the gastrointestinal (GI) tract and skin, which generally responds rapidly to a short course of prednisone.[16] By far the most frequent reason for treatment failure is disease recurrence, usually thought due to persistence of disease despite the preparative regimen. There is also a risk of contamination of the infused product with the patient's underlying disease. However, studies looking at removing malignant cells from the stem cell product have not shown a benefit in disease-free survival (DFS) or overall survival (OS).[17] Increasingly patients undergoing auto-HCT receive maintenance therapy starting approximately 1 to 3 months after HCT to decrease the risk of disease relapse. Maintenance therapy has been shown to prolong progression-free survival (PFS) following autotransplant in randomized studies of multiple myeloma and Hodgkin lymphoma and PFS and OS in mantle cell lymphoma.[18-20]

Syngeneic HCT

A syngeneic transplant refers to transplantation between identical twins. Syngeneic transplants are uncommon (only about 1 in 100 patients has an identical twin) but have the advantage over autologous transplantation in that the stem cell product cannot be contaminated by tumor. The choice of syngeneic vs allogeneic donor is more difficult; while use of syngeneic stem cells is clearly safer, they lack a graft versus leukemia effect.

Allogeneic HCT

When the BM of the patient is clearly abnormal such as in diseases like myelofibrosis, myelodysplastic syndrome, and acute and chronic leukemia, allo-HCT rather than auto-HCT is preferred. There are multiple sources of allo stem cells: HLA-matched sibling donor, HLA-matched and HLA-mismatched unrelated donor, HLA-mismatched related donor, and umbilical CB. Peripheral blood stem cells (PBSCs) can usually be collected using peripheral venous access, but if the peripheral veins are inadequate, a large bore double lumen catheter may need to be placed. In a large study of safety done by the NMDP (National Marrow Donor Program) (n = 2408 donors), collection of PBSCs was found to be safe but nearly all donors experienced bone pain and 25% had headache, nausea, or citrate induced toxicity with hypocalcemia or thrombocytopenia.[21] In this same study, serious and unexpected toxicities were experienced by 0.6% of donors, all of whom had complete recovery.

INDICATIONS FOR TRANSPLANTATION (TABLE 104.1)

Malignant Diseases

The leading indication for allo-HCT is acute myeloid leukemia (AML), followed by myelodysplasia (MDS), and acute lymphoblastic leukemia (ALL). The leading indication for auto-HCT is multiple myeloma, followed by non-Hodgkin lymphoma, and Hodgkin lymphoma.

Acute Myeloid Leukemia

Allo-HCT for AML consistently achieves 5-year DFS rates of 50% to 70% when performed in first remission.[22] Meta-analysis of studies of outcomes of matched sibling allo-HCT compared with conventional chemotherapy for adult patients with AML in first remission

Table 104.1. Common Indications for Transplantation

Autologous
Multiple myeloma
Non-Hodgkin lymphoma
Hodgkin lymphoma
Amyloidosis
Autoimmune diseases
Allogeneic
Nonmalignant Disease
Severe immune deficiency syndromes
Severe aplastic anemia
Hemoglobinopathies
Enzymatic disorders
Malignant Disease
Acute myeloid leukemia
Acute lymphocytic leukemia
Myelodysplastic syndrome
Chronic myeloid leukemia
Myeloproliferative disease
Chronic lymphocytic leukemia
Non-Hodgkin lymphoma
Hodgkin lymphoma
Multiple myeloma

show improved OS with HCT.[23] The advantages of transplantation are seen in patients with unfavorable and intermediate-risk leukemia but not in those with favorable risk disease.[24] Cure rates decrease if patients are transplanted in second complete remission (CR2) but are still better than expected for chemotherapy alone.[25] Allogeneic HCT is also able to cure a small but significant proportion of patients who fail primary induction therapy.[26] Younger patients who can tolerate a high-intensity regimen benefit from more intense therapy compared to RIC.[27] Patients with minimal residual disease (MRD) are in morphologic remission (blasts <5%) but have evidence of disease by flow cytometry, cytogenetics, fluorescent in situ hybridization, or molecular markers. These patients are at higher risk for relapse following HCT than patients with no MRD.[28] Studies are ongoing to see if additional therapy attempting to achieve MRD negative remission prior to HCT improves DFS and OS.

Acute Lymphocytic Leukemia

Long-term survival is improved with allo-HCT for ALL patients with high-risk disease including those with mixed lineage leukemia, Philadelphia chromosome positive (Ph+) ALL, and patients who are delayed in achieving remission beyond the first cycle of induction chemotherapy. Results are mixed in those with standard risk disease, especially for patients who are MRD negative.[29,30] Results in patients with Ph+ ALL have improved with the availability of tyrosine kinase inhibitors (TKIs), but HCT remains superior to chemotherapy.[31] Post-HCT therapy with second- and third-generation TKIs has been associated in some studies with decreased relapse and improved PFS; duration of therapy ranges from 1 to 5 years.[32] Patients who are refractory to chemotherapy but achieve remission following blinatumomab or chimeric antigen receptor (CAR) T-cells are also transplant candidates.

Myelodysplastic Syndrome

MDS is generally incurable except with allo-HCT, which may cure 20% to 80% of patients depending on disease risk, age, and de novo vs treatment-related MDS.[33] Because patients with early stage MDS often live for long periods without treatment, HCT is generally reserved for patients with advanced stage disease.[34,35] Current guidelines recommend allo-HCT be considered for patients up to age 65 years and with intermediate 2 or high risk staging score according to the standard or revised international prognostic staging score (IPSS). It is unproven whether pretreatment of patients with MDS prior to HCT improves outcomes.[36] Patients who are MRD positive by cytogenetics or flow cytometry benefit from a higher intensity conditioning regimen.[37]

Chronic Myeloid Leukemia

Although HCT can cure the majority of patients with CML, it is now reserved for patients who fail two TKIs and those with accelerated or blast phase disease.[38] TKI maintenance posttransplant is generally well tolerated, although randomized trials testing efficacy have not been conducted.[39]

Myeloproliferative Disease

Allo-HCT can cure patients with primary or secondary myelofibrosis. HCT is recommended for patients who have a dynamic (D) IPSS or DIPSS plus score of intermediate 2 or high risk (<5-year OS). Three-year OS with HCT ranges from 50% to 80% with patients responding to JAK inhibitors being more likely to have superior outcomes.[40,41] Graft failure is uncommon but it may take many months or even years for the fibrosis to resolve. Allo-HCT for chronic myelomonocytic leukemia is curative in approximately 30% of patients.[42]

Chronic Lymphocytic Leukemia

Allo-HCT can cure patients with CLL but it has not been extensively studied due to the older age of patients and the indolent nature of the disease. In registry studies looking at patients who have progressed through multiple lines of therapy, 5-year survival rates of 40% to 50% were seen.[43] The many new treatments for CLL in recent years including CAR-T cell therapy result in only the most refractory patients being treated with HCT.

Multiple Myeloma

Randomized trials have demonstrated that following standard induction chemotherapy, auto-HCT for multiple myeloma improves survival in patients younger than 65 years with newly diagnosed multiple myeloma.[18,44] PFS is longer if patients have HCT earlier rather than waiting for first relapse. Maintenance with lenalidomide or bortezomib further improves PFS.[18] One risk of maintenance therapy is an increased incidence of secondary malignancy such as MDS. Allo-HCT is the only curative therapy for myeloma. However, the lack of consistent survival benefit has limited this modality to patients who are younger and have high-risk disease or those being treated on clinical trials.[45]

Hodgkin Lymphoma

High-dose therapy followed by auto-HCT results in 5-year DFS in about 40% in patients with primary progressive Hodgkin disease (HD) (progression of disease during initial treatment or within 90 days of completion of initial chemotherapy).[46] Randomized trials have shown an advantage for salvage treatment followed by auto-HCT vs second-line treatment alone for patients with recurrent HD.[46] Allo-HCT can result in PFS for patients who have failed a prior auto-HCT; PFS is improved if patients achieve a CR prior to proceeding with the allo-HCT.[47]

Non-Hodgkin Lymphoma

Similar to HD, patients who fail to respond to initial therapy or relapse shortly after achieving remission have improved survival with auto-HCT following salvage chemotherapy over second-line chemotherapy alone.[48,49] Recurrent indolent non-Hodgkin lymphoma appears sensitive to the graft vs tumor (GVT) effect and very high response rates are seen with RIC allo-HCT for follicular lymphoma.[49] Auto- and allo-HCT are both useful in mantle cell lymphoma (MCL); auto-HCT has been shown to be curative in MCL in CR1 for some patients.[50] With many new targeted agents and the emergence of CD19-directed immunotherapy, the timing of HCT in the disease course for patients with non-Hodgkin lymphoma is the subject of numerous studies.

Nonmalignant Diseases

Immunodeficiencies

HCT can establish a normal immune system for patients with immunodeficiency disorders. Survival at 5 years can be expected in greater than 85% of children with severe combined immune deficiency.[51] Similar cure rates are seen for patients with other primary immune deficiency states such as Wiskott-Aldrich syndrome.[52]

Aplastic Anemia

Ninety percent of patients with aplastic anemia can be cured with HCT from a matched sibling making this the first-line treatment for such patients. Historically, results were slightly less favorable with a matched unrelated donor or a haploidentical related donor but have greatly improved in recent years.[53,54]

Hemoglobinopathies

HCT cures 70% to 90% of patients with thalassemia major with better results seen in patients with younger age, matched sibling donors, and those who have not yet experienced complications of their disease such as iron overload, hepatomegaly, or portal vein fibrosis.[55,56] For sickle cell anemia, most experts currently recommend HCT for patients who have suffered complications including stroke, recurrent veno-occlusive pain crises, acute chest syndrome, or sickle nephropathy. Five-year DFS and OS of 85% to 95% are seen in patients with matched siblings.[55,56] Because many patients with hemoglobinopathies are minorities who may not have unrelated donor options, CB and haplo donors are being explored as potential donor sources for patients.[57,58] HCT is also curative for patients with other hematopoietic disorders including Fanconi anemia, Blackfan Diamond Syndrome, and chronic granulomatous disease.[23]

Enzymatic Disorders

Allo-HCT can replace the abnormal enzyme systems and result in cure for patients with enzymatic disorders such as mucopolysaccharidosis and Gaucher disease.[59,60] Prior damage from the enzyme abnormality is likely irreversible suggesting that earlier HCT for patients with these inherited syndromes may be prudent.

Autoimmune Diseases

High-dose chemotherapy followed by auto-HCT has been shown to slow down or halt the progression of autoimmune diseases such as systemic sclerosis, multiple sclerosis, and systemic lupus erythematosus. In a study of 900 patients with autoimmune disease undergoing auto-HCT, sustained remissions of 5 years or greater were seen in 43% of patients refractory to standard therapy.[61] A randomized study of cyclophosphamide vs auto-HCT for patients with severe scleroderma demonstrated an OS (86 vs 51%) and event-free survival (74 vs 47%) benefit for HCT.[62] Studies of auto-HCT in GI, neurogenic, and other autoimmune disease continue to be pursued.

STEM CELL SOURCES

Bone Marrow

Bone marrow, which is rich in hematopoietic stem cells, was the first source of stem cells used for clinical transplantation. Bone marrow is obtained from the donor while under anesthesia through multiple aspirations from the posterior iliac crest. Each aspirate is limited to 5 to 10 mL to reduce contamination by peripheral blood. The goal of collection is usually 1 to 1.5 L and is based on recipient weight with a target of nucleated cell count of at least 2.5×10^8/kg recipient weight.[63] Often an autologous unit of blood is collected prior to marrow donation and returned during or after the procedure to replace blood lost during the collection. Life-threatening complications from marrow harvesting, usually related to anesthesia, have been reported in 0.27% to 0.4% of donors.[21] The marrow product is prepared for infusion by filtering out osseous particles and fat globules. Further processing may be required in the setting of ABO incompatibility. Ideally, marrow is infused in the patient immediately after harvesting. Delays of several days may occur without adverse consequences.

Peripheral Blood

Using G-CSF mobilization followed by leukopheresis, it is possible to collect sufficient stem cells from the peripheral blood for autologous or allogeneic HCT in the majority of cases. Side effects of G-CSF including bone pain, myalgias, and flu-like symptoms can be managed by pretreatment with antihistamine, and the use of acetaminophen and low-dose narcotics. Plerixafor is an antagonist of CXCR4, which blocks its interaction with SCF-1 resulting in mobilization of CD34 cells from the marrow. The addition of plerixafor allows for successful stem cell collections in most patients who fail to mobilize sufficient stem cells using G-CSF alone. Side effects of plerixafor include diarrhea, nausea, fatigue, headaches, and arthralgias. The advantage of peripheral blood collection is that donors avoid general anesthesia and other complications of marrow harvesting.

Due to the ease of peripheral blood collection and the more rapid engraftment with peripheral blood (up to 1 week faster), use of mobilized peripheral blood has largely replaced marrow as a source of stem cells for autologous transplantation. When more than 5 million CD34+ PBSCs are infused, engraftment (absolute neutrophil count [ANC] > 500) is seen at approximately 2 weeks post HCT. Randomized trials in matched sibling HCT have confirmed that the use of PBSCs accelerates engraftment without increasing acute GVHD.[64] Because peripheral blood also has a higher proportion of T-cells than marrow, the incidence of chronic GVHD may be higher with peripheral blood stem cell transplantation (PBSCT) than BMT; but disease recurrence appears to be less and survival equivalent or higher in the HLA-matched sibling setting.[64] In the unrelated setting, a large randomized study comparing BMT with PBSCT following a myeloablative preparative regimen and MTX plus a calcineurin inhibitor for GVHD prophylaxis showed faster engraftment but more chronic GVHD with PBSCT.[65] Survival was equivalent, but given the higher incidence of chronic GVHD, this study would favor the use of marrow, at least when using conventional methods of GVHD prophylaxis. Despite these results, there has not been a shift away from the use of PBSCT. Bone marrow and PBSC products can be cryopreserved in DMSO for later use. This has been essential in the era of coronavirus-19 (COVID-19) in order to collect products and have them confirmed at the recipient center prior to starting conditioning therapy.

Umbilical CB

CB is rich in CD34+ cells. Compared with a usual peripheral blood collection, one CB unit contains about a log less CD34+ stem cells per kg; however, the stem cells have potential for rapid expansion. CB cells are routinely collected and cryopreserved for storage in CB banks. After separation from the placenta, CB cells are collected into a closed system using a sterile donor blood collection set. Collected CB units must meet criteria of viability, sterility, and cell dose to be frozen for clinical use in patients.[66] Since October 2011, CB units have been a licensed bioproduct by the FDA. At present there are hundreds of thousands of HLA typed CBs banked in more than 100 public banks and they are conceivably available within several days' notice. Many of the banked specimens are from underrepresented ethnic and racial groups, thus expanding the donor pool for individuals poorly served by the unrelated donor registry.

HUMAN LEUKOCYTE ANTIGEN

Immune reactivity between donor and recipient is mediated by immunocompetent cells that react with HLA, which are encoded by genes of the major histocompatibility complex on chromosome 6 (*Figure 104.2A*). HLA molecules display exogenous peptides (from a virus or bacteria) and endogenous peptides presenting them to T-cells to initiate an immune response. If two people are not HLA-identical, T-cells from one person will react vigorously with the mismatched HLA molecules on the surface of the cells of the other person. Even when individuals are HLA matched, they are only matched at the major HLA antigens (HLA class I HLA-A, HLA-B, HLA-C, and HLA class II HLA-DR, HLA-DP, HLA-DQ), and the endogenous peptides presented will differ resulting in T-cell responses against the minor HLA antigens. Genes encoding HLA class I and II are tightly linked and inherited together with low recombination frequency.[67]

ALLOGENEIC DONOR TYPES

Matched sibling—Siblings with the same mother and father have a 25% chance of matching one another (*Figure 104.2B*). The likelihood of finding a matched sibling donor for a patient can be calculated by the formula $x = 1$ to 0.75^n where n equals the number of siblings. Historically, the probability of finding a healthy matched sibling donor for any patient was about 30%, but this may be decreasing in the modern era as people have fewer children and patients are older when they undergo HCT. Matched sibling donors remain the preferred option if healthy enough to donate.

Unrelated donor—Since the formation of the NMDP and other international registries, more than 40 million healthy individuals have volunteered to serve as stem cell donors. Donors who are completely unrelated to the patient but are matched at HLA A, B, C, DR, DQ have been increasingly used with results similar to HLA-matched siblings.[68] HLA-DP has also been recently shown to have an impact on post-HCT outcomes.[69] The likelihood of finding a 10 of 10 (HLA-A, B, C, DR, and DQ) matched unrelated donor varies among racial and ethnic groups from 75% for Caucasians to 16% for blacks of South and Central American descent.[70] This is not only due to underrepresentation of minorities in registries but also because of greater HLA diversity in certain populations. On average it takes 49 days (range 32-293) from the time a formal search is initiated to clearance of an unrelated donor.[71]

When compared with the outcome of a matched sibling HCT, matched unrelated donor HCTs are associated with greater morbidity

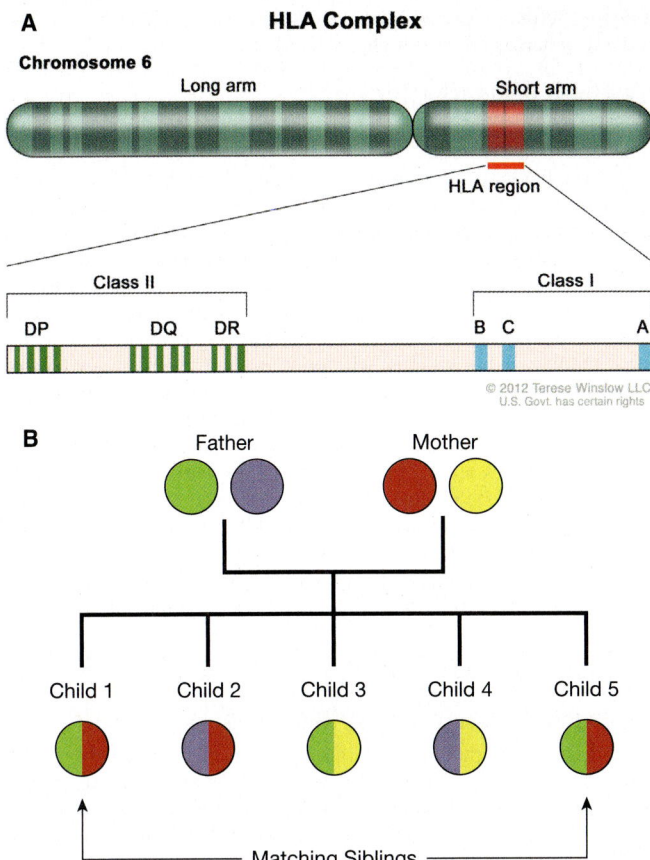

FIGURE 104.2 A, Human leukocyte antigen (HLA) complex. Human chromosome 6 with amplification of the HLA region. The locations of specific HLA loci for the class I B, C, and A alleles and the class II DP, DQ, and DR alleles are shown. B, Due to your genes being inherited from both parents, there is a 1 in 4 chance of finding a matched donor among siblings, because each parent pairing can have up to four different possible HLA combinations. However, in reality, only 30% of patients actually find a match within their family. Each child/parent is haploidentical matched and children have a 50% of having a haploidentical sibling. (A, National Cancer Institute: PDQ® Childhood Hematopoietic Cell Transplantation. Bethesda, MD: National Cancer Institute. https://www.cancer.gov/types/childhood-cancers/child-hct-hp-pdq#link/_21_toc. © 2012 Terese Winslow LLC, U.S. Govt. has certain rights.)

mostly from GVHD but survival at 3 to 5 years is similar.[68] Use of mismatched unrelated donors has historically been associated with more GVHD, higher nonrelapse mortality (NRM), and lower OS.[72] In a study of 3857 unrelated HCTs, which largely involved BM as a donor source, mismatches at A or DRBI were less well tolerated than mismatches at B or C; mismatching at 2 loci was associated with even greater risk.[73] If peripheral blood rather than marrow is the source of unrelated stem cells, mismatching for HLA-C appears to be less well tolerated.[74] Recently, it has been shown that certain HLA-C and HLA-DP mismatches are permissive and have survival outcomes identical to those expected with fully matched donor-recipient pairs.[75] Newer GVHD prophylaxis regimens, which include sirolimus as a third agent, T cell depletion, or post-HCT cyclophosphamide, may make the use of mismatched unrelated donors safer.[76]

Umbilical CB—The most common use of CBT is in the treatment of unrelated recipients who lack matched siblings or unrelated donor options. Because of the decreased number of mature T-cells in CB, matching criteria are less stringent, allowing treatment for patients with up to two mismatches (HLA 4 of 6 with antigen matches at A and B and allele match at DR); HLA 5 of 8 accounting for HLA C has been demonstrated to have lower NRM.[77] Advantages of CB as a donor source include allowing for greater HLA disparity, rapid availability, and possibly an increased GVT effect especially when two cords are used.[78-80] Furthermore, T-cells are more naïve and lower in number leading to less severe acute and chronic GVHD.[81,82] Disadvantages of CBT include slower engraftment and immune recovery, higher incidence of graft failure, and the inability to go back to the donor in the event of relapse. A threshold dose of 5×10^7 TNC (total nucleated cell) and 1.5×10^5 CD34+/kg is now recommended. Although most adult recipients receive two CB units to achieve an adequate cell dose, there may not be an advantage to the use of two cords in those cases where a single cord provides a sufficient number of cells.[83] Manipulation of CB units to expand the CD34+ fraction is being used as a strategy to avoid graft failure, decrease time to engraftment, and enhance GVT effects.[84,85]

Haploidentical family member—Mismatched related (haplo) donors share identity with the recipient for one HLA haplotype on chromosome 6 and are variably (1-6 antigen mismatched) matched for HLA on the unshared haplotype. As each individual inherits one HLA haplotype from each parent and passes on exactly one HLA haplotype to each child, any patient with a living parent or child has a potential haplo donor; each sibling or half-sibling has a 50% chance of sharing exactly one HLA haplotype with the patient.

The advantage of Haplo donors is that they can generally be identified quickly and the cost approximates that of a HLA-matched family donor.[86] The majority of haplo transplants performed world-wide take advantage of the PTCy strategy developed in the early 2000s at Johns Hopkins to control GVHD by eliminating rapidly dividing donor T cells.[87] The PTCy approach initially used nonmyeloablative conditioning and BM grafts.[88,89] Haplo donors have become the fastest growing donor source in recent years due to the ease of implementation and low rates of chronic GVHD. Adaptations to the initial schema have included the addition of myeloablative regimens, and more frequent use of PBSC as a donor source.[90-93]

With the availability of matched related, matched unrelated, haplo, and CB donors, almost every patient now has a donor (*Figure 104.3*). It has been difficult to compare donor sources prospectively. Retrospective data suggest similar survival between donor sources.[89,94-96]

Donor Characteristics

Once HLA is taken into account, other donor factors including age, sex, parity, and CMV serology have only minor effects on outcome. However, if a patient has many possible HLA-matched donors, preference is given to donors who are male, younger, ABO compatible, and sero-negative for CMV if the patient is CMV negative.

ABO Incompatibility

Since stem cells do not express ABO, HCT can be carried out across patient blood type. A major mismatch is considered to occur when the isohemagglutinins in the recipient plasma are directed against the donor red blood cell antigens (donor A, recipient O). This can result in immediate or delayed hemolysis of donor red cells and the need for prolonged red cell support post-HCT. A minor mismatch can result in immediate hemolysis of recipient RBCs by donor-derived hemagglutinins in the graft or delayed hemolysis of recipient RBCs by newly generated isohemagluttinins from the donor lymphocytes (recipient A, donor O). If the patient and donor are ABO incompatible and there are high anti-A or anti-B titers, the marrow can be red blood cell depleted or plasma depleted as necessary. Even after manipulating the graft by removing plasma or red blood cells, a major or minor ABO mismatch can result in life-threatening hemolysis. If there is continued production of antidonor isohemagluttinins in the recipient plasma after transplant, delayed erythropoiesis or even pure red cell aplasia may result. Having a major or minor mismatch has been associated with increased NRM in some studies.[80,97]

CONDITIONING REGIMENS

The choice of preparative regimen administered to patients prior to HCT depends on the disease being treated, the source of stem cells, and the age and comorbidities of the patient. The goals of the preparative regimen are to eliminate the abnormal or malignant cell population and in the setting of allogeneic HCT to suppress the immune system to prevent rejection.

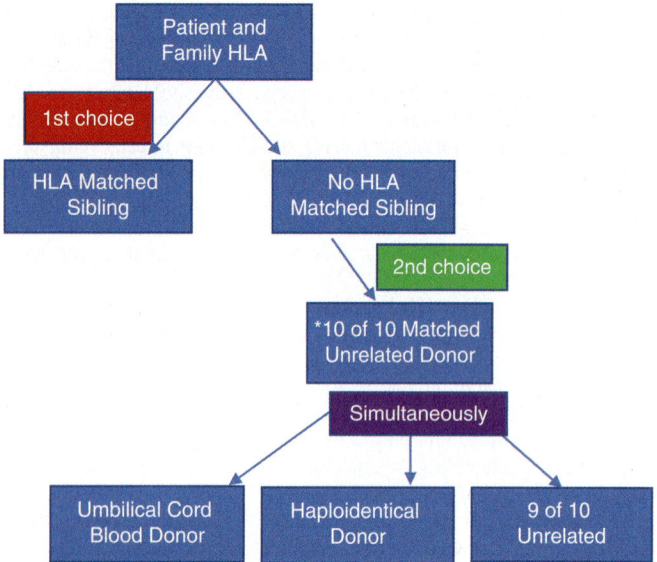

FIGURE 104.3 **Algorithm of donor search.** Matched sibling donors are most commonly the preference in any donor search. 10 of 10 matched unrelated donors are typically the second choice. With minimal prospective data available to choose alternative donor sources, one should consider the indication for the HCT, and features of the patient and possible donors. *In some cases and at some centers, haploidentical donors are being favored over 10 of 10 matched unrelated donors. Expertise of the center is very important.

Currently used preparative regimens can be placed into three general categories: myeloablative (MAC), non-myeloablative (NMA), and RIC (*Figure 104.4*). Regimens are considered NMA if, without transplantation they would cause only mild and quickly reversible myelosuppression. RIC regimens would be expected to produce significant cytopenias of some duration, while after myeloablative regimens hematopoietic recovery without stem cell rescue is unlikely.[98] Compared with high-dose preparative regimens, NMA and RIC regimens result in shorter duration of pancytopenias with reduced transfusion needs, fewer bacterial infections, and lower incidence of direct toxicities to the lungs and liver.[99] Relapse rates are higher with NMA and RIC whereas NRM is higher with MAC.[100]

NONMALIGNANT DISEASES

For patients undergoing HCT for most forms of severe combined immunodeficiency, no preparative regimen is needed because there are no cells to eliminate and no immune cells to mediate rejection. In patients with severe aplastic anemia (SAA), there is no population of hematopoietic cells to eliminate, but patients must be adequately immunosuppressed to prevent graft rejection. Immunosuppressive therapy such as antithymocyte globulin (ATG) plus high-dose cyclophosphamide is commonly used for transplanting younger patients for SAA and has been associated with primary graft rejection in <10% of cases and 5-year survival around 90%; age > 30 years was associated with inferior outcomes.[101,102] When using an unrelated donor, additional immune suppression such as low-dose radiation is often added to the regimen. Patients > 60 years of age are rarely transplanted for SAA and should be evaluated on a case-by-case basis. When transplanting patients for diseases such as sickle cell or thalassemia, the goal is to eliminate the disease and suppress the patient's immune system; in these cases busulfan is often added to the regimen in order to eradicate a highly proliferative host marrow population.

MALIGNANT DISEASES

Myeloablative Conditioning Regimens

High-dose chemotherapy and radiation regimens were the initial approach to HCT for malignant diseases. The first conditioning regimens consisted of TBI, alone or combined with cyclophosphamide.[103] TBI is an effective antineoplastic modality that is both cell cycle nonspecific and immunosuppressive. Cyclophosphamide is a chemotherapeutic agent with immunosuppressive properties that has few nonhematopoietic toxicities that overlap with TBI, and therefore can be used in combination. A common MAC regimen is Cytoxan 120 mg/kg + 1200 to 1320 cGy TBI. Doses up to 1600 cGy of TBI have been used with decreased relapse rates but with higher rates of regimen-related toxicity.[104] Another commonly used MAC regimen, busulfan 16 mg/kg + cyclophosphamide 120 mg/kg has been shown to be a good alternative to Cy/TBI in several studies.[105,106] Targeting busulfan levels in the plasma may decrease the risk of relapse and severe regimen-related toxicities such as sinusoidal obstruction syndrome (SOS).[107] The drug treosulfan has been shown to provide patients with similar incidence of DFS as comparable studies with busulfan but with less treatment-related toxicity; treosulfan has not been approved by the FDA in the United States.[108]

Nonmyeloablative/RIC Regimens

NMA and RIC regimens are generally selected for older patients, those with significant comorbidities, and those who have received prior therapy thought to limit their ability to tolerate high-dose regimens. RIC regimens fall between NMA and MAC and are associated with less toxicity than MAC but higher relapse rates. In general, after RIC regimens, recipients become aplastic and complete chimerism is established early after transplantation; however, recovery of hematopoiesis would be expected without the support of hematopoietic progenitor cells. Although reduced intensity, the regimen may contribute a substantial antitumor effect. RIC regimens include fludarabine 150 mg + melphalan 100 mg or fludarabine 90 mg + TBI 400 cGy. NMA regimens cause minimal marrow suppression and therefore depend on pre- and posttransplant immune suppression to prevent graft rejection. The conditioning regimen is not expected to have a substantial antitumor effect, so the efficacy of the treatment is largely from a GVT response. Evidence for the existence of a GVT effect includes the fact that relapse risk is lowest in patients who develop acute or chronic GVHD and highest in T-cell depleted HCT regimens.[109] Additional evidence for the GVT effect is the fact that donor lymphocyte infusions (DLIs) can eliminate post-HCT residual disease

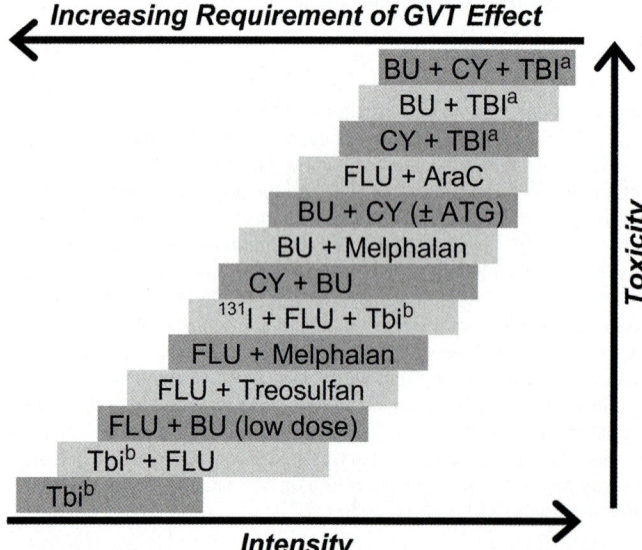

FIGURE 104.4 **Conditioning regimen intensity.** Selected conditioning regimens of different dose intensities. AraC, cytosine arabinoside; ATG, antithymocyte globulin (or thymoglobulin); ^{131}I, anti-CD45 antibody conjugated to ^{131}I. BU, busulfan; CY, cyclophosphamide; Flu, fludarabine (various dosing schedules). [a]High-dose TBI (800-1320 cGy). [b]Low-dose TBI (200-400 cGy). (Reprinted from Deeg HJ, Sandmaier BM. Who is fit for allogeneic transplantation? *Blood*. 2010;116(23):4762-4770. Copyright © 2010 American Society of Hematology. With permission.)

or relapse, especially in patients with CML but also in AML, MDS, and indolent lymphomas.[110] Examples of NMA conditioning include fludarabine 90 mg/m^2 + 200 cGy or 200 to 300 cGy TBI alone.

ENGRAFTMENT

Following administration of a MAC preparative regimen, a period of profound myelosuppression occurs. Stable engraftment of a hematopoietic cell graft requires the circulation, homing, and growth of hematopoietic stem cells. Engraftment is usually defined as the first of 3 days of ANC > 500 μL. When peripheral blood is the source of stem cells, this occurs at approximately day +14 post HCT. With marrow, it may take up to a week longer. If CB is the source, recovery may be further delayed by 4 to 6 days. The rate of myeloid recovery can be accelerated by 4 to 6 days with the use of G-CSF with marrow and CB, but G-CSF has less of an effect with the use of mobilized peripheral blood. The use of MTX as GVHD prophylaxis after allo-HCT also delays neutrophil recovery by an average of 4 days. Platelet and red cell counts usually recover shortly after recovery of neutrophils. Cryopreservation especially in the setting of unrelated donor PBSC grafts may also delay engraftment of both platelets and neutrophils.[111]

CHIMERISM

Engraftment of allo stem cells can be documented using fluorescence in situ hybridization of sex chromosomes if the donor and recipient are of opposite sex or DNA assays of short tandem repeat loci in same sex transplants. Chimerism is usually tested about 1 month after an NMA or RIC HCT and can provide early information about graft rejection. There are no data that testing chimerism routinely after myeloablative HCT guides therapy, but it is often examined around day 100 after HCT. Low chimerism values, specifically <50%, may warrant the administration of DLI to improve engraftment as long as the patient does not have active GVHD.

IMMUNE RECONSTITUTION

After myeloablative therapy and auto- or allo-HCT, both humoral and cellular immunity are impaired from months to years. The first phase of recovery is the increase in neutrophil counts, which occurs 2 to 3 weeks after transplant. Although the neutrophil function is intact for the most part, impaired chemotaxis persists for up to 4 months.[112] Monocyte recovery has been inversely correlated with infection rates between day 100 and 365 posttransplant.[113] Natural killer cells and other cell types capable of antibody-dependent cytotoxicity recover to normal levels by 1 month in both auto- and allo-HCT.[114]

Serum immunoglobulin levels typically fall to abnormally low levels initially after HCT. If serum IgG levels are below 400 g/L, patients are generally treated with intravenous immunoglobulin in the first 3 months following transplant. Serum IgG and IgM usually recover to normal levels by 1 year after HCT in the absence of chronic GVHD.

Although T-cell numbers may recover, diversity is initially limited in most recipients. Immune reconstitution may be slower in recipients of CB, haplo, and T-cell-depleted grafts and remains poor in those with chronic GVHD. CD8+ T-cells recover faster than CD4+ T-cells. Following auto-HCT, B- and CD8+ T cells recover by 3 to 6 months. However, CD4+ cells are not back to normal levels until 1 to 2 years after transplant.[115]

After allo transplant, recovery of the immune system from the donor graft occurs in phases over 1 to 2 years in patients who do not develop GVHD. There are significant delays in recovery of the immune system if GVHD develops. T cell recovery in younger patients is superior to older patients due to the persistence of thymic tissue.[116] Increased thymic output is associated with an increased number of naïve T-cells and broader T-cell repertoires while low T-cell receptor excision circle levels correlate with the presence of chronic GVHD and severe opportunistic infections.[117] Vaccination protocols may help improve cellular immunity against common communicable diseases.[118]

COMPLICATIONS OF HEMATOPOIETIC CELL TRANSPLANTATION

Predictors of Complications

The frequency of complications is higher and the rate of survival lower for patients with Karnofsky performance scores of less than 80% and for patients with significant comorbidities.[119] The hematopoietic cell HCT comorbidity index (HCT-CI) aids the provider in determining the risk of HCT-related mortality in individual patients. Initially published in 2005, the HCT-CI is a 12-point systematic quantification of a patient's cardiac, pulmonary, diabetes, hepatic, renal, and other functional status. The score is associated with posttransplant NRM and OS. If patients have a high HCT-CI score, consideration might be given to reduced intensity preparative regimens or alternative therapy.[120] The HCT-CI updated in 2014, to include age, assigns one additional point for patients older than 40 years.[121]

Regimen-Related Toxicities

Both the nature and degree of complications associated with HCT depend on the age and the health of the patient, the specific regimen used, and the source of stem cells. Early regimen-related toxicities depend on the regimen selected with fewer toxicities associated NMA and RIC regimens. MAC preparative regimens typically lead to nausea, vomiting, and diarrhea (up to 2-3 weeks); oral mucositis (5-7 days after HCT); alopecia (10-14 days after HCT); and cytopenias (5-7 days after HCT) leading to transfusion needs and increased risk for infection. The severity of the oral mucositis depends on the intensity of the MAC regimen and the use of MTX. Patients may require total parental nutrition (TPN) and narcotic analgesia during this time. Patient-controlled analgesia (PCA) provides the greatest patient satisfaction and results in lowest cumulative doses of narcotics. If high-dose cyclophosphamide is included, hemorrhagic cystitis can be seen. Mesna and/or continuous bladder irrigation can lower this risk. Keratinocyte growth factor (palifermin) can significantly shorten the duration of mucositis by up to 6 days following a myeloablative regimen and has been shown to decrease PCA and TPN use.[122,123]

SOS, previously termed veno-occlusive disease, can develop within 1 to 4 weeks following HCT and is more common with myeloablative regimens. SOS is characterized by weight gain, ascites, hepatomegaly, and jaundice. Histologic features of SOS include concentric narrowing or fibrous obliteration of terminal hepatic venules and sublobular veins and necrosis of zone 3 hepatocytes. The overall incidence of SOS is approximately 5% to 15% but incidence and severity vary by preparative regimen.[124] In general the risk of severe SOS is higher for patients with abnormal liver function tests before the HCT, pretransplant hepatitis, higher intensity conditioning regimens, and the use of busulfan.[125] SOS varies from a mild form that generally resolves in a few weeks to severe SOS, which is fatal in as many as 80% of cases.[124] Defibrotide may be effective both as prophylaxis and therapy.[126-129] Prophylaxis with ursodiol decreases the rates of hyperbilirubinemia and acute GVHD of the liver; some studies have demonstrated that ursodiol also decreases rates of SOS compared to controls.[130,131]

Most pneumonias that occur early after HCT are caused by bacteria and viruses but idiopathic pulmonary syndrome (IPS), which is thought to be a toxicity directly related to chemotherapy and/or radiation, occurs within 30 to 90 days after HCT in up to 4% to 12% of patients.[132,133] IPS occurs more frequently after high-dose TBI-containing regimens. Preexisting lung disease, older age and prior chest radiation are predisposing factors.[133] Fractionated radiation decreases this risk. Data suggest that occult infections may play a role in some cases of IPS.[134] The mortality rate with IPS is about 50% and no available treatments are clearly effective although tumor necrosis factor blockade and high-dose steroids are often used.[135]

Renal dysfunction is common after transplant. Some factors associated with the development of renal dysfunction include amphotericin B administration, hyperbilirubinemia, significant fluid retention, and pretransplant creatinine levels > 0.7.[136] Calcineurin inhibitors cause renal dysfunction that is reversible with aggressive hydration and eventual discontinuation of drug. Combining calcineurin inhibitors with sirolimus increases the risk of transplant-related microangiopathy (TMA). Mild TMA may have a benign course that requires no therapy or only modification of calcineurin inhibitor dosing. However, a proportion of cases develop a systemic vascular injury and these cases have mortality rates in excess of 80%. Elevated lactate dehydrogenase, proteinuria, and hypertension are the earliest signs of TMA and should trigger further evaluation including Complement 5b-9 levels.[137] Eculizumab is a treatment that can be used for patients with severe TMA.[138] Total hemolytic complement activity (CH50) levels should be followed and are expected to decrease in response to treatment.

Graft Rejection and Failure

Graft rejection is usually the result of residual host immune cells rejecting the donor marrow. In general, the greater the disparity between donor and recipient HLA-antigens, the greater the chance of rejection. Following transplantation from an HLA-identical donor, graft rejection occurs most commonly when the patient has received multiple transfusions and little chemotherapy prior to HCT such as in the case of aplastic anemia. Because donor T-cells react with and help eliminate host immune-competent cells not eradicated by the preparative regimen, T-depletion of donor marrow can lead to persistence of host immunity resulting in graft rejection. Increased incidence of graft rejection is also more frequently seen in NMA HCT due to persistence of host immunity and CBT due to decreased numbers of donor T-cells. If persistent host lymphocytes are detected, which documents immunologic graft rejection, a second HCT following an additional preparative regimen may be required.

Graft failure (as opposed to graft rejection) is defined as the achievement of full donor chimerism but poor count recovery. Risk factors for graft failure include low CD34+ cell dose in the graft and splenomegaly. In some instances, after functioning normally for a period of days or weeks marrow function is lost and myeloid elements are absent on marrow biopsy. This is considered secondary graft failure. Poor graft function is similar to graft failure and usually results in persistent cytopenias rather than aplasia. Patients with graft failure or poor graft function sometimes respond to G-CSF. Eltrombopag, which is a TPO agonist that stimulates platelet, red cell, and WBC growth in aplastic anemia, has been reported to improve counts in the post-HCT setting.[139,140] CD34+ cell boosts from the donor may also improve poor graft function in 60% to 90% of patients.[141]

Graft-vs-Host Disease

GVHD is the result of allo T-cells that were transfused with the graft reacting against targets on the genetically different host.[142,143] There are two categories of GVHD: acute and chronic; each has two subcategories: classic and delayed onset acute and classic and overlap chronic (*Figure 104.5*).[144]

GVHD Prevention

The two major approaches to the prevention of acute GVHD are pharmacologic immune suppression and T-cell depletion. The most commonly used pharmacologic regimens to prevent GVHD include a combination of MTX and a calcineurin inhibitor (cyclosporine [CSA] or TAC). In randomized controlled studies, the combination of TAC and MTX was associated with lower incidence of GVHD compared to CSA and MTX but there was no difference in chronic GVHD or survival between the two groups.[145,146] MTX delays but does not prevent engraftment and may worsen the mucositis associated with MAC regimens. Nephrotoxicity, neurotoxicity, and magnesium wasting are the most common complications associated with the calcineurin inhibitors. The costimulation blockade agent, cytotoxic lymphocyte four immunoglobulin, abatacept, in combination with TAC and MTX was recently FDA approved for acute GVHD prevention based on a randomized trial, which found that its addition resulted in a decreased risk

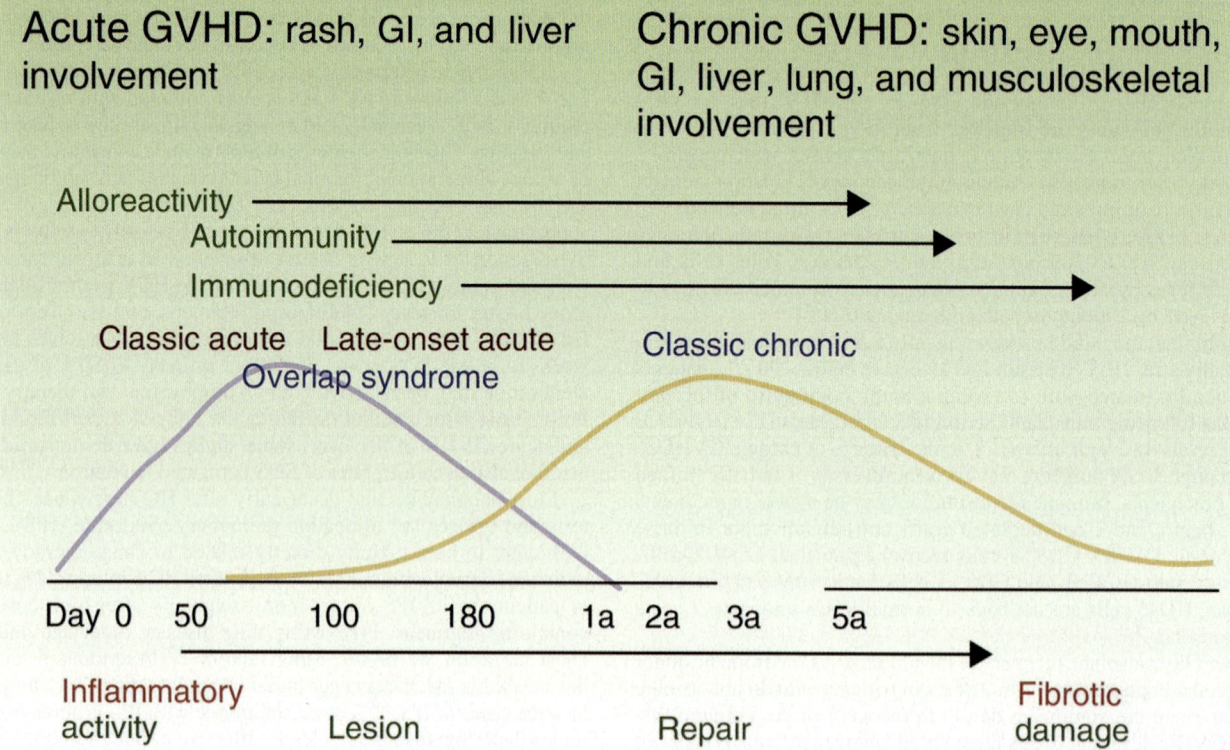

FIGURE 104.5 Acute and chronic graft-vs-host disease (GVHD). Acute GVHD can be divided into classic acute and late-onset acute GVHD. When acute and chronic features are both seen, GVHD is characterized as overlap. When the patient has chronic GVHD features only, they are considered to have classic chronic GVHD. GI, gastrointestinal. (Reprinted from Ballester-Sánchez R, Navarro-Mira M, Sanz-Caballer J, et al. Review of cutaneous graft-vs-host disease. *Actas Dermosifiliogr*. 2016;107(3):183-193. Copyright © 2015 AEDV. With permission.)

of severe acute GVHD in patients receiving either matched or mismatched unrelated donor HCT.[147]

Mycophenolate mofetil (MMF), a reversible inhibitor of inosine monophosphate dehydrogenase, has been successfully used in combination with CSA for the prevention of GVHD and graft rejection after NMA conditioning. The use of MMF instead of MTX results in similar rates of acute GVHD, less mucositis, and faster neutrophil engraftment.[148,149] Addition of sirolimus to TAC or to CSA and MMF may further reduce the incidence of acute GVHD in the NMA setting.[150,151] Other pharmaceuticals currently under investigation for use in combination with calcineurin inhibitors include ustekinumab, JAK inhibitors such as ruxolitinib and itacitanib, and alpha 1 antitrypsin.

The strategy of using PTCy given on days +3 and + 4 to eliminate activated T-cells that cause GVHD was initially pioneered for use in the HAPLO BM setting.[88,152] However, due to the profound reduction especially in chronic GVHD, the strategy is being used not only in the unrelated and matched sibling setting but also with peripheral blood grafts. A recent retrospective comparison study of PTCy in patients receiving matched unrelated donor vs HAPLO donor grafts demonstrated that patients who received matched unrelated donor grafts had superior survival and NRM but equivalent chronic GVHD solidifying that PTCy is not limited to only HAPLO donor transplants.[153]

Other approaches to prevent GVHD include removal of T-cells from the donor marrow or PBSCs using positive selection for CD34$^+$ or negative selection for CD3$^+$ cells, or the administration of horse or rabbit ATG in the peritransplant period.[154] Although reduction in acute and chronic GVHD has been seen with T-cell depleted marrow, there is also an associated increase in graft rejection, infections, posttransplant lymphoproliferative disease, and relapse. A randomized controlled trial did not demonstrate any survival benefit from ex vivo T-cell depletion compared to pharmacologic immune suppression in the matched unrelated donor setting.[155] Removal of CD45$^+$ RA naive T-cells have also been shown to prevent acute and chronic GVHD; in the matched related donor setting chronic GVHD was <10%.[156] In vivo T-cell depletion with ATG decreases acute and chronic GVHD and may lead to survival benefit in certain subsets of patients; however this may come at the cost of increase relapse.[157,158]

Acute GVHD

The skin, GI tract, and liver are the primary organs damaged by the GVH reaction. The cells targeted in the affected organs by the GVH reaction are the epithelial stem cells and their progeny.[159] In tissue involved with GVHD, a lymphoid infiltrate is present and cell death occurs by apoptosis. Acute GVHD typically develops within the first 3 months post-HCT and presents with a maculopapular or erythematous rash that can involve the palms and the soles and be pruritic or painful, nausea, vomiting, anorexia and diarrhea and/or with jaundice and hyperbilirubinemia. Late acute GVHD occurs after 3 months post HCT most commonly when immune suppression is withdrawn (late-onset acute GVHD) or in NMA or RIC HCT with later engraftment. Acute GVHD is usually graded by the Glucksberg Criteria (*Table 104.2*).[160] Grade I is mild and either does not require therapy or can be treated topically, Grade II is moderate and usually requires systemic therapy, and Grade III-IV is severe and can be life threatening. A biopsy of the involved organ may be required to confirm the diagnosis of GVHD and to distinguish it from other posttransplant complications. With standard regimens, such as MTX plus a calcineurin inhibitor, acute GVHD occurs in 30% of patients with HLA-matched siblings and 50% to 60% of patients with unrelated donors.[161] Factors associated with increased GVHD incidence include HLA mismatching, older age of patient, multiparous female donor, use of peripheral blood as the graft source, and more intensive conditioning.[162-164] In PBSC transplants, the CD34$^+$ dose has been reported to be an independent prognostic indicator of GVHD.[165]

Treatment of Acute GVHD

Standard treatment of acute GVHD is 2 mg/kg of prednisone, although a lower dose of 1 mg/kg may also be used for grade I-II GVHD.[166,167] Beclomethasone and budesonide added for acute GVHD of the upper and lower GI tract respectively has been shown to be effective in some clinical trials.[168-170] The optimal duration of steroid therapy is not known, but typically, therapy is given for 5 to 7 days and if a response is seen, a steroid taper is initiated. Forty to seventy percent of patients are initially steroid responsive, but GVHD sometimes flares during the taper requiring prolonged steroid treatment or alternative therapies (steroid dependent).[171] Patients who have steroid-refractory or steroid-dependent GVHD historically have very poor outcomes with median OS of approximately 6 months from diagnosis.[172,173]

Following the completion of the REACH1 and REACH2 trials, the drug ruxolitinib was shown to be superior to best available second-line therapies and approved for steroid-refractory or steroid-dependent acute GVHD.[174] Ruxolitinib is given orally at a dose of 5 mg BID and can be increased up to 10 mg BID as tolerated by side effects. Other possible treatments for steroid-refractory GVHD include ATG, tumor necrosis factor inhibitors, or extracorporeal photopheresis, which uses psoralen to denature T-cells and then give them back to the patient as an immunologic decoy.[172,175] Photopheresis is given to patients twice a week for the first 4 weeks and then twice a week every other week for at least another 8 weeks.[176]

Chronic GVHD

Chronic GVHD may develop as early as 50 to 60 days or as late as 400 days after transplantation. Chronic GVHD is seen in 30% to 70% of HCT recipients and is associated with increased NRM and decreased relapse.[177-179] Chronic GVHD is more frequent with unrelated donors, with the use of peripheral blood rather than marrow, in older patients, and in patients with a history of acute GVHD.[177,178,180] Chronic GVHD resembles an autoimmune disease in that its manifestations include oral and ocular sicca, serositis, fasciitis, esophageal and vaginal strictures, and systemic sclerosis. If generalized scleroderma occurs, it may lead to joint contractures and debility. The NIH Global

Table 104.2. Acute GVHD Scoring

	Extent of Organ Involvement		
Stage	Skin	Liver (Bilirubin)	Gut (Stool Output per day)
0	No GVHD rash	<2 mg/dL	<50 mL/d or persistent nausea (child: <10 mL/kg/d)
1	Maculopapular rash <25% BSA	2-3 mg/dL	500-999 mL/d (child: 10-19.9 mL/kg/d) or persistent nausea, vomiting, or anorexia, with a positive upper GI biopsy
2	Maculopapular rash 25%-50% BSA	3.1-6 mg/dL	1000-1500 mL/d (child: 20-30 mL/kg/d)
3	Maculopapular rash >50% BSA	6.1-15 mg/dL	Adult: >1500 mL/d (child: >30 mL/kg/d)
4	Generalised erythema plus bullous formation	>15 mg/dL	Severe abdominal pain with or without ileus
Grade	Skin	Liver (Bilirubin)	Gut (Stool Output per day)
I	Stages 1-2	None	None
II	Stage 3 or	Stage 1 or	Stage 1
III	-	Stage 2-3 or	Stages 2-4
IV	Stage 4 or	Stage 4	-

Abbreviations: BSA, body surface area; GI, gastrointestinal; GVHD, graft-vs-host disease
Reprinted by permission from Nature: Jacobsohn DA. Acute graft-versus-host disease in children. *Bone Marrow Transplant*. 2008;41(2):215-221. Copyright © 2007 Springer Nature.

Table 104.3. Example of Chronic GVHD Organ Scoring

	Score 0	Score 1	Score 2	Score 3
Lungs FEV_1 $DLCO$	No symptoms	Mild symptoms (shortness of breath after climbing one flight of steps)	Moderate symptoms (shortness of breath after walking on flat ground)	Severe symptoms (shortness of breath at rest; requiring O_2)
	$FEV_1 > 80\%$ **OR** LFS = 2	FEV_1 60%-79% **OR** LFS 3-5	FEV_1 40%-59% **OR** LFS 6-9	$FEV_1 \leq 39\%$ **OR** LFS 10-12
Joints and fascia	No symptoms	Mild tightness of arms and legs, normal or mild decreased range of motion (ROM) **AND** not affecting ADL	Tightness of arms and legs OR joint contractures, erythema thought due to fasciitis, moderate decrease of ROM **AND** mild to moderate limitation of ADL	Contractures **WITH** significant decrease of ROM **AND** significant limitation of ADL (unable to tie shoes, button shirts, dress self etc.)
Genital tract	No symptoms	Symptomatic with mild signs of examination **AND** no effect on coitus and minimal discomfort with gynecological examination	Symptomatic with moderate signs on examination **AND** with mild dyspareunia or discomfort with gynecological examination	Symptomatic **WITH** advanced signs (stricture, labial agglutination or severe ulceration) **AND** severe pain with coitus or inability to insert vaginal speculum

Abbreviations: ADL, activities of daily living; GVHD, graft-vs-host disease; LFS, lung function score.

Severity Score developed in 2005 and updated in 2014 has replaced limited and extensive designations with mild, moderate, and severe categories based on a 12 organ system evaluation.[144,181] A scoring system in which 0 = no symptoms and 3 = severe involvement is used to score each organ or site at any given time taking functional impairment into account (*Table 104.3*). A global assessment of chronic GVHD severity is then calculated based on the number of sites or organs involved and the degree of involvement of affected organs (*Table 104.4*). Identification of biomarkers that predict whether a patient is at risk of development of chronic GVHD is an area of active research but are not yet used in routine clinical care.

Bronchiolitis obliterans syndrome (BOS) is an obstructive lung disease characterized by nonproductive cough, progressive dyspnea, obstructive changes on pulmonary function tests (PFTs) including lowering of FEV1/FVC ratio < 70, and evidence of air trapping on a high-resolution inspiratory/expiratory CT scan.[182] Pathology shows increased deposition of collagen and granulation tissue in and around bronchial structures and eventual obliteration of small airways. BOS is highly associated with chronic GVHD.

Treatment of Chronic GVHD

Mild chronic GVHD can often be managed with local therapies including oral dexamethasone and eye drops such as preservative-free artificial tears and CSA eye drops (Restasis). More severe disease is frequently treated with prednisone alone or in combination with a calcineurin inhibitor, which can control GVHD in 50% to 70% of cases.[183] Three drugs have been FDA approved for the treatment of chronic GVHD since the last edition of this book. The first is ibrutinib, a B-cell modifier that results in higher response rates than previous standard approaches.[184] Ibrutinib is given orally at a standard dose of 480 mg. The package insert recommends that immune-compromised patients be treated with concurrent antifungal prophylaxis with voriconazole or posaconazole, in which case the dose needs to be reduced accordingly. The second approved drug is the JAK1 and 2 inhibitor ruxolitinib (Jakafi). The REACH3 trial showed that compared to physician's choice, 10 mg BID of ruxolitinib achieved a higher overall response and a prolonged duration of response.[185] The most recently approved drug for the treatment of chronic GVHD is belumosudil (Rezurock).[186] Belumosudil is a ROCK2 inhibitor that leads to the downstream inhibition of proinflammatory cytokines by blocking the activation of STAT 3. Belumosudil was notable for its effectiveness in sclerotic type GVHD. While these newly approved options are being integrated into the treatment algorithm for GVHD, treatments with sirolimus, MMF, weekly MTX, or photopheresis are still frequently used with reasonable effectiveness.[187]

Immune suppression can eventually be tapered and discontinued in 80% to 90% of patients with chronic GVHD, but it may be many months or several years of immune suppression before tolerance develops. The average duration of therapy is 2 to 3 years after peripheral blood transplantation, but is shorter with the use of BM or CB.[81,188] Patients with chronic GVHD are at increased risk of developing infections with encapsulated bacteria due to functional asplenia; therefore, these patients should be treated with PCN VK or daily Bactrim until they are off all immune suppression. Lung complications of chronic GVHD can be especially debilitating. There has been some evidence that treating BOS with a constellation of medications including fluticasone (a steroid) inhaler, azithromycin 250 mg, and Montelukast (FAM) ± a long-acting B-agonist daily can reduce steroid exposure and potentially slow or reverse progression of disease, which is usually followed by the FEV1/FVC level on the PFTs.[189] Steroids may be used in the management of BOS but they are not thought to be as effective as in cryptogenic organizing pneumonia (COP).

Infectious Complications

During the early posttransplant period, patients are at risk for infection (*Figure 104.6*), and are placed on prophylaxis for bacterial, fungal, and viral pathogens as well as *Pneumocystis jirovecii* pneumonia (PJP). Prophylaxis against fungal pathogens reduces the rate of fungal infections and improves OS.[190] Prophylaxis with fluconazole is routine for patients with standard risk, while prophylaxis with a mold-active agent such as voriconazole, posaconazole, or isavuconazonium is often used for patients at higher risk, such as those with prior fungal

Table 104.4. Chronic GVHD Global Severity Score

Mild chronic GVHD
Only 1-2 organs or sites involved (except lung) with no clinically significant functional impairment.

Moderate chronic GVHD
(1) At least 1 organ or site with clinically significant but no major disability (maximum score of 2 in any affected organ or site) or
(2) 3 or more organs or sites with no clinically significant functional impairment (max score of 1 in all affected areas or sites.). A lung score of 1 will also be considered moderate chronic GVHD.

Severe Chronic GVHD
Major disability caused by chronic GVHD (score of 3 in any organ or site). A lung score of 2 or greater will also be considered severe chronic GVHD.

Abbreviation: GVHD, graft-vs-host disease.

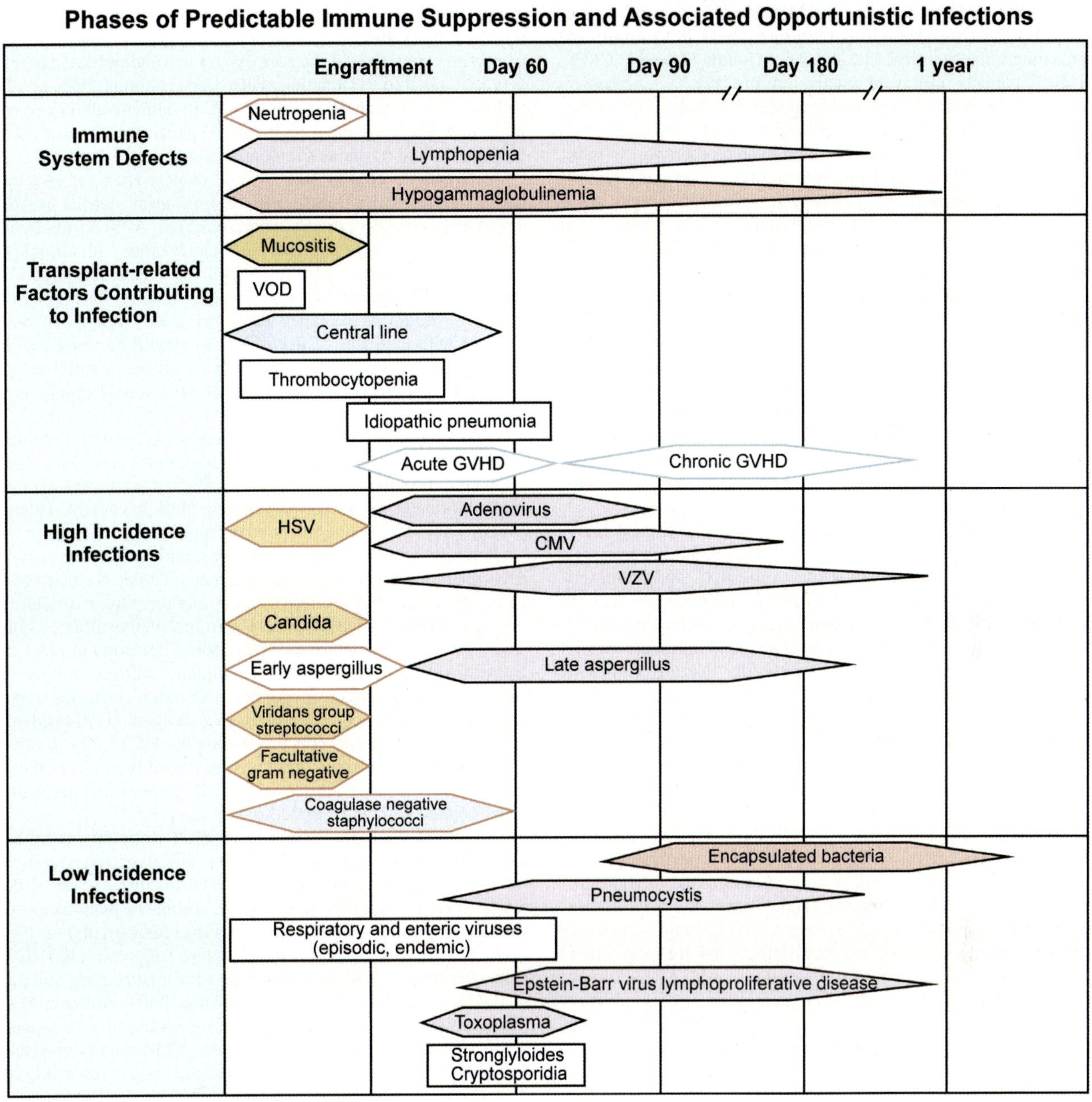

Phases of Predictable Immune Suppression and Associated Opportunistic Infections

[Figure showing timeline from Engraftment through Day 60, Day 90, Day 180, to 1 year with the following categories:]

Immune System Defects:
- Neutropenia
- Lymphopenia
- Hypogammaglobulinemia

Transplant-related Factors Contributing to Infection:
- Mucositis
- VOD
- Central line
- Thrombocytopenia
- Idiopathic pneumonia
- Acute GVHD
- Chronic GVHD

High Incidence Infections:
- HSV
- Adenovirus
- CMV
- VZV
- Candida
- Early aspergillus
- Late aspergillus
- Viridans group streptococci
- Facultative gram negative
- Coagulase negative staphylococci

Low Incidence Infections:
- Encapsulated bacteria
- Pneumocystis
- Respiratory and enteric viruses (episodic, endemic)
- Epstein-Barr virus lymphoproliferative disease
- Toxoplasma
- Stronglyloides
- Cryptosporidia

FIGURE 104.6 **Infectious complications following hematopoietic cell transplant (HCT)** Phases of predictable immune suppression with their opportunistic infections among allogeneic hematopoietic stem cell transplantation recipients. (PDQ® Pediatric Treatment Editorial Board. PDQ Complications, Graft-Versus-Host Disease, and Late Effects After Pediatric Hematopoietic Stem Cell Transplantation. Bethesda, MD: National Cancer Institute. https://www.cancer.gov/types/childhood-cancers/hp-stem-cell-transplant/gvhd. Adapted from Burik and Freifeld. Infection in the severely immunocompromised patient. In: Abeloff MD, Armitage JO, Niederhuber JE, eds. *Clinical Oncology*. 3rd ed. Churchill Livingstone; 2004:941-956. Copyright © 2004 Elsevier. With permission.)

infection or pulmonary nodules on pre-HCT CT scan.[191] All patients are given acyclovir or valacyclovir to prevent reactivation of herpes simplex virus and varicella zoster. Because late reactivations are possible, at many centers these antiviral agents are continued until at least a year post transplant. Patients who reactivate these viruses as localized disease should be treated with acyclovir to prevent disseminated disease, which can be fatal.

The drug of choice for PJP prophylaxis is Bactrim. With prophylaxis, the number of patients with post-HCT PJP is negligible; patients are treated for 1 week prior to HCT and then two times a week starting at the time of engraftment until at least 6 months posttransplant. Those who are allergic or have intolerable side effects to Bactrim receive dapsone (check G6PD) or atovaquone. Another agent less frequently used is inhaled or IV pentamidine. Levofloxacin is commonly started when the patient's neutrophil counts decrease below 500 µL to prevent aggressive bacterial infections.

Treatment of patients who develop a neutropenic fever despite prophylactic antibiotics is based on clinical judgment and hospital experience. In most cases, a broader spectrum antibiotic such as cefepime or piperacillin/tazobactam is added. If there is suspicion for a gram-positive infection due to severe mucositis or cellulitis, methicillin-resistant *Staphylococcus aureus* coverage such as vancomycin is often included. If anaerobic bacteria due to intra-abdominal infection are suspected, an agent such as meropenem or metronidazole can be added. If the fever persists for greater than 72 hours, additional antifungal coverage is often employed.

In the past, CMV infection (pneumonitis or colitis) frequently occurred after HCT leading to death in many patients. Greater than 50% of patients are CMV positive and NRM is higher in these patients than in recipients who are CMV negative.[192] Primary CMV infection can be prevented in seronegative patients by using CMV seronegative blood products and choosing a CMV negative donor if possible.

Patients who are CMV positive with CMV negative donors are the most likely to reactivate the virus. Letermovir was FDA approved based on a randomized clinical trial and is now routinely used in CMV positive HCT patients to prevent reactivation of CMV.[193] Letermovir is started as early as day 0 and as late as day 28 depending on the donor source and protocol. CMV blood levels are routinely monitored by PCR on a weekly or biweekly basis and treated preemptively with induction followed by maintenance ganciclovir or valganciclovir. Foscarnet can also be used but is usually reserved for patients with marrow suppression or those with virus resistant to ganciclovir.

Community acquired viral infections including respiratory syncytial virus (RSV), influenza virus, parainfluenza virus, and human metapneumovirus cause upper and lower respiratory infections and can be life threatening. These can be prevented by avoiding contact with visitors and staff who are exhibiting symptoms of infection, frequent hand washing, and mandating influenza vaccination of staff and caregivers. Patients who have upper respiratory symptoms pre-HCT should be screened by nasopharyngeal lavage for viral infections before proceeding to HCT. If RSV, influenza or parainfluenza virus is found, the HCT should be delayed. Inhaled or oral ribavirin may be effective for parainfluenza and RSV and Tamiflu has been shown to shorten the course of influenza.[194]

COVID-19 infection has been especially worrisome in post-HCT patients due to the higher associated risk of developing lower respiratory tract disease, requiring admission to the ICU, and increased mortality.[195,196] OS at 6 weeks from diagnosis has been reported to be around 70%, with children doing significantly better than adults.[195] Aggressive treatment with steroids, monoclonal antibodies, and available antivirals are warranted in this population. Patients who test COVID-19 positive prior to transplant should have their transplants delayed.

Human herpes virus six (HHV-6), a latent herpes virus found in immunocompromised hosts, may lead to graft failure, encephalitis, enteritis, and pneumonia. HHV-6 is more commonly seen in CB and T-cell-depleted transplant patients and should be suspected in patients with these clinical findings.[197] HHV-6 is treated similarly to CMV. High levels of BK virus in the blood and or urine can be associated with cystitis; treatment is with pyridium and oxybutinin. In severe cases patients develop hemorrhagic cystitis and may require continuous bladder irrigation. Adenovirus infections may be associated with pneumonia, hepatitis, and renal failure and are more often seen in patients on extended courses of steroids or ATG.[198] Cidofovir historically was the only treatment for uncontrolled or disseminated BK and adenovirus. Unfortunately cidofovir frequently causes renal failure in patients, some irreversible.[199] The drug Brincidofovir has been tested for this indication and is purported to be considerably less nephrotoxic.[200]

Antibody titers to vaccine preventable diseases decline after HCT. Therefore the transplant community has developed guidelines for revaccination.[118] Vaccination against tetanus/diphtheria/pertussis (TDAP), polio, *Haemophilus influenza*, pneumococcus, and meningococcus as well as hepatitis A and B is recommended starting at 1 year post-HCT.[118] Live vaccines such as MMR and Shingrix are not recommended until the patient is 2 years post HCT (5 years for Zostavax) and a least 1 year off of immune suppression. Revaccination with 3 monthly sequential doses of COVID-19 vaccine is recommended starting at 3 months post-HCT with the current guidelines suggesting a booster dose may be helpful as soon as 3 months following the third dose.

LATE EFFECTS

Late effects post HCT are common with at least 50% of long-term survivors reporting at least one late effect.[201] Commonly noted late effects are osteoporosis, hypothyroidism, cataracts, avascular necrosis (AVN), and iron overload. Bone mineral density loss occurs in 50% to 75% of patients post HCT.[202] To screen for osteoporosis, a bone density (Dexa) scan should be performed pre-HCT in high-risk patients and posttransplant in all patients, especially in those treated with corticosteroids. In addition to calcium and vitamin D, bisphosphonate therapy is indicated for patients with osteoporosis. Patients with osteopenia are treated if they are on steroids and/or have a high FRAX score.[202] Thyroid dysfunction is also very common (30% at >2 years) following HCT with an increased risk in patients who have received high-dose TBI-containing regimens.[203] Treatment is most commonly lifelong thyroid hormone supplementation.

Cataracts develop in 10% to 20% of post-HCT patients and may be secondary to high-dose TBI or long-term steroid use or both. Treatment is usually surgery when indicated. AVN occurs in as many as 5% to 19% of HCT patients, particularly those with chronic GVHD receiving long-term steroid treatment.[202,204] Patients diagnosed with AVN should be referred to an orthopedic surgeon for evaluation. Iron overload should be screened for starting at 1 year post transplant. Patients with evidence of iron overload should be treated with phlebotomy as first line if possible. Iron overload can be followed monthly by ferritin levels but T2-weighted liver MRI should also be evaluated intermittently if possible.[205]

Following allo-HCT, an autoimmune disorder may develop in 3% to 5% of patients, most commonly autoimmune hemolytic anemia or idiopathic thrombocytopenic purpura.[206,207] Risk factors include having an unrelated donor and developing chronic GVHD. Treatment is usually steroids first line followed by rituximab.[208]

Patients who are transplanted as children often suffer from decreased growth rate and delayed puberty. Children who have growth factor deficiency require replacement therapy. Ovarian failure develops in most postpubertal females who receive busulfan or high-dose TBI-containing regimens and azospermia develops in most men.[209] Because some postpediatric HCT recipients will regain their fertility, they should continue on pregnancy prevention strategies unless they wish to actively conceive children. In a study of 113 transplant recipients who were able to conceive following HCT, only 0.82% of the children had severe anomalies consistent with the rates in the general population.[210] It has been shown in CML patients that pregnancy may be associated with an increased risk of relapse.[211]

Among those living 5 years post HCT, mortality is higher than expected with an estimated 30% lower life expectancy compared to those in the general population.[212] The leading causes of death in 5-year survivors are recurrent disease, secondary malignancy, chronic GVHD, respiratory ailments, and cardiovascular events.

COP can be seen both early and late following HCT. COP is a restrictive lung disease characterized by fever, dry cough, and shortness of breath. Chest imaging shows a diffuse, fluffy infiltrate. Pathology shows patchy fibrosis, granulation tissue within alveolar spaces, and small airways with no infectious agent. COP usually responds well to a lengthy course of steroids (4-6 months) and is reversible but may have a relapsing and remitting course.[213] The most common cardiovascular events following transplant are acute coronary disease, which is most frequently seen in TBI-based regimens or in patients with a history of chest radiation.[214] Congestive heart failure and pulmonary hypertension are also side effects that may develop following transplant but are less common.[214]

Transplant patients are also at risk for developing secondary malignancies. Patients receiving high-dose chemotherapy or radiation are at the highest risk. Patients receiving T-cell-depleted grafts and those who develop chronic GVHD are also at risk of EBV-associated lymphoproliferative disease.[215] An increase in solid tumors of 6% to 11% at 15 years post HCT in children and adults is seen.[216,217] The incidence of MDS after auto-HCT for multiple myeloma is as high as 8% in patients receiving post-HCT lenalinomide and up to 10% in patients with non-Hodgkin lymphoma and HD.[218]

RELAPSE AFTER TRANSPLANT

There is a substantial risk of relapse after HCT, especially when the HCT is performed after failure of conventional chemotherapy rather than earlier in the disease course. Patients with Hodgkin and non-Hodgkin lymphoma who relapse after auto-HCT may respond to further conventional dose chemotherapy, particularly when the interval from transplantation to relapse is long.[219-221] CAR-T cell therapy following auto-HCT in patients with recurrent disease has also been found to be effective. RIC allo-HCT is also recommended for patients who are allo-HCT candidates and whose disease relapsed following an auto-HCT or CAR-T cell therapy; results are better in patients who are in remission or have low burden of disease.[222]

Patients who relapse after allo-HCT will sometimes have a complete response if immune suppression is discontinued prematurely albeit commonly accompanied by GVHD.[223] DLI can also result in CR for some patients. Without prior induction chemotherapy, complete responses can be seen in 60% of patients with CML (75% for those in chronic phase), 18% of patients with ALL, and 15% of patients with AML.[224] Most experts recommend patients with acute leukemia undergo reinduction chemotherapy prior to DLI. Complications of DLI include GVHD in about 60% of patients. Of those, 50% require therapy for GVHD and 15% experience life-threatening GVHD.[225] Myelosuppression occurs in 35% of patients and overall mortality associated with DLI is 20%. Starting the transfusion with a low cell number and then gradually increasing the dose can lessen the risk of severe toxicity.[226,227] CAR-T cells targeting CD19 have been shown to be effective in patients with ALL who have relapsed after allo-HCT.[228] AML CAR-T cells are currently under evaluation.

A second allo-HCT can occasionally be effective, particularly in younger patients and in patients who experience a longer interval from first HCT to relapse and who are able to achieve a CR prior to the second HCT.[222] There is debate over whether changing donor source for a second transplant matters. Retrospective studies report similar outcomes whether one uses the same donor as the first HCT or switches to an alternative.[229]

References

1. Jacobsen LO ME, Robeson MJ, Gaston EO, Zirkle RE. Effect of spleen protection on mortality following X-irradiation. *J Lab Clin Med.* 1949;34:1538-1543.
2. DE U. Genetic factors influencing irradiation protection by bone marrow. I. The Fl hybrid effect. *J Natl Cancer Inst.* 1957;19:123-130.
3. Storb R, Rudolph RH, Thomas ED. Marrow grafts between canine siblings matched by serotyping and mixed leukocyte culture. *J Clin Invest.* 1971;50(6):1272-1275.
4. Thomas ED, Collins JA, Herman EC, Jr, Ferrebee JW. Marrow transplants in lethally irradiated dogs given methotrexate. *Blood.* 1962;19:217-228.
5. Bach FH, AR, Joo P, Anderson JL, Bortin MM. Bone-marrow transplantation in a patient with Wiskott-Aldrich syndrome. *Lancet.* 1968;2:1366-1369.
6. Gatti RA, Meuwissen HJ, Allen HD, Hong R, Good RA. Immunological reconstitution of sex-linked lymphopenic immunological deficiency. *Lancet.* 1968;2(7583):1366-1369.
7. Thomas ED, Fefer A, Storb R, et al. Aplastic anaemia treated by marrow transplantation. *Lancet.* 1972;1(7745):284-289.
8. Thomas ED, Buckner CD, Banaji M, et al. One hundred patients with acute leukemia treated by chemotherapy, total body irradiation, and allogeneic marrow transplantation. *Blood.* 1977;49(4):511-533.
9. Hansen JA, Clift RA, Thomas ED, Buckner CD, Storb R, Giblett ER. Transplantation of marrow from an unrelated donor to a patient with acute-leukemia. *N Engl J Med.* 1980;303(10):565-567.
10. Weaver CH, Hazelton B, Birch R, et al. An analysis of engraftment kinetics as a function of the Cd34 content of peripheral-blood progenitor-cell collections in 692 patients after the administration of myeloablative chemotherapy. *Blood.* 1995;86(10):3961-3969.
11. Schmitz N, Dreger P, Suttorp M, et al. Primary transplantation of allogeneic peripheral-blood progenitor cells mobilized by Filgrastim (Granulocyte-Colony-Stimulating factor). *Blood.* 1995;85(6):1666-1672.
12. DiPersio JF, Stadtmauer EA, Nademanee A, et al. Plerixafor and G-CSF versus placebo and G-CSF to mobilize hematopoietic stem cells for autologous stem cell transplantation in patients with multiple myeloma. *Blood.* 2009;113(23):5720-5726.
13. Abbruzzese L, Agostini F, Durante C, et al. Long term cryopreservation in 5% DMSO maintains unchanged CD34+ cells viability and allows satisfactory hematological engraftment after peripheral blood stem cell transplantation. *Vox Sang.* 2013;105(1):77-80.
14. Gertz MA, Ansell SM, Dingli D, et al. Autologous stem cell transplant in 716 patients with multiple myeloma: low treatment-related mortality, feasibility of outpatient transplant, and effect of a multidisciplinary quality initiative. *Mayo Clin Proc.* 2008;83(10):1131-1138.
15. Jantunen E, Itala M, Lehtinen T, et al. Early treatment-related mortality in adult autologous stem cell transplant recipients: a nation-wide survey of 1482 transplanted patients. *Eur J Haematol.* 2006;76(3):245-250.
16. Batra A, Cottler-Fox M, Harville T, Rhodes-Clark BS, Makhoul I, Nakagawa M. Autologous graft versus host disease: an emerging complication in patients with multiple myeloma. *Biol Blood Marrow Transplant.* 2014;20:S261-S262.
17. Stewart AK, Vescio R, Schiller G, et al. Purging of autologous peripheral-blood stem cells using CD34 selection does not improve overall or progression-free survival after high-dose chemotherapy for multiple myeloma: results of a multicenter randomized controlled trial. *J Clin Oncol.* 2001;19(17):3771-3779.
18. Palumbo A, Cavallo F, Gay F, et al. Autologous transplantation and maintenance therapy in multiple myeloma. *N Engl J Med.* 2014;371(10):895-905.
19. Moskowitz CH, Nademanee A, Masszi T, et al. Brentuximab vedotin as consolidation therapy after autologous stem-cell transplantation in patients with Hodgkin's lymphoma at risk of relapse or progression (AETHERA): a randomised, double-blind, placebo-controlled, phase 3 trial. *Lancet.* 2015;385(9980):1853-1862.
20. Le Gouill S, Thieblemont C, Oberic L, et al. Rituximab after autologous stem-cell transplantation in mantle-cell lymphoma. *N Engl J Med.* 2017;377(13):1250-1260.
21. Pulsipher MA, Chitphakdithai P, Miller JP, et al. Adverse events among 2408 unrelated donors of peripheral blood stem cells: results of a prospective trial from the National Marrow Donor Program. *Blood.* 2009;113(15):3604-3611.
22. Armand P, Gibson CJ, Cutler C, et al. A disease risk index for patients undergoing allogeneic stem cell transplantation. *Blood.* 2012;120(4):905-913.
23. de Latour RP, Porcher R, Dalle JH, et al. Allogeneic hematopoietic stem cell transplantation in Fanconi anemia: the European Group for Blood and Marrow Transplantation experience. *Blood.* 2013;122:4279-4286.
24. Yanada M, Matsuo K, Emi N, Naoe T. Efficacy of allogeneic hematopoietic stem cell transplantation depends on cytogenetic risk for acute myeloid leukemia in first disease remission: a metaanalysis. *Cancer.* 2005;103:1652-1658.
25. Appelbaum FR. Hematopoietic cell transplantation beyond first remission. *Leukemia.* 2002;16(2):157-159.
26. Appelbaum FR. Indications for allogeneic hematopoietic cell transplantation for acute myeloid leukemia in the genomic era. *Am Soc Clin Oncol Educ Book.* 2014:e327-e333.
27. Scott BL, Pasquini MC, Logan BR, et al. Myeloablative versus reduced-intensity hematopoietic cell transplantation for acute myeloid leukemia and myelodysplastic syndromes. *J Clin Oncol.* 2017;35(11):1154-1161.
28. Walter RB, Buckley SA, Pagel JM, et al. Significance of minimal residual disease before myeloablative allogeneic hematopoietic cell transplantation for AML in first and second complete remission. *Blood.* 2013;122(10):1813-1821.
29. Yanada M, Matsuo K, Suzuki T, Naoe T. Allogeneic hematopoietic stem cell transplantation as part of postremission therapy improves survival for adult patients with high-risk acute lymphoblastic leukemia: a metaanalysis. *Cancer.* 2006;106(12):2657-2663.
30. Ribera JM. Allogeneic stem cell transplantation for adult acute lymphoblastic leukemia: when and how. *Haematologica.* 2011;96(8):1083-1086.
31. Brissot E, Labopin M, Beckers MM, et al. Tyrosine kinase inhibitors improve long-term outcome of allogeneic hematopoietic stem cell transplantation for adult patients with Philadelphia chromosome positive acute lymphoblastic leukemia. *Haematologica.* 2015;100(3):392-399.
32. Saini N, Marin D, Ledesma C, et al. Impact of TKIs post-allogeneic hematopoietic cell transplantation in Philadelphia chromosome-positive ALL. *Blood.* 2020;136(15):1786-1789.
33. Lindsley RC, Saber W, Mar BG, et al. Prognostic mutations in myelodysplastic syndrome after stem-cell transplantation. *N Engl J Med.* 2017;376(6):536-547.
34. Cutler CS, Lee SJ, Greenberg P, et al. A decision analysis of allogeneic bone marrow transplantation for the myelodysplastic syndromes: delayed transplantation for low-risk myelodysplasia is associated with improved outcome. *Blood.* 2004;104(2):579-585.
35. Koreth J, Pidala J, Perez WS, et al. Role of reduced-intensity conditioning allogeneic hematopoietic stem-cell transplantation in older patients with de novo myelodysplastic syndromes: an international collaborative decision analysis. *J Clin Oncol* 2013;31(21), 2662-2670.
36. Festuccia M, Baker K, Gooley TA, et al. Post-hematopoietic stem cell transplantation minimal residual disease and early relapses in MDS and AML evolving from MDS. *Blood.* 2015;126:2019.
37. Festuccia M, Deeg HJ, Gooley TA, et al. Minimal identifiable disease and the role of conditioning intensity in hematopoietic cell transplantation for myelodysplastic syndrome and acute myelogenous leukemia evolving from myelodysplastic syndrome. *Biol Blood Marrow Transplant.* 2016;22(7):1227-1233.
38. Baccarani M, Deininger MW, Rosti G, et al. European LeukemiaNet recommendations for the management of chronic myeloid leukemia: 2013. *Blood.* 2013;122(6):872-884.
39. Bar M, Radich J. Maintenance therapy with tyrosine kinase inhibitors after transplant in patients with chronic myeloid leukemia. *J Natl Compr Cancer Netw.* 2013;11(3):308-315.
40. Shanavas M, Popat U, Michaelis LC, et al. Outcomes of allogeneic hematopoietic cell transplantation in patients with myelofibrosis with prior exposure to Janus kinase 1/2 inhibitors. *Biol Blood Marrow Transplant.* 2016;22(3):432-440.
41. Kroger N, Sbianchi G, Sirait T, et al. Impact of prior JAK-inhibitor therapy with ruxolitinib on outcome after allogeneic hematopoietic stem cell transplantation for myelofibrosis: a study of the CMWP of EBMT. *Leukemia.* 2021;35(12):3551-3560.
42. Woo J, Choi DR, Storer BE, et al. Impact of clinical, cytogenetic, and molecular profiles on long-term survival after transplantation in patients with chronic myelomonocytic leukemia. *Haematologica.* 2020;105(3):652-660.
43. Sobecks RM, Leis JF, Gale RP, et al. Outcomes of human leukocyte antigen-matched sibling donor hematopoietic cell transplantation in chronic lymphocytic leukemia: myeloablative versus reduced-intensity conditioning regimens. *Biol Blood Marrow Transplant.* 2014;20(9):1390-1398.
44. Moreau P, Attal M, Facon T. Frontline therapy of multiple myeloma. *Blood.* 2015;125(20):3076-3084.
45. Dhakal B, Brazauskas R, Lara CA, Hari P, Pasquini M, D'Souza A. Monocyte recovery at day 100 is associated with improved survival in multiple myeloma patients who undergo allogeneic hematopoietic cell transplantation. *Bone Marrow Transplant.* 2016;51(2):297-299.
46. Schmitz N, Pfistner B, Sextro M, et al. Aggressive conventional chemotherapy compared with high-dose chemotherapy with autologous haemopoietic stem-cell transplantation for relapsed chemosensitive Hodgkin's disease: a randomised trial. *Lancet.* 2002;359(9323):2065-2071.

47. Salit RB, Bishop MR, Pavletic SZ. Allogeneic hematopoietic stem cell transplantation: does it have a place in treating Hodgkin lymphoma? *Curr Hematol Malig Rep.* 2010;5(4):229-238.
48. Gisselbrecht C, Glass B, Mounier N, et al. Salvage regimens with autologous transplantation for relapsed large B-cell lymphoma in the rituximab era. *J Clin Oncol.* 2010;28(27):4184-4190.
49. Stiff P. What is the role of autologous transplant for lymphoma in the current era? *Hematology Am Soc Hematol Educ Program.* 2015;2015:74-81.
50. Geisler CH, Kolstad A, Laurell A, et al. Nordic MCL2 trial update: six-year follow-up after intensive immunochemotherapy for untreated mantle cell lymphoma followed by BEAM or BEAC + autologous stem-cell support – still very long survival but late relapses do occur. *Br J Haematol.* 2012;158(3):355-362.
51. Pai SY, Logan BR, Griffith LM, et al. Transplantation outcomes for severe combined immunodeficiency, 2000-2009. *N Engl J Med.* 2014;371(5):434-446.
52. Mahlaoui N, Pellier I, Mignot C, et al. Characteristics and outcome of early-onset, severe forms of Wiskott-Aldrich syndrome. *Blood.* 2013;121(9):1510-1516.
53. Bacigalupo A, Socie G, Hamladji RM, et al. Current outcome of HLA identical sibling versus unrelated donor transplants in severe aplastic anemia: an EBMT analysis. *Haematologica.* 2015;100(5):696-702.
54. DeZern AE, Zahurak ML, Symons HJ, et al. Haploidentical BMT for severe aplastic anemia with intensive GVHD prophylaxis including posttransplant cyclophosphamide. *Blood Adv.* 2020;4(8):1770-1779.
55. King A, Shenoy S. Evidence-based focused review of the status of hematopoietic stem cell transplantation as treatment of sickle cell disease and thalassemia. *Blood.* 2014;123(20):3089-3094; quiz 3210.
56. Angelucci E, Matthes-Martin S, Baronciani D, et al. Hematopoietic stem cell transplantation in thalassemia major and sickle cell disease: indications and management recommendations from an international expert panel. *Haematologica.* 2014;99(5):811-820.
57. Ruggeri A, Eapen M, Scaravadou A, et al. Umbilical cord blood transplantation for children with thalassemia and sickle cell disease. *Biol Blood Marrow Transplant.* 2011;17(9):1375-1382.
58. Bolanos-Meade J, Fuchs EJ, Luznik L, et al. HLA-haploidentical bone marrow transplantation with posttransplant cyclophosphamide expands the donor pool for patients with sickle cell disease. *Blood.* 2012;120(22):4285-4291.
59. Somaraju UR, Tadepalli K. Hematopoietic stem cell transplantation for Gaucher disease. *Cochrane Database Syst Rev.* 2017;10:CD006974.
60. Tan EY, Boelens JJ, Jones SA, Wynn RF. Hematopoietic stem cell transplantation in inborn errors of metabolism. *Front Pediatr.* 2019;7:433.
61. Farge D, Labopin M, Tyndall A, et al. Autologous hematopoietic stem cell transplantation for autoimmune diseases: an observational study on 12 years' experience from the European Group for Blood and Marrow Transplantation Working Party on Autoimmune Diseases. *Haematologica.* 2010;95(2):284-292.
62. Sullivan KM, Goldmuntz EA, Keyes-Elstein L, et al. Myeloablative autologous stem-cell transplantation for severe scleroderma. *N Engl J Med.* 2018;378(1):35-47.
63. Goldman JM. A special report: bone marrow transplants using volunteer donors-recommendations and requirements for a standardized practice throughout the world-1994 update. The WMDA Executive Committee. *Blood.* 1994;84:2833-2839.
64. Bensinger WI. Allogeneic transplantation: peripheral blood vs. bone marrow. *Curr Opin Oncol.* 2012;24(2):191-196.
65. Anasetti C, Logan BR, Lee SJ, et al. Peripheral-blood stem cells versus bone marrow from unrelated donors. *N Engl J Med.* 2012;367(16):1487-1496.
66. Allan D, Petraszko T, Elmoazzen H, Smith S. A review of factors influencing the banking of collected umbilical cord blood units. *Stem Cell Int.* 2013;2013:463031.
67. Warren EH, Zhang XC, Li SY, et al. Effect of MHC and non-MHC donor/recipient genetic disparity on the outcome of allogeneic HCT. *Blood.* 2012;120(14):2796-2806.
68. Horowitz MM. Does matched unrelated donor transplantation have the same outcome as matched sibling transplantation in unselected patients? *Best Pract Res Clin Haematol.* 2012;25(4):483-486.
69. Pidala J, Lee SJ, Ahn KW, et al. Nonpermissive HLA-DPB1 mismatch increases mortality after myeloablative unrelated allogeneic hematopoietic cell transplantation. *Blood.* 2014;124(16):2596-2606.
70. Gragert L, Eapen M, Williams E, et al. HLA match likelihoods for hematopoietic stem-cell grafts in the US registry. *N Engl J Med.* 2014;371(4):339-348.
71. Barker JN, Krepski TP, DeFor TE, Davies SM, Wagner JE, Weisdorf DJ. Searching for unrelated donor hematopoietic stem cells: availability and speed of umbilical cord blood versus bone marrow. *Biol Blood Marrow Transplant.* 2002;8(5):257-260.
72. Spellman SR, Eapen M, Logan BR, et al. A perspective on the selection of unrelated donors and cord blood units for transplantation. *Blood.* 2012;120(2):259-265.
73. Lee SJ, Klein J, Haagenson M, et al. High-resolution donor-recipient HLA matching contributes to the success of unrelated donor marrow transplantation. *Blood.* 2007;110(13):4576-4583.
74. Woolfrey A, Klein JP, Haagenson M, et al. HLA-C antigen mismatch is associated with worse outcome in unrelated donor peripheral blood stem cell transplantation. *Biol Blood Marrow Transplant.* 2011;17(6):885-892.
75. Petersdorf EW, Gooley TA, Malkki M, et al. HLA-C expression levels define permissible mismatches in hematopoietic cell transplantation. *Blood.* 2014;124(26):3996-4003.
76. Mehta RS, Saliba RM, Chen J, et al. Post-transplantation cyclophosphamide versus conventional graft-versus-host disease prophylaxis in mismatched unrelated donor haematopoietic cell transplantation. *Br J Haematol.* 2016;173(3):444-455.
77. Oran B, Cao K, Saliba RM, et al. Better allele-level matching improves transplant-related mortality after double cord blood transplantation. *Haematologica.* 2015;100(10):1361-1370.
78. Scaradavou A, Brunstein CG, Eapen M, et al. Double unit grafts successfully extend the application of umbilical cord blood transplantation in adults with acute leukemia. *Blood.* 2013;121(5):752-758.
79. Delaney C, Gutman JA, Appelbaum FR. Cord blood transplantation for haematological malignancies: conditioning regimens, double cord transplant and infectious complications. *Br J Haematol.* 2009;147(2):207-216.
80. Milano F, Gooley T, Wood B, et al. Cord-blood transplantation in patients with minimal residual disease. *N Engl J Med.* 2016;375(10):944-953.
81. Newell LF, Flowers MED, Gooley T, et al. Characterization of chronic graft-versus-host disease and duration of immunosuppression after cord blood transplantation. *Blood.* 2011;118:1741.
82. Ponce DM, Gonzales A, Lubin M, et al. Graft-versus-Host disease after double-unit cord blood transplantation has unique features and an association with engrafting unit-to-recipient HLA match. *Biol Blood Marrow Transplant.* 2013;19(6):904-911.
83. Wagner JE, Eapen M, Carter S, et al. One-unit versus two-unit cord-blood transplantation for hematologic cancers. *N Engl J Med.* 2014;371(18):1685-1694.
84. Pineault N, Abu-Khader A. Advances in umbilical cord blood stem cell expansion and clinical translation. *Exp Hematol.* 2015;43(7):498-513.
85. Cohen S, Roy J, Lachance S, et al. Hematopoietic stem cell transplantation using single UM171-expanded cord blood: a single-arm, phase 1-2 safety and feasibility study. *Lancet Haematol.* 2020;7(2):e134-e145.
86. Debals-Gonthier M, Siani C, Faucher C, et al. Cost-effectiveness analysis of haploidentical vs matched unrelated allogeneic hematopoietic stem cells transplantation in patients older than 55 years. *Bone Marrow Transplant.* 2018;53(9):1096-1104.
87. Luznik L, Jalla S, Engstrom LW, Iannone R, Fuchs EJ. Durable engraftment of major histocompatibility complex-incompatible cells after nonmyeloablative conditioning with fludarabine, low-dose total body irradiation, and posttransplantation cyclophosphamide. *Blood.* 2001;98(12):3456-3464.
88. Luznik L, O'Donnell PV, Symons HJ, et al. HLA-haploidentical bone marrow transplantation for hematologic malignancies using nonmyeloablative conditioning and high-dose, posttransplantation cyclophosphamide. *Biol Blood Marrow Transplant.* 2008;14(6):641-650.
89. Brunstein CG, Fuchs EJ, Carter SL, et al. Alternative donor transplantation after reduced intensity conditioning: results of parallel phase 2 trials using partially HLA-mismatched related bone marrow or unrelated double umbilical cord blood grafts. *Blood.* 2011;118:282-288.
90. Solomon SR, Sizemore CA, Sanacore M, et al. Haploidentical transplantation using T cell replete peripheral blood stem cells and myeloablative conditioning in patients with high-risk hematologic malignancies who lack conventional donors is well tolerated and produces excellent relapse-free survival: results of a prospective phase II trial. *Biol Blood Marrow Transplant.* 2012;18(12):1859-1866.
91. Solomon SR, Jacobson S, Sanacore M, et al. Myeloablative conditioning with PBSC grafts for T-replete haploidentical donor hematopoietic cell transplantation using post-transplant cyclophosphamide results in universal engraftment, low rates of Gvhd, NRM and excellent survival outcomes: an analysis. *Blood.* 2013;122:3351.
92. Symons HJ, Chen AR, Luznik L, et al. Myeloablative haploidentical bone marrow transplantation with T cell replete grafts and post-transplant cyclophosphamide: results of a phase II clinical trial. *Blood.* 2011;118(21):4151. ASH.
93. Raj K, Pagliuca A, Bradstock K, et al. Peripheral blood hematopoietic stem cells for transplantation of hematological diseases from related, haploidentical donors after reduced-intensity conditioning. *Biol Blood Marrow Transplant.* 2014;20(6):890-895.
94. Granier C, Biard L, Masson E, et al. Impact of the source of hematopoietic stem cell in unrelated transplants: comparison between 10/10, 9/10-HLA matched donors and cord blood. *Am J Hematol.* 2015;90(10):897-903.
95. Atsuta Y, Morishima Y, Suzuki R, et al. Comparison of unrelated cord blood transplantation and HLA-mismatched unrelated bone marrow transplantation for adults with leukemia. *Biol Blood Marrow Transplant.* 2012;18(5):780-787.
96. Sakaguchi H, Watanabe N, Matsumoto K, et al. Comparison of donor sources in hematopoietic stem cell transplantation for childhood acute leukemia: a Nationwide retrospective study. *Biol Blood Marrow Transplant.* 2016;22(12):2226-2234.
97. Resnick IB, Tsirigotis PD, Shapira MY, et al. ABO incompatibility is associated with increased non-relapse and GVHD related mortality in patients with malignancies treated with a reduced intensity regimen: a single center experience of 221 patients. *Biol Blood Marrow Transplant.* 2008;14(4):409-417.
98. Bacigalupo A, Ballen K, Rizzo D, et al. Defining the intensity of conditioning regimens: working definitions. *Biol Blood Marrow Transplant.* 2009;15(12):1628-1633.
99. Storb R, Gyurkocza B, Storer BE, et al. Graft-versus-host disease and graft-versus-tumor effects after allogeneic hematopoietic cell transplantation. *J Clin Oncol.* 2013;31(12):1530-1538.
100. Ringden O, Labopin M, Ehninger G, et al. Reduced intensity conditioning compared with myeloablative conditioning using unrelated donor transplants in patients with acute myeloid leukemia. *J Clin Oncol.* 2009;27:4570-4577.
101. Champlin RE, Perez WS, Passweg JR, et al. Bone marrow transplantation for severe aplastic anemia: a randomized controlled study of conditioning regimens. *Blood.* 2007;109(10):4582-4585.
102. Bejanyan N, Kim S, Hebert KM, et al. Choice of conditioning regimens for bone marrow transplantation in severe aplastic anemia. *Blood Adv.* 2019;3(20):3123-3131.
103. Thomas ED, Storb R, Clift RA, et al. Bone-marrow transplantation 2. *New Engl J Med.* 1975;292:895-902.
104. Clift RA, Buckner CD, Appelbaum FR, et al. Allogeneic marrow transplantation in patients with chronic myeloid leukemia in the chronic phase: a randomized trial of two irradiation regimens. *Blood.* 1991;77(8):1660-1665.
105. Devergie A, Blaise D, Attal M, et al. Allogeneic bone-marrow transplantation for chronic myeloid-leukemia in first chronic phase—a randomized trial of busulfan-cytoxan versus cytoxan-total-body irradiation as preparative regimen—a report from the French-Society-of-Bone-Marrow-Graft (SFGM). *Blood.* 1995;85:2263-2268.
106. Blaise D, Maraninchi D, Archimbaud E, et al. Allogeneic bone marrow transplantation for acute myeloid leukemia in first remission: a randomized trial of a busulfan-cytoxan versus cytoxan-total body irradiation as preparative regimen – a report from the Group d'Etudes de la Greffe de Moelle Osseuse. *Blood.* 1992;79(10):2578-2582.

107. Deeg HJ, Storer B, Slattery JT, et al. Conditioning with targeted busulfan and cyclophosphamide for hemopoietic stem cell transplantation from related and unrelated donors in patients with myelodysplastic syndrome. *Blood.* 2002;100(4):1201-1207.
108. Nemecek ER, Guthrie KA, Sorror ML, et al. Conditioning with treosulfan and fludarabine followed by allogeneic hematopoietic cell transplantation for high-risk hematologic malignancies. *Biol Blood Marrow Transplant.* 2011;17(3):341-350.
109. Horowitz MM, Gale RP, Sondel PM, et al. Graft-versus-leukemia reactions after bone-marrow transplantation. *Blood.* 1990;75(3):555-562.
110. Kolb HJ, Schattenberg A, Goldman JM, et al. Graft-versus-leukemia effect of donor lymphocyte transfusions in marrow grafted patients. *Blood.* 1995;86(5):2041-2050.
111. Hsu JW, Farhadfar N, Murthy H, et al. The effect of donor graft cryopreservation on allogeneic hematopoietic cell transplantation outcomes: a center for international blood and marrow transplant research analysis. Implications during the COVID-19 pandemic. *Transplant Cell Ther.* 2021;27(6):507-516.
112. Clark RA, Johnson FL, Klebanoff SJ, Thomas ED. Defective neutrophil chemotaxis in bone-marrow transplant patients. *J Clin Invest.* 1976;58(1):22-31.
113. Storek J, Espino G, Dawson MA, Storer B, Flowers MED, Maloney DG. Low B-cell and monocyte counts on day 80 are associated with high infection rates between days 100 and 365 after allogeneic marrow transplantation. *Blood.* 2000;96(9):3290-3293.
114. Orrantia A, Terren I, Astarloa-Pando G, Zenarruzabeitia O, Borrego F. Human NK cells in autologous hematopoietic stem cell transplantation for cancer treatment. *Cancers.* 2021;13(7):1589.
115. Storek J, Dawson MA, Storer B, et al. Immune reconstitution after allogeneic marrow transplantation compared with blood stem cell transplantation. *Blood.* 2001;97(11):3380-3389.
116. Williams KM, Gress RE. Immune reconstitution and implications for immunotherapy following haematopoietic stem cell transplantation. *Best Pract Res Clin Haematol.* 2008;21(3):579-596.
117. Douek DC, Vescio RA, Betts MR, et al. Substantial thymic output occurs in adults after hematopoietic stem cell transplant and can predict T cell reconstitution. *Faseb J.* 2000;14:A1074-A.
118. Carpenter PA, Englund JA. How I vaccinate blood and marrow transplant recipients. *Blood.* 2016;127(23):2824-2832.
119. Sorror ML, Maris MB, Storb R, et al. Hematopoietic cell transplantation (HCT)-specific comorbidity index: a new tool for risk assessment before allogeneic HCT. *Blood.* 2005;106(8):2912-2919.
120. Sorror ML, Giralt S, Sandmaier BM, et al. Hematopoietic cell transplantation-specific comorbidity index as an outcome predictor for patients with acute myeloid leukemia in first remission: combined FHCRC and MDACC experiences. *Blood.* 2007;110:4606-4613.
121. Sorror ML, Storb RF, Sandmaier BM, et al. Comorbidity-age index: a clinical measure of biologic age before allogeneic hematopoietic cell transplantation. *J Clin Oncol.* 2014;32(29):3249-3256.
122. Spielberger R, Stiff P, Bensinger W, et al. Palifermin for oral mucositis after intensive therapy for hematologic cancers. *N Engl J Med.* 2004;351(25):2590-2598.
123. Hensley ML, Hagerty KL, Kewalramani T, et al. American Society of clinical Oncology 2008 clinical practice guideline update: use of chemotherapy and radiation therapy protectants. *J Clin Oncol.* 2009;27(1):127-145.
124. Mohty M, Malard F, Abecassis M, et al. Sinusoidal obstruction syndrome/veno-occlusive disease: current situation and perspectives-a position statement from the European Society for Blood and Marrow Transplantation (EBMT). *Bone Marrow Transplant.* 2015;50(6):781-789.
125. DeLeve LD, Shulman HM, McDonald GB. Toxic injury to hepatic sinusoids: sinusoidal obstruction syndrome (veno-occlusive disease). *Semin Liver Dis.* 2002;22(1):27-42.
126. Chao N. How I treat sinusoidal obstruction syndrome. *Blood.* 2014;123(26):4023-4026.
127. Richardson PG, Murakami C, Jin ZZ, et al. Multi-institutional use of defibrotide in 88 patients after stem cell transplantation with severe veno-occlusive disease and multisystem organ failure: response without significant toxicity in a high-risk population and factors predictive of outcome. *Blood.* 2002;100(13):4337-4343.
128. Richardson PG, Soiffer RJ, Antin JH, et al. Defibrotide for the treatment of severe hepatic veno-occlusive disease and multiorgan failure after stem cell transplantation: a multicenter, randomized, dose-finding trial. *Biol Blood Marrow Transplant.* 2010;16(7):1005-1017.
129. Corbacioglu S, Greil J, Peters C, et al. Defibrotide in the treatment of children with veno-occlusive disease (VOD): a retrospective multicentre study demonstrates therapeutic efficacy upon early intervention. *Bone Marrow Transplant.* 2004;33(2):189-195.
130. Ruutu T, Eriksson B, Remes K, et al. Ursodeoxycholic acid for the prevention of hepatic complications in allogeneic stem cell transplantation. *Blood.* 2002;100(6):1977-1983.
131. Tay J, Tinmouth A, Fergusson D, Huebsch L, Allan DS. Systematic review of controlled clinical trials on the use of ursodeoxycholic acid for the prevention of hepatic veno-occlusive disease in hematopoietic stem cell transplantation. *Biol Blood Marrow Transplant.* 2007;13(2):206-217.
132. Panoskaltsis-Mortari A, Griese M, Madtes DK, et al. An Official American Thoracic Society research statement: noninfectious lung injury after hematopoietic stem cell transplantation—idiopathic pneumonia syndrome. *Am J Respir Crit Care Med.* 2011;183(9):1262-1279.
133. Zhu KE, Hu JY, Zhang T, Chen J, Zhong J, Lu YH. Incidence, risks, and outcome of idiopathic pneumonia syndrome early after allogeneic hematopoietic stem cell transplantation. *Eur J Haematol.* 2008;81:461-466.
134. Seo S, Renaud C, Kuypers JM, et al. Idiopathic pneumonia syndrome after hematopoietic cell transplantation: evidence of occult infectious etiologies. *Blood.* 2015;125(24):3789-3797.
135. Yanik GA, Horowitz MM, Weisdorf DJ, et al. Randomized, double-blind, placebo-controlled trial of soluble tumor necrosis factor receptor: enbrel (etanercept) for the treatment of idiopathic pneumonia syndrome after allogeneic stem cell transplantation—blood and marrow transplant clinical trials network protocol. *Biol Blood Marrow Transplant.* 2014;20(6):858-864.
136. Zager RA, Oquigley J, Zager BK, et al. Acute renal-failure following bone-marrow transplantation - a retrospective study of 272 patients. *Am J Kidney Dis.* 1989;13(3):210-216.
137. Jodele S, Dandoy CE, Myers KC, et al. New approaches in the diagnosis, pathophysiology, and treatment of pediatric hematopoietic stem cell transplantation-associated thrombotic microangiopathy. *Transfus Apher Sci.* 2016;54(2):181-190.
138. Jodele S, Fukuda T, Vinks A, et al. Eculizumab therapy in children with severe hematopoietic stem cell transplantation-associated thrombotic microangiopathy. *Biol Blood Marrow Transplant.* 2014;20(4):518-525.
139. Marotta S, Marano L, Ricci P, et al. Eltrombopag for post-transplant cytopenias due to poor graft function. *Bone Marrow Transplant.* 2019;54(8):1346-1353.
140. Yuan C, Boyd AM, Nelson J, et al. Eltrombopag for treating thrombocytopenia after allogeneic stem cell transplantation. *Biol Blood Marrow Transplant.* 2019;25(7):1320-1324.
141. Shahzad M, Siddiqui RS, Anwar I, et al. Outcomes with CD34-selected stem cell boost for poor graft function after allogeneic hematopoietic stem cell transplantation: a systematic review and meta-analysis. *Transplant Cell Ther.* 2021;27(10):877.e1-e877.e8.
142. Markey KA, MacDonald KPA, Hill GR. The biology of graft-versus-host disease: experimental systems instructing clinical practice. *Blood.* 2014;124(3):354-362.
143. Holtan SG, Pasquini M, Weisdorf DJ. Acute graft-versus-host disease: a bench-to-bedside update. *Blood.* 2014;124(3):363-373.
144. Filipovich AH, Weisdorf D, Pavletic S, et al. National Institutes of Health consensus development project on criteria for clinical trials in chronic graft-versus-host disease: I. Diagnosis and staging working group report. *Biol Blood Marrow Transplant.* 2005;11(12):945-956.
145. Nash RA, Antin JH, Karanes C, et al. Phase 3 study comparing methotrexate and tacrolimus with methotrexate and cyclosporine for prophylaxis of acute graft-versus-host disease after marrow transplantation from unrelated donors. *Blood.* 2000;96(6):2062-2068.
146. Ratanatharathorn V, Nash RA, Przepiorka D, et al. Phase III study comparing methotrexate and tacrolimus (prograf, FK506) with methotrexate and cyclosporine for graft-versus-host disease prophylaxis after HLA-identical sibling bone marrow transplantation. *Blood.* 1998;92(7):2303-2314.
147. Watkins B, Qayed M, McCracken C, et al. Phase II trial of costimulation blockade with Abatacept for prevention of acute GVHD. *J Clin Oncol.* 2021;39(17):1865-1877.
148. Nash RA, Johnston L, Parker P, et al. A phase I/II study of mycophenolate mofetil in combination with cyclosporine for prophylaxis of acute graft-versus-host disease after myeloablative conditioning and allogeneic hematopoietic cell transplantation. *Biol Blood Marrow Transplant.* 2005;11(7):495-505.
149. Bolwell B, Sobecks R, Pohlman B, et al. A prospective randomized trial comparing cyclosporine and short course methotrexate with cyclosporine and mycophenolate mofetil for GVHD prophylaxis in myeloablative allogeneic bone marrow transplantation. *Bone Marrow Transplant.* 2004;34(7):621-625.
150. Cutler C, Logan BR, Nakamura R, et al. Tacrolimus/sirolimus vs. Tacrolimus/methotrexate for graft-vs.-host disease prophylaxis After HLA-matched, related donor hematopoietic stem cell transplantation: results of blood and marrow transplant clinical trials network trial 0402. *Blood.* 2012:120:739.
151. Perez-Simon JA, Martino R, Parody R, et al. The combination of sirolimus plus tacrolimus improves outcome after reduced-intensity conditioning, unrelated donor hematopoietic stem cell transplantation compared with cyclosporine plus mycofenolate. *Haematologica.* 2013;98(4):526-532.
152. O'donnell PV, Luznik L, Jones RJ, et al. Nonmyeloablative bone marrow transplantation from partially HLA-mismatched related donors using posttransplantation cyclophosphamide. *Biol Blood Marrow Transplant.* 2002;8(7):377-386.
153. Gooptu M, Romee R, St Martin A, et al. HLA-haploidentical vs matched unrelated donor transplants with posttransplant cyclophosphamide-based prophylaxis. *Blood.* 2021;138(3):273-282.
154. Pasquini MC, Devine S, Mendizabal A, et al. Comparative outcomes of donor graft CD34+ selection and immune suppressive therapy as graft-versus-host disease prophylaxis for patients with acute myeloid leukemia in complete remission undergoing HLA-matched sibling allogeneic hematopoietic cell transplantation. *J Clin Oncol.* 2012;30(26):3194-3201.
155. Wagner JE, Thompson JS, Carter SL, Kernan NA; Unrelated Donor Marrow Transplantation Trial. Effect of graft-versus-host disease prophylaxis on 3-year disease-free survival in recipients of unrelated donor bone marrow (T-cell Depletion Trial): a multi-centre, randomised phase II-III trial. *Lancet.* 2005;366(9487):733-741.
156. Bleakley M, Heimfeld S, Loeb KR, et al. Outcomes of acute leukemia patients transplanted with naive T cell-depleted stem cell grafts. *J Clin Invest.* 2015;125(7):2677-2689.
157. Soiffer RJ, LeRademacher J, Ho V, et al. Impact of immune modulation with anti-T-cell antibodies on the outcome of reduced-intensity allogeneic hematopoietic stem cell transplantation for hematologic malignancies. *Blood.* 2011;117(25):6963-6970.
158. Kroger N, Solano C, Wolschke C, et al. Antilymphocyte globulin for prevention of chronic graft-versus-host disease. *N Engl J Med.* 2016;374(1):43-53.
159. Sale GE, Anderson P, Browne M, Myerson D. Evidence of cytotoxic T-cell destruction of epidermal-cells in human graft-vs-host disease - immunohistology with monoclonal-antibody Tia-1. *Arch Pathol Lab Med.* 1992;116(6):622-625.
160. Glucksberg H, Storb R, Fefer A, et al. Clinical manifestations of graft versus host disease in human recipients of marrow from HL-A-matched sibling donors. *Transplantation.* 1974;18(4):295-304.
161. Saber W, Opie S, Rizzo JD, Zhang MJ, Horowitz MM, Schriber J. Outcomes after matched unrelated donor versus identical sibling hematopoietic cell transplantation in adults with acute myelogenous leukemia. *Blood.* 2012;119(17):3908-3916.

162. Weisdorf D, Hakke R, Blazar B, et al. Risk-factors for acute graft-versus-host disease in histocompatible donor bone-marrow transplantation. *Transplantation.* 1991;51(6):1197-1203.
163. Couriel DR, Saliba RM, Giralt S, et al. Acute and chronic graft-versus-host disease after ablative and nonmyeloablative conditioning for allogeneic hematopoietic transplantation. *Biol Blood Marrow Transplant.* 2004;10(3):178-185.
164. Eapen M, Logan BR, Confer DL, et al. Peripheral blood grafts from unrelated donors are associated with increased acute and chronic graft-versus-host disease without improved survival. *Biol Blood Marrow Transplant.* 2007;13(12):1461-1468.
165. Zaucha JM, Gooley T, Bensinger WI, et al. CD34 cell dose in granulocyte colony-stimulating factor-mobilized peripheral blood mononuclear cell grafts affects engraftment kinetics and development of extensive chronic graft-versus-host disease after human leukocyte antigen-identical sibling transplantation. *Blood.* 2001;98(12):3221-3227.
166. Bolanos-Meade J, Logan BR, Alousi AM, et al. Phase 3 clinical trial of steroids/mycophenolate mofetil vs steroids/placebo as therapy for acute GVHD: BMT CTN 0802. *Blood.* 2014;124(22):3221-3227; quiz 3335.
167. Mielcarek M, Furlong T, Storer BE, et al. Effectiveness and safety of lower dose prednisone for initial treatment of acute graft-versus-host disease: a randomized controlled trial. *Haematologica.* 2015;100(6):842-848.
168. McDonald GB, Bouvier M, Hockenbery DM, et al. Oral beclomethasone dipropionate for treatment of intestinal graft-versus-host disease: a randomized, controlled trial. *Gastroenterology.* 1998;115(1):28-35.
169. Bertz H, Afting M, Kreisel W, Duffner U, Greinwald R, Finke J. Feasibility and response to budesonide as topical corticosteroid therapy for acute intestinal GVHD. *Bone Marrow Transplant.* 1999;24(11):1185-1189.
170. Ibrahim RB, Abidi MH, Cronin SM, et al. Nonabsorbable corticosteroids use in the treatment of gastrointestinal graft-versus-host disease. *Biol Blood Marrow Transplant.* 2009;15(4):395-405.
171. Van Lint MT, Milone G, Leotta S, et al. Treatment of acute graft-versus-host disease with prednisolone: significant survival advantage for day+5 responders and no advantage for nonresponders receiving anti-thymocyte globulin. *Blood.* 2006;107(10):4177-4181.
172. Martin PJ, Rizzo JD, Wingard JR, et al. First- and second-line systemic treatment of acute graft-versus-host disease: recommendations of the American Society of Blood and Marrow Transplantation. *Biol Blood Marrow Transplant.* 2012;18(8):1150-1163.
173. Jagasia M, Zeiser R, Arbushites M, Delaite P, Gadbaw B, Bubnoff NV. Ruxolitinib for the treatment of patients with steroid-refractory GVHD: an introduction to the REACH trials. *Immunotherapy.* 2018;10(5):391-402.
174. Zeiser R, von Bubnoff N, Butler J, et al. Ruxolitinib for glucocorticoid-refractory acute graft-versus-host disease. *N Engl J Med.* 2020;382(19):1800-1810.
175. Foss FM, Gorgun G, Miller KB. Extracorporeal photopheresis in chronic graft-versus-host disease. *Bone Marrow Transplant.* 2002;29(9):719-725.
176. Abu-Dalle I, Reljic T, Nishihori T, et al. Extracorporeal photopheresis in steroid-refractory acute or chronic graft-versus-host disease: results of a systematic review of prospective studies. *Biol Blood Marrow Transplant.* 2014;20(11):1677-1686.
177. Atkinson K, Horowitz MM, Gale RP, et al. Risk-factors for chronic graft-versus-host disease after HLA-identical sibling bone-marrow transplantation. *Blood.* 1990;75(12):2459-2464.
178. Ochs LA, Miller WJ, Filipovich AH, et al. Predictive factors for chronic graft-versus-host disease after histocompatible sibling donor bone-marrow transplantation. *Bone Marrow Transplant.* 1994;13(4):455-460.
179. Lee SJ, Klein JP, Barrett AJ, et al. Severity of chronic graft-versus-host disease: association with treatment-related mortality and relapse. *Blood.* 2002;100(2):406-414.
180. Carlens S, Ringden O, Remberger M, et al. Risk factors for chronic graft-versus-host disease after bone marrow transplantation: a retrospective single centre analysis. *Bone Marrow Transplant.* 1998;22(8):755-761.
181. Jagasia MH, Greinix HT, Arora M, et al. National institutes of health consensus development project on criteria for clinical trials in chronic graft-versus-host disease: I. The 2014 diagnosis and staging working group report. *Biol Blood Marrow Transplant.* 2015;21(3):389-401.e1.
182. Barker AF, Bergeron A, Rom WN, Hertz MI. Obliterative bronchiolitis. *N Engl J Med.* 2014;370(19):1820-1828.
183. Jamil MO, Mineishi S. State-of-the-art acute and chronic GVHD treatment. *Int J Hematol.* 2015;101(5):452-466.
184. Miklos D, Cutler CS, Arora M, et al. Ibrutinib for chronic graft-versus-host disease after failure of prior therapy. *Blood.* 2017;130(21):2243-2250.
185. Zeiser R, Polverelli N, Ram R, et al. Ruxolitinib for glucocorticoid-refractory chronic graft-versus-host disease. *N Engl J Med.* 2021;385(3):228-238.
186. Cutler C, Lee SJ, Arai S, et al. Belumosudil for chronic graft-versus-host disease after 2 or more prior lines of therapy: the ROCKstar Study. *Blood.* 2021;138(22):2278-2289.
187. Socie G. Current challenges in chronic GVHD. *Onkologie.* 2010;33:214.
188. Stewart BL, Storer B, Storek J, et al. Duration of immunosuppressive treatment for chronic graft-versus-host disease. *Blood.* 2004;104(12):3501-3506.
189. Norman BC, Jacobsohn DA, Williams KM, et al. Fluticasone, azithromycin and montelukast therapy in reducing corticosteroid exposure in bronchiolitis obliterans syndrome after allogeneic hematopoietic SCT: a case series of eight patients. *Bone Marrow Transplant.* 2011;46(10):1369-1373.
190. Girmenia C, Barosi G, Piciocchi A, et al. Primary prophylaxis of invasive fungal diseases in allogeneic stem cell transplantation: revised recommendations from a consensus process by Gruppo Italiano Trapianto Midollo Osseo (GITMO). *Biol Blood Marrow Transplant.* 2014;20:1080-1088.
191. Wingard JR, Carter SL, Walsh TJ, et al. Randomized, double-blind trial of fluconazole versus voriconazole for prevention of invasive fungal infection after allogeneic hematopoietic cell transplantation. *Blood.* 2010;116(24):5111-5118.
192. Ljungman P, Hakki M, Boeckh M. Cytomegalovirus in hematopoietic stem cell transplant recipients. *Hematol Oncol Clin North Am.* 2011;25(1):151-169.
193. Marty FM, Ljungman P, Chemaly RF, et al. Letermovir prophylaxis for cytomegalovirus in hematopoietic-cell transplantation. *N Engl J Med.* 2017;377(25):2433-2444.
194. Casey J, Morris K, Narayana M, Nakagaki M, Kennedy GA. Oral ribavirin for treatment of respiratory syncitial virus and parainfluenza 3 virus infections post allogeneic haematopoietic stem cell transplantation. *Bone Marrow Transplant.* 2013;48(12):1558-1561.
195. Ljungman P, de la Camara R, Mikulska M, et al. COVID-19 and stem cell transplantation; results from an EBMT and GETH multicenter prospective survey. *Leukemia.* 2021;35(10):2885-2894.
196. Sharma A, Bhatt NS, St Martin A, et al. Clinical characteristics and outcomes of COVID-19 in haematopoietic stem-cell transplantation recipients: an observational cohort study. *Lancet Haematol.* 2021;8(3):e185-e193.
197. Ogata M, Satou T, Kadota Ji, et al. Human herpesvirus 6 (HHV-6) reactivation and HHV-6 encephalitis after allogeneic hematopoietic cell transplantation: a multicenter, prospective study. *Clin Infect Dis.* 2013;57(5):671-681.
198. La Rosa AM, Champlin RE, Mirza N, et al. Adenovirus infections in adult recipients of blood and marrow transplants. *Clin Infect Dis.* 2001;32:871-876.
199. Ljungman P, Ribaud P, Eyrich M, et al. Cidofovir for adenovirus infections after allogeneic hematopoietic stem cell transplantation: a survey by the infectious diseases working party of the European group for blood and marrow transplantation. *Bone Marrow Transplant.* 2003;31:481-486.
200. Perruccio K, Menconi M, Galaverna F, et al. Safety and efficacy of brincidofovir for Adenovirus infection in children receiving allogeneic stem cell transplantation: an AIEOP retrospective analyses. *Bone Marrow Transplant.* 2021;56(12):3104-3107.
201. Khera N, Storer B, Flowers MED, et al. Nonmalignant late effects and compromised functional status in survivors of hematopoietic cell transplantation. *J Clin Oncol.* 2012;30(1):71-77.
202. Bar M, Ott SM, Lewiecki EM, et al. Bone health management after hematopoietic cell transplantation: an expert panel opinion from the American Society for transplantation and cellular therapy. *Biol Blood Marrow Transplant.* 2020;26(10):1784-1802.
203. Farhadfar N, Stan MN, Shah P, et al. Thyroid dysfunction in adult hematopoietic cell transplant survivors: risks and outcomes. *Bone Marrow Transplant.* 2018;53(8):977-982.
204. Syrjala KL, Langer SL, Abrams JR, Storer BE, Martin PJ. Late effects of hematopoietic cell transplantation among 10-year adult survivors compared with case-matched controls. *J Clin Oncol.* 2005;23(27):6596-6606.
205. Majhail NS, DeFor T, Lazarus HM, Burns LJ. High prevalence of iron overload in adult allogeneic hematopoietic cell transplant survivors. *Biol Blood Marrow Transplant.* 2008;14(7):790-794.
206. Wang M, Wang WJ, Abeywardane A, et al. Autoimmune hemolytic anemia after allogeneic hematopoietic stem cell transplantation: analysis of 533 adult patients who underwent transplantation at King's college hospital. *Biol Blood Marrow Transplant.* 2015;21(1):60-66.
207. Sanz J, Arriaga F, Montesinos P, et al. Autoimmune hemolytic anemia following allogeneic hematopoietic stem cell transplantation in adult patients. *Bone Marrow Transplant.* 2007;39(9):555-561.
208. Holbro A, Abinun M, Daikeler T. Management of autoimmune diseases after haematopoietic stem cell transplantation. *Br J Haematol.* 2012;157(3):281-290.
209. Loren AW, Chow E, Jacobsohn DA, et al. Pregnancy after hematopoietic cell transplantation: a report from the late effects working committee of the Center for International Blood and Marrow Transplant Research (CIBMTR). *Biol Blood Marrow Transplant.* 2011;17(2):157-166.
210. Salooja N, Szydlo RM, Socie G, et al. Pregnancy outcomes after peripheral blood or bone marrow transplantation: a retrospective survey. *Lancet.* 2001;358(9278):271-276.
211. Schechter T, Finkelstein Y, Doyle J, Koren G. Pregnancy after stem cell transplantation. *Can Fam Physician.* 2005;51:817-818.
212. Martin PJ, Counts GW, Appelbaum FR, et al. Life expectancy in patients surviving more than 5 years after hematopoietic cell transplantation. *J Clin Oncol.* 2010;28:1011-1016.
213. Yoshihara S, Yanik G, Cooke KR, Mineishi S. Bronchiolitis obliterans syndrome (BOS), bronchiolitis obliterans organizing pneumonia (BOOP), and other late-onset noninfectious pulmonary complications following allogeneic hematopoietic stem cell transplantation. *Biol Blood Marrow Transplant.* 2007;13(7):749-759.
214. Chow EJ, Wong K, Lee SJ, et al. Late cardiovascular complications after hematopoietic cell transplantation. *Biol Blood Marrow Transplant.* 2014;20(6):794-800.
215. Rasche L, Kapp M, Einsele H, Mielke S. EBV-induced post transplant lymphoproliferative disorders: a persisting challenge in allogeneic hematopoetic SCT. *Bone Marrow Transplant.* 2014;49(2):163-167.
216. Ortega JJ, Olive T, de Heredia CD, Llort A. Secondary malignancies and quality of life after stem cell transplantation. *Bone Marrow Transplant.* 2005;35(suppl 1):S83-S87.
217. Favre-Schmuziger G, Hofer S, Passweg J, et al. Treatment of solid tumors following allogeneic bone marrow transplantation. *Bone Marrow Transplant.* 2000;25:895-898.
218. Metayer C, Curtis RE, Vose J, et al. Myelodysplastic syndrome and acute myeloid leukemia after autotransplantation for lymphoma: a multicenter case-control study. *Blood.* 2003;101(5):2015-2023.
219. Alinari L, Blum KA. How I treat relapsed classical Hodgkin lymphoma after autologous stem cell transplant. *Blood.* 2016;127(3):287-295.
220. Dietrich S, Tielesch B, Rieger M, et al. Patterns and outcome of relapse after autologous stem cell transplantation for mantle cell lymphoma. *Cancer.* 2011;117(9):1901-1910.

221. Kornacker M, Kornacker B, Schmitt C, Leo E, Ho AD, Hensel M. Commercial LightCycler-based quantitative real-time PCR compared to nested PCR for monitoring of Bcl-2/IgH rearrangement in patients with follicular lymphoma. *Ann Hematol*. 2009;88(1):43-50.
222. Baron F, Storb R, Storer BE, et al. Factors associated with outcomes in allogeneic hematopoietic cell transplantation with nonmyeloablative conditioning after failed myeloablative hematopoietic cell transplantation. *J Clin Oncol*. 2006;24(25):4150-4157.
223. Kekre N, Kim HT, Thanarajasingam G, et al. Efficacy of immune suppression tapering in treating relapse after reduced intensity allogeneic stem cell transplantation. *Haematologica*. 2015;100(9):1222-1227.
224. Collins RH, Jr, Shpilberg O, Drobyski WR, et al. Donor leukocyte infusions in 140 patients with relapsed malignancy after allogeneic bone marrow transplantation. *J Clin Oncol*. 1997;15(2):433-444.
225. Levine JE, Braun T, Penza SL, et al. Prospective trial of chemotherapy and donor leukocyte infusions for relapse of advanced myeloid malignancies after allogeneic stem-cell transplantation. *J Clin Oncol*. 2002;20(2):405-412.
226. Dazzi F, Szydlo RM, Cross NC, et al. Durability of responses following donor lymphocyte infusions for patients who relapse after allogeneic stem cell transplantation for chronic myeloid leukemia. *Blood*. 2000;96(8):2712-2716.
227. Frey NV, Porter DL. Graft-versus-host disease after donor leukocyte infusions: presentation and management. *Best Pract Res Clin Haematol*. 2008;21(2):205-222.
228. Maude SL, Frey N, Shaw PA, et al. Chimeric antigen receptor T cells for sustained remissions in leukemia. *N Engl J Med*. 2014;371(16):1507-1517.
229. Christopeit M, Kuss O, Finke J, et al. Second allograft for hematologic relapse of acute leukemia after first allogeneic stem-cell transplantation from related and unrelated donors: the role of donor change. *J Clin Oncol*. 2013;31(26):3259-3271.

Chapter 105 ■ Hematopoietic Cell Transplantation for Nonmalignant Disorders

MARK C. WALTERS • NAHAL ROSE LALEFAR

INTRODUCTION

Hematopoietic cell transplantation (HCT) has expanded over the past several decades with broader utilization in treating malignant and premalignant conditions such as acute leukemia and myelodysplastic syndrome (MDS), respectively.[1,2] A parallel expansion also has occurred in nonmalignant disorders such as hemoglobinopathies, primary immunodeficiency disorders (PIDs), inborn errors of metabolism, marrow failure syndromes, and other acquired and hereditary hematologic disorders, particularly among pediatric recipients.[3-6] Although supportive care for many of these conditions also has improved, long-term toxicity and morbidity of disease-modifying therapies (e.g., chronic blood transfusions and iron overload) can have a negative impact on the quality of life and can also contribute to a risk of early mortality.[7] Other newer therapies in sickle cell disease (SCD) have too short a period of follow-up to assess their long-term impact (voxelotor, crizanlumab, L-glutamine, and luspatercept).[8-10] Thus, HCT for nonmalignant disorders represents an alternative curative option for many patients who might otherwise succumb to complications of the underlying condition. More recently, the possibility of a curative outcome after gene therapy or genomic editing for several hereditary nonmalignant conditions has been suggested by results in recent clinical trials, which has the potential to widely broaden curative therapies for these disorders. In this chapter, we use representative hereditary hematologic diseases for which HCT is an option, to review outcomes in nonmalignant disorders after HCT and gene therapy, and outline the long-term effects of the therapy.

CONDITIONS SUITABLE FOR HEMATOPOIETIC CELL TRANSPLANTATION

A broad array of hereditary and acquired nonmalignant disorders derives from selected hematopoietic cell lineages, which by virtue of their origin in the hematopoietic stem cell (HSC), also are theoretically amenable to cure by successful allogeneic HCT. Rather than attempting to catalog all of these disorders, three broad categories have been selected to illustrate how and when to apply this therapeutic intervention.

The first of these are the PIDs, which classically are illustrated by the child with severe combined immunodeficiency syndrome (SCID) where there is absent B- and T-lymphocyte function. In these individuals, life-threatening infections occur in the first months of life and portend early mortality.[11] This category also includes hemophagocytic lymphohistiocytosis (HLH), which is a multisystemic inflammatory process that can either be inherited or acquired.

The next group of disorders is the hereditary bone marrow failure (BMF) syndromes, of which Fanconi anemia (FA) is a prototypic example. FA is caused by a heterogeneous collection of defects in genes that encode proteins involved in DNA repair.[12] This deficiency is associated with a variable phenotype that includes progressive aplastic anemia, musculoskeletal and other congenital defects, and cancer predisposition (particularly to MDS, acute myelogenous leukemia (AML), and carcinoma of the skin and oropharynx).[13] Although the hematologic manifestations of this condition are eliminated after successful HCT, donor selection, modulation of the conditioning regimen, and the possibility of malignant transformation in the marrow and after gene therapy together make this a challenging disease to treat by HCT.

Finally, the broad category of hemoglobin disorders is discussed. These disorders differ from the others because the immune and hematopoietic systems are intact before HCT, and a proliferative marrow develops as a consequence of chronic anemia and ineffective erythropoiesis. Thus, the conditioning regimen before HCT for the hemoglobin disorders typically requires a combination of ablative and immunosuppressive activities. In addition, there is a marked variability of clinical phenotype in SCD, which affects the decision-making about when and in whom to consider this aggressive therapy, particularly when there is a good response to disease modifying therapy.

Together, these broad examples of nonmalignant conditions illustrate the variety of clinical and genetic parameters one must consider in selecting appropriate transplantation candidates and regimens. These considerations are highlighted in the sections that follow.

HEMATOPOIETIC CELL TRANSPLANTATION FOR PRIMARY IMMUNODEFICIENCY DISORDERS

PIDs are classically associated with significant morbidity and early mortality caused by life-threatening infections in the first months and years of life. Before the availability of HCT, these infections invariably caused death in the vast majority of affected children. SCID is the most widely recognized manifestation of this group of disorders. SCID is a genetically heterogeneous group of more than 20 mutations in 13 genes identified to date that result in the common phenotype of impaired T-cell production and/or function. Some of the most common mutations are listed in *Table 105.1*. These mutations in target genes lead to impaired immunity as a consequence of absent T-cell function, but defects in B-cell and natural killer (NK) cell number or function often occur in parallel, as many of the genes affect all three lineages. However, the level of B- and NK-cell activity is highly variable.

Diagnosis of Primary Immunodeficiency Disorders

Newborn screening (NBS) and early referral to HCT are important to a successful outcome in SCID. An unbiased incidence of 1 in 58,000 births was established by population-based screening, which is higher than previous estimates.[14] NBS for T-cell receptor excision circles (TRECs) is performed in Guthrie card dried blood spots.[15-17] TRECs are circular DNA fragments formed upon rearrangement of the T-cell receptor genes during normal T-cell development. Very low TREC levels indicate T-lymphopenia. In addition, TRECs do not replicate during T-cell expansion and are thus a surrogate for the number of naive T-cells.[18] NBS program results compiled from 11 states showed that the most commonly affected SCID genes are interleukin-2 receptor common gamma chain (or X-SCID) (19%), RAG1 (15%), IL7 receptor (12%), and adenosine deaminase (ADA) (11%).[14] This contrasts with previous reports that almost 50% of SCID cases were X-SCID.

In a report from the Primary Immune Deficiency Treatment Consortium (PIDTC), retrospective data were analyzed from 240 infants with SCID and other PID from 25 transplant centers treated between 2000 and 2009.[19] The five-year survival was best if HCT was performed before 3.5 months of age (overall survival (OS), 94%), regardless of donor type (*Figure 105.1*). Survival was decreased in older infants who did not have a pre-HCT infection (90%) and also in those with an infection that resolved before HCT (82%). In contrast, survival decreased to 50% in infants older than 3.5 months who had an active infection during HCT, which highlights the importance of proceeding to HCT as soon as the diagnosis of SCID is established.[19] Among infants with an active infection who lacked a human leukocyte antigen identical (HLA-ID) sibling donor, survival was best among those who received a HLA-ID T-cell depleted HCT and no pretransplantation conditioning.

Table 105.1. Most Common Molecular Causes of SCID

Gene Defect	Defective Protein, Function, Features	Percentage of SCID[a] Cases	Lymphocyte Profile		
			T[b]	B	NK
IL2RG (X-linked)	Common γ-chain (γc) of receptors for IL-2, -4, -7, -9, -15, and -21	19 (only males)	–	+	–
ADA	Adenosine deaminase enzyme	9	–	–	–
IL7R	α-Chain of IL-7 receptor	11	–	+	+
JAK3	Janus kinase 3, activated by γc	5	–	+	–
RAG1, RAG2	Recombinase activating genes required for T- and B-cell antigen receptor gene rearrangement	15	–	–	+
DCLRE1C (Artemis)	Part of T- and B-cell antigen receptor gene rearrangement complex, also required for DNA repair	3	–	–	+
Currently unknown	Unknown defects, including SCID and congenital anomalies; SCID with multiple bowel atresias	~10	–/low	+/–	+/–

Abbreviations: –, indicates absent; +, indicates present; NK, natural killer; SCID, severe combined immunodeficiency.
Based on Kwan A, Abraham RS, Currier R, et al. Newborn screening for severe combined immunodeficiency in 11 screening programs in the United States. *JAMA*. 2014;312(7):729-738. Adapted from Puck JM. The case for newborn screening for severe combined immunodeficiency and related disorders. *Ann N Y Acad Sci*. 2011;1246(1):108-117. Copyright © 2011 New York Academy of Sciences. Reprinted by permission of John Wiley & Sons, Inc.
[a]Percentage of cases based upon data from 11 newborn screening programs in the United States.
[b]Some patients have substantial numbers of maternally derived T cells at the time of diagnosis; autologous T cells are shown.

Conditioning Regimens for Primary Immunodeficiency Disorders

The first transplant for SCID using an HLA-ID sibling bone marrow donor was performed in 1968 without pretransplant conditioning.[20] Unfortunately, most infants lack an HLA-ID sibling, and fatal graft-vs-host disease (GVHD) often occurred when donor/recipient pairs had a major HLA disparity. In animal models of SCID, it was determined that by using the technique of donor T-cell depletion, it was possible to eliminate GVHD after HLA-mismatched HCT if thorough T-cell depletion was accomplished.[21] However, even in the earliest clinical reports of HCT after T-cell depleted HLA-haploidentical HCT for SCID, B-cell engraftment was quite poor, and most patients required long-term immunoglobulin replacement after HCT.[19]

The patient's age, HLA donor matching, and the baseline immunologic function with regard to resistance to donor engraftment and the PID genotype all influence the selection of the conditioning regimen. Myeloablative conditioning [e.g., busulfan (BU)/cyclophosphamide (CY), BU/fludarabine + antithymocyte globulin (ATG), alemtuzumab, melphalan], reduced-intensity conditioning (e.g., fludarabine/ATG, moderate dose BU, treosulfan), and serotherapy alone (e.g., ATG, alemtuzumab) have been used.[22] Reduced intensity conditioning regimens are most appropriate in recipients with T-cell deficiency syndromes before unrelated donor (URD) HCT.[23-27] In addition, the selection of a preparative regimen will vary according to the level of baseline immune function. In an effort to optimize conditioning regimens, the European Society for Blood and Marrow Transplantation and European Society for Immunodeficiencies (EBMT/ESID) inborn errors working party created guidelines for six protocols, labeled A-F, which are recommended for the majority of immunodeficiency disorders shown in *Table 105.2*.[28]

Comparison of HLA-ID Sibling and Unrelated Donor HCT for PID

Patients with severe combined immunodeficiency disorder treated by HLA-ID sibling HCT do not require pre-HCT conditioning and experience 100% survival. In addition, donor B-cell functional recovery occurs in 40% to 50% of patients.[29] In the PIDTC study, most recipients received unmodified donor grafts and standard GVHD prophylaxis in URD and HLA-mismatched umbilical cord blood (UCB) donor transplantation. One hundred seventy-two patients (72%) had donor T-cell engraftment with or without donor B-cell recovery after transplant; infants who had graft rejection were treated by a second infusion of donor cells or a second transplant with conditioning.[19] At 2 years after HCT, HLA-ID sibling donor recipients were significantly more likely to have stopped intravenous immunoglobulin (IVIG) therapy and to have normal IgA levels than recipients of mismatched related or alternative donor HCT. Among children treated by HLA-mismatched related donor or other alternate donor HCT, those who received a reduced-intensity or myeloablative conditioning were more likely to have normal CD3+ T-cell levels, donor B-cell engraftment, and normal IgA levels without IVIG replacement therapy compared with those who received serotherapy alone or did not receive a conditioning regimen ($P = .005$).[19] Examples of donor and genotype related conditioning are shown in *Table 105.3*.

In a separate retrospective survey of transplant centers in North America, Europe, and Australia, HCT without conditioning before URD HCT ($n = 37$) was compared with HLA-ID sibling HCT ($n = 66$). Excellent donor T-cell engraftment was observed after URD HCT in the absence of conditioning therapy (92%), which was very similar to results after HLA-ID sibling HCT (97%).[30] However, the estimated five-year overall and event-free survival (EFS) probabilities were worse after URD HCT (71% and 60%, respectively) compared to HLA-ID sibling HCT (92% and 89%, respectively; $P < .01$ for both) (*Figure 105.2*). Poorer outcome was associated with a higher incidence of grade II to IV acute and chronic GVHD after URD (50% and 39%, respectively) compared with HLA-ID sibling HCT (22% and 5%, respectively) ($P < .01$ for both). Among survivors after HCT, there was no difference in T-cell reconstitution in the URD and HLA-ID sibling cohorts; however, B-cell reconstitution was more likely to occur after HLA-ID sibling HCT (72% vs 17%, $P < .001$).[30] URD recipients who received pre-HCT serotherapy (ATG or alemtuzumab) had a similar five-year OS probability (100%) to HLA-ID sib recipients (*Figure 105.3*). Thus, the negative outcome after URD HCT could be overcome by including serotherapy for GVHD prevention in the conditioning regimen.

Umbilical cord blood transplantation (UCBT) has a potential advantage over adult URDs because it is immediately available in infants at high-risk of infection. Fernandes et al compared results after HLA-mismatched related donor and UCBT.[31] There were 175 HLA-mismatched donor HCT recipients and 74 UCBT recipients who had SCID or Omenn syndrome. Most UCBT recipients received a myeloablative preparative regimen, whereas a larger fraction of the related donor recipients did not. UCBT recipients were more likely to have complete donor chimerism and faster lymphocyte recovery. T-cell engraftment was equivalent in the two groups, and immunoglobulin replacement was discontinued earlier after transplantation in the UCBT group. Although there was a significantly higher rate of chronic GVHD after UCBT, the five-year OS rates were equivalent. Other data suggest that B-cell engraftment may be better after UCBT.[32] Although

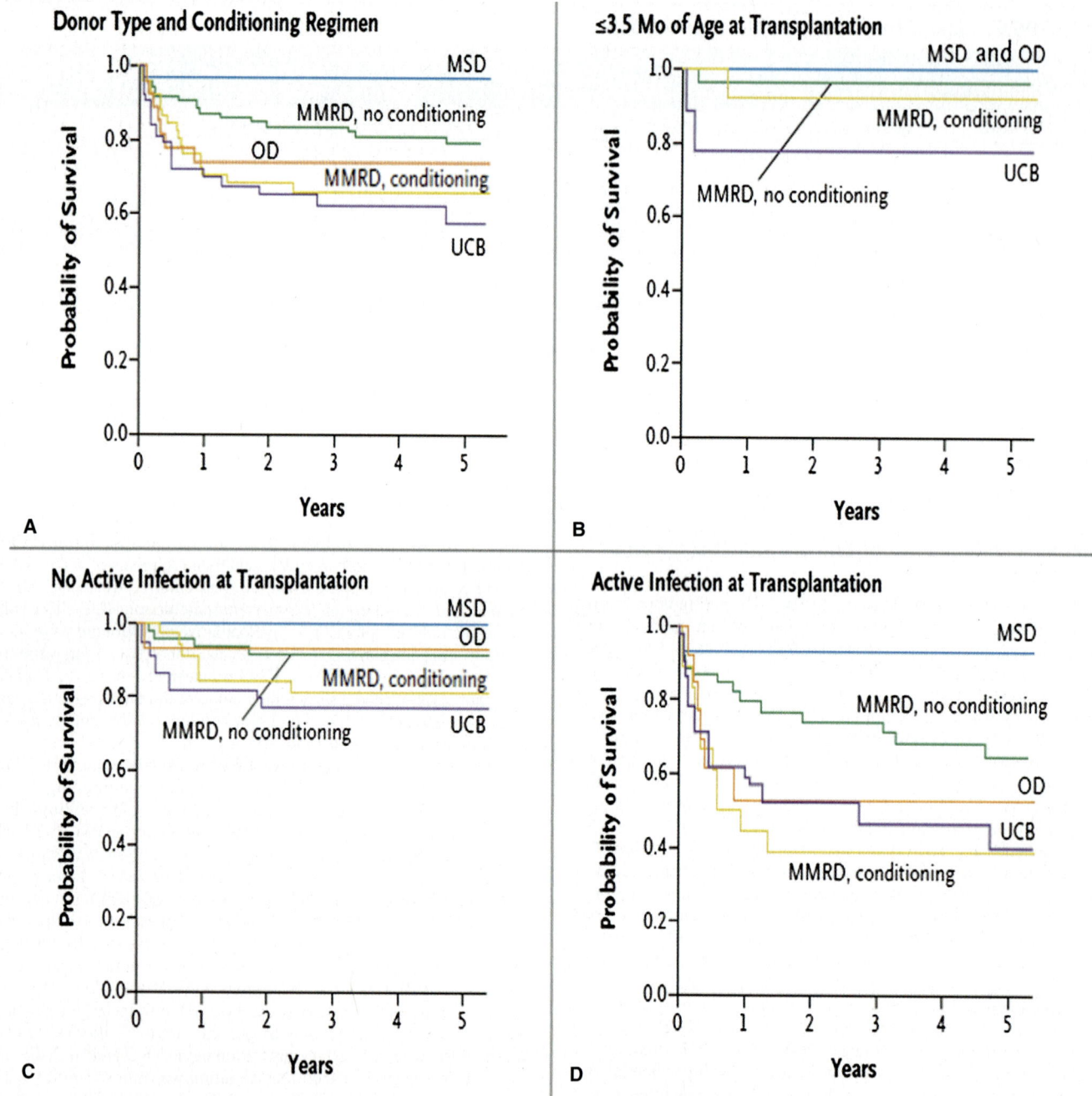

FIGURE 105.1 **Factors that affect survival after HCT for severe combined immunodeficiency syndrome.** Factors include donor type and conditioning regimen (A), age at the time of transplant (B), and infection status at the time of HCT (C and D). HCT, hematopoietic cell transplantation; MMRD, mismatched related donor; MSD, matched sibling donors; OD, unrelated donors; UCB, umbilical cord blood. (From Pai SY, Logan BR, Griffith LM, et al. Transplantation outcomes for severe combined immunodeficiency, 2000-2009. *N Engl J Med.* 2014;371(5):434-446. Copyright © 2014 Massachusetts Medical Society. Reprinted with permission from Massachusetts Medical Society.)

a randomized, prospective trial has not been performed, these data indicate that UCB appears to be a suitable alternative stem cell donor source for SCID.

HLA-Haploidentical HCT for PID

Long-term follow-up of the stability of donor T-cell engraftment after HLA-haploidentical HCT in the absence of a conditioning regimen showed mixed results. In a report by Buckley, 11 of 19 patients had normal T-cell function with no diminished T-cell repertoire diversity with follow-up extending through 25 years in some cases. However, most patients lacked donor B-cell engraftment and thus received long-term replacement immunoglobulin therapy.[11] In another series that included survivors with as many as 16 years follow-up, 35% of the patients had decreased TRECs and 27.5% of patients had a limited T-cell repertoire as evidenced by oligoclonality.[33] Based upon these observations, it has been suggested that the use of an ablative conditioning regimen before HCT may be required to ensure long-term T-cell engraftment in the setting of HLA-haploidentical donors. The EBMT/ESID group suggests that protocols A, B, C, or D (per *Table 105.2*) can be used with either ex vivo αβ+ T-cell and B-cell depletion or in vivo T-cell depletion by posttransplant CY in HLA-haploidentical HCT.[28]

Bertaina et al showed that a method of ex vivo αβ+ T-cell and B-cell depletion could promote recovery of adaptive immunity and protect from transplantation-related mortality (TRM) after HLA-haploidentical HCT for SCID.[34] Eight patients had SCID and received

Table 105.2. Chemotherapy Conditioning Regimens Before Allogeneic HCT for PID

Protocol	Days to HCT						
	−7	−6	−5	−4	−3	−2	−1
A							
Busulfan (AUC 85-95 mg/L × h)			x	x	x	x	
Fludarabine (4 × 40 mg/m²)			x	x	x	x	
B							
Treosulfan (3 × 10-14 g/m²)			x	x	x		
Fludarabine (5 × 30 mg/m²)		x	x	x	x	x	
Thiotepa (1 × 8 or 2 × 5 mg/kg)		x					
C							
Busulfan (AUC 60-70 mg/L × h)			x	x	x	(x)	
Fludarabine (5-6 × 30 mg/m²)	(x)	x	x	x	x	x	
D							
Treosulfan (3 × 10-14 g/m²)			x	x	x		
Fludarabine (5 × 30 mg/m²)		x	x	x	x	x	
E							
Melphalan (1 × 140 or 2 × 70 mg/m²)						x	
Fludarabine (5 × 30 mg/m²)		x	x	x	x	x	
F							
Cyclophosphamide (4 × 5 mg/kg)			x	x	x	x	
Fludarabine (5 × 30 mg/m²)		x	x	x	x	x	

Serotherapy is recommended in all alternative donor transplants and may be considered in HLA matched sibling HCT. HLA, human leukocyte antigen; HCT, hematopoietic cell transplantation.
Adapted from Lankester AC, Albert MH, Booth C, et al. EBMT/ESID inborn errors working party guidelines for hematopoietic stem cell transplantation for inborn errors of immunity. *Bone Marrow Transplantation.* 2021;56(9):2052-2062. https://creativecommons.org/licenses/by/4.0/

Table 105.3. Conditioning Regimen Protocols by SCID Genotype

	Conditioning Regimen Protocol	
SCID Subtypes	MSD/MRD	MUD/MMUD/MMFD
JAK3, IL2Rγ (TB⁺ NK⁻)	No conditioning	C/D
RAG1/2, DCLRE1C (TBNK⁺)	C/D	C/D
D IL7Rα, CD3 δ,ε,ζ, CD45 (T⁻, B⁺, NK⁺)	No conditioning/C/D	C/D
ADA	No conditioning/C/D	C/D
AK2	C/D	C/D

Refer to *Table 105.2* for descriptions of conditioning regimens "C" and "D". ADA, adenosine deaminase; MMFD: mismatched family donor; MMUD: mismatched unrelated donor; MRD: matched related donor, MSD: matched sibling donor; MUD: matched unrelated donor, SCID, severe combined immunodeficiency syndrome.
Adapted from Lankester AC, Albert MH, Booth C, et al. EBMT/ESID inborn errors working party guidelines for hematopoietic stem cell transplantation for inborn errors of immunity. *Bone Marrow Transplantation.* 2021;56(9):2052-2062. https://creativecommons.org/licenses/by/4.0/

treosulfan and fludarabine before HLA-haploidentical HCT after ex vivo elimination of αβ+ T-cells and CD19+ B-cells.[34] There was no additional GVHD prophylaxis. Four of 23 patients received a second allograft to treat graft failure, but all the other patients engrafted. There was limited acute GVHD (grade 1-2 skin GVHD) and no chronic GVHD. The cumulative incidence of TRM was 9.3%. With a median follow-up of 18 months, 21 of 23 children remained alive and disease-free, and the two-year probability of disease-free survival (DFS) was 91.1%. Recovery of γδ+ T-cells was prompt, with a longer time observed before recovery of αβ+ T-cells. Donor chimerism was 80% to 100%. Thus, the novel methodology of selective T-cell and B-cell depletion with a reduced intensity preparation before HCT appears very promising in HLA-mismatched HCT for PID.

B-Cell Recovery and Immune Reconstitution After HCT

In a compilation of 7 published studies, complete B-cell recovery was observed in 85% of patients when busulfan was administered before mismatched related donor HCT.[29] Recovery of B-cell function in the absence of B-cell engraftment occurs both in the absence or presence of a conditioning regimen, but it is much more likely to occur if there is donor B-cell engraftment (pooled odds ratio, 13.3; $P < .0001$). However, pretransplantation conditioning does not ensure B-cell functional recovery.[29]

Buckley et al showed that the most important determinant of B-cell function after HCT is the underlying molecular defect.[35] Overall,

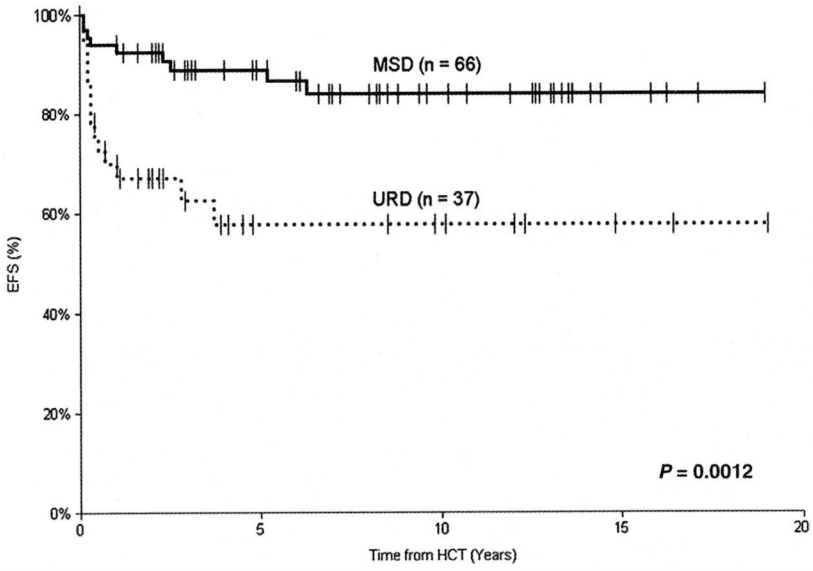

FIGURE 105.2 Event-free survival after HCT for severe combined immunodeficiency syndrome without conditioning in HLA-matched related and unrelated donors. Events were death and receiving a second HCT with conditioning therapy. EFS, event-free survival; HCT, hematopoietic cell transplantation; HLA, human leukocyte antigen; MSD, matched sibling donors; URD, unrelated donor. (Reprinted from Dvorak CC, Hassan A, Slatter MA, et al. Comparison of outcomes of hematopoietic stem cell transplantation without chemotherapy conditioning by using matched sibling and unrelated donors for treatment of severe combined immunodeficiency. *J Allergy Clin Immunol.* 2014;134(4):935.e15-943.e15. Copyright © 2014 American Academy of Allergy, Asthma & Immunology. With permission.)

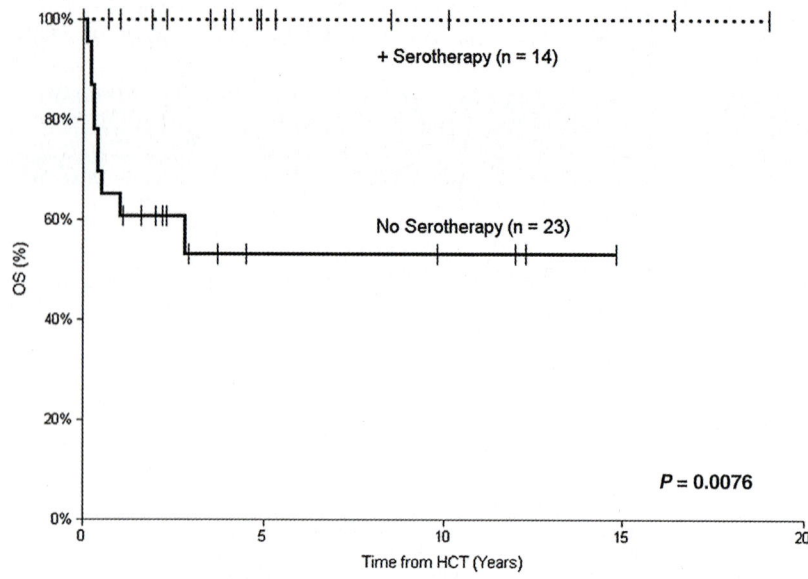

FIGURE 105.3 Overall survival after unrelated donor HCT for severe combined immunodeficiency syndrome with and without pre-HCT serotherapy for graft-vs-host-disease prophylaxis. HCT, hematopoietic cell transplantation; OS, overall survival. (Reprinted from Dvorak CC, Hassan A, Slatter MA, et al. Comparison of outcomes of hematopoietic stem cell transplantation without chemotherapy conditioning by using matched sibling and unrelated donors for treatment of severe combined immunodeficiency. *J Allergy Clin Immunol*. 2014;134(4):935.e15-943.e15. Copyright © 2014 American Academy of Allergy, Asthma & Immunology. With permission.)

donor B-cell engraftment occurred in 36 (29%) of 125 patients who received no pretransplantation chemotherapy. In selected PID genotypes such as the α chain of the IL-7 receptor (IL7Rα) deficiency, ADA deficiency and CD3 chain deficiency, host B-cells function normally, and myeloablative conditioning to ensure donor B-cell engraftment is not necessary. Only 1 of the 17 patients with IL7Rα deficiency, 6 of 18 patients with ADA deficiency, and none with CD3 chain–deficient SCID had donor B-cell engraftment. Nonetheless, residual host B-cells were for the most part, sufficient for normal B-cell function after HCT and 6% of patients with IL7Rα deficiency, 22% of patients with ADA-deficiency, and none with CD3-deficiency received IVIG posttransplant for hypogammaglobulinemia.

In contrast, donor B-cell engraftment after HCT is necessary for B-cell functional recovery after HCT in PID genotypes without endogenous host B-cell activity such as X-linked-SCID, Janus kinase 3 (Jak3)-deficiency and disorders with V-D-J recombination defects.[35] Sixty-two percent of X-linked SCID patients and 38% of Jak3-deficiency patients still received chronic IVIG therapy after HCT. In addition, patients with X-linked and Jak3-deficient SCID did not switch immunoglobulin isotype after immunization with bacteriophage ΦX174, in contrast to other genotypes immunized with this neoantigen.[29,35]

Late Effects and Future Directions in HCT for PID

There are limited series of HCT for SCID in which the follow-up period exceeds 10 years.[33,36] In several of these series, loss of T-cell diversity and autoimmune disorders was observed late after HCT, although follow-up through 25 years after HCT suggests expansion of the T-cell repertoire.[37] Patients with ADA deficiency have a high incidence of central nervous system abnormalities that include motor dysfunction, sensorineural hearing loss, and cognitive deficits that contribute to emotional and behavioral difficulties.[33] In addition, chronic infection by human papilloma virus has been reported.[33] It is unclear which, if any of these are related to pretransplant conditioning and GVHD prophylaxis or to the underlying genetic defect. Maternal T-cell engraftment and autologous autoreactive T-cells (described in Omenn syndrome) and SCID-related radiosensitivity (artemis and DNA protein kinase catalytic subunit defects) are unique comorbidities that must be accommodated in HCT for PID. If there is a DNA repair defect, standard myeloablative conditioning with alkylating agents can exert severe long-term toxicities such as growth failure.[22] In addition, information about BU pharmacokinetics in neonates and its long-term effects is not available.[29]

Finally, for those who lack an optimal donor, gene therapy may become an alternative therapy for some patients.[38] Recently, 50 patients with ADA deficiency (ADA-SCID) in the United States and United Kingdom were treated with autologous CD34+ hematopoietic stem and progenitor cells transduced ex vivo with a self-inactivating lentiviral vector encoding human ADA.[39] OS was 100% in all studies up to 24 and 36 months. EFS was greater than 95% up to 24 months for both countries. There was sustained ADA expression with functional immune reconstitution. In addition, there are ongoing gene therapy trials for X-linked SCID, chronic granulomatous disease (CGD), Wiskott-Aldrich syndrome, and leukocyte adhesion deficiency.[38]

HEMATOPOIETIC STEM CELL TRANSPLANTATION FOR HEMOPHAGOCYTIC LYMPHOHISTIOCYTOSIS

HLH is a multisystem inflammatory process caused by dysregulated activation of macrophages, histiocytes, and CD8+ T cells. HLH diagnostic criteria are shown in *Table 105.4*.[40-42] Primary HLH typically occurs in infants or younger children who have a history of familial inheritance or an identified genetic cause. Secondary HLH is more

Table 105.4. Diagnosis of HLH Can Be Made Established by Either A or B. HLH Criteria Adapted From HLH-2004[40]

A	Molecular/genetic diagnosis consistent with HLH such as: UNC13D (17q25), PRF1 (10q21-22), STXBP2 (19p13), STX11 (6q24), RAB271 (15q21), SH2D1A (Xq24-26), XIAP (Xq25)
	Or Five of the eight criteria below:
	Fever
	Splenomegaly
	Cytopenias (Affecting two of three Lineages in the Peripheral blood)
	Hemoglobin <90 g/L (Hemoglobin <100 g/L in Infants <4 wk)
	Platelets <100 × 10⁹/L
	Neutrophils <1.0 × 10⁹/L
	Hypertriglyceridemia or Hyperfibrinogenemia
	Fasting Triglycerides ≥3.0 mmol/L (i.e., ≥265 mg/dL)
	Fibrinogen <1.5 g/L
	Hemophagocytes in the bone Marrow Spleen or lymph Nodes in Absence of Malignancy
	Low or absent NK-Cell Activity
	Ferritin > 500 μg/L[a]
	Elevated Soluble CD25 (alpha-chain of sIL-2 Receptor) > 2400 U/mL[b]

Abbreviations: HLH, hemophagocytic lymphohistiocytosis; NK, natural killer.
Adapted from Henter JI, Horne A, Aricó M, et al. HLH-2004: Diagnostic and therapeutic guidelines for hemophagocytic lymphohistiocytosis. *Pediatr Blood Cancer*. 2007;48(2):124-131. Copyright © 2006 Wiley-Liss, Inc. Reprinted by permission of John Wiley & Sons, Inc.
[a]Ferritin levels above 10,000 μg/L appear to be specific and sensitive for HLH.[41]
[b]Two standard deviations above-age-adjusted, laboratory specific normal levels should be considered.[42]

often occurs in older children or adults without a known family history or genetic cause and is usually associated with a trigger such as Epstein-Barr virus (EBV) infection, malignancy, or rheumatologic disorder.

The Histiocyte Society HLH-94 protocol was developed to control T-cell proliferation and activation in order to induce remission. It specified eight-week induction course of combination etoposide-dexamethasone therapy. Those who had a hereditary cause, recurrent/refractory disease, CNS involvement, or persistent NK-cell dysfunction proceeded with continuation therapy followed by HCT as soon as possible pending identification of a donor.

Myeloablative HCT with BU, CY, and etoposide with or without ATG was previously considered standard for patients with HLH. However, this regimen was associated with high transplant–associated mortality.[42,43] In 124 patients who underwent HCT per HLH-1994 protocol, five-year survival rate was 66% ± 8%. Transplant outcomes were better in patients without active inflammatory marker elevation before HCT. Patients with familial disease had a five-year survival of 50% ± 13%; none survived without HCT.[44] The Center for International Blood and Marrow Transplant Research (CIBMTR) registry outcomes after URD HCT in the United States in 1989 to 2005 showed similar outcomes with five-year probability of OS rate of 53% in patients who received BU/CY/etoposide (compared with 24% in other regimens).[45] The early mortality rates were high (35% by day 100). The probabilities of grades 2 to 4 acute GVHD at day 100 and chronic GVHD at 5 years were 41% and 23%, respectively.

In the last 10 to 15 years, reduced intensity conditioning with fludarabine, melphalan and alemtuzumab has reduced TRM typical of myeloablative conditioning.[46-49] The improved survival there has been accompanied by loss of donor chimerism and primary graft failure. These complications can be managed by donor lymphocyte infusions or a second transplant. An initial approach to optimizing this regimen focused on the timing of alemtuzumab, distal (days -22 to -19) vs intermediate (days -14 to -10) vs proximal (days -9 to -5) dose schedules.[48] The intermediate timed conditioning showed better results with regard to mixed chimerism and acute GVHD compared with distal and proximal timing. There was no difference in OS between the different dose schedules.

The intermediate alemtuzumab approach was adopted in a multicenter phase 2 trial for the Blood and Marrow Transplant Clinical Trials Network (BMT-CTN 1204).[49] Transplant conditioning regimen included alemtuzumab days -14 through -10 (1 mg/kg subcutaneous with maximum cumulative dose 90 mg), fludarabine days 8 through 4 (30 mg/m^2/d or 5 mg/kg in patients weighing <10 kg), and melphalan on day 3 (140 mg/m^2 or 4.7 mg/kg in patients weighing <10 kg). GVHD prophylaxis was with cyclosporine (CSP) and prednisone. Thirty-four patients, ages 4 months-45 years, diagnosed with HLH and other primary immune deficiencies such as chronic active EBV disease, CGD, and immune dysregulation, polyendocrinopathy, enteropathy and X-linked syndrome were transplanted with HLA matched sibling or URDs (single mismatch HLA locus was acceptable). The one-year OS rate was 80.4%. However, at 1 year, the proportion of patients alive with sustained engraftment without donor lymphocyte infusions or a second HCT was only 39.1%. The incidence rates of acute grade II-IV GVHD and chronic GVHD were 17.4% and 26.7%, respectively. These results indicate that optimization with regard to mortality risk and sustained engraftment is needed in HLH and in similar disorders characterized by immune dysregulation.

HEMATOPOIETIC STEM CELL TRANSPLANTATION FOR BONE MARROW FAILURE: FANCONI ANEMIA

While FA is the most common hereditary cause of BMF, the application of HCT for marrow failure syndromes was pioneered in patients with acquired severe aplastic anemia (SAA). While the etiology of SAA is variable, and in many cases unknown, a therapeutic response to immunosuppressive therapy suggests that it is an autoimmune process often associated with an intercurrent infection.[50] Treatment of SAA has traditionally included immunosuppressive therapy with a combination of ATG and CSP,[51] or when there is a suitable donor, allogeneic HCT.[52] Allogeneic HCT relies on immunosuppressive condition therapy in lieu of myeloablation to overcome barriers to donor engraftment. The early allogeneic HCT experience was punctuated by difficulties with GVHD and graft rejection, and best results occurred after HLA-identical sibling HCT in patients who were <20 years of age and who were treated before administration of blood products.[53] More recent experience has shown similar results of HCT after HLA-ID and alternate donor HCT, with evidence to suggest that HLA-ID or well-matched URD HCT is a suitable front-line treatment for younger patients with SAA.[54] This advance followed optimization of a conditioning regimen that utilizes a combination of CY and fludarabine with low-dose total body irradiation (TBI) that is sufficient for engraftment yet spares most recipients from severe GVHD. These advances in patient outcomes after HCT for SAA have been mirrored in FA.

The genetic defects responsible for FA have been characterized in complementation groups, termed *FANC* genes, which are autosomal and recessive except FANCB (X-linked) and FANCR, which encodes RAD51 (autosomal dominant).[55,56] These gene products participate in a signal transduction pathway involved in DNA repair, called the FA/BRCA pathway (*Figure 105.4*).[57] The most common mutations occur in *FANCA, FANCC, FANCG*, and *FANCD2* genes.

Progressive marrow aplasia that causes cytopenias typically occurs in the first or second decade of life. Erythrocyte macrocytosis and elevated fetal hemoglobin (HbF) often are present. In some cases, the diagnosis of FA may not be established until after the patient has developed MDS or AML. Some patients never develop pancytopenia but do experience an increased risk of malignancy. Based upon the 15-year cohort follow-up of 163 FA patients at the National Cancer Institute, the cumulative incidence of severe BMF in FA has a peak hazard rate of 4% at ages 12 to 15 and the incidence of HCT for severe BMF or death without malignancy levels off at 70% by age 50 (*Figure 105.5A*).[58] The cumulative incidence of developing MDS is 50% by 50 years of age with a leukemia incidence of 5% by age 30 (*Figure 105.5B*). The median OS in this FA cohort is 39 years (*Figure 105.5C*).

The most common causes of death in FA are aplastic anemia and malignancy. Because of shortened survival, HCT was developed as a therapeutic measure to restore normal hematopoiesis and reduce or eliminate the risk of hematologic malignancy. There were several important observations generated in the early clinical trials. The first was that high-dose alkylating chemotherapeutic drugs at doses administered for severe aplastic anemia and gamma irradiation caused severe toxicity including mucositis and hemorrhagic cystitis as a consequence of the sensitivity to DNA damage in all tissues.[59,60] Second, the risk of acute GVHD was increased in comparison to other indications for HCT, presumably also as a consequence of impaired DNA repair and an extended duration of tissue injury eliciting an allogeneic reaction by donor T-cells.[61] The initial reports by Gluckman and her colleagues in 1984 showed that a reduced-dose regimen of CY 20 to 40 mg/kg and a single fraction of TBI or thoracoabdominal irradiation (400-450 cGy) effectively modulated the toxicity and was sufficient to ensure engraftment after HLA-ID sibling bone marrow transplantation with a long-term survival rate of 58.5%, although the rates of acute (55%) and chronic (70%) GVHD were quite elevated.[62] However, experience with this regimen in 35 patients was updated in 2007, and included ATG in the conditioning regimen.[63] These results showed a probability of survival of 89% at 10 years, with the incidence of acute and chronic GVHD at 23% and 12%, respectively.

HCT Conditioning Regimens for FA

Several notable improvements have occurred in the 3 decades since the initial results of HCT for FA were reported. Fludarabine-containing conditioning regimens with T-cell depleted marrow grafts have been established as a standard in HCT for FA. This approach reduces exposure to DNA cross-linking agents such as CY or irradiation, and thereby reduces the risk of GVHD.[64] It also effectively reduces the

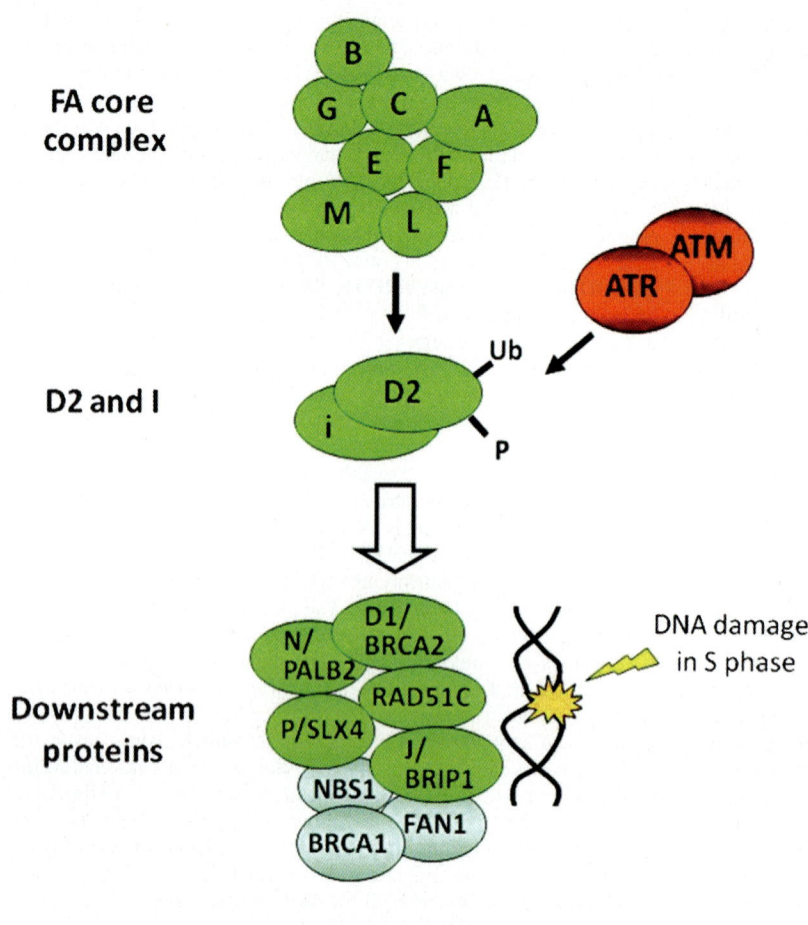

FIGURE 105.4 Fanconi anemia: FA/BRCA pathway. (Used with permission of American Society of Hematology from Soulier J. Fanconi anemia. *Hematol Am Soc Hematol Educ Program.* 2011;2011:492-497; permission conveyed through Copyright Clearance Center, Inc.)

rate of graft rejection, in particular after alternate donor HCT, without contributing significantly to toxicity.[65,66] A benefit after T-cell depletion of donor marrow has been observed after HLA-ID sibling and after unrelated HCT.[65,67,68] In the retrospective analysis noted above, the incidence of acute GVHD decreased from 71% to 21% in the T-cell depleted group and was decreased further to 16% if fludarabine and T-cell depletion were utilized together.

Radiation-containing HCT regimens for FA were associated with a significantly lower 10-year OS compared with nonradiation regimens (76% vs 91%, respectively; P = .005).[69] Investigators in Brazil observed that CY as a single agent (60 mg/kg) generated an overall five-year survival rate of 85% in 85 FA patients. Acute grade II-III and chronic GVHD rates were 21% and 29% of the evaluable patients, respectively, after HLA-ID sibling transplantation.[70,71] Patients <10 years of age had an OS rate of 95.6%. The major causes of death were related to GVHD/infections and graft rejection. Thus, in patients younger than age 10 who have an HLA-ID sibling donor and who have not yet progressed to MDS or AML, the results of the reduced intensity conditioning regimens are excellent.[72] Other risks factors for decreased survival include administration of androgens before HCT, cytomegalovirus (CMV) seropositivity in donor and/or recipient, and >20 blood product transfusions.[73] Examples of HCT regimens are shown in *Figure 105.6.*

Alternative Donor HCT for FA

The application of alternative donor HCT to FA is vital to expanding this treatment modality, as most individuals with FA lack an unaffected matched sibling donor. Initial trials of URD HCT in which the same regimen of low-dose CY and irradiation was used were characterized by high rates of graft rejection, organ toxicity, and GVHD, with OS in the 30% to 40% range.[74,75] The escalation of the dose of radiation to 600 cGy and the addition of ATG did little to improve OS.[76] However, in a retrospective analysis of the effect of fludarabine in the conditioning regimen, a significant impact was noted.[77] The probability of neutrophil and platelet recovery after HCT improved from 69% to 89% and from 23% to 74%, respectively, and this translated into a lower TRM (47% compared to 81%). The three-year OS rate was 52% in those who received a fludarabine-containing regimen compared to 13% in those who did not (*Figure 105.7*).

In the largest single-center experience of alternative donor HCT, 130 FA patients (ages 1-48) underwent alternative donor HCT between 1995 and 2012 at the University of Minnesota. Initially, patients received a combination of TBI (>450 cGy), CY (40 mg/kg), and horse ATG (150 mg/kg).[64] The conditioning regimen evolved over this era in an effort to improve results: fludarabine was added to the regimen, TBI dose was reduced to 300 cGy, thymic shielding during TBI was employed to minimize thymic damage and improve immune reconstitution after HCT, and mycophenolate mofetil (MMF) in lieu of methylprednisolone for GVHD prophylaxis were instituted. T-cell depletion was also instituted and ATG was eliminated to reduce the risk of post–transplant lymphoproliferative disorder. The five-year survival rate was 94%. The incidence of grades 2 to 4 acute and chronic GVHD was 20% and 10%, respectively. Two of 10 patients with advanced MDS or acute leukemia relapsed after transplant.

In a multi-institutional study designed to optimize outcomes of alternative donor HCT in patients with FA, BU was incorporated in lieu of TBI to reduce the risk of secondary solid tumors. Forty-five patients (11 of whom had MDS) received a preparative regimen of 4 doses of intravenous BU 0.8 to 1.0 mg/kg/dose (first 25 patients) and 0.6 to 0.8 mg/kg/dose (next 20 patients), CY, fludarabine, and rabbit

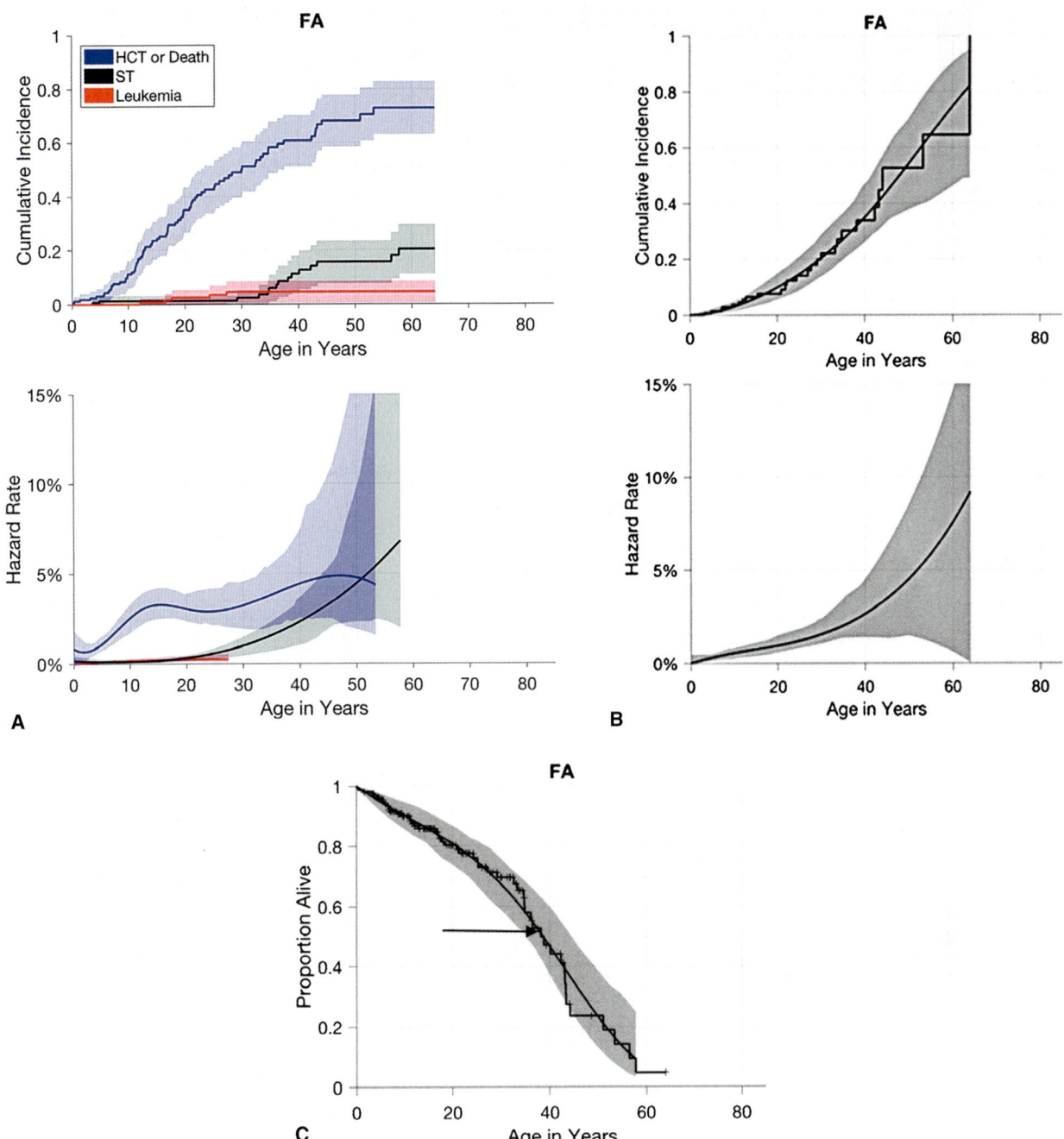

FIGURE 105.5 **Outcomes in Fanconi anemia.** A, Cumulative incidence and annual hazard rate of severe bone marrow failure leading to HCT or death (blue), acute leukemia (red), or solid tumors (/ST, black). B, Cumulative incidence and annual hazard rate of myelodysplastic syndrome by age in patients with Fanconi Anemia. C, Probability of survival in Fanconi anemia. Observed survival (stair-step lines) and smoothed survival (smooth curves) are shown. HCT, hematopoietic cell transplantation. (Reprinted with permission from Alter BP, Giri N, Savage SA, et al. Cancer in the National Cancer Institute inherited bone marrow failure syndrome cohort after fifteen years of follow-up. *Haematologica*. 2018;103(1):30-39. Copyright © 2018 Ferrata Storti Foundation.)

ATG. T-cell depletion was accomplished by CliniMacs CD34+ selection (Miltenyi). One-year probabilities of overall and DFS were 79.2% and 76.7%, respectively. Among patients <10 years of age, the EFS rate was 90%.[78]

In parallel, UCB was also tested in FA as a source of HSCs because it naturally contains fewer T-cells and is associated with a lower risk of GVHD after HCT. Of note, the first successful report of UCBT in 1989 was conducted in a patient with FA and who survives free of disease more than 20 years later.[79] A retrospective review of 93 cases of FA treated by URD UCBT showed acute and chronic GVHD rates of 32.5% and 16%, respectively, confirming a benefit.[80] Unfortunately, this benefit was balanced by high rate of graft rejection, with an OS rate of 40%. For this reason, the selection of UCB as a source for HCT is generally assigned a lower priority in patients with FA.[81]

HLA-Haploidentical HCT for FA

Many patients with FA will lack a well-matched related donor or URD. In these individuals, HLA-haploidentical HCT represents the only path to HCT. HLA-haploidentical HCT was investigated in 30 patients with FA. Posttransplant CY was administered (total dose, 50 mg/kg) on days 3 and 4 after transplant to accomplish in vivo T-cell depletion. A regimen of fludarabine 150 mg/m², 200 to 300 cGy TBI with or without CY 10 mg/kg, and with and without

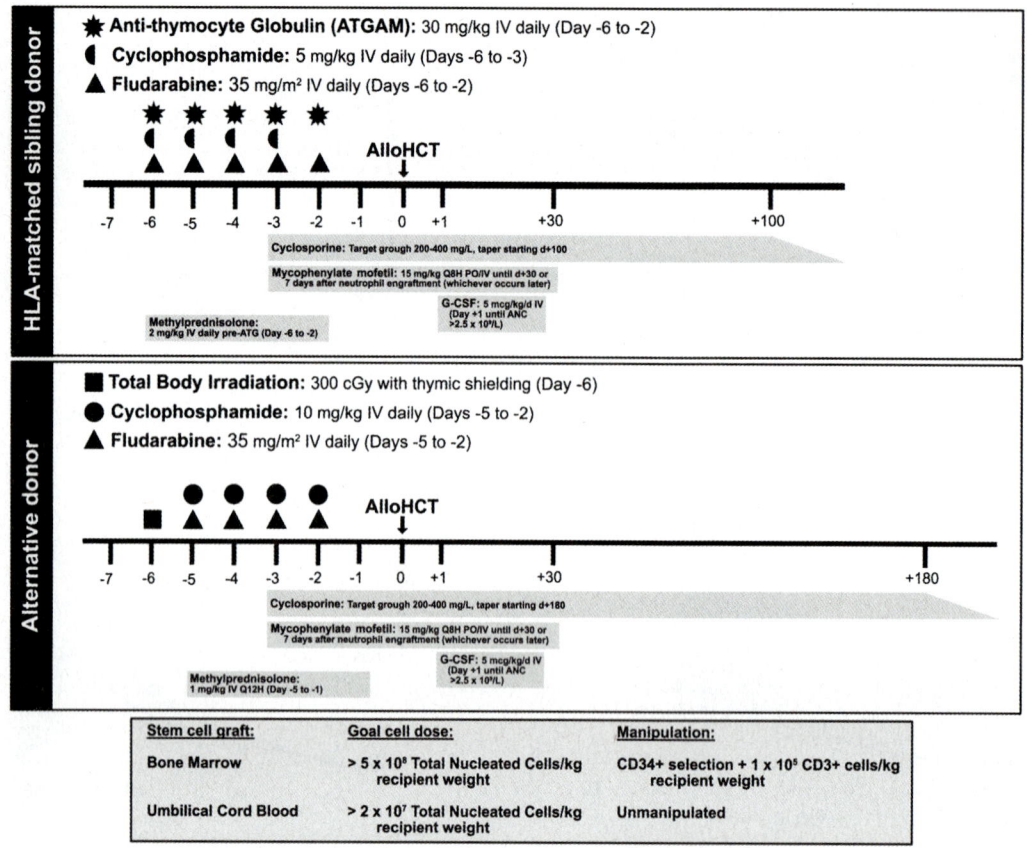

FIGURE 105.6 Conditioning regimens for HLA-matched sibling donor and alternative donor HCT for Fanconi anemia. HCT, hematopoietic cell transplantation; HLA human leukocyte antigen (From Ebens CL, MacMillan ML, Wagner JE. Hematopoietic cell transplantation in Fanconi anemia: current evidence, challenges and recommendations. *Expert Rev Hematol*. 2017;10(1):81-97. Reprinted by permission of Taylor & Francis Ltd. http://www.tandfonline.com)

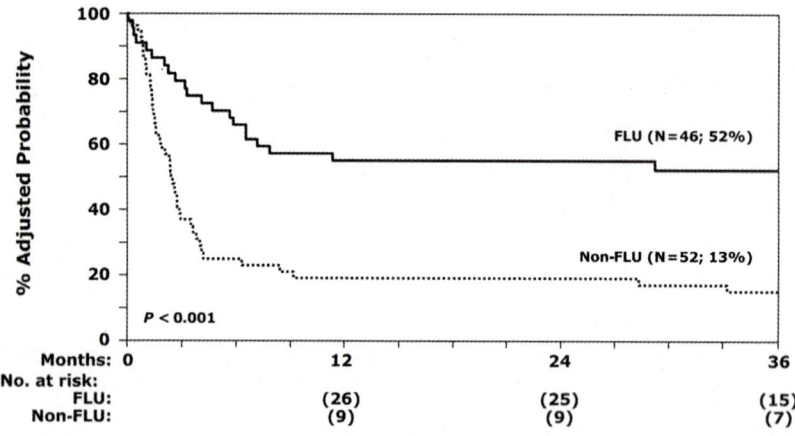

FIGURE 105.7 Effect of fludarabine in the preparative regimen after HCT for Fanconi anemia. Probability of overall survival is adjusted for pre–transplant red blood cell transfusion exposures and CMV serostatus. CMV, cytomegalovirus; HCT, hematopoietic cell transplantation. (Reprinted from Wagner JE, Eapen M, MacMillan ML, et al. Unrelated donor bone marrow transplantation for the treatment of Fanconi anemia. *Blood*. 2007;109(5):2256-2262. Copyright © 2007 American Society of Hematology. With permission.)

rabbit antithymocyte globulin (r-ATG) ($n = 14$) was investigated. In addition, patients received CSP and MMF to prevent GVHD. There was a high rate of hemorrhagic cystitis (50%) and CMV reactivation (75%) after haploidentical HCT. The one-year OS rate was 73% (95% CI, 64%-81%), and all surviving patients had full donor chimerism.[82,83] This regimen was also used to successfully rescue four patients who experienced primary or secondary graft failure after related or URD transplantation.

A similar experience was published in a smaller series of six patients treated by HLA-haploidentical HCT. Patients received CY (5 mg/kg) fludarabine (150 mg/m^2) and 200 cGy TBI before HCT. Posttransplantation CY was administered (25 mg/kg/d) as above. No r-ATG was given. Four patients survived free of FA, but two patients who had significant pretransplant comorbidities died of sepsis and one surviving patient developed severe acute GVHD.[84]

An Italian study reported a five-year OS, event-free survival, and DFS rates of 100% and 86%, respectively, of 24 pediatric and young adult FA patients who underwent HLA-haploidentical T-cell receptor αβ (TCRαβ+) and CD19$^+$ cell-depleted HCT from a haploidentical related donor.[85] The preparative regimen included fludarabine 120 mg/m^2, CY 1200 mg/m^2, single dose of TBI 200 cGy, and r-ATG. Sustained engraftment was achieved in 91% of the patients. The cumulative incidence of grade I to II acute and chronic GVHD was 17.4% and 5.5%, respectively.[85,86] Together, these results suggest that HLA-haploidentical HCT is a suitable option in selected patients with progressive marrow failure and FA.

FA and Myelodysplastic Syndrome/Leukemia

FA that progresses to MDS or acute leukemia is challenging to treat successfully because of an increased risk of relapse after HCT. Low-dose CY/fludarabine in the conditioning regimen alone may not be sufficiently intense to ablate residual host cells that can cause relapse. In a retrospective review of 21 FA patients with acute leukemia or advanced MDS treated at the University of Minnesota between 2008 and 2011, the five-year OS rate was 33% after HCT with a relapse rate of 24%.[87] The optimal intensity of pretransplant cytoreduction in FA patients with advanced MDS or leukemia is uncertain. Most patient series have applied modified dose CY in combination with TBI or BU. Patients with biallelic BRCA2/FAND1 mutations tend to develop MDS, AML, and/or solid tumors (such as Wilms tumor or medulloblastoma) very early in life and these patients in particular might benefit from a more aggressive conditioning regimen.[88]

Younger age at the time of HLA-ID HCT was associated with superior five-year OS (≤ vs > 14 years: 78% vs 34% respectively; $P < .001$) in a CIBMTR analysis of 113 FA patients with cytogenetic abnormalities, MDS or acute leukemia. Patients who had cytogenetic abnormalities but not MDS/leukemia also had an increased five-year OS compared with those with MDS/leukemia (67% vs 43%).[89] Having MDS had an adverse impact on survival, with an estimated five-year survival rate of 9%, compared with 92% for patients who had not developed MDS. Although patients with cytogenetic abnormalities, MDS, or acute leukemia may require more intensive preparative conditioning, this study did not show better outcomes following the use of radiation therapy or fludarabine.

Gene Therapy for FA

The phenomenon of spontaneous regression of the FA phenotype after reversion of the causative mutation in hematopoietic cells provides a rationale that gene therapy might exert a strong benefit on marrow aplasia.[67,90] The successful transfer and expression of a replacement gene has the potential to restore the proliferative potential and promote expansion of corrected HSCs. There are three gene therapy trials with nine patients that have been reported, all using lentiviral vectors carrying the FANCA gene. After collection, CD34+ hematopoietic cells were transduced with a lentiviral vector encoding the FANCA gene, and then infused back into the patients without any conditioning.[91-93] The mean age ranged from 5.85 to 16 years, and all but two had hematopoietic stem progenitor cells (HSPCs) collected by peripheral mobilization with granulocyte-colony stimulating factor alone or with plerixafor. In seven patients, no cytogenetic abnormalities were noted at 2 years follow-up, suggesting that there was no short-term risk of myeloid malignancy. However, clinical responses were transitory and gene marking assessments at 24 months in four patients showed 4% to 43.5% lentiviral vector positive cells in the marrow (reviewed in[94]). In a recent update of the trial by Rio et al, no serious adverse events were observed after up to 30 months follow-up, and three patients showed trends of stable neutrophil and hemoglobin levels at 6 months postinfusion.[91]

The isolation and manipulation of a sufficient quantity of true HSCs that can be efficiently transduced and subsequently expanded after reinfusion in the absence of chemotherapy or other selection of the transduced cells is the central challenge of gene therapy for FA. Recent observations that CRISPR-Cas9–induced double-stranded DNA breaks require rad51 and other FA pathway gene products to accomplish homology-directed repair (HDR) suggests that gene editing strategies also will have to take these constraints into account. The observations that correction of FANCD1, FANCC, and FANCI mutations in HSCs requires drug selection to expand rare gene editing events underlie this challenge.[95] Thus, it is unlikely that gene editing by CRISPR reagents that relies upon HDR will be sufficiently efficient for a clinical effect.

However, non–homologous end-joining occurs more frequently than HDR in FA HSCs, and naturally occurring somatic mosaic reversions in FANCA patients have been reported near a premature stop codon.[96] While most cases of mosaicism affect the T-cell lineage,[67] some patients have compensatory mutational events in the HSC that move the hematopoietic phenotype away from marrow failure. CRISPR/Cas9 ribonucleoprotein complex targeting a stop codon in the FANCA gene and frame-shift mutations in FANCB, FANCC, FANCD1, and FANCD2 was successfully accomplished in a small fraction of HSCs that expanded over several weeks in ex vivo culture indicating spontaneous expansion of the functionally restored HSCs. Corrected cells displayed increased protein levels and resistance to DNA-crosslinking agents.[97] Thus, the possibility of utilizing safe, efficient CRISPR reagents to correct selected frameshift or stop codon mutations in FA genes in autologous cells might represent a future strategy to expand a curative therapy for this disease.

Late Effects After HCT for FA

The most important late complication after HCT for FA is the development of cancer.[98,99] The most common forms of malignancies include squamous cell carcinomas of the head and neck, carcinoma of the esophagus, and gynecologic squamous cell carcinoma. Three percent of patients developed squamous cell carcinoma 9.4 to 13.3 years after HCT in one series.[69] The risk is increased fourfold and occurs earlier in those who undergo HCT compared to those who do not, and the cumulative incidence of a secondary cancer is 40% during the 15 to 20 years after HCT.[58,100] In addition, chronic GVHD is a key risk factor in developing a secondary cancer.[75,101,102]

While radiation exposure in the conditioning regimen may increase cancer risk, GVHD is also associated with cancer after HCT. Regardless, the risk of solid tumor is increased irrespective of transplant status. Therefore, cancer surveillance remains a high priority post-HCT with routine head and neck examinations by otolaryngology for leukoplakia or squamous cell carcinoma of the oral cavity/oropharynx. In addition, annual gynecologic examinations for females >16 years of age should be performed. Vaccination against HPV should be offered to FA patients after HCT.

Endocrinopathies also have been described after HCT. In a cohort of 44 patients with FA treated at the University of Minnesota, 86% had at least 1 endocrinopathy, and 11% had 3 or more.[103] Conditions included hypothyroidism, hypogonadism, short stature, dyslipidemia, insulin resistance, abnormalities in body composition, and bone health. Vitamin D deficiency (71%) and hypothyroidism (57%) were the most common endocrinopathies. Short stature was associated with younger age at HCT and gonadal failure was associated with older age at HCT.

In another retrospective analysis of 22 patients with FA and aplastic anemia, MDS, or AML who received either a TBI or BU-based regimen followed by T-cell–depleted transplants from alternative donors, persistent hemochromatosis, hypothyroidism, insulin resistance, and hypertriglyceridemia were noted posttransplant.[104]

HEMATOPOIETIC CELL TRANSPLANTATION FOR HEMOGLOBIN DISORDERS

With the institution of universal NBS programs in the United States and elsewhere, it is possible to identify patients with hemoglobin disorders shortly after birth and to institute comprehensive preventive care.[105] Together, thalassemia and SCD account for the most common hereditary disorders worldwide with broad distribution in regions of the world where malaria is endemic. The first case report of successful HCT for thalassemia occurred 40 years ago and has been followed by several thousand children with thalassemia who have been treated successfully.[106,107] The first reports of successful transplantation for SCD occurred somewhat later, and because of the variable clinical course many children experience, fewer individuals with SCD have been treated by HCT.[108,109] Nonetheless, outcomes after HLA-ID sibling donor bone marrow transplantation for the hemoglobin disorders are generally very good. The broader application of HCT is limited by its risks, which must be balanced by complications inherent to the underlying disease, for which significant progress in supportive care has occurred. The most common conditioning regimen used in hemoglobin disorders is a myeloablative combination BU, CY, and ATG, which is the same regimen pioneered in other non–malignant hematological disorders.[110,111]

HEMATOPOIETIC STEM CELL TRANSPLANTATION FOR THALASSEMIA

Pioneering studies for HCT in patients with thalassemia that span several decades were performed by the transplant team in Pesaro and later Rome, led by Lucarelli.[107] Using a backbone combination of BU and CY before transplantation and a standard combination of methotrexate and CSP to prevent GVHD, the majority of children were cured after an HLA-ID sibling bone marrow transplantation. Since these early reports, several thousand individuals with thalassemia major have received HCT, with most reports focused on results in children and young adults.[112,113] The likelihood of cure was highest in those recipients who had good-risk features, defined as having no hepatomegaly, no evidence of portal fibrosis by liver biopsy, and by having adhered to a regular program of iron chelation therapy. Alternatively, children who had one (risk class 2) and two or more prognostic features (risk class 3) fared worse. Class 3 patients who experienced a thalassemia-free survival probability of 50% and 30% had graft rejection with thalassemia recurrence.[114] Among 1493 consecutive transplant registry thalassemia major cases reported to the European Blood and Marrow Transplant Hemoglobinopathy database between 2000 and 2010, the two-year OS and EFS rates were 88% and 81%, respectively (*Figure 105*.8).[112] However, among children <2 years of age who received an HLA-ID sibling allograft, the OS and EFS rates at 2 years was 95% and 93%, respectively. Conversely, recipients >18 years of age had OS and EFS rates of 80% and 76%, respectively. Results after HLA-ID sibling UCB transplantation are very similar, with lower rates of acute and chronic GVHD after UCB compared to marrow transplantation.[115] A CIBMTR retrospective review of 1110 patients with β-thalassemia who received HLA-matched related, HLA-matched unrelated, and HLA-mismatched myeloablative transplants between 2000 and 2016 showed similar findings.[116] The five-year probabilities of OS for patients aged <6 years, 7 to 15 years, and 16 to 25 years, adjusted for donor type and conditioning regimen, were 90%, 84%, and 63%, respectively. The corresponding probabilities for EFS were 86%, 80%, and 63%, respectively. OS and EFS survival did not differ between HLA-matched related and HLA-matched URD transplantation. Thus, most clinicians agree that HCT for thalassemia should be considered in young patients with favorable risk profiles who have an HLA-ID sibling donor.[110]

Initially, attempts to reduce the toxicity of HCT in patients with high-risk features focused on modifications of the BU/CY backbone. In particular, it was possible to reduce the incidence of regimen-related toxicity by reducing the dose of CY. Unfortunately, this was accompanied by a higher incidence of graft rejection, so that the overall thalassemia-free survival rate did not improve after modifying the CY dose.[117] In response, a greater emphasis was placed on the role of immunosuppressive therapy before transplantation as a strategy

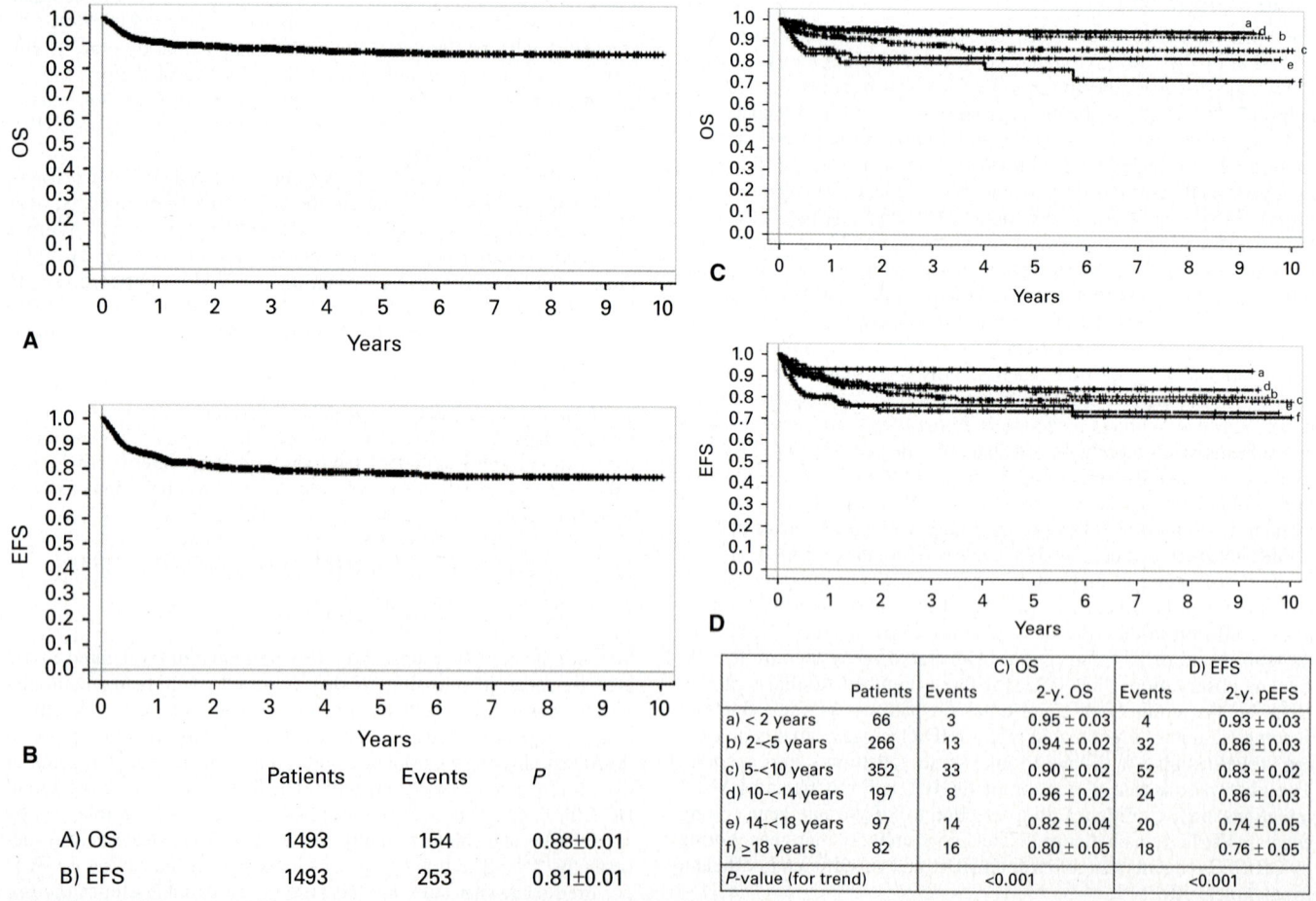

FIGURE 105.8 Overall survival (OS) (A) and event-free survival (EFS) (B) after human leukocyte antigen–identical sibling donor hematopoietic cell transplantation in 1493 patients with thalassemia major treated between 2000 and 2010. OS (C) and EFS (D) are shown by age group. (Reprinted by permission from Nature: Baronciani D, Angelucci E, Potschger U, et al. Hemopoietic stem cell transplantation in thalassemia: a report from the European Society for Blood and Bone Marrow Transplantation Hemoglobinopathy Registry, 2000-2010. *Bone Marrow Transplant*. 2016;51(4):536-541. Copyright © 2016 Springer Nature.)

for reducing graft rejection. Thus, Protocol 26 was established, which employed a combination of hydroxyurea, azathioprine, and hypertransfusion, with intensive iron chelation therapy that was commenced 6 weeks before transplantation to modulate the proliferative erythron and induce an immunosuppressive effect.[118] This was followed by a backbone of BU/CY with CY dosing that ranged from 120 to 160 mg/kg. This combination of changes resulted in a substantially improved outcome with an event-free probability of 85% and rejection incidence of 8% in class 3 recipients. However, the use of the BU/CY conditioning backbone was associated with a far inferior outcome in the high-risk category of patients older than 7 years who had hepatomegaly, where the thalassemia-free survival probability was 50%. This observation strengthened the conclusion that high-risk patients require a modified conditioning regimen for reasons of safety and efficacy. Protocol 26 was modified to include fludarabine 150 mg/m^2 and thiotepa. The problem of graft failure/rejection was eliminated by the modified protocol with no rejections observed and a five-year thalassemia-free survival rate of 92% compared to 73% with the previous regimen ($P = .047$) (*Figure 105.9*).[119] Both groups had similar rates of grades II to IV acute GVHD. These experiences suggest that risk category alone should not negatively impact the decision about whether or not to proceed to transplant when there is an HLA-ID sibling donor.

More recently, busulfan-fludarabine (BU-FLU) and treosulfan-fludarabine (TREO-FLU)–based regimens have been studied in an effort to reduce toxicity. In a retrospective review of 772 patients who underwent HCT for thalassemia major between 2010 and 2018, reported to the EBMT, the two-year OS rate was 92.7% after BU-FLU–based conditioning (median age 8.6 years) and 94.7% after TREO-FLU–based conditioning (median age 5.7 years) with low rates of severe GVHD and treatment-related mortality.[120] The two-year incidence of a second HCT was 4.6% in the BU-FLU group vs 9% in the TREO-FLU group.

Alternative Donor HCT for Thalassemia

As most individuals with thalassemia major lack a sibling donor, the development of URD transplantation and alternative donors has been pursued to broaden the availability of HCT. An early report from the Pesaro team showed that the use of HLA-mismatched related donors was associated with an inferior outcome, and in particular, a high rate of graft rejection.[121] Thus, it became apparent that additional modification of the conditioning regimen would be needed to ensure engraftment across a major histocompatibility complex barrier and that selecting donors with optimal HLA matching also was necessary. Several studies have shown similar EFS and OS after HCT with well-matched related donor and URD, with and without reduced toxicity regimens.[116,120,122-124] (*Table 105.5*). The addition of newer agents such as abatacept for GVHD prophylaxis has improved thalassemia-free survival.[125] Thus, incremental progress in URD transplantation shows the potential for outcomes that appear indistinguishable from those after HLA-ID sibling HCT.

HEMATOPOIETIC STEM CELL TRANSPLANTATION FOR SICKLE CELL DISEASE

The application of HCT for SCD has developed more slowly than in thalassemia, in part due to the heterogeneous phenotype of sickling syndromes and also from a lack of suitable donors. However, several clinical trials were conducted in the mid- to late-1990s in the United States and Europe and demonstrated very similar outcomes.[126-128] The aim of these early studies was to identify children who were at risk for early mortality or extensive morbidity from SCD, but to treat by HCT before organ damage had occurred that might increase the risk of transplant-related complications. Thus, patients were deemed eligible if they had a stroke and were receiving regular red blood cell (RBC) transfusion therapy to prevent another stroke, if they had recurrent painful episodes, or if there were recurrent episodes of acute chest syndrome. The current eligibility criteria are shown in *Table 105.6*.

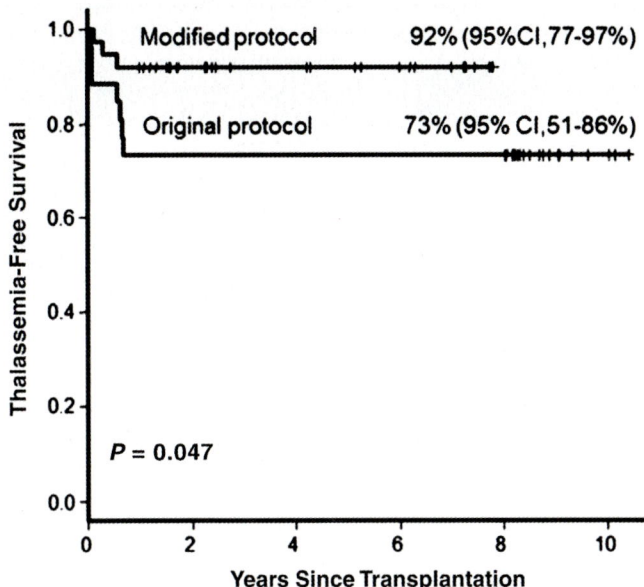

FIGURE 105.9 Cumulative incidence of graft failure/rejection in patients treated with original or modified protocol in class 3 patients with thalassemia. (Reprinted with permission from Gaziev J, Isgro A, Sodani P, et al. Optimal outcomes in young class 3 patients with Thalassemia undergoing HLA-ID sibling bone marrow transplantation. *Transplantation.* 2016;100(4):925-932.)

In most children with SCD, supportive care measures such as routine RBC transfusions or hydroxyurea and newer FDA-approved therapies such as voxelotor, crizanlizumab, and L-glutamine in children 12 years of age and older are safe in the short term, lessen anemia (voxelotor), pain (L-glutamine and crizanlizumab), and mitigate the risk of life-threatening events (hydroxyurea).[8-10,129] Unfortunately, the outlook for adults with SCD has not changed substantially since the 1980s, when a median survival in males of 42 years, and in females, of 48 years was observed in the Cooperative Study of Sickle Cell Disease (CSSCD).[130] As a consequence, although most children with sickle cell disease survive to age 20, the outlook for young adults remains unsatisfactory.[129,131,132] Thus, decisions about HCT for SCD are often driven by an individual's outlook in the long term and by donor availability. Summary of recent HSCT trials in SCD is summarized in *Table 105.7*.

HLA-ID Sibling HCT for SCD

Between 1988 and 2012, 234 patients <30 years of age with SCD in France were prepared with a myeloablative combination of BU, CY with or without r-ATG before HLA-ID sibling HCT.[139,140] The French investigators compared results before ($n = 38$) and after 2000 ($n = 196$) and showed significant improvement in the three-year EFS in the current era: the EFS rate was 73.3% before 2000 and 97.4% after 2000 (*Figure 105.10A*). Initially, patients were conditioned for transplantation with a BU/CY backbone alone, but after the initial 12 patients experienced a high rate of graft rejection, r-ATG was added to the conditioning regimen.[128] This strategy successfully reduced the rate of graft rejection from 20.0% to 1.4% (*Figure 105.10B*). A prospective clinical trial conducted by the French group investigated the effectiveness of HLA-ID sibling BMT in children at risk of stroke by transcranial Doppler ultrasound (TCD) screening. In a parallel comparative clinical trial study design with 28 children in the transplant arm and 32 controls receiving regular RBC transfusions for stroke prevention, this study showed protection from stroke. In addition, there was decreased TCD velocity and an improved brain magnetic resonance angiography stenosis score after HCT, and a normalized score was observed in 14 of 28 patients at 3 years posttransplant.[141,142]

Similar results were reported in an analysis of registry data from the CIBMTR and Eurocord/European Blood and Marrow Transplant.

Table 105.5. Summary of HCT Preparative Regimens and Outcomes for Patients With Thalassemia Major

Study	n = Number of Patient Dates of HCT if Available	Donor	Preparative Regimen	Outcomes
Li et al[116] (CIBMTR review)	n = 1110 patients 2000-2016	MRD MUD MMUD MMRD	BU/CY/TT/FLU BU/CY/FLU BU/CY TREO/TT/FLU	5-y EFS (OS): <6 y MRD 88% (92%) MMRD 73% (75%) MUD 89% (93%) MMUD 83% (89%) 7-15 y MRD 80% (84%) MMRD 56% (62%) MUD 89% (91%) MMUD 71% (79%)
Luftinger et al[120] (EBMT review)	N = 772 patients 2010-2018	MRD MUD MMUD MMRD	BU/FLU + CY + TT TREO/FLU + CY or TT	2-y OS BU/FLU: 92.7% BU/TREO 94.7%
Sheth et al[124]	n = 47 patients	MRD	BU/FLU/TT	10-y thalassemia-free survival 87%, 10-y OS 97%
Bernardo et al[122]	n = 60 patients 2005-2011	MRD MUD	TREO/FLU/TT	5-y thalassemia-free survival 84%, 5-y OS 93%
Anurathapan et al[123]	n = 98 1989-2013	MRD MUD	BU/CY (MAC) BU/FLU (RTC)	5-y EFS (OS) MRD 88% (94%) MUD 82% (94%) MAC 86% (95%) RTC 90% (90%)

Abbreviations: BU, Busulfan; CY, Cyclophosphamide; EFS, event-free survival; HCT, hematopoietic cell transplantation; MAC, myeloablative conditioning; MMRD, mismatched related donor; MMUD, mismatched unrelated donor; MRD, matched related donor; MUD, matched unrelated donor; OS, overall survival; RTC, reduced toxicity conditioning; TREO, Treosulfan; TRM, Treatment-related mortality; TT, Thiotepa.

Table 105.6. Hematopoietic Cell Transplantation Indications for Sickle Cell Disease

Patients With Sickle Cell Disease (HbSS or HbSβ⁰-Thalassemia Genotype)

One or more of the following complications:
Stroke or central nervous system event lasting longer than 24 h
Recurrent acute chest syndrome despite supportive care measures
Recurrent vaso-occlusive painful episodes or recurrent priapism
Impaired neuropsychologic function with abnormal cerebral magnetic resonance imaging and angiography
Administration of regular RBC transfusion therapy, defined as receiving 8 or more transfusions per year for >1 y to prevent vaso-occlusive clinical complications (i.e., pain, stroke, and acute chest syndrome)
An echocardiographic finding of tricuspid valve regurgitant jet >2.7 m/s

Other indications under consideration:
Elevated cerebral arterial velocity by transcranial Doppler with cerebral vasculopathy
Pulmonary hypertension by right heart catheterization
Silent cerebral infarction

Among 1000 individuals with SCD treated by HLA-ID sibling HCT between 1986 and 2013, the EFS and OS rates were 91.4% and 92.9%, respectively.[143] The median age at transplantation was 9 years and the median follow-up, longer than 5 years. Most patients received a myeloablative conditioning regimen (n = 873; 87%) and the remainder received reduced-intensity conditioning regimens (n = 125; 13%). OS was lower in peripheral blood stem cell recipients (*Figure 105.11*).[143] Twenty-three patients experienced graft failure; 70 patients (7%) died, most commonly related to infection.

Retrospective transplant registry data were analyzed to identify risk factors for outcomes after HCT.[144] A test cohort of 1425 transplant recipients treated between 2008 and 2017 was grouped by event-free probability that were judged good, intermediate, and poor. These risk groups were segregated by hazard ratios that included recipient age (greater than 13 years and less than or equal to 12 years) and donor type (HLA-ID sibling assigned best risk, HLA-matched URD, intermediate risk and HLA-mismatched related and URD, poor risk). The EFS rate was 92% after HLA-ID sibling in the youngest patients, intermediate EFS rate was 87% in older patients after HLD-ID sibling HCT, and EFS was 83% in younger patients after HLA-matched URD HCT. Of note, EFS in patients >13 years was judged poor with EFS that ranged from 49% to 52% after matched, mismatched URD, and mismatched related donor HCT. Outcomes were also poor after HLA-mismatched related and URD HCT in younger patients (62%-68%). Together, the registry data indicate that results of HCT are best in children, and the option of HCT is appropriate to consider in those with severe disease.

Myeloablative HCT for SCD

BU-based myeloablative transplant regimens are sufficient for engraftment of donor cells, but are toxic, particularly in high-risk and older patients. Dose adjustment and targeting an optimal exposure must be considered to ensure optimal drug exposure in hemoglobinopathy patients. Gaziev et al adapted a targeted BU exposure between 900 μM/min and 1350 μM/min to optimize outcomes. This strategy avoided dose adjustments after the initial dose and successfully targeted the therapeutic range.[145]

Alternate regimens have been explored as a strategy to improve the toxicity profile. The goal of a reduced intensity or nonmyeloablative conditioning regimen often is to establish mixed donor-host hematopoietic chimerism, an endpoint that retains the therapeutic effect of donor engraftment while improving the safety of HCT, particularly in high-risk patients. Stable donor mixed chimerism after HCT for thalassemia and SCD has been studied most extensively in the thalassemia cohort from Pesaro.[146-148] The cause of the phenomenon is uncertain, and it is associated with oligoclonal skewing of the T-cell repertoire, which is not associated with impaired immune function.[149] In the RBC lineage, there is a natural enrichment of donor cells in the blood, as a consequence of ineffective host erythropoiesis and longer RBC survival in donor erythrocytes. Most important, even when there

Table 105.7. Summary of Recent HCT Clinical Trials for Sickle Cell Disease

Study	n = Number of Patient Dates of HCT if Available Age (years)	Donor	Preparative Regimen	Outcomes
Gluckman et al[133]	n = 1000 1986-2013 Median age 9.4 (0.26-54.37)	MRD (PB, BM, CB)	MAC and RIC BU/CY BU/FLU + other	5-y OS 92.9%, 5-y EFS 91.4% GVHD free 86% (age <16 y) GVHD free 77% (age >15 y)
Bhatia et al[134]	n = 18 Median Age 8.9 (2.3-20)	MRD (BM, CB)	Busulfan Fludarabine Alemtuzumab	2-y OS 100% 2-y EFS 100% Grade II-IV acute GVHD 17% Mean whole blood and erythroid donor chimerism 91%(day +100) and 88 (day +365) Neurological, pulmonary, and cardiovascular functions were stable or improved at 2 y
Alzahrani at al[135]	n = 122 2004-2019 Median age 29 (10-65)	MRD (PBSC)	Alemtuzumab TBI 300cGY Sirolimus	5-y OS 93% Median 489 d until off IST
Shenoy et al[136]	n = 19 2008-2014 Age 4-19	MUD	Alemtuzumab Fludarabine Melphalan	1-y OS 86% 1-y EFS 76% 2-y OS 79% 2-y EFS 69% Chronic GVHD 62% PRES 34%
Krishnamurti et al[137]	n = 22 2012-2015 Median Age 22 (17-36)	MRD MUD	BU/FLU/r-ATG	1-y OS 91% 1-y EFS 86% 3-y EFS 82% 42% on IST at 1 y post BMT
Guilcher et al[138]	n = 16 2013-2017 Age 4-19	MRD (PBSC)	Alemtuzumab TBI 300cGY Sirolimus	OS, EFS 100% at 19.5 mo Median 14 mo until off IST

Abbreviations: BM, Bone Marrow; CB, Cord blood; EFS, Event-free survival; GVHD, graft-versus-host disease; HCT, Hematopoietic cell transplantation; IST, Immunesuppressive therapy; MRD, Matched related donor; MUD, Matched Unrelated Donor; OS, Overall survival; PBSC, Peripheral Blood Stem Cell; PRES, Posterior Reversible encephalopathy.

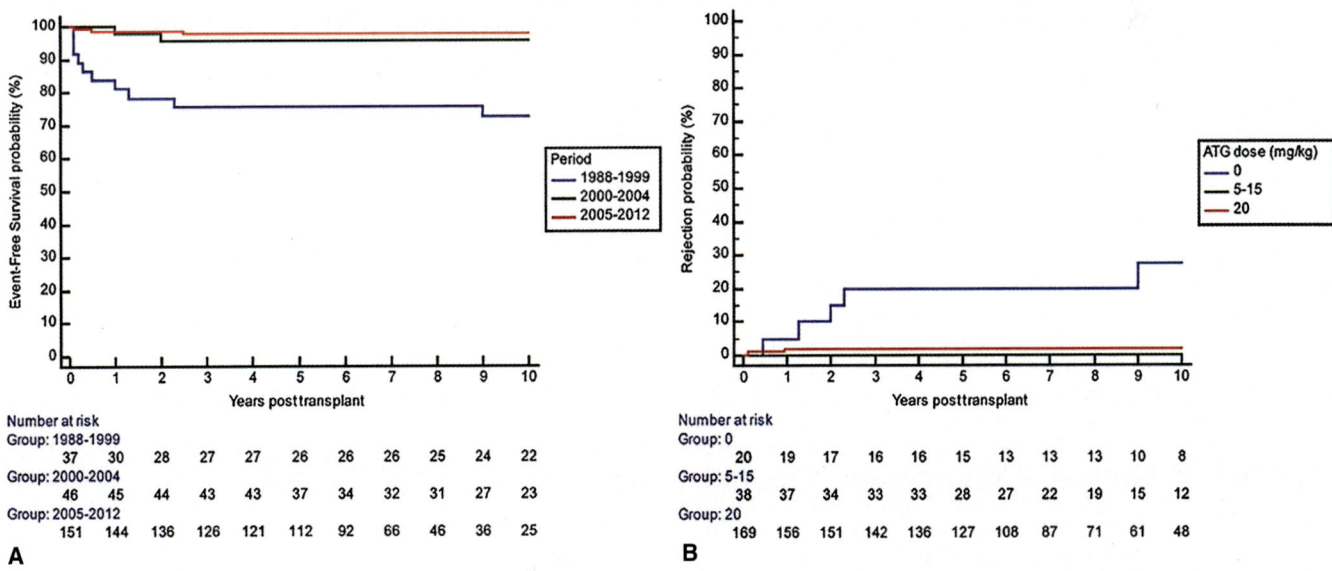

FIGURE 105.10 **A**, Event-free survival improved among in patients who received HLA–identical sibling hematopoietic cell transplantation for sickle cell disease depending on the period of transplant. It was only 73.3% before year 2000 and 97.4% after year 2000. **B**, The effect of rabbit antithymocyte globulin (ATG) on the cumulative incidence of graft rejection after sibling hematopoietic cell transplantation for sickle cell anemia. (Reprinted with permission from Bernaudin F, Dalle JH, Bories D, et al. Long-term event-free survival, chimerism and fertility outcomes in 234 patients with sickle-cell anemia younger than 30 years after myeloablative conditioning and matched-sibling transplantation in France. *Haematologica*. 2020;105(1):91-101. Copyright © 2020 Ferrata Storti Foundation.)

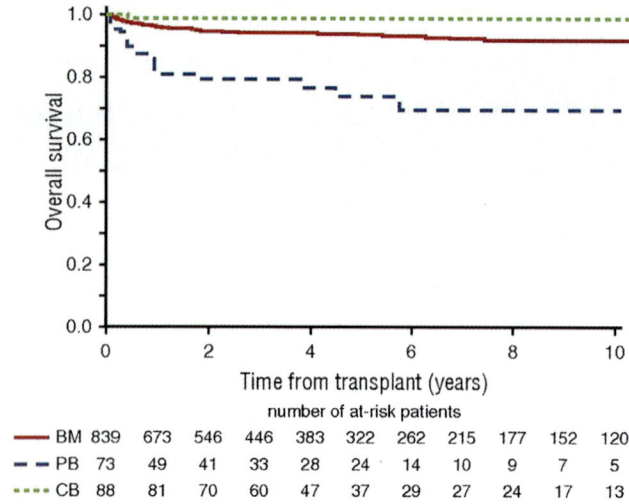

FIGURE 105.11 Overall survival in patients who received HLA–identical sibling hematopoietic cell transplantation for sickle cell disease according to stem cell source. BM, bone marrow; CB, cord blood; PB, peripheral blood. (Reprinted from Gluckman E, Cappelli B, Bernaudin F, et al. Sickle cell disease: an international survey of results of HLA-identical sibling hematopoietic stem cell transplantation. *Blood*. 2017;129(11):1548-1556. Copyright © 2017 American Society of Hematology. With permission.)

is a minority of donor cells, the patients who develop stable mixed chimerism do not experience symptoms of the underlying hemoglobinopathy and thus survive disease free; the threshold for a curative outcome appears to be 20% to 25% donor chimerism.[147,150]

Reduced Toxicity HCT for SCD

The initial minimal toxicity regimen tested in hemoglobinopathies consisted of fludarabine with a single fraction of TBI 200 cGy.[151] The results showed that transient donor engraftment was achieved in most patients. However, graft rejection occurred after postgrafting immune suppression was tapered and discontinued. The addition of r-ATG to a backbone of fludarabine and TBI did not improve the outcome.[152]

An alternative nonmyeloablative regimen was developed that centered on the observation that expanding a T-regulatory cell population after transplant promoted tolerance and thereby facilitated stable engraftment of donor cells. Based upon preclinical modeling, several groups have combined clinical trial results in 122 adult SCD patients with median age of 29 years who were treated by HLA-ID sibling HCT after receiving 300 cGy TBI and an anti-CD52 antibody, alemtuzumab. Sirolimus alone was given for posttransplantation immunosuppression.[135,153] With a median follow-up of 4 years (range, 0.6-15), 87% of recipients had long-term engraftment without acute or chronic GVHD and the OS rate was 93% at 5 years. At 5 years posttransplant CD3+ T-cell donor chimerism was >50%, and 83% of surviving patients were no longer receiving immunosuppressive therapy. Similar results have been observed in a smaller single-center pediatric study.[138] In addition, results from a retrospective registry data analysis study showed improved survival and decreased chronic GVHD after nonmyeloablative compared with reduced intensity and myeloablative conditioning regimens. However, conditioning regimen intensity was not associated with OS after HLA-identical sibling HCT.[144]

A BU-based reduced toxicity regimen was tested in a multicenter pilot clinical trial (STRIDE) to determine the feasibility, efficacy, and safety of HLA-matched related and URD HSCT in adults with severe SCD.[137] Twenty-two patients (ages 16-40 years) were enrolled and received a preparative regimen consisting of BU from day 8 to 5 (13.2 mg/kg), fludarabine (150 mg/m^2) and r-ATG (6 mg/kg). None of the patients had graft failure or SCD recurrence and the overall and EFS rates were 91% and 86%, respectively, at 12 months post-HSCT and EFS rate was 82% at 3 years post-HSCT. The overall incidence of acute GVHD was 18% and 20% for chronic GVHD. Full donor myeloid chimerism was observed after HCT. Statistically significant improvements in the pain interference and physical function domains of health-related quality of life were observed.

HLA-Haploidentical BMT and Gene Therapy for Hemoglobin Disorders

Clinical trial investigations aimed at expanding curative HCT for SCD and thalassemia have addressed the problems of limited donor selection and GVHD disease after alternate donor HCT by applying posttransplant CY to HLA-haploidentical HCT and autologous gene therapy with its promise of universal application. Advances in both technologies will be summarized.

HLA-haploidentical HCT for thalassemia has utilized either posttransplant cyclophosphamide (PT-CY) or TCRαβ+/CD19+-depleted transplantation to accomplished T-cell depletion to mitigate the risks of GVHD and graft rejection. A conditioning regimen with immunosuppressive and the absence of anti–donor-specific antibodies also appears necessary for reducing the risk of graft rejection. A limited cohort of five patients received rATG, fludarabine, and TBI 400cGY. All five remained transfusion-independent posttransplant with a median follow-up 705 days.[154] In another study that used a myeloablative conditioning regimen, 83 patients experienced a three-year EFS and OS rate of 96% after CY HLA-haploidentical HCT with PT-CY.[155] TCRαβ+/CD19+-depleted haploidentical transplantation for thalassemia is more limited.[156] In one study of 11 patients, the 5-year OS and DFS rates were 84% and 69%, respectively.[157] Graft failure is the most common obstacle with viral reactivation and post–transplant lymphoproliferative disorder as other potential complications.

In SCD, groups augmented the backbone of a reduced intensity conditioning regimen that was first investigated by a team of investigators at Johns Hopkins University.[158] By the addition of thiotepa or increasing the TBI dose from 200 to 400 cGy delivered in a single fraction, the incidence of graft rejection of HCT has improved from 43% to approximately 10% as observed in two studies of HLA-haploidentical HCT for SCD.[154] The overall EFS rate in the modified regimen studies has been approximately 85%, similar to outcomes after HLA-identical BMT in patients ≥13 years of age. A larger phase II study conducted by the BMT-CTN will test this approach in 40 adults and 40 children in separate strata with eligibility criteria that target individuals with a severe phenotype. If successfully completed, this study has the potential to widen the availability of allogeneic BMT in SCD.

Gene and Genomic Therapies for Hemoglobin Disorders

More recently, attention has focused on gene therapy for these disorders as another strategy to expand access to a curative therapy. Gene therapy relies upon the mobilization and collection of CD34+ HSPCs, isolation of the CD34+ cells followed by random genomic insertion of a gene addition lentiviral vector or modification of a targeted genomic sequence by gene editing reagents introduced by electroporation. The most common strategy utilizes expression of an antisickling globin that generates HbF-like properties. A second strategy targets inactivation of an erythroid-specific enhancer in BCL11a to induce high-level fetal globin expression. BCL11a is the master regulator of HbF repression that occurs at birth (reviewed in Ref. 159). Of interest, this approach has been applied to both SCD and transfusion–dependent β-thalassemia (TDT). Preliminary data and published reports strongly suggest that both strategies have been successful in either reducing or eliminating the need for RBC transfusions in TDT and in reducing episodes of severe vaso-occlusive pain and markers of hemolysis in SCD.[160,161] In these clinical trials, the typical toxicity profile mimics that predicted by administration of myeloablative BU that precedes infusion of the genome-modified HSPCs. There have been no reports of failure of the modified cells to engraft and no GVHD. A shift from relying upon a bone marrow harvest in SCD to using single-agent plerixafor-mobilized HSPCs also improved the therapeutic effect of the drug product.[162]

The initial report of patients from France (HGB 205 study), Australia, Thailand, and the United States (HGB 204 study) treated by lentiviral gene therapy in TDT included patients who had a more severe β°β° genotype in which very little or no endogenous hemoglobin is produced or a less severe β⁺β° genotype.[163] Of 22 patients who were treated, 15 of 22 patients stopped transfusions after infusion of the modified HSPCs. The average vector copy number (VCN) in drug product was 0.7 and 1.3 in the HGB 204 and HGB 205 studies, respectively, and was 0.3 and 2.0 in peripheral blood at 15 months postinfusion. This level of transduction was sufficient for transfusion independence in 12 of 13 patients with the β⁺β° genotype and 3 of 9 with the β°β° genotype. There was a direct relationship between the VCN and the level of the gene therapy hemoglobin (termed HbAT87Q) produced in the blood. For this reason, a modified manufacturing protocol for the gene therapy drug product was developed and results of a larger study restricted to patients with a β⁺β° genotype were recently reported.[164] Twenty-three were enrolled and 20 of 22 recipients (91%) experienced transfusion independence 20 of 22 patients (91%), and the median duration of RBC transfusion independence was 20.4 months (range, 15.7-21.6) (Figure 105.12). The average hemoglobin level was 11.7 g/dL (range, 9.5-12.8) compared with an average hemoglobin 11.2 g/dL (range, 8.2-13.7) in the earlier group. Notably, the optimized manufacturing protocol generated an average VCN in the drug product that was 3.3 and was 1.52 at 18 months postinfusion. The increased VCN appeared to overcome a reliance on endogenous hemoglobin production to accomplish transfusion independence.

The results of gene therapy in SCD using the same lentiviral vector also showed a significant clinical benefit.[165] Following the same optimized manufacturing protocol utilized in the thalassemia trial, 35 patients with severe SCD received autologous CD34⁺ HSPCs after transduction with a lentiviral vector that expresses the antisickling hemoglobin, HbA^{T87Q}. Postinfusion levels of the antisickling hemoglobin reached a plateau by 1 to 3 months postinfusion and were stable through 3 years median follow-up. These levels generated a median total hemoglobin value that increased from 8.5 g/dL at baseline to 11.0 g/dL or more at 6 months, and HbA^{T87Q} contributed to 40% or more of the total hemoglobin. Of interest, the HbA^{T87Q} in individual RBC had nearly pan-cellular distribution. There was a mean of 85 ± 8% of RBC with at least some HbA^{T87Q} at 24 months balanced by roughly 15% of RBC that contained only HbS, the latter of which would be at risk to sickle. In the Hb^{AT87Q}-containing RBC population, the median HbA^{T87Q} ranged from 11.7 to 22.7 pg per RBC, which approximates the range of 13 to 18 pg per RBC of HbA present in the sickle trait RBC. This distribution of the antisickling hemoglobin also would predict a clinical phenotype of sickle cell trait.

This prediction was illustrated by the clinical outcomes. Markers of hemolysis such as serum bilirubin, haptoglobin LDH, and reticulocyte count all approached normal levels or were improved compared with baseline postinfusion. There was cessation of severe vaso-occlusive painful events, defined as a hospitalization or administration of intravenous analgesics in an ambulatory setting in patients who had at least 6 months follow-up postinfusion. There was a median of 3.5 events per year (range, 2.0-13.5) 2 years before enrollment that declined to a median of 0 per year (range, 0-5.9) (Figure 105.13). There were no strokes reported in the follow-up period, which included patients at risk of stroke. In summary, the preliminary results showed near correction of the SCD phenotype after a one-time infusion of the lentiviral transduced autologous stem cells.

Parallel studies in gene therapy/gene editing aimed at inducing HbF also have shown a similar toxicity profile after myeloablative BU and infusion of the modified cells. One approach for HbF induction utilizes a lentiviral vector to express a short-hairpin inhibitory sequence embedded in a microRNA (shmiR) that targets BCL11a mRNA for posttranscriptional silencing.[160] Because expression of the shmiR is under control of erythroid-specific regulatory elements, BCL11a inhibition only occurs in the erythroid lineage. Six patients treated with the vector had high-level, sustained HbF expression postinfusion. The serum hemoglobin increased from 9.3 to 11.4 g/dL in the five patients not treated by RBC transfusions with an HbF percentage of 30.4% (range, 21.6-40.0). Markers of hemolysis also declined from baseline values but were not normalized. None of the six patients had a severe vaso-occlusive episode, acute chest syndrome or stroke postinfusion.

A second approach for inducing HbF utilizes engineered CRISPR gene editing reagents to inactivate an intronic erythroid-specific enhancer in BCL11a. In a case report, a patient with SCD and a patient with TDT had robust HbF induction and stable expression in the peripheral blood, with elimination of vaso-occlusive events and RBC transfusions in the SCD and TDT, respectively.[161] Together, both strategies for HbF induction by BCL11a inactivation in erythroid cells appear to be feasible and effective.

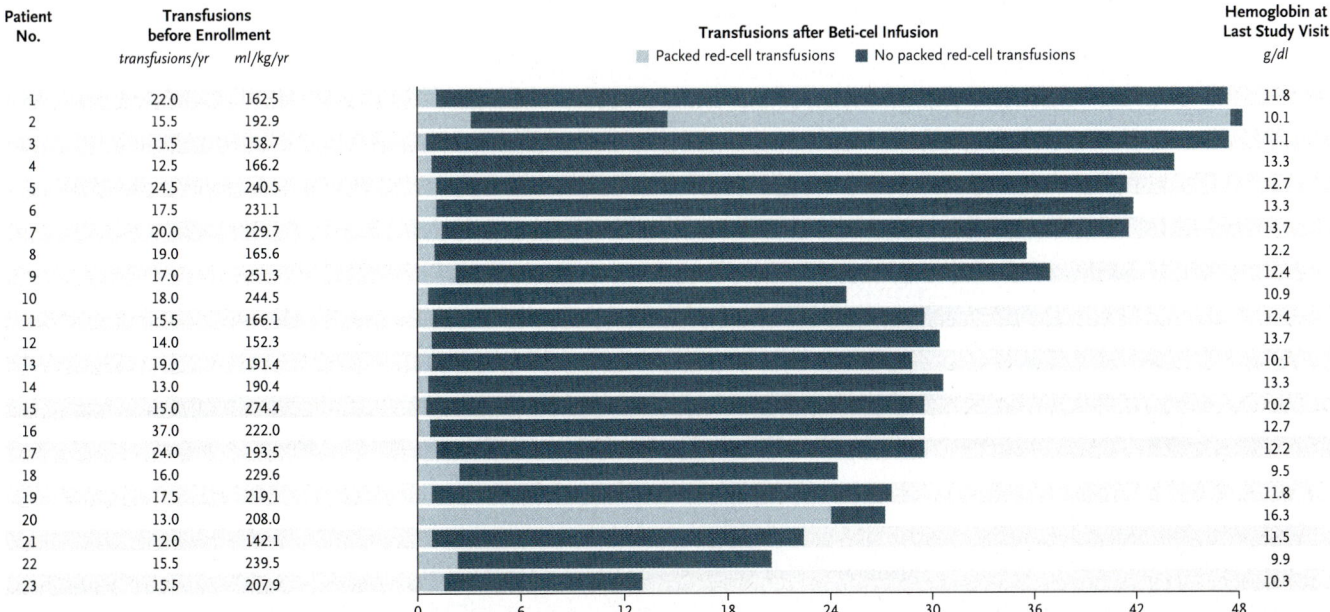

FIGURE 105.12 RBC transfusion independence after gene therapy for transfusion–dependent β-thalassemia (TDT). Twenty of 23 patients had transfusion independence, which was defined as a weighted average hemoglobin level of 9 g/dL or greater at least 12 months after drug product infusion. (From Locatelli F, Thompson AA, Kwiatkowski JL, et al. Betibeglogene autotemcel gene therapy for non-β(0)/β(0) genotype β-thalassemia. N Engl J Med. 2022;386(5):415-427. Copyright © 2022 Massachusetts Medical Society. Reprinted with permission from Massachusetts Medical Society.)

Acute Myelogenous Leukemia After Gene Therapy

While the long-term effectiveness and stability of gene therapy and gene editing for hemoglobinopathies still must be established, these preliminary results suggest that a universally available curative option might soon be available, with HLA-haploidentical allogeneic HCT, if the safety and efficacy are confirmed by ongoing clinical trials. This optimism is tempered, however, by the observation of MDS and AML that was observed in two participants with SCD in the lentiviral gene therapy trial with Lentiglobin.[166,167] In both cases, the bone marrow was used for CD34+ cell collections in lieu of mobilization and apheresis. Both patients developed monosomy 7 and the acquisition of driver mutations in Runx1 and PTPN11 in one case, and both died of AML. In the first case, no vector was detected in the leukemic blast population; thus, residual host cells exposed to the alkylating agent BU might have conferred treatment-related AML. In the second case, however, vector was present in leukemic blasts with integration near the VAMP-4 gene, which is not associated with acute leukemia. To investigate this association of AML with SCD, retrospective registry data have been analyzed to suggest an increased risk of AML in SCD. There is speculation that this association might be promoted by the inflammatory milieu and oxidative stress of hematopoiesis in the marrow niche that is characteristic of SCD. The selection of clonal hematopoiesis with driver mutations that exert a proliferative advantage in this milieu might also emerge after competitive repopulation of gene-modified HSCs following myeloablation and autologous HCT.[168] The basis for these observations is under investigation, and it will be important to better inform patients about the long-term risk of clonal hematopoiesis and AML after gene therapy, and more broadly after any curative therapy. This concern is warranted also by reports of MDS/AML after HLA-haploidentical HCT in which patients who experienced graft rejection developed treatment-related AML driven by host TP53 mutations that preceded transplantation.[169] There are efforts to incorporate genomic screening to assess risk before gene therapy.

LATE EFFECTS AFTER HCT FOR HEMOGLOBIN DISORDERS

DFS after HCT for hemoglobin disorders is defined as freedom from transfusions and iron loading in thalassemia, and in SCD, freedom from sickle-related clinical events and organ damage. However, the iron that accumulates as a consequence of RBC transfusions before and after HCT is not eliminated after successful HCT to any appreciable extent. If left untreated, iron overload causes significant morbidity and mortality with progressive liver disease and even cirrhosis after transplantation.[170] A prospective analysis of annual liver biopsies in thalassemia patients not treated by iron chelation and in whom thalassemia was cured by HCT demonstrated that iron overload and hepatitis C virus infection were independent risk factors for progressive liver fibrosis. Patients who had an active hepatitis C infection and also had very high levels of hepatic iron had an 80% risk of developing progressive hepatic fibrosis 10 to 12 years after successful transplantation.[171] Conversely, patients with a liver iron level less than 16 mg iron/g liver dry weight and who were also free of evidence of active hepatitis C virus infection showed no signs of progressive hepatic fibrosis.

Phlebotomy is safe, inexpensive, and highly efficient, and therefore, it is the treatment of choice to treat transfusion iron overload after HCT. Excess iron can be completely mobilized from the body by phlebotomy without any significant side effects. Following completion of a phlebotomy program, significant improvement in liver function was observed, particularly in patients infected with hepatitis C virus.[171] It is possible to reverse severe hepatic fibrosis and even early cirrhosis.[172] Patients with early cardiac involvement characterized by left ventricular diastolic dysfunction and impaired left ventricular contractility demonstrated regression of subclinical cardiac disease after phlebotomy.[173]

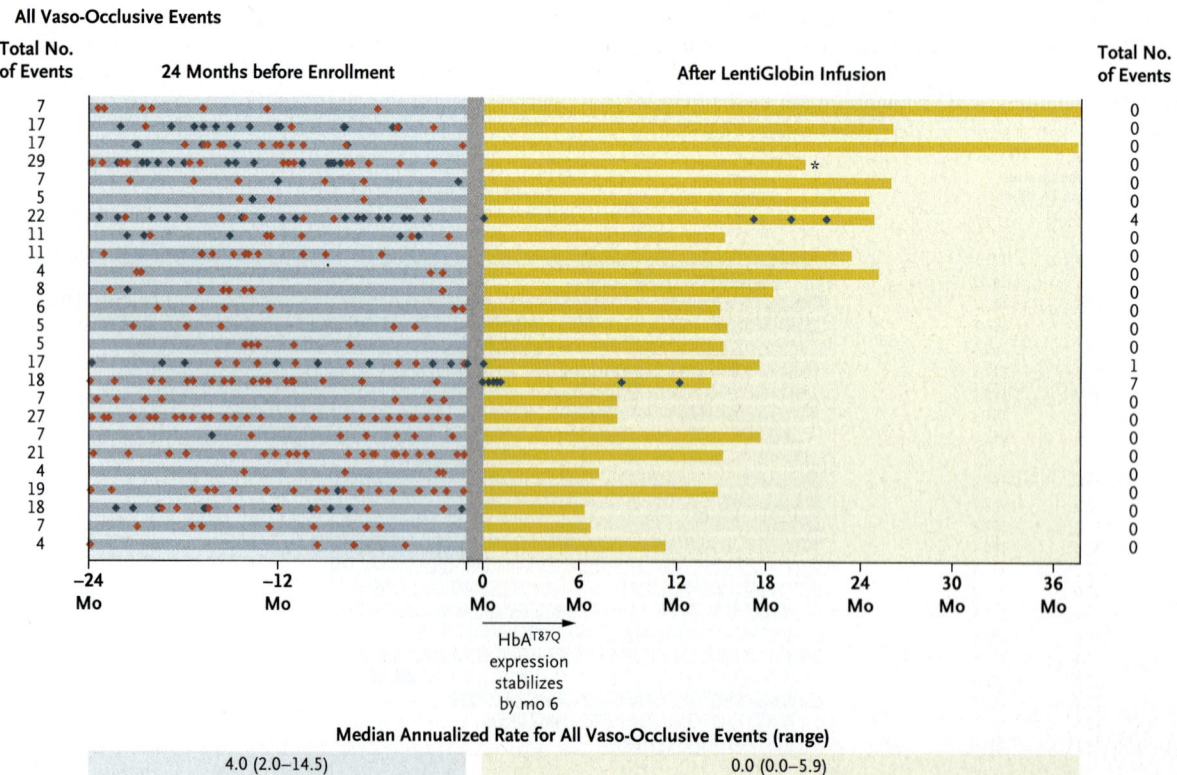

FIGURE 105.13 Changes in the rate of vaso-occlusive events before and after LentiGlobin infusion. All vaso-occlusive events after the LentiGlobin infusion are presented. The gray shaded area shows the period when preharvest transfusions were administered. Red and blue diamonds represent severe and non–severe vaso-occlusive pain events, respectively. (From Kanter J, Walters MC, Krishnamurti L, et al. Biologic and clinical efficacy of LentiGlobin for sickle cell disease. *N Engl J Med*. 2022;386(7):617-628. Copyright © 2022 Massachusetts Medical Society. Reprinted with permission from Massachusetts Medical Society.)

After successful HCT for SCD, patients with stable engraftment of donor cells do not experience sickle-related clinical complications, even if there is stable mixed donor-host hematopoietic chimerism.[128,147] With regard to target organs at risk for sickle-related damage, investigators have reported improvements in splenic function and osteonecrosis.[174-176] In addition, there is also improvement in selected domains of health-related quality of life instruments. Of interest, improvement in pain interference, physical functioning, and sleep have been observed, but sometimes little or no improvement in social and emotional domains noted by 1 year after reduced toxicity allogeneic HCT for SCD[177] (reviewed in[178]).

The incidence of secondary solid tumors in thalassemia and SCD after HCT is less than 10/100,000 patient-years, a rate that does not appear different compared to patients who receive supportive care treatment for β-thalassemia. More recently, a retrospective registry review of a cohort of nearly 1000 patients treated between 2008 and 2017 reported that 1% of patients with SCD developed malignant neoplasms after HCT, including AML and MDS. AML in SCD is often described as "therapy related," with complex cytogenetic abnormalities including monosomy 7, and mutations in drivers such as RUNX1.[179,180] There is also a possibility that individuals with SCD carry a high risk of AML that is related to stress hematopoiesis, which selects for clonal hematopoiesis associated with driver mutations that favor proliferation.[181,182]

Gonadotropin and sex hormone levels confirm the toxic effect of BU on gonadal function after HCT. In addition, hypogonadism is the most common endocrine disorder in medically treated patients with thalassemia major, affecting approximately half the patients.[183,184] In a study involving 68 children with thalassemia after HCT, 32% reached an advanced or complete puberty spontaneously (34% of girls and 63% of boys), despite clinical and hormonal evidence of gonadal impairment in most cases.[170] In this group, iron overload and the conditioning regimen were the major factors influencing endocrine function. In the cooperative study of HCT for SCD, follow-up gonadal function studies were performed in patients who were 21.6 (range, 16.1-28.5 years) and 21.7 (range, 14.1-27.8 years) years of age in males and females, respectively.[185] Among those evaluated, the luteinizing hormone (LH) and follicle-stimulating hormone (FSH) levels were normal in 9 males and less than normal in 4 after transplantation. However, only 3 of 13 had normal testosterone levels, consistent with hypogonadotrophic hypogonadism in most of the pubertal males. In contrast, 8 of 14 females had increased gonadotropin levels and/or below normal estradiol levels, a finding consistent with primary ovarian failure in the majority of postpubertal females. Only 4 of 14 females had normal estradiol levels. However, one female had a successful pregnancy 13 years after HCT and another female with graft rejection gave birth to a healthy baby following preimplantation genetic diagnosis 14 years after HCT, although she had experienced two previous spontaneous abortions several years earlier. Among six evaluable prepubertal girls in the Belgian cohort, five had primary amenorrhea with elevated serum LH and FSH.[127] Two postpubertal females developed secondary amenorrhea. Testicular function was also adversely affected in four of six evaluable boys who demonstrated decreased testosterone and elevated FSH levels. In the French series, seven postpubertal females, aged 13 to 22 years, developed amenorrhea after hematopoietic cell transplantation with decreased serum estradiol and elevated LH and FSH levels and received hormone replacement therapy.[128] It is anticipated that many, if not most, of the females will require hormonal replacement therapy after HCT. The development of reduced intensity conditioning regimens may reduce the late effect of gonadal toxicity.

Eggleston et al reported growth outcomes in children who were enrolled in a multicenter investigation of HCT for SCD.[186] The baseline height and weight and growth velocities after HCT were compared to children who were treated by HU and who were enrolled in the CSSCD, previous investigations of SCD during which prospective height and weight measurements were documented.[187,188] It was determined that growth after HCT was not impaired, except in older males, where data from the CSSCD showed a more rapid height and weight velocity after age 11.6 and 12.1 years, respectively. However, males grew 0.67 cm/year faster after HCT compared to males in the HU group before treatment with HU was initiated. Thus, the data showed that conventional myeloablative HCT generally had no adverse effect on height or weight gain in young children. However, diminished growth may occur in patients who undergo HCT at or near the growth spurt. This study emphasized the importance of treating children early in the course of their disease to minimize toxicity.

CONCLUSION

Allogeneic HCT has been the only treatment with curative potential for a number of non–malignant hematological disorders, as highlighted. The emergence of HLA-haploidentical donor HCT has the potential to broaden the availability of allogeneic HCT in those who lack a well-matched donor. A great deal of attention with new investigations has ushered in the era of autologous gene therapy for the primary immune deficiencies and hemoglobinopathies, which has the potential to be transformative. The further development of gene therapy will rest on a better understanding of durability of clinical benefit and safety over the long term. In addition, patient access to this intensive and expensive treatment will also affect the impact of gene therapy on these disorders.

References

1. Oran B, Weisdorf DJ. Allogeneic stem cell transplantation in first complete remission. *Curr Opin Hematol*. 2011;18(6):395-400.
2. Appelbaum FR. The role of hematopoietic cell transplantation as therapy for myelodysplasia. *Best Pract Res Clin Haematol*. 2011;24(4):541-547.
3. Shenoy S. Hematopoietic stem cell transplantation for sickle cell disease: current practice and emerging trends. *Hematology Am Soc Hematol Educ Program*. 2011;2011:273-279.
4. Batzios SP, Zafeiriou DI. Developing treatment options for metachromatic leukodystrophy. *Mol Genet Metabol*. 2012;105(1):56-63.
5. Sponzilli I, Notarangelo LD. Severe combined immunodeficiency (SCID): from molecular basis to clinical management. *Acta Biomed*. 2011;82(1):5-13.
6. Tolar J, Mehta PA, Walters MC. Hematopoietic cell transplantation for nonmalignant disorders. *Biol Blood Marrow Transplant*. 2012;18(1 suppl):S166-S171.
7. Rachmilewitz EA, Giardina PJ. How I treat thalassemia. *Blood*. 2011;118(13):3479-3488.
8. Niihara Y, Miller ST, Kanter J, et al. A phase 3 trial of l-glutamine in sickle cell disease. *N Engl J Med*. 2018;379(3):226-235.
9. Vichinsky E, Hoppe CC, Ataga KI, et al. A phase 3 randomized trial of voxelotor in sickle cell disease. *N Engl J Med*. 2019;381(6):509-519.
10. Ataga KI, Kutlar A, Kanter J, et al. Crizanlizumab for the prevention of pain crises in sickle cell disease. *N Engl J Med*. 2017;376(5):429-439.
11. Buckley RH. Transplantation of hematopoietic stem cells in human severe combined immunodeficiency: longterm outcomes. *Immunol Res*. 2011;49(1-3):25-43.
12. Kee Y, D'Andrea AD. Expanded roles of the Fanconi anemia pathway in preserving genomic stability. *Genes Dev*. 2010;24(16):1680-1694.
13. Bagby GC, Alter BP. Fanconi anemia. *Semin Hematol*. 2006;43(3):147-156.
14. Kwan A, Abraham RS, Currier R, et al. Newborn screening for severe combined immunodeficiency in 11 screening programs in the United States. *JAMA*. 2014;312(7):729-738.
15. Comeau AM, Hale JE, Pai SY, et al. Guidelines for implementation of population-based newborn screening for severe combined immunodeficiency. *J Inherit Metab Dis*. 2010;33(suppl 2):S273-S281.
16. Puck JM. The case for newborn screening for severe combined immunodeficiency and related disorders. *Ann N Y Acad Sci*. 2011;1246:108-117.
17. Verbsky JW, Baker MW, Grossman WJ, et al. Newborn screening for severe combined immunodeficiency; the Wisconsin experience (2008-2011). *J Clin Immunol*. 2012;32(1):82-88.
18. Buelow BJ, Routes JM, Verbsky JW. Newborn screening for SCID: where are we now? *Expert Rev Clin Immunol*. 2014;10(12):1649-1657.
19. Pai SY, Logan BR, Griffith LM, et al. Transplantation outcomes for severe combined immunodeficiency, 2000-2009. *N Engl J Med*. 2014;371(5):434-446.
20. Gatti RA, Meuwissen HJ, Allen HD, Hong R, Good RA. Immunological reconstitution of sex-linked lymphopenic immunological deficiency. *Lancet*. 1968;2(7583):1366-1369.
21. Buckley RH, Schiff SE, Sampson HA, et al. Development of immunity in human severe primary T cell deficiency following haploidentical bone marrow stem cell transplantation. *J Immunol*. 1986;136(7):2398-2407.
22. Kohn DB. Eliminating SCID row: new approaches to SCID. *Hematology Am Soc Hematol Educ Program*. 2014;2014(1):475-480.
23. DelToro G, Satwani P, Harrison L, et al. A pilot study of reduced intensity conditioning and allogeneic stem cell transplantation from unrelated cord blood and matched family donors in children and adolescent recipients. *Bone Marrow Transplant*. 2004;33(6):613-622.

24. Satwani P, Harrison L, Morris E, DelToro G, Cairo MS. Reduced-intensity allogeneic stem cell transplantation in adults and children with malignant and nonmalignant diseases: end of the beginning and future challenges. *Biol Blood Marrow Transplant*. 2005;11(6):403-422.
25. Satwani P, Morris E, Bradley MB, Bhatia M, van de Ven C, Cairo MS. Reduced intensity and non-myeloablative allogeneic stem cell transplantation in children and adolescents with malignant and non-malignant diseases. *Pediatr Blood Cancer*. 2008;50(1):1-8.
26. Veys P. Reduced intensity transplantation for primary immunodeficiency disorders. *Pediatr Rep*. 2011;3(suppl 2):e11.
27. Chiesa R, Veys P. Reduced-intensity conditioning for allogeneic stem cell transplant in primary immune deficiencies. *Expet Rev Clin Immunol*. 2012;8(3):255-266. quiz 267.
28. Lankester AC, Albert MH, Booth C, et al. EBMT/ESID inborn errors working party guidelines for hematopoietic stem cell transplantation for inborn errors of immunity. *Bone Marrow Transplant*. 2021;56(9):2052-2062.
29. Haddad E, Leroy S, Buckley RH. B-cell reconstitution for SCID: should a conditioning regimen be used in SCID treatment? *J Allergy Clin Immunol*. 2013;131(4):994-1000.
30. Dvorak CC, Hassan A, Slatter MA, et al. Comparison of outcomes of hematopoietic stem cell transplantation without chemotherapy conditioning by using matched sibling and unrelated donors for treatment of severe combined immunodeficiency. *J Allergy Clin Immunol*. 2014;134(4):935-943 e915.
31. Fernandes JF, Rocha V, Labopin M, et al. Transplantation in patients with SCID: mismatched related stem cells or unrelated cord blood? *Blood*. 2012;119(12):2949-2955.
32. Chan WY, Roberts RL, Moore TB, Stiehm ER. Cord blood transplants for SCID: better B-cell engraftment? *J Pediatr Hematol Oncol*. 2013;35(1):e14-8.
33. Mazzolari E, Forino C, Guerci S, et al. Long-term immune reconstitution and clinical outcome after stem cell transplantation for severe T-cell immunodeficiency. *J Allergy Clin Immunol*. 2007;120(4):892-899.
34. Bertaina A, Merli P, Rutella S, et al. HLA-haploidentical stem cell transplantation after removal of alphabeta+ T and B cells in children with nonmalignant disorders. *Blood*. 2014;124(5):822-826.
35. Buckley RH, Win CM, Moser BK, Parrott RE, Sajaroff E, Sarzotti-Kelsoe M. Post-transplantation B cell function in different molecular types of SCID. *J Clin Immunol*. 2013;33(1):96-110.
36. Patel NC, Chinen J, Rosenblatt HM, et al. Long-term outcomes of nonconditioned patients with severe combined immunodeficiency transplanted with HLA-identical or haploidentical bone marrow depleted of T cells with anti-CD6 mAb. *J Allergy Clin Immunol*. 2008;122(6):1185-1193.
37. Sarzotti-Kelsoe M, Win CM, Parrott RE, et al. Thymic output, T-cell diversity, and T-cell function in long-term human SCID chimeras. *Blood*. 2009;114(7):1445-1453.
38. Booth C, Romano R, Roncarolo MG, Thrasher AJ. Gene therapy for primary immunodeficiency. *Hum Mol Genet*. 2019;28(R1):R15-R23.
39. Kohn DB, Booth C, Shaw KL, et al. Autologous ex vivo lentiviral gene therapy for adenosine deaminase deficiency. *N Engl J Med*. 2021;384(21):2002-2013.
40. Henter JI, Horne A, Arico M, et al. HLH-2004: diagnostic and therapeutic guidelines for hemophagocytic lymphohistiocytosis. *Pediatr Blood Cancer*. 2007;48(2):124-131.
41. Allen CE, Yu X, Kozinetz CA, McClain KL. Highly elevated ferritin levels and the diagnosis of hemophagocytic lymphohistiocytosis. *Pediatr Blood Cancer*. 2008;50(6):1227-1235.
42. Jordan MB, Allen CE, Weitzman S, Filipovich AH, McClain KL. How I treat hemophagocytic lymphohistiocytosis. *Blood*. 2011;118(15):4041-4052.
43. Ouachee-Chardin M, Elie C, de Saint Basile G, et al. Hematopoietic stem cell transplantation in hemophagocytic lymphohistiocytosis: a single-center report of 48 patients. *Pediatrics*. 2006;117(4):e743-e750.
44. Trottestam H, Horne A, Arico M, et al. Chemoimmunotherapy for hemophagocytic lymphohistiocytosis: long-term results of the HLH-94 treatment protocol. *Blood*. 2011;118(17):4577-4584.
45. Baker KS, Filipovich AH, Gross TG, et al. Unrelated donor hematopoietic cell transplantation for hemophagocytic lymphohistiocytosis. *Bone Marrow Transplant*. 2008;42(3):175-180.
46. Shenoy S, Grossman WJ, DiPersio J, et al. A novel reduced-intensity stem cell transplant regimen for nonmalignant disorders. *Bone Marrow Transplant*. 2005;35(4):345-352.
47. Cooper N, Rao K, Goulden N, Webb D, Amrolia P, Veys P. The use of reduced-intensity stem cell transplantation in haemophagocytic lymphohistiocytosis and Langerhans cell histiocytosis. *Bone Marrow Transplant*. 2008;42(suppl 2):S47-S50.
48. Marsh RA, Kim MO, Liu C, et al. An intermediate alemtuzumab schedule reduces the incidence of mixed chimerism following reduced-intensity conditioning hematopoietic cell transplantation for hemophagocytic lymphohistiocytosis. *Biol Blood Marrow Transplant*. 2013;19(11):1625-1631.
49. Allen CE, Marsh R, Dawson P, et al. Reduced-intensity conditioning for hematopoietic cell transplant for HLH and primary immune deficiencies. *Blood*. 2018;132(13):1438-1451.
50. Young NS. Aplastic anemia. *N Engl J Med*. 2018;379(17):1643-1656.
51. Bacigalupo A. How I treat acquired aplastic anemia. *Blood*. 2017;129(11):1428-1436.
52. Dufour C, Pillon M, Sociè G, et al. Outcome of aplastic anaemia in children. A study by the severe aplastic anaemia and paediatric disease working parties of the European group blood and bone marrow transplant. *Br J Haematol*. 2015;169(4):565-573.
53. Storb R, Prentice RL, Thomas ED. Treatment of aplastic anemia by marrow transplantation from HLA identical siblings. Prognostic factors associated with graft versus host disease and survival. *J Clin Invest*. 1977;59(4):625-632.
54. Dufour C, Veys P, Carraro E, et al. Similar outcome of upfront-unrelated and matched sibling stem cell transplantation in idiopathic paediatric aplastic anaemia. A study on behalf of the UK Paediatric BMT Working Party, Paediatric Diseases Working Party and Severe Aplastic Anaemia Working Party of EBMT. *Br J Haematol*. 2015;171(4):585-594.
55. Wang W. Emergence of a DNA-damage response network consisting of Fanconi anaemia and BRCA proteins. *Nat Rev Genet*. 2007;8(10):735-748.
56. Hodson C, Walden H. Towards a molecular understanding of the fanconi anemia core complex. *Anemia*. 2012;2012:926787.
57. Soulier J. Fanconi anemia. *Hematology Am Soc Hematol Educ Program*. 2011;2011:492-497.
58. Alter BP, Giri N, Savage SA, Rosenberg PS. Cancer in the National Cancer Institute inherited bone marrow failure syndrome cohort after fifteen years of follow-up. *Haematologica*. 2018;103(1):30-39.
59. Gluckman E, Devergie A, Schaison G, et al. Bone marrow transplantation in Fanconi anemia. *Br J Haematol*. 1980;45(4):557-564.
60. Gluckman E, Devergie A, Dutreix J. Radiosensitivity in Fanconi anaemia: application to the conditioning regimen for bone marrow transplantation. *Br J Haematol*. 1983;54(3):431-440.
61. Berger R, Bernheim A, Gluckman E, Gisselbrecht C. In vitro effect of cyclophosphamide metabolites on chromosomes of Fanconi anaemia patients. *Br J Haematol*. 1980;45(4):565-568.
62. Gluckman E, Berger R, Dutreix J. Bone marrow transplantation for Fanconi anemia. *Semin Hematol*. 1984;21(1):20-26.
63. Farzin A, Davies SM, Smith FO, et al. Matched sibling donor haematopoietic stem cell transplantation in Fanconi anaemia: an update of the Cincinnati Children's experience. *Br J Haematol*. 2007;136(6):633-640.
64. MacMillan ML, DeFor TE, Young JA, et al. Alternative donor hematopoietic cell transplantation for Fanconi anemia. *Blood*. 2015;125(24):3798-3804.
65. Tan PL, Wagner JE, Auerbach AD, Defor TE, Slungaard A, Macmillan ML. Successful engraftment without radiation after fludarabine-based regimen in Fanconi anemia patients undergoing genotypically identical donor hematopoietic cell transplantation. *Pediatr Blood Cancer*. 2006;46(5):630-636.
66. Locatelli F, Zecca M, Pession A, et al. The outcome of children with Fanconi anemia given hematopoietic stem cell transplantation and the influence of fludarabine in the conditioning regimen: a report from the Italian pediatric group. *Haematologica*. 2007;92(10):1381-1388.
67. Gregory JJ, Jr, Wagner JE, Verlander PC, et al. Somatic mosaicism in Fanconi anemia: evidence of genotypic reversion in lymphohematopoietic stem cells. *Proc Natl Acad Sci U S A*. 2001;98(5):2532-2537.
68. Balci YI, Akdemir Y, Gumruk F, Cetin M, Arpaci F, Uckan D. CD-34 selected hematopoetic stem cell transplantation from HLA identical family members for fanconi anemia. *Pediatr Blood Cancer*. 2008;50(5):1065-1067.
69. Ayas M, Siddiqui K, Al-Jefri A, et al. Factors affecting the outcome of related allogeneic hematopoietic cell transplantation in patients with Fanconi Anemia. *Biol Blood Marrow Transplant*. 2014;20(10):1599-1603.
70. Bonfim CM, de Medeiros CR, Bitencourt MA, et al. HLA-matched related donor hematopoietic cell transplantation in 43 patients with Fanconi anemia conditioned with 60 mg/kg of cyclophosphamide. *Biol Blood Marrow Transplant*. 2007;13(12):1455-1460.
71. Bonfim CRL, Bitencourt M, Zanis-Neto J, et al. HLA matched related bone marrow transplantation in 85 patients with fanconi anemia: the Brazilian experience using cyclophosphamide 60Mg/kg. *Biol Blood Marrow Transplant*. 2012;18(2 suppl):S209.
72. Peffault de Latour R, Porcher R, Dalle JH, et al. Allogeneic hematopoietic stem cell transplantation in Fanconi anemia: the European Group for Blood and Marrow Transplantation experience. *Blood*. 2013;122(26):4279-4286.
73. Ebens CL, MacMillan ML, Wagner JE. Hematopoietic cell transplantation in Fanconi anemia: current evidence, challenges and recommendations. *Expet Rev Hematol*. 2017;10(1):81-97.
74. Gluckman E, Auerbach AD, Horowitz MM, et al. Bone marrow transplantation for Fanconi anemia. *Blood*. 1995;86(7):2856-2862.
75. Guardiola P, Pasquini R, Dokal I, et al. Outcome of 69 allogeneic stem cell transplantations for Fanconi anemia using HLA-matched unrelated donors: a study on behalf of the European Group for Blood and Marrow Transplantation. *Blood*. 2000;95(2):422-429.
76. MacMillan ML, Auerbach AD, Davies SM, et al. Haemopoietic cell transplantation in patients with Fanconi anaemia using alternate donors: results of a total body irradiation dose escalation trial. *Br J Haematol*. 2000;109(1):121-129.
77. Wagner JE, Eapen M, MacMillan ML, et al. Unrelated donor bone marrow transplantation for the treatment of Fanconi anemia. *Blood*. 2007;109(5):2256-2262.
78. Mehta PA, Davies SM, Leemhuis T, et al.. Radiation-free, alternative-donor HCT for Fanconi anemia patients: results from a prospective multi-institutional study. *Blood*. 2017;129(16):2308-2315.
79. Gluckman E, Broxmeyer HA, Auerbach AD, et al. Hematopoietic reconstitution in a patient with Fanconi's anemia by means of umbilical-cord blood from an HLA-identical sibling. *N Engl J Med*. 1989;321(17):1174-1178.
80. Gluckman E, Rocha V, Ionescu I, et al. Results of unrelated cord blood transplant in fanconi anemia patients: risk factor analysis for engraftment and survival. *Biol Blood Marrow Transplant*. 2007;13(9):1073-1082.
81. Gluckman E. Improving survival for Fanconi anemia patients. *Blood*. 2015;125(24):3676.
82. Bonfim C, Ribeiro L, Nichele S, et al. Haploidentical bone marrow transplantation with post-transplant cyclophosphamide for children and adolescents with fanconi anemia. *Biol Blood Marrow Transplant*. 2017;23(2):310-317.
83. Bonfim C, Ribeiro L, Nichele S, et al. Haploidentical bone marrow transplantation with post-transplant cyclophosphamide for children and adolescents with fanconi anemia. *Biol Blood Marrow Transplant*. 2016;23(2):310-317.

84. Thakar MS, Bonfim C, Sandmaier BM, et al. Cyclophosphamide-based in vivo T-cell depletion for HLA-haploidentical transplantation in Fanconi anemia. *Pediatr Hematol Oncol*. 2012;29(6):568-578.
85. Strocchio L, Pagliara D, Algeri M, et al. HLA-haploidentical TCRalphabeta+/CD19+-depleted stem cell transplantation in children and young adults with Fanconi anemia. *Blood Adv*. 2021;5(5):1333-1339.
86. Zecca M, Strocchio L, Pagliara D, et al. HLA-haploidentical T cell-depleted allogeneic hematopoietic stem cell transplantation in children with Fanconi anemia. *Biol Blood Marrow Transplant*. 2014;20(4):571-576.
87. Mitchell R, Wagner JE, Hirsch B, DeFor TE, Zierhut H, MacMillan ML. Haematopoietic cell transplantation for acute leukaemia and advanced myelodysplastic syndrome in Fanconi anaemia. *Br J Haematol*. 2014;164(3):384-395.
88. Peffault de Latour R, Soulier J. How I treat MDS and AML in Fanconi anemia. *Blood*. 2016;127(24):2971-2979.
89. Ayas M, Saber W, Davies SM, et al. Allogeneic hematopoietic cell transplantation for fanconi anemia in patients with pretransplantation cytogenetic abnormalities, myelodysplastic syndrome, or acute leukemia. *J Clin Oncol*. 2013;31(13):1669-1676.
90. Soulier J, Leblanc T, Larghero J, et al. Detection of somatic mosaicism and classification of Fanconi anemia patients by analysis of the FA/BRCA pathway. *Blood*. 2005;105(3):1329-1336.
91. Rio P, Navarro S, Wang W, et al. Successful engraftment of gene-corrected hematopoietic stem cells in non-conditioned patients with Fanconi anemia. *Nat Med*. 2019;25(9):1396-1401.
92. Kelly PF, Radtke S, von Kalle C, et al. Stem cell collection and gene transfer in Fanconi anemia. *Mol Ther*. 2007;15(1):211-219.
93. Adair JE, Becker PS, Chandrasekaran D, et al. Gene therapy for fanconi anemia in Seattle: clinical experience and next steps. *Blood*. 2016;128(22):3510.
94. Shafqat S, Tariq E, Parnes AD, Dasouki MJ, Ahmed SO, Hashmi SK. Role of gene therapy in Fanconi anemia: a systematic and literature review with future directions. *Hematology Oncol Stem Cell Ther*. 2021;14(4):290-301.
95. Richardson CD, Kazane KR, Feng SJ, et al. CRISPR-Cas9 genome editing in human cells occurs via the Fanconi anemia pathway. *Nat Genet*. 2018;50(8):1132-1139.
96. Waisfisz Q, Morgan NV, Savino M, et al. Spontaneous functional correction of homozygous fanconi anaemia alleles reveals novel mechanistic basis for reverse mosaicism. *Nat Genet*. 1999;22(4):379-383.
97. Roman-Rodriguez FJ, Ugalde L, Alvarez L, et al. NHEJ-mediated repair of CRISPR-cas9-induced DNA breaks efficiently corrects mutations in HSPCs from patients with fanconi anemia. *Cell Stem Cell*. 2019;25(5):607-621 e607.
98. Rosenberg PS, Alter BP, Ebell W. Cancer risks in fanconi anemia: findings from the German fanconi anemia registry. *Haematologica*. 2008;93(4):511-517.
99. Alter BP, Giri N, Savage SA, et al. Malignancies and survival patterns in the National Cancer Institute inherited bone marrow failure syndromes cohort study. *Br J Haematol*. 2010;150(2):179-188.
100. Rosenberg PS, Socie G, Alter BP, Gluckman E. Risk of head and neck squamous cell cancer and death in patients with Fanconi anemia who did and did not receive transplants. *Blood*. 2005;105(1):67-73.
101. Socie G, Devergie A, Girinski T, et al. Transplantation for Fanconi's anaemia: long-term follow-up of fifty patients transplanted from a sibling donor after low-dose cyclophosphamide and thoraco-abdominal irradiation for conditioning. *Br J Haematol*. 1998;103(1):249-255.
102. Ruggeri A, Peffault de Latour R, Carmagnat M, et al. Outcomes, infections, and immune reconstitution after double cord blood transplantation in patients with high-risk hematological diseases. *Transpl Infect Dis*. 2011;13(5):456-465.
103. Barnum JL, Petryk A, Zhang L, et al. Endocrinopathies, bone health, and insulin resistance in patients with Fanconi anemia after hematopoietic cell transplantation. *Biol Blood Marrow Transplant*. 2016;22(8):1487-1492.
104. Anur P, Friedman DN, Sklar C, et al. Late effects in patients with Fanconi anemia following allogeneic hematopoietic stem cell transplantation from alternative donors. *Bone Marrow Transplant*. 2016;51(7):938-944.
105. Hoppe CC. Newborn screening for hemoglobin disorders. *Hemoglobin*. 2011;35(5-6):556-564.
106. Thomas ED, Buckner CD, Sanders JE, et al. Marrow transplantation for thalassaemia. *Lancet*. 1982;2(8292):227-229.
107. Lucarelli G, Gaziev J. Advances in the allogeneic transplantation for thalassemia. *Blood Rev*. 2008;22(2):53-63.
108. Johnson FL, Look AT, Gockerman J, Ruggiero MR, Dalla-Pozza L, Billings FT,IIIrd. Bone-marrow transplantation in a patient with sickle-cell anemia. *N Engl J Med*. 1984;311(12):780-783.
109. Vermylen C, Fernandez Robles E, Ninane J, Cornu G. Bone marrow transplantation in five children with sickle cell anaemia. *Lancet*. 1988;1(8600):1427-1428.
110. Angelucci E, Matthes-Martin S, Baronciani D, et al. Hematopoietic stem cell transplantation in thalassemia major and sickle cell disease: indications and management recommendations from an international expert panel. *Haematologica*. 2014;99(5):811-820.
111. Horan JT, Haight A, Dioguardi JL, et al. Using fludarabine to reduce exposure to alkylating agents in children with sickle cell disease receiving busulfan, cyclophosphamide, and antithymocyte globulin transplant conditioning: results of a dose de-escalation trial. *Biol Blood Marrow Transplant*. 2015;21(5):900-905.
112. Baronciani D, Angelucci E, Potschger U, et al. Hemopoietic stem cell transplantation in thalassemia: a report from the European Society for Blood and Bone Marrow Transplantation Hemoglobinopathy Registry, 2000-2010. *Bone Marrow Transplant*. 2016;51(4):536-541.
113. Sabloff M, Chandy M, Wang Z, et al. HLA-matched sibling bone marrow transplantation for beta-thalassemia major. *Blood*. 2011;117(5):1745-1750.
114. Lucarelli G, Galimberti M, Polchi P, et al. Bone marrow transplantation in patients with thalassemia. *N Engl J Med*. 1990;322(7):417-421.
115. Locatelli F, Kabbara N, Ruggeri A, et al. Outcome of patients with hemoglobinopathies given either cord blood or bone marrow transplantation from an HLA-identical sibling. *Blood*. 2013;122(6):1072-1078.
116. Li C, Mathews V, Kim S, et al. Related and unrelated donor transplantation for beta-thalassemia major: results of an international survey. *Blood Adv*. 2019;3(17):2562-2570.
117. Manna M, Nesci S, Andreani M, Tonucci P, Lucarelli G. Influence of the conditioning regimens on the incidence of mixed chimerism in thalassemic transplanted patients. *Bone Marrow Transplant*. 1993;12(suppl 1):70-73.
118. Sodani P, Gaziev D, Polchi P, et al. New approach for bone marrow transplantation in patients with class 3 thalassemia aged younger than 17 years. *Blood*. 2004;104(4):1201-1203.
119. Gaziev J, Isgro A, Sodani P, et al. Optimal outcomes in young class 3 patients with thalassemia undergoing HLA-identical sibling bone marrow transplantation. *Transplantation*. 2016;100(4):925-932.
120. Luftinger R, Zubarovskaya N, Galimard JE, et al. Busulfan-fludarabine- or treosulfan-fludarabine-based myeloablative conditioning for children with thalassemia major. *Ann Hematol*. 2022;101(3):655-665.
121. Gaziev D, Galimberti M, Lucarelli G, et al. Bone marrow transplantation from alternative donors for thalassemia: HLA-phenotypically identical relative and HLA-nonidentical sibling or parent transplants. *Bone Marrow Transplant*. 2000;25(8):815-821.
122. Bernardo ME, Piras E, Vacca A, et al. Allogeneic hematopoietic stem cell transplantation in thalassemia major: results of a reduced-toxicity conditioning regimen based on the use of treosulfan. *Blood*. 2012;120(2):473-476.
123. Anurathapan U, Pakakasama S, Mekjaruskul P, et al. Outcomes of thalassemia patients undergoing hematopoietic stem cell transplantation by using a standard myeloablative versus a novel reduced-toxicity conditioning regimen according to a new risk stratification. *Biol Blood Marrow Transplant*. 2014;20(12):2066-2071.
124. Sheth V, Grisariu S, Avni B, et al. Fludarabine-based reduced toxicity yet myeloablative conditioning is effective and safe particularly in patients with high-risk thalassemia undergoing allogeneic transplantation. *Pediatr Blood Cancer*. 2018;65(11):e27312.
125. Khandelwal P, Yeh RF, Yu L, et al. Graft-versus-host disease prophylaxis with abatacept reduces severe acute graft-versus-host disease in allogeneic hematopoietic stem cell transplant for beta-thalassemia major with busulfan, fludarabine, and thiotepa. *Transplantation*. 2021;105(4):891-896.
126. Walters MC, Patience M, Leisenring W, et al. Bone marrow transplantation for sickle cell disease [see comments]. *N Engl J Med*. 1996;335(6):369-376.
127. Vermylen C, Cornu G, Ferster A, et al. Haematopoietic stem cell transplantation for sickle cell anaemia: the first 50 patients transplanted in Belgium. *Bone Marrow Transplant*. 1998;22(1):1-6.
128. Bernaudin F, Socie G, Kuentz M, et al. Long-term results of related myeloablative stem-cell transplantation to cure sickle cell disease. *Blood*. 2007;110(7):2749-2756.
129. Steinberg MH, McCarthy WF, Castro O, et al. The risks and benefits of long-term use of hydroxyurea in sickle cell anemia: a 17.5 year follow-up. *Am J Hematol*. 2010;85(6):403-408.
130. Platt OS, Brambilla DJ, Rosse WF, et al. Mortality in sickle cell disease. Life expectancy and risk factors for early death. *N Engl J Med*. 1994;330(23):1639-1644.
131. Wierenga KJ, Hambleton IR, Lewis NA. Survival estimates for patients with homozygous sickle-cell disease in Jamaica: a clinic-based population study. *Lancet*. 2001;357(9257):680-683.
132. DeBaun MR, Ghafuri DL, Rodeghier M, et al. Decreased median survival of adults with sickle cell disease after adjusting for left truncation bias: a pooled analysis. *Blood*. 2019;133(6):615-617.
133. Gluckman E, Cappelli B, Bernaudin F, et al. Sickle cell disease: an international survey of results of HLA-identical sibling hematopoietic stem cell transplantation. *Blood*. 2016;129(11):1548-1556.
134. Bhatia M, Jin Z, Baker C, et al. Reduced toxicity, myeloablative conditioning with BU, fludarabine, alemtuzumab and SCT from sibling donors in children with sickle cell disease. *Bone Marrow Transplant*. 2014;49(7):913-920.
135. Alzahrani M, Damlaj M, Jeffries N, et al. Non-myeloablative human leukocyte antigen-matched related donor transplantation in sickle cell disease: outcomes from three independent centres. *Br J Haematol*. 2021;192(4):761-768.
136. Shenoy S, Eapen M, Panepinto JA, et al. A trial of unrelated donor marrow transplantation for children with severe sickle cell disease. *Blood*. 2016;128(21):2561-2567.
137. Krishnamurti L, Neuberg DS, Sullivan KM, et al. Bone marrow transplantation for adolescents and young adults with sickle cell disease: results of a prospective multicenter pilot study. *Am J Hematol*. 2019;94(4):446-454.
138. Guilcher GMT, Monagel DA, Nettel-Aguirre A, et al. Nonmyeloablative matched sibling donor hematopoietic cell transplantation in children and adolescents with sickle cell disease. *Biol Blood Marrow Transplant*. 2019;25(6):1179-1186.
139. Bernaudin F, Robin M, Ferry C, et al. Related myeloablative stem cell transplantation (SCT) to cure sickle cell anemia (SCA): update of French results. *Blood*. 2010;116(21):3518.
140. Bernaudin F, Dalle JH, Bories D, et al. Long-term event-free survival, chimerism and fertility outcomes in 234 patients with sickle-cell anemia younger than 30 years after myeloablative conditioning and matched-sibling transplantation in France. *Haematologica*. 2020;105(1):91-101.

141. Bernaudin F, Verlhac S, Peffault de Latour R, et al. Association of matched sibling donor hematopoietic stem cell transplantation with transcranial Doppler velocities in children with sickle cell anemia. *JAMA*. 2019;321(3):266-276.
142. Verlhac S, Gabor F, Paillard C, et al. Improved stenosis outcome in stroke-free sickle cell anemia children after transplantation compared to chronic transfusion. *Br J Haematol*. 2021;193(1):188-193.
143. Gluckman E, Cappelli B, Bernaudin F, et al. Sickle cell disease: an international survey of results of HLA-identical sibling hematopoietic stem cell transplantation. *Blood*. 2017;129(11):1548-1556.
144. Brazauskas R, Scigliuolo GM, Wang HL, et al. Risk score to predict event-free survival after hematopoietic cell transplant for sickle cell disease. *Blood*. 2020;136(5):623-626.
145. Gaziev J, Isgro A, Mozzi AF, et al. New insights into the pharmacokinetics of intravenous busulfan in children with sickle cell anemia undergoing bone marrow transplantation. *Pediatr Blood Cancer*. 2015;62(4):680-686.
146. Andreani M, Testi M, Gaziev J, et al. Quantitatively different red cell/nucleated cell chimerism in patients with long-term, persistent hematopoietic mixed chimerism after bone marrow transplantation for thalassemia major or sickle cell disease. *Haematologica*. 2011;96(1):128-133.
147. Walters MC, Patience M, Leisenring W, et al. Stable mixed hematopoietic chimerism after bone marrow transplantation for sickle cell anemia. *Biol Blood Marrow Transplant*. 2001;7(12):665-673.
148. Andreani M, Manna M, Lucarelli G, et al. Persistence of mixed chimerism in patients transplanted for the treatment of thalassemia. *Blood*. 1996;87(8):3494-3499.
149. Battaglia M, Andreani M, Manna M, et al. Coexistence of two functioning T-cell repertoires in healthy ex-thalassemics bearing a persistent mixed chimerism years after bone marrow transplantation. *Blood*. 1999;94(10):3432-3438.
150. Fitzhugh CD, Cordes S, Taylor T, et al. At least 20% donor myeloid chimerism is necessary to reverse the sickle phenotype after allogeneic HSCT. *Blood*. 2017;130(17):1946-1948.
151. Iannone R, Casella JF, Fuchs EJ, et al. Results of minimally toxic nonmyeloablative transplantation in patients with sickle cell anemia and beta-thalassemia. *Biol Blood Marrow Transplant*. 2003;9(8):519-528.
152. Horan JT, Liesveld JL, Fenton P, Blumberg N, Walters MC. Hematopoietic stem cell transplantation for multiply transfused patients with sickle cell disease and thalassemia after low-dose total body irradiation, fludarabine, and rabbit anti-thymocyte globulin. *Bone Marrow Transplant*. 2005;35(2):171-177.
153. Hsieh MM, Fitzhugh CD, Weitzel RP, et al. Nonmyeloablative HLA-matched sibling allogeneic hematopoietic stem cell transplantation for severe sickle cell phenotype. *JAMA*. 2014;312(1):48-56.
154. Bolanos-Meade J, Cooke KR, Gamper CJ, et al. Effect of increased dose of total body irradiation on graft failure associated with HLA-haploidentical transplantation in patients with severe haemoglobinopathies: a prospective clinical trial. *Lancet Haematol*. 2019;6(4):e183-e193.
155. Anurathapan U, Hongeng S, Pakakasama S, et al. Hematopoietic stem cell transplantation for severe thalassemia patients from haploidentical donors using a novel conditioning regimen. *Biol Blood Marrow Transplant*. 2020;26(6):1106-1112.
156. Merli P, Pagliara D, Galaverna F, et al. TCRalphabeta/CD19 depleted HSCT from an HLA-haploidentical relative to treat children with different nonmalignant disorders. *Blood Adv*. 2022;6(1):281-292.
157. Gaziev J, Isgro A, Sodani P, et al. Haploidentical HSCT for hemoglobinopathies: improved outcomes with TCRalphabeta(+)/CD19(+)-depleted grafts. *Blood Adv*. 2018;2(3):263-270.
158. Bolaños-Meade J, Fuchs EJ, Luznik L, et al. HLA-haploidentical bone marrow transplantation with posttransplant cyclophosphamide expands the donor pool for patients with sickle cell disease. *Blood*. 2012;120(22):4285-4291.
159. Orkin SH, Bauer DE. Emerging genetic therapy for sickle cell disease. *Annu Rev Med*. 2019;70:257-271.
160. Esrick EB, Lehmann LE, Biffi A, et al. Post-transcriptional genetic Silencing of BCL11A to treat sickle cell disease. *N Engl J Med*. 2021;384(3):205-215.
161. Frangoul H, Altshuler D, Cappellini MD, et al. CRISPR-Cas9 gene editing for sickle cell disease and beta-thalassemia. *N Engl J Med*. 2021;384(3):252-260.
162. Tisdale JF, Pierciey FJ, Jr, Bonner M, et al. Safety and feasibility of hematopoietic progenitor stem cell collection by mobilization with plerixafor followed by apheresis vs bone marrow harvest in patients with sickle cell disease in the multi-center HGB-206 trial. *Am J Hematol*. 2020;95(9):E239-E242.
163. Thompson AA, Walters MC, Kwiatkowski J, et al. Gene therapy in patients with transfusion-dependent β-thalassemia. *N Engl J Med*. 2018;378(16):1479-1493.
164. Locatelli F, Thompson AA, Kwiatkowski JL, et al. Betibeglogene autotemcel gene therapy for non-β(0)/β(0) genotype β-thalassemia. *N Engl J Med*. 2022;386(5):415-427.
165. Kanter J, Walters MC, Krishnamurti L, et al. Biologic and clinical efficacy of LentiGlobin for sickle cell disease. *N Engl J Med*. 2022;386(7):617-628.
166. Goyal S, Tisdale J, Schmidt M, et al. Acute myeloid leukemia case after gene therapy for sickle cell disease. *N Engl J Med*. 2022;386(2):138-147.
167. Hsieh MM, Bonner M, Pierciey FJ, et al. Myelodysplastic syndrome unrelated to lentiviral vector in a patient treated with gene therapy for sickle cell disease. *Blood Adv*. 2020;4(9):2058-2063.
168. Jones RJ, DeBaun MR. Leukemia after gene therapy for sickle cell disease: insertional mutagenesis, busulfan, both, or neither. *Blood*. 2021;138(11):942-947.
169. Ghannam JY, Xu X, Maric I, et al. Baseline TP53 mutations in adults with SCD developing myeloid malignancy following hematopoietic cell transplantation. *Blood*. 2020;135(14):1185-1188.
170. Lucarelli G, Angelucci E, Giardini C, et al. Fate of iron stores in thalassaemia after bone-marrow transplantation. *Lancet*. 1993;342(8884):1388-1391.
171. Angelucci E, Muretto P, Nicolucci A, et al. Effects of iron overload and hepatitis C virus positivity in determining progression of liver fibrosis in thalassemia following bone marrow transplantation. *Blood*. 2002;100(1):17-21.
172. Muretto P, Angelucci E, Lucarelli G. Reversibility of cirrhosis in patients cured of thalassemia by bone marrow transplantation. *Ann Intern Med*. 2002;136(9):667-672.
173. Angelucci E, Muretto P, Lucarelli G, et al. Treatment of iron overload in the "ex-thalassemic". Report from the phlebotomy program. *Ann N Y Acad Sci*. 1998;850:288-293.
174. Hernigou P, Bernaudin F, Reinert P, Kuentz M, Vernant JP. Bone-marrow transplantation in sickle-cell disease. Effect on osteonecrosis: a case report with a four-year follow-up. *J Bone Joint Surg Am*. 1997;79(11):1726-1730.
175. Ferster A, Bujan W, Corazza F, et al. Bone marrow transplantation corrects the splenic reticuloendothelial dysfunction in sickle cell anemia. *Blood*. 1993;81(4):1102-1105.
176. Nickel RS, Seashore E, Lane PA, et al. Improved splenic function after hematopoietic stem cell transplant for sickle cell disease. *Pediatr Blood Cancer*. 2016;63(5):908-913.
177. Bhatia M, Kolva E, Cimini L, et al. Health-related quality of life after allogeneic hematopoietic stem cell transplantation for sickle cell disease. *Biol Blood Marrow Transplant*. 2015;21(4):666-672.
178. Badawy SM, Beg U, Liem RI, Chaudhury S, Thompson AA. A systematic review of quality of life in sickle cell disease and thalassemia after stem cell transplant or gene therapy. *Blood Adv*. 2021;5(2):570-583.
179. Li Y, Maule J, Neff JL, et al. Myeloid neoplasms in the setting of sickle cell disease: an intrinsic association with the underlying condition rather than a coincidence; report of 4 cases and review of the literature. *Mod Pathol*. 2019;32(12):1712-1726.
180. Eapen M, Brazauskas R, Walters MC, et al. Effect of donor type and conditioning regimen intensity on allogeneic transplantation outcomes in patients with sickle cell disease: a retrospective multicentre, cohort study. *Lancet Haematol*. 2019;6(11):e585-e596.
181. Brunson A, Keegan THM, Bang H, Mahajan A, Paulukonis S, Wun T. Increased risk of leukemia among sickle cell disease patients in California. *Blood*. 2017;130(13):1597-1599.
182. Seminog OO, Ogunlaja OI, Yeates D, Goldacre MJ. Risk of individual malignant neoplasms in patients with sickle cell disease: English national record linkage study. *J R Soc Med*. 2016;109(8):303-309.
183. De Sanctis V. Growth and puberty and its management in thalassaemia. *Horm Res*. 2002;58(suppl 1):72-79.
184. Raiola G, Galati MC, De Sanctis V, et al. Growth and puberty in thalassemia major. *J Pediatr Endocrinol Metab*. 2003;16(suppl 2):259-266.
185. Walters MC, Hardy K, Edwards S, et al. Pulmonary, gonadal, and central nervous system status after bone marrow transplantation for sickle cell disease. *Biol Blood Marrow Transplant*. 2010;16(2):263-272.
186. Eggleston B, Patience M, Edwards S, et al. Effect of myeloablative bone marrow transplantation on growth in children with sickle cell anaemia: results of the multicenter study of haematopoietic cell transplantation for sickle cell anaemia. *Br J Haematol*. 2007;136(4):673-676.
187. Wang WC, Helms RW, Lynn HS, et al. Effect of hydroxyurea on growth in children with sickle cell anemia: results of the HUG-KIDS Study. *J Pediatr*. 2002;140(2):225-229.
188. Platt OS, Rosenstock W, Espeland MA. Influence of sickle hemoglobinopathies on growth and development. *N Engl J Med*. 1984;311(1):7-12.

Chapter 106 ■ Hematopoietic Cell Transplantation for Hematologic Malignancies

BHAGIRATHBHAI DHOLARIA • JENNIFER MARVIN-PEEK • BIPIN N. SAVANI

INTRODUCTION

Allogeneic hematopoietic cell transplantation (allo-HCT) is the oldest and most widely used form of immunotherapy for many hematological diseases. Despite rapid improvement in non-transplant therapies, we are seeing more patients undergoing allo-HCT than ever before. Per the Center for International Blood and Marrow Transplant Research (CIBMTR) database, greater than 254,663 autologous, 251,053 allogeneic donor, and 15,057 cord blood transplantation have been reported through 2018.[1] Success of allo-HCT hinges on reducing the risk of disease relapse after transplant and minimizing transplant-related mortality (TRM) by improvement in prevention and management of short- and long-term transplant complications. Scientific and clinical advances in supportive care, donor selection, and conditioning regimens have resulted in lower TRM, extension of care to a wider population of patients and improvements in survival of transplant recipients. While graft-vs-host disease (GVHD) and relapse posttransplant remain profound challenges, the future holds great promise as the underlying molecular mechanisms of disease are unpicked to allow manipulation for therapeutic benefit.

Significant advances have been made in immunology and mechanisms of graft tolerance in recent years. Timely availability of an acceptable stem cell donor is a key consideration when planning allo-HCT. The prime considerations in donor selection are the degree of matching at the human leukocyte antigen (HLA) loci and the need to identify the best match for the patient within a clinically meaningful timeframe. Traditionally, an HLA-identical matched sibling donor (MSD) is preferred over an unrelated donor from the transplant registry. Finding a suitable donor remains an important challenge for racial and ethnic minorities. The use of posttransplant cyclophosphamide (PTCy) has significantly improved the outcomes of allo-HCT from a partially matched related (haploidentical) or unrelated donor.[2,3] PTCy use is rapidly expanding across donor types and malignancies with encouraging outcomes in recently completed prospective studies,[4,5] which has significantly expanded the potential donor pool.

Chronic GVHD (cGVHD) is a complication of HCT largely mediated by donor lymphocytes and may have profound effects on physical and mental health with a consequent reduction in quality of life (QoL) and survival.[6] Depletion of T lymphocytes in the donor graft may be achieved by ex vivo manipulation or by incorporation of antithymocyte globulin or alemtuzumab into the conditioning regimen. In practice, disease-free survival (DFS) is often similar in T-deplete or T-replete regimens as the reduction in cGVHD mortality is offset by increased relapse incidence (RI). Current trials are comparing outcomes using newer T-cell depletion approaches to those achieved using PTCy. We have also seen successful treatment options for steroid-refractory/dependent acute and chronic GVHD with approval of ruxolitinib, ibrutinib, and belumosudil.[7-10]

Disease relapse after transplant remains a major concern. Routine use of genomic sequencing and measurable residual disease (MRD) testing have allowed better pretransplant risk-stratification. Presence of MRD before or after transplant significantly increases the risk of disease relapse across hematological malignancies. Multiple strategies are being developed to deepen the disease control before conditioning therapy. Similarly, MRD-guided posttransplant therapies such has donor lymphocyte infusion (DLI), hypomethylating agents (HMAs), and targeted therapies are being studied as ways to reduce the relapse risk. Multiple prospective phase 3 studies are underway, which will better define posttransplant management in upcoming years.

The development of reduced-intensity (RIC) and nonmyeloablative (NMA) conditioning regimens has allowed transplant in older patients with comorbidities. Improved disease-related outcomes were seen in carefully selected patients above age 60 years who underwent transplant in prospective studies.[11,12] A widely applied method of assessing a patient's general health is the hematopoietic cell transplantation comorbidity index (HCT-CI).[13] The HCT-CI computes clinical data collected in the peritransplant timeframe to predict survival posttransplant. The index has a numerical scoring system with zero indicating the absence of significant comorbidity and values of one or more representing increasing degrees of comorbidity. Currently ongoing, bone marrow transplantation (BMT) CTN 1704 (CHARM) study is using composite heath assessment comprised of pre-HCT comorbidity, geriatric assessment, and biomarkers to predict non-relapse mortality (NRM) after allo-HCT in older patients.

Major advances in cellular engineering have resulted in the development of highly effective adoptive cellular therapies such as chimeric antigen receptor T cell (CAR T) therapy. Multiple CAR T agents have been approved by the regulatory agencies across the globe to treat relapsed/refractory hematological malignancies. These therapies are already changing the treatment landscape of non-Hodgkin lymphoma (NHL), acute lymphoblastic leukemia (ALL), and multiple myeloma (MM). The role of traditional auto-/allo-HCT in many hematological malignancies is being redefined by these novel therapies.

MYELOID MALIGNANCIES

Acute Myeloid Leukemia

Acute myeloid leukemia (AML) is the most common indication for allo-HCT worldwide.[14] Allo-HCT is curative for some patients with AML and assessment of the potential benefit to an individual patient needs to start at diagnosis so that HCT outcome is not compromised by undue delay. This assessment should integrate disease risk, patient's co-morbidities, and the wishes of the patient following counseling.

AML is a genetically heterogeneous disease with wide-ranging treatment outcomes. The 2017 European Leukemia Net (ELN) risk-stratification by genetics recognizes three categories of risk that predict outcome with long-term CR achieved in 60% to 70% of the favorable risk group but only 15% to 20% in the adverse risk group.[15] Treatment of newly diagnosed AML has recently seen significant advances with development of drugs targeting FMS-like tyrosine kinase 3 (*FLT3*), isocitrate dehydrogenase (*IDH*), and B-cell lymphoma 2 inhibitor (*BCL2*, venetoclax).[16] These therapies have enabled patients with high-risk AML to achieve complete remission (CR) and undergo subsequent all-HCT. Treatment response and MRD clearance have emerged as important prognostic makers regardless of cytogenetic risk group.[17-19] Patients with persistent or early recurrence of MRD despite apparent morphological CR after induction therapy should be offered salvage chemotherapy or intervene with allo-HCT.[20,21]

Acute Myeloid Leukemia in First Remission

Treatment of newly diagnosed AML consists of remission induction followed by various consolidation therapies. The decision for chemotherapy consolidation vs allo-HCT after achieving first complete remission (CR1) is based on probability of disease relapse and expected TRM from allo-HCT. A meta-analysis of 24 intent-to-treat trials showed significantly better relapse-free survival (RFS) with allo-HCT in CR1 in patients with adverse- and intermediate-risk compared to continued chemotherapy, whereas such a benefit was not obvious in patients with favorable-risk cytogenetics.[22] Several prospective studies have also shown a consistent benefit of allo-HCT in CR1 for adverse- and intermediate risk but no benefit for favorable-risk AML.[23-25] Patients with AML with a high risk of relapse (>40%) should generally be offered allo-HCT in an effort to improve their survival probabilities.[26] Delay until a CR2 is detrimental as a second CR is by no means assured and outcomes of allo-HCT in CR2 are generally poorer than CR1.[27] Decisions about HCT in intermediate-risk AML are less clear-cut and must consider patient fitness, availability of a sibling donor, or a well-matched unrelated donor (MUD) at high resolution and the availability of a clinical trial as well as the transplant center experience.[28,29] It is accepted that, in general, patients with favorable risk disease will not benefit from HCT in CR1 due to their relatively low risk of relapse of 10% to 35% balanced against the risk of TRM.[30] Such patients would be candidates for allo-HCT after relapse.[22,23] A subset of core-binding (transcription) factor-AML with high-risk features such as high white blood cell (WBC) at diagnosis[31,32] therapy-related disease,[33,34] associated mutations involving *KIT* or *FLT3-ITD* or *NRAS*,[35,36] and presence of MRD[37] might benefit from HCT in CR1.

Routine use of next-generation sequencing (NGS) has allowed better risk-stratification of AML and information on myeloid mutations is increasingly being used to guide therapeutic decisions. Per 2017 ELN stratification, AML with unmutated *NPM1* plus high-allelic ratio *FLT3-ITD*, *RUNX1*, *ASXL1*, or *TP53* mutations is considered adverse risk given poor outcomes with chemotherapy alone and allo-HCT in CR1 should be considered for these patients.[38,39] Initial studies showed very high relapse risk after allo-HCT resulting in long-term DFS of only 10% to 15% in AML with *TP53* mutation.[40] However, the interaction appears to be dependent on mono-/biallelic loss of TP53 gene, co-occurring mutations and cytogenetic abnormalities.[41-43] Complex interactions between myeloid mutations, chromosomal abnormalities, and patient-related factors make it difficult to accurately risk-stratify AML and larger prospective and registry-based studies are needed to determine the role of allo-HCT across various genomic sub-groups.

Allo-HCT may improve outcomes of patients with persistent MRD after induction therapy. In the AML17 trial, allo-HCT appeared to benefit standard-risk patients without *NPM1* who were mutations MRD$^+$ but not MRD negative (MRD$^-$) patients.[19] The GIMEMA AML1310 study utilized "MRD-guided risk-adapted" approach to assign allo-HCT vs auto-HCT in patients with intermediate-risk AML and showed comparable overall survival (OS) between MRD$^+$ and MRD$^-$ groups suggesting the benefit of allo-HCT in high-risk MRD$^+$ patients.[44] In a prospective study of AML with t(8;21), allo-HCT resulted in better DFS in the MRD$^+$ cohort compared to chemotherapy consolidation.[45]

Allogeneic Hematopoietic Cell Transplantation in Primary Refractory AML

About 8% to 20% of selected patients who fail to respond to induction therapy may be salvaged by early allo-HCT.[46,47] In a registry-based study, the following factors were associated with poor transplant outcomes of AML in relapse or with primary induction failure: first CR duration less than 6 months, donor other than HLA-identical sibling, circulating blasts, adverse-risk cytogenetics, and Karnofsky or Lansky score <90. In this study, 3-year OS ranged from 42% (score = 0) to 6% (score ≥ 3).[48] Attempt should be made to achieve some level of disease control before proceeding with allo-HCT. One such approach is using sequential chemotherapy as part of their conditioning regimen which may circumvent the need for multiple courses of chemotherapy to achieve remission prior to transplant.[49]

Allogeneic Hematopoietic Cell Transplantation in Relapsed, Therapy-Related, and Secondary AML

Relapse occurs in about half of patients with nonpromyelocytic AML under the age of 60 and 80% to 90% of those over 60 years.[50] Five-year OS for patients after first relapse is about 10%.[51] Advances in the understanding of the biology of the AML stem cell may eventually permit earlier and more accurate identification of patients destined to relapse. Ultimately, HCT will continue to be used more discriminately in CR1 for those who are most in need and are most likely to benefit. In the meantime, patients who relapse should be considered for allo-HCT. Survival rates after myeloablative (MA) allo-HCT for AML CR2 are about 40% to 50%.[52] However, CR2 and prolonged OS is often difficult to achieve and predicted by the duration of CR1, cytogenetics at diagnosis, age at relapse, prior HCT, and *FLT3-ITD* status.[53,54] Relapsed AML after allo-HCT carries a very poor prognosis with long-term survival less than 10%. Traditional salvage therapies are poorly tolerated in the post-allo setting given limited organ reserve and concurrent immunosuppression. These patients should be offered novel targeted or HMA-based therapies followed by consolidation of DLI or second allo-HCT. Outcomes were comparable between these two strategies in a registry-based observational study.[55]

Therapy-related (t-AML) and secondary AML (s-AML) arising from a previous myeloid malignancy have a significantly poorer prognosis compared to de novo AML. These AML subtypes are commonly associated with high-risk genomic profile characterized by poor response to standard induction therapy. These patients are less likely to receive allo-HCT due to early mortality during induction therapy, lower CR rates, and comorbidities from prior malignancy treatment. In a CIBMTR analysis, the 5-year outcomes were 48% NRM, 31% RI, 21% leukemia-free survival (LFS), and 22% OS after allo-HCT for t-AML and t-myelodysplastic syndrome (MDS). Lower OS was seen among patients with age > 35 years, adverse-risk cytogenetics, active disease at the time of allo-HCT, and transplant from an unrelated donor.[56] Preferential use of myeloablative (MAC) conditioning in eligible patient with s-AML may improve the outcomes of allo-HCT over RIC regimens.[57]

Autologous Hematopoietic Cell Transplantation in AML

Auto-HCT has been used infrequently in recent years but may be considered as postremission therapy in patients who are MRD negative and do not have high-risk disease.[58] Consolidation with auto-HCT may therefore be an option for patients in MRD-negative intermediate-risk AML in CR1 who do not have an HLA-matched sibling or in acute promyelocytic leukemia (APL) in CR2.[59,60] In a prospective randomized study, auto-HCT provided better DFS but similar OS compared to conventional chemotherapy consolidation.[61] In patients with relapsed APL (M3), consolidation with high-dose therapy and auto-HCT was associated with 5-year OS of 77% in a phase II study.[62] CIBMTR analysis showed improved 5-year OS with auto-HCT compared to allo-HCT in APL in CR2 mainly due to higher NRM after allo-HCT.[63]

Choice of Conditioning Regimen

Conditioning regimen intensity significantly impacts the outcomes of allo-HCT. Higher intensity regimens provide lower RI at the expense of TRM and the choice of MAC vs RIC/NMA regimen is guided by the risk of disease relapse vs TRM in an individual patient. Traditionally, high-dose intensity therapy has been the standard approach to eradicating AML in HCT. The standard MAC allo-HCT regimens used in AML are cyclophosphamide and total body irradiation (CyTBI) or cyclophosphamide and busulfan (CyBu).[64] The use of intravenous busulfan, pharmacokinetic monitoring of busulfan levels, and better understanding of the interaction with cyclophosphamide has caused a reassessment of the use of CyBu and it may be superior to CyTBI.[65,66] AML is predominantly a disease of the middle and later years, and many patients are ineligible or are not considered for MAC allo-HCT. RIC allo-HCT may offer a viable alternative to older or frailer patients.[67] Dose intensity is reduced to diminish TRM, while potent immunosuppression is exerted to aid engraftment and provide a launch pad for a graft vs AML effect.

In the phase 3 BMT CTN 0901 study, patients (age 18-65 years) with AML or MDS were randomized to receive allo-HCT after MAC vs RIC regimen. The study was closed after interim analysis showed significantly lower RI with MAC compared to RIC (15.9% vs 51%), resulting in higher 18-month OS (76.4% vs 63.4%).[68] Long-term follow-up of this study showed ongoing OS benefit with MAC (4-year OS: 65% vs 49%, P = .02) compared to RIC.[69] A posthoc analysis of BMT CTN 0901 stratified by pretransplant MRD status showed that benefit of MAC over RIC was greatest in the subgroup of patients with persistent pretransplant MRD, whereas there was less evidence of benefit in the 3-year OS between MAC vs RIC regimens among patients who were MRD- before allo-HCT.[70]

Use of Alternative Graft Source

The advent of high-resolution HLA typing has made selection of well-matched MUDs more accurate and outcomes are now similar to those seen with sibling donors.[67,71,72] Alternative donors such as umbilical cord blood (UCB) units and haploidentical family donors are widely used when no HLA-matched family or MUD is available. Although dependent upon cell doses, UCB HCT appears to yield equivalent survival in treatment of leukemia to conventional donors.[73] Haploidentical conditioning regimens have become very attractive in recent years due to reduction in TRM and rapid engraftment, but long-term outcomes are awaited.[74-76] A prospective BMT CTN 1101 study compared T cell replete haplo-related BMT with PTCy vs double CBU with RIC regimen. The study was closed early due to poor accrual. However, haplo-BMT was associated with lower NRM (11% vs 18%, $P = .04$) and better OS (57% vs 46%, $P = .04$) compared to CBU transplant.[77] A prospective randomized study based on donor availability showed similar transplant outcomes between haploidentical (Beijing approach) vs MSD allo-HCT in patients with AML in CR1.[78] Similar to haplo-HCT, allo-HCT outcomes using mismatched unrelated donor (MMUD) have also improved with incorporation of PTCy. In a National Marrow Donor Program–sponsored phase II study, BMT from a MMUD with PTCy resulted in encouraging 1-year OS of 76%[79] suggesting MMUD can be a safe alternative donor option.

Post-HCT Therapy to Reduce Relapse

Given the high rates of relapse post-HCT, especially when pre-/post-HCT MRD is present, a strategy of pre-emptive DLI may be adopted, particularly in the setting of a T lymphocyte depleted conditioning regimen pre-HCT.[80] *Table 106.1* summarized the published experience with the impact of MRD on allo-HCT outcomes. The proliferation of new agents has prompted exploration of maintenance therapy such as the FLT3 inhibitor sorafenib and epigenetic regulators.[104-106] A phase II SORMAIN trial showed improved 2-year RFS with sorafenib compared to placebo maintenance therapy after allo-HCT for AML with *FLT3-ITD*.[107] There was no benefit of RFS in a phase 3 study comparing 1-year of azacitidine maintenance vs no maintenance after allo-HCT.[108] Multiple ongoing studies are exploring various novel agents and cellular therapies to reduce relapses after allo-HCT.

Myelodysplastic Syndrome

MDS is a heterogeneous malignant hematopoietic clonal disorder whose incidence rises with age with median presentation in the 70s. MDS is characterized by chronic cytopenias and abnormal cellular maturation. Currently, the only therapy that is potentially curative in MDS is allo-HCT. Long-term survival in remission is reported in 30% to 40% of high-risk MDS with relapse risk posttransplant predicted by pretransplant bone marrow cytogenetics and myeloblast count.[109] (*Table 106.2*).

Since MDS is predominantly a disease of the elderly, each patient requires tailored assessment of the potential benefit of transplantation balanced against the natural history of the disease, any existing comorbidity, predictable toxicity of the transplant, availability of a donor, potential alternative therapies, and patient preferences. Existing tools to assist in the counseling of patients by transplant physicians are the World Health Organization Prognostic Scoring System, the International Prognostic Scoring System (IPSS), the Revised IPSS (IPSS-R) criteria, and the HCT-CI.[13,109,128] Advances in sequencing technology have led to rapid accrual of data about recurrent mutations that may in time be incorporated into existing scoring systems once their clinical impact is fully validated.[129]

Treatment Prior to Allogeneic Transplant

It is now common to offer patients whose marrow contains greater than 10% myeloblasts induction chemotherapy using similar regimens to AML although prospective clinical trials to formally assess this are lacking.[130] HMAs such as azacitidine and decitabine have also been used to try and achieve a better disease status pre-HCT as well as maintenance afterward and have been compared in retrospective studies with conventional induction chemotherapy. They appear less toxic than conventional chemotherapy regimens, but this requires further investigation in prospective studies.[131] Similar to AML, molecularly targeted therapies plus HMA strategies are being studied for better disease control before allo-HCT.[132]

Indications for Allogeneic Stem Cell Transplantation

Prior to HCT, a formal assessment of comorbidity should be made as this is a validated risk measure affecting transplant outcome.[133] An adverse comorbidity risk may negate the potential value of a transplant and reduce survival prematurely due to early TRM. Markov decision analysis has been influential in approaching the problem of optimal timing for allo-HCT.[134] Registry data were used to investigate the outcome of allo-HCT in patients up to the age of 60 years relative to IPSS stage. It was found that patients in the intermediate-2 or high IPSS risk category benefited from early transplant, whereas patients with low or intermediate-1 IPSS risk category had improved survival if transplant was delayed. A further Markov decision model with QoL utility estimates was developed in order to assess the value of transplantation in 514 patients with MDS aged 60 to 79 years.[135] Patients with IPSS low or intermediate-1 MDS derived little benefit from transplant since mean life expectancy was 38 months as opposed to 77 months in patients who were not transplanted. On the other hand, patients with intermediate-2 or high-risk MDS by IPSS criteria gained from transplant as their life expectancy improved from 28 to 36 months.

The strongest evidence supporting allo-HCT in intermediate-2 or high-risk de novo MDS comes from BMT CTM 1102 study. Patients aged 50 to 75 years were assigned RIC allo-HCT vs HMA or best supportive care based on HLA-matched donor availability. In an intention-to-treat analysis, OS at 3-year in the donor arm was 47.9% compared to 26.6% in the no-donor arm ($P = .0001$). The OS benefit was seen across all subgroups.[121] There was also no difference in patient-reported QoL outcomes at different time points between the study cohorts.

Patients with good risk disease as defined by existing staging schemes are therefore generally treated with nontransplant approaches such as HMAs.[134,135] Younger patients with low or intermediate-1 risk MDS whose normal life span is significantly limited by MDS may however benefit from allo-HCT.[135,136] The ELN recommends that patients with IPSS intermediate risk-1 with excess blasts or poor risk cytogenetics, IPSS intermediate-2 or high risk MDS, up to the age of 70 years, who are fit for the procedure, and are willing to accept the associated risks should be offered allo-HCT.[137]

Since the development of the IPSS-R, there has been interest in seeking a correlation with the outcome of allo-HCT for MDS. Outcomes of 519 allo-HCTs performed between 2000 and 2011 for MDS or AML with a blast count below 30% and reported to the Gruppo Italiano Trapianto di Midollo Osseo registry were studied retrospectively to evaluate the influence of IPSS-R and HCT-CI.[138] Survival at 5 years ranged from 0% to 94% and in multivariate analysis significant adverse factors included higher IPSS-R risk, monosomal karyotype, age of 50 years or more, an HLA mismatched donor and a high HCT-CI risk score. An increased relapse risk was significantly associated with higher IPSS-R risk, monosomal karyotype, and active disease at time of HCT and RIC. NRM was greater in those aged 50 years or more, higher HCT-CI scores, HLA-mismatched donors, and MAC regimens.

Similarly, the European Society for Blood and Marrow Transplantation (EBMT) studied a cohort of 903 patients transplanted for MDS or AML secondary to MDS and confirmed the importance of monosomal karyotype in predicting transplant outcome.[139] The CIBMTR developed a prognostic scoring tool to predict the outcome of transplant based on a retrospective review of 2133 patients with MDS.[140] Again the strong adverse impact of monosomal karyotype and age greater than 50 years was noted together with a moderately strong adverse impact of pre-HCT myeloblasts > 3%, platelets < 50 × 10^9/L, KPS < 90, age 30 to 49 years, and cytogenetics within the poor and very poor risk group of the MDS Comprehensive Cytogenetic Scoring System.[141] Genetic mutations play a key role in dictating the outcomes of allo-HCT in MDS. In a CIBMTR analysis of 1514 patients,

Table 106.1. Impact of MRD in HCT Outcomes in Acute Leukemia

Study	MRD Status	n	DFS	RR	OS	Follow-Up
AML						
Walter et al[81]	Negative	64	75%	18%	77%	2 y
	Positive	24	9%	65%	30%	
Grubovikj et al[82]	Negative	40	62%	15%	62%	3 y
	Positive	19	16%	58%	18%	
Wang et al[83]	Negative	110	76%	10%	78%	3 y
	Positive	20	52%	35%	57%	
Tian et al[84]	Negative	21	55%	21%	51%	5 y
	Positive	32	36%	29%	41%	
Walter et al[20]	Negative	190	61%	26%	64%	3 y
	Positive	51	21%	61%	28%	
Zhou et al[85]	Negative	216	70%	23%	75%	3 y
	Positive	63	17%	69%	27%	
Zheng et al[86]	Negative	40	63%	16%	69%	3 y
	Positive	32	53%	19%	58%	
Oran et al[87]	Negative	104	64%	14%	67%	1 y
	Positive	48	44%	33%	49%	
Baron et al[88]	Negative	66	58%	-	60%	2 y
	Positive	56	41%	-	48%	
Morsink et al[89]	Negative	596	60%	22%	64%	3 y
	Positive	147	19%	65%	32%	
Gilleece et al[90]	Negative	749	57%	24%	62%	2 y
	Positive	293	46%	40%	62%	
Paras et al[91]	Negative	649	62%	23%	66%	3 y
	Positive	161	21%	65%	33%	
Zhou et al[85,a]	Negative	263	61%	31%	67%	
	Positive	16	13%	81%	17%	
Shah et al[92,a]	Negative	232	-	29%		1 y
	Positive	9	-	78%	27%	
Paras et al[91,a]	Negative	749	58%	27%	64%	3 y
	Positive	61	2%	90%	13%	
ALL						
Knechtli et al[93]	Negative	33	73%	-	-	2 y
	Positive	23	17%	-	-	
Spinelli et al[94]	Negative	37	-	0%	80%	3 y
	Positive	6	-	46%	49%	
Bader et al[95]	Negative	46	60%	13%	-	5 y
	Positive	45	27%	57%	-	
Giebel et al[96]	Negative	77	57%	-	-	5 y
	Positive	26	17%	-	-	
Elorza et al[97]	Negative	21	74%	-	80%	2 y
	Positive	10	20%	-	20%	
Bachanova et al[98]	Negative	76	55%	16%	55%	2 y
	Positive	10	30%	30%	40%	
Ruggeri et al[99]	Negative	96	54%	39%	58%	4 y
	Positive	74	29%	24%	42%	
Lovisa et al[100]	Negative	51	73%	20%	-	10 y
	Positive	68	32%	57%	-	

Table 106.1. Impact of MRD in HCT Outcomes in Acute Leukemia (Continued)

Study	MRD Status	n	DFS	RR	OS	Follow-Up
Ifversen et al[101]	Negative	47	86%	5%	-	5.5 y
	Positive	22	67%	24%	-	
Pavlu et al[102]	Negative	1816	58%	24%	67%	2 y
	Positive	964	50%	32%	61%	
Baron et al[88]	Negative	34	55%	-	60%	2 y
	Positive	44	33%	-	47%	
Bader et al[103,a]	Negative	79	61%	27%	-	3 y
	Positive	14	36%	57%	-	
Lovisa et al[100,a]	Negative	71	63%	-	-	10 y
	Positive	27	30%	-	-	

[a]Indicates that MRD was measured post-HCT.
Abbreviations: ALL, acute lymphoblastic leukemia; AML, acute myeloid leukemia; DFS, disease free survival; HCT, hematopoietic cell transplantation; MRD, minimal residual disease; OS, overall survival; RR, relapse rate.

Table 106.2. Outcomes of Allogeneic HCT in MDS and MPN

Disease	Study	n	DFS	OS	NRM	Follow-Up
CML	Crawley et al[110]	186	37%	58%	23.3%	3 y
CML	Lubking et al[111]	118	-	65.4%	11.6%	5 y
CML	Warlick et al[112]	306	29.5%	50.2%	25.1%	3 y
aCML	Onida et al[113]	42	36%	51%	24%	5 y
CMML	Symeonidis et al[114]	513	27%	33%	41%	4 y
CMML	Sharma et al[115]	35	-	55%	25%	1.75 y
MDS/MPN-U		8	-	62%	14%	1.25 y
MDS/MPN-U	Kurosawa et al[116]	86	-	48.5%	26.3%	3 y
MDS + MDS/MF	Kroger et al[117]	721	40%	45%	-	3 y
MDS + CMML	Cao et al[118]	48	77%	86%	12%	1.5 y
MDS	Kroger et al[119]	81	30%	50%	19%	3 y
MDS	Platzbecker et al[120]	103	37%	39%	30%	2 y
MDS	Nakamura et al[121]	260	35.8%	47.9%	-	3 y
MDS	Shimomura et al[122]	645	-	71.2%	19%	3 y
MDS	Warlick et al[123]	84	38% 29%	48% 31%	39%	1 y 5 y
Primary and secondary MF	Gowin et al[124]	551	-	55% 47%	-	5 y 10 y
Primary MF	Kroger et al[125]	188	-	79.3% 48.4% 35.9%	-	1 y 5 y 10 y
Primary MF	Patriarca et al[126]	52	38%	44%	-	3 y
Secondary MF	Zeng et al[127]	141	61.8%	68.5%	25.0%	2 y

Abbreviations: CML, chronic myelogenous leukemia; CMML, chronic myelomonocytic leukemia; HCT, hematopoietic cell transplantation; MDS, myelodysplastic syndrome; MDS/MPN-U, myelodysplastic/myeloproliferative neoplasms, unclassified; MF, myelofibrosis; MPN, myeloproliferative neoplasm; n, number of patients; NRM, nonrelapse mortality; OS, overall survival; PFS, progression free survival.

presence of mutations involving *TP53* and *RAS* pathway was associated with increased relapse risk and poor OS after allo-HCT.[40]

Intensity of Conditioning Regimens

The success of RIC/NMA conditioning regimens in reducing early TRM, coupled with the advanced age of many patients with MDS, has led to a retreat from the use of MAC, although such an intense regimen may be appropriate in younger patients.[142,143] Around 20% of enrolled subjects in BMT CTN 0901 had MDS. The use of MAC was associated with lower RI compared to RIC (3.7% vs 37%), but 18 month OS was comparable between the study cohorts (81.5% vs 85.2%).[68] A subsequent analysis of NGS showed higher RI and poor OS when using RIC vs MAC among patients with detectable MRD before conditioning.[144]

A variety of RIC/NMA regimens are in use with none being clearly superior to another.[145,146] Many regimens incorporate busulfan, but treosulfan, a water-soluble prodrug of an alkylating agent, is now being tested in multicenter studies as a replacement drug with lower toxicity. In a multicenter phase 2 study of treosulfan combined with fludarabine and 2 Gy TBI in 90 patients with MDS and 60 patients with AML, all under the age of 60 years and with a median follow-up of 30 months, the estimated OS at 2 years was 77% in MDS and 71% in AML.[147] Interestingly, the RR of 28% in patients with unfavorable cytogenetics is similar to the 27% seen in intermediate risk cytogenetics.

The myeloablative conditioning is usually considered for younger fit patients and RIC for older frail patients, with 50 to 55 years often the age range separating the two groups, but paramount is an assessment of comorbidities and discussion with the patient.[148]

Myeloproliferative Neoplasms

Chronic Myeloid Leukemia

The success of tyrosine kinase inhibitors (TKIs) in the management of chronic myelogenous leukemia (CML) has had a profound impact on the use of transplantation. Most patients in chronic-phase CML can achieve deep and durable molecular remissions with TKI therapy. Among patients who relapse after initial TKI, a trial of later generation TKI should be considered. In patients with chronic-phase CML, allo-HCT is largely reserved for patients who are refractory or intolerant to multiple TKIs or who have advanced disease.[149] Compared to chronic-phase CML, patients with accelerated or blast-phase CML carry an inferior prognosis with a suboptimal response to TKI and allo-HCT should be considered in these patients after initial TKI-based induction therapy.[150]

Timing of HCT

Historically, in patients in chronic phase CML, sustained survival was seen in 50% to 85% of recipients of HLA-matched sibling stem cells following high-intensity conditioning (MAC) regimens.[151,152] However, those with accelerated phase or blast crisis fared worse with only 30% to 40% and 5% to 15% survival rates, respectively.[153,154] While the impact of disease status at transplant on survival is consistent,[155] the incorporation of TKIs into regimens used to treat advanced CML has increased the proportion achieving chronic phase before HCT. In a registry-based study of allo-HCT for blast-phase CML, 3-year OS was 38.5% and the presence of active blast-phase pretransplant was associated with poor LFS and OS.[156]

Prior use of TKIs does not have an adverse effect on survival post-HCT.[157] This may reflect a debulking effect of TKI therapy resulting in lower rates of TRM and relapse. Splenomegaly at the time of transplant may be associated with apparent delays in engraftment due to splenic sequestration. Splenectomy or splenic irradiation prior to transplant does not improve survival outcome and may be associated with morbidity.[158,159] The EBMT risk score was developed in the CML population and incorporates donor type, stage of disease at time of transplantation, age and sex of donor and recipient, and time from diagnosis to transplantation.[160] These parameters are weighted to result in an overall score that has been validated to predict 5-year survival and TRM post-HCT.[161]

Conditioning Regimen

Most studies comparing MAC vs RIC in CML were conducted in the pre-TKI era (*Table 106.2*). Young fit patients treated with high dose combinations of busulfan and cyclophosphamide or ablative doses of TBI combined with cyclophosphamide or busulfan were evaluated in initial studies with long-term remissions in 50% to 80% of CML transplanted in first or second chronic phase. Direct comparison of the two regimens suggests equivalence in OS but, in one study, reduced RI with BuCy.[162,163] Retrospective analyses suggest that the use of busulfan targeted to specific levels using patient-specific pharmacokinetic analyses reduces RI.[164]

The use of MAC regimens in patients over the age of 60, even when carefully selected, is associated with higher TRM rates than younger patients.[165] RIC and NMA conditioning regimens have permitted HCT to be offered to patients whose age or frailty might otherwise exclude them.[166,167] A CIBMTR study evaluated the impact of conditioning intensity in CML patients transplanted in the TKI-era from 2007 to 2014. There was no difference in LFS or OS between MAC and RIC/NMA. Pretransplant disease status being accelerated phase or second or more chronic phase was associated with higher RI and poor LFS regardless of conditioning regimen.[168]

Monitoring of Disease After HCT

Detection of CML-associated BCR-ABL transcripts by real-time quantitative reverse transcription polymerase chain reaction (qRT-PCR) in peripheral blood leukocytes after allo-HCT is a convenient way of monitoring disease activity. A reasonable monitoring approach is to measure levels at least every 3 months during the first 2 years post-HCT. The introduction of international standards for the performance of the assay will facilitate future comparisons of monitoring approaches between centers.[169] Transcripts may be detectable in the first 6 months post-HCT, particularly if a RIC/NMA conditioning regimen has been used. They usually decline, particularly once a taper of immunosuppression is underway. However, persistent or rising transcript levels after 6 months are likely to herald imminent relapse.[170] The role of post–transplant maintenance therapy with TKI in patients with chronic-phase CML who received MAC and achieved molecular remission remains unknown. A CIBMTR study showed no beneficial effect of TKI maintenance regardless of disease status pretransplant; however, it included a small number of patients in accelerated or blast phase CML. Given higher relapse risk in these patients, one can consider using TKI maintenance for the first 2 years after transplant with close MRD monitoring, but prospective data are lacking supporting such practice.

Management of Relapse After HCT

Early relapse or persistent MRD is usually detected by serial qRT-PCR assays.[170] Withdrawal of immunosuppression, reinstitution of a TKI, and DLI should all be considered. Choice of TKI will depend upon the nature of the patient's prior TKI exposure, the mutation profile of the disease, and the side effect profile of the available TKIs. Failure of the disease to respond to TKIs pre-HCT does not necessarily predict failure post-HCT. Imatinib has been used successfully post-HCT in patients who had previously not achieved a durable response, but TKIs may best be used together with DLI as therapy of relapse.[171] In post-HCT relapse of CML, DLIs can achieve durable remissions in 60% to 87%.[172,173] A strategy to reduce these risks is to use escalating doses spaced 2 to 3 months apart.[174] A registry based analysis showed no added benefit of DLI over TKI alone in management of relapsed CML post allo-HCT.[175]

Myelofibrosis

Primary or secondary myelofibrosis (MF) is a heterogeneous disease, which evolves over time with changing genomic alterations. The prognosis of MF varies widely where some patients have an indolent course for decades and others succumb to progressive marrow failure or transformed AML in a matter of months. Allo-HCT is the only potentially curative therapy for MF but is associated with relatively high NRM due to poor graft function secondary to a hostile marrow microenvironment and hypersplenism. Several prognostic scoring systems have been developed and all have been applied to define patient eligibility for transplant. The IPSS distinguished four groups of patients at diagnosis by virtue of age, hemoglobin level, leukocyte count, circulating blasts, and the presence of constitutional symptoms yielding low, intermediate-1, intermediate-2, and high-risk disease associated with median survivals of 135, 95, 48, and 27 months, respectively. Further iterations produced the Dynamic IPSS (DIPSS)[176] and the DIPSS Plus,[177] each of which may be used at time points beyond diagnosis. Presence of high-risk myeloid mutations such as *ASXL1*, *SRSF2*, and *U2AF1* is associated with rapid disease progression and poor response to systemic therapies. Genetically inspired international prognostic scoring system combines cytogenetic and mutational data to render a prognostic score that is comparable to more complex scoring systems such as MIPSS70.[178] In a retrospective analysis of 101 patients with MF, *ASXL1*, *SRSF2*, *IDH1/2*, *EZH2*, and *TP53* were associated with higher RI, whereas traditional DIPSS score did not influence the transplant outcomes.[179]

Although allo-HCT remains the only curative therapy for MF, whether primary or secondary, the substantial improvements in QoL achieved by the use of ruxolitinib, a JAK 1/2 inhibitor therapy, have added to the complexity of decision-making about the timing of transplantation.[180] However, ruxolitinib has variable effects on fibrosis and is discontinued in about half of patients by 2 to 3 years due to side effects or loss of response.[181,182]

Indications for HCT in Primary Myelofibrosis

There is no prospective study comparing allo-HCT vs palliative systemic therapies in MF. The evidence to support allo-HCT in MF is based on multiple retrospective studies suggesting long-term stable engraftment and potential cure. Compared to conventional care, allo-HCT was associated with improved OS in patients with intermediate-2 or high risk per DIPSS[125] (Table 106.2).

Selection of individual patients for allo-HCT requires assessment of disease status, comorbidities, and availability of a donor. Advanced disease has been associated with poorer survival post-HCT.[183,184] Splenectomy is not usually recommended prior to HCT and it has been associated with an increased risk of relapse, although it may lead to earlier engraftment without any impact upon survival.[185,186] HCT-CI scores greater than 4 together with older age groups have been predictive of poor outcomes after HCT.[187] However, careful selection of older patients can result in relatively good outcomes with a 3-year progression-free survival (PFS) of 40% reported in a small cohort of patients aged 60 to 78 years treated with a range of conditioning regimens of varying intensity.[184]

Pretreatment with JAK 1/2 inhibitors may enhance performance status and in responsive patients may improve post-HCT survival.[188] Careful titration of ruxolitinib in the week prior to conditioning HCT is essential to avoid rebound effects and a cytokine storm that might compromise HCT outcomes.[189] An EBMT study showed improved transplant outcomes among the recipients of pretransplant ruxolitinib and ongoing spleen response.[190] A phase 2 study (JAK ALO) tested role of pretransplant ruxolitinib for 6 months and showed a high rate of transplant (92%) with 1-year OS of 55%.[191]

Fully HLA-matched donors and higher cell doses are important in MF as mismatched donors and low cell doses increase the risk of graft failure.[185,192] Graft failure, reported in up to a quarter of cases, may necessitate a top-up dose of stem cells and is well recognized in MF, presumably attributable to the fibrotic marrow.[192,193] GVHD may also be particularly problematic after HCT for MF with 64% acute GVHD (aGVHD) grade II-IV and 59% extensive cGVHD.[194] T-cell depletion may reduce this since aGVHD grade II-IV and extensive cGVHD were seen in 27% and 25% of patients who had undergone T-cell depletion, with cGVHD associated with improved OS.[192] Encouraging outcomes were reported using PTCy and haploidentical related donor in a retrospective study. Use of marrow graft and spleen size ≥ 22 cm or prior splenectomy was associated with increased RI.[195]

Although patients may have a good QoL while on ruxolitinib, they are still at risk of leukemic transformation and this dilemma raises difficult questions about the timing of HCT. It is evident that counseling patients with MF about the possible benefits and timing of allo-HCT requires very careful consideration and attention to the patient's preferences.

LYMPHOID MALIGNANCIES

Acute Lymphoblastic Leukemia

Modern combination chemotherapy protocols have remarkably improved the outcomes of ALL. Compared to pediatric ALL, ALL in adults carries more high-risk mutations and a higher risk of relapse despite the majority achieving initial CR. Some 75% to 90% adult patients with ALL will achieve remission following induction, but many are destined to relapse with long-term survival seen in only 25% to 50%.[196] Philadelphia positive ALL (Ph+ ALL), associated with t(9;22), is seen in fewer than 5% of children but about 30% of adult cases.[197] The newly recognized entity of BCR-ABL1-like B cell ALL has a similar gene expression profile to that seen in Ph+ ALL, but without the t(9;22)/BCR-ABL fusion transcript. It has been described in 10% to 15% of pediatric and up to 27% of adult cases, and is associated with a poor prognosis.[198] Another important factor contributing to poor outcomes of adult ALL is an inability to tolerate pediatric-inspired chemotherapy regimens containing asparaginase. Consolidation with allo-HCT after achieving initial CR may overcome the negative impact of high-risk genomic features of adult ALL.

Indications for Hematopoietic Cell Transplantation in Acute Lymphoblastic Leukemia

Prognostic features have been identified that stratify patients by risk. Cytogenetic changes that are associated with very high risk disease and a poor prognosis include t(9;22) (q34;q11), t(4;11) (q21;q23), and t(8;14) (q24.1;q32), the presence of a complex karyotype (defined as ≥5 chromosomal abnormalities), or low hypodiploidy/near triploidy.[199] Better responses to chemotherapy and survival outcomes are seen in association with hyperdiploidy and t(12;21). In addition, quantitative MRD status in response to therapy has emerged as a key factor when assessing prognosis.[200]

Age is a risk factor and, overall, patients older than 55 have a DFS at 3 years of less than 20% without transplant.[201,202] A WBC at presentation that exceeds 30×10^9/L for B lineage ALL or 100×10^9/L for T lineage ALL is also a clinical parameter that has been used to identify high-risk disease.[200,203] Pro-B, pro-T, pre-T, and mature T sub-groups (European Group for Immunological Characterization of Acute Leukemias classification BI and TI/TII/TIV) are further high-risk groups that may be distinguished by immunophenotyping.[204]

Impact of Allogeneic Hematopoietic Cell Transplantation on Risk Groups of Acute Lymphoblastic Leukemia

The Leucémie Aiguës Lymphoblastique de l'Adulte LALA-94 study showed that patients with high-risk features benefitted from allo-HCT with 5-year DFS of 45% compared to 23% in those patients without a donor.[205,206] Similar results have been observed by other groups particularly if allo-HCT is offered in CR1 when survival ranges from 40% to 75%.[207-212] However, other studies were unable to show benefit to patients with high-risk ALL of allo-HCT over chemotherapy or autologous HCT (Auto-HCT).[201,213] The international prospective Medical Research Council UK ALL12/Eastern Co-operative Oncology Group ECOG E2993 study enrolled 1929 adult patients with ALL in the period 1993 to 2006.[202] In this study, allo-HCT offered a survival benefit to patients with standard risk with a 5-year OS of 62% vs 52% in a donor vs no donor analysis. High-risk Ph- ALL patients did not benefit, with a nonsignificant 5-year OS of 41% vs 35% in a donor vs no donor analysis and this was due to a 2-year TRM of 36%, mostly due to GVHD or infection. A meta-analysis of 2962 patients from 13 studies found a DFS and OS advantage for the donor vs no-donor arm when using MAC and MSD for adult ALL in CR1.[214] Pediatric-inspired protocols in adults have resulted in superior outcomes across multiple studies. A study compared the outcomes of CALGB10403 which treated adolescents and young adults with Ph- ALL with pediatric-inspired regimen vs a cohort of patients who received MAC allo-HCT in CR1 from CIBMTR. Allo-HCT was associated with poorer OS due to higher NRM compared to patients who received chemotherapy alone.[215] Major limitation of this analysis was its retrospective non-randomized nature and the lack of information on MRD.

MRD level at the end of induction/consolidation is an important risk-stratification tool when deciding about allo-HCT in CR1. Analysis of Ph- ALL patients from the GMALL study found that patients with persistent MRD who did not receive all-HCT had poor long-term OS.[216] The pediatric-inspired GRAALL protocol treated 522 adult patients with Ph- ALL. While there was no difference in RFS for the overall study population, participants with persistent MRD after induction derived RFS benefit from allo-HCT vs conventional therapy.[217] PETHEMA ALL-AR-03 trial assigned chemotherapy vs allo-HCT based on early cytogenetic response and flow MRD at the end of consolidation in patients aged 15 to 60 years with Ph- ALL. In this study, MRD clearance was the only factor predicting LFS and OS and outcomes were inferior in patients with persistent MRD. Five-year OS was 37% for allo-HCT cohort and 59% for chemotherapy cohort.[218] Patients with MRD at the time of allo-HCT do less well than their MRD negative counterparts due to higher rates of relapse and are candidates for therapy such as blinatumomab and other biological therapies prior to transplant.[219,220]

Adult patients with standard-risk Ph- ALL who are treated with pediatric-inspired regimens in MRD negative CR1 may achieve similar outcomes with conventional chemotherapy consolidation and maintenance compared to allo-HCT. Based on older studies (donor vs no donor), allo-HCT can be offered to fit patients with available MSD.[214,221] Patients with persistent MRD carry poor outcomes and consolidation with allo-HCT may improve outcomes of these patients.

Philadelphia Positive Acute Lymphoblastic Leukemia (Ph+ ALL)

Historically, Ph+ ALL has been associated with a poor prognosis with few survivors following conventional chemotherapy alone and potentially curative Allo-HCT possible for only a minority of patients.[221,222] However, this dismal outlook improved with the advent of TKI that targets the BCR-ABL fusion product. CR rates of over 90% have been obtained by incorporation of TKIs into induction regimens,[223,224] but almost all patients will relapse in the absence of further therapy. Patients who achieve CR and who are eligible for transplant will be spared further rounds of chemotherapy and the associated cumulative morbidity if a donor can be identified for allo-HCT and the procedure performed quickly.

At present, allo-HCT is the preferred postremission therapy for eligible patients to capitalize on the combined antileukemic effects of MAC and GVL as well as the high CR rates associated with TKI use during induction. Prior exposure to TKIs has been associated with improvements in survival after allo-HCT with up to 78% DFS at 3 years observed in preliminary reports.[225,226] A Japanese registry study of 738 patients transplanted between 1990 and 2010 reported 5-year OS of 59% in a cohort of patients pretreated with imatinib compared with 38% in an earlier group not exposed to pretransplant imatinib.[227] Perhaps the most significant impact of imatinib is the improved CR rates that allow more patients to proceed to allo-HCT in CR1.[228]

However, there have also been encouraging reports of prolonged survival in patients in complete molecular remission by using TKI maintenance without allo-HCT.[229-231] In summary, patients with Ph+ ALL with available HLA-matched donor should be offered allo-HCT in CR1. Outcomes of patients who can achieve molecular MRD clearance are favorable, and they may be able to avoid all-HCT and be treated with long-term TKI-based maintenance therapy.

Conditioning Regimen and Donor Type

Established MAC regimens for use in ALL are cyclophosphamide 120 mg/kg and fractionated TBI 12 to 13.2 Gy (CyTBI).[232-234] Multiple registry-based studies have shown reduced RI with TBI-based over non–TBI-containing MAC regimens.[235,236] FORUM was a phase 3 study comparing TBI12 Gy/etoposide vs fludarabine/thiotepa with busulfan or treosulfan in pediatric patients with ALL. TBI/etoposide resulted in improved OS and reduced RI compared to non–TBI-containing regimens.[237] Adult incidence of ALL peaks over the age of 40 years, an age range in which MAC regimens may be particularly hazardous and associated with substantial NRM and comorbidity. The outcomes of RIC/NMA allo-HCTs have been reported widely and it is possible to draw some conclusions about their use.[238-245] Predictably, they have been applied to older patients with median age at allo-HCT ranging from 38 to 50 years. They are effective when used in CR1 but have limited efficacy in more advanced disease, with no one regimen clearly superior to others.

The CIBMTR compared the outcomes of 93 RIC/NMA vs 1428 MAC allo-HCTs performed between 1995 and 2006 in patients with Ph- ALL.[246] In this retrospective study, the median age at transplant was 45 and 28 years and the median follow-up of survivors was 38 and 54 months in recipients of RIC/NMA and MAC regimens, respectively. Three-year TRM and RR were 33% and 26% in MAC allo-HCT compared to 32% and 35% in RIC/NMA allo-HCT. The 3-year DFS was statistically equivalent at 41% vs 32% in MAC and RIC/NMA transplants, respectively. Importantly, the use of RIC allo-HCT extends the access to HCT for patients who might otherwise be excluded because of comorbidity or age. Similar to BMT CTN 0901 in AML/MDS,[70] a prospective study is needed to determine the role of MAC over RIC/NMA among patients with ALL in MRD negative remission before transplant.

Only about 25% to 30% of patients will have a healthy HLA MSD and a MUD may be sought.[247] A CIBMTR study of allo-HCT performed between 1995 and 2004 found an equivalent incidence of NRM, RR, and LFS in recipients of sibling or MUD grafts.[248] Allo-HCT performed in 1139 patients between 1992 and 2007 was reported by Nishiwaki et al from the Japanese registry and this study found equivalent OS with an encouraging 65% and 62% OS at 4 years in related and MUD allo-HCT, respectively.[249] A CIBMTR analysis showed similar survival but less GVHD with haploidentical HCT using PTCy compared to traditional MSD and MUD allo-HCT. Cord blood transplants were associated with poorer OS and increased NRM compared to other graft sources.[250]

Posttransplant Management

Posttransplant maintenance with a TKI is frequently offered for 1 to 3 years. The EBMT retrospective study of 473 patients with de novo Ph+ ALL transplanted between 2000 and 2010 concluded that prophylactic TKI administration was a significant factor in improved DFS (HR = 0.44; P = .002) and OS (HR = 0.42; P = .004), and a lower relapse incidence (HR = 0.40; P = .01).[251] TKIs may be started early after transplant or delayed until serial monitoring of MRD reveals evidence of disease. A randomized phase II study showed no difference in outcomes between these two strategies, but maintenance TKI was associated with lower MRD recurrence.[252] Patients who do not achieve an MRD negative state in response to a TKI appear destined for hematological relapse.[252,253] More prospective studies are required to define the appropriate choice, dose, and duration of TKI maintenance in different allo-HCT platforms. Patients should also be monitored for MRD recurrence every 3 to 6 months for at least 2 years after allo-HCT. MRD following allo-HCT may herald relapse[254] (Table 106.1). A rational response to persistent MRD post–Allo-HCT would be reduction of immunosuppression, infusion of DLI, or targeted therapy, but the optimal strategy is still evolving.[255]

Allogeneic Hematopoietic Cell Transplant in the Management of Relapsed Acute Lymphoblastic Leukemia

Patients with ALL who relapse have poor survival rates but a minority may be rescued by HCT in CR2 with LFS of 18% to 45%.[196,256-258] In UKALL12/ECOG 2993 study, 120 patients with relapsed ALL who were not transplanted in CR1 went on to receive HCT with auto-HCT, MUD allo-HCT or sibling allo-HCT. The 5-year OS was 15%, 16%, and 23%, respectively, compared to 4% in a comparator chemotherapy only group. The benefit of HCT in CR2 was not affected by age or CR1 duration. A CIBMTR study reviewed the outcomes of 583 patients with relapsed or refractory ALL who were treated with MAC allo-HCT and found OS of 16%. High rates of GVHD were seen with 27% suffering grade III/IV aGVHD and a similar number with cGVHD.[48] In an EBMT analysis of patients with relapsed ALL after first allo-HCT, second allo-HCT resulted in 5-year OS of 14% with relapse being the major cause of transplant failure.[259]

One of the challenges in treating patients with primary refractory or relapsed ALL is achieving CR without inflicting further comorbidities that may compromise the delivery of a subsequent allo-HCT. Newer agents such as blinatumomab, inotuzumab, ponatinib, and nelarabine are all being studied to assess their potential for achieving CR and facilitating allo-HCT.[260-263] CD19-CAR T therapy (tisagenlecleucel and brexucabtagene autoleucel) has shown promising MRD-negative remissions in relapsed or refractory B cell ALL.[264,265] Data are conflicting on the need for a second allo-HCT once a patient has achieved CR using CAR T therapy and additional studies are needed.

Chronic Lymphocytic Leukemia

The last decade has seen an eruption of new agents offered for the treatment of chronic lymphocytic leukemia (CLL).[266,267] The resulting flow of drugs from clinical trials to clinical practice continues to change the therapeutic landscape in CLL.[268-271] This state of flux has prompted discussion about the timing and necessity of transplantation at a time when long-term outcome data associated with the newer agents are awaited. Retrospective data do support the value of RIC allo-HCT approaches in the setting of advanced refractory disease but precede the widespread use of novel agents.[272,273] While allo-HCT may cure some patients with CLL, it is associated with higher treatment-related mortality than the new agents and this has probably influenced patient and physician choices. Pertinently, CIBMTR data record a progressive reduction in allogeneic transplants performed in CLL with activity in 2015 being less than a third of that reported in 2011.

Currently available novel agents targeting Bruton tyrosine kinase (BTK), BCL2, and Pi3-kinase have profoundly changed the treatment landscape of newly diagnosed and relapsed CLL. These drugs when used as a single agent or in combination are well tolerated compared to traditional alkylator-based chemoimmunotherapy. These novel therapies can provide quite durable remissions. The European Research Initiative on CLL and the European Society for Blood and Marrow Transplantation have provided guidance in selecting high-risk patients who are nonresponsive or intolerant to prior BTK and/or BCL2 inhibitors.[274] In addition, there was a recommendation by the ASBMT to proceed to allo-HCT in patients with Richter transformation after an objective response to anthracycline-based chemotherapy was achieved.[275] Prior exposure to targeted therapies does not appear to impact outcomes of allo-HCT based on retrospective data.[276,277]

Diffuse Large B Lymphoma

Diffuse large B cell lymphoma (DLBCL) accounts for more than 30% of patients with NHL and is an aggressive disease.[278] The prognosis of DLBCL is based on multiple clinical and genomic factors. Around 30% to 40% of patients with DLBCL will relapse after first-line therapy chemoimmunotherapy[279] and their outcomes are poor despite salvage therapies.

Indications for Autologous Hematopoietic Transplantation

Currently, transplantation is not offered as part of routine therapy at first diagnosis. This reflects the findings of a meta-analysis of the outcomes of 3079 patients in 15 clinical trials that found toxicity but no evidence of survival benefit for high-dose therapy and auto-HCT given as consolidation of first CR with initial therapy.[280] More recent findings from prospective clinical trials confirm this approach for the present, although the question of whether particularly aggressive subgroups, such as the so-called "double hit" lymphoma with translocations affecting the MYC plus BCL2 or BCL6 genes, may benefit is still being investigated.[281] Patients who relapse after achieving CR or who do not achieve a CR after initial therapy are potentially eligible for salvage therapy followed by high-dose chemotherapy and auto-HCT. Randomized trials have demonstrated the efficacy of auto-HCT as consolidation of salvage therapy when reserved for the treatment of relapse.[282] The PARMA clinical trial compared the impact of salvage therapy with chemotherapy only vs chemotherapy and bone marrow auto-HCT and showed improvements in 5-year OS from 32% to 53% and event-free survival (EFS) from 12% to 46%.[283] The CORAL study compared two salvage regimens, rituximab, ifosfamide, carboplatin, etoposide (R-ICE) and R-dexamethasone, cytarabine, and cisplatin (DHAP), each followed by high-dose therapy and auto-HCT.[284] Multivariate analysis indicated that adverse factors for EFS were relapse less than 12 months vs more than 12 months after diagnosis (20% vs 45%, respectively), and international prognostic index (IPI) of 2 to 3 vs 0 to 1 (18% vs 40%), respectively. A subset analysis also showed that patients with DLBCL of germinal center cell origin had superior EFS if treated with R-DHAP rather than R-ICE, 100% vs 27%.[285]

Outcomes of primary refractory or relapsed disease within a year of treatment are poor with standard platinum-based chemotherapy and only a small proportion of these patients will be eligible for auto-HCT (SCHOLAR-1 study).[286] CD19 CAR T therapy is proven to be highly effective in relapsed or refractory high-grade B cell lymphoma. Three prospective phase 3 studies have compared CD19 CAR T therapies vs salvage chemotherapy plus auto-HCT in high-risk DLBCL. ZUMA-7 and TRANSFORM respectively used axicabtagene ciloleucel (axi-cel) and lisocabtagene maraleucel (liso-cel) and showed superior EFS compared to the control chemotherapy-auto-HCT arm.[287,288] On contrary, BELINDA study using tisagenlecleucel failed to show any meaningful advantage over the control arm. Based on the results of ZUMA 7, axi-cel was approved by the US FDA for DLBCL refractory to first-line chemoimmunotherapy or relapses within 12 months of first-line chemoimmunotherapy.

Indications for Allogeneic Hematopoietic Cell Transplantation

Allo-HCT may provide durable remissions in 30% to 40% of released DLBCL, but upfront NRM has limited its utilization. Patients having allo-HCT are often heavily pretreated with many having had a previous auto-HCT or chemorefractory disease.[289] Considerable toxicity has been reported following MAC allo-HCT due to TRM/NRM usually caused by direct toxicity of the regimen, sepsis, or GVHD and these have been reported to be as high as 28% to 53% at 3 years post-HCT.[290-295] There has been a trend in these early decades of the 21st century to move away from MAC in favor of RIC/NMA allo-HCT due to the reduced early toxicity as well as the opportunity to extend this therapy to older age groups. A CIBMTR analysis comparing various RIC regimens showed improved outcomes from fludarabine/busulfan compared to fludarabine/melphalan or BCNU/etoposide/cytarabine/melphalan (BEAM) due to lower NRM in less fit and heavily pretreated patients.[296]

CD19 CAR T therapy can provide durable remissions in around 40% even in heavily pretreated patients when used beyond second line. CIBMTR conducted a noncomparative cohort analysis of allo-HCT and CAR T therapy in patients relapsing after auto-HCT for DLBCL and showed comparable outcomes.[297] In practice, most clinicians and patients will choose CAR T over allo-HCT given its favorable toxicity profile and logistical simplicity. Allo-HCT may be reasonable in patients relapsing after CAR T therapy,[298] but additional studies are needed to determine the best transplant approach in this setting.

Hodgkin Lymphoma

About 10% to 15% of patients with Hodgkin lymphoma (HL) are refractory to initial therapy or progress during therapy. In addition, 10% to 20% of patients with stage I-III disease and 30% to 40% with advanced disease will relapse.

Indications for Autologous Hematopoietic Cell Transplantation

Primary Refractory Disease

Patients with primary refractory disease are usually offered salvage therapy and those who have a good performance status should be considered for auto-HCT as this yields better OS than conventional therapy alone, particularly in chemosensitive disease and in the absence of "B" symptoms.[299] Patients with chemosensitive disease have been reported to have 10-year PFS of 62% compared to 23% in poorly responsive disease.[300]

Relapsed Disease

Patients who relapse with recurrent nonlocalized disease should receive at least two cycles of salvage chemotherapy and then, if chemosensitive, have auto-HCT. Some patients may require alternative salvage therapy in order to demonstrate chemosensitivity prior to auto-HCT, preferably by positron emission tomography (PET)-computed tomography scan.[301] Two studies have demonstrated superior outcomes after auto-HCT compared to conventional chemotherapy. One study reported 3-year EFS of 53% vs 10%, while in the other study there was a 3-year freedom from treatment failure of 55 vs 34% although OS was not impacted due to further salvage.[302,303] A meta-analysis has endorsed the use of auto-HCT rather than conventional chemotherapy for refractory or relapsed HL.[304] Involved field radiotherapy may be used for residual disease demonstrated by fluorodeoxyglucose-PET scan and this may be delivered either pre- or post–Auto-HCT.[305]

The likelihood of relapse after auto-HCT is influenced by the presence at transplant of poor performance status, chemotherapy-resistant disease, more than 3 chemotherapy regimens pre-transplant, and extranodal disease. A prognostic index derived from the presence or absence of these features yields 4-year PFS of 71% in low risk and 42% in high risk.[306] Consolidation therapy with brentuximab vedotin after auto-HCT has been shown to provide PFS benefit and should be considered in high-risk HL (Phase III, AETHERA).[307] In a phase II study, consolidation with pembrolizumab after auto-HCT was feasible and resulted in 18-month PFS of 82%.[308]

Indications for Allogeneic Hematopoietic Cell Transplantation

Allo-HCT may provide durable remissions in patients with relapsed disease after auto-HCT. However, checkpoint inhibitors (CPI, nivolumab, pembrolizumab) have emerged as an effective therapeutic option in this setting providing durable remissions in subset of patients.[309] In absence of prospective data, decision to proceed with allo-HCT in patients responding to CPI depends on patient, provider preference, and expected NRM from transplant. Patients with exposure to CPI may be at increased risk for GVHD and non–infectious febrile illness after RIC allo-HCT.[310,311] Increasing the interval between the last CPI infusion and use of PTCy may mitigate these risks.[312,313]

RIC/NMA conditioning is preferred over MAC given higher NRM associated with the latter.[314,315] CIBMTR compared various RIC regimens and showed comparable outcomes between fludarabine/busulfan and fludarabine/melphalan140.[316] Marcais et al reported inferior outcomes associated with the use of UCB as a stem cell source.[315] In contrast, encouraging reports have been published for results of haploidentical transplantation.[317,318] The Seattle group observed significantly lower 2-year rates of relapse following haploidentical RIC HCT compared to matched related or MUD grafts.[317] EBMT analysis showed comparable survival with PTCy-based haploidentical-HCT vs traditional MSD and MUD allo-HCT with lower risk of chronic GVHD compared to MUD.[319]

Follicular Lymphoma

Follicular lymphoma (FL) is an indolent disease with a prognosis that may span many years. A Cochrane review concluded that in patients with relapsed disease there was a survival advantage to auto-HCT in comparison to standard chemotherapy or immunochemotherapy.[320] No survival advantage was seen with the use of auto-HCT as part of first-line therapy.[320]

FL relapsing within 24 months of initial therapy carries a poor long-term prognosis. A National LymphoCare/CIBMTR Study showed improved OS when receiving auto-HCT within 1 year of treatment failure.[321] Multiple registry studies have reported 10-year PFS in the 30 to 50 percent range on the long-term follow-up of auto-HCT for relapsed FL.[322,323]

The National Comprehensive Cancer Network (NCCN) reviewed 184 patients previously treated with rituximab and who had received an autologous or allogeneic HCT.[324] The two groups differed somewhat in age, prior therapy, and disease state, but there was clear evidence of excess NRM in the allo-HCT group, 24 vs 3% that translated into a significantly better survival at 3 years in the auto-HCT recipients of 87% vs 61%. Multivariate analysis confirmed the increased risk of death with an allo-HCT but in the Auto-HCT group identified age greater than 60 years or a history of three or more prior therapies as adverse factors.[324] MAC allo-HCT has been confirmed as offering lower RR than auto-HCT but at a cost of excess TRM.[325] RIC allo-HCT is associated with less toxicity than MAC Allo-HCT and is an option in older patients. Currently, allo-HCT is reserved for patients whose disease is multiply relapsed and refractory to other agents or shows evidence of histological transformation to a more aggressive phase.

CD19 CAR T therapy provides high overall response rates and durable remission in heavily pretreated FL.[326] Given the excellent safety profile of CAR T therapy, utilization of auto- or allo-HCT in relapsed FL in the future may be restricted to CAR T failures.

Mantle Cell Lymphoma

Mantle cell lymphoma is an uncommon NHL subtype that was originally distinguished by the presence of t(11;14) (q13;q32) and overexpression of cyclin D1. The disease has become better characterized at the molecular level with the SOX11 transcription factor used to identify cyclin D1 negative cases and also to define two variants of MCL. The median age at presentation is in the sixties and the median survival 4 to 5 years, since most patients will present with an advanced lymphoma that is predisposed to relapse despite initial responses to therapy.[278]

However, the last decade has seen progress in understanding the heterogeneity of the disease, the associated prognostic markers, the role of cytarabine and rituximab during induction therapy, the probable value of monitoring of MRD, and the potential of multiple new agents currently being studied in prospective clinical trials.

Prognostic Scores

Prognostic indicators have been recognized that enhance the understanding of the biological behavior of MCL. The MCL International Prognostic Index (MIPI) incorporates age, Eastern Cooperative Oncology Group (ECOG) performance status, *lactate dehydrogenase*, and WBC count.[327] Tumor Ki-67 proliferation index is also a very strong indicator of outcome.[328] High-risk disease with poor outcome may be identified by Ki-67 of 30% or more, deletions in *CDKN2A* and *TP53*, and high levels of expression of SOX11.[328-330] Genomic screening has illuminated a microRNA signature associated with poor-risk disease and a MIPI-B-miR prognostic index incorporating miR-18b has been validated.[331] Although patients with the low-risk disease may be identified, treatment algorithms do not yet support the notion of therapy de-escalation in such groups.

Indications for Autologous Hematopoietic Cell Transplant

The current standard of care for patients who are deemed fit for intensive chemotherapy is to give initial chemotherapy based on a high-dose cytarabine (HDAC) regimen combined with rituximab.[332] The recent EBMT/European MCL Network (EMCL) consensus project advocates that auto-HCT is used to consolidate response to induction in fit patients who have achieved at least a partial remission (PR) with induction therapy.[332]

Hyper-CVAD (hypofractionated cyclophosphamide, vincristine, doxorubicin, and dexamethasone alternating with cytarabine and methotrexate) induces a high CR rate of 87% and prolonged remissions but has been difficult to deliver in multicenter studies due to toxicity.[333] Alternatives include CHOP (cyclophosphamide, doxorubicin, vincristine, prednisolone) alternating with DHAP and the Nordic regimen R-Maxi-CHOP alternating with HDAC and these are generally consolidated with an auto-HCT.[329,334] The addition of rituximab prolongs EFS.[335]

A phase 3 randomized study conducted by the European Mantle Cell Lymphoma Network has confirmed the value of HDAC prior to auto-HCT.[336] In this study, 497 patients aged up to 65 years with untreated MCL stage II-IV were randomized to a control or HDAC group. The control group received six courses of R-CHOP (rituximab added to CHOP) followed by stem cell mobilization using Dexa-BEAM (dexamethasone, carmustine, etoposide, cytarabine and melphalan), MA CyTBI, and auto-HCT.[337,338] The HDAC group received six courses of R-CHOP alternating with R-DHAP (rituximab added to DHAP) followed by an MA TBI, HDAC, and melphalan conditioning regimen and auto-HCT. Median follow-up was 6.1 years and time to treatment failure was longer in the HDAC group with a median of 9.1 compared to 3.9 years in the control group. Almost twice as many patients achieved an MRD negative status prior to auto-HCT in the HDAC group, but nevertheless there were still late relapses. As yet there is no significant difference in OS but longer follow-up is necessary.

A recent update of the Nordic MCL2 regimen reported the outcomes of 160 patients aged less than 66 years, diagnosed with stage II-IV mantle cell lymphoma between 2000 and 2006.[334] They were treated with alternating maxi-CHOP and HDAC, three courses of each with rituximab also given during 3 to 5 courses. High-dose therapy prior to auto-HCT comprised BEAM (carmustine, etoposide, cytarabine, and melphalan) or BEAC (carmustine, etoposide, cytarabine, and cyclophosphamide). Median follow-up was 11.4 years and median OS and PFS were 12.7 and 8.5 years, respectively.[334] Survival outcomes validated the use of the MIPI, KI-67, and miR-18b to define risk groups. However, late relapses occurred in all risk groups and overall results were comparable to other recently updated studies.[333,335]

A better understanding of the underlying molecular pathophysiology of MCL facilitates rational choices of therapies. Bortezomib, temsirolimus, lenalidomide, and ibrutinib are among a plethora of newer agents being studied in MCL that may be incorporated into first-line care in the future and may even supplant the role of autologous transplantation. ECOG4151 is designed to test an MRD-guided transplant strategy and the study is currently enrolling patients.

Maintenance Treatment After Autologous Transplant

Given the prevalence of late relapse following auto-HCT, there has been considerable interest in the use of posttransplant maintenance. Agents chosen for investigation include rituximab and bortezomib as single agents or in combination.[339-341] The phase 3 Lymphoma Study Association (LYSA) trial showed PFS and OS benefit with maintenance rituximab for 3 years after auto-HCT.[342] A similar phase III study (MCL0208) showed better PFS and similar OS from maintenance lenalidomide vs observation alone after auto-HCT.[343]

Management of Relapse

Treatment of relapsed MCL has significantly improved with development of targeted therapies such as ibrutinib, venetoclax, and CD19 CAR T therapy. Brexucabtagene autoleucel is effective in relapsed MCL and may provide durable remissions. In a phase II trial, it resulted in 1-year EFS of 61% and OS of 83% in heavily pretreated MCL including prior BTK inhibitor failure.[344]

Auto-HCT has limited efficacy beyond CR1 although a recent CIBMTR registry study did identify some patients who will benefit with a 5-year OS of 44% for selected patients receiving auto-HCT in heavily pretreated disease.[345] Prognostic scores can identify patients with high-risk disease, but as yet there is no proof that such patients will benefit from early allogeneic HCT, in light of the risk of associated TRM. While allogeneic HCT is not routinely offered as part of first-line therapy, it may be considered as a consolidation of salvage therapy, preferably as part of a clinical trial.[332] Results to date have been conflicting. Patients and physicians may well opt for competing non–transplant clinical trials that use one or more of the newer agents. NMA or RIC regimens are preferred to MA regimens due to the lower early TRM. The use of assessments such as the HCT comorbidity index is advisable as the patient population is likely to be older and frailer than the average transplant candidate.[346] There is no one NMA/RIC approach superior to others.

Newer immunotherapies may provide a safer alternative to RIC allo-HCT in the future. Allo-HCT may be considered in fit patients with relapsed MCL after BTK inhibitor and CAR T therapy.

Mature T-/Natural Killer-Cell Malignancies

Peripheral T cell lymphoma (PTCL) accounts for about 10% to 20% of lymphomas, contains more than 20 distinct entities, and is more prevalent in Asia.[278] The largest single subgroup is PTCL not otherwise specified (NOS) and is itself a heterogeneous group of mature T cell lymphomas that do not satisfy the criteria for the remaining subgroups.[347] PTCL (NOS) together with anaplastic large cell lymphoma (ALCL) anaplastic lymphoma kinase (ALK)–positive, ALCL ALK–negative, and angioimmunoblastic T-cell lymphoma (AITL) are the commonest PTCLs.

Patients with advanced stage disease and/or high IPI are usually recommended to have induction therapy with multiagent chemotherapy, preferably as part of a clinical trial and depending upon their comorbidity.[348] The IPI may be used to predict the response to initial combination chemotherapy.[349] Advanced disease at presentation is common and prognosis is poor in PTCLs with an overall 5-year survival of about 30% with an exception of ALK-positive ALCL.[349-352]

A meta-analysis of anthracycline-based initial therapy of PTCL reported overall CR rates of 30% to 76%, but relapse rate (RR) of 43% with 30% to 40% of patients suffering disease progression during chemotherapy.[353] While OS survival at 5 years was estimated as 35.5% to 41.6% for all PTCLs, it was better at 42.8% to 69.2% in ALCL.[353] ECHELON-2 was a phase III study, which showed superior PFS and OS when brentuximab vedotin was added to a frontline anthracycline-based regimen in CD30-positive PTCL.[354]

Indications for Autologous Hematopoietic Cell Transplant

High RI after frontline therapy in many subtypes of PTCL has led to exploration of consolidative auto-HCT as a strategy to improve outcomes. Given excellent outcomes in ALK-positive ALCL with chemotherapy only, auto-HCT is reserved for relapsed cases only. Among other PTCL subtypes, auto-HCT in CR1 is shown to improve RI and provide PFS benefit based on retrospective and small prospective studies.[355-357] A recent systematic review/meta-analysis of the value of auto-HCT reviewed the outcomes of 1368 patients.[358] Where prospective studies had reported the use of auto-HCT as part of first-line therapy in 179 patients, PFS was 33% (95% confidence interval [CI], 14%-56%), OS of 54% (95% CI, 32%-75%), relapse/progression of 26% (95% CI, 20%-33%), and TRM of 2% (95% CI, 0%-5%).[358,359] Subgroup analysis by histological subgroup in one prospective study reported 5-year OS and PFS of 47% and 38% in PTCL NOS, 70% and 61% in ALCL ALK negative, and 52% and 49% in AITL, respectively.[355] Only retrospective study results were available for the interpretation of the value of auto-HCT in relapsed or refractory disease and these showed PFS of 36% (95% CI, 32%-40%), OS of 47% (95% CI, 43%-51%), relapse/progression of 51% (95% CI, 39% to 62%), and TRM of 10% (95% CI, 5%-17%).[358]

Indications for Allogeneic Hematopoietic Cell Transplant

The use of allo-HCT is generally limited to relapsed or refractory PTCL. AATT (Autologous or Allogeneic Transplantation in T-cell lymphoma) was a prospective randomized study that showed no difference in outcomes between consolidation with allo-HCT and auto-HCT after frontline therapy.[360] Outcomes of allo-HCT, in general, have improved due in large part to better supportive care, and in the case of PTCL, there has been a trend over time to use RIC/NMA regimens rather than MAC.[361] In terms of donors, haploidentical and unrelated donors as well as HLA-matched siblings have proved effective.[362,363] A CIBMTR retrospective analysis of 119 patients who had allo-HCT in PTCL beyond CR1 reported a 3-year PFS and OS of 37% and 46%, respectively, with no discernible impact of conditioning intensity.[361] In this study, multivariate analysis showed that in comparison to auto-HCT there was an increased TRM after allo-HCT that was balanced by a reduction in RR of approximately 50%. Such a reduction in RR as well as reported efficacy of DLI in reversing relapse substantiates the graft-versus-malignancy (GVM) effect in PTCL.[361,362] This study also confirmed that chemotherapy resistance is a poor prognostic factor even after allo-HCT.[361,362]

It is apparent that patients who benefit from high-dose therapy with auto-HCT are a highly selected subgroup and it may therefore be necessary in future prospective studies to define disease status stringently at the end of conventional therapy to address the real need for high-dose therapy. Conversely, patients with refractory disease or in PR may benefit from novel agents to optimize their response prior to high-dose therapy and these are candidates for allo-HCT.[347]

PLASMA CELL DISORDERS

Multiple Myeloma

MM is a hematological malignancy commonly affecting the bone marrow, bones, and kidneys resulting in pathological fractures, hypercalcemia, cytopenia, and renal failure. Recent advances in therapeutics have allowed rapid disease control and durable remissions in many patients with newly diagnosed and relapsed MM.[364] However, treatment resistant is common and most patients ultimately succumb to their disease after initial response to systemic therapies. Prognosis of MM is largely dependent on baseline genomic characteristics, response to therapy, and patients' comorbidities. High-risk abnormalities on FISH such as t(4;14), t(14;16), t(14;20), del17p13, or gain 1q found in approximately 25% of newly diagnosed MM are associated with early treatment failure and shortened survival.[365] Recently, MRD has emerged as an important prognostic and predictive marker across different settings. Recent meta-analysis of three prospective phase 3 trials that included patients treated with novel daratumumab-based regimens showed better PFS in patients in CR and undetectable MRD (estimated 48-month PFS 70 vs 52%) over patients with detectable MRD.[366] High-dose therapy followed by auto-HCT remains the most effective therapy for MM providing improved depth of response and duration of remissions.

Indications for Autologous Hematopoietic Cell Transplant

Upfront auto-HCT in fit patients with newly diagnosed MM after initial induction therapy for 3 to 4 months has been standard of care for decades. Studies in late 90s and early 2000 have confirmed PFS and OS benefit from auto-HCT compared to traditional chemotherapy-based induction regimens.[367,368] Since these initial studies were completed, proteosome inhibitor, immunomodulatory drugs, and monoclonal antibodies such as daratumumab (anti-CD39 mAb) have become part of standard induction regimens. Routine use of novel induction regimens has resulted in a better overall response rate in high-risk and unfit patients with newly diagnosed MM. Several studies have re-evaluated the role of upfront consolidative auto-HCT after modern induction regimens and show a consistent PFS benefit[369-373] (Table 106.3). IFM-2003 was a phase 3 study that showed superior PFS and MDS negativity in patients who received upfront auto-HCT after lenalidomide and bortezomib-based triplet induction therapy. There was no OS difference between the study cohorts; however, most patients in the control arm eventually received auto-HCT at relapse.[369,383] Benefit of upfront auto-HCT in patients ≥70 years of age is unknown as these patients were included in prospective studies. However, the feasibility and safety of auto-HCT in this age group have been shown in retrospective and registry-based observational studies.[384,385] Preplanned tandem auto-HCT and additional posttransplant consolidation therapies have been studied to deepen the response and allow durable remissions in multiple prospective studies with mixed results. BMT CTN 0702, STaMINA was a three-arm study that randomized patients to receive second auto-HCT followed by maintenance lenalidomide vs four cycles of consolidation (bortezomib, lenalidomide, and dexamethasone) followed by maintenance lenalidomide vs maintenance lenalidomide only. All three arms resulted in similar PFS and OS at 38 months.[386] There might be some benefit of tandem auto-HCT in patients with high-risk MM who fail to achieve CR after first auto-HCT.[373] Long-term post–transplant maintenance therapy is considered standard in most situations as it has shown consistent PFS benefit across multiple studies.[376,387] Patient–level meta-analysis of three prospective studies also showed OS benefit with lenalidomide maintenance after auto-HCT.[388] As induction and maintenance therapies improve with novel agents, additional prospective studies are needed to re-evaluate the role of tandem auto-HCT, consolidation therapies, and MRD–based transplant decision-making. In contrast to upfront auto-HCT, the role of transplant for relapsed or refractory MM is not clear given continuously evolving therapeutic armamentarium. In IFM-2009, 79% of patients received auto-HCT at first relapse.[369] Since there was no OS benefit between early vs delayed auto-HCT approach, transplant should be considered in MM at first relapse.

Indications for Allogeneic Hematopoietic Cell Transplant

Allo-HCT is the only potentially curative therapy for MM, but its role remains controversial given high NRM and RR. Multiple studies have used biological randomization (allo-HCT based on availability of MSD) to compare upfront tandem auto-HCT vs RIC allo-HCT after auto-HCT. The results varied across studies and PFS benefit of allo-HCT was offset by NRM in most situations. A meta-analysis of four studies showed improved PFS and OS at the expense of NRM with auto-allo compared to auto-auto approach.[389] Safety and efficacy of allo-HCT in MM may be improved with incorporation of novel agents during conditioning and posttransplant maintenance.[390]

Systemic Amyloidosis, POEMS
Indications for Autologous Hematopoietic Cell Transplant

Immunoglobulin light chain (AL) amyloidosis is a systemic clonal plasma cell disorder characterized by extracellular tissue deposition of fragments of monoclonal light chains. The goal of therapy is to eliminate production of light chains by plasma cell–directed therapies and allow improvement in organ function. The prognosis is mainly driven by degree of cardiac involvement as incorporated in various staging systems.[391,392] High-dose therapy and auto-HCT can result in deep hematological remissions allowing improvement in organ function and

Table 106.3. Outcomes in Autologous HCT for Multiple Myeloma

Study	n	PFS	OS	NRM	Follow-Up	Maintenance Therapy	Notes
Gay et al[374]	102	43%	63%	8%	5 y	R	New diagnosis; patients ≥ 65 y
Palumbo et al[375]	195	60%	-	-	3 y	R ± RP	New diagnosis
Palumbo et al[376]	273	65%	81.6%	-	4 y	± R	New diagnoses
Cavo et al[377]	208 207	60% 73%	-	12%	3 y	R	Single autologous HCT Double autologous HCT New diagnosis
Neukirchen et al[378]	437	70%	87%	-	4 y	± R	New diagnosis; patients ≥ 65 y
Attal et al[369]	350	50%	82%	1.7%	4 y	VRD	New diagnosis
Veltri et al[379]	233	38%	74%	2%	2 y	Many	Relapsed/refractory
Gagelmann et al[380]	202 286	29% 49%	54% 78%	2%	4 y	Unknown	High risk cytogenetics Normal risk cytogenetics New diagnosis
Moreau et al[381]	543	93%	97%	8.5%	1.5 y	D-VTd or VTd	New diagnosis
Cavo et al[373]	702	51%	75.1%	12%	5 y	±VRD	New diagnosis
Nishimura et al[382]	4329	-	62%	-	5 y	Many	New diagnosis Survival improved with year of HCT

Abbreviations: D-VTd, daratumumab + bortezomib/thalidomide/dexamethasone; HCT, hematopoietic cell transplantation; OS, overall survival; PFS, progression-free survival; R, lenalidomide; RCT, randomized control trial; RP, lenalidomide + prednisone; VRD, bortezomib, lenalidomide, dexamethasone; VTd, bortezomib/thalidomide/dexamethasone.

QoL. The evidence to support the use of auto-HCT on AL amyloidosis is based on retrospective and observational studies.[393,394] Compared to MM, patients undergoing auto-HCT for AL amyloidosis are at higher risk for TRM due to cardiac arrhythmia, sepsis, hypotension, and renal dysfunction. Careful patient selection by comprehensive multidisciplinary evaluation is key to minimize the risk of early complications after high-dose melphalan. Improved efficacy of upfront therapy with incorporation of daratumumab[395] has challenged the role of consolidative auto-HCT and prospective studies are needed to better define transplants role. Recently, a CIBMTR study showed feasibility of second auto-HCT for relapsed AL amyloidosis in carefully selected patients.[396]

POEMS syndrome (Polyneuropathy, Organomegaly, Endocrinopathy, Monoclonal protein, Skin changes) is a systemic inflammatory disorder driven by chronically elevated cytokine production and associated monoclonal gammopathy. Given the rarity of the diagnosis, there are no prospective studies guiding treatment recommendations. Multiple retrospective studies have shown improved organ function, neuropathy, and endocrinopathy among patients with advanced POEMS syndrome who underwent high-dose melphalan and auto-HCT.[397,398] The responses appear to be durable in a majority of patients with TRM comparable to patients with MM undergoing auto-HCT.[399]

References

1. D'Souza A, Fretham C, Lee SJ, et al. Current use of and trends in hematopoietic cell transplantation in the United States. *Biol Blood Marrow Transplant*. 2020;26(8):e177-e182.
2. Bracci L, Moschella F, Sestili P, et al. Cyclophosphamide enhances the antitumor efficacy of adoptively transferred immune cells through the induction of cytokine expression, B-cell and T-cell homeostatic proliferation, and specific tumor infiltration. *Clin Cancer Res*. 2007;13(2 pt 1):644-653.
3. Kanakry CG, Fuchs EJ, Luznik L. Modern approaches to HLA-haploidentical blood or marrow transplantation. *Nat Rev Clin Oncol*. 2016;13(1):10-24.
4. Fuchs EJ, O'Donnell PV, Eapen M, et al. Double unrelated umbilical cord blood vs HLA-haploidentical bone marrow transplantation: the BMT CTN 1101 trial. *Blood*. 2021;137(3):420-428.
5. Bolanos-Meade J, Reshef R, Fraser R, et al. Three prophylaxis regimens (tacrolimus, mycophenolate mofetil, and cyclophosphamide; tacrolimus, methotrexate, and bortezomib; or tacrolimus, methotrexate, and maraviroc) versus tacrolimus and methotrexate for prevention of graft-versus-host disease with haemopoietic cell transplantation with reduced-intensity conditioning: a randomised phase 2 trial with a non-randomised contemporaneous control group (BMT CTN 1203). *Lancet Haematol*. 2019;6(3):e132-e143.
6. Cooke KR, Luznik L, Sarantopoulos S, et al. The biology of chronic graft-versus-host disease: a task force report from the National Institutes of health consensus development project on criteria for clinical trials in chronic graft-versus-host disease. *Biol Blood Marrow Transplant J Am Soc Blood Marrow Transplant*. 2016;23(2):211-234.
7. Zeiser R, von Bubnoff N, Butler J, et al. Ruxolitinib for glucocorticoid-refractory acute graft-versus-host disease. *N Engl J Med*. 2020;382(19):1800-1810.
8. Zeiser R, Polverelli N, Ram R, et al. Ruxolitinib for glucocorticoid-refractory chronic graft-versus-host disease. *N Engl J Med*. 2021;385(3):228-238.
9. Miklos D, Cutler CS, Arora M, et al. Ibrutinib for chronic graft-versus-host disease after failure of prior therapy. *Blood*. 2017;130(21):2243-2250.
10. Jagasia M, Lazaryan A, Bachier CR, et al. ROCK2 inhibition with belumosudil (KD025) for the treatment of chronic graft-versus-host disease. *J Clin Oncol Off J Am Soc Clin Oncol*. 2021;39(17):1888-1898.
11. Devine SM, Owzar K, Blum W, et al. Phase II study of allogeneic transplantation for older patients with acute myeloid leukemia in first complete remission using a reduced-intensity conditioning regimen: results from cancer and leukemia group B 100103 (alliance for clinical trials in oncology)/blood and marrow transplant clinical trial Network 0502. *J Clin Oncol*. 2015;33(35):4167-4175.
12. Niederwieser D, Al-Ali HK, Krahl R, et al. Hematopoietic stem cell transplantation (HSCT) compared to consolidation chemotherapy (CT) to increase leukemia free survival (LFS) in acute myelogenous leukemia (AML) patients between 60 and 75 years irrespective of genetic risk: report from the AML 2004 of the East German Study Group (OSHO). *J Clin Oncol*. 2016;34(15_suppl):e18501.
13. Sorror ML, Maris MB, Storb R, et al. Hematopoietic cell transplantation (HCT)-specific comorbidity index: a new tool for risk assessment before allogeneic HCT. *Blood*. 2005;106(8):2912-2919.
14. Niederwieser D, Baldomero H, Szer J, et al. Hematopoietic stem cell transplantation activity worldwide in 2012 and a SWOT analysis of the Worldwide Network for Blood and Marrow Transplantation Group including the global survey. *Bone Marrow Transplant*. 2016;51(6):778-785.
15. Döhner H, Estey E, Grimwade D, et al. Diagnosis and management of AML in adults: 2017 ELN recommendations from an international expert panel. *Blood*. 2016;129(4):424-447.
16. Daver N, Wei AH, Pollyea DA, Fathi AT, Vyas P, DiNardo CD. New directions for emerging therapies in acute myeloid leukemia: the next chapter. *Blood Cancer J*. 2020;10(10):1-12.
17. Schuurhuis GJ, Heuser M, Freeman S, et al. Minimal/measurable residual disease in AML: a consensus document from the European LeukemiaNet MRD Working Party. *Blood*. 2018;131(12):1275-1291.
18. Kongtim P, Hasan O, Perez JMR, Varma A, Wang SA, Patel KP, et al. Novel disease risk model for patients with acute myeloid leukemia receiving allogeneic hematopoietic cell transplantation. *Biol Blood Marrow Transplant*. 2019;26(1):197-203.
19. Freeman SD, Hills RK, Virgo P, et al. Measurable residual disease at induction redefines partial response in acute myeloid leukemia and stratifies outcomes in patients at standard risk without NPM1 mutations. *J Clin Oncol*. 2018;36(15):1486-1497
20. Walter RB, Gyurkocza B, Storer BE, et al. Comparison of minimal residual disease as outcome predictor for AML patients in first complete remission undergoing myeloablative or nonmyeloablative allogeneic hematopoietic cell transplantation. *Leukemia*. 2015;29(1):137-144.
21. Ivey A, Hills RK, Simpson MA, et al. Assessment of minimal residual disease in standard-risk AML. *N Engl J Med*. 2016;374(5):422-433.
22. Koreth J, Schlenk R, Kopecky KJ, et al. Allogeneic stem cell transplantation for acute myeloid leukemia in first complete remission: systematic review and meta-analysis of prospective clinical trials. *JAMA*. 2009;301(22):2349-2361.
23. Cornelissen JJ, van Putten WLJ, Verdonck LF, et al. Results of a HOVON/SAKK donor versus no-donor analysis of myeloablative HLA-identical sibling stem cell transplantation in first remission acute myeloid leukemia in young and middle-aged adults: benefits for whom? *Blood*. 2007;109(9):3658-3666.
24. Yanada M, Matsuo K, Emi N, Naoe T. Efficacy of allogeneic hematopoietic stem cell transplantation depends on cytogenetic risk for acute myeloid leukemia in first disease remission: a metaanalysis. *Cancer*. 2005;103(8):1652-1658.
25. Schetelig J, Schaich M, Schafer-Eckart K, et al. Hematopoietic cell transplantation in patients with intermediate and high-risk AML: results from the randomized Study Alliance Leukemia (SAL) AML 2003 trial. *Leukemia*. 2015;29(5):1060-1068.
26. Cornelissen JJ, Gratwohl A, Schlenk RF, et al. The European LeukemiaNet AML Working Party consensus statement on allogeneic HSCT for patients with AML in remission: an integrated-risk adapted approach. *Nat Rev Clin Oncol*. 2012;9(10):579-590.
27. Paun O, Lazarus HM. Allogeneic hematopoietic cell transplantation for acute myeloid leukemia in first complete remission: have the indications changed? *Curr Opin Hematol*. 2012;19(2):95-101.
28. Passweg JR, Labopin M, Cornelissen J, et al. Conditioning intensity in middle-aged patients with AML in first CR: no advantage for myeloablative regimens irrespective of the risk group-an observational analysis by the Acute Leukemia Working Party of the EBMT. *Bone Marrow Transplant*. 2015;50(8):1063-1068.
29. Russell NH, Kjeldsen L, Craddock C, et al. A comparative assessment of the curative potential of reduced intensity allografts in acute myeloid leukaemia. *Leukemia*. 2015;29(7):1478-1484.
30. Cornelissen JJ, Blaise D. Hematopoietic stem cell transplantation for patients with AML in first complete remission. *Blood*. 2016;127(1):62-70.
31. Appelbaum FR, Gundacker H, Head DR, et al. Age and acute myeloid leukemia. *Blood*. 2006;107(9):3481-3485.
32. Frohling S, Schlenk RF, Kayser S, et al. Cytogenetics and age are major determinants of outcome in intensively treated acute myeloid leukemia patients older than 60 years: results from AMLSG trial AML HD98-B. *Blood*. 2006;108(10):3280-3288.
33. Borthakur G, Lin E, Jain N, et al. Survival is poorer in patients with secondary core-binding factor acute myelogenous leukemia compared with de novo core-binding factor leukemia. *Cancer*. 2009;115(14):3217-3221.
34. Gustafson SA, Lin P, Chen SS, et al. Therapy-related acute myeloid leukemia with t(8;21) (q22;q22) shares many features with de novo acute myeloid leukemia with t(8;21)(q22;q22) but does not have a favorable outcome. *Am J Clin Pathol*. 2009;131(5):647-655.
35. Ishikawa Y, Kawashima N, Atsuta Y, et al. Prospective evaluation of prognostic impact of KIT mutations on acute myeloid leukemia with RUNX1-RUNX1T1 and CBFB-MYH11. *Blood Adv*. 2020;4(1):66-75.
36. Paschka P, Du J, Schlenk RF, et al. Secondary genetic lesions in acute myeloid leukemia with inv(16) or t(16;16): a study of the German-Austrian AML Study Group (AMLSG). *Blood*. 2013;121(1):170-177.
37. Schlenk RF, Pasquini MC, Perez WS, et al. HLA-identical sibling allogeneic transplants versus chemotherapy in acute myelogenous leukemia with t(8;21) in first complete remission: collaborative study between the German AML Intergroup and CIBMTR. *Biol Blood Marrow Transplant*. 2008;14(2):187-196.
38. Schlenk RF, Kayser S, Bullinger L, et al. Differential impact of allelic ratio and insertion site in FLT3-ITD-positive AML with respect to allogeneic transplantation. *Blood*. 2014;124(23):3441-3449.
39. Dohner H, Estey E, Grimwade D, et al. Diagnosis and management of AML in adults: 2017 ELN recommendations from an international expert panel. *Blood*. 2017;129(4):424-447.
40. Lindsley RC, Saber W, Mar BG, et al. Prognostic mutations in myelodysplastic syndrome after stem-cell transplantation. *N Engl J Med*. 2017;376(6):536-547.
41. Yoshizato T, Nannya Y, Atsuta Y, et al. Genetic abnormalities in myelodysplasia and secondary acute myeloid leukemia: impact on outcome of stem cell transplantation. *Blood*. 2017;129(17):2347-2358.
42. Badar T, Atallah E, Shallis RM, et al. Outcomes of TP53-mutated AML with evolving frontline therapies: impact of allogeneic stem cell transplantation on survival. *Am J Hematol*. 2022;97(7):E232-E235.
43. Grob T, Al Hinai AS, Sanders MA, et al. Molecular characterization of mutant TP53 acute myeloid leukemia and high-risk myelodysplastic syndrome. *Blood*. 2022;139(15):2347-2354.
44. Venditti A, Piciocchi A, Candoni A, et al. GIMEMA AML1310 trial of risk-adapted, MRD-directed therapy for young adults with newly diagnosed acute myeloid leukemia. *Blood*. 2019;134(12):935-945.

45. Zhu HH, Zhang XH, Qin YZ, et al. MRD-directed risk stratification treatment may improve outcomes of t(8;21) AML in the first complete remission: results from the AML05 multicenter trial. *Blood*. 2013;121(20):4056-4062.
46. Nagler A, Savani BN, Labopin M, et al. Outcomes after use of two standard ablative regimens in patients with refractory acute myeloid leukaemia: a retrospective, multicentre, registry analysis. *Lancet Haematol*. 2015;2(9):e384-e392.
47. Ferguson P, Hills RK, Grech A, et al. An operational definition of primary refractory acute myeloid leukemia allowing early identification of patients who may benefit from allogeneic stem cell transplantation. *Haematologica*. 2016;101(11):1351-1358.
48. Duval M, Klein JP, He W, et al. Hematopoietic stem-cell transplantation for acute leukemia in relapse or primary induction failure. *J Clin Oncol Off J Am Soc Clin Oncol*. 2010;28(23):3730-3738.
49. Schmid C, Schleuning M, Schwerdtfeger R, et al. Long-term survival in refractory acute myeloid leukemia after sequential treatment with chemotherapy and reduced-intensity conditioning for allogeneic stem cell transplantation. *Blood*. 2006;108(3):1092-1099.
50. Burnett A, Wetzler M, Löwenberg B. Therapeutic advances in acute myeloid leukemia. *J Clin Oncol*. 2011;29(5):487-494.
51. Rowe JM, Li X, Cassileth PA, , et al. Very poor survival of patients with AML who relapse after achieving a first complete remission: the eastern cooperative oncology group experience. *Blood*. 2005;106(11):546. [Internet]. Accessed December 11, 2016. http://www.bloodjournal.org/content/106/11/546
52. Forman SJ, Rowe JM. The myth of the second remission of acute leukemia in the adult. *Blood*. 2013;121(7):1077-1082.
53. Breems DA, Van Putten WLJ, Huijgens PC, et al. Prognostic index for adult patients with acute myeloid leukemia in first relapse. *J Clin Oncol*. 2005;23(9):1969-1978.
54. Chevallier P, Labopin M, Turlure P, et al. A new Leukemia Prognostic Scoring System for refractory/relapsed adult acute myelogeneous leukaemia patients: a GOELAMS study. *Leukemia*. 2011;25(6):939-944.
55. Kharfan-Dabaja MA, Labopin M, Polge E, et al. Association of second allogeneic hematopoietic cell transplant vs donor lymphocyte infusion with overall survival in patients with acute myeloid leukemia relapse. *JAMA Oncol*. 2018;4(9):1245-1253.
56. Litzow MR, Tarima S, Perez WS, et al. Allogeneic transplantation for therapy-related myelodysplastic syndrome and acute myeloid leukemia. *Blood*. 2010;115(9):1850-1857.
57. Sengsayadeth S, Gatwood KS, Boumendil A, et al. Conditioning intensity in secondary AML with prior myelodysplastic syndrome/myeloproliferative disorders: an EBMT ALWP study. *Blood Adv*. 2018;2(16):2127-2135.
58. Keating A, DaSilva G, Pérez WS, et al. Autologous blood cell transplantation versus HLA-identical sibling transplantation for acute myeloid leukemia in first complete remission: a registry study from the Center for International Blood and Marrow Transplantation Research. *Haematologica*. 2013;98(2):185-192.
59. Cornelissen JJ, Breems D, van Putten WLJ, et al. Comparative analysis of the value of allogeneic hematopoietic stem-cell transplantation in acute myeloid leukemia with monosomal karyotype versus other cytogenetic risk categories. *J Clin Oncol Off J Am Soc Clin Oncol*. 2012;30(17):2140-2146.
60. Gorin N-C, Giebel S, Labopin M, Savani BN, Mohty M, Nagler A. Autologous stem cell transplantation for adult acute leukemia in 2015: time to rethink? Present status and future prospects. *Bone Marrow Transplant*. 2015;50(12):1495-1502.
61. Vellenga E, van Putten W, Ossenkoppele GJ, et al. Autologous peripheral blood stem cell transplantation for acute myeloid leukemia. *Blood*. 2011;118(23):6037-6042.
62. Yanada M, Tsuzuki M, Fujita H, et al. Phase 2 study of arsenic trioxide followed by autologous hematopoietic cell transplantation for relapsed acute promyelocytic leukemia. *Blood*. 2013;121(16):3095-3102.
63. Holter Chakrabarty JL, Rubinger M, Le-Rademacher J, et al. Autologous is superior to allogeneic hematopoietic cell transplantation for acute promyelocytic leukemia in second complete remission. *Biol Blood Marrow Transplant*. 2014;20(7):1021-1025.
64. Nagler A, Rocha V, Labopin M, et al. Allogeneic hematopoietic stem-cell transplantation for acute myeloid leukemia in remission: comparison of intravenous busulfan plus cyclophosphamide (Cy) versus total-body irradiation plus Cy as conditioning regimen – a report from the acute leukemia working party of the European group for blood and marrow transplantation. *J Clin Oncol*. 2013;31(28):3549-3556.
65. Copelan EA, Hamilton BK, Avalos B, et al. Better leukemia-free and overall survival in AML in first remission following cyclophosphamide in combination with busulfan compared with TBI. *Blood*. 2013;122(24):3863-3870.
66. Bredeson C, LeRademacher J, Kato K, et al. Prospective cohort study comparing intravenous busulfan to total body irradiation in hematopoietic cell transplantation. *Blood*. 2013;122(24):3871-3878.
67. Savani BN, Labopin M, Kröger N, et al. Expanding transplant options to patients over 50 years. Improved outcome after reduced intensity conditioning mismatched-unrelated donor transplantation for patients with acute myeloid leukemia: a report from the Acute Leukemia Working Party of the EBMT. *Haematologica*. 2016;101(6):773-780.
68. Scott BL, Pasquini MC, Logan BR, et al. Myeloablative versus reduced-intensity hematopoietic cell transplantation for acute myeloid leukemia and myelodysplastic syndromes. *J Clin Oncol*. 2017;35(11):1154-1161. doi:10.1200/jco.2016.70.7091
69. Scott BL. Long-term follow up of BMT CTN 0901, a randomized phase III trial comparing myeloablative (MAC) to reduced intensity conditioning (RIC) prior to hematopoietic cell transplantation (HCT) for acute myeloid leukemia (AML) or myelodysplasia (MDS) (MAvRIC trial). *Biol Blood Marrow Transplant*. 2020;26(3):S11.
70. Hourigan CS, Dillon LW, Gui G, et al. Impact of conditioning intensity of allogeneic transplantation for acute myeloid leukemia with genomic evidence of residual disease. *J Clin Oncol*. 2020;38(12):1273-1283.
71. Appelbaum FR. Alternative donor transplantation for adults with acute leukemia. *Best Pract Res Clin Haematol*. 2014;27(3-4):272-277.
72. Bacigalupo A. Matched and mismatched unrelated donor transplantation: is the outcome the same as for matched sibling donor transplantation? *Hematol Am Soc Hematol Educ Program*. 2012;2012:223-229.
73. Eapen M, Rocha V, Sanz G, et al. Effect of graft source on unrelated donor haemopoietic stem-cell transplantation in adults with acute leukaemia: a retrospective analysis. *Lancet Oncol*. 2010;11(7):653-660.
74. Wang Y, Liu DH, Xu L-P, et al. Haploidentical/mismatched hematopoietic stem cell transplantation without in vitro T cell depletion for T cell acute lymphoblastic leukemia. *Biol Blood Marrow Transplant*. 2012;18(5):716-721.
75. Federmann B, Bornhauser M, Meisner C, et al. Haploidentical allogeneic hematopoietic cell transplantation in adults using CD3/CD19 depletion and reduced intensity conditioning: a phase II study. *Haematologica*. 2012;97(10):1523-1531.
76. Ma YR, Huang XJ, Xu ZL, et al. Transplantation from haploidentical donor is not inferior to that from identical sibling donor for patients with chronic myeloid leukemia in blast crisis or chronic phase from blast crisis. *Clin Transplant*. 2016;30(9):994-1001.
77. Brunstein C, O'Donnell P, Eapen M, et al. *Results of Blood and Marrow Transplant Clinical Trials Network Protocol 1101 a Multicenter Phase III Randomized Trial of Transplantation of Double Umbilical Cord Blood vs. HLA-Haploidentical -Related Bone Marrow for Hematologic Malignancy*. 2020. Accessed June 29, 2020. https://tct.confex.com/tct/2020/meetingapp.cgi/Session/5289
78. Wang Y, Liu QF, Xu LP, et al. Haploidentical vs identical-sibling transplant for AML in remission: a multicenter, prospective study. *Blood*. 2015;125(25):3956-3962.
79. Shaw BE, Jimenez-Jimenez AM, Burns LJ, et al. National marrow donor program–sponsored multicenter, phase II trial of HLA-mismatched unrelated donor bone marrow transplantation using post-transplant cyclophosphamide. *J Clin Oncol*. 2021;39(18):1971-1982.
80. de Lima M, Porter DL, Battiwalla M, et al. Proceedings from the National Cancer Institute's second international workshop on the biology, prevention, and treatment of relapse after hematopoietic stem cell transplantation: part III. Prevention and treatment of relapse after allogeneic transplantation. *Biol Blood Marrow Transplant*. 2014;20(1):4-13.
81. Walter RB, Gooley TA, Wood BL, et al. Impact of pretransplantation minimal residual disease, as detected by multiparametric flow cytometry, on outcome of myeloablative hematopoietic cell transplantation for acute myeloid leukemia. *J Clin Oncol*. 2011;29(9):1190-1197.
82. Grubovikj RM, Alavi A, Koppel A, Territo M, Schiller GJ. Minimal residual disease as a predictive factor for relapse after allogeneic hematopoietic stem cell transplant in adult patients with acute myeloid leukemia in first and second complete remission. *Cancers*. 2012;4(2):601-617.
83. Wang Y, Liu DH, Liu KY, et al. Impact of pretransplantation risk factors on post transplantation outcome of patients with acute myeloid leukemia in remission after haploidentical hematopoietic stem cell transplantation. *Biol Blood Marrow Transplant*. 2013;19(2):283-290.
84. Tian H, Chen GH, Xu Y, et al. Impact of pre-transplant disease burden on the outcome of allogeneic hematopoietic stem cell transplant in refractory and relapsed acute myeloid leukemia: a single-center study. *Leuk Lymphoma*. 2015;56(5):1353-1361.
85. Zhou Y, Othus M, Araki D, et al. Pre- and post-transplant quantification of measurable ('minimal') residual disease via multiparameter flow cytometry in adult acute myeloid leukemia. *Leukemia*. 2016;30(7):1456-1464.
86. Zheng C, Zhu X, Tang B, et al. The impact of pre-transplant minimal residual disease on outcome of intensified myeloablative cord blood transplant for acute myeloid leukemia in first or second complete remission. *Leuk Lymphoma*. 2016;57(6):1398-1405.
87. Oran B, Jorgensen JL, Marin D, et al. Pre-transplantation minimal residual disease with cytogenetic and molecular diagnostic features improves risk stratification in acute myeloid leukemia. *Haematologica*. 2017;102(1):110-117.
88. Baron F, Labopin M, Ruggeri A, et al. Impact of detectable measurable residual disease on umbilical cord blood transplantation. *Am J Hematol*. 2020;95:1057-1065.
89. Morsink LM, Sandmaier BM, Othus M, et al. Conditioning intensity, pre-transplant flow cytometric measurable residual disease, and outcome in adults with acute myeloid leukemia undergoing allogeneic hematopoietic cell transplantation. *Cancers*. 2020;12(9):2339.
90. Gilleece MH, Shimoni A, Labopin M, et al. Measurable residual disease status and outcome of transplant in acute myeloid leukemia in second complete remission: a study by the acute leukemia working party of the EBMT. *Blood Cancer J*. 2021;11(5):88.
91. Paras G, Morsink LM, Othus M, et al. Conditioning intensity and peri-transplant flow cytometric MRD dynamics in adult AML. *Blood*. 2022;139(11):1694-1706.
92. Shah MV, Jorgensen JL, Saliba RM, et al. Early post-transplant minimal residual disease assessment improves risk stratification in acute myeloid leukemia. *Biol Blood Marrow Transplant*. 2018;24(7):1514-1520.
93. Knechtli CJ, Goulden NJ, Hancock JP, Grandage VL, Harris EL, Garland RJ. Minimal residual disease status before allogeneic bone marrow transplantation is an important determinant of successful outcome for children and adolescents with acute lymphoblastic leukemia. *Blood*. 1998;92(11):4072-4079.
94. Spinelli O, Peruta B, Tosi M, et al. Clearance of minimal residual disease after allogeneic stem cell transplantation and the prediction of the clinical outcome of adult patients with high-risk acute lymphoblastic leukemia. *Haematologica*. 2007;92(5):612-618.
95. Bader P, Kreyenberg H, Henze GHR, et al. Prognostic value of minimal residual disease quantification before allogeneic stem-cell transplantation in relapsed childhood acute lymphoblastic leukemia: the ALL-REZ BFM study group. *J Clin Oncol*. 2009;27(3):377-384.
96. Giebel S, Stella-Holowiecka B, Krawczyk-Kulis M, et al. Status of minimal residual disease determines outcome of autologous hematopoietic SCT in adult ALL. *Bone Marrow Transplant*. 2010;45(6):1095-1101.

97. Elorza I, Palacio C, Dapena JL, Gallur L, Sánchez de Toledo J, Díaz de Heredia C. Relationship between minimal residual disease measured by multiparametric flow cytometry prior to allogeneic hematopoietic stem cell transplantation and outcome in children with acute lymphoblastic leukemia. *Haematologica*. 2010;95(6):936-941.
98. Bachanova V, Burke MJ, Yohe S, et al. Unrelated cord blood transplantation in adult and pediatric acute lymphoblastic leukemia: effect of minimal residual disease on relapse and survival. *Biol Blood Marrow Transplant*. 2012;18(6):963-968.
99. Ruggeri A, Michel G, Dalle JH, et al. Impact of pretransplant minimal residual disease after cord blood transplantation for childhood acute lymphoblastic leukemia in remission: an Eurocord, PDWP–EBMT analysis. *Leukemia*. 2012;26(12):2455-2461.
100. Lovisa F, Zecca M, Rossi B, et al. Pre- and post-transplant minimal residual disease predicts relapse occurrence in children with acute lymphoblastic leukaemia. *Br J Haematol*. 2018;180(5):680-693.
101. Ifversen M, Turkiewicz D, Marquart HV, et al. Low burden of minimal residual disease prior to transplantation in children with very high risk acute lymphoblastic leukaemia: the NOPHO ALL2008 experience. *Br J Haematol*. 2019;184(6):982-993.
102. Pavlů J, Labopin M, Niittyvuopio R, et al. Measurable residual disease at myeloablative allogeneic transplantation in adults with acute lymphoblastic leukemia: a retrospective registry study on 2780 patients from the acute leukemia working party of the EBMT. *J Hematol OncolJ Hematol Oncol*. 2019;12(1):108.
103. Bader P, Kreyenberg H, von Stackelberg A, et al. Monitoring of minimal residual disease after allogeneic stem-cell transplantation in relapsed childhood acute lymphoblastic leukemia allows for the identification of Impending relapse: results of the ALL-BFM-SCT 2003 trial. *J Clin Oncol*. 2015;33(11):1275-1284.
104. Brunner AM, Li S, Fathi AT, et al. Haematopoietic cell transplantation with and without sorafenib maintenance for patients with FLT3-ITD acute myeloid leukaemia in first complete remission. *Br J Haematol*. 2016;175(3):496-504.
105. Schiller GJ, Tuttle P, Desai P. Allogeneic hematopoietic stem cell transplantation in FLT3-ITD-positive acute myelogenous leukemia: the role for FLT3 tyrosine kinase inhibitors post-transplantation. *Biol Blood Marrow Transplant*. 2016;22(6):982-990.
106. Craddock C, Jilani N, Siddique S, et al. Tolerability and clinical activity of post-transplantation azacitidine in patients allografted for acute myeloid leukemia treated on the RICAZA trial. *Biol Blood Marrow Transplant*. 2016;22(2):385-390.
107. Burchert A, Bug G, Fritz LV, et al. Sorafenib maintenance after allogeneic hematopoietic stem cell transplantation for acute myeloid leukemia with FLT3-Internal tandem duplication mutation (SORMAIN). *J Clin Oncol*. 2020;38(26):2993-3002.
108. Oran B, de Lima M, Garcia-Manero G, et al. A phase 3 randomized study of 5-azacitidine maintenance vs observation after transplant in high-risk AML and MDS patients. *Blood Adv*. 2020;4(21):5580-5588.
109. Greenberg PL, Tuechler H, Schanz J, et al. Revised international prognostic scoring system for myelodysplastic syndromes. *Blood*. 2012;120(12):2454-2465.
110. Crawley C, Szydlo R, Lalancette M, et al. Outcomes of reduced-intensity transplantation for chronic myeloid leukemia: an analysis of prognostic factors from the Chronic Leukemia Working Party of the EBMT. *Blood*. 2005;106(9):2969-2976.
111. Lübking A, Dreimane A, Sandin F, et al. Allogeneic stem cell transplantation for chronic myeloid leukemia in the TKI era: population-based data from the Swedish CML registry. *Bone Marrow Transplant*. 2019;54(11):1764-1774.
112. Warlick E, Ahn KW, Pedersen TL, et al. Reduced intensity conditioning is superior to nonmyeloablative conditioning for older chronic myelogenous leukemia patients undergoing hematopoietic cell transplant during the tyrosine kinase inhibitor era. *Blood*. 2012;119(17):4083-4090.
113. Onida F, de Wreede LC, van Biezen A, et al. Allogeneic stem cell transplantation in patients with atypical chronic myeloid leukaemia: a retrospective study from the Chronic Malignancies Working Party of the European Society for Blood and Marrow Transplantation. *Br J Haematol*. 2017;177(5):759-765.
114. Symeonidis A, van Biezen A, de Wreede L, et al. Achievement of complete remission predicts outcome of allogeneic haematopoietic stem cell transplantation in patients with chronic myelomonocytic leukaemia. A study of the Chronic Malignancies Working Party of the European Group for Blood and Marrow Transplantation. *Br J Haematol*. 2015;171(2):239-246.
115. Sharma P, Shinde S, Damlaj M, et al. Allogeneic hematopoietic stem cell transplant in adult patients with myelodysplastic syndrome/myeloproliferative neoplasm (MDS/MPN) overlap syndromes. *Leuk Lymphoma*. 2016;58:1-10.
116. Kurosawa S, Shimomura Y, Tachibana T, et al. Outcome of allogeneic hematopoietic stem cell transplantation in patients with myelodysplastic/myeloproliferative neoplasms-unclassifiable: a retrospective Nationwide study of the Japan society for hematopoietic cell transplantation. *Biol Blood Marrow Transplant*. 2020;26(9):1607-1611.
117. Kröger N, Zabelina T, van Biezen A, et al. Allogeneic stem cell transplantation for myelodysplastic syndromes with bone marrow fibrosis. *Haematologica*. 2011;96(2):291-297.
118. Cao YG, He Y, Zhang SD, et al. Conditioning regimen of 5-day decitabine administration for allogeneic stem cell transplantation in patients with myelodysplastic syndrome and myeloproliferative neoplasms. *Biol Blood Marrow Transplant*. 2020;26(2):285-291.
119. Kröger N, Sockel K, Wolschke C, et al. Comparison between 5-azacytidine treatment and allogeneic stem-cell transplantation in elderly patients with advanced MDS according to donor availability (VidazaAllo study). *J Clin Oncol*. 2021;39(30):3318-3327.
120. Platzbecker U, Schetelig J, Finke J, et al. Allogeneic hematopoietic cell transplantation in patients age 60-70 years with de novo high-risk myelodysplastic syndrome or secondary acute myelogenous leukemia: comparison with patients lacking donors who received azacitidine. *Biol Blood Marrow Transplant*. 2012;18(9):1415-1421.
121. Nakamura R, Saber W, Martens MJ, et al. Biologic assignment trial of reduced-intensity hematopoietic cell transplantation based on donor availability in patients 50-75 Years of age with advanced myelodysplastic syndrome. *J Clin Oncol*. 2021;39(30):3328-3339.
122. Shimomura Y, Hara M, Konuma T, et al. Allogeneic hematopoietic stem cell transplantation for myelodysplastic syndrome in adolescent and young adult patients. *Bone Marrow Transplant*. 2021;56(10):2510-2517.
123. Warlick ED, Cioc A, DeFor T, Dolan M, Weisdorf D. Allogeneic stem cell transplantation for adults with myelodysplastic syndromes: importance of pretransplant disease burden. *Biol Blood Marrow Transplant*. 2009;15(1):30-38.
124. Gowin K, Ballen K, Ahn KW, et al. Survival following allogeneic transplant in patients with myelofibrosis. *Blood Adv*. 2020;4(9):1965-1973.
125. Kröger N, Giorgino T, Scott BL, et al. Impact of allogeneic stem cell transplantation on survival of patients less than 65 years of age with primary myelofibrosis. *Blood*. 2015;125(21):3347-3350. quiz 3364.
126. Patriarca F, Bacigalupo A, Sperotto A, et al. Outcome of allogeneic stem cell transplantation following reduced-intensity conditioninig regimen in patients with idiopathic myelofibrosis: the g.I.T.m.o. Experience. *Mediterr J Hematol Infect Dis*. 2010;2(2):e2010010.
127. Zeng X, Xuan L, Fan Z, et al. Allogeneic stem cell transplantation may overcome the adverse impact of myelofibrosis on the prognosis of myelodysplastic syndrome. *Exp Hematol Oncol*. 2021;10(1):44.
128. Malcovati L, Porta MGD, Pascutto C, et al. Prognostic factors and life expectancy in myelodysplastic syndromes classified according to WHO criteria: a basis for clinical decision making. *J Clin Oncol*. 2005;23(30):7594-7603.
129. Gangat N, Patnaik MM, Tefferi A. Myelodysplastic syndromes: contemporary review and how we treat. *Am J Hematol*. 2016;91(1):76-89.
130. Fukumoto JS, Greenberg PL. Management of patients with higher risk myelodysplastic syndromes. *Crit Rev Oncol Hematol*. 2005;56(2):179-192.
131. Potter VT, Iacobelli S, van Biezen A, et al. Comparison of intensive chemotherapy and hypomethylating agents before allogeneic stem cell transplantation for advanced myelodysplastic syndromes: a study of the myelodysplastic syndrome subcommittee of the chronic malignancies working party of the European society for blood and marrow transplant research. *Biol Blood Marrow Transplant*. 2016;22(9):1615-1620.
132. Swoboda DM, Gesiotto Q, Sallman DA. Novel therapies in myelodysplastic syndromes. *Curr Opin Hematol*. 2020;27(2):58-65.
133. ElSawy M, Storer BE, Pulsipher MA, et al. Multi-centre validation of the prognostic value of the haematopoietic cell transplantation- specific comorbidity index among recipient of allogeneic haematopoietic cell transplantation. *Br J Haematol*. 2015;170(4):574-583.
134. Cutler CS, Lee SJ, Greenberg P, et al. A decision analysis of allogeneic bone marrow transplantation for the myelodysplastic syndromes: delayed transplantation for low-risk myelodysplasia is associated with improved outcome. *Blood*. 2004;104(2):579-585.
135. Koreth J, Pidala J, Perez WS, et al. Role of reduced-intensity conditioning allogeneic hematopoietic stem-cell transplantation in older patients with de novo myelodysplastic syndromes: an international collaborative decision analysis. *J Clin Oncol Off J Am Soc Clin Oncol*. 2013;31(21):2662-2670.
136. McClune BL, Weisdorf DJ, Pedersen TL, et al. Effect of age on outcome of reduced-intensity hematopoietic cell transplantation for older patients with acute myeloid leukemia in first complete remission or with myelodysplastic syndrome. *J Clin Oncol Off J Am Soc Clin Oncol*. 2010;28(11):1878-1887.
137. Malcovati L, Hellström-Lindberg E, Bowen D, et al. Diagnosis and treatment of primary myelodysplastic syndromes in adults: recommendations from the European LeukemiaNet. *Blood*. 2013;122(17):2943-2964.
138. Della Porta MG, Alessandrino EP, Bacigalupo A, et al. Predictive factors for the outcome of allogeneic transplantation in patients with MDS stratified according to the revised IPSS-R. *Blood*. 2014;123(15):2333-2342.
139. Koenecke C, Göhring G, de Wreede LC, et al. Impact of the revised International Prognostic Scoring System, cytogenetics and monosomal karyotype on outcome after allogeneic stem cell transplantation for myelodysplastic syndromes and secondary acute myeloid leukemia evolving from myelodysplastic syndromes: a retrospective multicenter study of the European Society of Blood and Marrow Transplantation. *Haematologica*. 2015;100(3):400-408.
140. Shaffer BC, Ahn KW, Hu Z-H, et al. Scoring system prognostic of outcome in patients undergoing allogeneic hematopoietic cell transplantation for myelodysplastic syndrome. *J Clin Oncol*. 2016;34(16):1864-1871.
141. Schanz J, Tüchler H, Solé F, et al. New comprehensive cytogenetic scoring system for primary myelodysplastic syndromes (MDS) and oligoblastic acute myeloid leukemia after MDS derived from an international database merge. *J Clin Oncol*. 2012;30(8):820-829.
142. Deeg HJ, Sandmaier BM. Who is fit for allogeneic transplantation? *Blood*. 2010;116(23):4762-4770.
143. Sorror ML, Sandmaier BM, Storer BE, et al. Long-term outcomes among older patients following nonmyeloablative conditioning and allogeneic hematopoietic cell transplantation for advanced hematologic malignancies. *JAMA*. 2011;306(17):1874-1883.
144. Dillon LW, Gui G, Logan BR, et al. Impact of conditioning intensity and genomics on relapse after allogeneic transplantation for patients with myelodysplastic syndrome. *JCO Precis Oncol*. 2021;5:265-274.
145. Martino R, Iacobelli S, Brand R, et al. Retrospective comparison of reduced-intensity conditioning and conventional high-dose conditioning for allogeneic hematopoietic stem cell transplantation using HLA-identical sibling donors in myelodysplastic syndromes. *Blood*. 2006;108(3):836-846.
146. Lim Z, Brand R, Martino R, et al. Allogeneic hematopoietic stem-cell transplantation for patients 50 years or older with myelodysplastic syndromes or secondary acute myeloid leukemia. *J Clin Oncol*. 2010;28(3):405-411.

147. Gyurkocza B, Gutman J, Nemecek ER, et al. Treosulfan, fludarabine, and 2-Gy total body irradiation followed by allogeneic hematopoietic cell transplantation in patients with myelodysplastic syndrome and acute myeloid leukemia. *Biol Blood Marrow Transplant*. 2014;20(4):549-555.
148. Kindwall-Keller T, Isola LM. The evolution of hematopoietic SCT in myelodysplastic syndrome. *Bone Marrow Transplant*. 2009;43(8):597-609.
149. Baccarani M, Deininger MW, Rosti G, et al. European LeukemiaNet recommendations for the management of chronic myeloid leukemia: 2013. *Blood*. 2013;122(6):872-884.
150. Visani G, Rosti G, Bandini G, et al. Second chronic phase before transplantation is crucial for improving survival of blastic phase chronic myeloid leukaemia. *Br J Haematol*. June 2000;109(4):722-728.
151. Goldman JM, Apperley JF, Jones L, et al. Bone marrow transplantation for patients with chronic myeloid leukemia. *N Engl J Med*. 1986;314(4):202-207.
152. Gratwohl A, Hermans J, Niederwieser D, et al. Bone marrow transplantation for chronic myeloid leukemia: long-term results. Chronic leukemia working party of the European group for bone marrow transplantation. *Bone Marrow Transplant*. 1993;12(5):509-516.
153. Biggs JC, Szer J, Crilley P, et al. Treatment of chronic myeloid leukemia with allogeneic bone marrow transplantation after preparation with BuCy2. *Blood*. 1992;80(5):1352-1357.
154. Clift RA, Buckner CD, Thomas ED, et al. Marrow transplantation for patients in accelerated phase of chronic myeloid leukemia. *Blood*. 1994;84(12):4368-4373.
155. Weisser M, Schleuning M, Ledderose G, et al. Reduced-intensity conditioning using TBI (8 Gy), fludarabine, cyclophosphamide and ATG in elderly CML patients provides excellent results especially when performed in the early course of the disease. *Bone Marrow Transplant*. 2004;34(12):1083-1088.
156. Radujkovic A, Dietrich S, Blok HJ, et al. Allogeneic stem cell transplantation for blast crisis chronic myeloid leukemia in the era of tyrosine kinase inhibitors: a retrospective study by the EBMT chronic malignancies working party. *Biol Blood Marrow Transplant*. 2019;25(10):2008-2016.
157. Jabbour E, Cortes J, Kantarjian H, et al. Novel tyrosine kinase inhibitor therapy before allogeneic stem cell transplantation in patients with chronic myeloid leukemia: no evidence for increased transplant-related toxicity. *Cancer*. 2007;110(2):340-344.
158. Gratwohl A, Hermans J, von Biezen A, et al. No advantage for patients who receive splenic irradiation before bone marrow transplantation for chronic myeloid leukaemia: results of a prospective randomized study. *Bone Marrow Transplant*. 1992;10(2):147-152.
159. Kalhs P, Schwarzinger I, Anderson G, et al. A retrospective analysis of the long-term effect of splenectomy on late infections, graft-versus-host disease, relapse, and survival after allogeneic marrow transplantation for chronic myelogenous leukemia. *Blood*. 1995;86(5):2028-2032.
160. Gratwohl A, Hermans J, Goldman JM, et al. Risk assessment for patients with chronic myeloid leukaemia before allogeneic blood or marrow transplantation. Chronic Leukemia Working Party of the European Group for Blood and Marrow Transplantation. *Lancet Lond Engl*. 1998;352(9134):1087-1092.
161. Passweg JR, Walker I, Sobocinski KA, et al. Validation and extension of the EBMT Risk Score for patients with chronic myeloid leukaemia (CML) receiving allogeneic haematopoietic stem cell transplants. *Br J Haematol*. 2004;125(5):613-620.
162. Clift RA, Buckner CD, Thomas ED, et al. Marrow transplantation for chronic myeloid leukemia: a randomized study comparing cyclophosphamide and total body irradiation with busulfan and cyclophosphamide. *Blood*. 1994;84(6):2036-2043.
163. Devergie A, Blaise D, Attal M, et al. Allogeneic bone marrow transplantation for chronic myeloid leukemia in first chronic phase: a randomized trial of busulfan-cytoxan versus cytoxan-total body irradiation as preparative regimen – a report from the French Society of Bone Marrow Graft (SFGM). *Blood*. 1995;85(8):2263-2268.
164. Radich JP, Gooley T, Bensinger W, et al. HLA-matched related hematopoietic cell transplantation for chronic-phase CML using a targeted busulfan and cyclophosphamide preparative regimen. *Blood*. 2003;102(1):31-35.
165. Wallen H, Gooley TA, Deeg HJ, et al. Ablative allogeneic hematopoietic cell transplantation in adults 60 years of age and older. *J Clin Oncol*. 2005;23(15):3439-3446.
166. Giralt S, Ballen K, Rizzo D, et al. Reduced-intensity conditioning regimen workshop: defining the dose spectrum. Report of a workshop convened by the center for international blood and marrow transplant research. *Biol Blood Marrow Transplant*. 2009;15(3):367-369.
167. Uzunel M, Mattsson J, Brune M, Johansson J-E, Aschan J, Ringdén O. Kinetics of minimal residual disease and chimerism in patients with chronic myeloid leukemia after nonmyeloablative conditioning and allogeneic stem cell transplantation. *Blood*. 2003;101(2):469-472.
168. Chhabra S, Ahn KW, Hu ZH, et al. Myeloablative vs reduced-intensity conditioning allogeneic hematopoietic cell transplantation for chronic myeloid leukemia. *Blood Adv*. 2018;2(21):2922-2936.
169. Branford S, Fletcher L, Cross NCP, et al. Desirable performance characteristics for BCR-ABL measurement on an international reporting scale to allow consistent interpretation of individual patient response and comparison of response rates between clinical trials. *Blood*. 2008;112(8):3330-3338.
170. Kaeda J, O'Shea D, Szydlo RM, et al. Serial measurement of BCR-ABL transcripts in the peripheral blood after allogeneic stem cell transplantation for chronic myeloid leukemia: an attempt to define patients who may not require further therapy. *Blood*. 2006;107(10):4171-4176.
171. Weisser M, Tischer J, Schnittger S, Schoch C, Ledderose G, Kolb HJ. A comparison of donor lymphocyte infusions or imatinib mesylate for patients with chronic myelogenous leukemia who have relapsed after allogeneic stem cell transplantation. *Haematologica*. 2006;91(5):663-666.
172. Kolb HJ, Schattenberg A, Goldman JM, et al. Graft-versus-leukemia effect of donor lymphocyte transfusions in marrow grafted patients. *Blood*. 1995;86(5):2041-2050.
173. Dazzi F, Szydlo RM, Cross NC, et al. Durability of responses following donor lymphocyte infusions for patients who relapse after allogeneic stem cell transplantation for chronic myeloid leukemia. *Blood*. 2000;96(8):2712-2716.
174. Guglielmi C, Arcese W, Dazzi F, et al. Donor lymphocyte infusion for relapsed chronic myelogenous leukemia: prognostic relevance of the initial cell dose. *Blood*. 2002;100(2):397-405.
175. Schmidt S, Liu Y, Hu ZH, et al. The role of donor lymphocyte infusion (DLI) in post-hematopoietic cell transplant (HCT) relapse for chronic myeloid leukemia (CML) in the tyrosine kinase inhibitor (TKI) era. *Biol Blood Marrow Transplant*. 2020;26(6):1137-1143.
176. Passamonti F, Cervantes F, Vannucchi AM, et al. A dynamic prognostic model to predict survival in primary myelofibrosis: a study by the IWG-MRT (International Working Group for Myeloproliferative Neoplasms Research and Treatment). *Blood*. 2010;115(9):1703-1708.
177. Gangat N, Caramazza D, Vaidya R, et al. DIPSS plus: a refined Dynamic International Prognostic Scoring System for primary myelofibrosis that incorporates prognostic information from karyotype, platelet count, and transfusion status. *J Clin Oncol*. 2011;29(4):392-397.
178. Tefferi A, Guglielmelli P, Nicolosi M, et al. GIPSS: genetically inspired prognostic scoring system for primary myelofibrosis. *Leukemia*. 2018;32(7):1631-1642.
179. Tamari R, Rapaport F, Zhang N, et al. Impact of high molecular risk mutations on transplant outcomes in patients with myelofibrosis. *Biol Blood Marrow Transplant J Am Soc Blood Marrow Transplant*. June 2019;25(6):1142-1151.
180. Harrison CN, Vannucchi AM, Kiladjian JJ, et al. Long-term findings from COMFORT-II, a phase 3 study of ruxolitinib vs best available therapy for myelofibrosis. *Leukemia*. 2016;30(8):1701-1707.
181. Breccia M, Molica M, Colafigli G, Alimena G. Improvement of bone marrow fibrosis with ruxolitinib: will this finding change our perception of the drug? *Expert Rev Hematol*. 2015;8(4):387-389.
182. Pardanani A, Tefferi A. Definition and management of ruxolitinib treatment failure in myelofibrosis. *Blood Cancer J*. 2014;4:e268.
183. Ciurea SO, de Lima M, Giralt S, et al. Allogeneic stem cell transplantation for myelofibrosis with leukemic transformation. *Biol Blood Marrow Transplant*. 2010;16(4):555-559.
184. Samuelson S, Sandmaier BM, Heslop HE, et al. Allogeneic haematopoietic cell transplantation for myelofibrosis in 30 patients 60-78 years of age. *Br J Haematol*. 2011;153(1):76-82.
185. Ballen KK, Shrestha S, Sobocinski KA, et al. Outcome of transplantation for myelofibrosis. *Biol Blood Marrow Transplant*. 2010;16(3):358-367.
186. Bacigalupo A, Soraru M, Dominietto A, et al. Allogeneic hemopoietic SCT for patients with primary myelofibrosis: a predictive transplant score based on transfusion requirement, spleen size and donor type. *Bone Marrow Transplant*. 2010;45(3):458-463.
187. Abelsson J, Merup M, Birgegård G, et al. The outcome of allo-HSCT for 92 patients with myelofibrosis in the Nordic countries. *Bone Marrow Transplant* [Internet]. 2011;47(3):380-386. Accessed August 2, 2011. http://www.ncbi.nlm.nih.gov/pubmed/21552298
188. Shanavas M, Popat U, Michaelis LC, et al. Outcomes of allogeneic hematopoietic cell transplantation in patients with myelofibrosis with prior exposure to janus kinase 1/2 inhibitors. *Biol Blood Marrow Transplant*. 2016;22(3):432-440.
189. Ballinger TJ, Savani BN, Gupta V, Kroger N, Mohty M. How we manage JAK inhibition in allogeneic transplantation for myelofibrosis. *Eur J Haematol*. 2015;94(2):115-119.
190. Kröger N, Sbianchi G, Sirait T, et al. Impact of prior JAK-inhibitor therapy with ruxolitinib on outcome after allogeneic hematopoietic stem cell transplantation for myelofibrosis: a study of the CMWP of EBMT. *Leukemia*. 2021;35(12):3551-3560.
191. Robin M, Porcher R, Orvain C, et al. Ruxolitinib before allogeneic hematopoietic transplantation in patients with myelofibrosis on behalf SFGM-TC and FIM groups. *Bone Marrow Transplant*. 2021;56(8):1888-1899.
192. Kröger N, Holler E, Kobbe G, et al. Allogeneic stem cell transplantation after reduced-intensity conditioning in patients with myelofibrosis: a prospective, multicenter study of the Chronic Leukemia Working Party of the European Group for Blood and Marrow Transplantation. *Blood*. 2009;114(26):5264-5270.
193. Slot S, Smits K, van de Donk NWCJ, et al. Effect of conditioning regimens on graft failure in myelofibrosis: a retrospective analysis. *Bone Marrow Transplant*. 2015;50(11):1424-1431.
194. Kerbauy DMB, Gooley TA, Sale GE, et al. Hematopoietic cell transplantation as curative therapy for idiopathic myelofibrosis, advanced polycythemia vera, and essential thrombocythemia. *Biol Blood Marrow Transplant*. 2007;13(3):355-365.
195. Kunte S, Rybicki L, Viswabandya A, et al. Allogeneic blood or marrow transplantation with haploidentical donor and post-transplantation cyclophosphamide in patients with myelofibrosis: a multicenter study. *Leukemia*. 2022;36(3):856-864.
196. Oliansky DM, Larson RA, Weisdorf D, et al. The role of cytotoxic therapy with hematopoietic stem cell transplantation in the treatment of adult acute lymphoblastic leukemia: update of the 2006 evidence-based review. *Biol Blood Marrow Transplant*. 2012;18(1):16-17.
197. Moorman AV, Chilton L, Wilkinson J, Ensor HM, Bown N, Proctor SJ. A population-based cytogenetic study of adults with acute lymphoblastic leukemia. *Blood*. 2010;115(2):206-214.
198. Roberts KG, Li Y, Payne-Turner D, et al. Targetable kinase-activating lesions in Ph-like acute lymphoblastic leukemia. *N Engl J Med*. 2014;371(11):1005-1015.
199. Rowe JM. Prognostic factors in adult acute lymphoblastic leukaemia. *Br J Haematol*. 2010;150(4):389-405.

200. Bassan R, Spinelli O, Oldani E, et al. Improved risk classification for risk-specific therapy based on the molecular study of minimal residual disease (MRD) in adult acute lymphoblastic leukemia (ALL). *Blood.* 2009;113(18):4153-4162.
201. Ribera JM, Oriol A, Bethencourt C, et al. Comparison of intensive chemotherapy, allogeneic or autologous stem cell transplantation as post-remission treatment for adult patients with high-risk acute lymphoblastic leukemia. Results of the PETHEMA ALL-93 trial. *Haematologica.* 2005;90(10):1346-1356.
202. Goldstone AH, Richards SM, Lazarus HM, et al. In adults with standard-risk acute lymphoblastic leukemia, the greatest benefit is achieved from a matched sibling allogeneic transplantation in first complete remission, and an autologous transplantation is less effective than conventional consolidation/maintenance chemotherapy in all patients: final results of the International ALL Trial (MRC UKALL XII/ECOG E2993). *Blood.* 2008;111(4):1827-1833.
203. Huguet F, Leguay T, Raffoux E, et al. Pediatric-inspired therapy in adults with Philadelphia chromosome-negative acute lymphoblastic leukemia: the GRAALL-2003 study. *J Clin Oncol.* 2009;27(6):911-918.
204. Chiaretti S, Zini G, Bassan R. Diagnosis and subclassification of acute lymphoblastic leukemia. *Mediterr J Hematol Infect Dis.* 2014;6(1):e2014073.
205. Thomas X, Boiron JM, Huguet F, et al. Outcome of treatment in adults with acute lymphoblastic leukemia: analysis of the LALA-94 trial. *J Clin Oncol.* 2004;22(20):4075-4086.
206. Sebban C, Lepage E, Vernant JP, et al. Allogeneic bone marrow transplantation in adult acute lymphoblastic leukemia in first complete remission: a comparative study. French Group of Therapy of Adult Acute Lymphoblastic Leukemia. *J Clin Oncol.* 1994;12(12):2580-2587.
207. Hunault M, Harousseau J-L, Delain M, et al. Better outcome of adult acute lymphoblastic leukemia after early genoidentical allogeneic bone marrow transplantation (BMT) than after late high-dose therapy and autologous BMT: a GOELAMS trial. *Blood.* 2004;104(10):3028-3037.
208. Attal M, Blaise D, Marit G, et al. Consolidation treatment of adult acute lymphoblastic leukemia: a prospective, randomized trial comparing allogeneic versus autologous bone marrow transplantation and testing the impact of recombinant interleukin-2 after autologous bone marrow transplantation. *Blood.* 1995;86(4):1619-1628.
209. Doney K, Fisher LD, Appelbaum FR, et al. Treatment of adult acute lymphoblastic leukemia with allogeneic bone marrow transplantation. Multivariate analysis of factors affecting acute graft-versus-host disease, relapse, and relapse-free survival. *Bone Marrow Transplant.* 1991;7(6):453-459.
210. Blume KG, Forman SJ, Snyder DS, et al. Allogeneic bone marrow transplantation for acute lymphoblastic leukemia during first complete remission. *Transplantation.* 1987;43(3):389-392.
211. Chao NJ, Forman SJ, Schmidt GM, et al. Allogeneic bone marrow transplantation for high-risk acute lymphoblastic leukemia during first complete remission. *Blood.* 1991;78(8):1923-1927.
212. Jamieson CHM, Amylon MD, Wong RM, Blume KG. Allogeneic hematopoietic cell transplantation for patients with high-risk acute lymphoblastic leukemia in first or second complete remission using fractionated total-body irradiation and high-dose etoposide: a 15-year experience. *Exp Hematol.* 2003;31(10):981-986.
213. Labar B, Suciu S, Zittoun R, et al. Allogeneic stem cell transplantation in acute lymphoblastic leukemia and non-Hodgkin's lymphoma for patients <or=50 years old in first complete remission: results of the EORTC ALL-3 trial. *Haematologica.* July 2004;89(7):809-817.
214. Gupta V, Richards S, Rowe J; Acute Leukemia Stem Cell Transplantation Trialists' Collaborative Group. Allogeneic, but not autologous, hematopoietic cell transplantation improves survival only among younger adults with acute lymphoblastic leukemia in first remission: an individual patient data meta-analysis. *Blood.* 2013;121(2):339-350.
215. Wieduwilt MJ, Stock W, Advani A, et al. Superior survival with pediatric-style chemotherapy compared to myeloablative allogeneic hematopoietic cell transplantation in older adolescents and young adults with Ph-negative acute lymphoblastic leukemia in first complete remission: analysis from CALGB 10403 and the CIBMTR. *Leukemia.* 2021;35(7):2076-2085.
216. Gökbuget N, Kneba M, Raff T, et al. Adult patients with acute lymphoblastic leukemia and molecular failure display a poor prognosis and are candidates for stem cell transplantation and targeted therapies. *Blood.* 2012;120(9):1868-1876.
217. Dhédin N, Huynh A, Maury S, et al. Role of allogeneic stem cell transplantation in adult patients with Ph-negative acute lymphoblastic leukemia. *Blood.* 2015;125(16):2486-2496. quiz 2586.
218. Ribera JM, Oriol A, Morgades M, et al. Treatment of high-risk Philadelphia chromosome-negative acute lymphoblastic leukemia in adolescents and adults according to early cytologic response and minimal residual disease after consolidation assessed by flow cytometry: final results of the PETHEMA ALL-AR-03 trial. *J Clin Oncol.* 2014;32(15):1595-1604.
219. Bar M, Wood BL, Radich JP, et al. Impact of minimal residual disease, detected by flow cytometry, on outcome of myeloablative hematopoietic cell transplantation for acute lymphoblastic leukemia. *Leuk Res Treat.* 2014;2014:421723.
220. Huguet F, Tavitian S. Emerging biological therapies to treat acute lymphoblastic leukemia. *Expert Opin Emerg Drugs.* 2016;22(1):107-121.
221. Fielding AK, Rowe JM, Richards SM, et al. Prospective outcome data on 267 unselected adult patients with Philadelphia chromosome-positive acute lymphoblastic leukemia confirms superiority of allogeneic transplantation over chemotherapy in the pre-imatinib era: results from the International ALL Trial MRC UKALLXII/ECOG2993. *Blood.* 2009;113(19):4489-4496.
222. Bassan R, Hoelzer D. Modern therapy of acute lymphoblastic leukemia. *J Clin Oncol.* 2011;29(5):532-543.
223. Daver N, Thomas D, Ravandi F, et al. Final report of a phase II study of imatinib mesylate with hyper-CVAD for the front-line treatment of adult patients with Philadelphia chromosome-positive acute lymphoblastic leukemia. *Haematologica.* 2015;100(5):653-661.
224. Lim SN, Joo YD, Lee KH, et al. Long-term follow-up of imatinib plus combination chemotherapy in patients with newly diagnosed Philadelphia chromosome-positive acute lymphoblastic leukemia. *Am J Hematol.* 2015;90(11):1013-1020.
225. de Labarthe A, Rousselot P, Huguet-Rigal F, et al. Imatinib combined with induction or consolidation chemotherapy in patients with de novo Philadelphia chromosome-positive acute lymphoblastic leukemia: results of the GRAAPH-2003 study. *Blood.* 2007;109(4):1408-1413.
226. Lee S, Kim YJ, Min CK, et al. The effect of first-line imatinib interim therapy on the outcome of allogeneic stem cell transplantation in adults with newly diagnosed Philadelphia chromosome-positive acute lymphoblastic leukemia. *Blood.* 2005;105(9):3449-3457.
227. Mizuta S, Matsuo K, Nishiwaki S, et al. Pretransplant administration of imatinib for allo-HSCT in patients with BCR-ABL-positive acute lymphoblastic leukemia. *Blood.* 2014;123(15):2325-2332.
228. Fielding AK, Rowe JM, Buck G, et al. UKALLXII/ECOG2993: addition of imatinib to a standard treatment regimen enhances long-term outcomes in Philadelphia positive acute lymphoblastic leukemia. *Blood.* 2014;123(6):843-850.
229. Short NJ, Jabbour E, Sasaki K, et al. Impact of complete molecular response on survival in patients with Philadelphia chromosome-positive acute lymphoblastic leukemia. *Blood.* 2016;128(4):504-507.
230. Schultz KR, Carroll A, Heerema NA, et al. Long-term follow-up of imatinib in pediatric Philadelphia chromosome-positive acute lymphoblastic leukemia: children's Oncology Group study AALL0031. *Leukemia.* July 2014;28(7):1467-1471.
231. Jabbour E, Short NJ, Ravandi F, et al. Combination of hyper-CVAD with ponatinib as first-line therapy for patients with Philadelphia chromosome-positive acute lymphoblastic leukaemia: long-term follow-up of a single-centre, phase 2 study. *Lancet Haematol.* 2018;5(12):e618-e627.
232. Thomas ED, Lochte HL, Lu WC, Ferrebee JW. Intravenous infusion of bone marrow in patients receiving radiation and chemotherapy. *N Engl J Med.* 1957;257(11):491-496.
233. Thomas E, Storb R, Clift RA, et al. Bone-marrow transplantation (first of two parts). *N Engl J Med.* 1975;292(16):832-843.
234. Thomas ED, Storb R, Clift RA, et al. Bone-marrow transplantation (second of two parts). *N Engl J Med.* 1975;292(17):895-902.
235. Kebriaei P, Anasetti C, Zhang M-J, et al. Intravenous busulfan compared with total body irradiation pretransplant conditioning for adults with acute lymphoblastic leukemia. *Biol Blood Marrow Transplant.* 2018;24(4):726-733.
236. Pavlu J, Labopin M, Niittyvuopio R, et al. The role of Measurable Residual Disease (MRD) at time of allogeneic hematopoietic cell transplantation in adults with acute lymphoblastic leukemia transplanted after myeloablative conditioning. A study on behalf of the acute leukemia working party of the European society for blood and marrow transplantation. *Biol Blood Marrow Transplant.* 2019;25(3):S7.
237. Peters C, Dalle J-H, Locatelli F, et al. Total body irradiation or chemotherapy conditioning in childhood ALL: a multinational, randomized, Noninferiority phase III study. *J Clin Oncol.* 2021;39(4):295-307.
238. Mohty M, Labopin M, Tabrizzi R, et al. Reduced intensity conditioning allogeneic stem cell transplantation for adult patients with acute lymphoblastic leukemia: a retrospective study from the European Group for Blood and Marrow Transplantation. *Haematologica.* 2008;93(2):303-306.
239. Bachanova V, Verneris MR, DeFor T, Brunstein CG, Weisdorf DJ. Prolonged survival in adults with acute lymphoblastic leukemia after reduced-intensity conditioning with cord blood or sibling donor transplantation. *Blood.* 2009;113(13):2902-2905.
240. Stein AS, Palmer JM, O'Donnell MR, et al. Reduced-intensity conditioning followed by peripheral blood stem cell transplantation for adult patients with high-risk acute lymphoblastic leukemia. *Biol Blood Marrow Transplant.* 2009;15(11):1407-1414.
241. Ram R, Storb R, Sandmaier BM, et al. Non-myeloablative conditioning with allogeneic hematopoietic cell transplantation for the treatment of high-risk acute lymphoblastic leukemia. *Haematologica.* 2011;96(8):1113-1120.
242. Burke MJ, Trotz B, Luo X, et al. Allo-hematopoietic cell transplantation for Ph chromosome-positive ALL: impact of imatinib on relapse and survival. *Bone Marrow Transplant.* 2009;43(2):107-113.
243. Mohty M, Labopin M, Volin L, et al. Reduced-intensity versus conventional myeloablative conditioning allogeneic stem cell transplantation for patients with acute lymphoblastic leukemia: a retrospective study from the European Group for Blood and Marrow Transplantation. *Blood.* 2010;116(22):4439-4443.
244. Marks DI, Wang T, Pérez WS, et al. The outcome of full-intensity and reduced-intensity conditioning matched sibling or unrelated donor transplantation in adults with Philadelphia chromosome-negative acute lymphoblastic leukemia in first and second complete remission. *Blood.* 2010;116(3):366-374.
245. Cho BS, Lee S, Kim YJ, et al. Reduced-intensity conditioning allogeneic stem cell transplantation is a potential therapeutic approach for adults with high-risk acute lymphoblastic leukemia in remission: results of a prospective phase 2 study. *Leukemia.* 2009;23(10):1763-1770.
246. Marks DI, Pérez WS, He W, et al. Unrelated donor transplants in adults with Philadelphia-negative acute lymphoblastic leukemia in first complete remission. *Blood.* 2008;112(2):426-434.
247. Cornelissen JJ, Carston M, Kollman C, et al. Unrelated marrow transplantation for adult patients with poor-risk acute lymphoblastic leukemia: strong graft-versus-leukemia effect and risk factors determining outcome. *Blood.* 2001;97(6):1572-1577.
248. Ringdén O, Pavletic SZ, Anasetti C, et al. The graft-versus-leukemia effect using matched unrelated donors is not superior to HLA-identical siblings for hematopoietic stem cell transplantation. *Blood.* 2009;113(13):3110-3118.

249. Nishiwaki S, Inamoto Y, Sakamaki H, et al. Allogeneic stem cell transplantation for adult Philadelphia chromosome-negative acute lymphocytic leukemia: comparable survival rates but different risk factors between related and unrelated transplantation in first complete remission. *Blood*. 2010;116(20):4368-4375.
250. Wieduwilt MJ, Metheny L, Zhang MJ, et al. Haploidentical vs sibling, unrelated, or cord blood hematopoietic cell transplantation for acute lymphoblastic leukemia. *Blood Adv*. 2022;6(1):339-357.
251. Brissot E, Labopin M, Beckers MM, et al. Tyrosine kinase inhibitors improve long-term outcome of allogeneic hematopoietic stem cell transplantation for adult patients with Philadelphia chromosome positive acute lymphoblastic leukemia. *Haematologica*. 2015;100(3):392-399.
252. Pfeifer H, Wassmann B, Bethge W, et al. Randomized comparison of prophylactic and minimal residual disease-triggered imatinib after allogeneic stem cell transplantation for BCR-ABL1-positive acute lymphoblastic leukemia. *Leukemia*. 2013;27(6):1254-1262.
253. Carpenter PA, Snyder DS, Flowers MED, et al. Prophylactic administration of imatinib after hematopoietic cell transplantation for high-risk Philadelphia chromosome-positive leukemia. *Blood*. 2007;109(7):2791-2793.
254. Ding Z, Han MZ, Chen SL, et al. Outcomes of adults with acute lymphoblastic leukemia after autologous hematopoietic stem cell transplantation and the significance of pretransplantation minimal residual disease: analysis from a single center of China. *Chin Med J (Engl)*. 2015;128(15):2065-2071.
255. Dominietto A, Pozzi S, Miglino M, et al. Donor lymphocyte infusions for the treatment of minimal residual disease in acute leukemia. *Blood*. 2007;109(11):5063-5064.
256. Reman O, Buzyn A, Lhéritier V, et al. Rescue therapy combining intermediate-dose cytarabine with amsacrine and etoposide in relapsed adult acute lymphoblastic leukemia. *Hematol J*. 2004;5(2):123-129.
257. Fielding AK, Richards SM, Chopra R, et al. Outcome of 609 adults after relapse of acute lymphoblastic leukemia (ALL); an MRC UKALL12/ECOG 2993 study. *Blood*. 2007;109(3):944-950.
258. Kozlowski P, Åström M, Ahlberg L, et al. High curability via intensive reinduction chemotherapy and stem cell transplantation in young adults with relapsed acute lymphoblastic leukemia in Sweden 2003-2007. *Haematologica*. 2012;97(9):1414-1421.
259. Nagler A, Labopin M, Dholaria B, et al. Second allogeneic stem cell transplantation in patients with acute lymphoblastic leukaemia: a study on behalf of the Acute Leukaemia Working Party of the European Society for Blood and Marrow Transplantation. *Br J Haematol*. 2019;186(5):767-776.
260. Gökbuget N, Basara N, Baurmann H, et al. High single-drug activity of nelarabine in relapsed T-lymphoblastic leukemia/lymphoma offers curative option with subsequent stem cell transplantation. *Blood*. 2011;118(13):3504-3511.
261. Topp MS, Gökbuget N, Zugmaier G, et al. Long-term follow-up of hematologic relapse-free survival in a phase 2 study of blinatumomab in patients with MRD in B-lineage ALL. *Blood*. 2012;120(26):5185-5187.
262. Kantarjian H, Thomas D, Jorgensen J, et al. Results of inotuzumab ozogamicin, a CD22 monoclonal antibody, in refractory and relapsed acute lymphocytic leukemia. *Cancer*. 2013;119(15):2728-2736.
263. Gökbuget N, Kelsh M, Chia V, et al. Blinatumomab vs historical standard therapy of adult relapsed/refractory acute lymphoblastic leukemia. *Blood Cancer J*. 2016;6(9):e473.
264. Shah BD, Ghobadi A, Oluwole OO, et al. KTE-X19 for relapsed or refractory adult B-cell acute lymphoblastic leukaemia: phase 2 results of the single-arm, open-label, multicentre ZUMA-3 study. *Lancet*. 2021;398(10299):491-502.
265. Maude SL, Laetsch TW, Buechner J, et al. Tisagenlecleucel in children and young adults with B-cell lymphoblastic leukemia. *N Engl J Med*. 2018;378(5):439-448.
266. Morabito F, Gentile M, Seymour JF, Polliack A. Ibrutinib, idelalisib and obinutuzumab for the treatment of patients with chronic lymphocytic leukemia: three new arrows aiming at the target. *Leuk Lymphoma*. 2015;56(12):3250-3256.
267. Robak P, Smolewski P, Robak T. Emerging immunological drugs for chronic lymphocytic leukemia. *Expert Opin Emerg Drugs*. 2015;20(3):423-447.
268. Byrd JC, Furman RR, Coutre SE, et al. Targeting BTK with ibrutinib in relapsed chronic lymphocytic leukemia. *N Engl J Med*. 2013;369(1):32-42.
269. Furman RR, Sharman JP, Coutre SE, et al. Idelalisib and rituximab in relapsed chronic lymphocytic leukemia. *N Engl J Med*. 2014;370(11):997-1007.
270. Goede V, Fischer K, Busch R, et al. Obinutuzumab plus chlorambucil in patients with CLL and coexisting conditions. *N Engl J Med*. 2014;370(12):1101-1110.
271. Stilgenbauer S, Eichhorst B, Schetelig J, et al. Venetoclax in relapsed or refractory chronic lymphocytic leukaemia with 17p deletion: a multicentre, open-label, phase 2 study. *Lancet Oncol*. 2016;17(6):768-778.
272. Herth I, Dietrich S, Benner A, et al. The impact of allogeneic stem cell transplantation on the natural course of poor-risk chronic lymphocytic leukemia as defined by the EBMT consensus criteria: a retrospective donor versus no donor comparison. *Ann Oncol*. 2014;25(1):200-206.
273. Poon ML, Fox PS, Samuels BI, et al. Allogeneic stem cell transplant in patients with chronic lymphocytic leukemia with 17p deletion: consult-transplant versus consult-no-transplant analysis. *Leuk Lymphoma*. 2015;56(3):711-715.
274. Dreger P, Ghia P, Schetelig J, et al. High-risk chronic lymphocytic leukemia in the era of pathway inhibitors: integrating molecular and cellular therapies. *Blood*. 2018;132(9):892-902.
275. Kharfan-Dabaja MA, Kumar A, Hamadani M, et al. Clinical practice recommendations for use of allogeneic hematopoietic cell transplantation in chronic lymphocytic leukemia on behalf of the guidelines committee of the American society for blood and marrow transplantation. *Biol Blood Marrow Transplant*. 2016;22(12):2117-2125.
276. Kim HT, Shaughnessy CJ, Rai SC, et al. Allogeneic hematopoietic cell transplantation after prior targeted therapy for high-risk chronic lymphocytic leukemia. *Blood Adv*. 2020;4(17):4113-4123.
277. Roeker LE, Dreger P, Brown JR, et al. Allogeneic stem cell transplantation for chronic lymphocytic leukemia in the era of novel agents. *Blood Adv*. 2020;4(16):3977-3989.
278. Swerdlow SH, Campo E, Harris NL, et al. *WHO Classification of Tumours of Haematopoietic and Lymphoid Tissues*. 4th ed. IARC; 2016.
279. Tilly H, Gomes da Silva M, Vitolo U, et al. Diffuse large B-cell lymphoma (DLBCL): ESMO Clinical Practice Guidelines for diagnosis, treatment and follow-up. *Ann Oncol*. 2015;26(suppl 5):v116-v125.
280. Greb A, Bohlius J, Schiefer D, Schwarzer G, Schulz H, Engert A. High-dose chemotherapy with autologous stem cell transplantation in the first line treatment of aggressive non-Hodgkin lymphoma (NHL) in adults. *Cochrane Database Syst Rev*. 2008;2008(1):CD004024.
281. Coiffier B, Sarkozy C. Diffuse large B-cell lymphoma: R-CHOP failure-what to do? *Hematol Am Soc Hematol Educ Program*. 2016;2016(1):366-378.
282. Stiff PJ, Unger JM, Cook JR, et al. Autologous transplantation as consolidation for aggressive non-Hodgkin's lymphoma. *N Engl J Med*. 2013;369(18):1681-1690.
283. Philip T, Guglielmi C, Hagenbeek A, et al. Autologous bone marrow transplantation as compared with salvage chemotherapy in relapses of chemotherapy-sensitive non-Hodgkin's lymphoma. *N Engl J Med*. 1995;333(23):1540-1545.
284. Gisselbrecht C, Glass B, Mounier N, et al. Salvage regimens with autologous transplantation for relapsed large B-cell lymphoma in the rituximab era. *J Clin Oncol*. 2010;28(27):4184-4190.
285. Thieblemont C, Briere J, Mounier N, et al. The germinal center/activated B-cell subclassification has a prognostic impact for response to salvage therapy in relapsed/refractory diffuse large B-cell lymphoma: a bio-CORAL study. *J Clin Oncol*. 2011;29(31):4079-4087.
286. Crump M, Neelapu SS, Farooq U, et al. Outcomes in refractory diffuse large B-cell lymphoma: results from the international SCHOLAR-1 study. *Blood*. 2017;130(16):1800-1808.
287. Locke FL, Miklos DB, Jacobson CA, et al. Axicabtagene ciloleucel as second-line therapy for large B-cell lymphoma. *N Engl J Med*. 2022;386(7):640-654.
288. Kamdar M. Lisocabtagene maraleucel (liso-cel), a CD19-directed Chimeric Antigen Receptor (CAR) T cell therapy, versus Standard of Care (SOC) with salvage chemotherapy (CT) followed by autologous stem cell transplantation (ASCT) as second-line (2L) treatment in patients (pts) with relapsed or refractory (R/R) large B-cell lymphoma (LBCL): results from the randomized phase 3 transform study. *ASH*. 2021;138(1):1-5044. Accessed April 3, 2022. https://ash.confex.com/ash/2021/webprogram/Paper147913.html
289. Fenske TS, Ahn KW, Graff TM, et al. Allogeneic transplantation provides durable remission in a subset of DLBCL patients relapsing after autologous transplantation. *Br J Haematol*. 2016;174(2):235-248.
290. Lazarus HM, Zhang MJ, Carreras J, et al. A comparison of HLA-identical sibling allogeneic versus autologous transplantation for diffuse large B cell lymphoma: a report from the CIBMTR. *Biol Blood Marrow Transplant*. 2010;16(1):35-45.
291. van Kampen RJW, Canals C, Schouten HC, et al. Allogeneic stem-cell transplantation as salvage therapy for patients with diffuse large B-cell non-Hodgkin's lymphoma relapsing after an autologous stem-cell transplantation: an analysis of the European Group for Blood and Marrow Transplantation Registry. *J Clin Oncol*. 2011;29(10):1342-1348.
292. Rigacci L, Puccini B, Dodero A, et al. Allogeneic hematopoietic stem cell transplantation in patients with diffuse large B cell lymphoma relapsed after autologous stem cell transplantation: a GITMO study. *Ann Hematol*. 2012;91(6):931-939.
293. Bacher U, Klyuchnikov E, Le-Rademacher J, et al. Conditioning regimens for allotransplants for diffuse large B-cell lymphoma: myeloablative or reduced intensity? *Blood*. 2012;120(20):4256-4262.
294. Hamadani M, Saber W, Ahn KW, et al. Impact of pretransplantation conditioning regimens on outcomes of allogeneic transplantation for chemotherapy-unresponsive diffuse large B cell lymphoma and grade III follicular lymphoma. *Biol Blood Marrow Transplant*. 2013;19(5):746-753.
295. Fenske TS, Hamadani M, Cohen JB, et al. Allogeneic hematopoietic cell transplantation as curative therapy for patients with non-hodgkin lymphoma: increasingly successful application to older patients. *Biol Blood Marrow Transplant*. 2016;22(9):1543-1551.
296. Epperla N, Ahn KW, Khanal M, et al. Impact of reduced-intensity conditioning regimens on outcomes in diffuse large B cell lymphoma undergoing allogeneic transplantation. *Transplant Cell Ther*. 2021;27(1):58-66.
297. Hamadani M, Gopal AK, Pasquini M, et al. Allogeneic transplant and CAR-T therapy after autologous transplant failure in DLBCL: a noncomparative cohort analysis. *Blood Adv*. 2022;6(2):486-494.
298. Locke FL, Ghobadi A, Jacobson CA, et al. Long-term safety and activity of axicabtagene ciloleucel in refractory large B-cell lymphoma (ZUMA-1): a single-arm, multicentre, phase 1-2 trial. *Lancet Oncol*. 2019;20(1):31-42.
299. Nieto Y, Popat U, Anderlini P, et al. Autologous stem cell transplantation for refractory or poor-risk relapsed Hodgkin's lymphoma: effect of the specific high-dose chemotherapy regimen on outcome. *Biol Blood Marrow Transplant*. 2013;19(3):410-417.
300. Moskowitz CH, Kewalramani T, Nimer SD, Gonzalez M, Zelenetz AD, Yahalom J. Effectiveness of high dose chemoradiotherapy and autologous stem cell transplantation for patients with biopsy-proven primary refractory Hodgkin's disease. *Br J Haematol*. 2004;124(5):645-652.
301. Perales M-A, Ceberio I, Armand P, et al. Role of cytotoxic therapy with hematopoietic cell transplantation in the treatment of Hodgkin lymphoma: guidelines from the American Society for Blood and Marrow Transplantation. *Biol Blood Marrow Transplant*. 2015;21(6):971-983.

302. Linch DC, Winfield D, Goldstone AH, et al. Dose intensification with autologous bone-marrow transplantation in relapsed and resistant Hodgkin's disease: results of a BNLI randomised trial. *Lancet Lond Engl*. 1993;341(8852):1051-1054.
303. Schmitz N, Pfistner B, Sextro M, et al. Aggressive conventional chemotherapy compared with high-dose chemotherapy with autologous haemopoietic stem-cell transplantation for relapsed chemosensitive Hodgkin's disease: a randomised trial. *Lancet Lond Engl*. 2002;359(9323):2065-2071.
304. Rancea M, Monsef I, von Tresckow B, Engert A, Skoetz N. High-dose chemotherapy followed by autologous stem cell transplantation for patients with relapsed/refractory Hodgkin lymphoma. *Cochrane Database Syst Rev*. 2013;(6):CD009411. doi:10.1002/14651858.CD009411.
305. Kahn S, Flowers C, Xu Z, Esiashvili N. Does the addition of involved field radiotherapy to high-dose chemotherapy and stem cell transplantation improve outcomes for patients with relapsed/refractory Hodgkin lymphoma? *Int J Radiat Oncol Biol Phys*. 2011;81(1):175-180.
306. Hahn T, McCarthy PL, Carreras J, et al. Simplified validated prognostic model for progression-free survival after autologous transplantation for hodgkin lymphoma. *Biol Blood Marrow Transplant*. 2013;19(12):1740-1744.
307. Moskowitz CH, Walewski J, Nademanee A, et al. Five-year PFS from the AETHERA trial of brentuximab vedotin for Hodgkin lymphoma at high risk of progression or relapse. *Blood*. 2018;132(25):2639-2642.
308. Armand P, Chen YB, Redd RA, et al. PD-1 blockade with pembrolizumab for classical Hodgkin lymphoma after autologous stem cell transplantation. *Blood*. 2019;134(1):22-29.
309. Kuruvilla J, Ramchandren R, Santoro A, et al. Pembrolizumab versus brentuximab vedotin in relapsed or refractory classical Hodgkin lymphoma (KEYNOTE-204): an interim analysis of a multicentre, randomised, open-label, phase 3 study. *Lancet Oncol*. 2021;22(4):512-524.
310. Ijaz A, Khan AY, Malik SU, et al. Significant risk of graft-versus-host disease with exposure to checkpoint inhibitors before and after allogeneic transplantation. *Biol Blood Marrow Transplant* [Internet]. 2018;25(1):94-99. doi:10.1016/j.bbmt.2018.08.028
311. Dada R, Usman B. Allogeneic hematopoietic stem cell transplantation in r/r Hodgkin lymphoma after treatment with checkpoint inhibitors: feasibility and safety. *Eur J Haematol*. 2019;102(2):150-156.
312. Herbaux C, Merryman R, Devine S, et al. Recommendations for managing PD-1 blockade in the context of allogeneic HCT in Hodgkin lymphoma: taming a necessary evil. *Blood*. 2018;132(1):9-16.
313. Merryman RW, Castagna L, Giordano L, et al. Allogeneic transplantation after PD-1 blockade for classic Hodgkin lymphoma. *Leukemia*. 2021;35(9):2672-2683.
314. Sureda A, Robinson S, Canals C, et al. Reduced-intensity conditioning compared with conventional allogeneic stem-cell transplantation in relapsed or refractory Hodgkin's lymphoma: an analysis from the Lymphoma Working Party of the European Group for Blood and Marrow Transplantation. *J Clin Oncol*. 2008;26(3):455-462.
315. Marcais A, Porcher R, Robin M, et al. Impact of disease status and stem cell source on the results of reduced intensity conditioning transplant for Hodgkin's lymphoma: a retrospective study from the French Society of Bone Marrow Transplantation and Cellular Therapy (SFGM-TC). *Haematologica*. 2013;98(9):1467-1475.
316. Ahmed S, Ghosh N, Ahn KW, et al. Impact of type of reduced-intensity conditioning regimen on the outcomes of allogeneic haematopoietic cell transplantation in classical Hodgkin lymphoma. *Br J Haematol*. 2020;190(4):573-582.
317. Burroughs LM, O'Donnell PV, Sandmaier BM, et al. Comparison of outcomes of HLA-matched related, unrelated, or HLA-haploidentical related hematopoietic cell transplantation following nonmyeloablative conditioning for relapsed or refractory Hodgkin lymphoma. *Biol Blood Marrow Transplant*. 2008;14(11):1279-1287.
318. Gayoso J, Balsalobre P, Pascual MJ, et al. Busulfan-based reduced intensity conditioning regimens for haploidentical transplantation in relapsed/refractory Hodgkin lymphoma: Spanish multicenter experience. *Bone Marrow Transplant*. 2016;51(10):1307-1312.
319. Martinez C, Gayoso J, Canals C, et al. Post-transplantation cyclophosphamide-based haploidentical transplantation as alternative to matched sibling or unrelated donor transplantation for hodgkin lymphoma: a registry study of the lymphoma working party of the European society for blood and marrow transplantation. *J Clin Oncol*. 2017;35(30):3425-3432.
320. Schaaf M, Reiser M, Borchmann P, Engert A, Skoetz N. High-dose therapy with autologous stem cell transplantation versus chemotherapy or immuno-chemotherapy for follicular lymphoma in adults. *Cochrane Database Syst Rev*. 2012;1:CD007678.
321. Casulo C, Friedberg JW, Ahn KW, et al. Autologous transplantation in follicular lymphoma with early therapy failure: a National LymphoCare study and center for international blood and marrow transplant research analysis. *Biol Blood Marrow Transplant*. 2018;24(6):1163-1171.
322. Rohatiner AZS, Nadler L, Davies AJ, et al. Myeloablative therapy with autologous bone marrow transplantation for follicular lymphoma at the time of second or subsequent remission: long-term follow-up. *J Clin Oncol*. 2007;25(18):2554-2559.
323. Metzner B, Pott C, Müller TH, et al. Long-term clinical and molecular remissions in patients with follicular lymphoma following high-dose therapy and autologous stem cell transplantation. *Ann Oncol*. 2013;24(6):1609-1615.
324. Evens AM, Vanderplas A, LaCasce AS, et al. Stem cell transplantation for follicular lymphoma relapsed/refractory after prior rituximab: a comprehensive analysis from the NCCN lymphoma outcomes project. *Cancer*. 2013;119(20):3662-3671.
325. van Besien K, Loberiza FR, Bajorunaite R, et al. Comparison of autologous and allogeneic hematopoietic stem cell transplantation for follicular lymphoma. *Blood*. 2003;102(10):3521-3529.
326. Jacobson CA, Chavez JC, Sehgal AR, et al. Axicabtagene ciloleucel in relapsed or refractory indolent non-Hodgkin lymphoma (ZUMA-5): a single-arm, multicentre, phase 2 trial. *Lancet Oncol*. 2022;23(1):91-103.
327. Hoster E, Dreyling M, Klapper W, et al. A new prognostic index (MIPI) for patients with advanced-stage mantle cell lymphoma. *Blood*. 2008;111(2):558-565.
328. Hoster E, Rosenwald A, Berger F, et al. Prognostic value of Ki-67 index, cytology, and growth pattern in mantle-cell lymphoma: results from randomized trials of the European Mantle Cell Lymphoma Network. *J Clin Oncol*. 2016;34(12):1386-1394.
329. Delfau-Larue MH, Klapper W, Berger F, et al. High-dose cytarabine does not overcome the adverse prognostic value of CDKN2A and TP53 deletions in mantle cell lymphoma. *Blood*. 2015;126(5):604-611.
330. Nordström L, Sernbo S, Eden P, et al. SOX11 and TP53 add prognostic information to MIPI in a homogenously treated cohort of mantle cell lymphoma--a Nordic Lymphoma Group study. *Br J Haematol*. 2014;166(1):98-108.
331. Husby S, Ralfkiaer U, Garde C, et al. miR-18b overexpression identifies mantle cell lymphoma patients with poor outcome and improves the MIPI-B prognosticator. *Blood*. 2015;125(17):2669-2677.
332. Robinson S, Dreger P, Caballero D, et al. The EBMT/EMCL consensus project on the role of autologous and allogeneic stem cell transplantation in mantle cell lymphoma. *Leukemia*. 2015;29(2):464-473.
333. Chihara D, Cheah CY, Westin JR, et al. Rituximab plus hyper-CVAD alternating with MTX/Ara-C in patients with newly diagnosed mantle cell lymphoma: 15-year follow-up of a phase II study from the MD Anderson Cancer Center. *Br J Haematol*. 2016;172(1):80-88.
334. Eskelund CW, Kolstad A, Jerkeman M, et al. 15-year follow-up of the Second Nordic Mantle Cell Lymphoma trial (MCL2): prolonged remissions without survival plateau. *Br J Haematol*. 2016;175(3):410-418.
335. Delarue R, Haioun C, Ribrag V, et al. CHOP and DHAP plus rituximab followed by autologous stem cell transplantation in mantle cell lymphoma: a phase 2 study from the Groupe d'Etude des Lymphomes de l'Adulte. *Blood*. 2013;121(1):48-53.
336. Hermine O, Hoster E, Walewski J, et al. Addition of high-dose cytarabine to immunochemotherapy before autologous stem-cell transplantation in patients aged 65 years or younger with mantle cell lymphoma (MCL Younger): a randomised, open-label, phase 3 trial of the European Mantle Cell Lymphoma Network. *Lancet Lond Engl*. 2016;388(10044):565-575.
337. Dreyling M, Lenz G, Hoster E, et al. Early consolidation by myeloablative radiochemotherapy followed by autologous stem cell transplantation in first remission significantly prolongs progression-free survival in mantle-cell lymphoma: results of a prospective randomized trial of the European MCL Network. *Blood*. 2005;105(7):2677-2684.
338. Hoster E, Metzner B, Forstpointner R, et al. Autologous stem cell transplantation and addition of rituximab Independently prolong response duration in advanced stage mantle cell lymphoma. *Blood*. 2009;114(22):880-880.
339. Graf SA, Stevenson PA, Holmberg LA, et al. Maintenance rituximab after autologous stem cell transplantation in patients with mantle cell lymphoma. *Ann Oncol*. 2015;26(11):2323-2328.
340. Kaplan LD, Jung S-H, Stock W, et al. Bortezomib maintenance (BM) versus consolidation (BC) following aggressive immunochemotherapy and autologous stem cell transplant (ASCT) for untreated mantle cell lymphoma (MCL): CALGB (alliance) 50403. *Blood*. 2015;126(23):337.
341. Chen R, Palmer J, Holmberg L, et al. Interim analysis of a phase 2 study of bortezomib plus rituximab maintenance therapy in patients with mantle cell lymphoma status post autologous stem cell transplantation. *Blood*. 2015;126(23):1961.
342. Le Gouill S, Thieblemont C, Oberic L, et al. Rituximab after autologous stem-cell transplantation in mantle-cell lymphoma. *N Engl J Med*. 2017;377(13):1250-1260.
343. Ladetto M, Cortelazzo S, Ferrero S, et al. Lenalidomide maintenance after autologous haematopoietic stem-cell transplantation in mantle cell lymphoma: results of a Fondazione Italiana Linfomi (FIL) multicentre, randomised, phase 3 trial. *Lancet Haematol*. 2021;8(1):e34-e44.
344. Wang M, Munoz J, Goy A, et al. KTE-X19 CAR T-cell therapy in relapsed or refractory mantle-cell lymphoma. *N Engl J Med*. 2020;382(14):1331-1342.
345. Fenske TS, Zhang MJ, Carreras J, et al. Autologous or reduced-intensity conditioning allogeneic hematopoietic cell transplantation for chemotherapy-sensitive mantle-cell lymphoma: analysis of transplantation timing and modality. *J Clin Oncol*. 2014;32(4):273-281.
346. Sorror ML, Storb RF, Sandmaier BM, et al. Comorbidity-age index: a clinical measure of biologic age before allogeneic hematopoietic cell transplantation. *J Clin Oncol*. 2014;32(29):3249-3256.
347. Schmitz N, de Leval L. How I manage peripheral T-cell lymphoma, not otherwise specified and angioimmunoblastic T-cell lymphoma: current practice and a glimpse into the future. *Br J Haematol*. 2016;176(6):851-866.
348. d'Amore F, Gaulard P, Trümper L, et al. Peripheral T-cell lymphomas: ESMO Clinical Practice Guidelines for diagnosis, treatment and follow-up. *Ann Oncol*. 2015;26(suppl 5):v108-v115.
349. Gutiérrez-García G, García-Herrera A, Cardesa T, et al. Comparison of four prognostic scores in peripheral T-cell lymphoma. *Ann Oncol*. 2011;22(2):397-404.
350. Ansell SM, Habermann TM, Kurtin PJ, et al. Predictive capacity of the international prognostic factor index in patients with peripheral T-cell lymphoma. *J Clin Oncol*. 1997;15(6):2296-2301.
351. Went P, Agostinelli C, Gallamini A, et al. Marker expression in peripheral T-cell lymphoma: a proposed clinical-pathologic prognostic score. *J Clin Oncol*. 2006;24(16):2472-2479.
352. Simon A, Peoch M, Casassus P, et al. Upfront VIP-reinforced-ABVD (VIP-rABVD) is not superior to CHOP/21 in newly diagnosed peripheral T cell lymphoma. Results of the randomized phase III trial GOELAMS-LTP95. *Br J Haematol*. 2010;151(2):159-166.
353. Abouyabis AN, Shenoy PJ, Sinha R, Flowers CR, Lechowicz MJ. A systematic review and meta-analysis of front-line anthracycline-based chemotherapy regimens for peripheral T-cell lymphoma. *ISRN Hematol*. 2011;2011:623924.

354. Horwitz S, O'Connor OA, Pro B, et al. Brentuximab Vedotin with Chemotherapy for CD30-Positive Peripheral T-cell Lymphoma (ECHELON-2): a global, double-blind, randomised, phase 3 trial. *Lancet Lond Engl.* 2019;393(10168):229-240.

355. d'Amore F, Relander T, Lauritzsen GF, et al. Up-front autologous stem-cell transplantation in peripheral T-cell lymphoma: NLG-T-01. *J Clin Oncol.* 2012;30(25):3093-3099.

356. Corradini P, Tarella C, Zallio F, et al. Long-term follow-up of patients with peripheral T-cell lymphomas treated up-front with high-dose chemotherapy followed by autologous stem cell transplantation. *Leukemia.* 2006;20(9):1533-1538.

357. Rodríguez J, Conde E, Gutiérrez A, et al. Prolonged survival of patients with angioimmunoblastic T-cell lymphoma after high-dose chemotherapy and autologous stem cell transplantation: the GELTAMO experience. *Eur J Haematol.* 2007;78(4):290-296.

358. El-Asmar J, Reljic T, Ayala E, et al. Efficacy of high-dose therapy and autologous hematopoietic cell transplantation in peripheral T cell lymphomas as front-line consolidation or in the relapsed/refractory setting: a systematic review/meta-analysis. *Biol Blood Marrow Transplant.* 2016;22(5):802-814.

359. Wilhelm M, Smetak M, Reimer P, et al. First-line therapy of peripheral T-cell lymphoma: extension and long-term follow-up of a study investigating the role of autologous stem cell transplantation. *Blood Cancer J.* 2016;6(7):e452.

360. Schmitz N, Truemper L, Ziepert M, et al. First-line therapy of T-cell lymphoma: allogeneic or autologous transplantation for consolidation—final results of the AATT study. *J Clin Oncol.* 2019;37:7503.

361. Smith SM, Burns LJ, van Besien K, et al. Hematopoietic cell transplantation for systemic mature T-cell non-Hodgkin lymphoma. *J Clin Oncol Off.* 2013;31(25):3100-3109.

362. Dodero A, Spina F, Narni F, et al. Allogeneic transplantation following a reduced-intensity conditioning regimen in relapsed/refractory peripheral T-cell lymphomas: long-term remissions and response to donor lymphocyte infusions support the role of a graft-versus-lymphoma effect. *Leukemia.* 2012;26(3):520-526.

363. Kanate AS, Mussetti A, Kharfan-Dabaja MA, et al. Reduced-intensity transplantation for lymphomas using haploidentical related donors vs HLA-matched unrelated donors. *Blood.* 2016;127(7):938-947.

364. Moore DC, Oxencis CJ, Shank BR. New and emerging pharmacotherapies for management of multiple myeloma. *Am J Health-Syst Pharm AJHP.* 2022;79(14):1137-1145.

365. Sonneveld P, Avet-Loiseau H, Lonial S, et al. Treatment of multiple myeloma with high-risk cytogenetics: a consensus of the International Myeloma Working Group. *Blood.* 2016;127(24):2955-2962.

366. Cavo M, San-Miguel J, Usmani SZ, et al. Prognostic value of minimal residual disease negativity in myeloma: combined analysis of POLLUX, CASTOR, ALCYONE, and MAIA. *Blood.* 2022;139(6):835-844.

367. Child JA, Morgan GJ, Davies FE, et al. High-dose chemotherapy with hematopoietic stem-cell rescue for multiple myeloma. *N Engl J Med.* 2003;348(19):1875-1883.

368. Attal M, Harousseau JL, Stoppa AM, et al. A prospective, randomized trial of autologous bone marrow transplantation and chemotherapy in multiple myeloma. Intergroupe Français du Myélome. *N Engl J Med.* 1996;335(2):91-97.

369. Attal M, Lauwers-Cances V, Hulin C, et al. Lenalidomide, bortezomib, and dexamethasone with transplantation for myeloma. *N Engl J Med.* 2017;376(14):1311-1320.

370. Dhakal B, Szabo A, Chhabra S, et al. Autologous transplantation for newly diagnosed multiple myeloma in the era of novel agent induction: a systematic review and meta-analysis. *JAMA Oncol.* 2018;4(3):343-350.

371. Gay F, Oliva S, Petrucci MT, et al. Chemotherapy plus lenalidomide versus autologous transplantation, followed by lenalidomide plus prednisone versus lenalidomide maintenance, in patients with multiple myeloma: a randomised, multicentre, phase 3 trial. *Lancet Oncol.* 2015;16(16):1617-1629.

372. Gay F, Musto P, Rota-Scalabrini D, et al. Carfilzomib with cyclophosphamide and dexamethasone or lenalidomide and dexamethasone plus autologous transplantation or carfilzomib plus lenalidomide and dexamethasone, followed by maintenance with carfilzomib plus lenalidomide or lenalidomide alone for patients with newly diagnosed multiple myeloma (FORTE): a randomised, open-label, phase 2 trial. *Lancet Oncol.* 2021;22(12):1705-1720.

373. Cavo M, Gay F, Beksac M, et al. Autologous haematopoietic stem-cell transplantation versus bortezomib-melphalan-prednisone, with or without bortezomib-lenalidomide-dexamethasone consolidation therapy, and lenalidomide maintenance for newly diagnosed multiple myeloma (EMN02/HO95): a multicentre, randomised, open-label, phase 3 study. *Lancet Haematol.* 2020;7(6):e456-e468.

374. Gay F, Magarotto V, Crippa C, et al. Bortezomib induction, reduced-intensity transplantation, and lenalidomide consolidation-maintenance for myeloma: updated results. *Blood.* 2013;122(8):1376-1383.

375. Palumbo A, Gay F, Spencer A, et al. A phase III study of ASCT Vs cyclophosphamide-lenalidomide-dexamethasone and lenalidomide-prednisone maintenance Vs lenalidomide alone in newly diagnosed myeloma patients. *Blood.* 2013;122(21):763.

376. Palumbo A, Cavallo F, Gay F, et al. Autologous transplantation and maintenance therapy in multiple myeloma. *N Engl J Med.* 2014;371(10):895-905.

377. Cavo M, Petrucci MT, Di Raimondo F, et al. Upfront single versus double autologous stem cell transplantation for newly diagnosed multiple myeloma: an Intergroup, multicenter, phase III study of the European myeloma Network (EMN02/HO95 MM trial). *Blood.* 2016;128(22):991.

378. Neukirchen J, Arat P, Teutloff C, et al. Favourable outcome of elderly patients with multiple myeloma treated with tandem melphalan 100 high-dose therapy, autologous stem cell transplantation and novel agents: a single center experience. *Blood.* 2016;128(22):3460.

379. Veltri LW, Milton DR, Delgado R, et al. Outcome of autologous hematopoietic stem cell transplantation in refractory multiple myeloma. *Cancer.* 2017;123(18):3568-3575.

380. Gagelmann N, Eikema DJ, Koster L, et al. Tandem autologous stem cell transplantation improves outcomes in newly diagnosed multiple myeloma with extramedullary disease and high-risk cytogenetics: a study from the chronic malignancies working party of the European society for blood and marrow transplantation. *Biol Blood Marrow Transplant.* 2019;25(11):2134-2142.

381. Moreau P, Attal M, Hulin C, et al. Bortezomib, thalidomide, and dexamethasone with or without daratumumab before and after autologous stem-cell transplantation for newly diagnosed multiple myeloma (CASSIOPEIA): a randomised, open-label, phase 3 study. *Lancet.* 2019;394(10192):29-38.

382. Nishimura KK, Barlogie B, van Rhee F, et al. Long-term outcomes after autologous stem cell transplantation for multiple myeloma. *Blood Adv.* 2020;4(2):422-431.

383. Perrot A, Lauwers-Cances V, Cazaubiel T, et al. Early versus late autologous stem cell transplant in newly diagnosed multiple myeloma: long-term follow-up analysis of the IFM 2009 trial. *Blood.* 2020;136(suppl 1):39.

384. Munshi PN, Vesole D, Jurczyszyn A, et al. Age no bar: a CIBMTR analysis of elderly patients undergoing autologous hematopoietic cell transplantation for multiple myeloma. *Cancer.* 2020;126(23):5077-5087.

385. Kumar SK, Dingli D, Lacy MQ, et al. Autologous stem cell transplantation in patients of 70 years and older with multiple myeloma: results from a matched pair analysis. *Am J Hematol.* 2008;83(8):614-617.

386. Stadtmauer EA, Pasquini MC, Blackwell B, et al. Autologous transplantation, consolidation, and maintenance therapy in multiple myeloma: results of the BMT CTN 0702 trial. *J Clin Oncol.* 2019;37(7):589-597.

387. Jackson GH, Davies FE, Pawlyn C, et al. Lenalidomide maintenance versus observation for patients with newly diagnosed multiple myeloma (Myeloma XI): a multicentre, open-label, randomised, phase 3 trial. *Lancet Oncol.* 2019;20(1):57-73.

388. McCarthy PL, Holstein SA, Petrucci MT, et al. Lenalidomide maintenance after autologous stem-cell transplantation in newly diagnosed multiple myeloma: a meta-analysis. *J Clin Oncol.* 2017;35(29):3279-3289.

389. Costa LJ, Iacobelli S, Pasquini MC, et al. Long-term survival of 1338 MM patients treated with tandem autologous vs. autologous-allogeneic transplantation. *Bone Marrow Transplant.* 2020;55(9):1810-1816.

390. Reinoso-Segura M, Caballero-Velázquez T, Herrera P, et al. Phase II trial of allogeneic transplantation plus novel drugs in multiple myeloma: effect of intensifying reduced-intensity conditioning and adding maintenance treatment. *Transplant Cell Ther.* 2022;28(5):258.e1-258.e8.

391. Kumar S, Dispenzieri A, Lacy MQ, et al. Revised prognostic staging system for light chain amyloidosis incorporating cardiac biomarkers and serum free light chain measurements. *J Clin Oncol.* 2012;30(9):989-995.

392. Lilleness B, Ruberg FL, Mussinelli R, Doros G, Sanchorawala V. Development and validation of a survival staging system incorporating BNP in patients with light chain amyloidosis. *Blood.* 2019;133(3):215-223.

393. Sanchorawala V, Sun F, Quillen K, Sloan JM, Berk JL, Seldin DC. Long-term outcome of patients with AL amyloidosis treated with high-dose melphalan and stem cell transplantation: 20-year experience. *Blood.* 2015;126(20):2345-2347.

394. D'Souza A, Dispenzieri A, Wirk B, et al. Improved outcomes after autologous hematopoietic cell transplantation for light chain amyloidosis: a center for international blood and marrow transplant research study. *J Clin Oncol.* 2015;33(32):3741-3749.

395. Palladini G, Kastritis E, Maurer MS, et al. Daratumumab plus CyBorD for patients with newly diagnosed AL amyloidosis: safety run-in results of ANDROMEDA. *Blood.* 2020;136(1):71-80.

396. Tan CR, Estrada-Merly N, Landau H, et al. A second autologous hematopoietic cell transplantation is a safe and effective salvage therapy in select relapsed or refractory AL amyloidosis patients. *Bone Marrow Transplant.* 2022;57(2):295-298.

397. D'Souza A, Lacy M, Gertz M, et al. Long-term outcomes after autologous stem cell transplantation for patients with POEMS syndrome (osteosclerotic myeloma): a single-center experience. *Blood.* 2012;120(1):56-62.

398. Karam C, Klein CJ, Dispenzieri A, et al. Polyneuropathy improvement following autologous stem cell transplantation for POEMS syndrome. *Neurology.* 2015;84(19):1981-1987.

399. Kawajiri-Manako C, Sakaida E, Ohwada C, et al. Efficacy and long-term outcomes of autologous stem cell transplantation in POEMS syndrome: a Nationwide survey in Japan. *Biol Blood Marrow Transplant.* 2018;24(6):1180-1186.

Chapter 107 ■ Graft-vs-Host Disease and Graft-vs-Tumor Response

JOSEPH PIDALA • BRIAN C. BETTS • FREDERICK L. LOCKE • CLAUDIO ANASETTI

INTRODUCTION

Graft-vs-host disease (GVHD) is the most common treatment complication following allogeneic hematopoietic stem cell transplantation (HCT) and is a major cause of recipient morbidity and mortality. GVHD results from the recognition of recipient tissue antigens by immune competent T cells transplanted with the graft. There is an acute form of GVHD with a rapid onset, usually early after transplantation, and a chronic form of GVHD with late onset. These two GVHD syndromes are largely distinct in pathogenesis, clinical manifestations, prevention, and treatment, and therefore are presented separately in this chapter. Donor cells in the graft also produce an immune response against targets in the recipient malignant cells, through a reaction that contributes substantially to the antitumor activity of HCT. Such a graft-vs-tumor (GVT) response is presented in the third section of this chapter.

ACUTE GRAFT-VS-HOST DISEASE

Pathophysiology

The requirements for the development of GVHD were recognized over 50 years ago by Billingham: (1) the inclusion of immune competent cells in the graft, (2) the inability of the recipient to reject the graft, and (3) the presence of recipient tissue antigens foreign to the donor. Animal model studies led to a three-step model of GVHD pathophysiology that emphasized cellular interactions and cytokines: (1) host antigen-presenting cell (APC) activation, (2) donor T-cell activation, and (3) pathogenic effector cells and inflammatory mediators producing the disease.[1,2] GVHD biology is complex, involving positive and negative signals at multiple levels including the cell surface, signaling protein networks, transcription promoters, mRNA, posttranslational modification, and cellular trafficking of immune cells into and out of lymphoid and visceral organs, driven by cytokine and chemokine signals. In addition to histocompatibility antigen disparities between donor and recipients, genetic polymorphisms at any of these immune checkpoints may promote or prevent GVHD. Paczesny and Reddy created a comprehensive model of GVHD pathophysiology. This proposed nonlinear model consists of four interrelated elements to describe the role of immune system recognition and activation at the genetic, cellular, and cytokine level: triggers, sensors, mediators, and effectors of GVHD (Table 107.1).[3] Critical to acute GVHD onset is the degree of genetic variability between donor and host, the level and site of tissue damage set forth by the conditioning regimen, the ability of host or donor cells to present antigen, the cellular and cytokine mediators of response, and the nature and degree of the immune effector activity.

Triggers

Human leukocyte antigens (HLAs) are encoded by the major histocompatibility gene complex (MHC) on chromosome 6p and function as major histocompatibility antigens in transplantation. The natural function of HLA is to present antigenic peptides to specific T cells. Exogenous and endogenous proteins present within human cells are continually broken down into peptides. HLA molecules on professional APCs bind those peptides within their groove and present them from the cell surface to the T-cell receptors on T lymphocytes. Inasmuch as the human genome includes greater than 10^7 polymorphic sequences, there is great likelihood that donor and recipient differ for one or more of the proteins that are presented as HLA:peptide complexes to T cells. These polymorphic proteins function as minor histocompatibility antigens (mHAs) in transplantation. Autoreactive T-cell recognition of "self" peptides in the thymus leads to negative selection (death), so that the probability of an individual developing autoimmunity is minimized. After transplantation, this delicate balance of self and nonself is perturbed. Donor and recipient may differ for HLA molecules or mHA. Each peripheral T cell harbors a unique T-cell antigen receptor; therefore, the human repertoire for recognition of foreign antigens is enormous. Donor and recipient *HLA* mismatching plays a critical role in the development of GVHD, because each type of HLA presents a unique repertoire of antigenic peptides. When recipient cells are mismatched at an *HLA* locus, the donor T cells have not undergone thymic deletion to avoid recognizing those HLA:peptide complexes. Therefore, the degree of *HLA* disparity directly increases the probability and severity of acute GVHD following transplantation.[4,5] For umbilical cord blood donors a greater degree of *HLA* mismatch is tolerated presumably due to the small number of T cells within the cord blood (~10^4 per kg recipient weight) as compared to adult donor blood (~10^8) or marrow (~10^7).

mHAs are polymorphic proteins genetically encoded anywhere outside *HLA*. Host mHA proteins are presented as HLA:peptide complexes to donor T cells and elicit an immune response even when presented via a matched HLA molecule. mHA mismatches are only partially characterized for the ability to affect acute GVHD. Some mHA have broad tissue expression such as the male-associated H-Y antigen.[6] Alternatively, HA-1 and HA-2, for example, have their expression restricted to hematopoietic cells, including leukemia, and immune cells.[7] It is this variability of tissue mHA expression that may allow for tailoring therapy toward hematopoietic-restricted mHA to promote GVT response without GVHD. Efforts to prevent GVHD would have to target immune responses against the ubiquitously expressed mHA.[6,8,9]

Other triggers of GVHD include molecules that activate the innate immune system. Pretransplant radiation or chemotherapy damages host cells and enteric microbes that contain damage-associated molecular patterns (DAMPs) or pathogen-associated molecular patterns (PAMPs), respectively. DAMPs such as proteases or ions released from damaged epithelial cells and PAMPs such as lipopolysaccharide within common bacteria can activate Toll-like receptors setting off a cascade of immune events characterized by proinflammatory cytokine secretion.[10] To a large degree these processes are responsible for initiation of the "cytokine storm" described as critical in earlier models of acute GVHD.[11] Loss of enteric flora diversity is relevant to acute GVHD risk.[12] Patients who lose Clostridiales bacteria from the gut and have a significant increase of Lactobacillales rapidly develop acute GVHD. Reduced intestinal microbial diversity represents an independent risk for posttransplant mortality.[13] Conversely, an increase in enteric *Blautia*, a normal host commensal bacterium, appears to reduce the risk of death from acute GVHD.[14] The microbial metabolite, butyrate, is involved in the maintenance of intestinal epithelial cell integrity and offers immune suppressive effects.[15]

The lack of enteric interleukin (IL)-22 is a unique GVHD trigger. IL-22 is produced by gut-resident, group 3 innate lymphoid cells (ILC3).[16] Innate lymphoid cells (ILC) are derived from the common lymphoid progenitor but do not express the recombination activating gene, or B or T cell receptors. ILC3 are dependent on transcription factor RORγt and produce IL-22 and IL-17A. They have an important role in protective immunity and inflammation, and their dysregulation can lead to autoimmune disease.[17] In rodents, recipients deficient for IL-22 succumb to severe acute GVHD.[16] Histologically, the lack of IL-22 leads to loss of crypt and epithelial architecture and decreased enteric epithelial progenitors.[16] Recombinant IL-22 can rescue intestinal stem

Table 107.1. Summary of Acute Graft vs Host Disease Pathogenesis

Key Elements	Physiologic Role	Aberrant Process in Graft-vs-Host Disease
Triggers		
HLA molecules	Present antigen to T cells	Mismatches in HLA molecules from donor to host lead to recognition of the cell as foreign by T cells.
mHA	Normal variability of protein within genome	mHA are recognized as foreign by MHC:T-cell interactions.
DAMPs and PAMPs	Common organic patterns originating from damaged cells or pathogens triggering innate immunity	DAMP release after cell death due to conditioning therapy or PAMP presence via pathogens triggers innate immunity and cytokine cascade.
Sensors		
Antigen-presenting cells	Present antigens to effectors	Present exogenous and endogenous protein sequences to T cells via direct, indirect, or cross presentation.
Mediators		
CD4 T helper subsets	Skew effector responses to the appropriate degree	Effects of T-cell subsets on graft-vs-host disease incompletely understood.
Regulatory T cells	T-cell subset which acts to prevent untoward autoimmunity	Donor regulatory T cells play a role in reducing graft-vs-host disease.
Inhibitory signals	Signals provided in concert with antigen presentation to decrease the immune response	
Co-stimulatory signals	Signals provided by professional antigen-presenting cells to initiate immune response	
Effectors		
Activated CD4 and CD8 T cells	Lead to killing or neutralization of foreign cells or debris via IFNγ, perforin, or granzyme secretion	Donor cells act to damage host cells and organs leading to manifestations of graft-vs-host disease.

Abbreviations: DAMPs, damage-associated molecular patterns; HLA, human leukocyte antigen; IFNγ, interferon gamma; mHA, minor histocompatibility antigen; MHC, major histocompatibility complex; PAMPs, pathogen-associated molecular patterns.
Adapted from Paczesny S, Hanauer D, Sun Y, Reddy P. New perspectives on the biology of acute GVHD. *Bone Marrow Transplant*. 2010;45:1-11.

cell development and expansion, thus significantly reducing acute GVHD mortality in mice.[18] A translational trial of IL-22 has been conducted in human acute GVHD, where IL-22 in combination with corticosteroids was well tolerated and the 70% lower gastrointestinal (GI) acute GVHD response rate met the primary efficacy endpoint.[19]

Sensors

Sensors of GVHD refer to the cells and processes that recognize the mHA or HLA mismatches as foreign, thereby setting the immune response in motion. Antigens are presented by host professional APCs such as dendritic cells, macrophages, or Langerhans cells. Host dendritic cells may be primed for antigen presentation via the cytokine storm accompanying the conditioning therapy. The nature of antigen presentation interactions includes *direct presentation*, which mimics physiologic APC-T-cell interactions. Specifically, direct presentation consists of host APC presenting endogenous (cytosolic) host peptide to donor CD8 T cells, and exogenous (extracellular, endocytosed peptide, processed in lysosomes) antigens are presented to donor CD4 T cells. *Indirect presentation* specifies exogenous antigen presented from donor APC to donor CD4 cells. Cross-presentation refers to exogenous antigen (derived from host cells) presented to donor T cells from donor APC. Over time APCs change from primarily host origin to donor origin. It is likely that direct presentation by host APCs is predominant during early stages of acute GVHD, whereas indirect or cross-presentation by donor APC is predominant in chronic GVHD. APC-T-cell interaction involves not only interaction between HLA plus cognate antigen with T cell receptor, but co-stimulatory and inhibitory signals at the immune synapse, secondary signals from cell subsets, and paracrine or autocrine mediators. APCs provide necessary co-stimulatory signals directly when activating T cells, such as CD28, CD40, and ICOS as well as inhibitory signals such as CTLA-4 and PD-1. Manipulation of these signals via antibody interference or small molecule blockade of downstream signaling events remains a field ripe for modulation of GVHD. Exogenous cell types critical to inhibition of APC include regulatory T cells, gamma-delta T cells in the GI tract, ILC, natural killer (NK) cells, and host NKT cells. T-cell response is an adaptive immune response that is often triggered by the innate immune response. As described, Toll-like receptors are sensors of the DAMP and PAMP release precipitated by the condition regimen. These Toll-like receptor interactions lead to release of proinflammatory cytokines such as tumor necrosis factor alpha (TNFα) and IL-6, which contribute to the inflammatory milieu surrounding T-cell-mediated GVHD damage.

Mediators

GVHD is primarily mediated by donor T cells, and differing subsets that have normal physiologic activities outside the framework of transplant act at different capacities to induce or inhibit GVHD development. Most animal models point to the relevance of naïve T cells, rather than memory T cells, in the induction of GVHD. The process of homeostatic proliferation in the lymphoablated host causes brisk clonal expansion of the transferred donor T cells and plays an important role for the initiation of acute GVHD. Donor regulatory T cells (Tregs) repress the GVHD responses. Tregs are CD4 T cells that express the FOXP3 transcription factor, high levels of the alpha chain of the IL-2 receptor, but no IL-7 receptor and function as a natural suppressor to maintain peripheral tolerance. These donor-derived regulatory T cells inhibit the activation and proliferation of donor T cells implicated in the pathogenesis of acute GVHD and may spare the GVT effect.[20] Low-dose IL-2 expands regulatory T cells in vivo and may be effective therapy for established GVHD,[21] whereas anti-IL-2 receptor antibodies, tested before Treg importance and biology were recognized, appear to accelerate GVHD.[22]

Additional CD4 T-cell subsets are critical. It is Th1 cells, characterized by TNFα and interferon gamma (IFNγ) secretion, that are the likely main T-cell mediators of acute GVHD. Th2 T cells have been linked to protection against acute GVHD. Murine transplant models provide evidence that Th17 can cause GVHD.[23,24] Human Th17 CD4 cells secrete IL-17 and seem to contribute to both acute and chronic human GVHD. T-cell trafficking is another important step in GVHD pathogenesis. Differential expression of chemokines on GVHD target organs and draining lymph nodes mediate differential trafficking of T-cell subsets expressing different chemokine receptors.

Effectors

The effectors of acute GVHD are the cytolytic cellular elements and inflammatory cytokines. Activated CD4 and CD8 cytotoxic T lymphocytes are the primary effectors of GVHD. Upon interaction with their cognate HLA:peptide they act to lyse or cause apoptosis of target cells via secretion of perforin and granzyme or binding of FAS, respectively. IFNγ and TNFα are both critical to the inflammatory process of GVHD. Inflammatory cytokines induce and amplify cellular damage.

Epidemiology

GVHD is the major source of transplant-related morbidity and mortality. The incidence of clinically relevant (grade II-IV) acute GVHD ranges from 35% to 80%, with a higher incidence reported for recipients of *HLA* mismatched and unrelated donors compared to matched related donors.[25] The day 100 incidence of severe acute GVHD (grades III-IV) is approximately 15%, but may be higher depending upon risk factors such as *HLA* disparity.[4]

Risk Factors

Risk factors for the development of acute GVHD include T-replete transplant, recipient and donor *HLA* disparity, female donor for a male recipient, donor and recipient age, hematopoietic stem cell source (peripheral blood progenitor cells [PBPCs] > marrow > cord blood), graft cellular composition (worse with higher T-cell and CD34 cell numbers), higher conditioning intensity, diagnosis (worse with chronic myeloid leukemia), and immune response gene polymorphisms.[26-28] Predictive factors are of great interest to stratify patients prior to development of serious morbidity or mortality and to focus prevention.

HLA matching is critical to prevent acute GVHD. A single allele mismatch at *HLA-A*, *HLA-B*, *HLA-C*, or *HLA-DRB1* increases the likelihood of acute GVHD development, and mismatch for multiple alleles compounds the risk.[4,29] The functional relevance of *HLA-A*, *HLA-B*, or *HLA-C* mismatch between donor and recipient varies according to the nature of the peptide-binding residues: for example, mismatch at *HLA-C* position 116 is associated with increased risk for severe acute GVHD.[30] *HLA-DPB1* and *HLA-DQB1* mismatches are associated with increased acute GVHD, and *HLA-DPB1* mismatch is associated with decreased risk of malignancy relapse.[31] Donor and recipient mismatch for certain types of nonpermissive *HLA-DPB1* disparities is associated with higher overall mortality compared with permissive *HLA-DPB1* disparities or donor match.[31]

Female donor for a male recipient and donor parity are risk factors for the development of acute GVHD. The increased risk for male recipients of female as opposed to male donors is attributed to the recognition of H-Y mHAs by female donor T cells.[32,33] During pregnancy, female donors develop an immune response to the paternal mHAs of the fetus and mount a secondary, augmented T-cell alloimmune response against the same mHAs if expressed in the recipient.[34] Increasing donor age is associated with increased risk for the development of severe acute and chronic GVHD, and worse mortality.[35] Age of the recipient is also important with higher rates of acute GVHD in older compared to younger cohorts.[28,36] Unrelated cord blood transplant is associated with a low rate of acute GVHD when compared to transplant with similarly *HLA* mismatched adult donors.[37,38] Multiple factors may contribute to this effect; however, the low number of T cells in the graft likely plays a protective role.

The conditioning regimen affects the incidence of acute GVHD. With high-dose intensity conditioning the incidence of acute GVHD is higher. For example, increasing doses of radiation can double the incidence of acute GVHD.[39] Several large retrospective studies showed that reduced-intensity regimens lead to reduced rates of grade II-IV acute GVHD when compared to higher-intensity regimens.[40,41] Animal models suggest the correlation of the incidence of GVHD with intensity may be due to increased damage to host tissue and amplified release of cytokines followed by activation of APC.[42] In addition, higher-intensity regimens decrease the fraction of recipient T cells that persist after the regimen, leading to a lower barrier to donor engraftment and greater homeostatic re-population by donor T cells, which is associated with worse acute GVHD.[43,44]

The cellular composition of the graft may be linked to the incidence of GVHD. The preponderance of evidence suggests that there is no correlation between CD34 cell dose and the incidence of acute GVHD, whether the progenitor source is marrow or PBPC,[45-47] although in patients given cyclosporine as prophylaxis, there was a positive association of CD34 dose with acute GVHD.[48]

Genetic polymorphisms of immune response genes are associated with an increased incidence of acute GVHD. Single nucleotide polymorphisms (SNPs) can alter cytokine binding domains, thereby altering affinity in a functional or nonfunctional way. Particular SNPs in genes coding IL-10, IL-6, IL-2, heparinase gene, CTLA-4, and MTHFR (methylenetetrahydrofolate reductase) have been identified as increasing the risk of clinically relevant or severe acute GVHD, likely via increased level or activity of these cytokines or their receptors.[49]

Clinical Manifestations of Acute Graft-vs-Host Disease

The most common sites of involvement are skin, GI tract, and liver. Additional organ sites may be involved and clinicians should maintain a high degree of suspicion for acute GVHD as a cause for any unexplained abnormalities in the eyes, buccal mucosa, and lung. A biopsy of the presumptive site should be attempted whenever possible to confirm diagnosis, although histological manifestations can overlap with many inflammatory conditions confounding histological results. A pathologist familiar with acute GVHD is preferable, and appropriate immunohistochemical stains should be employed to rule out viral infection, particularly of the GI tract.

The onset and natural history of acute GVHD is variable depending on organ site, nature, and severity of disease. A hyperacute form, occurring in the first 14 days after transplant,[50] is characterized by early onset of typical signs and symptoms, with a preponderance of patients, 90%, exhibiting skin involvement. In addition, a higher percentage of patients are likely to experience stage III-IV disease (88% vs 66%).[51,52]

Most cases of acute GVHD manifest within the first 100 days following transplant. With the use of modern prophylaxis regimens including cyclosporine or tacrolimus, the onset is typically 20 to 30 days after cell infusion. With T-cell depletion, average onset is typically at 30 days, although it can be delayed several months as T cells reconstitute.[53] NIH consensus criteria for chronic GVHD include classification of acute GVHD occurring after day 100 (late-onset acute GVHD) and for patients manifesting signs and symptoms of both acute GVHD and chronic GVHD (overlap subtype of chronic GVHD).[54] The severity of acute GVHD is assessed by organ staging and summarized as overall grading. The most current proposed acute GVHD grading system largely recapitulates previous consensus grading,[55] but also includes lower GI staging according to either diarrhea volume or number of diarrhea episodes, which facilitates GI staging of outpatients (*Table 107.2*).[56]

Skin

Skin is the most commonly involved site of acute GVHD, being present 80% of the time at onset. A maculopapular rash is characteristic and may be described as a painful or pruritic sunburn. Characteristically involved sites include the back of the neck, palms, soles, dorsal surfaces of the extremities, and ears, although the rash can spread quickly to include the entire body. Although many cases are mild, severe manifestations can include bullous lesions and a clinical picture consistent with toxic epidermal necrolysis. Full-body examination allows for staging of acute GVHD based upon percentage of body surface area (BSA) involvement. Grade I acute GVHD may require no more than topical steroids and frequent monitoring of symptoms (see "Primary and Secondary Therapy of Acute Graft-versus-host Disease"). A biopsy of the skin can help to solidify the diagnosis; however, treatment is usually based on the clinical assessment.

Table 107.2. Acute GVHD Organ Staging and Overall Grading

Stage	Skin (Active Erythema Only)	Liver (Bilirubin)	Upper GI	Lower GI (stool Output/day)
0	No active (erythematous) GVHD rash	<2 mg/dL	No or intermittent nausea, vomiting, or anorexia	Adult: <500 mL/d or <3 episodes/d Child: <10 mL/kg/d or <4 episodes/d
1	Maculopapular rash <25% BSA	2-3 mg/dL	Persistent nausea, vomiting, or anorexia	Adult: 500-999 mL/d or 3-4 episodes/d Child: 10-19.9 mL/kg/d or 4-6 episodes/d
2	Maculopapular rash 25%-50% BSA	3.1-6 mg/dL		Adult: 1000-1500 mL/d or 5-7 episodes/d Child: 20-30 mL/kg/d or 7-10 episodes/d
3	Maculopapular rash >50% BSA	6.1-15 mg/dL		Adult: >1500 mL/d or >7 episodes/d Child: >30 mL/kg/d or >10 episodes/d
4	Generalized erythroderma (>50% BSA) *plus* bullous formation and desquamation >5% BSA	>15 mg/dL		Severe abdominal pain with or without ileus or grossly bloody stool (regardless of stool volume)

Overall clinical grade (based on most severe target organ involvement):
Grade 0: No stage 1 to 4 of any organ.
Grade I: Stage 1 to 2 skin without liver, upper GI, or lower GI involvement.
Grade II: Stage 3 rash and/or stage 1 liver and/or stage 1 upper GI, and/or stage 1 lower GI.
Grade III: Stage 2 to 3 liver and/or stage 2 to 3 lower GI, with stage 0 to 3 skin and/or stage 0 to 1 upper GI.
Grade IV: Stage 4 skin, liver, or lower GI involvement, with stage 0 to 1 upper GI.
Abbreviations: BSA, body surface area; GI, gastrointestinal.
Adapted from Harris AC, Young R, Devine S, et al. International, multicenter standardization of acute graft-versus-host disease clinical data collection: A report from the Mount Sinai Acute GVHD International Consortium. *Biol Blood Marrow Transplant.* 2016;22(1):4-10. Copyright © 2016 American Society for Blood and Marrow Transplantation. With permission.

Hepatic

Liver acute GVHD is typically characterized by involvement of the bile duct epithelium, resulting in cholestasis. Bilirubin and alkaline phosphatase elevation, accompanied by cholestatic jaundice, are the typical manifestations. Direct hepatocyte damage is rare, absent a more chronic fibrosis, although transaminitis often occurs. Hyperbilirubinemia must be distinguished from other common posttransplant complications such as toxicity from preparative chemotherapeutics, sinusoidal obstructive syndrome (hepatic veno-occlusive disease), and occasionally viral hepatitis. Sinusoidal obstructive syndrome is characterized by hyperbilirubinemia, portal hypertension, and weight gain due to third spacing of fluids. Doppler assessment of portal hypertension, measurement of the hepatic vein occlusive pressure, and if necessary histological examination are critical in resolving the differential diagnosis. A transjugular liver biopsy is preferable to transcutaneous biopsy, as portal pressures can be measured. Acute GVHD produces cholestatic hepatitis, with histology showing frequent acidophilic bodies evolving to bile duct exocytosis and disruption. As the disease progresses beyond day 100 posttransplant, portal fibrosis is seen with increasing bile duct dropout.[57] This is in contrast to sinusoidal obstructive syndrome, which is characterized by occluded hepatic venules, sinusoidal fibrosis, and hepatocyte necrosis.[58]

Gastrointestinal Tract

Anorexia, nausea, and vomiting are the most common symptoms of GI acute GVHD, but diarrhea, abdominal pain, and hemorrhage are symptoms of serious lower-tract disease. Almost any site along the tract can be involved. Unexplained GI symptoms such as mouth ulcers or ileus can be caused by acute GVHD. Persistent symptoms should prompt upper and lower endoscopy, which affords both a visual examination of the mucosa, which may exhibit edema, erythema, ulceration, and mucosal sloughing, as well as the opportunity to obtain tissue for histology. Classic microscopic findings include epithelial crypt apoptotic bodies and lymphocytic infiltration. Involved mucosa can be noncontinuous and a lack of findings or a low degree of severity at one level does not rule out other areas or degrees of involvement.[59] The differential diagnosis of upper-tract GVHD includes herpes simplex, cytomegalovirus, or candida esophagitis, stomach ulcer, peptic gastritis, or duodenitis. The differential diagnosis of lower tract disease includes enteritis from *Clostridioides difficile*, cytomegalovirus, Norfolk viruses, cryptosporidium, giardia, or enteric pathogens such as *Salmonella*, and side effects of irradiation or medications including cytotoxic chemotherapy, tacrolimus, and mycophenolate mofetil (MMF), among others. Radiologic findings by computed tomography (CT) scan can include thickening of the esophageal, small, or large bowel wall; adjacent vasa recta engorgement; mesenteric fat stranding; or mucosal enhancement.[60]

Lung

Lung complications following allogeneic transplant can be of cardiac, infectious, vascular, or immune nature. Immune-mediated processes should be entertained when infectious workup is negative, or CT scanning is not consistent with infectious processes. Diffuse alveolar hemorrhage has long been recognized as a posttransplant complication and occurs in up to 10% of patients, with myeloablative regimens associated with a higher incidence. Diagnosis is typically made following bronchoscopy. Patients often require ventilatory support and mortality rates can reach 70%.[61] Bronchiolitis obliterans with organizing pneumonia (BOOP) is seen in up to 2% of patients at a median of 108 days after transplant. BOOP can display a wide range of severity and reversibility and is typically a restrictive lung disease with radiographic findings showing peripheral patchy consolidation, ground glass infiltrates, and nodular opacities. Although not considered a manifestation of GVHD, BOOP is associated with GVHD and steroid therapy affords a chance for improvement.[62] However, none of these pulmonary complications are considered definitive manifestations of acute GVHD.

Central Nervous System

Animal studies from the van den Brink Lab first revealed the potential for acute GVHD to manifest as neurologic symptoms: Donor T cells were found in the host brain with associated tissue damage. Recipient mice also demonstrated severe cognitive and behavioral sequelae from acute GVHD.[63] The Kean Lab was able to replicate these findings in nonhuman primates subjected to acute GVHD. Interestingly, recipient brain pathology was mediated by alloreactive $CD8^+$ T cells and acute GVHD of the central nervous system was reduced with tacrolimus and methotrexate or sirolimus.[64] Despite clear evidence that acute GVHD can impact recipient neurologic function, clinical documentation of the syndrome has yet to be established.

Prevention

To facilitate donor engraftment and to prevent serious and potentially fatal acute GVHD, immune suppressive therapy is standardly given in the setting of allogeneic HCT. Initial work demonstrated that the immunosuppressive agent methotrexate could mitigate or prevent the onset of acute GVHD, when applied shortly after transplantation.

Although oral mucositis and liver toxicity can be severe and preclude up to 40% of patients from receiving a full course of therapy, methotrexate remains widely in use, now typically in combination with a calcineurin inhibitor (CNI).[65-72] CNIs, cyclosporine or tacrolimus, act to inhibit secretion of IL-2 that mediates T-cell expansion. The combination of tacrolimus and methotrexate is considered a standard of care, as supported by randomized phase III trials in the matched sibling and matched unrelated donor setting.[66,68] These trials demonstrated that the use of tacrolimus and methotrexate reduced the incidence of acute GVHD compared to cyclosporine and methotrexate. While these trials support this standard of care to the present time, prevention of acute GVHD is incomplete, chronic GVHD remains common, and complete discontinuation of immune suppressive therapy after HCT is not possible in many patients.

Given these challenges and toxicity associated with methotrexate, investigators have examined alternative agents instead of methotrexate in combination with tacrolimus. The most thoroughly studied include the use of MMF or sirolimus. MMF is a prodrug of mycophenolic acid, an inhibitor of de novo synthesis of purines in lymphocytes required for lymphocyte proliferation. MMF has been examined in combination with cyclosporine or tacrolimus. Single-center randomized studies and registry studies of MMF suggest greater safety but not greater efficacy over methotrexate.[65,67,73] Data from the Center for International Blood and Marrow Transplant Research (CIBMTR) suggest cyclosporine/MMF results in worse acute GVHD (grades 3-4) and survival outcomes compared to cyclosporine/methotrexate or tacrolimus/methotrexate.[74]

Sirolimus is an mTOR inhibitor that has complex immunomodulatory properties affecting T cells and APC. The drug requires therapeutic monitoring and is affected by inhibitors or inducers of *CYP3A4*. Sirolimus is associated with the risk of endothelial damage such as in sinusoidal obstructive syndrome.[75] Initially shown to be safe in combination with tacrolimus and methotrexate,[76] sirolimus has now been tested in phase II and III studies in combination with tacrolimus and the two agents likely synergize to reduce acute GVHD rates.[72] In particular, sirolimus supports regulatory T-cell reconstitution posttransplant, which are protective against acute GVHD after transplantation.[72] Based on similar long-term outcomes, more rapid engraftment, and less oropharyngeal mucositis, the combination of tacrolimus/sirolimus is an acceptable alternative to tacrolimus/methotrexate after *HLA* matched related or unrelated HCT.[77]

T cell co-stimulation (CD28-CD80/CD86) blockade using abatacept has been studied in two sequential trials, given in combination with CNI/methotrexate[78,79] after *HLA* matched or mismatched unrelated donor HCT. The first small trial demonstrated safety and preliminary efficacy. The second (ABA2) was a large phase II trial enrolling patients onto two strata: an 8/8 matched unrelated HCT stratum where patients were randomized to CNI/methotrexate plus abatacept vs CNI/methotrexate plus placebo, and separately a 7/8 matched unrelated HCT stratum comparing CNI/methotrexate plus abatacept vs CNI/methotrexate CIBMTR controls. CNI included either tacrolimus or cyclosporine, and graft source included either PBSC or bone marrow. CNI/methotrexate was given together with four doses of abatacept. Improvements in both grade III-IV acute GVHD and severe-acute GVHD-free survival were observed in the abatacept treated subjects with effects more prominent in the 7/8 *HLA* matched cohort vs CIBMTR controls, and led to the FDA approval of abatacept for the prevention of acute GVHD after 8/8 or 7/8 unrelated donor transplants in 2021. As the first FDA approval of a regimen for GVHD prevention, the development of abatacept represents a major milestone; however, several other approaches continue to be pursued.

Among these alternatives, at least five major approaches with varied level of evidence to date have aimed to minimize donor alloreactive T cells' ability to induce GVHD through in vivo T cell depletion by antithymocyte globulin (ATG) or alemtuzumab, ex vivo T cell depletion by CD34+ selection, deletion of alloreactive T cells by posttransplant cyclophosphamide (PTCy), removal of naïve T cells, or through graft manipulation to deliver defined ratios of conventional and regulatory T cells. Among these, the use of ATG for GVHD prevention has the greatest evidence base including high-quality randomized trials,[80-84] both in the sibling and unrelated donor transplantation. While individual findings of these trials differ, the overall evidence supports that ATG reduces risk of both acute and chronic GVHD and facilitates long-term immune suppression discontinuation. Some transplant centers routinely use this approach outside of clinical trials. Infusion-related side effects and risk of viral reactivation (including Epstein-Barr virus reactivation and posttransplant lymphoproliferative disease) are notable issues that require monitoring and possible treatment.

CD34+ selection is a potent ex vivo means of T cell depletion and has been studied extensively in single centers,[85] as well as prior national BMT CTN trials.[86] These studies suggest that CD34+ selection alone (without additional post-HCT immune suppression) can effectively prevent acute and chronic GVHD. In the BMT CTN 1301 trial, however, CD34+ selected PBSC grafts had inferior survival to conventional tacrolimus/methotrexate given with bone marrow grafts.[87]

PTCy administered 3 to 4 days following transplantation effectively depletes alloreactive T-cell numbers, yet spares stem cells and regulatory T cells, which are critical for engraftment and the prevention of GVHD.[88,89] This strategy can result in low rates of severe acute GVHD, even when used as a single prophylactic agent.[90-92] PTCy is potent enough to prevent acute and chronic GVHD after T-replete marrow transplants from related donors mismatched for an entire *HLA* haplotype.[93] PTCy in combination with sirolimus/MMF appears to provide good outcomes even for those patients transplanted from a <7/8 *HLA* mismatched unrelated donor.[94]

The mounting evidence in support of PTCy as GVHD prophylaxis led to its inclusion in several major BMT CTN national trials. BMT CTN 1203 was a randomized phase II trial comparing (1) tacrolimus, MMF, and PTCy; (2) tacrolimus, methotrexate, and bortezomib; or (3) tacrolimus, methotrexate, and maraviroc against tacrolimus and methotrexate. BMT CTN 1203 was restricted to reduced-intensity conditioning and included HLA-matched related or 7 to 8/8 HLA-matched unrelated donors. BMT CTN 1203 demonstrated the superiority of the PTCy-based regimen in improving the primary endpoint of GVHD-free, relapse-free survival, a composite outcome measure including grade III-IV acute GVHD, chronic GVHD requiring systemic immunosuppression, disease relapse, and death.[95] PTCy was primarily associated with less grade III-IV acute GVHD, while relapse was similar across the study arms. As a follow-up to BMT CTN 1203, the ongoing BMT CTN 1703 phase III trial compares tacrolimus, MMF, and PTCy against tacrolimus and methotrexate after HLA-matched PBSC allografts and reduced-intensity conditioning.

BMT CTN 1301 compared CNI-free regimens, CD34-selected peripheral blood stem cell grafts or single-agent PTCy with an HLA-matched marrow graft, to tacrolimus and methotrexate with an HLA-matched marrow graft after myeloablative conditioning. The CNI-free regimens failed to improve chronic GVHD-free relapse-free survival compared to tacrolimus plus methotrexate and were associated with higher rates of infection. Further, CD34-selection was associated with worse overall survival.

Other approaches including removal of naïve T cells,[96] or graft manipulation to deliver defined ratio of conventional and regulatory T cells,[97] have promise and are being explored currently. Multiple other investigational approaches are underway, with focus on inhibitors of T cell signaling,[98] or neutralization of cytokines associated with pathogenic Th1/Th17 differentiation.[99,100]

Primary and Secondary Therapy of Acute Graft-vs-Host Disease

While patients may be initially treated with topical agents for low stage skin involvement, or minimally absorbed oral agents for upper GI symptoms,[101] systemic therapy is often needed either up front or after failure of topical agents. The current standard primary systemic therapy for acute GVHD consists of glucocorticoids, most commonly agreed upon as starting dose of 1 to 2 mg/kg/d prednisone (or prednisone equivalent) with subsequent taper based on GVHD treatment response. This standard is based upon historical empirical evidence and randomized controlled data that suggest no advantage to prednisone-equivalent steroid doses of >2.5 mg/kg/d and no disadvantage for 1 mg/kg/d for grade II acute GVHD.[102] Response to initial therapy (defined as complete response [CR]or partial response [PR] by day 28 of therapy) is an important determinant of subsequent mortality.[103]

Two other major research questions have been addressed regarding primary steroid therapy, namely risk-stratified treatment, and intensified multiple-agent therapy: First, a prior trial demonstrated that lower dose (0.5 mg/kg) prednisone could be used for lower-risk cases, while in high-risk cases 1 mg/kg or 2 mg/kg initial dosing provided similar outcomes, albeit with greater likelihood for second-line therapy in the 1 mg/kg group.[104] Second, several agents have been added to steroids to determine if augmented multiple-agent therapy could improve treatment response rates. The combination of MMF and glucocorticoids provided the most encouraging 28-day CR rate compared to other agents (etanercept, denileukin diftitox, and pentostatin) combined with steroids[105]; however, this apparent activity was not confirmed in a subsequent phase III trial.[106] Thus, currently there is no evidence in support of multiple-agent primary therapy for acute GVHD.

Allied investigation in the field has aimed to refine clinical- and biomarker-based tools for risk stratification of acute GVHD. These criteria have begun to be employed in clinical trials, with the overarching goals of minimizing treatment toxicity and maximizing GVHD control. The clinical risk model developed at the University of Minnesota examined combinations of GVHD organ involvement and severity to ultimately distinguish a standard risk vs high-risk group. Those in the high-risk group had significantly lower likelihood of treatment response by day 28 and suffered higher mortality.[107] Others (MAGIC Consortium) have identified and validated plasma biomarkers of acute GVHD treatment response and mortality. Plasma TNFR1, ST2, and Reg3α have been validated to define clinically meaningful risk strata for patients with newly diagnosed acute GVHD. In three independent datasets, the biomarker score increased as the response to primary GVHD treatment decreased and 6-month nonrelapse mortality increased.[108] In addition, a 2-biomarker model using ST2 and REG3α concentrations in a blood sample taken 7 days after HCT can identify a group of patients at high risk for lethal GVHD.[109] The BMT CTN developed an acute GVHD therapy clinical trial portfolio leveraging these risk assessment tools: In the BMT CTN 1501 study, patients with Minnesota standard risk were randomized to sirolimus vs prednisone, with the goal of confirming activity of sirolimus as a sole, steroid-free initial therapy approach in a multicenter context. The trial demonstrated that sirolimus achieved similar day 28 CR/PR rates as prednisone, was superior in a composite outcome of day 28 CR/PR with prednisone ≤ 0.25 mg/kg/d, and had improved patient-reported quality of life.[110] An ongoing trial (BMT CTN 1705) is testing the combination of prednisone and alpha-1-antitrypsin for therapy of high-risk acute GVHD.

Failure of initial therapy is termed steroid-refractory acute GVHD, and this is most commonly defined in clinical trials and routine clinical care as progression within 3 days or failure to demonstrate any improvement within 7 days. Failure of initial therapy has poor prognosis overall, both due to organ damage from GVHD and serious infectious complications due to profound immune compromise in this treatment setting. Multiple agents have been studied for steroid-refractory acute GVHD, and none appear to be superior to the others in prior analyses.[102] Some commonly used examples include ATG,[111] denileukin diftitox,[109,110] antibodies against TNFα,[112,113] MMF,[114,115] sirolimus,[116] pentostatin,[117] and extracorporeal photopheresis (ECP).[118]

In a randomized phase III trial, ruxolitinib was compared to investigator's choice of alternative therapy in a total of 309 patients with steroid-refractory acute GVHD.[119] The most commonly used agents in the control arm included ECP, MMF, etanercept, and ATG. CR or PR at day 28, durable overall response at day 56, and failure-free survival were all significantly improved in the ruxolitinib arm. Common toxicities of ruxolitinib included thrombocytopenia, anemia, and cytomegalovirus infection. This trial led to FDA approval of ruxolitinib for steroid-refractory acute GVHD, thus now constituting a standard therapy outside of clinical trials.

Supportive Care

Clinicians should pay special attention to the immunocompromised state of the patients with active acute GVHD. Understanding the hospital and community bacterial resistance patterns is essential to select appropriate prophylactic antibiotics. Patients on high-dose steroids are at high risk for fungal pneumonia and appropriate coverage with antifungal medication is warranted. A large randomized trial showed that the antifungal agent posaconazole is superior to fluconazole at preventing invasive aspergillus when used as prophylaxis in patients with GVHD requiring high-dose steroids.[120] A comparison of transplant outcomes between the time period of 1993 to 1997 and 2003 to 2007 at a large single center revealed significant reduction in mortality. Although this change is due to many factors including the advent of reduced-intensity regimens, decreased infection-related deaths, and decreased severe GVHD, improved supportive care plays a key role.[121] CIBMTR data also support improved survival after acute GVHD diagnosis in more recent time periods.[122]

Conclusion

Acute GVHD remains a significant source of morbidity and mortality after allogeneic transplant. The advent of improved prophylactic regimens has led to decreases in the rates and severity, although the most effective primary therapy remains steroids. Future directions should focus on genetic risk factors for the development of disease, ways to predict which patients will not respond to steroids as primary therapy, and agents or cellular therapies that will prevent the development or stop the progression of acute GVHD.

CHRONIC GRAFT-VS-HOST DISEASE

Introduction

Major efforts in basic, translational, and clinical research in chronic GVHD are underway, and promise to improve outcomes of patients affected by chronic GVHD. The following sections review major progress in our understanding of the pathobiology, clinical advances in the management of the syndrome, and remaining challenges for future research.

Biology

Preclinical models have suggested several areas for ongoing investigation and potential avenues for novel therapeutic approaches.

CD4 T-Cell Subsets

Clinical observations support the role of alloreactive donor T cells: peripheral blood mobilized stem cell products, which contain greater numbers of donor T cells compared to bone marrow harvested stem cells, impose a greater risk for chronic GVHD and prolonged duration of immune suppression.[123,124] Ex vivo T-cell depletion strategies,[125] as well as in vivo strategies such as ATG, ATG-Fresenius, or alemtuzumab, are associated with decreased risk of chronic GVHD.[126,127] Selective depletion of alloreactive T cells using PTCy has similarly reduced the incidence of chronic GVHD.[128] Additional efforts have focused on selective depletion of naïve T cells,[96,129] or Th17/Tc17 cells.[99,130] Ongoing investigation aims to discern the relationship between regulatory T cells and chronic GVHD. Use of sirolimus in GVHD prevention was associated with improved Treg reconstitution after HCT and reduction in chronic GVHD.[72] Exogenous low-dose IL-2 therapy has demonstrated activity in therapy of advanced chronic GVHD.[131] Taken together, total or selective T cell depletion approaches and efforts to augment regulatory T cells have potential to ameliorate clinical chronic GVHD.

Loss of Central Tolerance

Negative selection of autoreactive T cells naturally constitutes a major mechanism of immune tolerance. Immature T cells are positively selected first in the thymic cortex through recognition of class I or class II MHC. In the thymic medulla, T cells engage marrow-derived APCs bearing self-antigens. Strongly self-reactive T cells suffer negative selection through apoptosis. Thus, in normal immunity, naïve T cells are educated in the thymus, and autoreactive cells are deleted. Dysregulation of central tolerance due to thymic epithelial damage, which may result from transplantation conditioning therapy or prior GVHD, leads to impaired generation of tolerogenic Treg[132] and to failure to delete self-reactive T cells.[133] A murine model of thymic dysfunction largely recapitulates a chronic GVHD phenotype. Here, lethally irradiated C3H/HeN recipients receive T-cell-depleted bone marrow from MHC-mismatched B6 mice deficient in MHC class II antigens ($B6\ H2\text{-}Ab1^{-/-}$).[133] Thus, thymic negative selection is compromised by lack of MHC class II in thymic dendritic cells. The resulting phenotype includes sclerodermatous (Scl) skin changes, weight loss, bile duct loss, mononuclear cell infiltration of the salivary glands, and mortality. The clinical relevance of these findings has also been challenged, as thymic function declines with age and may not be relevant to development of GVHD in adult recipients of HSCT. Experimental models have suggested a benefit for keratinocyte growth factor to prevent thymic injury; however, this strategy was not successful in human clinical investigation.[134]

Altered B-Cell Homeostasis

Basic and clinical observations support the role of loss of B-cell tolerance and altered B-cell homeostasis following transplantation in chronic GVHD pathogenesis. B cells have multiple functions, including antibody production, immune regulation, antigen presentation, and cytokine production, all of which may have relevance to chronic GVHD pathogenesis.[135] A systemic lupus erythematosus–chronic GVHD murine model supports the coordination of CD4 T and B cells for antigen presentation and antibody production responsible for the chronic GVHD phenotype. In this model, both class I and class II MHC mismatched immune cells are adoptively transferred into nonirradiated mice, resulting in autoantibody production and immune-complex glomerulonephritis. In this model, B cells present antigen to CD4 T cells, leading to activation and production of Th2 cytokines including IL-4 and IL-10. These cytokines activate B cells, which produce autoantibodies. B-cell stimulatory signals, including B-cell-activating factor (BAFF), have a key role in B-cell reconstitution and homeostasis. In such models, B-cell survival is dependent on B-cell receptor and BAFF signaling, and B-cell homeostasis is dependent on soluble BAFF concentration.[136,137]

Human clinical evidence supports the role of B cells in chronic GVHD: Autoantibodies have been detected in patients with chronic GVHD. After sex mismatched HCT, alloantibodies directed against the Y chromosome-associated mHAs, or H-Y antibodies, have been detected and correlate with the occurrence of chronic GVHD.[138] In the setting of cutaneous sclerosis of chronic GVHD, activating anti-platelet-derived growth factor receptor (PDGFR) antibodies have been detected. As well, reduced levels of immature B cells in patients with chronic GVHD support altered B-cell homeostasis.[139] Investigators have demonstrated aberrant B-cell homeostasis and elevated BAFF levels in human HCT recipients with chronic GVHD. A consolidative model suggests that, in patients who develop chronic GVHD, high BAFF levels and decreased numbers of naïve B cells (high BAFF/B-cell ratio) support alloreactive pre- and postgerminal center CD27+ B cells that contribute to chronic GVHD development.[140-142] This mounting basic and clinical evidence has informed allied clinical investigation: clinical trials have demonstrated activity of B cell depletion through anti-CD20 monoclonal antibodies in the treatment of chronic GVHD that has failed standard glucocorticoid therapy,[143-145] primary therapy,[146] and prevention of chronic GVHD.[147,148]

Profibrotic Pathways

Clinical and basic evidence suggest that profibrotic pathways play a role in chronic GVHD development. In particular, the coordination of Th2 CD4 cells, TGF-β, IL-13, and potentially stimulatory anti-PDGFR antibodies affect fibroblast production of collagen and lead to fibrosis. The Scl-chronic GVHD murine model has provided mechanistic insight into the pathogenesis of fibrotic chronic GVHD phenotypes. In this model, B10.D2 ($H\text{-}2^d$) into BALB/c ($H\text{-}2^d$), donor immune cells (bone marrow and splenocytes) are adoptively transferred into sublethally irradiated mice that are matched at MHC, but mismatched for mHAs. The resulting phenotype includes fibrosis in multiple organs (skin, GI tract, liver, lung, and parotid salivary gland), mononuclear cell infiltration, collagen deposition, and mortality. In this model, inflammatory signals lead to activation of donor and host APC, recruiting CD4 T cells, which in turn produce TGF-β and IL-13. These signals drive fibroblast collagen synthesis and resultant fibrosis.[149] Activating anti-PDGFR antibodies have been detected in cutaneous sclerosis of chronic GVHD, and agents such as imatinib with activity against PDGFR have demonstrated activity in this condition.[150] In contrast to initial reports, a randomized trial comparing imatinib and rituximab achieved disappointingly low significant clinical response rates in patients with cutaneous sclerosis.[151] Based on evidence supporting the role of donor macrophages in chronic GVHD pathogenesis, CSF-1R targeting with the monoclonal antibody axatilimab has demonstrated promise in clinical investigation.

Diagnosis of Chronic Graft-vs-Host Disease

The syndrome of chronic GVHD is characterized by diverse manifestations, and formal NIH diagnosis and staging criteria have been developed.[152] The most commonly occurring manifestations arise in the skin, eyes, mouth, and liver. Common skin manifestations include pigmentation changes, lichen planus-like changes, poikiloderma, as well as more advanced cutaneous and subcutaneous sclerosis. Cutaneous erythema is a manifestation shared by acute GVHD and overlap subtype of chronic GVHD (when present together with other diagnostic findings of chronic GVHD). Oral findings include lichen planus-like changes, hyperkeratotic plaques, or decreased oral range of motion. Patients can suffer from oral and ocular sicca symptoms, including dry mouth and dry or gritty eyes. Hepatic involvement with chronic GVHD results in a cholestatic pattern of elevated alkaline phosphatase and bilirubin. In the GI tract, diagnostic chronic GVHD features include esophageal web, stricture, or concentric rings on endoscopic or radiographic study. Other manifestations such as anorexia, nausea/vomiting, and diarrhea are shared between acute and overlap subtype of chronic GVHD. Bronchiolitis obliterans represents a diagnostic manifestation of chronic GVHD and is characterized by clinical symptoms and respiratory physiologic abnormalities (forced expiratory volume in 1 second [FEV1]/forced vital capacity ratio <0.7, FEV1 <75% predicted value with ≥10% decline over less than 2 years, presence of another chronic GVHD manifestation, absence of infectious etiology, and supporting features of bronchiolitis obliterans syndrome (BOS)—air trapping, small airway thickening, or bronchiectasis by chest CT, or evidence of air trapping by pulmonary function test with residual volume >120% predicted value). Tissue biopsy is not required for BOS diagnosis. Biomarkers associated with chronic GVHD diagnosis have been identified and some verified in independent populations, yet none have been fully developed for clinical use.[153] Future research efforts have also been proposed for earlier diagnosis, acknowledging that patients at full diagnosis may already have significant morbidity and organ damage.[154]

In a prospective national Chronic GVHD Consortium study, 911 patients were enrolled and followed for the development of late post-HCT immune-mediated disorders (*Table 107.3*). Chronic GVHD overall was observed in 47% of patients by 2 years post-HCT with a median time to onset of 7.4 months. Specific chronic GVHD subtypes were also studied: Bronchiolitis obliterans at 2 years was 3% (median onset of 12.2 months), and cutaneous sclerosis occurred in 8% (median onset 14 months). Late acute GVHD occurred in 10% at a median of 5.5 months.[155] Accurate recognition and management of the syndrome is important, as it is a major source of late HCT-related morbidity and mortality,[156,157] an important determinant of overall health, functional ability, and quality of life,[158-160] as well as prolonged immune suppressive therapy after HCT.[161-163]

Table 107.3. Current Estimates of Late Immune-Mediated Disorders After Allogeneic Hematopoietic Cell Transplantation

Syndrome	N	2yr CI % (95% CI)	Median Time to Onset (months)	NRM at 2 y after Onset (95% CI)
Late acute GVHD	92	10 (8-12)	5.5 (0.9-24)	23 (15-35)
Chronic GVHD	428	47 (44-51)	7.4 (0.8-45.1)	12 (9-16)
BOS	30	3 (2-5)	12.2 (2.8-24.3)	32 (18-57)
Cutaneous sclerosis	68	8 (6-10)	14.0 (4-36.9)	20 (10-39)

Abbreviation: NRM, nonrelapse mortality.
Adapted from Arora M, Cutler CS, Jagasia MH, et al. Late acute and chronic graft-versus-host disease after allogeneic hematopoietic cell transplantation. *Biol Blood Marrow Transplant.* 2016;22(3):449-455. Copyright © 2016 American Society for Blood and Marrow Transplantation. With permission.

Classification and Severity Grading

The NIH Chronic GVHD Consensus Conference has made major changes in the classification and severity grading of the syndrome.[152] The new guidelines define chronic GVHD according to the diagnostic manifestations of the syndrome, rather than the time of onset following HCT. Manifestations of acute GVHD occurring before day 100 are defined as acute GVHD, and sole acute GVHD manifestations occurring after day 100 are considered persistent, recurrent, or late acute GVHD based on the prior occurrence of acute GVHD. The clinical features of late acute GVHD have been described.[164] Classic chronic GVHD is defined based on diagnostic manifestations of the syndrome in the absence of concurrent acute GVHD. The concurrent presentation of both chronic GVHD and acute GVHD manifestations defines the overlap subtype of chronic GVHD. Prospective data from the chronic GVHD Consortium demonstrate that patients with overlap have greater symptom burden, worse quality of life, impaired function, and inferior survival compared to classic chronic GVHD.[165]

Consensus guidelines for chronic GVHD severity grading were proposed to replace the previously accepted scheme based on limited vs extensive involvement. Chronic GVHD severity according to the NIH Chronic GVHD Consensus is scored according to objective criteria for each organ involved, with attention to the functional implications of the degree of involvement.[166] Individual organ scores are then utilized to formulate an overall global severity score of mild, moderate, or severe. A global severity score of mild encompasses no more than 2 organs, with severity of 1 each; moderate global severity indicates any organ site with a score of 2 (or lung score of 1), or involvement of 3 or more organ sites; finally, the severe category results from either any individual organ site score of 3, or a lung score of 2. The NIH Consensus severity criteria are prognostic: global severity scores are associated with nonrelapse mortality and survival; 2-year overall survival was 62% (severe), 86% (moderate), and 97% (mild).[167]

Risk Factors for Chronic GVHD Development

Clinical and laboratory predictors for the development of chronic GVHD may facilitate identification of patients at risk and could provide a rationale for risk-adapted strategies for prevention,[168] as well as preemptive therapy of the syndrome.[169] The most consistently reported risk factors for development of chronic GVHD have included increasing age of the donor or recipient, donor/recipient *HLA* disparity, donor relation, male recipients of allografts from female donors, prior occurrence of acute GVHD, and the use of peripheral blood mobilized stem cells vs bone marrow.[166,170,171]

Prognostic Variables

Previously reported prognostic variables include extensive vs limited involvement, progressive onset of chronic GVHD from acute GVHD, platelet count less than 100,000/μL at chronic GVHD diagnosis, impaired performance status, and failure to respond to therapy.[172-174] In a large CIBMTR analysis, investigators developed a chronic GVHD risk score in a sample of 5343 chronic GVHD patients. By multivariate analysis, 10 variables were significantly associated with overall survival and nonrelapse mortality: age, prior acute GVHD, time from transplantation to chronic GVHD, donor type, disease status at

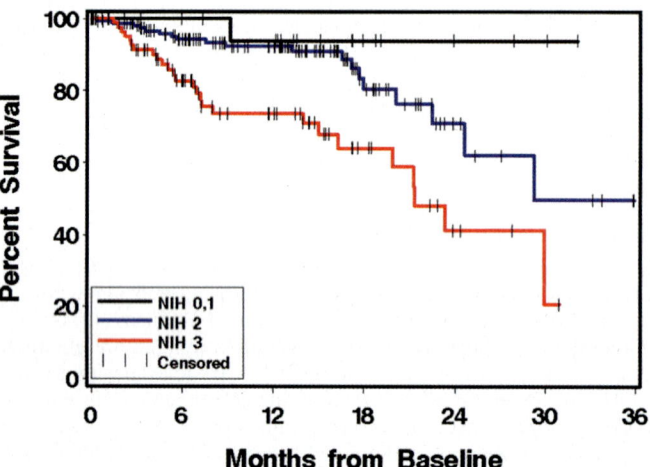

FIGURE 107.1 Survival outcomes per NIH chronic GVHD overall severity. (Adapted from Arai S, Jagasia M, Storer B, et al. Global and organ-specific chronic graft-versus-host disease severity according to the 2005 NIH consensus criteria. *Blood.* 2011;118(15):4242-4249. Copyright © 2011 American Society of Hematology. With permission.)

transplantation, GVHD prophylaxis, gender mismatch, serum bilirubin, Karnofsky performance status, and platelet count. From these data, six risk groups were identified based on the number of risk factors present. Nonrelapse mortality at 5 years ranged from 5% in the lowest risk group to 72% in those with greatest risk. Similarly, 5-year overall survival ranged from 91% in the lowest risk group down to 4% in the greatest risk group ($P < .01$).[175] This risk score has been subsequently validated.[176] Analyses performed to date from the Chronic GVHD Consortium support both the NIH overall severity (*Figure 107.1*), and the overlap subtype of chronic GVHD as significant determinants of overall survival and nonrelapse mortality, yet question the impact of prior acute GVHD.[177]

Prevention of Chronic Graft-vs-Host Disease

Successive advances in pharmacologic prophylaxis strategies for acute GVHD prevention have led to more effective reduction in grade II-IV and grade III/IV acute GVHD. Randomized phase III trials in matched sibling and unrelated donor HCT supported the superiority of tacrolimus/methotrexate over cyclosporine/methotrexate for prevention of acute GVHD, but did not result in reduction of the incidence of chronic GVHD.[66,68] Similarly, single-center phase II trials examining the combination of sirolimus/tacrolimus,[72] as well as a comparative trial of MMF/tacrolimus vs methotrexate/tacrolimus,[67] suggest that alternative strategies beyond conventional pharmacologic prophylaxis are needed to effectively reduce the burden of chronic GVHD.

Given that chronic GVHD can occur during immune suppression taper or after discontinuation, investigators have explored the relationship between immune suppression duration post-HCT and chronic GVHD risk. Some reports indicated decreased risk with prolonged administration of cyclosporine; however, a prospective trial did not demonstrate benefit.[178] Other conflicting data exist, and the ideal duration of immune suppression after HCT is not known. More recent work has explored determinants of successful immune suppression discontinuation and suggests avenues for future research.[163]

Details of chronic GVHD etiology and prevention have been recently reviewed.[168] Among possible prevention strategies, currently available evidence suggests more potent chronic GVHD prevention can be achieved using ex vivo or in vivo T cell depletion approaches, as well as depletion of alloreactive T cells through post-HCT cyclophosphamide. However, these strategies carry increased risks including infectious complications,[179,180] and more work is needed to apply personalized prevention approaches based on inherent chronic GVHD risk.

Memorial Sloan Kettering Cancer Center published a phase II trial of ex vivo T-cell depletion employing CD34 enrichment by the Miltenyi device in unrelated donor transplants.[125] The median CD3+ cell dose was 1.52×10^3/kg. With no pharmacologic prophylaxis, the incidence of chronic GVHD was only 29%. With intense conditioning, the relapse incidence was low, 6% at 4 years, despite a largely advanced disease cohort. The BMT CTN 0303 trial confirmed the efficacy of this protocol in HLA-matched sibling donor transplantation for acute myeloid leukemia in first or second complete remission.[86] T-cell-depleted allografts contained a median CD3+ dose of 6.6×10^3/kg. Without pharmacologic prophylaxis, extensive chronic GVHD was 6.8% (0%-14.4%) at 24 months. With median follow-up of 34 months, the 36-month leukemia-free survival was 58%. These results demonstrate that subtotal depletion of donor T cells provides protection against chronic GVHD. A more recent BMT CTN 1301 trial, however, suggested that CD34+ selection had greater infectious complications and increased mortality compared to standard tacrolimus/methotrexate prophylaxis.[87]

In vivo strategies for T-cell depletion, including antilymphocyte antibodies such as ATG or alemtuzumab, have promise to reduce risk for chronic GVHD as well. Long-term follow-up from a randomized phase III trial comparing ATG-Fresenius vs placebo alongside cyclosporine/methotrexate standard prophylaxis demonstrated cumulative incidence of extensive chronic GVHD after 3 years of 12% in the ATG-Fresenius group vs 45% in the control group ($P < .0001$), with comparable incidence of primary disease relapse and nonrelapse mortality. The 3-year probability of survival free of immune suppression was 53% and 17% in the ATG-Fresenius vs control.[126] Additional randomized trials employing ATG have consistently demonstrated benefit in chronic GVHD prevention.[80-84,181]

Investigators from Johns Hopkins have pioneered GVHD prophylaxis with PTCy based on its selective activity against alloactivated donor T cells.[92] In a recent phase I/II Bayesian design trial ($n = 117$) including grafts from HLA-matched related or unrelated donors, T replete marrow was transplanted following myeloablative doses of busulfan and cyclophosphamide. With sole PTCy prophylaxis, chronic GVHD incidence was 10% with median follow-up of 26 months. These data suggest that targeting alloreactive donor T cells may reduce chronic GVHD risk and facilitate transplantation tolerance. Use of PTCy-based prophylaxis has become standard in related haploidentical HCT and is increasingly used after matched sibling or matched unrelated donor HCT. This approach appeared promising in the BMT CTN 1203 trial[95] and is currently being studied in a randomized phase III trial, the BMT CTN 1703 trial.

Finally, based on preclinical insights supporting the role of B cells in chronic GVHD pathogenesis, as well as activity of anti-CD20 therapy in steroid-refractory chronic GVHD, rituximab has been studied in chronic GVHD prevention,[148] and a trial of obinutuzumab as chronic GVHD prevention is underway.

Treatment of Chronic Graft-vs-Host Disease

Mild chronic GVHD may be amenable to topical therapies and not require systemic immune suppressive therapy. For example, ocular sicca may be managed with artificial tears, topical medications, or occluding lenses to retain moisture. As well, steroid rinses for oral lesions and sensitivity, and topical steroid agents for skin involvement or vaginal dryness may all confer benefit and minimize symptoms.

However, many patients will require systemic immune suppressive therapy due to either lack of control with topical agents, or NIH-defined moderate to severe chronic GVHD. In total, the diverse manifestations of the syndrome require a tailored approach.

For those patients requiring systemic therapy, the accepted standard primary therapy for chronic GVHD includes 1 mg/kg/d or greater of prednisone or equivalent with or without a CNI.[182,183] A randomized trial comparing prednisone vs prednisone plus cyclosporine for primary therapy of extensive chronic GVHD showed less prednisone side effects in the combination arm.[183] Based on the limited durable response rates observed with standard primary therapy, several trials have aimed to determine whether combined therapy (i.e., steroids + additional systemic immune suppressive agent) improves response. The addition of other systemic immune suppressive agents has not provided benefit, as evidenced by trials employing azathioprine, thalidomide, hydroxychloroquine, or MMF.[184-187]

The best current estimates of NIH-defined, partial or complete overall response arise from the BMT CTN 0801 trial,[188] which examined sirolimus with prednisone vs sirolimus/tacrolimus with prednisone as initial therapy for chronic GVHD. These two- and three-drug approaches both provided approximately 50% overall response rate by 6 months of therapy, and CR was infrequent at approximately 15%. The two-drug approach resulted in less renal toxicity and improved quality of life. To assess long-term outcomes after initial systemic therapy for chronic GVHD, investigators have utilized failure-free survival, a composite outcome measure including death, malignancy relapse, and requirement for additional lines of systemic immune suppressive therapy for chronic GVHD. In the BMT CTN 0801 trial, failure-free survival was 68% at 6 months, and 54% by 12 months. The largest contribution to treatment failure in this trial was requirement for additional lines of systemic immune suppressive treatment,[189] thus highlighting the inadequacy of standard first-line therapy. Major considerations and future directions for chronic GVHD therapy have been recently reviewed[190] and include emphasis on developing more effective therapy for highly morbid forms of chronic GVHD.[191]

Based on limited response to primary therapy, many patients will require additional immune-suppressive agents for chronic GVHD control. Steroid-refractory chronic GVHD management was recently reviewed comprehensively.[192] Multiple immune-suppressive agents, including MMF, sirolimus, pentostatin, tacrolimus, and thalidomide, monoclonal antibodies including rituximab, and strategies such as ECP have demonstrated moderate activity in this setting, both ameliorating objective chronic GVHD manifestations, as well as facilitating decrease in systemic steroid exposure. Their activity is incomplete, however, and many patients with steroid-refractory chronic GVHD require multiple agents to achieve disease control. Failure-free survival after secondary therapy for chronic GVHD is 56% at 6 months and 45% at 12 months. As is true for primary therapy, treatment change constitutes the major source of failure.[193] Major recent clinical trials have led to FDA approvals for ibrutinib,[194] ruxolitinib,[195] and belumosudil[196] for steroid-refractory chronic GVHD treatment. Multiple additional agents are currently being tested in clinical trials. Thus, the landscape of treatment options for advanced chronic GVHD continues to expand, yet future investigation is needed to determine which patients will benefit from which of these available agents.

Chronic GVHD is associated with requirement for prolonged immune suppressive therapy after HCT (*Figure 107.2*). Current estimates indicate that 32% of patients will have discontinued all systemic immune suppressive therapy by 5 years after chronic GVHD diagnosis, while 35% remain alive under continued immune suppressive therapy, and the remainder have died or suffered malignancy relapse.[162] These data recapitulate a previous similar analysis,[161] and complement a larger analysis focused on immune suppression discontinuation from time of HCT.[163]

Assessment of Therapeutic Response

The method for response determination in routine clinical practice, as well as historic clinical trials, has been that of clinician-determined response. This method relies on the clinician's integration of dynamic

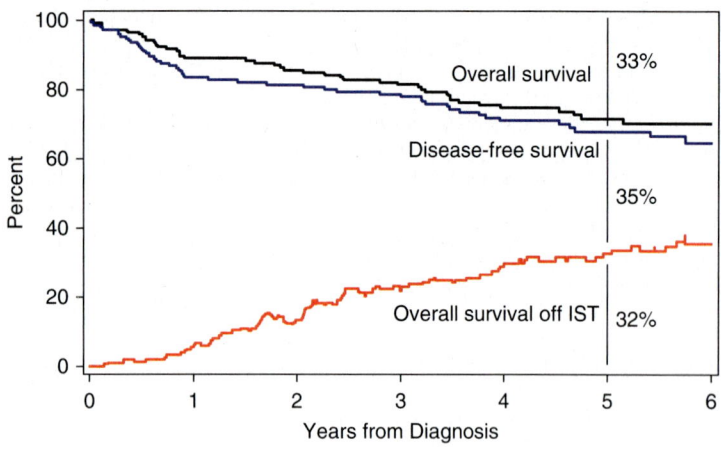

FIGURE 107.2 Discontinuation of immune suppression following chronic GVHD diagnosis. (Reprinted from Lee SJ, Nguyen TD, Onstad L, et al. Success of immunosuppressive treatments in patients with chronic graft-versus-host disease. *Biol Blood Marrow Transplant.* 2018;24(3):555-562. Copyright © 2017 American Society for Blood and Marrow Transplantation. With permission.)

chronic GVHD manifestations for a summary response categorization. CR indicates complete resolution of all chronic GVHD manifestations, PR signifies reduction in disease activity at response assessment compared to pretreatment levels but without complete resolution, stable disease indicates no response and no progression, and progressive disease indicates progressive chronic GVHD manifestations from baseline to response assessment. Limited agreement between clinician-assessed response and NIH response has been demonstrated,[197] and legitimate concerns exist regarding interrater reliability. However, clinician-assessed response at 6 months has been shown to associate with subsequent failure-free survival and overall survival.[198]

Formal objective response criteria for use in clinical trials have been developed through the NIH Consensus Conference for Chronic GVHD.[199,200] These response criteria are based on changes in NIH organ severity scores over time, and benefit from a structured objective response determination. These response criteria were originally proposed in 2005, and then were revised in 2014 based on evidence accumulated in the interim. Individual organ response criteria are described, and an overall response category is derived from these organ responses. Three major overall response categories are proposed for use in clinical trials, namely CR, PR, and lack of response (composite of unchanged, mixed response, and progression).[200] More recently designed chronic GVHD therapy trials have successfully employed these response criteria.

Supportive Care

Patients with chronic GVHD require careful supportive care and infectious prophylaxis. Prophylactic antimicrobials should be utilized to prevent *Pneumocystis jiroveci*, encapsulated bacterial infections such as *Streptococcus pneumoniae, Haemophilus influenzae*, and *Neisseria meningitides*, and *Varicella zoster*.[201] Systematic monitoring and preemptive therapy for *cytomegalovirus* reactivation are also important. The routine use of antifungal agents as prophylaxis beyond 75 days after transplantation has not been proven to be effective in preventing invasive fungal infections; however, many administer these agents for prophylaxis, particularly in those patients on prolonged courses of glucocorticoids. The use of intravenous immunoglobulin following HCT may be used for replacement therapy in those patients with hypogammaglobulinemia and recurrent infection. Other important components of supportive care include vaccination after transplantation, skin care, oral cavity health and symptom control, management of ocular sicca symptoms, supportive care for vulvovaginal manifestations of GVHD, physical therapy for musculoskeletal impairment, prevention and management of osteopenia and osteoporosis, management of fatigue, and psychosocial support. A comprehensive review of appropriate, evidence-based ancillary care has been published.[201]

Conclusion

Investigation into chronic GVHD pathogenesis, diagnosis and classification, and therapy offers promise for improved patient outcomes. Insights into chronic GVHD biology have provided novel strategies for prevention and therapy and will continue to advance the field. Validation of the proposed NIH Consensus diagnostic and severity classification criteria, as well as determination of best-response criteria, has moved the state of chronic GVHD clinical trials forward. Following the accomplishments of the 2005 and 2014 NIH Consensus meetings, investigators have articulated future directions for the field in 2020, with attention to early diagnosis and preemptive therapy, innovative treatment approaches, and management of highly morbid forms of chronic GVHD.[154,168,169,190,191]

GRAFT-VS-TUMOR RESPONSE

Evidence for Graft vs Tumor in Animals and Humans

Multiple lines of evidence point to a powerful immune response of donor immune cells against tumor cells after allogeneic HCT (*Table 107.4*). Initial proof of principle for an allogenic graft vs tumor effect (GVT)—or graft vs leukemia (GVL) effect—was established in rodents.[202,203] Single-center and registry studies found an inverse correlation between acute and chronic GVHD and relapse of malignancy after human marrow transplantation.[204,205] The probability of relapse was higher after twin compared to *HLA*-identical sibling transplants, pointing to disparate mHA as the target of the GVT effect. Similarly high was the probability of relapse after a T-depleted allogeneic transplant, pointing to mature donor T cells as GVT effectors. There was protection from relapse after a T-replete allogeneic HCT in patients without history of GVHD, indicating that GVHD is not required for the GVT effect. Lower relapse rates, however, were in patients who had experienced acute GVHD, and the lowest in those with chronic GVHD. As shown in *Figure 107.3*, the GVT effect in allogeneic recipients with GVHD did account for about half of the total antitumor activity of the transplant procedure, thus GVT was as effective as the high-dose chemoradiotherapy administered before the transplant. Allogeneic HCT after safer, low-intensity conditioning regimens is also associated with durable responses in some

Table 107.4. Evidence for a Graft-vs-Tumor Response

1. Allogeneic but not syngeneic marrow transplants can cure mice with leukemia.
2. Allogeneic marrow transplants are more effective than twin transplants in preventing leukemia relapse in humans.
3. Patients with graft-vs-host disease are more likely to be cured from leukemia than those without graft-vs-host disease.
4. Spontaneous remissions occur after stopping immune suppression in patients with relapsed malignancy after allogeneic marrow transplantation.
5. Donor lymphocyte infusions induce remission in patient with relapsed malignancy after allogeneic marrow transplantation.

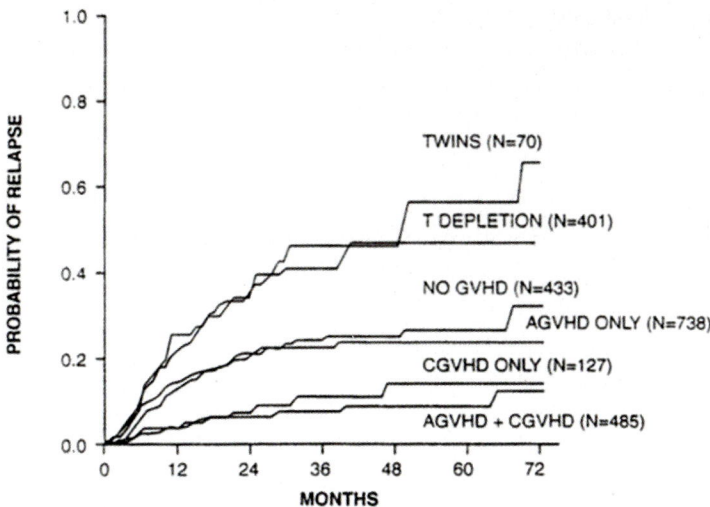

FIGURE 107.3 Actuarial probability of relapse after bone marrow transplantation for early leukemia according to type of graft and development of graft-vs-host disease (GVHD). AGVHD, acute GVHD; CGVHD, chronic GVHD. (Reprinted from Horowitz MM, Gale RP, Sondel PM, et al. Graft-versus-leukemia reactions after bone marrow transplantation. *Blood*. 1990;75(3):555-562. Copyright © 1990 American Society of Hematology. With permission.)

malignancies.[206] As immune-suppressive therapy to prevent or treat GVHD also affects GVT responses, spontaneous remissions have been observed after stopping immune suppression in a variety of hematologic malignancies that had relapsed after allogeneic HCT.[207] Direct evidence for a GVT effect was provided by infusion of donor lymphocytes for sole treatment of relapse after allogeneic HCT.[208] Response to donor lymphocyte infusions occurs after allogeneic transplants but not twin transplants, as disparate histocompatibility antigens are the GVT targets, and require stable donor engraftment, although it does not help patients who have rejected the graft. Donor lymphocytes are most effective in patients who have received a T-depleted graft, in those who have not already experienced GVHD, in chronic more than acute leukemia, and in patients with minimal tumor burden.[209]

T-Cell–Mediated Graft vs Tumor
Unmodified T Cells

Infusions of isolated CD4 or CD8 donor T cells for treatment of relapse have demonstrated that each of these cell types can mediate GVT.[210,211] The predominant GVT targets are mHA expressed in the recipient's malignant cells. As discussed under the "Acute Graft-versus-Host Disease" section, mHAs can be expressed ubiquitously (including, e.g., skin and leukemia) and are therefore targets for both GVHD and GVT (i.e., the H-Y associated male antigens), or their expression can be restricted to one or more hematopoietic lineages so they are targets for GVT but not GVHD (e.g., HA-1 and HA-2 antigens). Little is known about most mHAs, because diversity assessment of the human genome predicts over 10^7 polymorphisms that can function as mHAs in transplantation. A variety of genetic techniques have sped up the discovery of functional mHAs, and investigators hope to find a relatively small number of dominant mHAs that can be targeted for prevention of GVHD and exploitation of GVT.[212,213] Weaker immune targets are a variety of tumor-associated antigens that by themselves are not sufficiently immunogenic to elicit a protecting immune response, but in conjunction with the adjuvant effect of an allogeneic transplant can contribute to the GVT effect. These include the following: (1) tumor-specific antigens that result from the oncogenic mutations such as the Bcr/Abl tyrosine kinase in chronic myeloid leukemia, and the promyelocytic leukemia/retinoic acid receptor-α transcription factor in promyelocytic leukemia; (2) viral proteins, such as those from human papilloma virus in cervical cancer; (3) tissue-specific proteins, such as prostate-specific antigen in prostate cancer and proteinase-3 in myeloid leukemias; (4) germ-cell antigens, such as the melanoma-associated antigen family; (5) tumor-selective overexpressed self-proteins, such as WT1 in Wilms tumor or acute myeloid leukemia. Proteinase-3-derived PR1 peptide and WT1 are the best characterized tumor-associated antigens in patients after allogeneic HCT.[214,215] Initial attempts have been made to amplify tumor immunity after allogeneic HCT by vaccines.[216]

Future Approaches to Enhance T-Cell Immunity Against Tumors

Clinical strategies are needed to optimize immunological reconstitution after allogeneic HCT. Insulin-like growth factor 1, androgen blockade, and keratinocyte growth factor are candidates for clinical interventions to enhance thymopoiesis.[217,218] T cell progenitor subsets with enriched memory stem cell function may provide enhanced immune reconstitution upon adoptive transfer.[219,220] IL-7 and IL-15 have the potential for enhancing peripheral T-cell expansion in response to tumor antigens. Homeostatic peripheral expansion of adoptively transferred T-cells occurs after lymphodepletion and can be exploited to enhance proliferation of adoptively transferred T cells in response to tumor antigens.[221] IL-2 or IL-2 receptor blockade with neutralizing antibodies inhibit Tregs thereby providing the opportunity for relapse prevention.[222] Inhibition of negative checkpoint CTLA-4 and PD-1 are promising strategies to prevent or treat relapsed malignancy.[223,224]

Natural Killer Cell–Mediated Graft vs Tumor

As disparate HLA molecules are strong GVHD targets, one may expect that they would also be GVT targets for T cells. In contrast, most studies have failed to detect a GVT effect of *HLA* mismatch in T-replete transplants.[225,226] One hypothesis is that GVHD is so forceful after T-replete transplants from *HLA*-incompatible donors, that the required immune suppression may diminish any possible GVT. In contrast, a growing body of evidence supports the role of NK cell alloreactivity in GVL effects after transplant.

Several biological models suggest that alloreactive NK cells are responsible for favorable transplantation outcomes. Transfer of human alloreactive NK cells into immune-deficient mice eradicated human myeloid leukemia.[227] The basis for NK allorecognition resides primarily in a bi-allelic system of inhibitory killer-cell Ig-like receptors (*KIR*) that silence NK effector function after recognition of their cognate ligands encoded by *HLA-C* alleles.[228] KIR2DL1 recognizes HLA-C molecules characterized by a Lys80 residue (i.e., HLA-Cw4), and KIR2DL2 and KIR2DL3 recognize HLA-C with an Asn80 residue (i.e., HLA-Cw3). Also, KIR3DL1 is the receptor for HLA-B alleles that include a Bw4 domain and the CD94/NKG2A heterodimer (encoded by the *KLRD1/KLRC1* genes) is an inhibitory receptor for HLA-E. During development, HLA class I molecules select for a self-tolerant *KIR* repertoire so that every mature NK cell expresses at least one inhibitory receptor for self-HLA. NK cells that express a KIR for the class I group absent on allogeneic targets sense the missing expression of self-class I HLA and kill the allogenic target ("missing self" model). This was first demonstrated in HLA-incompatible related haploidentical donor transplants performed using potent T cell-depleting approaches (ex vivo T cell depletion, use of ATG). Here, NK-cell alloreactivity has been related to a reduced risk of leukemia relapse, no GVHD, and markedly improved survival in *HLA* disparate transplants.[227,229] For patients with acute myeloid leukemia in remission, the cumulative incidence of relapse was significantly lower after transplantation from NK alloreactive donors (3% vs 47%; $P < .003$), and this translated into an improved event-free survival (67% vs 18%; $P = .02$). For patients in relapse at the time of HCT, donor NK-cell alloreactivity was not protective. Based on these data, donor NK alloreactivity against recipient cells is a potential selection criterion for *HLA*-disparate donors when a T-depleted protocol is employed. In the present era, related haploidentical transplants commonly employ PTCy including those using unmanipulated T cell replete grafts. Use of PTCy may eliminate most mature donor NK cells infused, blunting effect of predicted NK alloreactivity.[230] Studies of KIR alloreactivity in the setting of umbilical cord blood transplantation have had mixed results.[231-234]

HLA matched transplants in contrast are KIR-ligand matched, thus NK alloreactivity should not be driven by missing-self activation. The alternative "missing ligand" model has been proposed to predict protection from relapse after HLA-matched transplants.[235] When KIR ligand-matched donors possess anergic NK cells with an "extra" KIR for which neither donor nor recipient has an HLA ligand, upon transfer into the recipient, those uneducated NK cells may regain competency and produce a GVT effect.[236] In support of this model, several large observational studies demonstrated that transplant recipients with acute myeloid leukemia missing one of the KIR ligands (HLA-C1, HLA-C2, HLA-Bw4) had reduced relapse risk after HLA-matched transplant.[235,237,238]

Specific focus on the inhibitory KIR, KIR3DL1, and Bw4 ligand interactions suggests possible donor selection strategies to reduce post-transplant relapse risk. KIR3DL1 subtypes have been characterized with varied cell surface expression and HLA-Bw4 binding affinity. In at least one large observational study, KIR3DL1-Bw4 interactions were associated with acute myelogenous leukemia (AML) relapse protection after transplant,[239] while not all studies support this conclusion.[240] HLA-A allotypes exhibiting the Bw4 epitope also have association with AML relapse posttransplant.[241]

Activating *KIR*s regulate both NK and T-cell functions. Unlike inhibitory *KIR*s, activating *KIR*s exhibit extensive population variation in gene number and content. Donor KIR haplotype groups vary (haplotype A vs B), where the KIR haplotype B group has greater possible activating KIR genes (KIR3DS1, KIR2DS1, KIR2DS2, KIR2DS3, KIR2DS4, KIR2DS5). Transplant from donors with B haplotypes may support an NK repertoire with lower threshold for activation, and more potent GVL, as supported by observational studies in AML.[242,243] KIR2DS1 in transplant donors protected from AML relapse after transplant, except in the setting of HLA-C2 homozygous donors.[244]

In total, observational studies have largely demonstrated beneficial reduction in AML relapse after transplant when KIR-advantageous donors are used, and prospective KIR typing for donor selection is feasible.[245] Several translational opportunities exist: Donor selection based on KIR/HLA genotype considerations is being tested in a prospective observational cohort study (NCT02450708), with potential promise to reduce relapse risk. As well, clinical trials testing benefit of NK cell therapy posttransplant are underway, with a phase I-II trial suggesting significant relapse protection.[246]

Conclusions

HCT from allogeneic donors provide powerful GVT effects, via innate and adaptive immunity. The most recent effects of these findings have been: (1) decreased reliance on the use of toxic conditioning regimens to control leukemia; (2) use of donor lymphocyte infusion for prevention or treatment of relapse; and (3) implementation of donor selection strategies leveraging KIR and HLA genotypes to potentially decrease AML relapse risk, as well as expanded NK cell adoptive therapy after transplant.

References

1. Billingham R. The biology of graft versus host reactions. *Harvey Lecture Series*. 1967;62:21-78. 1966-1967.
2. Ferrara JL, Levine JE, Reddy P, Holler E. Graft-versus-host disease. *Lancet*. 2009;373(9674):1550-1561.
3. Paczesny S, Hanauer D, Sun Y, Reddy P. New perspectives on the biology of acute GVHD. *Bone Marrow Transplant*. 2010;45(1):1-11.
4. Lee SJ, Klein J, Haagenson M, et al. High-resolution donor-recipient HLA matching contributes to the success of unrelated donor marrow transplantation. *Blood*. 2007;110(13):4576-4583.
5. Loiseau P, Busson M, Balere ML, et al. HLA Association with hematopoietic stem cell transplantation outcome: the number of mismatches at HLA-A, -B, -C, -DRB1, or -DQB1 is strongly associated with overall survival. *Biol Blood Marrow Transplant*. 2007;13(8):965-974.
6. Wang W, Meadows LR, den Haan JM, et al. Human H-Y: a male-specific histocompatibility antigen derived from the SMCY protein. *Science*. 1995;269(5230):1588-1590.
7. Goulmy E, Schipper R, Pool J, et al. Mismatches of minor histocompatibility antigens between HLA-identical donors and recipients and the development of graft-versus-host disease after bone marrow transplantation. *N Engl J Med*. 1996;334(5):281-285.
8. Goulmy E, Gratama JW, Blokland E, Zwaan FE, van Rood JJ. A minor transplantation antigen detected by MHC-restricted cytotoxic T lymphocytes during graft-versus-host disease. *Nature*. 1983;302(5904):159-161.
9. Marijt WA, Heemskerk MH, Kloosterboer FM, et al. Hematopoiesis-restricted minor histocompatibility antigens HA-1- or HA-2-specific T cells can induce complete remissions of relapsed leukemia. *Proc Natl Acad Sci U S A*. 2003;100(5):2742-2747.
10. Cooke KR, Hill GR, Crawford JM, et al. Tumor necrosis factor- alpha production to lipopolysaccharide stimulation by donor cells predicts the severity of experimental acute graft-versus-host disease. *J Clin Invest*. 1998;102(10):1882-1891.
11. Ferrara JL. Cytokine dysregulation as a mechanism of graft versus host disease. *Curr Opin Immunol*. 1993;5(5):794-799.
12. Jenq RR, Ubeda C, Taur Y, et al. Regulation of intestinal inflammation by microbiota following allogeneic bone marrow transplantation. *J Exp Med*. 2012;209(5):903-911.
13. Taur Y, Jenq RR, Perales MA, et al. The effects of intestinal tract bacterial diversity on mortality following allogeneic hematopoietic stem cell transplantation. *Blood*. 2014;124(7):1174-1182.
14. Jenq RR, Taur Y, Devlin SM, et al. Intestinal Blautia is associated with reduced death from graft-versus-host disease. *Biol Blood Marrow Transplant*. 2015;21(8):1373-1383.
15. Mathewson ND, Jenq R, Mathew AV, et al. Gut microbiome-derived metabolites modulate intestinal epithelial cell damage and mitigate graft-versus-host disease. *Nat Immunol*. 2016;17(5):505-513.
16. Hanash AM, Dudakov JA, Hua G, et al. Interleukin-22 protects intestinal stem cells from immune-mediated tissue damage and regulates sensitivity to graft versus host disease. *Immunity*. 2012;37(2):339-350.
17. Spits H, Cupedo T. Innate lymphoid cells: emerging insights in development, lineage relationships, and function. *Annu Rev Immunol*. 2012;30:647-675.
18. Lindemans CA, Calafiore M, Mertelsmann AM, et al. Interleukin-22 promotes intestinal-stem-cell-mediated epithelial regeneration. *Nature*. 2015;528(7583):560-564.
19. Ponce DM. A Phase 2 study of F-652, a novel tissue-targeted recombinant human interleukin-22 (IL-22) dimer, for the treatment of newly diagnosed acute GVHD of the lower GI tract. *Biol Blood Marrow Transplant*. 2020;26(suppl 3):S51-S52.
20. Edinger M, Hoffmann P, Ermann J, et al. CD4+CD25+ regulatory T cells preserve graft-versus-tumor activity while inhibiting graft-versus-host disease after bone marrow transplantation. *Nat Med*. 2003;9(9):1144-1150.
21. Koreth J, Matsuoka K, Kim HT, et al. Interleukin-2 and regulatory T cells in graft-versus-host disease. *N Engl J Med*. 2011;365(22):2055-2066.
22. Lee SJ, Zahrieh D, Agura E, et al. Effect of up-front daclizumab when combined with steroids for the treatment of acute graft-versus-host disease: results of a randomized trial. *Blood*. 2004;104(5):1559-1564.
23. Betts BC, Sagatys EM, Veerapathran A, et al. CD4+ T cell STAT3 phosphorylation precedes acute GVHD, and subsequent Th17 tissue invasion correlates with GVHD severity and therapeutic response. *J Leukoc Biol*. 2015;97(4):807-819.
24. Yu Y, Wang D, Liu C, et al. Prevention of GVHD while sparing GVL effect by targeting Th1 and Th17 transcription factor T-bet and RORγt in mice. *Blood*. 2011;118(18):5011-5020.
25. Castro-Malaspina H, Harris RE, Gajewski J, et al. Unrelated donor marrow transplantation for myelodysplastic syndromes: outcome analysis in 510 transplants facilitated by the National Marrow Donor Program. *Blood*. 2002;99(6):1943-1951.
26. Bensinger WI, Martin PJ, Storer B, et al. Transplantation of bone marrow as compared with peripheral-blood cells from HLA-identical relatives in patients with hematologic cancers. *N Engl J Med*. 2001;344(3):175-181.
27. Hahn T, McCarthy PL, Jr, Zhang MJ, et al. Risk factors for acute graft-versus-host disease after human leukocyte antigen-identical sibling transplants for adults with leukemia. *J Clin Oncol*. 2008;26(35):5728-5734.
28. Weisdorf D, Hakke R, Blazar B, et al. Risk factors for acute graft-versus-host disease in histocompatible donor bone marrow transplantation. *Transplantation*. 1991;51(6):1197-1203.
29. Morishima Y, Sasazuki T, Inoko H, et al. The clinical significance of human leukocyte antigen (HLA) allele compatibility in patients receiving a marrow transplant from serologically HLA-A, HLA-B, and HLA-DR matched unrelated donors. *Blood*. 2002;99(11):4200-4206.

30. Pidala J, Wang T, Haagenson M, et al. Amino acid substitution at peptide-binding pockets of HLA class I molecules increases risk of severe acute GVHD and mortality. *Blood.* 2013;122(22):3651-3658.
31. Pidala J, Lee SJ, Ahn KW, et al. Nonpermissive HLA-DPB1 mismatch increases mortality after myeloablative unrelated allogeneic hematopoietic cell transplantation. *Blood.* 2014;124(16):2596-2606.
32. Miklos DB, Kim HT, Zorn E, et al. Antibody response to DBY minor histocompatibility antigen is induced after allogeneic stem cell transplantation and in healthy female donors. *Blood.* 2004;103(1):353-359.
33. Randolph SSB, Gooley TA, Warren EH, Appelbaum FR, Riddell SR. Female donors contribute to a selective graft-versus-leukemia effect in male recipients of HLA-matched, related hematopoietic stem cell transplants. *Blood.* 2004;103(1):347-352.
34. Flowers ME, Pepe MS, Longton G, et al. Previous donor pregnancy as a risk factor for acute graft-versus-host disease in patients with aplastic anaemia treated by allogeneic marrow transplantation. *Br J Haematol.* 1990;74(4):492-496.
35. Kollman C, Spellman SR, Zhang MJ, et al. The effect of donor characteristics on survival after unrelated donor transplantation for hematologic malignancy. *Blood.* 2016;127(2):260-267.
36. Nash RA, Pepe MS, Storb R, et al. Acute graft-versus-host disease: analysis of risk factors after allogeneic marrow transplantation and prophylaxis with cyclosporine and methotrexate. *Blood.* 1992;80(7):1838-1845.
37. Laughlin MJ, Barker J, Bambach B, et al. Hematopoietic engraftment and survival in adult recipients of umbilical-cord blood from unrelated donors. *N Engl J Med.* 2001;344(24):1815-1822.
38. Rocha V, Labopin M, Sanz G, et al. Transplants of umbilical-cord blood or bone marrow from unrelated donors in adults with acute leukemia. *N Engl J Med.* 2004;351(22):2276-2285.
39. Clift RA, Buckner CD, Appelbaum FR, et al. Allogeneic marrow transplantation in patients with acute myeloid leukemia in first remission: a randomized trial of two irradiation regimens. *Blood.* 1990;76(9):1867-1871.
40. Aoudjhane M, Labopin M, Gorin NC, et al. Comparative outcome of reduced intensity and myeloablative conditioning regimen in HLA identical sibling allogeneic haematopoietic stem cell transplantation for patients older than 50 years of age with acute myeloblastic leukaemia: a retrospective survey from the Acute Leukemia Working Party (ALWP) of the European group for Blood and Marrow Transplantation (EBMT). *Leukemia.* 2005;19(12):2304-2312.
41. Perez-Simon JA, Diez-Campelo M, Martino R, et al. Influence of the intensity of the conditioning regimen on the characteristics of acute and chronic graft-versus-host disease after allogeneic transplantation. *Br J Haematol.* 2005;130(3):394-403.
42. Hill GR, Crawford JM, Cooke KR, Brinson YS, Pan L, Ferrara JL. Total body irradiation and acute graft-versus-host disease: the role of gastrointestinal damage and inflammatory cytokines. *Blood.* 1997;90(8):3204-3213.
43. Hill RS, Petersen FB, Storb R, et al. Mixed hematologic chimerism after allogeneic marrow transplantation for severe aplastic anemia is associated with a higher risk of graft rejection and a lessened incidence of acute graft-versus-host disease. *Blood.* 1986;67(3):811-816.
44. Petz LD, Yam P, Wallace RB, et al. Mixed hematopoietic chimerism following bone marrow transplantation for hematologic malignancies. *Blood.* 1987;70(5):1331-1337.
45. Baron F, Maris MB, Storer BE, et al. High doses of transplanted CD34+ cells are associated with rapid T-cell engraftment and lessened risk of graft rejection, but not more graft-versus-host disease after nonmyeloablative conditioning and unrelated hematopoietic cell transplantation. *Leukemia.* 2005;19(5):822-828.
46. Bittencourt H, Rocha V, Chevret S, et al. Association of CD34 cell dose with hematopoietic recovery, infections, and other outcomes after HLA-identical sibling bone marrow transplantation. *Blood.* 2002;99(8):2726-2733.
47. Ringden O, Barrett AJ, Zhang MJ, et al. Decreased treatment failure in recipients of HLA-identical bone marrow or peripheral blood stem cell transplants with high CD34 cell doses. *Br J Haematol.* 2003;121(6):874-885.
48. Przepiorka D, Smith TL, Folloder J, et al. Risk factors for acute graft-versus-host disease after allogeneic blood stem cell transplantation. *Blood.* 1999;94(4):1465-1470.
49. Chien JW, Zhang XC, Fan W, et al. Evaluation of published single nucleotide polymorphisms associated with acute GVHD. *Blood.* 2012;119(22):5311-5319.
50. Powles RL, Morgenstern GR, Kay HE, et al. Mismatched family donors for bone-marrow transplantation as treatment for acute leukaemia. *Lancet.* 1983;1(8325):612-615.
51. Saliba RM, de Lima M, Giralt S, et al. Hyperacute GVHD: risk factors, outcomes, and clinical implications. *Blood.* 2007;109(7):2751-2758.
52. Sullivan KM, Deeg HJ, Sanders J, et al. Hyperacute graft-v-host disease in patients not given immunosuppression after allogeneic marrow transplantation. *Blood.* 1986;67(4):1172-1175.
53. Antin JH, Bierer BE, Smith BR, et al. Selective depletion of bone marrow T lymphocytes with anti-CD5 monoclonal antibodies: effective prophylaxis for graft-versus-host disease in patients with hematologic malignancies. *Blood.* 1991;78(8):2139-2149.
54. Filipovich AH, Weisdorf D, Pavletic S, et al. National Institutes of Health consensus development project on criteria for clinical trials in chronic graft-versus-host disease: I. Diagnosis and staging working group report. *Biol Blood Marrow Transplant.* 2005;11(12):945-956.
55. Przepiorka D, Weisdorf D, Martin P, et al. 1994 consensus conference on acute GVHD grading. *Bone Marrow Transplant.* 1995;15(6):825-828.
56. Harris AC, Young R, Devine S, et al. International, multicenter standardization of acute graft-versus-host disease clinical data collection: a report from the Mount Sinai acute GVHD International consortium. *Biol Blood Marrow Transplant.* 2016;22(1):4-10.
57. Shulman HM, Sharma P, Amos D, Fenster LF, McDonald GB. A coded histologic study of hepatic graft-versus-host disease after human bone marrow transplantation. *Hepatology.* 1988;8(3):463-470.
58. Shulman HM, Fisher LB, Schoch HG, Henne KW, McDonald GB. Veno-occlusive disease of the liver after marrow transplantation: histological correlates of clinical signs and symptoms. *Hepatology.* 1994;19(5):1171-1181.
59. Ponec RJ, Hackman RC, McDonald GB. Endoscopic and histologic diagnosis of intestinal graft-versus-host disease after marrow transplantation. *Gastrointest Endosc.* 1999;49(5):612-621.
60. Kalantari BN, Mortele KJ, Cantisani V, et al. CT features with pathologic correlation of acute gastrointestinal graft-versus-host disease after bone marrow transplantation in adults. *AJR Am J Roentgenol.* 2003;181(6):1621-1625.
61. Wanko SO, Broadwater G, Folz RJ, Chao NJ. Diffuse alveolar hemorrhage: retrospective review of clinical outcome in allogeneic transplant recipients treated with aminocaproic acid. *Biol Blood Marrow Transplant.* 2006;12(9):949-953.
62. Freudenberger TD, Madtes DK, Curtis JR, Cummings P, Storer BE, Hackman RC. Association between acute and chronic graft-versus-host disease and bronchiolitis obliterans organizing pneumonia in recipients of hematopoietic stem cell transplants. *Blood.* 2003;102(10):3822-3828.
63. Hartrampf S, Dudakov JA, Johnson LK, et al. The central nervous system is a target of acute graft versus host disease in mice. *Blood.* 2013;121(10):1906-1910.
64. Kaliyaperumal S, Watkins B, Sharma P, et al. CD8-predominant T-cell CNS infiltration accompanies GVHD in primates and is improved with immunoprophylaxis. *Blood.* 2014;123(12):1967-1969.
65. Bolwell B, Sobecks R, Pohlman B, et al. A prospective randomized trial comparing cyclosporine and short course methotrexate with cyclosporine and mycophenolate mofetil for GVHD prophylaxis in myeloablative allogeneic bone marrow transplantation. *Bone Marrow Transplant.* 2004;34(7):621-625.
66. Nash RA, Antin JH, Karanes C, et al. Phase 3 study comparing methotrexate and tacrolimus with methotrexate and cyclosporine for prophylaxis of acute graft-versus-host disease after marrow transplantation from unrelated donors. *Blood.* 2000;96(6):2062-2068.
67. Perkins J, Field T, Kim J, et al. A randomized phase II trial comparing tacrolimus and mycophenolate mofetil to tacrolimus and methotrexate for acute graft-versus-host disease prophylaxis. *Biol Blood Marrow Transplant.* 2010;16(7):937-947.
68. Ratanatharathorn V, Nash RA, Przepiorka D, et al. Phase III study comparing methotrexate and tacrolimus (prograf, FK506) with methotrexate and cyclosporine for graft-versus-host disease prophylaxis after HLA-identical sibling bone marrow transplantation. *Blood.* 1998;92(7):2303-2314.
69. Storb R, Deeg HJ, Farewell V, et al. Marrow transplantation for severe aplastic anemia: methotrexate alone compared with a combination of methotrexate and cyclosporine for prevention of acute graft-versus-host disease. *Blood.* 1986;68(1):119-125.
70. Storb R, Deeg HJ, Whitehead J, et al. Methotrexate and cyclosporine compared with cyclosporine alone for prophylaxis of acute graft versus host disease after marrow transplantation for leukemia. *N Engl J Med.* 1986;314(12):729-735.
71. Koreth J, Stevenson KE, Kim HT, et al. Bortezomib, tacrolimus, and methotrexate for prophylaxis of graft-versus-host disease after reduced-intensity conditioning allogeneic stem cell transplantation from HLA-mismatched unrelated donors. *Blood.* 2009;114(18):3956-3959.
72. Pidala J, Kim J, Jim H, et al. A randomized phase II study to evaluate tacrolimus in combination with sirolimus or methotrexate after allogeneic hematopoietic cell transplantation. *Haematologica.* 2012;97(12):1882-1889.
73. Eapen M, Logan BR, Horowitz MM, et al. Bone marrow or peripheral blood for reduced-intensity conditioning unrelated donor transplantation. *J Clin Oncol.* 2015;33(4):364-369.
74. Hamilton BK, Liu Y, Hemmer MT, et al. Inferior outcomes with cyclosporine and mycophenolate mofetil after myeloablative allogeneic hematopoietic cell transplantation. *Biol Blood Marrow Transplant.* 2019;25(9):1744-1755.
75. Cutler C, Stevenson K, Kim HT, et al. Sirolimus is associated with veno-occlusive disease of the liver after myeloablative allogeneic stem cell transplantation. *Blood.* 2008;112(12):4425-4431.
76. Antin JH, Kim HT, Cutler C, et al. Sirolimus, tacrolimus, and low-dose methotrexate for graft-versus-host disease prophylaxis in mismatched related donor or unrelated donor transplantation. *Blood.* 2003;102(5):1601-1605.
77. Cutler C, Logan B, Nakamura R, et al. Tacrolimus/sirolimus vs tacrolimus/methotrexate as GVHD prophylaxis after matched, related donor allogeneic HCT. *Blood.* 2014;124(8):1372-1377.
78. Watkins B, Qayed M, McCracken C, et al. Phase II trial of costimulation blockade with abatacept for prevention of acute GVHD. *J Clin Oncol.* 2021;39(17):1865-1877.
79. Koura DT, Horan JT, Langston AA, et al. In vivo T cell costimulation blockade with abatacept for acute graft-versus-host disease prevention: a first-in-disease trial. *Biol Blood Marrow Transplant.* 2013;19(11):1638-1649.
80. Chang YJ, Wu DP, Lai YR, et al. Antithymocyte globulin for matched sibling donor transplantation in patients with hematologic malignancies: a multicenter, open-label, randomized controlled study. *J Clin Oncol.* 2020;38(29):3367-3376.
81. Walker I, Panzarella T, Couban S, et al; Canadian Blood and Marrow Transplant Group. Pretreatment with anti-thymocyte globulin versus no anti-thymocyte globulin in patients with haematological malignancies undergoing haemopoietic cell transplantation from unrelated donors: a randomised, controlled, open-label, phase 3, multicentre trial. *Lancet Oncol.* 2016;17(2):164-173.
82. Soiffer RJ, Kim HT, McGuirk J, et al. Prospective, randomized, double-blind, phase III clinical trial of anti-T-lymphocyte globulin to assess impact on chronic graft-versus-host disease-free survival in patients undergoing HLA-matched unrelated myeloablative hematopoietic cell transplantation. *J Clin Oncol.* 2017;35(36):4003-4011.

83. Finke J, Bethge WA, Schmoor C, et al. Standard graft-versus-host disease prophylaxis with or without anti-T-cell globulin in haematopoietic cell transplantation from matched unrelated donors: a randomised, open-label, multicentre phase 3 trial. *Lancet Oncol.* 2009;10(9):855-864.
84. Kroger N, Solano C, Wolschke C, et al. Antilymphocyte globulin for prevention of chronic graft-versus-host disease. *N Engl J Med.* 2016;374(1):43-53.
85. Barba P, Hilden P, Devlin SM, et al. Ex vivo CD34(+)-selected T cell-depleted peripheral blood stem cell grafts for allogeneic hematopoietic stem cell transplantation in acute leukemia and myelodysplastic syndrome is associated with low incidence of acute and chronic graft-versus-host disease and high treatment response. *Biol Blood Marrow Transplant.* 2017;23(3):452-458.
86. Devine SM, Carter S, Soiffer RJ, et al. Low risk of chronic graft-versus-host disease and relapse associated with T cell-depleted peripheral blood stem cell transplantation for acute myelogenous leukemia in first remission: results of the blood and marrow transplant clinical trials network protocol 0303. *Biol Blood Marrow Transplant.* 2011;17(9):1343-1351.
87. Luznik L, Pasquini MC, Logan B, et al. Randomized phase III BMT CTN trial of calcineurin inhibitor-free chronic graft-versus-host disease interventions in myeloablative hematopoietic cell transplantation for hematologic malignancies. *J Clin Oncol.* 2022;40(4):356-368. JCO2102293.
88. Ganguly S, Ross DB, Panoskaltsis-Mortari A, et al. Donor CD4+ Foxp3+ regulatory T cells are necessary for posttransplantation cyclophosphamide-mediated protection against GVHD in mice. *Blood.* 2014;124(13):2131-2141.
89. Kanakry CG, Ganguly S, Zahurak M, et al. Aldehyde dehydrogenase expression drives human regulatory T cell resistance to posttransplantation cyclophosphamide. *Sci Transl Med.* 2013;5(211):211ra157.
90. Kanakry CG, Bolanos-Meade J, Kasamon YL, et al. Low immunosuppressive burden after HLA-matched related or unrelated BMT using posttransplantation cyclophosphamide. *Blood.* 2017;129(10):1389-1393.
91. Kanakry CG, O'Donnell PV, Furlong T, et al. Multi-institutional study of posttransplantation cyclophosphamide as single-agent graft-versus-host disease prophylaxis after allogeneic bone marrow transplantation using myeloablative busulfan and fludarabine conditioning. *J Clin Oncol.* 2014;32(31):3497-3505.
92. Luznik L, Bolanos-Meade J, Zahurak M, et al. High-dose cyclophosphamide as single-agent, short-course prophylaxis of graft-versus-host disease. *Blood.* 2010;115(16):3224-3230.
93. Ciurea SO, Zhang MJ, Bacigalupo AA, et al. Haploidentical transplant with posttransplant cyclophosphamide vs matched unrelated donor transplant for acute myeloid leukemia. *Blood.* 2015;126(8):1033-1040.
94. Shaw BE, Jimenez-Jimenez AM, Burns LJ, et al. National marrow donor program-sponsored multicenter, phase II trial of HLA-mismatched unrelated donor bone marrow transplantation using post-transplant cyclophosphamide. *J Clin Oncol.* 2021;39(18):1971-1982.
95. Bolanos-Meade J, Reshef R, Fraser R, et al. Three prophylaxis regimens (tacrolimus, mycophenolate mofetil, and cyclophosphamide; tacrolimus, methotrexate, and bortezomib; or tacrolimus, methotrexate, and maraviroc) versus tacrolimus and methotrexate for prevention of graft-versus-host disease with haemopoietic cell transplantation with reduced-intensity conditioning: a randomised phase 2 trial with a non-randomised contemporaneous control group (BMT CTN 1203). *Lancet Haematol.* 2019;6(3):e132-e143.
96. Bleakley M, Heimfeld S, Loeb KR, et al. Outcomes of acute leukemia patients transplanted with naive T cell-depleted stem cell grafts. *J Clin Invest.* 2015;125(7):2677-2689.
97. Meyer EH, Laport G, Xie BJ, et al. Transplantation of donor grafts with defined ratio of conventional and regulatory T cells in HLA-matched recipients. *JCI Insight.* 2019;4(10):127244.
98. Pidala J, Walton K, Elmariah H, et al. Pacritinib combined with sirolimus and low-dose tacrolimus for GVHD prevention after allogeneic hematopoietic cell transplantation: preclinical and phase I trial results. *Clin Cancer Res.* 2021;27(10):2712-2722.
99. Pidala J, Beato F, Kim J, et al. In vivo IL-12/IL-23p40 neutralization blocks Th1/Th17 response after allogeneic hematopoietic cell transplantation. *Haematologica.* 2018;103(3):531-539.
100. Kennedy GA, Varelias A, Vuckovic S, et al. Addition of interleukin-6 inhibition with tocilizumab to standard graft-versus-host disease prophylaxis after allogeneic stem-cell transplantation: a phase 1/2 trial. *Lancet Oncol.* 2014;15(13):1451-1459.
101. Frairia C, Nicolosi M, Shapiro J, et al. Sole upfront therapy with beclomethasone and budesonide for upper gastrointestinal acute graft-versus-host disease. *Biol Blood Marrow Transplant.* 2020;26(7):1303-1311.
102. Martin PJ, Rizzo JD, Wingard JR, et al. First- and second-line systemic treatment of acute graft-versus-host disease: recommendations of the American Society of Blood and Marrow Transplantation. *Biol Blood Marrow Transplant.* 2012;18(8):1150-1163.
103. Levine JE, Logan B, Wu J, et al; Blood and Marrow Transplant Clinical Trials Network. Graft-versus-host disease treatment: predictors of survival. *Biol Blood Marrow Transplant.* 2010;16(12):1693-1699.
104. Mielcarek M, Storer BE, Boeckh M, et al. Initial therapy of acute graft-versus-host disease with low-dose prednisone does not compromise patient outcomes. *Blood.* 2009;113(13):2888-2894.
105. Alousi AM, Weisdorf DJ, Logan BR, et al; Blood and Marrow Transplant Clinical Trials Network. Etanercept, mycophenolate, denileukin, or pentostatin plus corticosteroids for acute graft-versus-host disease: a randomized phase 2 trial from the Blood and Marrow Transplant Clinical Trials Network. *Blood.* 2009;114(3):511-517.
106. Bolanos-Meade J, Logan BR, Alousi AM, et al. Phase 3 clinical trial of steroids/mycophenolate mofetil vs steroids/placebo as therapy for acute GVHD: BMT CTN 0802. *Blood.* 2014;124(22):3221-3227; quiz 3335. quiz 335.
107. MacMillan ML, Robin M, Harris AC, et al. A refined risk score for acute graft-versus-host disease that predicts response to initial therapy, survival, and transplant-related mortality. *Biol Blood Marrow Transplant.* 2015;21(4):761-767.
108. Levine JE, Braun TM, Harris AC, et al; Blood and Marrow Transplant Clinical Trials Network. A prognostic score for acute graft-versus-host disease based on biomarkers: a multicentre study. *Lancet Haematol.* 2015;2(1):e21-e29.
109. Hartwell MJ, Ozbek U, Holler E, et al. An early-biomarker algorithm predicts lethal graft-versus-host disease and survival. *JCI Insight.* 2018;3(16):124015.
110. Pidala J, Hamadani M, Dawson P, et al. Randomized multicenter trial of sirolimus vs prednisone as initial therapy for standard-risk acute GVHD: the BMT CTN 1501 trial. *Blood.* 2020;135(2):97-107.
111. Arai S, Margolis J, Zahurak M, Anders V, Vogelsang GB. Poor outcome in steroid-refractory graft-versus-host disease with antithymocyte globulin treatment. *Biol Blood Marrow Transplant.* 2002;8(3):155-160.
112. Couriel D, Saliba R, Hicks K, et al. Tumor necrosis factor-alpha blockade for the treatment of acute GVHD. *Blood.* 2004;104(3):649-654.
113. Pidala J, Kim J, Field T, et al. Infliximab for managing steroid-refractory acute graft-versus-host disease. *Biol Blood Marrow Transplant.* 2009;15(9):1116-1121.
114. Baudard M, Vincent A, Moreau P, Kergueris MF, Harousseau JL, Milpied N. Mycophenolate mofetil for the treatment of acute and chronic GVHD is effective and well tolerated but induces a high risk of infectious complications: a series of 21 BM or PBSC transplant patients. *Bone Marrow Transplant.* 2002;30(5):287-295.
115. Pidala J, Kim J, Perkins J, et al. Mycophenolate mofetil for the management of steroid-refractory acute graft vs host disease. *Bone Marrow Transplant.* 2010;45(5):919-924.
116. Hoda D, Pidala J, Salgado-Vila N, et al. Sirolimus for treatment of steroid-refractory acute graft-versus-host disease. *Bone Marrow Transplant.* 2010;45(8):1347-1351.
117. Ragon BK, Mehta RS, Gulbis AM, et al. Pentostatin therapy for steroid-refractory acute graft versus host disease: identifying those who may benefit. *Bone Marrow Transplant.* 2018;53(3):315-325.
118. Abu-Dalle I, Reljic T, Nishihori T, et al. Extracorporeal photopheresis in steroid-refractory acute or chronic graft-versus-host disease: results of a systematic review of prospective studies. *Biol Blood Marrow Transplant.* November 2014;20(11):1677-1686.
119. Zeiser R, von Bubnoff N, Butler J, et al; REACH2 Trial Group. Ruxolitinib for glucocorticoid-refractory acute graft-versus-host disease. *N Engl J Med.* 2020;382(19):1800-1810.
120. Ullmann AJ, Lipton JH, Vesole DH, et al. Posaconazole or fluconazole for prophylaxis in severe graft-versus-host disease. *N Engl J Med.* 2007;356(4):335-347.
121. Gooley TA, Chien JW, Pergam SA, et al. Reduced mortality after allogeneic hematopoietic-cell transplantation. *N Engl J Med.* 2010;363(22):2091-2101.
122. Khoury HJ, Wang T, Hemmer MT, et al. Improved survival after acute graft-versus-host disease diagnosis in the modern era. *Haematologica.* 2017;102(5):958-966.
123. Anasetti C, Logan BR, Lee SJ, et al. Peripheral-blood stem cells versus bone marrow from unrelated donors. *N Engl J Med.* 2012;367(16):1487-1496.
124. Stem Cell Trialists' Collaborative Group. Allogeneic peripheral blood stem-cell compared with bone marrow transplantation in the management of hematologic malignancies: an individual patient data meta-analysis of nine randomized trials. *J Clin Oncol.* 2005;23(22):5074-5087.
125. Jakubowski AA, Small TN, Kernan NA, et al. T cell-depleted unrelated donor stem cell transplantation provides favorable disease-free survival for adults with hematologic malignancies. *Biol Blood Marrow Transplant.* 2011;17(9):1335-1342.
126. Socie G, Schmoor C, Bethge WA, et al. Chronic graft-versus-host disease: long-term results from a randomized trial on graft-versus-host disease prophylaxis with or without anti-T-cell globulin ATG-Fresenius. *Blood.* 2011;117(23):6375-6382.
127. van Besien K, Kunavakkam R, Rondon G, et al. Fludarabine-melphalan conditioning for AML and MDS: alemtuzumab reduces acute and chronic GVHD without affecting long-term outcomes. *Biol Blood Marrow Transplant.* 2009;15(5):610-617.
128. Kanakry CG, Tsai HL, Bolanos-Meade J, et al. Single-agent GVHD prophylaxis with posttransplantation cyclophosphamide after myeloablative, HLA-matched BMT for AML, ALL, and MDS. *Blood.* 2014;124(25):3817-3827.
129. Bleakley M. Naive T-cell depletion in stem cell transplantation. *Blood Adv.* 2020;4(19):4980.
130. Forcade E, Paz K, Flynn R, et al. An activated Th17-prone T cell subset involved in chronic graft-versus-host disease sensitive to pharmacological inhibition. *JCI Insight.* 2017;2(12);2(12):e92111.
131. Koreth J, Kim HT, Jones KT, et al. Efficacy, durability, and response predictors of low-dose interleukin-2 therapy for chronic graft-versus-host disease. *Blood.* 2016;128(1):130-137.
132. Matsuoka KI, Kim HT, McDonough S, et al. Altered regulatory T cell homeostasis in patients with CD4+ lymphopenia following allogeneic hematopoietic stem cell transplantation. *J Clin Invest.* 2010;120(5):1479-1493.
133. Sakoda Y, Hashimoto D, Asakura S, et al. Donor-derived thymic-dependent T cells cause chronic graft-versus-host disease. *Blood.* 2007;109(4):1756-1764.
134. Blazar BR, Weisdorf DJ, Defor T, et al. Phase 1/2 randomized, placebo-control trial of palifermin to prevent graft-versus-host disease (GVHD) after allogeneic hematopoietic stem cell transplantation (HSCT). *Blood.* 2006;108(9):3216-3222.
135. Shimabukuro-Vornhagen A, Hallek MJ, Storb RF, von Bergwelt-Baildon MS. The role of B cells in the pathogenesis of graft-versus-host disease. *Blood.* 2009;114(24):4919-4927.
136. Lesley R, Xu Y, Kalled SL, et al. Reduced competitiveness of autoantigen-engaged B cells due to increased dependence on BAFF. *Immunity.* 2004;20(4):441-453.
137. Thien M, Phan TG, Gardam S, et al. Excess BAFF rescues self-reactive B cells from peripheral deletion and allows them to enter forbidden follicular and marginal zone niches. *Immunity.* 2004;20(6):785-798.

138. Miklos DB, Kim HT, Miller KH, et al. Antibody responses to H-Y minor histocompatibility antigens correlate with chronic graft-versus-host disease and disease remission. *Blood*. 2005;105(7):2973-2978.
139. Storek J, Ferrara S, Ku N, Giorgi JV, Champlin RE, Saxon A. B cell reconstitution after human bone marrow transplantation: recapitulation of ontogeny? *Bone Marrow Transplant*. 1993;12(4):387-398.
140. Sarantopoulos S, Stevenson KE, Kim HT, et al. Altered B-cell homeostasis and excess BAFF in human chronic graft-versus-host disease. *Blood*. 2009;113(16):3865-3874.
141. Allen JL, Tata PV, Fore MS, et al. Increased BCR responsiveness in B cells from patients with chronic GVHD. *Blood*. 2014;123(13):2108-2115.
142. Allen JL, Fore MS, Wooten J, et al. B cells from patients with chronic GVHD are activated and primed for survival via BAFF-mediated pathways. *Blood*. 2012;120(12):2529-2536.
143. Cutler C, Miklos D, Kim HT, et al. Rituximab for steroid-refractory chronic graft-versus-host disease. *Blood*. 2006;108(2):756-762.
144. Kharfan-Dabaja MA, Mhaskar AR, Djulbegovic B, Cutler C, Mohty M, Kumar A. Efficacy of rituximab in the setting of steroid-refractory chronic graft-versus-host disease: a systematic review and meta-analysis. *Biol Blood Marrow Transplant*. 2009;15(9):1005-1013.
145. Zaja F, Bacigalupo A, Patriarca F, et al; GITMO Gruppo Italiano Trapianto Midollo Osseo. Treatment of refractory chronic GVHD with rituximab: a GITMO study. *Bone Marrow Transplant*. 2007;40(3):273-277.
146. Lazaryan A, Lee SJ, Arora M, et al. Phase 2 multicenter trial of ofatumumab and prednisone as initial therapy of chronic graft-vs-host disease. *Blood Adv*. 2021;6(1):259-269.
147. Arai S, Sahaf B, Narasimhan B, et al. Prophylactic rituximab after allogeneic transplantation decreases B-cell alloimmunity with low chronic GVHD incidence. *Blood*. 2012;119(25):6145-6154.
148. Cutler C, Kim HT, Bindra B, et al. Rituximab prophylaxis prevents corticosteroid-requiring chronic GVHD after allogeneic peripheral blood stem cell transplantation: results of a phase 2 trial. *Blood*. 2013;122(8):1510-1517.
149. McCormick LL, Zhang Y, Tootell E, Gilliam AC. Anti-TGF-beta treatment prevents skin and lung fibrosis in murine sclerodermatous graft-versus-host disease: a model for human scleroderma. *J Immunol*. 1999;163(10):5693-5699.
150. Olivieri A, Locatelli F, Zecca M, et al. Imatinib for refractory chronic graft-versus-host disease with fibrotic features. *Blood*. 2009;114(3):709-718.
151. Arai S, Pidala J, Pusic I, et al. A randomized phase II crossover study of imatinib or rituximab for cutaneous sclerosis after hematopoietic cell transplantation. *Clin Cancer Res*. 2016;22(2):319-327.
152. Jagasia MH, Greinix HT, Arora M, et al. National institutes of health consensus development project on criteria for clinical trials in chronic graft-versus-host disease: I. The 2014 diagnosis and staging working group report. *Biol Blood Marrow Transplant*. 2015;21(3):389-401 e1.
153. Paczesny S, Hakim FT, Pidala J, et al. National institutes of health consensus development project on criteria for clinical trials in chronic graft-versus-host disease: III. The 2014 biomarker working group report. *Biol Blood Marrow Transplant*. 2015;21(5):780-792.
154. Kitko CL, Pidala J, Schoemans HM, et al. National institutes of health consensus development project on criteria for clinical trials in chronic graft-versus-host disease: IIa. The 2020 clinical implementation and early diagnosis working group report. *Transplant Cell Ther*. 2021;27(7):545-557.
155. Arora M, Cutler CS, Jagasia MH, et al. Late acute and chronic graft-versus-host disease after allogeneic hematopoietic cell transplantation. *Biol Blood Marrow Transplant*. 2016;22(3):449-455.
156. Lee SJ, Klein JP, Barrett AJ, et al. Severity of chronic graft-versus-host disease: association with treatment-related mortality and relapse. *Blood*. 2002;100(2):406-414.
157. Socie G, Stone JV, Wingard JR, et al. Long-term survival and late deaths after allogeneic bone marrow transplantation. Late effects working committee of the International bone marrow transplant registry. *N Engl J Med*. 1999;341(1):14-21.
158. Flowers MED, Parker PM, Johnston LJ, et al. Comparison of chronic graft-versus-host disease after transplantation of peripheral blood stem cells versus bone marrow in allogeneic recipients: long-term follow-up of a randomized trial. *Blood*. 2002;100(2):415-419.
159. Pidala J, Anasetti C, Jim H. Quality of life after allogeneic hematopoietic cell transplantation. *Blood*. 2009;114(1):7-19.
160. Pidala J, Kurland B, Chai X, et al. Patient-reported quality of life is associated with severity of chronic graft-versus-host disease as measured by NIH criteria: report on baseline data from the Chronic GVHD Consortium. *Blood*. 2011;117(17):4651-4657.
161. Stewart BL, Storer B, Storek J, et al. Duration of immunosuppressive treatment for chronic graft-versus-host disease. *Blood*. 2004;104(12):3501-3506.
162. Lee SJ, Nguyen TD, Onstad L, et al. Success of immunosuppressive treatments in patients with chronic graft-versus-host disease. *Biol Blood Marrow Transplant*. 2018;24(3):555-562.
163. Pidala J, Martens M, Anasetti C, et al. Factors associated with successful discontinuation of immune suppression after allogeneic hematopoietic cell transplantation. *JAMA Oncol*. 2020;6(1):e192974.
164. Holtan SG, Khera N, Levine JE, et al. Late acute graft-versus-host disease: a prospective analysis of clinical outcomes and circulating angiogenic factors. *Blood*. 2016;128(19):2350-2358.
165. Pidala J, Vogelsang G, Martin P, et al. Overlap subtype of chronic graft-versus-host disease is associated with an adverse prognosis, functional impairment, and inferior patient-reported outcomes: a Chronic Graft-versus-Host Disease Consortium study. *Haematologica*. 2012;97(3):451-458.
166. Atkinson K, Horowitz MM, Gale RP, et al. Risk factors for chronic graft-versus-host disease after HLA-identical sibling bone marrow transplantation. *Blood*. 1990;75(12):2459-2464.
167. Arai S, Jagasia M, Storer B, et al. Global and organ-specific chronic graft-versus-host disease severity according to the 2005 NIH Consensus Criteria. *Blood*. 2011;118(15):4242-4249.
168. Williams KM, Inamoto Y, Im A, et al. National institutes of health consensus development project on criteria for clinical trials in chronic graft-versus-host disease: I. The 2020 etiology and prevention working group report. *Transplant Cell Ther*. 2021;27(6):452-466.
169. Pidala J, Kitko C, Lee SJ, et al. National institutes of health consensus development project on criteria for clinical trials in chronic graft-versus-host disease: IIb. The 2020 preemptive therapy working group report. *Transplant Cell Ther*. 2021;27(8):632-641.
170. Ochs LA, Miller WJ, Filipovich AH, et al. Predictive factors for chronic graft-versus-host disease after histocompatible sibling donor bone marrow transplantation. *Bone Marrow Transplant*. 1994;13(4):455-460.
171. Przepiorka D, Anderlini P, Saliba R, et al. Chronic graft-versus-host disease after allogeneic blood stem cell transplantation. *Blood*. 2001;98(6):1695-1700.
172. Akpek G, Lee SJ, Flowers ME, et al. Performance of a new clinical grading system for chronic graft-versus-host disease: a multicenter study. *Blood*. 2003;102(3):802-809.
173. Arora M, Burns LJ, Davies SM, et al. Chronic graft-versus-host disease: a prospective cohort study. *Biol Blood Marrow Transplant*. 2003;9(1):38-45.
174. Pavletic SZ, Smith LM, Bishop MR, et al. Prognostic factors of chronic graft-versus-host disease after allogeneic blood stem-cell transplantation. *Am J Hematol*. 2005;78(4):265-274.
175. Arora M, Klein JP, Weisdorf DJ, et al. Chronic GVHD risk score: a center for International blood and marrow transplant research analysis. *Blood*. 2011;117(24):6714-6720.
176. Arora M, Hemmer MT, Ahn KW, et al. Center for International Blood and Marrow Transplant Research chronic graft-versus-host disease risk score predicts mortality in an independent validation cohort. *Biol Blood Marrow Transplant*. 2015;21(4):640-645.
177. Arora M, Pidala J, Cutler CS, et al. Impact of prior acute GVHD on chronic GVHD outcomes: a chronic graft versus host disease consortium study. *Leukemia*. 2013;27(5):1196-1201.
178. Kansu E, Gooley T, Flowers ME, et al. Administration of cyclosporine for 24 months compared with 6 months for prevention of chronic graft-versus-host disease: a prospective randomized clinical trial. *Blood*. 2001;98(13):3868-3870.
179. Goldsmith SR, Abid MB, Auletta JJ, et al. Posttransplant cyclophosphamide is associated with increased cytomegalovirus infection: a CIBMTR analysis. *Blood*. 2021;137(23):3291-3305.
180. Singh A, Dandoy CE, Chen M, et al. Post-transplantation cyclophosphamide is associated with an increase in non-cytomegalovirus herpesvirus infections in patients with acute leukemia and myelodysplastic syndrome. *Transplant Cell Ther*. 2021;28(1):48.e1-48.e10.
181. Walker I, Panzarella T, Couban S, et al; Cell Therapy Transplant Canada. Addition of anti-thymocyte globulin to standard graft-versus-host disease prophylaxis versus standard treatment alone in patients with haematological malignancies undergoing transplantation from unrelated donors: final analysis of a randomised, open-label, multicentre, phase 3 trial. *Lancet Haematol*. 2020;7(2):e100-e111.
182. Sullivan KM, Shulman HM, Storb R, et al. Chronic graft-versus-host disease in 52 patients: adverse natural course and successful treatment with combination immunosuppression. *Blood*. 1981;57(2):267-276.
183. Koc S, Leisenring W, Flowers MED, et al. Therapy for chronic graft-versus-host disease: a randomized trial comparing cyclosporine plus prednisone versus prednisone alone. *Blood*. 2002;100(1):48-51.
184. Arora M, Wagner JE, Davies SM, et al. Randomized clinical trial of thalidomide, cyclosporine, and prednisone versus cyclosporine and prednisone as initial therapy for chronic graft-versus-host disease. *Biol Blood Marrow Transplant*. 2001;7(5):265-273.
185. Gilman AL, Schultz KR, Goldman FD, et al. Randomized trial of hydroxychloroquine for newly diagnosed chronic graft-versus-host disease in children: a Children's Oncology Group study. *Biol Blood Marrow Transplant*. 2012;18(1):84-91.
186. Martin PJ, Storer BE, Rowley SD, et al. Evaluation of mycophenolate mofetil for initial treatment of chronic graft-versus-host disease. *Blood*. 2009;113(21):5074-5082.
187. Sullivan KM, Witherspoon RP, Storb R, et al. Prednisone and azathioprine compared with prednisone and placebo for treatment of chronic graft-v-host disease: prognostic influence of prolonged thrombocytopenia after allogeneic marrow transplantation. *Blood*. 1988;72(2):546-554.
188. Carpenter PA, Logan BR, Lee SJ, et al; BMT CTN. A phase II/III randomized, multicenter trial of prednisone/sirolimus versus prednisone/sirolimus/calcineurin inhibitor for the treatment of chronic graft-versus-host disease: BMT CTN 0801. *Haematologica*. 2018;103(11):1915-1924.
189. Inamoto Y, Flowers MED, Sandmaier BM, et al. Failure-free survival after initial systemic treatment of chronic graft-versus-host disease. *Blood*. 2014;124(8):1363-1371.
190. DeFilipp Z, Couriel DR, Lazaryan A, et al. National institutes of health consensus development project on criteria for clinical trials in chronic graft-versus-host disease: III. The 2020 treatment of chronic GVHD report. *Transplant Cell Ther*. 2021;27(9):729-737.
191. Wolff D, Radojcic V, Lafyatis R, et al. National institutes of health consensus development project on criteria for clinical trials in chronic graft-versus-host disease: IV. The 2020 highly morbid forms report. *Transplant Cell Ther*. 2021;27(10):817-835.

192. Sarantopoulos S, Cardones AR, Sullivan KM. How I treat refractory chronic graft-versus-host disease. *Blood.* 2019;133(11):1191-1200.
193. Inamoto Y, Storer BE, Lee SJ, et al. Failure-free survival after second-line systemic treatment of chronic graft-versus-host disease. *Blood.* 2013;121(12):2340-2346.
194. Miklos D, Cutler CS, Arora M, et al. Ibrutinib for chronic graft-versus-host disease after failure of prior therapy. *Blood.* 2017;130(21):2243-2250.
195. Zeiser R, Polverelli N, Ram R, et al; REACH3 Investigators. Ruxolitinib for glucocorticoid-refractory chronic graft-versus-host disease. *N Engl J Med.* 2021;385(3):228-238.
196. Cutler CS, Lee SJ, Arai S, et al. Belumosudil for chronic graft-versus-host disease after 2 or more prior lines of therapy: the ROCKstar Study. *Blood.* 2021;138(22):2278-2289.
197. Palmer JM, Lee SJ, Chai X, et al. Poor agreement between clinician response ratings and calculated response measures in patients with chronic graft-versus-host disease. *Biol Blood Marrow Transplant.* 2012;18(11):1649-1655.
198. Palmer J, Chai X, Pidala J, et al. Predictors of survival, nonrelapse mortality, and failure-free survival in patients treated for chronic graft-versus-host disease. *Blood.* 2016;127(1):160-166.
199. Pavletic SZ, Martin P, Lee SJ, et al; Response Criteria Working Group. Measuring therapeutic response in chronic graft-versus-host disease: national institutes of health consensus development project on criteria for clinical trials in chronic graft-versus-host disease—IV. Response criteria working group report. *Biol Blood Marrow Transplant.* 2006;12(3):252-266.
200. Lee SJ, Wolff D, Kitko C, et al. Measuring therapeutic response in chronic graft-versus-host disease. National Institutes of Health consensus development project on criteria for clinical trials in chronic graft-versus-host disease: IV. The 2014 Response Criteria Working Group report. *Biol Blood Marrow Transplant.* 2015;21(6):984-999.
201. Couriel D, Carpenter PA, Cutler C, et al. Ancillary therapy and supportive care of chronic graft-versus-host disease: national institutes of health consensus development project on criteria for clinical trials in chronic Graft-versus-host disease—V. Ancillary Therapy and Supportive Care Working Group Report. *Biol Blood Marrow Transplant.* 2006;12(4):375-396.
202. Barnes DW, Corp MJ, Loutit JF, Neal FE. Treatment of murine leukaemia with X rays and homologous bone marrow; preliminary communication. *Br Med J.* 1956;2(4993):626-627.
203. Barnes DW, Loutit JF. Treatment of murine leukaemia with x-rays and homologous bone marrow. II. *Br J Haematol.* 1957;3(3):241-252.
204. Horowitz MM, Gale RP, Sondel PM, et al. Graft-versus-leukemia reactions after bone marrow transplantation. *Blood.* 1990;75(3):555-562.
205. Weiden PL, Flournoy N, Thomas ED, et al. Antileukemic effect of graft-versus-host disease in human recipients of allogeneic-marrow grafts. *N Engl J Med.* 1979;300(19):1068-1073.
206. Sorror ML, Storer BE, Sandmaier BM, et al. Five-year follow-up of patients with advanced chronic lymphocytic leukemia treated with allogeneic hematopoietic cell transplantation after nonmyeloablative conditioning. *J Clin Oncol.* 2008;26(30):4912-4920.
207. Odom LF, August CS, Githens JH, et al. Remission of relapsed leukaemia during a graft-versus-host reaction. A "graft-versus-leukaemia reaction" in man? *Lancet.* 1978;2(8089):537-540.
208. Kolb HJ, Mittermuller J, Clemm C, et al. Donor leukocyte transfusions for treatment of recurrent chronic myelogenous leukemia in marrow transplant patients. *Blood.* 1990;76(12):2462-2465.
209. Kolb HJ. Graft-versus-leukemia effects of transplantation and donor lymphocytes. *Blood.* 2008;112(12):4371-4383.
210. Giralt S, Hester J, Huh Y, et al. CD8-depleted donor lymphocyte infusion as treatment for relapsed chronic myelogenous leukemia after allogeneic bone marrow transplantation. *Blood.* 1995;86(11):4337-4343.
211. Warren EH, Fujii N, Akatsuka Y, et al. Therapy of relapsed leukemia after allogeneic hematopoietic cell transplantation with T cells specific for minor histocompatibility antigens. *Blood.* 2010;115(19):3869-3878.
212. Bleakley M, Riddell SR. Molecules and mechanisms of the graft-versus-leukaemia effect. *Nat Rev Cancer.* 2004;4(5):371-380.
213. Ehx G, Larouche JD, Durette C, et al. Atypical acute myeloid leukemia-specific transcripts generate shared and immunogenic MHC class-I-associated epitopes. *Immunity.* 2021;54(4):737-752.e10.
214. Kohrt HE, Muller A, Baker J, et al. Donor immunization with WT1 peptide augments antileukemic activity after MHC-matched bone marrow transplantation. *Blood.* 2011;118(19):5319-5329.
215. Molldrem JJ, Lee PP, Wang C, et al. Evidence that specific T lymphocytes may participate in the elimination of chronic myelogenous leukemia. *Nat Med.* 2000;6(9):1018-1023.
216. Ho VT, Vanneman M, Kim H, et al. Biologic activity of irradiated, autologous, GM-CSF-secreting leukemia cell vaccines early after allogeneic stem cell transplantation. *Proc Natl Acad Sci U S A.* 2009;106(37):15825-15830.
217. Alpdogan O, Muriglan SJ, Kappel BJ, et al. Insulin-like growth factor-I enhances lymphoid and myeloid reconstitution after allogeneic bone marrow transplantation. *Transplantation.* 2003;75(12):1977-1983.
218. Kelly RM, Highfill SL, Panoskaltsis-Mortari A, et al. Keratinocyte growth factor and androgen blockade work in concert to protect against conditioning regimen-induced thymic epithelial damage and enhance T-cell reconstitution after murine bone marrow transplantation. *Blood.* 2008;111(12):5734-5744.
219. Gattinoni L, Klebanoff CA, Restifo NP. Paths to stemness: building the ultimate antitumour T cell. *Nat Rev Cancer.* 2012;12(10):671-684.
220. Zhang Y, Joe G, Hexner E, Zhu J, Emerson SG. Host-reactive CD8+ memory stem cells in graft-versus-host disease. *Nat Med.* 2005;11(12):1299-1305.
221. Greenberg PD, Cheever MA, Fefer A. Eradication of disseminated murine leukemia by chemoimmunotherapy with cyclophosphamide and adoptively transferred immune syngeneic Lyt-1+2- lymphocytes. *J Exp Med.* 1981;154(3):952-963.
222. Locke FL, Pidala J, Storer B, et al. CD25 blockade delays regulatory T cell reconstitution and does not prevent graft-versus-host disease after allogeneic hematopoietic cell transplantation. *Biol Blood Marrow Transplant.* 2017;23(3):405-411.
223. Bashey A, Medina B, Corringham S, et al. CTLA4 blockade with ipilimumab to treat relapse of malignancy after allogeneic hematopoietic cell transplantation. *Blood.* 2009;113(7):1581-1588.
224. Davids MS, Kim HT, Bachireddy P, et al; Leukemia and Lymphoma Society Blood Cancer Research Partnership. Ipilimumab for patients with relapse after allogeneic transplantation. *N Engl J Med.* 2016;375(2):143-153.
225. Anasetti C, Beatty PG, Storb R, et al. Effect of HLA incompatibility on graft-versus-host disease, relapse, and survival after marrow transplantation for patients with leukemia or lymphoma. *Hum Immunol.* 1990;29(2):79-91.
226. Szydlo R, Goldman JM, Klein JP, et al. Results of allogeneic bone marrow transplants for leukemia using donors other than HLA-identical siblings. *J Clin Oncol.* 1997;15(5):1767-1777.
227. Ruggeri L, Capanni M, Urbani E, et al. Effectiveness of donor natural killer cell alloreactivity in mismatched hematopoietic transplants. *Science.* 2002;295(5562):2097-2100.
228. Parham P, McQueen KL. Alloreactive killer cells: hindrance and help for haematopoietic transplants. *Nat Rev Immunol.* 2003;3(2):108-122.
229. Aversa F, Terenzi A, Tabilio A, et al. Full haplotype-mismatched hematopoietic stem-cell transplantation: a phase II study in patients with acute leukemia at high risk of relapse. *J Clin Oncol.* 2005;23(15):3447-3454.
230. Russo A, Oliveira G, Berglund S, et al. NK cell recovery after haploidentical HSCT with posttransplant cyclophosphamide: dynamics and clinical implications. *Blood.* 2018;131(2):247-262.
231. Brunstein CG, Wagner JE, Weisdorf DJ, et al. Negative effect of KIR alloreactivity in recipients of umbilical cord blood transplant depends on transplantation conditioning intensity. *Blood.* 2009;113(22):5628-5634.
232. Tanaka J, Morishima Y, Takahashi Y, et al. Effects of KIR ligand incompatibility on clinical outcomes of umbilical cord blood transplantation without ATG for acute leukemia in complete remission. *Blood Cancer J.* 2013;3:e164.
233. Rocha V, Ruggeri A, Spellman S, et al; Eurocord, Cord Blood Committee Cellular Therapy Immunobiology Working Party of the European Group for Blood and Marrow Transplantation, Netcord, and the Center for International Blood and Marrow Transplant Research. Killer cell immunoglobulin-like receptor-ligand matching and outcomes after unrelated cord blood transplantation in acute myeloid leukemia. *Biol Blood Marrow Transplant.* 2016;22(7):1284-1289.
234. Willemze R, Rodrigues CA, Labopin M, et al; Eurocord-Netcord and Acute Leukaemia Working Party of the EBMT. KIR-ligand incompatibility in the graft-versus-host direction improves outcomes after umbilical cord blood transplantation for acute leukemia. *Leukemia.* 2009;23(3):492-500.
235. Hsu KC, Keever-Taylor CA, Wilton A, et al. Improved outcome in HLA-identical sibling hematopoietic stem-cell transplantation for acute myelogenous leukemia predicted by KIR and HLA genotypes. *Blood.* 2005;105(12):4878-4884.
236. Yu J, Venstrom JM, Liu XR, et al. Breaking tolerance to self, circulating natural killer cells expressing inhibitory KIR for non-self HLA exhibit effector function after T cell-depleted allogeneic hematopoietic cell transplantation. *Blood.* 2009;113(16):3875-3884.
237. Hsu KC, Gooley T, Malkki M, et al; International Histocompatibility Working Group. KIR ligands and prediction of relapse after unrelated donor hematopoietic cell transplantation for hematologic malignancy. *Biol Blood Marrow Transplant.* 2006;12(8):828-836.
238. Miller JS, Cooley S, Parham P, et al. Missing KIR ligands are associated with less relapse and increased graft-versus-host disease (GVHD) following unrelated donor allogeneic HCT. *Blood.* 2007;109(11):5058-5061.
239. Boudreau JE, Giglio F, Gooley TA, et al. KIR3DL1/HLA-B subtypes govern acute myelogenous leukemia relapse after hematopoietic cell transplantation. *J Clin Oncol.* 2017;35(20):2268-2278.
240. Schetelig J, Baldauf H, Heidenreich F, et al. External validation of models for KIR2DS1/KIR3DL1-informed selection of hematopoietic cell donors fails. *Blood.* 2020;135(16):1386-1395.
241. van der Ploeg K, Le Luduec JB, Stevenson PA, et al. HLA-A alleles influencing NK cell function impact AML relapse following allogeneic hematopoietic cell transplantation. *Blood Adv.* 2020;4(19):4955-4964.
242. Cooley S, Trachtenberg E, Bergemann TL, et al. Donors with group B KIR haplotypes improve relapse-free survival after unrelated hematopoietic cell transplantation for acute myelogenous leukemia. *Blood.* 2009;113(3):726-732.
243. Cooley S, Weisdorf DJ, Guethlein LA, et al. Donor selection for natural killer cell receptor genes leads to superior survival after unrelated transplantation for acute myelogenous leukemia. *Blood.* 2010;116(14):2411-2419.
244. Venstrom JM, Pittari G, Gooley TA, et al. HLA-C-dependent prevention of leukemia relapse by donor activating KIR2DS1. *N Engl J Med.* 2012;367(9):805-816.
245. Shaffer BC, Le Luduec JB, Park S, et al. Prospective KIR genotype evaluation of hematopoietic cell donors is feasible with potential to benefit patients with AML. *Blood Adv.* 2021;5(7):2003-2011.
246. Ciurea SO, Kongtim P, Soebbing D, et al. Decrease post-transplant relapse using donor-derived expanded NK-cells. *Leukemia.* 2022;36(1):155-164.

Chapter 108 ■ Late Effects After Hematopoietic Cell Transplantation

PAUL A. CARPENTER

INTRODUCTION

Half a million hematopoietic cell transplantation (HCT) survivors are estimated by 2030 due to improvements in HLA typing and supportive care,[1] but among those surviving at 2 years without recurrence of their original disease indication for transplant, there is a 4- to 9-fold increased mortality rate for 5-year survivors relative to an age- and sex-matched general population.[2-5] This is attributed to an increased cumulative incidence (CI) of chronic health conditions; in one study 66% of survivors had at least one chronic health condition and the 10-year CI for severe/life-threatening conditions or death as result was 35% (95% confidence interval [C.I.], 32%-39%). Survivors were 3.5 times as likely as siblings to develop a severe/life-threatening condition, further amplified among survivors with chronic graft-vs-host disease (cGVHD).[6] A recent study reported late mortality after allo-HCT declined over the past 40 years but was not restored to rates comparable with the general US population. Decline in late mortality appeared limited to transplants performed in childhood or with marrow as a stem cell source, without meaningful declines for adults or those transplanted with peripheral blood stem cells.[7] Further efforts to mitigate chronic health conditions may be useful in this population.

All HCT late effects result from varying degrees of interaction between the negative influences of pretransplant exposures, posttransplant complications, and positive or negative influences of age, gender, genetics, and lifestyle (*Figure 108.1A*; *Table 108.1*). The graft-vs-host disease (GVHD) burden cannot be overemphasized given its potential for protean manifestations over several years, especially with morbid cGVHD forms that can include tissue sclerosis, joint contractures, bronchiolitis obliterans, and failure to thrive. Given that clinical immunological tolerance may take years rather than months,[41,42] toxicities arising from immunosuppressive therapies (ISTs) and medications used to treat side effects of ISTs can contribute to chronic health conditions per se, for example, hypertension, dyslipidemia, and chronic renal insufficiency to name a few.

Systematic long-term follow-up (LTFU) recognizes these complex interactions, but a major barrier to early detection and preventive efforts is premature LTFU termination that manifests with extended follow-up and is greatest for 15- to 29-year-olds, standard risk malignancy or nonmalignant underlying diseases, and those without cGVHD (*Figure 108.1B*).[43] LTFU termination was mainly physician directed when patients appeared in good medical condition. These observations, together with the fact that late effects often have 7- to 20-year latencies, mandate counter approaches and highlight a need for education of stakeholders to emphasize adherence to LTFU regardless of good clinical appearance.

There are few large-scale studies or randomized trials to guide LTFU recommendations. Those published are categorized by organ system or exposures and based on expert opinion or limited high-quality evidence. Some are relatively concise and HCT-focused but for any complication often lack granularity regarding pretransplant treatment exposures and/or age,[44] while others focus on exposures but not exclusive to HCT.[45] A Children's Oncology Group (COG) HCT Task Force did develop organ-system categorized HCT guidance.[46] Some international groups developed harmonized, color-coded, evidence-based, and topic-focused surveillance recommendations for breast cancer, cardiomyopathy, premature ovarian insufficiency, male gonadal toxicity, thyroid cancer, and ototoxicity.[47] Recognizing that general oncology guidelines often lack sufficient detail regarding high-dose conditioning, effects of GVHD and its management, and nonmalignant diseases (NMDs), HCT-specific guidelines have been developed for hemoglobinopathies, severe combined immunodeficiency (SCID), and bone marrow failure syndrome.[48-50]

One organized way to consider late effects is sequentially, "head-to-toe," drawing from organ, systems, and problem-based categories, lastly overlaying the HCT diagnosis-based lens to come up with an individualized LTFU evaluation (*Figure 108.1C*; *Table 108.2*).

ENGRAFTMENT

Definitions based on early neutrophil and platelet recovery are insufficient to address late graft failure and rejection because nonmyeloablative and reduced intensity conditioning may result in mixed donor chimerism in one or more leukocyte lineages. This is rarely an issue in heavily pretreated malignancies, although falling chimerism is followed closely by some centers with the goal of preemptive intervention for impending relapse. Beyond this rationale, chimerism monitoring during LTFU is of questionable value for malignant diseases unless confirmation of residual donor hematopoiesis is necessary before donor lymphocyte infusion.

By contrast, mixed chimerism is essential to LTFU for NMDs, albeit dynamic patterns of lineage-specific chimerism over years of follow-up, and their meaning, remain to be firmly established for individual NMDs. What level of lineage-specific chimerism is critical for durable correction of the underlying disease phenotype is also unclear for the full portfolio of NMDs.[48-50,55,56] Studies are first needed to determine if complete donor chimerism is maintained in individual NMDs during extended LTFU. When mixed chimerism is present initially, or emerges over time, does the underlying disease phenotype, and/or autoimmunity, eventually return? These unanswered questions prompted the Primary Immunodeficiency Disease Transplant Consortium to recommend lifelong, systematic, and comprehensive assessment of lineage-specific chimerism, plus numeric and functional immune reconstitution data, even if the patient is well and without signs of infection, to allow early detection and trajectory of possible declines in chimerism and immune function and so that intervention can occur before clinical complications of recurrent SCID emerge.[49] Testing begins no later than 3 months after HCT.

IRON OVERLOAD

Iron overload occurs frequently after HCT,[9,57] usually resulting from red blood cell (RBC) transfusions before and after HCT, in the context of ineffective erythropoiesis with intestinal hyperabsorption and, rarely, underlying hereditary hemochromatosis (HH). Thalassemia and sickle cell disease (SCD) exemplify ineffective erythropoiesis pretransplant, whereas marrow failure syndromes (Fanconi anemia [FA], Diamond-Blackfan anemia [DBA], aplastic anemia) or relapsed hematological malignancies intrinsically necessitate RBC transfusions. With eventual posttransplant discontinuation of RBC transfusions, body iron stores decline spontaneously over several years,[58] but accumulated iron may be high enough to warrant intervention to prevent liver and cardiac failure.

Liver and marrow iron content correlates poorly with number of transfused RBC units. Likewise, because elevated serum ferritin can be seen with active GVHD, recurrent malignancy or infection, it is challenging to determine who needs simple observation vs aggressive intervention for iron overload. The most accepted way to accurately quantify tissue iron overload is by T2*magnetic resonance imaging (MRI).[59,60] For patients without significant RBC transfusion history (or HH), T2*MRI is an unnecessary expense; elevated serum ferritin with normal transferrin saturation can be managed by avoidance of

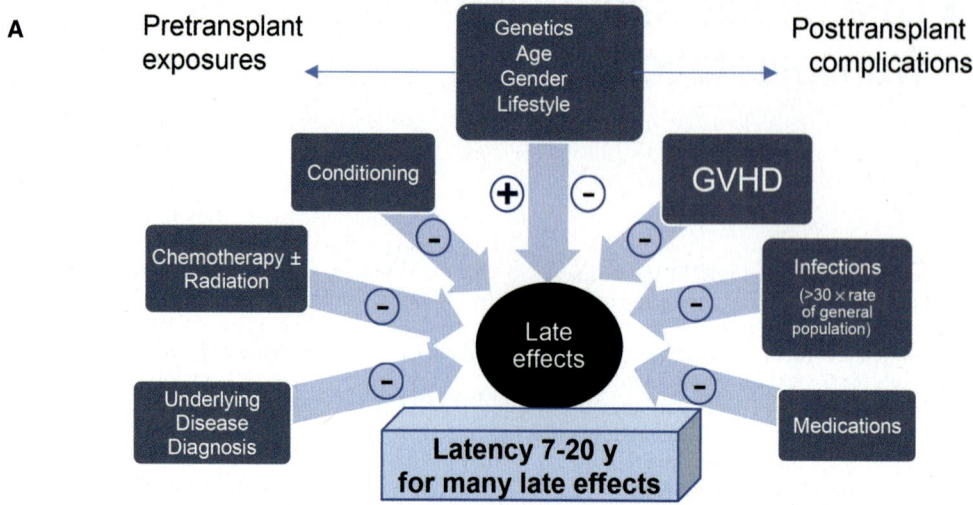
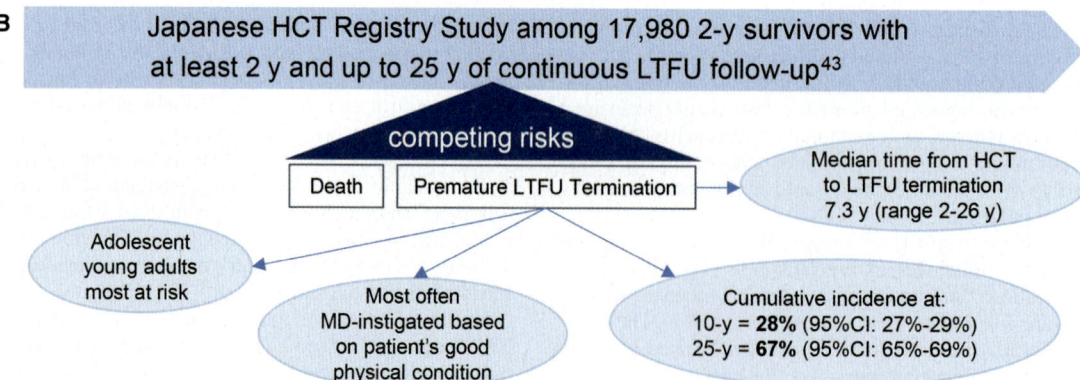
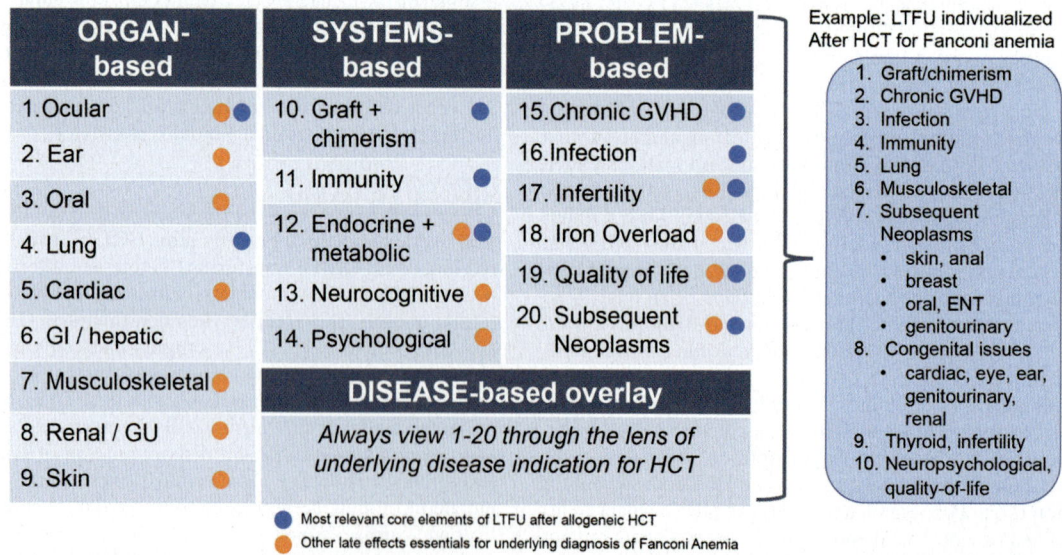

FIGURE 108.1 **HCT late effects.** A, latency and relationship to genetics, demographics, pre- and post-HCT exposures; (B) real-world problem of premature LTFU termination, and (C) individual comprehensive approach to sequential "head-to-toe" long-term follow-up (LTFU) evaluation.

iron-containing multivitamin ± simple phlebotomy, until serum ferritin has normalized. T2*MRI testing is best utilized for survivors with a lifetime history of ≥20 RBC units (often >50), thalassemia, SCD, DBA, HH, a need for iron chelation before HCT, or chronic hepatitis C where iron overload may accelerate cirrhosis.

Extreme iron overload (T2*MRI liver iron content [LIC] >15 mg/g dry) is treated with monthly phlebotomy ± an iron chelator to mitigate risks for dysrhythmias and cardiac failure, portal fibrosis and cirrhosis, diabetes mellitus, and other endocrinopathies. Iron overload also increases susceptibility to infections.[9,57] LIC 7

Table 108.1. Magnitude of Late Effects After Hematopoietic Cell Transplantation

Late Effect	Magnitude	Citation
Overall health		
Life expectancy decrement	20.8%	7
A chronic health condition: 2-y CI, 10-y CI	32%, 59%	6
Grades 3-5 chronic health condition, 10-y CI	35%	6
Iron overload		
5-y CI: auto, allo	0.7%, 25.4%	8
Prevalence rate liver iron content ≥1.8 mg/g	32%	9
Chronic GVHD sequelae		
Keratoconjunctivitis sicca	53%	10
Esophageal webs/strictures	~4%[a]	11
Bronchiolitis obliterans syndrome: prevalence	5.5%-14%[b]	12
Joint/fascia: point prevalence	24%-29%	13,14
Deep or superficial sclerosis: 3-5 y CI	15.5%-20%	15,16
Infection		
Vaccine-preventable late infections vs general population	30-fold higher	17
Infection-related mortality: 30-y CI, SMR	10.7%, 52.0	7
Lung		
Deaths due to pulmonary disease: 30-y CI, SMR	2.7%, 13.9	7
Bronchiolitis obliterans syndrome: prevalence	5.5%-14%[b]	12
Organizing pneumonia (COP) incidence proportion	2%	18,19
Pulmonary hypertension incidence proportion	2.4%	20
Late interstitial lung disease incidence proportion	<2%	21
Cardiovascular		
Deaths due to CVD: 10-y CI, 30-y CI	3.7%,[c] 4.1%	7
Congestive heart failure: 10-y CI, 15-y CI	6.0%, 9.1%[d]	22,23
Coronary artery disease: 10-y CI	3.8%[c]	23
Stroke: 10-y CI	3.5%	23
Renal		
AKF, 10-y CI in >2y survivors	9.4%	24
CKD, 10-y CI in >2y survivors	5.7%	24
Nephrotic syndrome incidence proportion	1%-4.3%	25,26
Thrombotic microangiopathy, 3-y CI	3%[e]	27
Liver		
Focal nodular hyperplasia incidence proportion	5.2%-12%	28,29
Cirrhosis, 20-y CI in >1 y survivors	3.8%[f]	30
Eyes		
Cataracts incidence proportions (adults, children)	11%-100%[g], 4%-76%[g]	31
Dry eyes point prevalence	35%-62%	14,32
Bone		
Bone loss incidence proportion: auto, allo	20%-65%, 50%-75%	33
Avascular necrosis incidence proportion: auto, allo	2%-4%, 5%-19%	33
Metabolic syndrome		
1-y period prevalence MS	37.5%[c]	34
Hypertension: 1-y period prevalence, 10-y CI	61%, 38%	34,35
Fasting hyperglycemia: 1-y period prevalence	47%	34
Dyslipidemia: 1-y period prevalence, 10-y CI	51%, 47%	34,35
Elevated waist circumference 1-y period prevalence	67%	34
Endocrine		
Thyroid dysfunction 5-y CI: auto, allo	14.2%, 13.3%[h]	8
Diabetes 5-y CI: auto, allo	3%, 22.9%	8
Adrenal insufficiency 5-y CI: auto, allo	1.3%, 13.4%	8
Hypogonadism prevalence: males, females	6.9%-84%,[i] na[j]	36
Infertility prevalence: males, females	20%-90%,[i] na[j]	36

(Continued)

Table 108.1. Magnitude of Late Effects After Hematopoietic Cell Transplantation (Continued)

Late Effect	Magnitude	Citation
Subsequent neoplasms		
Infection related mortality: 30-y CI, SMR	7.0%, 4.8	7
Neuropsychological, quality of life		
Depression: 1-y period prevalence	13%[c]	37
Fatigue: 1-y period prevalence	43%[c]	

[a]4% of those with cGVHD.
[b]14% in patients with cGVHD.
[c]Auto-HCT similar as allo-HCT.
[d]Increases in higher-risk groups (age, anthracycline dose, chest radiation, hypertension, diabetes, smoking).
[e]Higher rates reported by others, especially in children.[27,38,39]
[f]Almost all cases attributable to hepatitis C infection.
[g]Lowest rates when TBI absent, highest rates with unfractionated 10 Gy TBI.
[h]15%-25% 5-y CI if age < 18 y.[40]
[i]Varies widely by age and preparative regimen intensity (TBI dose, targeted busulfan).
[j]Not available given that starting pool of pretransplant oocytes depends on age and the lethal dose at which 50% of oocytes are lost decreases with increasing age, infertility is near 100% after myeloablative busulfan or high-dose TBI.
Abbreviations: AKF, acute kidney failure; CI, cumulative incidence; CKD, chronic kidney disease; CVD, cardiovascular disease (heart failure, coronary artery disease, arrhythmia, stroke); SIR, standardized incidence ratio; SMR, standardized mortality ratio vs general population.

Table 108.2. LTFU Recommendations for Survivors

Organ System or Late Effect	Recommendation	Qualifiers and Other Comments
Graft and chimerism	Annual CBC, MCV ± reticulocytes	• More frequently if persistent or progressive abnormalities that may be due to medications, infection, GVHD, relapse
	Flow cytometry–sorted donor chimerisms for T cells (CD3), granulocytes (usually CD33), plus B cells (usually CD19) and NK cells (CD56) as applicable in nonmalignant diseases or primary immunodeficiency diseases	• Usually unnecessary in malignant diseases except as a baseline before donor lymphocyte infusion • At least annual in nonmalignant diseases when long-term graft stability is unclear especially after NMT or RIC • SCD: check myeloid chimerism every 3-6 mo for 2 y, then yearly with HbS level • Thalassemia: if microcytic anemia recurs check chimerism as for SCD • Mixed chimerism undesirable for DBA and WAS because of risk MDS or AML
Iron overload	Ferritin, transferrin saturation (TS) at day 80-100, 1 y, then annually until normal	• Be mindful of ferritin as an acute phase reactant • Consider HFE gene testing if a family member has been diagnosed with HH or TS >45% in a patient of Northern or Western European ethnicity • FA, DC, DBA, hemoglobinopathies require more aggressive management beginning at 6 months
	Consider T2*MRI at baseline before starting phlebotomy ± iron chelation therapy and once ferritin <500 ng/mL to determine when to stop therapy	• Gold standard to quantify tissue iron burden in patients transplanted for hemoglobinopathies or otherwise heavily transfused • Annual for DBA until resolved
Chronic GVHD	Screen for cGVHD manifestations monthly while on IST, then every 3 mo until 2 y after stopping IST	• Screening includes GVHD-focused history and physical[51] directed at skin, mouth, eyes, GI tract, genitalia, lungs (Figure 108.2), LFTs and P-ROM
Infection and immunity	IgG, IgA, IgM at day 80-100, 1 y and otherwise as clinically appropriate	• If history of chronic conjunctivitis, sinopulmonary infections, other recurrent, unusual, or severe infections • Normalization of IgA, IgM plus increasing trough IgG levels before next IgG-replacement dose due tracks with humoral recovery, especially in primary immunodeficiency diseases where replacement is routine
	Peripheral blood T- and B-lymphocyte counts at 1 y and then as clinically appropriate	• Some centers use arbitrary cutoffs (CD4 >200 per microliter, CD19 >20 per microliter) for early vaccination beginning at day 180[52]
	Routine vaccinations	• See Table 108.3
	Serum viral PCR testing as clinically indicated	• May include serum PCR for CMV, EBV, HHV6, hepatitis B, C, HIV (HIV, HCV if exposed to blood products prior to universal testing)
	Pitted RBC score and liver-spleen scan (periodic) in certain disease indications	• SCD: ECO prophylaxis until splenic regeneration proven by liver-spleen scan, pitted RBC score < 1.5% and PCV13 and PPSV23 vaccinations complete • Thalassemia: If splenectomized need ECO prophylaxis life-long[48]
	Antimicrobial prophylaxis for patients during cGVHD therapy	• Directed against shingles, encapsulated organisms, and molds

Table 108.2. LTFU Recommendations for Survivors *(Continued)*

Organ System or Late Effect	Recommendation	Qualifiers and Other Comments
Pulmonary	Screen for airflow obstruction: *Figure 108.2*	• Spirometry alone is usually feasible age > 6 y • PFTs at cGVHD diagnosis, then every 3 mo for 1 y, then at least annually while on IST
	If detect restrictive rather than obstructive pattern PFTs, obtain HRCT to rule out COP, ILD, or pulmonary fibrosis	• DC: lifelong lung symptom screening and annual PFTs because high risk for pulmonary fibrosis and pulmonary arteriovenous malformation (see also Cardiovascular)
	Check TRJV by echocardiography in SCD or thalassemia to rule out pulmonary hypertension	• Cardiology should measure pulmonary arterial pressure if TRJV > 3 m/s to confirm pulmonary hypertension • Patients with pulmonary hypertension should be referred to a pulmonologist
Cardiovascular or metabolic	Blood pressure each visit, at least annual fasting blood glucose, HbA1c, fasting cholesterol (LDL, HDL) and triglycerides, while on IST, then at least every 5 y	• Early treatment of CVS risk factors like diabetes hypertension, dyslipidemia • Cardiovascular risk assessment tools: https://ccss.stjude.org/cvcalc
	Risk-based ECG with echocardiogram	• Use COG risk assessment tool to determine frequency: http://www.survivorshipguidelines.org/pdf/2018/COG_LTFU_Guidelines_v5.pdf • Referral to cardiology for abnormal declining of cardiac function. FA and DBA may also have congenital cardiac anomalies and cardiac iron overload (may need T2*MRI)
Musculoskeletal	Serum CPK, aldolase, CRP, ESR	• If investigating cGVHD-associated myositis/myopathy, or following myopathy/myositis while on tapered IST
	Spine x-ray	• FA: screen for scoliosis
Bone health	DEXA to evaluate BMD at 1 y then annually if abnormal	• DBA: can have significantly poor bone health (iron overload, endo, steroids) • DC: commonly have osteoporosis
	Vitamin D level annual while on IST or in growing child	• Optimize calcium + vitamin D intake
	MRI to rule out or stage AVN	• Refer to Orthopedics if MRI confirms AVN findings
Endocrine	*Adults*: Monitor height, weight, BMI annually *Children*: monitor height, weight, growth velocity, BMI at least annually. Check bone age (left wrist radiograph) peripubertally and before final adult height	• Evaluate suspected nutritional deficiency, obesity, or sarcopenic obesity • *Children*: refer to Pediatric Endocrinology if suspect GH deficiency via reduced height velocity > 1 y post HCT • Thalassemia: hypogonadism is common due to iron overload and busulfan or treosulfan-based conditioning
	Free T4, TSH annually	• Full-dose TBI, and to lesser extent high-dose targeted BU particularly at risk for thyroid dysfunction • If high TSH and normal free T4, repeat in 2 mo • Thyroid hormone replacement if high TSH/low T4 or persistently very high or progressively elevated TSH. Use lowest dose to achieve a mid-normal range TSH
	Annual Tanner stage (until adult) From age 11 y, serum FSH, LH, estradiol (girls), free serum testosterone (boys) annually	• Full-dose TBI, high-dose targeted busulfan, at higher risk for delayed puberty as well as patients with FA, DBA, DC and those with severe iron overload • Refer to endocrinologist, gynecologist, or urologist with abnormal pubertal timing or gonadal dysfunction • Treat ovarian failure with hormone replacement therapy generally until reach the expected age of menopause
	Cortisol-stimulation testing	• To rule out suspected adrenal insufficiency
Infertility	Consider anti-Mullerian hormone level	• As a surrogate to assess ovarian reserve if age > 25 y
	Consider semen analysis	• If age-appropriate older male seeks fertility potential
Liver	ALT, bilirubin (direct and indirect), alkaline phosphatase, albumin PT/INR, albumin to assess liver synthesis as needed Liver biopsy (selective)	• DC: surveillance for liver fibrosis and gastrointestinal bleeding, ulceration, telangiectasias, varices as clinically indicated • Thalassemia or SCD: Consider liver biopsy at 2 y if bridging fibrosis present before HCT • Consider liver biopsy at 2 y for patients who had hepatitis B or HCV before HCT • Refer patients with HCV or HBV infection to gastroenterologist or infectious disease specialist for consideration of antiviral therapy
Renal or genitourinary	Blood pressure at each visit Serum creatinine, BUN at least annual, at least monthly if on nephrotoxic medication	• FA, DC, DBA: follow-up congenital genitourinary anomalies with a urologist and renal abnormalities and renal function with a nephrologist • DC: examination for urethral stenosis
	Urine microalbumin: creatinine ratio at day 80-100, then minimum of annually	• If >30 mg/g and <300 mg/g, repeat with at least two tests in 3-6 mo • If >300 mg/g repeat every 3-6 mo • If >300 mg/g on 1 occasion or if >30 mg on 3 occasions within 6 mo and has hypertension, consider treatment with an ACEI or ARB (refer to Nephrology)
	Renal biopsy	• If suspect TMA or unexplained kidney disease

(Continued)

Table 108.2. LTFU Recommendations for Survivors (Continued)

Organ System or Late Effect	Recommendation	Qualifiers and Other Comments
Ocular	Annual full eye examination to screen for dry eyes, cataracts, retinal infections	• Cataracts most often due to TBI and steroids • Retinal examination essential for late CMV staging • FA: screen for vision, cataracts. DC: screen for vision, lacrimal duct stenosis, retinal pathology, and cataracts
Hearing	Consider annual audiology or per audiologist recommendations	• If platinum exposure or had >30 Gy cranial radiation: testing advised through age 10 y or 5 y post HCT whichever occurs later • If underlying HCT indication is FA or DC
Oral	Dental examinations and cleanings every 6 mo; educate on routine dental hygiene	• Ask about xerostomia, chewing difficulties, swallowing, and speaking • Antimicrobial endocarditis prophylaxis per AHA guidelines
	Children: Baseline panorex	• Special pediatric risks in the developing mandible, especially below age 6 y, include hypodontia, microdontia, enamel hypoplasia, and root malformation
	Cancer screening and prevention counseling	• Table 108.4 • Increased risk for oral cancers if received TBI, had oral GVHD, or underlying FA or DC
Skin	Examination for GVHD and neoplasms	• See also "Chronic GVHD" and Table 108.4 • Alopecia may be a sequela of TBI/cranial irradiation of high-dose targeted busulfan
Neurocognitive	Annual screen for educational or vocational progress	• Includes developmental milestone screen in children
	Consider neuropsychological testing at 1 y or later	Especially if >12 Gy TBI ± cranial radiation, FA, DC, DBA with craniofacial abnormalities and large ribosomal protein gene deletions, ALD, Hurler syndrome, SCD, and some forms of SCID. Results can inform individualized educational plans (IEP)
	Consider brain MRA/MRI at 1 y	• If SCD and pre-HCT moyamoya or stroke; repeat every 2 y as clinically indicated
	Ask about neuropathy symptoms	• Gabapentin, pregabalin therapy might be indicated
Psychological, quality of life	At least annually screen for pain, fatigue, sleep disturbance, anxiety, depression, social reintegration (return to work), nonadherence to health recommendations and medications, and high-risk behaviors	• If positive depression screen, ask about suicidal ideation • FA, DC, DBA: genetic counseling for patient and family, assistance with family planning • Counseling about living with chronic conditions • Return-to-work standardized guidance and programs are an unmet need[53,54]
Subsequent neoplasms	At least annual health care provider full physical examination and urinalysis for hematuria	• See Table 108.4

Abbreviations: AHA, American Heart Association; ALD, adrenoleukodystrophy; ALT, alanine transaminase; AML, acute myelogenous leukemia; AVN, avascular bone necrosis; BCC, basal cell carcinoma; BMD, bone mineral density; BMI, body mass index; BOS, bronchiolitis obliterans syndrome; CBC, complete blood count; cGVHD, chronic graft-vs-host disease; COP, cryptogenic organizing pneumonia; CPK, creatine phosphokinase; CRP, C-reactive protein; DBA, Diamond-Blackfan anemia; DC, dyskeratosis congenita; DTaP, diphtheria-tetanus-acellular pertussis; ECG, electrocardiogram; ECO, encapsulated organism; ESR, erythrocyte sedimentation rate; FA, Fanconi anemia; Free T4, free thyroxine; FSH, follicle stimulating hormone; GH, growth hormone; GVHD, graft-vs-host disease; HDL, high-density lipoprotein; HH, hereditary hemochromatosis; HFE, high ferrous gene; HPV9, 9-valent human papilloma virus vaccine; HRCT, high-resolution chest CT, IGF-1, insulin-like growth factor 1; IGFB3, insulin-like growth factor binding protein 3; ILD, interstitial lung disease; INR, international normalized ratio; IPV, inactivated polio vaccine; IST, systemic immunosuppressive therapy; LDL, low-density lipoprotein, LFT, liver function tests; LH, luteinizing hormone; MCV, mean corpuscular volume; MDS, myelodysplastic syndrome; MenB, Group B meningococcal vaccine; NMT, nonmyeloablative transplantation; PCR, polymerase chain reaction; PCV13, 13-valent pneumococcal-conjugated vaccine; PFT, pulmonary function tests; PPSV23, 23-valent pneumococcal-polysaccharide vaccine; P-ROM, photographic range of motion assessment; PT, prothrombin time; RBC, red blood cell; RIC, reduced intensity conditioning; SCC, squamous cell carcinoma; SCD, sickle cell disease; SCID, severe combined immunodeficiency disease; TSH, thyroid stimulating hormone; TRJV, tricuspid regurgitation jet velocity; WAS, Wiskott-Aldrich syndrome.

to 15 is treated with phlebotomy alone. For LIC 2 to 7, observation is acceptable unless the patient has HH in which case phlebotomy until ferritin <100 ng/mL is the goal. Phlebotomy is generally safe and cost-effective but requires venous access and normal hematopoiesis (hematocrit ≥ 35%), or hematopoiesis that can respond to every-other-week darbepoetin. A typical phlebotomy regimen is 3 to 5 mL/kg/month as tolerated until LIC < 7 (non-HH patient) or ferritin < 500 ng/mL (<100 ng/mL if HH). If phlebotomy is unfeasible 3 to 6 months post HCT but iron mobilization is indicated, iron chelator therapy can be used but with caution due to potential added toxicities of currently available chelators. Mobilization of iron in heavily overloaded patients improves cardiac function, normalizes serum alanine aminotransferase levels, and results in improved liver histology.[61,62]

CHRONIC GVHD

Late effects attributed to cGVHD and its treatment are discussed in the context of individual organ complications whenever applicable; for in-depth cGVHD discussion, see Chapter 107. The lower rates of cGVHD that children experience compared with adults[32,63-65] nonetheless vary widely with stem cell source, graft manipulations (antithymocyte globulins, various forms of T-cell depletion), and post-transplant cyclophosphamide. A prospective multicenter pediatric study reported a 21% incidence of cGVHD and 24.7% incidence of late acute GVHD.[65] While frequency of organ involvement appears to parallel that seen in adults, the intersection of normal childhood development with morbid forms of cGVHD can contribute to failure to thrive, linear growth delay, skeletal deformities, and increased risk for late infectious deaths even after IST has been discontinued.[66] Sclerotic forms of GVHD occur in 7% of children, but it is unclear if this is truly lower than in adults given shorter follow-up in the pediatric study,[65] and heterogeneities in the incidence of peripheral blood grafts and total body irradiation (TBI) >450 cGy between adult and pediatric studies[15,32,65] given that these were the two major risk factors for sclerosis established from an earlier study.[15] Because this form of cGVHD is difficult to treat when advanced, early detection of joint limitation may be screened and ultimately followed for response using the validated, easy to administer, and very sensitive, Photographic Range of Motion (P-ROM) scale.[13,67]

INFECTION AND IMMUNITY

Many patients without GVHD and off all ISTs after allogeneic HCT respond to vaccines and pathogens, but a large registry study found infection to be a primary or contributing factor for almost 30% of late deaths.[66] Older adults and anyone with cGVHD on IST at 2 years post HCT had the highest risk for late fatal infections. However, children had a 2.7-fold risk even if off IST. A large adult study found vaccine-preventable late infections to be >30-fold more frequent than in the general population.[17] These data emphasize the importance of infection prevention. Numeric and functional immune reconstitution are delayed when cGVHD is present or when HCT results in mixed T- and B-cell lineage chimerism, especially if the underlying diagnosis was a primary immunodeficiency disease (PID); functional asplenism is presumed whenever cGVHD is active. Antimicrobial prophylaxis directed against shingles, *Pneumocystis jirovecii* pneumonia (PJP), encapsulated organisms, and often molds is administered during cGVHD therapy.[68] In patients without cGVHD (often those with PID), if CD4 counts remain <200 per microliter or phytohemagglutinin proliferation is <50% lower limit of normal, PJP prophylaxis continues. Routine posttransplant vaccinations are detailed in *Table 108.3*,[69-73] detailed further by Carpenter and Englund.[52] Immunoglobulin replacement therapy is prescribed judiciously per American Society of Transplantation and Cellular Therapy "Choosing Wisely" unless profoundly low IgG (often with immeasurable IgA),[74] but children transplanted for PID have variable B-cell immune reconstitution and continue immunoglobulin therapy until functional B-cell reconstitution is documented.

Table 108.3. Recommended Vaccinations After Hematopoietic Cell Transplantation (HCT)

Vaccine	Months From HCT to First Vaccine	Total Doses in Primary Series	Comments and Qualifiers
Inactivated vaccines PCV13 (pneumococcal conjugate)	3-6	3-4	Although single-dose PCV15 and PCV20 were FDA approved in 2021 for age ≥18 y, it is unknown if one dose of either will be sufficient post HCT. Therefore, standard remains 3 doses of PCV13 plus a 4th dose given if GVHD is active and immune reconstitution is delayed
PPSV23 (23-valent polysaccharide pneumococcal vaccine)	Not applicable	1	If vaccine titers suggest good response to primary series of PCV13, then give PPSV23 6-12 mo (minimum 8 wk) after last dose of PCV13
DTaP (Diphtheria, tetanus, pertussis)	6-12	3	FDA approved for age <7 y but off-label use at all ages preferred by HCT consensus guidelines (higher antigen content, greater immunogenicity than adult options of Tdap or Td)
Hib (*Haemophilus influenzae* conjugate)	6-12	3	
MCV4 (meningococcal conjugate)	6-12	2	For all age >9 mo
MenB (group B meningococcal)	6-12	2 or 3 depending on brand	ACIP advises for high-risk age ≥10 y in addition to MCV4. Also offered on an individual basis to any adolescent or young adult (ideally age 16-18 y). Consider off-label use for >25-year-olds with anatomic asplenia or cGVHD, or workplace risks
IPV (inactivated polio vaccine)	6-12	3	
HBV (hepatitis B)	6-12	3	Double dose (40 µg) advised in HCT
HAV (hepatitis A)	6-12	2	Can be given separately or as combination (HAV + HBV) with dose 1 and dose 3 of HBV vaccination
HPV9 (human papilloma virus)	6-12	3	Recommended for all ages 9-26 y. ACIP advises shared clinical decision making for age 27-45 y
IIV (inactivated influenza vaccine)	4-6	1-2	Second dose 1 mo after first dose for age <9 y if was first ever IIV. Also consider second dose for any age if dose 1 given <4 mo post HCT during influenza epidemic
COVID-19 (SARS-CoV-2) vaccination	3	3	3 doses of mRNA vaccines preferred each 28 d apart with a bivalent dose (4th dose) given at least 2 mo after 3rd dose of primary series[69,70]
Zoster vaccine recombinant adjuvanted (SHINGRIX)	24	2	Although SHINGRIX has been given safely between 9 and 24 mo after HCT,[71] lack of efficacy data means vaccination does not mitigate the need to continue zoster prophylaxis while still on immunosuppressive therapy for cGVHD
Live vaccines MMR (measles-mumps-rubella)	24	2	Generally, should not be given <1 y after stopping immunosuppression and >8 mo after IVIG therapy. Recent local epidemics measles outbreaks due to falling herd immunity have led ASTCT to relax this rule to 12 mo post HCT if on no or low dose immunosuppression[72]
MMRV (measles-mumps-rubella-varicella)	24	2	Varicella seronegative patients get MMVR but seropositive patients get MMR plus SHINGRIX if age ≥ 50 y (FDA approved for age ≥ 18 y if immune compromised but see SHINGRIX comment above)

Abbreviations: ACIP, Advisory Committee on Immunization Practices; FDA, Food and Drug Administration; GVHD, graft-vs-host disease.

PULMONARY COMPLICATIONS

In terms of frequency, late noninfectious pulmonary complications (>3 months post HCT) are led by the cGVHD-associated bronchiolitis obliterans syndrome (BOS), followed by cryptogenic organizing pneumonia (COP), late interstitial lung disease (ILD), and likely underreported pulmonary hypertension (PH, Table 108.1). In practice, the associated pulmonary function test (PFT) abnormalities are airflow obstruction (AFO), restrictive lung disease, diffusion abnormality or combinations of all three.

Airflow Obstruction and BOS

Around one-third of patients with cGVHD develop AFO,[75] and up to 1 in 7 patients develop irreversible AFO[12] as the hallmark of BOS. BOS may present insidiously as nonproductive cough, wheeze, and dyspnea or be asymptomatic for long periods despite a rapid decline in FEV1, which has been observed in the 6 months preceding a diagnosis of BOS, then stabilization, if a patient survives.[76] Treating established BOS with systemic IST is often unsuccessful, and worse survival is seen among those with forced vital capacity <67% at time of BOS diagnosis. Taken together, early diagnosis and therapy are current strategies to avoid extensive irreversible damage of small airways. Standardized posttransplant PFT testing, further augmented upon a cGVHD diagnosis, can help identify early AFO/BOS (Figure 108.2). In children aged <6 years PFTs are unreliable and National Institutes of Health (NIH) consensus criteria for diagnosing BOS are difficult to satisfy. Multiple breath washout testing[78] and parametric response mapping from high-resolution inspiration plus expiration computed tomography (CT) images are promising diagnostic alternatives but require larger validation.[79] For early intervention, a double-blind randomized controlled study of inhaled corticosteroids plus long-acting beta agonist showed that inhaled combination therapy significantly improved FEV1 in moderate to severe BOS without changing systemic IST.[80] Based on prospective data, combining inhaled fluticasone twice daily, azithromycin 250 mg orally three times weekly, plus oral montelukast 10 mg once daily ("FAM" regimen) is standard for newly diagnosed BOS.[81] However, inclusion and/or duration of azithromycin are now more carefully considered given the increased risk for subsequent neoplasms.[82]

Restrictive Lung Disease

Restrictive-pattern PFTs can be seen with pulmonary fibrosis caused by pretransplant exposures to bleomycin, busulfan, carmustine, and lomustine. Other etiologies include COP, chest wall restriction from chest wall or total body irradiation, or cGVHD-associated sclerosis. COP is diagnosed after autologous or allogeneic HCT when a patient who may have fever also has solitary or multifocal pulmonary infiltrates on chest CT, and bronchoalveolar lavage testing has ruled out bacterial, viral, fungal, and other opportunistic pathogens. Unlike BOS, prognosis is generally favorable with 74% 5-year survival[18] after starting prednisone treatment at 0.75 to 1 mg/kg. Relatively fast tapering is reasonable for rapid responders, but because recurrences are common, subsequent tapering is usually over several months, guided by PFT monitoring.

Late ILDs besides COP are even less frequent after allo-HCT and usually present with rapid-onset dyspnea, cough, and sometimes fever, more often after peripheral blood HCT and when cGVHD is present.[21] High-resolution CT shows alveolar consolidations or ground glass opacities; PFTs show restrictive pattern in >80% of cases and universally reduced diffusing capacity. Biopsies may show nonspecific interstitial pneumonia, lymphocytic interstitial pneumonitis, and diffuse alveolar damage. Broad, empiric antimicrobial therapy is often administered while attempts to rule out infection are made. ILD is treated with high-dose steroids, often plus additional agents, and outcomes are variable.

Pulmonary Hypertension

Information about posttransplant PH is limited, but it should be considered whenever patients have hypoxemia, respiratory failure, or symptoms of transplant-associated thrombotic microangiopathy (TA-TMA), thrombosis, and especially in those who are critically ill. Although reported more often in children, PH is likely underdiagnosed because routine echocardiography can miss PH, which requires detailed assessment of tricuspid regurgitant jet velocity and/or dedicated PH protocols; treatment usually involves close collaboration with a cardiologist and may include treatment of TA-TMA.[20]

CARDIOVASCULAR COMPLICATIONS AND METABOLIC SYNDROME

The major cardiovascular complications (CVCs) are congestive heart failure (mainly anthracycline related) and radiation-induced structural abnormalities of the heart valves, coronary arteries, or cardiac conduction system. The risk for CVC is cumulative and represents an interplay of genetics, pretransplant exposures, and later side effects of prolonged cGVHD therapies (glucocorticoids, calcineurin inhibitors [CNIs]) with most patients taking >2 years to discontinue all IST after an initial diagnosis of cGVHD and 10% taking >5 years.

Metabolic Syndrome and Related Cardiovascular Disease

International diabetes federation defines metabolic syndrome (MS) risk factor cluster as >3 of 5 of the following: hyperglycemia, hypertriglyceridemia, low high-density lipoprotein cholesterol, hypertension, and obesity. Relative to siblings, allogeneic HCT survivors were 3 to 4 times more likely to report diabetes mellitus and twice as likely to report hypertension[83] and more likely to develop hypertension than autologous recipients. TBI exposure was associated with higher risk for diabetes mellitus (odds ratio [OR] = 3.42, 95% C.I.: 1.55-7.52). Compared with a well-matched general population, children (>70% allogeneic recipients) had higher rates of cardiomyopathy, stroke,

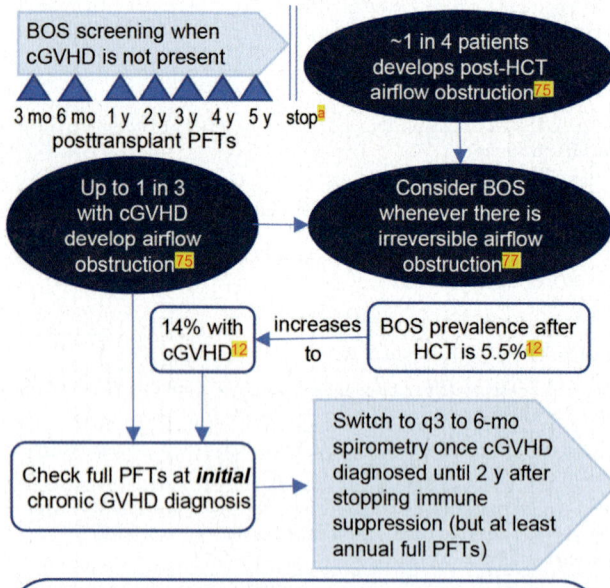

FIGURE 108.2 Approach to screening, diagnosis, and monitoring of bronchiolitis obliterans syndrome.

dyslipidemia, and diabetes,[84] in an analysis that adjusted for sex, race, age, body mass index (BMI), current smoking, daily fruit/vegetable intake, and recreational physical activity time. MS increases the risk for type 2 diabetes and atherosclerotic cardiovascular disease (CVD) (myocardial infarction, vascular disease, and stroke).[85,86] Another large study highlighted the importance of chest irradiation and comorbidities in the genesis of late CVD with >2 of obesity, diabetes, dyslipidemia, or hypertension being associated with a 5.2-fold increased risk of late CVD ($P < .01$) and pretransplant chest irradiation being associated with a 9.5-fold greater risk of coronary artery disease ($P = .03$).[87] Elegant studies recently teased out a ~25% polygenic contribution by established blood pressure gene loci to hypertension among 3572 childhood cancer survivors with other contributors being cancer therapies, obesity, and HP-axis irradiation.[88]

An analysis of potential risk reduction for ischemic heart disease, cardiomyopathy, or stroke found that controlling dyslipidemia was most helpful, followed by controlling hypertension, diabetes, and smoking.[84] Obesity was a risk factor for posttransplant hypertension, dyslipidemia, and diabetes. Lower fruit/vegetable intake was associated with more dyslipidemia and diabetes; lower physical activity level was associated with more hypertension and diabetes. Healthier survivor lifestyle characteristics attenuated the risk for all cardiovascular conditions assessed.

Congestive Heart Failure

A study of 2938 >1-year adult survivors reported 2% with congestive heart failure (CHF) (median ejection fraction 36.9%) at a median of 3.0 years (range 1-19 years) after allogeneic (32%) or autologous (68%) HCT. Previous anthracycline exposure and comorbidities (hypertension, chronic renal or lung disease, diabetes) primarily accounted for CHF risks without significant contribution from conditioning,[89] including posttransplant cyclophosphamide.[90] An analysis by the same group in auto-HCT showed a 4.8% CI of CHF at 5 years and 9.1% at 15 years or a 4.5-fold increased risk for CHF compared with the general population. Female lymphoma survivors were most at risk (14.5% CI at 15 years). This risk increased among those with >250 mg/m^2 cumulative anthracycline exposure (OR 9.9) and when hypertension (OR 35.3) or diabetes (OR 26.8) were additionally present.[22] Childhood cancer survivors have a 5- to 15-fold increased CHF risk compared with the general population; risk factors mirror those in adults, including female gender, but notably also age <5 years.[91] Potentiation of anthracycline-associated CHF risks by other comorbidities, especially hypertension, cannot be underestimated and informs prevention approaches. Although a dose relationship exists, there is no safe dose of anthracycline because interpatient variability is unaccounted for by clinical parameters alone. Elegant studies reviewed by Armenian and Bhatia[91] revealed strong contributions of functional polymorphisms within susceptibility genes relevant not only to hypertension but also to the biology of anthracycline metabolism, including, for example, increased oxidative stress (HAS3, RARG), reduced cellular drug efflux (ABC transporters, some of which have gender-dependent associations in females, like ABCB4 [rs4148808]), and variants relevant only to younger children like HNMT (rs17583889). No safe dose of anthracycline was identifiable among children homozygous for the V244M G allele of the CBR3 gene, which catalyzes reduction of anthracyclines to cardiotoxic alcohol, in an analysis that adjusted for age at diagnosis, gender, and chest irradiation. Posttransplant CHF predictive models in adults had the highest area under the curve when clinical parameters were combined with risk factors informed by gene polymorphisms relevant to free-radical metabolism (increased oxidative stress) or doxorubicin efflux.[92]

Recommendations to Address CVC and MS

Annual history and physical (dyspnea, chest pain, palpitations, exertional intolerance, edema) and calculating anthracycline and radiation exposures are essentials. Because imaging studies can detect negative functional or structural abnormalities of asymptomatic cardiac dysfunction (e.g., left ventricle remodeling) as a precursor to CHF, 2D echocardiography every 1 to 5 years is advised depending on age plus exposures.[45] Because beta-blockers might be able to reverse chronic cardiac remodeling, a randomized control trial (NCT0271750) is evaluating carvedilol therapy in patients treated with >250 mg/m^2 anthracyclines. Ideally intervention would begin before there is CHF. However, a study of 10-year childhood cancer survivors highlighted that left ventricular ejection fraction (LVEF) measurement alone missed 3 to 4 times as many additional cases of cardiac dysfunction as otherwise detected by reduced exercise capacity in a 6-minute walk test or more sensitive echocardiography measures of global longitudinal strain and left ventricle thickness/dimension ratio.[91] A recent study of a handheld wireless sensor device placed over the carotid pulse measured and streamed carotid wall displacement waveform data to an iPhone (for example). LVEF estimates then determined by an "Intrinsic Frequency" algorithm were more accurate than standard-of-care 2D echocardiography and comparable with gold-standard cardiac MRI.[93] If validated, this mobile platform could facilitate real-time monitoring of cardiac dysfunction by also confronting the problem of compliance with routine risk-based hospital-based echocardiographic screening among at-risk survivors. A pursuit of prognostic biomarkers led to studying abnormal N-terminal pro-B-type natriuretic peptide (NT-proBNP) levels, which are released in response to myocardial wall stretch and remodeling. NT-proBNP levels were highly prevalent among survivors previously exposed to anthracyclines or chest irradiation in a dose-dependent manner. Elevated NT-proBNP was associated with an increased risk for cardiac mortality and future cardiomyopathy among exposed survivors with normal baseline LVEF by echocardiography and without history of cardiomyopathy.[94] If confirmed, these results could prompt more frequent structural imaging if NT-proBNP is abnormal.

Susceptibility gene testing is currently not a standard of care. Variables used for COG's risk algorithm are doxorubicin-equivalent dose conversions, recognizing that total cumulative lifetime doses of anthracycline are multiplied by 4.0 (mitoxantrone), 5.0 (idarubicin), 0.5 (daunorubicin), or 0.67 (epirubicin), due to potency differences. The Childhood Cancer Survivorship Study Cardiovascular Risk Calculator[95] uses information about exposures (anthracycline, alkylator, platinum, and radiation) and also demographics (gender, current age, age at HCT, use of medications for diabetes, dyslipidemia, or hypertension) to predict incidence of heart failure, ischemic heart disease, and stroke. Prevention of obesity, avoidance of smoking, exercise, and healthy dietary choices are all important as discussed above. It is also reasonable after HCT to use medications to lower blood pressure and statins to target lower low-density lipoprotein cholesterol when therapeutic lifestyle modifications are ineffective or unfeasible, extrapolating from improved survival and other benefits observed when MS components were addressed in solid organ transplantation.[46,96-99] Lowest doses possible are used to minimize potential adverse drug interactions. Pleiotropic benefits of statins may extend to renal function, hypertension, bone mineral density (BMD), avascular bone necrosis (AVN), and even GVHD control.[100-107]

RENAL COMPLICATIONS

In order of frequency these include acute kidney injury (AKI), chronic kidney disease (CKD), TA-TMA, and nephrotic syndrome (NS). Many earlier scenarios that cause AKI early after HCT can also occur in LTFU. Knowledge of the interplay of prerenal (dehydration, fever, sepsis), postrenal (clots, stones), and direct renal insults (medications, adenovirus/BK virus, sepsis/shock, contrast dyes, TA-TMA) should inform preemptive planning and/or aggressive management to avoid cumulative renal injury leading to CKD.[24,25,38,39,108-110] Major risks for CKD include acute renal failure, previous autologous HCT, relevant exposures including alkylators, fludarabine, radiation, CNIs, nephrotoxic antimicrobials, BK viremia or adenoviremia, and acute and chronic GVHD. CKD and nonrelapse mortality rates at 1-year are 4- to 6-fold higher among those with proteinuria at day 100; acute kidney failure and CKD rates are severalfold higher at 2 to 10 years when hypertension is present <2 years posttransplant,[25] helping to inform LTFU monitoring (Table 108.2).

NS occurs after allogeneic HCT in up to 6% of patients with a median onset of 20 months, usually but not always associated with GVHD, and often after CNI therapy has been tapered.[108,111,112] If patients have edema or anasarca, a diagnosis of NS can be supported by hypoalbuminemia <2.5 g/dL, marked hyperlipidemia, and >3 to 2.5 g protein from a 24-hour urine collection (or spot urine protein-to-creatinine ratio >3-3.5 mg/mg creatinine). Renal biopsy is indicated to confirm diagnosis and direct therapy. Approximately 80% of minimal change NS (~20% of cases) is responsive to prednisone 1 mg/kg/d alone (used <20% of the time) or plus steroid-sparing agent(s), CNIs just over half the time. By contrast, membranous NS (~65% of cases) will often be refractory and so often treated also with rituximab or mycophenolate mofetil. Urine protein-to-creatinine ratio can be monitored serially to help guide prednisone taper and duration of immune suppressive therapies. Anticoagulation is considered for hypoalbuminemia <2.0 g/dL or in those with known prothrombotic tendency. Angiotensin-converting enzyme inhibitors (ACEIs) or angiotension II receptor blocker (ARBs) have been used in selected cases for their antiproteinuric effects.

Earlier retrospective studies reported TA-TMA prevalence at 10% to 25%,[27,39] but in a recent Center for International Blood and Marrow Transplant Research (CIBMTR) analysis of 23,665 allo-HCT recipients the 3-year CI was 3%.[113] A prospective multi-institutional study identified 16% with TA-TMA from 614 children screened systemically using set diagnostic criteria and reported greater morbidity and mortality compared with children without TA-TMA.[38] Although the CIMBTR study's provider-reported incidence is much lower than estimates using laboratory-detected TA-TMA, it does reflect real-world clinical severity. Importantly, the registry study found independent associations of increased TA-TMA with female sex, prior autologous transplant, acute lymphoblastic leukemia and severe aplastic anemia, mismatched or unrelated donor, myeloablative conditioning, GVHD prophylaxis with sirolimus plus CNI, pretransplant renal dysfunction, and acute GVHD (especially grade 3-4). There was a 3-fold increased risk of death and >7-fold higher risk for renal replacement therapy among those with TA-TMA compared with those without. Variability in TA-TMA reported prevalence reflects differing levels of awareness, diagnostic uncertainty, and limited single-institution data; harmonization of diagnostic criteria is a current international focus of ASTCT and European Society for Blood and Marrow Transplantation. Until then, diagnostic criteria suggested by Jodele et al are commonly used and include histological evidence in the affected organ (most commonly kidney or intestine) or at least four of seven laboratory markers (abnormal lactate dehydrogenase, schistocytes, each of de novo thrombocytopenia or red cells requiring transfusions, hypertension, elevated random urine protein-to-creatinine ratio, or elevated sC5b-9).[39] Treatment includes discontinuing offending medications, sometimes augmenting non-CNI therapy for underlying GVHD, and tailored eculizumab therapy when sC5b-9 levels are elevated as carefully detailed by the Cincinnati group.[114]

Renal LTFU Recommendations

Annual urinalysis for proteinuria (microalbuminuria), serum blood urea nitrogen (BUN), creatinine, and electrolytes is standard, with reflexive nephrology consultation when abnormalities are found. Survivors should be screened for hypertension defined as average systolic and/or diastolic blood pressure ≥95th percentile for gender, age, and height on ≥3 occasions.[108,109] Although hypertension after HCT has most commonly been treated with a long-acting calcium channel blocker, blockade of the renin-angiotensin axis using ACEIs alone or in combination with ARBs may be a better choice in patients with idiopathic CKD. This concept is based upon studies using ACEI and ARBs in animal models of radiation-induced injury and recent clinical experience.[115] In addition to controlling blood pressure, ACEI and ARB might exert additional positive affects by reducing inflammation and inflammatory markers.[116,117] Extrapolating from studies in diabetes, it is hoped that these agents might slow progression of CKD in patients with albuminuria after HCT. Controlled trials using ACEI or ARB after HCT are needed.

MUSCULOSKELETAL COMPLICATIONS

In practice these are low BMD and AVN, detailed comprehensively by Bar et al for the interested reader,[33] and more rarely myopathy/myositis.

Low Bone Mineral Density

Bone loss tends to peak 3 to 12 months post HCT followed by improvement (mainly trabecular) at spine, whereas femoral neck deficits (mainly cortical) may persist 4 to 10 years.[118,119] Prednisone >5 mg/d for >3 months is the strongest risk factor for bone loss, but others include dysregulated cytokines and hormones (hypogonadism, human growth hormone deficiency), vitamin D deficiency, CNI therapy, inactivity, and muscle weakness. Low BMD associates with significantly higher fragility fracture rates compared with age- and sex-matched general populations.[120] Dual-energy x-ray absorptiometry (DEXA) is commonly used to measure BMD. For adults age ≥40 years, T-scores report the standard deviations (SDs) from the average BMD of sex-matched 30-year-olds, *osteoporosis* being <2.5 SD and *osteopenia* being −1.0 to −2.4 SD. For adults age <40 years Z-scores that report SDs referenced to age- and sex-matched reference populations are preferred; for children, T-scores should never be used. In pediatric DEXA reports, "low BMD" (not osteopenia) is used when BMD Z-scores are ≤−2.0. Osteoporosis in children requires a clinically significant fracture history and BMD Z-score ≤−2.0, adjusted for height-age to avoid over- (short children) or under- (tall children) estimation. Posttransplant, up to 21% of children have BMD Z-scores <−2.0. If DEXA scan and fracture risk assessment (by DEXA or plain radiography) were not done pretransplant, this is advised at 3 months, especially if there was intervening glucocorticoid therapy. Follow-up DEXAs depend on the type of therapy offered and ongoing risks for bone loss, glucocorticoids or hypogonadism being key. Baseline preventive therapy includes vitamin D, calcium supplementation, and lifestyle modifications. Pharmacologic bone therapy is added when risk for fragility fractures outweighs treatment risks as reviewed elsewhere.[33] Limited adult data suggest utility of an online FRAX risk assessment algorithm, adjusting for glucocorticoid dose.[121] Managing hypogonadism can be sufficient for younger adults, but bisphosphonates are the usual first-line pharmacotherapy in adults but generally paused after 3 to 5 years given associations with atypical femur fractures. Alternative agents (calcitonin, denosumab, teriparatide, romosozumab, raloxifene) require careful consideration (reviewed elsewhere, 33). In children, the emphasis is on gonadal HRT and/or growth hormone if clinically appropriate, supervised by a pediatric endocrinologist to avoid compromising final adult height. There are limited pediatric data for newer alternative agents, and bisphosphonate therapy is usually reserved for osteoporosis. One retrospective study showed that pamidronate can improve BMD in children after HCT.[122]

Avascular Bone Necrosis

AVN occurs in 2% to 4% of autologous recipients and 5% to 19% of allogeneic recipients,[33] and risk factors include advanced age, TBI-based conditioning, cGVHD, duration of steroids, and female gender. The femoral head is the most common site, followed by knee, vertebral column, and ankle. Although poorly understood, potential causative mechanisms include local vascular insults leading to marrow edema and ischemia, ineffective osteoblastic repair due to metabolic factors, and increases in adipocyte size and number within the marrow compartment of convex joints, contributing to venous outflow obstruction. MRI is sensitive and an appropriate next step once AVN is suspected based on presence of risk factors and functional joint pain and stiffness. Consultation with an orthopedic surgeon is essential. Nonsurgical approaches (medications, hyperbaric oxygen, extracorporeal shock-wave therapy) have been tried for "precollapse" AVN lesions, but reported benefits have been mixed, without a standard of care consensus. Early bisphosphonate studies showed reduced incidence of joint collapse and improved function for up to 10 years, but for femoral head AVN a meta-analysis failed to demonstrate improvement in hip dysfunction, progression-free interval, or need for hip replacement.[123] Core decompression surgery for precollapse AVN involves removing the necrotic segment, which reduces intraosseous pressure to allow healing. Core decompression can relieve pain rapidly and is successful in ~65% but is usually more successful in younger patients with lower BMI[124,125]; it is unclear if natural progression of AVN is altered. Once collapse occurs, surgical options are osteotomy, designed to rotate necrotic bone away from weight-bearing surfaces and allow for healing of the involved segment; total hip resurfacing (metal-on-metal cup); or total joint replacement for skeletally mature patients. Medications like high-dose glucocorticoids or sirolimus can impede wound healing. While there is no consensus as to a safe dose of glucocorticoids, sirolimus may be held perioperatively or switched to another agent. Risks for impaired wound healing, fractures, and friability of connective tissues must be weighed against benefits of surgery.

Muscle or Connective Tissue

Myopathy and/or myositis may be cGVHD related. The differential diagnosis includes acute glucocorticoid-induced myopathy and often painful statin-associated myopathy. Serum CPK or aldolase can be helpful in diagnosing GVHD-associated myositis and then followed serially for trends to help guide the pace of immunosuppressive tapers.

ENDOCRINE COMPLICATIONS

These include disturbances of the hypothalamic-pituitary adrenal axis and end organ damage to thyroid and/or gonads mainly from alkylating agents and radiation exposures but are often multifactorial.

Insulin Resistance and Diabetes Mellitus

Two large studies suggest that the prevalence of diabetes after HCT is 7%–9%, which is higher than in the general population and 3-fold that of matched siblings.[83,126] Reported risk factors include a diagnosis of leukemia, non-Hispanic white ethnicity, family history of diabetes, TBI, and asparaginase toxicity. Patients with diabetes need to be monitored for microvascular complications (nephropathy, neuropathy, retinopathy) and managed with insulin or oral hypoglycemic agents. They are at risk for CVC, in part due to MS, discussed earlier.

Thyroid Dysfunction

This is most often associated with radiation and/or busulfan-based conditioning, causing compensated or overt hypothyroidism that develops more commonly in children than in adults.[8,40] By contrast, transient sick euthyroid syndrome (SES) is more common in adults vs children, more common in those receiving higher glucocorticoid doses, and is possibly an adaptive response to severe posttransplant systemic nonthyroidal illness. SES is recognized by low free T3 or T4, reduced total thyroxine, and a normal thyroid stimulating hormone and does not require treatment.[127] Isolated case reports and small case series have documented "auto"-immune hyperthyroidism and hypothyroidism after allogeneic HCT, and adoptive transfer of abnormal donor lymphocyte clones has been suggested as a possible mechanism, but immune dysregulation associated with concomitant cGVHD might be a contributing factor.[128,129] Treatment of overt hypothyroidism or hyperthyroidism is identical to nontransplant situations. Although the clinical significance of antithyroid microsomal antibodies is unclear, it is of interest that these have been detected in 5%–40% of patients with cGVHD.[130,131]

Iatrogenic Cushing Syndrome and Adrenal Insufficiency

Cushingoid appearance most often results from prolonged prednisone therapy; cosmetic changes are troubling for patients, and especially for teenagers who are often already dealing with major changes of body image. Divided-dose prednisone regimens should be avoided for cGVHD due to greater adrenal suppression than daily or alternating-day regimens. Abrupt withdrawal of steroids may provoke symptoms of secondary adrenal insufficiency (AI), which should be anticipated in any patient treated >3 weeks with daily doses >7.5 mg of prednisone or equivalent. Blunted cortisol response may be life threatening when stress responses are needed. AI symptoms are usually dominated by fatigue and weakness but may be difficult to distinguish from GVHD flare or steroid withdrawal syndrome; the latter is dominated by arthralgias and myalgias and tends to stabilize if taper decrements are smaller. AI may be confirmed by a serum cortisol <3.6 μg/dL at 07:00 to 09:00 hours or not >19 μg/dL at 30 or 60 minutes after a 250 μg intravenous cosyntropin test dose.[132-134] Hydrocortisone 8 mg/m^2 to 12 mg/m^2/d is the preferred adrenal cortisol replacement therapy, usually divided as two to three daily doses, with half to two-thirds of the daily dose administered at 08:00 h to mimic physiological cortisol secretion pattern and lower doses at 12:00 h and 17:00 h (or just 17:00 h). Dose regimens are individualized according to symptoms and signs suggestive of over- or underreplacement. Stress dose steroids should be considered for illnesses that include fever, vomiting, diarrhea, major surgery, or trauma. Hypothalamic pituitary adrenal axis recovery varies from days to months, which must be considered when tapering replacement therapy.

Hypogonadism, Pubertal Delay, and Infertility

Exposure-related gonadal toxicity may cause infertility. However, gonadal hormonal insufficiency causes premature menopause and less commonly early andropause, whereas children can experience delayed puberty, failure to develop secondary sexual characteristics, and failure to achieve normal adult bone mass. Underlying diagnoses like thalassemia, sickle cell disease, FA, DBA, and dyskeratosis congenita (DC) are at greater risk due to endocrinopathies associated with iron overload. In boys, Leydig cells are less sensitive to damage than spermatogonia. In prepubertal girls, hormonal function and fertility are equally impaired, and primary ovarian insufficiency is near universal after myeloablative busulfan in postpubertal girls. Age-appropriate monitoring of gonadotropin and gonadal hormone levels is standard; some providers find serial anti-Mullerian hormone levels to be helpful indicators of ovarian reserve.

Growth Hormone Deficiency

Growth in children and attainment of normal adult height is a complex process that requires balanced nutritional, genetic, endocrine, and other physical and psychosocial factors. During infancy, growth is highly dependent on nutrition and thyroid hormone. During childhood, hGH predominates, and in puberty the synergistic interplay of hGH and sex steroids is critical for attainment of final adult height. During all stages, any prolonged disturbance of physical or psychosocial well-being may adversely impact growth and development.[135,136] For a child these may include delayed hormonal and direct skeletal effects of pretransplant TBI ± cranial irradiation, chronic glucocorticoid therapy >5 mg/m^2/d,[135-137] and phases when GVHD activity is inadequately controlled. LTFU must include systematic plotting of height, height-velocity, weight annually on age/gender-appropriate (and sometimes disease-specific) growth charts, along with Tanner staging to assess pubertal status. Bone age is followed to assess skeletal maturity and growth potential until final adult height. Referral to pediatric endocrinology is advised if a child is falling off their height percentile channel and/or not entering puberty at the usual time. Coordination of gonadal hormone therapy for pubertal delay must be coordinated with hGH therapy so that final adult height is not compromised by premature epiphyseal closure. Although there is no threshold glucocorticoid dose above which growth response to hGH clearly and predictably declines, best responses to hGH generally occur when prednisone is ≤0.5 mg/kg once daily on alternate days.[138-140] A reasonable approach is to defer hGH testing and/or replacement therapy until prednisone therapy is at every-other-day dosing or at least <5 mg/m^2/d. Survivors who received TBI ± central nervous system (CNS) radiation showed an unfavorable profile of inflammation (higher IL-6), adipokines (higher leptin and lower adiponectin), and sarcopenic obesity (higher percent fat mass and lower lean body mass) compared with sibling controls despite having similar BMI.[141,142] Increasing lean body mass may represent a tangible target for mitigating high cardiometabolic risks of HCT survivors. Interestingly, obese prepubertal boys who received 6 months of hGH, without additional dietary or exercise modifications, experienced a 5% increase in lean body mass, which lends support to the hypothesis that hGH may provide other benefits in addition to promoting height growth.[143]

GASTROINTESTINAL COMPLICATIONS

Late acute or chronic GVHD of the overlap subtype (discussed in Chapter 107) should always be included in the differential diagnosis of nausea, early satiety, abdominal cramping, or diarrhea. Important other "rule-out" diagnoses include medication toxicity (oral magnesium supplements, mycophenolate mofetil, narcotic bowel with pain cramping, and fecal overflow incontinence), opportunistic infections, or pancreatic insufficiency when failure to thrive and steatorrhea are present. A low fecal elastase or increased fecal fat favor a trial of pancreatic enzyme supplementation with meals and snacks. Progressive dysphagia can be caused by cGVHD (webs and strictures) or strictures caused by gastroesophageal reflux disease, or radiation >30 Gy; symptoms may include dysphagia and heartburn. Infectious esophagitis (cytomegalovirus [CMV], varicella zoster virus [VZV], herpes simplex virus [HSV], or candida) generally needs to be excluded in patients on prednisone or other systemic immunosuppression. Serum liver function test (LFT) abnormalities during LTFU are commonly due to medications, GVHD, and hepatotropic viruses. Chronic hepatitis B and C can lead to cirrhosis, portal hypertension, and hepatocellular carcinoma and are discussed elsewhere (Chapter 70). If GVHD is not present at other sites, liver biopsy might be indicated to confirm a liver GVHD diagnosis. Iron overload may exacerbate any LFT abnormality, and so persistent elevation of serum ferritin might warrant checking transferrin saturation and possibly T2*MRI imaging to quantitate liver iron. Patients with significant LFT abnormalities should limit alcohol intake and avoid other hepatotoxins.

Focal nodular hyperplasia is often an incidental benign finding, best diagnosed on gadolinium-enhanced MRI, and usually just needs to be monitored to avoid unnecessary invasive procedures.[28,29]

OCULAR AND ORAL/DENTAL COMPLICATIONS

Cataracts and cGVHD-associated keratoconjunctivitis sicca are common. Other eye exposure-based complications for which ophthalmological evaluations are indicated include ischemic microvascular retinopathy (TBI, CNI, carmustine, busulfan), central retinal vein occlusion (MS or hypercoagulability), and ocular infections (late CMV disease, HSV, VZV, bacterial, fungal, and toxoplasmosis). Thus, history should ask about impaired vision, dry or gritty eyes, frequency of artificial tear usage, diplopia, halos, and history of opportunistic infections. Lens cataracts may be not visually significant when first detected; relevant prior exposures are TBI, cranial irradiation, busulfan, and glucocorticoids. Using NIH consensus criteria at least 50% of adults and 30% of children with cGVHD developed dry eyes; prior cranial/eye radiation can increase this risk. Eye examinations are advised at 1 year post HCT, then yearly if abnormal or symptomatic.

Xerostomia is common, caused by cGVHD, TBI, or other local radiation and medications and can result in dental decay, infections, periodontal disease, and difficulties with chewing, swallowing, and speaking. Unique problems below age 6 years include hypodontia, microdontia, enamel hypoplasia, and root malformation. A baseline panorex is advised to evaluate root development before dental procedures. LTFU recommendations include regular dental examinations and cleanings, antimicrobial endocarditis prophylaxis per American Heart Association (AHA) guidelines, dental hygiene education, avoidance of oral tobacco, and human papillomavirus (HPV) vaccination to prevent oral cancers. Annual oral examinations include screening for subsequent neoplasms, especially after TBI or persistent oral cGVHD, and are critical in FA or DC.

NEUROCOGNITIVE COMPLICATIONS

These include cognitive deficits with or without leukoencephalopathy, peripheral neuropathies, CNS GVHD, and CNS infections. Risk factors for cognitive deficits include high-dose TBI ± additional cranial irradiation; CNS-penetrant chemotherapies including busulfan, fludarabine, cytarabine, methotrexate, thiotepa, and intrathecal agents; and CNI therapy for GVHD. Irradiation can be very consequential in young children. As a rule of thumb ≥12 Gy TBI in a child <4 years old will lower IQ by ~10 points. If a child had *average* IQ before HCT, they could drop to *low average* IQ (with vocational limitations), whereas a child starting at low average might drop to *borderline* and then be suited for manual labor or have no job options. Cranial boost irradiation amplifies risk for cognitive impairment. Glucocorticoids may cause a variety of cognitive effects including sometimes major mood disturbances. Underlying diseases like FA, DC, Hurler syndrome, adrenoleukodystrophy, SCID, and SCD may have pretransplant neurological deficits that either stabilize or progress after HCT.

Painful peripheral neuropathy is a chief complaint for some survivors. Etiologies include neurotoxic chemotherapies (vincristine, platinum, brentuximab) that posttransplant CNI therapy can exacerbate. Management can be difficult but often includes gabapentin or pregabalin.

Although understudied, evidence for CNS GVHD is accumulating in murine models and humans with activated microglia, cytokines, and effector memory T cells thought to play central roles.[144-146] Unlike in controlled murine experiments, etiology of CNS damage in patients is difficult to attribute to GVHD vs infections, vascular events, or medication-induced toxicity. Infections with HHV6, HSV, VZV, CMV toxoplasmosis, and JC virus generally need exclusion in cases of post-HCT cognitive decline.

Psychological and Quality of Life

Survivors are at risk for depression, fatigue, pain, social withdrawal, educational problems, and vocational problems including unemployment and dependent living. Younger and non-college-educated survivors are less likely to report risky health behaviors like alcohol and smoking.[146] Among autologous recipients, younger age and current chronic pain were independently associated with more depression and fatigue. Among allogeneic recipients, cGVHD severity, being female, and having current pain were associated with depression and fatigue.[37] A registry study showed that the return to work of adolescent young adults improved over time but many became or remained unemployed or on medical disability.[53] Return to work programs are unavailable at most centers despite 87% endorsing this as a problem.[54]

SUBSEQUENT NEOPLASMS

These are secondary leukemias and lymphomas including myelodysplastic syndrome (MDS)/acute myelogenous leukemia (AML), Epstein Barr Virus (EBV)-mediated posttransplant lymphoproliferative disease (PTLD), as well as solid tumors, malignant and benign. Latency is shorter for lymphomas and leukemias but several years for most solid tumors. In the largest studies so far, the posttransplant subsequent neoplasm (SN) rate exceeded twice that of the general population[148] and was ~30-fold higher for EBV-mediated PTLD.[149] Cumulative incidence helps convey the clinical burden of SN, but heterogeneities in sample size and population demographics hamper CI comparisons in different reports. Standardized incidence ratios (SIRs) that compare observed numbers to expected age-, sex-, calendar-year-matched US (SEER) population rates may also vary widely (*Table 108.4*)[150]; large-scale, long-term (<10 years), systematic, and well annotated LTFU will be needed to better define magnitude of risks for common and rarer SNs, as well as risk factors including intensity of pre- and posttransplant exposures plus genetic susceptibilities.[152] A recent study of >4900 survivors had well annotated exposure data and interrogated age and conditioning intensity contributions. The 20-year CI of SN was 8.1% among patients transplanted before age 20 years, 13.5% for ages 20 to 50 years, and 23.6% for age >50 years.[153] The 2.8 SIR for this 76% adult study was comparable with the study mentioned above.[148] Children had SIRs of 12.5, attenuating over time but remaining 5-fold higher at >30 years post HCT; thus, lifetime monitoring is imperative. Notably, SN risk is not significantly different for 2 to 4.5 Gy TBI compared with chemotherapy alone, but still 2-fold higher than general population (SIR 1.9). SN

Table 108.4. Recommended Cancer Screening After Hematopoietic Cell Transplantation (HCT)

Subsequent Neoplasms	SIR[150]	Recommendations	Higher-Risk Scenarios[a]
Skin: BCC, SCC Melanoma	na 1.4-8.3	At least annual provider skin examination, but every 6 mo in those at higher risk. Photoprotection	Age <18 y at HCT, TBI >6 Gy, cGVHD, FA or DC
Oral: Mouth, pharynx Lip Tongue	7.3-17 19-27 9.3-20	At least annual dental examination but every 6 mo for those at higher risk. Nasolaryngoscopy for FA or DC, annually. HPV vaccination age 9 to 45 y.	Age <10 y at HCT, history of local irradiation, persistent cGVHD, IST >24 mo, FA or DC
Female breast	0.3-2.0	Breast awareness counseling for all. **Average risk:** *age 25-40 y*, clinical breast examination every 1-3 y; *age >40 y*, annual clinical breast examination and mammogram. **High-risk:** *age <25 y*, annual clinical breast examination from 8 to 10 y post radiation; *age ≥25 y*, annual mammogram (or MRI in some) starting 8-10 y post radiation but not later than age 40 y	Prior chest wall or total body irradiation (especially age <18 y), BRCA 1/2, ATM gene mutations, or positive family history
Thyroid	5.8-6.6	Annual neck palpation	Age ≤20 y at HCT, female, TBI conditioning, cGVHD
Gastrointestinal: Esophagus	8.5-11	Upper GI endoscopy if persistent GERD, dysphagia, especially if history of cGVHD	Barrett esophagus
Stomach	0.6	No specific general population guidelines	
Colon	0.5-1.2	Follow general population guidelines with full surveillance colonoscopy starting age 45 y for average risk.[b] Consider annual occult blood stool testing. For DBA, start age 20-29 y	Diamond-Blackfan anemia
Hepatocellular carcinoma	6.3-28	Follow general population guidelines but if high risk then consider serum AFP and liver ultrasound every 6-12 mo	History of chronic hepatitis B or C, or cirrhosis from any cause, possibly iron overload
Gynecological: Cervix	0.7-2.3	Annual PAP test and HPV DNA test for immunocompromised woman from age 18-21 y but start in early teens if FA	
Endometrium	1.1-1.4	No specific general population guidelines	
Ovary	0.8	Follow general population guidelines unless higher risk; consider screening every 6 mo with CA-125 and transvaginal ultrasound starting at age 30 y or 5-10 y earlier than the earliest diagnosis of ovarian cancer in the family	BRCA1/2 mutation or positive family history; FA
Lung	0.7-2.6	Follow general population guidelines with low-dose CT screening for higher risk (does not apply if quit smoking >15 y ago)	>55 y + smoking ≥30 pack-years or 50 y + ≥20 pack-years + 1 additional risk factor (radon, asbestos, family history of lung cancer)
Kidney/Bladder	0.5-2.5	Annual urinalysis for hematuria	Wilms tumor or neuroblastoma in FA with mutations of FANCN/PALB2 or FANCD1/BRCA2
Male genital: Prostate	0.5-0.7	PSA digital rectal examination after informed decision making	
Testis	0.9-1.2	No specific general population guidelines	
Brain/CNS	3.8-9.5	No specific general population guidelines	Prior history of CNS irradiation
Sarcoma	6.5-8.0	No specific general population guidelines	
Bone	8.5-13	No specific general population guidelines	DBA at risk for osteosarcoma

[a]Underlying disease indication for HCT may include additional cancer predisposition risks like Fanconi anemia (FA), dyskeratosis congenita (DC), Diamond-Blackfan anemia (DBA), and Li Fraumeni syndrome (TP53 mutation); aggressive monitoring in Li Fraumeni syndrome includes complete physical examination every 3 to 4 months with blood pressure, anthropometry, evaluation for precocious puberty, full neurological examination; imaging with abdominal and pelvic ultrasound (± serum testosterone, DHEA, and androstenedione) every 3 to 4 months, annual whole-body MRI including brain (initially with contrast and thereafter without contrast if previous MRI normal and no new abnormality).[151]
[b]Subsequent colonoscopies is at 10 years for negative initial surveillance, but 1 to 5 years depending on nature of abnormal study.
Abbreviations: AFP; alpha fetoprotein; BCC, basal cell carcinoma; CNS, central nervous system; GERD, gastroesophageal reflux disease; GI, gastrointestinal; GVHD, graft-vs-host disease; HPV, human papilloma virus; na, not available; PSA, prostate specific antigen; SCC, squamous cell carcinoma; TBI, total body irradiation.

risk escalated with 6 to 14 Gy fractionated TBI (SIR 3.1-3.3), and 14.4 to 17.5 Gy TBI (SIR 5.7). The highest excess absolute risks per 1000 patient years were for breast cancer (EAR 2.2) and oral (EAR 1.5) and nonsquamous or basal cell skin cancers (EAR 1.5).

Lymphoma or leukemia SIRs were 2.4 to 2.6 (95% C.I.: 1.5, 4.5) with corresponding EAR 0.2 to 0.3 cases per 1000 person years. After autologous HCT, secondary MDS/AML arises latently after DNA-damaging chemotherapy or radiation marrow exposures or in the reinfused stem cells. The same may apply in allogeneic HCT, particularly if residual host chimerism persists, which is especially concerning in Wiskott-Aldrich syndrome, DC, FA, or DBA.

Certain heritable conditions have an increased risk for solid tumors independent of HCT that warrant more detailed subspecialist SN screening consultation (see *Table 108.4*). Examples are DBA, certain phenotypes of FA, and DC. In patients with Li Fraumeni syndrome, HCT does not correct the underlying germline TP53 mutation and posttransplant SN risk is extremely high; cancer surveillance protocols are intense[151]; through age 18 years, surveillance focuses on "core" cancers: brain tumors, adrenocortical carcinoma, soft tissue sarcomas, bone tumors, and early-onset breast cancer.

Multiple melanocytic nevi can develop after high-dose chemotherapy exposures[154] and are best monitored periodically by a dermatologist with mole mapping. Osteochrondromas may appear incidentally on plain radiographs after an average of 4.6 years in up to a quarter of children who received TBI before age 5 years; they rarely become malignant.[155]

SURVIVORSHIP CARE PLANS

The Institute of Medicine has recommended that all survivors receive treatment summaries with individualized care plans[156] that appear to improve quality of life among HCT survivors.[157] A major barrier is that LTFU attenuates over time and compliance with LTFU guidelines is suboptimal by survivors and health care providers (HCPs) especially when patients are perceived to be doing well.[43,147,158] Given the latency of late effects, education of survivors, their families, plus their future HCPs is a critical starting place. An ASTCT survey found that respondents agreed that allo-HCT survivors have needs separate from GVHD and that complications can arise during transitions of care from pediatric to adult or from transplant center to primary care provider. However, only 45% had dedicated LTFU clinics; 84% of individual practitioners prefer to provide their own survivorship care. Other barriers include a lack of subspecialty LTFU expertise, logistics of the LTFU model of care, and financial issues.[159,160] Clearly much work is needed to optimize LTFU particularly for young adult survivors who are more prone to becoming lost to follow up.

References

1. Majhail NS, Tao L, Bredeson C, et al. Prevalence of hematopoietic cell transplant survivors in the United States. *Biol Blood Marrow Transplant*. 2013;19(10):1498-1501.
2. Martin PJ, Counts GW Jr, Appelbaum FR, et al. Life expectancy in patients surviving more than 5 years after hematopoietic cell transplantation. *J Clin Oncol*. 2010;28(6):1011-1016.
3. Majhail NS, Bajorunaite R, Lazarus HM, et al. Long-term survival and late relapse in 2-year survivors of autologous haematopoietic cell transplantation for Hodgkin and non-Hodgkin lymphoma. *Br J Haematol*. 2009;147(1):129-139.
4. Bhatia S, Francisco L, Carter A, et al. Late mortality after allogeneic hematopoietic cell transplantation and functional status of long-term survivors: report from the Bone Marrow Transplant Survivor Study. *Blood*. 2007;110(10):3784-3792.
5. Wingard JR, Majhail NS, Brazauskas R, et al. Long-term survival and late deaths after allogeneic hematopoietic cell transplantation. *J Clin Oncol*. 2011;29(16):2230-2239.
6. Sun CL, Francisco L, Kawashima T, et al. Prevalence and predictors of chronic health conditions after hematopoietic cell transplantation: a report from the Bone Marrow Transplant Survivor Study. *Blood*. 2010;116(17):3129-3139.
7. Bhatia S, Dai C, Landier W, et al. Trends in late mortality and life expectancy after allogeneic blood or marrow transplantation over 4 decades: a blood or marrow transplant survivor study report. *JAMA Oncol*. 2021;7(11):1626-1634.
8. Khera N, Storer B, Flowers MED, et al. Nonmalignant late effects and compromised functional status in survivors of hematopoietic stem cell transplantation. *J Clin Oncol*. 2012;30(1):71-77.
9. Majhail NS, DeFor T, Lazarus HM, Burns LJ. High prevalence of iron overload in adult allogeneic hematopoietic cell transplant survivors. *Biol Blood Marrow Transplant*. 2008;14(7):790-794.
10. Allan EJ, Flowers MED, Lin MP, et al. Visual acuity and anterior segment findings in chronic graft-versus-host disease. *Cornea*. 2011;30(12):1392-1397.
11. McDonald GB, Sullivan KM, Plumley TF. Radiographic features of esophageal involvement in chronic graft-vs.-host disease. *AJR Am J Roentgenol*. 1984;142(3):501-506.
12. Au BKC, Au MA, Chien JW. Bronchiolitis obliterans syndrome epidemiology after allogeneic hematopoietic cell transplantation. *Biol Blood Marrow Transplant*. 2011;17(7):1072-1078.
13. Inamoto Y, Pidala J, Chai X, et al. Assessment of joint and fascia manifestations in chronic graft-versus-host disease. *Arthritis Rheumatol*. 2014;66(4):1044-1052.
14. Carpenter PA, Logan BR, Lee SJ, et al. A phase II/III randomized, multicenter trial of prednisone/sirolimus versus prednisone/sirolimus/calcineurin inhibitor for the treatment of chronic graft-versus-host disease: BMT CTN 0801. *Haematologica*. 2018;103(11):1915-1924.
15. Inamoto Y, Storer BE, Petersdorf EW, et al. Incidence, risk factors and outcomes of sclerosis in patients with chronic graft-versus-host disease. *Blood*. 2013;121(25):5098-5103.
16. Skert C, Patriarca F, Sperotto A, et al. Sclerodermatous chronic graft-versus-host disease after allogeneic hematopoietic cell transplantation incidence, predictors and outcome. *Haematologica*. 2006;91(2):258-261.
17. Foord AM, Cushing-Haugen KL, Boeckh MJ, et al. Late infectious complications in hematopoietic cell transplantation survivors: a population-based study. *Blood Adv*. 2020;4(7):1232-1241.
18. Jinta M, Ohashi K, Ohta T, et al. Clinical features of allogeneic hematopoietic stem cell transplantation-associated organizing pneumonia. *Bone Marrow Transplant*. 2007;40(5):465-472.
19. Palmas A, Tefferi A, Myers JL, et al. Late-onset noninfectious pulmonary complications after allogeneic hematopoietic cell transplantation. *Br J Haematol*. 1998;100(4):680-687.
20. Dandoy CE, Hirsch R, Chima R, et al. Pulmonary hypertension after hematopoietic stem cell transplantation. *Biol Blood Marrow Transplant*. 2013;19(11):1546-1556.
21. Schlemmer F, Chevret S, Lorillon G, et al. Late-onset noninfectious interstitial lung disease after allogeneic hematopoietic stem cell transplantation. *Respir Med*. 2014;108(10):1525-1533.
22. Armenian SH, Sun CL, Shannon T, et al. Incidence and predictors of congestive heart failure after autologous hematopoietic cell transplantation. *Blood*. 2011;118(23):6023-6029.
23. Chow EJ, Wong K, Lee SJ, et al. Late cardiovascular complications after hematopoietic cell transplantation. *Biol Blood Marrow Transplant*. 2014;20(6):794-800.
24. Hingorani S. Kidney and bladder complications of hematopoietic cell transplantation. In: Forman SJ, Negrin RS, Antin JH, Appelbaum FR, eds. *Thomas' Hematopoietic Cell Transplantation*. 5th ed. John Wiley & Sons, Ltd; 2016:1131-1141.
25. Wu NL, Hingorani S, Cushing-Haugen KL, et al. Late kidney morbidity and mortality in hematopoietic cell transplant survivors. *Transplant Cell Ther*. 2021;27(5):434.e1-434.e6.
26. Reddy P, Johnson K, Uberti JP, et al. Nephrotic syndrome associated with chronic graft-versus-host disease after allogeneic hematopoietic cell transplantation. *Bone Marrow Transplant*. 2006;38(5):351-357.
27. Laskin BL, Goebel J, Davies SM, Jodele S. Small vessels, big trouble in the kidneys and beyond: hematopoietic cell transplantation-associated thrombotic microangiopathy. *Blood*. 2011;118(6):1452-1462.
28. Sudour H, Mainard L, Baumann C, et al. Focal nodular hyperplasia of the liver following hematopoietic SCT. *Bone Marrow Transplant*. 2009;43(2):127-132.
29. Pillon M, Carucci NS, Mainardi C, et al. Focal nodular hyperplasia of the liver: an emerging complication of hematopoietic SCT in children. *Bone Marrow Transplant*. 2015;50(3):414-419.
30. Strasser SI, Sullivan KM, Myerson D, et al. Cirrhosis of the liver in long-term marrow transplant survivors. *Blood*. 1999;93(10):3259-3266.
31. Inamoto Y, Petricek I, Burns L, et al. Non-graft-versus-host disease ocular complications after hematopoietic cell transplantation: expert review from the Late Effects and Quality of Life Working Committee of the CIBMTR and the Transplant Complications Working Party of the ESBMT. *Bone Marrow Transplant*. 2019;25(5):145-154.
32. Arora M, Cutler CS, Jagasia MH, et al. Late acute and chronic graft-versus-host disease after allogeneic hematopoietic cell transplantation. *Biol Blood Marrow Transplant*. 2016;22(3):449-455.
33. Bar M, Ott SM, Lewiecki EM, et al. Bone health management after hematopoietic cell transplantation: an expert panel opinion from the American Society for Transplantation and Cellular Therapy. *Biol Blood Marrow Transplant*. 2020;26(10):1784-1802.
34. Greenfield DM, Salooja N, Peczynski C, et al. Metabolic syndrome and cardiovascular disease after hematopoietic cell transplantation in adults: an EBMT cross-sectional non-interventional study. *Bone Marrow Transplant*. 2021;56(11):2820-2825.
35. Armenian SH, Cun CL, Vase T, et al. Cardiovascular risk factors in hematopoietic cell transplantation survivors: role in development of subsequent cardiovascular disease. *Blood*. 2012;120(23):4505-4512.
36. Phelan R, Im A, Hunter RL, et al. Male-specific late effects in adult hematopoietic cell transplantation recipients: a systematic review from the late effects and quality of life working committee of the CIBMTR and transplant complications working party of the ESBMT. *Transplant Cell Ther*. 2021;57(7):1150-1163.
37. Jim HS, Sutton SK, Jacobsen PB, et al. Risk factors for depression and fatigue among survivors of hematopoietic cell transplantation. *Cancer*. 2016;122(8):1290-1297.
38. Dandoy CE, Rotz S, Alonso PB, et al. A pragmatic multi-institutional approach to understanding transplant-associated thrombotic microangiopathy after stem cell transplant. *Blood Adv*. 2021;5(1):1-11.
39. Jodele S, Laskin BL, Dandoy CE, et al. A new paradigm: diagnosis and management of HSCT-associated thrombotic microangiopathy as multi-system endothelial injury. *Blood Rev*. 2015;29(3):191-204.
40. Sanders JE, Hoffmeister PA, Woolfrey AE, et al. Thyroid function following hematopoietic cell transplantation in children: 30-years experience. *Blood*. 2009;113(2):306-308.
41. Stewart BL, Storer B, Storek J, et al. Duration of immunosuppressive treatment for chronic graft-versus-host disease. *Blood*. 2004;104(12):3501-3506.
42. Newell LF, Flowers ME, Gooley TA, et al. Characteristics of chronic GVHD after cord blood transplantation. *Bone Marrow Transplant*. 2013;48(10):1285-1290.
43. Miyamura K, Yamashita T, Atsuta Y, et al. High probability of follow-up termination among AYA survivors after allogeneic hematopoietic cell transplantation. *Blood Adv*. 2019;3(3):397-405.
44. Center for International Blood and Marrow Transplant Research (CIBMTR). *Post-Transplant Guidelines*; 2012. Accessed January 7, 2023. https://www.cibmtr.org/ReferenceCenter/Patient/Guidelines/pages/index.aspx
45. Children's Oncology Group. *Long-Term Follow-Up Guidelines for Survivors of Childhood, Adolescent, and Young Adult Cancers*. Accessed January 7, 2023. http://www.survivorshipguidelines.org/
46. Chow EJ, Anderson L, Baker KS, et al. Late effects surveillance recommendations among survivors of childhood hematopoietic cell transplantation: a children's oncology group report. *Biol Blood Marrow Transplant*. 2016;22(5):782-795.
47. International Guideline Harmonization Group for Late Effects of Childhood Cancer. Accessed January 7, 2023. https://www.ighg.org/international-guideline-harmonization-group/

48. Shenoy S, Gaziev J, Angelucci E, et al. Late effects screening guidelines after hematopoietic cell transplantation (HCT) for hemoglobinopathy: consensus statement from the second pediatric blood and marrow transplant consortium international conference on late effects after pediatric HCT. *Biol Blood Marrow Transplant.* 2018;24(7):1313-1321.
49. Heimall J, Buckley RH, Puck J, et al. Recommendations for screening and management of late effects in patients with severe combined immunodeficiency after allogenic hematopoietic cell transplantation: a consensus statement from the second pediatric blood and marrow transplant consortium international conference on late effects after pediatric HCT. *Biol Blood Marrow Transplant.* 2017;23(8):1229-1240.
50. Dietz AC, Savage SA, Vlachos A, et al. Late effects screening guidelines after hematopoietic cell transplantation for inherited bone marrow failure syndromes: consensus statement from the second pediatric blood and marrow transplant consortium international conference on late effects after pediatric HCT. *Biol Blood Marrow Transplant.* 2017;23(9):1422-1428.
51. Carpenter PA. How I conduct a comprehensive chronic graft-versus-host disease assessment. *Blood.* 2011;118(10):2679-2687.
52. Carpenter PA, Englund JA. How I vaccinate blood and marrow transplant recipients. *Blood.* 2016;127(23):2824-2832.
53. Bhatt NS, Brazauskas R, Salit R, et al. Return to work among young adult survivors of allogeneic hematopoietic cell transplantation in the United States. *Transplant Cell Ther.* 2021;27(8):679.e1-679.e8.
54. Salit RB, Lee SJ, Burns LJ, et al. Return-to-work guidelines and programs for post-hematopoietic cell transplantation survivors: an initial survey. *Biol Blood Marrow Transplant.* 2020;26(8):1520-1526.
55. Kharfan-Dabaja MA, Kumar A, Ayala E, et al. Standardizing definitions of hematopoietic recovery, graft rejection, graft failure, poor graft function, and donor chimerism in allogeneic hematopoietic cell transplantation: a report on behalf of the American Society for Transplantation and Cellular Therapy. *Transplant Cell Ther.* 2021;27(8):642-649.
56. Hartz B, Marsh R, Rao K, et al. The minimum required level of donor chimerism in hereditary hemophagocytic lymphohistiocytosis. *Blood.* 2016;127(25):3281-3290.
57. Altes A, Remacha AF, Sarda P, et al. Frequent severe liver iron overload after stem cell transplantation and its possible association with invasive aspergillosis. *Bone Marrow Transplant.* 2004;34(6):505-509.
58. Lucarelli G, Angelucci E, Giardini C, et al. Fate of iron stores in thalassemia after bone marrow transplantation. *Lancet.* 1993;342:1388-1391.
59. Trottier BJ, Burns LJ, Defor TE, et al. Association of iron overload with allogeneic hematopoietic cell transplantation outcomes: a prospective cohort study using R2-MRI-measured liver iron content. *Blood.* 2013;122:1678-1684.
60. St Pierre TG, Clark PR, Chua-anusorn W, et al. Noninvasive measurement and imaging of liver iron concentrations using proton magnetic resonance. *Blood.* 2005;105(2):855-861.
61. Angelucci E, Muretto P, Lucarelli G, et al. Phlebotomy to reduce iron overload in patients cured of thalassemia by bone marrow transplantation. Italian Cooperative Group for Phlebotomy Treatment of Transplanted Thalassemia Patients. *Blood.* 1997;90(3):994-998.
62. Mariotti E, Angelucci E, Agostini A, Baronciani D, Sgarbi E, Lucarelli G. Evaluation of cardiac status in iron-loaded thalassaemia patients following bone marrow transplantation: improvement in cardiac function during reduction in body iron burden. *Br J Haematol.* 1998;103(4):916-921.
63. Baird K, Cooke K, Schultz KR. Chronic graft-versus-host disease (GVHD) in children. *Pediatr Clin North Am.* 2010;57(1):297-322.
64. Zecca M, Prete A, Rondelli R, et al. Chronic graft-versus-host disease in children: incidence, risk factors, and impact on outcome. *Blood.* 2002;100(4):1192-1200.
65. Cuvelier GDE, Nemecek ER, Wahlstrom JT, et al. Benefits and challenges with diagnosing chronic and late acute GVHD in children using the NIH consensus criteria. *Blood.* 2019;134(3):304-316.
66. Norkin M, Shaw BE, Brazauskas R, et al. Characteristics of late fatal infections after allogeneic hematopoietic cell transplantation. *Biol Blood Marrow Transplant.* 2019;25(2):362-368.
67. Inamoto Y, Lee SJ, Onstad LE, et al. Refined National Institutes of Health response algorithm for chronic graft-versus-host disease in joints and fascia. *Blood Adv.* 2020;4(1):40-46.
68. Carpenter PA, Kitko CL, Elad S, et al. National institutes of health consensus development project on criteria for clinical trials in chronic graft-versus-host disease: V. The 2014 ancillary therapy and supportive care working group report. *Biol Blood Marrow Transplant.* 2015;21(7):1167-1187.
69. Interim clinical considerations for use of COVID-19 vaccines currently approved or authorized in the United States. Accessed January 7, 2023. https://www.cdc.gov/vaccines/covid-19/clinical-considerations/covid-19-vaccines-us.html
70. Recommendations of the National Comprehensive Cancer Network® (NCCN®) Advisory Committee on COVID-19 Vaccination and Pre-exposure Prophylaxis* Version 5.0 01/04/2022. Accessed January 7, 2023. https://www.nccn.org/docs/default-source/covid-19/2021_covid_19_vaccination_guidance_v5-0.pdf?sfvrsn=b483da2b_74
71. Baumrin E, Izaguirre NE, Bausk B, et al. Safety and reactogenicity of the recombinant zoster vaccine after allogeneic hematopoietic cell transplantation. *Blood Av.* 2021;5(6):1585-1593.
72. Pergam SA, Englund JA, Kamboj, et al. Preventing measles in immunosuppressed cancer and hematopoietic cell transplantation patients: a position statement by the ASTCT. *Biol Blood Marrow Transplant.* 2019;25(11):321-330.
73. Rubin LG, Levin MJ, Ljungman P, et al. IDSA clinical practice guideline for vaccination of the immunocompromised host. *Clin Infect Dis.* 20132014;58(3):e44-e100.
74. Five things physicians and patients should question. Choosing Wisely - An initiative of the ABIM Foundation [Internet]. Accessed January 7, 2023. https://www.choosingwisely.org/wp-content/uploads/2018/01/ASTCT-CTTC-Choosing-Wisely-List_2019.pdf
75. Chien JW, Martin PJ, Gooley TA, et al. Airflow obstruction after myeloablative allogeneic hematopoietic stem cell transplantation. *Am J Respir Crit Care Med.* 2003;168(2):208-214.
76. Cheng GS, Storer B, Chien JW, et al. Lung function trajectory in bronchiolitis obliterans syndrome after allogeneic hematopoietic cell transplant. *Ann Am Thorac Soc.* 2016;13(11):1932-1938.
77. Jagasia M, Greinix HT, Arora M, et al. National institutes of health consensus development project on criteria for clinical trials in chronic graft-versus-host disease: I. The 2014 diagnosis and staging working group report. *Biol Blood Marrow Transplant.* 2015;21(3):389-401.
78. Rayment JH, Sandoval RA, Roden JP, Schultz KR. Multiple breath washout testing to identify pulmonary chronic graft versus host disease in children after haematopoietic stem cell transplantation. *Transplant Cell Ther.* 2022;28(6):328.e1-328.e7.
79. Galbán CJ, Boes JL, Bule M, et al. Parametric response mapping as an indicator of bronchiolitis obliterans syndrome after hematopoietic stem cell transplantation. *Biol Blood Marrow Transplant.* 2014;20(10):1592-1598.
80. Bergeron A, Chevret S, Chagnon K, et al. Budesonide/Formoterol for bronchiolitis obliterans after hematopoietic stem cell transplantation. *Am J Respir Crit Care Med.* 2015;191(11):1242-1249.
81. Williams KM, Cheng GS, Pusic I, et al. Fluticasone, azithromycin, and montelukast treatment for new-onset bronchiolitis obliterans syndrome after hematopoietic cell transplantation. *Biol Blood Marrow Transplant.* 2016;22(4):710-716.
82. Cheng GS, Bondeelle L, Gooler T, et al. Azithromycin use and increased cancer risk among patients with bronchiolitis obliterans after hematopoietic cell transplantation. *Biol Blood Marrow Transplant.* 2020;26(2):393-400.
83. Baker KS, Ness KK, Steinberger J, et al. Diabetes, hypertension, and cardiovascular events in survivors of hematopoietic cell transplantation: a report from the bone marrow transplantation survivor study. *Blood.* 2007;109(4):1765-1772.
84. Chow EJ, Baker KS, Lee SJ, et al. Influence of conventional cardiovascular risk factors and lifestyle characteristics on cardiovascular disease after hematopoietic cell transplantation. *J Clin Oncol.* 2014;32(3):191-198.
85. Baker KS, Chow E, Steinberger J. Metabolic syndrome and cardiovascular risk in survivors after hematopoietic cell transplantation. *Bone Marrow Transplant.* 2012;47(5):619-625.
86. Meacham LR, Chow EJ, Ness KK, et al. Cardiovascular risk factors in adult survivors of pediatric cancer--a report from the childhood cancer survivor study. *Cancer Epidemiol Biomarkers Prev.* 2010;19(1):170-181.
87. Armenian SH, Sun CL, Mills G, et al. Predictors of late cardiovascular complications in survivors of hematopoietic cell transplantation. *Biol Blood Marrow Transplant.* 2010;16(8):1138-1144.
88. Sapkota Y, Li N, Pierzuynski J, et al. Contribution of polygenic risk to hypertension among long-term survivors of childhood cancer. *JACC CardioOncol.* 2021;3(1):76-84.
89. Armenian SH, Sun CL, Francisco L, et al. Late congestive heart failure after hematopoietic cell transplantation. *J Clin Oncol.* 2008;26(34):5537-5543.
90. Yeh J, Whited L, Saliba RM, et al. Cardiac toxicity after matched allogeneic hematopoietic cell transplantation in the posttransplant cyclophosphamide era. *Blood Adv.* 2021;5(24):5599-5607.
91. Armenian S, Bhatia S. Predicting and preventing anthracycline-related cardiotoxicity. *Am Soc Clin Oncol Educ Book.* 2018;38:3-12.
92. Armenian SH, Ding Y, Mills G, et al. Genetic susceptibility to anthracycline-related congestive heart failure in survivors of hematopoietic cell transplantation. *Br J Haematol.* 2013;163(2):205-213.
93. Armenian SH, Rinderknecht D, Au K, et al. Accuracy of a novel handheld wireless platform for detection of cardiac dysfunction in anthracycline-exposed survivors of childhood cancer. *Clin Cancer Res.* 2018;24(13):3119-3125.
94. Dixon SB, Howell CR, Lu L, et al. Cardiac biomarkers and association with subsequent cardiomyopathy and mortality among adult survivors of childhood cancer: a report from the St. Judes Lifetime Cohort. *Cancer.* 2021;127(3):458-466.
95. The Childhood Cancer Survivor Study. CCSS Cardiovascular Risk Calculator. St. Jude Childrens' Research Hospital. Accessed January 7, 2023. https://ccss.stjude.org/cvcalc
96. Kobashigawa JA, Katznelson S, Laks H, et al. Effect of pravastatin on outcomes after cardiac transplantation. *N Engl J Med.* 1995;333(10):621-627.
97. Mahle WT, Vincent RN, Berg AM, Kanter KR. Pravastatin therapy is associated with reduction in coronary allograft vasculopathy in pediatric heart transplantation. *J Heart Lung Transplant.* 2005;24(1):63-66.
98. Argent E, Kainer G, Aitken M, et al. Atorvastatin treatment for hyperlipidemia in pediatric renal transplant recipients. *Pediatr Transplant.* 2003;7(1):38-42.
99. Cosio FG, Pesavento TE, Pelletier RP, et al. Patient survival after renal transplantation III: the effects of statins. *Am J Kidney Dis.* 2002;40(3):638-643.
100. Wang GJ, Cui Q, Balian G. The Nicolas Andry award. The pathogenesis and prevention of steroid-induced osteonecrosis. *Clin Orthop Relat Res.* 2000;(370):295-310.
101. Pritchett JW. Statin therapy decreases the risk of osteonecrosis in patients receiving steroids. *Clin Orthop Relat Res.* 2001;(386):173-178.
102. Prasad GV, Ahmed A, Nash MM, Zaltzman JS. Blood pressure reduction with HMG-CoA reductase inhibitors in renal transplant recipients. *Kidney Int.* 2003;63(1):360-364.
103. Prasad GV, Chiu R, Nash MM, Zaltzman JS. Statin use and bone mineral density in renal transplant recipients. *Am J Transplant.* 2003;3(10):1320-1321.

104. Tsiara S, Elisaf M, Mikhailidis DP. Early vascular benefits of statin therapy. *Curr Med Res Opin.* 2003;19(6):540-556.
105. Fehr T, Kahlert C, Fierz W, et al. Statin-induced immunomodulatory effects on human T cells in vivo. *Atherosclerosis.* 2004;175(1):83-90.
106. Mach F. Statins as immunomodulatory agents. *Circulation.* 2004;109(21 suppl. 1):II15-II17.
107. Pritchett JW. Statins and dietary fish oils improve lipid composition in bone marrow and joints. *Clin Orthop Relat Res.* 2007;456:233-237.
108. Hingorani S. Renal complications after hematopoietic-cell transplantation. *N Engl J Med.* 2016;374(23):2256-2267.
109. Hingorani S, Guthrie KA, Schoch G, et al. Chronic kidney disease in long-term survivors of hematopoietic cell transplant. *Bone Marrow Transplant.* 2007;39:223-229.
110. Hingorani SR, Seidel K, Lindner A, et al. Albuminuria in hematopoietic cell transplantation patients: prevalence, clinical associations, and impact on survival. *Biol Blood Marrow Transplant.* 2008;14(12):1365-1372.
111. Beyar-Katz O, Davila EK, Zucjerman T, et al. Adult nephrotic syndrome after hematopoietic cell transplantation; renal pathology is the best predictor of response to therapy. *Biol Blood Marrow Transplant.* 2016;22(6):975-981.
112. Srinivasan R, Balow JE, Sabnis S, et al. Nephrotic syndrome: an under-recognised immune-mediated complication of non-myeloablative allogeneic haematopoietic cell transplantation. *Br J Haematol.* 2005;131(1):7-79.
113. Epperla N, Li A, Logan B, et al. Incidence, risk factors for and outcomes of transplant-associated thrombotic microangiopathy. *Br J Haematol.* 2020;189(6):1171-1181.
114. Jodele S, Dandoy CE, Lane A, et al. Complement blockade for TA-TMA: lessons learned from a large pediatric cohort treated with eculizumab. *Blood.* 2020;135(13):1049-1057.
115. Vincent F, Costa MA, Rondeau E. Chronic renal failure: a nonmalignant late effect of allogeneic stem cell transplantation. *Blood.* 2003;102(7):2695-2696
116. Barnett AH, Bain SC, Bouter P, et al. Angiotensin-receptor blockade versus converting-enzyme inhibition in type 2 diabetes and nephropathy. *N Engl J Med.* 2004;351(19):1952-1961.
117. Strippoli GF, Craig M, Deeks JJ, Schena FP, Craig JC. Effects of angiotensin converting enzyme inhibitors and angiotensin II receptor antagonists on mortality and renal outcomes in diabetic nephropathy: systematic review. *Br Med J.* 2004;329(7470):828.
118. Schulte CMS, Beelen DW. Bone loss following hematopoietic stem cell transplantation; a long-term follow-up. *Blood.* 2004;103(10):3635-3643.
119. Tauchmanova L, Colao A, Lombardi G, et al. Bone loss and its management in long-term survivors from allogeneic stem cell transplantation. *J Clin Endocrinol Metab.* 2007;92(12):4536-4545.
120. Pundole XN, Barbo AG, Lin H, et al. Increased incidence of fractures in recipients of hematopoietic stem-cell transplantation. *J Clin Oncol.* 2015;33(12):1364-1370.
121. Pundole X, Murphy WA, Ebede CC, et al. Fracture risk prediction using FRAX in patients following hematopoietic stem cell transplantation. *Arch Osteoporos.* 2018;13(1):38.
122. Carpenter PA, Hoffmeister P, Chesnut CH III, et al. Bisphosphonate therapy for reduced bone mineral density in children with chronic graft-versus-host disease. *Biol Blood Marrow Transplant.* 2007;13:683-690.
123. Li D, Yang Z, Wei Z, Kang P. Efficacy of bisphosphonates in the treatment of femoral head osteonecrosis: a PRISMA-compliant meta-analysis of animal studies and clinical trials. *Sci Rep.* 2018;8(1):1450.
124. Mont MA, Cherian JJ, Sierra RJ, et al. Nontraumatic osteonecrosis of the femoral head: where do we stand today? A ten-year update. *J Bone Joint Surg Am.* 2015;97(19):1604-1627.
125. Hua KC, Yang XG, Feng JT, et al. The efficacy and safety of core decompression for the treatment of femoral head necrosis: a systematic review and meta-analysis. *J Orthop Surg Res.* 2019;14(1):306-31511030.
126. Hoffmeister PA, Storee BE, Sanders JE. Diabetes mellitus in long-term survivors of pediatric hematopoietic stem cell transplantation. *J Pediatr Hematol Oncol.* 2004;26(2):81-90.
127. Vexiau P, Perez-Castiglioni P, Socié G, et al. The 'euthyroid sick syndrome': incidence, risk factors and prognostic value soon after allogeneic bone marrow transplantation. *Br J Haematol.* 1993;85(4):778-782.
128. Lee V, Cheng PS, Chik KW, et al. Autoimmune hypothyroidism after unrelated haematopoietic stem cell transplantation in children. *J Pediatr Hematol Oncol.* 2006;28(5):293-295.
129. Karthaus M, Gabrysiak T, Brabant G, et al. Immune thyroiditis after transplantation of allogeneic CD34+ selected peripheral blood cells. *Bone Marrow Transplant.* 1997;20(8):697-699.
130. Patriarca F, Skert C, Sperotto A, et al. The development of autoantibodies after allogeneic stem cell transplantation is related with chronic graft-vs-host disease and immune recovery. *Exp Hematol.* 2006;34(3):389-396.
131. Lortan JE, Rochfort NC, el Tumi M, Vellodi A. Autoantibodies after bone marrow transplantation in children with genetic disorders: relation to chronic graft-versus-host disease. *Bone Marrow Transplant.* 1992;9(5):325-330.
132. Arlt W, Allolio B. Adrenal insufficiency. *Lancet.* 2003;361(9372):1881-1893.
133. Krasner AS. Glucocorticoid-induced adrenal insufficiency. *JAMA.* 1999;282(7):671-676.
134. Oelkers W. Adrenal insufficiency. *N Engl J Med.* 1996;335(16):1206-1212.
135. Powell GF, Brasel JA, Blizzard RM. Emotional deprivation and growth retardation simulating idiopathic hypopituitarism. I. Clinical evaluation of the syndrome. *N Engl J Med.* 1967;276(23):1271-1278.
136. Powell GF, Brasel JA, Raiti S, Blizzard RM. Emotional deprivation and growth retardation simulating idiopathic hypopituitarism. II. Endocrinologic evaluation of the syndrome. *N Engl J Med.* 1967;276(23):1279-1283.
137. Allen DB, Julius JR, Breen TJ, Attie KM. Treatment of glucocorticoid-induced growth suppression with growth hormone. National Cooperative Growth Study. *J Clin Endo Metabol.* 1998;83(8):2824-2829.
138. Tejani A, Butt KM, Rajpoot D, et al. Strategies for optimizing growth in children with kidney transplants. *Transplantation.* 1989;47(2):229-233.
139. Broyer M, Guest G, Gagnadoux MF. Growth rate in children receiving alternate-day corticosteroid treatment after kidney transplantation. *J Pediatr.* 1992;120(5):721-725.
140. Reimer LG, Morris HG, Ellis EF. Growth of asthmatic children during treatment with alternate-day steriods. *J Allergy Clin Immunol.* 1975;55(4):224-231.
141. Ketterl TG, Chow EJ, Leisenring WM, et al. Adipokines, inflammation, and adiposity in hematopoietic cell transplantation survivors. *Biol Blood Marrow Transplant.* 2018;24(3):622-626.
142. Armenian SH, Chemaitilly W, Chen M, et al. National Institutes of Health hematopoietic cell transplantation late effects initiative: the cardiovascular disease and associated risk factors working group report. *Biol Blood Marrow Transplant.* 2017;23(2):201-210.
143. Kamel A, Norgren S, Elimam A, et al. Effects of growth hormone treatment in obese prepubertal boys. *J Clin Endo Metabol.* 2000;85(4):1412-1419.
144. Grauer O, Wolff D, Betz H, et al. Neurological manifestations of chronic graft-versus-host disease after allogeneic haematopoietic stem cell transplantation: report from the Consensus Conference on Clinical Practice in chronic graft-versus-host disease. *Brain.* 2010;133(10):2852-2865.
145. Vinnakota JM, Zeiser R. Acute graft-versus-host disease, infections, vascular events and drug toxicities affecting the central nervous system. *Front Immunol.* 2021;12:748019.
146. Saad AG, Alyea EP, Wen PY, et al. *J Clin Oncol.* 2009;27(30):e147-e149.
147. Armenian SH, Sun CL, Francisco L, et al. Health behaviors and cancer screening practices in long-term survivors of hematopoietic cell transplantation (HCT): a report from the BMT Survivor Study. *Bone Marrow Transplant.* 2012;47(2):283-290.
148. Rizzo JD, Curtis RE, Socie G, et al. Solid cancers after allogeneic hematopoietic cell transplantation. *Blood.* 2009;113(5):1175-1183.
149. Curtis RE, Travis LB, Rowlings PA, et al. Risk of lymphoproliferative disorders after bone marrow transplantation: a multi-institutional study. *Blood.* 1999;94(7):2208-2216.
150. Inamoto Y, Shah NN, Savani BN, et al. Secondary solid cancer screening following hematopoietic cell transplantation. *Bone Marrow Transplant.* 2015;50(8):1013-1023.
151. Kratz CP, Achatz MI, Brugières L, et al. Cancer screening recommendations for individuals with Li-Fraumeni syndrome. *Clin Cancer Res.* 2017;23(11):e38-e45.
152. Morton LM, Saber W, Baker KS, et al. National Institutes of Health hematopoietic cell transplantation late effects initiative: the subsequent neoplasms working group report. *Biol Blood Marrow Transplant.* 2017;23(3):367-378.
153. Baker KS, Leisenring WM, Goodman PJ, et al. Total body irradiation dose and risk of subsequent neoplasms following allogeneic hematopoietic cell transplantation. *Blood.* 2019;133(26):2790-2799.
154. Naldi L, Adamoli L, Fraschini D, et al. Number and distribution of melanocytic nevi in individuals with a history of childhood leukemia. *Cancer.* 1996;77(7):1402-1408.
155. Taitz J, Cohn RJ, White L, et al. Osteochondroma after total body irradiation: an age-related complication. *Pediatr Blood Cancer.* 2004;42(3):225-229.
156. Van de Poll-Franse LV, Nicolaije KA, Ezendam NP. The impact of cancer survivorship care plans on patient and health care provider outcomes: a current perspective. *Acta Oncol.* 2017;56(2):134-138.
157. Majhail NS, Murphy E, Laud P, et al. Randomized controlled trial of individualized treatment summary and survivorship care plans for hematopoietic cell transplantation survivors. *Haematologica.* 2019;104(5):1084-1092.
158. Khera N, Chow EJ, Leisenring WM, et al. Factors associated with adherence to preventive care practices among hematopoietic cell transplantation survivors. *Biol Blood Marrow Transplant.* 2011;17(7):995-1003.
159. Hashmi SK, Lee SJ, Savani BN, et al. ASBMT practice guidelines committee survey on long-term follow-up clinics for hematopoietic cell transplant survivors. *Biol Blood Marrow Transplant.* 2018;24(6):1119-1124.
160. Hashmi S, Carpenter P, Khera N, et al. Lost in transition: the essential need for long-term follow-up clinic for blood and marrow transplantation survivors. *Biol Blood Marrow Transplant.* 2014;21(2):225-232.

Index

Note: Page numbers followed by *f* and *t* indicates figures and tables respectively.

A

Abciximab, 1291
Abdominal infections, 1480
Abdominal pain, 816, 840, 1144, 2245
   crampy, 1169
Abdominal trauma, 1432
Abelson murine leukemia virus (A-MuLV), 1782
Aberrant erythropoietin secretion, 1076
Aberrant T-cell population detection, 22, 25–26*f*
Abetalipoproteinemia, 743–744, 743*f*
ABL kinase inhibitors, 1458
Abruptio placentae, 1252
Abscesses, 1437–1438
Absolute eosinophil count (AEC), 1836
Absolute lymphocyte count (ALC), 1461
Absolute neutrophil count (ANC), 1331, 1468, 2300
Absorption, inherited disorders of, 963
Acalabrutinib, 1459, 1970, 2032, 2036, 2272
Acanthocytic disorders, 622, 742–743
   abetalipoproteinemia, 743–744
   McLeod phenotype, 744
   neuroacanthocytosis syndromes, 744
Accelerated adenosine triphosphate (ATP), 730
Accelerated erythropoiesis, 620
Acetaminophen, 753, 1109, 1387
Acetylation, 363, 370
Acetylcholinesterase, 796
Acetylsalicylic acid, 1289
Achlorhydria, 638
Achromobacter xylosoxidans, 1950
Acid citrate dextrose, 22
Acid hydrolases, 363
Acid phosphatase, 13
Acid sphingomyelinase deficiency (ASMD), 1362
aCL antibodies, high-titer, 1264
Acquired immunodeficiency syndrome (AIDS), 1233, 1409, 1944, 1951–1952
Actin cytoskeleton, 364
Actin-depolymerizing protein (ADP), 1189, 1346
   ADP-induced platelet aggregation, 1289
α-Actinin 1, 364
Actinomycin, 1108
Actinopathies, 1346–1347
Activated B-cell (ABC), 1908
Activated B-cell-type DLBCL (ABC-type DLBCL), 1877
Activated clotting time (ACT), 1087
Activated partial thromboplastin time (aPTT), 428, 1084–1085, 1085*f*, 1279, 1723
Activated protein C (APC), 441, 535, 1248, 1276
   clinical aspects, 1283
   laboratory diagnosis, 1283
   pathophysiology and genetics, 1283
   resistance, 1283
   treatment, 1284
Activating transcription factor 4 (ATF4), 98
Activation-induced cytidine deaminase (AID), 1397, 2152
Activator protein 1 (AP-1), 301, 1498
Activin receptor–like kinase gene (*ALK*1 gene), 1162
*ACTN*1 genes, 1153, 1960
Actual erythrocytosis, 1071
Actual iron deficiency anemia, 1048
Acute altitude disease, 1074
Acute blood loss, 601, 636
Acute chest syndrome (ACS), 838, 844–845
   causes of, 844*f*
Acute disseminated intravascular coagulation, 1250
Acute erythroleukemia, 1602
Acute febrile illnesses, 1169

Acute graft-*vs*-host disease (aGVHD), 1002, 1476, 2304–2305, 2341, 2355, 2362, 2365, 2382
   acute GVHD scoring, 2305*t*
   clinical manifestations of, 2357
      central nervous system, 2358
      gastrointestinal tract, 2358
      hepatic, 2358
      lung, 2358
      organ staging and overall grading, 2358*t*
      skin, 2357–2358
   epidemiology, 2357
      risk factors, 2357
   pathophysiology, 2355
      acute graft *vs*. host disease pathogenesis, 2356*t*
      effectors, 2357
      mediators, 2356–2357
      sensors, 2356
      triggers, 2355
   prevention, 2358–2359
   primary and secondary therapy of acute graft-*vs*-host disease, 2359–2360
   secondary therapy of, 2359–2360
   supportive care, 2360
   treatment of, 2305
Acute hemarthroses, 1205
Acute hemolytic anemia, 752–753, 824, 827
   drug-induced hemolysis, 753
   hemolysis associated with diabetic acidosis, 754
   infection-induced hemolysis, 753
Acute hemolytic transfusion reaction (AHTR), 570, 581
Acute hemorrhage, 1071
Acute hepatic porphyrias (AHPs), 702, 704, 709, 719
   acute intermittent porphyria, 704–708
   ALAD deficiency porphyria, 711–712
   diagnosis and treatment of, 719
   hereditary coproporphyria, 710–711
   variegate porphyria, 708–710
Acute infantile hemorrhagic edema, 1168
Acute intermittent porphyria (AIP), 704
   clinical description, 704–705, 705*t*
   homozygous dominant AIP, 708
   laboratory findings, 706–707
   long-term complications, 705
   long-term management, 708
   molecular basis and pathogenesis, 705–706
   treatment, 707
      emerging therapies, 708
      prevention, of acute attacks, 707–708
      treatment, of ongoing attack, 707
Acute intravascular hemolysis, 754
Acute iron intoxication, 649
Acute kidney injury (AKI), 853, 2379
Acute leukemia, 602, 804, 1102, 1441, 1562, 1595, 1596*f*, 1638, 1645, 1721, 1866, 1900, 2220, 2314
   acute lymphoblastic leukemia, 1602–1604
   acute myeloid leukemia, 1566–1580, 1600–1602
   of ambiguous lineage, 1604–1605, 1604*t*–1605*t*
   B-lymphoblastic leukemia/lymphoma, 1580–1585
   clonal cytopenia of undetermined significance, potential pre-MDS condition, 1600
   diagnostic evaluation, 1595–1596
   genomic perspective of, 1564–1566, 1565*t*, 1566*f*
   immunophenotyping of, 35–37, 36*f*
   multiple hit model of leukemia, 1562–1564
   myelodysplastic syndromes (MDSs), 1596–1600
   reasons for studying molecular genetics of, 1562
      pediatric B-ALL based on cytogenetic and molecular analysis, 1563*t*

      risk groups in adult AML based on cytogenetic and molecular analysis, 1563*t*
   T-lymphoblastic leukemia/lymphoma, 1585–1587
Acute lymphoblastic leukemia (ALL), 37, 272, 330, 1468, 1504, 1509–1511, 1595, 1602–1604, 1608, 1627, 1667, 1694, 1782, 1840, 1942, 1991, 2298–2299, 2335, 2341
   allogeneic hematopoietic cell transplant in management of relapsed ALL, 2342
   children with, 1677
   clinical features, 1611
   conditioning regimen and donor type, 2342
   differential diagnosis, 1612–1613
   health disparities and inequities in ALL, 1685
   hematopoietic stem cell transplantation, 1679–1680
   historical background, 1608–1609
   indications for, 2341–2342
   laboratory features, 1611–1612
   in older patients, 1619–1620
      B-lymphoblastic leukemia cytogenetic subtypes, 1604*t*
      with blasts containing scant, agranular cytoplasm, 1603*f*
      WHO classification of precursor lymphoid neoplasms, 1603*t*
   overall survival, in successive ALL patient cohorts, 1609*f*
   pathophysiology, 1609
      epidemiology, 1609
      etiology, 1609
      molecular pathogenesis, 1610
      percent of new cases by age group, 1609*f*
   Philadelphia positive acute lymphoblastic leukemia (Ph+ ALL), 2342
   precision medicine for, 1680
      BCL-2 family inhibitors, 1680
      current immunotherapeutic approaches, 1681*f*
      epigenetic regulators, 1680
      failure and relapse after T-cell–based immunotherapies, 1682*f*
      immunotherapies, 1680–1683
      kinase inhibitors, 1680
      proteasome inhibitors, 1680
   presenting clinical features, 1668–1669
      germline risk factors for development of ALL, 1668*t*
   presenting laboratory and radiographic features, 1669
   primary therapy, 1614–1620
   prognostic factors, 1613–1614
   risk factors and risk stratification, for treatment allocation, 1669
      clinical features and immunophenotype, 1669–1670
      early treatment response, 1671–1672
      EFS by EOI and end-of-consolidation MRD, 1671*f*
      recurrent sentinel genetic lesions in B-ALL, 1670*t*
      sentinel cytogenetic and molecular genetic alterations, 1670–1671
   risk factors for development of childhood ALL, 1667–1668
      ALL incidence by age, sex, and race/ethnicity, 1668*f*
      improvements in ALL survival over time, 1667*f*
   salvage therapy, 1620
   toxicities and late effects of therapy for, 1683
      cardiac toxicity, 1685
      endocrinologic late effects, 1685
      neuropsychologic sequelae, 1683
      osteonecrosis, 1684–1685
      quality of life, 1683

Acute lymphoblastic leukemia (ALL) (continued)
  secondary malignant neoplasms (SMN), 1683–1684
  treatment, 1672
    BFM and COG-based pediatric ALL chemotherapy, 1672–1673
    maintenance therapy, 1674
    postinduction intensification, 1673–1674
    presymptomatic central nervous system therapy, 1673
    primary treatment, 1672
    remission induction, 1672
  treatment after relapse, 1677
    biology of relapse, 1677
    relapse risk stratification, 1677–1678
    relapse risk stratification by study group, 1678t
    treatment of bone marrow relapse, 1678
    treatment of isolated extramedullary relapse, 1678–1679
  treatment outcome in elderly patients with ALL, 1620t
  unique patient subgroups, 1674
    adolescents and young adults with ALL, 1676
    children with down syndrome and ALL, 1677
    infants with ALL, 1676–1677
    Philadelphia chromosome-positive ALL, 1674–1675
    Philadelphia chromosome–like ALL, 1675
    T-lymphoblastic leukemia/lymphoma, 1675–1676
Acute megakaryoblastic leukemia (AMKL), 361, 1572, 1696
Acute monocytic leukemia, 1364
Acute mountain sickness, 1074
Acute myelogenous leukemia, allogeneic hematopoietic cell transplantation in primary refractory, 2336
Acute myeloid leukemia (AML), 35–37, 55, 57, 63, 316, 976, 1014, 1028, 1468, 1495, 1530, 1562, 1566, 1595, 1600–1602, 1611, 1627, 1667, 1694, 1721, 1737, 1755, 1821, 1928, 1946, 2022, 2122, 2298–2299, 2335
  biologic features, 1632–1633
  cellular and molecular origins of AML, 1694–1696
    survival curves from Children's Oncology Group and St. Jude Consortium, 1695f
  CHIP and AML risk in population studies, 1755–1757
  classification, 1566–1569
    mutations in MDS, secondary AML, and treatment-related AML, 1568f
    stem cells during progression of MDS to s-AML, 1567f
    WHO classification of, 1566t
  classification of, 1638
  clinical presentation, 1630–1631
  cohesins, 1578–1579
  criteria for diagnosis of AML with myelodysplasia-related changes, 1602t
  cytogenetic abnormalities, 1602t, 1633–1634
  diagnostic workup, 1698–1699
  distinctive clinical, morphologic, and immunophenotypic features of, 1601t
  dyspoietic changes in MDSs and AML, 1597f
  epidemiology, 1627, 1694
  epigenetic factors modifying chromatin and DNA, 1572
    ASXL1, 1575
    DNMT3A, 1573–1574
    epigenome in normal and cancer cells, 1572f
    EZH2, 1575
    IDH1/IDH2 and TET2 mutations, 1573
    KMT2A, 1574–1575
    overview of epigenetic factors, 1572–1573
  erythroid-rich myelodysplastic syndrome, 1602f
  European LeukemiaNet AML risk stratification by genetics, 1602t
  in first remission, 2335–2336
    allogeneic hematopoietic cell transplantation in primary refractory AML, 2336
    allogeneic hematopoietic cell transplantation in relapsed, therapy-related, and secondary AML, 2336
    autologous hematopoietic cell transplantation in AML, 2336
  granulocytic sarcoma, 1706
  hematopoietic stem cell transplantation, 1653–1656
  kinases, 1575
    C-KIT mutations, 1576
    FLT3 mutations, 1575–1576
  laboratory findings, 1631–1632
    gingival hypertrophy in patient with AML, 1632f
    leukemia cutis manifesting as subcutaneous nodules, 1631f
  late effects of therapy, 1704
  mixed phenotype acute leukemia (MPAL), 1706
  molecular abnormalities, 1634–1637
  morphologic features of common AML types with recurrent cytogenetic abnormalities, 1601f
  not otherwise specified (NOS), 1599
  nuclear pore proteins, 1576–1578
  predisposing factors and pathophysiology, 1696
    acquired predisposition, 1697
    environmental factors, 1697–1698
    inherited predisposition syndromes, 1696–1697
  prognosis, 1638
    AML deaths by age in United States, 1639f
    AML in pregnancy, 1645
    BCL-2 inhibitor, 1647–1648
    cytarabine, 1643f
    cytogenetic and molecular prognostic factors, 1639–1640
    disease-specific prognostic factors, 1640
    ELN risk stratification by genetics, 1638t
    endpoints of AML treatment, 1641–1642
    FLT3 inhibitors, 1648–1650
    gemtuzumab ozogamicin (GO), 1651–1652
    hedgehog pathway inhibitor, 1651
    IDH inhibitors, 1650–1651
    immunotherapy, 1652–1653
    initial treatment of AML in patients unfit for cytotoxic chemotherapy, 1647
    Kaplan-Meier curve, 1649f, 1651f
    main genomic subtypes of AML, 1639t
    measurable (minimal) residual disease as a prognostic factor, 1640
    overview of treatment, 1642–1643
    patient-specific prognostic factors, 1638–1639
    phases of therapy, 1643f
    postremission therapy, 1645–1646
    presence or absence of FLT3-ITD or NRAS codon 12/13 mutations, 1640t
    relapsed and refractory AML, 1653
    remission induction chemotherapy, 1643–1645
    survival of patients with AML, 1640f
    targeted therapies, 1647
    types of failure in therapy for acute myeloid leukemia, 1642t
  prognostic factors, 1706–1707
    comprehensive genomic profiling, 1710–1711
    disease-associated characteristics, 1709–1710
    disease-associated factors, 1709
    future therapeutic challenges, 1711–1713
    host factors, 1707–1708
    novel cryptic age-specific distributions of validated gene fusions, 1713f
    pie chart representations of cytogenetic abnormalities and gene mutations, 1707f
    therapeutic targets being tested in AML, 1711f
    treatment outcomes from selected pediatric group trials, 1708t
  risk factors, 1627
    age at exposure and temporal pattern effect of developing leukemia, 1629f
    clonal hematopoiesis, 1630
    environmental factors, 1629
    heritable genetic factors, 1629–1630
    lifestyle-related factors, 1629
    myeloid neoplasms with germ line predisposition, 1630t
    occupational exposures, 1629
    therapy-related AML, 1627–1629
  risk stratification of, 1579–1580
  secondary AML, 1706
  spliceosome proteins, 1578
  subtypes, 1699
  supportive care, 1703–1704
  therapy for patients with newly diagnosed AML, 1699
    background, 1699–1700
    induction therapy, 1700–1701
    key characteristics of AML in pediatric vs. adult patients, 1699t
    leukemia cutis in infant with congenital leukemia, 1700f
    postremission therapy, 1701–1703
    therapy for patients with newly diagnosed AML, 1703
  therapy for patients with relapsed/refractory disease, 1703
  therapy-related AML (t-AML), 1706
  transcription factors, 1569
    CCAAT/enhancer binding protein-α (CEBPA), 1571
    core binding factor translocations, 1570–1571
    GATA1/GATA2, 1571–1572
    model for role of nuclear corepressors and RARa fusion proteins, 1569f
    PML::RARA, 1569–1570
  WHO classification of AML and related precursor neoplasms, 1600t
Acute nonlymphocytic leukemia, 1627, 1694
Acute normovolemic hemodilution (ANH), 565
Acute pain crisis episodes in sickle cell disease, 840
Acute panmyelosis with myelofibrosis (APMF), 1595
Acute posthemorrhagic anemia, approach to, 624–625
  clinical features of acute hemorrhage in healthy young adults, 624t
Acute porphyria attacks, 704, 710, 719
  pathogenesis of, 705–706, 706f
  prevention of, 707–708
Acute promyelocytic leukemia (APL), 66, 1253, 1569, 1627, 1694, 1721, 2336
  approach to patients with suspected APL, 1721
  central nervous system prophylaxis (CNS prophylaxis), 1729
  coagulopathy and bleeding, 1723–1724
  epidemiology, 1721
  management of, 1705–1706, 1729–1731
  morphology, 1722f
    and diagnostic approach, 1721–1722
  pathophysiology, 1722–1723
  treatment of, 1724–1726, 1726f–1727f
    clinical trials in treatment of APL, 1725t
    common adverse events associated with agents used in treatment of APL, 1728t
    maintenance therapy, 1728–1729
    optimal dose and schedule for ATRA, 1728
    supportive care, 1729
Acute undifferentiated leukemias, 1604
Acyclovir, 1387, 1389
ADAMTS13 recombinant, 1137
A Disintegrin And Metalloprotease with ThromboSpondin type 1 repeats, member 13 (ADAMTS13), 351, 1124, 1216, 1413
  activity level assists management of TTP, 1137t
  antibody test, 1132
  antigen test, 1131
  autoimmunity, 1133
  causes of, 1124
    ADAMTS13 mutations, 1127
    animal models of ADAMTS13 deficiency, 1127
    characteristics of inhibitors, 1125
    inhibitory antibodies of ADAMTS13, 1124–1125
    pathogenic mechanisms of thrombotic thrombocytopenic purpura, 1127
    targets of ADAMTS13 inhibitors, 1125–1127
  conformation of von Willebrand factor and interaction with, 1128–1129
  gene, 1211, 1429
  GoF variant, 1126
  inhibitors
    domain structures of vWF and ADAMTS13 and interactions, 1126f
    targets of, 1125–1127
    tests, 1132
  mutations, 1127
  role of, 532
  tests, 1131, 1137, 1147
    activity level distinguishes TTP from causes of MAHA and thrombocytopenia, 1131f
Adaptive immunity, 225
  against tumors, 1496–1498
Adaptor protein 3 complex (AP-3), 1190
ADAR1 gene, 2155
Additional sex comb-like 1 (ASXL1), 1636, 1821
Additional X chromosome, 1974
Adenine base editors (ABEs), 1549
Adenine nucleotides, 395
Adeno-associated viruses (AAVs), 708, 1526
Adenosine deaminase (ADA), 763, 1402, 1530, 1541, 1546–1547

deficiency, 763
excess, 764
Adenosine diphosphate (ADP), 362, 394, 404, 534, 1083, 1278, 1402
   nucleotide metabolism and nonmetabolic role for, 395, 396f
   platelet $P2Y_1$ and $P2Y_{12}$ receptor roles in, 408
   receptor signaling, 408–409
Adenosine kinase (ADK), 764
Adenosine triphosphate (ATP), 96, 394, 560, 1059, 1278, 1402, 1784
   energy metabolism and generation of, 395
Adenoviral vectors, 1528
Adenoviruses, 1528
   infections, 2308
Adenylate cyclase 9 (ADCY9), 841
Adenylate kinase deficiency (AK deficiency), 763–765
Adhesive protein receptors
   22q112 deletion syndrome (22q11DS), 1188–1189
   abnormalities of, 1183
   Bernard-Soulier syndrome (BSS), 1184–1188
   defects of collagen receptors, 1189
   Ephrin type B receptor 2 defect (EPHB2 defect), 1189
   Glanzmann thrombasthenia (GT), 1183–1184
   platelet-type von Willebrand disease (PT-VWD), 1188
Adjuvant therapy, 1337
Adoptive cellular immunotherapy, 1508
Adoptive T cell therapy (ACT), 1499, 2126
Adrenal insufficiency (AI), 2381
α-Adrenergic agents, 845
$α_2$-Adrenergic receptors, 409, 1189
Adrenoleukodystrophy (ALD), 1538
Adriamycin, bleomycin, vinblastine, and dacarbazine (ABVD), 2122
Adult T-cell leukemia/lymphoma (ATLL), 34, 1502, 1888, 1931–1932, 1945, 2075
Advanced-stage Hodgkin lymphoma
   adriamycin, bleomycin, vinblastine, and dacarbazine (ABVD), 2122
   autologous transplant as consolidation in stage III-IV Hodgkin lymphoma, 2123–2124
   bleomycin, etoposide, doxorubicin, cyclophosphamide, vincristine, procarbazine, and prednisone, 2122–2123
   brentuximab vedotin, doxorubicin, vinblastine, and dacarbazine, 2123
   initial therapy for, 2122
   radiation therapy as consolidation in stage III-IV classic Hodgkin lymphoma, 2123
   risk-adapted treatment strategies in advanced Hodgkin lymphoma, 2123
   therapy of classic Hodgkin lymphoma, 2124
Aedes aegypti mosquito, 587
Aedes albopictus, 587
Aeromonas hydrophila, 899
AF9 gene, 1574, 1634
AF10 gene, 1634
Afadin gene (*AFDN*), 1634
Afamelanotide, 718
Afibrinogenemia, 474, 1217
   congenital, 474, 1217
   differential diagnosis and therapy of afibrinogenemia, 1217–1218
   laboratory diagnosis, 1217
Age-related chronic gastritis, 960
Age-related clonal hematopoiesis (ARCH), 1697
Age-related enzyme instability, 752
Age-related macular degeneration (AMD), 351, 1143
Agglutinins, incomplete, 571
Aggregation, impaired, 1189
Aggressive lymphomas, 1964
   diffuse large B-cell lymphomas, 1964–1968
Aggressive NK-cell leukemia, 35
Aggressive systemic mastocytosis (ASM), 1771–1772, 1854
Aggressive systemic mastocytosis/mast cell leukemia (ASM/MCL), 1850
Agranulocytosis, 906
AIDS-related lymphoma (ARL), 1415, 1951
   classification of human immunodeficiency virus–associated lymphomas, 1417t
   clinical manifestations, 1416
      Burkitt lymphoma, 1417
      plasmablastic lymphoma, 1418
      primary central nervous system lymphoma, 1417
      primary effusion lymphoma (PEL), 1417

therapy, 1416
   HIV-associated lymphomas, 1416f
   Hodgkin lymphoma (HL), 1418
   non-Hodgkin lymphoma incidence and incidence-based mortality, 1415f
AIDS-related malignancies, 1414–1415
AIHA, idiopathic, 787
Alanine transaminase (ALT), 907
Albumin, 362, 774
   diuresis, 2258
Alcohol, 962–963, 1040, 2119
   abuse, 1028
   consumption, 2176
   intake, 695
Alcohol-induced thrombocytopenia, 1157
Alcoholism, 668–669
Aldehyde dehydrogenase 2 (ALDH2), 978
Alder-Reilly anomaly, 1353
   neutrophils with Alder-Reilly bodies, 1354f
Aldolase, 757
   deficiency, 762
Alemtuzumab, 784, 1455, 1469, 1500–1501, 1845, 1977, 2029, 2101, 2319
Alkaline phosphatase, 1853
   serum, 2244
Alkylating agents, 1370, 1816, 2028
   alkylating agent–associated t-AML, 1628
   chemotherapy, 2140
   combining nucleoside analogs with, 2028
Alkylators, 2270
   alkylator-based therapy, 2249–2250
      alkylator-based chemotherapy for AL, 2250t
      maintenance with, 2209
   doxorubicin-based combination chemotherapy, 2193
All-*trans* retinoic acid (ATRA), 1462, 1569, 1698, 1721
   optimal dose and schedule for ATRA, 1728
Allele-specific oligonucleotide (ASO), 1901
Allele-specific oligonucleotide real-time PCR (ASO–PCR), 65, 1614
   clonality analysis and design, 65f
Alleles, 323
Allelic exclusion, 270–271
Allelic intensity ratio, 54
Allergic diseases, 199–200
Allergic reactions, 584
Allo stem cells, 2303
Alloantibodies, 591, 898, 1113
   in hemophilia A, 1255
      frequency of inhibitors, 1255
      induced antibody titer, 1255
Allogeneic donor blood
   alternatives to, 565
   directed donation (DD), 565–566
Allogeneic donor types, 2300–2301
   ABO incompatibility, 2301
   algorithm of donor search, 2302f
   donor characteristics, 2301
   HLA complex, 2301f
Allogeneic hematopoietic cell transplantation (allo-HCT), 2298, 2335
   impact of allogeneic hematopoietic cell transplantation on risk groups of ALL, 2341–2342
   indications, 2343
      Hodgkin lymphoma, 2344
      mantle cell lymphoma, 2345
      multiple myeloma, 2346
   in management of relapsed ALL, 2342
   in primary refractory AML, 2336
   in relapsed, therapy-related, and secondary AML, 2336
Allogeneic hematopoietic stem cell transplantation (allo-HSCT), 1616, 1627, 1832
Allogeneic stem cell transplantation (allo-SCT), 1800, 1845, 2102, 2184, 2203–2204, 2207, 2257, 2272
   allogeneic stem cell transplantation in patients with high-risk fluorescence in situ hybridization, 2206
   donor lymphocyte infusions, 2206
   European blood and marrow transplantation registry data, 2205f
   HLA-identical reduced-intensity allogeneic SCT, 2205t
   indications for, 2337–2339

myeloablative allogeneic stem cell transplantation, 2204
   nonrandomized comparisons of, 2204t
   reduced-intensity conditioning allo-SCT as part of first-line therapy, 2204–2206
   reduced-intensity conditioning allo-SCT in relapsed setting, 2206
Allogeneic transplant/transplantation, 327, 1522
   relapsed or refractory Hodgkin lymphoma, 2126
   treatment prior to, 2337
Alloimmune thrombocytopenia, 1111
   neonatal alloimmune thrombocytopenia (NAIT), 1111–1113
   posttransfusion purpura (PTP), 1113–1114
Alloimmunization, 898, 1111
   diagnosis and management of, 577
   to transfused antigens, 580
      alloantibodies reacting with leukocyte antigens, 580–581
      alloantibodies reacting with plasma proteins, 581
      alloantibodies reacting with red cell antigens, 580
Alloreactive T cells, 326
Alopecia, 603
Alpha heavy-chain disease, 1950
Alpha-1-antitrypsin inhibitor deficiency, 1528
Alpha-hemoglobin stabilizing protein (AHSP), 102
Altitude sickness, 1074
Alveolar hemorrhage, 639
Alveolar macrophages, 213
Alzheimer disease, 2238
Amegakaryocytic thrombocytopenia, 1157
Amegakaryocytic thrombocytopenia with radioulnar synostosis (ATRUS), 986
   syndrome in association with HOXA11 and MECOM mutation, 1156
American College of Chest Physicians Guidelines, The (ACCP Guidelines), 1288
Amino phospholipids, 726
Aminocaproic acid, 975, 987
ε-Aminocaproic acid (EACA), 1086, 1196, 1228, 1252
5-Aminolevulinic acid (ALA), 98, 656, 702–703
Aminolevulinic acid dehydratase (ALAD)-deficient porphyria (ADP), 704, 711–712
Aminolevulinic acid (ALA) synthase, 100
Aminopterin, 1608
Aminoptyrine, 753
AML1 gene, 1570, 1633
Amniotic fluid embolism, 1252
Amniotic fluid, human, 1053
Amorph type, 742
Amphotropic receptor, 1526
Amplification-refractory mutation system (ARMS), 61, 62f
Amyloid, 2238
   echocardiographic image of concentric thickening of wall of LV due to amyloid, 2243f
   myocardial wall diffusely thickened with, 2243f
   subcutaneous fat aspirate showing amyloid deposits, 2241f
Amyloid deposits, 2259
β-Amyloid fibrils, 338
Amyloid involvement, 2244
Amyloid light-chain (AL chain), 2276
Amyloid neuropathy, 2260
Amyloid proteins, 2238, 2246
Amyloidosis (AL), 1165, 2238, 2244, 2246
   alkylator-based chemotherapy for AL, 2250t
   ATTR, 2260–2261
   cutaneous, 2260
   diagnosis of, 2239–2241
   findings of biopsies among patients with, 2241t
   idiopathic, 2238
   initial treatment for newly diagnosed AL, 2249f
   light chain class usage in, 2240t
   nomenclature of most common forms of, 2239t
   overall survival of patients with AL, 2255f
   periorbital purpura in, 1166f
   positive special protein results in patients with newly diagnosed AL, 2240f
   rare forms of, 2261
   serum monoclonal protein in patients with, 2239f
   subcutaneous fat aspirate showing amyloid deposits, 2241f
   supportive therapy for, 2257
      amyloidosis involving autonomic nervous system, 2258–2259

Amyloidosis (AL) (*continued*)
    amyloidosis involving peripheral nervous system, 2258
    cardiac amyloidosis, 2257–2258
    factor X deficiency, 2259
    gastrointestinal tract amyloidosis, 2259
    hepatic amyloidosis, 2259
    renal amyloidosis, 2258
    respiratory amyloidosis, 2259
    solid organ transplant in patients with AL, 2258t
  syndromes in patients with, 2240t
  systemic senile, 2260
Amyloidosis, systemic, 2346–2347
  AA amyloidosis, 2260
  AL amyloidosis, 2248–2254
  ATTR amyloidosis, 2260–2261
  rare forms of amyloidosis, 2261
  types of, 2260
Amyloidosis, systemic AL, nontransplant therapies, 2249
  alkylator-based therapy, 2249–2250
    initial treatment for newly diagnosed AL, 2249f
    mSMART eligibility criteria for autologous stem cell transplant for patients with AL, 2250f
  antibodies, 2253–2254
    trials and case series of daratumumab to treat immunoglobulin light chain amyloidosis, 2253t
  BCL2 inhibitors, 2254
  immune modulatory drug–based therapy, 2250–2252
  proteasome inhibitor–based therapy, 2252–2253
Anabolic steroids, 1077
Anagrelide, 1179
Anaphylatoxins, 201, 349–350
Anaplastic large cell lymphoma (ALCL), 1463, 1866–1869, 1887, 1887f, 1908, 1925–1927, 1926f, 1961, 1972–1973, 1991, 1999
  ALK-1–positive anaplastic large cell lymphoma, 1973f
  anaplastic lymphoma kinase-negative anaplastic large cell lymphoma, 1887
  anaplastic lymphoma kinase-positive anaplastic large cell lymphoma, 1887
  breast implant–associated anaplastic large cell lymphoma, 1887–1888
  clinical presentation and management, 2000–2001
    FDG-PET anaplastic large cell lymphoma, 2000f
  guidelines for molecular testing in, 1927
  histology ALCL, 2000f
  pathology and molecular characteristics, 1999–2000
  primary cutaneous anaplastic large cell lymphoma, 1887
Anaplastic lymphoma kinase (ALK), 1463, 1957
  ALK gene, 1965, 1997, 2000
  ALK-1, 2084
  ALK-positive histiocytosis, 1380
  anaplastic lymphoma kinase-negative ALCLs (ALK-negative ALCLs), 1887, 1925–1927
  anaplastic lymphoma kinase-positive ALCLs (ALK-positive ALCLs), 1887, 1925–1927
  anaplastic lymphoma kinase–positive histiocytosis (ALK-positive histiocytosis), 1380
Ancillary testing in diagnosis, 10
  considerations for, 1325
    cytogenetics, 1325–1327
    immunophenotype, 1325
    molecular genetics, 1327–1328
Ancylostoma duodenale, 638
Androgen blockade, 2365
Androgenic steroids, 812–813, 1077
Androgens, 1827
Anemia, 600, 628, 639, 667, 669, 690, 715, 731–732, 753–754, 821, 829, 861, 868–869, 891, 895, 1033, 1061–1062, 1102, 1410–1411, 1632, 1740, 1976, 2177
  abnormal iron metabolism, 1035
  anemia in patients with cancer, 1035
  approach to acute posthemorrhagic anemia, 624–625
  approach to hemolysis, 616–624
  approach to macrocytic anemia, 608–611
  approach to microcytic anemia, 611–614
  approach to normocytic anemia, 614–616
  associated with endocrine disorders, 1041
    β-thalassemia, 691
    adrenal insufficiency, 1041
    androgen deficiency, 1041
    anorexia nervosa, 1042
    atherosclerosis, 692
    cardiomyopathy, 692
    diabetes mellitus, 1042
    hereditary spherocytosis, 691
    hyperparathyroidism, 1042
    hyperthyroidism, 1041
    hypopituitarism, 1042
    hypothyroidism, 1041
    infections in hemochromatosis patients, 691
    refractory anemia with ringed sideroblasts, 691
    subnormal immunoglobulins, 691–692
    X-linked sideroblastic anemia, 691
  chronic, 566, 757
  clinical effects of, 602
    cardiovascular and pulmonary features of, 602
    gastrointestinal changes, 603
    neuromuscular features, 603
    ophthalmologic findings, 603
    pallor, 602
    skin and mucosal changes, 602–603
  cytokines, 1034
  development and severity, 1033
  diagnosis, 1035–1036
  erythrocyte survival, 1034
  evaluation and classification of, 603–607, 604t, 604f–607f
  exacerbation of, 845
  general diagnostic approach to hemoglobinopathies and thalassemias, 614
  hematologic toxicities of antiretroviral drugs, 1411t
  impaired marrow response, 1035
  laboratory markers of iron status, 1034
  of liver disease, 1039
  in malaria, 821
  management of anemia of PNH, 809–811
    information useful for managing anemia in patients with PNH, 811t
    impact of phenotype and degree of mosaicism on hemolytic anemia of PNH, 810f
  morphologic features, 1033–1034
  pathogenesis, 1034
    schematic diagram representing contributing mechanisms in pathogenesis of anemia of inflammation, 1034f
  in PK deficiency, 759
  of prematurity, 1063
    terminal T½ of darbepoetin in adults, children, and neonates after subcutaneous or intravenous dosing, 1063t
  role of hepcidin, 1035
  shortened erythrocyte survival, 1035
  splenic infantum, 894
  treatment, 1036
  treatment of, 1827–1829
Anemia of chronic disease (ACD), 605, 613, 1033
Anergy, 770
Angioedema, 2282
Angioendotheliomatosis, malignant, 1965
Angiogenesis in normal and malignant hematopoiesis, 532–533
  hypothesis for role of angiogenesis in leukemia, 533f
Angiohemophilia, 1209
Angioimmunoblastic T-cell lymphoma (AITL), 34, 255, 1389, 1884–1885, 1886f, 1929, 1953
  genetics, 1886
  guidelines for molecular testing in, 1929–1930
  immunophenotype, 1886
  morphology, 1885–1886
  nodal lymphomas of T_{FH} origin, 1886–1887
Angiopoietin-1 (Ang1), 531
Angiopoietin-2 (Ang2), 531
Angiopoietins, 531
  activators and inhibitors of, 532t
Angiosarcoma of spleen, 1439
Angiotensin receptor blockers (ARBs), 853
Angiotensin-converting enzyme inhibitors (ACEIs), 853, 2380
Angiotension II receptor blocker (ARBs), 2380
Aniline-induced methemoglobinemia, 940
Animal models of ADAMTS13 deficiency, 1127
Anion exchanger-1 (AE1), 96
Anisocytosis, 643, 715, 952, 1020
ANKRD26 mutation, 1630
Ankyrin defects, 730
Annexin A1, 2058
Annexin I, 147, 154
Annexin II, 1723
Anopheles mosquito, 821
Anorexia nervosa, 1042
Anthracenediones, 1685
Anthracyclines, 1370, 1685, 1700, 1705, 1724, 2175
  therapy, 2139
Anti-A antibodies, 540
Anti-B antibodies, 540
Anti-C5 antibody, 812
Anti-CD20, 2028
  antibodies, 2212
    bendamustine/rituximab, 2029–2030
    chlorambucil with obinutuzumab or ofatumumab, 2030
    combinations with, 2029–2030
    first-line chemoimmunotherapy, 2029t
    fludarabine with rituximab and cyclophosphamide, 2029
  monoclonal antibody, 1417
  therapies, 1468
Anti-CD52, 2029
Anti-D therapy, 1106
Anti-Epo antibody–induced PRCA, 1013
Anti-idiotype therapy, 1502
Anti-idiotypic antibodies, 777
Anti-IL-5 clinical trials, 186–187
Anti-inflammatory agents, 864
Anti-inflammatory drugs, 1232
Anti-M, 547
Anti-VEGF therapy, 854
Anti-β$_2$gpI–dependent assay systems, 1264
Antibiotics, 1000–1001
Antibody drug conjugate (ADC), 1454
Antibody-dependent cell-mediated cytotoxicity (ADCC), 302, 1500, 1680
Anticancer therapy, 2276
Anticardiolipin antibodies (aCL antibodies), 1260–1266
Anticoagulants, 1, 1251
  drugs, 1291
    heparin, 1291–1293
    heparinoids, 1293
    low-molecular-weight heparins (LMWH), 1293
    parenteral direct thrombin inhibitors (Parenteral DTI), 1295
    pentasaccharides, 1293–1294
    warfarin, 1296–1301
  process, 427
  strategies, 1254
Anticomplement therapy, 1144–1147
Antidiuretic hormone (ADH), 705
Antieosinophil strategies in human asthma, 185–187
Antieosinophil treatment strategies, 187
Antifibrinolytic agents, 1196–1197, 1254
Antifibrinolytic drugs, 577, 1219
Antifibrinolytic medications, 987
Antifibrinolytic proteins, 1276
Antifibrinolytic therapy, 1230
Antigen, 458
  analysis of antigen-specific T cells, 42
  binding, 14
  presentation process, 330
  processing and presentation, 225, 1496–1497
Antigen-presenting cells (APCs), 161, 240, 288, 324, 356, 1494, 2355
Antigenic determinates, 327
Antigenic stimulation, chronic, 2176
Antiglobulin test, 572
  direct antiglobulin test with anti-IgG and anti-C3d, 572f
  indirect antiglobulin test, 572f
Anti–graft-*vs*-host disease therapy (anti-GVHD therapy), 1147
Antihuman globulin (AHG), 572, 773
Anti–human leukocyte antigen antibodies, 327
Anti-myelin-associated glycoprotein antibodies, 2268
Antineoplastic therapy, 1627
Antineutrophil antibodies, 1337
Anti–neutrophil cytoplasmic antibodies (ANCAs), 1168
Antiphospholipid antibodies (aPL antibodies), 1259
  syndrome, 1262
Antiphospholipid antibody syndrome (APS), 1260
Antiphospholipid-protein antibody (APA), 1255, 1260
  clinical manifestations, 1262, 1262t
    arterial and venous thromboembolic disease, 1262–1263
    cardiac disorders, 1263

catastrophic antiphospholipid-antibody syndrome, 1264
  clinical manifestations of antiphospholipid antibodies, 1263t
    dermatologic disorders, 1263
    neurologic syndromes, 1263
    obstetric aspects, 1263–1264
    pulmonary disorders, 1263
    seronegative antiphospholipid-antibody syndrome, 1264
    thrombocytopenia, 1263
  epidemiology and clinical associations, 1261–1262
    clinical diagnoses associated with antiphospholipid-protein antibodies, 1262t
  epitope specificity, 1260, 1261f
  laboratory diagnosis of antiphospholipid-protein antibodies, 1264–1265
    comparison of Factor VIII antibodies and antiphospholipid-protein antibodies, 1265t
    laboratory diagnosis of lupus anticoagulant, 1265t
  mechanism of thrombosis, 1261
  primary prevention, 1265
  thrombosis treatment, 1265
    obstetric treatment, 166
α_2-Antiplasmin, 491
  biochemistry, 492
  deficiency, 1224
  function, 493
  gene structure and expression, 491–492
  schematic of, 492f
Antiplatelet agents, 1814–1815
Antiplatelet antibodies, 1102
  diagnosis, 1102
Antiplatelet drugs, 1137, 1289
  aspirin, 1289–1291
  integrin $\alpha_{IIb}\beta_3$ receptor antagonists, 1291
  thienopyridines, 1291
Antithrombin, human, 467
Antiretroviral therapy (ART), 1388, 1944
  effect of antiretroviral therapy on anemia, 1411–1412
Antisickling agents, 861
  targeting Hb S polymerization, 863–864
Anti–staphylococcal β-lactams, 1473
Antithrombin (AT), 427, 467, 1086, 1248, 1276
  acquired antithrombin deficiency, 1281
  biochemistry, 467
  clinical aspects, 1280
    clinical presentations of venous thromboembolism suggest certain hypercoagulable states, 1280t
  deficiency, 1279
  function, 467–468
  gene structure and expression, 467
  laboratory diagnosis, 1280–1281
  pathophysiology and genetics, 1280
  treatment, 1281
Antithrombin–heparin cofactor, 467
Antithrombotic therapy, 1288
  anticoagulant drugs, 1291–1301
  antiplatelet drugs, 1289–1291
  thrombolytic agents, 1301–1303
Antithymocyte globulin (ATG), 585, 1013, 1157, 1746, 2302, 2315, 2359
Antithymocyte globulin and cyclosporine (ATG/CsA), 1001
Anti–TNF therapy, 664
α_1-Antitrypsin, 466, 1225
Antiviral agents, 1387
Antiviral therapy, 1417, 2288
ANXA1 gene, 2050
Aorta/gonadal/mesodermal region (AGM region), 71, 1570
Aortic valve stenosis, 1148
Apheresis, 558–559
  platelets, 561
Apixaban, 1300
Aplasia, 602, 845
Aplastic anemia (AA), 803, 955, 974, 998–999, 1000, 1028, 1050, 1331, 2299
Aplastic anemia, acquired (AA), 1760
  acquired vs. constitutional aplastic anemia, 995
  clinical features and diagnosis, 999–100
    bone marrow findings help to discriminate aplastic anemia from myelodysplasia, 1000t
    classification, 1000

differential diagnosis of pancytopenia with hypocellular bone marrow, 999t
  definitive treatment, 1001–1004
  epidemiology, 995
    benzene and environmental toxins, 997
    drugs and chemicals, 995–997
    evaluation of patient with suspected aplastic anemia to encompass risk of inherited disorders, 996t
    incidence, age, and geographic distribution, 995
    pregnancy, 998
    radiation, 997
    viruses, 997
  pathophysiology, 998
    autoimmunity, 998
    clonality and aplastic anemia, 998
    stem cells, 998
  supportive care, 1000
    antibiotics, 1000–1001
    growth factors, 1001
    transfusions, 1000
Aplastic anemia, severe (SAA), 997, 1000, 1697, 2302, 2319, 1001–1003
Aplastic crises, 617, 997
  severe aplastic crisis in patient with hereditary spherocytosis, 617f
Apnea-hypopnea index (AHI), 852
Apolactoferrin, 143, 158
Apolipoprotein A1 (ApoA1), 708, 2238
Apolipoprotein A2, 2238
Apolipoprotein B-100 (apo B-100), 1287
Apolipoprotein CII, 2238
Apolipoprotein CIII, 2238
Apoptosis, 43–44, 150
  abnormalities in, 2012
  role in regulation of platelet production, 365
Apoptotic pathways, 2133
Apple domains, 434–435
Aquaporin 1, 1027
Arachnidism, necrotic, 826
Ara-C triphosphate (ara-CTP), 1643
Arachidonic acid (AA), 178, 409–410, 1189, 1857
  cascade of metabolism of, 409f
  lipid composition and metabolism and generation of, 395–396
ARAF gene mutation, 1377, 1380
Arcanobacterium haemolyticum, 1386
Area under the curve concentrations (AUC), 1473
Arg-isoleucine (Ile), 338
Argatroban, 1295, 1309
Arginine, 865
L-Arginine derivative, 1295
Arginyl bonds, 338
Argon plasma coagulation, 1164
ARID1A, 1920
Array comparative genomic hybridization (aCGH), 1905, 1327
  schematic of, 1907f
Array single nucleotide polymorphisms (aSNP), 1905
Array-based karyotyping, 999
Arsenic trioxide (ATO), 1462–1463, 1705, 1721
Arsenicals, 1782
Arsenous acid (AA), 1463
Arsine (AsH_3), 825
Arterial thromboembolic disease, 1262–1263
Arteriolar stenosis, 1123
Arteriovenous malformation (AVM), 1164
Arthrocentesis, 1232
Arthrogryposis, renal dysfunction and cholestasis syndrome (ARC syndrome), 1192
Arthropathy, 687–688, 906
Arthropod disease
  babesiosis, 588
  infections transmitted by, 586–587
  malaria, 587
  transfusion-associated adverse events, 587t
  Trypanosoma cruzi, 588
  West Nile virus (WNV), 587
  Zika Virus (ZIKV), 587
Aryl hydrocarbon receptor (AHR), 317
Arylsulfatase A (ARSA), 1545
Ascaris infestations, 1242
Asciminib, 1796–1797
Ascorbate, 907
Ascorbic acid deficiency, 899
Asian tick typhus, 1170

Asparaginase, 1462, 1608, 1673
  activity, serum, 1673
L-Asparaginase, 1975, 1266
Aspartate aminotransferase (AST), 1049
Aspartic acid, 1635
ASPEN syndrome, 845
Aspergillosis, 1476–1477, 1476f
Aspergillus, 1350–1351, 1396, 1476, 1481, 1704
  IgE, 1837
  pneumonia, 1350
Aspiration cytology, 1866
Aspirin, 753, 1137, 1179, 1815, 1859
  resistance, 1291
Associated hematologic neoplasm (AHN), 1850
  systemic mastocytosis with, 1854
Asthma, 184
ASXL1 gene, 370, 1565, 1568, 1575, 1630, 1638, 1738, 1755, 1825, 1760, 1763, 1764, 1768, 1809, 1822, 1825, 1838, 1840, 1849, 1850, 1854, 1857, 1931, 2336
Ataxia, X-linked sideroblastic anemia with, 664
Ataxia telangiectasia (AT), 272, 976, 1403
  AT-deficient pregnant patients, 1281
Ataxia telangiectasia mutation (ATM), 2012
Ataxia telangiectasia-like disorder, 272
Atezolizumab, 2102
Atherogenesis, role of platelets in, 419–420
Atherosclerosis, 227, 692
Atherosclerotic cardiovascular disease (ASCVD), 638
Atherothrombosis, role of platelets in, 419–420
ATP-binding cassette transporter (ABC transporter), 99
  ABC-me, 99
  ABCB10, 99–100
ATPase inhibitory factor 1 (ATPIF1), 658
ATR gene, 2155
ATRA/idarubicin based therapy, 1727
Atransferrinemia, 636
Atrial arrhythmias, 2258
Atrial thrombi, 2243
Atrophic gastritis, 959–960
ATRX gene, 894
Atypical hemolytic uremic syndrome (aHUS), 351, 1050, 1123, 1130, 1141–1147
  clinical features, 1144
    abnormal vascular permeability, 1144
    anticomplement therapy, 1144–1146
    hypertension, 1144
    long-term management, 1146, 1146t
    MAHA and thrombocytopenia, 1144
    renal injury, 1144
    renal transplantation, 1146
  crisis, 1144
  pathogenesis, 1141
    complement system and regulation, 1142f
  pathophysiology, 1142
    pathophysiology of atypical hemolytic-uremic syndrome, 1143f
    retinopathy and abnormal vascular permeability in atypical hemolytic-uremic syndrome, 1143f
  patients, 1144
  phenotypes of complement dysregulation, 1142–1144
  prognosis, 1147
Australian Eastern Brown snake (Pseudonaja textilis), 456
Autism with platelet dense granule defect, 1191
Autoadsorption, 776
Autoagglutination test, 573
Autoantibodies, 548–549, 776
  to factor VIII in nonhemophilic patient, 1255
    characteristics of factor VIII inhibitory antibodies, 1256
    clinical manifestations, 1256
    laboratory evaluation, 1256
    pathophysiology of development of antibodies to factor VIII, 1255
    soft-tissue hemorrhage, 1256f
    strategy for management of factor VIII inhibitors in hemophilic and nonhemophilic patients, 1257f
    treatment, 1256
Autoerythrocyte sensitization, 1171–1172
Autographa californica, 1529
Autoimmune acquired pure red cell aplasia, 1008
Autoimmune disorders (ADs), 1952–1953, 2022–2023, 2054, 2308
  autoimmune disorders/collagen vascular disease, 1010

Autoimmune gastritis, 960
Autoimmune hemolytic anemia (AIHA), 770, 1010, 2022
  classification, 770t, 770–773
  cold-active antibodies, 776–780
  drug-induced immune hemolytic anemia, 784–787
  laboratory diagnosis, 773–776
    common laboratory features, 773
    direct antiglobulin test, 774–775
    elution, 776
    indirect antiglobulin test, 775
    serologic investigation, 773–774
    serologic techniques, 776
  mixed cold-and warm-active antibodies, 780
  during pregnancy, 1049
  transplant-associated immune hemolytic anemias, 787–788
  warm-active antibodies, 780–784
Autoimmune hemolytic anemia, warm (Warm AIHA), 780–781
  management of, 782
    first-linetreatment, 783
    immunosuppressive therapy, 783–784
    second-line treatment, 783
    therapies, 784
    transfusion, 784
Autoimmune hemolytic process, 787
Autoimmune lymphoproliferative syndrome (ALPS), 784, 1405, 1946
Autoimmune mechanism, 785–786
Autoimmune neutropenia of infancy (AIN), 552
Autoimmune PolyEndocrinopathy, Candidiasis, Ectodermal Dystrophy (APECED), 1404
Autoimmunity, 227, 998
  aplastic anemia vs. hypoplastic myelodysplastic syndrome, 999f
  factors affecting initiation of, 770
Autoimmunization, 898
Autologous donations, 565–566
Autologous hematopoietic cell transplant, 2124, 2125t, 2346
Autologous hematopoietic cell transplantation
  indications for, 2346–2347
    Hodgkin lymphoma, 2343
    mantle cell lymphoma, 2344
    primary refractory disease, 2343
    relapsed disease, 2343–2344
  toxicity of, 2124
Autologous hematopoietic transplantation, indications for, 2343
Autologous platelets, 1114
Autologous stem cell transplantation (ASCT), 1760, 1963, 1999, 2206–2207, 2120, 2138, 2182, 2245, 2254–2256, 2272
  bortezomib-based induction prior to ASCT, 2256–2257
  consolidation post, 2257
  induction before, 2256
    induction and consolidation pre and post-ASCT overall outcomes, 2256t
  non-bortezomib induction prior to, 2257
  overall survival of patients with AL, 2255f
  toxic responses post autologous stem cell transplantation, 2256t
  trials and case series of ASCT for immunoglobulin light chain amyloidosis, 2255t
  effect of troponin T on transplant-related mortality, 2255f
Autologous transplant, 2199
  autologous hematopoietic stem cell transplantation in special populations, 2202–2203
  conditioning therapy for stem cell transplantation, 2203
  as consolidation in stage III-IV Hodgkin lymphoma, 2123–2124
  conventional chemotherapy vs. autologous hematopoietic stem cell transplantation, 2201f
  hematopoietic stem cell collection, 2199
  nonrandomized comparisons of, 2204t
  nontransplant approach vs. autologous hematopoietic stem cell transplantation, 2200t
  salvage hematopoietic stem cell transplant, 2202
  single autologous stem cell transplantation, 2199–2201
  single autologous vs. double hematopoietic stem cell transplantation, 2202
  single vs. double transplantation, 2201, 2201t

Automated coagulation methods, 1086–1087
Automated decision support, 1329
Automated digital image analysis, 5
Automated hematology analyzers, 1–2
  advantages and sources of error with, 5
  histograms and printout generated by Coulter, 2f
  optical flow-cytometric technology used in, 2f
Autophagy, 225
Autosomal recessive mutations, 1397
Autotaxin (ATX), 253
Autotransplantation of splenic tissue, 1435
Avapritinib, 1861
Avascular bone necrosis, 2380–2381
Avascular necrosis (AVN), 921, 2308
Avidin-biotin techniques, 14
Avidity modulation, 414
Axicabtagene ciloleucel, 303
5-Azacytidine, 861, 911
Azanucleosides, 1832
Azathioprine, 1108, 1628
Azurophilic granules, 143, 158

B

B acute lymphoblastic leukemia (B-ALL), 302–303
B allele frequency, 54
B and T lymphocyte associated (BTLA), 301
B cell maturation antigen (BCMA), 2155
B cells, 29, 1396, 1496, 1943, 1949, 2049, 2072, 2314
  aplasia, 1513
  chronic lymphocytic leukemia, 31–33
  clinical presentation, 1396
  congenital sideroblastic anemia with B-cell immunodeficiency, 664
  diagnosis, 1398
  disorders, 2144
  lymphoma, 2117
  malignancies, 281–282
  non-Hodgkin lymphoma, 1468, 2062
    chemotherapy, 2002
  phenotype, 1608
  recovery and immune reconstitution after HCT, 2317–2318
  specific disorders, 1396
    common variable immunodeficiency syndromes (CVID syndromes), 1397–1398
    hyperimmunoglobulin M syndromes, 1397
    selective immunoglobulin A deficiency, 1398
    transient hypogammaglobulinemia, 1398
    X-Linked agammaglobulinemia (XLA), 1396–1397
  treatment, 1398–1398
  tumors, 2153
B lymphocytes, 267, 324, 326, 2010, 2152
  antibody effector functions, 278–280
  B-cell differentiation, 267f
  B-cell receptor signaling, 276–278
  cell interactions in early B-cell development, 273–274
  cytokine stimulation of B cells, 278
  early stages of B-cell development, 272
  generation of diverse lymphocyte repertoire, 267
  genetic defects in V(D) J recombination, 271–272
  genetic defects of early B-cell development, 274–275
  genetic profiles of B-cell activation and differentiation, 281–282
  immunoglobulin gene assembly, 267–271
  mature B lymphocytes and surface immunoglobulin, 275–276
  ontogeny, 267
  pro-B cell to immature B cell, 274
  stem cell to progenitor B cell, 272–273
  terminal stages of B-cell differentiation, 280–281
B miR-17, 371
B regulatory cells (Breg cells), 2020
B-1 B cells, 280–281
B-cell activating factor (BAFF), 2155, 2361
B-cell activation and differentiation, genetic profiles of, 281–282
B-cell acute lymphoblastic leukemia (B-ALL), 29, 54, 1454, 1504, 1562, 1580, 1608, 1617–1618, 1669, 1901
B-cell antigen receptor (BCR), 1458
B-cell lymphoma 2 inhibitor (BCL2), 1446, 1461, 1680, 1832, 1875, 2335
  amplification, 1878
  BCL2/IGH gene, 1943, 2017

family inhibitors, 1680
  gene, 1871, 1912, 1915, 1920, 1960, 1968, 2074
  inhibitors, 1647–1648, 2033, 2254
    toxicity with, 2034
  rearrangement, 1878
B-cell lymphoma-2 homology 3 (BH3), 1461
B-cell lymphoma/leukemia 1 region (BCL1), 1910
B-cell lymphomas (BCL), 1595, 1869, 1880, 1915, 1943, 1954, 1991, 2081, 2089
  analysis using Navios flow cytometer and Kaluza software, 22, 24f
  $BCL-X_L$, 376, 1463
  BCL10 overexpression, 1922
  BCL11A, 866, 884
  BCL6
    gene, 1871, 1922, 1965, 1968
    mutations, 1922
    rearrangement, 1878
    translocations, 1878
  Burkitt lymphoma, 1882
  chronic lymphocytic leukemia/small lymphocytic lymphoma, 1872–1873
  diffuse large B-cell lymphoma (DLBCLs), 1876–1882
  extranodal marginal zone B-cell lymphoma of mucosa-associated lymphoid tissue, 1875–1876
  follicular lymphoma (FL), 1869–1872, 1959–1961
    clinical schema for lymphoid neoplasms, 1960t
    therapeutic options for indolent lymphoma, 1960t
  frontline treatment options, 1962–1963
  median progression-free survival, 1962f
  immunotherapy, 1964
  lymphoplasmacytic lymphomas (LPLs), 1873, 1961
  mantle cell lymphoma (MCL), 1873–1874
  marginal zone lymphoma (MZL), 1961
  nodal marginal zone lymphomas (NMZLs), 1874–1875
  relapsed and refractory treatment options, 1963–1964
  small B lymphocytic lymphoma (SLL), 1961
  special clinicopathologic features, 1961
  splenic marginal zone B-cell lymphoma (SMZL), 1875
  treatment options, 1961–1962
B-cell lymphoproliferative disorders, 2146
B-cell maturation antigen (BCMA), 1456, 1511, 2218
B-cell neoplasms, 776
  chromosomal translocations in, 1909t
  mature neoplasms of, 1910
    Burkitt lymphoma (BL), 1923–1925
    chronic lymphocytic leukemia/small lymphocytic lymphoma (CLL/SLL), 1912–1914
    diffuse large B-cell lymphoma (DLBCL), 1921–1923
    extranodal marginal zone lymphoma, 1915–1916
    follicular lymphoma (FL), 1919–1921
    hairy cell leukemia (HCL), 1919
    high-grade B-cell lymphomas, 1921–1923
    lymphoplasmacytic lymphoma (LPL), 1918
    mantle cell lymphoma (MCL), 1910–1912
    mucosa-associated lymphoid tissue (MALT), 1915–1916
    nodal marginal zone lymphoma (NMZL), 1916–1917
    splenic marginal zone lymphoma (SMZL), 1917–1918
    Waldenström Macroglobulinemia (WM), 1918
  mature neoplasms of T cells, 1925–1932
  recurrent molecular aberrancies in, 1909–1910
B-cell prolymphocytic leukemia (B-PLL), 2018, 2058
B-cell receptor (BCR), 267, 276, 276f, 1900, 2010
  complex, 275
  signaling, 276–278, 277f
    adapter molecules, 277
    coreceptor complexes, 277–278
    initiation pathway, 276
    phosphoinositide pathways, 276
    RAS pathway, 276–277
B-lymphocytes, marure, 275–276
B-lymphoblastic leukemia/lymphoma, 1580
  B-lineage transcription factors affected in B-ALL, 1582f
  epigenetic regulators, 1584
    IDH1/IDH2 mutations, 1584–185
    nuclear protein in testis midline carcinoma family 1 (NUTM1), 1584
  kinases, 1583–1584
  transcription factors, 1580

*CDX*2, 1583
  core binding factors, 1582–1583
  *DUX*4, 1583
  *IKZF*1, 1580–1581
  myocyte enhancer factor 2D (*MEF2D*), 1583
  *PAX*5, 1580
  *TCF*3 translocations, 1581–1582
  zinc-finger protein 384 (*ZNF*384), 1583
  WHO classification, 1580, 1580*t*
B-lymphocyte activator of TNF-family (BAFF), 1952
B-lymphoid cells, 2133
B5 formalin, 12
Babesiosis, 588, 823–824
Bacille Calmette-Guérin vaccination (BCG vaccination), 1350, 1399
Bacterial artificial chromosomes (BACs), 54
Bactericidal permeability-increasing protein (BPI), 143
Baculovirus (BV), 1529
Band neutrophils, 139
Barcoding technique, 359
Bariatric surgery, 960
Bartonella bacilliformis, 824
Bartonellosis, 824
Basal cell carcinoma (BCC), 2095
Basal serum tryptase (BSL), 1853
Basic fibroblast growth factor (bFGF), 2051
Basic helix-loop-helix (bHLH), 1581
Basic leucine zipper (bZIP), 1582
Basophil differentiation-inducing cytokines, 199
Basophilic stippling, 715, 1020
Basophils, 1, 5, 29, 81, 196, 197*f*
  characteristics, 200
    inhibition, 202*t*, 202–203
    mediators, 201*t*, 202
    surface phenotype and activation, 200–202
  clinical relevance, 199–200
  environmental activation, 199
  expression of selected surface markers, 200*t*
  factors, 201*t*
  functions, 203
    containment of injury, initiation of repair, remodeling, and normal function, 204
    dynamic equilibrium and homeostasis, 204–205
    inflammatory injury and host defenses, 203–204
  and lineages from adult HSC and committed progenitors, 198*f*
  mediator secretion, 196–197
  mediators, 201*t*
  model of activities, 203*f*
  morphology, 196
  ontogeny and developmental biology, 198–200
  recovery after activation, 197
BATF3, 220
BCOR gene, 1568, 1638, 1760
*BCORL*1 gene, 1630
Beclomethasone, 2305
Bee stings, 827
Belantamab-mafodotin, 2212
Belinostat, 2099
Bence Jones proteins, 2148, 2238
Bence Jones proteinuria, idiopathic, 2170
Bendamustine, 1969, 1976, 2028, 2029–2030, 2032, 2127, 2138, 2175, 2217, 2270
Bendamustine plus obinutuzumab (BO), 1963
Benign monoclonal light chain proteinuria (BMPC), 2170
Benralizumab, 1845
Benzylpenicilloyl determinant, 785
BERK sickle cell mouse, 850
Berlin-Frankfurt-Münster (BFM), 1667, 1700, 1995
Bernard-Soulier syndrome (BSS), 38, 403, 986, 1100, 1154, 1184–1188, 1214
  monoallelic, 1184
Best available therapy (BAT), 1830
Best supportive care (BSC), 1504, 1652
Bexarotene, 2096
Biclonal gammopathy, 2170
Bictegravir (BIC), 1410
Biexponential, 26
Birefringence, apple green, 2238
Bile pigments, 127
Bilirubin, 778
  catabolism, 126–127
  formation, 124–125
  IXα, 124, 124*f*
  normal and abnormal pathways of bilirubin excretion by hepatic cell, 126*f*

serum, 618, 755
transport, 125
Biliverdin reductase (BVR), 97
Bing-Neel syndrome, 2268
Biogenesis of lysosome related organelle complexes (BLOCS), 1190
Biological assays, 359
Biopsy techniques, invasive, 1445
Birbeck granules, 1365
Birtamimab, 2254
Bispecific antibodies, 1504–1505, 2218
Bispecific T cell engagers (BiTE), 1456–1457, 1681
Bivalirudin, 1295, 1309
Blackfan Diamond Syndrome, 2299
Blast cell, 1600
Blast phase CML (BP-CML), 1765, 1782
Blast-phase primary myelofibrosis, management of, 1831–1832
Blastic plasmacytoid dendritic cell neoplasm (BPDCN), 1378–1379, 1379*f*, 1455
Blautia, 2355
Bleeding disorders, 1162, 1216
  acquired, 1082
  caused by vascular abnormalities
    bleeding due to disorders of perivascular tissue, 1166–1167
    clinical approach to patient, 1162
    mechanical purpura, 1162
    psychogenic purpura, 1171–1172
    purpura associated with infection, 1169–1170
    purpura associated with skin diseases, 1171
    purpura associated with vascular obstruction, 1170–1171
    structural malformations of vessels, 1162–1166
    vasculitis, 1167–1169
  clinical evaluation of, 1080
  clinical features of acquired bleeding disorders, 1081–1082
  confirmatory tests, 1087
    disorders in results of primary screening tests, 1089
    disorders of common pathway of coagulation, 1088–1089
    disorders of extrinsic pathway of coagulation, 1089
    disorders of intrinsic pathway of coagulation, 1087–1088
    qualitative platelet disorders, 1087
    thrombocytopenia, 1087
    von Willebrand Disease (vWD), 1087
  evaluation of neonate, 1091–1092
  initial laboratory evaluation, 1087, 1088*t*
    primary screening tests, 1087
  laboratory methods for study of hemostasis and blood coagulation, 1082–1087
  manifestations of disordered hemostasis, 1080–1081
  preoperative hemostasis evaluation, 1089–1091
Bleeding phenotype, autosomal recessive, 1195
Bleeding time, idiopathic prolonged, 1209
Blinatumomab (BLINCYTO), 1456–1457, 1504, 1616, 1619–1621, 1681, 1683, 2299
Blister cells, 623
BLNK mutation, 275
BLOC1S3, 1190
BLOC1S5, 1190
Blood components
  modification, 564
    closed *vs.* open systems, 564
    irradiation of blood products, 564–565
    leukocyte reduction, 564
    washed products, 564
  use of, 566
    patient blood management, 566, 567*f*
    patient informed consent, 566
Blood DC antigen (BDCA), 30
Blood filtration
  circulating, 1426
  clearance of particulate matter, 1426
  culling, 1426
  pitting, 1426
    schematic representation of process of pitting by spleen, 1427*f*
Blood transfusion, 779–780, 813, 860, 897–898, 1951
  adverse effects of, 579–580
    immunologic transfusion reactions, 580–585
    iron overload, 585
    massive transfusion, 585

metabolic effects and hypothermia, 585
nonimmunologic adverse effects of, 585
transfusion-associated circulatory load (TACO), 585
transfusion-associated graft-*vs*-host disease, 585*t*
indications for transfusions, 861
infectious complications of, 586
  bacterial contamination, 589
  blood donor screening for infectious diseases, 586
  COVID-19, 588–589
  cytomegalovirus (CMV), 589–590
  human immunodeficiency virus type 1 and type 2, 586
  infections transmitted by arthropods, 586–588
  pathogen-reduction technology (PRT), 590
  potential emerging infections, 588
  transfusion-associated hepatitis (TAH), 586
  transmissible spongiform encephalopathies, 588
Blood urea nitrogen (BUN), 2380
Blood-filled pseudosinuses, 2056
Blood-forming system, 1522
Bloodstream infections, 846, 1473
  candidemia, 1475
  catheter-related bloodstream infection (CRBSIs), 1474–1475
  gram-negative bacteremia, 1474
  gram-positive bacteremia, 1473–1474
Bloom syndrome (*BLM* gene), 976, 1629, 1737
Blunt trauma, 1162
Body iron, 628, 640
Body surface area (BSA), 2357
Bohr effect, 116
Bone age, 2381
Bone deformities, 895, 895*f*, 918
Bone disease, 2179
Bone lesions, 2054–2055
Bone marrow (BM), 22, 213, 233–234, 645–646, 702, 732, 734, 806, 824, 1011, 1037, 1102, 1322, 1369, 1595, 1608, 1668, 1721, 1764, 1808, 1811, 1891, 1992, 2020, 2093, 2148, 2152, 2267, 2276, 2297, 2300
  angiogenesis, 2163
  aplasia, 1610
  aspirates, 51, 1837
    and biopsy, 1445, 1791
    differential counts, 11*t*
    smear stained with Wright-Giemsa stain, 9, 10*f*
    specimens, 1445
  biopsy, 977, 1741, 1811*f*, 1855, 2144, 2166, 2277, 2279
  bone marrow aspirate and core biopsy, 1322*t*
  characteristic bone marrow biopsy from a patient with pure red cell aplasia, 1011*f*
  core biopsy, 9, 10*f*
    specimens, 1322
  disorders, 656
    PNH in setting of another specified, 809
  endogenous erythropoietin-mediated erythropoiesis or ESA–mediated erythropoiesis on iron saturation, 645*f*
  evaluation of bone marrow iron stores, 613
  extent of bone marrow involvement, 2167–2168
  histology, 2056
  karyotyping, 1791
  mapping with polychromatic flow cytometry, 22, 23*f*
  megaloblastic anemias, 610
  microenvironment, 2177
    changes in, 2163
    megakaryocyte and, 365–366
  normoblasts, 845
  pathophysiology of bone marrow suppression in HIV infection, 1413–1414
  of thalassemic patients, 909
  treatment of bone marrow relapse, 1678
Bone marrow evaluation, 1096, 1611
  cytogenetics, 1611
  detects disease, 1955
  immunophenotype, 1612
    WHO classification for precursor leukemia/lymphoma, 1612*t*
  next-generation sequencing, 1612
Bone marrow examination, 9, 1023
  bone marrow aspiration and biopsy, 9–10
  changes in differential counts of bone marrow with age, 12*t*
  histologic sections, 12

Index

Bone marrow examination (*continued*)
  in HIV-1 infection, 1414
  needed to clarify cause of anemia, 607–608
    peripheral blood smear, 607f
  special stains, 12–14
  staining and evaluation of bone marrow aspirates and touch preparations, 10–12
Bone marrow failure (BMF), 792, 974, 1410, 1630–1631
  hematopoietic stem cell transplantation for, 2319–2323
  syndromes, 66, 1339, 2314
    aplastic anemia/pure red cell aplasia, 1050
    associated with pregnancy, 1050
    sideroblastic anemia, 1050
Bone marrow mast cells (BMMCs), 29–30
Bone marrow mastocytosis (BMM), 1852
Bone marrow plasma cells (BMPCs), 2160, 2165
Bone marrow stromal cells (BMSCs), 2013
Bone marrow transplantation (BMT), 663, 813, 865–866, 955, 1001, 2064, 2297, 2335
  representative results from large mature studies, 1001t
  risk factors affecting survival before availability of eculizumab, 814t
Bone mineral density (BMD), 2379
Bone morphogenetic protein (BMP), 630
  BMP-2, 678
  BMP-6, 678
  Bmp4, 71
Bordetella pertussis, 348, 1386
Borrelia burgdorferi, 1949, 2076
Bortezomib, 784, 1134, 1460, 1680, 1963, 1970, 2100, 2175, 2184, 2191–2192, 2194, 2196–2198, 2211–2217, 2253, 2270, 2281, 2288, 2292
  bortezomib-based induction prior to ASCT, 2256–2257
  post-ASCT, 2255
Bortezomib, dexamethasone, and rituximab (BDR), 2270
Bortezomib-dexamethasone (BD), 2193, 2196
Bosutinib, 1458, 1782, 1796
Bovine spongiform encephalopathy (BSE), 588
Bovine thrombin–induced factor V inhibitors, 1259
Bowel dysfunction in AL, 2245
Bradykinin, 434
Brain natriuretic peptide (BNP), 2247
Branch-point sequence (BPS), 1578
Breakpoint cluster region (*BCR*), 1583, 1782
  BCR V gene repertoire, 271
  BCR-ABL gene, 1611
  BCR::ABL1, 1776, 1783, 1787
    BCR-ABL1-negative MPNs, 372
    fusion gene, 1583–1584
    kinase domain mutants to approved tyrosine kinase inhibitors, 1799t
    kinase domain mutations, 1798
    mRNA, 1789, 1792
    mutation, 1798, 1800
    mutation testing, 1793
    translocation and fusion gene, 1783
  BCR1, 1721
  BCR3, 1721
  constitutive kinase activation in BCR-ABL1 fusion protein, 1784–1785
  structural domains and signaling motifs in BCR, ABL1, and BCR-ABL1 proteins, 1785f
  gene, 1610–1611
  pathway
    effectors of, 2031
    inhibitors, 2033
  proteins and contribution to cellular transformation, 1783–1784
  signaling pathways in BCR-ABL1 transformed cells, 1785
    cytoskeletal proteins, 1786
    DNA damage surveillance and repair pathways, 1786–1787
    Janus kinase/signal transducer and activator of transcription pathway, 1786
    phosphatidylinositol-3 kinase (PI3K), 1785
    RAS/mitogen-activated protein kinase pathways, 1785–1786
Breast cancer, 690, 1628, 2129
  resistance protein, 951
Breast implant–associated anaplastic large cell lymphoma, 1887–1888
Breast lymphoma, 1955
Brentuximab, 2127

Brentuximab vedotin (BV), 1455, 1504, 1973, 2101, 2120, 2124–2125, 2137
Brexucabtagene autoleucel, 303
Brilliant cresyl blue, 8
Broad-spectrum antibiotics, 1266
5-Bromo-2-deoxyuridine (BrdU), 43
Bromodomain containing 9 (BRD9), 667
Bromodomain inhibitors, 1463
Bronchiolitis obliterans syndrome (BOS), 2306, 2361, 2378
Bronchiolitis obliterans with organizing pneumonia (BOOP), 2358
Bronchoalveolar lavage (BAL), 171, 1472
Bronchus-associated lymphoid tissue (BALT), 248, 1955
Bronze pigmentation, 684
Brown recluse spider (*Loxosceles reclusa*), 826
Bruises, 603
Bruton agammaglobulinemia, 275
Bruton tyrosine kinase (BTK), 1351, 1913, 1961, 2012, 2049, 2059, 2270, 2343
Bruton tyrosine kinase gene (*BTK* gene), 1396
Bruton tyrosine kinase inhibitors, 1458, 1468, 2271–2272
  acalabrutinib, 1459
  ibrutinib, 1458
  outcome after treatment with, 2033
  toxicity with, 2033
  zanubrutinib, 1459
Budd-Chiari syndrome, 808
Budesonide, 2305
Bulk tumor cell analysis, 1567
"Bulk-lyse-stain wash" methods, 22
Burkholderia, 1350
Burkitt leukemia, 1608, 1613
Burkitt lymphoma (BL), 33–34, 1323, 1382, 1388, 1885f, 1900, 1923–1925, 1943, 1970–1971, 1991, 1995–1998
  clinical features and management, 1997–1998
    mature B-NHL in children, 1998t
  guidelines for molecular testing in, 1925
  histology BL, 1996f
  pathology and molecular characteristics, 1996–1997
Burkitt-like lymphoma, 1996
Burns, 827
Burr cells, 1037
Burst-forming unit-MKs, 360
Burst-forming unit erythroid (BFU-E), 77, 93–94, 1008
Buschke disease, 2171
Busulfan (BU), 1179, 1793, 2315, 2340
Busulfan exposure, chronic, 1793
Busulfan-fludarabine (BU-FLU), 2325
Busulfan/melphalan (Bu-Mel), 2203
Butyrate, 911

C

C-reactive protein (CRP), 838, 2181, 2240, 2244, 2268, 2282
^{14}C-serotonin release assay (^{14}C-SRA), 1309
C-terminal Src kinase (Csk), 413
C-type lectin-like receptor (CLEC), 246
C-type lectins receptors (CLRs), 222
C-X-C motif ligand 4 (CXCL4), 419
C/EBP members, 168
Ca^{2+} release-activated Ca^{2+} (CRAC), 1195
CAAT enhancer binding protein α (C/EBPα), 1789
Cabotegravir (CAB), 1410
Caenorhabditis elegans, 955
Calcineurin inhibitors (CNIs), 2359, 2378
Calcium, 760
Calcium elevated, renal failure, anemia, lytic bone lesions (CRAB), 2179
Calcium ionophore, 176
Calcium-activated K^+ channel, 112
Calcium and DAG-regulated guanine exchange factor-1 defect (CalDAG-GEFI defect), 1193
Calicheamicin, 1484
Calnexin, 332
Caloric deficits, 707
CALR gene, 1177
CALR mutation, 1176, 1763, 1768, 1770, 1822–1823, 1826
Calreticulin (CALR), 332, 341, 373, 1821
Campylobacter jejuni, 1949
Candida spp., 1347, 1351, 1475
  C. parapsilosis, 1475
    chorioretinitis and endophthalmitis, 1475

Candidemia, 1475
Canine autologous transplantation model, 1537
Capillary zone electrophoresis (CZE), 114, 2146
Caplacizumab, 1136–1137, 1139
Caprini score, 1197
Carbamazepine, 1950
Carbapenem-resistant Enterobacterales (CRE), 1474
Carbapenems, 1471, 1474
Carbohydrate, 454, 707
Carbohydrate-rich polymers, 347
Carbon dioxide transport, 117, 117f
Carbon monoxide, 704
  poisoning, 942
    acute CO intoxication, 942
    chronic CO intoxication, 942
    treatment, 942
  rate of carbon monoxide production, 619
γ-Carboxyglutamic acid (Gla), 1298
Carboxyhemoglobin (CO hemoglobin), 3, 941–943
Carboxyhemoglobinemia, 942
Carboxylation and vitamin K–dependent carboxylase, 439–441
γ-Carboxylation reaction, 439
Carboxypeptidase U, 459
Carcinoembryonic antigen cell adhesion molecule-1 (CEACAM-1), 406
Carcinoembryonic antigen cell adhesion molecule-2 (CEACAM-2), 406
Carcinogenesis, 48
Carcinoma, 642, 1252–1253
CARD11 gene, 1928
CARD11 mutations, 1878, 1920, 1922
Cardiac abnormalities, 1631
Cardiac amyloidosis, 2257–2258
Cardiac arrhythmias, 662
Cardiac disease, 920–921
Cardiac disorders, 1263
Cardiac morbidity, 2128
Cardiac response, 2249
Cardiac surgery, 1845
Cardiac transplant, 550
Cardiac vessel abnormalities, 827
Cardiac-associated mechanical anemias, 966
Cardiomyopathy, 692, 696, 2260
Cardiopulmonary bypass surgery, 830, 1148
Cardiopulmonary disease, 1074
  acquired heart disease, 1075
  chronic cor pulmonale, 1075
  cyanotic heart disease, 1075
  hypoventilation syndromes, 1075
Cardiovascular complications (CVCs), 2378
  congestive heart failure (CHF), 2379
  metabolic syndrome and related cardiovascular disease, 2378–2379
  recommendations to address CVC and MS, 2379
Cardiovascular disease (CVD), 567, 1288, 1620, 1754–1755, 1797, 2379
Cardiovascular events, 1814
Cardiovascular risk factors, 1814
Cardiovascular system, 1809, 2144
Carfilzomib, 1460, 1680, 1963, 2175, 2184, 2191, 2196–2198, 2212–2215, 2253, 2270
Carmustine, 2175
Carmustine-cyclophosphamide-prednisone, 2193
Carpal tunnel syndrome, 2242
Carrier detection methods, 913
Carrion Disease, 824
Cartilage-hair hypoplasia (CHH), 984, 1403, 1335–1336, 1339
Casein kinase 1a1 (CK1a), 1745
Casitas B-lineage lymphoma (CBL), 373, 1821
Caspase 8 (*CASP8*), 1405
Caspase recruitment domain family member 11 (CARD11), 2074
Caspase recruitment domain–containing protein 9 (CARD9), 1347
Caspofungin, 1703
Castleman disease (CD), 1949, 2260, 2277–2279
Catalase, 119
  deficiency, 1351
Cataracts, 2308
Catastrophic antiphospholipid-antibody syndrome, 1260, 1264
CATCH22 syndrome, 1399
Cathepsin D, 363
Cathepsin E, 363

Catheter-assisted thrombolysis, 1306
Catheter-based therapy, 1306
C6 deficiency, homozygous, 352
CD30+ lymphoproliferative diseases, 2083
  lymphomatoid papulosis, 2083–2084
  lymphomatoid papulosis, 2084f
  primary cutaneous anaplastic large cell lymphoma (PCALCL), 2084–2085
  primary cutaneous CD30+ lymphoproliferative disorders, 2084t
CD4 T lymphocytes, 297
  differentiation of CD4+ T cells, 297f
  plasticity of CD4 T-cell subsets, 299
  regulatory T cells (Tregs), 298
  Th1 CD4+ T Cells, 297
  Th17 CD4+ T Cells, 298
  Th2 CD4+ T Cells, 297–298
  Th22 CD4+ T Cells, 298
  Th9 CD4+ T Cells, 298
CD4/CD8 lineage commitment, 289
CD4+ T cells, 288, 1401
CD40 gene, 2050
CD40 ligand (CD40L), 1397, 2133
CD40 stimulation, 278
CD40LG gene, 1397
CD8+ T cells, 288
CD8+ T lymphocytes, 299
  death receptor pathway, 300
  granzymes, 300
  inhibitory receptors and corresponding ligands, 301f
  perforin, 299–300, 299f
  T-cell exhaustion, 300–301
*CD8B*1 genes, 1960
CD94/NKG2A, 312, 314
Cefaclor, 1169
Cefazolin, 1473
Cefotetan, 787
Ceftazidime, 1471
Ceftazidime-avibactam, 1474
Cell adhesion, 338
Cell adhesion molecule-31 (CD31), 155
Cell counts, 1–2
Cell cycle analysis, 42–43
Cell destruction, 121
  extravascular hemolysis, 121
  intravascular hemolysis, 121
  mechanisms and site of RBC destruction, 121
Cell fusion, 226
Cell interactions in early B-cell development, 273–274
Cell transfusions, inadequate, 895
Cellular approaches, 1506
  acute lymphoblastic leukemia (ALL), 1509–1511
  adoptive cellular immunotherapy, 1508
  checkpoint blockade, 1513–1514
  chimeric antigen receptors (CAR), 1508–1509
  chronic lymphocytic leukemia (CLL), 1509
  diffuse large B-cell lymphoma (DLBCL), 1511
  donor lymphocyte CARs, 1512
  donor lymphocyte infusions, 1507–1508
  graft-*vs*-leukemia effect (GVL effect), 1506–1507
  lymphocyte-activated killer cells (LAK cells), 1508
  multiple myeloma, 1511
  neurologic toxicity grading and management guidance, 1514t
  "off-the-shelf" CAR immune cells, 1512
  placenta-derived NK cells, 1513
  side effects of CAR T therapy, 1512
    B-cell aplasia, 1513
    cytokine release syndrome (CRS), 1512–1513, 1512t
    future directions, 1513
    mechanisms of resistance to CAR T cells, 1513
    neurologic events, 1513
  tumor-infiltrating lymphocytes (TILs), 1508
  viral antigen–specific T cells, 1508
Cellular dehydration, 837
Cellular DNA content, 42–43
Cellular immunity, defects in, 1468–1469
Cellular immunotherapy for lymphomas, 1964
Cellular injury due to iron overload, 682–683
Cellular iron, 13
Cellular mechanisms, 1063
Cellular proliferation, 635
Cellular reservoir function, 1427–1428

Central nervous system (CNS), 123, 212, 744, 955–956, 1101, 1218, 1324, 1347, 1360, 1366, 1382, 1410, 1480–1481, 1513, 1544, 1608, 1631, 1667, 1698, 1880, 1945, 1992, 2268, 2283, 2287, 2358, 2381
  events, 840–843
    recommended TCD screening schedule in children with sickle cell disease, 842t
    studies investigating role of hydroxyurea in primary and secondary stroke prevention in sickle cell anemia, 843f
    vaso-occlusive effects in the central nervous system, 841f
  leukemia, 1631
  primary diffuse large B-cell lymphoma of 1880
  prophylaxis, 1729
  therapy, 1616
  thrombosis, 1810
  toxoplasmosis, 1481f
  vascular lesions, 1165
Central supramolecular activation cluster (cSMAC), 293
Central tolerance, 770
Central venous catheters (CVCs), 1470
Centrifugation techniques, 6
Centroblasts, 242–243, 1870
Centrocytes, 242–243
Cerebral amyloid angiopathy, 1166
Cerebral autosomal dominant arteriopathy with stroke and ischemic leukoencephalopathy (CADASIL), 1166
Cerebral blood flow (CBF), 840
Cerebral cavernous malformations (CCMs), 1165
Cerebral edema, 942
Cerebral malformations, 986
Cerebral small vessel disease, 1166
Cerebral thrombosis, 1262
Cerebrospinal fluid (CSF), 22, 706, 955, 1053, 1324, 1545, 1611, 1669, 1698, 1729, 2003
  pressure, 1810
Ceruloplasmin, 629, 634, 686
Cervical cancer, 1415
*CFHR*1, genomic deletion of, 1142
Chédiak-Higashi neutrophils, 1349
Chediak-Higashi syndrome (CHS), 363, 1191, 1335, 1347, 1404
  characteristic silver-gray hair of child with Chédiak-Steinbrink-Higashi anomaly, 1348f
  clinical features and course, 1349
  etiology and pathogenesis, 1347–1349
  inclusion bodies in Chédiak-Steinbrink-Higashi anomaly, 1348f
  inheritance, 1349
  laboratory findings, 1349
  management, 1349
Chelation therapy, 904
Chemoattractants, 153, 156
Chemoimmunotherapy, 1963, 2010, 2028–2029
  combinations with anti-CD20 antibodies, 2029–2030
Chemokine receptor 4 (CCR4), 1977
Chemokines, 153, 168, 197, 220, 419
  and receptors, 221f, 254–255
Chemoprophylaxis, 823
Chemorefractory disease, 2206
Chemotactic cytokines, 709
Chemotactins, 220
Chemotaxis, 157–158, 172, 220–221
  abnormal specific granule formation, 1347
  actinopathies and "lazy-leukocyte syndrome", 1346–1347
  autosomal dominant hyperimmunoglobulin E syndrome (AD-HIES), 1346
  CARD9 deficiency, 1347
  defects impacting, 1346–1347
  localized juvenile periodontitis, 1347
  Rac2 GTPase mutation, 1347
Chemotherapy, 1266, 1621, 1629, 1632, 1645, 1668, 1697, 1711, 2028, 2064, 2121, 2127
  alkylating agents, 2028
  approaches, 1992
  combining nucleoside analogs with alkylating agents, 2028
  nucleoside analogs, 2028
  regimen, 1608
  toxicity, 2128

Chest radiograph (CXR), 1837, 2134
Chimeric antigen receptor T cells (CARTs), 1713, 2335
  in CLL, 2035–2036t
  therapy, 1461, 1461t
Chimeric antigen receptors (CAR), 302, 318, 1508–1509, 1608, 1652, 1998–1999, 2035, 2126, 2138, 2299
  CAR-directed T cells, 1964
  components of first-, second-, and third-generation, 1509f
  early clinical trials in CD19 CART, 1510t
Chimerism, 2303
Chlamydia pneumoniae, 844
Chlamydia psittaci, 1949
Chlorambucil, 2028, 2032, 2064
Chloramphenicol, 669, 1157
Chlorella pyrenoidosa, 967
Chloride shift, 117
2-Chlorodeoxyadenosine (CdA), 1844, 1860, 2049, 2059
Chloroma, 1631, 1706, 2090
Chloroquine-porphyrin complexes, 714
Chlorosis, 628
Chlorothiazides, 1157
Chlorpromazine, 1262
Cholecystectomy, 760
Cholelithiasis, 617–618, 716, 732, 757, 896
Cholesterol, 109
  abnormalities, 1362
  embolization syndrome, 1171
Choline magnesium trisalicylate, 1232
Choline phospholipids, 726
Choline transporter-like protein 2 molecule (CTL2 molecule), 553
Chorea-acanthocytosis (ChAc), 744
Chromatin, epigenetic factors modifying, 1572–1575
Chromogenic substrate assays, 1207
Chromogenic techniques, 1087
Chromosomal aberrations, 1639
Chromosomal abnormalities, 48, 979
Chromosomal microarray analysis (CMA), 48, 54–55
  detection of 5q deletion and 11q copy-neutral loss of heterozygosity, 55f
Chromosomal translocations, 1709
Chromosome 17p loss and abnormalities of *TP*53, 2155
Chromosome 1q and loss of chromosome 1p, gain of, 2155
Chromosome content associated with different oncogenic pathways, 2153
Chromosome genomic array testing (CGAT), 54–55
Chromosome genomic array testing/chromosome microarray (CGAT/CMA), 56f
Chromosome instability syndromes, 1696–1697
Chromosomes 5 and/or 7, 1628
Chromosome vectors, artificial, 1526
Chronic ataxic neuropathy, 2281
Chronic B-cell disorder, 2049
Chronic eosinophilic leukemia (CEL), 1763, 1770–1771, 1771f, 1836, 1854
  treatment of HES and, 1844–1845
Chronic graft-*vs*-host disease (cGVHD), 909–910, 1476, 2203, 2305–2306, 2335, 2360, 2362–2363, 2371, 2374, 2376–2377, 2382
  assessment of therapeutic response, 2363–2364
    immune suppression following chronic GVHD diagnosis, 2364f
  biology, 2360
    altered B-cell homeostasis, 2361
    CD4 T-cell subsets, 2360
    loss of central tolerance, 2360–2361
    profibrotic pathways, 2361
  chronic GVHD global severity score, 2306f
  classification and severity grading, 2362
  diagnosis of, 2361–2362
  example of chronic GVHD organ scoring, 2306t
  late immune-mediated disorders after allogeneic hematopoietic cell transplantation, 2362t
  prevention of, 2362–2363
  prognostic variables, 2362
  survival outcomes per NIH chronic GVHD overall severity, 2362f
  risk factors for, 2362
  supportive care, 2364
  treatment of, 2306
  treatment of, 2363

Chronic granulomatous disease (CGD), 1346, 1349,
    1395–1396, 1536–1538, 1541, 2318
  catalase deficiency, 1351
  clinical and laboratory features, 1350
  cystic fibrosis (CF), 1351
  glucose-6-phosphate dehydrogenase deficiency, 1351
  glutathione peroxidase deficiency, 1351
  glutathione synthetase (GSS), 1351
  history and molecular genetics, 1349–1350
  immunodeficiency states and neutrophil dysfunction,
    1351
  lipochrome histiocytosis, 1350
  myeloperoxidase deficiency, 1351
  Papillon-Lefèvre syndrome, 1352
  reductase deficiency, 1351
  treatment, 1350
  variants and additional conditions associated with
    defective respiratory burst, 1350
Chronic hepatic porphyria, 719
Chronic hepatitis, 1337
Chronic hypoplastic neutropenia, 1332
Chronic inflammatory polyradiculoneuropathy (CIDP),
  2277
Chronic kidney disease (CKD), 632, 705, 853, 1036,
  2379
  anemia of, 1036–1039
Chronic lymphocytic leukemia (CLL), 31, 56–58, 271,
    781, 1009, 1102, 1430, 1454, 1468, 1499,
    1509, 1628, 1869, 1872, 1901, 1950, 2010,
    2011f, 2049, 2053, 2150, 2268, 2286, 2299,
    2342–2343
  and chronic B-cell disorders, 2018t
  clinical findings, 2019
    bone marrow and lymph nodes, 2020
    immunoglobulin production and light chain ratio,
      2020
    immunophenotyping, 2020
    peripheral blood, 2019–2020
  diagnosis, 2016–2017
    differential diagnosis, 2017, 2017t
      B cell–associated causes, 2017–2018
      benign causes, 2017
      malignant causes, 2017
      T cell–associated causes, 2017
  immune dysfunction in, 2020–2023
    autoimmune disorders, 2022–2023
    infections, COVID-19, and immunization, 2021
    second malignancies, 2022
  investigations, 2018
    additional tests for clinical trials and specific
      clinical situations, 2019
    bone marrow, 2019
    laboratory measurements, 2018
    physical assessment, 2018
    radiology, 2019
    standard tests for general practice, 2018
  management of immune dysfunction in CLL, 2037
    immune cytopenias, 2038–2039
    infections, 2037–2038
    second malignancies, 2038
  management of Richter syndrome and
    transformations, 2039–2040
  mixed cell type, 2020
  pathophysiology, 2010
    abnormalities in apoptosis, 2012
    age distribution of males and females, 2010f
    analysis by FISH, 2014–2015
    cell of origin, 2010–2011
    cell proliferation, 2014
    cellular features of microenvironment, 2014
    clonal evolution in CLL, 2016
    conventional cytogenetics, 2015–2016
    FISH abnormalities and gene expression, 2016
    GC reaction, 2011f
    genomic abnormalities, 2014
    microenvironment, 2012–2013
    modulators of apoptotic pathway in CLL, 2012
    molecular interactions in CLL, 2013f
    predisposing factors including familial CLL,
      2011–2012
    whole-genome and whole-exome sequencing, 2016
  prognostic and predictive markers, 2023
    age and sex, 2023
    gene mutation distribution, 2025f
    lymphocyte characteristics, 2023–2025
    marrow histology, 2025–2026
    plasma markers, 2026
    prognostic index, 2026
    Rai and Binet staging, 2023
    time to first therapy according to CLL, 2026f
  prognostic markers in CLL including those used in
    CLL-IPI, 2023t
  prolymphocytic transformation, 2040
  serum immunoglobulin levels in patients with CLL,
    2021f
  staging, 2019
    Binet staging, 2019t
    Rai staging, 2019t
  suggested algorithm for management of CLL, 2037f
  suggested algorithm for management of frontline
    CLL, 2037f
  treat CLL outside of clinical trials, 2036–2037
  treatment of, 2027
    acalabrutinib, 2032
    BCR pathway inhibitors, 2033
    chemoimmunotherapy, 2029–2030
    chemotherapy, 2028
    chimeric antigen receptor T cells in CLL,
      2035–2036
    combination therapy with novel agents, 2034
    criteria for response in, 2027t
    effectors of BCR pathway, 2031
    hematopoietic stem cell transplantation (HCT),
      2034–2035
    ibrutinib, 2031–2032
    idelalisib, 2033
    immunotherapy, 2028–2029
    indications for treatment, 2027
    inhibitors of Bcl-2, 2033
    major randomized studies with novel agents in
      frontline therapy of CLL, 2031t
    novel agents, 2030
    outcome after treatment with BTK inhibitors, 2033
    pirtobrutinib and nemtabrutinib, 2032
    radiotherapy, 2036
    resistance to ibrutinib, 2033
    resistance to venetoclax, 2034
    response criteria, resistance, and minimal residual
      disease, 2027
    signaling pathways in CLL cell, 2030f
    splenectomy, 2036
    steroids, 2028
    toxicity with BCL2 inhibitors, 2034
    toxicity with BTK inhibitors, 2033
    zanubrutinib, 2032
  and variants, 2010t
Chronic lymphocytic leukemia/small lymphocytic
  lymphoma (CLL/SLL), 1323, 1912–1914
  CLL biology, 1912f
  guidelines for molecular testing in, 1914t
  pathways with genomic alterations in CLL, 1914f
Chronic mast cell leukemia, 1852
Chronic mountain sickness, 1074
Chronic mucocutaneous candidiasis syndromes (CMC
  syndromes), 1404
Chronic myelogenous leukemia (CML), 1458, 1505,
  1530, 1627, 2340
  conditioning regimen, 2340
  management of relapse after HCT, 2340
  monitoring of disease after HCT, 2340
  timing of HCT, 2340
Chronic myeloid leukemia (CML), 48, 66, 1176, 1328,
    1562, 1674, 1695, 1763–1766, 1765f, 1782,
    1821, 2241, 2299
  allogeneic stem cell transplantation, 1800
    AlloHSCT risk factors and EBMT risk score,
      1800t
  approach to newly diagnosed chronic phase patient,
    1797
    BCR-ABL1 response milestones in chronic phase
      CML patients treated with TKIs, 1798t
    monitoring patients on therapy, 1797–1798
    selection of frontline tyrosine kinase inhibitor,
      1797
  approach to patient presenting in accelerated phase/
    blast phase, 1798
  approach to patient with tyrosine kinase inhibitor
    resistance, 1798–1800
  atypical, 1776, 1776f
  clinical features, 1789
    bone marrow aspirate in chronic phase chronic
      myeloid leukemia, 1789f
    clinical presentation, 1789
    definition of accelerated phase, 1790t
    disease phases, 1790–1791
    epidemiology, 1789
    risk scores, 1791
    signs and symptoms, 1789–1790
  diagnosis and initial workup, 1791
    bone marrow aspirate and biopsy, 1791
    bone marrow karyotyping, 1791
    clinical evaluation, 1791
    complete blood count (CBC), 1791
    differential diagnosis, 1791–1792
    fluorescence in situ hybridization (FISH),
      1791
    laboratory tests, 1791
    reverse transcription polymerase chain reaction,
      1791
  future perspectives, 1800–1801
  lymphoid blast phase of, 1766f
  monitoring response to therapy, 1792
    BCR-ABL1 mutation testing, 1793
    complete hematologic response (CHR), 1792
    cytogenetic response (PCyR), 1792
    leukemia burden with increasing depth of
      response, 1792f
    molecular response, 1792–1793
  myeloid blast phase of, 1765f
  pathophysiology, 1783
    BCR and ABL1 proteins and contribution to
      cellular transformation, 1783–1784
    BCR-ABL1 translocation and fusion gene, 1783
    CML hematopoiesis, 1787–1788
    constitutive kinase activation in BCR-ABL1 fusion
      protein, 1784–1785
    DNA repair pathways in cycling and quiescent
      HSCs and LSCs, 1787f
    metaphase karyogram of newly diagnosed man
      with CML, 1784f
    pathways implicated in survival of CML stem
      cells, 1788f
    signaling pathways in BCR-ABL1 transformed
      cells, 1785–1787
    simplified representation of signaling pathways
      activated in CML cells, 1786f
    somatic mutations associated with blast phase
      CML, 1789f
    transformation to blast phase, 1788–1789
  resistance to tyrosine kinase inhibitors, 1798
  therapy, 1793
    cytotoxic agents and interferon, 1793
    TKIs approved for first-line treatment of CML,
      1794t
    TKIs approved for salvage treatment of CML,
      1795t
    tyrosine kinase inhibitors (TKIs), 1793–1797
  treatment-free remission (TFR), 1800
  WHO criteria for accelerated phase of, 1765t
Chronic myelomonocytic leukemia (CMML), 37–38,
    378, 1763, 1774–1776, 1775f, 1838, 1854
  differential diagnosis of chronic-phase CML, atypical
    CML, and CMML in adults, 1775t
  WHO criteria for, 1775t
Chronic neutrophilic leukemia (CNL), 1763, 1771
Chronic NK-Cell proliferations, 34–35
Chronic nonspherocytic hemolytic anemia, 755
Chronic obstructive pulmonary disease (COPD), 316,
  1074
Chronic organ damage, 847
  bones and joints, 847–849
    long bones in sickle cell anemia, 849f
  cognitive function, 849–850
  eyes, 850
  growth and development, 847
    sex differences in height-for-age and TBLH
      aBMD-for-age curves in SCCRIP pediatric
      cohort, 848f
  heart, 850–851
  hepatobiliary and gastrointestinal systems, 852
  kidneys, 852–853
  lungs, 851–852
  pregnancy, 855–856
  skin ulcers, 855
  sleep disorders, 852
Chronic pulmonary disease, 851, 1620
Chronic recurrent multifocal nonbacterial osteomyelitis
  (CRMO), 1028

Chronically transfused populations, prophylactic antigen matching in, 548
Churg-Strauss disease, 1168
Cigarette smoking, 1629, 2176
Ciltacabtagene autoleucel, 2218
Circulating blood granulocyte pool (CGP), 150
Circulating immature myeloid cells, 1823
Circulating tumor DNA (ctDNA), 66, 1901, 1923
Cirrhose pigmentaire, 678
Cirrhosis, 688, 695
   anemia in, 1039–1041
Cirrhotic patients, 1039
Cisplatin, 2175
Citrate-based anticoagulants, 560
Citrate-phosphate-dextrose (CPD), 560
Citrate-phosphate-dextrose-adenine (CPDA-1), 560
Cladribine, 784, 1371, 1703, 1860, 2028, 2059, 2065, 2270
   in HCL, 2061–2062
     long-term responses to treatment with nucleoside analogs, 2061f
     toxicity, 2062
   monotherapy, 1371
Cladribine, high-dose cytarabine, filgrastim, and mitoxantrone (CLAG-M), 1653
Clarkson disease, 2292
Class switch recombination (CSC), 278, 279f
Class switch recombination (CSR), 270, 1918, 2152
Classic Gr1^{hi} subset, 81–82
Clindamycin, 1474
Clofarabine, 1371, 1621, 1703, 1971
Clonal anomalies, 49–50
Clonal cytogenetic abnormalities in Ph$^+$ cells (CCA/Ph$^+$), 1791
Clonal cytopenia of undetermined significance (CCUS), 1600, 1754
Clonal cytopenias uncertain significance, 1759
Clonal deletion by activation-induced cell death, 771
Clonal DNA (cDNA), 1903
Clonal expansion, 802, 1754
Clonal hematological disorders, 1176
Clonal hematopoiesis (CH), 1565, 1600, 1630, 1697, 1754, 1759
   in acquired and inherited bone marrow failure syndromes, 1760
     acquired aplastic anemia (AA), 1760
     inherited bone marrow failure syndromes, 1760
   and AML outcomes, 1759–1760
     CH and impact on HSCT outcomes, 1759t
   biology of, 1755
   CHIP and AML risk in population studies, 1755–1756
     biological and clinical impact of CH in patients, 1756f
     CH and myeloid cancer risk, 1757t
     clonal complexity, 1756
     clone size, 1757
     mutation-specific risk, 1756
   CHIP and hematopoietic stem cell transplant outcomes, 1760
   CHIP and inflammation, 1755
   clonal hematopoiesis and clonal cytopenias uncertain significance, 1759
   definitions, 1754–1755
   MCA and myeloid cancer risk, 1758
   and myeloproliferative neoplasms, 1759
   as risk factor for therapy-related myeloid neoplasm, 1757–1758
     studies of association of CH, cytopenia, and myeloid cancer risk, 1758f
   role of inflammation and aging in, 1754f
Clonal hematopoiesis of indeterminate potential (CHIP), 1565, 1600, 1627, 1697, 1738, 1754, 1809
   and AML risk in population studies, 1755–1756
   biology of, 1755
   and hematopoietic stem cell transplant outcomes, 1760
   and inflammation, 1755
Clonal myelopathies, 817
Clonal plasma cells, 1873
   disorders, 2148
Clonal stem cell disorders, 1737
Clonality, 998
   analysis, 64–65
Clone directed therapy, 2291
Clopidogrel, 1291
Clostridial sepsis, 824

Clostridioides difficile, 1470, 2358
Clostridium difficile, 1480
Clostridium perfringens, 824
Clot formation
   factor XIII, 471–472
   fibrinogen (Factor I) and fibrin, 472–479
   proteins of, 471
Clot retraction, 397, 1182
Cloud-like hyperchromatic nuclei, 1824
Clusterin, 349
Coagulation disorders, acquired, 1088, 1241t, 1267
   deficiencies of vitamin K–dependent factors, 1241
   disseminated intravascular coagulation, 1246–1254
   liver disease, 1244
   pathologic inhibitors of coagulation, 1254–1267
   primary fibrinolysis, 1254
   vitamin K deficiency bleeding in infancy (VKDB in infancy), 1241–1244
Coagulation disorders, inherited, 1202t, 1224, 1242
   abnormalities of protease inhibitors, 1224–1225
   clinical disorders of fibrinogen molecule, 1217–1219
   combined defects, 1224
   deficiency of factors V and VIII, 1224
   factor V deficiency, 1220–1221
   factor VII deficiency, 1221–1222
   factor X deficiency, 1222
   factor XI deficiency, 1222–1223
   factor XII deficiency, 1223
   factor XIII deficiency, 1219–1220
   hemophilia A, 1203–1208
   hemophilia B, 1208–1209
   high-molecular-weight Kininogen deficiency, 1224
   inherited coagulation disorders, 1224
   major and minor bleeding, 1228
     factor VII deficiency, 1230–1231
     factor XIII deficiency Treatment, 1231
     gene therapy for hemophilia, 1230
     Hemophilia A Major Bleeding, 1229
     Hemophilia A Minor Bleeding, 1229
     hemophilia B treatment, 1230
     treatment considerations for miscellaneous disorders, 1231–1232
     von Willebrand Disease, 1229
   prekallikrein deficiency, 1223
   principles of pathophysiology, 1202–1203
   prothrombin deficiency, 1220
   special aspects of treatment, 1232
     antibodies to coagulation factors, 1233
     hemarthrosis, 1232
     hemophilic cysts, 1232
     home treatment programs, 1233
     intracranial bleeding, 1232–1233
     viral transmission from past factor concentrates, 1233
   treatment of, 1225
     adjunctive therapies, 1228
     biodynamic properties of coagulation factors of concern in replacement therapy, 1225t
     hemostatic levels, 1225
     products, 1226–1228
     replacement therapy, 1225
     in vivo recovery and survival of infused coagulation factors, 1225–1226
   von Willebrand disease (vWD), 1209–1217
Coagulation factor replacement products
   comparison of miscellaneous antihemophilic agents, 1226t
   inherited coagulation disorders, 1226
   plasma, 1226
   plasma-derived factor VIII and IX products, 1226t
   prothrombin complex concentrates, Factor IX, and Factor VII, 1227–1228
   purified factor VIII, 1227
   purified or concentrated coagulation factors, 1227
   recombinant factor VIII and IX products, 1226t
Coagulation factor replacement therapy, 1225, 1228, 1246
   with platelets and coagulation factors, 1251–1252
   replacement therapy in hemophilia A and hemophilia B, 1226t
Coagulation factors, purified, 1227
Coagulation, initiation of, 427
Coagulopathy, 1723
   of COVID-19 infection, 1253
Cobalamin (Cbl), 945
   homocysteine testing in, 958
   issues of nutrition, 950

   and methionine metabolism, 946–947
   propionyl-CoA metabolism, 946
   replacement in infants and children, 965
   structure of cobalamin, 945f
Cobalamin absorption, 948–950
   cobalamin binding proteins, 949t
   inborn errors of cobalamin absorption and metabolism, 963
   processes of absorption of cobalamin by gastrointestinal tract, 949f
Cobalamin deficiency, 959
   age-related chronic gastritis, 960
   clinical manifestations of, 956
   cobalamin deficiency in infants and children, 961
   drug-induced cobalamin deficiency, 961
   gastric surgery, 960
   ileal resections and reconstruction surgery, 960–961
   methylmalonic acid testing in, 957–958
   neurologic abnormalities in, 954–956
   neurological aspects of cobalamin deficiency in infants, 956
   pernicious anemia and atrophic gastritis, 959–960
   small intestinal bacterial overgrowth and parasites, 960
   treatment, 964
     cobalamin replacement in infants and children, 965
     cobalamin replacement in vegetarians, 965
     megaloblastic anemia and myeloneuropathy, 964–965
     treatment considerations in seniors, 965
   vegetarianism, 961
CO intoxication, chronic, 942
Colchicine, 97
Cold agglutinin disease (CAD), 776
   antibody characteristics, 777
   clinical manifestations, 778
   functional characteristics, 778
   I/i blood group system specificity, 777–778
   immunochemistry and origin, 777
   laboratory features, 778
   management, 778
     B Cell–directed regimens, 778
     immunosuppressive and steroid therapy, 778–779
     primary cold agglutinin disease, 778
     secondary cold agglutinin disease, 779
   primary *vs.* secondary cold agglutinin disease, 776–777
   secondary cold agglutinin disease, 777t
   secondary, 777
   serologic overview of hemolytic anemias, 776t
   temperature ranges for cold agglutinin fixation and lytic complement action, 776f
Cold-active antibodies, 770
   immune hemolytic anemias caused by, 776
Cold-agglutinin disease (CAD), 351–352
Cold-stored platelets, 562
Collagen receptors, defects of, 1189
   $\alpha_2\beta_1$ defect, 1189
   GPIV defect, 1189
   GPVI defect, 1189
Collagen type I gene (*COL1A1*), 896
Collagen vascular diseases, 1010, 1102
Collagen-related peptide (CRP), 1189
Collagenase, 158
Collagens, 366, 404
Colon cancer, 2094
Colony-forming cell (CFC), 1529
Colony-forming unit (CFU), 356
   assays, 77–78
Colony-forming unit megakaryocyte (CFU-MK), 77
Colony-forming unit-erythroid (CFU-E), 93–94, 1008
Colony-stimulating factor 1 (CSF1), 256
Colony-stimulating factors (CSFs), 1472
Colorectal cancer, 689–690
Colorectal polyps, 689–690
Combination chemotherapy, 1974, 2100
Combined defects, 1287
Combined hydroxyurea groups, 868
Combined immunodeficiency disorders, 1403
   cartilage-hair hypoplasia (CHH), 1403
   chronic mucocutaneous candidiasis syndromes (CMC syndromes), 1404
   mammalian susceptibility to mycobacterial disease, 1404
   radiation sensitive disorders, 1403
   toll-like receptors and innate signaling pathway defects, 1404
   Wiskott-Aldrich syndrome (WAS), 1403

Combined α and δ-granules deficiency (αδ-SPD), 1190
Combined-modality therapy, 2100–2101
Committed erythroid progenitors, 93
  BFU-E, 94
  CFU-E, 93–94
Committed hematopoietic progenitor cells, 75–76
Common dendritic cell progenitor (CDP), 216
Common helper innate lymphoid progenitor (CHILP), 310
Common lymphoid progenitors (CLPs), 77, 233, 359
Common myeloid progenitor (CMP), 77, 359
Common region of amplification (CRA), 1583
Common variable immunodeficiency syndromes (CVID syndromes), 1397–1398
Comparative genomic hybridization (CGH), 50, 1326, 1564
Competitive binding luminescence assays (CBLAs), 956
Competitive repopulation assay, 78
Complement C1r/Cr1s, Uegf, and human bone morphogenetic protein (CUB), 338
  module, 338
Complement control protein (CCP), 338
Complement factor H (CFH), 1141
Complement factor I (CFI), 1141
Complement inhibition, 779
Complement inhibitory therapy, 811
Complement proteins, 172, 346
Complement receptor 1 (CR1), 346–347, 351
  cellular distribution and function of receptors for complement components, 347t
Complement receptors (CRs), 143, 222, 772
Complement regulatory proteins, 796
Complement system, 1141, 1393
  activation, 1394f
  alternative pathway, 342
  anaphylatoxins, 349–350
  classical pathway, 338–341
  clinical presentation, 1393
  complement component deficiencies, 350–352
    age-related macular degeneration (AMD), 351
    atypical hemolytic uremic syndrome (aHUS), 351
    C1 esterase inhibitor, 350
    cold-agglutinin disease (CAD), 351–352
    COVID-19, 352
    deficiencies of terminal complement components, 352
    deficiency of early complement components, 350
    hemolysis, elevated liver enzymes, and low platelets syndrome (HELLP syndrome), 351
    paroxysmal nocturnal hemoglobinuria, 350–351
    Shiga toxin–associated hemolytic uremic syndrome, 351
  diagnosis, 1394
  lectin complement pathway, 343
  membrane attack complex, 343–344
  membrane attack complex formation, 344–345
  regulation of complement activation, 345
    C1 inhibitor, 345
    C4b-binding protein (C4BP), 348
    control of C3 and C5 convertases, 346
    control of deposited MAC, 349
    control of initiation step, 345
    control of membrane attack complex assembly, 349
    factor I, 348–349
    regulators in body fluids, 347–348
    regulators on cell surfaces, 346–347
    regulatory proteins of complement, 345t
  specific disorders, 1394
    C1 esterase inhibitor deficiency, 1394
    C2 deficiency, 1394
  treatment, 1394
Complement-dependent cytotoxicity (CDC), 1501
Complement-insensitive cells, 797
Complement-mediated hemolytic uremic syndrome (cmHUS), 347
Complement-mediated lysis
  analysis of GPI-AP on erythrocytes and granulocytes from patient with PN, 794f
  complement-mediated lysis of PNH erythrocytes, 795f
  phenotypic mosaicism in PNH, 793f
  PNH phenotypes, 793t

sensitivity to, 792–796
Complement-mediated process, 822
Complement-sensitive cells, 797
Complementarity-determining regions (CDR), 291, 998
Complete blood count (CBC), 2, 605, 773, 979, 1138, 1321, 1595, 1791, 2165
Complete hematologic response (CHR), 1792
Complete molecular response (CMR), 1793
Complex immunodeficiency disorders, 1403
  cartilage-hair hypoplasia (CHH), 1403
  chronic mucocutaneous candidiasis syndromes (CMC syndromes), 1404
  mammalian susceptibility to mycobacterial disease, 1404
  radiation sensitive disorders, 1403
  toll-like receptors and innate signaling pathway defects, 1404
  Wiskott-Aldrich syndrome (WAS), 1403
Complex karyotypes (CKs), 57, 2015
Complex rearrangements involving MYC (c-MYC), 2153
Compound heterozygosity, 922, 1287
Compound heterozygotes, 916
Computed tomography (CT), 1132, 1163, 1305, 1367, 1425, 1470, 1611, 1827, 1955, 2016, 2092, 2119, 2134, 2148, 2179, 2241, 2245, 2378
  scanning, 687, 1208, 1233, 2343
Computer crossmatch, 573
Concentrated coagulation factors, 1227
Concordance, 2012
Confidence interval (CI), 568, 1630, 1755, 1963, 2075, 2188
Conformational alteration, 329
Congenital amegakaryocytic thrombocytopenia (CAMT), 372, 974, 986, 1153
  CAMT group I, 986
  CAMT group II, 986
  clinical features, 986
  differential diagnosis, 986
  laboratory findings, 986
  pathophysiology, 986–987
  supportive care, 987
  treatment, 987
Congenital anomalies, 976, 986
Congenital dyserythropoietic anemia type I (CDA-I), 1020
  clinical features, 1020
  laboratory features, 1020–1021
    electron microscopy of CDA-I binucleated erythroblast, 1022f
    macrophage in bone marrow, 1022f
    peripheral blood smear of patient with CDA-I, 1022f
  management, 1021–1022
  molecular biology of CDA-I, 1022–1023
Congenital dyserythropoietic anemia type II (CDA-II), 1023
  clinical features, 1023
  laboratory features, 1023–1024
    electron microscopy of binucleated erythroblast, 1024f
    peripheral blood smear of patient with CDA-II, 1023f
  management, 1024
  molecular biology of CDA-II, 1024–1025
Congenital dyserythropoietic anemia type III (CDA-III), 1025
  clinical features, 1025
  laboratory features, 1025
    erythroblast from case of CDA-III showing stellate intracytoplasmic inclusions, 1026f
    giant erythroblasts with multiple nuclei and additional karyorrhexis, 1026f
    multinucleate erythroblasts from bone marrow of a patient with CDA-IIIa, 1025f
    peripheral blood smear of patient with CDA-III, 1025f
  molecular biology of CDA III, 1026
Congenital dyserythropoietic anemia type IV, 1026
  clinical features, 1027
  laboratory features, 1027
    peripheral blood smear images of patient with CDA-IV, 1027f
  molecular biology of congenital dyserythropoietic anemia type IV, 1027–1028

Congenital dyserythropoietic anemias (CDAs), 611, 1020
  clinical presentation, 1020
    types of congenital dyserythropoietic anemias, causative genes, and bone marrow pathology findings, 1021t
  subtypes, 1020
    congenital dyserythropoietic anemia type I (CDA-I), 1020–1023
    congenital dyserythropoietic anemia type II (CDA-II), 1023–1025
    congenital dyserythropoietic anemia type III (CDA-III), 1025–1026
    congenital dyserythropoietic anemia variants, 1028
  variants, 1028
    bone marrow aspirate smear of patient with VPS4A-associated CDA, 1028f
    bone marrow aspirate smears resembling those of congenital dyserythropoietic anemia, 1029f
Congenital dyserythropoietic disorders, 1028
Congenital erythropoietic porphyria (CEP), 714, 719
  clinical description, 714, 715f
  diagnosis and treatment of, 720
  laboratory findings, 715
  molecular basis and pathogenesis, 714–715
  treatment 715
Congenital immune defects with associated neutropenia, 1334–1335
Congenital infection, fetal anemia owing to, 1062–1063
Congenital neutropenia, 1339, 1395
Congestive heart failure (CHF), 662, 1698, 2379
Congestive splenomegaly, 1040
Conotruncal anomaly face syndrome, 1399
Consensus sequence mutants, 887
Conservative prenatal treatment, 1062
Constitutive exocytosis, 197
Constitutive-specific transgene expression, 1524
Contact activation, 1085
Continuous erythropoietin activator (CERA), 1038
Continuous intravenous infusion (CIVI), 1456
Conventional care regimens (CCRs), 1647
Conventional cytogenetics, 2015–2016
Convertin, 445–446
Convoluted lymphocytic lymphoma, 1942
Convulsive seizures, 142
Coombs-negative hemolytic anemia, 809
Cooperative Study of Sickle Cell Disease (CSSCD), 839, 2325
Copanlisib, 1459
Copper, 825
  deficiency, 638, 669–670
Coproporphyrin, 98
Coproporphyrinogen I, 98
Coproporphyrinogen III, 98
Coproporphyrinogen oxidase (CPOX), 704
Copy number variations (CNVs), 61, 1564, 1903
  adult T-cell leukemia/lymphoma, 1931
  anaplastic large cell lymphoma, ALK positive and ALK negative, 1927
  angioimmunoblastic T-cell lymphoma, 1929
  chronic lymphocytic leukemia/small lymphocytic lymphoma, 1912
  enteropathy-associated T-cell lymphoma, 1931
  extranodal marginal zone lymphoma, 1916
  follicular lymphoma, 1920
  hairy cell leukemia, 1919
  lymphoplasmacytic lymphoma/Waldenström macroglobulinemia, 1918
  mantle cell lymphoma, 1911
  monomorphic epitheliotropic intestinal T-cell lymphoma, 1931
  mucosa-associated lymphoid tissue lymphoma, 1916
  nodal marginal zone lymphoma, 1917
  peripheral T-cell lymphoma, not otherwise specified, 1928
  T-prolymphocytic leukemia, 1930
Copy-neutral loss of heterozygosity (cnLOH), 54
Cord aneurysms, 1062
Core binding factor (CBF), 1568, 1633, 1699
  B-lymphoblastic leukemia/lymphoma, 1582–1583
  translocations, 1570–1571
    mutational landscape of RUNX1::RUNX1T1 AML and CBFB::MYH11 AML, 1571f
Core needle biopsy (CNB), 2093
Core-binding factor (CBF), 367

Coronary arterial thrombosis, 1276
Coronary artery blockage, 1631
Coronary artery bypass surgery, 779
Coronary atherosclerosis, 692
Coronary stents, 1148
Coronavirus disease 2019 (COVID-19), 352, 588–589, 777, 1159, 1478, 2021, 2300
    infection, 2308
        coagulopathy of, 1253
    pandemic, 2038, 2066
    pharmacologic complement inhibitors, 352
    PNH and, 816
Cor pulmonale, chronic, 1075
Corrected count increment (CCI), 575
Corrected QT (QTc), 1727
Cortical steroids, 812–813
Cortical thymic endothelial cells (cTECs), 236, 290
Cortical thymic epithelium development, 236
Cortical thymocytes, 234
Corticosteroids, 585, 813, 1012–1013, 1049, 1105, 1266, 1387, 1478, 1672, 1674, 1684, 1843, 1859, 2175, 2208, 2220
    administration, 1331
    role of corticosteroid prophylaxis, 1731
    therapy, 1827
    treatment, chronic, 1105
Corynebacterium diphtheriae, 1386
Costimulatory domains (CD), 1508
Cranial nerve palsies, 1386
Cranial radiation therapy (CRT), 1673
Cranial trauma, 1233
Crizanlizumab, 2325
Crizotinib, 1463, 1973
Crohn disease, 2260
Cryofibrinogenemia, 1170
Cryofibrinogens, 1170
Cryofiltration apheresis, 779
Cryoglobulinemia, 1168, 1277, 2054, 2146, 2220, 2246, 2284, 2290
    clinical features of cryoglobulinemia at diagnosis, 2285*t*
    clinical presentation of, 2286
        cryoglobulin-associated physical findings, 2287*f*
        dermatologic and joint manifestations of, 2286–2287
        liver manifestations of, 2287
        manifestations of, 2287
        nervous system manifestations of, 2287
        renal manifestations of, 2287
    diagnosis of, 2287–2288
    epidemiology, 2284–2285
    etiology, 2285
        connective tissue disease, 2286
        hepatitis C Virus, 2286
        lymphoproliferative disorders, 2286
        relationship among underlying diseases, 2285*f*
    treatment of, 2288, 2288*f*
        antiviral therapy, 2289
        rituximab therapy, 2289
        therapies for, 2289
        treatment of life-threatening disease, 2288–2289
        treatments for symptomatic mixed cryoglobulinemia, 2288*t*
    type I, 2286
Cryoglobulins, 1168, 2284–2285, 2287
Cryohemolysis test, 734
Cryohydrocytosis, 742
Cryopyrin-associated periodic syndromes (CAPS), 2282
Cryptic site mutants in introns and exons, 887
Cryptic splice sites, activation of, 888
Cryptococcal meningitis, 1480
Cryptogenic organizing pneumonia (COP), 2306, 2378
Cutaneous erythema, 2361
Cutaneous leukocytoclastic vasculitis, 1167–1168
    etiologies of leukocytoclastic vasculitis, 1168*t*
Cutaneous lymphocyte antigen (CLA), 254, 2072
Cutaneous mastocytosis (CM), 1850, 1852
Cutaneous T-cell lymphoma (CTCL), 1502, 2072, 2076
    classification of, 2076
    clinical presentation, 2076
    diagnostic evaluation, 2076
        blood involvement, 2080–2081
        bone marrow involvement, 2080
        cutaneous features of MF/SS, 2077–2079
        cutaneous phases of mycosis fungoides, 2077*f*
        extracutaneous MF/SS, 2079–2080
        extracutaneous sites, 2080
        frozen section immunohistochemistry of cutaneous plaque, 2081*f*
        histopathology, 2077
        immunophenotyping studies, 2081–2082
        large cell transformation of MF/SS, 2079
        lymph node pathology, 2080
        Sézary syndrome, 2081*f*
        tissue handling, 2076–2077
    differential diagnosis, 2082
        benign conditions, 2082–2083
        CD30$^+$ lymphoproliferative diseases, 2083–2085
        hematopoietic neoplasms with similar cutaneous presentations, 2089–2090
        primary cutaneous T-cell lymphomas, 2085–2089
    early CTCL, 2073*f*
    epidemiology, 2075–2076
    historical perspective and pathophysiology, 2072
        clinical description, 2072
        histopathology, 2072
        immunology, 2072–2074
        molecular genetics, 2074–2075
    late CTCL, 2073*f*
    membrane proteins of malignant T cell, 2073*f*
    NCI-VA grading scheme for lymph node histology in CTCL, 2080*t*
    prognosis, 2093–2094
    staging, 2090–2091
        bone marrow, 2093
        imaging, 2091–2092
        ISCL/EORTC staging of mycosis FUNGOIDES/Sézary syndrome, 2091*t*
        lymph nodes, 2092–2093
        recommended initial staging evaluation of mycosis Fungoides/Sézary syndrome, 2092*t*
    therapy, 2094
        combined-modality therapy, 2100–2101
        electron beam radiotherapy and photon beam irradiation, 2097–2098
        extracorporeal photochemotherapy (EC), 2098
        hematopoietic stem cell transplantation (HCT), 2102
        immunotherapy, 2101–2102
        interferons (IFNs), 2096–2097
        MF/SS treatment algorithm, 2094*f*
        photopheresis photochemotherapy, 2098
        phototherapy, 2095–2096
        retinoids, 2096
        systemic chemotherapy, 2098–2100
        topical chemotherapy, 2094–2095
Cyanmethemoglobin, 3
Cyanosis, 935, 939
Cyanotic heart disease, 1075
CYBB gene, 1396
Cyclic AMP response element binding protein (CREB), 1948
Cyclic guanosine monophosphate (cGMP), 411, 863
Cyclic hematopoiesis, 1334
Cyclic neutropenia (CN), 1334
Cyclin-dependent kinase (CDK), 361
    inhibitors, 1463
Cyclobutane pyrimidine dimer (CPD), 2095
Cyclooxygenase (COX), 1189
Cyclooxygenase-1 (COX-1), 1193
Cyclooxygenase-2, 534
Cyclophosphamide, 784, 1108, 1417, 1608, 1844, 1962, 2002, 2028, 2100, 2190, 2196–2198, 2216, 2220, 2251, 2270, 2302, 2340
Cyclosporine (CSP), 585, 1012, 1017, 1402, 2038, 2319
    response of PRCA to various immunosuppressive therapies, 1012*t*
    time course of response of patient 9 to cyclosporine A, 1012*f*
Cyclosporine A, 784, 1258
Cytochrome P-450 complex (CYP2C9), 1296–1297
Cytochrome P450 (CYP), 713, 840
Cytogenetic abnormalities, 1633–1634, 1709, 1741
    wright-stained bone marrow smear, 1633*f*
Cytogenetics, 48, 1325–1327, 1598, 1741, 1771, 1811–1812, 2051, 2181–2182
    chromosome genomic array testing nomenclature, 55
    CMA, 54–55
    comparison of cytogenetic analysis methods, 50*t*
    cytogenetics/molecular diagnostics, 1011
    diagnostic and prognostic impact of chromosomal abnormalities, 55–58
    fluorescence in situ hybridization analysis, 50–51
    fluorescence in situ hybridization nomenclature, 51–54
    frequency of abnormal cytogenetics by polycythemia vera disease stage in two series, 1812*t*
    history, 48
        fluorescence in situ hybridization, 49*f*
        t(9;22), 48*f*
        unbanded metaphase spread from bone marrow cells, 48*f*
    ideogram of normal G-banded chromosomes, 53*f*
    ISCN symbols and abbreviated terms, 52*t*
    methods for analysis of hematologic malignancies, 48
        karyotype analysis, 49–50
        specimens, 48–49
    methods of cytogenetic analysis, 1326*t*
    next-generation sequencing, 58
    nomenclature, 50
    studies on marrow cells, 1011
Cytokine receptor homology module (CRMs), 373
Cytokine release syndrome (CRS), 303, 1456–1457, 1505, 1512–1513, 1512*t*, 1622, 1730, 1964, 2035, 2218
Cytokine-induced killer cells (CIK cells), 1507–1508
Cytokines, 168, 197, 288, 371, 1034, 1505–1506, 2051–2053, 2279, 2282
    disseminated intravascular coagulation, 1247–1250
        chronic or "compensated" disseminated intravascular coagulation, 1249–1250
        consumption of coagulation factors and impaired anticoagulant pathways, 1248
        consumption of platelets, 1248
        fibrin degradation products (FDPs), 1248–1249
        fibrinolysis, 1248
        impairment of clearance mechanisms, 1249
        infections, 1247–1248
        intravascular fibrin formation, 1248
        pathophysiology of disseminated intravascular coagulation, 1249*f*
        shock, hypoperfusion, and hypoxemia, 1248
        stimuli, 1248
    domain, 371
    of IL-6 family, 378
    monitoring of cytokine profiles, 43
    and pathways, 378–379
    RAS-RAF-MEK-ERK signalling pathway, 2052*f*
    regulation of megakaryopoiesis and signaling, 371
        cytokines involved in positive or negative regulation of platelet production, 378–379
        thrombopoietin/myeloproliferative leukemia axis, 371–378
    signaling, 310–313
    stimulation of B cells, 278
    storm, 1501, 1529, 2355
Cytolysis, 175
Cytomegalovirus (CMV), 560, 589–590, 898, 1000, 1064, 1098, 1157, 1386, 1399, 1411, 1478–179, 1479*f*, 1668, 2017, 2285, 2298, 2320, 2382
Cytometry, 18
Cytopenias, 907, 1595, 1632, 1797, 1823–1824, 2287
Cytoreductive therapy, 1179, 1815, 1859–1860
    agents, 1862
    agents/modalities, 1179
    anagrelide, 1179
    avapritinib, 1861
    cladribine, 1860
    dasatinib and nilotinib, 1861–1862
    hematopoietic stem cell transplantation (HSCT), 1862
    hydroxyurea, 1179
    imatinib, 1861
    interferon, 1179
    interferon-α (IFN-α), 1860
    masitinib, 1861
    tyrosine kinase inhibitors, 1861
Cytosine arabinoside, 1643
Cytosine base editors (CBEs), 1549
Cytosine-cytosine-adenosine (CCA), 664
Cytoskeletal proteins, 111, 1786
    ADAP defect, 1194
    defects of, 1194
    filamin A defects, 1195
    Wiskott-Aldrich syndrome (WAS) and X-linked thrombocytopenia (XLT), 1195
Cytoskeleton, 363–365
Cytosolic phospholipase $A_{2\alpha}$ defect (cPLA$_{2\alpha}$ defect), 1192–1193

Cytostatic-hypomethylating compounds, 911
Cytotoxic agents, 1013
Cytotoxic CD8+ T cells, 1468
Cytotoxic chemotherapy
  DNA methyltransferase inhibitor therapy, 1647
  initial treatment of AML in patients unfit for, 1647
Cytotoxic T lymphocyte-associated antigen (CTLA-4), 2102, 2138
Cytotoxic T lymphocytes (CTLs), 1383, 1496
Cytotoxin-associated gene A (CagA), 1949

D

Dabrafenib, 1370–1371, 2064
Dacarbazine, 2127
Dacryocytosis, 1823
Dactylitis, 839
Damage-associated molecular patterns (DAMPs), 153, 176, 1495, 2355
Danaparoid sodium, 1293
Danazol, 1004, 1108–1109
Dapsone, 940
Dapsone-induced methemoglobinemia, 940
Daptomycin, 1473
Daratumumab, 775, 1456, 1502, 1622, 1683, 2175, 2184, 2190, 2192, 2197, 2212–2214, 2249, 2253, 2292
  maintenance, 2209
Dasatinib, 1458, 1613, 1619, 1782, 1794–1795, 1861–1862
Daunomycin, 1608
Daunorubicin, 1645, 1700, 1724
Deep venous thrombosis (DVT), 1276, 2186
  catheter-directed thrombolysis of, 1306
  isolated distal of leg, 1305
Defensins, 160
Deferasirox (DFX), 694, 906, 899
  toxicity, 906–907
    rash appearing in patients on deferasirox therapy, 906f
Deferiprone (DFP), 899, 905
Deferoxamine (DFO), 861, 895, 904
Defibrination syndrome and consumption coagulopathy (DIC), 1246
Delayed hemolytic transfusion reaction (DHTR), 571, 581–582, 860
  investigation of, 582
  management of, 582
  pseudohemolytic transfusion reactions, 582
Dendritic cells (DC), 27, 30, 208, 209f, 214, 233, 310, 324, 418, 1376, 1495, 2098
  in adult, 216–218
    AXL+ SIGLEC6+ DC, 215
    DC1, 214–215
    DC2, 215
    DC3, 215
  deficiency, 226
  discovery, 208–209
  growth factors, 218
  historical perspective, 208–209
    Langerhans cells, 215
  migratory DC, 215
  molecular and cellular functions, 220–226
  morphology and distribution, 214
  origin, 216–220, 217f
  plasmacytoid dendritic cells (pDC), 214
  regulation of development by transcription factors, 219, 219f
    ID2-ZEB2-TCF4 axis, 220
    IRF4, IRF8, and BATF3, 220
    pioneer factors in early stem cell compartment, 219–220
    terminal differentiation factors, 220
  role in disease, 226–227
    sarcomas, 1378
    tumors, 1378
Denileukin diftitox (DD), 1504, 2101
Denosumab, 2220
2-Deoxy-2-[fluorine-18] fluoro-D-glucose (18F-FDG), 2019
Deoxyadenosine, 2059
Deoxyadenosine triphosphate (dATP), 1402, 2059
Deoxycoformycin (dCF), 2059
2-Deoxycoformycin (DCF), 2099
Deoxygenated Hb S polymer, 834
Deoxyribonucleic acid (DNA), 833

Dermato-neuro syndrome, 2284
Dermoid cysts, 1431
1-Desamino-8-D-arginine vasopressin (DDAVP), 1196, 1246
Desmopressin, 1196
Desmopressin acetate (DDAVP), 987
Determinants of severity, 856–857
Dexamethasone (DEX), 1417, 1615, 1672, 2184, 2186, 2190–2194, 2196–2198, 2210, 2212–2217, 2251, 2253, 2255, 2270
Dexamethasone/prednisone, 2216
Dextran, 774, 1137
Diabetes, 903, 1620, 1797
  type 1, 330
  type 2, 688
Diabetes insipidus (DI), 1364
Diabetes mellitus, 688, 695, 903, 1042, 2381
Diabetic acidosis, hemolysis associated with, 754
Diacylglycerol (DAG), 276, 1193, 1498
Diacylglycerol kinase epsilon (*DGKE*), 1143
1,2-Diacylglycerol (DAG), 406
Diamond-Blackfan anemia (DBA), 96, 974, 1008, 1014, 1696, 1737, 1760, 2371
  clinical presentation, 1014
    physical abnormalities in patients with Diamond-Blackfan Anemia, 1014t
  differential diagnosis, 1016
    differential diagnosis of DBA *vs.* TEC, 1016t
    displaced and "trigger" thumbs in a patient with Diamond-Blackfan anemia, 1014f
  genetics, 1014–1015
  laboratory evaluation, 1015–1016
  pathogenesis, 1015
  prognosis, 1017–1018
  treatment, 1016–1017
Diamond-Blackfan syndrome, 615
Diarrhea, 2245
Diastolic dysfunction, 850
Didanosine (ddI), 1410
Dideoxynucleotides (ddNTPs), 61
Diepoxybutane (DEB), 974
Diffuse large B-cell lymphoma (DLBCL), 34, 281, 1415, 1455, 1458, 1511, 1866, 1872, 1876–1882, 1887f, 1901, 1921–1923, 1945–1946, 1964–1966, 1991, 1995–1996, 2039, 2117, 2343
  clinical features and management, 1997–1998
    mature B-NHL in children, 1998t
  cytologic variability in diffuse large B-cell lymphoma, 1877f
  frontline therapy for DLBCL, 1966–1967
  germinal center B-cell lymphoma phenotype, 1878f
  histology DLBCL, 1996f
  indications for allogeneic hematopoietic cell transplantation, 2343
  indications for autologous hematopoietic transplantation, 2343
  large B-cell lymphomas, 1965t
  management of relapsed/refractory disease, 1967–1968
  not otherwise specified (NOS), 1876–1878
  pathology and molecular characteristics, 1996–1997
  primary mediastinal large B-cell lymphoma, 1968–1969
    large B-cell lymphoma of mediastinum, 1968f
  proposed molecular classification of, 1924t
  uncommon types of, 1884f
Diffuse lymphangiomatosis, 1438
Diffuse pulmonary infiltrates, 1074
DiGeorge syndrome (DGS), 1156, 1399–1400
Digoxin, 1109
Dihydrofolate reductase (DHFR), 948, 1538
  homozygous mutation in, 963
Dihydrorhodamine (DHR), 1350, 1396, 1547
Dilute Russell viper venom time (DRVVT), 1260
Dilutional thrombocytopenia, 576
Dimethyl sulfoxide, 2259
Dimethylsulfoxide (DMSO), 100, 2298
Dimorphic anemia, 647
Dipeptidylpeptidase IV (DPPIV), 2072
Dipyridamole, 1137
Direct antiglobulin test (DAT), 547, 572, 774–775, 2018
  flowchart suggesting rational clinical laboratory approach for investigating positive direct antiglobulin test, 775f
  and indirect antiglobulin test (IAT), 774f

Direct Coombs test, 774–775
Direct nucleotide sequencing, 777
Direct oral anticoagulants (DOACs), 1264, 1291, 1298
  reversal of, 1301
Direct thrombin inhibitor (DTI), 1293
Direct-acting antivirals (DAAs), 1949
Directed differentiation protocols, 1550
Directed donation (DD), 565–566
  acute normovolemic hemodilution, 565
  intraoperative and postoperative salvage and reinfusion, 565–566
  preoperative autologous donation (PAD), 565
Direct thrombin inhibitors, parenteral, 1295
  argatroban, 1295
  bivalirudin, 1295
  comparison of parenteral direct thrombin inhibitors, 1295t
  hirudins, 1295
Disease progression, 1913
Disease severity, 761
Disease-causative variants, 1184
Disease-modifying antirheumatic drugs (DMARDs), 1432
Disialosyl antibodies, 2281
Disintegrin (Dis), 1126
Disseminated intravascular coagulation (DIC), 428, 581, 1081, 1158, 1242, 1246, 1279, 1630, 1698, 1723
  chronic, 1249–1250
  clinical features, 1250
    acute disseminated intravascular coagulation, 1250
    basic blood examinations, 1250
    chronic disseminated intravascular coagulation, 1250
    coagulation defect, 1250
    laboratory diagnosis, 1250
    laboratory findings, 1251
    tests for fibrinolysis, 1250
  compensated, 1249–1250
  differential diagnosis, 1251
  emerging therapies for, 1254
  emerging therapies for disseminated intravascular coagulation, 1254
  etiology and incidence, 1246
    etiologies of disseminated intravascular coagulation, 1246
  hemolysis due to, 829
  mechanisms by disseminated intravascular coagulation initiated, 1246–1247, 1247f
    tissue factor, 1247
    vascular endothelium, 1247
  pathology, 1253–1254
  pathophysiology, 1246
    mechanisms by disseminated intravascular coagulation initiated, 1246–1247
    role of cytokines, 1247–1250
  specific features of various forms of, 1252
    coagulopathy of COVID-19 infection, 1253
    disseminated intravascular coagulation in neonates and infants, 1252
    hemolytic transfusion reactions, 1253
    Kasabach-Merritt syndrome, 1253
    neoplastic disorders, 1252–1253
    obstetric disorders, 1252
    purpura fulminans, 1252
    snakebite, 1253
  treatment, 1251
    anticoagulants, 1251
    replacement therapy with platelets and coagulation factors, 1251–1252
    therapeutic measures, 1252
Disseminated juvenile xanthogranuloma (JXG), 1379
Distal, acquired, demyelinating, symmetric neuropathy with M-protein (DADS-M), 2276
Distal ischemia, 1177
Dithiothreitol (DTT), 755
Diuretic therapy, 2257
Divalent metal ion transporter 1 (DMT1), 628–629, 633
Diverse assay systems, 1261
Dizziness, 2245
DLBCL, frontline therapy for, 1966–1967
DNA methylation, 362

DNA methyltransferase (DNMT), 1636
DNA methyltransferase 1 (DNMT1), 2074
DNA methyltransferase 1-dependent DNA methylation
 (DNMT1-dependent DNA methylation), 1629
DNA methyltransferase 3A (*DNMT3A*), 1630, 1755
DNA methyltransferase inhibitor (DNMTi), 1647
 therapy, 1647
*DNAJC*21, 985
DNA microinjection, direct, 1524
Down syndrome (DS), 48, 1571, 1595, 1600, 1609, 1667,
 1696, 1737
 children with, 1677
 management of patients with, 1704
Down syndrome–associated transient myeloproliferative
 disorder (DS–TMD), 367
Doxil-vincristine-dexamethasone (DVD), 2198
Doxorubicin, 1417, 2002, 2099, 2100, 2122, 2128, 2197
Doxorubicin, bleomycin, vinblastine, and dacarbazine
 (ABVD), 1418, 2133
Doxoribicin pegylated liposomal, 2099, 2194, 2198, 2216
Doxycycline, 1474
Drug-induced immune hemolytic anemia (DI-IHA), 770,
 784–787
 clinical manifestations, 786
 drugs associated with immune hemolysis or
 autoantibodies, 785t
 laboratory features, 786
 management, 787
 mechanisms, 784
  autoimmune mechanism, 786
  drug adsorption mechanism, 785
  mechanisms of drug-induce hemolysis or positive
   direct antiglobulin test, 786t
  multiple mechanisms-unifying hypothesis, 786
  neoantigen mechanism, 785–786
  nonimmunologic protein adsorption mechanism,
   786
  proposed theory of drug-induced antibody
   reactions, 786f
Drugs, 669
Dysfibrinogenemia, 474, 1218–1219, 1259, 1287
 laboratory diagnosis of, 1218–1219
 molecular basis of, 1218
 therapy, 1219
Dyshemoglobinemias, 941–942
 carbon monoxide poisoning, 942
 SARS-CoV2 and dyshemoglobinemia, 942
 sulfhemoglobinemia, 942
Dyskeratosis congenita (DC), 955, 974, 980–984, 1335,
 1737, 2381
Dysmyelopoetic syndromes, 1737
Dysphagia, 649, 805, 816, 1790
Dysprothrombinemia, 1220, 1286

E

EBV infection, susceptibility to hemophagocytic
 lymphohistiocytosis and, 1404–1405
Echinocandins, 1475
Echinocytic disorders, 622 744
Echocardiography, 1809
Eculizumab, 350, 352, 779, 811, 815, 817, 1004, 1145,
 2303
Eculizumab/ravulizumab, 811–812, 812f
Eczematoid-like purpura, 1171
Electrophoresis, serum, 2175, 2239
ELISA systems, commercial, 1264
Elliptocytosis, spherocytic, 739
Emicizumab, 1228
Enasidenib, 1460, 1650
Encephalitis, 1386
Encephalopathy, 707
Encode unique housekeeping isozymes (ALAS1
 isozymes), 703
End-of-induction (EOI), 1671
End-stage renal disease (ESRD), 705
Endocrine disorders, 1041–1042
Endocrine glands, 902
 adrenal, 903
 diabetes, 903
 growth impairment, 902
 hypogonadism, 902–903
 hypoparathyroidism, 903
 hypothyroidism, 903
 pregnancy, 903
Endothelial P-selectin, 416

Endothelin receptor (ET$_A$), 853
 antagonists, 921
Endothelium, 416–418
 angiopoietins and receptors, 531
 normal angiogenesis, 531
 NOTCH signaling, 531–532
 role of ADAMTS13, 532
 vascular endothelial growth factor and receptors, 531
Endotoxin, 1344
Energy metabolism, 120–121
 and generation of adenosine triphosphate, 395
Energy producing pathway, 749
Enzyme-linked immunosorbent assay (ELISA), 1131,
 1202, 1260, 1280
Eosinophilia, 1772
 definition of, 1836
 eosinophilia-associated leukemias, 1836
 eosinophilia-myalgia syndrome, 1837
 myeloid and lymphoid neoplasms with, 1772
Eosinophilic esophagitis (EE), 168, 187
Eosinophilic granuloma, 1364, 1366
Eosinophilic granulomatosis with polyangiitis (eGPA),
 178
Eosinophilic lung diseases, 1837
Eosinophilic neoplasms, 1836
 biology of FIP1L1-PDGFRA, 1839–1840
 clinical presentation and prognosis, 1840
  allogeneic stem cell transplantation, 1845
  antibody approaches, 1845
  cardiac surgery, 1845
  clinical presentation, 1840
  clinicopathologic features, 1840
  fusion tyrosine kinase genes associated with
   myeloid/lymphoid neoplasms and eosinophilia,
   1842f
  organ manifestations of eosinophilic neoplasms/
   hypereosinophilic syndromes, 1842t
  prognosis, 1840–1842
  treatment of HES and chronic eosinophilic
   leukemia, 1844–1845
  treatment of patients with genetically defined
   neoplasms, 1843–1844
 definition of eosinophilia, 1836
 diagnostic evaluation for hypereosinophilia,
  1837–1839
 eosinophil physiology, 1836–1837
 epidemiology, 1836
 modern classification, 1837
 modern classification and clinicopathologic landmarks
  in eosinophilic disorders, 1836t
 primary eosinophilic neoplasms in international
  consensus classification, 1837t
Eosinophils, 1, 5, 29, 81, 168, 2283
 and allergic disease, 184–187
 and asthma, 184
 in autoimmune diseases, 187–188
 controversy, 185
 crystalloid granule, 173
 cytokines, chemokines, and growth factors, 182–183t
 cytolysis, 177–178
 degranulation, 174–178
  content of human eosinophil granules and
   secretory vesicles, 175t
  mechanisms, 177
  molecular regulation of secretory vesicle-plasma
   membrane fusion, 177f
  putative physiological modes, 176f
  receptors expressed by eosinophils, 176
  triggers, 176–177
 differentiation, 168–170
 effector role of eosinophil in worm infections, 188
 eosinophil-based treatment strategies using
  corticosteroids, 186
 eosinophil-derived cytokines, chemokines, and growth
  factors, 181–184
 granule proteins, 173–174
 hypersegmentation of eosinophils and negative
  staining for peroxidase and phospholipids, 1354
 immunological and physiological roles of, 184
 as immunoregulatory cells, 180–181
 mediators, 172–184, 173f
 membrane-derived mediators, 178
 migration, 1836
 morphology, 1840
 peripheral blood eosinophil
  electron photomicrographs, 169f

  stained with May-Grünwald-Giemsa, 168f
 production and survival in peripheral tissue, 170
 relative risk reduction of asthma exacerbations with
  monoclonal antibodies, 187t
 respiratory burst, 178–179
 signaling pathway leading from binding of IL-5, 170f
 tissue accumulation, 170–172
 translocation of chemokine CCL5/RANTES, 183f
EP300, 1920
Ephrin type B receptor 2 defect (EPHB2 defect), 1189
Epidemiologic data, 1246
Epidermal growth factor (EGF), 338
 EGF-like domains, 430
 module, 338
Epidermoid cysts, 1431
Epigenetic regulation of megakaryopoiesis, 369–371
Epigenetic regulators, 370
EpiLymph, 1950
Epinephrine, 394, 409, 1859
Episodic angioedema, 1837
Episodic hemolysis, 805, 1039
Episomal self-replicating Systems, 1526
Episomal vectors, integrating and, 1524
Epistaxis, 1101, 1163, 1220, 1245
 bleeding, 1220
Epitope spread, 1099
Epo receptors (EpoRs), 94, 633
Epratuzumab, 1501, 1680
Epstein syndrome, 1354
Epstein-Barr virus (EBV), 34, 997, 1336, 1378, 1382,
 1399, 1414, 1482, 1504, 1872, 1923, 1945,
 1991, 2076, 2133, 2285, 2319
 EBV-associated subtypes, 2116
 EBV-encoded small RNAs in situ hybridization, 1387
 EBV-mediated PTLD, 2382
 EBV–based vector plasmids, 1526
 Epstein-Barr Virus–associated hemophagocytic
  lymphohistiocytosis, 1387
 Epstein-Barr virus–associated lymphoma, 1388
 immune response to, 1383–1385
Epstein-Barr virus–positive diffuse large B-cell
 lymphoma, 1880–1881, 1881f
 considerations, 1881
 genetics, 1881
 immunophenotype, 1881
 morphology, 1881
Epstein-Barr virus–related disorders
 EBV–associated disorders in primary
  immunodeficiency, 1389–1390
 Epstein-Barr virus–associated lymphoma, 1388
  Burkitt Lymphoma, 1388
  EBV-associated lymphomas and lymphoid lesions,
   1389
  Epstein-Barr virus in people living with HIV, 1389
  Hodgkin lymphoma, 1388
  natural killer/T-Cell Lymphoma, 1389
  posttransplant Lymphoproliferative disease
   (PTLD), 1388–1389
 historical background, 1382
 immune response to Epstein-Barr virus infection,
  1383–1385
 infectious mononucleosis, 1385–1387
 other Epstein-Barr virus–related hematologic diseases,
  1387–1388
  chronic active EBV infection (CAEBV), 1387
  Epstein-Barr Virus–associated hemophagocytic
   lymphohistiocytosis, 1387
 viral biology/lymphocyte immortalization/viral gene
  expression, 1382–1383
  EBV latency gene patterns, 1384f
  schematic depicting EBV infection and antiviral
   immune response, 1383f
Erwinia caratovora, 1462
Erwinia chrysanthemi, 1673
Erythroblastic differentiation, stages of, 94–95
Erythroblasts, 77, 93, 94f
 iron metabolism within, 634
Erythrocytapheresis, 592, 694
Erythrocyte 2, 3-diphosphoglycerate (DPG), 761, 1074
Erythrocyte adenosine deaminase (eADA), 1009, 1014
Erythrocyte, human, 540
Erythrocyte membranes, 726–728, 727f, 742
 abnormal cells associated with alterations in
  erythrocyte membrane, 727f
 acanthocytic disorders, 742–744
 and cytoskeleton, 108, 111f

Erythrocyte membranes (*continued*)
  band 3 in anion and CO_2 transport, 112*f*
  lipid composition, 108–109
  lipid turnover and acquisition, 109
  membrane and membrane-associated enzymes, 112
  membrane proteins, 109–112
  membrane transport proteins and membrane permeability, 111–112
  metabolic pathways in erythrocyte, 120*f*
 echinocytic disorders, 744
 hereditary elliptocytosis syndromes, 735–740
 hereditary spherocytosis, 728–735
 human erythrocyte membrane proteins, genes, and associated disorders, 728*t*
 protein deficiencies, 796
  acetylcholinesterase, 796
  basis of protein deficiencies in PNH, 796
  decay accelerating factor, 796
  membrane inhibitor of reactive lysis (MIRL), 796
 skeleton protein interactions, 737
 stomatocytic disorders, 740–742
 sulfatide, 837
 target cell disorders, 744–745
Erythrocyte protoporphyrin, 662, 667, 713
Erythrocyte sedimentation rate (ESR), 2119
Erythrocytes, 1, 22, 729, 620, 773, 821, 1033, 1037, 1248, 1810, 1812
 abnormalities, 730
 function, 112–121
Erythrocytopheresis, 759
Erythrocytosis, 934, 1073
 chronic relative, 1072
 classification and approach to patient with erythrocytosis, 1071–1072
  approach to patients with erythrocytosis, 1073*f*
  classification of erythrocytosis, 1072*t*
  World Health Organization criteria for diagnosis of polycythemia vera, 1073*t*
 definitions and terminology, 1070
 hereditary, 1071, 1073
 idiopathic erythrocytosis, 1072, 1077
 with inappropriate increased erythropoietin secretion, 1076
  disorders associated with normoxic secondary erythrocytosis, 1076*t*
 pathologic physiology, 1070
  blood viscosity and oxygen transport, 1070–1071
  relation to treatment of erythrocytosis, 1071
 primary erythrocytosis, 1073–1074
 primary proliferative, 1072–1074
 relative erythrocytosis, 1072–1073
 secondary erythrocytosis, 1074–1077
  aberrant erythropoietin secretion 1076
  abnormal hemoglobins, 1075
  cardiopulmonary disease, 1074–1075
  drug-induced erythrocytosis, 1077
  familial secondary erythrocytosis due to abnormalities of Hb/oxygen affinity, 1075
  high-altitude erythrocytosis, 1074
 spurious 1072
Erythroderma, 2083
Erythroferrone (ERFE), 631, 690, 891, 1023
Erythroid ALAS2 regulation, 100–101
Erythroid cells, 11, 93, 736
 committed erythroid progenitors, 93–94
 differentiation, 93*f*
 erythroid precursors, 94
 flow cytometric analysis of erythroid precursors, 96
 heme synthesis in, 656–659
  pathways of regulation of erythroid 5-aminolevulinate synthase, 659*f*
 lineages, 1849
 proliferation and maturation of erythron, 96–97
 stages of erythroblastic differentiation, 94–95
Erythroid growth factors, 82–83
Erythroid heme synthesis, 656
Erythroid hyperplasia, 656, 662, 667
 chronic, 846
Erythroid niches in bone marrow, 84
Erythroid precursors, 634
 iron delivery to, 633–634
Erythroid-myeloid progenitors (EMPs), 70
Erythroid-predominant MDS (MDS-E), 1599
Erythroid-specific isozymes (ALAS2 isozymes), 703

Erythroid-stimulating agents (ESAs), 1827
Erythrokinetic studies, 857
Erythroleukemias, 13, 1599, 1694
Erythromyeloid progenitors (EMPs), 216
 from yolk sac, 216
Erythron, proliferation and maturation of, 96–97
Erythropoiesis, 93, 923
 control, 102–107
  abnormal Epo/EpoR signaling, 106
  action of erythropoietin, 103–106
  erythropoietin, 103
  mechanism of action, 106–107
  tissue oxygen, 102–103
 impaired, 1040–1041
Erythropoiesis-maturing agent (EMA), 1745
Erythropoiesis-stimulating agents (ESAs), 560, 640, 1037–1038, 1066, 1737, 1745
 causes of erythropoietin resistance, 1038*t*
 erythropoietin resistance, 1038
 side effects/adverse reactions, 1038
Erythropoietic activity, 690
Erythropoietic cells, 38
Erythropoietic cutaneous porphyrias, 714
 congenital erythropoietic porphyria (CEP), 714–715
 erythropoietic protoporphyria and X-linked protoporphyria, 716–718
Erythropoietic differentiation, 28
Erythropoietic hemochromatosis, 656
Erythropoietic protoporphyria (EPP), 714, 716–719, 717*f*
 clinical description, 716
 laboratory findings, 718
 late-onset protoporphyria, 718
 long-term management, 718
 molecular basis and pathogenesis, 716
 sideroblastic anemia in, 661–662
 treatment, 718
Erythropoietin (Epo), 11, 71, 103, 371, 378, 600, 631, 911, 966, 1017, 1053, 1175, 1538, 1695, 1745, 1827
 action, 103–106
 assays for erythropoietin and erythropoietin levels in health and disease, 107
 biology in fetus and neonate, 1053
 concentration, serum, 1811
 erythropoietin-independent colony formation, 1812
 in human fetus, 1053*t*
 structure, 103
 therapy, 734, 863
Erythropoietin receptor (EpoR), 103–106, 1675
 signaling pathways, 104*f*
Erythropoietin receptor gene (*EPOR*), 1074
Erythropoietin, recombinant human (rh Epo), 1051, 1035, 1077
 administration, 1048
 recombinant Epo-induced immune pure red cell aplasia, 1009
 therapy, 1035
Erythropoietin resistance (Epo resistance), 1038
Escherichia coli, 346, 348, 691, 709, 753, 846, 1332, 1434, 1438, 1462, 1673, 2221
Essential cryoglobulinemic vasculitis, 1168
Essential hyperglobulinemia, 2160
Essential thrombocythemia (ET), 375, 1175–1176, 1763, 1770, 1770*f*, 1811, 1821
 clinical and laboratory features, 1177
  characteristic megakaryocyte proliferation in marrow specimen from essential thrombocythemia patient, 1178*f*
  clinical and laboratory features of essential thrombocythemia patients from three series, 1177*t*
 clonal thrombocytosis, 1176
 diagnostic criteria, 1177
  2016 WHO diagnostic criteria for essential thrombocythemia, 1178*t*
 epidemiology, 1177
 natural history and prognosis, 1178–1178
  risk categories and treatment recommendations based on revised IPSET-Thrombosis, 1179*t*
 pathophysiology, 1177
 treatment, 1179
  aspirin, 1179
  cytoreductive therapy, 1179
  post–essential thrombocythemia myelofibrosis, 1179
Esterase, 138

Estimated glomerular filtration rate (eGFR), 853, 1036, 1143, 2244
Estrogenic hormones, 1157
Estrogens, 1157, 1165
Etanercept, 1371
Ethanol, 1157
Ethylenediaminetetraacetic acid (EDTA), 1, 22, 581
Etoposide, 1370, 1417, 1703, 1844, 2100, 2175
Etoposide, methylprednisolone, cytarabine, cisplatin (ESHAP), 2124
Etoposide, prednisone, vincristine, cyclophosphamide, doxorubicin (EPOCH), 2100
Etoposide and DAP (EDAP), 2217
Exosomes, 196, 225, 334
 uptake, 333–334
Exportin 1 (XPO1), 1462
Extended-spectrum-β-lactamase (ESBL), 1471
Extended-spectrum-β-lactamase-producing Enterobacterales (ESBL-E), 1474
Extensive replacement therapy, 1252
External pressure, 1162
External quality assurance (EQA), 27
Extracellular domain, MPL, 373
Extracellular matrix (ECM), 361, 531
Extracellular molecules, 363
Extracellular proteins, 331
Extracellular signal-regulated kinase pathway (ERK pathway), 43, 2049
Extracellular vesicles, 225, 333
Extracorporeal circulation, bleeding associated with, 1266
Extracorporeal membrane oxygenator, 1123
Extracorporeal photochemotherapy (ECP), 2096, 2098
Extracutaneous mastocytoma, 1855
Extracutaneous MF/SS, 2079–2080
Extraembryonic hematopoiesis, 70–71
Extrahepatic biliary tract obstruction, 1242
Extramedullary AML, 1631
Extramedullary disease (EMD), 1843
Extramedullary hematopoiesis (EMH), 70, 1821
Extramedullary leukemia, 1631
Extramedullary myeloid tumor (EMT), 2089
Extramedullary relapse, treatment of isolated, 1678–1679
Extranodal marginal zone B-cell lymphoma of mucosa-associated lymphoid tissue, 1875
 extranodal marginal zone B-cell lymphoma of mucosa-associated lymphoid tissue, 1876*f*
 genetics, 1876
 immunophenotype, 1876
 morphology, 1875–1876
 risk factors for extranodal marginal zone B-cell lymphomas of MALT lymphomas, 1876*t*
Extranodal marginal zone lymphoma, 1915–1916
 biology of translocations common in, 1915*f*
 guidelines for molecular testing in, 1916*t*
 translocations in, 1915*t*
Extranodal natural killer/T-cell lymphoma, 1889
Extranodal NK/T-cell lymphoma (ENKTL), 1974
Extranodal T-cell lymphomas, 1974–1975
Extrarenal complications, 1140
Extrasplenic tissue, 1424, 1435
Extravasated red blood cells, 1171
Extravascular hemoglobin degradation, 124
 alternate pathways of heme and bilirubin catabolism, 126–127
 bilirubin transport, 125
 heme oxygenase system and bilirubin formation, 124–125
 hepatic bilirubin metabolism, 125–126
 intestinal bile pigment metabolism, 126
 laboratory evaluation of hemoglobin catabolism and bile pigments, 127
Extravascular hemolysis, 121, 837
Extravascular matrix, 531
Extravascular overload, 2278–2279
Extremely low-birth-weight (ELBW), 1065
Extrinsic apoptotic pathway, 2012
Extrinsic pathway inhibitor, 464
Extrinsic pathway of coagulation, disorders of, 1089
Eyes, 853–855, 903–904
 ocular abnormalities in sickle cell anemia, 854*f*
EZH2 gene, 1568, 1630, 1638, 1738, 1825, 1838, 1857, 1871, 1920
EZH2 mutation, 1575, 1587, 1758, 1764, 1825, 1849, 1931

F

Fabry disease, 1546
Facial hypertrichosis, 712
Factitious anemia, 639
Factitious purpura, 1172
Factor H–related proteins (FHR proteins), 348
Factor V deficiency
   congenital, 454
   inherited, 1220
Factor VII recombinant activated (rFVIIa), 1197, 1227, 1228, 1246
Factor VIII autoantibodies in nonhemophilic patient, 1255–1258
Factor VIII recombinant (r-FVIII), 1208
Factor X deficiency, inherited, 1222
Factor XIII deficiency, congenital, 1219, 1231
Factor XIII quanitative assay method, 1086
Familial erythrocytosis, secondary, 1074
Fanconi anemia (FA), 955, 974–975, 1335, 1536, 1547, 1629, 1696, 1737, 2314, 2319, 2320f, 2371
   alternative donor HCT for FA, 2320–2321
   clinical features, 975–976
      physical findings associated with Fanconi anemia, 976t
   diagnostic testing, 975
      chromosomal breakage in Fanconi anemia, 975f
   differential diagnosis, 976
   FA and myelodysplastic syndrome/leukemia, 2323
   fludarabine in preparative regimen after HCT for, 2322f
   gene therapy for FA, 2323
   HCT conditioning regimens for FA, 2319–2320
   HLA-haploidentical HCT for FA, 2321–2323
   laboratory features, 976–977
   late effects after HCT for FA, 2323
   outcomes in, 2321f
   pathophysiology, 977–979
      Fanconi anemia genes, 977t
   supportive care, 979
   treatment, 979
Fanconi complementation group C gene (*FANCC*), 1536
Fanconi syndrome, 906
Farnesoid X receptor (FXR), 413
FAS gene, 2074
FAS mutations, 2074
Fas-associated death domain (FADD), 300
Fat cells, 11
Fatal neurodegenerative form (NPD-A), 1362
Fatty acid–binding protein 4 (FABP4), 1629
Fava bean (*Vicia fava*, broad bean), 754
Favism, 752, 754
FBXW7 gene, 1585, 1995
FBXW7 mutations, 1604, 1604, 1913
Fc receptor γ chain (FcR γ chain), 404
Fc receptors, 222
Fc-receptor-mediated phagocytosis, 770
FCM cross-match (FCXM), 40
Febrile nonhemolytic transfusion reactions (FNHTRs), 565, 582, 898
   management of, 582
   prevention of, 582
Fecal protoporphyrin excretion, 718
FECH cDNA, 718
FECH gene, 716
FECH mutation, 718
Fechtner syndrome, 1155, 1354
Fedratinib, 1459–1460, 1831
Feline leukemia virus, subgroup C receptor 1 (FLVCR1), 628, 658
Feline leukemia virus subgroup C (FeLV-C), 101
Feline leukemia virus subgroup C receptor (FLVCR), 101
Felty syndrome, 1337, 1432
Female embryo, 751
Fenton reaction, 891
FERMT3, 1346
Ferric citrate, 646
Ferric-transferrin (Fe-Tf), 101
Ferritin, 13, 634–635, 899, 1011, 1015
   serum, 612–613, 643, 858, 1034, 1037
Ferrochelatase (FECH), 98, 703
Ferrokinetic analysis, 890
Ferroportin, 629, 678, 681, 899
Ferroportin hemochromatosis (SLC40A1 hemochromatosis), 681
Ferroportin mutations, 681

Ferroportin transcript (FPN1B), 632
Ferroprotoporphyrin IX, 113
Ferroptosis, 683
Ferrylhemoglobin, 118
Fetal anemias
   anemia of prematurity, 1063
   characteristics of fetal/neonatal red blood cells, 1059t
   erythropoietin biology in, 1053
   fetal and neonatal erythrocyte membrane and metabolism, 1058–1059
   fetal anemia owing to congenital infection, 1062–1063
   iron deficiency in fetus and newborn infant, 1063–1064
   owing to hemolysis, 1059–1061
   owing to hemorrhage, 1061–1062
   reference intervals for erythrocyte values during human fetal development, 1054–1058
Fetal development, human, reference intervals for erythrocyte values during, 1054–1058
Fetal erythrocytes, 1061
   membrane and metabolism, 1058–1059
   oxygen dissociation curves of blood from term infants at different postnatal ages, 1060f
Fetal Hb carriers, δβ and hereditary persistence of, 913
Fetal hemoglobin (HbF), 856, 1014–1015, 1055
   hereditary persistence of, 868
   hereditary persistence of, 868
Fetal liver hematopoiesis, 216
Fetal macrophages and dendritic cells, 216
Fetal-like erythropoiesis, 1014
Fetal-like red cells, 1015
Fetoplacental hemorrhage, 1062
Fever, 1469–1470, 1630, 1668, 1703, 2053
   congenital sideroblastic anemia with, 664
   empiric approach to, 1470f
   lower risk patients with, 1470
   management of, 847
Fibrillin, 1166
Fibrin, 472–479, 493
   assembly, 477–478
      schematic representation of whole blood fibrin formation, 477f
   cross-linking, 478
   formation, 475–478
   intravascular, 1248
   monomers, 477, 1250
   regulation of fibrin lysis, 478
      fibrinogenolysis, 478
      fibrinolysis, 478–479
   stabilizing factor, 471
Fibrin degradation products (FDPs), 1085, 1244, 1248–1250, 1723
Fibrin-platelet thrombi, 1139
Fibrin-specific therapy, 1303
Fibrinogen, congenital quantitative defects in, 1218
Fibrinogen (factor I), 397, 402, 472–473, 858, 1217, 1247, 1259
   A-α chain, 2238
   biochemistry and activation, 474–475
   clinical disorders of fibrinogen molecule, 1217–1219
   dysfunction, 1218
   function, 478
   gene structure and expression, 473–474
      afibrinogenemia, 474
      biosynthesis, 474
      hereditary dysfibrinogenemias, 474
   human fibrinogen chains, 475t
   polymerization, 475–478
   regulation of fibrin lysis, 478–479
   replacement, 1252
   schematic and crystal structure of human fibrinogen, 476f
Fibrinogen-420, 473
Fibrinogen, Hall model of, 475
Fibrinogen quanitative disorders, pathogenesis of, 1217
Fibrinogenolysis, 478, 1244, 1254
   chronic, 1251
   intermittent, 1251
   secondary, 1248
Fibrinolysis, 478–479, 1244, 1248
   dynamic inhibitory system, 460–463
   essential features of coagulation, 427–428
   fibrinogenolysis and fibrinolysis, 479f
   impaired endogenous, 1285–1287
   inhibitors of fibrinolytic system, 486–493
   overview of procoagulant pathways, 428–429

   physiologic regulation of, 493
      cellular regulation of, 493
      role of platelets in regulation of, 494
      tissue-type plasminogen activator receptors, 493–494
      urokinase-type plasminogen activator receptor, 493
   procoagulant cofactor proteins, 451–458
   procoagulant proteins, 430–436
   proteinase inhibitors, 463–466
   proteins of clot formation, 471–479
   proteins of fibrinolytic system, 479–486
   serine protease inhibitor superfamily (SERPIN), 466–471
   tests for, 1086, 1250
   thrombin, 458–460
   vitamin K–dependent protein family, 436–451
Fibrinolytic process, 427
Fibrinolytic proteins, 1276
Fibrinolytic system, 1301
   inhibitors of, 486
      α_2-Antiplasmin, 491–493
      plasminogen activator inhibitor-1 (PAI-1), 488–490
      plasminogen activator inhibitor-2 (PAI-2), 490–491
      thrombin-activatable fibrinolysis inhibitor (TAFI), 486–488
   proteins of, 479
      dynamic interaction between proteins and inhibitors of fibrinolysis, 480f
      plasminogen, 479–480
      plasminogen activators, 480–486
Fibrinopeptide A (FPA), 459
Fibrinopeptide B (FPB), 459
Fibrinopeptides, 471
   release, 476
Fibroblast growth factor receptor 1 (*FGFR1*), 1772, 1836
   myeloid and lymphoid neoplasms with, 1774
      eosinophilia and rearrangement of, 1772–1774
Fibroblast growth factor receptor 3 genes, 1791
Fibroblastic dendritic cell sarcoma, 1378
Fibroblastic reticular cells (FRCs), 242, 246
Fibroelastography, 2244
Fibronectin, 366, 406, 2285
Ficolin-1–rich granules, 143
Ficolins, 160
Filamin A (FLNa), 1195
   defects, 1195
Fip1-like-1-platelet-derived growth factor receptor-α (FIP1L1-PDGFRA), 1850
FIP1L1-PDGFRA
   biology of, 1839–1840
   histopathology of, 1841f
   laboratory findings in lymphocyte-variant hypereosinophilia, 1839t
Fish-mouth deformity, 849
Fixed dosing (FD), 1674
FK506, 1402
Flaming cells, 2178
Flavin adenine dinucleotide (FAD), 755
Flavivirus, 587
Fletcher factor deficiency, 1223
Flexed-tail mouse (f/f mouse), 665
Flotetuzumab, 1653
Flow cytometry (FCM), 2, 18, 954, 1322, 1324–1325, 1401, 1446, 1741–1743, 1954, 2148
   analysis of erythroid precursors, 96
   analysis of maturation in granulopoiesis, 29f
   applications, 40–42
   cellular DNA content and cell cycle analysis, 42–43
   detection of HLA-B27, 40
   in diagnosis of major primary immune deficiency, 42t
   functional assays, 43–44
   in hematology, 38–40
   historical background, 18
   multicolor analysis of hematologic malignancies, 31–38
   normal hematopoiesis, 27–31
   principles, 18
      cell sorting, 19–20
      data analysis and reporting, 22–27
      fluorochromes and panels, 22
      monoclonal antibodies (MAbs), 20
      sample preparation, 22
      validation of assays and quality assurance, 27
   stem cell transplantation, 40
   technologies, 2
   testing, 1398

Flt-1 receptor, 531
*FLT*3 gene, 1636, 2050
FLT3 inhibitors (FLT3i), 1460, 1648–1650
  gilteritinib, 1460
  midostaurin, 1460
FLT3 ligand (FL), 74, 1575
*FLT*3 mutations, 1575–1576, 1604, 1636, 1641, 1680, 1710
  interaction of normal and mutant *FLT*3, 1575f
*FLT*3-ITD gene, 1640
*FLT*3-ITD mutations, 1655, 1709–1710, 2336
Fluconazole, 1483
Fludarabine, 784, 1644, 1650, 1703, 1963, 1976, 2028, 2032, 2062, 2099, 2270
  in chronic lymphocytic leukemia, 1628
Fludarabine, idarubicin, and cytarabine (FLAG-Ida), 1703
Fludarabine and rituximab (FR), 2029
Fludarabine monophosphate (FAMP), 2099
Fludarabine with rituximab (FR), 2270
  and cyclophosphamide, 2029
Fludarabine/cyclophosphamide/rituximab (FCR), 2022
Fludrocortisone, 2259
Fluorescence detection, 2
Fluorescence in situ hybridization (FISH), 27, 48, 66, 1321, 1445, 1564, 1595, 1611, 1721, 1765, 1791, 1869, 1900, 1903, 1957, 2014, 2024, 2148, 2181–2182, 2239
  abnormalities and gene expression, 2016
    del 11q, 2016
    del 13q, 2016
    del 17p, 2016
    translocations of 14q32, 2016
    trisomy 12q, 2016
  analysis, 50–51
  analysis by, 2014–2015
  examples of, 1905f
  incidence of genomic abnormalities by Döhner hierarchical classification, 2014t
  nomenclature, 51–54
  time to first treatment and OS by, 2015f
Fluorescence microscopy, 718
Fluorescent aerolysin (FLAER), 807
Fluorescent spot test, 755
Fluorochromes, 18, 19t, 22, 42
Fluorodeoxyglucose (FDG), 1991, 2134
^{18}Fluorodeoxyglucose positron emitting tomography/CT (FDG-PET/CT), 2179
Fluorometric techniques, 1087
Fluoroquinolones, 1470–1471
Fluticasone inhaler, azithromycin and Montelukast (FAM), 2306
Fms-like tyrosine kinase 3 (*FLT*3), 1460, 1627, 1634–1635, 2335
  genes with recurrent mutations in AML, 1634t
  simplified diagram of, 1635f
Fms-like tyrosine kinase-3 ligand (FLT3LG), 218, 273
Foamy viral vectors, 1528
Focal adhesion kinase (FAK), 376
Focal nodular hyperplasia, 2382
Folate, 813, 947, 962, 1015, 1028
  in cells, 951
  malabsorption, hereditary, 963
  reactions and interrelationships between cobalamin, folate, and methionine metabolism, 947f
  structure of folate, 948f
  transmethylation and transsulfuration, 948
Folate deficiency, 1016
  causes of, 961–963
    alcohol, 962–963
    dietary, 961
    drug interference with folate metabolism, 962
    increased cellular folate requirements, 962
    malabsorption, 962
    renal dialysis, 962
  clinical manifestations of, 956
  homocysteine testing in, 958
  during pregnancy, 1048
  serum, 959
  treatment of, 965–966
Folate metabolism
  drug interference with, 962
  megaloblastic anemias not related to, 964
    drugs inducing macrocytosis, 964
    hereditary orotic acidemia, 964

Lesch-Nyhan Disease, 964
  thiamine responsive megaloblastic anemia, 964
Folate physiology, 950
  nutrition, 950–951
Folate uptake and metabolism, megaloblastic anemia due to disorders of, 963
Folic acid, 734, 965, 1011
  antagonist, 1608
  deficiency, 921
  supplementation, 1284
Folinic acid, 965
Follicle-stimulating hormone (FSH), 903, 2331
Follicular dendritic cells (FDCs), 240, 244–246, 1376–1377, 1378f, 2014, 2152
Follicular lymphoma (FL), 33, 255, 1323, 1869–1870, 1900, 1919–1921, 1943, 1959–1961, 1997, 2344
  and diffuse large B-cell lymphoma, 1921f
  duodenal-type follicular lymphoma, 1872
  genetics, 1871
  guidelines for molecular testing in, 1921
  immunophenotype, 1871
  location of breakpoint clusters in *BCL*2 gene, 1919f
  morphology, 1870–1871
    lymph node, 1871f
  pediatric-type follicular lymphoma, 1872
  primary cutaneous follicle center lymphoma (PCFCL), 1872
  revised edition World Health Organization classification of lymphoid neoplasms, 1870t
  in situ follicular neoplasia, 1872
  transformation, 1872
Follicular mucinosis (FM), 2084
Follicular T-cell lymphoma, 1886, 1929
Folliculotropic mycosis fungoides (FMF), 2085–2087
  with follicular mucinosis, 2087f
Fondaparinux, 1293, 1309
Food folates, 951
Food folic acid fortification program, 959, 961
Forced expiratory volume in 1 second (FEV1), 2361
Forkhead box 3P (FOXP3), 2072
Forkhead O transcription factors (FOXO), 1785
Formalin, 112
Formalin-fixed paraffin–embedded tissue specimen (FFPE tissue specimen), 51, 1901
Formalin-fixed tissue, 1445
Formyl peptides, 153
Forodesine, 2099
Forward grouping, 570
Forward scatter (FS), 18
Forward typing, 570
Foscarnet, 1387
Fostamatinib, 1107–1108
Fragmentation hemolysis, 827
  cardiac and large vessel abnormalities, 827
    clinical manifestations, 828
    etiology, 827–828, 828t
    incidence, 828
    laboratory findings, 828
    treatment, 828
  giant hemangiomas and hemangioendotheliomas, 829
  hemolysis due to disseminated intravascular coagulation, 829
  hemolysis due to malignant hypertension, 829
  with immune disorders, 829
  march hemoglobinuria, 829
  schistocytes in patients, 827f
  small vessel disease, 828–829
Fragmented cells, 936
Frameshift mutations, 888
Francisella tularensis, 162
Fred Hutchinson Cancer Research Center, The, 1001
Free iron, 891
Freedom from progression (FFP), 2120
Freedom from treatment failure (FFTF), 2121
Free light chain assay, serum, 2168
Fresh frozen plasma (FFP), 562–563, 1220
Friend leukemia integration 1 defect (FLI1 defect), 1194
Friend leukemia virus–induced erythroleukemia-1 (FLI1), 361
Friend of GATA-1 (FOG-1), 366
Frontline tyrosine kinase inhibitor, selection of, 1797
Frozen red cells, 561
Frozen-thawed plasma products (FFP), 584
Fucosyltransferase (FUT3), 547
Full-scale IQ (FSIQ), 843

Fulminant hemolysis, 781
Functional asplenia, 869
Functional assays, 1282, 1309
Functional Assessment of Cancer Therapy Fatigue Scale (FACT Scale), 1827
Functional Outcomes in Cardiovascular Patients Undergoing Surgical Hip Fracture Repair (FOCUS), 569
Fungal infections, 1000, 1350
Fusarium spp., 1481
Fusion toxins, 1503–1504

G

G protein–coupled receptors (GPCRs), 253, 406, 1189
  α_2-adrenergic receptor, 1189
  abnormalities of, 1189
  thromboxane A_2 receptor, 1189
GA-binding protein α (GAPBα), 368
Gadolinium-diethylenetriamine pentaacetic acid (Gadolinium-DTPA), 850
Gaisböck syndrome, 1072
Gamma chain (γc), 1401
Gamma-glutamyl-cysteine synthetase (GCS), 756
Gamma-retroviral vectors, 1526–1527
Ganciclovir, 1387, 1389
Gadolinium enhancement, late, 2244
Gantrisin, 753
Gas chromatography/mass spectrometry (MS), 958
Gas exchange, 2246
Gastric IF-Cbl complex (GIF-Cbl complex), 963
Gastric lymphoma, 1949
Gastric surgery, 960
Gastrins, 690
Gastritis, 1245
Gastroesophageal reflux disease (GERD), 184
Gastrointestinal disorders, chronic, 1242
GATA binding factor 1 (GATA1), 658
GATA-1 transcription factor, 1156
GATA-binding protein 1 (GATA-1), 366
GATA-binding protein 3 (GATA3), 2002, 2074
*GATA*1 gene, 168, 370, 1153, 1696
*GATA*1 mutation, 986, 1027, 1571–1572
*GATA*2 alterations, 987
*GATA*2 deficiency, 988
*GATA*2 gene, 71–72, 988
*GATA*2 mutation, 987, 1571–1572, 1630
GATA syndromes, 974, 987
  clinical features, 987–988
    clinical features of patients with GATA2 deficiency, 987f
  differential diagnosis, 988
  laboratory findings, 988
  pathophysiology, 988
  supportive care, 988
  treatment, 988
Gaucher disease, 1359, 1536, 2172
  clinical manifestations, 1360
    type 1 disease, 1360–1361
    type 2 disease, 1361
    type 3 disease, 1361
  definition and history, 1359
  diagnosis, 1361
  etiology and pathogenesis, 1359
    schematic structures of globoside, 1360f
  pathology, 1359
    splenic histopathology in Gaucher disease, 1361f
  treatment, 1361
Gaucher-like cells, 2178
Gaussian distribution, 1901
GB virus C, 902
gC1q-binding protein (gC1qR), 341
GCLC genes, 756
GCLM genes, 756
G-CSF therapy, chronic, 1334
Gel solin gene (*GSN* gene), 1175
Gelatinase granules, 143
Gelsolin, 2238
Gemcitabine, 1978, 2099, 2138
Gemfibrozil, 2096
Gemtuzumab ozogamicin (GO), 1455, 1504, 1651–1652, 1700, 1707, 1726, 1731
Gene addition, 1522
Gene clusters, 883
Gene delivery systems in HSCs, 1524
  nonviral vectors, 1524–1526

vectors, 1529
viral vectors, 1526–1529
Gene editing
　strategies, 987
　therapy, 1522
Gene expression, 362
　in HCL, 2050–2051
　and methylation profiling
　　mantle cell lymphoma, 1912
Gene expression profiling (GEP), 1877, 1918, 1957, 2168, 2183
　anaplastic large cell lymphoma, ALK positive and ALK negative, 1927
　angioimmunoblastic T-cell lymphoma, 1929
　Burkitt lymphoma, 1925
　diffuse large B-cell lymphoma and other high-grade B-cell lymphomas, 1922
　follicular lymphoma, 1920
　lymphoplasmacytic lymphoma/waldenström macroglobulinemia, 1918
　MM, 2182–2183
　peripheral T-cell lymphoma, not otherwise specified, 1928
Gene marking trials, 1530
Gene profiling, 366
Gene therapy, 866, 911–912, 1156, 1522
　approaches, 860
　constitutive or tissue-specific transgene expression, 1524
　ex vivo vs. in vivo gene therapy, 1522
　for FA, 2323
　gene addition vs. gene editing therapy, 1522
　gene transfer vectors and transduction, 1522–1524
　genotoxicity and insertional mutagenesis, 1524
　for hemoglobin disorders, 2328
　for hemoglobin disorders, 2328–2330
　for hemophilia, 1230
　integrating and episomal vectors, 1524
　multiplicity of infection (MOI), 1524
　replication-defective vectors, 1524
　in SCD, 2329
　somatic vs. germ cell gene therapy, 1522
　transductional targeting by pseudotyping, 1524
　trials with therapeutic intent, 1530
　　chronic granulomatous disease (CGD), 1536–1537
　　Fanconi anemia (FA), 1536
　　first-, second-, and third-generation HSC gene therapy clinical trials, 1531–1535t
　　Gaucher disease, 1536
　　severe combined immunodeficiency disease (SCID), 1536
Gene transfer into human HSCs, preclinical assays to investigate, 1537–1538
Gene transfer methods, 1522
Genetic disarray, 1028
Genetic disorders, 1346, 1738
Genetic manipulation approaches, 866
Genetic mutations, 435, 1141
Genetic sex, as indicated by leukocytes, 147–148
Genetic syndromes, 1667, 1737
Genitourinary tract, 213, 1101
Genome editing, 1522, 1547
　approaches for, 1547–1548
　　genome editing with CRISPR/Cas9, 1548f
　challenges and new advances to genome editing in HSCs, 1548–1549
　clinical applications of genome editing in HSCs, 1549
　technologies, 1549
Genome-wide association studies (GWASs), 857, 1667
Genome-wide gene expression arrays, 1610
Genome-wide sequencing, 1696
Genomic DNA (gDNA), 1904
Germ cell gene therapy, 1522
Gestation, 1337
Gestational hypertension, 1144
Gestational thrombocytopenia, 1108
GF1B genes, 1153
GFI1, 1333
GFI1B, 366, 368, 1153
Giant cell formation, 226
Giant hemangiomas, 1253
　and hemangioendotheliomas, 829
Giardia, 1396
Gibbon-ape leukemia virus (GALV), 1527
Giemsa stain, 49

Gigantocytes, 1025
Gilbert syndrome (GS), 126, 624, 732
Gilteritinib, 1460, 1648, 1650
Gingival bleeding, 1101
Givosiran, 708, 710
Glanzmann thrombasthenia (GT), 39, 398, 986, 1182–1184
Glasdegib, 1462, 1651
Global marrow defects, 1331
Globin genes, functional, 886
Glomerular function, 2180
Glomerular hyperfiltration, 853
Glomerular microthrombi, 1123
Glomerulonephritis, 2023
Glomerulosclerosis, 352
Glossitis of tongue, 956
GLRX5 gene, 661
Glucocerebrosidase (GC), 1530
Glucocorticoids, 783
Glucose, 395, 710, 749
Glucose 6-phosphate, 755, 761
Glucose phosphate isomerase deficiency (GPI deficiency), 761
Glucose transporter 1 (GLUT1), 742
Glucose-6-phosphate dehydrogenase (G6PD), 93, 616, 749, 821, 841, 937
　acute hemolytic anemia, 752–754
　clinical and hematologic features, 752
　congenital nonspherocytic hemolytic anemia, 754
　deficiency, 749–750, 1351
　diagnosis, 754–755
　enzyme abbreviations, 750f
　enzyme and variants, 751
　favism, 754
　genetics, 751–752
　　biochemical, epidemiological, and clinical features of select G6PD variants, 752t
　isozymes, 1812
　neonatal hyperbilirubinemia, 754
　pathophysiology, 752
　prevalence and geographic distribution, 750–751
　primaquine-induced hemolysis in G6PD A-variant, 750f
　screening, 755
　treatment, 755
Glutamic acid (Gla), 441
L-Glutamine, 2325
γ-Glutamyl-cysteine, 756
Glutamylation, 363
γ-Glutamyltransferase level, 2244
Glutaredoxin 5 (GLRX5), 636
Glutathione (GSH), 118, 749
　oxidized, 120
Glutathione metabolism, 119–120
　disorders of, 749
　related disorders of HMP shunt and, 755
　　6-phosphogluconate dehydrogenase deficiency, 755
　　defects in glutathione synthesis, 756
　　glutathione peroxidase deficiency, 756
　　glutathione reductase deficiency, 755–756
Glutathione peroxidase (GPx), 119, 749
　deficiency, 756, 1351
Glutathione reductase (GSR), 120, 749
　deficiency, 755–756
Glutathione S-transferases (GSTs), 1630
Glutathione synthetase (GS), 756, 1351
Glyceraldehyde 3-phosphate dehydrogenase (G3PD), 112
Glycogen, 395
Glycogen storage disease Ib, 1335
Glycolysis, 749
　genetic testing in evaluating disorders of, 757–758
　glycolytic and nucleotide enzymopathies, 758t
Glycolytic defect, 757
Glycolytic enzymes abnormalities, 756–757
　glycolysis in erythrocyte, 757f
Glycolytic enzymopathies, 761
　aldolase deficiency, 762
　glucose phosphate isomerase deficiency (GPI deficiency), 761
　glycolytic enzymopathies of doubtful clinical significance, 763
　hexokinase deficiency, 761
　phosphofructokinase deficiency, 761–762
　phosphoglycerate kinase deficiency, 763
　triose phosphate isomerase deficiency, 762

Glycolytic pathway, 749
Glycolytic shunt enzymes, 1015
Glycophorin A (GPA), 28, 96
Glycophorin C (GPC), 726
　deficiency, 738
Glycophorins, 110
　glycophorins A and B, 110
　glycophorins C and D, 110
Glycoprotein (GP), 38, 398, 402, 1153, 1183, 1278
β_2-Glycoprotein I ($\beta_2$gpI), 1260
Glycoprotein Ib complex
　interaction with thrombin, 403–404
　signaling, 404
Glycoprotein IIb/IIIa receptor antagonists, 1291
Glycoprotein VI receptor, 405
Glycoprotein-1 domains, 471
Glycoproteins (GPs), 391, 1111, 1182
Glycosaminoglycans (GAGs), 436, 533, 1353, 1545, 2284
Glycosylation, 441
Glycosylation-dependent cell adhesion molecule-1 (Gly-CAM-1), 154
Glycosylphosphatidylinositol (GPI), 465, 792, 998
Golgi enzymes, 1024
Gonadal radiation, 2140
Gonadotropin, 2331
　treatment, 903
Gonadotropin-releasing hormone (GnRH), 707, 902
　analogues, 2128
Goodpasture syndrome, 591
GPI-AP synthesis, congenital abnormalities of genes involved in, 799
Graft-vs-host disease (GVHD), 218, 318, 327, 865, 976, 1000, 1399, 1470, 1505, 1507f, 1653, 1679, 1760, 1832, 2034, 2126, 2297, 2304, 2315, 2335, 2371
　acute graft-vs-host disease, 2355–2360
　chronic graft-vs-host disease, 2360–2364
　prevention, 2304–2305
Graft-vs-leukemia effect (GVL effect), 1506–1507, 1507f, 1653, 1679, 2364
Graft-vs-malignancy (GVM), 2345
Graft-vs-tumor effect (GVT effect), 1505, 2355, 2364
　actuarial probability of relapse after bone marrow transplantation, 2365f
　acute graft-vs-host disease, 2355–2360
　chronic graft-vs-host disease, 2360–2364
　evidence for graft vs. tumor in animals and humans, 2364–2365, 2364t
　graft-vs-tumor response, 2364–2366
　natural killer cell–mediated graft vs. tumor, 2365–2366
　T-cell-mediated graft vs. tumor, 2365
Granulocyte colony-stimulating factor (G-CSF), 150, 578, 975, 2298, 1332, 1395, 1412, 1522, 1569, 1628, 1650, 1695, 2128
Granulocyte colony-stimulating factor receptors (G-CSFRs), 1332, 1569
Granulocyte colony–stimulating factor–mobilized peripheral blood (G-CSF–MPB), 1522
Granulocyte growth factors, 81
Granulocyte-macrophage progenitor fractions, 218
Granulocyte transfusions, 578–579, 1472
　administration of, 579
　clinical indications and efficacy, 579
　donor preparation/selection, 579
　granulocyte collection/storage, 579
Granulocyte turnover rate (GTR), 161
Granulocyte-macrophage colony-stimulating factor (GM-CSF), 79, 94, 150, 168, 199, 1334, 1366, 1412
Granulocyte-macrophage progenitor (GMP), 77, 136, 216, 359
Granulocytes and sex chromatin patterns, 147, 147f
Granulocytic differentiation, 27
Granulocytic sarcoma, 1631, 1706, 2090
Granuloma formation, 227
Granulomatous slack skin disease (GSS), 2085, 2087, 2087f
Granulopoiesis, 136
Granzyme A, 300
Granzyme B, 300
Gray pigmentation, 684
Gray platelet syndrome (GPS), 362, 1100, 1156, 1190–1191
Gray zone lymphoma (GZL), 1880, 1953

Green fluorescent protein (GFP), 78, 1538
Green-sickness, 628
Griscelli syndrome type II (GS2), 1335
Griscelli syndromes (GS syndromes), 1404
Group 2 innate lymphoid cells (ILC2), 196
Group A beta-hemolytic streptococcal infection, 1386
Group A pharyngitis, 1386
Group A streptococci, 1386
Group C streptococci, 1386
Group for Research on Adult Acute Lymphoblastic Leukemia (GRAALL), 1613
Group G streptococci, 1386
Growth arrest specific 6 (GAS6), 978
Growth differentiation factor 15 (GDF15), 690, 1020
Growth factor independent-1 (Gfi-1), 136
Growth factors, 152, 585
Growth hormone (GH), 902
    deficiency, 2381–2382
Gruppo Italiano Malattie Ematologiche dell'Adulto (GIMEMA), 2194
Gruppo Italiano Studio Policitemia (GISP), 1809
Guanine nucleotide exchange factors (GEFs), 276
Guanosine (G), 1636
Guanosine diphosphate (GDP), 153, 276, 395, 1402, 1783
Guanosine triphosphatases (GTPases), 172, 277, 1777
Guanosine triphosphate (GTP), 376, 395, 1402
Guillain-Barré syndrome, 587, 591
Gum bleeding, 1196
Gynecomastia, 2279
H
Haemophilus influenzae, 735, 780, 847, 908, 1106, 1145, 1169, 1393, 1434, 2036, 2124, 2221, 2308, 2364
Haemophilus vaccination, 1434
Hageman factor deficiency, 1223
Hairy cell leukemia (HCL), 33, 1430, 1441, 1910, 1919, 2049
    bone marrow trephine biopsy, 2057f
    BRAF inhibition in, 2053f
    clinical findings, 2053
        autoimmune disorders, 2054
        bone lesions, 2054–2055
        COVID-19, 2054
        infections, 2053–2054
        organ dysfunction, 2055
        skin involvement, 2055
        splenic rupture, 2055
        unusual manifestations, 2054
    clinical manifestations, 2053t
    differential diagnosis, 2056t, 2057–2059
    guidelines for molecular testing in, 1919
    hairy cells from peripheral blood smear, 2056f
    HCL and differential, 2058t
    immune suppression in, 2054f
    incidence and etiology, 2049
    indications for therapy and types of treatment, 2059
        bone marrow transplantation, 2064
        BRAF and MEK inhibition, 2063–2064
        Bruton tyrosine kinase inhibition (BTK inhibition), 2064
        chemotherapy, 2064
        cladribine in HCL, 2061–2062
        interferon-α, 2062–2063
        leukapheresis, 2064
        minimal residual disease (MRD), 2064
        moxetumomab pasudotox, 2063
        new therapies, 2063–2064
        pentostatin in HCL, 2059–2061
        purine nucleoside analogs, 2059–2062
        radiation therapy, 2064
        rituximab, 2063
        splenectomy, 2059
        treatment of hairy cell leukemia variant, 2064–2065
        treatment of patients with active infections, 2064
        treatments of historical interest, 2064
    laboratory findings, 2055
    laboratory manifestations, 2055t
    long-term follow-up of patients with, 2060f
    mechanisms for, 2052t
    pathogenesis, 2049
        cytogenetics, 2051
        cytokines, 2051–2053
        GC reaction key event in adaptive immunity, 2050f
        gene expression in HCL, 2050–2051
        Ig VH family and gene usage in HCL, 2051f
        molecular genetics, 2049–2050
    pathologic diagnosis, 2055
        bone marrow histology, 2056
        cytology, 2055–2056
        detection of residual disease, 2056–2057
        immunophenotype and molecular pathology, 2056
        minimal residual disease (MRD), 2056–2057
        spleen and liver involvement, 2056
    recommended treatment schema for HCL, 2065f
    relapse-free survival after first-line purine analog therapy, 2061f
    response rates using different agents and treatment schedules for, 2060f
    unusual clinical manifestations, 2055t
Hairy cell leukemia variant (HCLv), 33, 1919, 2057
Hairy cells, 2055
Hallervorden-Spatz syndrome, 744
Ham test, 792, 806
Hämochromatose, 678
HAMP gene, 678
Hand-Schüller-Christian disease, 1364, 1366
Hantavirus, 2285
Haplo donors, 2301
Haploidentical family member 2301
Haploidentical grafts, 1703
Haptocorrin (HC), 948
Haptoglobin (Hp), 121–123, 773
    serum, 618–619
Haptoglobin-hemoglobin complex (Hp-Hb complex), 122
Harderoporphyria, 711
Hashimoto thyroiditis, 1952
Hashimoto-Pritzker syndrome, 1364, 1367
Hassall corpuscles, 181, 234
*HAX*1 mutation, 1630
Hazard ratio (HR), 1630
HbI/α-thalassemia, 894
Health care providers (HCPs), 2384
Health-related quality of life (HRQOL), 1683
Healthy controls (HCs), 1182
Heart failure, 2246
Heart Outcomes Prevention Evaluation 2 (HOPE-2), 1285
Heat shock protein (Hsp), 102
    Hsp60, 102
    Hsp70, 102
    Hsp90, 102
Heat-stable antigen (HSA), 1538
Heated fluids, 827
Heavy and light chain deposition disease (LHCDD), 2290
Heavy chain deposition disease (HCDD), 2290
Heavy metal toxicity, 825
Heavy-chain variable-region genes, 777
Hedgehog signaling pathway (Hh signaling pathway), 1462
Heinz bodies, 9, 118, 752, 754, 936, 1426
    formation
        process, 935
        tests for hemolytic disorders associated with, 623, 623f
    preparation, 936
Helicobacter pylori, 547, 638, 960, 1098, 1809, 1858, 1872, 1876, 1916, 1946, 1949, 2002, 2286
Helmet cells, 623
Helminthiases in humans and nonhuman primates, 188
Helper CD4+ T cells, 1468
Hemangioblasts, 71
Hemangiomas, 1438
Hemarthrosis, 1080–1081, 1205, 1220, 1224, 1232
    clinical presentation, 1205–1206
    hemophilic arthropathy, 1205f
    pathophysiology, 1205
        scoring system for hemophilic arthropathy using magnetic resonance imaging, 1205t
Hematocrit (Hct), 2–3, 560, 600, 647, 1070, 1809
    limitations in use of, 601–602
Hematologic abnormalities, anemia associated with, 604
Hematologic disorders, 1321, 1410, 1445, 2172
Hematologic malignancies (HMs), 1009, 2084
    applications of molecular genetic testing in, 61–66
    DMT, 1330
Hematologic malignancies, infectious complications in
    approach to infection in neutropenic host, 1469
        colony-stimulating factors (CSFs), 1472
        combination therapy, 1471
        duration of antimicrobial therapy and common modifications, 1472f
        fever and neutropenia, 1469–1470
        granulocyte transfusions, 1472
        initial antimicrobial therapy, 1470
        initial treatment for high-risk patients, 1470–1471
        lower risk patients with fever and neutropenia, 1470
        modification of initial empirical therapy, 1471–1472
        penicillin-allergic patients, 1471
    deficits in host defense mechanisms, 1468–1469
        immune deficits and examples of associated infections, 1469t
    hematopoietic cell transplantation (HCT), 1481–1483
    prevention of infection, 1483
        infection prevention practices, 1483
        prophylaxis to reduce infection risks, 1483–1486
    specific infectious syndromes, pathogens, and treatments, 1473–1481
Hematomas, 1206
Hematopoiesis, 69–70, 233, 1740
    branch points, 80
    common critical genes in independent origins of, 71–72
    origins and development, 70–72
    sites of and timing of, 70f
    vascular origins, 71
Hematopoietic cell transplantation (HCT), 318, 1388, 1396, 1468, 1481, 1503, 1699, 1701–1702, 1743, 1748–1749, 2028, 2116, 2314, 2371
    allogeneic donor types, 2300–2301
    allogeneic HCT in MDS and MPN, 2339t
    alternative donor HCT for thalassemia, 2325
    B-cell recovery and immune reconstitution after HCT, 2317–2318
    event-free survival after HCT, 2317f
    overall survival after unrelated donor HCT, 2318f
    cardiovascular complications and metabolic syndrome, 2378–2379
    chemotherapy conditioning regimens before allogeneic HCT for PID, 2317t
    chimerism, 2303
    chronic GVHD, 2376–2377
    comparison of HLA-ID sibling and unrelated donor HCT for PID, 2315–2316
    complications of, 2303
        acute and chronic GVHD, 2304f
        acute GVHD, 2305
        chronic GVHD, 2305–2306
        graft rejection and failure, 2304
        graft-*vs*-host disease (GVHD), 2304
        GVHD prevention, 2304–2305
        infectious complications, 2306–2308
        predictors of complications, 2303
        regimen-related toxicities, 2303–2304
        treatment of acute GVHD, 2305
        treatment of chronic GVHD, 2306
    conditioning regimen protocols by SCID genotype, 2317t
    conditioning regimens, 2301–2302
        conditioning regimen intensity, 2302f
    conditions suitable for, 2314
    donor sources, 2298
        allogeneic HCT, 2298
        autologous HCT, 2298
        syngeneic HCT, 2298
    early postengraftment, 1481–1482
    endocrine complications, 2381
        growth hormone deficiency, 2381–2382
        hypogonadism, pubertal delay, and infertility, 2381
        iatrogenic Cushing syndrome and adrenal insufficiency, 2381
        insulin resistance and diabetes mellitus, 2381
        thyroid dysfunction, 2381
    engraftment, 2303
    engraftment, 2371
    factors that affect survival after HCT for severe combined immunodeficiency syndrome, 2316f
    gastrointestinal complications, 2382
    HCT for hemoglobin disorders, 2323–2324
    HCT for primary immunodeficiency disorders, 2314–2318
    HCT late effects, 2372f
    hematopoietic stem cell transplantation for bone marrow failure, 2319–2323

alternative donor HCT for FA, 2320–2321
FA and myelodysplastic syndrome/leukemia, 2323
HCT conditioning regimens for FA, 2319–2320
HLA-haploidentical HCT for FA, 2321–2323
late effects after HCT for FA, 2323
hematopoietic stem cell transplantation for hemophagocytic lymphohistiocytosis, 2318–2319
hematopoietic stem cell transplantation for sickle cell disease, 2325–2330
  acute myelogenous leukemia after gene therapy, 2330
  event-free survival improved among in patients, 2327f
  gene and genomic therapies for hemoglobin disorders, 2328–2330
  HCT indications for sickle cell disease, 2326t
  HCT preparative regimens and outcomes for patients with thalassemia major, 2326t
  HLA-haploidentical BMT and gene therapy for hemoglobin disorders, 2328
  HLA-ID Sibling HCT for SCD, 2325–2326
  myeloablative HCT for SCD, 2326–2328
  overall survival in patients, 2328f
  recent HCT clinical trials for sickle cell disease, 2327t
  reduced toxicity HCT for SCD, 2328
hematopoietic stem cell transplantation for thalassemia, 2324–2325
history of, 2297–2298
  historical timeline, 2297f
HLA-haploidentical HCT for PID, 2316–2317
human leukocyte antigen, 2300
immune reconstitution, 2303
indications for HCT in primary myelofibrosis, 2341
indications for hematopoietic cell transplantation in ALL, 2341–2342
indications for transplantation, 2298, 2298t
  malignant diseases, 2298–2299
  nonmalignant diseases, 2299–2300
infection and immunity, 2377–2378
infectious complications following HCT, 2307f
iron overload, 2371–2376
late effects, 2308
late effects after HCT for hemoglobin disorders, 2330–2331
late effects and future directions in HCT for PID, 2318
late postengraftment, 1483
lymphoid malignancies, 2341–2345
magnitude of late effects after HCT, 2373–2374t
malignant diseases, 2302–2303
management of relapse after HCT, 2340
monitoring of disease after HCT, 2340
MRD in HCT outcomes in acute leukemia, 2338–2339t
musculoskeletal complications, 2380
  avascular bone necrosis, 2380–2381
  low bone mineral density, 2380
  muscle or connective tissue, 2381
myeloid malignancies, 2335–2341
neurocognitive complications, 2382
  psychological and quality of life, 2382
nonmalignant diseases, 2302
ocular and oral/dental complications, 2382
phases of predictable immune suppression and timing of common opportunistic infections, 1482f
plasma cell disorders, 2345–2347
pre-engraftment period, 1481
pulmonary complications, 2378
  airflow obstruction and BOS, 2378
  approach to screening, diagnosis, and monitoring of bronchiolitis obliterans syndrome, 2378f
  pulmonary hypertension, 2378
  restrictive lung disease, 2378
recommended cancer screening after HCT, 2383t
recommended vaccinations after HCT, 2377t
relapse after transplant, 2308–2309
renal complications, 2379–2380
  renal LTFU recommendations, 2380
stem cell sources, 2300
subsequent neoplasms, 2382
survivorship care plans, 2382
timing of HCT, 2340
Hematopoietic cell transplantation comorbidity index (HCT-CI), 2335

Hematopoietic cells, 373, 801
Hematopoietic cytokines, 80–81
Hematopoietic differentiation, 366
Hematopoietic engraftment, 77
Hematopoietic growth factors, 975, 980
  deficiency, 1001
  and hematopoiesis, 1812
Hematopoietic microenvironments, 83
  hematopoietic stem cell niches in bone marrow, 83
    adhesion molecules in hematopoietic niche, 84
    candidates for cellular identity of hematopoietic stem and progenitor cell niche, 84t
    erythroid niches in bone marrow, 84
    lymphoid niches in bone marrow, 85
  stroma of hematopoietic organs, 83
Hematopoietic neoplasms, 1444
  ancillary methods, 1446
  diagnostic report, 1446
    International Consensus Classification of classic Hodgkin lymphoma, 1448t
    International Consensus Classification of histiocytic and dendritic cell neoplasms, 1450–1474
    International Consensus Classification of immunodeficiency-associated lymphoproliferative disorders, 1449t
    International Consensus Classification of lymphoblastic leukemia/lymphoma, 1452t
    International Consensus Classification of mature B-cell neoplasms, 1447–1448t
    International Consensus Classification of mature T and NK-cell neoplasms, 1448–1449t
    International Consensus Classification of myeloid neoplasms and acute leukemias myeloproliferative, 1451–1452t
  genetic testing, 1446
  immunophenotyping, 1445–1446
  preoperative considerations, 1444
    schematic of protocol for processing lymph node biopsies from patients, 1444f
  sampling methods and limitations, 1445
  with similar cutaneous presentations, 2089–2090
    immunohistochemistry pattern of primary cutaneous B-cell lymphomas, 2090t
    leukemia cutis, 2090f
    primary cutaneous follicle center lymphoma, 2089f
  specimen processing, 1445
    tissue fixation and processing, 1445
    triaging protocols, 1445
Hematopoietic progenitor cells (HPC), 27, 69, 75, 982
  colony-forming capacity of hematopoietic progenitors assayed in vitro, 76t
  committed hematopoietic progenitor cells, 75–76
  multilineage progenitors, 76
  single-lineage progenitors, 76–77
  terminal phases of differentiation, 77
  trafficking of hematopoietic stem and progenitor cells, 79–80
Hematopoietic proliferations, 14
Hematopoietic stem and progenitor cells (HSPCs), 79, 911, 1754
Hematopoietic stem cell transplant(ation) (HSCT), 327, 715, 787–788, 865–866, 894, 909, 974, 1024, 1371, 1402, 1509, 1576, 1609, 1616–1617, 1635, 1653–1656, 1669, 1679–1680, 1731, 1843, 1862, 1995, 2034–2035, 2102, 2199, 2355
  for AL amyloidosis, 2254
  allogeneic stem cell transplantation, 2203–2206
  autologous transplant, 2199–2203
  Center for International Blood and Marrow Transplant Research data (CIBMTR data), 1656f
  chip and hematopoietic stem cell transplant outcomes, 1760
  diagram showing intensity of different regimens, 1655t
  few conventional salvage chemotherapy regimens and reported CR rates, 1654t
  and gene therapy, 1197
  RBC antigens in, 549–550
  trends in survival after allogeneic HSCTs, 1617f
Hematopoietic stem cells (HSCs), 69, 93, 216, 233, 356–360, 804, 979, 998, 1197, 1522, 1563, 1737, 1754, 1783, 2314
  conception and discovery, 72
    advent of transplantation, 72

age of morphologists, 72
definitive evidence for HSCs, 72–73
in culture, 74–75
different models of hematopoietic hierarchy and megakaryocyte commitment, 359f
first-generation HSC gene therapy trials, 1530–1540
flow cytometric definitions, 73t
gene delivery systems IN HSCs, 1524–1530
gene therapy, 1522–1524
genesis, 71
identification and isolation, 73
mobilization, 79–80
new perspectives and ongoing challenges, 1547
  derivation of genetically corrected HSCs from iPSCs, 1550
  expansion of genetically modified HSCs, 1549–1550
  genome editing, 1547–1549
  immune responses to vectors and transgenes, 1550–1551
  novel pretransplant conditioning regimens, 1550
  use of purified HSCs, 1550
  in vivo gene therapy, 1550
niche, 74f
polyclonal contribution, 73
quiescence, 73–74
second-generation HSC gene therapy trials, 1540–1543
third-generation gene therapy clinical trials, 1543–1547
tracking hematopoietic stem cells and progeny, 78–79
trafficking of hematopoietic stem and progenitor cells, 79–80
Hematopoietic system, 982, 2144
Hematopoietic transcription factors (Hematopoietic TFs), 1194
Hematopoietic tumors, 2089
Hematopoietic-specific depletion of Srsf2, 370
Hematoxylin and eosin–stained sections (H&E–stained sections), 1595, 1885
Hematuria, 853, 1131–1132, 1144
Heme biosynthesis, 98
  critical balance between iron assimilation, heme, and globin synthesis, 101–102
  erythroid ALAS2 regulation, 100–101
  heme biosynthetic pathway, 99f
  regulation, 100
  non-erythroid ALAS1 regulation, 100
Heme iron (Fe^{2+}) 628, 936, 938–939
Heme oxygenases (HOs), 101, 704
  antioxidative function, 124–125
  iron reutilization function of, 125
  system, 124–125
Heme-regulated eIF2α kinase (HRI), 98, 635
Heme-regulated inhibitor (HRI), 101–102, 658
Hemichromes, 118, 936
Hemighosts, 623
Hemin, 710
Hemochromatosis, 678, 689–690, 692
  β-thalassemia, 691
  in African Americans, 693
  anemias, hemochromatosis, and iron overload, 690–692
  arthropathy, 688
  atherosclerosis, 692
  cardiomyopathy, 692
  clinical features of, 683
    laboratory abnormalities, 684–686
    liver abnormalities, 687
    observations in 97 Utah hemochromatosis, 684t
    physical examination abnormalities, 684
    prevalence of hemochromatosis in men and women, 683
    radiography, 686–687
    self-reported health problems and *HFE* genotypes, 686t
    symptoms, 683–684
    transferrin saturation and serum ferritin in California screening study, 686t
    transferrin saturation and serum ferritin values of Utah Hemochromatosis Homozygotes, 684t
  colorectal polyps and colorectal cancer, 689–690
  diagnosis, 692
    evaluation of relatives, 692
    H-ferritin hemochromatosis, 693
    hemochromatosis in African Americans, 693

Hemochromatosis (*continued*)
    heterozygous relatives, 692–693
    history and physical examination findings, 692
    homozygous relatives, 693
    laboratory findings, 692
  differential diagnosis of iron overload, 678
  effects of hepcidin, 681
  expression of *HFE* protein, 681
  ferroportin hemochromatosis, 681
  hemochromatosis, iron, and cancer risk, 689–690
  hepatocellular carcinoma, 689
  hepcidin function in, 681
  hepcidin function in hemochromatosis, 681
  hereditary spherocytosis, 691
  HFE hemochromatosis, 678
  HFE mutations and conditions, 687–689
  history, 678
  homozygotes, 688
    as blood donors, 695
  infections in hemochromatosis patients, 691
  interaction of *HFE* and non-*HFE* iron-related mutations, 681
  intestinal mucosal iron uptake in *HFE* hemochromatosis, 682
  iron absorption and toxicity in *HFE* hemochromatosis, 682–683
  iron overload, 678
  juvenile hemochromatosis, 678–680
  management, 693
    alcohol intake, 695
    changes expected after phlebotomy therapy, 694*t*
    clinical changes after iron depletion, 695
    dietary recommendations, 695
    hemochromatosis homozygotes as blood donors, 695
    initial weekly phlebotomy schedule, 693–694
    lifelong maintenance phlebotomy, 694–695
    phlebotomy therapy, 693
    vitamins, 695
  porphyria cutanea tarda (PCT), 690
  prognosis, 695–696
  proportions of *HFE* p. C282Y homozygotes in hemochromatosis cohorts, 683
  protein effects of *HFE* gene mutations, 682
  refractory anemia with ringed sideroblasts, 691
  subnormal immunoglobulins, 691–692
  surveillance for hepatocellular carcinoma, 689
  types of cancer, 690
  X-linked sideroblastic anemia, 691
Hemochromatosis and Iron Overload Screening (HEIRS), 681
Hemoconchus contortus, 178
Hemodialysis, 853
  chronic renal failure treated with, 639
  inadequate, 1038
Hemodynamic instability, 1698
Hemoglobin (Hb), 1, 112, 558, 659, 752, 833, 883, 1792, 1808, 2319
  acquired abnormalities of, 1075
  with altered oxygen affinity, 933–935
  assembly, 115–116
  biosynthesis, 97
    globin biosynthesis, 97–98
    heme biosynthesis, 98–102
  concentration, 3, 600, 1054, 1070
    limitations in use of, 601–602
  disorders
    gene and genomic therapies for, 2328–2330
    HCT for, 2323–2324
    HLA-haploidentical BMT and gene therapy for, 2328
  dyshemoglobinemias, 941–943
  evolution and structure, 113
  fetal, neonatal, and adult erythropoiesis and hemoglobin production, 113*f*
  HPLC, 937
  and kidney, 123
  laboratory analysis, 114
  laboratory evaluation of hemoglobin catabolism, 127
  level, 2243
  met hemoglobins (M hemoglobins), 938–939
  methemoglobinemia unrelated to globin gene mutations, 939–940
  modifications of normal hemoglobin, 114
  ontogeny, 113–114
  oxidative denaturation, 118–119
  oxygen affinity, 933
  pathways for disposal of hemoglobin in plasma, 122*f*
  pulse oximetry, 941
  subunit interaction, 117*f*
  unstable hemoglobins, 935–938
Hemoglobin A (HbA), 933
Hemoglobin C disease (Hb CC), 869
Hemoglobin C disorders, 869
  hemoglobin C disease, 869
  hemoglobin C trait, 869
Hemoglobin E, 915–916
  syndromes, 894, 922
    asymptomatic forms, 922
    clinical picture, 923
    symptomatic forms, 922–923
Hemoglobin F (HbF), 38, 116, 1027
  effect of hydroxyurea on red blood cells, 863*f*
  inducers, 861–863
Hemoglobin H, 8
  disease, 892–893
    hemoglobin H inclusion bodies, 893
Hemoglobin M variants, 941
Hemoglobin S, 868
  structure of hemoglobin S polymer, 834
Hemoglobin SC disease, 867
  clinical features, 867–868
  laboratory features, 868
  treatment, 868
Hemoglobin SD disease, 868
Hemoglobin SE disease, 868
Hemoglobin SO-Arab disease, 868–869
Hemoglobin SS, 839
Hemoglobin stability tests, 937
Hemoglobin S thalassemia syndromes, 921
  HbS-hereditary persistence of fetal Hb, 922
  HbS-β-Thalassemia, 921–922
  HbS-δβ-Thalassemia, 922
Hemoglobin synthesis, disorders of, 613
Hemoglobin Sβ-Thalassemia, 868
Hemoglobin Zurich, 8
Hemoglobinemia, 619, 640, 773, 825, 827
Hemoglobinopathies, 883, 1544, 2314
  β-thalassemia, 1544
  general diagnostic approach to, 614
    sideroblastic anemias, 614
  screening, 867
  sickle cell disease (SCD), 1544–1545
Hemoglobinuria, 123, 619–620, 639–640, 804–805, 825, 827, 829
  chronic, 813
  presenting features in 80 patients with PNH, 804*t*
Hemojuvelin gene (*HJV*), 681
Hemojuvelin hemochromatosis (*HJV* hemochromatosis), 678–680
Hemolysis, Elevated Liver enzymes, and Low Platelets syndrome (HELLP syndrome), 351, 1049, 1139
  clinical characteristics of HELLP syndrome, TTP, and aHUS, 1050*t*
  pregnancy-associated thrombotic thrombocytopenic purpura and atypical hemolytic-uremic syndrome, 1050
Hemolysis (H), 733, 753, 763, 779, 826–828, 1040, 1049
  in AIHA, 773
  approach to, 616–624
  associated with diabetic acidosis, 754
  chronic, 857, 937
  classification of, 616*t*
  clinical features of acquired hemolytic anemia, 618
  clinical features of congenital hemolytic anemia, 617–618
  determining specific cause of, 624
  diagnostic strategy in patient with hemolytic anemia, 623–624
  due to disseminated intravascular coagulation, 829
  due to drugs and chemicals, 824
    heavy metal toxicity, 825
    oxidant drugs and chemicals, 824–825
    water, 825
  fetal and neonatal anemia owing to, 1059
    ABO hemolytic disease, 1061
    causes of hemolytic disease in newborns, 1060*t*
    hemolytic disease owing to non-Rh, non-ABO antigens, 1061
    Rh hemolytic disease, 1060–1061
  hemolytic anemias characterized by significant intravascular red cell destruction, 616*t*
  due to infection, 821
    babesiosis, 823–824
    bacterial infections, 824
    bartonellosis, 824
    clostridial sepsis, 824
    malaria, 821–823
    trypanosomiasis, 824
    visceral leishmaniasis, 824
  laboratory features of, 618
    methemalbumin and hemopexin, 620
    morphologic abnormalities in hemolytic anemia, 620*t*
    signs of accelerated erythropoiesis, 620
    signs of increased red blood cell destruction, 618–619
    signs of intravascular hemolysis, 619–620
  laboratory signs of, 618*t*
  laboratory tests useful in differential diagnosis of, 620
    direct antiglobulin test, 623
    osmotic fragility test, 623
    red blood cell abnormalities associated with, 621*f*
    sickle cell anemia, 622*f*
    specific morphologic abnormalities, 620–623
    tests for hemolytic disorders associated with Heinz body formation, 623
  due to malignant hypertension, 829
  other causes of, 829
    hypersplenism, 829
    hypophosphatemia, 830
    liver disease, 829
    renal disease, 830
  pathogenetic role of, 837–838
  with thermal injury, 827
    burns, 827
    heated fluids and blood, 827
  with venoms, 825
    bee stings, 827
    snake bites, 826–827
    spider bites, 825–826
Hemolytic anemia, 570, 616, 739, 756, 821, 825, 827, 829–830, 1039, 1386
  diagnostic strategy in patient with, 623
    conditions sometimes mistaken for, 623–624
    conditions sometimes mistaken for, 624*t*
    determining specific cause of hemolysis, 624
    establishing presence of, 623
  chronic, 760, 778
  in pregnancy, 1049
    autoimmune hemolytic anemia during pregnancy, 1049
    hemolysis, elevated liver enzymes, and low platelets syndrome (HELLP syndrome), 1049
    pregnancy-induced hemolytic anemia, 1049
  syndromes, 1049
Hemolytic anemia, congenital
  aplastic crises, 617
  cholelithiasis, 617–618
  clinical features of, 617
  degree of anemia, 617
  jaundice, 617
  leg ulcers, 618
  skeletal abnormalities, 618
  splenomegaly, 617
Hemolytic crises, 846
Hemolytic disease, 741, 761, 1059
  late anemia following hemolytic disease of fetus and neonate, 1061
  owing to non-Rh, non-ABO antigens, 1061
Hemolytic disease of fetus and newborn (HDFN), 542
  prenatal testing to determine risk of, 549
Hemolytic disorders, 616, 728
  acquired nonimmune
    fragmentation hemolysis, 827
    hemolysis due to drugs and chemicals, 824–825
    hemolysis due to infection, 821–824
    hemolysis with thermal injury, 827
    hemolysis with venoms, 825–827
    other causes of hemolysis, 829–830
    postperfusion syndrome, 830
    tests for hemolytic disorders associated with Heinz body formation, 623
Hemolytic episodes, 825
Hemolytic hereditary elliptocytosis, 735, 739
Hemolytic process, 828, 830
Hemolytic transfusion reactions, 581, 1253

acute (intravascular) hemolytic transfusion reactions, 581
Hemolytic uremic syndrome (HUS), 351, 828, 1102, 1139, 1251, 1454
Hemopexin, 123–124, 620
Hemophagocytic lymphohistiocytosis (HLH), 212, 226, 1349, 1380, 1382, 1404, 2000, 2314
   hematopoietic stem cell transplantation for, 2318–2319
      diagnosis of HLH, 2318t
   susceptibility to severe EBV infection and, 1404–1405
Hemophagocytic syndrome (HPS), 208, 8
Hemophilia, 67, 1528
   autosomal, 1216
   in female, 1204
   gene therapy for, 1230
Hemophilia A, 428, 1203
   alloantibodies in, 1254
   carrier detection, 1204
      coagulation-based assays, 1204
      DNA-based assays, 1204
   clinical manifestations of hemophilia, 1204–1205
      clinical aspects, 1206
      hemarthrosis, 1205–1206
      prevalence and severity of hemophilia A and hemophilia B in United States, 1204t
      psoas and retroperitoneal hematomas, 1206
      subcutaneous and intramuscular hematomas, 1206
      traumatic bleeding, 1206
   course and prognosis, 1206
   differential diagnosis, 1207–1208
   elbow and knee joints in patient with, 1205f
   genetics, 1203–1204
      inheritance of hemophilia A and hemophilia B, 1203f
   hemophilia in female, 1204
   incidence, 1203
   laboratory diagnosis, 1206
      Factor VIIIc Assays, 1207
      screening tests of hemostasis and coagulation, 1207
   pathophysiology, 1203
   variants, 1204
Hemophilia B, 428, 1208
   clinical features, 1208
   detection of carriers, 1208
   genetics, 1208
   laboratory diagnosis, 1208–1209
   treatment, 1230
Hemophilia B Leyden, 447, 1208
Hemophilia treatment centers (HTCs), 1202
Hemophilic arthropathy, chronic, 1205
Hemophilic cysts, 1232
Hemophilic pseudotumors, 1232
Hemopoietic stem cell transplant (HSCT), 760
Hemorrhage, 569, 1080, 1252
   fetal and neonatal anemia owing to, 1061
      causes of fetal or neonatal hemorrhage, 1061t
      perinatal hemorrhage, 1062
      postnatal hemorrhage, 1062
      prenatal hemorrhage, 1061–1062
Hemorrhagic disorder, inherited, 1081
Hemorrhagic fever viruses, 1170
Hemorrhagic manifestations of ITP, 1101
Hemosiderin, 13
Hemosiderosis, 899–900
   assessment of iron stores, 899
Hemostasis, 427, 533
   laboratory methods for study of, 1082–1084
   in MM, 2181
   screening tests of, 1207
   secondary, 1276
Hemostatic disorders, 66–67
Hemostatic system, 1276
Hemostatic thromboses, 1276
Henna, 940
Henoch-Schönlein purpura (HSP), 1168–1169
   lower extremity palpable purpura in a patient with Henoch-Schönlein purpura, 1169f
Heparin, 1, 1251, 1253, 1291
   cofactor, 467
   inhibition of thrombin activity by heparin-antithrombin mechanism, 1292f
   sodium 22

structure of common active saccharide moieties found in commercial unfractionated heparin, 1292f
therapy, 1253
weight-based nomogram of UFH in treatment of venous thromboembolism, 1292t
Heparin cofactor II (HCII), 468, 1086
   biochemistry, 468
   deficiency, 1281
   function, 468–469
   gene structure and expression, 468
   schematic of, 468f
Heparin-based anticoagulant, 1303
Heparin-induced skin lesions, 1308
Heparin-induced thrombocytopenia (HIT), 40, 1278, 1307–1310
Heparin-like anticoagulants, 1267
Heparinoids, 1293
Hepatic bilirubin metabolism, 125–126
Hepatic disease, 1244
Hepatic involvement, 1164
Hepatic iron pathogenesis, mechanism of, 713
Hepatic nuclear factor-4 (HNF-4), 445, 1053
Hepatic siderosis, 901
Hepatic vein thrombosis, 805, 814
Hepatitis A, 563
Hepatitis A virus (HAV), 564, 586, 852, 2285
Hepatitis B, 586
Hepatitis B core antigen (HBc antigen), 560
Hepatitis B surface antigen (HBsAg), 560
Hepatitis B virus (HBV), 560, 898, 1481, 1949, 2018, 2285
Hepatitis C, 586, 2172
   autoimmune thrombocytopenia in, 1111
   infection, 690
Hepatitis C virus (HCV), 330, 560, 712, 898, 1111, 1949, 2284, 2286, 2330
Hepatitis G virus, 2285
Hepatobiliary systems, 852
Hepatocellular carcinoma (HCC), 689, 705, 714, 902, 920
   surveillance for, 689
Hepatocutaneous porphyria, 702, 712
   porphyria cutanea tarda, 712–741
Hepatocytes, 682
Hepatoerythropoietic porphyria (HEP), 714
Hepatomegaly, 2244
Hepatosplenic T-cell lymphoma (HSTCL), 1884, 1888, 2001–2002
Hepatosplenic T-cell lymphoma, 35, 1323, 1440
Hepatosplenic γ/δ T-cell lymphoma (HSTL), 1974
Hepatosplenic γδ TCL, 1953
Hepatosplenomegaly, 1023, 1349, 1705, 1953
Hepatotropic viruses, 902
Hepcidin gene (HAMP), 681
Hepcidin, 678, 899, 1041
   effects of, 681
   function in hemochromatosis, 681
   of iron metabolism, 630–632
      hepcidin regulation by iron, 631f
      systemic iron homeostasis by hepcidin, 630f
Hereditary alpha-tryptasemia (HaT), 1852
Hereditary anemias, 1429–4130
Hereditary angioedema (HAE), 350, 1394
Hereditary coproporphyria (HCP), 704, 710
   clinical description, 710
   homozygous dominant HCP, 711
   laboratory findings, 710
   molecular basis and pathogenesis, 710
   treatment, 710
Hereditary dysfibrinogenemias, 474
Hereditary elliptocytosis syndromes (HE syndromes), 726, 735, 736f
   classification of, 736t
   clinical features, 738
      common hereditary elliptocytosis, 738
      hemolytic hereditary elliptocytosis, 739
      hereditary pyropoikilocytosis, 739
      Southeast Asian Ovalocytosis, 739
      spherocytic elliptocytosis, 739
   laboratory evaluation, 739–740
   membrane abnormalities leading to elliptocyte formation, 738
   pathogenesis of, 735
      membrane protein defects, 735–737
      spectrin abnormalities, 737–738
   prevalence of, 735

treatment, 740
Hereditary erythroblastic multinuclearity with positive acidified serum test (HEMPAS), 1023
Hereditary giant neutrophilia, 1354
Hereditary hemochromatosis (HH), 2371
Hereditary hemorrhagic telangiectasia (HHT), 639, 1082, 1162
   clinical manifestations, 1162–1164
      Curacao criteria for diagnosis of HHT, 1164t
      physical findings and associations of vascular disorders, 1163t
      telangiectases in hereditary hemorrhagic telangiectasia, 1164f
   management, 1164–1165
   medical therapy, 1165
Hereditary persistence of fetal hemoglobin (HPFH), 114, 868, 889–890, 913, 1549
Hereditary pyropoikilocytosis (HPP), 735, 739
Hereditary spherocytosis (HS), 691, 728, 1429
   classification of, 729t
   clinical features, 731–732
      complications, 732
      hereditary spherocytosis in infancy, 732
   diagnosis, 734
   laboratory features, 732–733
      Eosin-5-Maleimide Binding (EMA binding), 733–734
      molecular studies, 734
      osmotic fragility, 733
   pathogenesis, 728
      erythrocyte abnormalities, 730
      membrane protein defects, 729–730
      role of spleen, 730–731
   pathophysiology of, 731f
   prevalence and genetics, 728
   syndromes, 726
   treatment, 734
Hereditary stomatocytosis syndromes, 740, 741f
Hereditary thrombocytopenia, 1096, 1153–1156
Hereditary thrombotic thrombocytopenic purpura (hTTP), 1124, 1137–1138
Hereditary tyrosinemia type 1 (HT1), 706
Hereditary xerocytosis (HX), 734, 741–742
Hermansky-Pudlak syndrome (HPS), 363, 1190–1191, 1354
Hermansky-Pudlak syndrome II (HPSII), 1335
Herpes simplex virus (HSV), 2382
Herpes zoster (HZ), 1729
Herpesviruses, 1469, 1529
Heterochromatin, 1023
Heterochromatin protein 1 (HP1α), 1023
Heterogeneous nuclear ribonucleoprotein E2 (hnRNP-E2), 1789
Heterotrimers of protein domains, 338
Heterozygosity, copy neutral loss of, 1755
Hexagonal-phase configuration concept, 1261
Hexokinase (HK), 760
   deficiency, 761
Hexose monophosphate (HMP), 749, 1015
   related disorders of HMP shunt and glutathione metabolism, 755–756
      6-Phosphogluconate dehydrogenase deficiency, 755
      defects in glutathione synthesis, 756
      glutathione peroxidase deficiency, 756
      glutathione reductase deficiency, 755–756
   shunt, 121
   disorders of, 749
High-throughput sequencing (HTS), 1671
High-throughput techniques, 1328
High-throughput technology (HTS), 1612
Hirudins, 1295
   domains, 468
HIST1H1E mutation, 1931
Histiocyte Society, The, 1371
Histiocyte Society's LCH II trial, The, 1371
Histiocytes, 1376
Histiocytic neoplasms, 226
Histiocytic sarcoma (HS), 1379, 1379f
Histiocytosis
   congenital self-healing, 1367
   malignant, 1364
Histiocytosis X, 1364
Histograms, 26
Histologic transformation (HT), 1949
Histone acetyltransferase (HAT), 369, 1920

Histone acetyltransferases and histone deacetylases (HDACs), 1573, 2213
Histone deacetylase inhibitor (HDACi), 370, 1977, 2099, 2212–2213
Histone H1, 300
Histone H3 lysine (H3K4), 1574
Histone H3 lysine 79 (H3K79), 1574
Histone-lysine N-methyltransferase 2A gene (KMT2A gene), 1628
Histopathology, 2177–2179
HK isozyme, type I, 761
Hodgkin lymphoma (HL), 1323–1324, 1326, 1382, 1388, 1415, 1418, 1430, 1500, 1612, 1628, 1899, 1907, 1912, 1923, 1946, 1991, 2039–2040, 2081, 2084, 2094, 2116, 2133, 2260, 2299, 2308, 2343
  adverse long-term outcomes of therapy, 2138–2140
    general guidelines for risk and surveillance for adverse long-term outcomes, 2139t
  classic Hodgkin lymphoma (CHL), 1889–1892
  clinical considerations, 2134
    clinical and staging criteria for, 2135t
    diagnostic evaluation, 2134
    presentation and staging, 2134
    prognostic factors, 2134–2135
  clinical evaluation, 2118
    initial evaluation of Hodgkin lymphoma patient, 2119–2120
    Lugano classification for Hodgkin lymphoma, 2119t
    physical examination, 2118–2119
  clinical history, 2119
  epidemiology, 2116, 2133
    biology, 2133–2134
    common first-line chemotherapy protocols and acronyms, 2134t
    histology, 2134
    incidence, 2133
    risk factors, 2133
  favorable early stage, 2121
    treatment of, 2121–2122
  follow-up of patients with, 2129
  histopathology, 2116–2118
    lymphocyte-depleted type Hodgkin lymphoma, 2118f
    lymphocyte-rich "classic" Hodgkin lymphoma, 2118f
    mixed cellularity-type Hodgkin lymphoma, 2118f
    nodular sclerosing Hodgkin lymphoma, 2117–2118f
    relative incidence of histopathologic subtypes of Hodgkin lymphoma, 2117t
  history, 2116
  indications for allogeneic hematopoietic cell transplantation, 2344
  indications for autologous hematopoietic cell transplantation, 2343–2344
  initial evaluation of Hodgkin lymphoma patient, 2119
  initial therapy for advanced-stage Hodgkin lymphoma, 2122–2124
  initial treatment for pediatric Hodgkin lymphoma, 2135–2137
  long-term treatment-related toxicity, 2128–2129
  Lugano staging system, 2119
  mixed cellularity, 1889
    subtype, 1890, 1890f
    mixed cellularity HL (MCHL), 2116
  nodular lymphocyte predominant Hodgkin lymphoma (NLPHL), 1892–1894, 2126–2127
    associated conditions, 2127
    clinical features, 2127
    epidemiology and pathobiology, 2126
    genetics, 1894
    immunoarchitecture of, 1893f
    immunophenotype, 1893–1894
    lymphocyte-predominant Hodgkin lymphoma, 2126f
    morphology, 1892–1893
    therapy for, 2127
  nodular sclerosis, 1880, 1889-1890, 1890f, 1998, 2116, 2241
  pathogenesis, 2116
  pediatric initial treatment for, 2135–2137
    radiotherapy for Hodgkin lymphoma, 2137
    risk stratification for, 2136t
    timeline of Hodgkin lymphoma upfront therapy, 2136f
  prognostic indicators, 2120
  radiotherapy for, 2137
  required and suggested studies for initial evaluation, 2119–2120
    recommended initial evaluation for patients with Hodgkin lymphoma, 2120t
  risk factors, 2116
  special considerations in management of, 2127
    chemotherapy toxicity, 2128
    classic HL and human immunodeficiency virus, 2128
    in elderly, 2127
    HL and pregnancy, 2128
    infertility, 2128
  therapy for relapsed or refractory Hodgkin lymphoma, 2124–2126
  therapy of early-stage classic Hodgkin lymphoma, 2121–2122
  transplantation for Hodgkin lymphoma and non-Hodgkin Lymphoma, 1418
  treatment for relapsed Hodgkin lymphoma, 2137–2138
    treatment options for recurrent Hodgkin lymphoma, 2138t
  treatment of classic Hodgkin lymphoma, 2120–2121
Hodgkin lymphoma, classic (CHL), 256, 1866, 1889, 1899f, 2001, 2116, 2128, 2133
  bone marrow, 1891f
  cHL-derived cell lines, 1908
  extranodal involvement, 1891
  genetics, 1892
  immunophenotype, 1891–1892
  lymphocyte depleted subtype, 1890–1891
  lymphocyte-rich subtype, 1890
  mixed cellularity subtype, 1890
  morphology, 1889
  nodular sclerosis subtype, 1889–1890
  phenotypic features of RS cells in classic Hodgkin lymphoma, 1892f
  therapy of, 2124
  treatment of, 2120
    chemotherapy, 2121
    progression-free survival and survival, 2120f
    radiotherapy, 2120–2121
    unfavorable characteristics for stage I and II HL, 2120t
Hodgkin lymphoma, treatment of relapsed/refractory disease
  brentuximab vedotin (BV), 2124–2125
  PD-1 inhibitors, 2125–2126
  salvage therapy and autologous hematopoietic cell transplant, 2124
  therapeutic options for patients relapsing after autologous hematopoietic cell transplantation, 2124
  therapy for, 2124
  toxicity of autologous hematopoietic cell transplant, 2124
  treatment options, 2126
    adoptive T-cell therapy, 2126
    allogeneic transplant, 2126
Homozygotes, 916
  for α-globin variants, 933
  for β-globin high-oxygen-affinity variants, 933
Homozygous deficiencies, 350
Horiba, 2
Human B19 parvovirus, 1009
Human cell differentiation molecules (HCDM), 20
Human cytomegalovirus (HCMV), 316
Human elongation factor-1α, 1527
Human genome, 1564
Human granulocytic anaplasmosis, 161
Human hemostatic system, 1276
Human herpes virus 8 (HHV8), 1414, 1946
Human herpesvirus 6 (HHV-6), 1386, 1481, 2308
Human immunodeficiency virus (HIV), 34, 558, 1009, 1227, 1352, 1409, 1755, 1951, 2017, 2116
  AIDS-related lymphoma, 1415–1418
  AIDS-related malignancies, 1414–1415
  background, 1409
  clinical features of HIV-1 infection, 1410
  diagnosis, 1409
  hematologic complications of HIV infection, 1411
    anemia, 1411
    effect of antiretroviral therapy on anemia, 1411–1412
    bone marrow examination in HIV-1 infection, 1414
    coagulation abnormalities, 1414
    lymphopenia, 1413
    neutropenia, 1412–1413
    pathophysiology of bone marrow suppression in HIV infection, 1413–1414
    red blood cell destruction, 1412
    thrombocytopenia, 1412
    thrombotic thrombocytopenic purpura (TTP), 1413
  HIV-related autoimmune thrombocytopenia, 1097
  HIV–positive, 1882
  infection, 40–42
  pathophysiology, 1409
  treatment, 1410
    human immunodeficiency virus life cycle, 1410f
  type 1 and type 2, 586
Human leukocyte antigen (HLA), 322, 540, 678, 1109, 1196, 1255, 1337, 1495, 1522, 1611, 1679, 2075, 2300, 2335, 2355
  antibody detection, 40
  antigens and antibodies, 552–553
  cellular responses to, 326–327
  class II, 1376
  gene polymorphism and nomenclature, 322–323
  haplotypes and inheritance, 323–324
    HLA haplotype segregation in family, 325f
  HLA-identical sibling donors, 2297
  presentation, 330
    cross-dressing, 333–334
    cross-presentation, 331–333
    endogenous pathway, 330–331
    exogenous Pathway, 331
  structure and function of human leukocyte antigen molecules, 324–326
    schematic structure of human leukocyte antigen molecules, bound peptides, and T cell–antigen receptor interactions, 326f
Human leukocyte antigen identical (HLA-ID), 2314
  comparison of HLA-ID sibling and unrelated donor HCT for PID, 2315–2316
  HLA-ID Sibling HCT for SCD, 2325–2326
Human leukocyte antigen-DR (HLA-DR), 27, 1009, 1721
Human leukocyte differentiation antigen (HLDA), 20
Human mast cells normally, 1849
Human metapneumovirus (hMPV), 1478, 2308
Human myeloma cell lines (HMCLs), 2153
Human neutrophil antigens (HNAs), 147, 552
HNA-1, 1337
Human papilloma virus (HPV), 979, 1414, 2382
Human parvovirus B19, 563
Human phosphoglycerate kinase (PGK), 1527
Human plasma prekallikrein, 434
Human platelet antigen-1a (HPA-1a), 1111
Human platelet antigens (HPAs), 553, 576
Human prekallikrein gene, 432
Human retroviruses, 2075
Human T cell lymphotropic virus-1 (HTLV-1), 1010, 1888, 1931, 1945, 1948, 2075, 2285
  course of, 1948f
  geographic distribution of HTLV-1 infection, 1948f
Human umbilical vein endothelial cells (HUVECs), 171
Human Urea Transporter 11 (HUT11), 546
Humoral immunity, defects in, 1468
Hunter syndrome, 1353
Huntington Disease-Like 2 (HDL2), 744
Hurler syndrome, 1353, 1545–1546
Hydralazine, 1169, 1262
Hydroa vacciniforme (HV), 1387
Hydroa vacciniforme-like LPD (HV-like LPD), 2088
Hydrogen peroxide (H_2O_2), 749, 756
Hydroxycarbamide, 1650
Hydroxychloroquine, 713, 1265
12-Hydroxyeicosatetraenoic acid (12-HETE), 396
2-Hydroxyglutarate (2-HG), 1460, 1573
Hydroxyl radicals, 119, 683
Hydroxylation, 441
5-Hydroxymethyl cytosine (5hmC), 1573
Hydroxymethylbilane (HMB), 703
Hydroxymethylbilane synthase (HMBS), 656, 704
Hydroxyurea, 618, 856, 861, 863, 1179, 1729, 1815, 1817, 1843–1844, 1862
  alkylating agents, 1816
  interferon, 1815–1816

JAK2 inhibitors, 1816
   therapy, 848, 861
Hyper-cyclophosphamide, 1417
Hyper-IgD syndrome, 2282
Hyperalimentation hypophosphatemia, 1352
Hyperbilirubinemia, 618, 754–755, 2244
Hypercalcemia, 1955, 2177, 2179, 2220
Hypercoagulability, 1278–1279
Hypercoagulable states, 1276, 1278
Hyperdiploidy, 43, 2153
Hypereosinophilia (HE), 1771, 1836–1837
   diagnostic evaluation for, 1837–1839
      diagnostic algorithm for hypereosinophilia, 1839f
      international consensus classification diagnostic criteria for CEL, NOS and idiopathic HES, 1838t
Hypereosinophilic syndrome (HES), 1771, 1836
   biology of FIP1L1-PDGFRA, 1839–1840
   clinical presentation and prognosis, 1840
      allogeneic stem cell transplantation, 1845
      antibody approaches, 1845
      cardiac surgery, 1845
      clinical presentation, 1840
      clinicopathologic features, 1840
      fusion tyrosine kinase genes associated with myeloid/lymphoid neoplasms and eosinophilia, 1842f
      organ manifestations of eosinophilic neoplasms/hypereosinophilic syndromes, 1842t
      prognosis, 1840–1842
      treatment of HES and chronic eosinophilic leukemia, 1844–1845
      treatment of patients with genetically defined neoplasms, 1843–1844
   definition of eosinophilia, 1836
   diagnostic evaluation for hypereosinophilia, 1837–1839
   eosinophil physiology, 1836–1837
   epidemiology, 1836
Hyperfibrinolysis, 1244
Hypergammaglobulinemic purpura (HP), 1168
Hyperglobulinemia, 859
Hyperglycemia, 1352
   asymptomatic, 903
Hyperhemolysis, 838
Hyperhemolytic crises, 846
Hyperhomocysteinemia (HHcy), 708, 956, 962, 1284
   acquired, 1284
   clinical aspects, 1285
   laboratory diagnosis, 1285
   pathophysiology and genetics, 1284
   treatment, 1285
   treatment of, 966
      lowering homocysteine for prevention or treatment of vascular disease, 966
Hyperimmunoglobulin E syndrome (HIES), 1346
   autosomal dominant (AD-HIES), 1346
Hyperimmunoglobulin M syndromes, 1397
Hyperimmunoglobulinemia-D syndrome, 2260
Hyperimmunoglobulins, 564, 1837
Hyperleukocytosis, 1631–1633
Hypernephroma, 2260
Hyperparathyroidism, 1042
   secondary, 1038, 1042
Hyperphosphatemia, 1614
Hypersegmentation, 954
   of eosinophils and negative staining for peroxidase and phospholipids, 1354
   of neutrophil nuclei, hereditary, 1354
      hypersegmented neutrophil, 1354f
Hypersegmented granulocytes, 953
Hypersensitive sites (HSs), 886
Hypersensitivity, 662
Hypersensitivity vasculitis, 1167
Hypersplenism, 829, 918
   neutropenia due to increased, 1337
Hypertension, 1144, 1277
Hyperthyroidism, 1041, 1337, 2139
Hyperunstable globins, 888
Hyperunstable hemoglobin, 937
   variants, 936
Hyperuricemia, 1614, 1632, 1811, 1817, 1992
Hyperviscosity, 2220, 2268
Hypobromous acid (HOBr), 174
Hypocalcemia, secondary, 1614

Hypochlorous acid (HOCl), 158
Hypocholesterolemia, 2055
Hypochromia, 8, 1033
   anemia, chronic, 628
Hypochromic microcytic anemia, 1041
Hypodiploid MM, 2182
Hypodysfibrinogenemia, 1218
Hypofibrinogenemia, 474, 1217, 1244
   acquired, 1218, 1259
Hypogonadism, 902–903, 2331, 2381
Hypogonadotropic hypogonadism, 903
Hypohaptoglobinemia, 122
Hypokalemia, 1632
Hypomethylating agents (HMAs), 1738, 1747–1748, 2335
Hyponatremia, 707
Hypoparathyroidism, 903
Hypoperfusion, 1248, 1254
Hypophosphatemia, 830
Hypopituitarism, 1042
Hypoplastic myelodysplastic syndromes (hMDS), 999, 1599
Hypoprothrombinemia, 1220, 1266
Hyposegmented nuclei, 977
Hyposplenism, functional, 1468
Hyposthenuria, 852
Hypotension, hemoconcentration, and hypoalbuminemia (3 Hs), 2292
Hypothermia, 585, 670
   diagnostic evaluation of patients with sideroblastic anemia, 671f
Hypothyroidism, 903, 1041, 2129, 2308
   autoimmune, 1010
   pathogenesis, 1041
Hypoventilation syndromes, 1075
Hypoxemia, 1248
Hypoxia, 1254
Hypoxia inducible factor (HIF), 82, 103, 1035, 1053, 1074
Hypoxia-inducible factor-2α (HIF-2α), 632
Hypoxia-inducing factor1α (HIF1α), 1076

I

I/i blood group system specificity, 777–778
iAMP21. *See* Intrachromosomal amplification of chromosome 21 (iAMP21)
Ibrutinib, 1458, 1469, 1963, 1970, 2010, 2013, 2031–2032, 2036, 2064, 2271
   monotherapy, 2032
   resistance to, 2033
Idarubicin, 1650, 1729
Idecabtagene vicleucel, 2184, 2218
Idelalisib, 1459, 1469, 2013, 2033
Idiopathic MCD (iMCD), 1952
Idiopathic pulmonary syndrome (IPS), 2303
Idiopathic thrombocytopenic purpura (ITP), 1097, 1412, 1158
Idrabiotaparinux, 1293
Idraparinux, 1293
α-L-Iduronidase (IDUA), 1545
IFN-regulatory factor-4 (*IRF*4), 1972
IFNs, type I, 1505
IFNs, type II, 1505
Ifosfamide, 1417, 2138
Ifosfamide, carboplatin, etoposide (ICE), 2124
Ifosfamide, gemcitabine, vinorelbine, prednisolone (IGEV), 2124
IKAROS family zinc finger-1 (*IKZF1*), 1580–1581, 1610, 1671, 1675, 1677, 1821
IL-12 receptor β1 chain (IL12RB1), 1404
IL-2 receptor antagonists (IL-2RAs), 1506
IL-2-inducible T-cell kinase (ITK), 1972
IL-5 receptor (IL-5R), 168
IL-5receptor-a (*IL5RA*), 1839
IL-7 receptor (IL-7R), 273, 1402, 1586–1587, 1675
IL-7 receptor deficiency (IL7Rα deficiency), 2318
Ileal resections and reconstruction surgery, 960–961
Ileum, distal, 960
Imatinib, 1458, 1613, 1619, 1763, 1793–1794, 1797, 1861, 964
Imerslund-Gräsbeck syndrome, 963
Imipenem-relebactam, 1474
Imiquimod, 1370
Immature B cells, 29
Immature cells of normal bone marrow, 27

Immature myeloid cells, 1597
Immature progenitors, 373
Immature reticulocyte fraction (IRF), 4, 604
Immune activation, 2285
Immune antibody drug conjugates, 1454–1456
Immune cells, 418
Immune complex mechanism, 338, 785–786
Immune disorders, fragmentation hemolysis with, 829
Immune dysregulation, polyendocrinopathy, enteropathy, X-linked syndrome (IPEX syndrome), 1404
Immune effector cell–associated neurotoxicity syndrome (ICANS), 1964, 1622
Immune effector functions, 225
Immune evasion by tumors, 1499
Immune hemolytic anemias
   caused by cold-active antibodies, 776
      cold agglutinin disease, 776–779
      cold autoantibodies, 776t
      paroxysmal cold hemoglobinuria, 779–780
   caused by mixed cold- and warm-active antibodies, 780
   caused by warm-active antibodies, 780
   primary *vs.* secondary autoimmune hemolytic anemia, 781–784, 781t–782t
Immune modulatory drugs (IMiDs), 2250-2252
Immune neutropenia, 1337, 1339
Immune reconstitution, hematopoietic cell transplantation, 2303
Immune regulatory disorders, 1404–1405
Immune regulatory molecules, 225
Immune response
   etiology of immune response in autoimmune hemolytic anemia, 770
      central tolerance, 770
      factors affecting initiation of autoimmunity, 770–771
      peripheral tolerance, 770
   immune response to Epstein-Barr virus infection, 1383–1385
      schematic depicting development of humoral response to Epstein-Barr virus, 1384f
   against tumors, 1496, 1496f
   to vectors and transgenes, 1550–1551
Immune sculpting of tumors, 1499
Immune synapse (IS), 293–295, 294f
Immune thrombocytopenic purpura (ITP), 377, 576, 772, 1097, 1410, 1425, 1428, 2022
   in adults, 1100–1101
   bleeding manifestations, 1101
      bleeding after trauma, 1101
      central nervous system, 1101
      skin and mucous membranes, 1101
   in children, 1099–1100
   clinical picture, 1099
      immune thrombocytopenia in adults, 1100–1101
      immune thrombocytopenia in children, 1099–1100
   differential diagnosis, 1102
      adults, 1103
      children, 1103
   features of acute and chronic immune thrombocytopenia, 1097t
   first-line treatment, 1103–1106
   incidence, 1097
   laboratory findings, 1101
      antiplatelet antibodies, 1102
      blood, 1101–1102
      bone marrow, 1102
   nomenclature, 1097
   pathophysiology, 1097
      pathogenesis of immune thrombocytopenia, 1098f
      platelet antibodies, 1098–1099
   in pregnancy, 1108–1109
   treatment of chronic primary immune thrombocytopenia, 1106–1109
Immune tolerance (IT), 1256
Immune-mediated hemolytic anemia, 770, 782
Immune-mediated neutropenia, 1336
Immune-mediated process, 2358
Immune-mediated red blood cell lysis mechanism, 772
   immunoglobulin G–mediated red blood cell destruction, 772
   immunoglobulin M–mediated red blood cell destruction, 772
   red cell destruction by IgM and IgG antibodies, 772t
Immune-mediated thrombocytopenia, 986

Immune thrombocytopenia, chronic primary, treatment of, 1106
    fostamatinib, 1107–1108
    immune thrombocytopenia in pregnancy, 1108–1109
    immunosuppressive drugs, 1108
    proposed therapies, 1108
    rituximab, 1107
    splenectomy, 1106–1107
    supportive measures, 1108
    thrombopoiesis-stimulating agents, 1107
Immunization, 1485–1486, 2021–2022
Immunoalkaline phosphatase, 14
Immunoassays, 107
Immunochemistry and origin, 781
Immunocytochemical stains, 13–14
Immunodeficiencies, 1546, 2299
    adenosine deaminase-severe combined immunodeficiency disease, 1546–1547
    congenital, 1951
    disorders, 1383
    secondary, 1951
    states, 1351
    Wiskott-Aldrich syndrome (WAS), 1546
    X-chronic granulomatous disease, 1547
    X-linked SCID, 1546
Immunodeficient mouse model, 1537
Immunofixation electrophoresis, 2147
Immunofluorescence microscopy, 14, 2171
Immunoglobulin by immunohistochemistry (Ig-MPGN), 1143
Immunoglobulin, intramuscular (IMIg), 1398
Immunoglobulin E (IgE), 180, 196, 1849, 2222
Immunoglobulin G (IgG), 394, 890, 1008, 1125, 1255, 1495, 2160
    IgG-coated RBCs, 772
    IgG–mediated red blood cell destruction, 772
        characteristics of Fcγ Receptors, 773t
    replacement therapy, 1397
Immunoglobulin heavy chain (IgH), 65, 267, 275, 1900, 1995, 2002, 2062, 2166
    IGH-CRLF2, 1675
Immunoglobulin heavy chain variable region gene (*IGHV* gene), 1913 2010, 2012, 2017, 2024, 2027, 2032, 2036, 2039, 2049
    IGHV 2 points, 2026
    IGHV$_{3-21}$ usage and stereotypy, 2024
    IGLV1 gene, 2277
Immunoglobulin light chains (IGL), 65, 267, 2346
    amyloidosis, 2160
    classification, 2238–2239
    diagnosis of amyloidosis, 2239–2241
    presentation and clinical features, 2241–2242
        coagulation system, 2246
        gastrointestinal tract, 2245
        heart, 2243–2244
        kidney, 2244
        liver, 2244–2245
        nervous system, 2245–2246
        respiratory tract, 2246
        symptoms and signs, 2242–2243
    prognostic features, 2246–2248, 2247f-2248f
        improving overall survival over three time periods, 2247f
        interaction between biomarker stage and ultrahigh levels of NT-proBNP, 2248f
        overall survival of patients with AL, 2247f
    treatment, 2248, 2248t
        localized amyloidosis, 2259–2260
        measuring responses in systemic AL amyloidosis, 2248–2249
        nontransplant systemic therapies for systemic Al amyloidosis, 2249–2254
        stem cell transplantation, 2254–2257
        supportive therapy for amyloidosis, 2257–2259
        types of systemic amyloidosis, 2260–2261
Immunoglobulin M (IgM), 617, 770, 1251, 1384, 1426, 2222, 2267
    mediated red blood cell destruction, 772
    monoclonal gammopathy, 2146
    paraprotein, 2281
Immunoglobulin-E (IgE), 2072
Immunoglobulins (Igs), 564, 617, 1098, 1168, 1277, 1334, 1669, 1866, 1900, 1907, 1942, 2144, 2152, 2160
    allelic exclusion, 270–271
    free kappa and lambda, 2148
    gene, 1998, 2133
    light, 2147
    production and light chain ratio, 2020
    quantitation of, 2147
    replacement, 1398–1399
    secretion, 2178
    serum, 2303
    superfamily molecules, 221, 222f
Immunohistochemistry (IHC), 123, 1325, 1886, 1955, 1965
    staining, 1919
Immunologic abnormalities, 981
Immunologic disorders, 1952–1953
Immunologic method, 1085
Immunologic tolerance, 770
Immunologic transfusion reactions, 580
    allergic reactions, 584
    alloimmunization to transfused antigens, 580–581
    delayed hemolytic transfusion reactions, 581–582
    febrile nonhemolytic transfusion reactions, 582
    hemolytic transfusion reactions, 581
    posttransfusion purpura, 584
    transfusion-related acute lung injury, 582–584
    transfusion-related immunomodulation, 584
Immunomodulation, functional, 333
Immunomodulatory drugs (IMiDs), 1461, 1827, 2154, 2184, 2210–2211
Immunomodulatory modalities, 1013
Immunomodulatory therapy, 1012–1013
Immunoperoxidase, 14
Immunophenotypic analysis, 1866–1869
Immunophenotyping, 20, 22, 1325, 1445, 2020, 2056, 2083
    of acute leukemia, 35–37, 36f
    of B-Cell lymphoproliferative disorders, 31–34
    flow cytometry, 1446
    immunohistochemistry, 1446
    of plasma cell myeloma, 35
    of T-cell lymphoproliferative disorders, 34–35
Immunoreceptor tyrosine-based activation motifs (ITAMs), 278, 290, 301, 310, 313, 1497
Immunoreceptor tyrosine-based inhibitory motif-containing receptor (ITIM-containing receptor), 377
Immunoreceptor tyrosine-based switch motif (ITSM), 301
Immunoreceptors, 405
Immunosubtraction, 2147
Immunosuppression, 1551, 2162, 2171–2172
Immunosuppressive therapy (IST), 778–779, 783–784, 812–813, 955, 1000, 1002–1003, 1012–1013, 1133–1134, 1258, 1405, 1746–1747, 1760, 2371
    relapse-free survival after plasma exchange for an acute episode of TTP, 1134f
    survival after, 1013–1014
Immunosuppressive treatment (IST), 1746
Immunotherapy, 1494, 1652–1653, 1713, 1942, 1959, 1964, 2028, 2101–2102, 2335
    adaptive immunity against tumors, 1496–1498
    anti-CD20, 2028
    anti-CD52, 2029
    approaches to, 1499
    historical perspective, 1494–1495
    innate immunity against tumors, 1495–1496
    Kaplan-Meier curve of event-free survival, 1652f
    prognostic scoring systems for patients with refractory/relapsed AML, 1653t
    timeline of major advances in cancer immunology and immunotherapy, 1494f
    tumor-associated antigens, 1498–1499
    tumor-host interactions, 1499–1515
Immunotoxins, 1503–1504
Impaired anticoagulant pathways, consumption of coagulation factors and, 1248
Impaired bacterial killing, acquired conditions of, 1352
    desensitization, 1352
    hyperalimentation hypophosphatemia, 1352
    hyperglycemia, 1352
    neutrophil dysregulation in systemic inflammatory response syndrome, 1352
    viral infection, 1352
In situ follicular neoplasia (ISFN), 1870, 1872
In situ hybridization, 50–51
In situ mantle cell neoplasia, 1874
In vitro, 371, 836
    diagnostic assays for HIT, 1308
    infection of B lymphocytes, 1382
    and mouse parasitic helminth studies, 188
In vivo
    gene therapy, 1522, 1550
    hematopoietic assays, 77–78
    stored red cells, 561
    survival of infused coagulation factors, 1225–1226
Inab, 796
Inborn errors
    of cobalamin absorption and metabolism, 963
    of intracellular cobalamin metabolism with megaloblastic anemia, 963
    of metabolism, 2314
    of pyrimidine metabolism, 964
Indeterminate dendritic cell tumors, 1378
Index of Variant Human Fibrinogen, 474
Indian blood group antigens (In blood group antigens), 1027
Indinavir (IDV), 1410
Indirect antiglobulin test (IAT), 572, 775
Indirect Coombs Test, 775
Indirect presentation, 2356
Individual donor nucleic acid test (ID-NAT), 587
Indomethacin, 1371
Induced antibody titer, 1255
Induced pluripotent stem cell (iPSC), 75, 366, 1522
Inducible costimulator (ICOS), 295, 1929
Induction therapy, 1700–1701
Ineffective erythropoiesis, 608, 891, 1020
Ineffective thrombopoiesis, 1157
Infancy
    blood loss in, 640
    diet in, 640
    vitamin K deficiency bleeding, 1241–1244
Infantile monosomy 7 syndrome, 1776
Infants, 856, 1065, 1206, 1361
    cobalamin deficiency in, 961
    cobalamin replacement in, 965
    disseminated intravascular coagulation in, 1252
    neurological aspects of cobalamin deficiency in, 956
    of vitamin B$_{12}$-deficient mothers, 1048
Infarcts, 840
Infection(s), 227, 923, 1331
    in CLL, 2021
    hemolysis due to, 821–824
    infection-induced hemolysis, 753
    prevention practices, 846, 1483
    purpura associated with, 1169–1171
    risk postsplenectomy, 1434
    thrombocytopenia associated with, 1158–1159
Infectious agents, 1169
Infectious diseases, 1946
    blood donor screening for, 586
        residual risks of infection, 586
        testing strategy, 586
Infectious Diseases Society of America (IDSA), 1470
Infectious mononucleosis (IM), 777, 1010, 1382, 1385–1387
    clinical features, 1385
    complications, 1386–1387
    diagnosis, 1386
    differential diagnosis, 1386
    epidemiology, 1385
    Epstein-Barr virus–associated disorders in primary immunodeficiency, 1389–1390
    Epstein-Barr virus–associated lymphoma, 1388
    histologic findings, 1385–1386
    historical background, 1382
    immune response to Epstein-Barr virus infection, 1383–1385
    infectious mononucleosis, 1385–1387
    laboratory findings, 1385
    other Epstein-Barr virus–related hematologic diseases, 1387–1388
    treatment, 1387
    viral biology/lymphocyte immortalization/viral gene expression, 1382–1383
Inferior vena cava (IVC), 1305
Infertility, 2128, 2381
Inflammatory bowel disease (IBD), 298, 1010
Inflammatory cytokines, 378
Inflammatory markers, 858
Inflammatory pseudotumor-like follicular, 1378, 1441
Influenza virus, 1478, 2308

Infused coagulation factors, in vivo recovery and survival of, 1225–1226
Inherited abnormalities of hemoglobin, erythrocytosis due to, 1075
Inherited afibrinogenemia, 474, 1217
Inherited amegakaryocytic thrombocytopenia, 955
Inherited aplastic anemia syndromes germline
    approach to clinical management, 974–975
    congenital amegakaryocytic thrombocytopenia (CAMT), 986–987
    diagnostic approach, 974
    Fanconi anemia (FA), 975–980
    GATA2 syndromes, 987–988
    Shwachman-Diamond syndrome, 984–986
    telomere biology disorders (TBD)/dyskeratosis congenita, 980–984
Inherited bleeding disorders, 1081
    age at onset, 1081–1082
    drug history, 1082
    family history, 1082
Inherited bone marrow failure syndromes (IBMFS), 66, 974, 985, 1547
Inherited chromosomal instability syndrome, 975
Inherited disorders, 1088
    of absorption, 963
Inherited predisposition syndromes, 1696
    abnormal chromosomal number, 1696
    inherited marrow failure and chromosome instability syndromes, 1696–1697
    photomicrograph of peripheral blood smear, 1696f
    twins and familial cases, 1697
Inherited risk factors, 1278
Inherited thrombocytopenia, classic, 1153
    Bernard-Soulier syndrome, 1154
    classification of congenital thrombocytopenia based on pathogenic mechanism with selected genes involved, 1154t
    classification of inherited thrombocytopenia by platelet size, 1154t
    congenital amegakaryocytic thrombocytopenia, 1153
    familial platelet disorder with predisposition to myeloid malignancy, 1155
    gray platelet syndrome, 1156
    mediterranean macrothrombocytopenia, 1155
    MYH9-related disorders, 1154–1155
    Paris-Trousseau syndrome (PTS), 1155
    thrombocytopenia with absent radius syndrome (TAR syndrome), 1154
    X-linked microthrombocytopenia, 1156
Inhibitor of apoptosis proteins (IAPs), 1463
Inhibitor of DNA binding (ID), 220
Inhibitor of κB (IκB), 1498
Inhibitor(s)
    of fibrinolysis, 1228
    screens, 1086
    tests for inhibitors of coagulation, 1086
Inhibitors of apoptosis (IAP), 1915, 2062
Initiation codon mutations, 888
Initiator codon ATG, 888
Innate lymphoid cell (ILC), 233, 309
    clinical relevance and applications, 317–318
    development, human, 310
    models, 309f
    type 1, 316
    type 2, 316–317
    type 3, 317
Innate signaling pathway defects, 1404
Inosine 5′-monophosphate dehydrogenase, 784
Inositol 1, 4, 5-trisphosphate, 406, 1193
Inositol triphosphate (IP$_3$), 276, 1498
Inotuzumab, 1621, 1680
    ozogamicin, 1504
Insertional mutagenesis
    approaches to decrease risk of, 1542–1543
    in patient with ADA-SCID treated by HSC gene therapy, 1541
    in SCID-X1 patients treated by HSC gene therapy, 1540–1541
Inside-out signaling, 414
Institute of Medicine, The, 951
Institutional formulary committees, 1330
Instructive signals, 83
Insulin resistance, 2381
Insulin-like growth factor 1 (IGF-1), 83, 2365
Insulin-responsive aminopeptidase (IRAP), 333
Integrase defective lentiviral vectors (IDLVs), 1548

Integrated stress response (ISR), 98
Integration patterns, 1542
α,β2-Integrin dimer, 155, 155f
Integrin α$_{IIb}$β$_3$ receptor antagonists, 1291
Integrin-linked kinase (ILK), 405
Integrins, 79, 155, 221, 221f
Intellectual disability syndromes, 891
Intensive care unit (ICU), 639
Intensive chelation, 903
Intensive induction chemotherapy, 1748
Intensive therapies, 1417
Inter lymph, 1950
Intercellular adhesion molecule (ICAM), 155
Interdigitating dendritic cells (IDCs), 1376
Interferon (IFN), 273, 310, 1948, 1035, 1179, 1505–1506, 1815–1816, 1829–1830, 2096–2097
    maintenance with, 2209
    pegylated, 1817
Interferon alpha (IFNα), 377, 1253, 1782, 1843, 1860, 2175, 2049, 2062–2063
    combination chemotherapy with interferon-α for induction, 2193
    interferon-α2a, 2101
    monotherapy, 2289
Interferon regulatory factor 8 (Irf8), 137, 220
Interferon regulatory factor-4 gene (IRF4 gene), 220, 1878, 1931, 2001, 2155
α-interferon, 1370
γ-interferon, 978
Interferon-γ (IFNγ), 94, 170, 998, 1175, 1396, 1404, 1414, 1496, 2072
Intergroupe Français du Myélome (IFM), 2184
Interim maintenance (IM), 1672
Interleukin (IL), 288, 858
    IL-1, 432, 837, 1034–1035, 1247, 1344, 1366, 2177
    IL-11, 378
    IL-1β, 2277
    IL-1α-IL-1R1, 364
    IL-2, 770, 1401, 1411, 1498, 1506, 1850, 2051
    IL-2R, 2101
    IL-3, 74, 94, 168, 218, 371–372, 378, 1017, 1539, 1570
    IL-4, 218, 379, 2072
    IL5R, 1836
    IL-6, 74, 94, 372, 1034, 1175, 1383, 2163
        cytokines of IL-6 family, 378
    IL7, 1675
        IL7 receptor–deficient SCID, 1402
    IL7RA, 1402
    IL-8, 379
    IL-10, 771, 1946
    IL-22, 2355
    IL-33, 1035
    IL-34, 218
    IL2RG gene, 1401, 1927
Intermediate monocytes (iMo), 27, 212
Intermediate risk (IR), 1669
INT-1, 1858
INT-2, 1858
Intermountain Healthcare series, 1062
Internal tandem duplication (ITD), 1460, 1627, 1722
Internal tandem repeat (ITD), 1575
International Aplastic Anemia and Agranulocytosis Study, 1336
International Bone Marrow Transplant Registry (IBMTR), 813, 998, 1001, 1616, 2184
International Consensus Classification (ICC), 1446, 1638, 1837
International Fanconi Anemia Registry, The, 975–976
International Immune Tolerance Study, The, 1258
International Kidney and Monoclonal Gammopathy Research Group (IKMG), 2289
International Lymphoma Classification Project, 1943
International mortality data, 2176
International Myeloma Working Group (IMWG), 2148, 2168, 2184
International normalized ratio (INR), 578, 1133, 1245, 1281
International pediatric NHL staging system (IPNHLSS), 1992
International Peripheral T cell Lymphoma Project (IPTL), 1973
International prognostic index (IPI), 1955
International Prognostic Score (IPS), 2120

International Prognostic Score for Essential Thrombocythemia-thrombosis (IPSET-thrombosis), 1178
International Prognostic Scoring System (IPSS), 668, 1825, 2299, 2337
International prognostic scoring system for mastocytosis (IPSM), 1858
International Prognostic Staging System for Waldenström Macroglobulinemia (IPSSWM), 2269
International Randomized Study of Interferon and STI571 (IRIS), 1793
International scale (IS), 1792
International sensitivity index (ISI), 1297
International Society for Cutaneous Lymphomas (ISCL), 2080
International Society on Thrombosis and Haemostasis (ISTH), 1080, 1084, 1182, 1251, 1276
International Society on Thrombosis and Haemostasis Bleeding Assessment Tool (ISTH-BAT), 1182
International Staging System (ISS), 2181
International System for Human Cytogenomic Nomenclature (ISCN), 50
International Working Group for Myelofibrosis Research and Treatment (IWG-MRT), 1821
International Working Group in Myeloproliferative Neoplasms and Treatment (IWG-MRT), 1862
International Workshop of Chronic Lymphocytic Leukemia (iwCLL), 2016
Internationalized normal ratio (INR), 1723
Intestinal bile pigment metabolism, 126
Intestinal macrophages, 213
Intestinal T-cell lymphoma (ITL), 1888–1889
Intra-abdominal bleeding, 1208
Intracardiac patch repairs, 828
Intracellular adhesion molecule 1 (ICAM-1), 240
Intracellular cobalamin metabolism with megaloblastic anemia, inborn errors of, 963
Intracellular cytokine assays, 43
Intracellular DNA sensors, 223
Intracellular metabolism, 950–951
Intracellular organisms, 1321
Intracellular trafficking of MPL, 373–374
Intrachromosomal amplification of chromosome 21 (iAMP21), 1582, 1667, 1670
Intraclonal tumor heterogeneity associated with high-risk MM, 2156
Intracranial bleeding, 1232–1233
Intrahepatic biliary tract obstruction, 1242
Intrahepatic shunting, 1164
Intralesional histiocytes of LCH, 1365
Intraluminal crawling and transmigration, 253
Intramuscular hematomas, 1206
Intraperitoneal hemorrhage, 1208
Intrathecal chemotherapy (IT chemotherapy), 1706
Intrauterine fetal death, 1252
Intravascular coagulation, 1245
Intravascular hemoglobin, fate of, 122
Intravascular hemolysis, 121, 806, 827, 830, 864, 1025, 1148
    chronic, 792
    hemoglobinemia, 619
    hemoglobinuria, 619–620
    urine hemosiderin and urinary iron excretion, 620
Intravascular hemolytic transfusion reactions, 581
Intravascular plasminogen, 1285
Intravenous (IV), 2186
    currently available intravenous iron preparations, 648t
    hypotonic fluids, 840
    iron therapy, 641, 647–648, 1165
    MTX, 1673
    Rho (D) immune globulin, 1106
    side effects of, 648
Intravenous immune globulin (IVIG), 550, 558, 772, 1049, 1102, 1105, 1258, 1334, 1368, 1398, 1412, 1477, 2221, 2281, 2315
    IVIG-mediated hemolysis, 550
Intraventricular hemorrhage (IVH), 1055
Intrinsic apoptotic pathway, 2012
Intrinsic tenase, 436
Intrinsic pathway, 428
Introns, cryptic site mutants in and, 887
Invaginated membrane system (IMS), 360, 362
Invariant natural killer T cells (iNKT cells), 236, 1390, 1495
Invasive fungal infections (IFIs), 1471
Inverted terminal repeat (ITR), 1528

Involved field radiotherapy (IFRT), 2121, 2135
Involved-node radiotherapy (INRT), 2121
Iodine 131 (I-131), 1502
Iodine-labeled SAP scanning, 2241
Ionizing radiation, 997, 1629
Ipilimumab, 2102
iPSCs, derivation of genetically corrected HSCs from, 1550
Iron, 13, 658, 688–689, 704, 760, 813
  absorption and toxicity in *HFE* hemochromatosis, 682
    abnormal iron absorption, 682
    organ and cellular injury due to iron overload, 682–683
    postscreening evaluation of *HFE* p. C282Y homozygotes in HEIRS study, 683
    prevalence of *HFE* p. C282Y homozygosity in different populations, 683
    proportions of *HFE* p. C282Y homozygotes in hemochromatosis cohorts, 683
  bone marrow, 2371
  chelation therapy, 842, 861, 911, 919, 1747
  clinical changes after iron depletion, 695
  colorectal polyps and colorectal cancer, 689–690
  deposition, 902
  exporter ferroportin, 629
  hepatocellular carcinoma, 689
  iron-restricted erythropoiesis, 647
  metabolism, 635, 1428
    systemic regulation of, 630–632
  non-transferrin bound, 635, 681 899
  overload, organ injury, 682–683
  oxidation and spectral characteristics, 938–939
  pigment, 1811
  reutilization function of heme oxygenases, 125
  serum, 1011, 1015, 1037
  supplementation, 649
  surveillance for hepatocellular carcinoma, 689
  types of cancer, 690
Iron deficiency, 379, 1038, 1040
  biochemical, 1063
  clinical features of, 636
    blood loss, 638–639
    blood loss in infancy, 640
    chronic renal failure treated with hemodialysis, 639
    copper deficiency, 638
    decreased total body iron at birth, 640
    diet, 637–638
    diet in infancy and childhood, 640
    epithelial lesions associated with, 642*t*
    epithelial tissues, 641
    fatigue and nonspecific symptoms, 641
    genitourinary system, 643
    growth, 640
    impaired absorption, 638
    iron balance in pregnancy, 641*t*
    koilonychia, 641*f*
    neuromuscular system, 641
    pica, 643
    pregnancy and lactation, 640–641
    prevalence, 637
    runner anemia, 640
    signs and symptoms of, 641
    skeletal system, 643
    stages in development of, 636, 636*t*
    tongue of patient with iron-deficiency anemia, 642*f*
  erythropoiesis, 612
  in fetus and newborn infant, 1063–1064
  iron deficiency anemia, 635
    etiologic factors in, 637*t*
    genes involved in hereditary iron deficiency anemia, 635*t*
    genetic forms of, 635–636, 636*t*
    pathogenesis of, 635
  laboratory evaluation, 643
    blood smear from patient with microcytic anemia, 645*f*
    bone marrow, 645–646
    complete blood count and peripheral smear, 643
    iron deficiency states, 645*f*
    iron-related indices, 643–645
    leukocytes and platelets, 645
    potential role of hepcidin in diagnosis and management, 645*t*
    screening, evaluation, and management of anemia, 644*f*

  management of, 646
    acute iron intoxication, 649
    algorithm for treatment of, 646*f*
    intravenous iron therapy, 647–648
    oral iron therapy, 646–647
    preventive treatment, 649
    response to therapy, 648–649
  normal iron physiology, 628
    cellular uptake of iron-transferrin, 633*f*
    hepcidin and systemic regulation of iron metabolism, 630–632
    important Fe-containing compounds in humans, 629*t*
    intestinal absorption, 628
    iron balance, 628
    iron cycle, 632, 632*f*
    iron delivery to erythroid precursors, 633–634
    iron metabolism in tissues, 635
    iron metabolism within erythroblasts, 634
    macrophage iron recycling, 634–635
    molecular mechanisms of iron absorption, 628–629
    nonheme iron absorption in intestine, 629*f*
    plasma transport, 633
    regulation of iron absorption, 630
    regulation of iron absorption by intracellular mechanisms, 632
    total body iron, 628
  during pregnancy, 1047–1048
  and related disorders, 628
Iron deficiency anemia (IDA), 628
Iron overload, 585, 662, 678, 690, 2308, 2371–2376
  β-thalassemia, 691
  atherosclerosis, 692
  cardiomyopathy, 692
  clinical manifestations of, 900–908
    chelation, 904
    deferasirox, 906–907
    deferiprone, 905–906
    deferoxamine, 904–905
    endocrine glands, 902–903
    exocrine glands, 903
    eye, 903–904
    heart, 900–901
    kidney, 902
    liver, 901–902
    pulmonary problems, 904
    splenectomy, 907–908
    vitamin supplementation, 907
  differential diagnosis of, 678
  HCT late effects, 2372*f*
  hereditary spherocytosis, 691
  heritable and acquired disorders associated with, 679*t*
  infections in hemochromatosis patients, 691
  LTFU recommendations for survivors, 2374–2376*t*
  magnitude of late effects after HCT, 2373–2374*t*
  organ and cellular injury due to, 682–683
  recommended vaccinations after HCT, 2377*t*
  refractory anemia with ringed sideroblasts, 691
  subnormal immunoglobulins, 691–692
  X-linked sideroblastic anemia, 691
Iron pathway disorders, 612
  evaluation of bone marrow iron stores, 613
  measurement of serum iron and iron-binding capacity, 612
  serum ferritin, 612–613
  soluble transferrin receptors, 613
  tests to assess iron metabolism, 613
    disorders of hemoglobin synthesis, 613
    erythrocyte zinc protoporphyrin, 613
    liver iron stores, 613
Iron regulatory elements (IREs), 632
Iron regulatory proteins (IRP), 632, 657
Iron-refractory iron deficiency anemia (IRIDA), 636
Iron-responsive element (IRE), 657
Iron-sulfur (Fe-S), 656
Iron therapy, oral, 646
  failure of, 646
  side effects of, 646
Irradiation, 2382
Irreversible sickle cells (ISCs), 835
Isatuximab, 2184, 2215
Isavuconazole, 1477, 1483
Ischemia-reperfusion injury, 838
Ischemic disease, 1263
Ischemic-dermatologic syndromes, 1263
Isochromosome 17q, 1778

Isocitrate dehydrogenase (*IDH*), 1710, 1756, 1821, 1825, 1978, 2335
  differentiation syndrome, 1650
  *IDH*1 gene, 1460, 1565, 1573, 1584–1585, 1573, 1573*f*, 1636, 1648, 1710, 1738, 1756, 1812, 1825, 1857, 1929, 1931
  *IDH*2 gene, 1460, 1573, 1573*f*, 1584–1585, 1636, 1648, 1650, 1710, 1738, 1755–1756, 1768, 1812, 1825, 1840, 1857, 1928–1929, 1978
  inhibitors, 1650–1651
Isohemagglutinins, 540
Isolated histiocytosis of skin, 1370
Isolated lymphoid follicles (ILFs), 249
Isolated red cell membranes, 890
Isoleucine, 946
Isoniazid (INH), 665
Isopropanol test, 937
Isoschizomer restriction enzyme–based methods, 1909
ISTH-BAT. *See* International Society on Thrombosis and Haemostasis Bleeding Assessment Tool (ISTH-BAT)
Italian Gruppo Italiano Malattie Ematologiche dell' Adulto (GIMEMA), 1615
Italian Society for Haemostasis and Thrombosis (SISET), 1197
ITGA2B gene, 1156
ITGB2 gene, 1344
ITIM-containing receptor. *See* Immunoreceptor tyrosine-based inhibitory motif-containing receptor (ITIM-containing receptor)
ITK. *See* IL-2-inducible T-cell kinase (ITK)
ITL. *See* Intestinal T-cell lymphoma (ITL)
Ivosidenib, 1460
Ixazomib, 1460, 2175, 2184, 2192, 2197, 2212, 2213, 2253
IκB. *See* Inhibitor of κB (IκB)
IκB kinase (IKK), 2133

J

Jacobsen syndrome (JS), 1192, 1194
JAK. *See* Janus kinase (JAK)
Jamaican Cohort Study, 839
Jamshidi bone marrow aspiration and biopsy needle, 9, 9*f*
Janus kinase (JAK), 1505
  inhibitors, 1459–1460
    fedratinib, 1459–1460
    pacritinib, 1460
    ruxolitinib, 1459
  *JAK*1 gene, 1603, 1610, 1675, 1927, 2074
  *JAK*2 gene, 104, 356, 375, 1176, 1178, 1603, 1610, 1630, 1675, 1677, 1740, 1755, 1758, 1763, 1766, 1768, 1770, 1812, 1816, 1823, 1840, 1849–1850, 1857
    approved JAK inhibitors and those in late-stage development, 1830*t*
    inhibitors, 1830–1831
  JAK2V617F, 374–375, 1177
  JAK3 gene, 2074
  JAK3-deficient SCID, 1402
  V617F, 933, 1822, 2279, 1821
  V617F mutation-negative polycythemia vera, 1072
  V617F-negative patients, 1813
Janus kinase/signal transducers and activators of transcription pathway (JAK/STAT pathway), 1459, 1786, 1821, 2072, 2116
Japan Childhood Aplastic Anemia Study Group, 1004
Japanese atomic bomb survivors, 2176
Japanese Infant Leukemia/Lymphoma Study Group (JILSG), 1676
Japanese PRCA Consortium, 1013
JARID1A, 1710
Jaundice, 617, 731, 754, 1020
Job syndrome, 1346
Jordan anomaly, 1354
JS. *See* Jacobsen syndrome (JS)
Junctional adhesion molecule A (JAM-A), 413
Juvenile hemochromatosis, 678
  hemojuvelin hemochromatosis (*HJV* hemochromatosis), 678–680
  hepcidin hemochromatosis (*HAMP* hemochromatosis), 680
  transferrin receptor-2 hemochromatosis (*TFR2* hemochromatosis), 680
Juvenile idiopathic arthritis (JIA), 1668

Juvenile myelomonocytic leukemia (JMML), 1697, 1763, 1776–1777, 1777f
    WHO criteria for, 1777t

K

K-Cl cotransport channel (KCC), 112, 835–836
Kala-Azar, 824, 1028
Kallikrein, 434
Kaluza software, B-cell lymphoma analysis using, 22, 24f
Kaplow procedure, 13
Kaposi sarcoma (KS), 1410
Kappa (κ), 2160
Karyograms, 50
Karyotype analysis, 49–50, 1446, 1765
Karyotyping, 1322
Kasabach-Merritt syndrome, 986, 1253
KB test. *See* Kleihauer-Betke test (KB test)
KCC. *See* K-Cl cotransport channel (KCC)
KDH. *See* α-ketoglutarate dehydrogenase (KDH)
Kell antigens (K antigens), 860
Keratinocyte growth factor, 2303, 2365
α-ketoglutarate dehydrogenase (KDH), 658
α-ketoglutarate (α-KG), 1573, 1636
Ketron-Goodman disease, 2085
Kidd antigens and antibodies, 546–547
Kidney, 902, 852–853, 2244
    biopsy, 1144
    total protein excreted in urine, 2244f
    transplantation, 2291
Kidney Disease: Improving Global Outcomes Guideline (2012) (KDIGO Guideline), 1038
KIF23 mutation, 1025
Killer cell immunoglobulin-like receptors (KIR), 310, 311f, 326, 1888, 2081, 2365
    haplotypes, 326
    KIR2DL3, 328
Killer inhibitory receptors, 31
Kinase, 1401
Kinase domain receptor, 531
Kinase inhibitors (KIs), 2013
KIND3, 1346
Kindlin-3 CalDAG-GEFI, 1193
Kinetic techniques, 1085
KIT genes, 1840, 1849, 1570, 1602, 1857, 1861
    KIT p. D816V variant, 1853
    ligand, 378
Klebsiella, 899, 908
    K. pneumoniae, 899
Kleihauer-Betke test (KB test), 1059
KLF1 gene, 884, 914, 1027
KLF2 mutation, 1875
Klinefelter syndrome, 1696
Klotho gene, 855
KLRD1/KLRC1 genes, 2365
KMT2A gene, 1574–1575, 1638, 1699, 1709, 1931
KMT2A gene. *See* Histone-lysine N-methyltransferase 2A gene (*KMT2A* gene)
KMT2A rearrangements (KMT2A-R), 1670
KMT2A-R. *See* KMT2A rearrangements (KMT2A-R)
KMT2C gene, 1928
KMT2D gene, 1871, 1920
Knee arthroplasty, 688
Knudson's two-hit mutational hypothesis, 48
Koilonychia, 641
Kostmann syndrome, 1696, 1704
KRAS gene, 1380, 1680, 1850, 1857
KS. *See* Kaposi sarcoma (KS)
Kupffer cells, 213, 682, 852
Kyphoscoliosis, 1074

L

Labile factor deficiency. *See* Inherited factor V deficiency
β-Lactam antibiotics, 1266
β-Lactamase inhibitors, 784
Lactate dehydrogenase (LDH), 1049, 1132, 1413, 1823, 1954, 1991, 2018, 2091, 2181, 618, 755, 773, 805, 838, 952, 2344
    serum, 1632
Lactation, 640–641
Lactic acid, 562
Lactic acidosis, 664–665
Lactobacillus
    L. casei, 959
    L. delbrueckii, 967

L. lactis, 945
Lactoferrin, 152, 160
    deficiency, 1347
Lacunar cells, 1889
Lambda (λ), 2160
Lamellipodium, 157
Lamin B receptor (*LBR*), 146
Laminin, 406
Lamivudine, 964
Langerhans cell histiocytosis (LCH), 1364, 1366, 1376
    anaplastic lymphoma kinase–positive histiocytosis (ALK-positive histiocytosis), 1380
    blastic plasmacytoid dendritic cell neoplasm (BPDCN), 1378–1379
    clinical features, 1366
    dendritic cell sarcomas, 1378
    diagnosis, 1369
    disseminated juvenile xanthogranuloma (JXG), 1379
    epidemiology, 1365
    Erdheim-Chester disease (ECD), 1379–1380
    follicular dendritic cell sarcoma (FDC sarcoma), 1377
    hemophagocytic lymphohistiocytosis (HLH), 1380
    and histiocytic disorders, 1376t
    histiocytic sarcoma (HS), 1379
    history, 1364–1365
    interdigitating dendritic cell sarcoma (IDC sarcoma), 1378
    Langerhans cell sarcoma (LCS), 1376–1377
    LCH-associated neurodegenerative disease, 1368
    management and treatment, 1370–1371
    pathology and pathophysiology, 1365
    prognosis, 1369
    Rosai-Dorfman disease (RDD), 1380
Langerhans cell sarcoma (LCS), 1376–1377, 1377f
Langerhans cells (LC), 208, 215, 1365
Lanoteplase (nPA), 1302
Laparoscopic biopsy, 1445
Large cephalohematomas, 1082
Large plaque parapsoriasis (LPP), 2082
Large vessel abnormalities, 827
Large-animal models, 1537
Laryngeal amyloidosis, 2259
Laser light scattering, 2
Late complications, pathogenesis of, 706
Latent membrane protein 1 (LMP1), 256, 1881, 1382, 1388, 2116, 2133
Lazy-leukocyte syndrome, 1346–1347
Lecithin-cholesterol acyltransferase (LCAT), 109, 744
LECs. *See* Lymphatic endothelial cells (LECs)
LECT2. *See* Leukocyte chemotactic factor 2 (LECT2)
Lectin complement pathway, 343
Lectin mannose–binding type 1 (LMAN1). *See* Endoplasmic reticulum–Golgi intermediate compartment protein 53
Leder stain. *See* Specific (naphthol AS-D chloroacetate) esterase stain
Lef-1. *See* Lymphoid enhancer binding factor 1 (Lef-1)
LEF1 genes, 1960
Left ventricular (LV), 850
    diastolic dysfunction, 850
    LV-based vectors, 1538
    septum, 2243
Left ventricular assist device (LVAD), 1148, 2257
Left ventricular ejection fraction (LVEF), 2379
Leg
    isolated distal deep venous thrombosis of, 1305
    ulcers, chronic, 603, 618, 920
Legionella, 2053
Leiden Open Variation Database (LOVD), 454
Leishmania donovani, 824
Lenalidomide, 1461, 1745–1746, 1827, 1829, 1963, 1970, 2175, 2184, 2186, 2190–2194, 2196–2198, 2210, 2213, 2216–2217, 2251, 2253, 2281, 2284, 2292
    bortezomib, 2251
    maintenance, 2207
Lentiviral approaches for gene addition, 912
Lentiviral vectors (LV vectors), 1527
Lepirudin, 1295
Leptin receptor (lepR), 84
Lesch-Nyhan Disease, 964
Letermovir, 2308
Lethal midline granuloma, 1889
Letterer-Siwe disease, 1364, 1366
Leucine-rich repeat 5 (LRR-5), 1188

Leucine-rich repeat motifs (LRG motifs), 403
Leucyl-tRNA synthetase (LARS2), 665
Leukapheresis, 2064
Leukemia, 974, 1331, 1430, 1694, 1782, 1992–1995
    blasts, 1709
    congenital, 1704
    cutis, 1631, 1669, 2090
    multiple hit model of, 1562–1564
        multiple mutations are necessary for development of AML, 1564f
    SIRs, 2383
    therapy, 1614
Leukemia stem cells (LSCs), 1632
Leukemia-associated immunophenotype (LAIP), 37, 1640
Leukemia-initiating cell (LIC), 1632, 1695
Leukemic blast clearance, early, 1614
Leukemic cells extracts, 1248
Leukemic myeloblasts, 138
Leukemic promyelocytes, 1721
Leukemic reticuloendotheliosis, 2049
Leukemic skin infiltration, 1631
Leukemic stem cells, 1695
Leukhemia, 1627
Leukocyte adhesion defects (LADs), 156
Leukocyte adhesion deficiency (LAD), 1344, 1395, 1528, 2318
Leukocyte immunoglobulin-like receptor 2 (LIR1/ILT2), 328
Leukocyte transcript 1 (LST1), 2051
Leukocyte(s), 1, 136, 645, 804, 1810
    alloantibodies reacting with leukocyte antigens, 580–581
    analysis, 4–5
    differentials, 4–5
    familial vacuolization of, 1354
    inclusions in, 1354
    kinetics, 149
    morphologic characteristics, 138t
    normal blood leukocyte concentrations, 142t
    normal values for, 141
    qualitative disorders of
        defects affecting adhesion and/or margination, 1344–1346
        defects affecting phagocytosis and degranulation, 1347–1349
        defects impacting chemotaxis, 1346–1347
        disorders of bacterial killing and respiratory burst, 1349–1352
        frequency of identifiable qualitative neutrophil disorders, 1352
        functional neutrophil disorders, 1344
        morphologic changes in phagocytic leukocytes, 1352
        select qualitative disorders of leukocytes, 1344f
Leukocytoclastic vasculitis, 1170
Leukocytosis, 3, 141–142, 1650, 2282
    management of leukocytosis during induction in low-risk APL, 1729
    response criteria and monitoring, 1730
    corticosteroid prophylaxis, 1731
    treatment-related complications, 1730
Leukopenia, 792, 806, 1331, 1410
Leukopoiesis, 610
Leukotriene B$_4$ (LTB4), 150, 153, 161
Leuserpin 2. *See* Heparin cofactor II
Levofloxacin, 2307
Lewis antigens and antibodies, 547
Leydig cells, 2381
Li-Fraumeni syndrome, 1609, 1635, 1739
Lichen aureus, 2082
Ligand-receptor interactions, 402
Ligase IV (LIG4), 272
Ligases, defects of, 272
Light chain, 482
Light chain deposition disease (LCDD), 2290
Light chain MGUS (LC-MGUS), 2160
Light chain proximal tubulopathy (LCPT), 2289
Light microscopy, 391
Light transmission aggregometry (LTA), 1182
Light transmission platelet aggregation, 1083
Light zone (LZ), 245, 246f
Light-chain deposition disease (LCDD), 2177, 2222
LIM domain–binding protein 1 (LDB1), 1586
Limiting dilution assay, 78

Lineage assignment, 35–36
Lineage commitment, 80
    branch points of hematopoiesis, 80
    erythroid growth factors, 82–83
    factors act on multilineage progenitors, 81
    granulocyte growth factors, 81
    hematopoietic cytokines, 80–81
    hematopoietic factors based on receptor types, 81t
    lymphocyte growth factors, 83
    mast cell growth factors, 81
    megakaryocyte growth factors, 82
    micro-RNAs, 80
    monocyte/macrophage growth factors, 81–82
    phenotypes caused by nonfunctional mutations, 82t
    supportive vs. instructive signals, 83
    transcription factors, 80
Lineage priming in hematopoiesis, 216
Lineage-associated antigens, 22
Linear amplification–mediated PCR, 1542
Linezolid, 669, 1473–1474
Linkage disequilibrium, 323
Linker of activated T cells (LAT), 1498
Lipid nanoparticle-mediated delivery (LNP-mediated delivery), 708
Lipid-lowering agent (LLA), 2096
Lipid(s), 726
    bilayer hypothesis, 108
    bodies, 173
    chemical structure of heme and manner of union with globin to form hemoglobin, 110f
    chemoattractants, 153
    composition, 108–109
    composition and metabolism and generation of arachidonic acid, 395–396
    of normal human erythrocyte membrane, 108t
    pathways of lipid acquisition and turnover in mature red cell membrane, 109f
    rafts, 147, 276, 726
    turnover and acquisition, 109
Lipochrome histiocytosis, 1350
Lipocortin I, 147
Lipopolysaccharide (LPS), 152, 176, 211
Lipoprotein receptor-related protein (LRP), 464
Lipoproteins, 2285
Liposomal Doxil, 2099
Liposomes, 1525
Liquid chromatography-MS (LC-MS), 707, 958
Liquid plasma, 563
LIR1/ILT2. See Leukocyte immunoglobulin-like receptor 2 (LIR1/ILT2)
Lisocabtagene maraleucel (liso-cel), 303, 1511
Listeria monocytogenes, 1469, 2053
Live cells, 18
Live gate method, 22
Livedo reticularis, 778, 1171
Liver, 2244–2245, 2371
    abnormalities, 687
    acute GVHD, 2358
    biopsy, 662, 713, 2244
    manifestations of cryoglobulinemia, 2287
    primary NHL of, 1954
Liver disease, 611, 688, 829, 901, 920, 1028, 1242, 1244
    abnormalities of hemostasis and coagulation in liver disease, 1244
    anemia in, 1039–1041
    autoimmune, 1010
    clinical manifestations, 1245
    involvement, 2056
    iron stores, 613
    laboratory diagnosis, 1245
    pathophysiology, 1244
        deficient or aberrant synthesis of coagulation factors, 1244
        fibrinogenolysis and fibrinolysis, 1244
        intravascular coagulation, 1245
        prothrombotic changes, 1245
        thrombocytopenia, 1244
    treatment, 1245
Liver function test (LFT), 2382
Liver iron concentration (LIC), 860, 899, 2371
Liver X receptor (LXR), 413, 2096
Localized amyloidosis syndrome, 2259
    localized cutaneous amyloidosis, 2260
    localized laryngeal amyloidosis, 2259
    localized ocular amyloidosis, 2260
    localized pulmonary amyloidosis, 2259

localized ureterovesicular amyloidosis, 2259–2260
Locus control region (LCR), 884
Loeys-Dietz syndrome, 1167
Log$_2$ R intensity ratio, 54
Logarithmic amplification, 22, 27
Lon peptidase 1 (LONP1), 704
Loncastuximab tesirine, 1967
Long homologous repeats, 347
Long noncoding RNAs (lncRNAs), 371
Long terminal repeats (LTRs), 1526, 1948
Loss of heterozygosity (LOH), 51, 1905
Low bone disease (LB), 2182
Low bone mass density, 849
Low bone mineral density, 2380
Low molecular weight heparin (LMWH), 1197, 1305
Low von Willebrand Factor, 1215
Low-density lipoprotein (LDL),535, 592, 744, 912, 1284
Low-density lipoprotein receptor (LDLR), 343
Low-density microarray approach (LDA), 1584
Low-molecular-weight kininogen (LMWK), 434
Low-molecular-weight tcu-PA, 485
Low-oxygen-affinity hemoglobins, 935. See also High-oxygen-affinity hemoglobins
    clinical features, 935
    diagnosis, 935
    pathophysiology, 935
    treatment, 935
Low–molecular-weight heparin (LMWH), 815, 1253, 1280, 1293, 2219
Lugano staging system, 2119
Lumbar puncture (LP), 1324, 1698
Luminex platform, 40
Luminex SAB assay, 327
Luminex single antigen (SAB), 327
Lung(s), 851–852, 1955, 2358
Lupus anticoagulant (LA), 1259–1266
Luspatercept, 1745, 1829
Luteinizing hormone (LH), 2331
LV. See Left ventricular (LV)
Lyme disease, 2285
Lymph nodes (LNs), 22, 213–214, 233, 239, 239f, 241f, 1323–1324, 1853, 1866, 1879, 2020, 2077, 2080, 2092–2093, 2117, 2278
    alterations in lymphoma, 255–257
        spectrum, 256f
    architecture in SLL, 1872
    biopsy, 1378, 2091
    core biopsy, 1323
    cortex, 242–243
    methods for lymph node examination, 1323t
    normal, 240f
    ontogeny of secondary lymphoid tissue, 242
    paracortex, 243
    pathology, 2080
    stroma, 244–246
    stromal cell subtypes, 244f
    vasculature and conduit system, 243–244
Lymphadenopathic mastocytosis with eosinophilia, 1772
Lymphadenopathy, 1853, 2282, 2286
Lymphangiomatosis, 1438, 1439f
Lymphatic endothelial cells (LECs), 242
Lymphatics, 1424
Lymphoblastic lymphoma (LBL), 1612, 1942, 1971, 1992–1995
Lymphocyte activation gene 3 protein (LAG3), 301
Lymphocyte adaptor protein (LNK), 377, 1074
Lymphocyte depleted HL subtype (LD subtype), 1889–1891, 1891f
Lymphocyte doubling time (LDT), 2023
Lymphocyte function–associated antigen-1 (LFA-1), 314, 2072
Lymphocyte-activated killer cells (LAK cells), 1508
Lymphocyte-predominant cells (LP cells), 1879, 2117
Lymphocyte-predominant HL (LPHL), 1953
Lymphocyte-rich classic HL (LRCHL), 2117
Lymphocyte-rich HL subtype (LR subtype), 1889–1890, 1890f
Lymphocyte-specific adaptor protein (LNK), 1178
Lymphocyte(s), 1, 5, 11, 233, 1873, 1942, 2072
    characteristics, 2023
    differentiation, 28–29
    doubling time, 2023–2024
    egress from lymphoid tissues, 255
    flow cytometry, 2024
    functional studies, 2053
    genetics, 2024

growth factors, 83
immortalization, 1382–1383
large granular (LGL), 1009, 1337, 1975
lymph node alterations in lymphoma, 255–257
lymph nodes (LNs), 239–246
lymph nodes and lymphoid tissue, 233
lymphocyte-depleted HL, 2116, 2118
lymphocyte-variant HE, 1837
MicroRNA expression, 2025
morphology, 2023
mucosa-associated lymphoid tissue (MALT), 248–249
mutations of IGHV, IGHV$_{3-21}$ usage and stereotypy, 2024
NOTCH, SF3B1, and novel mutations, 2025
number, 2023
primary (central) lymphoid tissues, 233–239
spleen, 246–248
telomere length and telomerase activity, 2024
tertiary lymphoid organs (TLOs), 249–255
transcriptional remodeling of FL-associated lymph node stromal cells, 257f
Lymphocytic exocytosis, 2082
Lymphocytosis, 1976
Lymphoepithelioid lymphoma, 1885
Lymphoid blast crises, 1765
Lymphoid cells, 38, 2133
Lymphoid enhancer binding factor 1 (Lef-1), 136
Lymphoid lesions, EBV-associated lymphomas and, 1389
Lymphoid lineage, 69
Lymphoid malignancies, 2341–2345
Lymphoid neoplasms with eosinophilia, 1772–1774
Lymphoid niches in bone marrow, 85
Lymphoid proliferations, 1439–1441
Lymphoid tissue, 233
Lymphoid tissue inducer (LTi), 237, 309
Lymphoid tissue organizer, 242, 246
Lymphoid tissue, primary (central), 233
    bone marrow, 233–234
    early T-cell development and migration in cortex, 236
    medulla migration and emigration of thymocytes, 238
    mTEC development, 237–238
    mTEC-DC interactions for central tolerance, 238
    negative selection in cortex, 237
    positive selection in cortex, 236–237
    thymic involution, 239
    thymic nurse cells (TNCs), 237
    thymus, 234–236
    unconventional T-cell development in medulla, 238–239
Lymphoid-primed multipotent progenitors (LMPPs), 216
Lymphokine-activated killer (LAK), 313
Lymphoma(s), 1324, 1430, 1445, 1854, 1888, 1900, 1928, 1942, 1944, 1952, 1977, 2093, 2125t
    associations between, 2286
    B-cell lymphomas, 1869–1882
    breast primary, 1955
    cells, 1876
    cutaneous, 2072, 2075
    diagnosis and classification of, 1866
    of extraocular space, 1954
    follicular, pediatric, 919, 1872, 2001
    Hodgkin lymphoma, 1899–1894
    indolent B-cell lymphoma, 1961–1962, 1959
        follicular lymphoma (FL), 1959–1961
        frontline treatment options, 1962–1963
        immunotherapy, 1964
        lymphoplasmacytic lymphoma (LPL), 1961
        marginal zone lymphoma (MZL), 1961
        relapsed and refractory treatment options, 1963–1964
        small B lymphocytic lymphoma (SLL), 1961
        special clinicopathologic features, 1961
        treatment options, 1961–1962
    large cell (LCL), 2074
    natural killer cell lymphomas, 1882–1885
        adult T-cell leukemia/lymphoma (ATLL), 1888
        anaplastic large cell lymphoma (ALCL), 1887–1888
        angioimmunoblastic T-cell lymphoma, 1885–1887
        extranodal natural killer/t-cell lymphoma, nasal type, 1889
        hepatosplenic T-cell lymphoma (HSTCL), 1888
        intestinal T-cell lymphoma (ITL), 1888–1889
        peripheral T-cell lymphoma, not otherwise specified, 1885

subcutaneous panniculitis–like T-cell lymphoma, 1888
occular primary, 1954
pulmonary primary, 1955
specimen evaluation, 1866
  classification of non-Hodgkin lymphomas, 1869
  cytogenetic and molecular studies, 1869
  immunophenotypic analysis, 1866–1869
  immunophenotypic markers used in diagnosis of malignant lymphomas, 1867–1868t
  malignant lymphomas in lymph node according, 1866f
  morphologic examination, 1866
  pathologic features in differential diagnosis of small B-cell lymphomas, 1868t
  tissue sampling and processing, 1866
splenic primary, 1953
T-cell and natural killer cell lymphomas, 1882–1899
tumors, 2089
Lymphomatoid papulosis (LyP), 1887, 2079, 2083–2084
Lymphomatous meningeal infiltration, 1954
Lymphomyeloid clonal hematopoiesis, 1630
Lymphomyeloid progenitors, 216–218
Lymphopenia, 1413, 1860
Lymphoplasmacytic lymphoma (LPL), 33, 1873, 1917–1918, 1949, 1961, 2058
  genetics, 1873
  guidelines for molecular testing in, 1918
  immunophenotype, 1873
  morphology, 1873
Lymphoproliferative disorders (LPDs), 781–782, 1009, 1102, 2075, 2286
Lymphosarcoma cell leukemia, 2018
Lymphotoxin β receptor (LTβR), 237
Lymphotoxins (LTs), 237
Lymphotropic viruses, 1946
Lysine methyltransferase 2A gene (*KMT2A* gene), 1634
Lysine-binding sites, 480
Lysophosphatidic acid (LPA), 253
Lysosomal sphingomyelin accumulation, 1362
Lysosomal storage diseases (LSDs), 227, 1543–1545
  Fabry disease, 1546
  Hurler syndrome, 1545–1546
  metachromatic leukodystrophy (MLD), 1545
  pathophysiology of, 1359
Lysosomal traffic regulator gene (*LYST* gene), 1191, 1336, 1380
Lysosome-associated membrane proteins (LAMP-1/LAMP-2), 395
  LAMP1–3, 363
Lysosomes, 363, 395
Lysozyme, 160, 2238
Lytic bone disease, 2239

M

Macrocytes, 8, 606
Macrocytic anemia, 1025
  approach to, 608
    megaloblastic anemias, 608–610
    nonmegaloblastic macrocytic anemias, 610–611
  of pregnancy, 1048
Macrocytic pancytopenia anemia, 966
Macrocytosis, 611, 952
  drugs inducing, 964
α_2-Macroglobulin, 464
  biochemistry, 464
  function, 464
  gene structure and expression, 464
Macroglossia, 2242
Macrophage colony–stimulating factor (M-CSF), 81, 218
Macrophage inhibitory protein (MIP), 172, 315
Macrophage-dendritic cell progenitor (MDP), 216
Macrophage(s), 11, 208, 324, 829, 1247, 1468, 1495
  in adult, 216–218
  differentiation of resident, 212
  diversity and classification, 212–214
  growth factors, 218
  historical perspective, 208–209
  iron, 645
  lineages, 1849
  molecular and cellular functions, 220–226
  origin, 216–220, 217f
  regulation of development by transcription factors, 219, 219f
    ID2-ZEB2-TCF4 axis, 220
    IRF4, IRF8, and BATF3, 220
    pioneer factors in early stem cell compartment, 219–220
    terminal differentiation factors, 220
Macropinocytosis by dendritic cells, 224–225
Macropolycytes, 147
Macrothrombocytopenias, autosomal dominant, 1154
Maculopapular cutaneous mastocytosis (MPCM), 1849
Mad cow disease, 588
Magnetic resonance imaging (MRI), 687, 707, 758, 805, 840, 896, 954, 1132, 1164, 1205, 1367, 1827, 2003, 2134, 2145, 2166, 2179, 2243, 2371
Magnetic susceptometry, 899
Majeed syndrome, 1028
Major basic protein (MBP), 168, 173–174
Major BCR (M-BCR), 1782
Major breakpoint cluster region (M-bcr), 1583
Major breakpoint region (MBR), 1920
Major hematologic response, 1792
Major histocompatibility complex (MHC), 31, 174, 288, 309, 322, 363, 630, 1494, 1880, 2355
  alleles, 322
  anti–human leukocyte antigen antibodies, 327
  cellular responses to human leukocyte antigen alloantigens, 326–327
  genes, 322
  genetics of, 322
    human leukocyte antigen gene polymorphism and nomenclature, 322–323
    human leukocyte antigen haplotypes and inheritance, 323–324
  human leukocyte antigen presentation, 330–334
  nonclassical human leukocyte antigen class I genes and molecules, 327–329
  nonclassical major histocompatibility complex class II molecules, 329–330
  structure and function of human leukocyte antigen molecules, 324–326
Major molecular response (MMR), 1793
Major response (MR), 1860
Major translocation cluster (MTC), 1910
Malabsorption syndromes, 962, 1242, 1859
Malaria, 587, 821, 1028, 1049, 2238
  clinical manifestations, 821
  diagnosis, 822–823
  malarial pigment hemozocin, 822
  management, 823
  pathogenesis, 821–822
  prevalence, geographic distribution, and role of, 883
Malayan pit viper (*Calloselasma rhodostoma*), 1248
Male impotence, 805, 816
Malignancy, 200, 976, 1267, 1337
Malignant diseases, 1612, 2298, 2302. *See also* Nonmalignant diseases
  acute lymphocytic leukemia (ALL), 2299
  acute myeloid leukemia (AML), 2298–2299
  chronic lymphocytic leukemia, 2299
  chronic myeloid leukemia, 2299
  Hodgkin lymphoma, 2299
  multiple myeloma, 2299
  myeloablative conditioning regimens, 2302
  myelodysplastic syndrome, 2299
  myeloproliferative disease, 2299
  non-Hodgkin lymphoma, 2299
  nonmyeloablative/RIC regimens, 2302–2303
Malignant hypertension, hemolysis due to, 829
Malignant neoplasms secondary (SMN), 1683–1684
Malignant transformation, replication-defective gene transfer vectors contribute to, 1542
Mammalian Hb transitions, 834
Mammalian heme biosynthesis and regulation, 703–704
Mammalian MHC, 322
Mammalian susceptibility to mycobacterial disease, 1404
Mammalian target of rapamycin (mTOR), 2272
Mandibular lesions, 1366
Mannose-6-phosphate receptor (MPR), 299
Mannose-binding lectin (MBL), 341
Mantle cell lymphoma (MCL), 33, 1458, 1500, 1511, 1866, 1873, 1908, 1910–1912, 1943, 1969–1970, 2299, 2344
  genetics, 1874
  guidelines for molecular testing in, 1912t
  immunophenotype, 1873–1874
  indications for allogeneic hematopoietic cell transplant, 2345
  indications for autologous hematopoietic cell transplant, 2344–2345
  mantle cell international prognostic index and Ki67, 1969f
  morphology, 1873
  prognostic scores, 2344
  in situ mantle cell neoplasia, 1874
Mantle cell lymphoma IPI (MIPI), 1955
Manual donation, 558
MAP. *See* Melphalan-doxorubicin-prednisone (MAP)
MAP2K1 gene, 1380, 2001
MAP2K1 mutations, 1376–1377, 1919
March hemoglobinuria, 640, 829
Marchiafava-Micheli syndrome, 792
Marfan syndrome, 1166–1167
Marginal granulocyte pool (MGP), 150
Marginal reticular cells (MRCs), 242, 246
Marginal sinus, 1425
Marginal zone lymphoma (MZL), 33, 1949, 1961, 2001–2002, 2150
Marginating pool, 154
Marijuana, 1697
Markov decision model, 2337
Maroteaux-Lamy polydystrophic syndrome, 1353
Marrow cell subsets, minor, 29–31
Marrow environment role in platelet production, 364
Marrow failure syndromes, 2314
  inherited, 974
Marrow fibrosis, 1042, 1763
Marrow hypoplasia, 805, 1025
Marrow injury, drug-induced neutropenia and neutropenia due to, 1336–1337
Marrow response, impaired, 1035
Marrow stromal function, 1413
Marrow Transplant Clinical Trials Network, 2206
Mas-related G-protein–coupled receptor (MRGPR), 196
Masitinib, 1861
Masked hypodiploidy, 43
Mass cytometry, 1326
Mass spectrometry, 2147, 2261
Massive blood transfusion, thrombocytopenia after, 1159
Mast cell (MC), 11, 27, 196, 1771, 1849, 1852, 2056
  activation syndrome, 1855
  characteristics, 200
    inhibition, 202t, 202–203
    mediators, 201t, 202
    surface phenotype and activation, 200–202
  clinical relevance, 199–200
  environmental activation, 199
  expression of selected surface markers, 200t
  factors, 201t
  functions, 203
    containment of injury, initiation of repair, remodeling, and normal function, 204
    dynamic equilibrium and homeostasis, 204–205
    inflammatory injury and host defenses, 203–204
  growth and differentiation, 199
  growth factors, 81
  infiltration of liver, 1853
  mediator secretion, 196–197
  model of activities, 203f
  morphology, 196
  ontogeny and developmental biology, 198–200
  recovery after activation, 197
Mast cell activation syndrome (MCAS), 1855
Mast cell leukemia (MCL), 1772, 1854
Mast cell proteinase 8 (MCP8), 202
Mast cell sarcoma (MCS), 1855
Mastermind-like family (MAML), 1585
Mastocytomas, isolated cutaneous, 1852
Mastocytosis, 1849–1850, 1854–1855
Mastocytosis, global prognostic score for (GPSM), 1858
Mastocytosis, smoldering systemic (SSM), 1771
Mastoid ecchymosis, 1162
Matched sibling donor (MSD), 1001, 1679, 2300, 2335
Matched unrelated donor (MUD), 1701, 2206, 2336
Mate-pair sequencing (MPseq), 58
Maternal anemia associated with prenatal infections, 1048–1049
Maternal diabetes, 1063
Maternal erythrocytes, 1061
Maternal iron, 640
Maternal obesity, 1063
Maternal plasma volume, 1047
Maternal smoking, 1063
Matriptase-2 (MT-2), 630, 636

Matrix-assisted laser desorption/ionization (MALDI), 2147
Maturing myeloid compartment, 37–38
Maximal vertical fluid pocket (MVP), 1062
Maximal-tolerated doses (MTD), 1454, 1502, 2198
May-Hegglin anomaly, 394, 1154, 1353–1354
May-Hegglin disease, 986
Mayo Alliance Prognostic Scoring System (MAPS), 1858
Mayo Medical Index, 2170
McLeod phenotype, 744
MD Anderson Cancer Center (MDACC), 1616
Mean cell hemoglobin concentration (MCHC), 912
Mean corpuscular hemoglobin (MCH), 2–3, 600, 1054
Mean corpuscular hemoglobin concentration (MCHC), 2–3, 600, 732, 837, 856
Mean corpuscular volume (MCV), 2–3, 107, 600, 656, 683, 890, 732, 778, 856, 1033, 1054, 1070, 1133
Mean platelet volume (MPV), 5, 1082, 1101
Measurable residual disease (MRD), 63, 1608, 1613–1614, 1630, 1694, 1901, 1923, 2027, 2335
Mechlorethamine, 1628
　hydrochloride, 2094
*MED*12 mutation, 1931
Median RFS, 1646
Mediastinal disease, 2118
Mediastinal gray zone lymphoma (MGZL), 1998
Mediastinal GZL, 1953
Mediastinal radiotherapy, 2139
Medullary thymic epithelial cells (mTECs), 234
　development, 237–238
　mTEC-DC interactions for central tolerance, 238
　TRA expression by, 238
Medullary thymocytes, 234
Megakaryoblastic leukemia, 1694
Megakaryocyte-erythroid progenitor (MEP), 359, 645
Megakaryocyte(s) (MKs), 11, 77, 361–365, 356, 407, 1102, 1011, 1191, 1412
　and bone marrow microenvironment, 365–366
　commitment, 356–360
　cytokine regulation of megakaryopoiesis and signaling, 371–379
　cytoplasmic maturation, 362
　　cytoskeleton, 363
　　demarcation membranes or invaginated membrane system, 362
　　granules and mitochondria, 362–363
　different steps of megakaryopoiesis, 356–365
　drugs that selectively suppress, 1157
　epigenetic regulation of megakaryopoiesis, 369–371
　growth factors, 82
　as immune cells, 366
　inherited thrombocytopenia, 357–358t
　later steps of megakaryocyte differentiation and differentiation markers, 360–361
　　schematic illustration of megakaryocyte differentiation, 360f
　mass, 1156
　megakaryocyte-derived TGF β1, 1823
　morphology, 1595
　ontogeny, 366
　primary thrombocytosis, 357t
　principal pathologies associated with primary defect in megakaryopoiesis, 379
　progenitors, 360
　TPO/MPL and signaling cascade in, 375
　　Janus Kinase 2, 375
　　PI3K pathway, 376
　　Protein kinase C, 377
　　RAS-RAF-MEK-ERK pathway, 376
　　SRC Family Kinases and SYK Kinase, 376–377
　　STATS, 375–376
　transcriptional regulation of megakaryopoiesis, 366–369
Megakaryocytic dysplasia, 1597
Megakaryocytic-erythroid differentiation (MegE differentiation), 80
Megakaryopoiesis, 356
　cytokine regulation of, 371–379
　different steps of, 356
　epigenetic regulation of, 369–371
　hematopoietic stem cell and megakaryocyte commitment, 356–360
　later steps of megakaryocyte differentiation and differentiation markers, 360–361

megakaryocyte and platelet formation, 363
　proplatelet formation and MK Rupture, 363–364
　role of apoptosis in regulation of platelet production, 365
　role of cytoskeleton in regulation of platelet production, 364–365
　role of marrow environment in platelet production, 364
megakaryocyte and polyploidization, 361–362
megakaryocyte cytoplasmic maturation, 362–363
megakaryocyte progenitors, 360
principal pathologies associated with primary defect in, 379
transcriptional regulation of, 366–369
Megaloblastic abnormalities, 954
Megaloblastic anemia(s), 608, 945, 963–965, 1048
　bone marrow, 610
　causes of, 959
　　cobalamin deficiency, 959–961
　　disorders of cobalamin transport, 963
　　folate deficiency, 961–963
　　inherited disorders of absorption, 963
　clinical and laboratory features of, 951
　　clinical chemistry of, 954
　　laboratory evaluation of, 954
　　macrocytosis, 952
　　pathology of, 952–954, 953f, 955t
　　pathophysiology of, 952
　diagnostic testing for, 956–959
　of folate deficiency, 954
　hematologic features of, 609–610
　history of, 945
　management of causes of deficiency, 966
　management of nonresponding patient, 966
　neurologic abnormalities in cobalamin deficiency, 954–956
　normal physiology and pathophysiology, 945–951
　　cobalamin (Cbl), 945–947
　　cobalamin physiology, 948
　　folate, 947–948
　　folate physiology, 950–951
　prevention of cobalamin and folate deficiency worldwide, 966–967
　treatment of cobalamin deficiency, 964–965
　treatment of folate deficiency, 965–966
　treatment of hyperhomocysteinemia, 966
　vitamin B_{12} and folate levels in serum and erythrocytes, 610
Megaloblastic crises, 846
Megaloblastic red cell precursors, 952
MegE differentiation. *See* Megakaryocytic-erythroid differentiation (MegE differentiation)
MEITL. *See* Monomorphic epitheliotropic intestinal T-cell lymphoma (MEITL)
Meizothrombin, 450
Melanomas, 2022
Melanosomes, 363
Melphalan, 1628, 2184, 2190–2192, 2250
Melphalan and dexamethasone (MDex), 2249–2250
Melphalan and prednisone (MP), 2249, 2184
Melphalan-cyclophosphamide-carmustine-prednisone (MCBP), 2193
Melphalan-cyclophosphamide-prednisone, 2193
Melphalan-doxorubicin-prednisone (MAP), 2193
Membrane attack complex (MAC), 338, 343, 796, 1142, 1393
　C5, 343
　C6, 343–344
　C7, 344
　C8, 344
　C9, 344
　clusterin, 349
　control of membrane attack complex assembly, 349
　formation, 344–345
　protein S, 349
Membrane attack complex perforin (MACPF), 343–344
Membrane cofactor protein (MCP), 346, 1141
Membrane inhibitor of reactive lysis (MIRL), 792, 796
Membrane phospholipids, abnormalities of, 1195–1196
　Scott syndrome, 1195
　Stormorken syndrome, 1195–1195
Membrane protein defects, 729, 735–737
　αβ-spectrin self-association site in HE and HPP, 737f
　ankyrin defects, 730
　band 3 deficiency, 730
　protein 4.2 deficiency, 730

protein composition of RBC membrane skeleton, 729f
spectrin deficiency, 729–730
Membranoproliferative glomerulonephropathy (MPGN), 1142, 2171
Memorial Sloan Kettering Clinical Center (MSKCC), 1544
Memory B cell, 280
Men who have sex with men (MSM), 586
Menarche, 1197
Meningitis, 1386
Meningococcemia, 1158
Menorrhagia, 1220
Menstrual blood flow, 603, 639
Mepolizumab, 186, 1845
6-mercaptopurine (6-MP), 1370, 1608, 1628, 1673
Merkel cell tumors, 2022
Meropenem-vaborbactam, 1474
Mesenchymal stromal cells (MSCs), 75
Messenger RNA (mRNA), 80, 273, 434, 656, 1015
Meta-analyses, 1629
Metabolic syndrome (MS), 2378–2379
　congestive heart failure (CHF), 2379
　metabolic syndrome and related cardiovascular disease, 2378–2379
　recommendations to address CVC and MS, 2379
Metabolism regulation, 226
Metacarpal bones, 895
Metacarpophalangeal joints (MCP joints), 683
Metachromatic leukodystrophy (MLD), 1545
Metal ion–dependent adhesion site (MIDAS), 341
Metalloprotease (MP), 366, 1126
Metamyelocytes, 1764
Metaphase cytogenetics (MC), 1900, 1903
Metastatic cells, 418
Metastatic tumors, 1445
Metatarsal bones, 895
Metformin, 961
Methemalbumin, 123–124, 620
Methemoglobin, 3, 118, 938
　reductases, 119
　reduction test, 119, 755
Methemoglobinemia, 939
　acquired, 940
　cyanosis, 939
　cytochrome b5 reductase deficiency, 939–940
　diagnosis, 940
　treatment, 940
Methicillin-resistant *Staphylococcus aureus* (MRSA), 1471
Methionine, 946, 948
Methionine synthase (MTR), 946
Methotrexate (MTX), 962, 1370, 1417, 1432, 1671, 1950, 2297
Methotrexate, bleomycin, Adriamycin, cyclophosphamide, Oncovin, and dexamethasone (m-BACOD), 1966
Methotrexate, bleomycin, Adriamycin, cyclophosphamide, Oncovin, and prednisone (MACOP-B), 1966
8-methoxypsoralen (8-MOP), 2095
Methyl trap concept, 946
2-methyl-1,4-naphthoquinones, 436, 439
Methylation, 370
MethylCbl, 965, 967
Methylcholanthrene (MCA), 1495
2-methylcitric acid, 958
Methylcobalamin, 945
Methylene blue, 755
Methylenetetrahydrofolate dehydrogenase (MTHFD1), 963
Methylenetetrahydrofolate reductase (MTHFR), 948, 1284, 2357
L-Methylfolate, 965
5,10-methylenetetrahydrofolate reductase enzyme polymorphism, 959
Methylmalonic acid (MMA), 946, 957, 961
　cobalamin deficiency testing, 957–958
Methylmalonic aciduria Cbl C type with homocystinuria (MMACHC), 950
L-Methylmalonyl-CoA, 946
Methylmalonyl-CoA epimerase (MCE), 946
Methylmalonyl-CoA metabolism, 946
Metoclopramide, 1017
Mevalonate kinase deficiency syndrome, 2282
MHC alleles, 323
MHC class I chain–related A (*MICA*), 329

Index I-33

MHC class I chain–related B (*MICB*), 329
MHC class I chain–related genes (MIC genes), 329
MHC class I genes, 322
MHC class II compartment (MIIC), 329, 331
    defects in antigen presentation by, 1401–1402
MHC class II genes, 322
MHC class III genes, 322
MHC polymorphism, 322
M hemoglobins, 938
    clinical features and diagnosis, 938
    pathophysiology, 938
        iron oxidation and spectral characteristics, 938–939
        oxygen-binding properties and R → T transition of M hemoglobins, 938
    treatment, 939
Mice, 348
Micro-MKs, 361
Microalbuminuria, 2380
Microangiopathic hemolytic anemia (MAHA), 828–829, 1123, 1130, 1144, 1147, 1251
    causes of, 1147
        clinical conditions and mechanisms of MAHA and thrombocytopenia, 1147
        comorbid conditions with more than one potential mechanism of maha and thrombocytopenia, 1148t
    diagnosis, 1144
        diagnosis of atypical hemolytic-uremic syndrome, 1145
    management, 1144
Microarrays, 55
Microbiological assays, 956
Microclots, 1248
Microcytes, 8, 606
Microcytic anemia, 605
    approach to, 611–612
        diagnostic approach to patient with microcytic anemia, 612f
        iron pathway disorders, 612–614
        pathogenic classification of, 611t
        typical hemoglobin and mean corpuscular volume values in adults, 611t
Microcytic red blood cells, anemia associated with low reticulocyte response and, 605
Microcytosis, 1033, 1595
Microglia, 212–213
β2-microglobulin (β2M), 2181
Microparticles, 396, 418–419
Microperoxisomes, 395
MicroRNAs (miRNAs), 80, 97, 370–371, 419, 1908, 1922, 2074
    epigenetics, 1908–1909
    expression, 2025
Microscopy, 1782
    polyangiitis, 1167
Microsomal triglyceride transfer protein (MTP), 743
Microspherocytes, 936
Microtubule elongation, 363
Microtubule organizing center (MTOC), 314
Microtubules, 363, 393–394
Microvesiculation cell microabscesses, 2078
Midodrine, 2258
Midostaurin, 1460, 1649, 1861
Miglustat, 1363
Migration into tissues and sites of destruction, 150
Migratory DC, 215
Milatuzumab, 1501
Milder gene defects, 1208
Mineral density, 896
Minimal disseminated disease (MDD), 1995
Minimal residual disease (MRD), 22, 63, 1457, 1504, 1630, 1671, 1722, 1995, 2056–2057, 2063–2064, 2075, 2249, 2299
    monitoring of lymphoproliferative disorders, 64–65
    as prognostic factor, 1640
Minimally invasive splenectomy, 1433
Minor histocompatibility antigens (mHAs), 2355
miRNA transfer, 418–419
miRNome sequencing (miRNA-seq), 1907
Mismatched unrelated donor (MMUD), 2337
Missense mutations, 1208
Missing ligand model, 2366
Missing self model, 2366
Mitochondria, 138, 362–363, 395, 666
Mitochondria-mediated apoptosis, 1632

Mitochondrial ATPase 6 (MT-ATP6), 665
Mitochondrial carrier protein SLC25A38 deficiency, 661
Mitochondrial methylmalonic aciduria type B protein, 950
Mitochondrial myopathy, lactic acidosis, and SA (MLASA), 664–665
Mitochondrion, 658
Mitogen-activated protein kinase (MAPK), 104, 172, 277, 290, 1376, 1785–1786
Mitogen-activated protein-ERK kinase (MEK), 2049
Mitomycin C (MMC), 974
Mitotic kinesin-like protein 1 (MKLP1), 1026
Mitoxantrone, Ara-C, etoposide (MAE), 1700
Mitoxantrone, etoposide, and cytarabine (MEC), 1649
Mixed cold-and warm-active antibodies, immune hemolytic anemias caused by, 780
Mixed connective tissue disease, 1010
Mixed lineage leukemia (MLL), 1574–1575, 1628, 1669
Mixed phenotype acute leukemias (MPALs), 35–36, 1583, 1604, 1706
Mixed-phenotype acute leukemia (MPAL), 1612
Mixing studies, 1086
MK progenitor (MK-P), 359
*MLH*1 genes, 2074
MLL gene, 1612–1613, 1634, 1709
MLL-PTD gene, 1857
*MLL*3 gene, 1912
MM-020, 2188
MNS antigens and antibodies, 547
Mogamulizumab, 1502, 1977, 2102
MOI. *See* Multiplicity of infection (MOI)
Molecular abnormalities, 1634, 1639
    DNA methylation–related genes, 1636
    *FLT*3 mutations, 1634–1635
    mutations, 1636
    *NPM*1 mutation, 1635
    *TP*53 mutations, 1635–1636
Molecular biology, 751, 759
Molecular CR (CRm), 1642
Molecular diagnostics, 61
    applications of molecular genetic testing in hematologic malignancies, 61–66
    applications of molecular genetic testing in nonmalignant hematologic disorders, 66–67
    commonly used methodologies in, 61
        amplification-refractory mutation system (ARMS), 61, 62f
        multiplex ligation-dependent probe amplification (MLPA), 61
        next-generation sequencing (NGS), 61
        nucleic acids, extraction of, 61
        polymerase chain reaction (PCR), 61, 62f
        restriction enzyme digestion, 61
        sanger sequencing, 61
        SNaPshot genotyping, 61, 63f
    future directions, 67
    techniques, 1386
    tools, 1020
Molecular genetics, 14, 1327–1328
    alterations, 1670–1671
    methods for molecular genetic analysis, 1327t
    technology, 1446
Molecular immunohematology (MIH), 549
Molecular prognostic factors, 1639–1640
Molecular remission, 1730
Molecular response, 1792–1793
Molecular studies, 14, 802
Molecular tests, 14, 757
Molecular weight (MW), 103
Molecularly targeted therapies, 1711
Molnupiravir, 1478
Moloney murine leukemia virus (MMLV), 1526
Monge disease, 1074
Monoallelic variants, 1191
Monoclonal antibodies (MAbs), 2, 20, 1454–1456, 1494
Monoclonal B-cell lymphocytosis (MBL), 31, 33, 343, 1566, 2010, 2017–2018
Monoclonal gammopathies, 2144, 2171
    associated peripheral neuropathy, 2160
    association of monoclonal gammopathy with diseases, 2170
        connective tissue disorders, 2172
        dermatologic diseases, 2171
        disorders, 2172
        hematologic disorders, 2172
        hepatitis C, 2172

        immunosuppression, 2171–2172
        M proteins with antibody activity, 2172
        monoclonal gammopathy of renal significance, 2170–2171
        monoclonal gammopathy–associated neuropathy, 2170
        neurologic disorders, 2172
        systemic capillary leak syndrome, 2172
    classification of monoclonal immunoglobulin disorders, 2144
    diagnostic algorithm, 2144
    differential diagnosis of, 2144–2146
        simple diagnostic algorithm for patients with, 2145f
    distribution of, 2144f
    history and physical evaluation, 2150
    imaging, 2148–2150
        abnormal and normal plasma cells by flow cytometry, 2149f
        radiographic imaging in plasma cell disorders, 2149f
    initial evaluation, 2146
    laboratory evaluation, 2146
        bone marrow and tissue evaluation, 2148
        Congo red stain, 2148
        free light chain assay, 2148
        identification of type of monoclonal protein, 2147
        protein electrophoresis, 2146–2147
        quantitation of immunoglobulins, 2147
        urine evaluation, 2148
Monoclonal gammopathies of clinical significance (MGCS), 2276, 2291
    idiopathic systemic capillary leak syndrome, 2292
    monoclonal gammopathies of dermatologic significance, 2281–2289
        cryoglobulinemia, 2284–2289
        necrobiotic xanthogranuloma (NXG), 2284
        Schnitzler syndrome, 2281–2283
        scleromyxedema, 2283–2284
    monoclonal gammopathies of neurological significance, 2276
        chronic ataxic neuropathy, ophthalmoplegia, IgM paraprotein, cold agglutinins, and disialosyl antibodies, 2281
        distal, acquired demyelinating, symmetric neuropathy with M-protein, 2281
        POEMS syndrome, 2276–2281
        sporadic late-onset nemaline myopathy, 2281
    monoclonal gammopathies of renal significance (MGRS), 2289–2291
    TEMPI syndrome, 2291–2292
Monoclonal gammopathies of renal significance (MGRS), 2160, 2289
    classification of MGRS disorders, 2289
        MGRS with nonimmunoglobulin deposits, 2290–2291
        nonorganized monoclonal deposits, 2290
        organized monoclonal deposits, 2289–2290
    with nonimmunoglobulin deposits, 2290–2291
    treatment of, 2291
        clone directed therapy, 2291
        kidney transplantation, 2291
    workup of, 2291
Monoclonal gammopathy of undetermined significance (MGUS), 1566, 2144, 2160, 2175, 2238, 2276
    approach to MGUS, 2167f
    clinical features, 2163
    definition and terminology, 2160
    disease associations previously reported in literature in which significant disease association with, 2171t
    epidemiology, 2160
        incidence, 2162
        prevalence, 2160–2162
        risk factors, 2162
    International Myeloma Working Group diagnostic criteria for, 2161–2162t
    life expectancy and cause of death, 2165
    management, 2165–2166
    MGUS-associated peripheral neuropathy, 2160, 2276
    pathophysiology, 2162–2163
        alterations in bone turnover and new bone formation, 2163
        changes in bone marrow microenvironment, 2163
    prevalence of, 2163t
    prognosis, 2163–2164

Monoclonal gammopathy of undetermined significance (MGUS) (continued)
    follow-up in series, 2164
    probability of disease progression among residents of Southeastern Minnesota in MGUS, 2164f
    risk and pattern of progression MGUS, 2164t
    risk of progression among residents of Southeastern Minnesota in, 2164t
    prognostic factors, 2164
        abnormal serum-FLC ratio, 2164–2165
        bone marrow plasma cells, 2165
        risk of progression to myeloma or related disorder, 2165f
        size of monoclonal protein, 2164
        suppression of uninvolved immunoglobulins, 2165
        type of monoclonal protein, 2164
    progression of, 2165f
    risk-stratification, 2165
    risk-stratification model to predict progression of, 2166t
    secondary oncogenic events associated with progression of MGUS to MM, 2153
        activating mutations of NFkB pathway, 2155
        activating mutations of RAS/MAPK pathway, 2155
        chromosome 13 deletion, 2155
        chromosome 17p loss and abnormalities of *TP53*, 2155
        gain of chromosome 1q and loss of chromosome 1p, 2155
        light chain rearrangements, 2155
        mutations in significant pathways, 2155
        MYC dysregulation, 2153–2155
    variants of, 2169
        benign monoclonal light chain proteinuria (BMPC), 2170
        biclonal and triclonal gammopathy, 2170
        idiopathic Bence Jones proteinuria, 2170
        IgD MGUS, 2170
        secondary MGUS, 2169–2170
Monoclonal IgMκ antibody, 776
Monoclonal immunoglobulin, 2160
Monoclonal immunoglobulin deposition disease (MIDD), 2289
Monoclonal plasma cell disorder, 2279
Monoclonal protein (M protein), 2144, 2146, 2177, 2160, 2166
    change in, 2168
    detection of, 2160
    identification of type of, 2147
        serum protein electrophoresis and immunofixation electrophoresis, 2147f
    size of, 2164, 2167
    type of, 2164, 2167
Monocyte chemoattractant protein-3 (MCP-3), 172
Monocyte(s), 1, 5, 38, 77, 208, 209f, 1247. *See also* Lymphocytes
    in adult, 216–218
    deficiency, 226
    diversity and classification, 209–212, 211t
    growth factors, 218
        Fms-like tyrosine kinase-3 ligand (FLT3LG), 218
        GM-CSF, 218
        interleukin 34, 218
        interleukin 4, 218
        interleukin-3, 218
        M-CSF, 218
        RANK ligand, 218–219
        stem cell factor (SCF), 218
        thrombopoietin (TPO), 218
    historical perspective, 208–209
    molecular and cellular functions, 220–226
    monocyte-derived cells in steady-state tissues, 212
    monocyte-derived macrophages, 212
    monocyte-macrophage system, 1359
    monocyte/macrophage growth factors, 81–82
    origin, 216–220, 217f
    regulation of development by transcription factors, 219, 219f
        ID2-ZEB2-TCF4 axis, 220
        IRF4, IRF8, and BATF3, 220
        pioneer factors in early stem cell compartment, 219–220
        terminal differentiation factors, 220
    role in disease, 226–227
Monocytopenia, 2055
MonoMAC syndrome, 987

Monomethyl auristatin E (MMAE), 1455
Monomorphic B-cell lymphomas, 1951
Monomorphic epitheliotropic intestinal T-cell lymphoma (MEITL), 1888, 1931
Mononeuropathies, 1386
Mononuclear phagocyte system (MPS), 208
Monophasic hemolysins, 780
Monosomal karyotype (MK), 57, 364, 1634
    differentiation, 361, 370
    endomitosis, 371
    genes, 370
    lineages, 378
    maturation, 371
    MK-CSF, 371
    MK-specific proteins, 367
    MK-specific TF, 368
    MK/platelet lineage, 356
    MK/platelet-restricted proteins, 359
    rupture, 363–364
Monospecific antibodies, 1258–1259. *See also* Antiphospholipid antibodies
    acquired disorders associated with deficiency of single coagulation factor, 1258t
    factor IX, 1258
    factor V, 1258
    factor VII, 1259
    factor X, 1259
    factor XI, 1259
    factor XIII, 1259
    fibrinogen and prothrombin, 1259
    tissue factor, 1259
    von Willebrand factor, 1259
Mosaic chromosomal alterations (mCAs), 1754
    myeloid cancer risk, 1758
Mosaic chromosomal alterations, 1755
Mosse syndrome, 1809
Mosunetuzumab, 1964
Mott cells, 2178
Mouse knockout model, 1221
Mouse models, 374
Moxetumomab pasudotox, 1454, 1504, 2063
Moyamoya disease, 1165
MP and thalidomide (MPT), 2188
MPCM monomorphic (MPCM-m), 1852
MPCM polymorphic (MPCM-p), 1852
Mpl (*c-mpl* product), 371
MPL antagonists, 378
MPL gene, 370, 1156, 1821
MPL mutation, 1154, 1630, 1758, 1763, 1768, 1823, 1175–1176
MPN mutation, 1770
M-protein, 2144, 2172
    with antibody activity, 2172
    distal, acquired demyelinating, symmetric neuropathy with, 2281
MRD negative patients (MRD–patients), 2336
MRI-DTPA technique, 850
mSMART, 2184
MTCP1 gene, 1930
Mucha-Habermann disease, 2082
Muckel-Wells syndrome, 2282
Mucopolysaccharides, 1545
Mucopolysaccharidoses, 1353
Mucor, 1477
Mucorales, 1477, 1481
Mucormycosis, 1477
Mucosa-associated lymphoid tissue (MALT), 248–249, 1872, 1915–1916, 1949, 2286
Mucosal addressin, cell adhesion molecule-1 (MAdCAM-1), 222
Mucosal barrier injury laboratory-confirmed bloodstream infections (MBI-LCBIs), 1474
Mucosal changes, 602–603
Mucosal vascular addressin cell adhesion molecule 1 (MAdCAM-1), 242
Mucosal γδ T Cells, 1495–1496
Mucous membranes, 1101, 1809
    hemorrhages, 1808
        petechiae. pinpoint, nonblanching erythematous capillary bleeding sites, 1101f
Multi-parameter flow cytometry (MFC), 1614, 1671
    absence of normal plasma cells on, 2168
Multicenter Study of Hydroxyurea (MSH), 856
Multicentric CD (MCD), 1952
Multicolor analysis of hematologic malignancies, 31
    flow cytometry immunophenotypic findings, 35t

immunophenotyping of acute leukemia, 35–37
immunophenotyping of B-cell lymphoproliferative disorders, 31–34
immunophenotyping of plasma cell myeloma, 35
immunophenotyping of T-cell lymphoproliferative disorders, 34–35
myelodysplastic syndromes and chronic myelomonocytic leukemia, 37–38
myeloproliferative neoplasm (MPN), 38
Multicolor flow cytometry, principles of, 18, 18f
Multidrug resistance protein-1 (MDR-1), 1538
Multidrug resistance proteins, 951
Multilineage progenitors, 76
Multilocalized cutaneous mastocytomas, 1852
Multimeric analysis of von Willebrand Factor, 1214
Multimolecular complex, 338
Multinational Association for Supportive Care in Cancer index (MASCC), 1469, 1469t
Multinucleate cells, 1378
Multinucleated erythroblasts, 1023
Multiorgan surveillance, 982
Multiple coagulation factor deficiency-2 (MCFD2), 1224
Multiple endocrine gland insufficiency, 1010
Multiple genetic mechanisms, 1209
Multiple HSC gene therapy strategies, 1547
Multiple mechanisms-unifying hypothesis, 786
Multiple melanocytic nevi, 2383
Multiple myeloma (MM), 35, 1456, 1468, 1511, 2152, 2160, 2175, 2238, 2268, 2299, 2277, 2335, 2345–2346
    clinical manifestations, 2177
        acute terminal phase of plasma cell myeloma and cause of death, 2181
        anemia, 2177
        bone disease, 2179
        hemostasis in MM, 2181
        histopathology, 2177–2179
        hypercalcemia, 2179
        infection, 2181
        laboratory findings in patients with multiple myeloma, 2178f
        monoclonal proteins, 2177
        myeloma bone disease, 2180f
        renal insufficiency, 2179–2181
        signs and symptoms of newly diagnosed myeloma patients, 2177f
    combination therapy for induction, 2184–2199
    defing events, 2145, 2160
    diagnosis, 2176–2177, 2176t
    differential diagnosis, 2177
    early genetic abnormalities in, 2153
        chromosome content associated with different oncogenic pathways, 2153
        seven primary IgH translocations early oncogenic event in, 2153
    hematopoietic stem cell transplantation, 2199–2206
        allogeneic stem cell transplantation, 2203–2206
        autologous transplant, 2199–2203
    high-resolution sequencing studies and additional complexity of MM genomes, 2155–2157
    history, 2175
    incidence and epidemiology, 2176
        chronic antigenic stimulation, 2176
        cigarette smoking, alcohol consumption, and diet, 2176
        radiation exposure, 2176
        socioeconomic status, 2176
        workplace exposures, 2176
    indications for allogeneic hematopoietic cell transplant, 2346
    indications for autologous hematopoietic cell transplant, 2346
    interpreting treatment response, 2184
    intraclonal tumor heterogeneity associated with high-risk MM, 2156
    landmark therapeutic innovations, 2175f
    maintenance therapy, 2206
        allogeneic stem cell transplantation, 2207
        autologous stem cell transplantation, 2206–2207
        maintenance daratumumab, 2209
        maintenance lenalidomide in non–stem cell transplantation setting, 2207
        maintenance strategies incorporating proteasome inhibitors, 2207–2209
        maintenance thalidomide, 2207

maintenance with alkylators, steroids, or
interferon, 2209
management of relapsed or refractory disease, 2209
bispecific antibodies, 2218
cellular therapies, 2217
combinations of novel agents, 2213–2216
combinations of novel agents with conventional
agents, 2216–2217
conventional drug combinations for relapsed or
refractory disease, 2217
histone deacetylase inhibitors, 2212–2213
immunomodulatory drugs, 2210–2211
monoclonal antibodies, 2212
prognostic factors in relapsed disease, 2210
proteasome inhibitors, 2211–2212
targeted therapies with promising single-agent
activity, 2213
treatment of relapsed disease, 2210
MM plasma cell tumor of postgerminal center B cells,
2152–2153
molecular classification of, 2157
nonsecretory, 2222
prognosis, 2181
cytogenetics, fluorescence in situ hybridization,
and genetic abnormalities, 2181–2182
gene expression profiling, 2182–2183
immunophenotype of myeloma cells, 2183–2184
International Staging System and Revised
International Staging System, 2181t
plasma cell proliferative rate, 2183
relationship between genetic abnormalities among
patients with MM, 2182f
Revised International Staging System, 2183f
radiation therapy, 2218–2219
secondary oncogenic events associated with
progression of MGUS to MM, 2153–2155
comparison of different molecular classifications
in, 2154t
multistep molecular pathogenesis of MM, 2154f
special cases of
concurrent AL amyloidosis, 2221
immunoglobulin M, D, and E multiple myeloma,
2222
light-chain deposition disease (LCDDs), 2222
nonsecretory multiple myeloma, 2222
osteosclerotic myeloma, 2222
plasma cell leukemia (PCL), 2221–2222
solitary extramedullary plasmacytoma, 2223
solitary plasmacytoma of bone, 2222–2223
systemic therapy for diagnosed multiple myeloma,
2184–2218
treatment of complications and supportive care, 2219
complications specific to immunomodulatory
drugs, 2219
cryoglobulinemia and hyperviscosity, 2220
hypercalcemia, 2220
infection management, 2221
nonpharmacologic treatment of myeloma bone
disease, 2220
pharmacologic therapy of myeloma bone disease,
2219–2220
renal failure, 2220–2221
secondary myelodysplasia and acute leukemia,
2220
spinal cord compression, 2220
Multiple myeloma oncogene 1 (*MUM*1), 1972
Mutiple myeloma, smoldering (SMM), 2145, 2160, 2166
clinical features, 2166
definition, 2166
definition of high-risk smoldering multiple myeloma,
2169t
epidemiology, 2166
management, 2168–2169
drug therapy, 2169
management of smoldering multiple myeloma, 2169f
pathophysiology, 2166
prognosis, 2166–2167
prognostic factors, 2167
abnormalities on magnetic resonance imaging,
2168
abnormalities on positron emission tomography-
computed tomography, 2168
absence of normal plasma cells on multiparametric
flow cytometry, 2168
change in monoclonal protein level, 2168
circulating plasma cells, 2168

cytogenetic abnormalities, 2168
extent of bone marrow involvement, 2167
serum free light chain assay, 2168
size and type of monoclonal protein, 2167
suppression of uninvolved immunoglobulins,
2167–2168
risk-stratification of SMM, 2168
Multiple pulmonary emboli, 1074
Multiple sclerosis (MS), 1382
Multiple testing modalities, 1328
Multiplex cytokine bead arrays, 43
Multiplex ligation-dependent probe amplification
(MLPA), 61
Multiplicity of infection (MOI), 1524
Multipotent progenitors (MPPs), 356
Multispecies conserved sequences (MCSs), 885
Multivesicular bodies (MVBs), 362
*MUM*1. See Multiple myeloma oncogene 1 (*MUM*1)
Murine cytomegalovirus (MCMV), 316
Murine innate lymphoid cell development, 309–310
Murine multipotent progenitors (MPPs), 73
Murine stem cell virus, 1527
Murine transplantation models, preclinical, 1536
Muscle cells, 762
Muscle hematomas, 1220
Muscle metabolism, 641
Muscle tissue, 2381
Musculoskeletal symptoms, 2282
Mustargen, oncovin, procarbazine, and prednisone
(MOPP), 2121
Mutant prothrombins, 1220
Mutated murine protein, 1538
Mutation analysis, detection of, 937
λ5 mutation, 274
Mutation-adjusted risk score (MARS), 1858
Mutational Significance in Cancer (MuSiC), 1565
Mutations, 370
affecting mRNA processing, 887
cryptic site mutants in introns and exons, 887
frameshift mutations, 888
β-globin gene deletions, 888
initiation codon mutations, 888
poly (A) and 3′-UTR mutants, 887
splice junction and consensus sequence mutants, 887
β-thalassemic hemoglobinopathies, 888
MYC gene, 1878, 1912, 1925, 1943, 1949,
Mycobacterial disease, mammalian susceptibility to,
1404
Mycophenolate mofetil (MMF), 782, 784, 1108, 2305,
2320, 2358
Mycosis fungoides (MF), 2072
classification of, 2076
clinical presentation, 2076
cutaneous features of, 2077–2079
MF, patch stage, 2079f
survival for subtypes of cutaneous lymphoma,
2078t
diagnostic evaluation, 2076
blood involvement, 2080–2081
bone marrow involvement, 2080
cutaneous features of MF/SS, 2077–2079
cutaneous phases of mycosis fungoides, 2077f
extracutaneous MF/SS, 2079–2080
extracutaneous sites, 2080
frozen section immunohistochemistry of cutaneous
plaque, 2081f
histopathology, 2077
immunophenotyping studies, 2081–2082
large cell transformation of MF/SS, 2079
lymph node pathology, 2080
Sézary syndrome, 2081f
tissue handling, 2076–2077
differential diagnosis, 2082
benign conditions, 2082–2083
CD30+ lymphoproliferative diseases, 2083–2085
hematopoietic neoplasms with similar cutaneous
presentations, 2089–2090
primary cutaneous T-cell lymphomas, 2085–2089
early CTCL, 2073f
epidemiology, 2075–2076
extracutaneous MF/SS, 2079–2080
large cell transformation of MF, 2080f
historical perspective and pathophysiology, 2072
clinical description, 2072
histopathology, 2072
immunology, 2072–2074

molecular genetics, 2074–2075
large cell transformation of, 2079
late CTCL, 2073f
membrane proteins of malignant T cell, 2073f
NCI-VA grading scheme for lymph node histology in
CTCL, 2080t
prognosis, 2093–2094
staging, 2090–2091
bone marrow, 2093
imaging, 2091–2092
ISCL/EORTC staging of Mycosis Fungoides/
Sézary syndrome, 2091t
lymph nodes, 2092–2093
recommended initial staging evaluation of Mycosis
Fungoides/Sézary syndrome, 2092t
therapy, 2094
combined-modality therapy, 2100–2101
electron beam radiotherapy and photon beam
irradiation, 2097–2098
extracorporeal photochemotherapy (EC), 2098
hematopoietic stem cell transplantation (HCT),
2102
immunotherapy, 2101–2102
interferons (IFNs), 2096–2097
MF/SS treatment algorithm, 2094f
photopheresis photochemotherapy, 2098
phototherapy, 2095–2096
retinoids, 2096
systemic chemotherapy, 2098–2100
topical chemotherapy, 2094–2095
*MYD*88 mutations, 1878, 1913, 1917, 2271
Myelin and lymphocyte (MAL), 1998
Myelin-associated glycoprotein (MAG), 2281
Myeloablative allo-HCT (MA allo-HCT), 2336
Myeloablative allogeneic stem cell transplantation, 2204
Myeloablative autologous transplants, 1418
Myeloablative conditioning (MAC), 2035
Myeloablative HCT, 2319
Myeloablative regimens (MAC regimens), 2302
Myeloblastoma, 1631
Myeloblasts, 137–139, 139f
Myelocytes, 77, 1764
Myelodysplasia, 1331
secondary, 2220
Myelodysplastic disorders, 8
Myelodysplastic syndrome (MDS), 27, 37–38, 54, 63,
378, 602, 666, 715, 792, 894, 976, 998,
805, 974, 966, 1008, 1011, 1028, 1102, 1176,
1194, 1333, 1468, 1507, 1566, 1596–1600,
1627, 1696, 1737, 1774, 1763, 1821, 1849,
1946, 2022, 2123, 2298–2299, 2314, 2337,
2382
acute leukemias of ambiguous lineage, 1604–1605
acute lymphoblastic leukemia, 1602–1604
acute myeloid leukemia, 1600–1602
acute panmyelosis with myelofibrosis illustrating use
of immunohistochemistry in diagnosis, 1596f
allogeneic HCT in MDS and MPN, 2339t
anemia management, 1745
atypical chronic myeloid leukemia, 1776
chronic myelomonocytic leukemia, 1774–1776
clinical presentation of, 1740
clonal cytopenia of undetermined significance,
potential pre-MDS condition, 1600
comprehensive cytogenetic scoring system, 2337
diagnosis and classification of MDS, 1741
diagnostic evaluation, 1595–1596
dyspoietic changes in MDSs and AML, 1597f
elements of diagnostic evaluation, 1741
classification of MDS, 1742t
cytogenetics, 1741, 1742f
evaluation of cytopenias, 1741
flow cytometry, 1741–1743
minimal diagnostic criteria for MDS, 1741t
molecular analysis, 1743
morphologic evaluation, 1741
erythropoiesis-maturating agent (EMA), 1745
erythropoiesis-stimulating agents (ESAs), 1745
with excess blasts, 1568, 1598
with fibrosis, 1598
hypomethylating agents, 1747
immunosuppressive therapies, 1746–1747
indications for allogeneic stem cell transplantation,
2337–2339
integration of genetics into prognostic systems, 1743
comorbidities and frailty, 1743

Myelodysplastic syndrome (MDS) (continued)
  prognostic factors in MDS, 1744f
    Revised International Prognostic Scoring System (IPSS-R), 1743t
  intensity of conditioning regimens, 2339–2340
  juvenile myelomonocytic leukemia, 1776–1777
  lenalidomide, 1745–1746
  leukemia, FA and, 2323
  luspatercept, 1745
  MDS epidemiology and risk factors, 1737–1738
  MDS-RS-SLD, 667
  MRD in HCT outcomes in acute leukemia, 2338–2339t
  multilineage dysplasia, 1598
  myelodysplastic neoplasm with proliferative evolution and neutrophilia, 1776
  myelodysplastic/myeloproliferative neoplasm, unclassifiable, 1778
  myelodysplastic/myeloproliferative neoplasm with ring sideroblasts and thrombocytosis (MDS/MPN-RS-T), 1777–1778, 1777f
  neutropenia management, 1746
  pathogenesis of MDS, 1738, 1740f
    cohesin complex, 1740
    common mutations in MDS, 1739t
    epigenetic regulators, 1738
    key factors in MDS pathogenesis, 1740
    molecular pathogenesis of MDS, 1738
    RNA-splicing machinery, 1738–1739
    signaling pathway, 1740
    transcriptional factors, 1739
    tumor suppressors, 1739–1740
  pathogenesis of ring sideroblasts in, 666–667
  patients, 1748
  and PNH, 803–804
  prognostic assessment, 1743
  with proliferative evolution, 1774–1778
  recurrent chromosomal abnormalities and frequency in, 1598t
  with ring sideroblasts, 1745
  thrombocytopenia management, 1746
  thrombopoietin growth factors, 1746
  treatment of, 1744
    antimicrobial prophylaxis, 1747
    hematopoietic cell transplantation (HCT), 1748–1749
    higher risk MDS, 1747–1748
    iron chelation, 1747
    lower risk MDS (LR-MDS), 1744–1747
    MDS supportive interventions, 1747
    MDS treatment algorithm, 1744f
    platelet transfusion support, 1747
    PRBC transfusion support, 1747
  treatment prior to allogeneic transplant, 2337
  WHO classification of MDS, 1599t
Myelodysplastic/myeloproliferative neoplasm with ring sideroblasts and thrombocytosis (MDS/MPN-RS-T), 1777–1778, 1777f
Myelodysplastic/myeloproliferative neoplasms, 1599, 1763
Myelofibrosis (MF), 1430, 1694, 1768, 1810, 1821, 2340–2341
  clinical features, 1823
    splenomegaly due to extramedullary hematopoiesis, 1823f
  diagnosis, 1823–1824
    bone marrow in myelofibrosis, 1824f
  disease course, 1824–1825
    differential diagnosis for bone marrow fibrosis, 1824t
    WHO criteria for diagnosis of primary and post-ET/PV MF, 1825t
  epidemiology, 1821
  indications for HCT in primary myelofibrosis, 2341
  management, 1827
    allogeneic hematopoietic stem cell transplantation, 1832
    emerging therapies, 1832
    management of blast-phase primary myelofibrosis, 1831–1832
    myeloproliferative neoplasms research and treatment and European LeukemiaNet response criteria for, 1828t
    primary myelofibrosis and risk of thrombosis, 1831
    suggested algorithm for management of, 1829f
    treatment of anemia, 1827–1829
    treatment of splenomegaly and/or constitutional symptoms, 1829–1831
  pathogenesis, 1821–1823
    JAK-STAT signalling pathway, 1822
  risk stratification and prognosis, 1825–1826, 1827t
    response criteria and assessment tools, 1826–1827
    survival data of patients with primary myelofibrosis, 1826f
Myelofibrosis secondary to PV and ET-prognostic model (MYSEC-PM), 1826
Myelofibrosis Symptom Assessment Form (MFSAF), 1827
Myeloid blast phase, 1765
Myeloid cancer risk, MCA and, 1758
Myeloid cells, 11, 227, 1011, 1763
Myeloid colony-stimulating factors, 1472
Myeloid disorders, 1759
Myeloid growth factors, 1746
Myeloid leukemia, 1694
Myeloid lineage, 69
Myeloid malignancies, 1737, 1838, 2335
  acute myeloid leukemia (AML), 2335–2336
  choice of conditioning regimen, 2336–2337
  familial platelet disorder with predisposition to, 1155
  myelodysplastic syndrome (MDS), 2337–2340
  myelofibrosis, 2340–2341
  myeloproliferative neoplasms, 2340
Myeloid neoplasms, 1759
  associated with Down syndrome, 1601
  genes with recurrent genetic alterations detected in, 63, 64t
Myeloid neoplasms post cytotoxic therapy (MN-pCT), 1627
Myeloid proliferations of Down syndrome (MPDS), 1696
Myeloid sarcoma, 1631
Myeloid to erythroid (M:E) tio, 1015
Myeloid-derived suppressor cells (MDSCs), 318, 2020
Myeloid-to-erythroid ratio, 1767
Myeloid/lymphoid neoplasms, 1837
Myeloid homodimeric type I receptors, 375
Myelokathexis, 1335
Myelomastocytic leukemia (MML), 1855, 1858
Myeloneuropathy, 670, 964–965
Myeloperoxidase (MPO), 12, 35, 138, 2090
  deficiency, 1351
  MPO-deficient neutrophils, 1351
  MPO-positive primary granules, 1347
Myeloproliferation, 2279
Myeloproliferative Disease Research Consortium (MPD-RC), 1815
Myeloproliferative diseases, 1763, 2299
Myeloproliferative disorder (MPD), 1194, 1331, 1821
Myeloproliferative leukemia (MPL), 356, 367, 1821
  intracellular trafficking, 373
Myeloproliferative leukemia axis (MPL axis), 371
  expression and function, 373
  intracellular trafficking of, 373–374
  negative regulation of TPO/MPL/JAK2 signaling, 377
  schematic illustration of MPL activation by TPO and downstream signaling, 372f
  schematic illustration of MPL trafficking, 374f
  structure/function, 372–373
  TPO/MPL and signaling cascade in megakaryocytes, 375–377
  TPO/MPL axis and therapy, 377–378
Myeloproliferative leukemia virus (MPL), 1178
Myeloproliferative neoplasms (MPNs), 38, 54, 63, 374, 1175–1176, 1441, 1459, 1627, 1740, 1755, 1763–1764, 1784, 1821, 1837, 1849, 2340
  CH and, 1759
  chronic eosinophilic leukemia, 1770–1771
  chronic myelogenous leukemia (CML), 2340
  chronic myeloid leukemia (CML), 1764–1766
  chronic neutrophilic leukemia, 1771
  essential thrombocythemia, 1770
  myelodysplastic neoplasms, 1774–1778
  myeloid and lymphoid neoplasms with eosinophilia and rearrangement of *PDGFRA*, *PDGFRB*, or *FGFR*1 or with *PCM1::JAK2*, 1772–1774
  myeloid neoplasms with associated tyrosine kinases and genetic abnormalities, 1763
  polycythemia vera, 1766–1767
  primary myelofibrosis, 1767–1769
  with ring sideroblasts and thrombocytosis, 1777–1778
  select molecular genetic, morphologic, laboratory, and clinical findings in, 1764t
  systemic mastocytosis, 1771–1772
  unclassifiable, 1778
Myeloproliferative subtypes, 1774
Myeloproliferative syndromes, 1277
Myelosuppression, 1457
*MYH*10 gene, 361
*MYH*9 gene, 364, 1153–1154, 1570, 1633, 1697
*MYH*9 macrothrombocytopenias, 1100
*MYH*9-related disorders, 1154–1155
Myocardial fibrosis, 850
Myocardial infarction (MI), 402, 2124, 2244
Myocardial iron, 906
Myocardial ischemia, 850, 2244
Myocardial Ischemia and Transfusion (MINT), 569
Myocyte enhancer factor 2D (*MEF2D*), 1583
Myoepithelial sialoadenitis (MESA), 1952
Myoglobin, 619–620

N

N-acetyl-D-galactosamine, 540
N-acetylcysteine, 1137
N-benzoylstaurosporine, 1861
N-ethylmaleimide-sensitive factor attachment protein (SNAP), 414
N-finger, 1156
N-terminal activation domain (NAD), 367
N-terminal domain, 371
N-terminal pro-B-type natriuretic peptide (NT-proBNP), 851, 2247, 2379
Nasal NK/T-cell lymphomas, 1889
Nasal-associated lymphoid tissue (NALT), 249
Nasopharyngeal carcinoma, 1382
National Cancer Institute (NCI), 1417, 1565, 1608, 1669, 1923, 1999, 2099
National Cancer Institute Veterans Affairs (NCI-VA), 2080
National Collegiate Athletic Association (NCAA), 867
National Comprehensive Cancer Network (NCCN), 54, 648, 1329, 1471, 1727, 1793, 1815, 1857, 1955, 2128, 2344
National Health and Nutrition Examination Surveys (NHANES), 637, 2160
National Hemophilia Foundation's website, 1228
National Institutes of Health (NIH), 1699, 2378
National Marrow Donor Program (NMDP), 2298
Natural killer cell (NK cell), 26, 31, 233, 288, 309, 326, 346, 1383, 1389, 1400, 1468, 1495, 2014, 2303, 2314, 2356, 2365–2366, 1975–1978
  activating, inhibitory, and cytokine receptors and ligands, 311f
  activating receptors, 313
  activation, 312f
  clinical relevance and applications, 317–318
  cytokine production, 314–315
  cytokine receptors, 313
  cytotoxicity, 314
  development and tissue localization, 309–310
  functional immune cross talk, 315
  functions, 314–316
  inhibitory receptors, 310–312
  lymphomas, 1882–1885, 1974–1975
    adult T-cell leukemia/lymphoma (ATLL), 1888
    anaplastic large cell lymphoma (ALCL), 1887–1888
    angioimmunoblastic T-cell lymphoma, 1885–1887
    extranodal natural killer/t-cell lymphoma, nasal type, 1889
    hepatosplenic T-cell lymphoma (HSTCL), 1888
    intestinal T-cell lymphoma (ITL), 1888–1889
    mature T/NK leukemias, 1977f
    peripheral T-cell lymphoma, not otherwise specified, 1885
    subcutaneous panniculitis–like T-cell lymphoma, 1888
    therapy for T/NK neoplasms, 1978
  memory, 315–316, 315f
  NK-cell lymphoproliferative disorders, 1382
  NKp30, 313
  NKp44, 313
  NKp46, 313
  NKp80, 313
  receptors on, 310–313
  self tolerance via education, 313–314
  strategies to enhance, 319f

and tumor target cell cytotoxic synapse, 314f
Nausea, 1144
Navios flow cytometer, B-cell lymphoma analysis using, 22, 24f
Navitoclax, 1463
Necator americanus, 638
Necrobiotic xanthogranuloma (NXG), 2146, 2284
　clinical features, 2284
　therapy, 2284
Necroptosis, 150
Necrotizing enterocolitis (NEC), 1064
Needle biopsy, 1866
Nemtabrutinib, 2032
Neoantigen, 785–786
Neodymium:yttrium-aluminum-garnet (Nd:YAG), 1164
Neonatal alloimmune neutropenia (NAIN), 552, 1337
Neonatal alloimmune thrombocytopenia (NAIT), 553, 1111
　clinical features, 1112
　laboratory diagnosis, 1112
　pathophysiology, 1111–1112
　　pathophysiology of antibody development, 1111f
　prevention of, 1112
　treatment, 1112–1113
Neonatal anemias
　anemia of prematurity, 1063
　erythrocyte membrane and metabolism, 1058–1059
　erythrocyte transfusions in neonatal period, 1064–1066
　erythropoietin biology in, 1053
　iron deficiency in fetus and newborn infant, 1063–1064
　owing to hemolysis, 1059–1061
　owing to hemorrhage, 1061–1062
Neonatal bacterial sepsis, 1062
Neonatal erythrocyte membrane and metabolism, 1058–1059
　characteristics of fetal/neonatal red blood cells, 1059t
　decline in fetal hemoglobin synthesis as function of gestational age, 1059f
Neonatal hemolysis, 755
Neonatal hyperbilirubinemia, 752, 754
Neonatal intensive care unit (NICU), 1064
Neonatal neutropenia, 1337
Neonatal period, erythrocyte transfusions in, 1064–1066
Neonatal purpura fulminans, 1281
Neonatal red blood cells, 1057
Neonatal transfusion
　special considerations in, 574
　　exchange transfusion, 574
　　pretransfusion testing, 574
　　selection of products for, 574
Neonate(s), 1056, 1059
　bleeding in, 1081–1082
　disseminated intravascular coagulation in, 1252
　evaluation of, 1091–1092
　late anemia following hemolytic disease of, 1061
Neoplasms, 1247
Neoplastic cells, 1875, 1995, 1998
　of AITL, 1886
　in EBV-positive DLBCL, 1881
　of JXG, 1379
　of MCL, 1873
　in MF and SS, 2081
Neoplastic disease, 1608
Neoplastic disorders, 1252, 1364
　acute promyelocytic leukemia, 1253
　carcinoma, 1252–1253
Nephrectomy, 2259
Nephrogenic fibrosing dermopathy, 2283
Nephrotic syndrome, 853, 2379
Nerve biopsy, 2278
Nervous system, 2144, 2245–2246
NETosis, 150–151
Neulasta, 1339
Neuroacanthocytosis syndromes, 744
Neurobeachin (NBEA), 1191
Neurobeachin-like 2 gene (*NBEAL2* gene), 362, 1191
Neurodegenerative disease, 1368
Neurodevelopmental impairment (NDI), 1065
Neurofibromatosis type I (NF1), 1697
Neurogenic vasodilation, 201
Neurolymphomatosis, 1954
Neuromuscular system, 1810
Neurotoxicity, 1457
Neutral lipid storage disorders (NLSDs), 1354

Neutralization, 775
Neutropenia, 906, 984, 1412, 1468–1470, 1595, 1632, 1703
　autoimmune, 1337
　clinical presentation and diagnostic approach to neutropenia, 1337–1338
　　diagnostic approach to neutropenia in adult, 1339f
　　diagnostic approach to neutropenia in infant, 1338f
　definition and classification of, 1331
　differential diagnosis, 1331
　　congenital immune defects with associated neutropenia, 1334–1335
　　congenital syndromes with associated neutropenia, 1335–1336
　　cyclic neutropenia (CN), 1334
　　differential diagnosis and features of acquired neutropenias, 1333t
　　drug-induced neutropenia and neutropenia due to marrow injury, 1336–1337
　　Duffy null phenotype, 1331
　　and features of congenital neutropenia, 1332t
　　immune neutropenia, 1337
　　neutropenia due to increased margination and hypersplenism, 1337
　　neutropenia due to nutritional deficiency, 1337
　　nonfamilial chronic benign and idiopathic chronic severe neutropenia, 1331–1332
　　postinfectious neutropenia, 1336
　　primary causes of neutropenia, 1331
　　pseudoneutropenia, 1331
　　secondary causes of neutropenia, 1336
　　severe congenital neutropenia (SCN), 1332–1334
　empiric approach to, 1470f
　idiopathic chronic severe, 1331–1332
　lower risk patients with, 1470
　management of, 1746, 1338–1339
　　G-CSF biosimilars, 1339
　normal neutrophil kinetics, 1331
　treatment, 1412–1413
Neutropenic HIV-positive patients, 1412
Neutrophil abnormalities, congenital, 1347
Neutrophil elastase (*ELANE*), 1333–1334
Neutrophil extracellular traps (NETs), 150
Neutrophil granules, 143
　azurophilic granules, 143
　ficolin-1-rich granules, 143
　gelatinase granules, 143
　granule formation in neutrophil precursors viewed by electron microscopy, 144f
　secretory vesicles, 143–145
　specific granules, 143
Neutrophil kinetics, 149, 149f
　circulating and marginating pools, 151
　in fetus and newborn, 151–152
　kinetics in blood, 150
　migration, 152
　migration into tissues and sites of destruction, 150
　neutrophil death, 150–151
　neutrophil mitotic and maturation compartments, 149
　neutrophil release from bone marrow into blood, 149–150
　production and storage, 151
Neutrophil structure, 143
　CD antigens expressed on neutrophils, 146t
　cytosolic contents, 147
　genetic sex as indicated by leukocytes, 147–148
　human neutrophil granules, 145t
　lipid rafts, 147
　macropolycytes, 147
　membrane receptors and neutrophil antigens, 146–147
　neutrophil antigens, 147t
　neutrophil granules and secretory vesicles, 143–145
　neutrophil heterogeneity, 148
　nucleus, 145–146
　Pelger-Huët anomaly, 146
Neutrophil(s), 1, 5, 81, 136, 418, 1344, 1348, 1354, 1495, 1812
　adhesion to inflamed endothelium, 156f
　adhesion to vascular wall at site of inflammation, 157f
　aggregation, 156–157
　antigens, 146–147
　antimicrobial systems, 159t
　chemoattractants, 153
　contents of human neutrophil granules, 145t

　control mechanisms regulating neutrophil production, 152
　death, 150–151
　defects, 1468
　desensitization, 154
　development, 136–143
　dysfunction, 1351–1352
　dysregulation in systemic inflammatory response syndrome, 1352
　feedback mechanisms, 157f
　function, 152–162
　hereditary hypersegmentation of neutrophil nuclei, 1354
　heterogeneity, 148
　history, 136
　hypersegmentation, 609
　infections exhibit tropism for, 161–162
　kinetics, 149–152, 149f
　lineages, 1849
　maturation, 137f
　metamyelocytes, 139, 141f
　mitotic and maturation compartments, 149
　myelocytes, 139
　neutrophil-endothelial cell adhesion, 154–156, 155t
　PFK, 762
　physiologic variation in neutrophil values, 141–143
　priming, 154
　promyelocytes, 139
　release from bone marrow into blood, 149–150
　scanning electron micrograph of moving, 158f
　stages of neutrophil differentiation, 137–141
　structure, 143–148
　subsets and nomenclature, 138f
Neutrophilia, 1207
New methylene blue, 8
Newborn infants, 940
Newborn iron levels, 640
Newborn screening (NBS), 2314
Next-generation sequencing (NGS), 61, 323, 1327, 1562, 1564, 1698, 1788, 1869, 1900, 2336
Next-generation sequencing, 58
NF-E2 TF, 368
NF-E2. *See* Nuclear factor erythroid 2 (NF-E2)
NF-κB essential modulator deficiency (NEMO deficiency), 1351
Nicotinamide adenine dinucleotide (NAD$^+$), 864
Nicotinamide adenine dinucleotide phosphate (NADPH), 154, 749, 1351
　oxidase, 1349, 1396
Nicotinamide adenine dinucleotide–nicotinamide adenine dinucleotide system (NAD-NADH system), 395
Nicotinamide dinucleotide phosphate, 1349
NICU. *See* Neonatal intensive care unit (NICU)
Niemann-Pick cell, 1362–1363
Niemann-Pick disease (NPD), 1362
　clinical manifestations, 1362
　　types A and B Niemann-pick disease, 1362
　diagnosis, 1362
　etiology and pathogenesis, 1362
　pathology, 1362
　　splenic histology in Niemann-Pick disease type B, 1362f
　　types A and B Niemann-Pick disease, 1362
　treatment, 1362
Niemann-Pick types A disease, 1359
Niemann-Pick types B disease, 1359
NIH. *See* National Institutes of Health (NIH)
Nijmegen breakage syndrome (NBS), 272, 1403
Nilotinib, 1458, 1613, 1619, 1782, 1795–1796, 1861–1862
Nirmatrelvir-ritonavir, 1478
NIRS monitoring. *See* Near-infrared spectroscopic monitoring (NIRS monitoring)
NIRS sensor, 1064
Nitric oxide (NO), 117, 406, 531, 816, 838, 937
　modification of nitric oxide metabolism, 864
Nitric oxide-cGMP pathway (NO-cGMP pathway), 411
Nitrite (NO_2^-), 160, 940
Nitroblue tetrazolium (NBT), 1346
Nitrogen mustard (HN_2), 1370, 2094
Nitrosohemoglobins (NO hemoglobins), 941–943
Nitrous oxide (N_2O), 954
Nitryl chloride (NO_2Cl), 160
Nivestym, 1339
Nivolumab, 1456, 2040, 2102
NMMHC-A, 1354

Nodal marginal zone lymphomas (NMZLs), 1874, 1915–1917
   genetics, 1875
   guidelines for molecular testing in, 1917
   immunophenotype, 1874–1875
Nodal peripheral T-cell lymphoma, 1973–1974
Non-Hodgkin lymphomas (NHLs), 1414, 1500, 1612, 1900, 1942, 1991, 2049, 2072, 2117, 2299, 2308, 2335. See also Hodgkin lymphoma (HL)
   age-adjusted incidence and mortality rates of, 1946f
   age-specific incidence rates of, 1945f
   aggressive lymphomas, 1964–1969
   anaplastic large cell lymphoma (ALCL), 1999–2001
   Burkitt lymphoma (BL), 1995–1998
   cellular origins of, 1944f
   classification, 1991
   classification of, 1869
   clinical features at presentation, 1953–1955
      mantle cell lymphoma, 1953f
      primary central nervous system lymphoma, 1954f
   clinicopathologic differences between childhood and adult NHL, 1946t
   diagnostic workup, staging, and initial management, 1991–1992
      subtypes of NHLs most commonly encountered in children, 1992t
   diffuse large B-cell lymphoma (DLBCL), 1995–1998
   epidemiologic factors that associated with an increased risk of, 1945t
   epidemiology, 1943–1944
      age, race, sex, and familial differences, 1944–1946
      Burkitt lymphoma involving mandible, maxilla, and orbit, 1947f
      course of human T-lymphotropic virus type 1, 1948f
      environmental factors, 1950–1951
      geographic distribution of HTLV-1 infection, 1948f
      infections and associations with lymphoma, 1947t
      infectious agents, 1946–1950
      MALToma of stomach, 1950f
   epidemiology, 1991
   highly aggressive lymphomas, 1970
      anaplastic large cell lymphoma (ALCL), 1972–1973
      Burkitt lymphoma (BL), 1970–1971
      extranodal T-cell and natural killer-cell lymphomas, 1974–1975
      extranodal T-cell lymphomas, 1974
      lymphoblastic lymphoma, 1971
      management issues for extranodal lymphomas, 1975t
      mature T-cell and natural killer-cell leukemias, 1975–1978
      mature T/NK lymphoma/leukemia, 1972t
      nodal peripheral T-cell lymphoma, 1973–1974
      peripheral T-and NK-cell lymphomas, 1971–1972
   history of diagnosis and classifications of, 1942–1943t
   immunophenotypic features of most common pediatric NHLs, 1993t
   indolent B-cell lymphomas, 1959–1964
   leukemic phase of, 2018
   lymphoblastic lymphomas, 1992–1995
   mantle cell lymphoma (MCL), 1969–1970
   mature B-NHL in children, 1998t
   methodologies, 1900
      analytical sensitivity of immunoglobulin gene rearrangement studies, 1904f
      array comparative genomic hybridization (aCGH), 1905
      array single nucleotide polymorphisms (aSNP), 1905
      characteristics of different genome-wide studies, 1906t
      clonality testing, 1900
      commonly used techniques, 1900
      examples of FISH patterns, 1905f
      fluorescent in situ hybridization (FISH), 1903
      immunoglobulin gene rearrangements, 1900–1902
      immunoglobulin genes and chromosomal organization, 1902f
      metaphase cytogenetics (MC), 1903
      microRNAs, epigenetic changes, 1908–1909
      next-generation sequencing, 1905–1907
      next-generation sequencing using dye-labeled nucleotides, 1908f
      polymerase chain reaction (PCR), 1903
      SEER data, 1901f
      somatic hypermutation (SHM), 1903–1905
      T-cell gene rearrangements (TCR), 1902–1903
      T-cell receptor genes, 1905f
      transcriptional profiling, 1907–1908
   posttransplantation lymphoproliferative disorders (PTLDs), 2001
   prelymphomatous conditions, 1951–1953
   primary mediastinal B-cell lymphoma (PMBCL), 1998–1999
   recurrent molecular aberrancies in B-cell and T-cell neoplasms, 1909–1932
   response criteria for, 1959t
   staging and prognosis, 1955
      functional imaging, 1957–1958
      immunophenotypic and molecular markers, 1955–1957
      progression-free survival according to revised IPI, 1958f
   staging and prognostic indexes of, 1956–1957t
   staging classification for BM and CNS involvement from IPNHLSS, 1994t
   staging of NHLs in children, 1994t
   staging studies in, 1957t
   temporal trends in age-adjusted incidence rates, 1945f
   therapeutic principles, 1958–1959
      follicular lymphoma international prognostic index 2, 1958f
      gene expression arrays, 1959f
      prognostic biomarkers by immunohistochemistry in aggressive lymphoma, 1958t
   therapy, 1387
   transplantation for, 1418
   uncommon pediatric lymphomas, 2001
      hepatosplenic T-cell lymphoma (HSTCL), 2002
      marginal zone B-cell lymphoma (MZL), 2002
      pediatric follicular lymphoma, 2001–2002
      peripheral T-cell lymphoma not otherwise specified (PTCL-NOS), 2002
      primary CNS lymphoma (PCNSL), 2002–2003
Nonclassical human leukocyte antigen class I genes and molecules, 327–329
   HLA-E, -F, -G, -H, 327–239
   MHC class I chain–related A (MICA), 329
   MHC class I chain–related B (MICB), 329
   nonclassical HLA-E, -F, -G and MHC class I chain–related protein A/B, 328f
Nonclassical major histocompatibility complex class II molecules, 329
   HLA-DM, 329–330
   HLA-DO, 330
Nonclassical MHC I genes, 327
Nonclassical monocytes (ncMo), 27, 211–212
Noncrystalline acute tubular injury, 2290
Nondeletion HPFH, 889
Nondeletional α-thalassemia, 885–886
Nondeletional β-thalassemia, 886–887
Non–Down syndrome inherited syndromes, management of patients with, 1704
Non–DS-associated ALL (non–DS-ALL), 1677
Nonerythroid cells, 1600
Nonfamilial chronic benign neutropenia, 1331–1332
Non–Helicobacter pylori Helicobacter, 1396
Nonheparin anticoagulant, 1309
Nonhomologous end joining (NHEJ), 270, 373, 978, 1548, 1786
Nonhotspot genes, 1328
Non–human marker genes, 1550
Nonhyperdiploid (NHRD), 2153
Nonimmunoglobulin deposits, MGRS with, 2290–2291
Nonimmunologic platelet destruction, 1149
Nonimmunologic protein adsorption mechanism, 786
Nonlymphoid cell migration across HEVs, 253–254
Nonlymphoid tissue, 1324
Nonmalignant diseases (NMDs), 2299, 2302, 2314, 2371. See also Malignant diseases
   aplastic anemia, 2299
   autoimmune diseases, 2300
   enzymatic disorders, 2300
   hemoglobinopathies, 2299
   immunodeficiencies, 2299
Nonmalignant hematologic disorders, applications of molecular genetic testing in, 66
   bone marrow failure syndromes, 66
   hemostatic disorders, 66–67
   thalassemias, 66
Nonmegaloblastic macrocytic anemias, 610, 611t
   accelerated erythropoiesis, 610–611
   chronic alcohol use, 611
   liver disease, 611
Nonmetabolic role for adenosine diphosphate, 395
Nonmuscle myosin heavy chain II (NMMHCII), 394
Nonmuscle myosin heavy chain IIB, 1192
Nonmyeloablative (NMA) em cell transplantation, 2335
   allogeneic transplantation, 1418
   HSCT, 988
   regimens, 2302–2303
Nonorganized monoclonal deposits, 2290
Nonparasitic primary cysts, 1431
Nonperfused organ, 1423
Nonrelapse mortality (NRM), 2034, 2301, 2335
Non–risk organ disease, 1366
Nonselective proteinuria, 2145
Nonsense mutations, 888
Nonspecific esterase stains, 13
Nonspherocytic hemolytic anemia (NSHA), 1027
   congenital, 754
Non–stem cell transplantation setting, 2207
Nonsteroidal anti-inflammatory drugs (NSAIDs), 638, 688, 1169, 1387
Nonsteroidal inflammatory drugs, 840
Nonthymic solid tumors, 1010
Nonviral vectors, 1524
   chemical delivery methods, 1525
   episomal self-replicating systems, 1526
   physical delivery methods, 1524
   schematic representation of transduction of generic target cell by four major gene transfer vector systems, 1525f
   transposon systems, 1526
Noonan syndrome (NS), 1697, 1737
NOPHO. See Nordic Society for Pediatric Hematology and Oncology (NOPHO)
Nordic Society for Pediatric Hematology and Oncology (NOPHO), 1677, 1701
Nori (Edible purple laver porphyra species), 967
Normal bone marrow, 1035
Normal compensatory processes, 1247
Normal hematopoiesis, 27
   average relative frequency of major lymphoid cell subsets in normal tissues, 30t
   erythropoietic differentiation, 28
   granulocytic differentiation, 27
   immature cells of normal bone marrow, 27
   immunophenotypic changes, 31t
   lymphocyte differentiation, 28–29
   minor bone marrow cell subsets, 29–31
   monocytic differentiation, 28
   surface marker expression during maturation of granulopoietic precursors in bone marrow, 30t
Normal hemostasis, 1276
Normal neutrophil kinetics, 1331
Normal plasma cells on multiparametric flow cytometry, absence of, 2168
Normal platelet physiology, 398
Normal saline (NS), 840
Normal type enzyme, 751
Normoblastic hyperplasia, 806
Normoblasts, 806
Normocytic anemia, 824
   approach to, 614–616
      classification of, 615t
   diagnostic approach to patient with, 615f
Normocytic red blood cells, anemia associated with low reticulocyte response and, 605
North American Pediatric Transplant Cooperative Society, 853
North American Shwachman-Diamond Syndrome Registry, 985–986
Norwegian Vitamin (NORVIT), 1285
Nose bleeding, 1196
Novel therapeutic approaches, 911
   gene therapy, 911–912
   modulators of ineffective erythropoiesis, 911
   pharmacologic HbF reactivation, 911
Novel vectors, 1543
*NPM*1 gene, 1636, 1640, 1857, 1926
*NPM*1 mutation (*NPM*1^{mut}), 1635–1636, 1644, 1655, 1577, 1601–1602, 1710, 1759
NRAS gene, 1380, 1640, 1677, 1850, 1857

Nuclear factor kappa B (NFkB), 237, 270, 290, 419, 1876, 1948, 2074, 2133
Nuclear factor of activated T cells (NFAT), 290, 1498, 2074
Nuclear factor-erythroid 2, 884
Nuclear lobulation, 145
Nuclear magnetic resonance spectroscopy (NMR spectroscopy), 938
Nuclear pore complex (NPC), 1577
Nuclear pore proteins, 1576
    nucleophosmin (NPM1), 1576–1577
    *NUP*214, 1577–1578
    *NUP*98, 1578
Nuclear protein in testis midline carcinoma family 1 (*NUTM*1), 1584
Nucleated erythrocytes, 715
Nucleated red blood cells (NRBCs), 1, 4, 936, 1055
Nucleic acid amplification technology (NAT), 898
Nucleic acid extraction, 61
Nucleic acid testing (NTA), 560
Nucleophosmin (NPM), 1635, 1972
Nucleophosmin member 1 mutations (*NPM*1 mutations), 1702
Nucleoside analogs, 1411
Nucleoside analogues, 1628
Nucleosome and histone deacetylase (NuRD), 367
Nucleosome Remodeling and Deacetylation complex (NuRD complex), 1587
5′nucleotidase (P5′N), 764
Nucleotide metabolism and nonmetabolic role for adenosine diphosphate, 395
Nucleotide-binding domain leucine-rich repeats (NLR), 1495
Nucleus, 145–146
*NUDT*15 variants, 1674
*NUDT*6 gene, 2050
Null alleles, 323
NUP genes, 1709
*NUP*214 genes, 1577–1578, 1709
*NUP*98 genes, 1578, 1638, 1709
Nutrients deficiency during pregnancy, 1048
Nutrition, 948–950
    cobalamin absorption, 948–950
    cobalamin issues of, 950
    folate absorption and intracellular metabolism, 951
    intracellular metabolism, 950
Nutritional deficiencies, 1028
    neutropenia due to, 1337

O

O^6-benzylguanine, 2095
O^6-methylguanine-DNA methyltransferase (MGMT), 1538
Obesity, 688, 1629, 2162, 2176, 2379
Obinutuzumab (G), 1966, 2028, 2032, 2034
    chlorambucil with, 2030
    obinutuzumab-based frontline chemoimmunotherapy, 1963
    obinutuzumab-chemotherapy, 1963
Obstetric disorders, 1252
    abruptio placentae, 1252
    amniotic fluid embolism, 1252
    intrauterine fetal death, 1252
Obstructive sleep apnea, 1075
Occasional blood transfusions, 893
Octreotide, 2259
Ocular amyloidosis, 2260
Ocular lesions, 853
Odd chain fatty acids, 946
Odds ratio (OR), 1281
Ofatumumab, 2028, 2272
Off-the-shelf CAR immune cells, 1512
Oligo arrays, 54
Oligonucleotides, 54
Omacetaxine, 1798
Omenn syndrome, 271, 1837, 2315
Omic technology, 1907
Oncovirinae, 1526
One-carbon reactions, 947
Open circulation, 1426
Open-heart surgery, 827
Open-label EXTEND study, 1107
Ophthalmoplegia, 2281
Opportunistic infections (OIs), 1409
Optic neuropathy, 954

Optical density (OD), 1309, 1477
Optical genomic mapping (OGM), 58, 58f
OPTIMAL CARE study, 918
Optimal delivery of thromboprophylaxis, 1307
Optimized gene therapy protocols, 1539–1540
Optimizing drug therapy, 1797
Orbitopathy, 855
Organ Procurement and Transplantation Network, The, 327
Organ transplants, 1951
Organic hydroperoxides, 756
Organized monoclonal deposits, 2289–2290
Origin of replication (oriP), 1526
Ornithine transcarbamoylase (OTC)-deficiency, 1528
Orotic aciduria, hereditary, 964
Orthochromatic erythroblast, 95
Orthotopic cardiac transplant, 2258
Orthotopic liver transplantation, 707, 1363
Osler-Weber-Rendu syndrome, 1162
Osmotic fragility (OF), 733
Osmotic gradient ektacytometry, 734
Osmotic hemolysis, 825
Osteoclasts, 213
Osteogenesis imperfecta (OI), 1167
Osteonecrosis (ON), 1672, 1684–1685
Osteonecrosis of jaw (ONJ), 2219
Osteopenia, 2380
Osteoporosis, 896, 918, 1859, 2308, 2380
Osteoprotegerin (OPG), 237, 896
Osteosclerotic myeloma, 2222, 2277
Outside-in signaling, 414
Ovalbumin-related serpins, 490
Ovalocytosis, Southeast Asian (SAO), 735, 739
Oxacillin, 1473
Oxaliplatin, 1149, 1967
Oxidant drugs and chemicals, 824–825
Oxidative burst, 159, 642
Oxidative denaturation of hemoglobin, 118–119, 118f
Oxidative stress, 864
5-oxoproline, 756
Oxygen
    bridge, 566
    carriers, artificial, 566
    dissociation curve of hemoglobin, 116, 116f
    enzymes react with products of oxygen reduction, 119
    oxygen-dependent antimicrobial systems, 159–160
    oxygen-independent antimicrobial systems, 160
    regulation of oxygen affinity, 116–117
    saturation, 941
    therapy, 840
    transport, 116, 1070–1071
Oxygen extraction fraction (OEF), 841
Oxyhemoglobin, 3, 118
Oxymetholone, 1004

P

P antigen, 547, 779
P-glycoprotein (P-GP), 1299
P-selectin, 79, 154, 362
P-selectin glycoprotein ligand-1 (PSGL-1), 154, 222, 416
P1PK blood group system, 547
P2 receptors defects, 1190
p21-activated kinase (PAK1), 295
$P2X_1$ receptor, 408
$P2Y_{12}$ receptor (P2Y12R), 1190
PA inhibitor-1 (PAI-1), 1276
    deficiency, congenital, 489
Packed cell volume (PCV), 600
Packed red blood cells (pRBCs), 1745
Pacritinib, 1460, 1831
Pagetoid reticulosis, 2085, 2085f
Pagophagia, 642
Painful neuropathy, 2128
Paired box 5 (PAX5), 1610
Paired box domain (PRD), 1580
Paired immunoglobulin-like receptor B (PIRB), 406
PAK1. See p21-activated kinase (PAK1)
*PALB*2 gene, 978
Palliative therapy, 1620
Pallor, 602
Palpable purpura, 1167

Pan-cancer panels, 1907
Pan-histone deacetylase (HDAC), 365
Pancreatitis, 1797
Panels, 22, 26t
Panobinostat, 2184, 2214
Pantothenate kinase 2 (PANK2), 744
Paper electrophoresis, 2175
Papilledema, 2278–2279
Papillon-Lefèvre syndrome, 1352
Pappenheimer bodies, 1426
Papular-purpuric "gloves and socks" syndrome, 1169
Para-aortic splanchnopleura (P-Sp), 71
Paracoagulation techniques, 1086, 1251
Paracortex, 243
Paradoxic bleeding, 1170
Paradoxic emboli, 1163
Parahemophilia, 454, 1220
Paraimmunoblasts, 1872
Parainfluenza virus, 2308
Parallel-plate flow cytometer, 402
Paraprotein, 2238
Parasites, 960
Parasitic cysts, 1431
Parathyroidectomy, 1038
Parenchymal cells, 688
Parenteral anticoagulant overlap, 1296
Paris-Trousseau syndrome (PTS), 986, 1155, 1194
Paris-Trousseau thrombocytopenia, 1192
Paris-Trousseau-Jacobsen syndrome, 1192
Paroxysmal cold hemoglobinuria (PCH), 772, 779
    antibody characteristics, 779
        clinical manifestations, 780
        functional characteristics, 779–780
        immunochemistry and origin, 779
        laboratory features, 780
        P antigen specificity, 779
    management of, 780
Paroxysmal nocturnal hemoglobinuria (PNH), 27, 38, 112, 349–351, 639, 792, 804, 998, 1023, 1133
    clinical manifestations, 804
        dysphagia and male impotence, 805
        episodic hemolysis, 805
        hemoglobinuria, 804–805
        infections, 805–806
        marrow hypoplasia, 805
        physical examination, 806
        renal abnormalities, 805
        thromboembolic complications, 805
    differential diagnosis, 808–809
    disease course and prognosis, 816
    future directions for clinical and basic research, 817
    enumeration of blood for markers associated with, 39f
    etiology and pathogenesis, 792
        aplastic anemia and PNH, 803
        diagram of human PIGA gene and locations of somatic mutations reported in patients with PNH, 800f
        erythrocyte membrane protein deficiencies, 796–797
        hematopoietic stem cells, 804
        leukocytes and platelets, 804
        molecular basis of PNH, 797, 799f
        myelodysplastic syndrome and PNH, 803–804
        origin of PIGA-mutant stem cells, 801
        pathophysiology of PNH, 801
        PIGA genotype determines PNH phenotype, 800f
        sensitivity to complement-mediated lysis, 792–796
        structure of glycosyl phosphatidylinositol–anchored proteins, 798f
        two-step model of PNH pathogenesis, 801–803
    laboratory findings, 806
        blood, 806
        bone marrow, 806
        cytogenetic studies, 806
        diagnostic tests, 806, 807–808f
        plasma, 806
        urine, 806
    treatment, 809
        androgenic steroids, cortical steroids, and immunosuppressive therapy, 812–813
        bone marrow transplantation, 813
        clinical classification, 809, 809f, 810f
        complement inhibitory therapy, 811
        dysphagia, male impotence, abdominal pain, 816
        folate, 813

Paroxysmal nocturnal hemoglobinuria (PNH) (continued)
  geographic/ethnic differences, 816
  iron, 813
  management of anemia of PNH, 809–811
  pediatric PNH, 816
  PNH and COVID-19, 816
  pregnancy and PNH, 815–816
  prevention and treatment of thrombosis, 814–815
  reasons for eculizumab/ravulizumab failure, 811–812
  splenectomy, 813
  transfusions, 813
Partial albinism, 1349
Partial phagocytosis, 772
Partial pressure of oxygen (pO$_2$), 935
Partial resistance, 1283
Partial splenectomy, 735, 846, 1433
Partial thromboplastin time (PTT), 1082, 1207
  and factor VIIIc assay, 1213
Partially activated platelets, 1248
Parvovirus, 1412
  parvovirus-associated pure red cell aplasia, 1009, 1013
  pure red cell aplasia with infections other than, 1010
  serology, 1011
Parvovirus B19, 844, 1009, 1158, 2285
Passenger lymphocyte syndrome, 788
Past factor concentrates, viral transmission from, 1233
Paterson-Kelly syndrome, 642
Pathogen-associated molecular patterns (PAMPs), 153, 1495, 2355
Pathogen-reduction technology (PRT), 590
Pathologic fibrinolysis, 1254
Pathologic inhibitors of coagulation, 1254–1267
Pathologic thromboses, 1276
Pathological process, 801
Pathophysiologic mechanisms, 1099
Patient blood management (PBM), 565
Patient self-management (PSM), 1297
Patient self-testing (PST), 1297
Patient-controlled analgesia (PCA), 2303
Patient-specific prognostic factors, 1638–1639
Pattern recognition receptors (PRRs), 223, 1495
*PBRM*1 mutation, 1931
PCFT, 951
*PCM*1-*FGFR*1 fusion, 1844
*PCM*1, 1763
PD-1 ligands (PD-L1), 2134
*PDCD*1 gene, 1929
PDGFRA gene, 1763, 1837
PDGFRA variants, 1843
PDGFRB genes, 1763, 1675, 1680, 1837
PDGFRB variants, 1843
Pearson marrow-pancreas syndrome, 664, 984
PEBP2αB gene, 1633
PEBP2β. *See* CBFβ
Pediatric ALCL, 2000
Pediatric follicular lymphoma, 2001–2002
Pediatric ITP, 1099
Pediatric Oncology Group (POG), 1678, 2135
Pediatric patients, 567–568
PEG-IFN-α-2b. *See* Polyethylene glycol-IFN-α-2b (PEG-IFN-α-2b)
PEG-rHuMGDF, 377
Pegcetacoplan, 351, 812
Pegylated cytokine domain, 377
Pel-Ebstein fever, 2119
Pelger-Huët Anomaly, 146, 1352–1353
  acquired, 1353
Pelger-Huët heterozygote, 1353
Pelger-Huët cells, 1353
Pembrolizumab 1(PD-1 inhibitor), 1456, 2040, 2125–2126
Penicillin, 1169, 1262
  hypersensitivity, 785
  penicillin-allergic patients, 1471
  penicillin-type drug absorption mechanism, 785
  prophylaxis, 846
Penicillium molds, 1426
Pentasaccharides, 1293–1294
Pentostatin, 784, 1976, 2028, 2059
Pentraxin (PTX3), 156
Peptic ulcer, 1245
  disease, 1850
Peptide editing, 330
Peptide loading
  of class I molecule, 333
  in cross-presentation, 332–333
Peptide major histocompatibility complex (pMHC), 236
Peptide repertoire, 332
Peptide transporter 2 (PEPT2), 706
Peptide-bound HLA molecules, 333
Peptides, 1496
  artificial, 1087
Percutaneous coronary intervention (PCI), 1291
Perforin, 299–300, 299*f*
Performance IQ, 843
Performance status (PS), 1955
Periarteriolar lymphatic sheath (PALS), 247
Pericytes, 531
Perinatal hemorrhage, 1062
Periodic acid-Schiff (PAS), 110
Perioperative Autologous Blood Collection and Administration, standards for, 566
Peripartum hemolysis, 1050
Peripartum hemorrhage, 1050
Peripheral blood (PB), 22, 51, 1321, 1386, 1595, 2297, 2300
  counts, 1011
  lymphocytosis, 1386
  reticulocytes, 845
  smear, 1027–1028
Peripheral blood blasts rate of clearance (PBB-RC), 1641
Peripheral blood mononuclear cells (PBMCs), 1850
Peripheral blood progenitor cells (PBPCs), 2357
Peripheral blood stem cell transplantation (PBSCT), 910, 2298
Peripheral blood stem cells (PBSCs), 40, 1800, 2298
Peripheral neuropathy, 2278, 2287, 2382
Peripheral node addressins (PNAds), 222, 253
Peripheral smear, 782, 825
Peripheral supramolecular activation cluster (pSMAC), 293
Peripheral T-and NK-cell lymphomas, 1971–1972
Peripheral T-cell lymphoma (PTCL), 1382, 1884–1885, 1951, 2088
Peripheral T-cell lymphoma, not otherwise specified (PTCL, NOS), 1927–1928, 2001–2002
Peripheral tolerance, 770
Peritoneal dialysis, 853
Perivascular tissue, bleeding due to disorders of, 1166
  Ehlers-Danlos syndromes (EDSs), 1166
  Loeys-Dietz syndrome, 1167
  Marfan syndrome, 1166–1167
  osteogenesis imperfecta (OI), 1167
  pseudoxanthoma elasticum, 1167
  scurvy, 1167
  solar purpura, 1167
  steroid-induced purpura, 1167
Pernicious anemia, 954, 959–961, 966, 1010
  patients, 957
Peroxidase, hypersegmentation of eosinophils and negative staining for, 1354
Peroxisomal disorders, 1543–1544
Peroxisome proliferator-activating receptor (PPAR), 412
Peroxisomes, 395
Peroxynitrate (ONOO−), 160
Persistent mixed chimerism, 909
Petechiae, 603, 1080, 1082, 1852
Peyer patches (PPs), 233
*PF*4 gene, 362, 367, 379, 1156
Ph-like B-ALL, 1584
Phagocytes, 1395
  clinical presentation, 1395
  diagnosis, 1396
  specific disorders, 1395
    chronic granulomatous disease (CGD), 1395–1396
    congenital neutropenia and severe congenital neutropenia, 1395
    leukocyte adhesion deficiency (LAD), 1395
    Warts, Hypogammaglobulinemia, recurrent bacterial Infections, and Myelokathexis syndrome (WHIM syndrome), 1395
  treatment, 1396
Phagocytic cells, 1395, 1495
Phagocytic leukocytes, morphologic changes in, 1352
  Alder-Reilly anomaly, 1353
  familial vacuolization of leukocytes, 1354
  hereditary giant neutrophilia, 1354
  hereditary hypersegmentation of neutrophil nuclei, 1354
  hypersegmentation of eosinophils and negative staining for peroxidase and phospholipids, 1354
  inclusions in leukocytes, 1354
  May-Hegglin anomaly, 1353–1354
  Pelger-Huët Anomaly, 1352–1353
  pseudo–or acquired Pelger-Huët anomaly, 1353
  pseudo–Pelger-Huët cells, 1353*f*
Phagocytic oxidase (phox), 179
Phagocytic receptors, 224
Phagocytosis, 223–225, 224*f*, 158
Phagosome, 224
Phagosome to cytosol (P2C), 331
Pharmacokinetic studies, 904
Pharmacologic complement inhibitors, 352
Pharmacologic HbF reactivation, 911
Pharmacologic therapy for VTE, 1303
Pharyngitis, 1385
Phase 3 open label randomized trial, 2102
Phenothiazines, 1262
Phenotypic mosaicism, 792
Phenylalanine, 1785
Phenylhydroxylamine, 940
Phenytoin, 1950
Pheresis platelets, 561
Phialophora infections, 1347
Philadelphia chromosome (Ph chromosome), 48, 1458, 1603, 1608, 1611
Philadelphia positive acute lymphoblastic leukemia (Ph+ ALL), 2341, 2342
Phlebotomus. *See* Sand fly (Phlebotomus)
Phlebotomy, 1074, 1814–1815, 2330, 2376
Phorbol myristate acetate (PMA), 176
Phosphatases, 377
Phosphatidyl serine (PS), 835
Phosphatidylcholine (PC), 108, 726
Phosphatidylethanolamine, 108, 726
Phosphatidylinositol 3-kinases (PI3K), 104–105, 270, 404, 1459, 1576, 1785, 1839, 1963, 1978, 2272
Phosphatidylinositol 4, 5-bisphosphate (PIP2), 411, 153, 1193, 1459
Phosphatidylinositol-3, 4, 5-triphosphate (PIP$_3$), 275, 1459
Phosphatidylserine (PS), 108, 391, 442, 726, 1195, 1527
Phosphodiesterase-5 inhibitors, 921
Phosphoenolpyruvate, 1059
Phosphoflow method, 43
Phosphoglycerate kinase deficiency (PGK deficiency), 757, 763
Phosphoinositide 3-kinase delta inhibitors (PI3Kδ inhibitors), 2031
Phosphoinositides (PIP), 395
Phospholipase A$_2$ (PLA$_2$), 178
Phospholipase C gamma 1 (PLGC1), 2074
Phospholipase C γ2 (PlC γ2), 404, 406, 2033
Phospholipase C-β2 (PLC-β$_2$), 1193
Phospholipase Cγ1 (PLCγ1), 1498
Phospholipase Cγ2 (PLCG2), 1458
Phospholipids, 108, 726
Phosphorylation, 43, 112, 370
Photochemotherapy, 1859
Photographic Range of Motion (P-ROM), 2377
Photomultiplier tubes (PMTs), 18
Photon beam irradiation, 2097–2098
Photopheresis photochemotherapy, 2098
Phototherapy, 1370, 2095–2096
phox. *See* Phagocytic oxidase (phox)
PHT. *See* Pulmonary hypertension (PHT)
Physical delivery methods, 1524
Physiologic anemia, 1058
Physiologic fibrinolysis, 1254
Physiologic thrombocytopenia, 1108
Physiologically appropriate secondary erythrocytosis, 1074–1075
Physiologically inappropriate secondary erythrocytosis, 1075–1077
Phytohemagglutinin (PHA), 49
Phytosterolemia. *See* Sitosterolemia
Pickwickian syndrome, 1075
Piece-meal degranulation (PMD), 174, 197
PIEZO1 protein, 741
PIGA gene, 350, 792, 998
PIGA mutations, 799, 801, 804, 1760
PIGA-mutant, 803, 806
  cells, 802–803
  hematopoietic stem cells, 801

stem cells, 801, 814
  origin of, 801
Pigment stones, 617–618
Pigmented purpuric dermatitis, 1171
Pigmented purpuric dermatoses (PPDs), 2082
Pigmented purpuric eruptions, 1171
PIGT gene, 798
*PIM*1 mutations, 376, 1878
Pirtobrutinib, 2032
Pityriasis lichenoides chronica (PLC), 2082
Pityriasis lichenoides et varioliformis acuta (PLEVA), 2082
Placenta, 1062
Placenta previa, 1062
Placenta-derived NK cells, 1513
Placental-type PAI, 490
Plant homeodomain (PHD), 270, 1578
Plant homeodomain finger protein 6 gene (*PHF6* gene), 1587
Plasma, 806, 1226
  β2-microglobulin, 2026
  cryoprecipitate reduced, 563
  euglobulin fraction, 1086
  fluorescence scanning, 709
  heme, 123–124
  IL-6 levels, 1857
  infusion, 1133
  iron-binding protein, 633
  membrane, 391–392
  porphyrin, 719
  potassium, 561
  proenzyme plasminogen, 427
  proteins, 402
    alloantibodies reacting with, 581
    platelet forms of, 397
  therapeutic adsorption of plasma constituents, 592
  therapy, 1133
  transfusion, 578
    efficacy of, 578
    use of plasma components, 578
  transport, 633
  vitamin D, 2026
Plasma carboxypeptidase B, 459
Plasma cell dyscrasia (PCD), 2175, 1277
Plasma cell labeling index (PCLI), 2183
Plasma cell leukemia (PCL), 2175, 2221–2222
Plasma cells (PCs), 11, 1876, 1952, 2056, 2146, 2148, 2152, 2177, 2240, 2247, 2279
  bone marrow, 2178
  circulating, 2168
  differentiation, 280
    histology of plasma cells, 280*f*
    morphology of endoplasmic reticulum in plasma cell, 281*f*
  directed therapy, 2292
  disorders, 2276, 2345
    autologous HCT for multiple myeloma, 2346*t*
    indications for autologous hematopoietic cell transplant, 2346–2347
    multiple myeloma (MM), 2345–2346
    systemic amyloidosis, POEMS, 2346–2347
  DNA, 2157
  early genetic abnormalities in multiple myeloma, 2153
  high-resolution sequencing studies and additional complexity of MM genomes, 2155
  genetic changes in myeloma as result of therapy, 2157
  intraclonal tumor heterogeneity associated with high-risk MM, 2156
  mechanisms of mutagenesis in PC neoplasms, 2155–2156, 2156*f*
  malignancies, 2175
  MM plasma cell tumor of postgerminal center B cells, 2152–2153
  myelomas, 1910
    immunophenotyping of, 35
  neoplasm, 54, 1866
  normal and malignant plasma cell development, 2152*f*
  plasma cell development, 2152
  in POEMS syndrome, 2277
  process, 2239
  proliferative rate, 2183
  secondary oncogenic events associated with progression of MGUS to MM, 2153–2155
Plasma cell myeloma, acute terminal phase and cause of death, 2181

Plasma components, preparation of, 562
  plasma-derived therapeutics, 563–564
    coagulation factor concentrates, 564
    immunoglobulins, 564
    solvent/detergent-treated plasma (S/D plasma), 564
  for transfusion, 562
    cryoprecipitated antihemophilic factor, 563
    fresh frozen plasma, plasma frozen within 24 hours, 562–563
    liquid plasma, thawed plasma, 563
    plasma, cryoprecipitate reduced, 563
Plasma exchange, 1133
  therapy, 1138, 1231
Plasma frozen within 24 hours (PF24), 562–563
Plasma prekallikrein, 432
  activation, 434
  biochemistry, 434
  function, 434
  gene structure and expression, 432–434
    schematic representation of intrinsic pathway proteins, 433*f*
  regulation, 434
Plasma thromboplastin antecedent. See Factor XI
Plasma thromboplastin antecedent deficiency. See Factor XI deficiency
Plasma thromboplastin component. See Factor IX
Plasmablastic lymphoma (PBL), 1418, 1947
Plasmacytoid DCs (pDCs), 30, 214, 253
Plasmacytoid lymphocytes, 1873, 2267
Plasmacytomas, 2222
Plasmapheresis, 590, 779, 784, 1013, 2281
Plasmin, 494, 1301, 1723
α2-plasmin inhibitor, 1723
Plasminogen, 479
  biochemistry, 479–480
  deficiency, 1286
  function, 480
  gene structure and expression, 479
  proteins and inhibitors of fibrinolytic system, 481*t*
Plasminogen activator inhibitor-1 (PAI-1), 432, 488–489
  biochemistry, 489
  biochemistry, 489–490
  deficiency, 1224
  gene structure and expression, 489
  levels, 1286–1287
  schematic of, 490*f*
Plasminogen activator inhibitor-2 (PAI-2), 490
  biochemistry and function, 490
  gene structure and expression, 490
  schematic of, 491*f*
Plasminogen activator inhibitor-3. See Protein C inhibitor
Plasminogen activator, recombinant tissue (rt-PA), 1301
Plasminogen activators (PAs), 480–481, 1301–1302
  factor VII–activating protease, 485–486
  intrinsic activators, 481
  molecular forms of plasmin, 483*f*
  proteins and inhibitors of fibrinolytic system, 481*t*
  schematic of plasminogen, 482*f*
  tissue plasminogen activator, 481–484
  urokinase plasminogen activator, 484–485
Plasmodia, 821
Plasmodium, 821, 824, 1321
  infection, 742
  P. berghei, 1158
  P. falciparum, 547, 587, 739, 821, 883
  P. knowlesi, 547
  P. malariae, 821
  P. ovale, 821
  P. vivax, 547, 821, 1331
Plasmodium falciparum reticulocyte binding homolog (PfRh), 821
Plastic "nonwettable" coverslips, 6
Plasticity of CD4 T-cell subsets, 299
Platelet activation, 921
  key regulators of, 41
  physiologic inhibition of, 411–412
    inhibitory processes of, 413
    inhibitory prostaglandins, 412–413
    pleckstrin and protein kinase C inhibition, 413
    platelet activation and thrombus formation, 412*f*
    platelet secretion, 413–414
    role of cytoskeletal rearrangement in, 416
Platelet additive solutions (PASs), 562
Platelet alloantibodies, acquired, 1111

Platelet antibodies, 1098
  cell-mediated immunity, 1099
  characteristics of platelet autoantibodies in primary immune thrombocytopenia, 1099*t*
  impaired platelet production, 1099
Platelet disorders, inherited (IPDs), 67, 1182
Platelet disorders, quantitative, 1087
Platelet endothelial cell adhesion molecular-1 (PECAM-1), 394
Platelet factor 4 (PF4), 1191, 1307
Platelet function
  aggregation, impaired, 1192
  assays, 1083
    interpretation of aggregometer tracings, 1084*f*
    new assays of platelet function, 1084
  in hemostasis and thrombosis
    model for platelet adhesion to subendothelial matrix at sites of vascular injury and subsequent thrombus formation, 402*f*
    platelet adhesion and activation, 402
    platelet glycoprotein Ib complex-von Willebrand factor interaction and signaling, 402–40
  hereditary disorders of, 1183–1196
  key regulators of platelet activation, 411–414
  physiologic inhibition of platelet adhesion, 406
  platelet activation by soluble agonists, 409–410
  platelet adenosine diphosphate receptors and signaling, 407–408
    adenosine diphosphate receptor signaling, 408–409
    $P2X_1$ receptor, 408
    platelet $P2Y_1$ and $P2Y_{12}$ receptor roles in adenosine diphosphate, 408
  platelet adhesion receptors, 406
  platelet aggregation, 414–416
    and arterial shear flow, 415–416
  platelet signaling as a global interlinked network, 416
  platelet thrombin receptors and signaling, 406–407
    GPCRs signaling networks in human platelets, 407*f*
  platelet-cell interactions, 416
    complexity of platelet signaling networks, 417*f*
    platelet RNA transfer, microparticles, and miRNA transfer, 418–419
    platelets and endothelium, 416–418
    platelets and immune cells, 418
    platelets and metastatic cells, 418
    role of platelets in inflammation, 418
  platelet-collagen interaction and signaling, 404–405
    $\alpha_2\beta_1$ receptor, 405
    glycoprotein VI receptor, 405
    platelet-collagen signaling, 405–406
  production, 1099
  prophylaxis and treatment of platelet function disorders, 1196–1197
  qualitative disorders of
    diagnostic approach to inherited platelet function disorders, 1182–1183
    hereditary disorders of platelet function, 1183–1196
    management of thrombotic risk in patients with IPFD, 1197
    prophylaxis and treatment of platelet function disorders, 1196–1197
    timeline of IPFD discovery, 1183*f*
  regional architecture of platelet plug and regulation of platelet activation in vivo, 410–411
    regional architecture of hemostatic plug, 410*f*
  role of cytoskeletal rearrangement in platelet activation, 416
  role of platelets in atherogenesis and atherothrombosis, 419–420
    platelet adherence to endothelium, 419*f*
Platelet Function Analyzer-100 (PFA-100), 1213
Platelet Function Disorders of European Hematology Association, 1197
Platelet function disorders, inherited (IPFDs), 1182–1183
  diagnostic approach to, 1182–1183
  management of thrombotic risk in patients with, 1197
Platelet glycoprotein Ib complex-von Willebrand factor interaction and signaling, 402
  glycoprotein Ib complex interaction with thrombin, 403–404
  glycoprotein Ib complex signaling, 404
  schematic illustration of glycoprotein Ib/V/IX complex and associated proteins, 403*f*

Platelet granules, abnormalities of, 1190
  arthrogryposis, renal dysfunction and cholestasis syndrome (ARC syndrome), 1192
  autism with platelet dense granule defect, 1191
  Chediak-Higashi syndrome (CHS), 1191
  gray platelet syndrome (GPS), 1191
  Hermansky-Pudlak syndrome (HPS), 1190–1191
  Paris-Trousseau-Jacobsen syndrome, 1192
  SLFN14-related thrombocytopenia, 1191
  α, δ-storage pool deficiency, 1192
  δ-storage pool disease (δ-SPD), 1190
Platelet microparticles (PMPs), 396, 1195
Platelet P2 purinergic receptors, 1189
  P2 receptors defects, 1190
  $P2Y_{12}$ Defect, 1190
  protease-activated receptor-1 (PAR-1), 1190
Platelet preparation and storage, 561
  apheresis (pheresis) platelets, 561
  platelet storage and functional integrity, 561–562
    cold-stored platelets, 562
    platelet additive solutions (PASs), 562
    preparation of components from whole blood donation, 562f
  preparation of platelet concentrates, 561
Platelet production
  cytokines involved in positive or negative regulation of, 378–379
  role of apoptosis in regulation of, 365
  role of cytoskeleton in regulation of, 364–365
  role of marrow environment in, 364
Platelet structure
  biochemistry and metabolism, 395
    composition, 395
    energy metabolism and generation of adenosine triphosphate, 395
    lipid composition and metabolism and generation of arachidonic acid, 395–396
    nucleotide metabolism and nonmetabolic role for adenosine diphosphate, 395
  interactions beyond platelets, 397
    clinical impacts, 398
    clot retraction, 397
    platelet forms of plasma proteins, 397
    platelet interactions with plasma coagulation system, 397
    platelet-associated coagulation factors, 397–398, 398t
    protease inhibitors, 397
  microparticles and kinetics, 396
    distribution, 397
    lifespan, 397
    platelet distribution and survival kinetics, 397
    platelet heterogeneity, 396–397
  structural and functional anatomy, 391
    α-Granules, 394–395
    cytoplasmic actin and intermediate filaments, 393
    dense bodies, 395
    dense tubules, 392
    electron microscopy and subcellular features, 391
    Human platelet cytoskeletons, 393f
    light microscopy, 391
    lysosomes, 395
    membrane skeleton, 393
    microtubules, 393–394
    organelles, 395
    plasma membrane, 391–392
    platelet cytoskeleton, 392
    platelet granules and organelles, 394
    platelet membranous systems, 392
    platelet surface, 391
    surface-connected canalicular system, 392
Platelet transfusion, 575, 1197, 1723
  administration of, 575
  cold-stored platelets, 578
  dosage and expected response, 575
  indications for, 575
    prophylactic platelet transfusion, 575–576
    therapeutic platelet transfusion, 576
  platelet refractoriness and alloimmunization, 576
    diagnosis and management of alloimmunization, 577
    factors reported to be associated with platelet refractoriness, 576t
    immune causes of refractoriness and prevention of HLA alloimmunization, 576
    nonimmune causes of refractoriness, 576–577

  platelet transfusions for patients refractory to HLA-matched platelet transfusions, 577
  selection of platelet products, 577
    ABO group, 577
    RhD type, 577
  support, 1747
Platelet-derived growth factor (PDGF), 362
Platelet-derived growth factor receptor (PDGFR), 1782, 2361
Platelet-derived growth factor receptor-α (*PDGFRA*), 1772
  chronic eosinophilic leukemia with, 1773f
  myeloid and lymphoid neoplasms with, 1772–1773
  eosinophilia and rearrangement of, 1772–1774
Platelet-derived growth factor receptor-α/β (PDGFRA/B), 1836
Platelet-derived growth factor receptor-β (*PDGFRB*), 1649, 1772
  myeloid and lymphoid neoplasms with eosinophilia and rearrangement of, 1772–1774
  myeloid neoplasm with eosinophilia with, 1774f
  myeloid neoplasms with PDGFRB rearrangement, 1773–1774
Platelet-derived microparticles (PMPs), 40
Platelet-type bleeding disorder-22 (BDPLT22), 1189
Platelet-type von Willebrand disease (PT-VWD), 1155, 1188, 1216–1217
Platelet–activating factor (PAF), 150, 202, 1193
Platelet–endothelial cell adhesion molecule-1 (PECAM-1), 406
Platelets (PLTs), 1, 356, 366, 391, 416–418, 540, 645, 804, 858, 864, 1111, 1182, 1192–1193, 1230, 1276, 1810–1812
Pleckstrin, 413
Pleckstrin homology (PH), 376, 404
Plerixafor, 2199, 2300
Plumbo porphyria. See ALAD deficiency porphyria
Plummer-Vinson syndrome, 642
Pluripotent stem cells, 152, 267
PML gene, 1709, 1721
PML nuclear bodies (PNBs), 1723
PML oncogenic domains, 1723
PML-RARA gene, 1569–1570, 1709
PML-RARα fusion
  protein, 1721, 1723
  transcript, 1722
Pneumococcal conjugate vaccines (PCVs), 1485
  PCV13, 1485
  PCV15, 1485
  PCV20, 1485
Pneumococcal serotypes, 847
Pneumococcal vaccines, 844
Pneumocystis, 1397, 1469, 1477
  P. carinii, 1477
  P. carinii pneumonia, 1000
  P. jirovecii, 982, 1397, 1410, 1615, 1704, 2029, 2053, 2065, 2364
Pneumocystis jirovecii pneumonia (PJP), 1397, 1476, 2306, 2377
Pneumonia due to viral pathogens, 1478
PNH, subclinical (PNH-sc), 808–809
PNP–deficient SCID. See Purine nucleotide phosphorylase–deficient SCID (PNP–deficient SCID)
POC INR devices, 1297
POG. See Pediatric Oncology Group (POG)
Poikilocytosis, 715, 1020
Poikiloderma vasculare atrophicans (PVA), 2082
Point mutations, 886, 1219
Poiseuille law, The, 1070
Polatuzumab, 1967
  vedotin, 1455
POLE2 gene, 1912
Poloxamer-188, 864
Poly(A) mutants, 887
Poly(rC)-binding protein 1 (PCBP1), 634
Polyagglutination test, 573
Polychromasia, 715
Polychromatic flow cytometry, bone marrow mapping with, 22, 23f
Polyclonal activation, 270
Polycomb repressive complex 2 (PRC2), 370, 1572, 1587, 1789
Polycomb repressive complexes 1 (PRCs 1), 370
Polycystic ovary syndrome, 689
Polycytes, 147

Polycythemia, 3, 1070
Polycythemia rubra vera, 1277, 2241
Polycythemia vera (PV), 375, 711, 1071, 1073, 1176, 1763, 1766–1767, 1767f, 1808, 1821
  blood and laboratory findings, 1810
    bone marrow, 1811
    cytogenetics, 1811–1812
    hematologic findings, 1810–1811
    laboratory findings, 1811
    World Health Organization for diagnosis of polycythemia Vera, 1811t
  clinical features, 1808–1809
    cardiovascular system, 1809
    gastrointestinal system, 1809
    genitourinary system, 1809
    neuromuscular system, 1810
    respiratory system, 1809
    skin and mucous membranes, 1809
    splenomegaly, 1809
  definition and history, 1808
  diagnosis, 1813
  epidemiology, 1808
  key events in history of PV, 1808t
  natural history, 1813
    causes of death in polycythemia vera patients, 1813t
    risk stratification, 1813–1814
  pathogenesis, 1812
    clonality, 1812
    hematopoietic growth factors and hematopoiesis, 1812
    molecular genetic features, 1812
  physical findings and symptoms in, 1809t
  post-polycythemic phase of, 1767–1768f
  transformation of, 1768f
  treatment, 1814
    approach to treatment, 1816–1817
    cytoreductive therapy, 1815–1816
    phlebotomy and antiplatelet agents, 1814–1815
    special topics, 1817
    treatment algorithm for polycythemia vera patients, 1816t
  WHO criteria for diagnosis of, 1766t
Polycythemic phase, 1766
Polyethylene glycol-IFN-α-2b (PEG-IFN-α-2b), 1844
Polyglutamated folate, 951
Polymerase chain reaction (PCR), 14, 61, 62f, 1011, 1133, 1327, 1412, 1446, 1476, 1595, 1699, 1850, 1900, 1903, 2000, 2075
  PCR-based B-cell and T-cell receptor, 1869
  PCR-based laboratory test, 1611
  PCR-based methods, 914
  PCR-mediated detection of EBV DNA, 1386
Polymerization, 475–476
  fibrin assembly, 477–478
  fibrin cross-linking, 478
  fibrinopeptide release, 476
  physiologic determinants of, 834
Polymorphic B-cell hyperplasia, 1951
Polymorphic reticulosis, 1889
Polymorphisms, 678, 1630
Polymorphonuclear neutrophils, 139–141, 140f, 141f
Polymyalgia rheumatic, 2172
Polymyositis, 2172
Polyneuropathy, 2023
Polyneuropathy, organomegaly, endocrinopathy, M-protein, and skin changes syndrome (POEMS syndrome), 2170, 2177, 2222, 2246, 2276–2277, 2292, 2346–2347
  activity of therapy for treatment of, 2280f
  classic findings of, 2278f
  clinical presentation of, 2278
    elevated VEGF and cytokines, 2279
    monoclonal plasma cell disorder, sclerotic bone lesions, and myeloproliferation, 2279
    organomegaly, endocrinopathy, skin changes, papilledema, and extravascular overload, 2278–2279
    polyradiculoneuropathy, 2278
    pulmonary and coagulation abnormalities, 2279
  diagnosis of, 2277–2278
  diagnostic criteria for five selected syndromes, 2277t
  etiology of, 2277
  organ involvement and diseases, 2276f
  treatment of, 2279–2281, 2280f

without disseminated bone marrow involvement, 2280
with disseminated bone marrow involvement, 2280–2281
managing symptoms of disease, 2281
monitoring response, 2281
Polyoma Merkel cell virus, 2075
Polyploidization, 361–362
mechanism, 356
Polyradiculoneuropathy, 2278
Polyvinylpyrrolidone (PVP), 774
Pomalidomide, 1461, 1829, 2175, 2184, 2210, 2214–2216, 2251
Pomalidomide and dexamethasone (Pd), 2210
Ponatinib, 1458, 1613, 1619, 1782, 1796
Ponatinib Ph+ ALL and CML Evaluation (PACE), 1796
Popcorn cell, 2117
Population-based study of erythrocytosis, 934
Porphobilinogen (PBG), 703
Porphobilinogen deaminase (PBGD), 704
Porphyria cutanea tarda (PCT), 690, 702, 712, 719
clinical description, 712
diagnosis and treatment of, 719–720
hepatocellular carcinoma, 714
hepatoerythropoietic porphyria (HEP), 714
laboratory findings, 713
molecular basis and pathogenesis, 712
mechanism of hepatic iron pathogenesis, 713
precipitating factors, 713
renal dialysis, 713
toxic, 714
toxic porphyria cutanea tarda, 714
treatment, 713
Porphyrias, 702
acute hepatic porphyrias, 704–712
classification of, 703t
dual porphyrias, 719
erythropoietic cutaneous porphyrias, 714–718
genetic and key metabolic features of, 703t
heme biosynthetic pathway, 702f
hepatocutaneous porphyria, 712–714
key clinical summary points, 719
broad definitions of eight major porphyrias, 719
diagnosis and treatment of acute hepatic porphyrias, 719
diagnosis and treatment of congenital erythropoietic porphyria, 720
diagnosis and treatment of porphyria cutanea tarda, 719–720
diagnosis and treatment of protoporphyrias, 720
mutation analysis, 720
late-onset, 702
mammalian heme biosynthesis and regulation, 703–704
South African geneticv, 708
treatment of ongoing attack, 707
Porphyrinogens, 98
Porphyrins, 98, 709, 715
7 carboxylate, 719
Portal hypertension, 2244
Portal vein thrombosis, 1245
Posaconazole, 1350, 1477, 1483
Positive regulation of platelet production cytokines involved in, 378–379
positive regulators, 378
cytokines and pathways, 378–379
Cytokines of IL-6 Family, 378
Erythropoietin, 378
GM-CSF and IL-3, 378
SDF1/CXCL12, 378
Stem Cell Factor/KIT Ligand, 378
Positive selection (PS), 288–290
Positron emission tomography (PET), 1367, 1611, 1954, 1991, 2019, 2092, 2134, 2241, 2343
Positron emission tomography-computed tomography (PET-CT), 2119, 2168
abnormalities on, 2168
Post hoc analysis, 1066
Post splenectomy, 735
Post-HCT therapy to reduce relapse, 2337
Post-polycythemic myelofibrosis phase of PV, 1767
Posterior reversible encephalopathy syndrome (PRES), 1140, 1144
Posteroanterior (PA), 2134
Post–essential thrombocythemia myelofibrosis, 1179
Postgerminal center 2152

Postgerminal center B cells, MM plasma cell tumor of, 2152–2153
Postinduction intensification, 1673–1674
Postinduction treatment intensity, 1672
Postinfectious neutropenia, 1336
Postmarathon leukocytosis, 142
Postnatal hemorrhage, 1062
Postoperative thrombocytosis, 1434
Postpartum anemia, 1050–1051
Postpartum hemorrhage (PPH), 1197
secondary, 1050
Postremission intensification or consolidation therapy, 1615
Postremission therapy, 1643, 1645, 1701
consolidation therapy, 1645–1646
dose and duration, 1701
hematopoietic cell transplantation, 1701–1702
maintenance therapy, 1646
risk groups defined by cytogenetic, molecular alterations, and MRD, 1702t
Post-splenectomy infection, 1434–1435
Postsplenectomy sepsis, 734, 760, 907
Postsplenectomy thrombocytosis, 1176
Postthrombotic syndrome (PTS), 1289
Posttransfusion purpura (PTP), 584, 1111, 1113–1114
Posttransfusion thrombocytopenia, 584
Posttranslational modifications, 370
Posttransplant cyclophosphamide (PTCy), 2298, 2321, 2328, 2335, 2359
Posttransplantation lymphoproliferative disorders (PTLDs), 1382, 1388–1389, 1482, 1508, 1951, 2001, 2382
clinical presentation and management 2001
pathology and molecular characteristics, 2001
Posttraumatic bleeding, 1220
*POT*1 gene, 1912
*POT*1 mutation, 2012
Potassium, 561, 742
Potransferrinemia, 636
pP7 protein, 2267
Pragmatic, Randomized Optimal Platelet and Plasma Ratios (PROPPR), 569
Pralatrexate, 2099
Prasugrel, 1291
Pre-B cell receptor (pre-BCR), 273, 274, 274f
Pre-B cells, 29
Pre-B-cell leukemic homeoboX 1 (PBX1), 1582
Precursor mRNA (pre-mRNA), 1578
Prednisone, 784, 1962, 2184, 2190–2192
Prednisone-derived chemotherapy, 2002
Preeclampsia, 1049
Prefibrotic phase of PMF, 1767
Pregnancy, 640–641, 708, 760, 855–856, 903, 998, 1010, 1139, 1197, 1230
anemias during
maternal anemia associated with prenatal infections, 1048–1049
overview/epidemiology, 1047
physiologic anemia of pregnancy, 1047
postpartum anemia, 1050–1051
bone marrow failure syndromes associated with, 1050
deficiency of folate and nutrients during, 1048
hemolytic anemia in, 1049–1050
HL and, 2128
immune thrombocytopenia in, 1108–1109
iron deficiency during, 1047–1048
physiologic anemia of, 1047
and PNH, 815–816
pregnancy-associated aplastic anemia, 998
pregnancy-associated thrombotic thrombocytopenic purpura, 1050
pregnancy-induced hemolytic anemia, 1049
features of idiopathic pregnancy-induced hemolytic anemia, 1049t
Preimplantation genetic diagnosis (PGD), 916
Prekallikrein, 434, 1223
Preleukemia, 1696
Preliminary laboratory tests, 1182
Prelymphomatous conditions in NHL, 1951–1953, 1951t
Premalignant stem cells (pre-MDS-SC), 1567
Premature Infants in Need of Transfusion (PINT), 567
Prematurity, 1063
Prenatal hemorrhage, 1061–1062
Prenatal infections, maternal anemia associated with, 1048–1049
Prenatal macrophage populations, 216

Preoperative autologous donation (PAD), 565
Preoperative hemostasis
evaluation, 1089–1091
screening tests, 1089
Preplatelets, 363
Presymptomatic central nervous system therapy, 1673
Preterm Epo for Neuroprotection (PENUT), 1053
Prethrombin 1, 450
Pretransplant sperm banking, 910
*PRF*1 gene, 1380
Priapism, 845
stuttering, 845
Primaquine, 753, 755
Primary cardiac lymphoma, 1955
Primary central nervous system lymphoma (PCNSL), 1417, 1880, 1954, 2001–2003
Primary cold agglutinin disease, 776–778
Primary cutaneous acral CD8+ T-cell lymphoma (PCATCL), 2085, 2089
Primary cutaneous aggressive epidermotropic CD8+ cytotoxic T-cell lymphoma (PC8TCL), 2088
Primary cutaneous ALCL (PCALCL), 2079, 2083
Primary cutaneous anaplastic large cell lymphoma (PCALCL), 1887, 2084–2085
Primary cutaneous B-cell lymphomas, 2089
Primary cutaneous CD30-positive T-cell lymphoproliferative disorders, 1887
Primary cutaneous CD4+small/medium-sized pleomorphic T-cell lymphoproliferative disorder (PCSMPTCLPD), 2085, 2088–2089
Primary cutaneous diffuse large B-cell lymphoma (PCDLBCL), 2089
Primary cutaneous FL (PCFL), 1919
Primary cutaneous follicle center lymphoma (PCFCL), 1870, 1872, 2089
Primary cutaneous marginal zone B-cell lymphoma (PCMZL), 2089
Primary cutaneous T-cell lymphomas, 2085
EBV+ lymphoproliferative disorders, 2088
folliculotropic mycosis fungoides (FMF), 2085–2087
granulomatous slack skin disease (GSS), 2087
MF variants, 2085t
pagetoid reticulosis, 2085
primary cutaneous acral CD8+ T-cell lymphoma (PCATCL), 2089
primary cutaneous aggressive epidermotropic CD8+ cytotoxic T-cell lymphoma (PC8TCL), 2088
primary cutaneous CD4+ small/medium-sized pleomorphic T-cell lymphoproliferative disorder (PCSMPTCLPD), 2088–2089
primary cutaneous γδ T-cell lymphoma (PCGDTCL), 2088
rare CTCL variants, 2086t
subcutaneous panniculitis-like T-cell lymphoma (SPTL), 2087–2088
Primary cutaneous γ/δ T-cell lymphoma (PCGDTCL), 1974, 2088
Primary cysts, 1430, 1437–1438
Primary defect in megakaryopoiesis, principal pathologies associated with, 379
Primary diffuse large B-cell lymphoma of central nervous system, 1880
genetics, 1880
immunophenotype, 1880
morphology, 1880
Primary effusion lymphoma (PEL), 1382, 1415, 1417
Primary erythrocytosis, 1072–1074. *See also* Secondary erythrocytosis
mutations, 1074
polycythemia vera, 1073
primary familial/primary proliferative erythrocytosis, 1073–1074
Primary fibrinolysis, 1254
clinical features and laboratory diagnosis 1254
etiology, 1254
pathophysiology, 1254
treatment, 1254
Primary granules, 173
Primary hemostasis, 402, 1276
abnormalities of, 1212
Primary HP, 1168
Primary human HSCs, 1548
Primary IgH translocations, role of genes dysregulated by, 2157
Primary Immune Deficiency Treatment Consortium (PIDTC), 2314

Primary immune neutropenia, 1337
Primary immunodeficiencies, 1951
Primary immunodeficiency, EBV–associated disorders in, 1389–1390
Primary immunodeficiency diseases (PIDs), 40, 1389, 2377
   B cells/antibodies, 1396–1399
   basic laboratory workup for immune deficiency, 1405
      lab tests for basic evaluation of each compartment of the immune system, 1405f
      presentations associated with defects in each of four major immune compartments, 1405f
   complement, 1393–1395, 1393f
   complex or combined immunodeficiency disorders, 1403–1404
   immune regulatory disorders, 1404–1405
   major compartments of immune system, 1393
   phagocytes, 1395–1396
   T cells, 1399–1403
Primary immunodeficiency disorders (PIDDs), 1393, 2314
   B-cell recovery and immune reconstitution after HCT, 2317–2318
   chemotherapy conditioning regimens before allogeneic HCT for PID, 2317t
   comparison of HLA-ID sibling and unrelated donor HCT for PID, 2315–2316
   conditioning regimens for, 2315
   diagnosis of, 2314–2315
      common molecular causes of SCID, 2315t
   HCT for, 2314–2318
   HLA-haploidentical HCT for PID, 2316–2317
   late effects and future directions in HCT for PID, 2318
Primary mediastinal B-cell lymphoma (PMBCL), 1880, 1991, 1957, 1968–1969, 1998
   clinical presentation and management, 1999
   immunophenotype, 1880
   morphology, 1880
   pathology and molecular characteristics, 1998–1999
   PET/CT primary mediastinal B-cell lymphoma, 1999f
Primary messenger RNA (Primary mRNA), 884
Primary screening tests, 1087
   disorders in results of, 1089
Primary Secretion Defect (PSD), 1196
Primary therapy, 1609
   of acute graft-vs-host disease, 2359–2360
      ALL, 1614
         acute lymphoblastic leukemia in older patients, 1619–1620
         B-cell acute lymphoblastic leukemia, 1617–1618
         central nervous system therapy, 1616
Prime editing (PE), 1549
Priming, 154
Primitive hematopoiesis, 70
Primitive hemolytic jaundice, 895
Primitive origin macrophages, 216
Pro-B cell to immature B cell, 274
Proangiogenic cytokines, 854
Proangiogenic placental growth factor (PlGF), 1049
Probes, 51
Procainamide, 1262
Procoagulant cofactor proteins, 451–458
   factor V, 454–457
   factor VIII, 453–454
   tissue factor, 451–453
   von Willebrand Factor, 458
Procoagulant pathways
   hemostasis, 429f
   overview of, 428–429
Procoagulant plasma protein "factors", 1276
Procoagulant process, 427
Procoagulant proteins, 430, 436–451
   factor XI, 435–436
   factor XII, 430–432
   high-molecular-weight kininogen (HMWK), 434–435
   plasma prekallikrein, 432–434
Proerythroblasts, 94, 1023
Profilin 1 (PFN1), 365
Progenitor B cell (pro-B cell), 267
Progenitor cells, 37, 77, 1767
   mature, 360
Programmed cell death protein-1 (PD-1), 301, 2134
Programmed death-ligand 1 (PD-L1), 2102

Progressive transformation of germinal centers (PTGCs), 1871, 2127
Proinflammatory cytokines, 1248
Proliferation (PR), 2182
Proliferative glomerulonephritis and monoclonal immunoglobulin deposits (PGNMID), 2289
Proliferative retinal disease, 854
Proliferator-activated receptor γ coactivator 1α (PGC-1α), 100
Proline-rich motif (PXXPXP), 372
Prolyl 4-hydroxylase domain (PHD), 103
Prolyl hydroxylase domain-containing protein-2 (PHD-2), 1076
Prolymphocytes (PL), 1872, 2016
Prolymphocytic leukemia (PLL), 1910
Prolymphocytic transformation of CLL, 2040
Promiscuous gene expression (pGE), 290
Promoter activity regulation, 369–370
Promoter mutations, 887
Promyelocytes, malignant, 1247
Promyelocytic leukemia (PML), 1569, 1721
Promyelocytic leukemia zinc finger (PLZF), 1723
Promyelocytic zinc finger (PLZF), 1570
Propagation of α-thrombin formation, 427
Properdin, 342, 1427
Prophase of prednisone (PRED), 1671
Prophylactic antibiotics, 2038
Prophylactic anticoagulation, 815, 1197
Prophylactic G-CSF, algorithm for use of, 1472, 1473f
Prophylactic platelet transfusion, 575–576
Prophylactic therapy, 1218, 1231–1232
Prophylaxis to reduce infection risk
   to reduce infection risks, 1483, 1484t
      antibacterial, 1483
      antifungal, 1483–1485
      antiviral, 1485
      immunization, 1485–1486
Prophylaxis for surgery in patients with coagulopathy and treatment of platelet function disorders, 1196
      activated recombinant factor VIIa, 1197
      antifibrinolytic agents, 1196
      desmopressin, 1196
      general prophylaxis measures, 1196
      hematopoietic stem cell transplantation and gene therapy, 1197
      hormonal treatment, 1197
      local measures, 1196
      management of delivery, 1197
      management of surgery, 1197
      platelet transfusions, 1197
Propidium iodide (PI), 42
Propionyl-CoA metabolism, 946
Proplatelets, 363
Propolycytes, 147
PROPPR. See Pragmatic, Randomized Optimal Platelet and Plasma Ratios (PROPPR)
Propranolol, 707
Prostacyclin (PGI$_2$), 533
Prostaglandin H synthase 1, 1289
Prostaglandin H synthase 2, 1289
Prosthetic heart valves, 1123
Protease inhibitors, 397
   α1-antitrypsin Pittsburgh, 1225
   α2-antiplasmin deficiency, 1224
   abnormalities of, 1224
   plasminogen activator inhibitor-1 deficiency (PAI-1 deficiency), 1224–1225
   tissue factor deficiency, 1225
Protease nexin-2 (PN2), 436
Protease-activated receptor-1 (PAR-1), 460, 535, 1190
Protease-activated receptors (PARs), 176, 1247
Proteasome inhibitor–based therapy, 1460, 2252–2253, 2270–2271
Protein 4.1R defects, 737–738
Protein 4.2 deficiency, 730
Protein C, 460, 470–471, 535–536, 1086
   acquired protein C deficiency, 1282
   activation, 461
   biochemistry, 461
   clinical aspects, 1281
   deficiency, Type I, 1281
   function, 461
   gene structure and expression, 461
   laboratory diagnosis, 1281–1282
   pathophysiology and genetics, 1281

   regulation, 461
   treatment, 1282
Protein conjugate vaccines (PCV), 2021
Protein deficiencies in PNH, basis of, 796
Protein electrophoresis, 2144, 2146–2147
Protein kinase A (PKA), 1193–1194
Protein kinase B (PKB), 405
Protein kinase C (PKC), 153, 179, 377, 404, 1498
Protein kinase C-ε (PKCε), 364
Protein kinase G (PKG), 404
Protein kinases, 112
Protein phosphorylation, 43
Protein protoporpyrinogen oxidase (PPOX), 666
Protein quality control mechanisms, 102
Protein S, 349, 461, 1086
   biochemistry, 461–462
   deficiency, 1282
      clinical aspects, 1282
      laboratory diagnosis, 1282
      pathophysiology and genetics, 1282
      treatment, 1283
   function, 462
   gene structure and expression, 461
   regulation, 462
Protein tyrosine phosphatases, 153
Protein Z, 462
   biochemistry, 462
   deficiency, 1283
   function, 463
   gene structure and expression, 462
Protein-arginine deiminase type 4 (PAD4), 151
α$_1$-Proteinase inhibitor, 469
   biochemistry, 469
   function, 469
   gene structure and expression, 469
   schematic of, 469f
Proteinase inhibitors, 463–464
   α$_2$-Macroglobulin, 464
   tissue factor pathway inhibitor, 464–466
Proteins, 341, 362, 371, 786
   antigens, 330
Proteinuria, 1132, 2244, 2260, 2380
Proteolysis-targeting chimera (PROTAC), 1463
Proteolytic enzymes, 176
Proteostasis, 102
Prothrombin, 427, 1259, 1810–1811, 2259
   C20209T mutations, 1284
   deficiency, 1220
      clinical features, 1220
      inherited, 1220
      laboratory diagnosis, 1220
      pathophysiology, 1220
   fragment, 449
      schematic representation of pathways for prothrombin activation, 450f
   G20210A mutations, 1284
   mutations, 1284
      clinical aspects, 1284
      laboratory diagnosis, 1284
      pathophysiology and genetics, 1284
      treatment, 1284
Prothrombin complex concentrates (PCCs), 1220, 1227–1228, 1243, 1279
Prothrombin time (PT), 428, 1085, 1208, 1279, 1723
Prothrombinase, 436
Proto-oncogene (c-mpl), 371
Proton beam radiotherapy, 2137
Proton pump inhibitors, 961, 1859
Protoporphyria, 718
   diagnosis, 720
   follow-up, 720
   treatment, 720
Protoporphyrin, 98, 718
Protoporphyrinogen IX oxidase, 98
Protoporphyrinogen oxidase (PPOX), 704
Protospacer adjacent motif (PAM), 1548
Protozoal infections, thrombocytopenia associated with, 1158–1159
Prourokinase, 484
Proximal tubule (PT), 123
PRPF8 mutation, 1738
Pruritus, 1817, 1852, 2119
PRV1 gene, 1812
Pseudo Pelger-Huët anomaly, 1353
Pseudo Pelger-Huët cells, 146, 146f

Pseudo von Willebrand Disease, 1216–1217
Pseudoagglutination test, 573
Pseudocyanosis, 939
Pseudocysts, 1430
Pseudohemolytic transfusion reactions, 582
Pseudohemophilia, 1209
Pseudokinase domain, 375
Pseudomonas aeruginosa, 1332, 1404, 1470, 2094
Pseudoneutropenia, 1331
Pseudopodium, 157
Pseudotyping, transductional targeting by, 1524
Pseudouridylate synthase 1 (PUS1), 664
Pseudoxanthoma elasticum, 897, 921, 1167
Pseudoxanthoma elasticum-like syndrome (PXE-like syndrome), 897
Psoralen photochemotherapy, 2095
Psychogenic purpura, 1171–1172
   autoerythrocyte sensitization, 1171–1172
     Factitious purpura, 1172
     religious stigmata, 1172
PU. 1, 80, 168, 273
Pubertal delay, 2381
Public health programs, 883
Pulmonary amyloidosis, 2259
Pulmonary arteriovenous malformations (PAVMs), 1163
Pulmonary disorders, 1263
Pulmonary embolism (PE), 1276, 2188
   isolated subsegmental, 1305
   thrombolysis for, 1306
Pulmonary Embolism Prevention trial, 1290
Pulmonary function abnormalities, 851
Pulmonary function tests (PFTs), 844, 2119, 2306, 2378
Pulmonary hypertension (PHT), 838, 921, 937, 2378
Pulmonary infections, 1475–1479
Pulmonary problems, 904
Pulmonary venous hypertension (PVH), 850
Pulseless disease, 1262
Pure cutaneous histiocytosis, 1364
Pure red cell aplasia (PRCA), acquired, 1008
   ABO-incompatible stem cell transplantation, 1010
   anti-Epo antibody–associated pure red cell aplasia, 1013
   autoimmune disorders/collagen vascular disease, 1010
   classification of PRCA, 1009*t*
   clinical presentation, 1011
   drugs and chemicals, 1010, 1010*t*
   evaluation and treatment, 1011–1012
   hematologic malignancies, 1009
   immunosuppressive/immunomodulatory therapy, 1012–1013
   laboratory evaluation, 1011
   lymphoproliferative disorders, 1009
   myelodysplastic primary pure red cell aplasia, 1009
   nonthymic solid tumors, 1010
   parvovirus-induced pure red cell aplasia, 1009, 1013
   pregnancy, 1010
   primary acquired pure red cell aplasia, 1008
   pure red cell aplasia with infections other than parvovirus, 1010
   recombinant Epo-induced immune pure red cell aplasia, 1009
   refractory pure red cell aplasia, 1013
   thymoma-associated pure red cell aplasia, 1013
   transient erythroblastopenia of childhood (TEC), 1008–1009
Purine nucleoside analogs, 784, 2059–2062
Purine nucleotide metabolism
   abnormalities of, 763
   adenosine deaminase excess, 764
   adenylate kinase deficiency, 764–765
   in mature erythrocytes, 763*f*
   pyrimidine 5′ nucleotidase deficiency, 764
Purpura, 1158, 1162
   associated with infection, 1169
     acute febrile illness with petechiae, 1169
     hemorrhagic fever viruses, 1170
     papular-purpuric gloves and socks syndrome, 1169
     Rickettsial diseases, 1169–1170
     skin lesions of hands and feet associated with papular-purpuric gloves and socks syndrome, 1171*f*
   associated with skin diseases, 1171
     drug reactions, 1171
     pigmented purpuric dermatitis, 1171
   associated with vascular obstruction, 1170
     cholesterol embolization syndrome, 1171
     classification of bleeding disorders associated with vascular obstruction, 1171*t*
     cryofibrinogenemia, 1170–1171
     senile, 1167
Purpura fulminans, 1252
Purpuric religious stigmata, 1172
*Pus*1 gene, 665
Pyelonephritis
   acute, 2179
   chronic, 2179
Pyemia, 1694
Pyoderma gangrenosum, 1010
Pyridoxal 5′-phosphate (PLP), 657
Pyridoxine, 659, 662, 668
Pyrimidine 5′ nucleotidase deficiency, 763–764
Pyrimidine nucleotide metabolism
   abnormalities of, 763
   adenosine deaminase excess, 764
   adenylate kinase deficiency, 764–765
   in mature erythrocytes, 763*f*
   pyrimidine 5′ nucleotidase deficiency, 764
Pyroptosis, 150
Pyruvate kinase deficiency (PK deficiency), 756, 758
   biochemical genetics, 758–759
   clinical features, 759–760
   diagnosis, 760
   geographic distribution, 758
   pathophysiology, 759
   treatment, 760–761

Q

22q11 deletion syndrome, 1399
22q11.2 deletion syndrome (22q11DS), 1156, 1188–1189
14q32, translocations of, 2016
QT prolongation, 1797
Qualitative abnormalities, 1217
Qualitative detection methods, 1903
Qualitative PCR, 1791
Quality of life (QOL), 705, 1823, 2335, 2382
Quantitative detection methods, 1903
Quantitative polymerase chain reaction (qPCR), 980, 1791, 1900
Quantitative reverse transcription polymerase chain reaction (qRT-PCR), 2340
Quebec platelet disorder (QPD), 1182, 1196
Queensland tick typhus, 1170
Quinidine, 1109, 1262
Quinidine/Stibophen Type neoantigen mechanism, 785–786
Quinine, 1109, 1262
Quizartinib, 1648–1650

R

*RAB*27A gene, 1380
Rabbit antithymocyte globulin (r-ATG), 2322
Rac1, 179
Rac2 GTPase mutation, 1347
Rac2, 179
Raccoon eyes, 1162
*RACGAP*1 mutations, 1025
RAD21 protein, 1740
RAD51, 370
RAD51C gene, 978
Radiation chemotherapy, 2002
Radiation regimens, 2302
Radiation sensitive disorders, 1403
Radiation therapy (RT), 1629, 1694, 1706, 1831, 1962, 1999, 2064, 2128, 2133, 2218–2219
Radiation toxicity, 2128–2129
Radiation-containing HCT, 2320
Radiation-induced marrow aplasia, 2297
Radio-ulnar synostosis associated with amegakaryocytic thrombocytopenia (RUSAT), 368
Radioactive iodine (RAI), 1629
Radiofrequency conductivity, 2
Radioimmunoassays, 107
Radioimmunotherapy (RIT), 1502–1503
Radioisotopic synovectomy, 1232
Radionuclide bone scans, 2282
Radiotherapy, 1859, 2036, 2120–2121, 2126, 2138
Radixin (RDX), 2016
*RAG*1 gene, 1402
RAG1 mutations, 271
RAG1 proteins, 268–270
*RAG*2 gene, 1402
RAG2 mutations, 271
RAG2 proteins, 268–270
RAI. *See* Radioactive iodine (RAI)
RAN gene, 1912
Randomization, 1646
Randomized clinical trials (RCTs), 1063
RANK ligand, 218
RAR-related orphan receptor (ROR), 316
Rare bleeding disorders, 1221
Rare chemotherapy-resistant LSCs, 1632
Rare large B-cell lymphoma types, 1882, 1882–1883*t*
RAS-RAF-MEK-ERK pathway, 376
Rasburicase, 1992
Ravulizumab, 350, 352, 1004, 1145
Rb protein. *See* Retinoblastoma protein (Rb protein)
*RB*1 gene, 1610, 1912
RBM15, 370
RBM8A mutation, 1630
Reactive eosinophilias, 1836
Reactive nitrogen species, 225
Reactive oxygen species (ROS), 101, 151, 225, 363, 952, 1786
Reagin, 1260
Real-time PCR, 61
Real-time quantitative-PCR (RQ-PCR), 1614
Realgar-Indigo naturalis formula (RIF), 1732
$\alpha IIb\beta 3$ receptor and signaling mechanisms, 414–416
γ receptor chain (γc), 1401
Receptor for activating NF-κB (RANK), 237
$\alpha_2\beta_1$ receptor, 405
Receptors, 341
Recipient APCs, 334
Recipient platelets, 1114
RECK gene, 2050
Recognition unit, 338
Recombinant AAV (rAAV), 1529
Recombinant glycosylated prourokinase, 1302
Recombinant growth factors, 1412
Recombinant human activated factor VIIa (rFVIIa), 1228
Recombinant human C1-esterase (rhC1INH), 350, 352
Recombinant retroviral vectors, 1526
Recombination signal sequences (RSS), 268, 268*f*
RECQL4 gene, 1630
Red blood cell destruction, 1412
   erythrocyte survival, 619
   rate of carbon monoxide production, 619
   serum bilirubin, 618
   serum haptoglobin, 618–619
   serum LDH, 618
   signs of increased, 618
Red blood cell enzyme disorders
   abnormalities of purine and pyrimidine nucleotide metabolism, 763–765
   disorders of hexose monophosphate shunt and glutathione metabolism, 749
   genetic testing in evaluating disorders of glycolysis, 757–758
   glucose-6-phosphate dehydrogenase deficiency, 749–755
   glycolytic enzymes abnormalities, 756–757
   other glycolytic enzymopathies, 761–763
   overview of erythrocyte metabolism, 749
   pyruvate kinase deficiency, 758–761
   related disorders of HMP shunt and glutathione metabolism, 755–756
Red blood cell preservation and storage, 560
   anticoagulant/preservative solutions, 560
   changes in red cells during storage, 560
     biochemical changes, 561
     red cell 2, 3-diphosphoglycerate, 561
     structural changes, 560–561
   clinical implications of stored blood, 561
   frozen red cells, 561
   packed red cells *vs.* red cells in additive solutions, 560
   in vivo recovery of stored red cells, 561
   whole blood (WB), 560
Red blood cell transfusions, 566, 1641
   administration of blood, 574–575
   alloantibody to high-incidence antigens, 574
   clinical practice guidelines, 569
   drugs, 574
   indications for, 567
     adult patients, 568–569
     clinical trials of blood transfusion in adults, 568*t*
     pediatric patients, 567–568

Red blood cell transfusions (continued)
    pretransfusion testing of red cells, 570
        ABO grouping, 570t
        antibody identification tests, 572
        antiglobulin test, 572
        blood typing, 570–571
        compatibility testing process, 570
        media that enhance agglutination, 572
        significance of certain blood group antibodies, 571t
        testing for red cell antibodies, 571
    red cell autoantibodies, 573–574
        blood and plasma by ABO type, 573t
    red cell transfusion in specific settings, 569
        elective surgery, 569–570
        hemolytic anemias, 570
        hereditary red cell disorders, 570
        nutritional deficiencies, 570
        trauma, 569
    selection of red cells for transfusion, 572
        crossmatch, 573
        crossmatching problems, 573
        donor, 572
        recipient, 572
        type and screen, 573
        uncrossmatched blood for emergency transfusion, 573
    special considerations in neonatal transfusion, 574
Red blood cells (RBCs), 1, 66, 93, 540, 558, 600, 628, 656, 686, 726, 749, 770, 792, 821, 833, 857, 883, 936, 1008, 1411, 1049, 1070, 1747, 1808, 1823, 2056, 2325, 2371
    analysis, 38
    antigens and antibodies, 540
    assays for erythropoietin and erythropoietin levels in health and disease, 107
    blood smears of patients with hemoglobin Hb SS and Hb SC disease, 857f
    cell destruction, 121
    control of erythropoiesis, 102–107
    erythrocyte membranes and cytoskeleton, 108–112
    erythroid cells, 93–97
    erythropoiesis, 93
    extravascular hemoglobin degradation, 124–127
    fate of intravascular hemoglobin, 122–124
    hemoglobin and erythrocyte function, 112–121
    hemoglobin biosynthesis, 97–102
    IVIG-mediated hemolysis, 550
    limitations in use of, 601–602
    major RBC antigens, 540
        ABO blood group antigens, 541f
        Bombay and Para-Bombay, 542
        expected serologic reactions for, 541t
        expression of major RBC antigens on organs and tissues, 540–542
        important subtypes of blood group A and blood group B, 542t
        secretors, 542
        serology, 540
    mature RBC, 107
    minor RBC antigens and antibodies, 542
        antigen systems, 548
        autoantibodies, 548–549
        differences between ABO and lewis, 543f
        Duffy antigens and antibodies, 547
        I and i antigens and antibodies, 548
        International Society for Blood Transfusion Schematic of blood group systems, 544–545t
        Kell antigens and antibodies, 546
        Kidd antigens and antibodies, 546–547
        Lewis antigens and antibodies, 547
        MNS antigens and antibodies, 547
        P antigens and antibodies, 547
        prophylactic antigen matching in chronically transfused populations, 548
        relationship among ABO, P, and Ii blood group systems, 548f
        Rh antigens and antibodies, 542–546
        terminology used to describe Rh blood group antigens, 546t
    novel cancer drugs impact on transfusion compatibility testing, 550–552
    parameters, 2–4
        hematocrit (Hct), 2–3
        hemoglobin concentration, 3
        mean corpuscular hemoglobin (MCH), 3
        mean corpuscular hemoglobin concentration (MCHC), 3
        mean corpuscular volume (MCV), 3
        nucleated red blood cell counts, 4
        red cell count, 3
        red cell distribution width (RDW), 3–4
        reticulocyte counts, 4
    RBC antigens in hematopoietic stem cell transplantation, 549–550
    RBC transfusion independence after gene therapy for TDT, 2329f
    red blood cell antigens and solid organ transplantation, 550
    structural features, 107
        deformability, 108
        frequency distribution curve of erythrocyte volume, 107f
        normal mature erythrocyte, 107f
        shape and dimensions, 107
    use of genetic testing in blood bank, 549
Red cell distribution width (RDW), 3–4, 107, 600, 643, 656, 733, 1759
Red cell mass (RCM), 1070
Red cells, 733, 751, 763, 827
    additive, 898
    adenine nucleotide content, 764
    age, 752
    alloantibodies reacting with red cell antigens, 580
    anion transport, 730
    aplasia
        acquired pure red cell aplasia, 1008–1014
        Diamond-Blackfan anemia (DBA), 1014–1018
    count, 3
    damage by abnormal vascular surfaces, 1147–1149
    destruction, 936
    of different size, anemia associated with populations of, 605
    enzymopathies, 749
    folate, 959
    fragmentation, 828, 1148
    genotyping, 574
    glycolysis, 757
    integrity, 749
    membranes, 729, 891
        proteins, 729
    morphology, 739, 761
    PFK, 762
    PK, 761
    production, 610
    purine and pyrimidine enzyme disorders, 763
    sickling, 835
    size, 600
    sodium content, 741
    sparing/enhancing strategies, 1066
    underproduction, 604
Red pulp, 247–248
Reduced-intensity conditioning (RIC), 1503, 1748, 1832, 2035, 2126, 2203, 2272, 2297, 2335
Reductase deficiency, 1351
Reed-Sternberg cell (RS cell), 1872, 2040, 2116, 2133
Refractory anemia, 656, 1598
Refractory cytopenia of childhood (RCC), 1598
Regulated exocytosis, 196
Regulated upon Activation, Normal T cell Expressed and Secreted (RANTES), 172
Regulatory Factor X (RFX-5), 329
Regulatory receptors, 222–223
Regulatory T cells (Tregs), 298, 1404
Relative erythrocytosis, 1072–1073
Reliability of tests, 1
Religious stigmata, 1172
Remdesivir, 1478
Renal abnormalities, 805
Renal amyloidosis, 2258
Renal biopsy, 2379
Renal dialysis, 962
Renal disease, 830, 1036, 1809
Renal dysfunction, 2303
Renal failure, 2220–2221
Renal function impairment, 1142
Renal injury, 1144
Renal insufficiency, 2179–2181, 2239
    acute, 805
Renal manifestations of cryoglobulinemia, 2287
Renal replacement therapy, 1038–1039
Renal significance, monoclonal gammopathy of, 2170–2171
Renal system, 2144
Renal transplantation, 2258
Repetitive probes, 51
Replication-defective gene transfer vectors contribute to malignant transformation, 1542
Replication-defective vectors, 1524
Residual disease, detection of, 2056–2057
Resimmune, 1504, 2101
Reslizumab, 186
Resolving Infection in Neutropenia with Granulocytes trial (RING trial), 579, 1472
Respiratory burst, 159, 178–179
    assembly and activation of NADPH oxidase complex during, 179f
    disorders of, 1349–1352
Respiratory syncytial virus (RSV), 1478, 2308
Respiratory tract, 2246
Restriction enzyme digestion, 61
Restrictive lung disease, 2378
Reteplase (r-PA), 1302
Reticulated platelets, 5
Reticulin fibrosis, 1764, 1824
Reticulocyte counts, 1, 4
Reticulocyte enumeration, 38
Reticulocyte hemoglobin cellular content (RHCc), 604
Reticulocyte hemoglobin content (CHr), 604, 1034
Reticulocyte hemoglobin equivalent (RET-He), 604, 1034
Reticulocyte production index (RPI), 4
Reticulocytes, 8–9, 95, 95f, 822
Reticulocytopenia, 669, 780, 1632
Reticulocytosis, 620, 939
Reticuloendothelial system (RES), 208, 571
Retinoblastoma protein (Rb protein), 1910
Retinoic acid (RA), 1569
Retinoic acid receptor (RAR), 2096
Retinoic acid receptor-α gene (*RARα*), 1569, 1698, 1721
Retinoic acid response elements (RAREs), 1569
Retinoid X receptor (RXR), 413, 1569, 2096
Retinoids, 2096
Retroperitoneal hematomas, 1206, 1208
Retroviral vectors, 1538
γ-retroviral (γ-RV), 1526
Retroviridae, 1526
Retrovirus epidemiology donor iron status evaluation (RISE), 639
Revascularization surgery, 842
Reverse grouping, 570
Reverse transcriptase (RT), 1549
Reverse transcription polymerase chain reaction (RT-PCR), 1634, 1721, 1791, 1854
Reverse typing, 570
Reversible permeability pathways, 835–836
Revised European American Lymphoma (REAL) classification, 1869, 1943
Revised International Prognostic Scoring System (IPSS-R), 1738, 2337
Revised International Staging System (R-ISS), 2181
Revised IPI (R-IPI), 1955
rFVIIa. *See* Recombinant activated factor VII (rFVIIa); Recombinant human activated factor VIIa (rFVIIa)
RFX-5. *See* Regulatory Factor X (RFX-5)
Rh antigens and antibodies, 542–546
Rh hemolytic disease, 1060–1061
Rh-associated glycoprotein (RhAG), 742
*RH*30, 742
Rhabdomyolysis, 2096
RhAG. *See* Rh-associated glycoprotein (RhAG)
rhC1INH. *See* Recombinant human C1-esterase (rhC1INH)
RHCc. *See* Reticulocyte hemoglobin cellular content (RHCc)
RHCE genes, 543, 549
RHCE variants, 548
RHD genes, 543, 549
RheothRx. *See* Poloxamer-188
rhEpo, 1036–1038
Rheumatoid arthritis (RA), 330, 1010, 1337, 1950, 2172
Rhizomucor, 1477
Rhizopus, 1477
RHOA G17V mutations, 1886
RHOA mutation, 1929
Rhodobacter capsulatus, 660

Ribonucleic acid (RNA), 833, 1738
Ribose phosphate pyrophosphate (PRPP), 764
Ribosomal RNA, 764
Ribosomes, 749
Richter syndrome (RS), 1961, 2023
    Hodgkin lymphoma (HL), 2040
    management of Richter syndrome and transformations, 2039
    Richter syndrome, 2039–2040
Rickets-like bone abnormalities, 905
Rickettsial diseases, 1169–1170
Rickettsial infection, 1169
Rifampin, 1109
RIG-I-like receptors (RLRs), 223
Right ventricular dysfunction, 900
Rilpivirine (RPV), 1410
Ring sideroblasts, 614, 656
Ring sideroblasts as MDS with ring sideroblasts and multilineage dysplasia (RCMD-RS//MDS-RS-MLD), 666
Risk organ disease, 1366
Risk-adapted therapy, 1614
Risk-stratified approach, 1113
Ristocetin, 1149
    cofactor activity, 458, 1213–1214
Ristocetin–induced platelet aggregation (RIPA), 1213–1214
Ritonavir (RTV), 1410
Rituximab, 352, 778, 783, 1013, 1106–1107, 1133–1134, 1139, 1258, 1429, 1500, 1621, 1680, 1949, 1962–1963, 1966–1967, 1970, 2028–2030, 2032, 2063, 2253, 2270
    enhancing response by repeating treatment with purine nucleoside analog or adding rituximab, 2063
    maintenance, 1958
    as single agent, 2270
    therapy, 2289
    treatment, 1103
Rituximab plus CHOP (R-CHOP), 1500, 1966
Rivaroxaban, 1300
RNA expression studies, 2157
RNA interference (RNAi), 706
RNA polymerase, 887
RNA processing, 887
RNA sequencing (RNA-seq), 66, 1578
RNA-splicing machinery, 1738
Rocky Mountain spotted fever, 1170
Roentgen irradiation of spleen, 895
Rogers syndrome, 665
Role of FDG-PET imaging in clinical stages IA/IIA Hodgkin disease (RAPID), 2121
Rolling, 171
Romanowsky stains, 6
Rombocytosis, reactive, 1175–1176
Romidepsin, 2099
Romiplostim, 378, 1746
roPEG-IFN. *See* Ropeginterferon-Alfa-2b-njft (roPEG-IFN)
Ropeginterferon-Alfa-2b-njft (roPEG-IFN), 1815
Rosai-Dorfman disease (RDD), 1380, 1380*f*
Rotational thromboelastometry (ROTEM), 1266
Rouleaux, 8
RP genes, 1014
*RPL*10, 1014
*RPL*11 genes, 1015
*RPL*22, 1014
*RPL*23A, 1014
*RPL*5 genes, 1014–1015
*RPS*15, 1014
*RPS*19 gene, 1015
*RPS*24 gene, 1015
Rubella, congenital, 1154
Ruminants, 948
Runner anemia, 640
Runt homology domain (RHD), 1570
Runt-related transcription factor 1 (RUNX1), 71–72, 367–368, 1153, 1194, 1696
*RUNX*1 gene, 5, 370, 1570, 1630, 1633, 1637, 1857
*RUNX*1 mutation, 1578, 1600, 1630, 1739, 1775, 1849, 1854, 2336
*RUNX*1/*CEPB*-alpha gene, 1697
RUNX1::RUNX1T1 protein, 1570
*RUNX*1T1 gene, 1570
Russell bodies, 2178
Russell viper (*Daboia russelli*), 826
Ruxolitinib, 1459, 1769, 1830–1831, 1844, 2305

S

S-adenosylhomocysteine, 958
S-nitrosothiols (SNOs), 117
Saccharomyces cerevisiae, 660
Saline washing, 564
Salmonella, 846, 1350, 1438, 2358
Salsalate, 1232
Salvage hematopoietic stem cell transplant, 2202
Salvage therapy, 2124
    ALL, 1620
        additional agents/novel therapies, 1621–1622
        antibodies, 1621
        CD19-directed chimeric antigen receptor T-cell therapy, 1622
        chemotherapy, 1621
        treatment outcome in elderly patients with ALL, 1620*t*
    salvage combination chemotherapy regimens utilized for relapsed or refractory Hodgkin
Sample core stream, 18
Sampling methods and limitations, 1445
    bone marrow aspirate and biopsy, 1445
    fine-needle aspirate and core biopsy, 1445
    laparoscopic biopsy, 1445
    open biopsy, 1445
    peripheral blood, 1445
Sand fly (*Phlebotomus*), 824
Sanger sequence–based typing, 323
Sanger sequencing, 61, 64*f*
Sanger-based methods, 1907
SBDS gene, 955, 985, 1335
SBDS mutations, 984
Scavenger receptors, 222, 223*f*
Scedosporium spp., 1481
Schistocyte-like cells, 1132
Schistocytes, 623
Schistosoma haematobium, 639
Schistosoma mansoni, 639
Schlafen 14 (SLFN14), 1191
Schnitzler syndrome, 2146, 2171, 2281–2283
    clinical features, 2281–2282
    differential diagnosis, 2282
    histopathology, 2283
    imaging abnormalities, 2282
    laboratory features, 2282
    pathophysiology, 2282
    prognosis and long-term complications, 2283
    therapy, 2283
Schulman-Upshaw syndrome, 1137
Scid-repopulating cells (SRCs), 1537
Scientific and Standardization Committee on Genetics in Thrombosis and Haemostasis, The, 1183
Scientific Subcommittee on Standards of the International Society of Thrombosis and Haemostasis, The, 1207
Scientific Working Group on Thrombocytopenias, 1197
Sclerodermatous skin changes (Scl skin changes), 2361
Scleromyxedema, 2146, 2283
    cutaneous manifestations, 2283
    differential diagnosis, 2283
    extracutaneous features, 2283
    pathogenesis, 2283–2284
    therapy, 2284
Sclerosing angiomatoid nodular transformation (SANT), 1439
Sclerotic bone lesions, 2279
Scoring systems, 1133, 1213
Scott syndrome, 1195
Screening coagulation tests, 1217
Screening method, 1446
Screening programs, 867
Screening tests, 755, 1213
    of hemostasis and coagulation, 1207
    laboratory findings in common inherited coagulation disorders, 1207*t*
Scrotal ecchymosis, 1162
*SDC*3 gene, 2050
Sebastian syndrome, 1154, 1354
SEC23B gene, 1024
SEC23B hypomorphic genotypes, 1024
Second-generation HSC gene therapy trials, 1540–1541
    approaches to decrease risk of insertional mutagenesis, 1542–1543
    chronic granulomatous disease (CGD), 1541
    lessons from, 1541
    replication-defective gene transfer vectors contribute to malignant transformation, 1542
    severe combined immunodeficiency disease (SCID), 1540–1541
    Wiskott-Aldrich syndrome (WAS), 1541
Secondary AML (s-AML), 1566, 1706, 2336
Secondary amyloidosis, 2260
Secondary autoimmune hemolytic anemia, 781
Secondary autoimmune thrombocytopenic purpura, 1109
    autoimmune thrombocytopenia in hepatitis C, 1111
    autoimmune thrombocytopenia in systemic lupus erythematosus, 1110
    autoimmune thrombocytopenia secondary to drugs, 1109–1110
    immune thrombocytopenia in other disorders, 1111
Secondary cold agglutinin disease, 776–777, 779
Secondary granule formation, 1347
Secondary type mutations, 1568
Secreted antibodies, 280
Secreted exosomes, 334
Secretion of antidiuretic hormone (SIADH), 987
Secretory functions of neutrophil, 160–161
Secretory IgA (sIgA), 175
Secretory leukocyte protease inhibitor (SLPI), 1334
Secretory phospholipase A2 (sPLA$_2$), 838
Secretory vesicles, 143–145, 173
L-Selectin, 79, 154
Selectins, 154, 155*f*
Selective immunoglobulin A deficiency, 1398
Selective inhibitors of nuclear export (SINE), 711
Selenium (Se), 756
Self-inactivating feature (SIN feature), 1527
Self-major histocompatibility complex (Self-MHC), 770
Self-renewal, 69
Self-renewing leukemia-initiating cells, 1695
Self-tolerance, 770
Selinexor, 1462, 2184, 2213
Semiliquid aspirate material, 1322
Senicapoc, 864
Sensitive next-generation sequencing, 999
Sentinel cytogenetic alterations, 1670–1671
Septic transfusion reactions, 589
Sequence-specific oligonucleotide probes (SSO probes), 323
Sequence-specific priming (SSP), 323
Sequencing, 1328
Serial analysis, 1133
Serial transplantation assay, 78
Serine protease inhibitor superfamily (SERPIN), 466–467
    α$_1$-Proteinase inhibitor, 469
    antithrombin, 467–468
    C1 esterase inhibitor, 469–470
    heparin cofactor II, 468–469
    inhibitors, 467*t*
    protein C inhibitor, 470–471
Serious Hazards of Transfusion (SHOT), 585
Serologic microcytotoxicity techniques, 323
Serologic techniques, 776
Seronegative antiphospholipid-antibody syndrome, 1264
Seronegative erosive arthritis, 2172
Seronegative hepatitis, 997
Serotonin, 362–363
Serotype O157:H7, 1139
Serratia, 1350
Serratia marcescens, 1396
Serum, 2146
Serum M-protein, 2281–2282
Serum protease domain, 338–339
Serum protein electrophoresis, 2170
Serum prothrombin conversion accelerator deficiency, 1221
Serum Response Factor (SRF), 369, 1948
Serum sickness, 1169
*SETBP*1 gene, 1838, 1857
*SETBP*1 mutation, 1764
*SETD*1B gene, 1928
*SETD*2 genes, 1677
Severe acute respiratory syndrome coronavirus-2 (SARS-CoV-2), 352, 777, 1158, 1478, 2021
Severe combined immunodeficiency disease (SCID), 75, 269, 271, 1393, 1400, 1536, 1540, 2314, 2371
    caused by metabolic defects, 1402
        adenosine deaminase (ADA), 1402
        purine nucleotide phosphorylase–deficient SCID (PNP–deficient SCID), 1402

Severe combined immunodeficiency disease (SCID) *(continued)*
　CD3 component and CD45-deficient SCID, 1401
　common molecular causes, 2315t
　defects in antigen presentation by MHC I or MHC II, 1401–1402
　first clinical successes, 1540
　insertional mutagenesis in patient with ADA-SCID treated by HSC gene therapy, 1541
　insertional mutagenesis in SCID-X1 patients treated by HSC gene therapy, 1540–1541
　interleukin-7 receptor–deficient SCID, 1402
　JAK3-deficient SCID, 1402
　molecular defects associated with specific cellular phenotypes in SCID, 1400t
　SCID caused by defective cytokine signaling in T cells, 1401
　SCID caused by defective T-cell receptor structure, function, or activation, 1401
　SCID caused by defects in DNA recombination, 1402
　X-linked SCID, 1401
　Zap-70 and CD45-deficient SCID, 1401
Severe combined immunodeficiency syndromes, treatment of, 1402–1403
Severe congenital neutropenia (SCN), 1332–1334, 1395
Severity, determinants of, 856–857
Sex hormone, 2331
Sézary syndrome (SS), 2072
　classification of, 2076
　clinical presentation, 2076
　diagnostic evaluation, 2076
　　blood involvement, 2080–2081
　　bone marrow involvement, 2080
　　cutaneous features of MF/SS, 2077–2079
　　cutaneous phases of mycosis fungoides, 2077f
　　extracutaneous MF/SS, 2079–2080
　　extracutaneous sites, 2080
　　frozen section immunohistochemistry of cutaneous plaque, 2081f
　　histopathology, 2077
　　immunophenotyping studies, 2081–2082
　　large cell transformation of MF/SS, 2079
　　lymph node pathology, 2080
　　Sézary syndrome, 2081f
　　tissue handling, 2076–2077
　differential diagnosis, 2082
　　benign conditions, 2082–2083
　　CD30+ lymphoproliferative diseases, 2083–2085
　　hematopoietic neoplasms with similar cutaneous presentations, 2089–2090
　　primary cutaneous T-cell lymphomas, 2085–2089
　early CTCL, 2073f
　epidemiology, 2075–2076
　historical perspective and pathophysiology, 2072
　　clinical description, 2072
　　histopathology, 2072
　　immunology, 2072–2074
　　molecular genetics, 2074–2075
　late CTCL, 2073f
　membrane proteins of malignant T cell, 2073f
　NCI-VA grading scheme for lymph node histology in CTCL, 2080t
　prognosis, 2093–2094
　staging, 2090–2091
　　bone marrow, 2093
　　imaging, 2091–2092
　　ISCL/EORTC staging of mycosis Fungoides/Sézary syndrome, 2091t
　　lymph nodes, 2092–2093
　　recommended initial staging evaluation of mycosis Fungoides/Sézary syndrome, 2092t
　therapy, 2094
　　combined-modality therapy, 2100–2101
　　electron beam radiotherapy and photon beam irradiation, 2097–2098
　　extracorporeal photochemotherapy (EC), 2098
　　hematopoietic stem cell transplantation (HCT), 2102
　　immunotherapy, 2101–2102
　　interferons (IFNs), 2096–2097
　　MF/SS treatment algorithm, 2094f
　　photopheresis photochemotherapy, 2098
　　phototherapy, 2095–2096
　　retinoids, 2096
　　systemic chemotherapy, 2098–2100
　　topical chemotherapy, 2094–2095

SF3B1 gene, 1568, 1630, 1638, 1840, 1850, 1857
SF3B1 mutation, 666, 1578, 1738, 1743, 1745, 1755–1756, 1763, 1913, 2025
SF3B1 spliceosome gene, 1777
SH2D1A gene, 1380
Sheath fluid, 18
Shiga toxin molecule, 1139
Shiga toxin–associated hemolytic-uremic syndrome (STX-HUS), 351, 1123, 1139–1141
　clinical presentation, 1140
　diagnosis, management, and prognosis, 1140–1141
　etiology, 1139
　laboratory findings, 1140
　pathology, 1139
　pathophysiology, 1139–1140
　pathophysiology of STX-HUS, 1140f
Shiga toxin–associated HUS (STEC HUS), 351
Shiga toxin–producing *Escherichia coli* (STEC), 1139
Shigella dysenteriae serotype I, 1139
SHM. *See* Somatic hypermutation (SHM)
Shock, 1248
Short disease-free (DFS), 1628
Short telomere syndromes (STSs), 955
Short-term anticoagulation, 1291
Short-term reconstitution HSC (ST-HSC), 356
Shortened erythrocyte survival, 1035
Shwachman-Bodian-Diamond syndrome (SBDS), 984, 1333
Shwachman-Diamond syndrome (SBDS), 955, 974, 984, 1014, 1333, 1630, 1697, 1737, 1760
　clinical features, 984
　diagnostic testing, 984
　differential diagnosis, 984
　laboratory findings, 984–985
　pathophysiology, 985
　supportive care, 985
　treatment, 985
Sialoglycoproteins, 110
Sick euthyroid syndrome (SES), 2381
Sickle cell anemia (SCA), 622, 838–866, 1430
　clinical features, 839
　　acute events, 839
　　chronic organ damage, 847–856
　　hemoglobin concentration as function of age in infants with sickle cell anemia, 839f
　diagnosis, 858
　　neonatal diagnosis, 859–860, 859f
　　newborn and adult hemoglobin fractionation patterns of sickle hemoglobinopathies, 848f
　　prenatal diagnosis, 860
　epidemiology, 833
　　global distributions of Hb S and malaria, 835f
　　prevalence of sickle cell trait and disease, 834t
　laboratory features, 857
　　laboratory tests, 858
　　platelets and coagulation, 858
　　red blood cells, 857
　　white blood cells, 857
　pathophysiology, 833
　　molecular basis of sickling, 833–837
　　pathogenesis of vaso-occlusion, 838
　prognosis, 856–857
　　determinants of severity, 856–857
　sickle cell trait, 866–868
　treatment, 860
　　blood transfusion, 860
　　bone marrow transplantation, 865–866
　　gene therapy, 866
　　pharmacotherapy, 861–863
　　preventive measures, 860
Sickle cell disease (SCD), 833, 857–858, 1544–1545, 2314, 2371
　acute myelogenous leukemia after gene therapy, 2330
　cumulative incidence of graft failure/rejection, 2325f
　gene and genomic therapies for hemoglobin disorders, 2328–2330
　hematopoietic stem cell transplantation for, 2325
　HLA-haploidentical BMT and gene therapy for hemoglobin disorders, 2328
　HLA-ID Sibling HCT for SCD, 2325–2326
　myeloablative HCT for SCD, 2326–2328
　patients, 864
　reduced toxicity HCT for SCD, 2328
Sickle cells
　crisis, 839
　rheology of, 837

　trait, 866
　　clinical features, 866–867
　　diagnosis, 867
　　screening programs, 867
　　sickling syndromes, 867–868
　transgenic mice, 838
Sickle Hb (Hb S), 833
Sickle hepatopathy, 852
Sickle red cells, 836
Sickled red cell membranes, 837
Sickling
　erythrocytes from patient with sickle cell anemia examined with scanning electron microscopy, 836f
　kinetics of, 834–835
　membrane alterations, 835
　　adhesion, 836
　　dehydration, 835–836
　　pathogenetic role of hemolysis, 837–838
　　rheology of sickle cells, 837
　molecular basis of, 833
　physiologic determinants of polymerization, 834
　red cell sickling, 835
　structure of hemoglobin S polymer, 834
　electron photomicrographs of cell-free pellets of deoxyhemoglobin S, 837
Sickling phenomenon, 859
Sickling syndromes, 847, 867
　hemoglobin C disorders, 869
　hemoglobin S/hereditary persistence of fetal hemoglobin, 868
　hemoglobin SC disease, 867
　hemoglobin SD disease, 868
　hemoglobin SE disease, 868
　hemoglobin SO-Arab disease, 868–869
　hemoglobin Sβ-Thalassemia, 868
Sickling-induced pathway, 836
Side scatter (SS), 18
Sideroblastic anemias (SAs), 614, 656, 1028, 1050
　acquired clonal sideroblastic anemia, 666–668
　　clinical and laboratory features, 667, 667f
　　etiology and pathogenesis, 666–667
　　natural history, 667–668
　　treatment, 668, 668f
　classification of, 648t
　clinical and laboratory features of XLSA and SLC25A38 deficiency, 662
　congenital sideroblastic anemias, 659–666
　　animal models of, 665
　　animal models of congenital sideroblastic anemia, 665–666
　　with B-cell immunodeficiency, fevers, and developmental delay, 664
　　genetic and hematologic features of, 660t
　　mitochondrial myopathy, lactic acidosis, and sideroblastic anemia and related phenotypes, 664–665
　　nonsyndromic congenital sideroblastic anemias, 659–664
　　Pearson marrow-pancreas syndrome, 664
　　syndromic congenital sideroblastic anemias, 664
　　thiamine-responsive megaloblastic anemia, 665
　　undefined congenital sideroblastic anemia, 665
　in erythropoietic protoporphyria, 661–662
　heme synthesis in erythroid cells, 656–659
　historical aspects, 656
　inheritance patterns, molecular basis, and pathogenesis, 659
　　iron-sulfur cluster biogenesis deficiency, 661
　　mitochondrial carrier protein SLC25A38 deficiency, 661
　　sideroblastic anemia in erythropoietic protoporphyria, 661–662
　　X-linked sideroblastic anemia, 659–661
　morphologic features of, 647f
　and related phenotypes, 664–665
　reversible sideroblastic anemias, 668–670
　treatment and prognosis, 662–664
　　dimorphic red cell distribution in female patient, 664f
　　iron overload in congenital sideroblastic anemia, 663f
Sideroblasts, 634
Siderocytes, 634
Sideroflexin 1 (*Sfxn1*), 665

sIg. *See* Surface immunoglobulin (sIg)
sIgA. *See* Secretory IgA (sIgA)
Siglecs, 222
Signal regulatory protein alpha (SIRPA), 222–223
Signal transducer and activator of transcription 3 gene (*STAT*3 gene), 1346, 1500
Signal transducer and activator of transcription 5 (STAT5), 1786
Signal transduction inhibitors (STI), 1457–1458
    ABL kinase inhibitors, 1458
    BTK inhibitors, 1458–1459
    FLT3 inhibitors (FLT3i), 1460
    isocitrate dehydrogenase1 and 2 inhibitors (IDH 1 and 2 inhibitors), 1460
    JAK inhibitors, 1459–1460
    phosphatidylinositol 3-kinases inhibitors (PI3K inhibitors), 1459
    therapeutic targeting of intracellular signaling pathways, 1457f
Signal transduction proteins
    calcium- and DAG-regulated guanine exchange factor-1 defect (CalDAG-GEFI) defect, 1193
    cyclooxygenase-1 defect, 1193
    cytosolic phospholipase $A_{2\alpha}$ defect (cPLA$_{2\alpha}$ defect), 1192–1193
    defects of, 1192
    G-protein defects, 1192
    leukocyte adhesion deficiency-III (LAD-III), 1193
    phospholipase C-β2 (PLC-β$_2$), 1193
    Protein Kinase A Defect, 1193–1194
    Src defect, 1193
    thromboxane synthase defect, 1193
Signal-transducing activator of transcription 5 pathway (STAT5 pathway), 104–105
Signaling, cytokine regulation of, 371–379
Signaling cascade in megakaryocytes, 375–377
Signaling lymphocyte activating molecule family receptors (SFRs), 313
Signaling lymphocyte activation molecule (SLAM), 73, 313, 1389
Signaling lymphocyte activation molecule-associated protein (SLAM-SAP), 1389
Signaling-lymphocytic activation-molecule (SLAMF7), 1456
Sildenafil, 845, 852
Silent Cerebral Infarct Transfusion trial, The, 843
Silk, 2238
Simple mixing techniques, 1256
Simple necrosis, 150
Simpler ELISA-based methods, 1213
Single autologous stem cell transplantation, 2199–2201
Single cell transcriptomics, 212
Single coagulation factors, acquired deficiencies of, 1266–1267
Single glycoproteins, 339
Single molecule real-time (SMRT), 1576
Single nucleotide mutations, 885
Single nucleotide substitutions, 888
Single-agent and combination chemotherapy, 2098
Single-cell RNA sequencing (scRNA-seq), 181
Single-chain variable fragment (scFv), 1508
Single-chain u-PA (scu-PA), 484
Single-copy probes, 51
Single-lineage progenitors, 76–77
Single-nucleotide polymorphisms (SNPs), 54, 330, 356, 680, 842, 885, 1141, 1331, 1564, 1710, 1946, 2012, 2051, 2357
Single-nucleotide variants (SNVs), 58, 61, 1193, 1758, 1907
Single-platform technology (SPT), 42
Single-site LCH, 1376
Single-stranded DNA (ssDNA), 1529
Sinus histiocytosis, 1380
Sinus infections, 1480
Sinusoidal obstruction syndrome (SOS), 2302
Sirolimus, 782, 784, 1013, 2359
Sitosterolemia, 742
Sjögren syndrome (SS), 1010, 1168, 1952
Skeletal abnormalities, 618
Skeletal lesions, 1367
Skeletal system, 643, 2144
Skin, 1954, 2022, 2298, 2357–2358
    biopsy, 1379
    bleeding into, 1080
    cancers, 2022, 2094
    capillaries, 1809

    changes, 602–603, 2278–2279
    conditions, 2146
    diseases, 2093
    disorders, 1953
    hyperpigmentation, 662
    infections, 1480
    involvement, 1367, 2055
    lesions, 712, 1165, 1172, 2055
    manifestations, 2283
    membranes, 1101, 1809
    tumors, 2075
    ulcers, 855
SLAM-associated protein (SAP), 313
Slayter model of fibrinogen, 475
*SLC*19A2 gene, 665
SLC25A38 deficiency, clinical and laboratory features of, 662
*SLC*29A2 gene, 1912
*SLC*40A1 p. Q248H, 693
Sleep disorders, 852
Sleep-disordered breathing, 852
Sleeping Beauty transposon. (SB transposon), 1526
Sliding process, 363
Slight leukocytosis, 142
Slow early responders (SERs), 2136
Small B lymphocytic lymphoma, 1950, 1961
Small cephalohematomas, 1082
Small circular vectors, 1526
Small granules, 173
Small insertion/deletion detection, 63–64
Small intestinal angiodysplastic lesions, 1165
Small intestinal bacterial overgrowth, 960
Small lymphocytic lymphoma (SLL), 1511, 1866, 1872, 1903, 2010, 2150
    genetics, 1873
    immunophenotype, 1873
    morphology, 1872
        chronic lymphocytic leukemia/small lymphocytic lymphoma, 1873f
Small Maf proteins (sMaf), 635
Small noncoding RNAs, 370
Small nuclear ribonucleoproteins (snRNPs), 1578
Small vessel disease, 828–829
Small-field megavoltage photon beam irradiation, 2097–2098
Small-vessel thrombosis, 805
*SMARCA*4 gene, 1912
*SMARCB*1 mutation, 1931
SMC1A protein, 1740
SMC3 protein, 1740
Smoking, 1629
Smooth muscle cells, 531
Smooth muscle myosin heavy-chain protein (SMMHC), 1570
Smudge cells, 2020
Snake bites, 826–827
Snake venoms. 1248
Snakebite, 1253
SNaPshot Genotyping, 61, 63f
Social determinants of health (SDOH), 1685
Society for Hematopathology, 1446
Socks syndrome, 1169
Sodium, 742
Sodium dodecyl sulfate (SDS), 110
Sodium dodecyl sulfate–polyacrylamide gel electrophoresis (SDS-PAGE), 434, 1024
Sodium glucose cotransporter-2 (SGLT-2), 1072
Soft tissues
    bleeding into, 1080
    infections, 1480
    swelling, 1144
Solar purpura, 1167
Solid organ transplantation (SOT), 550, 1388, 1996
Solid tumors, 2022, 2323, 2331
Solid-phase immunobinding assays, 40
Solid-phase tests, 327
Solitary extramedullary plasmacytoma, 2223
Solitary plasmacytoma, 2145, 2175
Solitary plasmacytoma of bone, 2222–2223
Soluble agonists
    α$_2$-Adrenergic receptors and epinephrine, 409
    arachidonic acid, thromboxane A$_2$, and thromboxane receptors, 409–410
    coordination between platelet adhesion events and soluble agonist stimulation in thrombus growth, 410

    platelet activation by, 409
Soluble fms-like tyrosine kinase-1 (sFlt-1), 1049
Soluble forms of MICA or MICB (sMICA/sMICB), 329
Soluble platelet agonists, 1189
Soluble proteins, 362
Soluble stimuli, 176–177
Soluble transferrin receptors (sTfR), 613, 633, 643, 1034
Solvent/detergent-treated plasma (S/D plasma), 564
Solvents and detergents (S/D), 563
Somatic cell gene therapy, 1522
Somatic hypermutation (SHM), 279, 1901, 1903–1905, 1913, 2152
Somatic mosaicism, 974
Somatic *MPLW*515*L/K* mutation, 1177
Somatic mutations in *CALR* gene, 1177
Somatic single-nucleotide variant, 63–64
Somatic variants
    adult T-cell leukemia/lymphoma, 1931
    anaplastic large cell lymphoma, ALK positive and ALK negative, 1927
    angioimmunoblastic T-cell lymphoma, 1929
    Burkitt lymphoma, 1925
    chronic lymphocytic leukemia/small lymphocytic lymphoma, 1913
    diffuse large B-cell lymphoma and other high-grade B-cell lymphomas, 1922
    enteropathy-associated T-cell lymphoma, 1931
    extranodal marginal zone lymphoma, 1916
    follicular lymphoma, 1920
    hairy cell leukemia, 1919
    lymphoplasmacytic lymphoma/Waldenström macroglobulinemia, 1918
    mantle cell lymphoma, 1912
    monomorphic epitheliotropic intestinal T-cell lymphoma, 1931
    mucosa-associated lymphoid tissue lymphoma, 1916
    peripheral T-cell lymphoma, not otherwise specified, 1928
    splenic marginal zone lymphoma, 1917
    T-cell large granular lymphocytic leukemia, 1930
    T-prolymphocytic leukemia, 1930
Sonography, 1208
Sorafenib, 1649
Southern blot techniques, 14
Southwest Oncology Group (SWOG), 2184
Spacer (Spa), 1126
Sparing Conversion to Abnormal TCD Elevation (SCATE), 843
Special stains, 12
    acid phosphatase, 13
    cytochemical stains, 12
    immunocytochemical stains, 13–14
    iron, 13
    leukocyte alkaline phosphatase (LAP), 13
    myeloperoxidase, 12
    nonspecific esterase stains, 13
    periodic acid-Schiff stain (PAS stain), 13
    specific (naphthol AS-D chloroacetate) esterase stain, 13
    Sudan black B stains, 12–13
    terminal deoxynucleotidyl transferase (TdT), 13
    toluidine blue, 13
Specific (naphthol AS-D chloroacetate) esterase stain, 13
Specific antibody deficiency, 1398
Specific granule deficiency (SGD), 1347
Specific granules, 143
Specimen collection, 1
Specimens for hematologic cytogenetic analysis, 48–49
Spectral flow cytometry, 1326
Spectral karyotyping, 51
Spectrin, 726
    abnormalities, 737
        glycophorin C deficiency, 738
        protein 4. 1R defects, 737–738
    deficiency, 729–730
    proteins, 111
    spectrin/actin/myosin cytoskeleton, 364
    tetramers, 737
α-spectrin, 729, 737
αβ-Spectrin, 726
SPEN mutation, 1931
Spent phase of PV, 1767
Spherocytes, 8, 620, 733
Spherocytosis, 729
Sphingomyelin, 108, 726
Sphingomyelinase gene (*SMPD*1 gene), 1359

Sphingosine kinase 2 (Sphk2), 376
Sphingosine-1 phosphate (S1P), 238, 376
Spider bites, 825–826
Spinal compression fractures, 2239
Spinal cord compression, 1954, 2220
Spinner systems, 4
Spirochetes, 8
sPLA2, 858
Splanchnic venous thrombosis (SVT), 1809
Spleen, 213–214, 246, 247f, 1875
   complications of splenectomy, 1433
      infection risk postsplenectomy, 1434
      overwhelming postsplenectomy infection (OPSI), 1434–1435
   development and anatomy, 1423
      benign anatomic variants, 1424–1425
      gross anatomy, 1423
      innervations, 1424
      location and relationships, 1423, 1423f
      lymphatics, 1424
      marginal zone, 1425, 1425f
      microscopic anatomy, 1425
      microvasculature, 1425
      red pulp, 1425
      vascular supply, 1424
      white pulp, 1425
   involvement, 2056
   malignant tumors of, 1430
   ontogeny, 248
   partial embolization, 908
   primary tumors, 1430
   red pulp, 247–248
   role of, 730
      splenic conditioning, 731
      splenic entrapment, 731
   splenectomy, 1433
   splenic disorders and indications for splenectomy, 1428–1433
   splenic function, 1426–1428
   white pulp, 246–247
Spleen colony-forming units (CFUs-S), 72
Spleen focus-forming virus (SFFV), 1527
Spleen organizer (SPo), 248
Spleen tyrosine kinase (SYK), 1929, 2002, 2012
Splenectomy, 662, 734–735, 740, 760–761, 764, 779, 783, 813, 895, 907–908, 1013, 1021, 1106, 1134, 1433, 1831, 2036, 2059
   complications of, 1433–1435
   cumulative proportion of splenectomy-free survival, 907f
   minimally invasive splenectomy, 1433
   open splenectomy, 1433
   splenic disorders and indications for, 1428–1433
   surgical, 846
Splenic abscess, 1432
Splenic artery, 1424
   approaches, 1425
Splenic cords, 1425
Splenic cysts, 1430, 1437
Splenic diffuse red pulp lymphoma (SDRPL), 2056, 2058
Splenic disorders and indications for splenectomy, 1428
Splenic entrapment, 731
Splenic function, 1426
   cellular reservoir function, 1427–1428
   circulating blood filtration, 1426
   erythropoietic function, 1428
   immune function, 1426
   iron metabolism, 1428
Splenic hamartomas, 1441
Splenic injury, 1432
Splenic marginal zone lymphoma (SMZL), 33, 1439, 1874–1875, 1910, 1917–1918, 1953, 2058
   differential diagnosis of splenic small B cell lymphomas, 1875t
   genetics, 1875
   guidelines for molecular testing in, 1917–1918
   immunophenotype, 1875
   morphology, 185
Splenic pool, 1157
Splenic preservation, 1432
Splenic rupture, 2055, 2244
Splenic sequestration, 1040
   acute, 845–846
Splenic sinuses, 1425
Splenic tissue, 1425
   autotransplantation of, 1435

Splenomas. See Splenic hamartomas
Splenomegaly, 617, 731–732, 741, 921, 1020, 1428, 1437, 1441, 1809, 1823, 1853, 2118
   abdominal trauma and splenic injury, 1432
      AAST Grades of splenic injury, 1432t
   classification of splenomegaly by mechanism, 1429t
   delayed splenic rupture, 1433
   etiology of splenomegaly and cytopenia in selected disease states, 1429t
   Felty syndrome, 1432
   in HCL, 2053
   hereditary anemias, 1429–1430
   Hodgkin lymphoma, 1430
   immune thrombocytopenic purpura (ITP), 1428
   leukemia, 1430
   lymphoma, 1430
   malignant tumors of spleen, 1430
   massive, 829, 1433
   myelofibrosis, 1430
   reduction, 1829
   splenic abscess, 1432
   splenic cysts, 1430–1432
   spontaneous splenic rupture, 1433
   thrombotic thrombocytopenic purpura (TTP), 1429
   treatment of splenomegaly symptoms, 1829–1831
Splenosis, 1424–1425, 1435
Splice junction, 887
3′ splice sites (3′SS), 1578
Splice-site mutations, 1208
Spliceosome mutations, 1756
Spliceosome proteins, 1578
Splicing factor gene B1 (SF3B1), 1178
SPMs. See Second primary malignancies (SPMs)
SPo. See Spleen organizer (SPo)
Spontaneous remission, 817
Spontaneous splenic rupture, 1433
Sporadic late-onset nemaline myopathy (SLONM), 2146, 2281
Sporadic PCT, 712
Spur cell anemia, 742–743, 1040
Sputum analysis, 184
Squamous cell carcinoma (SCC), 2095
Src defect, 1193
SRC Family Kinases and SYK Kinase, 376–377
SRC family of tyrosine kinases (SFK), 1576
Src homology 2 (SH2), 104, 1850
Src Homology 2-like domain (SH2-like domain), 375
Src kinase (SFK), 376
SRC-like adaptor protein (SLAP), 290
SRP54, 985
SRP72 mutation, 1630
SRSF2 gene, 1568, 1638, 1825, 1850, 1857
SRSF2 mutation, 1738, 1755–1756, 1764, 1768, 1822, 1825, 1849, 1854
SRSF2/ASXL1/RUNX1 (S/A/R), 1857
St. Jude Children's Research Hospital (SJCRH), 1673
St. Jude Lifetime Cohort Study (SJLIFE), 2139
Stable isotope dilution, 958
STAG2 gene, 1568, 1638
STAG2 protein, 1740
Stain-lyse-wash methods, 22
Staining techniques, 136
Standard deviations (SDs), 2380
Standard ordering protocols (SOPs), 1330
Standardized incidence ratios (SIRs), 2382
Standardized uptake value (SUV), 2039, 2092
Staphylococci, 1350, 1434
Staphylococcus, 846, 1349, 1432, 1438
Staphylococcus aureus, 844, 1302, 1332, 1344, 1404, 1434, 2094, 2307
STAT3, 2074
STAT3 gene. See Signal transducer and activator of transcription 3 gene (STAT3 gene)
STAT3 mutations, 1008, 1931
STAT4 genes, 1960
STAT5, 1786
STAT5B gene, 2074
Statins, 864
Stavudine, 964
Steatorrhea, 2245
Stem cell factor (SCF), 74, 94, 198, 218, 1527, 1576, 1849
Stem cell leukemia (SCL), 366
Stem cell transplant(ation) (SCT), 40, 585, 784, 1339, 2254, 2270, 2272
   allogeneic stem cell transplantation, 2257

   autologous stem cell transplantation, 2254–2257
   conditioning therapy for, 2203
   side effects of, 910
      chronic graft-vs-host disease (cGVHD), 910
      growth, development, and fertility, 910
      malignancies, 910
      normalization of iron status, 910–911
      quality of life after HSCT, 911
   treatment of relapse and role of, 1731
Stem cells, 998, 2301
   disorders, 666
   donor, 2335
   marker CD34, 1721
   mobilization, 79
   to progenitor B cell, 272–273
   sources, 2300, 2371
      bone marrow, 2300
      peripheral blood, 2300
      umbilical CB, 2300
Stem-cell factor (SCF), 273
Steroids, 1104–1105, 1827, 2028
   maintenance with, 2209
   refractory, 1017
   steroid-induced purpura, 1167
   steroid-related side effects, 1017
   therapy, 778–779
STIM1 gene, 1195
Stimulation of platelets, 393
Stimuli, 1248
Stomatocytes, 622, 740
Stomatocytic disorders, 740–742. See also Acanthocytic disorders
   familial deficiency of high-density lipoproteins, 742
   features of hereditary stomatocytosis syndromes, 740t
   hereditary stomatocytosis, 741
   hereditary xerocytosis, 741–742
   intermediate stomatocytic syndromes, 742
   Rh-null disease, 742
   sitosterolemia, 742
Stomatocytosis, 740
Stool cultures, 1133
Stop Imatinib (STIM), 1782, 1800
α,δ-storage pool deficiency, 1192
Storage pool disease (SPD), 1190
α-storage pool disease (α-SPD), 1191
Stored blood, clinical implications of, 561
Stored red cells, in vivo recovery of, 561
Stormorken syndrome, 1195–1195
Streptococcus, 1432, 1438
Streptococcus pneumoniae, 734, 908, 1106, 1145, 1393, 1434, 2037, 2221, 2364
Streptococcus pyogenes, 346, 348, 1548
Streptococcus viridans, 1703–1704
Streptokinase (SK), 1301–1302
Streptomyces pilosus, 904
Stress erythrocytosis, 1072
Stress erythropoiesis, 1054
Stroke with Transfusions Changing to Hydroxyurea (SWiTCH), 842
Strokes, 840, 842
Stroma of hematopoietic organs, 83
Stromal cell–derived factor-1 (SDF-1), 234, 1140
Stromal cells, 11
Stromal interaction molecule 1 (STIM1), 1195
Strongyloides stercoralis, 1482
Structural Maintenance of Chromosome genes (SMC3), 1578
Stuart factor, 447–449
Stunted growth bone abnormalities, 905
STX11 gene, 1380
STXBP2 gene, 1380
Subclinical hepatitis, 1385
Subcutaneous hematomas, 1206
Subcutaneous panniculitis-like T-cell lymphoma (SPTL), 1888, 1974, 2085, 2087–2088
Subcutaneous γ-globulin, 2038
Subcutaneously immunoglobulin (SCIg), 1398
Subnormal immunoglobulins, 691–692
Subtotal nodal irradiation (STNRT), 2121
Suction purpura, 1162
Sudan black B stains, 12–13
Sulfamethoxazole, 753
Sulfasalazine, 962
Sulfhemoglobin, 3, 118, 941–943
Sulfhemoglobinemia, 942
Sulfhydryl containing tripeptide, 749

Index I-51

Sulfhydryl groups on hemoglobin, 752
Sulfisoxazole, 753
6-sulfo LacNAc (SLAN), 211
Sulfonamides, 1169
Sunitinib, 964
Superconducting quantum interference device (SQUID), 899
Superoxide anions (O_2^-), 119, 749
Superoxide dismutase, 119
Supine hypertension, 2259
Supportive signals, 83
Suppression by regulatory T cells, 770–771
Suppressor of cytokine signaling (SOCS), 105
Supravital staining, 8
Sural nerve biopsy, 956, 2246
Surface immunoglobulin (sIg), 22, 257, 275–276, 275f
Surface receptors, 221–223
Surface-connected canalicular system (SCCS), 391–392
Surgery, 625, 861, 1817
Surrogate light chains (SLCs), 274
Surveillance, Epidemiology, and End Results (SEER), 1609, 1627, 1737, 1836, 1943, 2010, 2152
Sustained engraftment of engineered HSCs, 1540
*SUZ*12 mutation, 1587
Swedish porphyria. *See* Acute intermittent porphyria (AIP)
Sweet syndrome, 2055
Symptomatic episodes, 796
Symptomatic syndromes, 923
Syndrome of inappropriate ADH (SIADH), 707
Syndromic congenital sideroblastic anemias, 664
Synergistic factor, 371
Syngeneic HCT, 2298
Syngeneic transplants, 2298
Synovectomy, 1232
Synovial biopsy, 2242
Synovial fluid aspiration, 2242
Syphilis, 2238
Sysmex, 2
Systemic capillary leak syndrome (SCLS), 2172, 2292
Systemic chemotherapy, 2002, 2098–2100
Systemic infections, 1337
Systemic inflammatory response syndrome, neutrophil dysregulation in, 1352
Systemic lupus erythematosus (SLE), 780, 1010, 1102, 1168, 1255, 1337, 1394, 1952, 2172
 autoimmune thrombocytopenia in, 1110
Systemic mastocytosis (SM), 1771–1772, 1849
 aggressive systemic mastocytosis, 1773f
 clinical features, 1850–1852
  aggressive systemic mastocytosis (ASM), 1854
  consensus criteria for variants of, 1851t
  cutaneous mastocytosis (CM), 1852
  extracutaneous mastocytoma, 1855
  indolent systemic mastocytosis (ISM), 1852–1853
  mast cell leukemia and MCL variants, 1854–1855
  mast cell sarcoma (MCS), 1855
  primary (clonal) mast cell activation syndrome, 1855
  secondary and idiopathic MCAS, 1855
  smoldering systemic mastocytosis (SSM), 1853–1854
  systemic mastocytosis with AHN, 1854
  World Health Organization diagnostic criteria for cutaneous and, 1851t
 development of clinical response criteria and biologic correlates to assess therapeutic efficacy, 1862
 differential diagnosis, 1858–1859
 future therapeutic directions, 1862
 indolent, 1771, 1850, 1852–1853
  morphologic features of mast cells from normal *vs.* mastocytosis bone marrow aspirate, 1853t
 laboratory findings, 1855–1857
  bone marrow histopathology showing focal mast cell infiltrates, 1856f
  immunohistochemical staining of lymphoid aggregates, 1856f
 management, 1859–1860
  cytoreductive therapy, 1860–1862
  suggested therapy for mastocytosis, 1860t
 Modified WHO criteria for, 1772f
 pathophysiology, 1849–1850
 prognostication using genetic and clinical variables, 1857–1858
  Global prognostic score for mastocytosis (GPSM), 1858

International Prognostic Scoring System for Mastocytosis (IPSM), 1858
Mayo Alliance Prognostic Scoring system (MAPS), 1858
Mutation-Adjusted Risk Score (MARS), 1858
WHO B and C findings in, 1772t
WHO classification of mastocytosis, 1771t
Systemic sclerosis (SS), 2283
Systemic symptoms, 1953
Systolic dysfunction, 850

T

T cell immunoreceptor with immunoglobulin and ITIM domains (TIGIT), 301
T cell receptor constant α chain (TRAC), 1512
T cells, 29, 1399, 1943, 2072, 2116
 abnormalities, 2020
 clinical presentation, 1399
 commitment, 288
 depletion techniques, 910
 exhaustion, 300–301
 immunophenotyping of T-cell lymphoproliferative disorders, 34–35
 and natural killer cell lymphomas, 1885
  lymphoepithelioid lymphoma, 1885
 neoplasms, 1945
  adult T-cell leukemia/lymphoma (ATLL), 1931–1932
  anaplastic large cell lymphoma (ALCLs), 1925–1927
  anaplastic lymphoma kinase-negative ALCLs (ALK-negative ALCLs), 1925–1927
  anaplastic lymphoma kinase-positive ALCLs (ALK-positive ALCLs), 1925–1927
  angioimmunoblastic T-cell lymphoma (AITL), 1929–1930
  chromosomal translocations in T-cell NHL, 1910t
  enteropathy-associated T-cell lymphoma (EATL), 1931
  follicular T-cell lymphomas (Tfh lymphomas), 1929
  mature neoplasms of B cells, 1910–1925
  mature neoplasms of T cells, 1925
  monomorphic epitheliotropic intestinal T-cell lymphoma (MEITL), 1931
  pathways with genomic alterations in several T-cell lymphomas, 1926f
  peripheral T-cell lymphoma, not otherwise specified, 1927–1928
  recurrent molecular aberrancies in, 1909
  T-cell large granular lymphocytic leukemia (T-LGL), 1930–1931
  T-prolymphocytic leukemia (T-PLL), 1930
 numbers, 2303
 polarization, 225
 polarizing signals, 225
 progenitors, 288
 SCID caused by defective cytokine signaling in, 1401
 specific disorders, 1399
  22q11 deletion syndrome, 1399–1400
  SCID caused by metabolic defects, 1402
  severe combined immune deficiency (SCID), 1400–1402
 T cell–associated causes, 2017
T-cell-based immunotherapy for AML, 1652
T-cell-directed immunosuppression, 1402
T-cell-mediated graft *vs.* tumor, 2365
 future approaches to enhance T-cell immunity against tumors, 2365
 unmodified T cells, 2365
T-cell–αβ selection, 288–289
T-cell–γδ selection, 288–289
T-cell–mediated inflammatory process, 1368
 treatment of severe combined immunodeficiency syndromes, 1402–1403
γδ T cells, 301–302
T helper type I cells (Th1 cells), 1404
T lymphocytes, 288, 326, 564–565, 1468, 1494, 1496, 1746, 2014, 2056, 2335
 γδ T cells, 301–302
 activation, 1497–1498
  signal transduction events involved in, 1498f
 CD4 T lymphocytes, 297–299
 CD8+ T lymphocytes, 299–301
 development, 288–290

morphology, 288
T-cell activation, 293–296
T-cell adoptive transfer for cancer immunotherapy, 302–303
T-cell receptor (TCR), 291–293
T regulatory cells (Treg cells), 2020
T-ALL. *See* T-cell lymphoblastic leukemia (T-ALL); T-cell precursor lymphoblastic leukemia (T-ALL)
T-cell gene rearrangements (TCR), 1902–1903
 immunoglobulin gene rearrangement assay, 1902f
 immunoglobulin gene rearrangement studies, 1903t
T-cell gene rearrangements γ (TRG), 1902
T-cell gene rearrangements δ (TRD), 1902
T-cell histiocyte-rich large B-cell lymphoma (THRLBCL), 1923
T-cell intracellular antigen-1 (TIA-1), 2082
T-cell kinase (ITK), 1929, 2021
T-cell large granular lymphocyte (T-LGL), 34
 leukemia, 1930–1931
  guidelines for molecular testing in, 1931
T-cell lymphoblastic leukemia (T-ALL), 1014
T-cell lymphoblastic lymphoma (T-LBL), 1991
T-cell lymphoma (TCL), 1389, 1882–1885, 1900, 1943, 2074, 2081
 adult T-cell leukemia/lymphoma (ATLL), 1888
 anaplastic large cell lymphoma (ALCL), 1887–1888
 angioimmunoblastic T-cell lymphoma, 1885–1887
 extranodal natural killer/t-cell lymphoma, nasal type, 1889
 hepatosplenic T-cell lymphoma (HSTCL), 1888
 intestinal T-cell lymphoma (ITL), 1888–1889
 peripheral T-cell lymphoma, not otherwise specified, 1885
 subcutaneous panniculitis–like T-cell lymphoma, 1888
T-cell precursor lymphoblastic leukemia (T-ALL), 1903
T-cell prolymphocytic leukemia (T-PLL), 34, 1459
T-cell protein tyrosine phosphatase (TCPTP), 377
T-cell receptor (TCR), 34, 65, 288, 291, 1390, 1401, 1495, 1900, 1943, 1994, 2074
 α/β T-cell-receptor complex, 291–292, 291f
 interaction with HLA-peptide complex, 293f
 signal transduction component, 292–293
 signaling, 295
 TCR-major histocompatibility complex coreceptor interaction, 292f
T-cell receptor constant β chain-1 (TRBC1), 2081
T-cell receptor excision circles (TRECs), 2314
T-cell rich large B-cell lymphoma (TCRLBL), 1893
α/β T-cell-receptor complex, 291–292, 291f
T-cell-rich B-cell lymphoma (TCRBCL), 2117
T-cell/histiocyte-rich large B-cell lymphoma (THRLBCL), 1879, 1879f, 1965
 genetics, 1879
 immunophenotype, 1879
 morphology, 1879
T-helper cell type 17 (Th17), 1346
T-large granular lymphocyte leukemia, 1952
T-lymphoblastic leukemia/lymphoma, 1675–1666, 1763, 1585. *See also* B-lymphoblastic leukemia/lymphoma
 epigenetic factors modifying chromatin and DNA, 1587
  DNMT3A and *PRC*2 complex, 1587
  plant homeodomain finger protein 6 gene (*PHF*6 gene), 1587
 ETP-ALL, 1587
 functional classes of genes mutated in, 1585t
 IL7R gene, 1586–1587
 kinases, 1586
 transcription factors, 1585
  homeodomain proteins, 1586
  LMO factors, 1585–1586
  *NOTCH*1, 1585
  T-cell acute lymphoblastic leukemia 1/stem cell leukemia (TAL1/SCL), 1585–1586
T-prolymphocytic leukemia (T-PLL), 1911, 1930, 1976
T-zone reticular cells (TRCs), 246
T315I mutation, 1621
Tacrolimus (TAC), 2298
Tafasitamab, 1967
Takatsuki syndrome, 2277
*TAL*1 gene, 370, 1604
*TAL*2 genes, 1971
TAP. *See* Transporter associated with antigen processing (TAP)

TARGET. *See* Therapeutically applicable research to generate effective treatments (TARGET)
Target cells, 622
  disorders, 744
    familial lecithin-cholesterol acyltransferase deficiency, 744–745
Target joint, 1205
TCD. *See* Transcranial Doppler (TCD)
T-cell acute lymphoblastic leukemia (T-ALL), 1668, 1942
TCF3, 273
  translocations, 1581–1582
TCL1A gene, 1930
TCL1B gene, 1930
TCR gene, 1902, 1907, 1932, 2075, 2081–2083, 2091
TCR γ-chain gene, 2075
TCR-γ gene, 2075
Tear duct-associated lymphoid tissue (TALT), 249
Teardrop-shaped RBCs, 1823
Telangiectasias, 1403, 1852
Telomerase reverse transcriptase (*TERT*), 995
Telomere biology disorders (TBD) /dyskeratosis congenita, 980
  clinical features, 980
    physical findings associated with telomere biology disorders, 981*t*
  diagnostic testing, 980
  differential diagnosis, 981
  laboratory findings, 981
  pathophysiology, 981–982
    clinical features of inherited aplastic anemia syndromes, 983*t*
  supportive care, 982
  treatment, 982–984
Telomere biology disorders (TBDs), 974
Telomeres, 981
Temozolomide, 2100
TEMPI syndrome, 2291–2292
Temporal arteritis, 1033
Temsirolimus, 1970
Ten-eleven translocation oncogene family member 2 (TET2), 370, 1177
  CH mutations, 1756
  gene, 1565, 1630, 1636, 1738, 1812, 1825, 1838, 1840, 1850, 1857, 1928
  knock-out mice, 1755
  mutation, 1573, 1754–1755, 1758, 1763–1764, 1809, 1849, 1929, 1931, 1978
Ten-eleven-translocation-2 (TET2), 1821
Tenecteplase (TNK), 1302
Tenofovir, 1410
Tenofovir alafenamide (TAF), 1410
Tenofovir disoproxil fumarate (TDF), 1410
Terminal complement components, deficiencies of, 352
Terminal deoxynucleotidyl transferase (TdT), 13, 234, 273, 1992
Terminal differentiation factors, 220
Terminal stages of B-cell differentiation, 280–281
Termination of procoagulant response, 427
Tertiary lymphoid organs (TLOs), 249
  chemokine-guided migration and positioning in spleen, 250*f*
  chemokines in TLO dynamics, 251*f*
  initiation and formation, 251*f*
  lymph node leukocyte traffic mediated by lymphatic endothelial cells, 252*f*
  lymphocyte egress from lymphoid tissues, 255
  lymphocyte migration across lymphoid tissue parenchyma, 255
  lymphocyte migration into lymphoid tissues, 251–253
  molecules regulating DC migration into lymphatics, 254–255
  molecules regulating lymphocyte migration, 253–254
TET methylcytosine dioxygenase 2, 1755
Tetanus/diphtheria/pertussis (TDAP), 2308
Tethering, 171
  tethering/rolling, 253
Tetrahydrofolate (THF), 946
Tetramer technology, 42
Tfh lymphomas. *See* follicular T-cell lymphomas (Tfh lymphomas)
TGF-β. *See* Transforming growth factor beta (TGF-β)
TGF-β1, 379
Th1 CD4$^+$ T cells, 297
Th17 CD4$^+$ T cells, 298
Th2 CD4$^+$ T cells, 297–298
Th22 CD4$^+$ T cells, 298
Th9 CD4$^+$ T cells, 298
Thalassemia, 66, 1028, 1430, 2331, 2371
  gene mutations, 883
  general diagnostic approach to, 614
    sideroblastic anemias, 614
  genotype-phenotype correlation in, 892
  hematopoietic stem cell transplantation for, 2324–2325
    alternative donor HCT for thalassemia, 2325
    overall survival and event-free survival, 2324*f*
  heterozygote, 883
  intermedia, 894, 916–921
  major, 895
  minor, 894–895, 912
    α-Thalassemia, 915
    β-Thalassemia and δβ-Thalassemia, 913–915
    δβ and hereditary persistence of fetal Hb carriers, 913
    atypical carriers, 913
    carrier detection, 913
    classic form, 912
    effect of coinheritance of different α-thalassemia alleles in β-thalassemia carriers, 914*f*
    genotype and phenotype of atypical β-Thalassemia carriers, 913*t*
    hemoglobin E, 915–916
    laboratory features, 912–913
    main hematologic parameters of β-Thalassemia carriers according to age, 912*t*
  molecular pathology, 883–885
  syndromes, 883
    α-and β-globin gene clusters and hemoglobins produced during development, 884*f*
    α-thalassemia, 885–886, 891–892
    β-thalassemia, 886–887, 890–891
    δ-thalassemia, 889
    clinical and laboratory features, 892
    current hemoglobin switching model, 884*f*
    genetic mechanisms and molecular pathology, 883–885
    Hb Barts hydrops fetalis syndrome, 893–894
    HbC Thalassemia, 922
    HbE syndromes, 922
    HbH disease, 892–893
    HbS thalassemia syndromes, 921–922
    HbS-Hb Lepore, 922
    hereditary persistence of fetal hemoglobin (HPFH), 889–890
    hyperunstable globins, 888
    non-transfusion-dependent thalassemia (NTDT), 916–921
    pathophysiology, 890–892
    prenatal diagnosis, 916
    prevalence, geographic distribution, and role of malaria, 883
    prognosis with conventional therapy, 908–912
    thalassemia minor, 912–916
    transcription mutations, 887
    transfusion-dependent thalassemia, 894–908
    unknown mechanisms, 888–889
    unusual causes of β-Thalassemia, 890
    unusual forms of α-Thalassemia, 894
  trait, 894
  α-Thalassemia, 883, 885, 891, 892, 915
    deletional α-Thalassemia, 885
    genotype-phenotype correlation in thalassemia, 892
    nondeletional α-Thalassemia, 885–886
    silent carrier, 892
    syndromes, 613
    trait, 614
    trait, 892
    unusual forms of, 894
      α-Thalassemia in association with structural variants, 894
      α-Thalassemia/myelodysplasia syndrome, 894
      and intellectual disability syndromes, 891
  β-Thalassemia, 617, 691, 886–887, 890–891, 894, 911, 913–915, 1538, 1544
    in association with β-chain structural variants, 921
    common silent and mild β-thalassemia mutations, 915*f*
    flowchart for diagnosis of thalassemia syndromes, 924*f*
    genotypes, 914
    mutations occurring in specific populations with high frequency, 915*t*
    nondeletional β-Thalassemia, 886–887
    syndromes, 894
    trait, 614
    unusual causes of, 890
  Thalassemia, nontransfusion dependent, 887, 916, 919
    genetic determinants, 916
      clinical features, 917–918
        CT scan of spine of thalassemia intermedia patient, 918*f*
        extramedullary erythropoiesis manifesting as bulky space-occupying masses in chest, 919*f*
        mechanisms of β-thalassemia intermedia, 917*f*
        transfusion therapy, 918–919
    iron overload, 919
      cardiac disease, 920–921
      complications, 921
      endocrine complications and pregnancy, 919
      iron chelation, 919
      leg ulcers, 920
      liver disease, 920
      pseudoxanthoma elasticum, 921
      pulmonary hypertension, 921
      thromboembolic disease, 920
  Thalassemia, transfusion dependent (TDT), 890, 894
    clinical features, 895
      anemia, 895
      bone deformities, 895
      cholelithiasis, 896
      osteoporosis, 896
      pseudoxanthoma elasticum, 897
      thromboembolic complications, 896–897
    history, 894
    laboratory findings and diagnosis, 897
      blood transfusion, 897–898
      clinical manifestations of iron overload, 900–908
      complications of transfusions, 898–899
      medical interventions, 897
      peripheral blood smears in β-thalassemia, 897*f*
Thalidomide, 1461, 1827, 2175, 2190, 2192, 2194, 2197–2198, 2210, 2251, 2255, 2281, 2284
  maintenance, 2207
Thalidomide and dexamethasone (TD), 2188, 2194
Thawed plasma, 563
The Cancer Genome Atlas (TCGA), 1565
Therapeutic apheresis, 590
  adverse effects, 592
  category and grade recommendations for TPE category i indications, 591*t*
  pathogen reduction technologies for transfusable blood components, 591*t*
  therapeutic adsorption of plasma constituents, 592
  therapeutic cytapheresis, 592
  therapeutic plasma exchange (TPE), 591–592
Therapeutic cytapheresis, 592
Therapeutic genome-editing strategies, 1549
Therapeutic leukapheresis, 592
Therapeutic plasma exchange (TPE), 578, 591
  indications, 591
  technical considerations, 592
Therapeutic platelet pheresis, 592
Therapeutic platelet transfusion, 576
Therapeutic regimens, 1231
Therapeutically applicable research to generate effective treatments (TARGET), 1699
Therapy-related AML (t-AML), 1568, 1627–1629, 1706, 2336
  AML incidence and mortality in United States, 1628*f*
Therapy–related myeloid neoplasms (T-MN), 1566, 1601, 1770, 1627, 1724, 1757
  CH as risk factor for, 1757–1758
    PPM1D and t-MN risk, 1758
    TP53 CH and t-MN risk, 1758
Thermal amplitude, 776, 778
Thermal injury, hemolysis with, 827
Thermolabile variant of MTHFR (tlMTHFR), 1284
Thiamine, 659
Thiazide diuretics, 1169
Thienopyridines, 1291
Thioguanine nucleotides (TGN), 1674
Thiopurine methyltransferase (TPMT), 1674
Thiopurine methyltransferase deficiency (TPMT), 997
Third National Health and Nutrition Examination Survey (NHANES III), 600
Third-generation gene therapy clinical trials, 1543

hemoglobinopathies, 1544–1545
immunodeficiencies, 1546–1547
inherited bone marrow failure syndromes, 1547
lysosomal storage diseases, 1545–1546
peroxisomal disorders, 1543–1544
THPO. See Thrombopoietin gene (THPO)
Three-dimensional genome (3D genome), 1565
THRLBCL. See T-cell histiocyte-rich large B-cell lymphoma (THRLBCL); T-cell/histiocyte-rich large B-cell lymphoma (THRLBCL)
Thrombin, 450, 458, 1189, 1247
 generation, 397
 regulation, 460
 roles in anticoagulation, 459
 roles in coagulation, 458–459
 roles in tissue repair and regeneration, 459–460
 structure/function relationships, 460
 thrombin receptors, 460
 thrombin-mediated platelet activation, 404
 time and related techniques, 1085–1086
Thrombin glycoprotein Ib complex interaction with, 403–404
α-Thrombin, 427, 451, 456, 458–459, 460
Thrombin-activatable fibrinolysis inhibitor (TAFI), 427, 486, 536, 1244
 activation, 487–488
 biochemistry, 487
 function, 488
 gene structure and expression, 486–487
 mechanism of, 487f
 regulation, 488
 schematic of, 488f
α-Thrombin-antithrombin (TAT), 460
Thrombocytopenia, 792, 806, 986, 1049, 1080, 1087, 1095, 1110–1111, 1142, 1144, 1147, 1149, 1153t, 1154, 1192, 1244, 1263, 1412, 1595, 1632, 1698, 1776, 1823, 1976
 acquired thrombocytopenia, 1156–1159
 approach for evaluation of thrombocytopenia, 1089f
 artifactual, 1095
 associated with infections, 1158
  thrombocytopenia after massive blood transfusion, 1159
  thrombocytopenia associated with bacterial and protozoal infections, 1158–1159
  thrombocytopenia associated with viral infections, 1158
 caused by abnormal platelet pooling, 1157–1158
 caused by immunologic platelet destruction
  alloimmune thrombocytopenia, 1111–1113
  immune thrombocytopenia, 1097t
  primary immune thrombocytopenia (primary ITP), 1097–1099
  secondary autoimmune thrombocytopenic purpura, 1109–1111
 classification, 1096
  pathophysiologic classification of thrombocytopenia, 1096t
 congenital/hereditary thrombocytopenia, 1153–1156
  classic inherited thrombocytopenia, 1153–1156
  classification of inherited thrombocytopenia by platelet size, 1154f
  others, 1156
  22q112 deletion syndrome, 1156
 diagnosis, 1144
 management, 1746
 pathophysiology, 1095, 1095f
  abnormal pooling, 1096
  accelerated platelet destruction, 1096
  artifactual thrombocytopenia, 1095
  deficient platelet production, 1096
  thrombokinetic patterns in various forms of thrombocytopenia, 1095t
 profiles of hemostasis screening tests in patients with bleeding disorders, 1088t
 treatment, 1412
Thrombocytopenia with absent radius syndrome (TAR syndrome), 1154
Thrombocytopenia-absent radii syndrome (TAR syndrome), 986
Thrombocytopenia, autoimmune, 1109
 in hepatitis C, 1111
 secondary to drugs, 1109
  clinical features, 1109–1110
  diagnosis, 1110
  pathophysiology, 1109

  treatment, 1110
Thrombocytopenia, inherited (IT), 1182
Thrombocytopenic disorders, congenital, 1100
Thrombocytosis, 908, 1632
 clonal, 1176
 classification of, 1175t
 differential diagnosis and clinical approach to, 1176
 approach to evaluating thrombocytosis, 1176f
 in ET, 1770
 inherited, 1175–1176
 secondary thrombocytosis, 1175–1176
  clonal thrombocytosis other than essential thrombocythemia, 1176
  epidemiology and pathophysiology, 1175
  inherited thrombocytosis, 1175–1176
  treatment, 1175
Thromboelastography (TEG), 1087, 1266
Thromboelastometry, 1087
Thromboembolic complications, 805, 896
Thromboembolic disease, 920, 2172
Thromboembolism, intrapulmonary, 852
β-thromboglobulin, 367
Thrombolysis for pulmonary embolism, 1306
Thrombolytic agents, 1301–1302
 other plasminogen activators, 1302
 properties of currently available and investigational thrombolytic agents, 1301t
 streptokinase, 1302
 thrombolytic fibrin specificity and hemorrhagic risk, 1302–1303
 thrombolytic therapy–associated bleeding, 1302
 tissue-type plasminogen activator variants, 1302
 urokinase-type plasminogen activator, 1302
Thrombolytic fibrin specificity and hemorrhagic risk, 1302–1303
Thrombolytic therapy, 1306
 for DVT, 1306
 thrombolytic therapy–associated bleeding, 1302
Thrombomodulin, 463, 535–536
 biochemistry, 463
 deficiency, 1287
 function, 463
 gene structure and expression, 463
  molecular genetics of human anticoagulant proteins and inhibitors, 462t
 regulation, 463
Thrombopathy, constitutional, 1209
Thrombophilia, 792, 1278
 of PNH, 817
Thromboplastins, 1085
Thrombopoiesis-stimulating agents, 1107
Thrombopoietin (TPO), 74, 94, 986, 218, 356, 1153, 1175, 1527, 1746, 1823
 growth factors, 1746
 mimetics, 1107
 receptor, 1812
 receptor MPL genes, 1191
 thrombopoietin-mimetic agents, 1246
 thrombopoietin/MPL axis, 371
  and biological effects, 371
  and identification, 371
  LNK, 377
  negative regulation of TPO/MPL/JAK2 signaling, 377
  phosphatases, 377
  regulation of plasma TPOlevel by synthesis and clearance, 375f
  regulation of thrombopoietin plasma level, 374–375
  and signaling cascade in megakaryocytes, 375–377
  SOCS Family, 377
  and therapy, 377–378
Thrombopoietin gene (THPO), 986, 1153, 1175
Thrombopoietin receptor gene (c-mpl/MPL), 1153
Thrombosis, 428, 792, 935, 1276, 1724, 2219
 activation of coagulation, 1279
 antithrombotic therapy, 1288–1303
 heparin-induced thrombocytopenia (HIT), 1307–1310
 inherited thrombotic disorders, 1279–1288
 physiology and pathophysiology of, 1276
 of portal venous system, 1434
 prevention and treatment of, 814–815
  thrombosis and PNH, 815t
 prevention of venous thromboembolic disease, 1306–1307
 primary myelofibrosis and risk of, 1831

 thrombosis-free cumulative survival, 1814
 venous thromboembolic disease, 1303–1306
 Virchow triad, 1276–1279
Thrombospondin type 1 repeats (TSRs), 343, 1126
Thrombotic disorders, inherited, 1279
 activated protein C resistance (APC resistance), 1283–1284
 antithrombin deficiency, 1279–1281
 combined defects, 1287
 dysfibrinogenemia, 1287
 heparin cofactor II deficiency (HCII deficiency), 1281
 hyperhomocysteinemia, 1284–1285
 impaired endogenous fibrinolysis, 1285–1287
 increased factor VIII activity, 1285
 increased levels of factors IX, X, XI, and XIII, 1285
 inherited risk factors in childhood venous thrombosis, 1287–1288
 laboratory testing for prethrombotic state, 1288
 lipoprotein(a) (Lp(a)), 1287
 perspective on laboratory testing for inherited thrombotic disorders, 1288
 prevalence of selected inherited and acquired hypercoagulable states in different patient populations, 1280t
 protein C deficiency, 1281–1282
 protein S deficiency, 1282–1283
 protein Z deficiency, 1283
 prothrombin mutations, 1284
 thrombomodulin deficiency, 1287
 tissue factor pathway inhibitor (TFPI), 1287
Thrombotic events, 391, 1814
Thrombotic microangiopathy (TMA), 351, 828, 1050, 1123, 1141, 2291
Thrombotic pulmonary disease, 1263
Thrombotic thrombocytopenia, 1410
Thrombotic thrombocytopenic purpura (TTP), 351, 563, 828, 1049, 1102, 1123, 1139, 1251, 1412–1413, 1429
 acquired thrombotic thrombocytopenic purpura, 1123
 alteration of von Willebrand Factor Multimers in, 1129–1130
 arteriolar and capillary stenosis pathologic basis for syndrome of microangiopathic hemolytic anemia and thrombocytopenia, 1123f
 atypical hemolytic-uremic syndrome (AHUS), 1141–1147
 causes of microangiopathic hemolytic anemia, 1147
 chronic relapsing, 1137
 diagnosis of thrombotic thrombocytopenic purpura, 1131–1133
 distinction between TTP disease and complications, 1130–1131
 management of, 1137
 nonimmunologic platelet destruction, 1149
 pathogenic mechanisms of, 1127
 platelet and red cell damage by abnormal vascular surfaces, 1147–1149
 Shiga toxin–associated hemolytic-uremic syndrome (STX-HUS), 1139–1141
 symptoms, 1138
 treatment, 1413
 TTP-related symptoms, 1138
Thrombotic thrombocytopenic purpura, acquired (acquired TTP), 1123, 1130, 1133
 causes of, ADAMTS13 deficiency, 1124–1127
 clinical features, 1130, 1131f
 diagnosis of, 1131–1133
  ADAMTS13 tests, 1131
  differential diagnosis, 1134
  laboratory findings, 1131–1133
  principles of, 1131t
 hereditary thrombotic thrombocytopenic purpura, 1137–1138
 management and prognosis, 1133
  ADAMTS13 tests and management of TTP, 1137
  ADAMTS13-guided rituximab therapy prevents relapse of TTP, 1136f
  caplacizumab, 1136–1137
  immunosuppressive therapy, 1133
  plasma therapy, 1133
  preventing relapse and death from TTP, 1137
  principles of managing acquired thrombotic thrombocytopenic purpura, 1135t
  therapeutic targets and treatment options for TTP, 1134t
  treatment options, 1137

Thrombotic thrombocytopenic purpura, acquired (acquired TTP) (*continued*)
  pathogenesis, 1123, 1126*t*, 1124*t*
  pathology, 1123
    histopathology and histochemistry of TTP and disorders associated with MAHA, 1125*f*
  pathophysiology, 1127
    ADAMTS13 and generation of vWF multimers, 1128*f*
    ADAMTS13 deficiency leads to vWF-platelet aggregation and thrombosis in TTP, 1129*f*
    alteration of von Willebrand factor multimers in TTP, 1129–1130
    conformation of von Willebrand factor and interaction with ADAMTS13, 1128–1129
    distinction between TTP disease and complications, 1130–1131
  thrombotic thrombocytopenic purpura and pregnancy, 1139
Thromboxane A$_2$ (TXA$_2$), 404, 409–410, 1278
  receptor, 369, 1189
Thromboxane receptors, 409–410
Thromboxane synthase defect, 1193
Thrombus growth, coordination between platelet adhesion events and soluble agonist stimulation in, 410
Thymic epithelium, 236
  generation, 236
Thymic involution, 239
Thymic microenvironment, 288
  migrants from bone marrow arrive and settle in corticomedullary junction, 289*f*
Thymic nurse cells (TNCs), 237
Thymic stromal lymphopoietin (TSLP), 181, 199, 273, 290, 2072
Thymic stromal lymphopoietin receptor (TSLPR), 1584
Thymic T-cell development, 234–236
Thymidine kinase (tk), 1543
Thymidylate synthase (TYMS), 948
Thymine, 946
Thymoma, 1009
Thymus, 214, 234–236, 235*f*
Thymus epithelial cells (TECs), 288
Thymus-specific serine protease (TSSP), 237
Thyroid, 1369
  cancer, 2129, 2139
  disorders, autoimmune, 689
  dysfunction, 2139, 2381
  function, 689
  ultrasonography, 903
Ticagrelor, 1291
Ticlopidine, 1124, 1291
Tie tyrosine kinase receptors, 531
Timber rattlesnake (*Crotalus horridus horridus*), 1253
Time in therapeutic range (TTR), 1296
*TIMP*1 gene, 2050
*TIMP*4 gene, 2050
*TINF*2 mutations, 955
Tisagenlecleucel, 303
Tissue
  damage by neutrophils, 161
  evaluation, 2148
  examination and testing
    approaches to test ordering improvement, 1329
    confirming likely diagnosis, 1328–1329
    considerations for ancillary testing, 1325–1328
    importance of clinical setting, 1328
    monitoring disease, 1329
    systems for ordering and coordinating testing, 1329
    tissue-based approach, 1321–1324
    uncertain new diagnosis, 1328
  homeostasis, repair, and fibrosis, 225–226
  hypoxia, 102–103
  iron metabolism in, 635
  macrophages, 634
  oxygen, 102–103
  repair, 427
    roles in tissue repair and regeneration, 459–460
  sampling and processing, 1866
  tissue-based approach, 1321
    body fluid, 1324
    bone marrow, 1322–1323
    lymph nodes, 1323–1324
    nonlymphoid tissue, 1324

  peripheral blood, 1321
  tissue-specific transgene expression, 1524
  tissue-type plasminogen activator, 1302
    receptors, 493–494
    variants, 1302
Tissue factor (TF), 428, 451, 533, 1247, 1259, 1278, 1698, 1723
  biochemistry, 451
  deficiency, 1225
  function, 451–453
    transmembrane cofactors, 452*f*
  gene structure and expression, 451
  pathway inhibitor, 464
    biochemistry, 465–466
    function, 466
    gene structure and expression, 464–465
    regulation, 466
    soluble stoichiometric inhibitors, 465*f*
  regulation, 453
Tissue factor pathway inhibitor (TFPI), 427, 446, 1287
Tissue Oxygenation by Transfusion in Severe Anemia with Lactic Acidosis (TOTAL), 567
Tissue plasminogen activator (t-PA), 430, 481–482, 533
  biochemistry, 482–483
  deficiency, 1286
  fibrinolytic proteins tissue-type plasminogen activator, 484*t*
  gene structure and expression, 482
  regulation, 483–484
*TLX*1 gene, 1604, 1971
*TLX*3 gene, 1604
*TMPRSS*6 gene, 636
*TNFAIP*3 mutations, 1878, 1922
*TNFRAF*5 gene, 2050
*TNFRSF*10*B* gene, 1912
*TNFRSF*14 gene, 1871, 2001
*TNFRSF*14 mutations, 1920
*TNFSF*3*B* genes, 1960
Tobacco, 1697, 2075
Tocilizumab, 2035
α-Tocopherol, 907
Toll-like receptor (TLR), 176, 197, 213, 223, 289, 366, 1404, 1495, 1878, 2097
Toluidine blue, 13
Topoisomerase I inhibitors, 1698
Topoisomerase II inhibitors, 1627–1628, 1698
Topologically associated domains (TADs), 1565
Total blood volume, 1811
Total body irradiation (TBI), 1679, 2199, 2297, 2319, 2377
Total cobalamin testing; specificity and sensitivity, 958–959
Total gastrectomy, 960
Total iron-binding capacity (TIBC), 612, 633
Total nucleated cell (TNC), 2301
Total parental nutrition (TPN), 2303
Total serum mast cell tryptase, 1857
Total-skin electron beam radiotherapy (TSEBRT), 2097
Toxic granulation, 8
Toxic porphyria cutanea tarda, 714
Toxoplasma gondii, 1386, 1481, 2053
Toxoplasmosis, 1482
Toxoplasmosis, rubella, cytomegalovirus, herpes simplex virus (TORCH simplex virus), 986
*TP*53 gene, 1328, 1610, 1630, 1634, 1677, 1825, 1840, 1857, 1965, 2012, 2074, 2210
  chromosome 17p loss and abnormalities of, 2155
  dysfunction, 2039
  *TP*53 CH, 1758
*TP*53 mutation, 1568, 1755–1756, 1758, 1912, 2015, 2024, 2036, 1609, 1628, 1635–1636, 1670, 1813, 1874, 1913, 1930, 2059, 2336
  *TP*53-*mutated* AML, 1636
*TPM*4, 1153
*TPSAB*1 gene, 1857
TRA/D gene, 1930
Trace minerals, 907
Trametinib, 1370–1371
Tranexamic acid, 975, 987, 1196, 1228, 1258
Transcatheter aortic-valve replacement (TAVR), 1300
Transcobalamin (TC), 948
Transcranial Doppler (TCD), 568
  ultrasound, 568
Transcription activator–like effector nucleases (TALENs), 1547

Transcription factors (TFs), 80, 219, 366, 369, 2133
  defects, 1194
    familial platelet disorder with associated myeloid malignancy (FPD/MM), 1194
    friend leukemia integration 1 defect (FLI1defect), 1194
    GATA-1 defect, 1194
    GFI1B-related defect, 1194
Transcription mutations, 887–888
Transcriptional regulation, 272, 356
  of megakaryopoiesis, 366
    ETS family, 368
    GATA-1and FOG-1, 367
    GATA-2, 367
    GFI1B, 368
    MYB, 368
    NF-E2, 368
    RUNX1, 367–368
    serum response factor and coactivator MKL1, 369
    T-cellacute lymphoblastic leukemia 1 (TAL1), 367
    transcription factors, 369
  of neutrophil development, 136–137
Transduction, 1522–1524
Transferrin, 633
Transferrin receptor (TfR), 94, 613, 633
  serum, 636
Transferrin receptor 1 (TfR1), 678
Transferrin receptor 2 (TfR2), 633, 678
  hemochromatosis, 680
Transferrin receptor-2gene (*TFR*2), 681
Transferrin saturation (TSAT), 633, 1011, 1015
  serum, 667
Transforming growth factor beta (TGF-β), 84, 94 236, 379, 461, 667–668, 771, 911, 1162, 1499
Transforming growth factor-β1 (TGF-β1), 394, 1823
Transfused red cells, 813
Transfusion and Anemia Expertise Initiative (TAXI), 567
Transfusion Indication Threshold Reduction (TITRe2), 569
Transfusion medicine, 558
  additional blood center activities, 565
  adverse effects of blood transfusion, 579–585
  alternatives to allogeneic donor blood, 565–566
  blood collection and processing, 558–559
  blood component modification, 564–565
  blood donor evaluation, 558
  donor testing, 559
  granulocyte transfusions, 578–579
  infectious complications of blood transfusion, 586–590
  plasma transfusion, 578
  platelet preparation and storage, 561–562
  platelet transfusion, 575–578
  preparation of plasma components, 562–564
  red blood cell preservation and storage, 560–561
  red blood cell transfusion, 566–575
  therapeutic apheresis, 590–592
  use of blood components, 566
  whole blood transfusion, 578
Transfusion of Prematures trial (TOP trial), 567, 1065
Transfusion Requirements in Cardiac Surgery (TRICS), 568–569
Transfusion Requirements in Septic Shock (TRISS), 568
Transfusion-associated circulatory load (TACO), 585
Transfusion-associated hepatitis (TAH), 586
  hepatitis A virus, 586
  hepatitis B, 586
  hepatitis C, 586
Transfusion-related acute lung injury (TRALI), 147, 552, 560, 582–584
  transfusion reaction decision tree, 583*f*
Transfusion-transmitted Babesia (TTB), 588
Transfusions, 784, 813, 1000, 1066
  complications of, 898–899
    alloimmunization, 898
    febrile nonhemolytic transfusion reactions, 898
    hemosiderosis, 899–900
    infections, 898
  therapy, 585, 860, 918–919, 1230
  transfusion-associated coagulation abnormalities, 1266
  transfusion-related immunomodulation, 584
  transfusion-transmitted viral infections, 898

transfusion-transmitted virus, 902
transfusion–dependent β-thalassemia, 2328
    RBC transfusion independence after gene therapy for TDT, 2329f
Transfusions Changing to Hydroxyurea (TWiTCH), 842
Transgenes, immune responses to vectors and, 1550–1551
Transgenic mouse model, 665
Transient abnormal myelopoiesis (TAM), 1571, 1696
Transient aplastic crises, 845
Transient elastography, 902
Transient erythroblastopenia of childhood (TEC), 615, 1008–1009
Transient hypogammaglobulinemia, 1398
Transient hypogammaglobulinemia of infancy (THI), 1398
Transient myeloproliferative disorder (TMD), 367
Transient risk factors, 1278
Transient transgene expression, 1528
Transitory coagulation disorder, 1245
Translational initiation factor 2-α (eIF2α), 658
Translocation-ETS-leukemia (TEL), 1582
Translocation-specific PCR, 1328
Translocation/fusion detection, 65–66
Transmembrane activator and CAML interactor (TACI), 2155
Transmembrane domain, 373
Transmembrane glycoprotein chains, 325
Transmembrane protease serine 6 (TMPRSS6). See Matriptase-2 (MT-2)
Transmembrane proteins, 110–111
Transmethylation, 948
Transmigration, 172
Transmission electron microscopy (TEM), 391, 1182
Transplant patients, 2308
Transplant-associated immune hemolyticanemias, 787
    hematopoietic stem cell transplants, 787–788
    solid organ transplants and passenger lymphocyte syndrome, 788
    timing of posttransplant immune hemolytic anemia, 787t
Transplant-associated thrombotic microangiopathy (TA-TMA), 2378
Transplant-eligible patients, 2186, 2193
    alkylator combinations, 2193
    combination chemotherapy with interferon-α for induction, 2193
    doublets, 2186–2190
    doublets, 2193–2194
    induction regimens among patients destined for ASCT, 2195t
    induction regimens of interest, 2198–2199
    quadruplets, 2192–2193
    quadruplets, 2197–2198
    selected phase II induction regimens, 2194t
    triplets, 2190–2192
    triplets, 2194–2197
Transplant-related microangiopathy (TMA), 2303
Transplant-related mortality (TRM), 1617, 2035, 2335
Transplantation, 227
Transplantation-related mortality (TRM), 2315
Transporter associated with antigen processing (TAP), 330, 1497
Transposon systems, 1526
Transsulfuration, 948
Transthyretin (TTR), 2238
Trauma, 569
    bleeding after, 1101
Traumatic bleeding, 1081, 1206
Traumatic injury, 569
Treacher Collins syndrome, 1737
Treatment-emergent adverse event (TEAE), 1844
Treatment-free remission (TFR), 1782, 1800
Treatment-related mortality (TRM), 1676, 2203
TREM, 222–223
Treosulfan-fludarabine (TREO-FLU), 2325
Trephine biopsy, 1837
Trial to Reduce Alloimmunization to Platelets (TRAP), 576
Trichostatin A (TSA), 1570
Trichuris, 639
    T. trichiura, 638
Triclonal gammopathy, 2170
Tricuspid regurgitant jet velocity (TRV), 850
Triggering receptor expressed on myeloid cells (TREM1–4), 222

Trimethoprim, 962
Trimethoprim–sulfamethoxazole (TMP-SMX), 1109, 1474
Triose phosphate isomerase (TPI), 757
    deficiency, 762
Triphosphate, 362
Triple-negative ET, 374, 1178
Triple-negative patients, 1825
Tripotassium salts, 1
Trisodium citrate, 1
Trisodium salts, 1
Trisomy, 2182
Trisomy 12, 1913, 2024
Trisomy 12q, 2016
Trisomy 21, 1696
Trisomy 3, 1974
Trisomy 5, 1974
Trithorax, 1574
tRNA genes, 664
Trogocytosis, 333
Trophic leg ulcers, 920
Tropical sprue, 961
Trousseau syndrome, 1252
TRPM7, 1153
True histiocytic lymphoma, 1364
True stem cells, 1787
Trypanosoma brucei gambiense, 824
Trypanosoma brucei rhodesiense, 824
Trypanosoma cruzi, 341, 560, 587–588, 898
Trypanosomes, 8
Trypanosomiasis, 824
Trypsinogen, serum, 985
Trypsin stain, 49
TTR gene, 2260–2261
TUBB1, 369, 1153
Tuberculosis, 2238
Tubular aggregate myopathy (TAM), 1195
Tubulin isoforms, 363
Tumor lysis syndrome (TLS), 1461, 1669, 1992
Tumor necrosis factor (TNF), 42, 150, 202, 237, 290, 314, 771, 955, 998, 1033, 1035, 1247, 1950, 2260
    therapy, 664
Tumor necrosis factor alpha (TNF-α), 94, 451, 631, 841–842, 858, 978, 1124, 1366, 1411, 1495, 2051, 1344, 2356
Tumor necrosis factor receptor (TNFR), 2012, 2074
Tumor necrosis factor receptor 2 (TNFR2), 2074
Tumor necrosis factor receptor superfamily member 1B (TNFRSF1B), 2074
Tumor necrosis factor receptor-associated factor 1 (TRAF1), 301
Tumor necrosis factor receptor-associated periodic syndrome (TRAPS), 2260
Tumor necrosis factor receptor–associated factor 6 (TRAF6), 1915
Tumor necrosis factor receptor–associated factor-1 (TRAF1), 2133
Tumor necrosis factor superfamily (TNFSF), 237
Tumor necrosis factor-receptor associated periodic syndrome (TRAPS), 2282
Tumor necrosis factor-related apoptosis-inducing ligand (TRAIL), 314, 2012
Tumor-associated antigens (TAAs), 1498–1499
Tumor-associated macrophages (TAMs), 227
Tumor-infiltrating lymphocytes (TILs), 302, 1499, 1508
Tumor-node-metastasis (TNM), 2090
Tumor(s), 1885
    cells, 1711, 1875–1876, 1880, 1952, 2049
        in ALCL, 1887
            express CD30, 2000
        in HL, 1388
        in HS, 1379
    fever, 2177
    heterogeneity, 1484
    mast cell, 1850
    microemboli, 1247
    microenvironment, 2116
    phase, 2075
    of spleen
        acute leukemia and myeloproliferative neoplasms, 1441
        chronic myeloid leukemia involving spleen, 1441f
        cysts and abscesses, 1437–1438
        lymphoid proliferations, 1439–1441
        patterns of tumorous spleen proliferations, 1437

        primary cysts, 1438f
        tumorous proliferations, 1441–1442
        vascular proliferations, 1438–1439
    suppressors, 1739–1740
    tissues, 1248
    tumor-host interactions, 1499
        antibody approaches, 1499–1505
        approaches to immunotherapy, 1499
        cellular approaches, 1506–1515
        cytokines, 1505–1506
        immune evasion by tumors, 1499
        immune sculpting of tumors, 1499
        tumor-promoting immune responses, 1499
    tumor-promoting immune responses, 1499
    tumor-specific antigens, 1680
    tumor-stage MF, 2078
    vesicles, 1247
Tumorous proliferations, 1441
Tumorous spleen proliferations, patterns of, 1437
Tunneling nanotubes (TNTs), 333–334
Turbulent blood flow, 1277
Turner syndrome, 1696
Twin-twin transfusion, 1061
    acute, 1062
    chronic, 1062
Twisted gastrulation protein homolog 1 (TWSG1), 690
TWiTCH. See Transfusions Changing to Hydroxyurea (TWiTCH)
Two-hit model, 1696
Two-parameter dot plots, 26
Two-step model of PNH pathogenesis, 801–803
TXA_2 receptor (TXR), 410
$TxA2$, 1189
TYK2 tyrosine kinase (TYK2), 1404
TYK2, 375
Tylenol, 753
Type III PCT, 712
Typical one-stage PTT assays, 1207
Typical unstable hemoglobinopathies, 938
Tyrosination, 363
Tyrosine 177 (Y177), 1785
Tyrosine kinase domain (TKD), 1460, 1576, 1611, 1648
Tyrosine kinase inhibitors (TKI), 1458, 1670, 1763, 1782, 1793, 1861, 2299, 2340
    approach to patient with tyrosine kinase inhibitor resistance, 1798–1800
        BCR-ABL1 kinase domain mutants to approved tyrosine kinase inhibitors, 1799t
    asciminib, 1796–1797
    BCR-ABL1 response milestones in chronic phase CML patients treated with TKIs, 1798t
    bosutinib, 1796
    dasatinib, 1794–1795
    drug combinations, 1797
    imatinib, 1793–1794
    nilotinib, 1795–1796
    overall survival of patients treated on international randomized study, 1796f
    ponatinib, 1796
    resistance to, 1798
        activation of alternative signaling pathways, 1798
        BCR-ABL1 kinase domain mutations, 1798
        TKI therapy in major front-line studies, 1795t
    TKIs approved for first-line treatment of CML, 1794t
    TKIs approved for salvage treatment of CML, 1795t
    tyrosine kinase inhibitor toxicity, 1797
Tyrosines (Y), 375
    phosphorylation, 153

U

U-MRD. See Undetectable-MRD (U-MRD)
U-STAT5, 376
U-STATs. See Unphosphorylated STATs (U-STATs)
U2AF1 mutation, 1738, 1755–1756, 1825
U2AF1 gene, 1568, 1638, 1857
UAMS. See University of Arkansas for Medical Sciences (UAMS)
Ubiquitin proteosome system (UPS), 102
UGT. See Uridineglucuronyl transferase (UGT)
Ulcerations, chronic, 618
Ulcers, 855
Ultra-large multimers, 1130
Ultrastructural analysis of cutaneous HHT lesions, 1162
Ultraviolet A (UVA), 2083
Ultraviolet B (UVB), 2083

Ultraviolet light exposure (UV light exposure), 1950
Ultraviolet radiation, 2075
Umbilical cord blood (UCB), 74, 910, 1679, 2315, 2337, 2300–2301
    clinical trials assessing strategies for ex vivo expansion of UCB units, 75t
Umbilical cord blood transplantation (UCBT), 2315
Umbilical cord RBC screening cells, 775
Umbilical stump bleeding, 1219
UNC13D gene, 1380
Unclassifiable B-celllymphomas, 1965
Unconjugated antibodies, 1500–1502
Unconventional T-cell development in medulla, 238–239
Uncrossmatched blood for emergency transfusion, 573
Undetectable-MRD (U-MRD), 2028
Unfavorable early-stage HL, 2121
Unfavorable early-stage Hodgkin lymphoma, treatment of, 2122
Unfractionated heparin (UFH), 1280, 1303
    molecules, 1292
Unicentric Castleman Disease (UCD), 1952
Unifocal bone disease, 1370
Unifocal LCH of bone, 1366
Uninvolved immunoglobulins, suppression of, 2167
United Kingdom (UK), 1048
    United Kingdom Haemophilia Centre Doctors' Organisation, 1231
    United Kingdom Acute Lymphoblastic Leukemia (UKALL), 1608, 1672
    United Kingdom National External Quality Assessment Service (UK NEQAS), 27
    United States Cutaneous Lymphoma Consortium (USCLC), 2080
    United States Food and Drug Administration (FDA), 303, 350, 558, 694, 811, 849, 901, 1004, 761, 774, 827, 1103, 1339, 1504, 1614, 1627, 1674, 1738, 1816, 1821, 1843, 1861, 1952, 1967, 1999, 2096, 2175, 2297–2298
    FDA-approved indications, 1293
    United States Preventative Services Task Force (USPSTF), 637
University of Arkansas for Medical Sciences (UAMS), 2157
Unphosphorylated STATs (U-STATs), 375
Unpolymerized fibrin monomer, 1086
Unrelated donor (URD), 1679, 2300, 2315
Unstable hemoglobins, 935, 937, 1028
    clinical features, 937
        hyperunstable hemoglobin, 937
        pulmonary hypertension, 937
    diagnosis, 936
        blood smear, 936
        detection of variant hemoglobin and mutation analysis, 937
        Heinz body preparation, 936
        hemoglobin HPLC, 937
        hemoglobin stability tests, 937
    Heinz body formation, 936
    mutations alter heme-globin interaction, 936
    pathophysiology, 935–936
    red cell destruction, 936
    treatment, 938
    variants, 937
5'untranslated region (UTR), 1155
3'untranslated regions (3'-UTR), 802, 887, 1908
Ureaplasma urealyticum, 1397
Uremia, 1087
Ureterovesicular amyloidosis, 2259–2260
Uridine diphosphate (UDP), 124
Uridineglucuronyl transferase (UGT), 124
Urinary acidification, 852
Urinary iron excretion, 620
Urinary protein loss, 2244
Urine, 806, 2146
    evaluation, 2148
    hemosiderin, 620
    protein-to-creatinine ratio, 2380
    tests, 780
    uroporphyrin, 719
UROD cDNA, 712
UROD mutation. *See* Uroporphyrinogen decarboxylase mutation (UROD mutation)
Urokinase plasminogen activator, 484
    activation, 485
    biochemistry, 485
    function, 485
    gene structure and expression, 484–485
Urokinase-type plasminogen activator (uPA), 430, 490, 1196, 1302
    receptor, 493
Uroporphyrin, 98, 713
Uroporphyrinogen, 98
    uroporphyrinogen I, 98
    uroporphyrinogen III synthase, 658
Uroporphyrinogen synthase gene (*UROS* gene), 714–715
Uroporphyrinogendecarboxylase mutation (UROD mutation), 712
Uroporphyrinuria, 714
UROS gene. *See* Uroporphyrinogen synthase gene (*UROS* gene)
Urticaria, 785
Urticaria pigmentosa (UP), 1849
Urticarial eruption, 2281
Urticarial vasculitis, 1168
US CALGB 8811 trial, 1618
US Centers for Disease Control and Prevention (CDC), 1409
US intergroup study, 1418
US Orphan Drug Act, 707
US Preventive Services Task Force, 1409
USCLC. *See* United States Cutaneous Lymphoma Consortium (USCLC)
USH2A genes, 1677
USPSTF. *See* United States Preventative Services Task Force (USPSTF)
5'-UTR mutations, 887
UV light exposure. *See* Ultraviolet light exposure (UV light exposure)
UVA. *See* Ultraviolet A (UVA)
UVB. *See* Ultraviolet B (UVB)

V

v-SNAREs. *See* Vesicular SNAREs (v-SNAREs)
V(D)J recombination, 269f, 270
Vaccines, 1434
Vaccinia virus, 1529
VACTERL-H, 976
Vacuolar pathway, 332
Vacuolar protein sorting 13 homolog A (VPS13A), 744
Valacyclovir, 1387
23-valent polysaccharide vaccine (PPSV23), 847
13-valent protein-conjugated pneumococcal vaccine, 847
Valine, 946
Vampire bat (*Desmodus rotundus*), 1302
Vancomycin, 1473
Vancomycin-resistant enterococci (VRE), 1471
Vanin-2 (VNN2), 143
Variant allele fraction (VAF), 1600, 1754–1755
Variant Creutzfeldt-Jakob disease (vCJD), 588
Variant hemoglobin, detection of, 937
Variants, 751, 1204
Varicella-zoster virus (VZV), 1480–1481, 2364, 2382
Varices, 1062
Variegate porphyria (VP), 704, 708
    clinical description, 708–709
    cutaneous manifestations of, 709f
    homozygous dominant VP, 710
    laboratory findings, 709–710
    molecular basis and pathogenesis, 709
    pathogenesis, 709
    treatment, 710
Vascular cell adhesion molecule 1 (VCAM-1), 236, 273, 837, 841, 2024
Vascular cells, 427
Vascular disease, 956
Vascular endothelial growth factor (VEGF), 72, 394, 531, 2277
Vascular endothelial growth factor C (VEGF-C), 242
Vascular endothelium, 1247, 1276, 1278
Vascular hemophilia, 1209
Vascular injury, 1278
Vascular macrophages, 213
Vascular malformations, 1075, 1165
Vascular model, 536
Vascular network, 531
Vascular obstruction, purpura associated with, 1170–1171
Vascular proliferations, 1438–1439
Vascular spasm, 816
Vascular tumors, 1438
Vasculitis, 1167
    acute infantile hemorrhagic edema 1168
    antineutrophil cytoplasmic antibody (ANCA), 1168
    cryoglobulinemia, 1168
    cutaneous leukocytoclastic vasculitis, 1167–1168
    Henoch-Schönlein Purpura (HSP), 1169
    hypergammaglobulinemic purpura (HP), 1168
    serum sickness, 1169
    urticarial vasculitis, 1168
Vasculogenesis, 531
Vasculopathies, 1165
    amyloidosis, 1165
    cerebral small vessel disease, 1166
    Moyamoya disease, 1165–1166
Vaso-occlusion
    multicellular and multistep model of sickle cell vaso-occlusion, 838f
    pathogenesis of, 838
Vaso-occlusive disease of retina, 853
Vaso-occlusive events, 839–840
Vaso-occlusive process, 855
Vasomotor phenomena, 780
VAV1 gene, 1928
Vector copy numbers (VCNs), 1544, 2329
Vectors, 1528–1529
    immune responses to, 1550–1551
    preparations, high-titer, 1524
Vegetarianism, 961
Vegetarians, cobalamin replacement in, 965
VEGF, 2279
Velamentous insertion of umbilical cord, 1062
Velocardiofacial syndrome (VCF syndrome), 1188–1189, 1399
Veltuzumab, 1501
Vemurafenib, 1370–1371, 2049–2050, 2064
Vena caval filter, 1305–1306
Venereal Disease Research Laboratory (VDRL), 1260
Venetoclax, 1461, 1463, 1621, 1648, 1704, 1832, 2034, 2213, 2272
Veno-occlusive disease (VOD), 1454, 1651, 1703
Venoms, hemolysis with, 825–827
Venous drainage, 1424
Venous thrombi, 1277
Venous thromboembolic disease, 1262–1263, 1303
    advanced therapies for venous thromboembolism, 1305
        catheter-directed thrombolysis of deep venous thrombosis, 1306
        thrombolysis for pulmonary embolism, 1306
        vena caval filter, 1305–1306
    extended treatment of venous thromboembolism, 1304–1305
        duration of anticoagulation in venousthromboembolic disease, 1304t
    initial treatment considerations in special populations with venous thromboembolism, 1304
        isolated distal deep venous thrombosis of leg, 1305
        isolated subsegmental pulmonary embolism, 1305
    management of venous thromboembolism, 1303
        initial treatment of venous thromboembolism, 1303
    prevention of, 1306
        general approach to VTE prophylaxis in hospitalized patients, 1308f
        individualized venous thromboembolism risk assessment models, 1307f
Venous thromboembolism (VTE), 784, 1175, 1279, 1283
Venous thrombosis, 808, 1277
Venous thrombotic events, 1288
Ventricular assist devices (VADs), 828, 1123
Ventricular thrombi, 2243
Verruca peruviana, 824
Vertebral bodies, 895
Vertebrate hemoglobin, 113
Very late antigen-4 (VLA-4), 273
Very severe aplastic anemia (VSAA), 1000
Very-low-birth-weight (VLBW), 1058
Vesicle-associated membrane protein (VAMP), 177, 414
Vesicle-associated membrane protein 4 (VAMP4), 1545
Vesicular monoamine transporter (VMAT2), 363
Vesicular SNAREs (v-SNAREs), 177
Vesicular stomatitis virus-G protein (*VSV-G*), 1527
Vessel wall, 533
Vessels, structural malformations of, 1162–1166
VEXAS syndrome, 2146
V_H4 family genes, 777
VHL protein. *See* von Hippel Lindau protein (VHL protein)

Vibrio cholera, 691
Vibrio vulnificus, 691
Vinblastine, 1108, 1370
Vincristine, 1108, 1370, 1412, 1417, 1608, 1672, 1674, 1844, 1962, 2002, 2100
Vincristine, doxorubicin, and dexamethasone (VAD), 2257
Vincristine, doxorubicin, methotrexate, and prednisone (VAMP), 2136
Vincristine and CAP (VCAP), 2193
Vincristine-BCNU-doxorubicin-prednisone (VBAP), 2193
Vincristine-melphalan-cyclophosphamide-prednisone (VMCP), 2193
Vinorelbine, 2099, 2138
Viral antigen–specific T cells, 1508
Viral biology, 1382–1383
Viral capsid antigen (VCA), 1384
Viral encephalitis, 1480
Viral gene expression, 1382–1383
Viral genomes, 1382
Viral hepatitis, 1010
Viral infection, 997, 1352
    thrombocytopenia associated with, 1158
Viral replication, 1547
Viral transmission from past factor concentrates, 1233
Viral vectors, 1526
    adeno-associated virus vectors (AA*vs*. vectors), 1529
    adenoviral vectors, 1528–1529
    foamy viral vectors, 1528
    gamma-retroviral vectors, 1526–1527
    lentiviral vectors (LVvectors), 1527
Virchow triad, 1276
    abnormalities of blood, 1278
        coagulation abnormalities, 1278–1279
        platelet abnormalities, 1278
    abnormalities of blood flow, 1277
    pathophysiology of thrombosis, 1277*f*
    vascular injury, 1278
Viridans group streptococci, 1474
Virions, 1382
Virus, 997, 1158
    particles, 1526
Visceral leishmaniasis, 824
Vital NETosis, 151
Vitamin A, 2096
Vitamin B_{12}, 1011, 1015, 1028, 1811, 1823
Vitamin B_6 metabolism, 668–669
Vitamin D, 760, 1950
    deficiency, 2323
    Vitamin D3, 1950
Vitamin E, 743, 755
Vitamin K, 439, 753
    deficiency, 1243
    Vitamin K_1, 439, 1241, 1246
    Vitamin K_2, 439
Vitamin K antagonists (VKAs), 1298
    VKA-based treatment, 1303
Vitamin K deficiency bleeding in infancy (VKDB in infancy), 1241
    causes of vitamin K deficiency, 1242
        treatment, 1243
    clinical features and laboratory diagnosis, 1241
        laboratory findings in acquired coagulation disorders, 1243*t*
    etiologies of vitamin K deficiency, 1241*f*
    pathophysiology, 1241
    treatment, 1241
Vitamin K epoxide reductase complex subunit 1 (VKORC1), 1296–1297
Vitamin K–dependent factors, 1224
    deficiencies of, 1241
Vitamin K–dependent protein family, 436
    factor IX, 446–447
    factor VII, 445–446
    factor X, 447–449
    gene structure and expression, 436–438
    general structure/function features, 441–442
        biochemical properties of human anticoagulant proteins and inhibitors, 441*t*
        epidermal growth factor domain, 444
        gla domain, 442–444
        highest resolution structures of human procoagulant, anticoagulant, fibrinolytic proteins, and inhibitors, 442–444*t*
        serine protease domain, 444
    posttranslational processing, 438–439
    proteolytic maturation, 439
        carboxylation and vitamin K–dependent carboxylase, 439–441
        glycosylation, 441
        hydroxylation, 441
    rate enhancement by vitamin K–dependent complexes, 439*t*
    schematic representation of, 437–438*f*
    vitamin K–dependent complexes, 439*f*
    vitamin K–dependent processes, 440*f*
Vitamins, 695, 907
    supplementation, 907
Volume packed red blood cells (vPRC), 600, 647, 1070
von Hippel Lindau protein (VHL protein), 1076
von Willebrand collagen–binding activity, 1214
von Willebrand disease (vWD), 67, 1081, 1087, 1202, 1209, 1229
    clinical manifestations, 1212–1213
    genetic testing in, 1214–1215
    genetics, 1209–1211
        features of common variants of von Willebrand Disease, 1211*t*
        pedigree of patients described by von Willebrand, 1211*f*
        structure and functional domains of von Willebrand factor, 1210*f*
    genetics of Type 1 and Type 3 vWD, 1215
    incidence, 1209
    laboratory diagnosis, 1213
        assay of von Willebrand factor's ability to bind factor VIII, 1214
        bleeding time and platelet function analyzer-100(PFA-100), 1213
        genetic testing in von Willebrand Disease, 1214–1215
        Multimeric Analysis of von Willebrand Factor, 1214
        partial thromboplastin time and factor VIIIc assay, 1213
        ristocetin cofactor activity and ristocetin-induced plateletaggregation, 1213–1214
        von Willebrand Collagen–Binding Activity, 1214
        von Willebrand factor functional assays, 1213
        von Willebrand factor immunoassay, 1213
        von Willebrand factor propeptide assay, 1214
    laboratory diagnosis of von Willebrand disease and platelet dysfunction, 1089*f*
    nomenclature, 1209
        revised classification of von Willebrand disease, 1209*t*
    pathophysiology, 1211
        abnormalities of primary hemostasis, 1212
        abnormalities of secondary hemostasis, 1212
    platelet-typevon Willebrand Disease, 1216–1217
    qualitative defects of von Willebrand factor, 1215–1216
    response to transfusion, 1212
        phenomenon of new factor VIII synthesis in patients with von Willebrand disease, 1212*f*
    Type 1 von Willebrand Disease and "Low von Willebrand Factor", 1215
    Type 2, 1210
    Type 2A, 1215–1216
    Type 2B, 1216
    Type 2M, 1216
    Type 2N, 1216
    Type 3 von Willebrand Disease, 1215
    von Willebrand disease type 1, 1182
von Willebrand factor (vWF), 341, 359, 362, 394, 397, 402–403, 451, 458, 532, 563, 1084, 1123, 1127, 1154, 1182, 1203, 1245, 1277, 1259
    alteration of vWF multimers in TTP, 1129–1130
        multimers in TTP, 1130*f*
    angiogenesis in normal and malignant hematopoiesis, 532–533
    antigen-II, 458
    antithrombotic properties of unperturbed endothelium, 533
        anticoagulant activities, 534–535
        antiplatelet activities, 533–534
        fibrinolytic activities, 535
    assay of von Willebrand factor's ability to bind factor VIII, 1214
    biochemistry, 458
    conformation of vWF and interaction with ADAMTS13, 1128–1129
    endothelial cell structure, 533
    functional assays, 1213
    gene structure and expression, 458
    hemostatic properties of perturbed endothelium, 535–536
        diversity of endothelial cell hemostatic properties, 536–537
        vessel wall prothrombotic properties, 536*f*
    immunoassay, 1213
    propeptide assay, 1214
    prothrombotic properties of unperturbed endothelium, 535
    qualitative defects of, 1215
        type 2A von Willebrand Disease, 1215–1216
        type 2B von Willebrand Disease, 1216
        type 2M von Willebrand Disease, 1216
        type 2N von Willebrand Disease, 1216
    vessel wall and hemostasis, 533
    vWF-platelet aggregation, 1137
    vWF-platelet thrombosis, 1131, 1138
von Willebrand factor propeptide (vWFpp), 1211
Vorapaxar, 1291
Voriconazole, 1350, 1477
Vorinostat, 2099
Voxelotor, 864, 2325

W

Waldenström macroglobulinemia (WM), 33, 776, 1918, 1951, 2150, 2282, 2160, 2267
    BTK inhibitors in symptomatic WM, 2271*t*
    clinical presentation, 2268
    diagnosis, 2267–2268
    diagnostic criteria for, 2268*t*
    epidemiology, 2267
    guidelines for molecular testing in, 1918
    mayo clinicmSMART, 2273*f*
    prognostic factors, 2269
    risk stratification, 2269–2270
        mayo clinic mSMART, 2269*f*
    start treatment, 2269
    therapeutic alternatives, 2272
        novel agents, 2272
        overall approach for relapsed and refractory WM, 2272
        stem cell transplant (SCT), 2272
    therapeutic options, 2270
        alkylators and bendamustine, 2270
        Bruton tyrosine kinase inhibitors, 2271–2272
        goals of therapy, 2270
        nucleoside analogs, 2270
        proteasome inhibitors, 2270–2271
        rituximab as single agent, 2270
Wandering spleen, 1425
Warfarin, 1296
    adverse effects of warfarin therapy, 1297–1299
    apixaban, 1300
    dabigatran etexilate, 1299–1300
    drugs and medical conditions affecting warfarin potency, 1296*t*
    edoxaban, 1300–1301
    effects of standard warfarin therapy on plasma vitamin K–dependent procoagulant coagulation proteins, 1296*f*
    laboratory monitoring of warfarin therapy, 1297
        method for determination of ISI value for laboratory thromboplastin preparation, 1297*f*
        relationship between patient's PT ratio on warfarin therapy and corresponding INR value, 1297*f*
    resistance, 1297
    reversal of direct oral anticoagulants, 1301
    rivaroxaban, 1300
    special populations, 1301
    therapy, moderate intensity, 1297
    warfarin-induced skin necrosis, 1298
Warm AIHA. *See* Warm autoimmune hemolytic anemia (Warm AIHA)
Warts, hypogammaglobulinemia, immunodeficiency, myelokathexis syndrome (*WHIM* syndrome), 1335–1336, 1395, 1918

Water, 825
    water channel-forming protein, 1027
    water-soluble vitamins, 962
Wegener granulomatosis, 1168, 1337
Weibel-Palade bodies, 533
Weisses blut, 1627
West Nile virus (WNV), 560, 587
Western blotting, 20
Western diets, 813
Wet purpura, 1101
White blood, 1694, 1782
White blood cell (WBC), 1, 564, 778, 838, 857, 1599, 1611, 1631, 1669, 1694, 1722, 1837, 2336. *See also* Red blood cells (RBCs)
    antigens and antibodies, 552
        HLA antigens and antibodies, 552–553
        platelet antigens and antibodies, 553–554
    counts, 4, 782
    differentials, 1
White clot syndrome, 1307
White pulp, 246–247
White thrombi, 1277
Whole blood (WB), 560
Whole exome sequencing (WES), 1694, 2016
Whole-body CT skeletal surveys, 2179
Whole-chromosome paint probes, 51
Whole-genome sequencing (WGS), 58, 1694, 1905, 2016, 2153
WHSC1 genes, 1677
Wide-band ultraviolet B phototherapy (WBUVB), 2095
Wild-type ADAMTS13, 1126
Wild-type enzyme, 751
Wild-type HIV-1 virions, 1527
Wilms tumor 1 gene (*WT1* gene), 1637, 1702
Wilson disease, 825
Wiskott-Aldrich syndrome (WAS), 1096, 1100, 1156, 1195, 1333, 1346, 1403, 1538, 1546, 1991, 2318, 2299
    gene, 1403
    mutation, 1156
Wiskott-Aldrich syndrome protein (WASp), 1403, 1541, 1333
Wnt pathway, 379
Wolffia globosa, 967
Working Formulation (WF), 1869, 1943

World Health Organization (WHO), 61, 600, 667, 751, 883, 909, 1060, 1072, 1176, 1207, 1297, 1366, 1387, 1446, 1562, 1595, 1611, 1627, 1694, 1721, 1737, 1763, 1791, 1809, 1813, 1821, 1837, 1849, 1869, 1900, 1915, 1942, 1991, 2075, 2117, 2267
    classification, 1446, 1638
    system, 2175
    prognostic scoring system, 2337
Wright or May-Grünwald-Giemsa stain, 6, 10
WRN gene, 1630
WT1 gene, 1710
WT1/FLT3-ITD mutations, 1710

X

X chromosome, 751 763, 660, 666, 1754, 1782, 1203
X-chronic granulomatous disease (CGD), 1528, 1547
X-linked agammaglobulinemia (XLA), 275, 1393, 1396–1397
X-linked gene *GATA*-1, 1156
X-linked hereditary disorder, 1156
X-linked inheritance, 1349
X-linked lymphoproliferative (XLP), 1387, 1951
X-Linked macrothrombocytopenia with dyserythropoiesis associated with GATA-1 mutation, 1156
X-linked microthrombocytopenia, 1156
X-linked neutropenia, 1346
X-linked protoporphyria (XLP), 702, 714, 716
    clinical description, 716
    laboratory findings, 718
    late-onset protoporphyria, 718
    long-term management, 718
    molecular basis and pathogenesis, 716
    treatment, 718
X-linked sideroblastic anemia (XLSA), 656, 659–661, 691
    with ataxia, 664
    human erythroid 5-aminolevulinate synthase gene and location, 661f
X-linked thrombocytopenia (XLT), 1195, 1403, 1195
X-linked thrombocytopenia with or without dyserythropoietic anemia (XLTDA), 1020
X-linked traits, 1082
X-ray, 704

Xenograft models, hematopoietic stem cell studies in, 78–79
Xeroderma pigmentosum group D (XPD), 1630
Xerostomia, 2240, 2382
XIAP gene, 1380
XK gene, 744
XLP1 immunodeficiency, 1389
XLSA deficiency, clinical and laboratory features of, 662

Y

Y. *See* Tyrosines (Y)
Y chromosome, 2002
Yersinia, 582, 662, 899
    Y. enterocolitica, 691, 899, 905
    Y. pseudotuberculosis, 691
Young adults, 2133
    with acute lymphoblasticleukemia, 1676
Yttrium 90 (Y-90), 1502

Z

Zanubrutinib, 1963, 1970, 2032, 2036, 2272
Zap-70, 290, 1401, 2024
Zarxio, 1339
ZBTB16 gene, 1570
Z-dependent protease inhibitor (ZPI), 462
Zebrafish, 661, 665
Zidovudine (ZDV), 964, 1387, 1410–1411, 1977
Zieve syndrome, 1039
Zika virus (ZIKV), 560, 587
Zinc, 670, 907
    deficiency, 855
    formalin, 12
Zinc finger (ZF), 366, 1156
Zinc finger E-box-binding homeobox 1 (*ZEB1*), 2074
Zinc finger nucleases (ZFNs), 1547
Zinc protoporphyrin (ZPP), 613
Zinc-finger protein 384 (*ZNF384*), 1583
ZMYM2 gene, 1774
ZMYM2-FGFR1 fusion, 1843
Zoledronic acid (ZA), 2219
ZRSR2 gene, 1568, 1638
ZRSR2 mutation, 1738, 1756
Zymogen factor X, 447–449